The Use of Antibiotics

A Clinical Review of Antibacterial, Antifungal and Antiviral Drugs

The Use of Antibiotics
A Clinical Review of Antibacterial, Antifungal and Antiviral Drugs

Fifth Edition

A Kucers MB BS FRACP Dr med hc (Latvian Academy of Sciences)
Infectious Diseases Physician,
Royal Melbourne Hospital, Victorian Infectious Diseases Service,
Victoria, Australia

S M Crowe MB BS FRACP
Head, AIDS Pathogenesis Research Unit,
MacFarlane Burnet Centre for Medical Research;
Associate Professor of Medicine, Monash University;
Infectious Diseases Physician, Alfred Hospital, Victoria, Australia

M L Grayson MB BS MD MSc FRACP FAFPHM
Director, Infectious Disease and Clinical Epidemiology Department,
Monash Medical Centre;
Associate Professor of Epidemiology and Preventive Medicine,
Monash University, Victoria, Australia

J F Hoy MB BS FRACP
Head, Clinical Research Section,
Infectious Diseases Physician,
Microbiology and Infectious Diseases Department,
Alfred Hospital;
Senior Lecturer, Department of Medicine,
Monash University, Victoria, Australia

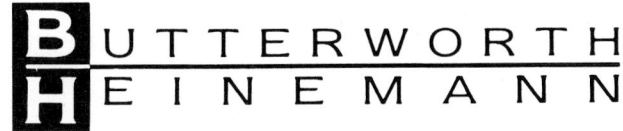
BUTTERWORTH
HEINEMANN

Butterworth-Heinemann
Linacre House, Jordan Hill, Oxford OX2 8DP
A division of Reed Educational and Professional Publishing Ltd

 A member of the Reed Elsevier plc group

OXFORD   BOSTON   JOHANNESBURG
MELBOURNE   NEW DELHI   SINGAPORE

First published 1972
Second edition 1975
Reprinted 1977
Third edition 1979
Reprinted 1982
Fourth edition 1987
Reprinted 1988, 1989
Fifth edition 1997

British Library Cataloguing in Publication Data
The use of antibiotics: a clinical review of
    antibacterial, antifungal and antiviral drugs. – 5th ed.
    1. Antibiotics
    I. Kucers, A. (Alvis), *1933–*
    615.3'29

Library of Congress Cataloging in Publication Data
The use of antibiotics: a clinical review of antibacterial, antifungal, and antiviral drugs/
    A. Kucers . . . [et al.]. – 5th ed.
    p.   cm.
    Rev. ed. of: The use of antibiotics/A. Kucers, N. McK. Bennett, with the assistance of
    R. J. Kemp, 4th ed. c1987.
    Includes bibliographical references and index.
    ISBN 0-7506-0155-8
    1. Anti-infective agents. I. Kucers, A.
    [DNLM: 1. Antibiotics – therapeutic use. QV 350 U835 1997]
    RM267.K8 1997
    615'.329—DC21
    DNLM/DLC
    for Library of Congress   97–21384
                                                                              CIP

ISBN 0 7506 0155 8

Composition by Genesis Typesetting, Rochester, Kent
Printed and bound in Great Britain by The Bath Press, Avon

Contents

Preface to Fifth Edition

Although I retired from my position at Fairfield Infectious Diseases Hospital in 1993 and thereafter worked only part-time at the Royal Melbourne Hospital, I still felt unable to tackle the task of the fifth edition alone. It was unfortunate that Dr N McK Bennett, my coauthor of the previous editions of this book, felt unable to continue the work; his contributions are gratefully acknowledged.

Three of my distinguished former pupils, namely Drs Suzanne M Crowe, M Lindsay Grayson and Jennifer F Hoy, volunteered to help. In the early to mid-1980s each of them spent two years at Fairfield Hospital as a Medical Registrar. These were advanced training positions for Infectious Disease Physicians, and other hospitals in Melbourne had very few such positions at that time. I was the Director of Medical Services at Fairfield in those years. Subsequently each of them secured a position in the USA for two to three years to continue Infectious Diseases physician training and also to acquire skills in research. Since they returned to Australia, they have held important Infectious Diseases posts. Our respective contributions to the fifth edition are indicated in the table of contents.

We have continued to provide the same systematic and concise presentation of the text, which was the case in previous editions. Obviously the size of the book has enlarged. Many new drugs, such as cephalosporins, macrolides, quinolones, antifungals and, especially, antivirals have been developed. Drug resistance is now a very serious problem in many parts of the world and new information has been included in chapters on older drugs such as penicillin G, third-generation cephalosporins, drugs for tuberculosis and many others. We have omitted or condensed the information on some older cephalosporins, quinolones and other drugs.

I would like to thank Dr Alan Street, Deputy Director, Royal Melbourne Hospital, Victorian Infectious Diseases Service, for revising the chapter on vancomycin. I am also very grateful to my secretary, Mrs Nellie Edmonds for typing and retyping my contribution to this volume. She also gave me much moral support. Ms Kathy Tolli provided invaluable secretarial and organizational assistance to Drs Crowe and Grayson, whilst Dr Hoy typed everything herself. The Medical Library of Fairfield Hospital was very helpful to us all in obtaining references.

Our publishers have waited rather patiently for our finished text. I would particularly like to thank Dr Geoffrey Smaldon, Ms Cathie Staves and Ms Jane Duncan for much practical and helpful support. Again I am grateful to many colleagues throughout the world who have expressed appreciation of the previous editions of this book. I hope that my new coauthors will receive similar appreciation once the fifth edition is published.

Alvis Kucers
Bulleen, Victoria, Australia, July 1997

Abbreviations

A.	*Aspergillus, Aeromonas, Acinetobacter, Actinomadura*	ID$_{50}$	Inhibitory dose (50%)
ADP	Adenosine diphosphate	IgA	Immunoglobulin A
AIDS	Aquired immunodeficiency syndrome	IgG	Immunoglobulin G
ALT	Alanine aminotransferase	IgM	Immunoglobulin M
AMB	Amphotericin B	i.m.	Intramuscular(ly)
AST	Aspartate aminotransferase	*I.*	*Isospora*
AUC	Area-under-the-(concentration-time)-curve	i.v.	Intravenous(ly)
B.	*Bacillus, Bacteroides, Bartonella, Blastomyces, Bordetella, Borrelia*	*Kl.*	*Klebsiella*
		kDa	kiloDalton
BCG	Bacille Calmette-Guerin	kg	kilogram
Br.	*Brucella*	*L.*	*Legionella, Leptospira, Listeria*
C.	*Campylobacter, Candida, Chlamydia, Coccidioides, Corynebacterium, Cryptococcus*	LDH	Lactic dehydrogenase
		m	meter
C	Degrees centigrade	M	mole
CAPD	Continuous ambulatory peritoneal dialysis	*M.*	*Microsporum, Moraxella, Mycobacterium, Mycoplasma*
CAVH	Continuous arteriovenous hemofiltration		
CDC	Centers for Disease Control	MBC	Minimum bactericidal concentration
CDI	Communicable Disease Report	mEq	milliequivalent
CDS	Communicable Diseases Scotland	MFC	Minimum fungicidal concentration
Cl.	*Clostridium*	mg	milligram
CLB	Coccidian-like bodies	MIC	Minimum inhibitory concentration
C$_{max}$	Steady-state peak serum concentration	min	minute
CSF	Cerebrospinal fluid	ml	milliliter
CVVH	Continuous venovenous hemofiltration	mm	millimeter
DHFR	Dehydrofolate reductase	mmol	millimole
DMSO	Dimethyl-sulfoxide	MRSA	Methicillin-resistant *Staphylococcus aureus*
DNA	Deoxyribonucleic acid	MRSE	Methicillin-resistant *Staphylococcus epidermidis*
DS	Double strength		
E.	*Enterobacter, Enterococcus, Epidermophyton, Escherichia*	MSSA	Methicillin-sensitive *Staphylococcus aureus*
		N.	*Naegleria, Neisseria, Nocardia*
F.	*Flavobacterium, Fusobacterium*	*P.*	*Paracoccidioides, Pasteurella, Plasmodium, Pneumocystis, Prevotella*
g	gram		
GABA	Gamma-aminobutyric acid	PABA	Para-aminobenzoic acid
GFR	Glomerular filtration rate	PAS	para-aminosalicylic acid
GM-CSF	Granulocyte macrophage colony stimulating factor	PBP	Penicillin binding protein
		PCP	*Pneumocystis carinii* pneumonia
H.	*Haemophilus, Herpes, Histoplasma*	PCR	Polymerase chain reaction
h	hour(s)	PHA	Phytohemagglutination
HEPA	High efficiency particle air	PPD	Purified protein derivative
HIV	Human immunodeficiency virus	PPL	Penicilloyl-polylysine
HPLC	High-performance liquid chromatography	*Ps.*	*Pseudomonas*
HLA	Human leukocyte antigen	*Pr.*	*Proteus, Providencia*
IC$_{50}$	Inhibitory concentration (50%)	*R.*	*Rhodococcus*
		RIF	Relative inhibition factor

RNA	Ribonucleic acid	SSD	Silver sulfadiazine
s	second(s)	*T.*	*Torulopsis, Toxoplasma, Trichomonas,*
S.	*Serratia, Stenotrophomonas, Streptomyces*		*Trichophyton*
Salm.	*Salmonella*	TK	Thymidine kinase
Sh.	*Shigella*	TPHA	*Treponema pallidum* hemagglutinating
Staph.	*Staphylococcus*		antibody
Strep.	*Streptococcus*	*U.*	*Ureaplasma*
SCID	Severe combined immunodeficiency	*u*	micro
SD	Standard deviation	UK	United Kingdom
SEM	Standard error of the mean	USA	United States of America
SGOT	Serum glutamic oxaloacetic transaminase	*V.*	*Vibrio*
SGPT	Serum glutamic pyruvic transaminase	VDRL	Venereal Disease Research Laboratory
spp.	Species	WHO	World Health Organisation
SS	Single strength	*Y.*	*Yersinia*

Part I

Antibiotics

Penicillin G (Pen G)

Description

Despite the availability of many new antibiotics, and the progressive development of resistance in bacterial species, penicillin G (Pen G) still remains a very useful agent.

Penicillin was isolated from *Penicillium notatum* by Fleming in 1929 and introduced into clinical medicine in 1941 by Florey, Chain and associates (Fleming, 1929; Chain *et al.*, 1940; Abraham, 1980). The history of penicillin is recorded in a number of monographs (Hare, 1970; Bickel, 1972).

The penicillin used initially was an amorphous compound containing impurities, which were introduced during the fermentative process; its activity and dosage were expressed in units. Early penicillin was also a mixture of several penicillin compounds, designated as F, G, X and K. Pen G (benzylpenicillin) was the most satisfactory and this is now used in a purified and crystalline form for clinical purposes. Pen G, similar to all penicillins and cephalosporins, is a beta-lactam antibiotic. Such compounds possess a beta-lactam ring which incorporates a beta-lactam bond. The penicillin nucleus, 6-aminopenicillanic acid (6-APA), consists of three components – a thiazolidine ring, the beta-lactam ring and a side-chain. The cephalosporin nucleus, 7-aminocephalosporanic acid (7-ACA), is similar, but the five-member thiazolidine ring characteristic of the penicillins is replaced by a six-member dihydrothiazide ring (Waldvogel, 1982). Both 6-APA and 7-ACA were isolated some 30 years ago and they have provided convenient starting points for the synthesis of other penicillins and cephalosporins which are described later in this book.

Pen G is a rather unstable acid and the following relatively stable salts are used clinically:

1 Sodium Pen G or sodium benzylpenicillin

This is a highly soluble salt, and a dose can be dissolved completely in a few ml of water prior to administration. The dosages of this and other Pen G preparations were previously expressed in units. One unit of activity is equivalent to $0.6\,\mu g$ of pure sodium Pen G.

2 Potassium Pen G

One unit of activity of this very soluble salt is equivalent to $0.625\,\mu g$ of pure potassium Pen G.

The terms 'crystalline penicillin G' or 'crystalline penicillin' are often used as synonyms for either of the above highly soluble Pen G salts. But all other penicillins in use are also crystalline, unlike the early impure amorphous compound.

3 Procaine Pen G (procaine benzylpenicillin or procaine penicillin)

This is a much less soluble salt. It is administered i.m. as a suspension of crystal particles which dissolve slowly, so that absorption of liberated Pen G takes place over a prolonged period. One unit of activity is equivalent to $1.0\,\mu g$ of pure procaine penicillin.

4 Benzathine Pen G (di-benzyl-ethylene-diamine penicillin or DBED penicillin)

An even less soluble salt than procaine penicillin, it is more slowly absorbed from an i.m. injection site producing prolonged serum levels of Pen G. One unit of activity is equivalent to $0.75\,\mu g$ of the pure substance.

Procaine and benzathine salts of Pen G are known as 'long-acting', 'depot' or 'repository' forms.

Sensitive Organisms

Since the introduction of Pen G into clinical use, many organisms which were originally highly sensitive to it, are no longer so.

1 Gram-positive cocci

a Streptococcus pyogenes (Group A beta-hemolytic streptococcus This has remained very sensitive and routine sensitivity testing is not required (Burkart and Watanakunakorn, 1992; Chow and Muder, 1992; Betriu et al., 1993). There has been no shift towards higher MIC levels of Pen G for natural isolates (Coonan and Kaplan, 1994), but less sensitive mutants (MIC 0.2 µg per ml compared with 0.006 µg per ml for susceptible strains) can be produced in the laboratory (Gutmann and Tomasz, 1982). Penicillin binding proteins (PBPs) 2 and 3 (p. 27) of such mutants have a decreased affinity for Pen G.

Penicillin-tolerant strains (p. 27) of Strep. pyogenes with MBC/MIC ratios greater than 32, can be produced experimentally. These organisms have also been isolated from clinical specimens (Gutmann and Tomasz, 1982; Dagan et al., 1987; Grahn et al., 1987). Their clinical significance remains uncertain (Woolfrey et al., 1988). The PBPs in tolerant strains differ from those in non-tolerant ones (Van Asselt et al., 1995). Pen G induces a significant post-antibiotic effect (PAE) on Strep. pyogenes in vitro and in vivo. This means that there is a persisting suppression of bacterial growth after short exposure to Pen G (Odenholt et al., 1989, 1990; Winstanley, 1990).

b Group B beta-hemolytic streptococcus (Strep. agalactiae) This organism is usually carried in the lower intestinal tract by both males and females; its common carriage in the urethral orifice, periurethral area and vagina, by both pregnant and non-pregnant women, appears to reflect secondary contamination (Anthony, 1982; Dillon et al., 1982; Easmon, 1986; Persson et al., 1987). Since about 1960 Group B streptococci have been recognized increasingly as an important cause of neonatal infections (McCracken, 1973; Berg et al., 1977; Cowen, 1979; Hamoudi and Hamoudi, 1981). The presence of these organisms in urine of the mothers at delivery results in frequent colonization of the babies, which may constitute a risk for a neonatal infection (Persson et al., 1986). Group B streptococci have been also implicated in certain adult infections (Anthony and Concepcion, 1975; Gallagher and Watanakunakorn, 1986; Verghese et al., 1986; Aharoni et al., 1990; Back et al., 1990, Dunne and Quagliarello, 1993; Sarmiento et al., 1993). In adults there is some 30-fold increased risk of infection by this organism in patients with diabetes mellitus, cancer and HIV infection (Farley et al., 1993; Wessels and Kasper, 1993). A 27-year-old woman who was reported with classical toxic shock-like syndrome (p. 35), was not bacteremic, but her urine and vaginal cultures grew Group B streptococci, which elaborated a pyrogenic toxin (Schlievert et al., 1993).

Group B streptococci are quite susceptible to Pen G, but their sensitivity is about 10-fold less than that of Group A streptococci (Table I.1). This sensitivity to Pen G has remained unchanged over the years and resistant strains had not been isolated from humans (Baker et al., 1981; Bayer et al., 1982; Verghese et al., 1986). Group B streptococci displaying resistance to penicillins, cephalosporins and several other antibiotics were isolated from the udders of dairy cattle which had received antibiotic chemoprophylaxis. Resistance appeared to be due to alteration of PBPs (p. 27) (Berghash and Dunny, 1985). More recently Betriu et al. (1994) tested 100 Group B streptococcal isolates from humans in Spain. Two of the strains had only intermediate susceptibility to Pen G (MICs 0.25–2.0 µg per ml).

Some strains of Group B streptococci may be penicillin-tolerant (p. 27), with their MBCs greatly exceeding their MICs (Kim and Anthony, 1981). This phenomenon can be more marked at a lower pH, which could be of clinical significance (Horne and Tomasz, 1981). In vitro and animal studies indicate that combinations of Pen G with an aminoglycoside, such as gentamicin (p. 455), are usually synergistic against Group B streptococci (Deveikis et al., 1977; Baker et al., 1981). In vitro, even the addition of low concentrations of gentamicin (0.1 µg or 0.5 µg per ml) to Pen G accelerates killing of Group B streptococci. This provides a rationale for the initial use of a combination of Pen G plus gentamicin in the treatment of Group B streptococcal meningitis (p. 36) or endocarditis (Swingle et al., 1985; Gallagher and Watanakunakorn, 1986). In vitro studies have shown that killing of Group B streptococci is enhanced if an opsonic i.v. immunoglobulin mixture is combined with Pen G, suggesting that this combination has potential for use in the treatment of neonatal Group B streptococcal infections (Miller et al., 1990).

c Groups C, G, F and R (Strep. suis) beta-hemolytic streptococci These are less common human pathogens. Group C (Arditi et al., 1989; Bradley et al., 1991), Group G (Craven et al., 1986; Venezio et al., 1986), Group F (Libertin et al., 1985) and Group R streptococci (Arends and Zanen, 1988) are consistently sensitive to Pen G. Strains of Group C streptococci can exhibit penicillin tolerance (p. 27) (Arditi *et al.* 1989); this was demonstrated in 16 of 17 clinical isolates tested by Portnoy *et al.* (1981). Pen G and gentamicin synergism occurred against all of the 17 strains. Clinical isolates of Group G streptococci also often show tolerance to Pen G and other antibiotics which act on the bacterial cell wall (Finch and Aveline, 1984; Ashkenazi *et al.*, 1988). Pen G plus gentamicin usually exhibits *in vitro* synergism against Group G streptococci (Lam and Bayer, 1984).

d Streptococcus pneumoniae This remained Pen G-sensitive until 1967 after which strains with intermediate resistance were isolated with increasing frequency from patients with pneumococcal infections or carriers of the organism. In 1977 highly resistant pneumococcal strains appeared in South Africa; initially their spread was minimal to other parts of the world, but now they have been detected in many other countries. Pneumococcal strains with MICs of 0.06 µg per ml or less are regarded as susceptible, those with MICs of 0.1–1.0 µg per ml as intermediately resistant and those with MICs of higher than 1.0 µg per ml are designated as highly resistant or simply resistant (Jacobs, 1992).

Streptococcus pneumoniae strains with intermediate resistance to Pen G were first detected in Australia and Papua New Guinea (Hansman *et al.*, 1971, 1974). The prevalence of such pneumococcal strains in Papua New Guinea soon rose to greater than 10% (Gratten *et al.*, 1980). Small numbers of such *Strep. pneumoniae* strains were also detected in other countries such as New Mexico (Tempest *et al.*, 1974), the UK (Howes and Mitchell, 1976), Spain (Liñares *et al.*, 1983) and North America (Naraqi *et al.*, 1974; Lauer and Reller, 1980; Maki *et al.*, 1980). These pneumococcal strains soon become more prevalent in the USA. Of 103 pneumococcal isolates from patients in Oklahoma, 16 had intermediate resistance to Pen G (Saah *et al.*, 1980); in Houston, this was also detected in 13 (5.9%) of 222 clinical isolates (Krause *et al.*, 1982).

Pneumococci highly resistant to Pen G and to many other antibiotics, were detected in South Africa in 1977 (Appelbaum *et al.*, 1977; Jacobs and Koornhof, 1978). Type 19a pneumococci, resistant to Pen G (MICs 4–8 µg per ml), cephalothin (MICs 4–15), chloramphenicol (MICs 9–37) and less resistant to ampicillin (MICs 1–4) were isolated from five children in a Durban hospital. Subsequently carriers of the same resistant strain were discovered in several Durban hospitals. Other pneumococci, with a wider spectrum of resistance were found in Johannesburg during the same period. A child with pneumococcal pneumonia following cardiac surgery recovered after treatment with cephalothin and ampicillin. The type 19 pneumococcus isolated from his sputum was relatively resistant to both of these drugs, and it was resistant to Pen G (MIC 4–8 µg per ml), methicillin, erythromycin, clindamycin, tetracycline, chloramphenicol, co-trimoxazole and the aminoglycosides. It was fully sensitive only to rifampicin, vancomycin and bacitracin and moderately sensitive to sodium fusidate (MIC 2 µg per ml). Many carriers of this multiply-resistant pneumococcus were detected among both patients and staff in the same hospital, and a few serious infections such as septicemia occurred, which were difficult to treat. In Johannesburg, some patients were also found to harbor pen G- and tetracycline-resistant type 6 pneumococci.

Subsequent surveys in South Africa showed pneumococci with at least five patterns of resistance; Pen G only; Pen G and tetracycline; Pen G, tetracycline and chloramphenicol; Pen G and chloramphenicol and Pen G, tetracycline, chloramphenicol, erythromycin and clindamycin. Some strains from the last group (referred to as 'multiply-resistant') also developed resistance to other antibiotics such as rifampicin. Pneumococci with these various resistance patterns were either type 6 or type 19a (CDC, 1978a).

In South Africa the problem of pneumococcal resistance has gradually increased (Oppenheim *et al.*, 1986; Klugman and Koornhof, 1988). Nationwide surveys have shown that either intermediate or high-level resistance to Pen G among South African strains of *Strep. pneumoniae* increased from 4.9% in 1979 to 14.4% in 1990 (Appelbaum, 1992; Koornhof *et al.*, 1992). Except for resistance to co-trimoxazole (44%), resistance to other antibiotics remained relatively low. Multiply-resistant strains belonged mainly to serotypes 6B, 19A, 14 and, more recently, 23F.

Streptococcus pneumoniae with both intermediate and high-level Pen G resistance also greatly increased in Spain. Otin *et al.* (1988) tested 91 strains from pediatric patients; only 43 were fully sensitive, 21 and 27 showing intermediate and high-level resistance, respectively. Fenoll *et al.* (1991) determined antibiotic susceptibilities for 2197 *Strep. pneumoniae* strains isolated from patients over an 11-year period in Spain. The prevalence of Pen G-resistant pneumococci rose from 6% in 1979 to 44% in 1989, and the degree of Pen G-resistance also increased throughout the study. In 1989, the last year of study, 521 strains were tested; 151 and 80 strains showed intermediate and high-level Pen G-resistance, respectively. Similarly, Garcia-Leoni *et al.* (1992) studied *Strep. pneumoniae* strains during a 22-month period in a hospital in Spain. From a total of 163 strains 42.5% showed either intermediate or high-level resistance to Pen G. Liñares *et al.* (1992) studied the susceptibility of 1492 pneumococcal strains from 1979 to 1990. The incidence of Pen G-resistant strains increased from 4.3 in 1979 to 40% in 1990. In Spain the infection with high-level Pen G-resistant strains was associated with the previous use of beta-lactam antibiotics (Nava *et al.*, 1994).

In France Pen G-resistant pneumococci remained infrequent until 1986, but then increased to 12% in 1990. The frequency of high-level resistance to Pen G among Pen G-resistant isolates increased from 13% in 1988 to 48% in 1990 (Geslin *et al.*, 1992). Pneumococci, mainly with low-level resistance, have also been detected in Israel (Dagan *et al.*, 1994).

There was a very high level of pneumococcal resistance to Pen G in Hungary. A total of 135 isolates were tested. Overall as many as 58% from children were Pen G-resistant. Among the resistant strains isolated from children, highly resistant strains predominated, whilst the resistant strains from adults were mostly with an intermediate level of resistance. Most of the Pen G-resistant isolates were also resistant to tetracycline, erythromycin and co-trimoxazole and 30% of them also to chloramphenicol (Marton *et al.*, 1991; Marton, 1992). In Romania about 30% of pneumococcal strains were Pen G-resistant, but in Poland this percentage was apparently only 3% (Hryniewicz, 1994). There may be more foci of pneumococcal resistance in other countries of Eastern Europe and the former Soviet Union. In Hungary apparently the percentage of Pen G-resistant pneumococci had decreased somewhat in recent years because of more prudent use of the penicillins (Nowak, 1994).

In the UK and West European countries, other than Spain, resistant pneumococci have been detected, but their prevalence has been relatively low (Appelbaum, 1992; Nielsen and Henrichsen, 1993). In a survey in Australia only 1% of isolates had intermediate degree of resistance and none were highly resistant (Collignon and Bell, 1992). In a survey in Pakistan 11.1% of pneumococcal isolates showed intermediate Pen G-resistance (Mastro *et al.*, 1993). In many other developing countries the position is not known (Appelbaum, 1992). A 6% prevalence of Pen G-resistant strains has been reported from Uruguay (Hortal *et al.*, 1994). In Turkey low-level resistance was found in 30% of strains and high-level resistance in 17% (Gür *et al.*, 1994).

In the USA, when first surveyed, some 5% of pneumococci were Pen G-resistant, but most belonged to the intermediate category, highly resistant strains being less common. Thirty-five hospitals submitted 5459 *Strep. pneumoniae* strains to CDC; 274 (5%) of the isolates had an MIC for Pen G $\geq 0.1 \mu g$ per ml, but only one was highly resistant with an MIC of 4 (Spika *et al.*, 1991). However, highly resistant pneumococci were soon identified in the USA. Ten serotype 19A strains with Pen G MICs of 1.0–2.0 μg per ml were isolated in Brooklyn, New York. These isolates came from nasopharyngeal cultures of patients without pneumococcal disease (Simberkoff *et al.*, 1986). In a day-care center in Ohio, *Strep. pneumoniae* type 23F, resistant to Pen G (MIC 2 μg per ml) and other antimicrobial agents, was isolated from the middle ear fluid of a child with otitis media. In the subsequent survey of other children, 52 nasopharyngeal carriers of this resistant pneumococcus were found at that day-care center attended by 250 children. A few staff members also carried this organism (Reichler *et al.*, 1992). Pneumococci, mainly with intermediate degree of resistance have also been detected in the nasopharynx of children in other day-care centers in the USA (Henderson *et al.*, 1988; Rauch *et al.*, 1990; Musher, 1992). In a children's hospital in Texas 95 pneumococcal isolates were surveyed; 34 were Pen G-sensitive, 42 had intermediate resistance, and 19 were highly resistant. Fifteen of the 19 highly resistant strains were recovered from the middle ear of children (Mason *et al.*, 1992). Two patients in Oklahoma, USA had invasive pneumococcal disease due to *Strep. pneumoniae* with high-level Pen G-resistance (Haglund *et al.*, 1993).

In the USA 2–5% of isolates in general hospitals and 10–12% in tertiary care pediatric facilities soon showed some degree of Pen G-resistance (Mason *et al.*, 1992; Musher, 1992). Invasive disease such as meningitis or septicemia due to Pen G-resistant pneumococci appeared to be more prevalent in children under 4 years of age and elderly persons over 70 years old (Istre *et al.*, 1987). A more recent survey of 13 USA hospitals detected Pen G-resistance in 6.6% of isolates, including 1.3% of them with MICs of 2.0 μg per ml or more (Breiman *et al.*, 1994). The exact percentage of resistant pneumococcal strains in the USA is not known, but Jacoby (1994) estimated that in 1990–1991 some 15–20% of pneumococcal isolates showed some degree of Pen G-resistance and 2–3% of these had high-level resistance. In Alaska during 1986–1990, intermediate Pen G-resistance was found in 3.8% of isolates but high-level resistance was not encountered (Parkinson *et al.*, 1994). In a survey in Southwest Virginia 6% of isolates had an intermediate level of resistance, but 10% of the total were highly resistant (Evans *et al.*, 1995).

Resistant pneumococci can spread within one institution, from center to center within one country and also intercontinentally. Isolates of serotype 23F *Strep. pneumoniae* with high level resistance to Pen G were common in Spain. The same pneumococcus was identified in children in Cleveland USA. The Spanish and Cleveland isolates were compared by electrophoretic analysis of PBP profiles and other tests. All strains were identical suggesting that this antibiotic resistant clone of serotype 23F *Strep. pneumoniae* had spread from Spain to the USA (Muñoz *et al.*, 1991). Investigators at CDC found that a multiresistant clone of *Strep. pneumoniae* serotype 23F that was related to multiresistant isolates from Spain and South Africa became disseminated in the USA (McDougal *et al.*, 1992). A single multiresistant clone of pneumococci was introduced into Iceland from Spain in the late 1980s (Soares *et al.*, 1993).

Pneumococcal strains with intermediate or high-level Pen G-resistance also show elevated MICs to other beta-lactam antibiotics such as cloxacillin, cephalothin, piperacillin, and cefamandole. They may show less decrease in sensitivity to ampicillin. Cefotaxime, ceftriaxone and imipenem are usually more active than Pen G against these pneumococci and have been useful to treat infections due to such strains, but compared with their activity against Pen G-susceptible strains, their activity is reduced 50- to 150-fold (Landesman *et al.*, 1981; Ward and Moellering, 1981; Jacobs, 1992 (see below). New cephalosporins such as cefpirome, and cefpodoxime also show good activity against these strains (Appelbaum *et al.*, 1989; Mason *et al.*, 1992; Goldstein and Garau, 1994).

Most human infections caused by pneumococcal strains of intermediate resistance (but not necessarily those caused by highly resistant strains) usually respond to Pen G, provided that sufficiently large doses are used (Hansman, 1976; Ward, 1981). But the response of serious infections, especially meningitis, caused by these pneumococci, has been poor after standard Pen G regimens (Howes and Mitchell, 1976; Gartner and Michaels, 1979; Caputo *et al.*, 1983; Collignon *et al.*, 1988; de Sousa Marques *et al.*, 1988; Weingarten *et al.*, 1990). A poor response has also been observed in some patients with severe pneumococcal pneumonia (Devitt *et al.*, 1977).

As both intermediate and highly resistant pneumococci are also resistant to other unrelated antibiotics, treatment of infections by these strains is difficult. Many Pen G-resistant pneumococci are also resistant to erythromycin, tetracycline and co-trimoxazole and less commonly chloramphenicol (Jorgensen *et al.*, 1990; Schwartz *et al.*, 1991; Musher, 1992). Erythromycin- and clindamycin-resistance among these strains is quite common in Spain (Latorre *et al.*, 1985). Most strains so far have remained sensitive to rifampicin and vancomycin, similar to multiply-resistant strains in South Africa (p. 5).

As the MICs of cefotaxime (p. 320) and ceftriaxone (p. 352) are usually lower than those of Pen G, and as these drugs penetrate well into the CSF, they have been used with success to treat pneumococcal meningitis, even if the MIC for Pen G has been as high as 1.0 μg per ml. Vancomycin has also been used to treat meningitis with differing results. Some cases have failed to respond to chloramphenicol even when the strain has been chloramphenicol-sensitive. Four epidemiologically unrelated cases of pneumococcal meningitis due to organisms that were also highly resistant to ceftriaxone (MIC≥ 8 μg per ml) have been reported; these patients failed to respond to ceftriaxone, although vancomycin with or without chloramphenicol did succeed. There are now also other reports of strains of Pen G-resistant pneumococci, whose MICs of cefotaxime (p. 320) and ceftriaxone (p. 352) were higher than those of Pen G. It now seems that some of the newer quinolones, such as sparfloxacin (p. 1141) will have to be investigated for the treatment of Pen G-resistant pneumococcal infections (Jacobs, 1992; Musher, 1992; Spangler *et al.*, 1992, 1993).

Original studies with multiply-resistant South African pneumococci failed to demonstrate beta-lactamases, or plasmids (p. 549) suggesting intrinsic resistance. The mechanism by which these pneumococci acquire resistance is by the development of specific, stepwise and cumulative alterations in four of their six PBPs (p. 27) (Zighelboim and Tomasz, 1980; Tomasz, 1982). Sensitive strains of *Strep. pneumoniae* contain six PBPs – 1a, 1b, 2x, 2a, 2b and 3. The PBPs in *Strep. pneumoniae* are somewhat complicated. Characterization of PBP profiles has revealed a considerable degree of antigenic variation among PBPs of Pen G-sensitive strains (Hakenbeck *et al.*, 1991a). In Pen G-resistant strains there is a cumulative stepwise change in the PBPs as the Pen G MIC of that strain increases. As the MIC of the strain reaches 0.4 μg per ml, four of the pneumococcal PBPs undergo changes in their Pen G affinity. At the higher levels of resistance (MIC> 0.4 μg per ml), the *Strep. pneumoniae* cell no longer contains PBPs 1a and 1b, but it now has a new PBP 1c which has an extremely low affinity to Pen G; PBP 2b is also altered (Smith and Klugman, 1995). With selective pressure, pneumococci with low-level resistance represent a reservoir from which highly resistant strains may emerge during clinical therapy (Handwerger and Tomasz, 1986a,b; Malouin and Bryan, 1986; Tomasz, 1986; Chalkley and Koornhof, 1988).

Multiply-resistant clinical isolates of *Strep. pneumoniae* from South Africa exhibited penicillin tolerance (p. 27). Exposing these strains to Pen G concentrations above their MICs did not induce cell wall degradation, lysis or leakage of intracellular components. Their cell walls contained less autolytic enzyme (p. 27), but they were not completely deficient of this enzyme which was usually the case with other tolerant organisms (p. 27). Pen G tolerance of these pneumococcal strains may be related to some alteration in the control of autolysin activity (Liu and Tomasz, 1985). Subsequently Moreillon and Tomasz (1988) demonstrated that treatment of pneumococcal cultures with cycles of high Pen G concentration selected lysis-defective mutants, whilst exposure to sustained low levels of pen G produced resistant mutants. As both types of exposure occur clinically, defective lysis and Pen G-resistance will often co-exist.

Pneumococcal resistance to Pen G is chromosomal, plasmids are not involved and this resistance is not transferable by conjugation (Murray, 1989). Yet Pen G-resistance in pneumococci can result not only by exposing the organisms to Pen G, but transfer of a resistance gene (DNA) from a resistant pneumococcal strain to a sensitive one. Transfer of Pen G-resistance determinants may also occur from resistant viridans streptococci (such as *Strep. sanguis* and *Strep. mitior*) to sensitive *Strep. pneumoniae* (Chalkley and Koornhof, 1990; Potgieter and Chalkley, 1991). There is some evidence that transposons (p. 550), in the chromosome of a *Strep. pneumoniae* could facilitate the dissemination of Pen G-resistance in the absence of plasmids (Cooksey *et al.*, 1989).

Examination of several hundred Pen G-resistant clinical isolates of *Strep. pneumoniae* revealed extensive strain-to-strain variation in the number and molecular size of their PBPs. Resistant isolates can be classified into groups, and it appears that each group or clone is prevalent in a specific geographic area. Resistant strains have emerged independently in different locations (Jabes *et al.*, 1983; Hakenbeck *et al.*, 1991b; Muñoz *et al.*, 1992a; Waltman *et al.* 1992; Smith *et al.*, 1993; Versalovic *et al.*, 1993).

Sensitivity tests should be performed on at least all pneumococcal isolates implicated in serious infections. Where practicable all pneumococcal isolates should be tested. Relatively resistant strains may not be recognized unless special laboratory methods are used (Swenson *et al.*, 1986; Jacobs, 1992). For routine testing of penicillin susceptibility of *Strep. pneumoniae*, 1-μg oxacillin discs have been widely used. However, strains of *Strep. pneumoniae* have been detected with intermediate resistance to oxacillin (MIC 1 μg per ml). These isolates showed similar low grade resistance to methicillin, cloxacillin and cefotaxime. Surprisingly they were completely sensitive to Pen G. Such strains may be wrongly regarded as having intermediate Pen G-resistance, unless Pen G itself is used in sensitivity testing. Such oxacillin-resistance is due to acquisition of a gene encoding an altered PBP, PBP2X (Dowson *et al.*, 1994).

e Streptococcus viridans (alpha-hemolytic streptococci) These streptococci may be further subdivided into species, such as *Strep. sanguis*, *Strep. mitior* (*mitis*), *Strep. mutans*, *Strep. milleri*, *Strep. salivarius* and *Strep. constellatus*. This subdivision has relatively little clinical significance. *Streptococcus viridans* is a common cause of bacterial endocarditis (Rapeport *et al.*, 1986; Shulman, 1986; Stein and Nelson, 1987), but *Strep. milleri* is also implicated in serious suppurative infections in various parts of the body (Gossling, 1988; Gelfand *et al.*, 1991; Jacobs *et al.*, 1994) (p. 40).

Streptococcus viridans is usually Pen G-sensitive (Bourgault *et al.*, 1979; Little *et al.*, 1979). Resistant variants may be found in the pharynx and teeth cavities of patients who have been treated by a penicillin, or who have received oral penicillin V for prolonged periods to prevent rheumatic fever (p. 75) (Phillips *et al.*, 1976). In contrast, patients treated with monthly i.m. benzathine penicillin have had little, if any, increase in resistant *Strep. viridans* strains.

Pen G-resistant viridans streptococci have been isolated from the oral flora (Hess *et al.*, 1983a) and from the blood (Rahman, 1982), from patients who have not received prior penicillin therapy. Venditti *et al.* (1989) studied 63 streptococcal isolates (most *Strep. viridans*) obtained from blood cultures of neutropenic patients; 80% were Pen G-sensitive and the others showed varying degrees of resistance. Wilcox *et al.* (1993) tested 44 *Strep. viridans* strains collected from patients with endocarditis; 20% of them were Pen G- resistant. Another study demonstrated that Pen G-resistant viridans streptococci resided more commonly in the mouths of children (both healthy ones and those suffering from leukemia), compared with adults (Guiot *et al.*, 1994). Highly resistant viridans streptococci were detected initially in South Africa in association with

Pen G-resistant pneumococci (p. 5). Later they appeared also in other countries. These strains were resistant to Pen G, penicillinase-resistant penicillins, cephalosporins, piperacillin, azlocillin and mezlocillin, but susceptible to vancomycin. They had altered PBPs (p. 7), similar to the Pen G-resistant pneumococci (Farber *et al.*, 1983a; Quinn *et al.*, 1988).

Frequently, *Strep. viridans* strains are Pen G tolerant (p. 27) (Dankert and Hess, 1982; James 1990). In particular, *Strep. sanguis* appears to be an inherently Pen G-tolerant organism; although its cell growth is inhibited by very low concentrations, Pen G is not bactericidal. *Streptococcus sanguis* is defective in autolysins which are essential for the irreversible bactericidal effect of Pen G (Horne and Tomasz, 1977) (p. 27). 'Nutritionally variant' streptococci have been isolated from 5–10% of patients with viridans streptococcal endocarditis (Gephart and Washington, 1982). These require supplemental media for isolation and sensitivity testing, and they may be Pen G-sensitive, resistant or tolerant (Feder *et al.*, 1980; Stein and Nelson, 1987). Eleven such strains tested by Holloway and Dankert (1982) were all tolerant to Pen G.

Tolerant *Strep. viridans* strains may possibly be responsible for failures of Pen G to protect against bacterial endocarditis (Holloway *et al.*, 1980). It is not known whether a synergistic Pen G/streptomycin combination would be more effective in this situation (Hess *et al.*, 1983a). In experimental endocarditis in rabbits, Pen G therapy was more effective if the infecting *Strep. viridans* strain was non-tolerant rather than tolerant (Meeson *et al.*, 1990). Pen G/streptomycin combination was more effective than Pen G alone in preventing endocarditis due to a tolerant *Strep. sanguis* strain (Hess *et al.*, 1983b). In induced endocarditis in rabbits due to tolerant strains, a Pen G/streptomycin combination was effective, but Pen G alone was also curative if a high-dose regimen was used (Brennan and Durack, 1983; Lowy *et al.*, 1983; Wilson *et al.*, 1985). In humans, occasionally the therapeutic failure of Pen G alone in viridans endocarditis has been attributed to 'tolerance' (Anderson and Cruickshank, 1982). Nevertheless, in general, Pen G alone has been as effective as Pen G/streptomycin regimen for *Strep. viridans* endocarditis (p. 41). If a patient is responsive both clinically and bacteriologically, despite a demonstration of Pen G tolerance for the infecting organism, it is unnecessary to alter antimicrobial therapy on the basis of this *in vitro* observation (Kim, 1988). The MBCs determined by conventional methods are often inaccurate and so a non-tolerant *Strep. viridans* strains may be labeled incorrectly as tolerant (James, 1990).

In vitro synergy between Pen G (or other penicillins, cephalosporins and vancomycin) and any of the aminoglycosides usually occurs with virtually all *Strep. viridans* strains, unlike *Enterococcus faecalis* (p. 455) (Sande and Scheld, 1980). Some *Strep. viridans* clinical isolates have exhibited high-level streptomycin-resistance (MICs > 2000 μg per ml). Pen G and streptomycin were not synergistic against these strains, but a combination of pen G and gentamicin was (Farber *et al.*, 1983b).

f Enterococci   *Enterococcus faecalis* and *E. faecium* are now classified in their own genus, the *Enterococcus* (Herman and Gerding, 1991). Less commonly encountered members of the enterococci include *E. durans*, *E. raffinosus* and *E. avium* (Grayson *et al.*, 1991b). Compared with streptococci, described in previous sections, *E. faecalis* is much less sensitive to Pen G and *E. faecium* is even less so (Table I.1) (Moellering *et al.*, 1979; Murray, 1991).

Enterococci were considered to be naturally occurring tolerant organisms (p. 27); penicillins and other drugs which act on the cell wall (e.g. vancomycin, cycloserine and bacitracin) have a MBC/MIC ratio of >32 for enterococci (Krogstad and Parquette, 1980). But it has now been shown that tolerance is an acquired characteristic and not necessarily intrinsic. The MICs of Pen G for enterococci from an antibiotic virgin area of the Solomon Islands were similar to those of strains isolated in the USA. However, the organisms from the Solomon Islands rapidly lyzed and were killed by concentrations of Pen G just above the MIC. After short exposure to Pen G *in vitro*, these organisms, like strains in the USA, rapidly became tolerant to beta-lactams (Moellering, 1991). Clinical isolates of enterococci often exhibit a peculiar type of tolerance to beta-lactams, in that these bacteria may be killed by relatively low antibiotic concentrations (2x to 4x MIC), but the percentage of survivors increases at increasing antibiotic concentrations (Shah, 1982; Fontana *et al.*, 1990a). When studying 50 clinical isolates of *E. faecalis*, Fontana *et al.* (1990b) found that this paradoxical response and tolerance were not exhibited by all strains. Some 22% of the strains were paradoxically responding but not tolerant, 65% were paradoxically responding and tolerant, 12% were neither paradoxically responding nor tolerant and only 2% were tolerant but not paradoxically responding.

The reason why enterococci have relatively high MICs to Pen G and several other penicillins such as ampicillin (p. 115) and are completely resistant to other penicillins such as methicillin, and to all cephalosporins is due to diminished affinity of their PBPs for these drugs; PBP 5 is of special importance. This PBP has low affinity for penicillins and is responsible for the relatively high MICs of *E. faecalis* and *E. faecium* to Pen G. If enterococcal cells manufacture more PBP 5, they develop intrinsic resistance to Pen G and ampicillin (p. 108). This indicates that PBP 5 has the potential capacity to take over the functions of all other PBPs and therefore can fully compensate for their activity in cells overproducing PBP 5 (Al Obeid *et al.*, 1990a,b; Moellering, 1991; Fontana *et al.*, 1992, 1994). In one experiment *in vitro* it was possible to derive an *E. faecium* strain which had no PBP 5. This strain could function normally and was very sensitive to all penicillins and cephalosporins (Fontana *et al.*, 1985).

Enterococci with this intrinsic Pen G-resistance have caused outbreaks in hospitals (Oster *et al.*, 1990). In one hospital the Pen G susceptibility of *E. faecium* was studied from strains isolated for 22 years starting in 1968. From 1969 to 1988 the geometric mean MIC was 14 μg per ml, whereas this was 123 μg per ml from 1989 to 1990. In the more recently isolated resistant strains, the penicillin-binding affinity of PBP 5 was notably lower (Grayson *et al.*, 1991a). Two *E. faecium* isolates were described which had high-level resistance to Pen G due to altered PBP 5, and these strains were also resistant to vancomycin (Handwerger *et al.*, 1992). Nosocomial outbreaks due to *E. faecium* have been reported where the strains had a high intrinsic resistance to Pen G, and they were also resistant to gentamicin and vancomycin (Handwerger *et al.*, 1993; Landman *et al.*, 1993). Experimental endocarditis in animals due to such strains partially responded to a ciprofloxacin, rifampicin and gentamicin combination, but the infection was not eradicated in 5 days (Whitman *et al.*, 1993). If the strain of *E. faecium* is not gentamicin-resistant, then if the Pen G MIC is lower than 200 μg per ml, Pen G and gentamicin combination is synergistic. It may be possible to treat infections by such strains with high-dose Pen G plus gentamicin (Torres *et al.*, 1993).

In vitro experiments have shown that increase in Pen G-resistance of *E. faecalis* with changes in PBPs can be obtained by exposure of the strain to stepwise increasing concentrations of Pen G or, to a lesser extent, by exposure to unchanging concentrations for a prolonged time. Pulsed administration of Pen G did not select intrinsic resistance (Hodges *et al.*, 1992).

The uncommon enterococci, *E. avium* and raffinosus have different Pen G susceptibilities. The MIC range for the former is 0.5–2 μg per ml, and for the latter 4–64 μg per ml. *Enterococcus raffinosus* appears to have a PBP 7 which is a low affinity PBP and this may play a role in the relative Pen G-resistance of this species (Grayson *et al.*, 1991b; Patel *et al.*, 1993).

Klare *et al.* (1992) considered that the overproduction of PBP 5 is not the only intrinsic resistance mechanism for enterococci. These authors found that overproduction of PBP 5 occurred in *E. faecium* strains, which were moderately Pen G-resistant, but when MICs were 128 μg per ml, this was no longer so and other so far unknown mechanisms were presumably involved.

Another mechanism of Pen G-resistance in the enterococci is beta-lactamase production. This was first described by Murray and Mederski-Samoray (1983) for one strain of *E. faecalis*. Soon such strains were found in other areas in the USA and also elsewhere in the world (George and Uttley, 1989; Murray, 1989, 1991; Moellering, 1992). There was one large outbreak of colonization with beta-lactamase producing enterococci in a children's hospital in Boston (Rhinehart *et al.*, 1990). Another study found evidence for clonal spread of a single strain of beta-lactamase-producing *E. faecalis* to six hospitals in five states in the USA (Murray *et al.*, 1991).

The beta-lactamase produced by some *E. faecalis* strains is similar to that produced by *Staph. aureus* (p. 11) and it is encoded on plasmids, which can be transferred by conjugation (Murray *et al.*, 1986; Zscheck *et al.*, 1988; Patterson *et al.*, 1990; Murray, 1992). One *E. faecalis* strain was found to contain three conjugative plasmids and a conjugative transposon (p. 549). These encoded beta-lactamase production, gentamicin-resistance and also resistance to other antibiotics (Murray *et al.*, 1988). All such *E. faecalis* strains have not arisen from a single strain, as there is significant variation in the plasmids which encode beta-lactamase (Smith and Murray, 1992). By contrast, other authors have found that in *E. faecalis* strains producing beta-lactamase, the beta-lactamase gene was integrated into the bacterial chromosome (Rice *et al.*, 1991b; Chow *et al.*, 1993; Rice and Marshall, 1994).

Similar to *Staph. aureus* beta-lactamase, the enzyme produced by *E. faecalis* can be inhibited by beta-lactamase inhibitors such as clavulanic acid (p. 192) (Murray, 1991). This can be utilized in treatment. Patterson *et al.* (1988b) reported two strains of *E. faecalis* which produced beta-lactamase. One also had high-level gentamicin-resistance (p. 456), but the other did not. With the latter it was possible to demonstrate synergistic killing with a combination of Pen G, clavulanic acid and gentamicin, but not with the former. Unfortunately the majority of beta-lactamase-producing strains of *E. faecalis* also show high-level gentamicin-resistance (Patterson *et al.*, 1988a; Murray, 1989; Rice *et al.*, 1991a; Chow *et al.*, 1993).

At least one *E. faecalis* strain has been reported which produced beta-lactamase and was also resistant to vancomycin (p. 765) (Handwerger *et al.*, 1992). Beta-lactamase production has been largely reported in *E. faecalis* and not with other enterococcal species. Coudron *et al.* (1992) reported one isolate of *E. faecium* which produced beta-lactamase. This was plasmid mediated and transferable into other plasmid-free *E. faecium* strains. The strain also showed high-level aminoglycoside-resistance.

g   Non-enterococcal Group D streptococci   Unlike the enterococci, these organisms, such as *Strep. bovis*, which may cause endocarditis, are nearly always highly sensitive to Pen G (Tuazon *et al.*, 1986). Similar to *Strep. viridans* (p. 9), Pen G acts synergistically with any of the aminoglycosides against non-enterococcal Group D streptococci (Moellering *et al.*, 1974; Sande and Scheld, 1980).

h   Rare human pathogens   Leuconostoc species are members of the family Streptococcaceae, and they only rarely cause infections, mainly in compromised hosts. These bacteria are moderately susceptible to Pen G, MICs ranging from 0.25 to 1.0 µg per ml (Handwerger *et al.*, 1990). *Stomatococcus mucilaginosus* (*Micrococcus mucilaginosus*) rarely causes septicemia in neutropenic patients. Its sensitivity to Pen G is variable, but the organism is always susceptible to vancomycin (McWhinney *et al.*, 1992; Henwick *et al.*, 1993; Tan *et al.*, 1994). *Micrococcus* is usually Pen G-sensitive (Von Eiff *et al.*, 1995).

i   Staphylococcus aureus   Originally this was very sensitive to Pen G, but the prevalence of Pen G-resistant *Staph. aureus* strains in hospitals increased during the period 1942–1958 reaching a value of >70% of all isolates. Resistance was due to the production of beta-lactamases (penicillinases) which rapidly hydrolyze Pen G (Richmond, 1979), and this was mediated by conjugative plasmids (Kaplan and Tenenbaum, 1982). A variety of beta-lactamase plasmids were been found in naturally occurring strains of Pen G-resistant *Staph. aureus*. In addition an increasing number of strains were described in which the genes for beta-lactamase production were apparently located on the chromosome. A beta-lactamase transposon (p. 550) may also be present in some strains (Lyon and Skurray, 1987; Weber and Goering, 1988).

Staphylococcus aureus produces four types of beta-lactamase (A, B, C, and D). Types A, B, and C exhibit comparable activity against Pen G, but type D hydrolyzes the drug less rapidly. These four beta-lactamases vary as to how rapidly they hydrolyze other beta-lactams, e.g. the cephalosporins (Zygmunt *et al.*, 1992).

Over the years, the majority of *Staph. aureus* strains, even outside hospitals, became beta-lactamase producers and resistant to Pen G (Bengtsson *et al.*, 1977; Helling *et al.*, 1980). One survey in Denmark showed that 86–87% of isolates were Pen G-resistant, and this percentage was the same with strains isolated in the community as those isolated in hospitals (Rosdahl *et al.*, 1990). Another Danish survey showed that during the period 1977–1990 the frequency of Pen G-resistance increased from 78.7 to 87.5% among a total of 278 193 *Staph. aureus* strains isolated from hospitalized patients (Renneberg and Rosdahl, 1992).

Resistance of *Staph. aureus* can also be intrinsic due to a cell wall change which renders them resistant to Pen G and to all other penicillins, including the penicillinase-resistant penicillins and cephalosporins (methicillin-resistant staphylococci, p. 77). This is never the sole mechanism whereby *Staph. aureus* is resistant to Pen G, because all strains with intrinsic resistance also produce beta-lactamases.

Staphylococcus aureus may also be Pen G-tolerant. Staphylococci exhibiting this phenomenon have deficient cell wall autolytic enzyme activity. This enzyme augments bacterial cell wall damage initiated by Pen G and the combined action produces a lethal effect on bacteria (Sabath *et al.*, 1977) (p. 27). Although the penicillins inhibit these organisms in usual concentrations, they are not bactericidal. Further aspects of tolerance of *Staph. aureus* to the penicillin group of drugs are discussed on pp. 81, 91.

j   Coagulase-negative staphylococci   These constitute a heterogenous group of organisms among which 15 different species are recognized (Parisi, 1985). Three, *Staph. epidermidis* (*Staph. albus*), *Staph. haemolyticus* and *Staph. saprophyticus*, are common pathogens particularly associated with the use of indwelling foreign devices and urinary tract infections. *Staph. epidermidis* may be Pen G-sensitive, but the majority of strains are resistant (>80% of isolates in the UK) because, similar to *Staph. aureus* (see above), they produce plasmid-mediated beta-lactamases (Price and Flournoy, 1982; Richardson and Marples, 1982). Exchange of plasmids may occur *in vivo* between *Staph. epidermidis* and *Staph. aureus* (Totten *et al.*, 1981).

Also *Staph. epidermidis* may possess intrinsic resistance to the penicillins, rendering them methicillin-resistant (p. 81). Originally *Staph. saprophyticus* was regarded as being always Pen G-sensitive (Wallmark *et al.*, 1978). Subsequently, an intermediate level of resistance for these organisms was described, but the distinction of sensitive and resistant strains by usual laboratory tests was difficult. Resistance appeared to be due to a beta-lactamase but its activity and quantity was much less than that produced by *Staph. epidermidis*. The clinical significance of this resistance in *Staph. saprophyticus* is uncertain (Price and Flournoy, 1982; Richardson and Marples, 1980). Usually *Staph. haemolyticus* is Pen G-resistant; many strains are also methicillin-resistant and some are now also vancomycin-resistant (p. 766) (Isaac *et al.*, 1993).

k Staphylococcus lugdunensis This is an uncommon pathogen which has caused endocarditis, septicemia, deep tissue infections and osteomyelitis. Of 59 strains tested by Herchline *et al.* (1990), 76% were beta-lactamase-negative and Pen G-sensitive, but 24% produced beta-lactamase and were Pen G-resistant. All strains were susceptible to oxacillin and to vancomycin.

l Anaerobic Gram-positive cocci These organisms which include *Peptococcus* and *Peptostreptococcus* spp. and anaerobic streptococci, are nearly always highly susceptible to Pen G (Sutter and Finegold, 1976).

2 Gram-positive bacilli

Corynebacterium diphtheriae is consistently sensitive to Pen G (Maple *et al.*, 1994). Other corynebacteria vary in sensitivity. Usually *C. pseudodiphthericum*, which may cause pneumonia or endocarditis, is susceptible (Colt *et al.*, 1991; Morris and Guild, 1991; Manzella *et al.*, 1995); *C. kerosis* may also be Pen G-sensitive (Booth *et al.*, 1991); *C. striatum* is usually Pen G-sensitive (Watkins *et al.*, 1993) and so is CDC Coryneform Group ANF-3 (Petit *et al.*, 1994); *C. bovis* varies in its sensitivity, whereas corynebacteria of Group JK (*C. jeikeium*) are always Pen G-resistant (Lipsky *et al.*, 1982). *Arcanobacterium* (formerly *Corynebacterium*) *haemolyticum*, which causes pharyngitis, is Pen G-sensitive (Carlson *et al.*, 1995).

Bacillus anthracis is susceptible to Pen G (Doganay and Aydin, 1991). Other *Bacillus* spp. can also cause serious infections in humans such as endocarditis, meningitis and surgical wound infections. Weber *et al.* (1988) studied 89 strains, all isolated from blood cultures of patients: *B. cereus* (54 strains) was the most common species and this was Pen G-resistant, but susceptible to imipenem (p. 228), vancomycin (p. 764), chloramphenicol, gentamicin (p. 457) and ciprofloxacin (p. 985). The rarer species such as *B. megaterium*, *B. polymyxa*, *B. pumilus* and *B. subtilis* were in general Pen G-sensitive but there was variability among the species.

Listeria monocytogenes is usually Pen G sensitive (Prichard *et al.*, 1983; Larsson *et al.*, 1985). This organism has five PBPs and PBP3 is an essential protein which is able to support normal growth of *L. monocytogenes* by itself and therefore becomes the lethal target for beta-lactams. Cephalosporins, unlike Pen G, interact poorly with PBP 3, so *L. monocytogenes* is resistant to cephalosporins. The organism is sensitive to imipenem (p. 228). In a laboratory an imipenem-resistant mutant of *L. monocytogenes* was produced and this mutant had altered PBP 3, which also had reduced affinity for Pen G (Vicente *et al.*, 1990).

Listeria monocytogenes may show tolerance (p. 27) to Pen G and sometimes this may be to a very high degree (Stamm *et al.*, 1982). But if subcultures are performed after 48 h rather than 24 h incubation, Pen G is bactericidal to most strains of *L. monocytogenes*. In this respect. *L. monocytogenes* is similar to *Staph. aureus* (p. 91) because the detection of tolerance depends on the laboratory test used and may be of marginal clinical significance (Winslow *et al.*, 1983). Pen G and gentamicin (p. 456) act synergistically against *L. monocytogenes* both *in vitro* and in experimental animal infections (Edmiston and Gordon, 1979; Scheld *et al.*, 1979). *Nocardia* spp. are Pen G-resistant (Gutmann *et al.*, 1983). *Rhodococcus equi* is a Gram-positive aerobic coccobacillus. It was previously known only as an animal pathogen, but now it has been added to the list of opportunistic pathogens in patients with AIDS in whom it usually causes a necrotizing pneumonia. *Rhodococcus equi* is Pen G-resistant, but it is generally susceptible to vancomycin (p. 764), erythromycin (p. 607), aminoglycosides and chloramphenicol (p. 555) (Emmons *et al.*, 1991). *Erysipelothrix rhusopathiae* is sensitive to Pen G (Gransden and Eykyn, 1988; Venditti *et al.*, 1990). A rare human pathogen, *Rothia dentocariosa*, is usually Pen G-sensitive (Anderson *et al.*, 1993; Sudduth *et al.*, 1993).

Anaerobic Gram-positive sporing bacilli, such as *Clostridium tetani*, *Cl. perfringens* (*welchii*), *Cl. septicum*, *Cl. botulinum*, *Cl. innocum* and *Cl. ramosum* are nearly always Pen G-sensitive (Swenson *et al.*, 1980; Gabay *et al.*, 1981; Dyewski *et al.*, 1989; Finegold, 1989; Nord and

Hedberg, 1990). Resistant strains of *Cl. perfringens* and other *Clostridium* spp. have been detected (Silpa *et al.*, 1982; Finegold, 1989). Relatively resistant strains of *Cl. perfringens* have also been reported. Brown and Waatti (1980) tested 44 *Cl. perfringens* strains; only 68% were inhibited by < 0.25 μg per ml of Pen G, the remainder requiring either 0.5, 1.0, or even 4.0 μg per ml for inhibition. The MICs of 45 *Cl. perfringens* strains tested by Marrie *et al.* (1981) were in the range of 0.15–9.0 μg per ml;, half were inhibited by 0.15 μg per ml and 90% by 5.0 μg per ml. Therefore routine sensitivity testing of clinical isolates of *Cl. perfringens* is advisable; *Cl. perfringens* contains six PBPs. Resistance to Pen G in *Cl. perfringens* is mediated by a decreased affinity of the largest PBP 1 for the antibiotic (Finegold, 1989; Nord and Hedberg, 1990). Possibly *Cl. butyricum* may be Pen G-resistant due to beta-lactamase production (Finegold, 1989); *Cl. tertium* is only moderately Pen G-susceptible, the MICs ranging from 0.25 to 8 μg per ml (Speirs *et al.*, 1988). Nearly always *Cl. sordellii* is Pen G-sensitive (Spera *et al.*, 1992); nearly always *Cl. difficile* isolates from patients with antibiotic-associated colitis (p. 594) are sensitive to Pen G (Dzink and Bartlett, 1980; Levett, 1988).

Pen G is active against nearly all strains of anaerobic Gram-positive asporogenous bacilli, such as the *Actinomyces*, *Eubacterium*, *Propionibacterium*, *Bifidobacterium* and *Lactobacillus* spp. (Sutter and Finegold, 1976; Holmberg *et al.*, 1977; Denys *et al.*, 1983; Fife *et al.*, 1991; Brook and Frazier, 1991; 1993). Lactobacilli are being recognized increasingly as important pathogens causing infections such as bacterial endocarditis and neonatal meningitis (Griffiths *et al.*, 1992). Their MICs for Pen G are quite low (0.3–1.0 μg per ml), but MBCs for about 75% of strains are high (Bayer *et al.*, 1978), indicating tolerance (p. 27). Pen G (or ampicillin) combined with either streptomycin or gentamicin are synergistic *in vitro* against tolerant *Lactobacillus* spp. strains (Bayer *et al.*, 1980; Griffiths *et al.*, 1992).

3 Gram-negative cocci

Neisseria meningitidis has been sensitive to Pen G for many years, but now a few reports of resistant strains have appeared. The organism is occasionally isolated from the genitourinary tract and/or anal canal of patients tested for gonorrhea (William *et al.*, 1979), so it is possible that plasmids can be transferred from gonococci to meningococci. A strain of *N. meningitidis* was isolated in Canada which harbored the 4.5 megadalton beta-lactamase-producing plasmid and the transfer factor, which were present in beta-lactamase-producing gonococci (p. 15) (Dillon *et al.*, 1983). It was then demonstrated by Roberts and Knapp (1988) *in vitro* that beta-lactamase-producing *N. gonorrhoeae* could easily transfer resistance plasmids to *N. meningitidis*. Thereafter Botha (1988) from South Africa described three patients with clinical meningococcal meningitis. Two had organisms with MICs to Pen G greater than 256 μg per ml and these produced beta-lactamase. The third had an MIC of 0.25 μg per ml and this had relative intrinsic resistance. A further report of beta-lactamase-producing *N. meningitidis* came from Spain (Fontanals *et al.* 1989), but other reports from Spain mainly described isolates, relatively resistant to Pen G due to intrinsic resistance.

Van Esso *et al.* (1987) reported four clinical isolates of meningococci whose MICs ranged from 0.25 to 0.5 μg per ml. They did not produce beta-lactamase, and intrinsic resistance due to altered PBPs appeared likely. Ten similar clinical isolates were reported from Spain by Uriz *et al.* (1991). The frequency of this type of meningococcal strain in Spain increased from 0.4% in 1985 to 41.6% in 1991 and these relatively resistant strains were found among both serogroup B and C isolates (Berrón and Vásquez, 1994). Meningitis caused by these strains still responded to Pen G, but defervescence was slower. If the MIC of the meningococcus is higher than 0.5 μg per ml, the disease may not respond to Pen G and alternative therapy, such as chloramphenicol, cefotaxime or ceftriaxone, may be needed (Buck, 1994; Woods *et al.*, 1994). All the Pen G-resistant strains were sensitive to chloramphenicol, rifampicin, cefotaxime and ceftriaxone. Relatively Pen G-insensitive meningococci have also been reported from the UK (Sutcliffe *et al.*, 1988), from Argentina (Lopardo *et al.*, 1993), from Israel (Block *et al.*, 1993) and from the USA (Buck, 1994; Jackson *et al.*, 1994; Woods *et al.*, 1994). Twelve of 43 *N. meningitidis* isolates from genital and anorectal sites, tested at CDC USA, were relatively resistant to Pen G (MIC range 0.125–0.5 μg per ml) (Winterscheid *et al.*, 1994). Special disc susceptibility tests should be used to detect these relatively resistant meningococci (Campos *et al.*, 1987; 1992b).

This relative resistance is due, at least in part, to a decreased affinity of PBP 2 for Pen G. Similar low-affinity forms of PBP 2 are also found in Pen G-resistant isolates of *N. lactamica* (p. 16), *N. polysacharea* and *N. gonorrhoeae* (Saez-Nieto *et al.*, 1992). There is great genetic diversity in Pen G-resistant *N. meningitidis*. Campos *et al.* (1992a) studied 42 Pen G-resistant strains obtained in Spain. Since Pen G-resistant meningococci have been isolated only relatively recently, it might be expected that they would be derived from one or a few original resistant isolates. But these studies showed considerable diversity in the PBP 2 genes and in the overall genetic relatedness of Pen G-resistant meningococci isolated from one hospital in 2 years. This suggested that horizontal spread of altered PBP 2 genes, along with clonal spread, is important in the epidemiology of Pen G-resistant meningococci. Zhang *et al.* (1990), who also found similar genetic diversity among Pen G-resistant meningococci, noted that some strains isolated in the UK and others in Spain were similar and appeared to belong to the same Pen G-resistant clone.

Originally *N. gonorrhoeae* was always sensitive to Pen G (Table I.1) (Catlin and Reyn, 1982), but this has changed drastically. Relatively resistant gonococcal variants appeared about 30 years ago, and not only has their degree of resistance slowly increased, but they have become more frequent (Gords *et al.*, 1982; Rice *et al.*, 1986). Their MICs vary, the majority of strains requiring at least 0.08 μg per ml for inhibition (Gords *et al.*, 1982; Ison *et al.*, 1987) whilst the remainder require 0.12–2.0 μg per ml (Rodriguez and Saz, 1975; Dowsett, 1980). Relatively resistant gonococci have been detected in most countries including the USA (Thornsberry *et al.*, 1978b; Rice *et al.* 1986), the UK (Ison *et al.*, 1987), Australia (Australian Gonococcal Surveillance Programme, 1988), Japan (Yoshida *et al.*, 1982), South Africa (Liebovitz *et al.* 1982), Taiwan (Chu *et al.*, 1992), Philippines (Clendennen *et al.*, 1992a), Thailand (Clendennen *et al.*, 1992b) and Germany (Abeck *et al.*, 1988). In the USA relatively resistant gonococci were more common in black patients, in patients who had received antimicrobials within the previous 2 weeks and in men with symptomatic urethritis (Thornsberry *et al.*, 1978b). There was no difference in the sensitivity of strains isolated from white patients or Carribean immigrants in the UK (Rodin *et al.*, 1980).

Relatively resistant gonococcal strains were often relatively resistant to other unrelated antibiotics, such as tetracyclines, erythromycin, chloramphenicol, streptomycin, rifampicin and less commonly spectinomycin. These organisms were usually sensitive to newer cephalosporins, such as cefotaxime (p. 320), ceftriaxone (p. 352) and fluoroquinolones such as ciprofloxacin (p. 983) (Ison *et al.*, 1987; Abeck *et al.*, 1988; Van Klingeren *et al.*, 1988; Clendennen *et al.*, 1992a). Resistance to such chemically diverse drugs, may be caused by the mutation of a single gene (Maness and Sparling, 1973; Powell and Bond, 1976) (p. 724). It can be transferred in mixed gonococcal cultures but it is not mediated by plasmids (p. 549). Transfer of genes amongst gonococci may take place similarly in nature (Sarubbi and Sparling, 1974). This intrinsic resistance of relatively resistant strains to Pen G is chromosomally mediated (Hook and Holmes, 1985). Their PBP 2 and to a lesser extent PBP 1 bind less Pen G (Dougherty *et al.*, 1980; Dougherty, 1985; Garcia-Bustos and Dougherty, 1987; Spratt and Cromie, 1988).

Soon gonococcal stains with chromosomally mediated Pen G resistance with higher MICs than 2 μg per ml were isolated and these were completely resistant to this drug. Two gonococcal strains with such resistance to Pen G (MIC 30 μg per ml) were isolated in Toronto, Canada, and these did not produce beta-lactamase (see below) (Shtibel, 1980). Similar gonococci were then detected in the UK (Copley and Egglestone, 1982). In 1983, an outbreak of Pen G-resistant gonococcal infection was reported in North Carolina, USA, in which more than 200 cases were detected. Since then 22 other states in the USA have reported cases due to such strains. By September 1984, a total of 446 cases were reported to CDC, USA. The MICs of these gonococci were in the range of 2–4 μg per ml. This intrinsic resistance to Pen G was chromosomally mediated, similar to the main resistance mechanism of relatively resistant gonococcal strains (see above). Their PBPs were again modified (Dougherty, 1986). These gonococci were also moderately resistant to tetracycline and erythromycin and their sensitivity to cefoxitin and trimethoprim was variable (p. 724). Most isolates were sensitive to spectinomycin, cefuroxime, cefotaxime and ceftriaxone (CDC, 1984; Rice *et al.*, 1984).

In 1984, of 200 non-penicillinase-producing gonococcal isolates tested in one London hospital, 5.5% were resistant to >9.5 μg per ml of cefuroxime (p. 296). These cefuroxime-resistant strains were highly resistant to Pen G, erythromycin and tetracyclines. Although all were sensitive to cefotaxime some strains had MICs as high as 0.125 μg per ml (Easmon, 1985). Gonococcal infections caused by these strains may prove to be a more difficult therapeutic problem than infections caused by beta-lactamase-producing strains (see below), as intrinsic resistance to Pen G may be accompanied by similar resistance to many beta-lactam antibiotics, including the enzyme-stable members of this group. Fortunately most gonococcal strains intrinsically resistant to Pen G have remained sensitive to cefotaxime (p. 320), ceftriaxone (p. 352) and to quinolones such as ciprofloxacin (p. 983) (Clendennen *et al.*, 1992a,b). Interestingly some strains of *N. gonorrhoeae* were isolated in the USA in 1985, which were resistant to tetracycline, but sensitive to Pen G (CDC, 1985).

It was reported that gonococcal strains, relatively resistant to Pen G, although capable of causing uncomplicated gonorrhea, may have a decreased capacity to cause disseminated infection (Handsfield *et al.*, 1976; Eisenstein *et al.*, 1977). But other investigators have now refuted this (Sackel *et al.*, 1977; Pinon *et al.*, 1981; Bohnhoff *et al.*, 1986).

Beta-lactamase-producing strains of *N. gonorrhoeae*, conferring complete resistance to Pen G, were first recognized during late 1975 in the Philippines. Soon after, they were detected in the USA (Ashford *et al.*, 1976), the UK (Percival *et al.*, 1976), Australia (Lindon and Handke, 1976), Holland (Blog *et al.*, 1977) and Africa (Hallett *et al.*, 1977). By 1977, these resistant gonococci had been identified in 16 countries, and in the USA they had become a significant cause of infection in civilian and military personnel (CDC, 1977; Siegel *et al.*, 1978).

Beta-lactamase-producing strains of *N. gonorrhoeae* soon became highly prevalent in the Philippines, in South-East Asian countries, such as Singapore and Thailand, and in West Africa. They comprised 30–50% of all isolates in some South-East Asian countries (Brown *et al.*, 1982; CDC, 1982; McCormack, 1982). In the USA, their incidence increased from 400 cases yearly during 1976–1979 to 1099 in 1980, to 2734 in 1981 and to 3424 during the first 9 months of 1982. Nevertheless, beta-lactamase-producing isolates still only accounted for less than 0.5% of the approximately one million cases of gonorrhea reported annually (McCormack, 1982; CDC, 1983). By 1982, beta-lactamase-producing gonococci had spread to most countries in the world, where they had usually increased 2- to 6-fold during the preceding 18–24 months (CDC, 1982).

Most of the early cases in the UK were due to importation of the disease from endemic areas, but in 1981, and even more so in 1982, disease caused by beta-lactamase-producing strains became endemic. At first the prevalence of these strains in the UK was relatively low (0.76% in 1981) but it reached about 2% in 1982 with a prevalence of 5% in some urban clinics (McCutchan *et al.*, 1982; PHLSCDSC, 1983; Thin *et al.*, 1983). These gonococci also reached a prevalence of 10% in the Netherlands (Van Embden *et al.*, 1981; Van Klingeren *et al.*, 1983). In Australia 3.65% of gonococci were beta-lactamase-producing in 1982 (CDI, 1982).

Gonococci producing beta-lactamase were also resistant to other penicillins which are beta-lactamase labile such as ampicillin and amoxycillin. Cefoxitin and especially cefuroxime were quite active against these organisms (Sparling *et al.*, 1977). They were often moderately resistant to the tetracyclines and erythromycin but usually sensitive to kanamycin, gentamicin, spectinomycin and co-trimoxazole (CDC, 1978b; Siegel *et al.*, 1978). Cephalosporins, such as cefotaxime, ceftazidime and ceftriaxone, were quite active against these strains (Khan *et al.*, 1981; Kerbs *et al.*, 1983). This also applies to quinolones such as ciprofloxacin (p. 983).

The production of beta-lactamase in gonococci is plasmid mediated (Elwell *et al.*, 1977; Roberts and Falkow, 1977; Handsfield *et al.*, 1989) (p. 549). This plasmid is like the TEM plasmid of ampicillin-resistant *H. influenzae* (p. 113), and it codes for the production of a cell-bound beta-lactamase, which is similar to the TEM-1 enzyme produced by many Gram-negative bacilli (Bergström *et al.*, 1978). Moreover, it can be transferred between gonococci and *E. coli* (Kirven and Thornsberry, 1977; Sparling *et al.*, 1977). Plasmid-containing gonococcal strains can lose their plasmids and revert to Pen G susceptibility. Initially there were two distinct types of beta-lactamase-producing *N. gonorrhoeae*. Most strains isolated in, or epidemiologically linked to, the Far East were relatively tetracycline-resistant *in vitro* and they carried a plasmid with a molecular weight of 4.5 megadaltons. Beta-lactamase-producing gonococci linked with West Africa and Europe were tetracycline-sensitive and they contained a smaller 3.2 megadalton plasmid. Over 50% of Far Eastern strains, but initially none of those from West Africa, also contained a 24.5 megadalton conjugative plasmid (p. 549), which could transfer plasmids to other gonococci and to some other Gram-negative bacilli (Van Embden *et al.*, 1980; Handsfield *et al.*, 1982). This conjugative plasmid may have conferred a selective advantage to Far Eastern strains, and initially they probably spread more readily than those from West Africa (Perine *et al.*, 1977). In 1980, there was a sharp increase in prevalence of infections caused by beta-lactamase-producing gonococci in the Netherlands; these were West Africa-type gonococci, which now contained the 24.5 megadalton conjugative plasmid, in addition to the 3.2 megadalton plasmid (Van Klingeren *et al.*, 1983).

Later, another type of penicillinase-producing gonococcus was identified. This was called the Toronto type which carried a 3.05 megadalton plasmid. This was first detected in several Canadian cities and provinces. Later it was also found in Taiwan and other Asian countries and it might have originated there (Yeung *et al.*, 1986; Chu *et al.*, 1992). Furthermore, at least three more plasmids were detected which were involved with beta-lactamase production in gonococci. These were the 2.9 megadalton Rio type, the 4.0 megadalton Nimes type and the 6.0 megadalton New Zealand type (Van Embden *et al.*, 1985; Brett 1989; Chu *et al.*, 1992). More recent evidence from CDC in USA indicated that most gonococci belonged to one of five categories: Pen G-sensitive gonococci; beta-lactamase-producing *N. gonorrhoeae* strains possessing 2.9, 3.05, 3.2 or 4.4 megadalton beta-lactamase plasmids; strains with high-level plasmid-mediated tetracycline-resistance; strains with plasmid-mediated resistance to Pen G and tetracycline; and strains with chromosomally mediated resistance to Pen G and tetracycline. Ceftriaxone, cefixime, and ciprofloxacin were the most active agents against all these strains (Rice and Knapp, 1994a).

In some cities and countries the prevalence of infections caused by beta-lactamase-producing gonococcal strains has decreased in recent years. This has been documented in one hospital in London (Ison *et al.*, 1986) and in Denmark, where the proportion of beta-lactamase-producing strains had increased, but the prevalence of gonorrhea had decreased markedly since 1986 (Lind, 1990). In Australia during the 5 years to end of June 1986 an increasing resistance of gonococci to Pen G was noted, this being both due to an increase in strains with chromosomal resistance and strains which produced beta-lactamase (AGSP, 1988). A slow but steady increase in the prevalence of beta-lactamase-producing gonococcal infections was reported from the USA until 1979, but after that only local outbreaks continued (Whittington and Knapp, 1988). In most Asian countries the prevalence of beta-lactamase-producing gonococci remained at a high level, e.g. in one survey in Thailand they accounted for 28% of total isolates (Clendennen *et al.*, 1992b). In Taiwan they comprised over 50% of isolates (Chu *et al.*, 1992), and a survey in Philippines showed that 55 % of gonococcal isolates produced this enzyme (Clendennen *et al.*, 1992a).

The use of Pen G, even in large doses, is quite ineffective for the treatment of gonorrhea caused by beta-lactamase-producing strains. Because of beta-lactamase production, an inoculum effect occurs when their sensitivity to Pen G is tested; MICs may be low if a small inoculum is used, but very high (>250 μg per ml) with a large inoculum (Percival *et al.*, 1976). Beta-lactamase-producing gonococci are quite virulent and can cause salpingitis, disseminated infections (Leftik *et al.*, 1978; Rinaldi *et al.*, 1982), and gonococcal ophthalmia neonatorum (Pang *et al.*, 1979). More recently 84 clinical isolates of *N. gonorrhoeae*, obtained from women with pelvic inflammatory disease in the USA were tested;14 were Pen G-resistant because of beta-lactamase production and 13 others were intrinsically resistant (Rice and Knapp, 1994b).

Neisseria mucosa, usually a saprophytic organism, can occasionally cause human infections such as meningitis and endocarditis. It may be sensitive to Pen G, but some strains need as much as 4 μg per ml for inhibition. Others are completely resistant as they contain a plasmid which codes for the production of beta-lactamase (Pintado *et al.*, 1985; Stotka *et al.*, 1991; Ingram *et al.*, 1992). The rare human pathogen, *N. lactamica* is usually Pen G-sensitive (Denning and Gill, 1991), but some strains may be relatively or completely resistant due to an altered PBP 2 (Lujan *et al.*, 1991). Other unusual pathogens, *N. elongata* (Struillou *et al.*, 1993) and *N. sicca* (Heiddal *et al.*, 1993) are usually Pen G-sensitive.

Kingella kingae is a Gram-negative coccobacillus which rarely causes human infections such as endocarditis and septic arthritis. This is always Pen G-sensitive (Morrison and Wagner, 1989; Meis *et al.*, 1992). Gram-negative anaerobic cocci such as *Veillonella* spp. are sensitive to Pen G (Sutter and Finegold, 1976). *Actinobacillus actinomycetemcomitans*, a rod shaped anaerobic coccobacillus, a human pathogen in peridental disease and also a rare cause of other infections such as endocarditis, is generally Pen G-sensitive, but some strains have rather high MICs and some are completely resistant (Kaplan *et al.*, 1989b; Pavicic *et al.*, 1992; Collazos *et al.*, 1994).

4 Gram-negative bacilli

The Enterobacteriaceae, such as *Escherichia coli* and the *Salmonella, Shigella, Enterobacter, Klebsiella, Proteus, Serratia, Citrobacter, Providencia, Yersinia, Hafnia, Edwardsiella* and *Arizona* spp., are resistant to Pen G. The same applies to most other Gram-negative bacilli, such as the *Brucella* spp., *Vibrio cholerae, Burkholderia* (previously *Pseudomonas*) *pseudomallei* and *Pseudomonas aeruginosa. Acinetobacter* spp. is Pen G-resistant. *Moraxella catarrhalis* may be Pen G-sensitive, but most strains are Pen G-resistant due to beta-lactamase production (Jorgensen *et al.*, 1990). Other *Moraxella* spp. are usually Pen G-susceptible (Graham *et al.*, 1990).

These Gram-negative bacilli are resistant to Pen G and certain other beta-lactam antibiotics either because they possess intrinsic resistance and/or they produce beta-lactamases. Intrinsic resistance is often due to the inability of the antibiotic to penetrate the bacterial cell envelope (p. 26). This is one mechanism of resistance to Pen G with some Enterobacteriaceae such as *E. coli* and in particular with *Ps. aeruginosa* (Godfrey and Bryan, 1987; Hancock and Woodruff, 1988; Livermore, 1988). Impermeability is more pronounced in *Ps. aeruginosa* than in *E. coli* (Curtis *et al.*, 1979 a,b; Hancock, 1986). Intrinsic resistance of *Serratia marcescens* to Pen G, like *Ps. aeruginosa*, is mainly due to a permeability barrier (Takata *et al.*, 1981). With *Proteus mirabilis*, *Pr. vulgaris*, *Morganella morganii*, *Providencia rettgeri* and *Providencia alkalifaciens*, difficulty to penetrate their outer membrane also plays a significant role in their resistance to Pen G and other beta-lactam antibiotics (Mitsuyama *et al.*, 1987). Recent evidence indicates that with *Ps. aeruginosa* the intrinsic resistance to beta-lactam antibiotics is not only due to the permeability barrier, but also due to an efflux pump, which actively removes these antibiotics from the periplasmic space of bacteria (Li *et al.*, 1994).

Intrinsic resistance of Gram-negative bacilli to Pen G, other penicillins and cephalosporins also reflects the affinity of these compounds for PBPs (Curtis *et al.*, 1979c; Livermore, 1987; Nicholas and Strominger, 1988). Resistance to beta-lactam antibiotics attributable to changes in PBPs of *Ps. aeruginosa* has been described (Godfrey *et al.*, 1981); but with most strains there is no difference in PBPs between highly Pen G-resistant and more sensitive strains (Zimmerman, 1980; Curtis *et al.*, 1981).

The second reason for resistance in Gram-negative bacilli is the production of beta-lactamase enzymes which are found in the periplasmic space of their bacterial cell walls (p. 26). These beta-lactamases are either chromosomally or plasmid controlled. All Gram-negative bacilli, including anaerobes such as *Bacteroides* spp. (see below), produce beta-lactamases (Sykes, 1982; Acar and Minozzi, 1986; Bush, 1988).

Haemophilus influenzae and *Bordetella pertussis* are usually regarded as Pen G-resistant, but they are inhibited by relatively low Pen G concentrations (Table I.1). Beta-lactamase-producing strains of *H. influenzae* (p. 112) are highly resistant to Pen G. The same applies to *H. influenzae* strains which have high-level intrinsic resistance to ampicillin (p. 114). Possibly, *H. ducreyi* may be susceptible, but the majority of strains now produce plasmid-mediated beta-lactamases and are Pen G-resistant (Dangor *et al.*, 1990). *Pasteurella multocida* is usually Pen G-sensitive (Raffi *et al.*, 1987; Kumar *et al.*, 1990), but strains isolated from septic arthritis or osteomyelitis tend to have higher MICs (0.02–0.7 µg per ml) compared with MICs of 0.02–0.08 µg per ml found in isolates obtained from superficial wounds (Spagnuolo and Friedman, 1979). Resistant strains of *P. multocida* occur but are rare (Stevens *et al.*, 1979). One *P. multocida* human isolate was Pen G-resistant because it produced a plasmid-mediated beta-lactamase (Rosenau *et al.*, 1991). *Capnocytophaga canimorsus* (formerly DF-2), a Gram-negative rod which has been associated with severe septicemia following dog bites, particularly in patients who have undergone prior splenectomy, is Pen G-sensitive (Butler *et al.*, 1977; Kalb *et al.*, 1985; Westerink *et al.*, 1987).

Legionella pneumophila appears 'sensitive' to Pen G *in vitro* (MIC 0.5–2.0 µg per ml), but the drug does not prevent death of guinea pigs inoculated with this bacterium (Fraser *et al.*, 1978; Thornsberry *et al.*, 1978a). *Legionella pneumophila* produces a beta-lactamase which is primarily a cephalosporinase, but it also slowly inactivates Pen G (Fu and Neu, 1979). *Legionella micdadei* (*Tatlockia micdadei* or *Pittsburg pneumonia* agent) does not produce beta-lactamase and is quite sensitive to Pen G *in vitro*, yet surprisingly Pen G is relatively ineffective *in vivo* (Dowling *et al.*, 1982). *Campylobacter fetus* is resistant to Pen G (Chow *et al.*, 1978), as is *Campylobacter coli* (Lachance *et al.*, 1993) and *Campylobacter jejuni* (Karmali *et al.*, 1981). *Helicobacter pylori* is quite sensitive to Pen G *in vitro*, but the drug is not useful clinically for treatment of infection by this organism (McNulty *et al.*, 1985).

Cardiobacterium hominis, an opportunistic Gram-negative bacillus, which has been implicated in diseases such as endocarditis, is Pen G-sensitive (Rechtman and Nadler, 1991). *Flavimonas oryzihabitans*, another opportunistic Gram-negative bacillus is Pen G-sensitive, but *Chryseomonas luteola* is not (Hawkins *et al.*, 1991).

Anaerobic Gram-negative bacilli vary in their sensitivity. Normal inhabitants of the oropharynx, such as *Prevotella* (previously *Bacteroides*) *melaninogenica*, *P. oralis*, *P. disiens*, *Fusobacterium nucleatum* and *F. necrophorum* and bacteria of the genus *Capnocytophaga*, are usually Pen G-sensitive (Sutter *et al.*, 1981; 1983; Seidenfeld *et al.*, 1982; Lewis *et al.*, 1989; Bilgrami *et al.*, 1992; Iralu *et al.*, 1993). *Prevotella* spp., *Fusobacterium* spp. and *Capnocytophaga* strains can produce beta-lactamase and thereby become Pen G-resistant (Tuner *et al.*, 1985; Finegold, 1989; Foweraker *et al.*, 1990). *Eikenella corrodens* is an anaerobic Gram-negative rod which is a normal inhabitant of human oral cavity; it may cause peridontidis, human bite wound infections or more serious infections such as endocarditis. Most strains are sensitive to Pen G, but some strains produce a constitutive beta-lactamase and are Pen G-resistant. Plasmids have not been detected in the strains producing the enzyme (Joshi *et al.*, 1991; Lacroix and Walker, 1991).

Bacteroides fragilis and other members of the *B. fragilis* group, habitually present in the gastrointestinal tract, are usually Pen G-resistant due to a permeability barrier (p. 26) and the production of beta-lactamases (Timewell *et al.*, 1981; Finegold, 1989; Nord and Hedberg, 1990).

Highly Pen G-resistant strains (MIC > 128 μg per ml) produce about 10-fold more beta-lactamase than less resistant strains (MIC 4–64 μg per ml) (Olsson *et al.*, 1979). *Bacteroides bivius* and *B. disiens*, which are frequently encountered in endometrial specimens, are usually beta-lactamase producers and resistant to Pen G (Snydman *et al.*, 1980). Other *Bacteroides* spp., less well known Fusobacterium spp. and other Gram-negative anaerobic bacteria may be Pen G-sensitive, but many strains are resistant (Kirby *et al.*, 1980; George *et al.*, 1981; Finegold, 1989).

5 Other bacteria

Treponema pallidum and the Leptospirae are consistently sensitive to Pen G (Johnson, 1989). *Borrelia hermsii*, the etiological agent of relapsing fever, is sensitive (MIC 0.15 μg per ml) (Barbour *et al.*, 1982). The same is true for *Streptobacillus moniliformis* and *Spirrillum minus*, the causes of rat-bite fever. *Borrelia burgdorferi*, the spirochete which causes Lyme disease, is sensitive to Pen G *in vivo*, but *in vitro* antibiotic sensitivity testing initially was not possible (Benach *et al.*, 1983; Steere *et al.*, 1983a). Now it has been established that this organism is not highly Pen G-sensitive, the MBC being 6.4 μg per ml, and ceftriaxone (p. 353), erythromycin (p. 609) and tetracycline (p. 726) are more active against this spirochete *in vitro* (Johnson *et al.*, 1987).

Mycobacteria are Pen G-resistant, except that some strains of the *Mycobacterium avium* complex (p. 644) are sensitive to relatively low Pen G concentrations (1.0–10 μg per ml) (Kasik *et al.*, 1980), but this has no clinical significance.

6 Chlamydia

Organisms of this genus are relatively resistant. For instance, Pen G interferes with the normal growth of *C. trachomatis* as evidenced by the production of abnormal non-fluorescent inclusions, but normal growth pattern returns when Pen G is removed (Johnson and Hobson, 1977).

7 Rickettsiae

These are Pen G-resistant. *Rickettsia prowazeki* may be inhibited by 20 μg per ml of Pen G, but other *Rickettsia* spp. need much higher concentrations for inhibition (Wisseman *et al.*, 1982).

8 Mycoplasmas, fungi and protozoa

These are all completely Pen G-resistant.

9 Minimum inhibitory concentrations

The MICs of Pen G against some selected bacterial species are shown in Table I.1. Pen G is still occasionally prescribed in units, and MICs expressed in units per ml are about 1.7 times higher than those shown in this table (one unit is equivalent to 0.6 μg of pure sodium Pen G).

Mode of Administration and Dosage

Pen G is destroyed by acid in the stomach and absorption after oral administration is variable. All Pen G preparations can be injected i.m. and its two highly soluble salts can also be given i.v. Procaine Pen G and benzathine Pen G can only be given i.m.

1 Crystalline Pen G

The common mode of administration was by the i.m. route, but in recent years in hospitals it has often been given i.v.. The i.v. method is preferable for shocked patients, in whom the absorption of Pen G from i.m. sites may be inadequate. In addition, i.v. administration is desirable for patients with a hemorrhagic diathesis. The i.v. route is often used for patients requiring large doses of parenteral Pen G for prolonged periods, to avoid frequent i.m. injections. However, i.m. administration may be preferable in some circumstances (p. 39).

Crystalline Pen G is usually administered every 4–6 h, but intervals of 3 hours between doses may be necessary in severe infections. A common adult dosage is 0.6 g (1 million units) i.m. or i.v. every 4–6 h. For serious infections (e.g. bacterial meningitis) higher doses can be given; a common dosage for adults is 1.2–1.8 g (2–3 million units) 4-hourly. Doses higher than this are usually unnecessary for infections, however severe, caused by Pen G-sensitive organisms. In the past 'massive' Pen G doses of up to 60 g (100 million units) daily, i.v. were occasionally used for serious infections due to relatively resistant organisms, such as the Gram-negative bacilli (Weinstein *et al.*, 1964). Conversely, some authors considered that a dose of 0.6 g 6-hourly, was unnecessarily high for many infections of moderate severity. For instance, Anderson *et al.* (1968)

Organism	MIC (µg per ml)
Gram-positive bacteria	
Staphylococcus aureus (non-penicillinase producer)	0.03
Streptococcus pyogenes (Group A)	≤0.01
Streptococcus pneumoniae	0.015
Streptococcus pneumoniae (relatively resistant)	0.1–1.0
Streptococci, Group B	0.06
Streptococci, Group C	0.015–0.1
Streptococci, Group G	0.02–0.5
Streptococcus viridans	0.01
Enterococcus faecalis	2.0
Enterococcus faecium	2.0–9.0
Streptococcus bovis (Group D)	0.024
Bacillus anthracis	0.015
Corynebacterium diphtheriae	0.062
Listeria monocytogenes	0.1
Clostridium tetani	0.06
Clostridium perfringens	0.06–0.25
Actinomyces israelii	0.05
Gram-negative bacteria	
Neisseria meningitidis	0.03
Neisseria gonorrhoeae:	
(a) sensitive strains	0.007
(b) relatively resistant strains	0.125–2.0
(c) penicillinase-producing strains	2.0–>250
Haemophilus influenzae	1.0
Bordetella pertussis	0.5
Brucella abortus	6.0
Salmonella typhi	4.0
Shigella spp.	16.0
Escherichia coli	64.0
Proteus mirabilis	32.0
Bacteroides fragilis	≥32.0
Prevotella melaninogenica	0.1–0.5

Table I.1

Compiled from data published by Garrod (1960a,b), Knox (1960), Barber and Waterworth (1962), Sutherland *et al.* (1970), Watanakunakorn (1974), Rodriguez and Saz (1975), Tally *et al.* (1975), Percival *et al.* (1976), Mohan *et al.* (1977), Moellering *et al.* (1979), Noble *et al.* (1980) and Portnoy *et al.* (1981)

regarded an adult dose of crystalline Pen G as low as 0.18 g (300 000 units) i.m. 12-hourly, as satisfactory for the treatment of pneumococcal pneumonia, a disease in which the blood supply to all diseased areas is good. This dosage would not be sufficient to treat infections caused by relatively resistant pneumococcal strains (p. 37).

Brewin *et al.* (1974) reported that procaine Pen G (see below) in a dose of 0.6 g (600 000 units) i.m. 12-hourly, was as satisfactory as a daily i.v. dose of 12 g (20 million units) crystalline Pen G, for the treatment of pneumococcal pneumonia. This procaine Pen G regimen may be inadequate for pneumonia caused by a relatively Pen G-resistant pneumococci (p. 5), whereas crystalline Pen G in a dosage of 0.6 g (1 million units) 6-hourly, may succeed (Hansman, 1976). Procaine Pen G i.m. in a dose as low as 1.2 g (1.2 million units) every 6 h is considered adequate for the treatment of *Strep. viridans* endocarditis provided that it is used in combination with streptomycin or gentamicin (p. 41). If Pen G is used as a single drug for this disease, crystalline Pen G in daily doses of 6–12 g (10–20 million units) is advocated. For *E. faecalis* endocarditis, crystalline Pen G in a dose of 12 g (20 million units) daily, combined with an aminoglycoside is always necessary (Kaye, 1980) (p. 42).

2 Method of i.v. administration

Crystalline Pen G may be administered i.v. by either continuous infusion or by intermittent injections or infusions. In emergency treatment of serious infections, an initial direct injection of Pen G should be given i.v. to achieve a high serum level quickly. This can then be followed by either continuous Pen G infusion or intermittent i.v. injections. Continuous infusion was considered the preferred method, because of the drug's rapid renal excretion and the presumed increased hazard of thrombophlebitis with intermittent administration. However, problems may arise if Pen G is added to i.v. fluid bottles. It is unstable in solution at room temperature or even at 4°C. Its activity therefore may be progressively lost, and furthermore, its degradation products may be more potent antigens than Pen G itself and cause sensitization (p. 29). This can be avoided if Pen G solutions are always freshly prepared and given i.v. as bolus doses (Neftel *et al.*, 1982). In addition, Pen G may be incompatible with additives to i.v. solutions. For example, Pen G and other penicillins are almost completely inactivated within a few hours in dextrose solutions containing sufficient bicarbonate to elevate the pH level above 8.0, and penicilloic acid (p. 29) is a major degradation product (Simberkoff *et al.*, 1970). Pen G and other penicillins are also unstable at room temperature in amino acid mixtures used for hyperalimentation (Feigin *et al.*, 1973), and in solutions of plasma expanders such as dextran (Koshiro and Fujita, 1983).

To avoid the problems associated with continuous infusion, most clinicians prefer either intermittent i.v. injections or intermittent rapid infusions of high concentration Pen G solutions via a secondary i.v. bottle or a buretrol. Each dose can be dissolved in 10–20 ml of sterile water in a syringe, and this is injected directly into the i.v. tubing over a period of 5 min. Alternatively, the drug can be given via a pediatric buretrol which is incorporated in the i.v. set. When a dose of the drug is due, 20–30 ml of i.v. fluid is delivered into the buretrol to which a dissolved dose of Pen G is added; this concentrated drug solution is then infused over a period of 10–15 min. An added advantage of this method is that the buretrol filter removes a proportion of particulate matter, which is commonly present in the syringe when antibiotics are withdrawn from ampoules or vials. For babies and young children, i.v. infusion pumps which can deliver both i.v. fluids and antibiotics intermittently at a desired rate, are advantageous (Leff and Roberts, 1981).

The therapeutic superiority of intermittent versus continuous i.v. Pen G administration, is still controversial. In animals, intermittent therapy may result in greater drug levels in interstitial fluid and fibrin clots (Barza, 1981; Bergeron *et al.*, 1981). In another animal study, a daily methicillin dose was more effective for the treatment of experimental *Staph. aureus* endocarditis when administered in divided doses 4- or 8-hourly, than by 12-hourly dosing or by continuous infusion (Gengo *et al.*, 1984b).

In recent years there has been a renewed interest in beta-lactam antibiotic administration by continuous infusion. The availability of improved i.v. drug delivery systems has overcome some of the problems associated with this method of administration. Most of the studies here have been done with newer beta-lactams such as ceftazidime (p. 372) for *Ps. aeruginosa* infections, rather than with Pen G. Pharmacokinetic studies have shown that lower daily dose of ceftazidime would be needed if the drug was given by continuous i.v. infusion. Significant data from clinical trials in humans are not yet available (Drusano, 1988; Craig and Ebert, 1992).

3 Procaine Pen G

During the later stages of treatment of many infections such as pneumonia, procaine Pen G can be substituted for crystalline Pen G. This penicillin is useful because absorption of an i.m. injected dose continues for up to 24 h, so that injections may be separated by this interval, but lower serum levels are obtained. These injections are less painful than crystalline Pen G. A common adult dosage for procaine Pen G is 1.0 g (1 million units) i.m. once or twice per day. In milder infections procaine Pen G may be satisfactory for initial treatment. This compound must not be given i.v. (p. 31).

4 Benzathine Pen G

This preparation, when injected i.m. in doses of 0.45–0.9 g (600 000 to 1 200 000 units) maintains a low serum concentration of Pen G for a period of 1–3 weeks (p. 23). Single injections of benzathine Pen G have been used for treatment of *Strep. pyogenes* infections (Ginsburg *et al.*, 1982), diphtheria carriers (McCloskey *et al.*, 1974) and syphilis (McCracken, 1974), while monthly injections are used for rheumatic fever prophylaxis (p. 51). This compound must not be given i.v.

5 Children

Dosages of crystalline, procaine or benzathine Pen G should be adjusted to the age and weight of the patient. In general, one-quarter of the adult dose is suitable for children under 3 years of age, and half the adult dose for older children.

6 Newborn and premature infants

Renal clearance of crystalline Pen G in this age group is reduced. The mean half-life value in infants under 6 days of age is 3.2 h; in those aged 7–13 days it is 1.7 h and in infants 14 days of age and older, it is 1.4 h (McCracken, 1974). The half-life in normal adults, is only 30 min (p. 22). Therefore, small doses of crystalline Pen G given at 8- or 12-hourly intervals are recommended for infants. For infants 0–7 days old, a total daily dosage of 30 mg (50 000 units) per kg body weight, administered in two divided doses is usually adequate for most infections caused by highly susceptible bacteria (McCracken et al., 1973). However, infants suffering from Group B streptococcal infections (p. 36), should receive 60 mg (100 000 units) per kg per day, given in two or three divided doses (McCracken, 1974). For serious infections such as meningitis, infants younger than 7 days may be prescribed 60–90 mg (100 000–150 000 units) per kg per day, given in two divided doses. For infants older than 7 days the usual dosage is 45 mg (75 000 units) per kg per day, given in three divided doses. For serious infections (e.g. meningitis) the dosage should be 120–180 mg (200 000–300 000 units) per kg per day, given in four divided doses. Preferably individual doses should be administered i.v. as 15–30 min infusions (McCracken and Nelson, 1983).

Procaine Pen G in a single daily i.m. dose of 50 mg (50 000 units) per kg, appears suitable for the treatment of milder infections. The drug is well tolerated in this age group and local reactions are uncommon (McCracken and Nelson, 1983). Benzathine Pen G, if indicated in neonates, is given in a single i.m. dose of 37.5 mg (50 000 units) per kg body weight (McCracken, 1974).

7 Elderly patients

These patients eliminate Pen G and many other antibiotics more slowly via the kidney. If large doses are used, serum level monitoring and appropriate dosage reduction may be needed (Ljungberg and Nilsson-Ehle, 1987).

8 Patients with renal failure

Pen G is often administered in the usual dosage to these patients, because with small doses there is no great risk of toxicity. Moderately large i.v. doses may yield high toxic serum levels (p. 32), necessitating dosage reduction. If a crystalline Pen G dose of 0.6–1.2 g (1–2 million units) 6-hourly is normally indicated, then in anuric or severely uremic patients, the intervals between the doses should be increased to 8–10 h (Kunin, 1967). If high dose i.v. Pen G therapy is contemplated, such as a dose of 14.4 g (24 million units) daily for patients with normal renal function, more meticulous dosage adjustment is necessary for those with renal failure. Table I.2 shows a dosage schedule for the administration of large doses of Pen G, given intermittently i.v., for patients with various degrees of renal failure. This aims to achieve a mean serum Pen G concentration of approximately 20 μg per ml (Bryan and Stone, 1975).

These authors suggested that a loading dose of 0.45–0.72 g (750 000–1 200 000 units) should be given initially to patients with severe renal failure. If hemodialysis is required, an additional dose of 0.3 g (500 000 units) is necessary 6-hourly during this procedure. The Pen G dose recommended in Table I.2 should be further reduced to 0.3 g (300 000 units) 8-hourly if advanced liver disease is associated with severe renal failure (p. 24).

Table I.2
Dosage schedule for intermittent i.v. penicillin G therapy for patients with renal failure. (After Bryan and Stone, 1975, with permission.)

Creatine clearance (ml per min)		Dose (g)	Dose (units)	Interval (h)
125		1.2	2 million	2
	or	1.8	3 million	3
60		1.2	2 million	4
40		0.9	1.5 million	4
20		0.6	1.0 million	4
10		0.6	1.0 million	6
Nil		0.3	0.5 million	6
	or	0.6	1.0 million	8

9 Intraperitoneal administration

Crystalline Pen G may be added to peritoneal dialysis fluid either to treat or to prevent intraperitoneal infection. Usually a dose of 30 mg (50 000 units) is added to each liter of dialysate resulting in a Pen G concentration of 30 μg per ml. If this concentration is maintained continuously, the drug is absorbed from the peritoneum, and Pen G serum levels of about 25–30% of the concentrations in the dialysate, are attained in patients with renal failure (Bulger et al., 1965).

10 Oral forms of potassium and benzathine Pen G

These have been used in children, but the acid stable phenoxypenicillins (p. 71) are preferred for oral therapy. The loose term 'oral penicillin' now usually applies to one of the phenoxypenicillins such as penicillin V or phenethicillin.

Serum Levels in Relation to Dosage

1 Intravenous crystalline Pen G

Immediate high serum levels are attained after rapid i.v. injection of this preparation. If a dose of 1.2 g (2 million units) is administered intermittently i.v. every 2 h, or 1.8 g (3 million units) every 3 h, a mean serum concentration of approximately 20 μg per ml is attained (Bryan and Stone, 1975). This is adequate for the treatment of severe infections (p. 39).

Plaut et al. (1969) studied serum levels in 10 patients with normal renal function, who received an i.v. injection of 3 g (5 million units) of sodium Pen G, during a 3–5 min period. The resulting mean serum concentration after 5 min was 400 μg per ml and after 10 min, 273 μg per ml. During the first hour there was a rapid decrease in the serum concentrations (due to both distribution and elimination of the drug), after which the mean serum level was 45 μg per ml. The subsequent fall in serum levels was slower, and this was mainly due to Pen G elimination; at 4 h the mean serum level was 3.0 μg per ml. When the same dose of Pen G was administered by continuous infusion over a 6-h period, 2 h were required to achieve a serum level of 12–20 μg per ml, which then could only be maintained by the use of a constant infusion pump. If the infusion was given by an ordinary i.v. drip, large fluctuations of serum levels were observed, despite close supervision.

2 Intramuscular crystalline Pen G

With this method of administration a peak serum level is obtained within 30 min. After 0.6 g (1 million units) this is usually 12 μg per ml; the level then falls rapidly, but detectable serum levels remain for 4–6 h. The usual half-life of the drug is only 30 min. The height of the peak and persistence of serum levels depend on the dose, but the relation is not always linear. There is also an individual variation, and even in the same subject the response may vary under different conditions. For instance, the period of sustained therapeutic levels is shorter in healthy ambulatory volunteers, than in patients confined to bed. Diabetic patients may absorb Pen G relatively poorly from i.m. sites (Weinstein and Dalton, 1968).

With an i.m. dose of 21 mg (approx. 32 000 units) per kg in children, a peak serum level of 10–15 μg per ml is attained in 30 min. The level then falls to zero in 4–6 h (Shann et al., 1987).

In newborn infants, after an i.m. dose of 15 mg (25 000 units) per kg body weight of crystalline Pen G, the mean peak serum level after 30–60 min, is approximately 22 μg per ml; this level falls to 1.0–2.0 μg per ml after 12 h. Pen G does not accumulate if this dose is given every 12 h. Following a dose of 30 mg (50 000 units) per kg, a peak level of approximately 40 μg per ml occurs, but the level at 12 h is similar to that resulting from a dose of 15 mg per kg. There is also no accumulation of Pen G when a dose of 30 mg per kg is given every 12 h (McCracken et al., 1973). In general, Pen G serum levels are independent of birth weight, except that in infants with a birth weight less than 2000 g, peak serum levels are slightly lower, possibly due to more of the drug being distributed in extracellular fluid (McCracken, 1974). With older infants, mean serum levels after these doses become lower, because the Pen G half-life decreases as postnatal age increases (p. 21).

3 Procaine Pen G

After i.m. injection of an aqueous suspension of procaine Pen G (Fig. I.1), a peak serum level is reached in about 2–3 h and in adults given 0.6 g (600 000 units) or more, detectable levels are

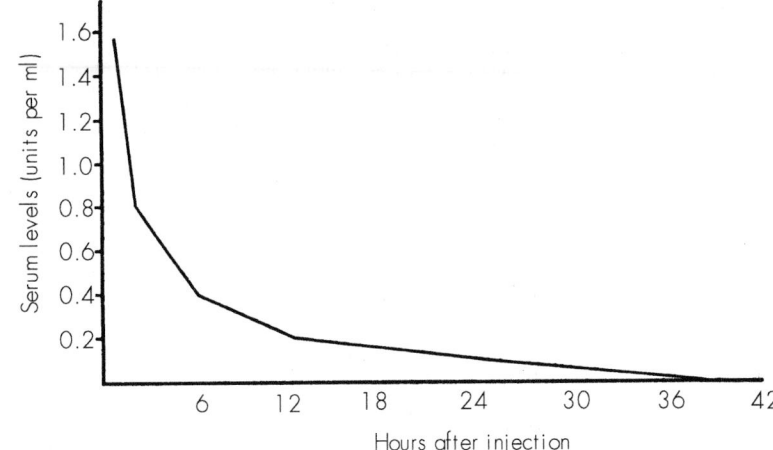

Fig. I.1. Serum levels after 300 000 units aqueous suspension of procaine penicillin i.m. (Redrawn from Welch, 1954, with permission.)

usually maintained for at least 24 h. When i.m. procaine penicillin in a dose of 50 mg per kg is given to children, the peak serum level 3–6 h later is 4–6 μg per ml and the serum level remains above 1 μg per ml for 26 h (Shann *et al.*, 1987).

In infants aged less than 1 week, following i.m. procaine Pen G in a dose of 50 mg (50 000 units) per kg body weight, the mean serum level 2–12 h later is 7 μg per ml, and the level at 24 h is 1.5 μg per ml. Pen G does not accumulate in the body if this dose is repeated every 24 h. Lower serum levels (5–6 μg per ml) during the first 4 h and 0–0.4 μg per ml at 24 h occur if this dose is given to infants older than 1 week (McCracken *et al.*, 1973; McCracken and Nelson, 1983).

4 Benzathine Pen G

This produces more prolonged therapeutic serum levels after i.m. injection. In young adults, after a single injection of 1.8 g (2.4 million units) of benzathine Pen G, the mean serum Pen G concentration was 0.2 μg per ml after 48 h, 0.05 μg per ml at 6 days, and 0.02 μg per ml at 13 days. At 13 days, 33% of subjects already had negligible serum Pen G concentrations, and thereafter no subjects had significant serum levels. After the same dose was given to elderly subjects, mean serum levels of 0.37, 0.1, 0.05, and 0.04 μg per ml occurred at 48 h, 6, 13 days and 20 days, respectively. Thereafter, serum Pen G levels became undetectable (Collart *et al.*, 1980). Prolonged and higher serum levels in elderly subjects are due to delayed renal excretion of Pen G. Kaplan *et al.* (1989a) administered 0.9 g (1.2 million units) of benzathine penicillin to young adults. Mean serum Pen G levels remained ≥0.02 μg per ml for 21 days, but by 28 days only 44% of the serum samples had detectable levels of Pen G. It was concluded that more frequent than 4-weekly i.m. injections are needed for rheumatic fever chemoprophylaxis (p. 51).

Ginsburg *et al.* (1982) studied serum levels of Pen G after i.m. benzathine Pen G administration to children aged 1.8–10.7 years. Seven children who weighed less than 27 kg, received a single dose of 0.45 g and six who weighed 27 kg or more were given a dose of 0.9 g. Serum level-time curves were similar for the two groups for the entire study period of 30 days. The mean peak serum concentration attained at 24 h, was 0.16 μg per ml and subsequent mean serum levels were 0.075, 0.04, and 0.01 μg per ml on days 5, 10, and 18, respectively. On day 30 Pen G was undetectable in serum of all children. Results of some clinical studies (p. 35) plus the findings of Pen G serum levels of 0.01 μg per ml or greater at day 10 in this study, indicates that benzathine Pen G may be effective for therapy of Group A streptococcal pharyngitis (p. 35). But this study again indicated that monthly administration of this preparation may not be adequate for rheumatic fever chemoprophylaxis (p. 51), or for the prevention of pneumococcal infections (p. 51).

In newborn infants, after an i.m. dose of 37.5 mg (50 000 units) per kg body weight, a mean peak serum level of 1.20 μg per ml was attained 12–24 h after administration, which fell to 0.65–0.90 μg per ml at 4 days, and concentrations of 0.07–0.09 μg per ml were still detectable at 12 days (Klein *et al.*, 1973; Kaplan and McCracken, 1973).

5 Pregnant patients

Serum Pen G levels are likely to be lower in pregnant than in non-pregnant patients after the same dose of the drug. This is because both the distribution volume and the renal clearance of Pen G increase during pregnancy. This phenomenon has been best studied with ampicillin (p. 117), but it is likely to apply to most other penicillins and cephalosporins (Chow and Jewesson, 1985).

Excretion

1 Urine

If renal function is normal, over 70% of an injected dose of Pen G is excreted within 6 hours, mainly as the active drug, and high urinary concentrations are attained. In healthy adults, only about 10% of an injected dose of Pen G is excreted by glomerular filtration, the remainder predominantly by tubular secretion (McCracken et al., 1973). Animal experiments indicated that this secretion takes place in the proximal tubules, and that a small amount (about 10% of the administered dose) was then reabsorbed in the collecting ducts (Bergeron et al., 1975). After this rapid elimination phase of Pen G, there follows a slow elimination phase (Ebert et al., 1988). In human volunteers they showed that the serum levels were still approximately 0.01 µg per ml 9 h after administration of 0.6 g Pen G i.v.. In newborn infants excretion is predominantly by glomerular filtration, because of the immaturity of tubular function at that age (McCracken et al., 1973); this results in a prolonged Pen G serum half-life (p. 22).

Renal tubular secretion can be partly blocked by probenecid , and if it is used with Pen G, serum concentrations are approximately doubled. Nauta et al. (1974) studying the effect of probenecid on the distribution of cloxacillin (p. 95) in anephric patients, and Barza et al. (1975) performing animal experiments, showed that probenecid did not confine Pen G to the vascular space and limit its access to organs and tissues, as originally postulated. Therefore, probenecid can be used to enhance serum levels of penicillins or cephalosporins and this will not lower the antibiotic concentration at the site of infection. The adult dosage of probenecid for this purpose is 2.0 g daily. The daily doses for children are 0.5–0.75, 0.75–1.25, and 1.25–1.5 g for children aged 2–4, 5–9, and 10–14 years, respectively. This is administered orally, usually in four divided doses.

Various other drugs, especially organic acids, may compete with Pen G for renal tubular secretion, similar to probenecid. In this way, the Pen G half-life may be prolonged by aspirin, phenylbutazone, sulfonamides, indomethacin, thiazide diuretics, furosemide and ethacrynic acid (Leading article, 1975).

In patients with impaired renal function, the Pen G serum half-life increases as renal function deteriorates (Plaut et al., 1969), but the drug still disappears from the blood at a significant but reduced rate in anuric patients (see below). Elderly subjects also have a diminished renal tubular secretory ability and are liable to Pen G neurotoxicity, if large doses are given i.v. (p. 32).

2 Bile

Some active Pen G is eliminated by this route. In animals, the drug is actively secreted into the bile and amounts to about 4.5% of the administered dose. Probenecid may reduce biliary secretion and possibly also interfere with Pen G inactivation in the liver (see below), because it significantly prolongs the cloxacillin half-life in anephric patients (Nauta et al., 1974).

3 Inactivation in body

The remainder of an administered dose of Pen G which is not excreted in urine or bile (usually less than 30%), is inactivated in the liver producing mainly penicilloic acid (Cole et al., 1973). Inactivation of Pen G is more rapid than that of other penicillins, such as ampicillin (p. 117) and carbenicillin (p. 152), so that in anuric patients, the serum half-life of Pen G is only 3 h, but with ampicillin and carbenicillin it is 7–8 h and 15 h, respectively. Serum levels of Pen G decline very slowly in patients with severe hepatic and renal dysfunction (Bryan and Stone, 1975).

Distribution of the Drug in Body

Pen G penetrates into bronchial secretions to a modest degree; peak sputum concentrations are only 5–20% of those in serum (Symonds, 1987). Pen G diffuses quite readily into lung empyemas, uncomplicated parapneumonic effusions (Taryle et al., 1981) and ascitic fluid (Gerding et al., 1977). Similarly, the drug penetrates well into pericardial and synovial fluids. Pen G easily diffuses into inflamed tissues where it persists longer than in normal tissues (Florey et al., 1946). Pen G concentrations in purulent saliva of patients with bacterial parotitis are considerably higher than in non-purulent saliva of healthy patients (Eneroth et al., 1978). The drug's passage into hematomas is quite good (Bergman, 1979), but it is poor into non-inflamed bone (Smilack et al., 1976), avascular areas and abscesses.

Penetration of Pen G into the CSF of patients with non-inflamed meninges is poor. Hieber and Nelson (1977) studied serial CSF Pen G concentrations in children with bacterial meningitis, who were treated by i.v. Pen G in a dosage of 0.15 g per kg per day. Mean CSF Pen G concentrations on days 1, 5 and 10 of therapy were 0.8, 0.7, and 0.3 μg per ml, respectively. These decreasing CSF levels correlated with the return of CSF protein concentrations towards normal. In adult patients with secondary, latent and central nervous system syphilis, Pen G usually cannot be detected in the CSF after administration of i.m. benzathine Pen G in doses of 1.8 or 5.4 g. The same is true if i.m. procaine Pen G is used in a daily dose of 2.4 g. Treponemicidal CSF Pen G concentrations (0.06–1.0 μg per ml) are usually attained by three other treatment regimens: (1) crystalline Pen G, 2.4 g i.v. 4-hourly, (2) crystalline Pen G, 0.3 g i.v. or i.m. 6-hourly plus oral probenecid 0.5 g 6-hourly, and (3) procaine Pen G, 2.4 g i.m. daily plus 0.5 g oral probenecid 6-hourly (Dunlop et al., 1979, 1981; Polnikorn et al., 1980; Ducas and Robson, 1981). After i.m. administration of 50 mg per kg body weight of procaine Pen G to neonates, the drug can always be detected in the CSF; mean peak CSF levels of 0.7 ± 0.35 (SEM) μg per ml occur 12 h after administration (Speer et al., 1981). In animal experiments, Pen G penetrates to some extent into inflamed brain tissue and brain abscesses where its concentration is reduced by concomitant administration of corticosteroids. By contrast, corticosteroids do not reduce penetration into brain tissue of lipophilic drugs, such as chloramphenicol (p. 561) or metronidazole (p. 943) (Kourtópoulos et al., 1983a).

When parenteral Pen G is administered to subjects with normal meninges, CSF Pen G levels are kept low, not only by passive CSF flow into the venous system via the arachnoid villi, but also by an active transport system localized in the choroid plexus, which specifically excretes Pen G and other organic acids from the CSF (Hieber and Nelson, 1977; Norrby, 1978). In patients with meningitis, there is increased vascular permeability allowing more Pen G to enter the CSF, and also a decreased clearance from the CSF by partial inhibition of the organic acid pump. In normal animals and in those with experimental bacterial meningitis, CSF Pen G levels increase two to three times if probenecid is also given. This increase is greater than can be expected from the associated serum level increase (p. 24). Probenecid elevates the CSF Pen G concentration by directly inhibiting excretion of organic acids from the CSF (Dacey and Sande, 1974). This probenecid effect may precipitate encephalopathy (p. 32) if Pen G is used in large doses. Probenecid has the same effect on CSF concentrations of other penicillins and cephalosporins. Occasionally this action may be useful therapeutically to increase CSF antibiotic levels, for instance, in the treatment of neurosyphilis (p. 47). In animals, Pen G CSF levels are considerably increased if the drug is given approximately 1 week after whole brain irradiation. Paradoxically, if probenecid is also given, CSF Pen G levels in irradiated animals are lower than in animals receiving irradiation alone. The mode of action of probenecid in this situation is not understood (Kourtopoulos et al., 1983b).

Pen G enters erythrocytes. If it is given by a direct i.v. injection followed by a constant Pen G infusion, the red blood cell Pen G concentration equals or exceeds the serum concentration after 2 h. If Pen G administration is then ceased, the erythrocytic Pen G concentration is only halved in 50–60 min, whereas the serum Pen G half-life is 30 min (p. 22). This slower rate of efflux of Pen G from erythrocytes probably helps to maintain high initial drug levels for a longer period (Kornguth and Kunin, 1976). Pen G, unlike antibiotics with good lipid solubility, such as chloramphenicol (p. 561) and rifampicin (p. 685), penetrates poorly into human polymorphonuclear leukocytes and into enucleated human polymorphonuclear leukocytes (cytoplasts) (Prokesch and Hand, 1982; Hand and King-Thompson, 1990). The drug crosses the placenta, producing adequate concentrations in both the fetus and amniotic fluid, except that fetal levels are low during the first trimester (Chow and Jewesson, 1985). Pen G is 46–58% protein bound (Kunin, 1967).

Mode of Action

1 Structure of bacterial cell envelope

The cell wall is complex and unique to bacteria. Being relatively inelastic, it confers shape on the organism and protects it against damage due to osmotic pressure differences between the cell cytoplasm and the external environment (Koch, 1988). The cytoplasmic membrane lies immediately beneath the cell wall and is pressed up against it by osmotic forces within the cell.

The cell wall and the cytoplasmic membrane together form the cell envelope. These component structures are interdependent and alterations in one may render the other ineffective. The composition of the cell envelope, the complexity of which varies with different bacterial species, has an important role in modifying the action of antibiotics (Costerton and Cheng, 1975). Antibiotics act on protein synthesis within the cell or at a site within the envelope, so that they must pass through part or all of the envelope to reach their target.

In Gram-positive bacteria the major portion of the cell wall consists of a mucopeptide layer (also known as murein or peptidoglycan), which supports the cytoplasmic membrane. This mucopeptide layer consists of a giant molecule, constructed in the form of a net of polysaccharide strands, which are interlinked by short peptide bonds. In the resting cell, this molecule is apparently united in every direction over the cell's surface and there are no free ends available for further growth (Tomasz, 1981). For cell growth to proceed, this mucopeptide lattice must be broken to enable new cell wall material to be inserted. In the dividing cell, there is the additional complex process of the formation of a septum or cross-wall (consisting of cytoplasmic membrane and wall), which splits in a special way to produce progeny identical to the parent cell. Lytic enzymes (autolysins) are involved in both of these processes (see below). In the normal growing cell, synthesis and lysis must be balanced to allow cell division, without cell destruction. In Gram-positive bacteria the interstices within the mucopeptide net, communicating as they do with the cytoplasmic membrane, constitute a periplasmic space. A number of degradative enzymes may be located in this space, which are capable of destroying a variety of antibiotics; these include beta-lactamases (penicillinases and cephalosporinases), which hydrolyze the beta-lactam ring (p. 3) of susceptible penicillins and cephalosporins. The type and amount of the enzymes present in the periplasmic space depends on the bacterial species. In pathogenic Gram-positive bacteria, the bacterial envelope is usually completed by a third component, a protein coat or a carbohydrate capsule, exterior to the mucopeptide layer.

In Gram-negative bacteria, the envelope is more complex and consists of four layers. A mucopeptide net again is exterior to, and supports the cytoplasmic membrane, but the periplasmic space formed by the niches in the mucopeptide, is extended out beyond the mucopeptide layer, by protruding lipoprotein bundles which meet an extra outer membrane (Nikaido and Vaara, 1985; Nikaido, 1988, 1989). Exterior to this outer membrane there is also usually a protein or a carbohydrate capsule. The periplasmic space of Gram-negative bacteria therefore consists of an area spreading from the cytoplasmic membrane through the mucopeptide net, to the outer membrane. This outer membrane plays a specific role in permeability since it contains several porin proteins with pores that allow small molecules to diffuse into the periplasmic space (Jaffe et al., 1982; Piddock and Wise, 1985, Nikaido 1988, 1989). Mutants of E. coli lacking one or more of these proteins have increased resistance to some antibiotics, although these drugs may utilize other pathways to enter the bacterial cell (Mortimer and Piddock, 1993).

The outer membrane normally has selective permeability and thereby preserves the microenvironment of the periplasmic space. For instance, it prevents the outward passage of periplasmic enzymes and prevents the inward passage of some antibiotics (p. 16). The penetrability of the outer membrane to various antibiotics is often specific for particular bacterial species, but may be altered by a number of factors, including the acquisition of plasmids (p. 549). Inability to penetrate the various layers of the envelope, is one explanation for intrinsic resistance of Gram-negative bacteria to antibiotics (p. 16). The effect of beta-lactamase activity (see below) and the outer membrane barrier on the elevation of MICs is also synergistic; the contribution of beta-lactamase is more effectively expressed in the bacterial cells with higher outer membrane barrier (Sawai et al., 1988). But the bacteria cannot make their outer membrane completely impenetrable; this then would exclude all essential nutrients as well. In an organism like Ps. aeruginosa in addition to the permeability barrier there is also the membrane-associated energy-driven efflux. This actively pumps antibiotics out of the periplasmic space and so prevents their access to their target proteins (Nikaido, 1994).

Degradative enzymes in the periplasmic space which are confined within the cell by the outer membrane of Gram-negative bacteria, are also very important in determining antibiotic resistance. Of special importance are the beta-lactamases which confer resistance to beta-lactam antibiotics (Sykes, 1982; Bush and Sykes, 1986; Bauernfeid, 1986; Bush, 1988, 1989a,b,c; Sanders, 1992). A number of factors influence the efficacy of beta-lactam antibiotics. These include the amount of the beta-lactam antibiotic which has penetrated through into the space, the amount of enzyme present, the affinity or specificity of the enzyme for the particular beta-lactam antibiotic involved, and its 'efficiency' in hydrolyzing the antibiotic. In addition, the amount of beta-lactamase present in the periplasmic space can be altered in many Gram-negative bacteria, by chromosomal mutation, induction or by the acquisition of plasmids. Beta-lactamase inhibitors have been developed to overcome the destruction of beta-lactam antibiotics by these enzymes.

2 Penicillin binding proteins in bacteria

Most, if not all, of the penicillin molecules which have diffused through the outer boundaries of the bacterial cell, and have not been destroyed by beta-lactamases in the periplasmic space, become strongly bound by the plasma membrane. The components of the membrane responsible for this binding are PBPs. There is a wide variation in both the number and the amount of PBPs in different bacteria, but related bacteria tend to have similar patterns of PBPs (Tomasz, 1982; 1986). The PBPs are proteins which normally play essential roles in a variety of physiological functions in the bacterial cell, such as maintenance of structural integrity, shape and cell division (Tomasz, 1979; Tuomanen et al., 1986; Georgopapadakou, 1993). For instance, in E. coli PBPs 1a, 1b, 2, 3, 4, 5 and 6 have been identified; PBPs 1a and 1b are jointly concerned in cell elongation, PBP2 in shape determination and PBP3 in cell division (Curtis, 1981). Pen G and other beta-lactam antibiotics mainly bind to PBPs 1a, 1b, 2 and 3 of E. coli. Rapid lysis of the cell is caused by beta-lactams which bind to PBP1 e.g. cephaloridine (p. 251). Inhibition of PBP 2 in E. coli results in the generation of stable round forms and not spheroplasts (p. 28) associated with exposure to some beta-lactams. These continue to grow for several generations before further aberrations occur and lysis ensures. Mecillinam (p. 186) binds exclusively to PBP2 and causes these changes. Most beta-lactam antibiotics inhibit PBP3, the protein concerned in cell division of E. coli. By inhibition of PBP3 cell division, and in particular cross-wall synthesis, is prevented resulting initially in production of filamentous forms; these continue to grow for some four to six generations, but then they become further deformed and cell death occurs (Curtis et al., 1979c; Curtis, 1981). The singular inhibition of PBP 3 is bactericidal in E. coli, even though standard bacteriological testing in broth culture may suggest bacteriostasis (Curtis et al., 1985). These authors showed that filament formation is accompanied by disruption of outer membrane barrier function, as witnessed by a rapid leakage of periplasmic beta-lactamase. Also human polymorphs kill bacterial filaments more efficiently than they kill a comparable mass of bacilli, so that filaments may be a favorable consequence of treatment of infection in immunocompetent patients with beta-lactam antibiotics (Lorian and Atkinson, 1984).

Different PBP patterns are found in other bacteria; PBPs of a particular bacterium are assigned serial numbers (PBP1, PBP2 etc) which indicate decreasing molecular weight. Thus the PBP1 of E. coli need not have anything in common with a PBP1 of another bacterium (Tomasz, 1982). Intrinsic resistance to beta-lactam antibiotics including Pen G, in many instances, is due to complex alterations in several PBPs, usually resulting in one or more PBPs with lower affinity for Pen G (p. 7) (Bryan, 1988). In addition PBP 5 in E. coli has been shown to have a weak beta-lactamase activity as well (Nicholas and Strominger, 1988).

3 Action of beta-lactam antibiotics

Pen G and other beta-lactam antibiotics interfere with biosynthesis of the bacterial cell wall and this eventually causes lysis and death. It was thought that Pen G selectively inhibited a Pen G-sensitive enzyme transpeptidase, which is involved in transpeptidation i.e. assembly of an intact, insoluble protective peptidoglycan in the bacterial cell wall (Shockman et al., 1979). Bacteria with weak cell walls were presumably produced, which then ruptured under the mechanical pressure of normally increasing cytoplasmic mass. But the set of events is much more complex. Bacteria contain a number of distinct Pen G-sensitive targets, PBPs (see above), but the functions of most of these proteins is unknown. Also the enzymatic and physiological processes inhibited by beta-lactam antibiotics vary widely, depending on their structure and the type of bacterial species (Tipper, 1979; Tomasz, 1979). Inhibition of bacterial growth seems to be elicited by direct interaction of beta-lactam antibiotics with their PBPs; subsequent bactericidal or lytic effects are triggered by this initial reaction (Ogawara, 1981).

The fact that Pen G and most other beta-lactam antibiotics inhibit cell wall growth does not account for their rapid lethality to many bacteria (Shockman et al., 1979; Tomasz, 1979). Important mediators of cell death after exposure to beta-lactam antibiotics, are the endogenous peptidoglycan (murein) hydrolases (autolysins) (Kitano and Tomasz, 1979; Handwerger and Tomasz, 1985). Bacterial cells contain enzymes which synthesize peptidoglycan and autolytic enzymes which break it down (p. 26). Organisms defective in autolysins are inhibited by Pen G, but not killed by it, a phenomenon called tolerance. Streptococcus pneumoniae defective in murein hydrolase was first described by Tomasz et al. (1970). In 1977 Sabath et al. described the same phenomenon in Staph. aureus, and subsequently Pen G-tolerant variants have been detected among many bacterial species (p. 91). In non-tolerant bacterial strains, initial interference with cell wall synthesis caused by Pen G, appears to upset the cellular control of endogenous autolysins, which then cause autolysis and death of bacteria (Tomasz, 1979). How Pen G causes this autolytic enzyme disturbance is unknown. It may be because antibiotics make cell walls more porous by inhibition of cross-linkages, thereby allowing leakage of autolysin inhibitors from cells (Tipper, 1979).

Mechanisms by which different beta-lactam antibiotics cause irreversible effects vary among bacterial species. In *E. coli* beta-lactams with high affinity for PBP1, such as cephalothin (p. 256), are the most effective triggers of autolysis, but this is not the case in other bacterial species (Kitano and Tomasz, 1979). Group A streptococci rapidly lose viability in the presence of Pen G, but there is no evidence of autolysis (Kessler and Van de Rijn, 1981). In these organisms Pen G induces a rapid specific loss of total cellular RNA in the absence of hydrolysis of the cell wall, and this leads to cell death (McDowell and Reed, 1989). *Streptococcus pneumoniae* is rapidly killed by Pen G, and it undergoes cell lysis. A pneumococcal isolate which caused relapsing meningitis in a patient infected with HIV was found to display an unusual response to Pen G. There was rapid death but a striking lack of cellular lysis. It is possible that defective lysis may adversely affect the course of pneumococcal meningitis (Tuomanen *et al.*, 1988). It appears that pneumococci can be killed by Pen G by two mechanisms: one is autolysis dependent and the other one is not (Moreillon *et al.*, 1990).

Pen G may also inhibit RNA and thereby protein synthesis, as well as peptidoglycan synthesis, in Pen G-tolerant *Strep. mutans* strains (Mychajlonka *et al.*, 1980, 1981). That Pen G-tolerant *Strep. sanguis* strains (p. 9) can be made to respond to Pen G in a manner similar to non-tolerant strains (which possess autolysins) by addition of heterologous autolysins to the growth medium, raises the possibility that Pen G may act synergistically with various host enzymes during infections (Horne and Tomasz, 1980).

In vitro, differing morphological changes may be induced when bacteria are exposed to beta-lactam antibiotics in varying concentrations. For instance, low concentrations of Pen G and the cephalosporins produce filamentous changes (see above) in *E. coli* (Hartmann *et al.*, 1972; Greenwood and O'Grady, 1973a,b). Subinhibitory concentrations of Pen G prevents normal cell division of *Staph. aureus* (Lorian, 1975). These effects are presumed to be due to inhibition of wall autolysins by antibiotics in low concentrations. That Pen G inhibits cell wall autolytic enzymes provides an explanation of bacterial persisters in the presence of beta-lactam antibiotics. Persisters are morphologically normal bacteria which survive lethal concentrations of an antibiotic, but whose progeny are fully sensitive to these agents. Pen G is only lethal to growing cells in which autolysins have already initiated cell wall growth points. The small percentage of bacteria which are not growing at the time become persisters, because they have an intact bacterial cell wall. Pen G prevents autolysins from forming growing-points in these cells and they become 'frozen in suspended animation'. Once the antibiotic is removed persisters revert to normal growth patterns.

Cell wall deficient variants of many bacterial species can be produced by Pen G and other antibiotics which inhibit bacterial cell wall synthesis. These have been named variously as protoplasts, spheroplasts and L-phase variants, between which there are only slight differences e.g. protoplasts have absent and spheroplasts have defective cell walls. By using hypertonic media, cell wall defective microbial variants can be easily induced in the laboratory. It has been postulated that these variants may occur and persist during Pen G treatment of infections, in areas where the surrounding medium is hypertonic e.g. the renal medulla or purulent accumulations. Subsequently they may revert to normal bacteria and cause persistence or relapse of the infection. There is no evidence that cell wall deficient variants have any role in pathogenesis, persistence, recurrence or relapse of human infections. Their pathogenic potential may deserve further study, particularly in patients with defective immunological or phagocytic function. Special hypertonic culture media are needed to detect wall-defective microbial variants (Palmer, 1979; Watanakunakorn, 1979).

Toxicity

1 Hypersensitivity reactions

These are common and sensitization is usually the result of previous treatment with a penicillin, but some subjects have had immediate reactions to the drug when first treated. In these cases, it is postulated that a 'hidden contact', such as consumption of milk containing Pen G resulting from veterinary treatment, has occurred. Penicillin hypersensitivity has resulted from blood transfusion; the transfused blood contained some Pen G, which was missed by the usual questioning procedure for drug intake prior to blood donation (Michel and Sharon, 1980).

Allergic phenomena were more common with early amorphous Pen G preparations because they contained impurities (p. 3), including high molecular weight proteins. The Pen G molecule may also evoke allergy by acting as a hapten and combining with body proteins to form an antigenic compound. Various derivatives of the penicillin nucleus, 6-APA (p. 3), often share cross-sensitivity demonstrating that it also plays an important role. It was predicted that all penicillins derived from 6-APA would cross-react in sensitized individuals, but this is not invariable (p. 83). The Pen G molecule does not combine readily with protein to produce an antigen and the actual haptens are various penicillin break-down products. The most important of these is the penicilloyl derivative, which is formed by breaking of the beta-lactam ring (p. 3) this may become stably attached to protein via an amino group. The penicilloyl derivative can arise directly from Pen G or through an intermediary, penicillenic acid, which is another penicillin degration product. The conjugate of the penicilloyl derivative with body proteins is commonly called the 'major antigenic determinant' (Idsøe et al., 1972). Other penicillin degradation products, such as penicilloic acid (p. 24), and penilloic acid, which are also involved in allergy, are grouped together and called 'minor antigenic determinants'. The major antigenic determinant cannot be used for skin-testing procedures, because it is itself a potent sensitizing agent. When the penicilloyl derivative is conjugated with polymerized lysine, penicilloyl-polylysine (PPL) results, which appears to be much safer as a skin-test reagent (p. 30).

Pen G can become more allergenic after a period in solution, either because it is degraded to more allergenic substances (p. 20), or because of the formation of high molecular weight Pen G polymers (Dewdney et al., 1971). It is therefore always wise to use freshly prepared Pen G solutions (p. 20).

Penicillin hypersensitivity may be broadly divided in the following forms:

a Anaphylactic reactions Occurring in previously sensitized patients, these are rare, but they may result in death within minutes. Features are nausea, vomiting, abdominal pain, pallor, tachycardia, severe dyspnea due to bronchospasm, rigors, loss of consciousness and peripheral circulatory failure due to vasodilation and loss of plasma volume into the tissues. Acute urticaria and angioneurotic edema which may affect the larynx, can also occur (Austen, 1974). Anaphylactic reactions are largely mediated by IgE (reaginic) antibodies, but certain IgG subclass antibodies may also play a part (Parker, 1975). In large-scale surveys, anaphylactic reactions have occurred in approximately 0.05% of Pen G treated patients (Idsøe et al., 1968; Holgate, 1988; Lin, 1992). Thus anaphylaxis to Pen G has been estimated to occur in about one to five per 10 000 patients treated, with fatalities in as many as one to five of 100 000 treated patients (Lin, 1992). Thus about 10% of anaphylactic reactions may be fatal (Polk, 1982). Parenteral Pen G accounts for nearly all cases of anaphylaxis but there are occasional reports following the use of oral potassium Pen G (Spark, 1971). 'Accelerated' reactions, occurring within 2–48 h may sometimes happen in previously sensitized patients and take the form of urticaria, but laryngeal edema may also ensue (Idsøe et al., 1972). Accelerated reactions may also result in anaphylaxis and may be fatal. These reactions are also mediated by IgE antibodies (Lin, 1992).

Treatment of anaphylaxis should include immediate i.m. administration of 500–1000 μg (0.5–1.0 ml of a 1 : 1000 solution) of adrenaline, (epinephrine), which is repeated every 15 min until improvement occurs (Leading article, 1981). Intramuscular injection is preferred because absorption of adrenaline from subcutaneous injection is too slow. Adrenaline may be given i.v. in the same dose, but this may cause ventricular premature beats and other arrhythmias (Sullivan, 1982). A slow i.v. injection of an antihistamine (such as 10–20 mg chlorpheniramine) should be given after i.m. adrenaline, and repeated over the next 24–48 h, to prevent relapse. Although histamine is only one of the mediators concerned in anaphylaxis, it may be an important one, as its increased serum concentrations appear to correlate with the degree of hypotension. Intravenous corticosteroids (such as 100–200 mg hydrocortisone) have little place in emergency resuscitation because their beneficial effects are delayed for several hours. Nevertheless, it is advisable to administer them early, as this will help to prevent deterioration after primary treatment has been given (Leading article, 1981). If possible, a tourniquet should be applied proximal to the site of the Pen G i.m. injection (which should be released at regular intervals thereafter). Other resuscitative measures, such as provision of a clear airway, positive pressure oxygen, continuous cardiographic monitoring and treatment of arrhythmias may be required (Sullivan, 1982). Rapid infusion of saline or plasma expanders may be necessary to combat shock (American Academy of Pediatrics, 1973). If hypotension persists i.v. metaraminol (aramine) can be tried. Penicillinase has little, if any place, in the emergency treatment of anaphylactic reactions. It rapidly breaks down circulating Pen G, but has no effect on preformed antigen–antibody complexes; also penicillinase itself may provoke sensitivity reactions (Idsøe *et al.*, 1968).

b Serum sickness (late reactions)   These have occurred in approximately 2% of patients treated with Pen G (Polk, 1982). They usually appear 7–10 days after primary administration of the drug. They are produced by circulating immune complexes, the formation of which is possible because intravascular antigen is still present when antibody is first produced (Parker, 1975). Serum sickness is characterized by fever, malaise, urticaria, joint pains, lymphadenopathy and occasionally angioneurotic edema. Erythema nodosum is less common. Exfoliative dermatitis (which may be serious or even fatal) and Stevens–Johnson syndrome may rarely occur.

Drug fever may be the sole manifestation of Pen G-induced serum sickness (Young *et al.*, 1982a). Other authors consider that the mechanisms by which drugs induce fever have not been well delineated and that this reaction may not have an allergic basis (Mackowiak and Le Maistre, 1987).

Serum sickness is usually not serious and it subsides when Pen G is withdrawn. Antihistamines are helpful but in severe cases corticosteroids are necessary. Penicillinase is effective in severe cases, but as this product can cause sensitivity reactions (see above), corticosteroids are preferable.

c Contact dermatitis   This results from topical Pen G application or exposure to Pen G aerosol; it is an occupational disease of nurses.

d Local reactions   Swelling and redness at the site of Pen G injection may occur.

A careful clinical history still remains the main indicator of possible reactors to Pen G. Idsøe *et al.* (1968) analyzed 151 deaths due to Pen G, reported from 1951 to 1965; 38 had a history of previous reaction and in 74 others, the previous drug history was not recorded. Some authors considered that patients with a history of asthma, hay fever and other allergies were more likely to react to Pen G (Smith, 1974), but others found no correlation with family or personal history of other allergies (Horowitz, 1975). In any case, the increased risk of Pen G reactions in patients with other allergies, appears to be small and the drug may be given to them whenever it is indicated.

Routine testing for sensitive individuals prior to Pen G administration is not practicable. Skin tests using Pen G as antigen are inadvisable, because even the small doses used may cause serious reactions or sensitize some patients. Moreover, this method of testing is unreliable for detecting the rare patient liable to anaphylaxis. Other tests may be performed in special instances, if the reagents are available. The PPL skin test (p. 29) is considerably safer, in spite of occasional reports of anaphylaxis. But this test does not detect all potential reactors to Pen G, particularly those who are more prone to anaphylaxis. The predictive value of skin testing is increased if the PPL test is combined with another test employing a 'minor determinant mixture' containing various penicillin metabolites (p. 29), and some crystalline Pen G (Levine and Zolov, 1969; Lin, 1992). Combined use of these two skin tests is helpful. If both tests are negative in a patient with a history of possible Pen G allergy, risk of an immediate reaction to the drug is very low (Levine and Zolov, 1969; Adkinson *et al.*, 1971; Saxon, 1983; Lin, 1992) and the frequency of late reactions to Pen G are not much greater than those in patients with no history of previous Pen G hypersensitivity (Levine, 1972). If skin tests without the minor determinant antigens are carried out, approximately 3% of Pen G-allergic patients will be missed, and these patients are more likely to have severe reactions. Using both reagents for skin testing in the USA since 1969, has shown that approximately 75% of patients who think that they are allergic to Pen G, have negative skin tests, and they can safely receive the drug. Pen G allergy may be lost after some years, but in others it persists for a long time, possibly for life (Lin, 1992).

In the USA, PPL is available commercially ('Pre-Pen'), and it was thought that this could be useful to screen patients without a history of Pen G allergy (Parker, 1975). Unfortunately, testing of patients with a history of Pen G allergy is still unsatisfactory, as a suitable preparation of the more important antigen, the 'minor determinant mixture' (see above), is not available for general use. Both reagents are being further assessed for commercial availability (De Swarte, 1982; Saxon, 1983; Lin, 1992). It is likely that their use will be restricted to special units. For most clinicians, the selection of a suitable alternate antibiotic to Pen G, will be an easier solution, than subjecting patients to these testing procedures.

In vitro tests were tried during the 1960s to investigate Pen G hypersensitivity. Serological tests only estimated IgM and IgG antibodies, and not reaginic (IgE) antibodies, which mediate anaphylaxis. Radioimmunoassay was then employed to demonstrate circulating IgG and IgE antibodies, specific for a Pen G antigen (Parker, 1975). Other tests which were tried included indirect basophil degranulation, lymphocyte transformation and the use of bacteriophages. None of these were suitable for routine clinical use.

Desensitization of Pen G-allergic patients may be practicable, but usually effective alternative antibiotics can be selected. It may be required on rare occasions because allergy poses an occupational hazard, or because the patient has a serious infection unresponsive to other antibiotics. Desensitization has its risks despite the development of a safer 4-h method using oral doses of penicillin (Holgate, 1988; Lin 1992).

2 Reactions peculiar to procaine Pen G

Occasionally severe reactions and even death, occurring during or shortly after an 'i.m.' injection of procaine Pen G, may result from accidental i.v. injection. These reactions are partly caused by microembolization of procaine Pen G particles to the lungs and brain, which produces hyperventilation, dilatation of pupils, convulsions and coma. Toxicity due to the procaine component of the drug is contributory. Early manifestations include marked anxiety, fever, hypertension, tachycardia, vomiting and audiovisual hallucinations. In severe cases, there may be convulsions, abrupt hypotension and cardiorespiratory arrest which may simulate anaphylaxis. Galpin *et al.* (1974) recorded three patients to whom procaine Pen G was administered inadvertently by i.v. infusion. Within 15 min, one patient developed a generalized seizure and cardiorespiratory arrest with slow idioventricular rhythm, but recovered with resuscitation. The other two patients had acute anxiety, tachypnea, dizziness and tinnitus.

Procaine Pen G may cause less severe side-effects. Some patients experience extreme anxiety and a sensation of impending death after an i.m. injection, but show no abnormal physical signs, such as shock or bronchospasm. Hallucinations, disorientation or psychotic behavior may occur. Minor physical abnormalities, such as tachycardia, hypertension or twitchings of extremities are sometimes observed. Attacks usually subside after 15–30 min, but some patients may exhibit mental lability for several months (Silber and D'Angelo, 1985). These side-effects may occur more commonly in patients with a past history of mental instability (Menke and Pepplinkhuizen, 1974). Minor reactions to procaine Pen G develop in about 0.1–0.3% of treated patients, and probably result from direct procaine toxicity. *In vivo*, procaine is quickly liberated from procaine Pen G; it can be detected in the serum immediately after an i.m. injection, and measurable levels persist for about 30 min (Green *et al.*, 1974). Accidental i.v. injection of part of the dose may sometimes be a factor. Patients exhibiting this side-effect may be regarded as hysterical by those who are unaware of this clinical entity.

3 Jarisch-Herxheimer reaction

This may be evoked when patients with syphilis are treated with Pen G (p. 46). It was thought to be due to release of endotoxins (lipopolysaccharides) from large numbers of killed treponemas (Gelfand *et al.*, 1976). This was not borne out by studies in animals. Other possible causes were considered to be the formation of immune complexes with treponemal antigens or the release of a non-endotoxin pyrogen from *T. pallidum* (Young *et al.*, 1982b). It now appears that the reaction is mediated by the action of cytokines released into the circulation (Griffin, 1992). The reaction usually occurs 6–8 h after commencement of Pen G and subsides within 12–24 h. Features include malaise, chills, fever, sore throat, myalgia, headache and tachycardia; there may be an exacerbation of existing syphilitic lesions, e.g. flaring of the rash of secondary syphilis (Bryceson, 1976; Gelfand *et al.*, 1976). Reactions in early syphilis are unpleasant but not serious. In late cardiovascular or neurosyphilis, serious reactions, although rare, are possible due to aggravation of local lesions. For instance, patients with late cardiovascular disease may die during a reaction, and those with cerebral syphilis may develop increased mental disturbance (Bryceson, 1976).

The Jarisch-Herxheimer reaction may occur in about 50% of patients treated with Pen G for primary syphilis, 75% of those with secondary syphilis and 30% of those with neurosyphilis (Gelfand *et al.*, 1976). Corticosteroids may modify this reaction, especially in early syphilis. Even large doses do not abolish all clinical and pathological changes, so their role in treatment is controversial and probably minimal (Teklu *et al.*, 1983). All patients with early syphilis and most with late cardiovascular and neurosyphilis, can be treated from the outset with therapeutic doses of Pen G. Initial treatment with small doses or the concomitant use of corticosteroids is only indicated in patients in whom there is a serious risk of increased local damage, e.g. syphilitic optic atrophy (Idsøe et al., 1968).

Jarisch-Herxheimer reactions occur when certain other infections are treated by Pen G. They are frequent in leptospirosis (p. 48), and result in fever, hypotension and precipitation or aggravation of the features of the disease. The reaction may even precipitate the need for hemodialysis and artificial respiration (Friedland and Warrell, 1991; Emmanouilides et al., 1994). It may follow the use of Pen G for the treatment of yaws (p. 48), rat-bite fever (p. 48), anthrax (p. 49) and rarely meningococcal meningitis (Berkowitz et al., 1983). A Jarisch-Herxheimer reaction can complicate the treatment of some infections by other antibiotics. A severe form may be provoked by tetracyclines in louse-borne relapsing fever (p. 736), which may be fatal (Bryceson, 1976). High dose corticosteroids, given before, or at the time of tetracycline treatment, does not alter the reaction, but it is diminished by meptazinol (a partial opioid antagonist), given i.v. in a dose of 300–500 mg to adults (Teklu et al., 1983). The reaction occasionally follows tetracycline treatment of brucellosis and tularemia (p. 736) and chloramphenicol use in typhoid fever (p. 567).

4 Direct Pen G toxicity

Pen G is of very low toxicity to humans but when 'massive doses' of 60 g daily or more are given i.v., encephalopathy with drowsiness, hyper-reflexia, myoclonic twitches, convulsions and coma may result (Nicholls, 1980; Snavely and Hodges, 1984). These very high doses of Pen G are not used nowadays. Toxicity is more likely to occur in patients with impaired renal function and in the elderly (Manian et al., 1990). In one patient who developed convulsions, the serum Pen G concentration was 433 μg per ml, 2 h after i.v. administration of 6 g (Weinstein et al., 1964). Pen G levels in CSF appear to be more important than serum levels; there is little danger of convulsions unless CSF Pen G levels exceed 5 μg per ml (Lerner et al., 1967). Animal studies have shown that the brain tissue concentrations, rather than CSF concentrations of Pen G are decisive for neurotoxicity (Schliamser et al., 1988a,b; 1989, 1991).

Since the permeability of the 'blood–brain barrier' to Pen G increases in meningitis (p. 25), smaller doses may precipitate encephalopathy in patients with this disease. Cardiopulmonary bypass may in some way predispose patients to Pen G neurotoxicity. Convulsions, apparently due to i.v. Pen G, were observed in patients undergoing open heart surgery (Seamans et al., 1968). If massive doses of Pen G are administered, probenecid should not be given (Lerner et al., 1967). Apart from its action of blocking renal tubular secretion (p. 24), probenecid also inhibits efflux of Pen G from the CSF where it accumulates (p. 25). Administration of much smaller doses of Pen G intrathecally can cause encephalopathy. The intrathecal dose for adults must not exceed 6–12 mg daily. In infants a daily intraventricular dose of 3 mg Pen G has been used without side-effects (Lee et al., 1977). Such forms of treatment for meningitis are unnecessary (p. 39). Pen G can be removed from the body by hemodialysis, but carbon hemoperfusion is far more efficient and is probably the treatment of choice for Pen G intoxication (Wickerts et al., 1980). Status epilepticus in Pen G overdosage is the usual immediate life-threatening complication. Marks and Cummins (1981) reported a 56-year-old woman who received 1.2 g of crystalline Pen G intrathecally by mistake. Status epilepticus was treated for several days by curarization, infused thiopentone and controlled ventilation; CSF lavage was also performed to reduce the toxic Pen G concentration, and she subsequently recovered. In animals Pen G encephalopathy can be reversed by systemically administered penicillinase (Raichle et al., 1971).

5 Nephropathy

Interstitial nephritis, which occurs with many antibiotics, particularly methicillin (p. 84), can complicate i.v. administration of large doses of Pen G (12–36 g daily) (Baldwin et al., 1968; Roxe, 1980). This usually ensues after about 8 days' treatment, and is manifested by fever, eosinophilia, occasional rashes, albuminuria and a rise in blood urea. Renal biopsy shows interstitial nephritis without glomerular abnormalities or arteritis. Most patients recover when Pen G is stopped. A hypersensitivity mechanism is probably involved (p. 84). There is no evidence that patients with renal impairment are more likely than patients with normal renal function to develop this complication when treated with appropriately adjusted doses of Pen G. If too high doses are used renal function may be aggravated (Manian et al., 1990).

Milder forms of Pen G hypersensitivity nephritis may present with features of dysuria, pyuria, proteinuria and eosinophilia suggesting a urinary tract infection, there usually being no azotemia. It rapidly resolves when Pen G is withdrawn, but promptly recurs on readministration of the drug (Orchard and Rooker, 1974). Rarely, renal disease characterized by glomerulonephritis or periarteritis, has been associated with the administration of relatively low doses of Pen G. The causal role of Pen G in these cases is doubtful (Baldwin *et al.*, 1968).

6 Hemolytic anemia

This uncommon complication may happen when i.v. Pen G in a dose usually greater than 6 g per day, is given to patients who have previously received large doses of the drug (White *et al.*, 1968). Characteristic of hemolysis, the hemoglobin level falls and the reticulocyte count rises. Pen G-induced hemolytic anemia is of the hapten type, i.e. the antibody produced is directed to the drug (hapten). A strongly positive direct antiglobulin reaction (Coombs' test) is the main diagnostic feature, which is due to induced IgG antibody reacting with Pen G coated red cells (Garratty and Petz, 1975; Axelson and Lo Buglio, 1980). Erythrocytes not coated with Pen G may also be destroyed because they may bind activated complement components, and thereby be susceptible to premature destruction by the reticuloendothelial system (Kerr *et al.*, 1972).

Pen G-induced hemolytic anemia should be suspected in patients who develop anemia while receiving high doses of Pen G. Patients with severe infections such as bacterial endocarditis, often develop anemia due to infection and the hemolytic component may be overlooked. On withdrawing Pen G, the hemoglobin value usually rises quickly, and the direct antiglobulin test becomes negative in 1–3 months. In most cases Pen G-induced hemolysis is not very severe; occasionally rapid intravascular hemolysis, followed by renal failure or even circulatory collapse and death may ensue (Jackson and Jaffe, 1979). Often IgG antibody to Pen G cross-reacts with red cells sensitized with the semisynthetic penicillins and cephalosporins, so that these drugs are not safe alternatives (White *et al.*, 1968).

It is much less common for Pen G administered in ordinary therapeutic doses to cause hemolytic anemia. In these cases, IgG antibody cannot be detected but an IgM antibody is present (Dove *et al.*, 1975). Pen G has been suggested as a possible cause of microangiopathic hemolytic syndrome (thrombotic thrombocytopenic purpura) in one patient (Parker and Barrett, 1971). Pen G-associated hemolytic anemia occurred in another patient who had postpartum disseminated intravascular coagulation and microangiopathy, and was receiving Pen G in a daily dose of 3 g for infection. Hemolysis occurred when her coagulation disorder had been controlled by 9 days' treatment with heparin (McPherson *et al.*, 1976).

7 Other hematological side-effects

Pen G, in large doses, can rarely cause pancytopenia due to apparent blockade of the release of mature cells from the bone marrow (Joorabchi and Kohout, 1973). Severe neutropenia, usually resulting from the use of high doses of Pen G i.v. for several weeks, is another complication, which usually resolves when Pen G is stopped (Corbett *et al.*, 1982; Al-Hadramy *et al.*, 1986). This neutropenia appears to be dose-related. Olaison and Alestig (1990) found neutropenia to be a common complication when Pen G in a dose of 18 g i.v. was used to treat bacterial endocarditis, whilst this complication was uncommon with a dose of 12 g i.v. cloxacillin daily. Patients with initial low neutrophil counts had an increased risk of developing neutropenia. Pre-existing liver disease also predisposes patients to Pen G-induced leukopenia. Pen G and other beta-lactam antibiotics when administered in usually recommended dosages can induce leukopenia in these patients. The more severe the hepatic dysfunction the greater the risk. Doses of beta-lactams may need to be reduced in these patients (Singh *et al.*, 1993).

When Pen G-induced neutropenia resolves after cessation of the drug it may recur if another beta-lactam is used. In one case neutropenia recurred when cefuroxime (p. 291), was given in high doses i.v. as a substitute for Pen G in the treatment of gonococcal endocarditis. The neutropenia resolved when i.v. erythromycin was substituted for cefuroxime (Timmis *et al.*, 1981). Severe neutropenia is a well known complication of high-dose therapy with most beta-lactam antibiotics. Secondary infection, related to this neutropenia has only been observed in a few cases and no fatalities have been reported. Treatment with high doses of beta-lactams in granulocytopenic patients receiving cytotoxic therapy simultaneously, may prolong the episode of granulocytopenia. It is not yet known how this effect can be recognized clinically and whether this may have an adverse effect on therapeutic outcome (Neftel *et al.*, 1985).

If administered in large doses of 6 g daily to uremic patients, or 24 g daily to those with normal renal function, Pen G can induce coagulation disorders. These may appear soon after Pen G administration and persist for about 4 days after it is stopped. Factors involved are platelet dysfunction (p. 153), disturbed conversion of fibrinogen to fibrin and increased antithrombin-III activity (Andrassy *et al.*, 1976; Manian *et al.*, 1990). Pen G therapy can also be associated with the development of acquired inhibitors of blood coagulation, particularly blocking inhibitors. These are proteins but not necessarily antibodies, which can interfere with many aspects of the coagulation reaction, but they are rarely, if ever, associated with overt bleeding. The prothrombin time is normal, but the activated partial thromboplastin time is usually prolonged. Uncommonly, Pen G hypersensitivity may be associated with the presence of specific clotting factor inhibitors which inactivate single factors. Inhibitors specifically directed against factors V, VIII, IX and XI have been described, factor VIII inhibitors being the most common. These factor inhibitors appear to be antibodies and their presence may be associated with severe bleeding (Orris *et al.*, 1980).

8 Cation intoxication

A 0.625 g dose of the potassium salt of crystalline Pen G contains 1.5 mEq of potassium ion (0.066 g potassium). If 'massive doses' of this preparation are given i.v., potassium intoxication may occur. The sodium salt, which contains 1.7 mEq (or 0.039 g sodium) in 0.6 g is unlikely to cause complications, unless 'massive doses' are used in patients with renal or cardiac failure. Brunner and Frick (1968) described hypokalemia, metabolic alkalosis and hypernatremia in a few patients treated with 60 g of sodium Pen G daily. Hypernatremia was probably aggravated by insufficient fluid intake. Despite this, their daily urine output exceeded 1 liter, due to the osmotic diuretic action of 60 g of Pen G (equivalent to about 600 ml of 10% mannitol). Pen G probably induces excessive renal potassium loss by direct action on distal renal tubules, thereby producing hypokalemia and metabolic alkalosis. Antibiotics, such as Pen G, may also cause a redistribution of potassium within the body (Tattersall *et al.*, 1972).

9 Other rare side-effects

Pen G has occasionally been reported as the cause of pericarditis, myocarditis, intestinal hemorrhage, liver necrosis and gangrene (Idsøe *et al.*, 1968). It may cause hypersensitivity vasculitis (Hannedouche and Fillastre, 1987). It has been tenuously associated with drug-induced lupus syndromes. Pen G therapy can cause eosinophilia and pulmonary infiltration, but this is a rare association compared with that of other chemotherapeutic agents, such as nitrofurantoin (p. 927) and the sulfonamides (p. 819) (Schatz *et al.*, 1981). Benign intracranial hypertension may occur rarely due to vasculitis caused by Pen G hypersensitivity (Schmitt and Krivit, 1969). One patient who experienced a severe serum sickness following Pen G, later developed increased intracranial pressure due to pachymeningitis which responded to corticosteroids (Farmer *et al.*, 1960). Intravenous Pen G is said to be a rare cause of colicky abdominal pain (Davies *et al.*, 1974).

10 Nerve and muscle injury

The danger of sciatic nerve injury from i.m. Pen G injections in the buttock is well known, , and in most hospitals the drug is given in the lateral aspect of the thigh. Muscle necrosis and abscess formation can occur after i.m. injection, and rarely, muscle contractures may be a sequel to repeated i.m. injections in the thigh.

11 Intra-arterial injection of Pen G

This is an uncommon but very serious complication of i.m. injections of procaine or benzathine penicillin. Atkinson (1969) described a 7-month-old girl in whom procaine-benzathine Pen G was accidentally injected into the gluteal artery, causing transverse myelopathy with permanent paraplegia. This was presumably due to retrograde distribution to the vessels supplying the spinal cord, when the drug was injected under pressure, resulting in occlusive vascular disease; the injection was given in the upper and outer quadrant of the buttock. Weir and Fearnow (1983), collected seven published cases of transverse myelitis due to i.m. viscous benzathine or procaine penicillin. These occurred in young children and the authors suggested that procaine or benzathine Pen G injections are unsafe in the gluteal musculature of children aged less than 2–3 years.

A similar catastrophe occurred in two young children in whom a procaine benzathine Pen G mixture was injected in the outer aspect of the thigh. The disposable syringes used were so constructed that it was impossible to create a negative pressure and to ascertain whether the needle was in muscle or in a blood vessel. One child developed severe ischemic changes in the lower extremity which recovered in 2 weeks, but the other developed gangrene of the toes and muscle contractures in the leg (Schanzer *et al.*, 1979). Irreversible ischemic gangrene of the upper limb has been reported in a child after an unintentional intra-arterial injection of procaine Pen G (Sengupta, 1976).

Clinical Uses of the Drug

1 *Streptococcus pyogenes* infections

Pen G remains effective treatment for infections caused by Group A beta-hemolytic streptococci, such as pharyngitis, scarlet fever, cellulitis, septic arthritis, pelvic infection (p. 45) and septicemia. In recent years septicemia in children and young adults has often been very severe with multisystem involvement and shock (Jackson *et al.*, 1991; Stevens, 1992; Demers *et al.*, 1993). A changing nature of septicemia has also been observed since 1988. A toxic shock-like syndrome occurred in 8% of invasive infections since that time. Adults with this syndrome were younger than patients with other invasive infections. These patients were similar in some ways to those with *Staph. aureus* toxic shock syndrome (p. 98). Both bacteremia and endotoxins caused this illness. Patients showed hypotension, erythematous rash, desquamation and renal and gastrointestinal manifestations and septic thrombophlebitis. Severe manifestations also included necrotizing fasciitis and gangrenous myositis, which resembled clostridial myonecrosis, but there was no crepitus. These two entities need early radical surgical debridement plus Pen G therapy (Yoder *et al.*, 1987; Roggiani and Schlievert, 1994). The blood cultures were positive in some 60% of cases and the mortality was approximately 30% (Cohen-Abbo and Harper, 1993; Shulman, 1993; Jevon *et al.*, 1994). In general there was a lower rate of streptococcal toxic shock syndrome and lower mortality in children with invasive Group A streptococcal infections, compared with young adults (Davies *et al.*, 1994).

Occasionally *Strep. pyogenes* causes bacterial meningitis (approximately 0.5% of cases) in neonates, older children and adults. In most patients an associated illness is present such as otitis media or pharyngitis (Murphy, 1983; Chow and Muder, 1992). In one 12-year-old girl *Strep. pyogenes* meningitis was complicated by a brain abscess (Jagdis, 1988).

For severe infections i.m. or i.v. crystalline Pen G in a dosage of 0.6–1.8 g (1–3 million units) every 3–6 h is required for adults. Mild to moderate streptococcal pharyngitis in children and adults can be treated satisfactorily by a single i.m. injection of benzathine Pen G (adult dose 1.2 million units or 0.9 g). When shorter acting preparations are used, treatment should be for at least 10 days in an endeavor to eradicate the organisms from the pharynx, and to prevent subsequent rheumatic fever (Peter and Smith, 1977; Peter, 1992). Although clinical resolution of streptococcal pharyngitis is always satisfactory, in some 10% of patients a 10–day course of either parenteral Pen G (including therapy with benzathine Pen G) or oral penicillin V (p. 74), fails to eradicate organisms from the pharynx (Peter, 1992). Some authors have found that this happens in as many as 20% (Gastanaduy *et al.*, 1980). A second course of therapy is unsuccessful in 30–50% of these patients. Clinical, epidemiological and serological (streptococcal antibody) data suggest that most patients designated as 'bacteriological treatment failures' are actually long-term streptococcal carriers. It is often extremely difficult to eradicate streptococci from carriers, so that a third course of treatment is rarely justified. An asymptomatic carrier of *Strep. pyogenes* identified by a routine throat swab, does not require antibiotic treatment, except if there are special circumstances, e.g. if a family member has had rheumatic fever or if there is a community epidemic of rheumatic fever (Kaplan, 1980; Ferrieri, 1981). A regimen of i.m. benzathine penicillin plus rifampicin (10 mg per kg twice a day for eight doses) is effective for the eradication of the pharyngeal *Strep. pyogenes* carrier state (Gerber and Markowitz, 1985; Tanz *et al.*, 1985).

Failure to eradicate Pen G-sensitive *Strep. pyogenes* from the pharynx may be due to the presence of anaerobes or *Staph. aureus* producing beta-lactamases, which 'shield' streptococci from the activity of Pen G (Brook, 1982; 1984; Lundberg and Nord, 1988; Brook and Gilmore, 1993). Gram-negative anaerobes, such as *Prevotella melaninogenica*, originally very sensitive to Pen G, are now often resistant because of beta-lactamase production (p. 17). Gram-negative anaerobes have no etiological role in pharyngitis, but they are pathogens in periapical and peridontal infections. Pen G has been satisfactory for such infections, but with the increasing resistance of anaerobes which normally populate the oropharynx, other chemotherapeutic agents, such as clindamycin (p. 597) or metronidazole (p. 948), may become necessary (Von Konow and Nord, 1983). Data are still conflicting whether beta-lactamase-producing organisms play a significant role in producing treatment failures when Pen G is used for streptococcal pharyngitis (Kaplan, 1985).

Some reports link the failure of Pen G treatment of *Strep. pyogenes* pharyngitis to the fact that the streptococcal strain is Pen G-tolerant (Kim and Kaplan, 1985, Dagan *et al.*, 1987; Grahn *et al.*, 1987). At present it seems unlikely that this is the correct explanation for such treatment failures (Kim, 1988). Stevens *et al.* (1993b) demonstrated a striking reduction in the effectiveness of Pen G *in vitro* and *in vivo* as the inoculum size of *Strep. pyogenes* was increased. They felt that this apparent reduction in the activity of Pen G was due to the slower growth of bacteria as the inoculum size was increased. It was further postulated that this at least in part was caused by variation in the expression of PBPs as the state of *Strep. pyogenes* changes during its growth cycle. By contrast, the activity of clindamycin, which does not depend on PBPs, was not adversely affected by inoculum size. Thus Pen G therapy may fail in deep seated *Strep. pyogenes* infections, especially if treatment is delayed.

2 Group B streptococcal infections

Since about 1960, these organisms have been recognized as an important cause of neonatal infections, and also of adult infections (p. 4). In infants, they may cause an acute disease presenting with sepsis, acute respiratory distress, pneumonia, apnea, shock, meningitis and septicemia; this is of 'early onset' and usually presents within 24 h of delivery or within the first 5 days of birth (Cowen, 1979; Van Oppen and Feldman, 1993). Many infants are already ill at birth, indicating that the infection had commenced during labor (Gotoff and Boyer, 1981; Hamoudi and Hamoudi, 1981). Mortality of this disease may be 20–50% (Siegel *et al.*, 1980; Van Oppen and Feldman, 1993). Other infants can develop a disease of later onset and present with meningitis with or without septicemia, usually after the age of 10 days. Mortality in this group is 14–18%. In adults, Group B streptococci commonly cause postpartum infections (p. 45), urinary tract infections in pregnant women, non-pregnant women and occasionally men (Muñoz *et al.*, 1992b), pneumonia and septicemia, but meningitis, endocarditis, osteomyelitis, septic arthritis, peritonitis, skin and wound infections, also occur (Verghese *et al.*, 1982, 1986; Aharoni *et al.*, 1990; Belfrage *et al.*, 1990; Sarmiento *et al.*, 1993).

Pen G is the drug of choice for treatment of all of these infections, and most cases require parenteral therapy with crystalline Pen G. In neonates, the high dose as recommended for meningitis, should be used (p. 21). Combination therapy using Pen G plus an aminoglycoside, such as gentamicin, may be more effective (p. 455), but one study in animals showed that Pen G plus gentamicin was about as effective as Pen G alone (Kim, 1987). However, this combination is necessary for all severe neonatal infections before the organism is identified (Leading article, 1979) (p. 473). On theoretical grounds, combination therapy should be valuable if the infecting organism is a Pen G-tolerant Group B streptococcus (p. 4), but this has not been studied by controlled trials (Siegel *et al.*, 1981).

The role of Pen G in chemoprophylaxis of neonatal infections is not well defined. Approximately 10–25% of pregnant women at term have Group B streptococci in their vaginal flora (Dillon *et al.*, 1982; Hoogkamp-Korstanje *et al.*, 1982), and this is the main source for sepsis in neonates. Neonatal colonization by these organisms is quite common but only a small proportion develop invasive infection (Baker, 1977; Anthony, 1982). Unfortunately, the eradication of genital Group B streptococci during pregnancy, is not only impracticable but difficult to attain (Anthony, 1982). This is not surprising because primary colonization is in the lower intestine (p. 4). Pen G treatment of all colonized infants is not recommended. It often fails to eradicate organisms from sites such as the throat, umbilicus and rectum (Paredes *et al.*, 1976). Routine prophylaxis for neonates is also not advocated. In a prospective controlled study involving 18 738 neonates, the administration of a single i.m. dose of crystalline Pen G at birth resulted in a decrease of diseases caused by all Pen G-susceptible organisms. Disease caused by Pen G-resistant pathogens, was increased in the Pen G treated group during the first year of study but unaffected during the second year (Siegel *et al.*, 1980). There is also concern that routine Pen G prophylaxis for neonates may mask but not cure early onset disease in those who are already symptomatic at birth (Gotoff and Boyer, 1981). This was the case in a study by Pyati *et al.* (1983). Pen G, given at birth to neonates weighing 2000 g or less, did not prevent early-onset disease or reduce its mortality; early onset disease appeared to be well established by the time of Pen G administration.

Another approach is to screen all obstetric patients for vaginal carriage of Group B streptococci. A single dose of Pen G is then administered as prophylaxis, both to maternal carriers during labor, and to their infants at birth (Gilbert and Garland, 1983). This appears to reduce vertical transmission of Group B streptococci and to prevent both maternal and neonatal disease (Fischer *et al.*, 1983). Similarly, ampicillin or Pen G administered selectively during labor to women with prenatal Group B streptococcal colonization and perinatal risk factors, resulted in a reduction of vertical transmission of these organisms to newborn infants (Boyer *et al.*, 1983). Therefore to be effective, antibiotic therapy should be given to the mother prior to the development of the disease *in utero*; to be practical, therapy must be limited to those at relatively high risk of infection (Dillon *et al.*, 1987; Schuchat *et al.*, 1994; Isaacs *et al.*, 1995)). In one prospective randomized study women were selected if they had a prenatal culture positive for Group B streptococci and if they had premature labor or prolonged rupture of n.embranes. Chemoprophylaxis with parenteral ampicillin was given intrapartum. After birth infants in the treatment group received additional antibiotic therapy until their blood culture results become available. There were no Group B streptococcal infections among 83 infants in the treatment group compared with five infections in the 77 control infants (Boyer and Gotoff, 1986). The intrapartum prophylaxis strategy, also significantly reduced maternal puerperal sepsis (Dillon *et al.*, 1987). Universal prenatal screening for Group B streptococci and chemoprophylaxis of colonized women with labor complications has also been advocated by Mohle-Boetani *et al.* (1993). An alternate strategy, which is also effective, is not to screen pregnant women for Group B streptococcal carriage, but give intrapartum chemoprophylaxis to all women with obstetric risk factors (Garland and Kelly, 1995).

3 Group C, G, F and R streptococcal infections

These are less common human pathogens. Group C streptococci occasionally cause pharyngitis, skin and wound infections, female genital tract infections, endocarditis and septicemia (Bradley *et al.*, 1991). Group G streptococci may cause infections such as endocarditis, septicemia, meningitis, cellulitis, septic arthritis, wound infections, cholangitis, pneumonia and peritonitis (Fujita *et al.*, 1982; Auckenthaler *et al.*, 1983; Craven *et al.*, 1986; Venezio *et al.*, 1986; Ashkenazi *et al.*, 1988). Infections by these two pathogens have often occurred in patients with underlying debilitating conditions such as alcoholism, drug abuse and malignancy. Pen G is the optimal treatment for Groups C and G streptococcal infections. For severe Group G streptococcal infections, such as endocarditis, a Pen G/aminoglycoside combination may be superior (Vartian *et al.*, 1985). Group F streptococci rarely cause abscesses and septicemia. Pen G again is the treatment of choice (Libertin *et al.*, 1985).

Group R streptococcus (*Strep. suis*) is an animal pathogen and rarely causes disease in humans working with animals, such as pigs. Twort (1981) reported five cases of meningitis due to these streptococci in the UK. Chau *et al.* (1983) described six in Hong Kong, and Arends and Zanen (1988) reported 30 in Netherlands. Nearly all patients had occupational exposure to pigs or pork products. All strains of *Strep. suis* were highly susceptible to Pen G (MIC 0.03 μg per ml), and it appears to be the best drug for treatment of this infection.

4 Respiratory infections in adults

For pneumococcal lobar pneumonia, Pen G is still the best treatment, even when pneumococcal strains with high degree of resistance to Pen G are encountered (p. 5). Provided that crystalline Pen G in a dose of 1.2 g (2 million units) 4-hourly (or more) is given i.v., pneumonia due to Pen G-resistant strains with MICs of 2.0 μg per ml or even higher will respond to Pen G (Klugman, 1994; Pallares *et al.*, 1995; Jernigan *et al.*, 1996; Plouffe *et al.*, 1996). In an animal model pneumonia due to such strains responded better to i.v. ceftriaxone, because its MICs for these strains were usually, but not invariably, lower (Moine *et al.*, 1994). This contrasts with pneumococcal meningitis, a disease in which Pen G usually fails even if organisms with only intermediate type of Pen G resistance are involved (p. 39). But sometimes treatment of pneumococcal pneumonia caused by *Strep. pneumoniae* with high degree of Pen G-resistance may be difficult. These strains may be resistant to many other antibiotics (p. 5). Vancomycin at present is the most reliable drug (Musher, 1992). Several new drugs may prove useful such as cefpirome (p. 398), cefpodoxime (p. 423), clarithromycin (p. 643), and sparfloxacin (p. 1140) (Mason *et al.*; 1992, Neal *et al.*, 1992; Spangler *et al.*, 1992, 1993).

Pneumococcal infection is still the commonest form of community-acquired pneumonia (Holmberg, 1987; Davies and Jolley, 1992; Marrie, 1994). Other bacterial causes of such pneumonia are *L. pneumoniae* (p. 618). *H. influenzae* (p. 338), *Staph. aureus* (p. 97) and *E. coli* (p. 338). Non-bacterial causes of community-acquired pneumonia are *M. pneumoniae*, *C. psittaci*, *C. pneumoniae*, *Coxiella burnetti* and viruses, mainly influenza (Lode, 1986). Every effort should be made to make an immediate diagnosis of pneumococcal pneumonia, so that monotherapy with Pen G can be given and the administration of multiple antibiotics avoided. The distinctive signs and symptoms of pneumococcal pneumonia are sudden onset of fever, cough and some sputum, the patient appears ill and has a greyish appearance. Pleuritic pain is often present. Crackling sounds are usually audible in the chest and X-rays show an area of infiltration, involving less than a full segment. Sputum microscopy is often helpful if a good specimen of sputum is collected (Musher, 1992). For treatment we usually advocate crystalline Pen G in a dose of 0.6 g i.v. or i.m. 6-hourly, so that the dose is high enough to cover pneumococcal strains with intermediate type of resistance (p. 5). Other authors consider that procaine penicillin 1.2 g i.m. once or preferably twice a day may be sufficient for this purpose (Brewin *et al.*, 1974; Musher, 1992). Treatment will usually be necessary for 7–10 days.

Certainly on occasions it may be impossible to distinguish pneumococcal pneumonia from *L. pneumonia* in which case a combination of Pen G and erythromycin (p. 618) will have to be given. Sometimes *M. pneumonia* may be severe and the distinction may be difficult in which case the combination of Pen G/doxycycline may be appropriate. In life-threatening pneumonia, where immediate diagnosis cannot be made, flucloxacillin (p. 97) or nafcillin (p. 105) should also be used to cover *Staph. aureus* pneumonia and one of the third-generation cephalosporins such as cefotaxime (p. 338) or ceftriaxone (p. 360) to cover Gram-negative organism etiology. The usual pathogens causing hospital-acquired pneumonia are *Staph. aureus*, Gram-negative rods and *Legionella*, and Pen G is not appropriate for the treatment of any of these.

In acute bronchitis, the pneumococcus may be the major pathogen necessitating the use of Pen G. In chronic bronchitis, *H. influenzae* may be an important cause, and Pen G is usually not satisfactory. Other drugs, such as ampicillin (p. 123), amoxycillin (p. 140), a tetracycline (p. 741) or co-trimoxazole (p. 863) may be needed.

In lung abscess the most frequent pathogens are Pen G-sensitive anaerobes, such as the *Peptococcus* and *Peptostreptococcus* spp. and *Prevotella melaninogenica*. Pen G-sensitive aerobes, such as *Strep. pyogenes* and *Strep. viridans*, may also be involved. Sometimes Pen G-resistant bacteria, such as *B. fragilis*, *E. coli* and *Kl. pneumoniae*, may be present (Brook and Finegold, 1979). For most cases of lung abscess Pen G has been the preferred antibiotic. Over the years more and more strains of *Prevotella melaninogenica* have become beta-lactamase producers and thus resistant to Pen G. In a controlled study Levison *et al.* (1983) first showed that clindamycin (p. 597) alone was superior to Pen G for treatment of community-acquired lung abscess. In a later randomly controlled study, Gudiol *et al.* (1990) clearly showed that clindamycin was superior to Pen G for the treatment of this disease and they also demonstrated that the presence of Pen G-resistant Gram-negative anaerobes were the main reason for Pen G treatment failures.

In aspiration pneumonia, Pen G-sensitive anaerobes are the most common pathogens, but sometimes the other bacterial species as in lung abscess, may be present. The initial result of pulmonary aspiration is chemical pneumonitis, and bacterial infection follows in 25–45% of cases. Infection typically occurs during the first week after aspiration, not uncommonly as the patient is recovering from chemical pneumonitis. Antibiotics may be used prophylactically immediately after the aspiration, but some clinicians prefer to delay chemotherapy until clinical and microbiological findings indicate infection (Murray, 1979). Pen G has been the mainstay of treatment, but in severe cases a combination such as Pen G/gentamicin/metronidazole (or clindamycin) can be used. As in lung abscess (see above), clindamycin alone may prove to be the best treatment (Lode, 1988). Combination chemotherapy as above is best used for aspiration-related chest infections acquired in hospitals and if the patient develops necrotizing pneumonia, lung abscess or empyema.

5 Childhood respiratory infections

Most childhood community-acquired bacterial pneumonias are pneumococcal and respond well to Pen G. However, in children many radiologically confirmed pneumonias are caused by viruses or *M. pneumoniae*. In one study of radiologically confirmed pneumonias, *Strep. pneumoniae* caused 38%, respiratory syncytial virus 30% and *M. pneumoniae* 20% (Ruuskanen *et al.*, 1992).

Therefore all modern diagnostic techniques should be used at the outset, so that Pen G is not used for viral infections, and erythromycin (p. 619) is correctly prescribed for *M. pneumonia*. Rarer bacterial causes of pneumonia in this age group are *H. influenzae* type b (p. 338) and *Staph. aureus* (p. 97) and drugs other than Pen G are necessary for these. For bronchitis, either ampicillin (p. 123), amoxycillin (p. 140) or co-trimoxazole (p. 863) are more satisfactory than Pen G. In lung abscess and aspiration pneumonia, antibiotics similar to those recommended for adults should be used (see above).

6 Otitis media and sinusitis

For otitis media in adults, Pen G is usually satisfactory because *Strep. pneumoniae* or occasionally *Strep. pyogenes* is responsible for the majority. In children, additionally *H. influenzae* (mainly non-typable strains) is frequently involved, and therapy with either ampicillin (p. 123), amoxycillin (p. 140), co-trimoxazole (p. 864), or erythromycin alone (p. 617) or combined with a sulfonamide (p. 821), is recommended. Acute sinusitis in adults and children is caused either by pneumococci or *H. influenzae* (p. 123), so one of the drugs used for treatment of otitis media in children should be employed. Less commonly other organisms may be involved (p. 123).

7 Bacterial meningitis and brain abscess

Despite the availability of several third-generation cephalosporins, which are effective for the treatment of bacterial meningitis, Pen G still remains an important antibiotic for this disease. With the exception of neonatal meningitis, a combination of Pen G and chloramphenicol (p. 568) was used for initial treatment (before the organism was identified) of acute bacterial meningitis since about 1955. This initial therapy covered nearly all causal organisms, but once the organism was identified, Pen G alone was the drug of choice for meningococcal and pneumococcal meningitis (Geiseler *et al.*, 1980; Sangster *et al.*, 1982) and chloramphenicol for *H. influenzae* meningitis. Indeed, chloramphenicol alone may be used for initial therapy as it is equally effective to Pen G for treatment of meningococcal and pneumococcal meningitis. This classical chemotherapy is still preferred by many physicians, and is used widely in developing countries where the third-generation cephalosporins are too expensive. It would only be inappropriate to use it in areas where chloramphenicol-resistant *H. influenzae* strains are prevalent.

Now there is a choice for initial therapy. The third-generation cephalosporins cefotaxime (p. 336) and ceftriaxone (p. 359) are effective as single drugs for initial treatment as they are active against all three major meningeal pathogens (McCracken *et al.*, 1987; Committee on Infectious Diseases, 1988). They are not effective as single drugs for children under 12 weeks of age. In these Pen G or ampicillin should be added because of possibility of *Listeria* or *Enterococcus* spp. as causative agents.

Once the organism is identified the cephalosporin should be continued in *H. influenzae* meningitis and in the rare cases of Gram-negative meningitis, but it is best to revert to Pen G for continuation treatment of meningococcal and pneumococcal meningitis. The adult dosage of Pen G is 9.6–14.4 g (16–24 million units) daily, given i.v. or i.m. in six or eight divided doses. Cases of pneumococcal meningitis caused by strains with an intermediate type of resistance to Pen G usually fail to respond to these doses. The dose should not be increased further, but treatment changed to chloramphenicol (p. 569) or vancomycin (p. 779) (Committee on Infectious Diseases, 1988). Cefotaxime (p. 336) and ceftriaxone (p. 359) may be effective for treatment of meningitis caused by these strains (McCracken *et al.*, 1987; Weingarten *et al.*, 1990; Jacobs, 1992). If the strain has a cefotaxime or ceftriaxone MIC equal or greater than 0.5 μg per ml, then as a rule one of these cephalosporins cannot be used alone. Some authors feel that the MIC of these cephalosporins should be even lower for these drugs to succeed (p. 359), but combination therapy by one of these cephalosporins with vancomycin may be satisfactory or alternatively vancomycin plus rifampicin can be tried (Friedland *et al.*, 1993; Quagliarello and Scheld, 1993). For meningitis due to highly resistant pneumococcal strains, vancomycin (p. 779), and perhaps added rifampicin (p. 700) appears to be the only effective treatment. Dexamethasone may be beneficial as an adjunct to therapy of bacterial meningitis (p. 360), but this drug reduces the penetration of vancomycin into the CSF. So if vancomycin has to be used for treatment of pneumococcal meningitis, it is best not to use dexamethasome (Friedland and McCracken, 1994; Paris *et al.*, 1994).

For meningococcal meningitis a 7-day course of treatment is usually used, but some authors have produced evidence that 4–5 days therapy with Pen G may be sufficient (Viladrich *et al.*, 1986; Isaacs *et al.*, 1988). Partially or completely Pen G-resistant meningococci now have been encountered in some countries, and especially if one of the latter strains are involved, drugs other than Pen G are needed for treatment (p. 336). Usually *H. influenzae* meningitis is treated for 10 days, and pneumococcal disease for 10–14 days (Committee on Infectious Diseases, 1988; Radetsky, 1990).

Most patients with bacterial meningitis do not need i.v. fluids except those in circulatory failure. The i.m. administration of Pen G is easier and cheaper, and perhaps there might be less risk of cerebral edema. During the period 1955–1965, almost all patients with bacterial meningitis at Fairfield Hospital were treated by i.m. antibiotics. Subsequently, mainly for the patient's comfort, i.v. administration of Pen G became customary, but there was no obvious change in the mortality of the disease. Nevertheless, large and frequent doses of Pen G, similar to those used i.v. nowadays, were required in the i.m. regimen used in the past. A new approach was tried in Papua New Guinea (Shann and Germer, 1981, 1983). Satisfactory results were achieved in bacterial meningitis by using oral probenecid (p. 24) with smaller doses of Pen G i.m. at 6-hourly intervals. Doses of crystalline Pen G used were 0.3 g and 0.6 g i.m. 6-hourly for children weighing less than 10 kg and 10–29 kg, respectively. The use of probenecid thereby allowed the usual Pen G dosage to be reduced by half or more in bacterial meningitis. The value of this form of treatment needs confirmation, and studies are required to investigate the reliability of oral absorption of probenecid and its effects on central nervous system pharmacokinetics of Pen G in patients with bacterial meningitis (p. 32).

For neonatal meningitis, preferred initial chemotherapy is Pen G or ampicillin combined with an aminoglycoside, such as gentamicin or amikacin. Cephalosporins, such as cefotaxime (p. 336) or ceftazidime (p. 378) may be substituted for the aminoglycoside. In the hospitalized premature infant in whom nosocomial *Ps. aeruginosa* infection is a possibility, ceftazidime is preferred over cefotaxime. Pen G (or ampicillin) should be used as continuation therapy if the organism is Group B streptococcus, *L. monocytogenes*, or an enterococcus (Committee on Infectious Diseases, 1988; Dobson and Baker, 1990). Rarely, *Strep. mitis* may also be involved, and for this Pen G is the drug of choice (Bignardi and Isaacs, 1989). For neonatal meningitis caused by Gram-negative enteric bacilli, specific therapy by an aminoglycoside plus/or a third-generation cephalosporin should be based on results of susceptibility studies.

Pen G or ampicillin are also the best drugs for the treatment of *L. monocytogenes* meningitis and other severe *Listeria* infections such as septicemia, endocarditis, pneumonia, pleural effusion, brainstem encephalitis, liver abscess and spontaneous peritonitis in patients with cirrhosis (Gallagher and Watanakunakorn, 1988; Kluge, 1990; Mazzulli and Salit, 1991; Armstrong and Fung, 1993; Braun *et al.*, 1993; Kent *et al.*, 1994). The manifestations of listeriosis in patients with AIDS are similar to those in other patients, and response to Pen G treatment is usually satisfactory (Kales and Holzman, 1990). For listeriosis the synergistic Pen G/gentamicin combination (p. 12) may have advantages compared with Pen G therapy alone (Stamm *et al.*, 1982; Gallagher and Watanakunakorn, 1988; Paul *et al.*, 1994).

Listeria monocytogenes is a food-borne pathogen. The association of this organism with several large food-borne outbreaks suggests that contaminated food may be the primary source of this bacterium (Farber and Peterkin, 1991; Büla *et al.*, 1995). *Listeria monocytogenes* is an opportunistic pathogen and risk factors include pregnancy, neonatal status, organ transplantation, renal failure, malignancy, systemic lupus, steroid therapy and HIV infection (Beninger *et al.*, 1988; Enocksson *et al.*, 1990; Skogberg *et al.*, 1992; Jurado *et al.*, 1993; Jensen *et al.*, 1994).

Hospital-acquired meningitis is now not rare. In a study of 493 episodes of acute bacterial meningitis in adults in one large USA general hospital, Durand *et al.* (1993) found that nosocomial meningitis accounted for 39% of patients with this disease. Gram-negative meningitis was frequent among these, and they needed antibiotics other than Pen G. In the same series recurrent meningitis occurred in 9% of patients.

One HIV-infected patient developed *Strep. bovis* septicemia and meningitis associated with *Strongyloides stercoralis* colitis. High-dose Pen G was the appropriate treatment for the *Strep. bovis* infection (Jain *et al.*, 1994). Enterococcal meningitis is rare, but it has occurred in neonates and adults who were immunosuppressed or had coexistent chronic illness. Therapy with Pen G/gentamicin combination was successful in most cases, unless there was resistance to one or both of these drugs (p. 10) (Stevenson *et al.*, 1994).

Mixed bacterial meningitis may also occur. Approximately 1% of all cases of meningitis may be caused by more than one bacterial species. This is mainly seen in adults with predisposing factors such as infection at contiguous foci, tumors in proximity to brain or fistuli to the CSF. One of the organisms is often a Gram-negative rod. Failure to recognize one of the organisms may lead to failure of therapy (Downs *et al.*, 1987).

The administration of dexamethasone as an adjunct to chemotherapy in bacterial meningitis may reduce the degree of inflammation and its associated morbidity. Most studies have been done in children. At present the routine use of dexamethasone is advocated in children with meningitis, but in adults only if there is impaired mental status or intracranial hypertension (Tarlow, 1991). In children, dexamethasone in a dose of 0.15 mg per kg body weight is given 15–20 min before the first antibiotic dose, and this is then continued every 6 h for 4 days (Odio *et al.*, 1991; Townsend and Scheld, 1993). More recent evidence indicates that dexamethasone administration for 2 days only is optimal (Syrogiannopoulos *et al.*, 1994).

Pen G is an important antibiotic for the treatment of cerebral abscess. Frontal lobe abscesses arising from the sinuses may respond to Pen G alone, as they are usually caused by various types of Pen G-sensitive streptococci, such as *Strep. milleri*. Abscesses of otitic origin which occur in the temporal lobe, usually yield a mixed flora often including anaerobic bacteria. For these Pen G should be combined with chloramphenicol (p. 569) or metronidazole (p. 948). Metastatic abscesses which occur anywhere within the brain, can be caused by streptococci, staphylococci or by a variety of other bacteria. Combination therapy, including an effective anti-staphylococcal drug is necessary until bacteriological results are available. Spinal and post-traumatic intracranial abscesses are usually caused by *Staph. aureus*. Initial combination treatment by Pen G and chloramphenicol may be effective, but specific anti-staphylococcal therapy with cloxacillin may be advisable before the bacteriological diagnosis is confirmed (de Louvois, 1978). Because of the seriousness of the disease, it is advisable to use combination chemotherapy for most cerebral abscesses initially (pp. 569, 948) (Donald, 1990; Seydoux and Francioli, 1992).

8 Meningococcal and pneumococcal septicemia

Pen G is the best drug for treatment of meningococcal septicemia, which can either be mild with good prognosis or fulminant with shock. In the latter group, the mortality is still 25–50% (Peltola, 1983; Halstensen et al., 1987a,b). In fulminant meningococcal septicemia as well as in severe meningococcal meningitis, prompt Pen G administration is life-saving. This means that primary care physicians should give empiric Pen G before the patient is sent to hospital. Similarly in hospital if lumbar puncture has to be delayed because a CT scan is done first, i.v. antibiotics are warranted before CSF is obtained (Talan et al., 1988; Cartwright et al., 1992; Strang and Pugh, 1992; Hart and Rogers, 1993). This not only applies to severe meningococcal infections, but also to other types of severe meningitis. Pneumococcal septicemia may occur in all age groups, including neonates (Jacobs et al., 1990), and again Pen G is the best treatment (Shanks et al., 1982). Patients who have had a splenectomy are prone to fulminant septicemia, and although other organisms may be involved, *Strep. pneumoniae* is responsible for the majority (Dickerman, 1979). Experiments with splenectomized animals, indicate that prompt high dosage Pen G treatment may be important in humans with post-splenectomy pneumococcal infections (Bakker-Woudenberg et al., 1982). If pneumococcal septicemia is caused by a strain resistant to penicillin G, it may respond to i.v. ceftriaxone. Some strains also have high MICs for ceftriaxone and then i.v. vancomycin is necessary (Leggiadro et al., 1994).

9 Bacterial endocarditis

Three different regimens are effective for the treatment of endocarditis caused by streptococci highly sensitive to Pen G, such as *Strep. viridans* (p. 8), and non-enterococcal Group D streptococci such as *Strep. bovis* and *Strep. equinus* (p. 11). Intravenous crystalline Pen G alone for 4 or sometimes 6 weeks, in doses of 6–12 g daily has given very satisfactory results. Two other regimens utilize Pen G/streptomycin synergism against these organisms (p. 429). A 2-week course of procaine Pen G, 1.2 g i.m. every 6 h plus streptomycin, 7.5 mg per kg i.m. every 12 h gave good results in 91 patients treated at the Mayo Clinic (Wilson et al., 1981). In this regimen, 6–12 g of crystalline Pen G i.v. daily could be used as an alternative to i.m. procaine Pen G. The advantage of this treatment schedule is that it shortens the period of hospitalization. The third regimen which has been very effective, is a combination of i.v. or i.m. Pen G with streptomycin in doses as above, for the first 2 weeks of treatment, and then continuation with Pen G alone for another 2 weeks (Sande and Scheld, 1980). It may be necessary to administer Pen G for a total of 6 weeks in severe cases of endocarditis. Clinical circumstances may dictate the regimen selected. The 2-week regimen can be used for patients who are unlikely to develop streptomycin ototoxicity, and who have had symptoms for less than 3 months. Pen G alone could be used for patients with renal insufficiency, for those with previous VIIIth nerve toxicity and for elderly patients. The regimen using Pen G for 4 weeks or longer, combined with streptomycin for the first 2 weeks, is preferable in patients with a long period of symptoms, and probably for those with large vegetations. In all the combination regimens streptomycin can be replaced by gentamicin in a dose of 3 mg per kg once-daily (p. 458). Although the clinical significance of Pen G-tolerant *Strep. viridans* strains (p. 9) is still uncertain, the third regimen may be optimal for infections caused by tolerant strains or nutritionally deficient variants of viridans streptococci (Rapeport et al., 1986; Shulman 1986; Scheld, 1987; Wilson, 1987; Karchmer, 1988). Endocarditis caused by nutritionally deficient variants of viridans streptococci still responds poorly to the combination therapy; in one series 38% of patients failed to respond to the antibiotics and required surgery (Stein and Nelson, 1987). It has been suggested that patients with endocarditis due to these organisms should be treated by a Pen G/aminoglycoside combination for at least 4 weeks (Wilson, 1987).

For endocarditis caused by other *Strep. viridans* strains, some authors have found no advantage of the addition of aminoglycoside to the third regimen; there was no difference in outcome in the two groups when patients were randomized to receive Pen G plus aminoglycoside or Pen G alone (Tuazon et al., 1986). Pen G alone or in combination with an aminoglycoside is also effective therapy for Group B streptococcal endocarditis (Backes et al., 1985). Preferably these patients should be treated by combined Pen G/aminoglycoside therapy for 2 weeks, and then another 2 weeks by Pen G alone (Wilson, 1987).

Patients in whom endocarditis is caused by relatively resistant *Strep. viridans* strains (MIC 0.1–1.0 μg per ml) should be treated with a regimen identical to that for patients with enterococcal endocarditis (see below), i.e. Pen G in high dosage combined with aminoglycoside administered for 4–6 weeks (Wilson, 1987; Boenning *et al.*, 1988). However, some authors have found Pen G alone satisfactory for these patients (Di Nubile, 1990). If endocarditis is caused by a *Strep. viridans* strain with a higher degree of Pen G resistance (p. 8), Pen G is not suitable for treatment, and the most likely antibiotic which will succeed is vancomycin (p. 778) (Quinn *et al.*, 1988).

Streptococcus viridans bacteremia can also occur in many patients without endocarditis. Pen G again is the treatment of choice in most cases (Watanakunakorn and Pantelakis, 1993). If bacteremia develops in a neutropenic cancer patient who has been on penicillin and quinolone chemoprophylaxis, the *Strep. viridans* strain may be Pen G-resistant and vancomycin (p. 781) may be needed for therapy (Bochud *et al.*, 1994).

For the treatment of enterococcal (*E. faecalis*, *E. faecium* and *E. durans*) endocarditis, a synergistic Pen G/aminoglycoside combination is always necessary. Standard treatment has been i.v. crystalline Pen G 12.0–14.4 g daily for 6 weeks plus i.m. streptomycin 7.5 mg per kg body weight i.m. 12-hourly (maximum 500 mg per dose) (Wilson, 1987; Megran, 1992). Modifications of this regimen have also produced satisfactory results. The total course of treatment may be reduced to 4 weeks (Kaye, 1980). Others have administered Pen G for 4 weeks, and have shortened the duration of concomitant aminoglycoside therapy, usually to 3 weeks (Herztein *et al.*, 1984).

Approximately 40% of clinical enterococcal isolates showed 'high-level' streptomycin resistance; Pen G/streptomycin did not show synergism against these, but a Pen G/gentamicin combination nearly always did (p. 455). If the MIC of streptomycin for the enterococcus is 2000 μg per ml or greater, gentamicin in a dosage of 1.0 mg per kg body weight i.m. or i.v. every 8 hours, should be substituted for streptomycin. Once-daily gentamicin dosing is not advocated. In theory it is inadvisable to use the Pen G/gentamicin combination for all patients with enterococcal endocarditis, as gentamicin (p. 469) is more nephrotoxic than streptomycin (p. 433) (Sande and Scheld, 1980). However, if gentamicin is used in a dose of only 3 mg per kg per day, nephrotoxicity is infrequent. This lower gentamicin dosage has now been shown to be effective. In practice therefore most physicians now use the Pen G/gentamicin regimen for all patients with enterococcal endocarditis (Wilson *et al.*, 1984; Report, 1985; Wilson, 1987; Megran, 1992). Pen G combined with gentamicin was not synergistic against a small number of *E. faecalis* strains (p. 455). A Pen G/tobramycin combination (p. 455) may be effective against these and can be used clinically. Pen G and tobramycin are not synergistic against *E. faecium* (Eliopoulos and Moellering, 1982).

In recent years enterococci with high level gentamicin-resistance have emerged in many parts of the world (p. 456); these strains are not killed synergistically by Pen G/gentamicin and usually not by Pen G combined with any other aminoglycoside. Against a small percentage of these strains Pen G/streptomycin combination is synergistic (Noskin *et al.*, 1993) (p. 429). Treatment of endocarditis caused by strains with no Pen G/aminoglycoside synergism is difficult. High-dose Pen G or vancomycin alone are unsatisfactory. Animal studies have shown that high-dose i.v. ampicillin, given by continuous infusion, may be marginally more bactericidal to these *E. faecalis* strains (Moellering, 1991). At present it seems that most patients with endocarditis caused by such *E. faecalis* strains will need a valve replacement. Beta-lactamase-producing enterococci have also emerged (p. 10). If this was the only problem endocarditis caused by these could be treated by ampicillin/sulbactam (p. 215) plus gentamicin. Unfortunately most strains which produce beta-lactamase also exhibit high-level gentamicin-resistance (p. 10) (Patterson *et al.*, 1988a).

Enterococcus faecalis has now become a more common nosocomial pathogen and septicemia without endocarditis is not rare. The most common entry sites are the urinary tract, the intra-abdominal cavity and burn and decubitus wounds. This septicemia responds to Pen G and the addition of gentamicin does not result in a better survival rate (Gullberg *et al.*, 1989; Graninger and Ragette, 1992; Watanakunakorn and Patel, 1993).

Pen G is effective in *Staph. aureus* endocarditis if the organism does not produce beta-lactamase. Against beta-lactamase-producing strains it is quite unreliable even if massive doses are used, and one of the penicillinase-resistant penicillins is indicated (p. 97). Pneumococcal endocarditis responds well to Pen G, provided the *Strep. pneumoniae* strain is fully Pen G-sensitive (Powderly *et al.*, 1986). Two pneumococcal strains, whose MICs for Pen G were 1 (intermediate resistance) and 4 (high-level resistance) μg per ml were used to induce experimental endocarditis in animals. Pen G alone could cure this, but it was essential to have a regimen which provided serum Pen G levels above the MICs throughout the intervals between doses. Cefotaxime (p. 339) and teicoplanin (p. 797) were also curative (Guerrero *et al.*, 1994).

Prosthetic valve endocarditis is commonly caused by *Staph. epidermidis*, which is usually resistant to Pen G and often to methicillin, so that drugs other than Pen G are required (p. 778). Diphtheroids are the next most common cause of prosthetic valve endocarditis. Most strains of these organisms show intermediate or high-level resistance to Pen G. Provided they are sensitive to gentamicin, which is usually the case, a Pen G/gentamicin combination is synergistic and useful clinically. The survival rate of patients treated in this way has been about 60%, the duration of parenteral chemotherapy among survivors was in the range of 33–55 days; some patients also required prosthetic valve replacement (Murray *et al.*, 1980). Alternatively vancomycin (p. 779) can be used to treat these patients. The JK diphtheroids are always highly resistant to Pen G, and prosthetic valve endocarditis due to these should be treated by vancomycin (p. 779). Now when *Enterococcus faecalis* has become a significant nosocomial pathogen, in addition to native valve endocarditis, it also causes prosthetic valve disease, and most of these patients can be cured by some 6 weeks course of Pen G/gentamicin combination and valve replacement is necessary in only a few patients (Rice *et al.*, 1991a). Also *E. faecalis* and *Staph. aureus* are the most common organisms which cause hospital-acquired infectious endocarditis not associated with cardiac surgery; the infection with *E. faecalis* follows urinary tract instrumentation and that with *Staph. aureus* intravenous catheterization (Fernández-Guerrero *et al.*, 1995).

Several rarer forms of endocarditis respond well to Pen G. These include gonococcal endocarditis, provided the *N. gonorrhoeae* strain involved is Pen G-sensitive (Timmis *et al.*, 1981), *Corynebacterium diphtheriae* endocarditis, which is usually caused by non-toxigenic strains (Love *et al.*, 1981; Tiley *et al.*, 1993) and *C. psuedodiphteriticum* endocarditis, this organism normally being a commensal in the human nasopharynx (Morris and Guild, 1991). *Erysipelothrix rhusiopathiae* endocarditis also responds well to Pen G (Gorby and Peacock, 1988; Gransden and Eykyn, 1988) as does endocarditis caused by *Rothia dentocariosa*, an aerophilic Gram-negative coccobacillus normally present in the oral cavity (Pape *et al.*, 1979; Schafer *et al.*, 1979; Sudduth *et al.*, 1993).

Listeria monocytogenes also rarely causes endocarditis and Pen G combined with gentamicin is probably the best treatment (Carvajal and Frederiksen, 1988; Gallagher and Watanakunakorn, 1988). Similarly the synergistic Pen G/gentamicin therapy appears to be the best for the rare cases of *Lactobacillus* spp. endocarditis (Sussman *et al.*, 1986; Griffiths *et al.*, 1992). Pen G either alone or in combination with gentamicin also appears to be the best treatment for the rare cases of *Neisseria mucosa* and *N. sicca* endocarditis; these organisms are saprophytic and are frequently found in the human nasopharynx and they only occasionally cause human infections (Stotka *et al.*, 1991; Ingram *et al.*, 1992; Heiddal *et al.*, 1993). Pen G alone is also the treatment of choice for *Streptobacillus moniliformis* endocarditis (Rupp, 1992).

Measurement of serum inhibitory and/or bactericidal concentration titers in patients during therapy for bacterial endocarditis has been a common practice; it was recommended that a peak serum bactericidal concentration titer of 1:8, or higher, should be maintained in streptococcal endocarditis (Sande and Scheld, 1980). Methods used to measure serum bactericidal concentrations have varied, and there has been no association between serum bactericidal titers of 1:8 or more, and the therapeutic outcome (Coleman *et al.*, 1982). In a multicentre evaluation of a standardized serum bactericidal test as a prognostic indicator of infective endocarditis, peak serum bactericidal titers of 1:64 or more and trough titers of 1:32 or more predicted bacteriological cure in all patients. However, the serum bactericidal test was a poor predictor of bacteriological failure or the ultimate clinical outcome, which depended on many factors (Weinstein *et al.*, 1985).

According to Reller (1986), more rigorous attempts have been made to standardize all the relevant variables that affect results of serum bactericidal titers. A defined SBT method is necessary for additional multicenter clinical trials to assess the value of these tests.

10 Endocarditis chemoprophylaxis

Pen G was recommended for this purpose in the past. In patients at risk, a mixture of crystalline Pen G 0.6 g plus procaine Pen G 0.6 g i.m. was recommended 30 min before dental procedures; this was then followed by oral penicillin V in a dosage of 0.5 g 6-hourly for 2 days. In the current British and US recommendations oral amoxycillin is substituted for Pen G, because the administration of injectable antibiotics is difficult in dental surgeries. In the USA the recommendations are made by The American Heart Association. The standard regimen of chemoprophylaxis suggested by this Association during dental, oral or upper gastrointestinal procedures consists of 3 g of oral amoxycillin 1 h before the procedure with a single follow-up dose of 1.5 g 6h later (Dajani *et al.*, 1990; Durack, 1995). One animal experiment suggested that it was important to maintain an effective amoxycillin serum level for at least 10 h for effective prophylaxis, so this study supported the above recommendations (Fluckiger *et al.*, 1994). But after further pharmacokinetic studies Dajani *et al.* (1994) found that a single 2 g dose of oral amoxycillin, although giving lower serum levels than the 3 g dose, still produced adequate levels to inhibit viridans streptococci for at least 6 h. The lower dose was better tolerated.

The regimen recommended for high-risk patients (e.g. those with prosthetic valves) who undergo dental or respiratory tract surgery consists of parenteral antibiotics, with ampicillin (2 g) plus gentamicin (1.5 mg per kg) given i.m. or i.v. 30 min prior to the procedure and followed by either a single 1.5 g dose of oral amoxycillin 6 h later or by repeat parenteral ampicillin and gentamicin once 8 h later. For penicillin-allergic individuals at standard risk, erythromycin stearate 1.0 g orally 2h before the procedure and 0.5 g 6 h later is suggested. Alternatively clindamycin 300 mg orally 1 h before the procedure and 150 mg 6 h after initial dose may be used. For penicillin-allergic higher risk individuals with prosthetic valves the recommendation is vancomycin 1 g given i.v. over 1 h, starting 1 h before the procedure, without a repeat dose. In patients who are taking prophylactic penicillin, penicillin-resistant *Strep. viridans* strains are often present in oral cavity. For these patients the erythromycin regimen or one of the parenteral regimens should be chosen (Dajani *et al.*, 1990; Petersen, 1990). Sensitivity testing of organisms obtained from dental plaques may be of assistance in planning prophylaxis in such patients (MacFarlane *et al.*, 1983), but this is not practical in most cases. Pen G-resistant *Strep. viridans* strains can also be detected in the oral flora of patients who had not been exposed recently to any form of penicillin. Also in several of these, post-dental extraction bacteremia with resistant organisms has occurred, despite prophylactic administration of i.m. Pen G. It is not known whether a Pen G/gentamicin combination would be more effective in preventing such bacteremia (Hess *et al.*, 1983a).

In the USA it is recommended that chemoprophylaxis should also be given for at-risk patients who are undergoing the following genitourinary and/or gastrointestinal procedures: cystoscopy, prostatic surgery, urethral catheterization (with infected urine), urinary tract surgery, vaginal hysterectomy, gallblader surgery, colonic surgery, esophageal dilatation, colonoscopy, procto-sigmoidoscopic biopsy and vaginal delivery in the presence of infection.

For high-risk patients prophylaxis is advised also for low-risk procedures such as liver biopsy, barium enema, uncomplicated vaginal delivery and others.

The regimen recommended for all these patients is parenteral ampicillin 2.0 g plus gentamicin 1.5 mg per kg given 30 min before the procedure. Another dose of both drugs 8 h later is optional. Penicillin-allergic patients should receive 1 g of i.v. vancomycin (infused over 1 h) plus parenteral gentamicin 1.5 mg per kg 1 h before the procedure with an optional second dose of each drug (Dajani *et al.*, 1990).

The British and European recommendations mainly differ from the above in that for standard low-risk patients a single 3 g dose of amoxycillin is suggested 1 h before dental work, but no follow-up dose is given. The other difference is that for patients with native valves no prophylaxis is recommended for patients undergoing endoscopy, colonoscopy, proctoscopy, sigmoidoscopy or Ba enema, but prophylaxis is recommended for those with prosthetic valves undergoing these procedures (Shanson, 1987; Recommendations, 1990). Instead of vancomycin/gentamicin, teicoplanin 400 mg i.v. (p. 798) and gentamicin 120 mg i.v. is advocated. In penicillin-allergic patients unable to take oral medications, i.v. clindamycin 300 mg (diluted in 50 ml and given over 10 min) is preferred. This is given just before the procedure, and a 150 mg dose, similarly administered, 6 h later (Simmons *et al.*, 1992).

Each of these regimens have advantages and disadvantages, and it is clear that clinical trials are not possible to evaluate these recommendations. Another approach is to analyze endocarditis prophylaxis failures. Fifty-two cases of apparent endocarditis prophylaxis failure were analyzed by Durack *et al.* (1983). Most of these patients had received oral penicillin as prophylaxis, and only six (12%) had received earlier regimens recommended by the American Heart Association, which involved the use of parenteral Pen G and later oral penicillin V. There have been other reports of endocarditis apparently developing despite 2 days of Pen G chemoprophylaxis in the recommended doses (Durack and Littler, 1974; McGowan, 1978). But there is little doubt that endocarditis chemoprophylaxis is effective. In one study among patients with high-risk cardiac lesions who developed endocarditis after dental procedures, only 13% had used antibiotic prophylaxis, whilst among a control group with no endocarditis, 63% had used chemoprophylaxis when indicated (Imperiale, 1990).

There is also evidence that clinicians frequently do not administer prophylactic antibiotics as recommended. One retrospective survey in the USA showed that for patients with prosthetic heart valves the compliance with American Heart Association's guidelines was only 30% (Brooks *et al.*, 1988). A similar study in the Netherlands showed that only 22% of patients in whom prophylaxis was indicated, actually received it (Van der Meer *et al.*, 1992). Although the value of chemoprophylaxis is generally accepted, in one study 2 g penicillin V or 3 g amoxycillin did not diminish post-dental extraction bacteremia and it was concluded that the protective effects of prophylactically administered penicillins must be due to interference with other steps in the development of endocarditis (Hall *et al.*, 1993).

11 Pelvic inflammatory disease

Many organisms can be involved but the exact bacteriological etiology is often difficult to determine. *N. gonorrheae*, *Strep. pyogenes*, Group B streptococci and anaerobic streptococci are important pathogens which are all, except *N. gonorrhoeae*, usually Pen G-sensitive. Others such as *C. trachomatis*, certain anaerobes including *B. fragilis*, and Enterobacteriaceae such as *E. coli* and *Klebsiella* spp., are Pen G-resistant (Goodrich, 1982). Seriously ill patients in whom bacteriological diagnosis has not been established, require combination chemotherapy. Crystalline Pen G in a dose of 12 g i.v. daily may be combined with a tetracycline (p. 747) and an aminoglycoside such as gentamicin (p. 471). This still does not provide cover for *B. fragilis* so the use of clindamycin (p. 597) or metronidazole (p. 947) should be considered (Burnakis and Hildebrandt, 1986).

The Centers for Disease Control in the USA have recommended one of two preferred regimens for the treatment of pelvic inflammatory disease. The first is cefoxitin 2 g i.v. every 6 h or cefotetan 2 g i.v. every 12 h combined with doxycycline 100 mg every 12 h orally or i.v. The second regimen is clindamycin 900 mg i.v. every 8 h plus gentamicin i.v., leading dose 2 mg per kg followed by a maintenance dose of 1.5 mg per kg every 8 h (CDC, 1993). Both regimens are equally effective and safe (Hemsell *et al.*, 1994). Clindamycin probably has some activity against *Chlamydia*, but when this infection is strongly suspected, doxycycline can be added to the second regimen. If patients quickly improve with these regimens, they can be discharged home from hospital on oral doxycycline 100 mg twice-daily for 10–14 days. Two outpatient regimens have also been suggested: regimen 1, ofloxacin (400 mg twice-daily) plus either clindamycin (450 mg four times daily) or metronidazole (500 mg twice-daily) for 14 days; regimen 2, cefoxitin (2 g i.m.) plus probenecid (1 g orally) concurrently once only plus doxycycline (100 mg orally twice-daily for 14 days (Walker *et al.*, 1993).

12 Gonorrhea

Since its discovery and until recently, Pen G was the preferred drug for treatment of this disease. But now because of the emergence of strains with chromosomally mediated resistance to Pen G and other antibiotics (p. 14) and beta-lactamase-producing *N. gonorrhoeae* (p. 15), Pen G is no longer used in most countries throughout the world. In the USA a single dose of ceftriaxone 125 or 250 mg i.m. (p. 361) or cefixime 400 mg orally once (p. 412) or ciprofloxacin 500 mg orally once (p. 1022) or ofloxacin 400 mg orally once (p. 1122) is recommended along with doxycycline 100 mg orally twice-daily for 7 days (p. 747). The latter drug is used to eradicate a coexistent *Chlamydia* infection which may be present in up to 50% of patients with gonorrhea (Handsfield *et al.*., 1989; CDC, 1993). The same now applies to several areas of Australia (Mashford *et al.*, 1994), Mexico City (Conde-Glez *et al.*, 1988), Taiwan (Chu *et al.*, 1992) and Thailand (Clendennen *et al.*, 1992b). An alternative to ceftriaxone is a single 2 g i.m. dose of spectinomycin (p. 717), but in some countries, spectinomycin is now also less useful because of increasing resistance of *N. gonorrhoeae* to this drug (Clendennen *et al.*, 1992b). Other alternatives are norfloxacin 800 mg orally once (p. 1067) and cefotaxime 0.5 g i.m. once (p. 338). All of these have to be combined with 7 days oral doxycyline (CDC, 1993).

Pen G-resistant gonococci are also common in many developing countries, such as the Far East and Africa, so that Pen G can no longer be used for treatment of gonorrhea (Lind, 1990).

In contrast, in the UK and in Scandinavian countries, the prevalence, particularly of beta-lactamase-producing strains, increased in the early 1980s, but then showed a decrease in the mid 1980s (Ison *et al.*, 1986; Jephcott, 1986; Lind, 1990). If in any area the prevalence of Pen G-resistant gonococci is still low, Pen G can still be used for treatment, although amoxycillin (p. 141) or ampicillin plus probenecid (p. 125) would usually be preferred. With the latter two regimens the disadvantages of a large Pen G injection, possible procaine reactions (p. 31) or Pen G anaphylaxis (p. 29) can be avoided.

The recommended dosage of Pen G was procaine Pen G 4.8 g injected i.m. in two divided doses plus 1.0 g of oral probenecid. Coexistent *Chlamydia* infection again had to be treated by a 7-day course of doxycycline (Washington, 1982). This Pen G regimen was effective for anorectal gonorrhea in females and males but 'single-session' amoxycillin or ampicillin was not satisfactory for males. Gonococcal pharyngitis was also not reliably cured by single-session Pen G, and a 5- to 7-day course of Pen G was recommended (Lebedeff and Hochman, 1980; Washington, 1982). Anorectal infections in both sexes and pharyngeal infections are best treated by a single dose of ceftriaxone 250 mg i.m., even if the strain is Pen G-sensitive, as the response to ceftriaxone is always good (CDC, 1993).

Gonorrhea during pregnancy is treated by single-dose ceftriaxone 250 mg i.m. (or amoxycillin 3.0 g orally for Pen G-sensitive strains) plus erythromycin ethylsuccinate 400 mg orally four times-daily for 14 days (CDC, 1993).

Infants with gonococcal infections (e.g. ophthalmia neonatorum or disseminated gonococcal infections should be treated by ceftriaxone 25–50 mg per kg per day i.v. or i.m. in a single daily dose for 7 days. Alternatively cefotaxime 25 mg per kg i.v. or i.m. every 12 h may be used. If the gonococcal isolate is Pen G-sensitive, crystalline Pen G may be given in a dose of 30–60 mg per kg per day administered in two equal doses i.v. or i.m. In infants with ophthalmia neonatorum, eyes should be irrigated with saline, but topical antibiotic treatment alone is inadequate (Washington, 1982; CDC, 1993). Epidemic gonococcal conjunctivitis in children is easier to treat than ophthalmia neonatorum, and if the strain is Pen G-sensitive, the disease usually responds to a single-dose of this drug (Merianos *et al.*, 1995). Chlamydial ophthalmia (p. 746) may be clinically indistinguishable from gonococcal ophthalmia and is the commoner infection in the USA (Washington, 1982). Silver nitrate drops (1%) are useful for the prevention of gonococcal ophthalmia neonatorum, but not for chlamydial conjunctivitis. Both infections can be prevented by 1% tetracycline ophthalmic ointment or drops and 0.5% erythromycin ophthalmic ointment or drops. Povidone-iodine eye drops have also been used for chemoprophylaxis (p. 746).

Disseminated gonococcal infections or pelvic infections nowadays are usually treated by i.v. cefotaxime 1 g every 8 h or ceftriaxone 1 g every 24 h. Cefuroxime axetil 500 mg twice-daily (p. 310) or amoxycillin 500 mg with clavulanic acid three times daily (p. 200) may be substituted for the parenteral drug if response is good in 2–3 days time. Total duration of therapy should be at least 7 days. For gonococcal meningitis or endocarditis the doses of the parenteral drugs may be doubled and treatment with these continued for 10–14 days (CDC, 1993). If the *N. gonorrhoeae* strain is Pen G-sensitive, a satisfactory treatment for gonococcal pelvic infection is a 10–14 day course of crystalline Pen G, in a dosage of 6–12 g daily (p. 18). In patients who respond well, oral amoxycillin may be substituted for Pen G after 2–3 days and then be continued to complete the 7–10 days course. Disseminated gonococcal infection, commonly manifested by arthritis, tenosynovitis and dermatitis, has been cured with only 3 days of parenteral Pen G in high dosage (Thompson *et al.*, 1980). However, a 7–14 day course, similar to that used for pelvic infection, is recommended (Handsfield *et al.*, 1976). For the less common gonococcal endocarditis or meningitis, prolonged treatment for at least 2 weeks with i.v. crystalline Pen G 6–12 g daily is necessary (Handsfield *et al.*, 1976).

13 Syphilis

Pen G remains an excellent drug for the treatment of this disease. *Treponema pallidum* has not become increasingly resistant to Pen G, being immobilized *in vitro* at a maximal rate by only 0.1 µg per ml. Lesions of experimental syphilis resolve most readily in the presence of serum Pen G levels of only 0.4 µg per ml. It is commonly stated that the aim of treatment is to maintain sustained comparatively low Pen G serum and tissue levels for 7–10 days. *Treponema pallidum* is sensitive to such levels, it multiplies slowly by dividing once every 30–33 h, and only actively dividing organisms are susceptible to Pen G (Willcox, 1981; Zenker and Rolfs, 1990). But to attain such levels in tissues, much higher serum levels of Pen G may be necessary, and so the treatment schedules for the various stages of syphilis have remained controversial. As with gonorrhea (see above), 'single-session' treatment has been extensively used for treatment of syphilis. It is still recommended that primary, secondary and latent syphilis of less than 1 year duration can be treated with a single dose of benzathine Pen G 2.4 million units (1.8 g) i.m. (CDC, 1993). Failures have occurred with such treatment (Brown, 1982; Zenker and Rolfs, 1990). Good results have been obtained in both primary and secondary syphilis by using two doses of 2.4 million units (1.8 g) benzathine Pen G, i.m. separated by 1 week (Fiumara, 1980, 1986). Another recommendation is a minimum of 0.6 g of procaine Pen G i.m. daily for 10 days (Willcox, 1981; Thin, 1989). Because of the possible long-term catastrophic sequeli of inadequately treated syphilis, where possible we prefer to use a 10- to 14-day course of procaine Pen G in daily i.m. doses of 1.0 g for early syphilis. Some patients with secondary syphilis, especially those with early central nervous system involvement evidenced by meningitis, are best treated by i.v. crystalline Pen G in a dose of 6–12 g daily, for 2 weeks (Zenker and Rolfs, 1990). Treatment of latent syphilis of more than 1 year duration is controversial (Brown, 1982). Most clinicians believe that neurosyphilis should be managed differently from syphilis of more than 1 year duration without central nervous system involvement. For this reason, a lumbar puncture should be performed on all patients with latent syphilis, irrespective of whether they have clinical neurological abnormalities or not; if the CSF is abnormal, this should be re-examined after treatment (Jaffe and Kabins, 1982). For patients with latent syphilis of more than 1 year duration, who have no clinical or CSF evidence of neurosyphilis, benzathine Pen G 7.2 million units (5.4 g) total, administered as three doses of 2.4 million units (1.8 g) i.m., given 1 week apart for 3 consecutive weeks, is recommended (CDC, 1993). Such treatment has failed in both early and latent syphilis during the second and third trimesters of pregnancy (Reyes et al., 1993). We feel that a more satisfactory treatment for all patients with latent syphilis of more than 1 year duration would be daily i.m. injections of 1.0 g of procaine Pen G for 2 weeks. Patients with neurosyphilis should receive crystalline Pen G in a daily dose of 7.2–14.4 g i.v. (in six divided doses) for 2 weeks (CDC, 1993). Some recommended that this 2 weeks i.v. Pen G should be followed by benzathine penicillin G 2.4 million units i.m weekly for 3 weeks (Scheck and Hook, 1994). Adequate CSF levels of Pen G are attained only with i.v. crystalline Pen G and not with other Pen G regimens (Mohr et al., 1976).

Treponemicidal Pen G concentrations in CSF are not reached in all patients with neurosyphilis if an i.m. procaine penicillin regimen is used for treatment (Van der Valk et al., 1988). Treponema pallidum has been isolated from the CSF of patients treated by high dosage of benzathine Pen G i.m. but they were eliminated after re-treatment with large doses of i.v. crystalline Pen G (Tramont, 1976). Despite the widespread use of a 10-day i.m. procaine Pen G regimen for neurosyphilis in the UK, there appears to be only one report of progressive neurosyphilis after such treatment (Giles, 1980).

The above Pen G regimens are satisfactory for the treatment of syphilis during pregnancy (CDC, 1993). Congenital neurosyphilis should be treated by i.m. or i.v. crystalline Pen G, for 10–14 days. Procaine Pen G i.m. daily for 10–14 days also may be satisfactory (Stoll, 1994). In newborn infants adequate CSF levels of Pen G cannot be achieved after benzathine Pen G administration (Lane and Oates, 1988). It appears that single-dose treatment with 4.8 million units (4.8 g) of procaine Pen G i.m. for gonorrhea is also effective therapy for incubating syphilis (Schroeter et al., 1971). For the treatment of syphilis in Pen G-allergic patients, tetracyclines are indicated, except that pregnant patients should be desensitized to Pen G or, if really necessary, receive the less reliable erythromycin.

Syphilis in patients with HIV infection poses problems. First of all diagnosis may be delayed or not made because serological response to syphilis in some patients may be absent or delayed. If clinical findings suggest syphilis, but serological tests are negative, other tests such as dark fluid microscopy or direct fluorescent antibody test for T. pallidum should be performed (Hook, 1989a). In patients with early syphilis, HIV may also alter the serological response to therapy (Telzak et al., 1991). Patients with HIV infection also present more often in the secondary stage and those with secondary syphilis often still have chancres (Hutchinson et al., 1994).

It also appears that neurosyphilis is more common in the early stages of syphilis in HIV-infected patients, and a CSF examination may be wise in every HIV-positive patient in whom syphilis is diagnosed in any stage of this disease (Lukehart et al., 1988). If there is CSF pleocytosis, elevated CSF protein and positive CSF Venereal Disease Research Laboratory (VDRL) test, neurosyphilis is very likely. If there are CSF abnormalities, but the VDRL test is negative, these CSF abnormalities may be due to neurosyphilis or due to HIV infection itself. Tomberlin et al. (1994) suggested that the accuracy of diagnosis of neurosyphilis may be improved if the patients are also evaluated for production of intrathecal treponemal antibody with the use of TPHA index. This test needs further evaluation. Hook (1994) suggested that every presumed case of neurosyphilis, who is treated by high doses of i.v. Pen G, should be re-evaluated some time after the treatment. If the CSF abnormalities resolve after treatment, the diagnosis was very likely neurosyphilis. Often HIV-infected patients with syphilis, and especially those with neurosyphilis, relapse after adequate courses of Pen G, and so long-term follow-up of these patients is necessary (Malone et al., 1995).

Any patient who has presumptive evidence of neurosyphilis should be treated preferably by crystalline Pen G 7.2–14.4 g daily i.v. for 10–14 days (Musher, 1988, 1991). As it is difficult to admit all patients to hospital, in the USA it is proposed to investigate therapy consisting of benzathine Pen G supplemented by high-dosage oral amoxycillin (2.0 g orally three times daily) plus probenecid (Hook, 1989a). But home administration of i.v. Pen G may be preferable. Patients with syphilis but no central nervous system involvement also probably need more Pen G, but special regimens have not yet been established (Hook, 1989b). Destructive bone disease can occur in congenital or tertiary syphilis, but one HIV-infected patient developed this as the initial manifestation of secondary syphilis. High-dose i.v. Pen G was curative (Kastner *et al.*, 1994).

14 Yaws

Similar to syphilis, Pen G is the recommended treatment for this disease (Taber and Feigin, 1979). In countries where the prevalence of active yaws is over 10%, the whole population is often given a single i.m. injection of 1.2 or 2.4 million units (0.9 or 1.8 g) of benzathine Pen G. Alternatively, this treatment may only be given to active cases and all their contacts (Brown, 1985; Willcox, 1985).

15 Leptospirosis

This acute disease is often mild and self-limited, so that the efficacy of antibiotic treatment is difficult to assess. Although leptospirae are sensitive to Pen G *in vitro*, some consider that this drug (or any other antibiotic) is of little value for treatment of human infections. Most authors believe that Pen G is beneficial provided it is started early in the course of the disease (Taber and Feigin, 1979). A 5- to 10-day course of crystalline Pen G 2.4–6.0 g daily should be given; this usually reduces the duration of pyrexia and also reduces the frequency of jaundice and renal involvement in severe cases, such as those caused by *Leptospira icterohaemorrhagiae* (Kennedy *et al.*, 1979; Tennent, 1980; Watt *et al.*, 1988). It is important to administer Pen G to pregnant women with this disease as this usually prevents fetal infection (Shaked *et al.*, 1993).

16 Lyme disease

Described in 1976, this disease presents with skin lesions (erythema chronicum migrans) and often headache, fever, malaise and fatigue. Some patients develop recurrent arthritis, and occasionally neurological and cardiac complications occur (Steere *et al.*, 1987; Dekonenko *et al.*, 1988; Williams *et al.*, 1990; Motiejunas *et al.*, 1994). In the first empirical antibiotic trial Steere *et al.* (1980) used oral Pen G for 7–10 days to treat this disease. This shortened early manifestations and fewer patients developed arthritis, but subsequent neurological and cardiac abnormalities were unaffected. Tetracycline was also helpful, but erythromycin had no significant effect. The discovery that this disease was caused by a spirochete *Borrelia burgdorferi*, transmitted by the tick *Ixodes dammini* (Harris, 1983), explains why Pen G treatment was effective. Three antibiotic regimens were compared in 108 adult patients with early manifestations of Lyme disease. Oral tetracycline was the most effective, then oral penicillin V, while erythromycin was the least effective (Steere *et al.*, 1983b). High dose i.v. crystalline Pen G of 12 g daily for 10 days) was effective therapy for the neurological abnormalities of Lyme disease (Steere *et al.*, 1983c; Vikerfors and Rudback, 1987; Halperin, 1989). The same high-dose Pen G regimen is often but not always effective for established Lyme arthritis or myositis (Steere *et al.*, 1985; Horowitz *et al.*, 1994). Ceftriaxone is more effective against this spirochete *in vitro*, and in a dose of 2–4 g daily appears to be more effective than large doses of crystalline Pen G for neurological manifestations, chronic arthritis and myositis (Halperin, 1989; Cryan and Wright, 1990; Philipson, 1991; Rahn and Malawista, 1991; Horowitz *et al.*, 1994).

One controlled trial using amoxicillin prophylaxis for Lyme disease after deer-tick bites showed that even in an area in which Lyme disease was endemic, the risk of infection with *B. burgdorferi* after a recognized deer-tick bite was so low that prophylactic antimicrobial treatment was not routinely indicated (Shapiro *et al.*, 1992). One study in a rodent model showed that infection by this spirochete can be aborted by topical application of an antibiotic (either tetracycline, Pen G, amoxycillin, erythromycin, ceftriaxone or doxycycline) to the site of the tick attachment (Shih and Spielman, 1993). Empirical antibiotic treatment is not advocated for patients who are seropositive for Lyme disease, but who lack clinical features of this infection and who only have fatigue (Luft *et al.*, 1994).

17 Rat-bite fever

Pen G is effective for both *Streptobacillus moniliformis* (*Actinobacillus muris*) and *Spirillum minus* infections (Raffin and Freemark, 1979). If endocarditis is present, 4–6 weeks chemotherapy is advisable (Rupp, 1992).

18 Clostridium perfringens (welchii) infections

For treatment of gas gangrene, postpartum infection with *Cl. perfringens* and post-abortal *Cl. perfringens* septicemia, Pen G has been regarded as the best antibiotic (Dylewski *et al.*, 1989). Large doses of crystalline Pen G are recommended, such as 1.2 g i.v. every 2 h, with appropriate dosage reduction in children, elderly patients and in those with impaired renal function (Deveridge and Unsworth, 1973). The use of polyvalent gas gangrene antitoxin, as an adjunct to Pen G has been controversial; but most authorities advise against its use (Dylewski *et al.*, 1989). Gas gangrene may occur in patients with occlusive arterial disease undergoing lower limb amputation, and prophylactic Pen G for 2 days, starting immediately before the operation, should be used (Brumfitt and Hamilton-Miller, 1975; Mashford *et al.*, 1994). For Pen G-allergic patients, either chloramphenicol (p. 555) or erythromycin (p. 620) are suitable alternatives. Pen G-resistant *Cl. perfringens* strains have been reported (p. 13).

Studies in experimental animals have shown that clindamycin (p. 597) and metronidazole (p. 949) are superior to Pen G for the treatment of *Cl. perfringens* infection. Hyperbaric oxygen, if given early, improved the results of Pen G and metronidazole therapy, but not that of clindamycin, which had a superior efficacy compared with the other two drugs (Stevens *et al.*, 1987, 1993b).

19 Tetanus

Pen G is used in conjunction with antitoxin in the treatment of tetanus. Although *Cl. tetani* is sensitive to Pen G, the nature of the infected wound is often such that the organism is inaccessible to antibiotics. The main principles in the treatment of a tetanus wound are surgical debridement and prevention or treatment of associated infection. The latter may lead to activation of spores and create an anaerobic environment (particularly if an undetected foreign body is present) for the proliferation of *Cl. tetani*. Pen G is unreliable for tetanus prophylaxis, and in previously non-immunized patients, human tetanus hyperimmune immunoglobulin should be used. Metronidazole has also been used for treatment of tetanus.

20 Anthrax

Pen G is the mainstay of treatment for this disease (La Force, 1994). Pen G therapy is usually sufficient for cases of cutaneous anthrax, but in severe cases, such as pulmonary, intestinal or throat anthrax, it may be worth adding anti-anthrax serum, but its efficacy is controversial (Doganay *et al.*, 1986). *Bacillus anthracis* can rarely cause bacterial meningitis, which should be treated by large doses of Pen G, possibly combined with streptomycin (Tabatabaie and Syadati, 1993).

21 Diphtheria

Pen G is used to eradicate organisms in this disease, but the timely administration of diphtheria antitoxin remains the essential measure. Pen G can also be used to eradicate the diphtheria carrier state. McCloskey *et al.* (1974) found that a single i.m. injection of benzathine penicillin was effective in 84% of carriers, but oral erythromycin (p. 620) or clindamycin (p. 597) were superior.

22 Actinomycosis

Pen G is the drug of choice, but owing to the fibrotic, necrotic and avascular nature of the lesions, large doses for several months are necessary (Spinola *et al.*, 1981). Thoracic involvement occurs in 15–34% of cases; cardiac involvement is rare, but if this occurs pericardium is usually involved. Treatment consists of high-dose, long-term Pen G therapy as well as drainage of the pericardial space (Fife *et al.*, 1991). Endocarditis is rare, and Pen G again is the treatment of choice (Lam *et al.*, 1993). Actinomyces can also cause liver abscess. Treatment is usually successful with prolonged administration of Pen G and drainage is needed only in some cases (Mijamoto and Fang, 1993). Actinomyces can also involve the central nervous system causing brain abscess, meningitis, meningoencephalitis, subdural empyema and epidural abscess. Optimal management involves combined adequate surgical drainage with prolonged Pen G therapy (Smego, 1987). Uterine actinomycosis infection can occur in association with intrauterine contraceptive devices. Infection is usually superficial and relatively harmless, but it may become invasive and fatalities have occurred (de la Monte *et al.*, 1982; Perlow *et al.*, 1991).

23 Pasteurella multocida infections

This organism may cause wound infections following animal bites such as those inflicted by dogs and cats. Other organisms, such as various types of staphylococci, alpha-hemolytic streptococci and anaerobic bacteria may also cause infections following animal bites (Goldstein,

1992). Less commonly *Pasteurella multocida* can cause septic arthritis, osteomyelitis, septicemia, meningitis, endocarditis, puerperal sepsis, renal infection, acute epiglotittis or pleuropulmonary infections (Johnson and Rumans, 1977; Lehmann *et al.*, 1977; Mitchell *et al.*, 1982; Raffi *et al.*, 1987; Kumar *et al.*, 1990; Leung and Jassal, 1994). Septicemia is more likely to occur in patients with severe underlying diseases, such as advanced hepatic disease or neoplasms. Pen G is indicated for all of these infections, as this Gram-negative bacillus is usually highly sensitive to Pen G (p. 17) (Weber *et al.*, 1984). Resistant strains occur, but are rare.

24 Capnocytophaga canimorosus (DF-2) infections

Infections by this organism are usually acquired from dog bites (p. 17). In splenectomized patients often a fulminant septicemia with shock results; in patients with intact spleens the illness is usually milder, but septicemia and endocarditis may occur. Crystalline Pen G, given i.v., is the treatment of choice, but other antibiotics, such as clindamycin (p. 598), are also effective (Findling *et al.*, 1980; Kalb *et al.*, 1985; Westerink *et al.*, 1987).

25 Lactobacillus infections

These respond to Pen G or to Pen G/gentamicin combination (p. 13). *Lactobacillus* septicemia has occurred after liver transplantation; the strains were usually sensitive to Pen G, but resistant to vancomycin (p. 767). Some of the patients responded to i.v. Pen G therapy (Patel *et al.*, 1994).

26 Infections caused by miscellaneous opportunistic pathogens

Stomatococcus mucilaginosus is a Gram-positive coagulase-negative coccus which forms part of the normal mouth flora. It can cause endocarditis, catheter-related infection, septicemia and septicemia in neutropenic patients. Pen G is the best drug for the treatment of infections, but a few strains of this organism are Pen G-resistant (Ascher *et al.*, 1991; McWhinney *et al.*, 1992). *Kingella kingae* normally colonizes the mucous membranes of the upper gastrointestinal tract and it is a Gram-negative coccobacillus. It has been increasingly recognized as a cause of human infections, particularly in children. It can cause arthritis, osteomyelitis, diskitis, endocarditis and pulmonary infections. The treatment of choice is Pen G, to which all strains are sensitive (de Groot *et al.*, 1988; Morrison and Wagner, 1989; Meis *et al.*, 1992).

Eikenella corrodens is a slowly growing anaerobic Gram-negative rod which is a normal inhabitant of the human oral cavity. It most commonly causes pleuropulmonary infections in patients with underlaying malignancy. Rarely it can cause a pancreatic abscess. Pen G is the best treatment although a few strains may be Pen G-resistant (Joshi *et al.*, 1991; Stein *et al.*, 1993). *Capnocytophaga* is an anaerobic Gram-negative bacillus that normally inhabits the oral cavity. It can cause bacteremia in immunocompromised patients and this is usually associated with severe oral pathology and neutropenia. Pen G is usually a satisfactory treatment, but some strains produce beta-lactamase and are Pen G-resistant (Bilgrami *et al.*, 1992). *Actinobacillus actinomycetemcomitans* is a small anaerobic Gram-negative coccobacillus. It can cause serious infections in humans, such as peridontal infection, soft tissue abscess and endocarditis. Pen G is usually effective treatment, but some strains are resistant (Kaplan *et al.*, 1989b; Van Winkelhoff *et al.*, 1993). *Neisseria lactamica* is a rare cause of meningitis, usually in children, but one adult developed this following skull trauma. Pen G is the best treatment (Denning and Gill, 1991). *Neisseria sicca* is a rare cause of endocarditis; Pen G is the best treatment (Heiddal *et al.*, 1993).

Bacteria of the *Leuconostoc* species are Gram-positive cocci which are normally found in dairy products or vegetable matter. These organisms rarely cause septicemia, mainly in hospitalized patients with underlying diseases. Pen G in high doses is probably the best treatment (Handwerger *et al.*, 1990). *Cardiobacterium hominis*, an opportunistic Gram-negative bacillus has been implicated as a cause of endocarditis. Rechtman and Nadler (1991) have described a patient with abdominal abscess due to this organism plus *Clostridium bifermentans*. Pen G is usually the best treatment.

Chryseomones luteola and *Flavimonas oryzihabitans* are similar Gram-negative bacilli and they can rarely cause bacteremia in otherwise critically ill patients and peritonitis in patients undergoing continuous ambulatory peritoneal dialysis. *Chryseomonas luteola* isolates are often Pen G-resistant and other drugs such as ceftazidime (p. 371) are necessary for treatment. By contrast, *F. oryzihabitans* is usually Pen G-sensitive and this drug is suitable for treatment (Hawkins *et al.*, 1991). *Propionibacterium* spp. are anaerobic Gram-positive bacilli which normally inhabit the mouth and upper respiratory tract. Occasionally they can cause brain abscess, parotid and dental infections, pulmonary infections and peritonitis. The patients usually have a predisposing condition. These organisms are susceptible to Pen G, which in most cases is the antibiotic of choice (Brook and Frazier, 1991).

27 Infections due to other Gram-negative bacilli

Serious infections such as *E. coli* septicemia, have been treated successfully with 'massive' doses of Pen G (up to 36 g per day) i.v. (Weinstein *et al.*, 1964). There are dangers associated with such high doses, and other drugs are now preferred for such infections.

Pen G in commonly prescribed doses, can often be used successfully for the treatment of urinary tract infections, because it is excreted in high concentrations in the urine; in one trial, even potassium Pen G given in an oral dosage of 500 mg 6-hourly, was as satisfactory as other established regimens (Hulbert, 1972).

28 Chemoprophylaxis of rheumatic fever

For this indication benzathine Pen G in a dosage of 600 000 to 1 200 000 units (0.45–0.9 g) i.m., once a month has been used. However, pharmacokinetic data indicate that this dose should be given once every 2 weeks. Currie *et al.* (1994) studied 4-weekly i.m. doses of 1 200 000 units (0.9 g), 1 800 000 units (1.35 g) and 2 400 000 units (1.8 g). Proportion of patients who had adequate serum levels of Pen G at 4 weeks increased with each increasing benzathine Pen G dose. The authors suggested that further studies are needed to find the ideal 4-weekly dose of benzathine Pen G. Where patient compliance can be assured, one of the oral acid-stable phenoxypenicillins can be used.

In the USA armed forces i.m. benzathine Pen G has been used to prevent Group A streptococcal infections and acute rheumatic fever since the mid-1950s. Streptococcal infection has been a significant problem in military recruit camps in the USA for a long time. Some recent terminations of benzathine Pen G prophylaxis programs have been followed by epidemics of Group A streptococcal infections. Treatment options should be tailored to each specific training area. In areas with high rates of infection, i.m. benzathine Pen G should be given monthly all year whilst seasonal administration of benzathine Pen G from October to April may suffice if surveillance data suggest a low summer rate, or in some situations benzathine Pen G may be given even less frequently (Thomas *et al.*, 1988; Heggie *et al.*, 1992). The regimen of monthly doses of 0.9 g appears to be effective despite the fact that serum levels of Pen G which inhibit *Strep. pyogenes* in these trainees persist for only 1–2 weeks after this dose (Bass *et al.*, 1996). In the army camp situation there is also evidence that benzathine Pen G in addition to controlling Group A streptococcal infections, has a broad effect in the prevention of acute respiratory disease in general (Gunzenhauser *et al.*, 1992).

Despite the fact that benzathine Pen G has a long half-life, and thus if a severe allergic reaction starts early after the injection, there will be further absorption of Pen G from the injection site, there is no evidence that its regular use for rheumatic fever prophylaxis is associated with more frequent anaphylaxis and other allergic reactions compared with the administration of other forms of Pen G (International Rheumatic Fever Study Group, 1991).

29 Prevention of pneumococcal infections

Benzathine Pen G, in a dosage of 600 000 units (0.45 g) i.m. monthly, has proved superior to pneumococcal vaccine for the prevention of pneumococcal infection in children with homozygous sickle cell disease (John *et al.*, 1984).

30 Whipple's disease

Bacterial infection with an atypical bacillary organism, *Tropheryma whippelii* is involved in the etiology of this disease (Dobbins, 1995). For this reason Pen G has been advocated for treatment. Usually there is a good clinical response and the bacillary organisms (seen most easily on electron microscopy) disappear from the small bowel rapidly. A 2-week course of crystalline Pen G followed by oral phenoxymethylpenicillin for 3 months, has been recommended. Despite this treatment, some patients still develop central nervous system disease, or this may occur on withdrawal of penicillin therapy. One of the penicillins has been preferred for treatment of Whipple's disease but the tetracyclines, chloramphenicol and erythromycin are also effective (Feldman *et al.*, 1980). After a long-term follow-up of 88 patients, Keinath *et al.* (1985) suggested that Pen G or tetracycline alone is not adequate as initial therapy for Whipple's disease. They recommended initial therapy by parenteral Pen G plus streptomycin followed by 1 year of oral co-trimoxazole or oral co-trimoxazole alone for 1 year as initial therapy. Another recommendation is i.m. procaine penicillin 1.2 g and 1 g i.m. streptomycin daily for 10–14 days, followed by tetracycline 1 g daily for 10–12 months (Maizel *et al.*, 1970). In one patient in whom the Whipple's bacillus caused uveitis, the diagnosis was confirmed by polymerase-chain-reaction assay, which detected 16S ribosomal RNA gene sequences corresponding to *Tropheryma whippelii*. The patient responded to a 14-day course of i.v. Pen G (14.4 g per day) and i.m. streptomycin (1.0 g per day) (Rickman *et al.*, 1995).

31 Botulism

Pen G therapy has been suggested as an adjunct to other treatment in this disease, to prevent *Clostridium* spore germination and release of more toxin in the bowel (Eisenberg and Bender, 1976). Similarly Pen G has been used as an adjunct to other treatment in wound botulism, but it is not clear whether this treatment promotes recovery (Weber *et al.*, 1993).

32 Chemoprophylaxis in acute myeloid leukemia

In some units there has been a high prevalence of streptococcal septicemia in patients with this disease undergoing cytotoxic chemotherapy. In these circumstances Pen G chemoprophylaxis has been of value (de Jong *et al.*, 1993). In patients undergoing high-dose chemotherapy and bone marrow transplantation it is worth adding crystalline Pen G 0.6 g i.v. 6-hourly to the standard chemoprophylaxis with norfloxacin, fluconazole and acyclovir. Pen G prevents streptococcal infections in these patients (Broun *et al.*, 1994).

33 Louse-borne relapsing fever

For this disease one of the tetracyclines has been regarded as the treatment of choice. However, Seboxa and Rahlenbeck (1995) found that single low doses of procaine Pen G i.m. (100 000–400 000 units) were also effective, but there were more relapses after the Pen G treatment than after a single 250-mg tetracycline dose. Severe Jarisch-Herxheimer reactions were less common after Pen G and therefore the authors considered Pen G preferable to tetracycline for the treatment of this disease.

References

Abeck D, Johnson AP, Alexander F *et al.* (1988). *In vitro* activity of eight antimicrobial agents against non-penicillinase-producing gonococci isolated in Munich. *Genitourin Med* **64**: 233.

Abraham EP (1980). Fleming's discovery. *Rev Infect Dis* **2**: 140.

Acar JF, Minozzi C (1986). Role of beta-lactamases in the resistance of Gram-negative bacilli to beta-lactam antibiotics. *Rev Infect Dis* **8**(Suppl 5): 482.

Adkinson NF Jr, Thompson WL, Maddrey WC, Lichtenstein LM (1971). Routine use of penicillin skin testing on an inpatient service. *New Engl J Med* **285**: 22.

Aharoni A, Potasman I, Levitan Z *et al.* (1990). Postpartum maternal Group B streptococcal meningitis. *Rev Infect Dis* **12**: 273.

Al-Hadramy MS, Aman H, Omer A, Khan MA(1986). Benzylpenicillin-induced neutropenia. *J Antimicrob Chemother* **17**: 251.

Al-Obeid S, Gutmann L, Williamson R (1990a). Correlation of penicillin-induced lysis of *Enterococcus faecium* with saturation of essential penicillin-binding proteins and release of lipoteichoic acid. *Antimicrob Ag Chemother* **34**: 1901.

Al-Obeid S, Gutmann L, Williamson R (1990b). Modification of penicillin-binding proteins of penicillin-resistant mutants of different species of enterococci. *J Antimicrob Chemother* **26**: 613.

American Academy of Pediatrics (1980). Prophylaxis and treatment of neonatal gonococcal infections. *Pediatrics* **65**: 1047.

American Academy of Pediatrics Committee on Drugs (1973). Anaphylaxis. *Pediatrics* **51**: 136.

Anderson AW, Cruickshank JG (1982). Endocarditis due to viridans-type streptococci tolerant to beta-lactam antibiotics: therapeutic problems. *Brit Med J* **285**: 854.

Anderson MD, Kennedy CA, Walsh TP, Bowler WA (1993). Prosthetic valve endocarditis due to *Rothia dentocariosa*. *Clin Infect Dis* **17**: 945.

Anderson R, Bauman M, Austrian R (1968). Lincomycin and penicillin G in the treatment of mild and moderately severe pneumococcal pneumonia. *Amer Rev Respir Dis* **97**: 914.

Andrassay K, Scherz M, Ritz E *et al.* (1976). Penicillin-induced coagulation disorder. *Lancet* **ii**: 1039.

Anthony BF (1982). Carriage of Group B streptococci during pregnancy: a puzzler. *J Infect Dis* **145**: 789.

Anthony BF, Concepcion NF (1975). Group B streptococcus in a general hospital. *J Infect Dis* **132**: 561.

Appelbaum PC (1992). Antimicrobial resistance in *Streptococcus pneumoniae*: an overview. *Clin Infect Dis* **15**: 77.

Appelbaum PC, Scragg JN, Bowen AJ *et al.* (1977). *Streptococcus pneumoniae* resistant to penicillin and chloramphenicol. *Lancet* **ii**: 995.

Appelbaum PC, Spangler SK, Crotty E, Jacobs MR (1989). Susceptibility of penicillin-sensitive and -resistant strains of *Streptococcus pneumoniae* to new antimicrobial agents, including daptomycin, teicoplanin, cefpodoxime and quinolones. *J Antimicrob Chemother* **23**: 509.

Arditi M, Shulman ST, Davis AT, Yogev R (1989). Group C beta hemolytic streptococcal infections in children: nine pediatric cases and review (1989). *Rev Infect Dis* **11**: 34.

Arends JP, Zanen HC (1988). Meningitis caused by *Streptococcus suis* in humans. *Rev Infect Dis* **10**: 131.

Armstrong RW, Fung PC (1993). Brainstem encephalitis (rhombencephalitis). due to *Listeria monocytogenes*: case report and review. *Clin Infect Dis* **16**: 689.

Ascher DP, Zbick C, White C, Fischer GW (1991). Infection due to *Stomatococcus mucilaginosus*: 10 cases and review. *Rev Infect Dis* **13**: 1048.

Ashford WA, Golash RG, Hemming VG (1976). Penicillinase-producing *Neisseria gonorrhoeae*. *Lancet* **ii**: 657.

Ashkenazi S, Franck R, Wanger A *et al.* (1988). Group G. streptococcal meningitis in childhood. *Pediatr Infect Dis J* **7**: 522.

Atkinson JP (1969). Transverse myelopathy secondary to injection of penicillin. *J Pediatr* **75**: 867.

Auckenthaler R, Hermans PE, Washington JA II (1983). Group G streptococcal bacteremia: clinical study and review of the literature. *Rev Infect Dis* **5**: 196.

Austen KF (1974). Current concepts. Systemic anaphylaxis in the human being. *New Engl J Med* **291**: 661.

AGSP (Australian Gonococcal Surveillance Programme) (1988). Penicillin sensitivity of gonococci isolated in Australia 1981–6. *Genitourin Med* **64**: 147.

Axelson JA, Lo Buglio AF (1980). Immune hemolytic anemia. *Med Clin North Amer* **64**: 597.

Back SA, O'Neill T, Fishbein G, Gwinup G (1990). A case of Group B streptococcal pyomyositis. *Rev Infect Dis* **12**: 784.

Backes RJ, Wilson WR, Geraci JE (1985). Group B streptococcal infective endocarditis. *Arch Intern Med* **145**: 693.

Baker CJ (1977). Summary of the workshop on perinatal infections due to Group B streptococcus. *J Infect Dis* **136**: 137.

Baker CN, Thornsberry C, Facklam RR (1981). Synergism, killing kinetics and antimicrobial susceptibility of Group A and B streptococci. *Antimicrob Ag Chemother* **19**: 716.

Bakker-Woudenberg IAJM, de Bos P, van Gerwen ALEM *et al.* (1982). Effect of splenectomy upon the course of experimental pneumococcal bacteraemia in rats and the efficacy of penicillin therapy. *J Infect* **4**: 17.

Baldwin DS, Levine BB, McClusky RT, Gallo GR (1968). Renal failure and interstitial nephritis due to penicillin and methicillin. *New Engl J Med* **279**: 1245.

Barber M, Waterworth PM (1962). Antibacterial activity of the penicillins. *Brit Med J* **1**: 1159.

Barbour AG, Todd WJ, Stoenner HG (1982). Action of penicillin on *Borrelia hermsii*. *Antimicrob Ag Chemother* **21**: 823.

Barza M (1981). Principle of tissue penetration of antibiotics. *J Antimicrob Chemother* **8** (Suppl C): 7.

Barza M, Brusch J, Bergeron MG *et al.* (1975). Extraction of antibiotics from the circulation by liver and kidney: effect of probenecid. *J Infect Dis* **131** (Suppl): 86.

Bass JW, Longfield JN, Jones RG, Hartmann RM (1996). Serum levels of penicillin in basic trainees in the US army who received intramuscular penicillin G benzathine. *Clin Infect Dis* **22**: 727.

Bauernfeind A (1986). Classification of beta-lactamases. *Rev Infect Dis* **8** (Suppl 5): 470.

Bayer AS, Chow AW, Anthony BF, Guze LB (1976). Serious infections in adults due to Group B streptococci. Clinical and serotypic characterization. *Amer J Med* **61**: 498.

Bayer AS, Chow AW, Concepcion N, Guze LB (1978). Susceptibility of 40 lactobacilli to six antimicrobial agents with broad Gram-positive anaerobic spectra. *Antimicrob Ag Chemother* **14**: 720.

Bayer AS, Chow AW, Morrison JO, Guze LB (1980). Bactericidal synergy between penicillin or ampicillin and aminoglycosides against anitbiotic-tolerant lactobacilli. *Antimicrob Ag Chemother* **17**: 359.

Bayer AS, Morrison JO, Kim K-S (1982). Comparative *in vitro* bactericidal activity of cefonicid, ceftizoxime, and penicillin against Group B streptococci. *Antimicrob Ag Chemother* **21**: 344.

Belfrage E, Anzén B, Jörbeck H *et al.* (1990). Streptococcal infections in late pregnancy and labor. *Scand J Infect Dis* (Suppl 71): 79.

Benach JL, Bosler EM, Hanrahan JP *et al.* (1983). Spirochetes isolated from the blood of two patients with Lyme disease. *New Engl J Med* **308**: 740.

Bengtsson S, Forsgren A, Mellbin T (1977). Penicillinase production in community strains of *Staphylococcus aureus*. *Scand J Infect Dis* **9**: 23.

Beninger PR, Savoia MC, Davis CE (1988). *Listeria monocytogenes* meningitis in a patient with AIDS-related complex. *J Infect Dis* **158**: 1396.

Berenguer J, Solera J, Diaz MD *et al.* (1991). Listeriosis in patients infected with human immunodeficiency virus. *Rev Infect Dis* **13**: 115.

Berg T, Hallander HO, Nathorst-Windahl G, Nordlander I-M (1977). Group B beta-hemolytic streptococci as an important cause of perinatal mortality. *Scand J Infect Dis* **9**: 19.

Bergeron MG, Gennari FJ, Barza M *et al.* (1975). Renal tubular transport of penicillin G and carbenicillin in the rat. *J Infect Dis* **132**: 374.

Bergeron MG, Beauchamp D, Poirier A, Bastille A (1981). Continuous vs intermittent administration of antimicrobial agents: tissue penetration and efficacy *in vivo*. *Rev Infect Dis* **3**: 84.

Berghash SR, Dunny GM (1985). Emergence of a multiple beta-lactam-resistance phenotype in Group B streptococci of bovine origin. *J Infect Dis* **151**: 494.

Bergman BR (1979). Concentration of dicloxacillin and benzylpenicillin in fracture haematoma. *Scand J Infect Dis* **11**: 225.

Bergström S, Norlander L, Norqvist A, Normark S (1978). Contribution of a TEM-1-like beta-lactamase to penicillin resistance in *Neisseria gonorrhoeae*. *Antimicrob Ag Chemother* **13**: 618.

Berkowitz FE, Vallabh P, Altman DI *et al.* (1983). Jarisch-Herxheimer reaction in meningococcal meningitis. *Amer J Dis Child* **137**: 599.

Berrón S, Vázquez JA (1994). Increase in moderate penicillin resistance and serogroup C in meningococcal strains isolated in Spain. Is there any relationship? *Clin Infect Dis* **18**: 161.

Betriu C, Sanchez A, Gomez M *et al.* (1993). Antibiotic susceptibility of Group A streptococci: a 6-year follow-up study. *Antimicrob Ag Chemother* **37**: 1717.

Betriu C, Gomez M, Sanchez A *et al.* (1994). Antibiotic resistance and penicillin tolerance in clinical isolates of Group B streptococci. *Antimicrob Ag Chemother* **38**: 2183.

Bickel L (1972). *Rise up to Life. A Biography of Howard Walter Florey who gave Penicillin to the World.* London: Angus and Robertson.

Bignardi GE, Isaacs D (1989). Neonatal meningitis due to *Streptococcus mitis*. *Rev Infect Dis* **11**: 86.

Bilgrami S, Bergstrom SK, Peterson DE *et al.* (1992). *Capnocytophaga* bactremia in a patient with Hodgkins disease following bone marrow transplantation: case report and review. *Clin Infect Dis* **14**: 1045.

Block C, Davidson Y, Melamed E, Keller N (1993). Susceptibility of *Neisseria meningitidis* in Israel to penicillin and other drugs of interest. *J Antimicrob Chemother* **32**: 166.

Blog FB, Chang A, DeKoning GAJ *et al.* (1977). Penicillinase-producing strains of *Neisseria gonorrhoeae* isolated in Rotterdam. *Brit J Vener Dis* **53**: 98.

Bochud P-Y, Eggiman Ph, Calandra Th *et al.* (1994). Bacteremia due to viridans streptococcus in neutropenic patients with cancer: clinical spectrum and risk factors. *Clin Infect Dis* **18**: 25.

Boenning DA, Nelson LP, Campos JM (1988). Relatively penicillin-resistant *Streptococcus sanguis* endocarditis in an adolescent. *Pediatr Infect Dis J* **7**: 205.

Bohnhoff M, Morello JA, Lerner SA (1986). Auxotypes, penicillin susceptibility, and serogroups of *Neisseria gonorrhoeae* from disseminated and uncomplicated infections. *J Infect Dis* **154**: 225.

Booth LV, Richards RH, Chandran DR (1991). Septic arthritis caused by *Corynebacterium xerosis* following vascular surgery. *Rev Infect Dis* **13**: 548.

Botha P (1988). Penicillin-resistant Neisseria meningitidis in Southern Africa. *Lancet* **i**: 54.

Bourgault A-M, Wilson WR, Washington JA II (1979). Antimicrobial susceptibilities of species of viridans streptococci. *J Infect Dis* **140**: 316.

Boyer KM, Gotoff SP(1986). Prevention of early onset neonatal group B streptococcal disease with selective intrapartum chemoprophylaxis. *New Engl J Med* **314**: 1665.

Boyer KM, Gadzala CA, Kelly PD, Gotoff SP (1983). Selective intrapartum chemoprophylaxis of neonatal Group B streptococcal early-onset disease. III Interruption of mother-to-infant transmission. *J Infect Dis* **148**: 810.

Bradley SF, Gordon JJ, Baumgartner DD *et al.* (1991). Group C streptococcal bacteremia: analysis of 88 cases. *Rev Infect Dis* **13**: 270.

Braun TI, Travis D, Dee RR, Nieman RE (1993). Liver abscess due to

Listeria monocytogenes: case report and review. *Clin Infect Dis* **17**: 267.

Breiman RF, Butler JC, Tenover FC *et al.* (1994). Emergence of drug-resistant pneumococcal infections in the United States. *JAMA* **271**: 1831.

Brennan RO, Durack DT (1983). Therapeutic significance of penicillin tolerance in experimental streptococcal endocarditis. *Antimicrob Ag Chemother* **23**: 273.

Brett M (1989). A novel gonococcal beta-lactamase plasmid. *J Antimicrob Chemother* **23**: 653.

Brewin A, Arango L, Hadley WK, Murray JF (1974). High-dose penicillin therapy and pneumococcal pneumonia. *JAMA* **230**: 409.

Brook I (1982). Treatment of Group A streptococcal pharyngo-tonsillitis. *JAMA* **247**: 2496.

Brook I (1984). The role of beta-lactamase-producing bacteria in the persistence of streptococcal tonsillar infection. *Rev Infect Dis* **6**: 601.

Brook I, Finegold SM (1979). Bacteriology and therapy of lung abscess in children. *J Pediatr* **94**: 10.

Brook I, Frazier EH (1991). Infections caused by *Propionibacterium* species. *Rev Infect Dis* **13**: 819.

Brook I, Frazier EH (1993). Significant recovery of nonsporulating anaerobic rods from clinical specimens. *Clin Infect Dis* **16**: 476.

Brook I, Gilmore JD (1993). Evaluation of bacterial interference and beta-lactamase production in management of experimental infection with Group A beta-hemolytic streptococci. *Antimicrob Ag Chemother* **37**: 1452.

Brooks RG, Notario G, McCabe RE (1988). Hospital survey of anti-microbial prophylaxis to prevent endocarditis in patients with prosthetic heart valves. *Amer J Med* **84**: 617.

Broun ER, Wheat JL, Kneebone PH *et al.* (1994). Randomized trial of the addition of Gram-positive prophylaxis for patients undergoing autologous bone marrow transplantation. *Antimicrob Ag Chemother* **38**: 576.

Brown S, Warnnissorn T, Biddle J *et al.* (1982). Antimicrobial resistance of *Neisseria gonorrhoeae* in Bangkok: is single drug treatment passé. *Lancet* **2**: 1366.

Brown ST (1982). Update on recommendations for the treatment of syphilis. *Rev Infect Dis* **4** (Suppl): 837.

Brown ST (1985). Therapy for nonvenereal trepanematoses: review of the efficacy of penicillin and consideration of alternatives. *Rev Infect Dis* **7** (Suppl 2): 318.

Brown WJ, Waatti PE (1980). Susceptibility testing of clinically isolated anaerobic bacteria by an agar dilution technique. *Antimicrob Ag Chemother* **17**: 629.

Brumfitt W, Hamilton-Miller JMT (1975). The place of antibiotic prophylaxis in medicine. *J Antimicrob Chemother* **1**: 163.

Brunner FP, Frick PG (1968). Hypokalaemia, metabolic alkalosis, and hypernatraemia due to 'massive' sodium penicillin therapy. *Brit Med J* **4**: 550.

Bryan CS, Stone WJ (1975). Comparably massive penicillin G therapy in renal failure. *Ann Intern Med* **82**: 189.

Bryan LE (1988). General mechanisms of resistance to antibiotics. *J Antimicrob Chemother* **22** (Suppl A): 1.

Bryceson ADM (1976). Clinical pathology of the Jarisch-Herxheimer reaction. *J Infect Dis* **133**: 696.

Buck GE (1994). Meningococcus with reduced susceptibility to penicillin isolated in the United States. *Pediatr Infect Dis J* **13**: 156.

Büla CJ, Bille J, Glauser MP (1995). An epidemic of food-borne listeriosis in Western Switzerland: description of 57 cases involving adults. *Clin Infect Dis* **20**: 66.

Bulger RJ, Bennett JV, Boen ST (1965). Intraperitoneal administration of broad-spectrum antibiotics in patients with renal failure. *JAMA* **194**: 1198.

Burkart T, Watanakunakorn C (1992). Group A streptococcal bacteremia in a community teaching hospital – 1980–1989. *Clin Infect Dis* **14**: 29.

Burnakis TG, Hildebrandt NB (1986). Pelvic inflammatory disease: a review with emphasis on antimicrobial therapy. *Rev Infect Dis* **8**: 86.

Bush K (1988). Recent developments in beta-lactamase research and their

implications for the future. *Rev Infect Dis* **10**: 681.

Bush K (1989a). Characterization of beta-lactamases. *Antimicrob Ag Chemother* **33**: 259.

Bush K (1989b). Classification of beta-lactamases: groups 1, 2a, 2b and 2 b[1]. *Antimicrob Ag Chemother* **33**: 264.

Bush K (1989c). Classification of beta-lactamases: groups 2c, 2d, 2e, 3, and 4. *Antimicrob Ag Chemother* **33**: 271.

Bush K, Sykes RB (1986). Methodology for the study of beta-lactamases. *Antimicrob Ag Chemother* **30**: 6.

Butler T, Weaver RE, Ramani TKV *et al.* (1977). Unidentified Gram-negative rod infection. A new disease in man. *Ann Intern Med* **86**: 1.

Campos J, Mendelman PM, Sako MU *et al.* (1987). Detection of relatively penicillin G-resistant *Neisseria meningitidis* by disk susceptibility testing. *Antimicrob Ag Chemother* **31**: 1478.

Campos J, Fusté MC, Trujillo G *et al.* (1992a). Genetic diversity of penicillin-resistant *Neisseria meningitidis*. *J Infect Dis* **166**: 173.

Campos J, Trujillo G, Seuba T, Rodriguez A (1992b). Discriminative criteria for *Neisseria meningitidis* that are moderately susceptible to penicillin and ampicillin. *Antimicrob Ag Chemother* **36**: 1028.

Caputo GM, Sattler FR, Jacobs MR, Appelbaum PC (1983). Penicillin-resistant pneumococcus and meningitis. *Ann Intern Med* **98**: 416.

Carlson P, Kontianinen S, Renkonen O-V *et al.* (1995). *Arcanobacterium haemolyticum* and streptococcal pharyngitis in army conscripts. *Scand J Infect Dis* **27**: 17.

Cartwright K, Reilly S, White D, Stuart J (1992). Early treatment with parenteral penicillin in meningococcal disease. *Brit Med J* **305**: 143.

Carvajal A, Frederiksen W (1988). Fatal endocarditis due to *Listeria monocytogenes*. *Rev Infect Dis* **10**: 616.

Catlin BW, Reyn A (1982). Neisseria gonorrhoeae isolated from dis-seminated and localised infections in prepenicillin era. Auxotypes and antibacterial drug resistances. *Brit J Vener Dis* **58**: 158.

CDC (Center for Disease Control) (1977). Follow-up on penicillinase-producing *Neisseria gonorrhoeae* – worldwide. *MMWR* **26**: 153.

CDC (Center for Disease Control) (1978a). Follow-up on multiple-antibiotic-resistant pneumococci – South Africa. *MMWR* **27**: 1.

CDC (Center for Disease Control) (1978b). Penicillinase-(beta-lactamase-). producing *Neisseria gonorrhoeae* – worldwide. *MMWR* **27**: 10.

CDC (Centers for Disease Control) (1982). Global distribution of penicillinase-producing *Neisseria gonorrhoeae* (PPNG). *MMWR* **31**: 1.

CDC (Centers for Disease Control) (1983). Penicillinase-producing Neis-seria gonorrhoeae – Los Angeles. *MMWR* **32**: 181.

CDC (Centers for Disease Control) (1984). Chromosomally mediated resistant Neisseria gonorrhoeae – United States. *MMWR* **33**: 408.

CDC (Centers for Disease Control) (1985). Tetracycline-resistant *Neisseria gonorrhoeae* – Georgia, Pennsylvania, New Hampshire. *MMWR* **34**: 563.

CDC (Centers for Disease Control) (1993). Sexually transmitted diseases treatment guidelines. *MMWR* **42** (No RR-14): 27, 56.

Chain E, Florey HW, Gardner AD *et al.* (1940). Penicillin as a chemotherapeutic agent. *Lancet* **ii**: 226.

Chalkley LJ, Koornhof HJ (1988). Penicillin-binding proteins of *Strepto-coccus pneumoniae*. *J Antimicrob Chemother* **22**: 791.

Chalkley LJ, Koornhof HJ (1990). Intra- and inter-specific transformation of *Streptococcus pneumoniae* to penicillin resistance. *J Antimicrob Chemother* **26**: 21.

Chau PY, Huang CY, Kay R (1983). *Streptococcus suis* meningitis. An important under-diagnosed disease in Hong Kong. *Med J Aust* **1**: 414.

Cherubin CE, Appleman MD, Heseltine PNR *et al.* (1991). Epidemiological spectrum and current treatment of listeriosis. *Rev Infect Dis* **13**: 1108.

Chow AW, Jewesson PJ (1985). Pharmacokinetics and safety of anti-microbial agents during pregnancy. *Rev Infect Dis* **7**: 287.

Chow AW, Patten V, Bednorz D (1978). Susceptibility of *Campylobacter fetus* to twenty-two antimicrobial agents. *Antimicrob Ag Chemother* **13**: 416.

Chow JW, Muder RR(1992). Group A streptococcal meningitis. *Clin Infect Dis* **14**: 418.

Chow JW, Perri MB, Thal LA, Zervos MJ (1993). Mobilization of the penicillin gene in *Enterococcus faecalis. Antimicrob Ag Chemother* **37**: 1187.

Chu M-L, Ho L-J, Lin H-C, Wu Y-C (1992). Epidemiology of penicillin-resistant *Neisseria gonorrhoeae* isolated in Taiwan, 1960–1990. *Clin Infect Dis* **14**: 450.

Clendennen TE III, Hames CS, Kees ES *et al.* (1992a). *In vitro* antibiotic susceptibilities of *Neisseria gonorrhoeae* isolates in the Phillipines. *Antimicrob Ag Chemother* **36**: 277.

Clendennen TE, Eschevarria P, Saengeur S *et al.* (1992b). Antibiotic susceptibility survey of *Neisseria gonorrhoeae* in Thailand. *Antimicrob Ag Chemother* **36**: 1682.

Cohen-Abbo A, Harper MB (1993). Case report: streptococcal toxic shock syndrome presenting as septic thrombophlebitis in a child with varicella. *Pediatr Infect Dis J* **12**: 1033.

Cole M, Kenig MD, Hewitt VA (1973). Metabolism of penicillins to penicilloic acids and 6-aminopenicillanic acid in man and its significance in assessing penicillin absorption. *Antimicrob Ag Chemother* **3**: 463.

Coleman DL, Horwitz RI, Andriole VT (1982). Association between serum inhibitory and bactericidal concentrations and therapeutic outcome in bacterial endocarditis. *Amer J Med* **73**: 260.

Collart P, Poitevin M, Milovanovic A *et al.* (1980). Kinetic study of serum penicillin concentrations after single doses of benzathine and bene-thamine penicillins in young and old people. *Brit J Vener Dis* **56**: 355.

Collazos J, Diaz F, Ayarza R, de Miguel J (1994). *Actinobacillus actinomycetemcomitans*: a cause of pulmonary-valve endocarditis of 18 months' duration with unusual manifestations. *Clin Infect Dis* **18**: 115.

Collignon PJ, Bell JM (1992). *Streptococcus pneumoniae*: how common is penicillin resistance in Australia? *Aust NZJ Med* **22**: 473.

Collignon PJ, Bell J, Hufton IW, Mitchell D (1988). Meningitis caused by a penicillin- and chloramphenicol-resistant *Streptococcus pneumoniae Med J Aust* **149**: 497.

Colt HG, Morris JF, Marston BJ, Sewell DL (1991). Necrotizing tracheitis caused by *Corynebacterium pseudodiphtherieum*: unique case and review. *Rev Infect Dis* **13**: 73.

Committee on Infectious Diseases (1988). Treatment of bacterial meningitis. *Pediatrics* **81**: 904.

Communicable Diseases Intelligence (1982). Gonococcal surveillance in Australia (July-September 1982); **82**: 2.

Conde-Glez CJ, Calderon E, Echaniz G *et al.* (1988). Serogroup specificity and antimicrobial susceptibilities of *Neisseria gonorrhoeae* isolated in Mexico City. *J Antimicrob Chemother* **21**: 413.

Cooksey RC, Swenson JM, Clark NC, Thornsberry C (1989). DNA hybridization studies of a nucleotide sequence homologous to transposon Tn 1545 in the 'Minnesota' strain of multiresistant *Streptococcus pneumoniae* isolated in 1977. *Diagn Microbiol Infect Dis* **12**: 13.

Coonan KM, Kaplan EL (1994). *In vitro* susceptibility of recent North American Group A streptococcal isolates to eleven oral antibiotics. *Pediatr Infect Dis J* **13**: 630.

Copley CG, Egglestone I (1982). Gonococci without plasmids. *Lancet* **i**: 1133.

Corbett GM, Perry DJ, Shaw TRD (1982). Penicillin-induced leukopenia. *New Engl J Med* **307**: 1642.

Costerton J, Cheng K-J (1975). The role of bacterial cell envelope in antibiotic resistance. *J Antimicrob Chemother* **1**: 363.

Coudron PE, Markowitz SM, Wong ES (1992). Isolation of beta-lactamase-producing, aminoglycoside-resistant strain of *Enterococcus faecium. Antimicrob Ag Chemother* **36**: 1125.

Cowen J (1979). Clinical observations on group-B streptococcal infections. *J Antimicrob Chemother* **5** (Suppl A): 39.

Craig WA, Ebert SC(1992). Continuous infusion of beta-lactam antibiotics. *Antimicrob Ag Chemother* **36**: 2577.

Craven DE, Rixinger AI, Bisno AL (1986). Bacteremia caused by Group G streptococci in parenteral drug abusers: epidemiological and clinical aspects. *J Infect Dis* **153**: 988.

Cryan B, Wright DJM (1990). Antimicrobial agents in Lyme disease. *J Antimicrob Chemother* **25**: 187.

Currie BJ, Burt T, Kaplan EL (1994). Penicillin concentrations after

increased doses of benzathine penicillin G for prevention of secondary rheumatic fever. *Antimicrob Ag Chemother* **38**: 1203.

Curtis NAC (1981). Penicillin-binding proteins in theory and practice. *J Antimicrob Chemother* **8: 85.**

Curtis NAC, Brown C, Boxall M, Boulton MG (1979a). Inhibition of *Escherichia coli* K-12 by beta-lactam antibiotics with poor antibacterial activity: interaction of permeability and intrinsic activity against penicillin-binding proteins. *Antimicrob Ag Chemother* **15**: 332.

Curtis NAC, Orr D, Ross GW, Boulton MG (1979b). Competition of beta-lactam antibiotics for the penicillin-binding proteins of *Pseudomonas aeruginosa, Enterobacter cloacae, Klebsiella aerogenes, Proteus rettgeri*, and *Escherichia coli*: comparison with antibacterial activity and effects upon bacterial morphology. *Antimicrob Ag Chemother* **16**: 325.

Curtis NAC, Orr D, Ross GW, Boulton MG (1979c). Affinities of penicillins and cephalosporins for the penicillin-binding proteins of *Escherichia coli* K-12 and their antibacterial activity. *Antimicrob Ag Chemother* **16**: 533.

Curtis NAC, Orr D, Boulton MG, Ross GW (1981). Penicillin-binding proteins of *Pseudomonas aeruginosa*. Comparison of two strains differing in their resistance to beta-lactam antibiotics. *J Antimicrob Chemother* **7**: 127.

Curtis NAC, Eisenstadt RL, Turner KA, White AJ (1985). Inhibition of penicillin-binding protein 3 of *Escherichia coli* K-12. Effects upon growth, viability and outer membrane barrier function. *J Antimicrob Chemother* **16**: 287.

Dacey RG, Sande MA (1974). Effect of probenecid on cerebrospinal fluid concentrations of penicillin and cephalosporin derivatives. *Antimicrob Ag Chemother* **6**: 437.

Dagan R, Ferne M, Sheinis M *et al.* (1987). An epidemic of penicillin-tolerant Group A streptococcal pharyngitis in children living in a closed community: mass treatment with erythromycin. *J Infect Dis* **156**: 514.

Dagan R, Yagupsky P, Goldbart A *et al.* (1994). Increasing prevalence of penicillin-resistant pneumococcal infections in children in southern Israel: implications for future immunization policies. *Pediatr Infect Dis J* **13**: 782.

Dajani AS, Bisno AL, Chung KJ *et al.* (1990). Prevention of bacterial endocarditis. Recommendations by the American Heart Association. *JAMA* **264**: 2919.

Dajani AS, Bawdon RE, Berry MC (1994). Oral amoxicillin as prophylaxis for endocarditis: what is the optimal dose? *Clin Infect Dis* **18**: 157.

Dankert J, Hess J (1982). Penicillin-sensitive streptococcal endocarditis. *Lancet* **ii**: 1219.

Dangor Y, Ballard RC, Miller SD, Koornhof HJ (1990). Antimicrobial susceptibility of *Haemophilus ducreyi. Antimicrob Ag Chemother* **34**: 1303.

Davies AJ, Jolley A (1992). Antibacterial therapy of community-acquired chest infections. *J Antimicrob Chemother* **29**: 1.

Davies GK, Turner P, Spencer BT (1974). Abdominal pain after intravenous benzylpenicillin. *Lancet* **ii**: 167.

Davies HD, Matlow A, Scriver SR *et al.* (1994). Apparent lower rates of streptococcal toxic shock syndrome and lower mortality in children with invasive Group A streptococcal infections compared with adults. *Pediatr Infect Dis J* **13**: 49.

de Groot R, Glover D, Clausen C *et al.* (1988). Bone and joint infections caused by *Kingella kingae*: six cases and review of the literature. *Rev Infect Dis* **10**: 998.

de Jong P, de Jong M, Kuijper E, van der Lelie J (1993). Evaluation of penicillin G in the prevention of streptococcal septicemia in patients with acute myeloid leukaemia undergoing cytoxic chemotherapy. *Eur J Clin Microbiol Infect Dis* **12**: 750.

Dekonenko EJ, Steere AC, Berardi VP, Kravchuk LN (1988). *Lyme borreliosis* in the Soviet Union: a cooperative US-USSR report. *J Infect Dis* **158**: 748.

de la Monte SM, Gupta PK, White CL (1982). Systemic *Actinomyces* infection A potential complication of intrauterine contraceptive devices. *JAMA* **248**: 1876.

de Louvois J (1978). The bacteriology and chemotherapy of brain abscess. *J Antimicrob Chemother* **4**: 395.

Demers B, Simor AE, Vellend H *et al.* (1993). Severe invasive Group A streptococcal infections in Ontario, Canada: 1987–1991. *Clin Infect Dis* **16**: 792.

Denning DW, Gill SS (1991). *Neisseria lactamica* meningitis following skull trauma. *Rev Infect Dis* **13**: 216.

Denys GA, Jerris RC, Swenson JM, Thornsberry C (1983). Susceptibility of *Propionibacterium acnes* clinical isolates to 22 antimicrobial agents. *Antimicrob Ag Chemother* **23**: 335.

de Sousa Marques HH, Yamamoto M, Sakane PT *et al.* (1988). Relatively penicillin-resistant pneumococcal meningitis in a Brazilian infant. *Pediatr Infect Dis J* **7**: 433.

de Swarte RD (1982). Penicillin allergy skin tests. *JAMA* **247**: 1745.

Deveikis A, Schauf V, Mizen M, Riff L (1977). Antimicrobial therapy of experimental Group B streptococcal infection in mice. *Antimicrob Ag Chemother* **11**: 817.

Deveridge RJ, Unsworth IP (1973). Gas gangrene. *Med J Aust* **1**: 1106.

Devitt L, Riley I, Hansman D (1977). Human infection caused by penicillin-insensitive pneumococci. *Med J Aust* **1**: 586.

Dewdney JM, Smith H, Wheeler AW (1971). The formation of antigenic polymers in aqueous solutions of β-lactam antibiotics. *Immunology* **21**: 517.

Dickerman JD (1979). Splenectomy and sepsis: a warning. *Pediatrics* **63**: 938.

Dillon HC Jr, Gray E, Pass MA, Gray BM (1982). Anorectal and vaginal carriage of Group B streptococci during pregnancy. *J Infect Dis* **145**: 794.

Dillon HC Jr, Khare S, Gray BM (1987). Group B streptococcal carriage and disease: a 6-year prospective study. *J Pediatr* **110**: 31.

Dillon JR, Pauzé M, Yeung K-H (1983). Spread of penicillinase-producing and transfer plasmids from the gonococcus to *Neisseria meningitidis*. *Lancet* **i**: 799.

Di Nubile MJ (1990). Treatment of endocarditis caused by relatively resistant nonenterococcal streptococci: is penicillin enough? *Rev Infect Dis* **12**: 112.

Dobbins WO III (1995). The diagnosis of Whipple's disease. *New Engl J Med* **332**: 390.

Dobson SRM, Baker CJ (1990). Enterococcal sepsis in neonates: features by age at onset and occurrence of focal infection. *Pediatrics* **85**: 165.

Doganay M, Aydin N (1991). Antimicrobial susceptibility of *Bacillus anthracis*. *Scand J Infect Dis* **23**: 333.

Doganay M, Almac A, Hanagasi R (1986). Primary throat anthrax. *Scand J Infect Dis* **18**: 415.

Donald FE (1990). Treatment of brain abscess. *J Antimicrob Chemother* **25**: 310.

Dougherty TJ (1985). Involvement of a change in penicillin target and peptidoglycan structure in low-level resistance to beta-lactam antibiotics in *Neisseria gonorrhoeae*. *Antimicrob Ag Chemother* **28**: 90.

Dougherty TJ (1986). Genetic analysis and penicillin-binding protein alterations in *Neisseria gonorrhoeae* with chromosomally mediated resistance. *Antimicrob Ag Chemother* **30**: 649.

Dougherty TJ, Koller AE, Tomasz A (1980). Penicillin-binding proteins of penicillin-susceptible and intrinsically resistant *Neisseria gonorrhoeae*. *Antimicrob Ag Chemother* **18**: 730.

Dove AF, Thomas DJB, Aronstam A, Chant RD (1975). Haemolytic anaemia due to penicillin. *Brit Med J* **3**: 684.

Dowling JN, Weyant RS, Pasculle AW (1982). Bactericidal activity of antibiotics against *Legionella micdadei* (Pittsburgh pneumonia agent). *Antimicrob Ag Chemother* **22**: 272.

Downs NJ, Hodges GR, Taylor SA (1987). Mixed bacterial meningitis. *Rev Infect Dis* **9**: 693.

Dowsett EG (1980). Penicillin-resistant gonococci. *Lancet* **ii**: 202.

Dowson CG, Johnson AP, Cercenado E, George RC (1994). Genetics of oxacillin resistance in clinical isolates of *Streptococcus pneumoniae* that are oxacillin resistant and penicillin susceptible. *Antimicrob Ag Chemother* **38**: 49.

Drusano GL (1988). Role of pharmacokinetics in the outcome of infections. *Antimicrob Ag Chemother* **32**: 289.

Ducas J, Robson HG (1981). Cerebrospinal fluid penicillin levels during therapy for latent syphilis. *JAMA* **246**: 2583.

Dunlop EMC, Al-Egaily SS, Houang ET (1979). Penicillin levels in blood and CSF achieved by treatment of syphilis. *JAMA* **241**: 2538.

Dunlop EMC, Al-Egaily SS, Houang ET (1981). Production of treponemicidal concentrations of penicillin in cerebrospinal fluid. *Brit Med J* **283**: 646.

Dunne DW, Quagliarello V (1993). Group B streptococcal meningitis in adults. *Medicine* **72**: 1.

Durack DT (1995). Prevention of infective endocarditis. *New Engl J Med* **332**: 38.

Durack DT, Littler WA (1974). Failure of 'adequate' penicillin therapy to prevent bacterial endocarditis after tooth extraction. *Lancet* **ii**: 846.

Durack DT, Kaplan EL, Bisno AL (1983). Apparent failures of endocarditis prophylaxis Analysis of 52 cases submitted to a National Registry. *JAMA* **250**: 2318.

Durand ML, Calderwood SB, Weber DJ *et al.* (1993). Acute bacterial meningitis in adults. A review of 493 episodes. *New Engl J Med* **328**: 21.

Dylewski J, Wiesenfeld H, Latour A (1989). Postpartum uterine infection with *Clostridium perfringens*. *Rev Infect Dis* **11**: 470.

Dzink J, Bartlett JG (1980). *In vitro* susceptibility of *Clostridium difficile* isolates from patients with antibiotic-associated diarrhea or colitis. *Antimicrob Ag Chemother* **17**: 695.

Easmon CSF (1985). Leading article. Gonococcal resistance to antibiotics. *J Antimicrob Chemother* **16**: 409.

Easmon CSF (1986). The carrier state: Group B streptococcus. *J Antimicrob Chemother* **18** (Suppl A): 59.

Ebert SC, Leggett J, Vogelman B, Craig WA (1988). Evidence for a slow elimination phase for penicillin G. *J Infect Dis* **158**: 200.

Edmiston CE Jr, Gordon RC (1979). Evaluation of gentamicin and penicillin as a synergistic combination in experimental murine listeriosis. *Antimicrob Ag Chemother* **16**: 862.

Eisenberg MS, Bender TR (1976). Botulism in Alaska, 1947 through 1974. *JAMA* **235**: 35.

Eisenstein BI, Lee TJ, Sparling PF (1977). Penicillin sensitivity and serum resistance are independent attributes of strains of *Neisseria gonorrhoeae* causing disseminated gonococcal infection. *Infect Immun* **15**: 834.

Eliopoulos GM, Moellering RC Jr (1982). Antibiotic synergism and antimicrobial combinations in clinical infections. *Rev Infect Dis* **4**: 282.

Elwell LP, Roberts M, Mayer LW, Falkow S (1977). Plasmid-mediated beta-lactamase production in *Neisseria gonorrhoeae*. *Antimicrob Ag Chemother* **11**: 528.

Emmanouilides CE, Kohn OF, Garibaldi R (1994). Leptospirosis complicated by a Jarisch-Herxheimer reaction and adult respiratory distress syndrome: case report. *Clin Infect Dis* **18**: 1004.

Emmons W, Reichwein B, Winslow DL (1991). Rhodococcus equi infection in the patient with AIDS: literature review and report of an unusual case. *Rev Infect Dis* **13**: 91.

Eneroth C-M, Lundberg C, Malmström L, Ramström G (1978). Antibiotic concentrations in saliva of purulent parotitis. *Scand J Infect Dis* **10**: 219.

Enocksson E, Wretlind B, Sterner G, Anzen B (1990). Listeriosis during pregnancy and in neonates. *Scand J Infect Dis* (Suppl 71): 89.

Evans TG, Kamara A, Minnich K *et al.* (1995). Pneumococcal resistance in Southwest Virginia. *Antimicrob Ag Chemother* **39**: 985.

Farber BF, Eliopoulos GM, Ward JI *et al.* (1983a). Multiply resistant viridans streptococci: susceptibility to beta-lactam antibiotics and comparison of penicillin-binding protein patterns. *Antimicrob Ag Chemother* **24**: 702.

Farber BF, Eliopoulos GM, Ward JI *et al.* (1983b). Resistance to penicillin-streptomycin synergy among clinical isolates of viridans streptococci. *Antimicrob Ag Chemother* **24**: 871.

Farber JM, Peterkin PI (1991). *Listeria monocytogenes*, a food-borne pathogen. *Microbiol Rev* **55**: 476.

Farley MM, Harvey RC, Stull T *et al.* (1993). A population-based assessment of invasive disease due to Group B streptococcus in nonpregnant adults. *New Engl J Med* **328**: 1807.

Farmer L, Echlin FA, Loughlin WC *et al.* (1960). Pachymeningitis apparently due to penicillin hypersensitivity. *Ann Intern Med* **52**: 910.

Feder HM Jr, Olsen N, McLaughlin JC *et al.* (1980). Bacterial endocarditis caused by vitamin B6-dependent viridans group streptococcus. *Pediatrics* **66**: 309.

Feigin RD, Moss KS, Shackleford PG (1973). Antibiotic stability in solutions used for intravenous nutrition and fluid therapy. *Pediatrics* **51**: 1016.

Feldman M, Hendler RS, Morrison EB (1980). Acute meningo-encephalitis after withdrawal of antibiotics in Whipple's disease. *Ann Intern Med* **93**: 709.

Fenoll A, Bourgon CM, Muñóz R *et al.* (1991). Serotype distribution and antimicrobial resistance of *Streptococcus pneumoniae* isolates causing systemic infections in Spain, 1979–1989. *Rev Infect Dis* **13**: 56.

Fernández-Guerrero ML, Verdejo C, Azofra J, de Górgolas M (1995). Hospital-acquired infectious endocarditis not associated with cardiac surgery: an emerging problem. *Clin Infect Dis* **20**: 16.

Ferrieri P (1981). Editorial Treatment of Group A streptococcal pharyngitis: reflections on glue and other things. *JAMA* **246**: 1813.

Fife TD, Finegold SM, Grennan T (1991). Pericardial actinomycosis: case report and review. *Rev Infect Dis* **13**: 120.

Finch RG, Aveline A (1984). Group G streptococcal septicaemia: clinical observations and laboratory studies. *J Infect* **9**: 126.

Findling JW, Pohlman GP, Rose HD (1980). Fulminant Gram-negative bacillemia (DF-2). following a dog bite in an asplenic woman. *Amer J Med* **68**: 154.

Finegold SM (1989). Mechanisms of resistance in anaerobes and new developments in testing. *Diagn Microbiol Infect Dis* **12**: 117S.

Fiumara NG (1980). Treatment of primary and secondary syphilis Serologica response. *JAMA* **243**: 2500.

Fiumara NJ (1986). Failure of recommended treatment for secondary syphilis. *JAMA* **256**: 1443.

Fischer G, Horton RE, Edelman R (1983). Summary of the National Institutes of Health Workshop on Group B streptococcal infection. *J Infect Dis* **148**: 163.

Fleming A (1929). On the antibacterial action of cultures of a penicillium with special reference to their use in the isolation of *B influenzae*. *Brit J Exp Path* **10**: 226; quoted by Welch (1954).

Florey ME, Turton EC, Duthrie ES (1946). Penicillin in wound exudates. *Lancet* **ii**: 405.

Fluckiger U, Francioli P, Blaser J *et al.* (1994). Role of amoxicillin serum levels for successful prophylaxis of experimental endocarditis due to tolerant streptococci. *J Infect Dis* **169**: 1397.

Fontana R, Grossato A, Rossi L *et al.* (1985). Transition from resistance to hypersusceptibility to beta-lactam antibiotics associated with loss of a low-affinity penicillin-binding protein in a *Streptococcus faecium* mutant highly resistant to penicillin. *Antimicrob Ag Chemother* **28**: 678.

Fontana R, Boaretti M, Grossato A *et al.* (1990a). Paradoxical response of *Enterococcus faecalis* to the bactericidal activity of penicillin is associated with reduced activity of one autolysin. *Antimicrob Ag Chemother* **34**: 314.

Fontana R, Grossato A, Ligozzi M, Tonin EA (1990b). *In vitro* response to bactericidal activity of cell wall-active antibiotics does not support the general opinion that Enterococci are naturally tolerant to these antibiotics. *Antimicrob Ag Chemother* **34**: 1518.

Fontana R, Amalfitano G, Rossi L, Satta G (1992). Mechanisms of resistance to growth inhibition and killing by beta-lactam antibiotics in enterococci. *Clin Infect Dis* **15**: 486.

Fontana R, Aldegheri M, Ligozzi M *et al.* (1994). Overproduction of a low-affinity penicillin-binding protein and high-level ampicillin resistance in *Enterococcus faecium*. *Antimicrob Ag Chemother* **38**: 1980.

Fontanals D, Pineda V, Pons I, Rojo JC (1989). Penicillin-resistant beta-lactamase producing *Neisseria meningitidis* in Spain. *Eur J Clin Microbiol* **8**: 90.

Foweraker JE, Hawkey PM, Heritage J, Van Landuyt HW (1990). Novel beta-lactamase from *Capnocytophaga* sp. *Antimicrob Ag Chemother* **34**: 1501.

Fraser DW, Wachsmuth IK, Bopp C *et al.* (1978). Antibiotic treatment of guinea-pigs infected with agent of legionnaires' disease. *Lancet* **i**: 175.

Friedland IR, McCracken GH Jr (1994). Management of infections caused by antibiotic-resistant *Streptococcus pneumoniae*. *New Engl J Med* **331**: 377.

Friedland IR, Paris M, Ehrett S *et al.* (1993). Evaluation of antimicrobial regimens for treatment of experimental penicillin- and cephalosporin-resistant pneumococcal meningitis. *Antimicrob Ag Chemother* **37**: 1630.

Friedland JS, Warrell DA (1991). The Jarisch-Herxheimer reaction in leptospirosis: possible pathogenesis and review. *Rev Infect Dis* **13**: 207.

Fu KP, Neu HC (1979). Inactivation of beta-lactam antibiotics by *Legionella pneumophilia*. *Antimicrob Ag Chemother* **16**: 561.

Fujita NK, Lam K, Bayer AS (1982). Septic arthritis due to Group G streptococcus. *JAMA* **247**: 812.

Gabay EL, Rolfe RD, Finegold SM (1981). Susceptibility of *Clostridium septicum* to 23 antimicrobial agents. *Antimicrob Ag Chemother* **20**: 852.

Gallagher PG, Watanakunakorn C (1986). Group B streptococcal endocarditis: report of seven cases and review of the literature, 1962–1985. *Rev Infect Dis* **8**: 175.

Gallagher PG, Watanakunakorn C (1988). *Listeria monocytogenes* endocarditis: a review of the literature 1950–1986. *Scand J Infect Dis* **20**: 359.

Galpin JE, Chow AW, Yoshikawa TT, Guze LB (1974). Pseudoanaphylactic reactions from inadvertent infusion of procaine penicillin G. *Ann Intern Med* **81**: 358.

Garcia-Bustos JF, Dougherty TJ (1987). Alterations in peptidoglycan of *Neisseria gonorrhoeae* induced by sub-MICs of beta-lactam antibiotics. *Antimicrob Ag Chemother* **31**: 178.

Garcia-Leoni ME, Cercenado E, Rodeno P *et al.* (1992). Susceptibility of *Streptococcus pneumoniae* to penicillin: a prospective microbiological and clinical study. *Clin Infect Dis* **14**: 427.

Garland SM, Kelly N (1995). Early-onset neonatal group B streptococcal sepsis: economics of various prevention strategies. *Med J Aust* **162**: 413.

Garratty G, Petz LD (1975). Drug-induced immune hemolytic anemia. *Amer J Med* **58**: 398.

Garrod LP (1960a). Relative antibacterial activity of three penicillins. *Brit Med J* **1**: 527.

Garrod LP (1960b). The relative antibacterial activity of four penicillins. *Brit Med J* **2**: 1695.

Gartner C, Michaels RH (1979). Meningitis from a pneumococcus moderately resistant to penicillin. *JAMA* **241**: 1707.

Gastanaduy AS, Kaplan EL, Huwe BB *et al.* (1980). Failure of penicillin to eradicate Group A streptococci during an outbreak of pharyngitis. *Lancet* **ii**: 498.

Geiseler PJ, Nelson KE, Levin S *et al.* (1980). Community-acquired purulent meningitis: A review of 1316 cases during the antibiotic era, 1954–1976. *Rev Infect Dis* **2**: 725.

Gelfand JA, Elin RJ, Berry FW Jr, Frank MM (1976). Endotoxemia associated with the Jarisch-Herxheimer reaction. *New Engl J Med* **295**: 211.

Gelfand MS, Bakhtian BJ, Simmons BP (1991). Spinal sepsis due to Streptococcus milleri: two cases and review. *Rev Infect Dis* **13**: 559.

Genco CA, Knapp JS, Clark VL (1984). Conjugation of plasmids of *Neisseria gonorrhoeae* to other *Neisseria* species: potential reservoirs for the beta-lactamase plasmid. *J Infect Dis* **150**: 397.

Gengo FM, Mannion TW, Nightingale CH, Schentag JJ (1984). Integration of pharmacokinetics and pharmacodynamics of methicillin in curative treatment of experimental endocarditis. *J Antimicrob Chemother* **14**: 619.

George RC, Uttley AHC (1989). Susceptibility of enterococci and epidemiology of enterococcal infection in the 1980s. *Epidem Inf* **103**: 403.

George WL, Kirby BD, Sutter VL *et al.* (1981). Gram-negative anaerobic bacilli: their role in infection and patterns of susceptibility to antimicrobial agents. II Little-known *Fusobacterium* species and miscellaneous genera. *Rev Infect Dis* **3**: 599.

Georgopapadakou NH (1993). Penicillin-binding proteins and bacterial resistance to beta-lactams. *Antimicrob Ag Chemother* **37**: 2045.

Gephart JF, Washington JA II (1982). Antimicrobial susceptibilities of nutritionally variant streptococci. *J Infect Dis* **146**: 536.

Gerber MA, Markowitz M (1985). Management of streptococcal pharyngitis reconsidered. *Ped Infect Dis* **4**: 518.

Gerding DN, Hall WH, Schierl EA (1977). Antibiotic concentrations in ascitic fluid of patients with ascites and bacterial peritonitis. *Ann Intern Med* **86**: 708.

Geslin P, Buu-Hoi A, Fremaux A, Acar JF (1992). Antimicrobial resistance in *Streptococcus penumoniae*: an epidemiological survey in France, 1970–1990. *Clin Infect Dis* **15**: 95.

Gilbert GL, Garland SM (1983). Perinatal group B streptococcal infections. *Med J Aust* **1**: 566.

Giles AJH (1980). Tabes dorsalis progressing to general paresis after 20 years despite routine penicillin therapy. *Brit J Vener Dis* **56**: 368.

Ginsburg CM, McCracken GH Jr, Zweighaft TC (1982). Serum penicillin concentrations after intramuscular administration of benzathine penicillin G in children. *Pediatrics* **69**: 452.

Godfrey AJ, Bryan LE (1987). Penetration of beta-lactams through *Pseudomonas aeruginosa* porin channels. *Antimicrob Ag Chemother* **31**: 1216.

Godfrey AJ, Bryan LE, Rabin HR (1981). Beta-lactam-resistant *Pseudomonas aeruginosa* with modified penicillin-binding proteins emerging during cystic fibrosis treatment. *Antimicrob Ag Chemother* **19**: 705.

Goldstein EJC (1992). Bite wounds and infection. *Clin Infect Dis* **14**: 633.

Goldstein FW, Garau J (1994). Resistant pneumococci: a renewed threat in respiratory infections. *Scand J Infect Dis* (Suppl 93): 55.

Goodrich JT (1982). Pelvic inflammatory disease: considerations related to therapy. *Rev Infect Dis* **4** (Suppl): 778.

Gorby GL, Peacock JE Jr (1988). *Erysipelothrix rhusiopathiae* endocarditis: microbiologic, epidemiological and clinical features of an occupational disease. *Rev Infect Dis* **10**: 317.

Gordts B, Vanhoof R, Hubrechts JM *et al.* (1982). *In vitro* activity of 21 antimicrobial agents against *Neisseria gonorrhoeae* in Brussels. *Brit J Vener Dis* **58**: 23.

Gossling J (1988). Occurrence and pathogenicity of the *Streptococcus milleri* group. *Rev Infect Dis* **10**: 257.

Gotoff SP, Boyer KM (1981). Penicillin prophylaxis against neonatal streptococcal infections. *New Engl J Med* **304**: 484.

Graham DR, Band JD, Thornsberry C *et al.* (1990). Infections caused by *Moraxella*, *Moraxella urethralis*, *Moraxella*-like groups M-5 and M-6, and *Kingella kingae* in the United States, 1953–1980. *Rev Infect Dis* **12**: 423.

Grahn E, Holm SE, Roos K (1987). Penicillin tolerance in beta-streptococci isolated from patients with tonsillitis. *Scand J Infect Dis* **19**: 421.

Graninger W, Ragette R (1992). Nosocomial bacteremia due to *Enterococcus faecalis* without endocarditis. *Clin Infect Dis* **15**: 49.

Gransden WR, Eykyn SJ (1988). *Erysipelothrix rhusiopathiae* endocarditis. *Rev Infect Dis* **10**: 1228.

Gratten M, Naraqi S, Hansman D (1980). High prevalence of penicillin-insensitive pneumococci in Port Moresby, Papua New Guinea. *Lancet* **ii**: 192.

Grayson ML, Eliopoulos GM, Wennersten CB *et al.* (1991a). Increased resistance to beta-lactam antibiotics among clinical isolates of *Enterococcus faecium*: a 22-year review at one institution. *Antimicrob Ag Chemother* **35**: 2180.

Grayson ML, Eliopoulos GM, Wennersten CB *et al.* (1991b). Comparison of *Enterococcus raffinosus* with *Enterococcus avium* on the basis of penicillin susceptibility penicillin-binding protein analysis and high-level aminoglycoside resistance. *Antimicrob Ag Chemother* **35**: 1408.

Green RL, Lewis JE, Kraus SJ, Frederickson EL (1974). Elevated plasma procaine concentrations after administration of procaine penicillin G. *New Engl J Med* **291**: 223.

Greenwood D, O'Grady F (1973a). Comparison of the responses of *Escherichia coli* and *Proteus mirabilis* to seven beta-lactam antibiotics. *J Infect Dis* **128**: 211.

Greenwood D, O'Grady F (1973b). The two sites of penicillin action in *Escherichia coli*. *J Infect Dis* **128**: 791.

Griffin GE (1992). New insights into the pathophysiology of the Jarisch-Herxheimer reaction. *J Antimicrob Chemother* **29**: 613.

Griffiths JK, Daly JS, Dodge RA (1992). Two cases of endocarditis due to *Lactobacillus* species: antimicrobial susceptibility, review, and discussion of therapy. *Clin Infect Dis* **15**: 250.

Gudiol F, Manresa F, Pallares R *et al.* (1990). Clindamycin vs penicillin for anaerobic lung infections. *Arch Intern Med* **150**: 2525.

Guerrero MLF, Arbol F, Verdejo C *et al.* (1994). Treatment of experimental endocarditis due to penicillin-resistant *Streptococcus pneumoniae*. *Antimicrob Ag Chemother* **38**: 1103.

Guiot HFL, Corel LJA, Vossen JMJJ (1994). Prevalence of penicillin-resistant-viridans streptococci in healthy children and in patients with malignant haematological disorders. *Eur J Clin Microbiol Infect Dis* **13**: 645.

Gullberg RM, Homann SR, Phair JP (1989). Enterococcal bacteremia: analysis of 75 episodes. *Rev Infect Dis* **11**: 74.

Gunzenhauser JD, Brundage JF, McNeil JG, Miller RN (1992). Broad and persistent effects of benzathine penicillin G in the prevention of febrile, acute respiratory disease. *J Infect Dis* **166**: 365.

Gür D, Tanckanat F, Sener B *et al.* (1994). Penicillin resistance in *Streptococcus pneumoniae* in Turkey. *Eur J Clin Microbiol Infect Dis* **13**: 440.

Gutmann L, Tomasz A (1982). Penicillin-resistant and penicillin-tolerant mutants of Group A streptococci. *Antimicrob Ag Chemother* **22**: 128.

Gutmann L, Goldstein FW, Kitzis MD *et al.* (1983). Susceptibility of *Nocardia asteroides* to 46 antibiotics, including 22 beta-lactams. *Antimicrob Ag Chemother* **23**: 248.

Haglund LA, Istre GR, Pickett DA *et al.* (1993). Invasive pneumococcal disease in central Oklahoma: emergence of high-level penicillin resistance and multiple antibiotic resistance. *J Infect Dis* **168**: 1532.

Hakenbeck R, Briese T, Chalkley L *et al.* (1991a). Variability of penicillin-binding proteins from penicillin-sensitive *Streptococcus pneumoniae*. *J Infect Dis* **164**: 307.

Hakenbeck R, Briese T, Chalkley L *et al.* (1991b). Antigenic variation of penicillin-binding proteins from penicillin-resistant clinical strains of *Steptococcus pneumoniae*. *J Infect Dis* **164**: 313.

Hall G, Hedström SÅ, Hermdahl A, Nord CE (1993). Prophylactic administration of penicillins for endocarditis does not reduce the incidence of postextraction bacteremia. *Clin Infect Dis* **17**: 188.

Hallett AF, Appelbaum PC, Cooper R *et al.* (1977). Penicillinase-producing *Neisseria gonorrhoeae* from South Africa. *Lancet* **i**: 1205.

Halperin JJ (1989). Abnormalities of the nervous system in Lyme disease: response to antimicrobial therapy. *Rev Infect Dis* **11** (Suppl 6): 1499.

Halstensen A, Vollset SE, Haneberg B *et al.* (1987a). Antimicrobial therapy and case fatality in meningococcal disease. *Scand J Infect Dis* **19**: 403.

Halstensen A, Pedersen SHJ, Haneberg B *et al.* (1987b). Case fatality of meningococcal disease in Western Norway. *Scand J Infect Dis* **19**: 35.

Hamoudi AC, Hamoudi AB (1981). Fatal Group B streptococcal pneumonia in neonates: effects of antibiotics. *Amer J Clin Path* **76**: 823.

Hancock REW (1986). Intrinsic antibiotic resistance of *Pseudomonas aeruginosa*. *J Antimicrob Chemother* **18**: 653.

Hancock REW, Woodruff WA (1988). Roles of porin and beta-lactamase in beta-lactam resistance of *Pseudomonas aeruginosa*. *Rev Infect Dis* **10**: 770.

Hand WL, King-Thompson NL (1990). Uptake of antibiotics by human polymorphonuclear leukocyte cytoplasts. *Antimicrob Ag Chemother* **34**: 1189.

Handsfield HH, Wiesner PJ, Holmes KK (1976). Treatment of the gonococcal arthritis-dermatitis syndrome. *Ann Intern Med* **84**: 661.

Handsfield HH, Sandström EG, Knapp JS *et al.* (1982). Epidemiology of penicillinase-producing *Neisseria gonorrhoeae* infections Analysis by auxotyping and serogrouping. *New Engl J Med* **306**: 950.

Handsfield HH, Rice RJ, Roberts MC, Holmes KK (1989). Localized outbreak of penicillinase-producing *Neisseria gonorrhoeae*. Paradigm for introduction and spread of gonorrhea in a community. *JAMA* **261**: 2357.

Handwerger S, Tomasz A (1985). Antibiotic tolerance among clinical isolates of bacteria. *Rev Infect Dis* **7**: 368.

Handwerger S, Tomasz A (1986a). Alterations in kinetic properties of penicillin-binding proteins of penicillin-resistant *Streptococcus pneumoniae*. *Antimicrob Ag Chemother* **30**: 57.

Handwerger S, Tomasz A (1986b). Alterations in penicillin-binding proteins of clinical and laboratory isolates of pathogenic *Streptococcus pneumoniae* with low levels of penicillin resistance. *J Infect Dis* **153**: 83.

Handwerger S, Horowitz H, Coburn K *et al.* (1990). Infection due to *Leuconostoc* species: six cases and review. *Rev Infect Dis* **12**: 602.

Handwerger S, Perlman DC, Altarac D, McAuliffe V (1992). Concomitant high-level vancomycin and penicillin resistance in clinical isolates of enterococci. *Clin Infect Dis* **14**: 655.

Handwerger S, Raucher B, Altarac D *et al.* (1993). Nosocomial outbreak due to *Enterococcus faecium* highly resistant to vancomycin, penicillin, and gentamicin. *Clin Infect Dis* **16**: 750.

Hannedouche T, Fillastre JP (1987). Penicillin-induced hypersensitivity vasculitides. *J Antimicrob Chemother* **20**: 3.

Hansman D (1976). Penicillin-insensitive pneumococci and pneumococcal infections. *Med J Aust* **1**: 132.

Hansman D, Glasgow H, Sturt J *et al.* (1971). Increased resistance to penicillin of pneumococci isolated from man. *New Engl J Med* **284**: 175.

Hansman D, Devitt L, Miles H, Riley I (1974). Pneumococci relatively insensitive to penicillin in Australia and New Guinea. *Med J Aust* **2**: 353.

Hare R (1970). *The Birth of Penicillin and the Disarming of Microbes*. London: George Allen and Unwin.

Harris ED Jr (1983). Lyme disease – success for academia and the community. *New Engl J Med* **308**: 773.

Hart CA, Rogers TRF (1993). Meningococcal disease. *J Med Microbiol* **39**: 3.

Hartmann R, Höltje J, Schwarz U (1972). Targets of penicillin action in Escherichia coli. *Nature* **235**: 426.

Hawkins RE, Moriarty RA, Lewis DE, Oldfield EC (1991). Serious infections involving the CDC group Ve bacteria *Chryseomonas luteola* and *Flavimonas oryzihabitans*. *Rev Infect Dis* **13**: 257.

Heggie AD, Jacobs MR, Linz PE *et al.* (1992). Prevalence and characteristics of pharyngeal Group A beta-hemolytic streptococci in US navy recruits receiving benzathine penicillin prophylaxis. *J Infect Dis* **166**: 1006.

Heiddal S, Sverrisson JT, Yngvason FE *et al.* (1993). Native-valve endocarditis due to *Neisseria sicca*: case report and review. *Clin Infect Dis* **16**: 667.

Helling DK, Jones ME, Masjanovich JJ, Massad S (1980). Antibiotic sensitivity of penicillin-resistant *Staphylococcus aureus* in three midwestern family practice populations. *Drug Intell Clin Pharm* **14**: 851.

Hemsell DL, Little BB, Faro S *et al.* (1994). Comparison of three regimens recommended by the Centers for Disease Control and Prevention for the treatment of women hospitalized with acute pelvic inflammatory disease. *Clin Infect Dis* **19**: 720.

Henderson FW, Gilligan PH, Wait K, Goff DA (1988). Nasopharyngeal carriage of antibiotic-resistant pneumococci in children in group day care. *J Infect Dis* **157**: 256.

Henwick S, Koehler M, Patrick CC (1993). Complications of bacteremia due to *Stomatococcus mucaliginosus* in neutropenic patients. *Clin Infect Dis* **17**: 667.

Herchline TE, Barnishan J, Ayers LW, Fass RJ (1990). Penicillinase production and *in vitro* susceptibilities of *Staphylococcus lugdunensis*. *Antimicrob Ag Chemother* **34**: 2434.

Herman DJ, Gerding DN (1991). Antimicrobial resistance among enter-

ococci. *Antimicrob Ag Chemother* **35**: 1.

Herztein J, Ryan JL, Mangi RJ *et al.* (1984). Optimal therapy for enterococcal endocarditis. *Amer J Med* **76**: 186.

Hess J, Holloway Y, Dankert J (1983a). Penicillin prophylaxis in children with cardiac disease: postextraction bacteremia and penicillin-resistant strains of viridans streptococci. *J Infect Dis* **147**: 133.

Hess J, Dankert J, Durack D (1983b). Significance of penicillin tolerance *in vivo*: prevention of experimental *Streptococcus sanguis* endocarditis. *J Antimicrob Chemother* **11**: 555.

Hieber JP, Nelson JD (1977). A pharmacologic evaluation of penicillin in children with purulent meningitis. *New Engl J Med* **297**: 410.

Hodges TL, Zighelboim-Daum S, Eliopoulos GH *et al.* (1992). Antimicrobial susceptibility changes in *Enterococcus faecalis* following various penicillin exposure regimens. *Antimicrob Ag Chemother* **36**: 121.

Hoge CW, Schwartz B, Talkington DF *et al.* (1993). The changing epidemiology of invasive Group A streptococcal infections and the emergence of streptococcal toxic shock-like syndrome. *JAMA* **269**: 384.

Holgate ST (1988). Penicillin allergy: how to diagnose and when to treat. *Brit Med J* **296**: 1213.

Holloway Y, Dankert J (1982). Penicillin tolerance of nutritionally variant streptococci. *Antimicrob Ag Chemother* **22**: 1073.

Holmberg H (1987). Aetiology of community-acquired pneumonia in hospital treated patients. *Scand J Infect Dis* **19**: 491.

Holmberg K, Nord CE, Dornbusch K (1977). Antimicrobial *in vitro* susceptibility of *Actinomyces israelii* and *Archnia propionica*. *Scand J Infect Dis* **9**: 40.

Hoogkamp-Korstanje JAA, Gerards LJ, Cats BP (1982). Maternal carriage and neonatal acquisition of Group B streptococci. *J Infect Dis* **145**: 800.

Hook EW, Homes KK (1985). Gonococcal infections. *Ann Intern Med* **102**: 229.

Hook EWIII (1989a). Syphilis and HIV infection. *J Infect Dis* **160**: 530.

Hook EWIII (1989b). Treatment of syphilis: current recommendations, alternatives, and continuing problems. *Rev Infect Dis* **11** (Suppl 6): 1511.

Hook EWIII (1994). Editorial response: diagnosing neurosyphilis. *Clin Infect Dis* **18**: 295.

Horne D, Tomasz A (1977). Tolerant response of *Streptococcus sanguis* to beta-lactams and other cell wall inhibitors. *Antimicrob Ag Chemother* **11**: 888.

Horne D, Tomasz A (1980). Lethal effect of a heterologous murein hydrolase on penicillin-treated *Streptococcus sanguis*. *Antimicrob Ag Chemother* **17**: 235.

Horne D, Tomasz A (1981). pH Dependent penicillin tolerance of Group B streptococci. *Antimicrob Ag Chemother* **20**: 128.

Horowitz HW, Sanghera K, Goldberg N *et al.* (1994). Dermatomyositis associated with Lyme disease: case report and review of Lyme myositis. *Clin Infect Dis* **18**: 166.

Horowitz L (1975). Atopy as factor in penicillin reactions. *New Engl J Med* **292**: 1243.

Hortal M, Palacio R, Camou T, Mogdasy C (1994). Antimicrobial resistance in *Streptococcus pneumoniae* strains from Uruguay. *Pediatr Infect Dis J* **13**: 542.

Howes VJ, Mitchell RG (1976). Meningitis due to relatively penicillin-resistant pneumococcus. *Brit Med J* **1**: 996.

Hryniewicz W (1994). Bacterial resistance in Eastern Europe – selected problems. *Scand J Infect Dis* (Suppl 93): 33.

Hulbert J (1972). Gram-negative urinary infection treated with oral penicillin G. *Lancet* **ii**: 1216.

Hutchinson CM, Hook EW III, Shepherd M *et al.* (1994). Altered clinical presentation of early syphilis in patients with human immunodeficiency virus infection. *Ann Intern Med* **121**: 94.

Idsøe O, Guthe T, Willcox RR, de Weck AL (1968). Nature and extent of penicillin side-reactions, with particular reference to fatalities from anaphylactic shock. *Bull Wld Hlth Org* **38**: 159.

Idsøe O, Guthe T, Willcox RR (1972). Penicillin in the treatment of syphilis. The experience of three decades. *Bull Wld Hlth Org* **47** (Suppl): 1.

Imperiale TF (1990). Does prophylaxis prevent postdental infective endocarditis? A controlled evaluation of protective efficacy. *Amer J Med* **88**: 131.

Ingram RJH, Cornere B, Ellis-Pegler RB (1992). Endocarditis due to *Neisseria mucosa*: two case reports and review *Clin Infect Dis* **15**: 321.

International Rheumatic Fever Study Group (1991). Allergic reactions to long-term benzathine penicillin prophylaxis for rheumatic fever. *Lancet* **337**: 1308.

Iralu JV, Roberts D, Kazanjian PH (1993). Chorioamnionitis caused by *Capnocytophaga*: case report and review. *Clin Infect Dis* **17**: 457.

Isaac DW, Pearson TA, Hurwitz CA, Patrick CC (1993). Clinical and microbiologic aspects of *Staphylococcus haemolyticus* infections. *Pediatr Infect Dis J* **12**: 1018.

Isaacs RD, Howden CW, Lang WR, Ellis-Pegler RB (1988). Short course chemotherapy for meningococcal meningitis. *Aust NZ J Med* **18**: 731.

Isaacs RD, Barfield CP, Grimwood K *et al.* (1995). Systemic bacterial and fungal infections in infants in Australian neonatal units. *Med J Aust* **162**: 198.

Ison CA, Gedney J, Harris JRW, Easmon CSF (1986). Penicillinase producing gonococci: a spent force? *Genitourin Med* **62**: 302.

Ison CA, Gedney J, Easmon CSF (1987). Chromosomal resistance of gonococci to antibiotics. *Genitourin Med* **63**: 239.

Istre GR, Tarpay M, Anderson M *et al.* (1987). Invasive disease due to *Streptococcus pneumoniae* in an area with a high rate of relative penicillin resistance. *J Infect Dis* **156**: 732.

Jabes D, Nachman S, Tomasz A (1989). Penicillin binding protein families: evidence for the clonal nature of penicillin resistance in clinical isolates of pneumococci. *J Infect Dis* **159**: 16.

Jackson FN, Jaffe JP (1979). Fatal penicillin-induced hemolytic anemia. *JAMA* **242**: 2286.

Jackson LA, Tenover FC, Baker C *et al.* (1994). Prevalence of *Neisseria meningitidis* relatively resistant to penicillin in the United States, 1991. *J Infect Dis* **169**: 438.

Jackson MA, Burry VF, Olson LC (1991). Multisystem Group A beta-hemolytic streptococcal disease in children. *Rev Infect Dis* **13**: 783.

Jacobs J, Garmyn K, Verhaegen J *et al.* (1990). Neonatal sepsis due to *Streptococcus pneumoniae*. *Scand J Infect Dis* **22**: 493.

Jacobs JA, Pietersen HG, Stobberingh EE, Soeters PB (1994). Bacteremia involving the 'Streptococcus milleri' Group: analysis of 19 cases. *Clin Infect Dis* **19**: 704.

Jacobs MR (1992). Treatment and diagnosis of infections caused by drug-resistant *Streptococcus pneumoniae*. *Clin Infect Dis* **15**: 119.

Jacobs MR, Koornhof HJ (1978). Multiple-antibiotic resistance – now the pneumococcus. *J Antimicrob Chemother* **4**: 481.

Jacobs MR, Gaspar MN, Robins-Browne RM, Koornhof HJ (1980). Antimicrobial susceptibility testing of pneumococci. *J Antimicrob Chemother* **6**: 53.

Jacoby GA (1994). Prevalence and resistance mechanisms of common bacterial respiratory pathogens. *Clin Infect Dis* **18**: 951.

Jaffe A, Chabbert YA, Semonin O (1982). Role of porin proteins Omp F and Omp C in the permeation of beta-lactams. *Antimicrob Ag Chemother* **22**: 942.

Jaffe HW, Kabins SA (1982). Examination of cerebrospinal fluid in patients with syphilis. *Rev Infect Dis* **4** (Suppl): 842.

Jagdis F (1988). Group A streptococcal meningitis and brain abscess. *Pediatr Infect Dis J* **7**: 885.

Jain AK, Agarwal SK, El-Sadr W (1994). *Streptococcus bowis* bacteremia and meningitis associated with *Strongyloides stercoralis* colitis in a patient infected with human immunodeficiency virus. *Clin Infect Dis* **18**: 253.

James PA (1990). Comparison of four methods for the determination of MIC and MBC of penicillin for viridans streptococci and the implications for penicillin tolerance. *J Antimicrob Chemother* **25**: 209.

Jensen A, Frederiksen W, Gerner-Smidt P (1994). Risk factors for listeriosis in Denmark, 1989–1990. *Scand J Infect Dis* **26**: 171.

Jephcott AE (1986). Epidemiology of resistance in *Neisseria gonorrhoeae*. *J Antimicrob Chemother* **18** (Suppl C): 199.

Jernigan DB, Cetron MS, Breiman RF (1996). Minimizing the impact of drug-resistant *Streptococcus pneumoniae* (DRSP). *JAMA* **275**: 206.

Jevon GP, Dunne WM Jr, Hawkins HK *et al.* (1994). Fatal Group A streptococcal meningitis and toxic shock-like syndrome: case report. *Clin Infect Dis* **18**: 91.

John AB, Ramlal A, Jackson H *et al.* (1984). Prevention of pneumococcal infection in children with homozygous sickle cell disease. *Brit Med J* **288**: 1567.

Johnson FWA, Hobson D (1977). The effect of penicillin on genital strains of *Chlamydia trachomatis* in tissue culture. *J Antimicrob Chemother* **3**: 49.

Johnson, RC (1989). Isolation techniques for spirochetes and their sensitivity to antibiotics *in vitro* and *in vivo*. *Rev Infect Dis* **11** (Suppl 6): 1505.

Johnson, RC, Kodner C, Russell M (1987). *In vitro* and *in vivo* susceptibility of the Lyme disease spirochete *Borrelia burgdorferi* to four antimicrobial agents. *Antimicrob Ag Chemother* **31**: 164.

Johnson RH, Rumans LW (1977). Unusual infections caused by *Pasteurella multocida*. *JAMA* **237**: 146.

Joorabchi B, Kohout E (1973). Apparent penicillin-induced arrest of mature bone marrow element. *Brit Med J* **2**: 26.

Jorgensen JH, Doern GV, Maher LA *et al.* (1990). Antimicrobial resistance among respiratory isolates of *Haemophilus influenzae*, *Moraxella catarrhalis*, and *Streptococcus pneumoniae* in the United States. *Antimicrob Ag Chemother* **34**: 2075.

Joshi N, O'Bryan T, Appelbaum PC (1991). Pleuropulmonary infections caused by *Eikenella corrodens*. *Rev Infect Dis* **13**: 1207.

Jurado RL, Farley MM, Pereira E *et al.* (1993). Increased risk of meningitis and bacteremia due to *Listeria monocytogenes* in patients with human immunodeficiency virus infection. *Clin Infect Dis* **17**: 224.

Kalb R, Kaplan MH, Tenenbaum MJ *et al.* (1985). Cutaneous infection at dog bite wounds associated with fulminant DF-2 septicemia. *Amer J Med* **78**: 687.

Kales CP, Holzman RS (1990). Listeriosis in patients with HIV infectin: clinical manifestations and response to therapy. *J AIDS* **3**: 139.

Kalish SB, Sands ML (1983). *Pasteurella multocida* infection of a prosthetic vascular graft. *JAMA* **249**: 514.

Kaplan EL (1980). The Group A streptococcal upper respiratory tract carrier stage: an enigma. *J Pediatr* **97**: 337.

Kaplan EL (1985). Benzathine penicillin G for treatment of Group A streptococcal pharyngitis: a reappraisal in 1985. *Ped Infect Dis* **4**: 592.

Kaplan EL, Berrios X, Speth J *et al.* (1989a). Pharmacokinetics of benzathine penicillin G: serum levels during the 28 days after intramuscular injection of 1 200 000 units. *J Pediatr* **115**: 146.

Kaplan AH, Weber DJ, Oddone EZ, Perfect JR (1989b). Infection due to *Actinobacillus actinomycetemcomitans*: 15 cases and review. *Rev Infect Dis* **11**: 46.

Kaplan JM, McCracken GH Jr (1973). Clinical pharmacology of benzathine penicillin G in neonates with regard to its recommended use in congenital syphilis. *J Pediatr* **82**: 1069.

Kaplan MH, Tenenbaum MJ (1982). *Staphylococcus aureus*: cellular biology and clinical application. *Amer J Med* **72**: 248.

Karchmer AW (1988). Antibiotic therapy for nonenterococcal streptococcal and staphylococcal endocarditis: current regimens and some future considerations. *J Antimicrob Chemother* **21** (Suppl C): 91.

Karmali MA, De Grandis S, Fleming PC (1981). Antimicrobial susceptibility of *Campylobacter jejuni* with special reference to resistance patterns of Canadian isolates. *Antimicrob Ag Chemother* **19**: 593.

Kasik JE, Monick M, Schwarz B (1980). Beta-lactamase activity in slow-growing nonpigmented mycobacteria and their sensitivity to certain beta-lactam antibiotics. *Tubercle* **61**: 213.

Kastner RJ, Malone JL, Decker CF (1994). Syphilitic osteitis in a patient with secondary syphilis and concurrent human immunodeficiency virus infection. *Clin Infect Dis* **18**: 250.

Kaye D (1980). Antibiotic treatment of streptococcal endocarditis. *Amer J Med* **69**: 650.

Keinath RD, Merrell DE, Vlietstra R, Dobbins WO III (1985). Antibiotic treatment of relapse in Whipple's disease. Long-term follow-up of 88 patients. *Gastroenterology* **88**: 1867.

Kennedy ND, Pusey CD, Rainford DJ, Higginson A (1979). Leptospirosis and acute renal failure – clinical experiences and a review of the literature. *Postgrad Med J* **55**: 176.

Kent SJ, Van Scoy MS, Skerrett S (1994). *Listeria monocytogenes* peritonitis with review of literature. *Aust NZ J Med* **24**: 405.

Kerbs SB, Stone JR Jr, Berg SW, Harrison WO (1983). *In vitro* antimicrobial activity of eight new beta-lactam antibiotics against penicillin-resistant *Neisseria gonorrhoeae*. *Antimicrob Ag Chemother* **23**: 541.

Kerr RO, Cardamone J, Dalmasso AP, Kaplan ME (1972). Two mechanisms of erythrocyte destruction in penicillin-induced hemolytic anemia. *New Engl J Med* **287**: 1322.

Kessler RE, Van de Rijn I (1981). Effect of penicillin on Group A streptococcus: loss of viability appears to precede stimulation of release of lipoteichoic acid. *Antimicrob Ag Chemother* **19**: 39.

Khan MY, Siddiqui Y, Simpson ML, Gruninger RP (1981). Comparative *in vitro* activity of cefmenoxime, cefotaxime, cefuroxime, cefoxitin, and penicillin against *Neisseria gonorrhoeae*. *Antimicrob Ag Chemother* **20**: 681.

Kim KS (1987). Effect of antimicrobial therapy for experimental infections due to Group B streptococcus on mortality and clearance of bacteria. *J Infect Dis* **155**: 1233.

Kim KS (1988). Clinical perspectives on penicillin tolerance. *J Pediatrics* **112**: 509.

Kim KS, Anthony BF (1981). Penicillin tolerance in Group B streptococci isolated from infected neonates. *J Infect Dis* **144**: 411.

Kim KS, Kaplan EL (1985). Association of penicillin tolerance with failure to eradicate group A streptococci from patients with pharyngitis. *J Pediatrics* **107**: 681.

Kirby BD, George WL, Sutter VL *et al.* (1980). Gram-negative anaerobic bacilli: their role in infection and patterns of susceptibility of antimicrobial agents. I Little-known *Bacteroides* species. *Rev Infect Dis* **2**: 914.

Kirven LA, Thornsberry C (1977). Transfer of beta-lactamase genes of *Neisseria gonorrhoeae* by conjugation. *Antimicrob Ag Chemother* **11**: 1004.

Kitano K, Tomasz A (1979). Triggering of autolytic cell wall degradation in *Escherichia coli* by beta-lactam antibiotics. *Antimicrob Ag Chemother* **16**: 838.

Klare I, Rodloff AC, Wagner J *et al.* (1992). Overproduction of penicillin-binding protein is not the only mechanism of penicillin resistance in *Enterococcus faecium*. *Antimicrob Ag Chemother* **36**: 783.

Klein JO, Schaberg MJ, Buntin M, Gezon HM (1973). Levels of penicillin in serum of newborn infants after single intramuscular doses of benzathine penicillin G. *J Pediatr* **82**: 1065.

Kluge RM (1990). Listeriosis-problems and therapeutic options. *J Antimicrob Chemother* **25**: 887.

Klugman KP (1994). Management of antibiotic-resistant pneumococcal infections. *J Antimicrob Chemother* **34**: 191.

Klugman KP, Koornhof HJ (1988). Drug resistance patterns and serogroups or serotypes of pneumococcal isolates, from cerebrospinal fluid or blood, 1979–1986. *J Infect Dis* **158**: 956.

Knox R (1960). A new penicillin (BRL 1241). active against penicillin-resistant staphylococci. *Brit Med J* **2**: 690.

Koch AL (1988). Biophysics of bacterial walls viewed as stress-bearing fabric. *Microbiol Rev* **52**: 337.

Koornhof HJ, Wasas A, Klugman K (1992). Antimicrobial resistance in *Streptococcus pneumoniae*: a South African perspective. *Clin Infect Dis* **15**: 84.

Kornguth ML, Kunin CM (1976). Uptake of antibiotics by human erythrocytes. *J Infect Dis* **133**: 175.

Koshiro A, Fujita T (1983). Interaction of penicillins with the components of plasma expanders. *Drug Intell Clin Pharm* **17**: 351.

Kourtópoulos H, Holm SE, Norrby SR (1983a). The influence of steroids on the penetration of antibiotics into brain tissue and brain abscess. An experimental study in rats. *J Antimicrob Chemother* **11**: 245.

Kourtópoulos H, Holm SE, Norrby SR (1983b). The effects of irradiation and probenecid on cerebrospinal fluid transport of penicillin. *J Antimicrob Chemother* **11**: 251.

Krause KL, Stager C, Gentry LO (1982). Prevalence of penicillin-resistant pneumococci in Houston, Texas. *Amer J Clin Pathol* **77**: 210.

Krogstad DJ, Parquette AR (1980). Defective killing of enterococci: a common property of antimicrobial agents acting on the cell wall. *Antimicrob Ag Chemother* **17**: 965.

Kumar A, Devlin HR, Vellend H (1990). *Pasteurella multocida* meningitis in an adult: case report and review. *Rev Infect Dis* **12**: 440.

Kunin CM (1967). A guide to use of antibiotics in patients with renal disease. *Ann Intern Med* **67**: 151.

Lachance N, Gaudreau C, Lamothe F, Turgeon F (1993). Susceptibilities of beta-lactamase-positive and -negative strains of *Campylobacter coli* to beta-lactam agents. *Antimicrob Ag Chemother* **37**: 1174.

Lacroix J-M, Walker C (1991). Characterization of a beta-lactamase found in *Eikenella corrodens*. *Antimicrob Ag Chemother* **35**: 886.

La Force FM (1994). Anthrax. *Clin Infect Dis* **19**: 1009.

Lam K, Bayer AS (1984). *In vitro* bactericidal synergy of gentamicin combined with penicillin G., vancomycin, or cefotaxime against Group G streptococci. *Antimicrob Ag Chemother* **26**: 260.

Lam S, Samray J, Rahman S, Hilton E (1993). Primary actinomycotic endocarditis: case report and review. *Clin Infect Dis* **16**: 481.

Landesman SH, Cummings M, Gruarin A, Bernheimer H (1981). Susceptibility of multiply antibiotic-resistant pneumococci to the new beta-lactam drugs and rosaramicin. *Antimicrob Ag Chemother* **19**: 675.

Landman D, Mobarakai NK, Quale JM (1993). Novel antibiotic regimens against *Enterococcus faecium* resistant to ampicillin, vancomycin, and gentamicin. *Antimicrob Ag Chemother* **37**: 1904.

Lane GK, Oates RK (1988). Congenital syphilis has not disappeared. *Med J Aust* **148**: 171.

Larsson S, Walder MH, Cronberg SN *et al.* (1985). Antimicrobial susceptibilities of *Listeria monocytogenes* strains isolated from 1958 to 1982 in Sweden. *Antimicrob Ag Chemother* **28**: 12.

Latorre C, Juncosa T, Sanfeliu I (1985). Antibiotic resistance and serotypes of 100 *Streptococcus pneumoniae* strains isolated in a children's hospital in Barcelona, Spain. *Antimicrob Ag Chemother* **28**: 357.

Lauer BA, Reller LB (1980). Serotypes and penicillin susceptibility of pneumococci isolated from blood. *J Clin Microbiol* **11**: 242.

Leading Article (1975). Drug interactions. *Lancet* **i**: 904.

Leading Article (1979). Neonatal bacteraemia: diagnosis and management. *Brit Med J* **ii**: 1385.

Leading Article (1981). Treatment of anaphylactic shock. *Brit Med J* **282**: 1011.

Lebedeff DA, Hochman EB (1980). Rectal gonorrhea in men: diagnosis and treatment. *Ann Intern Med* **92**: 463.

Lee EL, Robinson MJ, Thong ML *et al.* (1977). Intraventricular chemotherapy in neonatal meningitis. *J Pediatr* **91**: 991.

Leff RD, Roberts RJ (1981). Methods for intravenous drug administration in the pediatric patient. *J Pediatr* **98**: 631.

Leftik MI, Miller JW, Brown JD (1978). Penicillin-resistant gonococcal polyarthritis. *JAMA* **239**: 134.

Leggiadro RJ, David Y, Tenover FC (1994). Outpatient drug-resistant pneumococcal bacteremia. *Pediatr Infect Dis J* **13**: 1144.

Lehmann V, Knutsen SB, Ragnhildstveit E *et al.* (1977). Endocarditis caused by *Pasteurella multocida*. *Scand J Infect Dis* **9**: 247.

Lerner PI, Smith H, Weinstein L (1967). Penicillin neurotoxicity. *Ann NY Acad Sci* **145**: 310.

Leung R, Jassal J (1994). *Pasteurella* epiglottitis. *Aust NZ J Med* **24**: 218.

Levett PN (1988). Antimicrobial susceptibility of *Clostridium difficile* determined by disc diffusion and breakpoint methods. *J Antimicrob Chemother* **22**: 167.

Levine BB (1972). Editorial. Skin rashes with penicillin therapy: current management. *New Engl J Med* **286**: 42.

Levine BB, Zolov DM (1969). Prediction of penicillin allergy by immunological tests. *J Allergy* **43**: 231.

Levison ME, Mangura CT, Lorber B *et al.* (1983). Clindamycin compared with penicillin for the treatment of anaerobic lung abscess. *Ann Intern Med* **98**: 466.

Lewis MAO, McFarlane TW, McGowan DA (1989). Antibiotic susceptibilities of bacteria isolated from acute dentoalveolar abscesses. *J Antimicrob Chemother* **23**: 69.

Li X-Z, Ma D, Livermore DM, Nikaido H (1994). Role of efflux pump(s). in intrinsic resistance of *Pseudomonas aeruginosa*: active efflux as a contributing factor to beta-lactam resistance. *Antimicrob Ag Chemother* **38**: 1742.

Libertin CR, Hermans PE, Washington JA II (1985). Beta-hemolytic Group F streptococcal bacteremia: a study and review of the literature. *Rev Infect Dis* **7**: 498.

Liebowitz LD, Ballard RC, Koornhof HJ (1982). *In vitro* susceptibility and cross-resistance of South African isolates of *Neisseria gonorrhoeae* to 14 antimicrobial agents. *Antimicrob Ag Chemother* **22**: 598.

Liñares J, Garau J, Domînguez C, Perez JL (1983). Antibiotic resistance and serotypes of *Streptococcus pneumoniae* from patients with community-acquired pneumococcal disease. *Antimicrob Ag Chemother* **23**: 545.

Liñares J, Pallares R, Alonso T *et al.* (1992). Trends in antimicrobial resistance in clinical isolates of *Streptococcus pneumoniae* in Bellvitge hospital, Barcelona, Spain (1979–1990). *Clin Infect Dis* **15**: 99.

Lin RY (1992). A perspective on penicillin allergy. *Arch Intern Med* **152**: 930.

Lind I (1990). Epidemiology of antibiotic resistant *Neisseria gonorrhoeae* in industrialized and developing countries. *Scand J Infect Dis* (Suppl 69): 77.

Lindon M, Handke G (1976). Penicillinase-producing *Neisseria gonorrhoeae* in Adelaide. *Med J Aust* **2**: 660.

Lipsky BA, Goldberger AC, Tompkins LS, Plorde JJ (1982). Infections caused by nondiphtheria *Corynebacteria*. *Rev Infect Dis* **4**: 1220.

Little WA, Thomson LA, Bowen WH (1979). Antibiotic susceptibility of *Streptococcus mutans*: comparison of serotype profiles. *Antimicrob Ag Chemother* **15**: 440.

Liu HH, Tomasz A (1985). Penicillin tolerance in multiply drug-resistant natural isolates of *Streptococcus pneumoniae*. *J Infect Dis* **152**: 365.

Livermore DM (1987). Radiolabelling of penicillin-binding proteins (PBPs). in intact *Pseudomonas aeruginosa* cells: consequences of beta-lactamase activity by PBP-5. *J Antimicrob Chemother* **19**: 733.

Livermore DM (1988). Permeation of beta lactam antibiotics into *Escherichia coli*, *Pseudomonas aeruginosa*, and other Gram-negative bacteria. *Rev Infect Dis* **10**: 691.

Ljungberg B, Nilsson-Ehle I (1987). Pharmacokinetics of antimicrobial agents in the elderly. *Rev Infect Dis* **9**: 250.

Lode H (1986). Initial therapy of pneumonia. Clinical, radiographic, and laboratory data important for the choice. *Amer J Med* **80** (5C): 70.

Lode H (1988). Microbiological and clinical aspects of aspiration pneumonia. *J Antimicrob Chemother* **21** (Suppl C): 83.

Lopardo HA, Santander C, Ceinos M, Rubeglio EA (1993). Isolation of moderately penicillin-susceptible strains of *Neisseria meningitidis* in Argentina. *Antimicrob Ag Chemother* **37**: 1728.

Lorian V (1975). Some effects of subinhibitory concentrations of penicillin on the structure and division of staphylococci. *Antimicrob Ag Chemother* **7**: 864.

Lorian V, Atkinson B (1984). Bactericidal effect of polymorphonuclear neutrophils on antibiotic-induced filaments of Gram-negative bacilli. *J Infect Dis* **149**: 719.

Love JW, Medina D, Anderson S, Braniff B (1981). Infective endocarditis due to *Corynebacterium diphtheriae*: report of a case and review of the literature. *John Hopkins Med J* **148**: 41.

Lowy FD, Neuhaus EG, Chang DS, Steigbigel NH (1983). Penicillin therapy of experimental endocarditis induced by tolerant *Streptococcus sanguis* and non-tolerant *Streptococcus mitis*. *Antimicrob Ag Chemother* **23**: 67.

Luft BJ, Gardner P, Lightfoot RW Jr *et al.* (1994). Empiric antibiotic treatment of patients who are seropositive for Lyme disease but lack classic features. *Clin Infect Dis* **18**: 112.

Lujan R, Zhang Q-Y, Saez Nieto JA *et al.* (1991). Penicillin-resistant isolates of *Neisseria lactamica* produce altered forms of penicillin-binding protein 2 that arose by interspecies horizontal gene transfer *Antimicrob Ag Chemother* **35**: 300.

Lukehart SA, Hook EW, Baker-Zander SA *et al.* (1988). Invasion of central nervous system by *Treponema pallidum*: implications for diagnosis and treatment. *Ann Intern Med* **109**: 855.

Lundberg C, Nord C-E (1988). Streptococcal throat infections: still a complex clinical problem. *Scand J Infect Dis* (Suppl 57): 7.

Lyon BR, Skurray R (1987). Antimicrobial resistance of *Staphylococcus aureus*: genetic basis. *Microbiol Rev* **51**: 88.

Macfarlane TW, McGowan DA, Hunter K, Mackenzie D (1983). Prophylaxis for infective endocarditis: antibiotic sensitivity of dental plaque. *J Clin Pathol* **36**: 459.

Mackowiak PA, Le Maistre CF (1987). Drug fever: a critical appraisal of convential concepts. *Ann Intern Med* **106**: 728.

Maisel H, Ruffin JM, Dobbins WO (1970). Whipple's disease: a review of 19 patients from one hospital and a review of the literature since 1950. *Medicine* **49**: 175.

Maki DG, Helstad AG, Kimball JL (1980). Penicillin susceptibility of *Streptococcus pneumoniae* in 1978. Screening for resistance by disc testing. *Amer J Clin Pathol* **73**: 177.

Malone JL, Wallace MR, Hendrick BB *et al.* (1995). Syphilis and neurosyphilis in human immunodeficiency virus type-1 seropositive population: evidence for frequent serologic relapse after therapy. *Amer J Med* **99**: 55.

Malouin F, Bryan LE (1986). Modification of penicillin-binding proteins as mechanisms of beta-lactam resistance. *Antimicrob Ag Chemother* **30**: 1.

Maness MJ, Sparling PF (1973). Multiple antibiotic resistance due to a single mutation in *Neisseria gonorrhoeae*. *J Infect Dis* **128**: 321.

Manian FA, Stone WJ, Alford RH (1990). Adverse antibiotic effects associated with renal insufficiency. *Rev Infect Dis* **12**: 236.

Manzella JP, Kellogg JA, Parsey KS (1995). *Corynebacterium psuedodiphthericum*: a respiratory tract pathogen in adults. *Clin Infect Dis* **20**: 37.

Maple PAC, Efstratiou A, Tseneva G *et al.* (1994). The *in-vitro* susceptibilities of toxigenic strains of *Corynebacterium diphtheriae* isolated in northwestern Russia and surrounding areas to ten antibiotics. *J Antimicrob Chemother* **34**: 1037.

Marks C, Cummins BH (1981). Rescue after 2 megaunits of intrathecal penicillin. *Lancet* **i**: 658.

Marrie TJ (1994). Community-acquired pneumonia. *Clin Infect Dis* **18**: 501.

Marrie TJ, Haldane EV, Swantee CA, Kerr EA (1981). Susceptibility of anaerobic bacteria to nine antimicrobial agents and demonstration of decreased susceptibility of *Clostridium perfringens* to penicillin. *Antimicrob Ag Chemother* **19**: 51.

Marton A (1992). Pneumococcal antimicrobial resistance: the problem in Hungary. *Clin Infect Dis* **15**: 106.

Marton A, Gulyas M, Munoz R, Tomasz A (1991). Extremely high incidence of antibiotic resistance in clinical isolates of *Streptococcus pneumoniae* in Hungary. *J Infect Dis* **163**: 542.

Mashford ML *et al.* (1994). *Antibiotic Guidelines* 8th edn. Victorian Drug Usage Advisory Committee. Moorabin, Victoria, Australia: Interprint Services Ltd.

Mason EO Jr, Kaplan SL, Lamberth LB, Tillman J (1992). Increased rate of isolation of penicillin-resistant *Streptococcus pneumoniae* in a children's hospital and *in vitro* susceptibilities to antibiotics of potential therapeutic use. *Antimicrob Ag Chemother* **36**: 1703.

Mastro TD, Nomani NK, Ishaq Z *et al.* (1993). Use of nasopharyngeal isolates of *Streptococcus pneumoniae* and *Haemophilus influenzae* from children in Pakistan for surveillance for antimicrobial resistance. *Pediatr Infect Dis J* **12**: 824.

Mazzulli T, Salit IE (1991). Pleural fluid infection caused by *Listeria monocytogenes*: case report and review. *Rev Infect Dis* **13**: 564.

McCloskey RV, Green MJ, Eller J, Smilack J (1974). Treatment of diphtheria carriers: benzathine penicillin, erythromycin and clindamycin. *Ann Intern Med* **81**: 788.

McCormack WM (1982). Penicillinase-producing *Neisseria gonorrhoeae* – a retrospective. *New Engl J Med* **307**: 438.

McCracken GH Jr (1973). Group B streptococci: the new challenge in neonatal infections. *J Pediatr* **82**: 703.

McCracken GH Jr (1974). Pharmacological basis for antimicrobial therapy in newborn infants. *Amer J Dis Child* **128**: 407.

McCracken GH Jr, Nelson JD (1983). *Antimicrobial Therapy for Newborns* 2nd edn, p 8. New York: Grune and Stratton.

McCracken GH Jr, Ginsberg C, Chrane DF et al. (1973). Clincal pharmacology of penicillin in newborn infants. *J Pediatr* **82**: 692.

McCracken GH Jr, Nelson JD, Kaplan SL et al. (1987). Consensus report: antimicrobial therapy for bacterial meningitis in infants and children. *Pediatr Infect Dis J* **6**: 501.

McCutchan JA, Adler MW, Berrie JRH (1982). Penicillinase-producing *Neisseria gonorrhoeae* in Great Britain, 1977–81: alarming increase in incidence and recent development of endemic transmission. *Brit Med J* **285**: 337.

McDougal LK, Facklam R, Reeves M et al. (1992). Analysis of multiply antimicrobial-resistant isolates of *Streptococcus pneumoniae* from the United States. *Antimicrob Ag Chemother* **36**: 2176.

McDowell TD, Reed KE (1989). Mechanism of penicillin killing in the absence of bacterial lysis. *Antimicrob Ag Chemother* **33**: 1680.

McGowan DA (1978). Failure of prohylaxis of infective endocarditis following dental treatment. *J Antimicrob Chemother* **4**: 486.

McManus TJ, Harris JRW, Ison CA, Easmon CSF (1982). Penicillinase-producing *Neisseria gonorrhoeae*. *New Engl J Med* **307**: 1706.

McNulty CAM, Dent J, Wise R (1985). Susceptibility of clinical isolates of *Campylobacter pyloridis* to 11 antimicrobial agents. *Antimicrob Ag Chemother* **28**: 837.

McPherson AJ, Parkin JD, Hope R (1976). Penicillin-induced haemolytic anaemia associated with microangiopathy. *Aust NZ J Med* **6**: 152.

McWhinney PHM, Kibbler CC, Gillespie SH et al. (1992). *Stomatococcus mucilaginosus*: an emerging pathogen in neutropenic patients. *Clin Infect Dis* **14**: 641.

Mederski-Samoraj BD, Murray BE (1983). High-level resistance to gentamicin in clinical isolates of enterococci. *J Infect Dis* **147**: 751.

Meeson J, McColm AA, Acred P, Greenwood D (1990). Differential response to benzylpenicillin *in vivo* of tolerant and non-tolerant variants of *Streptococcus sanguis* II. *J Antimicrob Chemother* **25**: 103.

Megran DW (1992). Enterococcal endocarditis. *Clin Infect Dis* **15**: 63.

Meis JF, Sauerwein RW, Gyssens IC et al. (1992). *Kingella kingae* intervertebral diskitis in an adult. *Clin Infect Dis* **15**: 530.

Menke HE, Pepplinkhuizen L (1974). Acute non-allergic reaction to aqueous procaine penicillin. *Lancet* **ii**: 723.

Merianos A, Condon RJ, Tapsall JW et al. (1995). Epidemic gonococcal conjunctivitis in central Australia. *Med J Aust* **162**: 178.

Michel J, Sharon R (1980). Non-haemolytic adverse reaction after transfusion of a blood unit containing penicillin. *Brit Med J* **280**: 152.

Mijamoto MI, Fang FC (1993). Pyogenic liver abscess involving Actinomyces: case report and review. *Clin Infect Dis* **16**: 303.

Miller PS, Schauf V, Salo RJ (1990). Enhanced killing of Group B streptococci *in vitro* by penicillin and opsonophagocytosis with intravenous immunoglobulin. *J Infect Dis* **161**: 1225.

Mitchell H, Travers R, Barraclough D (1982). Septic arthritis caused by *Pasteurella multocida*. *Med J Aust* **1**: 137.

Mitsuyama J, Hiruma R, Yamaguchi A, Sawai T (1987). Identification of porins in outer membrane of *Proteus*, *Morganella* and *Providencia* spp and their role in outer membrane permeation of beta-lactams. *Antimicrob Ag Chemother* **31**: 379.

Moellering RC Jr (1991). The enterococcus: a classic example of the impact of antimicrobial resistance on therapeutic options. *J Antimicrob Chemother* **28**: 1.

Moellering RC Jr (1992). Emergence of Enterococcus as a significant pathogen. *Clin Infect Dis* **14**: 1173.

Moellering RC Jr, Watson BK, Kunz LJ (1974). Endocarditis due to Group D streptococci Comparison of disease caused by *Streptococcus bovis* with that produced by the enterococci. *Amer J Med* **57**: 239.

Moellering RC Jr, Korzeniowski OM, Sande MA, Wennersten CB (1979). Species-specific resistance to antimicrobial synergism in *Streptococcus faecium* and *Streptococcus faecalis*. *J Infect Dis* **140**: 203.

Mohan K, Gordon RC, Beaman TC et al. (1977). Synergism of penicillin and gentamicin against *Listeria monocytogenes* in *ex vivo* hemodialysis culture. *J Infect Dis* **135**: 51.

Mohle-Boetani JC, Schuchat A, Plikaytis BD et al. (1993). Comparison of prevention strategies for neonatal Group B streptococcal infection. A population-based economic analysis. *JAMA* **270**: 1442.

Mohr JA, Griffiths W, Jackson R et al. (1976). Neurosyphilis and penicillin levels in cerebrospinal fluid. *JAMA* **236**: 2208.

Moine P, Valée E, Azoulay-Dupuis E et al. (1994). *In vivo* efficacy of a broad spectrum cephalosporin, ceftriaxone, against penicillin-susceptible and -resistant strains of *Streptococcus pneumoniae* in a mouse pneumonia model. *Antimicrob Ag Chemother* **38**: 1953.

Moreillon P, Tomasz A (1988). Penicillin resistance and defective lysis in clinical isolates of pneumococci: evidence for two kinds of antibiotic pressure operating in the clinical environment. *J Infect Dis* **157**: 1150.

Moreillon P, Markiewicz Z, Nachman S, Tomasz A (1990). Two bactericidal targets for penicillin in pneumococci: autolysis-dependent and autolysis-independent killing mechanisms. *Antimicrob Ag Chemother* **34**: 33.

Morris A, Guild I (1991). Endocarditis due to *Corynebacterium pseudodiphthericum*: five case reports, review, and antibiotic susceptibilities of nine strains. *Rev Infect Dis* **13**: 887.

Morrison VA, Wagner KF (1989). Clinical manifestations of *Kingella kingae* infections: case report and review. *Rev Infect Dis* **11**: 776.

Mortimer PGS, Piddock LJV (1993). The accumulation of five antibacterial agents in porin-deficient mutants of *Escherichia coli*. *J Antimicrob Chemother* **32**: 195.

Motiejunas L, Bunikis J, Barbour AG, Sadziene A (1994). Lyme borreliosis in Lithuania. *Scand J Infect Dis* **26**: 149.

Muñoz R, Coffey TJ, Daniels M et al. (1991). Intercontinental spread of multiresistant clone of serotype 23F *Streptococcus pneumoniae*. *J Infect Dis* **164**: 302.

Muñoz R, Musser JM, Crain M (1992a). Geographic distribution of penicillin-resistant clones of *Streptococcus pneumoniae*: characterization by penicillin-binding protein profile, surface protein A typing, and multilocus enzyme analysis. *Clin Infect Dis* **15**: 112.

Muñoz R, Coque T, Creixems MR et al. (1992b). Group B streptococcus: a cause of urinary tract infection in nonpregnant adults. *Clin Infect Dis* **14**: 492.

Murphy DJ Jr (1983). Group A streptococcal meningitis. *Pediatrics* **71**: 1.

Murray BE (1989). Problems and mechanisms of antimicrobial resistance. *Infect Dis Clin North Amer* **3**: 423.

Murray BE(1991). New aspects of antimicrobial resistance and the resulting therapeutic dilemmas. *J Infect Dis* **163**: 1185.

Murray BE (1992). Beta lactamase-producing enterococci. *Antimicrob Ag Chemother* **36**: 2355.

Murray BE, Mederski-Samoray B (1983). Transferable beta-lactamase: a new mechanism for *in vitro* penicillin resistance in *Streptococcus faecalis*. *J Clin Invest* **72**: 1168.

Murray BE, Karchmer AW, Moellering RC Jr (1980). Diphtheroid prosthetic valve endocarditis. A study of clinical features and infecting organisms. *Amer J Med* **69**: 838.

Murray BE, Tsao J, Panida J (1983). Enterococci from Bangkok, Thailand, with high-level resistance to currently available aminoglycosides. *Antimicrob Ag Chemother* **23**: 799.

Murray BE, Church DA, Wanger A et al. (1986). Comparison of two beta-lactamase-producing strains of *Streptococcus faecalis*. *Antimicrob Ag Chemother* **30**: 861.

Murray BE, An FY, Clewell DB(1988). Plasmids and pheromone response of the beta-lactamase producer *Streptococcus* (*Enterococcus*) *faecalis* HH22. *Antimicrob Ag Chemother* **32**: 547.

Murray BE, Singh KV, Markowitz SM et al. (1991). Evidence for clonal spread of a single strain of beta-lactamase-producing *Enterococcus* (*Streptococcus*) *faecalis* to six hospitals in five states. *J Infect Dis* **163**: 780.

Murray HW (1979). Antimicrobial therapy in pulmonary aspiration. *Amer J Med* **66**: 188.

Musher DM (1988). How much penicillin cures early syphilis? *Ann Intern Med* **109**: 849.

Musher DM (1991). Syphilis, neurosyphilis, penicillin, and AIDS. *J Infect Dis* **163**: 1201.

Musher DM (1992). Infections caused by *Streptococcus pneumoniae*: clinical spectrum, pathogenesis, immunity, and treatment *Clin Infect Dis* **14**: 801.

Mychajlonka M (1981). Effects of low penicillin concentrations on cell morphology and on peptidoglycan and protein synthesis in a tolerant *Streptococcus* strain. *Antimicrob Ag Chemother* **19**: 972.

Mychajlonka M, McDowell TD, Shockman GD (1980). Inhibition of peptidoglycan ribonucleic acid and protein synthesis in tolerant strains of *Streptococcus mutans*. *Antimicrob Ag Chemother* **17**: 572.

Naraqi S, Kirkpatrick GP, Kabins S (1974). Relapsing pneumococcal meningitis: isolation of an organism with decreased susceptibility to penicillin G. *J Pediatr* **85**: 671.

Nauta EH, Mattie H, Goslings WRO (1974). Effect of probenecid on the apparent volume of distribution and elimination of cloxacillin. *Antimicrob Ag Chemother* **6**: 300.

Nava JM, Bella F, Garau J *et al.* (1994). Predictive factors for invasive disease due to penicillin-resistant *Streptococcus pneumoniae*: a population-based study. *Clin Infect Dis* **19**: 884.

Neal TJ, O'Donoghue MAT, Ridgway EJ, Allen KD (1992). *In-vitro* activity of ten antimicrobial agents against penicillin-resistant *Streptococcus pneumoniae*. *J Antimicrob Chemother* **30**: 39.

Neftel KA, Wälti M, Spengler H, de Weck AL (1982). Effect of storage of penicillin-G solutions on sensitisation to penicillin-G intravenous administration. *Lancet* **i**: 986.

Neftel KA, Hauser SP, Müller MR (1985). Inhibition of granulopoiesis *in vivo* and *in vitro* by beta-lactam antibiotics. *J Infect Dis* **152**: 90.

Nicholas RA, Strominger JL (1988). Relations between beta-lactamases and penicillin-binding proteins: beta-lactamase activity of penicillin-binding protein 5 from *Escherichia coli*. *Rev Infect Dis* **10**: 733.

Nicholls PJ (1980). Leading article. Neurotoxicity of penicillin. *J Antimicrob Chemother* **6**: 161.

Nielsen SV, Henrichsen J (1993). Capsular types and susceptibility to penicillin of pneumococci isolated from cerebrospinal fluid or blood in Denmark, 1983–1988. *Scand J Infect Dis* **25**: 165.

Nikaido H (1988). Structure and functions of the cell envelope of Gram-negative bacteria. *Rev Infect Dis* **10** (Suppl 2): 279.

Nikaido H (1989). Outer membrane barrier as a mechanism of antimicrobial resistance. *Antimicrob Ag Chemother* **33**: 1831.

Nikaido H (1994). Prevention of drug access to bacterial targets: permeability barriers and active efflux. *Science* **264**: 362.

Nikaido H, Vaara M (1985). Molecular basis of bacterial outer membrane permeability. *Microbiol Rev* **49**: 1.

Noble JT, Tybuarski MB, Berman M *et al.* (1980). Antimicrobial tolerance in Group G streptococci. *Lancet* **ii**: 982.

Nord CE, Hedberg M (1990). Resistance to beta-lactam antibiotics in anaerobic bacteria. *Rev Infect Dis* **12** (Suppl 2): 231.

Norrby R (1978). A review of the penetration of antibiotics into CSF and its clinical significance. *Scand J Infect Dis* (Suppl 14): 296.

Noskin GA, Till M, Patterson BK *et al.* (1993). High-level gentamicin resistance in *Enterococcus faecalis* bacteremia. *J Infect Dis* **164**: 1212.

Nowak R (1994). Hungary sees an improvement in penicillin resistance. *Science* **264**: 364.

Odenholt I, Holm SE, Cars O (1989). Effects of benzylpenicillin on *Streptococcus pyogenes* during the postantibiotic phase *in vitro*. *J Antimicrob Chemother* **24**: 147.

Odenholt I, Holm SE, Cars O (1990). Effects of supra- and sub-MIC benzylpenicillin concentrations on group A β-haemolytic streptococci during the postantibiotic phase *in vivo*. *J Antimicrob Chemother* **26**: 193.

Odio CM, Faingezicht I, Paris M *et al.* (1991). The beneficial effects of early dexamethasone administration in infants and children with acute bacterial meningitis. *New Engl J Med* **324**: 1525.

Ogawara H (1981). Antibiotic resistance in pathogenic and producing bacteria, with special resistance to beta-lactam antibiotics. *Microbiol Rev* **45**: 591.

Olaison L, Alestig K (1990). A prospective study of neutropenia induced by high doses of beta-lactam antibiotics. *J Antimicrob Chemother* **25**: 449.

Olsson B, Dornbusch K, Nord CE (1979). Factors contributing to resistance to beta-lactam antibiotics in *Bacteroides fragilis*. *Antimicrob Ag Chemother* **15**: 263.

Oppenheim B, Koornhof HJ, Austrian R (1986). Antibiotic-resistant pneumococcal disease in children at Baragwanath Hospital, Johannesburg. *Pediatr Infect Dis* **5**: 520.

Orchard RT, Rooker G (1974). Penicillin-hypersensitivity nephritis. *Lancet* **i**: 689.

Orris DJ, Lewis JH, Spero JA, Hasiba U (1980). Blocking coagulation inhibitors in children taking penicillin. *J Pediatr* **97**: 426.

Oster SE, Chirurgi VA, Goldberg AA *et al.* (1990). Ampicillin-resistant enterococcal species in an acute-care hospital. *Antimicrob Ag Chemother* **34**: 1821.

Otin CL, Morros TJ, Sala IS (1988). Antibiotic susceptibility of *Streptococcus pneumoniae* isolates from paediatric patients. *J Antimicrob Chemother* **22**: 659.

Pallares R, Liñares J, Vadillo M *et al.* (1995). Resistance to penicillin and cephalosporin and mortality from severe pneumococcal pneumonia in Barcelona, Spain. *New Engl J Med* **333**: 474.

Palmer DW (1979). Inadequate response to 'adequate' treatment of bacterial infection: L forms and 'bactericidal antibiotic activity'. *J Infect Dis* **139**: 725.

Pang R, Teh LB, Rajan VS, Sng EH (1979). Gonococcal ophthalmia neonatorum caused by beta-lactamase-producing *Neisseria gonorrhoeae*. *Brit Med J* **1**: 380.

Pape J, Singer C, Kiehn TE *et al.* (1979). Infective enocarditis caused by *Rothia dentocariosa*. *Ann Intern Med* **91**: 746.

Paredes A, Wong P, Yow MD (1976). Failure of penicillin to eradicate the carrier stage of Group B streptococcus in infants. *J Pediatr* **89**: 191.

Paris MM, Hickey SM, Uscher MI *et al.* (1994). Effect of dexamethasone on therapy of experimental penicillin- and cephalosporin -resistant pneumococcal meningitis. *Antimicrob Ag Chemother* **38**: 1320.

Parisi JT (1985). Coagulase-negative staphylococci and the epidemiological typing of *Staphylococcus epidermidis*. *Microbiol Rev* **49**: 126.

Parker CW (1975). Drug allergy. *New Engl J Med* **292**: 511, 732, 957.

Parker JC, Barrett DA II (1971). Microangiopathic hemolysis and thrombocytopenia related to penicillin drugs. *Arch Intern Med* **127**: 474.

Parkinson AJ, Davidson M, Fitzgerald MA *et al.* (1994). Serotype distribution and antimicrobial resistance patterns of invasive isolates of *Streptococcus pneumoniae*: Alaska 1986–1990. *J Infect Dis* **170**: 461.

Patel R, Keating MR, Cockerill FR III, Steckelberg JM (1993). Bacteremia due to *Enterococcus avium*. *Clin Infect Dis* **17**: 1006.

Patel R, Cockerill FR, Porayko MK *et al.* (1994). Lactobacillemia in liver transplant patients. *Clin Infect Dis* **18**: 207.

Patterson JE, Colodny SM, Zervos MJ (1988a). Serious infection due to beta-lactamase-producing *Streptococcus faecalis* with high-level resistance to gentamicin. *J Infect Dis* **158**: 1144.

Patterson JE, Masecar BL, Zervos MJ (1988b). Characterization and comparison of two penicillinase-producing strains of *Streptococcus* (*Enterococcus*) *faecalis*. *Antimicrob Ag Chemother* **32**: 122.

Patterson JE, Wanger A, Zscheck KK *et al.* (1990). Molecular epidemiology of beta-lactamase-producing enterococci. *Antimicrob Ag Chemother* **34**: 302.

Paul ML, Dwyer DE, Chow C *et al.* (1994). Listeriosis – a review of eighty-four cases. *Med J Aust* **160**: 489.

Pavicic MJAMP, Van Winkelhoff AJ, de Graaff J (1992). *In vitro* susceptibilities of *Actinobacillus actinomycetemcomitans* to a number of antibiotic combinations. *Antimicrob Ag Chemother* **36**: 2634.

Peltola H (1983). Meningococcal disease: still with us. *Rev Infect Dis* **5**: 71.

Percival A, Rowlands J, Corkill JE *et al.* (1976). Penicillinase-producing gonococci in Liverpool. *Lancet* **ii**: 1379.

Perine PL, Schalla W, Siegel MS *et al.* (1977). Evidence for two distinct types of penicillinase-producing *Neisseria gonorrhoeae*. *Lancet* **ii**: 993.

Perlow JH, Wigton T, Yordan EL *et al.* (1991). Disseminated pelvic actinomycosis presenting as metastatic carcinoma: associated with the progestasert intrauterine device. *Rev Infect Dis* **13**: 1115.

Persson K, Bjerre B, Elfstrom L, *et al.* (1986). Group B streptococci at delivery: high count in urine increases risk for neonatal colonization. *Scand J Infect Dis* **18**: 525.

Persson K, Bjerre B, Elfstrom L, Forsgren A (1987). Longitudinal study of Group B streptococcal carrige during late pregnancy. *Scand J Infect Dis* **19**: 325.

Peter G (1992). Streptococcal pharyngitis: current therapy and criteria for evaluation of new agents. *Clin Infect Dis* **14** (Suppl 2): 218.

Peter G, Smith AL (1977). Group A streptococcal infections of the skin and pharynx (Second of two parts). *New Engl J Med* **297**: 365.

Petersen EA (1990). Prevention of bacterial endocarditis. *Arch Intern Med* **150**: 2447.

Petit PLC, Bok JW, Thompson J *et al.* (1994). Native-valve endocarditis due to CDC Coryneform Group ANF-3: report of a case and review of *Corynebacterium endocarditis*. *Clin Infect Dis* **19**: 897.

Philipson A (1991). Antibiotic treatment of Lyme borreliosis. *Scand J Infect Dis* (Suppl 77): 145.

Phillips I, Warren C, Harrison JM *et al.* (1976). Antibiotic susceptibilities of streptococci from the mouth and blood of patients treated with penicillin or lincomycin and clindamycin. *J Med Microbiol* **9**: 393.

Piddock LJV, Wise R (1985). Newer mechanisms of resistance to beta-lactam antibiotics in Gram-negative bacteria. *J Antimicrob Chemother* **16**: 279.

Pinon G, Quentin R, Laudat P, Vargues R (1981). Beta-lactam susceptibility of *Neisseria gonorrhoeae*: isolates from pelvic inflammatory disease. *Antimicrob Ag Chemother* **20**: 260.

Pintado C, Salvador C, Rotger R, Nombela C (1985). Multiresistance plasmid from commensal *Neisseria* strains. *Antimicrob Ag Chemother* **27**: 120.

Plaut ME, O'Connell CJ, Pabico RC, Davidson D (1969). Penicillin handling in normal and azotemic patients. *J Lab Clin Med* **74**: 12.

Plouffe JF, Breiman RF, Facklam RR for the Franklin County Pneumonia Study Group (1996). Bacteremia with *Streptococcus pneumoniae*. Implications for therapy and prevention. *JAMA* **275**: 194.

Polk IJ (1982). Penicillin allergy skin tests. *JAMA* **247**: 1745.

Polnikorn N, Witoonpanich R, Vorachit M *et al.* (1980). Penicillin concentrations in cerebrospinal fluid after different treatment regimens for syphilis. *Brit J Vener Dis* **56**: 363.

Portnoy D, Prentis J, Richards GK (1981). Penicillin tolerance of human isolates of Group C streptococci. *Antimicrob Ag Chemother* **20**: 235.

Potgieter E, Chalkley LJ (1991). Reciprocal transfer of penicillin resistance genes between *Streptococcus pneumoniae*, *Streptococcus mitior* and *Streptococcus sanguis*. *J Antimicrob Chemother* **28**: 463.

Powderly WG, Stanley SL Jr, Medofff G (1986). Pneumococcal endocarditis: report of a series and review of the literature. *Rev Infect Dis* **8**: 786.

Powell JT, Bond JH (1976). Multiple antibiotic resistance in clinical strains of *Neisseria gonorrhoeae* isolated in South Carolina. *Antimicrob Ag Chemother* **10**: 639.

Price SB, Flournoy DJ (1982). Comparison of antimicrobial susceptibility patterns among coagulase-negative staphylococci. *Antimicrob Ag Chemother* **21**: 436.

Prichard MG, Miles HM, Pavillard ER (1983). *Listeria meningitis – in vitro* sensitivities to co-trimoxazole, penicillins and gentamicin. *Aust NZ J Med* **13**: 76.

Prokesch RC, Hand WL (1982). Antibiotic entry into human polymorphonuclear leukocytes. *Antimicrob Ag Chemother* **21**: 373.

Public Health Laboratory Service Communicable Diseases Surveillance Centre (1983). Penicillinase-producing *Neisseria gonorrhoeae* in Britain 1982. *Brit Med J* **286**: 1628.

Pyati SP, Pildes RS, Jacobs NM *et al.* (1983). Penicillin in infants weighting two kilograms or less with early-onset Group B streptococcal disease. *New Engl J Med* **308**: 1383.

Quagliarello VJ, Scheld WM (1993). New perspectives on bacterial meningitis. *Clin Infect Dis* **17**: 603.

Quinn JP, Di Vincenzo CA, Lucks DA *et al.* (1988). Serious infections due to penicillin-resistant strains of viridans streptococci with altered penicillin-binding proteins. *J Infect Dis* **157**: 764.

Radetsky M (1990). Duration of treatment in bacterial meningitis: a historical inquiry. *Pediatr Infect Dis J* **9**: 2.

Raffi F, Barrier J, Baron D *et al.* (1987). *Pasteurella multocida* bacteremia: report of thirteen cases over twelve years and review of the literature. *Scand J Infect Dis* **19**: 385.

Raffin BJ, Freemark M (1979). Streptobacillary rat-bite fever: a pediatric problem. *Pediatrics* **64**: 214.

Rahman M (1982). Penicillin resistance in viridans streptococci. *J Infect* **4**: 89.

Rahn DW, Malawista SE (1991). Lyme disease: recommendations for diagnosis and treatment. *Ann Intern Med* **114**: 472.

Raichle ME, Kutt H, Louis S, McDowell F (1971). Neurotoxicity of intravenously administered penicillin G. *Arch Neurol* **25**: 232.

Rapeport KB, Giron JA, Rosner F (1986). *Streptococcus mitis* endocarditis. Report of 17 cases. *Arch Intern Med* **146**: 2361.

Rauch AM, O'Ryan M, Van R, Pickering LK (1990). Invasive disease due to multiply resistant *Streptococcus pneumoniae* in a Houston, Texas, day-care center. *Amer J Dis Child* **144**: 923.

Rechtman DJ, Nadler JP (1991). Abdominal abscess due to *Cardiobacterium hominis* and *Clostridium bifermentans*. *Rev Infect Dis* **13**: 418.

Recommendations from the Endocarditis Working Party of the British Society for Antimicrobial Chemotherapy (1990). Antibiotic prophylaxis of infective endocarditis. *Lancet* **335**: 88.

Reichler MR, Allphin AA, Breiman RF *et al.* (1992). The spread of multiply resistant *Streptococcus pneumoniae* at a day care center in Ohio. *J Infect Dis* **166**: 1346.

Reller LB (1986). The serum bactericidal test. *Rev Infect Dis* **8**: 803.

Renneberg J, Rosdahl VT (1992). Epidemiological studies of penicillin resistance in Danish *Staphylococcus aureus* strains in the period 1977–1990. *Scand J Infect Dis* **24**: 401.

Report of a Working Party of the British Society for Antimicrobial Chemotherapy (1985). Antibiotic treatment of streptococcal and staphylococcal endocarditis. *Lancet* **ii**: 815.

Reyes MP, Hunt N, Ostrea EMJr, George D (1993). Maternal/congenital syphilis in a large tertiary-care urban hospital. *Clin Infect Dis* **17**: 1041.

Rhinehart E, Smith NE, Wennersten C *et al.* (1990). Rapid dissemination of beta-lactamase-producing aminoglycoside-resistant *Enterococcus faecalis* among patients and staff on an infant-toddler surgical ward. *New Engl J Med* **323**: 1814.

Rice LB, Marshall SH (1994). Insertion of IS256-like element flanking the chromosomal beta-lactamase gene of *Enterococcus faecalis* CX19. *Antimicrob Ag Chemother* **38**: 693.

Rice LB, Calderwood SB, Eliopoulos GM *et al.* (1991a). Enterococcal endocarditis: a comparison of prosthetic and native valve disease. *Rev Infect Dis* **13**: 1.

Rice LB, Eliopoulos GM, Wennersten C *et al.* (1991b). Chromosomally mediated beta-lactamase production and gentamicin resistance in *Enterococcus faecalis*. *Antimicrob Ag Chemother* **35**: 272.

Rice RJ, Knapp JS (1994a). Antimicrobial susceptibilities of *Neisseria gonorrhoeae* strains representing five distinct resistance phenotypes. *Antimicrob Ag Chemother* **38**: 155.

Rice RJ, Knapp JS (1994b). Susceptibility of *Neisseria gonorrhoeae* associated with pelvic inflammatory disease to cefoxitin, ceftriaxone, clindamycin, gentamicin, doxycycline, azithromycin and other antimicrobial agents. *Antimicrob Ag Chemother* **38**: 1688.

Rice RJ, Blount JH, Biddle JW *et al.* (1984). Changing trends in gonococcal antibiotic resistance in the United States, 1983–1984. Centers for Disease Control Surveillance Summaries **33** (no. 4ss): 11ss.

Rice RJ, Biddle JW, Jean Louis YA et al. (1986). Chromosomally mediated resistance in *Neisseria gonorrhoeae* in the United States: results of surveillance and reporting, 1983–1984. *J Infect Dis* **153**: 340.

Richardson JF, Marples RR (1982). Changing resistance to antimicrobial drugs, and resistance typing in clinically significant strains of *Staphylococcus epidermidis*. *J Med Microbiol* **15**: 475.

Richmond MH (1979). Beta-lactam antibiotics and beta-lactamases: two sides of a continuing story. *Rev Infect Dis* **1**: 30.

Rickman LS, Freeman WR, Green WR et al. (1995). Brief report: uveitis caused by *Tropheryma whippelii* (Whipple's bacillus). *New Engl J Med* **332**: 363.

Rinaldi RZ, Harrison WO, Fan PT (1982). Penicillin-resistant gonococcal arthritis. A report of four cases. *Ann Intern Med* **97**: 43.

Roberts M, Falkow S (1977). Conjugal transfer of R plasmids in *Neisseria gonorrhoeae*. *Nature* **266**: 630.

Roberts MC, Knapp JS (1988). Transfer of beta-lactamase plasmids from *Neisseria gonorrhoeae* to *Neisseria meningitidis* and commensal *Neisseria* species by the 252-megadalton conjugative plasmid. *Antimicrob Ag Chemother* **32**: 1430.

Rodin P, Seth AD, King DM, Wilkinson AE (1980). Sensitivity to penicillin of gonococci in different racial groups. *Brit J Vener Dis* **56**: 308.

Rodriguez W, Saz AK (1975). Possible mechanism of decreased susceptibility of *Neisseria gonorrhoeae* to penicillin. *Antimicrob Ag Chemother* **7**: 788.

Roggiani M, Schlievert PM (1994). Streptococcal toxic shock syndrome, including necrotizing fasciitis and myositis. *Curr Opin Infect Dis* **7**: 423.

Rosdahl VT, Westh H, Jensen K (1990). Antibiotic susceptibility and phage-type pattern of *Staphylococcus aureus* strains isolated from patients in general practice compared to strains from hospitalized patients. *Scand J Infect Dis* **22**: 315.

Rosenau A, Labigne A, Escande F et al. (1991). Plasmid-mediated ROB-1 beta-lactamase in *Pasteurella multocida* from a human specimen. *Antimicrob Ag Chemother* **35**: 2419.

Rupp ME (1992). *Streptobacillus moniliformis* endocarditis: case report and review. *Clin Infect Dis* **14**: 769.

Ruuskanen O, Nohynek H, Ziegler T et al. (1992). Pneumonia in childhood: etiology and response to antimicrobial therapy. *Eur J Clin Microbiol Infect Dis* **11**: 217.

Saah AJ, Mallonee JP, Tarpay M et al. (1980). Relative resistance to penicillin in the pneumococcus. A prevalence and case-control study. *JAMA* **243**: 1824.

Sabath LD, Wheeler N, Laverdiere M et al. (1977). A new type of penicillin resistance of *Staphylococcus aureus*. *Lancet* **i**: 433.

Sackel SG, Alpert S, Rosner B et al. (1977). *In vitro* activity of p-hydroxybenzyl penicillin (penicillin X). and five other penicillins against *Neisseria gonorrhoeae*: comparisons of strains from patients with uncomplicated infections and from women with pelvic inflammatory disease. *Antimicrob Ag Chemother* **12**: 31.

Saez-Nieto JA, Lujan R, Berrón S et al. (1992). Epidemiology and molecular basis of penicillin-resistant *Neisseria meningitidis* in Spain: a 5-year history (1985–1989). *Clin Infect Dis* **14**: 394.

Sande MA, Scheld WM (1980). Combination antibiotic therapy of bacterial endocarditis. *Ann Intern Med* **92**: 390.

Sanders CC (1992). Beta-lactamases of Gram-negative bacteria: new challenges for new drugs. *Clin Infect Dis* **14**: 1089.

Sangster G, Murdoch J, McC, Gray JA (1982). Bacterial meningitis 1940–79. *J Infect* **5**: 245.

Sarmiento R, Wilson FM, Khatib R (1993). Group B streptococcal meningitis in adults: case report and review of the literature. *Scand J Infect Dis* **25**: 1.

Sarubbi FA Jr, Sparling PF (1974). Transfer of antibiotic resistance in mixed cultures of *Neisseria gonorrhoeae*. *J Infect Dis* **130**: 660.

Sawai T, Yamaguchi A, Hiruma R (1988). Effect of interaction between outer membrane permeability and beta-lactamase production on resist-

ance to beta-lactam agents in Gram-negative bacteria. *Rev Infect Dis* **10**: 761.

Saxon A (1983). Immediate hypersensitivity reactions to beta-lactam antibiotics. *Rev Infect Dis* **5** (Suppl 2): 368.

Schafer FJ, Wing EJ, Norden CW (1979). Infectious endocarditis caused by *Rothia dentocariosa*. *Ann Intern Med* **91**: 747.

Schanzer H, Gribetz I, Jacobson JH II (1979). Accidental intra-arterial injection of penicillin G. A preventable catastrophe. *JAMA* **242**: 1289.

Schatz M, Wasserman S, Patterson R (1981). Eosinophils and immunologic lung disease. *Med Clin North Amer* **65**: 1055.

Scheck DN, Hook EW (1994). Neurosyhphilis. *Inf Dis Clin North Amer* **8**: 769.

Scheld WM (1987). Therapy of streptococcal endocarditis: correlation of animal model and clinical studies. *J Antimicrob Chemother* **20** (Suppl A): 71.

Scheld WM, Fletcher DD, Fink FN, Sande MA (1979). Response to therapy in an experimental rabbit model of meningitis due to *Listeria monocytogenes*. *J Infect Dis* **140**: 287.

Schliamser SE, Bolander H, Kourtopoulos H, Norrby SR (1988a). Neurotoxicity of benzylpenicillin: correlation to concentrations in serum, cerebrospinal fluid and brain tissue fluid in rabbits. *J Antimicrob Chemother* **21**: 365.

Schliamser SE, Bolander H, Kortopoulos H et al. (1988b). Neurotoxicity of benzylpenicillin in experimental *Escherichia coli* meningitis. *J Antimicrob Chemother* **22**: 521.

Schliamser SE, Bolander H, Broholm K-A et al. (1989). Neurotoxicity of benzylpenicillin in experimental renal failure and *Enterobacter cloacae* meningitis. *J Antimicrob Chemother* **24**: 215.

Schliamser SE, Cars O, Norrby SR (1991). Neurotoxicity of beta-lactam antibiotics: predisposing factors and pathogenesis. *J Antimicrob Chemother* **27**: 405.

Schlievert PM, Gocke JE, Deringer JR (1993). Group B streptococcal toxic shock-like syndrome: report of a case and purification of an associated pyrogenic toxin. *Clin Infect Dis* **17**: 26.

Schmitt BD, Krivit W (1969). Benign intracranial hypertension associated with a delayed penicillin reaction. *Pediatrics* **43**: 50.

Schroeter AL, Turner RH, Lucas JB, Brown WJ (1971). Therapy for incubating syphilis. Effectiveness of gonorrhea treatment. *JAMA* **218**: 711.

Schuchat A, Deaver-Robinson K, Plikaytis BD et al. (1994). Multistate case-control study of maternal risk factors for neonatal Group B streptococcal disease. *Pediatr Infect Dis J* **13**: 623.

Schwartz RH, Khan WN, Akram S (1991). Penicillin and trimethoprim-sulfamethoxazole-resistant pneumococci isolated from blood cultures of three infants in metropolitan Washington DC: a harbinger of serious future problems. *Pediatr Infect Dis J* **10**: 782.

Seamans KB, Gloor P, Dobell ARC, Wyant JD (1968). Penicillin-induced seizures during cardio-pulmonary bypass. *New Engl J Med* **278**: 861.

Seboxa T, Rahlenbeck SI (1995). Treatment of louse-borne relapsing fever with low dose penicillin or tetracycline: a clinical trial. *Scand J Infect Dis* **27**: 29.

Seidenfeld SM, Sutker WL, Luby JP (1982). *Fusobacterium necrophorum* septicemia following oropharyngeal infection. *JAMA* **248**: 1348.

Sengupta S (1976). Gangrene following intra-arterial injection of procaine penicillin. *Aust NZ J Med* **6**: 71.

Seydoux Ch, Francioli P (1992). Bacterial brain abscesses: factors influencing mortality and sequelae. *Clin Infect Dis* **15**: 394.

Shah PM (1982). Paradoxical effect of antibiotics. I. The 'Eagle effect'. *J Antimicrob Chemother* **10**: 259.

Shaked Y, Shpilberg O, Samra D, Samra Y (1993). Leptospirosis in pregnancy and its effect on the fetus: case report and review. *Clin Infect Dis* **17**: 241.

Shanks G, Turnidge J, Marshall P, McDonald P (1982). Pneumococcal sepsis in a neonate. *Aust NZ J Med* **12**: 185.

Shann F, Germer S (1981). Treatment of bacterial meningitis in children without intravenous fluids. *Med J Aust* **1**: 577.

Shann F, Germer S (1983). Treatment of bacterial meningitis without intravenous fluids. *Med J Aust* **1**: : 305.

Shann F, Linnemann V, Gratten M (1987). Serum concentrations of penicillin after intramuscular administrtion of procaine, benzyl and benethamine penicillin in children with pneumonia. *J Pediatr* **110**: 299.

Shanson DC (1987). Antibiotic prophylaxis of infective endocarditis in the United Kingdom and Europe. *J Antimicrob Chemother* **20**: (Suppl A): 119.

Shapiro ED, Gerber MA, Holabirol NB et al. (1992). A controlled trial of antimicrobial prophylaxis for Lyme disease after deer-tick bites. *New Engl J Med* **327**: 1769.

Shih C-M, Spielman A (1993). Topical prophylaxis for Lyme disease after tick bite in a rodent model. *J Infect Dis* **168**: 1042.

Shockman GD, Daneo-Moore L, Cornett JB, Mychajlonka M (1979). Does penicillin kill bacteria? *Rev Infect Dis* **1**: 787.

Shtibel R (1980). Non-beta-lactamase producing *Neisseria gonorrhoeae* highly resistant to penicillin. *Lancet* **ii**: 39.

Shulman ST (1986). Infective endocarditis: 1986. *Pediatr Infect Dis J* **5**: 691.

Shulman ST (1993). Invasive Group A streptococcal infections and streptococcal toxic shock syndrome. *Pediatr Infect Dis J* **12**: S21.

Siegel JD, McCracken GH Jr, Threlkeld N et al. (1980). Single-dose penicillin prophylaxis against neonatal Group B streptococcal infections. *New Engl J Med* **303**: 769.

Siegel JD, Shannon KM, de Passe BM (1981). Recurrent infection associated with penicillin-tolerant Group B streptococci: a report of two cases. *J Pediatr* **99**: 920.

Siegel MS, Thornsberry C, Biddle JW et al. (1978). Penicillinase-producing *Neisseria gonorrhoeae*: results of surveillance in the United States. *J Infect Dis* **137**: 170.

Silber TJ, D'Angelo L (1985). Psychosis and seizures following the injection of penicillin G procaine. *Amer J Dis Child* **139**: 335.

Silpa DE, Bulloch GF, Silverman ME, Kenny WR (1982). *Clostridium perfringens* empyema unresponsive to penicillin. *JAMA* **247**: 2568.

Simberkoff MS, Thomas L, McGregor D et al. (1970). Inactivation of penicillins by carbohydrate solutions at alkaline pH. *New Engl J Med* **283**: 116.

Simberkoff MS, Lukaszewski M, Cross A et al. (1986). Antibiotic-resistant isolates of *Streptococcus pneumoniae* from clinical specimens: a cluster of serotype 19A organisms in Brooklyn, New York. *J Infect Dis* **153**: 78.

Simmons NA, Ball AP, Cawson RA et al. (1992). Antibiotic prophylaxis and infective endocarditis. *Lancet* **339**: 1292.

Singh N, Yu VL, Mieles LA, Wagener MM (1993). Beta-lactam antibiotic-induced leukopenia in severe hepatic dysfunction: risk factors and implications for dosing in patients with liver disease. *Amer J Med* **94**: 251.

Skogberg K, Syrjänen J, Jahkola M et al. (1992). Clinical presentation and outcome of listeriosis in patients with and without immunosupressive therapy. *Clin Infect Dis* **14**: 815.

Smego RA Jr (1987). Actinomycosis of the central nervous system. *Rev Infect Dis* **9**: 855.

Smilak JD, Flittie WH, Williams TW Jr (1976). Bone concentrations of antimicrobial agents after parenteral administration. *Antimicrob Ag Chemother* **9**: 169.

Smith AM, Klugman KP (1995). Alterations in penicillin-binding protein 2B from penicillin-resistant wild-type strains of *Streptococcus pneumoniae*. *Antimicrob Ag Chemother* **39**: 859.

Smith AM, Klugman KP, Coffey TJ, Spratt BG (1993). Genetic diversity of penicillin-binding protein 2B and 2X genes from *Streptococcus pneumoniae* in South Africa. *Antimicrob Ag Chemother* **37**: 1938.

Smith JM (1974). Incidence of atopic disease. *Med Clin North Amer* **58**: 3.

Smith MC, Murray BE(1992). Comparison of enterococcal and staphylococcal beta-lactamase-encoding fragments. *Antimicrob Ag Chemother* **36**: 273.

Snavely SR, Hodges GR (1984). The neurotoxicity of antibacterial agents. *Ann Intern Med* **101**: 92.

Snydman DR, Tally FP, Knuppel R et al. (1980). *Bacteroides bivius* and *Bacteroides disiens* in obstetrical patients: clinical findings and antimicrobial susceptibilities. *J Antimicrob Chemother* **6**: 519.

Soares S, Kristinsson KG, Musser JH, Tomasz A (1993). Evidence for the introduction of a multiresistant clone of serotype 6B *Streptococcus pneumoniae* from Spain to Iceland in late 1980s. *J Infect Dis* **168**: 158.

Spagnuolo PJ, Friedman RI (1979). Penicillin sensitivity of invasive and non-invasive. *Pasteurella multocida. J Antimicrob Chemother* **5**: 324.

Spangler SK, Jacobs MR, Appelbaum PC (1992). Susceptibilities of penicillin-susceptible and -resistant strains of *Streptococcus pneumoniae* to RP 59500, vancomycin, erythromycin, PD131628, sparfloxacin, temafloxacin, Win 57273, ofloxacin, and ciprofloxacin. *Antimicrob Ag Chemother* **36**: 856.

Spangler SK, Jacobs MR, Pankuch GA, Appelbaum PC (1993). Susceptibility of 170 penicillin-susceptible and penicillin-resistant pneumococci to six oral cephalosporins, four quinolones, desacetylcefotaxime, Ro 23–9424 and RP 67829. *J Antimicrob Chemother* **31**: 273.

Spark RP (1971). Fatal anaphylaxis due to oral penicillin. *Amer J Clin Path* **56**: 407.

Sparling PF, Holmes KK, Wiesner PJ, Puziss M (1977). Summary of the conference on the problem of penicillin-resistant gonococci. *J Infect Dis* **135**: 865.

Speer ME, Mason EO, Scharnberg JT (1981). Cerebrospinal fluid concentrations of aqueous procaine penicillin G in the neonate. *Pediatrics* **67**: 387.

Speirs G, Warren RE, Rampling A (1988). *Clostridium tertium* septicemia in patients with neutropenia. *J Infect Dis* **158**: 1336.

Spera RV Jr, Kaplan MH, Allen SL (1992). *Clostridium sordelli* bacteremia: case report and review. *Clin Infect Dis* **15**: 950.

Spika JS, Facklam RR, Plikaytis BD et al. (1991). Antibiotic resistance of *Streptococcus pneumoniae* in the United States (1979–1987). *J Infect Dis* **163**: 1273.

Spinola SM, Bell RA, Henderson FW (1981). Actinomycosis. A cause of pulmonary and mediastinal mass lesions in children. *Amer J Dis Child* **135**: 336.

Spratt BG, Cromie KD (1988). Penicillin-binding proteins of Gram-negative bacteria. *Rev Infect Dis* **10**: 699.

Stamm AM, Dismukes WE, Simmons BP et al. (1982). Listeriosis in renal transplant recipients: report of an outbreak and review of 102 cases. *Rev Infect Dis* **4**: 665.

Steere AC, Malawista SE, Newman JH et al. (1980). Antibiotic therapy of Lyme disease. *Ann Intern Med* **93**: 1.

Steere AC, Grodzicki RL, Kornblatt AN et al. (1983a). The spirochetal etiology of Lyme disease. *New Engl J Med* **308**: 733.

Steere AC, Hutchinson GJ, Rahn DW et al. (1983b). Treatment of early manifestations of Lyme disease. *Ann Intern Med* **99**: 22.

Steere AC, Pachner AR, Malawista SE (1983c). Neurologicai abnormalities of Lyme disease: successful treatment with high-dose intravenous penicillin. *Ann Intern Med* **99**: 767.

Steere AC, Green J, Schoen RT et al. (1985). Successful parenteral penicillin therapy of established Lyme arthritis. *New Engl J Med* **312**: 869.

Steere AC, Schoen RT, Taylor E (1987). The clinical evolution of Lyme arthritis. *Ann Intern Med* **107**: 725.

Stein A, Teysseire N, Capobianco C et al. (1993). *Eikenella corrodens*, a rare cause of pancreatic abscess: two case reports and review. *Clin Infect Dis* **17**: 273.

Stein AA, Fialk MA, Blevins A, Armstrong D (1983). *Pasteurella multocida* septicemia. Experience at a cancer hospital. *JAMA* **249**: 508.

Stein DS, Nelson KE (1987). Endocarditis due to nutritionally deficient streptococci: theapeutic dilemma. *Rev Infect Dis* **9**: 908.

Stevens DL (1992). Invasive Group A streptococcal infections. *Clin Infect Dis* **14**: 2.

Stevens DL, Higbee JW, Oberhofer TR, Everett ED (1979). Antibiotic susceptibilities of human isolates of *Pasteurella multocida*. *Antimicrob Ag Chemother* **16**: 322.

Stevens DL, Maier KA, Mitten JE (1987). Effect of antibiotics on toxin production and viability of *Clostridium perfringens*. *Antimicrob Ag Chemother* **31**: 213.

Stevens DL, Yan S, Bryant AE (1993a). Penicillin-binding protein expression at different growth stages determines penicillin efficacy *in vitro* and *in vivo*: an explanation for the inoculum effect. *J Infect Dis* **167**: 1401.

Stevens DL, Bryant AE, Adams K, Mader JT (1993b). Evaluation of therapy with hyperbaric oxygen for experimental infection with *Clostridium perfringens*. *Clin Infect Dis* **17**: 231.

Stevenson KB, Murray EW, Sarubbi FA (1994). Enterococcal meningitis: report of four cases and review. *Clin Infect Dis* **18**: 233.

Stoll BJ (1994). Congenital syphilis: evaluation and management of neonates born to mothers with reactive serologic tests for syphilis. *Pediatr Infect Dis J* **13**: 845.

Stotka JL, Rupp ME, Meier FA, Markowitz SM (1991). Meningitis due to *Neisseria mucosa*: case report and review. *Rev Infect Dis* **13**: 837.

Strang JR, Pugh EJ (1992). Meningococcal infections: reducing the case fatality rate by giving penicillin before admission to hospital. *Brit Med J* **305**: 141.

Struillou L, Raffi F, Barrier JH (1993). Endocarditis caused by *Neisseria elongata* subspecies nitroreducens: case report and literature review. *Eur J Clin Microbiol Infect Dis* **12**: 625.

Sudduth EJ, Rozich JD, Farrar WE (1993). *Rothia dentocariosa* endocarditis complicated by perivalvular abscess. *Clin Infect Dis* **17**: 772.

Sullivan TJ (1982). Cardiac disorders in penicillin-induced anaphylaxis. Association with intravenous epinephrine therapy. *JAMA* **248**: 2161.

Sussman JI, Baron EJ, Goldberg SM *et al.* (1986). Clinical manifestations and therapy of *Lactobacillus endocarditis*: report of a case and review of the literature. *Rev Infect Dis* **8**: 771.

Sutcliffe EM, Jones DM, El Sheikh S, Percival A (1988). Penicillin insensitive meningococci in the UK. *Lancet* **i**: 657.

Sutherland R, Croydon EAP, Rolinson GN (1970). Flucloxacillin, a new isoxazolyl penicillin, compared with oxacillin, cloxacillin and dicloxacillin. *Brit Med J* **4**: 455.

Sutter VL, Finegold SM (1976). Susceptibility of anaerobic bacteria to 23 antimicrobial agents. *Antimicrob Ag Chemother* **10**: 736.

Sutter VL, Pyeatt D, Kwok YY (1981). *In vitro* susceptibility of *Capnocytophaga* strains to 18 antimicrobial agents. *Antimicrob Ag Chemother* **20**: 270.

Sutter VL, Jones MJ, Ghoneim ATM (1983). Antimicrobial susceptibilities of bacteria associated with peridontal disease. *Antimicrob Ag Chemother* **23**: 483.

Swenson JM, Thornsberry C, McCrosckey LM *et al.* (1980). Susceptibility of *Clostridium botulinum* to thirteen antimicrobial agents. *Antimicrob Ag Chemother* **18**: 13.

Swenson JM, Hill BC, Thornsberry C (1986). Screening pneumococci for penicillin resistance. *J Clin Microbiol* **24**: 749.

Swingle HM, Bucciarelli RL, Ayoub EM (1985). Synergy between penicillins and low concentrations of gentamicin in the killing of Group B streptococci. *J Infect Dis* **152**: 515.

Sykes RB (1982). The classification and terminology of enzymes that hydrolyze beta-lactam antibiotics. *J Infect Dis* **145**: 762.

Symonds J (1987). Penetration of antibiotics into the respiratory tract. *Brit Med J* **294**: 1181.

Syrogiannopoulos GA, Lourida AN, Theodoridou MC *et al.* (1994). Dexamethasone therapy for bacterial meningitis in children: 2- versus 4-day regimen. *J Infect Dis* **169**: 853.

Tabatabaie P, Syadati A (1993). Bacillus anthracis as a cause of bacterial meningitis. *Pediatr Infect Dis J* **12**: 1035.

Taber LH, Feigin RD (1979). Spirochetal infections. *Ped Clin North Amer* **26**: 377.

Takata N, Suginaka H, Kotani S *et al.* (1981). Beta-lactam resistance in *Serratia marcescens*: comparison of action of benzylpenicillin, apalcillin, cefazolin and ceftizoxime. *Antimicrob Ag Chemother* **19**: 397.

Talan DA, Hoffman JR, Yoshikawa TT, Overturf GD (1988). Role of empiric parenteral antibiotics prior to lumbar puncture in suspected bacterial meningitis: state of the art. *Rev Infect Dis* **10**: 365.

Tally FP, Jacobus NV, Bartlett JG, Gorbach SL (1975). *In vitro* activity of penicillins against anaerobes. *Antimicrob Ag Chemother* **7**: 413.

Tan R, White V, Servais G, Bryce EA (1994). Postoperative endophthalmitis caused by *Stomatococcus mucilaginosus*. *Clin Infect Dis* **18**: 492.

Tanz RR, Shulman ST, Barthel MJ *et al.* (1985). Penicillin plus rifampin eradicates pharyngeal carriage of Group A streptococci. *J Pediatr* **106**: 876.

Tarlow MJ (1991). Adjunct therapy in bacterial meningitis. *J Antimicrob Chemother* **28**: 329.

Taryle DA, Good JT Jr, Morgan EJ III *et al.* (1981). Antibiotic concentrations in human parapneumonic effusions. *J Antimicrob Chemother* **7**: 171.

Tattersall MHN, Battersby G, Spiers ASD (1972). Antibiotics and hypokalaemia. *Lancet* **i**: 630.

Teklu B, Habte-Michael A, Warrell DA *et al.* (1983). Meptazinol diminishes the Jarisch-Herxheimer reaction of relapsing fever. *Lancet* **i**: 835.

Telzak EE, Greenberg MSZ, Harrison J *et al.* (1991). Syphilis treatment response in HIV-infected individuals. *AIDS* **5**: 591.

Tempest B, Carney JP, Eberle B (1974). Distribution of the sensitivities to penicillin of types of *Diplococcus pneumoniae* in an American Indian population. *J Infect Dis* **130**: 67.

Tennent RB (1980). Diagnosis and treatment of leptospirosis. *New Ethic* Oct issue: 77.

Thin RN (1989). Treatment of venereal syphilis. *J Antimicrob Chemother* **24**: 481.

Thin RN, Barlow D, Eykyn S, Phillips I (1983). Imported penicillinase producing *Neisseria gonorrhoeae* becomes endemic in London. *Brit J Vener Dis* **59**: 364.

Thomas RJ, Conwill DE, Morton DE *et al.* (1988). Penicillin prophylaxis for streptococcal infections in United States Navy and marine corps recruit camps, 1951–1985. *Rev Infect Dis* **10**: 125.

Thompson SE III, Jacobs NF Jr, Zacarias F *et al.* (1980). Gonococcal tenosynovitis – dermatitis and septic arthritis. Intravenous penicillin vs oral erythromycin. *JAMA* **244**: 1101.

Thornsberry C, Baker CN, Kirven LA (1978a). *In vitro* activity of antimicrobial agents on Legionnaires' Disease bacterium. *Antimicrob Ag Chemother* **13**: 78.

Thornsberry C, Jaffe HW, Reynolds GH *et al.* (1978b). Patient variables associated with penicillin resistance in *Neisseria gonorrhoeae*. *Antimicrob Ag Chemother* **14**: 327.

Tiley SM, Kociuba KR, Heron LG, Munro R (1993). Infective endocarditis due to nontoxigenic *Corynebacterium diphtheriae*: report of seven cases and review. *Clin Infect Dis* **16**: 271.

Timmis AD, Crofts MA, Metcalfe J *et al.* (1981). Gonococcal endocarditis with penicillin-induced bone marrow hypoplasia. *JAMA* **246**: 672.

Timewell R, Taylor E, Phillips I (1981). The beta-lactamases of *Bacteroides* species. *J Antimicrob Chemother* **7**: 137.

Tipper DJ (1979). Mode of action of beta-lactam antibiotics. *Rev Infect Dis* **1**: 39.

Tomasz A (1979). From penicillin-binding proteins to the lysis and death of bacteria. A 1979 view. *Rev Infect Dis* **1**: 434.

Tomasz A (1981). Surface components of *Streptococcus pneumoniae*. *Rev Infect Dis* **3**: 190.

Tomasz A (1982). Penicillin-binding proteins in bacteria. *Ann Intern Med* **96**: 502.

Tomasz A (1986). Penicillin-binding proteins and the antibacterial effectiveness of beta-lactam antibiotics. *Rev Infect Dis* **8** (Suppl 3): 260.

Tomasz A, Albino A, Zanati E (1970). Multiple antibiotic resistance in a bacterium with suppressed autolytic system. *Nature* **227**: 138.

Tomberlin MG, Holtom PD, Owens JL, Larsen RA (1994). Evaluation of neurosyphilis in human immunodeficiency virus-infected individuals. *Clin Infect Dis* **18**: 288.

Torres C, Tenorio C, Lantero M *et al.* (1993). High-level penicillin resistance and penicillin-gentamicin synergy in *Enterococcus faecium*. *Antimicrob Ag Chemother* **37**: 2427.

Totten PA, Vidal L, Baldwin JN (1981). Penicillin and tetracycline resistance plasmids in *Staphylococcus epidermidis*. *Antimicrob Ag Chemother* **20**: 359.

Townsend GC, Scheld WM (1993). Adjunctive therapy for bacterial meningitis: rationale for use, current status, and prospects for the future. *Clin Infect Dis* **17** (Suppl 2): 537.

Tramont EC (1976). Persistence of *Treponema pallidum* following penicillin G therapy. Report of two cases. *JAMA* **236**: 2206.

Tuazon CU, Gill V, Gill F (1986). Streptococcal endocarditis: single vs combination antibiotic therapy and role of various species. *Rev Infect Dis* **8**: 54.

Tunér K, Lindqvist L, Nord CE (1985). Purification and properties of a novel beta-lactamase from *Fusobacterium nucleatum*. *Antimicrob Ag Chemother* **27**: 943.

Tuomanen E, Gilbert K, Tomasz A (1986). Modulation of bacteriolysis by cooperative effects of penicillin-binding proteins 1a and 3 in *Escherichia coli*. *Antimicrob Ag Chemother* **30**: 659.

Tuomanen E, Pollack H, Parkinson A *et al.* (1988). Microbiological and clinical significance of a new property of defective lysis in clinical strains of pneumococci. *J Infect Dis* **158**: 36.

Twort CHC (1981). Group R streptococcal meningitis (*Streptococcus suis* type 11): a new industrial disease? *Brit Med J* **282**: 523.

Uriz S, Pineda V, Grau M *et al.* (1991). *Neisseria meningitidis* with reduced sensitivity to penicillin: observations in 10 children. *Scand J Infect Dis* **23**: 171.

Van Asselt GJ, de Kort G, van de Klundert JAM (1995). Differences in penicillin-binding protein patterns of penicillin tolerant and non-tolerant Group A streptococci. *J Antimicrob Chemother* **35**: 67.

Van der Meer JTM, van Wijk W, Thompson J *et al.* (1992). Awareness of need and actual use of prophylaxis: lack of patient compliance in the prevention of bacterial endocarditis. *J Antimicrob Chemother* **29**: 187.

Van der Valk PGM, Kraai EJ, Van Voorst Vader PC *et al.* (1988). Penicillin concentrations in cerebrospinal fluid (CSF). during repository treatment regimen for syphilis. *Genitourin Med* **64**: 223.

Van Embden JDA, Van Klingeren B, Dessens-Kroon M, Van Wijngaarden LJ (1980). Penicillinase-producing *Neisseria gonorrhoeae* in the Netherlands: epidemiology and genetic and molecular characterization of their plasmids. *Antimicrob Ag Chemother* **18**: 789.

Van Embden JDA, Van Klingeren B, Dessens-Kroon M, Van Wijngaarden LJ (1981). Emergence in the Netherlands of penicillinase-producing gonococci carrying 'Africa' plasmid in combination with transfer plasmid. *Lancet* **i**: 938.

Van Embden JDA, Dessens-Kroon M, Van Klingeren B (1985). A new beta-lactamase plasmid in *Neisseria gonorrhoeae*. *J Antimicrob Chemother* **15**: 247.

Van Esso D, Fontanals D, Uriz S *et al.* (1987). *Neisseria meningitidis* strains with decreased susceptibility to penicillin. *Pediatr Infect Dis J* **6**: 438.

Van Klingeren B, Van Wijngaarden LJ, Dessens-Kroon M, Van Embden JDA (1983). Penicillinase-producing gonococci in the Netherlands in 1981. *J Antimicrob Chemother* **11**: 15.

Van Klingeren B, Ansink-Schipper MC, Doornbos L *et al.* (1988). Surveillance of the antibiotic susceptibility of non-penicillinase producing *Neisseria gonorrhoeae* in the Netherlands from 1983–1986. *J Antimicrob Chemother* **21**: 737.

Van Oppen C, Feldman R (1993). Antibiotic prophylaxis of neonatal group B streptococcal infections. *Brit Med J* **306**: 411.

Van Winkelhoff AJ, Overbeek BP, Pavicic MJAMP *et al.* (1993). Long-standing bacteremia caused by oral *Actinobacillus actinomycetemcomitans* in a patient with a pacemaker. *Clin Infect Dis* **16**: 216.

Vartian C, Lerner PI, Schlaes DM, Gopalakrishna KV (1985). Infections due to Lancefield Group G streptococci. *Medicine* **64**: 75.

Venditti M, Baiocchi P, Santini C *et al.* (1989). Antimicrobial susceptibilities of *Streptococcus* species that cause septicemia in neutropenic patients. *Antimicrob Ag Chemother* **33**: 580.

Venditti M, Gelfusa V, Torasi A *et al.* (1990). Antimicrobial susceptibilities of *Erysipelothrix rhusiopathiae*. *Antimicrob Ag Chemother* **34**: 2038.

Venezio FR, Gullberg RM, Westenfelder GO *et al.* (1986). Group G streptococcal endocarditis and bacteremia. *Amer J Med* **81**: 29.

Verghese A, Berk SL, Boelen LJ, Smith JK (1982). Group B streptococcal pneumonia in the elderly. *Arch Intern Med* **142**: 1642.

Verghese A, Mireault K, Arbeit RD (1986). Group B streptococcal bacteremia in men. *Rev Infect Dis* **8**: 912.

Versalovic J, Kapur V, Mason EO *et al.* (1993). Penicillin-resistant *Streptococcus pneumoniae* strains recovered in Houston: identification and molecular characterizations of multiple clones. *J Infect Dis* **167**: 850.

Vicente MF, Pérez-Diaz JC, Baquero F *et al.* (1990). Penicillin-binding protein 3 of *Listeria monocytogenes* as the primary lethal target for beta-lactams. *Antimicrob Ag Chemother* **34**: 539.

Vikerfors T, Rudback N (1987). *Borrelia* meningoradiculitis with severe pain. *Scand J Infect Dis* **19**: 701.

Viladrich PF, Pallares R, Ariza J *et al.* (1986). Four days of penicillin therapy for meningococcal meningitis. *Arch Intern Med* **146**: 2380.

Von Eiff C, Herrmann M, Peters G (1995). Antimicrobial susceptibilities of *Stomatococcus mucilaginosus* and of *Micrococcus* spp. *Antimicrob Ag Chemother* **39**: 268.

Von Konow L, Nord CE (1983). Ornidazole compared to phenoxymethyl-penicillin in the treatment of orofacial infections. *J Antimicrob Chemother* **11**: 207.

Waldvogel FA (1982). The future of beta-lactam antibiotics. *Rev Infect Dis* **4** (Suppl): 491.

Walker CK, Kahn JG, Washington AE *et al.* (1993). Pelvic inflammatory disease: metaanalysis of antimicrobial regimen efficacy. *J Infect Dis* **168**: 969.

Wallmark GI, Aremark I, Telander B (1978). *Staphylococcus saprophyticus*: a frequent cause of acute urinary tract infection among female outpatients. *J Infect Dis* **138**: 791.

Waltman WDII, Talkington DF, Lipinski AE *et al.* (1992). Evidence for a clonal origin of relative penicillin resistance among type 9L pneumococci in Northwestern Canada. *J Infect Dis* **165**: 671.

Ward J (1981). Antibiotic-resistant *Streptococcus pneumoniae*: clinical and epidemiologic aspects. *Rev Infect Dis* **3**: 254.

Ward JI, Moellering RC Jr (1981). Susceptibility of pneumococci to 14 beta-lactam agents: comparison of strains resistant, intermediate-resistant, and susceptible to penicillin. *Antimicrob Ag Chemother* **20**: 204.

Washington AE (1982). Update on treatment recommendations for gonococcal infections. *Rev Infect Dis* **4** (Suppl): 758.

Watanakunakorn C (1974). Streptococcus bovis endocarditis. *Amer J Med* **56**: 256.

Watanakunakorn C (1979). Are wall-defective microbial variants important in clinical infectious diseases? *J Antimicrob Chemother* **5**: 239.

Watanakunakorn C, Pantelakis J (1993). Alpha-hemolytic streptococcal bacteremia: a review of 203 episodes during 1980–1991. *Scand J Infect Dis* **25**: 403.

Watanakunakorn C, Patel R (1993). Comparison of patients with enterococcal bacteremia due to strains with and without high-level resistance to gentamicin. *Clin Infect Dis* **17**: 74.

Watkins DA, Chahine A, Creger RJ *et al.* (1993). *Corynebacterium striatum*: a diphtheroid with pathogenic potential. *Clin Infect Dis* **17**: 21.

Watt G, Padre LP, Tuazon ML *et al.* (1988). Placebo-controlled trial of intravenous penicillin for severe and late leptospirosis. *Lancet* **i**: 433.

Weber DA, Goering RV (1988). Tn 4201, a beta-lactamase transposon in *Staphylococcus aureus*. *Antimicrob Ag Chemother* **32**: 1164.

Weber DJ, Wolfson JS, Swartz MN, Hooper DC (1984). *Pasteurella multocida* infections. Report of 34 cases and review of the literature. *Medicine* **63**: 133.

Weber DJ, Saviteer SM, Rutala WA, Thomann C (1988). *In vitro* susceptibility of *Bacillus* spp. to selected antimicrobial agents. *Antimicrob Ag Chemother* **32**: 642.

Weber JT, Goodpasture HC, Alexander H *et al.* (1993). Wound botulism in a patient with a tooth abscess: case report and review. *Clin Infect Dis* **16**: 635.

Weingarten RD, Markiewicz Z, Gilbert DN (1990). Meningitis due to penicillin-resistant *Streptococcus pneumoniae* in adults. *Rev Infect Dis* **12**: 118.

Weinstein L, Dalton AC (1968). Host determinants of response to antimicrobial agents. *New Engl J Med* **279**: 524.

Weinstein L, Lerner PI, Chew WH (1964). Clinical and bacteriologic studies of the effect of 'massive' doses of penicillin G on infections caused by Gram-negative bacilli. *New Engl J Med* **271**: 525.

Weinstein MP, Stratton CW, Ackley A *et al.* (1985). Multicenter collaborative evaluation of a standardized serum bactericidal test as a prognostic indicator in infective endocarditis. *Amer J Med* **78**: 262.

Weir MR, Fearnow RG (1983). Transverse myelitis and penicillin. *Pediatrics* **71**: 988.

Welch H (1954). *Principles and Practice of Antibiotic Therapy* pp. 46, 66, 74. New York: Medical Encyclopedias Inc.

Wessels MR, Kasper DL (1993). The changing spectrum of Group B streptococcal disease. *New Engl J Med* **328**: 1843.

Westerink MAJ, Amsterdam D, Petell RJ *et al.* (1987). Septicemia due to DF-2 Cause of false-positive cryptococcal latex agglutination result. *Amer J Med* **83**: 155.

White JM, Brown DL, Hepner GW, Worlledge SM (1968). Penicillin induced haemolytic anaemia. *Brit Med J* **3**: 26.

Whitman MS, Pitsakis PG, Zausner A *et al.* (1993). Antibiotic treatment of experimental endocarditis due to vancomycin- and ampicillin-resistant *Enterococcus faecium*. *Antimicrob Ag Chemother* **37**: 2069.

Whittington WL, Knapp JS (1988). Trends in resistance of *Neisseria gonorrhoeae* to antimicrobial agents in the United States. *Sex Transm Dis* **15**: 202.

Wickerts CJ, Asaba H, Gunnarsson B *et al.* (1980). Combined carbon haemoperfusion and haemodialysis in treatment of penicillin intoxication. *Brit Med J* **280**: 1254.

Wilcox MH, Winstanley TG, Douglas CWI, Spencer RC (1993). Susceptibility of alpha-haemolytic streptococci causing endocarditis to benzylpenicillin and ten cephalosporins. *J Antimicrob Chemother* **32**: 63.

Wilcox RR (1981). Treatment of syphilis. *Bull Wld Hlth Org* **59**: 655.

Wilcox RR (1985). Mass treatment campaigns against the endemic treponematoses. *Rev Infect Dis* **7** (Suppl 2): 278.

William DC, Felman YM, Corsaro MC (1979). *Neisseria meningitidis.* Probable pathogen in two related cases of urethritis, epididymitis and acute pelvic inflammatory disease. *JAMA* **242**: 1653.

Williams CL, Strobino B, Lee A *et al.* (1990). Lyme disease in childhood: clinical and epidemiological features of ninety cases. *Pediatr Infect Dis J* **9**: 10.

Wilson WR (1987). Antimicrobial therapy of streptococcal endocarditis. *J Antimicrob Chemother* **20** (Suppl A): 147.

Wilson WR, Thompson RL, Wilkowske CJ *et al.* (1981). Short-term therapy for streptococcal infective endocarditis. Combined intramuscular administration of penicillin and streptomycin. *JAMA* **245**: 360.

Wilson WR, Wilkowske CJ, Wright AJ *et al.* (1984). Treatment of streptomycin-susceptible and streptomycin-resistant enterococcal endocarditis. *Ann Intern Med* **100**: 816.

Wilson WR, Zak O, Sande MA (1985). Penicillin therapy for treatment of experimental endocarditis caused by viridans streptococci in animals. *J Infect Dis* **151**: 1028.

Winslow DL, Damme J, Dieckman E (1983). Delayed bactericidal activity of betalactam antibiotics against *Listeria monocytogenes*: antagonism of chloramphenicol and rifampin. *Antimicrob Ag Chemother* **23**: 555.

Winstanley TG (1990). Penicillin-induced post-antibiotic effects on streptococci *in vitro* and *in vivo*. *J Antimicrob Chemother* **26**: 165.

Winterscheid KK, Whitington WL, Roberts MC *et al.* (1994). Decreased susceptibility to penicillin G and Tet M plasmids in genital and anorectal isolates of *Neisseria meningitidis*. *Antimicrob Ag Chemother* **38**: 1661.

Wisseman CL Jr, Silverman DJ, Waddell A, Brown DT (1982). Penicillin-induced unstable intracellular formation of spheroplasts by rickettsiae. *J Infect Dis* **146**: 147.

Woods CR, Smith AL, Wasilauskas BL *et al.* (1994). Invasive disease caused by *Neisseria meningitidis* relatively resistant to penicillin in North Carolina. *J Infect Dis* **170**: 433.

Woolfrey BF, Lally RT, Gresser-Burns M (1988). Penicillin tolerance in Group A streptococci. *J Infect Dis* **158**: 487.

Word BM, Klein JO (1988). Current therapy of bacterial sepsis and meningitis in infants and children: a poll of directors of programs in pediatric infectious diseases. *Pediatr Infect Dis J* **7**: 267.

Yeung K-H, Dillon JR, Pauze M, Wallace E (1986). A novel 49 – kilobase plasmid associated with an outbreak of penicillinase-producing *Neisseria gonorrhoeae*. *J Infect Dis* **153**: 1162.

Yoder EL, Mendez J, Khatib R (1987). Spontaneous gangrenous myositis induced by *Streptococcus pyogenes*: case report and review of the literature. *Rev Infect Dis* **9**: 382.

Yoshida S-I, Urabe S, Mizuguchi Y (1982). Antibiotic sensitivity patterns of penicillinase-positive and penicillinase-negative strains of *Neisseria gonorrhoeae* isolated in Fukuoka, Japan. *Brit J Vener Dis* **58**: 305.

Young EJ, Fainstein V, Musher DM (1982a). Drug-induced fever: cases seen in the evaluation of unexplained fever in a general hospital population. *Rev Infect Dis* **4**: 69.

Young EJ, Weingarten NM, Baughn RE, Duncan WC (1982b). Studies on the pathogenesis of the Jarisch-Herxheimer reaction: development of an animal model and evidence against a role for classical endotoxin. *J Infect Dis* **146**: 606.

Zenker PN, Rolfs RT(1990). Treatment of syphilis, 1989. *Rev Infect Dis* **12** (Suppl 6): 590.

Zhang Q-Y, Jones DM, Saez Nieto JA *et al.* (1990). Genetic diversity of penicillin-binding protein 2 genes of penicillin-resistant strains of *Neisseria meningitidis* revealed by fingerprinting of amplified DNA. *Antimicrob Ag Chemother* **34**: 1523.

Zighelboim S, Tomasz A (1980). Penicillin-binding proteins of multiply antibiotic-resistant South African strains of *Streptococcus pneumoniae*. *Antimicrob Ag Chemother* **17**: 434.

Zighelboim S, Tomasz A (1981). Multiple antibiotic resistance in South African strains of *Streptococcus pneumoniae*: mechanisms of resistance to beta-lactam antibiotics. *Rev Infect Dis* **3**: 267.

Zimmerman W (1980). Penetration of beta-lactam antibiotics into their target enzymes in *Pseudomonas aerguinosa*: comparison of a highly sensitive mutant with its parent strain. *Antimicrob Ag Chemother* **18**: 94.

Zscheck KK, Hull R, Murray BE (1988). Restriction mapping and hybridization studies of a beta-lactamase-encoding fragment from *Streptococcus (Enterococcus) faecalis*. *Antimicrob Ag Chemother* **32**: 768.

Zygmunt DJ, Stratton CW, Kernodle DS (1992). Characterization of four beta-lactamases produced by *Staphylococcus aureus*. *Antimicrob Ag Chemother* **36**: 440.

Phenoxypenicillins

Description

Four acid-stable phenoxypenicillins have been developed, which are all suitable for oral administration. In general, their clinical use is restricted for the treatment of minor infections and chemoprophylaxis.

1 Phenoxymethylpenicillin (penicillin V)

This was introduced in 1953 (Spitzy, 1953), and has been widely used as an 'oral penicillin'. Penicillin V, like G, is a natural penicillin produced biosynthethically. It is obtained if the precursor, phenoxyacetic acid, is added to the fermentation medium, while addition of phenylacetic acid results in production of penicillin G.

2 Phenoxyethylpenicillin (phenethicillin)

With the discovery of the penicillin nucleus, 6-APA (Batchelor *et al.*, 1959) (p. 3), it became possible to synthesize new penicillins by the introduction of side-chains. Phenoxyethylpenicillin, an oral penicillin analogous to penicillin V was the first penicillin produced semisynthetically. It was introduced by Beecham Research Laboratories in 1959 (Rolinson, 1979).

3 Phenoxypropylpenicillin and phenoxybenzylpenicillin (propicillin and phenbenicillin)

These semisynthetic penicillins, analogous to penicillin V, were introduced in the early 1960s. Although they are better absorbed from the gastrointestinal tract (Fig. I.2), overall they are inferior to phenoxymethylpenicillin and phenoxyethylpenicillin because of their lower antibacterial activity (Bond *et al.*, 1963). They are therefore no longer used.

Penicillin V and phenethicillin are very similar, but differ slightly in their antibacterial activity and absorption from the gastrointestinal tract. They are both marketed as potassium salts.

Sensitive Organisms

The range of antimicrobial activity of the phenoxypenicillins is generally similar to that of penicillin G (p. 4).

These compounds are active against Gram-positive cocci, such as *Streptococcus pyogenes*, *Strep. pneumoniae*, non-penicillinase (beta-lactamase)-producing *Staphylococcus aureus*, *Strep. viridans* and anaerobic streptococci. Beta-lactamase-producing *Staph. aureus* strains are resistant. Gram-positive bacilli, such as *Clostridium tetani*, *Cl. perfringens*, *Cl. diphtheriae* and *Bacillus anthracis*, are also sensitive.

Among Gram-negative bacteria, both *Neisseria meningitidis* and Pen G-sensitive *N. gonorrhoeae* (p. 14) are susceptible to a degree, *Haemophilus influenzae* is moderately resistant, and all other aerobic Gram-negative bacilli are highly resistant. Anaerobic Gram-negative bacilli which reside in the upper respiratory tract, may be sensitive to these penicillins, but some of these have become beta-lactamase producers (p. 17) and are therefore resistant; *Bacteroides fragilis* is always resistant (Busch *et al.*, 1976).

There are some important differences between the activity of penicillin G (p. 4) and these compounds and also some slight differences between the two phenoxypenicillins. Their activity against streptococci, pneumococci and non-beta-lactamase-producing staphylococci, decreases in the order penicillin G, penicillin V and phenethicillin. Penicillin G is about 4-fold more active than penicillin V against meningococci and gonococci and phenethicillin is even less active than penicillin V (Garrod, 1960b). The activity of penicillin G against *H. influenzae* is 4- to 8-fold greater than that of penicillin V or phenethicillin (Table I.3).

Table I.3 shows the MICs of penicillin G and the two phenoxypenicillins against some selected bacteria.

Organism	MIC (μg per ml)		
	Penicillin G	Penicillin V	Phenethicillin
Gram-positive bacteria			
Staphylococcus aureus (non- penicillinase producer)	0.03	0.03	0.03
Streptococcus pyogenes	0.007	0.015	0.03
Streptococcus pneumoniae	0.015	0.03	0.06
Enterococcus faecalis	2.0	4.0	4.0
Bacillus anthracis	0.015	0.015	0.06
Corynebacterium diphtheriae	0.06	0.03	0.12
Gram-negative bacteria			
Escherichia coli	64.0	128.0	512.0
Salmonella typhi	4.0	64.0	256.0
Neisseria gonorrhoeae	0.007	0.03	0.12
Neisseria meningitidis	0.03	0.25	1.0
Haemophilus influenzae	1.0	4.0	4.0

Table I.3
Compiled from data published by Garrod (1960a,b) and Barber and Waterworth (1962)

Mode of Administration and Dosage

These drugs are administered by the oral route. The dosage for children under 5 years is 125 mg, and for children over 5 years and adults, 250–500 mg, administered 6-hourly. These drugs should be given when fasting, preferably about 1 h before meals. Higher doses may be used for the treatment of more serious infections.

Several studies have shown that oral penicillin V is effective in streptococcal pharyngitis and bacterial upper respiratory tract infections if the total daily dose is administered in two divided doses instead of three or four divided doses (Gerber and Markowitz, 1985; Fyllingen *et al.*, 1991a,b). In another study in children 250 mg of penicillin V given twice-daily was found to be equally effective as 250 mg given three times daily for the treatment of streptococcal pharyngitis (Gerber *et al.*, 1985).

Serum Levels in Relation to Dosage

After oral administration of these compounds (Fig. I.2), peak serum levels are obtained within 30–60 min. Phenethicillin produces higher and more prolonged levels than penicillin V. Doubling the usual doses of these two penicillins, approximately doubles the serum concentrations.

There is considerable variation in the absorption of oral phenoxypenicillins, and some patients for reasons unexplained, absorb them poorly. Diarrhea of short duration does not influence the absorption of oral penicillins, but if diarrhea persists for a week, absorption is usually reduced (Bolme and Eriksson, 1975). Similarly, oral penicillin absorption is reduced in patients with celiac disease and other malabsorption states (Prescott, 1974; Bolme and Eriksson, 1978). Peak serum levels may be three times higher and the total amount of a phenoxypenicillin absorbed about doubled, if the dose is taken 1 h before meals rather than with food (Bell, 1970; Welling and Tse, 1982). This also applies to the absorption of penicillin V suspensions in children (McCracken *et al.*, 1978).

Excretion

1 Urine

About 20–40% of a given dose can be recovered from urine during the first 6 h. The drugs are mainly excreted unchanged, but small amounts of antibacterially active breakdown products are also present in the urine (Bond *et al.*, 1963). Renal tubular secretion of the phenoxypenicillins can be partially blocked by probenecid (p. 24).

2 Bile

Only small amounts are excreted in the bile, mainly in the unchanged form.

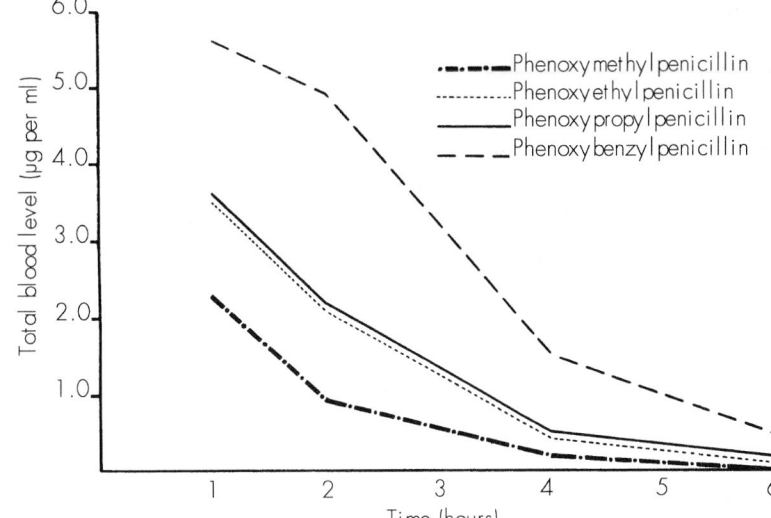

Fig. I.2. Mean blood levels of total antibiotic after a single oral dose of 250 mg in 19 subjects. (After Bond *et al.*, 1963, with permission from the BMJ Publishing Group.)

Distribution of the Drugs in Body

Phenoxypenicillins, like penicillin G, diffuse readily into pleural, pericardial, ascitic and synovial fluids and pass into the fetal circulation. There is very little penetration of the phenoxypenicillins into the CSF if the meninges are uninflamed. Penicillin V penetrates poorly into maxillary sinus secretions (Lundberg and Malmborg, 1973). In inflamed tonsillar tissue the concentration is about 20% of the serum level at that time (Roos *et al.*, 1986).

Penicillin V is 80% and phenethicillin is 75% bound to serum proteins (Bond *et al.*, 1963). These values are higher than other reported figures, but in this study human sera with low penicillin concentrations, similar to those which would be found *in vivo*, were used. If serum protein binding is estimated at a very high penicillin concentration, lower percentages of serum binding are obtained. The clinical significance of protein binding of these and other penicillins is discussed on p. 95.

Mode of Action

The mode of action of phenoxypenicillins is similar to penicillin G (p. 25).

Toxicity

1 Gastrointestinal side-effects

Transient disturbances, such as nausea and diarrhea, can follow administration of these drugs. Moniliasis may also occur. Pseudomembranous colitis (p. 594) developed in one 12-year-old girl following a 4-day course of oral phenoxymethylpenicillin (Larson *et al.*, 1977). Transient right-sided colitis occurred in two young female patients after ingestion of these drugs (Barrison and Kane, 1978).

2 Hypersensitivity reactions

These may occur in penicillin-sensitive patients. Phenoxypenicillins may be cross-allergenic with penicillin G and also with all other penicillins.

a Anaphylaxis This is much less common with the oral phenoxypenicillins than with parenteral penicillin G (p. 29). In one patient symptoms started 30 min after ingestion of 500 mg of penicillin V (Coates, 1963). In another patient generalized pruritus and flushing commenced within 3 min of ingestion of a tablet of penicillin V. This was followed by abdominal cramps, nausea and vomiting; she received medical treatment 30 min after the dose when she was semiconscious, cyanosed with tachycardia and hypotension. She responded to standard resuscitative measures (p. 29) (Simmonds *et al.*, 1978).

b Serum sickness This is quite common, and reactions are similar to those which occur after penicillin G (p. 30).

3 Direct toxicity

Oral penicillins are of low toxicity, but massive doses, like those used with penicillin G (p. 32), have not been administered to humans. Penicillin V and phenethicillin are well tolerated orally in doses of 6 g per day.

4 Hemolytic anemia

One case has been reported in a 3-year-old boy who was treated by penicillin V in a dose of 125 mg 6-hourly (Bird et al., 1975). This was an immune hemolytic anemia due to a penicillin antibody of the IgM class. Antibodies of the IgM class may also be implicated in hemolytic anemias following penicillin G administration in ordinary doses, but more commonly hemolytic anemia induced by penicillin G is a sequel to large doses and antibody of the IgG class is involved (p. 33).

5 Jaundice

Beeley et al. (1976) reported one adult patient, who developed liver damage as part of a severe hypersensitivity reaction to penicillin V.

6 Cation toxicity

All the phenoxypenicillins are marketed as potassium salts. Doses employed (up to 8 g per day) would not cause potassium intoxication, unless there is serious renal insufficiency.

Clinical uses of the Drugs

1 Streptococcus pyogenes and Strep. pneumoniae infections

Phenoxypenicillins are suitable for the oral treatment of mild or convalescent infections due to Strep. pyogenes, such as pharyngitis, scarlet fever and cellulitis. Mild or moderate acute streptococcal pharyngitis in children can usually be successfully treated by one of these drugs, provided that parents are instructed on the importance of regular medication (Colcher and Bass, 1972). Despite some previous doubts, it has been demonstrated that oral penicillin V therapy has a definite beneficial impact on the clinical course of Strep. pyogenes pharyngitis (Randolph et al., 1985). Patients with streptococcal pharyngitis should be treated for 10 days. A randomized trial of a 7- versus 10-day therapy of streptococcal pharyngitis with penicillin V showed that 31% of patients who received the shorter course compared with 18% of those receiving the 10-day course, had positive post-treatment cultures (Schwartz et al., 1981). The appreciable failure rate after even 10 days of oral penicillin is of some concern. At times when Strep. pyogenes infections are prevalent, some so-called treatment failures may well be reinfections (Roos et al., 1985). In one study it was demonstrated that relapses or reinfections were significantly fewer in children in whom penicillin V treatment for streptococcal pharyngitis was delayed until day 3 of symptoms, compared with those in whom treatment was started immediately. Early treatment apparently diminishes immunity to this organism and so increases the risk of recurrences. The authors also found that the delay in initiating penicillin treatment resulted in persistent acute symptoms (Pichichero et al., 1987). The clinician thus has to consider both the beneficial and the adverse consequences of delaying penicillin treatment in this disease. Despite the fact that in recent trials, some oral cephalosporins (p. 416) appeared better than penicillin V for this disease, penicillin still remains the drug of choice (Shulman et al., 1994).

The management of the Group A streptococcal carrier state is discussed on p. 35. An epidemic of streptococcal pharyngitis in a closed community may be hard to control by treatment of cases and carriers alone, and full penicillin prophylaxis to all subjects on entry may be essential (Colling et al., 1982).

Phenoxypenicillins are suitable for the treatment of mild or convalescent pneumococcal infections, such as bronchitis, pneumonia, sinusitis and otitis media. In young children, bronchitis and especially otitis media is frequently caused by H. influenzae, and in these, results of treatment with oral phenoxypenicillins are poor, as serum levels attained following usual doses are rarely high enough to inhibit this pathogen (Kamme and Lundgren, 1971; Laurin et al., 1985).

Although some authors have obtained satisfactory results with oral penicillin V in patients with community acquired pneumococcal pneumonia (Fredlund et al., 1987), parenteral penicillin G is a more reliable drug for the treatment of severe pneumococcal infections, as absorption of oral phenoxypenicillins is variable (p. 72). Oral therapy with penicillin V or phenethicillin is therefore only recommended for relatively mild infections, or for late treatment of more severe infections, after a favorable clinical response has been obtained with parenteral penicillin G.

Long-term penicillin prophylaxis may be useful in some patients who are prone to recurrent streptococcal cellulitis, such as those with lymphedema of the arms or legs. Similar chemoprophylaxis is useful to prevent overwhelming pneumococcal sepsis in children and adults who have had a splenectomy. It is even more important in children with sickle cell disease who have a defective splenic function. In these children prophylaxis should be initiated at 4 months of age; its optimal duration is not known but it should continue beyond the age of 3 (Buchanan *et al.*, 1982; Gaston *et al.*, 1986; Powars and Overturf, 1987; Wong *et al.*, 1992; Read and Finch, 1994). This chemoprophylaxis can also be carried out by i.m. benzathine penicillin G, (p. 51). Similar chemoprophylaxis with oral penicillin V has also been successful in preventing pneumococcal septicemia in children with HIV infection (Peters *et al.*, 1994). But this adds yet another medication to the regimen, and the difficulties include problems with compliance, drug interactions and antibiotic resistance (Gesner *et al.*, 1994).

2 Bacterial meningitis

Oral phenoxypenicillins are not recommended for treatment of any stage of this disease. It appears that recurrent pneumococcal meningitis related to a previous head injury, can be prevented by long-term oral penicillin prophylaxis (Levin *et al.*, 1972). Data from controlled studies on the efficacy of such chemoprophylaxis are not available. Some authors advise against such oral penicillin use, as administration of prophylactic antibiotics may be associated with a greater incidence of infection due to resistant organisms (Pappas *et al.*, 1993).

3 Rheumatic fever chemoprophylaxis

Long-term administration of one of the penicillins, is recommended for patients who have had prior rheumatic fever to prevent recurrence of the disease (Leading article, 1982). Monthly i.m. injections of 1.2 million units (0.9 g) of benzathine penicillin G can be used for this purpose (p. 51). If compliance can be assured oral chemotherapy is often preferred, in which case penicillin V or phenethicillin is recommended (Garrod, 1975). The usual adult dosage is 0.5 g daily given in two divided doses. In patients receiving long-term penicillin chemoprophylaxis, oral *Strep. viridans* strains often become penicillin-resistant (Parillo *et al.*, 1979), and drugs other than one of the penicillins should be used for short-term endocarditis prophylaxis (p. 44).

Individuals who have reached their early 20s, with their most recent attack being more than 5 years previously, and who did not have carditis with their previous attack(s), and are free from rheumatic heart disease, can discontinue their rheumatic fever prophylaxis with relative safety (Berrios *et al.*, 1993).

4 Endocarditis chemoprophylaxis

Oral penicillin V was used for this purpose, but because of its better absorption from the gastrointestinal tract, oral amoxycillin is now preferred (p. 43).

5 Whipple's disease and Lyme disease

One of the oral phenoxypenicillins is useful for the long-term treatment of Whipple's disease (p. 51). They are also useful for the treatment of early manifestations of Lyme disease (Strle *et al.*, 1992) (p. 48).

6 Comparative efficacy of penicillin V and phenethicillin

This has not been determined by clinical trials, but many years' experience indicates that they are of about the same value. Phenethicillin is better absorbed than penicillin V (p. 72), but it has lower intrinsic antibacterial activity (p. 71). An *in vitro* comparison of these compounds by Bond *et al.* (1963) predicted that they would be about equally effective.

References

Barber M, Waterworth PM (1962). Antibacterial activity of the penicillins. *Brit Med J* 1: 1159.

Barrison IG, Kane SP (1978). Penicillin-associated colitis. *Lancet* ii: 843.

Batchelor FR, Doyle FP, Nayler JHC, Rolinson GN (1959). Synthesis of penicillin: 6-aminopenicillanic acid in penicillin fermentation. *Nature (Lond)* 183: 257.

Beeley L, Gourevitch A, Kendall MJ (1976). Jaundice after oral penicillin. *Lancet* ii: 1297.

Bell SM (1970). Supervision of antibiotic treatment – an important medical responsibility. *Aspects of Infection*, p. 107. Auckland, Sydney and Melbourne: Proc Symp.

Berrios X, del Campo E, Guzman B, Bisno AL (1993). Discontinuing rheumatic fever prophylaxis in selected adolescents and young adults. *Ann Intern Med* 118: 401.

Bird GWG, McEvoy MW, Wingham J (1975). Acute haemolytic anaemia due to IgM penicillin antibody in a 3-year-old child: a sequel to oral penicillin. *J Clin Path* 28: 321.

Bolme P, Eriksson M (1975). Influence of diarrhoea on the oral absorption of penicillin V and ampicillin in children. *Scand J Infect Dis* 7: 141.

Bolme P, Eriksson M (1978). Absorption of phenoxymethylpenicillin in children The influence of age, state of disease and pharmaceutical preparation. *Scand J Infect Dis* 10: 223.

Bond JM, Lightbown JW, Barber M, Waterworth PM (1963). A comparison of four phenoxypenicillins. *Brit Med J* 2: 956.

Buchanan GR, Siegel JD, Smith SJ, De Passe BM (1982). Oral penicillin prophylaxis in children with impaired splenic function: a study of compliance. *Pediatrics* 70: 926.

Busch DF, Kureshi LA, Sutter VL, Finegold SM (1976). Susceptibility of respiratory tract anaerobes to orally administered penicillins and cephalosporins. *Antimicrob Ag Chemother* 10: 713.

Coates WH (1963). Anaphylactic shock following the administration of oral penicillin. *Med J Aust* 1: 967.

Colcher IS, Bass JW (1972). Penicillin treatment of streptococcal pharyngitis. *JAMA* 222: 657.

Colling A, Kerr I, Maxted WR, Widdowson JP (1982). Minimum amount of penicillin prophylaxis required to control *Streptococcus pyogenes* epidemic in closed community. *Brit Med J* 285: 95.

Fredlund H, Bodin L, Back E et al. (1987). Antibiotic therapy in pneumonia: a comparative study of parenteral and oral administration of penicillin. *Scand J Infect Dis* 19: 459.

Fyllingen G, Arnesen AR, Biermann C et al. (1991a). Phenoxymethylpenicillin two or three times daily for tonsillitis with beta-haemolytic streptococci Group A: a blinded, randomized and controlled clinical sudy. *Scand J Infect Dis* 23: 553.

Fyllingen G, Arnesen AR, Ronnevig J (1991b). Phenoxymethylpenicillin two or three times daily in bacterial upper respiratory tract infections: a blinded, randomized and controlled clinical study. *Scand J Infect Dis* 23: 755.

Garrod LP (1960a). Relative antibacterial activity of three penicillins. *Brit Med J* 1: 527.

Garrod LP (1960b). The relative antibacterial activity of our penicillins. *Brit Med J* 2: 1695.

Garrod LP (1975). Chemoprophylaxis. *Brit Med J* 4: 561.

Gaston MH, Verter JI, Woods G et al. (1986). Prophylaxis with oral penicillin in children with sickle cell anemia. A randomized trial. *New Engl J Med* 314: 1593.

Gerber MA, Markowitz M. (1985). Management of streptococcal pharyngitis reconsidered. *Pediatr Infect Dis* 4: 518.

Gerber MA, Spadaccini LJ, Wright LL et al. (1985). Twice-daily penicillin in the treatment of streptococcal pharyngitis. *Amer J Dis Child* 139: 1145.

Gesner M, Desiderio D, Kim M et al. (1994). *Streptococcus pneumoniae* in human immunodeficiency virus type 1-infected children. *Pediatr Infect Dis J* 13: 697.

Kamme C, Lundgren K (1971). Frequency of typable and non-typable *Haemophilus influenzae* strains in children with acute otitis media and results of penicillin V treatment. *Scand J Infect Dis* 3: 225.

Larson HE, Parry JV, Price AB et al. (1977). Undescribed toxin in pseudomembranous colitis. *Brit Med J* 1: 1246.

Laurin L, Prellner K, Kamme C (1985). Phenoxymethylpenicillin and therapeutic failure in acute otitis media. *Scand J Infect Dis* 17: 367.

Leading Article (1982). Prevention of rheumatic heart disease. *Lancet* i: 143.

Levin S, Nelson KE, Spies HW, Lepper MH (1972). Pneumococcal meningitis: the problem of the unseen cerebrospinal fluid leak. *Amer J Med Sci* 264: 319.

Lundberg C, Malmborg AS (1973). Concentration of penicillin V and tetracycline in maxillary sinus secretion after repeated doses. *Scand J Infect Dis* 5: 123.

McCracken GH Jr, Ginsburg CM, Clahsen JC, Thomas ML (1978). Pharmacologic evaluation of orally administered antibiotics in infants and children: effect of feeding on bioavailability. *Pediatrics* 62: 738.

Pappas DGJr, Hammerschlag PE, Hammerschlag M (1993). Cerebrospinal fluid rhinorrhea and recurrent meningitis. *Clin Infect Dis* 17: 364.

Parrillo JE, Borst GC, Mazur MH et al. (1979). Endocarditis due to resistant viridans streptococci during oral penicillin chemoprophylaxis. *New Engl J Med* 300: 296.

Peters VB, Hyatt AC, Schechter C et al. (1994). Evaluation of prophylaxis against invasive pneumococcal infections in human immunodeficiency virus-infected children. *Pediatr Infect Dis J* 13: 667.

Pichichero ME, Disney FA, Talpey WB et al. (1987). Adverse and beneficial effects of immediate treatment of Group A beta-hemolytic streptococcal pharyngitis with penicillin. *Pediatr Infect Dis J* 6: 635.

Powars D, Overturf G (1987). Penicillin in sickle cell anemia. *Amer J Dis Child* 141: 250.

Prescott LF (1974). Gastrointestinal absorption of drugs. *Med Clin North Amer* 58: 907.

Randolph MF, Gerber MA, De Meo KK, Wright L (1985). Effect of antibiotic therapy on the clinical course of streptococcal pharyngitis. *J Pediatr* 106: 870.

Read RC, Finch RG (1994). Prophylaxis after splenectomy. *J Antimicrob Chemother* 33: 4.

Rolinson GN (1979). 6-APA and the development of the beta-lactam antibiotics. *J Antimicrob Chemother* 5: 7.

Roos K, Holm SE, Ekedahl C (1985). Treatment failure in acute streptococcal tonsillitis in children over the age of 10 and in adults. *Scand J Infect Dis* 17: 357.

Roos K, Grahn E, Ekedahl C, Holm SE (1986). Pharmacokinetics of phenoxymethylpenicillin in tonsils. *Scand J Infect Dis* 18: 125.

Schwartz RH, Wientzen RL Jr, Pedreira F et al (1981). Penicillin V for Group A streptococcal pharyngotonsillitis. A randomized trial of seven vs ten days' therapy. *JAMA* 246: 1790.

Shulman ST, Gerber MA, Tanz RR, Markowitz M (1994). Streptococcal pharyngitis: the case for penicillin therapy. *Pediatr Infect Dis J* 13: 1.

Simmonds J, Hodges S, Nicol F, Barnett D (1978). Anaphylaxis after oral penicillin. *Brit Med J* 2: 1404.

Spitzy KH (1953). *Wein Klin Wschr* 65: 583; quoted by Bond et al. (1963).

Strle F, Ruzic E,Cimperman J (1992). *Erythema migrans*: comparison of treatment with azithromycin, doxycycline and phenoxymethyl-penicillin. *J Antimicrob Chemother* 30: 543.

Welling PG, Tse FLS (1982). The influence of food on the absorption of antimicrobial agents. *J Antimicrob Chemother* 9: 7.

Wong W-Y, Overturf GD, Powars DR (1992). Infection caused by *Streptococcus pneumoniae* in children with sickle cell disease: epidemiology, immunological mechanisms, prophylaxis, and vaccination. *Clin Infect Dis* 14: 1124.

Methicillin

Description

Methicillin was the first penicillinase-resistant semisynthetic penicillin to be derived from the penicillin nucleus, 6-APA (p. 3) (Knudsen and Rolinson, 1960). The drug was discovered at Beecham Research Laboratories. Initially it was used widely, but because of its toxicity (p. 84), it was gradually superseded by other penicillinase-resistant penicillins, such as nafcillin (p. 102), cloxacillin and flucloxacillin (p. 102).

Sensitive Organisms

1 Antibacterial spectrum

This is similar to that of penicillin G. Methicillin is active against Gram-positive bacteria, and also against Gram-negative cocci such as meningococci and gonococci. It is some 20- to 50-fold less active than penicillin G against bacteria sensitive to both drugs (Table I.4, p. 81). Being both stable and active in the presence of staphylococcal beta-lactamase (Rolinson et al., 1960), methicillin is active against penicillin G-resistant staphylococci. Stability of the penicillinase-resistant penicillins in the presence of the enzyme is one of degree. Methicillin and nafcillin are the most stable and they are followed closely in descending order of stability by dicloxacillin, oxacillin, cloxacillin and flucloxacillin (Sabath et al., 1975; Basker et al., 1980). Reported results on such stability are conflicting, and this property is of doubtful clinical significance.

2 Methicillin-resistant Staphylococcus aureus (MRSA)

Staphylococcal resistance to methicillin is not due to the destruction of the antibiotic by a bacterial enzyme such as a beta-lactamase (p. 26), but it is intrinsic. There is no penetration barrier to methicillin in MRSA strains, but there is a marked decrease in the affinity of penicillin binding proteins (PBPs 1, 2 and 3) of MRSA for methicillin, compared with methicillin-sensitive strains (Hartman and Tomasz, 1981). In addition, in the presence of methicillin MRSA, strains synthesize a novel 78-kilodalton penicillin binding protein (PBP 2a) located between PBP 2 and PBP 3 and also synthesize a greater amount of PBP 3.

In MRSA strains both PBP 2a and PBP 3 show very low affinity for methicillin. Methicillin-resistance in MRSA strains is not only due to decreased affinity for methicillin of existing PBPs, but it is also due to synthesis of an extra PBP with very low affinity for methicillin. It may be that PBP 2a is involved in peptidoglycan synthesis, which can proceed normally in presence of methicillin (Rossi et al., 1985; Ubukata et al., 1985; Lyon and Skurray, 1987; Hackbarth and Chambers, 1989a, 1993; Hürlimann-Dalel et al., 1992). In MRSA strains this novel PBP with low affinity for methicillin probably takes over all the PBP functions; it is also produced in increased amounts under particular growth conditions such as the presence of sodium chloride and 30°C (see below) (Fontana, 1985; Chambers and Hackbarth, 1987). Strains of MRSA have a methicillin-resistant septal peptidoglycan synthetic system, and cell lysis does not occur upon treatment of MRSA with the drug (Wilkinson and Nadakavukaren, 1983). When methicillin is added even at relatively low concentrations (e.g. 5 μg per ml) to the medium, MRSA cells start producing a new peptidoglycan with an abnormal muropeptide composition. This is probably the synthetic product of PBP 2a (de Jonge and Tomasz, 1993). Also, MRSA strains are always beta-lactamase producers, thereby being penicillin G-resistant (p. 11) by two separate mechanisms (Franciolli et al., 1991).

The genes coding for the altered PBPs, the additional PBP 2a and methicillin-resistance in MRSA strains are sited on the chromosome (Lyon *et al.*, 1983; Berger-Bächi, 1989; Hackbarth and Chambers, 1989a). The gene which codes for PBP 2a production is referred to as mec A gene and this resides on the methicillin-resistance determinant (mec), which is located on a fragment of the *Staph. aureus* chromosome (Patel *et al.*, 1989; Berger-Bächi *et al.*, 1992; Ryffel *et al.*, 1992). This mec A gene was probably transferred to *Staph. aureus* from coagulase-negative staphylococci (Archer *et al.*, 1994). But at least 10–12 additional new genetic determinants, which are sited on the chromosome, are also needed for the optimal expression of methicillin-resistance (de Lencestre and Tomasz, 1994; Hackbarth *et al.*, 1994). Several additional chromosomal sites have been identified outside the mec A gene in which transposon inactivation reduced the level of beta-lactam resistance. It appeared that these determinants, rather than the quantity of PBP 2a in the bacterial cells determined the MIC value of an MRSA isolate (de Lencestre *et al.*, 1994; Sumita *et al.*, 1995). In addition beta-lactamase plasmids, which are present in most MRSA strains, play a role in the stability of the mec A gene. If plasmids are eliminated from MRSA cells, they gradually also lose the mec A gene and PBP 2a production, and thus become methicillin-susceptible (Hiramatsu *et al.*, 1990). Even though the mec A gene, which codes for PBP 2a, is located on the chromosome, it has been shown to be regulated by the penicillinase plasmid which is present in most MRSA cells (Ubukata *et al.*, 1985; Suzuki *et al.*, 1993). Plasmid-derived genes regulate the production of both PBP 2a and beta-lactamase (Boyce and Medeiros, 1987; Hackbarth and Chambers, 1993).

The MRSA strains show intrinsic resistance to all other penicillinase-resistant penicillins, such as the isoxazolyl penicillins and nafcillin, all cephalosporins, such as cephalothin and cephalexin, and also to other beta-lactam antibiotics, such as cefamandole, cefotaxime, cefoperazone, cefsulodin and moxalactam (Thompson and Wenzel, 1982; Thompson *et al.*, 1982; Hirschl *et al.*, 1984). Imipenem (p. 227) has somewhat better *in vitro* activity against MRSA strains with MICs of 1–8 μg per ml (Verbist and Verhagen 1981; Thompson *et al.*, 1982).

Methicillin-resistance in any given *Staph. aureus* culture is heterogeneous, and it is present in only a small percentage of a given *Staph. aureus* inoculum (Ryffel *et al.*, 1994). This is particularly so in cultures incubated at 37°C, so that methicillin-resistance can be overlooked by routine laboratory sensitivity tests. The MRSA component of a heterogeneous culture grows much better at 30°C, and incubation for 18 h at this temperature is the best method for its detection (Figueiredo *et al.*, 1991). The disc diffusion method is reliable for detection of methicillin-resistance if the correct antibiotic and temperature are used. Resistance is readily detected for oxacillin (1-μg disk), nafcillin (1-μg disk), and methicillin (5-μg disk) at 30 and 35°C, but may be missed at 37°C (Hackbarth and Chambers, 1989b). The pH of the medium is important for the sensitivity testing of MRSA strains, because acidity (pH 5.2) abolishes methicillin-resistance. Resistance is enhanced and more easily detected if 5% sodium chloride is added to the testing medium (Boyce *et al.*, 1982; Chambers and Hackbarth, 1987).

In MRSA strains a greater proportion of the organisms are sensitive to methicillin at 37°C than at 30°C (Parker and Hewitt, 1970) (see above), and this phenomenon is more marked with other penicillinase-resistant penicillins such as cloxacillin and flucloxacillin (p. 91). Many MRSA isolates have been reported to be 'sensitive' to cephalosporins, such as cephalothin, but this is due to the fallibility of cephalosporin disc susceptibility testing of MRSA at an incubation temperature of 35°C (Canawati *et al.*, 1982). Automated systems which use very short incubation periods also may fail to detect MRSA strains. Despite the fact that MRSA cultures, being heterogeneous, may appear more 'sensitive' to cloxacillin, flucloxacillin or cephalothin at 37°C, compared with methicillin at 30°C, this has no clinical significance. Cephalothin is ineffective for the treatment of MRSA infections in animals, when the strains have appeared 'cephalothin-sensitive' as tested by standard disc diffusion tests (Chambers *et al.*, 1984, 1990). Extensive clinical experience has also confirmed that serious infections in humans, caused by MRSA strains, do not respond to any of the penicillinase-resistant penicillins or cephalosporins (Richmond *et al.*, 1977; Peacock *et al.*, 1980; Myers and Linnemann, 1982; Harvey and Pavillard, 1982; Hackbarth and Chambers, 1989b).

Rarely, clinical isolates of MRSA are homogeneously resistant and these also produce little or no beta-lactamase. This finding suggests that sequences present on beta-lactamase coding plasmids might alter expression of methicillin-resistance by regulating the amount of PBP 2a produced (Boyce and Medeiros, 1987; Opal *et al.*, 1989). Strains of MRSA all of which posses the mec gene and PBP 2a can vary greatly in their degree of methicillin-resistance. Some of them have a methicillin MIC as low as 1.5–3.0 μg per ml; in others the MIC ranges from 6.0 to 12.0 μg per ml, whilst in others this may be 50–200 μg per ml. These classes may represent stages in an evolutionary sequence leading to progressively increased methicillin-resistance in staphylococci (Tomasz *et al.*, 1991).

Rare MRSA strains have also been identified, where the resistance mechanism is different. These strains lack the PBP 2a gene and contain just the usual PBPs. It appears that the PBPs here are altered in some way in a manner similar to penicillin-resistance in pneumococci (p. 7). These *Staph. aureus* strains only exhibit a low degree of methicillin-resistance (MICs 2–4 µg per ml). PBPs 1 and 2 of these strains appear to have lower penicillin binding capacities (Tomasz *et al.*, 1989; de Lencastre *et al.*, 1991).

Another variant of resistant *Staph. aureus* is the 'borderline methicillin-resistant *Staph. aureus*' or 'borderline oxacillin-resistant *Staph. aureus*' (BORSA). The MICs of these strains are only 4 µg per ml for methicillin and 2 µg per ml for oxacillin. They are not intrinsically resistant to methicillin and they do not have PBP 2a. The beta-lactamase inhibitors clavulanic acid (p. 192) and sulbactam (p. 209) reduce the MICs of methicillin and oxacillin and therefore it has been postulated that in these strains the borderline resistance is due to hyperproduction of beta-lactamase (Chambers *et al.*, 1989; Liu *et al.*, 1990; Montanari *et al.*, 1990; Liu and Lewis, 1992). The clinical significance of these strains is uncertain. Hirano and Bayer (1991) found that ampicillin plus sulbactam was active for treatment of experimental endocarditis caused by these *Staph. aureus* strains. Chambers *et al.* (1989) found that methicillin itself or nafcillin were fully effective against experimental *Staph. aureus* endocarditis regardless of whether the infecting strain was fully susceptible or borderline resistant.

Other authors have found that 'borderline susceptibility' is not solely due to hyperproduction of beta-lactamase, and that it may be due to beta-lactamase plus a small increase in intrinsic resistance (Barg *et al.*, 1991). The MICs of these strains to methicillin are very similar to those where the intrinsic resistance is caused by alteration of the usual PBPs and not by PBP 2a (see above), so that wrong identification of such strains may occur. There may well be different classes of the 'borderline sensitive *Staph. aureus*'. They may have different meanings and different mechanisms and might need to be dealt with differently both in laboratory and in clinical practice (Varaldo, 1993; Varaldo *et al.*, 1993).

Of some interest is the finding that classical MRSA strains which possess PBP 2a are more sensitive to beta-lactamase labile penicillins such as penicillin G, ampicillin and amoxicillin, provided that the beta-lactamase can be neutralized, which can be done by inhibitors of the enzyme such as clavulanic acid or sulbactam. Apparently PBP 2a has much greater affinity for penicillin G, amoxycillin and ampicillin than for methicillin and all other penicillinase-resistant penicillins and cephalosporins. Both penicillin G and amoxycillin MIC for MRSA strains in presence of clavulanic acid is 8 µg per ml, which is much lower than that of methicillin. Results of *in vivo* studies in animals with amoxycillin/clavulanic acid and with ampicillin/sulbactam have been conflicting and it appears that these penicillin/beta-lactamase inhibitor combinations will not be useful for treatment of MRSA infections in humans (Chambers *et al.*. 1990; Franciolli *et al.*, 1991). Mainly MRSA strains produce types A and C beta-lactamases (p. 193) (Norris *et al.*, 1994).

When methicillin was first introduced, resistant staphylococcal strains appeared to be rare; about 5000 strains were examined in the UK before a naturally occurring resistant one was found (Jevons, 1961). In subsequent surveys in London, the percentage of resistant strains rose from 0.06 in 1960 to 0.97 in 1964 (Dyke *et al.*, 1966). The prevalence of MRSA strains in different parts of the world was variable. Initially they were common in some hospitals in the UK and in certain European countries (Parker and Hewitt, 1970; Kayser and Mak, 1972). Before the mid 1970s MRSA strains were uncommon in the USA; thereafter they were isolated more frequently from patients in hospitals (Blackwell and Feingold, 1975; Klimek *et al.*, 1976; Richmond *et al.*, 1977). The occurrence of MRSA strains appeared to be related to the use of all penicillins and perhaps other antibiotics, and not specifically to the use of penicillinase-resistant penicillins (Parker and Hewitt, 1970; Klimek *et al.*, 1976).

In Australia, MRSA strains caused nosocomial infections in Sydney as early as 1966 (Bell, 1982). Initially it was thought that MRSA strains may be less pathogenic (Rountree and Beard, 1968), but further experience in Australia (Rountree and Vickery, 1973) and in the USA (Klimeck *et al.*, 1976) indicated that they were equally capable of producing serious diseases, such as pneumonia, empyema, osteomyelitis, enterocolitis and septicemia. The MRSA cells resist destruction by human polymorphonuclear leukocytes to the same extent as virulent methicillin-sensitive *Staph. aureus* cells (Vaudaux and Waldvogel, 1979). Clinical studies at that time also confirmed the virulence of MRSA strains (Crossley *et al.*, 1979a; Peacock *et al.*, 1981; McDonald *et al.*, 1981; Saravolatz *et al.*, 1982). However, MRSA differs from the beta-lactamase-producing *Staph. aureus* strains which caused hospital outbreaks in the late 1940s and

1950s (p. 11); the latter had a predilection to cause overt infections in healthy hospital staff and family contacts of infected patients (McDonald, 1982).

In the 1960s and early 1970s MRSA was also often found to be resistant to unrelated antibiotics, such as streptomycin, tetracyclines, chloramphenicol, erythromycin, lincomycin, clindamycin and kanamycin (Rountree and Vickery, 1973; Jordan and Hoeprich, 1977). Initially MRSA was usually sensitive to gentamicin and amikacin (Jordan and Hoeprich, 1977). A hospital outbreak of infection with a MRSA strain, resistant also to gentamicin was described by Shanson et al. (1976). Since then hospital outbreaks of MRSA infections and colonizations have been increasingly associated with MRSA multiply-resistant to most other antibiotics, except vancomycin (p. 763), rifampicin (p. 676), sodium fusidate (p. 580) and sometimes co-trimoxazole (p. 836), (Thompson and Wenzel, 1982). The MRSA strains from the UK and Australia have been predominantly resistant to trimethoprim, whereas many strains from other areas in Europe and the USA have been sensitive (Maple et al., 1989). Since the late 1970s there has been an increasing prevalence of these infections in hospitals in the USA, UK and Australia (Thompson and Wenzel, 1982; McDonald, 1982; de Saxe et al., 1983; Keane and Cafferkey, 1984; Schaefler et al., 1984; Bradley et al., 1985). Hospital outbreaks reported from the affected countries have usually been caused by strains with the classical pattern of multiple antibiotic-resistance (see above). Resistant isolates have generally been more prevalent in large metropolitan hospitals, where they have accounted for 20–40% of all Staph. aureus isolates. In surgical and burns patients MRSA infections have been common (Crossley et al., 1979b; Craven et al., 1981; Myers and Linnemann, 1982; Boyce et al., 1983), intensive care, immunocompromised and debilitated patients (Peacock et al., 1980; Pavillard et al., 1982) and in newborn nurseries (Gilbert et al., 1982). Spread of MRSA has occurred more readily where intensive medical and nursing care was practised, and where there was overcrowding (Aeilts et al., 1982; Haley and Bregman, 1982). These infections usually became endemic in affected institutions, and complete eradication of MRSA from a hospital was unusual (Boyce, 1981). Spread of MRSA strains into the community usually did not occur.

Since the mid-1980s MRSA has remained a significant nosocomial pathogen in the USA (McGowan, 1988), in the UK (Kerr et al., 1990; Marples and Reith, 1992) in most states in Australia (Turnidge et al., 1989), in Southern Europe (Voss et al., 1994), in Poland (Hryniewicz, 1994) and in many other countries. But during the years much has been learned about how to contain hospital outbreaks of MRSA infections and colonizations. In MRSA-free institutions systems have been devised for immediate recognition of new importations of MRSA, and then institution of barrier precautions before the organism spreads to critical care areas. In institutions where MRSA is entrenched, much can be done by culturing of patients and personnel and then setting up MRSA isolation wards (Haley, 1991). Guidelines for the control of epidemic methicillin-resistant Staph. aureus have been published in many countries e.g. the UK (Report, 1986). By using these principles Brady et al. (1990) successfully controlled endemic MRSA in a cardiothoracic surgical unit in Australia. Duckworth et al. (1988) controlled an outbreak of MRSA in a London hospital with the combination of screening patients and staff, mupirocin (p. 545) for treatment of carriers and the use of an isolation ward. Similarly a report from South Africa (Blumberg and Klugman, 1994) and several reports from the USA documented the control of MRSA infections and colonizations in large acute hospitals (Murray-Leisure et al., 1990; Reboli et al., 1990; Boyce et al., 1993). Molecular epidemiologic methods can be used in the analysis of nosocomial MRSA outbreaks, and these are helpful in addition to traditional infection control measures (Fang et al., 1993; Boyce, 1994). Outbreaks of MRSA have also been controlled in a nursing facility (Thomas et al., 1989), and a long-term care facility (Muder et al., 1991). In another USA long-term-care facility mupirocin ointment was extensively used to eradicate MRSA carriage, but long-term use of this ointment led to mupirocin-resistant MRSA strains. It was concluded that mupirocin should be saved for short-term use in outbreak situations and it should not be used for prolonged periods in facilities with endemic MRSA colonizations (Kauffman et al., 1993).

Simple measures, as outlined above, were successful in containing an outbreak of MRSA infections in an intensive care unit in France (Guiguet et al., 1990). In some countries such as Denmark (Rosdahl and Knudsen, 1991) and New Zealand (Heffernan et al., 1993) MRSA has been quite uncommon and it is not posing problems to their hospitals. Studies by Inglis et al. (1993) indicated that the methicillin-resistance gene, i.e. the mec region of the chromosome (p. 78), is quite unstable and Staph. aureus strains can lose this and revert to methicillin sensitivity under certain laboratory conditions. This has also been seen in clinical isolates of MRSA. Limitations on the administration of antibiotics may induce MRSA to loose the mec gene. This may be important for devising future strategies for control of resistant microorganisms.

3 Methicillin-resistant coagulase-negative staphylococci

There are many members of this group, *Staph. epidermidis* being the most important. Some of the other species include *Staph. haemolyticus*, *Staph. hominis* and *Staph. simulans*. These, in particular *Staph. epidermidis*, have become important causes of nosocomial infections; infections occur in neonatal intensive-care units (Lyytikäinen *et al.*, 1995), in patients with compromised resistance to microbial disease, such as those with prosthetic heart valves, central nervous system ventricular shunts, indwelling peritoneal or vascular catheters (Archer, 1978; John and McNeill, 1980; Moller, 1988). Similarly patients with granulocytopenia are vulnerable to these infections (Wade *et al.*, 1982). A large number of hospital staff may be colonized by methicillin-resistant coagulase-negative staphylococci (John *et al.*, 1993). Many strains of *Staph. epidermidis* produce an extracellular polysaccharide matrix, called glycocalyx or slime, which is associated with adherence and growth on smooth surfaces, such as i.v. catheters and artificial heart valves, and which inhibit host defences (Mempel *et al.*, 1994). Transposon mutants of *Staph. epidermidis* have been developed, which do not produce this capsular polysaccharide and slime. These mutants are much less pathogenic in experimental animals, and unlike wild strains, they rarely cause endocarditis (Shiro *et al.*, 1994).

Methicillin-resistance of coagulase-negative staphylococci is intrinsic, similar to *Staph. aureus* (p. 77). The resistance mechanism is also the same. They have the mec A gene in the chromosome which codes for the production PBP 2a (p. 77) which has low affinity for methicillin and all penicillinase-resistant penicillins and cephalosporins. These strains are resistant to all penicillinase-resistant penicillins and cephalosporins (John and McNeill, 1980; Karchmer *et al.*, 1983; Menzies *et al.*, 1987; Tesch *et al.*, 1988; Pierre *et al.*, 1990; Ubukata *et al.*, 1990; Suzuki *et al.*, 1992). Similar to *Staph aureus*, the methicillin-resistance of coagulase-negative staphylococci is heterogeneous and special testing methods should be used to detect it (p. 78).

Some 50% of hospital strains of coagulase-negative staphylococci are now methicillin-resistant and most of them are also multiresistant; many strains now are only sensitive to vancomycin and rifampicin (Price and Flournoy, 1982; Richardson and Marples; 1982; Moller, 1988). Some strains of *Staph. haemolyticus* also have elevated MICs for vancomycin (p. 766) (Froggatt *et al.*, 1989). Otherwise vancomycin-resistance is rare and it remains the mainstay for treatment of serious hospital-acquired, methicillin-resistant coagulase-negative staphylococcal infections (Baumgart *et al.*, 1983) (p. 777).

There is some evidence that *Staph. epidermidis* may serve as a repository for the various genes encoding antimicrobial resistance, and that these genes may subsequently be passed to *Staph. aureus* (Blanchard *et al.*, 1986; Archer, 1988).

4 Methicillin-tolerant Staph. aureus

These strains have a deficiency of autolytic enzymes in their cell walls, the presence of which is necessary for the penicillins to exert a bactericidal effect (p. 91). The MICs of methicillin against these strains are in the usual low (sensitive) range, but MBCs are high (Sabath *et al.*, 1977). The clinical significance of these strains is discussed on p. 91.

5 Minimum inhibitory concentrations

The MICs of methicillin and penicillin G against some bacteria are listed in Table I.4. Methicillin inhibits the growth of both penicillin-sensitive and penicillinase-producing staphylococci. The activity of penicillin G is approximately 20- to 50-fold greater than methicillin against penicillin G-sensitive staphylococci and streptococci.

Organism	MIC (µg per ml)	
	Penicillin G	Methicillin
Gram-positive bacteria		
Staphylococcus aureus (non-penicillinase-producer)	0.02	1.0
Staphylococcus aureus (penicillinase-producer)	>125.0	2.0
Staphylococcus epidermidis (penicillinase-producer)	Resistant	2.0
Streptococcus pyogenes (Group A)	0.005	0.2
Streptococcus viridans	0.01	0.1

Table I.4
Compiled from data published by Knox (1960) and John and McNeill (1980)

Mode of Administration and Dosage

Methicillin is unstable in acids, so it is ineffective if given orally. It can be administered i.m. or i.v., and the i.v. route is useful to avoid frequent painful i.m. injections.

1 Dosage

This can be varied widely according to the site and severity of infection. For infections of moderate severity, a commonly used adult dosage is 1 g 4-hourly. The corresponding dosage for children is 100 mg per kg body weight per day, given in four or six divided doses.

2 Serious infections

For these the dose can be doubled or increased even further. Daily doses of up to 25 g have been given i.v. for several weeks without toxic effect.

3 Patients with renal failure

Methicillin, being relatively non-toxic, is often administered in the normal dosage to patients with mild to moderate renal failure. Because its serum half-life is prolonged by profound renal failure, the dosage should be reduced and an adult dose of 1–2 g administered every 8–12 h, has been recommended (Bulger et al., 1964). If a patient with renal failure requires i.v. methicillin in large doses (equivalent to 16 g daily for an adult with normal renal function), this dosage can be adjusted in a similar manner to that of penicillin G. Dosage can be estimated by using Table I.2 (p. 21), and substituting 0.6 g of methicillin for 0.6 g of penicillin G.

4 Newborn and premature infants

Renal excretion of methicillin in these patients is decreased. A dose of 25 mg per kg body weight every 12 h should be given to infants weighing less than 2000 g and who are 0–7 days old. For infants still weighing less than 2000 g but who are 8–30 days old, the dose of 25 mg per kg should be given 8-hourly. For infants weighing more than 2000 g, the dose is 25 mg per kg given 8-hourly to those aged 0–7 days, and the same dose 6-hourly to those aged 8–30 days (McCracken, 1974; McCracken and Nelson, 1983). After the age of 1 month methicillin should be administered in doses recommended for older children (see above).

Serum Levels in Relation to Dosage

1 Intramuscular administration

After a 1 g dose, a mean peak serum level of 18 μg per ml is reached after 30 min (Fig. I.3), and this level falls to 3–4 μg per ml after 3 h (Knudsen and Rolinson, 1960). Probenecid, by slowing the rate of renal tubular secretion of methicillin, can enhance the peak serum level and prolong the serum half-life, as with penicillin G (p. 24).

2 Intravenous administration

After an i.v. injection of 1 g methicillin over a 5-min period, a peak serum level of about 60 μg per ml is reached. This peak level is doubled by doubling the dose. Subsequently, there is a rapid fall in the serum level to about 7 μg per ml after 1 h, and in 2–3 h the level is usually less than 1 μg per ml, a therapeutically ineffective concentration. Usually methicillin cannot be detected in the serum after 4 h.

3 Newborn infants

After a single i.m. dose of 25 mg per kg, the peak serum levels are 47, 41, 35 and 25 μg per ml in infants aged 4–5, 8–9, 13–15 and 25–30 days, respectively (McCracken, 1974).

4 Patients with cystic fibrosis

These patients eliminate methicillin (and dicloxacillin, p. 94) much faster than normal subjects due to an increase in their tubular secretory capacity. Thus, serum levels attained are lower, and these patients may need larger methicillin doses, especially when serious infections are treated (Yaffe et al., 1977).

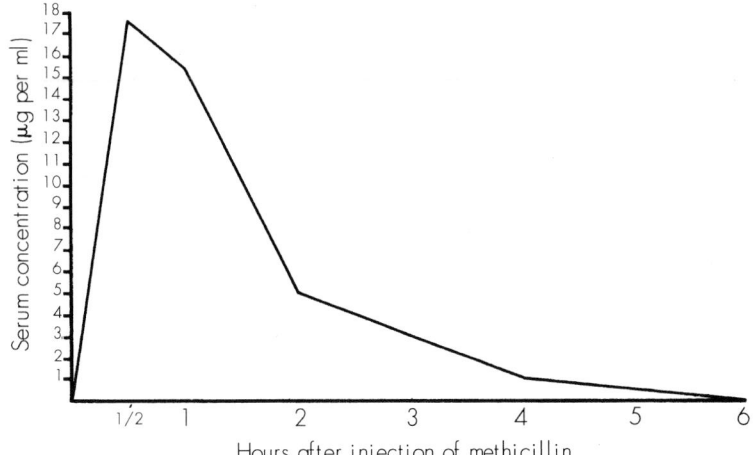

Fig. I.3.
Mean serum concentration in 12 subjects after i.m. injection of 1 g methicillin. (Redrawn from Knudsen and Rolinson, 1960, with permission from the BMJ Publishing Group.)

Excretion

1 Urine

The drug is excreted in urine in an unchanged active form (Stewart *et al.*, 1960). Very high urine concentrations of methicillin are attained, provided renal function is normal. It is excreted by both glomerular filtration and tubular secretion, and up to 80% of an injected dose can be recovered from urine. Probenecid delays renal tubular secretion (p. 24).

2 Bile

Some 2–3% of an injected dose is excreted in bile. This is not reabsorbed, and is subsequently destroyed in the gut.

3 Inactivation in body

The fraction of methicillin which is not excreted, is inactivated in the body. Like penicillin G, it still disappears from the blood at a significant, but reduced rate in anuric patients. The liver is an important extrarenal site for inactivation of the penicillins, including methicillin (p. 24).

Distribution of the Drug in Body

Methicillin is widely distributed in various body fluids. Antibacterial levels which equate with those in serum, occur in pleural, pericardial and ascitic fluids (White and Varga, 1961), and in septic joint effusions (Nelson, 1971). The drug reaches high concentrations in pus and bone of patients with acute osteomyelitis (Tetzlaff *et al.*, 1978). As with other penicillins, only low methicillin concentrations are attained in normal CSF but these may be moderately high in patients with meningitis (p. 25).

Methicillin is one of the penicillins which is least bound to serum proteins. Serum protein binding values ranging from 17 to 43% have been reported (46–58% for penicillin G). The clinical significance of antibiotic protein binding is discussed on p. 95.

Mode of Action

Methicillin acts on bacteria in a similar manner to penicillin G (p. 25).

Toxicity

1 Hypersensitivity reactions

These should be anticipated in patients known to be sensitive to the penicillins. However, not all patients allergic to penicillin G react to methicillin. In a study of eight consecutive patients with histories of penicillin G anaphylaxis, Luton (1964) showed that all tolerated usual i.m. doses of methicillin without reaction. Antecedent skin testing with penicillin G in these patients gave positive reactions, while similar tests with methicillin were negative. Skin testing by these reagents is not recommended (p. 30). Severe allergic reactions to methicillin and to other semisynthetic penicillins may be less common than to penicillin G. Nevertheless, it should be assumed that patients allergic to other penicillins will be sensitized to methicillin, and it should be avoided in such subjects. All hypersensitivity reactions which occur with penicillin G, can be provoked by methicillin (p. 28). In a study of 124 children who received methicillin for 10 days or longer, the frequency of skin rashes, either maculopapular or urticarial, was 6% (Yow *et al.*, 1976).

2 Drug fever

This can occur with methicillin; it is abrupt in onset and the patient usually appears otherwise relatively well. It rapidly resolves when the drug is stopped, and may recur later if another penicillin analog is administered (Yow *et al.*, 1976).

3 Nephropathy and cystitis

An interstitial nephritis can be caused by large i.v. doses of methicillin (Baldwin *et al.*, 1968; Woodroffe *et al.*, 1974; Galpin *et al.*, 1978). This is characterized by fever, rash, eosinophilia, hematuria, proteinuria, sterile pyuria, marked eosinophiluria and renal insufficiency. Microscopic changes in the kidneys consist of patchy but usually heavy interstitial infiltrate with lymphocytes, plasma cells and eosinophils i.e. interstitial changes without glomerular abnormalities. Cogan and Arieff (1978) reported a patient in whom methicillin-induced interstitial nephritis also resulted in functional impairment specific for the distal tubule. The patient developed dehydration due to a sodium-losing nephropathy, renal tubular acidosis and hyperkalemia due to impaired ability to excrete potassium. Sometimes hematuria may be the sole manifestation of nephropathy, and in such cases it may be difficult to distinguish whether this is due to the drug or to the patient's disease such as staphylococcal septicemia (Gallagher and Wayne, 1971). Hematuria and dysuria may also result in some methicillin-treated patients because the drug occasionally causes a hemorrhagic cystitis, possibly by direct chemical irritation (Yow *et al.*, 1976; Bracis *et al.*, 1977; Godin *et al.*, 1980). This complication is distinct from methicillin-induced interstitial nephritis, and its presence can be confirmed by cystoscopy. In methicillin cystitis, hematuria may disappear when a few doses of the drug are omitted, and therapy is resumed with a lower daily dose in association with an increase in fluid intake. As in the case of methicillin-induced interstitial nephritis, it is preferable to discontinue methicillin when this complication occurs.

Most patients recover slowly and completely from methicillin interstitial nephritis after cessation of the drug. Corticosteroid therapy should be considered for severe cases. Eight of 14 patients reported by Galpin *et al.* (1978) received prednisolone therapy. The period for maximal serum creatinine levels to fall to stable lower levels in convalescence was less in the prednisolone-treated, compared with the non-treated patients. Jensen *et al.* (1971) reported one patient with this complication, who still had evidence of impaired renal function 2 years later. The substitution of another penicillin such as oxacillin in these patients is not recommended because of possible cross-sensitization (Yow *et al.*, 1976). A cephalosporin may also not always be a safe substitute. Sanjad *et al.* (1974) described 13 children with methicillin nephritis whose renal abnormalities disappeared when the drug was ceased; in two later treated by cephalothin, an identical renal disease recurred.

The clinical picture suggests that a delayed hypersensitivity reaction may be involved in methicillin nephritis (Linton *et al.*, 1980). Immunofluorescent studies in one patient showed that dimethoxphenyl-penicilloyl, the hapten group of methicillin (p. 29) was firmly bound to kidney tissue together with immunoglobulin (Baldwin *et al.*, 1968). In another patient a methicillin antigen, assumed to be dimethoxyphenyl-penicilloyl, was fixed in a linear pattern along the renal tubular basement membrane together with IgG and the C3 component of complement. This patient also had a serum autoantibody, which was reactive with tubular basement membranes of normal human and monkey kidneys (Border *et al.*, 1974). Methicillin nephritis therefore may be an example of drug-induced autoimmunity; methicillin acts as a hapten and alters the antigenicity of the tubular basement membrane; resultant autoantibodies react not only against the drug but also against the tissue antigen (Flax, 1974).

Methicillin nephritis appears to be a common complication when large doses of the drug are given for extended periods (Sanjad *et al.*, 1974; Linton *et al.*, 1980). Over 100 cases of this complication were reported (Graber and Gluckin, 1977). This side-effect was more common with methicillin than with other penicillins (pp. 32, 120) (Neu, 1982).

4 Hematological side-effects

Leukopenia is fairly common during methicillin therapy. It was observed in 16 of 124 children who received methicillin for 10 days or longer, and it usually occurred 10–20 days after starting treatment (Yow *et al.*, 1976). Some patients developed a decrease in both neutrophils and lymphocytes, others an absolute neutropenia (less than 500 per mm^3). The white cell count usually reverted to normal in a few days after cessation of methicillin. The leukopenia may worsen if another penicillin, such as oxacillin, is substituted for methicillin. No serious problems resulting from leukopenia have been encountered.

Thrombocytopenia caused by methicillin is rare. Schiffer *et al.* (1976) described a patient with leukemia who developed a thrombocytopenia during methicillin treatment and again later when the drug was readministered. Methicillin-dependent anti-platelet antibodies were demonstrated.

5 Transaminase elevation

As with the isoxazolyl penicillins (p. 96), elevation of the SGOT has been occasionally observed during methicillin therapy (Berger and Potter, 1977).

6 Encephalopathy

This complication, similar to that seen after 'massive' doses of penicillin G (p. 32), would be expected if very large doses (50–100 g daily) were given i.v., and it could arise with smaller doses in patients with renal failure.

7 Coombs' positive hemolytic anemia

This side-effect, similar to that described with penicillin G (p. 33), can also be caused by methicillin.

Clinical Use of the Drug

1 Methicillin is useful for the treatment of *Staph. aureus* infections (proven or suspected), due to beta-lactamase-producing staphylococci which are resistant to penicillin G. Originally this antibiotic was regarded as the drug of first choice for severe staphylococcal infections, such as septicemia, endocarditis, pneumonia, meningitis, osteomyelitis and septic arthritis.

It is effective for the treatment of penicillin-resistant staphylococcal infections (White and Varga, 1961), including staphylococcal septicemia and endocarditis (Allen *et al.*, 1962). It was extensively used for these infections for some years after its discovery. All other parenteral beta-lactamase-resistant penicillins, such as oxacillin (p. 97), cloxacillin (p. 98), flucloxacillin (p. 98) and nafcillin (p. 105), have the same therapeutic efficacy as methicillin (Neu, 1982). The drug which is selected is therefore usually the one with which the clinician is most familiar.

Nowadays most clinicians, including ourselves, prefer one of the isoxazolyl penicillins, such as flucloxacillin, or nafcillin to methicillin. Methicillin seems to cause nephritis (p. 84) more commonly than the other penicillins and it can only be administered parenterally. It is virtually never used today.

2 Methicillin was used for severe hospital-acquired *Staph. epidermidis* infections, such as prosthetic valve endocarditis, provided that the strain was sensitive. For the reasons given above, one of the isoxazolyl penicillins or nafcillin are now preferred for these infections. Methicillin, other penicillinase-resistant penicillins and cephalosporins are no longer suitable for immediate emergency treatment of severe hospital-acquired *Staph. epidermidis* infections, as over 50% of hospital strains may be methicillin-resistant (p. 81). Vancomycin (p. 778) is the drug of choice, perhaps combined with rifampicin (p. 696) (Karchmer *et al.*, 1983).

References

Aeilts GD, Sapico FL, Canawati HN *et al.* (1982). Methicillin-resistant *Staphylococcus aureus* colonization and infection in a rehabilitation facility. *J Clin Microbiol* **16**: 218.

Allen JD, Roberts CE, Kirby WMM (1962). Staphylococcal septicaemia treated with methicillin: report of twenty-two cases. *New Engl J Med* **266**: 111.

Archer GL (1978). Antimicrobial susceptibility and selection of resistance among *Staphylococcus epidermidis* isolates recovered from patients with infections of indwelling foreign devices. *Antimicrob Ag Chemother* **14**: 353.

Archer GL (1988). Molecular epidemiology of multiresistant *Staphylococcus epidermidis*. *J Antimicrob Chemother* **21** (Suppl C): 133.

Archer GL, Niemeyer DM, Thanassi JA, Pucci MJ (1994). Dissemination among staphylococci of DNA sequences associated with methicillin resistance. *Antimicrob Ag Chemother* **38**: 447.

Baldwin DS, Levine BB, McCluskey RT, Gallo RR (1968). Renal failure and interstitial nephritis due to penicillin and methicillin. *New Engl J Med* **279**: 1245.

Barg N, Chambers H, Kernodle D(1991). Borderline susceptibility to antistaphylococcal penicillins is not conferred exclusively by the hyperproduction of beta-lactamase. *Antimicrob Ag Chemother* **35**: 1975.

Basker MJ, Edmondson RA, Sutherland R (1980). Comparative stabilities of penicillins and cephalosporins to staphylococcal beta-lactamase and activities against *Staphylococcus aureus*. *J Antimicrob Chemother* **6**: 333.

Baumgart S, Hall SE, Campos JM, Polin RA (1983). Sepsis with coagulase-negative staphylococci in critically ill newborns. *Amer J Dis Child* **137**: 461.

Bell SM (1982). Recommendations for control of the spread of methicillin-resistant *Staphylococcus aureus* infection. Based on 18 years' experience in a group of teaching hospitals. *Med J Aust* **1**: 472.

Berger-Bächi B (1989). Genetics of methicillin resistance in *Staphylococcus aureus*. *J Antimicrob Chemother* **23**: 671.

Berger-Bächi B, Strässle A, Gustafson JE, Kayser FH (1992). Mapping and characterization of multiple chromosomal factors involved in methicillin resistance in *Staphylococcus aureus*. *Antimicrob Ag Chemother* **36**: 1367.

Berger M, Potter DE (1977). Pitfall in diagnosis of viral hepatitis on haemodialysis unit. *Lancet* **ii**: 95.

Blackwell CC, Feingold DS (1975). Frequency and some properties of clinical isolates of methicillin-resistant *Staphylococcus aureus*. *Amer J Clin Path* **64**: 372.

Blanchard TJ, Poston SM, Reynolds PJ (1986). Recipient characteristics in the transduction of methicillin resistance in *Staphylococcus epidermidis*. *Antimicrob Ag Chemother* **29**: 539.

Blumberg LH, Klugman KP (1994). Control of methicillin-resistant *Staphylococcus aureus* bacteraemia in high-risk areas. *Eur J Clin Microbiol Infect Dis* **13**: 82.

Border WA, Lehman DH, Egan JD *et al.* (1974). Antitubular basement-membrane antibodies in methicillin-associated interstitial nephritis. *New Engl J Med* **291**: 381.

Boyce JM (1981). Nosocomial staphylococcal infections. *Ann Intern Med* **95**: 241.

Boyce JM (1994). Methicillin-resistant *Staphylococcus aureus*: a continuing infection control challenge. *Eur J Clin Microbiol Infect Dis* **13**: 45.

Boyce JM, Medeiros AA (1987). Role of beta-lactamase in expression of resistance by methicillin-resistant *Staphylococcus aureus*. *Antimicrob Ag Chemother* **31**: 1426.

Boyce JM, White RL, Bonner MC, Lockwood WR (1982). Reliability of the MS-2 stystem in detecting methicillin-resistant *Staphylococcus aureus*. *J Clin Microbiol* **15**: 220.

Boyce JM, White RL, Causey WA, Lockwood WR (1983). Burn units as a source of methicillin-resistant *Staphylococcus aureus* infections. *JAMA* **249**: 2803.

Boyce JM, Opal SM, Potter-Bynol G, Medeiros AA (1993). Spread of methicillin-resistant *Staphylococcus aureus* in a hospital after exposure to a health care worker with chronic sinusitis. *Clin Infect Dis* **17**: 496.

Bracis R, Sanders CV, Gilbert DN (1977). Methicillin hemorrhagic cystitis. *Antimicrob Ag Chemother* **12**: 438.

Bradley JM, Noone P, Townsend DE, Grubb WB (1985). Methicillin-resistant *Staphylococcus aureus* in a London hospital Lancet **1**: 1493.

Brady LM, Thomson M, Palmer MA, Harkness JL (1990). Successful conrol of endemic MRSA in a cardiothoracic surgical unit. *Med J Aust* **152**: 240.

Bran JL, Levison ME, Kaye D (1972). Survey for methicillin-resistant staphylococci. *Antimicrob Ag Chemother* **1**: 235.

Bulger RJ, Lindholm DD, Murray JS, Kirby WMM (1964). Effect of uremia on methicillin and oxacillin blood levels. *JAMA* **187**: 319.

Canawati HN, Witte JL, Sapico FL (1982). Temperature effect on the susceptibility of methicillin-resistant *Staphylococcus aureus* to four different cephalosporins. *Antimicrob Ag Chemother* **21**: 173.

Chambers HF, Hackbarth CJ (1987). Effect of NaCl and nafcillin on penicillin-binding protein 2a and heterogeneous expression of methicillin resistance in *Staphylococcus aureus*. *Antimicrob Ag Chemother* **31**: 1982.

Chambers HF, Hackbarth CJ, Drake TA *et al.* (1984). Endocarditis due to methicillin-resistant *Staphylococcus aureus* in rabbits: expression of resistance to beta-lactam antibiotics *in vivo* and *in vitro*. *J Infect Dis* **149**: 894.

Chambers HF, Archer G, Matsuhashi M (1989). Low-level methicillin resistance in strains of *Staphylococcus aureus*. *Antimicrob Ag Chemother* **33**: 424.

Chambers HF, Sachdeva M, Kennedy S (1990). Binding affinity for penicillin-binding protein 2a correlates with *in vivo* activity of beta-lactam antibiotics against methicillin-resistant *Staphylococcus aureus*. *J Infect Dis* **162**: 705.

Cogan MC, Arieff AI (1978). Sodium wasting, acidosis and hyperkalemia induced by methicillin interstitial nephritis Evidence for selective distal tubular dysfunction. *Amer J Med* **64**: 500.

Craven DE, Reed C, Kollisch N *et al.* (1981). A large outbreak of infections caused by a strain of *Staphylococcus aureus* resistant to oxacillin and aminoglycosides. *Amer J Med* **71**: 53.

Crossley K, Loesch D, Landesman B *et al.* (1979a). An outbreak of infections caused by strains of Staphylococcus aureus resistant to methicillin and aminoglycosides. I. Clinical studies. *J Infect Dis* **139**: 273.

Crossley K, Landesman B, Zaske D (1979b). An outbreak of infections caused by strains of Staphylococcus aureus resistant to methicillin and aminoglycosides. II. Epidemiologic studies. *J Infect Dis* **139**: 280.

De Jonge BLM, Tomasz A (1993). Abnormal peptidoglycan produced in a methicillin-resistant strain of Staphylococcus aureus grown in the presence of methicillin: functional role for penicillin-binding protein 2A in cell wall synthesis. *Antimicrob Ag Chemother* **37**: 342.

de Lencastre H, Tomasz A (1994). Reassessment of the number of auxillary genes essential for expression of high-level methicillin resistance in *Staphylococcus aureus*. *Antimicrob Ag Chemother* **38**: 2590.

de Lencastre H, Figueiredo AMS, Urban C *et al.* (1991). Multiple mechanisms of methicillin resistance and improved methods for detection in clinical isolates of *Staphylococcus aureus*. *Antimicrob Ag Chemother* **35**: 632.

de Lencastre H, de Jonge BLM, Matthews PR, Tomasz A (1994). Molecular aspects of methicillin resistance in *Staphylococcus aureus*. *J Antimicrob Chemother* **33**: 7.

de Saxe M, Mayon-White R, Galbraith NS, Casewell M (1983). Methicillin-resistant *Staphylococcus aureus* in the UK. *CDR* **36**.

Duckworth GJ, Lothian JLE, Williams JD (1988). Methicillin-resistant *Staphylococcus aureus*: report of an outbreak in a London teaching hospital. *J Hosp Infect* **11**: 1.

Dyke KGH, Jevons P, Parker MT (1966). Penicillinase production and intrinsic resistance to penicillins in *Staphylococcus aureus*. *Lancet* **i**: 835.

Fang FC, McClelland M, Guiney DG *et al* (1993). Value of molecular epidemiologic analysis in a nosocomial methicillin-resistant. *Staphylococcus aureus* outbreak. *JAMA* **270**: 1323.

Figueiredo AMS, Ha E, Kreiswirth BN *et al.* (1991). *In vivo* stability of heterogeneous expression classes in clinical isolates of methicillin-resistant staphylococci. *J Infect Dis* **164**: 883.

Flax MH (1974). Editorial Drug-induced autoimmunity. *New Engl J Med* **291**: 414.

Fontana R (1985). Leading article Penicillin-binding proteins and the intrinsic resistance to beta-lactams in Gram-positive cocci. *J Antimicrob Chemother* **16**: 412.

Franciolli M, Bille J, Glauser MP, Moreillon P (1991). Beta-lactam resistance mechanisms of methicillin-resistant *Staphylococcus aureus*. *J Infect Dis* **163**: 514.

Froggatt JW, Johnston JL, Galetto DW, Archer GL (1989). Antimicrobial resistance in nosocomial isolates of *Staphylococcus haemolyticus*. *Antimicrob Ag Chemother* **33**: 460.

Gallagher PJ, Wayne DJ (1971). Haematuria during methicillin therapy. *Postgrad Med J* **47**: 511.

Galpin JE, Shinaberger JH, Stanley TM *et al.* (1978). Acute interstitial nephritis due to methicillin. *Amer J Med* **65**: 756.

Giamarellou H, Papapetropoulou M, Daikos GK (1981). Methicillin-resistant *Staphylococcus aureus* infections during 1978–79: clinical and bacteriologic observations. *J Antimicrob Chemother* **7**: 649.

Gilbert GL, Asche V, Hewstone AS, Mathiesen JL (1982). Methicillin-resistant *Staphylococcus aureus* in neonatal nurseries. Two years' experience in special-care nurseries in Melbourne. *Med J Aust* **1**: 455.

Godin M, Deshayes P, Ducastelle T *et al.* (1980). Agranulocytosis, haemorrhagic cystitis and acute interstitial nephritis during methicillin therapy. *J Antimicrob Chemother* **6**: 296.

Graber ML, Gluckin DS (1977). Antimicrobials and the kidney. *New Engl J Med* **297**: 224.

Guiguet M, Rekacewicz C, Leclercq B *et al.* (1990). Effectiveness of simple measures to control an outbreak of nosocomial methicillin-resistant *Staphylococcus aureus* infections in an intensive care unit. *Infect Control Hosp Epidemiol* **11**: 23.

Hackbarth CJ, Chambers HF (1989a). Methicillin-resistant staphylococci: genetics and mechanisms of resistance. *Antimicrob Ag Chemother* **33**: 991.

Hackbarth CJ, Chambers HF (1989b). Methicillin-resistant staphylococci: detection methods and treatment of infections. *Antimicrob Ag Chemother* **33**: 995.

Hackbarth CJ, Chambers HF (1993). blaI and blaRI regulate beta-lactamase and PBP 2a production in methicillin-resistant *Staphylococcus aureus*. *Antimicrob Ag Chemother* **37**: 1144.

Hackbarth CJ, Miich C, Chambers HF (1994). Altered production of penicillin-binding protein 2a can affect phenotypic expression of methicillin resistance in *Staphylococcus aureus*. *Antimicrob Ag Chemother* **38**: 2568.

Haley RW (1991). Methicillin-resistant *Staphylococcus aureus*: do we just have to live with it? *Ann Intern Med* **114**: 162.

Haley RW, Bregman DA (1982). The role of understaffing and overcrowding in recurrent outbreaks of staphylococcal infection in a neonatal special-care unit. *J Infect Dis* **145**: 875.

Hartman B, Tomasz A (1981). Altered penicillin-binding proteins in methicillin-resistant strains of *Staphylococcus aureus*. *Antimicrob Ag Chemother* **19**: 726.

Hartman BJ, Tomasz A (1986). Expression of methicillin resistance in heterogeneous strains of *Staphylococcus aureus*. *Antimicrob Ag Chemother* **29**: 85.

Harvey K, Pavillard R (1982). Methicillin resistance in *Staphylococcus aureus* with particular reference to Victorian strains. *Med J Aust* **1**: 465.

Heffernan H, Stehr-Green J, Davies H *et al.* (1993). Methicillin-resistant *Staphylococcus aureus* (MRSA). in New Zealand 1988–90. *NZ Med J* **106**: 72.

Hiramatsu K, Suzuki E, Takayama H *et al* (1990). Role of penicillinase plasmids in the stability of the mec A gene in methicillin-resistant *Staphylococcus aureus*. *Antimicrob Ag Chemother* **34**: 600.

Hirano L, Bayer AS (1991). Beta-lactam-beta-lactamase-inhibitor combinations are active in experimental endocarditis caused by beta-lactamase-producing oxacillin-resistant staphylococci. *Antimicrob Ag Chemother* **35**: 685.

Hirschl A, Stanek G, Rotter M (1984). Effectiveness of cefamandole against methicillin-resistant strains of *Staphylococcus aureus in vitro* and in experimental infections. *J Antimicrob Chemother* **13**: 429.

Hrynicwicz W (1994). Bacterial resistance in Eastern Europe – selected problems. *Scand J Infect Dis* (Suppl 93): 33.

Hürlimann-Dalel RL, Ryffel C, Kayser FH, Berger-Bächi B (1992). Survey of the methicillin resistance-associated genes mec A, mec RI-mec I, and fem A-fem B in clinical isolates of methicillin-resistant *Staphylococcus aureus*. *Antimicrob Ag Chemother* **36**: 2617.

Inglis B, El-Adhami W, Stewart PR (1993). Methicillin-sensitive and -resistant homologues of *Staphylococcus aureus* occur together among clinical isolates. *J Infect Dis* **167**: 323.

Jensen HA, Halveg AB, Saunamki KI (1971). Permanent impairment of renal function after methicillin nephropathy. *Brit Med J* **4**: 406.

Jevons MP (1961). 'Celbenin'-resistant staphylococci. *Brit Med J* **1**: 124.

John JF Jr, McNeill WF (1980). Activity of cephalosporins against methicillin-susceptible and methicillin-resistant, coagulase-negative staphylococci: minimal effect of beta-lactamase. *Antimicrob Ag Chemother* **17**: 179.

John JF Jr, Grieshop TJ, Atkins LM, Platt CG (1993). Widespread colonization of personnel at a Veterans Affairs Medical Center by methicillin-resistant coagulase-negative staphylococcus. *Clin Infect Dis* **17**: 380.

Jordan GW, Hoeprich PD (1977). Susceptibility of three groups of *Staphylococcus aureus* to newer antimicrobial agents. *Antimicrob Ag Chemother* **11**: 7.

Karchmer AW, Archer GL, Dismukes WE (1983). *Staphylococcus epidermidis* causing prosthetic valve endocarditis: microbiologic and clinical observations as guides to therapy. *Ann Intern Med* **98**: 447.

Kayser FH, Mak TM (1972). Methicillin-resistant staphylococci. *Amer J Med Sci* **264**: 197.

Kauffman CA, Terpenning MS, He X *et al.* (1993). Attempts to eradicate methicillin-resistant *Staphylococcus aureus* from a long-term-care facility with the use of mupirocin ointment. *Amer J Med* **94**: 371.

Keane CT, Cafferkey MT (1984). Re-emergence of methicillin-resistant *Staphylococcus aureus* causing severe infection. *J Infect* **9**: 6.

Kerr S, Kerr GE, Mackintosh CA, Marples RR (1990). A survey of methicillin-resistant *Staphylococcus aureus* affecting patients in England and Wales. *J Hosp Infect* **16**: 35.

Klimek JJ, Marsik FJ, Bartlett RC *et al.* (1976). Clinical, epidemiologic and bacteriologic observations of an outbreak of methicillin-resistant *Staphylococcus aureus* at a large community hospital. *Amer J Med* **61**: 340.

Knox R (1960). A new penicillin (BRL 1241). active against penicillin-resistant staphylococci. *Brit Med J* **2**: 690.

Knudsen ET, Rolinson GN (1960). Absorption and excretion of a new antibiotic (BRL. 1241). *Brit Med J* **2**: 700.

Laverdiere M, Welter D, Sabath LD (1978). Use of a heavy inoculum in the *in vitro* evaluation of the anti-staphylococcal activity of 19 cephalosporins. *Antimicrob Ag Chemother* **13**: 669.

Linton AL, Clark WF, Driedger AA *et al.* (1980). Acute interstitial nephritis due to drugs. Review of the literature with a report of nine cases. *Ann Intern Med* **93**: 735.

Liu H, Lewis N (1992). Comparison of ampicillin/sulbactam and amoxicillin/clavulanic acid for detection of borderline oxacillin-resistant *Staphylococcus aureus*. *Eur J Clin Microbiol Infect Dis* **11**: 47.

Liu H, Buescher G, Lewis N *et al.* (1990). Detection of borderline oxacillin-resistant *Staphylococcus aureus* and differentiation from methicillin-resistant strains. *Eur J Clin Microbiol Infect Dis* **9**: 717.

Luton EF (1964). Methicillin tolerance after penicillin G anaphylaxis. *JAMA* **190**: 39.

Lyon BR, Skurrray R (1987). Antimicrobial resistance of *Staphylococcus aureus*: genetic basis. *Microbiol Rev* **51**: 88.

Lyon BR, May JW, Skurray RA (1983). Analysis of plasmids in nosocomial strains of multiple-antibiotic-resistant *Staphylococcus aureus*. *Antimicrob Ag Chemother* **23**: 817.

Lyytikäinen O, Saxén H, Ryhänen R *et al.* (1995). Persistence of a multiresistant clone of *Staphylococcus epidermidis* in a neonatal intensive-care unit for a four-year period. *Clin Infect Dis* **20**: 24.

Maple PAC, Hamilton-Miller JMT, Brumfitt W (1989). World-wide antibiotic resistance in methicillin-resistant *Staphylococcus aureus*. *Lancet* **i**: 537.

Markowitz N, Pohlod DJ, Saravolatz LD, Quinn EL (1983). *In vitro* susceptibility patterns of methicillin-resistant and -susceptible *Staphylococcus aureus* strains in a population of parenteral drug abusers from 1972 to 1981. *Antimicrob Ag Chemother* **23**: 450.

Marples RR, Reith S (1992). Methicillin-resistant *Staphylococcus aureus* in England and Wales. *CDR Review* **2**: R25.

McCracken GH Jr (1974). Pharmacological basis for antimicrobial therapy in newborn infants. *Amer J Dis Child* **128**: 407.

McCracken GH Jr, Nelson JD (1983). *Antimicrobial Therapy for Newborns* p. 24. New York: Grune and Stratton.

McDonald M, Hurse A, Sim KN (1981). Methicillin-resistant *Staphylococcus aureus* bacteraemia. *Med J Aust* **2**: 191.

McDonald PJ (1982). Leading article. Methicillin-resistant staphylococci. *Med J Aust* **1**: 445.

McGowan JE, Jr (1988). Gram-positive bacteria: spread and antimicrobial resistance in university and community hospitals in the USA. *J Antimicrob Chemother* **21**(Suppl C): 49.

Mempel M, Feucht H, Ziebuhr W *et al.* (1994). Lack of mec A transcription in slime-negative phase variants of methicillin-resistant *Staphylococcus epidermidis*. *Antimicrob Ag Chemother* **38**: 1251.

Menzies RE, Cornere BM, MacCulloch D (1987). Cephalosporin susceptibility of methicillin-resistant, coagulase-negative staphylococci. *Antimicrob Ag Chemother* **31**: 42.

Moller JK (1988). Observations on multiple drug resistance in coagulase-negative staphylococci isolated in hospitals from 1975 to 1985. *J Hosp Infect* **11**: 26.

Montanari MP, Tonin E, Biavasco F, Varaldo PE (1990). Further characterization of borderline methicillin-resistant *Staphylococcus aureus* and analysis of penicillin-binding proteins. *Antimicrob Ag Chemother* **34**: 911.

Muder RR, Brennen C, Wagener M *et al.* (1991). Methicillin-resistant staphylococcal colonization and infection in a long-term care facility. *Ann Intern Med* **114**: 107.

Munson DP, Thompson TR, Johnson DE *et al.* (1982). Coagulase-negative staphylococcal septicemia: experience in a newborn intensive care unit. *J Pediatr* **101**: 602.

Murray-Leisure KA, Geib S, Graceley D *et al.* (1990). Control of epidemic methicillin-resistant *Staphylococcus aureus*. *Infect Control Hosp Epidemiol* **11**: 343.

Mutton KJ, Andrew JH (1982). Antibiotic susceptibility of *Staphylococcus aureus*. Community acquired strains. *Med J Aust* **1**: 459.

Myers JP, Linnemann CC Jr (1982). Bacteremia due to methicillin-resistant *Staphylococcus aureus*. *J Infect Dis* **145**: 532.

Nelson JD (1971). Antibiotic concentrations in septic joint effusions. *New Engl J Med* **284**: 349.

Neu HC (1982). Antistaphylococcal penicillins. *Med Clin N Amer* **66**: 51.

Norris SR, Stratton CW, Kernodle DS (1994). Production of A and C variants of staphylococcal beta-lactamase by methicillin-resistant strains of *Staphylococcus aureus*. *Antimicrob Ag Chemother* **38**: 1649.

Opal SM, Boyce JM, Medeiros AA *et al.* (1989). Modification of homogeneous resistance in a methicillin-resistant strain of *Staphylococcus aureus* by acquisition of a beta-lactamase encoding plasmid. *J Antimicrob Chemother* **23**: 315.

Parker MT, Hewitt JH (1970). Methicillin resistance in *Staphylococcus aureus*. *Lancet* **i**: 800.

Patel AH, Foster TJ, Pattee PA (1989). Physical and genetic mapping of the protein A gene in the chromosome of *Staphylococcus aureus* 8325–4. *J Gen Microbiol* **135**: 1799.

Pavillard R, Harvey K, Douglas D *et al.* (1982). Epidemic of hospital-acquired infection due to methicillin-resistant *Staphylococcus aureus* in major Victorian hospitals. *Med J Aust* **1**: 451.

Peacock JE Jr, Marsik FJ, Wenzel RP (1980). Methicillin-resistant *Staphylococcus aureus*: introduction and spread within a hospital. *Ann Intern Med* **93**: 526.

Peacock JE Jr, Moorman DR, Wenzel RP, Mandell G L (1981). Methicillin-resistant *Staphylococcus aureus*: microbiological characteristics, antimicrobial susceptibilities, and assessment of virulence of an epidemic strains. *J Infect Dis* **144**: 575.

Pierre J, Williamson R, Barnet M, Gutmann L (1990). Presence of an additional penicillin-binding protein in methicillin-resistant *Staphylococcus epidermidis*, *Staphylococcus haemolyticus*, *Staphylococcus hominis*, and *Staphylococcus simulans* with a low affinity for methicillin, cephalothin, and cefamandole. *Antimicrob Ag Chemother* **34**: 1691.

Price SB, Flournoy DJ (1982). Comparison of antimicrobial susceptibility patterns among coagulase-negative staphylococci. *Antimicrob Ag Chemother* **21**: 436.

Reboli AC, John JF Jr, Platt GG, Cantey JR (1990). Methicillin-resistant *Staphylococcus aureus* outbreak at a veterans' affairs medical center: importance of carriage of the organism by hospital personnel. *Infect Control Hosp Epidemiol* **11**: 291.

Report of a Combined Working Party of the Hospital Infection Society and British Society for Antimicrobial Chemotherapy (1986). Guidelines for the control of epidemic methicillin-resistant *Staphylococcus aureus*. *J Hosp Infect* **7**: 193.

Richardson JF, Marples RR (1982). Changing resistance to antimicrobial durgs, and resistance typing in clinically significant strains of *Staphylococcus epidermidis*. *J Med Microbiol* **15**: 475.

Richmond AS, Simberkoff MS, Schaefler S, Rahal JJ Jr (1977). Resistance of *Staphylococcus aureus* to semisynthetic penicillins and cephalothin. *J Infect Dis* **135**: 108.

Rolinson GN, Stevens S, Batchelor FR *et al.* (1960). Bacteriological studies on a new penicillin – BRL 1241. *Lancet* **ii**: 564.

Rosdahl VT, Knudsen AM (1991). The decline of methicillin resistance among Danish *Staphylococcus aureus* strains. *Infect Control Hosp Epidemiol* **12**: 83.

Rossi L, Tonin E, Cheng YR, Fontana R (1985). Regulation of penicillin-binding protein activity: description of a methicillin-inducible penicillin-binding protein in *Staphylococcus aureus*. *Antimicrob Ag Chemother* **27**: 828.

Rountree PM, Beard MA (1968). Hospital strains of *Staphylococcus aureus*, with particular reference to methicillin-resistant strains. *Med J Aust* **2**: 1163.

Rountree PM, Vickery AM (1973). Further observations on methicillin-resistant staphylococci. *Med J Aust* **1**: 1030.

Ryffel C, Kayser FH, Berger-Bächi B (1992). Correlation between regulation of mecA transcription and expression of methicillin resistance in staphylococci. *Antimicrob Ag Chemother* **36**: 25.

Ryffel C, Strässle A, Kayser FH, Berger-Bächi B (1994). Mechanisms of heteroresistance in methicillin-resistant *Staphylococcus aureus*. *Antimicrob Ag Chemother* **38**: 724.

Sabath LD, Garner C, Wilcox C, Finland M (1975). Effect of inoculum and of beta-lactamase on the anti-staphylococcal activity of thirteen penicillins and cephalosporins. *Antimicrob Ag Chemother* **8**: 344.

Sabath LD, Wheeler N, Laverdiere M *et al.* (1977). A new type of penicillin resistance of *Staphylococcus aureus*. *Lancet* **i**: 443.

Sanjad S, Haddad GG, Nassar VH (1974). Nephropathy, an underestimated complication of methicillin therapy. *J Pediatr* **84**: 873.

Saravolatz LD, Markowitz N, Arking L *et al.* (1982). Methicillin-resistant *Staphylococcus aureus*. Epidemiological observations during a community-acquired outbreak. *Ann Intern Med* **96**: 11.

Schaefler S, Jones D, Perry W *et al.* (1984). Methicillin-resistant *Staphylococcus aureus* strains in New York City hospitals: inter-hospital spread of resistant strains of type 88. *J Clin Microbiol* **20**: 536.

Schiffer CA, Weinstein HJ, Wiernik PH (1976). Methicillin-associated thrombocytopenia. *Ann Intern Med* **85**: 338.

Shanson DC (1981). Antibiotic-resistant *Staphylococcus aureus*. *J Hosp Infect* **2**: 11.

Shanson DC, Kensit JG, Duke R (1976). Outbreak of hospital infection with a strain of *Staphylococcus aureus* resistant to gentamicin and methicillin. *Lancet* **ii**: 1347.

Shiro H, Muller E, Gutierrez N *et al.* (1994). Transposon mutants of *Staphylococcus epidermidis* deficient in elaboration of capsular polysaccharide/adhesion and slime are avirulent in a rabbit model of endocarditis. *J Infect Dis* **169**: 1042.

Stewart GT, Harrison PM, Holt RJ (1960). Microbiological studies on sodium 6-(2,6-dimethoxybenzamido). penicillanate monohydrate (BRL 1241) *in vitro* and in patients. *Brit Med J* **2**: 694.

Sumita Y, Fukasawa M, Mitsuhashi S, Inoue M (1995). Binding affinities of beta-lactam antibodies for penicillin-binding protein 2^1 in methicillin-resistant *Staphylococcus aureus*. *J Antimicrob Chemother* **35**: 473.

Suzuki E, Hiramatsu K, Yokota T (1992). Survey of methicillin-resistant clinical strains of coagulase-negative staphylococci for mecA gene distribution. *Antimicrob Ag Chemother* **36**: 429.

Suzuki E, Kuwahara-Arai K, Richardson JF, Hiramatsu K (1993). Distribution of mec regulator genes in methicillin-resistant *Staphylococcus* clinical strains. *Antimicrob Ag Chemother* **37**: 1219.

Tesch W, Strassle A, Berger-Bachi B *et al.* (1988). Cloning and expression of methicillin resistance from *Staphylococcus epidermidis* in *Staphylococcus carnosus. Antimicrob Ag Chemother* **32**: 1494.

Tetzlaff TR, Howard JB, McCracken GH Jr *et al.* (1978). Antibiotic concentrations in pus and bone of children with osteomyelitis. *J Pediatr* **92**: 135.

Thomas JC, Bridge J, Waterman S *et al.* (1989). Transmission and control of methicillin-resistant *Staphylococcus aureus* in a skilled nursing facility. *Infect Control Hosp Epidemiol* **10**: 106.

Thompson RL, Wenzel RP (1982). International recognition of methicillin-resistant strains of *Staphylococcus aureus. Ann Intern Med* **97**: 925.

Thompson RL, Fisher KA, Wenzel RP (1982). *In vitro* activity of N-formimidoyl thienamycin and other beta-lactam antibiotics against methicillin-resistant *Staphylococcus aureus. Antimicrob Ag Chemother* **21**: 341.

Tomasz A, Drugeon HB, de Lencastre HM *et al.* (1989). New mechanism for methicillin resistance in *Staphylococcus aureus*: clinical isolates that lack the PBP 2a gene and contain normal penicillin-binding proteins with modified penicillin-binding capacity. *Antimicrob Ag Chemother* **33**: 1869.

Tomasz A, Nachman S, Leaf H (1991). Stable classes of phenotypic expression in methicillin-resistant clinical isolates of staphylococci. *Antimicrob Ag Chemother* **35**: 124.

Turnidge J, Lawson P, Munro R, Benn R (1989). A national survey of antimicrobial resistance in *Staphylococcus aureus* in Australian teaching hospitals. *Med J Aust* **150**: 65.

Ubukata K, Yamashita N, Konno M (1985). Occurrence of a beta-lactam-inducible penicillin-binding protein in methicillin-resistant staphylococci. *Antimicrob Ag Chemother* **27**: 851.

Ubukata K, Nonoguchi R, Song MD *et al.* (1990). Homology of mec A gene in methicillin-resistant *Staphylococcus haemolyticus* and *Staphylococcus simulans* to that of *Staphylococcus aureus. Antimicrob Ag Chemother* **34**: 170.

Varaldo PE (1993). The 'borderline methicillin-susceptible' *Staphylococcus aureus. J Antimicrob Chemother* **31**: 1.

Varaldo PE, Montanari MP, Biavasco F *et al.* (1993). Survey of clinical isolates of *Staphylococcus aureus* for borderline susceptibility to antistaphylococcal penicillins. *Eur J Clin Microbiol Infect Dis* **12**: 677.

Vaudaux P, Waldvogel FA (1979). Methicillin-resistant strains of *Staphylococcus aureus*: relation between expression of resistance and phagocytosis by polymorphonuclear leukocytes. *J Infect Dis* **139**: 547.

Verbist L, Verhagen J (1981). *In vitro* activity of N-formimidoyl thienamycin in comparison with cefotaxime, moxalactam and ceftazidime. *Antimicrob Ag Chemother* **19**: 402.

Voss A, Milatovic D, Wallrauch-Schwarz C *et al.* (1994). Methicillin-resistant staphylococcus in Europe. *Eur J Clin Microbiol Infect Dis* **13**: 50.

Wade JC, Schimpff SC, Newman KA, Wiernick PH (1982). *Staphylococcus epidermidis*: an increasing cause of infection in patients with granulocytopenia. *Ann Intern Med* **97**: 503.

White A, Varga DT (1961). Antistaphylococcal activity of sodium methicillin. *Arch Intern Med* **108**: 671.

Wilkinson BJ, Nadakavukaren MJ (1983). Methicillin-resistant septal peptidoglycan synthesis in a methicillin-resistant *Staphylococcus aureus* strain. *Antimicrob Ag Chemother* **23**: 610.

Woodroffe AJ, Thomson NM, Meadows R, Lawrence JR (1974). Nephropathy associated with methicillin administration. *Aust NZ J Med* **4**: 256.

Yaffe SJ, Gerbracht LM, Mosovich LL *et al.* (1977). Pharmacokinetics of methicillin in patients with cystic fibrosis. *J Infect Dis* **135**: 828.

Yow MD, Taber LH, Barrett FF *et al.* (1976). A ten-year assessment of methicillin-associated side-effects. *Pediatrics* **58**: 329.

Isoxazolyl Penicillins
Oxacillin, Cloxacillin, Dicloxacillin and Flucloxacillin

Description

These semisynthetic compounds, derived from the penicillin nucleus, 6 APA (p. 3), are all closely related, being 3:5 disubstituted 4-isoxazolyl penicillins. They combine the property of resistance to beta-lactamase with resistance to gastric acidity. Similar to methicillin (p. 77) and nafcillin (p. 102), they are effective antistaphylococcal agents, but they may be administered orally. Four such penicillins are available:

1 Oxacillin

Chemically this is 3-methyl-5-phenyl-4-isoxazolyl penicillin, it was synthesized in 1961 and has been extensively used in North America.

2 Cloxacillin

The chemical formula of this is 3-0-chlorophenyl-5-methyl-4-isoxazolyl penicillin (Knudsen *et al.*, 1962); this only differs from oxacillin by an additional chlorine atom.

3 Dicloxacillin

This is chemically 3(2,6-dichlorophenyl)-5-methyl-4-isoxazolyl penicillin. It differs from cloxacillin by having two chloride ions attached to the phenyl group.

4 Flucloxacillin

Chemically 3(2-chloro-6-fluorophenyl)-5-methyl-4-isoxazolyl penicillin, this only differs from dicloxacillin by the substitution of a fluorine for a chlorine atom (Sutherland *et al.*, 1970).

Sensitive Organisms

1 Antibacterial spectrum

This is similar to that of methicillin; isoxazolyl penicillins are active against Gram-positive cocci, such as *Staphylococcus aureus*, *Staph. epidermidis*, *Strep. pyogenes*, *Strep. pneumoniae*, *Strep. viridans* and the Gram-positive bacilli, but *Enterococcus faecalis* is relatively resistant. The *Neisseria* spp. are the only Gram-negative bacteria sensitive to these drugs.

2 Staphylococcus aureus and Staph. epidermidis

The isoxazolyl penicillins are primarily of interest because, being beta-lactamase-resistant, they are active against staphylococci resistant to penicillin G. Resistance to this enzyme varies, some beta-lactamase-resistant penicillins being more resistant than others (p. 102) (Frimodt-Moller *et al.*, 1986; Jarlov *et al.*, 1988; Rennenberg and Forsgren, 1989). The clinical significance of this remains uncertain. The less common human pathogen *Staph. lagdunensis* may be penicillin G-sensitive, as many strains do not produce penicillinase. Penicillinase-producing strains are sensitive to isoxazolyl penicillins (Herchline *et al.*, 1990; Vandenesch *et al.*, 1993).

Cross-resistance occurs between methicillin and all other penicillinase-resistant penicillins, so that methicillin-resistant strains of *Staph. aureus* (p. 77) and *Staph. epidermidis* (p. 81) are also resistant to isoxazolyl penicillins (Sutherland *et al.*, 1970; Richmond *et al.*, 1977). This resistance is one of degree, because cultures of *Staph. aureus* are heterogeneous; the proportion of organisms sensitive to methicillin and the isoxazolyl penicillins varies according to the temperature at which the test is performed (p. 78). All evidence, however, indicates that patients with methicillin-resistant staphylococcal infections do not respond to other penicillinase-resistant penicillins or cephalosporins (p. 78).

Synergism between one of the isoxazolyl penicillins or nafcillin (p. 102) and an aminoglycoside, such as gentamicin, against sensitive *Staph. aureus* strains, can usually be demonstrated *in vitro* and in animal experiments. Clinically, it is still uncertain whether combination therapy has any advantages compared with single drug therapy with an appropriate penicillinase-resistant penicillin (Abrams *et al.*, 1979; Kaplan and Tenenbaum, 1982) (p. 105).

3 Borderline oxacillin-resistant Staph. aureus (BORSA)

These *Staph. aureus* strains appear to hyperproduce beta-lactamase, but other mechanisms may also be involved (p. 79). Woods and Yam (1988) found that the MICs of oxacillin against these strains were 1–2 μg per ml. The MBCs were higher, but the bactericidal testing results were markedly influenced by the technique employed. Sierra-Madero *et al.* (1988) found that the MICs of these strains varied from 1 to 4 μg per ml and considered that oxacillin may well be less effective clinically for treatment of infections caused by these strains. Animal studies performed by Pefanis *et al.* (1993) suggested that oxacillin would be clinically effective in the treatment of infections caused by borderline oxacillin-susceptible strains of *Staph. aureus*. This has also been confirmed by clinical studies (Massanari *et al.*, 1988).

4 Penicillin-tolerant Staph. aureus

These strains have a deficiency in an autolytic enzyme on their cell surface, which appears to be necessary before any penicillins, including penicillinase-resistant penicillins, can exert a bactericidal effect (p. 11). Oxacillin tolerance in *Staph. aureus* can also be due to enhanced secretion of an autolysin inhibitor, such as lipoteichoic acid (Raynor *et al.*, 1979). Tolerance seems to be quite common, and was found in 30–60% of strains isolated from blood cultures (Watanakunakorn, 1978; Hilty *et al.*, 1980). With regard to tolerance *Staph. aureus* cultures are heterogeneous; the majority of cells are not tolerant to the antibiotic tested, and the remainder are tolerant to varying degrees (Watanakunakorn, 1978; Kim, 1981; Holzhoffer *et al.*, 1985). Tolerance of *Staph. aureus* strains to oxacillin, may disappear after storage of the organism in the laboratory (Mayhall and Apollo, 1980). With many strains tolerance may only be demonstrable in the laboratory at an acid pH of 6.22 but not at pH of 7.15 (Venglarcik *et al.*, 1983). It is uncertain whether such pH-induced tolerance has any clinical relevance. The whole question of tolerance is further complicated by inconsistent laboratory techniques; the MBC/MIC ratio used for defining tolerance (p. 81) has varied 10- to 100-fold from study to study and no standardized method has been used for measuring antibiotic MBCs (Kim, 1981). Numerous variables can influence MBC determination, especially if this is performed by the usual broth dilution plate count method (Woolfrey *et al.*, 1985). Perhaps MBC testing should be an experimental laboratory test which should not be done by clinical microbiology laboratories (Pelletier and Baker, 1988). Also Handwerger and Tomasz (1985) considered that the MBC/MIC ratio is not reliable and may only serve as a first hint of tolerance in a clinical specimen. This test should be followed by time-kill studies and confirmed by more detailed microbiological tests using genetically and physiologically homogeneous cultures of the isolate. Furthermore, genetically non-tolerant bacteria, which possess autolysins in their cell walls, may be modified by low pH, composition of growth medium and other factors in their environment. Under certain growth conditions both *in vitro* and *in vivo* such genetically non-tolerant bacteria may become tolerant; this may happen in certain sites of infection such as the heart valves *in vivo*. This is referred to as phenotypic tolerance.

Some animal studies suggested that *Staph. aureus* tolerance may be clinically significant. Endocarditis in rats, caused by a tolerant *Staph. aureus* strain responded better to cloxacillin/gentamicin combination than to cloxacillin alone (Voorn *et al.*, 1991). Similarly cloxacillin/gentamicin was more effective in prophylaxis of experimental *Staph. aureus* endocarditis than cloxacillin alone when a tolerant strain was used in these experiments. Cloxacillin alone, however, was effective when a non-tolerant *Staph. aureus* strain was used (Voorn *et al.*, 1992). The clinical significance of staphylococcal tolerance to penicillinase-resistant penicillins is discussed on p. 105.

Table I.5

Compiled from data published by Hammerstrom *et al.* (1967) and Sutherland *et al.* (1970)

Organism	MIC (μg per ml)				
	Penicillin G	Oxacillin	Cloxacillin	Dicloxacillin	Flucloxacillin
Staphylococcus aureus (non-penicillinase producer)	0.02	0.35	0.1–0.25	0.06	0.1–0.25
Staphylococcus aureus (penicillinase producer)	50.0	0.4	0.25–0.5	0.12	0.25–0.5
Streptococcus pyogenes	0.01	0.05–0.1	0.05–0.1	0.05	0.05–0.1
Streptococcus pneumoniae	0.01	0.5	0.25–0.5	0.15	0.25
Enterococcus faecalis	5.0	>12.5	25.0	>12.5	25.0

5 Comparative antibacterial activity of isoxazolyl penicillins

Cloxacillin is considerably less active than penicillin G against bacteria which are sensitive to penicillin G. However, it is 4- to 8-fold more active than methicillin against *Staph. aureus*. Oxacillin has about the same activity as cloxacillin against *Staph. aureus* but dicloxacillin s slightly more active (Gravenkemper *et al.*, 1965). The activity of flucloxacillin is similar to oxacillin and cloxacillin (Sutherland *et al.*, 1970; Bergeron *et al.*, 1976).

6 Minimum inhibitory concentrations

Table I.5 shows the MICs of the four isoxazolyl penicillins against some selected bacteria, compared with those of penicillin G. The MICs of cloxacillin, oxacillin and flucloxacillin against staphylococci are increased 10-fold if the test is performed in 95% human serum instead of nutrient broth (Barber and Waterworth, 1964; Sutherland *et al.*, 1970). Dicloxacillin is more protein bound than cloxacillin, and its MICs increase 20- to 25-fold in 95% serum (Hammerstrom *et al.*, 1967).

Mode of Administration and Dosage

1 Oral administration

Isoxazolyl penicillins are acid stable and can be administered orally. The usual oral adult dosage of these drugs is 0.5 g 6-hourly and for children 50 mg per kg body weight per day, given in four divided doses. The dose should be administered about 1 h before meals for optimal absorption (Sutherland *et al.*, 1970) (p. 93). In severe infections the dose can be doubled or even further increased. Bell (1968; 1976) obtained good results in chronic osteomyelitis by using oral cloxacillin in a dosage of 1 g 4-hourly for prolonged periods; oral probenecid 2 g daily, was used to produce higher serum levels. A regimen of dicloxacillin or flucloxacillin 1–2 g orally twice-daily with probenecid, also has been satisfactory for long-term therapy of chronic osteomyelitis (Hedström and Kahlmeter, 1980).

2 Parenteral administration

Oxacillin, cloxacillin and flucloxacillin can be administered i.m. or i.v.. A dosage as small as 250 mg 6-hourly may suffice for mild infections, but for those of moderate severity the usual adult parenteral dose is 1 g every 4 h. This may be doubled or even further increased for severe infections. Oxacillin in a dosage of up to 18 g daily i.v. has been used to treat seriously ill patients (Klein *et al.*, 1963). Comparable i.v. doses for children are 100–300 mg per kg per day. When these drugs are administered i.v., the techniques recommended for penicillin G, should be used (p. 20).

3 Patients with renal failure

In the presence of severe renal impairment, the dosage of cloxacillin, dicloxacillin or flucloxacillin should be reduced as for methicillin (p. 82), especially if high parenteral doses are used. Compared with methicillin, the serum half-life of oxacillin in such patients is much shorter, so that a high parenteral dosage of oxacillin (1 g every 4–6 h) has been recommended for the treatment of severe infections in anuric patients (Bulger *et al.*, 1964).

4 Newborn and premature infants

Renal excretion of oxacillin in these patients is slower (Axline *et al.*, 1967), and this probably applies to all isoxazolyl penicillins. During the first 7 days of life an oxacillin dosage of 25 mg per kg, administered every 12 h, is recommended for infants weighing less than 2000 g; for those weighing more than 2000 g this dose should be given 8-hourly. Infants aged 8–30 days require 25 mg per kg 8-hourly if weighing less than 2000 g, and the same dose 6-hourly if weighing over 2000 g (McCracken and Nelson, 1983).

5 Patients with massive bleeding

In some surgical operations blood loss may even exceed the blood volume, and in these the loss of an antibiotic such as cloxacillin may be similar in extent to loss of blood. Therefore a more frequent dosing interval or priming of all replacement fluids with the drug may be required to maintain a therapeutic level(Levy *et al.*, 1990).

Serum Levels in Relation to Dosage

1 Oral administration

When a 0.5 g oral dose of oxacillin is given, a peak serum level of about 4 μg per ml is reached in 30–60 min (Hammerstrom *et al.*, 1967). Thereafter, the serum concentration falls, but significant levels are maintained for 4–6 h. Serum levels after cloxacillin are about twice as high as those obtained with oxacillin (Fig. I.4) (Turck *et al.*, 1965; Sutherland *et al.*, 1970). Oral dicloxacillin produces serum levels approximately twice as high as cloxacillin (Gravenkemper *et al.*, 1965), as does flucloxacillin (Fig. I.5).

The differing serum levels obtained with oral administration of these antibiotics, are not solely due to differences in their absorption. If they are administered by continuous i.v. infusion, the clearance of dicloxacillin and flucloxacillin from the body is slower than that of cloxacillin, which in turn is slower than that of oxacillin (Rosenblatt *et al.*, 1968; Nauta and Mattie, 1975).

Doubling the dose of all of these penicillins doubles serum concentrations. The presence of food in the stomach interferes with their absorption. The peak serum level of cloxacillin can be 4-fold higher if it is given whilst fasting (Bell, 1970). Flucloxacillin serum levels also are higher if it is given in the fasting state (Kamme and Ursing, 1974).

Fig. I.4.
Serum levels after oral and i.m. cloxacillin. (Redrawn from Sutherland *et al.*, 1970, with permission from the BMJ Publishing Group.)

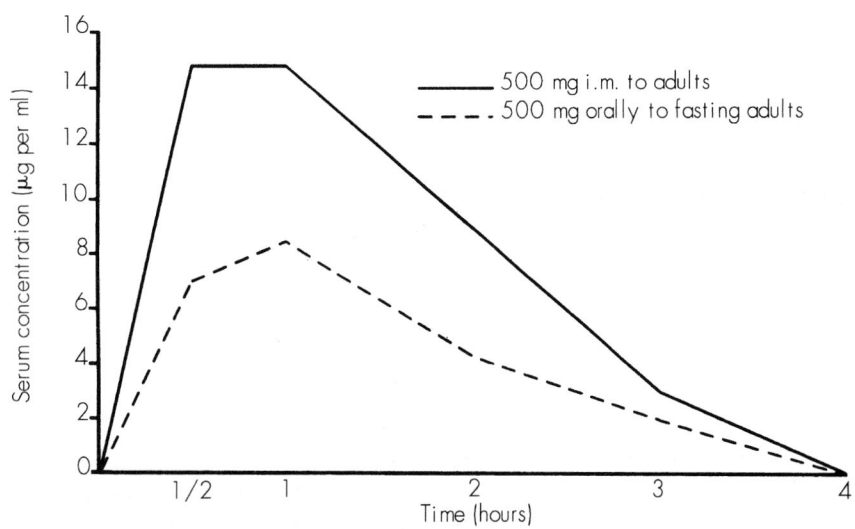

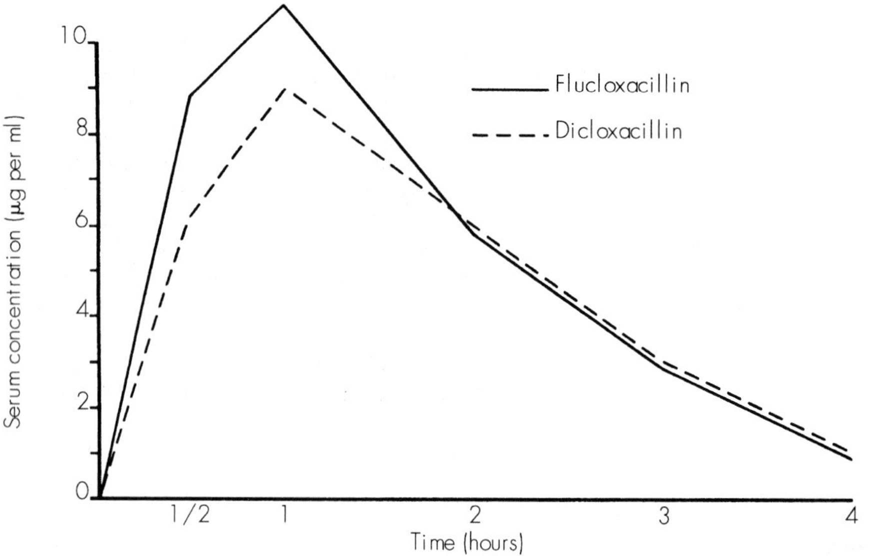

Fig. I.5.
Serum concentrations of flucloxacillin and dicloxacillin after a single 250 mg oral dose to fasting subjects. (Redrawn from Sutherland *et al.*, 1970, with permission from the BMJ Publishing Group.)

2 Parenteral administration

The serum level after i.m. oxacillin is 3- to 4-fold higher than that obtained, when the same dose is given orally. Similarly, i.m. cloxacillin produces higher serum concentrations than the orally administered drug (Fig. I.4). Peak serum levels of oxacillin, cloxacillin, dicloxacillin and flucloxacillin after a single i.m. injection of 0.5 g are similar (14–16 μg per ml). Flucloxacillin levels are considerably more prolonged than those of oxacillin and slightly more prolonged than those of cloxacillin (Sutherland *et al.*, 1970). This is because flucloxacillin, like dicloxacillin (see above), is cleared more slowly from the body than cloxacillin.

As with other penicillins, concurrent administration of probenecid enhances serum concentrations (p. 24).

3 Newborn and premature infants

After a single i.m. injection of oxacillin in a dose of 20 mg per kg to newborn infants (aged 8–15 days), the mean peak serum concentration was 51.5 μg per ml and the mean serum half-life 1.6 h. In infants aged 20–21 days, the peak level was 47 μg per ml and the mean serum half-life 1.2 h (Axline *et al.*, 1967).

Schwartz *et al.* (1976) studied a neonate in whom therapeutic levels were not achieved after oral administration of dicloxacillin, even when the dosage was as high as 175 mg per kg per day. Intestinal absorption appeared normal, but there was an abnormally high urinary excretion rate. It was postulated that the renal tubular secretion of the drug was stimulated by the penicillin derivative itself, or by phenobarbital which was used concurrently. Phenobarbital is also known to induce the metabolism of some antibiotics (p. 568). Where possible antibiotic serum level monitoring should be carried out in neonates.

4 Patients with cystic fibrosis

These patients eliminate cloxacillin and dicloxacillin three times faster than normal subjects. While increase in their tubular secretory capacity may account for some of this (Jusko *et al.*, 1975), this is mainly due to increased biotransformation (Spino *et al.*, 1984). Other isoxazolyl penicillins may be handled in a similar manner. Therefore, when patients with cystic fibrosis are treated with these drugs, larger doses and serum level monitoring is necessary (p. 82).

Excretion

1 Urine

Isoxazolyl penicillins are mainly excreted in the urine. After oral administration of cloxacillin about 30% of the dose is excreted in this way (Stewart, 1965); a higher percentage of the dose is recoverable when it is administered i.m. Compared with cloxacillin, oral oxacillin is excreted to a lesser extent via the kidney, partly because of its poorer absorption, and partly because more oxacillin is cleared by other mechanisms (see below). Larger amounts of dicloxacillin and flucloxacillin are excreted in urine after oral administration, because the absorption of these drugs is better than cloxacillin (Sutherland *et al.*, 1970).

Antibacterially active metabolites of the isoxazolyl penicillins exist in serum and are excreted in urine (Thijssen and Mattie, 1976). Under normal conditions serum levels of these metabolites are low, representing only 9% of the total antibiotic serum concentration. In patients with markedly impaired renal function, metabolites may represent up to 50% of the total serum level. In healthy subjects, 10–23% of these penicillins excreted in urine is in the form of metabolites; higher percentages occur with oxacillin and the lowest with flucloxacillin. Because only small amounts of active metabolites are formed from the isoxazolyl penicillins, and these have similar activity to the parent drugs, they have no clinical significance.

Isoxazolyl penicillins are excreted by both glomerular filtration and tubular secretion. Probenecid can delay their excretion by partly blocking renal tubular secretion (p. 24). Nauta *et al.* (1974) showed that the volume of distribution of cloxacillin in anephric patients was not significantly affected by probenecid, but it reduced its elimination. This indicates that probenecid does not limit the access of penicillins to tissues, but it diminishes the extrarenal elimination of the penicillin via the liver (see below).

2 Bile

These penicillins are eliminated by the biliary tract to some extent; this is more marked with oxacillin than cloxacillin.

3 Inactivation in body

This occurs with all the isoxazolyl penicillins, and probably takes place in the liver. Oxacillin is more rapidly destroyed in the body than the others, and therefore has little tendency to accumulate in patients with renal failure (Bulger *et al.*, 1964).

Distribution of the Drugs in Body

Cloxacillin and dicloxacillin, which are highly serum protein bound (see below), when compared with drugs with a low degree of protein binding such as methicillin (p. 83) and ampicillin (p. 118), penetrate equally well into pus and bone of patients with acute osteomyelitis and into septic joint effusions (Nelson *et al.*, 1978; Tetzlaff *et al.*, 1978). Isoxazolyl penicillins penetrate into normal bone and synovial fluid to a lesser extent; 1 h after an i.v. dose of 1 g of oxacillin or 0.5 g of flucloxacillin, the tissue levels in the synovial capsule and cortical bone may just reach the MICs of these drugs against staphylococci (Fitzgerald *et al.*, 1978; Pollard *et al.*, 1979). Therapeutic concentrations of oxacillin (Taryle *et al.*, 1981) and cloxacillin (Stewart, 1962) have been detected in pleural fluid. Cloxacillin penetrates well into cardiac tissue (Bergeron *et al.*, 1985). In one study 37 patients were given a single 2 g i.v. bolus injection of flucloxacillin prior to open-heart surgery. Within 12 h, flucloxacillin serum and heart valve concentrations declined from 125.2 to 4.4 µg per ml and from 16.5 to 3.7 µg per g, respectively. Concentrations in the subcutaneous tissue and muscle were almost identical, declining from 14.7 or 14.2 µg per g to undetectable levels after 8–10 h (Frank *et al.*, 1988).

Oxacillin, like other penicillins (p. 25), does not penetrate into human polymorphonuclear leukocytes (Lorian and Atkinson, 1980). These drugs are excreted in breast milk and cross the placenta (Neu, 1982). They do not pass into normal CSF, but both oxacillin and methicillin reach therapeutic concentrations in the CSF of rabbits with experimental staphylococcal meningitis (Strausbaugh *et al.*, 1980). After subconjunctival injection of 100 mg of oxacillin in the infected eyes of rabbits, tissue concentrations are high in the cornea, iris and anterior chamber fluid, and these concentrations are higher than those achieved with methicillin (p. 83). Oxacillin, like methicillin, penetrates poorly into the vitreous humor (Barza *et al.*, 1982).

Protein binding of all these penicillins is extensive *in vitro*. Oxacillin is 93% serum protein bound, cloxacillin and flucloxacillin 94% and dicloxacillin at 97% is the most highly bound of all penicillins (Rolinson and Sutherland, 1965; Sutherland *et al.*, 1970; Bergeron *et al.*, 1976). Slightly differing figures have been reported, results varying according to methodology (Neu, 1982).

The percentage of any drug bound to serum proteins is less when high serum levels are attained, because the binding capacity of serum protein is exceeded. *In vitro*, with penicillin G and cloxacillin the percentage of the unbound drug is only significantly increased when a total serum concentration of 200 µg per ml or higher, is attained (Rolinson and Sutherland, 1965). In patients with hypoalbuminemia the unbound fraction of the drug is increased. In those with renal failure, binding of drugs to albumin is inhibited by accumulated endogenous metabolites and possibly also by changes in the structure of albumin (Lindup and Orme, 1981). Binding of one drug can be inhibited by the presence of another, when both compete for the same albumin binding site. Another drug can inhibit binding indirectly e.g. heparin inhibits the protein binding of other drugs by raising the serum concentrations of free fatty acids, which reduce protein binding of some antibiotics such as dicloxacillin, but increase binding of others such as penicillin G (Suh *et al.*, 1981). In the past the binding of any penicillin to serum protein was believed to be a passive chemical process, but now it appears that this is facilitated by some serum factors. The extent of penicillin binding to proteins in serum is much higher than with solutions having comparable concentrations of purified albumin (Di Piro *et al.*, 1993).

It has been suggested that the protein-bound part of an antibiotic has little or no antibacterial activity (Rolinson and Sutherland, 1965; Merrikin *et al.*, 1983). The greater intrinsic activity of cloxacillin compared with methicillin, may thereby be compromised *in vivo* by its higher protein binding. Antibiotics which are highly protein-bound, are known to have diminished activity *in vitro* in the presence of serum (Merrikin *et al.*, 1983).

Serum protein binding of the penicillins may not have any clinical significance, because this binding may be loose and rapidly reversible *in vivo* (Barza *et al.*, 1972; Mattie *et al.*, 1973). Protein-bound drug may serve as a circulating drug reservoir, which releases more drug as the free drug is excreted or metabolized (Koch-Weser and Sellers, 1976). This may increase the duration of action of many drugs. Antibiotics such as flucloxacillin which are highly protein-bound, diffuse poorly into human interstitial fluid (Wise *et al.*, 1980; Wise, 1983) and into fibrin clots in experimental animals (Barza *et al.*, 1974). In the latter, their penetration is enhanced by probenecid (Lee *et al.*, 1975). The relevance of these experimental findings to human inflammatory disease is uncertain. Highly protein-bound antibiotics may have a therapeutic advantage in large-volume, high protein-containing spaces, such as ascitic or pleural fluid, by acting as a reservoir for replacement of free drug that diffuses slowly back into the vascular system (Peterson and Gerding, 1980). Isoxazolyl penicillins, despite their high degree of serum binding, and also two other antibiotics which are even more protein-bound, sodium fusidate (97.3%) and novobiocin (99.2%), are all effective in clinical practice. One reason for this may be that the peak serum level of 'free antibiotic' after usual therapeutic doses, still exceeds the concentration necessary to inhibit highly sensitive bacteria (Rolinson, 1980; Gerding and Peterson, 1985).

Serum protein binding does diminish the extravascular penetration of antibiotics. The degree of penetration ranges from 100% for an antibiotic with the lowest level of serum protein binding (e.g. gentamicin – no drug-bound) to 20% for that with high level of protein binding (flucloxacillin). The concentrations of flucloxacillin in extravascular fluids and tissues are still high enough to make the drug clinically effective. The major impacts of high protein binding are slightly slower passage into extravascular space, slightly later peak concentrations, and levels in extravascular fluid which are persistently below those in serum (Bergan *et al.*, 1986; 1987). In an *in vitro* model Dudley *et al.* (1990) found that the bactericidal activity of a highly protein-bound drug (dicloxacillin) was reduced in protein-containing extravascular spaces. But the findings by Perl *et al.* (1990) were different. Their results suggested that the addition of serum, even with the most highly protein-bound antibiotics, resulted in few changes in the *in vitro* susceptibility of Gram-negative nosocomial blood stream isolates.

Toxicity

1 Hypersensitivity reactions

These drugs are contraindicated in penicillin-allergic patients, because they may evoke all the hypersensitivity reactions caused by penicillin G (p. 28).

2 Gastrointestinal side-effects

Oral administration of isoxazolyl penicillins may cause nausea and diarrhea, which only occasionally necessitates cessation of treatment. Antibiotic-associated colitis due to *Clostridium difficile* (p. 594) can be caused by these drugs; toxin producing *Cl. difficile* was isolated from the feces of one child who developed watery diarrhea with i.v. oxacillin therapy, and from another child who developed diarrhea following 4 days of oral dicloxacillin (Brook, 1980).

3 Hepatotoxicity

Oxacillin occasionally causes fever, nausea and vomiting associated with abnormal liver function tests, mainly elevated SGOT levels (Dismukes, 1973; Onorato and Axelrod, 1978). Liver biopsy may show a non-specific hepatitis (Bruckstein and Attia, 1978). Some patients remain asymptomatic and anicteric, the only abnormalities being elevated serum enzymes and sometimes eosinophilia (Olans and Weiner, 1976). Reversible cholestatic hepatitis occurred in one patient (Ten Pas and Quinn, 1965). Liver function abnormalities rapidly disappeared when oxacillin was ceased. Hepatotoxicity due to oxacillin appears to be common in HIV-infected patients. In one series 81% of such patients receiving oxacillin developed liver damage (Saliba and Herbert, 1994)

Hepatotoxicity may be more common with oxacillin than other isoxazolyl penicillins, because it is cleared to a greater extent through the liver and biliary tract (p. 95). Penicillin G, nafcillin or cephalothin can be safe substitutes, because liver dysfunction rapidly resolves when they replace oxacillin (Olans and Weiner, 1976; Bruckstein and Attia, 1978; Taylor et al., 1979). Another isoxazolyl penicillin such as cloxacillin may not be a safe substitute. Elevation of SGOT levels has been noted rarely with cloxacillin and dicloxacillin (Yow, 1964; Berger and Potter, 1977). Severe cholestatic hepatitis caused by cloxacillin has been reported (Lotric-Furlan et al., 1994). Severe intrahepatic cholestasis also occurred in a patient after taking nitrofurantoin, ampicillin and cloxacillin; cholestasis reappeared at once when cloxacillin alone was administered 2 years later (Enat et al., 1980).

Flucloxacillin also causes rather severe cholestatic hepatitis from which patients usually take over 2 months to recover. The risk of this has been estimated to be in the range of 7.6 per 100 000 users (Derby et al., 1993; Jick et al., 1994). Miros et al. (1990) also reported four patients with severe flucloxacillin-induced cholestatic hepatitis. These patients presented with deep jaundice and pruritus which developed soon after ceasing flucloxacillin. Symptoms only resolved in 6 weeks, but abnormal liver function tests persisted in two patients for over 6 months.

4 Neurotoxicity

This may occur if very large doses are given i.v., especially to patients with renal failure. Conway et al. (1968) reported a patient who convulsed whilst receiving 18 g of i.v. cloxacillin per day, but who also had renal functional impairment and was concurrently receiving cephaloridine in a dose of 2 g daily. Malone et al. (1977) described a patient with acute bacterial endocarditis and impaired renal function, who convulsed while receiving 16 g oxacillin i.v. per day. This patient's pre-dose oxacillin serum level was 270 µg per ml, 1 h after a dose it was 340 µg per ml, and the CSF level was 70 µg per ml (p. 32).

5 Neutropenia

This has been noted particularly with oxacillin, but it can occur with the other isoxazolyl penicillins, and with all beta-lactam antibiotics (p. 33). Leventhal and Silken (1976) described four children who developed marked neutropenia during the third week of treatment with i.v. oxacillin in a dose of 200 mg or more, per kg per day. In all cases the white cell count returned to normal when the drug was stopped (p. 33). Oxacillin and other beta-lactam antibiotics (p. 84) probably exert a toxic effect on the maturation of neutrophils (Chu et al., 1977), but antibody-mediated suppression of granulopoiesis may also be a factor, at least in some patients (Murphy et al., 1985). Acute agranulocytosis has been described in two patients receiving oxacillin therapy; both recovered when the drug was withdrawn (Scalley and Roark, 1977; Kahn, 1978). Agranulocytosis associated with fever and pharyngitis, has been described in one adult patient receiving cloxacillin; resolution occurred after withdrawal of the drug (Westerman et al., 1978).

6 Kernicterus

Animal studies suggested that flucloxacillin, similar to sulfonamides (p. 819), may displace bilirubin from its binding sites on albumin. It is possible that this drug, if used in the jaundiced neonate, may cause kernicterus (Hanefeld and Ballowitz, 1976).

Clinical Uses of the Drugs

Isoxazolyl penicillins are used primarily for treatment of penicillin-resistant staphylococcal infections. Results comparable with those obtained with methicillin (p. 85) or nafcillin (p. 105), have been obtained with oxacillin administered in large doses parenterally (6–18 g daily for adults), for the treatment of severe staphylococcal infections, including severe pneumonia, meningitis and endocarditis (Klein et al., 1963; Abrams et al., 1979; Rajashekaraiah et al., 1980; Watanakunakorn, 1987; Quintiliani and Cooper, 1988). Despite the availability of good medical treatment, many patients with Staph. aureus endocarditis still need emergency valve replacement during the acute phase of their illness (Mullany et al., 1989).

It is still uncertain whether patients with staphylococcal endocarditis due to either tolerant or non-tolerant strains, would benefit from the addition of gentamicin to the treatment regimen (p. 81) (Karchmer, 1988). Some clinical studies suggested that oxacillin/rifampicin combination may be slightly superior than oxacillin therapy alone for patients severely ill with *Staph. aureus* sepsis (Van der Auwera *et al.*, 1983; 1985). Further studies are needed to confirm this. Parenteral cloxacillin and flucloxacillin are also satisfactory for the treatment of severe staphylococcal infections (Williams, 1982; Lacey, 1983; Eykyn, 1987).

All the penicillinase-resistant penicillins which can be administered parenterally, are about equally effective for the treatment of severe staphylococcal diseases. Nafcillin (p. 105) or one of the isoxazolyl penicillins are now preferred to methicillin because of the latter's toxicity (p. 84). Parenteral flucloxacillin has a slight pharmacological advantage over cloxacillin, but some clinicians prefer cloxacillin to flucloxacillin because the former is somewhat more resistant to staphylococcal beta-lactamase (p. 77) and less frequently it may cause jaundice.

For oral administration, cloxacillin is superior to oxacillin because of its better gastrointestinal absorption. Oral cloxacillin is effective for treatment of staphylococcal infections of moderate severity (Stewart, 1962; Turck *et al.*, 1965), and also for prolonged outpatient treatment of chronic infections such as osteomyelitis (Bell, 1968; 1976; Black *et al.*, 1987).

Dicloxacillin being well absorbed, also gives satisfactory results in staphylococcal infections such as osteomyelitis, when administered by the oral route (Hammerstrom *et al.*, 1967; Hedström, 1975; Parker and Fossieck, 1980). Dicloxacillin may supersede flucloxacillin for oral therapy because it appears to cause jaundice less frequently than the latter drug. Oral flucloxacillin has been used with success for the treatment of staphylococcal skin and soft tissue infections, as well as for deeper infections, such as osteomyelitis, empyema and postoperative abscesses (Price and Harding, 1975; Hedström and Kahlmeter, 1980). Chronic osteomyelitis is sometimes a polymicrobial disease, involving in addition to *Staph. aureus*, organisms such as *Staph. epidermidis*, *E. faecalis*, *E. coli*, *Proteus* spp. and various anaerobes; in such infections standard treatment with any of the penicillinase-resistant penicillins will be unsatisfactory (Pichichero and Friesen, 1982).

Isoxazolyl penicillins are sometimes employed for surgical chemoprophylaxis in situations predisposed to postoperative *Staph. aureus* or *Staph. epidermidis* infections. Flucloxacillin alone has been recommended as chemoprophylaxis for open heart surgery; a 2-g i.v. dose is given at the beginning of surgery and this dose repeated again at end of operation (Farrington *et al.*, 1985, 1986). Some advocate continuing chemoprophylaxis afterwards; a dose of 500 mg flucloxacillin is given 6-hourly until the centrally placed postoperative i.v. catheters are removed, usually within 24–48 h (Freeman, 1990). Some authors advocate adding gentamicin or tobramycin as a second drug to this prophylactic regimen (Wilson, 1988; Wilson *et al.*, 1988), but most consider that flucloxacillin alone is sufficient. The use of flucloxacillin aims to prevent early onset prosthetic valve endocarditis in patients undergoing valve replacement and staphylococcal sternotomy infections after coronary artery bypass graft surgery (Freeman, 1990).

In orthopedic surgery (hip replacement and internal fixation of some fractures), flucloxacillin or cloxacillin in doses of 1–2 g given 1–2 h preoperatively i.m. or just before the operation i.v., have been recommended. Some clinicians give repeated doses of these drugs postoperatively, but a single dose probably suffices and prophylaxis should not exceed a three-dose course (Unsworth *et al.*, 1978; Hirschmann and Inui, 1980; Norden, 1983). Some authors consider that cloxacillin or flucloxacillin alone may not be sufficient in this situation, as Gram-negative organism infection and even anaerobic infections are being encountered more commonly after orthopedic operations. Therefore the triple-drug regimen of flucloxacillin, gentamicin and metronidazole has been proposed for prophylaxis in this situation (Sanderson, 1989; Court-Brown, 1990).

A prospective, double-blind, placebo-controlled study was performed to assess the value of perioperative cloxacillin (first dose of 1 g at the start of anesthesia and then the same dose 6-hourly up to a total of four doses) prophylaxis in patients who were about to undergo a craniotomy. Significantly fewer neurosurgical infections occurred in the cloxacillin group. A 1-year follow-up study also confirmed that cloxacillin had been beneficial to the patients and it also had reduced the costs of health care (Van Ek *et al.*, 1988, 1991a,b). A combination of ampicillin (2 g), oxacillin (2 g) and gentamicin (1.5 mg per kg body weight), has been given i.v. once at the time of induction of anesthesia, prior to renal transplantation (Tilney *et al.*, 1978). Cloxacillin alone or combined with gentamicin also appears to be effective prophylaxis for placement of CSF shunts (Langley *et al.*, 1993).

The clinical entity of the toxic shock syndrome results from a toxin or toxins elaborated by *Staph. aureus*, the infection commonly being in the vagina. Bacteremia is absent in most cases (Eykyn, 1982; Chesney, 1989). A penicillinase-resistant antibiotic, such as flucloxacillin, should be given parenterally to these patients, in addition to general supportive measures to combat shock. In some cases toxic shock syndrome has been associated with *Staph. aureus* septicemia and endocarditis (Whitby *et al.*, 1983; Crowther and Ralph, 1993).

A variant of the toxic shock syndrome has been described in patients with AIDS. Cone *et al.* (1992) described five such patients. They had prolonged erythema, extensive cutaneous desquamation, hypotension, tachycardia and multiple organ involvement. Toxin-producing *Staph. aureus* was isolated from blood or other body tissues. Three of the five patients died of renal failure and central nervous system abnormalities. Appropriate antimicrobial treatment such as cloxacillin or nafcillin (p. 105) should be used in all of these patients. Isoxazolyl penicillins are suitable for the treatment of hospital-acquired coagulase-negative staphylococcal infections only if the strain involved is methicillin-sensitive (p. 81).

References

Abrams B, Sklaver A, Hoffman T, Greenman R (1979). Single or combination therapy of staphylococcal endocarditis in intravenous drug abusers. *Ann Intern Med* **90**: 789.

Axline SG, Yaffe SJ, Simon HJ (1967). Clinical pharmacology of antimicrobials in premature infants. II Ampicillin, methicillin, oxacillin, neomycin and colistin. *Pediatrics* **39**: 97.

Barber M, Waterworth PM (1964). Penicillinase-resistant penicillins and cephalosporins. *Brit Med J* **2**: 344.

Barza M, Vine H, Weinstein L (1972). Reversibility of protein binding of penicillins: an *in vitro* study employing a rapid diafiltration process. *Antimicrob Ag Chemother* **1**: 427.

Barza M, Samuelson T, Weinstein L (1974). Penetration of antibiotics into fibrin loci *in vivo*. II Comparison of nine antibiotics; effect of dose and degree of protein binding. *J Infect Dis* **129**: 66.

Barza M, Kane A, Baum J (1982). Ocular penetration of subconjunctival oxacillin, methicillin and cefazolin in rabbits with staphylococcal endophthalmitis. *J Infect Dis* **145**: 899.

Bell SM (1968). Oral penicillins in the treatment of chronic staphylococcal osteomyelitis. *Lancet* **ii**: 295.

Bell SM (1970). Supervision of antibiotic treatment – an important medical responsibility. *Aspects of Infection.* Proc Symp Auckland, Sydney and Melbourne, p 107.

Bell SM (1976). Further observations on the value of oral penicillins in chronic staphylococcal osteomyelitis. *Med J Aust* **2**: 591.

Bergan T, Engeset A, Olszewski W *et al* (1986). Extravascular penetration of highly protein-bound flucloxacillin. *Antimicrob Ag Chemother* **30**: 729.

Bergan T, Engeset A, Olszewski W (1987). Does serum protein binding inhibit tissue penetration of antibiotics? *Rev Infect Dis* **9**: 713.

Berger M, Potter DE (1977). Pitfall in diagnosis of viral hepatitis on haemodialysis unit. *Lancet* **ii**: 95.

Bergeron MG, Brusch JL, Barza M, Weinstein L (1976). Bactericidal activity and pharmacology of flucloxacillin. *Amer J Med Sci* **271**: 13.

Bergeron MG, Desaulniers D, Lessard C *et al.* (1985). Concentrations of fusidic acid, cloxacillin and cefamandole in sera and atrial appendages of patients undergoing cardiac surgery. *Antimicrob Ag Chemother* **27**: 928.

Black J, Hunt TL, Godley PG, Matthew E (1987). Oral antimicrobial therapy for adults with osteomyelitis or septic arthritis. *J Infect Dis* **155**: 968.

Brook I (1980). Isolation of toxin producing *Clostridium difficile* from two children with oxacillin- and dicloxacillin-associated diarrhea. *Pediatrics* **65**: 1154.

Bruckstein AH, Attia AA (1978). Oxacillin hepatitis. Two patients with liver biopsy, and review of the literature. *Amer J Med* **64**: 519.

Bulger RJ, Lindholm DD, Murray JS, Kirby WMM (1964). Effect of uremia on methicillin and oxacillin blood levels. *JAMA* **187**: 139.

Chesney PJ (1989). Clinical aspects and spectrum of illness of TSS: overview (1989). *Rev Infect Dis* **11** (Suppl 1): 1.

Chu J-Y, O'Connor DM, Schmidt RR (1977). The mechanism of oxacillin-induced neutropenia. *J Pediatr* **90**: 668.

Cone LA, Woodard DR, Byrd RG *et al.* (1992). A recalcitrant, erythematous, desquamating disorder associated with toxin-producing staphylococci in patients with AIDS. *J Infect Dis* **165**: 638.

Conway N, Beck E, Somerville J (1968). Penicillin encephalopathy. *Postgrad Med J* **44**: 891.

Court-Brown CM (1990). Antibiotic prophylaxis in orthopaedic surgery. *Scand J Infect Dis* (Suppl 70): 74.

Crowther MA, Ralph ED (1993). Menstrual toxic shock syndrome complicated by persistent bacteremia: case report and review. *Clin Infect Dis* **16**: 288.

Derby LE, Jick H, Henry DA, Dean AD (1993). Cholestatic hepatitis associated with flucloxacillin. *Med J Aust* **158**: 596.

Di Piro JT, Adkinson NF Jr, Hamilton RG (1993). Facilitation of penicillin haptenation to serum proteins. *Antimicrob Ag Chemother* **37**: 1463.

Dismukes WE (1973). Oxacillin-induced hepatic dysfunction. *JAMA* **226**: 861.

Dudley MN, Blaser J, Gilbert D, Zinner SH (1990). Significance of 'extravascular' protein binding for antimicrobial pharmacodynamics in an *in vitro* capillary model of infection. *Antimicrob Ag Chemother* **34**: 98.

Enat R, Pollack S, Ben-Arieh Y *et al.* (1980). Cholestatic jaundice caused by cloxacillin: macrophage inhibition factor test in preventing rechallenge with hepatotoxic drugs. *Brit Med J* **280**: 982.

Eykyn SJ (1982). Toxic shock syndrome: some answers but questions remain. *Brit Med J* **284**: 1585.

Eykyn SJ (1987). The treatment of staphylococcal endocarditis. *J Antimicrob Chemother* **20** (Suppl A): 161.

Farrington M (1986). The prevention of wound infection after coronary bypass surgery. *J Antimicrob Chemother* **18**: 656.

Farrington M, Fenn A, Phillips I (1985). Flucloxacillin concentration in serum and wound exudate during open heart surgery. *J Antimicrob Chemother* **16**: 253.

Fitzgerald RH Jr, Kelly PJ, Snyder RJ, Washington JA II (1978). Penetration of methicillin, oxacillin and cephalothin into bone and synovial tissues. *Antimicrob Ag Chemother* **14**: 723.

Frank U, Schmidt-Eisenlohr E, Schlosser V, *et al.* (1988). Concentration of flucloxacillin in heart valves and subcutaneous and muscle tissue of patients undergoing open-heart surgery. *Antimicrob Ag Chemother* **32**: 930.

Freeman R (1990). Antimicrobial prophylaxis in cardiovascular surgery. *Scand J Infect Dis* (Suppl 70): 80.

Frimodt-Moller N, Rosdahl VT, Sorensen G et al. (1986). Relationship between penicillinase production and the in vitro activity of methicillin, oxacillin, cloxacillin, dicloxacillin, flucloxacillin, and cephalothin against strains of Staphylococcus aureus of different phage patterns and penicillinase activity. J Antimicrob Chemother 18: 27.

Gerding DN, Peterson LR (1985). Serum protein binding and extravascular distribution of antimicrobials. J Antimicrob Chemother 15: 136.

Gravenkemper CF, Bennett JV, Brodie JL, Kirby WMM (1965). Dicloxacillin. In vitro and pharmacologic comparisons with oxacillin and cloxacillin. Arch Intern Med 116: 340.

Hammerstrom CF, Cox F, McHenry MC, Quinn EL (1967). Clinical, laboratory, and pharmacological studies of dicloxacillin. Antimicrob Ag Chemother 1966: 69.

Handwerger S, Tomasz A (1985). Antibiotic tolerance among clinical isolates of bacteria. Rev Infect Dis 7: 368.

Hanefeld F, Ballowitz L (1976). Flucloxacillin and bilirubin binding. Lancet i: 433.

Hedström SÅ (1975). Treatment of chronic staphylococcal osteomyelitis with cloxacillin and dicloxacillin – a comparative study in 12 patients. Scand J Infect Dis 7: 55.

Hedström SÅ, Kahlmeter G (1980). Dicloxacillin and flucloxacillin twice daily with probenecid in staphylococcal infections. Scand J Infect Dis 12: 221.

Herchline TE, Barnishan J, Ayers LW, Fass RJ (1990). Penicillinase production and in vitro susceptibilities of Staphylococcus lugdunensis. Antimicrob Ag Chemother 34: 2434.

Hilty MD, Venglarcik JS, Best GK (1980). Oxacillin-tolerant staphylococcal bacteremia in children. J Pediatr 96: 1035.

Hirschmann JV, Inui TS (1980). Antimicrobial prophylaxis: a critique of recent trials. Rev Infect Dis 2: 1.

Holzhoffer S, Süssmuth R, Haag R (1985). Oscillating tolerance in synchronized cultures of Staphylococcus aureus. Antimicrob Ag Chemother 28: 456.

Jarlov JO, Rosdahl VT, Mortensen I, Bentzon MW (1988). In vitro activity and beta-lactamase stability of methicillin, isoxazolyl penicillins and cephalothin against coagulase-negative staphylococci. J Antimicrob Chemother 22: 119.

Jick H, Derby LE, Dean AD, Henry DA (1994). Flucloxacillin and cholestatic hepatitis. Med J Aust 160: 525.

Jusko WJ, Mosovich LL, Gerbracht LM et al (1975). Enhanced renal excretion of dicloxacillin in patients with cystic fibrosis. Pediatrics 56: 1038.

Kahn JB (1978). Oxacillin-induced agranulocytosis. JAMA 240: 2632.

Kamme C, Ursing B (1974). Serum levels and clinical effect of flucloxacillin in patients with staphylococcal infections. Scand J Infect Dis 6: 273.

Kaplan MH, Tenenbaum MJ (1982). Staphylococcus aureus: cellular biology and clinical application. Amer J Med 72: 248.

Karchmer AW (1988). Antibiotic therapy of nonenterococcal streptococcal and staphylococcal endocarditis: current regimens and some future considerations. J Antimicrob Chemother 21 (Suppl C): 91.

Kim KS (1981). Oxacillin-tolerant staphylococcal bacteremia in children. J Pediatr 98: 170.

Klein JO, Sabath LD, Steinhauer BW, Finland M (1963). Oxacillin treatment of severe staphylococcal infections. New Engl J Med 269: 1215.

Knudsen ET, Brown DM, Rolinson GN (1962). A new orally effective penicillinase-stable penicillin – BRL. 1621 Lancet ii: 632.

Koch-Weser J, Sellers EM (1976). Binding of drugs to serum albumin (first of two parts). New Engl J Med 294: 311.

Lacey RW (1983). Treatment of staphylococcal infections. J Antimicrob Chemother 11: 3.

Langley JM, Le Blanc JC, Drake J, Milner R (1993). Efficacy of antimicrobial prophylaxis in placement of cerebrospinal fluid shunts: meta-analysis. Clin Infect Dis 17: 98.

Lee RD, Brusch JL, Barza MJ, Weinstein L (1975). Effect of probenecid on penetration of oxacillin into fibrin clots in vitro. Antimicrob Ag Chemother 8: 105.

Leventhal JM, Silken AB (1976). Oxacillin-induced neutropenia in children. J Pediatr 89: 769.

Levy M, Egersegi P, Strong A et al (1990). Pharmacokinetic analysis of cloxacillin loss in children undergoing major surgery with massive bleeding. Antimicrob Ag Chemother 34: 1150.

Lindup WE, Orme MCLE (1981). Clinical pharmacology: plasma protein binding of drugs. Brit Med J 282: 212.

Lorian V, Atkinson B (1980). Killing of oxacillin-exposed staphylococci in human polymorphonuclear leukocytes. Antimicrob Ag Chemother 18: 807.

Lotric-Furlan S, Lejko Zupanc T, Jereb M (1994). Cloxacillin-induced cholestasis. Clin Infect Dis 19: 981.

Malone AJ Jr, Field S, Rosman J, Shemerdiak WP (1977). Neurotoxic reaction to oxacillin. New Engl J Med 296: 453.

Massanari RM, Pfaller MA, Wakefield DS, et al. (1988). Implications of acquired oxacillin resistance in the management and control of Staphylococcus aureus infections. J Infect Dis 158: 702.

Mattie H, Goslings WRO, Noach EL (1973). Cloxacillin and nafcillin: serum binding and its relationship to antibacterial effect in mice. J Infect Dis 128: 170.

Mayhall CG, Apollo E (1980). Effect of storage and changes in bacterial growth phase and antibiotic concentrations on anti-microbial tolerance in Staphylococcus aureus. Antimicrob Ag Chemother 18: 784.

McCracken GH Jr, Nelson JD (1983). Antimicrobial Therapy for Newborns, 2nd edn, p. 27. New York: Grune and Stratton.

Merrikin DJ, Briant J, Rolinson GN (1983). Effect of protein binding on antibiotic activity in vivo. J Antimicrob Chemother 11: 233.

Miros M, Walker N, Kerlin P, Harris O (1990). Flucloxacillin induced delayed cholestatic hepatitis. Aust NZ J Med 20: 251.

Mullany CJ, McIsaacs AI, Rowe MH, Hale GS (1989). The surgical treatment of infective endocarditis. World J Surg 13: 132.

Murphy MF, Chapman JF, Metcalfe P, Waters AH (1985). Antibiotic-induced neutropenia. Lancet ii: 1306.

Nauta EH, Mattie H (1975). Pharmacokinetics of flucloxacillin and cloxacillin in healthy subjects and patients on chronic intermittent haemodialysis. Brit J Clin Pharmac 2: 111.

Nauta EH, Mattie H, Goslings WRO (1974). Effect of probenecid on the apparent volume of distribution and elimination of cloxacillin. Antimicrob Ag Chemother 6: 300.

Nelson JD, Howard JB, Shelton S (1978). Oral antibiotic therapy for skeletal infections of children I Antibiotic concentrations in suppurative synovial fluid. J Pediatr 92: 131.

Neu HC (1982). Antistaphylococcal penicillins. Med Clin N Amer 66: 51.

Norden CW (1983). A critical review of antibiotic prophylaxis in orthopedic surgery. Rev Infect Dis 5: 928.

Olans RN, Weiner LB (1976). Reversible oxacillin hepatotoxicity. J Pediatr 89: 835.

Onorato IM, Axelrod JL (1978). Hepatitis from intravenous high-dose oxacillin therapy. Ann Intern Med 89: 497.

Parker RH, Fossieck BE Jr (1980). Intravenous followed by oral antimicrobial therapy for staphylococcal endocarditis. Ann Intern Med 93: 832.

Pefanis A, Thauvin-Eliopoulos C, Eliopoulos GM, Moellering RCJr (1993). Activity of ampicillin-sulbactam and oxacillin in experimental endocarditis caused by beta-lactamase-hyperproducing Staphylococcus aureus. Antimicrob Ag Chemother 37: 507.

Pelletier LL Jr, Baker CB (1988). Oxacillin, cephalothin, and vancomycin tube macrodilution MBC result reproducibility and equivalence to MIC results for methicillin-susceptible and reputedly tolerant Staphylococcus aureus isolates. Antimicrob Ag Chemother;32: 374.

Perl TM, Pfaller MA, Houston A, Wenzel RP (1990). Effect of serum on the in vitro activities of 11 broad-spectrum antibiotics. Antimicrob Ag Chemother 34: 2234.

Peterson LR, Gerding DN (1980). Influence of protein binding of antibiotics on serum pharmacokinetics and extravascular penetration: clinically useful concepts. Rev Infect Dis 2: 340.

Pichichero ME, Friesen HA (1982). Polymicrobial osteomyelitis: report of three cases and review of the literature. *Rev Infect Dis* **4**: 86.

Pollard JP, Hughes SPF, Evans MJ *et al.* (1979). Concentration of flucloxacillin in femoral head and joint capsule in total hip replacement. *J Antimicrob Chemother* **5**: 721.

Price JD, Harding JW (1975). Flucloxacillin in the treatment of infectious conditions in children. *Curr Med Res Opin* **3**: 77.

Quintiliani R, Cooper BW (1988). Current concepts in the treatment of staphylococcal meningitis. *J Antimicrob Chemother* **21** (Suppl C): 107.

Rajashekaraiah KR, Rice T, Rao VS *et al.* (1980). Clinical significance of tolerant strains of *Staphylococcus aureus* in patients with endocarditis. *Ann Intern Med* **93**: 796.

Raynor RH, Scott DF, Best GK (1979). Oxacillin-induced lysis of *Staphylococcus aureus*. *Antimicrob Ag Chemother* **16**: 134.

Rennenberg J, Forsgren A (1989). The activity of isoxazolyl penicillins in experimental staphylococcal infection. *J Infect Dis* **159**: 1128.

Richmond AS, Simberkoff MS, Schaefler S, Rahal JJ Jr (1977). Resistance of *Staphylococcus aureus* to semisynthetic penicillins and cephalothin. *J Infect Dis* **135**: 108.

Rolinson GN (1980). The significance of protein binding of antibiotics in antibacterial chemotherapy. *J Antimicrob Chemother* **6**: 311.

Rolinson GN, Sutherland R (1965). The binding of antibiotics to serum proteins. *Brit J Pharmacol* **25**: 638.

Rosenblatt JE, Kind AC, Brodie JL, Kirby WMM (1968). Mechanisms responsible for the blood level differences of isoxazolyl penicillins, oxacillin, cloxacillin and dicloxacillin. *Arch Intern Med* **121**: 345.

Saliba B, Herbert PN (1994). Oxacillin hepatotoxicity in HIV-infected patients. *Ann Intern Med* **120**: 1048.

Sanderson PJ (1989). Preventing infection in orthopaedic implants. *J Antimicrob Chemother* **24**: 277.

Scalley RD, Roark RD (1977). Oxacillin-induced agranulocytosis. *Drug Intellig Clin Pharm* **2**: 420.

Schwartz GJ, Hegyi T, Spitzer A (1976). Subtherapeutic dicloxacillin levels in a neonate: possible mechanisms. *J Pediatr* **89**: 310.

Sierra-Madero JG, Knapp C, Karaffa C, Washington JA (1988). Role of beta-lactamase and different testing conditions in oxacillin-borderline-susceptible staphylococci. *Antimicrob Ag Chemother* **32**: 1754.

Spino M, Chai RP, Isles AF *et al.* (1984). Cloxacillin absorption and disposition in cystic fibrosis. *J Pediatr* **105**: 829.

Stewart GT (ed). (1962). A report from six hospitals. Clinical and laboratory results with BRL. 1621. *Lancet* **ii**: 634.

Stewart GT (1965). *The Penicillin Group of Drugs*, p. 41. Amsterdam, London, New York: Elsevier Publishing Company.

Strausbaugh LJ, Murray TW, Sande MA (1980). Comparative penetration of six antibiotics into the cerebrospinal fluid of rabbits with experimental staphylococcal meningitis. *J Antimicrob Chemother* **6**: 363.

Suh B, Craig WA, England AC, Elliott RL (1981). Effect of free fatty acids on protein binding of antimicrobial agents. *J Infect Dis* **143**: 609.

Sutherland R, Croydon EAP, Rolinson GN (1970). Flucloxacillin, a new isoxazolyl penicillin, compared with oxacillin, cloxacillin and dicloxacillin. *Brit Med J* **4**: 455.

Taryle DA, Good JT Jr, Morgan EJ Jr III *et al.* (1981). Antibiotic concentrations in human parapneumonic effusions. *J Antimicrob Chemother* **7**: 171.

Taylor C, Corrigan K, Steen S, Craig C (1979). Oxacillin and hepatitis. *Ann Intern Med* **90**: 857.

Ten Pas A, Quinn EL (1965). Cholestatic hepatitis following the administration of sodium oxacillin. *JAMA* **191**: 674.

Tetzlaff TR, Howard JB, McCracken GH Jr *et al.* (1978). Antibiotic concentrations in pus and bone of children with osteomyelitis. *J Pediatr* **92**: 135.

Thijssen HHW, Mattie H (1976). Active metabolites of isoxazolylpenicillins in humans. *Antimicrob Ag Chemother* **10**: 441.

Tilney NL, Strom TB, Vineyard GC, Merrill JP (1978). Factors contributing to the declining mortality rate in renal transplantation. *New Engl J Med* **299**: 1321.

Turck M, Ronald A, Petersdorf RG (1965). Clinical studies with cloxacillin. A new antibiotic. *JAMA* **192**: 961.

Unsworth PF, Heatley FW, Phillips I (1978). Flucloxacillin in bone. *J Clin Pathol* **31**: 705.

Vandenesch F, Etienne J, Reverdy E, Eykyn SJ (1993). Endocarditis due to *Staphylococcus lugdunensis*: report of 11 cases and review. *Clin Infect Dis* **17**: 871.

Van der Auwera P, Meunier-Carpentier F, Klastersky J (1983). Clinical study of combination therapy with oxacillin and rifampin for staphylococcal infections. *Rev Infect Dis* **5** (Suppl 3): 515.

Van der Auwera P, Klastersky J, Thys JP *et al.* (1985). Double-blind, placebo-controlled study of oxacillin combined with rifampin in the treatment of staphylococcal infections. *Antimicrob Ag Chemother* **28**: 467.

Van Ek B, Dijkmans BAC, Van Dulken H, Van Furth R (1988). Antibiotic prophylaxis in craniotomy: a prospective double-blind placebo-controlled study. *Scand J Infect Dis* **20**: 633.

Van Ek B, Dijkmans BAC, Van Dulken H *et al.* (1991a). Efficacy of cloxacillin prophylaxis in craniotomy: a one year follow-up study. *Scand J Infect Dis* **23**: 617.

Van Ek B, Dijkmans BAC, Van Dulken H, Van Furth R (1991b). Cloxacillin prophylaxis in craniotomies reduces costs of health care. *J Infect Dis* **164**: 1243.

Venglarcik JS III, Blair LL, Dunkle LM (1983). pH-dependent oxacillin tolerance of *Staphylococcus aureus*. *Antimicrob Ag Chemother* **23**: 232.

Voorn GP, Thompson J, Goessens WHF *et al.* (1991). Role of tolerance in cloxacillin treatment of experimental *Staphylococcus aureus* endocarditis. *J Infect Dis* **163**: 640.

Voorn GP, Thompson J, Goessens WHF *et al.* (1992). Role of tolerance in cloxacillin prophylaxis of experimental *Staphylococcus aureus* endocarditis. *J Infect Dis* **166**: 169.

Watanakunakorn C (1978). Antibiotic-tolerant *Staphylococcus aureus*. *J Antimicrob Chemother* **4**: 561.

Watanakunakorn C (1987). Bacteremic *Staphylococcus aureus* pneumonia. *Scand J Infect Dis* **19**: 623.

Westerman EL, Bradshaw MW, Williams TW Jr (1978). Agranulocytosis during therapy with orally administered cloxacillin. *Amer J Clin Pathol* **69**: 559.

Whitby M, Fraser S, Gemmell CG, Wright PA (1983). Toxic shock syndrome and endocarditis. *Brit Med J* **286**: 1613.

Williams RF (1982). Choice of chemotherapy for infection by *Staphylococcus aureus*. *J Antimicrob Chemother* **9**: 1.

Wilson APR (1988). Antibiotic prophylaxis in cardiac surgery. *J Antimicrob Chemother* **21**: 522.

Wilson APR Taylor B, Treasure T *et al.* (1988). Antibiotic prophylaxis in cardiac surgery: serum and tissue levels of teicoplanin, flucloxacillin and tobramycin. *J Antimicrob Chemother* **21**: 201.

Wise R (1983). Protein binding of beta-lactams: the effects on activity and pharmacology particularly tissue penetration. II Studies in man. *J Antimicrob Chemother* **12**: 105.

Wise R, Gillett AP, Cadge B *et al.* (1980). The influence of protein binding upon tissue fluid levels of beta-lactam antibiotics. *J Infect Dis* **142**: 77.

Woods GL, Yam P (1988). Bactericidal activity of oxacillin against beta-lactamase-hyperproducing *Staphylococcus aureus*. *Antimicrob Ag Chemother* **32**: 1614.

Woolfrey BF, Lally RT, Ederer MN (1985). Evaluation of oxacillin tolerance in *Staphylococcus aureus* by a novel method. *Antimicrob Ag Chemother* **28**: 381.

Yow MD, South MA, Hess CG (1964). The use of the penicillinase-resistant penicillin in the pneumonias of children. *Postgrad Med J* (Suppl) **40**: 127.

Nafcillin

Description

Nafcillin, 6-(2-ethoxy-1-naphthamido) penicillanic acid, is another semisynthetic penicillin derived from the penicillin nucleus, 6 APA (p. 3). Similar to methicillin (p. 77) and the isoxazolyl penicillins (p. 90), it is penicillinase-resistant. Developed in 1961, it has since been widely used in the USA for the parenteral treatment of serious beta-lactamase-producing staphylococcal infections.

Sensitive Organisms

Nafcillin has a similar antibacterial spectrum to the isoxazolyl penicillins (p. 90). It is about as active as oxacillin against both penicillin G-sensitive and penicillin G-resistant *Staphylococcus aureus* strains (Klein *et al.*, 1963). Stability of nafcillin in the presence of staphylococcal beta-lactamase (penicillinase) is comparable with that of methicillin (p. 77) and greater than that of the isoxazolyl penicillins (p. 77). Methicillin-resistant *Staph. aureus* strains are resistant to all penicillinase-resistant penicillins, including nafcillin (Barber and Waterworth, 1964; Richmond *et al.*, 1977) (p. 78). Both penicillin G-sensitive and beta-lactamase-producing strains of coagulase-negative staphylococci are nafcillin-sensitive. In some hospitals over 50% of coagulase-negative staphylococci are methicillin-resistant (p. 81), and these are resistant to nafcillin (Karchmer *et al.*, 1983). Penicillin-tolerant *Staph. aureus* and coagulase-negative staphylococci are usually also tolerant to nafcillin, but this varies according to the laboratory technique used (Norden and Keleti, 1981; Arthur *et al.*, 1982). As with isoxazolyl penicillins (p. 91), this may vary *in vivo* in different parts of body. Thus in the presence of polyvinylchloride catheters, the MBCs of nafcillin for coagulase-negative staphylococci are considerably higher than in the absence of such catheters (Sheth *et al.*, 1985). Clinical significance of staphylococcal tolerance is discussed on p. 91. Nafcillin and gentamicin are synergistic *in vitro* against most *Staph. aureus* strains (Eliopoulos and Moellering, 1982); the therapeutic advantage of this combination is uncertain (p. 105).

Nafcillin has a higher degree of activity than methicillin and the isoxazolyl penicillins against pneumococci and hemolytic streptococci. *Enterococcus faecalis* is relatively resistant (Table I.6). A nafcillin/ampicillin combination is synergistic *in vitro* against ampicillin-resistant *Haemophilus influenzae* strains (p. 112); these strains are inhibited when both drugs are used in a concentration of 0.78 μg per ml. The combination is effective for the treatment of experimental *H. influenzae* sepsis in animals, and it was used to treat successfully a child with osteomyelitis due to an ampicillin-resistant *H. influenzae* strain (Yogev and Kabat, 1980; Yogev *et al.*, 1980).

Table I.6
Compiled from data published by Barber and Waterworth (1964) and Arthur *et al.* (1982)

Organism	MIC (μg per ml)
Staphylococcus aureus (non-penicillinase producer)	0.25–0.5
Staphylococcus aureus (penicillinase producer)	0.25–1.0
Staphylococcus epidermidis (penicillinase producer)	1.5
Streptococcus pyogenes	0.03–0.06
Streptococcus pneumoniae	0.03–0.06
Enterococcus faecalis	8.0

The MICs of nafcillin against some selected bacteria are shown in Table I.6. If activity against *Staph. aureus* is tested in 95% human serum instead of nutrient broth, extensive protein binding occurs, and MICs are increased about 10-fold (Barber and Waterworth, 1964).

Mode of Administration and Dosage

1 Oral administration

Because it is poorly absorbed from the gastrointestinal tract, oral administration of nafcillin is not recommended (Klein *et al.*, 1963; Watanakunakorn, 1977).

2 Parenteral administration

Nafcillin can be given either i.m. or i.v.. The usual adult dosage is 1 g 4-hourly, but this can be doubled for the treatment of severe infections. Doses of up to 18 g i.v. daily have been given to adults with no ill effects (Eickhoff *et al.*, 1965). The drug should be given i.v. using techniques as described for penicillin G (p. 20).

3 Children

The usual dosage is 100–200 mg per kg body weight per day i.m. or i.v., given in four or six divided doses.

4 Newborn and premature infants

The recommended dosage for severe infection is 100 mg per kg per day, given in two divided doses for infants less than 7 days of age, and in three divided doses for those older than 7 days. This dose is safe for all newborns, but in those with birth weights less than 2000 g unnecessarily high serum levels are obtained. A dose of 20 mg per kg body weight, administered 8-hourly, is probably sufficient for those with low birth weights (Banner *et al.*, 1980).

5 Patients with renal failure

Nafcillin is eliminated from the body rapidly by non-renal mechanisms (Kind *et al.*, 1970), so that dosage reduction is not needed in such patients. The serum nafcillin half-life is unaltered in anuric patients during hemodialysis and in the interval between dialyses, so that they can be treated by a nafcillin dosage used for patients with normal renal function (Diaz *et al.*, 1977).

Serum Levels in Relation to Dosage

Following i.v. infusion of a 0.5 g dose of nafcillin over 15 min to adults, the serum level is 11 μg per ml at the end of the infusion and 0.5 μg per ml at 6 h (Neu, 1982). After an i.m. injection of 1 g, a peak serum level of about 8 μg per ml is reached 1 h later; it falls to about 0.5 μg per ml at 6 h (Whitehouse *et al.*, 1963). Concomitant oral administration of probenecid increases and prolongs nafcillin levels, similar to other penicillins (Klein *et al.*, 1963) (p. 24). Nafcillin serum levels are lower than those attained with equal doses of i.m. oxacillin (p. 94), because it is distributed in a larger volume in the body, and it is more rapidly inactivated by the liver (Kind *et al.*, 1970). Serum levels following oral nafcillin are low and irregular. If the drug is taken with food, its absorption is even more impaired (Klein *et al.*, 1963; Whitehouse *et al.*, 1963).

Excretion

1 Urine

About 30% of an i.m. administered dose of nafcillin can be recovered from the urine where concentrations reach as high as 1000 μg per ml. A considerably smaller amount of active nafcillin (about 19% of the administered dose) is recovered from the urine after i.m. administration if it is given with probenecid (Klein *et al.*, 1963).

2 Bile

A small amount, probably only about 8% of an i.m. dose is eliminated via the bile (Kind *et al.*, 1970).

3 Inactivation in body

The remainder of administered nafcillin appears to be inactivated in the liver (Kind *et al.*, 1970). This inactivation takes place even more rapidly than in the case of oxacillin (p. 95).

Distribution of the Drug in Body

Tissue penetration of nafcillin is probably similar to the isoxazolyl penicillins (p. 95). It penetrates into the CSF of rabbits with experimental staphylococcal meningitis to about the same extent as oxacillin, producing CSF concentrations which are 1.4–2% of simultaneous serum levels (Strausbaugh *et al.*, 1980). Higher nafcillin CSF concentrations have been detected in patients with and without meningitis. In seven patients with normal meninges who receive an i.v. nafcillin dose of 40 mg per kg infused over 30 min, mean CSF concentrations were 0.05, 0.12, 0.09 and 0.03 µg per ml, 1, 2, 3 and 4 h after infusion, respectively (Fossieck *et al.*, 1977). Ruiz and Warner (1976) treated an adult patient with staphylococcal meningitis using a nafcillin dose of 200 mg per kg per day; a high CSF concentration of 9.5 µg per ml was reached 45 min after a 3 g i.v. dose, administered over 5 min. Kane *et al.* (1977) studied nine patients with severe staphylococcal infections who were treated by i.v. nafcillin. High CSF levels (7.5–88.0 µg per ml) were found in three patients with purulent meningitis and in two with staphylococcal septicemia who only had a CSF pleocytosis; lower CSF levels (0.13–2.7 µg per ml) occurred in patients without a CSF pleocytosis. Penetration of i.v. administered nafcillin into the ventricular fluid of hydrocephalic children has been studied; in seven with bacterial ventriculitis, concentrations of nafcillin in ventricular fluid were 0.8–20.4% of the peak serum level, whilst in seven others without bacterial ventriculitis, these levels were <0.02–4% of peak serum concentrations (Yogev *et al.*, 1981).

Mode of Action

The mode of action of nafcillin on bacteria is similar to penicillin G (p. 25).

Toxicity

1 Hypersensitivity reactions

Nafcillin, like other penicillins, may cause the same hypersensitivity reactions that occur with penicillin G (p. 28). The drug is contraindicated in any patient with a history of penicillin sensitivity.

2 Nephrotoxicity

Parry *et al.* (1973) described a patient who developed renal damage due to methicillin, which resolved when lincomycin was substituted. Later when therapy was changed to nafcillin, the 'hypersensitivity nephritis' recurred. Nephropathy has been reported on many occasions with methicillin (p. 84), but less commonly with other penicillinase-resistant penicillins. If nephropathy develops after the use of one penicillin analog, it is likely to recur if any other penicillin is subsequently used.

Nafcillin administered in large doses i.v. (200 mg per kg per day) can cause hypokalemia and associated alkalosis. Nafcillin acts as a non-reabsorbable anion and increases passive renal distal tubular potassium excretion. This is similar to what occurs with other penicillins used in large doses, such as penicillin G (p. 34). Hypokalemia may resolve when the nafcillin dose is reduced (Andreoli *et al.*, 1980).

Nafcillin in the urine can cause a false-positive urine reaction for protein, when the sulfasalicylic test is used, but not with the dipstick test. Unrecognized, this may lead to unnecessary cessation of the drug and even renal biopsy (Line *et al.*, 1976). Penicillin G and oxacillin can also cause false-positive urine protein determinations, but to a lesser degree.

3 Hematological side-effects

Neutropenia with concomitant fever, occurred in one patient receiving a daily dose of 12 g i.v. nafcillin. This complication resolved when the drug was stopped (Sandberg *et al.*, 1975). In another patient, i.v. nafcillin therapy (12 g daily) was associated with the development of agranulocytosis, which only improved after the drug was discontinued (Markowitz *et al.*, 1975). Greene and Cohen (1978) described neutropenia in three children receiving i.v. nafcillin, which resolved when nafcillin was ceased. All beta-lactam antibiotics can cause neutropenia (p. 33).

Two patients treated by high daily doses of nafcillin i.v. (12–14 g) developed abnormal bleeding times and one had a bleeding episode. This was due to platelet dysfunction, similar to that described with penicillin G (p. 33) (Alexander *et al.*, 1983).

4 Skin and tissue necrosis

This can occur after accidental subcutaneous extravasation of i.v. nafcillin, and may necessitate multiple tissue debridement and skin grafting. In animals, tissue necrosis occurs after subcutaneous inoculation of nafcillin, but not with oxacillin, methicillin and cephalothin (Tilden et al., 1980). In humans, nafcillin-induced tissue injury can be prevented by prompt administration of hyaluronidase into the site of extravasation (Zenk et al., 1981).

Clinical uses of the Drug

1 Staphylococcus aureus infections

Parenteral nafcillin has been used successfully for the treatment of severe Staph. aureus infections, such as septicemia, endocarditis, osteomyelitis, septic arthritis, pneumonia, meningitis and pyomyositis (Eickhoff et al., 1965; Goldenberg and Cohen 1976; Parker and Fossieck, 1980; Carney et al., 1982; Watanakunakorn, 1987; Kim et al., 1989; Walling and Kaelin, 1991; Givner and Kaplan, 1993). In the USA nafcillin is usually preferred for treatment of Staph. aureus endocarditis (Masur et al., 1978; Sande and Scheld, 1980). Severe Staph. aureus septicemia only slowly responds to treatment, and if a patient on day 3 or 4 of treatment is still febrile and still has a positive blood culture, this in itself does not mean that the chemotherapy should be changed (Eng et al., 1987).

Although the synergistic combination of nafcillin plus gentamicin has usually demonstrated a superior therapeutic effect, compared with nafcillin alone, in experimental animals (Fantin and Carbon, 1992), it is still uncertain whether the synergistic nafcillin/gentamicin combination is clinically superior to nafcillin alone, for the treatment of human endocarditis caused by tolerant or non-tolerant Staph. aureus strains (p. 91). The USA National Collaborative Endocarditis Study Group compared a regimen of nafcillin alone for 6 weeks with one in which gentamicin was added for the first 2 weeks for the treatment of Staph. aureus endocarditis patients, a proportion of whom were parenteral drug addicts. With the combination regimen there was a slightly more rapid clinical response (defervescence and normalization of leukocyte count) and somewhat more rapid clearance of bacteremia. In the non-addict group there was a higher frequency of nephrotoxicity with the combination therapy. The addition of gentamicin did not alter morbidity or mortality in either group. The authors suggested that it may be reasonable to initiate combination therapy in patients with Staph. aureus endocarditis, but the aminoglycoside should be stopped after clearance of bacteremia (3–5 days) and that nafcillin alone be continued for a total of 6 weeks (Korzeniowski et al., 1982). In another study, patients with Staph. aureus septicemia (with or without endocarditis) were treated by nafcillin alone. Patients infected with tolerant organisms (p. 91) remained febrile longer than those infected by non-tolerant strains, but they did not require additional antibiotics for cure (Rahal et al., 1986). Selected i.v. drug abusers with uncomplicated right-sided endocarditis have been treated successfully with only a 2-week course of nafcillin plus tobramycin (Chambers et al., 1988). A 2-week treatment with cloxacillin 2 g 4-hourly plus amikacin 7.5 mg per kg 12-hourly was also successful for the treatment of Staph. aureus right-sided endocarditis in these patients, provided they appeared to have good prognosis initially (Torres-Tortosa et al., 1994).

A rifampicin/nafcillin combination has been used to treat chronic staphylococcal osteomyelitis (p. 695). Nafcillin is now preferred to methicillin, mainly because of the latter's greater propensity to cause nephropathy (p. 84). In Australia and in Europe one of the parenteral isoxazolyl penicillins such as cloxacillin or flucloxacillin (p. 97) are commonly used. The response obtained in severe staphylococcal infections is about the same with all of these drugs, provided they are given parenterally in appropriate doses.

Because of its better penetration into the CSF (p. 104), some authors regard nafcillin as the drug of choice for staphylococcal meningitis (Ruiz and Warner, 1976; Fossieck et al., 1977). If nafcillin is used for this purpose, the parenteral dose should be at least 2 g 4-hourly for adults (Kane et al., 1977; Quintiliani and Cooper, 1988). For the treatment of staphylococcal meningitis a nafcillin/rifampicin combination may prove to be more effective (Gordon et al., 1985) (p. 695).

There is some evidence that beta-lactam antibiotics such as nafcillin are more effective than vancomycin (p. 777) for the treatment of severe methicillin-sensitive Staph. aureus infections such as endocarditis. Therefore the use of vancomycin for such infections should be avoided as far as possible (Wood and Wisniewski, 1994).

2 Infections due to coagulase-negative staphylococci

Nafcillin can be used to treat severe hospital-acquired infections caused by these organisms, such as prosthetic valve endocarditis, provided the strain is methicillin-sensitive (p. 81). The addition of either gentamicin (p. 474) or rifampicin (p. 696) or both to the nafcillin regimen may improve the results of treatment (Sande and Scheld, 1980). If the strain is methicillin-resistant, which is often so if the infection is hospital-acquired, vancomycin should be used and the addition of either rifampicin or gentamicin or both, may be of benefit (Karchmer *et al.*, 1983; Caputo *et al.*, 1987). Chemoprophylaxis with nafcillin plus rifampicin has been used for patients undergoing cardiac valve surgery. But in one study more than half of the patients receiving such chemoprophylaxis became colonized by *Staph. epidermidis* strains resistant to methicillin, gentamicin and rifampicin (Archer and Armstrong, 1983). Antibiotic prophylaxis is therefore an important factor in perpetuating the hospital reservoir for antibiotic-resistant staphylococcal strains.

References

Alexander DP, Russo ME, Fohrman DE, Rothstein G (1983). Nafcillin-induced platelet dysfunction and bleeding. *Antimicrob Ag Chemother* **23**: 59.

Andreoli SP, Kleiman MB, Glick MR, Bergstein JM (1980). Nafcillin, pseudo-proteinuria and hypokalemic alkalosis. *J Pediatr* **97**: 841.

Archer GL, Armstrong BC (1983). Alteration of staphylococcal flora in cardiac surgery patients receiving antibiotic prophylaxis. *J Infect Dis* **147**: 642.

Arthur JD, Bass JW, Keiser JF *et al.* (1982). Nafcillin-tolerant *Staphylococcus epidermidis* endocarditis. *JAMA* **247**: 487.

Banner W Jr, Gooch WM, Burckart G, Korones SB (1980). Pharmacokinetics of nafcillin in infants with low birth weights. *Antimicrob Ag Chemother* **17**: 691.

Barber M, Waterworth PM (1964). Penicillinase-resistant penicillins and cephalosporins. *Brit Med J* **2**: 344.

Caputo GM, Archer GL, Calderwood SB *et al.* (1987). Native valve endocarditis due to coagulase-negative staphylococci. Clinical and microbiological features. *Amer J Med* **83**: 619.

Carney DN, Fossieck BE Jr, Parker RH, Minna JD (1982). Bacteremia due to *Staphylococcus aureus* in patients with cancer: report on 45 cases in adults and review of the literature. *Rev Infect Dis* **4**: 1.

Chambers HF, Miller RT, Newman MD (1988). Right-sided *Staphylococcus aureus* endocarditis in intravenous drug abusers; two-week combination therapy. *Ann Intern Med* **109**: 619.

Diaz CR, Kane JG, Parker RH, Pelsor FR (1977). Pharmacokinetics of nafcillin in patients with renal failure. *Antimicrob Ag Chemother* **12**: 98.

Eickhoff TC, Kislak JW, Finland M (1965). Clinical evaluation of nafcillin in patients with severe staphylococcal disease. *New Engl J Med* **272**: 699.

Eliopoulos GM, Moellering RC Jr (1982). Antibiotic synergism and antimicrobial combinations in clinical infections. *Rev Infect Dis* **4**: 282.

Eng RHK, Bishburg E, Smith SM, Scadutto P (1987). *Staphylococcus aureus* bacteremia during therapy. *J Infect Dis* **155**: 1331.

Fantin B, Carbon C (1992). *In vivo* antibiotic synergism: contribution of animal models. *Antimicrob Ag Chemother* **36**: 907.

Fossieck BE Jr, Kane JG, Diaz CR, Parker RH (1977). Nafcillin entry into human cerebrospinal fluid. *Antimicrob Ag Chemother* **11**: 965.

Givner LB, Kaplan SL (1993). Meningitis due to *Staphylococcus aureus* in children. *Clin Infect Dis* **16**: 766.

Goldenberg DL, Cohen AS (1976). Acute infectious arthritis A review of patients with nongonococcal joint infections (with emphasis on therapy and prognosis). *Amer J Med* **60**: 369.

Gordon JJ, Harter DH, Phair JP (1985). Meningitis due to *Staphylococcus aureus*. *Amer J Med* **78**: 965.

Greene GR, Cohen E (1978). Nafcillin-induced neutropenia in children. *Pediatrics* **61**: 94.

Kane JG, Parker RH, Jordan GW, Hoeprich PD (1977). Nafcillin concentration in cerebrospinal fluid during treatment of staphylococcal infections. *Ann Intern Med* **87**: 309.

Karchmer AW, Archer GL, Dismukes WE (1983). *Staphylococcus epidermidis* causing prosthetic valve endocarditis: microbiologic and clinical observations as guides to therapy. *Ann Intern Med* **98**: 447.

Kim JH, van der Horst C, Mulrow CD, Corey GR (1989). *Staphylococcus aureus* meningitis: review of 28 cases. *Rev Infect Dis* **11**: 698.

Kind AC, Tupasi TE, Standiford HC, Kirby WMM (1970). Mechanisms responsible for plasma levels of nafcillin lower than those of oxacillin. *Arch Intern Med* **125**: 685.

Klein JO, Finland M, Wilcox C (1963). Nafcillin. Antibacterial action *in vitro* and absorption and excretion in normal young men. *Amer J Med Sci* **246**: 10.

Korzeniowski O, Sande MA The National Collaborative Endocarditis Study Group (1982). Combination antimicrobial therapy for *Staphylococcus aureus* endocarditis in patients addicted to parenteral drugs and in nonaddicts. *Ann Intern Med* **97**: 496.

Line DE, Adler S, Fraley DS, Burns FJ (1976). Massive pseudoproteinuria caused by nafcillin. *JAMA* **235**: 1259.

Markowitz SM, Rothkopf M, Holden FD *et al.* (1975). Nafcillin-induced agranulocytosis. *JAMA* **232**: 1150.

Masur H, Murray HW, Roberts RB (1978). Nafcillin therapy for *Staphylococcus aureus* endocarditis. *Antimicrob Ag Chemother* **14**: 457.

Neu HC (1982). Antistaphylococcal penicillins. *Med Clin N Amer* **66**: 51.

Norden CW, Keleti E (1981). Antibiotic tolerance in strains of *Staphylococcus aureus*. *J Antimicrob Chemother* **7**: 599.

Parker RH, Fossieck BE Jr (1980). Intravenous followed by oral antimicrobial therapy for staphylococcal endocarditis. *Ann Intern Med* **93**: 832.

Parry MF, Ball WD, Conte JE Jr, Cohen SN (1973). Nafcillin nephritis. *JAMA* **225**: 178.

Quintiliani R, Cooper BW (1988). Current concepts in the treatment of staphylococcal meningitis. *J Antimicrob Chemother* **21** (Suppl C): 107.

Rahal JJ Jr, Chan Y-K, Johnson G (1986). Relationship of staphylococcal tolerance, teichoic acid antibody and serum bactericidal activity to therapeutic outcome in *Staphylococcus aureus* bacteremia. *Amer J Med* **81**: 43.

Richmond AS, Simberkoff MS, Schaefler S, Rahal JJ Jr (1977). Resistance of *Staphylococcus aureus* to semisynthetic penicillin and cephalothin. *J Infect Dis* **135**: 108.

Rolinson GN, Sutherland R (1965). The binding of antibiotics to serum proteins. *Brit J Pharmacol* **25**: 638.

Ruiz DE, Warner JF (1976). Nafcillin treatment of *Staphylococcus aureus* meningitis. *Antimicrob Ag Chemother* **9**: 554.

Sandberg M, Tuazon CU, Sheagren JM (1975). Neutropenia probably resulting from nafcillin. *JAMA* **232**: 1152.

Sande MA, Scheld WM (1980). Combination antibiotic therapy of bacterial endocarditis. *Ann Intern Med* **92**: 390.

Sheth NK, Franson TR, Sohnle PG (1985). Influence of bacterial adherence to intravascular catheters on in-vitro antibiotic susceptibility. *Lancet* **ii**: 1266.

Strausbaugh LJ, Murray TW, Sande MA (1980). Comparative penetration of six antibiotics into the cerebrospinal fluid of rabbits with experimental staphylococcal meningitis. *J Antimicrob Chemother* **6**: 363.

Tilden SJ, Craft JC, Cano R, Daum RS (1980). Cutaneous necrosis associated with intravenous nafcillin therapy. *Amer J Dis Child* **134**: 1046,.

Torres-Tortosa M, de Cueto M, Vergara A *et al.* (1994). Prospective evaluation of two-week course of intravenous antibiotics in intravenous drug addicts with infective endocarditis. *Eur J Clin Microbiol Infect Dis* **13**: 559.

Walling DM, Kaelin WGJr (1991). Pyomyositis in patients with diabetes mellitus. *Rev Infect Dis* **13**: 797.

Watanakunakorn C (1977). Absorption of orally administered nafcillin in normal healthy volunteers. *Antimicrob Ag Chemother* **11**: 1007.

Watanakunakorn C (1987). Bacteremic *Staphylococcus aureus* pneumonia. *Scand J Infect Dis* **19**: 623.

Whitehouse AC, Morgan JG, Schumacher J, Hamburger M (1963). Blood levels and anti-staphylococcal titers produced in human subjects by a penicillinase-resistant penicillin, nafcillin, compared with similar penicillins. *Antimicrob Ag Chemother* **1962**: 384.

Wood CA, Wisniewski RM (1994). Beta-lactams versus glycopeptides in treatment of subcutaneous abscesses infected with *Staphylococcus aureus*. *Antimicrob Ag Chemother* **38**: 1023.

Yogev R, Kabat WJ (1980). Synergistic action of nafcillin and ampicillin against ampicillin-resistant *Haemophilus influenzae*. Type B bacteremia and meningitis in infant rats. *Antimicrob Ag Chemother* **18**: 122.

Yogev R, Burkholder E, Davis AT (1980). Synergistic action of ampicillin and nafcillin against ampicillin-resistant *Haemophilus influenzae*. *Antimicrob Ag Chemother* **17**: 461.

Yogev R, Schultz WE, Rosenman SB (1981). Penetrance of nafcillin into human ventricular fluid: correlation with ventricular pleocytosis and glucose levels. *Antimicrob Ag Chemother* **19**: 545.

Zenk KE, Dungy CI, Greene GR (1981). Nafcillin extravasation injury. *Amer J Dis Child* **135**: 1113.

Ampicillin (AMP)

Description

Ampicillin (AMP) is a semisynthetic penicillin derived from the penicillin nucleus, 6 APA (p. 3). It was developed at the Beecham Research Laboratories and it is chemically alpha-aminophenylacetamido-penicillanic acid (Rolinson and Stevens, 1961).

Sensitive Organisms

Not only is AMP active against most of the bacteria sensitive to penicillin G, but in addition, it is active against some Gram-negative bacilli, which are penicillin G-resistant. It has been referred to loosely as a 'broad spectrum penicillin', a somewhat misleading term which is better avoided.

1 Gram-positive cocci

It is known that AMP is active against many of the Gram-positive cocci, such as *Streptococcus pyogenes*, *Strep. pneumoniae* and *Strep. viridans*. Pneumococcal strains which are relatively resistant to penicillin G, are also usually relatively resistant to AMP to the same degree (p. 7) (Jorgensen *et al.*, 1990; Powell *et al.*, 1991). Completely penicillin G-resistant pneumococcal strains are also completely AMP-resistant (p. 7). Group B streptococci are always AMP-sensitive (Bayer *et al.*, 1976); in addition AMP combined with aminoglycosides, such as kanamycin, gentamicin, tobramycin or amikacin, acts synergistically against these organisms resulting in accelerated streptococcal killing (Cooper *et al.*, 1979). This effect has also been demonstrated in experimental Group B streptococcal meningitis of animals (Scheld *et al.*, 1982). Cephalosporins such as cefotaxime (p. 320) neither enhance nor decrease the activity of AMP or penicillin G against Group B streptococci *in vitro* (Landesman *et al.*, 1981). By contrast, chloramphenicol (Weeks *et al.*, 1981) and rifampicin (Smith *et al.*, 1982) inhibit the bactericidal activity of AMP for Group B streptococci *in vitro*.

Enterococcus faecalis is usually sensitive to AMP and often slightly more so than to penicillin G (p. 9). Strains resistant to penicillin G, e.g. those that produce beta-lactamase (p. 10) are also AMP-resistant. Other enterococci such as *E. faecium*, *E. raffinosus*, *E. durans* and *E. gallinarum* are usually sensitive, but many strains have acquired resistance to both penicillin G and ampicillin due to altered PBPs (Rupar *et al.*, 1989; Grayson *et al.*, 1991; Boyce *et al.*, 1992) (p. 10). Strains of *E. faecium* have also emerged which were resistant to vancomycin, AMP and to all aminoglycosides (Montecalvo *et al.*, 1994).

The combination of AMP with either streptomycin (p. 429) or kanamycin (p. 440) was synergistic against 50–75% of *E. faecalis* strains, whereas AMP plus gentamicin (p. 455) was synergistic against nearly all such strains. But now high-level gentamicin-resistant *E. faecalis* strains have emerged and with these AMP/aminoglycoside synergism cannot be obtained with any of the aminoglycosides, except occasionally with streptomycin, similar to penicillin G (p. 455). (Cercenado *et al.*, 1992). Also AMP plus ciprofloxacin are not synergistic against these strains (Smith and Eng, 1988). Anaerobic Gram-positive cocci, such as the *Peptococcus* and *Peptostreptococcus* spp. and anaerobic streptococci, are nearly always AMP-sensitive (Sutter and Finegold, 1976). With the exception of *E. faecalis*, penicillin G is more active against all of the above Gram-positive cocci, but its superiority to AMP is not great.

Because AMP is destroyed by staphylococcal beta-lactamase, most *Staphylococcus aureus* and hospital-acquired *Staph. epidermidis* strains are AMP-resistant, just as they are to penicillin G (p. 11). Usually *Staph. saprophyticus* which may be isolated from the urethra of young females, is AMP-sensitive (Marrie and Kwan, 1982; Hovelius and Mårdh, 1984). An intermediate type resistance for *Staph. saprophyticus* has been described for penicillin G, possibly due to production of small amounts of a beta-lactamase (p. 12).

2 Gram-positive bacilli

Corynebacterium diphtheriae and *Bacillus anthracis* are sensitive to AMP. *Listeria monocytogenes* is also usually sensitive to a degree comparable with that of penicillin G (p. 12). Whether these drugs are bactericidal to *L. monocytogenes* depends on the conditions under which the test is performed; with normal subculture after 24 h incubation, MICs of AMP are low (0.24 μg per ml), but MBCs are high (15.6–125.0 μg per ml) (Penn *et al.*, 1982); if subcultures are performed after 48 h incubation, AMP is bactericidal to most strains in low concentrations (Winslow *et al.*, 1983). Serum from AMP-treated patients is nearly always bactericidal to *L. monocytogenes*. It appears that human serum proteins, lysozyme and beta-lysin, are synergistic with AMP against this organism, so they probably contribute to the effectiveness of AMP *in vivo* (Asensi and Fierer, 1991). *In vitro* synergism against most strains of *L. monocytogenes* occurs with an AMP/gentamicin combination (Wiggins *et al.*, 1978). Liposomal encapsulation of AMP results in an increased availability of the drug for *L. monocytogenes* which is an intracellular organism (Bakker-Woudenberg *et al.*, 1986; Fattal *et al.*, 1991). The lipid composition of the liposome is important. All lipid capsules, carrying AMP, rapidly enter cells, but the more solid liposomes degrade slowly and result in slow release of AMP. The 'fluid type' liposomes degrade in cells more rapidly, release AMP without delay and this results in rapid killing of *L. monocytogenes* (Bakker-Woudenberg *et al.*, 1988).

Nocardia asteroides strains are AMP-resistant. In one study 27% and 62% of strains were susceptible to 3.1 and 25 μg per ml of AMP, respectively; beta-lactamase was detected in most isolates; and *in vitro* synergism between AMP and cloxacillin occurred with many AMP-resistant *Nocardia* strains (Wallace *et al.*, 1978).

Anaerobic Gram-positive sporing bacilli, such as *Clostridium tetani*, *Cl. perfringens*, *Cl. botulinum* and other *Clostridium* spp., are usually AMP-sensitive. Nearly always AMP is active against anaerobic Gram-positive asporogenous bacilli, such as the *Actinomyces*, *Eubacterium*, *Propionibacterium*, *Bifidobacterium* and *Lactobacillus* spp. (Sutter and Finegold, 1976).

3 Enterobacteriaceae

In contrast with penicillin G, AMP is active against some of these bacteria (Rolinson and Stevens, 1961). *Escherichia coli* may be sensitive, but many strains are resistant. This is particularly so in hospitals where more than 50% of *E. coli* strains can be AMP-resistant (Yoshioka *et al.*, 1977; Cooksey *et al.*, 1990; Gransden *et al.*, 1990; Spencer *et al.*, 1990; Burman *et al.*, 1992). Also AMP-resistant *E. coli* strains occur in community-acquired infections (Søgaard, 1975; Levy *et al.*, 1988; Chamberland *et al.*, 1992), and they are present in stools of normal volunteers (London *et al.*, 1993). A survey of 232 enteropathic *E. coli* strains from community-acquired infections during 1980–81 in the UK, showed that 37% were resistant to AMP (Gross *et al.*, 1982). Nearly always AMP-resistance of *E. coli* is due to beta-lactamase production. Often AMP-resistance genes and those producing resistance to gentamicin are found together in plasmids (Martin *et al.*, 1987; Ling *et al.*, 1994).

Enterobacter, *Klebsiella*, *Serratia*, *Citrobacter*, *Hafnia*, *Edwardsiella* and *Providencia* spp. are nearly always AMP-resistant (Eickhoff *et al.*, 1966). *Arizona* spp., which cause human disease similar to that produced by the salmonellae, are usually AMP-sensitive (Johnson *et al.*, 1976). Similarly, *Proteus mirabilis* is usually sensitive unless it is a beta-lactamase-producer. Other *Proteus* spp. are resistant. *Yersinia enterocolitica* is also usually resistant (Raevuori *et al.*, 1978; Baker and Farmer, 1982).

Salmonella spp. were usually susceptible to AMP but resistant strains, particularly of *Salm. typhimurium* have been reported increasingly since about 1967 (Bissett *et al.*, 1974; Grant *et al.*, 1976). In a survey of 718 *Salmonella* strains isolated from humans in North-Eastern USA, AMP resistance was detected in 36.9% of *Salm. typhimurium*; this resistance was less common among other *Salmonella* spp. On testing 688 *Salmonella* isolates from animal sources, AMP-resistant *Salm. typhimurium* was slightly less common (31%), but the reverse was true for most of the other *Salmonella* spp. tested (Neu *et al.*, 1975a). A change occurred in this area of the USA in 1975, when there was a decline in AMP-resistance of *Salm. typhimurium*; only 5.0–7.9% of human isolates were resistant compared with 75% resistant isolates obtained from farm animals (Cherubin *et al.*, 1980). It was concluded from this and other epidemiological observations, that antibiotic-resistant *Salmonella* strains which cause human infections, were usually not derived from animal sources in the USA (Cherubin, 1981). Other authors in the USA disputed this

(Bennett, 1980). In the UK, multiresistant *Salm. typhimurium* strains appeared in calves in 1977 and then spread to cattle; food poisoning was regarded as the main way humans acquired antibiotic-resistant *Salmonella* infections (Leading article, 1982). Use of antimicrobial drugs for the treatment and prophylaxis of disease in cattle was implicated in the occurrence of these resistant strains. Threlfall *et al.* (1980) studied 187 human isolates of resistant *Salm. typhimurium* strains in the UK; these were not only resistant to AMP, but also resistant to chloramphenicol, kanamycin, streptomycin, sulfonamides and tetracyclines; during 1979, 20 strains were isolated which were resistant to trimethoprim as well. During 1989–90, 14% of *Salmonella* spp. strains in the USA were AMP-resistant (Lee *et al.*, 1994).

Multiple antibiotic-resistance in salmonellae is usually mediated by plasmids (p. 549). By comparing the molecular structure of plasmids derived from multiresistant *Salmonella* strains of human and animal origin, O'Brien *et al.* (1982) showed that such strains were spread from animals to humans in the USA, as observed in the UK. This was confirmed in the USA when antimicrobial-resistant *Salm. newport* of animal origin caused serious human disease (Holmberg *et al.*, 1984). This conclusion was criticized by others (Du Pont and Steele, 1987). In the USA, AMP-resistant *Salm. typhimurium* increased in frequency from 1970, reaching about 40% by 1975, when about 10% of other *Salmonella* spp. had also become AMP-resistant. Associated resistance to streptomycin, tetracyclines and sulfonamides was quite common, but chloramphenicol-resistance was rare. Trimethoprim-resistant *Salm. krefeld* with plasmid-mediated multiple antibiotic-resistance was isolated from clinically ill animals in Texas, USA (Mathewson and Murray, 1983).

Multiple drug-resistant *Salmonella* strains have been implicated in nosocomial infections. In a South African hospital, *Salm. typhimurium* was isolated from 487 patients (many asymptomatic) over a 23-month period; the organism was resistant to AMP, chloramphenicol, kanamycin, streptomycin, spectinomycin, sulfonamides, tetracyclines, trimethoprim, and nalidixic acid (Robins-Browne *et al.*, 1983).

Multiply-resistant salmonellae have been a problem in developing countries. *Salmonella wien*, resistant to AMP and most other antibiotics except trimethoprim, caused a large prolonged epidemic in North Africa and Southern Europe (McConnell *et al.*, 1979). Multiresistant *Salm. typhimurium* was responsible for a large outbreak starting in 1977 in the Middle East and India. The majority of strains were resistant to AMP, chloramphenicol, kanamycin, streptomycin, sulfonamides, tetracyclines, gentamicin and trimethoprim. Most patients presented with gastroenteritis, but cases of septicemia occurred, and in some areas there was a high mortality (Rowe *et al.*, 1980). Multiresistant *Salm. typhimurium* has also caused outbreaks in South America, and other resistant *Salmonella* spp. have been causing disease in Hong Kong and Indonesia (Leading article, 1982). In Bombay, India, *Salm. typhimurium* was isolated from feces of 145 patients with gastroenteritis and from CSF, feces or blood of 42 patients with systemic salmonellosis; multiple antibiotic-resistance was encountered in 88.9% of isolates from the first group and in all the isolates from the second group. Resistance occurred to many antibiotics including AMP and chloramphenicol, but only in a proportion of isolates to trimethoprim and gentamicin (Rangnekar *et al.*, 1983). At any one time the prevalence of AMP-resistant salmonellae varied widely from country to country. For example in Thailand in the 1980s there was a nationwide outbreak of *Salmonella krefeld* infections and the strain was resistant to AMP, chloramphenicol and co-trimoxazole, yet in Sri Lanka and Mexico resistant salmonellae were rare at that time (Murray, 1986). In developing countries the main method of spread of *Salmonella* infection seems to have been from person to person, and resistance has probably arisen due to antibiotic use in humans (Rowe and Threlfall, 1981; Leading article, 1982). In most cases AMP-resistance is plasmid-mediated, but occasionally other resistance mechanisms, such as permeability change (p. 26) or PBPs alterations (p. 27) have been detected (Bellido *et al.*, 1989).

Ampicillin-resistant *Salmonella* spp. strains are usually susceptible to amoxycillin/clavulanic acid, cefotaxime, ceftriaxone, aztreonam and ciprofloxacin (Alos *et al.*, 1992).

Usually *Salm. typhi* is still susceptible to AMP. In the USA there were 2666 cases of acute typhoid fever between 1975 and 1984; 62% of them were imported, mainly from Mexico and India. Antimicrobial resistance was a minor problem, only 3% of the strains being resistant to AMP (Ryan *et al.*, 1989). Also during the 1972 chloramphenicol-resistant typhoid fever epidemic in Mexico (p. 550), when AMP was extensively used for treatment of the disease, a few *Salm. typhi* strains resistant to AMP and to chloramphenicol, were isolated from patients (Olarte and Galindo, 1973). These resistant strains did not become widespread in Mexico at that time. Since then *Salm. typhi* strains resistant to both AMP and chloramphenicol have been encountered in South-East Asia and India (Lampe *et al.*, 1975; Herzog, 1976), but were uncommon elsewhere

(Barros *et al.*, 1977; Chun *et al.*, 1977). Chloramphenicol-resistant *Salm. typhi* strains became endemic in some countries in South-East Asia, but AMP-resistant strains were still uncommon (Leading article, 1982; Murray, 1986).

The prevalence of multiresistant *Salm. typhi* strains increased more recently in Calcutta, India. They were resistant to chloramphenicol, AMP and co-trimoxazole; the disease caused by them responded to treatment with ciprofloxacin (p. 1016) (Dutta *et al.*, 1993). Strains of *Salm. typhi* which had acquired-resistance to AMP, chloramphenicol, co-trimoxazole and gentamicin following multiple antibiotic therapy have been recovered from stools. From the same stool sample, *E. coli* and *Klebsiella pneumoniae* isolates were obtained which had the same resistance patterns, and all these bacteria contained a high-molecular-weight plasmid, which coded for the multiple antibiotic-resistance (Schwalbe *et al.*, 1990). Similar *Salm. typhi* strains, resistant to chloramphenicol, AMP and co-trimoxazole have been reported from North-Eastern Africa (Mourad *et al.*, 1993).

Salmonellae resistant to AMP (including *Salm. typhi*) were also resistant to mecillinam (p. 182), but to a lesser degree. Although the same plasmid mediated resistance to both drugs, it is possible that the beta-lactamase produced was highly active against AMP but only mildly so against mecillinam (Chau *et al.*, 1981).

Some *Shigella* spp. strains were sensitive to low AMP concentrations *in vitro*, but the sensitivity of these organisms has varied widely both geographically and temporally (Murray, 1986). Soon after the discovery of AMP, resistant *Sh. sonnei* strains were reported. In one early survey of 1102 *Sh. sonnei* strains in London, over 80% were AMP-resistant (Davies *et al.*, 1970). Later surveys in the UK showed increasing resistance to AMP of other *Shigella* spp. such as *Sh. dysenteriae*, *Sh. flexneri* and *Sh. boydii*; the majority of infections due to these species were acquired abroad, particularly in the Indian subcontinent and North Africa; in addition to AMP-resistance, most strains were often multiply-resistant to sulfonamides, streptomycin, tetracyclines and chloramphenicol. In contrast, there was a decreasing incidence of AMP-resistance among indigenous *Sh. sonnei* in the UK (Gross *et al.*, 1981; Frost and Rowe, 1983).

Originally infrequent, AMP-resistant *Shigella* strains (mainly *Sh. sonnei*) rose to over 80% in some areas of the USA (Ross *et al.*, 1972; Tilton *et al.*, 1972). During the 1970s AMP-resistant shigellae became prevalent in many cities of the USA. Neu *et al.* (1975b) investigated AMP sensitivity of 102 *Sh. sonnei* and 14 *Sh. flexneri* strains isolated from patients in the New York City Hospital; *Sh. flexneri* strains were sensitive, but resistance was present in 60% of *Sh. sonnei* strains. Of isolates from patients in Houston, Texas, 55% of *Sh. sonnei* (113 strains) and 7% of *Sh. flexneri* (56 strains), were AMP-resistant (Byers *et al.*, 1976). These shigellae were also usually resistant to sulfonamides, streptomycin and tetracyclines. This multiple resistance was plasmid-mediated (Prince and Neu, 1976).

In 1987 an outbreak of shigellosis occurred in North Carolina, USA following an annual gathering of people. The *Sh. sonnei* strain was resistant to AMP, tetracycline and co-trimoxazole. Later in the year clusters of this multiply-resistant *Sh. sonnei* infection occurred in other states in the USA, (CDC, 1987). A nationwide survey of *Shigella* isolates showed that 32% were resistant to AMP, 7% to co-trimoxazole and 0.4% to nalidixic acid. Fifty (20%) of the 252 isolates were associated with foreign travel. Co-trimoxazole resistance was found in 20% of isolates from foreign travellers compared with only 4% of isolates from those without history of travel (Tauxe *et al.*, 1990). In Israel during the period 1984 to 1992 AMP-resistant *Sh. sonnei* strains increased from 13% to 86% (Ashkenazi *et al.*, 1995).

Shigella dysenteriae, type 1 (Shiga's bacillus) causes the most severe form of *Shigella* dysentery. Its resistance to AMP was first reported from Bangladesh (Rahaman *et al.* 1974). Between 1968 and 1970 there was an extensive epidemic of dysentery in Central America and a smaller one in Mexico. The Shiga's bacillus strain responsible was resistant to chloramphenicol, tetracyclines, streptomycin and sulfonamides, but sensitive to AMP. Later, AMP-resistant *Sh. dysenteriae*, type 1 strains were isolated, from one child in Costa Rica and from five others in Mexico city (Olarte *et al.*, 1976). Determinants for this AMP-resistance were carried on one plasmid, whilst the determinants for resistance to chloramphenicol, tetracycline, sulfonamides and streptomycin were carried on another plasmid (Crosa *et al.*, 1977). *Shigella dysenteriae* type 1 resistant to chloramphenicol, streptomycin, sulfonamides and tetracyclines caused an outbreak in Bangladesh during 1972–73, and some of the strains were resistant to AMP as well (Crossa *et al.*, 1977; Yunus *et al.*, 1982). Since 1976 Shiga's bacillus strains with multiple antibiotic-resistance sometimes including resistance to AMP, became prevalent in India (Frost *et al.*, 1981). In some outbreaks of dysentery in India and Bangladesh the *Sh. dysenteriae*, type 1 strains were also resistant to co-trimoxazole (p. 842). An extensive epidemic of shigellosis, associated with many deaths, began in Central Africa in 1979; the strain of *Sh.*

dysenteriae type 1 was resistant to AMP, chloramphenicol, streptomycin, sulfonamides and tetracyclines. The plasmid in this epidemic strain was different from those found in the strains implicated in Central America and South-East Asia. A single plasmid conferred resistance to AMP, chloramphenicol and tetracyclines, but resistance to streptomycin and sulfonamides was not transferable (Frost *et al.*, 1981).

In Bangladesh antimicrobial sensitivities of *Shigella* isolates were monitored from 1983 through 1990. By 1990 51.2% of isolates were resistant to AMP, 47.7% to co-trimoxazole, and 40.5% were resistant to both of these drugs. Resistance to nalidixic acid was 20.2% in 1990. In 1990 71.5% of *Shigella dysenteriae* type 1 isolates were resistant to AMP, 68.5% to co-trimoxazole, 67.7% to both drugs and 57.9% to nalidixic acid (Bennish *et al.*, 1992). In the developing countries there was a great variation in the prevalence of resistant shigellae in various locations around the world. For example the incidence of resistance to AMP in 1980 was as low as 7% in Dacca and as high as 87% in Bangkok in 1982–83 (Murray, 1986). In Burundi, Africa, *Sh. dysenteriae* type 1 appeared in epidemic form in 1990; all isolates were resistant to AMP, chloramphenicol, nalidixic acid, tetracycline and co-trimoxazole. The MICs of these strains for ciprofloxacin (p. 982) were 0.25 μg per ml, whilst the MICs of this drug for *Sh. sonnei* and *Sh. flexneri* strains were ≥0.06 μg per ml (Ries *et al.*, 1994). Similar multiresistant strains of *Sh. dysenteriae* type 1 caused an epidemic in Zambia, which started in 1990 (Tuttle *et al.*, 1995).

4 Other Gram-negative aerobic bacteria

The Brucella spp. and *Bordetella pertussis* are sensitive to AMP (Bannatyne and Cheung, 1982). The same is true for *Neisseria meningitidis*, except that strains resistant to penicillin G (p. 13) are also AMP-resistant. It is possible that *N. gonorrhoeae* may be AMP-sensitive but gonococcal strains with chromosomally mediated resistance to penicillin G (p. 14) also show similar resistance to AMP. Beta-lactamase-producing gonococcal strains (p. 15) are always AMP-resistant (Elmros *et al.*, 1979). *Moraxella catarrhalis* may be AMP-sensitive, but the majority of strains produce beta-lactamase and these are resistant (Kovatch *et al.*, 1983; Powell *et al.*, 1991). About 93% of beta-lactamase producers produce a BRO-1 enzyme and 7% a BRO-2 enzyme. The MICs of AMP for BRO-1 producers were 25-fold higher than for non-producers, but those for BRO-2 producers were raised only 4-fold. *Neisseria elongata* subsp. *nitroreducens* is AMP-sensitive. It is a Gram-negative rod which rarely causes endocarditis or septicemia in humans (Grant *et al.*, 1990). *Acinetobacter johnsonii* (formerly a subset of *A. calcoaceticus* var. *lwoffii*) is usually AMP-sensitive (Seifert *et al.*, 1993).

Vibro cholerae (serogroup 01) is usually AMP-sensitive. Multiply-resistant strains (El Tor biotype) have been responsible for two outbreaks of cholera. In a Tanzanian epidemic, the strain involved was resistant to AMP, chloramphenicol, kanamycin, streptomycin, sulfonamides and tetracyclines (Rowe and Threlfall, 1981). In an epidemic in Bangladesh the strain was resistant to AMP, tetracycline, kanamycin, streptomycin, sulfonamides and trimethoprim (Glass *et al.*, 1983). Resistance in both epidemics was plasmid-mediated. Most strains of *V. parahaemolyticus* are AMP-resistant because they produce a beta-lactamase (Joseph *et al.*, 1978). *Legionella pneumophila* is sensitive to AMP *in vitro* (MIC 0.25–2.0 μg per ml) (Thornsberry *et al.*, 1978) (p. 17). *Campylobacter jejuni* is usually resistant (Karmali *et al.*, 1981). Between 83 and 92% of the strains produce a beta-lactamase, which only hydrolyzes AMP, amoxicillin and ticarcillin. The beta-lactamase-positive strains are significantly more resistant to these three drugs, compared with beta-lactamase-negative strains. By contrast, resistance to penicillin G is similar for both beta-lactamase-positive and -negative strains (p. 17) (Lachance *et al.*, 1991). Most strains of *C. fetus* are moderately sensitive to AMP (Chow *et al.*, 1978). Ampicillin in combination with either cefazolin and gentamicin acts synergistically against this organism (Goossens *et al.*, 1989). *Campylobacter coli*, which is resistant to penicillin G, is usually AMP-susceptible. More than half of the strains of this organism produce a beta-lactamase and these are less sensitive to AMP than beta-lactamase-negative strains. Clavulanic acid improves the susceptibility of the enzyme producing strains to AMP (Lachance *et al.* 1993). *Helicobacter pylori* is sensitive to AMP *in vitro* (Loo *et al.*, 1992).

The rare opportunistic human pathogen *Kingella indologenes* is AMP-sensitive (Jenny *et al.*, 1987). It is probably also sensitive to penicillin G, as is the more common pathogen of this genus, *K. kingae* (p. 16). Another rare human pathogen *Agrobacterium tumefaciens*, which caused peritonitis in a patient with alcoholic cirrhosis, is AMP-sensitive (Ramirez *et al.*, 1992). Both *Pseudomonas aeruginosa* and *Burkholderia* (previously *Pseudomonas*) *pseudomallei* are always highly AMP-resistant.

All strains of *Haemophilus influenzae* type b were considered to be AMP-sensitive until 1974, when reports of highly resistant strains (MIC often higher than 50 μg per ml) originated from the

USA. Resistant strains were isolated from the CSF of children with *H. influenzae* meningitis (Thomas *et al.*, 1974) and from the nasopharynx of healthy children (Schiffer *et al.*, 1974). Subsequently, resistant strains were detected in geographically widespread areas in the USA (Jacobson *et al.*, 1976). They were also reported from many other countries including the UK (Fallon, 1976), Sweden (Biörklund *et al.*, 1975) and Australia (Bell and Smith, 1975). Strains of AMP-resistant *H. influenzae* type b were isolated from children with septicemia, meningitis, epiglottitis, otitis media and other severe childhood infections. There were also healthy nasopharyngeal carriers of the organism. Sometimes AMP-resistant strains emerged *in vivo* during AMP treatment of a severe infection such as meningitis, and this was associated with recrudescence of the infection (Albritton *et al.*, 1977; Granoff *et al.*, 1978). Some clinical isolates from severe infections were heterogeneous, consisting of both AMP-sensitive and AMP-resistant populations. Sometimes the sensitivity of simultaneous isolates from blood and CSF have differed (Jubelirer and Yeager, 1979; MacMahon and Ramberan, 1980), whilst in others resistant and sensitive strains were isolated from the same specimen (Beckwith, 1980; Stewardson-Krieger and Naidu, 1981).

This resistance of *H. influenzae* type b to AMP was mediated by a plasmid (p. 549), which coded for the production of beta-lactamase (Eickhoff *et al.*, 1976; Brunton *et al.*, 1986). This beta-lactamase was of the TEM-1 type which is commonly produced by, and widely transferred amongst Gram-negative bacilli (Matthew, 1979). Transfer of AMP-resistance from a resistant to a sensitive *H. influenzae* type b strain can occur by conjugation *in vitro* (Thorne and Farrar, 1975). Resistance can also be transferred from an AMP-resistant *H. influenzae* type b strain to other organisms such as *H. parainfluenzae* and *E. coli* (Eickhoff *et al.*, 1976; Saunders and Sykes, 1977). Attempts to transfer conjugally the resistance plasmid from *H. influenzae* to *N. gonorrhoeae* met only with limited success. However, this transfer did occur if the commensal, *N. cinerea* was used as a transfer intermediate (Brunton *et al.*, 1986; McNicol *et al.*, 1986).

A second beta-lactamase enzyme, designated Rob or ROB-1 was found in a small number of *H. influenzae* strains. In *H. influenzae* AMP resistance was also mediated by this enzyme (Rubin *et al.*, 1981; Daum *et al.*, 1988; Scriver *et al.*, 1994). The Rob beta-lactamase differs from the TEM-1 enzyme as it has a different isoelectric point. The Rob and TEM-1 beta lactamase genes are not related. An animal pathogen, *Actinobacillus pleuropneumoniae* is often AMP-resistant because it produces Rob beta-lactamase. The animal reservoir of this gene may play a role in the spread of this resistance to human pathogens (Medeiros *et al.*, 1986; Juteau *et al.*, 1991).

There was a gradual increase in the frequency of AMP-resistant *H. influenzae* strains in the USA. An 18% prevalence was detected in a nationwide survey carried out in 1978 (CDC, 1979). In the 1980s three more nationwide surveys were carried out. In the survey performed during 1983–1984 21% of *H. influenzae* type b were AMP-resistant. More than half of the isolates reported in this study came from children younger than 6 years (Doern *et al.*, 1986). The second study was performed in 1986, and 31.7% of *H. influenzae* type b were beta-lactamase producers. Slightly more than 40% of specimens in this study came from children aged less than 6 years. Once again beta-lactamase production was more common in isolates obtained from young children (Doern *et al.*, 1988). The third study in the USA was performed in 1987–1988 and employed primarily respiratory isolates from adults. Despite this as many as 29.5% of *H. influenzae* type b were beta-lactamase producers (Jorgensen *et al.*, 1990).

In the UK during 1981, 11.4% of *H. influenzae* type b strains were beta-lactamase producers (Philpott-Howard and Williams, 1982). In a European study including the UK, performed in 1986, the prevalence of beta-lactamase-producing strains varied widely from country to country, the highest prevalence being in Spain. Overall, 17% of the isolates were AMP-resistant (Jorgensen, 1992). In a study in the UK of *H. influenzae* isolated from sputa, 9.4% of *H. influenzae* were beta-lactamase producers, but another 5.2% were AMP-resistant but were beta-lactamase-negative (see below) (Powell *et al.*, 1991). In a nationwide survey in Australia, 21.6% of H. influenzae type b strains produced beta-lactamase (Collignon *et al.*, 1992). By contrast, in the Scandinavian countries less than 5% of *H. influenzae* type b strains were beta-lactamase producers (Peltola *et al.*, 1990). In Finland some 10% of type b *H. influenzae* strains produced beta-lactamase in early 1980s and by 1990, this percentage had not increased (Nissinen *et al.*, 1995). In a survey in Canada of 1688 *H. influenzae* strains, 28.4% were beta-lactamase positive (Scriver *et al.*, 1994). Beta-lactamase-producing *H. influenzae* strains were also detected in several Asian countries (Jorgensen, 1992).

Strains of AMP-resistant *H. influenzae* type b are highly resistant to penicillin G and amoxycillin. Originally these strains were sensitive to chloramphenicol, erythromycin, rifampicin, gentamicin, co-trimoxazole and less consistently tetracycline (Emerson *et al.*, 1975; McGowan *et al.*, 1976). They were also sensitive to cephalosporins such as cefuroxime and cefoxitin (Kammer *et al.*, 1975), and very sensitive to third-generation cephalosporins such as cefotaxime and ceftriaxone (Baker *et al.*, 1980).

Gradually beta-lactamase-producing strains of *H. influenzae* have acquired resistance to other antibiotics and some strains now show multiple antibiotic-resistance. Some are now resistant to one or more of the following – tetracycline, erythromycin, co-trimoxazole, rifampicin and chloramphenicol. Some strains are also resistant to cefuroxime. Only resistance to third-generation cephalosporins such as cefotaxime and ceftriaxone and to fluoroquinolones such as ciprofloxacin has not yet been documented (Simasathien *et al.*, 1980; MacMahon *et al.*, 1982; Doern *et al.*, 1988; Howard and Williams, 1988; Campos *et al.*, 1989; Jorgensen *et al.*, 1990; Jorgensen, 1992; Levy *et al.*, 1993).

Strains of AMP-resistant *H. influenzae* type b occur without detectable beta-lactamase activity and their MICs are in the range of 4–8 μg per ml. This resistance is intrinsic (p. 27) and the major mechanism of resistance in these strains is altered PBPs (p. 27) (Philpott-Howard and Williams, 1982; Reid *et al.*, 1987; Clairoux *et al.*, 1992; Mendelman, 1992). Altered penicillin binding proteins (PBPs) 3, 4, and 5 appear to be associated with AMP-resistance of *H. influenzae*. These PBPs may be the major targets for the beta-lactam antibiotics in *H. influenzae* (Mendelman *et al.*, 1990). Other resistance mechanisms may also be involved, as some of these strains have exhibited outer membrane protein profiles which differed from those of sensitive strains (Reid *et al.*, 1987).

These strains probably still represent less than 1% of all *H. influenzae* isolates in the USA (Barry *et al.*, 1993), and Canada (Scriver *et al.*, 1994), but they are becoming more prevalent in the UK (Powell *et al.*, 1991). The concern here is that these strains show some degree of resistance to most beta-lactam antibiotics. For instance the MICs of cefotaxime for these strains were at least 10-fold greater than those for susceptible strains. However, all the AMP-resistant strains were still inhibited by ≥1.0 μg of cefotaxime per ml, so it is still likely to be useful clinically. On the other hand the MICs of ceftibuten, cefixime, cefaclor and cefuroxime were such that these drugs would be unlikely to be useful clinically (Barry *et al.*, 1993). In these strains the susceptibility to carbapenems such as imipenem was not altered (Powell and Livermore, 1990).

Non-typable strains of *H. influenzae* are pathogens in respiratory tract infections in adults. Otitis media in children may be caused either by these strains (Shurin *et al.*, 1976) or by *H. influenzae* type b (Crosson *et al.*, 1976). AMP-resistant strains of these non-encapsulated *H. influenzae* strains have been isolated from the sputum of patients with chronic bronchitis (Kauffman *et al.*, 1979; Ling *et al.*, 1983). They have been isolated also from patients, mainly children, with otitis media (Schwartz *et al.*, 1978; Jokipii and Jokipii, 1980) and from healthy nasopharyngeal carriers (Lerman *et al.*, 1979). In one early survey of non-typable *H. influenzae* strains in the UK, 10 (1.1%) of 889 isolates were AMP-resistant (Howard *et al.*, 1978); in 1981, when 1762 strains were examined, AMP-resistance had increased to approximately 6% (Philpott-Howard and Williams, 1982). The majority of these strains, similar to those of AMP-resistant *H. influenzae* type b, produce beta-lactamase (Malmvall and Branefors-Helander, 1978). The few non-typable *H. influenzae* strains which are AMP-resistant but do not produce beta-lactamase, possess intrinsic resistance, similar to *H. influenzae* type b (see above) (Bell and Plowman, 1980).

Cefuroxime is quite active against beta-lactamase-producing strains but it is less active against beta-lactamase-negative AMP-resistant strains. Cefotaxime and ceftriaxone are quite active against all AMP-resistant strains (Newsom and Matthews, 1982; Jorgensen, 1992). Surveys in the USA have shown that non-typable *H. influenzae* are less commonly AMP-resistant than strains of *H. influenzae* type b. In the 1983–1984, 1986 and 1987–1988 surveys, 12.1%, 15.6% and 15.0% of non-b strains were AMP-resistant, respectively (Doern *et al.*, 1986; Jorgensen *et al.*, 1990). Some of the non-b *H. influenzae* strains also have shown multiple drug-resistance e.g. they have been also resistant to tetracycline, chloramphenicol and co-trimoxazole (Doern *et al.*, 1988; Jorgensen *et al.*, 1990; Jorgensen, 1992).

A small proportion of ampicillin-sensitive *H. influenzae* strains, exhibit tolerance to the drug (MBC/MIC > 32.0) (p. 27), but the clinical significance of this is uncertain (Bergeron and Lavoie, 1985).

Usually *H. parainfluenzae* is AMP-sensitive but beta-lactamase-producing AMP-resistant strains occur (Auten *et al.*, 1991). Some surveys have shown that carriage of resistant strains in the throat of children is quite common. Simultaneous colonization with AMP-resistant *H. parainfluenzae*, has been found in over 80% of subjects who are carriers of AMP-resistant or AMP-sensitive *H. influenzae* strains. Possibly *H. parainfluenzae* may be a vector for spread of plasmids coding for the production of TEM-1 beta-lactamase to *H. influenzae* (Scheifele and Fussell, 1981; Scheifele *et al.*, 1982). As with resistant *H. influenzae* (see above), an AMP-resistant *H. parainfluenzae* strain (MIC 32 μg per ml) has been isolated from blood cultures,

Organism	MIC (μg per ml
Gram-positive bacteria	
Staphylococcus aureus (non-penicillinase producer)	0.05
Streptococcus pyogenes	0.05–0.1
Streptococcus pneumoniae	0.02–0.05
Streptococci, Group B	0.06
Streptococcus viridans	0.04–1.6
Enterococcus faecalis	1.0–5.0
Listeria monocytogenes	0.08–0.32
Gram-negative bacteria	
Escherichia coli	5.0
Enterobacter spp.	250.0
Klebsiella pneumoniae	1.25
Proteus mirabilis	1.25
Proteus vulgaris	5.0
Salmonella typhi	0.25
Salmonella typhimurium	1.0–5.0
Shigella sonnei	1.0–10.0
Shigella flexneri	1.25
Neisseria gonorrhoeae	0.02–0.6
Neisseria meningitidis	0.05
Haemophilus influenzae	0.05
Bacteroides fragilis	4.0–256.0
Prevotella melaninogenica	0.5–4.0

Table I.7
Compiled from data published by Rolinson and Stevens (1961), Stewart *et al.* (1961), Bass *et al.* (1969), Bear *et al.* (1970), Smith (1976), Sutter and Finegold (1976), and Schauf *et al.* (1976)

which did not produce beta-lactamase and which was presumably intrinsically resistant (Needham Walker and Smith, 1980).

It may be that *H. ducreyi* is AMP-sensitive but many strains produce a beta-lactamase and are resistant (Brunton *et al.*, 1979; Totten *et al.*, 1982). *Gardnerella vaginalis* is AMP-sensitive, most strains being inhibited by 1 μg per ml or less (McCarthy *et al.*, 1979).

5 Gram-negative anaerobic bacteria

Some of these, such as *Prevotella* (previously *Bacteroides*) *melaninogenica* and the *Fusobacterium* spp., may be AMP-sensitive unless they produce beta-lactamase (p. 17), but *B. fragilis* is resistant. Other *Bacteroides* spp. vary in sensitivity but less than 50% of isolates are inhibited by low AMP concentrations (Sutter and Finegold, 1976; Stark *et al.*, 1993).

6 Other organisms

The Leptospirae are AMP-sensitive (Oie *et al.*, 1983). Mycoplasmas and Rickettsiae are resistant. Mycobacteria are also resistant.

7 Minimum inhibitory concentrations

Table I.7 lists MICs of AMP against various bacteria. In this table the MICs are those of fully AMP-sensitive strains. As has been described above AMP-resistance is now common with many bacterial species.

Mode of Administration and Dosage

1 Oral administration

Acid stable AMP can be given orally. The usual oral dosage for children and adults to treat mild to moderate infections is 50–100 mg per kg body weight per day, given in four divided doses. A common adult dosage is 0.5 g 6-hourly, though 250 mg 6-hourly may suffice for mild infections due to highly susceptible organisms.

2 Parenteral administration

This drug, in the form of the sodium salt, can also be given either i.m. or i.v. For serious infections, high parenteral doses are often necessary; in children a daily dose of 150–200 mg per kg is recommended, but up to 400 mg per kg per day has been given occasionally (Fleming *et al.*, 1967). A comparable high dosage for adults is 1–2 g every 4–6 h.

Intramuscularly, AMP is usually given every 4–6 h. Unless the patient has circulatory failure or a hemorrhagic diathesis, i.m. AMP, given in the same dosage, is as effective as i.v. AMP for the treatment of severe infections such as bacterial meningitis (Girgis *et al.*, 1982). The only advantage of i.v. administration is the avoidance of frequent painful i.m. injections. Intravenous administration is usually by intermittent injections into the i.v. tubing or by intermittent infusions, similar to penicillin G (p. 20). AMP can be added to i.v. fluid bottles for continuous infusion, provided incompatibilities and drug inactivation on prolonged standing in solution are avoided (Colding and Andersen, 1982). Some antibiotic solutions, including sodium ampicillin, can be prepared and kept frozen in plastic bags; these are then thawed in a microwave oven before use (Holmes *et al.*, 1982). Because so many variables are involved, ideally, the preparation of AMP or other antibiotic solutions in an i.v. flask or bag, should be carried out under pharmaceutical supervision.

3 Newborn and premature infants

In this age group the drug should be given either i.m. or i.v. For infants less than 7 days old, a dosage of 25 mg per kg body weight 12-hourly is recommended for mild to moderate infections. With serious infections, such as meningitis, this dosage should be doubled to 50 mg per kg, given 12-hourly. For infants older than 7 days, a dosage of 25 mg per kg 8-hourly is sufficient for infections of mild to moderate severity; with serious infections such as meningitis, 50 mg per kg 6-hourly is recommended (total daily dose 200 mg per kg body weight) (Kaplan *et al.*, 1974; McCracken and Nelson, 1983).

4 Patients with renal failure

As AMP is relatively non-toxic it is often given in the usual doses to patients with renal failure. If high parenteral doses are used, appropriate dosage reduction is necessary. In anuric patients the AMP serum half-life is prolonged to 8.5 h (p. 117). In patients with severe renal failure it has been suggested that the total daily dose should be halved and given in two divided doses (Bennett *et al.*, 1970). Others consider that an AMP dose of 0.5 g daily may be sufficient for patients with a creatinine clearance of 10 ml per min or less (Lee and Hill, 1968).

5 Intraperitoneal administration

In a dose of 50 mg to each liter AMP can be added to peritoneal dialysate. A variable amount of the drug is absorbed from the peritoneal cavity and if this dose is continuously added to the dialysate, a steady serum AMP concentration of around 9 µg per ml is attained (Bulger *et al.*, 1965).

Serum Levels in Relation to Dosage

After oral administration of AMP to adults, peak serum concentrations are obtained at about 2 h, and the drug is still detectable in the serum at 6 h (Fig. I.6). Doubling the dose virtually doubles the serum concentration. The absorption of AMP is reduced by about 50% if it is administered with food (Welling and Tse, 1982). Concurrent administration of cimetidine does not diminish AMP absorption (Rogers *et al.*, 1980), but co-administration with chloroquine does (Ali, 1985). The drug is absorbed normally in patients with celiac disease (Parsons *et al.*, 1975). The concomitant use of *Lactobacillus* preparation does not interfere with the absorption of ampicillin (Yost and Gotz, 1985). Animal experiments show that morphine administration elevates serum levels of AMP after its administration i.v. Morphine appears to impair both renal and hepatobiliary elimination of AMP. In contrast, morphine markedly reduces the levels of the drug in serum, when it is given by gastric intubation. This results from delayed absorption because of retardation of gastric emptying by morphine (Garty and Hurwitz, 1985).

With i.m. administration, a much higher peak level is achieved within 30 min (Fig. I.6). Compared with penicillin G, AMP produces considerably higher serum levels after parenteral administration; this is chiefly due to its slower renal clearance (Kirby and Kind, 1967).

In newborn and premature infants, after an i.m. dose of 10 mg per kg, a peak serum level of about 20 µg per ml is reached 1 h later. With a dose of 25 mg per kg, the peak level is approximately 60 µg per ml. Detectable serum levels persist for at least 12 h after injection. The serum half-life of AMP in infants declines with increasing postnatal age; it is 4 h in infants aged

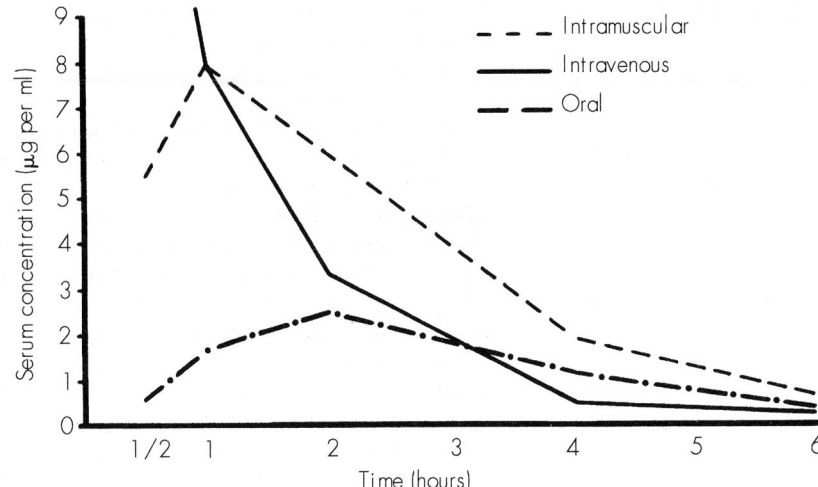

Fig. I.6. Comparative serum levels of ampicillin after 0·5 g with three routes of administration. (Redrawn after Kirby and Kind, 1967, with permission.)

2–7 days, 2.8 h in those aged 8–14 days and 1.7 h in infants 15–30 days of age (Axline *et al.*, 1967; McCracken, 1974).

During pregnancy, AMP serum levels are lower than those attained in the same women after pregnancy. This appears to be due to increased plasma volume and body water during pregnancy which results in an increase in the drug's distribution volume. In addition, during pregnancy the renal plasma clearance of AMP is increased. Pregnant women may require higher doses of AMP than non-pregnant patients (Philipson, 1977; Jeffries and Bochner, 1988).

Excretion

1 Urine

Some 30% of an oral dose of AMP is excreted in urine during the first 6 h. High concentrations of the active drug are attained in urine; after a 0.5 g oral dose urinary concentrations range from 250 to 1000 μg per ml. There are no active AMP metabolites formed in the body prior to excretion (Cole and Ridley, 1978). The AMP is excreted partly by glomerular filtration and partly by tubular secretion. Probenecid slows excretion by partial blockage of tubular secretion (p. 24). After parenteral administration, about 75% of the dose is excreted in urine. Compared with penicillin G, AMP is cleared at a slower rate by the kidney, its serum half-life in normal adults being 1.5 h, compared with 0.5 h for penicillin G (p. 22). Therefore, the action of probenecid in lowering renal clearance and elevating serum levels is more marked with penicillin G (Kirby and Kind, 1967; Bennett *et al.*, 1974).

2 Bile

Also AMP is excreted unchanged in bile. In patients with T-tube drainage after cholecystectomy, only 0.1% of an i.v. or oral dose of AMP was excreted via the bile. In these patients biliary concentrations varied from 0.4 to 6.5 μg per ml during a 12-h period after an oral AMP dose of 0.5 g (Pinget *et al.*, 1976). These concentrations are higher than the MICs of AMP for highly susceptible pathogens (p. 108). Some of the drug excreted in bile is reabsorbed from the gut, but recycling through the liver is probably only a minor factor in maintaining serum levels (Kirby and Kind, 1967). Data on biliary excretion, obtained from patients with free biliary drainage, are not applicable to patients with obstructive biliary tract disease. For instance, AMP concentrations obtained in a non-functioning gall bladder are low, and therapeutic levels are only present in the common bile duct if it is not obstructed (Mortimer *et al.*, 1969).

3 Inactivation in body

Unexcreted AMP is inactivated chiefly in the liver, but at a slower rate than penicillin G. In anuric patients, the average serum half-life for AMP is 8.5 h compared with 4 h for penicillin G (Kirby and Kind, 1967).

Distribution of the Drug in Body

Throughout most body tissues AMP is evenly distributed. With the exception of the kidney and liver, tissue concentrations are lower than simultaneous serum levels. In healthy humans the intra-renal tissue concentration is about eight times higher than the concomitant serum level. By contrast, the AMP concentration in chronic glomerulonephritic kidneys is only about half the serum level at the time. In such severe kidney disease, urinary concentration of AMP is greatly reduced, and the serum rather than urinary concentration more closely reflects the AMP renal tissue level (Whelton *et al.*, 1972). Animal studies show that AMP renal tissue levels are also significantly reduced in acute pyelonephritis (Trottier and Bergeron, 1981).

Adequate AMP concentrations are attained in septic joint effusions (Nelson, 1971), in ascitic fluid of patients with ascites and bacterial peritonitis (Gerding *et al.*, 1977) and in human parapneumonic effusions (Taryle *et al.*, 1981). AMP penetrates poorly into bronchial secretions, though this may be increased 2- to 3-fold with inflammation and marked sputum purulence. In bronchial secretions from patients with moderate pulmonary infection, the AMP concentration is usually only about 10% of the simultaneous serum level (Wong *et al.*, 1975). Peak interstitial tissue fluid concentrations of AMP are lower than those attained in serum, but the drug persists in tissue fluid for a longer period; AMP does not accumulate in tissue fluid with repeated doses (Chisholm *et al.*, 1973; Cars, 1981). In pancreatic secretions AMP concentrations are low in normal animals, but they are quite high in those with induced pancreatitis (Rubinstein *et al.*, 1980). Similar to penicillin G (p. 25), AMP does not readily enter human polymorphonuclear leucocytes (Jacobs *et al.*, 1982), and it is usually undetectable in saliva, sweat and tears (Philipson *et al.*, 1975).

Only minute amounts of AMP can be detected in normal CSF, but in patients with bacterial meningitis higher levels occur. In such patients following an i.v. dose of 150 mg per kg per day, a mean CSF AMP level of 2.9 μg per ml was detected during the first 3 days of treatment, but this level fell during convalescence (Thrupp *et al.*, 1966). In another study of patients with bacterial meningitis, AMP was given either i.v. or i.m. in a dose of 160 mg per kg per day in six divided doses. Comparable CSF concentrations of about 1 μg per ml, were attained 1 h after i.m. or i.v. administrations on days 1 and 2 of treatment; 4 h after administration, CSF concentrations were higher in patients receiving i.m. therapy (2.94–3.64 μg per ml) than in those treated by i.v. AMP (0.67–1.02 μg per ml) but clinical response was the same in both groups (Mikhail *et al.*, 1981). In experimental meningitis in animals, pretreatment with methylprednisolone reduced the CSF AMP concentration, but this did not have a deleterious effect on the course of the meningitis (Scheld and Brodeur, 1983). In animals with experimental meningitis, the concomitant administration of AMP and ceftazidime, reduced the CSF AMP concentration; but when ceftriaxone was combined with AMP, there was no change of the CSF penetration of either drug (Okura *et al.*, 1988).

It is known that AMP crosses the placenta. In pregnant women given an oral dosage of 0.5 g 6-hourly, AMP levels in amniotic fluid at delivery ranged from 0.42 to 4.1 μg per ml. Concentrations in cord blood were lower, being in the range of 0.24–2.0 μg per ml (Blecher *et al.*, 1966). The drug did not reach therapeutic concentrations in amniotic fluid during the first trimester (Wasz-Höckert *et al.*, 1970).

The binding of AMP to serum proteins (18%) is the lowest of all the penicillins (Rolinson and Sutherland, 1965).

Mode of Action

The action of AMP is similar to that of penicillin G (p. 25). Its differences in antibacterial spectrum, compared with penicillin G, can be explained by its greater ability to penetrate the outer membrane of the cell wall of some Gram-negative bacilli (p. 26).

Toxicity

1 Hypersensitivity reactions and rashes

It may be that AMP is 'cross-allergenic' with other penicillins, and in sensitized patients it may evoke any of the hypersensitivity reactions caused by penicillin G (p. 28). Patients allergic to penicillin G do not always react to AMP, but because of this possibility AMP is contraindicated in such patients. Despite this, on rare occasions AMP has been used, when it has been the drug of choice for the treatment of a severe infection. Petheram and Boyce (1976) used i.v. AMP plus gentamicin successfully for the treatment of *Enterococcus faecalis* endocarditis in a penicillin-allergic patient; prednisolone and an antihistamine were administered concomitantly and full resuscitation facilities were immediately available.

Rashes due to AMP are more common than with other penicillins, but most of these may not be due to true penicillin hypersensitivity (see below). In two large surveys, the risk of an AMP rash was estimated as 7.7% and 7.3%, compared with 2.75% with other penicillins (Shapiro *et al.*, 1969; Report, 1973). The Boston Collaborative Drug Surveillance Program detected a somewhat lower occurrence of rashes (5.2% of 2988 patients), but other possible causes of rashes in AMP-treated patients were more carefully excluded (Arndt and Jick, 1976). The frequency of these rashes may be related to the dose of the drug (Bass *et al.*, 1973; Report 1973). About 20% of patients developed a rash when large doses of AMP were used for treatment of *Salmonella* infections (Sleet *et al.*, 1964). Also rashes are more common in patients with renal failure treated by usual AMP doses, which result in high serum concentrations of the drug (Lee and Hill, 1968).

All AMP rashes are not always urticarial, but may be macular resembling measles or rubella. They frequently appear 4–5 days after starting therapy (Stevenson and Mandal, 1966), usually without other associated signs of allergy, and they may intensify, but often subside if treatment is continued. Patients with macular rashes have negative skin tests to AMP and to the major and minor penicillin antigenic determinants (Kerns *et al.*, 1973) (p. 29). These rashes appear to be 'AMP-specific' and do not indicate true penicillin hypersensitivity (Report, 1973).

Rashes are very common in patients with glandular fever who are given AMP. A small percentage of glandular fever patients develop a rash without a history of prior drug therapy, but it has been estimated that 65–95% of them will develop a rash if they are given AMP (Pullen *et al.*, 1967; Lund and Bergan, 1975). It has been prescribed frequently for pharyngitis, a condition for which other forms of penicillins are indicated (p. 74). This 'sensitivity' to AMP of patients with glandular fever is temporary, because rashes do not recur if patients are given AMP when they have recovered from the disease (Nazareth *et al.*, 1972; Lund and Bergan, 1975). The glandular fever-like disease due to *Cytomegalovirus* also predisposes patients to AMP rashes (Klemola, 1970). The risk of developing an AMP rash is very high (90%) in patients with lymphatic leukemia, and it is also increased in those with reticulosarcoma and other lymphomas (Potter, 1972). Because of these associations, AMP rashes may be due to a 'toxic' mechanism associated with abnormal lymphocytes, rather than due to hypersensitivity. Patients with infectious mononucleosis do not produce AMP-specific IgM, IgG or IgE antibodies after intradermal testing with AMP, which is further evidence that these rashes are not due to hypersensitivity (Kluge *et al.* 1982). There are other interesting associations with AMP rashes; they are more common in females and in patients with hyperuricemia receiving concurrent allopurinol therapy, and also if the drug is given for a viral rather than a bacterial infection (Report, 1972, 1973).

It is clear that AMP has a greater predilection to cause rashes than other penicillins, mainly of the benign macular variety, which are unrelated to true penicillin allergy. Thus the occurrence of an AMP rash during or after treatment, should not be considered necessarily as a contra-indication to future treatment with one of the penicillins (Report, 1973).

Ampicillin can cause serious allergic reactions, such as anaphylaxis and urticaria but the frequency of these is probably no higher than with other penicillins (Shapiro *et al.*, 1969) (p. 29).

2 Gastrointestinal side-effects

Oral or less commonly parenteral AMP therapy, can cause nausea and diarrhea but these are usually not serious (Bass *et al.*, 1973). In one study of children, the severity of diarrhea was such that 85 of all orally and 3% of all i.v. treated patients, required discontinuation of AMP or the use of anti-diarrhea drugs (Phillips *et al.*, 1976). Diarrhea induced by AMP appeared to be more common in younger children. In another study of children treated for otitis media, AMP oral suspension caused diarrhea more frequently than amoxycillin (p. 139) or co-trimoxazole suspensions (Feder, 1982). In adults, diarrhea may occur in 5–20% of treated patients and is probably more common in older age groups (Gurwith *et al.*, 1977; Lusk *et al.*, 1977).

Antibiotic-associated diarrhea can result from the production of toxin by *Cl. difficile* in the bowel, the most severe form of which is pseudomembranous colitis. This was first described with lincomycin and clindamycin therapy (p. 594), but AMP (and many other antibiotics) can also cause the same illness (Keating *et al.*, 1974; Fekety and Shah, 1993). In one study, diarrhea was noted in 62 (18%) of 343 clindamycin-treated patients, but only in 16 (5%) of 315 AMP-treated patients, pseudomembranous colitis occurred in seven (2%) of the clindamycin-treated patients, but only in one (0.3%) of those treated with AMP (Gurwith *et al.*, 1977). In one child with AMP-associated colitis a toxigenic *Cl. perfringens* type C strain was implicated (Schwartz *et al.*, 1980).

It seems anomalous that AMP is a cause of *Cl. difficile*-associated colitis, when the organism is usually AMP-sensitive. This may be because AMP is inactivated by beta-lactamases produced by other organisms of the bowel flora, thereby permitting AMP-sensitive *Cl. difficile* to multiply and produce disease. Concomitant administration of a non-absorbable beta-lactamase inhibitor such as sulbactam (p. 209) with AMP, therefore may prevent AMP-associated colitis (Rolfe and Finegold, 1983). Some patients taking AMP or other penicillins develop bloody diarrhea, without characteristic changes of pseudomembranous colitis (Toffler, 1978) (p. 594).

Gastrointestinal moniliasis may be caused by AMP therapy, but as in the case of tetracyclines (p. 735), it is usually not a causative factor in AMP-induced diarrhea.

3 Nephropathy

A number of anecdotal case reports indicate that AMP is an uncommon cause of renal damage. One case of interstitial nephritis, which immediately followed a small dose of AMP, has been reported (Tannenberg *et al.*, 1971). Azotemia did not occur, but the other clinical, histological and immunological features were similar to those of methicillin nephritis (p. 84). Maxwell *et al.* (1974) described another patient with AMP-induced interstitial nephritis in whom the large dose of the drug used (200 mg per kg per day) was a probable factor. Lee and Hill (1968) observed three patients with renal failure, who, following a severe cutaneous AMP hypersensitivity reaction, developed further permanent deterioration in renal function. Two other patients developed acute renal failure due to interstitial nephritis in association with a hypersensitivity reaction to AMP (Ruley and Lisi, 1974; Woodroffe *et al.* 1975). One patient developed severe dysentery, polyarthritis, purpuric rash and glomerulonephritis, characteristic of the Henoch-Schönlein purpura syndrome while taking oral AMP. He slowly recovered after the drug was stopped (Beeching *et al.*, 1982).

Crystalluria has been observed in patients treated with large doses of i.v. AMP (Potter *et al.*, 1971). It appears that high urinary AMP levels and an acid urine (pH 5), favour crystallization of this drug. The site of crystal formation is unknown, but it may well be intrarenal, as concentration and acidification of urine occurs in the distal tubule. It is uncertain whether nephrotoxicity is associated with AMP crystalluria.

4 Hematological side-effects

Similar to penicillin G, AMP, if administrated in large doses i.v., can cause neutropenia and this is more likely to occur in patients with pre-existing liver disease (p. 33). Agranulocytosis with monohistiocytosis has been described in one patient in association with AMP therapy (Graf and Tarlov, 1968). Severe acute thrombocytopenia with bleeding occurred in one patient receiving AMP and no other agents could be implicated (Brooks, 1974). With high doses of the drug there is a tendency for red cells to become coated with AMP and a Coombs' positive hemolytic anemia may be a sequel, as with penicillin G (p. 33).

5 Encephalopathy

Convulsions may be anticipated with very large doses of i.v. AMP, particularly if serum levels reach 800 µg per ml. This threshold concentration for convulsions is higher than that for penicillin G. Also AMP may cause convulsions when administered in ordinary does, such as 2 g daily, if it is given to patients prone to seizures, such as those with head injuries or idiopathic epilepsy (Serdaru *et al.*, 1982).

6 Elevated SGOT levels

Elevated SGOT levels have been reported after AMP given i.m. This may be due to muscle irritation rather than hepatotoxicity (Knirsch and Gralla, 1970).

7 Benign intracranial hypertension

Bhowmick (1972) described one patient with this complication, who had severe headache and papilledema, which was apparently provoked by AMP and then perpetuated by tetracycline therapy (p. 740).

8 Drug interactions

Because AMP can impair the absorption of oral contraceptives, treatment with AMP occasionally results in breakthrough bleeding or pregnancy in patients who are reliable oral contraceptive users. In pregnant women, AMP decreases the amount of urinary estriol excretion, but levels of estrogens in the blood are largely unaffected. The reason for this is that AMP interferes with the normal enterohepatic circulation of estrogens; estrogen conjugates normally excreted in the bile are not hydrolyzed by intestinal bacteria, reconjugated and absorbed. These changes have no effect on the pregnancy, but are important when interpreting urinary estriol levels as an index of feto–placental function (Roberton and Johnson, 1976, True, 1982).

Clinical Uses of the Drug

1 Urinary tract infections

Acute and uncomplicated urinary tract infections caused by *E. coli* and *Pr. mirabilis* usually respond to AMP. The drug is also useful for the treatment of *Enterococcus faecalis* infections. High concentrations of AMP are attained in urine (p. 117), and treatment is sometimes successful despite the demonstration of *in vitro* resistance of the causative organism. Treatment of patients with chronic bacteriuria or underlaying renal disease is often unsuccessful, and they either relapse or become re-infected with AMP-resistant *E. coli* or other resistant bacteria such as *Klebsiella* or *Enterobacter* spp. (Turck, 1967). Amoxycillin (p. 139) has largely replaced AMP for the treatment of urinary tract infections.

2 Septicemia due to Gram-negative bacilli

Some patients with septicemia due to AMP-sensitive strains of *Pr. mirabilis* or *E. coli*, can be managed successfully by large doses of AMP given parenterally. Treatment with AMP alone, prior to sensitivity testing of the causative organism, is inadvisable. It is commonly used for the treatment of suspected neonatal septicemia, as it is active against Group B streptococci, *L. monocytogenes*, *E. faecalis* and *Pr. mirabilis*. In neonates, it is usually combined with either gentamicin (p. 473) or amikacin (p. 514), to provide cover for AMP-resistant Gram-negative bacilli, such as *E. coli*, *Klebsiella* spp. and *Ps. aeruginosa* (Kaplan *et al.*, 1974; McCracken and Eichenwald, 1974).

3 Typhoid fever and other Salmonella infections

Salmonella typhi strains resistant to chloramphenicol and sometimes also to AMP have been detected (p. 109). If sensitive strains are involved, AMP is not as effective as chloramphenicol for the treatment of typhoid fever; defervescence is slower and some severe cases fail to respond to AMP, whilst response to chloramphenicol is uniformly good (Sanders, 1965; Manriquez *et al.*, 1965; Snyder *et al.*, 1976). In addition, positive stool cultures persist longer in AMP-treated patients, compared with those treated by chloramphenicol (Snyder *et al.*, 1976). Chloramphenicol is also superior to AMP for the treatment of paratyphoid fever, even when relatively large doses of AMP (6 g per day in adults) are used (Sleet *et al.*, 1964). Therefore, in most parts of the world, chloramphenicol (p. 568) was preferred to AMP for the treatment of typhoid and paratyphoid fevers (Svenungsson, 1982). Nowadays many clinicians prefer to use ciprofloxacin (p. 1016) for these diseases, even if sensitive strains are involved. In developing countries, there has been an emergence of resistant strains to chloramphenicol, AMP and amoxycillin (p. 136) and in some parts of the world also to co-trimoxazole (p. 841). In such cases one of the quinolones such as ciprofloxacin (p. 1016) or a third-generation cephalosporin, such as ceftriaxone (p. 360), is the treatment of choice.

For the treatment of severe septicemia due to other *Salmonella* spp., chloramphenicol was preferred to AMP. In infants younger than 3 months, *Salmonella* sepsis associated with meningitis responded poorly to AMP but chloramphenicol was effective (Davis, 1981). Also AMP-resistant salmonellae, particularly *Salm. typhimurium*, are now common in all parts of the world (p. 109). Rather than chloramphenicol, AMP or amoxycillin (p. 141) may be adequate for milder *Salmonella* infections caused by AMP-sensitive strains, such as enteritis associated with transient septicemia, focal *Salmonella* infection such as osteomyelitis, and uncomplicated enteritis in compromised hosts (Nelson, 1981). For seriously ill patients chloramphenicol is preferable. Patients with AIDS are predisposed to serious *Salmonella* infections and HIV infection also compromises their ability to eradicate these bacteria. Such compromised hosts with chronic bacteremia may be best treated with AMP or amoxycillin, rather than chloramphenicol. Co-trimoxazole is also best avoided for this indication in AIDS patients (Jacobs *et al.*, 1985; Fischl *et al.*, 1986; Sperber and Schleupner, 1987). One of the 4-fluoroquinolones such as ciprofloxacin (p. 1016) will probably be the best drug for both short-term treatment and prolonged prophylaxis for salmonellosis in AIDS patients (Asperilla *et al.*, 1990).

Patients with underlying abnormalities of the urinary tract with chronic *Salmonella* bacteriuria are also best treated by AMP, amoxycillin (p. 141) or co-trimoxazole (p. 867) or if necessary ciprofloxacin (p. 1016) rather than chloramphenicol (Bassily *et al.*, 1981). For the treatment of endocarditis and other endovascular infections such as *Salmonella* aortitis, AMP or amoxycillin appear to be more effective than chloramphenicol (Parsons *et al.*, 1983; Ljungberg and Braconier, 1986; Aguado *et al.*, 1987).

In uncomplicated *Salmonella* enteritis in normal hosts, AMP or any other antibiotic is unwarranted. In prospective studies, oral antibiotic therapy with drugs such as AMP, amoxycillin (p. 141) and co-trimoxazole (p. 868), had no effect on the duration of symptoms or on the duration of the resultant asymptomatic *Salmonella* carrier state (Kazemi *et al.*, 1973; Nelson *et al.*, 1980; Yamamoto and Ashton, 1988). In addition, in one of these studies, approximately half of the children treated by either AMP or amoxycillin had a bacteriological relapse; this occasionally occurred during treatment, but was more common during the post-treatment period; about one-third of these had a concomitant recurrence of diarrhea. Bacteriological and clinical relapses were not observed in placebo-treated patients. Unlike neomycin (p. 538), AMP treatment did not prolong the asymptomatic excretion of salmonellae (Nelson *et al.*, 1980). Some authors have reported that in patients with uncomplicated *Salmonella* enteritis the use of one of the quinolones, such as ciprofloxacin (p. 1016), shortened the duration of clinical symptoms and terminated the excretion of organisms in the stool (Asperilla *et al.*, 1990). However, in one controlled study, ciprofloxacin was no better than placebo for this disease (Sánchez *et al.*, 1993).

Some success has been obtained in the treatment of the prolonged *Salm. typhi* carrier state, by using large doses of AMP plus probenecid for 1–3 months, or longer (Simon and Miller, 1966). In carriers who have gallstones, the best results have been obtained by a combination of biliary surgery and prolonged AMP administration (Dinbar *et al.*, 1969). Short-term chemotherapy with AMP or another suitable antibiotic (p. 141), is advisable for all typhoid or paratyphoid carriers undergoing biliary surgery, to prevent possible exacerbations of these chronic infections. Despite reported successes, treatment aimed at eradicating the carrier state of *Salm. typhi* was still unsatisfactory. Some carriers remained refractory to all forms of treatment and results had to be critically assessed over a prolonged period, because some subjects were intermittent excretors, and clearance of feces was only temporary. It appeared that patients who were regularly followed, and who did not excrete typhoid bacilli within 2 years of stopping AMP, were probably cured of their carrier state (Johnson *et al.*, 1973). Quinolones such as ciprofloxacin (p. 1018) may be more effective in eradicating intestinal and biliary reservoirs in chronic carriers compared with previously used drugs (Asperilla *et al.*, 1990).

4 Shigella infections

Shigella sonnei dysentery is often an acute self-limiting disease, for which rehydration is the most important measure. In these cases AMP treatment may only be of practical value under certain circumstances. Possibly the clinical status, as well as the social and physical environment of the patient, should be taken into consideration when deciding whether to use this drug (Weissman *et al.*, 1974). In contrast with *Salmonella* enteritis (see above), provided the strain is sensitive, AMP is of clinical benefit in shigellosis, both in milder cases treated as outpatients (Haltalin *et al.*, 1972), and in severe *Sh. flexneri* infections in hospitalized children (Haltalin *et al.*, 1967). The drug also reduces the duration of fecal excretion of shigellae (McCracken and Eichenwald, 1974). Children with shigellosis who are treated with ampicillin also absorb nutrients more efficiently from the bowel during the acute stage of the disease, compared with untreated controls (Molla and Molla, 1991).

During the large Central American epidemic AMP was extensively used for the treatment of dysentery due to *Sh. dysenteriae* type 1 (Shiga's bacillus) (Olarte *et al.*, 1976) and also in other developing countries. In a prospective study in Bangladesh, low-dose AMP therapy (50 mg per kg body weight per day) was compared with 150 mg per kg per day, both given for 5 days; this trial was carried out in both children and adults suffering from Shiga's dysentery. There were no clinical failures in either group, but among children younger than 3 years, bacteriological relapses were more frequent in the low-dose group. The authors recommended that an AMP dose of 50 mg per kg per day is usually sufficient, but younger children should be treated with a dose of 100 mg per kg per day (Gilman *et al.*, 1980). In a subsequent study in Bangladesh, a single AMP dose of 100 mg per kg was effective clinically for shigellosis in adults and children older than 4 years of age, but many patients remained *Shigella* carriers (Gilman *et al.*, 1981). A comparison of AMP with co-trimoxazole for treatment of *Shigella* dysentery in Bangladesh has been made; most infections were due to either *Sh. dysenteriae* type 1 or *Sh. flexneri*. Both drugs were effective, but symptoms such as abdominal pain, tenesmus and stool blood and mucus improved more rapidly with co-trimoxazole (Yunus *et al.*, 1982).

Owing to the emergence of AMP-resistant strains among all *Shigella* spp. in various parts of the world (p. 111), AMP has become unsuitable for the treatment of shigellosis. Co-trimoxazole is the best alternative, but unfortunately resistance to this drug has also emerged (p. 842). The quinolone drugs such as ciprofloxacin (p. 1016) are of value for the treatment of patients with shigellosis caused by multiresistant strains.

5 Respiratory tract infections

Pneumococcal lobar pneumonia responds to AMP, but penicillin G is preferable (p. 37); AMP should not be used alone for life-threatening forms of pneumonia, in which the bacteriological etiology cannot be immediately determined (p. 38). It is ineffective for *Mycoplasma* pneumonia. In chronic bronchitis, it is one of several effective drugs (p. 140).

Also AMP should not be used for acute bacterial tonsillitis, which is usually due to *Strep. pyogenes* infection; penicillin G or one of the phenoxypenicillins are preferred (p. 74). This is because AMP has a greater potential to cause rashes, particularly if the diagnosis of glandular fever is overlooked (p. 119).

6 Otitis media and sinusitis

For otitis media in adults, penicillin G (p. 38) is suitable as pneumococci are the most frequent pathogens; if as sometimes occurs, *H. influenzae* is implicated, other drugs are required (Paradise, 1980). In children, in addition to pneumococci, *H. influenzae* (mainly non-typable strains) are frequently involved (Paradise, 1980). Therefore, AMP or amoxycillin (p. 140) have been regarded as the drugs of choice in this age group (Bosso and Jackman, 1977). The emergence of AMP-resistant *H. influenzae* strains is now a problem (p. 113). Nevertheless, it is still reasonable to use AMP (or amoxycillin) for childhood otitis media in areas where AMP-resistant *H. influenzae* strains are not very prevalent. If infection by an AMP-resistant *H. influenzae* strain is suspected or confirmed, then co-trimoxazole (p. 864), an erythromycin/sulfisoxazole combination (p. 617), cefaclor (p. 278) or cefixime (p. 412) may be used (Michaels, 1981; Bluestone, 1982). A small proportion of cases of otitis media in children are caused by *Moraxella catarrhalis*; many strains are beta-lactamase producers (p. 112), and infection by these do not respond to AMP (Kovatch *et al.*, 1983).

Causative agents in acute maxillary sinusitis are *Strep. pneumoniae* and *H. influenzae* with other bacteria such as *Neisseria* spp., *Strep. pyogenes*, *Strep. viridans*, *Staph. aureus* and Gram-negative bacilli, being involved only occasionally (Hamory *et al.*, 1979). Sinusitis usually responds well to treatment with AMP, amoxycillin or co-trimoxazole (p. 863). *Moraxella catarrhalis* has been increasingly implicated as a cause of respiratory infections, including sinusitis; because many strains produce beta-lactamase, AMP may be ineffective therapy (Brorson *et al.*, 1981).

7 Pertussis

It may be useful to prescribe AMP for the treatment and prevention of secondary pulmonary infection in pertussis. The main factor in reducing the once-large mortality in pertussis has probably been the use of antibiotics to prevent and treat bronchopneumonia, particularly in young babies (Bennett, 1973). Similar to other antibiotics, AMP does not shorten the clinical course of whooping cough. Erythromycin, oxytetracycline and chloramphenicol eliminate *B. pertussis* within a few days (presumably rendering patients non-infectious), whereas AMP-treated patients have positive cultures for periods comparable with those of untreated patients (Bass *et al.*, 1969). For this reason, erythromycin is generally regarded as the drug of choice for treatment of patients with pertussis (Bass, 1973; Zackrisson *et al.*, 1983).

8 Bacterial meningitis

In children *H. influenzae* type b meningitis was successfully treated by using large doses (150–200 mg per kg per day) of parenteral AMP (Barrett *et al.*, 1966). Some authors found AMP equally effective to chloramphenicol (p. 569) for the treatment of this disease (Barrett *et al.*, 1972; Feigin *et al.*, 1976). Others noted that in AMP-treated patients, the duration of fever was more prolonged (Schulkind *et al.*, 1971), bacteriological responses were slower and some bacteriological relapses occurred, compared with uniformly good results obtained with chloramphenicol (Shackelford *et al.*, 1972).

After 1974 AMP-resistant strains of *H. influenzae* were isolated in many parts of the world (p. 113). Moreover, AMP-resistant strains of *H. influenzae* occasionally emerged during the treatment of meningitis (p. 113). For these reasons, chloramphenicol was the preferred antibiotic for the treatment of *H. influenzae* meningitis in many parts of the world. In some countries, particularly in North America, AMP was still used successfully for this disease. It was recommended that initially combination therapy with either penicillin G/chloramphenicol or

AMP/chloramphenicol should be used, and only when the sensitivity of the organism to AMP was confirmed, could AMP be continued as a single drug (McCracken, 1979; Koo *et al.*, 1982).

Chloramphenicol or AMP are no longer used for the treatment of *H. influenzae* meningitis in developed countries. Chloramphenicol-resistant strains are also emerging (p. 552) (Mackenzie and Chan, 1986). Parenteral third-generation cephalosporins such as cefotaxime (p. 336) and ceftriaxone (p. 359) are very safe and effective for the treatment of this disease (Powell, 1991). Treatment with AMP has been given for chemoprophylaxis of severe *H. influenzae* infections such as meningitis. In children *H. influenzae* meningitis is a contagious disease; the risk of spread to unvaccinated household contacts under 5 years of age is about 2.3%, some 800 times higher than the endemic attack rate for *H. influenzae* meningitis (Glode *et al.*, 1980) (p. 698). Theoretically, AMP may abort incipient attacks of invasive disease in contacts, but it does not dependably eradicate the *H. influenzae* carrier state (Ginsburg *et al.*, 1977). Rifampicin (p. 698) is recommended for this purpose.

9 Other severe *H. influenzae* type b infections

Given in high doses parenterally, AMP may be effective in epiglottitis, osteomyelitis, septic arthritis, cellulitis, pneumonia or septicemia (McCracken and Eichenwald, 1974). Nowadays for severe and especially life-threatening infections, cefotaxime or ceftriaxone is usually used. Severe *H. influenzae* infections including meningitis are nowadays frequently encountered in adults (Simon *et al.*, 1980; Whitby *et al.*, 1982). If treatment with AMP is contemplated for severely ill patients, initial treatment with either penicillin G/chloramphenicol or AMP/chloramphenicol, as in the case of meningitis (see above), is necessary, until the sensitivity of the strain is determined. Murphy and Todd (1979) reported six children with soft tissue infections caused by AMP-resistant *H. influenzae* strains, who responded satisfactorily to high doses of AMP (200–400 mg per kg per day i.v.). Such treatment of severe infections entails risks and it cannot be recommended (McCracken, 1979). In fact *H. influenzae* endocarditis is uncommon, and the best chemotherapy has not been determined. If the strain is AMP-sensitive, an AMP/gentamicin combination may be effective (Parker *et al.*, 1983). Cephalosporins, such as cefotaxime or ceftriaxone, may be more satisfactory.

Haemophilus parainfluenzae is an infrequent cause of invasive disease (Auten *et al.*, 1991). If sensitivity to AMP is confirmed, it can be used for treatment but other antibiotics such as cefotaxime are also available.

10 *Listeria monocytogenes* infections

For the treatment of these infections AMP is about equally effective as penicillin G (p. 40) (Nieman and Lorber, 1980; Cherubin *et al.*, 1981; Stamm *et al.*, 1982). It has been used with success to treat *Listeria* meningitis (Lavetter *et al.*, 1971; Hansen *et al.*, 1987), and it is also valuable for treatment of listeriosis in the neonatal age group (Visintine *et al.*, 1977). Results of animal experiments indicate that an AMP/gentamicin combination is more effective *in vivo* for *Listeria* infections than AMP therapy alone (Scheld *et al.*, 1979). Data in humans comparing this combination with AMP or penicillin G therapy alone, are not available. Use of AMP alone or combined with gentamicin is also suitable for the treatment of listeriosis in AIDS patients (Decker *et al.*, 1991). Combined with arterial surgery AMP has also been successful in treatment of *L. monocytogenes* infections of abdominal aortic aneurisms (Gauto *et al.*, 1992).

11 Bacterial endocarditis

It is known that AMP is slightly more active than penicillin G against most strains of *E. faecalis*, and it can be used instead of penicillin G for the treatment of this disease. Nevertheless a synergistic combination of AMP/gentamicin should be used, as AMP alone is unreliable (Mandell *et al.*, 1970). Recently *E. faecalis* strains with high-level gentamicin-resistance are posing new problems (p. 455). One animal experiment indicated that AMP alone, given as continuous infusion, may be more bactericidal for such strains, but this has not been confirmed in humans (Thauvin *et al.*, 1987). By contrast, Hellinger *et al.* (1992) in another animal study did not find AMP given by continuous infusion any better than the drug given by intermittent injections. One patient with *E. faecalis* endocarditis due to a strain with high-level gentamicin-resistance, recovered after a 6-week course of AMP 1.5 g i.v. 4-hourly (Lipman and Silva, 1989). Enterococcal bacteremia without endocarditis responds more satisfactorily to AMP monotherapy (Boulanger *et al.*, 1991).

Bacterial endocarditis due to Gram-negative bacilli is uncommon. One would not expect AMP alone to be reliable, but AMP combined with kanamycin has been successful in treating endocarditis due to *E. coli* (Hansing *et al.*, 1967). Cephalosporins, such as cefotaxime (p. 338) or ceftriaxone (p. 360), combined with an aminoglycoside, such as gentamicin (p. 471) or amikacin (p. 514), are usually preferred for this disease. Occasionally AMP has been used for other rare forms of endocarditis. It was successful in a case of *N. mucosa* endocarditis in a 30-year-old i.v. drug abuser (Davis *et al.*, 1983). This infection also responds to penicillin G (p. 16). *Neisseria elongata* endocarditis may also respond to AMP (Grant *et al.*, 1990). Several other *Neisseria* spp. (other than meningococci and gonococci) may rarely cause endocarditis (Johnson, 1983); these are not necessarily sensitive to AMP or penicillin G, so that sensitivities should be determined in each case.

12 Biliary infections

If the infecting organism is AMP-sensitive AMP is useful for the treatment of cholangitis. Most frequently *E. coli* is involved but others include *Enterococcus faecalis* and the *Klebsiella*, *Proteus* and *Clostridium* spp. (Kune and Burdon, 1975). Sometimes *B. fragilis* is involved, especially in elderly patients with bile duct obstruction (Shimada *et al.*, 1977). In general, a combination of AMP with gentamicin, is satisfactory for the treatment of these infections, before the causal organism is identified (p. 475). In very ill patients, the addition of clindamycin (p. 597) or metronidazole (p. 946) may be prudent to cover the possibility of a *B. fragilis* infection (Munro and Sorrell, 1986). It is often stressed that antibiotics which are excreted and concentrated in the bile (including AMP), are preferable for treatment of biliary infections. Mortimer *et al.* (1969) demonstrated that therapeutic concentrations of AMP were not attained in the bile of patients with obstructive biliary tract disease. In these patients, preoperative control of the septicemia which usually complicates cholangitis, is more important than sterilization of the bile (Van den Hazel *et al.*, 1994).

In the treatment of patients with acute cholecystitis, unlike cholangitis, chemotherapy is not always indicated. In cholecystitis the administration of an antibiotic such as AMP does not decrease the frequency of local septic complications. It does decrease the number of wound infections and the frequency of septicemia in high-risk patients, such as those over 60 years of age or those with debilitating diseases (Kune and Burdon, 1975). In such patients, chemoprophylaxis with a single i.v. dose of 1 g AMP, given just before surgery, may be sufficient. Patients without acute cholangitis, but who are undergoing biliary tract surgery involving the common bile duct, particularly in the presence of obstruction, may also warrant antibiotic prophylaxis. In this group Gram-negative anaerobes may be present and a single i.v. dose of 1 g cefoxitin (p. 308), given just before the operation, may be more suitable.

13 Other surgical infections

There is little if any place for AMP alone in the treatment or prophylaxis of other surgical infections such as peritonitis. A combination of AMP, oxacillin and gentamicin has been given as a single dose prophylaxis just before renal transplantation (p. 98).

14 Gonorrhea

This disease was treated by AMP in the past. A dose of 3.5 g plus 1 g oral probenecid was recommended (Washington, 1982). Because of the emergence of penicillin G- and AMP-resistant gonococci (p. 112), AMP is virtually no longer used for this disease, the preferred drugs being ceftriaxone (p. 361), other newer cephalosporins (p. 412), spectinomycin (p. 717) and quinolones such as ciprofloxacin (p. 1022).

15 Brucellosis

Although all *Brucella* spp. are sensitive to AMP *in vitro*, the drug is not useful clinically in *Br. abortus* and *Br. melitensis* infections. For infections by *Br. canis*, an uncommon human pathogen, AMP has been used in conjunction with other drugs, such as tetracycline and streptomycin, but optimal therapy for this infection has not been defined (Blankenship and Sanford, 1975).

16 Infections caused by some opportunistic bacteria

Therapy with AMP, initially combined with tobramycin, was successful in the treatment of prosthetic valve endocarditis caused by *Kingella indologenes* (Jenny *et al.*, 1987). Also AMP was useful for the treatment of peritonitis caused by *Agrobacterium tumefaciens* in a patient with alcoholic cirrhosis (Ramirez *et al.*, 1992).

17 Diarrhea due to verotoxin-producing E. coli 0157:H7

It does not seem that treatment with AMP or any other antibiotics is effective in this disease and antibiotic therapy in children does not prevent the development of hemolytic uremic syndrome (Orr *et al.*, 1994; Tarr, 1995).

References

Aguado JM, Fernandez-Guerrero ML, La Banda F, Garces JLG (1987). *Salmonella* infections of the abdominal aorta cured with prolonged antibiotic treatment. *J Infect* **14**: 135.

Albritton WL, Hammond G, Hoban S, Ronald AR (1977). Ampicillin-resistant *H influenzae* subdural empyema following successful treatment of apparently ampicillin-sensitive *H. influenzae* meningitis. *J Pediatr* **90**: 320.

Ali HM (1985). Reduced ampicillin bioavailability following oral coadministration with chloroquine. *J Antimicrob Chemother* **15**: 781.

Alos JI, Gomez-Garces JL, Cogollos R *et al.* (1992). Susceptibilities of ampicillin-resistant strains of *Salmonella* other than *S. typhi* to 10 antimicrobial agents. *Antimicrob AgChemother* **36**: 1794.

Arndt KA, Jick H (1976). Rates of cutaneous reactions to drugs A report from the Boston Collaborative Drug Surveillance Program. *JAMA* **235**: 918.

Asensi V, Fierer J (1991). Synergistic effect of human lysozyme plus ampicillin or beta-lysin on the killing of *Listeria monocytogenes*. *J Infect Dis* **163**: 574.

Ashkenazi S, May-Zahav M, Sulkes J *et al.* (1995). Increasing antimicrobial resistance of *Shigella* isolates in Israel during the period 1984 to 1992. *Antimicrob Ag Chemother* **39**: 819.

Asperilla MO, Smego RA Jr, Scott LK (1990). Quinolone antibiotics in the treatment of salmonella infections. *Rev Infect Dis* **12**: 873.

Auten GM, Levy CS, Smith MA (1991). *Haemophilus parainfluenzae* as a rare cause of epidural abscess: case report and review. *Rev Infect Dis* **13**: 609.

Axline SG, Yaffe SJ, Simon HJ (1967). Clinical pharmacology of antimicrobials in premature infants: II Ampicillin, methcillin, oxacillin, neomycin and colistin. *Pediatrics* **39**: 97.

Baker CN, Thornsberry C, Jones RN (1980). *In vitro* antimicrobial activity of cefoperazone, cefotaxime, moxalactam (LY 127935), azlocillin, mezlocillin, and other beta-lactam antibiotics against *Neisseria gonorrhoeae* and *Haemophilus influenzae*, including beta-lactamase-producing strains. *Antimicrob Ag Chemother* **17**: 757.

Baker PM, Farmer JJ III (1982). New bacteriophage typing system for *Yersinia enterocolitica, Yersinia kristenseni, Yersinia frederiksenii*, and *Yersinia intermedia*: correlation with serotyping, biotyping and antibiotic susceptibility. *J Clin Microbiol;* **15**: 491.

Bakker-Woudenberg IAJM, Lokerse AF, Vink-van den Berg JC *et al.* (1986). Effect of liposome-entrapped ampicillin on survival of *Listeria monocytogenes* in murine peritoneal macrophages. *Antimicrob Ag Chemother* **30**: 295.

Bakker-Woudenberg IAJM, Lokarse AF, Roerdink FH (1988). Effect of lipid composition on activity of liposome-entrapped ampicillin against intracellular *Listeria monocytogenes*. *Antimicrob Ag Chemother* **32**: 1560.

Bannatyne RM, Cheung R (1982). Antimicrobial susceptibility of *Bordetella pertussis* strains isolated from 1960 to 1981. *Antimicrob Ag Chemother* **21**: 666.

Barrett FF, Eardley WA, Yow MD, Leverett HA (1966). Ampicillin in the treatment of acute suppurative meningitis. *J Pediatr* **69**: 343.

Barrett FF, Taber LH, Morris CR *et al.* (1972). A 12 year review of the antibiotic management of *Haemophilus influenzae* meningitis. *J Pediatr* **81**: 370.

Barros F, Korzeniowski OM, Sande MA *et al.* (1977). *In vitro* antibiotic susceptibility of salmonellae. *Antimicrob Ag Chemother* **11**: 1071.

Barry AL, Fuchs PC, Pfaller MA (1993). Susceptibilities of beta-lactamase-producing and -nonproducing ampicillin-resistant strains of *Haemophilus influenzae* to ceftibuten, cefaclor, cefuroxime, cefixime, cefotaxime, and amoxicillin-clavulanic acid. *Antimicrob Ag Chemother* **37**: 14.

Bass JW (1973). The role of antimicrobial agents in the treatment of pertussis. *J Pediatr* **83**: 891.

Bass JW, Klenk EL, Kotheimer JB *et al.* (1969). Antimicrobial treatment of pertussis. *J Pediatr* **75**: 768.

Bass JW, Crowley DM, Steele RW *et al.* (1973). Adverse effects of orally administered ampicillin. *J Pediatr* **83**: 106.

Bassily SB, Kilpatrick ME, Farid Z *et al.* (1981). Chronic salmonella bacteriuria with intermittent bacteremia treated with low doses of amoxicillin or ampicillin. *Antimicrob Ag Chemother* **20**: 630.

Bayer AS, Chow AW, Anthony BF, Guze LB (1976). Serious infections in adults due to Group B streptococci. Clinical and serotypic characterization. *Amer J Med* **61**: 498.

Bayer AS, Chow AW, Concepcion N, Guze LB (1978). Susceptibility of 40 lactobacilli to six antimicrobial agents with broad Gram-positive anaerobic spectra. *Antimicrob Ag Chemother* **14**: 720.

Bear DM, Turck M, Petersdorf RG (1970). Ampicillin. *Med Clin N Amer* **54**: 1145.

Beckwith DG (1980). Simultaneous recovery of ampicillin-sensitive and ampicillin-resistant *H influenzae* from blood. *J Pediatr* **96**: 954.

Beeching NJ, Gruer LD, Findlay CD, Geddes AM (1982). A case of Henoch-Schönlein purpura syndrome following oral ampicillin. *J Antimicrob Chemother* **10**: 479.

Bell SM, Smith DD (1975). Ampicillin-resistant *Haemophilus influenzae*, type b. *Med J Aust* **1**: 517.

Bell SM, Plowman D (1980). Mechanisms of ampicillin resistance in *Haemophilus influenzae* from respiratory tract. *Lancet* **i**: 279.

Bellido F, Vladoianu IR, Auckenthaler R *et al.* (1989). Permeability and penicillin-binding protein alterations in *Salmonella muenchen*: stepwise resistance acquired during beta-lactam therapy. *Antimicrob Ag Chemother* **33**: 1113.

Bennett JV (1980). Editorial. Antibiotic use in animals and human salmonellosis. *J Infect Dis* **142**: 631.

Bennett N McK (1973). Whooping cough in Melbourne. *Med J Aust* **2**: 481.

Bennett WM, Singer I, Coggins CJ (1970). A practical guide to drug usage in adult patients with impaired renal function. *JAMA* **214**: 1468.

Bennett WM, Singer I, Coggins CJ (1974). A guide to drug therapy in renal failure. *JAMA* **230**: 1544.

Bennish ML, Salam MA, Hossain MA *et al.* (1992). Antimicrobial resistance of *Shigella* isolates in Bangladesh, 1983–1990: increasing frequency of strains multiply resistant to ampicillin, trimethoprim-sulfamethoxazole, and nalidixic acid. *Clin Infect Dis* **14**: 1055.

Bergeron MG, Lavoie GY (1985). Tolerance of *Haemophilus influenzae* to beta-lactam antibiotics. *Antimicrob Ag Chemother* **28**: 320.

Bhowmick BK (1972). Benign intracranial hypertension after antibiotic therapy. *Brit Med J* **3**: 30.

Biörklund A, Dahlquist E, Kamme C, Nilsson NI (1975). Ampicillin-resistant *Haemophilus influenzae* in otitis media. *Lancet* **i**: 1135.

Bissett ML, Abbot SL, Wood RM (1974). Antimicrobial resistance and R factors in salmonella isolated in California (1971–1972). *Antimicrob Ag Chemother* **5**: 161.

Black CT, Kupfershmid JP, West KW, Grosfeld JL (1988). *Haemophilus parainfluenzae* infections in children, with the report of a unique case. *Rev Infect Dis* **10**: 342.

Blankenship RM, Sanford JP (1975). *Brucella canis*. A cause of undulant fever. *Amer J Med* **59**: 424.

Blecher TE, Edgar WM, Melville HAH, Peel KR (1966). Transplacental passage of ampicillin. *Brit Med J* **1**: 137.

Bluestone CD (1982). Otitis media in children: to treat or not to treat? *New Engl J Med* **306**: 1399.

Bosso JA, Jackman JR (1977). Acute otitis media. *Drug Intel Clin Pharm* **11**: 665.

Boulanger JM, Ford-Jones EL, Matlow AG (1991). Enterococcal bacteremia in a pediatric institution: a four-year review. *Rev Infect Dis* **13**: 847.

Boyce JM, Opal SM, Potter-Bynoe G *et al.* (1992). Emergence and nosocomial transmission of ampicillin-resistant enterococci. *Antimicrob Ag Chemother* **36**: 1032.

Brooks AP (1974). Thrombocytopenia during treatment with ampicillin. *Lancet* **ii**: 723.

Brorson J-E, Martinell J, Wilske H (1981). *Branhamella catarrhalis*: antibiotic susceptibility and beta-lactamase production. *J Antimicrob Chemother* 7: 208.

Brunton JL, Maclean I, Ronald AR, Albritton WL (1979). Plasmid-mediated ampicillin resistance in *Haemophilus ducreyi*. *Antimicrob Ag Chemother* 15: 294.

Brunton J, Clare D, Meier MA (1986). Molecular epidemiology of antibiotic resistance plasmids of *Haemophilus* species and *Neisseria gonorrhoeae*. *Rev Infect Dis* 8: 713.

Bulger RJ, Bennett JV, Boen ST (1965). Intraperitoneal administration of broad-spectrum antibiotics in patients with renal failure. *JAMA* 194: 1198.

Burman LG, Haeggman S, Kuistila M *et al.* (1992). Epidemiology of plasmid-mediated beta-lactamases in enterobacteria in Swedish neonatal wards and relation to antimicrobial therapy. *Antimicrob Ag Chemother* 36: 989.

Byers PA, Dupont HL, Goldschmidt MC (1976). Antimicrobial susceptibilities of shigellae isolated in Houston, Texas, in 1974. *Antimicrob Ag Chemother* 9: 288.

Campos J, Chanyangam M, de Groot R *et al.* (1989). Genetic relatedness of antibiotic resistance determinants in multiply resistant *Haemophilus influenzae*. *J Infect Dis* 160: 810.

Cars O (1981). Tissue distribution of ampicillin: assays in muscle tissue and subcutaneous tissue cage fluid from normal and nephrectomized rabbits. *Scand J Infect Dis* 13: 283.

CDC (Center for Disease Control) (1979). Bacterial meningitis and meningococcemia – United States, 1978. *MMWR* 28: 277.

CDC (Centers for Disease Control) (1987). Nationwide dissemination of multiply resistant *Shigella sonnei* following a common-source outbreak. *MMWR* 36: 633.

Cercenado E, Eliopoulos GM, Wennersten CB, Moellering RC Jr (1992). Influence of high-level gentamicin resistance and beta-hemolysis on susceptibility of enterococci to the bactericidal activities of ampicillin and vancomycin. *Antimicrob Ag Chemother* 36: 2526.

Chamberland S, L'Ecuyer J, Lessard C *et al.* (1992). Antibiotic susceptibility profiles of 941 Gram-negative bacteria isolated from septicemic patients throughout Canada. *Clin Infect Dis* 15: 615.

Chau PY, Ng WS, Ling J, Arnold K (1981). Plasmid-mediated partial cross-resistance between ampicillin, mecillinam and cefamandole in *Salmonella johannesburg* and *Salmonella typhimurium*. *J Antimicrob Chemother* 7: 245.

Cherubin CE (1981). Antibiotic resistance of *Salmonella* in Europe and the United States. *Rev Infect Dis* 3: 1105.

Cherubin CE, Timoney JF, Sierra MF *et al.* (1980). A sudden decline in ampicillin resistance in *Salmonella typhimurium*. *JAMA* 243: 439.

Cherubin CE, Marr JS, Sierra MF, Becker S (1981). *Listeria* and Gram-negative bacillary meningitis in New York City, 1972–1979. *Amer J Med* 71: 199.

Chisholm GD, Waterworth PM, Calnan JS, Garrod LP (1973). Concentration of antibacterial agents in interstitial tissue. *Brit Med J* 1: 569.

Chow AW, Patten V, Bednorz D (1978). Susceptibility of *Campylobacter fetus* to twenty-two antimicrobial agents. *Antimicrob Ag Chemother* 13: 416.

Chun D, Seol SY, Cho DT, Tak R (1977). Drug resistance and R plasmids in *Salmonella typhi* isolated in Korea. *Antimicrob Ag Chemother* 11: 209.

Clairoux N, Picard M, Brochu A *et al.* (1992). Molecular basis of the non-beta-lactamase-mediated resistance to beta-lactam antibiotics in strains of *Haemophilus influenzae* isolated in Canada. *Antimicrob Ag Chemother* 36: 1504.

Clay J (1981). Non-specific vaginitis: its diagnosis and treatment. *J Antimicrob Chemother* 7: 501.

Colding H, Andersen GE (1982). Administration of gentamicin and ampicillin by continuous intravenous infusion to newborn infants during parenteral nutrition. *Scand J Infect Dis* 14: 61.

Cole M, Ridley B (1978). Absence of bioactive metabolites of ampicillin and amoxycillin in man. *J Antimicrob Chemother* 4: 580.

Collignon PJ, Bell JM, MacInnes SJ *et al.* (1992). A national collaborative study of resistance to antimicrobial agents in Haemophilus influenzae in Australian hospitals *J Antimicrob Chemother* 30: 153.

Cooksey R, Swenson J, Clark N *et al.* (1990). Patterns and mechanisms of beta-lactam resistance among isolates of *Escherichia coli* from hospitals in the United States. *Antimicrob Ag Chemother* 34: 739.

Cooper MD, Keeney RE, Lyons SF, Cheatle EL (1979). Synergistic effects of ampicillin-aminoglycoside combinations on Group B streptococci. *Antimicrob Ag Chemother* 15: 484.

Crosa JH, Olarte J, Mata LJ *et al.* (1977). Characterization of an R-plasmid associated with ampicillin resistance in *Shigella dysenteriae* type 1 isolated from epidemics. *Antimicrob Ag Chemother* 11: 553.

Crosson FJ Jr, Watson C III, Bailey DW, MacLowry JD (1976). Acute otitis media caused by ampicillin-resistant *Haemophilus influenzae* type B. *JAMA* 236: 2778.

Daum RS, Murphey-Corb M, Shapira E, Dipp S (1988). Epidemiology of Rob beta-lactamase among ampicillin-resistant *Haemophilus influenzae* isolates in the United States. *J Infect Dis* 157: 450.

Davis CL, Towns M, Henrich WL, Melby K (1983). *Neisseria mucosa* endocarditis following drug abuse. Case report and review of the literature. *Arch Intern Med* 143: 583.

Davies JR, Farrant WN, Uttley AHC (1970). Antibiotic resistance of *Shigella sonnei*. *Lancet* ii: 1157.

Davis RC (1981). Salmonella sepsis in infancy. *Amer J Dis Child* 135: 1096.

Decker CF, Simon GL, DiGioia RA, Tuazon CU (1991). *Listeria monocytogenes* infections in patients with AIDS: report of five cases and review. *Rev Infect Dis* 13: 413.

Dinbar A, Altmann G, Tulcinsky DB (1969). The treatment of chronic biliary salmonella carriers. *Amer J Med* 47: 236.

Doern GV, Jorgensen JH, Thornsberry C *et al.* (1986). Prevalence of antimicrobial resistance among clinical isolates of *Haemophilus influenzae*: a collaborative study. *Diagn Microbiol Infect Dis* 4: 95.

Doern GV, Jorgensen JH, Thornsberry C *et al.* (1988). National collaborative study of the prevalence of antimicrobial resistance among clinical isolates of *Haemophilus influenzae*. *Antimicrob Ag Chemother* 32: 180.

Dorman DC, Kilham HA (1976). Meningitis and ampicillin-resistant *Haemophilus influenzae*. *Med J Aust* 2: 359.

Du Pont HL, Steele JH (1987). Use of antimicrobial agents in animal feeds: implications for human health. *Rev Infect Dis* 9: 447.

Dutta P, Rasaily R, Saha MR *et al.* (1993). Ciprofloxacin for treatment of severe typhoid fever in children. *Antimicrob Ag Chemother* 37: 1197.

Eickhoff TC, Steinhauer BW, Finland M (1966). The *Klebsiella-Enterobacter-Serratia* division. Biochemical and serologic characteristics and susceptibility to antibiotics. *Ann Intern Med* 65: 1163.

Eickhoff TC, Ehret JM, Baines RD (1976). Characterization of an ampicillin-resistant *Haemophilus influenzae* type B. *Antimicrob Ag Chemother* 9: 889.

Elmros T, Holm S, Kjellberg E *et al.* (1979). Effects of low ampicillin concentrations on penicillin sensitive and beta-lactamase producing strains of *Neisseria gonorrhoeae*. *J Antimicrob Chemother* 5: 555.

Emerson BB, Smith AL, Harding AL, Smith DH (1975). *Haemophilus influenzae* type B susceptibility to 17 antibiotics. *J Pediatr* 86: 617.

Fallon RJ (1976). Leading article. Haemophilus influenzae meningitis. *J Antimicrob Chemother* 2: 3.

Fattal E, Rojas J, Youssef M *et al.* (1991). Liposome-entrapped ampicillin in the treatment of experimental murine listeriosis and salmonellosis. *Antimicrob Ag Chemother* 35: 770.

Feder HM Jr (1982). Comparative tolerability of ampicillin, amoxicillin, and trimethoprim-sulfamethoxazole suspensions in children with otitis media. *Antimicrob Ag Chemother* 21: 426.

Feigin RD, Stechenberg BW, Chang MJ *et al.* (1976). Prospective evaluation of treatment of *Haemophilus influenzae* meningitis. *J Pediatr* 88: 542.

Fekety R, Shah AB (1993). Diagnosis and treatment of *Clostridium difficile* colitis *JAMA* 269: 71.

Fischl MA, Dickinson GM, Sinave C *et al.* (1986). *Salmonella* bacteremia as manifestation of acquired immunodeficiency syndrome. *Arch Intern Med* **146**: 113.

Fleming PC, Murray JDM, Fujiwara MW *et al.* (1967). Ampicillin in the treatment of bacterial meningitis. *Antimicrob Ag Chemother* **1966**: 47.

Frost JA, Rowe B (1983). Plasmid-determined antibiotic resistance in *Shigella flexneri* isolated in England and Wales between 1974 and 1978. *J Hyg Camb* **90**: 27.

Frost JA, Rowe B, Vandepitte J, Threlfall EJ (1981). Plasmid characterization in the investigation of an epidemic caused by multiply resistant *Shigella dysenteriae* type 1 in Central Africa. *Lancet* **ii**: 1074.

Fung C-P, Yeo S-F, Livermore DM (1994). Susceptibility of *Moraxella catarrhalis* isolates to beta lactam antibiotics in relation to beta-lactamase pattern. *J Antimicrob Chemother* **33**: 215.

Garty M, Hurwitz A (1985). Effects of morphine on the disposition of ampicillin in mice. *Antimicrob Ag Chemother* **28**: 489.

Gauto AR, Cone LA, Woodard DR (1992). Arterial infections due to *Listeria monocytogenes*: report of four cases and review of world literature. *Clin Infect Dis* **14**: 23.

Gerding DN, Hall WH, Schierl EA (1977). Antibiotic concentrations in ascitic fluid of patients with ascites and bacterial peritonitis. *Ann Intern Med* **86**: 708.

Gilman RH, Koster F, Islam S *et al.* (1980). Randomized trial of high- and low-dose ampicillin therapy for treatment of severe dysentery due to *Shigella dysenteriae* type 1. *Antimicrob Ag Chemother* **17**: 402.

Gilman RH, Spira W, Rabbani H *et al.* (1981). Single-dose ampicillin therapy for severe shigellosis in Bangladesh. *J Infect Dis* **143**: 164.

Ginsburg CM, McCracken GH Jr, Rae S, Parke JC Jr (1977). *Haemophilus influenzae* type B disease incidence in a day-care center. *JAMA* **238**: 604.

Girgis NI, Yassin W, Sippel JE, Farid Z (1982). Intramuscular compared with intravenous ampicillin in the treatment of meningococcal meningitis. *Scand J Infect Dis* **14**: 239.

Glass RI, Huq MI, Lee JV *et al.* (1983). Plasmid-borne multiple drug resistance in *Vibrio cholerae* serogroup 01, biotype E1 Tor: evidence for a point-source outbreak in Bangladesh. *J Infect Dis* **147**: 204.

Glode MP, Daum RS, Goldman DA *et al.* (1980). *Haemophilus influenzae* type B meningitis: a contagious disease in children. *Brit Med J* **280**: 899.

Goossens H, Coignau H, Vlaes L, Butzler J-P (1989). *In vitro* evaluation of antibiotic combinations against *Campylobacter fetus*. *J Antimicrob Chemother* **24**: 195.

Graf M, Tarlov A (1968). Agranulocytosis with monohistiocytosis associated with ampicillin therapy. *Ann Intern Med* **69**: 91.

Granoff DM, Sargent E, Jolivette D (1978). *Haemophilus influenzae* type B osteomyelitis. *Amer J Dis Child* **132**: 488.

Gransden WR, Eykyn SJ, Phillips I, Rowe B (1990). Bacteremia due to *Escherichia coli*: a study of 861 episodes. *Rev Infect Dis* **12**: 1008.

Grant PE, Brenner DJ, Steigerwalt AG *et al.* (1990). *Neisseria elongata* subsp *nitroreducens* subsp nov, formerly CDC Group M-6, a Gram-negative bacterium associated with endocarditis. *J Clin Microbiol* **28**: 2591.

Grant RB, Bannatyne RM, Shapley AJ (1976). Resistance to chloramphenicol and ampicillin of *Salmonella typhimurium* in Ontario, Canada. *J Infect Dis* **134**: 354.

Grayson ML, Eliopoulos GM, Wennersten CB *et al.* (1991). Increasing resistance to beta-lactam antibiotics among clinical isolates of *Enterococcus faecium*: a 22-year review at one institution. *Antimicrob Ag Chemother* **35**: 2180.

Gross RJ, Rowe B, Cheasty T, Thomas LV (1981). Increase in drug resistance among *Shigella dysenteriae*, *Sh. flexneri*, and *Sh. boydii*. *Brit Med J* **283**: 575.

Gross RJ, Ward LR, Threlfall EJ *et al.* (1982). Drug resistance among infantile enteropathogenic *Escherichia coli* strains isolated in the United Kingdom. *Brit Med J* **285**: 472.

Gurwith MJ, Rabin HR, Love K, Co-operative Antibiotic Diarrhea Study Group (1977). Diarrhea associated with clindamycin and ampicillin therapy: preliminary results of a co-operative study. *J Infect Dis* **135** (Suppl): 104.

Haltalin KC, Nelson JD, Ring R *et al.* (1967). Double-blind treatment study of shigellosis comparing ampicillin sulfadiazine and placebo. *J Pediatr* **70**: 970.

Haltalin KC, Kusmiesz HT, Hinton LV, Nelson JD (1972). Treatment of acute diarrhoea in outpatients. Double-blind study comparing ampicillin and placebo. *Amer J Dis Child* **124**: 554.

Hamory BH, Sande MA, Sydnor A Jr *et al.* (1979). Etiology and antimicrobial therapy of acute maxillary sinusitis. *J Infect Dis* **139**: 197.

Hansen PB, Jensen TH, Lykkegaard S, Kristensen HS (1987). *Listeria monocytogenes* meningitis in adults. Sixteen consecutive cases 1973–1982. *Scand J Infect Dis* **19**: 55.

Hansing CE, Allen VD, Cherry JD (1967). *Escherichia coli* endocarditis A review of the literature and a case study. *Arch Intern Med* **120**: 472.

Hellinger WC, Rouse MS, Rabadan PM *et al.* (1992). Continuous intravenous versus intermittent ampicillin therapy of experimental endocarditis caused by aminoglycoside-resistant enterococci. *Antimicrob Ag Chemother* **36**: 1272.

Herzog CH (1976). Drug treatment of typhoid fever. *Brit Med J* **2**: 941.

Holmberg SD, Osterholm MT, Senger KA, Cohen ML (1984). Drug-resistant salmonella from animals fed antimicrobials. *New Engl J Med* **311**: 617.

Holmes CJ, Ausman RK, Kundsin RB, Walter CW (1982). Effect of freezing and microwave thawing on the stability of six antibiotic admixtures in plastic bags. *Amer J Hosp Pharm* **39**: 104.

Hovelius B, Mårdh P-A (1984). *Staphylococcus saprophyticus* as a common cause of urinary tract infections. *Rev Infect Dis* **6**: 328.

Howard AJ, Williams HM, (1988). The prevalence of antibiotic resistance in *Haemophilus influenzae* in Wales. *J Antimicrob Chemother* **21**: 251.

Howard AJ, Hince CJ, Williams JD (1978). Antibiotic resistance in *Streptococcus pneumoniae* and *Haemophilus influenzae*. Report of a study group on bacterial resistance. *Brit Med J* **1**: 1657.

Jacobs JL, Gold JWM, Murray HW et al. (1985). Salmonella infections in patients with acquired immunodeficiency syndrome. *Ann Intern Med* **102**: 186.

Jacobs RF, Wilson CB, Laxton JG *et al.* (1982). Cellular uptake and intracellular activity of antibiotics against *Haemophilus influenzae* type B. *J Infect Dis* **145**: 152.

Jacobson JA, McCormick JB, Hayes P *et al.* (1976). Epidemiologic characteristics of infections caused by ampicillin-resistant *Haemophilus influenzae*. *Pediatrics* **58**: 388.

Jenny DB, Letendre PW, Iverson G (1987). Endocarditis caused by *Kingella indologenes*. *Rev Infect Dis* **9**: 787.

Jeffries WS, Bochner F (1988). The effect of pregnancy on drug pharmacokinetics. *Med J Aust* **149**: 675.

Johnson AP (1983). The pathogenic potential of commensal species of *Neisseria*. *J Clin Pathol* **36**: 213.

Johnson RH, Lutwick LI, Huntley GA, Vosti KL (1976). *Arizona hinshawii* infections. New cases, antimicrobial sensitivities and literature review. *Ann Intern Med* **85**: 587.

Johnson WD Jr, Hook EW, Lindsey E, Kaye D (1973). Treatment of chronic typhoid carriers with ampicillin. *Antimicrob Ag Chemother* **3**: 439.

Jokipii L, Jokipii AMM (1980). Emergence and prevalence of beta-lactamase producing *Haemophilus influenzae* in Finland and susceptibility of 102 respiratory isolates to eight antibiotics. *J Antimicrob Chemother* **6**: 623.

Jorgensen JH (1992). Update on mechanisms and prevalence of antimicrobial resistance in *Haemophilus influenzae*. *Clin Infect Dis* **14**: 1119.

Jorgensen JH, Doern GV, Maher LA *et al.* (1990). Antimicrobial resistance among respiratory isolates of *Haemophilus influenzae, Moraxella catarrhalis*, and *Streptococcus pneumoniae* in the United States. *Antimicrob Ag Chemother* **34**: 2075.

Joseph SW, DeBell RM, Brown WP (1978). *In vitro* response to chloramphenicol, tetracycline, ampicillin, gentamicin, and beta-lactamase production by halophilic vibrious from human and environmental sources. *Antimicrob Ag Chemother* **13**: 244.

Jubelirer DP, Yeager AS (1979). Simultaneous recovery of ampicillin-sensitive and ampicillin-resistant organisms in *Haemophilus influenzae* type B meningitis. *J Pediatr* **95**: 415.

Juteau J-M, Sirois M, Medeiros AA, Levesque RC (1991). Molecular distribution of ROB-1 beta-lactamase in *Actinobacillus pleuropneumoniae*. *Antimicrob Ag Chemother* **35**: 1397.

Kammer RB, Preston DA, Turner JR, Hawley LC (1975). Rapid detection of ampicillin-resistant *Haemophilus influenzae* and their susceptibility to sixteen antibiotics. *Antimicrob Ag Chemother* **8**: 91.

Kaplan JM, McCracken GH Jr, Horton LJ *et al.* (1974). Pharmacologic studies in neonates given large dosages of ampicillin. *J Pediatr* **84**: 571.

Karmali MA, De Grandis S, Fleming PC (1981). Antimicrobial susceptibility of *Campylobacter jejuni* with special reference to resistance patterns of Canadian isolates. *Antimicrob Ag Chemother* **19**: 593.

Kauffman CA, Bergman AG, Hertz CS (1979). Antimicrobial resistance of *Haemophilus* species in patients with chronic bronchitis. *Amer Rev Respir Dis* **120**: 1382.

Kazemi M, Gumpert TG, Marks MI (1973). A controlled trial comparing sulfamethoxazole-trimethoprim, ampicillin and no therapy in the treatment of salmonella gastro-enteritis in children. *J Pediatr* **83**: 646.

Keating JP, Frank AL, Barton LL, Tedesco FJ (1974). Pseudomembranous colitis associated with ampicillin therapy. *Amer J Dis Child* **128**: 369.

Kerns DL, Shira JE, Go S *et al.* (1973). Ampicillin rash in children Relationship to penicillin allergy and infectious mononucleosis. *Amer J Dis Child* **125**: 187.

Kirby WMM, Kind AC (1967). Clinical pharmacology of ampicillin and hetacillin. *Ann NY Acad Sci* **145**: 291.

Klemola E (1970). Hypersensitivity reactions to ampicillin in *Cytomegalovirus mononucleosis*. *Scand J Infect Dis* **2**: 29.

Kluge RM, Waldman RH, Delafuente JC, Slavin RG (1982). Ampicillin-specific antibody and delayed hypersensitivity skin tests to ampicillin in patients with acute infectious mononucleosis. *J Infect Dis* **145**: 397.

Knirsch AK, Gralla EJ (1970). Serum transaminase levels after parenteral ampicillin and carbenicillin. *New Engl J Med* **282**: 1081.

Koo W, Oley C, Munro R, Tomlinson P (1982). Systemic *Haemophilus influenzae* infection in childhood. *Med J Aust* **2**: 77.

Kovatch AL, Wald ER, Michaels RH (1983). β-Lactamase-producing *Branhamella catarrhalis* causing otitis media in children. *J Pediatr* **102**: 261.

Kune GA, Burdon JGW (1975). Are antibiotics necessary in acute cholecystitis? *Med J Aust* **2**: 627.

Lachance N, Gaudreau C, Lamothe F, Lariviere LA (1991). Role of the beta-lactamase of *Campylobacter jejuni* in resistance to beta-lactam agents. *Antimicrob Ag Chemother* **35**: 813.

Lachance N, Gaudreau C, Lamothe F, Turgeon F (1993). Susceptibilities of beta-lactamase -positive and -negative strains of *Campylobacter coli* to beta-lactam agents. *Antimicrob Ag Chemother* **37**: 1174.

Lampe RM, Duangmani C, Mansuwan P (1975). Chloramphenicol- and ampicillin-resistant typhoid fever. *JAMA* **233**: 768.

Landesman SH, Corrado ML, Cherubin CE, Sierra MF (1981). Activity of moxalactam and cefotaxime alone and in combination with ampicillin or penicillin against Group B streptococci. *Antimicrob Ag Chemother* **19**: 794.

Lavetter A, Leedom JM, Mathies AW Jr *et al.* (1971). Meningitis due to *Listeria monocytogenes*. A review of 25 cases. *New Engl J Med* **285**: 598.

Leading Article (1982). Drug resistance in salmonellas. *Lancet* **i**: 1391.

Lee HA, Hill LF (1968). The use of ampicillin in renal disease. *Brit J Clin Pract* **22**: 354.

Lee LA, Puhr ND, Maloney EK *et al.* (1994). Increase in antimicrobial-resistant *Salmonella* infections in the United States, 1989–1990. *J Infect Dis* **170**: 128.

Lerman SJ, Kucera JC, Brunken JM (1979). Nasopharyngeal carriage of antibiotic-resistant *Haemophilus influenzae* in healthy children. *Pediatrics* **64**: 287.

Levy J, Verhaegen G, De Mol P *et al.* (1993). Molecular characterization of

resistance plasmids in epidemiologically unrelated strains of multi-resistant *Haemophilus influenzae*. *J Infect Dis* **168**: 177.

Levy SB, Marshall B, Schluederberg S *et al.* (1988). High frequency of antimicrobial resistance in human fecal flora. *Antimicrob Ag Chemother* **32**: 1801.

Ling J, Chau PY, Leung YK *et al.* (1983). Antibiotic susceptibility of pneumococci and *Haemophilus influenzae* isolated from patients with acute exacerbations of chronic bronchitis: prevalence of tetracycline-resistant strains in Hong Kong. *J Infect* **6**: 33.

Ling TKW, Lyon DJ, Cheng AFB, French GL (1994). In-vitro antimicrobial susceptibility and beta-lactamases of ampicillin-resistant *Escherichia coli* in Hong Kong. *J Antimicrob Chemother* **34**: 65.

Ljungberg B, Braconier JH (1986). Abdominal aortitis and infected aneurysms due to *Salmonella*. *Scand J Infect Dis* **18**: 401.

Lipman ML, Silva J Jr (1989). Endocarditis due to *Streptococcus faecalis* with high-level resistance to gentamicin. *Rev Infect Dis* **11**: 325.

London N, Nijsten R, Bogaard AVD, Stobberingh E (1993). Antibiotic resistance of faecal Enterobacteriaceae isolated from healthy volunteers, a 15-week follow-up study. *J Antimicrob Chemother* **32**: 83.

Loo VG, Sherman P, Matlow AG (1992). *Helicobacter pylori* infection in a pediatric population: *in vitro* susceptibilities to omeprazole and eight antimicrobial agents. *Antimicrob Ag Chemother* **36**: 1133.

Lund BMA, Bergan T (1975). Temporary skin reactions to penicillins during the acute stage of infectious mononucleosis. *Scand J Infect Dis* **7**: 21.

Lusk RH, Fekety FR Jr, Silva J Jr *et al.* (1977). Gastrointestinal side effects of clindamycin and ampicillin therapy. *J Infect Dis* **135** (Suppl): 111.

MacKenzie AMR, Chan FTH (1986). Combined action of chloramphenicol and ampicillin on chloramphenicol-resistant *Haemophilus influenzae*. *Antimicrob Ag Chemother* **29**: 565.

MacMahon P, Ramberan P (1980). Potential hazard of discontinuing chloramphenicol once sensitivity results are available in *Haemophilus meningitis*. *Lancet* **i**: 1080.

MacMahon P, Sills J, Hall E, Fitzgerald T (1982). *Haemophilus influenzae* type b resistant to both chloramphenicol and ampicillin in Britain. *Brit Med J* **284**: 1229.

Malmvall B-E, Branefors-Helander P (1978). R-factor involvement in a local outbreak of ampicillin-resistant *Haemophilus influenzae* infections. *Scand J Infect Dis* **10**: 53.

Mandell GL, Kaye D, Levison ME, Hook EW (1970). Enterococcal endocarditis. *Arch Intern Med* **125**: 258.

Manriquez L, Salcedo M, Borgoño JM *et al.* (1965). Clinical trials with ampicillin in typhoid fever and paratyphoid A. *Brit Med J* **2**: 152.

Marrie TJ, Kwan C (1982). Antimicrobial susceptibility of *Staphylococcus saprophyticus* and urethral staphylococci. *Antimicrob Ag Chemother* **22**: 395.

Martin C, Gomez-Lus R, Ortiz JM, Garcia-Lobo JM (1987). Structure and mobilization of an ampicillin and gentamicin resistance determinant. *Antimicrob Ag Chemother* **31**: 1266.

Matthew M (1979). Plasmid-mediated beta-lactamases of Gram-negative bacteria: properties and distribution. *J Antimicrob Chemother* **5**: 349.

Mathewson JJ, Murray BE (1983). Plasmid-mediated resistance to trimethoprim-sulfamethoxazole in *Salmonella krefeld* strains isolated in the United States. *Antimicrob Ag Chemother* **23**: 495.

Maxwell D, Szwed JJ, Wahle W, Kleit SA (1974). Ampicillin nephropahty. *JAMA* **230**: 586.

McCarthy LR, Mickelson PA, Smith EG (1979). Antibiotic susceptibility of *Haemophilus vaginalis* (*Corynebacterium vaginale*). to 21 antibiotics. *Antimicrob Ag Chemother* **16**: 186.

McConnell MM, Smith HR, Leonardopoulous J, Anderson ES (1979). The value of plasmid studies in the epidemiology of infections due to drug resistant *Salmonella wien*. *J Infect Dis* **139**: 178.

McCracken GH Jr (1974). Pharmacological basis for antimicrobial therapy in newborn infants. *Amer J Dis Child* **128**: 407.

McCracken GH Jr (1979). Resistant *H influenzae* and high-dose ampicillin Commentary. *J Pediatr* **94**: 987.

McCracken GH Jr, Eichenwald HF (1974). Antimicrobial therapy: therapeutic recommendations and review of newer drugs. Part 1. Therapy of infectious conditions. *J Pediatr* **85**: 297.

McCracken GH Jr, Nelson JD (1983). *Antimicrobial Therapy for Newborns* 2nd edn, p. 13. New York: Grune and Stratton.

McGowan JE Jr, Terry PM, Nahmias AJ (1976). Susceptibility of *Haemophilus influenzae* isolates from blood and cerebrospinal fluid to ampicillin, chloramphenicol and trimethoprim-sulfamethoxazole. *Antimicrob Ag Chemother* **9**: 137.

McNicol PJ, Albritton WL, Ronald AR (1986). Transfer of plasmid-mediated ampicillin resistance from *Haemophilus* to *Neisseria gonorrhoeae* requires an intervening organism. *Sex Transm Dis* **13**: 145.

Medeiros AA, Levesque R, Jacoby GA (1986). An animal source for the ROB-1 beta-lactamase of *Haemophilus influenzae* type b. *Antimicrob Ag Chemother* **29**: 212.

Mendelman PM (1992). Targets of the beta-lactam antibiotics, penicillin-binding proteins, in ampicillin-resistant non-beta-lactamase-producing *Haemophilus influenzae*. *J Infect Dis* **165** (Suppl 1): 107.

Mendelman PM, Chaffin DO, Stull TL et al. (1984). Characterization of non-beta-lactamase-mediated ampicillin resistance in *Haemophilus influenzae*. *Antimicrob Ag Chemother* **26**: 235.

Mendelman PM, Chaffin DO, Kalaitzoglou G (1990). Penicillin-binding proteins and ampicillin resistance in *Haemophilus influenzae*. *J Antimicrob Chemother* **25**: 525.

Michaels RH (1981). Ampicillin-resistant *Haemophilus influenzae* and otitis media. *Amer J Dis Child* **135**: 403.

Mikhail IA, Sippel JE, Girgis NI, Yassin MW (1981). Cerebrospinal fluid and serum ampicillin levels in bacterial meningitis patients after intravenous and intramuscular administration. *Scand J Infect Dis* **13**: 237.

Molla AM, Molla AM (1991). Effect of antibiotics on food intake and absorption of nutrients for children with diarrhea due to shigella. *Rev Infect Dis* **13** (Suppl 4): 347.

Montecalvo MA, Horowitz H, Gedris C et al. (1994). Outbreak of vancomycin-, ampicillin-, and aminoglycoside-resistant *Enterococcus faecium* bacteremia in an adult oncology unit. *Antimicrob Ag Chemother* **38**: 1363.

Mortimer PR, Mackie DB, Haynes S (1969). Ampicillin levels in human bile in the presence of biliary tract disease. *Brit Med J* **3**: 88.

Mourad AS, Metwally M, El Deen AN et al. (1993). Multiple-drug-resistant *Salmonella typhi*. *Clin Infect Dis* **17**: 135.

Munro R, Sorrell TC (1986). Biliary sepsis Reviewing treatment options *Drugs* **31**: 449.

Murphy D, Todd J (1979). Treatment of ampicillin-resistant *Haemophilus influenzae* in soft tissue infections with high doses of ampicillin. *J Pediatr* **94**: 983.

Murray BE (1986). Resistance of *Shigella*, *Salmonella* and other selected enteric pathogens to antimicrobial agents. *Rev Infect Dis* **8** (Suppl 2): 172.

Nazareth I, Mortimer P, McKendrick GDW (1972). Ampicillin sensitivity in infectious mononucleosis – temporary or permanent? *Scand J Infect Dis* **4**: 229.

Needham Walker C, Smith PW (1980). Ampicillin resistance in *Haemophilus parainfluenzae*. *Amer J Clin Pathol* **74**: 229.

Nelson JD (1971). Antibiotic concentrations in septic joint effusions. *New Engl J Med* **284**: 349.

Nelson JD (1981). Antibiotic therapy for *Salmonella* syndromes. *Amer J Dis Child* **135**: 1093.

Nelson JD, Kusmiesz H, Jackson LH, Woodman E (1980). Treatment of *Salmonella gastroenteritis* with ampicillin, amoxicillin or placebo. *Pediatrics* **65**: 1125.

Neu HC, Cherubin CE, Longo ED et al. (1975a). Antimicrobial resistance and R-factor transfer among isolates of salmonella in the Northeastern United States: a comparison of human and animal isolates. *J Infect Dis* **132**: 617.

Neu HC, Cherubin CE, Longo ED, Winter J (1975b). Antimicrobial resistance of shigella isolated in New York City in 1973. *Antimicrob Ag Chemother* **7**: 833.

Newsom SWB, Matthews J (1982). Ampicillin resistance in *Haemophilus influenzae*-test methods for the activity of acylureidopenicillins, cephamycins and new cephalosporins. *J Antimicrob Chemother* **10**: 527.

Nieman RE, Lorber B (1980). Listeriosis in adults: a changing pattern. Report of eight cases and review of the literature, 1968–1978. *Rev Infect Dis* **2**: 207.

Nissinen A, Herva E, Katila M-L et al. (1995). Antimicrobial resistance in *Haemophilus influenzae* isolated from blood, cerebrospinal fluid, middle ear fluid and throat samples of children. A nationwide study in Finland in 1988–1990 *Scand. J Infect Dis* **27**: 57.

O'Brien TF, Hopkins JD, Gilleece ES et al. (1982). Molecular epidemiology of antibiotic resistance in *Salmonella* from animals and human beings in the United States. *New Engl J Med* **307**: 1.

Oie S, Hironaga K, Koshiro A et al. (1983). *In vitro* susceptibilities of five *Leptospira* strains to 16 antimicrobial agents. *Antimicrob Ag Chemother* **24**: 905.

Okura K, Haruta T, Kobayashi Y (1988). Drug transfer into cerebrospinal fluid after simultaneous administration of ampicillin with ceftriaxone or ceftazidime in rabbits with *Staphylococcus aureus* meningitis. *J Antimicrob Chemother* **22**: 207.

Olarte J, Galindo E (1973). *Salmonella typhi* resistant to chloramphenicol, ampicillin, and other antimicrobial agents: strains isolated during an extensive typhoid fever epidemic in Mexico. *Antimicrob Ag Chemother* **4**: 597.

Olarte J, Filloy L, Galindo E (1976). Resistance of *Shigella dysenteriae* type 1 to ampicillin and other antimicrobial agents: strains isolated during a dysentery outbreak in a hospital in Mexico City. *J Infect Dis* **133**: 572.

Orr P, Lorencz B, Brown R (1994). An outbreak of diarrhea due to verotoxin-producing *Escherichia coli* in the Canadian Northwest Territories. *Scand. J Infect Dis* **26**: 675.

Paradise JL (1980). Otitis media in infants and children. *Pediatrics* **65**: 917.

Parker SW, Apicella MA, Fuller CM (1983). Haemophilus endocarditis. Two patients with complications. *Arch Intern Med* **143**: 48.

Parr TR Jr, Bryan LE (1984). Mechanism of resistance of an ampicillin-resistant, beta-lactamase-negative clinical isolate of *Haemophilus influenzae* type b to beta-lactam antibiotics. *Antimicrob Ag Chemother* **25**: 747.

Parsons R, Gregory J, Palmer DL (1983). *Salmonella* infections of the abdominal aorta. *Rev Infect Dis* **5**: 227.

Parsons RL, Hossack G, Paddock G (1975). The absorption of antibiotics in adult patients with coeliac disease. *J Antimicrob Chemother* **1**: 39.

Peltola H, Rod TO, Jonsdottir K et al. (1990). Life-threatening *Haemophilus influenzae* infections in Scandinavia: a five-country analysis of the incidence and the main clinical and bacteriologic characteristics. *Rev Infect Dis* **12**: 708.

Penn RL, Ward TT, Steigbigel RT (1982). Effects of erythromycin in combination with penicillin, ampicillin or gentamicin on the growth of *Listeria monocytogenes*. *Antimicrob Ag Chemother* **22**: 289.

Petheram IS, Boyce JMH (1976). Prosthetic endocarditis treated with ampicillin and gentamicin in a penicillin-hypersensitive patient. *Brit Med J* **2**: 851.

Philipson A (1977). Pharmacokinetics of ampicillin during pregnancy. *J Infect Dis* **136**: 370.

Philipson A, Sabath LD, Rosner B (1975). Sequence effect on ampicillin blood levels noted in an amoxicillin, ampicillin, and epicillin triple crossover study. *Antimicrob Ag Chemother* **8**: 311.

Phillips JA, Lovejoy FH Jr, Matsumiya Y (1976). Ampicillin-associated diarrhoea: effect of dosage and route of administration. *Pediatrics* **58**: 869.

Philpott-Howard J, Williams JD (1982). Increase in antibiotic resistance in *Haemophilus influenzae* in the United Kingdom since 1977: report of study group. *Brit Med J* **284**: 1597.

Pinget M, Brogard JM, Dauchel J, Lavillaureix J (1976). Biliary excretion of ampicillin, metampicillin and carbenicillin. *J Antimicrob Chemother* **2**: 195.

Potter JL, Weinberg AG, West R (1971). Ampicillinuria and ampicillin crystalluria. *Pediatrics* **48**: 636.

Powell M (1991). Chemotherapy for infections caused by *Haemophilus influenzae*: curent problems and future prospects. *J Antimicrob Chemother* **27**: 3.

Powell M, Livermore DM (1990). Selection and transformation of non-beta-lactamase-mediated insusceptibility to beta-lactams in *Haemophilus influenzae*: lack of cross-resistance between carbapenems and other agents. *J Antimicrob Chemother* **26**: 741.

Powell M, McVey D, Kassim MH *et al.* (1991). Antimicrobial susceptibility of *Streptococcus pneumoniae*, *Haemophilus influenzae* and *Moraxella (Branhamella) catarrhalis* isolated in the UK from sputa. *J Antimicrob Chemother* **28**: 249.

Prince A, Neu HC (1976). Beta-lactamase activity in *Shigella sonnei*. *Antimicrob Ag Chemother* **9**: 776.

Pullen H, Wright N, Murdoch J McC (1967). Hypersensitivity reactions to anti-bacterial drugs on infectious mononucleosis. *Lancet* **ii**: 1176.

Raevuori M, Harvey SM, Pickett MJ, Martin WJ (1978). *Yersinia enterocolitica*; *in vitro* antimicrobial susceptibility. *Antimicrob Ag Chemother* **13**: 888.

Rahaman MM, Huq I, Dey CR et al. (1974). Ampicillin-resistant shiga bacillus in Bangladesh. *Lancet* **i**: 406.

Ramirez FC, Saeed ZA, Darouiche RO *et al.* (1992). *Agrobacterium tumefaciens* peritonitis mimicking tuberculosis. *Clin Infect Dis* **15**: 938.

Rangnekar VM, Banker DD, Jhala HI (1983). Antimicrobial resistance and incompatibility groups of R plasmids in *Salmonella typhimurium* isolated from human sources in Bombay from 1978 to 1980. *Antimicrob Ag Chemother* **23**: 54.

Reid AJ, Simpson IN, Harper PB, Amyes SGB (1987). Ampicillin resistance in *Haemophilus influenzae*: identification of resistance mechanisms. *J Antimicrob Chemother* **20**: 645.

Report from the Boston Collaborative Drug Surveillance Program, Boston University Medical Center (1972). Excess of ampicillin rashes associated with allopurinol or hyperuricaemia. *New Engl J Med* **286**: 505.

Report of a Collaborative Study Group (1973). Prospective study of ampicillin rash. *Brit Med J* **1**: 7.

Ries AA, Wells JG, Olivola D (1994). Epidemic *Shigella dysenteriae* type 1 in Burundi: panresistance and implications for prevention. *J Infect Dis* **169**: 1035.

Roberton YR, Johnson ES (1976). Interactions between oral contraceptives and other drugs: a review. *Curr Med Res Opin* **3**: 647.

Robins-Browne RM, Rowe B, Ramsaroop R *et al.* (1983). A hospital outbreak of multiresistant *Salmonella typhimurium* belonging to phage type 193. *J Infect Dis* **147**: 210.

Rogers HJ, James CA, Morrison PJ, Bradbrook ID (1980). Effect of cimetidine on oral absorption of ampicillin and cotrimoxazole. *J Antimicrob Chemother* **6**: 297.

Rolfe RD, Finegold SM (1983). Intestinal beta-lactamase activity in ampicillin-induced, *Clostridium difficile*-associated ileocecitis. *J Infect Dis* **147**: 227.

Rolinson GN, Stevens S (1961). Microbiological studies on a new broad-spectrum penicillin, 'Penbritin'. *Brit Med J* **2**: 191.

Rolinson GN, Sutherland R (1965). The binding of antibiotics to serum proteins. *Brit J Pharmacol* **25**: 638.

Ross S, Controni G, Khan W (1972). Resistance of shigellae to ampicillin and other antibiotics. *JAMA* **221**: 45.

Rowe B, Threlfall EJ (1981). Multiple antimicrobial drug resistance in enteric pathogens. *J Antimicrob Chemother* **7**: 1.

Rowe B, Frost JA, Threlfall EJ, Ward LR (1980). Spread of multiresistant clone of *Salmonella typhimurium* phage type 66/122 in South-East Asia and the Middle East. *Lancet* **i**: 1070.

Rubin LG, Medeiros AA, Yolken RH, Moxon ER (1981). Ampicillin treatment failure of apparently beta-lactamase-negative *Haemophilus influenzae* type b meningitis due to novel beta-lactamase. *Lancet* **ii**: 1008.

Rubinstein E, Haspel J, Klein E *et al.* (1980). Effect of pancreatitis in ampicillin excretion in pancreatic fluid of dogs. *Antimicrob Ag Chemother* **17**: 905.

Ruley EJ, Lisi LM (1974). Interstitial nephritis and renal failure due to ampicillin. *J Pediatr* **84**: 878.

Rupar DG, Fisher MC, Fletcher H, Mortensen J (1989). Emergence of isolates resistant to ampicillin. *Amer J Dis Child* **143**: 1033.

Ryan CA, Hargrett-Bean NT, Blake PA (1989). *Salmonella typhi* infections in the United States, 1975–1984: increasing role of foreign travel. *Rev Infect Dis* **11**: 1.

Sánchez C, Garcia-Restoy E, Garau J *et al.* (1993). Ciprofloxacin and trimethoprim-sulfamethoxazole versus placebo in acute uncomplicated *Salmonella enteritis*: a double blind trial. *J Infect Dis* **168**: 1304.

Sanders WL (1965). Treatment of typhoid fevers: a comparative trial of ampicillin and chloramphenicol. *Brit Med J* **2**: 1226.

Saunders JR, Sykes RB (1977). Transfer of a plasmid-specified beta-lactamase gene from *Haemophilus influenzae*. *Antimicrob Ag Chemother* **11**: 339.

Schauf V, Deveikis A, Riff L, Serota A (1976). Antibiotic-killing kinetics of Group B streptococci. *J Pediatr* **89**: 194.

Scheifele DW, Fussell SJ (1981). Frequency of ampicillin-resistant *Haemophilus parainfluenzae* in children. *J Infect Dis* **143**: 495.

Scheifele DW, Fussell SJ, Roberts MC (1982). Characterization of ampicillin-resistant *Haemophilus parainfluenzae*. *Antimicrob Ag Chemother* **21**: 734.

Scheld WM, Brodeur JP (1983). Effect of methylprednisolone on entry of ampicillin and gentamicin into cerebrospinal fluid in experimental pneumococcal and *Escherichia coli* meningitis. *Antimicrob Ag Chemother* **23**: 108.

Scheld WM, Fletcher DD, Fink FN, Sande MA (1979). Response to therapy in an experimental rabbit model of meningitis due to *Listeria monocytogenes*. *J Infect Dis* **140**: 287.

Scheld WM, Alliegro GM, Field MR, Brodeur JP (1982). Synergy between ampicillin and gentamicin in experimental meningitis due to Group B streptococci. *J Infect Dis* **146**: 100.

Schiffer MS, MacLowry J, Schneerson R, Robbins JB (1974). Clinical bacteriological and immunological characterization of ampicillin-resistant *Haemophilus influenzae* type B. *Lancet* **ii**: 257.

Schulkind ML, Altemeier WA, Ayoub EM (1971). A comparison of ampicillin and chloramphenicol therapy in *Haemophilus influenzae* meningitis. *Pediatrics* **48**: 411.

Schwalbe RS, Hoge CW, Morris JGJr (1990). *In vivo* selection for transmissible drug resistance in *Salmonella typhi* during antimicrobial therapy. *Antimicrob Ag Chemother* **34**: 161.

Schwartz JN, Hamilton JP, Fekety R *et al.* (1980). Ampicillin-induced enterocolitis: implication of toxigenic *Clostridium perfringens* type C. *J Pediatr* **97**: 661.

Schwartz R, Rodriguez W, Khan W, Ross S (1978). The increasing incidence of ampicillin-resistant *Haemophilus influenzae* A cause of otitis media. *JAMA* **239**: 320.

Scriver SR, Walmsley SL, Kau CL *et al.* (1994). Determination of antimicrobial susceptibilities of Canadian isolates of *Haemophilus influenzae* and characterization of their beta-lactamases. *Antimicrob Ag Chemother* **38**: 1678.

Seifert H, Strate A, Schulze A, Pulverer G (1993). Vascular catheter-related bloodstream infection due to *Acinetobacter johnsonii* (formerly *Acinetobacter calcoaticus* var *lwoffi*): report of 13 cases. *Clin Infect Dis* **17**: 632.

Serdaru M, Diquet B, Lhermitte F (1982). Generalised seizures and ampicillin. *Lancet* **ii**: 617.

Shackelford PG, Bobinski JE, Feigin RD, Cherry JD (1972). Therapy of *Haemophilus influenzae* meningitis reconsidered. *New Engl J Med* **287**: 634.

Shapiro S, Slone D, Siskind V *et al.* (1969). Drug rash with ampicillin and other penicillins. *Lancet* **ii**: 969.

Shimada J, Inamatus T, Yamashiro M (1977). Anaerobic bacteria in biliary disease in elderly patients. *J Infect Dis* **135**: 850.

Shurin PA, Pelton SI, Scheifele D, Klein JO (1976). Otitis media caused by non-typable, ampicillin-resistant strains of *Haemophilus influenzae*. *J Pediatr* **88**: 646.

Simasathien S, Duangmani C, Echeverria P (1980). *Haemophilus influenzae* type b resistant to ampicillin and chloramphenicol in an orphanage in Thailand. *Lancet* ii: 1214.

Simon HB, Southwick FS, Moellering RC Jr, Sherman E (1980). *Haemophilus influenzae* in hospitalized adults: current perspectives. *Amer J Med* 69: 219.

Simon HJ, Miller RC (1966). Ampicillin in the treatment of chronic typhoid carriers. Report on fifteen treated cases and a review of the literature. *New Engl J Med* 274: 808.

Sleet RA, Sangster G, Murdoch JMcC (1964). Comparison of ampicillin and chloramphenicol in treatment of paratyphoid fever. *Brit Med J* 1: 148.

Smith AL (1976). Current concepts. Antibiotics and invasive *Haemophilus influenzae*. *New Engl J Med* 294: 1329.

Smith SM, Eng RHK, (1988). Interaction of ciprofloxacin with ampicillin and vancomycin for *Streptococcus faecalis*. *Diagn Microbiol Inect Dis;9*: 239.

Smith SM, Eng RHK, Landesman S (1982). Effect of rifampin on ampicillin killing of Group B streptococci. *Antimicrob Ag Chemother* 22: 522.

Snyder MJ, Perroni J, Gonzalez O et al. (1976). Comparative efficacy of chloramphenicol, ampicillin, and co-trimoxazole in the treatment of typhoid fever. *Lancet* ii: 1155.

Søgaard H (1975). Incidence of antibiotic resistance and transmissible R factors in the Gram-negative bowel flora of hospital patients on admission. *Scand J Infect Dis* 7: 253.

Spencer RC, Wheat PF, Magee JT, Brown EH (1990). A three year survey of clinical isolates in the United Kingdom and their antimicrobial susceptibility. *J Antimicrob Chemother* 26: 435.

Sperber SJ, Schleupner CJ (1987). Salmonellosis during infection with human immunodeficiency virus. *Rev Infect Dis* 9: 925.

Stamm AM, Dismukes WE, Simmons BP et al. (1982). Listeriosis in renal transplant recipients: report of an outbreak and review of 102 cases. *Rev Infect Dis* 4: 665.

Stark CA, Edlund C, Sjostedt S et al. (1993). Antimicrobial resistance in human oral and intestinal anaerobic microfloras. *Antimicrob Ag Chemother* 37: 1665.

Stevenson J, Mandal BK (1966). Ampicillin and the fifth-day rash. *Brit Med J* 1: 1359.

Stewardson-Krieger P, Naidu S (1981). Simultaneous recovery of beta-lactamase-negative and beta-lactamase-positive *Haemophilus influenzae* type b from cerebrospinal fluid of a neonate. *Pediatrics* 68: 253.

Stewart GT, Coles HMT, Nixon HH, Holt RJ (1961). 'Penbritin': an oral penicillin with broad-spectrum activity. *Brit Med J* 2: 200.

Sutter VL, Finegold SM (1976). Susceptibility of anaerobic bacteria to 23 antimicrobial agents. *Antimicrob Ag Chemother* 10: 736.

Svenungsson B (1982). Typhoid fever in a Swedish hospital for infectious diseases – a 20-year review. *J Infect* 5: 139.

Tannenberg AM, Wicher KJ, Rose NR (1971). Ampicillin nephropathy. *JAMA* 218: 449.

Tarr PI (1995). *Escherichia coli* 0157: H7: clinical, diagnostic, and epidemiological aspects of human infection. *Clin Infect Dis* 20: 1.

Taryle DA, Good JT Jr, Morgan EJ III et al. (1981). Antibiotic concentrations in human parapneumonic effusion. *J Antimicrob Chemother* 7: 171.

Tauxe RV, Puhr ND, Wells JG et al. (1990). Antimicrobial resistance of *Shigella* isolates in the USA: the importance of international travelers. *J Infect Dis* 162: 1107.

Thauvin C, Eliopoulos GM, Willey S et al. (1987). Continuous-infusion ampicillin therapy of enterococcal endocarditis in rats. *Antimicrob Ag Chemother* 31: 139.

Thomas WJ, McReynolds JW, Mock CR, Bailey DW (1974). Ampicillin-resistant *Haemophilus influenzae* meningitis. *Lancet* i: 313.

Thorne GM, Farrar WE Jr (1975). Transfer of ampicillin resistance between strains of Haemophilus influenzae type B. *J Infect Dis* 132: 276.

Thornsberry C, Baker CN, Kirven LA (1978). *In vitro* activity of antimicrobial agents on Legionnaires' disease bacterium. *Antimicrob Ag Chemother* 13: 78.

Threlfall EJ, Ward LR, Ashley AS, Rowe B (1980). Plasmid-encoded trimethoprim resistance in multiresistant epidemic *Salmonella typhimurium* phage types 204 and 193 in Britain. *Brit Med J* 280: 1210.

Thrupp LD, Leedom JM, Ivler D et al. (1966). Ampicillin levels in the cerebrospinal fluid during treatment of bacterial meningitis. *Antimicrob Ag Chemother* 1965: 206.

Tilton RC, Corcoran L, Newberg L, Sedgwick AK (1972). Ampicillin-resistant *Shigella sonnei*. *JAMA* 222: 487.

Toffler RB (1978). Acute colitis related to penicillin and penicillin derivatives. *Lancet* ii: 707.

Totten PA, Handsfield HH, Peters D et al. (1982). Characterization of ampicillin resistance plasmids from *Haemophilus ducreyi*. *Antimicrob Ag Chemother* 21: 622.

Trottier S, Bergeron MG (1981). Intrarenal concentrations of ampicillin in acute pyelonephritis. *Antimicrob Ag Chemother* 19: 761.

True RJ (1982). Interactions between antibiotics and oral contraceptives. *JAMA* 247: 1408.

Turck M (1967). Broad-spectrum penicillins and other antibiotics in the treatment of urinary tract infections. *Ann NY Acad Sci* 145: 344.

Tuttle J, Ries AA, Chimba RM et al. (1995). Antimicrobial resistant epidemic *Shigella dysenteriae* type 1 in Zambia: modes of transmission. *J Infect Dis* 171: 371.

Van den Hazel SJ, Speelman P, Tytgat GNJ et al. (1994). Role of antibiotics in the treatment and prevention of acute and recurrent cholangitis. *Clin Infect Dis* 19: 279.

Visintine AM, Oleske JM, Nahmias AJ (1977). *Listeria monocytogenes* infection in infants and children. *Amer J Dis Child* 131: 393.

Wallace RJ Jr, Vance P, Weissfeld A, Martin RR (1978). Beta-lactamase production and resistance to beta-lactam antibiotics in nocardia. *Antimicrob Ag Chemother* 14: 704.

Washington AE (1982). Update on treatment recommendations for gonococcal infections. *Rev Infect Dis* 4 (Suppl): 758.

Wasz-Höckert O, Nummi S, Vuopala S, Järvinen PA (1970). Transplacental passage of azidocillin, ampicillin and penicillin G during early and late pregnancy. *Scand J Infect Dis* 2: 125.

Weeks JL, Mason EO Jr, Baker CJ (1981). Antagonism of ampicillin and chloramphenicol for meningeal isolates of Group B streptococci. *Antimicrob Ag Chemother* 20: 281.

Weissman JB, Gangarosa EJ, Dupont HL et al. (1974). Shigellosis. To treat or not to treat? *JAMA* 229: 1215.

Welling PG, Tse FLS (1982). The influence of food on the absorption of antimicrobial agents. *J Antimicrob Chemother* 9: 7.

Whelton A, Sapir DG, Carter GG et al. (1972). Intrarenal distribution of ampicillin in the normal and diseased human kidney. *J Infect Dis* 125: 466.

Whitby M, Nimmo GR, Rao A (1982). *Haemophilus influenzae* meningitis in adults. *Aust NZ J Med* 12: 182.

WHO (1981). Nongonococcal urethritis and other selected sexually transmitted diseases of public health importance. *Tech Rep Ser* 660: 75.

Wiggins GL, Albritton WL, Feeley JC (1978). Antibiotic susceptibility of clinical isolates of *Listeria monocytogenes*. *Antimicrob Ag Chemother* 13: 854.

Winslow DL, Damme J, Dieckman E (1983). Delayed bactericidal activity of beta-lactam antibiotics against *Listeria monocytogenes*: antagonism of chloramphenicol and rifampin. *Antimicrob Ag Chemother* 23: 555.

Wong GA, Peirce TH, Goldstein E, Hoeprich PD (1975). Penetration of antimicrobial agents into bronchial secretions. *Amer J Med* 59: 219.

Woodroffe AJ, Weldon M, Meadows R, Lawrence JR (1975). Acute interstitial nephritis following ampicillin hypersensitivity. *Med J Aust* 1: 65.

Yamamoto LG, Ashton MJ (1988). *Salmonella* infections in infants in Hawaii. *Pediatr Infect Dis J* 7: 48.

Yogev R (1981). Soft-tissue infections of ampicillin-resistant *Haemophilus influenzae* type b The use of ampicillin and nafcillin in their treatment. *Amer J Dis Child* 135: 410.

Yoshioka H, Rudoy P, Riley HD Jr, Yoshida K (1977). Antimicrobial susceptibility of Escherichia coli isolated at a children's hospital. *Scand J Infect Dis* **9**: 207.

Yost RL, Gotz VP (1985). Effect of a Lactobacillus preparation on the absorption of oral ampicillin. *Antimicrob Ag Chemother* **28**: 727.

Yunus M, Mizanur Rahman ASM, Farooque ASG, Glass RI (1982). Clinical trial of ampicillin v trimethoprim-sulphamethoxazole in the treatment of *Shigella* dysentery. *J Trop Med Hyg* **85**: 195.

Zackrisson G, Brorson J-E, Krantz I, Trollfors B (1983). *In-vitro* sensitivity of Bordetella pertussis. *J Antimicrob Chemother* **11**: 407

Ampicillin-like Penicillins
Amoxycillin, Epicillin, Cyclacillin, Hetacillin, Pivampicillin, Talampicillin, Bacampicillin and Metampicillin

Description

Ampicillin has been modified chemically in various ways in an attempt to produce an improved compound; eight such modifications have been available. Amoxycillin, epicillin and cyclacillin have intrinsic antibacterial activity, but the other five antibiotics are hydrolyzed in the body to ampicillin after administration. Most of these compounds exhibit no, or only marginal, superiority over ampicillin (Dyas and Wise, 1983). Amoxycillin has advantages over ampicillin and probably will gradually replace it, at least for oral administration.

1 Amoxycillin

Chemically alpha-amino-p-hydroxybenzyl-penicillin, it is also known as amoxicillin. Developed by Beecham Research Laboratories (Sutherland et al., 1972), its main advantage over ampicillin is its better absorption from the gastrointestinal tract (p. 136). It is available as amoxycillin trihydrate for oral administration and sodium amoxycillin, for parenteral use.

2 Epicillin

Chemically this is 6-[D2-amino-2-(1,4-cyclohexadienyl) acetamido]-penicillanic acid (Basch et al., 1971).

3 Cyclacillin

This is a partially penicillinase-resistant penicillin with a chemical formula of 6-(1-aminocyclo-hexanecarboxamide)-penicillanic acid (Gonzaga et al., 1974).

4 Hetacillin

Developed by Bristol Laboratories in 1965 by reacting ampicillin with acetone, this is also referred to as phenazacillin. Hetacillin hydrolyzes in solution to form ampicillin both in vitro and in vivo, therefore its ultimate active component is mainly ampicillin (Sutherland and Robinson, 1967; Kahrimanis and Pierpaoli, 1971).

5 Pivampicillin

This is the hydrochloride salt of pivaloyl-oxymethyl D-alpha-aminobenzyl-penicillinate, which is an ampicillin ester. It is better absorbed from the gastrointestinal tract than ampicillin, to which after absorption it is rapidly and completely hydrolyzed in the tissues and blood (Daehne et al., 1971).

6 Talampicillin

Chemically this is a thiazolide carboxylic ester of ampicillin. It has no antibacterial activity until it is hydrolyzed by tissue esterases in the intestinal wall to form ampicillin, which is then rapidly absorbed. Serum levels after administration of this drug, are approximately twice those attained with an equivalent dose of ampicillin (Clayton et al., 1974; Leigh et al., 1976).

7 Bacampicillin

Similarly, this is another ester of ampicillin which is chemically 1'-ethoxycarbonyloxy-ethyl 6-(D-alpha-aminophenylacetamido) penicillinate. After absorption, it is rapidly hydrolyzed to ampicillin by esterases present in the serum and in the intestinal wall. Serum levels achieved are 2- to 3-fold higher than those after equivalent doses of ampicillin (Bodin *et al.*, 1975; Neu, 1981).

8 Metampicillin

This is produced by combining ampicillin with formaldehyde. When administered orally, it is rapidly hydrolyzed to ampicillin in the gut and administered in this way it has no advantages over ampicillin. After parenteral administration, some of the drug apparently circulates as unchanged metampicillin, because it has a greater stability in serum than in aqueous acid solutions. It is excreted into the bile in a greater concentration than ampicillin (Neu, 1975).

The last seven compounds have no special advantages and in recent years they have been used very little if at all in most countries. They will therefore not be described any further in this edition, and the details given below will only apply to amoxycilllin.

Sensitive Organisms

In vitro amoxycillin is much the same as ampicillin (p. 108), although it has its own intrinsic activity and it is not converted to ampicillin in the body (Sutherland *et al.*, 1972; Cole and Ridley, 1978). There are only a few differences between the antibacterial actions of these drugs. Amoxycillin is about twice as active as ampicillin against *Enterococcus faecalis* and *Salmonella* spp., but 2-fold less active against *Shigella* spp. (Sabto *et al.*, 1973; Neu, 1974). *Haemophilus influenzae* also appears to be slightly less sensitive to amoxycillin than to ampicillin (Kosmidis *et al.*, 1972); the same is true for Gram-positive and Gram-negative anaerobic bacteria (Sutter and Finegold, 1976). In one USA study 64.7% of *Prevotella* (previously *Bacteroides*) spp. and 41.1% of *Fusobacterium* spp. were beta-lactamase producers and therefore amoxycillin-resistant (Appelbaum *et al.*, 1990). Similar to penicillin G and ampicillin, amoxycillin when combined with an aminoglycoside usually acts synergistically against *E. faecalis* (Basker and Sutherland, 1977) (p. 455). *Brucella* spp. are more sensitive to amoxycillin than to ampicillin, and marked *in vitro* synergy can occur when amoxycillin, gentamicin and rifampicin are combined against *Br. melitensis* (Gwynn and Rolinson, 1980). Unlike ampicillin, amoxycillin is effective in experimental *Chlamydia trachomatis* infections in mice (Kramer *et al.*, 1979). *Helicobacter pylori* is sensitive to many antibiotics *in vitro*, but amoxycillin with an MIC of 0.06 µg per ml is one of the most active antibiotics against this organism (Garcia-Rodriguez *et al.*, 1989). It also attains high concentrations in gastric mucosa and shows bactericidal activity against slowly growing *H. pylori*; these properties may explain why amoxycillin (combined with other drugs) has shown activity against this organism *in vivo* (McNulty *et al.*, 1988; Millar and Pike, 1992) (p. 142).

Amoxycillin is inactive against all bacteria which have developed either intrinsic resistance or resistance due to beta-lactamase production to penicillin G or ampicillin. It has no activity against beta-lactamase-producing *Staphylococcus aureus* (p. 11) and *E. faecalis* strains (p. 10). Strains of pneumococci and *E. faecium* which either have intermediate or high-level intrinsic

Organism	MIC (µg per ml)
Gram-positive bacteria	
Streptococcus pyogenes	0.01
Streptococcus pneumoniae	0.02
Enterococcus faecalis	0.5
Gram-negative bacteria	
Escherichia coli	5.0
Proteus mirabilis	2.5
Haemophilus influenzae	0.25
Helicobacter pylori	0.06
Bacteroides fragilis	32.0–64.0
Prevotella melaninogenica	0.5–1.0

Table I.8
Compiled from data published by Sutherland *et al.* (1972), Sutter and Finegold (1976) and Garcia-Rodriguez *et al.* (1989)

resistance to penicillin G, show similar resistance to amoxycillin (pp. 5, 10). Amoxycillin also has reduced activity against strains of meningococci and gonococci with intermediate intrinsic resistance to penicillin G (p. 13, 14). Strains of gonococci with high-level intrinsic resistance to penicillin G or resistance due to beta-lactamase production, are amoxycillin-resistant. The drug also has no activity against any strains of Gram-negative bacilli, such as *H. influenzae* (p. 112) (George *et al.*, 1991), the *Salmonella* spp. (p. 109), *Shigella* spp. (p. 111) or *Escherichia coli* (p. 109), which have developed resistance to ampicilin.

The MICs of amoxycillin against some selected sensitive bacterial species are shown in Table I.8. For practical purposes, there is no difference between this drug and ampicillin (Table I.7, p. 115).

Mode of Administration and Dosage

1 Oral administration

The usual oral dosage of amoxycillin is 50–100 mg per kg body weight per day, administered in three or four divided doses. The usual adult dosage of this drug is 250–500 mg, given 6- or 8-hourly.

2 Parenteral administration

Sodium amoxycillin is suitable for both i.m. and i.v. use. For mild infections the dosage can be the same as recommended for oral use (see above). For serious infections the dosage is 150–200 mg per kg body weight per day, given in six divided doses. An usual adult dosage is 1 g 4-hourly, but this can be doubled if necessary. These dosages are similar to those of parenteral ampicillin (p. 116). Amoxycillin sodium should be administered i.v. in a manner similar to penicillin G (p. 20). In an animal study amoxycillin given subcutaneously in a dose of 10 mg per kg 12-hourly for two doses could cure pneumococcal otitis media when the strain involved was moderately penicillin G-resistant (MIC 2.0 µg per ml for penicillin G and 1.0 µg per ml for amoxycillin). A higher dose of 25 mg per kg 12-hourly for two doses cured the otitis when the strain was more highly penicillin G-resistant (MIC 4–8 µg per ml for penicillin G and 2–4 µg per ml for amoxycillin) (Barry *et al.*, 1993). These data should be interpreted cautiously in terms of their clinical relevance.

3 Newborn and premature infants

In this age group dosage reduction of amoxycillin, similar to ampicillin (p. 116), is advocated. It is preferable to use the more familiar ampicillin for the treatment of these patients. In one study, oral amoxycillin was found to be safe and effective in a dosage of 50 mg per kg body weight 12-hourly for newborn infants aged 6–13 days (Lönnerholm *et al.*, 1982). For pre-term infants in the first week of life with gestational ages of less than 32 weeks, a dosage of 25 mg per kg every 12 h is recommended (Huisman-de Boer *et al.*, 1995).

4 Patients with renal failure

Amoxycillin is relatively non-toxic and may be given in the usual recommended dosage to patients with mild renal failure. In patients with moderate to severe renal failure, as in the case of ampicillin (p. 116), the dose should be reduced (Sabto *et al.*, 1973). With amoxycillin, dosage adjustment is unnecessary if the patient's creatinine clearance exceeds 30 ml per min; with creatinine clearance of 10–30 ml per min and <10 ml per min, the dose should be halved or quartered, respectively. Amoxycillin is removed from the body by hemodialysis, but removal by peritoneal dialysis is slow. In anuric or end-stage renal failure patients, who are treated by regular hemodialysis, a 1 g i.v. dose of amoxycillin should be given at the end of dialysis, and then be repeated once every 24 h (Chelvan *et al.*, 1979; Humbert *et al.*, 1979).

Serum Levels in Relation to Dosage

Amoxycillin is well absorbed after oral administration (Sutherland *et al.*, 1972; Verbist, 1976). After a 0.5 g dose in adults, a peak serum level of 8–10 µg per ml is reached 2 h later (Fig. I.7). Doubling the dose doubles the peak serum level. Thereafter, serum concentrations fall, and reach zero after 6–8 h. These serum levels are about twice as high as those produced by an equivalent dose of oral ampicillin, and about the same as those attained when this dose of ampicillin or

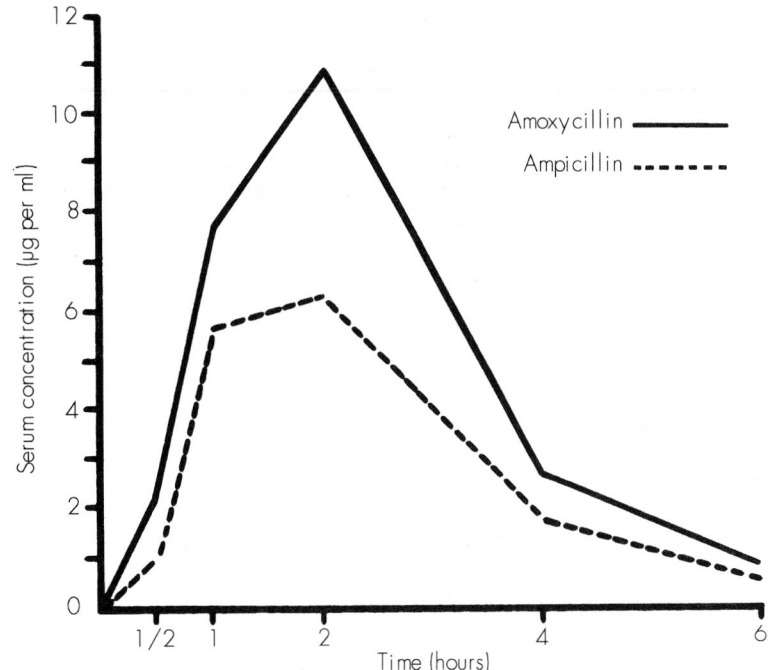

Fig. I.7.

Mean serum concentrations of amoxycillin and ampicillin after a single 500-mg oral dose in a cross-over study in 12 fasting subjects. (Redrawn after Sutherland *et al.*, 1972, with permission.)

amoxycillin is given i.m. (p. 116) (Hill *et al.*, 1980). The absorption of amoxycillin appears to be an active process. There is evidence for a saturable carrier-mediated uptake of this antibiotic and a dipeptide carrier system is probably the most likely transport mechanism (Westphal *et al.*, 1991). Food in the stomach impairs ampicillin absorption (p. 116), but has a lesser effect on amoxycillin. In one study in adults, amoxycillin was equally well absorbed in the fasting and non-fasting state (Eshelman and Spyker, 1978), but others have recorded some reduction of the drug's absorption when it is taken with food (Welling *et al.*, 1977). In children, after a 15 mg per kg oral dose, mean peak serum levels of amoxycillin were reduced from 5.4 μg per ml in the fasting state, to 3.2 μg per ml in the non-fasting state (Ginsburg *et al.*, 1979). Amoxycillin absorption is satisfactory in patients with achlorhydria (Lawson *et al.*, 1974), but it is impaired in those with celiac disease (Parsons *et al.*, 1975). The concomitant administration of aluminum magnesium hydroxide, pirenzepine or ranitidine does not impair amoxycillin absorption (Deppermann *et al.*, 1989).

After a single 3 g oral dose of amoxycillin is given to non-fasting adults, a peak serum level of about 24 μg per ml is reached at 2 h, and the levels are 7.8, 3.6 and 1.4 μg per ml at 4, 6 and 8 h, respectively (Shanson *et al.*, 1980). If this dose is given with 1 g of oral probenecid, higher and more prolonged amoxycillin serum levels are obtained; in one study, mean serum levels were 30.51, 34.96, 28.42 and 10.31 μg per ml at 2,3, 4 and 8 h after administration, respectively (Barbhaiya *et al.*, 1979).

After a rapid i.v. injection of 0.5 g sodium amoxycillin to adults, the serum level ranges from 83 to 112 μg per ml, 1 min after injection. Thereafter, there is a rapid decline, and the level falls to about 1 μg per ml, 3.5 h after administration. After i.m. injection of 0.5 g, a mean peak serum level of approximately 10 μg per ml is attained at 1 h, which falls to zero after 6–8 h. Doubling the i.m. dose doubles the serum concentrations. Serum levels of amoxycillin are similar after i.m. and oral administration, except that the peak is reached earlier with the former. The pharmacokinetics of ampicillin and amoxycillin are essentially similar if the drugs are administered by the i.m. or i.v. routes (Spyker *et al.*, 1977; Rudoy *et al.*, 1979; Hill *et al.*, 1980).

Excretion

1 Urine

About 58–68% of an orally administered dose of amoxycillin is excreted in the urine in an unchanged active form, during the first 6 h (Sutherland *et al.*, 1972). High amoxycillin urinary levels of 115–1850 μg per ml occur after a 0.5 g oral dose to adults. Like ampicillin (p. 117), this drug is excreted by both glomerular filtration and tubular secretion; the latter can be reduced by concomitant administration of probenecid (Neu, 1979).

2 Bile

Amoxycillin is probably excreted in the bile, similar to ampicillin (p. 117). In animals amoxycillin is concentrated in bile (Acred *et al.*, 1971).

3 Inactivation in body

Amoxycillin is probably inactivated in the body to some extent, chiefly in the liver, similar to ampicillin (p. 117).

Distribution of the Drug in Body

Amoxycillin is probably largely distributed similarly to ampicillin (p. 118) but some minor differences have been described.

In a comparison with ampicillin, May and Ingold (1974) found that both drugs produced similar concentrations in purulent sputum, but amoxycillin had higher levels in mucoid sputum. Law *et al.* (1983) used amoxycillin in a dosage of 0.5 g three times daily to treat infective exacerbations of chronic bronchitis in adults. The mean amoxycillin concentration in purulent sputum was 1 μg per ml, but a much lower value of 0.2 μg per ml was obtained in mucoid sputum. Penetration of amoxycillin in purulent sputum was confirmed by Cole *et al.* (1983). It was given in a dosage of 3 g orally twice-daily to 17 patients with bronchiectasis, most of whom had purulent sputum; on day 7 mean peak and trough sputum levels were 1.7 (range 0.2–3.7) and 0.25 (range 0.2–0.3) μg per ml, respectively. Lovering *et al.* (1990) gave simultaneous single i.v. injections of both amoxycillin and ampicillin (500 mg of each) to five patients with exacerbations of chronic bronchitis. Concentrations of both drugs in sputum were estimated separately. Mean sputum levels after dosing were 2.7 μg per ml for amoxycillin and 1.4 μg per ml for ampicillin.

Brun *et al.* (1981) found a mean tissue level of 3.05 μg per g in normal lung of patients who were undergoing thoracic surgery receiving amoxycillin in a dosage of 0.5 g twice-daily. Amoxycillin lung tissue concentrations were usually about 40% of the simultaneous serum levels (Baldwin *et al.*, 1992). The drug penetrates into pleural fluid to about the same extent as ampicillin, but it enters and leaves the pleural cavity at a faster rate (Dashner *et al.*, 1981). Amoxycillin is only excreted in small amounts in breast milk. Saliva, sweat and tears also contain very small amounts of amoxycillin, while ampicilin is usually undetectable in these secretions (Philipson *et al.*, 1975). Like ampicillin, amoxycillin crosses the placenta and levels in cord blood are about one-quarter to one-third of those in maternal blood (Furuya *et al.*, 1973). Amoxycillin, similar to ampicillin (p. 118), only attains low levels in the CSF of patients with normal meninges (Clumeck *et al.*, 1978). Higher amoxycillin CSF levels are reached in patients with meningitis (Strausbaugh *et al.*, 1978). The CSF levels have been studied in children with bacterial meningitis who were treated by i.v. amoxycillin, 200 mg per kg per day, given as rapid i.v. infusions in six divided doses. Mean peak CSF concentrations on days 1 and 5 were similar, but day 1 concentrations remained 2–5 μg per ml for 4 h after a dose, whereas the corresponding value on day 5 decreased to a mean of 0.6 μg per ml. On day 10, the mean peak level was 1.6 μg per ml 0.5 h after the dose and this decreased to 0.6 and 0.7 μg per ml at 1 h and 4 h after the dose; 24 h prior to this day half the children received oral probenecid, and their corresponding CSF values were 1.1, 2.3 and 1.0 μg per ml (Craft *et al.*, 1979). Thus probenecid was effective in increasing the CSF concentrations of amoxycillin (and other beta-lactam antibiotics, (p. 25) but whether this is of any practical value is unknown.

Cooreman *et al.* (1993) measured amoxycillin levels in gastric mucosa after giving amoxycillin in tablet form or as water-dissolved fizzing. Biopsies were taken from antrum, corpus and fundus of stomach. The dissolved form of amoxycillin was superior to the tablet form with regard to drug concentrations in the antrum. With the tablet form, given as single 1 g dose, subbactericidal levels with respect to *H. pylori* were attained in antral mucosa. With both amoxycillin forms, with a dose of 1 g, concentrations were far below the required bactericidal levels in the mucosa of the corpus and fundus. This makes a reservoir function of these parts of the stomach for *H. pylori* likely and probably explains why amoxycillin monotherapy usually fails for *H. pylori* infections (p. 142).

Protein binding of amoxycillin (17%) is similar to that of ampicillin (Sutherland *et al.*, 1972).

Mode of Action

The action of amoxycillin on bacteria is similar to penicillin G (p. 28).

Toxicity

1 Hypersensitivity reactions

Amoxycillin may be 'cross-allergenic' with other penicillins, and is therefore contraindicated in penicillin-allergic patients. Amoxycillin has had widespread use and large surveys show that its propensity to cause rashes is the same as ampicillin (ADRAC, 1978; Porter and Jick, 1980). The maculopapular eruptions produced by amoxycillin are similar to those seen with ampicillin (p. 119). Rashes due to amoxycillin have been reported in patients with glandular fever, and in this respect the drug appears to have the same predilection to cause rashes as ampicillin (Mulroy, 1973; ADRAC, 1978). The side-chain of amoxycillin, and other semi-synthetic penicillins, can also rarely provoke severe amoxycillin hypersensitivity. Martin et al. (1992) reported six patients who experienced anaphylactic reactions after treatment and challenge with amoxycillin, but who tolerated parenteral challenges with penicillin G, aztreonam, and ceftazidime. Results of skin tests for amoxycillin were positive in four of the six patients. Skin tests for penicillin G (p. 30) were negative in all.

2 Gastrointestinal side-effects

Oral administration of amoxycillin can cause nausea, epigastric discomfort and diarrhea. As with ampicillin (p. 119), these are not usually severe. Amoxycillin, because of its better absorption appears to cause these side-effects less commonly than ampicillin; the reported frequency of diarrhea following amoxycillin treatment is about 2% (Knudsen, 1977). In one study of 263 children with otitis media, ampicillin produced diarrhea more frequently than amoxycillin (Feder, 1982). Pseudomembranous colitis (p. 594) was described in one 10-year-old boy, who received amoxycillin for an upper respiratory tract infection (Similä et al., 1976), and this complication was fatal in a 5-week-old infant who had been treated by oral amoxycillin (Richardson et al., 1981).

3 Encephalopathy

This complication, which occurs with ampicillin (p. 120), may occur if large doses of amoxycillin are given i.v.

4 Pancytopenia

This has been described in one elderly man who was treated by amoxycillin and co-trimoxazole (p. 855). Results of bone marrow culture studies indicated that amoxycillin was directly toxic to the bone marrow (Irvine et al., 1985). Large doses of i.v. amoxycillin similar to other beta-lactam antibiotics, can cause neutropenia (p. 33).

Clinical Uses of the Drug

1 Urinary tract infections

Amoxycillin has been used to treat urinary tract infections, and results of treatment have been about the same as with ampicillin (Sabto et al., 1973). In women with infections restricted to the bladder, a single amoxycillin dose of 3 g appeared to be just as effective as a 14-day course of 250 mg given three times daily (Fang et al., 1978; Savard-Fenton et al., 1982; Tolkoff-Rubin et al., 1984). Failure to eradicate a urinary tract infection after single-dose therapy may be because of resistant organisms, or if the infection is more invasive, perhaps in the kidney, which warrants more prolonged chemotherapy and/or further investigation (Souney and Polk, 1982). Low cure rates and progression to acute pyelonephritis may occur following ineffective single-dose amoxycillin therapy if patients are not properly selected (Hooton et al., 1985). If antibody-coated bacteria in the urine are absent it is more likely that bladder infection alone is present, and that response to single-dose amoxycillin therapy will be good (Rubin et al., 1980). The single-dose regimen has the advantage of being cheaper, it has fewer side-effects and patient cooperation is better. A single-dose amoxycillin regimen also has little effect on fecal flora, whilst a 7-day course selects resistant fecal organisms (Souney and Polk, 1982). Similarly, conventional courses of amoxycillin alter peri-urethral flora, producing one with either resistant aerobic Gram-negative rods or *Candida albicans*, which may be involved in future recurrences of urinary tract infections (Ronald *et al.*, 1977). This is likely to be a lesser problem with single-dose amoxycillin.

However, when Philbrick and Bracikowski (1985) reviewed the pooled results of therapy, they found that single-dose amoxycilin (3 g) was significantly less effective than conventional multi-dose therapy (cure rates of 69% v. 84%), while single-dose and multidose therapy with co-trimoxazole (p. 860) were equally effective.

In asymptomatic bacteriuria in pregnancy, in one trial, amoxycillin as single dose of 3 g was found to be equally effective as the same drug in a dosage of 250 mg 8-hourly, given for 4 days (Gerstner *et al.*, 1989).

Nowadays amoxycillin-resistant *E. coli* strains and also other resistant Enterobacteriaceae are prevalent, even in community-acquired infections (p. 136), and therefore many prefer drugs other than amoxycillin for single-dose therapy. Many suitable drugs are available such as trimethoprim (p. 884), co-trimoxazole (p. 860), aminoglycosides such as gentamicin (p. 473) and quinolones such as ciprofloxacin (p. 1014) (Ronald, 1987; Johnson and Stamm, 1989; Naber, 1989, Tan and File, 1990; Stamm and Hooton, 1993).

A 2-week course, now most commonly co-trimoxazole, rather than amoxycillin, appears to be the optimal treatment for women with renal infections. A 6-week course is appropriate for men, particularly if the prostate is the probable focus of infection. Acutely ill patients with pyelonephritis should be admitted to hospital and treated by i.v. ampicillin/gentamicin or i.v. cefotaxime (p. 338). Once their fever and other acute symptoms have subsided, a single oral antibiotic can be substituted. This can be amoxycillin if the infecting organism is amoxycillin-sensitive (Ronald, 1987; Johnson and Stamm, 1989).

Single-dose regimens are not recommended for presumed uncomplicated urinary infections in children. Many children will respond satisfactorily to such therapy, but the recurrence rate is unacceptably large (Avner *et al.*, 1983; Madrigal *et al.*, 1988; Jones, 1990). In particular single-dose therapy is unsuitable in infants younger than 4 months. These are best managed in hospital, as their infections are often more severe and in some, especially neonates, septicemia may be present. For these initial chemotherapy with an ampicillin/gentamicin or amoxycillin/gentamicin combination is often necessary (Ginsburg and McCracken, 1982). After improvement an oral single drug can be substituted and this could be amoxycillin if the infecting organism is amoxycillin-sensitive (McCracken, 1989). Treatment should usually continue for 14 days.

A methodological review of the literature performed by Moffatt *et al.* (1988) showed that short-course antibiotic therapies (4 days or less) were less effective for the treatment of urinary tract infections in children, than conventional 7- to 10-day long courses of therapy.

2 Respiratory tract infections

For the treatment of chronic bronchial infections, amoxycillin has been regarded as superior to ampicillin because it penetrates into bronchial secretions to a greater extent (May and Ingold, 1972, 1974) (p. 138). But it also has been shown that some amoxycillin may be inactivated in the bronchial secretions, probably by beta-lactamases and that doses higher than 0.5 g 8-hourly may sometimes be necessary for successful therapy (Hill *et al.*, 1992). A regimen of amoxycillin 3 g orally twice-daily, has been advocated for patients producing large volumes of purulent sputum, especially if *H. influenzae* is involved (Cole *et al.*, 1983). In a trial in patients with chronic bronchitis, treatment with 3 g twice-daily for 3 days was compared with 0.5 g 8-hourly for 7 days. The outcome in the two groups was similar (Bennett *et al.*, 1988). In patients in whom beta-lactamase-producing strains of *H. influenzae* are involved, the results of amoxycillin treatment may be poor and other drugs such as amoxycillin/clavulanate (p. 200) or co-trimoxazole may be indicated (Pedersen *et al.*, 1986).

For most patients, however the lower dose of 250 mg three or four times daily is sufficient (Anthonisen *et al.*, 1987) and others also have found that amoxycillin and ampicillin are about equally effective to treat exacerbations of chronic bronchitis (Mackay, 1980).

Amoxycillin is one of several satisfactory drugs for treatment of acute otitis media in children. Most authors advocate a 10- to 14-day course of chemotherapy for this disease (Bluestone, 1982; Feder, 1982; Kaleida *et al.*, 1991). In general, despite the availability of many other drugs, amoxycillin is still the drug of first choice in most cases (Klein, 1994; McCracken, 1994).

For treatment of streptococcal pharyngitis Shvartzman *et al.* (1993) found oral amoxycillin, administered in one daily dose (50 mg per kg or adults 750 mg) equal in efficacy to oral penicillin V administered in usual doses three or four times daily. In view of the greater rash potential of amoxycillin (p. 139) it would seem prudent to use either parenteral penicillin G or oral penicillin V for the treatment of this disease.

3 Bacterial endocarditis

A 6-week course of oral amoxycillin 1 g every 4 h, combined with i.m. gentamicin, was successful in one patient with *E. faecalis* endocarditis (Seligman, 1974). This treatment was instituted after the patient had relapsed following therapy with i.v. penicillin G plus i.m. streptomycin and then i.v. vancomycin, and at a time further i.v. chemotherapy was difficult to maintain.

In the USA, UK and Australia, amoxycillin is now recommended for endocarditis chemoprophylaxis. The regimens for amoxycillin and other drugs for this purpose are described on p. 43. Bacterial endocarditis supervened in a patient after total dental clearance of his 12 remaining teeth, despite the prophylactic administration of 3 g oral amoxycillin (Denning *et al.*, 1984). Such patients may also pose a higher risk, thereby warranting parenteral amoxycillin or an amoxycillin/gentamicin combination for chemoprophylaxis. In patients who receive two doses of 3 g amoxycillin at weekly intervals for repeated dental procedures, amoxycillin-resistant streptococci may emerge in their mouth flora; but these become undetectable 13 weeks after the last dose of amoxycillin. It has been suggested therefore that if further dental treatment is required within 6 weeks of double-dose amoxycillin prophylaxis, an alternative regimen should be used (Southall *et al.*, 1983). From animal experiments, there is evidence that amoxycillin, like vancomycin (p. 781), may protect against endocarditis not only by bacterial killing but also by inhibiting adherence of streptococci to sterile vegetations (Glauser *et al.*, 1983). Also if amoxycillin-resistant strains of *Strep. sanguis* enter the circulation, amoxycillin prophylaxis can still be effective (Longman *et al.*, 1992).

4 Typhoid fever and salmonellosis

Amoxycillin, in an oral dose of 100 mg per kg per day, or 1.0 g (occasionally 1.5 g) 6-hourly for adults, is a satisfactory treatment for typhoid fever. It cures patients with disease due to chloramphenicol-resistant strains, and in this respect it is about as effective as co-trimoxazole (p. 867) (Gilman *et al.*, 1975). Amoxycillin was used for 14 days to treat 30 typhoid fever patients who had hematological contraindications to chloramphenicol. Response to treatment was satisfactory and comparable with that of 30 other patients treated with chloramphenicol (Afifi *et al.*, 1976). In a randomized clinical trial involving 124 adults with typhoid fever, amoxycillin in a dosage of 1.0 g 6-hourly for 14 days, was as effective as treatment with chloramphenicol (Pillay *et al.*, 1975). In a trial involving 155 African children with typhoid fever, oral amoxycillin was slightly superior to chloramphenicol when assessed by clinical response, relapse rate and subsequent carrier state (Scragg, 1976). Another 30 African children were treated by i.m. amoxycillin 100 mg per kg per day for the first 3 days, and then the drug was given orally; all responded satisfactorily, and the availability of parenteral amoxycillin made it possible to treat critically ill patients (Scragg and Robinson, 1980). Patients with *Salm. typhi* or *Salm. paratyphi* A bacteriuria and recurrent septicemia associated with schistosomiasis, have responded to amoxycillin in a dosage of 250 mg four times a day for 4 weeks (Farid *et al.*, 1975). But in recent years *Salm. typhi* strains resistant to chloramphenicol, amoxycillin and co-trimoxazole have emerged in some parts of the world (p. 550) and typhoid fever caused by such strains needs treatment either by one of the quinolones such as ciprofloxacin (p. 1017) or a third-generation cephalosporin such as ceftriaxone (p. 360). Amoxycillin is also suitable for the treatment of neonatal typhoid fever, provided the *Salm. typhi* is susceptible (Reed and Klugman, 1994).

Amoxycillin, in a dose of 2 g three times daily for 28 days, has eradicated the chronic typhoid carrier state in a proportion of patients (Nolan and White, 1978) (p. 122). For the treatment of uncomplicated *Salmonella* gastroenteritis, amoxycillin, similar to ampicillin (p. 122), is contraindicated. Compromised hosts, such as children with chronic granulomatous disease, who can suffer from recurrent attacks of *Salmonella* septicemia, may benefit from long-term amoxycillin prophylaxis (Burniat *et al.*, 1980).

5 Shigellosis

In one trial, amoxycillin, unlike ampicillin (p. 122), was ineffective in shigellosis (Nelson and Haltalin, 1974). This is difficult to understand. Amoxycillin is slightly less active than ampicillin against shigellae *in vitro* (p. 135); also the lack of response to amoxycillin may be in part due to its ineffective intraluminal colinic concentrations (McCracken, 1979).

6 Gonorrhea

Amoxycillin in a single-dose of 3 g plus 1 g probenecid orally was widely recommended as a suitable 'single-dose' regimen for treatment of this disease. It is ineffective for the disease caused by penicillin G-resistant strains which are either intrinsically resistant (p. 136), or beta-lactamase producers (p. 136). Such strains are now common in the USA, most states in Australia, and in many other countries, including the UK (Lewis *et al.*, 1995). Ceftriaxone, given i.m. (p. 361) or oral ciprofloxacin are now most commonly recommended for treatment of gonorrhea. In areas where penicillin G-resistant strains of gonococci are still uncommon, amoxycillin can be used.

7 Helicobacter pylori disease

In one trial amoxycillin plus metronidazole was more successful in eradication of *H. pylori* and in prevention of recurrences of duodenal ulcer than placebo (Hentschel *et al.*, 1993). For eradication of *H. pylori* most commonly bismuth subcitrate is combined with metronidazole and tetracycline (p. 743). In patients who cannot tolerate tetracycline, amoxycillin can be substituted, but another, almost equally effective regimen is amoxycillin 750 mg orally 12-hourly for 2 weeks plus omeprazole 20 mg orally, twice-daily for 2 weeks, then 20 mg orally, daily for a further 2 weeks. This is better tolerated (Fennerty, 1994).

8 Other infections

Parenteral amoxycillin has been used for severe infections in hospitalized patients, such as pyelonephritis, pneumonia or septicemia due to susceptible pathogens (Leigh and Nash, 1979; Francke *et al.*, 1980). In children *H. influenzae* meningitis due to non-beta-lactamase-producing strains has also been treated successfully (Nolan *et al.*, 1979). In all of these infections i.m. or i.v. amoxycillin provides therapy comparable with that of parenteral ampicillin.

Certain infections caused by beta-lactamase producing organisms may respond to amoxycillin and clavulanic acid used in combination (p. 200). One controlled trial showed that amoxycillin was effective for treatment of genital chlamydial infections in pregnancy, and it was suggested that this drug should be used for those pregnant women who do not tolerate erythromycin (p. 619) (Alary *et al.*, 1994).

References

Acred P, Hunter PA, Mizen L, Rolinson GN (1971). X-amino-p-hydroxybenzyl-penicillin (BRL 2333), a new broad-spectrum semisynthetic penicillin: *in vivo* evaluation. *Antimicrob Ag Chemother* **1970**: 416.

ADRAC (Adverse Drug Reactions Advisory Committee) (1978). Ampicillin and amoxycillin – identical twins. *Asut Presc* **2**: 81.

Afifi AM, Adnan M, El Garf AA (1976). Amoxycillin in treatment of typhoid fever in patients with haematological contraindications to chloramphenicol. *Brit Med J* **2**: 1033.

Alary M, Joly JR, Moutquin J-M *et al.* (1994). Randomized comparison of amoxycillin and erythromycin in treatment of genital chlamydial infection in pregnancy. *Lancet* **344**: 1461.

Anthonisen NR, Manfreda J, Warren CPW *et al.* (1987). Antibiotic therapy in exacerbations of chronic obstructive pulmonary disease. *Ann Intern Med* **106**: 196.

Appelbaum PC, Spangler SK, Jacobs MR (1990). Beta-lactamase production and susceptibilities to amoxicillin, amoxicillin-clavulanate, ticarcillin, ticarcillin-clavulanate, cefoxitin, imipenem and metronidazole of 320 non-*Bacteroides fragilis Bacteroides* isolates and 129 *Fusobacteria* from 28 US centers. *Antimicrob Ag Chemother* **34**: 1546.

Avner ED, Ingelfinger JR, Herrin JT *et al.* (1983). Single-dose amoxicillin therapy of uncomplicated pediatric urinary tract infections. *J Pediatr* **102**: 623.

Baldwin DR, Honeybourne D, Wise R (1992). Pulmonary disposition of antimicrobial agents: *in vivo* observations and clinical relevance. *Antimicrob Ag Chemother* **36**: 1176.

Barbhaiya R, Thin RN, Turner P, Wadsworth J (1979). Clinical pharmacological studies of amoxicillin: effect of probenecid. *Brit J Vener Dis* **55**: 211.

Barry B, Muffat-Joly M, Gehanno P, Pocidalo J-J (1993). Effect of increased dosages of amoxicillin in treatment of experimental middle ear otitis due to penicillin-resistant *Streptococcus pneumoniae*. *Antimicrob Ag Chemother* **37**: 1599.

Basch H, Erickson R, Gadebusch H (1971). Epicillin: *in vitro* laboratory studies. *Infect Immun* **4**: 44.

Basker MJ, Sutherland R (1977). Activity of amoxicillin, alone, and in combination with aminoglycoside antibiotics against streptococci associated with bacterial endocarditis. *J Antimicrob Chemother* **3**: 273.

Bennett JB, Crook SJ, Shaw EJ, Davies RJ (1988). A randomized double blind controlled trial comparing two amoxicillin regimens in the treatment of acute exacerbations of chronic bronchitis. *J Antimicrob Chemother* **21**: 225.

Bluestone CD (1982). Otitis media in children: to treat or not to treat? *New Engl J Med* **306**: 1399.

Bodin N-O, Ekström B, Forsgren U *et al.* (1975). Bacampicillin: a new orally well-absorbed derivative of ampicillin. *Antimicrob Ag Chemother* **8**: 518.

Brun Y, Forey F, Gamondes JP *et al.* (1981). Levels of erythromycin in pulmonary tissue and bronchial mucus compared to those of amoxicillin. *J Antimicrob Chemother* **8**: 459.

Burniat W, Toppet M, De Mol P (1980). Acute and recurrent salmonella infections in three children with chronic granulomatous disease. *J Infect* **2**: 263.

Chelvan P, Hamilton-Miller JMT, Brumfitt W (1979). Pharmacokinetics of parenteral amoxicillin, biliary excretion and effect of renal failure. *J Antimicrob Chemother* **5**: 232.

Clayton JP, Cole M, Elson SW, Ferres H (1974). BRL 8988 (talampicillin)., a well-absorbed oral form of ampicillin. *Antimicrob Ag Chemother* **5**: 670.

Clumeck N, Thys JP, Vanhoof R *et al.* (1978). Amoxicillin entry into human cerebrospinal fluid: comparison with ampicillin. *Antimicrob Ag Chemother* **14**: 531.

Cole M, Ridley B (1978). Absence of bioactive metabolites of ampicillin and amoxicillin in man. *J Antimicrob Chemother* **4**: 580.

Cole PJ, Roberts DE, Davies SF, Knight RK (1983). A simple oral antimicrobial regimen effective in severe chronic bronchial suppuration associated with culturable *Haemophilus influenzae*. *J Antimicrob Chemother* **11**: 109.

Cooreman MP, Krausgrill P, Hengels KJ (1993). Local gastric and serum amoxicillin concentrations after different oral application forms. *Antimicrob Ag Chemother* **37**: 1506.

Craft JC, Feldman WE, Nelson JD (1979). Clinicopharmacological evaluation of amoxicillin and probenecid against bacterial meningitis. *Antimicrob Ag Chemother* **16**: 346.

Daehne W, von, Godtfredsen WO, Roholt K, Tybring L (1971). Pivampicillin, a new orally active ampicillin ester. *Antimicrob Ag Chemother* **1970**: 431.

Daschner FD, Gier E, Lentzen H *et al.* (1981). Penetration into the pleural fluid after bacampicillin and amoxicillin. *J Antimicrob Chemother* **7**: 585.

Denning DW, Cassidy M, Dougall A, Hillis WS (1984). Failure of single dose amoxycillin as prophylaxis against endocarditis. *Brit Med J* **289**: 1499.

Deppermann K-M, Lode H, Hoffken G *et al.* (1989). Influence of ranitidine, pirenzepine, and aluminum magnesium hydroxide on the bioavailability of various antibiotics, including amoxicillin, cephalexin, doxycycline and amoxicillin-clavulanic acid. *Antimicrob Ag Chemother* **33**: 1901.

Dyas A, Wise R (1983). Leading article. Ampicillin and alternatives. *Brit Med J* **286**: 583.

Eshelman FN, Spyker DA (1978). Pharmacokinetics of amoxycillin and ampicillin: crossover study of the effect of food. *Antimicrob Ag Chemother* **14**: 539.

Fang LST, Tolkoff-Rubin NE, Rubin RH (1978). Efficacy of single-dose and conventional amoxicillin therapy in urinary-tract infection localized by the antibody-coated bacteria technic. *New Engl J Med* **298**: 413.

Farid Z, Bassily S, Mikhail IA *et al.* (1975). Treatment of chronic enteric fever with amoxicillin. *J Infect Dis* **132**: 698.

Feder HM Jr (1982). Comparative tolerability of ampicillin, amoxicillin, and trimethoprim-sulfamethoxazole suspensions in children with otitis media. *Antimicrob Ag Chemother* **21**: 426.

Fennerty MB (1994). *Helicobacter pylori*. *Arch Intern Med* **154**: 721.

Francke EL, Pancoast SJ, Neu HC (1980). Parenteral amoxicillin in the treatment of infections in hospitalized patients. *J Antimicrob Chemother* **6**: 683.

Furuya H, Matsuda S, Mori S *et al.* (1973). Clinical application of amoxycillin in the field of obstetrics and gynaecology. *Chemotherapy (Tokyo)* **21**: 1752.

Garcia-Rodriguez JA, Garcia Sanchez JE, Garzia Garcia MI *et al.* (1989). *In vitro* activities of new oral beta-lactams and macrolides against *Campylobacter pylori*. *Antimicrob Ag Chemother* **33**: 1650.

George MJ, Kitch B, Henderson FW, Gilligan PH (1991). *In vitro* activity of orally administered antimicrobial agents against *Haemophilus influenzae* recovered from children monitored longitudinally in a group day-care center. *Antimicrob Ag Chemother* **35**: 1960.

Gerstner GJ, Muller G, Nahler G (1989). Amoxicillin in the treatment of asymptomatic bacteriuria in pregnancy: a single dose of 3 g amoxicillin versus a 4-day course of 3 doses 750 mg amoxicillin. *Gynecol Obstet Invest* **27**: 84.

Gilman RH, Terminel M, Levine MM *et al.* (1975). Comparison of trimethoprim-sulfamethoxazole and amoxicillin in therapy of chloramphenicol-resistant and chloramphenicol-sensitive typhoid fever. *J Infect Dis* **132**: 630.

Ginsburg CM, McCracken GH Jr (1982). Urinary tract infections in young infants. *Pediatrics* **69**: 409.

Ginsburg CM, McCracken GH Jr, Thomas ML, Clahsen JC (1979). Comparative pharmacokinetics of amoxicillin and ampicillin in infants and children. *Pediatrics* **64**: 627.

Glauser MP, Bernard JP, Moreillon P, Francioli P (1983). Successful single-dose amoxicillin prophylaxis against experimental streptococcal endocarditis: evidence for two mechanisms of protection. *J Infect Dis* **147**: 568.

Gonzaga AJ, Antonio-Velmonte M, Tupasi TE (1974). Cyclacillin: a clinical and *in vitro* profile. *J Infect Dis* **129**: 545.

Gwynn MN, Rolinson GN (1980). Bactericidal action of amoxicillin alone and in combination with gentamicin and rifampicin against *Brucella melitensis*. *J Infect* **2**: 61.

Hentschel E, Brandstatter G, Dragosics B *et al.* (1993). Effect of ranitidine and amoxicillin plus metronidazole on the eradication of *Helicobacter pylori* and the recurrence of duodenal ulcer. *New Engl J Med* **328**: 308.

Hill SA, Jones KH, Lees LJ (1980). Pharmacokinetics of parenterally administered amoxicillin. *J Infect* **2**: 320.

Hill SL, Burnett D, Lovering AL, Stockley RA (1992). Use of enzyme-linked immunosorbent assay to assess penetration of amoxicillin into lung secretions. *Antimicrob Ag Chemother* **36**: 1545.

Hooton TM, Running K, Stamm WE (1985). Single-dose therapy for cystitis in women. A comparison of trimethoprim-sulfamethoxazole, amoxillin and cyclacillin. *JAMA* **253**: 387.

Huisman-de Boer JJ, Van den Anker JN, Vogel M *et al.* (1995). Amoxicillin pharmacokinetics in preterm infants with gestational ages of less than 32 weeks. *Antimicrob Ag Chemother* **39**: 431.

Humbert G, Spyker DA, Fillastre JP, Leroy A (1979). Pharmacokinetics of amoxicillin: dosage nomogram for patients with impaired renal function. *Antimicrob Ag Chemother* **15**: 28.

Irvine AE, Agnew AND, Morris TCM (1985). Amoxicillin induced pancytopenia. *Brit Med J* **290**: 968.

Johnson JR, Stamm WE (1989). Urinary tract infections in women: diagnosis and treatment. *Ann Intern Med* **111**: 906.

Jones KV (1990). Antimicrobial treatment for urinary tract infections. *Arch Dis Child* **65**: 327.

Kahrimanis R, Pierpaoli P (1971). Hetacillin vs ampicillin. *New Engl J Med* **285**: 236.

Kaleida PH, Casselbrant ML, Rockette HE *et al.* (1991). Amoxicillin or myringotomy or both for acute otitis media: results of a randomized clinical trial. *Pediatrics* **87**: 466.

Klein JO (1994). Otitis media. *Clin Infect Dis* **19**: 823.

Knudsen ET (1977). Amoxil and talpen. *Brit Med J* **1**: 442.

Kosmidis J, Williams JD, Andrews J *et al.* (1972). Amoxicillin – pharmacology, bacteriology and clinical studies. *Brit J Clin Pract* **26**: 341.

Kramer MJ, Cleeland R, Grunberg E (1979). Activity of oral amoxicillin, ampicillin and oxytetracycline against infections with *Chlamydia trachomatis* in mice. *J Infect Dis* **139**: 717.

Law MR, Holt HA, Reeves DS, Hodson ME (1983). Cefaclor and amoxicillin in the treatment of infective exacerbations of chronic bronchitis. *J Antimicrob Chemother* **11**: 83.

Lawson DH, Anderson AK, McGeachy RR (1974). Amoxycillin: pharmacokinetic studies in normal subjects, patients with pernicious anaemia and those with renal failure. *Postgrad Med J* **50**: 500.

Leigh DA, Nash JG (1979). Parenteral amoxicillin treatment of severe infections in hospitalized patients. *J Antimicrob Chemother* **5**: 109.

Leigh DA, Reeves DS, Simmons K *et al.* (1976). Talampicillin: a new derivative of ampicillin. *Brit Med J* **1**: 1378.

Lewis PA, Ison CA, Livermore DM *et al.* (1995). A one-year survey of *Neisseria gonorrhoeae* isolated from patients attending an east London genitourinary medicine clinic: antibiotic susceptibility patterns and patients' characteristics. *Genitourin Med* **71**: 13.

Longman LP, Marsh PD, Martin MV (1992). Amoxicillin-resistant oral streptococci and experimental infective endocarditis in the rabbit. *J Antimicrob Chemother* **30**: 349.

Lönnerholm G, Bengtsson S, Ewald U (1982). Oral pivampicillin and amoxicillin in newborn infants. *Scand J Infect Dis* **14**: 127.

Lovering AM, Pycock CJ, Harvey JE, Reeves DS (1990). The pharmacokinetics and sputum penetration of ampicillin and amoxycillin following simultaneous iv administration. *J Antimicrob Chemother* **25**: 385.

Mackay AD (1980). Amoxycillin versus ampicillin in treatment of exacerbations of chronic bronchitis. *Brit J Dis Chest* **74**: 379.

Madrigal G, Odio CM, Mohs E *et al.* (1988). Single dose antibiotic therapy is not as effective as conventional regimens for management of acute urinary tract infections in children. *Pediatr Infect Dis J* **7**: 316.

Martin JA, Igea JM, Fraj J *et al.* (1992). Allergy to amoxicillin in patients who tolerated benzylpenicillin, aztreonam, and ceftazidime. *Clin Infect Dis* **14**: 592.

May JR, Ingold A (1972). Amoxycillin in the treatment of chronic non-tuberculous bronchial infections. *Brit J Dis Chest* **66**: 185.

May JR, Ingold A (1974). Amoxycillin in the treatment of infections of the lower respiratory tract. *J Infect Dis* **129** (Suppl): 189.

McCracken GH Jr (1979). Antibiotic treatment of shigellosis. *J Pediatr* **95**: 334.

McCracken GHJr (1989). Options in antimicrobial management of urinary tract infections in infants and children. *Pediatr Infect Dis J* **8**: 552.

McCracken GHJr (1994). Considerations in selecting an antibiotic for treatment of acute otitis media. *Pediatr Infect Dis J* **13**: 1054.

McNulty CAM, Dent JC, Ford GA, Wilkinson SP (1988). Inhibitory antimicrobial concentrations against *Campylobacter pylori* in gastric mucosa. *J Antimicrob Chemother* **22**: 729.

Millar MR, Pike J (1992). Bactericidal activity of antimicrobial agents against slowly growing *Helicobacter pylori*. *Antimicrob Ag Chemother* **36**: 185.

Moffatt M, Embree J, Grimm P, Law B (1988). Short-course antibiotic therapy for urinary tract infections in children. *Am J Dis Child* **142**: 57.

Mulroy R (1973). Amoxycillin rash in infectious mononucleosis. *Brit Med J* **1**: 554.

Naber KG (1989). Single-dose therapy of uncomplicated urinary tract infections in females – treatment of choice? *Infection* **17**: 119.

Nelson JD, Haltalin KC (1974). Amoxicillin less effective than ampicillin against *Shigella in vitro* and *in vivo*: relationship of efficacy to activity in serum. *J Infect Dis* **129** (Suppl): 222.

Neu HC (1974). Antimicrobial activity and human pharmacology of amoxicillin. *J Infect Dis* **129** (Suppl): 123.

Neu HC (1975). Aminopenicillins – clinical pharmacology and use in disease states. *Int J Clin Pharmacol* **11**: 132.

Neu HC (1979). Amoxicillin. *Ann Intern Med* **90**: 356.

Neu HC (1981). The pharmacokinetics of bacampicillin. *Rev Infect Dis* **3**: 110.

Nolan CM, White PC Jr (1978). Treatment of typhoid carriers with amoxicillin. Correlates of successful therapy. *JAMA* **239**: 2352.

Nolan CM, Chalhub EG, Nash DG, Yamauchi T (1979). Treatment of bacterial meningitis with intravenous amoxicillin. *Antimicrob Ag Chemother* **16**: 171.

Parsons RL, Hossack G, Paddock G (1975). The absorption of antibiotics in adult patients with coeliac disease. *J Antimicrob Chemother* **1**: 39.

Pedersen M, Stovring S, Morkassel E *et al.* (1986). A comparative study of amoxycillin and pivampicillin in persistent *Haemophilus influenzae* infection of the lower respiratory tract in children with chronic lung disease. *Scand. J Infect Dis* **18**: 245.

Philbrick JT, Bracikowski JP (1985). Single-dose antibiotic treatment for uncomplicated urinary tract infections. Less for less? *Arch Intern Med* **145**: 1672.

Philipson A, Sabath LD, Rosner B (1975). Sequence effect on ampicillin blood levels noted in an amoxicillin, ampicillin, and epicillin triple crossover study. *Antimicrob Ag Chemother* **8**: 311.

Pillay N, Adams EB, North-Coombes D (1975). Comparative trial of amoxycillin and chloramphenicol in treatment of typhoid fever in adults. *Lancet* **ii**: 333.

Porter J, Jick H (1980). Amoxicillin and ampicillin: rashes equally likely. *Lancet* **i**: 1037.

Reed RP, Klugman KP (1994). Neonatal typhoid fever. *Pediatr Infect Dis J* **13**: 774.

Richardson SA, Brookfield DSK, French TA, Gray J (1981). Pseudomem-branous colitis in a 5-week-old infant. *Brit Med J* **283**: 1510.

Ronald AR (1987). Optimal duration of treatment for kidney infection. *Ann Intern Med* **106**: 467.

Ronald AR, Jagdis FA, Harding GKM *et al.* (1977). Amoxicillin therapy of acute urinary tract infections in adults. *Antimicrob Ag Chemother* **11**: 780.

Rubin RH, Fang LST, Jones SR (1980). Single-dose amoxicillin therapy for urinary tract infection. Multicenter trial using antibody-coated bacteria localization technique. *JAMA* **244**: 561.

Rudoy RC, Goto N, Petit D, Uemura H (1979). Pharmacokinetics of intravenous amoxicillin in pediatric patients. *Antimicrob Ag Chemother* **15**: 628.

Sabto J, Carson P, Morgan T (1973). Evaluation of amoxycillin – a new semisynthetic penicillin. *Med J Aust* **2**: 537.

Savard-Fenton M, Fenton BW, Reller LB *et al.* (1982). Single-dose amoxicillin therapy with follow-up urine culture. *Amer J Med* **73**: 808.

Scragg JN (1976). Further experience with amoxycillin in typhoid fever in children. *Brit Med J* **2**: 1031.

Scragg JN, Robinson OPW (1980). Parenteral and oral amoxycillin therapy in paediatric typhoid. *J Antimicrob Chemother* **6**: 156.

Seligman SJ (1974). Treatment of enterococcal endocarditis with oral amoxicillin and intramuscular gentamicin. *J Infect Dis* **129** (Suppl): 213.

Shanson DC, Ashford RFU, Singh J (1980). High-dose oral amoxycillin for preventing endocarditis. *Brit Med J* **280**: 446.

Shvartzman P, Tabenkin H, Rosentzwaig A, Dolginov F (1993). Treatment of streptococcal pharyngitis with amoxycillin once a day. *Brit Med J* **306**: 1170.

Similä S, Kouvalainen K, Mäkelä P (1976). Pseudomembranous colitis after amoxycillin. *Lancet* **ii**: 317.

Souney P, Polk BF (1982). Single-dose antimicrobial therapy for urinary tract infections in women. *Rev Infect Dis* **4**: 29.

Southall PJ, Mahy NJ, Davies RM, Speller DCE (1983). Resistance in oral streptococci after repeated two-dose amoxycillin prophylaxis. *J Antimicrob Chemother* **12**: 141.

Spyker DA, Rugloski RJ, Vann RL, O'Brien WM (1977). Pharmacokinetics of amoxicillin: dose dependence after intravenous, oral and intramuscular administration. *Antimicrob Ag Chemother* **11**: 132.

Stamm WE, Hooton TM (1993). Management of urinary tract infections in adults. *New Engl J Med* **329**: 1328.

Strausbaugh LJ, Girgis NI, Mikhail IA *et al.* (1978). Penetration of amoxicillin into cerebrospinal fluid. *Antimicrob Ag Chemother* **14**: 899.

Sutherland R, Robinson OPW (1967). Laboratory and pharmacological studies in man with hetacillin and ampicillin. *Brit Med J* **2**: 804.

Sutherland R, Croydon EAP, Rolinson GN (1972). Amoxicillin: a new semi-synthetic penicillin. *Brit Med J* **3**: 13.

Sutter VL, Finegold SM (1976). Susceptibility of anaerobic bacteria to 23 antimicrobial agents. *Antimicrob Ag Chemother* **10**: 736.

Tan JS, File TMJr (1990). Urinary tract infections in obstetrics and gynecology. *J Reprod Med* **35** (Suppl 3): 339.

Tolkoff-Rubin NE, Wilson ME, Zuromskis P *et al.* (1984). Single-dose amoxicillin therapy of acute uncomplicated urinary tract infections in women. *Antimicrob Ag Chemother* **25**: 626.

Verbist L (1976). Triple crossover study on absorption and excretion of ampicillin, talampicillin and amoxycillin. *Antimicrob Ag Chemother* **10**: 173.

Welling PG, Huang H, Koch PA *et al.* (1977). Bioavailability of ampicillin and amoxicillin in fasted and non-fasted subjects. *J Pharm Sci* **66**: 549.

Westphal JF, Deslandes A, Brogard JM, Carbon C (1991). Reappraisal of amoxycillin absorption kinetics. *J Antimicrob Chemother* **27**: 647.

Carbenicillin, Carindacillin, Carfecillin and Ticarcillin

Description

Carbenicillin (disodium alpha-carboxybenzyl-penicillin) is a semisynthetic penicillin derived from the penicillin nucleus, 6 APA (p. 3), and can only be administered parenterally (Knudsen *et al.*, 1967). Two carbenicillin esters, carbenicillin indanyl sodium (carindacillin) and a phenyl ester of carbenicillin (carfecillin) were also developed. These are absorbed after oral administration and rapidly hydrolyzed in the body to produce carbenicillin (p. 151).

Ticarcillin, which has the chemical formula of alpha-carboxyl-3-thienylmethyl penicillin, is very similar to carbenicillin but is more active against *Pseudomonas aeruginosa* (Sutherland *et al.*, 1971). It has now replaced carbenicillin for clinical use.

Sensitive Organisms

1 *Pseudomonas aeruginosa*

Activity against this organism, although of a relatively low order, is the most important feature of carbenicillin. It can be administered parenterally in sufficient dosage to obtain serum concentrations exceeding 50–60 μg per ml, which inhibit most *Ps. aeruginosa* strains. Some strains are not inhibited by concentrations as high as 200 μg per ml. Strains of *Ps. aeruginosa* with increased resistance can emerge in patients treated with carbenicillin (Darrell and Waterworth, 1969). There was a progressive increase in these strains in a burns unit in the UK between 1966 and 1969, when highly resistant strains suddenly displaced all other *Ps. aeruginosa* strains from the unit (Lowbury *et al.*, 1969). Resistance of *Ps. aeruginosa* can be due to either production of beta-lactamases (carbenicillinases) or intrinsic. Virtually all *Ps. aeruginosa* isolates produce a chromosomally mediated beta-lactamase, which destroys many beta-lactam antibiotics, such as the older cephalosporins, which normally have no activity against *Ps. aeruginosa* (Richmond, 1980). Carbenicillin is not inactivated by this particular beta-lactamase. Strains of *Ps. aeruginosa* can acquire plasmids (p. 549) which code for the production of beta-lactamases that destroy carbenicillin. These plasmids can be transferred from certain Enterobacteriaceae to *Ps. aeruginosa* and *vice versa* (Roe *et al.*, 1971; Labia *et al.*, 1977). At least 14 different types of plasmid-mediated beta-lactamases can be encountered in *Ps. aeruginosa*, most of which can destroy carbenicillin (Philippon *et al.*, 1986).

In other strains of *Ps. aeruginosa*, resistance to carbenicillin is intrinsic. This may result from an alteration of cell wall permeability (Livermore *et al.*, 1981; Livermore, 1984) or a marked decrease in the affinity of penicillin-binding proteins (p. 27) for carbenicillin (Godfrey *et al.*, 1981). In some highly carbenicillin-resistant *Ps. aeruginosa* strains both of these mechanisms of intrinsic resistance may be involved, together with the production of beta-lactamases mediated by plasmids (Rodriguez-Tebar *et al.*. 1982).

Strains of *Ps. aeruginosa* isolated from cystic fibrosis patients may be very heterogeneous and contain populations with differing antimicrobial susceptibility patterns (Thomassen *et al.*, 1979). In particular, mucoid strains isolated from such patients contain resistant and normally sensitive populations plus others which are hyper-susceptible to carbenicillin (MIC <1 μg per ml) (Irvin *et al.*, 1981). The existence of such hyper-susceptible strains in patients receiving antibiotic therapy may suggest that they were not exposed to a significant antibiotic concentration. Some very susceptible *Ps. aeruginosa* strains (MIC 0.7–6.0 μg per ml) have been isolated from sputum of patients with other chronic respiratory infections (May and Ingold, 1973; Duncan, 1974). In these patients interference with antibiotic activity by the extracellular alginate slime may afford the bacteria some degree of protection (Bolister *et al.*, 1989).

In most hospitals strains of *Ps. aeruginosa* resistant to carbenicillin did not emerge rapidly. Two large surveys in the early 1970s in North America, showed that over 90% of isolates from hospitalized patients were carbenicillin-sensitive (Duncan, 1974; Gaman *et al.*, 1976). Similarly, Baird *et al.* (1976) isolated *Ps. aeruginosa* from 535 hospital patients in the USA during an 11-month period; 85 of these patients were colonized or infected with strains resistant to both carbenicillin and gentamicin (p. 451). Resistant strains were isolated mainly from the urinary tract of patients who had recently received gentamicin and other antibiotics; their pathogenicity appeared unaltered; they did not spread rapidly and only rarely caused infections in the general hospital population, where only a minority of patients were highly vulnerable e.g. immunosuppressed. Of 650 *Ps. aeruginosa* strains isolated from Australian hospital patients, only 16 were carbenicillin-resistant (Dean *et al.*, 1977). A survey from 24 hospitals in UK in 1982 showed that only 9.6% of *Ps. aeruginosa* strains were carbenicillin-resistant (Williams *et al.*, 1984), and this percentage only increased to 11.7 by 1993 (Chen *et al.*, 1995). It appears that carbenicillin-resistant *Ps. aeruginosa* strains are still relatively uncommon in hospitals, except in special areas, such as intensive care and burns units, where carbenicillin (or ticarcillin) has been used extensively.

A carbenicillin and gentamicin combination may exhibit *in vitro* synergism against strains of *Ps. aeruginosa* sensitive to both drugs, and also against strains which are carbenicillin-sensitive and which have only a low level of gentamicin-resistance (MIC $< 40 \mu g$ per ml) (Kluge *et al.*, 1974a; Reyes *et al.*, 1979). With gentamicin-resistant and carbenicillin-sensitive strains, there may sometimes be *in vitro* synergism between carbenicillin and one of the other aminoglycosides such as tobramycin (p. 490) or amikacin (p. 504), even if the strain is not susceptible to a clinically attainable concentration of the aminoglycoside (Kluge *et al.*, 1974b; Marks *et al.*, 1976). The aminoglycoside which will be synergistic is not always predictable from its MIC against *Ps. aeruginosa* (Anderson *et al.*, 1975; Marks *et al.*, 1976).

Ticarcillin is consistently at least twice, and sometimes four times, as active as carbenicillin against *Ps. aeruginosa* (Sutherland *et al.*, 1971; Prior and Fass, 1978) (Table I.9). Strains of all bacteria, including *Ps. aeruginosa*, which have become resistant to carbenicillin, are also ticarcillin-resistant (Kalkani and Marketos, 1976; McGowan and Terry, 1979). In most hospitals the majority of *Ps. aeruginosa* strains are still ticarcillin-sensitive (Smith and Henry, 1988). Similar to carbenicillin, ticarcillin combined with an aminoglycoside, such as gentamicin, tobramycin or amikacin, exhibits *in vitro* synergism against some strains of *Ps. aeruginosa*. The degree of synergy, as with carbenicillin, varies with the *Ps. aeruginosa* strain tested and with the particular aminoglycoside used. The MICs of individual drugs are not predictive of the degree of synergism, and *in vitro* testing of drug combinations is necessary (Comber *et al.*, 1977; Heineman and Lofton, 1978). The mechanism of carbenicillin or ticarcillin synergism with aminoglycosides is not understood. The possibility that the beta-lactam antibiotic increases the permeability of the outer membrane of the bacterial cell to the aminoglycoside, has been refuted by Scudamore and Goldner (1982).

2 Other Gram-negative aerobic bacteria

These exhibit similar susceptibility to carbenicillin and ticarcillin (Sutherland *et al.*, 1971). Compared with ampicillin, carbenicillin and ticarcillin have a relatively high activity against *Proteus vulgaris*, *Providencia rettgeri* and *Morganella morganii*. Their activity against other Gram-negative bacteria is comparable with that of ampicillin (p. 109); they are effective to a degree against *Escherichia coli*, *Proteus mirabilis*, salmonellae, shigellae and also *Haemophilus influenzae*, *Neisseria meningitidis* and *N. gonorrhoeae*. Ampicillin is preferred for treatment of infections due to these bacteria because it is the more active drug. Carbenicillin and ticarcillin have some activity against ampicillin-resistant *H. influenzae* strains (p. 113), but this activity is less (MIC $4-32 \mu g$ per ml) than their activity against ampicillin-sensitive strains (MIC $0.25-1.0 \mu g$ per ml) (Kammer *et al.*, 1975; Thornsberry *et al.*, 1976). *Klebsiella* spp. are almost invariably resistant to carbenicillin and ticarcillin but some strains of *Enterobacter* spp. are relatively sensitive (Standford *et al.*, 1969; Sutherland *et al.*, 1971). Some *Serratia marcescens* strains are susceptible to these drugs in relatively low concentrations ($25 \mu g$ per ml), others are either highly resistant (MIC $>8000 \mu g$ per ml) or moderately resistant (MIC $<2000 \mu g$ per ml) (Sutherland *et al.*, 1971; Hewitt and Winters, 1973).

Carbenicillin in inhibitory or subinhibitory concentrations, potentiates the action of the aminoglycosides gentamicin, tobramycin, amikacin and netilmicin, against *Serratia marcescens* strains, which are either sensitive or only moderately resistant to carbenicillin (Lin *et al.*, 1979). Carbenicillin or ticarcillin combined with an aminoglycoside, such as gentamicin or tobramycin, also exhibits *in vitro* synergism against some strains of other Enterobacteriaceae such as *E. coli* and *Enterobacter* spp. (Comber *et al.*, 1977; White *et al.*, 1979). Most *Acinetobacter* spp. strains are inhibited by 62.5 μg per ml of carbenicillin, and this drug often acts synergistically with an aminoglycoside, such as kanamycin, gentamicin or tobramycin, against this organism. Such synergy is unlikely if the *Acinetobacter* strain is highly resistant to the aminoglycoside concerned (Glew *et al.*, 1977). Most strains of *Ps. putida*, *Burkholderia* (previously *Pseudomonas*) *cepacia* and *Stenotrophomonas* (previously *Xanthomonas*) *maltophilia* are usually resistant to carbenicillin and ticarcillin (Appelbaum *et al.*, 1982; Khardori *et al.*, 1990). Triple combinations of either gentamicin/carbenicillin/rifampicin or co-trimoxazole/carbenicillin/rifampicin are synergistic against *S. maltophilia* (Yu *et al.*, 1980). *Yersinia enterocolitica* is carbenicillin-resistant (Gaspar and Soriano, 1981), but *Achromobacter xylosoxidans* is usually sensitive to carbenicillin and ticarcillin (Legrand and Anaissie, 1992).

3 Gram-negative anaerobic bacteria

Most strains of *Prevotella* (previously *Bacteroides*) *melaninogenica* and *Fusobacterium* spp., are sensitive to carbenicillin and ticarcillin, with MICs in the range of 0.1–8.0 μg per ml. *Bacteroides fragilis* is more resistant, but 80% of strains can be inhibited by 64 μg per ml and 95% by 128 μg per ml of carbenicillin, both of which are clinically attainable concentrations (p. 150) (Sutter and Finegold 1975, 1976). Ticarcillin may be slightly more active than carbenicillin against *B. fragilis* (Roy *et al.*, 1977; Monif *et al.*, 1978). Other *Bacteroides* spp. vary in their sensitivity, some strains being inhibited by low carbenicillin concentrations, others showing marked resistance (Kirby *et al.*, 1980; Appelbaum *et al.*, 1990). A carbenicillin/cefoxitin combination is usually synergistic against *B. fragilis in vitro* (Bansal and Thadepalli, 1983) but this combination may be antagonistic against other organisms. Carbenicillin has a slightly higher activity than penicillin G (p. 17) against *Bacteroides* spp. but otherwise these two penicillins have a similar activity against Gram-negative anaerobic bacteria (Sutter and Finegold, 1975, 1976).

4 Gram-positive bacteria

Carbenicillin and ticarcillin are active against *Staphylococcus aureus* (non-penicillinase producers), *Streptococcus pyogenes* and *Strep. pneumoniae*. *Enterococcus faecalis* and *Listeria monocytogenes* are not so sensitive and usually need quite high carbenicillin and ticarcillin concentrations for inhibition (Table I.9) (Sutherland *et al.*, 1971; McCracken *et al.*, 1973). Penicillin G and ampicillin have a higher degree of activity against all of these organisms. *Nocardia brasiliensis* may be susceptible to 100 μg per ml of carbenicillin or less, but other *Nocardia* spp. are carbenicillin-resistant (Wallace *et al.*, 1983). Beta-lactamase-producing staphylococci are resistant to these drugs.

Anaerobic Gram-positive bacteria, such as *Peptococcus* and *Peptostreptococcus* spp., anaerobic streptococci, *Clostridium*, *Lactobacillus*, *Actinomyces* and *Propionibacterium* spp. are all usually sensitive to low carbenicillin and ticarcillin concentrations (Sutter and Finegold, 1976; Monif *et al.*, 1978; Denys *et al.*, 1983). *Clostridium difficile* is also ticarcillin-sensitive (Chow *et al.*, 1985).

5 Minimum inhibitory concentrations

Table I.9 shows the *in vitro* activity of carbenicillin and ticarcillin, compared with that of ampicillin, against some selected bacterial species. The MICs of carbenicillin and ticarcillin are lower than those of ampicillin for *Ps. aeruginosa*, *Serratia marcescens*, *Proteus* spp. (other than *Pr. mirabilis*), *Morganella morganii* and *B. fragilis*.

Mode of Administration and Dosage

Carbenicillin and ticarcillin are not absorbed from the gastrointestinal tract and must be administered either i.m. or i.v. The dosage used can be varied widely depending on the nature of the infection and the sensitivity of the organism. Carindacillin and carfecillin are well absorbed from the gastrointestinal tract but they are not suitable for the treatment of systemic infections because therapeutic serum levels are not attained. They are useful for oral treatment of certain urinary tract infections because adequate urine concentrations of carbenicillin are achieved.

Organism	MIC (μg per ml)		
	Carbenicillin	Ticarcillin	Ampicillin
Gram-positive bacteria			
Staphylococcus aureus (non-penicillinase producer)	1.25	1.25	0.06
Streptococcus pyogenes	0.15	0.5	0.008
Streptococcus pneumoniae	0.15	1.25	0.008
Enterococcus faecalis	25.0	125.0	1.0–5.0
Listeria monocytogenes	10.0	–	0.08–0.32
Clostridium tetani	0.25	0.5	–
Clostridium perfringens	0.25	0.5	–
Gram-negative bacteria			
Escherichia coli	12.5	5.0	5.0
Enterobacter spp.	50.0	5.0	100.0
Klebsiella pneumoniae	>250.0	500.0	1.56
Serratia marcescens	12.5	12.5	200.0
Proteus mirabilis	3.12	1.25	1.25
Proteus vulgaris	25.0	2.5	100.0
Providencia rettgeri	0.78	2.5	25.0
Morganella morganii	6.25	2.5	200.0
Neisseria gonorrhoeae	0.3	0.02	0.02–0.6
Neisseria meningitidis	0.1	0.25	–
Haemophilus influenzae	0.5	0.25	0.05
Haemophilus influenzae (ampicillin-resistant)	4.0–32.0	4.0–32.0	3.0–500
Pseudomonas aeruginosa	50.0	25.0	500.0
Prevotella melaninogenica	0.1–4.0	0.1–4.0	0.1–4.0
Bacteroides fragilis	4.0–128.0	4.0–128.0	4.0–256

Table 1.9
Compiled from data published by Knudsen *et al.* (1967), Butler *et al.* (1970), Smith *et al.* (1970), Adler *et al.* (1971), Sutherland *et al.* (1971), McCracken *et al.* (1973) Kammer *et al.* (1975) and Sutter and Finegold (1976)

1 Parenteral carbenicillin and ticarcillin for systemic Ps. aeruginosa infections

An adult dose of 24–40 g of carbenicillin per day, given i.v. is necessary for the treatment of these infections. The corresponding high dosage for children is 400–600 mg per kg body weight per day. The adult dose of ticarcillin for these infections is 18–24 g per day and the corresponding schedule for children is 300–400 mg per kg per day. Both carbenicillin and ticarcillin are best given in six to eight divided doses. For instances, if a total daily dose of 30 g carbenicillin or 18 g of ticarcillin is to be administered, doses of 5 g or 3 g, respectively, can be given every 4 h; each dose can be dissolved in 50–100 ml of i.v. fluid in a pediatric buretrol for infusion over 30–60 min (Neu and Garvey, 1975). Alternatively, the drugs may be already dispensed in a secondary i.v. bottle. These doses can be infused at a faster rate but, similar to penicillin G (p. 20), the infusion rate does not appear to influence their clinical efficiency. Probenecid in doses of 1–2 g orally per day, may be administered to delay the excretion of either carbenicillin or ticarcillin (p. 24).

Carbenicillin, ticarcillin or any other systemically administered antibiotic is not indicated for the treatment of mild or superficial *Ps. aeruginosa* infections, unless other factors suggest that the infection is potentially dangerous, in which case these drugs should be given in full dosage as for septicemia. The isolation of *Ps. aeruginosa* from the trachea or a wound may only indicate colonization, and, in itself, is not sufficient reason for treatment. Furthermore, treatment of such infections by small doses of carbenicillin or ticarcillin will not benefit the patient and may encourage emergence of resistant *Ps. aeruginosa* strains.

2 Systemic Ps. aeruginosa infections in patients with renal failure

The half-lives of both drugs, normally about 1 h (p. 152), are prolonged to 13–14 h in patients with severe renal failure, so that dosage reduction is necessary. All patients with any degree of renal failure should be given an initial loading dose of 5 g carbenicillin or 3 g ticarcillin i.v. Thereafter, patients with a creatinine clearance >60 ml per min may be treated with usual doses of both drugs. If the creatinine clearance is 30–60 ml per min, 3 g carbenicillin or 2 g ticarcillin should be given 4-hourly, and if it is 10–30 ml per min, the dose is 3 g carbenicillin or 2 g ticarcillin every 8 h. Dosages for patients with severe renal failure (creatinine clearance <10 ml per min), are carbenicillin 2 g every 8–12 h and ticarcillin 2 g every 12 h (Eastwood and Curtis, 1968; Parry and Neu, 1976a).

Both drugs are removed by hemodialysis but removal with peritoneal dialysis is slow. During hemodialysis a carbenicillin dosage of 2 g i.v. 4-hourly is recommended; during peritoneal dialysis a smaller carbenicillin dosage of 2 g every 6 h is appropriate (Eastwood and Curtis, 1968). A ticarcillin dosage of 1 g 4-hourly may be given during hemodialysis (Wise et al., 1974); alternatively an extra 3 g may be given i.v. after each dialysis, followed by the standard dosage for patients with severe renal failure (2 g 12-hourly) between dialyses (Parry and Neu, 1976a).

Further dosage reduction to 2 g per day for both carbenicillin and ticarcillin is recommended for patients with severe renal failure who have concomitant severe liver disease (Hoffman et al., 1970; Parry and Neu, 1976a).

3 Systemic Ps. aeruginosa infections in severely burned patients

The renal clearance, total clearance and the volume of distribution of ticarcillin is increased in these patients. Whilst the maximum recommended dosage of ticarcillin will suffice in most of these patients, serum level monitoring and appropriate dosage adjustment seems advisable (Adam et al., 1989; Boucher et al., 1992).

4 Systemic Ps. aeruginosa infections in newborn and premature infants

a Carbenicillin In older children and adults the serum half-life of carbenicillin is 1 h. During the first week of life this is prolonged to 2.7 h in normal birth weight infants and to 4.0 h in low birth weight infants. The initial dose of carbenicillin for these infections in the newborn is 100 mg per kg body weight. Neonates with a birth weight higher than 2000 g should then receive 75 mg per kg every 6 h (total daily dose 300 mg per kg) until 7 days of age, followed by 100 mg per kg 6-hourly (total daily dose 400 mg per kg). For neonates with a birth weight lower than 2000 g, the maintenance dosage is 75 mg per kg 8-hourly (total daily dose 225 mg per kg) until 7 days of age and thereafter a dosage of 100 mg per kg 6-hourly (the normal dosage for older children). Either i.m. or i.v. carbenicillin administration is suitable. Therapeutic non-toxic serum levels of 150–200 µg per ml are achieved with these dosage schedules (Morehead et al., 1972; Nelson and McCracken, 1973).

b Ticarcillin In the first week of life, a dose of 75 mg per kg should be given every 12 h to infants weighing less than 2000 g (total daily dose 150 mg per kg) and 75 mg per kg is administered every 8 h to those weighing more than 2000 g (total daily dose 225 mg per kg). For babies who still weigh less than 2000 g after 1 week of age, the dosage should be increased to 75 mg per kg 8-hourly (total daily dose 225 mg per kg), and for those who weigh more than 2000 g after 1 week of age, the dosage should be increased to 100 mg per kg 8-hourly (total daily dose 300 mg per kg). The drug can be administered either i.m. or i.v., usually by intermittent 30 min infusions. With these dosage schedules, serum levels 30 min after the completion of the infusion are approximately 150 µg per ml, and trough levels just before the next dose are 25–50 µg per ml (Nelson et al., 1978; Nelson, 1979).

5. Systemic infections due to more sensitive organisms

Some Gram-negative bacteria, such as *Proteus* spp., may be more susceptible to both carbenicillin and ticarcillin (MICs 5 µg per ml or less, Table I.9). Intramuscular or i.v. carbenicillin or ticarcillin, in a dosage of 1–2 g given every 4–6 h, may be adequate for the treatment of infections caused by these bacteria (Neu and Garvey, 1975). If the organism is less sensitive, as may be the case with *Enterobacter* and *Serratia* spp. and *B. fragilis*, or if the precise sensitivity is unknown, higher doses given i.v., as for *Ps. aeruginosa* septicemia, are necessary (see above).

6 Parenteral carbenicillin and ticarcillin for urinary tract infections

An adult dosage as low of 1 g i.m. every 6 h of either drug may suffice for these, because resultant urine concentrations are usually higher than the MICs for most *Ps. aeruginosa* strains. The corresponding low dosage schedule for children is 50–100 mg per kg per day (Turck et al., 1970; Parry and Neu, 1976b). When treating infections confined to the urinary tract, probenecid should not be administered.

7 Oral carindacillin

The adult dosage is 0.5 or 1 g orally every 6 h (Turck, 1973). The same doses can be used to treat certain urinary tract infections in patients with mild to moderate degrees of renal failure. The drug is unsuitable for patients with severe renal failure (creatinine clearance <14 ml per min) because very low carbenicillin concentrations are attained in the urine (Cox, 1973). Carindacillin therapy is not recommended for children.

8 Oral carfecillin

The usual adult dosage is 0.5 g 8-hourly (Leigh and Simmons, 1976). This dosage is also satisfactory for the treatment of urinary tract infections in patients with mild to moderate degrees of renal failure, because adequate urinary levels of active carbenicillin are attained. Serum levels resulting from a higher oral dosage of 1 g 4-hourly are still inadequate for the treatment of systemic infections, even in patients with severe renal failure (Wilkinson *et al.*, 1975).

Serum Levels in Relation to Dosage

1 Carbenicillin

After i.m. administration of this drug, a peak serum concentration is obtained about 1 h after injection (Fig. I.8). Doubling the dose doubles the serum level.

Figure I.9 shows the serum levels achieved with the usual large doses of i.v. carbenicillin; administered at a rate of 1 g per h would just achieve adequate serum levels (100 μg per ml) for treatment of systemic *Ps. aeruginosa* infections. Enhancement of serum levels with concomitant oral probenecid is also demonstrated.

2 Ticarcillin

Serum levels after both i.m. and i.v. administration are comparable with those of carbenicillin, and its serum half-life (70 min) is only slightly longer than that of carbenicillin (60 min) (Neu and Garvey, 1975; Meyers *et al.*, 1980). After administration of 1 g of ticarcillin i.m. to adults, a mean peak serum level of 35 μg per ml is reached in 1 h; thereafter, it falls and at 6 h it is only about 6 μg per ml (Rodriguez *et al.*, 1973a).

Following a rapid 5 min i.v. infusion of 3 g ticarcillin, the mean serum level 15 min later is 257 μg per ml; this falls to 218 at 30 min, 119 at 1 h, 70 at 2 h and after 4 h it is 30 μg per ml (Neu and Garvey, 1975). If a 3 g i.v. ticarcillin dose is infused slowly over 90–120 min, every 4 h, the mean peak serum level at the end of the infusion is 239 μg per ml and the mean trough level at the end of the 4 h interval is 94 μg per ml (Parry and Neu, 1976b). When ticarcillin is administered i.v. at either of these rates in a dose of 3 g every 4 h, serum levels are adequate for the treatment of systemic *Ps. aeruginosa* infections (Neu and Garvey, 1975). As with other penicillins, probenecid increases both serum levels and the half-life of ticarcillin.

Fig. I.8.
Serum concentration in human volunteers after i.m. and i.v. administration of 1 g of carbenicillin. (Redrawn after Knudsen *el al.*, 1967, with permission from the BMJ Publishing Group.)

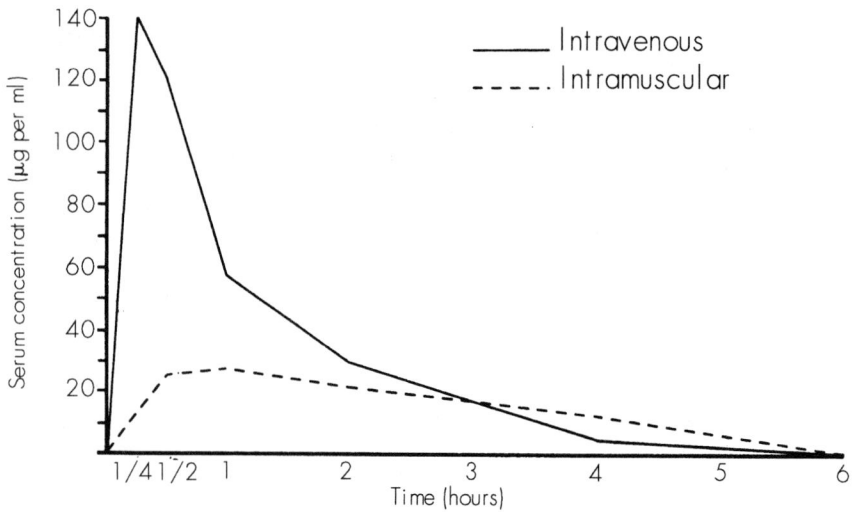

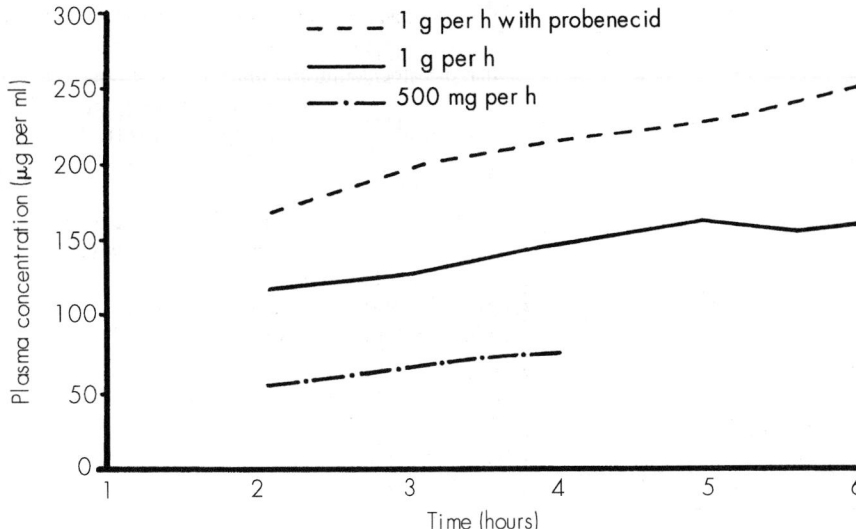

Fig. I.9.
Average serum concentrations of carbenicillin in four healthy volunteers given a continuous i.v. infusion. (Redrawn after Standiford *et al.*, 1970, with permission from the University of Chicago Press.)

3 Carindacillin

This ester, being acid stable, is well absorbed when administered orally. After absorption, it is rapidly hydrolyzed to carbenicillin plus indanol, probably either in the intestinal mucosa or in the liver (Butler *et al.*, 1973). Following an oral dose of 0.5 g of carindacillin to adults, a peak serum level of about 10 μg per ml of carbenicillin is reached in 1.0–1.5 h. Thereafter, the serum level falls and usually reaches zero at 6 h. Doubling the dose to 1 g only raises the peak serum level to 15–17 μg per ml. Simultaneous administration of probenecid results in higher serum levels but they are still inadequate for treatment of systemic *Ps. aeruginosa* infections. With dosages larger than 1 g 6-hourly, higher serum levels can be obtained but doubling the dose does not double the serum concentrations. In patients treated with doses greater than 4 g per day, diarrhea is common because a large proportion of the dose is unabsorbed (Knirsch *et al.*, 1973).

4 Carfecillin

Also being acid stable, this ester is well absorbed after oral administration. It is then rapidly hydrolyzed to carbenicillin and phenol, the phenol moiety being quickly detoxicated by conjugation (Wilkinson *et al.*, 1975). After a 0.5 g dose to adults, a mean peak serum level of approximately 3 μg per ml is attained in 1–2 h and at 6 h the drug is undetectable in serum. Levels after a 1.0 g dose are higher but not doubled. Serum levels attained by different individuals are also very variable (Wilkinson *et al.*, 1975; Leigh and Simmons, 1976).

Excretion

1 Urine

Carbenicillin and ticarcillin are excreted in urine by glomerular filtration and tubular secretion. Probenecid (p. 24) reduces their rate of excretion by partially blocking renal tubular secretion. High urinary concentrations of active carbenicillin or ticarcillin are obtained after the administration of the usual i.m. or i.v. doses; urinary levels of 65–2475 μg per ml are reached during the first 3 h after a single 3 g i.v. dose of ticarcillin (Knudsen *et al.*, 1967; Neu and Garvey, 1975). When ticarcillin is given in appropriate doses to patients with renal failure (p. 148), urinary concentrations are high irrespective of the degree of renal impairment. Even in patients with a creatinine clearance of 10 ml per min, urinary ticarcillin concentrations are in the range 250–3900 μg per ml (Parry and Neu, 1976a). The same probably applies to carbenicillin.

Approximately 80% of an i.v. administered dose of ticarcillin can be recovered from the urine as the active drug during the first 6 h after administration. This is less than the comparable figure for carbenicillin (95%), because more ticarcillin is inactivated before renal excretion. Approximately 10% of the administered dose of ticarcillin is excreted in the urine as penicilloic acid (Neu and Garvey, 1975).

In animals with comparable serum levels, the renal tubular secretion of carbenicillin is only approximately half that which occurs with penicillin G (Bergeron *et al.*, 1975). This is the reason why the renal clearance of carbenicillin is slower than that of penicillin G (Standiford *et al.*, 1970). The same is probably true for ticarcillin, which has a similar serum half-life (70 min) to that of carbenicillin (60 min).

In the first 3 h after an oral dose of 1 g carindacillin, urine carbenicillin concentrations exceed 1000 µg per ml (Knirsch *et al.*, 1973). After a 1 g dose of carfecillin, maximal urinary carbenicillin excretion occurs during the first 4 h, with urinary concentrations ranging from 52 to 1120 µg per ml (mean 434 µg per ml) (Wilkinson *et al.*, 1975). All the indanol, which is formed when carindacillin is hydrolyzed *in vivo*, is eliminated in the urine as glucuronide and sulfate conjugates (Knirsch *et al.*, 1973). Phenol resulting from carfecillin hydrolysis, is also rapidly excreted in urine as glucuronide and sulfate conjugates (Wilkinson *et al.*, 1975).

2 Bile

Small amounts of carbenicillin and ticarcillin are eliminated via the bile; in patients after cholecystectomy with T-tube drainage, about 0.19% of an i.v. administered carbenicillin dose is excreted this way (Pinget *et al.*, 1976).

3 Inactivation in body

A small amount of carbenicillin is inactivated in the liver but this is slower than with other penicillins. Some ticarcillin is metabolized in the liver to produce antibacterially inactive penicilloic acid. In severely uremic or anuric patients the serum half-life of carbenicillin and ticarcillin are 13–14 h (p. 148), compared with about 3 h for penicillin G (p. 24) and 8 h for ampicillin (p. 116).

Distribution of the Drugs in Body

Carbenicillin and ticarcillin are probably distributed in body fluids and tissues similarly to penicillin G (p. 24). Both drugs diffuse well into human interstitial fluid (Tan and Salström, 1977). Insignificant amounts of carbenicillin and ticarcillin appear in the CSF of patients with uninflamed meninges, but higher and sometimes therapeutically effective CSF levels against *Ps. aeruginosa* occur in patients with meningitis treated by large doses i.v. (Parry and Neu, 1976b).

These drugs penetrate into bronchial secretions but concentrations reached are usually lower than those needed for inhibition of *Ps. aeruginosa*. In one animal experiment the bronchial secretion concentration was only 11% of the simultaneous peak serum level 30 min after a carbenicillin injection, and after 2 h it was only 18% of the serum level (Pennington and Reynolds, 1973). A mean peak sputum concentration of 78 µg per ml was attained in such patients when massive carbenicillin doses (600 mg per kg every 4 h) were administered for a short period of time (Marks *et al.*, 1971). In cystic fibrosis patients, sputum levels of ticarcillin ranged from 2.8 to 12 µg per ml, when the drug was given i.v. in the usual dosage (Parry and Neu, 1976b).

Levels of carbenicillin in healthy renal cortical tissue may be three times higher than serum levels at the time. Tissue concentrations in the renal papillae may be 17 times higher than those in the serum if the patient is dehydrated, but this gradient decreased with rehydration. In severe renal disease due to chronic pyelonephritis or glomerulonephritis, penetration of carbenicillin into renal parenchyma is markedly decreased; carbenicillin concentrations in the cortex, medulla and papillae being only about half the serum levels at the time (Whelton *et al.*, 1973).

Ticarcillin penetrates into peritoneal and pleural fluids, where the average concentrations are 34% and 22% of simultaneous serum levels, respectively (Parry and Neu, 1976b). After a single i.v. dose of 5 g of ticarcillin, mean concentrations in serum, muscle and fat were 185, 18 and 32 µg per ml, respectively, 1.0–1.5 h after the injection (Daschner *et al.*, 1980). Significant ticarcillin concentrations are not attained in normal bone after usual i.v. doses (Summersgill *et al.*, 1982).

Carbenicillin is about 50% and ticarcillin 45% bound to serum proteins (Standiford *et al.*, 1970; Sutherland *et al.*, 1971).

Mode of Action

Carbenicillin and ticarcillin, like penicillin G, inhibit the synthesis of bacterial cell walls (p. 25). Their increased activity against organisms, such as *Ps. aeruginosa* and *Morganella morganii*, is mainly due to their superior ability to penetrate the outer cell membrane of these Gram-negative bacilli (p. 26). These drugs are also less susceptible than penicillin G and many other beta-lactam antibiotics, to at least one beta-lactamase produced by *Ps. aeruginosa* (p. 145).

Toxicity

1 Hypersensitivity reactions

Carbenicillin and ticarcillin may provoke any of the reactions which occur with penicillin G in penicillin-sensitive subjects (p. 28). Anaphylaxis due to carbenicillin has been reported (Silverblatt and Turck, 1969). These drugs are contraindicated in patients with a history of penicillin hypersensitivity. Eosinophilia has been fairly frequently noted during ticarcillin therapy (Parry and Neu, 1976b; Lang *et al.*, 1991), and occasionally this has been associated with an urticarial rash (Ervin and Bullock, 1976). Carbenicillin can also cause drug fever (Lang *et al.*, 1991).

2 Neurotoxicity

High doses of i.v. carbenicillin and ticarcillin, similar to 'massive' doses of penicillin G (p. 32), may cause neurotoxicity. This is more likely to occur in patients with renal failure. Hoffman and Bullock (1970) reported two patients with severe renal failure, who developed convulsions whilst receiving a daily i.v. carbenicillin dose of only 4 g. In one of these the carbenicillin CSF level was 37 μg per ml during the fits, and the serum level was only about 320 μg per ml. By contrast, Whelton *et al.* (1971) described another patient with moderately severe renal failure who convulsed on the 13th day of carbenicillin therapy (20 g daily) and the serum level was high at 1860 μg per ml, 3 h after the seizure. One patient with end-stage renal failure receiving maintenance hemodialysis who was treated by ticarcillin 8 g i.v. daily, developed severe neurotoxicity after 23 days of therapy. However, 12 h after discontinuation of ticarcillin, the serum level was 850 μg per ml and CSF level 120 μg per ml (Kallay *et al.*, 1979). It is possible that relatively low serum and CSF carbenicillin or ticarcillin levels may provoke convulsions in some uremic patients. Patients with underlying central nervous system disease may also be more prone to convulsions with high serum levels of any of the penicillins.

3 Bleeding disorders

These have been noted in association with carbenicillin and ticarcillin given i.v. Lurie *et al.* (1970) described three patients in whom carbenicillin appeared to act as an anticoagulant by interfering with the conversion of fibrinogen to fibrin; these patients had severe renal failure and the dosage used (24 g daily) exceeded that recommended for such patients. Waisbren *et al.* (1971) reported another five patients (two with renal failure), who developed bleeding associated with the administration of moderately high carbenicillin doses; the nature of the bleeding disorder was not elucidated.

McClure *et al.* (1970) first observed purpura and mucosal bleeding in six patients with fibrocystic disease, who were given carbenicillin in a dose of 500–750 mg per kg body weight daily, and whose serum levels were in the range of 200–400 μg per ml. These six patients and 24 others receiving carbenicillin without overt bleeding, were shown to have a disturbance of platelet function. Subsequently, Brown *et al.* (1974) performed detailed studies on 17 volunteers given doses of either 300, 400 or 600 mg per kg per day of carbenicillin and on five patients receiving the drug for Gram-negative infections. Some defect in platelet function was demonstrated in all subjects; in addition, in 14 there was prolongation of the bleeding time, in seven reduced clot retraction and in eight decreased prothrombin consumption. Severity of these disturbances appeared to be dose-dependent, and abnormal platelet function persisted for as long as 12 days after the drug was stopped. This suggested that not only circulating platelets but also megakaryocytes were affected, so that newly formed platelets were defective even though the drug was no longer present. Three of the volunteers given 600 mg per kg per day, and two of the patients given 340 and 375 mg per kg, respectively, experienced bleeding during carbenicillin administration. There was no evidence of any disturbance of coagulation. Life-threatening hemorrhage, attributable to carbenicillin-induced platelet dysfunction, has been described in a patient receiving the drug in a dose of 500 mg per kg per day (Woodruff *et al.*, 1976).

Because of this carbenicillin effect on platelet function, Brown *et al.* (1975) studied 17 volunteers who received i.v. ticarcillin for periods of 3–10 days, in doses of 100, 200 or 300 mg per kg per day (7–21 g per day). Blood coagulation was unaffected but platelet function was impaired in all subjects. Lower doses produced only mild defects in platelet function, but with a dose of 300 mg per kg per day hemostasis was more seriously impaired and the defects were similar in degree to those produced by the same dose of carbenicillin. It is possible that bleeding disorders may be less common with ticarcillin because clinically it is used in lower doses than carbenicillin. Ervin and Bullock (1976) described two patients in whom prolongation of the bleeding time appeared to be caused by ticarcillin; one had received a high dose of 400 mg per kg per day but the other only 275 mg per kg per day. Another patient who had renal failure and inadvertently received a full dosage of ticarcillin, developed a bleeding disorder characterized by petechiae, ecchymoses and epistaxis; the serum ticarcillin level 9 h after the last dose was 1050 μg per ml (Schimpff *et al.*, 1976). In another study 156 adult patients were treated with either ticarcillin, piperacillin, mezlocillin, or cefotaxime. Increases in bleeding times occurred in 73% of patients receiving ticarcillin, 43% of those treated with piperacillin, 25% of patients receiving mezlocillin and 17% of those receiving cefotaxime. Significant bleeding occurred in 34% of patients treated with ticarcillin, 17% of those receiving piperacillin, 2% with mezlocillin and 5% with cefotaxime (Fass *et al.*, 1987). Platelet dysfunction may be caused by virtually all penicillins, but it is more severe with carbenicillin and ticarcillin. The penicillins disturb platelet membrane function by interfering with ADP receptors and leaving them unavailable for agonists to induce aggregation (Ferres and Nunn, 1983; Fass *et al.*, 1987).

It appears that carbenicillin and ticarcillin usually only affect the platelet component of hemostasis, and other causes for bleeding, although reported (see above), must be rare.

4 Neutropenia

Reyes *et al.* (1973) described reversible neutropenia in two patients, which appeared to be dose-related. In one with normal renal function who was treated with 50 g of carbenicillin i.v. per day, neutropenia recurred twice on readministration of the drug; neutropenia appeared after about 16 days of therapy and on each occasion resolved within about 1 week of the drug being ceased. In both patients bone marrow showed depression of myeloid precursors. There was no evidence that an immunological mechanism was involved, and it was concluded that this was probably due to a direct toxic effect of carbenicillin. Lang *et al.* (1991) reported neutropenia in two patients treated by i.v. carbenicillin. This side-effect can occur with all beta-lactam antibiotics if they are administered i.v. in large doses (p. 33). Severe neutropenia in one adult patient occurred in association with i.v. ticarcillin therapy; it resolved when the drug was stopped and recurred on re-exposure to ticarcillin (Gastineau *et al.*, 1981). Ticarcillin-associated neutropenia was also reported in a child with cystic fibrosis (Ohning *et al.*, 1982). In this case the authors favored an immunological basis because the time for onset of neutropenia was rapid (4 days) and there were other features suggestive of an allergic reaction such as fever, diarrhea, SGOT elevation and eosinophilia.

5 Hepatotoxicity

Elevated SGOT levels have been observed during carbenicillin therapy. Knirsch and Gralla (1970) noted these elevations only in patients receiving i.m. carbenicillin and concluded that they were due to muscle irritation. Other authors have observed raised SGOT levels during i.v. carbenicillin administration, suggesting that the source of the enzyme is the liver, though the degree of hepatotoxicity is usually slight and rapidly reversible after cessation of the drug (Boxerbaum *et al.*, 1970; Gump, 1970). Four other patients who collectively had eight episodes of a mild reversible anicteric hepatitis associated with i.v. carbenicillin therapy, have been reported (Wilson *et al.*, 1975). Hepatitis was characterized by nausea, vomiting, a tender slightly enlarged liver, raised serum transaminases and alkaline phosphatase, but a normal serum bilirubin level. Liver biopsies showed spotty liver cell necrosis without cholestasis. A toxic mechanism was postulated because skin rashes and other hypersensitivity manifestations were usually absent. Other penicillins could be given to these patients without ill effects but on readministration of carbenicillin, hepatotoxicity recurred.

There has generally been a lower frequency of hepatic injury with ticarcillin compared with carbenicillin (Neu, 1982). In three patients reported by Graft and Chesney (1982), increases in SGPT developed during treatment with carbenicillin; these decreased after carbenicillin was stopped and they rose minimally or not at all during subsequent therapy with ticarcillin.

6 Electrolyte and acid-base disturbances

In 1 g of carbenicillin there is 4.7 mEq of sodium. The sodium load could, therefore, be significant in patients receiving large doses of i.v. carbenicillin. This may cause hypernatremia and pulmonary edema, particularly in patients with cardiac failure or impaired renal function. Some patients receiving large doses of i.v. carbenicillin developed hypokalemia, which was associated with metabolic alkalosis (Cabizuca and Desser, 1976). Hypokalemia probably occurs because carbenicillin promotes potassium loss via the renal tubules but it may also cause a redistribution of potassium within the body (p. 34). Hypokalemia usually responds to oral or i.v. potassium chloride administration and carbenicillin need not be discontinued.

Carbenicillin being a weak acid, can cause acute acidosis if excessively high serum levels are reached, particularly in patients with renal disease and pre-existing acidosis (Whelton *et al.*, 1971). High carbenicillin urine concentrations which result when large i.v. doses are given, produce a high urine specific gravity. For instance, one adult patient with normal renal function receiving carbenicillin in a dose of 30 g i.v. daily, had a sustained high urine specific gravity of 1042 (Deziel *et al.*, 1977). This finding should not be misinterpreted to mean that the patient is dehydrated.

Electrolyte disturbances similar to those caused by i.v. carbenicillin may occur with ticarcillin therapy. Hypokalemia has been observed in several patients treated by high doses i.v. (Schimpff *et al.*, 1976; Parry *et al.*, 1977).

7 Other side-effects

Pseudomembranous colitis (p. 594) has rarely been associated with i.v. carbenicillin therapy (Saadah, 1980). One case report described carbenicillin-induced hemorrhagic cystitis (Møller, 1978), a complication more commonly noted with methicillin (p. 84). Carbenicillin and ticarcillin can inactivate aminoglycosides (see below). Animal studies show that ticarcillin has an *in vivo* protective effect on experimental tobramycin nephrotoxicity (p. 497) (English *et al.*, 1985).

8 Carindacillin side-effects

This drug tastes very bitter and although the tablets have a special coating, many patients complain of an unpleasant after-taste and nausea. It can also cause diarrhea, especially if the dosage of 1 g 6-hourly is exceeded (Knirsch *et al.*, 1973).

9 Carfecillin side-effects

Some patients have developed diarrhea while taking this drug, but the after-taste associated with carindacillin has not been noted (Wilkinson *et al.*, 1975). Nausea and vomiting also appeared to be less common than with carindacillin.

Clinical Uses of the Drugs

A Parenteral carbenicillin

1 Pseudomonas aeruginosa infections

The main use of carbenicillin was for the treatment of systemic *Ps. aeruginosa* infections, provided that the MIC of the strain was not higher than 120 µg per ml. It was effective for these infections, despite the fact that they were usually associated with serious underlying diseases. Carbenicillin, either used alone, or combined with aminoglycosides, such as gentamicin, tobramycin or amikacin, was useful for the treatment of *Ps. aeruginosa* septicemia, (including septicemia in neutropenic patients), endocarditis, meningitis, pneumonia, endophthalmitis or external otitis (Mombelli *et al.*, 1982; Bodey *et al.*, 1983; Reyes and Lerner, 1983). Ticarcillin (see below) is now preferred for the treatment of these diseases. Carbenicillin, ticarcillin and other penicillins, which are used in large doses can inactivate aminoglycosides, such as kanamycin, gentamicin, tobramycin, netilmicin and amikacin both *in vitro* and *in vivo* (Davies *et al.*, 1975; Pickering and Gearhart, 1979; Pieper *et al.*, 1980; Farchione, 1981). The rate of inactivation of a given aminoglycoside depends on the concentration of the penicillin. Amikacin is less susceptible to inactivation than kanamycin, gentamicin and tobramycin, and netilmicin is affected to an intermediate degree. Inactivation is most likely to occur if the two antibiotics are mixed together in the same i.v. fluid container and administered by continuous infusion. Originally it was thought that significant aminoglycoside inactivation would be unlikely in patients with normal renal function, if the two drugs were given separately by intermittent i.v. injections or the gentamicin was administered i.m. (Riff and Jackson, 1971). However, under these conditions, Murillo *et al.* (1979) noted reduced gentamicin serum levels in patients with normal renal function, when the drug was used with ticarcillin, and surprisingly ticarcillin levels were also slightly reduced. It was uncertain whether this resulted from increased renal excretion or drug interaction. Other authors have confirmed significant tobramycin inactivation by carbenicillin in patients with normal renal function (Konishi *et al.*, 1983).

When carbenicillin/aminoglycoside combinations are used, it is advisable to estimate aminoglycoside serum levels to ensure that they are adequate, particularly in patients with renal failure. In such patients these drugs are usually administered less frequently, and they both may have high sustained circulating levels, allowing ample time for significant gentamicin inactivation. This effect of carbenicillin on gentamicin has been confirmed in patients with end-stage renal failure. The half-life of gentamicin in these patients of 61.6 h was reduced to 19.4 h in the presence of carbenicillin (Thompson *et al.*, 1982). Patients with renal failure, therefore, required an increased dosage of gentamicin to compensate for inactivation when carbenicillin was administered concurrently. By contrast, the half-life of amikacin in the presence of carbenicillin *in vitro* and *in vivo* was not greatly altered (Pieper *et al.*, 1980), and in both situations the drug retained greater than 75% of its activity in the presence of carbenicillin after 48 h (Farchione, 1981). Therefore, amikacin has an advantage over other aminoglycosides for inclusion in combination therapy with carbenicillin or ticarcillin, for the treatment of seriously ill patients and for those with renal failure (Pickering and Gearhart, 1979; Farchione, 1981).

2 Other Gram-negative aerobic bacterial infections

Carbenicillin was satisfactory for treatment of *Proteus* infections, particularly those caused by ampicillin-resistant species (Ross *et al.*; 1970). Carbenicillin was also useful for the treatment of infections due to *E. coli* and *Enterobacter* spp. on rare occasions, if indicated by sensitivity tests (Standiford *et al.*, 1969).

B Ticarcillin

1 Pseudomonas aeruginosa infections

Ticarcillin is a useful and preferable alternative to carbenicillin (p. 155) for the treatment of these infections. It has been used with success in *Ps. aeruginosa* septicemia (Parry and Neu, 1976b), including those occurring in patients with neutropenia and underlying neoplastic disease (Rodriguez *et al.*, 1973b; Korvick and Yu, 1991), *Ps. aeruginosa* pneumonia (Ervin and Bullock, 1976) and pulmonary infections in patients with cystic fibrosis (Parry *et al.*, 1977). *Pseudomonas* urinary tract infections may also respond to ticarcillin therapy (Parry and Neu, 1976b). Results of treatment of these diseases with ticarcillin has been comparable with those previously achieved with larger doses of carbenicillin. As ticarcillin is administered in a lower dosage, it probably causes less bleeding (p. 153), sodium overload and hypokalemia (p. 154) than carbenicillin. For these reasons, ticarcillin has largely replaced carbenicillin (Bodey *et al.*, 1983).

There may be *in vitro* synergism between ticarcillin and aminoglycosides, such as gentamicin, tobramycin and amikacin (Korvick and Yu, 1991). Such synergistic combinations have been extensively used, but the results have been usually about the same as those obtained by ticarcillin alone (Parry and Neu, 1976b; Parry *et al.*, 1977). Some authors consider that when serious *Pseudomonas* infections are treated, ticarcillin should always be combined with a second drug, such as gentamicin, to prevent emergence of ticarcillin-resistant *Ps. aeruginosa* strains during treatment (Peterson *et al.*, 1977). This is controversial, except for *Pseudomonas* meningitis (Rahal and Simberkoff, 1982) and *Pseudomonas* endocarditis, where it is generally agreed that treatment should be by a combination of ticarcillin with an aminoglycoside, such as gentamicin, tobramycin or amikacin. For *Ps. aeruginosa* endocarditis, a regimen of ticarcillin 18 g per day combined with tobramycin 8 mg per kg body weight per day, has been recommended (Reyes and Lerner, 1983). Right-sided *Pseudomonas* endocarditis in i.v. drug users may often be cured by such chemotherapy alone, but left-sided endocarditis usually needs 6 weeks chemotherapy and an early valve replacement (Komshian *et al.*, 1990). In one retrospective analysis of 410 episodes of *Pseudomonas* bacteremia, cure rates of patients who received an anti-pseudomonal beta-lactam antibiotic, such as carbenicillin or ticarcillin, with (72%) or without an aminoglycoside (71%), were higher than in patients who received an aminoglycoside alone (29%) (Bodey *et al.*, 1985). Treatment of *Ps. aeruginosa* septicemia with an aminoglycoside alone has also been found to be relatively ineffective by other authors (Chen *et al.*, 1993; Fergie *et al.*, 1994). Severe *Ps. aeruginosa* infections occur in patients infected with HIV; prolonged i.v. therapy with a combination such as ticarcillin/gentamicin is needed, followed by oral treatment with a drug such as ciprofloxacin to eradicate the infection (Kielhofner *et al.*, 1992).

Ticarcillin/gentamicin or ticarcillin/tobramycin combinations have been used with success as initial empiric chemotherapy for patients with granulocytopenia and neoplastic disease with a suspected severe infection (Klastersky *et al.*, 1975; Schimpff *et al.*, 1976; Murillo *et al.*, 1978). In one trial ticarcillin plus either gentamicin, amikacin or netilmicin, were all equally effective for this purpose (Love *et al.*, 1979). The neutropenic patient who becomes febrile has some 60% likelihood of being infected. If the absolute neutrophil count is ≤100 per mm^3, 20% or more of the febrile episodes will have an associated bacteremia. Gram-negative aerobes such as *E. coli*, *Klebsiella* spp. or *Ps. aeruginosa* are most often involved, but Gram-positive cocci such as coagulase-negative staphylococci, *Staph. aureus* and *Strep. viridans* may also cause infections in these patients. Fungi are common as secondary invaders in patients who already have had a course of broad-spectrum chemotherapy. Ticarcillin plus an aminoglycoside such as gentamicin, tobramycin or amikacin is suitable for initial therapy. Another anti-pseudomonal beta-lactam such as mezlocillin (p. 173), piperacillin (p. 174), azlocillin (p. 174), imipenem (p. 236), or ceftazidime (p. 377) may be substituted for ticarcillin. If Gram-positive cocci have been commonly involved in one hospital or unit, then vancomycin (p. 780) should also be added to the regimen. Sometimes a combination of two beta-lactams are also suitable e.g. piperacillin plus ceftazidime. Monotherapy also has been tried using drugs such as imipenem or ceftazidime. If after a week there is no response and blood cultures are negative for bacteria, amphotericin B may be added. At that stage it is best to cease the aminoglycoside and use perhaps ceftazidime instead to avoid the use of two nephrotoxic drugs (Klastersky, 1986; Schimpff, 1986; Rubin, 1988; Sage *et al.*, 1988; Hughes *et al.*, 1990; Pizzo, 1993; Aquino *et al.*, 1995; Martino *et al.*, 1995). The combination of ticarcillin and ceftizoxime is also a suitable double beta-lactam therapy for these patients (Rolston *et al.*, 1987).

An HIV-infected individual may develop fever and neutropenia either because they are receiving antineoplastic chemotherapy or later in the course of their disease neutropenia may occur due to HIV infection itself, due to other drugs or other factors. Many of these patients are already receiving antimicrobial drugs when fever and neutropenia develop, and blood cultures are often negative. There are no clear guidelines available for the management of febrile neutropenic HIV-infected patients (Hambleton *et al.*, 1995).

Ticarcillin in high concentrations, similar to carbenicillin (p. 155), can inactivate aminoglycosides *in vitro* and *in vivo*, particularly in patients with renal failure (Farchione, 1981; Chow *et al.*, 1982). Amikacin, and to a lesser extent netilmicin, are more resistant than gentamicin and tobramycin to this inactivation. Lower serum levels occur with ticarcillin because it is used in lower dosage than carbenicillin. Therefore, it usually inactivates gentamicin and tobramycin at a slower rate *in vivo* than carbenicillin (Ervin *et al.*, 1976; Pickering and Gearhart, 1979). Nevertheless, inactivation of gentamicin and tobramycin by ticarcillin may be significant in all patients, and especially in those with renal failure (Murillo *et al.*, 1979; Chow *et al.*, 1982). Serum level monitoring and dosage adjustment of the aminoglycoside, is necessary in patients with both normal and impaired renal function, when gentamicin or tobramycin are used with ticarcillin.

2 Other Gram-negative aerobic bacterial infections

Ticarcillin may be useful for *Proteus* infections (Rodriguez *et al.*, 1973b). It may on occasions also be suitable for the treatment of *E. coli*, *Enterobacter* spp. and *Serratia marcescens* infections (Parry and Neu, 1976b; Schimpff *et al.*, 1976). Bacteremia due to *Achromobacter xylosoxidans* rarely occurs in cancer patients. Ticarcillin may be suitable therapy, either alone or in combination with other drugs (Mandell *et al.*, 1987; Legrand and Anaissie, 1992).

3 Gram-negative anaerobic bacterial infections

Ticarcillin may be useful for the treatment of these infections (Nichols, 1983). Ticarcillin, chloramphenicol and clindamycin, each in combination with gentamicin were equally effective in therapy for intra-abdominal or female genital tract sepsis in one study (Harding *et al.*, 1980).

C Oral carindacillin and carfecillin

These drugs are mainly indicated for therapy of *Ps. aeruginosa* urinary tract infections. They may be useful occasionally for the treatment of similar infections caused by *Enterobacter* spp., *Pr. vulgaris*, *Pr. rettgeri* or *Morganella morganii* (Turck, 1973; Leigh and Simmons, 1976). Infections by these pathogens usually occur in patients with some underlying urinary tract pathology, and bacteriuria is often recurrent and difficult to eradicate. Furthermore, superinfection with carbenicillin-resistant organisms such as *Klebsiella* spp. may occur (Hodges and Perkins, 1973). Nevertheless, these oral carbenicillins have been used with some success either as short-term therapy (Leigh and Simmons, 1976), as a 6-week course of therapy in patients with chronic pyelonephritis (Michiels *et al.*, 1978), or as long-term suppressives in patients with chronic bacteriuria (Holloway and Taylor, 1973).

Carindacillin and carfecillin should not be used for the treatment of urinary tract infections caused by other bacterial species such as *E. coli*, which respond to many other drugs. Their widespread use may result in the spread of *Ps. aeruginosa* strains resistant to carbenicillin. These two drugs should only be used in outpatients in whom the use of the more effective parenteral ticarcillin is inconvenient. The need for these two oral drugs is now rather limited because more effective oral anti-pseudomonal drugs such as ciprofloxacin (p. 1014) are available.

References

Adam D, Zellner PR, Koeppe P, Wesch R (1989). Pharmacokinetics of ticarcillin/clavulanate in severely burned patients *J Antimicrob Chemother* **24** (Suppl B): 121.

Adler JL, Burke JP, Wilcox C, Finland M (1971). Susceptibility of *Proteus* species and *Pseudomonas aeruginosa* to penicillins and cephalosporins. *Antimicrob Ag Chemother* **1970**: 63.

Anderson EL, Gramling PK, Vestal PR, Farrar WE Jr (1975). Susceptibility of *Pseudomonas aeruginosa* to tobramycin or gentamicin alone and combined with carbenicillin. *Antimicrob Ag Chemother* **8**: 300.

Appelbaum PC, Tamim J, Stavitz J *et al.* (1982). Sensitivity of 341 non-fermentative Gram-negative bacteria to seven beta-lactam antibiotics. *Eur J Clin Microbiol* **1**: 159.

Appelbaum PC, Spangler SK, Jacobs MR (1990). Beta-lactamase production and susceptibilities to amoxicillin, amoxicillin-clavulanate, ticarcillin, ticarcillin-clavulanate, cefoxitin, imipenem, and metronidazole of 320 non-*Bacteroides fragilis Bacteroides* isolates and 129 *Fusobacteria* from 28 US centers. *Antimicrob Ag Chemother* **34**: 1546.

Aquino VM, Pappo A, Buchanan GR *et al.* (1995). The changing epidemiology of bacteremia in neutropenic children with cancer. *Pediatr Infect Dis J* **14**: 140.

Baird IM, Slepack JM, Kauffman CA, Phair JP (1976). Nosocomial infection with gentamicin-carbenicillin-resistant *Pseudomonas aeruginosa*. *Antimicrob Ag Chemother* **10**: 626.

Bansal MB, Thadepalli H (1983). Antimicrobial effect of beta-lactam antibiotic combinations against *Bacteroides fragilis in vitro*. *Antimicrob Ag Chemother* **23**: 166.

Bergeron MG, Gennari FJ, Barza M *et al.* (1975). Renal tubular transport of penicillin G and carbenicillin in the rat. *J Infect Dis* **132**: 374.

Bodey GP, Bolivar R, Fainstein V, Jadeja L (1983). Infections caused by *Pseudomonas aeruginosa*. *Rev Infect Dis* **5**: 279.

Bodey GP, Jadeja L, Elting L (1985). *Pseudomonas* bacteremia. Retrospective analysis of 410 episodes. *Arch Intern Med* **145**: 1621.

Bolister N, Basker M, Hodges N, Marriott C (1989). Reduced susceptibility of a mucoid strain of *Pseudomonas aeruginosa* to lysis by ticarcillin and piperacillin. *J Antimicrob Chemother* **24**: 619.

Boucher BA, Kuhl DA, Hickerson WL (1992). Pharmacokinetics of systemically administered antibiotics in patients with thermal injury. *Clin Infect Dis* **14**: 458.

Boxerbaum B, Doershuk CF, Matthews LW (1970). Use of carbenicillin in patients with cystic fibrosis. *J Infect Dis* **122** (Suppl): 59.

Brown CH III, Natelson EA, Bradshaw MW *et al.* (1974). The hemostatic defect produced by carbenicillin. *New Engl J Med* **291**: 265.

Brown CH III, Natelson EA, Bradshaw MW *et al.* (1975). Study of the effects of ticarcillin on blood coagulation and platelet function. *Antimicrob Ag Chemother* **7**: 652.

Butler K, English AR, Ray VA, Timreck AE (1970). Carbenicillin: chemistry and mode of action. *J Infect Dis* **122** (Suppl): 1.

Butler K, English AR, Briggs B *et al.* (1973). Indanyl carbenicillin: chemistry and laboratory studies with a new semisynthetic penicillin. *J Infect Dis* **127** (Suppl): 97.

Cabizuca SV, Desser KG (1976). Carbenicillin-associated hypokalemic alkalosis. *JAMA* **236**: 956.

Chen HY, Yuan M, Ibrahim-Elmagboul IB, Livermore DM (1995). National survey of susceptibility to antimicrobials amongst clinical isolates of *Pseudomonas aeruginosa*. *J Antimicrob Chemother* **35**: 521.

Chen SCA, Lawrence RH, Byth K, Sorrell TC (1993). *Pseudomonas aeruginosa* bacteraemia Is pancreatobiliary disease a risk factor? *Med J Aust* **159**: 592.

Chow AW, Cheng N, Bartlett KH (1985). *In vitro* susceptibility of *Clostridium difficile* to new beta-lactam and quinolone antibiotics. *Antimicrob Ag Chemother* **28**: 842.

Chow MSS, Quintiliani R, Nightingale CH (1982). *In vivo* inactivation of tobramycin by ticarcillin. A case report. *JAMA* **247**: 658.

Comber KR, Basker MJ, Osborne CD, Sutherland R (1977). Synergy between ticarcillin and tobramycin against *Pseudomonas aeruginosa* and enterobacteriaceae *in vitro* and *in vivo*. *Antimicrob Ag Chemother* **11**: 956.

Cox CE (1973). Pharmacology of carbenicillin indanyl sodium in renal insufficiency. *J Infect Dis* **127** (Suppl): 157.

Darrell JH, Waterworth PM (1969). Carbenicillin resistance in *Pseudomonas aeruginosa* from clinical material. *Brit Med J* **3**: 141.

Daschner FD, Thoma G, Langmaack H, Dalhoff A (1980). Ticarcillin concentrations in serum, muscle and fat after a single intravenous injection. *Antimicrob Ag Chemother* **17**: 738.

Davies M, Morgan JR, Anand C (1975). Interactions of carbenicillin and ticarcillin with gentamicin. *Antimicrob Ag Chemother* **7**: 431.

Dean HF, Morgan AF, Asche LV, Holloway BW (1977). Isolates of *Pseudomonas aeruginosa* from Australian hospitals having R-plasmid determined anitbiotic resistance. *Med J Aust* **2**: 116.

Denys GA, Jerris RC, Swenson JM, Thornsberry C (1983). Susceptibility of *Propionibacterium acnes* clinical isolates to 22 antimicrobial agents. *Antimicrob Ag Chemother* **23**: 335.

Deziel C, Daigneault B, Marc-Aurele J *et al.* (1977). High urine specific gravity induced by carbenicillin. *Lancet* **ii**: 980.

Duncan IBR (1974). Susceptibility of 1500 isolates of *Pseudomonas aeruginosa* to gentamicin, carbenicillin, colistin and polymyxin B. *Antimicrob Ag Chemother* **5**: 9.

Eastwood JB, Curtis JR (1968). Carbenicillin administration in patients with severe renal failure. *Brit Med J* **1**: 486.

English J, Gilbert DN, Kohlhepp S *et al.* (1985). Attenuation of experimental tobramycin nephrotoxicity by ticarcillin. *Antimicrob Ag Chemother* **27**: 897.

Ervin FR, Bullock WE Jr (1976). Clinical and pharmacological studies of ticarcillin in Gram-negative infections. *Antimicrob Ag Chemother* **9**: 94.

Ervin FR, Bullock WE Jr, Nuttall CE (1976). Inactivation of gentamicin by penicillins in patients with renal failure. *Antimicrob Ag Chemother* **9**: 1004.

Farchione LA (1981). Inactivation of aminoglycosides by penicillins. *J Antimicrob Chemother* **8** (Suppl A): 27.

Fass RJ, Copelan EA, Brandt JT *et al.* (1987). Platelet-mediated bleeding caused by broad-spectrum penicillins. *J Infect Dis* **155**: 1242.

Fergie JE, Shema SJ, Lott L *et al.* (1994). *Pseudomonas aeruginosa* bacteremia in immunocompromised children: analysis of factors associated with a poor outcome. *Clin Infect Dis* **18**: 390.

Ferres H, Nunn B (1983). Penicillin metabolites and platelet function. *Lancet* **ii**: 226.

Gaman W, Cates C, Snelling CFT *et al.* (1976). Emergence of gentamicin- and carbenicillin-resistant *Pseudomonas aeruginosa* in a hospital environment. *Antimicrob Ag Chemother* **9**: 474.

Gaspar MC, Soriano F (1981). Susceptibility of *Yersinia enterocolitica* to eight beta-lactam antibiotics and clavulanic acid. *J Antimicrob Chemother* **8**: 161.

Gastineau D, Spector R, Philips D (1981). Severe neutropenia associated with ticarcillin therapy. *Ann Intern Med* **94**: 711.

Glew RH, Moellering RC Jr, Buettner KR (1977). *In vitro* synergism between carbenicillin and aminoglycosidic aminocyclitols against *Acinetobacter calcoaceticus* var *anitratus*. *Antimicrob Ag Chemother* **11**: 1036.

Godfrey AJ, Bryan LE, Rabin HR (1981). Beta-lactam-resistant *Pseudomonas aeruginosa* with modified penicillin-binding proteins emerging during cystic fibrosis treatment. *Antimicrob Ag Chemother* **19**: 705.

Graft DF, Chesney PJ (1982). Use of ticarcillin following carbenicillin-associated hepatotoxicity. *J Pediatr* **100**: 497.

Gump DW (1970). Elevated SGOT levels after carbenicillin. *New Engl J Med* **282**: 1489.

Hambleton J, Aragón T, Modin G *et al.* (1995). Outcome for hospitalized patients with fever and neutropenia who are infected with the human immunodeficiency virus. *Clin Infect Dis* **20**: 363.

Harding GKM, Buckwold FJ, Ronald AR *et al.* (1980). Prospective randomized comparative study of clindamycin, chloramphenicol, and ticarcillin, each in combination with gentamicin in therapy for intra-abdominal and female genital tract sepsis. *J Infect Dis* **142**: 384.

Heineman HS, Lofton WM (1978). Unpredictable response of *Pseudomonas aeruginosa* to synergistic antibiotic combinations *in vitro*. *Antimicrob Ag Chemother* **13**: 827.

Hewitt WL, Winters RE (1973). The current status of parenteral carbenicillin. *J Infect Dis* **127** (Suppl): 120.

Hodges GR, Perkins RL (1973). Carbenicillin indanyl sodium oral therapy of urinary tract infections. *Arch Intern Med* **131**: 679.

Hoffman TA, Bullock WE (1970). Carbenicillin therapy of *Pseudomonas* and other Gram-negative bacillary infections. *Ann Intern Med* **73**: 165.

Hoffman TA, Cestero R, Bullock WE (1970). Pharmacokinetics of carbenicillin in patients with hepatic and renal failure. *J Infect Dis* **122** (Suppl): 75.

Holloway WJ, Taylor WA (1973). Long term oral carbenicillin therapy in complicated urinary tract infections. *J Infect Dis* **127** (Suppl): 143.

Hughes WT, Armstrong D, Bodey GP *et al.* (1990). Guidelines for the use of antimicrobial agents in neutropenic patients with unexplained fever. *J Infect Dis* **161**: 381.

Irvin RT, Govan JWR, Fyfe JAM, Costerton JW (1981). Heterogeneity of antibiotic resistance in mucoid isolates of *Pseudomonas aeruginosa* obtained from cystic fibrosis patients: role of outer membrane proteins. *Antimicrob Ag Chemother* **19**: 1056.

Kalkani E, Marketos N (1976). Comparative *in vitro* evaluation of the effects of ticarcillin and carbenicillin upon *Pseudomonas aeruginosa*. *Antimicrob Ag Chemother* **9**: 89.

Kallay MC, Tabechian H, Riley GR, Chessin LN (1979). Neurotoxicity due to ticarcillin in patient with renal failure. *Lancet* **i**: 608.

Kammer RB, Preston DA, Turner JR, Hawley LC (1975). Rapid detection of ampicillin-resistant *Haemophilus influenzae* and their susceptibility to sixteen antibiotics. *Antimicrob Ag Chemother* **8**: 91.

Khardori N, Elting L, Wong E *et al.* (1990). Nosocomial infections due to *Xanthomonas maltophilia* (*Pseudomonas maltophilia*). in patients with cancer. *Rev Infect Dis* **12**: 997.

Kielhofner M, Atmar RL, Hamill RJ, Musher DM (1992). Life threatening *Pseudomonas aeruginosa* infections in patients with human immunodeficiency virus infection. *Clin Infect Dis* **14**: 403.

Kirby BD, George WL, Sutter VL *et al.* (1980). Gram-negative anaerobic bacilli: their role in infection and patterns of susceptibility to antimicrobial agents. I. Little-known *Bacteroides* species. *Rev Infect Dis* **2**: 914.

Klastersky J (1983). Empiric treatment of infections in neutropenic patients with cancer. *Rev Infect Dis* **5** (Suppl 1): 21.

Klastersky J (1986). Concept of empiric therapy with antibiotic combinations. *Amer J Med* **80** (5C): 2.

Klastersky J, Hensgens C, Debusscher L (1975). Empiric therapy for cancer patients: comparative study of ticarcillin-tobramycin, ticarcillin-cephalothin, and cephalothin-tobramycin. *Antimicrob Ag Chemother* **7**: 640.

Kluge RM, Standiford HC, Tatem B *et al.* (1974a). The carbenicillin-gentamicin combination against *Pseudomonas aeruginosa*. *Ann Intern Med* **81**: 584.

Kluge RM, Standiford HC, Tatem B *et al.* (1974b). Comparative activity of tobramycin, amikacin and gentamicin alone and with carbenicillin against *Pseudomonas aeruginosa*. *Antimicrob Ag Chemother* **6**: 442.

Knirsch AK, Gralla EJ (1970). Serum transaminase levels after parenteral ampicillin and carbenicillin. *New Engl J Med* **282**: 1081.

Knirsch AK, Hobbs DC, Korst JJ (1973). Pharmacokinetics, toleration, and safety of indanyl carbenicillin in man. *J Infect Dis* **127** (Suppl): 105.

Knudsen ET, Rolinson GN, Sutherland R (1967). Carbenicillin: a new semisynthetic penicillin active against *Pseudomonas pyocyanea*. *Brit Med J* **3**: 75.

Komshian SV, Tablan OC, Palutke W, Reyes MP (1990). Characteristics of left-sided endocarditis due to *Pseudomonas aeruginosa* in the Detroit medical center. *Rev Infect Dis* **12**: 693.

Konishi H, Goto M, Nakamoto Y *et al.* (1983). Tobramycin inactivation by carbenicillin, ticarcillin, and piperacillin. *Antimicrob Ag Chemother* **23**: 653.

Korvick JA, Yu VL (1991). Antimicrobial agent therapy for *Pseudomonas aeruginosa*. *Antimicrob Ag Chemother* **35**: 2167.

Labia R, Guionie M, Masson J-M *et al.* (1977). Beta-lactamases produced by a *Pseudomonas aeruginosa* strain highly resistant to carbenicillin. *Antimicrob Ag Chemother* **11**: 785.

Lang R, Lishner M, Ravid M (1991). Adverse reactions to prolonged treatment with high doses of carbenicillin and ureidopenicillins. *Rev Infect Dis* **13**: 68.

Leading Article (1983). Antimicrobials and haemostasis. *Lancet* **i**: 510.

Legrand C, Anaissie E (1992). Bacteremia due to *Achromobacter xylosoxidans* in patients with cancer. *Clin Infect Dis* **14**: 479.

Leigh DA, Simmons K (1976). The treatment of simple and complicated urinary tract infections with carfecillin, a new oral ester of carbenicillin. *J Antimicrob Chemother* **2**: 293.

Lin MYC, Tuazon CU, Sheagren JN (1979). Synergism of aminoglycosides and carbenicillin against resistant strains of *Serratia marcescens*. *J Antimicrob Chemother* **5**: 37.

Livermore DM (1984). Penicillin-binding proteins, porins and outer membrane permeability of carbenicillin-resistant and -susceptible strains of *Pseudomonas aeruginosa*. *J Med Microbiol* **18**: 261.

Livermore DM, Williams RJ, Williams JD (1981). Comparison of the beta-lactamase stability and the *in-vitro* activity of cefoperazone, cefotaxime, cefsulodin, ceftazidime, moxalactam and ceftriaxone against *Pseudomonas aeruginosa*. *J Antimicrob Chemother* **8**: 323.

Love LJ, Schimpff SC, Hahn DM *et al.* (1979). Randomized trial of empiric antibiotic therapy with ticarcillin in combination with gentamicin, amikacin or netilmicin in febrile patients with granulocytopenia and cancer. *Amer J Med* **66**: 603.

Lowbury EJL, Kidson A, Lilly HA *et al.* (1969). Sensitivity of *Pseudomonas aeruginosa* to antibiotics: emergence of strains highly resistant to carbenicillin. *Lancet* **ii**: 448.

Lurie A, Ogilvie M, Townsend R *et al.* (1970). Carbenicillin-induced coagulopathy. *Lancet* **i**: 1114.

Mandell WF, Garvey GJ, Neu HC (1987). *Achromobacter xylosoxidans* bacteremia. *Rev Infect Dis* **9**: 1001.

Marks MI, Prentice R, Swarson R *et al.* (1971). Carbenicillin and gentamicin: pharmacologic studies in patients with cystic fibrosis and *Pseudomonas* pulmonary infections. *J Pediatr* **79**: 822.

Marks MI, Hammerberg S, Greenstone G, Silver B (1976). Activity of newer aminoglycosides and carbenicillin, alone and in combination, against gentamicin-resistant *Pseudomonas aeruginosa*. *Antimicrob Ag Chemother* **10**: 399.

Martino R, Subirá M, Manteiga R *et al.* (1995). Viridans streptococcal bacteremia and viridans streptococcal shock syndrome in neutropenic patients: comparison between children and adults receiving chemotherapy or undergoing bone marrow transplantation. *Clin Infect Dis* **20**: 476.

May JR, Ingold A (1973). Sensitivity of respiratory strains of *Pseudomonas aeruginosa* to carbenicillin. *J Med Microbiol* **6**: 77.

McClure PD, Casserly JG, Monsier C, Crozier D (1970). Carbenicillin induced bleeding disorder. *Lancet* **ii**: 1307.

McCracken GH Jr, Nelson JD, Thomas ML (1973). Discrepancy between carbenicillin and ampicillin activities against enterococci and *Listeria*. *Antimicrob Ag Chemother* **3**: 343.

McGowan JE Jr, Terry PM (1979). Susceptibility of Gram-negative aerobic bacilli resistant to carbenicillin in a general hospital to piperacillin and ticarcillin. *Antimicrob Ag Chemother* **15**: 137.

Meyers BR, Hirschman SZ, Strougo L, Srulevitch E (1980). Comparative study of piperacillin, ticarcillin and carbenicillin pharmacokinetics. *Antimicrob Ag Chemother* **17**: 608.

Michiels HGF, Debruyne FMJ, Moonen WA (1978). The treatment of chronic pyelonephritis with carindacillin. *Curr Med Res Opin* **5**: 394.

Møller NE (1978). Carbenicillin-induced haemorrhagic cystitis. *Lancet* **ii**: 946.

Mombelli G, Coppens L, Husson M *et al.* (1982). Carbenicillin in treatment of meningoventriculitis due to *Pseudomonas aeruginosa*. *J Antimicrob Chemother* **10**: 249.

Monif GRG, Clark PR, Shuster JJ, Baer H (1978). Susceptibility of the anaerobic bacteria, Group D streptococci, Enterobacteriaceae, and *Pseudomonas* to semisynthetic penicillins: carbenicillin, piperacillin, and ticarcillin. *Antimicrob Ag Chemother* **14**: 643.

Morehead CD, Shelton S, Kusmiesz H, Nelson JD (1972). Pharmacokinetics of carbenicillin in neonates of normal and low birth weight. *Antimicrob Ag Chemother* **2**: 267.

Murillo J, Standiford HC, Schimpff SC, Tatem BA (1978). Comparison of serum bactericidal activity among three antimicrobial combinations. *Antimicrob Ag Chemother* **13**: 992.

Murillo J, Standiford HC, Schimpff SC, Tatem B (1979). Gentamicin and ticarcillin serum levels. *JAMA* **241**: 2401.

Nelson JD (1979). Neonatal ticarcillin dosage. *Pediatrics* **64**: 549.

Nelson JD, McCracken GH (1973). Clinical pharmacology of carbenicillin and gentamicin in the neonate and comparative efficacy with ampicillin and gentamicin. *Pediatrics* **52**: 801.

Nelson JD, Kusmiesz H, Shelton S, Woodman E (1978). Clinical pharmacology and efficacy of ticarcillin in infants and children. *Pediatrics* **61**: 858.

Neu HC (1982). Carbenicillin and ticarcillin. *Med Clin N Amer* **66**: 61.

Neu HC, Garvey GJ (1975). Comparative *in vitro* activity and clinical pharmacology of ticarcillin and carbenicillin. *Antimicrob Ag Chemother* **8**: 457.

Nicholas E, Hess G, Coulten HR (1982). Degradation of penicillin, ticarcillin and carbenicillin resulting from storage of unit doses. *New Engl J Med* **306**: 547.

Nichols RL (1983). Empiric antibiotic therapy for intraabdominal infections. *Rev Infect Dis* **5** (Suppl 1): 90.

Ohning BL, Reed MD, Doershuk CF, Bulmer JL (1982). Ticarcillin-associated granulocytopenia. *Amer J Dis Child* **136**: 645.

Parry MF, Neu HC (1976a). Pharmacokinetics of ticarcillin in patients with abnormal renal function. *J Infect Dis* **133**: 46.

Parry MF, Neu HC (1976b). Ticarcillin for treatment of serious infections with Gram-negative bacteria. *J Infect Dis* **134**: 476.

Parry MF, Neu HC, Merlino M *et al.* (1977). Treatment of pulmonary infections in patients with cystic fibrosis: a comparative study of ticarcillin and gentamicin. *J Pediatr* **90**: 144.

Pennington JE, Reynolds HY (1973). Concentrations of gentamicin and carbenicillin in bronchial secretions. *J Infect Dis* **128**: 63.

Peterson CD, Kaatz BL, Angaran DM (1977). Drug evaluation data Ticarcillin and carbenicillin. A comparison. *Drug Intellig Clin Pharm* **11**: 482.

Philippon AM, Paul GC, Thabaut AP, Jacoby GA (1986). Properties of a novel carbenicillin-hydrolyzing beta-lactamase (CARB-4). specified by an IncP-2 plasmid from *Pseudomonas aeruginosa*. *Antimicrob Ag Chemother* **29**: 519.

Pickering LK, Gearhart P (1979). Effect of time and concentration upon interaction between gentamicin, tobramycin, netilmicin, or amikacin and carbenicillin or ticarcillin. *Antimicrob Ag Chemother* **15**: 592.

Pieper JA, Vidal RA, Schentag JJ (1980). Animal model distinguishing *in vitro* from *in vivo* carbenicillin-aminoglycoside interactions. *Antimicrob Ag Chemother* **18**: 604.

Pinget M, Brogard JM, Dauchel J, Lavillaureix J (1976). Biliary excretion of ampicillin, metampicillin and carbenicillin. *J Antimicrob Chemother* **2**: 195.

Pizzo PA (1993). Management of fever in patients with cancer and treatment-induced neutropenia. *New Engl J Med* **328**: 1323.

Prior RB, Fass RJ (1978). Comparison of ticarcillin and carbenicillin activity against random and select populations of *Pseudomonas aeruginosa*. *Antimicrob Ag Chemother* **13**: 84.

Rahal JJ, Simberkoff MS (1982). Host defense and antimicrobial therapy in adult Gram-negative bacillary meningitis. *Ann Intern Med* **96**: 468.

Reyes MP, Lerner AM (1983). Current problems in the treatment of infective endocarditis due to *Pseudomonas aeruginosa*. *Rev Infect Dis* **5**: 314.

Reyes MP, Palutke M, Lerner AM (1973). Granulocytopenia associated with carbenicillin. Five episodes in two patients. *Amer J Med* **54**: 413.

Reyes MP, El-Khatib MR, Brown WJ *et al.* (1979). Synergy between carbenicillin and an aminoglycoside (gentamicin or tobramycin). against *Pseudomonas aeruginosa* isolated from patients with endocarditis and sensitivity of isolates to normal human serum. *J Infect Dis* **140**: 192.

Richmond MH (1980). Resistance of *Pseudomonas aeruginosa* to anitbiotics. In *Pseudomonas aeruginosa*: The organism, diseases it causes, and their treatment (Sabath LD, ed), p. 176. Bern, Stuttgart, Vienna: Hans Huber Publishers.

Riff L, Jackson GG (1971). Gentamicin plus carbenicillin. *Lancet* **i**: 592.

Rodriguez V, Inagaki J, Bodey GP (1973a). Clinical pharmacology of ticarcillin (x-carboxyl-3-thienylmethyl penicillin, BRL 2288). *Antimicrob Ag Chemother* **4**: 31.

Rodriguez V, Bodey GP, Horikoshi N *et al.* (1973b). Ticarcillin therapy of infections. *Antimicrob Ag Chemother* **4**: 427.

Rodriguez-Tebar A, Rojo F, Dámaso D, Vazquez D (1982). Carbenicillin resistance of *Pseudomonas aeruginosa*. *Antimicrob Ag Chemother* **22**: 255.

Roe E, Jones RJ, Lowbury EJL (1971). Transfer of antibiotic resistance between *Pseudomonas aeruginosa*, *Escherichia coli*, and other Gram-negative bacilli in burns. *Lancet* **i**: 149.

Rolston KVI, Jones PG, Fainstein V *et al.* (1987). Ceftizoxime plus ticarcillin: double beta-lactam therapy for infections in cancer patients. *J Antimicrob Chemother* **19**: 367.

Ross S, Kraybill EN, Khan W (1970). Treatment of *Proteus* meningitis with carbenicillin: a report of four cases. *J Infect Dis* **122** (Suppl): 62.

Roy I, Bach V, Thadepalli H (1977). *In vitro* activity of ticarcillin against anaerobic bacteria compared with that of carbenicillin and penicillin. *Antimicrob Ag Chemother* **11**: 258.

Rubin RH (1988). Empiric antibacterial therapy in granulocytopenia induced by cancer chemotherapy. *Ann Intern Med* **108**: 134.

Saadah HA (1980). Carbenicillin and pseudomembranous enterocolitis. *Ann Intern Med* **93**: 645.

Sage R, Hann I, Prentice HG *et al.* (1988). A randomized trial of empirical antibiotic therapy with one of four beta-lactam antibiotics in combination with netilmicin in febrile neutopenic patients. *J Antimicrob Chemother* **22**: 237.

Schimpff SC (1986). Empiric antibiotic therapy for granulocytopenic cancer patients. *Amer J Med* **80** (5c): 13.

Schimpff SC, Landesman S, Hahn DM *et al.* (1976). Ticarcillin in combination with cephalothin or gentamicin as empiric antibiotic therapy in granulocytopenic cancer patients. *Antimicrob Ag Chemother* **10**: 837.

Scudamore RA, Goldner M (1982). Penetration of the outer membrane of *Pseudomonas aeruginosa* by synergistic combinations of beta-lactam and aminoglycoside antibiotics. *Antimicrob Ag Chemother* **21**: 1007.

Silverblatt F, Turck M (1969). Laboratory and clinical evaluation of carbenicillin (carboxybenzyl penicillin). *Antimicrob Ag Chemother* **1968**: 279.

Smith CB, Wilfert JN, Dans PE *et al.* (1970). *In vitro* activity of carbenicillin and results of treatment of infections due to *Pseudomonas* with carbenicillin singly and in combination with gentamicin. *J Infect Dis* **122** (Suppl): 14.

Smith JA, Henry DA (1988). Comparison of bactericidal activity of selected beta-lactam antimicrobials against *Pseudomonas aeruginosa*. *J Antimicrob Chemother* **22**: 849.

Standiford HC, Kind AL, Kirby WMM (1969). Laboratory and clinical studies of carbenicillin against Gram-negative bacilli. *Antimicrob Ag Chemother* **1968**: 286.

Standiford HC, Jordan MC, Kirby WMM (1970). Clinical pharmacology of carbenicillin compared with other penicillins. *J Infect Dis* **122** (Suppl): 9.

Summersgill JT, Schupp LG, Raff MJ (1982). Comparative penetration of metronidazole, clindamycin, choramphenicol, cefoxitin, ticarcillin and moxalactam into bone. *Antimicrob Ag Chemother* **21**: 601.

Sutherland R, Burnett J, Rolinson GN (1971). X-carboxy-3-thienylmethylpenicillin (BRL 2288), a new semisynthetic penicillin: *in vitro* evaluation. *Antimicrob Ag Chemother* **1970**: 390.

Sutter VL, Finegold SM (1975). Susceptibility of anaerobic bacteria to carbenicillin, cefoxitin, and related drugs. *J Infect Dis* **131**: 417.

Sutter VL, Finegold SM (1976). Susceptibility of anaerobic bacteria to 23 antimicrobial agents. *Antimicrob Ag Chemother* **10**: 736.

Tan JS, Salström SJ (1977). Levels of carbenicillin, ticarcillin, cephalothin, cefazolin, cefamandole, gentamicin, tobramycin and amikacin in human serum and interstitial fluid. *Antimicrob Ag Chemother* **11**: 698.

Thomassen MJ, Demko CA, Boxerbaum B *et al.* (1979). Multiple isolates of *Pseudomonas aeruginosa* with differing antimicrobial susceptibility patterns from patients with cystic fibrosis. *J Infect Dis* **140**: 873.

Thompson MIB, Russo ME, Saxon BJ *et al.* (1982). Gentamicin inactivation by piperacillin or carbenicillin in patients with end-stage renal disease. *Antimicrob Ag Chemother* **21**: 268.

Thornsberry C, Baker CN, Kirven LA, Swenson JM (1976). Susceptibility of ampicillin-resistant *Haemophilus influenzae* to seven penicillins. *Antimicrob Ag Chemother* **9**: 70.

Turck M (1973). The treatment of urinary-tract infections with an oral carbenicillin. *J Infect Dis* **127** (Suppl): 133.

Turck M, Silverblatt F, Clark H, Holmes K (1970). The role of carbenicillin in treatment of infections of the urinary tract. *J Infect Dis* **122** (Suppl): 29.

Waisbren BA, Evani SV, Ziebert AP (1971). Carbenicillin and bleeding. *JAMA* **217**: 1243.

Wallace RJ Jr, Wiss K, Curvey R et al. (1983). Differences among *Nocardia* spp in susceptibility to aminoglycosides and beta-lactam antibiotics and their potential use in taxonomy. *Antimicrob Ag Chemother* **23**: 19.

Whelton A, Carter GG, Barth MA *et al.* (1971). Carbenicillin-induced acidosis and seizures. *JAMA* **218**: 1942.

Whelton A, Carter GG, Bryant HH *et al.* (1973). Carbenicillin concentrations in normal and diseased kidneys. A therapeutic consideration. *Ann Intern Med* **78**: 659.

White GW, Malow JB, Zimelis VM *et al.* (1979). Comparative *in vitro* activity of azlocillin, ampicillin, mezlocillin, piperacillin and ticarcillin alone and in combination with an aminoglycoside. *Antimicrob Ag Chemother* **15**: 540.

Wilkinson PJ, Reeves DS, Wise R, Allen JT (1975). Volunteer and clinical studies with carfecillin: a new orally administered ester of carbenicillin. *Brit Med J* **2**: 250.

Williams RJ, Lindridge MA, Said AA *et al.* (1984). National survey of antibiotic resistance in *Pseudomonas aeruginosa*. *J Antimicrob Chemother* **14**: 9.

Wilson FM, Belamaric J, Lauter CB, Lerner AM (1975). Anicteric carbenicillin hepatitis. Eight episodes in four patients. *JAMA* **232**: 818.

Wise R, Reeves DS, Parker AS (1974). Administration of ticarcillin, a new anti-pseudomonal antibiotic, in patients undergoing dialysis. *Antimicrob Ag Chemother* **5**: 119.

Woodruff RK, Bell WR, Castaldi PA (1976). Carbenicillin danger. *Med J Aust* **1**: 278.

Yu VL, Felegie TP, Yee RB *et al.* (1980). Synergistic interaction *in vitro* with use of three antibiotics simultaneously against *Pseudomonas maltophilia*. *J Infect Dis* **142**: 602.

Mezlocillin, Azlocillin, Piperacillin and Apalcillin

Description

These semisynthetic penicillins are described together because they are often referred to as 'newer anti-pseudomonal penicillins'. They are all vulnerable to the action of many beta-lactamases, but most of them are considerably more active *in vitro* than carbenicillin and ticarcillin (p. 146) against *Pseudomonas aeruginosa*, other Gram-negative bacteria and some Gram-positive bacteria. These drugs are acylamino penicillins. Because mezlocillin and azlocillin each contain a ureido (-N-CO-N-) group, they are called ureido-penicillins (Slack, 1981; Selwyn, 1982).

1 Mezlocillin

This has the chemical formula of D-alpha (2-oxo-3-mesyl-imidazolidinyl)-carbonyl amino-benzyl-penicillin. It is an ureido-penicillin and resembles an alpha-amino-substituted ampicillin (Bodey and Pan, 1977; Wise and Andrews, 1982).

2 Azlocillin

Another ureido-substituted penicillin it has a chemical formula of 6D-2-(2-oxoimidazolidine-1-carboxamido-2-phenylacetamido)-penicillanic acid (Stewart and Bodey, 1977). Azlocillin can also be considered as an alpha-amino-substituted ampicillin (Wise and Andrews, 1982).

3 Piperacillin

This is an aminobenzyl-penicillin derivative with a chemical formula of sodium 6-(D(-)-alpha-(4-ethyl-2, 3-dioxo-1-piperazinylcarbonylamino-alpha-phenylacetamido) penicillinate. Its molecule contains a side-chain with an ureido group, but because of chemical differences arising from its terminal piperazine structure, it is often not classified as an ureido-penicillin like mezlocillin and azlocillin. Piperacillin has an *in vitro* antimicrobial spectrum qualitatively, but not quantitatively, similar to that of carbenicillin (Fu and Neu, 1978a; Selwyn, 1982).

4 Apalcillin (PC-904)

Chemically, this is sodium 6-(D(-)alpha-(4-hydroxy-1, 5-naphthyridine-3-carboxamido) phenyl-acetamido) penicillinate. It is active in quite low concentrations against a large proportion of Gram-negative organisms (Noguchi *et al.*, 1976).

Sensitive Organisms

The antibacterial spectra of these compounds are similar to those of carbenicillin and ticarcillin (p. 145), but there are differences between their degree of activity against various bacterial species.

1 Mezlocillin

This is more active than carbenicillin and ticarcillin against most *Eschericha coli*, *Enterobacter* spp, *Proteus vulgaris*, *Pr. rettgeri* and *Morganella morganii* strains. It is also more active than ticarcillin against *Klebsiella* spp.; more than 50% of strains can be inhibited by clinically achievable concentrations (Fu and Neu, 1978b; Wise and Andrews, 1982) (Table I.10). Activity of mezlocillin is about the same as that of ticarcillin against *Serratia* marcescens and *Ps. aeruginosa* (Parry and Folta, 1983). As with azlocillin (see below), the activity of mezlocillin against *Ps. aeruginosa* is markedly inoculum-dependent and MBCs are much higher than MICs, suggesting that each culture contains some highly mezlocillin-resistant *Ps. aeruginosa* cells (Bodey and Pan, 1977; Greenwood and Eley, 1982). *Providencia* alkalifaciens is quite sensitive (MIC 1–2 μg per ml), but *Pr. stuartii* is relatively mezlocillin-resistant (Hawkey *et al.*, 1983). Most strains of *Pseudomonas* spp. other than *Ps. aeruginosa*, such as *Burkholderia* (*Pseudomonas*) *cepacia* are inhibited by lower mezlocillin than carbenicillin concentrations. Mezlocillin and carbenicillin are equally active against *Acinetobacter* spp. (Fass and Barnishan, 1980). Salmonellae and shigellae are mezlocillin-sensitive, but ampicillin is slightly more active; ampicillin-resistant strains of both species (p. 110) are mezlocillin-resistant (Thadepalli *et al.*, 1979; Verbist, 1979). *Prevotella* (*Bacteroides*) *melaninogenica* is quite sensitive, but *B. fragilis* is variably so (Table I.10). Sutter and Finegold (1976) reported that the activity of mezlocillin against *B. fragilis* was similar to that of penicillin G (p. 17), ampicillin (p. 115) and carbenicillin (p. 147). Others have found mezlocillin more active against this organism (MICs of most strains 25–30 μg per ml) (Fu and Neu, 1978b;Wise and Andrews, 1982).

As mezlocillin is vulnerable to many beta-lactamases of Gram-negative bacteria, some isolates, especially hospital-associated strains, of all these bacteria may be highly mezlocillin-resistant (Ellis *et al.*, 1979; White *et al.*, 1979). Unfortunately, mezlocillin and other acylamino penicillin derivatives (p. 164) are not resistant to TEM beta-lactamases (p. 192), which are the most frequent plasmid-mediated beta-lactamases among resistant *Enterobacteriaceae* (Eliopoulos and Moellering, 1982). However, some *E. coli* isolates which produce TEM-1 beta-lactamase, remain relatively mezlocillin-sensitive, whilst they are resistant to ampicillin (Livermore *et al.*, 1986).

Mezlocillin is highly active against *Haemophilus influenzae*, its activity exceeding that of ampicillin (p. 112) (Sanders, 1982a). Meningococci and gonococci are quite sensitive. Strains of *Neisseria gonorrhoeae* highly susceptible to penicillin G are equally sensitive to mezlocillin. Strains with intermediate susceptibility to penicillin G (p. 14) (MICs 0.125–0.5 μg per ml), are much more sensitive to mezlocillin (MICs 0.0004–0.125). The same applies to gonococcal strains with even higher intrinsic resistance to penicillin G; for those with penicillin G MICs of 1–4 μg per ml, mezlocillin MICs are 0.06–0.5 μg per ml (Rodriguez *et al.*, 1983). Beta-lactamase-producing gonococci are mezlocillin-resistant.

Mezlocillin is highly active against Gram-positive bacteria, such as *Streptococcus pyogenes*, Group B streptococci, *Strep. pneumoniae* and *Strep. viridans*, but penicillin G (p. 4) and ampicillin (p. 108) are more active against these organisms. Mezlocillin is slightly less active than ampicillin, but equally active to penicillin G against *Enterococcus faecalis* (Sanders, 1981). Some authors have found that mezlocillin, unlike penicillin G and ampicillin, has identical MICs and MBCs against this organism (Moody *et al.*, 1984). *Listeria monocytogenes* is also mezlocillin-sensitive (Odio *et al.*, 1984b). It is moderately active against penicillin G-sensitive staphylococci, but beta-lactamase-producing strains are resistant (Sanders, 1982a). Similar to most other penicillins, mezlocillin is inactive against *Chlamydia trachomatis* (Hammerschlag and Gleyzer, 1983).

In combination with an aminoglycoside, such as gentamicin, tobramycin, amikacin or netilmicin, mezlocillin acts synergistically against many strains of Gram-negative bacilli, such as *Ps. aeruginosa*, *E. coli*, *Pr. vulgaris*, *Pr. rettgeri*, *Morganella morganii* and *Klebsiella*, *Citrobacter*, *Enterobacter* and *Serratia* spp. *In vitro* synergy occurs with mezlocillin-sensitive and -resistant strains of these bacteria (Neu and Fu, 1978; Perea *et al.*, 1980; Moody *et al.*, 1984; Lyon *et al.*, 1986).

Mezlocillin (and related penicillins) combined with some beta-lactamase-resistant cephalosporins, may be antagonistic against certain Gram-negative bacilli. When a mezlocillin/ cefoxitin combination was tested against *B. fragilis*, synergism was observed in 10 of 20 strains, but there was no antagonism (Bansal and Thadepalli, 1983). In studies where mezlocillin was combined with either cefoxitin, cefotaxime, cefoperazone or moxalactam, and tested against Enterobacteriaceae and *Ps. aeruginosa*, the most common result was indifference, but antagonism occurred occasionally with mezlocillin/cefoxitin (Neu and Labthavikul, 1982b). The effects of combining mezlocillin (or piperacillin) with cefoxitin, cefamandole or cephalothin, was studied by Kuck *et al.* (1981). Against most Gram-negative bacilli there was either synergy or indifference but with *Ps. aeruginosa*, *Pr. vulgaris*, *Pr. rettgeri*, *Serratia* and *Enterobacter* spp., antagonism was commonly observed, particularly with combinations containing cefoxitin. Animals infected with organisms showing this *in vitro* antagonism, required much higher doses of mezlocillin to control infection, when it was combined with a cephalosporin, than when it was used singly. Sanders *et al.* (1982) found that cefoxitin/ mezlocillin antagonism occurred with strains of Gram-negative bacilli which possessed inducible beta-lactamases. These chromosomally mediated enzymes are present in many Gram-negative bacteria, such as *Enterobacter*, *Serratia* and *Pseudomonas* spp. Tested against these strains, cefoxitin antagonized many other beta-lactam antibiotics. Antagonism between the enzyme-stable beta-lactams (e.g. cefoxitin) and mezlocillin and related drugs, occurs because the former antibiotics function as inducers of beta-lactamases (p. 295). The mechanism for antagonism is that the drug-induced beta-lactamase hydrolyzes the antagonized beta-lactam (p. 295). As a result, enzyme-stable beta-lactam antibiotics have the potential ability to antagonize many other antibiotics of this group. These types of beta-lactam antibiotics have been used together in certain clinical situations (p. 165), but there is little evidence that such combinations are advantageous, and because of potential antagonism, they should be avoided (Sanders, 1983; Gutmann *et al.*, 1986).

2 Azlocillin

The main advantage of this drug is that its activity against *Ps. aeruginosa* is superior to carbenicillin, ticarcillin and mezlocillin (Table I.10). It is also active against many carbenicillin-resistant strains of this organism (Stewart and Bodey, 1977; Coppens and Klastersky, 1979; Parry, 1983). Azlocillin-resistant *Ps. aeruginosa* strains are uncommon; in 24 UK hospitals only 3.9% of strains were resistant with MICs greater than 32 µg per ml (Williams *et al.*, 1984).

Superiority of azlocillin over other anti-pseudomonal penicillins has been disputed. When conventional MIC tests and small inocula are used, azlocillin has lower MICs than the other drugs against *Ps. aeruginosa* (Table I.10). When tests for bactericidal activity are done, using large inocula, the 'activities' of azlocillin, mezlocillin and piperacillin are inferior to those of carbenicillin and ticarcillin. These drugs, unlike carbenicillin and ticarcillin, are susceptible to chromosomally mediated pseudomonal beta-lactamase (p. 145), so that they are inactivated in dense bacterial populations during overnight incubation (White *et al.*, 1980; Greenwood and Eley, 1982; Livermore and Yang, 1987). Strains of *Ps. aeruginosa* can be produced *in vitro*, which as a result of enzyme induction or spontaneous chromosomal mutation, produce increased amounts of pseudomonal beta-lactamase. If high inocula are used for testing, sensitivities of these strains to azlocillin and piperacillin are reduced at least 10-fold, whilst those for carbenicillin and ticarcillin are reduced by only 2- to 5-fold (Gwynn and Rolinson, 1983). Estimates of the comparative activity of anti-pseudomonal beta-lactam antibiotics (including newer cephalosporins, pp. 324, 369) vary with the *in vitro* test used. With *Ps. aeruginosa* standard MIC tests may underestimate resistance to azlocillin, other ureido-penicillins and cephalosporins (Jacobs *et al.*, 1984).

Compared with mezlocillin, azlocillin has the same activity against *Bacteroides fragilis*, but it is somewhat less active against most other Gram-negative bacilli (Fu and Neu, 1978b; Ellis *et al.*, 1979) (Table I.10). Azlocillin is as active as mezlocillin against *H. influenzae*, *N. meningitidis*, *N. gonorrhoeae* and Gram-positive bacteria (Wise *et al.*, 1978; Reeves *et al.*, 1979). Its activity against *Enterococcus faecalis* is comparable with that of ampicillin (p. 108) (Tofte *et al.*, 1984). *Aeromonas* spp. is usually azlocillin-sensitive (Koehler and Ashdown, 1993).

Similar to mezlocillin, azlocillin combined with an aminoglycoside, such as gentamicin, tobramycin, amikacin or netilmicin, acts synergistically against many strains of *Ps. aeruginosa*, *E. coli*, *Pr. vulgaris*, *Pr. rettgeri*, *Morganella morganii*, the *Klebsiella*, *Citrobacter*, *Enterobacter* and *Serratia* spp. Synergy occurs with both azlocillin-sensitive and -resistant strains of these bacteria (Neu and Fu, 1978; Hoogkamp-Korstanje *et al.*, 1981; Chin and Neu, 1983). A combination of azlocillin with a beta-lactamase-resistant cephalosporin, such as cefoxitin or cefotaxime, may provide a broad initial cover for the treatment of serious undiagnosed infections (Ellis *et al.*, 1979). In one *in vitro* study, azlocillin plus cefotaxime complemented each other's spectrum and antagonism was not demonstrated (Fass, 1982a). Because beta-lactamase stable cephalosporins may act as enzyme inducers (p. 295), it is probably best to avoid using azlocillin with such beta-lactam antibiotics to treat infections caused by some Gram-negative bacilli, such as *Enterobacter*, *Serratia* and *Pseudomonas* spp.

3 Piperacillin

This drug is at least equally active, or with many strains twice as active, as azlocillin against *Ps. aeruginosa* (Table I.10). Similar to mezlocillin (p. 162) and azlocillin (see above), piperacillin is less bactericidal to this organism than carbenicillin (Milne and Waterworth, 1978; Watanakunakorn, 1986). Other *Pseudomonas* species, such as *Burkholderia* (*Pseudomonas*) *cepacia*, are more susceptible to piperacillin than to carbenicillin (Fass and Barnishan, 1980). Piperacillin has good activity against the *Enterobacteriaceae*. Most strains of *E. coli*, *Pr. mirabilis* and the *Klebsiella*, *Enterobacter*, *Serratia*, *Citrobacter*, *Salmonella* and *Shigella* spp. are inhibited by low concentrations, MICs being similar or sometimes lower than those of mezlocillin (Table

I.10) (Fass, 1983). Only about 50% of *Pr. vulgaris*, *Morganella morganii*, *Providencia* and *Acinetobacter* spp. strains are inhibited by low piperacillin concentrations (Ueo *et al.*, 1977; Fu and Neu, 1978a; Reeves *et al.*, 1982). Piperacillin is active against a proportion of cephalothin-resistant *Enterobacteriaceae* and aminoglycoside-resistant Gram-negative bacilli (George *et al.*, 1978; Winston *et al.*, 1978; Magnussen *et al.*, 1982). *Aeromonas* spp. is usually piperacillin-sensitive (Koehler and Ashdown, 1993), as are most isolates of *Achromobacter xylosoxidans* (Mandell *et al.*, 1987).

Similar to mezlocillin and azlocillin, piperacillin is susceptible to beta-lactamases, so that many Gram-negative bacteria with acquired resistance to ampicillin or carbenicillin, are also piperacillin-resistant (Verbist, 1978; Reeves *et al.*, 1982; Dornbusch *et al.*, 1990). With *Ps. aeruginosa*, intrinsic resistance to piperacillin due to changes in penicillin binding proteins (PBPs) (p. 27), particularly PBP3, has emerged *in vivo* during piperacillin treatment of *Ps. aeruginosa* infections in cystic fibrosis patients (Godfrey *et al.*, 1981). In an *in vitro* study piperacillin-resistant variants were detected in each of ten strains of *Ps. aeruginosa*. This resistance was due to an increased production of chromosomally mediated *Ps. aeruginosa* beta-lactamase (p. 145); the resistant strains remained stable on subculture and they arose as a result of chromosomal mutation and enzyme induction was not involved (Bell *et al.*, 1985). *Pseudomonas aeruginosa* can develop a biofilm and the bacteria are then enmeshed in a mucoid exopolysaccharide. In this biofilm *Ps. aeruginosa* cells are more resistant to aminoglycosides and beta-lactam antibiotics. This particularly happens in chronic infections, such as those due to *Ps. aeruginosa* of the urinary tract and pulmonary infections in patients with cystic fibrosis. Young bacteria of this type may be eradicated after a 2 h exposure to piperacillin concentration of 200 µg per ml plus tobramycin 10 µg per ml, but old sessile bacteria cannot be eradicated by concentrations of these antibiotics which can be obtained *in vivo*. Therefore biofilm-associated infections should be eradicated as early as possible (Anwar and Costerton, 1990; Hoyle *et al.*, 1992).

Piperacillin is moderately active against *B. fragilis*, most strains being inhibited by 25 µg per ml; in this respect it is about equally as active as mezlocillin (Robinson *et al.*, 1980; Cuchural *et al.*, 1981). Piperacillin-resistant variants of this organism have been detected (Tally *et al.*, 1983, 1985). The activity of piperacillin against other species of Gram-negative anaerobic bacteria is variable, some strains are quite sensitive but many are highly resistant (Goldstein *et al.*, 1993).

Although *H. influenzae* is very susceptible to piperacillin, beta-lactamase-producing strains (p. 113) are resistant. The drug is inactivated by the TEM-type beta-lactamase (p. 113) (Thornsberry *et al.*, 1979). It is as active as penicillin G (p. 14) and mezlocillin (p. 163) against penicillin G-susceptible *N. gonorrhoeae* strains (Table I.10). Like mezlocillin (p. 163), piperacillin exhibits increased activity against gonococcal strains with intrinsic type resistance to penicillin G (Rodriguez *et al.*, 1983). Beta-lactamase-producing gonococci (p. 15) are piperacillin-resistant (Gootz *et al.*, 1979).

Against Gram-positive bacteria, such as *Staphylococcus aureus* (non-beta-lactamase producers), *Staph. epidermidis*, *Strep. pyogenes*, *Strep. pneumoniae* and *Enterococcus faecalis*, the activity of piperacillin is comparable with that of mezlocillin and azlocillin (Table I.10) (Dickinson *et al.*, 1978; Gootz *et al.* 1979). *Clostridium difficile* is sensitive to piperacillin (Chow *et al.*, 1985). *Chlamydia trachomatis* is piperacillin-resistant (Bowie, 1982).

A combination of piperacillin with an aminoglycoside, such as gentamicin, tobramycin or amikacin, is synergistic *in vitro* against many strains of Enterobacteriaceae and *Ps. aeruginosa* (Kurtz *et al.*, 1981; Fass 1982b; McAllister, 1982). A piperacillin-amikacin combination is usually synergistic against strains of *Enterobacteriaceae* which are resistant to other aminoglycosides and beta-lactam antibiotics (Glew and Pavuk, 1984; Lyon *et al.*, 1986). The combination of piperacillin and amikacin is also more effective than piperacillin/pefloxacin in preventing the emergence of resistant mutants (Boisivon *et al.*, 1988). *In vitro* combinations of piperacillin with cephalosporins, such as cefoxitin, cefotaxime or moxalactam, may be synergistic but occasionally may be antagonistic against some Gram-negative bacilli (Kuck *et al.*, 1981). Imipenem was antagonistic to piperacillin with 28 of 35 strains of *Ps. aeruginosa* examined by Bertram and Young (1984). Antagonism occurred because imipenem induced a beta-lactamase (p. 229). For reasons applicable to mezlocillin (p. 164), the use of these combinations may be best avoided (Sanders, 1983).

4 Apalcillin

Pseudomonas aeruginosa is as sensitive to this drug as it is to piperacillin (Table I.10). Some authors have found apalcillin to be more active than piperacillin against this organism (Barry *et*

	MIC (μg per ml)				
Organism	Ticarcillin	Mezlocillin	Azlocillin	Piperacillin	Apalcillin
Gram-positive bacteria					
Staphylococcus aureus (non-penicillinase producer)	1.25	0.2	0.2	0.78	0.39
Streptococcus pyogenes	0.5	0.025	<0.1	0.1	0.1
Streptococcus pneumoniae	1.25	0.025	0.1	0.01	0.05
Enterococcus faecalis	125.0	1.0	0.5	0.4–1.6	12.5
Clostridium perfringens	0.5	0.07	0.04	0.06–4.0	1.56
Gram-negative bacteria					
Escherichia coli	5.0	1.0–2.0	1.0–8.0	0.8	0.39
Enterobacter spp.	5.0	2.0–8.0	12.5–100.0	1.6	3.1
Klebsiella spp.	500.0	12.5–100.0	12.5–>100.0	3.1	6.3
Serratia marcescens	12.5	12.5	12.5	0.8–>100.0	25.0
Proteus mirabilis	1.25	1.56	1.56	0.2	0.76
Proteus vulgaris[a]	2.5	1.56	12.5	0.78	12.5
Morganella morganii	2.5	1.56	12.5	0.78	3.1
Salmonella typhi	2.5	2.0	8.0	0.39	3.1
Neisseria gonorrhoeae	0.02	0.005	0.005	0.015–0.03	0.1
Haemophilus influenzae	0.25	0.15–0.25	0.06	0.015–0.03	–
Pseudomonas aeruginosa	25.0	25.0–50.0	12.5	6.5	6.3
Prevotella melanino-genica	0.1–4.0	0.5–4.0	–	–	–
Bacteroides fragilis	4.0–128.0	1.0–128.0	1.0–128.0	25.0	25.0

Table I.10
Compiled from data published by Adler *et al.* (1971), Sutherland *et al.* (1971), Noguchi *et al.* (1976), Sutter and Finegold (1976), Bodey and Pan (1977), Stewart and Bodey (1977), Ueo *et al.* (1977), Eickhoff and Ehret (1978), Fu and Neu (1978a,b), Wise *et al.* (1978), Reeves *et al.* (1979; 1982), Neu and Labthavikul (1982)

[a] Indole-positive *Proteus* species.

al., 1984; 1985). Against most Enterobacteriaceae, such as *E. coli* and the *Citrobacter*, *Klebsiella*, *Enterobacter*, *Proteus* and *Providencia* spp., it is similar to mezlocillin (p. 162) and piperacillin (p. 164). It is somewhat less inhibitory than these two drugs against *Serratia* spp., but *B. fragilis* is equally sensitive to apalcillin and piperacillin (Table I.10) (Noguchi *et al.*, 1976; Neu and Labthavikul, 1982; Wexler *et al.*, 1984). Other *Pseudomonas* species, such as *Ps. fluorescens*, *Ps. putida*, *Burkholderia* (*Ps.*) *cepacia* and *Stenotrophomonas maltophilia* may be apalcillin-sensitive (Noguchi *et al.*, 1978a). Strains of *Ps. aeruginosa* which are only moderately carbenicillin-resistant (MIC 400–1600 μg per ml) are apalcillin-sensitive; highly carbenicillin-resistant strains (MIC >3200 μg per ml) are moderately apalcillin-resistant (MIC 50–1600 μg per ml) (Noguchi *et al.*, 1978a). *Acinetobacter* spp. is quite sensitive (Allan *et al.*, 1985).

Haemophilus influenzae and *N. gonorrhoeae* are sensitive to apalcillin, but beta-lactamase-producing strains are resistant, as apalcillin is inactivated by TEM-like and other beta-lactamases produced by Gram-negative bacteria (Wretlind *et al.*, 1978). The drug is also active against Gram-positive bacteria, except beta-lactamase-producing strains of *Staph. aureus* (Table I.10) (Noguchi *et al.*, 1976).

5 Minimum inhibitory concentrations

The MICs of mezlocillin, azlocillin, piperacillin and apalcillin, compared with those of ticarcillin, are shown in Table I.10. We are aware of the possible shortcomings of pooling the results of MIC tests performed by many investigators, such as in this table and in others in this book because different laboratory methods are often used. Nevertheless, we believe these tables are useful for quick reference.

Mode of Administration and Dosage

1 Mezlocillin

The usual dosage for adults and children is 200–450 mg per kg body weight per day, given i.m. or more commonly i.v., in six divided doses. Each dose can be injected directly into the i.v. tubing, but it is preferable to give it as an infusion over 15–30 min, as described for penicillin G (p. 20). A common adult dosage for serious infections, is 3 g i.v. 4-hourly or 4 g 6-hourly (Pancoast *et al.*, 1979; Neu 1982; Colaizzi *et al.*, 1986b). Alternatively a dosage of 5 g every 8 h is satisfactory (Flaherty *et al.*, 1987; Janicke *et al.*, 1988). Higher dosages such as 5 g i.v. 6-hourly (Thadepalli and Rao, 1979) or 10 g i.v. 8-hourly (Meunier-Carpentier and Klastersky, 1982), have been used. Some authors have given adults doses as large as 36 g daily (600 mg per kg per day), usually in six divided doses (Parry and Neu, 1982), but this is unnecessary for infections, however severe, caused by sensitive microorganisms. The optimal dosage for children with serious infections is 450 mg per kg per day, given i.v. in six divided doses (Pickering *et al.*, 1982). Similar to piperacillin (p. 168), higher (usually doubled) mezlocillin doses are needed for patients with cystic fibrosis (Bergan, 1981).

For the treatment of uncomplicated urinary tract infections, smaller doses such as 2 g every 8 h, are sufficient (Cox, 1982). Such doses may be conveniently administered by the i.m. route, with or without the addition of lidocaine (Parry and Neu, 1982).

Recommended dosages for newborn infants are:

(a) Preterm infants (gestational age less than 38 weeks) who are 7 days old or younger – 75 mg mezlocillin per kg body weight 12-hourly (150 mg per kg per day).
(b) Preterm infants older than 7 days or term infants 7 days old or younger – 75 mg mezlocillin per kg 8-hourly (225 mg per kg per day).
(c) For term infants older than 7 days a dosage of 75 mg per kg 6-hourly (300 mg per kg per day) is appropriate (Rubio *et al.*, 1982; Janicke *et al.*, 1984).

Patients with renal failure only require slight modification of mezlocillin dosage provided they have normal liver function and relatively low doses are used; under these conditions the mean mezlocillin half-life in normal patients of 1.1 h is only prolonged to 1.6 h in patients with severe renal failure (Bergan *et al.*, 1979). With low mezlocillin dosage (2 g 6-or 8-hourly), dose reduction is only necessary in severe renal failure (creatinine clearance <10 ml per min), when the dosage should only be reduced by approximately 30%. Some mezlocillin is removed by hemodialysis, so that during this procedure the same dosage regimen as for patients with normal renal function can be used. Very little of the drug is removed during peritoneal dialysis, so that reduced dosage is necessary (Kampf *et al.*, 1980; Janicke *et al.*, 1981; Thorsteinsson *et al.*, 1981).

Mezlocillin clearance by both renal and non-renal mechanisms is dose-dependent, and there is a marked decrease of the clearance of the drug by both mechanisms over a 1–5 g dose range (Mangione *et al.*, 1982). According to these authors large mezlocillin dosages (5 g 6-hourly) should be adjusted for all degrees of renal functional impairment, by altering the intervals between the 5 g doses, as shown in Table I.11. Alternatively, the dosing interval may be left unchanged, and individual doses reduced accordingly (Drusano *et al.*, 1984b).

Table I.11
Intervals for 5 g doses of mezlocillin for adults (approx. weight 70 kg) with different degrees of renal failure. (After Mangione *et al.*, 1982, with permission.)

Creatinine clearance (ml per min)	Interval (h)
<10	48
11–25	36
26–40	24
41–80	12
81–120	10
>120	6

Mezlocillin dose should also be reduced in patients with moderate or severe hepatobiliary dysfunction (Meyers *et al.*, 1986). Mezlocillin pharmacokinetics is little altered in women in the postpartum period and a dose of 4–5 g every 8 h appears suitable (Martens *et al.*, 1987).

2 Azlocillin

This drug is given in a dosage of 100–300 mg per kg body weight per day, or occasionally for severe infections 450 mg per kg per day. This is usually administered in four or six divided doses; each dose is given i.v. by a rapid injection or as a 15–30 min infusion by method as described for penicillin G (p. 20). In adults, a dosage varying from 1 to 5 g i.v. 6-hourly may be used depending on the severity of the infection (Ellis *et al.*, 1979; Eykyn, 1982; Levy *et al.*, 1982). The usual adult dosage for severe infection is either 4 g every 6 h or 5 g every 8 h (Lander *et al.*, 1989). In patients with cystic fibrosis, the renal, and to some extent non-renal clearance of azlocillin is much increased, and similar to piperacillin (see below), much higher azlocillin doses (usually at least doubled) are necessary (Bergan, 1981). This recommendation conflicts with findings by Bosso *et al.* (1984), who reported that azlocillin elimination did not appear to be altered in cystic firbrosis patients.

In patients with severe renal failure azlocillin dosage should be reduced. The azlocillin serum half-life is normally 43.7 min, and this increases to 6.53 h in patients with end-stage renal failure. Similar to mezlocillin (see above), azlocillin clearance is dose-dependent. For severe systemic infections in patients with normal renal function, the azlocillin dosage is at least 5 g (80 mg per kg) i.v. every 8 h. This may also be used in patients with renal failure whose creatinine clearance exceeds 30 ml per min. In more severe renal failure (creatinine clearance 10–30 ml per min), dosage should be reduced to 5 g (80 mg per kg) every 12h. In those with a creatinine clearance below 10 ml per min, a loading dose of 5 g (80 mg per kg) can be given followed by 2.5 g (40 mg per kg) 12-hourly. Azlocillin is removed during hemodialysis, and in patients undergoing long-term hemodialysis, 5 g (80 mg per kg) can be given at the end of each dialysis, and then 2.5 g (40 mg per kg) 12-hourly between dialyses (Leroy *et al.*, 1980). During peritoneal dialysis the removal of azlocillin from the body is slow (Whelton *et al.*, 1983).

3 Piperacillin

Both i.m. and i.v. administrations are suitable, but the i.v. route is preferable when large doses are used. The usual dosage is 200–300 mg per kg body weight per day, given in six divided doses (Winston *et al.*, 1980, 1982). A low adult dosage suitable for milder infections, is 4–12 g daily, given in four divided doses; for more serious infections this may be increased to 12–24 g daily, administered in six divided doses (Lutz *et al.*, 1982). Each i.v. dose is usually infused over 15–30 min, as described for penicillin G (p. 20). In children an i.v. dose of 50 mg per kg body weight, administered every 4 h, is recommended (Thirumoorthi *et al.*, 1983). Patients with cystic fibrosis require higher doses to achieve serum levels comparable with those attained in normal patients of similar age; a dosage of 500–600 mg per kg per day, almost twice the normal dosage is required (Prince and Neu, 1980, 1983). Therefore, serum level monitoring and dosage adjustment is necessary in cystic fibrosis patients receiving piperacillin, mezlocillin (p. 167) or azlocillin (see above). Similarly, pregnant patients may require higher doses, as with the usual doses the serum levels of piperacillin are lower. This is because in pregnant patients there is a larger volume of distribution of the drug and also a higher clearance rate (Heikkilä and Erkkola, 1991).

In neonates 75 mg per kg i.v. every 12 h during the first week of life and every 8 h in the second week provide appropriate concentrations in those of less than 36 weeks gestational age. In full-term newborns 75 mg per kg i.v. every 8 h is appropriate during the first week of life, and the same dose 4 times daily should be given thereafter (Kacet *et al.*, 1992).

In patients with mild renal failure, usual piperacillin dosage can probably be used but in moderate renal failure (creatinine clearance 20–40 ml per min), dosage should not exceed 12 g daily (4 g 8-hourly). In patients with severe renal failure (creatinine clearance <20 ml per min) dosage should be reduced to 4 g 12-hourly. Some piperacillin is removed by hemodialysis, so that a 2–4 g i.v. piperacillin dose can be given after each hemodialysis, with a regimen of 4 g 12-hourly being used between dialyses (Francke *et al.*, 1979; Thompson *et al.*, 1981). Other authors recommend only approximately half of the above dosages for patients with both moderate and severe renal failure (Giron *et al.*, 1981a). By contrast, Welling *et al.* (1983) considered that dosage modification is only required in patients with severe renal failure in whom they recommend half the usual doses. In patients with combined severe renal and hepatic insufficiency, a further reduction of piperacillin dosage is necessary (DeSchepper *et al.*, 1982).

Compared with mezlocillin (p. 168), piperacillin has a shorter half-life and an increased clearance rate in postpartum women compared with those for non-pregnant patients (Martens *et al.*, 1987). Some dosage increase may be indicated in these patients.

4 Apalcillin

Daily doses ranging from 0.5 to 6 g, usually administered i.v., have been used in clinical trials in Japan (Miki *et al.*, 1978).

Serum Levels in Relation to Dosage

1 Mezlocillin

After i.v. administration of a 3 g dose given over a 15 min period, the mean peak serum level at the end of the infusion is 269 μg per ml. Thereafter, the serum level falls, and at 6 h it is less than 10 μg per ml. Its half-life (66 min) is similar to that of ampicillin (p. 117) and carbenicillin (p. 152). When 3 g of mezlocillin is given i.v. every 4 h as a 2 h infusion, the peak serum level just after the infusion is over 100 μg per ml, and levels are maintained above 50 μg per ml between infusions (Issell *et al.*, 1978).

If 1 g of mezlocillin is given as a 'bolus' injection i.v. over 4–5 min to normal adults, serum levels are 56.2, 17.2, 2.9 and 0.1 μg per ml at 5 min, 30 min, 2 h and 6 h, respectively. When a 5 g i.v. dose is administered in the same manner, serum levels are 383.5, 145.5, 26.9, 2.2 and 0.4 μg per ml at 5 min, 30 min, 2 h, 6 h and 8 h, respectively (Bergan, 1978). In this study and others, mezlocillin serum levels rose to a greater extent than expected, with increasing dosage. Moreover, its half-life was prolonged with increasing doses; for instance, after a 5 g i.v. dose it was 1.21 h. This occurs because with larger doses there is saturation of the drug's biotransformation in the liver and biliary excretion (p. 170). Renal clearance of the drug is also somewhat reduced when larger mezlocillin doses are used (Mangione *et al.*, 1982; Bergan, 1983).

2 Azlocillin

After a rapid i.v. injection of 1 g (15 mg per kg body weight), the peak serum level at 5 min is 92.93 μg per ml, and the drug is undetectable in the serum at 8 h. At the end of a 30 min infusion of 5 g azlocillin (80 mg per kg), the serum level is 409 μg per ml, and it is still 2.6 μg per ml 8 h after the infusion. Similar to mezlocillin (see above), the pharmacokinetics of azlocillin change when the dose is increased. With doses of 1–2 g, the serum half-life is 0.7–1.1 h, but with a 5 g dose this is prolonged to 1.2–1.8 h. As the azlocillin dose is increased, increases in serum levels are more than proportional to dose increments; the reasons for this are the same as for mezlocillin (see above). Azlocillin appears to be subject to dose-dependent pharmacokinetics to a higher degree than mezlocillin and piperacillin; with large doses serum levels of azlocillin are higher than those of the other two drugs. As with other penicillins, concomitant administration of probenecid increases and prolongs the serum levels of azlocillin (p. 24) (Fiegel and Becker, 1978; Bergan, 1981; Delgado *et al.*, 1983; Colaizzi *et al.*, 1986a).

3 Piperacillin

After administration of single i.m. doses of 0.5, 1 and 2 g to healthy adults, mean peak serum levels of 4.9, 13.3 and 30.2 μg per ml, respectively, occur at 30–50 min; measurable levels after these three doses are present up to 4, 6 and 8 h, respectively, after dosing. The serum half-life of this drug is 60–80 min after i.m. administration. Immediately after rapid ('bolus') i.v. injections of 1,2, 4 or 6 g of piperacillin, serum levels were 70.7, 199.5, 330.7 and 451.8 μg per ml, respectively. Thereafter, the decline of serum levels was slower after the larger doses (Fig. I.10). After rapid i.v. administration the drug's serum half-life varied from 36 to 63 min, depending on the dose (Tjandramaga *et al.*, 1978).

Similar to mezlocillin and azlocillin, pharmacokinetics of piperacillin are dose-dependent, i.e. increases in the serum level are more than proportional to increments in the dose (Bergan, 1981). The reasons for this are the same as with mezlocillin (see above).

If piperacillin is administered i.v. more slowly, as a 30 min or 2 h infusion, peak serum levels after the infusions are lower than after rapid i.v. injections, but the areas under the curve for each method of administration are the same with comparable doses. All of these methods of i.v. administration of piperacillin appear satisfactory clinically (Evans *et al.*, 1978; Wilson *et al.*, 1982). Like other penicillins, concomitant administration of probenecid (p. 24) increases and prolongs piperacillin serum levels (Tjandramaga *et al.*, 1978).

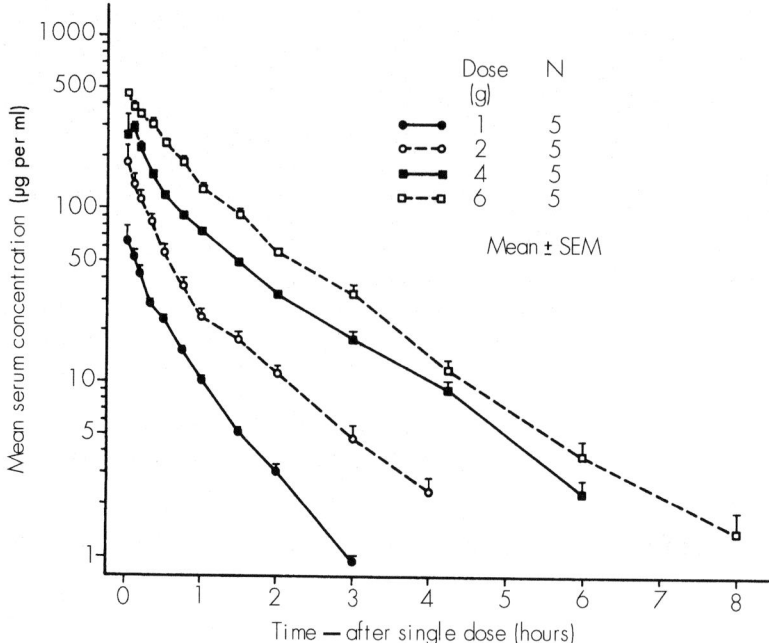

Fig. I.10. Mean serum concentrations of piperacillin after single i.v. injections of 1–6 g in normal volunteers. (Redrawn after Tjjandramaga *et al.*, 1978, with permission.)

4 Apalcillin

When a 2 g dose of apalcillin is infused i.v. over 15 min, the mean peak serum level 5 min after the infusion is 218.6 μg per ml. This level decreases to 59, 7.1 and 0.9 μg per ml after 1, 4 and 8 h after the infusion, respectively. When compared with piperacillin (p. 169), peak serum levels are the same, but apalcillin has a longer terminal half-life. Concentrations of piperacillin are below measurable levels 8 h after a 2 g i.v. infusion whereas concentrations of apalcillin are still measurable at 10 h (Lode *et al.*, 1984).

Excretion

1 Urine

Mezlocillin, azlocillin and piperacillin are excreted unchanged in the urine by both glomerular filtration and tubular secretion. Approximately 50–80% of an i.v. dose of these drugs is eliminated via the kidneys in an unchanged form (Bergan, 1978; Fiegel and Becker, 1978; Meyers *et al.*, 1980). With apalcillin only 18–20% of an administered dose is eliminated renally in the active form (Lode *et al.*, 1984).

With dose increments, an increasing proportion of all these drugs are recovered unchanged in the urine; for instance, with azlocillin 61% is recovered in the urine after a 1 g dose compared with 69% after a 5 g dose (Bergan, 1978). This is because with higher doses non-renal mechanisms for drug elimination are saturated (p. 169). Probenecid decreases renal excretion of these penicillins by partial blockage of renal tubular secretion (p. 24). High concentrations of the active form of all these drugs are attained in the urine after usual i.m. or i.v. doses.

2 Bile

Significant amounts of mezlocillin, azlocillin, piperacillin and apalcillin are eliminated via the bile. Provided the biliary tract is not obstructed, high biliary concentrations are attained. Piperacillin biliary concentrations in the common duct were in the range of 31–920 μg per ml, 35–90 min after an i.v. dose of 1 g, in postoperative patients after cholecystectomy (Giron *et al.*, 1981b). After i.v. administration of a 5 g dose of piperacillin to patients undergoing biliary tract surgery, peak levels in bile exceeded 4000 μg per ml, but in one patient with cystic duct obstruction, levels in the gall bladder bile were subtherapeutic (Russo *et al.*, 1982). In one study biliary excretion of piperacillin was assessed in 11 patients with obstructive jaundice due to cholangiocarcinoma. After a 1 g i.v. dose no drug was detected in bile in the majority of patients. In the others bile levels were much lower than serum levels. After a period of external biliary drainage of up to 28 days, levels of antibiotic in bile after i.v. administration were only minimally increased, although liver function was improved as judged by fall of serum bilirubin (Blenkharn *et al.*, 1985). With azlocillin in patients after biliary surgery, a mean peak biliary concentration of 1137 µg per ml occurred 1.0–1.5 h after a 2 g i.v. dose (Bergan, 1981). In ten patients after cholecystectomy with a T-tube *in situ*, i.m. injection of 1 g of mezlocillin resulted in a mean biliary peak concentration of 295.7 µg per ml (Brogard *et al.*, 1980). With apalcillin in patients with T-tube bile drainage and no biliary obstruction, high biliary concentrations were attained after the usual therapeutic doses, and biliary recovery over a 12 h period amounted to some 12% of the dose (Brogard *et al.*, 1984). The percentage of these drugs eliminated via bile may increase in patients with impaired hepatic function; this is probably because there is less biotransformation in the liver (see below). (Bergan, 1981).

The proportion of an administered dose, which is eliminated via the bile varies considerably from patient to patient. Gundert-Remy *et al.* (1982) found that biliary elimination of mezlocillin ranged from 26.65 to 0.05% of the administered dose, and this did not correlate with renal function. Biliary concentrations and clearance of mezlocillin were low in patients with cholelithiasis. In patients with T-tube drainage following cholecystectomy, after i.v. doses of 2 and 4 g, 22.1% and 14.2% of the administered doses, respectively, were excreted in the bile. These findings suggest a capacity limited, dose-dependent process of biliary excretion.

3 Inactivation in body

Unexcreted mezlocillin, azlocillin, piperacillin and apalcillin are probably inactivated in the body, presumably chiefly in the liver. Only small amounts of inactive metabolites such as penicilloate have been identified in the serum (Bergan, 1981).

Distribution of the Drugs in Body

Mezlocillin, azlocillin, piperacillin and apalcillin are distributed in the body in a similar manner. Mezlocillin levels were quite high in pleural and ascitic fluid (Pancoast *et al.*, 1979), but mezlocillin and piperacillin penetrated poorly into bronchial secretions, where concentrations of only 1–5 µg per ml were attained with usual doses (Pancoast *et al.*, 1979, 1981). Azlocillin may pass into these secretions better than mezlocillin (Bergan, 1981). Apalcillin penetrates into bronchial secretions; a mean peak value of 5.8 µg per ml was attained 2 h after an i.v. dose of 30 mg per kg body weight (Bergogne-Berezin *et al.*, 1984). Mezlocillin, azlocillin and piperacillin penetrated well into interstitial and wound fluids, but after usual doses only low levels were reached in normal bone (Bergan, 1981). Twenty-eight adult patients undergoing open heart surgery were given 4 g piperacillin i.v. preoperatively, which resulted in a serum level of 173.8 which declined to 14.4 µg per ml in 6 h. Mean concentrations in cardiac valvular tissue were 48 µg per g at 0.5–1.0 h, and 11.8 µg per g, 4–5 h after piperacillin administration; mean subcutaneous and muscle concentrations varied from 11.8 to 7.1 µg per g during this time (Daschner *et al.*, 1982). Mezlocillin also penetrated well into heart valves and papillary muscles (Bergan, 1981), and into human prostatic tissue (Naber and Adam, 1983). Azlocillin crossed the placenta and attained high concentrations in fetal tissues (Kafetzis *et al.*, 1983).

In animals these penicillins penetrate poorly into normal CSF. Mezlocillin and azlocillin penetrate much better when bacterial meningitis is induced, when CSF concentrations of 13.5% and 13.3%, of steady-state serum concentrations, respectively, can be attained (Hodges and Worley, 1982). Piperacillin was used to treat four patients with bacterial meningitis (three *Ps. aeruginosa*, one *Flavobacterium meningosepticum*) in a dosage ranging from 324 to 436 mg per kg body weight per day given by continuous i.v. infusion. This resulted in a mean CSF level of 23 µg per ml 24 h after starting therapy, which was 32% of the mean serum level at the time (Dickinson *et al.*, 1981). In another patient with *Ps. aeruginosa* meningitis treated by azlocillin 5 g 6-hourly i.v., CSF concentrations were 42–125 µg per ml, when serum levels were 137–460 µg per ml (Eykyn, 1982). Similarly, apalcillin penetrated poorly into the CSF of patients with normal meninges, but in patients with bacterial meningitis CSF levels of 5–30 µg per ml were reached after usual therapeutic doses (Raoult *et al.*, 1985).

The serum protein binding of these drugs, as in the case of all penicillins (p. 95), depends on their serum concentration. At concentrations of 200 µg per ml, mezlocillin is 27% and azlocillin 30% protein bound. For piperacillin the mean protein binding is 16% at concentrations in the range of 200–300 µg per ml (Bergan, 1981).

Mode of Action

The mode of action of these penicillins on bacteria is similar to that of penicillin G (p. 25). Their increased activity against *Ps. aeruginosa* and other Gram-negative bacilli, is mainly due to an ability to pass through the various layers of the cell envelope to reach their target PBPs (p. 27). Mezlocillin, azlocillin, piperacillin and apalcillin have an increased affinity for PBP3, and a lesser affinity for PBP 1 and 2 of both *E. coli* and *Ps. aeruginosa*. PBP3 is an enzyme, septal murein synthetase, which is responsible for septum formation during bacterial growth and cell division. Inhibition of this enzyme results in the formation of non-viable and readily lyzed filamentous bacteria (Noguchi *et al.*, 1978b; Neu, 1983; Prince and Neu, 1983). Piperacillin-resistant *Ps. aeruginosa* strains with modified PBP, particularly PBP3, have emerged *in vivo* during piperacillin treatment of *Pseudomonas* infections in patients with cystic fibrosis (p. 165).

Toxicity

1 Hypersensitivity reactions

Mezlocillin, azlocillin and piperacillin may provoke any of the reactions which occur with penicillin G (p. 28). These drugs are contraindicated in patients with a history of penicillin hypersensitivity. Parry and Neu (1982) evaluated 1148 mezlocillin treated patients for adverse reactions. Hypersensitivity, manifested by drug fever, skin rashes or eosinophilia occurred in 0.3%, 1.8% and 2.2% of treated patients, respectively. Eykyn (1982) reported one patient treated with azlocillin and tobramycin who had a severe hypersensitivity reaction after 18 days of therapy; she developed fever, malaise, rash, eosinophilia and leukopenia, and recovered rapidly when both antibiotics were ceased. In a survey of 485 hospitalized patients treated by piperacillin, the frequency of hypersensitivity reactions, such as drug fever, rashes, pruritus and eosinophilia, was approximately 4% (Gooding *et al.*, 1982). Among 63 patients whose chronic *Pseudomonas* osteomyelitis was treated with high doses of extended spectrum penicillins for prolonged periods, side-effects such as rash, drug fever and eosinophilia were more common in patients treated with ureidopenicillins than those treated with carbenicillin (Lang *et al.*, 1991).

2 Neurotoxicity

High doses of these drugs given i.v., similar to 'massive' doses of penicillin G (p. 32) and carbenicillin (p. 153), may have the propensity to cause neurotoxicity.

3 Bleeding disorders

Similar to carbenicillin and ticarcillin (p. 153), mezlocillin, azlocillin, piperacillin and apalcillin can cause a disturbance of platelet function (Dijkmans *et al.*, 1980; Gentry *et al.*, 1981). Mezlocillin, piperacillin and apalcillin have a lesser effect on platelet function than carbenicillin and ticarcillin at an equivalent dosage (Gentry *et al.*, 1981, 1985; Copelan *et al.*, 1983; Ballard *et al.*, 1984). A prolonged bleeding time has been observed in a few patients receiving azlocillin (Dijkmans *et al.*, 1980), but clinical bleeding has not been reported (Gooding *et al.*, 1982; Parry and Neu, 1982).

4 Neutropenia and thrombocytopenia

As with carbenicillin and ticarcillin (p. 154) and other beta-lactam antibiotics (p. 33), reversible neutropenia can occur during therapy with mezlocillin, azlocillin and piperacillin (Eykyn, 1982; Gooding *et al.*, 1982; Parry and Neu, 1982). This side-effect is more common with these penicillins compared with carbenicillin. Thrombocytopenia can also rarely occur (Lang *et al.*, 1991; Olivera *et al.*, 1992; Gharpure *et al.*, 1993).

5 Hepatotoxicity

Reversible hepatotoxicity, mainly manifested by elevated enzymes such as serum alkaline phosphatase, SGOT and SGPT, has been noted in 0.9% of mezlocillin-treated patients (Parry and Neu, 1982). One patient with severe cholestatic jaundice caused by mezlocillin has been reported (Hargreaves and Herchline, 1992). Elevations of hepatic enzymes and slight elevations of the serum bilirubin occurred in 3% of patients treated with piperacillin; one patient developed cholestatic hepatitis which reappeared with increased severity upon rechallenge with the drug (Gooding *et al.*, 1982).

6 Electrolyte and acid-base disturbance

An advantage of these penicillins is that their sodium content per gram is less than half that of carbenicillin and ticarcillin, thus decreasing the risk of fluid overload and hypokalemia when high doses are used (Eliopoulos and Moellering, 1982). The sodium contents per gram of mezlocillin and piperacillin are 1.8 and 1.98 mEq, respectively, compared with a value of 4.7 mEq for carbenicillin (p. 154). In one comparative study, antibiotic-related hypokalemia occurred less frequently in patients treated with combined piperacillin/amikacin than in those receiving carbenicillin/amikacin (Winston *et al.*, 1982), but in another trial, roughly equal proportions of patients treated by either piperacillin/gentamicin or carbenicillin/gentamicin developed hypokalemia (Kohler *et al.*, 1982).

7 Other side-effects

Some patients have developed nausea and diarrhea associated with parenteral use of these drugs. Azlocillin and probably also other drugs of this group induce marked changes in colon microflora (Nord *et al.*, 1986). A positive Coombs' test has developed in a few patients treated by either mezlocillin or piperacillin, but hemolytic anemia has not been observed. Renal function deteriorated in two patients during mezlocillin therapy, but this reverted to normal when the drug was ceased (Gooding *et al.*, 1982; Parry and Neu, 1982). Surprisingly, in one study, side-effects characteristic of gentamicin (p. 466), such as nephrotoxicity and ototoxicity, were more common when gentamicin was combined with mezlocillin, compared with a gentamicin/ticarcillin combination; these regimens were used to treat febrile episodes in neutropenic patients (Rankin *et al.*, 1984). By contrast, in a prospective randomized trial in which netilmicin (p. 527) was combined with either mezlocillin, piperacillin, ticarcillin or cefoperazone, cases of nephro- and ototoxicity were not correlated with any particular beta-lactam (Noone *et al.*, 1985). Two patients have been described who developed acute interstitial nephritis and mezlocillin alone was implicated as the cause (Cushner *et al.*, 1985).

Among 4000 patients treated by apalcillin, 18 developed increased creatinine levels; in five of these apalcillin was possibly responsible. When apalcillin was studied in normal volunteers, no nephrotoxicity was observed (Fillastre *et al.*, 1988).

In animals piperacillin appears to protect against gentamicin-induced nephrotoxicity (Hayashi *et al.*, 1988). Similarly the drug protects against cisplatin (an antitumour chemotherapeutic agent) induced renal damage in rats (Hayashi *et al.*, 1989).

Clinical Uses of the Drugs

1 Mezlocillin

This drug has no special advantages for the treatment of *Ps. aeruginosa* infections, but it has been used with success for the treatment of moderate and severe infections caused by other sensitive Gram-negative aerobic and anaerobic bacilli (Ellis *et al.*, 1979; Thadepalli and Rao, 1979). Mezlocillin is quite effective in the treatment of septicemia (Neu, 1982; Bjorvatn *et al.*, 1983), pneumonia, peritonitis and infections of the urinary tract, skin and soft tissue, bone and joint and the biliary tract caused by susceptible Gram-negative and Gram-positive aerobic and anaerobic bacteria (Pancoast *et al.*, 1979; Konopka *et al.*, 1982; Sanders, 1982b).

Mezlocillin is inadequate if used as a single drug in empiric therapy of granulocytopenic and other immunocompromised patients with fever (Issell and Bodey, 1980; Wade *et al.*, 1980). If it is combined with an aminoglycoside, such as gentamicin or netilmicin, it is more effective, but results are comparable with those obtained with ticarcillin plus an aminoglycoside (Melikian *et al.*, 1981; Hanson *et al.*, 1982; Sage *et al.*, 1988).

Mezlocillin, as a single preoperative dose of 5 g or three mezlocillin doses 8-hourly have been tried as prophylaxis of wound infection after appendicectomy, biliary and colorectal surgery. Some authors have found mezlocillin alone as good as cefuroxime plus metronidazole for the prevention of wound infection after large bowel surgery (Stubbs *et al.*, 1987; Diamond *et al.*, 1988). Others, whilst finding these two regimens equally satisfactory following appendicectomy, biliary and gastroesophageal surgery, found that in patients undergoing colorectal surgery, mezlocillin was inferior (wound infection rate 30.2%) to cefuroxime/metronidazole (wound infection rate 11.5%) (Cann *et al.*, 1988).

An infant with *Flavobacterium meningosepticum* meningitis and ventriculitis was cured by a synergistic combination of mezlocillin and cefoxitin, when previous therapy with erythromycin and rifampicin had failed (Kelsey *et al.*, 1982). *In vitro* and *in vivo* antagonism between mezlocillin and cefoxitin can occur with some Gram-negative bacilli (p. 164). Data from *in vitro* studies and animal experiments suggest that mezlocillin should be effective for the treatment of *Enterococcus faecalis* infections, and a mezlocillin/gentamicin combination may be effective for *E. faecalis* endocarditis (Fass and Wright, 1984). Mezlocillin is unlikely to be superior to penicillin G (p. 42) or ampicillin (p. 124) for this purpose. Animal experiments also indicate that mezlocillin may be about as effective as ampicillin (p. 124) for the treatment of serious *L. monocytogenes* infections such as meningitis (Odio *et al.*, 1984b).

2 Azlocillin

Being more active than ticarcillin and mezlocillin *in vitro* against *Ps. aeruginosa*, this drug has been mainly used for *Pseudomonas* infections. It is quite effective in serious *Ps. aeruginosa* infections, such as septicemia, meningitis, bronchopneumonia and urinary tract infections (Ellis and Walter, 1979; Eykyn, 1982; Vestin *et al.*, 1982; Neu *et al.*, 1983). Azlocillin plus an aminoglycoside such as tobramycin is synergistic *in vitro* against *Ps. aeruginosa* (p. 490) and *in vivo* it is satisfactory treatment for infections in neutropenic cancer patients (Klastersky *et al.*, 1986; Gibson *et al.*, 1989; Kibbler *et al.*, 1989). A double beta-lactam combination of azlocillin plus ceftazidime is also satisfactory for the treatment of these patients (Kibbler *et al.*, 1989).

Cystic fibrosis patients with acute exacerbations of pulmonary infection, were treated randomly with either ticarcillin/tobramycin, azlocillin/tobramycin or azlocillin alone, for 10 days. All three regimens had similar beneficial effects on pulmonary function and sputum bacterial concentration. Antibiotic resistance, particularly of *Ps. aeruginosa*, developed more frequently in patients treated by azlocillin alone (McLaughlin *et al.*, 1983). Others have noted the emergence of azlocillin-resistant *Ps. aeruginosa* in patients with cystic fibrosis, if the drug is used singly. When azlocillin is used for such patients it should be combined with an aminoglycoside (Michalsen and Bergan, 1981; Levy *et al.*, 1982).

Azlocillin is quite effective for the treatment of *Ps. aeruginosa* infections, but it has not been proved to be clinically superior to carbenicillin or ticarcillin (p. 156) (Bodey *et al.*, 1983). For the treatment of *Ps. aeruginosa* endocarditis ticarcillin plus an aminoglycoside is preferred (see below) (Reyes and Lerner, 1983). Azlocillin was also not superior to ticarcillin for the treatment of *Ps. aeruginosa* infections in irradiated neutropenic mice (Van der Voet *et al.*, 1985).

3 Piperacillin

Similar to mezlocillin, this has been used successfully to treat moderate and severe infections caused by sensitive Gram-negative aerobic and anaerobic bacteria e.g. septicemia, pneumonia, peritonitis and urinary tract, skin and soft tissue and bone and joint infections. It has been especially useful for patients with Gram-negative rod infections, for whom further aminoglycoside therapy was contraindicated (Winston *et al.*, 1980; Pancoast *et al.*, 1981; Gooding *et al.*, 1982). In an uncontrolled trial, Morris *et al.* (1983) found the drug satisfactory for chemoprophylaxis in patients undergoing elective biliary surgery. A dose of 2 g i.m. was given 2 h before surgery, followed by 2 g i.v. at the beginning of the operation. All patients undergoing biliary surgery do not warrant chemoprophylaxis, and other drugs are also suitable for this purpose (p. 125). Piperacillin can be used for the treatment of acute cholangitis, but if resistant strains of *E. coli* and *Klebsiella* spp. are likely to be present, an aminoglycoside such as gentamicin (p. 475), should be added (Van den Hazel *et al.*, 1994). In one trial postpartum endometritis, where facultative and anaerobic bacteria, genital *Mycoplasma* and *Chlamydia trachomatis* were involved, piperacillin proved to be an equally successful treatment to cefoxitin 2 g every 6 h (Rosene *et al.*, 1986). Aerobic Gram-negative bacilli including *Ps. aeruginosa* are involved in early infections after liver transplantation and a combination such as piperacillin plus an aminoglycoside is appropriate for chemoprophylaxis and early treatment (George *et al.*, 1991).

Piperacillin is suitable for initial empiric therapy of febrile granulocytopenic patients. As with mezlocillin (see above), it is preferable to combine it with an aminoglycoside; if piperacillin is used as a single agent for the treatment of serious infections of this type, emergence of resistant organisms during therapy may be a problem (Gribble *et al.*, 1983; Drusano *et al.*, 1984b). A piperacillin/amikacin combination is equally effective as a carbenicillin or ticarcillin/amikacin or ceftazidime/amikacin combination in febrile granulocytopenic patients (Klastersky, 1982; Winston *et al.*, 1982; Rawlinson *et al.*, 1988; Sage *et al.*, 1988; Feliu *et al.*, 1992). Piperacillin/gentamicin and carbenicillin/gentamicin combinations had similar efficacy in patients with serious Gram-negative infections (Kohler *et al.*, 1982). Use of piperacillin in such combinations may be associated with a lesser frequency of side-effects, such as bleeding, hepatotoxicity and hypokalemia (p. 172) (Gooding *et al.*, 1982; Marier *et al.*, 1982).

Piperacillin is useful for the treatment of *Ps. aeruginosa* infections (Tosolini *et al.*, 1985), but despite its superior *in vitro* activity (p. 164), it is not clinically superior to carbenicillin or ticarcillin (Bodey *et al.*, 1983). It has been used with some success to treat acute exacerbations of pulmonary disease in patients with cystic fibrosis (Prince and Neu, 1980). Some authors have found piperacillin alone as effective as ticarcillin/tobramycin for these patients (Jackson *et al.*,

1986); others considered piperacillin/tobramycin superior to piperacillin alone (Hoogkamp-Korstanje and Van der Laag, 1983). When piperacillin has been used to treat difficult *Ps. aeruginosa* infections such as pneumonia and those of the urinary tract, relapses accompanied by the development of piperacillin-resistant *Ps. aeruginosa* strains have been observed (Simon *et al.*, 1980). Therefore, combination therapy with piperacillin and an aminoglycoside is preferable for serious Gram-negative infections, especially if *Ps. aeruginosa* is the pathogen. Reyes and Lerner (1983) treated eight consecutive patients with *Ps. aeruginosa* endocarditis by a regimen of 24 g i.v. piperacillin plus tobramycin 8 mg per kg body weight daily; treatment was unsuccessful in all cases. *Ps. aeruginosa* isolates were initially beta-lactamase-negative, but strains recovered later from blood had higher MICs for piperacillin and produced beta-lactamases. Similar failure of *Ps. aeruginosa* endocarditis to piperacillin/tobramycin therapy has been recorded by others (Jimenez-Lucho *et al.*, 1986; Letendre *et al.*, 1988). Piperacillin is less stable to inducible chromosomally mediated beta-lactamase(s) than carbenicillin and ticarcillin (p. 145); it also may be a better enzyme inducer. As a result of this experience, Reyes and Lerner (1983) recommended a ticarcillin/tobramycin combination for treatment of *Ps. aeruginosa* endocarditis (p. 156).

4 Aminoglycoside inactivation

Mezlocillin, azlocillin and piperacillin, similar to carbenicillin (p. 155) and ticarcillin (p. 157), inactivate aminoglycosides *in vitro* and *in vivo* (Farchione, 1981). When carbenicillin and piperacillin are used in the same concentrations *in vivo*, the former inactivates aminoglycosides more rapidly. This is not so *in vitro,* where both drugs inactivate gentamicin to a similar degree. This is probably because gentamicin has less contact with high piperacillin serum concentrations due to the increased rate of non-renal elimination of piperacillin, especially in patients with renal failure (p. 168) (Thompson *et al.*, 1982). Tobramycin followed by gentamicin are the most rapidly inactivated aminoglycosides, but amikacin is quite resistant to effect by these penicillins (Hale *et al.*, 1980). Clinically, inactivation is most likely to occur when one of these drugs is combined with an aminoglycoside in patients with renal failure (Lau *et al.*, 1983). In one study, patients with end-stage renal failure were treated either by piperacillin 4 g i.v. 12-hourly, or by carbenicillin 2 g i.v. 8-hourly. When gentamicin in a single dose of 2 mg per kg body weight was added to these regimens, gentamicin half-lives were 37.7 h and 19.4 h, in patients receiving piperacillin or carbenicillin, respectively (Thompson *et al.*, 1982). When the same dose of gentamicin was given alone to these patients, its half-life was 61.6 h, indicating that piperacillin inactivated gentamicin *in vivo*, albeit more slowly than carbenicillin. Serum level monitoring and aminoglycoside dosage adjustment (except perhaps for amikacin), are necessary when these drug combinations are used in patients with renal failure (Walterspeel *et al.*, 1991; Halstenson *et al.*, 1992).

References.

Adler JL, Burke JP, Wilcox C, Finland M (1971). Susceptibility of *Proteus* species and *Pseudomonas aeruginosa* to penicillins and cephalosporins. *Antimicrob Ag Chemother* 1970: 63.

Allan JD, Eliopoulos GM, Ferraro MJ, Moellering RC Jr (1985). Comparative *in vitro* activities of cefpiramide and apalcillin individually and in combination. *Antimicrob Ag Chemother* 27: 782.

Anwar H, Costerton JW (1990). Enhanced activity of combination of tobramycin and piperacillin for eradication of sessile biofilm cells of *Psudomonas aeruginosa. Antimicrob Ag Chemother* 34: 1666.

Ballard JO, Barnes SG, Sattler FR (1984). Comparison of the effects of mezlocillin, carbenicillin, and placebo on normal hemostasis. *Antimicrob Ag Chemother* 25: 153.

Bansal MB, Thadepalli H (1983). Antimicrobial effect of beta-lactam antibiotic combinations against *Bacteroides fragilis* in vitro. *Antimicrob Ag Chemother* 23: 166.

Barry AL, Jones RN, Ayers LW *et al.* (1984). *In vitro* activity of apalcillin compared with those of piperacillin and carbenicillin against 6797 bacterial isolates from four separate medical centers. *Antimicrob Ag Chemother* 25: 669.

Barry AL, Jones RN, Thornsberry C (1985). Apalcillin (PC-904).: spectrum of activity and beta-lactamase hydrolysis/inhibition. *Diagn Microbiol Infect Dis* 3: 7.

Bell SM, Pham JN, Lanzarone JYM (1985). Mutation of *Pseudomonas aeruginosa* to piperacillin resistance mediated by beta-lactamase production. *J Antimicrob Chemother* 15: 665.

Bergan T (1978). Pharmacokinetics of mezlocillin in healthy volunteers. *Antimicrob Ag Chemother* 14: 801.

Bergan T (1981). Overview of acylureidopenicillin pharmacokinetics. *Scand J Infect Dis* (Suppl 29): 33.

Bergan T (1983). Review of the pharmacokinetics of mezlocillin. *J Antimicrob Chemother* 11 (Suppl C): 1.

Bergan T, Brodwall EK, Wiik-Larsen E (1979). Mezlocillin pharmacokinetics in patients with normal and impaired renal functions. *Antimicrob Ag Chemother* 16: 651.

Bergogne-Berezin E, Pierre J, Chastre J *et al.* (1984). Pharmacokinetics of apalcillin in intensive-care patients: study of penetration into the respiratory tract. *J Antimicrob Chemother* 14: 67.

Bertram MA, Young LS (1984). Imipenem antagonism of the *in vitro* activity of piperacillin against *Pseudomonas aeruginosa*. *Antimicrob Ag Chemother* **26**: 272.

Bjorvatn B, Schultz TB, Haug BI *et al.* (1983). Mezlocillin treatment of septicemia in general hospitals. *Scand J Infect Dis* **15**: 81.

Blenkharn JI, Habib N, Mok D *et al.* (1985). Decreased biliary excretion of piperacillin after percutaneous relief of extrahepatic obstructive jaundice. *Antimicrob Ag Chemother* **28**:778.

Bodey GP, Pan T (1977). Mezlocillin: *in vitro* studies of a new broad-spectrum penicillin. *Antimicrob Ag Chemother* **11**: 74.

Bodey GP, Bolivar R, Fainstein V, Jadeja L (1983). Infections caused by *Pseudomonas aeruginosa*. *Rev Infect Dis* **5**: 279.

Boisivon A, Guiomar C, Gutmann L (1988). Interaction between piper-acillin and pefloxacin or amikacin on the selection of resistant mutants of *Pseudomonas aeruginosa*. *J Antimicrob Chemother* **22**: 651.

Bosso JA, Saxon BA, Herbst JJ, Matsen JM (1984). Azlocillin pharmacokinetics in patients with cystic fibrosis. *Antimicrob Ag Chemother* **25**: 630.

Bowie WR (1982). Lack of *in vitro* activity of cefoxitin, cefamandole, cefuroxime and piperacillin against *Chlamydia trachomatis*. *Antimicrob Ag Chemother* **21**: 339.

Brogard J-M, Kopferschmitt J, Arnaud J-P *et al.* (1980). Biliary elimination of mezlocillin: an experimental and clinical study. *Antimicrob Ag Chemother* **18**: 69.

Brogard J-M, Arnaud J-P, Blickle JF, Lavillaureix J (1984). Biliary elimination of apalcillin in humans. *Antimicrob Ag Chemother* **26**: 428.

Cann KJ, Watkins RM, George C *et al.* (1988). A trial of mezlocillin versus cefuroxime with or without metronidazole for the prevention of wound sepsis after biliary and gastrointestinal surgery. *J Hosp Infect* **12**: 207.

Chin N-X, Neu HC (1983). Synergy of azlocillin with aminoglycosides. *J Antimicrob Chemother* **11** (Suppl B): 33.

Chow AW, Cheng N, Bartlett KH (1985). *In vitro* susceptibility of *Clostridium difficile* to new beta-lactam and quinolone antibiotics. *Antimicrob Ag Chemother* **28**: 842.

Collaizzi PA, Polk RE, Poynor WJ *et al.* (1986a). Comparative pharmacokinetics of azlocillin and piperacillin in normal adults. *Antimicrob Ag Chemother* **29**: 938.

Collaizzi PA, Coniglio AA, Poynor WJ *et al.* (1986b). Comparative pharmacokinetics of two multiple-dose mezlocillin regimens in normal volunteers. *Antimicrob Ag Chemother* **30**: 675.

Copelan EA, Kusumi RK, Miller L, Fass RJ (1983). A comparison of the effects of mezlocillin and carbenicillin on haemostasis in volunteers. *J Antimicrob Chemother* **11** (Suppl C): 43.

Coppens L, Klastersky J (1979). Comparative study of anti-*Pseudomonas* activity of azlocillin, mezlocillin and ticarcillin. *Antimicrob Ag Chemother* **15**: 396.

Cox CE (1982). Multi-institutional study of mezlocillin therapy of urinary tract infections. *J Antimicrob Chemother* **9** (Suppl A): 173.

Cuchural G, Jacobus N, Gorbach SL, Tally FP (1981). A survey of *Bacteroides* susceptibility in the United States. *J Antimicrob Chemother* **8** (Suppl D): 27.

Cushner HM, Copley JB, Bauman J, Hill SC (1985). Acute interstitial nephritis associated with mezlocillin, nafcillin, and gentamicin treatment for *Pseudomonas* infection. *Arch Intern Med* **145**: 1204.

Daschner FD, Just M, Spillner G, Schlosser V (1982). Penetration of piperacillin into cardiac valves, subcutaneous and muscle tissue of patients undergoing open-heart surgery. *J Antimicrob Chemother* **9**: 489.

Delgado FA, Stout RL, Whelton A (1983). Pharmacokinetics of azlocillin in normal renal function: single and repetitive dosing studies. *J Antimicrob Chemother* **11** (Suppl B): 79.

De Schepper PJ, Tjandramaga TB, Mullie A *et al.* (1982). Comparative pharmacokinetics of piperacillin in normals and in patients with renal failure. *J Antimicrob Chemother* **9** (Suppl B): 49.

Diamond T, Mullholland CK, Hanna WA, Parks TG (1988). A prospective randomized trial to compare triple dose mezlocillin with triple dose cefuroxime plus metronidazole as prophylaxis in colorectal surgery. *J Hosp Infect* **12**: 215.

Dickinson GM, Clearly TJ, Hoffman TA (1978). Comparative evaluation of piperacillin *in vitro*. *Antimicrob Ag Chemother* **14**: 919.

Dickinson GM, Droller DG, Greenman RL, Hoffman TA (1981). Clinical evaluation of piperacillin with observation on penetrability into cerebrospinal fluid. *Antimicrob Ag Chemother* **20**: 481.

Dijkmans BAC, Van der Meer JWM, Boekhout-Mussert MJ *et al.* (1980). Prolonged bleeding time during azlocillin therapy. *J Antimicrob Chemother* **6**: 554.

Dornbusch K and the European Study Group on Antibiotic Resistance (1990). Resistance to beta-lactam antibiotics and ciprofloxacin in Gram-negative bacilli and staphylococci isolated from blood: a European collaborative study. *J Antimicrob Chemother* **26**: 269.

Drusano GL, Forrest A, Fiore D *et al.* (1984a). Effect of saturable clearance during high-dose mezlocillin therapy. *Antimicrob Ag Chemother* **26**: 686.

Drusano GL, Schimpff SC, Hewitt WL (1984b). The acylampicillins: mezlocillin, piperacillin and azlocillin. *Rev Infect Dis* **6**: 13.

Eickhoff TC, Ehret JM (1978). *In vitro* studies of piperacillin, a new broad-spectrum penicillin. In *Current Chemotherapy*: *Proceedings of the 10th International Congress of Chemotherapy, Zurich/Switzerland, 1977* (Siegenthaler W, Lüthy R, eds), p. 598. Washington DC: American Society for Microbiology.

Eliopoulos GM, Moellering RG Jr (1982). Azlocillin, mezlocillin, and piperacillin: new broad-spectrum penicillins. *Ann Intern Med* **97**: 755.

Ellis CJ, Walter PH (1979). *Pseudomonas* meningitis treated with azlocillin. *Brit Med J* **2**: 767.

Ellis CJ, Geddes AM, Davey PG *et al.* (1979). Mezlocillin and azlocillin; an evaluation of two new beta-lactam antibiotics. *J Antimicrob Chemother* **5**: 517.

Evans MAL, Wilson P, Leung T, Williams JD (1978). Pharmacokinetics of piperacillin following intravenous administration. *J Antimicrob Chemother* **4**: 255.

Eykyn SJ (1982). Azlocillin in the treatment of serious infection with *Pseudomonas aeruginosa*. *J Antimicrob Chemother* **9**: 395.

Farchione LA (1981). Inactivation of aminoglycosides by penicillins. *J Antimicrob Chemother* **8** (Suppl A): 27.

Fass RJ (1982a). Comparative *in vitro* activities of azlocillin-cefotaxime and azlocillin-tobramycin combinations against blood and multidrug-resistant bacterial isolates. *Antimicrob Ag Chemother* **22**: 167.

Fass RJ (1982b). Comparative *in vitro* activities of beta-lactam-tobramycin combinations against *Pseudomonas aeruginosa* and multidrug-resistant Gram-negative enteric bacilli. *Antimicrob Ag Chemother* **21**: 1003.

Fass RJ (1983). Statistical comparison of the antibacterial activities of broad-spectrum penicillins against Gram-negative bacilli. *Antimicrob Ag Chemother* **24**: 156.

Fass RJ, Barnishan J (1980). *In vitro* susceptibilities of nonfermentative Gram-negative bacilli other than *Pseudomonas aeruginosa* to 32 antimicrobial agents. *Rev Infect Dis* **2**: 841.

Fass RJ, Wright CA (1984). Comparative efficacies of mezlocillin and ampicillin alone or in combination with gentamicin in the treatment of *Streptococcus faecalis* endocarditis in rabbits. *Antimicrob Ag Chemother* **25**: 408.

Feliu J, Artal A, Baron MG *et al.* (1992). Comparison of two antibiotic regimens (piperacillin plus amikacin versus ceftazidime plus amikacin). as empiric therapy for febrile neutropenic patients with cancer. *Antimicrob Ag Chemother* **36**: 2816.

Fiegel P, Becker K (1978). Pharmacokinetics of azlocillin in persons with normal and impaired renal functions. *Antimicrob Ag Chemother* **14**: 288.

Fillastre J-P, Moulin B, Godin M, Frelon J-H (1988). Is apalcillin nephrotoxic? *Antimicrob Ag Chemother* **32**: 942.

Flaherty JF, Barriere SL, Mordenti J, Gambertoglio JG (1987). Effect of dose on pharmacokinetics and serum bactericidal activity of mezlocillin. *Antimicrob Ag Chemother* **31**: 895.

Francke EL, Appel GB, Neu HC (1979). Pharmacokinetics of intravenous piperacillin in patients undergoing chronic hemodialysis. *Antimicrob Ag Chemother* **16**: 788.

Fu KP, Neu HC (1978a). Piperacillin, a new penicillin active against many bacteria resistant to other penicillins. *Antimicrob Ag Chemother* **13**: 358.

Fu KP, Neu HC (1978b). Azlocillin and mezlocillin: new ureido penicillins. *Antimicrob Ag Chemother* **13**: 390.

Gentry LO, Jamsek JG, Natelson EA (1981). Effect of sodium piperacillin on platelet function in normal volunteers. *Antimicrob Ag Chemother* **19**: 532.

Gentry LO, Wood BA, Natelson EA (1985). Effects of apalcillin on platelet function in normal volunteers. *Antimicrob Ag Chemother* **27**: 683.

George DL, Arnow PM, Fox AS *et al.* (1991). Bacterial infection as a complication of liver transplantation: epidemiology and risk factors. *Rev Infect Dis* **13**: 387.

George WL, Lewis RP, Meyer RD (1978). Susceptibility of cephalothin-resistant Gram-negative bacilli to piperacillin, cefuroxime, and other selected antibiotics. *Antimicrob Ag Chemother* **13**: 484.

Gharpure V, O'Connell B, Schiffer CA (1993). Mezlocillin-induced thrombocytopenia. *Ann Intern Med* **119**: 862.

Gibson J, Benn R, Date L *et al.* (1989). A randomised trial of empirical antibiotic therapy in febrile neutropenic patients with hematological disorders: ceftazidime versus azlocillin plus amikacin. *Aust NZ J Med* **19**: 417.

Giron JA, Meyers BR, Hirschman SZ, Srulevitch E (1981a). Pharmacokinetics of piperacillin in patients with moderate renal failure and in patients undergoing hemodialysis. *Antimicrob Ag Chemother* **19**: 279.

Giron JA, Meyers BR, Hirschman SZ (1981b). Biliary concentrations of piperacillin in patients undergoing cholecystectomy. *Antimicrob Ag Chemother* **19**: 309.

Glew RH, Pavuk RA (1984). Early synergistic interactions between amikacin and six beta-lactam antibiotics against multiply resistant members of the family *Enterobacteriaceae*. *Antimicrob Ag Chemother* **26**: 378.

Godfrey AJ, Bryan LE, Rabin HR (1981). Beta-lactam-resistant *Pseudomonas aeruginosa* with modified penicillin-binding proteins emerging during cystic fibrosis treatment. *Antimicrob Ag Chemother* **19**: 705.

Goldstein EJC, Citron DM, Cherubin CE, Hillier SL (1993). Comparative susceptibility of the *Bacteroides fragilis* group species and other anaerobic bacteria to meropenem, imipenem, piperacillin, cefoxitin, ampicillin/sulbactam, clindamycin and metronidazole. *J Antimicrob Chemother* **31**: 363.

Gooding PG, Clark BJ, Sathe SS (1982). Piperacillin: a review of clinical experience. *J Antimicrob Chemother* **9** (Suppl B): 93.

Gootz TD, Sanders CC, Sanders WE Jr (1979). *In vitro* activity of furazlocillin (Bay K 4999) compared with those of mezlocillin, piperacillin, and standard beta-lactam antibiotics. *Antimicrob Ag Chemother* **15**: 783.

Greenwood D, Eley A (1982). A turbidimetric study of the responses of selected strains of *Pseudomonas aeruginosa* to eight antipseudomonal beta-lactam antibiotics. *J Infect Dis* **145**: 110.

Gribble MJ, Chow AW, Naiman SC *et al.* (1983). Prospective randomized trial of piperacillin monotherapy versus carboxypenicillin-aminoglycoside combination regimens in the empirical treatment of serious bacterial infections. *Antimicrob Ag Chemother* **24**: 388.

Gundert-Remy U, Förster D, Schacht P, Weber E (1982). Kinetics of mezlocillin in patients with biliary t-tube drainage. *J Antimicrob Chemother* **9** (Suppl A): 65.

Gutmann L, Williamson R, Kitzis M-D, Acar JF (1986). Synergism and antagonism in double beta-lactam antibiotic combinations. *Amer J Med* **80(5c)**: 21.

Gwynn MN, Rolinson GN (1983). Selection of variants of Gram-negative bacteria with elevated production of type 1 beta-lactamase. *J Antimicrob Chemother* **11**: 577.

Hale DC, Jenkins R, Matsen JM (1980). *In vitro* inactivation of aminoglycoside antibiotics by piperacillin and carbenicillin. *Amer J Clin Path* **74**: 316.

Halstenson CE, Wong MO, Herman CS *et al.* (1992). Effect of concomitant administration of piperacillin on the disposition of isepamicin and gentamicin in patients with end-stage renal disease. *Antimicrob Ag Chemother* **36**: 1832.

Hammerschlag MR, Gleyzer A (1983). *In vitro* activity of a group of broad-spectrum cephalosporins and other beta-lactam antibiotics against *Chlamydia trachomatis*. *Antimicrob Ag Chemother* **23**: 493.

Hanson B, Coppens L, Klastersky J (1982). Comparative studies of ticarcillin and mezlocillin plus sisomicin in Gram-negative bacillary bacteraemia and broncho-pneumonia. *J Antimicrob Chemother* **10**: 335.

Hargreaves JE, Herchline TE (1992). Severe cholestatic jaundice caused by mezlocillin. *Clin Infect Dis* **15**: 179.

Hawkey PM, Pedler SJ, Turner A (1983). Comparative *in vitro* activity of semi-synthetic penicillins against Proteeae. *Antimicrob Ag Chemother* **23**: 619.

Hayashi T, Watanabe Y, Kumano K *et al.* (1988). Protective effect of piperacillin against nephrotoxicity of cephaloridine and gentamicin in animals. *Antimicrob Ag Chemother* **32**: 912.

Hayashi T, Watanabe Y, Kumano K *et al.* (1989). Protective effect of piperacillin against the nephrotoxicity of cisplatin in rats. *Antimicrob Ag Chemother* **33**: 513.

Heikkilä A, Erkkola R (1991). Pharmacokinetics of piperacillin during pregnancy. *J Antimicrob Chemother* **28**: 419.

Hodges GR, Worley SE (1982). Comparative penetration of azlocillin and mezlocillin into cerebrospinal fluid of normal rabbits and rabbits with experimentally induced *Pseudomonas aeruginosa* meningitis. *Antimicrob Ag Chemother* **22**: 909.

Høiby N, Bremmelgaard A, Schouenborg P (1981). *In vitro* activity of azlocillin, carbenicillin, mezlocillin and piperacillin against *Pseudomonas aeruginosa*. *Scand J Infect Dis* (Suppl 29): 27.

Hoogkamp-Korstanje JAA, Van der Laag J (1983). Piperacillin and tobramycin in the treatment of *Pseudomonas* lung infections in cystic fibrosis. *J Antimicrob Chemother* **12**: 175.

Hoogkamp-Korstanje JAA, Pot CM, Westerdaal NAC (1981). *In vitro* activity of cefoperazone and penicillins alone and in combination with aminoglycosides against *Pseudomonas aeruginosa*. *J Antimicrob Chemother* **8**: 101.

Hoyle BD, Alcantara J, Costerton JW (1992). *Pseudomonas aeruginosa* biofilm as a diffusion barrier to piperacillin. *Antimicrob Ag Chemother* **36**: 2054.

Issell BF, Bodey GP (1980). Mezlocillin for treatment of infections in cancer patients. *Antimicrob Ag Chemother* **17**: 1008.

Issell BF, Bodey GP, Weaver S (1978). Clinical pharmacology of mezlocillin. *Antimicrob Ag Chemother* **13**: 180.

Jackson MA, Kusmiesz H, Shelton S *et al.* (1986). Comparison of piperacillin vs ticarcillin plus tobramycin in the treatment of acute pulmonary exacerbations of cystic fibrosis. *Pediatr Infect Dis* **5**: 440.

Jacobs JY, Livermore DM, Davy KWM (1984). *Pseudomonas aeruginosa* beta-lactamase as a defence against azlocillin, mezlocillin and piperacillin. *J Antimicrob Chemother* **14**: 221.

Janicke DM, Mangione A, Schultz RW, Jusko WJ (1981). Mezlocillin disposition in chronic hemodialysis patients. *Antimicrob Ag Chemother* **20**: 590.

Janicke DM, Rubio TT, Wirth FH Jr *et al.* (1984). Developmental pharmacokinetics of mezlocillin in newborn infants. *J Pediatr* **104**: 773.

Janicke DM, Parker SW, Cafarell RF *et al.* (1988). Pharmacokinetics of two multiple dose mezlocillin regimens. *Antimicrob Ag Chemother* **32**: 777.

Jimenez-Lucho VE, Saravolatz LD, Medeiros AA, Pohlod D (1986). Failure of therapy in *Pseudomonas* endocarditis: selection of resistant mutants. *J Infect Dis* **154**: 64.

Kacet N, Roussel-Delvallez M, Gremillet C *et al.* (1992). Pharmacokinetic study of piperacillin in newborns relating to gestational and postnatal age. *Pediatr Infect Dis J* **11**: 365.

Kafetzis DA, Brater DC, Fanourgakis JE (1983). Materno-fetal transfer of azlocillin. *J Antimicrob Chemother* **12**: 157.

Kampf D, Schurig R, Weihermüller K, Förster D (1980). Effects of impaired renal function, hemodialysis, and peritoneal dialysis on the pharmacokinetics of mezlocillin. *Antimicrob Ag Chemother* **18**: 81.

Kelsey MC, Emmerson AM, Drabu Y (1982). *Flavobacterium meningosepticum* ventriculitis: *in vivo* and *in vitro* results with the combinations rifampicin-erythromycin and mezlocillin-cefoxitin. *Eur J Clin Microbiol* **1**: 138.

Kibbler CC, Prentice HG, Sage RJ et al. (1989). A comparison of double beta-lactam combinations with netilmicin/ureidopenicillin regimens in the empirical therapy of febrile neutropenic patients. *J Antimicrob Chemother* **23**: 759.

Klastersky J (1982). Treatment of severe infections in patients with cancer The role of new acyl-penicillins. *Arch Intern Med* **142**: 1984.

Klastersky J, Glauser MP, Schimpff SC et al. (1986). Prospective randomized comparison of three antibiotic regimens for empirical therapy of suspected bacteremic infection in febrile granulocytopenic patients. *Antimicrob Ag Chemother* **29**: 263.

Koehler JM, Ashdown LR (1993). *In vitro* susceptibilities of tropical strains of *Aeromonas* species from Queensland, Australia, to 22 antimicrobial agents. *Antimicrob Ag Chemother* **37**: 905.

Kohler RB, Foerster LA, Wheat LJ et al. (1982). Piperacillin and gentamicin v carbenicillin and gentamicin for treatment of serious Gram-negative infections. *Arch Intern Med* **142**: 1335.

Konopka CA, Arcieri G, Schacht P (1982). Clinical experience with mezlocillin in Europe – overview. *J Antimicrob Chemother* **9** (Suppl A): 267.

Kuck NA, Testa RT, Forbes M (1981). *In vitro* and *in vivo* antibacterial effects of combinations of beta-lactam antibiotics. *Antimicrob Ag Chemother* **19**: 634.

Kurtz TO, Winston DJ, Bruckner DA, Martin WJ (1981). Comparative *in vitro* synergistic activity of new beta-lactam antimicrobial agents and amikacin against *Pseudomonas aeruginosa* and *Serratia marcescens*. *Antimicrob Ag Chemother* **20**: 239.

Lander RD, Henderson RP, Pyszczynski DR (1989). Pharmacokinetic comparison of 5 g of azlocillin every 8 h and 4 g every 6 h in healthy volunteers. *Antimicrob Ag Chemother* **33**: 710.

Lang R, Lishner M, Ravid M (1991). Adverse reactions to prolonged treatment with high doses of carbenicillin and ureidopenicillins. *Rev Infect Dis* **13**: 68.

Lau A, Lee M, Flascha S et al. (1983). Effect of piperacillin on tobramycin pharmacokinetics in patients with normal renal function. *Antimicrob Ag Chemother* **24**: 533.

Leroy A, Humbert G, Godin M, Fillastre JP (1980). Pharmacokinetics of azlocillin in subjects with normal and impaired renal function. *Antimicrob Ag Chemother* **17**: 344.

Letendre ED, Mantha R, Turgeon PL (1988). Selection of resistance by piperacillin during *Pseudomonas aeruginosa* endocarditis. *J Antimicrob Chemother* **22**: 557.

Levy J, Baran D, Klastersky J (1982). Anti-*Pseudomonas* activity of azlocillin during pulmonary infection in patients with cystic fibrosis. *J Antimicrob Chemother* **10**: 235.

Livermore DM, Yang Y-J (1987). Beta-lactamase lability and inducer power of newer beta-lactam antibiotics in relation to their activity against beta-lactamase-inducibility mutants of *Pseudomonas aeruginosa*. *J Infect Dis* **155**: 775.

Livermore DM, Moosdeen F, Lindridge MA et al. (1986). Behaviour of TEM-1 beta-lactamase as a resistance mechanism to ampicillin, mezlocillin and azlocillin in *Escherichia coli*. *J Antimicrob Chemother* **17**: 139.

Lode H, Elvers A, Koeppe P, Borner K (1984). Comparative pharmacokinetics of apalcillin and piperacillin. *Antimicrob Ag Chemother* **25**: 105.

Lutz B, Mogabgab W, Holmes B et al. (1982). Clinical evaluation of the therapeutic efficacy and tolerability of piperacillin. *Antimicrob Ag Chemother* **22**: 10.

Lyon MD, Smith KR, Saag MS et al. (1986). *In vitro* activity of piperacillin, ticarcillin, and mezlocillin alone and in combination with aminoglycosides against *Pseudomonas aeruginosa*. *Antimicrob Ag Chemother* **30**: 25.

Magnussen CR, Sammartino MT, Ernest KD (1982). Aminoglycoside-resistant Gram-negative bacilin in a community hospital: comparative *in*

vitro activity of cefotaxime, moxalactam, cefoperazone, and piperacillin. *Antimicrob Ag Chemother* **22**: 154.

Mandell WF, Garvey GJ, Neu HC (1987). *Achromobacter xylosoxidans* bacteremia. *Rev Infect Dis* **9**: 1001.

Mangione A, Boudinot FD, Schultz RM, Jusko WJ (1982). Dose-dependent pharmacokinetics of mezlocillin in relation to renal impairment. *Antimicrob Ag Chemother* **21**: 428.

Marier RL, Sanders CV, Faro S et al. (1982). Piperacillin v carbenicillin in the therapy for serious infections. *Arch Intern Med* **142**: 2000.

Martens MG, Faro S, Feldman S et al. (1987). Pharmacokinetics of the acylureidopenicillins piperacillin and mezlocillin in the postpartum patient. *Antimicrob Ag Chemother* **31**: 2015.

McAllister TA (1982). Piperacillin against clinical isolates: antimicrobial profile and clinical role. *J Antimicrob Chemother* **9** (Suppl B): 75.

McLaughlin FJ, Matthews WJ Jr, Strieder DJ et al. (1983). Clinical and bacteriological responses to three antibiotic regimens for acute exacerbations of cystic fibrosis: ticarcillin-tobramycin, azlocillin-tobramycin, and azlocillin-placebo. *J Infect Dis* **147**: 559.

Melikian V, Wise R, Allum WH, Wells WD (1981). Mezlocillin and gentamicin in the treatment of infections in seriously ill and immunosuppressed patients. *J Antimicrob Chemother* **7**: 657.

Meunier-Carpentier F, Klastersky J (1982). Experience of mezlocillin in immuno-compromised patients. *J Antimicrob Chemother* **9** (Suppl A): 223.

Meyers BR, Hirschman SZ, Strougo L, Srulevitch E (1980). Comparative study of piperacillin, ticarcillin, and carbenicillin pharmacokinetics. *Antimicrob Ag Chemother* **17**: 608.

Meyers BR, Srulevitch ES, Sacks HS et al. (1986). Pharmacokinetics of mezlocillin in patients with hepatobiliary dysfunction. *J Antimicrob Chemother* **18**: 709.

Michalsen H, Bergan T (1981). Azlocillin with and without an aminoglycoside against respiratory tract infections in children with cystic fibrosis. *Scand J Infect Dis* (Suppl 29): 92.

Miki F, Shiota K, Hara K, Shibata K (1978). Clinical experience with PC-904, a new semisynthetic penicillin. In *Current Chemotherapy: Proceedings of the 10th International Congress of Chemotherapy, Zurich/Switzerland, 1977* (Siegenthaler W, Lüthy R, eds), p. 642. Washington, DC: American Society for Microbiology.

Milne SE, Waterworth PM (1978). Piperacillin, a new penicillin with high anti-pseudomonal activity. *J Antimicrob Chemother* **4**: 247.

Moody JA, Peterson LR, Gerding DN (1984). *In vitro* activities of ureidopenicillins alone and in combination with amikacin and three cephalosporin antibiotics. *Antimicrob Ag Chemother* **26**: 256.

Morris DL, Mojaddedi ZJ, Burdon DW, Keighley MRB (1983). Clinical and microbiological evaluation of piperacillin in elective biliary surgery. *J Hosp Infect* **4**: 159.

Naber KG, Adam D (1983). Tissue concentrations of mezlocillin in benign hypertrophy of the prostate following intravenous bolus injection versus infusion. *J Antimicrob Chemother* **11** (Suppl C): 17.

Neu HC (1982). The efficacy of mezlocillin in the therapy of bacteraemia. *J Antimicrob Chemother* **9** (Suppl A): 23.

Neu HC (1983). Structure-activity relations of new beta-lactam compounds and *in vitro* activity against common bacteria. *Rev Infect Dis* **5** (Suppl 2): 319.

Neu HC, Fu KP (1978). Synergy of azlocillin and mezlocillin combined with aminoglycoside antibiotics and cephalosporins. *Antimicrob Ag Chemother* **13**: 813.

Neu HC, Labthavikul P (1982). *In vitro* activity of apalcillin compared with that of other new penicillins and anti-*Pseudomonas* cephalosporins. *Antimicrob Ag Chemother* **21**: 906.

Neu HC, Francke EL, Ortiz-Neu C, Prince AS (1983). The use of azlocillin to treat serious infections. *J Antimicrob Chemother* **11** (Suppl B): 141.

Noguchi H, Eda Y, Tobiki H et al. (1976). PC-904, a novel broad-spectrum semi-synthetic penicillin with marked antipseudomonal activity: microbiological evaluation. *Antimicrob Ag Chemother* **9**: 262.

Noguchi H, Kubo M, Kurashige S, Mitsuhashi S (1978a). Antibacterial activity of apalcillin (PC-904). against Gram-negative bacilli, especially ampicillin-,carbenicillin-, and gentamicin-resistant clinical isolates. *Antimicrob Ag Chemother* **13**: 745.

Noguchi H, Matsuhashi M, Takaoka M, Mitsuhashi S (1978b). New antipseudomonal penicillin, PC-904: affinity to penicillin-binding proteins and inhibition of the enzyme cross-linking peptidoglycan. *Antimicrob Ag Chemother* **14**: 617.

Noone P, Prentice HG, Sage RJ (1985). Aminoglycoside toxicity. *J Antimicrob Chemother* **15**: 785.

Nord CE, Bergan T, Aase S (1986). Impact of azlocillin on the colon microflora. *Scand J Infect Dis* **18**: 163.

Odio C, Threlkeld N, Thomas ML, McCracken GH Jr (1984a). Pharmacokinetic properties of mezlocillin in newborn infants. *Antimicrob Ag Chemother* **25**: 556.

Odio C, Thomas ML, McCracken GH Jr (1984b). Pharmacokinetics and bacteriological efficacy of mezlocillin in experimental *Escherichia coli* and *Listeria monocytogenes* meningitis. *Antimicrob Ag Chemother* **25**: 427.

Olivera E, Lakhani P, Watanakunakorn C (1992). Isolated severe thrombocytopenia and bleeding caused by piperacillin. *Scand J Infect Dis* **24**: 815.

Pancoast SJ, Jahre JA, Neu HC (1979). Mezlocillin in the therapy of serious infections. *Amer J Med* **67**: 747.

Pancoast S, Prince AS, Francke EL, Neu HC (1981). Clinical evaluation of piperacillin therapy for infection. *Arch Intern Med* **141**: 1447.

Parry MF (1983). The *in-vitro* activity of azlocillin: a community hospital study of 1900 clinical isolates. *J Antimicrob Chemother* **11** (Suppl B): 15.

Parry MF, Folta D (1983). The *in-vitro* activity of mezlocillin against community hospital isolates in comparison to other penicillins and cephalosporins. *J Antimicrob Chemother* **11** (Suppl C): 97.

Parry MF, Neu HC (1982). The safety and tolerance of mezlocillin. *J Antimicrob Chemother* **9** (Suppl A): 273.

Perea EJ, Nogales MC, Anzar J *et al.* (1980). Synergy between cefotaxime, cefsulodin, azlocillin, mezlocillin and aminoglycosides against carbenicillin resistant or sensitive *Pseudomonas aeruginosa*. *J Antimicrob Chemother* **6**: 471.

Pickering LK, Kramer WG, Armes DA *et al.* (1982). Clinical pharmacology and efficacy of mezlocillin in paediatric patients with malignancy. *J Antimicrob Chemother* **9** (Suppl A): 245.

Prince AS, Neu HC (1980). Use of piperacillin, a semisynthetic penicillin, in the therapy of acute exacerbations of pulmonary disease in patients with cystic fibrosis. *J Pediatr* **97**: 148.

Prince AS, Neu HC (1983). New penicillins and their use in pediatrics. *Ped Clin N Amer* **30**: 3.

Rankin EM, Jones DM, Lawston FG *et al.* (1984). Observations on the toxicity of the combination of gentamicin and mezlocillin in the treatment of patients with acute leukaemia. *J Antimicrob Chemother* **14**: 411.

Raoult D, Gallias H, Casanova P *et al.* (1985). Meningeal penetration of apalcillin in man. *J Antimicrob Chemother* **15**: 123.

Rawlinson W, Sorrell T, Munro R, (1988). Bacteremia in neutropenic patients at a major teaching hospital – 1981 to 1987. *Aust NZ JMed* **18**: 815.

Reeves DS, Bywater MJ, Holt HA, Broughall JM (1979). Azlocillin and mezlocillin: laboratory studies of their properties, including comparison with the antibacterial activity of other antibiotics. *Arzneim-Forsch/Drug Res* **29** (11): 1920.

Reeves DS, Holt HA, Bywater MJ, Bidwell JL (1982). Comparative activity *in vitro* of piperacillin. *J Antimicrob Chemother* **9** (Suppl B): 59.

Reyes MP, Lerner AM (1983). Current problems in the treatment of infective endocarditis due to *Pseudomonas aeruginosa*. *Rev Infect Dis* **5**: 314.

Robinson RG, Saunders J, Cassel R *et al.* (1980). Comparative *in vitro* appraisal of piperacillin, including its activity against *Salmonella typhi*. *Antimicrob Ag Chemother* **18**: 493.

Rodriguez J, Fuxench-Chiesa Z, Ramirez-Ronda CH *et al.* (1983). *In vitro* susceptibility of 50 non-beta-lactamase-producing *Neisseria gonorrhoeae* strains in 12 antimicrobial agents. *Antimicrob Ag Chemother* **23**: 242.

Rosene K, Echenbach DA, Tompkins LS *et al.* (1986). Polymicrobial early postpartum endometritis with facultative and anaerobic bacteria, genital *Mycoplasma*, and *Chlamydia trachomatis*: treatment with piperacillin or cefoxitin. *J Infect Dis* **153**: 1028.

Rubio T, Wirth F, Karotkin E (1982). Pharmacokinetic studies of mezlocillin in newborn infants. *J Antimicrob Chemother* **9** (Suppl A): 241.

Russo J Jr, Thompson MIB, Russo ME *et al.* (1982). Piperacillin distribution into bile, gallbladder wall, abdominal skeletal muscle, and adipose tissue in surgical patients. *Antimicrob Ag Chemother* **22**: 488.

Sage R, Hann I, Prentice HG, *et al.* (1988). A randomized trial of empirical antibiotic therapy with one of four beta-lactam antibiotics in combination with netilmicin in febrile neutropenic patients. *J Antimicrob Chemother* **22**: 237.

Sanders CC (1981). Comparative activity of mezlocillin, penicillin, ampicillin, carbenicillin and ticarcillin against Gram-positive bacteria and *Haemophilus influenzae*. *Antimicrob Ag Chemother* **20**: 843.

Sanders CC (1982a). Mezlocillin: a broad spectrum penicillin highly active against Gram-positive organisms and *Haemophilus influenzae*. *J Antimicrob Chemother* **9** (Suppl A): 15.

Sanders WE Jr (1982b). Mezlocillin: role in management of infectious diseases. *J Antimicrob Chemother* **9** (Suppl A): 281.

Sanders CC (1983). Novel resistance selected by the new expanded-spectrum cephalosporins: a concern. *J Infect Dis* **147**: 585.

Sanders CC, Sanders WE Jr, Goering RV (1982). *In vitro* antagonism of beta-lactam antibiotics by cefoxitin. *Antimicrob Ag Chemother* **21**: 968.

Selwyn S (1982). The evolution of the broad-spectrum penicillins. *J Antimicrob Chemother* (Suppl B): 1.

Simon GL, Snydman DR, Tally FP, Gorbach SL (1980). Clinical trial of piperacillin with acquisition of resistance by *Pseudomonas* and clinical relapse. *Antimicrob Ag Chemother* **18**: 167.

Slack MPE (1981). Antipseudomonal beta-lactams. *J Antimicrob Chemother* **8**: 165.

Stewart D, Bodey GP (1977). Azlocillin: *in vitro* studies of a new semisynthetic penicillin. *Antimicrob Ag Chemother* **11**: 865.

Stubbs RS, Griggs NJ, Kelleher JP *et al.* (1987). Single dose mezlocillin versus three dose cefuroxime plus metronidazole for the prophylaxis of wound infection after large bowel surgery. *J Hosp Infect* **9**: 285.

Sutherland R, Burnett J, Rolinson GN (1971). x-Carboxy-3-thienylmethylpenicillin (BRL 2288)., a new semisynthetic penicillin: *in vitro* evaluation. *Antimicrob Ag Chemother* **1970**: 360.

Sutter VL, Finegold SM (1976). Susceptibility of anaerobic bacteria to 23 antimicrobial agents. *Antimicrob Ag Chemother* **10**: 736.

Tally FP, Cuchural GJ, Jacobus NV *et al.* (1983). Susceptibility of the *Bacteroidies fragilis* group in the United States in 1981. *Antimicrob Ag Chemother* **23**: 536.

Tally FP, Cuchural GJJr, Jacobus NV *et al.* (1985). Nationwide study of the susceptibility of the *Bacteroides fragilis* group in the United States. *Antimicrob Ag Chemother* **28**: 675.

Thadepalli H, Rao B (1979). Clinical evaluation of mezlocillin. *Antimicrob Ag Chemother* **16**: 605.

Thadepalli H, Roy I, Bach VT, Webb D (1979). *In vitro* activity of mezlocillin and its related compounds against aerobic and anaerobic bacteria. *Antimicrob Ag Chemother* **15**: 487.

Thirumoorthi MC, Asmar BI, Buckley JA *et al.* (1983). Pharmacokinetics of intravenously administered piperacillin in preadolescent children. *J Pediatr* **102**: 941.

Thompson MIB, Russo ME, Matsen JM, Atkin-Thor E (1981). Piperacillin pharmacokinetics in subjects with chronic renal failure. *Antimicrob Ag Chemother* **19**: 450.

Thompson MIB, Russo ME, Saxon BJ *et al.* (1982). Gentamicin inactivation by piperacillin or carbenicillin in patients with end-stage renal disease. *Antimicrob Ag Chemother* **21**: 268.

Thornsberry C, Baker CN, Jones RN (1979). *In vitro* antimicrobial activity of piperacillin and seven other beta-lactam antibiotics against *Neisseria gonorrhoeae* and *Haemophilus influenzae*, including beta-lactamase producing strains. *J Antimicrob Chemother* **5**: 137.

Thorsteinsson SB, Steingrimsson O, Asmundsson P, Bergan T (1981).

Pharmacokinetics of mezlocillin during haemodialysis. *Scand J Infect Dis* (Suppl 29): 59.

Tjandramaga TB, Mullie A, Verbesselt R *et al.* (1978). Piperacillin: human pharmacokinetics after intravenous and intramuscular administration. *Antimicrob Ag Chemother* **14**: 829.

Tofte RW, Solliday J, Crossley KB (1984). Susceptibilities of enterococci to twelve antibiotics. *Antimicrob Ag Chemother* **25**: 532.

Tosolini FA, Dawborn JK, Fensling B *et al.* (1985). Clinical, microbiological and pharmacokinetic assessment of piperacillin sodium. *Curr Ther Research* **37**: 9.

Ueo K, Fukuoka Y, Hayashi T *et al.* (1977). *In vitro* and in vivo antibacterial activity of T-1220, a new semisynthetic penicillin. *Antimicrob Ag Chemother* **12**: 455.

Van den Hazel SJ, Speelman P, Tytgat GNJ *et al.* (1994). Role of antibiotics in the treatment and prevention of acute and recurrent cholangitis. *Clin Infect Dis* **19**: 279.

Van der Voet GB, Mattie H, Van Furth R (1985). Comparison of the antibacterial activity of azlocillin and ticarcillin *in vitro* and in irradiated neutropenic mice. *J Antimicrob Chemother* **16**: 605.

Verbist L (1978). *In vitro* activity of piperacillin, a new semisynthetic penicillin with an unusually broad spectrum of activity. *Antimicrob Ag Chemother* **13**: 349.

Verbist L (1979). Comparison of the activities of the new ureido-penicillins piperacillin, mezlocillin, azlocillin and Bay K 4999 against Gram-negative organisms. *Antimicrob Ag Chemother* **16**: 115.

Vestin L, Burman LåA, Holm S, Sellers J (1982). Clinical experience with azlocillin in the treatment of urinary tract infections with *Pseudomonas aeruginosa*. *Scand J Infect Dis* **14**: 289.

Wade JC, Schimpff SC, Newman KA *et al.* (1980). Potential of mezlocillin as empiric single-agent therapy in febrile granulocytopenic cancer patients. *Antimicrob Ag Chemother* **18**: 299.

Walterspeel JN, Feldman S, Van R, Ravis WR (1991). Comparative inactivation of isepamicin, amikacin, and gentamicin by nine beta-lactams and two beta-lactamase inhibitors, cilastatin and heparin. *Antimicrob Ag Chemother* **35**: 1875.

Watanakunakorn C (1986). Effects of inoculum size on the activity of carboxy- and ureido-penicillins and effects of combinations of ureido-penicillins with aminoglycosides against resistant *Pseudomonas aeruginosa*. *J Antimicrob Chemother* **17**: 91.

Welling PG, Craig WA, Bundtzen RW *et al.* (1983). Pharmacokinetics of piperacillin in subjects with various degrees of renal function. *Antimicrob Ag Chemother* **23**: 881.

Wexler H, Carter WT, Harris B, Finegold SM (1984). Comparative *in vitro* activities of cefpiramide and apalcillin against anaerobic bacteria. *Antimicrob Ag Chemother* **25**: 162.

Whelton A, Stout RL Delgado FA (1983). Azlocillin kinetics during extracorporeal haemodialysis and peritoneal dialysis. *J Antimicrob Chemother* **11** (Suppl B): 89.

White AR, Comber KR, Sutherland R (1980). Comparative bactericidal effects of azlocillin and ticarcillin against *Pseudomonas aeruginosa*. *Antimicrob Ag Chemother* **18**: 182.

White GW, Malow JB, Zimelis VM *et al.* (1979). Comparative *in vitro* activity of azlocillin, ampicillin, mezlocillin, piperacillin and ticarcillin, alone and in combination with an aminoglycoside. *Antimicrob Ag Chemother* **15**: 540.

Williams RJ, Lindridge MA, Said AA *et al.* (1984). National survey of antibiotic resistance in *Pseudomonas aeruginosa*. *J Antimicrob Chemother* **14**: 9.

Wilson CB, Koup JR, Opheim KE *et al.* (1982). Piperacillin pharmacokinetics in pediatric patients. *Antimicrob Ag Chemother* **22**: 442.

Winston DJ, Wang D, Young LS *et al.* (1978). *In vitro* studies of piperacillin, a new semisynthetic penicillin. *Antimicrob Ag Chemother* **13**: 944.

Winston DJ, Murphy W, Young LS, Hewitt WL (1980). Piperacillin therapy for serious bacterial infections. *Amer J Med* **69**: 255.

Winston DJ, Ho WG, Young LS *et al.* (1982). Piperacillin plus amikacin therapy v carbenicillin plus amikacin therapy in febrile, granulocytopenic patients. *Arch Intern Med* **142**: 1663.

Wise R, Andrews JM (1982). Activity of mezlocillin against Gram-negative and Gram-positive organisms: comparison with other penicillins. *J Antimicrob Chemother* **9** (Suppl A): 1.

Wise R, Gillett AP, Andrews JM, Bedford KA (1978). Activity of azlocillin and mezlocillin against Gram-negative organisms: comparison with other penicillins. *Antimicrob Ag Chemother* **13**: 559.

Wretlind B, Gezelius L, Karlsson I, Hagberg R (1978). *In vitro* activity of a new semisynthetic penicillin, PC-904, against ampicillin-resistant Gram-negative bacteria. In *Current Chemotherapy*: *Proceedings of the 10th International Congress of Chemotherapy, Zurich/Switzerland, 1977* (Siegenthaler W, Lüthy R, eds), p. 638. Washington DC: American Society for Microbiology.

Mecillinam (Amdinocillin)

Description

Mecillinam, developed by Leo Pharmaceutical Laboratories, has a beta-lactam structure and is derived from the penicillin nucleus, 6 APA (p. 3). Natural and semisynthetic penicillins are acylamino-penicillinates, but mecillinam is a different penicillin being a 6-beta-amidinopenicillanic acid, which contains a substituted amidino group (Lund and Tybring, 1972; Matsuhashi *et al.*, 1974). Mecillinam, in its hydrochloride dihydrate form is suitable for i.m. or i.v. administration but it is not absorbed when given orally. A pivaloyloxymethyl ester of the drug, pivmecillinam hydrochloride, is readily absorbed from the gastrointestinal tract. After absorption it is hydrolyzed by enzymes with the liberation of active mecillinam (Roholt *et al.*, 1975).

Sensitive Organisms

1 Gram-negative bacteria

Mecillinam differs in its antibacterial activity from other penicillins, being much more active against Gram-negative than against Gram-positive organisms (Reeves *et al.*, 1975; Tybring, 1975; Neu 1976a). It is highly active against most Enterobacteriaceae, such as *Escherichia coli*, the *Enterobacter*, *Klebsiella*, *Salmonella*, *Shigella*, *Yersinia* and *Citrobacter* species. *Proteus mirabilis* and *Pr. vulgaris* are usually sensitive, but *Morganella morganii*, *Providencia rettgeri* and other *Providencia* spp. are less often so. *Serratia marcescens* may be mecillinam-sensitive but most strains are moderately or highly resistant (Neu, 1976a). *Pseudomonas aeruginosa*, *Acinetobacter* spp. and the anaerobic Gram-negative bacilli, such as *B. fragilis*, are mecillinam-resistant (Trestman *et al.*, 1979; Steinkraus and McCarthy, 1980).

Neisseria spp. are much less sensitive to mecillinam than to ampicillin (Table I.12). Gonococci are relatively resistant and beta-lactamase-producing strains are completely resistant (Khan *et al.*, 1982). *Haemophilus influenzae* is moderately resistant, and ampicillin-resistant strains (p. 113) are highly resistant (Neu, 1976a).

2 Gram-positive bacteria

Compared with ampicillin, the activity of mecillinam against these organisms is relatively low (Table I.12). All *Enterococcus faecalis* strains are highly resistant (Neu, 1976a). *Staphylococcus saprophyticus* (p. 12) is relatively resistant but sufficiently high concentrations may be attained in the urine to inhibit this bacterium (Anderson *et al.*, 1976a; Hovelius and Mårdh, 1984).

3 Chlamydia

Mecillinam has moderate activity against *C. trachomatis* (MIC 0.25–0.5 μg per ml) (Hammerschlag and Gleyzer, 1983).

4 Laboratory methodology and MIC values

In media with high osmolality and high conductivity, the MIC values of mecillinam for some organisms are markedly increased (Tybring and Melchior, 1975; Greenwood, 1976). As mecillinam has a place in the treatment of urinary tract infections, and as urine normally has a high osmolality and conductivity, this finding has clinical significance.

If large inocula of bacteria are used for *in vitro* sensitivity testing, the MICs of mecillinam are markedly increased for all bacteria. With many Gram-negative bacteria there is also a large difference (8- to 32-fold) between the MICs and MBCs of mecillinam (Neu, 1976a). Instability of mecillinam in the assay medium may account for these differences, and the drug probably has a bactericidal effect *in vivo*, similar to other penicillins. According to Tybring and Melchior (1975), the drug has a bactericidal effect but this is evident *in vitro* only after prolonged incubation of the culture. This is because growing cells of *E. coli* respond to the action of mecillinam by first forming swollen and then spherical cells, and lysis only occurs later. This effect is different to that of other penicillins (p. 186).

5 Acquired resistance and cross-resistance with ampicillin

Mecillinam-resistant strains of many bacterial species can be readily selected *in vitro* by repeated passage in the presence of the antibiotic (Matsuhashi *et al.*, 1974; Tybring, 1975). Emergence of resistant strains has not been a major problem when the drug has been used to treat urinary tract infections (Aaraas *et al.*, 1977; Damsgaard *et al.*, 1979). Short courses of treatment are unlikely to select resistant fecal organisms and lead to therapeutic failure (Anderson, 1977). Mecillinam-resistant variants can sometimes be demonstrated in urine containing therapeutic concentrations of the drug. The generation time of these resistant strains is 3.0–4.5 times as long as that of susceptible organisms, which may be why such resistant organisms do not usually colonize the urinary tract during chemotherapy (Anderson *et al.*, 1977).

Mecillinam-resistant strains have emerged during treatment of other infections. Jonsson and Tunevall (1975) treated 12 chronic *Salmonella* spp. carriers with mecillinam; eight were apparently cured but in four others mecillinam-resistant salmonellae emerged, and in three a plasmid was implicated (p. 549). A mecillinam-resistant mutant of *E. coli* was isolated from a patient who had relapse of *E. coli* bacteremia after mecillinam therapy (Barbour *et al.*, 1981). Mecillinam-resistant variants of *Klebsiella pneumoniae* were isolated from the blood of a neonate, who had been treated with mecillinam for 4 weeks (Verweij-van Vught *et al.*, 1982). These mecillinam-resistant variants were spherical in shape and most of them were unstable and readily reverted to their mecillinam-sensitive rod-shaped form. Stable mutants of *Kl. pneumoniae* and *E. coli* were also detected, which were identical to the unstable variants with regard to form, growth rate and sensitivity to mecillinam. The stable mutants were fully virulent when tested in mice and they were not easily phagocytosed and killed by human polymorphonuclear leukocytes. These mecillinam-resistant mutants, despite their lower growth rate, may be a problem in patients during mecillinam therapy, especially when host defence mechanisms are impaired.

Amongst Enterobacteriaceae isolated from patients in the community and hospitals, resistance to mecillinam has been much less common than to ampicillin (Anderson *et al.*, 1976b; Hassam, 1978). Most ampicillin-resistant Enterobacteriaceae isolated from fecal flora or infected urine have been mecillinam-sensitive. In Swedish surveys, all *Shigella* spp. strains (Hansson *et al.*, 1981) and all *Yersinia enterocolitica* strains (Juhlin and Winblad, 1981) were mecillinam-sensitive. Some ampicillin-resistant Gram-negative bacilli were also mecillinam-resistant (Greenwood *et al.*, 1974; Neu 1976a). Most ampicillin-resistant *Shigella* isolates (p. 111) were mecillinam-sensitive (Uwaydah and Osseiran, 1981), and only occasionally mecillinam-resistant *Sh. flexneri* and *Sh. boydii* strains were isolated, where the resistance appeared to be plasmid mediated (Haider *et al.*, 1991). Mecillinam-resistant *Shigella* spp. strains have been isolated in Bangladesh (Haider *et al.*, 1993). Ampicillin-resistant salmonellae (p. 109) showed partial resistance to mecillinam. The MICs of mecillinam for ampicillin-sensitive strains of salmonellae were 0.2 μg per ml or lower, but those for ampicillin-resistant strains were 0.8 μg per ml or higher (Chau *et al.*, 1981). Bacteria exhibiting cross-resistance between ampicillin and mecillinam were usually those which produced large amounts of beta-lactamases. Although mecillinam can be inactivated by beta-lactamases, it is generally more stable than ampicillin because of its relatively low affinity for them. The two drugs may also differ in their sensitivity to the various types of beta-lactamases produced by individual organisms (p. 26). Another reason why Enterobacteriaceae are more sensitive to mecillinam than to ampicillin, is the superior ability of mecillinam to penetrate through the outer layers of the bacterial cell envelope (Tybring, 1975; Richmond, 1977).

6 Synergy with other drugs

Because of their differing mechanisms of action (p. 186), mecillinam may be synergistic with other beta-lactam antibiotics. *In vitro* synergy occurs between mecillinam and ampicillin under certain conditions (Lorian and Atkinson, 1977). Large spherical forms of bacteria produced by pretreatment with mecillinam (p. 186), are more sensitive to ampicillin than normal cells (Van der Voet *et al.*, 1983a).

Synergistic action of mecillinam with other beta-lactam antibiotics is rather selective; it depends on the other antibiotic, the proportions of the antibiotics used, the bacterial species, and the individual strain within each species. For instance, bacterial isolates which are highly susceptible to mecillinam, are not synergistically inhibited by the addition of any beta-lactam antibiotic. Also, if media of low osmolality and conductivity are used, the activity of mecillinam may be too great for synergy to be apparent *in vitro* (Neu, 1976b). Otherwise synergy between mecillinam and beta-lactam antibiotics such as ampicillin, amoxycillin, carbenicillin, cephalothin, cefazolin, cephradine, cefamandole, cefoxitin and ceftriaxone can be demonstrated with selected isolates of most Enterobacteriaceae (Baltimore *et al.*, 1976; Chattopadhyay and Hall, 1979; Neu, 1983; Verbist, 1985; Yourassowsky *et al.*, 1986; Stobberingh *et al.*, 1987). *Enterobacter cloacae* strains readily acquire resistance to ceftazidime *in vitro*. This emergence of resistance is prevented by addition of mecillinam to the growth medium. Against strains sensitive to both drugs, ceftazidime and mecillinam also act synergistically (Yourassowsky *et al.*, 1988). Mecillinam may also potentiate the activity of some beta-lactam antibiotics not only by binding to a complimentary PBP, but also by causing leakage of beta-lactamase from the cell. Its ability to bind to PBP2 (p. 186) may produce changes of outer membrane permeability. Thus prior treatment of *E. cloacae* with mecillinam enhances the efficacy of azlocillin, an enzyme-labile drug, but not that of cefotaxime, which is relatively beta-lactamase-stable (Sanders *et al.*, 1987). In animals mecillinam combined with ampicillin acts synergistically against infections with most Enterobacteriaceae (Grunberg *et al.*, 1976; Scheld *et al.*, 1979; Van der Voet *et al.*, 1983b).

The *in vitro* interaction between mecillinam and the beta-lactamase-stable cephalosporin, moxalactam, against Enterobacteriaceae was variable; percentages of strains showing synergy, indifference, and antagonism were 11%, 76% and 13%, respectively (Fass, 1982). Antagonism may occur with this combination because moxalactam may act as an inducer of beta-lactamases, which then inactivate mecillinam.

Mecillinam-resistant beta-lactamase-producing strains of Enterobacteriaceae, such as *E. coli* and *Enterobacter*, *Klebsiella*, *Citrobacter*, *Serratia* and *Salmonella* spp. are synergistically inhibited by mecillinam combined with a beta-lactamase inhibitor, such as clavulanic acid (p. 192) or sulbactam (p. 209). But only a proportion of beta-lactamase containing *Pr. mirabilis*, *Morganella morganii* and *Providencia* spp. are synergistically inhibited by these combinations (Neu, 1982).

Neu (1976b) was unable to demonstrate synergy between mecillinam and aminoglycosides, chloramphenicol, tetracycline or polymyxins. Baltimore *et al.* (1976) had different results; mecillinam/amikacin was synergistic against 10 of 11 *Pr. mirabilis* strains, and gentamicin and tobramycin were also each synergistic with mecillinam against four of these strains; mecillinam combined with chloramphenicol or clindamycin acted synergistically against seven of 12 *Morganella morganii* strains.

Mecillinam does not increase the activity of beta-lactam antibiotics against Gram-positive bacteria (Neu, 1976b; Cleeland and Squires, 1983) (p. 186).

7 Minimum inhibitory concentrations

Table I.12 shows the comparative activity of mecillinam and ampicillin against various bacteria. Most of these values are expressed as the MIC_{50}, the concentration of the antibiotic necessary to inhibit 50% of strains of the bacterium concerned. Usually the term MIC equates with MIC_{90}, which is the concentration necessary to inhibit 90% of the strains.

Mode of Administration and Dosage

1 Parenteral administration

Mecillinam hydrochloride dihydrate is available as a powder, containing 82% anhydrous mecillinam, which when dissolved in sterile water is only suitable for i.m. or i.v. administration. This is administered i.v. in doses of 10 mg per kg (600 mg for adults), as a 15 min infusion every 4 h, for the treatment of severe systemic infections. For the treatment of urinary tract infections, 10 mg per kg administered i.v. 6-hourly, is sufficient. The i.m. dosage of the drug is the same (Gambertoglio *et al.*, 1980; Barriere *et al.*, 1982). In clinical trials, somewhat different dosages were used. Clarke *et al.* (1976) used 400 mg i.m. or i.v. every 6 h to treat adults with typhoid fever. Klastersky *et al.* (1980) prescribed mecillinam 600 mg i.v. 6-hourly for the treatment of Gram-negative septicemia, and McKendrick and Geddes (1979) used it i.v. in an adult dosage of 800 mg i.v. 6-hourly in combination with amoxycillin for the initial treatment of typhoid fever. In young children, 40 mg per kg body weight per day, was given i.m. to treat enteropathogenic *E. coli* gastroenteritis (Thorén *et al.*, 1980).

	MIC$_{50}$ (μg per ml)	
Organism	Mecillinam	Ampicillin
Gram-positive bacteria		
Staphylococcus aureus (non-penicillinase producer)	5.0	0.016
Streptococcus pyogenes	0.50	0.006
Streptococcus pneumoniae	1.60	0.016
Enterococcus faecalis	100.0	0.20
Staphylococcus saprophyticus	16.0–64.0[a]	–
Clostridium perfringens	8.0–64.0[a]	–
Gram-negative bacteria		
Neisseria gonorrhoeae	0.125–8.0[a]	0.005
Haemophilus influenzae	16.0	0.16
Escherichia coli	0.016	0.50
Enterobacter cloacae	0.16	100.0
Klebsiella pneumoniae	0.10	100.0
Proteus mirabilis	0.10	0.50
Proteus vulgaris	0.16	40.0
Morganella morganii	0.13	100.0
Salmonella typhimurium	0.10	1.0
Shigella dysenteriae	0.05	1.0
Serratia marcescens	12.5–100.0[a]	32.0
Pseudomonas aeruginosa	160.0	500.0
Prevotella melaninogenica	0.25–16.0[a]	0.5–4.0[a]
Bacteroides fragilis	1.0–64.0%	4.0–256.0[a]

[a] These values are expressed as the MIC

Table I.12
Compiled from data published by Lund and Tybring (1972), Greenwood *et al.* (1974), Neu (1976a), Steinkraus and McCarthy (1980) and Khan *et al.* (1982)

2 Oral administration

Pivmecillinam has been available in capsules of 150 or 200 mg, each containing 68% anhydrous mecillinam, suitable for oral administration. Depending on the nature and severity of the infection, pivmecillinam can be given in adult doses of 200 mg to 400 mg three or four times daily (Jonsson and Tunevall, 1975; Aaraas *et al.*, 1977; Limson *et al.*, 1982; Bruun *et al.*, 1983). Probenecid, in an adult dose of 1 g daily, can also be administered to augment serum levels, when systemic infections, such as typhoid fever, are treated by oral pivmecillinam (McKendrick and Geddes, 1979). In young children, oral pivmecillinam has been used in a dosage of 80 mg per kg per day (twice the parenteral dose), administered in four divided doses, to treat *E. coli* gastroenteritis (Thorén *et al.*, 1980).

3 Patients with renal failure

The serum half-life of mecillinam, normally 53 min (p. 185), is prolonged to some 334 min in patients with severe renal failure. When mecillinam was given in a dosage of 400 mg i.v. 6-hourly for 5 days to patients with severe renal failure, high serum concentrations were attained but there was no further accumulation of the drug after the first few days. Accordingly, it was recommended that mecillinam can be given safely and in normal doses for short-term treatment of patients with renal failure, even when renal function is severely reduced. For long-term treatment, the mecillinam dose should be reduced in patients with severe renal failure (Svarva and Wessell-Aas, 1980). Other authors recommend that the mecillinam dose should always be reduced in patients with severe renal failure (Ekberg *et al.*, 1978; Bailey *et al.*, 1980). In patients receiving treatment by chronic hemodialysis, the rate of removal of mecillinam is such that serum levels remain in the therapeutic range during the procedure. A booster dose of mecillinam is only necessary after dialysis for patients with severe infections. In between dialysis the intervals between standard doses of the drug should be prolonged to avoid high potentially toxic mecillinam serum levels (Bailey *et al.*, 1980; Patel *et al.*, 1985).

Serum Levels in Relation to Dosage

1 Intramuscular mecillinam

After i.m. injection of a 335 mg dose of mecillinam hydrochloride dihydrate (equivalent to 273 mg anhydrous mecillinam) to adults, a mean peak serum level of 4.5–5.0 μg per ml (expressed as anhydrous mecillinam) is reached 30–45 min later. This peak level is approximately double that attained after an equivalent dose of oral pivmecillinam (see below). Thereafter, the serum level falls more rapidly than that after oral pivmecillinam and the drug cannot be detected in the serum 6 h after the dose (Williams *et al.*, 1976). Doubling the dose, doubles both the peak serum concentration and the area-under-the-curve (AUC).

2 Intravenous mecillinam

If a 10 mg per kg dose (about 600 mg to adults and equivalent to 492 mg anhydrous mecillinam) is administered i.v. as an infusion over 15 min, the mean peak serum level, just after the infusion, is approximately 50 μg per ml; this falls to about 13 μg per ml 1 h after the infusion, and at 4 h it is 1.0–1.5 μg per ml. These values are expressed as anhydrous mecillinam. When this dose is administered 4-hourly to adults with normal renal function, there is no accumulation of the drug in the serum. The half-life of mecillinam is approximately 53 min (Gambertoglio *et al.*, 1980; Barriere *et al.*, 1982; Meyers *et al.*, 1983).

3 Oral pivmecillinam

This is well absorbed. After a 400 mg dose (equivalent to 273 mg anhydrous mecillinam) to adults, a mean peak serum level of 2.5 μg per ml (expressed as anhydrous mecillinam) is reached approximately 1.5 h after the dose. Thereafter, the serum level falls but some mecillinam is still detectable in the serum 6 h after administration. The serum half-life is approximately 1 h (Williams *et al.*, 1976; Mitchard *et al.*, 1977). Higher serum levels after oral administration have been reported. A mean peak serum level as high as 5 μg per ml was detected after a 400-mg dose in older ambulatory subjects (Roholt *et al.*, 1975; Roholt, 1977). Williams *et al.* (1976) and Mitchard *et al.* (1977) used younger subjects who remained supine throughout the study. Older patients are likely to have higher serum concentrations as renal excretion of the drug is slower, and physical activity after antibiotic administration also tends to produce higher serum levels (Mitchard *et al.*, 1977).

On doubling the oral pivmecillinam dose, peak serum concentrations increase by approximately 50%, but the AUC is doubled. If pivmecillinam is given with food, its bioavailability is much the same (Bornemann *et al.*, 1988). As with other penicillins, concurrent administration of probenecid (p. 24) produces higher and more prolonged mecillinam serum levels (Roholt, 1977).

Excretion

1 Urine

Mecillinam is excreted in the urine in an unchanged active form by both glomerular filtration and tubular secretion. Probenecid delays excretion by reducing renal tubular secretion (p. 24) (Roholt, 1977). After i.v. administration, as much as 67% of an administered dose is excreted in urine in the first 4 h; approximately 71% of the dose can be recovered within 24 h (Gambertoglio *et al.*, 1980). High urinary concentrations of active mecillinam, up to 3000 μg per ml during times of low urine flow, are attained after an i.v. dose of 10 mg per kg (Barriere *et al.*, 1982). Findings by Roholt *et al.* (1975) and Roholt (1977) were similar; approximately 60% of a parenterally administered dose and 40–45% of an oral pivmecillinam dose was recovered from the urine during the 24 h after administration. Most of this was excreted within the first 6 h.

2 Bile

Biliary levels are higher than those in the serum, provided that the biliary tract is not obstructed. Hares *et al.* (1982) investigated 53 patients undergoing biliary surgery, all of whom received a single i.m. dose of 800 mg mecillinam 1 h preoperatively; 11 patients were jaundiced. Serum and bile samples were obtained 1–3 h after the administration of the drug. In non-jaundiced patients, the mean concentration of mecillinam in gallbladder bile was 40 μg per ml in 26 patients with normal gallbladder function, compared with 12 μg per ml in 16 patients with a non-functioning gallbladder. Mean concentrations of mecillinam in the common bile duct bile were 49 and 8 μg per ml, in non-jaundiced and jaundiced patients, respectively. In patients with marked jaundice, the concentration of mecillinam in gall bladder bile was less than 1 μg per ml.

3 Inactivation in body

Unexcreted mecillinam is presumably inactivated in the body, similar to other penicillins (p. 24). Three antibacterially inactive metabolites of mecillinam have been identified (Roholt, 1977).

Distribution of the Drug in Body

Mecillinam penetrates into human CSF in only marginal amounts in the absence of meningeal inflammation, being 1–10% of the concomitant serum concentration (Gambertoglio et al., 1983). In animals, mecillinam is evenly distributed in body fluids and tissues and produces high concentrations in the kidneys, liver and lungs, but low concentrations in the fetus and breast milk (Roholt, 1977). Serum protein binding of mecillinam is relatively low (Bailey et al., 1980).

Mode of Action

Mecillinam acts on bacteria in a different way to other beta-lactam antibiotics (Braun and Wolff, 1975; Spratt, 1977a,b; Lorian and Atkinson, 1979). Escherichia coli, exposed to low mecillinam concentrations, forms large spherical bodies and not the spheroplasts associated with exposure to penicillin G (p. 28). Cell division is eventually inhibited and cell lysis occurs after several hours of growth in the presence of mecillinam (p. 27). This is very different from the rapid lysis caused by other beta-lactam antibiotics (Tybring and Melchior, 1975; Spratt 1977a). Enzymes known to be inhibited by other penicillins, are not inhibited by a lethal mecillinam concentration, and the drug does not affect proteins which are implicated in cell elongation and septum formation (p. 27).

With high affinity, mecillinam binds to one of six PBPs in the cytoplasmic membrane of E. coli. It exerts its effect by binding to PBP2, but a specific corresponding mecillinam-susceptible enzyme has not been identified. All other beta-lactam antibiotics have a low affinity for PBP2; they bind to most of the other PBPs, and bacterial lysis is caused by their specific binding to PBP1 (Spratt, 1977a) (p. 27). Mecillinam acts in the same way against a wide variety of Gram-negative bacilli including Salmonella typhimurium, Kl. aerogenes and S. marcescens. Some mecillinam-resistant mutants have been isolated which fail to bind mecillinam to their PBP2 (Spratt, 1977b).

Morphological effects produced by mecillinam on Bacillus subtilis are similar to those produced by penicillin G (p. 27). This organism has five PBPs, and mecillinam binds to all of these proteins. Against B. subtilis the drug acts as a typical but weak beta-lactam antibiotic. It may have a similar mode of action on some other Gram-positive bacteria, which may be why mecillinam and other beta-lactam antibiotics are not synergistic against them (Spratt, 1977b) (p. 183). With Clostridium perfringens, mecillinam acts somewhat differently to other beta-lactam antibiotics. This organism has six PBPs and most drugs, including penicillin G, saturate PBPs 3 and 4 at concentrations equal to their MICs. Mecillinam has a higher affinity for PBP5 than for other PBPs. Despite this, mecillinam in inhibitory concentrations, similar to other beta-lactam antibiotics, induces marked filament formation of Cl. perfringens, suggesting interference with septum formation. This is in contrast to the effect of mecillinam causing large spherical bodies in Gram-negative aerobic bacilli (see above) (Murphy et al., 1981). Subinhibitory concentrations of mecillinam also transform Fusobacterium nucleatum, a Gram-negative anaerobic bacillus, into a filament form, quite different from the spherical form demonstrated in E. coli (Onoe et al., 1981). In Streptococcus mutans, another Gram-positive organism, which has six PBPs, mecillinam seems to bind to PBPs 1 and 4; thereafter it primarily causes inhibition of peptidoglycan synthesis. This is followed rapidly and sequentially by substantial but less severe inhibition of RNA and protein synthesis (McDowell et al., 1983).

These examples emphasize that the mode of action of beta-lactam antibiotics often varies with different bacterial species (p. 27).

Toxicity

Mecillinam appears to have few toxic effects.

1 Gastrointestinal side-effects

Nausea, vomiting, upper gastrointestinal discomfort and diarrhea occur in some patients treated with oral pivmecillinam (Jonsson and Tunevall, 1975; Pines et al., 1977; Limson et al., 1982).

2 Hypersensitivity reactions

Maculopapular or urticarial skin rashes appear to be uncommon. Two patients developed erythematous rashes whilst receiving pivmecillinam, which subsided within a few days of cessation of treatment (Verrier-Jones and Asscher, 1975; Bresky, 1977). No rashes were encountered in several other clinical trials (Jonsson and Tunevall, 1975; Clarke et al., 1976; Limson et al., 1982). One patient who developed a skin rash after pivampicillin treatment, was treated 2 weeks later by pivmecillinam without recurrence of the rash (Aarass et al., 1977). Nevertheless, it is wise to assume that mecillinam is cross-allergenic with other penicillins, and to avoid its use in patients with a previous history of penicillin allergy.

Clinical Uses of the Drug

1 Urinary tract infections

Mecillinam has been extensively used for these. Infections caused by E. coli respond well, and those caused by other Enterobacteriaceae, such as the Klebsiella, Proteus and Enterobacter spp., also usually respond satisfactorily (Bentzen et al., 1975; Verrier-Jones and Asscher, 1975). As with other drugs, results of mecillinam treatment are superior in patients with uncomplicated infections, compared with those in patients with recurrent infection and structural abnormalities of the urinary tract. The efficacy of mecillinam in both uncomplicated and complicated infections is comparable with that of ampicillin or co-trimoxazole (Verrier-Jones and Asscher, 1975; Damsgaard et al., 1979; Cox, 1983). Bacteriological success rate in patients with bacteriuria in pregnancy was 87% in one study, and the drug appeared safe as there were no drug-related fetal abnormalities (Sanderson and Menday, 1984). Pivmecillinam was compared with pivampicillin (p. 134) in gynecological patients with bacteriuria at the time of removal of an indwelling catheter 3–4 days after surgery. After treatment all 17 patients in the pivmecillinam group, but only six of 14 patients in the pivampicillin group were cured (Aaraas et al., 1977).

Experiments with urine containing mecillinam suggest that uncomplicated urinary tract infections caused by Staph. saprophyticus (p. 181), may respond to pivmecillinam treatment, but the drug is unlikely to be effective in infections caused by Enterococcus faecalis (Anderson et al., 1976a). But Granlund et al. (1983), who treated 15 women with Staph. saprophyticus bacteriuria, found on review 2–4 weeks after treatment, that only 11 patients were cured. They suggested that mecillinam should not be used for treatment of urinary tract infections caused by this organism, which is resistant to mecillinam in vitro (p. 181).

Pivmecillinam or a pivmecillinam/pivampicillin combination have been compared for the treatment of urinary tract infections in patients with underlying urological abnormalities. Combination therapy was more successful in eradicating urinary pathogens (Igesund and Vorland, 1982; Multicenter Study, 1983; Eriksson et al., 1986). Combination mecillinam and cefoxitin therapy was efficacious for the treatment of complicated urinary tract infections caused by multiply-resistant S. marcescens strains (Ward et al., 1983).

Pivmecillinam in a single bed-time dose of 5–10 mg per kg body weight is also satisfactory as long-term prophylaxis in girls with recurrent bacteriuria (Jodal et al., 1989). Animal studies using rabbits with Foley catheters in situ showed that mecillinam in low doses could eliminate bacteria in bladder urine and also the bacterial population adherent to bladder mucosa. But the bacterial biofilm on the Foley catheter could be eradicated only by a very high dose of the antibiotic (400 mg per kg). The authors suggested that antibiotics used in short-term catheterization may reduce the serious sequeli associated with catheter-related infections by clearing the potentially dangerous bladder mucosal bacterial populations and the bacteria in the urine (Olson et al., 1989).

The markedly enhanced effect obtained when E. coli is exposed to mecillinam in conditions of low osmolality (p. 183), suggests that it may be advisable to reduce urine osmolality by increased fluid intake, when mecillinam is used to treat urinary tract infections (Greenwood, 1976).

2 Other infections caused by Gram-negative bacilli

Parenterally administered, mecillinam may be suitable for the treatment of septicemias and other systemic infections caused by E. coli and other sensitive Enterobacteriaceae. Addition of mecillinam to cefazolin/carbenicillin for early therapy of septicemia caused by Gram-negative organisms in patients with serious underlying diseases, did not improve results of treatment (Klastersky et al., 1980). In a controlled study of infantile gastroenteritis caused by enteropathogenic E. coli, one group received mecillinam, another received co-trimoxazole and a third group a placebo. Cure rates evaluated clinically on the third day, were 79% for mecillinam, 73% for co-trimoxazole, and 7% in control subjects. Organisms were eliminated from the bowel in 53% of patients who received either antibiotic, but from none of those who received a placebo (Thorén *et al.*, 1980).

3 Salmonella infections

Ball *et al.* (1979) used mecillinam to treat 26 patients with typhoid or paratyphoid fever; cure was obtained in 23 but the three others relapsed. Results in 21 other patients treated with co-trimoxazole, did not differ from the mecillinam treated group except in the frequency of convalescent excretion of salmonellae. Only three patients in the mecillinam-treated group had negative stool cultures following treatment, compared with 13 of 21 in the co-trimoxazole-treated group. Mandal *et al.* (1979) had less favorable results with only seven of 12 typhoid fever patients being cured by mecillinam. Two other patients with typhoid fever who were cured clinically by chloramphenicol, but had positive stool cultures after therapy, were given pivmecillinam 800 mg three times daily in an attempt to eradicate the organisms. Unexpectedly, while the patients were taking the drug, they had clinical relapses of the disease, confirmed by positive blood cultures (Jones *et al.*, 1982). This suggests that mecillinam alone is unreliable for the treatment of typhoid fever.

In vitro findings (p. 182) indicate that a mecillinam/ampicilin or a mecillinam/amoxycillin combination may be more effective in typhoid fever, although Butler *et al.* (1981) were unable to demonstrate mecillinam/ampicillin synergism in murine *Salm. typhimurium* infections. McKendrick and Geddes (1979) used mecillinam 800 mg with amoxycilin 750 mg both given i.v. 6-hourly, to treat seven patients with enteric fever; treatment was continued until 48 h after defervescence (4–10 days), when pivmecillinam 400 mg orally 6-hourly plus probenecid was used to complete a total of 14 days chemotherapy. All patients responded initially, but after treatment one patient relapsed 20 days later and only one patient had six sequentially negative stool cultures. It was considered that this combination had no advantage over conventional therapy of enteric fever (p. 568). Tanphaichitra *et al.* (1981) treated 12 patients with typhoid by a combination of pivmecillinam and pivampicillin for 10–14 days; all responded to treatment and stool cultures were negative in eight patients who were available for follow-up. In four patients the *Salm. typhi* strain was ampicillin-resistant, and as expected these strains showed relative resistance to mecillinam (MIC 1.3–2.5 μg per ml) (p. 182). Nevertheless, mecillinam and ampicillin were synergistic against these strains *in vitro*, which was compatible with the clinical outcome. Similarly, Limson *et al.* (1982) treated 15 enteric fever patients with fixed-dose combination tablets, each containing 100 mg pivmecillinam and 125 mg of pivampicillin; the dosage was two tablets four times daily, but six patients received i.v. chemotherapy initially. All patients responded satisfactorily, but they were not monitored for persistent fecal excretion of *Salm. typhi*. These authors also treated 12 enteric fever patients by mecillinam alone; clinical response was satisfactory in only eight.

Mecillinam may be suitable for the treatment of septicemias caused by other *Salmonella* spp.; a mecillinam/ampicillin combination was used successfully to control septicemia in a patient with *Salm.* enteritidis endocarditis associated with a prosthetic heart valve (Shanson *et al.*, 1977).

Jonsson and Tunevall (1975) treated 12 chronic *Salmonella* carriers (two *Salm. typhi*, two *Salm. paratyphi* B and eight other *Salmonella* spp.), with oral pivmecillinam 300 mg four times daily, for 28 days. The carrier state was eradicated in eight patients, but three of these also had a cholecystectomy. Mecillinam-resistant salmonellae emerged during treatment in the remaining four patients. In another study, a 6-week course of mecillinam eradicated the *Salmonella* carrier state from one of three long-term *Salmonella* carriers; a 6-week course of pivmecillinam and pivampicillin (plus oral probenecid in one patient) subsequently eliminated the carrier state in the other two patients (Bruun *et al.*, 1983).

4 Chronic bronchitis

An amoxycillin/mecillinam combination (either amoxycillin 250 mg and pivmecillinam 200 mg or double the dose of both drugs, three times daily) has been compared with amoxycillin alone 500 mg three times daily, in 10-day courses for the treatment of purulent exacerbations of chronic bronchitis (Pines *et al.*, 1977). By the 7th day of treatment, a greater improvement was noted in patients receiving the combination. At the end of treatment, results in patients receiving the lower dosage were the same as with amoxycillin, but clinical improvement was better in those receiving the higher doses of the combination; patients who were treated by amoxycillin alone, later relapsed more frequently. Combination of amoxycillin and pivmecillinam may be superior to amoxycillin alone in chronic bronchitis due to its synergy against *H. influenzae* and organisms such as *E. coli*, the latter being sometimes a respiratory tract pathogen in debilitated patients (p. 863). In another study of patients with acute exacerbations of chronic bronchitis, a pivmecillinam/pivampicillin combination was equally as effective as co-trimoxazole (p. 863) Lal *et al.*, 1984).

5 Systemic infections treated by mecillinam combined with other beta-lactam antibiotics

Some success has been obtained by combining mecillinam with other beta-lactam antibiotics, such as carbenicillin, ticarcillin, cephalothin, cefamandole or cefoxitin, for the treatment of severe infections such as pyelonephritis, septicemia and pneumonia caused by Gram-negative bacilli (King *et al.*, 1983; Rotstein and Farrar, 1983). A combination of mecillinam plus ticarcillin or carbenicillin was only moderately effective as initial therapy for neutropenic, febrile cancer patients (Lawson *et al.*, 1983).

6 Travelers' diarrhea

One study in tourists visiting Egypt and the Far East, showed that pivmecillinam in a dosage of 200 mg orally daily for 25 days, provided about the same prophylactic efficacy as doxycycline (p. 743) (Black *et al.*, 1983).

7 Vibrio cholerae and V. parahaemolyticus infections

In one trial either oral pivmecillinam or oral mecillinam (which is not absorbed) appeared to be equally as effective as co-trimoxazole in adults and children with these infections (Uylangco *et al.*, 1984).

8 Shigellosis

Oral pivmecillinam seems comparable with ampicillin (p. 122) and co-trimoxazole (p. 868) for the treatment of *Shigella* dysentery, and it may also be effective for the treatment of this disease caused by ampicillin-resistant strains (Kabir *et al.*, 1984; Prado *et al.*, 1993). The combination of pivampicillin and pivmecillinam also eradicates the organism from most *Shigella* spp. carriers (Ekwall and Svenungsson, 1990).

9 Chemoprophylaxis

In patients undergoing transurethral prostatic resection, a perioperative course of pivmecillinam plus pivampicillin, given until removal of the catheter, but for no longer than 1 week, was successful in eliminating bacteremia and acute urinary tract infections, and was comparable with cefotaxime 1 g daily i.v. given for the same period (Grabe *et al.*, 1986; Grabe and Forsgren, 1986).

References

Aaraas I, Skarsten KW, Neess HC (1977). Pivmecillinam in the treatment of post-operative bacteriuria in gynecological patients. A double-blind comparison with pivmecillinam and pivampicillin. *J Antimicrob Chemother* **3**: 227.

Anderson JD (1977). Mecillinam resistance in clinical practice – a review. *J Antimicrob Chemother* **3**: (Suppl B): 89.

Anderson JD, Adams MA, Wilson LC, Shepherd CA (1976a). Studies on the effect of mecillinam upon micrococcaceae and faecal streptococci under conditions simulating urinary tract infection. *J Antimicrob Chemother* **2**: 351.

Anderson JD, Adams MA, Barrington JC *et al.* (1976b). Comparison of the epidemiology of bacterial resistance to mecillinam and ampicillin. *Antimicrob Ag Chemother* **10**: 872.

Anderson JD, Adams MA, Webster HM, Smith L (1977). Growth properties of mecillinam-resistant bacterial variants in urine. *Antimicrob Ag Chemother* **12**: 559.

Bailey K, Cruickshank JG, Bisson PG, Radford BL (1980). Mecillinam in patients on haemodialysis. *Brit J Clin Pharmac* **10**: 177.

Ball AP, Farrell ID, Gillett AP *et al.* (1979). Enteric fever in Birmingham: clinical features, laboratory investigation and comparison of treatment with pivmecillinam and co-trimoxazole. *J Infect* **1**: 353.

Baltimore RS, Klein JD, Wilcox C, Finland M (1976). Synergy of mecillinam (FL 1060). with penicillins and cephalosporins against *Proteus* and *Klebsiella*, with observations on combinations with other antibiotics and against other bacterial species. *Antimicrob Ag Chemother* **9**: 701.

Barbour AG, Mayer LW, Spratt BG (1981). Mecillinam resistance in *Escherichia coli*: dissociation of growth inhibition and morphologic change. *J Infect Dis* **143**: 114.

Barriere SL, Gambertoglio JG, Lin ET, Conte JE Jr (1982). Multiple-dose pharmacokinetics of amdinocillin in healthy volunteers. *Antimicrob Ag Chemother* **21**: 54.

Bentzen AJ, Vejlsgaard R, Jacobsen J, Tybring L (1975). Clinical evaluation of a novel beta-lactam antibiotic: pivmecillinam (FL 1039). *Infection* **3**: 154.

Black FT, Gaarslev K, Ørskov F *et al.* (1983). Mecillinam, a new prophylactic for travellers' diarrhoea. *Scand J Infect Dis* **15**: 189.

Bornemann LD, Castellano S, Lin AH, et al. (1988). Influence of food on bioavailability of amdinocillin pivoxil. *Antimicrob Ag Chemother* **32**: 592.

Braun V, Wolff H (1975). Attachment of lipoprotein to murein (peptidoglycan). of *Escherichia coli* in the presence and absence of penicillin FL 1060. *J Bacteriol* **123**: 888.

Bresky B (1977). Controlled randomized study comparing amoxycillin and pivmecillinam in adult out-patients presenting with symptoms of acute urinary tract infection. *J Antimicrob Chemother* **3** (Suppl B): 121.

Bruun JN, Digranes A, Bøe J, Maeland A (1983). Treatment of *Salmonella* carriers with pivmecillinam alone or in combination with pivampicillin: experience with three patients. *Scand J Infect Dis* **15**: 21.

Butler T, Shuster CW, Dixon P (1981). Treatment of experimental *Salmonella typhimurium* infection with mecillinam and ampicillin. *Antimicrob Ag Chemother* **19**: 328.

Chattopadhyay B, Hall I (1979). *In vitro* combination of mecillinam with cephradine or amoxycillin for organisms resistant to single agents. *J Antimicrob Chemother* **5**: 549.

Chau PY, Ng WS, Ling J, Arnold K (1981). Plasmid-mediated partial cross-resistance between ampicillin, mecillinam and cefamandole in *Salmonella johannesburg* and *Salmonella typhimurium*. *J Antimicrob Chemother* **7**: 245.

Clarke PD, Geddes AM, McGhie D, Wall JC (1976). Mecillinam: a new antibiotic for enteric fever. *Brit Med J* **2**: 14.

Cleeland R, Squires E (1983). Enhanced activity of beta-lactam antibiotics with amdinocillin – *in vitro* and *in vivo*. *Amer J Med* (Amdinocillin symposium): 21.

Cox CE (1983). Parenteral amdinocillin for treatment of complicated urinary tract infections. *Amer J Med* (Amdinocillin symposium): 82.

Damsgaard T, Jacobsen J, Korner B, Tybring L (1979). Pivmecillinam and trimethoprim/sulfamethoxazole in the treatment of bacteriuria. *J Antimicrob Chemother* **5**: 267.

Ekberg M, Denneberg T, Larsson S, Juhlin I (1978). Pharmacokinetic and therapeutic studies of pivmecillinam in patients with normal and impaired renal function. *Scand J Infect Dis* **10**: 127.

Ekwall E, Swenungsson B (1990). Pivampicillin/pivmecillinam in the treatment of *Shigella* carriers. *Scand J Infect Dis* **22**: 623.

Eriksson S, Zbornick J, Dahnsjo H et al. (1986). The combination of pivampicillin and pivmecillinam versus pivampicillin alone in the treatment of acute pyelonephritis. *Scand J Infect Dis* **18**: 431.

Fass RJ (1982). In vitro activity of moxalactam and mecillinam, singly and in combination, against multi-drug-resistant Enterobacteriaceae and *Pseudomonas* species. *Antimicrob Ag Chemother* **21**: 188.

Gambertoglio JG, Barriere SL, Lin ET, Conte JE Jr (1980). Pharmacokinetics of mecillinam in healthy subjects. *Antimicrob Ag Chemother* **18**: 952.

Gambertoglio JG, Barriere SL, Lin ET, Conte JE Jr (1983). Amdinocillin pharmacokinetics. Simultaneous administration with cephalothin and cerebrospinal fluid penetration. *Amer J Med* (Amdinocillin symposium): 54.

Grabe M, Forsgren A (1986). The effectiveness of a short perioperative course with pivampicillin/pivmecillinam in transurethral prostatic resection: bacteriological results. *Scand J Infect Dis* **18**: 575.

Grabe M, Forsgren A, Hellsten S (1986). The effectiveness of a short perioperative course with pivampicillin/pivmecillinam in transurethral prostatic resection: clinical results. *Scand J Infect Dis* **18**: 567.

Granlund M, Landgren E, Henning C (1983). Pivmecillinam in treatment of *Staphylococcus saprophyticus* urinary tract infections. *Scand J Infect Dis* **15**: 65.

Greenwood D (1976). Effect of osmolality on the response of *Escherichia coli* to mecillinam. *Antimicrob Ag Chemother* **10**: 824.

Greenwood D, Brooks HL, Gargan R, O'Grady F (1974). Activity of FL 1060, a new beta-lactam antibiotic, against urinary tract pathogens. *J Clin Path* **27**: 192.

Grunberg E, Cleeland R, Beskid G, De Lorenzo WF (1976). *In vivo* synergy between 6-beta-amidinopenicillanic acid derivatives and other antibiotics. *Antimicrob Ag Chemother* **9**: 589.

Gutmann L, Vincent S, Billot-Klein D et al. (1986). Involvement of penicillin-binding protein 2 with other penicillin-binding proteins in lysis of *Escherichia coli* by some beta-lactam antibiotics alone and in synergistic lytic effect of amdinocillin (mecillinam). *Antimicrob Ag Chemother* **30**: 906.

Haider K, Albert MJ, Nahar S, Kibriya AKMG (1991). Plasmid-associated resistance to pivmecillinam in *Shigella flexneri* and *Shigella boydii*. *J Antimicrob Chemother* **28**: 599.

Haider K, Malek MA, Albert MJ (1993). Occurrence of drug resistance in *Shigella* species isolated from patients with diarrhoea in Bangladesh. *J Antimicrob Chemother* **32**: 509.

Hammerschlag MR, Gleyzer A (1983). *In vitro* activity of a group of broad-spectrum cephalosporins and other beta-lactam antibiotics against *Chlamydia trachomatis*. *Antimicrob Ag Chemother* **23**: 493.

Hansson HB, Walder M, Juhlin I (1981). Susceptibility of shigellae to mecillinam, nalidixic acid, trimethoprim, and five other antimicrobial agents. *Antimicrob Ag Chemother* **19**: 271.

Hares MM, Hegarty A, Tomkyns J et al. (1982). A study of the biliary excretion of mecillinam in patients with biliary disease. *J Antimicrob Chemother* **9**: 217.

Hassam Z (1978). Sensitivity of urinary-tract isolates to mecillinam and amoxycillin. *Lancet* **i**: 445.

Hovelius B, Mårdh P-A (1984). *Staphylococcus saprophyticus* as a common cause of urinary tract infection. *Rev Infect Dis* **6**: 328.

Igesund A, Vorland L (1982). A fixed combination of pivmecillinam and pivampicillin in complicated urinary tract infections. A double-blind comparison with pivmecillinam. *Scand J Infect Dis* **14**: 159.

Jodal U, Larsson P, Hansson S, Bauer C-A (1989). Pivmecillinam in long-term prophylaxis to girls with recurrent urinary tract infection. *Scand J Infect Dis* **21**: 299.

Jones DA, Kudlac H, Edwards IR (1982). Pivmecillinam and relapse of typhoid fever. *J Infect Dis* **145**: 773.

Jonsson M, Tunevall G (1975). FL 1039: a new beta-lactam derivative for the treatment of infections with Gram-negative bacteria. *Infection* **3**: 31.

Juhlin I, Winblad S (1981). Susceptibility to mecillinam and other anitbiotics of 28 O-serotypes of *Yersinia enterocolitica*. *J Antimicrob Chemother* **8**: 291.

Kabir I, Rahaman MM, Ahmed SM et al. (1984). Comparative efficacies of pivmecillinam and ampicillinam in acute shigellosis. *Antimicrob Ag Chemother* **25**: 643.

Khan MY, Siddiqui Y, Gruninger RP (1982). Comparative *in-vitro* activity of selected new beta-lactam antimicrobials against *Neisseria gonorrhoeae*. *Brit J Vener Dis* **58**: 228.

King JW, Beam TR Jr, Neu HC, Smith LG (1983). Systemic infections treated with amdinocillin in combination with other beta-lactam antibiotics. *Amer J Med* (Amdinocillin symposium): 90.

Klastersky J, Coppens L, Meunier-Carpentier F, Menday AP (1980). Carbenicillin plus cefazolin with or without mecillinam as an early treatment of bacteremia caused by Gram-negative organisms: randomized double-blind study. *Antimicrob Ag Chemother* **18**: 437.

Lal S, McGhie D, Kerfoot P (1984). A comparison of pivmecillinam/pivampicillin and co-trimoxazole in hospitalized patients with acute exacerbations of chronic bronchitis. *J Antimicrob Chemother* **14**: 179.

Lawson RD, Estey EH, Bodey GP (1983). Amdinocillin: use alone or in combination with cefoxitin or carbenicillin-ticarcillin. *Amer J Med* (Amdinocillin symposium): 113.

Limson BM, Mendoza MT, Liwanag E et al. (1982). Randomised, comparative trial of mecillinam, mecillinam/ampicillin and chloramphenicol in the treatment of enteric fever. *J Antimicrob Chemother* **9**: 405.

Lorian V, Atkinson B (1977). Comparison of the effects of mecillinam and 6-amino-penicillanic acid on *Proteus mirabilis*, *Escherichia coli*, and *Staphylococcus aureus*. *Antimicrob Ag Chemother* **11**: 541.

Lorian V, Atkinson BA (1979). Effect of serum and blood on Enterobacteriaceae grown in the presence of subminimal inhibitory concentrations of ampicillin and mecillinam. *Rev Infect Dis* **1**: 797.

Lund F, Tybring L (1972). 6-beta-amidinopenicillanic acids – a new group of antibiotics. *Nature New Biol* **236**: 135.

Mandal BK, Ironside AG, Brennand J (1979). Mecillinam in enteric fever. *Brit Med J* **1**: 586.

Matsuhashi S, Kamiryo T, Blumberg PM et al. (1974). Mechanism of action and development of resistance to a new amidino penicillin. *J Bacteriol* **117**: 578.

McDowell TD, Buchanan CE, Coyette J et al. (1983). Effects of mecillinam and cefoxitin on growth, macromolecular synthesis and penicillin-binding proteins in a variety of streptococci. *Antimicrob Ag Chemother* **23**: 750.

McKendrick MW, Geddes AM (1979). Mecillinam and amoxycillin in enteric fever. *J Antimicrob Chemother* **5**: 727.

Meyers BR, Jacobson J, Masci J et al. (1983). Pharmacokinetics of amdinocillin in healthy adults. *Antimicrob Ag Chemother* **23**: 827.

Mitchard M, Andrews J, Kendall MJ, Wise R (1977). Mecillinam serum levels following intravenous injection: a comparison with pivmecillinam. *J Antimicrob Chemother* **3** (Suppl B): 83.

Multicenter study from medical, surgical and bacteriological departments at Danish hospitals and the State Serum Institute, Copenhagen, Denmark (1983). A fixed combination of pivmecillinam and pivampicillin in complicated urinary tract infections. *Scand J Infect Dis* **15**: 195.

Murphy TF, Barza M, Park JT (1981). Penicillin-binding proteins in *Clostridium perfringens*. *Antimicrob Ag Chemother* **20**: 809.

Neu HC (1976a). Mecillinam, a novel penicillanic acid derivative with unusual activity against Gram-negative bacteria. *Antimicrob Ag Chemother* **9**: 793.

Neu HC (1976b). Synergy of mecillinam, a beta-amidinopenicillanic acid derivative, combined with beta-lactam antibiotics. *Antimicrob Ag Chemother* **10**: 535.

Neu HC (1982). Synergistic activity of mecillinam in combination with the beta-lactamase inhibitors clavulanic acid and sulbactam. *Antimicrob Ag Chemother* **22**: 518.

Neu HC (1983). Penicillin-binding proteins and role of amdinocillin in causing bacterial cell death. *Amer J Med* (Amdinocillin symposium): 9.

Olson ME, Nickel JC, Khoury AE et al. (1989). Amdinocillin treatment of catheter-associated bacteriuria in rabbits. *J Infect Dis* **159**: 1065.

Onoe T, Umemoto T, Sagawa H, Suginaka H (1981). Filament formation of *Fusobacterium nucleatum* cells induced by mecillinam. *Antimicrob Ag Chemother* **19**: 487.

Patel IH, Bornemann LD, Brocks VM et al. (1985). Pharmacokinetics of intravenous amdinocillin in healthy subjects and patients with renal insufficiency. *Antimicrob Ag Chemother* **28**: 46.

Pines A, Nandi AR, Raafat H, Rahman M (1977). Pivmecillinam and amoxycillin as combined treatment in purulent exacerbations of chronic bronchitis. *J Antimicrob Chemother* **3** (Suppl B): 141.

Prado D, Liu H, Velasquez T, Cleary TG (1993). Comparative efficacy of pivmecillinam and cotrimoxazole in acute shigellosis in children. *Scand J Infect Dis* **25**: 713.

Reeves DS, Wise R, Bywater MJ (1975). A laboratory evaluation of a novel beta-lactam antibiotic mecillinam. *J Antimicrob Chemother* **1**: 337.

Richmond MH (1977). *In vitro* studies with mecillinam on *Escherichia coli* and *Pseudomonas aeruginosa*. *J Antimicrob Chemother* **3** (Supp B): 29.

Roholt K (1977). Pharmacokinetic studies with mecillinam and pivmecillinam. *J Antimicrob Chemother* **3** (Suppl B): 71.

Roholt K, Nielsen B, Kristensen E (1975). Pharmacokinetic studies with mecillinam and pivmecillinam. *Chemother* **21**: 146; quoted by Aaraas et al. (1977).

Rotstein C, Farrar WE Jr (1983). Amdinocillin in combination with beta-lactam antibiotics for treatment of serious Gram-negative infections. *Amer J Med* (Amdinocillin symposium): 96.

Sanders CC, Sanders WE Jr, Goering RV, McCloskey RV (1987). Leakage of beta-lactamase: a second mechanism for antibiotic potentiation by amdinocillin. *Antimicrob Ag Chemother* **31**: 1164.

Sanderson P, Menday P (1984). Pivmecillinam for bacteriuria in pregnancy. *J Antimicrob Chemother* **13**: 383.

Scheld WM, Fink FN, Fletcher DD, Sande MA (1979). Mecillinam-ampicillin synergism in experimental Enterobacteriaceae meningitis. *Antimicrob Ag Chemother* **16**: 271.

Shanson DC, Brigden W, Weaver EJM (1977). *Salmonella enteritidis* endocarditis. *Brit Med J* **1**: 612.

Spratt BG (1977a). Comparison of the binding properties of two 6-beta-amidinopenicillanic acid derivatives that differ in their physiological effects on *Escherichia coli*. *Antimicrob Ag Chemother* **11**: 161.

Spratt BG (1977b). The mechanism of action of mecillinam. *J Antimicrob Chemother* **3** (Suppl B): 13.

Steinkraus GE, McCarthy LR (1980). *In vitro* activity of mecillinam against anaerobic bacteria. *Antimicrob Ag Chemother* **17**: 954.

Stobberingh EE, Houben AW, Van Boven CPA (1987). *In vitro* activity of ampicillin alone and in combination with different concentrations of 6 beta-bromopenicillanic acid, clavulanic acid and mecillinam. *Scand J Infect Dis* **19**: 105.

Svarva PL, Wessel-Aas T (1980). Serum levels of mecillinam in patients with severely impaired renal function. *Scand J Infect Dis* **12**: 303.

Tanphaichitra D, Bussayanond A, Christensen O (1981). The combination of pivmecillinam and pivampicillin in the treatment of acute enteric fever. *J Antimicrob Chemother* **8**: 23.

Thorén A, Wolde-Mariam T, Stintzing G et al. (1980). Antibiotics in the treatment of gastro-enteritis caused by enteropathogenic *Escherichia coli*. *J Infect Dis* **141**: 27.

Trestman I, Kaye D, Levison ME (1979). Activity of semisynthetic penicillins and synergism with mecillinam against *Bacteroides* species. *Antimicrob Ag Chemother* **16**: 283.

Tybring L (1975). Mecillinam (FL 1060)., a 6-beta-amidinopenicillanic acid derivative; *in vitro* evaluation. *Antimicrob Ag Chemother* **8**: 266.

Tybring L, Melchior NH (1975). Mecillinam (FL 1060)., a 6-beta-amidinopenicillanic acid derivative: bactericidal action and synergy *in vitro*. *Antimicrob Ag Chemother* **8**: 271.

Uwaydah M, Osseiran M (1981). Susceptibility of recent *Shigella* isolates to mecillinam, ampicillin, tetracycline, chloramphenicol and cotrimoxazole. *J Antimicrob Chemother* **7**: 619.

Uylangco C, Santiago L, Pescante M et al. (1984). Pivmecillinam, co-trimoxazole and oral mecillinam in gastroenteritis due to *Vibrio* spp. *J Antimicrob Chemother* **13**: 171.

Van der Voet GB, Mattie H, Van Furth R (1983a). Comparison of *in vitro* and in vivo ampicillin susceptibility of *Escherichia coli* pretreated with low concentrations of mecillinam and ampicillin. *Scand J Infect Dis* **15**: 97.

Van der Voet GB, Mattie H, Van Furth R (1983b). The antibacterial activity of combinations of mecillinam and ampicillin *in vitro* and in normal and granulopenic mice. *Scand J Infect Dis* **15**: 91.

Verbist L (1985). In-vitro activity of the combinations of ampicillin with mecillinam or with beta-lactamase inhibitors against stains resistant to ampicillin. *J Antimicrob Chemother* **16**: 719.

Verrier Jones ER, Asscher AW (1975). Treatment of recurrent bacteriuria with pivmecillinam (FL 1039). *J Antimicrob Chemother* **1**: 193.

Verweij-Van Vught AMJJ, Namavar F, Smit AM et al. (1982). Virulence of mecillinam-resistant spherical mutants of *Klebsiella pneumoniae* and *Escherichia coli*. *J Antimicrob Chemother* **9**: 379.

Ward TT, Amon MB, Krause LK (1983). Combination of amdinocillin and cefoxitin therapy of multiply-resistant *Serratia marcescens* urinary tract infections. *Amer J Med* (Amdinocillin symposium): 85.

Williams JD, Andrews J, Mitchard M, Kendall MJ (1976). Bacteriology and pharmacokinetics of the new amidinopenicillin-mecillinam. *J Antimicrob Chemother* **2**: 61.

Yourassowsky E, Van der Linden M-P, Lismont M-J et al. (1986). Efffect of mecillinam on *Escherichia coli* growth curves when given alone and associated with ampicillin. *Scand. J Infect Dis* **18**: 439.

Yourassowsky E, Van der Linden M-P, Lismont M-J et al. (1988). Protective effect of amdinocillin against emergence of resistance to ceftazidime in *Enterobacter cloacae*. *Antimicrob Ag Chemother* **32**: 1632.

Clavulanic Acid

Description

Beta-lactamases (p. 26) are responsible for the resistance of many bacteria to beta-lactam antibiotics. Many beta-lactamase inhibitors have been investigated, and the three which are most suitable for clinical use are clavulanic acid, sulbactam (p. 209) and tazobactam (p. 220).

Clavulanic acid is a naturally occurring beta-lactamase inhibitor, which was isolated from *Streptomyces clavuligerus* (Reading and Cole, 1977). It contains a beta-lactam ring, but unlike the penicillins and cephalosporins, it shows only a low level of antibacterial activity. Clavulanic acid is, however, a potent inhibitor of many beta-lactamases (Reading *et al.*, 1983). Initially it binds beta-lactamases and functions as a competitive inhibitor, then there is acylation of these enzymes through the beta-lactam carbonyl part of the clavulanic acid molecule. This reaction is much the same as that which occurs between a beta-lactamase and a labile beta-lactam antibiotic, such as penicillin G. In the latter case, the acyl enzyme undergoes rapid hydrolysis to release active enzyme again together with penicillin degradation products. By contrast, the acyl enzyme formed by reaction with clavulanic acid is hydrolyzed only very slowly, and therefore the enzyme is transiently inhibited (Rolinson, 1984). Beta-lactamases differ in their susceptibility to inhibition by clavulanic acid. Those which are readily inhibited include staphylococcal and *Enterococcus faecalis* (p. 11) beta-lactamases and the plasmid-mediated enzymes, including TEM (p. 15) which are widespread among the Enterobacteriaceae, *Pseudomonas aeruginosa*, *Haemophilus influenzae*, *Neisseria gonorrhoeae* and *Moraxella catarrahlis*. Clavulanic acid is a more potent inhibitor against the beta-lactamases of these organisms than sulbactam (p. 209). This also applies to the extended-spectrum beta-lactamases which are affected by the inhibitors (see below). But against all these enzymes clavulanic acid is about as potent as tazobactam (Payne *et al.*, 1994).

Rare *Escherichia coli* strains have been reported where the enzyme is not well inhibited, apparently because the TEM beta-lactamase is hyperproduced (Page *et al.*, 1989; Livermore and Seetulsingh, 1991; Reguera *et al.*, 1991). Furthermore, TEM-derived variant beta-lactamase with increased resistance to clavulanic acid and other beta-lactamase inhibitors can be selected *in vitro* by repeated subculture of *E. coli* in the presence of subinhibitory concentrations of amoxycillin plus clavulanic acid (Thomson and Amyes, 1993). Such *E. coli* strains, harboring clavulanic acid-resistant beta-lactamases, have also been found in clinical isolates. It appears that these have arisen *in vivo* during co-amoxiclav treatment of *E. coli* infections (Vedel *et al.*, 1992; Blazquez *et al.*, 1993; Henquell *et al.*, 1994; Sirot *et al.*, 1994; Zhou *et al.*, 1994).

Chromosomally mediated beta-lactamases of *Klebsiella pneumoniae*, *Proteus mirabilis*, *Pr. vulgaris* and *Bacteroides fragilis* are also readily inhibited by clavulanic acid, but chromosomally mediated beta-lactamases produced by *Morganella morganii*, *Pr. rettgeri*, *Serratia marcescens*, *Enterobacter* spp. and *Ps. aeruginosa* are poorly inhibited by this drug (Brown, 1981; Rolinson, 1984; Moellering, 1991; Rolinson, 1991). This latter group of enzymes are inducible and they are important causes of bacterial resistance to third-generation cephalosporins (p. 322).

Since about the mid-1980s several new plasmid-mediated beta-lactamases appeared in *Klebsiella* spp., *E. coli* and then also in other Enterobacteriaceae and *Ps. aeruginosa*. They were capable of hydrolyzing some third-generation cephalosporins such as cefotaxime, ceftriaxone, ceftazidime and aztreonam, but not cefoxitin, cefotetan, moxalactam and imipenem. These enzymes are collectively referred to as extended-spectrum beta-lactamases (p. 323). This group of enzymes is inhibited by clavulanic acid and other beta-lactamase inhibitors (Jarlier *et al.*, 1988; Kitzis *et al.*, 1988; Philippon *et al.*, 1989; Jacoby and Carreras, 1990; Murray, 1991).

However, another type of plasmid-mediated, extended-spectrum group of beta-lactamases have appeared in *Kl. pneumoniae*, some other Enterobacteriaceae and *Ps. aeruginosa*, which, in addition to above-mentioned third-generation cephalosporins, can also hydrolyze cefoxitin, cefotetan, moxalactam and rarely imipenem. This latter group of enzymes are not inhibited by clavulanic acid and other beta-lactamase inhibitors (Papanicolaou *et al.*, 1990; Jacoby and Archer, 1991; Jacoby and Medeiros, 1991; Horii *et al.*, 1993; Pörnull *et al.*, 1993).

Clavulanic acid is not used singly as a chemotherapeutic agent, but it is used with beta-lactamase-labile beta-lactam antibiotics, to prevent their destruction by various beta-lactamases. The drug acts in this way with many beta-lactam antibiotics, such as penicillin G, ampicillin, piperacillin and cephalothin (Reading and Cole, 1977; Neu and Fu, 1978; Dumon *et al.*, 1979). Commercially clavulanic acid has only been made available in two combinations, namely amoxycilin/clavulanic acid ('Augmentin') and ticarcillin/clavulanic acid ('Timentin').

Sensitive Organisms

Clavulanic acid exhibits a weak and usually clinically insignificant antibacterial activity against most bacterial species (Table I.13) (Neu and Fu, 1978; Slocombe *et al.*, 1984). By its action of inhibiting beta-lactamases, clavulanic acid in combination improves the antibacterial activity of amoxycillin and ticarcillin.

A Amoxycillin/ clavulanic acid (co-amoxiclav)

Clavulanic acid neither enhances nor diminishes the activity of amoxycillin against non-beta-lactamase-producing bacteria which are normally sensitive to amoxycillin (p. 135) (Slocombe *et al.*, 1984).

1 Gram-positive bacteria

Unlike amoxycillin alone, co-amoxiclav readily inhibits beta-lactamase-producing methicillin-sensitive *Staphylococcus aureus* and *Staph. epidermidis* strains (Bush, 1988; Goldstein and Citron, 1988), but MICs of amoxycillin in the presence of clavulanic acid for these strains are about 4-fold higher than those for enzyme-negative strains (Table I.13) (Fuchs *et al.*, 1983; Slocombe *et al.*, 1984). Co-amoxiclav shows greater *in vitro* activity than flucloxacillin (p. 90) against many beta-lactamase-producing strains; this *in vitro* advantage does not occur with *Staph. aureus* strains which produce large amounts of beta-lactamase (Thomas *et al.*, 1985). Strains of *Staph. aureus* may produce either type A, B, C, or D beta-lactamase. Strains which produce types A or C enzymes predominate. Organisms with type C beta-lactamase are less susceptible to co-amoxiclav and to piperacillin-tazobactam (Bonfiglio and Livermore, 1994). Methicillin-resistant strains of *Staph. aureus* and *Staph. epidermidis* (p. 77) are resistant to this combination (Graninger *et al.*, 1989). Beta-lactamase-producing strains of *E. faecalis* (p. 10) are sensitive to penicillin G/clavulanic acid and also to co-amoxiclav, provided this is the only resistance mechanism of the *E. faecalis* strain (Ingerman *et al.*, 1987). Intrinsically resistant *E. faecalis* strains are not sensitive to co-amoxiclav (p. 10). *Nocardia asteroides* and *N. brasiliensis*, usually penicillin G- and amoxycillin-resistant because of beta-lactamase production, are sensitive to co-amoxiclav (Kitzis *et al.*, 1985; Wallace *et al.*, 1987). Most *Clostridium* spp. strains do not produce beta-lactamase and are amoxycillin-sensitive. Some strains of *Cl. beijerinckii/butyricum* are amoxycillin-resistant because of beta-lactamase production, and are sensitive to co-amoxiclav (Brazier *et al.*, 1985).

2 Gram-negative aerobic bacteria

Beta-lactamase-producing strains of *N. gonorrhoeae* (p. 15), *H. influenzae* (p. 113), *H. ducreyi* (p. 115) and *M. catarrhalis* (p. 112) are all co-amoxiclav-sensitive (Girouard *et al.*, 1981; Farmer and Reading, 1982; Coovadia and Ramsaroop, 1984; Alvarez *et al.*, 1985; Lapointe and Lavallee, 1987; Dangor *et al.*, 1988; Cooper *et al.*, 1990). Strains of *N. gonorrhoea* with intrinsic resistance to penicillin G and amoxycillin (p. 14) are co-amoxiclav-resistant. The same is true for intrinsically resistant, beta-lactamase-negative *H. influenzae* strains (p. 114) (Powell *et al.*, 1991). Beta-lactamase-producing gonococcal strains possessing a 3.2 megadalton beta-lactamase plasmid (p. 15) are more sensitive to co-amoxiclav than strains possessing a 2.9, a 3.05 or a 4.4 megadalton plasmid (Rice and Knapp, 1994).

Co-amoxiclav inhibits some Enterobacteriaceae which produce beta-lactamases causing amoxycillin-resistance. Thus amoxycillin-resistant *E. coli*, *Kl. pneumoniae*, *Pr. mirabilis*, *Pr. vulgaris*, some *Citrobacter* spp., and to a lesser extent *Yersinia enterocolitica*, are co-amoxiclav-sensitive (Table I.13) (Gaspar and Soriano, 1981; Fuchs *et al.*, 1983; Slocombe *et al.*, 1984; Bush,

1988; Roy *et al.*, 1989). However, some strains of *E. coli* hyperproduce TEM-1 beta-lactamase; they may need higher concentrations of clavulanic acid to inhibit the enzyme, and they may be resistant to the standard co-amoxiclav formulation (Wu *et al.*, 1994). If some of the Enterobacteriaceae have acquired plasmids which code for the production of extended-spectrum beta-lactamases, which are not inhibited by clavulanic acid (p. 323), then they are co-amoxiclav-resistant. Beta-lactamase-producing *Salmonella* and *Shigella* strains are readily inhibited by amoxycillin in combination with clavulanic acid (Neu and Fu, 1978).

Amoxycillin-resistant Gram-negative bacteria, such as *Enterobacter*, *Providencia* and *Serratia* spp. and *Morganella morganii*, which produce chromosomally mediated inducible beta-lactamases (p. 322), are resistant to co-amoxiclav (Slocombe *et al.*, 1984; Weber and Sanders, 1990; Bush *et al.*, 1991). Clavulanic acid is a weak inducer of these beta-lactamases, but this appears to have little clinical significance as co-amoxiclav has no place in the treatment of infections produced by organisms which possess these inducible enzymes (Livermore *et al.*, 1989; Rolinson, 1989; Bush *et al.*, 1991).

Campylobacter jejuni is moderately sensitive to amoxycillin/clavulanic acid, which may be in part because this organism, unlike others, is particularly susceptible to clavulanic acid itself (Table I.13) (Slocombe *et al.*, 1984). Similar to ampicillin (p. 112), amoxycillin has moderate *in vitro* activity against *C. jejuni*. The moderate resistance of this organism to beta-lactam antibiotics is probably due to a combination of beta-lactamase production, permeability barrier and modification of penicillin-binding proteins. Gaudreau *et al.* (1987) found that the addition of clavulanic acid to amoxycillin made this organism amoxycillin-susceptible, but this did not occur with penicillin G/clavulanic acid combination. By contrast Van der Auwera and Scorneaux (1985) reported that the addition of clavulanic acid did not enhance the activity of amoxycillin or that of any other beta-lactam antibiotic against *C. jejuni*. Usually *C. coli* is sensitive to amoxycillin alone. A small number of strains produce a beta-lactamase and these are amoxycillin-resistant, but sensitive to co-amoxiclav (Lachance *et al.*, 1993). Most strains of *Plesiomonas shigelloides* produce a beta-lactamase and are amoxycillin-resistant, but sensitive to co-amoxiclav (Clark *et al.*, 1990).

In vitro data suggest that clavulanic acid inhibits the low potency beta-lactamase found in *Legionella pneumophila*. The MIC of amoxycillin for this organism is usually reduced only by one-half to one-third when the drug is combined with clavulanic acid. The clinical significance of this is uncertain (Pohlod *et al.*, 1980; Jones and Thornsberry 1984; Stokes *et al.*, 1989a,b). Clavulanic acid *per se* also has some activity against *Legionella* spp. (Smith *et al.*, 1991). *Pseudomonas aeruginosa* is co-amoxiclav-resistant (Comber *et al.*, 1980). *Burkholderia* (previously *Pseudomonas*) *pseudomallei* produces a beta-lactamase which is inhibited by clavulanic acid and co-amoxiclav; MICs of this organism may be in the range of 4–8 μg per ml which are clinically achievable concentrations (Livermore *et al.*, 1987; McEniry *et al.*, 1988). But the chromosomal beta-lactamase of this organism can change during treatment *in vivo* and organisms can become insensitive to inhibition by co-amoxiclav (Godfrey *et al.*, 1991).

3 Gram-negative anaerobic bacteria

Some of these, such as *Prevotella* (previously *Bacteroides*) *melaninogenica*, *Fusobacterium* spp. and *Capnocytophaga* spp. may be amoxycillin-sensitive, but in recent years many strains have become resistant because of beta-lactamase production (p. 17). The latter strains are quite sensitive to co-amoxiclav. Most members of the *B. fragilis* group are resistant to penicillin G (p. 17) and amoxycillin (p. 135) due to beta-lactamase production. These organisms are considerably more sensitive to amoxycillin in the presence of clavulanic acid and more than 90% of strains of the *B. fragilis* group are inhibited by clinically attainable concentrations of the combination. The same applies to other Gram-negative anaerobic bacteria such as *Prevotella intermedia*, *P. oralis* and *P. disiens* (Brown, 1984; Bourgault and Lamothe, 1986; Arlet *et al.*, 1987; Appelbaum *et al.*, 1990, 1991, 1992; Chen *et al.*, 1992).

4 Chlamydia trachomatis

Co-amoxiclav partially inhibits this organism *in vitro* and also *in vivo* in experimental animal infections (Bowie, 1986; Beale *et al.*, 1991). The clinical significance of this is uncertain.

5 Mycobacteria

The normally high MIC of amoxycillin for *Mycobacterium tuberculosis* and *M. bovis* are lowered by the addition of clavulanic acid and the MIC of co-amoxiclav may be as low as 4 μg per ml; *M. kansasii* and *M. fortuitum* are less sensitive to the combination. Apart from beta-lactamase production, Mycobacteria probably have other resistance mechanisms, such as cell wall permeability and decreased affinity for their PBPs, to beta-lactam antibiotics. It seems unlikely that co-amoxiclav could be useful clinically for the treatment of mycobacterial infections (Cynamon and Palmer, 1983; Wong *et al.*, 1988; Fattorini *et al.*, 1991; Wagner *et al.*, 1995). Co-amoxiclav also inhibits the multiplication of *M. leprae* in the footpads of mice (Gelber, 1991). The clinical significance of this is not known.

B Ticarcillin/clavulanic acid

Bacteria which are normally sensitive to ticarcillin (p. 146) are sensitive to this combination. In addition, many bacteria which are ticarcillin-resistant because of beta-lactamase production, are sensitive. These include beta-lactamase producing strains of *Staph. aureus*, *Staph. epidermidis*, *H. influenzae*, *N. gonorrhoeae* and *Moraxella catarrhalis*. Most strains of Enterobacteriaceae, which are ticarcillin-resistant, are susceptible to the combination. This embraces ticarcillin-resistant strains of *E. coli*, *Klebsiella* spp., *Pr. mirabilis* and *Pr. vulgaris*. Clavulanic acid does not inhibit the beta-lactamases of *Enterobacter* spp., *Morganella morganii*, *Serratia marcescens* and some strains of *Providencia* spp. However, *Enterobacter* spp. and *Morganella morganii* are normally sensitive to ticarcillin alone (Table I.13) (Clarke and Zemcov, 1984; Fuchs *et al.*, 1984; Knapp *et al.*, 1989; Murray *et al.*, 1993). Ticarcillin-resistant *E. cloacae* and *S. marcescens* are also resistant to the combination (Pulverer *et al.*, 1986).

Clavulanic acid usually has no effect on the MICs of ticarcillin against *Ps. aeruginosa*. This is because high-level resistance mediated by plasmids, is uncommon with this organism. Rare strains, where such resistance occurs are affected by clavulanic acid (Hunter *et al.*, 1980). Most ticarcillin-resistant strains of *Ps. aeruginosa* owe their resistance to a permeability barrier. These strains and ticarcillin-sensitive strains produce inducible chromosomally mediated beta-lactamase (p. 145) which is unaffected by clavulanic acid. Ticarcillin/clavulanic acid is usually active against other *Pseudomonas* spp. such as *Ps. acidovorans* and *Burkholderia* (*Pseudomo-*

Table I.13
Compiled from data published by Clarke and Zemcov (1984), Fuchs *et al.* (1984), Slocombe *et al.* (1984) and Khardori *et al.* (1990)

Organism	MIC (μg per ml)				
	Amoxycillin	Amoxycillin and clavulanic acid	Ticarcillin	Ticarcillin and clavulanic acid	Clavulanic acid
Gram-positive bacteria					
Staphylococcus aureus[a]	256.0	1.0	8.0	0.25–1.0	16.0
Streptococcus pyogenes	0.01	0.01	–	–	8.0
Gram-negative bacteria					
Haemophilus influenzae[a]	64.0	0.5	1.0–8.0	0.06–0.12	32.0
Neisseria gonorrhoeae[a]	128.0	1.0	32.0	0.5	4.0
Escherichia coli[a]	>512.0	8.0	>128.0	16.0	16.0
Klebsiella pneumoniae	64.0	2.0	>128.0	4.0	32.0
Proteus mirabilis[a]	>512.0	4.0	0.25–64.0	0.25–1.0	32.0
Yersinia enterocolitica	32.0	8.0	–	–	32.0
Enterobacter spp.	512.0	64.0	2.0–128.0	2.0–128.0	32.0
Providencia rettgeri	64.0	32.0	1.0–128.0	1.0–64.0	64.0
Morganella morganii	64.0	64.0	0.5–1.0	0.5–8.0	32.0
Serratia marcescens	64.0	64.0	>128.0	>128.0	32.0
Campylobacter jejuni	4.0	4.0	–	–	2.0
Pseudomonas aeruginosa	>512.0	512.0	8.0–>1024.0	8.0–64.0	128.0
Prevotella melaninogenica	16.0	0.1	–	–	32.0
Bacteroides fragilis	32.0	0.5	4.0–1024.0	0.008–8.0	32.0
Stenotrophomonas maltophilia	–	–	512.0	128.0	–

[a] Amoxycillin-resistant, beta-lactamase-producing strains

nas) *cepacia* and also *Acinetobacter* spp. (Fuchs *et al.*, 1984; Pulverer *et al.*, 1986; Knapp *et al.*, 1989; Murray *et al.*, 1993). Over 90% of strains of *Burkholderia* (*Pseudomonas*) *pseudomallei* are sensitive to ticarcillin/clavulanic acid (Sookpranee *et al.*, 1991). But as with co-amoxiclav, the beta-lactamase of this organism may become insensitive to clavulanic acid during treatment *in vivo* (p. 194). Clavulanic acid lowers the MIC of ticarcillin against *Stenotrophomonas maltophilia*, but for most strains the MIC is still too high to make this combination useful clinically to treat infections caused by this organism (Table I.13) (Khardori *et al.*, 1990; Pankuch *et al.*, 1994). In animal studies ticarcillin alone is ineffective against *L. pneumophila*, but clavulanic acid alone is active and ticarcillin/clavulanic acid even more so (Smith *et al.*, 1991). The clinical significance of this is not known.

Ticarcillin/clavulanic acid is very active against Gram-negative anaerobic bacteria. The organisms of the *B. fragilis* group are sensitive and in most studies only about 1% of the isolates have been resistant to ticarcillin/clavulanic acid (Cuchural *et al.*, 1988, 1990; Cornick *et al.*, 1990; Chen *et al.*, 1992). Isolatesof *B. fragilis*, which are resistant to cefoxitin (p. 295) may have higher ticarcillin/clavulanic acid MICs but most are still susceptible to the combination (Barry and Fuchs, 1991). Similarly other Gram-negative anaerobic bacteria such as *Prevotella* (*Bacteroides*) *melanogenica*, *P. disiens* and *P. oralis* are highly sensitive to ticarcillin/clavulanic acid. The same is true for *Fusobacterium* spp. (Appelbaum *et al.*, 1990, 1991; Chen *et al.*, 1992; Murray *et al.*, 1993).

Clavulanic acid lowers the MICs of ticarcillin against several Mycobacteria, but they are still 32 μg per ml or higher (Casal *et al.*, 1987; Wong *et al.*, 1988). This has no clinical significance.

C Minimum inhibitory concentrations

The MICs of amoxycillin and ticarcillin alone and when tested in the presence of clavulanic acid against some selected bacterial species, are shown in Table I.13. The MICs of clavulanic acid alone are also presented.

Mode of Administration and Dosage

A Amoxycillin/clavulanic acid

1 Oral administration for adults

Co-amoxiclav is available in tablets for oral administration in two formulations: 250 mg amoxycillin plus 125 mg clavulanic acid (375 mg co-amoxiclav) and 500 mg amoxycillin plus 125 mg clavulanic acid (625 mg co-amoxiclav). Mild infections may be treated by 375 mg co-amoxiclav 8-hourly and for more severe infections 625 mg co-amoxiclav 6- or 8-hourly is appropriate (Jackson *et al.*, 1984).

If a higher oral dose is required, 500 mg amoxycillin should be added to 625 mg co-amoxiclav which is then administered 6-hourly. This is because with increasing dosage of amoxycillin, there is no need to proportionally increase the dose of clavulanic acid. The adult dosage of 125 mg clavulanic acid three or four times daily provides adequate concentrations of the drug in the tissues to inhibit beta-lactamases (Rolinson, 1985). A dose of 125 mg clavulanic acid is even sufficient in combination with 3 g amoxycillin for single-dose therapy of gonorrhea caused by beta-lactamase-producing strains; 3 g amoxycillin plus 250 mg clavulanic acid is no more effective clinically and causes more gastrointestinal side-effects (Key *et al.*, 1985; Lawrence and Shanson, 1985).

2 Oral administration for children

Pediatric suspensions of amoxycillin/clavulanic acid are available in a 4:1 ratio. Amoxycillin 500 mg and potassium clavulanate 125 mg (625 mg co-amoxiclav) is available in either 10 ml or 20 ml of pediatric syrup (Jackson *et al.*, 1984). The daily dose of co-amoxiclav for children is 25–50 mg per kg body weight per day, administered in three divided doses (Dambro *et al.*, 1984; Gooch *et al.*, 1984). The lower dose is satisfactory for the treatment of urinary tract infections. For the treatment of systemic infections 8-hourly doses of 4 mg per kg of clavulanic acid are required to produce optimal serum concentrations of this drug. This is equivalent to 50–75 mg per kg of co-amoxiclav per day (40–60 mg amoxycillin plus 10–15 mg of clavulanic acid), given in three divided doses (Nelson *et al.*, 1982; Schaad *et al.*, 1986). Some authors have used higher doses for serious infections e.g. 40/10 mg per kg of co-amoxiclav, administered three times daily (Dagan and Bar-David, 1989). Also co-amoxiclav in a dosage of 50 mg amoxycillin plus 12.5 mg clavulanic acid, administered 12-hourly was satisfactory for treatment of children with acute otitis media (Jacobsson *et al.*, 1993).

3 Patients with renal failure

Currently available co-amoxiclav formulations are hard to use in these patients. Extrarenal elimination of clavulanic acid (p. 199) is much more rapid than that of amoxycillin (p. 138). Compared with normal patients, the elimination half-life of amoxycillin increases 6-fold in those with severe renal failure, whereas the corresponding increase for clavulanic acid is only 2.6-fold (Jackson *et al.*, 1984). Therefore, ideally the two drugs need independent dosage adjustment in renal failure, which is not possible with a fixed-drug combination. As a compromise all patients with renal failure should receive the normal initial dose of co-amoxiclav. If the patient with normal renal function is treated by 4-hourly doses of oral or i.v. co-amoxiclav, then patients with a glomerular filtration rate (GFR) of >75 ml per min per 1.75 m^2 can still receive the normal dose. However, patients with a GFR of between 35 and 75 ml per min per 1.73 m^2 should be given the standard dose every 8 h and patients with a GFR between 10 and 35 ml per min per 1.73 m^2 should be given the standard dose every 12 h (Horber *et al.*, 1986). These authors found that, despite the more rapid elimination of clavulanic acid, effective concentrations of this drug were still maintained in serum and urine when the above dosage regimen was used.

4 Intravenous amoxycillin/clavulanic acid

This is not generally available in the USA or Australia. An i.v. formulation of amoxycillin/clavulanic acid in a ratio of 5:1 is available in Europe. Each vial of 1.2 g 'co-amoxiclav injectable' contains 1 g amoxycillin and 200 mg clavulanic acid (1.2 g co-amoxiclav) (Schaad *et al.*, 1983; Hall *et al.*, 1989). The usual adult dose is 1.2 g co-amoxiclav i.v. 6-hourly (Obwegeser *et al.*, 1989). The usual pediatric dose of i.v. co-amoxiclav is 100 mg per kg per day, given in four divided doses, each dose administered as a 30 min infusion (Fischbach *et al.*, 1989). In a study by Schaad *et al.* (1987) co-amoxiclav vials of 1.0 g amoxycillin plus 100 clavulanic acid were used. Pediatric patients were given 110–220 mg per kg of co-amoxiclav per day i.v., divided into four equal doses.

B Ticarcillin/clavulanic acid

1 Intravenous administration to adults

This combination is available in a 30:1 ratio. Vials contain 3 g ticarcillin plus 0.1 g clavulanic acid (3.1 g 'Timentin'). These are suitable for i.v. use. For urinary tract infections 3.2 g vials (15:1 ratio) have been investigated (*Amer Soc Hosp Pharm*; 1986). The contents of each vial are dissolved in 20–30 ml of sterile water and then infused over a period of 20–30 min, every 4–6 h depending on the severity of the infection. The dosage of ticarcillin is similar to that recommended when the drug is used alone (p. 148) (File *et al.*, 1984; Roselle *et al.*, 1985; Faro *et al.*, 1991).

2 Intravenous administration to children

The usual dose of i.v. ticarcillin/clavulanic acid for children is 300/10 mg per kg per day, administered in four divided doses. The same dose can be given to full-term neonates. A reduced dose of 83.3/3.3 mg per kg ticarcillin/clavulanic acid, administered i.v. 8-hourly is appropriate for preterm neonates. For preterm neonates with a low birth weight (less than 1500 g) a further dose reduction to 83.3/3.3 mg per kg, given 12-hourly was recommended by Fricke *et al.* (1989). These authors used a 25/1 combination of ticarcillin and clavulanic acid. For this latter group, Burstein *et al.* (1994) suggested a slightly higher dose of 50 mg (48.3 mg ticarcillin and 1.7 mg clavulanic acid) per kg body weight of the usual formulation of 30 to 1 ratio of ticarcillin and clavulanic acid, administered every 6 h.

3 Patients with renal failure

In patients with creatine clearance >80 ml per min a dose of 3.1 g ticarcillin/clavulanic acid can be given 4–6 hourly. In those with creatinine clearance of 60–80 this dose can be given 6-hourly.

If the creatinine clearance is 30–60 ml per min, 3.1 g ticarcillin/clavulanic acid should be given every 8 h. If the creatinine clearance is 10–30, the 3.1 g dose should be given 12-hourly and if the creatinine clearance is <10 ml per min, the 3.1 g dose of ticarcillin/clavulanic acid should be given once every 24 h (Jungbluth *et al.*, 1986).

Serum Levels in Relation to Dosage

1 Amoxycillin and ticarcillin

The pharmacokinetics of amoxycillin are unaffected by the simultaneous administration of clavulanic acid (Jackson *et al.*, 1983). Serum levels attained after i.v. administration of ticarcillin are also unaffected (Bennett *et al.*, 1983).

2 Oral clavulanic acid

The bioavailability of the drug after oral administration averages some 60% of the administered dose, but this varies considerably (range 31.4–98.8%), indicating variable absorption from the gastrointestinal tract (Nilsson-Ehle *et al.*, 1985). After an oral dose of 625 mg co-amoxiclav (125 mg clavulanic acid), a mean peak serum level of 3.49 μg per ml is attained 45 min after the dose; this falls to 2, 1.4, and 0 μg per ml, at 1.5, 4 and 6 h, respectively. The elimination half-life of clavulanic acid is 59 min, whilst that of amoxycillin is 78 min. Doubling the dose of clavulanic acid to 250 mg, increases but does not double serum levels (Jackson *et al.*, 1983). Absorption of clavulanic acid is slightly better in the presence of amoxycillin (Adam *et al.*, 1982).

In children when co-amoxiclav in a dose of 25 mg per kg (20 mg amoxicillin and 5 mg clavulanic acid) body weight was administered on an empty stomach, the mean plasma concentrations 60–90 min after dosing were 7.2 μg per ml for amoxicillin and 2.0 μg per ml for clavulanic acid (Schaad *et al.*, 1986).

Serum levels of clavulanic acid are much the same when the drug is taken at the beginning of meals or in the fasting state (Staniforth *et al.*, 1982; Jackson *et al.*, 1984). As amoxycillin absorption is also only slightly affected by food (p. 137), co-amoxiclav should be taken just before meals, because the prevalence of gastrointestinal side-effects, such as nausea, vomiting and diarrhea, is less than when it is taken in the fasting state (Staniforth *et al.*, 1982). Administration of milk with co-amoxiclav produces a slight decrease in clavulanic acid absorption, but aluminum hydroxide has no significant effect. In contrast, when co-amoxiclav is administered together with cimetidine, absorption of clavulanic acid and to a lesser extent amoxycillin, is enhanced (Jackson *et al.*, 1984).

Probenecid has no effect on the serum levels of clavulanic acid, indicating that the drug is cleared by the kidney predominantly by glomerular filtration (p. 24). Probenecid enhances and prolongs serum levels of amoxycillin (p. 138) (Staniforth *et al.*, 1983; Jackson *et al.*, 1984).

3 Intravenous clavulanic acid

When a 2 mg per kg clavulanic acid dose is administered i.v. by a rapid injection, the serum level straight after injection is approximately 20 μg per ml, which falls to 4, 2 and 0 μg per ml at 1, 2 and 6 h, respectively (Jackson *et al.*, 1983). When a 50 mg per kg amoxicillin and 5 mg per kg clavulanic acid dose was given as a 30 min i.v. infusion in children, the mean peak concentrations at the end of the infusion were 121.0 μg per ml of amoxicillin and 12.0 μg per ml of clavulanic acid, falling to a mean of 15.8 and 1.92 μg per ml, respectively after 2 h (Jones *et al.*, 1990).

After an i.v. infusion over 30 min of a single 3.1 g dose of 'Timentin' (containing 3 g of ticarcillin and 0.1 g clavulanic acid) to adults, the peak serum levels of ticarcillin and clavulanic acid averaged 324 and 8 μg per ml, respectively, immediately after the infusion. At 1 and 5.5 h after the infusion, serum ticarcillin concentrations averaged 223 and 6 μg per ml, respectively and those of clavulanic acid were 4.6 and 0 μg per ml, respectively (*Amer Soc Hosp Pharm*, 1986).

Excretion

1 Urine

Some clavulanic acid is excreted in the urine in the active unchanged form. This occurs mainly by glomerular filtration and tubular secretion plays only a minor, if any, role (Staniforth *et al.*, 1983). Probenecid does not delay the excretion of clavulanic acid. The fraction of an i.v. administered dose which is excreted unchanged in urine approximates 50%. After oral administration, 18–38% of the dose is excreted unchanged in urine (Jackson *et al.*, 1984; Jacobs *et al.*, 1985; Nilsson-Ehle *et al.*, 1985).

2 Inactivation in body

Approximately half of the total dose of clavulanic acid appears to be metabolized in the body. Clavulanic acid is relatively unstable at 37°C and this may also contribute to the disappearance of the drug from the body (Jackson *et al.*, 1984).

Distribution of the Drug in Body

Clavulanic acid is well distributed in animals after administration of co-amoxiclav or ticarcillin/ clavulanic acid. Adequate concentrations occur in peritoneal and pleural fluid, lymph, pus and infected tissue homogenates. Sometimes amoxycillin concentrations measured after co-amoxiclav were higher than those after treatment with amoxycillin alone, presumably as a result of inhibition of bacterial beta-lactamases by clavulanic acid at the site of infection (Boon *et al.*, 1982; Woodnutt *et al.*, 1987, 1990).

In humans, clavulanic acid does not penetrate into normal CSF to any extent (Münch *et al.*, 1981). In one study in humans with acute bacterial meningitis, after a single 2/0.2-g dose of i.v. co-amoxiclav, the mean levels of amoxycillin and clavulanic acid in CSF were 2.25 and 0.25 µg per ml, and the CSF penetrations relative to plasma were 5.8 and 8.4% respectively (Bakken *et al.*, 1986). But in another investigation where adult patients with bacterial meningitis received i.v. co-amoxiclav in a dose of 200/20 mg per kg per day, divided in six doses, the CSF clavulanic levels were lower and variable. They ranged from undetectable to 0.8 µg per ml. The authors concluded that these results do not encourage investigation of co-amoxiclav therapy of meningitis caused by beta-lactamase-producing organisms (Decazes *et al.*, 1987).

After an i.v. dose of 3 g ticarcillin and 0.1 g of clavulanic acid to healthy volunteers, both agents penetrated blister fluid rapidly (Jaresko *et al.*, 1992). Clavulanic acid diffuses into normal human peritoneal fluid, where it reaches a concentration of 66% of the simultaneous serum level (Wise *et al.*, 1983; Houang *et al.*, 1985; Manek *et al.*, 1987). It also penetrates well into the ascitic fluid in patients with cirrhosis (Grange *et al.*, 1989) and in normal human bone (Adam *et al.*, 1987). Penetration in human lymph is also satisfactory. Clavulanic acid is 20% bound to serum proteins (Bergan *et al.*, 1986).

Mode of Action

Clavulanic acid is a beta-lactam compound and its weak antibacterial activity presumably results from a mode of action similar to penicillin G (p. 25). The mechanism for its inhibition of beta-lactamases is described on p. 192.

Toxicity

Clavulanic acid appears to be free of serious side-effects. Adverse reactions occurring in 9700 patients participating in clinical trials with oral co-amoxiclav were: diarrhea 398 (4.1%), nausea 294 (3%), vomiting 175 (1.8%), indigestion 158 (1.6%), rash 110 (1.1%), urticaria nine, anaphylaxis one, *Candida* superinfection 98 (1%), jaundice one and altered liver function tests in three (Croydon, 1984). The low frequency of rashes is surprising because amoxycillin alone is associated with a higher frequency of rashes. In one study in which 116 female patients were treated by co-amoxiclav, rashes were observed in 4.1% (Iravani and Richard, 1982). Rashes and fever occurred more frequently when HIV-infected patients were treated by co-amoxiclav (Van der Ven *et al.*, 1994). This drug can certainly cause jaundice and increasing age is a risk factor. From 1986 to 1993, 34 cases of co-amoxiclav-induced cholestatic jaundice were reported to the Australian Adverse Drug Reactions Advisory Committee (Thompson *et al.*, 1995). One death from this complication occurred in an 81-year-old man (Hebbard *et al.*, 1992).

Gastrointestinal side-effects, such as nausea, vomiting and diarrhea, seem to be more common with co-amoxiclav than with amoxycillin alone (Iravani and Richard, 1982; Pien, 1983; Conner, 1985). This difference is small when adults receive the usual 125 mg individual doses of clavulanic acid. When this dose is doubled to 250 mg, and combined with either the usual 0.5- or 3-g doses of amoxycillin (p. 115) gastrointestinal side-effects are more frequent and severe (Crokaert *et al.*, 1982; Lawrence and Shanson, 1985). In one study oral administration of co-amoxiclav caused motor disturbances in the small intestine (Caron *et al.*, 1991). The clinical significance of this is unclear.

Clavulanic acid administration can be associated with the development of a positive direct Coombs' test, but hemolysis has not been observed (Williams *et al.*, 1985). Ticarcillin/clavulanic acid has good activity against the normal anaerobic intestinal flora, so its administration is associated with yeast colonization of the gut in humans (Samonis *et al.*, 1993).

Clinical Uses of the Drug

A Amoxycillin/clavulanic acid

1 Urinary tract infections

Co-amoxiclav has been extensively used with good cure rates to treat infections caused by both beta-lactamase-producing and non-producing organisms. Often a 5–15 day course of 250 mg amoxycillin and 125 mg clavulanic acid 8-hourly has been used (Iravani and Richard, 1982; Snavely *et al.*, 1984). The combination has also been successful in patients with recurrent urinary tract infections (Brumfitt and Hamilton-Miller, 1984) and for this purpose in one trial it was comparable with cephradine (Brumfitt and Hamilton-Miller, 1990). Comparing co-amoxiclav and oral cefaclor, results have been much the same (Gurwith *et al.*, 1983; Iravani and Richard, 1986). Co-amoxiclav was comparable with cephalexin (p. 269) for the treatment of bacteriuria during pregnancy (Pedler and Bint, 1985). Unexpectedly, results were good in complicated urinary tract infections caused by *S. marcescens*, *Enterobacter cloacae* and *Citrobacter freundii*, bacteria which produce beta-lactamases that are not inhibited by clavulanic acid (p. 194). This may have occurred because urinary concentrations of clavulanic acid itself exceeded its MICs for these strains (Table I.13) (Nakazawa *et al.*, 1983).

Co-amoxiclav is probably about as useful for urinary tract infections as other effective agents such as co-trimoxazole (Smith and Le Frock, 1985). In uncomplicated urinary tract infections Bailey *et al.* (1983) found co-trimoxazole to be slightly superior, whilst results of Fancourt *et al.* (1984) and Karachalios (1985) suggested that co-amoxiclav gave marginally better results. Some authors consider co-amoxiclav preferable for 'blind' treatment of recurrent urinary tract infections because of high incidence both of a history of hypersensitivity reactions after taking co-trimoxazole and of trimethoprim resistance in their infecting bacteria (Brumfitt and Hamilton-Miller, 1985). For simple uncomplicated urinary tract infections in women a single-dose of co-amoxiclav (3 g amoxicillin plus 125 mg clavulanic acid) has been tried, but this treatment was inferior to a 3-day course of co-amoxiclav in a dose of 375 mg (250 mg amoxicillin plus 125 mg clavulanic acid) 8-hourly (Raz *et al.*, 1991).

2 Other Gram-negative aerobic and anaerobic infections

In animals, penicillin G plus clavulanic acid is quite effective for infections caused by *B. fragilis* alone and when there is associated infection due to beta-lactamase-producing Gram-negative aerobic bacteria (Brook *et al.*, 1983). In another animal study co-amoxiclav was quite effective for treatment of mixed *B. fragilis* and *E. coli* infection (Beale *et al.*, 1988). In countries where the i.v. preparation of co-amoxiclav is available, this can be used to treat quite severe infections of this type. The usual i.v. dosage for adults is 1.2 g co-amoxiclav (1.0 g amoxicillin plus 200 mg clavulanic acid) every 6 h. Mehtar and Ball (1985) used this i.v. formulation of co-amoxiclav to treat patients with severe Gram-negative bacillary infections, such as pneumonia, empyema, peritonitis and septicemia. Intravenous co-amoxiclav has also been satisfactory for treatment of perforated appendicitis in children (Schmitt *et al.*, 1989) and for pelvic inflammatory disease in women (Obwegeser *et al.*, 1989; Walker *et al.*, 1993). For the latter indication other treatment regimens (p. 45) are usually preferred.

Because salmonellae resistant to chloramphenicol, ampicillin and trimethoprim have emerged in various parts of the world co-amoxiclav may be valuable for treatment of systemic *Salmonella* infections caused by such strains. For this indication a quinolone such as ciprofloxacin (p. 1016) or a third-generation cephalosporin such as ceftriaxone (p. 360) are usually preferred.

3 Respiratory tract infections

An increasing number of respiratory tract pathogens have become beta-lactamase producers (Wallace, 1984). The prevalence of such strains of *H. influenzae* in the USA varies from 10% to 40% according to geographical area (p. 113). Either type b or non-typable *H. influenzae* is a major pathogen in otitis media and in sinusitis in children and adults. Non-typable *H. influenzae* has also long been associated with acute and chronic bronchitis. *Moraxella catarrhalis*, which often produces beta-lactamase, is an important pathogen in bronchitis, sinusitis and otitis media. The most common anaerobe causing pleuro-pulmonary disease, *Prevotella* (*Bacteroides*) *melaninogenica*, was formerly nearly always penicillin G-sensitive, but now it is often resistant due to beta-lactamase production (p. 17). Therefore, drugs other than penicillin G or amoxycillin alone are often necessary for the treatment of all these infections.

In many parts of the world where beta-lactamase-producing pathogens are still infrequent, penicillin G (p. 37) or amoxycillin (p. 140) are still satisfactory for the treatment of these infections. Co-amoxiclav is a suitable substitute if beta-lactamase producers are suspected or confirmed. Other alternatives are available, such as co-trimoxazole (p. 863), tetracyclines (p. 741), erythromycin (p. 617) cefaclor (p. 278), cefixime (p. 411) and others. Co-amoxiclav has no outstanding advantages over these alternatives. In clinical trials co-amoxiclav has been effective in lower respiratory tract infections due to *H. influenzae* (Tan and File, 1984; Jensen *et al.*, 1988), acute sinusitis (Wald *et al.*, 1984) and acute otitis media (Bluestone, 1988; Engelhard *et al.*, 1989). For treatment of this disease co-amoxiclav is about as effective as cefaclor (Kaleida *et al.*, 1987). Otitis media and purulent bronchial infections caused by *Moraxella catarrhalis* also responded to co-amoxiclav, although some bronchial infections caused by this organism relapsed when treatment was stopped (Maesen *et al.*, 1987; Van Hare *et al.*, 1987; Davies and Maesen, 1990). A proportion of children with acute otitis media, in whom amoxycillin treatment had failed, did respond to co-amoxiclav (Pichichero and Pichichero, 1995). Co-amoxiclav has also been curative in children and adults with pneumonia caused by *Strep. pneumoniae*, *H. influenzae* and *Moraxella catarrhalis* (Gooch *et al.*, 1984; Wallace *et al.*, 1985).

Co-amoxiclav has proved to be effective in some cases of nocardiosis (due to *N. asteroides*) in renal transplant patients (Arduino *et al.*, 1993). Co-trimoxazole (p. 871) remains the drug of choice, but if the *N. asteroides* strain is sensitive and co-trimoxazole is contraindicated, co-amoxiclav can be used for treatment of this disease. When penicillin V is used to treat Group A streptococcal pharyngitis, although there always is a clinical cure, in many patients the streptococci are not eradicated from the pharynx (p. 74) whilst with co-amoxiclav eradication is nearly always achieved (Kaplan and Johnson, 1988; Brook, 1989). It has been postulated that beta-lactamase (produced by normal upper respiratory tract flora) inactivates penicillin and leads to persistence of Group A streptococci, but this explanation remains controversial. Co-amoxiclav is active against *L. pneumophila* in experimental animals (Smith *et al.*, 1992), but there are no data indicating that it is effective for the treatment of *Legionella* pneumonia in humans.

4 Skin and soft tissue infections

In experimental surgical wounds in mice infected by both *Strep. pyogenes* and *Staph. aureus*, amoxycillin alone did not eliminate *Strep. pyogenes* in the presence of beta-lactamase-producing *Staph. aureus*, whilst co-amoxiclav eliminated both organisms (Boon and Beale, 1987). Abscesses, cellulitis and impetigo, particularly in children, are mainly caused by *Strep. pyogenes*, *Staph. aureus* or *H. influenzae*, and the latter two may be beta-lactamase producers. These pathogens are susceptible to co-amoxiclav. This combination is equally as effective as cefaclor (p. 278) for the treatment of these infections, but it produces mild gastrointestinal side-effects more commonly (Fleisher *et al.*, 1983; Pien, 1983; Dagan and Bar-David, 1989; Gentry, 1992). If the pathogen has been identified, older, cheaper and more narrow spectrum antibiotics are indicated, e.g. penicillin G or V for *Strep. pyogenes* infections and flucloxacillin (p. 98) for those caused by *Staph. aureus*.

5 Gonorrhea

Oral co-amoxiclav is effective for infections caused by beta-lactamase-producing gonococcal strains. Single-dose treatment is effective using 3 g of amoxycillin plus 125 mg clavulanic acid plus 1 g probenecid (Key *et al.*, 1985; Lawrence and Shanson, 1985). But this combination is not effective if the disease is caused by strains with intrinsic resistance to penicillin G (p. 14), and so nowadays other drugs such as ceftriaxone (p. 361) are preferred for treatment of gonorrhea.

6 Chancroid

Multiresistant strains of *H. ducreyi* are now prevalent in many parts of the world (p. 17). Co-amoxiclav was effective for this disease in Kenya, where tetracyclines and sulphonamides were no longer effective, and where most strains of *H. ducreyi* were beta-lactamase producers. After a 7-day course of treatment all but two of 56 patients had responded clinically and *H. ducreyi* had been eradicated from their ulcers (Fast *et al.*, 1982). Single-dose ceftriaxone is now usually preferred for the treatment of this disease (CDC, 1993).

7 Bacterial vaginosis

Co-amoxiclav is not as effective as metronidazole (p. 947) for treatment of this, but it appears more effective than amoxycillin alone (Van der Meijden *et al.*, 1987). It can be used for treatment of patients in whom metronidazole is contraindicated.

8 Methicillin-resistant Staph. aureus infections

Despite the fact that methicillin-resistant *Staph. aureus* strains are resistant to co-amoxiclav *in vitro*, in some animal infections the drug has proved to be effective against methicillin-resistant *Staph. aureus* and methicillin-resistant *Staph. epidermis* infections *in vivo* (Cantoni *et al.*, 1989; Chavanet *et al.*, 1993). This is because clavulanic acid inhibits the beta-lactamase which these strains produce, and furthermore amoxycillin apparently has a better affinity for PBP 2A (p. 77) of these strains than the penicillinase-resistant penicillins (p. 77) (Entenza *et al.*, 1994). The clinical significance of this is unknown.

9 Surgical chemoprophylaxis

Co-amoxiclav has been used for this but as here one or two i.v. injections are necessary (p. 287); this can only be done where the i.v. preparation of the drug is marketed. Hall *et al.* (1989) found i.v. co-amoxiclav equally as effective as gentamicin/metronidazole for prophylaxis in elective colorectal surgery. Dieterich *et al.* (1989) showed that co-amoxiclav was as effective as cefoxitin (p. 309) for prophylaxis in vascular surgery. In renal transplantation surgery, co-amoxiclav proved to be of value compared with patients not receiving any antibiotics (Evans *et al.*, 1988).

B Ticarcillin/clavulanic acid

This combination has a broad antimicrobial spectrum. It is active against most Gram-positive organisms, except for methicillin-resistant staphylococci. Most Gram-negative bacteria are also susceptible. Clavulanic acid does not improve the activity of ticarcillin against *Ps. aeruginosa*.

1 Fever in neutropenic patients

Ticarcillin/clavulanic acid can be used for the initial treatment, but as with most beta-lactam agents, results are better if an aminoglycoside such as gentamicin or amikacin, is also added (Schaison *et al.*, 1986; Meunier *et al.*, 1986; Armstrong, 1991). If in a given hospital or area Gram-positive infections (mainly due to staphylococci) are also common in these patients, then vancomycin should be added to the initial regimen (Shenep *et al.*, 1988; Bolton-Maggs *et al.*, 1991).

2 Nosocomial pneumonia

A regimen of ticarcillin plus clavulanic acid offers a wide spectrum, covering most etiological agents of this disease such as staphylococci (except methicillin-resistant strains), *Ps. aeruginosa* and other Gram-negative aerobes and anaerobes. The drug has proven efficacy in this disease, although alternatives are available such as imipenem (p. 236) and ceftazidime (p. 378). In severe cases or if *Ps. aeruginosa* is the pathogen, an aminoglycoside such as gentamicin should also be given, at least initially (Brittain *et al.*, 1985; Schwigon *et al.*, 1986; Finegold, 1991; Scheld and Mandell, 1991).

3 Intra-abdominal infections

Ticarcillin/clavulanic acid is quite active against most Gram-negative aerobes and anaerobes. It is satisfactory for the treatment of peritonitis such as that which follows a perforated viscus (Inthorn *et al.*, 1989). In another study it was comparable with a clindamycin/gentamicin combination (Fink *et al.*, 1989). Other treatments are available for this disease such as monotherapy with imipenem (p. 236) and various combination regimens (p. 947).

4 Skin and soft tissue infections

Acute skin infections in non-hospitalized patients are usually caused by *Strep. pyogenes* and/or *Staph. aureus* and for the treatment of these a drug like ticarcillin/clavulanic acid is not required. But in patients with chronic indolent infection, ulcers on the extremities, other pressure-induced infections and feet infections of diabetics a large number of pathogens may be involved, such as *Staph. aureus*, various streptococci, Enterobacteriaceae, *Ps. aeruginosa* and anaerobes. Some of these infections are polymicrobial. Ticarcillin/clavulanic acid has proved to be an effective chemotherapy for such infections (Pankey *et al.*, 1985; File and Tan, 1991).

5 Other infections

Ticarcillin/clavulanic acid has also been used with success in complicated urinary tract infections (Cox, 1986; Westenfelder *et al.*, 1986), in postpartum endometritis (Faro *et al.*, 1991; Pastorek and Sanders, 1991), and in various other nosocomial and polymicrobial infections such as septicemia, cellulitis, intra-abdominal abscess, osteomyelitis and others (Gentry *et al.*, 1985; Carlet *et al.*, 1986).

6 Bacterial meningitis

Studies in animals have shown that clavulanic acid penetrates into the CSF in concentrations which will potentiate the activity of ticarcillin against beta-lactamase-producing *E. coli* or *Kl. pneumoniae* (Syrogiannopoulos *et al.*, 1987; Mizen *et al.*, 1989). Because the third-generation cephalosporins such as cefotaxime (p. 336), ceftriaxone and ceftazidime (p. 378) are very successful in the treatment of bacterial meningitis caused by Gram-negative bacilli, clinical studies with ticarcillin/clavulanic acid have not been pursued in this disease.

7 Treatment of infections caused by Gram-negative bacilli harboring extended spectrum beta-lactamases

One group of extended spectrum beta-lactamases are inhibited by clavulanic acid and other beta-lactamase inhibitors, but others are not (p. 192). Ticarcillin/clavulanic acid has not been evaluated here, but there are reasons to think that it may not be very successful. The main organism harboring these beta-lactamases so far has been *Kl. pneumoniae* (Meyer *et al.*, 1993). Ticarcillin *per se* is not highly active against this organism (p. 146), so a combination such as cefotaxime/clavulanic acid would be more logical to employ, but such a combination is not commercially available. Furthermore extended spectrum beta-lactamases, susceptible to clavulanic acid, may become resistant to it during treatment *in vivo*, so the role of ticarcillin/clavulanic acid is likely to be limited for treatment of these infections (Medeiros, 1993).

8 Stenotrophomonas maltophilia infections

Although this organism is relatively resistant to ticarcillin/clavulanic acid, Vartivarian *et al.* (1994) recommended that this combination plus co-trimoxazole plus minocycline, all at or close to the maximum tolerated doses, could be used in the treatment for serious infections due to this organism.

References

Adam D, De Visser I, Koeppe P (1982). Pharmacokinetics of amoxicillin and clavulanic acid administered alone and in combination. *Antimicrob Ag Chemother* **22**: 353.

Adam D, Heilmann H-D, Weismeier K (1987). Concentrations of ticarcillin and clavulanic acid in human bone after prophylactic administration of 52 g of Timentin. *Antimicrob Ag Chemother* **31**: 935.

Alvarez S, Jones M, Holtsclaw-Berk S *et al.* (1985). *In vitro* susceptibilities and beta-lactamase production of 53 clinical isolates of *Branhammella catarrhalis*. *Antimicrob Ag Chemother* **27**: 646.

American Society of Hospital Pharmacists (1986). Ticarcillin disodium and clavulanate potassium. *AHFS Drug Information* 269.

Appelbaum PC, Spangler SK, Jacobs MR (1990). Beta-lactamase production and susceptibilities to amoxicillin-clavulanate, ticarcillin, ticarcillin-clavulanate, cefoxitin, imipenem and metronidazole of 320 non-*Bacteroides fragilis Bacteroides* isolates and 129 *Fusobacteria* from 28 US centers. *Antimicrob Ag Chemother* **34**: 1546.

Appelbaum PC, Spangler SK, Jacobs MR (1991). Susceptibilities of 394 *Bacteroides fragilis*, non-*B fragilis* group *Bacteroides* species and *Fusobacterium* species to newer antimicrobial agents. *Antimicrob Ag Chemother* **35**: 1214.

Appelbaum PC, Spangler SK, Shiman R, Jacobs MR (1992). Susceptibilities of 540 anaerobic Gram-negative bacilli to amoxicillin, amoxicillin-BRL 42715, amoxicillin-clavulanate, temafloxacin and clindamycin. *Antimicrob Ag Chemother* **36**: 1140.

Arduino RC, Johnson PC, Miranda AG (1993). Nocardiosis in renal transplant recipients undergoing immunosuppression with cyclosporine. *Clin Infect Dis* **16**: 505.

Arlet G, Sanson-Le Pors M-J, Casin IM *et al.* (1987). *In vitro* susceptibility of 96 *Capnocytophaga* strains, including a beta-lactamase producer, to new beta-lactam antibiotics and six quinolones. *Antimicrob Ag Chemother* **31**: 1283.

Armstrong D (1991). Empiric therapy for the immunocompromised host. *Rev Infect Dis* **13** (Suppl 9): 763.

Bailey RR, Bishop V, Peddie B *et al.* (1983). Comparison of augmentin with co-trimoxazole for treatment of uncomplicated urinary tract infections. *N Z Med J* **96**: 970.

Bakken JS, Bruun JN, Gaustad P, Tasker TCG (1986). Penetration of amoxicillin and potassium clavulanate into the cerebrospinal fluid of patients with inflamed meninges. *Antimicrob Ag Chemother* **30**: 481.

Barry AL, Fuchs PC (1991). *In vitro* activity of four penicillin/beta-lactamase inhibitor combinations against cefoxitin-susceptible and cefoxitin-resistant *Bacteroides fragilis* isolates. *J Antimicrob Chemother* **27**: 243.

Beale AS, Gisby J, Sutherland R (1988). Efficacy of amoxicillin/clavulanic acid in experimental *Bacteroides fragilis/Escherichia coli* mixed infections. *J Antimicrob Chemother* **21**: 451.

Beale AS, Faulds E, Hurn SE *et al.* (1991). Comparable activities of amoxycillin, amoxycillin/clavulanic acid and tetracycline against *Chla-*

mydia trachomatis in cell culture and in an experimental mouse pneumonitis. *J Antimicrob Chemother* **27**: 627.

Bennett S, Wise R, Weston D, Dent J (1983). Pharmacokinetics and tissue penetration of ticarcillin combined with clavulanic acid. *Antimicrob Ag Chemother* **23**: 831.

Bergan T, Olszewski W, Engeset A (1986). Penetration to peripheral human lymph of clavulanic acid and ticarcillin. *J Antimicrob Chemother* **17**: 97.

Blazquez J, Baquero M-R, Canton R et al. (1993). Characterization of new TEM-type beta-lactamase resistant to clavulanate, sulbactam, and tazobactam in a clinical isolate of *Escherichia coli*. *Antimicrob Ag Chemother* **37**: 2059.

Bluestone CD (1988). Management of otitis media in infants and children: current role of old and new antimicrobial agents. *Pediatr Infect Dis J* **7**: S129.

Bolton-Maggs PHB, van Saene HKF, McDowell HP, Martin J (1991). Clinical evaluation of ticarcillin, with clavulanic acid, and gentamicin in the treatment of febrile episodes in neutropenic children. *J Antimicrob Chemother* **27**: 669.

Bonfiglio G, Livermore DM (1994). Beta-lactamase types amongst *Staphylococcus aureus* isolates in relation to susceptibility to beta-lactamase inhibitor combinations. *J Antimicrob Chemother* **33**: 465.

Boon RJ, Beale AS (1987). Response of *Streptococcus pyogenes* to therapy with amoxicillin or amoxicillin-clavulanic acid in a mouse model of mixed infection caused by *Staphylococcus aureus* and *Streptococcus pyogenes*. *Antimicrob Ag Chemother* **31**: 1204.

Boon RJ, Beale AS, Comber KR et al. (1982). Distribution of amoxicillin and clavulanic acid in infected animals and efficacy against experimental infections. *Antimicrob Ag Chemother* **22**: 369.

Bourgault A-M, Lamothe F (1986). *In-vitro* activity of amoxycillin and ticarcillin in combination with clavulanic acid compared with that of new beta-lactam agents against species of the *Bacteroides fragilis* group. *J Antimicrob Chemother* **17**: 593.

Bowie WR (1986). *In vitro* activity of clavulanic acid, amoxicillin and ticarcillin against *Chlamydia trachomatis*. *Antimicrob Ag Chemother* **29**: 713.

Brazier JS, Levett PN, Stannard AJ et al. (1985). Antibiotic susceptibility of clinical isolates of *Clostridia*. *J Antimicrob Chemother* **15**: 181.

Brittain DC, Scully BE, Neu HC (1985). Ticarcillin plus clavulanic acid in the treatment of pneumonia and other serious infections. *Amer J Med* **79** (Suppl 5B): 81.

Brook I (1989). Treatment of patients with acute recurrent tonsillitis due to group A beta-haemolytic streptococci: a prospective randomized study comparing penicillin and amoxicillin/clavulanate potassium. *J Antimicrob Chemother* **24**: 227.

Brook I, Coolbaugh JC, Walker RI (1983). Antibiotic and clavulanic acid treatment of subcutaneous abscesses caused by *Bacteroides fragilis* alone or in combination with aerobic bacteria. *J Infect Dis* **148**: 156.

Brown AG (1981). New naturally occurring beta-lactam antibiotics and related compounds. *J Antimicrob Chemother* **7**: 15.

Brown EM (1984). The *in-vitro* susceptibility of the *Bacteroides fragilis* group to amoxycillin-clavulanic acid. *J Antimicrob Chemother* **14**: 367.

Brumfitt W, Hamilton-Miller JMT (1984). Amoxicillin plus clavulanic acid in the treatment of recurrent urinary tract infections. *Antimicrob Ag Chemother* **25**: 276.

Brumfitt W, Hamilton-Miller JMT (1985). Changing role of co-trimoxazole in the treatment of recurrent urinary infections: a comparison with augmentin. *Brit J Clin Pract* **39**: 346.

Brumfitt W, Hamilton-Miller JMT (1990). Comparative study of cephradine and amoxicillin-clavulanate in the treatment of recurrent urinary tract infections. *Antimicrob Ag Chemother* **34**: 1803.

Burstein AH, Wyble LE, Gal P et al. (1994). Ticarcillin-clavulanic acid pharmacokinetics in preterm neonates with presumed sepsis. *Antimicrob Ag Chemother* **38**: 2024.

Bush K (1988). Beta-lactamase inhibitors from laboratory to clinic. *Clin Microbiol Rev* **1**: 109.

Bush K, Flamm RK, Ohringer S et al. (1991). Effect of clavulanic acid on

activity of beta-lactam antibiotics in *Serratia marcescens* isolates producing both a TEM beta-lactamase and a chromosomal cephalosporinase. *Antimicrob Ag Chemother* **35**: 2203.

Cantoni L, Wenger A, Glauser MP, Bille J (1989). Comparative efficacy of amoxicillin-clavulanate, cloxacillin, and vancomycin against methicillin-sensitive and methicillin-resistant *Staphylococcus aureus* endocarditis in rats. *J Infect Dis* **159**: 989.

Carlet J, Goldstein FW, Bleriot JP et al. (1986). Timentin in the antimicrobial treatment of nosocomial and polymicrobial infection. *J Antimicrob Chemother* **17** (Suppl C): 149.

Caron F, Ducrotte P, Lerebours E et al. (1991). Effects of amoxicillin-clavulanate combination on the motility of the small intestine in human beings. *Antimicrob Ag Chemother* **35**: 1085.

Casal MJ, Rodriguez FC, Luna MD, Benavente MC (1987). *In vitro* susceptibility of *Mycobacterium tuberculosis*, *Mycobacterium africanum*, *Mycobacterium bovis*, *Mycobacterium avium*, *Mycobacterium fortuitum*, and *Mycobacterium chelonae* to ticarcillin in combination with clavulanic acid. *Antimicrob Ag Chemother* **31**: 132.

CDC (Centers for Disease Control) (1993). Sexually transmitted diseases treatment guidelines. *MMWR* **42** (No RR-14): 20.

Chavanet P, Collin F, Muggeo E et al. (1993). The *in-vivo* activity of co-amoxiclav with netilmicin against experimental methicillin and gentamicin-resistant *Staphylococcus epidermidis* infection in rabbits. *J Antimicrob Chemother* **31**: 129.

Chen SCA, Gottlieb T, Palmer JM et al. (1992). Antimicrobial susceptibility of anaerobic bacteria in Australia. *J Antimicrob Chemother* **30**: 811.

Clark RB, Lister PD, Arneson-Rotert L, Janda JM (1990). *In vitro* susceptibilities of *Plesiomonas shigelloides* to 24 antibiotics and antibiotic-beta-lactamase-inhibitor combinations. *Antimicrob Ag Chemother* **34**: 159.

Clarke AM, Zemcov SJV (1984). Clavulanic acid in combination with ticarcillin: an in-vitro comparison with other beta-lactams. *J Antimicrob Chemother* **13**: 121.

Comber KR, Horton R, Layte SJ et al. (1980). Augmentin: antibacterial activity *in vitro* and *in vivo*. In *Augmentin* (Rolinson GN, Watson A, eds), p. 19. Amsterdam: Excerpta Medica.

Conner C (1985). Beta-lactamase inhibitors. *Drug Intel Clin Pharm* **19**: 475.

Cooper CE, Slocombe B, White AR (1990). Effect of low concentrations of clavulanic acid on the *in-vitro* activity of amoxycillin against beta-lactamase-producing *Branhamella catarrhalis* and *Haemophilus influenzae*. *J Antimicrob Chemother* **26**: 371.

Coovadia YM, Ramsaroop U (1984). *In vitro* antimicrobial susceptibilities of penicillinase-producing and non-penicillinase-producing strains of *Neisseria gonorrhoeae* isolated in Durban, South Africa. *Antimicrob Ag Chemother* **26**: 770.

Cornick NA, Cuchural GJJr, Snydman DR et al. (1990). The antimicrobial susceptibility patterns of the *Bacteroides fragilis* group in the United States, 1987. *J Antimicrob Chemother* **25**: 1011.

Cox CE (1986). Timentin versus piperacillin in the treatment of hospitalized patients with urinary tract infections. *J Antimicrob Chemother* **17** (Suppl C): 93.

Crokaert F, van der Linden MP, Yourassowsky E (1982). Activities of amoxicillin and clavulanic acid combinations against urinary tract infections. *Antimicrob Ag Chemother* **22**: 346.

Croydon P (1984). Worldwide clinical review of augmentin. *Postgraduate Medicine, Progress and Perspectives on Beta-Lactamase Inhibition: A Review of Augmentin* p. 71. New York: Custom Communications.

Cuchural GJJr, Tally FP, Jacobus NV et al. (1988). Susceptibility of the *Bacteroides fragilis* Group in the United States: analysis by site of isolation. *Antimicrob Ag Chemother* **32**: 717.

Cuchural GJJr, Tally FP, Jacobus NV et al. (1990). Comparative activities of newer beta-lactam agents against members of the *Bacteroides fragilis* group. *Antimicrob Ag Chemother* **34**: 479.

Cynamon MH, Palmer GS (1983). *In vitro* activity of amoxicillin in combination with clavulanic acid against *Mycobacterium tuberculosis*. *Antimicrob Ag Chemother* **24**: 429.

Dagan R, Bar-David Y (1989). Comparison of amoxicillin and clavulanic acid (Augmentin). for the treatment of nonbullous impetigo. *Amer J Dis Child* **143**: 916.

Dambro N, Friedman AD, Alexander ER, Harrison HR (1984). Augmentin therapy for urinary tract infections in children. *Postgraduate Medicine, Progress and Perspectives on Beta-Lactamase Inhibition: A Review of Augmentin* p. 263. New York: Custom Communications.

Dangor Y, Miller SD, Exposto F da L, Koornhof HJ (1988). Antimicrobial susceptibilities of Southern African isolates of *Haemophilus ducreyi*. *Antimicrob Ag Chemother* **32**: 1458.

Davies BI, Maesen FPV (1990). Treatment of *Branhamella catarrhalis* infections. *J Antimicrob Chemother* **25**: 1.

Decazes JM, Bure A, Wolff M *et al.* (1987). Bactericidal activity against *Haemophilus influenzae* of cerebrospinal fluid of patients given amoxicillin-clavulanic acid. *Antimicrob Ag Chemother* **31**: 2018.

Dieterich H-J, Groh J, Behringer K *et al.* (1989). The prophylactic activity of amoxycillin/clavulanate and cefoxitin in vascular surgery – a randomized clinical study. *J Antimicrob Chemother* **24** (Suppl B): 209.

Dumon L, Adriaens P, Anné J Eyssen H (1979). Effect of clavulanic acid on the minimum inhibitory concentration of benzylpenicillin, ampicillin, carbenicillin, or cephalothin against clinical isolates resistant to beta-lactam antibiotics. *Antimicrob Ag Chemother* **15**: 315.

Engelhard D, Cohen D, Strauss N *et al.* (1989). Randomised study of myringotomy, amoxycillin/clavulanate, or both for acute otitis media in infants. *Lancet* **ii**: 141.

Entenza JM, Fluckiger U, Glauser MP, Moreillon P (1994). Antibiotic treatment of experimental endocarditis due to methicillin-resistant *Staphylococcus epidermidis*. *J Infect Dis* **170**: 100.

Evans CM, Purohit S, Colbert JW, *et al.* (1988). Amoxycillin – clavulanic acid (Augmentin). antibiotic prophylaxis against wound infections in renal failure patients. *J Antimicrob Chemother* **22**: 363.

Fancourt GJ, Flavell Matts SG, Mitchell CJ (1984). Augmentin (amoxycillin-clavulanic acid). compared with co-trimoxazole in urinary tract infections. *Brit Med J* **289**: 82.

Farmer T, Reading C (1982). Beta-lactamases of *Branhamella catarrhalis* and their inhibition by clavulanic acid. *Antimicrob Ag Chemother* **21**: 506.

Faro S, Hammill HA, Maccato M, Martens M (1991). Ticarcillin/clavulanate for treatment of postpartum endometritis. *Rev Infect Dis* **13** (Suppl 9): 758.

Fast MV, Nsanze H, D'Costa LJ *et al.* (1982). Treatment of chancroid by clavulanic acid with amoxycillin in patients with beta-lactamase-positive *Haemophilus ducreyi* infection. *Lancet* **ii**: 509.

Fattorini L, Scardaci G, Jin SH *et al.* (1991). Beta-lactamase of *Mycobacterium fortuitum*: kinetics of production and relationship with resistance to beta-lactam antibiotics. *Antimicrob Ag Chemother* **35**: 1760.

File TM Jr, Tan JS (1991). Ticarcillin-clavulanate therapy for bacterial skin and soft tissue infections. *Rev Infect Dis* **13** (Suppl 9): 733.

File TM Jr, Tan JS, Salstrom S-J *et al.* (1984). Timentin versus piperacillin or moxalactam in the therapy of acute bacterial infections. *Antimicrob Ag Chemother* **26**: 310.

Finegold SM (1991). Aspiration pneumonia. *Rev Infect Dis* **13** (Suppl 9): 737.

Fink MP, Helsmoortel CM, Arous EJ *et al.* (1989). Comparison of the safety and efficacy of parenteral ticarcillin/clavulanate and clindamycin/gentamicin in serious intra-abdominal infections. *J Antimicrob Chemother* **24** (Suppl B): 147.

Fischbach M, Simeoni U, Mengus L *et al.* (1989). Urinary tract infections with tissue penetration in children: cefotaxime compared with amoxycillin/clavulanate. *J Antimicrob Chemother* **24** (Suppl 5): 177.

Fleisher GR, Wilmott CM, Campos JM (1983). Amoxicillin combined with clavulanic acid for the treatment of soft tissue infections in children. *Antimicrob Ag Chemother* **24**: 679.

Franz P, von Rosen F, Garner C *et al.* (1989). Cerebrospinal fluid penetration after single or multiple dosage with ticarcillin/clavulanate. *J Antimicrob Chemother* **24** (Suppl B): 107.

Fricke G, Doerck M, Hafner D *et al.* (1989). The pharmacokinetics of ticarcillin/clavulanate acid in neonates. *J Antimicrob Chemother* **24** (Suppl B): 111.

Fuchs PC, Barry AL, Thornsberry C *et al.* (1983). *In vitro* evaluation of augmentin by broth microdilution an disk diffusion susceptibility testing: regression analysis, tentative interpretative criteria and quality control limits. *Antimicrob Ag Chemother* **24**: 31.

Fuchs PC, Barry AL, Thornsberry C, Jones RN (1984). *In vitro* activity of ticarcillin plus clavulanic acid against 632 clinical isolates. *Antimicrob Ag Chemother* **25**: 392.

Gaspar MC, Soriano F (1981). Susceptibility of *Yersinia enterocolitica* to eight beta-lactam antibiotics and clavulanic acid. *J Antimicrob Chemother* **8**: 161.

Gaudreau CL, Lariviere LA, Lauzer JC, Turgeon FF (1987). Effect of clavulanic acid on susceptibility of *Campylobacter jejuni* and *Campylobacter coli* to eight beta-lactam antibiotics. *Antimicrob Ag Chemother* **31**: 940.

Gelber RH (1991). The activity of amoxicillin plus clavulanic acid against *Mycobacterium leprae* in mice. *J Infect Dis* **163**: 1374.

Gentry LO (1992). Therapy with newer oral beta-lactam and quinolone agents for infections of the skin and skin structures: a review. *Clin Infect Dis* **14**: 285.

Gentry LO, Macko V, Lind R, Heilman AL (1985). Ticarcillin plus clavulanic acid (Timentin). therapy for osteomyelitis. *Amer J Med* **79** (Suppl 5B): 116.

Girouard YC, Maclean IW, Ronald AR, Albritton WL (1981). Synergistic antibacterial activity of clavulanic acid and amoxicillin against beta-lactamase-producing strains of Haemophilus ducreyi. *Antimicrob Ag Chemother* **20**: 144.

Godfrey AJ, Wong S, Dance DAB *et al.* (1991). *Pseudomonas pseudomallei* resistance to beta-lactam antibiotics due to alterations in the chromosomally encoded beta-lactamase. *Antimicrob Ag Chemother* **35**: 1635.

Goldstein EJC, Citron DM (1988). Comparative activities of cefuroxime, amoxicillin-clavulanic acid, ciprofloxacin, enoxacin, and ofloxacin against aerobic and anaerobic bacteria isolated from bite wounds. *Antimicrob Ag Chemother* **32**: 1143.

Gooch WM III, Swenson E, Congeni BL, Snellman LW III (1984). Oral Augmentin in the management of pediatric pneumonia. *Postgraduate Medicine. Progress and Perspectives on Beta-Lactamase Inhibition: A Review of Augmentin*, p. 187. New York: Custom Communications.

Grange JD, Gouyette A, Gutmann L *et al.* (1989). Pharmacokinetics of amoxycillin/clavulanic acid in serum and ascitic fluid in cirrhotic patients. *J Antimicrob Chemother* **23**: 605.

Graninger W, Leitha T, Griffin K *et al.* (1989). Activity of clavulanate-potentiated penicillins against methicillin-resistant *Staphylococcus aureus*. *J Antimicrob Chemother* **24** (Suppl B): 49.

Gurwith MJ, Stein GE, Gurwith D (1983). Prospective comparison of amoxicillin-clavulanic acid and cefaclor in treatment of uncomplicated urinary tract infections. *Antimicrob Ag Chemother* **24**: 716.

Hall C, Curran F, Burdon DW, Keighley MRB (1989). A randomized trial to compare amoxycillin/clavulanate with metronidazole plus gentamicin in prophylaxis in elective colorectal surgery. *J Antimicrob Chemother* **24** (Suppl B): 195.

Hebbard GS, Smith KGC, Gibson PR, Bhathal PS (1992). Augmentin-induced jaundice with a fatal outcome. *Med J Aust* **156**: 285.

Henquell C, Sirot D, Chanal C *et al.* (1994). Frequency of inhibitor-resistant TEM beta-lactamases in *Escherichia coli* isolates from urinary tract infections in France. *J Antimicrob Chemother* **34**: 707.

Horber FF, Frey FJ, Descoeudres C *et al.* (1986). Differential effect of impaired renal function on the kinetics of clavulanic acid and amoxicillin. *Antimicrob Ag Chemother* **29**: 614.

Horii T, Arakawa Y, Ohta M *et al.* (1993). Plasmid-mediated amp C-type beta-lactamase isolated from *Klebsiella pneumoniae* confers resistance to broad-spectrum beta-lactams, including moxalactam. *Antimicrob Ag Chemother* **37**: 984.

Houang ET, Colley N, Chapman M (1985). Penetration of sulbactam-ampicillin and clavulanic acid-amoxicillin into the pelvic peritoneum. *Antimicrob Ag Chemother* **28**: 165.

Hunter PA, Coleman K, Fisher J, Taylor D (1980). *In vitro* synergistic properties of clavulanic acid, with ampicillin, amoxycillin and ticarcillin. *J Antimicrob Chemother* **6**: 455.

Inthorn D, Mühlbayer D, Hartl WH (1989). Ticarcillin/clavulanate in the treatment of severe peritonitis. *J Antimicrob Chemother* **24** (Suppl B): 141.

Iravani A, Richard GA (1982). Treatment of urinary tract infections with a combination of amoxicillin and clavulanic acid. *Antimicrob Ag Chemother* **22**: 672.

Iravani A, Richard GA (1986). Amoxicillin-clavulanic acid versus cefaclor in the treatment of urinary tract infections and their effects on the urogenital and rectal flora. *Antimicrob Ag Chemother* **29**: 107.

Ingerman M, Pitsakis PG, Rosenberg A *et al.* (1987). Beta-lactamase production in experimental endocarditis due to aminoglycoside-resistant *Streptococcus faecalis*. *J Infect Dis* **155**: 1226.

Jackson D, Cooper DL, Horton R *et al.* (1983). Absorption, pharmacokinetic and metabolic studies with Augmentin. In *Augmentin* (Croydon EAP, Michel MF, eds), p. 83. Amsterdam: Excerpta Medica.

Jackson D, Filer CW, Cooper DL, Langley PF (1984). Augmentin: absorption, excretion and pharmacokinetic studies in man. *Postgraduate Medicine. Progress and Perspectives on Beta-Lactamase Inhibition: A Review of Augmentin* p. 51. New York: Custom Communications.

Jacobs RF, Trang JM, Kearns GL *et al.* (1985). Ticarcillin/clavulanic acid pharmacokinetics in children and young adults with cystic fibrosis. *J Pediatr* **106**: 1001.

Jacoby GA, Archer GL (1991). New mechanisms of bacterial resistance to antimicrobial agents. *New Engl J Med* **324**: 601.

Jacoby GA, Carreras I (1990). Activities of beta-lactam antibiotics against *Escherichia coli* strains producing extended spectrum beta-lactamases. *Antimicrob Ag Chemother* **34**: 858.

Jacoby GA, Medeiros AA (1991). More extended-spectrum beta-lactamases. *Antimicrob Ag Chemother* **35**: 1697.

Jacobsson S, Fogh A, Larsson P *et al.* (1993). Evaluation of amoxicillin clavulanate twice daily versus thrice daily in the treatment of otitis media in children. *Eur J Clin Microbiol Infect Dis* **12**: 319.

Jaresko GS, Barriere SL, Johnson BLJr (1992). Serum and blister fluid pharmacokinetics and bactericidal activities of ampicillin-sulbactam, cefotetan, cefoxitin, ceftizoxime, and ticarcillin-clavulanate. *Antimicrob Ag Chemother* **36**: 2233.

Jarlier J, Nicolas M-H, Fournier G, Phillipon A (1988). Extended broad-spectrum beta-lactamases conferring transferable resistance to newer beta-lactam agents in Enterobacteriaceae: hospital prevalence and susceptibility patterns. *Rev Infect Dis* **10**: 867.

Jensen T, Pedersen SS, Stafanger G *et al.* (1988). Comparison of amoxycillin/clavulanate with amoxycillin in children and adults with chronic obstructive pulmonary disease and infection with *Haemophilus influenzae*. *Scand J Infect Dis* **20**: 517.

Jones AE, Barnes ND, Tasker TCG, Horton R (1990). Pharmacokinetics of intravenous amoxycillin and potassium clavulanate in seriously ill children. *J Antimicrob Chemother* **25**: 269.

Jones RN, Thornsberry C (1984). Beta-lactamase studies of eight *Legionella* species: antibacterial activity of Augmentin compared to newer cephalosporins, erythromycin and rifampin. *Postgraduate Medicine. Progress and Perspectives on Beta-Lactamase Inhibition: A Review of Augmentin* p. 259. New York: Custom Communications.

Jungbluth GL, Cooper DL, Doyle GD *et al.* (1986). Pharmacokinetics of ticarcillin and clavulanic acid (Timentin). in relation to renal function. *Antimicrob Ag Chemother* **30**: 896.

Kaleida PH, Bluestone CD, Rockette HE *et al.* (1987). Amoxicillin-clavulanate potassium compared with cefaclor for acute otitis media in infants and children. *Pediatr Infect Dis J* **6**: 265.

Kaplan EL, Johnson DR (1988). Eradication of group A streptococci from the upper respiratory tract by amoxicillin with clavulanate after oral penicillin V treatment failure. *J Pediatr* **113**: 400.

Karachalios GN (1985). Randomized comparative study of amoxicillin-

clavulanic acid and co-trimoxazole in the treatment of acute urinary tract infections in adults. *Antimicrob Ag Chemother* **28**: 693.

Key PR, Azadian BS, Evans BA (1985). Augmentin compared with amoxycillin in treating uncomplicated gonorrhoea. *Genitourin Med* **61**: 165.

Khardori N, Elting L, Wong E *et al.* (1990). Nosocomial infections due to Xanthomonas maltophilia (*Pseudomonas maltophilia*). in patients with cancer. *Rev Infect Dis* **12**: 997.

Kitzis MD, Gutmann L, Acar JF (1985). *In-vitro* susceptibility of *Nocardia asteroides* to 21 beta-lactam antibiotics, in combination with three beta-lactamase inhibitors, and its relationship to the beta-lactamase content. *J Antimicrob Chemother* **15**: 23.

Kitzis MD, Billot-Klein D, Goldstein FW *et al.* (1988). Dissemination of the novel plasmid-mediated beta-lactamase CTX-1, which confers resistance to broad-spectrum cephalosporins, and its inhibition by beta-lactamase inhibitors. *Antimicrob Ag Chemother* **32**: 9.

Knapp CC, Sierra-Madero J, Washington JA (1989). Activity of ticarcillin/clavulanate and piperacillin/tazobactam (YTR 830; CL 298,741). against clinical isolates and against mutants derepressed for class 1 beta-lactamase. *Diagn Microbiol Infect Dis* **12**: 511.

Lachance N, Gaudreau C, Lamothe F, Turgeon F (1993). Susceptibilities of beta-lactamase-positive and -negative strains of *Campylobacter coli* to beta-lactam agents. *Antimicrob Ag Chemother* **37**: 1174.

Lapointe J-R, Lavallee C (1987). Antibiotic interaction of amoxycillin and clavulanic acid against 132 beta-lactamase positive *Haemophilus* isolates: a comparison with some other oral agents. *J Antimicrob Chemother* **19**: 49.

Lawrence AG, Shanson DC (1985). Single dose oral amoxicillin 3 g with either 125 mg or 250 mg clavulanic acid to treat uncomplicated anogenital gonorrhoea. *Genitourin Med* **61**: 168.

Livermore DM, Seetulsing P (1991). Susceptibility of *Escherichia coli* isolates with TEM-1 beta-lactamase to combinations of BRL42715, tazobactam or clavulanate with piperacillin or amoxycillin. *J Antimicrob Chemother* **27**: 761.

Livermore DM, Chau PY, Wong AIW, Leung YK (1987). Beta-lactamase of *Pseudomonas pseudomallei* and its contribution to antibiotic resistance. *J Antimicrob Chemother* **20**: 313.

Livermore DM, Akova M, Wu P, Yang Y (1989). Clavulanate and beta-lactamase induction. *J Antimicrob Chemother* **24** (Suppl B): 23.

Maesen FPV, Davies BI, Baur C (1987). Amoxycillin/clavulanate in acute purulent exacerbations of chronic bronchitis. *J Antimicrob Chemother* **19**: 373.

Manek N, Wise R, Donovan IA (1987). Intraperitoneal penetration of ticarcillin/clavulanic acid (Timentin). *J Antimicrob Chemother* **19**: 363.

McEniry DW, Gillespie SH, Felmingham D (1988). Susceptibility of *Pseudomonas pseudomallei* to new beta-lactam and aminoglycoside antibiotics. *J Antimicrob Chemother* **21**: 171.

Medeiros AA(1993). Nosocomial outbreaks of multiresistant bacteria: extended-spectrum beta-lactamases have arrived in North America. *Ann Intern Med* **119**: 428.

Mehtar S, Ball AP (1985). Intravenous augmentin in bacteraemia and severe invasive polymicrobial sepsis. *J Antimicrob Chemother* **15**: 765.

Meunier F, Snoack R, Lagost H *et al.* (1986). Empirical antimicrobial therapy with Timentin plus amikacin in febrile granulocytopenic cancer patients. *J Antimicrob Chemother* **17** (Suppl C): 195.

Meyer KS, Urban C, Eagan JA *et al.* (1993). Nosocomial outbreak of *Klebsiella* infection resistant to late-generation cephalosporins. *Ann Intern Med* **119**: 353.

Mizen L, Woodnutt G, Kernutt I, Catherall EJ (1989). Simulation of human serum pharmacokinetics of ticarcillin-clavulanic acid and ceftazidime in rabbits and efficacy against experimental *Klebsiella pneumoniae* meningitis. *Antimicrob Ag Chemother* **33**: 693.

Moellering RCJr (1991). Beta-lactamase inhibition: therapeutic implications in infectious diseases – an overview. *Rev Infect Dis* **13** (Suppl 9): 723.

Münch R, Lüthy R, Blaser J, Siegenthaler W (1981). Human pharmacokinetics and CSF penetration of clavulanic acid. *J Antimicrob Chemother* **8**: 29.

Murray BE (1991). New aspects of antimicrobial resistance and the resulting therapeutic dilemmas. *J Infect Dis* **163**: 1185.

Murray PR, Jones RN, Allen SD *et al.* (1993). Multilaboratory evaluation of the in vitro activity of 13 beta-lactam antibiotics against 1974 clinical isolates of aerobic and anaerobic bacteria. *Diagn Microbiol Infect Dis* **16**: 191.

Nakazawa H, Hashimoto T, Nishiura T, Mitsuhashi S (1983). Efficacy of BRL 25000 against *Serratia marcescens*, *Enterobacter cloacae*, and *Citrobacter freundii* in urinary tract infections. *Antimicrob Ag Chemother* **24**: 437.

Nelson JD, Kusmiesz H, Shelton S (1982). Pharmacokinetics of potassium clavulanate in combination with amoxicillin in pediatric patients. *Antimicrob Ag Chemother* **21**: 681.

Neu HC, Fu KP (1978). Clavulanic acid, a novel inhibitor of beta-lactamases. *Antimicrob Ag Chemother* **14**: 650.

Nilsson-Ehle I, Fellner H, Hedström S-Å *et al.* (1985). Pharmacokinetics of clavulanic acid, given in combination with amoxycillin in volunteers. *J Antimicrob Chemother* **16**: 491.

Obwegeser J, Kunz J, Wüst J *et al.* (1989). Clinical efficacy of amoxycillin/clavulanate in laparoscopically confirmed salpingitis. *J Antimicrob Chemother* **24** (Suppl B): 165.

Page JWJ, FarmerTH, Elson SW (1989). Hyperproduction of TEM-1 beta-lactamase by Escherichia coli strains. *J Antimicrob Chemother* **23**: 160.

Pankey GA, Katner HP, Valainis GT *et al.* (1985). Overview of bacterial infections of the skin and soft tissue and clinical experience with ticarcillin plus clavulanate potassium in their treatment. *Amer J Med* **79** (Suppl 5B): 106.

Pankuch GA, Jacobs MR, Rittenhouse SF, Appelbaum PC (1994). Susceptibilities of 123 strains of *Xanthomonas maltophilia* to eight beta-lactams (including beta-lactam-beta-lactamase inhibitor combinations). and ciprofloxacin tested by five methods. *Antimicrob Ag Chemother* **38**: 2317.

Papanicolaou GA, Medeiros AA, Jacoby GA (1990). Novel plasmid-mediated beta-lactamase (MIR-1). conferring resistance to oxymino- and alpha-methoxy beta-lactams in clinical isolates of *Klebsiella pneumoniae*. *Antimicrob Chemother* **34**: 2200.

Pastorek JGII, Sanders CVJr (1991). Antibiotic therapy for postcesarean endomyometritis. *Rev Infect Dis* **13** (Suppl 9): 752.

Payne DJ, Cramp R, Winstanley DJ, Knowles DJC (1994). Comparative activities of clavulanic acid, sulbactam, and tazobactam against clinically important beta-lactamases. *Antimicrob Ag Chemother* **38**: 767.

Pedler SJ, Bint AJ (1985). Comparative study of amoxicillin-clavulanic acid and cephalexin in the treatment of bacteriuria during pregnancy. *Antimicrob Ag Chemother* **27**: 508.

Philippon A, Labia R, Jacoby G (1989). Extended-spectrum beta-lactamases. *Antimicrob Ag Chemother* **33**: 1131.

Pichichero ME, Pichichero CL (1995). Persistent acute otitis media: II Antimicrobial treatment. *Pediatr Infect Dis J* **14**: 183.

Pien FD (1983). Double-blind comparative study of two dosage regimens of cefaclor and amoxicillin-clavulanic acid in the outpatient treatment of soft tissue infections. *Antimicrob Ag Chemother* **24**: 856.

Pohlod DJ, Saravolatz LD, Quinn EL, Somerville MM (1980). Effect of clavulanic acid on minimal inhibitory concentrations of 16 antimicrobial agents tested against *Legionella pneumophila*. *Antimicrob Ag Chemother* **18**: 353.

Pörnull KJ, Göransson E, Rytting A-S, Dornbusch K (1993). Extended-spectrum beta-lactamases in *Escherichia coli* and *Klebsiella* spp in European septicaemia isolates. *J Antimicrob Chemother* **32**: 559.

Powell M, McVey D, Kassim MH *et al.* (1991). Antimicrobial susceptibility of *Streptococcus pneumoniae*, *Haemophilus influenzae* and *Moraxella* (*Branhamella*) *catarrhalis* isolated in the UK from sputa. *J Antimicrob Chemother* **28**: 249.

Pulverer G, Peters G, Kunstmann G (1986). In-vitro activity of ticarcillin with and without clavulanic acid against clinical isolates of Gram-positive and Gram-negative bacteria. *J Antimicrob Chemother* **17** (Suppl C): 1.

Raz R, Rottensterich E, Boger S, Potasman I (1991). Comparison of single-

dose administration and three-day course of amoxicillin with those of clavulanic acid for the treatment of uncomplicated urinary tract infection in women. *Antimicrob Ag Chemother* **35**: 1688.

Reading C, Cole M (1977). Clavulanic acid: a beta-lactamase-inhibiting beta-lactam from *Streptomyces clavuligerus*. *Antimicrob Ag Chemother* **11**: 852.

Reading C, Farmer T, Cole M (1983). The beta-lactamase stability of amoxycillin with the beta-lactamase inhibitor, clavulanic acid. *J Antimicrob Chemother* **11**: 27.

Reguera JA, Baquero F, Perez-Diaz JC, Martinez JL (1991). Factors determining resistance to beta-lactam combined with beta-lactamase inhibitors in *Escherichia coli*. *J Antimicrob Chemother* **27**: 569.

Rice RJ, Knapp JS (1994). Antimicrobial susceptibilities of *Neisseria gonorrhoeae* strains representing five distinct resistance phenotypes. *Antimicrob Ag Chemother* **38**: 155.

Rolinson GN (1984). History and mode of action of augmentin. *Postgraduate Medicine. Progress and Perspectives on Beta-Lactamase Inhibition: A Review of Augmentin* p. 23. New York: Custom Communications.

Rolinson GN (1985). Clavulanic acid/antibiotic ratios. *J Antimicrob Chemother* **15**: 256.

Rolinson GN (1989). Beta-lactamase induction and resistance to beta-lactam antibiotics. *J Antimicrob Chemother* **23**: 1.

Rolinson GN (1991). Evolution of beta-lactamase inhibitors. *Rev Infect Dis* **13** (Suppl 9): 727.

Roselle GA, Bode R, Hamilton B *et al.* (1985). Clinical trial of the efficacy and safety of ticarcillin and clavulanic acid. *Antimicrob Ag Chemother* **27**: 291.

Roy C, Segura C, Torrellas A *et al.* (1989). Activity of amoxycillin/clavulanate against beta-lactamase-producing *Escherichia coli* and *Klebsiella* spp. *J Antimicrob Chemother* **24** (Suppl B): 41.

Samonis G, Gikas A, Anaissie EJ *et al.* (1993). Prospective evaluation of effects of broad-spectrum antibiotics on gastrointestinal yeast colonization of humans. *Antimicrob Ag Chemother* **37**: 51.

Schaad UB, Casey PA, Cooper DL (1983). Single-dose pharmacokinetics of intravenous clavulanic acid with amoxicillin in pediatric patients. *Antimicrob Ag Chemother* **23**: 252.

Schaad UB, Casey PA, Ravenscroft AT (1986). Pharmacokinetics of a syrup formulation of amoxycillin-potassium clavulanate in children. *J Antimicrob Chemother* **17**: 341.

Schaad UB, Pfenninger J, Wedgwood-Krucko J (1987). Sequential intravenous-oral amoxycillin/clavulanate (Augmentin). therapy in paediatric hospital practice. *J Antimicrob Chemother* **19**: 385.

Schaison G, Reinert Ph, Leverger G, Leaute JB (1986). Timentin (ticarcillin and clavulanic acid). in combination with aminoglycosides in the treatment of febrile episodes in neutropenic children. *J Antimicrob Chemother* **17** (Suppl C): 177.

Scheld WM, Mandell GL (1991). Nosocomial pneumonia: pathogenesis and recent advances in diagnosis and therapy. *Rev Infect Dis* **13** (Suppl 9): 743.

Schmitt M, Bondonny JM, Delmas P *et al.* (1989). Antibiotic therapy of perforated appendicitis in children: a comparison of amoxycillin/clavulanate with a combination of benzylpenicillin, netilmicin and metronidazole. *J Antimicrob Chemother* **24** (Suppl B): 157.

Schwigon CD, Hulla FW, Schulze B, Maslak A (1986). Timentin in the treatment of nosocomial bronchopulmonary infections in intensive care units. *J Antimicrob Chemother* **17** (Suppl C): 115.

Shenep JL, Hughes WT, Robertson PK *et al.* (1988). Vancomycin, ticarcillin, and amikacin compared with ticarcillin – clavulanate and amikacin in the empirical treatment of febrile, neutropenic children with cancer. *New Engl J Med* **319**: 1053.

Sirot D, Chanal C, Henquell C *et al.* (1994). Clinical isolates of *Escherichia coli* producing multiple TEM mutants resistant to beta-lactamase inhibitors. *J Antimicrob Chemother* **33**: 1117.

Slocombe B, Beale AS, Boon RJ *et al.* (1984). Antibacterial activity *in vitro* and *in vivo* of amoxicillin in the presence of clavulanic acid. *Postgraduate Medicine. Progress and Perspectives on Beta-Lactamase*

Inhibition: A Review of Augmentin p. 29. New York: Custom Communications.

Smith BR, Le Frock JL (1985). Amoxicillin-potassium clavulanate A novel beta-lactamase inhibitor. *Drug Intel Clin Pharm* **19**: 415.

Smith GM, Abbott KH, Wilkinson MJ (1991). Bactericidal effects of ticarcillin-clavulanic acid against *Legionella pneumophila* pneumonia in immunocompromised weanling rats. *Antimicrob Ag Chemother* **35**: 1423.

Smith GM, Abbott KH, Sutherland R (1992). Bactericidal effects of co-amoxiclav (amoxycillin clavulanic acid). against a *Legionella-pneumophila* pneumonia in the immunocompromised weanling rat. *J Antimicrob Ag Chemother* **30**: 525.

Snavely SR, Harms JL, Hinthorn DR, Liu C (1984). Efficacy of amoxicillin-potassium clavulanate in the treatment of urinary tract infections. *Postgraduate Medicine. Progress and Perspectives on Beta-Lactamase Inhibition: A Review of Augmentin* p. 213. New York: Custom Communications.

Sookpranee T, Sookpranee M, Mellencamp MA, Preheim LC (1991). *Pseudomonas pseudomallei*, a common pathogen in Thailand that is resistant to the bactericidal effects of many antibiotics. *Antimicrob Ag Chemother* **35**: 484.

Staniforth DH, Lillystone RJ, Jackson D (1982). Effect of food on the bioavailability and tolerance of clavulanic acid/amoxicillin combination. *J Antimicrob Chemother* **10**: 131.

Staniforth DH, Jackson D, Clarke HL, Horton R (1983). Amoxycillin/clavulanic acid: the effect of probenecid. *J Antimicrob Chemother* **12**: 273.

Stokes DH, Slocombe B, Sutherland R (1989a). Bactericidal effects of amoxycillin/clavulanic acid against *Legionella pneumophila*. *J Antimicrob Chemother* **23**: 43.

Stokes DH, Wilkinson MJ, Tyler J*et al.* (1989b). Bactericidal effects of amoxycillin/clavulanic acid against intracellular *Legionella pneumophila* in tissue culture studies. *J Antimicrob Chemother* **23**: 547.

Syrogiannopoulos GA, Al-Sabbagh A, Olsen KD, McCracken GHJr (1987). Pharmacokinetics and bacteriological efficacy of ticarcillin-clavulanic acid (Timentin). in experimental *Escherichia coli* K-1 and *Haemophilus influenzae* type b meningitis. *Antimicrob Ag Chemother* **31**: 1296.

Tan JS, File TM Jr (1984). Double blind efficacy and safety study of Augmentin versus cefaclor in the treatment of lower respiratory tract infections. *Postgraduate Medicine. Progress and Perspectives on Beta-Lactamase Inhibition: A Review of Augmentin* p. 129. New York: Custom Communications.

Thomas MG, Gillies M, Roberts S, Lang SDR (1985). Comparison of the anti-staphylococcal activity of serum from healthy subjects taking flucloxacillin or augmentin. *N Z J Med* **98**: 452.

Thomson CJ, Amyes SGB (1993). Selection of variants of the TEM-1 beta-lactamase, encoded by a plasmid of clinical origin, with increased resistance to beta-lactamase inhibitors. *J Antimicrob Chemother* **31**: 655.

Thomson JA, Fairley CK, Ugoni AM *et al.* (1995). Risk factors for the development of amoxycillin-clavulanic acid associated jaundice. *Med J Aust* **162**: 638.

Van Hare GF, Shurin PA, Marchant CD *et al.* (1987). Acute otitis media caused by *Branhamella catarrhalis*: biology and therapy. *Rev Infect Dis* **9**: 16.

Van der Auwera P, Scorneaux B (1985). *In vitro* susceptibility of *Campylobacter jejuni* to 27 antimicrobial agents and various combinations of beta-lactams with clavulanic acid or sulbactam. *Antimicrob Ag Chemother* **28**: 37.

Van der Meijden WI, Piot P, Loriaux SM, Stolz E (1987). Amoxycillin, amoxycillin-clavulanic acid and metronidazole in the treatment of clue cell-positive discharge. A comparative clinical and laboratory study. *J

Antimicrob Chemother* **20**: 735.

Van der Ven AJM, Koopmans PP, Vree TB, Van der Meer JWM (1994). Drug intolerance in HIV disease. *J Antimicrob Chemother* **34**: 1.

Vartivarian S, Anaissie E, Bodey G *et al.* (1994). A changing pattern of susceptibility of *Xanthomonas maltophilia* to antimicrobial agents: implications for therapy. *Antimicrob Ag Chemother* **38**: 624.

Vedel G, Belaaouaj A,Gilly L *et al.* (1992). Clinical isolates of *Escherichia coli* producing TRI beta-lactamases: novel TEM-enzymes conferring resistance to beta-lactamase inhibitors. *J Antimicrob Chemother* **30**: 449.

Wagner B, Fattorini L, Wagner M *et al.* (1995). Antigenic properties and immunoelectron microscopic localization of *Mycobacterium fortuitum* beta-lactamase. *Antimicrob Ag Chemother* **39**: 739.

Wald ER, Casselbrant MC, Reilly JS, Chiponis DM (1984). Treatment of acute sinusitis in children: Augmentin versus cefaclor. *Postgraduate Medicine. Progress and Perspectives on Beta-Lactamase Inhibition: A Review of Augmentin* p. 133. New York: Custom Communications.

Walker CK, Kahn JG, Washington AE *et al.* (1993). Pelvic inflammatory disease: metaanalysis of antimicrobial regimen efficacy. *J Infect Dis* **168**: 969.

Wallace RJ Jr (1984). The increasing role of beta-lactamase-producing organisms as causative agents of respiratory tract disease: the decline and fall of penicillin? *Postgraduate Medicine. Progress and Perspectives on Beta-Lactamase Inhibition: A Review of Augmentin* p. 121. New York: Custom Communications.

Wallace RJ Jr, Steele LC, Brooks DL *et al.* (1985). Amoxicillin-clavulanic acid in the treatment of lower respiratory tract infections caused by beta-lactamase-positive *Haemophilus influenzae* and *Branhamella catarrhalis*. *Antimicrob Ag Chemother* **27**: 912.

Wallace RJ Jr, Nash DR, Johnson WK *et al.* (1987). Beta-lactam resistance in Nocardia brasiliensis is mediated by beta-lactamase and reversed in the presence of clavulanic acid. *J Infect Dis* **156**: 959.

Weber DA, Sanders CC (1990). Diverse potential of beta-lactamase inhibitors to induce class I enzymes. *Antimicrob Ag Chemother* **34**: 156.

Westenfelder M, Pelz K, Hulla FW (1986). Clinical evaluation of Timentin in complicated urinary tract infections. *J Antimicrob Chemother* **17** (Suppl C): 97.

Williams ME, Thomas D, Harman CP *et al.* (1985). Positive direct antiglobulin tests due to clavulanic acid. *Antimicrob Ag Chemother* **27**: 125.

Wise R, Donovan IA, Drumm J *et al.* (1983). The penetration of amoxycillin/clavulanic acid into peritoneal fluid. *J Antimicrob Chemother* **11**: 57.

Wong CS, Palmer GS, Cynamon MH (1988). *In-vitro* susceptibility of *Mycobacterium tuberculosis*, *Mycobacterium bovis* and *Mycobacterium kansasii* to amoxycillin and ticarcillin in combination with clavulanic acid. *J Antimicrob Chemother* **22**: 863.

Woodnutt G, Kernutt I, Mizen L (1987). Pharmacokinetics and distribution of ticarcillin-clavulanic acid (Timentin). in experimental animals. *Antimicrob Ag Chemother* **31**: 1826.

Woodnutt G, Berry V, Kernutt I, Mizen L (1990). Penetration of amoxycillin, ticarcillin and clavulanic acid into lymph after intravenous infusion in rabbits to simulate human serum pharmacokinetics. *J Antimicrob Chemother* **26**: 695.

Wu P-J, Shannon K, Phillips I (1994). Effect of hyperproduction of TEM-1 beta-lactamase on *in vitro* susceptibility of *Escherichia coli* to beta-lactam antibiotics. *Antimicrob Ag Chemother* **38**: 494.

Zhou XY, Bordon F, Sirot D *et al.* (1994). Emergence of clinical isolates of *Escherichia coli* producing TEM-1 derivatives or an OXA-1 beta-lactamase conferring resistance to beta-lactamase inhibitors. *Antimicrob Ag Chemother* **38**: 1085.

Sulbactam

Description

Sulbactam (penicillanic acid sulfone) is a semisynthetic beta-lactamase inhibitor, which was derived from the penicillin nucleus, 6 APA (p. 3), at Pfizer Research Laboratories (English et al., 1978). It is active against the same range of beta-lactamases as clavulanic acid (p. 192), but in this respect it is less potent. Unlike clavulanic acid, it is also active against inducible chromosomally mediated enzymes which cause resistance to third-generation cephalosporins (p. 192) (Jacobs et al., 1986; Klastersky and Van der Auwera, 1989; Sawai and Yamaguchi, 1989). Sulbactam inhibits beta-lactamases by the same mechanism as clavulanic acid (p. 192) (Fu and Neu, 1979; Wise, 1982; Bush and Sykes, 1983; Labia et al., 1986).

Sulbactam itself exhibits a moderate antibacterial activity that is related to its affinity for penicillin-binding proteins (PBPs) (p. 211) of various bacterial strains. Therefore in some bacterial strains which produce no beta-lactamases, a minor synergistic effect can be observed with sulbactam and some beta-lactam antibiotics (Labia et al., 1986; Kazmierczak et al., 1989).

Sulbactam, like clavulanic acid, can be combined with one of many beta-lactamase-labile beta-lactam antibiotics, such as penicillin G, ampicillin, carbenicillin, or cefoperazone to prevent their destruction by beta-lactamases (Retsema et al., 1980; Wise et al., 1980; Crosby and Gump, 1982; Fu et al., 1984).

For clinical use sulbactam has been combined with ampicillin, and this combination is available in the USA. For oral administration a mutual pro-drug, sultamicillin, has been produced. It consists of esters of sulbactam and ampicillin linked via a methylene group. Following absorption, hydrolysis occurs, probably in the intestinal wall, and equimolar proportions of sulbactam and ampicillin are liberated into the systemic circulation. Ampicillin given in the form of sultamicillin, is absorbed more rapidly and efficiently to produce serum levels approximately double those achieved by an equivalent dosage of ampicillin alone. Sulbactam is poorly absorbed after oral administration, but its pivaloyloxy methyl ester is well absorbed. Sultamicillin, therefore, provides effective plasma concentrations of both ampicillin and sulbactam when administered orally (Wise, 1981; Hartley and Wise, 1982; Rogers et al., 1983). For i.v. use ampicillin/sulbactam is now available in vials containing 1 g of ampicillin and 0.5 g of sulbactam (Reinhardt et al., 1986; Chang et al., 1989).

The combination of cefoperazone and sulbactam has also been studied in vitro (Bodey et al., 1989). In clinical trials the two drugs have been used in a 1:1 ratio (Horiuchi et al., 1989) but others have used cefoperazone 2.0 g plus sulbactam 1.0 g 6-hourly i.v. (Bodey et al., 1993).

Sensitive Organisms

1 Ampicillin/sulbactam

Sulbactam itself has a low level of antibacterial activity against most bacterial species, but Neisseria gonorrhoeae (Table I.14) and N. meningitidis and a few other bacteria (p. 211) are exceptions (Retsema et al., 1986). Sulbactam may slightly improve the activity of ampicillin against ampicillin-sensitive strains of various bacterial species (p. 108), but this has little clinical significance. It never antagonizes the activity of ampicillin against these bacteria. When combined with ampicillin, sulbactam reduces the amount of ampicillin required to inhibit growth of beta-lactamase-producing organisms to a level encountered with susceptible bacteria. Consequently beta-lactamase-producing strains of Staphylococcus aureus, Enterococcus faecalis, N. gonorrhoeae, Haemophilus influenzae, H. ducreyi, Moraxella catarrhalis, Klebsiella *pneumoniae*, and the *Proteus*, *Salmonella* and *Shigella* spp. are usually ampicillin/sulbactam-sensitive (Jones *et al.*, 1986; Labia *et al.*, 1986; Ling *et al.*, 1988; Azimi and Dunphy, 1989; Markowitz *et al.*, 1991; Baddour *et al.*, 1992; Murray *et al.*, 1993). Unlike co-amoxiclav (p. 192), this combination is less effective against *Escherichia coli* strains producing plasmid-mediated TEM beta-lactamase (Jacobs *et al.*, 1986; Livermore, 1992).

In contrast with clavulanic acid, sulbactam is a better inhibitor of chromosomally mediated, inducible beta-lactamases (p. 322). However, these beta-lactamases produced by *Enterobacter* and *Citrobacter* spp. and *Pseudomonas aeruginosa* are poorly inhibited by sulbactam, and so these organisms are usually resistant to ampicillin/sulbactam combination (Table I.14) (English *et al.*, 1978; Fu and Neu, 1979; Yamaguchi *et al.*, 1983; Sawai *et al.*, 1988). The same enzymes produced by *Serratia marcescens*, *Morganella morganii* and *Providencia* spp. appear to be inhibited by sulbactam to a greater degree, so that these organisms may be sensitive to ampicillin/sulbactam concentrations attainable *in vivo* (Table I.14) (English *et al.*, 1978; Greenwood and Eley, 1982).

Anaerobic Gram-negative bacteria of the *Bacteroides fragilis* group are nearly always susceptible to ampicillin/sulbactam (Wexler *et al.*, 1985; 1991;Cornick *et al.*, 1990; Goldstein *et al.*, 1993). Similarly the *Prevotella* spp., *Fusobacteria* and Gram-positive anaerobes such as *Clostridium* and *Lactobacillus* spp. are also nearly always susceptible to this combination (Brown, 1988; Jones and Barry, 1988; Munro, 1989; Appelbaum *et al.*, 1991; Goldstein *et al.*, 1993).

Pseudomonas aeruginosa is ampicillin/sulbactam-resistant (Table I.14) (Aldridge *et al.*, 1986). Surprisingly most *Burkholderia* (previously *Pseudomonas*) *cepacia* strains are inhibited by sulbactam alone (usual MIC 2.5 µg per ml) (Jacoby and Sutton, 1989). Sulbactam also has activity as a single agent against many strains of *Acinetobacter* spp., and combined with ampicillin it inhibits some 90% of strains (Retsema *et al.*, 1986; Obana and Nishino, 1990; Urban *et al.*, 1993). Methicillin-resistant *Staph. aureus* strains are resistant to ampicillin/sulbactam, but methicillin-sensitive strains and those with borderline susceptibility to methicillin or oxacillin are susceptible to the combination (Barry and Jones, 1990; Murray *et al.*, 1993; Pefanis *et al.*, 1993).

In an *in vitro* model ampicillin/sulbactam appeared to have greater bactericidal activity against intracellular *L. pneumophila* than erythromycin (p. 000) (Ramirez *et al.*, 1993). The clinical significance of this is unknown. Ampicillin/sulbactam is bactericidal to *M. leprae* growing in the foot pads of mice. *In vitro* it also shows activity against *M. tuberculosis* (Randhawa *et al.*, 1994). The clinical significance of this is uncertain.

As with clavulanic acid, the appearance of extended spectrum beta-lactamases (p. 323), particularly in *Kl. pneumoniae* and *E. coli*, may make these organisms ampicillin/sulbactam-resistant. These organisms may produce beta-lactamase which hydrolyzes cefotaxime, ceftriaxone, ceftazidime, and aztreonam, but not cefoxitin, cefotetan, moxalactam or imipenem. Such enzymes are usually still inhibited by sulbactam (Jarlier *et al.*, 1988). In animal experiments some extended-spectrum beta-lactamase-producing *Klebsiella* spp. infections responded to ampicillin/sulbactam therapy (Rice *et al.*, 1994). But *E. coli* and *Kl. pneumoniae* may also produce enzymes with broader spectrum of activity, which are not inhibited by sulbactam, and so ampicillin/sulbactam no longer acts synergistically against these strains (Thomson *et al.*, 1990;Rice *et al.*, 1993).

2 Cefoperazone/sulbactam

Cefoperazone is a broad spectrum third-generation cephalosporin (p. 319). It is hydrolyzed by some beta-lactamases of Gram-negative bacilli. Combination of cefoperazone with sulbactam inhibited some strains of *E. coli*, *Klebsiella* spp. and *B. fragilis* which were resistant to cefoperazone alone. Sulbactam did not increase the activity of cefaperazone against *Pseudomonas* spp. (Fu and Neu, 1980). The MICs of organisms susceptible to cefoperazone are often reduced by the addition of sulbactam (Jones *et al.*, 1985). *Acinetobacter* spp. is susceptible to the combination, probably because sulbactam as a single agent has good activity against this organism (*see above*) (Bodey *et al.*, 1989). In a study by Wexler and Finegold (1988) cefoperazone/sulbactam was very active against *B. fragilis* and other anaerobes of the *B. fragilis* group, whilst cefoperazone without sulbactam was relatively inactive against these bacteria. Cefoperazone/sulbactam was also very active against *Prevotella* spp. and against *Fusobacteria*, although cefoperazone alone was also active against these anaerobes.

The MICs of ampicillin alone, and when tested in the presence of sulbactam, against some bacterial species, are shown in Table I.14. The concentration of sulbactam required to produce the lowest MIC of ampicillin against each of these organisms, was, in general, the same as the MIC of ampicillin so produced. The MICs of sulbactam alone are also presented.

	MIC (μg per ml)		
Organism	Sulbactam alone	Ampicillin alone	Sulbactam plus ampicillin
Gram-positive bacteria			
Streptococcus pyogenes	50	0.025	0.025 + 0.025
Staphylococcus aureus[a]	>200.0	>200.0	6.25 + 6.25
Staphylococcus epidermidis[a]	>50.0	>25.0	3.12 + 1.56
Enterococcus faecalis	>50.0	1.56	1.56 + 1.56
Gram-negative bacteria			
Neisseria gonorrhoeae[a]	1.2	>10.0	0.31 + 0.31
Haemophilus influenzae[a]	100.0	200.0	1.56 + 1.56
Escherichia coli[a]	50.0	100.0	12.5 + 25.0
Klebsiella pneumoniae[a]	50.0	50.0	6.25 + 6.25
Enterobacter cloacae	100.0	200.0	50.0 + 50.0
Proteus vulgaris	100.0	>200.0	3.12 + 3.12
Serratia marcescens	100.0	200.0	12.5 + 12.5
Morganella morganii	200.0	50.0	3.12 + 3.12
Pseudomonas aeruginosa	>400.0	1000.0	100.0 + 125.0
Bacteroides fragilis	25.0	200.0	0.78 + 3.12

Table I.14
(After English *et al.*, 1978)

[a] Ampicillin-resistant beta-lactamase-producing strains.

Mode of Administration and Dosage

1 Oral administration

Orally, ampicillin plus sulbactam are usually administered in the form of the mutual pro-drug, sultamicillin (p. 209). Sultamicillin is manufactured in 250 or 500 mg tablets, which contain 147 mg or 294 mg available ampicillin and 98 mg or 196 mg sulbactam, respectively (Hartley and Wise, 1982; Rogers *et al.*, 1983). In adults, sultamicillin is used in dosages of 500 mg 8-hourly, 750 mg 12-hourly or 1 g 12-hourly (Ball *et al.*, 1984; Davies *et al.*, 1984). For children the following sultamicillin schedule has been suggested: patients under 5 years of age, 250 mg 12-hourly; those over 5 years of age 500 mg 12-hourly; and those weighing more than 20 kg, 750 mg 12-hourly (Goldfarb *et al.*, 1987). For young children and babies a study by Ginsburg *et al.* (1985), suggested that 42.5 mg of sultamicillin per kg body weight (25 mg ampicillin plus 17.5 mg sulbactam), administered 8- or 12-hourly, may be suitable.

2 Intravenous administration of ampicillin/sulbactam

Intravenously ampicillin and sulbactam are administered in a 2:1 ratio by intermittent rapid i.v. injections or infusions, similar to penicillin G (p. 20). Doses used clinically have ranged from 1 g ampicillin plus 0.5 g sulbactam 8-hourly to 2 g ampicillin plus 1 g sulbactam 6-hourly (Foulds, 1986; Chang *et al.*, 1989; Martens *et al.*, 1989). The dose can be further increased for treatment of serious infections. Children are usually treated by 200 mg of ampicillin plus 100 mg of sulbactam per kg per day given i.v. in four divided doses. For severe infections the dose can be increased to 400 mg of ampicillin plus 200 mg of sulbactam per kg body weight per day (Kanra *et al.*, 1989).

In patients with renal failure, sulbactam is excreted from the body by a similar mechanism to ampicillin (p. 213). If the two agents are given together to patients with varying degrees of renal failure, the ratio of their serum concentrations remains constant whatever the renal function. Therefore, the dose of sulbactam should be reduced in these patients in a similar manner to ampicillin (p. 116) (Wright and Wise, 1983). In patients with a creatinine clearance higher than 30 ml per min, the usual ampicillin/sulbactam dose can be given. A reduction of the ampicillin (2 g) and sulbactam (1 g) dose to twice-daily is appropriate for patients with a creatinine clearance of between 7 and 30 ml per min. These doses should be given once every 24 h for those undergoing maintenance hemodialysis. On dialysis days, the dose should be given after hemodialysis (Blum *et al.*, 1989).

3 Intravenous administration of cefoperazone/sulbactam

In clinical trials cefoperazone/sulbactam has been given to adults i.v. by short i.v. infusions in doses of cefoperazone (2 g) plus sulbactam (1 g) 12-hourly (Schwartz *et al.*, 1988), or cefoperazone (3 g) plus sulbactam (1.5 g) i.v. 12-hourly (Reitberg *et al.*, 1988a). In patients with impaired renal function, cefoperazone is eliminated normally, so normal dosage can be used (p. 328). Sulbactam elimination is reduced in patients with severe renal failure. For patients with a creatinine clearance of less than 30 ml per min, one daily dose of the 2:1 combination product should be given, followed in 12 h by the usual dose of cefoperazone alone. During hemodialysis the same regimen can be used, as hemodialysis does not remove enough sulbactam to require a supplemental dose after the dialysis, but the daily cefaperazone/sulbactam dose should be given after hemodialysis (Reitberg *et al.*, 1988b; Rho *et al.*, 1992).

Serum Levels in Relation to Dosage

1 Oral sultamicillin

After administration of a 250-mg dose of sultamicillin (containing 147 mg ampicillin) to adults, a mean peak ampicillin concentration of 3.2 μg per ml is attained in 40 min. The 500-mg dose of sultamicillin (containing 294 mg ampicillin) results in a mean peak ampicillin concentration of 5.6 μg per ml, 60 min after administration. In contrast, a 250-mg dose of ampicillin alone produces a lower mean peak concentration of 2.1 μg per ml, 2 h after dosing (Hartley and Wise, 1982). Serum ampicillin levels achieved with sultamicillin are approximately double those following an equivalent oral dose of ampicillin.

Sulbactam as such, is poorly absorbed from the gastrointestinal tract, but when it is administered as sultamicillin, similar to ampicillin (*see above*), it is well absorbed. After a 250-mg dose of sultamicillin (containing 98 mg sulbactam) is administered to adults, a mean peak serum level of 2.2 μg per ml is attained after 1 h. After a 500-mg sultamicillin dose the mean peak serum level is 4.0 μg per ml, again attained at 1 h. The serum half-lives are 1.2 h following the 500-mg dose and 1.1 h following the 250-mg dose. Sulbactam is undetectable in serum 6–8 h after administration (Hartley and Wise, 1982). The half-lives and bioavailability (about 80%) for both ampicillin and sulbactam following oral sultamicillin administration, are similar (Rogers *et al.*, 1983).

Ginsburg *et al.* (1985) studied sulbactam serum concentrations after oral administration of 42.5 mg per kg body weight of sultamicillin (25 mg ampicillin and 17.5 mg of sulbactam) to children. The average peak serum levels of sulbactam in fasting children were 5.3 μg per ml after 60 min, 6.5 μg per ml after 90 min and 3.7 μg per ml after 120 min. Slightly higher serum levels were obtained in non-fasting children. Again ampicillin serum levels after administration of sultamicillin were about twice as high as those after administration of the same dose of ampicillin alone.

2 Intravenous ampicillin/sulbactam

After a single 2-g dose of ampicillin combined with 1 g of sulbactam in 60 ml of i.v. solution was administered i.v. to young adults over a 30-min period, the serum levels of sulbactam after 0.5 h, 1 h, 2 h, 3.5 h, 5.5 h and 8.5 h after the end of the infusion were 52.21, 24.95, 10.46, 3.46, 1.01 and 0.14 μg per ml, respectively. For ampicillin the corresponding serum levels were 99.79, 43.25, 15.96, 5.29, 1.60 and 0.25 μg per ml, respectively. In elderly subjects (65–85 years) the serum levels after 0.5 h were higher for both drugs than those in younger subjects. This is because the urinary excretion of both ampicillin and sulbactam was lower in the elderly subjects. When 2 g of ampicillin and 1 g of sulbactam was given to volunteers, the ratio of ampicillin to sulbactam (approximately 2:1) was maintained over 8 h (Rho *et al.*, 1989; Meyers *et al.*, 1991). The kinetics of ampicillin is not affected by co-administration of sulbactam. The half-life of both drugs is also prolonged during labor, in neonates and in patients with renal impairment (Foulds,

1986). The pharmacokinetics of sulbactam in young children is similar to that in young adults, but the mean terminal half-life of 1.75 h in children is significantly longer than the mean value of 0.93 h reported for young adult volunteers (Schaad *et al.*, 1986; Meyers *et al.*, 1991).

When 50 mg per kg body weight of both ampicillin and sulbactam was administered as an i.v. bolus injection to newborns every 12 h, the mean ampicillin and sulbactam serum levels were 87 and 110 μg per ml, respectively, 3 h after the injection. Mean elimination half-lives were 9.4 h for ampicillin and 7.9 h for sulbactam. There was no evidence of accumulation of the drug with this dosage in newborns (Sutton *et al.*, 1986).

3 Intramuscular administration of sulbactam to adults

After i.m. administration of 0.5 g sulbactam, the mean peak serum concentration of 13 μg per ml is attained in 30 min. Bioavailability of sulbactam after i.m. administration is the same as after i.v. dosing. Pharmacokinetics of sulbactam in humans are similar to those of ampicillin (p. 116) or amoxycillin (p. 136) (Foulds *et al.*, 1983).

4 Intravenous cefoperazone/ sulbactam

Co-administration of cefoperazone and sulbactam i.v. results in pharmacokinetic profiles which are very similar to those observed for each drug when they are administered as single agents. Cefoperazone is mainly excreted via the bile (p. 332), whilst sulbactam is eliminated via the kidney (see below). If a 3-g dose of cefoperazone plus a 1.5-g dose of sulbactam is given i.v. 12-hourly to volunteers for 7 days, for cefoperazone the maximal serum concentration is 430 μg per ml, the terminal elimination half-life is 1.8 and urinary excretion of total dose is 30%. For sulbactam these three measurements are 90 μg per ml, 1 h and 89%, respectively (Reitberg *et al.*, 1988a).

Excretion

1 Urine

The principal mode of elimination of sulbactam is renal by both glomerular filtration and tubular secretion. The elimination half-life of the drug is prolonged by about 40% if probenecid is also given (p. 24). Probenecid enhances and prolongs its serum levels, similar to those of ampicillin (p. 117). Renal clearance of sulbactam is approximately 204 ml per min, and about 70% of a parenteral dose is excreted in the urine within 6 h of administration, with an additional recovery of 5% between 6 and 12 h after the dose (Foulds *et al.*, 1983; Foulds, 1986). High sulbactam concentrations are attained in urine (Hartley and Wise, 1982; Meyers *et al.*, 1991).

2 Bile

Some sulbactam can be detected in the feces after i.v. administration, so like ampicilin (p. 117), a portion of the drug appears to be eliminated via the bile (Kager *et al.*, 1982).

3 Inactivation in body

Some sulbactam is probably inactivated in the liver, similar to ampicillin (p. 117).

Distribution of the Drug in Body

The total apparent volume of distribution of sulbactam in adults is between 19 and 28 liters, which is over half that of the total body fluid of approximately 40 liters in a person weighing 70 kg. This suggests that sulbactam is widely distributed into the tissues (Foulds *et al.*, 1983). Sulbactam penetrates well into normal peritoneal fluid, where concentrations as high as 96% of the simultaneous serum level are attained (Wise *et al.*, 1983). The drug penetrates well into human tissue blister fluid, where its concentration is 1.5-fold higher than that of ampicillin administered i.v. in the same dose (Brown *et al.*, 1982; Jaresko *et al.*, 1992).

Adequate concentrations of both ampicillin and sulbactam are also found in pus, middle ear fluid, sputum and alveolar lining fluid (Foulds, 1986; Valcke *et al.*, 1990). In patients with bacterial meningitis the CSF concentrations of sulbactam are approximately one-third of those in the serum. As meningitis resolves with therapy, the CSF concentrations of sulbactam decline (Stahl *et al.*, 1986; Foulds *et al.*, 1987). In animals sulbactam is well distributed to many tissues, highest concentrations, similar to ampicillin, are found in kidney and liver tissue and lesser concentrations in lung, spleen and muscle (English *et al.*, 1984).

Sulbactam is 38% serum protein bound (Kager *et al.*, 1982).

Mode of Action

Sulbactam is a beta-lactam compound and its weak antibacterial activity presumably results from a mode of action similar to penicillin G (p. 25). The mechanism for its inhibition of beta-lactamases is similar to that of clavulanic acid (p. 192).

Toxicity

1 Oral sultamicillin

Oral administration of this compound is associated with more gastrointestinal symptoms than the administration of ampicillin alone (Neu, 1984). Symptoms include nausea, vomiting and diarrhea; these have been quite frequent in some clinical studies, and in a number of patients have been severe enough to necessitate cessation of treatment (Davies *et al.*, 1982, 1984). In one pharmacokinetic study of sultamicillin, all six healthy male volunteers developed a change in bowel habit, ranging from just softer motions to severe diarrhea for 5 days. Severe symptoms were more common with a dosage of 500 mg 8-hourly, compared with a lower one of 250 mg 8-hourly (Hartley and Wise, 1982). Goldfarb *et al.* (1987) compared sultamicillin with cloxacillin for treatment of soft tissue infections in children; 21 children in each group. Diarrhea occurred in a few children only, and it was no more frequent nor severe with sultamicillin than with cloxacillin. Similarly, Chan *et al.* (1993) who compared sultamicillin with co-amoxiclav (p. 199) for treatment of acute otitis media in children, found that diarrhea was mild, relatively infrequent and equal in both groups.

2 Parenteral ampicilin/ sulbactam

Sulbactam, administered i.v., in a dosage of 0.5–1.0 g 6-hourly together with ampicillin to adults, has not shown additional side-effects unexpected from i.v. administration of ampicilin alone (Houang *et al.*, 1984; Neu, 1984). Intramuscular sulbactam causes pain at the site of injection, but no other adverse effects (Foulds *et al.*, 1983; Caine *et al.*, 1984). Changes of fecal flora have been studied after ampicillin 0.5 g plus sulbactam 0.5 g were given i.v. 8-hourly for 2 days prior to colorectal surgery. The numbers of streptococci, enterococci and Gram-negative aerobic bacteria were unchanged, but anaerobic bacteria were affected. Anaerobic cocci and Gram-positive rods such as eubacteria and lactobacilli, were decreased, as were *Bacteroides* spp. No overgrowth of anaerobes resistant to ampicillin plus sulbactam occurred (Kager *et al.*, 1982).

Ampicillin/sulbactam appears quite safe in patients with diabetes mellitus (Chiodini *et al.*, 1985) and in those with chronic liver disease (Galante *et al.*, 1987). It also has no effect on neutrophil function and host defences in general (Gunther *et al.*, 1993).

Clinical Uses of the Drug

1 Oral sultamicillin

The uses of this compound are similar to those of oral co-amoxiclav (p. 200). In patients who can tolerate sultamicillin without gastrointestinal side-effects (see above), results of treatment have been approximately the same as those achieved with co-amoxiclav. Reports include the successful use of sultamicillin in adults with urinary tract infections caused by ampicillin-resistant Gram-negative bacteria (Ball *et al.*, 1984), in adults with purulent exacerbations of chronic bronchitis (Davies *et al.*, 1982; 1984; Pressler *et al.*, 1986) and in children with otitis media (Chan *et al.*, 1993). Superficial skin and soft tissue infections also have been treated by this drug (Goldfarb *et al.*, 1987), and sometimes sultamicillin has been used to follow i.v. ampicillin/sulbactam in various more severe medical and surgical infections (Chang *et al.*, 1989).

2 Parenteral ampicillin/ sulbactam

a Intra-abdominal infections In animals infected by a mixed *E. coli* and *Bacteroides* group of organisms, ampicillin/sulbactam eliminated the *Bacteroides* more successfully than *E. coli*, especially if the *E. coli* produced large amounts of beta-lactamase. The combination of amoxycilin/clavulanic acid eliminated such *E. coli* more successfully (Gisby and Beale, 1988; Brook, 1989). Nevertheless, in clinical studies i.v. ampicillin/sulbactam has been as effective as cefoxitin alone (p. 308) or clindamycin/gentamicin for the treatment of peritonitis arising from a perforated viscus (Mehtar *et al.*, 1986; Study Group, 1986; Chang *et al.*, 1989; Nichols, 1989).

b   Complicated urinary tract infections   Ampicillin/sulbactam is effective in urinary tract infections in animals caused by ampicillin-resistant bacilli (English *et al.*, 1986). It is also clinically effective in pyelonephritis caused by ampicillin-resistant organisms (Syriopoulou *et al.*, 1986; Chang *et al.*, 1989; Lee *et al.*, 1989).

c   Gynecologic infections   Ampicillin/sulbactam has been used with success in various gynecologic infections such as pelvic cellulitis (Giamarellou *et al.*, 1986), post-cesarean section endometritis (Martens *et al.*, 1989) and pelvic inflammatory disease. In this group those infected with *Chlamydia trachomatis* may relapse after ampicillin/sulbactam therapy (Kosseim *et al.*, 1991).

d   Osteomyelitis, pneumonia and soft tissue infections   Experimental chronic *Staph. aureus* osteomyelitis in animals responds well to ampicillin/sulbactam (Norden and Budinsky, 1990). Clinically the combination also has been successful for the treatment of both children and adults with acute and chronic osteomyelitis, septic arthritis, cellulitis and more chronic skin and soft tissue infections such as feet infections in diabetics (Löffler *et al.*, 1986; Chang *et al.*, 1989; Kulhanjian *et al.*, 1989; Grayson *et al.*, 1994). Ampicillin/sulbactam is also effective for the treatment of community-acquired pneumonia (Williams *et al.*, 1994).

e   Bacterial meningitis   Rodriguez *et al.* (1986) demonstrated that ampicillin/sulbactam was equally efficacious in children with bacterial meningitis as chloramphenicol/ampicillin. In this study the majority of pathogens were *H. influenzae*, *N. meningitidis* and *Streptococcus pneumoniae*. In the ampicillin/sulbactam treated group only one strain of *H. influenzae* was ampicillin-resistant. Guerra-Romero *et al.* (1991) assessed ampicillin-sulbactam in a rabbit model of meningitis due to a beta-lactamase-producing strain of *E. coli*. These authors found that the combination was only of limited value. As the third-generation cephalosporins such as cefotaxime (p. 336) and ceftriaxone (p. 359) are very effective in meningitis caused by beta-lactamase-producing Gram-negative bacilli, it seems unlikely that ampicilin/sulbactam will be used for the treatment of this disease. Acute epiglottitis due to beta-lactamase-producing *H. influenzae* type b responds to ampicillin/sulbactam (Wald *et al.*, 1986).

f   Beta-lactamase-producing *Enterococcus faecalis* infections   Ampicilin/sulbactam is quite effective against such infections. Most beta-lactamase-producing strains also show high-level gentamicin resistance. Therefore there is no satisfactory therapy available at present for the treatment of endocarditis caused by such strains (Lavoie *et al.*, 1993; Thal *et al.*, 1993).

g   Infections caused by Enterobacteriaceae which produce extended broad-spectrum beta-lactamases   These plasmid-mediated beta-lactamases hydrolyze third-generation cephalosporins (p. 323). Some of them are inhibited by sulbactam and others are not (p. 323). They have mainly been found in *Klebsiella* spp. and *E. coli* to date. Fantin *et al.* (1990) studied ceftriaxone/sulbactam combination against *E. coli* (which produced such an enzyme) *in vitro* and *in vivo* in experimental animals. The results were promising as sulbactam enhanced the activity of ceftriaxone against this organism. By contrast, Caron *et al.* (1990) found poor activity of ceftriaxone/sulbactam in an animal model infected by *Kl. pneumoniae* with produced an extend-broad-spectrum beta-lactamase.

h   Chemoprophylaxis   Ampicillin/sulbactam has been used as chemoprophylaxis in general abdominal surgery, gynecologic surgery, colorectal surgery and termination of pregnancy. For these indications the combination was equally as effective as metronidazole/ampicillin or metronidazole/cefazolin (Lees *et al.*, 1986). As antimicrobial chemoprophylaxis for major head and neck surgery in cancer patients ampicillin/sulbactam was suboptimal, but no worse than clindamycin/amikacin combination (Phan *et al.*, 1992). Pharmacokinetic properties of ampicillin/sulbactam indicate that a 2/1-g dose of the combination, administered 8-hourly for 3–6 days may be suitable as perioperative prophylaxis of patients undergoing heart surgery (Wildfeuer *et al.*, 1991). In animal experiments vancomycin had superior prophylactic efficacy than ampicillin/sulbactam against endocarditis caused by beta-lactamase-producing, aminoglycoside-resistant enterococci, but this was due to superior pharmacokinetic profile of vancomycin (Bayer and Tu, 1990).

3 Parenteral cefoperazone/ sulbactam

In an animal study, cefoperazone/sulbactam proved superior to cefoperazone alone when the infecting organisms were beta-lactamase-producing *E. coli* and *Ps. aeruginosa* strains which were cefoperazone-resistant, but sensitive to the combination (Chandrasekar *et al.*, 1993). In clinical trials the combination has been used to treat infections in patients with hematological diseases and in cancer patients (Horiuchi *et al.*, 1989; Bodey *et al.*, 1993). Cefoperazone/ sulbactam has also been used to treat intra-abdominal infections (Jauregui *et al.*, 1990). In one trial it was about as effective and safe as a clindamycin/gentamicin combination for this indication (Greenberg *et al.*, 1994). It is doubtful whether this combination has any advantage over the many other available regimens for treatment of peritonitis.

4 Inactivation of aminoglycosides by sulbactam

At clinically achievable levels (e.g. 25 μg per ml), sulbactam does not inactivate any aminoglycosides *in vitro*. Sulbactam alone and in combination with ampicillin or cefoperazone inactivates tobramycin, gentamicin, netilmicin and amikacin *in vitro* when the sulbactam concentration is 200 μg per ml. At 75 μg per ml, sulbactam only inactivates tobramycin (Fuchs *et al.*, 1991).

References

Aldridge KE, Sanders CV, Marier RL (1986). Variation in the potentiation of beta-lactam antibiotic activity by clavulanic acid and sulbactam against multiply antibiotic-resistant bacteria. *J Antimicrob Chemother* **17**: 463.

Appelbaum PC, Spangler SK, Jacobs MR (1991). Susceptibilities of 394 *Bacteroides fragilis*, non-*B. fragilis* group *Bacteroides* species, and *Fusobacterium* species to newer antimicrobial agents. *Antimicrob Ag Chemother* **35**: 1214.

Azimi PH, Dunphy MG (1989). Susceptibility of *Haemophilus influenzae* type b to ampicillin-sulbactam. *Antimicrob Ag Chemother* **33**: 1620.

Baddour LM, Busby L, Shapiro E *et al.* (1992). Evaluation of treatment with single-dose ampicillin/sulbactam with probenecid or ceftriaxone in patients with uncomplicated gonorrhea. *Sex Transm Dis* **19**: 341.

Ball AP, Fox C, Ghosh D (1984). Sultamicillin (CP-49, 952).: evaluation of two dosage schedules in urinary infection. *J Antimicrob Chemother* **14**: 395.

Barry AL, Jones RN (1990). *In vitro* activities of ampicillin-sulbactam and cefoperazone-sulbactam against oxacillin-susceptible and oxacillin-resistant staphylococci. *Antimicrob Ag Chemother* **34**: 1830.

Bayer AS, Tu J (1990). Chemoprophylactic efficacy against experimental endocarditis caused by beta-lactamase-producing, aminoglycoside-resistant enterococci is associated with prolonged serum inhibitory activity. *Antimicrob Ag Chemother* **34**: 1068.

Blum RA, Kohli RK, Harrison NJ, Schentag JJ (1989). Pharmacokinetics of ampicillin (20 grams). and sulbactam (10 gram). coadministered to subjects with normal and abnormal renal function and with end-stage renal disease on hemodialysis. *Antimicrob Ag Chemother* **33**: 1470.

Bodey GP, Miller P, Ho DH (1989). *In vitro* assessment of sulbactam plus cefoperazone in the treatment of bacteria isolated from cancer patients. *Diagn Microbiol Infect Dis* **12**: 209S.

Bodey GP, Elting LS, Narro J *et al.* (1993). An open trial of cefoperazone plus sulbactam for the treatment of fever in cancer patients. *J Antimicrob Chemother* **32**: 141.

Brook I (1989). *In vitro* susceptibility and *in vivo* efficacy of antimicrobials in the treatment of *Bacteroides fragilis-Escherichia coli* infections in mice. *J Infect Dis* **160**: 651.

Brown R M, Wise R, Andrews JM, Hancox J (1982). Comparative pharmacokinetics and tissue penetration of sulbactam and ampicillin after concurrent intravenous administration. *Antimicrob Ag Chemother* **21**: 565.

Brown WJ (1988). National committee for clinical laboratory standards agar dilution susceptibility testing of anaerobic Gram-negative bacteria. *Antimicrob Ag Chemother* **32**: 385.

Bush K, Sykes RB (1983). Beta-lactamase inhibitors in perspective. *J Antimicrob Chemother* **11**: 97.

Caine VA, Foulds G, Handsfield HH (1984). Therapeutic trial and pharmacokinetics of sulbactam for uncomplicated gonorrhea in men. *Antimicrob Ag Chemother* **26**: 683.

Caron F, Gutmann L, Bure A *et al.* (1990). Ceftriaxone-sulbactam combination in rabbit endocarditis caused by a strain of *Klebsiella pneumoniae* producing extended-brood-spectram TEM-3 beta-lactamase. *Antimicrob Ag Chemother* **34**: 2070.

Chan KH, Bluestone CD, Tan LS *et al.* (1993). Comparative study of sultamicillin and amoxicillin-clavulanate: treatment of acute otitis media. *Pediatr Infect Dis J* **12**: 24.

Chandrasekar PH, Sluchak JA, Kruse JA (1993). Therapy with cefoperazone plus sulbactam against disseminated infection due to cefoperazone-resistant *Pseudomonas aeruginosa* and *Escherichia coli* in granulocytopenic mice. *Antimicrob Ag Chemother* **37**: 1927.

Chang ST, Chung HY, Pai SD, Lee JH (1989). Sulbactam/ampicillin followed by oral treatment with sultamicillin for medical and surgical infections. *Diagn Microbiol Infect Dis* **12**: 175S.

Chiodini PL, Toop MJ, Odugbesan O *et al.* (1985). Sulbactam/ampicillin: effects on glucose metabolism in diabetics with soft tissue infection. *J Antimicrob Chemother* **16**: 643.

Cornick NA, Cuchural GJJr, Snydman DR *et al.* (1990). The antimicrobial susceptibility patterns of the *Bacteroides fragilis* group in the United States, 1987. *J Antimicrob Chemother* **25**: 1011.

Crosby MA, Gump DW (1982). Activity of cefoperazone and two beta-lactamase inhibitors, sulbactam and clavulanic acid, against *Bacteroides* spp correlated with beta-lactamase production. *Antimicrob Ag Chemother* **22**: 398.

Davies BI, Maesen FPV, Jevons S, Brouwers J (1982). Combination of sulbactam pivoxyl and bacampicillin in acute exacerbations of chronic bronchitis. *J Antimicrob Chemother* **10**: 445.

Davies BI, Maesen FPV, Van Noord JA (1984). Clinical, bacteriological and pharmacokinetic results from an open trial of sultamicillin with acute exacerbations of chronic bronchitis. *J Antimicrob Chemother* **13**: 161.

English AR, Retsema JA, Girard AE *et al.* (1978). CP-45, 899, a beta-lactamase inhibitor that extends the antibacterial spectrum of beta-lactams: initial bacteriological characterization. *Antimicrob Ag Chemother* **14**: 414.

English AR, Girard D, Haskell SL (1984). Pharmacokinetics of sultamicillin in mice, rats, and dogs. *Antimicrob Ag Chemother* 25: 599.

English AR, Girard D, Cimochowski C et al. (1986). Activity of sulbactam/ampicillin in screening and discriminative animal models of infection. *Rev Infect Dis* 8 (Suppl 5): 535.

Fantin B, Pangon B, Potel G et al. (1990). Activity of sulbactam in combination with ceftriaxone in vitro and in experimental endocarditis caused by *Escherichia coli* producing SHV-2-like beta-lactamase. *Antimicrob Ag Chemother* 34: 581.

Foulds G (1986). Pharmacokinetics of sulbactam/ampicillin in humans: a review. *Rev Infect Dis* 8 (Suppl 5): 503.

Foulds G, Stankewich JP, Marshall DG et al. (1983). Pharmacokinetics of sulbactam in humans. *Antimicrob Ag Chemother* 23: 692.

Foulds G, McBride TJ, Knirsch AK et al. (1987). Penetration of sulbactam and ampicillin into cerebrospinal fluid of infants and young children with meningitis. *Antimicrob Ag Chemother* 31: 1703.

Fu KP, Neu HC (1979). Comparative inhibition of beta-lactamases by novel beta-lactam compounds. *Antimicrob Ag Chemother* 15: 171.

Fu KP, Neu HC (1980). Synergistic activity of cefoperazone in combination with beta-lactamase inhibitors. *J Antimicrob Chemother* 7: 287.

Fu KP, Kimble EF, Zoganas H, Konopka EA (1984). Synergistic activity of cefsulodin combined with cefoxitin and sulbactam against *Bacteroides* species. *J Antimicrob Chemother* 13: 257.

Fuchs PC, Stickel S, Anderson PH et al. (1991). *In vitro* inactivation of aminoglycosides by sulbactam, other beta-lactams and sulbactam-beta-lactam combinations. *Antimicrob Ag Chemother* 35: 182.

Galante D, Esposito S, Barba D, Ruffilli MP (1987). Clinical efficacy and safety of sulbactam/ampicillin in patients suffering from chronic liver disease. *J Antimicrob Chemother* 19: 527.

Giamarellou H, Trouvas G, Avlami A et al. (1986). Efficacy of sulbactam plus ampicillin in gynecologic infections. *Rev Infect Dis* 8 (Suppl 5): 579.

Ginsburg CM, McCracken GH Jr, Olsen K, Petruska M (1985). Pharmacokinetics and bactericidal activity of sultamicillin in infants and children. *J Antimicrob Chemother* 15: 345.

Gisby J, Beale AS (1988). Comparative efficacies of amoxicillin-clavulanic acid and ampicillin-sulbactam against experimental *Bacteroides fragilis-Escherichia coli* mixed infections. *Antimicrob Ag Chemother* 32: 1830.

Goldfarb J, Aronoff SC, Jaffe A et al. (1987). Sultamicillin in the tretment of superficial skin and soft tissue infections in childen. *Antimicrob Ag Chemother* 31: 663.

Goldstein EJC, Citron DM, Cherubin CE, Hillier SL (1993). Comparative susceptibility of the *Bacteroides fragilis* group species and other anaerobic bacteria to meropenem, imipenem, piperacillin, cefoxitin, ampicillin/sulbactam, clindamycin and metronidazole. *J Antimicrob Chemother* 31: 363.

Grayson ML, Gibbons GW, Habershaw GM et al. (1994). Use of ampicillin/sulbactam versus imipenem/cilastatin in the treatment of limb-threatening foot infections in diabetic patients. *Clin Infect Dis* 18: 683.

Greenberg RN, Cayavec P, Danko LS et al. (1994). Comparison of cefoperazone plus sulbactam with clindamycin plus gentamicin as treatment for intra-abdominal infections. *J Antimicrob Chemother* 34: 391.

Greenwood D, Eley A (1982). *In-vitro* evaluation of sulbactam, a penicillanic acid sulphone with beta-lactamase inhibitory properties. *J Antimicrob Chemother* 10: 117.

Guerra-Romero L, Kennedy SL, Fournier MA et al. (1991). Use of ampicillin-sulbactam for treatment of experimental meningitis caused by a beta-lactamase-producing strain of *Escherichia coli* K-1. *Antimicrob Ag Chemother* 35: 2037.

Gunther MR, Mao J, Cohen MS (1993). Oxidant-scavenging activities of ampicillin and sulbactam and their effects on neutrophil functions. *Antimicrob Ag Chemother* 37: 950.

Hartley S, Wise R (1982). A three-way crossover study to compare with pharmacokinetics and acceptability of sultamicillin at two dose levels with that of ampicillin. *J Antimicrob Chemother* 10: 49.

Horiuchi A, Hasegava H, Kageyama T et al. (1989). Efficacy of sulbactam/

cefoperazone for the treatment of infections in patients with hematologic diseases. *Diagn Microbiol Infect Dis* 12: 215S.

Houang ET, Watson C, Howell R, Chapman M (1984). Ampicillin combined with sulbactam or metronidazole for single-dose chemoprophylaxis in major gynaecological surgery. *J Antimicrob Chemother* 14: 529.

Jacobs MR, Aronoff SC, Johenning S et al. (1986). Comparative activities of the beta-lactamase inhibitors YTR 830, clavulanate, and sulbactam combined with ampicillin and broad-spectrum penicillins against defined beta-lactamase-producing aerobic Gram-negative bacilli. *Antimicrob Ag Chemother* 29: 980.

Jacoby GA, Sutton L (1989). *Pseudomonas cepacia* susceptibility to sulbactam. *Antimicrob Ag Chemother* 33: 583.

Jaresco GS, Barriere SL, Johnson BLJr (1992). Serum and blister fluid pharmacokinetics and bactericidal activities of ampicillin-sulbactam, cefotetan, cefoxitin, ceftizoxime and ticarcillin-clavulanate. *Antimicrob Ag Chemother* 36: 2233.

Jarlier V, Nicolas M-H, Fournier G, Phillipon A (1988). Extended broad-spectrum beta-lactamases conferring transferable resistance to newer beta-lactam agents in Enterobacteriaceae: hospital prevalence and susceptibility patterns. *Rev Infect Dis* 10: 867.

Jauregui LE, Appelbaum PC, Fabian TC et al. (1990). A randomized clinical study of cefoperazone and sulbactam versus gentamicin and clindamycin in the treatment of intra-abdominal infections. *J Antimicrob Chemother* 25: 423.

Jones BM, Hafiz S, Duerden BI (1986). Susceptibility of *Haemophilus ducreyi* to ampicillin and sulbactam *in vitro*. *Antimicrob Ag Chemother* 29: 1110.

Jones RN Barry AL, (1988). *In-vitro* activity of ampicillin/sulbactam against cefoxitin-resistant anaerobic bacteria. *J Antimicrob Chemother* 21: 135.

Jones RN, Wilson HW, Thornsberry C et al. (1985). *In vitro* antimicrobial activity of cefoperazone-sulbactam combinations against 554 clinical isolates including a review of beta-lactamase studies. *Diagn Microbiol Infect Dis* 3: 489.

Kager L, Liljeqvist L, Malmborg AS et al (1982). Effects of ampicillin plus sulbactam on bowel flora in patients undergoing colorectal surgery. *Antimicrob Ag Chemother* 22: 208.

Kanra G, Secmeer G, Akalin E et al. (1989). Sulbactam/ampicillin in the treatment of pediatric infections. *Diagn Microbiol Infect Dis* 12: 185S.

Kazmierczak A, Pechinot A, Siebor E et al. (1989). Sulbactam: secondary mechanisms of action. *Diagn Microbiol Infect Dis* 12: 139S.

Klastersky J, Van der Auwera P (1989). *In vitro* activity of sulbactam in combination with various beta-lactam antibiotics. *Diagn Microbiol Infect Dis* 12: 165S.

Kosseim M, Ronald A, Plummer FA et al. (1991). Treatment of acute pelvic inflammatory disease in the ambulatory setting: trial of cefoxitin and doxycycline versus ampicillin-sulbactam. *Antimicrob Ag Chemother* 35: 1651.

Kulhanjian J, Dunphy MG, Hamstra S et al. (1989). Randomized comparative study of ampicillin/sulbactam vs ceftriaxone for treatment of soft tissue and skeletal infections in children. *Pediatr Infect Dis J* 8: 605.

Labia R, Morand A, Lelievre V et al. (1986). Sulbactam: biochemical factors involved in its synergy with ampicillin. *Rev Infect Dis* 8 (Suppl 5): 496.

Lavoie SR, Wong ES, Coudron PE et al. (1993). Comparison of ampicillin-sulbactam with vancomycin for treatment of experimental endocarditis due to a beta-lactamase-producing, highly gentamicin-resistant isolate of *Enterococcus faecalis*. *Antimicrob Ag Chemother* 37: 1447.

Lee C-Y, Lin T-Y, Chu M-L et al. (1989). Intravenous sulbactam/ampicillin in the treatment of pediatric infections. *Diagn Microbiol Infect Dis* 12: 179S.

Lees L, Milson JA, Knirsch AK, Greenhalgh K (1986). Sulbactam plus ampicillin: interim review of efficacy and safety for therapeutic and prophylactic use. *Rev Infect Dis* 8 (Suppl 5): 644.

Ling J, Kam KM, Lam AW, French GL (1988). Susceptibilities of Hong

Kong isolates of multiply resistant *Shigella* spp to 25 antimicrobial agents, including ampicillin plus sulbactam and new 4-quinalones. *Antimicrob Ag Chemother* 32: 20.

Livermore DM (1992). Activity of sulbactam combinations against *Escherichia coli* isolates with known amounts of TEM-1 beta-lactamase. *J Antimicrob Chemother* 29: 222.

Löffler L, Bauernfeind A, Keyl W *et al.* (1986). An open, comparative study of sulbactam plus ampicillin vs cefotaxime as initial therapy for serious soft tissue and bone and joint infections. *Rev Infect Dis* 8 (Suppl 5): 593.

Markowitz SM, Wells VD, Williams DS *et al.* (1991). Antimicrobial susceptibility and molecular epidemiology of beta-lactamase-producing, aminoglycoside-resistant isolates of *Enterococcus faecalis. Antimicrob Ag Chemother* 35: 1075.

Martens MG, Faro S, Hammill HA *et al.* (1989). Sulbactam/ampicillin versus metronidazole/gentamicin in the treatment of post-cesarean section endometritis. *Diagn Microbiol Infect Dis* 12: 189S.

Mehtar S, Croft RJ, Hilas A (1986). A non-comparative study of parenteral ampicillin and sulbactam in intra-thoracic and intra-abdominal infections. *J Antimicrob Chemother* 17: 389.

Meyers BR, Wilkinson P, Mendelson MH *et al.* (1991). Pharmacokinetics of ampicillin-sulbactam in healthy elderly and young volunteers. *Antimicrob Ag Chemother* 35: 2098.

Munro R (1989). Patterns of resistance to anaerobic organisms in Australia. *Diagn Microbiol Infect Dis* 12: 159S.

Murray PR, Jones RN, Allen SD *et al.* (1993). Multilaboratory evaluation of the *in vitro* activity of 13 beta-lactam antibiotics against 1474 clinical isolates of aerobic and anaerobic bacteria. *Diagn Microbiol Infect Dis* 16: 191.

Neu HC (1984). Trends in the development of beta-lactam antibiotics. *Scand J Infect Dis* (Suppl 42): 7.

Nichols RL (1989). The treatment of intraabdominal infections in surgery. *Diagn Microbiol Infect Dis* 12: 195S.

Norden CW, Budinsky A (1990). Treatment of experimental chronic osteomyelitis due to *Staphylococcus aureus* with ampicillin/sulbactam. *J Infect Dis* 161: 52.

Obana Y, Nishino T (1990). *In-vitro* and *in-vivo* activities of sulbactam and YTR 830H against *Acinetobacter calcoaceticus. J Antimicrob Chemother* 26: 677.

Pefanis A, Thauvin-Eliopoulos C, Eliopoulos GM, Moellering RCJr (1993). Activity of ampicillin/sulbactam and oxacillin in experimental endocarditis caused by beta-lactamase-hyperproducing *Staphylococcus aureus. Antimicrob Ag Chemother* 37: 507.

Phan M, Van der Auwera P, Andry G *et al.* (1992). Antimicrobial prophylaxis for major head and neck surgery in cancer patients: sulbactam-ampicillin versus clindamycin-amikacin. *Antimicrob Ag Chemother* 36: 2014.

Pressler T, Pedersen SS, Christiansen L *et al.* (1986). Sultamicillin – a new antibiotic in the treatment of persistent lower respiratory tract infections caused by *Haemophilus influenzae. J Antimicrob Chemother* 17: 529.

Ramirez JA, Summersgill JT, Miller RD *et al.* (1993). Comparative study of the bactericidal activity of ampicillin/sulbactam and erythromycin against intracellular Legionella pneumophila. *J Antimicrob Chemother* 32: 93.

Randhawa B, Harris EB, Prabhakaran K, Hastings RC (1994). Bactericidal action of ampicillin/sulbactam against *Mycobacterium leprae. J Antimicrob Chemother* 33: 1035.

Reinhardt JF, Johnston L, Ruane P *et al.* (1986). A randomized, double-blind comparison of sulbactam/ampicillin and clindamycin for the treatment of aerobic and aerobic-anaerobic infections. *Rev Infect Dis* 8 (Suppl 5): 569.

Reitberg DP, Whall TJ, Chung M *et al.* (1988a). Multiple-dose pharmacokinetics and toleration of intravenously administered cefoperazone and sulbactam when given as single agents or in combination. *Antimicrob Ag Chemother* 32: 42.

Reitberg DP, Marble DA, Schultz RW *et al.* (1988b). Pharmacokinetics of cefoperazone (2.0g) and sulbactam (1.0g) coadministered to subjects with normal renal function, patients with decreased renal function, and patients with end-stage renal disease on hemodialysis. *Antimicrob Ag Chemother* 32: 503.

Retsema JA, English AR, Girard AE (1980). CP-45,899 in combination with penicillin or ampicillin against penicillin-resistant *Staphylococcus, Haemophilus influenzae* and *Bacteroides. Antimicrob Ag Chemother* 17: 615.

Retsema JA, English AR, Girard A *et al.* (1986). Sulbactam/ampicillin; *in vitro* spectrum, potency, and activity in models of acute infection. *Rev Infect Dis* 8 (Suppl 5): 528.

Rho JP, Jones A, Woo M *et al.* (1989). Single-dose pharmacokinetics of intravenous ampicillin plus sulbactam in healthy elderly and young adult subjects. *J Antimicrob Chemother* 24: 573.

Rho JP, Castle S, Smith K *et al.* (1992). Effect of impaired renal function on the pharmacokinetics of coadministered cefoperazone and sulbactam. *J Antimicrob Chemother* 29: 701.

Rice LB, Carias LL, Etter L, Shlaes DM (1993). Resistance to cefoperazone-sulbactam in *Klebsiella pneumoniae*: evidence for enhanced resistance resulting from the coexistence of two different resistance mechanisms. *Antimicrob Ag Chemother* 37: 1061.

Rice LB, Carias LL, Shlaes DM (1994). *In vivo* efficacies of beta-lactam-beta-lactamase inhibitor combinations against TEM-26-producing strain of *Klebsiella pneumoniae. Antimicrob Ag Chemother* 38: 2663.

Rodriguez WJ, Khan WN, Puig J *et al.* (1986). Sulbactam/ampicillin vs chloramphenicol/ampicillin for the treatment of meningitis in infants and children. *Rev Infect Dis* 8 (Suppl 5): 620.

Rogers HJ, Bradbrook ID, Morrison PJ *et al.* (1983). Pharmacokinetics and bioavailability of sultamicillin estimated by high performance liquid chromatography. *J Antimicrob Chemother* 11: 435.

Sawai T, Yamaguchi A (1989). Mechanism of beta-lactamase inhibition: differences between sulbactam and other inhibitors. *Diagn Microbiol Infect Dis* 12: 121S.

Sawai T, Yamaguchi A, Tsukamoto K (1988). Amino acid sequence, active-site residue, and effect of suicide inhibitors on cephalosporinase of *Citrobacter freundii* GN 346. *Rev Infect Dis* 10: 721.

Schaad UB, Guenin K, Straehl P (1986). Single-dose pharmacokinetics of intravenous sulbactam in pediatric patients. *Rev Infect Dis* 8 (Suppl 5): 512.

Schwartz JI, Jauregui LE, Bachmann KA *et al.* (1988). Multiple dose pharmacokinetics of intravenously administered cefoperazone and sulbactam when given in combination to infected, seriously ill, elderly patients. *Antimicrob Ag Chemother* 32: 730.

Stahl J-P, Bru J-P, Fredj G *et al.* (1986). Penetration of sulbactam into the cerebrospinal fluid of patients with meningitis receiving ampicillin therapy. *Rev Infect Dis* 8 (Suppl 5): 612.

Study Group of Intraabdominal Infections (1986). A randomized controlled trial of ampicillin plus sulbactam vs gentamicin plus clindamycin in the treatment of intraabdominal infections: a preliminary report. *Rev Infect Dis* 8 (Suppl 5): 583.

Sutton AM, Turner TL, Cockburn F, McAllister TA (1986). Pharmacokinetic study of sulbactam and ampicillin administered concomitantly by intraarterial or intravenous infusion in the newborn. *Rev Infect Dis* 8 (Suppl 8): 518.

Syriopoulou V, Bitsi M, Theodoridis C *et al.* (1986). Clinical efficacy of sulbactam/ampicillin in pediatric infections caused by ampicillin-resistant or penicillin-resistant organisms. *Rev Infect Dis* 8 (Suppl 5): 630.

Thal LA, Vazquez J, Perri MB *et al.* (1993). Activity of ampicillin plus sulbactam against beta-lactamase producing enterococci in experimental endocarditis. *J Antimicrob Chemother* 31: 182.

Thomson KS, Weber DA, Sanders CC, Sanders WEJr (1990). Beta-lactamase production in members of the family Enterobacteriaceae and resistance to beta-lactam-enzyme inhibitor combinations. *Antimicrob Ag Chemother* 34: 622.

Urban C, Go E, Mariano N *et al.* (1993). Effect of sulbactam on infections caused by imipenem-resistant *Acinetobacter calcoaceticus* biotype anitratus. *J Infect Dis* 167: 448.

Valcke YJ, Rosseel MT, Pauwels RA *et al.* (1990). Penetration of ampicillin and sulbactam in the lower airways during respiratory infections. *Antimicrob Ag Chemother* **34**: 958.

Wald E, Reilly JS, Bluestone CD, Chiponis D (1986). Sulbactam/ampicillin in the treatment of acute epiglottitis in children. *Rev Infect Dis* **8** (Suppl 5): 617.

Wexler HM, Finegold SM (1988). *In vitro* activity of cefoperazone plus sulbactam compared with that of other antimicrobial agents against anaerobic bacteria. *Antimicrob Ag Chemother* **32**: 403.

Wexler HM, Harris B, Carter WT, Finegold SM (1985). *In vitro* efficacy of sulbactam combined with ampicillin against anaerobic bacteria. *Antimicrob Ag Chemother* **27**: 876.

Wexler HM, Molitoris E, Finegold SM (1991). Effect of beta-lactamase inhibitors on the activities of various beta-lactam agents against anaerobic bacteria. *Antimicrob Ag Chemother* **35**: 1219.

Wildfeuer A, Muller V, Springsklee M, Sonntag H-G (1991). Pharmacokinetics of ampicillin and sulbactam in patients undergoing heart surgery. *Antimicrob Ag Chemother* **35**: 1772.

Williams D, Perri M, Zervos MJ (1994). Randomized comparative trial with ampicillin/sulbactam versus cefamandole in the therapy of community acquired pneumonia. *Eur J Clin Microbiol Infect Dis* **13**: 293.

Wise R (1981). After pro-drugs-mutual pro-drugs. *J Antimicrob Chemother* **7**: 503.

Wise R (1982). Beta-lactamase inhibitors. *J Antimicrob Chemother* **9** (Suppl B): 31.

Wise R, Andrews JM, Bedford KA (1980). Clavulanic acid and CP-45,899: a comparison of their *in vitro* activity in combination with penicillins. *J Antimicrob Chemother* **6**: 197.

Wise R, Donovan IA, Andrews JM *et al.* (1983). Penetration of sulbactam and ampicillin into peritoneal fluid. *Antimicrob Ag Chemother* **24**: 290.

Wright N, Wise R (1983). The elimination of sulbactam alone and combined with ampicillin in patients with renal dysfunction. *J Antimicrob Chemother* **11**: 583.

Yamaguchi A, Hirata T, Sawai T (1983). Kinetic studies on inactivation of *Citrobacter freundii* cephalosporinase by sulbactam. *Antimicrob Ag Chemother* **24**: 23.

Tazobactam and Brobactam

Description

1 Tazobactam (YTR 830)

This is a penicillinate sulfone, structurally related to sulbactam (p. 209). Being a beta-lactamase inhibitor, it is synergistic with many beta-lactamase-labile drugs, such as penicillin G, ampicillin or piperacillin against many bacterial species which produce beta-lactamases (Aronoff *et al.*, 1984; Akova *et al.*, 1990). For clinical use only tazobactam combined with piperacillin has been made available. Each adult dose contains 4 g piperacillin, and 0.5 g tazobactam (Eklund *et al.*, 1993). The combination of piperacillin/tazobactam may have some advantages over other beta-lactam/beta-lactamase inhibitor combinations such as co-amoxiclav (p. 200), ticarcillin/clavulanic acid (p. 202) and ampicillin/sulbactam (p. 214). First of all piperacillin is easier to protect against TEM beta-lactamases. This is probably because of the lower affinity of piperacillin for these enzymes (Livermore, 1993). Tazobactam inhibits all beta-lactamases inhibited by clavulanic acid (p. 192), but in addition it also has some activity against chromosomally mediated induced (or derepressed) enzymes of *Morganella morganii*, *Citrobacter freundii*, *Enterobacter cloacae*, *Serratia marcescens* and sometimes *Pseudomonas aeruginosa*. Some authors have not been able to demonstrate any synergy between tazobactam and piperacillin against *Ps. aeruginosa*, *Burkholderia* (*Pseudomonas*) *cepacia* and *Stenotrophomonas maltophilia* (Jacobs *et al.*, 1986a,b; Eliopoulos *et al.*, 1989; Kuck *et al.*, 1989; Akova *et al.*, 1990; Higashitani *et al.*, 1990; Bush *et al.*, 1993). Tazobactam also appears to be a weaker enzyme inducer than other beta-lactamase inhibitors. Whilst with a few organisms such as *E. cloacae* and *Ps. aeruginosa* it is sometimes possible to demonstrate *in vitro* antagonism between ticarcillin and clavulanic acid (presumably because of enzyme induction by clavulanic acid), this has not been demonstrated with tazobactam/piperacillin (Akova *et al.*, 1990).

2 Brobactam (6-beta-bromo penicillanic acid)

This is another beta-lactamase inhibitor, similar to clavulanic acid. It is a simple substituted compound of the penicillin nucleus, 6-APA (p. 3) (Wise *et al.*, 1981; Melchior and Keiding, 1991). For pharmacological studies 800 mg of pivampicillin has been combined with 200 mg of brobactam (Wise *et al.*, 1992).

The details below apply only to tazobactam/piperacillin.

Sensitive organisms

1 Gram-positive bacteria

Beta-lactamase-producing strains of *Staphylococcus aureus* and *Staph. epidermidis* are piperacillin/tazobactam sensitive, but methicillin-resistant strains are not (Fass and Prior, 1989; Acar *et al.*, 1993). As with amoxycillin/clavulanic acid, *Staph. aureus* strains which produce type C beta-lactamase are less susceptible to piperacillin/tazobactam, than type A enzyme producers (p. 193). Beta-lactamase-producing *E. faecalis* strains are also usually susceptible, but *E. faecium* strains with high level intrinsic resistance to penicillin G (p. 10) are also resistant to this combination (Jones *et al.*, 1989; Chen *et al.*, 1993; Okhuysen *et al.*, 1993).

The addition of tazobactam does not affect the activity of piperacillin against sensitive strains of streptococci, enterococci and *Listeria monocytogenes*. Tazobactam does not improve the action of piperacillin against penicillin G-resistant pneumococci (p. 5) or against resistant strains of *Corynebacterium jeikeium* (Jones and Barry, 1989). Only very few strains of Gram-positive anaerobes such as *Clostridium* spp. produce beta-lactamase and these are sensitive to piperacillin/tazobactam. All others are sensitive to piperacillin alone (Appelbaum *et al.*, 1993).

2 Gram-negative aerobic bacteria

Beta-lactamase-producing strains of *Neisseria gonorrhoeae*, *N. meningitidis*, *Haemophilus influenzae* and *Moraxella catarrhalis* are piperacillin/tazobactam-sensitive. Tazobactam also enhances the activity of piperacillin against most strains of *Escherichia coli*, *Klebsiella*, *Proteus* and *Providencia* spp., *Citrobacter diversus* and *Morganella morganii*. It only occasionally enhances the activity of piperacillin against *Enterobacter* spp., *Citrobacter freundii* and *S. marcescens*. Tazobactam usually does not enhance the activity of piperacillin against *Aeromonas hydrophila*, *Ps. aeruginosa*, *Burkholderia (Pseudomonas) cepacia*, *S. maltophilia* and *Acinetobacter* spp. (Fass and Prior, 1989; Jones and Barry, 1989; Kuck *et al.*, 1989; Acar *et al.*, 1993; Chen *et al.*, 1993; Stobberingh *et al.*, 1994). The activity of piperacillin/tazobactam is usually good against *Acinetobacter* spp., but this may be because this organism is unusually susceptible to tazobactam alone (Table I.15) (Obana and Nishino, 1990). With respect to *Ps. aeruginosa* Giwercman *et al.* (1990) found that in cystic fibrosis patients after treatment with beta-lactam antibiotics, *Ps. aeruginosa* strains which produced large quantities of chromosomal beta-lactamase were selected and these were resistant to piperacillin. Tazobactam restored their sensitivity to piperacillin. But most other authors have not been able to demonstrate any improvement of the activity of piperacillin against *Ps. aeruginosa* in the presence of tazobactam (Eliopoulos *et al.*, 1989; Fass and Prior, 1989; Acar *et al.*, 1993; Reeves *et al.*, 1993). Both as a single agent and in combination with piperacillin, tazobactam is active *in vitro* against *Legionella* spp. (Collins *et al.*, 1994). But piperacillin plus tazobactam, unlike erythromycin (p. 609), is not effective against intracellular *Legionella* organisms, and therefore it seems unlikely that this combination will be effective for the treatment of Legionnaire's disease in humans (Edelstein and Edelstein, 1994).

3 Gram-negative anaerobic bacteria

Bacteroides fragilis and other anaerobes of *B. fragilis* group, such as *B. vulgatus*, *B. distasonis* and indolo-positive *B. thetaiotaomicron* and *B. ovatus* are nearly always piperacillin/tazobactam-sensitive (Bourgault *et al.*, 1992; Namavar *et al.*, 1994). This also applies to cefoxitin-resistant strains (Aldridge, 1993). The *Prevotella* spp., such as *P. bivia*, *P. disiens* and *P. melaninogenica* and bacteria of the *Porphyromonas* and *Fusobacterium* spp. are also nearly always susceptible to piperacillin/tazobactam (Appelbaum *et al.*, 1986, 1993; Eliopoulos *et al.*, 1989; Appelbaum, 1993).

4 Piperacillin/tazobactam and Gram-negative bacteria harboring extended spectrum beta-lactamases

These beta-lactamases are mainly found in Enterobacteriaceae, in particular in *Klebsiella* spp. and *E. coli*. A piperacillin/tazobactam combination is effective against a higher proportion of *E. coli* and *Klebsiella* spp. strains (which produce these enzymes) than ticarcillin/clavulanic acid (p. 203). However, some 18% of *E. coli* and *Klebsiella* spp. strains are not inhibited by piperacillin/tazobactam (Kempers and MacLaren, 1990; Thomson *et al.*, 1990). The efficacy of tazobactam in combination with piperacillin was studied *in vitro* and in rabbit experimental endocarditis due to a *Kl. pneumoniae* strain producing an extended spectrum beta-lactamase, TEM 3. This strain was resistant to piperacillin. Tazobactam restored its sensitivity to piperacillin *in vitro* and *in vivo*, but *in vivo*, piperacillin/tazobactam combined with gentamicin was the most effective regimen which more rapidly produced sterilization of vegetations (Mentec *et al.*, 1992). Another *Kl. pneumoniae* strain producing TEM 3 extended-spectrum beta-lactamase was studied by Leleu *et al.* (1994). Piperacillin/tazobactam was able to cure experimental meningitis caused by this organism, but only when tazobactam dosage within the combination was increased to 80:25.

Organism	MIC (μg per ml)		
	Tazobactam alone	Piperacillin alone	Piperacillin in presence of tazobactam
Gram-positive bacteria			
Staphylococcus aureus[a]	64.0	>128.0	4.0
Enterococcus faecalis	>128.0	4.0	4.0
Gram-negative bacteria			
Haemophilus influenzae[a]	–	512.0	2.0
Moraxella catarrhalis[a]	–	8.0	0.125
Escherichia coli[a]	>128.0	>128.0	8.0
Klebsiella pneumoniae[a]	>128.0	>128.0	16.0
Proteus mirabilis	>128.0	2.0	2.0
Proteus vulgaris	>128.0	8.0	2.0
Enterobacter aerogenes	>128.0	32.0	8.0
Pseudomonas aeruginosa	>128.0	16.0	16.0
Stenotrophomonas maltophilia	>128.0	>128.0	>128.0
Acinetobacter spp.	16.0	128.0	32.0
Bacteroides fragilis	–	128.0	4.0

[a] Piperacillin-resistant beta-lactamase-producing strains.

Table I.15
Compiled from data published by Eliopoulos *et al.* (1989), Mehtar *et al.* (1990) and Bourgault *et al.* (1992)

5 Minimum inhibitory concentrations

The MICs of piperacillin alone, and when tested in the presence of tazobactam against some selected bacterial species, are shown in Table I.15. The MICs of tazobactam alone are also presented.

Mode of Administration and Dosage

1 Adults

Piperacillin/tazobactam has been most commonly administered in an individual dose of 4 g piperacillin plus 0.5 g tazobactam, both infused together i.v. over 5 or more commonly over 30 min, similar to penicillin G (p. 20). This dose is then administered 8-hourly (Brismar *et al.*, 1992; Eklund *et al.*, 1993; Strayer *et al.*, 1994). Some clinical investigators have used lower dosages for less severe infections e.g. 2 g piperacillin plus 0.5 g tazobactam 8-hourly or a higher dosage of 4 g piperacillin plus 0.5 g tazobactam 6-hourly for more severe infections (Wise, 1993). The pharmacokinetics of piperacillin and tazobactam differs slightly (see below), but this difference is not so great as to warrant independent dosage adjustment of both agents in patients with renal failure. In patients with creatinine clearance of less than 40 ml per min, extension of dosing interval by 2 h is recommended; in those with creatinine clearance of less than 20 ml per min, a further 2 h increase in the dosing interval is warranted. In patients undergoing hemodialysis about one-third of the dose should be replaced at the end of the procedure. Peritoneal dialysis removes very little piperacillin and tazobactam, so extra dosing is not required after this dialysis (Sörgel and Kinzig, 1993).

2 Children

Based on pharmacokinetic studies, one suggested dosage of piperacillin/tazobactam for children is 100 mg of piperacillin and 12.5 mg of tazobactam per kg body weight administered as a fixed-dose combination every 6–8 h i.v. This dosage should be effective for most infections arising outside the central nervous system (Reed *et al.*, 1994).

Serum Levels in Relation to Dosage

The serum levels of piperacillin administered as a single drug (p. 169) are the same as when the drug is given together with tazobactam (Sörgel and Kinzig, 1993). By contrast, piperacillin inhibits renal clearance of tazobactam leading to higher tazobactam serum levels and a prolongation of its elimination half-life. Piperacillin probably inhibits tubular secretion of tazobactam. When 0.5 g of tazobactam is infused over 30 min as a single drug, the maximal serum level after the infusion averages 27.1 μg per ml, the terminal half-life is 0.67 h and its renal clearance is 268 ml per min. About 75.8% of the administered dose is excreted by the kidney. When 0.5 g of tazobactam is infused i.v. over 5 min together with 4 g of piperacillin, the maximal average serum level is 35.3 μg per ml, the terminal half-life is 0.92 h and its renal clearance is only 188 ml per min. Only about 68.2% of the given dose is excreted by the kidney (Kinzig et al., 1992; Sörgel and Kinzig, 1993; Van der Auwera et al., 1993).

Excretion

Both piperacillin and tazobactam are mainly eliminated via the kidneys by both tubular secretion and glomerular filtration. Probenecid reduces the renal elimination of both drugs (Sörgel and Kinzig, 1993). Piperacillin's excretion is unaffected by tazobactam, but piperacillin slows the renal excretion of tazobactam (see above). Overall 50–60% of administered dose of both drugs is excreted via the kidneys.

Biliary excretion of both drugs is probably low (<5%) (Sörgel and Kinzig, 1993), although some authors have reported high levels of piperacillin in the biliary tract in patients with no bile duct obstruction (p. 170). The remainder of both drugs are inactivated, probably chiefly in the liver.

Distribution of the Drugs in Body

The distribution of piperacillin in the body is described on p. 171. After a single i.v. dose of 4 g piperacillin and 0.5 g tazobactam, the latter is well distributed in many body fluids and tissues. The concentrations in fatty tissue and muscle have been estimated to be 10–13 and 18–30% of the levels in plasma, respectively. Adequate tazobactam concentrations are also reached in normal human bone tissue (Incavo et al., 1994). High concentrations of tazobactam are reached in skin and gastrointestinal mucosa, where concentration of the drug exceeds the levels in plasma after 1 h (Kinzig et al., 1992). High tazobactam concentrations are also attained in lung tissue and bronchial secretions, but its concentration is lower in gall bladder wall. High piperacillin levels are usually found in bile (p. 170), but tazobactam concentrations there are lower (1.33–42.9 μg per ml). In blister fluid tazobactam reaches about half of the plasma concentration (Wise et al., 1991; Sörgel and Kinzig, 1993; Jehl et al., 1994).

Tazobactam is 20–23% bound to human serum protein ((Sörgel and Kinzig, 1993).

Mode of Action

Tazobactam inhibits beta-lactamases by a mechanism similar to that of clavulanic acid (p. 192).

Toxicity

In general piperacillin/tazobactam is a combination with low toxicity. All reported side-effects are those which could occur with piperacillin alone. Some 4.6% of 944 treated patients developed a gastrointestinal disturbance, usually diarrhea. Diarrhea was the only event reported more often after treatment with piperacillin/tazobactam than with piperacillin alone. Twenty-one patients (2.2%) had drug-related skin rash, erythema, or pruritus. Some patients developed abnormal liver function tests with elevated alkaline phosphatase, SGOT, SGPT and total bilirubin. This either resolved during treatment or after the cessation of the drug.

These adverse reactions were usually not severe and in most patients therapy could be continued (Kuye et al., 1993). During piperacillin/tazobactam administration there were changes in intestinal microflora. In one study the number of enterobacteria and enterococci slightly decreased. There was also a minor decrease in some anaerobic bacteria, such as eubacteria, lactobacilli and Clostridium spp. The numbers of Gram-positive cocci and Bacteroides spp. were unaffected. No patients developed diarrhea (Nord et al., 1992).

Clinical Uses of the Drug

1 Intra-abdominal infections

Piperacillin plus tazobactam in a dosage of 4 g piperacillin plus 0.5 g tazobactam i.v. 8-hourly appears effective and safe in the treatment of peritonitis, usually due to a perforated viscus. Clinical investigators have obtained slightly superior results with piperacillin/tazobactam compared with imipenem /cilastatin (p. 236) in the treatment of these infections (Brismar *et al.*, 1992; Eklund *et al.*, 1993). In a dosage of 3 g piperacillin plus 375 mg tazobactam every 6 h, this combination also was as efficacious and at least as safe as a clindamycin/gentamicin regimen for the treatment of peritonitis (Polk *et al.*, 1993).

2 Lower respiratory tract infections including nosocomial pneumonia

In an open non-comparative study, the majority of patients with pneumonia responded well to piperacillin 4 g plus tazobactam 0.5 g i.v. 8-hourly (Mouton *et al.*, 1993). The main causative organisms were *Streptococcus pneumoniae*, *Kl. pneumoniae* and *H. influenzae*. In one comparative trial piperacillin/tazobactam appeared superior to ticarcillin/clavulanic acid for the treatment of community-acquired bacterial lower respiratory tract infections (Shlaes *et al.*, 1994).

3 Bacteremia

Wise (1993) reported his experience with piperacillin/tazobactam in various types of bacteremia. Most of the patients had a bacteremia where the focus of infection was the urinary tract and the causative organisms were one of the Enterobacteriaceae such as *E. coli*, *Klebsiella* spp. and *Pr. mirabilis*. The results of treatment were good in this group. In this series there were also neutropenic patients and several of them cultured Gram-positive organisms such as *Staph. aureus*, *Staph. epidermidis*, *Strep. bovis* and *Strep. mitis*. A small number of these patients did not respond to piperacillin/tazobactam therapy.

4 Skin and soft tissue infections

The results of piperacillin/tazobactam treatment have been good and comparable with those obtained with ticarcillin/clavulanic acid (p. 202) in chronic and complicated skin and soft tissue infections, such as cellulitis with drainage, cutaneous abscesses, diabetic or ischemic foot infections and infected wounds and ulcers with drainage (Tan *et al.*, 1993; Tassler *et al.*, 1993).

5 Empiric treatment of fever in neutropenic patients

In one prospective randomized trial piperacillin/amikacin/teicoplanin was compared with piperacillin/amikacin/tazobactam. If there was persistence of fever, teicoplanin was also added to patients in group 2 on day 4. In a large proportion of the second group teicoplanin had to be added. It was concluded that piperacillin/amikacin/tazobactam may be a reasonable combination to use in these patients, provided that either vancomycin or teicoplanin is added in unresponsive cases (Micozzi *et al.*, 1993). In another comparative trial Cometta *et al.* (1995) found piperacillin/tazobactam plus amikacin slightly superior to ceftazidime plus amikacin for the initial empiric therapy for fever in neutropenic patients with cancer.

6 Pelvic infections in women

Piperacillin/tazobactam in a dose of piperacillin 3 g i.v. plus tazobactam 375 mg i.v. 6-hourly was equally satisfactory to clindamycin plus gentamicin in the treatment of hospitalized women with infections in the upper genital tract (Sweet *et al.*, 1994).

7 Bacterial meningitis

Kern *et al.* (1990) evaluated the therapeutic efficacy of piperacillin/tazobactam in animal experimental meningitis due to a beta-lactamase-producing strain of *E. coli*. Only at the relatively high doses of 160/20 and 200/25 mg of piperacillin/tazobactam per kg per h, the bactericidal activity of the combination was comparable with that of 10 and 25 mg of ceftriaxone per kg per h, respectively. As several of the third-generation cephalosporins (p. 336) are very effective for the treatment of bacterial meningitis caused by Gram-negative bacilli, it is unlikely that piperacillin/tazobactam will gain a place in the treatment of this disease.

References

Acar JF, Goldstein FW, Kitzis MD (1993). Susceptibility survey of piperacillin alone and in the presence of tazobactam. *J Antimicrob Chemother* **31** (Suppl A): 23.

Akova M, Yang Y, Livermore DM (1990). Interactions of tzobactam and clavulanate with inducibly-and constitutively-expressed class 1 beta-lactamases. *J Antimicrob Chemother* **25**: 199.

Aldridge KE (1993). Cross-resistance to beta-lactam-beta-lactamase inhibitor combinations and clindamycin among cefoxitin-resistant and cefoxitin-susceptible strains of the *Bacteroides fragilis* group. *Diagn Microbiol Infect Dis* **17**: 251.

Appelbaum PC (1993). Comparative susceptibility profile of piperacillin/tazobactam against anaerobic bacteria. *J Antimicrob Chemother* **31** (Suppl A): 29.

Appelbaum PC, Jacobs MR, Spangler SK, Yamabe S (1986). Comparative activity of beta-lactamase inhibitors YTR 830, clavulanate, and sulbactam combined with beta-lactams against beta-lactamase-producing anaerobes. *Antimicrob Ag Chemother* **30**: 789.

Appelbaum PC, Spangler SK, Jacobs MR (1993). Susceptibility of 539 Gram-positive and Gram-negative anaerobes to new agents, including RP 59500, biapenem, trospectinomycin and piperacillin/tazobactam. *J Antimicrob Chemother* **32**: 223.

Aronoff SC, Jacobs MR, Johenning S, Yamabe S (1984). Comparative activities of the beta-lactamase inhibitors YTR 830, sodium clavulanate, and sulbactam combined with amoxicillin or ampicillin. *Antimicrob Ag Chemother* **26**: 580.

Bourgault A-M, Lamothe F, Hoban DJ et al. (1992). Survey of *Bacteroides fragilis* group susceptibility patterns in Canada. *Antimicrob Ag Chemother* **36**: 343.

Brismar B, Malmborg AS, Tunevall G et al. (1992). Piperacillin-tazobactam versus imipenem-cilastatin for treatment of intra-abdominal infections. *Antimicrob Ag Chemother* **36**: 2766.

Bush K, Macalintal C, Rasmussen BA et al. (1993). Kinetic interactions of tazobactam with beta-lactamases from all major sructural classes. *Antimicrob Ag Chemother* **37**: 851.

Chen HY, Bonfiglio G, Allen M et al. (1993). Multicentre survey of the comparative *in-vitro* activity of piperacillin/tazobactam against bacteria from hospitalized patients in the British Isles. *J Antimicrob Chemother* **32**: 247.

Collins LA, Wennersten CB, Ferraro MJ et al. (1994). Comparative activities of piperacillin and tazobactam against clinical isolates of *Legionella* spp. *Antimicrob Ag Chemother* **38**: 144.

Cometta A, Zinner S, de Bock R et al. (1995). Piperacillin-tazobactam plus amikacin versus ceftazidime plus amikacin as empiric therapy for fever in granulocytopenic patients with cancer. *Antimicrob Ag Chemother* **39**: 445.

Edelstein PH, Edelstein MAC (1994). *In vitro* extracellular and intracellular activities of clavulanic acid and those of piperacillin and ceftriaxone alone and in combination with tazobactam against clinical isolates of *Legionella* species. *Antimicrob Ag Chemother* **38**: 200.

Eklund A-E, Nord CE and Swedish Study Group (1993). A randomized multicenter trial of piperacillin/tazobactam versus imipenem/cilastatin in the treatment of severe intra-abdominal infections. *J Antimicrob Chemother* **31** (Suppl A): 79.

Eliopoulos GM, Klimm K, Ferraro MJ et al. (1989). Comparative *in vitro* activity of piperacillin combined with the beta-lactamase inhibitor tazobactam (YTR 830). *Diagn Microbiol Infect Dis* **12**: 481.

Fass RJ, Prior RB (1989). Comparative *in vitro* activities of piperacillin-tazobactam and ticarcillin-clavulanate. *Antimicrob Ag Chemother* **33**: 1268.

Giwercman B, Lambert PA, Rosdahl VT et al. (1990). Rapid emergence of resistance in *Pseudomonas aeruginosa* in cystic fibrosis patients due to *in-vivo* selection of stable partially derepressed beta-lactamase producing strains. *J Antimicrob Chemother* **26**: 247.

Higashitani F, Hyodo A, Ishida N et al. (1990). Inhibition of beta-lactamases by tazobactam and *in-vitro* antibacterial activity of tazobactam combined with piperacillin. *J Antimicrob Chemother* **25**: 567.

Incavo SJ, Ronchetti PJ, Choi JH et al. (1994). Penetration of piperacillin-tazobactam into cancellous and cortical bone tissue. *Antimicrob Ag Chemother* **38**: 905.

Jacobs MR, Aronoff SC, Johenning S, Yamabe S (1986a). Comparative activities of the beta-lactamase inhibitors YTR 830, clavulanate and sulbactam combined with extended-spectrum penicillins against ticarcillin-resistant Enterobacteriaceae and pseudomonads. *J Antimicrob Chemother* **18**: 177.

Jacobs MR, Aronoff SC, Johenning S et al. (1986b). Comparative activities of the beta-lactamase inhibitors YTR 830, clavulanate and sulbactam combined with ampicillin and broad-spectrum penicillins against defined beta-lactamase-producing aerobic Gram-negative bacilli. *Antimicrob Ag Chemother* **29**: 980.

Jehl F, Muller-Serieys C, De Larminat V et al. (1994). Penetration of piperacillin-tazobactam into bronchial secretions after multiple doses to intensive care patients. *Antimicrob Ag Chemother* **38**: 2780.

Jones RN, Barry AL (1989). Studies to optimize the *in vitro* testing of piperacillin combined with tazobactam (YTR 830). *Diagn Microbiol Infect Dis* **12**: 495.

Jones RN, Pfaller MA, Fuchs PC et al. (1989). Piperacillin/tazobactam (YTR 830). combination Comparative antimicrobial activity against 5889 recent aerobic clinical isolates and 60 *Bacteroides fragilis* group strains. *Diagn Microbiol Infect Dis* **12**: 489.

Kempers J, MacLaren DM (1990). Piperacillin/tazobactam and ticarcillin/clavulanic acid against resistant Enterobacteriaceae. *J Antimicrob Chemother* **26**: 598.

Kern W, Kennedy SL, Sachdeva M et al. (1990). Evaluation of piperacillin-tazobactam in experimental meningitis caused by a beta-lactamase-producing strain of K1-positive *Echerichia coli*. *Antimicrob Ag Chemother* **34**: 697.

Kinzig M, Sörgel F, Brismar B, Nord CE (1992). Pharmacokinetics and tissue penetration of tazobactam and piperacillin in patients undergoing colorectal surgery. *Antimicrob Ag Chemother* **36**: 1997.

Kuck NA, Jacobus NV, Petersen PJ et al. (1989). Comparative *in vitro* and *in vivo* activities of piperacillin combined with the beta-lactamase inhibitors tazobactam, clavulanic acid, and sulbactam. *Antimicrob Ag Chemother* **33**: 1964.

Kuye O, Teal J, De Vries VG et al. (1993). Safety profile of piperacillin/tazobactam in phase I and III clinical studies. *J Antimicrob Chemother* **31** (Suppl A): 113.

Leleu G, Kitzis MD, Vallois JM et al. (1994). Different ratios of the piperacillin-tazobactam combination for treatment of experimental meningitis due to *Klebsiella pneumoniae* producing the TEM-3 extended-spectrum beta-lactamase. *Antimicrob Ag Chemother* **38**: 195.

Livermore DM (1993). Determinants of the activity of beta-lactamase inhibitor combinations. *J Antimicrob Chemother* **31** (Suppl A): 9.

Mehtar S, Drabu YJ, Blakemore PH (1990). The *in vitro* activity of piperacillin/tazobactam, ciprofloxacin, ceftazidime and imipenem against multiple resistant Gram-negative bacteria. *J Antimicrob Chemother* **25**: 915.

Melchior NH, Keiding J (1991). *In vitro* evaluation of ampicillin/brobactam and comparison with other beta-lactam antibiotics. *J Antimicrob Chemother* **27**: 29.

Mentec H, Vallois JM, Bure A et al. (1992). Piperacillin, tazobactam, and gentamicin alone or combined in an endocarditis model of infection by a TEM-3-producing strain of *Klebsiella pneumoniae* or its susceptible variant. *Antimicrob Ag Chemother* **36**: 1883.

Micozzi A, Nucci M, Venditti M et al. (1993). Piperacillin/tazobactam/amikacin versus piperacillin/amikacin/teicoplanin in the empirical treatment of neutropenic patients. *Eur J Clin Microbiol Infect Dis* **12**: 1.

Mouton Y, Leroy O, Beuscart C et al. (1993). Efficacy, safety and tolerance of parenteral piperacillin/tazobactam in the treatment of patients with lower respiratory tract infections. *J Antimicrob Chemother* **31** (Suppl A): 87.

Namavar F, Severin WPJ, Stobberingh E *et al.* (1994). The sensitivity of clinical isolates of anaerobic species to piperacillin-tazobactam and other antimicrobial agents. *J Antimicrob Chemother* **34**: 415.

Nord CE, Brismar B, Kasholm-Tengve B, Tunevall G (1992). Effect of piperacillin/tazobactam therapy on intestinal microflora. *Scand J Infect Dis* **24**: 209.

Obana Y, Nishino T (1990). *In-vitro* and *in-vivo* activities of sulbactam and YTR830H against *Acinetobacter calcoaceticus*. *J Antimicrob Chemother* **26**: 677.

Okhuysen PC, Singh KV, Murray BE (1993). Susceptability of beta-lactamase-producing enterococci to piperacillin with tazobactam. *Diagn Microbiol Infect Dis* **17**: 219.

Polk HC, Jr, Fink MP, Leverdiere M *et al.* (1993). Prospective randomized study of piperacillin/tazobactam therapy of surgically treated intra-abdominal infectin. *Amer Surg* **59**: 598.

Reed MD, Goldfarb J, Yamashita TS *et al.* (1994). Single-dose pharmacokinetics of piperacillin and tazobactam in infants and children. *Antimicrob Ag Chemother* **38**: 2817.

Reeves DS, Holt HA, Bywater MJ, MacGowan AP (1993). The activity of piperacillin/tazobactam against clinical isolates collected in 20 UK centres and the design of a disc test for susceptibility testing. *J Antimicrob Chemother* **32**: 51.

Shlaes DM, Baughman R, Boylen CT *et al.* (1994). Piperacillin/tazobactam compared with ticarcillin/clavulanate in community-acquired bacterial lower respiratory tract infectins. *J Antimicrob Chemother* **34**: 565.

Sörgel F, Kinzig M (1993). The chemistry, pharmacokinetics and tissue distribution of piperacillin/tazobactam. *J Antimicrob Chemother* **31** (Suppl A): 39.

Stobberingh EE, Maclaren DM, Schmitz PIM and the Multicentre Study Group (1994). Comparative *in-vitro* activity of piperacillin-tazobactam against recent clinical isolates, a Dutch national multicentre study. *J Antimicrob Chemother* **34**: 777.

Strayer AH, Gilbert DH, Pivarnik P *et al.* (1994). Pharmacodynamics of piperacillin alone and in combination with tazobactam against piperacillin-resistant and -susceptible organisms in an *in vitro* model of infection. *Antimicrob Ag Chemother* **38**: 2351.

Sweet RL, Roy S, Faro S *et al.* (1994). Piperacillin and tazobactam versus clindamycin and gentamicin in the treatment of hospitalized women with pelvic infection. *Obstet Gynecol* **83**: 280.

Tan JS, Wishnow RM, Talan DA *et al.* (1993). Treatment of hospitalized patients with complicated skin and skin structure infections: double-blind, randomized, multicenter study of piperacillin-tazobactam versus ticarcillin-clavulanate. *Antimicrob Ag Chemother* **37**: 1580.

Tassler H, Cullmann W, Elhardt D (1993). Therapy of soft tissue infections with piperacillin/tazobactam. *J Antimicrob Chemother* **31** (Suppl A): 105.

Thomson KS, Weber DA, Sanders CC, Sanders WEJr (1990). Beta-lactamase production in members of the family Enterobacteriaceae and resistance to beta-lactam-enzyme inhibitor combinations. *Antimicrob Ag Chemother* **34**: 622.

Van der Auwera P, Duchateau V, Lambert C *et al.* (1993). *Ex vivo* pharmacodynamic study of piperacillin alone and in combination with tazobactam, compared with ticarcillin plus clavulanic acid. *Antimicrob Ag Chemother* **37**: 1860.

Wise R (1993). The efficacy and safety of piperacillin/tazobactam in the therapy of bacteraemia. *J Antimicrob Chemother* **31** (Suppl A): 97.

Wise R, Andrews JM, Patel N (1981). 6-Beta-bromo and 6-beta-iodo penicillanic acid, two novel beta-lactamase inhibitors. *J Antimicrob Chemother* **7**: 531.

Wise R, Logan M, Cooper M, Andrews JM (1991). Pharmacokinetics and tissue penetration of tazobactam administered alone and with piperacillin. *Antimicrob Ag Chemother* **35**: 1081.

Wise R, O'Sullivan N, Johnson J, Andrews JM (1992). Pharmacokinetics and tissue penetratin of ampicillin and brobactam following oral administration of 2085P. *Antimicrob Ag Chemother* **36**: 1002.

Imipenem/Cilastatin

Description

The carbapenems are a group of bicyclic beta-lactam compounds with a common carbapenem nucleus. Imipenem is one of these and it has high activity against both aerobic and anaerobic bacteria.

In the 1970s Beecham Research Laboratories identified a carbapenem group, called olivanic acids, which were beta-lactamase inhibitors and broad spectrum antibiotics (Butterworth *et al.*, 1979). At about the same time, Merck, Sharp and Dohme Research Laboratories independently identified thienamycin, derived from *Streptomyces cattleya*. This had the same carbapenem nucleus but different side-chains which increased its antibacterial potency (Albers-Schonberg *et al.*, 1978). Its chemical instability in concentrated solution was overcome by crystallization of the N-formimidoyl derivative of thienamycin, called imipenem. Urinary recovery *in vivo* was less than expected due to extensive renal tubular metabolism by a brush border dipeptidase enzyme, dehydropeptidase I. A selective competitive antagonist of this enzyme was then developed and named cilastatin, which has similar pharmacokinetics to imipenem. Imipenem and cilastatin are marketed in combination in a 1:1 ratio (Kahan *et al.*, 1983). The abbreviation imipenem/c will be used for imipenem/cilastatin and the dosages stated for imipenem/c refer only to the imipenem component.

Sensitive Organisms

Imipenem has one of the widest spectrum of the beta-lactam antibiotics. It is active against nearly all common bacterial species, including those resistant to aminoglycosides and newer cephalosporins. There is usually no cross-resistance between imipenem and the penicillins and cephalosporins (Barry *et al.*, 1985; Geddes and Stille, 1985; Kropp *et al.*, 1985; Remington, 1985).

1 Gram-positive aerobic bacteria

Imipenem is very active against *Streptococcus pyogenes* and Group B, C and G streptococci (MICs 0.5 µg per ml). The same applies to streptococci of the viridans group and to non-enterococcal Group D streptococci such as *Strep. bovis* (Acar *et al.*, 1983; Barry *et al.*, 1985; Jones, 1985; Kropp *et al.*, 1985; Murray *et al.*, 1993). Some strains of *Strep. viridans* with high-level intrinsic resistance to penicillin G (p. 8), remain imipenem-sensitive (Carratalá and Gudiol, 1995). Penicillin G-sensitive *Staphylococcus aureus*, and beta-lactamase-producing, methicillin-susceptible *Staph. aureus* strains are imipenem-sensitive. The same applies to coagulase-negative staphylococci. But both methicillin-resistant *Staph. aureus* strains (MRSA) and coagulase-negative staphylococci are imipenem-resistant. Some laboratories have reported them to be imipenem-sensitive (Kropp *et al.*, 1985). Imipenem combined with a cephalosporin may act synergistically against MRSA (Matsuda *et al.*, 1991; Oka *et al.*, 1993). Similarly imipenem/vancomycin may show *in vitro* synergy against MRSA (Shlaes *et al.*, 1993). The clinical significance of this is not known. Imipenem may show low MICs for MRSA after only 18 h growth, but there is a marked increase in the MICs of imipenem after 48 h incubation. Imipenem therefore, similar to other beta-lactam antibiotics, is ineffective for treatment of MRSA infections (Markowitz *et al.*, 1983; Jones, 1985; Murray *et al.*, 1993).

Streptococcus pneumoniae is highly sensitive to imipenem. Strains with decreased penicillin G sensitivity have increased imipenem MICs, but they are lower than those of penicillin G. Strains with intermediate penicillin G-resistance (MIC 1 µg per ml) are inhibited by 0.25 µg of imipenem and strains with high degree of penicillin G-resistance (MIC 4 µg per ml) are inhibited by 0.5 μg of imipenem (Table I.16) (Otin *et al.*, 1988; Liñares *et al.*, 1992; Murray *et al.*, 1993; Spangler *et al.*, 1994). The drug has good bactericidal activity against these pneumococci (Barakett *et al.*, 1994).

Imipenem has good inhibitory activity against *Enterococcus faecalis*, but, similar to penicillin G (p. 9), it is not bactericidal (Eliopoulos and Moellering, 1981). Beta-lactamase-producing strains of *E. faecalis* are imipenem-sensitive, but as most of these strains also exhibit high-level gentamicin-resistance (p. 10), a synergistic imipenem/aminoglycoside combination usually cannot be obtained for the purpose of treating *E. faecalis* endocarditis (Hindes *et al.*, 1989; Markowitz *et al.*, 1991). Both *E. faecalis* and more commonly *E. faecium* strains which have high-level intrinsic resistance to penicillin G (p. 10) and ampicillin, are also imipenem-resistant (Acar *et al.*, 1983).

Listeria monocytogenes is sensitive to imipenem (Kropp *et al.*, 1985), but imipenem alone or combined with gentamicin is less effective than ampicillin or ampicillin/gentamicin against *L. monocytogenes* infections in experimental animals (Kim, 1986). Also *L. monocytogenes* mutants, resistant to imipenem and penicillin G can be selected *in vitro*. In these penicillin-binding protein (PBP) 3 was altered and this had decreased affinity for imipenem and penicillin G (Pierre *et al.*, 1990). Imipenem is one of the most active beta-lactam agents against *Nocardia asteroides*; some 90% of isolates are inhibited by clinically achievable concentrations (Dewsnup and Wright, 1984; Wallace *et al.*, 1988; Farina *et al.*, 1995). The most common other aerobic actinomycetes include *Actinomadura madurae*, *Streptomyces griseus*, and *Nocardia brasiliensis*. Although *A. madurae* is always imipenem-sensitive, and about 80% of *S. griseus* strains are sensitive, but the majority of strains of *N. brasiliensis* are resistant (McNeil *et al.*, 1990). *Rhodococcus equi*, a Gram-positive coccobacillus, is an opportunistic pathogen in immunocompromised patients, especially AIDS. It is usually susceptible to imipenem but the drug is not bactericidal. Imipenem/amikacin combination acts synergistically against *R. equi* (Nordmann and Ronco, 1992). *in vitro* mutants of *R. equi* have been selected with decreased susceptibility to imipenem. In these PBP3 was replaced by PBP3a. This change in PBP3 probably explains the resistance, but the exact mechanism has not been determined. (Nordmann *et al.*, 1993a). The *Corynebacterium* spp. are imipenem-sensitive with the exception of *C. jeikeium* (J.K. diphtheroids) which are resistant (Spitzer *et al.*, 1986; Vurma-Rapp *et al.*, 1986; Barnass *et al.*, 1991). The *Bacillus* spp., especially all *B. cereus* strains, are imipenem-sensitive (Weber *et al.*, 1988).

2 Gram-positive anaerobic bacteria

Anaerobes such as the *Peptococcus*, *Peptostreptococcus*, *Actinomyces*, *Clostridium*, *Propionibacterium* and *Lactobacillus* spp. are nearly always imipenem-sensitive (Kropp *et al.*, 1985; Goldstein and Citron, 1986; Höffler, 1986; Griffiths *et al.*, 1992). *Clostridium difficile* is less sensitive, most strains needing 8–16 μg per ml for inhibition (Chow *et al.*, 1985; Wexler and Finegold, 1985).

3 Gram-negative aerobic bacteria

Both *Neisseria meningitidis* and *N. gonorrhoeae* are very sensitive to imipenem. Beta-lactamase-producing strains are equally susceptible (Jones, 1985; Kropp *et al.*, 1985). *Haemophilus influenzae* and *H. parainfluenzae* are also imipenem-sensitive, including beta-lactamase producing strains (Kropp *et al.*, 1985; Cerami and Shungu, 1986). Ampicillin-resistant *H. influenzae* strains, which do not produce beta-lactamase, but where the resistance is intrinsic *and* chromosomally mediated (p. 114), usually have reduced susceptibility to other penicillins, cephalosporins and aztreonam. Such strains are usually sensitive to imipenem (Powell and Williams, 1987; Powell and Livermore, 1990; James *et al.*, 1993). But one more recent study showed that intrinsically resistant *H. influenzae* strains also had elevated MICs for imipenem (Yeo and Livermore, 1994). *Moraxella cattarrhalis* is imipenem-sensitive irrespective of beta-lactamase production (Murray *et al.*, 1993). *Campylobacter jejuni*, *C. fetus* (Kropp *et al.*, 1985; Farrugia *et al.*, 1994) and *Helicobacter pylori* (Shungu *et al.*, 1987) are imipenem-sensitive.

Imipenem is active against *Legionella pneumophila*; its MIC and MBC are both less than 0.02 μg per ml, which is much lower than values for aztreonam, mecillinam, cefotaxime and cefoxitin (Farrell *et al.*, 1985). Imipenem causes lysis of *L. pneumophila* without extensive cell wall degradation (Weisholtz and Tomasz, 1985). *Pasteurella multocida* is susceptible, but Flavobacterium spp. are imipenem-resistant (Jones, 1985). *Acinetobacter* and *Aeromonas* spp. and *Plesiomonas shigelloides* are all susceptible to imipenem (Kropp *et al.*, 1985; Gold and Salit, 1993; Murray *et al.*, 1993; Seifert *et al.*, 1993; Zemelman *et al.*, 1993). Inducible chromosomally mediated beta-lactamases normally do not hydrolyze imipenem (unlike the third-generation cephalosporins), but some enzymes of this type, produced by *Aeromonas* spp., can hydrolyze imipenem. The MICs of such strains are still relatively low, and they remain imipenem-sensitive. This may be because only a low level of enzyme is produced and there is rapid permeation of imipenem into the Gram-negative cell (Shannon *et al.*, 1986; Bakken *et al.*, 1988). Other authors have described *Aeromonas* spp. strains which possessed a beta-lactamase (carbapenemase) which hydrolyzed only carbapenems and penems. Penicillins and cephalosporins were unaffected. These strains were imipenem-resistant (Segatore *et al.*; 1993; Morita *et al.*, 1994; Rossolini *et al.*, 1995). *Acinetobacter* spp. strains can also become imipenem-resistant, particularly if the drug is extensively used in a hospital environment (Meyer *et al.*, 1993; Urban *et al.*, 1993; Wood and Reboli, 1993; Kuah *et al.*, 1994). The *Brucella* spp. are imipenem-sensitive (Kropp. *et al.*, 1985).

The Enterobacteriaceae, such as *Escherichia coli*, the *Enterobacter*, *Klebsiella*, *Proteus*, *Salmonella*, *Shigella*, *Providencia*, *Serratia*, *Citrobacter*, *Hafnia*, *Edwardsiella*, *Arizona* and *Yersinia* spp. are nearly always imipenem-sensitive (Kropp *et al.*, 1985; Vurma-Rapp *et al.*, 1986; Murray *et al.*, 1993). Aminoglycoside-resistant Enterobacteriaceae are usually imipenem-sensitive (Mayer and Zinner, 1985; Vurma Rapp *et al.*, 1986). Chromosomally mediated beta-lactamases produced by *Morganella morganii*, *Proteus rettgeri*, *Serratia marcescens* and *Enterobacter* spp. are inducible. Imipenem acts as an inducer of these enzymes, but it is not hydrolyzed by them. So these organisms, when the enzymes are induced, remain sensitive to imipenem, but they are resistant to most third-generation cephalosporins (Labia *et al.*, 1986; Ashby *et al.*, 1987). Enterobacteriaceae, in particular *E. coli* and *Klebsiella* spp., which produce extended-spectrum beta-lactamases (p. 323), may be resistant to a wide range of cephalosporins and cephamycins, but imipenem is usually not hydrolyzed by these enzymes and so these strains remain imipenem-sensitive (Jacoby and Carreras, 1990; Jacoby and Medeiros, 1991; Meyer *et al.*, 1993; Zemelman *et al.*, 1993).

Some Enterobacteriaceae, particularly *Enterobacter* spp. can produce beta-lactamases, usually inducible, which can slowly hydrolyze imipenem and meropenem (p. 246). Hydrolysis is slow and these *Enterobacter* strains remain imipenem-sensitive, but if the *Enterobacter* spp. strain develops a porin-deficient cell wall, then the combination of the beta-lactamase and decreased permeability of the antibiotic can make this strain imipenem-resistant (Lee *et al.*, 1991; Livermore, 1992b; Ehrhard *et al.*, 1993; Tzouvelekis *et al.*, 1994). In other studies it was possible to produce *E. cloacae* and *Pr. rettgeri* strains which were resistant to imipenem. Again they had the dual mechanism of resistance. Their chromosomal beta-lactamases were strongly derepressed (p. 322), and these strains were also deficient in the porins in their cell walls (Raimondi *et al.*, 1991; Cornaglia *et al.*, 1995). Rarely Enterobacteriaceae can acquire beta-lactamases, which in their own right hydrolyze imipenem. These enzymes have been usually chromosomally mediated (Livermore, 1992b). Two *S. marcescens* strains have been described which produced a beta-lactamase (carbapenemase), which hydrolyzed imipenem and made the strains imipenem-resistant. No other resistance mechanisms were involved. The beta-lactamase was not fully characterized, but it was not plasmid- or transposon-mediated (Yang *et al.*, 1990). Other *S. marcescens* strains have been detected, which produced chromosomally mediated beta-lactamases, which made these strains imipenem-resistant (Naas *et al.*, 1994; Osano *et al.*, 1994). In hospitals in Japan *S. marcescens* strains have been identified which produced plasmid-mediated metallo-beta-lactamases, which could hydrolyze imipenem and other broad-spectrum beta-lactams (Ito *et al.*, 1995).

A strain of *Enterobacter* spp., resistant to imipenem, which hyperproduced the group 1 chromosomally mediated beta-lactamase has been described. No other resistance mechanisms were detected (Thomson *et al.*, 1993). Another strain of *Enterobacter* spp. produced a novel chromosome-encoded beta-lactamase, which differed from all the previously described carbapenamases. The strain was imipenem-resistant (Nordmann *et al.*, 1993b). Other reports described imipenem-resistant *Enterobacter* spp. strains, where the resistance appeared to be solely due to a loss of porin proteins and so a decreased permeability of the bacterial cell wall. Only minor variations in beta-lactamase activity was observed in these organisms (Hopkins and Towner, 1990; Chow and Shlaes, 1991). A similar resistance mechanism was reported for one strain of imipenem-resistant *Pr. mirabilis* (Mehtar *et al.*, 1991).

Pseudomonas aeruginosa is normally highly sensitive to imipenem (Jones, 1985; Kropp *et al.*, 1985; Vurma-Rapp *et al.*, 1986). Imipenem-resistant strains develop quite readily and they often arise *in vivo* when imipenem is used to treat a *Ps. aeruginosa* infection. This often leads to treatment failure (Quinn *et al.*, 1986; Büscher *et al.*, 1987a; Ogle *et al.*, 1988; Quinn *et al.*, 1988). Resistant strains of *Ps. aeruginosa* may show cross-resistance to the related drug meropenem (p. 246), but there is no cross-resistance to the third-generation cephalosporins nor any other beta-lactam compounds (Neu, 1985; Quinn *et al.*, 1988; Bellido *et al.*, 1990; Vurma-Rapp *et al.*,

1990). This imipenem resistance of *Ps. aeruginosa* is due to a loss of a specific outer membrane porin protein (Opr D2), and this is associated with decreased penetration of the antibiotic across the outer membrane of *Ps. aeruginosa* cell (Büscher *et al.*, 1987b; Lynch *et al.*, 1987; Studemeister and Quinn, 1988; Trias *et al.*, 1989; Quinn *et al.*, 1991; Quinn, 1994). The *Ps. aeruginosa* gene which codes for the removal of the specific porin protein may reside on a plasmid or the chromosome (Yoneyama and Nakae, 1993). The synthesis of the outer membrane porin protein (Opr D2) is suppressed by salicylate. In the presence of salicylate *Ps. aeruginosa* can become less susceptible to imipenem. This resistance is transient and only exists whilst salicylate is present (Sumita and Fukasawa, 1993).

In patients with cystic fibrosis treated by imipenem, the organisms produce large amounts of chromosomally mediated beta-lactamase and in this situation with imipenem-resistant strains, the beta-lactamase production is the main mechanism of resistance (Giwercman *et al.*, 1992).

Some imipenem-resistant *Ps. aeruginosa* strains may be resistant because of both loss of membrane porin protein D_2 as well as excessive derepressed chromosomal beta-lactamase synthesis (Aronoff and Shlaes, 1987; Satake *et al.*, 1991; Livermore, 1992a). Another report described a strain of *Ps. aeruginosa*, in which one PBP, PBP4 bound less imipenem and the strain also had reduced permeability of its cell wall (Bellido *et al.*, 1990). One *Ps. aeruginosa* strain has been reported, which possessed an extended-spectrum beta-lactamase which hydrolyzed ceftazidime and imipenem (p. 369).

In chronic infections such as *Ps. aeruginosa* infections in cystic fibrosis and foreign device infections, there are biofilms present next to the foreign device. Also large amounts of chromosomal-beta lactamase may be produced which permeates in the biofilm. The presence of such levels of beta-lactam-degrading enzymes in a biofilm affords these *Ps. aeruginosa* cells a large measure of protection from imipenem and other beta-lactam antibiotics (Giwercman *et al.*, 1991), but despite these resistance mechanisms, a survey of 24 hospitals in the UK in 1993 showed that only 2.5% of *Ps. aeruginosa* strains were imipenem-resistant (Chen *et al.*, 1995).

In one study the combination of imipenem plus ciprofloxacin and imipenem plus amikacin was synergistic in 36% and 45%, respectively of imipenem-sensitive *Ps. aeruginosa* strains. The incidence of synergy against imipenem-resistant isolates was only 10% for both combinations (Bustamante *et al.*, 1987). Imipenem, but not ceftazidime or meropenem (p. 247) caused a significant post-antibiotic effect on *Ps. aeruginosa* after single or repeated dosage (Wu and Livermore, 1990; McGrath *et al.*, 1993b).

Burkholderia (previously *Pseudomonas*) *pseudomallei* is usually imipenem-sensitive (McEniry *et al.*, 1988; Dance *et al.*, 1989; Smith *et al.*, 1994). Imipenem-resistant variants of this organism can be selected during growth in media *in vitro* (Eng *et al.*, 1986). Some strains produce a chromosomal beta-lactamase, which hydrolyzes some cephalosporins but not imipenem (Livermore *et al.*, 1987). *Pseudomonas acidovorans*, *Ps. putida* and *Ps. stutzeri* are imipenem-sensitive. *Burkholderia* (previously *Pseudomonas*) *cepacia* and *Stenotrophomonas maltophilia* are resistant (Jones, 1985; Dufresne *et al.*, 1988; Kumar *et al.*, 1989; Victor *et al.*, 1994). The reason why *S. maltophilia* is consistently resistant is that it produces a special beta-lactamase (carbapenemase), which hydrolyzes imipenem (Livermore, 1992b). Other authors have reported that *S. maltophilia* produces at least four types of metallo- and serine- beta-lactamases most of which hydrolyze imipenem (Paton *et al.*, 1994; Payne *et al.*, 1994).

4 Gram-negative anaerobic bacteria

Bacteroides fragilis and other members of the *B. fragilis* group, such as *B. thetaiotaomicron*, *B. ovatus*, *B. vulgatus*, *B. distasonis*, *B. uniformis* and *B. caccae* are nearly always imipenem-sensitive. In large-scale surveys imipenem-resistant strains have been zero or less than 1% (Betriu *et al.*, 1990; Cuchural *et al.*, 1990; Bourgault *et al.*, 1992; Horn *et al.*, 1992; Turgeon *et al.*, 1994). Rare imipenem-resistant strains of this group have been identified. Cuchural *et al.* (1986) found two *B. fragilis* strains from over 350 which were capable of hydrolyzing imipenem as they produced a special beta-lactamase (carbapenamase). This novel beta-lactamase contained zinc as a cofactor. This has also been found in a few more strains of *B. fragilis* by other investigators (Lamothe *et al.*, 1986; Chen *et al.*, 1992; Hedberg *et al.*, 1992; Livermore, 1992b). Some *B. fragilis* strains contain silent metallo-beta-lactamase genes. One step mutation can lead to production of large amounts of these beta-lactamases, which can hydrolyze the carbapenems (including imipenem) and all other beta-lactam antibiotics (Rassmussen *et al.*, 1994).

Prevotella spp. such as *P. oris*, *P. melaninogenica*, *P. intermedia*, *P. oralis*, *P. bivia* and *P. disiens* are nearly always imipenem-sensitive. The same applies to the *Fusobacterium* spp. such as *F. nucleatum* and *F. necroforum* (Appelbaum *et al.*, 1990; Chen *et al.*, 1992; Goldstein *et al.*, 1993; Stark *et al.*, 1993). *Capnocytophaga* spp., normal inhabitants of oral cavity, are imipenem-

Organism	MICs (μg per ml)
Gram-positive bacteria	
Staphylococcus aureus (methicillin-sensitive)	0.03
Staphylococcus aureus (methicillin-resistant)	27.00
Streptococcus pneumoniae (Pen G sensitive)	0.06
Streptococcus pneumoniae (intermediate Pen G resistance)	0.25
Streptococcus pneumoniae (high Pen G resistance)	0.5
Enterococcus faecalis	2.0
Listeria monocytogenes	0.12
Nocardia asteroides	8.0
Actinomyces spp.	1.0
Clostridium perfringens	0.5
Clostridium difficile	8.0
Propionibacterium spp.	0.125
Gram-negative bacteria	
Escherichia coli	0.5
Klebsiella pneumoniae	0.5
Enterobacter spp.	1.0
Serratia marcescens	4.0
Proteus spp.	4.0
Yersinia enterocolitica	0.5
Acinetobacter spp.	0.125
Pseudomonas aeruginosa	4.0
Stenotrophomonas maltophilia	>32.0
Neisseria gonorrhoeae	2.0
Haemophilus influenzae	1.0
Bacteroides fragilis	0.5

Table I.16
Compiled from data published by Cherubin *et. al.* (1981), Cohn *et al.* (1982), Fernandes *et al.* (1983), Dewsnup and Wright (1984), Del Bene *et al.* (1985), Hornstein *et al.* (1985), Jones (1985), Shafran *et al.* (1985) and Liñares *et al.* (1992)

sensitive (Roscoe *et al.*, 1992). *Bilophila wadsworthia* is an anaerobic Gram-negative bacillus, commonly encountered in intra-abdominal infections. Initially many strains appeared imipenem-resistant. But susceptibility results were hard to interpret because many strains produced a heavy haze on agar dilution plates. It is now known that this growth on imipenem-containing plates consists of spheroplasts, which are capable of reverting back to normal morphology upon removal of the antibiotic. It is not yet clear whether these strains are imipenem-resistant or -sensitive (Summanen *et al.*, 1993). Anaerobic Gram-negative cocci such as *Veillonella* spp. are imipenem-sensitive (Chen *et al.*, 1992).

5 Mycobacteria

Imipenem has relatively low MICs for several *Mycobacterium* spp., e.g. *M. tuberculosis* 2 μg per ml, *M. avium* complex 4–8 μg per ml, *M. fortiutum* 2–4 μg per ml and *M. chelonae* 2 μg per ml (Yew *et al.*, 1990; Watt *et al.*, 1992).

6 Minimum inhibitory concentrations

The MICs of imipenem against some selected bacterial species are shown in Table I.16.

Mode of Administration and Dosage

Imipenem/c is not absorbed after oral administration. It can be administered i.m., but for this a special microcrystalline suspension is necessary (Signs *et al.*, 1992). The drug is usually administered i.v. Each dose can be given by rapid i.v. injection ('bolus') or a 30 min infusion, similar to penicillin G (p. 20). (Barza, 1985; Rogers *et al.*, 1985). Each i.v. dose of imipenem/c is best dissolved in 100–200 ml of isotonic saline and this delivered i.v. in 30 min (Standiford *et al.*, 1986; Signs *et al.*, 1992).

1 Adults

Imipenem/c is most commonly administered in a dosage of 0.5 g i.v. 6-hourly (Wang *et al.*, 1986; Liu and Wang, 1989; Gradon *et al.*, 1992). For milder infection a dosage of 250 mg 6-hourly may suffice (Wang *et al.*, 1986) although this drug is not normally used for the treatment of mild infections. For serious infections the dose can be increased to 1 g i.v. 6-hourly (Zajac *et al.*, 1985; Bodey *et al.*, 1986; MacGregor *et al.*, 1986; Janmohamed *et al.*, 1990).

As imipenem/c has a post-antibiotic effect with *Ps. aeruginosa* (p. 230) and also with most other Gram-negative and Gram-positive bacteria (Baquero *et al.*, 1986; Renneberg and Walder, 1989), other dosage schedules have been investigated. In an *in vitro* model of *Ps. aeruginosa* infection imipenem/c in a dosage of 1 g 8-hourly was adequate therapy, but 1 g 12-hourly was not (McGrath *et al.*, 1993a).

2 Children

The imipenem/c dose for these is 60–100 mg per kg per day, administered in four divided doses. Children older than 3 years should receive the smaller dose of 60 mg per kg per day (Alpert *et al.*, 1985; Baruchel *et al.*, 1986; Freij *et al.*, 1987).

3 Newborn and premature infants

The serum half-life of both imipenem and cilastatin is prolonged in these patients, but not to the same extent. The half-life of cilastatin is more prolonged and serum levels are higher than those of imipenem. The plasma clearance of cilastatin in neonates is only 20–30% of that for imipenem (Freij *et al.*, 1985). These authors suggested that it may be reasonable to use an imipenem-to-cilastatin ratio of 1:0.25 in these patients. Reed *et al.* (1990) found that the excess of cilastatin in serum was not harmful to neonates, and suggested that in premature infants during the first week of life the usual imipenem/c preparation can be used and that a dose of 20 mg per kg administered every 12 h is appropriate for the treatment of bacterial infections outside the central nervous system.

4 Elderly patients

In one study i.m. imipenem/c was given to patients older than 65 years. The dosage was 500 mg i.m. 12-hourly. Dosage reduction was not necessary, provided creatinine clearance was above 50 ml per min (Pietroski *et al.*, 1991). In another trial six patients aged between 68 and 83 years received i.v. imipenem/c 0.5 g 6-hourly. Dosage reduction was not necessary if their glomerular filtration rate (GFR) exceeded 30 ml per min (Finch *et al.*, 1986).

5 Patients with renal failure

It is recommended that 2–4 g per day, or 50 mg per kg per day, whichever is the less, be given to patients with a GFR exceeding 30 ml per min; the dose should be reduced by 50% for those with a GFR at or below 30 ml per min and when the GFR is below 10 ml per min, only 500 mg of imipenem/c should be given every 12 h. Hemodialysis removed 40–70% of imipenem and variable amounts of cilastatin depending upon the type of dialysis and coil employed. A supplementary dose should be administered at the end of each hemodialysis (Gibson *et al.*, 1985; Verbist *et al.*, 1986; Konishi *et al.*, 1991). Severe renal failure resulted in terminal half-lives of 4 h for imipenem and 16 h for cilastatin, but both drugs were well cleared by hemodialysis (Drusano, 1986). If a patient is treated by intermittent hemofiltration, a supplementary dose of imipenem/c 0.5 g is needed directly after this procedure. This dose should be the starting dose for a period of 12 h dosing intervals until the next hemofiltration is performed (Alarabi *et al.*, 1990). Much less imipenem/c is removed during peritoneal dialysis and a dose of 0.5 g i.v. 12-hourly is probably appropriate in patients with end-stage renal disease undergoing continuous ambulatory peritoneal dialysis (Somani *et al.*, 1988). Serum level monitoring is advisable in all of these patients.

Serum Levels in Relation to Dosage

1 Adults

When imipenem was administered as a 0.5 g 20 min i.v. infusion in conjunction with an equal amount of cilastatin, the mean peak plasma concentrations for imipenem and cilastatin were 35 and 42 μg per ml, respectively, straight after the infusion. The plasma levels thereafter fell and 6 h after the infusion the concentrations of both of them reached about 0. The mean terminal elimination half-life of both imipenem and cilastatin was approximately 1 h (Drusano, 1986).

The mean peak serum imipenem level immediately after an i.v. infusion of 1 g of imipenem/c, given over a period of 30 min to volunteers, was 52.1 µg per ml and after 1 h this fell to 18.7 µg per ml; the elimination serum half-life again was approximately 1 h, and the serum level was down to approximately 0 at 6 h (Drusano et al., 1984; Drusano and Standiford, 1985).

2 Neonates

When doses of 15 and 25 mg per kg of imipenem/c were given as 15 min i.v. infusions to neonates less than 8 days old, the serum levels reached 30 min after the infusion were 27.2 and 54.5 µg per ml for imipenem and cilastatin, respectively. Their mean serum half-lives were 1.8 h and 2.1 h, respectively (Gruber et al., 1985). Freij et al. (1985) gave 10, 15 and 20 mg per kg doses of imipenem/c to neonates by 60 min i.v. infusions and peak serum levels of imipenem immediately afterwards were 11.1, 20.7 and 31.6 µg per ml, respectively. The serum half-life of imipenem varied from 1.7 to 2.4 h. In five other babies given 12-hourly doses of 20 mg per kg of imipenem/c, no accumulation was observed after five to eight doses. Pharmacokinetics in neonates resembled those of adults with moderate to severe renal insufficiency (p. 232).

3 Patients with cystic fibrosis

Peak serum levels and serum half-lives in these patients were similar to those observed in normal adult volunteers (Reed et al., 1985).

4 Pregnant patients

As with other beta-lactam antibiotics (p. 24) the serum levels are often considerably lower in these patients, and an increased dosage may be needed when serious infections are treated (Heikkilä et al., 1992).

Excretion

1 Urine

Imipenem is predominantly excreted by glomerular filtration. Renal tubular secretion accounts for only a very small fraction of renal elimination (Kropp et al., 1982; Norrby et al., 1983b). Co-administration of probenecid or dehydropeptidase inhibitors have only a slight effect on imipenem pharmacokinetics and its serum half-life is unaltered (Norrby et al., 1983 a,b).

Urinary recovery of imipenem administered alone is low and variable (6–38% of the dose), because a renal tubular dipeptidase enzyme metabolizes the drug by opening its lactam ring. When cilastatin is administered alone, 68% of the dose is recovered in the urine. Concomitant i.v. administration of imipenem and cilastatin results in increased urinary excretion of imipenem; a maximal effect is achieved with an imipenem/cilastatin ratio of 1: 4, when renal clearance of imipenem is 70% of the plasma clearance. A ratio of imipenem to cilastatin of at least 1:1 is necessary to maintain effective antibacterial urinary levels if imipenem, and therefore this fixed ratio has been adopted for clinical use of imipenem/c. Urinary excretion of each entity then accounts for about 70% of the dose (Rogers et al., 1985). Doubling the dose of cilastatin to give a ratio of 1:2, produces a further 15% increase in the urinary recovery of imipenem, but such a combination would lead to unnecessary accumulation of cilastatin in patients with reduced renal function (Norrby, 1985).

Beta-lactam antibiotics that undergo minimal renal tubular secretion generally show no alteration in overall biodisposition in patients with cystic fibrosis. In cystic fibrosis patients, 50% and 78%, respectively, of administered doses of imipenem and cilastatin are recovered from the urine in the first 6 h. Renal clearance of each drug averages 54 and 88%, respectively, of the total serum clearance of each compound, suggesting extrarenal elimination or metabolism of imipenem (Reed et al., 1985).

2 Bile

A small amount of imipenem is excreted via the bile. In patients with common bile duct drainage, peak imipenem concentrations in the bile averaged 4.4 µg per ml and 8.6 µg per ml after 0.5 g and 1 g i.v. doses of imipenem/c, respectively. Slightly higher cilastatin concentrations were found in the bile, but there were large variations from patient to patient (Graziani et al., 1987). In patients in whom the common bile duct was obstructed no imipenem nor cilastatin could be detected in the bile (Leung et al., 1992).

3 Inactivation in the body

The portion of imipenem and cilastatin not excreted by the kidney is inactivated in the body. In the case of imipenem a portion of this non-renal clearance appears to be *in vivo* degradation of the drug in serum (Swanson *et al.*, 1986). The rest of imipenem and probably all of cilastatin is metabolized by the kidneys. Although most drugs are mainly metabolized in the liver, the kidneys are also metabolically quite active and possess drug-metabolizing capability which can contribute to non-renal clearance. A decline in renal function can presumably also be associated with reduction in renal metabolic clearance. Non-renal clearance of imipenem is reduced 58% in end-stage renal failure, but non-renal clearance of cilastatin is reduced by 87% in such patients (Gibson *et al.*, 1985; Drusano, 1986). This is why the terminal half-life of cilastatin is much more prolonged than that of imipenem in patients with end-stage renal disease (p. 232).

Distribution of the Drug in Body

Imipenem is widely distributed in the body. It has been found in adequate concentrations, to inhibit susceptible pathogens, in sputum, pus, pleural fluid, synovial fluid, bone, aqueous humor, interstitial fluid and in peritoneal fluid in patients undergoing elective abdominal surgery. Imipenem concentrations in ascitic fluid in patients with cirrhosis were lower, but still high enough to inhibit susceptible pathogens. The CSF concentrations in patients with uninflamed meninges were relatively low (0.8 μg per ml) and the level in saliva was also low (0.38 μg per ml) (MacGregor *et al.*, 1984, 1986; Jacobs, 1986; Wise *et al.*, 1986; Rolando *et al.*, 1994). Imipenem concentration in skin window fluid was also adequate (Signs *et al.*, 1992). In patients undergoing thoracotomy, imipenem concentration was 10.5 μg per ml in pericardial fluid, but only 0.28 μg per g in lung tissue, 2.25 h after administration of 1 g imipenem/c i.v. (Benoni *et al.*, 1987).

In patients with bacterial meningitis, the CSF imipenem and cilastatin concentrations are higher. Modai *et al.* (1985) studied this in 12 patients with bacterial meningitis treated with other drugs. Each patient received four 1.0 g doses of imipenem/c at 6-hourly intervals. Samples for estimation of imipenem/c CSF concentrations were taken at 60, 90 and 120 min after the fourth dose of imipenem/c. Concentrations of imipenem in CSF ranged from 0.5 to 11 μg per ml and those of cilastatin from 1.1 to 10.5 μg per ml. Jacobs *et al.* (1986) studied imipenem/c penetration into the CSF in children with bacterial meningitis. They found CSF imipenem concentrations of 15–27% of simultaneous serum levels and CSF cilastatin penetration of 16–66%. With multiple doses there was no accumulation of imipenem nor cilastatin in the CSF. In two neonates with no meningitis, CSF imipenem levels obtained 1.5 h after 15 min i.v. infusions of 15 and 25 mg per kg, were 1.1 and 5.6 μg per ml, respectively, representing 4 and 10% of the serum levels at 1 h (Gruber *et al.*, 1985).

Imipenem/c crosses the placenta and therapeutic concentrations are achieved in umbilical blood and amniotic fluid during late pregnancy (Heikkilä *et al.*, 1992).

The drug is approximately 20% serum protein bound (Wise *et al.*, 1981).

Mode of Action

Imipenem binds to all the PBPs of *E. coli* but has its greatest affinity for PBP 2 and PBP 1 (p. 27), the transpeptidases implicated in elongation of the bacterial cell wall. Binding to PBP 2 produces the 'lemon-shapes' which occur when *E. coli* is exposed to imipenem, in contrast to the long filaments that result from exposure to penicillins and cephalosporins, which seem to be consequent upon the binding of those drugs to PBP 3 (Spratt *et al.*, 1977; Majcherczyk and Livermore, 1990). When *Ps. aeruginosa* cultures were exposed to either ceftazidime, which induces filamentation, or to imipenem, ceftazidime treatment resulted in much more release of a lipopolysaccharide endotoxin than similar treatment with imipenem. Antibiotic-induced release of endotoxins may be harmful during the treatment of severe infections caused by Gram-negative bacilli (Jackson and Kropp, 1992).

In general a wide range of beta-lactam antibiotics which are highly bactericidal for rapidly growing bacteria, become bacteriostatic for slowly growing bacteria (Cozens *et al.*, 1986). However, imipenem seems to trigger autolysins and to produce a rapid bactericidal effect to both rapidly and slowly growing bacteria (Cozens *et al.*, 1989).

Other factors which contribute to the *in vitro* activity of imipenem are its high stability to beta-lactamases and its ability to permeate into most Gram-negative bacteria. Imipenem is highly resistant to attack by beta-lactamases of both Gram-positive and Gram-negative bacteria, whether the enzymes are of chromosomal origin or plasmid-mediated (Richmond, 1981; Neu and Labthavikul, 1982). The drug owes its their resistance to beta-lactamases to the unusual *trans*-conformation of its hydroxyethyl side-chain, as opposed to the *cis*-conformation of the acylamino substituent on the beta-lactam ring of penicillins and cephalosporins (Cassidy, 1981).

When Yoshimura and Nikaido (1985) compared diffusion rates of various beta-lactam antibiotics through porin channels (p. 26) of *E. coli*, imipenem had the highest permeability of the compounds tested, which included first-, second- and third-generation cephalosporins and early and late generation penicillins. Its faster diffusion was presumably due to its compact molecular structure. Although imipenem penetrated into *E. coli* twice as fast as meropenem, the latter was more active antibacterially (p. 246) (Cornaglia *et al.*, 1992). An outer membrane protein D2 especially facilitated the diffusion of imipenem into *Ps. aeruginosa* cells; when this protein was lost the *Ps. aeruginosa* strain became imipenem-resistant (p. 230) (Trias and Nikaido, 1990).

A combination of poor permeability and hydrolysis by beta-lactamases produced in the periplasmic space (p. 26) was responsible for the resistance of *Enterobacter* spp. to several later-generation beta-lactam antibiotics, whilst the better penetration of imipenem explained why the organism remained sensitive to this compound (Vu and Nikaido, 1985). But some imipenem-resistant strains have now been reported (p. 229).

Toxicity

1 Gastrointestinal side-effects

Nausea and or vomiting has occurred in some 3–4% of patients. In a few persistent vomiting necessitated stopping the drug. Slowing the rate of i.v. infusion appeared to lessen this side-effect in some patients (Calandra *et al.*, 1985, 1986; Zajac *et al.*, 1985; Report, 1987). When high doses of imipenem/c were given to patients with cystic fibrosis, nausea and vomiting were more common and more severe (Pedersen *et al.*, 1987). Diarrhea has been observed in some 3% of treated patients, and a small number of these had *Cl. difficile* in their stools. Pseudomembraneous colitis has been reported but appears to be rare (0.1% of all treated patients) (Callandra *et al.*, 1985; 1986; Wang *et al.*, 1985; Leyland *et al.*, 1992).

In patients given imipenem/c and who did not develop diarrhoea, there were changes in colonic microflora. Van der Leur *et al.* (1993) found that there was increase in yeasts and enterococci in such patients. Kager *et al.* (1989) gave i.v. imipenem/c as chemoprophylaxis to patients undergoing colorectal surgery. In these patients the aerobic bacteria – staphylococci, streptococci, enterococci and enterobacteria were suppressed for about 2 weeks. Among the anaerobic bacteria, cocci, eubacteria, lactobacilli, clostridia, fusobacteria and *Bacteroides* spp. also decreased markedly during the same time.

2 Central nervous system side-effects

In one animal study rabbits with normal meninges were given i.v. penicillin G or imipenem/c in various doses and it was found that imipenem/c was considerably more neurotoxic than penicillin G (Schliamser *et al.*, 1988). Grand mal seizures, focal seizures or myoclonus has also occurred in some patients, treated by imipenem/c, but most of these had either renal insufficiency and/or a background history of CNS lesions such as prior seizure focus, brain tumor, brain abscess or past cerebral infarct. In most patients the seizures responded readily to a decrease in dose or discontinuation of therapy (Barza, 1985; Callandra *et al.*, 1986; Smith *et al.*, 1988; Norrby *et al.*, 1993).

It has been presumed that there would be a greater risk of neurotoxicity if bacterial meningitis was treated with imipenem/c rather than with other beta-lactam antibiotics. Complete proof for this is not available as imipenem/c has been used very little for the treatment of this disease (Jacobs, 1992). Therefore for the treatment of pneumococcal meningitis caused by pneumococci with intermediate type resistance to penicillin G (p. 5), third-generation cephalosporins such as cefotaxime (p. 336) or ceftriaxone (p. 359) have been preferred to imipenem/c. One child with meningitis caused by such organism was successfully treated with large doses (100 mg per kg 6-hourly) of imipenem/c and neurotoxicity was not encountered (Asensi *et al.*, 1989), but in one trial where high dosage (1 g 8-hourly) imipenem/c was used to treat severe nosocomial pneumonia, seizures occurred in some patients (Fink *et al.*, 1994).

3 Hypersensitivity reactions

Some 2–3% of patients treated by imipenem/c have developed a rash, pruritus or urticaria. The incidence of allergic reactions to imipenem/c might have been higher as patients with known beta-lactam allergies are not usually treated by imipenem/c. Of 12 patients with a history of penicillin allergy, two developed allergic manifestations when treated with imipenem/c. The drug may be cross-allergenic with penicillins and cephalosporins and it should be avoided in patients with previous allergic reactions to these drugs, especially if the previous reaction was severe, (Barza, 1985; Wang et al., 1985; Callandra et al., 1986; Boguniewicz and Leung, 1995).

4 Hematological side-effects

Neutropenia, a known side-effect of beta-lactam antibiotics (p. 33) occurred in a small number of patients. This was usually reversible on ceasing the drug (Gentry, 1985; Callandra et al., 1986). Eosinophilia was more common, but it was not associated with clinical abnormalities. A small number of patients developed a positive Coombs' test, but there were no cases of hemolytic anemia. Changes in platelets and abnormal prothrombin times were rare (Calandra et al., 1986).

5 Hepatotoxicity

Abnormalities in liver function tests have been seen during imipenem/c therapy. These have been usually transient and without clinical signs of disease. Three patients during the early trials with imipenem/c developed jaundice, necessitating the discontinuation of the drug (Callandra et al., 1986).

6 Nephrotoxicity

In animals, concomitant administration of cilastatin eliminates the nephrotoxicity associated with high doses of imipenem (Kahan et al., 1983; Norrby, 1985). Daily doses of 4 g imipenem/c for up to 4 weeks have not been associated with nephrotoxicity in humans.

Clinical Uses of the Drug

1 Initial therapy for fever in neutropenic cancer patients

Imipenem/c, similar to antipseudomonal penicillins and cephalosporins, such as ticarcillin (p. 156), piperacillin (p. 174) and ceftazidime (p. 377) can be used with success in combination with an aminoglycoside, such as gentamicin (p. 471), to treat these patients (Baruchel et al., 1986). A number of studies have also shown that imipenem/c is also satisfactory as monotherapy, and that it compares favorably with ceftazidime (the other drug used as monotherapy) for the initial therapy of these patients (Bodey et al., 1986; Norrby et al., 1987; Liu and Wang, 1989; Liang et al., 1990; Cornelissen et al., 1992; Leyland et al., 1992; Petrilli et al., 1993). But for initial treatment, imipenem/c as a single drug should only be used for selected patients and in selected institutions. In recent years bacterial infections in these patients have been often caused not by Gram-negative rods, but by Gram-positive bacteria such as Staph. aureus, coagulase-negative staphylococci, Corynebacterium spp. and alpha-hemolytic streptococci. Most strains of these in hospitals are methicillin-resistant and so also imipenem-resistant. When a Gram-positive organism is isolated, vancomycin may be added, but at least if methicillin-resistant Staph. aureus is the pathogen, the results of treatment are better if vancomycin is included in the initial regimen. Therefore in institutions where Gram-positive infections, especially with Staph. aureus, are likely it may be wise to use imipenem/c plus vancomycin from the beginning. If Ps. aeruginosa infection is likely, it seems preferable to use imipenem/c plus an aminoglycoside, as this organism can become imipenem-resistant during treatment (p. 229) (Wade, 1989; Hughes et al., 1990).

2 Intra-abdominal infections

As imipenem has a broad spectrum of activity against aerobic and anaerobic bacteria, results of imipenem/c therapy of peritonitis, resulting from a perforated viscus, have been good, comparing favorably to other therapies available for this indication such as clindamycin/gentamicin (p. 598), metronidazole/gentamicin (p. 947), cefoxitin (p. 308), ticarcillin/clavulanic acid (p. 202), ampicillin/sulbactam (p. 214) and piperacillin/tazobactam (p. 224) (Kager and Nord, 1985; Leaper et al., 1987; de Groot et al., 1993; Gorbach, 1993).

3 Respiratory tract infections

Imipenem/c is particularly suitable for treatment of nosocomial pneumonia such as that arising after operations and in intensive care units. These pneumonias are often caused by Gram-negative bacilli all of which are normally imipenem-sensitive. Cure rates of approximately 80% have been obtained in these patients; the results being similar to those obtained with ceftazidime used as a single drug (p. 378). Imipenem/c is not suitable as a single drug if methicillin-resistant

Staph. aureus is a likely pathogen. Results of treatment of *Ps. aeruginosa* pneumonia have also been somewhat unsatisfactory, as in some patients the *Ps. aeruginosa* strain has become imipenem-resistant *in vivo* during treatment, with subsequent failure of therapy. If *Ps. aeruginosa* infection is suspected or proven, it may be best to use combination therapy with imipenem/c plus an aminoglycoside. But in one randomized study imipenem/c alone was as effective as its combination with netilmicin. The addition of netilmicin increased nephrotoxicity but did not prevent the emergence of imipenem-resistant *Ps. aeruginosa* strains (Cometta *et al.*, 1994). In another trial large doses of i.v. imipenem/c were compared with high-dosage i.v. ciprofloxacin for the treatment of severe pneumonia. Most of the patients had nosocomial pneumonia due to Gram-negative organisms. Ciprofloxacin eradicated Enterobacteriaceae more successfully than imipenem/c. When *Ps. aeruginosa* was recovered from initial respiratory tract cultures, development of resistance during treatment and treatment failures were common in both groups (Fink *et al.*, 1994).

In nosocomial pneumonias treated by imipenem/c, colonization of the respiratory tract with *S. maltophilia*, resistant *Ps. aeruginosa*, coagulase-negative staphylococci and various yeasts frequently occur during therapy. Sometimes these organisms may cause superinfections, which may be difficult to treat (Acar, 1985; Freimer *et al.*, 1985; Salata *et al.*, 1985; Lode *et al.*, 1987; Wathen *et al.*, 1988; Norrby *et al.*, 1993).

Imipenem/c therapy has also been tried for *Ps. aeruginosa* infections in patients with cystic fibrosis. Satisfactory improvement was often obtained if the drug was only used short-term (less than 14 days), but if imipenem/c was used for longer periods, the *Ps. aeruginosa* strains usually became imipenem-resistant. Combination therapy with tobramycin did not prevent the emergence of imipenem-resistance (Pedersen *et al.*, 1987; Strandvik *et al.*, 1988).

Community-acquired pneumonia caused by *Acinetobacter* spp. and that due to *Burkholderia* (*Pseudomonas*) *pseudomallei* may also respond well to imipenem/c, provided that the strain involved is imipenem-sensitive (Anstey *et al.*, 1992).

4 Osteomyelitis

Imipenem/c is suitable for the treatment of chronic osteomyelitis, which is often polymicrobial and may be caused by nosocomial bacteria, including *Staph. aureus* and Gram-negative bacteria. Such osteomyelitis often follows trauma or orthopedic surgical procedures and often there are predisposing host factors such as diabetes mellitus or peripheral vascular disease. Treatment for 6 weeks with single broad-spectrum antimicrobial agent such as imipenem/c can give a success rate similar to those obtained with combination therapy. Imipenem/c is not suitable as a single drug if methicillin-resistant *Staph. aureus* is one of the pathogens (Gentry, 1985; 1988; MacGregor and Gentry, 1985).

5 Bacterial endocarditis

A small number of patients with *Ps. aeruginosa* endocarditis have been cured by imipenem/c therapy, usually in combination with tobramycin. In many others this treatment has failed, usually due to emergence of imipenem-resistant *Ps. aeruginosa* strains. Combination therapy with an aminoglycoside such as tobramycin should always be used, although this does not always prevent the emergence of imipenem-resistant strains. Ticarcillin/tobramycin may be preferable for this disease (Donabedian and Freimer, 1985; Fichtenbaum and Smith, 1992) (p. 156).

Imipenem/c may also be used with success in endocarditis due to other Gram-negative bacilli which may be resistant to other drugs, such as *Acinetobacter* spp. (Gradon *et al.*, 1992). An animal study showed that imipenem/c plus gentamicin may be effective for the treatment of endocarditis caused by penicillin G-resistant *Strep. sanguis* (Martinez *et al.*, 1994).

6 Bacterial meningitis

Animal studies suggested that imipenem/c may be useful in the treatment of penicillin G-resistant pneumococcal meningitis (McCracken and Sakata, 1985). By contrast, useful bactericidal titers could not be demonstrated in CSF of animals with meningitis caused by *H. influenzae* which was resistant to both ampicillin and chloramphenicol (Sakata *et al.*, 1984). In an animal study of *E. coli* bacteremia and meningitis, imipenem/c was compared with ampicillin/ gentamicin combination; mean bactericidal titers in blood and CSF were greater with imipenem/ c, but the drug was no more effective *in vivo* than the combination of the two older drugs (Kim, 1985). Animal studies also indicated that imipenem/c may be effective therapy for *Salmonella* spp. meningitis (Bryan and Scheld, 1992). Clinical studies with imipenem/c in bacterial meningitis have not been pursued to any extent, as it is considered that this drug may cause convulsions more readily than other beta-lactams (p. 235). One child with meningitis due to *Strep. pneumoniae* with intermediate type of penicillin G-resistance was treated successfully with large doses of imipenem/c and there were no complications (p. 235).

7 Urinary tract infections

In a study of 43 patients, mostly males, with complicated urinary tract infections of which more than half were due to *Ps. aeruginosa*, 500 mg of imipenem/c i.v. 8-hourly produced clinical improvement and microbiological eradication in early follow-up; long-term results were unavailable (Cox and Corrado, 1985). There are other reports of the satisfactory use of imipenem/c for the treatment of difficult upper urinary tract infections, some of which have been associated with septicemia, (Brooks *et al.*, 1985; Norrby *et al.*, 1993).

8 Miscellaneous bacterial infections

Imipenem/c has been used with success in the treatment of severe Gram-negative bacterial infections in neonates and young infants. The most common pathogens were *Ps. aeruginosa* and *Klebsiella* spp. (Nalin and Jacobsen, 1987). Most patients with hospital-acquired septicemia due to Gram-negative rods responded well (Norrby *et al.*, 1993). One patient with multiple hepatic abscesses due to *Edwardsiella tarda* responded well to medical therapy alone with imipenem/c (Zighelboim *et al.*, 1992). The drug is also useful for the treatment of foot infections in diabetics (Grayson *et al.*, 1994). *Aeromonas hydrophila* infections of skin and soft tissues need a combination of medical and surgical treatment. Imipenem/c is one suitable antibiotic, but the infection also responds to third-generation cephalosporins (p. 321), co-trimoxazole (p. 837) and ciprofloxacin (p. 1019) (Gold and Salit, 1993). A single 0.5 g i.m. dose of imipenem/c cures uncomplicated gonorrhea in adults, but it has no advantages over other available regimens (Verdon *et al.*, 1988). One immunocompetent patient with blood transfusion-acquired *Rhodococcus* spp. septicemia responded to imipenem/c (de Clari *et al.*, 1992).

In animal studies imipenem/c was found to be effective for treatment of *N. asteroides* pneumonia (Gombert *et al.*, 1990). Although *Y. enterocolitica* is imipenem-sensitive *in vitro* (p. 229), in one animal study imipenem/c was ineffective against infection by this organism *in vivo* (Scavizzi *et al.*, 1987).

9 Mycobacterial infections

A few patients with *M. fortuitum* and *M. chelonae* infections have responded to imipenem/c (Yew *et al.*, 1992). A combination of amikacin, ciprofloxacin and imipenem/c has been used for the treatment of *M. avium* infections in AIDS patients (Young *et al.*, 1986). In an animal study imipenem/c was completely ineffective as a single drug and it also did not potentiate amikacin against *M. avium* infections (Inderlied *et al.*, 1989). Imipenem/c is not recommended for the inclusion in treatment regimens for this infection in patients with AIDS.

References

Acar JF (1985). Therapy for lower respiratory tract infections with imipenem/cilastatin: A review of worldwide experience. *Rev Infect Dis* **7** (Suppl 3): 513.

Acar JF, Goldstein FW, Kitzis MD, Gutmann L (1983). Activity of imipenem on aerobic bacteria. *J Antimicrob Chemother* **12** (Suppl D): 37.

Alarabi AA, Cars O, Danielson BG *et al.* (1990). Pharmacokinetics of intravenous imipenem/cilastatin during intermittent haemofiltration. *J Antimicrob Chemother* **26**: 91.

Albers-Schonberg G, Arison BH, Hensens OD *et al.* (1978). Structure and absolute configuration of thienamycin. *J Amer Chem Soc* **100**: 6491.

Alnor D, Frimodt-Møller N, Espersen F, Frederiksen W (1994). Infections with the unusual human pathogens *Agrobacterium* species and *Ochrobactrum anthropi*. *Clin Infect Dis* **18**: 914.

Alpert G, Dagan R, Connor E *et al.* (1985). Imipenem/cilastatin for the treatment of infections in hospitalized children. *Amer J Dis Child* **139**: 1153.

Anstey NM, Currie BJ, Withnall KM (1992). Community-acquired *Acinetobacter* pneumonia in the Northern Territory of Australia. *Clin Infect Dis* **14**: 83.

Appelbaum PC, Spangler SK, Jacobs MR (1990). Beta-lactamase production and susceptibilities to amoxicillin, amoxicillin-clavulanate, ticarcillin, ticarcillin-clavulanate, cefoxitin, imipenem and metronidazole of 320 non-*Bacteroides fragilis Bacteroides* isolates and 129 *Fusobacteria* from 28 US centers. *Antimicrob Ag Chemother* **34**: 1546.

Aronoff SC, Shlaes DM (1987). Factors that influence the evolution of beta-lactam resistance in beta-lactamase-inducible strains of *Enterobacter cloacae* and *Pseudomonas aeruginosa*. *J Infect Dis* **155**: 936.

Asensi F, Perez-Tamarit D, Otero MC *et al.* (1989). Imipenem-cilastatin therapy in a child with meningitis caused by a multiply resistant pneumococcus. *Pediatr Infect Dis J* **8**: 895.

Ashby J, Kirkpatrick B, Piddock LJV, Wise R (1987). The effect of imipenem on strains of Enterobacteriaceae expressing Richmond & Sykes Class I beta-lactamases. *J Antimicrob Chemother* **20**: 15.

Auckenthaler R, Wilson WR, Wright AJ et al. (1982). Lack of in vivo and in vitro bactericidal activity of N-formimidoyl thienamycin against enterococci. Antimicrob Ag Chemother 22: 448.

Bakken J, Sanders CC, Clark RB, Hori M (1988). Beta-lactam resistance in Aeromonas spp caused by inducible beta-lactamases active against penicillins, cephalosporins, and carbapenems. Antimicrob Ag Chemother 32: 1314.

Baquero F, Culebras E, Patron C et al. (1986). Postantibiotic effect of imipenem on Gram-positive and Gram-negative micro-organisms. J Antimicrob Chemother 18 (Suppl E): 47.

Barakett V, Lesage D, Delisle F et al. (1994). Killing kinetics of imipenem against penicillin-resistant Steptococcus pneumoniae. J Antimicrob Chemother 33: 1025.

Barnass S, Holland K, Tabaqchali S (1991). Vancomycin-resistant Corynebacterium species causing prosthetic valve endocarditis successfully treated with imipenem and ciprofloxacin. J Infect 22: 161.

Barry AL, Jones RN, Thornsberry C et al. (1985). Imipenem (N-Formimidoyl Thienamycin): in vitro antimicrobial activity and beta-lactamase stability. Diagn Microbiol Infect Dis 3: 93.

Baruchel A, Hartmann O, Andremont A, Tancrede C (1986). Severe Gram-negative infections in neutropenic children cured by imipenem/cilastatin in combination with an aminoglycoside. J Antimicrob Chemother 18 (Suppl E): 167.

Barza M (1985). Imipenem: first of a new class of beta-lactam antibiotics. Ann Intern Med 103: 552.

Bellido F, Veuthey C, Blaser J et al. (1990). Novel resistance to imipenem associated with an altered PBP-4 in a Pseudomonas aeruginosa clinical isolate. J Antimicrob Chemother 25: 57.

Benoni G, Cuzzolin L, Bertrand C et al. (1987). Imipenem kinetics in serum, lung tissue and pericardial fluid in patients undergoing thoracotomy. J Antimicrob Chemother 20: 725.

Betriu C, Campos E, Cabronero C et al. (1990). Susceptibilities of species of the Bacteroides fragilis group to 10 antimicrobial agents. Antimicrob Ag Chemother 34: 671.

Bodey GP, Alvarez ME, Jones PG et al. (1986). Imipenem-cilastatin as initial therapy for febrile cancer patients. Antimicrob Ag Chemother 30: 211.

Boguniewicz M, Leung DYM (1995). Hypersensitivity reactiion to antibiotics commonly used in children. Pediatr Infect Dis J 14: 221.

Bourgault A-M, Lamothe F, Hoban DJ et al. (1992). Survey of Bacteroides fragilis group susceptibility patterns in Canada. Antimicrob Ag Chemother 36: 343.

Brooks RG, McCabe RE, Vosit KL, Remington JS (1985). Open trial of imipenem/cilastatin therapy for serious bacterial infections. Rev Infect Dis 7 (Suppl 3): 496.

Bryan JP, Scheld WM (1992). Therapy of experimental meningitis due to Salmonella enteritidis. Antimicrob Ag Chemother 36: 949.

Büscher K-H, Cullmann W, Opperkuch W (1987a). Resistance of Pseudomonas aeruginosa to imipenem is independent of beta-lactamase production. J Antimicrob Chemother 19: 700.

Büscher K-H, Cullmann W, Dick W, Opferkuch W (1987b). Imipenem resistance in Pseudomonas aeruginosa resulting from diminished expression of outer membrane protein. Antimicrob Ag Chemother 31: 703.

Bustamante CI, Drusano GL, Wharton RC, Wade JC (1987). Synergism of the combinations of imipenem plus ciprofloxacin and imipenem plus amikacin against Pseudomonas aeruginosa and other bacterial pathogens. Antimicrob Ag Chemother 31: 632.

Butterworth D, Cole M, Hanscomb G, Rolinson GN (1979). Olivanic acids, a family of beta-lactam antibiotics with beta-lactamase inhibitory properties produced by Streptomyces species. I. Detection, properties and fermentation studies. J Antibiot 32: 287.

Calandra GB, Brown KR, Grad LC et al. (1985). Review of adverse experiences and tolerability in the first 2,516 patients treated with imipenem/cilastatin. Amer J Med 78 (6A): 73.

Calandra GB, Wang C, Aziz M, Brown KR (1986). The safety profile of imipenem/cilastatin: worldwide clinical experience based on 3470 patients. J Antimicrob Chemother 18 (Suppl E): 193.

Carratalá J, Gudiol F (1995). Life-threatening infections due to penicillin-resistant viridans streptococci. Curr Opin Infect Dis 8: 123.

Cassidy PJ (1981). Novel naturally occurring beta-lactam antibiotics – a review. Dev Ind Microbiol 22: 181.

Cerami AT, Shungu DL (1986). Comparative in vitro activity of imipenem against Haemophilus influenzae and Haemophilus parainfluenzae. Antimicrob Ag Chemother 30: 179.

Chen SCA, Gottlieb T, Palmer JM et al. (1992). Antimicrobial susceptibility of anaerobic bacteria in Australia. J Antimicrob Chemother 30: 811.

Chen HY, Yuan M, Ibrahim-Elmagboul IB, Livermore DM (1995). National survey of susceptibillity to antimicrobials amongst clinical isolates of Pseudomonas aeruginosa. J Antimicrob Chemother 35: 521.

Cherubin CE, Corrado ML, Sierra MF et al. (1981). Susceptibility of Gram-positive cocci to various antibiotics, including cefotaxime, moxalactam and N-formimidoyl thienamycin. Antimicrob Ag Chemother 20: 553.

Chow AW, Cheng N, Bartlett KH (1985). In vitro susceptibility of Clostridium difficile to new beta-lactam and quinolone antibiotics. Antimicrob Ag Chemother 28: 842.

Chow JW, Shlaes DM (1991). Imipenem resistance associated with the loss of a 40 KDa outer membrane protein in Enterobacter aerogenes. J Antimicrob Chemother 28: 499.

Cohn DL, Reimer LG, Reller LB (1982). Comparative in vitro activity of MK0787 (N-formimidoyl thienamycin). against 540 blood culture isolates. J Antimicrob Chemother 9: 183.

Cometta A, Baumgartner JD, Lew D et al. (1994). Prospective randomized comparison of imipenem monotherapy with imipenem plus netilmicin for treatment of severe infections in nonneutropenic patients. Antimicrob Ag Chemother 38: 1309.

Cornaglia G, Guan L, Fontana R, Satta G (1992). Diffusion of meropenem and imipenem through the outer membrane of Escherichia coli K-12 and correlation with their antibacterial activities. Antimicrob Ag Chemother 36: 1902.

Cornaglia G, Russell K, Satta G, Fontana R (1995). Relative importance of outer membrane permeability and Group 1 beta-lactamase as determinants of meropenem and imipenem activities against Enterobacter cloacae. Antimicrob Ag Chemother 39: 350.

Cornelissen JJ, de Graeff A, Verdonck LF et al. (1992). Imipenem versus gentamicin combined with either cefuroxime or cephalothin as initial therapy for febrile neutropenic patients. Antimicrob Ag Chemother 36: 801.

Cox CE, Corrado ML (1985). Safety and efficacy of imipenem/cilastatin in treatment of complicated urinary tract infections. Amer J Med 78 (6A): 92.

Cozens RM, Tuomanen E, Tosch W et al. (1986). Evolution of the bactericidal activity of beta-lactam antibiotics on slowly growing bacteria cultured in the chemostat. Antimicrob Ag Chemother 29: 797.

Cozens RM, Markiewicz Z, Tuomanen E (1989). Role of autolysins in the activities of imipenem and CGP 31608, a novel penem, against slowly growing bacteria. Antimicrob Ag Chemother 33: 1819.

Cuchural GJJr, Malamy MH, Tally FP (1986). Beta-lactamase-mediated imipenem resistance in Bacteroides fragilis. Antimicrob Ag Chemother 30: 645.

Cuchural GJJr, Tally FP, Jacobus NV et al. (1990). Comparative activities of newer beta-lactam agents against members of the Bacteroides fragilis Group. Antimicrob Ag Chemother 34: 479.

Cynamon MH, Palmer GS, Sorg TB (1987). Comparative in vitro activities of ampicillin, BMY 28142, and imipenem against Mycobacterium avium complex. Diagn Microbiol Infect Dis 6: 151.

Dance DAB, Wuthiekanun V, Chaewagul W, White NJ (1989). The antimicrobial susceptibility of Pseudomonas pseudomallei. Emergence of resistance in vitro and during treatment. J Antimicrob Chemother 24: 295.

de Groot HGW, Hustinx PA, Lampe AS, Oosterwijk WM (1993). Comparison of imipenem/cilastatin with the combination of aztreonam and clindamycin in the treatment of intra-abdominal infections. J Antimicrob Chemother 32: 491.

de Clari F, Menghini T, Biaggi G, Magnoli P (1992). Septicaemia due to a new species of *Rhodococcus* that contaminated closed system packed red blood cells – cure with imipenem monotherapy. *J Antimicrob Chemother* **30**: 729.

Del Bene VE, Carek PJ, Twitty JA, Burkey LJ (1985). *In vitro* activity of cefbuperazone compared with that of other new β-lactam agents against anaerobic Gram-negative bacilli and contribution of β-lactamase to resistance. *Antimicrob Ag Chemother* **27**: 817.

Dewsnup DH, Wright DN (1984). *In vitro* susceptibility of *Nocardia asteroides* to 25 antimicrobial agents. *Antimicrob Ag Chemother* **25**: 165.

Donabedian H, Freimer EH (1985). Pathogenesis and treatment of endocarditis. *Amer J Med* **78** (6A): 127.

Drusano GL (1986). An overview of the pharmacology of imipenem/cilastatin. *J Antimicrob Chemother* **18** (Suppl E): 79.

Drusano GL, Standiford HC (1985). Pharmacokinetic profile of imipenem/cilastatin in normal volunteers. *Amer J Med* **78** (6A): 47.

Drusano GL, Standiford HC, Bustamante C et al. (1984). Multiple-dose pharmacokinetics of imipenem-cilastatin. *J Antimicrob Chemother* **26**: 715.

Dufresne J, Vezina G, Levesque RC (1988). Cloning and expression of the imipenem-hydrolysing beta-lactamase operon from *Pseudomonas maltophilia* in *Escherichia coli*. *Antimicrob Ag Chemother* **32**: 819.

Ehrhard AF, Sanders CC, Thomson KS et al. (1993). Emergence of resistance to imipenem in *Enterobacter* isolates masquerading as *Klebsiella pneumoniae* during therapy with imipenem/cilastatin. *Clin Infect Dis* **17**: 120.

Eliopoulos GM, Moellering RC Jr (1981). Susceptibility of enterococci and *Listeria monocytogenes* to N-formimidoyl thienamycin alone and in combination with an aminoglycoside. *Antimicrob Ag Chemother* **19**: 789.

Eng RHK, Smith SM, Cherubin CE (1986). *In-vitro* emergence of beta-lactam-resistant variants of *Pseudomonas aeruginosa*. *J Antimicrob Chemother* **17**: 717.

Farina C, Boiron P, Goglio A et al. (1995). Human nocardiosis in Northern Italy from1982 to 1992. *Scand J Infect Dis* **27**: 23.

Farrell ID, Barker J, Chiodini PL et al. (1985). The activity of imipenem on *Legionella pneumophila*, with a note on the treatment of two cases. *J Antimicrob Chemother* **16**: 61.

Farrugia DC, Eykyn SJ, Smyth EG (1994). *Campylobacter fetus* endocarditis: two case reports and review. *Clin Infect Dis* **18**: 443.

Fernandes CJ, Stevens DA, Murray SI, Ackerman VP (1983). An evaluation of recently developed antibiotics. *J Antimicrob Chemother* **12**: 577.

Fichtenbaum CJ, Smith MJ (1992). Treatment of endocarditis due to *Pseudomonas aeruginosa* with imipenem. *Clin Infect Dis* **14**: 353.

Finch RG, Craddock C, Kelly J, Deaney NB (1986). Pharmacokinetic studies of imipenem/cilastatin in elderly patients. *J Antimicrob Chemother* **18** (Suppl E): 103.

Fink MP, Snydman DR, Niederman MS et al. (1994). Treatment of severe pneumonia in hospitalized patients: results of a multicenter, randomized, double-blind trial comparing intravenous ciprofloxacin with imipenem-cilastatin. *Antimicrob Ag Chemother* **38**: 547.

Freij BJ, McCracken GH Jr, Olsen KD, Threlkeld N (1985). Pharmacokinetics of imipenem-cilastatin in neonates. *Antimicrob Ag Chemother* **27**: 431.

Freij BJ, Kusmiesz H, Shelton S, Nelson JD (1987). Imipenem and cilastatin in acute osteomyelitis and suppurative arthritis. Therapy in infants and children. *Amer J Dis Child* **141**: 335.

Freimer EH, Donabedian H, Raeder R, Ribner BS (1985). Empirical use of imipenem as the sole antibiotic in the treatment of serious infections. *J Antimicrob Chemother* **16**: 499.

Geddes AM, Stille W (1985). Imipenem: The first thienamycin antibiotic. *Rev Infect Dis* **7** (Suppl 3): 353.

Gentry LO (1985). Role for newer beta-lactam antibiotics in treatment of osteomyelitis. *Amer J Med* **78** (6A): 134.

Gentry LO (1988). Osteomyelitis: options for diagnosis and management. *J Antimicrob Chemother* **21** (Suppl C): 115.

Gibson TP, Demetriades JL, Bland JA (1985). Imipenem/cilastatin: pharmacokinetic profile in renal insufficiency. *Amer J Med* **78** (6A): 54.

Giwercman B, Jensen ET, Hoiby N et al. (1991). Induction of beta-lactamase production in *Pseudomonas aeruginosa* biofilm. *Antimicrob Ag Chemother* **35**: 1008.

Giwercman B, Meyer C, Lambert PA et al. (1992). High-level beta-lactamase activity in sputum samples from cystic fibrosis patients during antipseudomonal treatment. *Antimicrob Ag Chemother* **36**: 71.

Gold WL, Salit IE (1993). Aeromonas hydrophila infections of skin and soft tissue: report of 11 cases and review. *Clin Infect Dis* **16**: 69.

Goldstein EJC, Citron DM (1986). Comparative *in vitro* activities of amoxicillin-clavulanic acid and imipenem against anaerobic bacteria isolated from community hospitals. *Antimicrob Ag Chemother* **29**: 158.

Goldstein EJC, Citron DM, Cherubin CE, Hillier SL (1993). Comparative susceptibility of the *Bacteroides fragilis* group species and other anaerobic bacteria to meropenem, imipenem, piperacillin, cefoxitin, ampicilin/sulbactam, clindamycin and metronidazole. *J Antimicrob Chemother* **31**: 363.

Gombert ME, Berkowitz LB, Aulicino TM, du Bouchet L (1990). Therapy of pulmonary nocardiosis in immunocompromised mice. *Antimicrob Ag Chemother* **34**: 1766.

Gorbach SL (1993). Intraabdominal infections. *Clin Infect Dis* **17**: 961.

Gradon JD, Chapnick EK, Lutwick LI (1992). Infective endocarditis of a native valve due to *Acinetobacter*: case report and review. *Clin Infect Dis* **14**: 1145.

Grayson ML, Gibbons GW, Habershaw GM et al. (1994). Use of ampicillin/sulbactam versus imipenem/cilastatin in the treatment of limb-threatening foot infections in diabetic patients. *Clin Infect Dis* **18**: 683.

Graziani AL, Gibson GA, MacGregor RR (1987). Biliary excretion of imipenem-cilastatin in hospitalized patients. *Antimicrob Ag Chemother* **31**: 1718.

Griffiths JK, Daly JS, Dodge RA (1992). Two cases of endocarditis due to Lactobacillus species: antimicrobial susceptibility, review and discussion of therapy. *Clin Infect Dis* **15**: 250.

Gruber WC, Rench MA, Garcia-Prats JA et al. (1985). Single-dose pharmacokinetics of imipenem-cilastatin in neonates. *Antimicrob Ag Chemother* **27**: 511.

Hedberg M, Edlund C, Lindqvist L et al. (1992). Purification and characterization of an imipenem hydrolyzing metallo-beta-lactamase from *Bacteroides fragilis*. *J Antimicrob Chemother* **29**: 105.

Heikkilä A, Renkonen O-V, Erkkola R (1992). Pharmacokinetics and transplacental passage of imipenem during pregnancy. *Antimicrob Ag Chemother* **36**: 2652.

Hindes RG, Willey SH, Eliopoulos GM et al. (1989). Treatment of experimental endocarditis caused by a beta-lactamase-producing strain of *Enterococcus faecalis* with high level resistance to gentamicin. *Antimicrob Ag Chemother* **33**: 1019.

Höffler U (1986). *In vitro* sensitivity of bacteroidaceae, clostridia and propionibacteria to newer antimicrobial agents. *J Antimicrob Chemother* **18** (Suppl E): 41.

Hopkins JM, Towner KJ (1990). Enhanced resistance to cefotaxime and imipenem associated with outer membrane protein alterations in *Enterobacter aerogenes*. *J Antimicrob Chemother* **25**: 49.

Horn R, Lavallee J, Robson HG (1992). Susceptibilities of members of the *Bacteroides fragilis* Group to 11 antimicrobial agents. *Antimicrob Ag Chemother* **36**: 2051.

Hornstein MJ, Jupeau AM, Scavizzi MR et al. (1985). *In vitro* susceptibilities of 126 clinical isolates of *Yersinia enterocolitica* to 21 β-lactam antibiotics. *Antimicrob Ag Chemother* **27**: 806.

Hughes WT, Armstrong D, Bodey GP et al. (1990). Guidelines for the use of antimicrobial agents in neutropenic patients with unexplained fever. *J Infect Dis* **161**: 381.

Hurblut S, Cuchural GJ, Tally FP (1990). Imipenem resistance in *Bacteroides distasonis* mediated by a novel beta-lactamase. *Antimicrob Ag Chemother* **34**: 117.

Inderlied CB, Kolonoski PT, Wu M, Young LS (1989). Amikacin, ciprofloxacin and imipenem treatment for disseminated *Mycobacterium avium* complex infection of beige mice. *Antimicrob Ag Chemother* **33**: 176.

Ito H, Arakawa Y, Ohsuka S *et al.* (1995). Plasmid-mediated dissemination of the metallo-beta-lactamase gene blaIMP among clinically isolated strains of *Serratia marcescens. Antimicrob Ag Chemother* **39**: 824.

Jacobs MR (1992). Treatment and diagnosis of infections caused by drug-resistant *Streptococcus pneumoniae. Clin Infect Dis* **15**: 119.

Jacobs RF (1986). Imipenem-cilastatin: the first thienamycin antibiotic. *Pediatr Infect Dis* **5**: 444.

Jacobs RF, Kearns GL, Brown AL, Longee DC (1986). Cerebrospinal fluid penetration of imipenem and cilastatin (Primaxin). in children with central nervous system infections. *Antimicrob Ag Chemother* **29**: 670.

Jacoby GA, Carreras I (1990). Activities of beta-lactam antibiotics against *Escherichia coli* strains producing extended spectrum beta-lactamases. *Antimicrob Ag Chemother* **34**: 858.

Jacoby GA, Medeiros AA (1991). More extended-spectrum beta-lactamases. *Antimicrob Ag Chemother* **35**: 1697.

Jackson JJ, Kropp H (1992). Beta-lactam antibiotic-induced release of free endotoxin: *in vitro* comparison of penicillin-binding protein (PBP). 2-specific imipenem and PBP 3-specific ceftazidime. *J Infect Dis* **165**: 1033.

James PA, Hossain FK, Lewis DA, White DG (1993). Beta-lactam susceptibility of *Haemophilus influenzae* strains showing reduced susceptibility to cefuroxime. *J Antimicrob Chemother* **32**: 239.

Janmohamed RMI, Leyland MJ, Kelly J, Farrell I (1990). Pharmacokinetics of imipenem/cilastatin in neutropenic patients with haematological malignancies. *J Antimicrob Chemother* **25**: 407.

Jones RN (1985). Review of the *in vitro* spectrum of activity of imipenem. *Amer J Med* **78** (6A): 22.

Kager L, Nord CE (1985). Imipenem/cilastatin in the treatment of intraabdominal infections: A review of worldwide experience. *Rev Infect Dis* (Suppl 3): 518.

Kager L, Brismar B, Malmborg A-S, Nord CE (1989). Imipenem concentrations in colorectal surgery and impact on the colonic microflora. *Antimicrob Ag Chemother* **33**: 204.

Kahan FM, Kropp H, Sundelof JG, Birnbaum J (1983). Thienamycin: development of imipenem-cilastatin. *J Antimicrob Chemother* **12** (Suppl D): 1.

Kim KS (1985). Comparison of cefotaxime, imipenem-cilastatin, ampicillin-gentamicin and ampicillin-chloramphenicol in the treatment of experimental *Escherichia coli* bacteremia and meningitis. *Antimicrob Ag Chemother* **28**: 433.

Kim KS (1986). *In vitro* and *in vivo* studies of imipenem-cilastatin alone and in combination with gentamicin against *Listeria monocytogenes. Antimicrob Ag Chemother* **29**: 289.

Konishi K, Suzuki H, Saruta T *et al.* (1991). Removal of imipenem and cilastatin by hemodialysis in patients with end-stage renal failure. *Antimicrob Ag Chemother* **35**: 1616.

Kropp H, Sundelof JG, Hajdu R, Kahan FM (1982). Metabolism of thienamycin and related carbapenem antibiotics by the renal dipeptidase, dehydropeptidase-I. *Antimicrob Ag Chemother* **22**: 62.

Kropp H, Gerckens L, Sundelof JG, Kahan FM (1985). Antibacterial activity of imipenem: the first thienamycin antibiotic. *Rev Infect Dis* **7** (Suppl 3): 389.

Kuah BG, Kumarasinghe G, Doran J, Chang HR (1994). Antimicrobial susceptibilities of clinical isolates of *Acinetobacter baumannii* from Singapore. *Antimicrob Ag Chemother* **38**: 2502.

Kumar A, Wofford-McQueen R, Gordon RC (1989). Ciprofloxacin, imipenem and rifampicin: *in-vitro* synergy of two and three drug combinations against Pseudomonas cepacia. *J Antimicrob Chemother* **23**: 831.

Labia R, Morand A, Guionie M (1986). Beta-lactamase stability of imipenem. *J Antimicrob Chemother* **18** (Suppl E): 1.

Lamothe F, Fijalkowski C, Malouin F *et al.* (1986). *Bacteroides fragilis* resistant to both metronidazole and imipenem. *J Antimicrob Chemother* **18**: 642.

Lariviere LA, Gaudreau CL, Turgeon FF (1986). Susceptibility of clinical isolates of *Campylobacter jejuni* to twenty five antimicrobial agents. *J Antimicrob Chemother* **18**: 681.

Leaper DJ, Kennedy RH, Sutton A *et al.* (1987). Treatment of acute bacterial peritonitis: a trial of imipenem/cilastatin against ampicillin-metronidazole-gentamicin. *Scand J Infect Dis* (Suppl 52): 7.

Lee EH, Nicolas MH, Kitzis MD *et al.* (1991). Association of two resistance mechanisms in a clinical isolate of *Enterobacter cloacae* with high-level resistance to imipenem. *Antimicrob Ag Chemother* **35**: 1093.

Leung JWC, Chan CY, Lai CW *et al.* (1992). Effect of biliary obstruction on the hepatic excretion of imipenem-cilastatin. *Antimicrob Ag Chemother* **36**: 2057.

Leyland MJ, Bayston KF, Cohen J *et al.* (1992). A comparative study of imipenem versus piperacillin plus gentamicin in the initial management of febrile neutropenic patients with haematological malignancies. *J Antimicrob Chemother* **30**: 843.

Liang R, Yung R, Chiu E *et al.* (1990). Ceftazidime versus imipenem-cilastatin as initial monotherapy for febrile neutropenic patients. *Antimicrob Ag Chemother* **34**: 1336.

Liñares J, Alonso T, Pèrez JL *et al.* (1992). Decreased susceptibility of penicillin-resistant pneumococci to twenty-four beta-lactam antibiotics. *J Antimicrob Chemother* **30**: 279.

Liu CY, Wang F-D (1989). A comparative study of ceftriaxone plus amikacin, ceftazidime plus amikacin and imipenem/cilastatin in the empiric therapy of febrile granulocytopenic cancer patients. *Chemotherapy* **35** (Suppl 2): 16.

Livermore DM (1992a). Interplay of impermeability and chromosomal beta-lactamase activity in imipenem-resistant *Pseudomonas aeruginosa. Antimicrob Ag Chemother* **36**: 2046.

Livermore DM (1992b). Carbapenemases. *J Antimicrob Chemother* **29**: 609.

Livermore DM, Chau PY, Wong AIW, Leung YK (1987). Beta-lactamase of *Pseudomonas pseudomallei* and its contribution to antibiotic resistance. *J Antimicrob Chemother* **20**: 313.

Lode H, Wiley R, Hoffken G *et al.* (1987). Prospective randomized controlled study of ciprofloxacin versus imipenem-cilastatin in severe clinical infections. *Antimicrob Ag Chemother* **31**: 1491.

Lynch MJ, Drusano GL, Mobley HLT (1987). Emergence of resistance to imipenem in *Pseudomonas aeruginosa. Antimicrob Ag Chemother* **31**: 1892.

MacGregor RR, Gentry LO (1985). Imipenem/cilastatin in the treatment of osteomyelitis. *Amer J Med* **78** (6A): 100.

MacGregor RR, Gibson GA, Bland JA (1984). Imipenem pharmacokinetics and body fluid levels in high dose patient treatment. In *Program and Abstracts of the 24th Interscience Conference on Antimicrobial Agents and Chemotherapy, Washington, DC* (Abstr. 597). Washington, DC: American Society for Microbiology.

MacGregor RR, Gibson GA, Bland JA (1986). Imipenem pharmacokinetics and body fluid concentrations in patients receiving high-dose treatment for serious infections. *Antimicrob Ag Chemother* **29**: 188.

Majcherczyk PA, Livermore DM (1990). Penicillin-binding protein (PBP)2 and the post-antibiotic effect of carbapenems. *J Antimicrob Chemother* **26**: 593.

Markowitz N, Pohlod DJ, Saravolatz LD, Quinn EL (1983). *In vitro* susceptibility patterns of methicillin-resistant and -susceptible *Staphylococcus aureus* strains in a population of parenteral drug abusers from 1972 to 1981. *Antimicrob Ag Chemother* **23**: 450.

Markowitz SM, Wells VD, Williams DS *et al.* (1991). Antimicrobial susceptibility and molecular epidemiology of beta-lactamase-producing aminoglycoside-resistant isolate of *Enterococcus faecalis. Antimicrob Ag Chemother* **35**: 1075.

Martínez F, Martin-Luengo F, Garcia A, Valdes M (1994). Treatment with imipenem of experimental endocarditis caused by penicillin-resistant *Streptococcus sanguis. J Antimicrob Chemother* **33**: 1201.

Matsuda K, Asahi Y, Sanada M *et al.* (1991). *In-vitro* activity of imipenem combined with beta-lactam antibiotics for methicillin-resistant *Staphylococcus aureus. J Antimicrob Chemother* **27**: 809.

Mayer KH, Zinner SH (1985). Bacterial pathogens of increasing significance in hospital-acquired infections. *Rev Infect Dis* **7** (Suppl 3): 371.

McCracken GH Jr, Sakata Y (1985). Antimicrobial therapy of experimental meningitis caused by *Streptococcus pneumoniae* strains with different susceptibilities to penicillin. *Antimicrob Ag Chemother* **27**: 141.

McEniry DW, Gillespie SH, Felmingham D (1988). Susceptibility of *Pseudomonas pseudomallei* to new beta-lactam and aminoglycoside antibiotics. *J Antimicrob Chemother* **21**: 171.

McGrath BJ, Lamp KC, Rybak MJ (1993a). Pharmacodynamic effects of extended dosing intervals of imipenem alone and in combination with amikacin against *Pseudomonas aeruginosa* in an *in vitro* model. *Antimicrob Ag Chemother* **37**: 1931.

McGrath BJ, Marchbanks CR, Gilbert D, Dudley MN (1993b). *In vitro* postantibiotic effect following repeated exposure to imipenem, temafloxacin, and tobramycin. *Antimicrob Ag Chemother* **37**: 1723.

McNeil MM, Brown JM, Jarvis WR, Ajello L (1990). Comparison of species distribution and antimicrobial susceptibility of aerobic actinomycetes from clinical specimens. *Rev Infect Dis* **12**: 778.

Mehtar S, Tsakris A, Pitt TL (1991). Imipenem resistance in *Proteus mirabilis*. *J Antimicrob Chemother* **28**: 612.

Meyer KS, Urban C, Eagan JA et al. (1993). Nosocomial outbreak of *Klebsiella* infection resistant to late generation cephalosporins. *Ann Intern Med* **119**: 353.

Modai J, Vittecoq D, Decazes JM, Meulemans A (1985). Penetration of imipenem and cilastatin into cerebrospinal fluid of patients with bacterial meningitis. *J Antimicrob Chemother* **16**: 751.

Morita K, Watanabe N, Kurata S, Kanamori M (1994). Beta-lactam resistance of motile *Aeromonas* isolates from clinical and environmental sources. *Antimicrob Ag Chemother* **38**: 353.

Murray PR, Jones RN, Allen SD et al. (1993). Multilaboratory evaluation of the *in vitro* activity of 13 beta-lactam antibiotics against 1474 clinical isolates of aerobic and anaerobic bacteria. *Diagn Microbiool Infect Dis* **16**: 191.

Naas T, Vandel L, Sougakoff W et al. (1994). Cloning and sequence analysis of the gene for a carbapenem-hydrolysing class A beta-lactamase, Sme-1, from *Serratia marcescens*. *Antimicrob Ag Chemother* **38**: 1262.

Nalin DR, Jacobsen CA (1987). Imipenem/cilastatin in therapy for serious infections in neonates and infants. *Scand J Infect Dis* (Suppl 52): 46.

Neu HC (1985). Carbapenems: special properties contributing to their activity. *Amer J Med* **78** (6A): 33.

Neu HC, Labthavikul P (1982). Comparative *in vitro* activity of N-formimidoyl thienamycin against Gram-positive and Gram-negative aerobic and anaerobic species and its beta-lactamase stability. *Antimicrob Ag Chemother* **21**: 180.

Nordmann P, Ronco E (1992). *In-vitro* antimicrobial susceptibility of *Rhodococcus equi*. *J Antimicrob Chemother* **29**: 383.

Nordmann P, Nicolas MH, Gutmann L (1993a). Penicillin-binding proteins of *Rhodococcus eqii*: potential role in resistance to imipenem. *Antimicrob Ag Chemother* **37**: 1404.

Nordmann P, Mariotte S, Naas T et al. (1993b). Biochemical properties of a carbapenem-hydrolysing beta-lactamase from *Enterobacter cloacae* and cloning of the gene into *Escherichia coli*. *Antimicrob Ag Chemother* **37**: 939.

Norrby SR (1985). Imipenem/cilastatin: rationale for a fixed combination. *Rev Infect Dis* **7** (Suppl 3): 447.

Norrby SR, Alestig K, Ferber F et al. (1983a). Pharmacokinetics and tolerance of N-formimidoyl thienamycin (MK0787). in humans. *Antimicrob Ag Chemother* **23**: 293.

Norrby SR, Alestig K, Björnegård B et al. (1983b). Urinary recovery of N-formimidoyl thienamycin (MK0787). as affected by coadministration of N-formimidoyl thienamycin dehydropeptidase inhibitors. *Antimicrob Ag Chemother* **23**: 300.

Norrby SR, Vandercam B, Louie T et al. (1987). Imipenem/cilastatin versus amikacin plus piperacillin in the treatment of infections in neutropenic patients: a prospective randomized multi-clinic study. *Scand J Infect Dis* (Suppl 52): 65.

Norrby SR, Finch RG, Glauser M, European Study Group (1993).

Monotherapy in serious hospital-acquired infections: a clinical trial of ceftazidime versus imipenem/cilastatin. *J Antimicrob Chemother* **31**: 927.

Ogle JW, Reller LB, Vasil ML (1988). Development of resistance in *Pseudomonas aeruginosa* to imipenem, norfloxacin, and ciprofloxacin during therapy: proof provided by typing with a DNA probe. *J Infect Dis* **157**: 743.

Oka S, Goto M, Kaji Y et al. (1993). Synergic activity of imipenem/cilastatin combined with cefotiam against methicillin-resistant *Staphylococcus aureus*. *J Antimicrob Chemother* **31**: 533.

Osano E, Arakawa Y, Wacharotayankun R et al. (1994). Molecular characterization of an enterobacterial metallo beta-lactamase found in a clinical isolate in *Serratia marcescens* that shows imipenem resistance. *Antimicrob Ag Chemother* **38**: 71.

Otin CL, Morros TJ, Sala IS (1988). Antibiotic susceptibility of *Streptococcus pneumoniae* isolates from paediatric patients. *J Antimicrob Chemother* **22**: 659.

Paton R, Miles RS, Amyes SGB (1994). Biochemical properties of inducible beta-lactamases produced from *Xanthomonas maltophilia*. *Antimicrob Ag Chemother* **38**: 2143.

Payne DJ, Cramp R, Bateson JH et al. (1994). Rapid identification of metallo- and serine beta-lactamases. *Antimicrob Ag Chemother* **38**: 991.

Pedersen SS, Pressler T, Jensen T et al. (1987). Combined imipenem/cilastatin and tobramycin therapy of multiresistant *Pseudomonas aeruginosa* in cystic fibrosis. *J Antimicrob Chemother* **19**: 101.

Petrilli AS, Melaragno R, Barros KVT et al. (1993). Fever and neutropenia in children with cancer: a therapeutic approach related to the underlying disease. *Pediatr Infect Dis J* **12**: 916.

Pierre J, Boisivon A, Gutmann L (1990). Alteration of PBP 3 entails resistance to imipenem in *Listeria monocytogenes*. *Antimicrob Ag Chemother* **34**: 1695.

Pietroski NA, Graziani AL, Lawson LA et al. (1991). Steady-state pharmacokinetics of intramuscular imipenem-cilastatin in elderly patients with various degrees of renal function. *Antimicrob Ag Chemother* **35**: 972.

Powell M, Livermore DM (1990). Selection and transformation on non-beta-lactamase-mediated insusceptibility to beta-lactams in *Haemophilus influenzae*: lack of cross-resistance between carbapenems and other agents. *J Antimicrob Chemother* **26**: 741.

Powell M, Williams JD (1987). *In vitro* activities of aztreonam, imipenem and amoxycillin-clavulanate against ampicillin-resistant *Haemophilus influenzae*. *Antimicrob Ag Chemother* **31**: 1871.

Quinn JP (1994). Imipenem resistance among Gram-negative bacilli. *Eur J Clin Microbiol Infect Dis* **13**: 203.

Quinn JP, Dudek EJ, Di Vincenzo CA et al. (1986). Emergence of resistance to imipenem during therapy for *Pseudomonas aeruginosa* infections. *J Infect Dis* **154**: 289.

Quinn JP, Studemeister AE, Di Vincenzo CA, Lerner SA (1988). Resistance to imipenem in *Pseudomonas aeruginosa*: clinical experience and biochemical mechanisms. *Rev Infect Dis* **10**: 892.

Quinn JP, Darzins A, Miyashiro D et al. (1991). Imipenem resistance in *Pseudomonas aeruginosa* PAO: mapping of the OprD$_2$ gene. *Antimicrob Ag Chemother* **35**: 753.

Raimondi A, Traverso A, Nikaido H (1991). Imipenem-and meropenem-resistant mutants of Enterobacter cloacae and *Proteus rettgeri* lack porins. *Antimicrob Ag Chemother* **35**: 1174.

Rassmussen BA, Yang Y, Jacobus N, Bush K (1994). Contribution of enzymatic properties, cell permeability, and enzyme expression to microbiological activities of beta-lactams in three *Bacteroides fragilis* isolates that harbor a metallo-beta-lactamase gene. *Antimicrob Ag Chemother* **38**: 2116.

Reed MD, Stern RC, O'Brien CA et al. (1985). Pharmacokinetics of imipenem and cilastatin in patients with cystic fibrosis. *Antimicrob Ag Chemother* **27**: 583.

Reed MD, Kliegman RM, Yamashita TS et al. (1990). Clinical pharmacology of imipenem and cilastatin in premature infants during the first week of life. *Antimicrob Ag Chemother* **34**: 1172.

Remington JS (1985). Introduction to a symposium on imipenem/cilastatin. *Amer J Med* **78** (6A): 1.

Renneberg J, Walder M (1989). Postantibiotic effects of imipenem, norfloxacin, and amikacin *in vitro* and *in vivo*. *Antimicrob Ag Chemother* **33**: 1714.

Report from a Norwegian Study Group (1987). Imipenem/cilastatin as monotherapy in severe infections: comparison with cefotaxime in combination with metronidazole and cloxacillin. *Scand J Infect Dis* **19**: 667.

Richmond MH (1981). The semi-synthetic thienamycin derivative MK0787 and its properties with respect to a range of beta-lactamases from clinically relevant bacterial species. *J Antimicrob Chemother* **7**: 279.

Rogers JD, Meisinger MAP, Ferber F *et al.* (1985). Pharmacokinetics of imipenem and cilastatin in volunteers. *Rev Infect Dis* **7** (Suppl 3): 435.

Rolando N, Wade JJ, Philpott-Howard JN *et al.* (1994). The penetration of imipenem/cilastatin into ascitic fluid in patients with chronic liver disease. *J Antimicrob Chemother* **33**: 163.

Roscoe DL, Zemcov JV, Thornber D *et al.* (1992). Antimicrobial susceptibilities and beta-lactamase characterization of *Capnocytophaga* species. *Antimicrob Ag Chemother* **36**: 2197.

Rossolini GM, Zanchi A, Chiesurin A *et al.* (1995). Distribution of cph. A. or related carbapenemase-encoding genes and production of carbapenemase activity in members of genus *Aeromonas*. *Antimicrob Ag Chemother* **39**: 346.

Sakata Y, McCracken GH Jr, Thomas ML, Olsen KD (1984). Pharmacokinetics and therapeutic efficacy of imipenem, ceftazidime, and ceftriaxone in experimental meningitis due to an ampicillin- and chloramphenicol-resistant strain of *Haemophilus influenzae* type b. *Antimicrob Ag Chemother* **25**: 29.

Salata RA, Gebhart RL, Palmer DL *et al.* (1985). Pneumonia treated with imipenem/cilastatin. *Amer J Med* **78** (6A): 104.

Satake S, Yoneyama H, Nakae T (1991). Role of Omp D2 and chromosomal beta-lactamase in carbapenem resistance in clinical isolates of *Pseudomonas aeruginosa*. *J Antimicrob Chemother* **28**: 199.

Scavizzi MR, Alonso J-M, Philippon AM *et al.* (1987). Failure of newer beta-lactam antibiotics for murine *Yersinia enterocolitica* infection. *Antimicrob Ag Chemother* **31**: 523.

Schliamser SE, Broholm K-A, Liljedahl A-L, Norrby SR (1988). Comparative neurotoxicity of benzylpenicillin, imipenem/cilastalin and FCE 22101, a new injectible penem. *J Antimicrob Chemother* **22**: 687.

Segatore B, Massidda O, Satta G *et al.* (1993). High specificity of cph A-encoded metallo-beta-lactamase from *Aeromonas hydrophila* AE 036 for carbapenems and its contribution to beta-lactam resistance. *Antimicrob Ag Chemother* **37**: 1324.

Seifert H, Baginski R, Schulze A, Pulverer G (1993). Antimicrobial susceptibility of *Acinetobacter* species. *Antimicrob Ag Chemother* **37**: 750.

Shafran SD, Wong J, Chow AW (1985). *In vitro* activity of Sch 34343 and cefbuperazone against anaerobic bacteria. *Antimicrob Ag Chemother* **27**: 749.

Shannon K, King A, Phillips I (1986). Beta-lactamases with high activity against imipenem and Sch 34343 from *Aeromonas hydrophila*. *J Antimicrob Chemother* **17**: 45.

Shlaes DM, Binczewski B, Rice LB (1993). Emerging antimicrobial resistance and the immunocompromised host. *Clin Infect Dis* **17** (Suppl 2): 527.

Shungu DL, Nalin DR, Gilman RH *et al.* (1987). Comparative susceptibilities of *Campylobacter pylori* to norfloxacin and other agents. *Antimicrob Ag Chemother* **31**: 949.

Signs SA, Tan JS, Salstrom S-J, File TM (1992). Pharmacokinetics of imipenem in serum and skin window fluid in healthy adults after intramuscular or intravenous administration. *Antimicrob Ag Chemother* **36**: 1400.

Smith MD, Bielawska C, Kelsey MC *et al.* (1988). Evaluation of imipenem/cilastatin for treatment of infection in an elderly population. *J Antimicrob Chemother* **21**: 481.

Smith MD, Wuthiekancin V, Walsh AL, White NJ (1994). Susceptibility of *Pseudomonas pseudomallei* to some newer beta-lactam antibiotics and antibiotic combinations using time-kill studies. *J Antimicrob Chemother* **33**: 145.

Somani P, Freimer EH, Gross ML, Higgins JTJr (1988). Pharmacokinetics of imipenem-cilastatin in patients with renal insufficiency undergoing continuous ambulatory peritoneal dialysis. *Antimicrob Ag Chemother* **32**: 530.

Spangler SK, Jacobs MR, Appelbaum PC (1994). Susceptibilities of 177 penicillin-susceptible and -resistant pneumococci to FK 037, cefpirome, cefepime, ceftriaxone, cefotaxime, ceftazidime, imipenem, biapenem, meropenem and vancomycin. *Antimicrob Ag Chemother* **38**: 898.

Spitzer PG, Eliopoulos GM, Karchmer AW, Moellering RCJr (1986). Activity of newer polypeptide antibiotics compared with other agents against pathogenic *Corynebacterium* species. In *Program and Abstracts of the 26th Interscience Conference on Antimicrobial Agents and Chemotherapy, New Orleans.* (Abstr. 904). Washington, DC: American Society for Microbiology.

Spratt BG, Jobanputra V, Zimmermann W (1977). Binding of thienamycin and clavulanic acid to the penicillin-binding proteins of *Escherichia coli* K-12. *Antimicrob Ag Chemother* **12**: 406.

Standiford HC, Drusano GL, Bustamante CI *et al.* (1986). Imipenem coadministered with cilastatin compared with moxalactam: integration of serum pharmacokinetics and microbiologic activity following single-dose administration to normal volunteers. *Antimicrob Ag Chemother* **29**: 412.

Stark CA, Edlund C, Sjöstedt S *et al.* (1993). Antimicrobial resistance in human oral and intestinal anaerobic microfloras. *Antimicrob Ag Chemother* **37**: 1665.

Strandvik B, Malmborg A-S, Bergan T *et al.* (1988). Imipenem/cilastatin, an alternative treatment of pseudomonas infection in cystic fibrosis. *J Antimicrob Chemother* **21**: 471.

Studemeister AE, Quinn JP (1988). Selective imipenem resistance in *Pseudomonas aeruginosa* associated with diminished outer membrane permeability. *Antimicrob Ag Chemother* **32**: 1267.

Sumita Y, Fukasawa M (1993). Transient carbapenem resistance induced by salicylate in *Pseudomonas aeruginosa* associated with suppression of outer membrane protein D_2 synthesis. *Antimicrob Ag Chemother* **37**: 2743.

Summanen P, Wexler HM, Lee K *et al.* (1993). Morphological response to *Bilophila wadsworthia* to imipenem: correlation with properties of penicillin-binding proteins. *Antimicrob Ag Chemother* **37**: 2638.

Swanson DJ, De Angelis C, Smith IL, Schentag JJ (1986). Degradation kinetics of imipenem in normal saline and in human serum. *Antimicrob Ag Chemother* **29**: 936.

Thomson KS, Sanders CC, Chmel H (1993). Imipenem resistance in *Enterobacter*. *Eur J Clin Microbiol Infect Dis* **12**: 610.

Trias J, Nikaido H (1990). Outer membrane protein D2 catalyzes faciliated diffusion of carbapenems and penems through the outer membrane of *Pseudomonas aeruginosa*. *Antimicrob Ag Chemother* **34**: 52.

Trias J, Dufresne J, Levesque RC, Nikaido H (1989). Decreased outer membrane permeability in imipenem-resistant mutants of *Pseudomonas aeruginosa*. *Antimicrob Ag Chemother* **33**: 1201.

Turgeon P, Turgeon V, Gordeau M *et al.* (1994). Longitudinal study of susceptibilities of species of the *Bacteroides fragilis* group to five antimicrobial agents in three medical centers. *Antimicrob Ag Chemother* **38**: 2276.

Tzouvelekis LS, Tzelepi E, Kaufmann ME, Mentis AF (1994). Consecutive mutations leading to the emergence *in vivo* of imipenem resistance in a clinical strain of *Enterobacter aerogenes*. *J Med Microbiol* **40**: 403.

Urban C, Go E, Mariano N *et al.* (1993). Effect of sulbactam on infections caused by imipenem-resistant *Acinetobacter calcoaceticus* biotype anitratus. *J Infect Dis* **167**: 448.

Van der Leur JJJPM, Thunnissen PLM, Clasener HAL *et al.* (1993). Effects of imipenem, cefotaxime and cotrimoxazole on aeobic microbial colonization of the digestive tract. *Scand J Infect Dis* **25**: 473.

Verbist L, Verpooten GA, Giuliano RA *et al.* (1986). Pharmacokinetics and tolerance after repeated doses of imipenem/cilastatin in patients with severe renal failure. *J Antimicrob Chemother* **18** (Suppl E): 115.

Verdon MS, Judson FN, Ehret JM *et al.* (1988). Treatment of uncomplicated gonorrhea with single dose imipenem-cilastatin. *Antimicrob Ag Chemother* **32**: 773.

Victor MA, Arpi M, Bruun B *et al.* (1994). *Xanthomonas maltophilia* bacteremia in immunocompromised hematological patients. *Scand J Infect Dis* **26**: 163.

Vu H, Nikaido H (1985). Role of beta-lactam hydrolysis in the mechanism of resistance of a beta-lactamase-constitutive *Enterobacter cloacae* strain to expanded-spectrum beta-lactams. *Antimicrob Ag Chemother* **27**: 393.

Vurma-Rapp U, Kayser FH, Barberis-Maino L (1986). Antibacterial properties of imipenem with special reference to the activity against methicillin-resistant staphylococci cefotaxime-resistant Enterobacteriaceae and *Pseudomonas aeruginosa*. *J Antimicrob Chemother* **18** (Suppl E): 27.

Vurma-Rapp U, Kayser FH, Hadorn K, Wiederkehr F (1990).Mechanism of imipenem resistance acquired by three *Pseudomonas aeruginosa* strains during imipenem therapy. *Eur J Clin Microbiol Infect Dis* **9**: 580.

Wade JC (1989). Antibiotic therapy for the febrile granulocytopenic cancer patient: combination therapy vs. monotherapy. *Rev Infect Dis* **11** (Suppl 7): 1572.

Wallace RJJr, Steele LC, Sumter G, Smith JM (1988). Antimicrobial susceptibility patterns of *Nocardia asteroides*. *Antimicrob Ag Chemother* **32**: 1776.

Wang C, Calandra GB, Aziz MA, Brown KR (1985). Efficacy and safety of imipenem/cilastatin: a review of worldwide clinical experience. *Rev Infect Dis* **7** (Suppl 3): 528.

Wang C, Pappas F, Cook T (1986). Imipenem/cilastatin: a multicentre international study of its clinical efficacy, safety and potential as empirical therapy. *J Antimicrob Chemother* **18** (Suppl E): 185.

Wathen CG, Carbarns NJ, Jones PA *et al.* (1988). Imipenem-cilastatin in the treatment of respiratory infections in patients with chronic airways obstruction. *J Antimicrob Chemother* **21**: 107.

Watt B, Edwards JR, Rayner A *et al.* (1992). *In vitro* activity of meropenem and imipenem against mycobacteria: development of a daily antibiotic dosing schedule. *Tubercle Lung Dis* **73**: 134.

Weber DJ, Saviteer SM, Rutala WA, Thomann CA (1988). *In vitro* susceptibility of *Bacillus* spp to selected antimicrobial agents. *Antimicrob Ag Chemother* **32**: 642.

Weisholtz S, Tomasz A (1985). Response of *Legionella pneumophila* to β-lactam antibiotics. *Antimicrob Ag Chemother* **27**: 695.

Wexler HM, Finegold SM (1985). *In vitro* activity of imipenem against anaerobic bacteria. *Rev Infect Dis* **7** (Suppl 3): 417.

Wise R, Andrews JM, Patel N (1981). N-formimidoyl-thienamycin a novel beta-lactam: an *in-vitro* comparison with other beta-lactam antibiotics. *J Antimicrob Chemother* **7**: 521.

Wise R, Donovan IA, Lockley MR *et al.* (1986). The pharmacokinetics and tissue penetration of imipenem. *J Antimicrob Chemother* **18** (Suppl E): 93.

Wood CA, Reboli AC (1993). Infections caused by imipenem-resistant *Acinetobacter calcoaceticus* biotype *anitratus*. *J Infect Dis* **168**: 1602.

Wu PJ, Livermore DM (1990). Response of chemostat cultures of *Pseudomonas aeruginosa* to carbapenems and other beta-lactams. *J Antimicrob Chemother* **25**: 891.

Yang Y, Wu P, Livermore DM (1990). Biochemical characterization of a beta-lactamase that hydrolyzes penems and carbapenems from two *Serratia marcescens* isolates. *Antimicrob Ag Chemother* **34**: 755.

Yeo S-F, Livermore DM (1994). Comparative *in-vitro* activity of biapenem and other carbapenems against *Haemophilus influenzae* isolates with known resistance mechanisms to ampicillin. *J Antimicrob Chemother* **33**: 861.

Yew WW, Kwan SYL, Wong PC, Lee J (1990). Ofloxacin and imipenem in the treatment of *Mycobacterium fortuitum* and *Mycobacterium chelonae* lung infections. *Tubercle* **71**: 131.

Yew WW, Lau KS, Tse WK, Wong CF (1992). Imipenem in the treatment of lung infections due to *Mycobacterium fortuitum* and *Mycobacterium chelonae*: further experience. *Clin Infect Dis* **15**: 1046.

Yoneyama H, Nakae T (1993). Mechanism of efficient elimination of protein D_2 in outer membrane of imipenem-resistant *Pseudomonas aeruginosa*. *Antimicrob Ag Chemother* **37**: 2385.

Yoshimura F, Nikaido H (1985). Diffusion of beta-lactam antibiotics through the porin channels of *Escherichia coli* K-12. *Antimicrob Ag Chemother* **27**: 84.

Young LS, Inderlied CB, Berlin OG, Gottlieb MS (1986). Mycobacterial infections in AIDS patients, with an emphasis on the *Mycobacterium avium* complex. *Rev Infect Dis* **8**: 1024.

Zajac BA, Fisher MA, Gibson GA, MacGregor RR (1985). Safety and efficacy of high-dose treatment with imipenem-cilastatin in seriously ill patients. *Antimicrob Ag Chemother* **27**: 745.

Zemelman R, Bello H, Dominguez M *et al.* (1993). Activity of imipenem, third generation cephalosporins, aztreonam and ciprofloxacin against multi-resistant Gram-negative bacilli isolated from Chilean hospitals. *J Antimicrob Chemother* **32**: 413.

Zighelboim J, Williams TWJr, Bradshaw MW, Harris RL (1992). Successful medical management of a patient with multiple hepatic abscesses due to *Edwardsiella tarda*. *Clin Infect Dis* **14**: 117.

Meropenem and Biapenem

Description

1 Meropenem (previously SM 7338)

This, similar to imipenem (p. 227) is a new parenteral synthesized carbapenem antimicrobial agent. Like imipenem, it is very stable to most beta-lactamases, but unlike imipenem, meropenem is also relatively stable to human renal dehydropeptidase-1. Therefore it does not require concomitant administration of an enzyme inhibitor such as cilastatin (Moellering et al., 1989; Sentochnik et al., 1989). The drug is more easily hydrolyzed by renal dehydropeptidase 1 of some animals such as mice, rabbits, and monkeys, but it is quite resistant to the human renal enzyme, so that about 60–80% of an administered dose is excreted in the urine in an unchanged active form (Bax et al., 1989; Fukasawa et al., 1992; Hikida et al., 1992). Meropenem is somewhat more active than imipenem against the Enterobacteriaceae, but less active than the latter against Gram-positive organisms (Jones et al., 1989a,b; Sentochnik et al., 1989). Meropenem may have advantages over imipenem for the treatment of infections caused by some microorganisms.

2 Biapenem (previously L-627)

This is another newer parenterally administered carbapenem, which is stable against hydrolysis by kidney dehydropeptidase 1. It is at least as active as imipenem against the Enterobacteriaceae, and more active against *Psendomonas aeruginosa* than meropenem and imipenem. Against *Bacteroides fragilis* and Gram-positive organisms it is approximately as active as imipenem (Catchpole et al., 1992; Appelbaum et al., 1993; Hoban et al., 1993; Malanoski et al., 1993; Aldridge et al., 1994). Like imipenem and meropenem, biapenem is largely unaffected by inducible chromosomally mediated beta-lactamases and also extended-spectrum enzymes (p. 229) (Chen and Livermore, 1994 a and b).

The details below only apply to meropenem.

Sensitive Organisms

1 Gram-positive bacteria

Most of these, such as *Staphylococcus aureus*, coagulase negative staphylococci, *Streptococcus pyogenes*, streptococci of groups B, C and G and *Strep. pneumoniae*, are some 2- to 4-fold less susceptible to meropenem than imipenem. Methicillin-resistant staphylococci are meropenem-resistant. Strains of *Strep. pneumoniae* with intermediate resistance to penicillin G have an increased susceptibility to meropenem, but imipenem is more active against these (Jones et al., 1989a,b; Sentochnik et al., 1989). Meropenem is also less active than imipenem against *Strep. viridans*, *Enterococcus faecalis* and *E. faecium*. Only two Gram-positive bacilli, *Bacillus* spp. and *Listeria monocytogenes* are more susceptible to meropenem than imipenem, although some authors have found the reverse to be true for *L. monocytogenes*. Meropenem inhibits the Gram-positive anaerobes such as the peptococci, peptostreptococci, *Propionibacterium acnes* and *Clostridium perfringens* at much the same concentrations as imipenem (Jones et al., 1989 a, b; Neu et al., 1989). *Corynebacterium jeikeium* is resistant to both meropenem and imipenem (Neu et al., 1989). Meropenem is slightly less active against *Nocardia asteroides* than imipenem. The reverse is true for *N. brasiliensis*, but even with meropenem most strains of this organism have MICs higher than clinically attainable concentrations (Yazawa et al., 1992).

2 Gram-negative bacteria

Neisseria gonorrhoeae, including beta-lactamase-producing strains and strains intrinsically resistant to penicillin G, are more sensitive to meropenem than imipenem. Meropenem is 8- to 32-fold more active than imipenem against *Haemophilus influenzae* and this applies also to strains which produce beta-lactamase and strains intrinsically resistant to ampicillin. Meropenem is also about twice as active as imipenem against *H. ducreyi*, including beta-lactamase-producing strains. *Moraxella* spp. strains, irrespective of beta-lactamase production, are also more susceptible to meropenem than imipenem (Neu *et al.*, 1989; Slaney *et al.*, 1989; Jorgensen *et al.*, 1991a; Yeo and Livermore, 1994).

Against most Enterobacteriaceae meropenem is some 2- to 8-fold more active than imipenem. This includes *E. coli*, the *Klebsiella*, *Enterobacter*, *Citrobacter*, *Proteus*, *Providencia*, *Salmonella* and *Shigella* spp., *Morganella morganii* and *Yersinia enterocolitica* (Edwards *et al.*, 1989; Jones *et al.*, 1989a,b; Neu *et al.*, 1989). Many strains of Enterobacteriaceae, highly resistant to other unrelated antibiotics are meropenem-sensitive (Jorgensen *et al.*, 1991b). Meropenem, like imipenem, retains full activity against most *E. coli* strains which produces plasmid-mediated beta-lactamases, including extended-spectrum enzymes (p. 323) (Chen and Livermore, 1994a).

Similar to imipenem (p. 229), some strains of Enterobacteriaceae have been detected which were resistant to meropenem. For instance, meropenem-resistant mutants of *Enterobacter cloacae* and *Providencia rettgeri* were deficient in the production of non-specific porins in their cell walls and they also produced excessive amounts of chromosomally mediated beta-lactamase. The synergism between the lowered outer membrane permeability and the slow but significant hydrolysis of meropenem by the overproduced enzymes probably explained why these strains were resistant (Raimondi *et al.*, 1991). In the case of meropenem, the lowered membrane permeability was the more important factor in the resistance of *E. cloacae*; the reverse was true for imipenem (p. 229) (Cornaglia *et al.*, 1995).

The activity of meropenem against *Ps. aeruginosa* is comparable with that of imipenem (Table I.17) (Jones *et al.*, 1989 b; Neu *et al.*, 1989). Some meropenem-resistant mutants of *Ps. aeruginosa* have been detected, and these, similar to imipenem-resistant organisms, most commonly lacked the specific channel porin protein D_2, yet retained the major non-specific porins (Livermore and Yang, 1989; Trias and Nikaido, 1990; Raimondi *et al.*, 1991). One strain of *Ps. aeruginosa* was also described where the main resistance mechanism was a plasmid-mediated beta-lactamase (carbapenamase), which hydrolyzed both imipenem and meropenem (Watanabe *et al.*, 1991; Livermore, 1992). Meropenem-resistant *Ps. aeruginosa* strains were also isolated which showed cross-resistance to cefsulodin, cefoperazone, ceftazidime, the quinolones, but not to imipenem. These strains appeared to have an increase of an outer membrane protein (designated Opr M). If the strain was also D_2 deficient, then the level of meropenem-resistance was higher and the strain was also resistant to imipenem (Masuda and Ohya, 1992).

Table I.17
Compiled from data published by Jones *et al.* (1989a,b), Neu *et al.* (1989), Jorgensen *et al.* (1991a) and Hoban *et al.* (1993)

Organism	MICs (μg per ml)	
	Imipenem	Meropenem
Gram-positive bacteria		
Staphylococcus aureus (methicillin-sensitive)	0.03	0.25
Streptococcus pneumoniae (Pen G-sensitive)	≤0.015	0.015
Clostridium perfringens	0.5	1.0
Gram-negative bacteria		
Haemophilus influenzae (ampicillin-sensitive)	1.0	0.125
Escherichia coli	0.5	0.03
Klebsiella pneumoniae	0.5	0.06
Serratia marcescens	4.0	0.5
Pseudomonas aeruginosa	4.0	8.0
Stenotrophomonas maltophilia	> 32.0	128.0
Acinetobacter spp.	0.125	4.0
Bacteroides fragilis	0.5	0.25

Most *Burkholderia* (previously *Pseudomonas*) *pseudomallei* strains are meropenem-sensitive (Yamamoto *et al.*, 1990). Some strains of *Burkholderia* (*Pseudomonas*) *cepacia* are meropenem-sensitive, but others are resistant. Strains isolated from patients with cystic fibrosis are usually more resistant to meropenem than those isolated from other sources. *Flavobacterium* spp. and *Stenotrophomonas maltophilia* are meropenem-resistant (Neu *et al.*, 1989; Hoban *et al.*, 1993; Lewin *et al.*, 1993). *Aeromonas* and *Acinetobacter* spp. are nearly always meropenem-sensitive (Neu *et al.*, 1989; Hoban *et al.*, 1993).

Among the Gram-negative anaerobic bacteria, *B. fragilis* and other organisms of the *B. fragilis* group are highly sensitive to meropenem, often slightly more so than to imipenem (Neu *et al.*, 1989; Garcia-Rodriguez *et al.*, 1991). The *Prevotella* and *Fusobacteria* spp. are also nearly always meropenem-sensitive (Nord *et al.*, 1989; Watt and Naden, 1989).

Meropenem, like imipenem (p. 230) may show a post-antibiotic effect with some strains of *Ps. aeruginosa*, but not with other Gram-negative organisms such as *E. coli* (Odenholt-Tornqvist, 1993).

3 Minimum inhibitory concentrations

The MICs of meropenem against some selected bacterial species are shown in Table I.17. Those for imipenem are included for comparison.

Mode of Administration and Dosage

1 Pharmacokinetic studies

The pharmacokinetic studies of meropenem have confirmed that this drug, unlike imipenem, can be administered to humans without the need for an inhibitor of renal dehydropeptidase- 1, such as cilastatin (Bax *et al.*, 1989; Wise *et al.*, 1990; Mouton and Michel, 1991).

2 Dosage schedules

The best dosage schedules of meropenem have not yet been formulated, but in one clinical trial 1 g of the drug, given i.v. by a 30 min infusion 8-hourly was found to be appropriate for the treatment of adults with intra-abdominal infections (Bedikian *et al.*, 1994). For bacterial meningitis adult doses of up to 6 g daily have been used (p. 249).

3 Patients with renal failure

As meropenem is predominantly excreted via the kidneys, and as the terminal half-life of unchanged meropenem is 1.2 h in those with normal renal function and as this increases to 10 h in those with end-stage renal disease, dosage adjustments are necessary for patients with severe renal impairment. A provisional recommendation is that in those with creatinine clearance of >80 ml per min one standard dose (0.5–1 g) can be given i.v. every 6–8 h. For those with creatinine clearance of 30–80 ml per min one dose can be given 8–12-hourly. If the creatinine clearance is 10–30 ml per min 0.5–1.0 g dose is given 12-hourly. If the creatinine clearance is <10, one dose once every 24 h should suffice (Christensson *et al.*, 1992; Leroy *et al.*, 1992). The drug is removed by hemodialysis, and a full dose of meropenem should be given after this procedure (Chimata *et al.*, 1993). As renal function slowly deteriorates in old age, elderly patients also may need dosage reduction, which should be based on their calculated creatinine clearance and not on their serum creatinine (Ljungberg and Nilsson-Ehle, 1992).

Serum Levels in Relation to Dosage

If a 0.5 g dose of meropenem is infused i.v. over 30 min to normal adults the peak serum level straight after the infusion is approximately 25 μg per ml. This then falls progressively and reaches zero in 7–8 h. The serum half-life of the drug is approximately 1 h. The area-under-the-curve averages some 30 μg per h per ml. If the dose is doubled to 1 g, the peak serum level is doubled to some 50 μg per ml and the area-under-the-curve is doubled to approximately 60 μg per h per ml. The serum half-life is the same i.e. approximately 1 h and the serum level returns to zero again in 7–8 h (Bax *et al.*, 1989; Leroy *et al.*, 1992).

Excretion

1 Urine

Most of the administered dose of meropenem (about 72% in normal subjects) is excreted in the urine in the active unchanged form by both glomerular filtration and tubular secretion. If probenecid is also given, tubular secretion is reduced and the plasma half-life of the drug increases by some 33% (Bax et al., 1989; Burman et al., 1991).

2 Bile

A small amount of unchanged meropenem is eliminated via the bile. In one study 1 g of i.v. meropenem was administered to patients undergoing endoscopic retrograde cholangiography. Bile was collected for assays of biliary concentrations of the drug. In patients with no obstruction to biliary tracts the biliary meropenem concentrations were some 50 μg per ml during the period of 1 and 3 h after the dose. The bile concentrations of meropenem were significantly lower in patients with obstructed biliary tracts (Granai et al., 1992).

3 Inactivation in body

Meropenem, which is not excreted as active drug via the kidney and bile is inactivated in the body and from this a ring-opened metabolite (ICA 213,689) results. This again is excreted in the urine. Similar to meropenem itself, the metabolite also accumulates in the serum in elderly or uremic patients (Leroy et al., 1992; Ljungberg and Nilsson-Ehle, 1992). Some of the metabolism of meropenem occurs in the kidneys and there is an individual variation as to how active this metabolism is. However, in all subjects, unlike imipenem (p. 227), there is enough excretion of unchanged meropenem in the urine, so that co-administration of a renal dehydropeptidase 1 inhibitor, such as cilastatin is unnecessary. It is possible that some meropenem may also be metabolized in the liver (Harrison et al., 1989; Burman et al., 1991; Ljungberg and Nilsson-Ehle, 1992).

Distribution of the Drug in Body

Meropenem penetrates well into human blister fluid (Wise et al., 1990; Mouton and Michel, 1991). It also attains concentrations about equal to serum levels in the peritoneal fluid when the peritoneum is not inflamed (Hextall et al., 1991). In general, beta-lactam antibiotics are not very active against intracellular bacteria. Easmon (1989) found that meropenem killed intracellular Staph. aureus at concentrations equal to eight times the MBC, while imipenem did not. Cuffini et al. (1993) reported that meropenem penetrated human macrophages achieving intracellular concentrations much higher than extracellular ones, and that this drug was very active in killing intraphagocytic pathogens.

Animal studies have shown that meropenem is rapidly distributed in most organs and tissues, with highest levels detected in kidney and other highly perfused organs. Only a trace of the drug penetrated uninflamed meninges and brain, but it did cross the placenta (Harrison et al., 1989). However, in patients with bacterial meningitis the range of meropenem concentrations in CSF was 0.9–6.5 μg per ml after usual doses (Dagan et al., 1994).

Mode of Action

This is presumably largely similar to that of imipenem/cilastatin (p. 234).

Toxicity

The adverse effects are likely to be similar to those observed with imipenem/cilastatin. In one clinical trial in which intra-abdominal infections were treated, the commonest side-effects were diarrhea and elevated liver enzymes (Bedikian et al., 1994). Animal studies have shown that meropenem is significantly less likely to induce convulsions than imipenem/cilastatin (Patel and Giles, 1989). One adult patient with Ps. aeruginosa meningitis was treated with meropenem 2 g i.v. 8-hourly for 20 days and seizures did not occur (Chmelik and Gutvirth, 1993). In an animal E. coli meningitis model the administration of meropenem (or other antibiotics) caused a 2- to 10-fold increase in CSF concentration of free endotoxin within 2 h of starting treatment. However, free endotoxin concentrations increased almost 100-fold in untreated animals 4 h later as bacteria continued to multiply (Friedland et al., 1993).

Clinical Uses of the Drug

Meropenem has similar efficacy to imipenem/cilastatin (p. 236) and other regimens such as cefotaxime/metranidazole for the treatment of intra-abdominal infections (Bedikian *et al.*, 1994; Brismar *et al.*, 1995; Huizinga *et al.*, 1995; Wilson, 1995). For treatment of febrile neutropenic patients, meropenem 1.0 g i.v. 8-hourly appears to be equally as effective as ceftazidime 2.0 g i.v. 8-hourly (Del Favero *et al.*, 1995).

Meropenem has an advantage over imipenem/cilastin for the treatment of bacterial meningitis because it does not cause convulsions as frequently as the latter drug (p. 235). In a trial in pediatric patients meropenem (40 mg per kg i.v. every 8 h) was equally as safe and effective as cefotaxime for treatment of bacterial meningitis caused by organisms susceptible to both drugs such as *H. influenzae* (Klugman *et al.*, 1995). Similarly, in adults, meropenem (maximum dose of 6 g daily i.v.) again was equally as safe and effective as either cefotaxime or ceftriaxone (Schmutzhard *et al.*, 1995). In certain clinical situations meropenem may have an advantage over these cephalosporins. This may be so with meningitis caused by cefotaxime-resistant Enterobacteraceae such as *Enterobacter spp.* (p. 322) or ceftazidime-resistant *Ps. aeruginosa* (Klugman and Dagan, 1995).

The other possible indication for meropenum may be pneumococcal meningitis when the strain involved is resistant to penicillin G and also to both cefotaxime and ceftriaxone, but sensitive to meropenem. Fuchs *et al.*, (1996) consider that *Strep. pneumoniae* meningitis would respond to meropenem if the strain's MIC is 0.25 µg per ml or lower, but this still needs clinical confirmation.

References

Aldridge KE, Morize N, Schiro DD (1994). *In vitro* activity of biapenem (L-627)., a new carbapenem, against anaerobes. *Antimicrob Ag Chemother* **38**: 889.

Appelbaum PC, Spangler SK, Jacobs MR (1993). Susceptibility of 539 Gram-positive and Gram-negative anaerobes to new agents, including RP 59500, biapenem, trospectomycin and piperacillin/tazobactam. *J Antimicrob Chemother* **32**: 223.

Bax RP, Bastain W, Featherstone A *et al* (1989). The pharmacokinetics of meropenem in volunteers. *J Antimicrob Chemother* **24** (Suppl A): 311.

Bedikian A, Okamoto MP, Nakahiro RK *et al.* (1994). Pharmacokinetics of meropenem in patients with intra-abdominal infections. *Antimicrob Ag Chemother* **38**: 151.

Brismar B, Malmborg AS, Tunevall G *et al.* (1995). Meropenem versus imipenem/cilastatin in the treatment of intra-abdominal infections. *J Antimicrob Chemother* **35**: 139.

Burman LåA, Nilsson-Ehle I, Hutchison M *et al.* (1991). Pharmacokinetics of meropenem and its metabolite ICI 213, 689 in healthy subjects with known renal metabolism of imipenem. *J Antimicrob Chemother* **27**: 219.

Catchpole CR, Wise R, Thornber D, Andrews JM (1992). *In vitro* activity of L-627, a new carbapenem. *Antimicrob Ag Chemother* **36**: 1928.

Chen HY, Livermore DM (1994a). Comparative *in-vitro* activity of biapenem against enterobacteria with beta-lactamase-mediated antibiotic resistance. *J Antimicrob Chemother* **33**: 453.

Chen HY, Livermore DM (1994b). *In vitro* activity of biapenem, compared with imipenem and meropenem, against *Pseudomonas aeruginosa* strains and mutants with known resistance mechanisms. *J Antimicrob Chemother* **33**: 949.

Chimata M, Nagase M, Suzuki Y *et al.* (1993). Pharmacokinetics of meropenem in patients with various degrees of renal function, including patients with end-stage renal disease. *Antimicrob Ag Chemother* **37**: 229.

Chmelik V, Gutvirth J (1993). Meropenem treatment of post-traumatic meningitis due to *Pseudomonas aeruginosa*. *J Antimicrob Chemother* **32**: 922.

Christensson BA, Nilsson-Ehle I, Hutchison M *et al.* (1992). Pharmacokinetics of meropenem in subjects with various degrees of renal impairment. *Antimicrob Ag Chemother* **36**: 1532.

Cornaglia G, Russell K, Satta G, Fontana R (1995). Relative importances of outer membrane permeability and Group 1 beta-lactamase as determinants of meropenem and imipenem activities against *Enterobacter cloacae*. *Antimicrob Ag Chemother* **39**: 350.

Cuffini AM, Tullio V, Allocco A *et al.* (1993). The entry of meropenem into human macrophages and its immunododulating activity. *J Antimicrob Chemother* **32**: 695.

Dagan R, Velghe L, Rodda JL, Klugman KP (1994). Penetration of meropenem in the cerebrospinal fluid in patients with inflamed meninges. *J Antimicrob Chemother* **34**: 175.

Del Favero A, Bucaneve G, Menichetti F (1995). Empiric monotherapy in neutropenia: a realistic goal? *Scand J Infect Dis* (Suppl 96): 34.

Easmon CSF (1989). Interactions of meropenem into humoral and phagocytic defences. *J Antimicrob Chemother* **24** (Suppl A):.259.

Edwards JR, Turner PJ, Wannop C *et al.* (1989). *In vitro* antibacterial activity of SM-7338, a carbapenem antibiotic with stability to dehydropeptidase. I. *Antimicrob Ag Chemother* **33**: 215.

Friedland IR, Jafari H, Ehret S *et al.* (1993). Comparison of endotoxin release by different antimicrobial agents and the effect of inflammation in experimental *Escherischia coli* meningitis. *J Infect Dis* **168**: 657.

Fuchs PC, Barry AL, Brown SD (1996). Pneumococcal susceptibility to meropenem. *J Antimicrob Chemother* **37**: 1036.

Fukasawa M, Sumita Y, Harabe ET *et al.* (1992). Stability of meropenem and effect of 1 beta-methyl substitution on its stability in the presence of renal dehydropeptidase 1. *Antimicrob Ag Chemother* **36**: 1577.

Garcia-Rodriguez JA, Garcia Sanchez JE, Trujillano I, Sanchez de San Lorenzo A (1991). Meropenem: *in vitro* activity and kinetics of activity against organisms of the *Bacteroides fragilis* group. *J Antimicrob Chemother* **27**: 599.

Granai F, Smart HL, Triger DR (1992). A study of the penetration of meropenem into bile using endoscopic retrograde cholangiography. *J Antimicrob Chemother* **29**: 711.

Harrison MP, Moss SR, Featherstone A *et al.* (1989). The disposition and metabolism of meropenem in laboratory animals and man. *J Antimicrob Chemother* **24** (Suppl A): 265.

Hextall A, Andrews JM, Donovan IA, Wise R (1991). Intraperitoneal penetration of meropenem. *J Antimicrob Chemother* **28**: 314.

Hikida M, Kawashima K, Yoshida M, Mitsuhashi S (1992). Inactivation of new carbapenem antibiotics by dehydropeptidase-1 from porcine and human renal cortex. *J Antimicrob Chemother* **30**: 129.

Hoban DJ, Jones RN, Yamane N *et al.* (1993). *In vitro* activity of three carbapenem antibiotics. Comparative studies with biapenem (L-627)., imipenem, and meropenem against aerobic pathogens isolated worldwide. *Diagn Microbiol Infect Dis* **17**: 299.

Huizinga WKJ, Warren BL, Baker LW *et al.* (1995). Antibiotic monotherapy with meropenem in the surgical management of intra-abdominal infections. *J Antimicrob Chemother* **36** (Supll A): 179.

Jones RN, Aldridge KE, Allen SD *et al.* (1989a). Multicenter *in vitro* evaluation of SM-7338, a new carbapenem. *Antimicrob Ag Chemother* **33**: 562.

Jones RN, Barry AL, Thornsberry C (1989b). *In-vitro* studies of meropenem. *J Antimicrob Chemother* **24** (Suppl A): 9.

Jorgensen JH, Maher LA, Howell AW (1991a). Activity of a new carbapenem antibiotic, meropenem, against *Haemophilus influenzae* strains with beta-lactamase-and non-enzyme-mediated resistance to ampicillin. *Antimicrob Ag Chemother* **35**: 600.

Jorgensen JH, Maher LA, Howell AW (1991b). Activity of meropenem against antibiotic-resistant or infrequently encountered Gram-negative bacilli. *Antimicrob Ag Chemother* **35**: 2410.

Klugman KP, Dagan R (1995). Carbapenem treatment of meningitis. *Scand J Infect Dis* (Suppl 96): 45.

Klugman KP, Dagan R and The Meropenem Meningitis Study Group (1995). Randomized comparison of meropenem with cefotaxime for treatment of bacterial meningitis. *Antimicrob Ag Chemother* **39**: 1140.

Leroy A, Fillastre JP, Borsa-Lebas F *et al.* (1992). Pharmacokinetics of meropenem (ICI 194,660). and its metabolite (ICI 213,689). in healthy subjects and in patients with renal impairment. *Antimicrob Ag Chemother* **36**: 2794.

Lewin C, Doherty C, Govan J (1993). *In vitro* activities of meropenem, PD 127391, PD 131628, ceftazidime, chloramphenicol, co-trimoxazole, and ciprofloxacin against *Pseudomonas cepacia*. *Antimicrob Ag Chemother* **37**: 123.

Livermore DM (1992). Carbapenemases. *J Antimicrob Chemother* **29**: 609.

Livermore DM, Yang Y (1989). Comparative activity of meropenem against *Pseudomonas aeruginosa* strains with well-characterized resistance mechanisms. *J Antimicrob Chemother* **24** (Suppl A): 149.

Ljungberg B, Nilsson-Ehle I (1992). Pharmacokinetics of meropenem and its metabolite in young and elderly healthy men. *Antimicrob Ag Chemother* **36**: 1437.

Malanoski GJ, Collins L, Wennersten C *et al.* (1993). *In vitro* activity of biapenem against clinical isolates of Gram-positive and Gram-negative bacteria. *Antimicrob Ag Chemother* **37**: 2009.

Masuda N, Ohya S (1992). Cross-resistance to meropenem, cephems and quinolones in *Pseudomonas aeruginosa*. *Antimicrob Ag Chemother* **36**: 1847.

Moellering RCJr, Eliopoulos GM, Sentochnick DE (1989). The carbapenems: new broad spectrum beta-lactam antibiotics. *J Antimicrob Chemother* **24** (Suppl A): 1.

Mouton JW, Michel MF (1991). Pharmacokinetics of meropenem in serum and suction blister fluid during continuous and intermittent infusion. *J Antimicrob Chemother* **28**: 911.

Neu HC, Novelli A, Chin N-X (1989). *In vitro* activity and beta-lactamase stability of a new carbapenem, SM-7338. *Antimicrob Ag Chemother* **33**: 1009.

Nord CE, Lindwork A, Persson I (1989). Susceptibility of anaerobic bacteria to meropenem. *J Antimicrob Chemother* **24** (Suppl A): 113.

Odenholt-Tornquist I (1993). Studies on the postantibiotic effect and the postantibiotic sub-MIC effect of meropenem. *J Antimicrob Chemother* **31**: 881.

Patel JB, Giles RE (1989). Meropenem: evidence of lack of proconvulsive tendency in mice. *J Antimicrob Chemother* **24** (Suppl A): 307.

Raimondi A, Traverso A, Nikaido H (1991). Imipenem-and meropenem-resistant mutants of *Enterobacter cloacae* and *Proteus rettgeri* lack porins. *Antimicrob Ag Chemother* **35**: 1174.

Schmutzhard E, Williams KJ, Vukmirovits G *et al.* (1995). A randomized comparison of meropenem with cefotaxime or ceftriaxone for the treatment of bacterial meningitis in adults. *J Antimicrob Chemother* **36** (Suppl A): 85.

Sentochnik DE, Eliopoulos GM, Ferraro MJ, Moellering RC Jr (1989). Comparative *in vitro* activity of SM 7338, a new carbapenem antimicrobial agent. *Antimicrob Ag Chemother* **33**: 1232.

Slaney L, Chubb H, Mohammed Z, Ronald A (1989). *In vitro* activity of meropenem against *Neisseria gonorrhoeae*, *Haemophilus influenzae* and *H ducreyi* from Canada and Kenya. *J Antimicrob Chemother* **24** (Suppl A): 183.

Trias J, Nikaido H (1990). Outer membrane proten D$_2$ catalyses facilitated diffusion of carbapenems and penems through the outer membrane of *Pseudomonas aeruginosa*. *Antimicrob Ag Chemother* **34**: 52.

Watanabe M, Iyobe S, Inoue M, Mitsuhashi S (1991). Transferable imipenem resistance in *Pseudomonas aeruginosa*. *Antimicrob Ag Chemother* **35**: 147.

Watt B, Naden M (1989). The growth-inhibitory properties of meropenem against anaerobes of clinical importance. *J Antimicrob Chemother* **24** (Suppl A): 119.

Wilson SE (1995). Carbapenems: monotherapy in intra-abdominal sepsis. *Scand J Infect Dis* (Suppl 96): 28.

Wise R, Logan M, Cooper M *et al.* (1990). Meropenem pharmacokinetics and penetration into an inflammatory exudate. *Antimicrob Ag Chemother* **34**: 1515.

Yamamoto T, Naigowit P, Deysirilert S *et al.* (1990). *In vitro* susceptibilities of *Pseudomonas pseudomallei* to 27 antimicrobial agents. *Antimicrob Ag Chemother* **34**: 2027.

Yazawa K, Mikami Y, Ohashi S *et al.* (1992). *In-vitro* activity of new carbapenem antibiotics: comparative studies with meropenem, L-627 and imipenem against pathogenic *Nocardia* spp. *J Antimicrob Chemother* **29**: 169.

Yeo SF, Livermore DM (1994). Comparative *in-vitro* activity of biapenem and other carbapenems against *Haemophilus influenzae* isolates with known resistance mechanisms to ampicillin. *J Antimicrob Chemother* **33**: 861.

Cephalothin and Cephaloridine

Description

Cephalothin and cephaloridine are semisynthetic cephalosporins derived from cephalosporin C, a natural antibiotic produced by a strain of the mould *Cephalosporium acremonium*. The cephalosporin C nucleus, 7-ACA, is closely related but not identical to the penicillin nucleus, 6-APA (p. 3). These were the first two cephalosporins introduced for clinical use. Together with the drugs described in the next three chapters, they are often referred to as first-generation cephalosporins.

1 Cephalothin

This parenteral cephalosporin is chemically 7-(thiophene-2-acetamido)-cephalosporanic acid (Griffith and Black, 1964). It is marketed as the sodium salt.

2 Cephaloridine

This was derived by adding two side-chains to the nucleus, and has a formula of 7-(2-thienyl) acetamido)-3-(1-pyridylmethyl)-3-cephem-4-carboxylic acid betaine (Muggleton *et al.*, 1964). Cephaloridine was initially widely used, but it had two main disadvantages. It was an unreliable anti-staphylococcal drug, as it was relatively easily hydrolyzed by *Staphylococcus aureus* beta-lactamase (Laverdiere *et al.*, 1978; Sabath, 1989). Secondly, cephaloridine was nephrotoxic (Foord, 1975; Appel and Neu, 1977). Nowadays this drug is used very rarely, if at all. Therefore further details about cephaloridine will not be given; full description is available in our fourth edition.

The text below only applies to cephalothin.

Sensitive Organisms

1 Staphylococcus aureus

Cephalothin is highly active against non-beta-lactamase-producing staphylococci. It is also highly active against beta-lactamase-producing strains, if sensitivity is tested by either disc diffusion methods or by dilution tests with low inocula (Bell, 1974). When large inocula are used, resistance of the strain to cephalothin is only increased approximately 4-fold (Sabath *et al.*, 1975; Laverdiere *et al.*, 1978) (Table I.18). This is because cephalothin is quite resistant to hydrolysis by staphylococcal beta-lactamase (Regamey *et al.*, 1975; Lacey and Stokes, 1977). It is in accord with clinical findings that cephalothin is a reliable anti-staphylococcal drug (p. 258).

Methicillin-resistant *Staph. aureus* strains (p. 77) are always resistant to cephalothin and all other cephalosporins; this resistance, as in the case of methicillin, is intrinsic and also both heterogeneous and temperature-dependent (p. 78) (Richmond *et al.*, 1977; Laverdiere *et al.*, 1978; Chambers *et al.*, 1984).

Penicillin-tolerant *Staph. aureus* strains (p. 91) also show tolerance to cephalothin. The MICs of cephalothin against these strains are in the usual low (sensitive) range, but MBCs are high (Sabath *et al.*, 1977). Clinical significance of tolerant *Staph. aureus* strains is discussed on p. 91.

2 Other Gram-positive cocci

Most of these, such as coagulase-negative staphylococci, *Streptococcus pyogenes*, *Strep. pneumoniae*, Group B streptococci, and alpha-hemolytic streptococci of the viridans group

(p. 8), are usually sensitive to cephalothin (Bayer *et al.*, 1976; Phillips *et al.*, 1976; Bourbeau and Campos, 1982). Methicillin-resistant coagulase-negative staphylococci (p. 81) are always resistant to all cephalosporins (John and McNeill, 1980; Karchmer *et al.*, 1983). Usually *Staph. saprophyticus* is moderately sensitive to cephalothin (MIC 0.5–2.0 μg per ml) (Bourgault and Gauvreau, 1983).

Enterococcus faecalis and other enterococci are usually cephalothin-resistant (Table I.18), but non-enterococcal group D streptococci, such as *Strep. bovis*, are usually sensitive (Moellering *et al.*, 1974). A cephalosporin antibiotic combined with an aminoglycoside, such as gentamicin, may act synergistically against *E. faecalis*, but these combinations are not useful for the treatment of *E. faecalis* endocarditis. For a synergistic and possibly therapeutic effect, cephalosporin serum levels several times in excess of the MIC of the *E. faecalis* strain are required; such levels cannot be achieved safely in patients (Weinstein and Moellering, 1975; Weinstein and Lentnek, 1976).

Anaerobic Gram-positive cocci, such as *Peptostreptococcus* spp. and anaerobic streptococci, are usually sensitive to cephalothin (Tally *et al.*, 1975; Sutter and Finegold, 1976).

3 Gram-positive bacilli

Bacillus anthracis and *Corynebacterium diphtheriae* are highly susceptible, but *Listeria monocytogenes* is usually only moderately so (MIC 2–4 μg per ml) (Kayser, 1971; Wiggins *et al.*, 1978). *Nocardia* are resistant (Gutmann *et al.*, 1983). Anaerobes, such as *Clostridium perfringens*, *Cl. tetani* and the *Lactobacillus* and *Actinomyces* spp., are usually cephalothin-sensitive (Sutter and Finegold 1976; Bayer *et al.*, 1978). Cephalothin-resistant strains of *Cl. perfringens* have been isolated from patients (Mohr *et al.*, 1978).

4 Gram-negative aerobic bacteria

The *Neisseria* spp. (meningococci and gonococci), *Salmonella* and *Shigella* spp., *Pasteurella multocida* and *Vibrio cholerae* (serogroup 01) are usually sensitive. *Haemophilus influenzae*, *Bordatella pertussis* and *Br. abortus* are only sensitive to a degree, and moderately high cephalothin concentrations are usually needed for inhibition (Waterworth, 1971; Williams and Andrews, 1974). *Moraxella catarrhalis* is usually sensitive to cephalothin. Most strains of this organism produce a beta-lactamase of chromosomal origin, which inactivates penicillins, such as penicillin G (p. 16) and ampicillin (p. 112), but it has no effect on cephalosporins (Doern *et al.*, 1980).

Escherichia coli is usually sensitive but resistant strains are not uncommon, especially in hospitals (Yoshioka *et al.*, 1977). *Proteus mirabilis* and *Providencia alcalifaciens* are usually sensitive. *Proteus vulgaris*, *Providencia rettgeri*, *Providencia stuartii* and *Morganella morganii* are resistant (Penner *et al.*, 1982). Cephalothin and aminoglycosides, such as gentamicin (p. 450), may act synergistically against these organisms. Even if isolates of these species are resistant to both cephalothin and the aminoglycoside, the MIC and MBC of either gentamicin or tobramycin may be reduced by the addition of cephalothin (Hyams *et al.*, 1974).

Susceptibility of the *Klebsiella* spp. varies; *Kl. pneumoniae* is usually sensitive, but *Kl. aerogenes* is less often so. *Klebsiella* spp. strains which are moderately resistant to ampicillin (MIC 32–500 μg per ml), are usually sensitive to cephalothin; but strains that are highly ampicillin-resistant, are also cephalothin-resistant (Greenwood and O'Grady, 1975). *In vitro* synergy can be demonstrated against most *Klebsiella* strains by using cephalothin in combination with an aminoglycoside, such as kanamycin (p. 439), gentamicin (p. 450) or amikacin (p. 504) (D'Alessandri *et al.*, 1976).

All strains of *Serratia* and *Enterobacter* spp., most strains of *Citrobacter*, *Edwardsiella* and *Arizona* spp. and *Yersinia enterocolitica* are highly resistant to cephalothin (Farrar and O'Dell, 1976; Gaspar and Soriano, 1981; Baker and Farmer, 1982). *Pseudomonas aeruginosa* and *Burkholderia* (*Pseudomonas*) *pseudomallei* are always resistant (Waterworth, 1971). *Campylobacter jejuni* is resistant to cephalothin. *Campylobacter fetus* is moderately resistant (MIC 16–32 μg per ml) (Karmali *et al.*, 1980). *Legionella pneumophila* is relatively resistant to cephalothin (MIC 4–32 μg per ml) (Thornsberry *et al.*, 1978). This organism produces a beta-lactamase which inactivates cephalothin, as well as penicillin G (p. 17) and ampicillin (p. 112) (Fu and Neu, 1979). *Legionella micdadei* (Pittsburg pneumonia agent) is moderately sensitive to cephalothin *in vitro* (MIC 2.5 μg per ml), but the drug, similar to penicillin G (p. 17), has poor *in vivo* activity against infections caused by this organism (Dowling *et al.*, 1982).

Organism	MIC (μg per ml)
Gram-positive bacteria	
Staphylococcus aureus (non-penicillinase producer)	0.2
Staphylococcus aureus (penicillinase producer, using light inoculum)	0.25–0.5
Staphylococcus aureus (penicillinase producer, using heavy heavy inoculum	0.8
Streptococcus pyogenes	0.06
Streptococcus pneumoniae	0.06–0.12
Enterococcus faecalis	32.0
Clostridium perfringens	1.0
Gram-negative bacteria	
Escherichia coli	2.0–8.0
Enterobacter spp.	128.0–256.0
Klebsiella aerogenes	2.0–32.0
Proteus mirabilis	4.0–8.0
Proteus vulgaris	64.0–256.0
Neisseria meningitidis	0.12–0.5
Haemophilus influenzae	2.0–8.0
Pseudomonas aeruginosa	Resistant
Bacteroides fragilis	64.0–>512.0
Prevotella melaninogenica	0.5–32.0

Table I.18
Compiled from data published by Barber and Waterworth (1964), Sabath *et al.* (1975), Sutter and Finegold (1976) and Lacey and Stokes (1977)

5 Gram-negative anaerobic bacteria

Bacteroides fragilis is resistant to cephalothin. *Prevotella melaninogenica* and some strains of other *Bacteroides* spp. may be inhibited by therapeutically achievable concentrations of the drug (Tally *et al.*, 1975; Sutter and Finegold, 1976).

6 Other organisms

Treponema pallidum and Leptospirae are sensitive to cephalothin. *Mycobacteria, Mycoplasma, Rickettsiae, Chlamydia, Fungi* and *Protozoa* are resistant (Thompson and Dretler, 1982).

7 Minimum inhibitory concentrations

The MICs of cephalothin against some bacterial species are shown in Table I.18. This antibiotic only has high activity against Gram-positive cocci. Gram-negative bacilli vary greatly in sensitivity; only 50–60% of both *E. coli* and *Pr. mirabilis* strains can be inhibited by relatively low concentrations.

Mode of Administration and Dosage

Cephalothin can only be given parenterally as absorption after oral administration is negligible.

1 Intramuscular and intravenous administration

The dosage by both of these routes is 50–100 mg per kg body weight per day for children, and 0.5–1 g every 4 or 6 h for adults. For serious infections, adult doses as high as 12 g daily have been used (Rahal *et al.*, 1968), but with these doses a serum sickness-like reaction may occur (p. 256). When large doses are used, i.v. administration is preferable because i.m. injections are painful. Cephalothin can be given i.v. by continuous infusion, but intermittent injections or intermittent i.v. infusions of a concentrated solution via a pediatric buretrol, as with penicillin G (p. 256), are preferred. Thrombophlebitis can sometimes be a problem when the drug is used i.v., and this may be reduced if the acid pH of the cephalothin solution is buffered by sodium bicarbonate (Bergeron *et al.*, 1976). Cephalothin sodium suitably buffered to produce a pH in the range of 6.0–8.5 is available commercially.

2 Patients with renal failure

Cephalothin has often been administered to patients with mild to moderate renal impairment with only minor modification of dosage. Venuto and Plaut (1971), studying hemodialysis patients, found that an i.v. dose of 1 g of cephalothin at the beginning of hemodialysis provided an adequate level throughout dialysis; the same dose after dialysis provided adequate serum levels for at least 48 h, indicating that prolonged cephalothin retention did occur in severely uremic patients. The drug itself does not accumulate to any great extent, but its breakdown product, desacetylcephalothin, does (p. 255). This metabolite also has antibacterial activity, which is 2- to 4-fold less than that of cephalothin against Gram-positive bacteria, and 8- to 16-fold less against Gram-negative bacteria (Kirby et al., 1971). Therefore, cephalothin dosage cannot be greatly reduced for the treatment of Gram-negative infections in uremic patients, because such therapy may be ineffective. In this situation, accumulation of therapeutically relatively inactive desacetylcephalothin in the serum, must be accepted. The toxicity of this metabolite is probably not great, but it is possible that this together with high serum levels of cephalothin may aggravate pre-existing renal failure (p. 256) and cause a Coombs' positive hemolytic anemia (p. 257). For these reasons, it is best not to use cephalothin for the treatment of severe Gram-negative infections in patients with severe renal failure (Venuto and Plaut, 1971). It is practicable to reduce the dose of cephalothin for the treatment of Gram-positive infections in such patients (Weinstein and Kaplan, 1970). If patients with normal renal function are given 1 g cephalothin 6-hourly, then those with moderate renal failure should receive this dose 6–8 hourly, and those with severe renal failure should be given 1 g 12-hourly (Kabins and Cohen, 1965; Perkins et al., 1969).

Cephalothin is removed during peritoneal dialysis, and during this procedure a dosage of 1 g 6 to 12-hourly is usually needed (Perkins et al., 1969).

3 Newborn and premature infants

A dosage of 20 mg per kg body weight, administered every 12h, is recommended for infants weighing less than 2000 g and aged less than 7 days; those weighing more than 2000 g but aged less than 7 days (and those weighing less than 2000 g but aged more than 7 days) should be given 20 mg per kg every 8 h; and the dosage for those weighing more than 2000 g and aged more than 7 days is 20 mg per kg every 6 h (McCracken and Nelson, 1983).

4 Intraperitoneal administration

Cephalothin can be added to peritoneal dialysis fluid, commonly in a concentration of 50 µg per ml. If this is used continuously during dialysis, some cephalothin is absorbed, and serum levels of about 10 µg per ml may be attained in patients with renal failure (Bulger et al., 1965).

Serum Levels in Relation to Dosage

After i.m. injection of 0.5 g to adults, the peak serum level of cephalothin is attained after 30 min, and it is about 10 µg per ml (Fig. I.11). Doubling the dose doubles its serum concentration. The cephalothin level with this dose falls below 2 µg per ml after 4 h, and at 6 h the drug is undetectable (Benner et al., 1966).

When a large dose of 12 g cephalothin is administered every 24 h by continuous i.v. infusion, serum levels fluctuate between 10 and 30 µg per ml. If the same daily dose is given by intermittent i.v. injections (3 g every 6 h), peak levels of 150–200 µg per ml are attained, but these fall to 0 before the next dose (Griffith and Black, 1971).

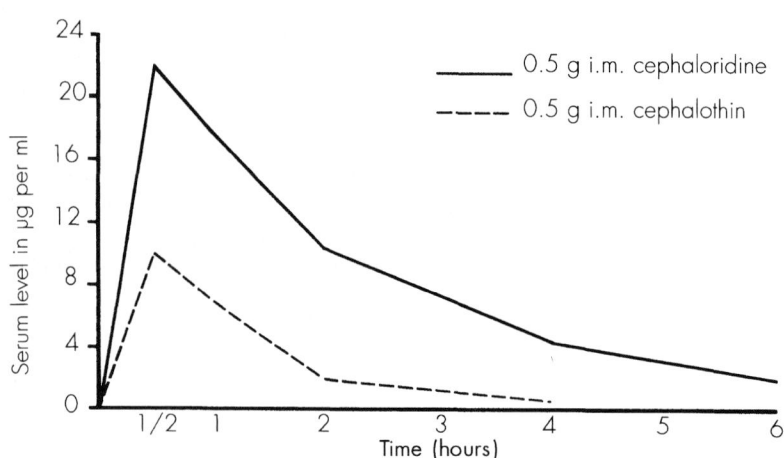

Fig. I.11.

Comparison of serum levels of cephaloridine and cephalothin in healthy male volunteers. (Redrawn after Benner et al., 1996, with permission.)

Excretion

1 Urine and Inactivation in body

Cephalothin is excreted in large amounts in the urine, primarily by tubular secretion, and its elimination is diminished by probenecid (Saslaw, 1970). Cephalothin is also rapidly deacetylated in the body, presumably mainly in the liver, producing the metabolite, desacetylcephalothin. Some cephalothin may be inactivated in the blood, because *in vitro* the drug is destroyed when incubated with human serum at body temperature (Pitkin *et al.*, 1977). About 65% of cephalothin is excreted unchanged and the remainder as its metabolite (Griffith and Black, 1971). Desacetylcephalothin also has antibacterial activity, but this is lower than that of cephalothin (p. 254). In some studies renal functional impairment only caused a slight decrease in the rate of disappearance of cephalothin from the serum; the normal half-life of 0.85 h was increased only to 2.9 h in patients with severe renal failure (Kunin and Atuk, 1966). Others confirmed that in uremic patients there was an early rapid decline in cephalothin serum levels with an apparent half-life of only about 2.8 h, but there was also subsequently a slower decline over the next 8 h resulting in a half-life of about 12 h (Kabins and Cohen, 1965). By using methods which measure cephalothin and desacetylcephalothin serum levels separately, the secondary slow decline in serum level was shown to be chiefly due to the metabolite. For instance, when a 1 g cephalothin dose was given to a uremic patient, the cephalothin level fell rapidly (half-life 2 h), but the desacetylcephalothin concentrations increased over the first 12 h, and then declined slowly with a half-life of 8 h (Kirby *et al.*, 1971). A high desacetylcephalothin serum level (177 µg per ml) was recorded in one uremic patient treated by cephalothin 1 g every 4 h, confirming that this metabolite, which is normally rapidly excreted via the kidney, accumulates in patients with renal failure (Kirby *et al.*, 1971).

2 Bile

Cephalothin is excreted in the bile; measurable concentrations usually occur in both gall bladder and common duct bile, provided that the biliary tract is not obstructed. This drug is not concentrated in the bile to any extent, and levels in the bile are usually lower than those in the serum at the time (Mendelson *et al.*, 1974; Ratzan *et al.*, 1974).

Distribution of the Drug in Body

Cephalothin penetrates very poorly into normal CSF. Even in patients with meningitis, CSF concentrations are only approximately 1% of serum levels at the time. One hour after a 2-g i.v. cephalothin dose to such patients, CSF levels were only 0.16 to 0.31 µg per ml (Vianna and Kaye, 1967). The drug's *in vivo* metabolite, desacetylcephalothin (see above), which has less antibacterial activity than the parent drug, reached higher concentrations in the CSF than cephalothin itself. This may be related to the higher serum level of the metabolite. In addition, cephalothin disappears much more rapidly than its desacetyl derivative from CSF, and some cephalothin is converted to desacetylcephalothin in CSF or its contiguous structures (Nolan and Ulmer, 1980). This intrathecal metabolism of cephalothin may contribute to the unsatisfactory performance of this drug in the therapy of bacterial meningitis. A measurable amount (1.6 µg per g) of cephalothin was found in brain tissue of a patient who had received 2 g of the drug parenterally, 2 to 4 h previously (Griffith and Black, 1971).

Cephalothin penetrated well into inflammatory exudate (Guerrero and McGregor, 1979), parapneumonic effusions (Taryle *et al.*, 1981), ascitic fluid and into the peritoneal fluid of patients with bacterial peritonitis (Gerding *et al.*, 1977; 1978). The concentration in bronchial secretions was usually about 25% of the simultaneous serum level (Wong *et al.*, 1975). Cephalothin concentrations were low in normal bone and synovial tissue. Cortical bone levels of cephalothin in 21 patients 1 h after i.v. administration of 1 g, were 0.9–17.5 µg per g (mean 3.9 µg per g); in 19 patients after the same dose, synovial tissue levels 1 h later were 0.9–5.6 µg per g (mean 2.4 µg per g) (Fitzgerald *et al.*, 1978). Cephalothin was detected in prostatic tissue in a concentration approximately 25% of the simultaneous serum level (Adam *et al.*, 1975). The drug was excreted in adequate concentrations in human pancreatic fluid, and these were higher than those found in animals with induced pancreatitis (Studley *et al.*, 1982). The drug was transferred across the placenta (Morrow *et al.*, 1968).

Perkins and Saslaw (1966) studied tissue levels of cephalothin after death in a patient who had received the drug in a dosage of 2 g 4-hourly. High levels were found in the renal cortex, pleural fluid, myocardium, striated muscle, skin and stomach wall.

Cephalothin is 50–60% serum protein bound (Kunin, 1967).

Mode of Action

Cephalosporins, being beta-lactam antibiotics, act on bacteria in a similar manner to penicillin G (p. 25) (Curtis *et al.*, 1976). There are some differences because structurally different beta-lactams cause different biochemical, morphological and antibacterial effects in the same or other bacterial species (Tomasz, 1979). The PBPs of various bacteria (p. 27) have different affinities to penicillins and cephalosporins, and this is the reason for some of the varying morphological effects on bacteria produced by different beta-lactam antibiotics (Georgopapadakou and Liu, 1980a). For instance, the penicillin-binding proteins of *E. faecalis* have very low affinity for cephalosporins, compared with penicillin G, which explains why this organism is resistant to the cephalosporins (Georgopapadakou and Liu, 1980b).

Toxicity

1 Hypersensitivity reactions

On the assumption that it is not cross-allergenic with the penicillins, cephalothin is frequently recommended for the treatment of infections in penicillin-allergic patients. In some clinical studies allergic reactions have not been observed in penicillin-allergic patients treated with cephalothin (Perkins and Saslaw, 1966; Rahal *et al.*, 1968). Occasionally penicillin-sensitive patients have reacted to cephalosporin C derivatives. Immediate severe reactions to cephalothin in penicillin-allergic patients have been described (Rothschild and Doty, 1966; Scholand *et al.*, 1968; Spruill *et al.*, 1974). A skin-sensitizing antibody to cephalothin and 7-ACA (p. 251) was demonstrated in one patient who had suffered an anaphylactic reaction to penicillin G 5 months previously (Grieco, 1967). This author suggested that cross-reactivity between penicillins and cephalosporins may be more common than is apparent from clinical data, as only 10% of patients with a past history of penicillin allergy exhibit recurrent reactions on readministration of penicillin. A small number of patients in whom the presence of IgE to penicillin was confirmed by positive skin tests to both major and minor penicillin determinants (p. 30), have been treated by one of the cephalosporins and no reactions were observed. The presence of IgE to penicillin determinants in these patients was not predictive of an IgE-mediated reaction to a cephalosporin. This requires further study in a large number of patients (Saxon, 1983; Anderson, 1986).

From large surveys, it appears that 93–97% of patients with a history of penicillin allergy do not react to cephalosporins (Dash, 1975; Boguniewicz and Leung, 1995). Therefore the risk seems small, and cephalosporins may be used in some patients with a past history of penicillin hypersensitivity. It is best to avoid their use in patients with a past history of anaphylaxis or other immediate-type penicillin hypersensitivity reactions (Petz, 1978). If their use in such patients is unavoidable, facilities for treatment of anaphylaxis should be readily available (p. 29).

Allergic manifestations due to cephalothin occur in the absence of a history of penicillin allergy, indicating that this drug itself is allergenic. Cephalothin was administered to 15 volunteers in increasing dosage of up to a maximum of 2 g four times daily, by intermittent rapid i.v. infusions. After 2–4 weeks therapy, they all developed a serum sickness-like illness consisting of malaise, weakness, arthralgia, myalgia, fever, lymphadenopathy and skin rashes. These symptoms appeared to be due to a hypersensitivity reaction (Sanders *et al.*, 1974). Similar reactions were also noted in volunteers treated with cephapirin (p. 282). The authors postulated that the use of large doses of these drugs by rapid i.v. infusion for prolonged periods, may have been responsible for the high rate of reactions. It is possible that similar side-effects have occurred in patients treated by cephalosporins in this way, but they may have been attributed to other causes. Antibodies to cephalosporins may be directed towards side-chain determinants rather than to the common beta-lactam ring (Boguniewicz and Leung, 1995).

As with penicillin G (p. 30), routine testing for possible cephalosporin hypersensitivity, is not practicable.

2 Nephrotoxicity

Cephalothin is much less nephrotoxic than cephaloridine (p. 251). Cephalothin, its metabolite desacetylcephalothin (p. 255), or both, may be responsible for this side-effect. Serum concentrations of the metabolite are very high in patients with renal failure, even when the cephalothin dose is suitably reduced (Nilsson-Ehle and Nilsson-Ehle, 1979). In most reports of nephrotoxicity, there was either evidence of pre-existing renal damage or the cephalothin dosage was unusually large, such as 8–24 g daily for 8–35 days (Rahal *et al.*, 1968; Benner, 1970; Hansten, 1973; Engle *et al.*, 1975; Barrientos *et al.*, 1976). Some instances of cephalothin nephrotoxicity appear to be due to direct toxicity of the drug and this has a histological picture of acute tubular necrosis. Pathology in other cases resembles hypersensitivity interstitial nephritis, similar to that caused by the penicillins (p. 84) (Barza, 1978; Durham and Ibels, 1981).

Acute, usually reversible renal failure, has occurred in patients receiving high doses of cephalothin in combination with gentamicin (Fillastre *et al.*, 1973; Kleinknecht *et al.*, 1973). Gentamicin alone can cause renal damage (p. 467), but this drug combination may be more nephrotoxic than either agent acting alone. Nephrotoxicity has been reported when cephalothin was combined with one of the other aminoglycosides or with one of the polymyxins (Hansten, 1973; Appel and Neu, 1977). In the Boston Collaborative Drug Surveillance Program, data from over 22 000 consecutive patients admitted to hospital were analyzed. A rise in the blood urea was attributed to antibiotic therapy in 8.6% of patients receiving gentamicin alone, 2.9% of those receiving cephalothin alone and 9.3% of those receiving the two drugs together. These data, therefore, did not demonstrate that cephalothin potentiated gentamicin nephrotoxicity (Fanning *et al.*, 1976). In a trial by Giamarellou *et al.* (1979), there was no significant difference in nephrotoxicity between gentamicin- and gentamicin/cephalothin-treated patients. By contrast, two small comparative trials showed that cephalothin potentiated nephrotoxicity of gentamicin to a greater extent than one of the penicillins, such as methicillin or carbenicillin (The EORTC, 1978; Wade *et al.*, 1978). Clinicians should assume that cephalothin may aggravate aminoglycoside nephrotoxicity, and use these combinations with caution (Mannion *et al.*, 1981; Brown *et al.*, 1982; Silverblatt, 1982).

Animal studies have shown that the nephrotoxicity of gentamicin is reduced by simultaneous administration of cephalothin (Dellinger *et al.*, 1976). This does not seem to apply to humans. In animals diuretics such as frusemide may potentiate cephalothin nephrotoxicity (Lawson *et al.*, 1972; Foord, 1975). These diuretics do not have a significant effect on renal clearance of cephalothin in humans (Tice *et al.*, 1975).

3 Hematological side-effects

A positive direct Coombs' test occurs in many patients receiving cephalothin (Molthan *et al.*, 1967). This may interfere with blood cross-matching procedures, but otherwise there are no ill effects. Only a few cases of Coombs' positive hemolytic anemia due to cephalothin have been reported; antibodies of the IgG class against cephalothin were present in the serum (Gralnick *et al.*, 1971; Rubin and Burka, 1977). In a patient with hemolytic anemia due to penicillin G, the disease worsened when cephalothin was substituted, but full recovery occurred 12 days after cephalothin was stopped (Medical News, 1968). Circulating antibodies in this patient were identical to those of another patient who had hemolysis caused by penicillin G only, in that the sera of both patients were equally reactive with penicillin and cephalothin coated red cells (p. 33). A severe cephalothin-induced hemolytic anemia occurred in a patient following aortic valve replacement (Lemole *et al.*, 1972). Cephalothin usually causes an aggregation type hemolytic anemia – it binds to the red cells, but during this process serum proteins are also aggregated. In this condition either the IgG Coombs' test, or the C3 Coombs' test, or both, may be positive (Garratty and Petz, 1975).

Other hematological effects due to cephalothin are rare. Natelson *et al.* (1976) demonstrated combined defects of platelet function and blood coagulation, in volunteers receiving cephalothin in a high dosage of 300 mg per kg per day. The platelet defect was similar to that seen with carbenicillin (p. 153). When cephalothin dosage was reduced to 200 mg per kg per day, platelet and coagulation defects disappeared. This suggests that patients with normal renal function are unlikely to develop bleeding problems due to cephalothin, even when maximum dosages are used. Bleeding may occur in those with impaired renal function or possibly if a cephalothin/carbenicillin combination is used. Thrombocytopenia caused by cephalothin, apparently due to the binding of a specific antibody to cephalothin-coated platelets, has been described (Gralnick *et al.*, 1972). There is a report of leukopenia due to cephalothin (Di Cato and Ellman, 1975). Eosinophilia can be associated with the administration of this drug. In one patient leukopenia and thrombocytopenia developed during cephalothin therapy, and both resolved after the drug was stopped. After 4 weeks when the patient had negative scratch and intradermal skin tests with cephalothin, the drug was readministered. Hematological abnormalities did not recur, suggesting that cephalothin was not the original cause (Naraqi and Raiser, 1982).

Cephalothin, in therapeutic concentrations, may inhibit optimal polymorphonuclear leukocyte microbicidal function (Welch *et al.*, 1981). Cephalothin also appears to suppress lymphocyte transformation, but it enhances production of the lymphokine leukocyte migration-inhibition factor by stimulated lymphocytes; this latter effect may explain some of the immunologic reactions caused by this antibiotic (p. 256) (Larson *et al.*, 1980).

4 Gastrointestinal side-effects

Diarrhea and pseudomembraneous colitis (p. 594) developed in one patient who had been treated successively for over 1 month with oral cephalexin, parenteral cephalothin and parenteral cefazolin (Tures *et al.*, 1976). According to Bartlett *et al.* (1979) both parenteral and oral cephalosporins are quite frequent causes of this complication. They reported 17 patients with pseudomembranous colitis associated with oral or parenteral cephalosporin use, two of whom died. In five of these i.v. cephalothin was involved.

In animals, poorly absorbed cephalosporins, such as cephalothin and cefazolin, administered orally, are effective in preventing clindamycin-induced colitis. The MICs of these cephalosporins for *Cl. difficile* are higher than those of vancomycin and metronidazole, so they are unsatisfactory antibiotics for treating human cases of pseudomembranous colitis (Ebright *et al.*, 1981); *Cl. difficile* is inhibited by 0.2 μg per ml of vancomycin and only by 6.3 μg per ml of cephalothin (Fekety *et al.*, 1979).

5 Other side-effects

Bacterial meningitis occurred in five patients receiving cephalothin for other severe infections (Mangi *et al.*, 1973). Two patients had pneumococcal meningitis and the other three were due to a meningococcus, a *Klebsiella* spp. and *L. monocytogenes*, respectively. Freij *et al.* (1975) reported another patient who developed pneumococcal meningitis during cephalothin treatment for pneumococcal septicemia. The occurrence of meningitis in these circumstances was erroneously described as a specific complication of cephalothin therapy. Meningitis is not an uncommon association of any septicemia. Furthermore, it may develop during treatment, particularly if the antibiotic used, such as cephalothin, does not easily pass into the CSF (p. 255) and the bacterial species involved is not highly susceptible. This has also occurred with other cephalosporins (p. 277).

Teratogenicity in humans due to cephalothin has not been described (Williams and Smith, 1973). Similar to penicillins, cephalosporins can probably be safely used during the first trimester of pregnancy. No adverse effects, such as hemolytic anemia in the newborn, have been detected due to cephalothin administration to mothers near term (Hirsch, 1971).

Clinical Uses of the Drugs

1 Streptococcal and pneumococcal infections

Cephalothin is an useful alternative to penicillin G for the treatment of these infections, but being less effective, it is mainly indicated for penicillin-allergic patients (p. 256) (Symonds and Geddes, 1987). *Streptococcus pyogenes* infections, such as pharyngitis, scarlet fever and cellulitis, and pneumococcal pneumonia respond well to cephalothin (Neu, 1980). Cephalothin alone is quite unsatisfactory for the treatment of pneumococcal and all other types of meningitis (Fisher *et al.*, 1975). Cephalothin is effective for the treatment of *Strep. viridans* or *Strep. bovis* endocarditis but ineffective, even in combination with aminoglycosides, for the treatment of *E. faecalis* endocarditis (Abrutyn *et al.*, 1978; Drake and Sande, 1983).

2 Staphylococcal infections

Cephalothin is a satisfactory anti-staphylococcal agent. Clinical efficacy of cephalothin in severe staphylococcal sepsis is probably about the same as that of the parenteral penicillinase-resistant penicillins (p. 97). Cephalothin is effective in experimental *Staph. aureus* endocarditis in animals (Carrizosa *et al.*, 1982). It may be used for the treatment of severe staphylococcal infections such as septicemia and endocarditis in penicillin-allergic patients, although some clinicians prefer vancomycin (p. 777) (Sande and Scheld, 1980; Kaplan and Tenenbaum, 1982).

Cephalothin is quite ineffective for the treatment of infections caused by methicillin-resistant *Staph. aureus* strains (p. 77). Cephalothin may be used for the treatment of severe *Staph. epidermidis* infections such as prosthetic valve endocarditis, provided the strain is methicillin-sensitive. For infections caused by methicillin-resistant *Staph. epidermidis* strains, cephalothin or any other cephalosporin, is ineffective, even if used in combination with gentamicin and/or rifampicin. For these infections, vancomycin (p. 778) often combined with gentamicin and rifampicin, should be used (Karchmer *et al.*, 1983).

3 Urinary tract infections

Cephalothin is effective in eradicating sensitive strains of *Eschericha coli* and *Pr. mirabilis* from urine, but results are less satisfactory with infections due to *Klebsiella* and *Enterobacter* spp. In chronic infections, associated with urinary tract abnormalities, results of treatment with cephalothin as with other antibiotics, are unsatisfactory.

4 Septicemias due to Gram-negative bacilli

These may be treated by cephalothin, provided the organism is sensitive to a concentration of the drug which is easily attainable *in vivo* (Benner *et al.*, 1966). Cephalothin is not reliable as single agent for initial emergency treatment of severe unidentified Gram-negative infections, but a combination of cephalothin and gentamicin was used successfully in the past. Nowadays cephalothin is no longer used for severe Gram-negative organism sepsis, and one of the more effective third-generation cephalosporins such as cefotaxime (p. 338) or ceftriaxone (p. 360) is usually selected.

5 Actinomycosis

A few patients with this disease have been successfully treated by cephalothin (Caldwell, 1971).

6 Chemoprophylaxis and treatment of Clostridium perfringens infections

It was suggested that cephalothin, administered i.v. in large doses, may be the best alternative drug to penicillin G for treatment of this infection in penicillin-allergic patients (Schwartzman *et al.*, 1977). But Mohr *et al.* (1978) described four cases of clostridial myonecrosis that developed in patients with open fractures, who had received i.v. cephalothin prophylactically. Subsequently, they found four of seven human isolates of *Cl. perfringens* to be cephalothin-resistant. This experience indicates that cephalothin should not be used for the prophylaxis or treatment of gas gangrene. Erythromycin (p. 620), clindamycin (p. 597), chloramphenicol (p. 555) and metronidazole (p. 949) are effective for this infection.

7 Chemoprophylaxis in surgical patients

Bain *et al.* (1977) used cephalothin for prophylaxis in 100 consecutive patients undergoing open heart surgery. It was given in a high dose of 28 g which was administered by continuous i.v. infusion over 48 h. The frequency of postoperative infections was low and drug toxicity was not encountered. Other regimens have been tried, such as 1–2 g cephalothin i.m. or i.v., given as a single intraoperative dose, or repeated 6-hourly for either 2 or 6 days. Available data indicate that prophylaxis for longer than 48 h is unnecessary, and that the 'single-dose' regimen may be sufficient (Archer *et al.*, 1978; Hirschmann and Inui, 1980). Penicillinase-resistant penicillins, such as nafcillin (p. 106), are also satisfactory for cardiac surgery chemoprophylaxis. It is possible that cephalothin and other cephalosporins (p. 287) have been extensively used in cardiac surgery on the erroneous assumption that methicillin-resistant *Staph. epidermidis* strains are cephalosporin-sensitive (p. 78) (Hirschmann and Inui, 1980). Nafcillin plus rifampicin chemoprophylaxis can result in many cardiac surgery patients being colonized with methicillin-resistant *Staph. epidermidis* strains (p. 106). This may also happen when cephalothin chemoprophylaxis is used; and presumably the risk of this would be less with short courses such as 'single-dose' chemoprophylaxis.

Cephalothin or other older cephalosporins, such as cefazolin (p. 287), have been used as chemoprophylactic agents in patients undergoing vascular grafts of the abdominal aorta or lower extremity, vaginal hysterectomy, abdominal hysterectomy and high-risk cesarean section. Clinical trials have established their value in these situations (Hirschmann and Inui, 1980; Neu, 1980). Short-course chemoprophylaxis is preferable, and often a single dose, given at the time of induction of anesthesia, is sufficient (Brennan *et al.*, 1982). Cephalothin has also been used with success in patients undergoing biliary surgery (Neu, 1980), but other antibiotics, such as ampicillin (p. 125), may be preferable. If cephalosporins are used to prevent surgical wound infections, cefazolin (p. 288) may be preferable to cephalothin; both drugs reach acceptable incisional concentrations rapidly in humans; cefazolin concentrations are then well maintained but cephalothin disappears very rapidly (Polk *et al.*, 1980). However, cefazolin may be less effective than cephalothin in preventing *Staph. aureus* infections (Sabath, 1989). These older cephalosporins, unlike some of the newer ones (p. 320), are not effective against Gram-negative anaerobic bacilli.

References

Abrutyn E, Lincoln L, Gallagher M, Weinstein AJ (1978). Cephalothin-gentamicin synergism in experimental enterococcal endocarditis. *J Antimicrob Chemother* **4**: 153.

Adam D, Hofstetter AG, Jacoby W, Reichardt B (1975). Studies on the diffusion of cephradine and cephalothin into human tissue. *Proceedings of 9th International Congress of Chemotherapy*, Abstract M-69.

Anderson JA (1986). Cross-sensitivity of cephalosporins in patients allergic to penicillin. *Pediatr Infect Dis* **5**: 557.

Appel GB, Neu HC (1977). The nephrotoxicity of antimicrobial agents (first of three parts). *New Engl J Med* **296**: 663.

Archer GL, Polk RE, Duma RJ, Lower R (1978). Comparison of cephalothin and cefamandole prophylaxis during insertion of prosthetic heart valves. *Antimicrob Ag Chemother* **13**: 924.

Bain WH, McGeachie J, Lindsay G, Underwood J (1977). The use of cephalothin sodium (Keflin). as the prophylactic antibiotic for open heart surgery. *J Antimicrob Chemother* **3**: 339.

Baker PM, Farmer JJ III (1982). New bacteriophage typing system for *Yersinia enterocolitica, Yersinia kristenseni, Yersinia frederiksenii* and *Yersinia intermedia*: correlation with serotyping, biotyping and antibiotic susceptibility. *J Clin Microbiol* **15**: 491.

Barber M, Waterworth PM (1964). Penicillinase-resistant penicillins and cephalosporins. *Brit Med J* **2**: 344.

Barrientos A, Bello I, Gutierrez-Millet V et al. (1976). Renal failure and cephalothin. *Ann Intern Med* **84**: 612.

Bartlett JG, Willey SH, Chang TW, Lowe B (1979). Cephalosporin-associated pseudomembranous colitis due to *Clostridium difficile*. *JAMA* **242**: 2683.

Barza M (1978). The nephrotoxicity of cephalosporins: an overview. *J Infect Dis* **137** (Suppl): 60.

Bayer AS, Chow AW, Anthony BF, Guze LB (1976). Serious infections in adults due to Group B streptococci. Clinical and serotypic characterization. *Amer J Med* **61**: 498.

Bayer AS, Chow AW, Concepcion N, Guze LB (1978). Susceptibility of 40 lacto-bacilli to six antimicrobial agents with broad Gram-negative anaerobic spectra. *Antimicrob Ag Chemother* **14**: 720.

Bell SM (1974). The significance of sensitivity tests of *Staphylococcus aureus* to cephaloridine. *Med J Aust* **2**: 902.

Benner EJ (1970). Renal damage associated with prolonged administration of ampicillin, cephaloridine and cephalothin. *Antimicrob Ag Chemother* **1969**: 417.

Benner EJ, Brodie JS, Kirby WMM (1966). Laboratory and clinical comparison of cephaloridine and cephalothin. *Antimicrob Ag Chemother* **1965**: 888.

Bergeron MG, Brusch JL, Barza M, Weinstein L (1976). Significant reduction in the incidence of phlebitis with buffered versus unbuffered cephalothin. *Antimicrob Ag Chemother* **9**: 646.

Boguniewicz M, Leung DYM (1995). Hypersensitivity reactions to antibiotics commonly used in children. *Pediatr Infect Dis J* **14**: 221.

Bourbeau P, Campos JM (1982). Current antibiotic susceptibility of Group A beta-hemolytic streptococci. *J Infect Dis* **145**: 916.

Bourgault A-M, Gauvreau L (1983). Antimicrobial susceptibilities of coagulase-negative staphylococci isolated from urinary infections. *Antimicrob Ag Chemother* **23**: 793.

Brennan SS, Pickford IR, Evans M, Pollock AV (1982). The prophylaxis of wound infection after abdominal operations: is one dose of antibiotic enough? *J Hosp Infect* **3**: 351.

Brown AE, Queseda O, Armstrong D (1982). Minimal nephrotoxicity with cephalosporin-aminoglycoside combinations in patients with neoplastic disease. *Antimicrob Ag Chemother* **21**: 592.

Bulger RJ, Bennett JV, Boen ST (1965). Intraperitoneal administration of broad-spectrum antibiotics in patients with renal failure. *JAMA* **194**: 1198.

Caldwell JL (1971). Actinomycosis treated with cephalothin. *South Med J* **64**: 987.

Carrizosa J, Kobasa WD, Snepar R et al. (1982). Cefazolin versus cephalothin in beta-lactamase-producing *Staphylococcus aureus* endocarditis in a rabbit experimental model. *J Antimicrob Chemother* **9**: 387.

Chambers HF, Hackbarth CJ, Drake TA et al. (1984). Endocarditis due to methicillin-resistant *Staphylococcus aureus* in rabbits: expression of resistance to beta-lactam antibiotics *in vivo* and *in vitro*. *J Infect Dis* **149**: 894.

Curtis NAC, Hughes JM, Ross GW (1976). Inhibition of peptidoglycan cross-linking in growing cells of *Escherichia coli* by penicillins and cephalosporins, and its prevention by R factor-mediated beta-lactamase. *Antimicrob Ag Chemother* **9**: 208.

D'Alessandri RM, McNeely DJ, Kluge RM (1976). Antibiotic synergy and antagonism against clinical isolates of *Klebsiella* species. *Antimicrob Ag Chemother* **10**: 889.

Dash CH (1975). Penicillin allergy and the cephalosporins. *J Antimicrob Chemother* **1** (Suppl): 107.

Dellinger P, Murphy T, Pinn V et al. (1976). Protective effect of cephalothin against gentamicin-induced nephrotoxicity in rats. *Antimicrob Ag Chemother* **9**: 172.

Di Cato M-A, Ellman L (1975). Cephalothin-induced granulocytopenia. *Ann Intern Med* **83**: 671.

Doern GV, Siebers KG, Hallick LM, Morse SA (1980). Antibiotic susceptibility of beta-lactamase-producing strains of *Branhamella (Neisseria) catarrhalis*. *Antimicrob Ag Chemother* **17**: 24.

Dowling JN, Weyant RS, Pasculle AW (1982). Bactericidal activity of antibiotics against *Legionella micdadei* (Pittsburg pneumonia agent). *Antimicrob Ag Chemother* **22**: 272.

Drake TA, Sande MA (1983). Studies of the chemotherapy of endocarditis: correlation of *in vitro*, animal model, and clinical studies. *Rev Infect Dis* **5** (Suppl 2): 345.

Durham DS, Ibels LS (1981). Cephalothin-induced acute allergic interstitial nephritis. *Aust NZ J Med* **11**: 266.

Ebright JR, Fekety R, Silva J, Wilson KH (1981). Evaluation of eight cephalosporins in hamster colitis model. *Antimicrob Ag Chemother* **19**: 980.

Engle JE, Drago J, Carlin B, Schoolwerth AC (1975). Reversible acute renal failure after cephalothin. *Ann Intern Med* **83**: 232.

Fanning WL, Gump D, Jick H (1976). Gentamicin- and cephalothin-associated rises in blood urea nitrogen. *Antimicrob Ag Chemother* **10**: 80.

Farrar WE Jr, O'Dell NM (1976). Beta-lactamases and resistance to penicillins and cephalosporins in *Serratia marcescens*. *J Infect Dis* **134**: 245.

Fekety R, Silva J, Toshniwal R et al. (1979). Antibiotic-associated colitis: effects of antibiotics on *Clostridium difficile* and the disease in hamsters. *Rev Infect Dis* **1**: 386.

Fillastre JP, Laumonier R, Humbert G et al. (1973). Acute renal failure associated with combined gentamicin and cephalothin therapy. *Brit Med J* **2**: 396.

Fisher LS, Chow AW, Yoshikawa TA, Guze LB (1975). Cephalothin and cephaloridine therapy for bacterial meningitis. An evaluation. *Ann Intern Med* **82**: 689.

Fitzgerald RH Jr, Kelly PJ, Snyder RJ, Washington JA II (1978). Penetration of methicillin, oxacillin, cephalothin into bone and synovial tissue. *Antimicrob Ag Chemother* **14**: 723.

Foord RD (1975). Cephaloridine, cephalothin and the kidney. *J Antimicrob Chemother* **1** (Suppl): 119.

Freij L, Hebelka M, Seeberg S (1975). Meningitis developing during cephalothin therapy of septicaemia. *Scand J Infect Dis* **7**: 153.

Fu KP, Neu HC (1979). Inactivation of beta-lactam antibiotics by *Legionella pneumophila*. *Antimicrob Ag Chemother* **16**: 561.

Garratty G, Petz LD (1975). Drug-induced immune hemolytic anemia. *Amer J Med* **58**: 398.

Gaspar MC, Soriano F (1981). Susceptibility of *Yersinia enterocolitica* to eight beta-lactam antibiotics and clavulanic acid. *J Antimicrob Chemother* **8**: 161.

Georgopapadakou NH, Liu FY, (1980a). Penicillin-binding protein in bacteria. *Antimicrob Ag Chemother* **18**: 148.

Georgopapdakou NH, Liu FY (1980b). Binding of beta-lactam antibiotics to penicillin-binding proteins of *Staphylococcus aureus* and *Streptococcus faecalis*: relation to antibacterial activity. *Antimicrob Ag Chemother* **18**: 834.

Gerding DN, Hall WH, Schierl EA (1977). Antibiotic concentrations in ascitic fluid of patients with ascites and bacterial peritonitis. *Ann Intern Med* **86**: 708.

Gerding DN, Peterson LR, Legler DC *et al.* (1978). Ascitic fluid cephalosporin concentrations: influence of protein binding and serum pharmacokinetics. *Antimicrob Ag Chemother* **14**: 234.

Giamarellou H, Metzikoff Ch, Papachristophorou S *et al.* (1979). Prospective comparative evaluation of gentamicin or gentamicin plus cephalothin in the production of nephrotoxicity in man. *J Antimicrob Chemother* **5**: 581.

Gralnick HR, McGinniss M, Elton W, McCurdy P (1971). Hemolytic anemia associated with cephalothin. *JAMA* **217**: 1193.

Gralnick HR, McGinniss M, Halterman R (1972). Thrombocytopenia with sodium cephalothin therapy. *Ann Intern Med* **77**: 401.

Greenwood D, O'Grady F (1975). Resistance categories of enterobacteria to beta-lactam antibiotics. *J Infect Dis* **132**: 233.

Grieco MH (1967). Cross-allergenicity of the penicillins and the cephalosporins. *Arch Intern Med* **119**: 141.

Griffith RS, Black HR (1964). Cephalothin – a new antibiotic. *JAMA* **189**: 823.

Griffith RS, Black HR (1971). Blood, urine and tissue concentrations of the cephalosporin antibiotics in normal subjects. *Postgrad Med J* **47** (Suppl): 32.

Guerrero IC, MacGregor RR (1979). Comparative penetration of various cephalosporins into inflammatory exudate. *Antimicrob Ag Chemother* **15**: 712.

Gutmann L, Goldstein FW, Kitzis MD *et al.* (1983). Susceptibility of *Nocardia asteroides* to 46 antibiotics, including 22 beta lactams. *Antimicrob Ag Chemother* **23**: 248.

Hansten PD (1973). Cephalothin, gentamicin, colistin hazards. *JAMA* **223**: 1158.

Hirsch HA (1971). The use of cephalosporin antibiotics in pregnant women. *Postgrad Med J* **47** (Suppl): 90.

Hirschmann JV, Inui TS (1980). Antimicrobial prophylaxis: a critique of recent trials. *Rev Infect Dis* **2**: 1.

Hymans PJ, Simberkoff MS, Rahal JJ Jr (1974). Synergy between cephalosporin and aminoglycoside antibiotics against *Providencia* and *Proteus*. *Antimicrob Ag Chemother* **5**: 571.

John JF Jr, McNeill WF (1980). Activity of cephalosporins against methicillin-susceptible and methicillin-resistant, coagulase-negative staphylococci: minimal effect of beta-lactamase. *Antimicrob Ag Chemother* **17**: 179.

Kabins SA, Cohen S (1965). Cephalothin serum levels in the azotemic patient. *Antimicrob Ag Chemother* **1964**: 207.

Kaplan MH, Tenenbaum MJ (1982). *Staphylococcus aureus*: cellular biology and clinical application. *Amer J Med* **72**: 248.

Karchmer AW, Archer GL, Dismukes WE (1983). *Staphylococcus epidermidis* causing prosthetic valve endocarditis: microbiologic and clinical observations as guides to therapy. *Ann Intern Med* **98**: 447.

Karmali MA, De Grandis S, Fleming PC (1980). Antimicrobial susceptibility of *Campylobacter jejuni* and *Campylobacter fetus* subs. *fetus* to eight cephalosporins with special reference to species differentiation. *Antimicrob Ag Chemother* **18**: 948.

Kayser FH (1971). *In vitro* activity of cephalosporin antibiotics against Gram-positive bacteria. *Postgrad Med J* **47** (Suppl): 14.

Kirby WMM, de Maine JB, Serrill WS (1971). Pharmacokinetics of the cephalosporins in healthy volunteers and uremic patients. *Postgrad Med J* **47** (Suppl): 41.

Kleinknecht D, Ganeval D, Droz D (1973). Acute renal failure after high doses of gentamicin and cephalothin. *Lancet* **i**: 1129.

Kunin CM (1967). A guide to use of antibiotics in patients with renal disease. *Ann Intern Med* **67**: 151.

Kunin CM, Atuk N (1966). Excretion of cephaloridine and cephalothin in patients with renal impairment. *New Engl J Med* **274**: 654.

Lacey RW, Stokes A (1977). Susceptibility of the 'penicillinase-resistant' penicillins and cephalosporins to penicillinase of *Staphylococcus aureus*. *J Clin Path* **30**: 35.

Larson SE, Damert GJ, Collins-Lech C, Sohnle PG (1980). Direct stimulation of lymphokine production by cephalothin. *J Infect Dis* **142**: 265.

Laverdiere M, Welter D, Sabath LD (1978). Use of a heavy inoculum in the *in vitro* evaluation of the anti-staphylococcal activity of 19 cephalosporins. *Antimicrob Ag Chemother* **13**: 669.

Lawson DH, Macadam RF, Singh H *et al.* (1972). Effect of furosemide on antibiotic-induced renal damage in rats. *J Infect Dis* **126**: 593.

Lemole GM, Fadali AMA, Molthan L (1972). Cephalothin-induced tachycardia following aortic valve replacement. *JAMA* **221**: 593.

Mangi RJ, Kundargi RS, Quintiliani R, Andriole VT (1973). Development of meningitis during cephalothin therapy. *Ann Intern Med* **78**: 347.

Mannion JC, Bloch R, Popovich NG (1981). Cephalosporin-aminoglycoside synergistic nephrotoxicity: fact or fiction? *Drug Intell Clin Pharm* **15**: 248.

McCracken GH Jr, Nelson JD (1983). *Antimicrobial Therapy for Newborns* 2nd edn, p. 31. New York: Grune and Stratton.

Medical News (1968). Reactions to cephalothin. *JAMA* **206**: 1701.

Mendelson J, Portnoy J, Sigman H, Dick V (1974). Pharmacology of cephalothin in the biliary tract of humans. *Antimicrob Ag Chemother* **6**: 659.

Moellering RC Jr, Watson BK, Kunz LJ (1974). Endocarditis due to Group D streptococci Comparison of disease caused by *Streptococcus bovis* with that produced by the enterococci. *Amer J Med* **57**: 239.

Mohr JA, Griffiths W, Holm R *et al.* (1978). Clostridial myonecrosis ('gas gangrene'). during cephalosporin prophylaxis. *JAMA* **239**: 847.

Molthan L, Reidenberg MM, Eichman MF (1967). Positive direct Coombs' tests due to cephalothin. *New Engl J Med* **277**: 123.

Morrow S, Palmisano P, Cassady G (1968). The placental transfer of cephalothin. *J Pediatr* **73**: 262.

Muggleton PW, O'Callaghan CH, Stevens WK (1964). Laboratory evaluation of a new antibiotic – cephaloridine (ceporan). *Brit Med J* **2**: 1234.

Naraqi S, Raiser M (1982). Nonrecurrence of cephalothin-associated granulocytopenia and thrombocytopenia. *J Infect Dis* **145**: 281.

Natelson EA, Brown CH III, Bradshaw MW *et al.* (1976). Influence of cephalosporin antibiotics on blood coagulation and platelet function. *Antimicrob Ag Chemother* **9**: 91.

Neu HC (1980). The place of cephalosporins in antibacterial treatment of infectious diseases. *J Antimicrob Chemother* **6** (Suppl A): 1.

Nilsson-Ehle I, Nilsson-Ehle P (1979). Pharmacokinetics of cephalothin: accumulation of its deacetylated metabolite in uremic patients. *J Infect Dis* **139**: 712.

Nolan CM, Ulmer WC Jr (1980). A study of cephalothin and desacetylcephalothin in cerebrospinal fluid in therapy for experimental pneumococcal meningitis. *J Infect Dis* **141**: 326.

Penner J L, Preston MA, Hennessy JN *et al.* (1982). Species differences in susceptibilities of *Proteeae* spp to six cephalosporins and three aminoglycosides. *Antimicrob Ag Chemother* **22**: 218.

Perkins RL, Saslaw S (1966). Experience with cephalothin. *Ann Intern Med* **64**: 13.

Perkins RL, Smith EJ, Saslaw S (1969). Cephalothin and cephaloridine: comparative pharmacodynamics in chronic uremia. *Amer J Med Sci* **257**: 116.

Petz LD (1978). Immunologic cross-reactivity between penicillins and cephalosporins: a review. *J Infect Dis* **137** (Suppl): 74.

Phillips I, Warren C, Harrison JM *et al.* (1976). Antibiotic susceptibilities of streptococci from the mouth and blood of patients treated with penicillin or lincomycin and clindamycin. *J Med Microbiol* **9**: 393.

Pitkin D, Actor P, Filan JJ *et al.* (1977). Comparative stability of cephalothin and cefazolin in buffer in human serum. *Antimicrob Ag Chemother* **12**: 284.

Polk HC Jr, Trachtenberg L, Finn MP (1980). Antibiotic activity in surgical incisions. The basis for prophylaxis in selected operations. *JAMA* **244**: 1353.

Rahal JJ Jr, Meyers BR, Weinstein L (1968). Treatment of bacterial endocarditis with cephalothin. *New Engl J Med* **279**: 1305.

Ratzan KR, Ruiz C, Irvin GL III (1974). Biliary tract excretion of cefazolin, cephalothin, and cephaloridine in the presence of biliary tract disease. *Antimicrob Ag Chemother* **6**: 426.

Regamey C, Libke RD, Engelking ER *et al.* (1975). Inactivation of cefazolin, cephaloridine and cephalothin by methicillin-sensitive and methicillin-resistant strains of *Staphylococcus aureus*. *J Infect Dis* **131**: 291.

Richmond AS, Simberkoff MS, Schaefler S, Rahal JJ Jr (1977). Resistance of *Staphylococcus aureus* to semisynthetic penicillins and cephalothin. *J Infect Dis* **135**: 108.

Rothschild PD, Doty DB (1966). Cephalothin reaction after penicillin sensitization. *JAMA* **196**: 372.

Rubin RN, Burka ER (1977). Anti-cephalothin antibody and Coombs'-positive hemolytic anemia. *Ann Intern Med* **86**: 64.

Sabath LD (1989). Reappraisal of the antistaphylococcal activities of first-generation (narrow spectrum). and second-generation (expanded spectrum). cephalosporins. *Antimicrob Ag Chemother* **33**: 407.

Sabath LD, Garner C, Wilcox C, Finland M (1975). Effect of inoculum and of beta-lactamase on the anti-staphylococcal activity of thirteen penicillins and cephalosporins. *Antimicrob Ag Chemother* **8**: 344.

Sabath LD, Wheeler N, Laverdiere M *et al.* (1977). A new type of penicillin resistance of *Staphylococcus aureus*. *Lancet* i: 443.

Sande MA, Scheld WM (1980). Combination antibiotic therapy of bacterial endocarditis. *Ann Intern Med* **92**: 390.

Sanders WE Jr, Johnson JE III, Taggart JG (1974). Adverse reactions to cephalothin and cephapirin. Uniform occurrence on prolonged intravenous administration of high doses. *New Engl J Med* **290**: 424.

Saslaw S (1970). Cephalosporins. *Med Clin N Amer* **54**: 1217.

Saxon A (1983). Immediate hypersensitivity reactions to beta-lactam antibiotics. *Rev Infect Dis* **5** (Suppl 2): 368.

Scholand JF, Tennenbaum JI, Cerilli GJ (1968). Anaphylaxis to cephalothin in a patient allergic to penicillin. *JAMA* **206**: 130.

Schwartzman JD, Reller LB, Wang W-LL (1977). Susceptibility of *Clostridium perfringens* isolated from human infections to twenty antibiotics. *Antimicrob Ag Chemother* **11**: 695.

Silverblatt F (1982). Pathogenesis of nephrotoxicity of cephalosporins and aminoglycosides: a review of current concepts. *Rev Infect Dis* **4** (Suppl): 360.

Spruill FG, Minette LJ, Sturner WQ (1974). Two surgical deaths associated with cephalothin. *JAMA* **229**: 440.

Studley JGN, Schentag JJ, Schenk WG Jr (1982). Excretion of cephalothin and cefamandole by the normal pancreas and in acute pancreatitis in dogs. *Antimicrob Ag Chemother* **22**: 262.

Sutter VL, Finegold SM (1976). Susceptibility of anaerobic bacteria to 23 anti-microbial agents. *Antimicrob Ag Chemother* **10**: 736.

Symonds J, Geddes AM (1987). Cephalosporins in Gram-positive infections *Drugs* **34** (Suppl 2): 121.

Tally FP, Jacobus NV, Bartlett JG, Gorbach SL (1975). Susceptibility of anaerobes to cefoxitin and other cephalosporins. *Antimicrob Ag Chemother* **7**: 128.

Taryle DA, Good JT Jr, Morgan EJ III *et al.* (1981). Antibiotic concentrations in human parapneumonic effusions. *J Antimicrob Chemother* **7**: 171.

The EORTC International Antimicrobial Therapy Project Group (1978). Three antibiotic regimens in the treatment of infection in febrile granulocytopenic patients with cancer. *J Infect Dis* **137**: 14.

Thompson SE III, Dretler RH (1982). Epidemiology and treatment of chlamydial infections in pregnant women and infants. *Rev Infect Dis* **4** (Suppl): 747.

Thornsberry C, Baker CN, Kirven LA (1978). *In vitro* activity of antimicrobial agents on Legionnaires disease bacterium. *Antimicrob Ag Chemother* **13**: 78.

Tice AD, Barza M, Bergeron MG *et al.* (1975). Effect of diuretics on urinary excretion of cephalothin in humans. *Antimicrob Ag Chemother* **7**: 168.

Tomasz A (1979). From penicillin-binding proteins to the lysis and death of bacteria: a 1979 view. *Rev Infect Dis* **1**: 434.

Tures JF, Townsend WF, Rose HD (1976). Cephalosporin-associated pseudomembranous colitis. *JAMA* **236**: 948.

Venuto RC, Plaut ME (1971). Cephalothin handling in patients undergoing hemodialysis. *Antimicrob Ag Chemother* **1970**: 50.

Vianna NJ, Kaye D (1967). Penetration of cephalothin into the spinal fluid. *Amer J Med Sci* **254**: 216, quoted by Fisher *et al.* (1975).

Wade JC, Smith CR, Petty GB *et al.* (1978). Cephalothin plus an aminoglycoside is more nephrotoxic than methicillin plus an aminoglycoside. *Lancet* ii: 604.

Waterworth PM (1971). The susceptibility of pathogenic Gram-negative bacilli to cephalosporins. *Postgrad Med J* **47** (Suppl): 25.

Weinstein L, Kaplan K (1970). The cephalosporins Microbiological, chemical and pharmacological properties and use in chemotherapy of infection. *Ann Intern Med* **72**: 729.

Weinstein AJ, Lentnek AL (1976). Cephalosporin-aminoglycoside synergism in experimental enterococcal endocarditis. *Antimicrob Ag Chemother* **9**: 983.

Weinstein AJ, Moellering RC Jr (1975). Studies of cephalothin: aminoglycoside synergism against enterococci. *Antimicrob Ag Chemother* **7**: 522.

Welch WD, Davis D, Thrupp LD (1981). Effect of antimicrobial agents on human polymorphonuclear leukocyte microbicidal function. *Antimicrob Ag Chemother* **20**: 15.

Wiggins GL, Albritton WL, Feeley JC (1978). Antibiotic susceptibility of clinical isolates of *Listeria monocytogenes*. *Antimicrob Ag Chemother* **13**: 854.

Williams JD, Andrews J (1974). Sensitivity of *Haemophilus influenzae* to antibiotics. *Brit Med J* **1**: 134.

Williams JD, Smith EK (1973). Antibiotic use in obstetric patients In *Current Antibiotic Therapy* (Geddes AM, Williams JD, eds), p. 71. Edinburgh and London: Churchill Livingstone.

Wong GA, Peirce TH, Goldstein E, Hoeprich PD (1975). Penetration of antimicrobial agents into bronchial secretions. *Amer J Med* **59**: 219.

Yoshioka H, Rudoy P, Riley HD Jr, Yoshida K (1977). Antimicrobial susceptibility of *Escherichia coli* isolated at a children's hospital. *Scand J Infect Dis* **9**: 207.

Cephalexin

Description

Cephalexin is a semisynthetic antibiotic derived from cephalosporin C (p. 251), but unlike cephalothin (p. 251), it is absorbed after oral administration.

Sensitive Organisms

The antibacterial spectrum of cephalexin resembles that of cephalothin (p. 251) but in general, its activity is of a lower order against most bacteria (Muggleton et al., 1969).

1 Gram-positive cocci

Similar to cephalothin (p. 251), cephalexin is relatively resistant to inactivation by staphylococcal beta-lactamase (Sabath et al., 1975). Nevertheless, only penicillin G-sensitive *Staphylococcus aureus* strains are uniformly cephalexin-sensitive; beta-lactamase-producing strains vary in their degree of susceptibility and their MICs are generally higher than those of penicillin G-sensitive strains (Braun et al., 1968) (Table I.19). Methicillin-resistant *Staph. aureus* strains (p. 77) are resistant to cephalexin (Kayser, 1971).

Most other aerobic Gram-positive cocci, such as coagulase-negative staphylococci; *Streptococcus pyogenes*, *Strep. pneumoniae* and *Strep. viridans* are cephalexin-sensitive. Methicillin-resistant coagulase-negative staphylococcal strains are resistant to cephalexin (p. 81). *Enterococcus faecalis* is resistant (Marrie and Kwan, 1982). Anaerobic Gram-positive cocci such as the *Peptococcus* and *Peptostreptococcus* spp. are usually moderately sensitive. Most strains recovered from airway associated infections are inhibited by 8–16 µg per ml. Other strains are resistant, needing 64 µg per ml or higher for inhibition (Tally et al., 1975; Busch et al., 1976).

2 Gram-positive bacilli

Corynebacterium diphtheriae is cephalexin-sensitive but *Listeria monocytogenes* is relatively resistant (Wick, 1967; Kayser, 1971). Anaerobic Gram-positive rods, such as *Clostridium perfringens*, *Cl. tetani* and other *Clostridium* spp., are relatively resistant. Some strains may be inhibited by 8–16 µg per ml of cephalexin but others need 32–64 µg per ml, or even higher, for inhibition (Tally et al., 1975).

3 Gram-negative aerobic bacteria

The *Neisseria* spp. (meningococci and gonococci) are sensitive. Cephalexin retains moderate *in vitro* activity against beta-lactamase-producing gonococci (p. 15); it inhibits large inocula of these strains at a concentration of 2.5 µg per ml (Selwyn and Bakhtiar, 1977).

Other Gram-negative bacteria vary in sensitivity. Some strains of *E. coli*, *Pr. mirabilis* and *Klebsiella*, *Salmonella* and *Shigella* spp., may be inhibited by concentrations of cephalexin that can be easily attained *in vivo*, but other strains require much higher concentrations (Braun et al., 1968; Konforti and Halperin, 1975). High concentrations of cephalexin can be attained in urine (p. 267). *Salmonella* spp. strains can become cephalexin-resistant not because of beta-lactamase production, but because of loss of certain porins in their cell wall (Medeiros et al., 1987). *Bordetella pertussis* and *H. influenzae* are both moderately resistant (Waterworth, 1971; Powell and Williams, 1988). *Proteus vulgaris*, *Morganella morganii*, *Enterobacter* spp. and especially *Pseudomonas aeruginosa* are always cephalexin-resistant. *Serratia marcescens* and the *Providencia*, *Hafnia*, *Citrobacter*, *Edwardsiella* and *Arizona* spp. are also usually not susceptible. *Campylobacter jejuni* is resistant (Karmali et al., 1980).

Organism	MIC (μg per ml)	
	Range	Median
Gram-positive bacteria		
Staphylococcus aureus (non-penicillinase producer)	1.6–12.5	3.1
Staphylococcus aureus (penicillinase producer)	1.6–>100	12.5
Streptococcus pyrogenes (Group A)	0.2–6.3	0.4
Streptococcus pneumoniae	1.6–6.3	3.1
Streptococcus viridans	0.8–12.5	6.3
Enterococcus faecalis	100–>100	100
Peptostreptococcus spp.	0.5–64.0	–
Clostridium perfringens	8.0–64.0	–
Gram-negative bacteria		
Escherichia coli	25–>100	>100
Enterobacter spp.	50 > 100	50
Klebsiella pneumoniae	50 > 100	> 100
Serratia marcescens	50–>100	100
Proteus mirabilis	>100	>100
Proteus vulgaris	25–>100	>100
Neisseria gonorhoeae	0.1–6.3	3.1
Neisseria meningitidis	1.6–6.3	3.1
Haemophilus influenzae	12.5–>100	>100
Pseudomonas aeruginosa	>100	>100
Bacteroides fragilis	>64.0	–

Table I.19
Compiled from data published by Braun *et al.* (1968) and Talley *et al.* (1975)

4 Gram-negative anaerobic bacteria

Bacteroides fragilis is cephalexin-resistant but other anaerobes, such as *Prevotella* spp., which populate the oropharynx, are sensitive. Similarly, *Fusobacterium* and *Veillonella* spp. are usually sensitive to cephalexin, especially strains recovered from airway-related infections, as opposed to those isolated from intra-abdominal infections (Tally *et al.*, 1975; Busch *et al.*, 1976).

5 Other organisms

Mycoplasma and Mycobacteria are cephalexin-resistant.

6 Minimum inhibitory concentrations

The MICs of cephalexin against some bacterial species are shown in Table I.19. Braun *et al.* (1968) found that most strains of Gram-negative aerobic bacilli were resistant to cephalexin at 100 μg per ml. More sensitive strains of *E. coli*, *Pr. mirabilis* and *Klebsiella* spp. have been reported by others as shown in Table I.20.

Mode of Administration and Dosage

1 Mild to moderate infections

The usual adult dosage for these infections is 250–500 mg four times a day, and for children 25–50 mg per kg body weight, per day, given in four divided doses. For milder infections cephalexin has also been given in an adult dose of 500 mg 12-hourly (Kumar *et al.*, 1988).

2 Severe systemic infections

Cephalexin has been tried in moderately severe systemic infections, in a higher dosage of 3–4 g daily (Bailey *et al.*, 1970). The corresponding dosage for children is up to 100 mg per kg per day.

Organism	MIC (μg per ml)
Escherichia coli	16.0
Proteus mirabilis	31.0
Klebsiella pneumoniae	16.0

Table I.20
After Muggleton *et al.* (1969)

For treatment of severe infections, an adult dose of 6 g daily has been occasionally used, sometimes with probenecid (Zabransky *et al.*, 1969).

3 Patients with renal failure

Cephalexin accumulates in these patients so that dosage modification with serum level estimations is necessary. Table I.21 shows a proposed dosage regimen for treatment of moderately severe systemic infections, in patients with various degrees of renal impairment. Oral cephalexin dosage schedules in this table are designed to produce sustained serum levels of 12 or 30 μg per ml. The former level is sufficient to inhibit staphylococci, the latter, the most susceptible Gram-negative bacilli. The drug is removed by hemodialysis, and an additional dose is needed following this procedure.

Cephalexin is suitable for treatment of urinary tract infections in azotemic patients, because it produces satisfactory and prolonged concentrations in the urine, even in presence of severe renal failure (Bailey *et al.*, 1970). Suitable dosage adjustments for this situation are shown in Table I.22. Alternatively, the appropriate daily dosage of cephalexin may be calculated by dividing the usual dosage of 2 g per day by the patient's serum creatinine level measured in mg % (Butcher *et al.*, 1972). For conversion from SI units to mg %, see gentamicin, p. 460.

4 Newborn infants

The dosage as for older children i.e. 25–50 mg per kg body weight per day, given in two or three divided doses, is usually recommended, but up to 100 mg per kg per day has been well tolerated (Marget, 1971).

5 Parenteral cephalexin

This is not generally available but it has been used for investigational purposes (Gower *et al.*, 1973; Hughes *et al.*, 1974). In patients with normal renal function, an i.m. or i.v. dosage of 1 g every 4–6 h is suitable, but for severe infections an i.v. dosage of up to 12 g per day can probably be used. In patients with severe renal failure a dose of 1 g every 8–12 h seems satisfactory. An i.v. dose of 1 g cephalexin maintains an adequate serum level for up to 8 h during hemodialysis (Davies and Holt, 1972).

Group	Creatinine clearance (ml per min)	For sustained levels				Loading dose (mg)
		12 μg per ml		30 μg per ml		
		Dose (mg)	Interval (hours)	Dose (mg)	Interval (hours)	
1	58–124	1000	4	–	–	–
2	33–48	250	12	250	8	1000
3	3–10	250	24	250	12	500
4	0–2.5	250	48	250	24	500
4 (on day of dialysis)	0–2.5	500	–	750	–	–

Table I.21
Proposed oral dose schedule of cephalexin. (After Kabins *et al.*, 1970, with permission.)

Table I.22
Recommended dosage of cephalexin for urinary tract infections in patients with impaired renal function. (After Bailey *et al.*, 1970, with permission.)

Creatinine clearance of glomerular filtration rate (ml per min)	Intervals for 500-mg dose
<20	daily
20–50	12-hourly
>50	8-hourly
Intermittent hemodialysis	daily plus 500 mg at end of each dialysis

Serum Levels in Relation to Dosage

1 Oral administration

Cephalexin is almost completely absorbed after oral administration, and doubling the usual dose doubles the serum concentration (Fig. I.12). These serum levels are higher than those after i.m. cephalothin (p. 254) (Meyers *et al.*, 1969). Food delays absorption, resulting in lower peak but more prolonged serum levels; the total amount of the drug absorbed is only slightly less when given with food (Tetzlaff *et al.*, 1978). In fasting patients 82% of orally administered cephalexin is found in urine, compared with 73% in those given food simultaneously (Griffith and Black, 1968). Probenecid prolongs and enhances serum levels (p. 24).

Cephalexin absorption is unimpaired in patients with obstructive jaundice, achlorhydria, partial gastrectomy and congestive cardiac failure. The same applies to elderly patients, who develop more sustained serum levels due to slower cephalexin excretion (Davies and Holt, 1975). There is improved absorption in patients with celiac disease, small bowel diverticulosis and fibrocystic disease, but absorption is slightly impaired in those with Crohn's disease. Concomitant administration of cholestyramine reduces cephalexin absorption, and therefore these two drugs should not be administered simultaneously (Parsons *et al.*, 1975; Parsons and Paddock, 1975).

The above serum levels are attained after oral administration of the usual cephalexin preparation, cephalexin monohydrate. Cephalexin hydrochloride has also been made available. This is more rapidly absorbed and serum levels at 15 and 30 min after dosing are higher than those attained by the monohydrate. The peak serum level and the area-under-the-curve is the same as those attained with the monohydrate. Clinically both preparations have the same efficacy (Kumar *et al.*, 1988).

Fig. I.12.
Cephalexin blood levels with increasing dosage in fasting adults. (Redrawn after Griffith and Black, 1968, with permission.)

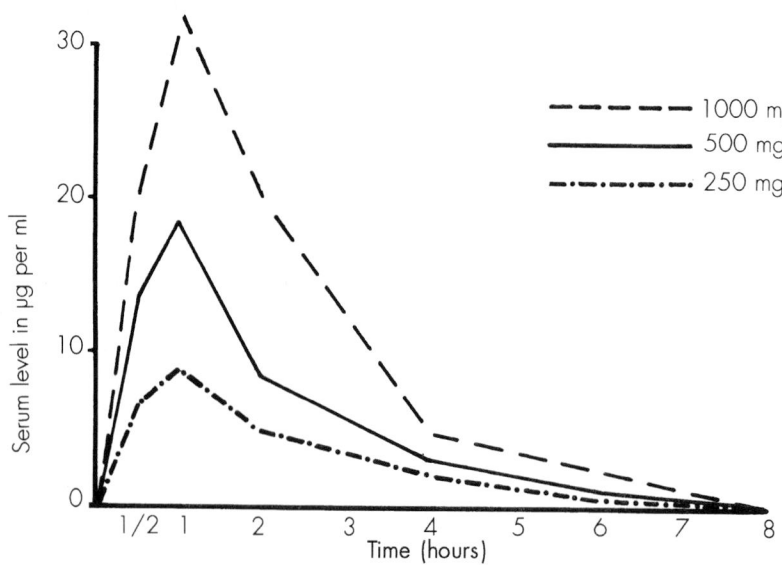

2 Parenteral administration

After an i.v. dose of 1 g administered over a period of 5 min, a serum level of about 60 μg per ml is attained 15 min later. Thereafter, this falls to 5–10 and to 1–4 μg per ml at 2 and 4 h, respectively. The serum half-life of i.v. cephalexin is 1.1 h, but this can be nearly doubled by concomitant administration of probenecid (Davies and Holt, 1972). Following an i.m. injection of 1 g cephalexin, a mean peak serum level of 10.6 μg per ml is reached 2 h later; at 6 h the level is down to 2.5 μg per ml, and at 12 h the drug is undetectable in serum (Nicholas *et al.*, 1973). These serum levels are lower than those obtained after equivalent doses of oral cephalexin (see above). Probably a local depot effect occurs with i.m. injections (Gower *et al.*, 1973).

Excretion

1 Urine

Cephalexin is excreted in urine in an active unchanged form by glomerular filtration and tubular secretion. High urinary concentrations are attained and 80% or more of an oral dose can be recovered from urine. Probenecid delays excretion by partially blocking renal tubular secretion (Braun *et al.*, 1968; Griffith and Black, 1971). Cephalexin accumulates in patients with impaired renal function. In normal subjects the mean serum half-life is 0.9 h but in patients with severe renal functional impairment it increases to 20–30 h (Kabins *et al.*, 1970).

2 Bile

Some cephalexin is excreted in bile. After repeated doses, moderately high cephalexin levels (15–90 μg per ml) are attained in gallbladder bile, provided that the gallbladder is functioning normally. Biliary levels are much lower in patients with non-functioning gallbladders, and in the presence of complete biliary obstruction no cephalexin is excreted in bile (Sales *et al.*, 1972).

3 Inactivation in body

Cephalexin is not metabolized in the body (Griffith and Black, 1971).

Distribution of the Drug in Body

Griffith and Black (1971) studied postmortem tissue levels of cephalexin in a patient who had received 2 g orally every 6 h, the last dose being 5.5 h prior to death. The level in heart blood was 1.9 μg per ml, and tissue levels in lung, spleen, liver, adrenals, pancreas, heart muscle and stomach ranged from 0.12 to 0.6 μg per g. A higher concentration of 4.05 μg per g was found in kidney tissue. Moderately high cephalexin concentrations were reached in purulent sputum of patients with inflamed bronchi, but this decreased as bronchial inflammation resolved (Halprin and McMahon, 1973). Therapeutic levels of cephalexin were achieved in amniotic fluid and cord blood, if the drug was given in late pregnancy (Goodspeed, 1975). Cephalexin is about 15% serum protein bound (Kind *et al.*, 1969).

Mode of Action

Cephalexin, similar to penicillin G (p. 25) and other cephalosporins (p. 256), inhibits the synthesis of bacterial cell walls. With *E. coli*, cephalexin has high affinity for PBP3, the protein concerned in cell division, and so initially it induces filament formation. Such filaments continue to grow for some four to six generations before cell death occurs (Curtis *et al.*, 1979).

Toxicity

1 Gastrointestinal side-effects

Diarrhea, vomiting and abdominal cramps occur in some patients receiving oral cephalexin therapy. Pruritus and candidiasis have been observed (Griffith and Black, 1970). According to Bartlett *et al.* (1979), pseudomembranous colitis (due to *Cl. difficile*) is not a rare complication of both oral or parenteral cephalosporin therapy (p. 258). They reported 17 patients with pseudomembranous colitis associated with cephalosporin use; in five oral cephalexin was implicated as a single drug, and two others had received cephalexin plus one of the parenteral cephalosporins.

2 Hypersensitivity reactions

Skin rashes and eosinophilia have been observed in cephalexin-treated patients. Serum sickness can also occur but seems relatively rare (Platt *et al.*, 1988). Cephalexin caused toxic epidermal necrolysis in one patient (Dave *et al.*, 1991). It has been assumed that cephalexin is not cross-allergenic with the penicillins, but as with cephalothin (p. 256), cross-allergy may sometimes be encountered. Published data indicate that 91–94% of patients with a history of penicillin allergy have not reacted to cephalexin or cephalothin (p. 256); therefore the risk appears to be small (Dash, 1975).

3 Nephrotoxicity

This has been rare with oral cephalexin (Kabins *et al.*, 1970). The drug does not aggravate pre-existing renal disease (Kunin and Finkelberg, 1970). Hematuria and eosinophilia occurred in two patients with bacterial endocarditis, who were treated with very high oral cephalexin doses (20 or 24 g per day plus probenecid); one patient also developed a transient elevation of serum creatinine. All abnormalities disappeared when cephalexin was ceased (Verma and Kieff, 1975).

4 Hematological side-effects

A positive Coombs' test has been reported with cephalexin therapy (Erikssen *et al.*, 1970). As with other cephalosporins (p. 257), the clinical significance of this is not clear. Coombs' positive hemolytic anemia is rare. Forbes *et al.* (1972) described a 14-year-old hemophiliac patient, who developed severe intravascular hemolysis 9 days after starting cephalexin in a dose of 2 g daily. Hemolysis ceased after cephalexin was stopped.

5 Neurotoxicity

Cephalexin may occasionally cause central nervous system disturbances. Diplopia, headache, tinnitus and ataxia occurred in one patient; these symptoms gradually disappeared within 2 weeks of cessation of the drug (Erikssen *et al.*, 1970). Similar symptoms were observed in another patient by Kind *et al.* (1969). If very high serum levels of cephalexin are reached, convulsions and coma may result. Saker *et al.* (1973) described a patient with severe renal disease treated by cephalexin, who developed a grand mal seizure which was followed by disorientation lasting for over 1 week. The drug was given in a dose of 2 g daily and its serum level prior to the seizure was 120 μg per ml.

6 Effects on fetus

Cephalexin has been administered as early as the second month of pregnancy without evidence of fetal damage (Goodspeed, 1975).

Clinical Uses of the Drug

A Oral cephalexin

This drug is satisfactory for some conditions in which parenteral cephalosporins (p. 258) are used, provided that the use of an oral antibiotic is not contraindicated. Compared with cephalothin, cephalexin has an inferior antibacterial activity against most bacterial species (p. 251).

1 Streptococcal and pneumococcal infections

Cephalexin is an alternative to the oral phenoxypenicillins (p. 74) for the treatment of relatively mild infections due to these organisms, possibly in penicillin-allergic patients. It has been used successfully for *Strep. pyogenes* throat and soft tissue infections (Stillerman *et al.*, 1972; Matsen *et al.*, 1974), and pneumococcal pneumonia (Rosenthal *et al.*, 1971).

2 Other respiratory tract infections

Cephalexin has been used for bronchitis, bronchopneumonia and otitis media (Nassar and Allen, 1974). The bacterial etiology of these infections cannot always be easily determined, especially in children, and poor results may occur if *H. influenzae* is the pathogen (Stechenberg *et al.*,

1977). One 20–month-old child developed *H. influenzae* meningitis whilst receiving cephalexin therapy for otitis media (Raucher *et al.*, 1982). In general, antibiotics other than cephalexin (pp. 140, 863) are preferable for the treatment of all of these infections.

3 Staphylococcal infections

Minor staphylococcal infections, such as skin and soft tissue sepsis, can be satisfactorily treated by cephalexin (Kind *et al.*, 1969; Kumar *et al.*, 1988). Chronic staphylococcal osteomyelitis has been managed by administering large doses of oral cephalexin for a prolonged period (Hedlund, 1970). One patient with endocarditis due to *Staph. epidermidis* was cured by oral cephalexin, given in a dosage of 6 g daily for 1 month (Zabransky *et al.*, 1969). Despite this success parenteral antibiotics should be used for bacterial endocarditis. Seventeen patients with mild to moderate pulmonary disease due to cystic fibrosis were treated by cephalexin, alternating 4-month treatment and 4-month placebo period for 2 years. This decreased the frequency of respiratory illness, and hospitalization for respiratory illness, in patients initially colonized with *Staph. aureus* and/or *H. influenzae*. Severity deteriorated in patients initially colonized by *Ps. aeruginosa*, and one patient acquired *Enterobacter* spp. in the sputum. Overall disease severity improved in patients who were not initially colonized with *Ps. aeruginosa* (Loening-Baucke *et al.*, 1979). Other antibiotics which are effective against *Ps. aeruginosa*, are necessary for the treatment of acute exacerbations of infection in cystic fibrosis patients (p. 378).

4 Urinary tract infections

The drug has been used extensively for these infections (Kind *et al.*, 1969; Glass, 1973). It is reasonably effective in eradicating relatively sensitive strains of *E. coli*, *Pr. mirabilis* and *Klebsiella* spp. (Clark and Turck, 1969). Cephalexin appears to be about as effective as ampicillin (Davies *et al.*, 1971). A single dose therapy with oral cephalexin of 3 g is also effective in women with uncomplicated lower urinary tract infections (Cardenas *et al.*, 1986), but such treatment is now not generally advocated. In a study of 100 women with urinary tract infections, cephalexin in a dosage of 1 g twice-daily, was found to be inferior to co-trimoxazole (p. 860), given as two standard tablets twice-daily, both regimens lasting 1 week (Gower and Tasker, 1976). Another trial demonstrated superiority of nalidixic acid (p. 975) over cephalexin for the treatment of bacteriuric women with both bladder and renal infections (Preksaitis *et al.*, 1981). Cephalexin is more slowly bactericidal to Enterobacteriaceae than other beta-lactam antibiotics, and it is also susceptible to beta-lactamases produced by Gram-negative bacilli. These and other factors (p. 860) may explain the superior performance of co-trimoxazole and nalidixic acid compared with cephalexin in urinary tract infections (Greenwood and O'Grady, 1976).

Relatively resistant strains of *E. coli*, *Pr. mirabilis* and *Klebsiella* spp. are often encountered in urinary tract infections, but urine levels inhibitory to the majority of these strains can be attained with usual oral doses of cephalexin (Levison *et al.*, 1969). Similar to the use of other chemotherapeutic agents, patients with a predisposition to urinary tract infections may benefit from long-term, low dose cephalexin administration. A dose as low as 125 mg nightly may be effective in preventing recurrent urinary tract infections (Gower, 1975). During pregnancy women with a history of recurrent urinary infections benefit by postcoital prophylaxis consisting of a single dose of 250 mg of oral cephalexin (Pfau and Sacks, 1992). Routine treatment with cephalexin of asymptomatic bacteriuria in long-term catheterized patients, even with susceptible organisms, is not warranted. In one controlled study, 10-day courses of cephalexin were given to such patients, whenever asymptomatic bacteriuria was detected; there was no benefit from this treatment. The frequency of fever was unchanged when cephalexin was being used, and more cephalexin-resistant bacteria were isolated from patients who received repeated cephalexin courses, compared with placebo treated patients (Warren *et al.*, 1982).

B Parenteral cephalexin

Hughes *et al.* (1974) treated 20 patients, the majority of whom had either urinary tract infections following prostatectomy or pulmonary infections, by i.m. or i.v. cephalexin in a dosage of 1.0 g every 6 h. Results of treatment were satisfactory in most patients. Svensson and Seeberg (1974) used parenteral cephalexin to treat staphylococcal infections such as chronic osteomyelitis, soft tissue and wound infections and septicemia. Clinical improvement occurred in most patients and side-effects of treatment were minimal.

References

Bailey RR, Gower PE, Dash CH (1970). The effect of impairment of renal function and haemodialysis on serum and urine levels of cephalexin. *Postgrad Med J* **46** (Suppl): 60.

Bartlett JG, Willey SH, Chang TW, Lowe B (1979). Cephalosporin-associated pseudomembranous colitis due to *Clostridium difficile*. *JAMA* **242**: 2683.

Braun P, Tillotson JR, Wilcox C, Finland M (1968). Cephalexin and cephaloglycin activity *in vitro* and absorption and urinary excretion of single oral doses in normal young adults. *Appl Microbiol* **16**: 1684.

Busch DF, Kureshi LA, Sutter VL, Finegold SM (1976). Susceptibility of respiratory tract anaerobes to orally administered penicillins and cephalosporins. *Antimicrob Ag Chemother* **10**: 713.

Butcher RH, Dawborn JK, Pattison G (1972). Blood and urine levels of cephalexin in patients with impaired renal function. *Med J Aust* **2**: 1282.

Cardenas J, Quinn EL, Rooker G *et al.* (1986). Single-dose cephalexin therapy for acute bacterial urinary tract infections and acute urethral syndrome with bladder bacteriuria. *Antimicrob Ag Chemother* **29**: 383.

Clark H, Turck M (1969). *In vitro* and *in vivo* evalution of cephalexin. *Antimicrob Ag Chemother* **1968**: 296.

Curtis NAC, Orr D, Ross GW, Boulton MG (1979). Affinities of penicillins and cephalosporins for the penicillin-binding proteins of *Escherichia coli* K-12 and their antibacterial activity. *Antimicrob Ag Chemother* **16**: 533.

Dash CH (1975). Penicillin allergy and the cephalosporins. *J Antimicrob Chemother* **1** (Supp): 107.

Dave J, Heathcock R, Fenelon L *et al.* (1991). Cephalexin induced toxic epidermal necrolysis. *J Antimicrob Chemother* **28**: 477.

Davies JA, Holt JM (1972). Clinical pharmacology of cephalexin administered by intravenous injection. *J Clin Path* **25**: 518.

Davies JA, Holt JM (1975). Absorption of cephalexin in diseased and aged subjects. *J Antimicrob Chemother* **1** (Suppl): 69.

Davies JA, Strangeways JEM, Mitchell RG *et al.* (1971). Comparative double-blind trial of cephalexin and ampicillin in treatment of urinary infections. *Brit Med J* **3**: 215.

Erikssen J, Midtvedt T, Bergan T (1970). Treatment of urinary tract infections with cephalexin. *Scand J Infect Dis* **2**: 53.

Forbes CD, Craig JA, Mitchell R, McNicol GP (1972). Acute intravascular haemolysis associated with cephalexin therapy. *Postgrad Med J* **48**: 186.

Glass RD (1973). Cephalexin in the treatment of urinary infection in childhood. *Med J Aust* **1**: 793.

Goodspeed AH (1975). Cephalexin in special cases. *J Antimicrob Chemother* **1**: (Suppl): 105.

Gower PE (1975). The use of small doses of cephalexin (125mg). in the management of recurrent urinary tract infection in women. *J Antimicrob Chemother* **1** (Suppl): 93.

Gower PE, Tasker PRW (1976). Comparative double-blind study of cephalexin and co-trimoxazole in urinary tract infections. *Brit Med J* **1**: 684.

Gower PE, Dash CH, O'Callaghan CH (1973). Serum and blood concentration of sodium cephalexin in man given single intramuscular and intravenous injections. *J Pharm Pharmac* **25**: 376.

Greenwood D, O'Grady F (1976). Co-trimoxazole and cephalexin in urinary tract infection. *Brit Med J* **1**: 1073.

Griffith RS, Black HR (1968). Cephalexin: a new antibiotic. *Clin Med* **75**: 14.

Griffith RS, Black HR (1970). Cephalexin. *Med Clin N Amer* **54**: 1229.

Griffith RS, Black HR (1971). Blood, urine and tissue concentrations of the cephalosporin antibiotics in normal subjects. *Postgrad Med J* **47** (Suppl): 32.

Halprin GM, McMahon SM (1973). Cephalexin concentrations in sputum during acute respiratory infections. *Antimicrob Ag Chemother* **3**: 703.

Hedlund P (1970). Clinical evaluation of cephalexin in staphylococcal infections. *Postgrad Med J* **46** (Suppl): 152.

Hughes SPF, Hurst L, Dash CH (1974). Parenteral cephalexin in a general surgical unit. *Brit J Clin Pract* **28**: 51.

Kabins SA, Kelner B, Waltone E, Goldstein E (1970). Cephalexin therapy as related to renal function. *Amer J Med Sci* **259**: 133.

Karmali MA, De Grandis S, Fleming PC (1980). Antimicrobial susceptibility of *Campylobacter jejuni* and *Campylobacter fetus* subsp. *fetus* to eight cephalosporins with special reference to species differentiation. *Antimicrob Ag Chemother* **18**: 948.

Kayser FH (1971). *In vitro* activity of cephalosporin antibiotics against Gram-positive bacteria. *Postgrad Med J* **47** (Suppl): 14.

Kind AC, Kestle DG, Standiford HC, Kirby WMM (1969). Laboratory and clinical experience with cephalexin. *Antimicrob Ag Chemother* **1968**: 361.

Konforti N, Halperin E (1975). Sensitivities of strains of enteropathogenic *Escherichia coli* to cephalexin and other antibiotics. *Amer J Clin Path* **64**: 121.

Kumar A, Murrray DL, Hanna CB *et al.* (1988). Comparative study of cephalexin hydrochloride and cephalexin monohydrate in the treatment of skin and soft tissue infections. *Antimicrob Ag Chemother* **32**: 882.

Kunin CM, Finkelberg Z (1970). Oral cephalexin and ampicillin: antimicrobial activity, recovery in urine, and persistence in blood of uremic patients. *Ann Intern Med* **72**: 349.

Levison ME, Johnson WD, Thornhill TS, Kaye D (1969). Clinical and *in vitro* evaluation of cephalexin. *JAMA* **209**: 1331.

Loening-Baucke VA, Mischler E, Myers MG (1979). A placebo-controlled trial of cephalexin therapy in the ambulatory management of patients with cystic fibrosis. *J Pediatr* **95**: 630.

Marget W (1971). Special aspects of cephalosporin therapy in infants and children. *Postgrad Med J* **47** (Suppl): 54.

Marrie TJ, Kwan C (1982). Antimicrobial susceptibility of *Staphylococcus saprophyticus* and urethral staphylococci. *Antimicrob Ag Chemother* **22**: 395.

Matsen JM, Torstenson O, Siegel SE, Bacaner H (1974). Use of available dosage forms of cephalexin in clinical comparison with phenoxymethyl penicillin and benzathine penicillin in the treatment of streptococcal pharyngitis in children. *Antimicrob Ag Chemother* **6**: 501.

Medeiros AA, O'Brien TF, Rosenberg EY, Nikaido H (1987). Loss of Omp C porin in a strain of *Salmonella typhimurium* causes increased resistance to cephalosporins during therapy. *J Infect Dis* **156**: 751.

Meyers BR, Kaplan K, Weinstein L (1969). Cephalexin: microbiological effects and pharmacologic parameters in man. *Clin Pharm Ther* **10**: 810.

Muggleton PW, O'Callaghan CH, Foord RD *et al.* (1969). Laboratory appraisal of cephalexin. *Antimicrob Ag Chemother* **1968**: 353.

Nassar WY, Allen BM (1974). A double-blind comparative clinical trial of cephalexin and ampicillin in the treatment of childhood acute otitis media. *Curr Med Res Opin* **2**: 198.

Nicholas P, Meyers BR, Hirschman SZ (1973). Cephalexin: pharmacologic evaluation following oral and parenteral administration. *J Clin Pharmacol* **13**: 463.

Parsons RL, Paddock GM (1975). Asborption of two antibacterial drugs, cephalexin and co-trimaxozole, in malabsorption syndromes. *J Antimicrob Chemother* **1** (Suppl): 59.

Parsons RL, Hossack G, Paddock G (1975). The absorption of antibiotics in adult patients with coeliac disease. *J Antimicrob Chemother* **1**: 39.

Pfau A, Sacks TG (1992). Effective prophylaxis for recurrent urinary tract infections during pregnancy. *Clin Infect Dis* **14**: 810.

Platt R, Dreis MW, Kennedy DL, Kuritsky JN (1988). Serum sickness-like reactions to amoxicillin, cefaclor, cephalexin and trimethoprim-sulfamethoxazole. *J Infect Dis* **158**: 474.

Powell M, Williams JD (1988). *In-vitro* activity of cefaclor, cephalexin and ampicillin against 2458 clinical isolates of *Haemophilus influenzae*. *J Antimicrob Chemother* **21**: 27.

Preksaitis JK, Thompson L, Harding GKM *et al.* (1981). A comparison of the efficacy of nalidixic acid and cephalexin in bacteriuric women and their effect on fecal and periurethral carriage of Enterobacteriaceae. *J Infect Dis* **143**: 603.

Raucher HS, Murphy RJC, Barzilai A (1982). Meningitis occurring during therapy for otitis media with cephalexin and cefaclor. *Amer J Dis Child* **136**: 745.

Rosenthal IM, Metzger WA, Laxminarayana MS (1971). Treatment of pneumonia in childhood with cephalexin. *Postgrad Med J* **47** (Suppl): 51.

Sabath LD, Garner C, Wilcox C, Finland M (1975). Effect of inoculum and of beta-lactamase on the anti-staphylococcal activity of thirteen penicillins and cephalosporins. *Antimicrob Ag Chemother* **8**: 344.

Saker BM, Musk AW, Haywood EF, Hurst PE (1973). Reversible toxic psychosis after cephalexin. *Med J Aust* **1**: 497.

Sales JEL, Sutcliffe M, O'Grady F (1972). Cephalexin levels in human bile in presence of biliary tract disease. *Brit Med J* **3**: 441.

Selwyn S, Bakhtiar M (1977). Penicillin-resistant gonococci. *Brit Med J* **2**: 118.

Stechenberg BW, Anderson D, Chang MJ *et al.* (1977). Cephalexin compared to ampicillin treatment of otitis media. *Pediatrics* **58**: 532.

Stillerman M, Isenberg HD, Moody M (1972). Streptococcal pharyngitis therapy Comparison of cephalexin, phenoxymethylpenicillin, and ampicillin. *Amer J Dis Child* **123**: 457.

Svensson R, Seeberg S (1974). Clinical evaluation of parenteral cephalexin sodium. *Scand J Infect Dis* **6**: 279.

Tally FP, Jacobus NV, Bartlett JG, Gorbach SL (1975). Susceptibility of anaerobes to cefoxitin and other cephalosporins. *Antimicrob Ag Chemother* **7**: 128.

Tetzlaff TR, McCracken GH Jr, Thomas ML (1978). Bioavailability of cephalexin in children: relationship to drug formulations and meals. *J Pediatr* **92**: 292.

Verma S, Kieff E (1975). Cephalexin-related nephropathy. *JAMA* **234**: 618.

Warren JW, Anthony WC, Hoopes JM, Muncie HL Jr (1982). Cephalexin for susceptible bacteriuria in afebrile, long-term catheterized patients. *JAMA* **248**: 454.

Waterworth PM (1971). The susceptibility of pathogenic Gram-negative bacilli to cephalosporins. *Postgrad Med J* **47** (Suppl): 25.

Wick WE (1967). Cephalexin, a new orally absorbed cephalosporin antibiotic. *Appl Microbiol* **15**: 765.

Zabransky RJ, Gardner MA, Geraci JE (1969). Cephalexin: preliminary *in vitro* studies of a new orally administered cephalosporin and report of a case of endocarditis cured with cephalexin. *Mayo Clin Proc* **44**: 876.

Cephradine, Cefadroxil, Cefaclor and Cefatrizine

Description

These four cephalosporins, similar to cephalexin (p. 263), are all suitable for oral administration. Cephradine and cefatrizine can also be administered parenterally.

1 Cephradine

This semisynthetic cephalosporin was developed at the Squibb Institute for Medical Research (Dolfini et al., 1971; Miraglia et al., 1973). It is very similar to cephalexin (p. 263) in its antimicrobial activity and in most other respects (Moellering and Swartz, 1976). Unlike cephalexin, for which a parenteral preparation is not generally available (p. 274), cephradine is marketed in some countries for both oral and parenteral use.

2 Cefadroxil*

Developed by Bristol Laboratories, its antibacterial activity is similar to that of cephalexin and cephradine. After oral administration its peak serum level is slightly lower than that of cephalexin, but it is excreted more slowly. Therefore, it can be used for oral administration at 8- or 12-hourly intervals (Buck and Price, 1977; Pfeffer et al., 1977).

3 Cefaclor

Although this drug is similar in many aspects to cephalexin and cephradine, it differs by being more active in vitro against a number of Gram-positive and Gram-negative bacteria (Bill and Washington, 1977).

4 Cefatrizine

This is slightly more active than cephalexin against most Gram-positive and Gram-negative bacteria (Leitner et al., 1975; Overturf et al., 1975). Peak serum levels obtained after oral cefatrizine are lower than those after cephalexin, but they decline at a slower rate (Del Busto et al., 1976). This drug can also be administered parenterally.

The following only applies to the first three of these cephalosporins.

Sensitive Organisms

1 Cephradine

Its spectrum is similar to that of cephalexin (p. 263) (Table I.23), with only minor differences (Moellering and Swartz, 1976). Like cephalexin, cephradine is less active against most bacterial species, compared with cephalothin (p. 252).

Gram-positive bacteria are usually sensitive. *Staphylococcus aureus*, including most penicillin-resistant, but not methicillin-resistant strains, is sensitive. Cephradine is about as resistant as cephalothin (p.251) to inactivation by staphylococcal beta-lactamase (Fong et al., 1976; Basker et al., 1980). Most other aerobic Gram-positive cocci, such as coagulase-negative staphylococci, *Streptococcus pyogenes*, *Strep. pneumoniae* and *Strep. viridans*, are susceptible. *Enterococcus faecalis* is resistant (Hamilton-Miller, 1974). Anaerobic Gram-positive cocci, such as the *Peptococcus* and *Peptostreptococcus* spp., are usually cephradine-sensitive. Most strains

---

*The letter 'f' replaced 'ph' in the spelling of cephalosporins named after 1975.

recovered from airway associated infections are relatively sensitive (MICs 8–16 μg per ml), but other strains are less so (Busch *et al.*, 1976). Against Gram-positive bacilli, cephradine has a similar inhibitory action to cephalexin (p. 263).

The activity of cephradine against Gram-negative bacteria is comparable with that of cephalexin, but it is slightly less active against *Escherichia coli*, *Proteus mirabilis* and *Klebsiella* spp. (McGowan *et al.*, 1974; Bill and Washington, 1977; Wise *et al.*, 1979). Both cephalexin (p. 263) and cephradine are only moderately active against *Neisseria gonorrhoeae* (Phillips *et al.*, 1976), but they retain this activity against beta-lactamase-producing strains (Selwyn and Bakhtiar, 1977). Like cephalexin (p. 263), cephradine is relatively inactive against *H. influenzae*, many strains of which are completely resistant to these drugs (Sinai *et al.*, 1978; Watanakunakorn and Glotzbecker, 1979). The drug is moderately active against *Gardnerella vaginalis* (Goldstein *et al.*, 1983).

2 Cefradroxil

For practical purposes, the antibacterial activity of this drug against both Gram-positive and Gram-negative bacteria, is identical to that of cephalexin (p. 263) and cephradine (Buck and Price, 1977; Leitner *et al.*, 1982) (Table I.23).

3 Cefaclor

This is more active than cephalexin and cephradine against Gram-positive bacteria, such as staphylococci and streptococci, but against *Staph. aureus* it is not as active as cephalothin. The drug is somewhat less resistant to staphylococcal beta-lactamase than cephalexin (p. 263), and so it may not be a reliable anti-staphylococcal agent (Bill and Washington, 1977; Tally *et al.*, 1979). *Enterococcus faecalis* is resistant (Preston, 1979).

Cefaclor is more active than cephalexin against many Gram-negative bacteria such as meningococci, gonococci, *E. coli*, *Klebsiella pneumoniae*, *Pr. mirabilis* and *Salmonella* and *Shigellae* spp. (Sanders, 1977; Scheld *et al.*, 1977; Gillett *et al.*, 1979). The drug is active against beta-lactamase-producing gonococci (Tupasi *et al.*, 1982). Ampicillin-sensitive strains of *H. influenzae* and most which are ampicillin-resistant because of beta-lactamase production (p. 113) are sensitive to cefaclor. Most strains which show intrinsic resistance to ampicillin, are cefaclor-resistant (Powell and Williams, 1988; Powell *et al.*, 1991; Picard and Malouin, 1992). *Moraxella catarrhalis* is also usually cefaclor-sensitive. Cefaclor is inactive against *Serratia*, *Providencia* and *Acinetobacter* spp. and *Pseudomonas aeruginosa*. Most strains of *Pr. vulgaris* and *Morganella morganii* are also resistant (Neu and Fu, 1978; Preston, 1979).

Table I.23
Compiled from data published by Hamilton-Miller (1974), Overturf *et al.* (1975), Leitner *et al.* (1975), Selwyn (1976), Buck and Price (1977), Bill and Washington (1977) and Preston (1979)

Organism	MIC (μg per ml)			
	Cephalexin	Cephradine	Cefadroxil	Cefaclor
Gram-positive bacteria				
Staphylococcus aureus (non-penicillinase producer)	1.6–12.5	4.0	2.0	2.0
Staphylococcus aureus (penicillinase producer)	1.6–>100.0	8.0	8.0	2.0
Streptococcus pyogenes	0.2–6.3	1.0	0.63	0.25
Enterococcus faecalis	200.0	100.0	57.0	64.0
Gram-negative bacteria				
Escherichia coli	25.0–>100.0	16.0–>125.0	16.0–>125.0	8.0
Enterobacter spp.	50.0–>100.0	>125.0	>125.0	>128.0
Klebsiella spp.	50.0–>100.0	4.0–125.0	4.0–125.0	8.0
Proteus mirabilis	25.0–>100.0	4.0–63.0	4.0–63.0	>128.0
Proteus vulgaris	>100.0	>125.0	>125.0	>128.0
Providencia spp.	>125.0	>125.0	>125.0	>128.0
Serratia spp.	>125.0	>125.0	>125.0	>128.0
Haemophilus influenzae	12.5–>100.0	4.0–63.0	8.0–63.0	2.0

Anaerobic Gram-positive cocci and most Gram-negative anaerobes, other than those of *Bacteroides fragilis* group (p. 295), are usually cefaclor-sensitive. The *Clostridium* spp. are usually resistant (Bach *et al.*, 1978).

4 Minimum inhibitory concentrations

The MICs of cephradine, cefadroxil and cefaclor against some selected bacteria are shown in Table I.23. Those for cephalexin are included for comparison.

Mode of Administration and Dosage

1 Cephradine

The usual oral adult dosage is 0.5 g every 6 h. For mild infections, 250 mg 6-hourly (or 500 mg 12-hourly) may suffice, and up to 1 g every 4 h may be given for severe or chronic infections (Klastersky *et al.*, 1973; Scholand *et al.*, 1974). The oral dosage for children is 60 mg per kg body weight per day, administered in four divided doses (Ginsburg and McCracken, 1979), but up to 100 mg per kg per day can be used for severe infections.

The parenteral dosage for adults is 2–4 g daily, given in four divided doses i.m. or i.v. (Caloza *et al.*, 1979). For treatment of severe infections, a total daily dose of up to 8 g can be used. The usual parenteral dosage for children is 50–100 mg per kg per day, given in four divided doses. For serious infections, up to 300 mg per kg has been given i.v. to children without toxicity (Macias and Eller, 1975; Mogabgab, 1976).

In patients with renal failure, cephradine accumulates if the usual doses are used, so that dosage reduction is necessary. The recommendations are: for moderate renal failure (creatinine clearance 10–50 ml per min), 50% of the usual daily dose; for severe renal failure (creatinine clearance <10 ml per min), 25% of the usual daily dose. The drug is removed by both peritoneal dialysis and hemodialysis, so that dose supplements are necessary during or after these procedures (Bennett *et al.*, 1977).

2 Cefadroxil

Having a longer serum half-life (p. 275), it can be administered orally 8- or 12-hourly or even once-daily (Pfeffer *et al.*, 1977; Brisson and Fourtillan, 1982; Gerber *et al.*, 1986). A dosage of 0.5 g two or three times a day, is suitable for mild to moderate infections in adults. A dosage regimen of 1 g twice-daily may be used for adults with more severe infections (Wilber *et al.*, 1982).Cefadroxil can be given to children in a dosage of 50 mg per kg per day in two divided doses (Windorfer and Bauer, 1982). In acute urinary tract infections once-daily cefadroxil administration is satisfactory; for adults the dose is usually 1 g (Henning *et al.*, 1982) and for children 30 mg per kg (Ginsburg *et al.*, 1982).

In patients with renal failure a loading dose of 1 g orally can be given. Thereafter, this dose should be given at intervals of 12, 24 or 48 h to patients with creatinine clearance values of 40–80, 20–40 and <20 ml per min, respectively. Cefadroxil is removed by hemodialysis; 1 g should be given at the end of each hemodialysis, and thereafter be repeated every 72 h in anephric patients (Leroy *et al.*, 1982).

3 Cefaclor

Oral doses of 250–500 mg 6-hourly are suitable for adults (Korzeniowski *et al.*, 1977). An adult dosage of 0.5 g 8-hourly is also satisfactory (Wernstedt *et al.*, 1979). In children the dosage is 40–50 mg per kg body weight per day, given in three or four divided doses (McCracken *et al.*, 1978; Rodriguez *et al.*, 1979). For the treatment of milder infections in children, a dosage of 40 mg per kg, given in two divided doses is also satisfactory (Edèn *et al.*, 1983).

Similar to amoxycillin (p. 139) and other drugs, cefaclor in a dose of 2 g, can be used for single-dose treatment of acute uncomplicated urinary tract infections in adults (Greenberg *et al.*, 1981).

Cefaclor's half-life in normal subjects of 40–60 min, only increases to 3 h in anephric patients (Levison *et al.*, 1979). As a result, its dose can be reduced in patients with renal failure to a lesser extent than cephalexin (p. 265). Patients with severe renal failure should receive 25% of the usual dose, and those with moderate renal failure 50% of the usual dose. In patients with mild renal failure (creatinine clearance >40 ml per min), modification of cefaclor dosage is unnecessary

(Bloch *et al.*, 1977; Santoro *et al.*, 1978). Cefaclor is removed from the body by hemodialysis (Gartenberg *et al.*, 1979). During this procedure its clearance is doubled and approximates to that which occurs in a patient with a creatinine clearance of about 20 ml per min; after hemodialysis the usual cefaclor dose should be repeated (Spyker *et al.*, 1982).

Serum Levels in Relation to Dosage

1 Cephradine

Serum levels after oral administration are similar to those after cephalexin (Fig. I.12, p. 266). After a 0.5 g oral dose to adults, a peak serum level of approximately 15 μg per ml is reached in 1 h, which falls to 6.5, 1, and 0.1 μg per ml at 2, 4 and 6 h, respectively. Doubling the dose to 1 g increases the peak serum level by over 50% but usually does not double it (Scholand *et al.*, 1974; Pfeffer *et al.*, 1977). In children the absorption of cephradine and cephalexin is reduced if they are given with milk (Ginsburg and McCracken, 1979; Ginsburg, 1982). Following i.v. or i.m. administration, serum levels attained are identical to those after parenteral cephalexin (p. 267). As with cephalexin, i.m. cephradine produces lower serum levels than equivalent oral doses.

2 Cefadroxil

The peak serum level attained 1 h after an oral dose is about the same or slightly lower than that after cephalexin (p. 266). Cefadroxil differs from cephalexin and cephradine by having a slower urinary excretion rate, and thereby a longer serum half-life and more sustained serum levels (Pfeffer *et al.*, 1977; Brisson and Fourtillan, 1982). After a 0.5-g oral dose to adults, the peak serum level in 1 h is about 15 μg per ml, which falls to 12.5, 4.5., 1.8, 1.1 and 0.65 μg per ml at 2, 4, 6, 8 and 12 h, respectively (Pfeffer *et al.*, 1977). The area-under-the-curve for cefadroxil is some 1.6 times greater than that for cephalexin.

Doubling the dose of cefadroxil results in doubling of its serum concentrations, but this relationship is only linear in the 250–500 mg dose range. With these doses the mean serum half-life is about 1.2 h, but after a 1 g dose, it is 1.6 h. This decrease in clearance in the dose range of 0.5–1.0 g, may be due to a saturation of mechanisms by which cefadroxil is secreted by renal tubules (La Rosa *et al.*, 1982). Bioavailability of the drug, therefore, is greater with a dose of 1 g 12-hourly than with 0.5 g every 6 h (Santella and Henness, 1982). If 1 g cefadroxil dose is given every 8 h, a slight increase in the peak levels from day 1 to day 8, has been observed (Hampel *et al.*, 1982). Others have failed to detect any accumulation of the drug, even with doses as high as 6 g daily for 7 days (Santella and Henness, 1982). The drug's absorption is not impaired by food in adults or children (Pfeffer *et al.*, 1977; Ginsburg, 1982).

3 Cefaclor

This drug is rapidly absorbed from the gastrointestinal tract, but its peak and subsequent serum levels are lower than with cephalexin (p. 266). After a 200-mg oral dose, the mean peak serum level at 1 h is 6 μg per ml (comparable level for cephalexin 9.4), which falls to 0.33 μg per ml (cephalexin 0.68) at 4 h. Cefaclor is more rapidly excreted than cephalexin, their half-lives being 0.58 and 0.8 h, respectively (Korzeniowski *et al.*, 1977). Concomitant administration of probenecid prolongs the serum levels of cefaclor. Food intake reduces the maximum concentration of the cefaclor in the serum and prolongs the time to attain this concentration. However, the area-under-the-concentration-time-curve and urinary recovery of the drug are unaffected (Oguma *et al.*, 1991). The serum half-life of cefaclor in patients with severe renal failure is only about 3 h, which suggests that it is also eliminated by non-renal mechanisms (Glynne *et al.*, 1978; Rotschafer *et al.*, 1982).

Excretion

1 Cephradine

Similar to cephalexin (p.267), this drug is excreted unchanged in urine by glomerular filtration and tubular secretion. Up to 30% of an orally administered dose is excreted during the first 6 h, resulting in high urine concentrations (Scholand *et al.*, 1974). Probenecid delays its excretion by partially blocking tubular secretion. Cephradine accumulates in patients with impaired renal function. Its serum half-life is 1.3 h in normal subjects, but this rises to 15 h in patients with end-stage renal disease (Bennett *et al.*, 1977). Like cephalexin, some cephradine is also excreted in bile, where its concentration may be about four times higher than the serum level at the time. Biliary excretion is reduced with biliary tract obstruction and jaundice (Maroske *et al.*, 1976).

2 Cefadroxil

This is excreted in the urine in the active form by both glomerular filtration and tubular secretion (Pfeffer *et al.*, 1977). Approximately 93% of a 0.5 g oral dose is excreted in the urine during the first 24 h; most of this occurs during the first 6 h, when urine concentrations are in the range 400–2400 µg per ml (Hartstein *et al.*, 1977). The tubular secretion rate of cefadroxil is less than that of cephalexin, so that urinary excretion of cefadroxil is of longer duration. This explains its more prolonged serum levels (p. 275). Initial urine concentrations of cefadroxil are lower than those of cephalexin, but during the period 3–12 h after a dose, they are higher (Pfeffer *et al.*, 1977; Santella and Henness, 1982).

3 Cefaclor

Approximately 70% of an orally administered dose can be recovered from urine as the active drug during the first 6 h. During this period, after a 250-mg oral dose, urine concentrations are in the range 50–1000 µg per ml. Urinary levels of cefaclor are adequate to inhibit susceptible pathogens even in patients with moderately severe renal failure (Santoro *et al.*, 1978). The serum half-life is only prolonged about 3-fold in patients with essentially no renal function. This indicates that cefaclor, unlike cephalexin (p. 267), has a major non-renal route of elimination. A considerable proportion of the drug is metabolized in the body (Levison *et al.*, 1979; Rotschafer *et al.*, 1982). In animals, cefaclor is also excreted via the bile, and biliary concentrations greatly exceed serum levels (Waterman and Scharfenberger, 1978).

Distribution of the Drugs in Body

1 Cephradine

This is well distributed into various body fluids and tissues. It does not penetrate into the CSF of patients with uninflamed meninges, but some cephradine has been found in human brain tissue after usual therapeutic doses (Adam *et al.*, 1975). Its concentration in liver tissue approximates to the serum level at the time (Maroske *et al.*, 1976), and satisfactory concentrations are also reached in heart muscle, uterine muscle, lung and prostatic tissue (Adam *et al.*, 1975; Kiss *et al.*, 1976). Cephradine also penetrates well into both normal and infected bone (Parsons *et al.*, 1976; Leigh, 1989), and crosses the placenta and is detectable in amniotic fluid (Craft and Forster, 1978). Its serum protein binding is only 10% (Bennett *et al.*, 1977).

2 Cefadroxil

This is distributed like cephalexin (p. 267), but as it is eliminated more slowly, it remains in body tissues for longer after single doses. It is 20% serum protein bound (Pfeffer *et al.*, 1977; Quintiliani, 1982).

3 Cefaclor

This drug diffuses readily into soft tissue interstitial fluid (Waterman and Scharfenberger, 1978). Its concentration in sputum is usually low, and it is not excreted in saliva (Levison *et al.*, 1979). Cefaclor attains therapeutically effective concentrations in middle ear fluid of patients with otitis media (Edèn *et al.*, 1983). The drug is approximately 50% serum protein bound (Tally *et al.*, 1979).

Mode of Action

These cephalosporins act on bacteria in a manner similar to cephalothin (p. 256).

Toxicity

1 Cephradine

This drug is well tolerated. Gastrointestinal symptoms after oral administration are probably similar, and as frequent, as those after oral cephalexin (p. 267). Pseudomembranous colitis after the use of oral cephradine has been reported (Bartlett *et al.*, 1979). Other side-effects include urticarial rashes, joint pains, headaches and dizziness, all of which are uncommon (Klastersky *et al.*, 1973; Scholand *et al.*, 1974; Mogabgab, 1976). Mild elevations of blood urea have been noted during cephradine therapy, but serious nephrotoxicity has not been reported (Macias and Eller, 1975; Mogabgab, 1976). Immunologically mediated neutropenia due to cephradine has been reported (Lawson *et al.*, 1984).

2 Cefadroxil

Side-effects with this drug are uncommon. A small number of patients develop nausea, vomiting, diarrhea, abdominal pain, pruritus, allergic rashes, vaginitis or drug fever (Rugendorff, 1982; Wilber *et al.*, 1982).

3 Cefaclor

Therapy with this drug has been associated with a low frequency of side-effects. Gastrointestinal symptoms, such as diarrhea and nausea, have occurred in some 2.6% of treated patients. Cefaclor only has a minor effect on the anaerobic intestinal microflora (Nord *et al.*, 1987). Hypersensitivity phenomena, such as allergic rashes, have been noted in 1.55% of patients (Kammer and Short, 1979). Eosinophilia, positive Coombs' test without hemolysis, reversible leukopenia and elevated SGOT levels have also been noted occasionally. Muray *et al.* (1980) reported eight children who developed a severe generalized rash and arthritis while taking oral cefaclor; six were taking the drug for the second time. Symptoms subsided within 4–5 days after cefaclor was stopped. Such serum sickness-like reactions appear to occur more commonly with cefaclor than with cephalexin (Platt *et al.*, 1988). These reactions occur with cefaclor because of the drugs' biotransformation in liver into immunogenic metabolites (Boguniewicz and Leung, 1995).

An elevated blood urea occurs occasionally during cefaclor therapy, but serious nephrotoxicity has not been observed (Kammer and Short, 1979). Animal experiments show that unilateral obstruction of the ureter increases the nephrotoxicity of cefaclor and of other cephalosporins which are rapidly secreted across renal tubular cells (Wang *et al.*, 1982). Cefaclor increases the rate of phagocytosis of staphylococci. In four patients with chronic bacterial infections who had low levels of neutrophil myeloperoxidase activity, these increased after cefaclor treatment, and the clinical response of three patients was satisfactory (Grant *et al.*, 1983). In the presence of cefaclor, there is an increase of phagocytosis of *E. coli* (Scheffer *et al.*, 1992).

Pneumococcal meningitis developed in a child, treated for otitis media by cefaclor (Raucher *et al.*, 1982). Thus cefaclor, like some other cephalosporins (p. 258), should be used with caution for infections which may be complicated by bacterial meningitis.

Clinical Uses of the Drugs

In general, the use of these oral cephalosporins, like cephalexin (p. 268) is limited to treatment of relatively mild infections.

1 Cephradine

The oral preparation is suitable for the same indications as oral cephalexin (p. 268). It has been used with success in pharyngeal, skin, soft tissue, respiratory and urinary tract infections (Klastersky *et al.*, 1973; Scholand *et al.*, 1974; Cooper *et al.*, 1980; Hart *et al.*, 1981). Results are similar to those obtained with cephalexin (p. 268). For the treatment of urinary tract infections, the drug is about as effective as amoxycillin (p. 139), but in one study cephradine treatment resulted in less resistance of *E. coli* in the saliva and intestine, than similar treatment with amoxycillin (Lacey *et al.*, 1983). In a daily dose of 250 mg cephradine is useful as a prophylactic antibiotic for patients with recurrent urinary tract infections (Brumfitt and Hamilton-Miller, 1990).

Parenteral cephradine has been advocated for some infections which would usually be treated by older parenteral cephalosporins such as cephalothin (p. 258) and cefazolin (p. 287). It has no definite place in severe infections such as pneumococcal pneumonia, *Strep. viridans* endocarditis and staphylococcal septicemia in penicillin-allergic patients. Some authors obtained good results by using i.v. cephradine for severe infections of this type (Macias and Eller, 1975; Caloza *et al.*, 1979). It was suggested that parenteral cephradine could replace cephalothin and cefazolin because of its possible lesser toxicity, low serum protein binding and good stability to staphylococcal beta-lactamase; the drug can be also administered orally, i.m. and i.v. (Selwyn, 1976). This view is not justified. Cephradine and cephalexin (Table I.23, p. 273) have a lesser intrinsic antibacterial activity than cephalothin and cefazolin (Tables I.18 and I.24, pp. 253, 284). In addition, compared with cephalothin (p. 258), experience with parenteral cephradine for serious infections is limited. Daggett and Nathan (1975) reported a case of *Strep. viridans* endocarditis which failed to respond to i.v. cephradine in a dosage of 0.5 g every 3 h; the MIC of cephradine for this organism was 0.312 μg per ml.

Oral or intraperitoneal cephradine has been used with success to treat peritonitis in continuous ambulatory peritoneal dialysis patients, but other antibiotics would be necessary if the pathogen was a methicillin-resistant *Staph. epidermidis* (Boeschoten *et al.*, 1985).

2 Cefadroxil

Indications for this oral cephalosporin are the same as those for cephalexin (p. 268). The advantage of cefadroxil is its twice-daily or once-daily dosage regimens (p. 274). The drug has been used with success, similar to that of cephalexin, for the treatment of urinary tract infections in children and adults (Ginsburg *et al.*, 1982; Henning *et al.*, 1982). In uncomplicated urinary tract infections, a cefadroxil regimen of 1 g daily is equally effective to 1 g 12-hourly (Rugendorff, 1982). The drug has also been used in children with otitis media (Puhakka *et al.*, 1982) and in lower respiratory tract infections in both children and adults (Kramer, 1982; Weingarten, 1982; Blaser *et al.*, 1983). In streptococcal pharyngitis cefadroxil, given once-daily, is at least as effective as penicillin V, administered in three daily doses (Gerber *et al.*, 1986; Pichichero *et al.*, 1987). Once-daily cefadroxil is also satisfactory for the treatment of impetigo, a disease in which both *Strep. pyogenes* and *Staph. aureus* may be involved (Hains *et al.*, 1989).

One trial with a small number of patients showed that cefadroxil was equally effective to metronidazole for the treatment of bacterial vaginosis (p. 947) (Wathne *et al.*, 1989).

3 Cefaclor

This drug has been satisfactory for the treatment of urinary tract infections, including cases of complicated and/or recurrent infections. Pyelonephritis caused by ampicillin-resistant organisms, such as *Klebsiella* spp., also responds to cefaclor (Kammer and Short, 1979; Lindan, 1979). Uncomplicated urinary tract infections in non-pregnant women may respond to 2 g single-dose cefaclor therapy (Greenberg *et al.*, 1981) (p. 139). A single daily dose of 250 mg cefaclor is satisfactory as prophylactic antibiotic for patients with recurrent urinary infections (Brumfitt and Hamilton-Miller, 1990).

Cefaclor has been curative for children and adults with acute streptococcal pharyngitis (Stillerman, 1986), otitis media and maxillary sinusitis. In children with acute otitis media it is about as good as amoxycillin (Giebink *et al.*, 1984; Mandel *et al.*, 1993). It is effective in otitis media and sinusitis caused by beta-lactamase-producing strains of *H. influenzae* and *Moraxella catarrhalis* (Bluestone *et al.*, 1979; McLinn, 1980; Ekedahl, 1983; Wald *et al.*, 1984). One child who received this drug for otitis media, developed pneumococcal meningitis (p. 277). Cefaclor is ineffective for eradicating *H. influenzae* from pharyngeal carriers (Horner *et al.*, 1980). It is about equally as effective as amoxycillin (p. 140) for the treatment of infective exacerbations of chronic bronchitis (Mattson *et al.*, 1979; Law *et al.*, 1983). In a small group of patients Maeson *et al.* (1990) found low dosage cefaclor unsatisfactory for chronic bronchitis. Oberlin and Hyslop (1990) analyzed data from 18 clinical studies and concluded that cefaclor had been successful as treatment of upper and lower respiratory tract infections caused by *Moraxella catarrhalis*.

References

Adam D, Hofstetter AG, Jacoby W, Reichardt B (1975). *Studies on the Diffusion of Cephradine and Cephalothin into Human Tissue: Proceedings of the 9th International Congress of Chemotherapy, London, 1975* (Abstr. M69). Washington, DC: American Society for Microbiology.

Bach VT, Khurana MM, Thadepalli H (1978). *In vitro* activity of cefaclor against aerobic and anaerobic bacteria. *Antimicrob Ag Chemother* 13: 210.

Bartlett JG, Willey SH, Chang TW, Lowe B (1979). Cephalosporin-associated pseudomembranous colitis due to *Clostridium difficile*. *JAMA* 242: 2683.

Basker MJ, Edmondson RA, Sutherland R (1980). Comparative stabilities of penicillins and cephalosporins to staphylococcal beta-lactamase and activities against *Staphylococcus aureus*. *J Antimicrob Chemother* 6: 333.

Bennett WM, Singer I, Golper T *et al.* (1977). Guidelines for drug therapy in renal failure. *Ann Intern Med* 86: 754.

Bill NJ, Washington JA II (1977). Comparison of *in vitro* activity of cephalexin, cephradine and cefaclor. *Antimicrob Ag Chemother* 11: 470.

Blaser MJ, Klaus BD, Jacobsen JA *et al.* (1983). Comparison of cefadroxil and cephalexin in the treatment of community-acquired pneumonia. *Antimicrob Ag Chemother* 24: 163.

Bloch R, Szwed JJ, Sloan RS, Luft FC (1977). Pharmacokinetics of cefaclor in normal subjects and patients with chronic renal failure. *Antimicrob Ag Chemother* 12: 730.

Bluestone CD, Beery QC, Michaels RH *et al.* (1979). Cefaclor compared with amoxycillin in acute otitis media with effusion: a preliminary report. *Postgrad Med J* **55** (Suppl 4): 42.

Boeschoten EW, Rietra PJGM, Krediet RT *et al.* (1985). CAPD peritonitis: a prospective randomized trial of oral versus intraperitoneal treatment with cephradine. *J Antimicrob Chemother* **16**: 789.

Boguniewicz M, Leung DYM (1995). Hypersensitivity reactions to antibiotics commonly used in children. *Pediatr Infect Dis J* **14**: 221.

Brisson AM, Fourtillan JB (1982). Pharmacokinetic study of cefadroxil following single and repeated doses. *J Antimicrob Chemother* **10** (Suppl B): 11.

Brumfitt W, Hamilton-Miller JMT (1990). Prophylactic antibiotics for recurrent urinary tract infections. *J Antimicrob Chemother* **25**: 505.

Buck RE, Price KE (1977). Cefadroxil, a new broad-spectrum cephalosporin. *Antimicrob Ag Chemother* **11**: 324.

Busch DF, Kureshi LA, Sutter VL, Finegold SM (1976). Susceptibility of respiratory tract anaerobes to orally administered penicillins and cephalosporins. *Antimicrob Ag Chemother* **10**: 713.

Caloza DL Jr, Semar RW, Bernfeld GE (1979). Intravenous use of cephradine and cefazolin against serious infections. *Antimicrob Ag Chemother* **15**: 119.

Cooper J, Brumfitt W, Hamilton-Miller JMT (1980). A comparative trial of cotrimoxazole and cephradine in patients with recurrent urinary infections. *J Antimicrob Chemother* **6**: 231.

Craft I, Forster TC (1978). Materno-fetal cephradine transfer in pregnancy. *Antimicrob Ag Chemother* **14**: 924.

Daggett PR, Nathan AW (1975). Failure of cephradine in infective endocarditis. *Lancet* **ii**: 877.

Del Busto R, Haas E, Madhavan T *et al.* (1976). *In vitro* and clinical studies of cefatrizine, a new semisynthetic cephalosporin. *Antimicrob Ag Chemother* **9**: 397.

Dolfini JE, Applegate HE, Bach G *et al.* (1971). A new class of semisynthetic penicillins and cephalosporins derived from D-2-(1, 4-cyclohexadienyl). glycine. *J Med Chem* **14**: 117.

Edén T, Anari M, Ernstson S, Sundberg L (1983). Penetration of cefaclor to adenoid tissue and middle ear fluid in secretory otitis media. *Scand J Infect Dis* (Suppl 39): 48.

Ekedahl C (1983). Treatment of maxillary sinusitis. *Scand J Infect Dis* (Suppl 39): 56.

Fong IW, Engelking ER, Kirby WMM (1976). Relative inactivation by *Staphylococcus aureus* of eight cephalosporin antibiotics. *Antimicrob Ag Chemother* **9**: 939.

Gartenberg G, Meyers BR, Hirschman SZ, Srulevitch E (1979). Pharmacokinetics of cefaclor in patients with stable renal impairment, and patients undergoing haemodialysis. *J Antimicrob Chemother* **5**: 465.

Gerber MA, Randolph MF, Chanatry J (1986). Once daily therapy for streptococcal pharyngitis with cefadroxil. *J Pediatr* **109**: 531.

Giebink GS, Batalden PB, Russ JN, Le CT (1984). Cefaclor v amoxicillin in treatment of acute otitis media. *Amer J Dis Child* **138**: 287.

Gillett AP, Andrews JM, Wise R (1979). Comparative *in vitro* microbiological activity and stability of cefaclor. *Postgrad Med J* **55** (Suppl 4): 9.

Ginsburg CM (1982). Comparative pharmacokinetics of cefadroxil, cefaclor, cephalexin and cephradine in infants and children. *J Antimicrob Chemother* **10** (Suppl B): 27.

Ginsburg CM, McCracken GH Jr (1979). Pharmacokinetics of cephradine suspension in infants and children. *Antimicrob Ag Chemother* **16**: 74.

Ginsburg CM, McCracken GH Jr, Petruska M (1982). Once-daily cefadroxil versus twice-daily cefaclor for treatment of acute urinary tract infections in children. *J Antimicrob Chemother* **10** (Suppl B): 53.

Glynne A, Goulbourn RA, Ryden R (1978). A human pharmacology study of cefaclor. *J Antimicrob Chemother* **4**: 343.

Goldstein EJC, Kwok YY, Sutter VL (1983). Susceptibility of *Gardnerella vaginalis* to cephradine. *Antimicrob Ag Chemother* **24**: 418.

Grant M, Raeburn JA, Sutherland R *et al.* (1983). Effect of two antibiotics on human granuloctye activities. *J Antimicrob Chemother* **11**: 543.

Greenberg RN, Sanders CV, Lewis AC, Marier RL (1981). Single-dose cefaclor therapy of urinary tract infection. Evaluation of antibody-coated bacteria test and C-reactive protein assay as predictors of cure. *Amer J Med* **71**: 841.

Hains CS, Johnson SE, Nelson KG (1989). Once daily cefadroxil therapy for pyoderma. *Pediatr Infect Dis J* **8**: 648.

Hamilton-Miller JMT (1974). Comparative activity of ampicillin and seven cephalosporins against Group D streptococci. *J Clin Path* **27**: 828.

Hampel B, Lode H, Wagner J, Koeppe P (1982). Pharmacokinetics of cefadroxil and cefaclor during an eight-day dosage period. *Antimicrob Ag Chemother* **22**: 1061.

Hart CA, Desmond AD, Percival A (1981). Treatment of gentamicin-resistant Klebsiella urinary tract infections with cephradine, augmentin, cefuroxime and amikacin. *J Antimicrob Chemother* **8**: 231.

Hartstein AI, Patrick KE, Jones SR *et al.* (1977). Comparison of pharmacological and antimicrobial properties of cefadroxil and cephalexin. *Antimicrob Ag Chemother* **12**: 93.

Henning C, Iwarson S, Paulsen O, Sandberg T (1982). Cefadroxil single-dose long and short therapy versus amoxicillin in female urinary tract infections. *J Antimicrob Chemother* **10** (Suppl B): 73.

Horner DB, McCracken GH Jr, Ginsburg CM, Zweighaft TC (1980). A comparison of three antibiotic regimens for eradication of *Haemophilus influenzae* type B from the pharynx of infants and children. *Pediatrics* **66**: 136.

Kammer RB, Short LJ (1979). Cefaclor-summary of clinical experience. *Postgrad Med J* **55** (Suppl 4): 93.

Kiss IJ, Faragó E, Pintér J (1976). Serum and lung tissue levels of cephradine in thoracic surgery. *Brit J Clin Pharmac* **3**: 891.

Klastersky J, Daneau D, Weerts D (1973). Cephradine antibacterial activity and clinical effectiveness. *Chemotherapy* **18**: 191.

Korzeniowski OM, Scheld WM, Sande MA (1977). Comparative pharmacology of cefaclor and cephalexin. *Antimicrob Ag Chemother* **12**: 157.

Kramer RI (1982). Comparison of cefadroxil and cephalexin therapies in the treatment of acute lower respiratory tract infections in children. *J Antimicrob Chemother* **10** (Suppl B): 105.

Lacey RW, Lord VL, Howson GL *et al.* (1983). Double-blind study to compare the selection of antibiotic resistance by amoxycillin or cephradine in the commensal flora. *Lancet* **ii**: 529.

La Rosa F, Ripa S, Prenna M *et al.* (1982). Pharmacokinetics of cefadroxil after oral administration in humans. *Antimicrob Ag Chemother* **21**: 320.

Law MR, Holt HA, Reeves DS, Hodson ME (1983). Cefaclor and amoxycillin in the treatment of infective exacerbations of chronic bronchitis. *J Antimicrob Chemother* **11**: 83.

Lawson AA, McArdle T, Ghosh S (1984). Cephradine-associated immune neutropenia. *New Engl J Med* **312**: 651.

Leigh DA (1989). Determination of serum and bone concentrations of cephradine and cefuroxime by HPLC in patients undergoing hip and knee joint replacement surgery. *J Antimicrob Chemother* **23**: 877.

Leitner F, Buck RE, Misiek M *et al.* (1975). BL-S 640, a cephalosporin with a broad spectrum of antibacterial activity: properties *in vitro*. *Antimicrob Ag Chemother* **7**: 298.

Leitner F, McGregor MC, Pursiano TA (1982). Comparative antibacterial spectrum of cefadroxil. *J Antimicrob Chemother* **10** (Suppl B): 1.

Leroy A, Humbert G, Godin M, Fillastre JP (1982). Pharmacokinetics of cefadroxil in patients with impaired renal function. *J Antimicrob Chemother* **10** (Suppl B): 39.

Levison ME, Santoro J, Agarwal BN (1979). *In vitro* activity and pharmacokinetics of cefaclor in normal volunteers and patients with renal failure. *Postgrad Med J* **55** (Suppl 4): 12.

Lindan R (1979). Comparison of cefaclor and amoxycillin in the treatment of urinary infections in a chronic disease hospital. *Postgrad Med J* **55** (Suppl 4): 67.

Macias EG, Eller JJ (1975). Intravenous cephradine in serious paediatric infections. *Lancet* **i**: 38.

Maeson FPV, Geraedts WH, Davies BI (1990). Cefaclor in the treatment of chronic bronchitis. *J Antimicrob Chemother* **26**: 456.

Mandel EM, Kardatzke D, Bluestone CD, Rockette HE (1993). A comparative evaluation of cefaclor and amoxicillin in the treatment of acute otitis media. *Pediatr Infect Dis J* **12**: 726.

Maroske D, Knothe H, Rox A (1976). Liver tissue concentration of cephradine and cephacetrile and their excretion in bile. *Infection* **4**: 159.

Mattson K, Renkonen O-V, Laitinen L, Nikander-Hurme R (1979). Treatment of acute bronchitis and pneumonia with cefaclor. *Postgrad Med J* **55** (Suppl 4): 59.

McCracken GH Jr, Ginsburg CM, Clahsen JC, Thomas ML (1978). Pharmacokinetics of cefaclor in infants and children. *J Antimicrob Chemother* **4**: 515.

McGowan JE Jr, Garner C, Wilcox C, Finland M (1974). Antibiotic susceptibility of Gram-negative bacilli isolated from blood cultures: results of tests with 35 agents and strains from 169 patients at Boston City Hospital during 1972. *Amer J Med* **57**: 225, quoted by Bill and Washington (1977).

McLinn SE (1980). Cefaclor in treatment of otitis media and pharyngitis in children. *Amer J Dis Child* **134**: 560.

Miraglia GJ, Renz KJ, Gadebusch HH (1973). Comparison of the chemotherapeutic and pharmacodynamic activities of cephradine, cephalothin and cephaloridine in mice. *Antimicrob Ag Chemother* **3**: 270.

Moellering RC Jr, Swartz MN (1976). Drug therapy The newer cephalosporins. *New Engl J Med* **294**: 24.

Mogabgab WJ (1976). Treatment of urinary tract infections with cephradine. *Curr Ther Res* **19**: 520.

Murray DL, Singer DA, Singer AB (1980). Cefaclor – a cluster of adverse reactions. *New Engl J Med* **303**: 1003.

Neu HC, Fu KP (1978). Cefaclor: *in vitro* spectrum of activity and beta-lactamase stability. *Antimicrob Ag Chemother* **13**: 584.

Nord CE, Heimdahl A, Lundberg C, Marklund G (1987). Impact of cefaclor on the normal human oropharyngeal and intestinal microflora. *Scand J Infect Dis* **19**: 681.

Oberlin JA, Hyslop DL (1990). Cefaclor treatment of upper and lower respiratory tract infections caused by *Moraxella catarrhalis*. *Pediatr Infect Dis J* **9**: 41.

Oguma T, Yamada H, Sawaki H, Narita N (1991). Pharmacokinetic analysis of the effects of different foods on absorption of cefaclor. *Antimicrob Ag Chemother* **35**: 1729.

Overturf GD, Ressler RL, Marengo PB, Wilkins J (1975). *In vitro* evaluation of BL-S640, a new oral cephalosporin antibiotic. *Antimicrob Ag Chemother* **8**: 305.

Parsons RL, Beavis JP, Paddock GM, Hossack GM (1976). Cephradine bone concentrations during total hip replacement. In *Chemotherapy* (Williams JD, Geddes AM, eds), Vol. 1, p. 201 New York: Plenum Press.

Pfeffer M, Jackson A, Ximenes J, De Menezes JP (1977). Comparative human oral clinical pharmacology of cefadroxil, cephalexin, and cephradine. *Antimicrob Ag Chemother* **11**: 331.

Phillips I, King A, Warren C et al. (1976). The activity of penicillin and eight cephalosporins on *Neisseria gonorrhoeae*. *J Antimicrob Chemother* **2**: 31.

Picard M, Malouin F (1992). Molecular basis of the efficacy of cefaclor against *Haemophilus influenzae*. *Antimicrob Ag Chemother* **36**: 2569.

Pichichero ME, Disney FA, Aronovitz GH et al. (1987). Randomized, single-blind evaluation of cefadroxil and phenoxymethyl penicillin in the treatment of streptococcal pharyngitis. *Antimicrob Ag Chemother* **31**: 903.

Platt R, Dreis MW, Kennedy DL, Kuritsky JN (1988). Serum sickness-like reactions to amoxicillin, cefaclor, cephalexin and trimethoprim-sulfamethoxazole. *J Infect Dis* **158**: 474.

Powell M, Williams JD (1988). *In-vitro* activity of cefaclor, cephalexin and ampicillin against 2458 clinical isolates of *Haemophilus influenzae*. *J Antimicrob Chemother* **21**: 27.

Powell M, McVey D, Kassim MH et al. (1991). Antimicrobial susceptibility of *Streptococcus pneumoniae*, *Haemophilus influenzae* and *Moraxella* (*Branhamella*) *catarrhalis* isolated in the UK from sputa. *J Antimicrob Chemother* **28**: 249.

Preston DA (1979). Summary of laboratory studies on the antibacterial activity of cefaclor. *Postgrad Med J* **55** (Suppl 4): 22.

Puhakka H, Virolainen E, Eskola J, Holm S (1982). Cefadroxil in the treatment of acute otitis media in children. *J Antimicrob Chemother* **10** (Suppl B): 99.

Quintiliani R (1982). A review of the penetration of cefadroxil into human tissue. *J Antimicrob Chemother* **10** (Suppl B): 33.

Raucher HS, Murphy RJC, Barzilai A (1982). Meningitis occurring during therapy for otitis media with cephalexin and cefaclor. *Amer J Dis Child* **136**: 745.

Rodriquez WJ, Ross S, Schwartz R et al. (1979). Cefaclor in the treatment of susceptible infections in infants and children. *Postgrad Med J* **55** (Suppl 4): 35.

Rotschafer JC, Crossley KB, Lesar TS et al. (1982). Cefaclor pharmacokinetic parameters: serum concentrations determined by a new high-performance liquid chromatographic technique. *Antimicrob Ag Chemother* **21**: 170.

Rugendorff EW (1982). Randomized, comparative, open study of cefadroxil administered once or twice daily in urinary tract infections. *J Antimicrob Chemother* **10** (Suppl B): 57.

Sanders CC (1977). *In vitro* studies with cefaclor, a new oral cephalosporin. *Antimicrob Ag Chemother* **12**: 490.

Santella PJ, Henness D (1982). A review of the bioavailability of cefadroxil. *J Antimicrob Chemother* **10** (Suppl B): 17.

Santoro J, Agarwal BN, Martinelli R et al. (1978). Pharmacology of cefaclor in normal volunteers and patients with renal failure. *Antimicrob Ag Chemother* **13**: 951.

Scheffer J, Knöller J, Cullmann W, König W (1992). Effects of cefaclor, cefatamet and Ro40-6890 on inflammatory responses on human granulocytes. *J Antimicrob Chemother* **30**: 57.

Scheld WM, Korzeniowski OM, Sande MA (1977). *In vitro* susceptibility studies with cefaclor and cephalexin. *Antimicrob Ag Chemother* **12**: 290.

Scholand JF, Hodges GR, Fass RJ, Saslaw S (1974). Clinical evaluation of cephradine, a new oral cephalosporin. *Amer J Med Sci* **267**: 111.

Selwyn S (1976). Rational choice of penicillins and cephalosporins based on parallel *in-vitro* and *in-vivo* tests. *Lancet* **ii**: 616.

Selwyn S, Bakhtiar M (1977). Penicillin-resistant gonococci. *Brit Med J* **2**: 118.

Sinai R, Hammerberg S, Marks MI, Pai CH (1978). *In vitro* susceptibility of *Haemophilus influenzae* to sulfamethoxazole-trimethoprim and cefaclor, cephalexin, and cephradine. *Antimicrob Ag Chemother* **13**: 861.

Spyker DA, Gober LL, Scheld WM et al. (1982). Pharmacokinetics of cefaclor in renal failure: effects of multiple doses and hemodialysis. *Antimicrob Ag Chemother* **21**: 278.

Stillerman M (1986). Comparison of oral cephalosporins with penicillin therapy for Group A streptococcal pharyngitis. *Pediatr Infect Dis* **5**: 649.

Tally FP, Jacobus NV, Barza M (1979). *In vitro* activity and serum protein-binding of cefaclor. *J Antimicrob Chemother* **5**: 159.

Tupasi TE, Calubiran OV, Torres CA (1982). Single oral dose of cefaclor for the treatment of infections with penicillinase-producing strains of *Neisseria gonorrhoeae*. *Brit J Vener Dis* **58**: 176.

Wald ER, Reilly JS, Casselbrant M et al. (1984). Treatment of acute maxillary sinusitis in childhood: a comparative study of amoxicillin and cefaclor. *J Pediatr* **104**: 297.

Wang PL, Prime DJ, Hsu C-Y, Tune BM (1982). Effects of ureteral obstruction on the toxicity of cephalosporins in the rabbit kidney. *J Infect Dis* **145**: 574.

Watanakunakorn C, Glotzbecker C (1979). Comparative susceptibility of *Haemophilus* species to cefaclor, cefamandole, and five other cephalosporins and ampicillin, chloramphenicol, and tetracycline. *Antimicrob Ag Chemother* **15**: 836.

Waterman NG, Scharfenberger LF (1978). Concentration relationships of cefaclor in serum, interstitial fluid, bile and urine of dogs. *Antimicrob Ag Chemother* **14**: 614.

Wathne B, Hovelius B, Holst E (1989). Cefadroxil as an alternative to metronidazole in the treatment of bacterial vaginosis. *Scand J Infect Dis* **21**: 585.

Weingarten C (1982). Randomized, comparative study of oral cefadroxil and cephalexin in lower respiratory infections in adults. *J Antimicrob Chemother* **10** (Suppl B): 109.

Wernstedt L, Berntsson E, Thiringer G (1979). Cefaclor therapy in acute exacerbations of chronic bronchitis. *Postgrad Med J* **55** (Suppl 4): 56.

Wilber RB, De Regis RG, Fox EJ (1982). The role of cefadroxil in the therapy of urinary tract infections. *J Antimicrob Chemother* **10** (Suppl B): 77.

Windorfer A, Bauer P (1982). Pharmacokinetics and clinical studies with cefadroxil in paediatrics. *J Antimicrob Chemother* **10** (Suppl B): 85.

Wise R, Andrews JM, Dean S *et al.* (1979). A pharmacological and *in vitro* comparison of three oral cephalosporins. *J Antimicrob Chemother* **5**: 601.

Cefazolin, Cephacetrile and Cephapirin

Description

Many compounds have been derived from the cephalosporin C nucleus (p. 251) in an attempt to produce antibiotics with advantages over the older parenteral cephalosporin, cephalothin (p. 251), or over the oral cephalosporin, cephalexin (p. 263).

The three cephalosporins described in this chapter are grouped together because they can only be administered parenterally, and their antibacterial spectrum is similar to that of cephalothin (Turck, 1982). Only cefazolin has some practical advantages over cephalothin.

1 Cefazolin

This has many similarities to cephalothin (Wick and Preston, 1972), but it produces higher serum levels, and its i.m. administration is less painful than that of cephalothin (Kirby and Regamey, 1973).

2 Cephacetrile

It is like cephalothin, but after i.v. administration higher peak serum levels are attained, and its serum half-life is longer (Brogard *et al.*, 1973a,b). Cephacetrile appears to have no clinical advantages over cephalothin as demonstrated in one comparative trial (Jackson *et al.*, 1974).

3 Cephapirin

This is very similar to cephalothin, and the pain produced by i.m. injection of both drugs is the same (Bran *et al.*, 1972). The initial impression that i.v. administration of cephapirin may cause less thrombophlebitis than cephalothin has not been confirmed (Robson and Bowmer, 1974).

In recent years cephacetrile and cefapirin have been used very little. The details below will only apply to cefazolin. A description of cephacetrile and cephapirin is available in the fourth edition of this book.

Sensitive Organisms

The antibacterial spectrum of cefazolin, in general, resembles that of cephalothin (p. 251).

1 Gram-positive cocci

Cefazolin is active against *Staphylococcus aureus* and coagulase-negative staphylococci, including penicillin-resistant, but not methicillin-resistant strains. However, cefazolin is somewhat vulnerable to staphylococcal beta-lactamase, but usually not to the same degree as cephaloridine (p. 251) (Sabath *et al.*, 1975; Farrar and Gramling, 1976). There are functionally important differences in beta-lactamase activities in different strains of *Staph. aureus*. Some beta-lactamases hydrolyze cephaloridine more easily than cefazolin, and others do the opposite (Sabath, 1989). In addition, some *Staph. aureus* beta-lactamases may even inactivate cefamandole (p. 292) more easily than cefazolin (Fields *et al.*, 1993). Bonfiglio and Livermore (1994) identified four different beta-lactamases, designated types A, B, C and D, produced by different strains of *Staph. aureus*. Types A and C predominated. Producers of type A enzyme were less susceptible to cefazolin than those with class C beta-lactamase.

Most other Gram-positive cocci, such as *Streptococcus pyogenes*, *Strep. pneumoniae* and the alpha-hemolytic streptococci of the 'viridans' group, are sensitive, but *Enterococcus faecalis* is usually moderately resistant (Wick and Preston, 1972; Hamilton-Miller, 1974; Motley and

Shadomy, 1974; Wilcox *et al.*, 1993). At clinically achievable concentrations, cefazolin acts synergistically with aminoglycosides, such as gentamicin or tobramycin, against *E. faecalis in vitro*; but similar to cephalothin (p. 252), these combinations are not effective for the treatment of *E. faecalis* endocarditis (Bourque *et al.*, 1976; Collins and Edwards, 1980). Anaerobic Gram-positive cocci, such as the *Peptococcus* spp., are usually sensitive to cefazolin (Sutter and Finegold, 1975; Tally *et al.*, 1975).

2 Gram-positive bacilli

Bacillus anthracis, *Corynebacterium diphtheriae* and *Listeria monocytogenes* are usually susceptible. Anaerobes, such as *Clostridium perfringens*, *Cl. tetani* and other *Clostridium* spp., are also sensitive (Sutter and Finegold, 1975; Tally *et al.*, 1975).

3 Gram-negative aerobic bacteria

The *Neisseria* spp. (meningococci and gonococci) are usually sensitive. Cefazolin may be quite active against gonococcal strains which are relatively resistant to penicillin G (p. 14) (Phillips *et al.*, 1976). Cefazolin is inactive against beta-lactamase-producing gonococci (p.15).

Salmonella and *Shigella* spp., *Haemophilus influenzae* and *Bordetella pertussis* are usually sensitive. *Escherichia coli*, *Klebsiella pneumoniae* and *Proteus mirabilis* are commonly sensitive unless they are derived from a hospital environment. A survey in UK showed that some 91% of *E. coli* strains isolated from both hospitals and community were cefazolin-sensitive (MacGowan *et al.*, 1993). Other species of *Klebsiella*, such as *Kl. aerogenes* are frequently resistant. *Proteus vulgaris*, *Morganella morganii*, *Enterobacter* and *Providencia* spp., *Serratia marcescens* and *Pseudomonas aeruginosa* are always resistant (Motley and Shadomy, 1974; Yourassowsky *et al.*, 1976). Cefazolin and amikacin often show *in vitro* synergism against *Klebsiella* spp. strains (Klastersky *et al.*, 1976). *Campylobacter* jejuni is cefazolin-resistant (Karmali *et al.*, 1980).

4 Gram-negative anaerobic bacteria

Bacteroides fragilis is resistant, but *Prevotella* spp., especially *P. melaninogenica*, and the *Fusobacterium* and *Veillonella* spp., are usually cefazolin-sensitive (Tally *et al.*, 1975). A combination of cefazolin with the beta-lactamase inhibitors, clavulanic acid (p. 193) or sulbactam (p. 209), is active against *B. fragilis*, but such combinations are not available commercially (Fekete *et al.*, 1987).

5 Differences in antibacterial activity with cephalothin

Cefazolin has much the same activity as cephalothin against Gram-positive cocci and *Pr. mirabilis*, but it is more active against *E. coli*, *Kl. pneumoniae* and *Salmonellae* spp. (Sabath *et al.*, 1973; Strausbaugh *et al.*, 1978).

6 Acquired resistance

There is almost complete cross-resistance between cefazolin and cephalothin (Phair *et al.*, 1972; Verbist, 1976). Occasionally, cephalothin-resistant *E. coli*, *Klebsiella* and *Enterobacter* spp. strains, may be sensitive to cefazolin (Jones and Fuchs, 1976; Kisch and Bartholomew, 1976).

7 Minimum inhibitory concentrations

The MICs of cefazolin against some selected bacterial species, are compared with those of cephalothin in Table I.24.

Mode of Administration and Dosage

Cefazolin can be administered i.m. and the usual adult dosage is 0.5 g every 8 h (Reller *et al.*, 1973). The total daily dose can be varied widely according to the nature and severity of the infection. Daily doses ranging from 1 to 4 g (occasionally up to 6 g) administered in two, three or four divided doses have been used (Reinarz *et al.*, 1973; Ries *et al.*, 1973). Cefazolin causes less pain on i.m. injection than cephalothin, and also thrombophlebitis is not a major problem when the drug is used i.v. (Shemonsky *et al.*, 1975).

Cefazolin can be administered i.v. by either continuous infusion, intermittent infusions (via a pediatric buretrol or separate secondary i.v. bottles), or by direct i.v. injections. The continuous infusion method may have some pharmacological advantages; when resultant serum levels are graphed, it produces a greater area under the curve and also biliary levels are more sustained (Thys *et al.*, 1976). Incompatibility and drug inactivation problems may arise if cefazolin is

Organism	MIC (μg per ml)	
	Cephalothin	Cefazolin
Gram-positive bacteria		
Staphylococcus aureus (non-penicillinase producer)	0.25	0.5
Staphylococcus aureus (penicillinase producer)	0.5	0.5
Staphylococcus epidermidis	0.12–0.5	0.25–0.5
Streptococcus pyogenes	0.06–0.12	0.12
Streptococcus pneumoniae	0.12–0.25	0.12–0.25
Streptococcus viridans	0.5	0.5–1.0
Enterococcus faecalis	16.0–32.0	32.0
Gram-negative bacteria		
Escherichia coli	4.0–32.0	2.0–4.0
Klebsiella spp.	1.0–2.0	1.0–2.0
Proteus mirabilis	4.0–8.0	8.0
Proteus vulgaris	>100.0	>100.0
Bacteroides fragilis	64.0	64.0

Table I.24
Compiled from data published by Wick and Preston (1972), Hamilton-Miller (1974) and Tally *et al.* (1975)

added to i.v. solution bottles. The intermittent infusion method, as with penicillin G (p. 200), is preferable.

Dosage for children is 25–50 mg per kg body weight per day, given in three or four divided doses (Pickering *et al.*, 1973). Total daily dosage may be increased to 100 mg per kg per day for the treatment of severe infections. For newborn and premature infants, aged 0–7 days and weighing less than 2000 g a dosage of 20 mg per kg every 12 h is recommended (total daily dose 40 mg per kg). For infants weighing more than 2000 g or who are older than 7 days, a dosage of 20 mg per kg 8-hourly (total daily dose 60 mg per kg) is recommended (McCracken and Nelson, 1983).

Patients with renal failure require dosage reduction and serum level monitoring (Levison et **al.**, 1973; Benner *et al.*, 1975). All adults with renal failure should receive an initial loading dose of 0.5 g. Thereafter, those with mild to moderate renal failure (creatinine clearance 40–60 ml per min), may be given 60% of the normal daily dose in two divided doses. The dose for patients with moderate renal failure (creatinine clearance 20–40 ml per min) is 25–35% of the normal daily dose, given in two divided doses. In severe renal failure (creatinine clearance 5–20 ml per min), a dose of approximately 10% of the normal daily one, administered as a single dose every 24 h, is recommended. For patients with essentially no renal function (creatinine clearance <5 ml per min), only 5% of the normal daily dose should be given, as a single dose once every 24 h.

Cefazolin is removed relatively slowly by hemodialysis; over 4 h about 46% of an administered dose is removed (Madhavan *et al.*, 1975). Therefore, for anephric patients undergoing twice-weekly hemodialysis, an extra dose of 250 mg at the end of each dialysis is recommended (Levison *et al.*, 1973; McCloskey *et al.*, 1973). Cefazolin is not removed by peritoneal dialysis so that additional dosing is not needed during this procedure (Madhavan *et al.*, 1975). Cefazolin can be added to peritoneal dialysis fluid and when administered by this route it is well tolerated. Kaye *et al.* (1978b) added cefazolin to make a concentration of 50 or 150 mg per liter in dialysis fluid. Some of the added drug was absorbed; after the 24th exchange with the 150 mg per liter concentration, the mean serum concentration was 71.9 μg per ml. When 1 g of cefazolin was given intraperitoneally and dialysis was ceased, serum concentrations rose by a mean of 62.5 μg per ml in 2 h.

Serum Levels in Relation to Dosage

A peak serum level as high as 34 μg per ml is attained 1 h after a 0.5 g i.m. dose of cefazolin and 6 h later the level is about 6 μg per ml (Ishiyama *et al.*, 1971). These levels are about four times as high as those after cephalothin (p. 254). In addition, measurable levels of cefazolin may still be present 12 h after this dose (Ries *et al.*, 1973). Doubling the dose usually doubles serum concentrations (Cahn *et al.*, 1974). After i.v. infusion of 0.5 g cefazolin over 20 min, a peak serum level of 118 μg per ml is obtained, and a detectable level is still present 8 h later (Kirby and Regamey, 1973). When a 1.5 g dose of cefazolin is injected i.v. over a 3-min period, the peak serum level 5-min later is 206 μg per ml. For a given i.v. dose, cefazolin serum concentrations are consistently higher than those of moxalactam (p. 330) (Polk *et al.*, 1981). If a 6-g dose of cefazolin is administered by continuous infusion over 24 h (using a constant infusion device), a serum level of 52 μg per ml is maintained. In one study, the resultant area-under-the-curve (graph of serum levels against time) after such a continuous infusion, was 24% greater than that obtained after rapid injections of 1.5 g doses every 6 h (Thys *et al.*, 1976). The serum half-life of cefazolin is 1.8 h.

Excretion

Cefazolin is rapidly excreted via the kidney in an unchanged form. High urinary concentrations (4000 μg per ml) of the active drug are attained, and about 60% of an i.m. administered dose is excreted in the urine during the first 6 h (Ishiyama *et al.*, 1971). Its renal clearance is about 80% of the simultaneous creatinine clearance, and nearly all of a given dose can be recovered from the urine in 24 h (Reller *et al.*, 1973; Rattie and Ravin, 1975). Cefazolin is excreted primarily by glomerular filtration and to a lesser degree by tubular secretion; its excretion can be reduced and serum levels elevated by concomitant administration of probenecid (Kirby and Regamey, 1975). Renal clearance of cefazolin is slower than that of cephalothin, and this explains its higher and more prolonged serum levels (p. 284).

In the presence of impaired renal function, excretion is delayed and serum concentrations are even more sustained (Ries *et al.*, 1973). In uremic patients with a creatinine clearance in excess of 10 ml per min, high cefazolin concentrations are still attained in the urine (Brodwall *et al.*, 1977). The serum half-life of cefazolin in anephric patients is approximately 42 h (Rein *et al.*, 1973).

Only small quantities are excreted via the bile, where the concentration is about the same or slightly in excess of the simultaneous serum level, provided that the biliary tract is not obstructed (Brogard *et al.*, 1975; Thys *et al.*, 1976). In patients with cystic duct obstruction, cefazolin, like other antibiotics (p. 117), cannot be detected in gall bladder bile. Cefazolin concentrations attained in bile after usual therapeutic doses, are higher (17–31 μg per ml) and more sustained than those attained by cephalothin (p. 255); this is entirely due to the higher serum levels which are attained with cefazolin (Ratzan *et al.*, 1974). Cefazolin is not inactivated in the body.

Distribution of the Drug in Body

Cefazolin is highly bound to serum proteins (approximately 80%) and the volume in which it is distributed in the body is one of the smallest among the cephalosporins. The 'apparent volume of distribution' has been estimated as 10 liters per 1.73 m² body surface area (average adult) (Kirby and Regamey, 1973). This, together with its low renal clearance, is partly responsible for its high serum levels (p. 284). Therefore, despite high cefazolin serum levels, concentrations of this drug may be low at the site of infection, at least in some tissues. Nadai *et al.* (1993) showed that in endotoxemic rats the protein binding of cefazolin was decreased and its renal excretion was also decreased. The clinical significance of this is uncertain.

Cefazolin does not penetrate into the CSF in the absence of meningeal inflammation (Thys *et al.*, 1976). It readily crosses inflamed synovial membranes, and penetrates into bone reaching considerably higher concentrations in acutely inflamed, compared with normal bone tissue (Reller *et al.*, 1973; Fass, 1978). In uninflamed muscle the levels closely resemble the free (non-protein bound) concentration of cefazolin in the serum at the time, but these levels are still high enough to inhibit sensitive pathogens such as *Staph. aureus* (Connors *et al.*, 1990).

The drug is present in the ascitic fluid and also if this is complicated by bacterial peritonitis (Gerding *et al.*, 1977). Cefazolin penetrates into pleural fluid in adequate concentrations, but these are lower than serum levels at the time (Cole and Pung, 1977). Concentrations of cefazolin in inflammatory exudate are almost identical to concomitant serum levels, but levels are lower in fluid aspirated from surgical wounds (Ellis *et al.*, 1975). Therapeutic concentrations are found in wound secretions of patients with toe or heel ulcers due to peripheral arterial circulatory insufficiency (Rylander *et al.*, 1979). In patients given 2 g i.v. cefazolin 30 min before open heart surgery, cefazolin concentrations above the usual MICs of sensitive strains of *Staph. aureus* and *Staph. epidermidis*, persist for 12.9 h in the right atrial appendage and for 9.8 h in the serum; adequate concentrations are also attained in pericardial fluid (Nightingale *et al.*, 1980). Cefazolin crosses the placenta, but concentrations are lower in fetal than in maternal serum; in one study the drug, while present in fetal body fluids, was undetectable in fetal tissues (Bernard *et al.*, 1977). Only minute amounts are excreted in breast milk (Yoshioka *et al.*, 1979).

In animals, cefazolin penetrates well into interstitial fluid, and it attains higher concentrations in extravascular fluid with a high protein content (Waterman *et al.*, 1976; Peterson and Gerding, 1978). Penetration into surgical wounds is also good (Rosin *et al.*, 1989). It reaches satisfactory concentrations in lung, heart, liver and kidney, but tissue concentrations in animals are somewhat lower in the spleen and much lower in the brain (Ishiyama *et al.*, 1971). Penetration in both normal and osteomyelitic bone in animals is good (Daly *et al.*, 1982). After a subconjunctival dose of 100 mg cefazolin to rabbits with staphylococcal endophthalmitis, drug concentrations were adequate in the cornea and aqueous humor, but penetration into the vitreous humor was poor (Barza *et al.*, 1982). In animal studies, Bamberger *et al.* (1993) showed that in *Staph. aureus* abscess cavities zinc concentrations were diminished. Supplementation with physiological concentrations of zinc was detrimental to the antibacterial properties of the abscess fluid, but this enhanced the killing effects of cefazolin within the fluid.

Mode of Action

Cefazolin inhibits bacterial cell wall synthesis similar to other cephalosporins (p. 256) and penicillin G (p. 25).

Toxicity

1 Hypersensitivity reactions

Eosinophilia commonly occurs in association with cefazolin therapy (Ries *et al.*, 1973). Allergic reactions occur in approximately 5% of patients treated with cephalothin (p. 256) and the prevalence with cefazolin is likely to be much the same. Drug fever alone has been occasionally observed with cefazolin (Ries *et al.*, 1973).

These cephalosporins, like cephalothin (p. 256), are probably only occasionally cross-allergenic with the penicillins (Levine, 1973). It is wise to avoid these drugs in patients with a past history of anaphylaxis or other immediate-type hypersensitivity to any of the penicillins. This stands despite the report that a small number of patients shown to possess IgE penicillin determinants by the use of special skin tests (p. 30), have received cefazolin and other cephalosporins without any reactions (Saxon, 1983). Like cephalothin (p. 256), these drugs may be used cautiously in patients with a history of less severe penicillin allergy.

2 Nephrotoxicity

This appears to be rare, mild and reversible with cefazolin (Moellering and Swartz, 1976). Cefazolin has been used in doses as high as 12 g daily, without evidence of nephrotoxicity (Reinarz *et al.*, 1973). Cefazolin produces renal tubular damage in experimental animals, but the lesions are relatively mild (Silverblatt *et al.*, 1973). In rabbits bilateral ureteral obstruction increases toxicity of cefaclor (p. 277), but not of cefazolin. Cefaclor unlike cefazolin is rapidly secreted across renal tubular cells (Wang *et al.*, 1982). In animals, transient renal ischemia seems to aggravate cephalosporin toxicity; this is particularly so with rapidly secreted cephalosporins, and it is not significant with cefazolin, which is slowly secreted (Browning *et al.*, 1983).

It is not known whether cefazolin enhances nephrotoxicity of aminoglycoside antibiotics; as with cephalothin (p.257), it seems prudent to use such combinations with caution and to monitor renal function.

3 Hematological side-effects

Bleeding occurred in one uremic patient who had high serum levels of cefazolin (Lerner and Lubin, 1974). High serum concentrations of cefazolin (as well as most other beta-lactam antibiotics), interfere with platelet function by suppressing ADP-induced platelet aggregation, similar to carbenicillin and ticarcillin (p. 153) (Bang and Kammer, 1983). Hypoprothrombinema and bleeding occurs with cephalosporins which contain a N-methyl-thiotetrazole side-chain, such as cefamandole (p. 306), cefoperazone (p. 335), and moxalactam (p. 350). Cefazolin contains a structurally similar but not identical side-chain. Both animal studies (Lipsky *et al.*, 1986) and one patient who developed hypoprothrombinemia and bleeding whilst treated by cefazolin (Kurz *et al.*, 1986) have shown that this side-effect can also occur with cefazolin.

4 Hepatotoxicity

Transient elevations of SGOT or serum alkaline phosphatase have been noted during treatment with cefazolin (Ries *et al.*, 1973). No cases of serious hepatotoxicity have been reported.

5 Encephalopathy

As with the penicillins (p. 32) and other beta-lactams, this may occur if very high serum levels of cefazolin are reached. A patient reported by Gardner *et al.* (1978), who had renal functional impairment, and who was initially treated with inappropriately high doses of cefazolin (12 g per day), developed repeated convulsions while undergoing hemodialysis. A post-dialysis serum cefazolin level was greater than 512 µg per ml. Animal studies have shown that the quinolones potentiate cefazolin-induced seizures (De Sarro *et al.*, 1993).

6 Other side-effects

Lorber *et al.* (1975) described one patient who developed *Listeria meningitis*, in whom treatment with cefazolin for 5 days for *Listeria septicemia* had been initially successful. Meningitis has also developed during cephalothin therapy (p. 258). Therefore, drugs like cephalothin and cefazolin, which penetrate poorly into the CSF, should be used with caution in infections which may be complicated by meningitis.

Clinical Uses of the Drug

Cefazolin may have some advantages over cephalothin because it produces higher serum levels and is well tolerated. It has been used with success in streptococcal cellulitis, pneumococcal pneumonia and staphylococcal infections, such as septicemia, pneumonia, osteomyelitis, septic arthritis and endocarditis (Reller *et al.*, 1973; Reinarz *et al.*, 1973; Fass, 1978). Children with soft tissue infections, pneumonia or osteomyelitis have been treated with cefazolin, and the response has been satisfactory, similar to that obtained with cephalothin (Pickering *et al.*, 1974). As cefazolin is somewhat less stable to staphylococcal beta-lactamase than cephalothin (p. 282), it may not be a good drug for the treatment of severe staphylococcal infections such as endocarditis. Data from animal studies are conflicting. Goldman and Petersdorf (1980) found cephalothin superior to cefazolin for the treatment of experimental *Staph. aureus* endocarditis in rabbits, while Carrizosa *et al.* (1978, 1982) showed that both drugs were equally effective. Successes and failures have been described when cefazolin was used for *Staph. aureus* endocarditis in humans, and its role for this infection remains controversial (Quinn *et al.*, 1973; Bryant and Alford, 1977, 1978; Kaye *et al.*, 1978a; Drake and Sande, 1983). These differing results may be explicable by the fact that different strains of *Staph. aureus* produce different beta-lactamases and some of them easily hydrolyze cefazolin whilst others do not (p. 282). In common with other cephalosporins, cefazolin is ineffective for the treatment of *E. faecalis* endocarditis.

The efficacy of cefazolin for the treatment of urinary tract infections is comparable with that of cephalothin (Ries *et al.*, 1973) or ampicillin (Benner *et al.*, 1975). Uncomplicated gonorrhea and gonococcal arthritis also respond to a course of cefazolin (Karney *et al.*, 1973). Single-dose treatment for uncomplicated gonorrhoea, using an i.m. dose of 2 g with or without probenecid, is unsatisfactory (Duncan, 1974).

Cefazolin has been used for surgical chemoprophylaxis in certain situations. It may be more suitable for this purpose than cephalothin as single i.m. or i.v. injections result in more prolonged serum levels (p. 284). In the past it was commonly given in three 1–2 g doses; the first just before surgery, and the others 6 and 12 h later (Polk *et al.*, 1980a,b; Gorbach, 1982). Nowadays in many cases a single dose of 1–2 g cefazolin, given i.v. at the time of induction of anesthesia is considered to be sufficient (Hirschmann and Inui, 1980; Hemsell, 1991). Cefazolin chemoprophylaxis has been used in cardiac surgery if the operation involves valve replacement or cardiopulmonary bypass (Gorbach, 1982). A penicillinase-resistant penicillin, such as nafcillin, (p. 106) is also suitable. Chemoprophylaxis may be associated with detrimental effects. In one study, 68% of cardiac surgery patients who received cefazolin prophylaxis, were colonized rapidly by methicillin- and gentamicin-resistant *Staph. epidermidis* strains (Archer and Armstrong, 1983). It is possible, that in institutions where methicillin-resistant *Staph. epidermidis* or *Staph. aureus* are prevalent, chemoprophylaxis by drugs such as nafcillin, cefazolin or rifampicin (p. 106) may help perpetuate the hospital reservoir of drug-resistant organisms.

In heart transplantation patients cefazolin (or cefamandole or cefuroxime) has been given at induction of anesthesia and then until 48 h postoperatively. These patients also received other chemoprophylaxis e.g. that directed against *Pneumocystis carinii* pneumonia and others against viral diseases and *Candida* infections (Petri, 1994). Perioperative antibiotic prophylaxis with cefazolin has also been used in breast surgery (Platt *et al.*, 1993). Cefazolin chemoprophylaxis is of value for vascular grafts of the abdominal aorta or lower extremity and total hip replacement, although for the latter one of the penicillinase-resistant penicillins is also satisfactory (Hirschmann and Inui, 1980; Earnshaw, 1989; Hopkins, 1991; Norden, 1991). Such prophylaxis is also effective in vaginal and abdominal hysterectomies and high-risk cesarean sections (Polk *et al.*, 1980b; Gorbach, 1982; Shapiro *et al.*, 1983; Brown, 1987; Hager *et al.*, 1991; Hemsell, 1991). Cefazolin has been advocated for the prevention of wound infections, because it reaches acceptable incisional concentrations which are more sustained than those of cephalothin (p. 259). Cefazolin has been used as prophylaxis during biliary endoscopic procedures (Alveyn, 1993). Cefazolin is not suitable for prophylaxis in colonic surgery where anaerobes are often involved (Neu, 1980). It may be used for biliary surgery but other antibiotics, such as ampicillin, (p. 125) are usually preferred. Cefazolin is of no proven value for prophylaxis in non-cardiac thoracic surgery (Truesdale *et al.*, 1979; Hopkins, 1991). In clean non-implant neurosurgery the data as to the value of chemoprophylaxis are inconclusive, but if chemoprophylaxis is given, cefazolin may be a suitable drug (Brown, 1993). In neurosurgical procedures where air sinuses are crossed in the absence of pre-existing infection (clean-contaminated procedures), it is recommended that metronidazole plus cefazolin (or cefuroxime) be used for chemoprophylaxis. In CSF shunt surgery the data are conflicting, but if chemoprophylaxis is used, cefazolin alone is reasonable. In patients with skull fractures and CSF leaks, prophylactic antibiotics are best withheld and the patients should be monitored closely for signs and symptoms of meningitis (Infection in Neurosurgery, 1994).

Sabath (1989) analyzed results of preoperative prophylaxis in situations where *Staph. aureus* or coagulase-negative staphylococci were the usual pathogens and prophylaxis failed. Such was the case in cardiothoracic surgery. In trials involving large numbers of patients, cefazolin failed more frequently than cefamandole (p. 308) or cefuroxime (p. 310). These findings are consistent with the *in vitro* evidence that cefazolin is more easily hydrolyzed by staphylococcal beta-lactamase than cephalothin and some second-generation cephalosporins.

References

Alveyn CG (1993). Antimicrobial prophylaxis during biliary endoscopic procedures. *J Antimicrob Chemother* **31** (Suppl B): 101.

Archer GL, Armstrong BC (1983). Alteration of staphylococcal flora in cardiac surgery patients receiving antibiotic prophylaxis. *J Infect Dis* **147**: 642.

Bamberger DM, Herndon BL, Suvarna PR (1993). The effect of zinc on microbial growth and bacterial killing by cefazolin in a *Staphylococcus aureus* abscess milieu. *J Infect Dis* **168**: 893.

Bang NU, Kammer RB (1983). Hematologic complications associated with beta-lactam antibiotics. *Rev Infect Dis* **5** (Suppl 2): 380.

Barza M, Kane A, Baum J (1982). Ocular penetration of subconjunctival oxacillin, methicillin and cefazolin in rabbits with staphylococcal endophthalmitis. *J Infect Dis* **145**: 899.

Benner EJ, Kranhold JF, Bush WG (1975). Cephazolin: a comparison to ampicillin in respiratory and urinary infections with dosage regulation by a nomogram. *Scot Med J* **20**: 244.

Bernard B, Barton L, Abate M, Ballard CA (1977). Maternal-fetal transfer of cefazolin in the first twenty weeks of pregnancy. *J Infect Dis* **136**: 377.

Bonfiglio G, Livermore DM (1994). Beta-lactamase types amongst *Staphylococcus aureus* isolates in relation to susceptibility to beta-lactamase inhibitor combinations. *J Antimicrob Chemother* **33**: 465.

Bourque M, Quintiliani R, Tilton RC (1976). Synergism of cefazolin-gentamicin against enterococci. *Antimicrob Ag Chemother* **10**: 157.

Bran JL, Levison ME, Kaye D (1972). Clinical and *in vitro* evaluation of cephapirin, a new cephalosporin antibiotic. *Antimicrob Ag Chemother* **1**: 35.

Brodwall EK, Bergan T, Ørjavik O (1977). Kidney transport of cefazolin in normal and impaired renal function. *J Antimicrob Chemother* **3**: 585.

Brogard JM, Kuntzmann F, Lavillaureix J (1973a). Blood levels, renal and biliary excretions of a new cephalosporin, cephacetrile (Ciba 36278 Ba). *Schweiz Med Wschr* **103**: 110.

Brogard JM, Haegele P, Dorner M, Lavillaureix J (1973b). Biliary excretion

of a new semisynthetic cephalosporin cephacetrile. *Antimicrob Ag Chemother* **3**: 19.

Brogard JM, Dorner M, Pinget M *et al.* (1975). The biliary excretion of cefazolin. *J Infect Dis* **131**: 625.

Brown EM (1987). Systemic antimicrobial prophylaxis in hysterectomy. *J Antimicrob Chemother* **20**: 143.

Brown EM (1993). Antibiotic prophylaxis in neurosurgery. *J Antimicrob Chemother* **31** (Suppl B): 49.

Browning MC, Hsu C-Y, Wang PL, Tune BM (1983). Interaction of ischemic and antibiotic-induced injury in rabbit kidney. *J Infect Dis* **147**: 341.

Bryant RE, Alford RH (1977). Unsuccessful treatment of staphylococcal endocarditis with cefazolin. *JAMA* **237**: 569.

Bryant RE, Alford RH (1978). Treatment of staphylococcal endocarditis. *JAMA* **239**: 1130.

Cahn MM, Levy EJ, Actor P, Pauls JF (1974). Comparative serum levels and urinary recovery of cefazolin, cephaloridine and cephalothin in man. *J Clin Pharmacol* **14**: 61.

Carrizosa J, Santoro J, Kaye D (1978). Treatment of experimental *Staphylococcus aureus* endocarditis; comparison of cephalothin, cefazolin, and methicillin. *Antimicrob Ag Chemother* **13**: 74.

Carrizosa J, Kobasa WD, Snepar R *et al.* (1982). Cefazolin versus cephalothin in beta-lactamase-producing *Staphylococcus aureus* endocarditis in a rabbit experimental model. *J Antimicrob Chemother* **9**: 387.

Cole DR, Pung J (1977). Penetration of cefazolin into pleural fluid. *Antimicrob Ag Chemother* **11**: 1033.

Collins RF, Edwards LD (1980). *In vitro* synergy of cefazolin-tobramycin against Gram-positive bacteria. *J Antimicrob Chemother* **6**: 323.

Connors JE, Di Piro JT, Hayter RG *et al.* (1990). Assessment of cefazolin and cefuroxime tissue penetration by using a continuous intravenous infusion. *Antimicrob Ag Chemother* **34**: 1128.

Daly RC, Fitzgerald RH Jr, Washington JA II (1982). Penetration of cefazolin into normal and osteomyelitic canine cortical bone. *Antimicrob Ag Chemother* 22: 461.

De Sarro A, Zappala M, Chimirri A *et al.* (1993). Quinolones potentiate cefazolin-induced seizures in DBA/² mice. *Antimicrob Ag Chemother* 37: 1497.

Drake TA, Sande MA (1983). Studies of the chemotherapy of endocarditis: correlation of *in vitro*, animal model, and clinical studies. *Rev Infect Dis* 5 (Suppl 2): 345.

Duncan WC (1974). Treatment of gonorrhea with cefazolin plus probenecid. *J Infect Dis* 130: 398.

Earnshaw JJ (1989). Prevention of infection after vascular reconstruction. *J Antimicrob Chemother* 23: 480.

Ellis BW, Standbridge RDeL, Sikorski JM *et al.* (1975). Penetration into inflammatory exudate and wounds of two cephalosporins for the prevention of surgical infections. *J Antimicrob Chemother* 1: 291.

Farrar WE Jr, Gramling PK (1976). Antistaphylococcal activity and beta-lactamase resistance of newer cephalosporins. *J Infect Dis* 133: 691.

Fass RJ (1978). Treatment of osteomyletis and septic arthritis with cefazolin. *Antimicrob Ag Chemother* 13: 405.

Fekete T, McGowen J, Cundy KR (1987). Activity of cefazolin and two beta-lactamase inhibitors, clavulanic acid and sulbactams against *Bacteroides fragilis*. *Antimicrob Ag Chemother* 31: 321.

Fields MT, Herndon BL, Bamberger DM (1993). Beta-lactamase-mediated inactivation and efficacy of cefazolin and cefmetazole in *Staphylococcus aureus* abscesses. *Antimicrob Ag Chemother* 37: 203.

Gardner ME, Fritz WL, Hyland RN (1978). Antibiotic-induced seizures. A case attributed to cefazolin. *Drug Intell Clin Pharm* 12: 268.

Gerding DN, Hall WH, Schierl EA (1977). Antibiotic concentrations in ascitic fluid of patients with ascites and bacterial peritonitis. *Ann Intern Med* 86: 708.

Goldman PL, Petersdorf RG (1980). Importance of beta-lactamase inactivation in treatment of experimental endocarditis caused by *Staphylococcus aureus*. *J Infect Dis* 141: 331.

Gorbach SL (1982). Prophylactic antibiotics – indications in surgical patients. *Scand J Infect Dis* (Suppl 36): 134.

Hager WD, Rapp RP, Billeter M, Bradley BB (1991). Choice of antibiotic in nonelective Cesarean section. *Antimicrob Ag Chemother* 35: 1782.

Hamilton-Miller JMT (1974). Comparative activity of ampicillin and seven cephalosporins against Group D streptococci. *J Clin Path* 27: 828.

Hemsell DL (1991). Prophylactic antibiotics in gynecologic and obstetric surgery. *Rev Infect Dis* 13 (Suppl 10): 821.

Hirschmann JV, Inui TS (1980). Antimicrobial prophylaxis: a critique of recent trials. *Rev Infect Dis* 2: 1.

Hopkins CC (1991). Antibiotic prophylaxis in clean surgery: peripheral vascular surgery, noncardiovascular thoracic surgery, herniorrhaphy, and mastectomy. *Rev Infect Dis* 13 (Suppl 10): 869.

Infection in Neurosurgery Working Party of the British Society for Antimicrobial Chemotherapy (1994). Antimicrobial prophylaxis in neurosurgery and after head injury. *Lancet* 344: 1547.

Ishiyama S, Nakayama I, Iwamoto H *et al.* (1971). Absorption, tissue concentration, and organ distribution of cefazolin. *Antimicrob Ag Chemother* 1970: 476.

Jackson GG, Riff LJ, Zimelis VM *et al.* (1974). Double-blind comparison of cephacetrile with cephalothin/cephaloridine. *Antimicrob Ag Chemother* 5: 247.

Jones RN, Fuchs PC (1976). Comparison of *in vitro* antimicrobial activity of cefamandole and cefazolin with cephalothin against over 8000 clinical bacterial isolates. *Antimicrob Ag Chemother* 9: 1066.

Karmali MA, De Grandis S, Fleming PC (1980). Antimicrobial susceptibility of *Campylobacter jejuni* and *Campylobacter fetus* subsp. fetus to eight cephalosporins with special reference to species differentiation. *Antimicrob Ag Chemother* 18: 948.

Karney WW, Turck M, Holmes KK (1973). Cefazolin in the treatment of gonorrhea. *J Infect Dis* 128 (Suppl): 399.

Kaye D, Hewitt W, Remington JS, Turck M (1978a). Treatment of staphylococcal endocarditis. *JAMA* 239: 1130.

Kaye D, Wenger N, Agarwal B (1978b). Pharmacology of intraperitoneal

cefazolin in patients undergoing peritoneal dialysis. *Antimicrob Ag Chemother* 14: 318.

Kirby WMM, Regamey C (1973). Pharmacokinetics of cefazolin compared with four other cephalosporins. *J Infect Dis* 128 (Suppl): 341.

Kisch AL, Bartholomew L (1976). Comparison of the *in vitro* activity of several cephalosporin antibiotics against Gram-negative and Gram-positive bacteria resistant to cephaloridine. *Antimicrob Ag Chemother* 10: 507.

Klastersky J, Meunier-Carpentier F, Prevost JM, Staquet M (1976). Synergism between amikacin and cefazolin against *Klebsiella*: in vitro studies and effect on the bactericidal activity of serum. *J Infect Dis* 134: 271.

Kurz RW, Wallner M, Graninger W, Tragl KH (1986). Hypoprothrombinaemia and bleeding associated with cefazolin. *J Antimicrob Chemother* 18: 772.

Lerner PI, Lubin A (1974). Coagulopathy with cefazolin in uremia. *New Engl J Med* 290: 1324.

Levine BB (1973). Antigenicity and cross-reactivity of penicillins and cephalosporins. *J Infect Dis* 128 (Suppl): 364.

Levison ME, Levison SP, Ries K, Kaye D (1973). Pharmacology of cefazolin in patients with normal and abnormal renal functions. *J Infect Dis* 128 (Suppl): 354.

Lipsky JJ, Lewis JC, Novick WJ, Jr (1986). Production of hypoprothrombinaemia by cefazolin and 2-methyl- 1, 3, 4 -thiadiazole – 5-thiol in the rat. *J Antimicrob Chemother* 18: 131.

Lorber B, Santoro J, Swenson RM 91975). *Listeria meningitis* during cefazolin therapy. *Ann Intern Med* 82: 226.

MacGowan AP, Brown NM, Holt HA *et al.* (1993). An eight-year survey of antimicoribal susceptibility patterns of 85,971 bacteria isolated from patients in a district general hospital and the local community. *J Antimicrob Chemother* 31: 543.

Madhavan T, Yaremchuk K, Levin N *et al.* (1975). Effects of renal failure and dialysis on cefazolin pharmacokinetics. *Antimicrob Ag Chemother* 8: 63,.

McCloskey RV, Forland MF, Sweeney MJ, Lawrence DN (1973). Hemodialysis of cefazolin. *J Infect Dis* 128 (Suppl): 358.

McCracken GH Jr, Nelson JD (1983). *Antimicrobial Therapy for Newborns* 2nd edn, p. 33. New York: Grune & Stratton.

Moellering RC Jr, Swartz MN (1976). Drug therapy: the newer cephalosporins. *New Engl J Med* 294: 24.

Motley M, Shadomy S (1974). *In vitro* studies with cefazolin. *Antimicrob Ag Chemother* 6: 856.

Nadai M, Hasegawa T, Kato K *et al.* (1993). Alterations in pharmacokinetics and protein binding behavior of cefazolin in endotoxemic rats. *Antimicrob Ag Chemother* 37: 1781.

Neu HC (1980). The place of cephalosporins in antibacterial treatment of infectious diseases. *J Antimicrob Chemother* 6 (Suppl A): 1.

Nightingale CH, Klimek JJ, Quintiliani R (1980). Effect of protein binding on the penetration of nonmetabolized cephalosporins into atrial appendage and pericardial fluids in open-heart surgical patients. *Antimicrob Ag Chemother* 17: 595.

Norden CW (1991). Antibiotic prophylaxis in orthopedic surgery. *Rev Infect Dis* 13 (Suppl 10): 842.

Peterson LR, Gerding DN (1978). Prediction of cefazolin penetration into high-and low-protein-containing extravascular fluid: new method for performing simultaneous studies. *Antimicrob Ag Chemother* 14: 533.

Petri WAJr (1994). Infections in heart transplant recipients. *Clin Infect Dis* 18: 141.

Phair JP, Carleton J, Tan JS (1972). Comparison of cefazolin, a new cephalosporin antibiotic, with cephalothin. *Antimicrob Ag Chemother* 2: 329.

Phillips I, King A, Warren C *et al.* (1976). The activity of penicillin and eight cephalosporins on *Neisseria gonorrhoeae*. *J Antimicrob Chemother* 2: 31.

Pickering LK, O'Connor DM, Anderson D *et al.* (1973). Clinical and pharmacologic evaluation of cefazolin in children. *J Infect Dis* 128 (Suppl): 407.

Pickering LK, O'Connor DM, Anderson D *et al.* (1974). Comparative evaluation of cefazolin and cephalothin in children. *J Pediatr* **85**: 842.

Platt R, Zucker JR, Zaleznik DF *et al.* (1993). Perioperative antibiotic prophylaxis and wound infection following breast surgery. *J Antimicrob Chemother* **31** (Suppl B): 43.

Polk BF, Tager IB, Shapiro M *et al.* (1980a). Randomised clinical trial of peri-operative cefazolin in preventing infection after hysterectomy. *Lancet* **i**: 437.

Polk HC Jr, Trachtenberg L, Finn MP (1980b). Antibiotic activity in surgical incisions. The basis for prophylaxis in selected operations. *JAMA* **244**: 1353.

Polk RE, Kline BJ, Markowitz SM (1981). Cefazolin and moxalactam pharmacokinetics after simultaneous intravenous infusion. *Antimicrob Ag Chemother* **20**: 576.

Quinn EL, Pohlod D, Madhavan T *et al.* (1973). Clinical experiences with cefazolin and other cephalosporins in bacterial endocarditis. *J Infect Dis* **128** (Suppl): 386.

Rattie ES, Ravin LJ (1975). Pharmacokinetic interpretation of blood levels and urinary excretion data for cefazolin and cephalothin after intravenous and intramuscular administration in humans. *Antimicrob Ag Chemother* **7**: 606.

Ratzan KR, Ruiz C, Irvin GL III (1974). Biliary tract excretion of cefazolin, cephalothin, and cephaloridine in the presence of biliary tract disease. *Antimicrob Ag Chemother* **6**: 426.

Rein MF, Westervelt FB, Sande MA (1973). Pharmacodynamics of cefazolin in the presence of normal and impaired renal function. *Antimicrob Ag Chemother* **4**: 366.

Reinarz JA, Kier CM, Guckian JC (1973). Evaluation of cefazolin in the treatment of bacterial endocarditis and bacteremia. *J Infect Dis* **128** (Suppl): 392.

Reller LB, Karney WW, Beaty HN *et al.* (1973). Evaluation of cefazolin, a new cephalosporin antibiotic. *Antimicrob Ag Chemother* **3**: 488.

Ries K, Levison ME, Kaye D (1973). Clinical and *in vitro* evaluation of cefazolin, a new cephalosporin antibiotic. *Antimicrob Ag Chemother* **3**: 168.

Robson HG, Bowmer MI (1974). Treatment of pneumonia and other serious bacterial infections with cephapirin. *Antimicrob Ag Chemother* **6**: 274.

Rosin E, Ebert S, Uphoff TS *et al.* (1989). Penetration of antibiotics into the surgical wound in a canine model. *Antimicrob Ag Chemother* **33**: 700.

Rylander M, Mannheimer C, Brorson J-E (1979). Penetration of cephradine and cefazolin into ulcers of patients suffering from peripheral arterial circulatory insufficiency. *Scand J Infect Dis* **11**: 281.

Sabath LD (1989). Reappraisal of the antistaphylococcal activities of first-generation (narrow spectrum) and second generation (expanded spectrum) cephalosporins. *Antimicrob Ag Chemother* **33**: 407.

Sabath LD, Wilcox C, Garner C, Finland M (1973). *In vitro* activity of cefazolin against recent clinical bacterial isolates. *J Infect Dis* **128** (Suppl): 320.

Sabath LD, Garner C, Wilcox C, Finland M (1975). Effect of inoculum and of beta-lactamase on the anti-staphylococcal activity of thirteen penicillins and cephalosporins. *Antimicrob Ag Chemother* **8**: 344.

Saxon A (1983). Immediate hypersensitivity reactions to beta-lactam antibiotics. *Rev Infect Dis* **5** (Suppl 2): 368.

Shapiro M, Schoenbaum SC, Tager IB *et al.* (1983). Benefit-cost analysis of anti-microbial prophylaxis in abdominal and vaginal hysterectomy. *JAMA* **249**: 1290.

Shemonsky NK, Carrizosa J, Kaye D, Levison ME (1975). Double-blind comparison of phlebitis produced by cefazolin versus cephalothin. *Antimicrob Ag Chemother* **7**: 481.

Silverblatt F, Harrison WO, Turck M (1973). Nephrotoxicity of cephalosporin antibiotics in experimental animals. *J Infect Dis* **128** (Suppl): 367.

Strausbaugh LJ, Mikhail IA, Edman DC (1978). Comparative *in vitro* activity of five cephalosporin antibiotics against salmonellae. *Antimicrob Ag Chemother* **13**: 134.

Sutter VL, Finegold SM (1975). Susceptibility of anaerobic bacteria to carbenicillin, cefoxitin, and related drugs. *J Infect Dis* **131**: 417.

Tally FP, Jacobus NV, Bartlett JG, Gorbach SL (1975). Susceptibility of anaerobes to cefoxitin and other cephalosporins. *Antimicrob Ag Chemother* **7**: 128.

Thys JP, Vanderkelen B, Klastersky J (1976). Pharmacological study of cefazolin during intermittent and continuous infusion: a crossover investigation in humans. *Antimicrob Ag Chemother* **10**: 395.

Truesdale R, D'Alessandri R, Manuel V *et al.* (1979). Antimicrobial vs. placebo prophylaxis in noncardiac thoracic surgery. *JAMA* **241**: 1254.

Turck M (1982). Cephalosporins and related anitbiotics: an overview. *Rev Infect Dis* **4** (Suppl): 281.

Verbist L (1976). Comparison of the antibacterial activity of nine cephalosporins against Enterobacteriaceae and nonfermentative Gram-negative bacilli. *Antimicrob Ag Chemother* **10**: 657.

Wang PL, Prime DJ, Hsu C-Y, Tune BM (1982). Effects of ureteral obstruction on the toxicity of cephalosporins in the rabbit kidney. *J Infect Dis* **145**: 574.

Waterman NG, Raff MJ, Scharfenberger L, Barnwell PA (1976). Protein binding and concentrations of cephaloridine and cefazolin in serum and interstitial fluid of dogs. *J Infect Dis* **133**: 642.

Wick WE, Preston DA (1972). Biological properties of three 3-heterocyclicthiomethyl cephalosporin antibiotics. *Antimicrob Ag Chemother* **1**: 221.

Wilcox MH, Winstanley TG, Douglas CWI, Spencer RC (1993). Susceptibility of alpha-haemolytic streptococci causing endocarditis to benzylpenicillin and ten cephalosporins. *J Antimicrob Chemother* **32**: 63.

Yoshioka H, Cho K, Takimoto M *et al.* (1979). Transfer of cefazolin into human milk. *J Pediatr* **94**: 151.

Yourassowsky E, Schoutens E, Vanderlinden MP (1976). Antibacterial activity of eight cephalosporins against *Haemophilus influenzae* and *Streptococcus pneumoniae*. *J Antimicrob Chemother* **2**: 55.

Cefamandole, Cefoxitin and Cefuroxime

Description

Having increased resistance to beta-lactamases produced by Gram-negative bacteria, these three compounds are active against many Gram-negative organisms, which are resistant to the older cephalosporins. These drugs are often referred to as the second-generation cephalosporins. Newer cephalosporins, referred to as extended spectrum or third-generation cephalosporins (Turck, 1982), have an even broader spectrum of activity, particularly against Gram-negative bacteria (p. 320).

The three antibiotics described in this chapter have many similarities but there are some important differences in their antimicrobial activities.

1 Cefamandole

Developed at Lilly Research Laboratories, this was shown by Wick and Preston (1972) to have good activity against Gram-negative bacteria, including beta-lactamase-producing strains of *Proteus* and *Enterobacter* species. Cefamandole is used clinically as the sodium salt of the O-formyl ester, cefamandole nafate. The independent antibacterial activity of cefamandole nafate is about 10-fold less than that of cefamandole, but after administration this ester is rapidly converted *in vivo* to cefamandole, which is the predominant circulating antibiotic (Wold *et al.*, 1978a). This occurs even in the presence of renal failure (Nielsen *et al.*, 1979).

2 Cefoxitin

This is a cephamycin. Cephamycins A, B and C are naturally occurring antibiotics which were obtained from several *Streptomyces* spp. at Merck Sharp and Dohme Research Laboratories (Stapley *et al.*, 1972). They are not cephalosporin antibiotics, but are structurally related to cephalosporin C (p. 251), and so they are included in this chapter. Cephamycin C has the greatest activity particularly against Gram-negative bacteria. It is more stable to beta-lactamases than earlier cephalosporins, and it is active *in vitro* against many cephalothin-resistant strains of Gram-negative bacilli (Miller *et al.*, 1972). Chemically modified semisynthetic cephamycins have been produced from cephamycin C. One of these is cefoxitin, a parenterally administered antibiotic, which is available for clinical use.

3 Cefuroxime

Research at Glaxo Laboratories led to the development of this cephalosporin with increased stability to beta-lactamases (O'Callaghan *et al.*, 1976). In addition to its activity against non-beta-lactamase-producing Gram-negative bacteria, cefuroxime is active against many beta-lactamase-producing strains of *Enterobacter*, *Klebsiella* and *Proteus* species. It is also highly active against *Neisseria gonorrhoeae* (including beta-lactamase-producing strains), *N. meningitidis* and *Haemophilus influenzae* (including ampicillin-resistant strains) (Norrby *et al.*, 1976; O'Callaghan *et al.*, 1976). Cefuroxime sodium is only suitable for parenteral administration (p. 299).

Cefuroxime axetil, an ester of the drug, is suitable for oral administration. The ester linkage is hydrolyzed in the intestinal mucosa after absorption, yielding cefuroxime. Compared with i.v. administered cefuroxime, the bioavailability of orally administered cefuroxime axetil is 35% in fasting volunteers. If the ester is given within 15 min of a meal, bioavailability is about 45%, indicating that it should be administered shortly after food. In children, bioavailability may be

25%–88% higher when cefuroxime axetil and milk are administered simultaneously than when the same dose is given in the fasting state. Cefuroxime axetil may be suitable for treatment of some infections for which parenteral cefuroxime is used, provided that oral chemotherapy is not contraindicated (Harding *et al.*, 1984; Sommers *et al.*, 1984; Williams and Harding, 1984; Wise *et al.*, 1984; Ginsburg *et al.*, 1985).

Sensitive Organisms

A Cefamandole

1 Gram-positive bacteria

Cefamandole is active against *Staphylococcus aureus* (non-beta-lactamase- and beta-lactamase-producing strains), coagulase-negative staphylococci, *Streptococcus pyogenes*, *Strep. pneumoniae*, Group B streptococci and alpha-hemolytic streptococci (*Strep. viridans*). *Enterococcus faecalis* is resistant. This activity against Gram-positive cocci is comparable with that of cephalothin (Table I.25), although cefamandole is marginally less active, particularly against *Staph. aureus* (Neu, 1974b; Bodey and Weaver, 1976; Dan *et al.*, 1983). It is slightly less resistant to inactivation by staphylococcal beta-lactamase than cephalothin (p. 251) but more resistant in presence of this enzyme than cefazolin (p. 282). It can be considered to be a reliable anti-staphylococcal drug (Fong *et al.*, 1976a; Chapman and Steigbigel, 1983; Sabath, 1989). Methicillin-resistant *Staph. aureus* and coagulase-negative staphylococci (p. 77) are cefamandole-resistant (Barry *et al.*, 1979).

Gram-positive bacilli, such as *Cl. tetani*, *Cl. perfringens* and *C. diphtheriae*, are sensitive to cefamandole (Wick and Preston, 1972). Most *Nocardia asteroides* strains are moderately sensitive, being inhibited by 6.3–12.5 μg per ml, but *N. caviae* and *N. brasiliensis* are completely cefamandole-resistant (Gutmann *et al.*, 1983; Wallace *et al.*, 1983).

2 Gram-negative cocci

Cefamandole is active against the *Neisseria* spp. (Table I.25). Against meningococci, it is more active than cephalothin and cefoxitin and about equally as active as cefuroxime. Its activity against gonococci is greater than that of cephalothin and cefoxitin but less than that of cefuroxime (Wick and Preston, 1972; Piot *et al.*, 1979). The drug is also active against beta-lactamase producing gonococci (Hall *et al.*, 1979), but *in vitro* activity is affected by the size of the inoculum (p. 16).

3 Gram-negative aerobic bacilli

As cefamandole is more stable to many beta-lactamases produced by these bacilli, it has greater activity than cephalothin, and it is active against some cephalothin-resistant species. But cefamandole is not as active against many Gram-negative aerobic bacilli as the third-generation cephalosporins such as cefotaxime (p. 320) or ceftriaxone (p. 353). Bacteria which are normally cephalothin-sensitive, such as *Escherichia coli*, *Proteus mirabilis* and the *Klebsiella* spp., are even more sensitive to cefamandole (Neu, 1974b; Barry *et al.*, 1979). Cefamandole is active against most cephalothin-resistant isolates of *E. coli*, but not against those of *Kl. pneumoniae* (Bodey and Weaver, 1976). Among bacteria which are normally cephalothin-resistant, such as *Morganella morganii*, *Providencia rettgeri* and other *Providencia* spp., cefamandole shows good activity, but *Pr. vulgaris* is usually resistant (Penner and Preston, 1980; Penner *et al.*, 1982). Many *Enterobacter* and *Citrobacter* spp. strains are cefamandole-sensitive (Neu, 1974b; Meyers and Hirschman, 1978). *Yersinia enterocolitica* is moderately cefamandole-sensitive (MIC 0.5–8.0 μg per ml) (Gaspar and Soriano, 1981).

Cefamandole is active, and considerably more so than cephalothin, against all *Salmonella* spp., including *Salm. typhi* (Barros *et al.*, 1977; Strausbaugh *et al.*, 1978). Ampicillin-resistant strains of *Salm. typhi* (p. 109) have been reported to be cefamandole-sensitive (Hirschman *et al.*, 1977), but Chau *et al.* (1981) found that ampicillin-resistant strains of *Salm. typhimurium* and *Salm. johannesburg*, exhibited partial resistance. *Shigella* spp. are only moderately sensitive to cefamandole (Wick and Preston, 1972). The drug is highly active against *H. influenzae*, to an extent greater than that of cephalothin and cefoxitin, but about equal to that of cefuroxime (Table I.25) (Kammer *et al.*, 1975; Meyers and Hirschman, 1978). However, in one study cefamandole had poor bactericidal activity against 11 of 75 ampicillin-sensitive strains, MBCs being much higher than the MICs. Cefamandole was also relatively inactive against beta-lactamase producing strains of *H. influenzae* (Table I.25) (Bergeron *et al.*, 1981). *Haemophilus ducreyi* strains which do not produce beta-lactamase are cefamandole-sensitive, but most strains are enzyme producers and are relatively resistant (MIC 0.25–8.0 μg per ml) (Sanson-Le Pors et al., 1983).

About 25% of *Serratia marcescens* isolates are inhibited by cefamandole concentrations of 12–50 μg per ml; others are completely resistant. *Acinetobacter* spp. are usually resistant, and *Pseudomonas aeruginosa* is always so (Neu, 1974b; Verbist, 1976; Fu and Neu, 1978).

4 Gram-negative anaerobic bacilli

The Prevotella spp. such as P. melaninogenica and Fusobacterium spp. are usually sensitive to cefamandole, but anaerobes of the *Bacteroides fragilis* group are resistant (Sutter and Finegold, 1976; Jenkins et al., 1982). Most *B. fragilis* strains produce beta-lactamase(s) and the genes coding for these appear to be located on the chromosome. These enzymes easily inactivate older cephalosporins such as cephalothin (p. 253) and cefazolin (p. 283). Whereas cefamandole is only slightly more resistant, cefoxitin (p. 295) is considerably more resistant to these enzymes (Tally et al., 1979a).

5 Other organisms

Cefamandole is inactive against *Chlamydia trachomatis* (Bowie, 1982).

6 Acquired resistance

Strains of *Enterobacter* spp. can be readily made resistant *in vitro*, by repeated passage in cultures containing cefamandole. Some of these resistant variants inactivate cefamandole enzymatically, others possess intrinsic resistance (Findell and Sherris, 1976). Several clinical reports of failure of cefamandole therapy in *Enterobacter* infections have been due to emergence of resistant strains during treatment (Sanders et al., 1982b; Murray et al., 1983; Olson et al., 1983). Acquired resistance to cefamandole by *Enterobacter* spp. and some other Enterobacteriaceae, such as *Pr. vulgaris*, *Morganella morganii*, *Providencia rettgeri* and other *Providencia* and *Serratia* spp., is usually caused by chromosomally mediated beta-lactamases. Beta-lactamases possessed by these and other Enterobacteriaceae and other Gram-negative bacilli, such as *Ps. aeruginosa* are inducible. Normally *Enterobacter* spp. and strains of other Enterobacteriaceae are cefamandole-sensitive because their beta-lactamase production is low (repressed). This enzyme production can become markedly increased (derepressed), leading to resistance to cefamandole. This can occur either by a reversible derepression by an enzyme inducer or by chromosomal mutation to a stably derepressed state. Beta-lactamase-resistant cephalosporins, such as cefoxitin (p. 295) and cefotaxime (p. 322), are good inducers of these enzymes (Aronoff and Shlaes, 1987). In this way, cefoxitin can induce cefamandole-resistance in *Enterobacter* spp. strains. When cefamandole-resistance is acquired during treatment, the mechanism involved is chromosomal mutation resulting in stably derepressed bacterial cells producing large amounts of beta-lactamase. Compared with cefoxitin, cefamandole is a poor enzyme inducer, because it is relatively unstable to hydrolysis by beta-lactamases (Sanders and Sanders, 1979; Gootz et al., 1982; Sanders, 1983). Resistance due to induction of beta-lactamases also occurs with third-generation cephalosporins (p. 322). Enterobacteriaceae, particularly *E. coli* and *Klebsiella* spp. strains, which have acquired plasmid-mediated extended-spectrum beta-lactamases (p. 323) are also cefamandole-resistant.

B Cefoxitin

1 Gram-positive bacteria

Most pyogenic cocci such as *Staph. aureus* (including those resistant to penicillin G), coagulase-negative staphylococci, *Strep. pyogenes*, *Strep. pneumoniae*, Group B streptococci and the alpha-hemolytic streptococci (*Strep. viridans*), are cefoxitin-sensitive (Neu, 1974a; Wallick and Hendlin, 1974). The activity of cefoxitin against these organisms is 5- to 10-fold less than that of cephalothin and cefamandole (Table I.25), and is comparable with that of cephalexin (Table I.19, p. 264). *Enterococcus faecalis* (MIC 800 μg per ml) is more resistant to cefoxitin than to most cephalosporins (Hamilton-Miller, 1974). Cefoxitin is as stable as cephalothin (p. 251) to inactivation by staphylococcal beta-lactamase (Fong et al., 1976a), so that except for its lesser intrinsic activity, it is a reliable anti-staphylococcal agent. Methicillin-resistant strains of *Staph. aureus* and coagulase-negative staphylococci are cefoxitin-resistant (Stapley et al., 1979).

Anaerobic Gram-positive cocci, such as the *Peptococcus* and *Peptostreptococcus* spp. and anaerobic streptococci, are nearly always cefoxitin-sensitive (Bach et al., 1977; Chow and Bednorz, 1978).

Some aerobic Gram-positive bacilli, such as *C. diphtheriae*, are cefoxitin-sensitive but *Listeria monocytogenes* is resistant (Moellering *et al.*, 1974; Stapley *et al.*, 1979). Cefoxitin is inactive against *N. asteroides*, most strains needing 50 μg per ml or more for inhibition (Cynamon and Palmer, 1981; Gutmann *et al.*, 1983). Gram-positive anaerobic bacilli, such as *Cl. perfringens*, *Cl. tetani*, other *Clostridium* spp., the *Actinomyces*, *Eubacterium* and *Propionibacterium* spp., are cefoxitin-sensitive. *Lactobacillus* spp. are less susceptible (MIC 16 μg per ml) (Chow and Bednorz, 1978; Sutter *et al.*, 1978).

2 Gram-negative cocci

Cefoxitin is active against meningococci but to a lesser extent than cefamandole or cefuroxime. It also has slightly less activity than cephalothin against these organisms (Eickhoff and Ehret, 1976; Norrby *et al.*, 1976) (Table I.25). The activity of cefoxitin against gonococci is marginally greater than that of cephalothin, but less than that of cefamandole, or especially cefuroxime. Like cefamandole and cefuroxime, cefoxitin is active against beta-lactamase-producing strains. Cefoxitin is stable in the presence of gonococcal beta-lactamase, so its activity against these strains is unaffected if the sensitivity test is done using a large inoculum. This is not the case with cefamandole, so its activity is inferior to that of cefoxitin against beta-lactamase-producing strains if a large inoculum is used. Cefuroxime is affected to a small degree by gonococcal beta-lactamase but as it has much higher intrinsic activity against gonococci, it still remains more active than cefoxitin against beta-lactamase-producing strains, even if large inocula are used (Phillips, 1978; Phillips and Shannon, 1978; Khan *et al.*, 1981).

3 Gram-negative aerobic bacilli

A feature of cefoxitin is its high stability to various types of beta-lactamases produced by Gram-negative organisms (Onishi *et al.*, 1974). The drug demonstrates almost no inoculum effect (p. 16) and a rapid bactericidal activity against most Enterobacteriaceae (Brook, 1989; Goldstein *et al.*, 1991a). As a result it is active against many of these bacteria which are normally cephalothin-resistant, or which have acquired resistance to this drug and other cephalosporins (Neu, 1974a; Stapley *et al.*, 1979). Against cephalothin-sensitive strains of *E. coli*, *Pr. mirabilis* and *Klebsiella* spp., cefoxitin is only slightly more active than cephalothin (Brumfitt *et al.*, 1974; Neu, 1974a) (Table I.25). Cefoxitin usually remains highly active against ampicillin-resistant *E. coli* strains (Norrby *et al.*, 1976), and against strains of *E. coli*, *Pr. mirabilis* and *Kl. pneumoniae* which have become cephalothin-resistant. Cephalothin and gentamicin-resistant *Kl. pneumoniae* isolates are usually cefoxitin-sensitive (Jackson *et al.*, 1977; Stapley *et al.*, 1979).

Cefoxitin is active against some bacterial species normally resistant to cephalothin, such as *Morganella morganii*, *Pr. vulgaris*, *Providencia rettgeri* and other *Providencia* spp. It is more active than both cefamandole and cefuroxime against *Serratia marcescens*, about 50% or more of all isolates being inhibited by low cefoxitin concentrations. Cefoxitin is not as active as cefamandole against *Enterobacter* spp., and approximately 50% of all strains are either completely resistant or need high concentrations for inhibition. Some strains of *Citrobacter* and *Acinetobacter* spp. are also sensitive to cefoxitin (Wallick and Hendlin, 1974; Stapley *et al.*, 1979; Vuye *et al.*, 1979).

The activity of cefoxitin against *Salmonella* and *Shigella* spp. is comparable with that of cephalothin but inferior to that of cefamandole (Moellering *et al.*, 1974; Neu, 1974a) (Table I.25). Against *H. influenzae*, it is considerably less active than cefamandole and cefuroxime, and slightly less active than cephalothin (Norrby *et al.*, 1976; Yourassowsky *et al.*, 1976). Cefoxitin is active against ampicillin-resistant strains of *H. influenzae*; although the drug's intrinsic activity against this organism is not very high, it is not diminished with beta-lactamase-producing strains when the sensitivity test is done with a large inoculum, indicating that cefoxitin is unaffected by this enzyme (Kammer *et al.*, 1975; Bulger and Washington, 1980). Similar to cefamandole and cefuroxime, *Ps. aeruginosa* is always highly cefoxitin-resistant (Wallick and Hendlin, 1974). *Legionella pneumophila* is sensitive to cefoxitin *in vitro* (MIC 0.06–0.25 μg per ml) (Thornsberry *et al.*, 1978). *Flavobacterium meningosepticum* is moderately susceptible (MIC 16 μg per ml) (Kelsey *et al.*, 1982). *Campylobacter jejuni* is resistant (Muytjens and Van der Ros-van de Repe, 1982), but *Helicobacter pylori* is cefoxitin-sensitive (McNulty *et al.*, 1985).

Klebsiella pneumoniae can become resistant to cefoxitin, if it is exposed to subinhibitory concentrations of the drug *in vitro*; this resistance appears to be intrinsic because beta-lactamase activity was not demonstrated (Hoeprich and Huston, 1976). In a study of organisms isolated from intra-abdominal abscesses, Saah *et al.* (1981) found that all anaerobes tested were susceptible to cefoxitin, but 19 of 57 (33%) of aerobic Gram-negative bacilli were resistant. Resistant organisms were not only those which are normally cefoxitin-resistant, such as *Ps.*

aeruginosa, but resistant *Enterobacter*, *Citrobacter* and *Klebsiella* spp. and *E. coli* and *Serratia marcescens* strains were also encountered.

In vitro, *Enterobacter* spp. strains become resistant to other cephalosporins in the presence of cefoxitin; these strains regain their sensitivity when cefoxitin is removed (Waterworth and Emmerson, 1979). Cefoxitin and other beta-lactamase-stable cephalosporins (p. 322) are potent inducers of chromosomally mediated beta-lactamases (Moritz and Carson, 1986). Some species of Gram-negative aerobic bacteria possess inducible enzymes (p. 322), which normally exist in a non-induced or repressed state. By beta-lactamase induction (derepression), cefoxitin can cause resistance in *Enterobacter* spp. strains. Furthermore, if cefoxitin is used with another beta-lactam antibiotic, such as carbenicillin or mezlocillin (p. 164), which is not stable to enzymes produced by Gram-negative bacilli, it can antagonize the other beta-lactam antibiotic. This antagonism with cefoxitin has been demonstrated *in vitro* and in animals (Kuck *et al.*, 1981; Goering *et al.*, 1982; Sanders *et al.*, 1982a; Miller *et al.*, 1983). Cefoxitin appears to cause antagonism more frequently than other beta-lactamase stable cephalosporins. This may be because its intrinsic activity against strains possessing inducible beta-lactamases is relatively low, compared with its inducer activity, so that beta-lactamase induction proceeds faster than its antibacterial effect. Other enzyme stable beta-lactams, such as cefotaxime (p. 320), differ from cefoxitin by having higher intrinsic antibacterial activity, and antagonism with them can only be easily demonstrated when subinhibitory concentrations are used (Sanders, 1983).

Enzyme induction or derepression (p. 322) may result in bacterial resistance to a drug such as cefoxitin, which acts as the enzyme inducer, despite the fact that it is resistant to enzyme hydrolysis. In the derepressed (beta-lactamase-induced) state, there are many more enzyme molecules in the bacterial periplasmic space (p. 322), and these normally hydrolyze substrate drugs like cefamandole (p. 293). Drugs which normally resist hydrolysis (non-substrate drugs), such as cefoxitin, may also be hydrolyzed by some of these chromosomal enzymes (p. 322). By this mechanism it is possible that cefoxitin-resistance may emerge during treatment of patients (Sanders, 1983; Seeberg *et al.*, 1983).

Strains of *Klebsiella* spp., *E. coli* and other Enterobacteriaceae which have acquired plasmid-mediated extended-spectrum beta-lactamases are often still cefoxitin-sensitive. This is generally so if the beta-lactamase is inhibited by beta-lactamase inhibitors. But other extended-spectrum beta-lactamases exist, which are not inhibited by beta-lactamase inhibitors and which hydrolyze cefoxitin. Strains possessing this latter type of extended-spectrum beta-lactamase are also cefoxitin-resistant (p. 323) (Jacoby and Archer, 1991; Meyer *et al.*, 1993).

4 Gram-negative anaerobic bacilli

An important property of cefoxitin is that, unlike cefamandole and cefuroxime, it has good activity against the *B. fragilis* group of anaerobic bacteria. Early studies showed that approximately 80% of isolates were inhibited by a concentration of 16 μg per ml or less (Sutter and Finegold, 1976; Bach *et al.*, 1977; Pollock *et al.*, 1983). In an early survey in the USA of 750 clinical isolates of the *B. fragilis* group of anaerobic bacteria, only eight (2%) were cefoxitin-resistant (Tally *et al.*, 1983). Because species within the *B. fragilis* group have different sensitivities to beta-lactam antibiotics, further subdivision of this group is of clinical interest. There are seven distinct species, four indole-positive (*B. thetaiotaomicron*, *B. ovatus*, *B. unformis*, and *B. eggerthii*) and three indole-negative (*B. fragilis*, *B. distasonis* and *B. vulgatus*). Indole-positive members are generally more resistant to beta-lactams than indole-negative species. In the case of cefoxitin, all but a few strains of the indole-negative species were inhibited by 16 μg per ml or less, but many indole-positive strains needed 16–32 μg per ml for inhibition (Nasu *et al.*, 1981; Jenkins *et al.*, 1982).

In later surveys there were a higher prevalence of cefoxitin-resistance among bacteria of the *B. fragilis* group. Cuchural *et al.* (1990) in a nationwide survey in the USA found that 11% of strains were resistant and Appelbaum *et al.* (1991) in the same country found 9% of strains to be cefoxitin-resistant. In the UK, Fox and Phillips (1987) found 16% of strains of bacteria of the *B. fragilis* group to be resistant, whereas in Bali the cefoxitin-resistance rate was only 2% (Suata *et al.*, 1993). In Korea the resistance rate to cefoxitin was also relatively low (6%) (Lee *et al.*, 1992). In Canada 2.9% of *B. fragilis* strains and 17.2% of other members of the *B. fragilis* group were cefoxitin-resistant (Turgeon *et al.*, 1994).

Cefoxitin is quite active against other Gram-negative anaerobes such as *Prevotella melaninogenica*, *P. disiens*, *P. oralis*, *P. intermedia* and *Fusobacterium* spp. (Sutter and Finegold, 1976; Snydman *et al.*, 1980; Appelbaum *et al.*, 1990). In surveys in the USA over 94% of these bacteria were cefoxitin-sensitive (Appelbaum *et al.*, 1991; Hill *et al.*, 1991).

Resistance to beta-lactamase hydrolysis is the main reason for the action of cefoxitin against *B. fragilis*. Darland and Birnbaum (1977) examined 79 strains of *B. fragilis*; several isolates were resistant to cefuroxime because they produced enzymes capable of hydrolyzing it, but cefoxitin was active against over 90% of strains, because of its beta-lactamase stability. All bacteria of the *B. fragilis* group possess a chromosomally mediated beta-lactamase, which inactivates earlier cephalosporins, such as cephalothin (p. 253), but not cefoxitin (Tally *et al.*, 1979a). Strains of *B. fragilis* group do not exhibit 'tolerance' (p. 81) to cefoxitin; the MBCs of the drug are equal or only slightly higher than its MICs against this organism (Goldstein *et al.*, 1981). Cefoxitin is bactericidal to the bacteria of *B. fragilis* group and it shows very small inoculum effect (Goldstein *et al.*, 1991b).

More recently cefoxitin-resistant strains of the *B. fragilis* group have appeared. Initially it was considered that this resistance was probably intrinsic (p. 27) because inactivating enzymes could not be demonstrated (Dornbusch *et al.*, 1979; 1980; Nord and Olsson-Liljequist, 1981). Some strains of *B. fragilis* appeared to be resistant to cefoxitin because of altered penicillin-binding proteins or decreased outer membrane permeability (Piddock and Wise, 1987; Wexler and Halebian, 1990), but it was also shown that cefoxitin-resistance could be transferred from *B. thetaiotaomicron* to other species of *Bacteroides* (Rashtchian *et al.*, 1982). In a survey of 1575 clinical isolates of *B. fragilis* in USA, 11 were found to be highly cefoxitin-resistant (MIC >64 μg per ml). Four of these were able to inactivate the drug in broth cultures (Cuchural *et al.*, 1983). Enzymes inactivating cefoxitin and even imipenem (p. 230) have now been isolated from *B. fragilis* group of organisms (Nord *et al.*, 1985; Cuchural *et al.*, 1986; Eley and Greenwood, 1986; Malouin *et al.*, 1986; Soriano *et al.*, 1991). Resistance of *B. fragilis* to most penicillins is largely due to production of chromosomal beta-lactamases. But the novel beta-lactamases, which can inactivate cefoxitin and imipenem are transferable. The presence of plasmids have not been demonstrated, but this resistance may be encoded on a transposon, similar to clindamycin resistance in *B. fragilis* (p. 589) (Tally and Cuchural, 1988; Parker and Smith, 1993).

5 Other organisms

Some strains (<50%) of *Mycobacterium fortuitum* and *M. chelonae* can be inhibited by 16 μg per ml of cefoxitin (Casal and Rodriguez, 1982; Cynamon and Palmer, 1982; Swenson *et al.*, 1985; Finch, 1986). *Chlamydia trachomatis* is cefoxitin-resistant (Bowie, 1982).

C Cefuroxime

1 Gram-positive bacteria

Staphylococcus aureus and coagulase-negative staphylococci, irrespective of beta-lactamase production, are cefuroxime-sensitive, but methicillin-resistant strains (p. 77) are resistant. *Streptococcus pyogenes*, *Strep. pneumoniae*, Group B streptococci and the alpha-hemolytic streptococci (*Strep. viridans*) are sensitive. *Enterococcus faecalis* is resistant (Eykyn *et al.*, 1976; O'Callaghan *et al.*, 1976; Mehtar, 1980). *Strep. pneumoniae* with intermediate resistance to penicillin G and those with high-level resistance, also show similar resistance to cefuroxime (Spangler *et al.*, 1993). The activity of cefuroxime against all of these organisms is similar to that of cephalothin, but *Staph. aureus* and coagulase-negative staphylococci are slightly less susceptible to cefuroxime than cephalothin, and the reverse is true for *Strep. viridans* (Eykyn *et al.*, 1976; Jones *et al.*, 1977). *Nocardia asteroides* is only moderately sensitive (MIC 1–16 μg per ml) (Gutmann *et al.*, 1983). The *Peptostreptococcus* and *Clostridium* spp. are usually sensitive (O'Callaghan *et al.*, 1976; Goldstein and Citron, 1988).

2 Gram-negative cocci

Cefuroxime is quite active against *N. meningitidis* (Brown and Fallon, 1980). It is especially active against *N. gonorrhoeae*, being more active than cefamandole, cefoxitin and cephalothin (O'Callaghan *et al.*, 1976; Piot *et al.*, 1979). It is also fully active against beta-lactamase producing strains (Hall *et al.*, 1979; Yoshikawa *et al.*, 1980). Gonococcal strains with intrinsic resistance to penicillin G are usually cefuroxime-sensitive (p. 4).

3 Gram-negative bacilli

Activity of cefuroxime against these bacteria is rather like that of cefamandole (p. 292), both drugs being relatively stable to most beta-lactamases produced by aerobic Gram-negative bacilli (Greenwood, 1977). Enterobacteriaceae which are usually cephalothin-susceptible, such as *E. coli*, *Pr. mirabilis* and *Kl. pneumoniae*, are even more sensitive to cefuroxime (Eykyn *et al.*, 1976). The drug is not as active as cefoxitin against ampicillin-resistant *E. coli* (Norrby *et al.*,

1976). Trimethoprim-resistant strains of *E. coli* are usually cefuroxime-sensitive (Singh *et al.*, 1990). Neonates treated by cefuroxime often develop cefuroxime-resistant strains of *E. coli* and *Klebsiella* spp. in their feces (Tullus *et al.*, 1990). In one study in Sweden there was a small increase in cefuroxime-resistant strains of *E. coli* isolated from blood cultures during 1980–1981, compared with similar strains isolated during 1973–1974 (Brorson and Larsson, 1982). Strains of *E. coli* and *Klebsiella* spp. which have acquired plasmid-mediated extended-spectrum beta-lactamases (p. 323), are cefuroxime-resistant.

In low concentrations, cefuroxime inhibits approximately 60% of Gram-negative bacilli which are normally cephalothin-resistant; these include *Morganella morganii*, *Pr. vulgaris*, *Pr. rettgeri* and other *Providencia*, *Enterobacter*, *Citrobacter* and *Hafnia* spp. (Greenwood *et al.*, 1976; O'Callaghan *et al.*, 1976; George *et al.*, 1978). A few *Serratia marcescens* strains are inhibited by cefuroxime in low concentrations, but the majority require either high concentrations or are completely resistant (O'Callaghan *et al.*, 1976; Neu and Fu, 1978) (Table I.25). Compared with cephalothin, cefuroxime is as active against the *Salmonella* spp., but slightly more active against *Shigella* spp. (O'Callaghan *et al.*, 1976).

Cefuroxime is very active against *H. influenzae*, and in this respect it is about the same as cefamandole but exceeds cephalothin and cefoxitin (Table I.25). Unlike cefamandole,

Table I.25

Compiled from data published by Wick and Preston (1972), Wallick and Hendlin (1974), Neu (1974a,b), Brumfitt *et al.* (1974), Kammer *et al.* (1975), O'Callaghan *et al.* (1976), Norrby *et al.* (1976), Phillips *et al.* (1976), Sutter and Finegold (1976), Verbist (1976), Report (1978), Berg *et al.* (1979) and Bergeron *et al.* (1981)

Organism	MIC (μg per ml)			
	Cephalothin	Cefamandole	Cefoxitin	Cefuroxime
Gram-positive bacteria				
Staphylococcus aureus (non-penicillinase-producer)	0.25	0.25–1.0	1.6–6.4	0.25
Staphylococcus aureus (penicillinase-producer)	0.5	0.5–1.0	1.6–6.4	0.25
Streptococcus pyogenes	0.06–0.12	0.03–0.06	<0.8–1.6	≤0.125
Streptococcus pneumoniae	0.12–0.25	0.12–0.25	1.6–6.4	≤0.125
Streptococcus viridans	0.5–1.0	0.5	<0.8–1.6	≤0.125
Enterococcus faecalis	16.0–32.0	32.0	200.0–800.0	>125.0
Clostridium perfringens	0.25–0.5	0.03–0.5	0.5–16.0	0.23
Gram-negative bacteria				
Escherichia coli	4.0–32.0	0.5–1.0	0.78–25.0	2.9
Enterobacter spp.	16.0–>128.0	1.0–8.0	1.56–100.0	10.2
Klebsiella spp.	2.0–32.0	0.5–1.0	0.78–50.0	8.2
Proteus mirabilis	4.0–8.0	1.0–2.0	0.25–4.0	2.2
Proteus vulgaris	>128.0	8.0–32.0	0.25–8.0	39.0
Morganella morganii	128.0	1.0	0.25–8.0	16.0
Providencia spp.	50.0–>100.0	1.63–100.0	3.1	11.5
Salmonella spp.	4.0	1.0	0.8–3.12	3.6
Shigella spp.	8.0	2.0	0.8–6.25	4.6
Serratia marcescens	>128.0	4.0–>100.0	12.5–>100.0	116.0
Neisseria gonorrhoeae	0.15	0.02	0.12	0.005
N. gonorrhoeae (beta-lactamase-producer)	Resistant	0.25–2.0	0.3–1.2	0.25–1.0
Neisseria meningitidis	0.5	0.125	0.25–4.0	0.125
Haemophilus influenzae	2.0–8.0	0.5	2.0–8.0	0.5
H. influenzae (beta-lactamase producer)	2.0–8.0	2.0–≥128.0	2.0–8.0	0.5
Pseudomonas aeruginosa	>128.0	>128.0	640.0–>1,000	>125.0
Bacteroides fragilis	64.0–>512.0	32.0–>512.0	0.5–32.0	53.0
Prevotella melaninogenica	0.5–32.0	0.1–8.0	0.1–8.0	0.5–8.0

cefuroxime remains active against ampicillin-resistant strains, because it is resistant to their specific beta-lactamase (p. 113) (O'Callaghan *et al.*, 1976; Sykes *et al.*, 1977; Geddes *et al.*, 1978). *Actinobacillus* and *Moraxella* spp. are usually sensitive, but *Flavobacterium* spp. are resistant. *Pasteurella multocida* is cefuroxime-sensitive (Goldstein and Citron, 1988).

Most strains of *Acinetobacter* spp. and all strains of *Ps. aeruginosa* are resistant. Some strains of *Burkholderia* (*Pseudomonas*) *cepacia*, may be sensitive to cefuroxime. Some Gram-negative anaerobic bacilli, such as *Prevotella melaninogenica*, are sensitive to cefuroxime but bacteria of the *B. fragilis* group usually need high concentrations for inhibition or are completely resistant (O'Callaghan *et al.*, 1976; Jones *et al.*, 1977).

4 Other organisms

Treponema palladium is sensitive *in vitro* and cefuroxime is effective in experimental infections in animals (Acred *et al.*, 1980). *Borrelia burgdorferi* is cefuroxime-sensitive (Johnson *et al.*, 1990; Agger *et al.*, 1992), but *Chlamydia trachomatis* is resistant (Bowie, 1982).

D Minimum inhibitory concentrations

The MICs of cefamandole, cefoxitin and cefuroxime compared with those of cephalothin, against some selected bacterial species are shown in Table I.25.

Mode of Administration and Dosage

1 Cefamandole

Cefamandole nafate can only be given parenterally and it is suitable for both i.m. and i.v. administration. Dosage can be varied widely in adults and children, according to the nature and severity of the infection. Total daily doses may be in the range of 1.5–12 g for adults and 22.5–200 mg per kg body weight for children. These may be given in three, four or six divided doses. The higher doses are usually given i.v. A common adult dosage for severe infections is 2 g i.v. 4-hourly (Griffith *et al.*, 1976; Walker and Gahol, 1978; Thirumoorthi *et al.*, 1981). Cefamandole is usually given i.v. by intermittent rapid infusions, similar to penicillin G. The i.v. dose, suitably diluted, can be administered over 5–30 min (Griffith *et al.*, 1976; Short *et al.*, 1976).

Patients with impaired renal function need a reduced dosage, because renal excretion is the main method for eliminating the drug (p. 303). The normal cefamandole half-life of 1.33 h is prolonged to 7–8 h in patients with end-stage renal failure (Appel *et al.*, 1976; Andriole, 1978). For patients with impaired renal function, Czerwinski and Pederson (1979) recommended that the normal dose of 8 g per day (2 g i.v. 6-hourly) should be modified as follows: for patients with creatinine clearance of 40, 20 and 6 ml per min, a 1 g dose should be administered every 6, 8 and 12 h, respectively. If smaller or larger doses than these are required, they should be modified proportionally. These dosage guidelines are less reliable in patients with severe renal failure (creatinine clearance 20 ml per min or less), so serum level monitoring for dosage adjustment is important.

Very little cefamandole is removed during peritoneal dialysis, and additional dosing is not necessary during this procedure. For patients treated with hemodialysis, which removes some cefamandole, several dosage regimens have been advocated. Appel *et al.* (1976) suggested that extra dosage is unnecessary, provided that the patient has received a dose just before dialysis. Ahern *et al.* (1976) found that the cefamandole half-life was shortened during hemodialysis (6.6 h), and advised that one-half or one-third of the dose should be administered at 6–7 h intervals during dialysis. Schwartz *et al.* (1978) confirmed that hemodialysis reduced the serum half-life by about 32%, and recommended a 1 g (15 mg per kg) loading dose followed by doses of 0.5 g (7.5 mg per kg) every 12 h thereafter, regardless of the interdialysis interval. They also identified a subpopulation of hemodialysis patients who eliminated cefamandole more rapidly, presumably via hepatobiliary clearance. Rapid eliminators can be detected by serum level monitoring, and they require larger doses.

2 Cefoxitin

Like cefamandole (see above), this can only be administered parenterally. Intravenous administration is preferred because i.m. injection is only slightly less painful than that of cephalothin (Brumfitt *et al.*, 1974) (p. 253). The adult dosage can be varied according to the nature and severity of the infection from 1 g 8-hourly to 2 g 6-hourly. Dosage as high as 2 g 4-hourly has been used (Geddes *et al.*, 1977; Heseltine *et al.*, 1977). Corresponding doses for children range from 15 mg per kg 8-hourly to 30 mg per kg 6- to 4-hourly. For the treatment of children aged 3–15 months with severe infections, Feldman *et al.* (1980) found a dose of 150 mg per kg per day (37.5 mg per kg 6-hourly) to be satisfactory.

Cefoxitin, similar to penicillin G (p. 20), can be administered satisfactorily i.v. by intermittent injections or intermittent infusions, over periods of 3–30 min or even 120 min (Goodwin *et al.*, 1974; Geddes *et al.*, 1977; Feldman *et al.*, 1980).

As cefoxitin is excreted almost entirely via the kidneys (p. 304), it accumulates in patients with impaired renal function if usual doses are given. Its serum half-life in patients with normal renal function of 39 min is prolonged to 23.5 h in those with virtually no renal function (Kampf *et al.*, 1981). One approximate dosage schedule for patients with renal failure is based on a normal dose of 1 g (15 mg per kg) every 3–6 h, according to the nature of the infection. For patients with creatinine clearance values of 30–60, 10–30 and <10 ml per min, this dose should be given at intervals of 8–12, 12–24 and 24–36 h, respectively. For hemodialysis patients, the same dose can be given at the end of each dialysis, and repeated at 72 h, i.e. the usual time interval between two dialysis sessions. Cefoxitin's clearance from serum may be increased 5-fold by hemodialysis in patients with end-stage renal disease (Humbert *et al.*, 1979). Very little cefoxitin is removed by peritoneal dialysis, so further dosage modification is unnecessary in patients undergoing this procedure (Greaves *et al.*, 1981).

3 Cefuroxime

a Parenteral cefuroxime This drug, in the form of cefuroxime sodium, is suitable for both i.v. and i.m. administration. The solubility of this sodium salt is only 1 g per 4 ml of sterile water, and i.m. injections are rather large and may be painful. For this reason, cefuroxime lysine was developed, which is more soluble (1 g in 3 ml) and less painful on i.m. injection. Pharmacokinetics, clinical efficacy and side-effects of i.m. cefuroxime lysine are identical to those of i.m. cefuroxime sodium (Havard *et al.*, 1981). Trollfors *et al.* (1980a) administered cefuroxime lysine by the i.v. route to 11 patients and there was a high frequency of side-effects: renal functional impairment (5), diarrhea (5) and skin rashes (2). Therefore, cefuroxime sodium is the preferred preparation for i.v. administration.

The i.m. or i.v. dose of cefuroxime can be varied widely, depending on the nature and severity of infection. Adult dosage in the range of 0.5–2.0 g 8-hourly can be used (Norrby *et al.*, 1977). For severe infections, such as bacterial meningitis, an adult dosage of 3 g i.v. 8-hourly has been used, and the corresponding high dosage for children is 60–75 mg per kg body weight, administered 8-hourly (Report, 1982). For i.v. administration, each dose suitably diluted, can be injected or infused over periods of 3–30 min (Foord, 1976; Goodwin *et al.*, 1977).

Cefuroxime is excreted almost entirely by the kidneys and patients with renal failure require a modified dosage. The normal cefuroxime serum half-life of 1.4–1.8 h is prolonged to approximately 20 h in anuric patients (Bundtzen *et al.*, 1981). An approximate dosage for use in patients with varying degrees of renal insufficiency, has been published by Van Dalen *et al.* (1979). Patients with a creatinine clearance of more than 60 ml per min should be given a normal dose of 1 g 8-hourly. For those with creatinine clearance values of 45–60, 30–45, 15–30, 4–15 and less than 4 ml per min, a 1-g dose should be given every 12, 18–24, 36–48, 60–72 or 72–96 h, respectively. If a patient with a creatinine clearance less than 4 ml per min is being treated by regular hemodialysis, a dose of 1 g cefuroxime i.v. after each dialysis, is sufficient. Hemodialysis is an effective means of eliminating cefuroxime from the body.

Pregnant women may need increased cefuroxime dosage. They usually have 30–50% lower serum levels and a shorter serum half-life during pregnancy than after delivery due to increased volume of distribution and increased renal excretion in pregnancy (Philipson, 1983).

b Oral cefuroxime axetil Food increases the absorption of this drug by some 50%, so it should be administered shortly after food (Emmerson, 1988; James *et al.*, 1991). A common adult dosage of this drug is 0.5 g 12-hourly; an increased dosage of 0.5 8-hourly gives inferior clinical results probably because of more frequent gastrointestinal side-effects with the larger dose (Cooper *et al.*, 1985; Emmerson, 1988). For sick elderly patients a dosage of 250 mg 12-hourly may be sufficient (Ridgway *et al.*, 1991). But Cowling *et al.* (1992) pointed out that absorption of this drug in these patients is highly variable and suggested that a dosage of 0.5 g 12-hourly should be used when treating bronchitis. The lower dosage of 250 mg 12-hourly suffices for the treatment of acute uncomplicated urinary tract infections (Emmerson, 1988). Oral cefuroxime axetil in a single dose of 1 g plus probenecid has been used for the treatment of gonorrhea (Gottlieb and Mills, 1986).

For infants and children 10–15 mg per kg, administered 12-hourly is the suggested dose (Powell *et al.*, 1991). This again should be administered together with milk (Ginsburg *et al.*, 1985).

In patients with renal failure, dosage modification is not necessary if creatinine clearance is above 50 ml per min per 1.73 m^2 and to adults a dose of cefuroxime axetil 250–500 mg 8-hourly can be given. This dose should be given every 12 h when creatinine clearance is 49–30 ml per min per 1.73 m^2, every 24 h when it is 29–10 ml per min per 1.73 m^2, and every 48 h when it is below 10 ml per min per 1.73 m^2 (Konishi *et al.*, 1993).

Serum Levels in Relation to Dosage

1   Cefamandole

After an i.m. injection of 1 g to adults, a peak serum level of approximately 20 μg per ml is reached 45 min after the dose (Fig. I.13). This peak level is similar to that attained after a 1-g i.m. cephalothin dose, but with cephalothin the peak occurs 30 min after the injection (p. 254).

Beginning at 45 min after i.m. administration, cefamandole serum levels are consistently higher than those of cephalothin, and its area under the serum level curve is about 25% larger (Fong *et al.*, 1976b). After a 1-g i.m. dose, cephalothin can be detected in the serum for only 5–6 h (Fig. I.13), but cefamandole activity is detectable for 6–8 h (Griffith *et al.*, 1976; Meyers *et al.*, 1976). The serum half-life of cefamandole after i.m. injection is approximately 1 h (Fong *et al.*, 1976b).

Immediately following a 1-g i.v. infusion of cefamandole over 20 min, the mean peak serum level is 88.0 μg per ml, the comparable value for cephalothin being 64.0 μg per ml (Fig. I.14). In addition, successive cefamandole levels are higher than those of cephalothin at all time intervals; at 2.5 h the cefamandole level is 3 μg per ml and that of cephalothin less than 1 μg per ml. Higher peaks are obtained if the dose is infused over a period of 3 or 5 min. Repeated i.v. dosing with 2 g of cefamandole every 6 h, has no effect on peak serum levels, half-life, serum clearance or apparent volume of distribution of the drug (Barza *et al.*, 1976). The serum half-life of cefamandole after i.v. administration is only 34 min (Fong *et al.*, 1976b).

With both i.m. and i.v. administration, doubling the dose of cefamandole approximately doubles peak serum levels, and prolongs but does not double the period during which the drug is detectable in the serum (Griffith *et al.*, 1976). Concomitant administration of probenecid (p. 24) increases and prolongs serum levels of cefamandole (Griffith *et al.*, 1977).

Fig. I.13.
Average serum levels after a 1-g i.m. injection showing consistently higher levels for cefamandole beginning at 45 min, and an area-under-the-curve about 25% greater than for cephalothin. (Redrawn after Fong *et al.*, 1976b, with permission.)

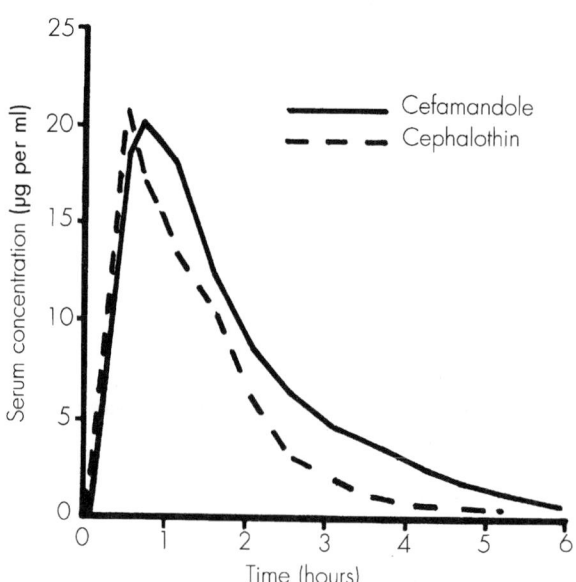

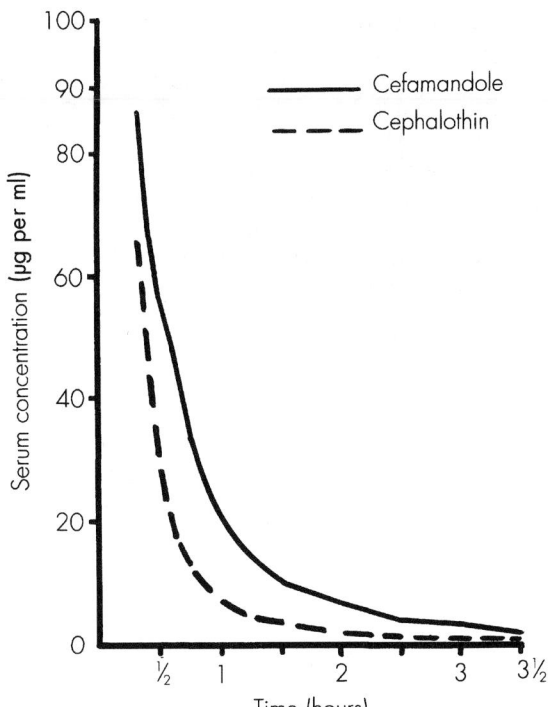

Fig. I.14.

Average serum cefamandole and cephalothin concentrations after a 1-g i.v. infusion given in 20 min. (Redrawn after Fong *et al.*, 1976b, with permission.)

2 Cefoxitin

Serum levels of cefoxitin after both i.m. and i.v. administration, like those of cefamandole, are higher than cephalothin levels (Brumfitt *et al.*, 1974). After a 1-g i.m. dose to adults, a mean peak serum level of 22.5 µg per ml is reached 20 min later (Fig. I.15). Thereafter, the level falls, but cefoxitin can be detected in the serum for at least 4 h.

If a 2-g dose of cefoxitin is administered i.v. over 3 min to adults, the mean peak serum level attained at approximately 5 min, is 222.6 µg per ml (Fig. I.16). This level falls more slowly than that of cephalothin, and a concentration of 3.4 µg per ml is still detectable at 3 h. When the same dose of cefoxitin is given as a 30-min i.v. infusion, the peak serum level (immediately after the infusion) is lower, but subsequent serum concentrations are slightly more sustained (Goodwin *et al.*, 1974).

Doubling the i.m. or i.v. dose of cefoxitin, virtually doubles serum concentrations (Brumfitt *et al.*, 1974; Geddes *et al.*, 1977). The mean cefoxitin serum half-life after either i.m. or i.v. administration is 45 min. Concomitant administration of probenecid greatly enhances and prolongs cefoxitin serum levels, so that its half-life is then 83 min (Goodwin *et al.*, 1974).

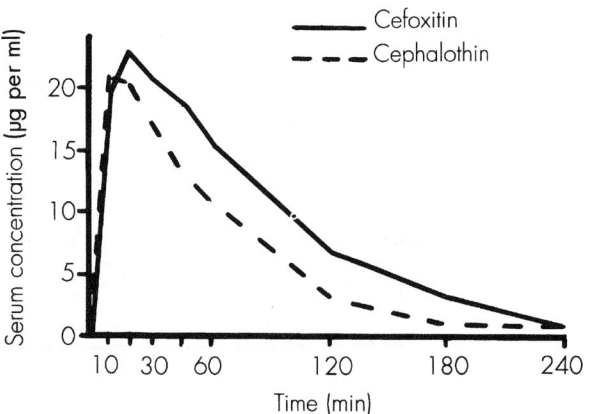

Fig. I.15.

Serum concentrations of cefoxitin and cephalothin after i.m. administration of 1 g. (Redrawn after Brumfitt *et al.*, 1974, with permission.)

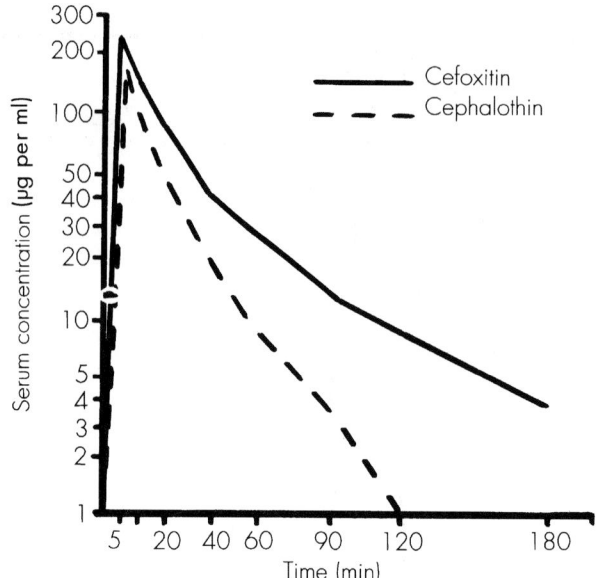

Fig. I.16.
Serum concentrations of cefoxitin and cephalothin after i.v. administration of 2 g. (Redrawn after Brumfitt *et al.*, 1974, with permission.)

3 Parenteral cefuroxime

After a 0.5-g i.m. dose to adults, a mean peak serum level of 25.3 µg per ml is reached in 30 min. Following a 1-g i.m. dose the peak is higher (39.1 µg per ml), but not doubled, and it is reached in 45–60 min (Fig. I.17). Serum levels after both doses are prolonged, and measurable concentrations of cefuroxime are still present 8 h after the injection. The area-under-the-serum concentration-time-curve increases, but does not double with the higher dose.

If a 0.5-g dose of cefuroxime is infused i.v. over 30 min into adults, the mean peak serum level immediately after the infusion is 37.8 µg per ml; this level falls to 5.1 µg per ml at 3 h and the drug is still detectable in serum for 5–6 h (Fig. I.18). If the same dose is given by rapid i.v. injection (over 3 min), the peak serum level is much higher (82.7 µg per ml), but at 3 h and thereafter the levels are slightly lower than after the 30 min infusion (Foord, 1976; Goodwin *et al.*, 1977).

The cefuroxime serum half-life after i.m. or i.v. administration is 1.4–1.8 h (Bundtzen *et al.*, 1981). Concomitant administration of probenecid increases the serum concentrations of cefuroxime the total area-under-the-curve, and its serum half-life (p. 24).

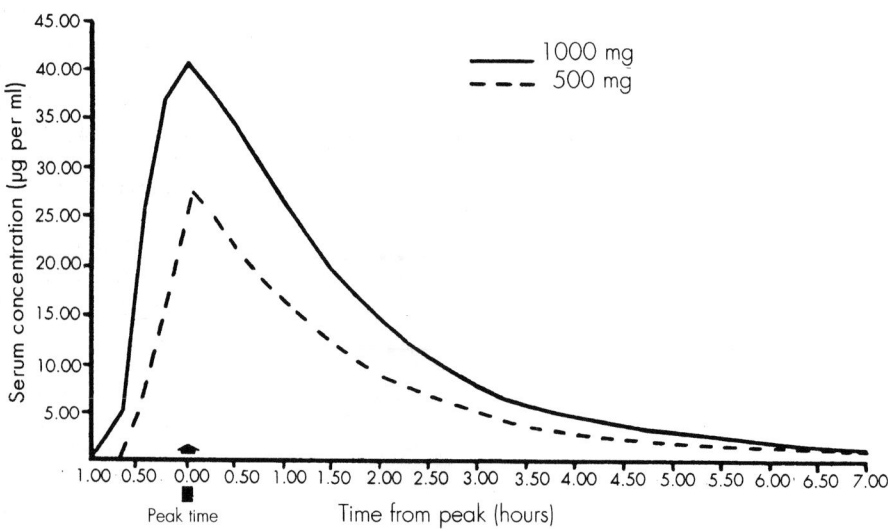

Fig. I.17.
Serum concentrations of cefuroxime after i.m. injections. (Redrawn after Foord, 1976, with permission.)

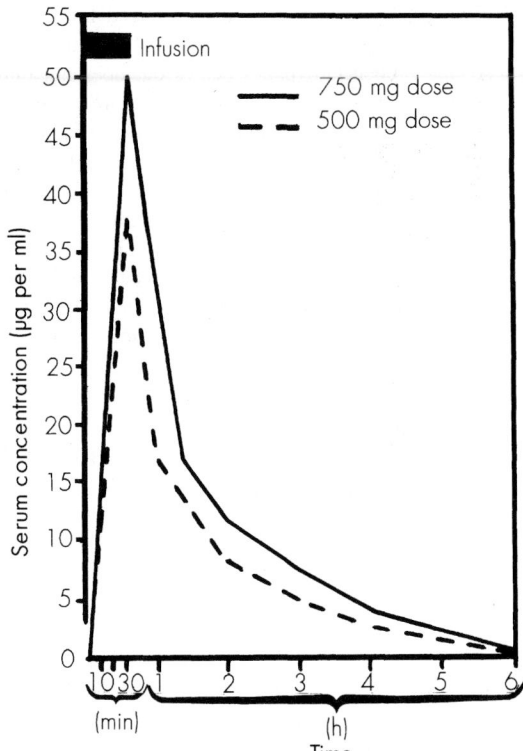

Fig. I.18.
Serum concentrations of cefuroxime: mean values during a 6-h period after the commencement of a 30-min infusion. (Redrawn after Goodwin *et al.*, 1977, with permission.)

4 Oral cefuroxime axetil

When a 250-mg dose is administered orally to adults together with food, the mean peak serum level is reached in 2.5 h and it is 4.63 μg per ml. The serum half-life thereafter is approximately 1 h and detectable serum concentrations are present for at least 8 h (James *et al.*, 1991). The serum levels are similar when a 15 mg per kg dose is administered to infants and children with milk (Powell *et al.*, 1991).

Excretion

1 Cefamandole

Unlike cephalothin (p. 255), cefamandole is not metabolized in the body (Barza *et al.*, 1976), and nearly all of a parenterally administered dose is excreted via the kidney in an unchanged active form (Griffith *et al.*, 1976). High concentrations are obtained in urine; mean urinary concentrations of 1633 and 3458 μg per ml after 0.5- and 1-g i.m. doses, respectively, can be detected during the first 8 h period (Meyers *et al.*, 1976).

The renal clearance of cefamandole is approximately 234 ml per min (per 1.72 m^2 of body surface area); this exceeds the creatinine clearance of patients with normal renal function (82 ml per min per 1.72 m^2). Therefore, cefamandole is not only excreted by glomerular filtration, but also by active tubular secretion (Mellin *et al.*, 1977) Probenecid delays the drug's excretion by partly blocking tubular secretion (Griffith *et al.*, 1977). The mean serum clearance of cefamandole (272 ml per min per 1.72 m^2) is similar to its renal clearance (see above), indicating that it is excreted mainly by the kidneys (Fong *et al.*, 1976b; Mellin *et al.*, 1977).

Some cefamandole is eliminated via the bile. In patients with a T-tube in the common bile duct, peak biliary levels after 1 g i.v., average 352 μg per ml. After the same dose of cefazolin and cephalothin, comparative biliary levels are only 46 and 12 μg per ml, respectively (Ratzan *et al.*, 1978). Also concentrations of cefamandole in the bile collected during operation are usually high in patients with hepatobiliary pathology. The drug is undetectable in gallbladder bile when there is complete cystic duct obstruction (Uwaydah *et al.*, 1982). Cefamandole has, therefore, some pharmacokinetic advantages for use in biliary sepsis (Lindahl *et al.*, 1980; Burns *et al.*, 1989).

2 Cefoxitin

Excretion in the urine in an unchanged form is virtually the only way this cephamycin is eliminated from the body. It is excreted by both glomerular filtration and active tubular secretion, so that probenecid (p. 24) delays but does not diminish its excretion (Vlasses *et al.*, 1980; Arvidsson *et al.*, 1981). About 90% or more of a parenterally administered dose can be recovered from the urine as active unchanged drug during the following 12 h (Brumfitt *et al.*, 1974). High cefoxitin concentrations are attained in urine; after a 0.5-g i.m. dose, these are 1000–3500 µg per ml during the first 3 h, and 22–350 µg per ml in the succeeding 9 h (Kosmidis *et al.*, 1973). The renal elimination of cefoxitin, is unaffected by concomitant administration of furosemide (frusemide) (Trollfors and Norrby, 1980).

In some subjects cefoxitin is deacylated in the body to detectable amounts of antibacterially inactive decarbamoyl-cefoxitin. This only occurs to a minor extent, as the metabolite can only be found in the urine after a delay of several hours, and it always accounts for less than 2% of the administered dose (Goodwin *et al.*, 1974; Schrogie *et al.*, 1979).

A small amount of cefoxitin may also be excreted in the bile; biliary levels in two patients with T-tube drainage after cholecystectomy were 4- to 12-fold higher than simultaneous serum levels (Geddes *et al.*, 1977). Cefoxitin enters the gall bladder bile via the gall bladder wall in patients with cystic duct obstruction, and therapeutically effective concentrations of the drug may be found in the common bile duct in patients with obstructive jaundice. However, in both of these situations, biliary levels are lower than serum levels at the time (Hansbrough and Clark, 1982). The amount of cefoxitin excreted in the bile is <1% of the administered dose (Schrogie *et al.*, 1979).

3 Cefuroxime

This drug also is not inactivated in the body; virtually all of a parenterally administered dose is excreted via the kidney, in an active unchanged form, by glomerular filtration and tubular secretion. The latter accounts for approximately 50% of the total drug excreted, so that concomitant administration of probenecid (p. 24) decreases cefuroxime clearance by about 40% (Foord, 1976).

Over 95% of i.m. or i.v. administered cefuroxime can be recovered from the urine during the first 24 h. High concentrations of the drug are attained in urine; after a 0.5-g i.m. dose, urinary concentrations are 300–3000 µg per ml during the first 6 h (Foord, 1976; Goodwin *et al.*, 1977). Like cefoxitin, simultaneous administration of furosemide has no effect on renal excretion of cefuroxime (Trollfors and Norrby, 1980).

Very little cefuroxime is excreted via the bile. Biliary levels are lower than simultaneous serum levels even if the biliary tract is not obstructed. Severn and Powis (1979) found that after an i.v. dose of 750 mg of cefuroxime, the mean biliary level in diseased gallbladders was 4.8 µg per ml, and the mean level was only 9 µg per ml in the common bile duct bile, in patients without biliary tract obstruction.

Some 38.65% of an administered dose of cefuroxime, given orally as cefuroxime axetil, can be recovered from the urine (Lang *et al.*, 1990).

Distribution of the Drugs in Body

1 Cefamandole

The drug, like other cephalosporins, such as cephalothin (p. 255) and cefazolin (p. 285), does not penetrate into normal CSF to any extent. It may reach inflamed meninges in significant concentrations. Steinberg *et al.* (1977) studied CSF cefamandole levels in 12 patients with bacterial meningitis, who had received a single i.v. cefamandole dose (33 mg per kg), 75–140 min before lumbar puncture. Most of these patients had a detectable CSF level which correlated with the CSF protein; in six with a CSF protein less than 100 mg per 100 ml (1000 mmol per liter), the cefamandole concentration was 0–0.62 µg per ml, and in the other six with a CSF protein greater than 100 mg per 100 ml, the range was 0.57–7.4 µg per ml.

Cefamandole diffuses well into human interstitial fluid (Tan and Salstrom, 1977). Four adult patients with pneumonia caused by Gram-negative organisms receiving a cefamandole dose of 6–8 g daily, had sputum cefamandole levels of 0.27–2.5 µg per ml (Minor *et al.*, 1976). In patients undergoing cardiac surgery, after a 1–2 g preoperative i.v. dose of cefamandole, adequate levels of the drug were attained in heart valve tissue, right atrial appendage, pericardial fluid, aortic wall and intercostal muscle, for 4–5 h after administration (Daschner *et al.*, 1980; Mullany *et al.*, 1982; Daschner and Frank, 1987).

In animals cefamandole reaches adequate concentrations in non-inflamed cortical bone (Lunke et al., 1981), but it penetrates poorly into experimental chronic *E. coli* abdominal abscesses (Gerding et al., 1980). Also in animals, cefamandole is secreted in adequate concentrations in pancreatic fluid and it penetrates into normal pancreatic tissue. Unlike cephalothin (p. 255), cefamandole penetration into pancreatic tissue is increased in animals with induced pancreatitis (Studley et al., 1982). Cefamandole is approximately 70% serum protein bound (Fong et al., 1976b).

2 Cefoxitin

Like penicillins (p. 25) and cephalosporins (p. 255), this cephamycin does not penetrate into normal CSF (Geddes et al., 1977). After large parenteral doses to patients with bacterial meningitis, moderate CSF concentrations of the drug are found, but these are not always high enough to inhibit susceptible strains of *H. influenzae* and *Strep. pneumoniae* (Nair et al., 1979; Humbert et al., 1980; Feldman et al., 1982).

Parenterally administered cefoxitin penetrates quite well into the peritoneal fluid of surgical patients (Wise et al., 1981), and into normal human interstitial fluid, where concentrations are very similar to serum levels (Gillett and Wise, 1978). It also reaches therapeutically effective levels in pelvic tissue of patients undergoing abdominal hysterectomy (Bawdon et al., 1982). Cefoxitin penetrates into normal lung and bone but these tissue levels are considerably lower than simultaneous serum levels (Summersgill et al., 1982; Perea et al., 1983). The cefoxitin concentration in breast milk of one patient collected 2 h after an i.v. dose of 1 g was 5.6 μg per ml (Geddes et al., 1977).

Cefoxitin diffuses poorly into experimental *B. fragilis* intra-abdominal abscesses in animals, producing a concentration of only 2% of the simultaneous serum level (O'Keefe et al., 1979). In animals, cefoxitin penetrates into brain, heart, kidney, liver, lung, muscle and spleen, where its concentration is greater than that of cephalothin (Miller et al., 1974). Binding of cefoxitin to serum proteins is approximately 20% (O'Callaghan, 1975).

3 Cefuroxime

CSF levels of this drug are low in patients with uninflamed meninges, but unlike cefamandole (p. 304) and cefoxitin (see above), therapeutically effective concentrations are attained after large parenteral doses, in patients with bacterial meningitis (Müller et al., 1980; De Los et al., 1982). With a dosage of 1.5 g cefuroxime i.v. every 6 h in adults, CSF levels were in the range 1.5–13.5 (mean 6) μg per ml, during the acute stage of bacterial meningitis (Netland et al., 1981). In 21 patients with bacterial meningitis treated by cefuroxime 60–75 mg per kg body weight i.v. every 8 h, CSF concentrations were high and in most cases therapeutic levels were maintained between doses (Report, 1982). In one study the penetration in ventricular fluid of i.v. cefuroxime, in a dose of 200–230 mg per kg body weight, was assessed in pediatric patients with ventriculoperitoneal shunt infections. Levels of cefuroxime in ventricular fluid ranged from 1.6 to 22.5 μg per ml (Edwards et al., 1989).

Cefuroxime penetrates well into pleural fluid (Hoffstedt et al., 1980) and into middle ear effusions of patients with chronic purulent otitis media (Martini and Xerri, 1982). Drug concentrations in bronchial secretions are relatively low, mean levels being 0.67 and 1.78 μg per ml after 750 mg and 1.5 g doses, respectively; but these levels exceed the MICs of susceptible pathogens (Peirce et al., 1980). Cefuroxime reaches therapeutically effective concentrations in muscle and fat tissue taken from proximal parts of ischemic amputated limbs (Bullen et al., 1981). In adults after a 750 mg dose of i.v. cefuroxime, tissue levels in normal bone averaged 8 μg per g (Leigh, 1989). Cefuroxime diffused easily into normal human interstitial fluid, where concentrations were similar to serum levels at the time (Gillett and Wise, 1978). Cefuroxime protein binding in adult serum is concentration-dependent with the percentage bound varying from 88% at 25 μg per ml to 8.8% at 700 μg per ml. Cefuroxime binding in neonatal serum is independent of concentration averaging 15.6% over the above concentration range (Benson et al., 1993).

After an oral dose of cefuroxime axetil (500 mg), the concentration of cefuroxime in bronchial mucosa ranged from 1.8 to 2.18 μg per g (Winter and Dhillon, 1991; Baldwin et al., 1992). After oral administration of cefuroxime axetil, the concentrations in normal human bone were 20–30% of serum concentrations (Renneberg et al., 1993).

Mode of Action

These cephalosporins and cefoxitin act on bacteria in a manner similar to penicillin G (p. 25), and cephalothin (p. 256).

Toxicity

1 Cefamandole

Relatively few side-effects have been observed with this drug. Urticarial rashes (Steinberg *et al.*, 1977; Azimi 1978) and eosinophilia (Perkins *et al.*, 1978) have been noted occasionally. Cefamandole, like cephalothin (p. 256), is probably only infrequently cross-allergenic with the penicillins. A positive Coombs' test without hemolysis can occur with cefamandole, as with other cephalosporins (p. 257) (Rodriguez *et al.*, 1978). Other side-effects are drug fever (Steinberg *et al.*, 1977) and transient SGOT elevations (Minor *et al.*, 1976). Diarrhea has been attributed occasionally to parenteral administration of the drug (Ekwall *et al.*, 1979).

Cefamandole nephrotoxicity is uncommon. In a survey of 2000 treated patients, two developed reversible nephropathy which might have been related to the drug, and a third patient died of infection associated with renal damage possibly due to cefamandole (Barza, 1978). In animals, cefamandole is less nephrotoxic than cefazolin (p. 286) (Wold *et al.*, 1978b), and high doses do not increase tobramycin nephrotoxicity but protect against aminoglycoside-induced renal injury, presumably by enhancing tobramycin excretion (Barza *et al.*, 1978). Nephrotoxicity has been uncommon in patients treated by cefamandole combined with one of the aminoglycosides, such as gentamicin or tobramycin (Brown *et al.*, 1982).

Similar to moxalactam (p. 350), cefamandole can cause hypoprothrombinemia and possibly bleeding. Parenteral vitamin K therapy rapidly reverses the abnormality, suggesting that cefamandole interferes with its synthesis or action. This is probably not due to antibiotic-induced killing of intestinal bacteria, because in man the production of vitamin K by these bacteria does not play any role in the synthesis of clotting factors (Smith and Lipsky, 1983). Data from animal studies do not suggest that cefamandole acts directly on vitamin K-dependent enzymes (Uotila and Suttie, 1983). In common with moxalactam and cefoperazone, cefamandole contains a N-methylthiotetrazole side-chain. This side-chain released by *in vivo* degradation of the drugs, inhibits gamma carboxylation of glutamic acid, which is necessary for the synthesis of prothrombin (p. 350). Patients with renal failure may be at more risk of bleeding, because in renal failure this side-chain accumulates to a greater degree than cefamandole itself (Aronoff *et al.*, 1986). Other factors are also involved in production of hypoprothrombinemia. Most reported cases of cefamandole-induced hypoprothrombinemia have occurred in elderly, debilitated and/or malnourished patients. This suggests that pre-existing vitamin K deficiency or some other factor, must be present in order for cefamandole to produce this effect. It is advisable to give prophylactic parenteral vitamin K when cefamandole is used in such patients (Bailey, 1983; Smith and Lipsky, 1983).

Cefamandole, similar to carbenicillin and ticarcillin (p. 153), can cause impaired platelet function, by suppressing ADP-induced platelet aggregation. This only occurs with abnormally high cefamandole serum levels, such as 3000–4000 µg per ml (Custer *et al.*, 1979; Bang and Kammer, 1983).

Cefamandole, cefoperazone (p. 335) and moxalactam (p. 350) all have a N-methylthiotetrazole side-chain, which can provoke a disulfiram-like reaction in patients ingesting ethanol (p. 335). Patients should avoid alcoholic beverages during, and for several days after, cefamandole treatment (Buening and Wold, 1982). One patient has been reported who developed a bad taste, apparently related to i.v. cefamandole therapy (Hodgson, 1981).

As with cephalothin (p. 258) and cefazolin (p. 287), several case reports have documented the development of meningitis during cefamandole therapy. Meningitis caused by *H. influenzae* type b developed in children, who were treated by cefamandole for severe non-meningeal *H. influenzae* infections such as cellulitis, septic arthritis or empyema; both beta-lactamase-producing and non-beta-lactamase-producing strains were involved (Aronoff *et al.*, 1981; Azimi and Chase, 1981; Chartrand *et al.*, 1981). Because cefamandole penetrates poorly into CSF, it should be avoided in infections which may be complicated by meningitis, particularly those due to *H. influenzae* (Marks, 1981).

2 Cefoxitin

Eosinophilia (Heseltine *et al.*, 1977) and rashes (McCloskey, 1977) can occur. Two patients developed a positive Coombs' test during therapy (Heseltine *et al.*, 1977), and rarely hemolytic anemia and pancytopenia have been reported in association with cefoxitin therapy (De Torres, 1983). Eight of 31 patients treated by Geddes *et al.* (1977), had transient slight rises in SGOT levels.

During initial pharmacological studies in human volunteers, cefoxitin appeared free from nephrotoxicity (Kosmidis *et al.*, 1973; Brumfitt *et al.*, 1974). Proteinuria without a rise in blood urea, was observed in two of 31 patients given cefoxitin by Geddes *et al.* (1977). Heseltine *et al.* (1977) treated 38 patients and four developed deterioration of renal function; two had pre-existing renal functional impairment, and the other two had hepatic failure and septicemia which may have contributed to renal failure. Subsequent large-scale clinical studies showed that cefoxitin nephrotoxicity was uncommon, as with cephalothin (p. 256) (Neu, 1979). It does not aggravate pre-existing renal failure, provided that appropriate doses are given, and it can be used with furosemide, which does not prolong its serum half-life (Trollfors *et al.*, 1978; Trollfors, 1980). In animals cefoxitin is not nephrotoxic, and does not potentiate aminoglycoside nephrotoxicity (Ormrod and Miller, 1981; Viotte *et al.*, 1981).

Cefoxitin has no hepatotoxicity (Van Winzum, 1978; Neu, 1979). Similar to cefamandole (p. 306), it may suppress ADP-induced platelet aggregation but this only occurs with abnormally high cefoxitin serum concentrations (Bang and Kammer, 1983). Surprisingly in a clinical study Brown *et al.* (1986) observed clinical bleeding in 8.2% of cefoxitin-treated patients. The exact cause for this was not determined. Some patients developed diarrhea due to i.v. cefoxitin, especially with large doses (Trollfors *et al.*, 1979). Intravenous cefoxitin produced quite marked alterations in fecal flora, such as acquisition of *E. faecalis*, *Staph. epidermidis*, *Cl. difficile*, cefoxitin-resistant Enterobacteriaceae and *Ps. aeruginosa* and concomitant eradication or decrease of cefoxitin-susceptible Enterobacteriaceae and *Bacteroides* spp. (Mulligan *et al.*, 1984; Barza *et al.*, 1987).

3 Cefuroxime

This drug is relatively free from side-effects. In one study, 18 of 60 treated patients developed slight reversible rises in SGOT levels and two a positive direct Coombs' test without hemolysis (Norrby *et al.*, 1977). Cefuroxime may have an immunosuppressant effect but the clinical relevance of this is not known (Manzella and Clark, 1983). Similar to cefamandole (p. 306) and cefoxitin (see above), it may interfere with platelet function but only when excessively high serum levels are attained (Bang and Kammer, 1983). Nephrotoxicity is uncommon, and cefuroxime can be administered safely with furosemide. Provided the dose is suitably reduced, the drug can be used in patients with pre-existing renal damage without further compromising renal function (Trollfors, 1980; Trollfors *et al.*, 1980b). Some patients treated by i.v. cefuroxime, especially by high doses, have developed diarrhea (Trollfors *et al.*, 1979). A psychotic reaction to i.v. cefuroxime has been reported in one patient (Vincken, 1984).

With oral cefuroxime axetil patients have experienced nausea, vomiting and diarrhea, but the incidence of these events did not differ significantly from those due to other oral antibiotics such as co-amoxiclav (p. 199) and cefaclor (p. 277) (Emmerson, 1988; McLinn *et al.*, 1994). The calculated incidence of antibiotic-associated colitis is approximately one in 2100 (Emmerson, 1988). Cefuroxime axetil had an effect on fecal flora of healthy volunteers; there was a reduction of anaerobes and more marked elimination of Enterobacteriaceae and increase in streptococci (Leigh *et al.*, 1990).

Clinical Uses of the Drugs

Cefamandole, cefoxitin and cefuroxime may be useful for the treatment of infections caused by Gram-negative bacteria, especially those which are resistant to cephalothin and other earlier cephalosporins. All three, under certain conditions, may be suitable for the treatment of infections such as pyelonephritis and septicemia caused by these organisms. Cefoxitin is valuable for treatment of sepsis following abdominal surgery, because it is active against both aerobic and anaerobic Gram-negative bacteria. Cefuroxime is suitable for treatment of *H. influenzae* infections, especially those due to ampicillin-resistant strains. Both cefoxitin and cefuroxime are suitable for the treatment of gonococcal infections due to beta-lactamase producing strains.

None of these three drugs are preferable to cephalothin for the treatment of infections caused by Gram-positive bacteria, such as staphylococcal septicemia or *Strep. viridans* endocarditis; cefamandole and cefuroxime are probably equally as effective as cephalothin, whereas cefoxitin although also clinically effective, is 5- to 10-fold less active *in vitro* than cephalothin in this respect (p. 293).

A Cefamandole

1 Urinary tract infections

This drug has been used with success for the treatment of these infections, mainly caused by cephalothin-sensitive *E. coli* and *Klebsiella* and *Proteus* spp. (Hoyme and Madsen, 1978). A single dose of 1 g i.m. cefamandole may be effective, even in complicated urinary tract infections provided the organism is cefamandole-sensitive (Shaw *et al.*, 1980). Complicated urinary tract and some systemic infections caused by cephalothin-resistant *Enterobacter*, *Pr. vulgaris*, *Pr. rettgeri* and *Morganella morganii* strains, may also respond to a course of cefamandole (Levine and McCain, 1978a). If a parenteral antibiotic is indicated nowadays one of the third-generation cephalosporins, such as cefotaxime (p. 338) or ceftriaxone (p. 360) would be used to treat these more difficult infections.

2 Other Gram-negative infections

Satisfactory results were obtained in a proportion of patients in whom cefamandole was used to treat pulmonary infections caused by a variety of Gram-negative bacilli (Delgado *et al.*, 1979; Clarke *et al.*, 1980). Cefamandole was also used with success for treatment of severe infections caused by Gram-negative rods, such as septicemia, but nowadays one of the third-generation cephalosporins (see above) would be used for this indication.

3 Streptococcal and staphylococcal infections

Results of cefamandole treatment of these infections are about the same as those obtained with cephalothin (p. 258). Cefamandole, like other beta-lactam drugs, has sometimes not been successful for the treatment of severe staphylococcal infections, such as endocarditis and septicemia (Eng *et al.*, 1985). The drug is satisfactory for the treatment of respiratory tract, skin, soft tissue, bone and joint infections (Levine and McCain, 1978b; Perkins *et al.*, 1978; Petty *et al.*, 1978).

4 Haemophilus influenzae infections

Cefamandole is not satisfactory for treatment for severe systemic *H. influenzae* type b infections in children. Steinberg *et al.* (1978) described three children with *H. influenzae* type b meningitis, in which cefamandole therapy was unsatisfactory. Rodriguez *et al.* (1978) reported one infant with periorbital cellulitis and *H. influenzae* septicemia who developed bacterial meningitis while receiving cefamandole; *H. influenzae* meningitis supervened in several other children, who were treated by cefamandole for other systemic *H. influenzae* type b infections (p. 306). Cefamandole should not be used for the treatment of these infections (Sanders *et al.*, 1985).

5 Salmonella infections

De Carvalho *et al.* (1982) treated 19 patients with *Salmonella* septicemia, eight due to *Salm. typhi*. Although all strains were highly susceptible to cefamandole *in vitro*, treatment failed in seven patients, including three with *Salm. typhi*. Cefamandole does not appear to be reliable for the treatment of systemic *Salmonella* infections.

6 Surgical chemoprophylaxis

Cefamandole has been used for surgical chemoprophylaxis, but for most indications where a cephalosporin is appropriate, earlier drugs such as cephalothin (p. 259) or cefazolin (p. 287) may be equally effective. Cefamandole may be superior to these cephalosporins for chemoprophylaxis in biliary surgery and for treatment of biliary tract infections (Lindahl *et al.*, 1980), but other drugs, such as ampicillin (p. 125), are also effective. In one randomized comparison of cefamandole, cefazolin, and cefuroxime prophylaxis in open heart surgery there were more infections in patients treated with cefazolin than in those treated with cefamandole or cefuroxime. Most of the infections in the cefazolin group were due to staphylococci (Slama *et al.*, 1986). This corresponds with the observation by Sabath (1989) that cefazolin is an inferior anti-staphylococcal drug (p. 288).

B Cefoxitin

1 Intra-abdominal sepsis and other anaerobic infections

As this drug is effective against most Gram-negative aerobic bacilli (except *Ps. aeruginosa*) and Gram-negative anaerobes including *B. fragilis*, it has been extensively used for intra-abdominal infections such as peritonitis. Clinical and experimental studies have shown that antibiotic(s) with this spectrum of activity are needed to treat intra-abdominal sepsis (Nichols, 1983). Many experiments with induced intra-abdominal sepsis in animals have shown that cefoxitin is effective and comparable with other useful drugs or drug regimens, such as clindamycin/gentamicin (p. 597), metronidazole/gentamicin (p. 947), chloramphenicol (p. 569) and imipenem (p. 236) (Bartlett *et al.*, 1981, 1983; Joiner *et al.*, 1982). Clinical studies have confirmed that cefoxitin, either used alone, or combined with an aminoglycoside, such as gentamicin, is effective in patients with intra-abdominal sepsis (Geddes *et al.*, 1977; Nair and Cherubin, 1978; Tally *et al.*, 1979b; Gorbach and McGowan, 1981), provided that the *Bacteroides* spp. strain involved is cefoxitin-sensitive (Snydman *et al.*, 1992).

Cefoxitin has been used with success for other patients with sepsis caused predominantly by Gram-negative anaerobes, such as *B. fragilis*. Examples include anaerobic infections in cancer patients (Klastersky *et al.*, 1979), infections of the female genital tract (Rosene *et al.*, 1986; Counts, 1988) and pleuropulmonary infections (Le Frock *et al.*, 1982). For the treatment of intra-abdominal and other anaerobic infections, cefoxitin is not clearly superior to other available alternative regimens (see above). Its toxicity, when used alone, may be less than that of some combination regimens such as clindamycin/gentamicin (Gorbach and McGowan, 1981). All of the above infections are polymicrobial, and in addition to *B. fragilis*, many aerobic Gram-negative bacilli are involved which may possess inducible chromosomally mediated beta-lactamases. Cefoxitin is an excellent inducer of these enzymes (p. 295), and this is a possible disadvantage when it is used for the treatment of these infections, especially in debilitated or otherwise compromised patients. Other disadvantages of cefoxitin are superinfections due to cefoxitin-resistant organisms such as *E. faecalis* or *Ps. aeruginosa* (Nordbring and Nord, 1982).

2 Surgical chemoprophylaxis

The drug has been used with success for chemoprophylaxis in large bowel surgery. For elective colon operations, 1 g doses i.v. before, during and 6 h after the operative incision, have been recommended. For this some now favor just a single dose of 2 g cefoxitin i.v. at the time of induction of anesthesia. For emergency colonic operations or for patients with bowel obstruction, 2 g i.v. doses prior to surgery, during operation, and then every 6 h for five doses, have been recommended (Gorbach, 1982; Lau *et al.*, 1986). Other drug regimens are available for chemoprophylaxis in large bowel surgery (p. 949). Cefoxitin prophylaxis has also been used for penetrating abdominal injuries (Dellinger, 1991) and for prophylaxis of obstetric and gynecologic infections (Counts, 1988). For the latter one of the first-generation cephalosporins such as cephalothin (p. 259) or cefazolin (p. 288) is usually adequate.

3 Gram-negative aerobic infections

Cefoxitin has been effective in infections, such as pyelonephritis, pneumonia and septicemia caused by Gram-negative aerobic bacilli, such as *E. coli*, *Enterobacter* and *Klebsiella* spp., which often were cephalothin-resistant (Heseltine *et al.*, 1977; Le Frock *et al.*, 1982). Soft tissue infections, such as cellulitis caused by *H. influenzae*, also respond to cefoxitin, but the drug is ineffective for *H. influenzae* meningitis (Santos *et al.*, 1981). There are alternate antibiotics available for the treatment of all of these Gram-negative infections (p. 338).

4 Streptococcal and staphylococcal infections

Gram-positive infections, such as those caused by *Staph. aureus* and *Strep. pyogenes*, also respond to cefoxitin (McCloskey, 1977; Perkins *et al.*, 1979). If a cephalosporin is indicated for one of these infections, cephalothin (p. 258) or cefazolin (p. 287) is preferred. Cefoxitin is safe and effective for the treatment of infections such as cellulitis, osteomyelitis, septic arthritis and pneumonia, in infants and children. In most reported cases the etiological agents were Gram-positive, such as *Strep. pyogenes*, *Strep. pneumoniae* and *Staph. aureus*, but some moderately severe *H. influenzae* infections were also treated, except meningitis (Jacobson *et al.*, 1979; Feldman *et al.*, 1980). As in adults, other antibiotics are usually preferred for these infections.

5 Gonorrhea

Cefoxitin 2 g i.m. plus 1 g probenecid orally, is a satisfactory single-dose treatment for uncomplicated genital gonorrhea. It is equally effective for gonorrhea caused by penicillin G-sensitive and beta-lactamase-producing strains (Berg *et al.*, 1979; Greaves *et al.*, 1983). For the treatment of gonorrhea, single-dose ceftriaxone (p. 361), cefixime (p. 412), ciprofloxacin (p. 1022) or ofloxacin (p.1122) are now preferred (CDC, 1993).

6 Mycobacterium fortuitum and Mycobacterium chelonae infections

Cefoxitin in a dose of 12 g i.v. daily plus 2–4 g oral probenecid is useful for the treatment of non-pulmonary infections by these organisms. For the initial 2–4 weeks the drug is often combined with amikacin (p. 516), and then cefoxitin therapy alone is continued for 10–12 weeks (Wallace *et al.*, 1985; Raad *et al.*, 1991). Pulmonary infection with *M. chelonae* has been treated successfully by i.v. cefoxitin and oral ciprofloxacin (p. 1032) (Singh and Yu, 1992).

C Parenteral cefuroxime

1 Gram-negative infections

This drug is effective for the treatment of urinary tract infections, pulmonary infections and septicemia, caused by Gram-negative aerobic bacilli, such as *E. coli* and the *Enterobacter*, *Klebsiella* and *Proteus* spp., many of which are resistant to cephalothin or aminoglycosides, such as gentamicin (Bint *et al.*, 1979; Hart *et al.*, 1981). Cefuroxime is quite useful for respiratory tract infections caused by *H. influenzae* (Geddes *et al.*, 1978; Mehtar *et al.*, 1982). Children with *H. influenzae* type b bacteremia, facial cellulitis or epiglottitis, respond satisfactorily to the drug (Barson *et al.*, 1985). For many of these infections nowadays a third-generation cephalosporin, such as cefotaxime (p. 338) or ceftriaxone (p. 360), is preferred by many clinicians.

Cefuroxime was compared with combined therapy with ampicillin and chloramphenicol to treat 50 consecutive patients with acute bacterial meningitis. Good results were obtained in 18 of 21 evaluable patients treated with cefuroxime; ten of these had *H. influenzae* meningitis, eight of whom were cured, including one with a beta-lactamase producing strain; the others had meningococcal (4), pneumococcal (4), *Strep. viridans* (1), and *Moraxella catarrhalis* meningitis (1). One patient with *Staph. aureus* meningitis, treated by cefuroxime, died. Overall results obtained with cefuroxime were comparable with those obtained by ampicillin plus chloramphenicol (Report, 1982). In another trial, five children with *H. influenzae* type b and two children with *Salmonella* meningitis were treated successfully by i.v. cefuroxime (Sirinavin *et al.*, 1984). But cefuroxime treatment failed in one case of non-typable *H. influenzae* meningitis, where the strain was relatively resistant to cefuroxime due to altered PBPs (p. 27) (Mendelman *et al.*, 1990). In a randomized controlled trial Marks *et al.* (1986) found cefuroxime generally as effective in bacterial meningitis as ampicillin plus chloramphenicol, but in some of the cefuroxime treated patients sterilization of the CSF was slower. In another study Schaad *et al.* (1990) found ceftriaxone superior to cefuroxime for the treatment of acute bacterial meningitis in children. In general most clinicians now prefer one of the third-generation cephalosporins such as cefotaxime (p. 336) or ceftriaxone (p. 359), rather than cefuroxime for the treatment of bacterial meningitis (McCracken *et al.*, 1987).

2 Streptococcal and staphylococcal infections

Cefuroxime is as effective as cephalothin (p. 258) for treatment of pneumonia, soft tissue infections, osteomyelitis and septic arthritis, covering as it does a spectrum of Gram-positive bacteria, such as *Strep. pyogenes*, *Strep. pneumoniae*, *Strep viridans* and *Staph. aureus* (Norrby *et al.*, 1977; Hugo *et al.*, 1980; Hedström *et al.*, 1984). According to Nelson (1983), cefuroxime is an effective initial empiric therapy for non-meningitic infections in children when the suspected bacterial pathogens are streptococci, staphylococci or *H. influenzae*.

3 Surgical chemoprophylaxis

Cefuroxime in a single-dose of 1.5 g i.v. has been used for chemoprophylaxis in patients undergoing elective operations on the stomach. In one trial cefuroxime chemoprophylaxis given as a single i.v. dose of 2 g proved to be superior to mezlocillin (p. 173) (Morris *et al.*, 1984). Cefuroxime chemoprophylaxis has also been used in open-heart surgery (Slama *et al.*, 1986). For prophylaxis of coronary artery bypass grafting a single-dose of 1.5 g i.v. at time of induction of anesthesia was as effective as 750 mg 8-hourly for 3 days (Nooyen *et al.*, 1994).

4 Gonorrhea

Similar to cefoxitin (p. 309), cefuroxime is a satisfactory drug for gonorrhea; it is effective for infections caused by both penicillin G-sensitive and beta-lactamase producing strains (Tupasi *et al.*, 1982; 1983). Cefuroxime is effective for uncomplicated genital gonorrhea in adults in a single i.m. dose of 1.5 g with or without oral probenecid (Lossick *et al.*, 1982; Chitwarakorn *et al.*, 1985). This single-dose therapy is not always successful for pharyngeal gonorrhea in adults (Graudal *et al.*, 1985). Gonorrhea in children has been treated successfully with a single i.m. dose of cefuroxime, 25 mg per kg body weight; this eliminated gonococci from genital, pharyngeal and anal sites in all cases (Patamasucon *et al.*, 1981).

D Oral cefuroxime axetil

1 Urinary tract infections

Leigh *et al.* (1989) found cefuroxime axetil, in a single daily dose of 250 mg for 10 days, a satisfactory treatment for women with acute uncomplicated urinary tract infections. In another study a single-dose of cefuroxime axetil 1 g was comparable with cefaclor 250 mg three times daily for 7 days for treatment of acute urinary tract infections in women (Iravani and Richard, 1989).

2 Respiratory tract infections

In one randomized trial in children with proven Group A streptococcal pharyngitis, cefuroxime axetil suspension (20 mg per kg body weight per day in two divided doses) was compared with that of penicillin V suspension (50 mg per kg per day in three divided doses), each administered for 10 days. In this study cefuroxime axetil demonstrated significantly greater bacteriological and clinical efficacies than penicillin V (Gooch et al., 1993). In another randomized trial cefuroxime axetil (30 mg per kg of body weight per day in two divided doses) was compared with amoxycillin/clavulanic acid (40 mg per kg per day in three divided doses), for the treatment of acute otitis media with effusion in children. Both treatments were given for 10 days. Both drugs were equally effective, but children treated with co-amoxiclav developed diarrhea or loose stools more frequently (McLinn et al., 1994). Cefuroxime axetil is likely to succeed in treatment of otitis media when the causative organism is a pneumococcus with intermediate resistance to penicillin G, but it will probably fail if the penicillin G MIC for the strain is higher than 2.0 µg per ml (Gehanno et al., 1995). For the treatment of bronchitis and pneumonia cefuroxime axetil was at least as effective as cefaclor (Carson et al., 1987; Schleupner et al., 1988).

3 Skin infections

These infections in children caused by *Staph. aureus* or *Strep. pyogenes* can be satisfactorily treated by cefuroxime axetil 30 mg per kg body weight per day, given in two divided doses. For this indication cefuroxime axetil proved to be at least as effective as cefadroxil (p. 278) (Jacobs et al., 1992). Cefuroxime axetil in a dose of 0.5 g 12-hourly may also be suitable for the treatment of similar infections in adults (Gentry, 1992).

4 Gonorrhea

Cefuroxime axetil in a single-dose of 1 or 1.5 g plus probenecid 1 g can cure uncomplicated urogenital and rectal gonorrhea in men and women (Gottlieb and Mills, 1986; Schift et al., 1986). This treatment for gonorrhea is probably less effective than oral cefixime (CDC, 1993).

5 Lyme disease

In one trial oral cefuroxime axetil 500 mg twice-daily was as effective as doxycycline 100 mg three times daily (both given for 20 days) for the treatment of patients with early Lyme disease associated with erythema migrans (Luger et al., 1995).

References

Acred P, Grujic P, Ryan DM et al. (1980). *In vitro* activity of cefuroxime against *Treponema pallidum* and *Neisseria gonorrhoeae*. *J Antimicrob Chemother* 6: 407.

Agger WA, Callister SM, Jobe DA (1992). *In vitro* susceptibilities of *Borrelia burgdorferi* to five oral cephalosporins and ceftriaxone. *Antimicrob Ag Chemother* 36: 1788.

Ahern MJ, Finkelstein FO, Andriole VT (1976). Pharmacokinetics of cefamandole in patients undergoing hemodialysis and peritoneal dialysis. *Antimicrob Ag Chemother* 10: 457.

Andriole VT (1978). Pharmacokinetics of cephalosporins in patients with normal or reduced renal function. *J Infect Dis* 137 (May Suppl): 88.

Appel GB, Neu HC, Parry MF et al. (1976). Pharmacokinetics of cefamandole in the presence of renal failure and in patients undergoing hemodialysis. *Antimicrob Ag Chemother* 10: 623.

Appelbaum PC, Spangler SK, Jacobs MR (1990). Beta-lactamase production and susceptibilities to amoxicillin, amoxicillin-clavulanate, ticarcillin, ticarcillin-clavulanate, cefoxitin, imipenem, and metronidazole of 320 non-*Bacteroides fragilis* Bacteroides isolates and 129 *Fusobacteria* from 28 US centers. *Antimicrob Ag Chemother* 34: 1546.

Appelbaum PC, Spangler SK, Jacobs MR (1991). Susceptibilities of 394 *Bacteroides fragilis*, non-*B fragilis* group *Bacteroides* species, and *Fusobacterium* species to newer antimicrobial agents. *Antimicrob Ag Chemother* 35: 1214.

Aronoff GR, Wolen RL, Obermeyer BD, Black HR (1986). Pharmacokinetics and protein binding of cefamandole and its 1-methyl-1 H-tetrazole-5-thiol side chain in subjects with normal and impaired renal function. *J Infect Dis* 153: 1069.

Aronoff SC, Shlaes DM (1987). Factors that influence the evolution of beta-lactam resistance in beta-lactamase-inducible strains of *Enterobacter cloacae* and *Pseudomonas aeruginosa*. *J Infect Dis* 155: 936.

Aronoff SC, Thomford W, Bertino JS, Speck WT (1981). Development of meningitis during therapy with cefamandole. *Pediatrics* 67: 727.

Arvidsson A, Borgå O, Kager L, Pieper R (1981). Renal elimination of cefoxitin and effect of probenecid after single and repeated doses. *J Antimicrob Chemother* 7: 423.

Azimi PH (1978). Clinical and laboratory investigation of cefamandole therapy of infections in infants and children. *J Infect Dis* 137 (Suppl): 155.

Azimi PH, Chase PA (1981). The role of cefamandole in the treatment of *Haemophilus influenzae* infections in infants and children. *J Pediatr* 98: 995.

Bach VT, Roy I, Thadepalli H (1977). Susceptibility of anaerobic bacteria to cefoxitin and related compounds. *Antimicrob Ag Chemother* 11: 912.

Bailey RR (1983). Bleeding tendency in patients on cephalosporins. *Lancet* i: 322.

Baldwin DR, Andrews JM, Wise R, Honeybourne D (1992). Bronchoalveolar distribution of cefuroxime axetil and in-vitro efficacy of observed concentrations against respiratory pathogens. *J Antimicrob Chemother* 30: 377.

Bang NU, Kammer RB (1983). Hematologic complications associated with beta-lactam antibiotics. *Rev Infect Dis* **5** (Suppl 2): 380.

Barros F, Korzeniowski OM, Sande MA *et al.* (1977). *In vitro* antibiotic susceptibility of salmonellae. *Antimicrob Ag Chemother* **11**: 1071.

Barry AL, Schoenknect FD, Shadomy S *et al.* (1979). *In-vitro* activities of cefamandole and cephalothin against 1881 clinical isolates. *Amer J Clin Path* **72**: 858.

Barson WJ, Miller MA, Marcon MJ *et al.* (1985). Cefuroxime therapy for bacteremic soft-tissue infections in children. *Amer J Dis Child* **139**: 1141.

Bartlett JG, Louie TJ, Gorbach SL, Onderdonk AB (1981). Therapeutic efficacy of 29 antimicrobial regimens in experimental intraabdominal sepsis. *Rev Infect Dis* **3**: 535.

Bartlett JG, Marien GJR, Dezfulilan M, Joiner KA (1983). Relative efficacy of beta-lactam antimicrobial agents in two animal models of infections involving *Bacteroides fragilis*. *Rev Infect Dis* **5** (Suppl 2): 338.

Barza M (1978). The nephrotoxicity of cephalosporins: an overview. *J Infect Dis* **137** (Suppl): 60.

Barza M, Melethil S, Berger S, Ernst EC (1976). Comparative pharmacokinetics of cefamandole, cephapirin and cephalothin in healthy subjects and effect of repeated dosing. *Antimicrob Ag Chemother* **10**: 421.

Barza M, Pinn V, Tanguay P, Murray T (1978). Nephrotoxicity of newer cephalosporins and aminoglycosides alone and in combination in a rat model. *J Antimicrob Chemother* **4** (Suppl): 59.

Barza M, Giuliano M, Jacobus NV, Gorbach SL (1987). Effect of broad-spectrum parenteral antibiotics on 'colonization resistance' of intestinal microflora of humans. *Antimicrob Ag Chemother* **31**: 723.

Bawdon RE, Hemsell DL, Gus SP (1982). Comparison of cefoperazone and cefoxitin concentrations in serum and pelvic tissue of abdominal hysterectomy patients. *Antimicrob Ag Chemother* **22**: 999.

Benson JM, Boudinot FD, Pennell AT *et al.* (1993). *In vitro* protein binding of cefonicid and cefuroxime in adult and neonatal sera. *Antimicrob Ag Chemother* **37**: 1343.

Berg SW, Kilpatrick ME, Harrison WO, McCutchan JA (1979). Cefoxitin as a single-dose treatment for urethritis caused by penicillinase-producing *Neisseria gonorrhoeae*. *New Engl J Med* **301**: 509.

Bergeron MG, Claveau S, Simard P (1981). Limited *in vitro* activity of cefamandole against 100 beta-lactamase and non-beta-lactamase-producing *Haemophilus influenzae* strains: comparison of moxalactam chloramphenicol and ampicillin. *Antimicrob Ag Chemother* **19**: 101.

Bint AJ, Bullock DW, Speller DCE *et al.* (1979). Cefuroxime therapy for urinary tract infections caused by a multi-resistant, epidemic *Klebsiella aerogenes*. *J Antimicrob Chemother* **5**: 189.

Bodey GP, Weaver S (1976). *In vitro* studies of cefamandole. *Antimicrob Ag Chemother* **9**: 452.

Bowie WR (1982). Lack of *in vitro* activity of cefoxitin, cefamandole, cefuroxime and piperacillin against *Chlamydia trachomatis*. *Antimicrob Ag Chemother* **21**: 339.

Brook I (1989). Inoculum effect. *Rev Infect Dis* **11**: 361.

Brorson J-E, Larsson P (1982). Increase in resistance to cefuroxime of *Escherichia coli* isolated from blood. *Scand J Infect Dis* **14**: 313.

Brown AE, Quesada O, Armstrong D (1982). Minimal nephrotoxicity with cephalosporin-aminoglycoside combinations in patients with neoplastic disease. *Antimicrob Ag Chemother* **21**: 592.

Brown RB, Klar J, Lemeshow S *et al.* (1986). Enhanced bleeding with cefoxitin or moxalactam Statistical analysis within a defined population of 1493 patients. *Arch Intern Med* **146**: 2159.

Brown W, Fallon RJ (1980). The sensitivity of strains of *N meningitidis* to cefuroxime, rifampicin and minocycline. *J Antimicrob Chemother* **6**: 91.

Brumfitt W, Kosmidis J, Hamilton-Miller JMT, Gilchrist JNG (1974). Cefoxitin and cephalothin: antimicrobial activity, human pharmacokinetics, and toxicology. *Antimicrob Ag Chemother* **6**: 290.

Buening MK, Wold JS (1982). Ethanol-moxalactam interactions *in vivo*. *Rev Infect Dis* **4** (Suppl): 555.

Bulger RR, Washington JA II (1980). Effect of inoculum size and beta-lactamase production on *in vitro* activity of new cephalosporins against *Haemophilus* species. *Antimicrob Ag Chemother* **17**: 393.

Bullen BR, Ramsden CH, Kester RC (1981). Cefuroxime levels attained in tissues and wound exudates from severely ischaemic limbs. *J Antimicrob Chemother* **7**: 163.

Bundtzen RW, Toothaker RD, Nielson OS *et al.* (1981). Pharmacokinetics of cefuroxime in normal and impaired renal function: comparison of high-pressure liquid chromatography and microbiological assays. *Antimicrob Ag Chemother* **19**: 443.

Burns GP, Stein TA, Cohen M (1989). Biliary and pancreatic excretion of cefamandole. *Antimicrob Ag Chemother* **33**: 977.

Carson JWK, Watters K, Taylor MRH, Keane CT (1987). Clinical trial of cefuroxime axetil in children. *J Antimicrob Chemother* **19**: 109.

Casal M, Rodriguez F (1982). *In vitro* susceptibility of *Mycobacterium fortuitum* and *Mycobacterium chelonei* to cefoxitin. *Tubercle* **63**: 125.

CDC (Centers for Disease Control) (1993). Sexually transmitted diseases treatment guidelines. *MMWR* **42** (No RR-14): 56.

Chapman SW, Steigbigel RT (1983). Staphylococcal beta-lactamase and efficacy of beta-lactam antibiotics: *in vitro* and *in vivo* evaluation. *J Infect Dis* **147**: 1078.

Chartrand SA, Marks MI, Roberts R *et al.* (1981). Development of *Haemophilus influenzae* meningitis in patients treated with cefamandole. *J Pediatr* **98**: 1003.

Chau PY, Ng WS, Ling J, Arnold K (1981). Plasmid-mediated partial cross-resistance between ampicillin, mecillinam and cefamandole in *Salmonella johannesburg* and *Salmonella typhimurium*. *J Antimicrob Chemother* **7**: 245.

Chitwarakorn A, Ariyarit C, Panikabutra K *et al.* (1985). Treating gonococcal infections resistant to penicillin in Bangkok: comparison of cefuroxime and spectinomycin. *Genitourin Med* **61**: 306.

Chow AW, Bednorz D (1978). Comparative *in vitro* activity of newer cephalosporins against anaerobic bacteria. *Antimicrob Ag Chemother* **14**: 668.

Clarke CW, Hannant CA, May CS, Rawal BD (1980). Cefamandole in the treatment of lower respiratory tract infections. *J Antimicrob Chemother* **6**: 723.

Cooper TJ, Ladusans E, Williams PEO *et al.* (1985). A comparison of oral cefuroxime axetil and oral amoxycillin in lower respiratory tract infections. *J Antimicrob Chemother* **16**: 373.

Counts GW (1988). Cefoxitin: its role in treatment and prophylaxis in obstetric and gynecologic infections. *Rev Infect Dis* **10**: 76.

Cowling P, Case CP, MacGowan AP *et al.* (1992). Cefuroxime axetil in the sick elderly patient. *J Antimicrob Chemother* **29**: 350.

Cuchural GJ Jr, Tally FP, Jacobus NV *et al.* (1983). Cefoxitin inactivation by *Bacteroides fragilis*. *Antimicrob Ag Chemother* **24**: 936.

Cuchural GJ,Jr, Tally FP, Storey JR, Malamy MH (1986). Transfer of beta-lactamase-associated cefoxitin resistance in *Bacteroides fragilis*. *Antimicrob Ag Chemother* **29**: 918.

Cuchural GJ,Jr, Tally FP, Jacobus NV *et al.* (1990). Comparative activities of newer beta-lactam agents against members of the *Bacteroides fragilis* group. *Antimicrob Ag Chemother* **34**: 479.

Custer GM, Briggs BR, Smith RE (1979). Effect of cefamandole nafate on blood coagulation and platelet function. *Antimicrob Ag Chemother* **16**: 869.

Cynamon MH, Palmer GS (1981). *In vitro* susceptibility of *Nocardia asteroides* to N-formimidoyl thienamycin and several cephalosporins. *Antimicrob Ag Chemother* **20**: 841.

Cynamon MH, Palmer GS (1982). *In vitro* susceptibility of *Mycobacterium fortuitum* to N-formimidoyl thienamycin and several cephamycins. *Antimicrob Ag Chemother* **22**: 1079.

Czerwinski AW, Pederson JA (1979). Pharmacokinetics of cefamandole in patients with renal impairment. *Antimicrob Ag Chemother* **15**: 161.

Dan M, Marien GJR, Sand C (1983). Susceptibility of group B streptococci to cloxacillin, methicillin and cefamandole. *J Antimicrob Chemother* **11**: 93.

Darland G, Birnbaum J (1977). Cefoxitin resistance to β-lactamase: a major factor for susceptibility of *Bacteroides fragilis* to the antibiotic. *Antimicrob Ag Chemother* **11**: 725.

Daschner FD, Frank U (1987). Antimicrobial drugs in human cardiac valves and endocarditic lesions. *J Antimicrob Chemother* **20**: 776.

Daschner FD, Metz B, Spillner G *et al.* (1980). Concentrations of cefamandole and cefsulodin in serum, heart valves, subcutaneous tissue and muscle of patients undergoing open-heart surgery. *J Infect Dis* **142**: 290.

De Carvalho EM, Martinelli R, De Oliveira MMG, Rocha H (1982). Cefamandole treatment of salmonella bacteremia. *Antimicrob Ag Chemother* **21**: 334.

Delgado DG, Brau CJ, Cobbs CG, Dismukes WE (1979). Clinical and laboratory evaluation of cefamandole in the therapy of *Haemophilus* spp bronchopulmonary infections. *Antimicrob Ag Chemother* **15**: 807.

Dellinger EP (1991). Antibiotic prophylaxis in trauma: penetrating abdominal injuries and open fractures. *Rev Infect Dis* **13** (Suppl 10): 847.

De Los A, Del Rio M, Chrane DF *et al.* (1982). Pharmacokinetics of cefuroxime in infants and children with bacterial meningitis. *Antimicrob Ag Chemother* **22**: 990.

De Torres OH (1983). Hemolytic anemia and pancytopenia induced by cefoxitin. *Drug Intell Clin Pharm* **17**: 816.

Dornbusch K, Nord CE, Olsson-Liljeqvist B (1979). Antibiotic susceptibility of anaerobic bacteria with special reference to *Bacteroides fragilis*. *Scand J Infect Dis* (Suppl 19): 17.

Dornbusch K, Olsson-Liljeqvist B, Nord CE (1980). Antibacterial activity of new beta-lactam antibiotics on cefoxitin-resistant strains of *Bacteroides fragilis*. *J Antimicrob Chemother* **6**: 207.

Edwards MS, Baker CJ, Butler KM *et al.* (1989). Penetration of cefuroxime into ventricular fluid in cerebrospinal fluid shunt infections. *Antimicrob Ag Chemother* **33**: 1108.

Eickhoff TC, Ehret JM (1976). *In vitro* comparison of cefoxitin, cefamandole, cephalexin and cephalothin. *Antimicrob Ag Chemother* **9**: 994.

Ekwall E, Homgren EB, Lundbergh P *et al.* (1979). Cefamandole nafate: an evaluation of antibacterial activity, serum levels, clinical effect, and incidence of side reactions in 58 patients. *Scand J Infect Dis* **11**: 135.

Eley A, Greenwood D (1986). Beta-lactamases of type culture strains of the *Bacteroides fragilis* group and of strains that hydrolyse cefoxitin, latamoxef and imipenem. *J Med Microbiol* **21**: 49.

Emmerson AM (1988). Cefuroxime axetil. *J Antimicrob Chemother* **22**: 101.

Eng RHK, Corrado ML, Tillotson J *et al.* (1985). Cefamandole for the therapy of serious *Staphylococcus aureus* infections. *J Antimicrob Chemother* **16**: 663.

Eykyn S, Jenkins C, King A, Phillips I (1976). Antibacterial activity of cefuroxime, a new cephalosporin antibiotic, compared with that of cephaloridine, cephalothin and cefamandole. *Antimicrob Ag Chemother* **9**: 690.

Feldman WE, Moffitt S, Sprow N (1980). Clinical and pharmacokinetic evaluation of parenteral cefoxitin in infants and children. *Antimicrob Ag Chemother* **17**: 669.

Feldman WE, Moffitt S, Manning NS (1982). Penetration of cefoxitin into cerebrospinal fluid of infants and children with bacterial meningitis. *Antimicrob Ag Chemother* **21**: 468.

Finch R (1986). Beta-lactam antibiotics and mycobacteria. *J Antimicrob Chemother* **18**: 6.

Findell CM, Sherris JC (1976). Susceptibility of *Enterobacter* to cefamandole: evidence for a high mutation rate to resistance. *Antimicrob Ag Chemother* **9**: 970.

Fong IW, Engelking ER, Kirby WMM (1976a). Relative inactivation by *Staphylococcus aureus* of eight cephalosporin antibiotics. *Antimicrob Ag Chemother* **9**: 939.

Fong IW, Ralph ED, Engelking ER, Kirby WMM (1976b). Clinical pharmacology of cefamandole as compared with cephalothin. *Antimicrob Ag Chemother* **9**: 65.

Foord RD (1976). Cefuroxime: human pharmacokinetics. *Antimicrob Ag Chemother* **9**: 741.

Fox AR, Phillips I (1987). The antibiotic sensitivity of *Bacteroides fragilis* group in the United Kingdom. *J Antimicrob Chemother* **20**: 477.

Fu KP, Neu HC (1978). A comparative study of the activity of cefamandole

and other cephalosporins and analysis of the β-lactamase stability and synergy of cefamandole with aminoglycosides. *J Infect Dis* **137** (Suppl): 38.

Gaspar MC, Soriano F (1981). Susceptibility of *Yersinia enterocolitica* to eight beta-lactam antibiotics and clavulanic acid. *J Antimicrob Chemother* **8**: 161.

Geddes AM, Schnurr LP, Ball AP *et al.* (1977). Cefoxitin: a hospital study. *Brit Med J* **1**: 1126.

Geddes AM, McGhie D, Ball AP, Gould I (1978). Studies with cefuroxime and cefoxitin. *Scand J Infect Dis* (Suppl 13): 78.

Gehanno P, Lenoir G, Berche P (1995). *In vivo* correlates for *Streptococcus pneumoniae* penicillin resistance in acute otitis media. *Antimicrob Ag Chemother* **39**: 271.

Gentry LO (1992). Therapy with newer oral beta-lactam and quinolone agents for infections of the skin structures: a review. *Clin Infect Dis* **14**: 285.

George WL, Lewis RP, Meyer RD (1978). Susceptibility of cephalothin-resistant Gram-negative bacilli to piperacillin, cefuroxime and other selected antibiotics. *Antimicrob Ag Chemother* **13**: 484.

Gerding DN, Kozak AJ, Peterson LR, Hall WH (1980). Failure of single doses of cefazolin and cefamandole to penetrate experimental chronic *Escherichia coli* abdominal abscesses. *Antimicrob Ag Chemother* **17**: 1023.

Gillett AP, Wise R (1978). Penetration of four cephalosporins into tissue fluid in man. *Lancet* **i**: 962.

Ginsburg CM, McCracken GH Jr, Petruska M, Olson K (1985). Pharmacokinetics and bactericidal activity of cefuroxime axetil. *Antimicrob Ag Chemother* **28**: 504.

Goering RV, Sanders CC, Sanders WE Jr (1982). Antagonism of carbenicillin and cefamandole by cefoxitin in treatment of experimental infections in mice. *Antimicrob Ag Chemother* **21**: 963.

Goldstein EJC, Citron DM (1988). Comparative activities of cefuroxime, amoxicillin-clavulanic acid, ciprofloxacin, enoxacin, and ofloxacin against aerobic and anaerobic bacteria isolated from bite wounds. *Antimicrob Ag Chemother* **32**: 1143.

Goldstein EJC, Kwok YY, Sutter VL (1981). Absence of tolerance to cefoxitin in anaerobic bacteria. *Antimicrob Ag Chemother* **20**: 146,.

Goldstein EJC, Citron DM, Cherubin CE (1991a). Comparison of the inoculum effects of members of the family Enterobacteriaceae on cefoxitin and other cephalosporins, beta-lactamase inhibitor combinations, and the penicillin-derived components of these combinations. *Antimicrob Ag Chemother* **35**: 560.

Goldstein EJC, Citron DM, Cherubin CE (1991b). Comparison of the inoculum effect of cefoxitin and other cephalosporins and of beta-lactamase inhibitors and their penicillin-derived components on the *Bacteroides fragilis group*. *Antimicrob Ag Chemother* **35**: 1868.

Gooch WM III, McLinn SE, Aronovitz GH *et al.* (1993). Efficacy of cefuroxime axetil suspension compared with that of penicillin V suspension in children with Group a streptococcal pharyngitis. *Antimicrob Ag Chemother* **37**: 159.

Goodwin CS, Raftery EB, Goldberg AD *et al.* (1974). Effects of rate of infusion and probenecid on serum levels, renal excretion, and tolerance of intravenous doses of cefoxitin in humans: comparison with cephalothin. *Antimicrob Ag Chemother* **6**: 338.

Goodwin CS, Dash CH, Hill JP, Goldberg AD (1977). Cefuroxime: pharmacokinetics after a short infusion, and *in vitro* activity against hospital pathogens. *J Antimicrob Chemother* **3**: 253.

Gootz TD, Sanders CC, Goering RV (1982). Resistance to cefamandole: derepression of beta-lactamases by cefoxitin and mutation in *Enterobacter cloacae*. *J Infect Dis* **146**: 34.

Gorbach SL (1982). Prophylactic antibiotics – indications in surgical patients. *Scand J Infect Dis* (Suppl 36): 134.

Gorbach SL, McGowan K (1981). Comparative clinical trials in treatment of intra-abdominal sepsis. *J Antimicrob Chemother* **8** (Suppl D): 95.

Gottlieb A, Mills J (1986). Cefuroxime axetil for treatment of uncomplicated gonorrhea. *Antimicrob Ag Chemother* **30**: 333.

Graudal C, Bollerup AC, Lange K *et al.* (1985). The outcome of single-dose cefuroxime treatment in patients with pharyngeal gonorrhea. *Sex Transm Dis* **12**: 49.

Greaves WL, Kreeft JH, Ogilview RI, Richards GK (1981). Cefoxitin disposition during peritoneal dialysis. *Antimicrob Ag Chemother* **19**: 253.

Greaves WL, Kraus SJ, McCormack WM *et al.* (1983). Cefoxitin vs penicillin in the treatment of uncomplicated gonorrhea. *Sex Transm Dis* **10**: 53.

Greenwood D (1977). Enterobacterial β-lactamases. *J Antimicrob Chemother* **3**: 7.

Greenwood D, Pearson NJ, O'Grady F (1976). Cefuroxime: a new cephalosporin antibiotic with enhanced stability to enterobacterial β-lactamases. *J Antimicrob Chemother* **2**: 337.

Griffith RS, Black HR, Brier GL, Wolny JD (1976). Cefamandole: *in vitro* and clinical pharmacokinetics. *Antimicrob Ag Chemother* **10**: 814.

Griffith RS, Black HR, Brier GL, Wolny JD (1977). Effect of probenecid on the blood levels and urinary excretion of cefamandole. *Antimicrob Ag Chemother* **11**: 809.

Gutmann L, Goldstein FW, Kitzis MD *et al.* (1983). Susceptibility of *Nocardia asteroides* to 46 antibiotics including 22 beta-lactams. *Antimicrob Ag Chemother* **23**: 248.

Hall WH, Schierl EA, Maccani JE (1979). Comparative susceptibility of penicillinase-positive and -negative *Neisseria gonorrhoeae* to 30 antibiotics. *Antimicrob Ag Chemother* **15**: 562.

Hamilton-Miller JMT (1974). Comparative activity of ampicillin and seven cephalosporins against Group D streptococci. *J Clin Path* **27**: 828.

Hansbrough JF, Clark JE (1982). Concentrations of cefoxitin in gallbladder bile of cholecystectomy patients. *Antimicrob Ag Chemother* **22**: 709.

Harding SM, Williams PEO, Ayrton J (1984). Pharmacology of cefuroxime as the 1-acetoxyethyl ester in volunteers. *Antimicrob Ag Chemother* **25**: 78.

Hart CA, Desmond AD, Percival A (1981). Treatment of gentamicin-resistant Klebsiella urinary tract infections with cephradine, augmentin, cefuroxime and amikacin. *J Antimicrob Chemother* **8**: 231.

Havard CWH, Fernando A, Bannister B *et al.* (1981). Clinical and pharmacokinetic comparison of cefuroxime sodium and cefuroxime lysine in the treatment of lower respiratory tract infections. *J Antimicrob Chemother* **8**: 401.

Hedström SÅ, Lindgren L, Nilsson-Ehle I (1984). Cefuroxime in acute septic arthritis. *Scand J Infect Dis* **16**: 79.

Heseltine PNR, Busch DF, Meyer RD, Finegold SM (1977). Cefoxitin: clinical evaluation in thirty-eight patients. *Antimicrob Ag Chemother* **11**: 427.

Hill GB, Ayers OM, Everett BQ (1991). Susceptibilities of anaerobic Gram-negative bacilli to thirteen antimicrobials and beta-lactamase inhibitor combinations. *J Antimicrob Chemother* **28**: 855.

Hirschman SZ, Meyers BR, Miller A (1977). Antimicrobial activity of cefamandole against *Salmonella typhi*. *Antimicrob Ag Chemother* **11**: 369.

Hodgson TG (1981). Bad taste from cefamandole. *Drug Intell Clin Pharm* **15**: 100.

Hoeprich PD, Huston AC (1976). Induction of resistance in *Staphylococcus aureus* and *Klebsiella pneumoniae* by exposure to cephalothin and cefoxitin. *J Infect Dis* **133**: 681.

Hoffstedt B, Ode B, Walder M *et al.* (1980). Penetration of cefuroxime and doxycycline into the pleural fluid. *J Antimicrob Chemother* **6**: 153.

Hoyme U, Madsen PO (1978). Cefamandole and cefazolin in the therapy of complicated urinary tract infections. *J Infect Dis* **137** (Suppl): 100.

Hugo H, Dornbusch K, Sterner G (1980). Cefuroxime in soft tissue infections and septicaemia. *Scand J Infect Dis* **12**: 227.

Humbert G, Fillastre JP, Leroy A *et al.* (1979). Pharmacokinetics of cefoxitin in normal subjects and in patients with renal insufficiency. *Rev Infect Dis* **1**: 118.

Humbert G, Leroy A, Rogez J-P, Cherubin C (1980). Cefoxitin concentrations in the cerebrospinal fluids of patients with meningitis. *Antimicrob Ag Chemother* **17**: 675.

Iravani A, Richard GA (1989). Single-dose cefuroxime axetil versus multiple-dose cefaclor in the treatment of acute urinary tract infections. *Antimicrob Ag Chemother* **33**: 1212.

Jackson RT, Thomas FE, Alford RH (1977). Cefoxitin activity against multiple antibiotic-resistant *Klebsiella pneumoniae in vitro*. *Antimicrob Ag Chemother* **11**: 84.

Jacobs RF, Brown WD, Chartrand S *et al.* (1992). Evaluation of cefuroxime axetil and cefadroxil suspensions for treatment of pediatric skin infections. *Antimicrob Ag Chemother* **36**: 1614.

Jacobson JA, Santos JI, Palmer WM (1979). Clinical and bacteriological evaluation of cefoxitin therapy in children. *Antimicrob Ag Chemother* **16**: 183.

Jacoby GA, Archer GL (1991). New mechanisms of bacterial resistance to antimicrobial agents. *New Engl J Med* **324**: 601.

James NC, Donn KH, Collins JJ *et al.* (1991). Pharmacokinetics of cefuroxime axetil and cefaclor: relationship of concentrations in serum to MICs for common respiratory pathogens. *Antimicrob Ag Chemother* **35**: 1860.

Jenkins SG, Birk RJ, Zabransky RJ (1982). Differences in susceptibilities of species of the *Bacteroides fragilis* group to several beta-lactam antiobiotics; indole production as an indicator of resistance. *Antimicrob Ag Chemother* **22**: 628.

Johnson RC, Kodner CB, Jurkovich PJ, Collins JJ (1990). Comparative *in vitro* and *in vivo* susceptibilities of the Lyme disease spirochete *Borrelia burgdorferi* to cefuroxime and other antimicrobial agents. *Antimicrob Ag Chemother* **34**: 2133.

Joiner K, Lowe B, Dzink J, Bartlett JG (1982). Comparative efficacy of 10 antimicrobial agents in experimental infections with *Bacteroides fragilis*. *J Infect Dis* **145**: 561.

Jones RN, Fuchs PC, Gavan TL *et al.* (1977). Cefuroxime, a new parenteral cephalosporin: collaborative *in vitro* susceptibility comparison with cephalothin against 5877 clinical bacterial isolates. *Antimicrob Ag Chemother* **12**: 47.

Kammer RB, Preston DA, Turner JR, Hawley LC (1975). Rapid detection of ampicillin-resistant *Haemophilus influenzae* and their susceptibility to sixteen antibiotics. *Antimicrob Ag Chemother* **8**: 91.

Kampf D, Schurig R, Korsukewitz I, Brückner O (1981). Cefoxitin pharmacokinetics: relation to three different renal clearance studies in patients with various degrees of renal insufficiency. *Antimicrob Ag Chemother* **20**: 741.

Kelsey MC, Emmerson AM, Drabu Y (1982). Flavobacterium meningo-septicum ventriculitis: *in vivo* and *in vitro* results with the combinations rifampicin-erythromycin and mezlocillin-cefoxitin. *Eur J Clin Microbiol* **1**: 138.

Khan MY, Siddiqui Y, Simpson ML, Gruninger RP (1981). Comparative *in vitro* activity of cefmenoxime, cefotaxime, cefuroxime, cefoxitin, and penicillin against *Neisseria gonorrhoeae*. *Antimicrob Ag Chemother* **20**: 681.

Klastersky J, Coppens L, Mombelli G (1979). Anaerobic infection in cancer patients: comparative evaluation of clindamycin and cefoxitin. *Antimicrob Ag Chemother* **16**: 366.

Konishi K, Suzuki H, Hayashi M, Saruta T (1993). Pharmacokinetics of cefuroxime axetil in patients with normal and impaired renal function. *J Antimicrob Chemother* **31**: 413.

Kosmidis J, Hamilton-Miller JMT, Gilchrist JNG *et al.* (1973). Cefoxitin, a new semi-synthetic cephamycin: an *in vitro* and *in vivo* comparison with cephalothin. *Brit Med J* **4**: 653.

Kuck NA, Testa RT, Forbes M (1981). *In vitro* and *in vivo* antibacterial effects of combinations of beta-lactam antibiotics. *Antimicrob Ag Chemother* **19**: 634.

Lang CC, Moreland TA, Davey PG (1990). Bioavailability of cefuroxime axetil: comparison of standard and abbreviated methods. *J Antimicrob Chemother* **25**: 645.

Lau WY, Fan ST, Chu KW *et al.* (1986). Cefoxitin versus gentamicin and metronidazole in prevention of post-appendicectomy sepsis: a randomized, prospective trial. *J Antimicrob Chemother* **18**: 613.

Lee K, Jang IH, Kim YJ, Chang Y (1992). *In vitro* susceptibilities of *Bacteroides fragilis* Group to 14 antimicrobial agents in Korea. *Antimicrob Ag Chemother* **36**: 195.

Le Frock JL, Schell RF, Carr BB *et al.* (1982). Cefoxitin therapy in aerobic, anaerobic, and mixed aerobic-anaerobic infections. *Drug Intell Clin Pharm* **16**: 306.

Leigh DA (1986). Serum and bone concentrations of cefuroxime in patients undergoing knee arthroplasty. *J Antimicrob Chemother* **18**: 609.

Leigh DA (1989). Determination of serum and bone concentrations of cephradine and cefuroxime by HPLC in patients undergoing hip and knee joint replacement surgery. *J Antimicrob Chemother* **23**: 877.

Leigh DA, Joy GE, Tait S *et al.* (1989). Treatment of acute uncomplicated urinary tract infections with single daily doses of cefuroxime axetil. *J Antimicrob Chemother* **23**: 267.

Leigh DA, Walsh B, Leung A *et al.* (1990). The effect of cefuroxime axetil on the faecal flora of healthy volunteers. *J Antimicrob Chemother* **26**: 261.

Levine LR, McCain E (1978a). Cefamandole in the treatment of infections due to Enterobacter and indole-positive *Proteus*. *J Infect Dis* **137** (Suppl): 125.

Levine LR, McCain E (1978b). Clinical experience with cefamandole for treatment of serious bone and joint infections. *J Infect Dis* **137** (Suppl): 119.

Lindahl F, Kjaer TB, Thomsen VF (1980). Excretion of cefamandole in the bile. *Scand J Infect Dis* (Suppl 25): 58.

Lossick JG, Thompson SE, Smeltzer MP (1982). Comparison of cefuroxime and penicillin in the treatment of uncomplicated gonorrhea. *Antimicrob Ag Chemother* **22**: 409.

Luger SW, Paparone P, Wormser GP *et al.* (1995). Comparison of cefuroxime axetil and doxycycline in treatment of patients with early Lyme disease associated with erythema migrans. *Antimicrob Ag Chemother* **39**: 661.

Lunke RJ, Fitzgerald RH Jr, Washington JA II (1981). Pharmacokinetics of cefamandole in osseous tissue. *Antimicrob Ag Chemother* **19**: 851.

Malouin F, Fijalkowski C, Lamothe F, Lacroix J-M (1986). Inactivation of cefoxitin and moxalactam by *Bacteroides bivius* beta-lactamase. *Antimicrob Ag Chemother* **30**: 749.

Manzella JP, Clark JK (1983). Effects of moxalactam and cefuroxime on mitogen-stimulated human mononuclear leukocytes. *Antimicrob Ag Chemother* **23**: 360.

Marks MI (1981). Editorial Antibiotic therapy of serious *Haemophilus* infections – a continuing problem. *J Pediatr* **98**: 910.

Marks WA, Stutman HR, Marks MI *et al.* (1986). Cefuroxime versus ampicillin plus chloramphenicol in childhood bacterial meningitis: a multicenter randomized controlled trial. *J Pediatrics* **109**: 123.

Martini A, Xerri L (1982). Study of diffusion of cefuroxime into middle ear effusions of patients with chronic purulent otitis media. *J Antimicrob Chemother* **10**: 197.

McCloskey RV (1977). Results of a clinical trial of cefoxitin, a new cephamycin antibiotic. *Antimicrob Ag Chemother* **12**: 636.

McCracken GH Jr, Nelson JD, Kaplan SL *et al.* (1987). Consensus report Antimicrobial therapy for bacterial meningitis in infants and children. *Pediatr Infect Dis J* **6**: 501.

McLinn SE, Moskal M, Goldfarb J *et al.* (1994). Comparison of cefuroxime axetil and amoxicillin-clavulanate suspensions in treatment of acute otitis media with effusion in childen. *Antimicrob Ag Chemother* **38**: 315.

McNulty CAM, Dent J, Wise R (1985). Susceptibility of clinical isolates of *Campylobacter pyloridis* to 11 antimicrobial agents. *Antimicrob Ag Chemother* **28**: 837.

Mehtar S (1980). The *in vitro* efficacy of cefuroxime against Group B streptococci. *J Antimicrob Chemother* **6**: 556.

Mehtar S, Parr JH, Morgan DJR (1982). A comparison of cefuroxime and cotrimoxazole in severe respiratory tract infections. *J Antimicrob Chemother* **9**: 479.

Mellin H-E, Welling PG, Madsen PO (1977). Pharmacokinetics of cefamandole in patients with normal and impaired renal function. *Antimicrob Ag Chemother* **11**: 262.

Mendelman PM, Chaffin DO, Krilov LR *et al.* (1990). Cefuroxime treatment failure of nontypable *Haemophilus influenzae* meningitis associated with alteration of penicillin-binding proteins. *J Infect Dis* **162**: 1118.

Meyer KS, Urban C, Eagan JA *et al.* (1993). Nosocomial outbreak of *Klebsiella* infection resistant to late-generation cephalosporins. *Ann Intern Med* **119**: 353.

Meyers BR, Hirschman SZ (1978). Antibacterial activity of cefamandole *in vitro*. *J Infect Dis* **137** (Suppl): 25.

Meyers BR, Ribner B, Yancovitz S, Hirschman SZ (1976). Pharmacological studies with cefamandole in human volunteers. *Antimicrob Ag Chemother* **9**: 140.

Miller AK, Celozzi E, Pelak BA *et al.* (1972). Cephamycins, a new family of β-lactam antibiotics III *In vitro* studies. *Antimicrob Ag Chemother* **2**: 281.

Miller AK, Celozzi E, Kong Y *et al.* (1974). Cefoxitin, a semisynthetic cephamycin antibiotic: *in vivo* evaluation. *Antimicrob Ag Chemother* **5**: 33.

Miller AK, Celozzi E, Pelak BA *et al.* (1980). *In vivo* inoculum effect and resistance selection with cefamandole and cefoxitin against *Enterobacter cloacae* in mice. *J Antimicrob Chemother* **6**: 804.

Miller MA, Finan M, Yousuf M (1983). *In-vitro* antagonism by N-formimidoyl thienamycin and cefoxitin of second and third generation cephalosporins in *Aeromonas hydrophila* and *Serratia marcescens*. *J Antimicrob Chemother* **11**: 311.

Minor MR, Sande MA, Dilworth JA, Mandell GL (1976). Cefamandole treatment of pulmonary infection caused by Gram-negative rods. *J Antimicrob Chemother* **2**: 49.

Moellering RC Jr, Dray M, Kunz LJ (1974). Susceptibility of clinical isolates of bacteria to cefoxitin and cephalothin. *Antimicrob Ag Chemother* **6**: 320.

Moritz VA, Carson PBD (1986). Cefoxitin sensitivity as a marker for inducible beta-lactamases. *J Med Microbiol* **21**: 203.

Morris DL, Young D, Burdon DW, Keighley MRB (1984). Prospective randomized trial of single dose cefuroxime against mezlocillin in elective gastric surgery. *J Hosp Infect* **5**: 200.

Mullany LD, French MA, Nightingale CH *et al.* (1982). Penetration of ceforanide and cefamandole into the right atrial appendage, pericardial fluid, sternum and intercostal muscle of patients undergoing open heart surgery. *Antimicrob Ag Chemother* **21**: 416.

Müller C, Netland A, Dawson AF, Andrew E (1980). The penetration of cefuroxime into the cerebrospinal fluid through inflamed and non-inflamed meninges. *J Antimicrob Chemother* **6**: 279.

Mulligan ME, Citron D, Gabay E *et al.* (1984). Alterations in human fecal flora, including ingrowth of *Clostridium difficile*, related to cefoxitin therapy. *Antimicrob Ag Chemother* **26**: 343.

Murray PR, Granich GG, Krogstad DJ, Niles AC (1983). *In vivo* selection of resistance to multiple cephalosporins by *Enterobacter cloacae*. *J Infect Dis* **147**: 590.

Muytjens HL, Van der Ros-Van de Repe J (1982). Comparative activities of 13 beta-lactam antibiotics. *Antimicrob Ag Chemother* **21**: 925.

Nair SR, Cherubin CE (1978). Use of cefoxitin, new cephalosporin-like antibiotic in the treatment of aerobic and anaerobic infections. *Antimicrob Ag Chemother* **14**: 866.

Nair SR, Cherubin CE, Weinstein M (1979). Penetration of cefoxitin into cerebrospinal fluid and treatment of meningitis caused by Gram-negative bacteria. *Rev Infect Dis* **1**: 134.

Nasu M, Maskell JP, Williams RJ, Williams JD (1981). *In vitro* activity of MK0787 (N-formimidoyl thienamycin) and other beta-lactam compounds against *Bacteroides* spp. *Antimicrob Ag Chemother* **20**: 433.

Nelson JD (1983). Cefuroxime: a cephalosporin with unique applicability to pediatric practice. *Pediatr Infect Dis* **2**: 394.

Netland A, Müller C, Andrew E (1981). Concentration of cefuroxime in cerebrospinal fluid in patients with bacterial meningitis. *Scand J Infect Dis* **13**: 273.

Neu HC (1974a). Cefoxitin, a semisynthetic cephamycin antibiotic: antibacterial spectrum and resistance to hydrolysis by Gram-negative β-lactamases. *Antimicrob Ag Chemother* **6**: 170.

Neu HC (1974b). Cefamandole, a cephalosporin antibiotic with an unusually wide spectrum of activity. *Antimicrob Ag Chemother* **6**: 177.

Neu HC (1979). Comparative studies of cefoxitin and cephalothin: an overview. *Rev Infect Dis* **1**: 144.

Neu HC, Fu KP (1978). Cefuroxime, a β-lactamase-resistant cephalosporin with a broad spectrum of Gram-positive and -negative activity. *Antimicrob Ag Chemother* **13**: 657.

Nichols RL (1983). Empiric antibiotic therapy for intraabdominal infections. *Rev Infect Dis* **5** (Suppl 1): 90.

Nielsen RL, Wolen R, Luft FC, Ozawa T (1979). Hydrolysis of cefamandole nafate in dialysis patients. *Antimicrob Ag Chemother* **16**: 683.

Nooyen SMH, Overbeek BP, de la Riviére AB *et al.* (1994). Prospective randomised comparison of single-dose versus multiple-dose cefuroxime for prophylaxis in coronary artery bypass grafting. *Eur J Clin Microbiol Infect Dis* **13**: 1033.

Nord CE, Olsson-Liljeqvist B (1981). Resistance to beta-lactam antibiotics in *Bacteroides* species. *J Antimicrob Chemother* **8** (Suppl D): 33.

Nord CE, Lindqvist L, Olsson-Liljeqvist B, Tuner K (1985). Beta-lactamases in anaerobic bacteria. *Scand J Infect Dis* (Suppl 46): 57.

Nordbring F, Nord CE (1982). Aspects of antibacterial treatment of anaerobic infections. *Scand J Infect Dis* (Suppl 35): 59.

Norrby R, Brorsson J-E, Seeberg S (1976). Comparative study of the *in vitro* antibacterial activity of cefoxitin, cefuroxime, and cephaloridine. *Antimicrob Ag Chemother* **9**: 506.

Norrby R, Foord RD, Hedlund P (1977). Clinical and pharmacokinetic studies on cefuroxime. *J Antimicrob Chemother* **3**: 355.

O'Callaghan CH (1975). Classification of cephalosporins by their antibacterial activity and pharmacokinetic properties. *J Antimicrob Chemother* **1** (Suppl): 1.

O'Callaghan CH, Sykes RB, Griffiths A, Thornton JE (1976). Cefuroxime, a new cephalosporin antibiotic: activity *in vitro*. *Antimicrob Ag Chemother* **9**: 511.

O'Keefe JP, Tally FP, Barza M, Gorbach SL (1979). Penetration of cephalothin and cefoxitin into experimental infections with *Bacteroides fragilis*. *Rev Infect Dis* **1**: 106.

Olson B, Weinstein RA, Nathan C, Kabins SA (1983). Broad spectrum beta-lactam resistance in *Enterobacter*: emergence during treatment and mechanisms of resistance. *J Antimicrob Chemother* **11**: 299.

Onishi HR, Daoust DR, Zimmerman SB *et al.* (1974). Cefoxitin, a semisynthetic cephamycin antibiotic: resistance to β-lactamase inactivation. *Antimicrob Ag Chemother* **5**: 38.

Ormrod DJ, Miller TE (1981). Evaluation of cefoxitin nephrotoxicity in experimentally induced renal failure. *Antimicrob Ag Chemother* **19**: 18.

Parker AC, Smith CJ (1993). Genetic and biochemical analysis of a novel ambler class A beta-lactamase responsible for cefoxitin resistance in *Bacteroides* species. *Antimicrob Ag Chemother* **37**: 1028.

Patamasucon P, Rettig PJ, Nelson JD (1981). Cefuroxime therapy of gonorrhea and coinfection with *Chlamydia trachomatis* in children. *Pediatrics* **68**: 534.

Peirce TH, Kenny RA, Dawson AF, Hobbs PM (1980). Levels of cefuroxime in bronchial secretion. *Curr Med Res Opin* **6**: 649.

Penner JL, Preston MA (1980). Differences among *Providencia* species in their *in vitro* susceptibilities to five antibiotics. *Antimicrob Ag Chemother* **18**: 868.

Penner JL, Preston MA, Hennessy JN *et al.* (1982). Species differences in susceptibilities of *Proteeae* spp to six cephalosporins and three aminoglycosides. *Antimicrob Ag Chemother* **22**: 218.

Perea EJ, Garcia-Iglesias MC, Ayarra J, Loscertales J (1983). Comparative concentrations of cefoxitin in human lungs and sera. *Antimicrob Ag Chemother* **23**: 323.

Perkins RL, Fass RJ, Warner JF *et al.* (1978). Cefamandole therapy of respiratory tract, skin, and soft tissue infections in 74 patients. *J Infect Dis* **137** (Suppl): 110.

Perkins RL, Slama TG, Fass RJ *et al.* (1979). Therapy of skin, soft tissue, and bone infections with cefoxitin sodium. *Rev Infect Dis* **1**: 165.

Petty BG, Smith CR, Wade JC *et al.* (1978). Double-blind comparison of cefamandole and penicillin in pneumococcal pneumonia. *Antimicrob Ag Chemother* **14**: 13.

Philipson A (1983). The use of antibiotics in pregnancy. *J Antimicrob Chemother* **12**: 101.

Phillips I (1978). The susceptibility of *Neisseria gonorrhoeae* to cefoxitin sodium. *J Antimicrob Chemother* **4** (Suppl B): 61.

Phillips I, Shannon K (1978). The activity of cephalosporins on beta-lactamase-producing *Neisseria gonorrhoeae*. *Scand J Infect Dis* (Suppl 13): 23.

Phillips I, King A, Warren C *et al.* (1976). The activity of penicillin and eight cephalosporins of *Neisseria gonorrhoeae*. *J Antimicrob Chemother* **2**: 31.

Piddock LJV, Wise R (1987). Cefoxitin resistance in *Bacteroides* species: evidence indicating two mechanisms causing decreased susceptibility. *J Antimicrob Chemother* **19**: 161.

Piot P, Van Dyck E, Colaert J *et al.* (1979). Antibiotic susceptibility of *Neisseria gonorrhoeae* strains from Europe and Africa. *Antimicrob Ag Chemother* **15**: 535.

Pollock HM, Holt J, Murray C (1983). Comparison of susceptibilities of anaerobic bacteria to cefmenoxime, ceftriaxone and other antimicrobial compounds. *Antimicrob Ag Chemother* **23**: 780.

Powell DA, James NC, Ossi MJ *et al.* (1991). Pharmacokinetics of cefuroxime axetil suspension in infants and children. *Antimicrob Ag Chemother* **35**: 2042.

Raad II, Vartivarian S, Khan A, Bodey GP (1991). Catheter-related infections caused by the *Mycobacterium fortuitum* complex: 15 cases and review. *Rev Infect Dis* **13**: 1120.

Rashtchian A, Dubes GR, Booth SJ (1982). Transferable resistance to cefoxitin in *Bacteroides thetaiotaomicron*. *Antimicrob Ag Chemother* **22**: 701.

Ratzan KR, Baker HB, Lauredo I (1978). Excretion of cefamandole, cefazolin and cephalothin into T-tube bile. *Antimicrob Ag Chemother* **13**: 985.

Renneberg J, Christensen OM, Thomsen NOB, Tørholm C (1993). Cefuroxime concentrations in serum, joint fluid and bone in elderly patients undergoing arthoplasty after administration of cefuroxime axetil. *J Antimicrob Chemother* **32**: 751.

Report from a Swedish Study Group (1982). Cefuroxime versus ampicillin and chloramphenicol for the treatment of bacterial meningitis. *Lancet* **i**: 295.

Report of a WHO Scientific Group (1978). *Neisseria gonorrhoeae* and gonococcal infections. *Wld Hlth Org Techn Rep Ser* **616**: 130.

Ridgway E, Stewart K, Rai G *et al.* (1991). The pharmacokinetics of cefuroxime axetil in the sick elderly patient. *J Antimicrob Chemother* **27**: 663.

Rodriguez WJ, Ross S, Khan WN, Goldenberg R (1978). Clinical and laboratory evaluation of cefamandole in infants and children. *J Infect Dis* **137** (Suppl): 150.

Rosene K, Eschenbach DA, Tompkins LS *et al.* (1986). Polymicrobial early postpartum endometritis with facultative and anaerobic bacteria, genital Mycoplasmas and *Chlamydia trachomatis*: treatment with piperacillin or cefoxitin. *J Infect Dis* **153**: 1028.

Saah AJ, Drusano GL, Warren JW *et al.* (1981). Cefoxitin-resistant facultative or aerobic Gram-negative bacilli in infections associated with the gastrointestinal tract. *Ann Intern Med* **94**: 487.

Sabath LD (1989). Reappraisal of the antistaphylococcal activities of first generation (narrow spectrum) and second-generation (expanded spectrum) cephalosporins. *Antimicrob Ag Chemother* **33**: 407.

Sanders CC (1983). Novel resistance selected by the new expanded-spectrum cephalosporins: a concern. *J Infect Dis* **147**: 585.

Sanders CC, Sanders WE Jr (1979). Emergence of resistance to cefamandole: possible role of cefoxitin-inducible beta-lactamases. *Antimicrob Ag Chemother* **15**: 792.

Sanders CC, Sanders WE Jr, Goering RV (1982a). *In vitro* antagonism of beta-lactam antibiotics by cefoxitin. *Antimicrob Ag Chemother* **21**: 968.

Sanders CC, Moellering RC Jr, Martin RR *et al.* (1982b). Resistance to cefamandole: a collaborative study of emerging clinical problems. *J Infect Dis* **145**: 118.

Sanders CV, Greenberg RN, Marier RL (1985). Cefamandole and cefoxitin. *Ann Intern Med* **103**: 70.

Sanson-Le Pors MJ, Casin I, Ortenberg M, Perol Y (1983). *In vitro* susceptibility of thirty strains of *Haemophilus ducreyi* to several antibiotics including six cephalosporins. *J Antimicrob Chemother* **11**: 271.

Santos JI, Jacobson JA, Swensen P, Palmer WM (1981). Cellulitis: treatment with cefoxitin compared with multiple antibiotic therapy. *Pediatrics* **67**: 887.

Schaad UB, Suter S, Gianella-Borradori A et al. (1990). A comparison of ceftriaxone and cefuroxime for the treatment of bacterial meningitis in children. *New Engl J Med* **322**: 141.

Schift R, Van Ulsen J, Ansink-Schipper MC (1986). Comparison of oral treatment of uncomplicated urogenital and rectal gonorrhoea with cefuroxime axetil ester or clavulanic acid potentiated amoxycillin (Augmentin). *Genitourin Med* **62**: 313.

Schleupner CJ, Anthony WC, Tan J et al. (1988). Blinded comparison of cefuroxime to cefaclor for lower respiratory tract infections. *Arch Intern Med* **148**: 343.

Schrogie JJ, Rogers JD, Yeh KC et al. (1979). Pharmacokinetics and comparative pharmacology of cefoxitin and cephalosporins. *Rev Infect Dis* **1**: 90.

Schwartz AR, Asper RF, Bekes C, Schwartz AB (1978). Cefamandole in chronic hemodialysis patients In *Current Chemotherapy: Proceedings of the 10th International Congress of Chemotherapy, Zurich/Switzerland, 1977* (Siegenthaler W, Lüthy R, eds), p. 798. Washington DC: American Society of Microbiology.

Seeberg AH, Tolxdorff-Neutzling RM, Wiedemann B (1983). Chromosomal beta-lactamases of *Enterobacter cloacae* are responsible for resistance to third-generation cephalosporins. *Antimicrob Ag Chemother* **23**: 918.

Severn M, Powis SJA (1979). Biliary excretion and tissue levels of cefuroxime A study in eleven patients undergoing cholecystectomy. *J Antimicrob Chemother* **5**: 183.

Shaw PG, Fairley KF, Whitworth JA (1980). Treatment of urinary tract infection wiht a single-dose intramuscular administration of ceph-amandole. *Med J Aust* **1**: 489.

Short HD, Gentry IO, Sessoms S (1976). Cefamandole nafate therapy in the treatment of acute urinary tract infections. *J Antimicrob Chemother* **2**: 345.

Singh KV, Reves RR, Pickering LK, Murray BE (1990). Comparative *in vitro* activities of amoxicillin-clavulanic acid, cefuroxime, cephalexin, and cephalothin against trimethoprim-resistant *Escherichia coli* isolated from stools of children attending day-care centers. *Antimicrob Ag Chemother* **34**: 2047.

Singh N, Yu VL (1992). Successful treatment of pulmonary infection due to *Mycobacterium chelonae*: case report and review. *Clin Infect Dis* **14**: 156.

Sirinavin S, Chiemchanya S, Visudhipan P, Lolekha S (1984). Cefuroxime treatment of bacterial meningitis in infants and children. *Antimicrob Ag Chemother* **25**: 273.

Slama TG, Sklar SJ, Misinski J, Fess SW (1986). Randomized comparison of cefamandole, cefazolin, and cefuroxime prophylaxis in open-heart surgery. *Antimicrob Ag Chemother* **29**: 744.

Smith CR, Lipsky JJ (1983). Hypoprothrombinemia and platelet dysfunction caused by cephalosporin and oxalactam antibiotics. *J Antimicrob Chemother* **11**: 496.

Snydman DR, Tally FP, Knuppel R et al. (1980). *Bacteroides bivius* and *Bacteroides disiens* in obstetrical patients: clinical findings and antimicrobial susceptibilities. *J Antimicrob Chemother* **6**: 519.

Snydman DR, Cuchural GJJr, McDermott L, Gill M (1992). Correlation of various *in vitro* testing methods with clinical outcomes in patients with *Bacteroides fragilis* Group infections treated with cefoxitin: a retrospective analysis. *Antimicrob Ag Chemother* **36**: 540.

Sommers D, Van Wyk M, Williams PEO, Harding SM (1984). Pharmacokinetics and tolerance of cefuroxime axetil in volunteers during repeated doses. *Antimicrob Ag Chemother* **25**: 344.

Soriano F, Edwards R, Greenwood D (1991). Comparative susceptibility of cefminox and cefoxitin to beta-lactamases of *Bacteroides* spp. *J Antimicrob Chemother* **28**: 55.

Spangler SK, Jacobs MR, Pankuch GA, Appelbaum PC (1993). Susceptibility of 170 penicillin-susceptible and penicillin-resistant pneumococci to six oral cephalosporins, four quinolones, desacetylcefotaxime, Ro 23–9424 and RP 67829. *J Antimicrob Chemother* **31**: 273.

Stapley EO, Jackson M, Hernandez S et al. (1972). Cephamycins, a new family of β-lactam antibiotics. *Antimicrob Ag Chemother* **2**: 122.

Stapley EO, Birnbaum J, Miller AK et al. (1979). Cefoxitin and cephamycins: microbiological studies. *Rev Infect Dis* **1**: 73.

Steinberg EA, Overturf GD, Baraff LJ, Wilkins J (1977). Penetration of cefamandole into spinal fluid. *Antimicrob Ag Chemother* **11**: 933.

Steinberg EA, Overturf GD, Wilkins J et al. (1978). Failure of cefamandole in treatment of meningitis due to *Haemophilus influenzae* type b. *J Infect Dis* (Suppl 157): 180.

Strausbaugh LJ, Mikhail IA, Edman DC (1978). Comparative *in vitro* activity of five cephalosporin antibiotics against salmonellae. *Antimicrob Ag Chemother* **13**: 134.

Studley JGN, Schentag JJ, Schenk WG Jr (1982). Excretion of cephalothin and cefamandole by the normal pancreas and in acute pancreatitis in dogs. *Antimicrob Ag Chemother* **22**: 262.

Suata K, Watanabe K, Ueno K, Homma M (1993). Antimicrobial susceptibility patterns and resistance transferability among *Bacteroides fragilis* group isolates from patients with appendicitis in Bali, Indonesia. *Clin Infect Dis* **16**: 561.

Summersgill JT, Schupp LG, Raff MJ (1982). Comparative penetration of metronidazole, clindamycin, chloramphenicol, cefoxitin, ticarcillin and moxalactam into bone. *Antimicrob Ag Chemother* **21**: 601.

Sutter VL, Finegold SM (1976). Susceptibility of anaerobic bacteria to 23 antimicrobial agents. *Antimicrob Ag Chemother* **10**: 736.

Sutter VL, Oberhammer I, Kwok Y-Y, Finegold SH (1978). Susceptibility of anaerobes to cefoxitin sodium and cephalothin. *J Antimicrob Chemother* **4** (Suppl B): 41.

Swenson JM, Wallace RJ Jr, Silcox VA, Thornsberry C (1985). Antimicrobial susceptibility of five subgroups of *Mycobacterium fortuitum* and *Mycobacterium chelonae*. *Antimicrob Ag Chemother* **28**: 807.

Sykes RB, Griffiths A, Ryan DM (1977). Comparative activity of ampicillin and cefuroxime against three types of *Haemophilus influenzae*. *Antimicrob Ag Chemother* **11**: 599.

Tally FP, Cuchural GJJr (1988). Antibiotic resistance in anaerobic bacteria. *J Antimicrob Chemother* **22** (Suppl A): 63.

Tally FP, O'Keefe JP, Sullivan NM, Gorbach SL (1979a). Inactivation of cephalosporins by bacteroides. *Antimicrob Ag Chemother* **16**: 565.

Tally FP, Miao PVM, O'Keefe JP, Gorbach SL (1979b). Cefoxitin therapy of anaerobic and aerobic infections. *J Antimicrob Chemother* **5**: 101.

Tally FP, Cuchural GJ Jr, Jacobus NV et al. (1983). Susceptibility of the *Bacteroides fragilis* group in the United States in 1981. *Antimicrob Ag Chemother* **23**: 536.

Tan JS, Salstrom SJ (1977). Levels of carbenicillin, ticarcillin, cephalothin, cefazolin, cefamandole, gentamicin, tobramycin, and amikacin in human serum and interstitial fluid. *Antimicrob Ag Chemother* **11**: 698.

Thirumoorthi MC, Dajani AS, Vincent CV, Maurer MJ (1981). Pharmacology, safety and efficacy of cefamandole in childhood infections. *Antimicrob Ag Chemother* **20**: 21.

Thornsberry C, Baker CN, Kirven LA (1978). *In vitro* activity of antimicrobial agents on Legionnaires' disease bacterium. *Antimicrob Ag Chemother* **13**: 78.

Trollfors B (1980). Quantitative studies on antibiotic nephrotoxicity. *Scand J Infect Dis* (Suppl 21): 1–46.

Trollfors B, Norrby R (1980). Effect of frusemide on the elimination of cefuroxime and cefoxitin. *J Antimicrob Chemother* **6**: 405.

Trollfors B, Norrby R, Kristianson K (1978). Effects on renal function of treatment with cefoxitin sodium alone or in combination with furosemide. *J Antimicrob Chemother* **4** (Suppl B): 85.

Trollfors B, Alestig K, Norrby R (1979). Local and gastrointestinal reactions to intravenously administered cefoxitin and cefuroxime. *Scand J Infect Dis* **11**: 315.

Trollfors B, Alestig K, Carlsten C, Norrby R (1980a). Unexpected side-effects of cefuroxime lysine, a new cefuroxime salt. *J Antimicrob Chemother* **6**: 558.

Trollfors B, Suurkula M, Price JD, Norrby R (1980b). Renal function during cefuroxime treatment in patients with pre-existing renal impairment. *J Antimicrob Chemother* **6**: 665.

Tupasi TE, Crisologo LB, Torres CA, Calubiran OV (1982). Comparison of spectinomycin, cefuroxime, thiamphenicol and penicillin G in the treatment of uncomplicated gonococcal infections in women. *J Infect Dis* **145**: 583.

Tupasi TE, Crisologo LB, Torres CA *et al.* (1983). Cefuroxime, thiamphenicol, spectinomycin, and penicillin G in uncomplicated infections due to penicillinase-producing strains of *Neisseria gonorrhoeae*. *Brit J Vener Dis* **59**: 172.

Turck M (1982). Cephalosporins and related antibiotics: an overview. *Rev Infect Dis* **4** (Suppl): 281.

Turgeon P, Turgeon V, Geurdeau M *et al.* (1994). Longitudinal study of susceptibilities of species of the *Bacteroides fragilis* group to five antimicrobial agents in three medical centers. *Antimicrob Ag Chemother* **38**: 2276.

Tullus K, Berglund B, Burman LG (1990). Emergence of cross-resistance to beta-lactam antibiotics in fecal *Escherichia coli* and *Klebsiella* strains from neonates treated with ampicillin or cefuroxime. *Antimicrob Ag Chemother* **34**: 361.

Uotila L, Suttie JW (1983). Inhibition of vitamin K-dependent carboxylase *in vitro* by cefamandole and its structural analogs. *J Infect Dis* **148**: 571.

Uwaydah M, Kantarjian H, Osseiran M, Bal'a F (1982). Cefamandole bile levels in patients with hepatobiliary disease. *Antimicrob Ag Chemother* **22**: 1087.

Van Dalen R, Vree TB, Hafkenscheid JCM, Gimbrère JSF (1979). Determination of plasma and renal clearance of cefuroxime and its pharmacokinetics in renal insufficiency. *J Antimicrob Chemother* **5**: 281.

Van Winzum C (1978). Clinical safety and tolerance of cefoxitin sodium: an overview. *J Antimicrob Chemother* **4** (Suppl B): 91.

Verbist L (1976). Comparison of the antibacterial activity of nine cephalosporins against Enterobacteriacea and nonfermentative Gram-negative bacilli. *Antimicrob Ag Chemother* **10**: 657.

Vincken W (1984). Psychotic reaction to cefuroxime. *Lancet* **i**: 965.

Viotte G, Morin JP, Godin M, Fillastre JP (1981). Changes in the renal function of rats treated with cefoxitin and a comparison with other cephalosporins and gentamicin. *J Antimicrob Chemother* **7**: 537.

Vlasses PH, Holbrook AM, Schrogie JJ *et al.* (1980). Effect of orally administered probenecid on the pharmacokinetics of cefoxitin. *Antimicrob Ag Chemother* **17**: 847.

Vuye A, Pijck J, Van Landuyt HW (1979). Comparative activity of two newer cephalosporins, cefoxitin and cephalothin against selected Enterobacteriaceae and correlation with enzymatic resistance mechanisms. *J Antimicrob Chemother* **5**: 293.

Walker SH, Gahol VP (1978). Pharmacokinetics of cefamandole in infants and children. *Antimicrob Ag Chemother* **14**: 315.

Wallace RJ Jr, Wiss K, Curvey R *et al.* (1983). Differences among *Nocardia* spp in susceptibility to aminoglycosides and beta-lactam antibiotics and their potential use in taxonomy. *Antimicrob Ag Chemother* **23**: 19.

Wallace RJ Jr, Swenson JM, Silcox VA, Bullen MG (1985). Treatment of nonpulmonary infections due to *Mycobacterium fortuitum* and *Mycobacterium chelonei* on the basis of *in vitro* susceptibilities. *J Infect Dis* **152**: 500.

Wallick H, Hendlin D (1974). Cefoxitin, a semisynthetic cephamycin antibiotic: susceptibility studies. *Antimicrob Ag Chemother* **5**: 25.

Waterworth PM, Emmerson AM (1979). Dissociated resistance among cephalosporins. *Antimicrob Ag Chemother* **15**: 497.

Wexler HM, Halebian S (1990). Alterations to the penicillin-binding proteins in the *Bacteroides fragilis* group: a mechanism for non-beta-lactamase mediated cefoxitin resistance. *J Antimicrob Chemother* **26**: 7.

Wick WE, Preston DA (1972). Biological properties of three 3-hetero-cyclicthiomethyl cephalosporin antibiotics. *Antimicrob Ag Chemother* **1**: 221.

Williams PEO, Harding SM (1984). The absolute bioavailability of cefuroxime axetil in male and female volunteers after fasting and after food. *J Antimicrob Chemother*: **13**: 191.

Winter J, Dhillon P (1991). Penetration of cefuroxime into bronchial mucosa following oral administration of cefuroxime axetil. *J Antimicrob Chemother* **27**: 556.

Wise R, Donovan IA, Ambrose NS, Allcock JE (1981). The penetration of cefoxitin into peritoneal fluid. *J Antimicrob Chemother* **8**: 453.

Wise R, Bennett SA, Dent J (1984). The pharmacokinetics of orally absorbed cefuroxime compared with amoxycillin/clavulanic acid. *J Antimicrob Chemother* **13**: 603.

Wold JS, Joost RR, Black HR, Griffith RS (1978a). Hydrolysis of cefamandole nafate to cefamandole *in vivo*. *J Infect Dis* **137** (Suppl): 17.

Wold JS, Welles JS, Owen NV *et al.* (1978b). Toxicologic evaluation of cefamandole nafate in laboratory animals. *J Infect Dis* **137** (Suppl): 51.

Yoshikawa TT, Shibata SA, Herbert P, Oill PA (1980). *In vitro* activity of Ro 13–9904, cefuroxime, cefoxitin and ampicillin against *Neisseria gonorrhoeae*. *Antimicrob Ag Chemother* **18**: 355.

Yourassowsky E, Schoutens E, Vanderlinden MP (1976). Antibacterial activity of eight cephalosporins against *Haemophilus influenzae* and *Streptococcus pneumoniae*. *J Antimicrob Chemother* **2**: 55.

Cefotaxime, Cefoperazone, Ceftizoxime and Cefsulodin

Description

These four cephalosporins and others described in sbsequent chapters, are referred to as extended-spectrum or third-generation cephalosporins. They were developed after the first-and second-generation drugs (p. 291). Most third-generation cephalosporins have some common characteristics. These include stability to beta-lactamases, particularly those produced by Gram-negative bacteria, high potency against all, or at least most Enterobacteriaceae and moderate to good activity against *Pseudomonas aeruginosa* (Dunn, 1982). Cefotaxime, cefoperazone and ceftizoxime have these characteristics, but cefsulodin has a narrow spectrum (p. 326).

1 Cefotaxime

Developed in the 1970s, this was stable in the presence of practically all beta-lactamases, both chromosomally and plasmid-mediated, which were produced by Gram-negative bacteria and *Staphylococcus aureus* (Richmond, 1980). Some of the drug is metabolized *in vivo* to desacetylcefotaxime, which has less antibacterial activity against most bacterial species (Schrinner *et al.*, 1980).

2 Cefoperazone

Good activity against *Ps. aeruginosa* is one of the main features of this drug. It has a similar antibacterial spectrum to cefotaxime, but it is less stable to some beta-lactamases (Jones and Barry, 1983a).

3 Ceftizoxime

This is a 7-aminothiazolyl alpha-methoxymino cephalosporin, which is structurally related to cefotaxime and its desacetyl metabolite (see above). Unlike cefotaxime, this drug is not deacetylated *in vivo*. It has similar activity to cefotaxime but it is less active against *Ps. aeruginosa* (Barry *et al.*, 1982).

4 Cefsulodin

Antibacterial activity of this is largely limited to *Ps. aeruginosa* and *Staph. aureus* (Barry *et al.*, 1981).

Sensitive Organisms

A Cefotaxime

1 Gram-positive bacteria

Both penicillin G-sensitive and beta-lactamase producing *Staph. aureus* and coagulase-negative staphylococci are cefotaxime-sensitive, but the drug is some 8-fold less active than cephalothin against these bacteria (p. 251) (Dornbusch *et al.*, 1990). *Staphylococcus aureus* is more susceptible (2- to 4-fold reduction of MICs) to a combination of cefotaxime with its metabolite desacetylcefotaxime (p. 323). On this basis cefotaxime appears to be one of the most active anti-staphylococcal compounds among the newer cephalosporins, being comparable with cefa-mandole (p. 292) and cefuroxime (p. 296) (Jones *et al.*, 1984; Jones and Barry, 1987).

Methicillin-resistant strains of *Staph. aureus* and coagulase-negative staphylococci are cefotaxime-resistant (Jones and Thornsberry, 1982). Against *Streptococcus pyogenes*, Group B streptococci and *Strep. pneumoniae*, cefotaxime is 2- to 8-fold more active than cephalothin (Table I.26) (Chabbert and Lutz, 1978; Jacobs *et al.*, 1982). The MICs of cefotaxime are usually lower than those of penicillin G (pp. 336, 359) against both relatively and highly penicillin G-resistant pneumococcal strains (Table I.26) (Spangler *et al.*, 1994). Based on *in vitro* studies, pneumococcal meningitis caused by either of these strains may respond to cefotaxime, ceftriaxone, or vancomycin (p. 779) (Ward and Moellering, 1981; Tweardy *et al.*, 1983; Bosley *et al.*, 1987; Liñares *et al.*, 1992). However, some *Strep. pneumoniae* clinical isolates, with intermediate or high resistance to penicillin G, have been detected for which the MICs of cefotaxime and ceftriaxone were even higher than those of penicillin G (Figueiredo *et al.*, 1992; Leggiadro *et al.*, 1994; Welby *et al.*, 1994).

Streptococcus viridans is cefotaxime-sensitive, but *Enterococcus faecalis* is resistant (Jones and Thornsberry, 1982). The MICs of cefotaxime against many enterococci are lower in the presence of serum. In one animal study, cefotaxime had anti-enterococcal activity within newly formed cardiac valve vegetations. Although cefotaxime is not useful for treatment of *E. faecalis* infections, its ability to inhibit enterococcal growth *in vivo* under certain conditions, may explain why *E. faecalis* superinfections have been uncommon during cefotaxime therapy (Sullam *et al.*, 1985).

Listeria monocytogenes is moderately sensitive to cefotaxime (Ahonkhai *et al.*, 1982). Most strains of *Nocardia asteroides* are inhibited by 8 μg per ml (Gutmann *et al.*, 1983; Wallace *et al.*, 1988), and the drug is effective in murine acute pulmonary nocardiosis (Sugar *et al.*, 1983).

Anaerobic Gram-positive bacteria such as the *Peptococcus*, *Peptostreptococcus*, *Actinomyces* and *Propionibacterium* spp. are susceptible to cefotaxime. *Clostridium perfringens* is sensitive but *Cl. difficile* is resistant (Rolfe and Finegold, 1981; Denys *et al.*, 1983).

2 Gram-negative cocci

Cefotaxime is highly active against *N. meningitidis* and *N. gonorrhoeae*, and it is equally active against beta-lactamase-producing gonococcal strains (Table I.26) (Kamimura *et al.*, 1979; Kerbs *et al.*, 1983). Cefotaxime is very active (MIC 0.004–0.03 μg per ml) against gonococci relatively resistant to penicillin G. Against gonococcal strains which are penicillin G-resistant and do not produce beta-lactamase (p. 4), cefotaxime is active (MIC 0.015–0.125 μg per ml), but about 16-fold less so than against sensitive strains (Cohen *et al.*, 1983; Rodrìguez *et al.*, 1983). A rare human pathogen, *N. flavescens* is cefotaxime-sensitive (Sinave and Ratzan, 1987).

3 Gram-negative aerobic bacilli

The drug is normally highly resistant to hydrolysis by both plasmid and chromosomal beta-lactamases (p. 319) of Gram-negative bacilli; it also has a great affinity for their penicillin-binding proteins (p. 334) (Richmond, 1980; Neu, 1983). Thus, cefotaxime has a good potency against all Enterobacteriaceae, such as *Escherichia coli*, the *Klebsiella* and *Enterobacter* spp., *Proteus mirabilis*, *Pr. vulgaris*, *Morganella morganii* and the *Providencia*, *Citrobacter*, *Salmonella* and *Shigella* spp. (Neu *et al.*, 1979; Muytjens and Van der Ros-van de Repe, 1982; Amyes *et al.*, 1994). Most strains of *Serratia marcescens* are also sensitive (Markowitz and Sibilla, 1980). The drug is quite active against *Yersinia enterocolitica* (Hornstein *et al.*, 1985; Gahrn-Hansen and Søgaard, 1990; Kwaga and Iversen, 1990). Cefotaxime shows paradoxical antibacterial activity against *Pr. vulgaris*; the organism is more sensitive to low-cefotaxime than high-cefotaxime concentrations. This is probably because with high concentrations more chromosomal beta-lactamase is induced (p. 322), which makes the organism resistant (Ikeda and Nishino, 1988). The combination of cefotaxime and its metabolite desacetylcefotaxime demonstrates partial synergy against *S. marcescens* and synergy against *E. coli* and *Pr. vulgaris* (Neu, 1982b; Mandell and Afnan, 1991).

Aminoglycoside (gentamicin and tobramycin)-resistant Enterobacteriaceae are usually as susceptible to cefotaxime as aminoglycoside-sensitive strains (Hall *et al.*, 1980; Magnussen *et al.*, 1982; Muytjens and Van der Ros-van de Repe, 1982). Inoculum size does not have a marked effect on the MICs of the drug for most Enteobacteriaceae, except for some strains of *Citrobacter* spp., *Enterobacter cloacae* and *Pr. vulgaris*. Cefotaxime is bactericidal at, or close to, its MICs (Neu *et al.*, 1979; Jones and Thornsberry, 1982).

Cefotaxime, combined with one of the aminoglycosides, such as gentamicin or amikacin, show *in vitro* synergism against some strains of the Enterobacteriaceae (Neu *et al.*, 1979;

Jorgensen *et al.*, 1980b; Jones and Packer, 1982). An amikacin/cefotaxime combination often exhibits *in vitro* synergism against Enterobacteriaceae resistant to other aminoglycosides and beta-lactams such as cephalothin (Glew and Pavuk, 1984; Maslow *et al.*, 1985). When cefotaxime is combined with another beta-lactam antibiotic, such as cefoxitin, antagonism against certain Gram-negative bacilli, such as *S. marcescens*, may result (Miller *et al.*, 1983). This is because of beta-lactamase induction (p. 322).

Haemophilus influenzae, including beta-lactamase producing strains, is highly sensitive to cefotaxime (Drasar *et al.*, 1978; Jorgensen *et al.*, 1980a). In one study 10 of 200 *H. influenzae* strains were cefotaxime-tolerant (MBC/MIC >32) (p. 9), but the clinical significance of this is uncertain (Bergeron and Lavoie, 1985). Chloramphenicol-resistant strains of this organism (p. 552) are inhibited by cefotaxime and other third-generation cephalosporins, such as cefoperazone and moxalactam (p. 324) (Campos *et al.*, 1984; Campos and Garcia-Tornel, 1987). The combination of ampicillin/cefotaxime may be synergistic against some strains of *H. influenzae* and the combination of ampicilin/chloramphenicol may be antagonistic for some, but for most strains these combinations exhibit neither synergism nor antagonism (Lapointe *et al.*, 1986). Accelerated killing of *H. influenzae* is observed in CSF if amikacin (p. 504) is added to cefotaxime, but this is not associated with an increase in endotoxin release. The clinical significance of this is uncertain (Bingen *et al.*, 1992). *Haemophilus influenzae* strains with intrinsic resistance to ampicillin are cefotaxime-sensitive, but the cefotaxime MICs for these strains are higher (up to 0.5 μg per ml) than those of ampicillin-sensitive strains or beta-lactamase producers (Yeo and Livermore, 1994).

Haemophilus ducreyi is also susceptible (Sanson-Le Pors *et al.*, 1983), but Sturm (1987) demonstrated that the MICs of this organism for cefotaxime slightly increased between the period 1978–1981 and 1982–1985 in Amsterdam. *Brucella melitensis* with MICs ranging from 0.5 to 2.0 μg per ml is moderately cefotaxime-sensitive (Palenque *et al.*, 1986). The drug is active against *Bordetella pertussis*, *Aeromonas hydrophila* and the *Moraxella*, *Pasteurella* and *Vibrio* species. *Acinetobacter Iwoffi* is also usually sensitive, but subspecies *anitratus* (now called *A. baumannii*) may be moderately resistant. The *Alcaligenes* spp. and *Campylobacter jejuni* are only inhibited to a degree, and the *Flavobacterium* spp. are cefotaxime-resistant (Appelbaum *et al.*, 1982; Jones and Thornsberry, 1982; Muytjens and Van der Ros-van de Repe, 1982; Van der Auwera and Scorneaux, 1985; Siegman-Igra *et al.*, 1993). A rare opportunistic human pathogen, *Agrobacterium radiobacter*, is usually cefotaxime-sensitive (Edmond *et al.*, 1993).

Most *Ps. aeruginosa* strains are moderately resistant (MICs 16–32 μg per ml), but about 20% are highly resistant (MICs 64 μg per ml or higher) (Fuchs *et al.*, 1980; Greenwood *et al.*, 1980; Livermore *et al.*, 1981). Others have found the majority of *Ps. aeruginosa* strains to be highly resistant (Kurtz *et al.*, 1980; Muytjens and Van der Ros-van de Repe, 1982). When combined with an aminoglycoside, such as tobramycin or amikacin, it often exhibits *in vitro* synergism against *Ps. aeruginosa* (Jorgensen *et al.*, 1980b; Mintz and Drew, 1981; Maslow *et al.*, 1985).

Some other *Pseudomonas* spp., such as *Ps. acidovorans*, *Ps. diminuta*, *Ps. pseudoalcaligenes*, *Ps. putrefaciens* and *Ps. stutzeri*, are cefotaxime-sensitive. *Burkholderia* (*Pseudomonas*) *cepacia* is usually resistant and *Ps. fluorescens*, *Ps. putida* and *Stenotrophomonas maltophilia* highly resistant (Appelbaum *et al.*, 1982; Jones and Thornsberry, 1982; Chen *et al.*, 1991); *B. cepacia* produces an inducible chromosomal beta-lactamase (Proenca *et al.*, 1993). *Stenotrophomonas maltophilia* owes its resistance to all beta-lactam antibiotics due to a combination of low outer membrane permeability and two inducible chromosomally mediated beta-lactamases (Mett *et al.*, 1988).

4 Gram-negative anaerobic bacteria

Some of these, such as *Prevotella* (*Bacteroides*) *melaninogenica* and *Fusobacterium* spp., are inhibited by low cefotaxime concentrations. Bacteria of the *Bacteroides fragilis* group are more resistant, against which cefotaxime is less active than cefoxitin (p. 295) and moxalactam (p. 350), but it is more active than cefoperazone (p. 325), cefamandole (p. 293) and carbenicillin (p. 147) (Rolfe and Finegold, 1981; Jones and Thornsberry, 1982; Ohm-Smith *et al.*, 1982). As with cefoxitin (p. 295), indole negative members of the *B. fragilis* group are more sensitive to cefotaxime; 90% of strains are inhibited by 8–32 μg per ml, whereas this is only accomplished for indole positive members by a concentration of 64 μg per ml (Jenkins *et al.*, 1982). In early surveys in 1981 and 1983 in the USA, 35% of isolates of the *B. fragilis* group were cefotaxime-resistant (MICs >32 μg per ml) (Tally *et al.*, 1983, 1985). Cefotaxime is inactivated by some beta-lactamases produced by *B. fragilis*, and its MICs and MBCs increase if high inocula are used in sensitivity testing (Yu and Washington, 1983). Most *B. fragilis* strains appear to be synergistically killed by a cefotaxime and desacetylcefotaxime (p. 323) combination. This may expand the spectrum of cefotaxime to include an increased percentage of *B. fragilis* group strains, a feature which would not be appreciated by *in vitro* testing of the parent compound alone (Aldridge *et al.*, 1984; Jones, 1984). But Cornick and Gorbach (1988) found that desacetylcefotaxime enhanced the *in vitro* activity of cefotaxime against cefotaxime-susceptible strains of the *B. fragilis* group and resistant strains were not significantly affected.

5 Other organisms

Chlamydie trachomatis is resistant to cefotaxime (Hammerschlag and Gleyzer, 1983). Leptospirae are sensitive and the MICs and MBCs of this drug against these organisms are lower than those of penicillin G (Oie *et al.*, 1983).

6 Acquired resistance

The prevalence of cefotaxime-resistant Enterobacteriaceae and *Ps. aeruginosa* has gradually increased over the years, particularly in hospitals and in special areas such as intensive care units. These organisms are often also resistant to other third-generation cephalosporins (Grayson and Eliopoulos, 1990; Pierson and Friedman, 1992). Some of them may have intrinsic resistance. For instance *Ps. aeruginosa* has low outer membrane permeability (Hancock and Woodruff, 1988). This can also be a factor in the cefotaxime-resistance of some Enterobacteriaceae such as *Enterobacter* spp. (Hopkins and Towner, 1990). In these instances beta-lactamase production also plays a part and so these organisms have a dual mechanism for their cefotaxime-resistance (Hancock and Woodruff, 1988; Grayson and Eliopoulos, 1990). It now seems that beta-lactamase production is the major mechanism for cefotaxime resistance. Initially cefotaxime and other third-generation cephalosporins were thought to be very stable to all beta-lactamases, but it was soon realized that some organisms possessed enzymes capable of hydrolyzing them (Neu 1982a; Curtis *et al.*, 1986). The beta-lactamases which inactivate cefotaxime and other third-generation cephalosporins are of two main types. First there are the chromosomally mediated inducible beta-lactamases (Vu and Nikaido, 1985; Sanders and Sanders, 1988) and second plasmid-mediated extended-spectrum beta-lactamases (Philippon *et al.*, 1989; Jacoby and Archer, 1991).

The chromosomally mediated enzymes are present in *Ps. aeruginosa*, *Pr. vulgaris*, *Morganella morganii* and the *Enterobacter*, *Serratia*, *Citrobacter* and *Providencia* spp. (Eliopoulos, 1988; Sanders and Sanders, 1988). Normally these organisms produce a low level of these enzymes and the bacteria are cefotaxime-sensitive. The enzymes in these organisms are said to be 'repressed', but they can start overproducing these beta-lactamases or become 'derepressed' by one of two mechanisms. The first involves exposure of wild type bacteria to an enzyme inducer, such as cefoxitin (p. 295), another beta-lactamase-stable cephalosporin, or some other beta-lactam antibiotic. The second mechanism involves spontaneous chromosomal mutation to a stably 'derepressed' state, when again these enzymes are overproduced. Once this happens the bacteria are resistant to cefotaxime and other third-generation cephalosporins (Lindberg and Normark, 1986; Sanders and Sanders, 1986; Yang and Livermore, 1988; Michéa-Hamzehpour and Pechere, 1989; Lodge and Piddock, 1991; Bennett and Chopra, 1993). This resistance can arise during cefotaxime (or other cephalosporin) use in treatment of infections caused by these bacteria, *in vivo*. Failed treatment with cefamandole of *Enterobacter* spp. infections can occur *in vivo* due to emergence of cefamandole-resistant Enterobacter spp. strains (p. 293). These resistant strains also show high level resistance to cefotaxime, cefoperazone (p. 325), and ceftriaxone (p. 354) (Murray *et al.*, 1983; Olson *et al.*, 1983; Andresen *et al.*, 1994). Therefore, the use of one cephalosporin may induce cross-resistance to other cephalosporins. This cross-resistance is due to induction (derepression) of chromosomally mediated beta-lactamases (Olson *et al.*, 1983; Seeberg *et al.*, 1983).

This form of resistance is probably fairly common in clinical practice. In one neonatal intensive care unit, where gentamicin-resistant *Klebsiella pneumoniae* infections had occurred, a regimen of cefotaxime plus ampicillin was begun as the standard initial treatment of all serious neonatal infections. Within 10 weeks an outbreak of serious infections due to cefotaxime-resistant *E. cloacae* occurred. This suggests that routine use of newer cephalosporins leads to emergence of drug resistant microorganisms more rapidly than with aminoglycosides (Bryan *et al.*, 1985). Some authors have estimated that the emergence of this type of resistance has been associated with clinical failure or relapse of infection in at least 25% or even 75% of patients infected by these organisms when treated by cefotaxime or another newer cephalosporin

(Sanders and Sanders, 1988). The more cefotaxime is used for an individual patient, the more likely it is that the patient will become colonized or infected by these resistant bacteria (Prevot *et al.*, 1986). The more cefotaxime and other third-generation cephalosporins are used in a hospital or a special unit the more of this resistance is encountered (Wiedemann, 1986; Andersen *et al.*, 1989; Sanders and Sanders, 1992).

Initially it was considered that when the chromosomally induced beta-lactamases were overproduced, the normally enzyme-stable drugs, such as cefotaxime, were bound to beta-lactamases by so called 'trapping' mechanism but not hydrolyzed by them (Sanders and Sanders 1985; Werner *et al.*, 1985), but it was soon established that when the amounts of these enzymes were increased after induction, most third-generation cephalosporins were actually inactivated by these beta-lactamases (Livermore, 1985; Towner and Massam, 1985; Vu and Nikaido, 1985; White and Curtis, 1985; Curtis *et al.*, 1986; Livermore *et al.*, 1986; Charnas and Then, 1988; Hiraoka *et al.*, 1988). Variants of *Ps. aeruginosa* and *Citrobacter* and *Enterobacter* spp., which produce elevated levels of inducible chromosomally mediated beta-lactamase(s), can be produced *in vitro*. These show marked increase in resistance to cefotaxime, and other related drugs, such as cefoperazone and moxalactam (Gwynn and Rolinson, 1983; Gootz *et al.*, 1984). Some strains of *B. fragilis* are cefotaxime-resistant because they possess a beta-lactamase which hydrolyzes cefotaxime, but not cefoxitin (Pechère *et al.*, 1980); others may possess intrinsic resistance (Dornbusch *et al.*, 1979).

Plasmid-mediated beta-lactamases which can hydrolyze cefotaxime, other third-generation cephalosporins and aztreonam, but not cefoxitin, cefotetan, moxalactam and imipenem, were first detected in the mid-1980s. Initially they were mainly found in *Kl. pneumoniae* and *E. coli*, but they later spread also to other Enterobacteriaceae, such as *S. marcescens* (Gianneli *et al.*, 1994) and *Pr. mirabilis* (Palzkill *et al.*, 1995). They were initially mainly found in France but soon spread to other European countries (Jarlier *et al.*, 1988; Sirot *et al.*, 1988; Paul *et al.*, 1989; Livermore, 1991; Sirot *et al.*, 1992), to the UK (Liu *et al.*, 1992) and the USA (Nicolas *et al.*, 1989; Sanders 1992; Medeiros, 1993; Meyer *et al.*, 1993). Collectively these plasmid-mediated enzymes are referred to as extended-spectrum beta-lactamases. This group of enzymes are still inhibited by beta-lactamase inhibitors (p. 192). These beta-lactamases are single mutations from the previously well known plasmid-mediated TEM-1, TEM-2, and SHV-1 enzymes, which did not hydrolyze cefotaxime etc. (Philippon *et al.*, 1989, Murray, 1991; Mariotte *et al.*, 1994). In 1993 four strains of cefotaxime- and ceftazidime-resistant *E. coli* were isolated in a nursing home in New York. They produced a novel extended-spectrum beta-lactamase, designated SHV-7 (Bradford *et al.*, 1995).

Soon other extended-spectrum beta-lactamases appeared, which not only hydrolyzed cefotaxime, ceftriaxone, ceftazidime etc., but also alpha-methoxy beta-lactams such as cefoxitin, cefotetan, moxalactam and rarely also imipenem (Papanicolaou *et al.*, 1990; Jacoby and Medeiros, 1991; Horii *et al.*, 1993; Pörnull *et al.*, 1993). These enzymes were usually not inhibited by beta-lactamase inhibitors such as clavulanic acid (p. 193) (Jacoby and Archer, 1991; Tzouvelekis *et al.*, 1993; Pörnull *et al.*, 1994).

It remains to be seen how extensive these two types of extended-spectrum beta-lactamases will become in various countries (Payne and Amyes, 1991). Being plasmid-mediated and therefore transferable both types of extended-spectrum beta-lactamases could easily spread to other Enterobacteriaceae and to organisms so far unaffected by them such as *H. influenzae* (Murray, 1991; Du Bois *et al.*, 1995).

7 Activity of desacetylcefotaxime

This metabolite of cefotaxime has independent antibacterial activity. It is about 10-fold less active than the parent compound against most Enterobacteriaceae, and it has no useful activity against *Ps. aeruginosa*. Gram-positive bacteria and *B. fragilis* are approximately 2-fold less susceptible to desacetylcefotaxime than to cefotaxime. Therefore, at clinically achievable concentrations, this metabolite does not inhibit some strains of *Serratia* and *Providencia* spp., many strains of *Morganella morganii* and all strains of *Ps. aeruginosa*. Cefotaxime and desacetylcefotaxime act synergistically against many bacteria, so that the presence of the metabolite often increases rather than decreases the activity of cefotaxime (Wise *et al.*, 1980a; Neu, 1982b). They are synergistic against *B. fragilis* (p. 322). This may also be the case with some Gram-positive bacteria, such as *E. faecalis*, which is cefotaxime-resistant (p. 320). Surprisingly, cefotaxime therapy has been infrequently associated with Gram-positive bacterial and other superinfections. Superinfections have been more common with other third-generation cephalosporins, such as cefoperazone (p. 335) and ceftazidime (p. 377) (Jones and Thornsberry, 1985).

B Cefoperazone

1 Gram-positive bacteria

Cefoperazone is about as active as cefotaxime against *Staph. aureus* and coagulase-negative staphylococci (Table I.26), but methicillin-resistant strains are resistant. *Streptococcus pneumoniae*, including strains relatively resistant and highly resistant to penicillin G, need slightly higher concentrations of cefoperazone than of cefotaxime for inhibition (Table I.26) (Ward and Moellering, 1981; Tweardy *et al.*, 1983). Compared with cefotaxime, its activity against *Strep. pyogenes* is similar (Table I.26), but Group B streptococci and most *Strep. viridans* strains are slightly less susceptible (Jacobs *et al.*, 1982; Jones and Barry, 1983a). *Enterococcus faecalis* is resistant and *L. monocytogenes* is moderately resistant. *Nocardia asteroides* is usually resistant (Gutmann *et al.*, 1983).

Some Gram-positive anaerobes, such as *Peptococcus* and *Propionibacterium* spp. and *Cl. perfringens*, are cefoperazone-sensitive; *Cl. difficile* is resistant (Rolfe and Finegold, 1981; Denys *et al.*, 1983).

2 Gram-negative cocci

Meningococci are quite sensitive to cefoperazone but slightly less so than to cefotaxime (Table I.26) (Scribner *et al.*, 1982). This also applies to gonococci including beta-lactamase-producing strains, but the reported degree of sensitivity of the latter has varied. Baker *et al.* (1980) noted about a 3-fold increase in the MICs of cefoperazone against beta-lactamase-producing strains, whilst Kerbs *et al.* (1983) reported identical MICs for penicillin G-sensitive and enzyme-producing strains. Gonococcal strains relatively resistant to penicillin G or completely resistant to penicillin G, which do not produce beta-lactamase (p. 14), are also cefoperazone-sensitive; MICs for these two types of strains are ≤0.004–0.5 and 0.125–0.5 μg per ml, respectively. Cefotaxime (p. 320) exhibits a higher degree of activity than cefoperazone against all gonococcal strains (Rodrìguez *et al.*, 1983).

3 Gram-negative aerobic bacilli

Similar to cefotaxime (p. 320), cefoperazone is active against nearly all Enterobacteriaceae, but against most species this is to a lesser degree (Table I.26). Cefoperazone is somewhat less stable than cefotaxime to beta-lactamases, so that the frequency of cefoperazone-resistant strains amongst Enterobacteriaceae is higher (5–10%) than with cefotaxime (p. 322) (Jones *et al.*, 1980; Jones and Barry, 1983a; Sykes and Bush, 1983). Strains of Enterobacteriaceae resistant to aminoglycosides, such as gentamicin and tobramycin, are usually cefoperazone-sensitive (Hall *et al.*, 1980; Magnussen *et al.*, 1982). Unlike cefotaxime (p. 320), MICs and MBCs of cefoperazone against many Enterobacteriaceae, are inoculum-dependent (Hinkle *et al.*, 1980; Lang *et al.*, 1980). This is due to a lesser stability of cefoperazone to some beta-lactamases (Jones and Barry, 1983a). Cefoperazone when combined with an aminoglycoside, such as amikacin, frequently exhibits *in vitro* synergism against many Enterobacteriaceae (Jones and Packer, 1982; Van Laethem *et al.*, 1983).

Against *H. influenzae*, cefoperazone is not quite as active as cefotaxime (Table I.26). Cefoperazone shows inoculum-dependent decreases in inhibitory and bactericidal activity when tested against beta-lactamase producing organisms (Bulger and Washington, 1980; Wise *et al.*, 1981a); *H. parainfluenzae* is also cefoperazone-susceptible.

Bordetella pertussis, *Pasteurella multocida*, *Aeromonas hydrophila* and the *Moraxella* spp. are usually sensitive. Some *Alcaligenes* spp. are susceptible but *Alcaligenes faecalis* is resistant. *Legionella pneumophila* is moderately resistant (MIC 16 μg per ml). *Flavobacterium* and *Acinetobacter* spp. are cefoperazone-resistant (Edelstein and Meyer, 1980; Fass, 1980; Jones and Barry, 1983a).

Cefoperazone has a moderately high degree of activity against *Ps. aeruginosa*. Approximately 50% of all isolates are inhibited by 4 μg per ml, and 90% by 32 μg per ml (Kurtz *et al.*, 1980; Mitsuhashi *et al.*, 1980; Gillett, 1982). Thereby, amongst beta-lactams the drug is more active against *Ps. aeruginosa* than cefotaxime (p. 321) and moxalactam (p. 350), and it has about the same potency as azlocillin (p. 164) and piperacillin (p. 164). Cefsulodin (p. 326) and ceftazidime (p. 369), however, have a higher activity against this organism. The MICs of cefoperazone against *Ps. aeruginosa* increase if the sensitivity tests are done with large inocula (Hinkle *et al.*, 1980).

Pseudomonas species other than *aeruginosa* vary in their susceptibility to cefoperazone. Usually *Ps. stutzeri* and *Ps. putrefaciens* are sensitive. *Burkholderia* (*Pseudomonas*) *cepacia* is moderately resistant, and *Ps. putida* and *Ps. vesicularis* usually resistant. *Stenotrophomonas maltophilia* is always resistant (Fass, 1980; Appelbaum *et al.*, 1982).

4 Gram-negative anaerobic bacteria

Some of these, such as *Prevotella melaninogenica*, *P. disiens* and *Fusobacterium* spp., are usually cefoperazone-sensitive. Organisms of the *B. fragilis* group are variable. Some strains are inhibited by low cefoperazone concentrations, but 50% and 90% require 64 and 128 μg per ml, respectively, for inhibition. The drug is about as active as cefotaxime (p. 321), but less active than cefoxitin (p. 295) against the *B. fragilis* group (Rolfe and Finegold, 1981; Muytjens and Van der Ross-van de Repe, 1982; Sutter, 1983).

5 Acquired resistance

In contrast to cefotaxime (p. 320), cefoperazone is more susceptible to ordinary beta-lactamases produced by Gram-negative bacilli, and therefore only has weak activity against some of these strains (Sykes and Bush, 1983). Enterobacteriaceae completely resistant to this drug, are more common than cefotaxime-resistant strains (p. 322). Similar to cefotaxime (p. 322), cefoperazone resistance in Enterobacteriaceae and *Ps. aeruginosa* can arise because of induction of chromosomally mediated beta-lactamases. Similarly any Enterobacteriaceae which have acquired plasmid-mediated extended-spectrum beta-lactamases (p. 323) are cefoperazone resistant.

Cefoperazone is easily destroyed by beta-lactamase(s) produced by the *B. fragilis* group of organisms (Sykes and Bush, 1983). The frequency of resistance to these organisms may increase with more widespread use of the drug. In an early survey in the USA, 33% of strains had MICs higher than 32 μg per ml, and these were considered to be cefoperazone-resistant (Tally *et al.*, 1983). Similar to cefotaxime (p. 321), MICs and MBCs of cefoperazone against *B. fragilis* increase markedly if high inocula are used in sensitivity testing (Yu and Washington, 1983).

C Ceftizoxime

1 Gram-positive bacteria

Staphylococcus aureus and coagulase-negative staphylococci are ceftizoxime-sensitive, except for methicillin-resistant strains. *Streptococcus pyogenes*, *Strep. pneumoniae*, Group B streptococci and *Strep. viridans* are sensitive, but *E. faecalis* is resistant. *Listeria monocytogenes* is only moderately sensitive; *Cl. perfringens* is sensitive but *Cl. difficile* is usually resistant. Activity of ceftizoxime against these organisms is identical to that of cefotaxime (p. 319) (Table I.26) (Fu and Neu, 1980; Greenwood *et al.*, 1980; Barry *et al.*, 1982).

2 Gram-negative cocci

Against *N. meningitidis* and *N. gonorrhoeae*, ceftizoxime is equally potent to cefotaxime. Beta-lactamase producing gonococcal strains are fully ceftizoxime-sensitive (Barry *et al.*, 1982). Non-beta-lactamase producing gonococci, relatively and completely penicillin G-resistant, are also ceftizoxime-sensitive; MICs (0.008–0.03 μg per ml) for completely resistant strains are slightly higher than those for penicillin G-sensitive strains (Table I.26) (Rodrìguez *et al.*, 1983).

3 Gram-negative aerobic bacilli

Ceftizoxime, similar to cefotaxime (p. 320), shows a high degree of stability to beta-lactamases produced by these bacteria (Simpson *et al.*, 1982; Sykes and Bush, 1983). It is highly active against all Enterobacteriaceae, and in this respect it is virtually identical to cefotaxime, there being only minor variations with some bacterial species. Ceftizoxime is slightly more active than cefotaxime against *Klebsiella*, *Enterobacter*, *Providencia* and *Serratia* spp., while *Morganella morganii* is more susceptible to cefotaxime (Fu and Neu, 1980; Greenwood *et al.*, 1980; Barry *et al.*, 1982; Muytjens and Van der Ros-van de Repe, 1982). Ceftizoxime, like cefotaxime, is quite active against *Y. enterocolitica* (Hornstein *et al.*, 1985).

Haemophilus influenzae, including beta-lactamase producing strains, is highly ceftizoxime-sensitive (Barry *et al.*, 1982). *Pasteurella multocida* is sensitive, *Acinetobacter* spp., *Alcaligenes faecalis* and *Moraxella* spp. are moderately sensitive, but *Flavobacterium* spp. are usually resistant (Yabuuchi *et al.*, 1981; Appelbaum *et al.*, 1982; Barry *et al.*, 1982).

Ceftizoxime is about 2-fold less active than cefotaxime against *Ps. aeruginosa* and over 50% of strains are not inhibited by clinically achievable concentrations (Kamimura *et al.*, 1979; Bodey *et al.*, 1981; Barry *et al.*, 1982). *Pseudomonas acidovorans* and *Ps. stutzeri* are ceftizoxime-sensitive, *Burkholderia* (*Pseudomonas*) *cepacia* and *Ps. putida* are relatively resistant and *Ps. fluorescens* and *S. maltophilia* are resistant (Yabuuchi *et al.*, 1981; Appelbaum *et al.*, 1982).

4 Gram-negative anaerobic bacteria

Some of these, such as *Prevotella melaninogenica* and *P. disiens*, are susceptible to low ceftizoxime concentrations. Those of the *B. fragilis* group need higher concentrations for inhibition, but against many strains ceftizoxime is about 2-fold more active than cefotaxime. Despite an enhanced stability to most beta-lactamases, some enzymes produced by *B. fragilis* can hydrolyze ceftizoxime. This is why MICs of ceftizoxime for *B. fragilis* are inoculum dependent. This does not occur with cefoxitin (p. 295), which is virtually resistant to hydrolysis by these beta-lactamases. Some *B. fragilis* strains are highly ceftizoxime-resistant because their beta-lactamases hydrolyze the drug (Eley and Greenwood, 1981; Rolfe and Finegold, 1981; Chow and Finegold, 1982; Neu, 1982c). Conversely, ceftizoxime is active against some cefoxitin-resistant strains of the *B. fragilis* group (Aldridge and Stratton, 1991).

5 Other organisms

Similar to cefotaxime (p. 322), ceftizoxime is highly active against leptospirae *in vitro* (Oie *et al.*, 1983).

D Cefsulodin

Activity against *Ps. aeruginosa* is the most important property of this cephalosporin; some 50% of strains are inhibited by 1 μg per ml or less, and about 90% by 4 μg per ml or less. An increase of inoculum has little effect on these MICs. Cefsulodin is more active than azlocillin (p. 164), piperacillin (p. 164), cefotaxime and cefoperazone against *Ps. aeruginosa*, but ceftazidime (p. 369) shows higher activity (Tsuchiya *et al.*, 1978; Neu and Fu, 1979; King *et al.*, 1980; Gillett, 1982). In a study in Belgium, 90% of *Ps. aeruginosa* strains isolated from cystic fibrosis patients and 90% of those from other chronically infected patients were inhibited by 8.2 and 3.1 μg per ml of cefsulodin, respectively (Gordts *et al.*, 1984). Cefsulodin is active against cefotaxime-resistant *Ps. aeruginosa* strains which harbor induced chromosomally mediated beta-lactamases. This is possibly because cefsulodin, unlike cefotaxime (p. 322), has a very low affinity for these enzymes (Livermore, 1983; Gould and Wise, 1985). However, Gwynn and Rolinson (1983) reported that these *Ps. aeruginosa* strains had reduced sensitivity to cefsulodin if high inocula were used for sensitivity testing.

When *Ps. aeruginosa* is grown in the presence of cefsulodin *in vitro*, resistant strains can be selected which show cross-resistance to carbenicillin and ticarcillin (p.145); this may be because their outer cell membrane has become less permeable to these drugs (Slack and Pitt, 1982). Some *Ps. aeruginosa* strains can become cefsulodin-resistant because they show a significant reduction in affinity for PBP3, which is the principal target for cefsulodin in *Ps. aeruginosa* (Gotoh *et al.*, 1990). Aminoglycoside-resistant strains of *Ps. aeruginosa* are usually cefsulodin-sensitive (Ullmann, 1979; Lerner *et al.*, 1984). When cefsulodin is combined with an aminoglycoside, such as gentamicin, tobramycin or amikacin, it may exhibit *in vitro* synergism against *Ps. aeruginosa* (Slack *et al.*, 1979; Perea *et al.*, 1980; Neu and Scully, 1984).

Cefsulodin is quite active against *Ps. diminuta*, *Ps. paucimobilis*, *Ps. pseudoalcaligenes* and even *S. maltophilia* (King *et al.*, 1980). It is not active against other *Pseudomonas* spp., and it has no clinically useful activity against Enterobacteriaceae and other Gram-negative bacteria (Neu and Fu, 1979; King *et al.*, 1980). Cefsulodin has poor activity against Gram-positive bacteria, and only the staphylococci are inhibited by relatively low concentrations (Tsuchiya *et al.*, 1978; Neu and Scully, 1984).

E Minimum inhibitory concentrations

The MICs of cefotaxime, cefoperazone and ceftizoxime against some selected bacterial species are shown in Table I.26.

Mode of Administration and Dosage

1 Cefotaxime

This is not absorbed after oral administration, and it is administered i.m. or i.v. To reduce pain, it can be administered i.m. with lignocaine which has no effect on its absorption (Esmieu *et al.*, 1980). Individual doses may be given by rapid (3–5 min) i.v. injections; a 1-g dose should be dissolved in 4 ml of sterile water for this purpose. Cefotaxime can be given also as a short

Table I.26

Compiled from data published by Kamimura *et al.* (1979), Neu *et al.* (1979), Neu and Fu (1979), Bulger and Washington (1980), Fu and Neu (1980), Nasu *et al.* (1981), Ahonkhai *et al.* (1982), Barry *et al.* (1982), Jones and Thornsberry (1982), Muytjens and Van der Ros-van de Repe (1982), and Tweardy *et al.* (1983)

Organism	MIC (μg per ml)		
	Cefotaxime	Cefoperazone	Ceftizoxime
Gram-positive bacteria			
Staphylococcus aureus	0.5–8.0	<0.1–>128.0	<0.5–128.0
Staphylococcus epidermidis	3.13–8.0	0.1–>128.0	0.5–>128.0
Streptococcus pyogenes	0.015–0.25	0.01–0.25	<0.01–0.1
Streptococcus pneumoniae	<0.01–0.25	0.12	<0.01–0.25
Streptococcus pneumoniae (relatively penicillin G-resistant)	0.25	1.0	–
Streptococcus pneumoniae penicillin G-resistant)	2.0	2.0	–
Streptococci, Group B	<0.01–0.1	0.01–0.25	<0.01–0.1
Streptococcus viridans	<0.12	0.1–32.0	0.5
Enterococcus faecalis	16.0–200.0	4.0–>128	8.0–>128
Listeria monocytogenes	8.0	16.0	1.6–>100.0
Clostridium perfringens	2.0–4.0	0.5–2.0	1.0–2.0
Gram-negative bacteria			
Escherichia coli	<0.1–8.0	<0.1–>128.0	<0.1–8.0
Enterobacter spp.	<0.01–4.0	0.1–16.0	<0.01–4.0
Klebsiella spp.	<0.1–2.0	<0.1–>128.0	<0.1–2.0
Proteus mirabilis	<0.001–0.5	<0.001–0.5	<0.001–0.5
Proteus vulgaris	<0.01–12.5	0.4–50.0	0.063–12.5
Morganella morganii	0.2–4.0	0.2–>128.0	0.2–4.0
Providencia spp.	<0.01–3.1	0.2–50.0	0.0063–0.05
Salmonella spp.	0.1–0.5	<0.1–128.0	0.1–0.5
Shigella spp.	<0.1–0.5	<0.1–64.0	<0.1–0.5
Serratia marcescens	0.2–>128.0	0.2–>128.0	0.2–>128.0
Neisseria gonorrhoeae	0.0006–0.08	0.005–0.3	0.006–0.08
Neisseria gonorrhoeae (beta-lactamase-producer)	0.0006–0.04	0.005–0.3	0.006–0.08
Neisseria meningitidis	<0.025	<0.01–0.1	<0.01–0.025
Haemophilus influenzae	0.008–0.064	<0.01–0.5	0.01–0.03
Haemophilus influenzae (beta-lactamase-producer)	0.008–0.064	0.03–16.0	<0.01–0.03
Pseudomonas aeruginosa	2.0–>128.0	0.1–50.0	2.0–>200.0
Bacteroides fragilis	2.0–>128.0	32.0–>128.0	0.1–50.0
Prevotella melaninogenica	<0.03–4.0	<0.03–8.0	<0.062–0.5

20–30 min infusion (1–2 g dissolved in 40 ml), or as a prolonged infusion over 4 h (2 g dissolved in 100 ml) (Esmieu *et al.*, 1980; Lüthy *et al.*, 1981; Doluisio, 1982). The drug is therefore given i.v. similarly to penicillin G (p. 20), and all of these methods appear satisfactory.

The total daily adult dose of cefotaxime (i.m. or i.v.) ranges from 2 to 8 g, depending on the nature and severity of the infection, and this is administered in three or four divided doses. For children the dosage is 100–150 mg per kg body weight per day, administered in three or four divided doses (Esmieu *et al.*, 1980; Kafetzis *et al.*, 1981; Kalager *et al.*, 1982). For serious infections, such as bacterial meningitis, the daily dose can be increased to 12 g for adults and to 150–200 mg per kg for children. These high daily dosages are usually given i.v. in four or six divided doses (Cherubin *et al.*, 1982; Corrado *et al.*, 1982; Trang *et al.*, 1985). For the newborn, 50 mg per kg of cefotaxime can be given every 12 h to infants 0–7 days of age and every 8 h to those 7–28 days of age (McCracken *et al.*, 1982b; Baird-Lambert *et al.*, 1984).

In patients with renal failure only minor modification of dosage is necessary. Cefotaxime is excreted in the urine as the active drug (p. 331), but in addition it is metabolized in the body to desacetylcefotaxime (p. 331), and two other metabolites designated M_2 and M_3. In patients with a creatinine clearance >20 ml per min, neither cefotaxime nor its metabolites accumulate in the body after repeated cefotaxime doses (Doluisio, 1982). When the creatinine clearance is <20 ml per min, cefotaxime itself does not accumulate in the serum, but the metabolites M_2 and M_3 show slight accumulation. These metabolites, unlike desacetylcefotaxime (p. 323), are biologically inactive (Reeves et al., 1980). In patients with a creatinine clearance of 5 ml per min, cefotaxime still does not accumulate after repeated doses, but metabolites M_2 and M_3 show significant accumulation, and desacetylcefotaxime (which has antibacterial activity) shows some accumulation. Standard doses of cefotaxime can be given to patients with creatinine clearance values >20 ml per min. Doluisio (1982) suggested that the dose should be halved in patients with a creatinine clearance of <20 ml per min, while Ings et al. (1982) considered that halving the usual dose was only necessary for patients whose creatinine clearance was <5 ml per min. Hemodialysis reduces the half-life of both cefotaxime and desacetylcefotaxime, so that a standard dose of the drug should be administered after this procedure (Todd and Brogden, 1990). In patients undergoing continuous ambulatory peritoneal dialysis, a dose of cefotaxime 2 g i.v. every 12 h or 2 g instillation in the peritoneum every 24 h may be used for the treatment of intraperitoneal infections with highly susceptible organisms (MIC <1.0 μg per ml) (Heim et al., 1986).

In patients over 65 years of age, the changes of pharmacokinetics are not substantive enough to warrant major alterations in either dose or dosing intervals of cefotaxime (Deeter et al., 1990).

Pregnant patients may need higher cefotaxime doses, as the serum levels in these patients of all beta-lactam antibiotics are lower compared with non-pregnant patients (p. 24). This altered pharmacokinetic behavior of cefotaxime and other antibiotics appears to persist into early puerperium (Charles and Larsen, 1986).

There is modest accumulation of cefotaxime in patients with severe liver disease, but this is unlikely to produce toxicity and dosage modification is not usually required (Ko et al., 1991). Prophylactic cefotaxime is often given to patients during and after liver transplantation. Burckart et al. (1987) found that cefotaxime clearance was reduced in these patients and therefore suggested a relatively low dose of 1 g 8-hourly for adults. However, Arnow et al. (1992) used a dose of 2 g i.v. 6-hourly during surgery and then 2 g i.v. 8-hourly thereafter for 48 h and found that this regimen produced serum levels appropriate for prophylaxis.

2 Cefoperazone

The usual adult dosage is 1–2 g, given i.m. or i.v. 12-hourly. For serious infections, the total daily adult dose can be increased to 6–12 g, given in two, three or four divided doses. The dosage for children is 50–100 mg per kg body weight per day, given in two divided doses; for serious infections up to 200 mg per kg per day has been used, administered in two, three or four divided doses. Cefoperazone can be given i.m. dissolved in a 0.5% lignocaine solution. Similar to cefotaxime (see above), individual i.v. doses can be administered over 3–5 min, or infused more slowly over intervals of 30–60 min (Balant et al., 1980; Gordon and Phyfferoen, 1983; Lyon, 1983).

In newborn infants aged 1–7 days, the cefoperazone half-life is prolonged about 3-fold, and a single dose of 50 mg per kg body weight produces high serum levels for 24 h. As cefoperazone is mainly eliminated via the liver (p. 332), prolongation of its half-life is probably due to immaturity of hepatic function in neonates (Rosenfeld et al., 1983). According to Bosso et al. (1983), a 50 mg per kg dose every 12 h may be safe and effective for the treatment of serious infections in newborn and premature infants.

As biliary excretion is the primary route of cefoperazone elimination (p. 332), dosage modification is unnecessary in patients with any degree of renal failure (Balant et al., 1980; Bolton et al., 1981). The serum half-life of cefoperazone is prolonged to 3.4–5.9 h in patients with liver disease compared with 1.6 h in normal subjects. Nevertheless, when cefoperazone is given in a dosage of 1 g 12-hourly to patients with liver disease, there is no accumulation after 3 days; this is because its half-life in such patients is still less than the dosage interval used. With dose intervals of 12 h, little, if any, dosage modification is required in patients with hepatic disease. Major dosage modification may be required only in the presence of concomitant renal and hepatic dysfunction (Boscia et al., 1983; Greenfield et al., 1983).

In pregnant patients and in those in early puerperium, serum levels of cefaperazone are not as low as those of other beta-lactam antibiotics (p. 24). This is because the drug is not primarily excreted by the kidney. Therefore cefoperazone dosage may not need to be greatly increased in these patients (Gonik et al., 1986).

3 Ceftizoxime

Like cefotaxime and cefoperazone, this can only be administered i.m. or i.v. A commonly used dosage for adults is 2–4 g daily, given in two, three or four divided doses. For serious infections a daily dose of 6–12 g has been used (Johnson and Smith, 1982; Parks et al., 1982). For children, the dosage is 50–150 mg per kg body weight per day, given in two, three or four divided doses (Parks et al., 1982; Shikuma et al., 1982). The drug is given i.v. in the same way as cefotaxime.

In clinical trials ceftizoxime was used to treat serious neonatal infections in dosages ranging from 100 to 400 mg per kg per day without encountering toxicity (Parks et al., 1982; Yamauchi et al., 1982). Unlike cefotaxime, ceftizoxime is not metabolized in the body, and its normal serum half-life of 1.4 h is prolonged to some 30 h in anephric patients (Ohkawa et al., 1982). Therefore, in patients with renal failure ceftizoxime dosage should be reduced. Assuming that the usual dosage for normal adults is 1 g 8-hourly, the following dosages have been recommended for patients with renal failure. Patients with mild renal failure (creatinine clearance 70 ml per min) can be given the usual individual 1 g dose 12-hourly. Those with moderately severe renal failure (creatinine clearance 20–30 ml per in) should receive such a dose every 36–48 h, while those with severe renal failure (creatinine clearance <1 ml per min) should be given the normal dose at a time interval greater than 48 h, depending on frequency of hemodialysis (Kowalsky et al., 1983). Ceftizoxime is removed by hemodialysis but supplemental dosage is not always necessary after this procedure (Cutler et al., 1982). Some ceftizoxime is also removed by peritoneal dialysis. In patients with end-stage renal disease undergoing continuous ambulatory peritoneal dialysis, a 3 g i.v. dose of ceftizoxime given once every 48 h is recommended (Burgess and Blair, 1983).

4 Cefsulodin

This can be administered i.m. or i.v. For treatment of *Ps. aeruginosa* urinary tract infections, a dosage of 1 g 12-hourly may suffice. For the treatment of severe systemic *Pseudomonas* infections, daily doses of 6–9 g (100–150 mg per kg body weight per day), administered in three divided doses i.v., have been used (Møller et al., 1982). The dosage given to children has been 60–100 mg per kg per day administered in three or four divided doses (Nishimura and Fujii, 1984). In patients with renal failure cefsulodin dosage should be reduced. There is a linear relationship between the serum clearances of cefsulodin and creatinine clearance. The normal intervals between usual doses of cefsulodin should be prolonged approximately 1.9, 2.5 and 3.7 times for patients with creatinine clearances of 50, 30 and 10 ml per min, respectively (Matzke and Keane, 1983). In anephric patients treated by hemodialysis, only 10% of the usual dose should be used. The drug is removed by hemodialysis, and 30% of a dose of cefsulodin is recovered in the dialysate over 5 h (Lecaillon et al., 1984). Sixty per cent of the usual dose has been recommended after each dialysis (Gibson et al., 1982; 1984). In patients with renal failure, non-renal mechanisms of cefsulodin clearance also seem to be decreased, but the reason for this is uncertain (Matzke and Keane, 1983).

Serum Levels in Relation to Dosage

1 Cefotaxime

After i.m. administration of 1 g to adults, the mean peak serum level of 20.5 μg per ml is reached in 30 min. This level falls to 3.36 μg per ml at 4 h and it still exceeds 1 μg per ml at 6 h. The mean serum half-life of cefotaxime after the administration of a 1-g dose i.m., is 1.34 h (Fu et al., 1979).

If a 1-g dose is given by a 'bolus' i.v. injection over 3 min to adults, the mean serum concentration 5 min after the injection is 86.1 μg per ml. The serum level thereafter falls and adequate therapeutic concentrations only persist for 4–6 h; the half-life after this dose is approximately 1.25 h. After the i.v. injection of 1 g cefotaxime, a maximal mean desacetylcefotaxime (p. 319) level of 16.6 μg per ml is already present 5 min after the injection; the level of this metabolite slowly decreases with a mean half-life of about 1.5 h. After 1–2 h desacetylcefotaxime serum concentrations are equal to, or above, corresponding cefotaxime concentrations (Kemmerich et al., 1983a). Serum levels of desacetylcefotaxime are higher and more prolonged in patients with renal failure due to its delayed renal excretion (p. 331). In patients with severe renal failure (creatinine clearance 3–10 ml per min) the cefotaxime serum half-life is 2.6 h, whilst that of the metabolite is 10 h (Wise et al., 1981b).

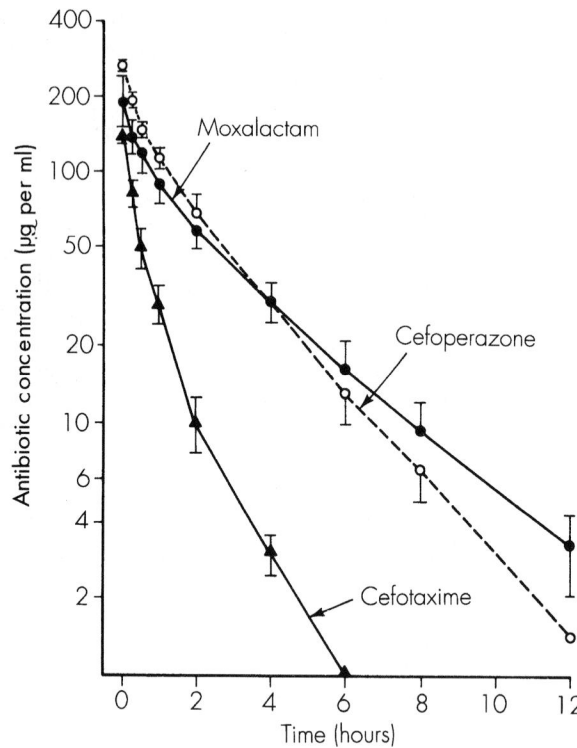

Fig. I.19.

Mean serum levels of moxalactam, cefoperazone and cefotaxime after i.v. doeses of 2 g infused over 30 min, in six normal volunteers. (Redrawn after Standiford *et al.*, 1982, with permission from the University of Chicago Press.)

Standiford *et al.* (1982) compared serum levels of cefotaxime with those of cefoperazone (see below) and moxalactam (p. 350); each drug was given as an i.v. infusion of 2 g over a period of 30 min to adults (Fig. I.19). The levels obtained immediately after the infusion were highest for cefoperazone and lowest for cefotaxime (about 150 μg per ml); 1, 2 and 4 h after the infusion mean serum cefotaxime levels were down to 29, 10 and 3 μg per ml, respectively. By 6 h cefotaxime was undetectable in the serum, its elimination half-life was 1.18 h. After this method of administration the desacetylcefotaxime peak of 10.1 μg per ml was reached between 30–40 min after parent drug administration, at 4 h it was equal to cefotaxime concentration and thereafter its level was slightly higher than that of cefotaxime (Vallee and Le Bel, 1991). Serum levels of cefoperazone and moxalactam were higher than those of cefotaxime at all times and more prolonged (Fig. I.19). The cefoperazone half-life was 1.87 h and that of moxalactam 2.51 h.

In newborn infants, at the completion of a 10 min i.v. infusion of 50 mg per kg body weight of cefotaxime, mean peak levels of 116 and 132 μg per ml occur in low and average birth weight infants, respectively (McCracken *et al.*, 1982b). In neonates, mean peak concentrations of desacetylcefotaxime are about a quarter of those of cefotaxime (Crooks *et al.*, 1984).

2 Cefoperazone

After a 1-g i.m. injection to adults, the mean peak serum level of 65 μg per ml is reached after 1 h; at 8 h the serum concentration falls to 7.2 μg per ml and it is still 1–2 μg per ml at 12 h. The mean half-life of cefoperazone, after a 1-g dose i.m. or i.v., is 1.6 h (Greenfield *et al.*, 1983).

Srinivasan *et al.* (1981) administered 2-g doses to volunteers as a 30 min i.v. infusion. At the end of infusion the mean serum level was 256 μg per ml, and at 1, 4, 6, 8 and 12 h after infusion levels were 108, 20, 11, 4.2 and 0.25 μg per ml, respectively. These results were similar to those obtained by Standiford *et al.* (1982) (Fig. I.19). Serum levels of cefoperazone were higher and more prolonged than those of cefotaxime. Initially, cefoperazone serum levels were also slightly higher than those of moxalactam but after 4 h they were exceeded by those of moxalactam. Cefoperazone produced higher serum levels early because of its smaller volume of distribution in the 'central compartment' of the body. Cefoperazone's smaller distribution may be related to its higher protein binding, which is 90% compared with 50% for moxalactam. Moxalactam had higher concentrations than those of cefoperazone after 4 h, because its longer half-life counterbalanced its larger volume of distribution.

3 Ceftizoxime

The elimination half-life of this drug is approximately 1.4 h, which is shorter than that of cefoperazone (see above), but somewhat longer than that of cefotaxime (p. 330). This means that serum levels of ceftizoxime reached after i.m. and i.v. administration are higher and more sustained than those of cefotaxime, but lower than those of cefoperazone (Quintiliani and Nightingale, 1982).

After i.m. administration of 0.5 g of ceftizoxime to adults, a mean peak serum level of 13.7 μg per ml is attained 1 h later. Thereafter, the level falls and it is 9.2, 4.8, 1.8 and 0.73 μg per ml at 2, 4, 6 and 8 h, respectively (Neu and Srinivasan, 1981). Doubling the i.m. dose to 1 g approximately doubles the serum concentrations (Le Bel et al., 1983).

If 2 g of ceftizoxime is infused i.v. over a 30-min period in adults, the mean peak serum level after the infusion is about 150 μg per ml. The level then falls to 30, 10, 4 and 0.3 μg per ml, at 2, 4, 6 and 8 h after infusion, respectively (Peterson et al., 1982; Quintiliani and Nightingale, 1982). These serum levels are higher and more sustained than those after i.v. infusion of a 2 g dose of cefotaxime (Vallee and Le Bel, 1991), but they are lower than those obtained with cefoperazone (Fig. I.19, p. 330).

4 Cefsulodin

After i.m. administration peak serum levels are attained at 1.5 h, and they are 5.6, 12.7 and 20.1 μg per ml, after doses of 250 mg, 500 mg and 1 g, respectively. Serum levels fall slowly and some cefsulodin (<1 μg per ml) is still detectable 12 h after administration of all three doses. Peak levels attained are approximately in proportion to the dose used. After i.v. infusion of 0.5-g and 1-g doses over 30 min to adults, mean peak serum levels after infusion are 32.7 and 65.5 μg per ml, respectively. Thereafter, levels fall but some cefsulodin is still detectable in the serum 12 h after administration. The cefsulodin half-life, after both i.m. and i.v. administration, is approximately 1.6 h (Granneman et al., 1982).

Excretion

1 Cefotaxime

This is excreted in urine in an active unchanged form by both glomerular filtration and tubular secretion. High levels of active cefotaxime are attained in urine; after a 1-g dose, urine levels in the first 2 h are in the range 150–2178 μg per ml. Probenecid decreases renal clearance by almost 50% by partially blocking tubular secretion. When probenecid is administered concomitantly, cefotaxime serum levels are nearly doubled and also prolonged (Fu et al., 1979; Lüthy et al., 1981).

Some cefotaxime is metabolized in the liver and the major metabolite is desacetylcefotaxime which is antibacterially active (p. 323). This is mainly excreted in urine where it attains high concentrations. In the first 24 h about 60% of an administered dose is excreted in the urine as unchanged cefotaxime, and about 29% as desacetylcefotaxime (Kemmerich et al., 1983a). A small amount of desacetylcefotaxime undergoes further transformation in the liver, prior to urinary excretion, producing in turn desacetylcefotaxime lactone and then two metabolites, designated M_2 and M_3, which do not possess antibacterial activity. In patients with normal renal function, M_2 and M_3 are excreted in urine and are undetectable in serum. They are probably cleared by the kidneys at a greater rate than they are formed. In the urine M_2 and M_3 metabolites each account for approximately 6% of an administered dose of cefotaxime (Reeves et al., 1980; Coombes, 1982), so that virtually all cefotaxime is excreted in the urine either in one form or another. Elimination of the drug via the bile is normally negligible (0.01–0.1%), and biliary levels are only about 2 μg per ml (Soussy et al., 1980). In rats subjected to nephrectomy, there is a slight increase in biliary levels (Coombes, 1982).

In patients with severe renal failure the metabolites of cefotaxime accumulate in serum (p. 328). When the creatinine clearance is <20 ml per min, metabolites M_2 and M_3, which are normally undetectable in serum, start to accumulate. When the creatinine clearance is <5 ml per min, desacetylcefotaxime also accumulates (Doluisio, 1982; Ings et al., 1982). The production of desacetylcefotaxime is reduced in liver disease, but this has only a minor effect on the elimination half-life of cefotaxime in patients with normal renal function, as the non-metabolized drug is quickly excreted by the kidneys (Wise et al., 1981b; Turnidge and Craig, 1983).

2 Cefoperazone

Only 20–30% of an administered dose is excreted in the urine as the unchanged drug. Nevertheless, therapeutic urinary levels of the active drug are achieved; they exceed 25 μg per ml during the first 8 h after a 2-g i.v. dose (Srinivasan *et al.*, 1981; Standiford *et al.*, 1982). Renal excretion of cefoperazone is mainly by glomerular filtration and tubular secretion appears to play a minor role. Concomitant administration of probenecid only causes slight elevation of the serum levels of cefoperazone, and prolongation of its half-life from 92 to 109 min (Shimizu, 1980).

Cefoperazone is metabolized in the body only to a minor extent. The principal metabolite is cefoperazone A, which has an antibacterial activity some 16-fold less than the parent drug. Small amounts of this metabolite are found in human bile (Jones and Barry, 1983b). The major excretory pathway for cefoperazone is via the bile in its active form. In animals, biliary recovery accounts for 79% of an administered dose (Greenfield *et al.*, 1983). In humans probably some 60–80% of the administered dose is excreted via the bile, a percentage higher than for any other available cephalosporin. This may be because cefoperazone has the highest molecular weight (Turnidge and Craig, 1983). It has been difficult to confirm that such a high percentage of the drug is eliminated by bile in humans. Kemmerich *et al.* (1983b) found that 18.5% (range 3.8%-37.5%) of an administered dose was excreted in bile, but these estimations were made in patients with T-tube drainage following biliary surgery, in whom there was still some element of hepatic dysfunction, which would affect biliary excretion. A prolonged half-life and compensatory increase in urine elimination of cefoperazone indicated significant hepatic dysfunction in these patients. Very high peak biliary concentrations of cefoperazone (481–6598 μg per ml) are attained in patients with T-tubes and relatively normal hepatic function (Shimizu, 1980; Greenfield *et al.*, 1983; Kemmerich *et al.*, 1983b). Biliary levels of cefoperazone are about 30-fold higher than those of cefazolin (p. 285). Although high biliary levels of cefoperazone imply significant biliary excretion, the total amount of the drug eliminated by this pathway has not been adequately determined for humans (Greenfield *et al.*, 1983). Biliary tract obstruction stops cefoperazone excretion via the bile, but 24 h after relief of obstruction, passive excretion of the drug in bile occurs, but the active excretion mechanism has not yet recovered (Leung *et al.*, 1990).

Similar to moxalactam (p. 350), cefotetan (p. 396) and cefamandole (p. 306), cefoperazone contains an N-methylthiotetrazole side-chain, which has been implicated as a cause of hypoprothrombinemia (p. 350). This side-chain is split from the antibiotic *in vivo* and cephalosporins which undergo extensive biliary excretion such as cefoperazone are associated with the greatest amount of *in vivo* release of this side-chain. The mechanism by which this side-chain is removed from the body remains unknown (Welage *et al.*, 1990).

3 Ceftizoxime

This drug, unlike cefotaxime (p. 331), is not metabolized in the body; most of an administered dose is excreted via the kidneys by both glomerular filtration and tubular secretion. Probenecid partially blocks renal tubular secretion, thereby delaying excretion and enhancing serum levels by about 50%. High urinary levels of the active drug are attained, which are 700–3200 μg per ml during the first 4 h after an i.m. dose of 0.5 g (Neu and Srinivasan, 1981; Cutler *et al.*, 1982; Le Bel *et al.*, 1983). Urinary recovery of ceftizoxime after parenteral administration, has been reported to be between 70% and 100% (Neu and Srinivasan, 1981; Peterson *et al.*, 1982; Le Bel *et al.*, 1983). Very little ceftizoxime is excreted by non-renal routes in humans. In animals, small amounts are excreted in bile, including an antimicrobially active metabolite, but no such metabolite has been detected in human bile (Murakawa *et al.*, 1980).

4 Cefsulodin

In animal studies, nearly all parenterally administered cefsulodin is excreted in urine within 24 h as the active unchanged drug, with only small amounts appearing in feces via the bile (Tanayama *et al.*, 1978). In humans after i.v. administration, only approximately 60% of the administered dose can be recovered from the urine. High (>100 μg per ml) urinary concentrations of the active drug are attained consistently with a dosage of 250 mg 6-hourly. Urinary clearance of cefsulodin in cystic fibrosis patients, unlike that of some other beta-lactam antibiotics (p. 374), is comparable with that in normal controls (Reed *et al.*, 1984).

Plasma clearance of cefsulodin after i.v. administration averages 140 ml per min, and this is lower than values for other cephalosporins which are partially secreted by renal tubules. Cefsulodin is excreted only by glomerular filtration. *in vitro*, cefsulodin degrades in plasma at room temperature, and *in vivo* a similar process may contribute to plasma clearance. Some degradation may also occur in bladder urine, so the 60% recovery of the administered dose in urine probably represents an underestimate of the total amount of cefsulodin excreted via the kidneys (Granneman *et al.*, 1982).

Distribution of the Drugs in Body

1 Cefotaxime

In animals this drug penetrates poorly into normal CSF, but therapeutically effective concentrations are attained in those with induced bacterial meningitis. In rabbits with meningitis, CSF levels of moxalactam (p. 350) and cefoperazone remain above the MICs for the majority of Gram-negative bacilli for some 5 h after a single dose of each drug; by comparison the CSF level of cefotaxime becomes low in less than 2 h. Of the three drugs, moxalactam produces the greatest concentration in the CSF. Similar to cephalothin (p. 255), it appears that cefotaxime is converted to the less active desacetylcefotaxime (p. 323) by the choroid plexus. But cefotaxime reaches higher CSF concentrations than cephalothin (p. 255). This is probably because cefotaxime and moxalactam, unlike cephalothin, are not removed from the CSF by the exit pump of the choroid plexus (p. 25) (Perfect and Durack, 1981; Schaad et al., 1981; Nolan and Ulmer, 1982). When rabbits with experimental E. coli meningitis were treated by cefotaxime or chloramphenicol both antibiotics reduced the bacterial counts about equally. But cefotaxime (and not chloramphenicol) induced a marked increase of endotoxin in the CSF and also caused an increase of brain water content. The clinical significance of this is not clear (Taüber et al., 1987).

In humans cefotaxime penetrates into uninflamed meninges, but the levels attained are relatively low. When 16 patients without meningitis were given 30 mg per kg cefotaxime i.v., CSF concentrations were in the range of 0.01–0.7 µg per ml (Karimi et al., 1980). When others gave 2 g cefotaxime as a 30-min i.v. infusion to adults with uninflamed meninges, higher CSF concentrations were obtained. Maximum levels were obtained 0.5–8 h after the infusion and ranged from 0.18 to 1.81 µg per ml (Nau et al., 1993). Concentrations of CSF were higher in patients with bacterial meningitis. Belohradsky et al. (1980) gave i.v. cefotaxime to 13 children with bacterial meningitis; CSF levels usually exceeded 1 µg per ml and reached 27.2 µg per ml in one patient. Corrado et al. (1982) successfully treated an adult man with S. marcescens meningitis using cefotaxime 12 g i.v. daily; a CSF level of 5 µg per ml was recorded. Other studies in patients with bacterial meningitis showed a wide range of cefotaxime CSF levels (0.3–30 µg per ml), but they were commonly 1–10 µg per ml, which is 10- to 100-fold greater than MBCs of highly sensitive meningeal pathogens (Cherubin et al., 1982, 1989; Peretti et al., 1984; Asmar et al., 1985). In patients with bacterial meningitis, a mean CSF concentration of desacetylcefotaxime was 5.4 µg per ml. Concentrations of both cefotaxime and this metabolite initially correlated with the degree of meningeal inflammation but the concentrations showed no marked decline by day 10 of treatment, when signs of inflammation had largely resolved (Humbert et al., 1984; Cherubin et al., 1989). Penetration of CSF by cefotaxime and desacetylcefotaxime was evaluated in 13 infants and children with meningitis after the sixth dose of the drug, given in a dosage of 50 mg per kg i.v. 6-hourly. The mean CSF cefotaxime concentration 1 h after the dose was 6.2 µg per ml. The CSF/serum ratios were variable (0–20%), with a mean penetration of 10.1%. The mean peak concentration of desacetylcefotaxime in CSF at the same time was 5.6 µg per ml; its CSF/serum ratios were extremely variable (0–103%), and the mean penetration was 28.8% (Trang et al., 1985). Both cefotaxime and its metabolite penetrated well into brain abscesses, reaching concentrations above MIC for the likely bacteria, except Gram-negative anaerobes (Sjölin et al., 1991).

Cefotaxime penetrates into pleural fluid; after a 1-g i.v. dose, a maximal concentration of abut 7 µg per ml was attained (Lode et al., 1980). Sputum concentrations are relatively low, being in the range 0.18–5.4 µg per ml after doses of 0.75–2.0 g (Lode et al., 1980; Morel et al., 1980). But desacetylcefotaxime concentrations in respiratory secretions are higher, reaching about 77% of mean levels of this metabolite in plasma (Fick et al., 1987). The drug reaches therapeutic concentrations in otitis media effusions (Danon, 1980) and ascitic fluid (Moreau et al., 1980). Cefotaxime attains adequate concentrations in tissue fluid (Wise et al., 1980b; Kalager et al., 1982), and in inflammatory exudates (Scaglione et al., 1990). It is excreted in breast milk and crosses the placenta (Kafetzis et al., 1980). After usual doses, therapeutic concentrations occur in the prostate, uterus, skin, bone, liver, lung and muscle (Novick, 1982). Cefotaxime is 35–40% serum protein bound (Esmieu et al., 1980).

2 Cefoperazone

Similar to cefotaxime this drug does not penetrate into normal CSF to any extent but it does in animals with induced bacterial meningitis (Perfect and Durack, 1981; Schaad et al., 1981; McCracken et al., 1982a). In neonates given a single i.v. dose of 50 mg per kg body weight, CSF levels in those with bacterial meningitis were in the range 2.8–9.5 µg per ml, whereas for those without meningitis this value was 1–7 µg per ml (Rosenfeld et al., 1983). Ten children and five adults with bacterial meningitis were given cefoperazone either as a single dose of 50 mg per kg, a single dose of 100 mg per kg, or three doses of 100 mg per kg 8-hourly. Of 44 CSF samples, only 26 had detectable cefoperazone levels (range <0.8–11.5 µg per ml). Cefoperazone may not reach the CSF of patients with bacterial meningitis as well as other third-generation cephalosporins (Cable et al., 1983).

Cefoperazone penetrates into other body fluids and tissues (Lyon, 1983). After usual therapeutic doses, adequate concentrations were attained in skeletal muscle and surgical wound drainage fluid (Muder et al., 1984). Mean sputum concentrations of 0.08–6.1 µg per ml were detected in patients treated for respiratory tract infections. Adequate levels were reached in ascitic fluid, and the drug crossed the placenta (Shimizu, 1980). After a 2-g i.m. dose, concentration of the drug in pelvic tissue was some 20 µg per g, approximately 3 h later (Bawdon et al., 1982). Cefoperazone is about 90% serum protein bound (Balant et al., 1980).

3 Ceftizoxime

Distribution of this drug in the body is probably similar to that of cefotaxime. It does not penetrate well into normal CSF, but therapeutic levels are found in most patients with bacterial meningitis. Cable et al. (1982) gave single doses of 30 mg per kg by i.v. infusion to 12 patients with bacterial meningitis. Concentrations of CSF 2 h later were 0–17 (mean 4.9) µg per ml. In animals, ceftizoxime reaches therapeutic levels in the kidney, liver, lungs, heart and tissue fluid (Murakawa et al., 1980; Gerding et al., 1982; Van Etta et al., 1983). Serum protein binding of ceftizoxime in humans is 31% (Cutler et al., 1982).

4 Cefsulodin

After a 5 min i.v. bolus administration of 2 g cefsulodin, concentrations greater than the MICs of 90% of Ps. aeruginosa strains are reached in serum, heart valves, subcutaneous tissue and muscle during the operative period in patients undergoing open heart surgery (Daschner et al., 1980). In animals therapeutic concentrations occur in kidney, adrenal gland, lung, heart and liver and interstitial fluid (Tanayama et al., 1978; Landau et al., 1981). Cefsulodin is only 15% bound to serum proteins (Matzke and Keane, 1983).

Mode of Action

This is similar to that of other cephalosporins (p. 256) and penicillin G (p. 25). Enhanced activity of some third-generation cephalosporins against Gram-negative bacteria is due to their resistance to destruction by beta-lactamases, and their high affinity for penicillin binding proteins (PBPs) (p. 27). For instance, cefotaxime and ceftizoxime bind to PBPs 1a, 1b and 3 of E. coli at lower concentrations than many other cephalosporins. Binding to PBP 3 causes filamentation prior to cell death, or alternatively binding to PBP 1a and 1b may lead to rapid lysis and death of bacteria (Curtis et al., 1979; Neu, 1982a and c; 1983). Bacteroides fragilis appears to have only three PBPs, and cefotaxime binds to all of them (Botta et al., 1983).

Cefoperazone induces filamentation and eventually cell death in E. coli and Ps. aeruginosa. This is consistent with its high affinity for PBP 3 in both of these organisms. It also has high affinities for PBPs 1b, 2 and 1a of E. coli and PBP 1a of Ps. aeruginosa. Cefoperazone has somewhat lower affinities for PBPs of Ps. aeruginosa than for PBPs of E. coli, except for PBP 3. The incubation time for cell lysis is longer with Ps. aeruginosa than with E. coli (Matsubara et al., 1980). Cefsulodin has a high affinity for PBPs of Ps. aeruginosa, but binds poorly to those of other bacteria (Neu and Scully, 1984).

Toxicity

1 Cefotaxime

Its side-effects are similar to those of other cephalosporins (p. 256). Maculopapular, and less commonly urticarial rashes, have occurred in about 2% of treated patients (Young et al., 1980; Kalager et al., 1982; Smith, 1982). Cefotaxime, like cephalothin (p. 256), is probably only infrequently cross-allergenic with the penicillins. Transient eosinophilia and/or a positive Coombs' test without hemolysis, may occur with cefotaxime as with other cephalosporins (p. 257) (Schleupner and Engle, 1982; Smith, 1982). Transient elevations of SGOT and/or serum alkaline phosphatase have been noted in a few patients (McKendrick et al., 1981; Smith, 1982). One patient developed possible drug-induced hepatitis (Keaney et al., 1982). Diarrhea has been attributed occasionally to parenteral use of the drug, and pseudomembranous colitis (p. 594) has been reported in a small number of patients (Karakusis *et al.*, 1982; Meyers, 1982; Smith, 1982; Golledge *et al.*, 1989). The third-generation cephalosporins, including cefotaxime, even when administered as short-term perioperative prophylaxis, are associated with *Cl. difficile*-related diseases (de Lalla *et al.*, 1989). Intravenous administration of cefotaxime changes the fecal flora in normal volunteers. There is usually an increase of enterococci and yeasts and sometimes also cefotaxime-resistant Gram-negative aerobic bacilli (Vollaard *et al.*, 1990).

In animals nephrotoxicity is minimal and it is not aggravated by frusemide and aminoglycosides, such as gentamicin (Doerr *et al.*, 1982; Luft *et al.*, 1982). Some deterioration of renal function, possibly related to cefotaxime, has only occurred in 1.4% of treated patients (Smith, 1982).

Hallucinations, vertigo, or disorientation occurred in 0.3% of 2,157 treated patients but epileptic seizures or myoclonus have not been reported. Other rare side-effects include reversible neutropenia and thrombocytopenia (Smith, 1982). Cefotaxime, like other beta-lactam antibiotics inhibits ADP-induced platelet aggregation (p. 153), but this only occurs with very high serum levels (Bang and Kammer, 1983). Hypoprothrombinemia, which occurs with cefamandole (p. 306), cefoperazone and moxalactam (p. 350), has not been reported with cefotaxime (Smith, 1982; Smith and Lipsky, 1983). The drug does not provoke a disulfiram-like reaction (see below) (Smith, 1982; Parker and Park, 1984). *In vitro* cefotaxime enhances the bactericidal activity of human neutrophils against *Staph. aureus*, but not phagocytosis (Labro *et al.*, 1986).

Jacobs *et al.* (1992) evaluated the safety profile of 2243 cases of hospitalized children treated with cefotaxime. Overall 57 (2.5%) of children experienced adverse reactions. There were local reactions in six (0.3%), rash in 28 (1.2%), diarrhea in 15 (0.97%), vomiting in ten (0.7%), headache in three (0.4%) and drug fever in one (0.1%). It was concluded that cefotaxime was a safe drug for children.

2 Cefoperazone

Similar to other cephalosporins (p. 256), allergic rashes occasionally occur (Gordon and Phyfferoen, 1983). Diarrhea follows parenteral cefoperazone therapy more commonly than after other parenteral cephalosporins (File *et al.*, 1982; 1983; Gordon and Phyfferoen, 1983). In one study, diarrhea occurred in 12 of 52 patients treated with cefoperazone, and in five *Cl. difficile* and its toxin was found in the feces; in another 11 stools were looser than normal and *Cl. difficile* and its toxin were present in three (Carlberg *et al.*, 1982). Cefoperazone therapy is associated with major changes in fecal flora. There is suppression of anaerobic cocci, Gram-negative anaerobes and Enterobacteriaceae, and acquisition of enterococci, *Candida* spp. and in some patients *Cl. difficile* (Mulligan *et al.*, 1982; Alestig *et al.*, 1983). This is because the drug is excreted mainly through the bile into the gut (p. 332).

Like cefotaxime (see above), the nephrotoxic potential of cefoperazone appears to be low, and it has been used with furosemide or aminoglycosides, such as gentamicin, without encountering renal toxicity (Trollfors *et al.*, 1982; Gordon and Phyfferoen, 1983). In common with cefamandole (p. 306) and moxalactam (p. 350), cefoperazone contains an N-methylthiotetrazole side-chain, and it may cause hypoprothrombinemia and bleeding, particularly in elderly malnourished, vitamin K-deficient patients. Administration of parenteral vitamin K may prevent this complication (Carlberg *et al.*, 1982; Smith and Lipsky, 1983; Gordon and Phyfferoen, 1983). In one patient reported by Parker *et al.* (1984), cefoperazone caused coagulopathy and clinical bleeding despite prior administration of i.v. vitamin K. Cefoperazone can inhibit ADP-induced platelet aggregation (p. 153), but this only occurs with very high serum levels (Bang and Kammer, 1983).

As cefoperazone, like cefamandole (p. 306) and moxalactam (p. 350), has a N-methylthiotetrazole side-chain, it can cause a disulfiram-like reaction (p. 306) if alcoholic beverages are ingested during, or several days after cessation of its administration (Buening and Wold, 1982). Mild elevations of SGOT levels have occasionally been noted (Carlberg *et al.*, 1982). Eosinophilia, reversible neutropenia and a positive direct Coombs' test have been reported (Strausbaugh and Llorens, 1983; Warren *et al.*, 1983). Cefoperazone inhibits neutrophil chemotaxis *in vitro*, but the clinical significance of this is not known (Fietta *et al.*, 1983). Cephalosporins with N-methylthiotetrazole side-chain, such as cefoperazone, have shown adverse effects in the testes of neonatal rats (Lipsky, 1986).

3 Ceftizoxime

In clinical trials side-effects have been mild and infrequent and are similar to those of most other cephalosporins (p. 256). These include hypersensitivity rashes, eosinophilia, drug fever and transient elevations of SGOT and serum alkaline phosphatase. Elevated platelet counts (thrombocytosis) occur not infrequently during ceftizoxime therapy. These are not associated with symptoms and counts revert to normal after the drug is stopped. Reversible thrombocytopenia and neutropenia are less frequent. Some patients develop a positive Coombs' test. Diarrhea, nausea and vomiting are infrequent. *Clostridium difficile* toxin was detected in the feces of one patient who developed diarrhea on day 14 of ceftizoxime treatment. Transient elevations of blood urea and serum creatinine levels occur in some patients, but serious nephrotoxicity has not been encountered (Counts *et al.*, 1982; Parks *et al.*, 1982).

4 Cefsulodin

Clinical experience with this drug is limited. Twenty patients with cystic fibrosis and chronic pulmonary *Ps. aeruginosa* infection, were given cefsulodin 100–150 mg per kg body weight per day i.v., in three divided doses. Most patients complained of dizziness, nausea and mild abdominal cramps which occurred at the time of i.v. administration. One patient developed impaired vestibular function, which was still present 11 weeks after cessation of treatment. Cefsulodin used singly was not associated with nephrotoxicity, but a few patients treated with a cefsulodin/tobramycin combination developed reversible rises in blood urea values (Møller *et al.*, 1982).

Clinical Uses of the Drugs

Third-generation cephalosporins with a broad spectrum of antimicrobial activity, such as cefotaxime, cefoperazone and ceftizoxime, are effective for a wide range of infections caused by both Gram-positive and Gram-negative bacteria. Nevertheless, they are not the drugs of choice for many of such infections, which respond to older, cheaper and more narrow-spectrum drugs. These include those caused by Gram-positive bacteria and common community-acquired Gram-negative infections, such as pyelonephritis and cholecystitis (Gleckman and Gantz, 1982).

A Cefotaxime

1 Bacterial meningitis

Cefotaxime and ceftriaxone (p. 359) are now prime drugs for the treatment of bacterial meningitis. Cefotaxime has achieved a cure rate of over 90% for meningitis due to *Strep. pneumoniae*, *N. meningitidis* and *H. influenzae* (Lapointe *et al.*, 1984; Jacobs *et al.*, 1985). For initial treatment before the organism is identified and also for continuation treatment for meningitis due to these pathogens cefotaxime is about as effective as penicillin G (or ampicillin) combined with chloramphenicol (Cherubin and Eng, 1986; Odio *et al.*, 1986; Feldstein *et al.*, 1987; Peltola *et al.*, 1989). Penicillin G (or ampicillin) plus chloramphenicol (conventional therapy) is now used less and less in developed countries and third-generation cephalosporins such as cefotaxime or ceftriaxone are regarded as the best drugs. Whilst in 1987 in the USA the use of conventional therapy was still extensively used (McCracken *et al.*, 1987); 2 years later cefotaxime was used more frequently (Word and Klein, 1989) and by 1992 cefotaxime (or ceftriaxone) had become the drugs of choice (Klass and Klein, 1992).

Cefotaxime alone is suitable for initial therapy for bacterial meningitis in children 3 months to 18 years old and for otherwise healthy adults 18–50 years old (Lecour *et al.*, 1984; Tunkel *et al.*, 1990; Klass and Klein, 1992). For meningococcal meningitis, once organism is identified, it is logical to change to penicillin G, but as the recommended treatment course is short (7 days or even less) many continue cefotaxime for the entire course. Meningococcal strains, moderately resistant to penicillin G (p. 13) are fully susceptible to cefotaxime, ceftriaxone and chloramphenicol (Blondeau and Yaschuk, 1995), so cefotaxime is a suitable drug if a strain of this type is involved. Cefotaxime is continued for the entire course for *H. influenzae* meningitis (usually 10 days), as it is the drug of choice and it is effective for infection by *H. influenzae* strains resistant to ampicillin and chloramphenicol (Givner *et al.*, 1989; Valleyo *et al.*, 1991; The Research Committee, 1995).

Pneumococcal meningitis should be treated for 14 days, so after identification of organism it is logical to change to the cheaper penicillin G, provided the pneumococcus is completely sensitive to it. Some cases of meningitis due to *Strep. pneumoniae* with intermediate degree of resistance to penicillin G (p. 5) can be treated by cefotaxime, but some strains of *Strep. pneumoniae* with this type of resistance, may have even higher MICs for cefotaxime (p. 320) and so vancomycin is the drug of choice. In one case in which the MIC of cefotaxime for the pneumococcus was 2 µg per ml, the treatment failed with this drug and 6 days later the MIC was >2 µg per ml; it is possible that with exposure to cefotaxime this organism's resistance increased *in vivo.* Cefotaxime or ceftriaxone (p. 359) treatment is only likely to succeed if the pneumococcal strain's MICs for these drugs is 0.5 μg per ml or less (John, 1994). Others have made different recommendations. Leggiadro *et al.* (1994) and Thompson *et al.* (1994) suggested that cefotaxime or ceftriaxone can only be used if their MICs for the pneumococcus are 0.25 μg per ml or less. Tan *et al.* (1994) considered that pneumococcal meningitis will respond to these cephalosporins if their MICs of the strain are 1.0 μg per ml or less. But Catalán *et al.* (1994) reported a patient where cefotaxime failed for the treatment of pneumococcal meningitis, when the MIC of cefotaxime for the pneumococcal strain was 1 μg per ml.

If very high doses of cefotaxime are used, such as 200–300 mg per kg per day (maximum 24 g daily), pneumococcal meningitis is usually cured even if the MIC of the *Strep. pneumoniae* strain is as high as 2.0 μg per ml. However, it is recommended that if the MIC is ≥2 μg per ml, cefotaxime should not be used alone (Jacobs *et al.*, 1996; Viladrich *et al.*, 1996). In such cases vancomycin (p. 779) should be added to cefotaxime therapy (Tunkel *et al.*, 1990; Weingarten *et al.*, 1990). High dosage cefotaxime, such as 24 g daily for adults may cause neurotoxicity (p. 32).

If patients in these age groups are immunosuppressed, at least penicillin G should be added to cefotaxime initially to cover the possibility of *L. monocytogenes* infection.

For neonates (first 4 weeks of age), the conventional therapy of penicillin G (or ampicillin) plus an aminoglycoside can be used, but most now favor ampicillin plus cefotaxime. The organisms to be covered initially include *E. coli* and other Gram-negative rods, Group B streptococci, *E. faecalis* and *L. monocytogenes* (McCracken *et al.*, 1987; Tunkel *et al.*, 1990; Klass and Klein, 1992). Some prefer adding an aminoglycoside also to the latter regimen initially, as some Gram-negative rods may be cefotaxime-resistant (Francis and Gilbert, 1992; De Louvois, 1994). Once the organism is identified cefotaxime is the treatment for Gram-negative bacillary meningitis and penicillin G or ampicillin for meningitis due to the Gram-positive bacteria. Neonatal meningitis should be treated for about 3 weeks.

In children 4–12 weeks of age, the commonest organisms causing meningitis are the classical *N. meningitidis*, *H. influenzae* and *Strep. pneumoniae*, but meningitis due to *L. monocytogenes* still occurs, so cefotaxime should not be used alone for initial therapy, but it should be combined with penicillin G or ampicillin (McCracken *et al.*, 1987; Tunkel *et al.*, 1990).

In adults older than 50 years *Strep. pneumoniae* and *N. meningitidis* are the usual causal organisms for meningitis, but *L. monocytogenes* and Gram-negative Enterobacteriaceae are causes in some cases, so cefotaxime should be combined with penicillin G or ampicillin for initial therapy (Tunkel *et al.*, 1990).

The third-generation cephalosporins such as cefotaxime or ceftriaxone (p. 359) have gradually replaced chloramphenicol for treatment of meningitis because they are equally effective. There are now also chloramphenicol-resistant *H. influenzae* strains in some parts of the world (p. 552) and chloramphenicol may have serious side-effects (p. 563). The second-generation cephalosporin, cefuroxime has been gradually used less and less, because it is marginally less effective than cefotaxime or ceftriaxone (p. 310). In developing countries chloramphenicol is still widely used because of cost considerations.

Cefotaxime or ceftriaxone now also have become prime drugs for treatment of Gram-negative bacillary meningitis e.g. that caused by Enterobacteriaceae. In neonates it is about equally as effective as ampicillin/aminoglycoside combination (McCracken, 1984; 1985; Naqvi *et al.*, 1985; Nelson, 1985). However, in adults and older children with Gram-negative meningitis, cefotaxime produces superior results than former regimens consisting of chloramphenicol or an aminoglycoside (Corrado *et al.*, 1982; Rahal and Simberkoff 1982; Mullaney and John, 1983). The results are always good in *E. coli* and *Klebsiella* spp. meningitis (Tunkel *et al.*, 1990; Tang and Chen, 1994). Results are also generally satisfactory in meningitis caused by other Enterobacteriaceae, but with those which possess inducible chromosomally mediated beta-lactamases (p. 322), *in vivo* development of resistance may occur with consequent treatment failure. This has happened in *S. marcescens* meningitis (Eng *et al.*, 1987), but most commonly with *Enterobacter* spp. meningitis (Eng *et al.*, 1987; Ralph and Behme, 1987). With Enterobacter spp. meningitis relapses have been so frequent that some authors now recommend the use of co-trimoxazole for this meningitis rather than cefotaxime (Wolff *et al.*, 1993).

Cefotaxime is not suitable for *Ps. aeruginosa* meningitis, for which ceftazidime/aminoglycoside combination may be satisfactory (Tunkel *et al.*, 1990), but cefotaxime with or without an aminoglycoside appears suitable for *Aeromonas* spp. meningitis (Parras *et al.*, 1993).

Cefotaxime plus metronidazole can also be used to treat a brain abscess (Sjölin *et al.*, 1993) but other regimens are available such as penicillin G/metronidazole (p. 948) and penicillin G/chloramphenicol (p. 569).

2 Other serious H. influenzae infections, such as septicemia, epiglottitis, pneumonia, septic arthritis and osteomyelitis

These all respond well to cefotaxime therapy. *H. influenzae* septicemia and pneumonia in AIDS patients also respond (Mullaney and John, 1982).

3 Gram-negative (usually nosocomial pneumonia)

Cefotaxime is valuable for this indication, especially if it is caused by organisms resistant to first-generation cephalosporins, amoxycillin and aminoglycosides (Scheld, 1989; Garber *et al.*, 1992). Nosocomial pneumonia in cancer patients with adequate granulocyte counts sometimes responds poorly especially if it is polymicrobial (Rolston *et al.*, 1985). Cefotaxime i.v. together with topically applied drugs such as endotracheal gentamicin, pharyngeal and tracheal polymyxin B and others has also been used to prevent pneumonia in critically ill patients, such as those in intensive care units. Routine clinical use of this probably should be discouraged, but further study is warranted, documenting carefully the emergence of drug-resistant organisms and cost-benefits (Hamer and Barza, 1993).

4 Gram-negative organism infection including septicemia in neutropenic patients

The drug has proved valuable for septicemia and endocarditis caused by these organisms in non-neutropenic patients. These infections are often hospital acquired (Armengaud *et al.*, 1980; Karakusis *et al.*, 1982; Meyers, 1982; Saito *et al.*, 1989; Watanakunakorn, 1989). Septicemia due to *Edwardsiella* spp. usually responds to cefotaxime (Janda and Abbott, 1993), but septicemia due to *Y. enterocolitica* does not respond to the drug in spite of the *in vitro* sensitivity of the organism (Scavizzi *et al.*, 1987). One case of endocarditis caused by a beta-lactamase-producing strain of *N. flavescens* responded to cefotaxime (Sinave and Ratzan, 1987). For febrile neutropenic patients a cefotaxime/amikacin regimen was unsatisfactory, compared with azlocillin/amikacin (Klastersky *et al.*, 1986). Given the frequency of *Ps. aeruginosa* septicemia in these patients, cefotaxime is not suitable for this indication, and a beta-lactam antibiotic with good antipseudomonal activity, such as ticarcillin (p. 156), piperacillin (p. 174), azlocillin (p. 174) or ceftazidime (p. 377) should be included in the regimen (Neu, 1987).

5 Systemic Salmonella spp. infections

Given that in some areas in the world salmonellae, including *Salm. typhi*, are now resistant to chloramphenicol (p. 550), amoxycillin (p. 136) and co-trimoxazole (p. 841), the third-generation cephalosporins have been investigated for the therapy of these infections (Bryan *et al.*, 1986; Cherubin *et al.*, 1986). In one trial cefotaxime cured 12 patients with typhoid/paratyphoid fever, nine with non-typhoid *Salmonella* bacteremia, and two with *Salmonella* meningitis (Soe and Overturf, 1987). Similarly Lepage *et al.* (1990) found cefotaxime to be satisfactory treatment for children with systemic infections by multiresistant *Salm. typhimurium*. Ceftriaxone is also satisfactory for these infections and there seems to be more clinical experience with this drug than with cefotaxime (p. 360). Quinolones such as ciprofloxacin (p. 1016) are also effective.

6 Pyelonephritis

If a Gram-negative bacillus causing this is resistant to older and cheaper drugs such as amoxycillin (p. 136) or co-trimoxazole (p. 540), cefotaxime may be useful for complicated upper urinary tract infections (Todd and Brogden, 1990).

7 Osteomyelitis and septic arthritis

Chronic osteomyelitis caused by Gram-negative bacilli responds satisfactorily to cefotaxime. Results are also usually satisfactory in mixed infections with Gram-positive cocci, provided one of the latter is not a methicillin-resistant *Staph. aureus* (Le Frock and Carr, 1982; Gentry, 1988; Gomis *et al.*, 1990). One patient with septic arthritis caused by *Corynebacterium xerosis* (penicillin G-sensitive) was treated successfully by cefotaxime. The patient was allergic to penicillin (Booth *et al.*, 1991).

8 Gonorrhea

A single-dose cefotaxime, 0.5 g i.m. is effective for the treatment of uncomplicated genital or anal gonococcal infections (Judson *et al.*, 1991; CDC, 1993; McCormack *et al.*, 1993). Centers for Disease control currently favor a single i.m. dose of 125 or 250 mg ceftriaxone for this disease (p. 361). A course of cefotaxime 1 g i.v. every 8 h is effective for disseminated gonococcal infections. This regimen should be continued for 24–48 h after improvement begins, then therapy can be changed to oral cefixime (p. 412) or ciprofloxacin (p. 1022) to complete 7 days of antimicrobial therapy (CDC, 1993).

9 Neonatal necrotizing enterocolitis

In one trial a cefotaxime/vancomycin regimen proved superior to ampicillin plus gentamicin for the treatment of this disease (Scheifele et al., 1987).

10 Lyme neuroborreliosis

The most frequent neurological manifestations of Lyme disease (p. 48) are meningitis, cranial neuritis, and painful radiculoneuritis. In addition there may be myelitis, encephalitis, cerebral arteritis or chronic peripheral neuropathy. A 10-day treatment by cefotaxime 2 g i.v. 8-hourly or ceftriaxone 2 g i.v. every 24 h was definitely beneficial to these patients, but some patients were still symptomatic at follow-up later, so prolongation of treatment may be necessary (Pfister et al., 1991; Weber and Pfister, 1994). Most now regard ceftriaxone as the drug of choice for this disease (p. 362).

11 Surgical chemoprophylaxis

Hargreave et al. (1982) used a 48 h course of cefotaxime to effectively reduce infective episodes after prostatic surgery. Cefotaxime was also satisfactory as a single-dose prophylaxis for vaginal hysterectomy (Bräutigam et al., 1988). A single-dose cefotaxime plus metronidazole was also efficacious as chemoprophylaxis in colorectal surgery (Rowe-Jones et al., 1990; Davey et al., 1992). Before broad spectrum third-generation cephalosporins, such as cefotaxime, are used for chemoprophylaxis, there should be convincing evidence that they are superior to older cheaper narrow spectrum first-generation cephalosporins, such as cephalothin (p. 259) or cefazolin (p. 287), or the second-generation cephalosporin cefamandole (p. 308). In general, prophylactic antibiotics should be inexpensive, non-toxic, and effective against major pathogens likely to be encountered in the operative area (Hirschmann and Inui, 1980). Broad spectrum third-generation cephalosporins are usually unnecessary for this purpose (Gleckman and Gantz, 1982). Seventeen published studies were surveyed to evaluate the use of parenteral prophylactic cephalosporins in surgery. The use of third-generation cephalosporins resulted in no less postoperative infections than prophylaxis with first-generation drugs (Di Piro et al., 1984).

12 Penicillin G-resistant pneumococcal endocarditis

In an animal experimental endocarditis two strains of Strep. pneumoniae were used. Their MICs for penicillin G were 1.0 and 4 µg per ml. Their corresponding MICs for cefotaxime were 0.01 and 0.5 µg per ml. Cefotaxime was successful in eradicating the endocarditis due to both strains, provided dosages used were high and serum levels achieved were similar to those normally attained in humans with i.v. cefotaxime. Such serum levels exceeded the MICs of these strains by more than 100-fold (Guerrero et al., 1994).

13 Inactivation of aminoglycosides

Cefotaxime, unlike carbenicillin (p. 155) and ticarcillin (p. 157), does not cause in vitro inactivation of the aminoglycosides, gentamicin, tobramycin and amikacin (Jorgensen and Crawford, 1982; Glew and Pavuk, 1983).

B Cefoperazone

Because better antibiotics are now available for treatment of Ps. aeruginosa infections and because cefotaxime and ceftriaxone are more effective for infections caused by Enterobacteriaceae, cefoperazone is now infrequently used. It also has the side-effect of hypoprothrombinemia (p. 335). Cefoperazone is effective in Ps. aeruginosa infections (File and Tan, 1983; Jewett et al., 1985), but more effective drugs such as ceftazidime (p. 377) are now preferred. Cefoperazone/netilmicin is not as effective treatment as mezlocillin/netilmicin for febrile neutropenic patients (Sage et al., 1988). In one trial cefoperazone was as effective as ceftriaxone for the treatment of nosocomial pneumonia (Mangi et al., 1992), but in general if a third-generation cephalosporin is needed for H. influenzae infections or infections caused by Enterobacteriaceae, the more effective cefotaxime or ceftriaxone are preferred.

High biliary concentrations attained with cefoperazone, suggested that it could be valuable for treatment of biliary tract infections. Mashimo (1981) obtained good results in 116 patients who had cholecystitis, cholangitis and liver abscess. Bergeron et al. (1988) found cefoperazone to be an excellent antibiotic in the therapy of biliary tract infections, but in patients with biliary tract obstruction, preoperative biliary levels of cefoperazone may be low (p. 322); in addition, the control of associated septicemia is more important than sterilization of bile in this situation (p. 125).

C Ceftizoxime

Clinical experience with this drug is more limited than that with cefotaxime (p. 336), but the two drugs are very similar and so the potential clinical uses of them may be much the same. Ceftizoxime has been used with success in severe hospital-acquired infections caused by the Enterobacteriaceae, such as pyelonephritis, pneumonia and septicemia (Bechard, 1982; Cohen and Mogabgab, 1982; Scully and Neu, 1982). Ceftizoxime is more active *in vitro* than cefotaxime against some Enterobacteriaceae (p. 325), and the drug has appeared especially useful for treatment of *Serratia* infections (Counts *et al.*, 1982).

Ceftizoxime has not been adequately evaluated for bacterial meningitis caused by Enterobacteriaceae. Adequate CSF concentrations of the drug are reached in patients with meningitis (p. 334). A small number of patients with meningitis caused by pneumococci, meningococci and *H. influenzae* type b have been cured by i.v. ceftizoxime in a dose of 200 mg per kg body weight per day (Cable *et al.*, 1982; Overturf *et al.*, 1984). Ceftizoxime has been quite effective in the treatment of other severe *H. influenzae* infections in both adults and children (Parks *et al.*, 1982).

Lou *et al.* (1982) found ceftizoxime satisfactory for the treatment of 119 patients with peritonitis. This drug is more active than cefotaxime against *B. fragilis* (p. 326), and it may have a place for the treatment of intra-abdominal sepsis. In one randomized study, ceftizoxime in large dosage (3 g i.v. 8-hourly) was equally effective to a clindamycin/tobramycin combination for the treatment of intra-abdominal and female genital tract infections (Harding *et al.*, 1984).

Uncomplicated genital gonorrhea responds well to a single 0.5–1.0 g i.m. dose of ceftizoxime without probenecid. It is effective for infections caused by beta-lactamase-producing strains (Lutz *et al.*, 1982; Spencer *et al.*, 1984). The value of ceftizoxime in gonorrhea is comparable with that of cefotaxime (p. 338).

D Cefsulodin

This is only potentially useful for the treatment of *Ps. aeruginosa* infections. Despite its low MIC against *Ps. aeruginosa* (p. 326), the drug was not superior to ticarcillin (p. 156) for the treatment of *Ps. aeruginosa* pneumonia in guinea pigs (Pennington *et al.*, 1982). Cefsulodin was tried in 20 patients with cystic fibrosis and chronic pulmonary *Ps. aeruginosa* infection, in an i.v. dosage of 100–150 mg per kg body weight per day given in three divided doses. Clinical improvement was marked in most patients, and in five, *Ps. aeruginosa* disappeared from bronchial secretions (Møller *et al.*, 1982). Other authors have also found cefsulodin clinically effective in these infections (Cabezudo *et al.*, 1984; Caplan and Buchanan, 1984). Cefsulodin has been used with some success for the treatment of other *Ps. aeruginosa* infections, such as chronic osteomyelitis (Pottage *et al.*, 1984), urinary tract infections (Elder and Roy, 1984) and *Ps. aeruginosa* infections in children, such as septicemia, pneumonia and pyelonephritis (Nishimura and Fujii, 1984).

References

Ahonkhai VI, Sierra MF, Cherubin CE, Shulman MA (1982). The comparative activities of N-formimidoyl thienamycin (MK 0787)., moxalactam, cefotaxime and cefoperazone against *Yersinia enterocolitica* and *Listeria monocytogenes*. *J Antimicrob Chemother* **9**: 411.

Aldridge KE, Stratton CW (1991). Bactericidal activity of ceftizoxime, cefotetan and clindamycin against cefoxitin-resistant strains of *Bacteroides fragilis* group. *J Antimicrob Chemother* **28**: 701.

Aldridge KE, Sanders CV, Marier RL (1984). *In vitro* synergy and potentiation between cefotaxime and desacetylcefotaxime against clinical isolates of *Bacteroides*. *Diagn Microbiol Infect Dis* **2**: 47S.

Alestig K, Carlberg H, Nord CE, Trollfors B (1983). Effect of cefoperazone on faecal flora. *J Antimicrob Chemother* **12**: 163.

Amyes SGB, Baird DR, Crook DW *et al.* (1994). A multicentre study of the *in-vitro* activity of cefotaxime, cefuroxime, ceftazidime, ofloxacin and ciprofloxacin against blood and urinary pathogens. *J Antimicrob Chemother* **34**: 639.

Andersen BM, Sørlie D, Hotvedt R *et al.* (1989). Multiply beta-lactam resistant *Enterobacter cloacae* infections linked to the environmental

flora in a unit for cardiothoracic and vascular surgery. *Scand J Infect Dis* **21**: 181.

Andresen J, Asmar BI, Dajani AS (1994). Increasing *Enterobacter* bacteremia in pediatric patients. *Pediatr Infect Dis J* **13**: 787.

Appelbaum PC, Tamim J, Stavitz J *et al.* (1982). Sensitivity of 341 non-fermentative Gram-negative bacteria to seven beta-lactam antibiotics. *Eur J Clin Microbiol* **1**: 159.

Armengaud M, Massip P, Aubertin J *et al.* (1980). Cefotaxime in the treatment of septicaemia and endocarditis. *J Antimicrob Chemother* **6** (Suppl A): 263.

Arnow PM, Furmaga K, Flaherty JP, George D (1992). Microbiological efficacy and pharmacokinetics of prophylactic antibiotics in liver transplant patients. *Antimicrob Ag Chemother* **36**: 2125.

Asmar BI, Thirumoorthi MC, Buckley JA *et al.* (1985). Cefotaxime diffusion into cerebrospinal fluid of children with meningitis. *Antimicrob Ag Chemother* **28**: 138.

Baird-Lambert J, Doyle PE, Thomas D *et al.* (1984). Pharmacokinetics of cefotaxime in neonates. *J Antimicrob Chemother* **13**: 471.

Baker CN, Thornsberry C, Jones RN (1980). *In vitro* antimicrobial activity of cefoperazone, cefotaxime, moxalactam (LY 127935)., azlocillin, mezlocillin, and other beta-lactam antibiotics against *Neisseria gonorrhoeae* and *Haemophilus influenzae*, including beta-lactamase-producing strains. *Antimicrob Ag Chemother* 17: 757.

Balant L, Dayer P, Rudhardt M et al. (1980). Cefoperazone: pharmacokinetics in humans with normal and impaired renal function and pharmacokinetics in rats. *Clin Ther* (Special issue) 3: 50.

Bang NU, Kammer RB (1983). Hematologic complications associated with beta-lactam antibiotics. *Rev Infect Dis* 5 (Suppl 2): 380.

Barry AL, Jones RN, Thornsberry C (1981). Cefsulodin: antibacterial activity and tentative interpretative zone standards for the disc susceptibility test. *Antimicrob Ag Chemother* 20: 525.

Barry AL, Jones RN, Thornsberry C et al. (1982). Ceftizoxime: collaborative multiphased *in-vitro* evaluation including tentative interpretative standards for disc susceptibility tests, beta-lactamase stability, and inhibition. *J Antimicrob Chemother* 10: (Suppl C): 25.

Bawdon RE, Hemsell DL, Guss SP (1982). Comparison of cefoperazone and cefoxitin concentrations in serum and pelvic tissue of abdominal hysterectomy patients. *Antimicrob Ag Chemother* 22: 999.

Bechard DL (1982). The efficacy of ceftizoxime in the therapy of bacteraemia. *J Antimicrob Chemother* 10 (Suppl C): 175.

Bégué P, Floret D, Mallet E et al. (1984). Pharmacokinetics and clinical evaluation of cefotaxime in children suffering with purulent meningitis. *J Antimicrob Chemother* 14 (Suppl B): 161.

Belohradsky BH, Bruch K, Geiss D et al. (1980). Intravenous cefotaxime in children with bacterial meningitis. *Lancet* i: 61.

Bennett PM, Chopra I (1993). Molecular basis of beta-lactamase induction in bacteria. *Antimicrob Ag Chemother* 37: 153.

Bergeron MG, Lavoie GY (1985). Tolerance of *Haemophilus influenzae* to beta-lactam antibiotics. *Antimicrob Ag Chemother* 28: 320.

Bergeron MG, Mendelson J, Harding GK et al. (1988). Cefoperazone compared with ampicillin plus tobramycin for severe biliary tract infections. *Antimicrob Ag Chemother* 32: 1231.

Bingen E, Goury V, Bennani H et al. (1992). Bactericidal activity of beta-lactams and amikacin against *Haemophilus influenzae*: effect on endotoxin release. *J Antimicrob Chemother* 30: 165.

Blondeau JM, Yaschuk Y (1995). *In vitro* activities of ciprofloxacin, cefotaxime, ceftriaxone, chloramphenicol, and rifampin against fully susceptible and moderately penicillin-resistant *Neisseria meningitidis*. *Antimicrob Ag Chemother* 39: 2577.

Bodey GP, Fainstein V, Hinkle AM (1981). Comparative *in vitro* study of new cephalosporins. *Antimicrob Ag Chemother* 20: 226.

Bolton WK, Scheld WM, Spyker DA, Sande MA (1981). Pharmacokinetics of cefoperazone in normal volunteers and subjects with renal insufficiency. *Antimicrob Ag Chemother* 19: 821.

Booth LV, Richards RH, Chandran DR (1991). Septic arthritis caused by *Corynebacterium xerosis* following vascular surgery. *Rev Infect Dis* 13: 548.

Boscia JA, Korzeniowski OM, Snepar R et al. (1983). Cefoperazone pharmacokinetics in normal subjects and patients with cirrhosis. *Antimicrob Ag Chemother* 23: 385.

Bosley GS, Elliott JA, Oxtoby MJ, Facklam RR (1987). Susceptibility of relatively penicillin-resistant *Streptococcus pneumoniae* to newer cephalosporin antibiotics. *Diagn Microbiol Infect Dis* 7: 21.

Bosso JA, Chan GM, Matsen J M (1983). Cefoperazone pharmacokinetics in pre-term infants. *Antimicrob Ag Chemother* 23: 413.

Botta GA, Privitera G, Menozzi MG (1983). Penicillin-binding proteins in *Bacteroides fragilis* and their affinities for several new cephalosporins. *J Antimicrob Chemother* 11: 332.

Bradford PA, Urban C, Jaiswal A et al. (1995). SHV-7, a novel cefotaxime-hydrolysing beta-lactamase, identified in *Escherichia coli* isolates from hospitalized nursing home patients. *Antimicrob Ag Chemother* 39: 899.

Bräutigam HH, Knothe H, Rangoonwala R (1988). Impact of cefotaxime and ceftriaxone on the bowel and vaginal flora after single dose prophylaxis in vaginal hysterectomy. *Drugs* 35 (Suppl 2): 163.

Bryan CS, John JF Jr, Pai MS, Austin TL (1985). Gentamicin vs cefotaxime for therapy of neonatal sepsis. Relationship to drug resistance. *Am J Dis Child* 139: 1086.

Bryan JP, Rocha H, Scheld WM (1986). Problems in salmonellosis: rationale for clinical trials with newer beta-lactam agents and quinolones. *Rev Infect Dis* 8: 189.

Buening MK, Wold JS (1982). Ethanol-moxalactam interactions *in vivo*. *Rev Infect Dis* 4 (Suppl): 555.

Bulger RR, Washington JA II (1980). Effect of inoculum size and beta-lactamase production on *in vitro* activity of new cephalosporins against *Haemophilus* species. *Antimicrob Ag Chemother* 17: 393.

Burckart GJ, Ptachcinski RJ, Jones DH et al. (1987). Impaired clearance of ceftizoxime and cefotaxime after orthotopic liver transplantation. *Antimicrob Ag Chemother* 31: 323.

Burgess ED, Blair AD (1983). Pharmacokinetics of ceftizoxime in patients undergoing continuous ambulatory peritoneal dialysis. *Antimicrob Ag Chemother* 24: 237.

Cabezudo I, Thompson RL, Selden RF et al. (1984). Cefsulodin sodium therapy in cystic fibrosis patients. *Antimicrob Ag Chemother* 25: 4.

Cable D, Edralin G, Overturf GD (1982). Human cerebrospinal fluid pharmacokinetics and treatment of bacterial meningitis with ceftizoxime. *J Antimicrob Chemother* 10 (Suppl C): 121.

Cable D, Overturf G, Edralin G (1983). Concentrations of cefoperazone in cerebrospinal fluid during bacterial meningitis. *Antimicrob Ag Chemother* 23: 688.

Campos J, Garcia-Tornel S (1987). Comparative susceptibilities of ampicillin and chloramphenicol resistant *Haemophilus influenzae* to fifteen antibiotics. *J Antimicrob Chemother* 19: 297.

Campos J, Garcia-Tornel S, Sanfeliu I (1984). Susceptibility studies of multiply resistant *Haemophilus influenzae* isolated from pediatric patients and contacts. *Antimicrob Ag Chemother* 25: 706.

Caplan DB, Buchanan CN (1984). Treatment of lower respiratory tract infections due to *Pseudomonas aeruginosa* in patients with cystic fibrosis. *Rev Infect Dis* 6: (Suppl 3): 705.

Carlberg H, Alestig K, Nord CE, Trollfors B (1982). Intestinal side-effects of cefoperazone. *J Antimicrob Chemother* 10: 483.

Catalán MJ, Fernández JM, Vasquez A et al. (1994). Failure of cefotaxime in the treatment of meningitis due to relatively resistant *Streptococcus pneumoniae*. *Clin Infect Dis* 18: 766.

CDC (Centers for Disease Control) (1993). Sexually transmitted diseases guidelines. *MMWR* 42 (No RR-14): 56.

Chabbert YA, Lutz AJ (1978). HR 756, the syn isomer of a new methoxyimino cephalosporin with unusual antibacterial activity. *Antimicrob Ag Chemother* 14: 749.

Charles D, Larsen B (1986). Pharmacokinetics of cefotaxime, moxalactam and cefoperazone in the early puerperium. *Antimicrob Ag Chemother* 29: 873.

Charnas RL, Then RL (1988). Mechanism of inhibition of chromosomal beta-lactamases by third generation cephalosporins. *Rev Infect Dis* 10: 752.

Chen SCA, Lawrence RH, Packham DR, Sorrell TC (1991). Cellulitis due to *Pseudomonas putrefaciens*: possible production of exotoxins. *Rev Infect Dis* 13: 642.

Cherubin CE, Eng RHK (1986). Experience with the use of cefotaxime in the treatment of bacterial meningitis. *Amer J Med* 80: 398.

Cherubin CE, Corrado ML, Nair SR et al. (1982). Treatment of Gram-negative bacillary meningitis: role of the new cephalosporin antibiotics. *Rev Infect Dis* 4 (Suppl): 453.

Cherubin CE, Eng RHK, Smith SM, Goldstein JC (1986). Cephalosporin therapy for salmonellosis Questions of efficacy and cross-resistance with ampicillin. *Arch Intern Med* 146: 2149.

Cherubin CE, Eng RHK, Norrby R et al. (1989). Penetration of newer cephalosporins into cerebrospinal fluid. *Rev Infect Dis* 11: 526.

Chow AW, Finegold SM (1982). *In-vitro* activity of ceftizoxime against anaerobic bacteria and comparison with other cephalosporins. *J Antimicrob Chemother* 10: (Suppl C): 45.

Cohen E, Mogabgab WJ (1982). Ceftizoxime therapy of infections in hospitalized patients and comparison with cefamandole for urinary tract infections. *J Antimicrob Chemother* **10** (Suppl C): 253.

Cohen MS, Cooney MH, Blackman E, Sparling PF (1983). *In vitro* antimicrobial susceptibility of penicillinase-producing and intrinsically resistant *Neisseria gonorrhoeae* strains. *Antimicrob Ag Chemother* **24**: 597.

Coombes JD (1982). Metabolism of cefotaxime in animals and humans. *Rev Infect Dis* **4** (Suppl): 325.

Cornick NA, Gorbach SL (1988). Synergistic activity of cefotaxime and desacetycefotaxime against the *Bacteroides fragilis* group. *Diagn Microbiol Infect Dis* **10**: 81.

Corrado ML, Gombert ME, Cherubin CE (1982). Designing appropriate therapy in the treatment of Gram-negative baciliary meningitis. *JAMA* **248**: 71.

Counts GW, Hill CD, Hooton TM, Turck M (1982). Ceftizoxime treatment of pneumonia, cellulitis and other infections in 120 hospitalized patients. *J Antimicrob Chemother* **10** (Suppl C): 201.

Crooks J, White LO, Burville LJ *et al.* (1984). Pharmacokinetics of cefotaxime and desacetyl-cefotaxime in neonates. *J Antimicrob Chemother* **14** (Suppl B): 97.

Curtis NAC, Orr D, Ross GW, Boulton MG (1979). Affinities of penicillins and cephalosporins for the penicillin-binding proteins of *Escherichia coli* K-12 and their antibacterial activity. *Antimicrob Ag Chemother* **16**: 533.

Curtis NAC, Eisenstadt RL, Rudd C, White AJ (1986). Inducible type 1 beta-lactamases of Gram-negative bacteria and resistance to beta-lactam antibiotics. *J Antimicrob Chemother* **17**: 51.

Cutler RE, Blair AD, Burgess ED, Parks D (1982). Pharmacokinetics of ceftizoxime. *J Antimicrob Chemother* **10** (Suppl C): 91.

Danon J (1980). Cefotaxime concentrations in otitis media effusions. *J Antimicrob Chemother* **6** (Suppl A): 131.

Daschner FD, Metz B, Spillner G *et al.* (1980). Concentrations of cefamandole and cefsulodin in serum, heart valves, subcutaneous tissue and muscle of patients undergoing open-heart surgery. *J Infect Dis* **142**: 290.

Davey P, Lynch B, Malek M *et al.* (1992). Cost-effectiveness of single dose cefoxime plus metronidazole compared with three doses each of cefuroxime plus metronidazole for the prevention of wound infection after colorectal surgery. *J Antimicrob Chemother* **30**: 855.

Deeter RG, Weinstein MP, Swanson KA *et al.* (1990). Crossover assessment of serum bactericidal activity and pharmacokinetics of five broad-spectrum cephalosporins in the elderly. *Antimicrob Ag Chemother* **34**: 1007.

de Lalla F, Privitera G, Ortisi G *et al.* (1989). Third generation cephalosporins as a risk factor for *Clostridium difficile*-associated disease: a four year survey in a general hospital. *J Antimicrob Chemother* **23**: 623.

de Louvois J (1994). Acute bacterial meningitis in the newborn. *J Antimicrob Chemother* **34** (Suppl A): 61.

Denys GA, Jerris RC, Swenson JM, Thornsberry C (1983). Susceptibility of *Propionibacterium acnes* clinical isolates to 22 antimicrobial agents. *Antimicrob Ag Chemother* **23**: 335.

Di Piro JT, Bowden TA Jr, Hocks VH III (1984). Prophylactic parenteral cephalosporins in surgery Are the newer agents better? *JAMA* **252**: 3277.

Doerr BI, Glomot R, Kief H *et al.* (1982). Cefotaxime toxicity studies: a review of preclinical studies and some clinical reports. *Rev Infect Dis* **4** (Suppl): 354.

Doluisio JT (1982). Clinical pharmacokinetics of cefotaxime in patients with normal and reduced renal function. *Rev Infect Dis* **4** (Suppl): 333.

Dornbusch K, Nord CE, Olsson-Liljeqvist B (1979). Antibiotic susceptibility of anaerobic bacteria with special reference to *Bacteroides fragilis*. *Scand J Infect Dis* (Suppl 19): 17.

Dornbusch K and the European Study Group on Antibiotic Resistance (1990). Resistance to beta-lactam antibiotics and ciprofloxacin in Gram-negative bacilli and staphylococci isolated from blood: a European collaborative study. *J Antimicrob Chemother* **26**: 269.

Drasar FA, Farrell W, Howard AJ *et al.* (1978). Activity of HR 756 against

Haemophilus influenzae, *Bacteroides fragilis* and Gram-negative rods. *J Antimicrob Chemother* **4**: 445.

Du Bois SK, Marriott MS, Amyes SGB (1995). TEM- and SHV-derived extended-spectrum beta-lactamases: relationship between selection, structure and function. *J Antimicrob Chemother* **35**: 7.

Dunn GL (1982). Ceftizoxime and other third-generation cephalosporins: structure-activity relationships. *J Antimicrob Chemother* **10** (Suppl C): 1.

Edelstein PH, Meyer RD (1980). Susceptibility of *Legionella pneumophila* to twenty antimicrobial agents. *Antimicrob Ag Chemother* **18**: 403.

Edmond MB, Riddler SA, Baxter CM *et al.* (1993). *Agrobacterium radiobacter*: a recently recognized opportunistic pathogen. *Clin Infect Dis* **16**: 388.

Elder HA, Roy I (1984). Treatment of urinary tract infections due to *Pseudomonas aeruginosa* with cefsulodin. *Rev Infect Dis* **6** (Suppl 3): 734.

Eley A, Greenwood D (1981). *In vitro* activity of ceftizoxime against *Bacteroides fragilis*: comparison with benzylpenicillin, cephalothin, and cefoxitin. *Antimicrob Ag Chemother* **20**: 332.

Eliopoulos GM (1988). Induction of beta-lactamases. *J Antimicrob Chemother* **22** (Suppl A): 37.

Eng RHK, Cherubin CE, Pechere J-C, Beam TRJr (1987). Treatment failures of cefotaxime and latamoxef in meningitis caused by *Enterobacter* and *Serratia* spp. *J Antimicrob Chemother* **20**: 903.

Esmieu F, Guibert J, Rosenkilde HC *et al.* (1980). Pharmacokinetics of cefotaxime in normal human volunteers. *J Antimicrob Chemother* **6** (Suppl A): 83.

Fass RJ (1980). *In vitro* activity of cefoperazone against nonfermenters and *Aeromonas hydrophila*. *Antimicrob Ag Chemother* **18**: 483.

Feldstein TJ, Uden DL, Larson TA (1987). Cefotaxime for treatment of Gram-negative bacterial meningitis in infants and children. *Pediatr Infect Dis J* **6**: 471.

Fick RB Jr, Alexander MR, Prince RA, Kasik JE (1987). Penetration of cefotaxime into respiratory secretions. *Antimicrob Ag Chemother* **31**: 815.

Fietta A, Sacchi F, Bersani C *et al.* (1983). Effect of beta-lactam antibiotics on migration and bactericidal activity of human phagocytes. *Antimicrob Ag Chemother* **23**: 930.

Figueiredo AMS, Connor JD, Severin A *et al.* (1992). A pneumococcal clinical isolate with high-level resistance to cefotaxime and ceftriaxone. *Antimicrob Ag Chemother* **36**: 886.

File TM Jr, Tan JS (1983). Cefoperazone for the treatment of acute urinary tract infection: multicentered comparative and non-comparative studies. *Rev Infect Dis* **5** (Suppl 1): 145.

File TM Jr, Tan JS, Baird I *et al.* (1982). Evaluation of cefoperazone in the therapy of urinary tract infections. *J Antimicrob Chemother* **9**: 223.

File TM Jr, Tan JS, Gardner WG, Baird I (1983). Cefoperazone versus cefamandole in the treatment of acute bacterial lower respiratory tract infections. *J Antimicrob Chemother* **11**: 75.

Francis BM, Gilbert GL (1992). Survey of neonatal meningitis in Australia: 1987–1989. *Med J Aust* **156**: 240.

Fu KP, Neu HC (1980). Antibacterial activity of ceftizoxime, a beta-lactamase-stable cephalosporin. *Antimicrob Ag Chemother* **17**: 583.

Fu KP, Aswapokee P, Ho I *et al.* (1979). Pharmacokinetics of cefotaxime. *Antimicrob Ag Chemother* **16**: 592.

Fuchs PC, Barry AL, Thornsberry C *et al.* (1980). Cefotaxime: *in vitro* activity and tentative interpretive standards for disc susceptibility testing. *Antimicrob Ag Chemother* **18**: 88.

Gahrn-Hansen B, Søgaard P (1990). *In-vitro* activity of cefotaxime against clinical isolates of *Yersinia enterocolitica*, biotype 4, serogroup 03. *J Antimicrob Chemother* **26**: 599.

Garber GE, Auger P, Chan RMT *et al.* (1992). A multicenter, open comparative study of paranteral cefotaxime and ceftriaxone in the treatment of nosocomial lower respiratory tract infections. *Diagn Microbiol Infect Dis* **15**: 85.

Gentry LO (1988). Osteomyelitis: options for diagnosis and management. *J Antimicrob Chemother* **21** (Suppl C): 115.

Gerding DN, Van Etta LL, Peterson LR (1982). Role of serum protein binding and multiple antibiotic doses in the extravascular distribution of ceftizoxime and cefotaxime. *Antimicrob Ag Chemother* 22: 844.

Gianneli D, Tzelepi E, Tzouvelekis LS *et al.* (1994). Dissemination of cephalosporin-resistant *Serratia marcescens* strains producing a plasmid SHV type beta-lactamase in Greek hospitals. *Eur J Clin Microbiol Infect Dis* 13: 764.

Gibson TP, Granneman GR, Kallal JE, Sennello LT (1982). Cefsulodin kinetics in renal impairment. *Clin Pharmacol Ther* 31: 602.

Gibson TP, Granneman GR, Kallal JE, Sennello LT (1984). Kinetics of cefsulodin in patients with renal impairment. *Rev Infect Dis* 6 (Suppl 3): 689.

Gillett AP (1982). Antibiotics against pseudomonas. *J Antimicrob Chemother* 9: (Suppl B): 41.

Givner LB, Abramson JS, Wasilauskas B (1989). Meningitis due to *Haemophilus influenzae* type b resistant to ampicillin and chloramphenicol. *Rev Infect Dis* 11: 329.

Gleckman R, Gantz NM (1982). The third-generation cephalosporins. A plea for restraint. *Arch Intern Med* 142: 1267.

Glew RH, Pavuk RA (1983). Stability of gentamicin, tobramycin, and amikacin in combination with four beta-lactam antibiotics. *Antimicrob Ag Chemother* 24: 474.

Glew RH, Pavuk RA (1984). Early synergistic interactions between amikacin and six beta-lactam antibiotics against multiply resistant members of the family *Enterobacteriaceae*. *Antimicrob Ag Chemother* 26: 378.

Golledge CL, McKenzie T, Riley TV (1989). Extended spectrum cephalosporins and *Clostridium difficile*. *J Antimicrob Chemother* 23: 929.

Gomis M, Herranz A, Aparicio P *et al.* (1990). Cefotaxime in the treatment of chronic osteomyelitis caused by Gram-negative bacilli. *J Antimicrob Chemother* 26 (Suppl A): 45.

Gonik B, Feldman S, Pickering LK, Doughtie CG (1986). Pharmacokinetics of cefoperazone in the parturient. *Antimicrob Ag Chemother* 30: 874.

Gootz TD, Jackson DB, Sherris JC (1984). Development of resistance to cephalosporins in clinical strains of *Citrobacter* spp. *Antimicrob Ag Chemother* 25: 591.

Gordon AJ, Phyfferoen M (1983). Cefoperazone sodium in the treatment of serious bacterial infections in 2100 adults and children: multicentered trials in Europe, Latin America and Australasia. *Rev Infect Dis* 5 (Suppl 1): 188.

Gordts B, Vandenborre C, Vander Auwera Ph, Butzler JP (1984). Comparison between the *in-vitro* activity of new agents on *Pseudomonas aeruginosa* isolates from cystic fibrosis patients and other chronic infections. *J Antimicrob Chemother* 14: 25.

Gotoh N, Nunomura K, NIshino T (1990). Resistance of *Pseudomonas aeruginosa* to cefsulodin: modification of penicillin-binding protein 3 and mapping of its chromosomal gene. *J Antimicrob Chemother* 25: 513.

Gould IM, Wise R (1985). *Pseudomonas aeruginosa*: clinical manifestations and management. *Lancet* ii: 1224.

Granneman GR, Sennello LT, Sonders RC *et al.* (1982). Cefsulodin kinetics in healthy subjects after intramuscular and intravenous injection. *Clin Pharmacol Ther* 31: 95.

Grayson ML, Eliopoulos GM (1990). Antimicrobial resistance in the intensive care unit. *Semin Resp Infec* 5: 204.

Greenfield RA, Gerber AU, Craig WA (1983). Pharmacokinetics of cefoperazone in patients with normal and impaired hepatic and renal function. *Rev Infect Dis* 5 (Suppl 1): 127.

Greenwood D, Pearson N, Eley A, O'Grady F (1980). Comparative *in vitro* activities of cefotaxime and ceftizoxime (FK 749): new cephalosporins with exceptional potency. *Antimicrob Ag Chemother* 17: 397.

Guerrero MLF, Arbol F, Verdeyo C *et al.* (1994). Treatment of experimental endocarditis due to penicillin-resistant *Streptococcus pneumoniae*. *Antimicrob Ag Chemother* 38: 1103.

Gutmann L, Goldstein FW, Kitzis MD *et al.* (1983). Susceptibility of *Nocardia asteroides* to 46 antibiotics including 22 beta-lactams. *Antimicrob Ag Chemother* 23: 248.

Gwynn MN, Rolinson GN (1983). Selection of variants of Gram-negative bacteria with elevated production of type 1 beta-lactamase. *J Antimicrob Chemother* 11: 577.

Hall WH, Opfer BJ, Gerding DN (1980). Comparative activities of the oxa-beta-lactam LY 127935, cefotaxime, cefoperazone, cefamandole and ticarcillin against multiply resistant Gram-negative bacilli. *Antimicrob Ag Chemother* 17: 273.

Hamer DH, Barza M (1993). Prevention of hospital-acquired pneumonia in critically ill patients. *Antimicrob Ag Chemother* 37: 931.

Hammerschlag MR, Gleyzer A (1983). *In vitro* activity of a group of broad spectrum cephalosporins and other beta-lactam antibiotics against *Chlamydia trachomatis*. *Antimicrob Ag Chemother* 23: 493.

Hancock REW, Woodruff WA (1988). Roles of porin and beta-lactamase in beta-lactam resistance of *Pseudomonas aeruginosa*. *Rev Infect Dis* 10: 770.

Harding GKM, Nicolle LE, Haase DA *et al.* (1984). Prospective, randomized, comparative trials in the therapy for intraabdominal and female genital tract infections. *Rev Infect Dis* 6 (Suppl 1): 283.

Hargreave TB, Hindmarsh JR, Elton R *et al.* (1982). Short-term prophylaxis with cefotaxime for prostatic surgery. *Brit Med J* 284: 1008.

Heim KL, Halstenson CE, Comty CM *et al.* (1986). Disposition of cefotaxime and desacetyl cefotaxime during continuous ambulatory peritoneal dialysis. *Antimicrob Ag Chemother* 30: 15.

Hinkle AM, Le Blanc BM, Bodey GP (1980). *In vitro* evaluation of cefoperazone. *Antimicrob Ag Chemother* 17: 423.

Hiraoka M, Inoue M, Mitsuhashi S (1988). Hydrolytic rate at low drug concentrations as a limiting factor in resistance to newer cephalosporins. *Rev Infect Dis* 10: 746.

Hirschmann JV, Inui TS (1980). Antibiotic prophylaxis: a critique of recent trials. *Rev Infect Dis* 2: 1.

Hopkins JM, Towner KJ (1990). Enhanced resistance to cefotaxime and imipenem associated with outer membrane protein alterations in *Enterobacter aerogenes*. *J Antimicrob Chemother* 25: 49.

Horii T, Arakawa Y, Ohta M *et al.* (1993). Plasmid-mediated AmC-type beta-lactamase isolated from *Klebsiella pneumoniae* confers resistance to broad-spectrum beta-lactams, including moxalactam. *Antimicrob Ag Chemother* 37: 984.

Hornstein MJ, Jupeau AM, Scavizzi MR *et al.* (1985). *In vitro* susceptibilities of 126 clinical isolates of *Yersinia enterocolitica* to 21 beta-lactam antibiotics. *Antimicrob Ag Chemother* 27: 806.

Ikeda Y, Nishino T (1988). Paradoxical antibacterial activities of beta-lactams against *Proteus vulgaris*: mechanism of the paradoxical effect. *Antimicrob Ag Chemother* 32: 1073.

Ings RMJ, Fillastre J-P, Godin M *et al.* (1982). The pharmacokinetics of cefotaxime and its metabolites in subjects with normal and impaired renal function. *Rev Infect Dis* 4 (Suppl): 379.

Jacobs MR, Kelly F, Speck WT (1982). Susceptibility of Group B streptococci to 16 beta-lactam antibiotics, including new penicillin and cephalosporin derivatives. *Antimicrob Ag Chemother* 22: 897.

Jacobs RF, Wells TG, Steele RW, Yamauchi T (1985). A prospective randomized comparison of cefotaxime vs. ampicillin and chloramphenicol for bacterial meningitis in children. *J Pediatr* 107: 129.

Jacobs RF, Darville T, Parks JA, Enderlin G (1992). Safety profile and efficacy of cefotaxime for the treatment of hospitalized children. *Clin Infect Dis* 14: 56.

Jacobs RF, Kaplan SL, Schutze GE *et al.* (1996). Relationship of MICs to efficacy of cefotaxime in treatment of *Streptococcus pneumoniae* infections. *Antimicrob Ag Chemother* 40: 895.

Jacoby GA, Archer GL (1991). New mechanisms of bacterial resistance to antimicrobial action. *New Engl J Med* 324: 601.

Jacoby GA, Medeiros AA (1991). More extended-spectrum beta-lactamases. *Antimicrob Ag Chemother* 35: 1697.

Janda JM, Abbott SL (1993). Infections associated with the genus *Edwardsiella*: the role of *Edwardsiella tarda* in human disease. *Clin Infect Dis* 17: 742.

Jarlier V, Nicolas M-H, Fournier G, Phillipon A (1988). Extended broad-spectrum beta-lactamases conferring transferable resistance to newer beta-lactam agents in Enterobacteriaceae: hospital prevalence and susceptibility patterns. *Rev Infect Dis* **10**: 867.

Jenkins SG, Birk RJ, Zabransky RJ (1982). Differences in susceptibilities of species of the *Bacteroides fragilis* Group to several beta-lactam antibiotics: indole production as an indicator of resistance. *Antimicrob Ag Chemother* **22**: 628.

Jewett CV, Ledbetter J, Lyrene RK *et al.* (1985). Comparison of cefoperazone sodium vs methicillin, ticarcillin, and tobramycin in treatment of pulmonary exacerbations in patients with cystic fibrosis. *J Pediatr* **106**: 669.

John CC (1994). Treatment failure with use of a third generation cephalosporin for penicillin-resistant pneumococcal meningitis; case report and review. *Clin Infect Dis* **18**: 188.

Johnson ES, Smith LG (1982). Ceftizoxime in moderate-to-severe infections. *J Antimicrob Chemother* **10** (Suppl C): 151.

Jones RN (1984). The activity of cefotaxime and desacetylcefotaxime against *Bacteroides* species compared to 7-methoxy cephems and other anti-anaerobe drugs. *J Antimicrob Chemother* **14** (Suppl B): 39.

Jones RN, Barry AL (1983a). Cefoperazone: a review of its antimicrobial spectrum, beta-lactamase stability, enzyme inhibition, and other *in vitro* characteristics. *Rev Infect Dis* **5** (Suppl 1): 108.

Jones RN, Barry AL (1983b). Antimicrobial activity and other *in vitro* properties of cefoperazone A, the principal metabolite of cefoperazone sodium. *Antimicrob Ag Chemother* **24**: 293.

Jones RN, Barry AL (1987). Antimicrobial activity of ceftriaxone, cefotaxime, desacetycefotaxime and cefotaxime-desacetylcefotaxime in the presence of human serum. *Antimicrob Ag Chemother* **31**: 818.

Jones RN, Packer RR (1982). Antimicrobial activity of amikacin combinations against Enterobacteriaceae moderately susceptible to third-generation cephalosporins. *Antimicrob Ag Chemother* **22**: 985.

Jones RN, Thornsberry C (1982). Cefotaxime: a review of *in vitro* antimicrobial properties and spectrum of activity. *Rev Infect Dis* **4** (Suppl): 300.

Jones RN, Thornsberry C (1985). Gram-positive superinfections: a consequence of modern beta-lactam chemotherapy. *Antimicrobic Newsletter* **2**: 17.

Jones RN, Fuchs PC, Barry AL *et al.* (1980). Cefoperazone (T-1551), a new semisynthetic cephalosporin: comparison with cephalothin and gentamicin. *Antimicrob Ag Chemother* **17**: 743.

Jones RN, Barry AL, Packer RR (1984). The activity of cefotaxime and desacetylcefotaxime alone and in combination against anaerobes and staphylococci. *Diagn Microbiol Infect Dis* **2**: 37S.

Jorgensen JH, Crawford SA (1982). Selective inactivation of aminoglycosides by newer beta-lactam antibiotics. *Curr Ther Res* **32**: 25.

Jorgensen JH, Crawford SA, Alexander GA (1980a). *In vitro* activities of cefotaxime and moxalactam (LY 127935). against *Haemophilus influenzae*. *Antimicrob Ag Chemother* **17**: 516.

Jorgensen JH, Crawford SA, Alexander GA (1980b). *In vitro* activities of moxalactam and cefotaxime against aerobic Gram-negative bacilli. *Antimicrob Ag Chemother* **17**: 937.

Judson FN, Eron LJ, Lutz FB *et al.* (1991). Multicenter study of a single 500 mg dose of cefotaxime for treatment of uncomplicated gonorrhea. *Sex Transm Dis* **18**: 41.

Kafetzis DA, Lazarides CV, Siafas CA *et al.* (1980). Transfer of cefotaxime in human milk and from mother to foetus. *J Antimicrob Chemother* **6** (Suppl A): 135.

Kafetzis DA, Brater DC, Kanarios J *et al.* (1981). Clinical pharmacology of cefotaxime in pediatric patients. *Antimicrob Ag Chemother* **20**: 487.

Kalager T, Digranes A, Bakke K *et al.* (1982). Cefotaxime in serious infections – a clinical and pharmacokinetic study. *J Antimicrob Chemother* **9**: 157.

Kamimura T, Matsumoto Y, Okada N *et al.* (1979). Ceftizoxime (FK 749)., a new parenteral cephalosporin; *in vitro* and *in vivo* antibacterial activities. *Antimicrob Ag Chemother* **16**: 540.

Karakusis PH, Feczko JM, Goodman LJ *et al.* (1982). Clinical efficacy of cefotaxime in serious infections. *Antimicrob Ag Chemother* **21**: 119.

Karimi A, Seeger K, Stolke D, Knothe H (1980). Cefotaxime concentration

in cerebrospinal fluid. *J Antimicrob Chemother* **6** (Suppl A): 119.

Keaney M, Caister H, Bax R, Noone P (1982). Clinical experience with cefotaxime in hospitalized patients. *J Antimicrob Chemother* **9**: 313.

Kemmerich B, Lode H, Belmega G *et al.* (1983a). Comparative pharmacokinetics of cefoperazone, cefotaxime and moxalactam. *Antimicrob Ag Chemother* **23**: 429.

Kemmerich B, Lode H, Borner K *et al.* (1983b). Biliary excretion and pharmacokinetics of cefoperazone in humans. *J Antimicrob Chemother* **12**: 27.

Kerbs SB, Stone JR Jr, Berg SW, Harrison WO (1983). *In vitro* antimicrobial activity of eight new beta-lactam antibiotics against penicillin-resistant *Neisseria gonorrhoeae*. *Antimicrob Ag Chemother* **23**: 541.

King A, Shannon K, Phillips I (1980). *In vitro* antibacterial activity and susceptibility of cefsulodin, an antipseudomonal cephalosporin, to beta-lactamases. *Antimicrob Ag Chemother* **17**: 165.

Klass PE, Klein JO (1992). Therapy of bacterial sepsis, meningitis and otitis media in infants and children: 1992 poll of directors of programs in pediatric infectious diseases. *Pediatr Infect Dis J* **11**: 702.

Klastersky J, Glauser MP, Schimpff SC *et al.* (1986). Prospective randomized comparison of three antibiotic regimens for empirical therapy of suspected bacteremic infection in febrile granulocytopenic patients. *Antimicrob Ag Chemother* **29**: 263.

Ko RJ, Sattler FR, Nichols S *et al.* (1991). Pharmacokinetics of cefotaxime and desacetylcefotaxime in patients with liver disease. *Antimicrob Ag Chemother* **35**: 1376.

Kowalsky SF, Echols RM, Venezia AR, Andrews EA (1983). Pharmacokinetics of ceftizoxime in subjects with various degrees of renal function. *Antimicrob Ag Chemother* **24**: 151.

Kurtz TO, Winston DJ, Hindler JA *et al.* (1980). Comparative *in vitro* activity of moxalactam, cefotaxime, cefoperazone, piperacillin and aminoglycosides against Gram-negative bacilli. *Antimicrob Ag Chemother* **18**: 645.

Kwaga J, Iversen JO (1990). *In vitro* antimicrobial susceptibilities of *Yersinia enterocolitica* and related species isolated from alaughtered pigs and pork products. *Antimicrob Ag Chemother* **34**: 2423.

Labro MT, Babin-Chevaye C, Hakim J (1986). Effects of cefotaxime and cefodizime on human granulocyte functions *in vitro*. *J Antimicrob Chemother* **18**: 233.

Landau Z, Halkin H, Rubinstein E (1981). Interstitial fluid concentrations of cefsulodin, azlocillin and carbenicillin. *Scand J Infect Dis* **13**: 227.

Lang SDR, Edwards DJ, Durack DT (1980). Comparison of cefoperazone, cefotaxime and moxalactam (LY 127935). against aerobic Gram-negative bacilli. *Antimicrob Ag Chemother* **17**: 488.

Lapointe J-R, Béliveau C, Chicoine L, Joncas JH (1984). A comparison of ampicillin-cefotaxime and ampicillin-chloramphenicol in childhood bacterial meningitis: an experience in 55 patients. *J Antimicrob Chemother* **14** (Suppl B): 167.

Lapointe J-R, Lavallee C, Michaud A *et al.* (1986). *In vitro* comparison of ampicillin-chloramphenicol and ampicillin-cefotaxime against 284 *Haemophilus* isolates. *Antimicrob Ag Chemother* **29**: 594.

Le Bel M, Paone RP, Lewis GP (1983). Effect of probenecid on the pharmacokinetics of ceftizoxime. *J Antimicrob Chemother* **12**: 147.

Lecaillon JB, Rouan MC, Binswanger U *et al.* (1984). Pharmacokinetics of cefotiam and cefsulodin after simultaneous administration to patients with impaired renal function. *Antimicrob Ag Chemother* **26**: 368.

Lecour H, Seara A, Miranda AM *et al.* (1984). Treatment of 160 cases of acute bacterial meningitis with cefotaxime. *J Antimicrob Chemother* **14** (Suppl B): 195.

Le Frock JL, Carr BB (1982). Clinical experience with cefotaxime in the treatment of serious bone and joint infections. *Rev Infect Dis* **4** (Suppl): 465.

Leggiadro RJ, Barrett FF, Chesney PJ *et al.* (1994). Invasive pneumococci with high level penicillin and cephalosporin resistance at a Mid-South childrens hospital. *Pediatr Infect Dis J* **13**: 320.

Lepage P, Bogaerts J, Van Goethem C *et al.* (1990). Multiresistant *Salmonella typhimurium* systemic infection in Rwanda Clinical features and treatment with cefotaxime. *J Antimicrob Chemother* **26** (Suppl A): 53.

Leung JWC, Chan RCY, Cheung SW *et al.* (1990). The effect of obstruction on the biliary excretion of cefoperazone and ceftazidime. *J Antimicrob Chemother* **25**: 399.

Liñares J, Alonso T, Perez JL *et al.* (1992). Decreased susceptibility of penicillin-resistant pneumococci to twenty-four beta-lactam antibiotics. *J Antimicrob Chemother* **30**: 279.

Lindberg F, Normark S (1986). Contribution of chromosomal beta-lactamases to beta-lactam resistance in enterobacteria. *Rev Infect Dis* **8** (Suppl 3): 292.

Lipsky JJ (1986). Testicular atrophy in animals – an effect of methylthiotetrazole-containing antibiotics. *J Antimicrob Chemother* **17**: 267.

Liu PYF, Gur D, Hall LMC, Livermore DM (1992). Survey of the prevalence of beta-lactamases amongst 1000 Gram-negative bacilli isolated consecutively at the Royal London Hospital. *J Antimicrob Chemother* **30**: 429.

Livermore DM (1983). Kinetics and significance of the activity of the Sabath and Abrahams' beta-lactamase of *Pseudomonas aeruginosa* against cefotaxime and cefsulodin. *J Antimicrob Chemother* **11**: 169.

Livermore DM (1985). Leading article Do beta-lactamases 'trap' cephalosporins? *J Antimicrob Chemother* **15**: 511.

Livermore DM (1991). Mechanisms of resistance to beta-lactam antibiotics *Scand J Infect Dis* (Suppl 78): 7.

Livermore DM, Williams RJ, Williams JD (1981). Comparison of the beta-lactamase stability and the *in-vitro* activity of cefoperazone, cefotaxime, cefsulodin, ceftazidime, moxalactam and ceftriaxone against *Pseudomonas aeruginosa*. *J Antimicrob Chemother* **8**: 323.

Livermore DM, Riddle SJ, Davy KWM (1986). Hydrolytic model for cefotaxime and ceftriaxone resistance in beta-lactamase-derepressed *Enterobacter cloacae*. *J Infect Dis* **153**: 619.

Lode H, Kemmerich B, Gruhlke G *et al.* (1980). Cefotaxime in bronchopulmonary infections – a clinical and pharmacological study. *J Antimicrob Chemother* **6**: (Suppl A): 193.

Lodge JM, Piddock LJV (1991). The control of class I beta-lactamase expression in Enterobacteriaceae and *Pseudomonas aeruginosa*. *J Antimicrob Chemother* **28**: 167.

Lou MA, Chen DF, Bansal M *et al.* (1982). Evaluation of ceftizoxime in acute peritonitis. *J Antimicrob Chemother* **10** (Suppl C): 183.

Luft FC, Aronoff GR, Evan AP *et al.* (1982). Effects of moxalactam and cefotaxime on rabbit renal tissue. *Antimicrob Ag Chemother* **21**: 830.

Lüthy R, Blaser J, Bonetti A *et al.* (1981). Comparative multiple-dose pharmacokinetics of cefotaxime, moxalactam and ceftazidime. *Antimicrob Ag Chemother* **20**: 567.

Lutz B, Mogabgab WJ, Parks D *et al.* (1982). Comparison of ceftizoxime and penicillin for the treatment of uncomplicated gonorrhoea. *J Antimicrob Chemother* **10** (Suppl C): 229.

Lyon JA (1983). Cefoperazone (Cefobid, Pfizer). *Drug Intel Clin Pharm* **17**: 7.

Magnussen CR, Sammartino MT, Ernest KD (1982). Aminoglycoside-resistant Gram-negative bacilli in a community hospital: comparative *in vitro* activity of cefotaxime, moxalactam, cefoperazone, and piperacillin. *Antimicrob Ag Chemother* **22**: 154.

Mandell LA, Afnan M (1991). Synergistic killing of Gram-negative bacilli by cefotaxime, its desacetyl metabolite and human polymorphonuclear neutrophils. *J Antimicrob Chemother* **27**: 817.

Mangi RJ, Peccerillo KM, Ryan J *et al.* (1992). Cefoperazone versus ceftriaxone monotherapy of nosocomial pneumonia. *Diagn Microbiol Infect Dis* **15**: 441.

Markowitz SM, Sibilla DJ (1980). Comparative susceptibilities of clinical isolates of *Serratia marcescens* to newer cephalosporins, alone and in combination with various aminoglycosides. *Antimicrob Ag Chemother* **18**: 651.

Marriotte S, Nordmann P, Nicholas MH (1994). Extended-spectrum beta-lactamase in *Proteus mirabilis*. *J Antimicrob Chemother* **33**: 925.

Mashimo K (1981). Clinical experience with cefoperazone in biliary tract infections. *Drugs* **22** (Suppl 1): 100.

Maslow MJ, Simberkoff MS, Rahal JJ (1985). Clinical efficacy of a synergistic combination of cefotaxime, and amikacin against multi-resistant *Pseudomonas* and *Serratia* infections. *J Antimicrob Chemother* **16**: 227.

Matsubara N, Minami S, Matsuhashi M *et al.* (1980). Affinity of cefoperazone for penicillin-binding proteins. *Antimicrob Ag Chemother* **18**: 195.

Matzke GR, Keane WF (1983). Cefsulodin pharmacokinetics in patients with various degrees of renal function. *Antimicrob Ag Chemother* **23**: 369.

McCormack WM, Mogabgab WJ, Jones RB *et al.* (1993). Multicenter, comparative study of cefotaxime and ceftriaxone for treatment of uncomplicated gonorrhea. *Sex Transm Dis* **20**: 269.

McCracken GH Jr (1984). Management of neonatal meningitis, 1984. *J Antimicrob Chemother* **14** (Suppl B): 23.

McCracken GH Jr (1985). Use of third-generation cephalosporins for treatment of neonatal infections. *Amer J Dis Child* **139**: 1079.

McCracken GH Jr, Nelson JD, Grimm L (1982a). Pharmacokinetics and bacteriological efficacy of cefoperazone, cefuroxime, ceftriaxone, and moxalactam in experimental *Streptococcus pneumoniae* and *Haemophilus influenzae* meningitis. *Antimicrob Ag Chemother* **21**: 262.

McCracken GH Jr, Threlkeld NE, Thomas ML (1982b). Pharmacokinetics of cefotaxime in newborn infants. *Antimicrob Ag Chemother* **21**: 683.

McCracken GH Jr, Nelson JD, Kaplan SL *et al.* (1987). Consensus report Antimicrobial therapy for bacterial meningitis in infants and children. *Pediatr Infect Dis J* **6**: 501.

McKendrick MW, Geddes AM, Wise R, Andrews JA (1981). Cefotaxime – a clinical study. *J Antimicrob Chemother* **7**: 405.

Medeiros AA (1993). Nosocomial outbreaks of multiresistant bacteria: extended-spectrum beta-lactamases have arrived in North America. *Ann Intern Med* **119**: 428.

Mett H, Rosta S, Schacher B, Frei R (1988). Outer membrane permeability and beta-lactamase content of *Pseudomonas maltophilia* clinical isolates and laboratory mutants. *Rev Infect Dis* **10**: 765.

Meyer KS, Urban C, Eagan JA *et al.* (1993). Nosocomial outbreak of *Klebsiella* infection resistant to late-generation cephalosporins. *Ann Intern Med* **119**: 353.

Meyers BR (1982). Clinical experience with cefotaxime in the treatment of patients with bacteremia. *Rev Infect Dis* **4** (Suppl): 411.

Michéa-Hamzehpour M, Pechere JC (1989). How predictible is development of resistance after beta-lactam therapy in *Enterobacter cloacae* infection?. *J Antimicrob Chemother* **24**: 387.

Miller MA, Finan M, Yousuf M (1983). *In vitro* antagonism by N-formimidoyl thienamycin and cefoxitin of second and third generation cephalosporins in *Aeromonas hydrophilia* and *Serratia marcescens*. *J Antimicrob Chemother* **11**: 311.

Mintz L, Drew WL (1981). Comparative synergistic activity of cefoperazone, cefotaxime, moxalactam and carbenicillin, combined with tobramycin, against *Pseudomonas aeruginosa*. *Antimicrob Ag Chemother* **19**: 332.

Mitsuhashi S, Minami S, Matsubara N *et al.* (1980). *In vitro* and *in vivo* antibacterial activity of cefoperazone. *Clin Ther* (Special issue) **3**: 1.

Møller NE, Koch C, Vesterhauge S, Jensen K (1982). Treatment of pulmonary *Pseudomonas aeruginosa* infection in cystic fibrosis with cefsulodin. *Scand J Infect Dis* **14**: 207.

Moreau L, Durand H, Biclet P (1980). Cefotaxime concentrations in ascites. *J Antimicrob Chemother* **6** (Suppl A): 121.

Morel C, Monrocq N, Besnard Y (1980). Concentrations of cefotaxime in bronchial secretions. *J Antimicrob Chemother* **6** (Suppl A): 123.

Muder RR, Yu VL, Johnson J *et al.* (1984). Penetration of cefoperazone into surgical wound drainage in patients undergoing head and neck surgery. *Antimicrob Ag Chemother* **25**: 473.

Mullaney DT, John JF Jr (1982). Cefotaxime therapy of serious bacterial infection in adults. *Antimicrob Ag Chemother* **21**: 421.

Mullaney DT, John JF (1983). Cefotaxime therapy Evaluation of its effect on bacterial meningitis, CSF drug levels, and bactericidal therapy. *Arch Intern Med* **143**: 1705.

Mulligan ME, Citron DM, McNamara BT, Finegold SM (1982). Impact of cefoperazone therapy on fecal flora. *Antimicrob Ag Chemother* **22**: 226.

Murakawa T, Sakamoto H, Fukada S *et al.* (1980). Pharmacokinetics of ceftizoxime in animals after parenteral dosing. *Antimicrob Ag Chemother* **17**: 157.

Murray BE (1991). New aspects of antimicrobial resistance and the resulting therapeutic dilemmas. *J Infect Dis* **163**: 1185.

Murray PR, Granich GG, Krogstad DJ, Niles AC (1983). *In vivo* selection of resistance to multiple cephalosporins by *Enterobacter cloacae*. *J Infect Dis* **147**: 590.

Muytjens HL, Van der Ros-van de Repe J (1982). Comparative activities of 13 beta-lactam antibiotics. *Antimicrob Ag Chemother* **21**: 925.

Naqvi SH, Maxwell MA, Dunkle LM (1985). Cefotaxime therapy of neonatal Gram-negative bacillary meningitis. *Pediatr Infect Dis* **4**: 499.

Nasu M, Maskell JP, Williams RJ, Williams JD (1981). *In vitro* activity of MK0787 (N-formimidoyl thienamycin). and other beta-lactam compounds against *Bacteroides* spp. *Antimicrob Ag Chemother* **20**: 433.

Nau R, Prange HW, Muth P *et al.* (1993). Passage of cefotaxime and ceftriaxone into cerebrospinal fluid of patients with uninflamed meninges. *Antimicrob Ag Chemother* **37**: 1518.

Nelson JD (1985). Emerging role of cephalosporins in bacterial meningitis. *Amer J Med* **79** (Suppl 2A): 47.

Neu HC (1982a). Mechanisms of bacterial resistance to antimicrobial agents, with particular reference to cefotaxime and other beta-lactam compounds. *Rev Infect Dis* **4** (Suppl): 288.

Neu HC (1982b). Antibacterial activity of desacetylcefotaxime alone and in combination with cefotaxime. *Rev Infect Dis* **4** (Suppl): 374.

Neu HC (1982c). Factors that affect the *in-vitro* activity of cephalosporin antibiotics. *J Antimicrob Chemother* **10** (Suppl C): 11.

Neu HC (1983). Structure-activity relations of new beta-lactam compounds and *in vitro* activity against common bacteria. *Rev Infect Dis* **5** (Suppl 2): 319.

Neu HC (1987). New antibiotics: areas of appropriate use. *J Infect Dis* **155**: 403.

Neu HC, Fu KP (1979). *In vitro* anti-bacterial activity and beta-lactamase stability of SCE-129, a new cephalosporin. *Antimicrob Ag Chemother* **15**: 646.

Neu HC, Scully BE (1984). Activity of cefsulodin and other agents against *Pseudomonas aeruginosa*. *Rev Infect Dis* **6** (Suppl 3): 667.

Neu HC, Srinivasan S (1981). Pharmacology of cefitzoxime compared with that of cefamandole. *Antimicrob Ag Chemother* **20**: 366.

Neu HC, Aswapokee N, Aswapokee P, Fu KP (1979). HR 756, a new cephalosporin active against Gram-positive and Gram-negative aerobic and anaerobic bacteria. *Antimicrob Ag Chemother* **15**: 273.

Nicolas M-H, Jarlier V, Honare N *et al.* (1989). Molecular characterization of the gene encoding SHV-3 beta-lactamase responsible for transferable cefotaxime resistance in clinical isolates of *Klebsiella pneumoniae*. *Antimicrob Ag Chemother* **33**: 2096.

Nishimura T, Fujii R (1984). Clinical and pharmacokinetic study of parenteral administration of cefsulodin in pediatric patients in Japan. *Rev Infect Dis* **6** (Suppl 3): 751.

Nolan CM, Ulmer C Jr (1982). Penetration of cefotaxime and moxalactam into cerebrospinal fluid of rabbits with experimentally induced *Escherichia coli* meningitis. *Rev Infect Dis* **4** (Suppl): 396.

Novick WJ Jr (1982). Levels of cefotaxime in body fluids and tissues: a review. *Rev Infect Dis* **4** (Suppl): 346.

Odio CM, Faingezich I, Salas JL *et al.* (1986). Cefotaxime vs. conventional therapy for the treatment of bacterial meningitis of infants and children. *Pediatr Infect Dis* **5**: 402.

Ohkawa M, Okasho A, Sugata T, Kuroda K (1982). Elimination kinetics of ceftizoxime in humans with and without renal insufficiency. *Antimicrob Ag Chemother* **22**: 308.

Ohm-Smith MJ, Hadley WK, Sweet RL (1982). *In vitro* activity of new beta-lactam antibiotics and other antimicrobial drugs against anaerobic isolates from obstetric and gynecological infections. *Antimicrob Ag Chemother* **22**: 711.

Oie S, Hironaga K, Koshiro A *et al.* (1983). *In vitro* susceptibilities of five *Leptospira* strains to 16 antimicrobial agents. *Antimicrob Ag Chemother* **24**: 905.

Olson B, Weinstein RA, Nathan C, Kabins SA (1983). Broad-spectrum beta-lactam resistance to *Enterobacter*: emergence during treatment and mechanisms of resistance. *J Antimicrob Chemother* **11**: 299.

Overturf GD, Cable DC, Forthal DN, Shikuma C (1984). Treatment of bacterial meningitis with cefitzoxime. *Antimicrob Ag Chemother* **25**: 258.

Palenque E, Otero JR, Noriega AR (1986). *In vitro* susceptibility of *Brucella melitensis* to new cephalosporins crossing the blood-brain barrier. *Antimicrob Ag Chemother* **29**: 182.

Palzkill T, Thomson KS, Sanders CC *et al.* (1995). New variant of TEM-10 beta-lactamase gene produced by a clinical isolate of *Proteus mirabilis*. *Antimicrob Ag Chemother* **39**: 1199.

Papanicolaou GA, Medeiros AA, Jacoby GA (1990). Novel plasmid-mediated beta-lactamase (MIR-1) conferring resistance to oxymino- and alpha-methoxy beta-lactams in clinical isolates of *Klebsiella pneumoniae*. *Antimicrob Ag Chemother* **34**: 2200.

Parker RH, Park S (1984). Safety of cefotaxime and other new beta-lactam antibiotics. *J Antimicrob Chemother* **14** (Suppl B): 331.

Parker SW, Baxter J, Beam TR Jr (1984). Cefoperazone-induced coagulopathy. *Lancet* **i**: 1016.

Parks D, Layne P, Uri J *et al.* (1982). Ceftizoxime; clinical evaluation of efficacy and safety in the USA. *J Antimicrob Chemother* **10** (Suppl C): 327.

Parras F, Diaz MD, Reina J *et al.* (1993). Meningitis due to *Aeromonas* species: case report and review. *Clin Infect Dis* **17**: 1058.

Paul GC, Gerbaud G, Bure A *et al.* (1989). TEM-4, a new plasmid-mediated beta-lactamase that hydrolyses broad spectrum cephalosporins in a clinical isolate of *Escherichia coli*. *Antimicrob Ag Chemother* **33**: 1958.

Payne DJ, Amyes SGB (1991). Transferable resistance to extended-spectrum beta-lactams: a major threat or a minor inconvenience. *J Antimicrob Chemother* **27**: 255.

Pechére JC, Guay R, Dubois J, Letarte R (1980). Hydrolysis of cefotaxime by a beta-lactamase from *Bacteroides fragilis*. *Antimicrob Ag Chemother* **17**: 1001.

Peltola H, Anttila M, Renkonen O-V and The Finnish Study Group (1989). Randomised comparison of chloramphenicol, ampicillin, cefotaxime and cefriaxone for childhood bacterial meningitis. *Lancet* **i**: 1281.

Pennington JE, Johnson CE, Platt R (1982). Third-generation cephalosporins in the treatment of pneumonia due to *Pseudomonas aeruginosa* in guinea pigs. *J Infect Dis* **146**: 567.

Perea EJ, Nogales MC, Aznar J *et al.* (1980). Synergy between cefotaxime, cefsulodin, azlocillin, mezlocillin and aminoglycosides against carbenicillin-resistant and sensitive *Pseudomonas aeruginosa*. *J Antimicrob Chemother* **6**: 471.

Peretti P, Sueri L, Tosi M *et al.* (1984). Cefotaxime in the cerebrospinal fluid and serum in patients with purulent meningitis. *J Antimicrob Chemother* **14** (Suppl B): 117.

Perfect JR, Durack DT (1981). Pharmacokinetics of cefoperazone, moxalactam, cefotaxime, trimethoprim and sulphamethoxazole in experimental meningitis. *J Antimicrob Chemother* **8**: 49.

Peterson LR, Gerding DN, Van Etta LL *et al.* (1982). Pharmacokinetics, protein binding and extravascular distribution of ceftizoxime in normal subjects. *Antimicrob Ag Chemother* **22**: 878.

Pfister H-W, Preac-Mursik V, Wilske B *et al.* (1991). Randomized comparison of ceftriaxone and cefotaxime in Lyme neuroborreliosis. *J Infect Dis* **163**: 311.

Philippon A, Labia R, Jacoby G (1989). Extended-spectrum beta-lactamases. *Antimicrob Ag Chemother* **33**: 1131.

Pierson CL, Friedman BA (1992). Comparison of susceptibility to beta-lactam antimicrobial agents among bacteria isolated from intensive care units. *Diagn Microbiol Infect Dis* **15**: 19S.

Pörnull KJ, Göransson E, Rytting A-S, Dornbusch K (1993). Extended-spectrum beta-lactamases in *Escherichia coli* and *Klebsiella* spp in

European septicaemia isolates. *J Antimicrob Chemother* **32**: 559.

Pörnull KJ, Rodrigo G, Dornbusch K (1994). Production of a plasmid-mediated ampC-like beta-lactamase by a *Klebsiella pneumoniae* septicaemia isolate. *J Antimicrob Chemother* **34**: 943.

Pottage JC, Jr, Karakusis PH, Trenholme GM (1984). Cefsulodin therapy for osteomyelitis due to *Pseudomonas aeruginosa*. *Rev Infect Dis* **6** (Suppl 3): 728.

Prevot M-H, Andremont A, Sancho-Garnier H, Tancrede C (1986). Epidemiology of intestinal coloniation by members of the family Enterobacteriaceae resistant to cefotaxime in a hematology-oncology unit. *Antimicrob Ag Chemother* **30**: 945.

Proenca R, Niu WW, Cacalano G, Prince A (1993). The *Pseudomonas cepacia* 249 chromosomal penicillinase is a member of the Amp C family of chromosomal beta-lactamases. *Antimicrob Ag Chemother* **37**: 667.

Quintiliani R, Nightingale CH (1982). Comparative pharmacokinetics of ceftizoxime and other third-generation cephalosporins in humans. *J Antimicrob Chemother* **10** (Suppl C): 99.

Rahal JJ, Simberkoff MS (1982). Host defense and antimicrobial therapy in adult Gram-negative bacillary meningitis. *Ann Intern Med* **96**: 468.

Ralph ED, Behme RJ (1987). Enterobacter meningitis treatment complicated by emergence of mutants resistant to cefotaxime. *Scand J Infect Dis* **19**: 577.

Reed MD, Stern RC, Yamashita TS *et al.* (1984). Single-dose pharmacokinetics of cefsulodin in patients with cystic fibrosis. *Antimicrob Ag Chemother* **25**: 579.

Reeves DS, White LO, Holt HA *et al.* (1980). Human metabolism of cefotaxime. *J Antimicrob Chemother* **6** (Suppl A): 93.

Richmond MH (1980). Beta-lactamase stability of cefotaxime. *J Antimicrob Chemother* **6** (Suppl A): 13.

Rodriguez J, Fuxench-Chiesa Z, Ramirez-Ronda CH *et al.* (1983). *In vitro* susceptibility of 50 non-beta-lactamase-producing *Neisseria gonorrhoeae* strains to 12 antimicrobial agents. *Antimicrob Ag Chemother* **23**: 242.

Rolfe RD, Finegold SM (1981). Comparative *in vitro* activity of new beta-lactam antibiotics against anaerobic bacteria. *Antimicrob Ag Chemother* **20**: 600.

Rolston K, Bolivar R, Fainstein V *et al.* (1985). Cefotaxime: single agent therapy for infections in cancer patients with adequate granulocyte counts. *J Antimicrob Chemother* **15**: 91.

Rosenfeld WN, Evans HE, Batheja R *et al.* (1983). Pharmacokinetics of cefoperazone in full-term and premature neonates. *Antimicrob Ag Chemother* **23**: 866.

Rowe-Jones DC, Peel ALG, Kingston RD *et al.* (1990). Single dose cefotaxime plus metronidazole versus three dose cefuroxime plus metronidazole as prophylaxis against wound infection in colorectal surgery: multicentre prospective randomized study. *Brit Med J* **300**: 18.

Sage R, Hann I, Prentice HG *et al.* (1988). A randomized trial of empirical antibiotic therapy with one of four beta-lactam antibiotics in combination with netilmicin in febrile neutropenic patients. *J Antimicrob Chemother* **22**: 237.

Saito H, Elting L, Bodey GP, Bergey P (1989). *Serratia* bacteremia: review of 118 cases. *Rev Infect Dis* **11**: 912.

Sanders CC (1992). Beta-lactamases of Gram-negative bacteria: new challenges for new drugs. *Clin Infect Dis* **14**: 1089.

Sanders CC, Sanders WE Jr (1985). Microbial resistance to newer generation beta-lactam antibiotics: clinical and laboratory implications. *J Infect Dis* **151**: 399.

Sanders CC, Sanders WE, Jr (1986). Type 1 beta-lactamases of Gram-negative bacteria: interactions with beta-lactam antibiotics. *J Infect Dis* **154**: 792.

Sanders WE Jr, Sanders CC (1988). Inducible beta-lactamases: clinical and epidemiologic implications for use of newer cephalosporins. *Rev Infect Dis* **10**: 830.

Sanders CC, Sanders WE Jr (1992). Beta-lactam resistance in Gram-negative bacteria: global trends and clinical impact. *Clin Infect Dis* **15**: 824.

Sanson-Le Pors MJ, Casin I, Ortenberg M, Perol Y (1983). *In vitro*

susceptibility of thirty strains of *Haemophilus ducreyi* to several antibiotics including six cephalosporins. *J Antimicrob Chemother* **11**: 271.

Scaglione F, Raichi M, Fraschini F (1990). Serum protein binding and extravascular diffusion of methoxyimino cephalosporins Time courses of free and total concentrations of cefotaxime and ceftriaxone in serum and pleural exudate. *J Antimicrob Chemother* **26** (Suppl A): 1.

Scavizzi MR, Alonso J-M, Philippon AM *et al.* (1987). Failure of newer beta-lactam antibiotics for murine *Yersinia enterocolitica* infection. *Antimicrob Ag Chemother* **31**: 523.

Schaad UB, McCracken GH Jr, Loock CA, Thomas ML (1981). Pharmacokinetics and bacteriologic efficacy of moxalactam, cefotaxime, cefoperazone and rocephin in experimental bacterial meningitis. *J Infect Dis* **143**: 156.

Scheld WM (1989). Third-generation cephalosporins in the treatment of severe infections: introduction to a workshop. *Chemotherapy* **35** (Suppl 2): 1.

Scheld WM, Brodeur JP, Sande MA, Alliegro GM (1982). Comparison of cefoperazone with penicillin, ampicillin, gentamicin and chloramphenicol in the therapy of experimental meningitis. *Antimicrob Ag Chemother* **22**: 652.

Scheifele DW, Ginter GL, Olsen E *et al.* (1987). Comparison of two antibiotic regimens for neonatal necrotising enterocolitis. *J Antimicrob Chemother* **20**: 421.

Schleupner CJ, Engle JC (1982). Clinical evaluation of cefotaxime for therapy of lower respiratory tract infections. *Antimicrob Ag Chemother* **21**: 327.

Schrinner E, Limbert M, Penasse L, Lutz A (1980). Antibacterial activity of cefotaxime and other newer cephalosporins (*in vitro* and *in vivo*). *J Antimicrob Chemother* **6** (Suppl A): 25.

Scribner RK, Wedro BC, Weber AH, Marks MI (1982). Activities of eight new beta-lactam antibiotics and seven antibiotic combinations against *Neisseria meningitidis*. *Antimicrob Ag Chemother* **21**: 678.

Scully BE, Neu HC (1982). The use of ceftizoxime in the treatment of critically ill patients infected with multiply antibiotic resistant bacteria. *J Antimicrob Chemother* **10** (Suppl C): 141.

Seeberg AH, Tolxdorff-Neutzling RM, Wiedemann B (1983). Chromosomal beta-lactamases of *Enterobacter cloacae* are responsible for resistance to third-generation cephalosporins. *Antimicrob Ag Chemother* **23**: 918.

Shikuma CM, Cable DC, Edralin G, Overturf GD (1982). Use of ceftizoxime in the treatment of pediatric infections. *J Antimicrob Chemother* **10** (Suppl C): 293.

Shimizu K (1980). Cefoperazone: absorption, excretion distribution and metabolism. *Clin Ther* (Special issue) **3**: 60.

Siegman-Igra Y, Bar-Yosef S, Gorea A, Avram J (1993). Nosocomial *Acinetobacter meningitis* secondary to invasive procedures: report of 25 cases and review. *Clin Infect Dis* **17**: 843.

Simpson IN, Plested SJ, Harper PB (1982). Investigation of the beta-lactamase stability of ceftazidime and eight other new cephalosporin antibiotics. *J Antimicrob Chemother* **9**: 357.

Simpson ML, Khan MY, Siddiqui Y *et al.* (1981). Treatment of gonorrhea: comparison of cefotaxime and penicillin. *Antimicrob Ag Chemother* **19**: 798.

Sinave CP, Ratzan KR (1987). Infective endocarditis caused by *Neisseria flavescens*. *Amer J Med* **82**: 163.

Sirot J, Chanal C, Petit A *et al.* (1988). *Klebsiella pneumoniae* and other Enterobacteraceae producing novel plasmid-mediated beta-lactamases markedly active against third generation cephalosporins: epidemiologic studies. *Rev Infect Dis* **10**: 850.

Sirot DL, Goldstein FW, Soussy CJ *et al.* (1992). Resistance to cefotaxime and seven other beta-lactams in members of the family Enterobacteriaceae: a 3-year survey in France. *Antimicrob Ag Chemother* **36**: 1677.

Sjölin J, Eriksson N, Arneborn P, Cars O (1991). Penetration of cefotaxime and desacetylcefotaxime into brain abscesses in humans. *Antimicrob Ag Chemother* **35**: 2606.

Sjölin J, Lilja A, Eriksson N *et al.* (1993). Treatment of brain abscess with cefotaxime and metronidazole: prospective study on 15 consecutive patients. *Clin Infect Dis* **17**: 857.

Slack MPE, Pitt TL (1982). Characterization of cefsulodin-resistant variants of *Pseudomonas aeruginosa*. *J Antimicrob Chemother* **9**: 111.

Slack MPE, Wheldon DB, Swann RA, Perks E (1979). Cefsulodin, a cephalosporin with specific antipseudomonal activity; *in vitro* studies of the drug alone and in combination. *J Antimicrob Chemother* **5**: 687.

Smith CR (1982). Cefotaxime and cephalosporins: adverse reactions in perspective. *Rev Infect Dis* **4** (Suppl): 481.

Smith CR, Lipsky JJ (1983). Hypoprothrombinemia and platelet dysfunction caused by cephalosporin and oxalactam antibiotics. *J Antimicrob Chemother* **11**: 496.

Smith CR, Ambinder R, Lipsky JJ *et al.* (1984). Cefotaxime compared with nafcillin plus tobramycin for serious bacterial infections. *Ann Intern Med* **101**: 469.

Soe GB, Overturf GD (1987). Treatment of typhoid fever and other systemic salmonelloses with cefotaxime, ceftriaxone, cefoperazone and other newer cephalosporins. *Rev Infect Dis* **9**: 719.

Soussy CJ, Deforges LP, Le Van Thoi J *et al.* (1980). Cefotaxime concentration in the bile and wall of the gallbladder. *J Antimicrob Chemother* **6** (Suppl A): 125.

Spangler SK, Jacobs MR, Appelbaum PC (1994). Susceptibilities of 177 penicillin-susceptible and -resistant pneumococci to FK 037, cefpirome, cefepime, ceftriaxone, cefotaxime, ceftazidime, imipenem, biapenem, meropenem and vancomycin. *Antimicrob Ag Chemother* **38**: 898.

Spencer RC, Smith T, Talbot MD (1984). Ceftizoxime in the treatment of uncomplicated gonorrhoea. *Brit J Vener Dis* **60**: 90.

Srinivasan S, Francke EL, Neu HC (1981). Comparative pharmacokinetics of cefoperazone and cefamandole. *Antimicrob Ag Chemother* **19**: 298.

Standiford HC, Drusano GL, McNamee WB *et al.* (1982). Comparative pharmacokinetics of moxalactam, cefoperazone, and cefotaxime in normal volunteers. *Rev Infect Dis* **4** (Suppl): 585.

Strausbaugh LJ, Llorens AS (1983). Cefoperazone therapy for obstetric and gynecologic infections. *Rev Infect Dis* **5** (Suppl): 154.

Sturm AW (1987). Comparison of antimicrobial susceptibility patterns of fifty-seven strains of *Haemophilus ducreyi* isolated in Amsterdam from 1978 to 1985. *J Antimicrob Chemother* **19**: 187.

Sugar AM, Chahal RS, Stevens DA (1983). A cephalosporin active *in vivo* against *Nocardia*: efficacy of cefotaxime in murine model of acute pulmonary nocardiosis. *J Hyg Camb* **91**: 421.

Sullam PM, Drake TA, Täuber MG *et al.* (1985). Influence of the developmental state of valvular lesions on the antimicrobial activity of cefotaxime in experimental enterococcal infections. *Antimicrob Ag Chemother* **27**: 320.

Sutter VL (1983). Frequency of occurrence and antimicrobial susceptibility of bacterial isolates from the intestinal and female genital tracts. *Rev Infect Dis* **5** (Suppl 1): 84.

Sykes RB, Bush K (1983). Interaction of new cephalosporins with beta-lactamases and beta-lactamase-producing Gram-negative bacilli. *Rev Infect Dis* **5** (Suppl 2): 356.

Tally FP, Cuchural GJ, Jacobus NV *et al.* (1983). Susceptibility of the *Bacteroides fragilis* group in the United States in 1981. *Antimicrob Ag Chemother* **23**: 536.

Tally FP, Cuchural GJ, Jr, Jacobus NV *et al.* (1985). Nationwide study of the susceptibility of the *Bacteroides fragilis* group in the United States. *Antimicrob Ag Chemother* **28**: 675.

Tan TQ, Schutze GE, Mason EOJr, Kaplan SL (1994). Antibiotic therapy and acute outcome of meningitis due to *Streptococcus pneumoniae* considered intermediately susceptable to broad-spectrum cephalosporins. *Antimicrob Ag Chemother* **38**: 918.

Tanayama S, Yoshida K, Kanai Y (1978). Metabolic fate of SCE-129, a new anti-pseudomonal cephalosporin, after parenteral administration in rats and dogs. *Antimicrob Ag Chemother* **14**: 137.

Tang L-M, Chen S-T (1994). *Klebsiella pneumoniae* meningitis: prognostic factors. *Scand J Infect Dis* **26**: 95.

Täuber MG, Shibl AM, Hackbarth CJ *et al.* (1987). Antibiotic therapy, endotoxin concentration in cerebrospinal fluid and brain edema in experimental *Escherichia coli* meningitis in rabbits. *J Infect Dis* **156**: 456.

The Research Committee of the BSSI (1995). Bacterial meningitis: causes for concern. *J Infect* **30**: 89.

Thompson JW, Lewno MJ, Schutze GE (1994). Antibiotic-resistant pneumococcal disease at Arkansas Childrens Hospital, 1990 to 1993. *Pediatr Infect Dis J* **13**: 408.

Todd PA, Brogden RN (1990). Cefotaxime An update of its pharmacology and theapeutic use. *Drugs* **40**: 608.

Towner KJ, Massam M (1985). Resistance to beta-lactamase-stable cephalosporin antibiotics in strains of Enterobacteriaceae and *Pseudomonas aeruginosa* isolated from blood cultures. *J Antimicrob Chemother* **16**: 699.

Trang JM, Jacobs RF, Kearns GL *et al.* (1985). Cefotaxime and desacetylcefotaxime pharmacokinetics in infants and children with meningitis. *Antimicrob Ag Chemother* **28**: 791.

Trollfors B, Ahlmen J, Alestig K (1982). Renal function during cefoperazone treatment. *J Antimicrob Chemother* **9**: 485.

Tsuchiya K, Kondo M, Nagatomo H (1978). SCE-129, antipseudomonal cephalosporin: *in vitro* and *in vivo* antibacterial activities. *Antimicrob Ag Chemother* **13**: 137.

Tunkel AR, Wispelwey B, Scheld WM (1990). Bacterial meningitis: recent advances in pathophysiology and treatment. *Ann Intern Med* **112**: 610.

Turnidge JD, Craig WA (1983). Beta-lactam pharmacology in liver disease. *J Antimicrob Chemother* **11**: 499.

Tweardy DJ, Jacobs MR, Speck WT (1983). Susceptibility of penicillin-resistant pneumococci to eighteen antimicrobials: implications for treatment of meningitis. *J Antimicrob Chemother* **12**: 133.

Tzouvelekis LS, Tzelepi E, Mentis AF, Tsakris A (1993). Identification of a novel plasmid-mediated beta-lactamase with chromosomal cephalosporinase characteristics from *Klebsiella pneumoniae*. *J Antimicrob Chemother* **31**: 645.

Ullmann U (1979). Bacteriological studies with cefsulodin (CGP 7174/E)., the first antipseudomonal cephalosporin. *J Antimicrob Chemother* **5**: 563.

Vallee F, Le Bel M (1991). Comparative study of pharmacokinetics and serum bactericidal activity of ceftizoxime and cefotaxime. *Antimicrob Ag Chemother* **35**: 2057.

Vallejo JG, Kaplan SL, Mason EOJr (1991). Treatment of meningitis and other infections due to ampicillin-resistant *Haemophilus influenzae* type b in children. *Rev Infect Dis* **13**: 197.

Van der Auwera P, Scorneaux B (1985). *In vitro* susceptibility of *Campylobacter jejuni* to 27 antimicrobial agents and various combinations of beta-lactams with clavulanic acid or sulbactam. *Antimicrob Ag Chemother* **28**: 37.

Van Etta LL, Fasching CE, Peterson LR, Gerding DN (1983). Comparison study of the kinetics of ceftizoxime penetration into extravascular spaces with known surface area/volume ratio *in vitro* and *in vivo* in rabbits. *Antimicrob Ag Chemother* **23**: 49.

Van Laethem Y, Lagast H, Klastersky J (1983). Serum bactericidal activity of ceftazidime and cefoperazone alone or in combination with amikacin against *Pseudomonas aeruginosa* and *Klebsiella pneumoniae*. *Antimicrob Ag Chemother* **23**: 435.

Viladrich PF, Cabellos C, Pallares R *et al.* (1996). High doses of cefotaxime in treatment of adult meningitis due to *Streptococcus pneumoniae* with decreased susceptibilities to broad-spectrum cephalosporins. *Antimicrob Ag Chemother* **40**: 218.

Vollaard EJ, Clasener HAL, Janssen AJHM, Wynne HJA (1990). Influence of cefotaxime on microbial colonization resistance in healthy volunteers. *J Antimicrob Chemother* **26**: 117.

Vu H, Nikaido H (1985). Role of beta-lactam hydrolysis in the mechanism of resistance of a beta-lactamase-constitutive *Enterobacter cloacae* strain to expanded-spectrum beta-lactams. *Antimicrob Ag Chemother* **27**: 393.

Wallace RJJr, Steele LC, Sumter G, Smith JM (1988). Antimicrobial susceptibility patterns of *Nocardia asteroides*. *Antimicrob Ag Chemother* **32**: 1776.

Ward JI, Moellering RC Jr (1981). Susceptibility of pneumococci to 14 beta-lactam agents: comparison of strains resistant, intermediate-resistant, and susceptible to penicillin. *Antimicrob Ag Chemother* **20**: 204.

Warren JW, Miller EH Jr, Fitzpatrick B *et al.* (1983). A randomized, controlled trial of cefoperazone vs cefamandole-tobramycin in the treatment of putative, severe infections with Gram-negative bacilli. *Rev Infect Dis* **5** (Suppl 1): 173.

Watanakunakorn C (1989). *Serratia* bacteremia: a review of 44 episodes. *Scand J Infect Dis* **21**: 477.

Weber K, Pfister H-W (1994). Clinical management of Lyme borreliosis. *Lancet* **343**: 1017.

Weingarten RD, Markiewicz Z, Gilbert DN (1990). Meningitis due to penicillin-resistant *Streptococcus pneumoniae* in adults. *Rev Infect Dis* **12**: 118.

Welage LS, Borin MT, Wilton JH *et al.* (1990). Comparative evaluation of the pharmacokinetics of N-methylthiotetrazole following administration of cefoperazone, cefotetan, and cefmetazole. *Antimicrob Ag Chemother* **34**: 2369.

Welby PL, Keller DS, Cromien JL *et al.* (1994). Resistance to penicillin and non-beta-lactam antibiotics of *Streptococcus pneumoniae* at a children's hospital. *Pediatr Infect Dis J* **13**: 281.

Wells TG, Trang JM, Brown AL *et al.* (1984). Cefotaxime therapy of bacterial meningitis in children. *J Antimicrob Chemother* **14** (Suppl B): 181.

Werner V, Sanders CC, Sanders WE Jr, Goering RV (1985). Role of beta-lactamases and outer membrane proteins in multiple beta-lactam resistance of *Enterobacter cloacae*. *Antimicrob Ag Chemother* **27**: 455.

White AJ, Curtis NAC (1985). Hydrolysis of beta-lactamase-stable beta-lactams by type I 'sponge' beta-lactamases. *J Antimicrob Chemother* **16**: 403.

Wiedemann B (1986). Selection of beta-lactamase producers during cephalosporin and penicillin therapy. *Scand J Infect Dis* (Suppl 49): 100.

Wise R, Wills PJ, Andrews JM, Bedford KA (1980a). Activity of the cefotaxime (HR 756). desacetylmetabolite compared with those of cefotaxime and other cephalosporins. *Antimicrob Ag Chemother* **17**: 84.

Wise R, Baker S, Livingstone R (1980b). Comparison of cefotaxime and moxalactam pharmacokinetics and tissue levels. *Antimicrob Ag Chemother* **18**: 369.

Wise R, Andrews JM, Bedford KA (1981a). Cefoperazone and cefotiam – two new cephalosporins: an *in vitro* comparison. *J Antimicrob Chemother* **7**: 343.

Wise R, Wright N, Wills PJ (1981b). Pharmacology of cefotaxime and its desacetyl metabolite in renal and hepatic disease. *Antimicrob Ag Chemother* **19**: 526.

Wolff MA, Young CL, Ramphal R (1993). Antibiotic therapy for *Enterobacter meningitis*: a retrospective review of 13 episodes and review of the literature. *Clin Infect Dis* **16**: 772.

Word BM, Klein JO (1989). Therapy of bacterial sepsis and meningitis in infants and children: 1989 poll of directors of programs in pediatric infectious diseases. *Pediatr Infect Dis J* **8**: 635.

Yabuuchi E, Ito T, Tanimura E *et al.* (1981). *In vitro* antimicrobial activity of ceftizoxime against glucose-nonfermentative Gram-negative rods. *Antimicrob Ag Chemother* **20**: 136.

Yamauchi T, Hill DE, Steele RW (1982). The use of ceftizoxime in neonates. *J Antimicrob Chemother* **10** (Suppl C): 297.

Yang Y, Livermore DM (1988). Chromosomal beta-lactamase expression and resistance to beta-lactam antibiotics in *Proteus vulgaris* and *Morganella morganii*. *Antimicrob Ag Chemother* **32**: 1385.

Yeo S-F, Livermore DM (1994). Comparative *in-vitro* activity of biapenem and other carbapenems against *Haemophilus influenzae* isolates with known resistance mechanisms to ampicillin. *J Antimicrob Chemother* **33**: 861.

Young JPW, Husson JM, Bruch K *et al.* (1980). The evaluation of efficacy and safety of cefotaxime: a review of 2500 cases. *J Antimicrob Chemother* **6** (Suppl A): 293.

Yu PKW, Washington JA II (1983). Bactericidal activities of new beta-lactam antibiotics against *Bacteroides fragilis*. *Antimicrob Ag Chemother* **24**: 1.

Moxalactam (Latamoxef)

Description

For practical purposes, moxalactam was regarded as one of the third-generation cephalosporins (p. 319). Its antimicrobial spectrum, resistance to bacterial beta-lactamases and clinical application, were similar to other members of this group. It differs chemically from true cephalosporins because in its nucleus, unlike 7-ACA (p. 3), sulfur is replaced by an oxygen atom (Webber and Yoshida, 1982).

The drug is now no longer used clinically, although initially it appeared quite promising, particularly for the treatment of *Haemophilus influenzae* meningitis and meningitis due to Enterobacteriaceae (Corrado *et al.*, 1982; Freedman *et al.*, 1983; Kaplan *et al.*, 1983; Rahal *et al.*, 1984). It achieved quite high CSF concentrations (McCracken and Schaad, 1982; Creger *et al.*, 1985) and results of treatment were much the same as those obtained with cefotaxime (p. 336) or ceftriaxone (p. 359), but moxalactam was considerably less active than cefotaxime (p. 319) against Gram-positive bacteria such as *Staphylococcus aureus*, *Streptococcus pyogenes* and *Strep. pneumoniae* (Neu *et al.*, 1979). Therefore moxalactam, unlike cefotaxime (p. 336) could not be used as a single-drug for initial treatment of bacterial meningitis in the age groups where there was only need to cover *N. meningitidis*, *H. influenzae* and *Strep. pneumoniae* infections (p. 336). Penicillin G or ampicillin always had to be used together with moxalactam to cover *Strep. pneumoniae* infection (Nelson, 1983). This was a disadvantage.

Against organisms of the *Bacteroides fragilis* group moxalactam was more active than cefotaxime (p. 321) and it was about as potent as cefoxitin (p. 295) (Jenkins *et al.*, 1982), but it did not have a place in the treatment of intra-abdominal infections, because of its side-effects (see below), and as many other drugs were available for this treatment.

The main disadvantage of moxalactam was that it caused bleeding. In common with cefamandole (p. 306) and cefoperazone (p. 335) it contains the N-methylthiotetraxole side-chain. This side-chain, released *in vivo*, inhibits gamma carboxylation of glutamic acid, which is necessary for the synthesis of prothrombin. Many other factors are usually also involved, including dietary intake, vitamin K turnover, hepatic and renal function and the status of the gastrointestinal tract (Lipsky, 1983; 1988; Brown *et al.*, 1986; Nichols *et al.*, 1987). The bleeding in most cases could be prevented by prophylactic administration of vitamin K (Panwalker and Rosenfeld, 1983; Shevchuk and Conly, 1990).

By 1987 moxalactam was no longer recommended for treatment of bacterial meningitis in infants and children in the USA (McCracken *et al.*, 1987) and it now seems that this drug is no longer used for any indication.

References

Brown RB, Klar J, Lemeshow S *et al.* (1986). Enhanced bleeding with cefoxitin or moxalactam. Statistical analysis within a defined population of 1493 patients. *Arch Intern Med* **146**:2159.

Corrado ML, Gombert ME, Cherubin CE (1982). Designing appropriate therapy in the treatment of Gram-negative bacillary meningitis. *JAMA* **248**: 71.

Creger RJ, Cowan RI, Nearman HS *et al.* (1985). Cerebrospinal fluid penetration of moxalactam in ventriculostomy patients. *Antimicrob Ag Chemother* **28**: 839.

Freedman JM, Hoffman SH, Scheld WM *et al.* (1983). Moxalactam for the treatment of bacterial meningitis in children. *J Infect Dis* **148**: 886.

Jenkins SG, Birk RJ, Zabransky RJ (1982). Differences in susceptibilities of species of the *Bacteroides fragilis* group to several beta-lactam antibiotics: indole production as an indicator of resistance. *Antimicrob Ag Chemother* **22**: 628.

Kaplan SL, Mason EO Jr, Kvernland SJ *et al.* (1983). Moxalactam treatment of serious infections primarily due to *Haemophilus influenzae* type b in children. *Pediatrics* **71**: 187.

Lipsky JJ (1983). N-methyl-thio-tetrazole inhibition of the gamma carboxylation of glutamic acid: possible mechanism for antibiotic-associated hypoprothrombinaemia. *Lancet* **ii**: 192.

Lipsky JJ (1988). Antibiotic-associated hypoprothrombinaemia. *J Antimicrob Chemother* **21**: 281.

McCracken GH Jr, Schaad UB (1982). The pharmacologic basis for moxalactam therapy for Gram-negative enteric bacillary meningitis of infancy. *Rev Infect Dis* **4** (Suppl): 603.

McCracken GH Jr, Nelson JD, Kaplan SL *et al.* (1987). Consensus report Antimicrobial therapy for bacterial meningitis in infants and children. *Pediatr Infect Dis J* **6**: 501.

Nelson JD (1983). A primer for pediatricians on new cephalosporin antibiotics. *Amer J Dis Child* **137**: 1041.

Neu HC, Aswapokee N, Fu KP, Aswapokee P (1979). Antibacterial activity of a new 1-oxa cephalosporin compared with that of other beta-lactam compounds. *Antimicrob Ag Chemother* **16**: 141.

Nichols RL, Wikler MA, McDevitt JT *et al.* (1987). Coagulopathy associated with extended-spectrum cephalosporins in patients with serious infections. *Antimicrob Ag Chemother* **31**: 281.

Panwalker AP, Rosenfeld J (1983). Hemorrhage, diarrhea and superinfection associated with the use of moxalactam. *J Infect Dis* **147**: 171.

Rahal JJ Jr, Simberkoff MS, Landesman SH, Metropolitan Meningitis Study Group (1984). Prospective evaluation of moxalactam therapy for Gram-negative bacillary meningitis. *J Infect Dis* **149**: 562.

Shevchuk YM, Conly JM (1990). Antibiotic-associated hypoprothrombinemia: a review of prospective studies. 1966–1988. *Rev Infect Dis* **12**: 1109.

Webber JA, Yoshida T (1982). Moxalactam: the first of a new class of beta-lactam antibiotics. *Rev Infect Dis* **4** (Suppl): 496.

Ceftriaxone

Description

Ceftriaxone is another third-generation cephalosporin, which is stable to beta-lactamases, particularly those produced by Gram-negative bacteria. It has high potency against all the Enterobacteriaceae, *Haemophilus influenzae*, the *Neisseria* and most Gram-positive cocci except Enterococcal spp. (Shannon *et al.*, 1980; Neu *et al.*, 1981). Ceftriaxone is unique because of its prolonged serum half-life, which permits once- or twice-daily dosing (Garzone *et al.*, 1983).

Sensitive Organisms

1 Gram-positive bacteria

In general, ceftriaxone has a similar activity to cefotaxime (p. 319) against Gram-positive cocci (Table I.27). *Staphylococcus aureus* and coagulase-negative staphylococci are somewhat less susceptible to ceftriaxone than to cefotaxime, and methicillin-resistant variants of these organisms are resistant to both drugs (Angehrn *et al.*, 1980; Shannon *et al.*, 1980). Against *Streptococcus pyogenes*, Group B streptococci and *Strep. pneumoniae*, the activity of ceftriaxone is similar to that of cefotaxime (Table I.27). The MICs of ceftriaxone may be lower than those of penicillin G against pneumococcal strains with intermediate type of resistance to penicillin G (Neal *et al.*, 1992). However, similar to cefotaxime (p. 320) sometimes the MICs of ceftriaxone are higher than those of penicillin G for these strains (Figueiredo *et al.*, 1992). Cefriaxone or cefotaxime may be useful for treatment of pneumococcal meningitis caused by these strains only if their MICs are sufficiently low (p. 359). This increased activity against penicillin G-resistant pneumococci does not occur with all third-generation cephalosporins. For instance, ceftizoxime is usually much less effective than cefotaxime or ceftriaxone against these strains (Haas *et al.*, 1995). *Streptococcus viridans* is sensitive but *Enterococcus faecalis* is resistant (Verbist and Verhaegen, 1981). *Listeria monocytogenes* is only moderately sensitive (Table I.27). *Nocardia asteroides* is moderately sensitive; some 80% of strains are inhibited by 8 μg per ml or less of ceftriaxone (Gombert *et al.*, 1987; Wallace *et al.*, 1988). All *Actinomadura madurae* isolates are sensitive and more than 80% of strains of *Streptomyces griseus* and *Nocardia brasiliensis* are ceftriaxone-sensitive (McNeil *et al.*, 1990). Anaerobic Gram-positive bacteria, such as the *Peptococcus*, *Peptostreptococcus*, *Actinomyces* and *Lactobacillus* spp., are usually sensitive. Most *Clostridium* spp., including *Cl. perfringens*, are sensitive, but *Cl. difficile* is resistant (Rolfe and Finegold, 1982).

2 Gram-negative cocci

Ceftriaxone is very active against *Neiseria meningitidis*, more so than cefotaxime (Table I.27). Beta-lactamase-producing meningococci (p. 13) and organisms with intrinsic resistance to penicillin G are also ceftriaxone-sensitive (Uriz *et al.*, 1991). The drug is equally active against both penicillin G-sensitive and beta-lactamase-producing strains of *N. gonorrhoeae* (Kerbs *et al.*, 1983; Ng *et al.*, 1983). Gonococci, relatively resistant to penicillin G, which do not produce beta-lactamase, are usually more sensitive to ceftriaxone than to penicillin G (Liebowitz *et al.*, 1982). Surveys in the Philippines (Clendennen *et al.*, 1992a), Thailand (Clendennen *et al.*, 1992b), Gambia (Ison *et al.*, 1992), Nicaragua (Castro *et al.*, 1993) and the USA (Rice and Knapp, 1994; Schwebke *et al.*, 1995) showed that all gonococcal strains, including those that were multiresistant, were still ceftriaxone-sensitive, but the MICs of ceftriaxone for strains with chromosomally mediated resistance to penicillin G (0.125 μg per ml) were slightly higher than for strains resistant to penicillin G because of beta-lactamase production (0.03 μg per ml).

3 Gram-negative aerobic bacilli

Similar to cefotaxime (p. 320), ceftriaxone is highly resistant to hydrolysis by both plasmid and chromosomally mediated beta-lactamases of Gram-negative bacilli. It has approximately equal potency to cefotaxime against Enterobacteriaceae, such as *Escherichia coli, Morganella morganii*, the *Klebsiella, Enterobacter, Providencia, Citrobacter, Salmonella* and *Shigella* spp. Against *Proteus* spp., the drug is more active than cefotaxime (Table I.27) (Shannon *et al.*, 1980; Neu *et al.*, 1981). Ceftriaxone is quite active against *Yersinia enterocolitica* (Scribner *et al.*, 1982). Aminoglycoside-resistant Enterobacteriaceae may be ceftriaxone-sensitive (Fass, 1982; Muytjens and Van der Ros-van de Repe, 1982). Ceftriaxone in combination with an aminoglycoside, such as gentamicin or amikacin, usually exhibits an enhanced bactericidal effect against most strains of Enterobacteriaceae (Bayer *et al.*, 1984).

Haemophilus influenzae, including beta-lactamase producing strains and chloramphenicol-resistant strains, is highly sensitive to ceftriaxone (Laferriere *et al.*, 1983; Campos and Garcia-Tornel, 1987). *Bordetella pertussis* (MIC 0.1 μg per ml) is also susceptible (Bannatyne and Cheung, 1984). *Haemophilus ducreyi* is highly sensitive (Dangor *et al.*, 1990; Knapp *et al.*, 1993). It has remained sensitive in various parts in the world (Abeck *et al.*, 1988; Dangor *et al.*, 1988; Motley *et al.*, 1992; Aldridge *et al.*, 1993). In Kenya the usually recommended dose of ceftriaxone (single-dose of 250 mg i.m.) failed in treatment, particularly in HIV-infected patients, yet the isolates remained highly susceptible to the drug *in vitro*) (Tyndall *et al.*, 1993). *Brucella melitensis* is also ceftriaxone-sensitive (MICs 0.25–1.0 μg per ml) (Bosch *et al.*, 1986; Palenque *et al.*, 1986).

Acinetobacter spp. and *Campylobacter jejuni* (Muytjens and Van der Ros-van de Repe, 1982) and *Pseudomonas aeruginosa* (Neu *et al.*, 1981) are moderately resistant. During ceftriaxone treatment *in vivo* of *Ps. aeruginosa* infections, this organism may become more highly resistant (Paull and Morgan, 1986). Ceftriaxone in combination with gentamicin, tobramycin or amikacin, shows *in vitro* synergy with some strains of *Ps. aeruginosa* but antagonism or indifference with others (Angehrn, 1983; Watanakunakorn, 1983). *Burkholderia (Pseudomonas) pseudomallei* may be sometimes sensitive to ceftriaxone (Shaefer *et al.*, 1983), whereas *Burkholderia cepacia*, *Ps. stutzeri* and *Ps. diminuta* are usually resistant and *Stenotrophomonas maltophilia* is always resistant (Neu *et al.*, 1981; Fass, 1983).

Kingella kingae is ceftriaxone-susceptible (Jensen *et al.*, 1994). Similarly *Bartonella* (previously *Rochalimaea*) *quintana, Bartonella vinsonii* and *Bartonella henselae* are quite sensitive to cefriaxone and cefotaxime (MICs <0.125 μg per ml). The *Bartonella* spp. often cause septicemia and other infections in immunocompromised patients such as those with HIV (Lucey *et al.*, 1992; Maurin and Raoult, 1993). *Pasteurella multocida* and *P. dagmatis* are ceftriaxone-sensitive (Noel and Teele, 1986; Sorbello *et al.*, 1994).

4 Gram-negative anaerobic bacteria

Some of these, such as *Prevotella (Bacteroides) melaninogenica, Fusobacterium* spp. and *Actinobacillus actinomycetemcomitans*, are inhibited by low ceftriaxone concentrations. *Bacteroides fragilis* is more resistant and the action of ceftriaxone against this species is comparable with that of cefotaxime (Table I.27). As with cefotaxime (p. 321), ceftriaxone is hydrolyzed by some *B. fragilis* beta-lactamases of chromosomal origin, (Neu *et al.*, 1981; Rolfe and Finegold, 1982; Pollock *et al.*, 1983; Grace *et al.*, 1988).

5 Other organisms

Chlamydia trachomatis is ceftriaxone-resistant (Hammerschlag and Gleyzer, 1983). The drug has some activity against *Coxiella burnetii*. One-third of isolates are inhibited by <4 μg per ml (Torres and Raoult, 1993). *Mycoplasma* and *Mycobacterium* spp. and fungi are resistant. *Treponema pallidum* is sensitive as the drug is effective against experimentally induced syphilis in rabbits, where although it has high anti-treponemal activity, this is lower than that of penicillin G (Johnson *et al.*, 1982; Johnson, 1989). *Borrelia burgdorferi* is ceftriaxone-sensitive (MICs 0.02–0.04 μg per ml) (Johnson *et al.*, 1987; Agger *et al.*, 1992). In *in vitro* studies human fibroblasts protect this organism from the lethal effect of ceftriaxone. *Borrelia burgdorferi* first infects the skin, where there is an abundance of fibroblasts. It is possible that these organisms may survive antibiotic treatment intracellularly in fibroblasts. *Borrelia burgdorferi* has been isolated from skin and other tissues after antibiotic treatment of Lyme disease (Georgilis *et al.*, 1992).

6 Acquired resistance

Enterobacteriaceae, which are normally highly ceftriaxone-sensitive, may become resistant. Resistant strains of *Enterobacter* spp., and other Gram-negative aerobic bacilli, may emerge during ceftriaxone treatment of patients, due to a mechanism similar to that which occurs with other third-generation cephalosporins, such as cefotaxime (p. 322). These strains possess an inducible chromosomally mediated beta-lactamase, which hydrolyzes these normally beta-lactamase-stable drugs (Sanders and Sanders, 1983; Marchou *et al.*, 1987a). In some organisms such as *Enterobacter cloacae* a decreased outer membrane permeability may contribute to the resistance (Marchou *et al.*, 1987b). With Enterobacteriaceae, especially *Klebsiella* spp., ceftriaxone-resistance may also occur due to the acquisition of plasmid-mediated extended-spectrum beta-lactamases, similar to cefotaxime (p. 323) (Goldstein *et al.*, 1993).

7 Minimum inhibitory concentrations

The MICs of ceftriaxome, compared with those of cefotaxime, against some selected bacterial species are shown in Table I.27.

Organism	MIC (µg per ml)	
	Cefotaxime	Ceftriaxone
Gram-positive bacteria		
Staphylococcus aureus	0.5–8.0	1.6–>50.0
Staphylococcus epidermidis	3.13–8.0	0.8–>50.0
Streptococcus pyogenes	0.015–0.25	0.012–0.25
Streptococcus pneumoniae	<0.01–0.25	0.012–0.1
Streptococci, Group B	<0.01–0.1	0.012–0.1
Streptococcus viridans	≤0.12	1.1–1.6
Enterococcus faecalis	>16.0–200.0	12.5–>100.0
Listeria monocytogenes	8.0	0.8–25.0
Clostridium perfringens	2.0–4.0	0.25–25.0
Gram-negative bacteria		
Escherichia coli	<0.1–8.0	0.0125–25.0
Enterobacter spp.	<0.01–4.0	0.006–3.1
Klebsiella spp.	<0.1–2.0	0.0125–0.4
Proteus mirabilis	<0.001–0.5	0.006–0.01
Proteus vulgaris	<0.01–12.5	≤0.03–0.13
Morganella morganii	0.2–4.0	≤0.03–1.0
Providencia spp.	<0.01–3.1	≤0.03–1.0
Salmonella spp.	0.1–0.5	<0.025–100.0
Shigella spp.	<0.1–0.5	<0.006–0.2
Serratia marcescens	0.2–>128.0	0.2–>100.0
Neisseria gonorrhoeae	0.0006–0.08	0.006–0.04
Neisseria gonorrhoeae (beta-lactamase-producer)	0.006–0.04	0.006–0.02
Neisseria meningitidis	≤0.025	0.0004–0.0016
Haemophilus influenzae	0.008–0.063	0.003
Haemophilus influenzae (beta-lactamase producer)	0.008–0.064	0.003
Pseudomonas aeruginosa	2.0–>128.0	0.8–100.0
Bacteroides fragilis	2.0–>128.0	0.8–>100.0
Prevotella melaninogenica	≤0.03–4.0	≤0.03–8.0

Table I.27
Compiled from data published by Angehrn *et al.* (1980), Neu *et al.* (1981), Verbist and Verhaegen (1981), Fass (1983) Kerbs *et al.* (1983) and Laferriere *et al.* (1983)

Mode of Administration and Dosage

1 Parenteral administration

Ceftriaxone is not absorbed after oral administration, and so it must be administered by either the i.m. or i.v. route. It is more suitable for i.m. administration than other third-generation cephalosporins because it has a prolonged serum half-life (p. 356), which allows administration at 12-hourly or 24-hourly intervals (Eron et al., 1983; Marks, 1983). When given i.m., the drug can be mixed with lignocaine (lidocaine) to reduce pain (Patel et al., 1982; Aronoff et al., 1983). Ceftriaxone is given i.v. either by direct intermittent injections over 2–5 min or by short 20–30 min infusions, similar to penicillin G (p. 20) (Schaad and Stoeckel, 1982; Steele and Bradsher, 1983b).

2 Adults

The usual adult dosage is 1–2 g daily i.m. or i.v., given once-daily, even in moderately serious infections (Eron et al., 1983; Rothwell et al., 1983). For the treatment of skin and soft tissue infections, an adult dosage of 1 g i.m. daily may suffice (Gordin et al., 1985). For the treatment of life-threatening infections, such as meningitis and septicemia in immunocompromised patients, the dosage was often increased to 2 g 12-hourly or even to 2 g 8-hourly in the past (Salvador et al., 1983; Tunkel et al., 1990). It is now accepted that a dosage of 2 g i.v. once every 24 h is sufficient for serious infections such as bacterial meningitis or septicemia (Garber et al., 1992; Marhoum et al., 1993; The Internat. Antimicrob. Therap. Coop. Group, 1993; Mashford et al., 1994), but a dose as high as 2 g 12-hourly is still occasionally used (p. 362).

3 Children

The dosage is 50–100 mg per kg body weight daily, given in one or two divided doses (Steele and Bradsher, 1983; Peltola et al., 1989). For the treatment of bacterial meningitis, a dosage of 50 mg per kg 12-hourly has been recommended, which could be preceded by an initial loading dose of 75 mg per kg (Schaad and Stoeckel, 1982; Del Rio et al., 1983; Steele and Bradsher, 1983a). Single daily doses of 50 mg per kg have been effective for the treatment of children with a variety of non-meningitic bacterial infections (Congeni et al., 1985). Single daily doses of 100 mg per kg have been used successfully in bacterial meningitis (Martin, 1983a,b; Bryan et al., 1985; Danker et al., 1988; Peltola et al., 1989; Schaad et al., 1990).

4 Newborn infants

Pharmacokinetic studies indicate that a single daily dose of 50 mg per kg body weight may be sufficient in this age group, even for severe infections such as bacterial meningitis (McCracken et al., 1983). Others have found that in neonates over 7 days of age, a dosage of 50 mg per kg every 12 h is safe and effective for the treatment of bacterial meningitis (Steele et al., 1983; Steele and Bradsher, 1983a).

5 Elderly patients

In patients over 65 years of age the ceftriaxone serum elimination half-life may be prolonged from the normal 6.5 h to 15 h. So dosing intervals greater than 24 h or a reduction of the dose without a change in dosing interval may be indicated (Deeter et al., 1990).

6 Pregnant patients

In contrast to other beta-lactam antibiotics (p. 117), a daily ceftriaxone dose of 2 g i.v. is sufficient in these patients and a loading dose or increase in maintenance dose is not necessary (Bourget et al., 1993).

7 Patients with renal failure

The normal ceftriaxone half-life of approximately 6 h is only prolonged to about 14 h in patients with end-stage renal failure. Dosage reduction is not required for the majority of renal failure patients, provided the dose is 2 g per day or less, because the drug has significant biliary excretion. For patients with essentially no renal function, receiving regular hemodialysis, a dosage of 1 g daily is usually sufficient. However, there may be considerable variation in the half-life of ceftriaxone in such patients (p. 356), so that serum level monitoring is advisable. Ceftriaxone is not removed during hemodialysis, and supplemental doses are not required after this procedure (Cohen *et al.*, 1983; Patel *et al.*, 1984; Patel and Kaplan, 1984). The clearance of ceftriaxone during peritoneal dialysis is also minimal. During continuous arterivenous hemofiltration also relatively little ceftriaxone is removed from the body (De'Clari, 1991).

8 Patients undergoing therapeutic plasmapheresis

Only some 11.5–24.5% of the ceftriaxone dose is removed during this procedure. Patients undergoing plasmapheresis for 150 min or less may safely be treated with ceftriaxone 2 g i.v. daily without risking periods of subtherapeutic plasma ceftriaxone levels. It is better to administer the drug after the plasmapheresis to ensure its therapeutic efficiency (Bakken *et al.*, 1990, 1993; Fauvelle *et al.*, 1994).

9 Patients with cirrhosis of liver

The usual ceftriaxone dosage can be given to these patients, provided that the renal function is normal (Westphal *et al.*, 1994).

Serum Levels in Relation to Dosage

After i.m. injection of a 1-g dose to adults, a mean peak serum level of 79.2 µg per ml is attained at 1.5 h; thereafter this level falls slowly, being 58.2, 35.5 and 7.8 µg per ml at 4, 12 and 24 h after the injection, respectively (Meyers *et al.*, 1983). The elimination half-life after i.m. injection is approximately 6 h.

If 1 g ceftriaxone is given i.v. to adults as a 30-min infusion, the mean peak serum level, attained immediately after infusion, is 123.2 µg per ml; this falls to 94.8, 57.8, 20.2 and 4.6 µg per ml at 1.5, 4, 12 and 24 h after commencement of the infusion, respectively (Meyers *et al.*, 1983). The elimination half-life of the drug is again about 6 h. Doubling the i.v. dose approximately doubles the above serum concentrations, but the elimination half-life remains unchanged (Patel *et al.*, 1981). When i.v. doses of 0.5, 1.0 and 2 g are given to adults every 12 h, some ceftriaxone accumulates in the serum. Assuming linear pharmacokinetics, a 40% accumulation of ceftriaxone in serum could be expected by the fourth day of these regimens. Observed serum accumulations of the drug were 35% with a 0.5 g 12-hourly regimen, but only 20% with the 1 g and 2 g 12-hourly regimens. The less than predicted accumulation of ceftriaxone with the higher dosage regimens, probably resulted from a concentration-dependent decrease in its plasma protein binding, which increased both its distribution and elimination (Pollock *et al.*, 1982).

In newborn infants, after a 15-min i.v. infusion of 50 mg per kg, the mean peak level after infusion increases with the age of the infant. In one study, the mean peak was 145 µg per ml in infants aged 3 days, and this increased to 173 µg per ml in those aged 22 days. This occurs because younger infants have larger distribution volumes. In both age groups, mean serum levels were about the same (66 µg per ml) 6 h after infusion, because older infants excrete the drug more rapidly; mean ceftriaxone half-lives being 7.7 and 5.2 h in those aged 3 and 22 days, respectively (McCracken *et al.*, 1983).

Excretion

1 Urine

Ceftriaxone is not metabolized in the body and 40–50% of a parenterally administered dose is excreted in urine within 48 h as the active drug (Patel *et al.*, 1981; Findlay *et al.*, 1982). High concentrations of the active drug are attained in urine. Compared with other cephalosporins, ceftriaxone is only slowly eliminated by the kidneys. Renal elimination is only about 7% of glomerular filtration rate and tubular secretion probably does not occur. High serum protein binding (about 95%) may partly explain its slow renal clearance (Wise and Andrews, 1983). Ceftriaxone is not reabsorbed by renal tubules (Arvidsson *et al.*, 1982).

2 Bile

The remainder of a dose of ceftriaxone appears to be excreted unchanged in bile; in human volunteers this is at least 11% of an administered dose. The degree of biliary excretion varies considerably between individuals; this explains the variable doses of ceftriaxone which may be required in patients with end-stage renal disease (p. 355). Following biliary excretion, the drug is probably gradually inactivated in the gut by fecal enzymes (Welling *et al.*, 1992). After i.v.

administration of radioactive-labeled ceftriaxone to human volunteers, 44% of the dose was recovered as microbiologically inactive material in the feces (Patel *et al.*, 1981; Patel and Kaplan, 1984). If ceftriaxone is administered together with diclofenac, a non-steroidal anti-inflammatory drug, there is a significant decrease in biliary excretion of ceftriaxone in animals (Merle-Melet *et al.*, 1989). In contrast, in humans, diclofenac causes an increase in ceftriaxone biliary excretion, and some decrease of the drug's urinary excretion (Merle-Melet *et al.*, 1992).

Distribution of the Drug in Body

In common with cefotaxime (p. 333) ceftriaxone penetrates poorly into CSF of animals with uninflamed meninges, but it reaches therapeutically effective concentrations in those with induced bacterial meningitis. In rabbits, ceftriaxone has the longest CSF half-life and duration of bactericidal activity (Schaad *et al.*, 1981; Täuber *et al.*, 1984). In rabbit meningitis due to *H. influenzae* type b or *Strep. pneumoniae* infection, CSF concentrations of ceftriaxone have reached 3–14% of serum levels (McCracken *et al.*, 1982). In humans, there has been only 1.5 % penetration of drug into the CSF in those with uninflamed meninges (Chandresekar *et al.*, 1984). In another study in humans with uninflamed meninges Nau *et al.* (1993) found that after a 2-g dose of ceftriaxone, infused i.v. over 30 min, the levels of ceftriaxone in the CSF ranged from 0.18 to 1.04 μg per ml and they were seen 1–16 h after the infusion, but the drug diffuses well into the CSF of patients with bacterial meningitis. Latif and Dajani (1983) gave single doses of 75 mg per kg body weight of ceftriaxone to children with bacterial meningitis; 3 h after the dose, the mean CSF level was 5.7 μg per ml during early stages of their infection and 2.1 μg per ml in later stages of meningitis. By 6 h after a dose, mean CSF levels in the early and late stage of meningitis were 7.2 and 2.5 μg per ml, respectively. In patients with bacterial meningitis CSF ceftriaxone concentrations exceeded by at least 10-fold MICs of susceptible pathogens, such as the Enterobacteriaceae, *H. influenzae* type b, meningococci, pneumococci and Group B streptococci. Ceftriaxone is effective for the treatment of meningitis caused by these organisms (p. 359). It is not likely to be of value for treatment of meningitis caused by less sensitive pathogens, such as *L. monocytogenes*, *E. faecalis*, *Staph. aureus* and *Ps. aeruginosa* (Del Rio *et al.*, 1982; Chadwick *et al.*, 1983; Steele and Bradsher, 1983a; Steele *et al.*, 1983; Martin *et al.*, 1984). In an animal study of penicillin G-resistant pneumococcal meningitis, the CSF ceftriaxone concentrations were slightly reduced if dexamethasone was given concurrently (Paris *et al.*, 1994). However, in children with bacterial meningitis, who were treated by ceftriaxone plus dexamethasone, the CSF ceftriaxone concentrations were about the same as those in children treated by ceftriaxone alone (Gaillard *et al.*, 1994).

The concentrations of beta-lactam antibiotics in the CSF and brain tissue depends on their passive diffusion there, which is counteracted by an active transport system in the choroid plexus which transfers these substances back into the blood (p. 25). Ceftriaxone and to a lesser extent cefotaxime are less affected by this transport system than penicillins and other cephalosporins, and are therefore pumped out from the CSF less efficiently (Spector, 1987). In one study patients received 2 g of ceftriaxone i.v. 2–13 h before brain samples were taken during neurosurgery for tumors. Cerebral ceftriaxone concentrations ranged from 0.3 to 12 μg per g (Lucht *et al.*, 1990).

Ceftriaxone penetrates well into extravascular spaces, tissue fluid and the synovial fluid of inflamed joints, where similar to serum, its half-life is longer than that of other cephalosporins (Kalager *et al.*, 1984; Morgan *et al.*, 1985). Animal studies have shown that the drug diffuses adequately into lung tissue (Cohen *et al.*, 1984). In humans ceftriaxone penetrates well into transudative and exudative pleural effusions (Benoni *et al.*, 1986; Kimura *et al.*, 1992). In ischaemic tissues in patients with peripheral arterial occlusive disease, the ceftriaxone concentrations were lower, but still high enough to inhibit sensitive pathogens (Hirschl *et al.*, 1995).

When 1 g of ceftriaxone was given i.v. to patients approximately 2 h before cardiopulmonary bypass surgery, adequate concentrations were attained in sternal bone and in the atrial appendage (Bryan *et al.*, 1984). During cardiopulmonary bypass surgery there was also diminished protein binding of the drug owing to low serum albumin. This lower binding increased the volume of distribution and extended the half-life of ceftriaxone to some 15 h. These changes may augment the effectiveness of the drug because of the increase in unbound drug concentrations (Jungbluth *et al.*, 1989). When a single dose of 1 g ceftriaxone was given to patients prophylactically just before thoracic surgery, at the operation average drug concentrations were 13.5 μg per g in thoracic wall fat and 27 μg per g in lung tissue (Martin *et al.*, 1992). When 1 g of ceftriaxone was given i.v. just before liver transplantation, the serum and tissue levels of ceftriaxone were adequate during the 440± 84 min of the operation to inhibit *E. coli* and *Klebsiella* spp., but prophylaxis against *Staph. aureus* and *E. faecalis* needed other antibiotics (Steib *et al.*, 1993).

Ceftriaxone crossed the placenta, and reached adequate levels in umbilical cord blood, amniotic fluid and placenta. Concentrations achieved in fetal tissues were sufficient for a therapeutic effect. It entered breast milk rapidly where its half-life was 12–17 h, but concentrations achieved were only 3–4% of those in serum (Kafetzis *et al.*, 1983). Ceftriaxone is 95% bound to serum proteins (Tawara *et al.*, 1992). The clinical significance of this high degree of protein binding is still controversial (p. 95). For most infections ceftriaxone is as effective clinically as cefotaxime (p. 336) which has a lesser degree of serum protein binding (Nath *et al.*, 1994). In addition to human serum albumin the drug also binds to immunoglobulin G (IgG). For patients with hypergammaglobulinemia or those receiving high doses of i.v. IgG, the unbound concentration of ceftriaxone may become subtherapeutic and higher doses, given 12-hourly may be needed (Sun *et al.*, 1991).

Mode of Action

The mode of action of ceftriaxone on bacteria is similar to that of other cephalosporins (p. 256) and penicillin G (p. 25). It has enhanced activity against Gram-negative bacteria for the same reasons as cefotaxime (p. 344). Ceftriaxone induces filamentation in *E. coli* and *Ps. aeruginosa*, suggesting that it binds primarily to the penicillin-binding protein PBP3 (p. 27) (Hall *et al.*, 1981).

Toxicity

Side-effects of ceftriaxone are like those of other cephalosporins (p. 256) (Moskovitz, 1984). Allergic rashes occur, but are uncommon (Marks, 1983). Diarrhea developed in some 10% of treated patients (Del Rio *et al.*, 1983; Marks, 1983; Chonmaitree *et al.*, 1984; Congeni, 1984). *Clostridium difficile* colitis has occurred in some patients but this has not been very common (Golledge *et al.*, 1989; Lejko-Zupanc *et al.*, 1992). A factor in this complication may be that the active drug is excreted via the bile (p. 356), and thereby affects fecal flora (Nilsson-Ehle *et al.*, 1985). Bodey *et al.* (1983) found that after administration of the drug there were no aerobic Gram-negative bacilli, and there were only 24% of aerobic Gram-positive bacilli and 10% of anaerobes still present in the bowel. De Vries-Hospers *et al.* (1991), after ceftriaxone treatment, reported suppression of aerobic Gram-negative bacilli with overgrowth of yeasts and enterococci. Samonis *et al.* (1993) also detected colonization by yeasts of the gastrointestinal tract in patients treated by ceftriaxone. Some ceftriaxone in the gut may be inactivated by fecal enzymes; this may minimize the effect of ceftriaxone on fecal flora, but the degree to which this happens varies greatly between volunteers or patients (Welling *et al.*, 1992).

Other unwanted effects noted include drug fever, eosinophilia, leukopenia, thrombocytosis and thrombocytopenia (Eron *et al.*, 1983; Marks, 1983; Aronoff *et al.*, 1984; Chonmaitree *et al.*, 1984). One patient developed severe but reversible neutropenia during ceftriaxone therapy (Tantawichien *et al.*, 1994). Transient elevations of SGOT, not necessitating cessation of treatment, have also been noted (Marks, 1983). In icteric neonates ceftriaxone may displace bilirubin from albumin and so increase the 'free' or unbound bilirubin and erythrocyte-bound bilirubin. The drug should be used with caution in high-risk jaundiced infants (Fink *et al.*, 1987; Gulian *et al.*, 1987). Ceftriaxone does not interfere with human polymorphonuclear neutrophil function, but synergy is seen between ceftriaxone and leucocytes in the killing of some microorganisms (Labro *et al.*, 1987a,b).

Borgna-Pignatti *et al.* (1995) reported a fatal case of ceftriaxone-induced hemolytic anemia in an 8-year-old HIV-infected boy. They also cite two other children and an adult, who had different immunodeficiencies, and who developed the same fatal ceftriaxone complication. This hemolytic anemia differed from that seen with penicillin G (p. 33). It occurred immediately after administration of ceftriaxone and the drug was not absorbed on the red blood cell membrane. The hemolysis was due to the 'immune complex mechanism', where the drug-antibody complex became bound to red blood corpuscle membrane, and this activated the complement cascade.

Some patients, who received ceftriaxone, have demonstrated abnormal sonograms of gallbladders. The shadows seen are not gall stones but probably precipitates of calcium ceftriaxone. They have usually been asymptomatic, except that a few patients reported vomiting. These opacities usually disappeared 9–26 days after cessation of ceftriaxone (Schaad *et al.*, 1986; Cometta *et al.*, 1990; Heim-Duthoy *et al.*, 1990), but Ettestad *et al.* (1995) noted a high prevalence of gall stones, often treated surgically, in patients treated with high i.v. doses of ceftriaxone for proven or only suspected late manifestations of Lyme disease (p. 362).

Clinical Uses of the Drug

In common with cefotaxime (p. 336) and other third-generation cephalosporins, ceftriaxone is effective for a wide range of infections caused by Gram-negative bacteria. Nevertheless, it is not the preferred drug for many of these infections, which respond to older, cheaper and more narrow spectrum antibiotics. The main advantage of ceftriaxone over other third-generation cephalosporins is its longer serum half-life, enabling it to be given once every 24 h. If i.v. administration is not practicable, this less frequent i.m. administration makes it more acceptable to patients.

1 Bacterial meningitis

Early studies showed that in induced bacterial meningitis in animals, ceftriaxone was effective for the treatment of meningitis due to Enterobacteriaceae such as *E. coli* (Schaad *et al.*, 1981) and *H. influenzae* type b, including strains resistant to ampicillin and/or chloramphenicol (McCracken *et al.*, 1982; Sakata *et al.*, 1984; Kim, 1988). The drug also cured experimental meningitis caused by pneumococci and Group B streptococci, but not that due to *E. faecalis* and *L. monocytogenes*, two organisms which are much less susceptible (p. 352) (Schaad *et al.*, 1981; McCracken *et al.*, 1982; Delaplane *et al.*, 1983). Ceftriaxone is effective against the same range of meningeal pathogens as cefotaxime. Results of studies in humans have confirmed predictions from animal experiments (McCracken, 1983, 1984). Ceftriaxone is as useful as cefotaxime (p. 336) for the treatment of Gram-negative meningitis caused by the Enterobacteriaceae (Aronoff *et al.*, 1983; Chadwick *et al.*, 1983; Martin, 1983a). Like cefotaxime, ceftriaxone can be regarded as a prime drug for the treatment of meningitis caused by these pathogens. Several studies have demonstrated the efficacy of ceftriaxone in *H. influenzae* type b meningitis in children, and results are comparable with those obtained with cefotaxime, ampicillin, or chloramphenicol (p. 568) (Del Rio *et al.*, 1983; Steele and Bradsher, 1983a; Aronoff *et al.*, 1984; Congeni, 1984; Barson *et al.*, 1985; Danker *et al.*, 1988; Peltola *et al.*, 1989). In one study ceftriaxone proved to be superior to cefuroxime (p. 310) for treatment of meningitis in children (Schaad *et al.*, 1990). In general, cefotaxime (p. 336) or ceftriaxone are now regarded as the best cephalosporins for treatment of meningitis; cefuroxime, although only slightly inferior, is no longer recommended. Ceftriaxone is also quite effective for treatment of meningococcal, pneumococcal and Group B streptococcal meningitis (Martin, 1983a,b; Steele and Bradsher, 1983a; Congeni, 1984; Scheld *et al.*, 1984; Barson *et al.*, 1985; Girgis *et al.*, 1988; Aharoni *et al.*, 1990; Marhoum *et al.*, 1993). Penicillin G remains the preferred drug for the treatment of these forms of meningitis, once the organism is identified (p. 39) but cefriaxone alone can be used initially.

Cefotaxime plus ampicillin is still the favored combination for initial treatment of neonatal bacterial meningitis but for children 4–12 weeks old ceftriaxone (or cefotaxime) plus penicillin G (or ampicillin) is now acceptable. For children aged 3 months to 18 years, initial treatment can be with ceftriaxone alone. After identification of the organism, ceftriaxone (or cefotaxime) is used alone for *H. influenzae* and Gram-negative bacillary meningitis, and penicillin G (or ampicillin) for Group B streptococcal, *Listeria*, *E. faecalis*, *N. meningitidis* and pneumococcal meningitis. For adults aged 18–50 years of age, some favor cefotaxime or ceftriaxone alone and others penicillin G or ampicillin alone. Perhaps it is best to use a third-generation cephalosporin plus penicillin G. The main causative organisms here are *N. meningitidis* and *Strep. pneumoniae*, but occasionally *H. influenzae* or *L. monocytogenes* meningitis may occur. In immunocompromised patients certainly ceftriaxone should be combined with penicillin G initially and perhaps other drugs added as well. In patients older than 50 years a ceftriaxone/penicillin G combination should be used initially because of the greater possibility of *Listeria* meningitis. Once the organism is identified, penicillin G is the best drug for meningococcal and pneumococcal meningitis (McCracken *et al.*, 1987; Tunkel *et al.*, 1990; Klass and Klein, 1992). An increasing number of meningitis, especially if this is acquired in hospital, in the older age groups are caused by Gram-negative enteric bacilli (Durand *et al.*, 1993). A ceftriaxone/penicillin G combination would be appropriate as initial therapy for most of these except if the causative organism is *Ps. aeruginosa*.

A special problem is posed by penicillin G-resistant pneumococci. Meningitis due to these organisms can be treated by ceftriaxone alone, but only if their MIC for ceftriaxone is sufficiently low. Recommendations as to how low they should be vary. Leggiadro *et al.* (1994) suggested that they should be 0.25 μg per ml or lower. John (1994) considered that ceftriaxone will succeed in treatment if its MIC was 0.5 μg per ml or less, but Tan *et al.* (1994) recommended that ceftriaxone could be used if its MIC for the strain was 1.0 μg per ml or lower. In general the ceftriaxone MICs are low enough to use it for treatment of meningitis caused by strains with intermediate type of penicillin G-resistance, but there are exceptions. Occasionally one of these strains may have a high MIC for ceftriaxone. Therefore until the MIC for ceftriaxone is known, the patient should be treated by vancomycin/ceftriaxone combination (John, 1994; Leggiadro et al., 1994). If the MIC for ceftriaxone is too high for it to be used as a single drug, vancomycin plus ceftriaxone may be used for the duration of treatment as these two drugs are still synergistic (Friedland et al., 1994). Alternately vancomycin plus rifampicin may be chosen (p. 700).

Ceftriaxone has an identical place to cefotaxime (p. 336) in the treatment of bacterial meningitis, except that in neonates, cefotaxime is favored. Which of these two drugs should be used in other age groups, will depend on individual considerations. For treatment of meningitis, ceftriaxone has been usually given i.v., but the same dose, given i.m., is equally effective, provided that peripheral circulation is normal (Bradley et al., 1994). Corticosteroids may be beneficial, along with the appropriate antibiotic in the treatment of acute bacterial meningitis (p. 40). Ceftriaxone therapy, in experimental H. influenzae meningitis, and treatment of this meningitis in children, initially leads to release of free endotoxins and exacerbation of the meningeal inflammatory response, which can be modulated by concurrent dexamethasone administration (Arditi et al., 1989; Mustafa et al., 1989), but because of vaccination, H. influenzae meningitis is now less common, and meningitis due to penicillin G-resistant pneumococci is becoming more prevalent. Corticosteroids may slightly decrease the CSF concentrations of ceftriaxone (p. 357) and they more markedly decrease vancomycin CSF levels (p. 779). A slight reduction of the CSF of ceftriaxone concentrations does not matter when H. influenzae (a highly sensitive organism) meningitis is treated by ceftriaxone, but this may matter when resistant pneumococcal meningitis is treated by the drug. Therefore the use of dexamethasone in bacterial meningitis remains controversial (Schaad et al., 1995).

Although rifampicin (p. 697) is considered to be the best drug for eradication of N. meningitidis from carriers, a single i.m. injection of 50 mg per kg ceftriaxone for children and 2 g i.m. for adults has also been effective (Schwartz et al., 1988; Wall, 1988; Cuevas and Hart, 1993; Cuevas et al., 1995). Ceftriaxone 1 g i.m. daily for 2 days also usually eliminates H. influenzae carrier state. Ceftriaxone, rather than rifampicin, is preferable for the eradication of these carrier states in pregnant women.

2 Other serious H. influenzae type b and other Haemophilus spp. infections such as septicemia, epiglottitis, pneumonia, osteomyelitis and endophthalmitis

Similar to cefotaxime, ceftriaxone is effective for all of these infections (Bradley et al., 1988; Frenkel et al., 1988; Barradas et al., 1989; Nahass et al., 1989; Garber et al., 1992; Mangi et al., 1992; Schmidt et al., 1993). Ceftriaxone treatment was also successful in a case of septic arthritis caused by the unusual pathogen, Haemophilus aphrophilus (Merino et al., 1994).

3 Serious infections by Enterobacteriaceae such as septicemia and nosocomial pneumonia

Ceftriaxone has the same efficacy as cefotaxime (p. 338) for the treatment of many infections caused by Gram-negative rods, such as septicemia, pneumonia, pyelonephritis and bone and joint infections (Aronoff et al., 1983; Rothwell et al., 1983; Steele and Bradsher, 1983b; Chonmaitree et al., 1984; Frenkel et al., 1988; Hoepelman et al., 1988; Mandell et al., 1989; Smith et al., 1989; Mangi et al., 1992; Nathoo et al., 1993). Similar to cefotaxime (p. 322), if an organism such as Enterobacter or Serratia spp. is involved, which possess inducible chromosomally mediated beta-lactamases, resistance to ceftriaxone may emerge during treatment with this drug in vivo (Eron et al., 1983; Spanish Ceftriaxone Study Group, 1989). However, the majority of these infections can be successfully cured by ceftriaxone (Barradas et al., 1989; Mermel and Spiegel, 1992).

4 Typhoid fever and other systemic Salmonella infections

These may respond to other third-generation cephalosporins, such as cefotaxime, but there has been more experience with ceftriaxone. This cephalosporin (or a quinolone such as ciprofloxacin, p. 1016) is especially indicated if the Salmonella spp. strain is resistant to chloramphenicol (p. 550), amoxycillin (p. 136) and co-trimoxazole (p. 841) (Soe and Overturf, 1987). It was predicted from in vitro studies that ceftriaxone should be effective for these infections (Cherubin et al., 1986). Also studies in animals confirmed this (Anton et al., 1982). We feel unhappy to treat a disease such as typhoid fever for a short time, but many clinical studies have confirmed that a 5- to 7-day course of ceftriaxone is as effective as a 14-day treatment with chloramphenicol (Ti et al., 1985; Bryan et al., 1986; Farid et al., 1987; Islam et al., 1988; Moosa and Rubidge, 1989; Islam et al., 1993). However, rather high ceftriaxone doses were often used e.g. once-daily 75 mg per kg of body weight for children and 4 g daily once for adults (Islam *et al.*, 1993). In one trial ceftriaxone, 3 or 4 g once-daily, was curative for typhoid, when administered for 3 days only (Lasserre *et al.*, 1991). Although the elimination half-life of ceftriaxone is shorter in typhoid fever patients, compared with normal volunteers, and the volume of distribution of the drug is increased in these patients, Acharya *et al.* (1994) still found ceftriaxone therapy, 3 g i.v. daily for 3 days only, satisfactory for the treatment of typhoid fever.

Good results have also been reported with ceftriaxone therapy in typhoid fever in children (Gupta, 1994) and in neonates (Reed and Klugman, 1994), but another study demonstrated that ciprofloxacin in a dosage of 0.5 g orally 12-hourly was superior to ceftriaxone 3 g daily i.m. or i.v., when both were given for 7 days for treatment of multiresistant typhoid fever (Wallace *et al.*, 1993). Similarly, ofloxacin (200 mg 12-hourly) given orally for 5 days was more effective than ceftriaxone 3 g once-daily i.v. for 3 days for the treatment of this disease (Smith *et al.*, 1994).

Ceftriaxone was successful for *Salmonella enterididis* meningitis in experimental animals (Bryan and Scheld, 1992). *Salmonella* meningitis and brain abscess in humans has been successfully cured by ceftriaxone (Kinsella *et al.*, 1987). *Salmonella* spp. endocarditis (Rodriguez *et al.*, 1990) and multidrug-resistant *Salmonella* osteomyelitis (Sherman and Conte, 1987) have also been cured by ceftriaxone. The drug is suitable for prolonged treatment of *Salmonella* septicemia in patients with neutropenia or immunosuppression (Galofré *et al.*, 1994). Salmonellosis and mycotic aneurysms of the aorta have been treated by ceftriaxone, although surgery was also usually required (Chan *et al.*, 1995). However, during an outbreak of *Salmonella enterididis* gastroenteritis in neonates, ceftriaxone failed to eradicate the organism from the gastrointestinal tract (Einhorn and Granoff, 1987).

5 Infections due to other Gram-negative bacilli

Ceftriaxone is ineffective for *Ps. aeruginosa* and *Acinetobacter* spp. infections (Gnann *et al.*, 1982). Ceftriaxone is curative of *Yersinia pestis* infections in experimental animals (Bonacorsi *et al.*, 1994). Ceftriaxone plus an aminoglycoside may be effective in endocarditis caused by *Actinobacillus actinomycetemcomitans*, but penicillin G or ampicillin plus an aminoglycoside (p. 50) are also effective (Grace *et al.*, 1988). *Bartonella* (*Rochalimaea*) *henselae* can cause septicemia in immunocompetent hosts and also in those with immunosuppression, particularly HIV infection. Ceftriaxone has been used in treatment, although other drugs such as erythromycin (p. 619), doxycycline (p. 744) and ciprofloxacin (p. 1031) are also effective (Lucey *et al.*, 1992). Most patients with *Y. enterocolitica* septicemia respond to ceftriaxone, but the quinolones such as ciprofloxacin (p. 1019) may be more effective (Gayraud *et al.*, 1993).

6 Initial therapy for fever in neutropenic patients

Some studies suggested that the combination of ceftriaxone/amikacin was equally efficaceous to ceftazidime/amikacin in the initial management of these patients (Liu and Wang, 1989; The Internat. Antimicrob. Ther. Coop. Group, 1993), but if a cephalosporin is included in these regimens, ceftazidime (p. 377) with its additional anti-pseudomonal activity may be preferable.

7 Gonorrhea

Ceftriaxone, given as a single dose of 125 mg, 250 mg or 500 mg i.m. is effective for the treatment of uncomplicated urethral or anorectal gonorrhea in men and women. It is equally effective for gonorrhea caused by penicillin G-sensitive, beta-lactamase-producing and intrinsically penicillin G-resistant strains (Judson *et al.*, 1983; Zajdowicz *et al.*, 1983; Panikabutra *et al.*, 1985; Le Saux and Ronald, 1989; Covino *et al.*, 1993). If an injectable antibiotic is needed, CDC (1993) recommended ceftriaxone 125 mg i.m. as a single-dose. Acceptable oral alternatives are cefixime (p. 412), ciprofloxacin (p. 1022) and ofloxacin (p. 1122). Neonatal gonococcal ophthalmia responds well to a single dose of 25–50 mg pr kg i.v. or i.m. The dose should not exceed 125 mg. There is no need for any topical therapy (Laga *et al.*, 1986; CDC, 1993). Gonococcal conjunctivitis in adults responds to 1 g i.m. ceftriaxone plus one lavage of the infected eye with saline solution (CDC, 1993). Disseminated gonococcal infections respond to ceftriaxone 1 g i.m. or i.v. every 24 h for 7 days (Bush and Boscia, 1987; CDC, 1993). Gonococcal meningitis and endocarditis can be treated with 1–2 g i.v. ceftriaxone every 12 h. Therapy for meningitis should extend for 10–14 days, and that for endocarditis for at least 4 weeks (Black *et al.*, 1988; CDC, 1993).

Similar to penicillin G (p. 47), ceftriaxone treatment may abort incubating syphilis (Sng *et al.*, 1984). Ceftriaxone does not cure concomitant *Chlamydia* infection, so patients with gonorrhea should receive in addition a 7-day course of doxycycline 100 mg 12-hourly (CDC, 1993).

8 Chancroid

Tetracycline (p. 725)- and co-trimoxazole (p. 842)- resistant strains of *H. ducreyi* have emerged in many parts of the world, and for many years now a single i.m. dose of 250 mg ceftriaxone has been effective for this disease (Taylor *et al.*, 1985; Bowmer *et al.*, 1987; Schmid, 1990); CDC (1993) also recommend this dose of ceftriaxone for the treatment of chancroid. However, one report from Kenya documented that 250 mg of i.m. ceftriaxone failed to cure chancroid in 35% of patients, mainly in those with HIV infection (Tyndall *et al.*, 1993). The *H. ducreyi* isolates from these patients were sensitive to ceftriaxone.

9 Syphilis

Ceftriaxone has shown some effect in experimental *T. pallidum* infections in animals (Marra *et al.*, 1992). It has also been tried in humans. Ceftriaxone in doses of 2 g i.m. daily for 2 or 5 days has cured primary syphilis, but a single 3-g dose was not effective. Some patients with primary or secondary syphilis were cured with 250 mg ceftriaxone administered i.m. daily for 10 days. The best dosage schedules for ceftriaxone for the treatment of syphilis have not been determined (Hook, 1989; Zenker and Rolfs, 1990). Penicillin G remains the drug of choice for the treatment of this disease (p. 46), and one of the tetracyclines (p. 747) and erythromycin (p. 621), are the only alternatives which have been sufficiently studied (CDC, 1993). However, ceftriaxone in doses of 1–2 g daily for 10–14 days, is currently being evaluated for treatment of neurosyphilis in HIV-infected patients (Scheck and Hook, 1994).

10 Lyme disease

In late disease in patients with neurologic or rheumatologic manifestations, ceftriaxone has been evaluated. Ceftriaxone in a dose of 1–2 g i.m. or i.v. 12-hourly for 14 days has proved to be superior to penicillin G (p. 48) for the treatment of these patients, but some failures of ceftriaxone therapy still occur (Dattwyler *et al.*, 1987, 1988; Halperin, 1989; Luft *et al.*, 1989; Weber and Pfister, 1994). It has been postulated that in some patients, despite adequate chemotherapy, degenerate products, such as granules and encysted *B. burgdorferi* persist and are responsible for chronic symptoms (Kersten *et al.*, 1995). One patient with Lyme disease, which had persisted for 53 years, responded to i.v. ceftriaxone 2 g daily for 14 days (Gasser *et al.*, 1994). Ceftriaxone also eliminates *B. burgdorferi* from experimental animals even if first administered 90 days after infection (Moody *et al.*, 1994). Another late manifestation of Lyme disease is multiple-site osteomyelitis and the drug of choice again is ceftriaxone (Oksi *et al.*, 1994). However, some authors have produced evidence that in patients with late disease the results of treatment are improved if the 14-day course of i.v. ceftriaxone is followed by 100 days of oral amoxycillin plus probenecid or 100 days of oral cefadroxil (Wahlberg *et al.*, 1994).

11 Nocardiosis

Some case reports suggest that ceftriaxone may have a place in combination with other antibiotics such as amikacin, in the treatment of *Nocardia asteroides* infections, especially if they involve the central nervous system (Braun *et al.*, 1991; Garlando *et al.*, 1992).

12 Tularemia

Single-dose ceftriaxone or a course of this drug for 7–8 days has proved to be ineffective for the treatment of this disease (Cross and Jacobs, 1993).

13 Home parenteral antibiotic therapy

Because of the convenience of once-daily i.m. or i.v. administration, ceftriaxone has been evaluated for home parenteral antibiotic therapy, mainly for *Strep. viridans* endocarditis. One daily dose of ceftriaxone plus single-daily dose of netilmicin proved successful for this disease in experimental animals (Blatter *et al.*, 1993; Francoli and Glauser, 1993). In humans ceftriaxone alone 2 g daily for 4 weeks has cured *Strep. viridans* endocarditis (Francioli *et al.*, 1992). Alternatively this dose of ceftriaxone has been given for *Strep. viridans* endocarditis for 2 weeks, followed by oral amoxycillin for another 2 weeks. This has also been successful (Stamboulian *et al.*, 1991). Home treatment with ceftriaxone has also been successful in some other infections, such as osteomyelitis and a few cases of *Staph. aureus* endocarditis (Russo *et al.*, 1988).

14 Granuloma inguinale

This infection, caused by the intracellular Gram-negative bacillus *Calymmatobacterium granulomatis*, often causes chronic genital ulceration in Aboriginal people in central Australia. The advanced lesions in these patients often respond poorly to conventional treatment regimens such as erythromycin and doxycycline. This infection responded well to i.m. ceftriaxone usually in a dosage of 1 g daily, administered for 10 days (Merianos *et al.*, 1994).

15 Actinomycosis

Thoracic actinomycosis responds to ceftriaxone therapy (Skoutelis *et al.*, 1994).

References

Abeck D, Johnson AP, Dangor Y, Ballard RC (1988). Antibiotic susceptibilities and plasmid profiles of *Haemophilus ducreyi* isolates from southern Africa. *J Antimicrob Chemother* **22**: 437.

Acharya G, Crevoisier C, Butler T *et al.* (1994). Pharmacokinetics of ceftriaxone in patients with typhoid fever. *Antimicrob Ag Chemother* **38**: 2415.

Agger WA, Callister SM, Jobe DA(1992). *In vitro* susceptibilities of *Borrelia burgdorferi* to five oral cephalosporins and ceftriaxone. *Antimicrob Ag Chemother* **36**: 1788.

Aharoni A, Potasman I, Levitan Z *et al.* (1990). Postpartum maternal Group B streptococcal meningitis. *Rev Infect Dis* **12**: 273.

Aldridge KE, Cammarata C, Martin DH (1993). Comparison of the *in vitro* activities of various parenteral and oral antimicrobial agents against endemic *Haemophilus ducreyi*. *Antimicrob Ag Chemother* **37**: 1986.

Angehrn P (1983). *In vitro* and *in vivo* synergy between ceftriaxone and aminoglycosides against *Pseudmononas aeruginosa*. *Eur J Clin Microbiol* **2**: 489.

Angehrn P, Probst PJ, Reiner R, Then RL (1980). RO 13–9904, a long-acting broad-spectrum cephalosporin: *in vitro* and *in vivo* studies. *Antimicrob Ag Chemother* **18: 913**.

Anton PA, Kemp JA, Butler T, Jacobs MR (1982). Comparative efficacies of ceftriaxone, moxalactam, and ampicillin in experimental *Salmonella typhimurium* infection. *Antimicrob Ag Chemother* **22**: 312.

Arditi M, Ables L, Yogev R (1989). Cerebrospinal fluid endotoxin levels in children with *H influenzae* meningitis before and after administration of intravenous ceftriaxone. *J Infect Dis* **160**: 1005.

Aronoff SC, Murdell D, O'Brien CA *et al.* (1983). Efficacy and safety of ceftriaxone in serious pediatric infections. *Antimicrob Ag Chemother* **24**: 663.

Aronoff SC, Reed MD, O'Brien CA, Blumer JL (1984). Comparison of the efficacy and safety of ceftriaxone to ampicillin/chloramphenicol in the treatment of childhood meningitis. *J Antimicrob Chemother* **13**: 143.

Arvidsson A, Alván G, Angelin B *et al.* (1982). Ceftriaxone: renal and biliary excretion and effect on the colon microflora. *J Antimicrob Chemother* **10**: 207.

Bakken JS, Cavalieri SJ, Gangeness D (1990). Influence of plasma exchange pheresis on plasma elimination of ceftriaxone. *Antimicrob Ag Chemother* **34**: 1276.

Bakken JS, Cavalieri SJ, Gangeness D *et al.* (1993). Influence of therapeutic plasmapheresis on elimination of ceftriaxone. *Antimicrob Ag Chemother* **37**: 1171.

Bannatyne RM, Cheung R (1984). Susceptibility of *Bordetella pertussis* to cephalosporin derivatives and imipenem. *Antimicrob Ag Chemother* **26**: 604.

Barradas P, Zamith M, Videira W *et al.* (1989). Therapy of lower respiratory tract infections: a comparison of ceftriaxone and cefotaxime. *Chemotherapy* **35** (Suppl 2): 33.

Barson WJ, Miller MA, Brady MT, Powell DA (1985). Prospective comparative trial of ceftriaxone vs conventional therapy for treatment of bacterial meningitis in children. *Pediatr Infect Dis* **4**: 362.

Bayer AS, Eisenstadt R, Morrison JO (1984). Enhanced *in vitro* bactericidal activity of amikacin or gentamicin combined with three new extended-spectrum cephalosporins against cephalosporin-resistant members of the family Enterobacteriaceae. *Antimicrob Ag Chemother* **25**: 725.

Benoni G, Arosio E, Cuzzolin L *et al.* (1986). Penetration of ceftriaxone into human pleural fluid. *Antimicrob Ag Chemother* **29**: 906.

Black JR, Brint JM, Reichart CA (1988). Successful treatment of gonococcal endocarditis with ceftriaxone. *J Infect Dis* **157**: 1281.

Blatter M, Fluckiger U, Entenza J *et al.* (1993). Simulated human serum profiles of one daily dose of ceftriaxone plus netilmicin in treatment of experimental streptococcal endocarditis. *Antimicrob Ag Chemother* **37**: 1971.

Bodey GP, Fainstein V, Garcia I *et al.* (1983). Effect of broad-spectrum cephalosporins on the microbial flora of recipients. *J Infect Dis* **148**: 892.

Bonacorsi SP, Scavizzi MR, Guiyoule A *et al.* (1994). Assessment of a fluoroquinolone, three beta-lactams, two aminoglycosides, and a cycline in treatment of murine *Yersinia pestis* infection. *Antimicrob Ag Chemother* **38**: 481.

Borgna-Pignatti C, Bezzi TM, Reverberi R (1995). Fatal ceftriaxone-induced hemolysis in a child with acquired immunodeficiency syndrome. *Pediatr Infect Dis J* **14**: 1116.

Bosch J, Liñares J, Lopez de Goicoechea MJ *et al.* (1986). *In-vitro* activity of ciprofloxacin, ceftriaxone and five other antimicrobial agents against 95 strains of *Brucella melitensis*. *J Antimicrob Chemother* **17**: 459.

Bourget P, Fernandez H, Quinquis V, Delouis C (1993). Pharmacokinetics and protein binding of ceftriaxone during pregnancy. *Antimicrob Ag Chemother* **37**: 54.

Bowmer MI, Nsanze H, D'Costa LJ *et al.* (1987). Single-dose ceftriaxone for chancroid. *Antimicrob Ag Chemother* **31**: 67.

Bradley JS, Ching DK, Phillips SE (1988). Outpatient therapy of serious pediatric infections with ceftriaxone. *Pediatr Infect Dis J* **7**: 160.

Bradley JS, Farhat C, Stamboulian D *et al.* (1994). Ceftriaxone therapy of bacterial meningitis: cerebrospinal fluid concentrations and bactericidal activity after intramuscular injection in children treated with dexamethasone. *Pediatr Infect Dis J* **13**: 724.

Braun TI, Kerson LA, Eisenberg FP (1991). Nocardial brain abscess in a pregnant woman. *Rev Infect Dis* **13**: 630.

Bryan CS, Morgan SL, Jordan AB *et al.* (1984). Ceftriaxone levels in blood and tissue during cardiopulmonary bypass surgery. *Antimicrob Ag Chemother* **25**: 37.

Bryan JP, Scheld WM (1992). Therapy of experimental meningitis due to *Salmonella* enteritidis. *Antimicrob Ag Chemother* **36**: 949.

Bryan JP, Rocha H, Da Silva HR *et al.* (1985). Comparison of ceftriaxone and ampicillin plus chloramphenicol for the therapy of acute bacterial meningitis. *Antimicrob Ag Chemother* **28**: 361.

Bryan JP, Rocha H, Scheld WM (1986). Problems in salmonellosis: rationale for clinical trials with newer beta-lactam agents and quinolones. *Rev Infect Dis* **8**: 189.

Bush LM, Boscia JA (1987). Disseminated multiple antibiotic-resistant gonococcal infection: needed changes in antimicrobial therapy. *Ann Intern Med* **107**: 692.

Campos J, Garcia-Tornel S (1987). Comparative susceptibilities of ampicillin and chloramphenicol resistant *Haemophilus influenzae* to fifteen antibiotics. *J Antimicrob Chemother* **19**: 297.

Castro I, Bergeron MG, Chamberland S (1993). Characterization of multiresistant strains of *Neisseria gonorrhoeae* isolated in Nicaragua. *Sex Transm Dis* **20**: 314.

CDC (Centers for Disease Control) (1993). Sexually transmitted diseases treatment guidelines. *MMWR* (No RR-14): **42**: 19, 56.

Chadwick EG, Connor EM, Shulman ST, Yogev R (1983). Efficacy of cetriaxone in treatment of serious childhood infections. *J Pediatr* **103**: 141.

Chan P, Tsai CW, Huang JJ *et al.* (1995). Salmonellosis and mycotic aneurysm of the aorta. A report of 10 cases. *J Infect* **30**: 129.

Chandrasekar PH, Rolston KVI, Smith BR, Le Frock JL (1984). Diffusion of ceftriaxone into the cerebrospinal fluid of adults. *J Antimicrob Chemother* **14**: 427.

Cherubin CE, Eng RHK, Smith SM, Goldstein EJC (1986). Cephalosporin therapy for salmonellosis. Questions of efficacy and cross-resistance with ampicillin. *Arch Intern Med* **146**: 2149.

Chonmaitree T, Congeni BL, Munoz J *et al.* (1984). Twice daily ceftriaxone therapy for serious bacterial infections in children. *J Antimicrob Chemother* **13**: 511.

Clendennen TEIII, Hames CS, Kees ES *et al.* (1992a). *In vitro* antibiotic susceptibilities of *Neisseria gonorrhoeae* isolates in the Phillipines. *Antimicrob Ag Chemother* **36**: 277.

Clendennen TE, Echeverria P, Saengeur S *et al.* (1992b). Antibiotic susceptibility survey of *Neisseria gonorrhoeae* in Thailand. *Antimicrob Ag Chemother* **36**: 1682.

Cohen D, Appel GB, Scully B, Neu HC (1983). Pharmacokinetics of ceftriaxone in patients with renal failure and in those undergoing hemodialysis. *Antimicrob Ag Chemother* **24**: 529.

Cohen SH, Hoeprich PD, Demling R *et al.* (1984). Entry of four cephalosporins into the ovine lung. *J Infect Dis* **149**: 264.

Cometta A, Gallot-Lavallee-Villars S, Iten A *et al.* (1990). Incidence of gallbladder lithiasis after ceftriaxone treatment. *J Antimicrob Chemother* **25**: 689.

Congeni BL (1984). Comparison of ceftriaxone and traditional therapy of bacterial meningitis. *Antimicrob Ag Chemother* **25**: 40.

Congeni BL, Chonmaitree T, Rakusan TA, Box QT (1985). Once-daily ceftriaxone therapy for serious bacterial infections in children. *Antimicrob Ag Chemother* **27**: 181.

Covino JM, Smith BL, Cummings MC *et al.* (1993). Comparison of enoxacin and ceftriaxone in the treatment of uncomplicated gonorrhea. *Sex Transm Dis* **20**: 227.

Cross JT, Jacobs RF (1993). Tularemia: treatment failures with outpatient use of ceftriaxone. *Clin Infect Dis* **17**: 976.

Cuevas LE, Hart CA (1993). Chemoprophylaxis of bacterial meningitis. *J Antimicrob Chemother* **31** (Suppl B): 79.

Cuevas LE, Kazembe P, Mughogho GK *et al.* (1995). Eradication of nasopharyngeal carriage of *Neisseria meningitidis* in children and adults in rural Africa: a comparison of ciprofloxacin and rifampicin. *J Infect Dis* **171**: 728.

Dangor Y, Miller SD, Exposto F da L, Koornhof HJ (1988). Antimicrobial susceptibilities of Southern African isolates of *Haemophilus ducreyi*. *Antimicrob Ag Chemother* **32**: 1458.

Dangor Y, Ballard RC, Miller SD, Koornhof HJ (1990). Antimicrobial susceptibility of *Haemophilus ducreyi*. *Antimicrob Ag Chemother* **34**: 1303.

Danker WM, Connor JD, Sawyer M *et al.* (1988). Treatment of bacterial meningitis with once daily ceftriaxone therapy. *J Antimicrob Chemother* **21**: 637.

Dattwyler RJ, Halperin JJ, Pass H, Luft BJ (1987). Ceftriaxone as effective therapy in refractory Lyme disease. *J Infect Dis* **155**: 1322.

Dattwyler RJ, Halperin JJ, Volkman DJ, Luft BJ (1988). Treatment of late Lyme borreliosis – randomised comparison of ceftriaxone and penicillin. *Lancet* **i**: 1191.

De'Clari F (1991). Ceftriaxone pharmacokinetics during continuous arteriovenous haemofiltration. *J Antimicrob Chemother* **27**: 394.

Deeter RG, Weinstein MP, Swanson KA *et al.* (1990). Crossover assessment of serum bactericidal activity and pharmacokinetics of five broad-spectrum cephalosporins in the elderly. *Antimicrob Ag Chemother* **34**: 1007.

Delaplane D, Yogev R, Shulman ST (1983). Ceftriaxone therapy of group B streptococcal bacteraemia and meningitis in infant rats. *J Antimicrob Chemother* **11**: 69.

Del Rio M, McCracken GH Jr, Nelson JD *et al.* (1982). Pharmacokinetics and cerebrospinal fluid bactericidal activity of ceftriaxone in the treatment of pediatric patients with bacterial meningitis. *Antimicrob Ag Chemother* **22**: 622.

Del Rio M, Chrane D, Shelton S *et al.* (1983). Ceftriaxone versus ampicillin and chloramphenicol for treatment of bacterial meningitis in children. *Lancet* **i**: 1241.

De Vries-Hospers HG, Tonk RHJ, Van der Waaij D (1991). Effect of intramuscular ceftriaxone on aerobic oral and faecal flora of 11 healthy volunteers. *Scand J Infect Dis* **23**: 625.

Durand ML, Calderwood SB, Weber DJ *et al.* (1993). Acute bacterial meningitis in adults. A review of 493 episodes. *New Engl J Med* **328**: 21.

Einhorn MS, Granoff DM (1987). Failure of ceftriaxone therapy to eradicate *Salmonella enteritidis* from the gastrointestinal tract of neonates. *Pediatr Infect Dis J* **6**: 1067.

Eron LJ, Park CH, Hixon DL *et al.* (1983). Ceftriaxone therapy of bone and soft tissue infections in hospital and outpatient settings. *Antimicrob Ag Chemother* **23**: 731.

Ettestad PJ, Campbell GL, Welbel SF *et al.* (1995). Biliary complications in the treatment of unsubstantiated Lyme disease. *J Infect Dis* **171**: 356.

Farid Z, Girgis N, El Ella AA (1987). Successful treatment of typhoid fever in children with parenteral ceftriaxone. *Scand J Infect Dis* **19**: 467.

Fass RJ (1982). Comparative *in vitro* activities of beta-lactam-tobramycin combinations against *Pseudomonas aeruginosa* and multidrug-resistant Gram-negative enteric bacilli. *Antimicrob Ag Chemother* **21**: 1003.

Fass RJ (1983). Comparative *in vitro* activities of third-generation cephalosporins. *Arch Intern Med* **143**: 1743.

Fauvelle F, Lortholary O, Tod M *et al.* (1994). Pharmacokinetics of ceftriaxone during plasma exchange in polyarteritis nodosa patients. *Antimicrob Ag Chemother* **38**: 1519.

Figueiredo AMS, Connor JD, Severin A *et al.* (1992). A pneumococcal clinical isolate with high-level resistance to cefotaxime and ceftriaxone. *Antimicrob Ag Chemother* **36**: 886.

Findlay CD, Brown RM, Allcock JE *et al.* (1982). A study of the relationship between dose and pharmacokinetics of ceftriaxone. *J Antimicrob Chemother* **9**: 57.

Francioli P, Etienne J, Hoigne R *et al.* (1992). Treatment of streptococcal endocarditis with a single daily dose of ceftriaxone sodium for 4 weeks. Efficacy and outpatient treatment feasibility. *JAMA* **267**: 264.

Francioli PB, Glauser MP (1993). Synergistic activity of ceftriaxone combined with netilmicin administered once daily for treatment of experimental streptococcal endocarditis. *Antimicrob Ag Chemother* **37**: 207.

Frenkel LD and the Multicenter Ceftriaxone Pediatric Study Group (1988). Once-daily administation of ceftriaxone for the treatment of selected serious bacterial infections in children. *Pediatrics* **82**: 486.

Fink S, Karp W, Robertson A (1987). Ceftriaxone effect on bilirubin-albumin binding. *Pediatrics* **80**: 873.

Friedland IR, Paris M, Shelton S, McCracken GH (1994). Time-kill studies of antibiotic combinations against penicillin-resistant and-susceptible *Streptococcus pneumoniae*. *J Antimicrob Chemother* **34**: 231.

Gaillard J-L, Abadie V, Cheron G *et al.* (1994). Concentrations of ceftriaxone in cerebrospinal fluid of children with meningitis receiving dexamethasone therapy. *Antimicrob Ag Chemother* **38**: 1209.

Galofré J, Moreno A, Mensa J *et al.* (1994). Analysis of factors influencing the outcome and development of septic metastasis or relapse in *Salmonella bacteremia*. *Clin Infect Dis* **18**: 873.

Garber GE, Auger P, Chan RMT *et al.* (1992). A multicenter, open comparative study of parenteral cefotaxime and ceftriaxone in the treatment of nosocomial lower respiratory tract infections. *Diagn Microbiol Infect Dis* **15**: 85.

Garlando F, Bodmer T, Lee C *et al.* (1992). Successful treatment of disseminated nocardiosis complicated by cerebral abscess with ceftriaxone and amikacin: case report. *Clin Infect Dis* **15**: 1039.

Garzone P, Lyon J, Yu VL (1983). Third generation and investigational cephalosporins: II. Microbiologic review and clinical summaries. *Drug Intell Clin Pharm* **17**: 615.

Gasser RNA, Dusleag J, Reisinger EC (1994). Treatment of long-standing Lyme disease with ceftriaxone. *Lancet* **343**: 1227.

Gayraud M, Scavizzi MR, Mollaret HH *et al.* (1993). Antibiotic treatment of *Yersinia enterocolitica* septicemia: a retrospective review of 43 cases. *Clin Infect Dis* **17**: 405.

Georgilis K, Peacoke M, Klempner MS (1992). Fibroblasts protect the Lyme disease spirochete, *Borrelia burgdorferi*, from ceftriaxone *in vitro*. *J Infect Dis* **166**: 440.

Girgis NI, Abu El Ella AH, Farid Z *et al.* (1988). Intramuscular ceftriaxone versus ampicillin-chloramphenicol in childhood bacterial meningitis. *Scand J Infect Dis* **20**: 613.

Gnann JW Jr, Goetter WE, Elliott AM, Cobbs CG (1982). Ceftriaxone: *in vitro* studies and clinical evaluation. *Antimicrob Ag Chemother* **22**: 1.

Goldstein FW, Pean Y, Rosato A *et al.* (1993). Characterization of ceftriaxone-resistant Enterobacteriaceae: a multicentre study in 26 French hospitals. *J Antimicrob Chemother* **32**: 595.

Gordin FM, Wofsy CB, Mills J (1985). Once daily ceftriaxone for skin and soft tissue infections. *Antimicrob Ag Chemother* **27**: 648.

Grace CJ, Levitz RE, Katz-Pollak H, Brettman LR (1988). Actinobacillus actinomycetemcomitans prosthetic valve endocarditis. *Rev Infect Dis* **10**: 922.

Golledge CL, McKenzie T, Riley TV (1989). Extended spectrum cephalosporins and *Clostridium difficile*. *J Antimicrob Chemother* **23**: 929.

Gombert ME, Aulicino TM, DuBouchet L, Berkowitz LR (1987). Susceptibility of *Nocardia asteroides* to new quinolones and beta-lactams. *Antimicrob Ag Chemother* **31**: 2013.

Gulian J-M, Gonard V, Dalmasso C, Palix C (1987). Bilirubin displacement by ceftriaxone in neonates: evaluation by determination of 'free' bilirubin and erythrocyte-bound bilirubin. *J Antimicrob Chemother* **19**: 823.

Gupta A (1994). Multidrug-resistant typhoid fever in children: epidemiology and therapeutic approach. *Pediatr Infect Dis J* **13**: 134.

Haas DW, Stratton CW, Griffin JP *et al.* (1995). Diminished activity of ceftizoxime in comparison to cefotaxime and ceftriaxone against *Streptococcus pneumoniae*. *Clin Infect Dis* **20**: 671.

Hall MJ, Westmacott D, Wong-Kai-In P (1981). Comparative *in vitro* activity and mode of action of ceftriaxone (RO 13–9904)., a new highly potent cephalosporin. *J Antimicrob Chemother* **8**: 193.

Halperin JJ (1989). Abnormalities of the central nervous system in Lyme disease: response to antimicrobial therapy. *Rev Infect Dis* **11** (Suppl 6): 1499.

Hammerschlag MR, Gleyzer A (1983). *In vitro* activity of a group of broad-spectrum cephalosporins and other beta-lactam antibiotics against *Chlamydia trachomatis*. *Antimicrob Ag Chemother* **23**: 493.

Heim-Duthoy KL, Caperton EM, Pollock R *et al.* (1990). Apparent biliary pseudolithiasis during ceftriaxone therapy. *Antimicrob Ag Chemother* **34**: 1146.

Hell K (1989). Ceftriaxone workshop: overview and conclusions. *Chemother* **35** (Suppl 2): 41.

Hirschl M, Kundi M, Hirschl AM, Georgopoulos A (1995). Effects of macro- and microcirculatory functions on ceftriaxone concentrations in tissues of patients with stage IV peripheral arterial occlusive disease. *Antimicrob Ag Chemother* **39**: 15.

Hoepelman IM, Rozenberg-Arska M, Verhoef J (1988). Comparison of once-daily ceftriaxone with gentamicin plus cefuroxime for treatment of serious bacterial infections. *Lancet* **i**: 1305.

Hook EW III (1989). Treatment of syphilis: current recommendations, alternatives, and continuing problems. *Rev Infect Dis* **11** (Suppl 6): 1511.

Islam A, Butler T, Nath SK *et al.* (1988). Randomized treatment of patients with typhoid fever by using ceftriaxone or chloramphenicol. *J Infect Dis* **158**: 742.

Islam A, Butler T, Kabir I, Alam NH (1993). Treatment of typhoid fever with ceftriaxone for 5 days or chloramphenicol for 14 days: a randomized clinical trial. *Antimicrob Ag Chemother* **37**: 1572.

Ison CA, Pepin J, Roope NS *et al.* (1992). The dominance of multiresistant strain of *Neisseria gonorrhoeae* among prostitutes and STD patients in the Gambia. *Genitourin Med* **68**: 356.

Jensen KT, Schonheyder H, Thomsen VF (1994). *In-vitro* activity of beta-lactam and other antimicrobial agents against *Kingella kingae*. *J Antimicrob Chemother* **33**: 635.

John CC (1994). Treatment failure with use of a third generation cephalosporin for penicillin-resistant pneumococcal meningitis: case report and review. *Clin Infect Dis* **18**: 188.

Johnson RC (1989). Isolation techniques for spirochetes and their sensitivity to antibiotics *in vitro* and *in vivo*. *Rev Infect Dis* **11** (Suppl 6): 1505.

Johnson RC, Bey RF, Wolgamot SJ (1982). Comparison of the activities of ceftriaxone and penicillin G against experimentally induced syphilis in rabbits. *Antimicrob Ag Chemother* **21**: 984.

Johnson RC, Kodner C, Russell M (1987). *In vitro* and *in vivo* susceptibility of the Lyme disease spirochete, *Borrelia burgdorferi*, to four antimicrobial agents. *Antimicrob Ag Chemother* **31**: 164.

Judson FN, Ehret JM, Root CJ (1983). Comparative study of ceftriaxone and aqueous procaine penicillin G in the treatment of uncomplicated gonorrhea in women. *Antimicrob Ag Chemother* **23**: 218.

Jungbluth GL, Pasko MT, Beam TR, Jusko WJ (1989). Ceftriaxone disposition in open-heart surgery patients. *Antimicrob Ag Chemother* **33**: 850.

Kafetzis DA, Brater DC, Fanourgakis JE *et al.* (1983). Ceftriaxone distribution between maternal blood and fetal blood and tissues at parturition and between blood and milk postpartum. *Antimicrob Ag Chemother* **23**: 870.

Kalager T, Digranes A, Bergan T, Solberg CO (1984). The pharmacokinetics of ceftriaxone in serum, skin blister and thread fluid. *J Antimicrob Chemother* **13**: 479.

Kerbs SB, Stone JR Jr, Berg SW, Harrison WO (1983). *In vitro* antimicrobial activity of eight new beta-lactam antibiotics against penicillin-resistant *Neisseria gonorrhoeae*. *Antimicrob Ag Chemother* **23**: 541.

Kersten A, Poitschek C, Rauch S, Aberer E (1995). Effects of penicillin, ceftriaxone, and doxycycline on morphology of *Borrelia burgdorferi*. *Antimicrob Ag Chemother* **39**: 1127.

Kim KS (1988). Therapeutic efficacy of chloramphenicol, co-trimoxazole (trimethoprim/sulphamethoxazole)., cefmenoxime and ceftriaxone in experimental bacteraemia and meningitis caused by ampicillin-resistant *Haemophilus influenzae* type b. *J Antimicrob Chemother* **22**: 697.

Kimura M, Matsushima T, Nakamura J, Kobashi Y (1992). Comparative study of penetration of lomefloxacin and ceftriaxone into transudative and exudative pleural effusion. *Antimicrob Ag Chemother* **36**: 2774.

Kinsella TR, Yogev R, Shulman ST *et al.* (1987). Treatment of *Salmonella* meningitis and brain abscess with the new cephalosporins: two case reports and review of the literature. *Pediatr Infect Dis J* **6**: 476.

Klass PE, Klein JO (1992). Therapy of bacterial sepsis meningitis and otitis media in infants and children 1992 poll of directors of programs in pediatric infectious diseases. *Pediatr Infect Dis J* **11**: 702.

Knapp JS, Back AF, Babst AF *et al.* (1993). *In vitro* susceptibilities of isolates of *Haemophilus ducreyi* from Thailand and the United States to currently recommended and newer agents for treatment of chancroid. *Antimicrob Ag Chemother* **37**: 1552.

Labro MT, Babin-Chevaye C, Pochet I, Hakim J (1987a). Interaction of ceftriaxone with human polymorphonuclear neutrophil functions. *J Antimicrob Chemother* **20**: 849.

Labro MT, Pochet I, Babin-Chevaye C, Hakim J (1987b). Effect of ceftriaxone-induced alterations of bacteria on neutrophil bactericidal function. *J Antimicrob Chemother* **20**: 857.

Laferriere C, Marks MI, Welch DF (1983). Effect of inoculum size on *Haemophilus influenzae* type b susceptibility to new and conventional antibiotics. *Antimicrob Ag Chemother* **24**: 287.

Laga M, Naamara W, Brunham RC *et al.* (1986). Single-dose therapy of gonococcal ophthalmia neonatorum with ceftriaxone. *New Engl J Med* **315**: 1382.

Lasserre R, Sangalang RP, Santiago L (1991). Three day treatment of typhoid fever with two different doses of ceftriaxone, compared to 14-day therapy with chloramphenicol: a randomized trial. *J Antimicrob Chemother* **28**: 765.

Latif R, Dajani AS (1983). Ceftriaxone diffusion into cerebrospinal fluid of children with meningitis. *Antimicrob Ag Chemother* **23**: 46.

Leggiadro RJ, Barrett FF, Chesney PJ *et al.* (1994). Invasive pneumococci with high level penicillin and cephalosporin resistance at Mid-South children's hospital. *Pediatr Infect Dis J* **13**: 320.

Lejko-Zupanc T, Zakelj J, Strle F *et al.* (1992). Influence of ceftriaxone on emergence of Clostridium difficile. *Antimicrob Ag Chemother* **36**: 2850.

Le Saux N, Ronald AR (1989). Role of ceftriaxone in sexually transmitted diseases. *Rev Infect Dis* **11**: 299.

Liebowitz LD, Ballard RC, Koornhof HJ (1982). *In vitro* susceptibility and cross-resistance of South African isolates of *Neisseria gonorrhoeae* to 14 antimicrobial agents. *Antimicrob Ag Chemother* **22**: 598.

Liu C-Y, Wang F-D (1989). A comparative study of ceftriaxone plus amikacin, ceftazidime plus amikacin and imipenem/cilastatin in the empiric therapy of febrile granulocytopenic cancer patients. *Chemotherapy* **35** (Suppl 2): 16.

Lucey D, Dolan MJ, Moss CW *et al.* (1992). Relapsing illness due to

Rochalimaea henselae in immunocompetent hosts: implication for therapy and new epidemiological associations. *Clin Infect Dis* **14**: 683.

Lucht F, Dorche G, Aubert G *et al.* (1990). The penetration of ceftriaxone into human brain tissue. *J Antimicrob Chemother* **26**: 81.

Luft BJ, Gorevic PD, Halperin JJ *et al.* (1989). A perspective in the treatment of Lyme borreliosis. *Rev Infect Dis* **11** (Suppl 6): 1518.

Mandell LA, Bergeron MG, Ronald AR *et al.* (1989). Once-daily therapy with ceftriaxone compared with daily multiple-dose therapy with cefotaxime for serious bacterial infections: a randomized, double-blind study. *J Infect Dis* **160**: 433.

Mangi RJ, Peccerillo KM, Ryan J *et al.* (1992). Cefoperazone versus ceftriaxone monotherapy of nosocomial pneumonia. *Diagn Microbiol Infect Dis* **15**: 441.

Marchou B, Michea-Hamzehpour M, Lucain C, Pechere J-C (1987a). Development of beta-lactam-resistant *Enterobacter cloacae* in mice. *J Infect Dis* **156**: 369.

Marchou B, Bellido F, Charnas R *et al.* (1987b). Contribution of beta-lactamase hydrolysis and outer membrane permeability to ceftriaxone resistance in *Enterobacter cloacea*. *Antimicrob Ag Chemother* **31**: 1589.

Marhoum K, Filali E, Noun M *et al.* (1993). Ceftriaxone versus penicillin G in the short-term treatment of meningococcal meningitis in adults. *Eur J Clin Microbiol Infect Dis* **12**: 766.

Marks MI (1983). Ceftriaxone – and more to come. *J Pediatr* **103**: 70.

Marra CM, Slatter V, Targaglione TA *et al.* (1992). Evaluation of aqueous penicillin G and ceftriaxone for experimental neurosyphilis. *J Infect Dis* **165**: 396.

Martin C, Ragni J, Lokiec F *et al.* (1992). Pharmacokinetics and tissue penetration of a single dose of ceftriaxone (1000 miligrams intravenously). for antibiotic prophylaxis in thoracic surgery. *Antimicrob Ag Chemother* **36**: 2804.

Martin E (1983a). Once-daily administration of ceftriaxone in the treatment of meningitis and other serious infections in children. *Eur J Clin Microbiol* **2**: 509.

Martin E (1983b). Ceftriaxone for meningitis. *Lancet* **ii**: 43.

Martin E, Koup JR, Paravicini U, Stoeckel K (1984). Pharmacokinetics of ceftriaxone in neonates and infants with meningitis. *J Pediatr* **105**: 475.

Mashford ML, Andrew JH, Christiansen K *et al.* (1994). *Antibiotic Guidelines* 8th edn p. 109. Antibiotic Guidelines Sub-Committee. Victorian Drug Usage Advisory Committee. Moorabin, Victoria, Australia: Interprint Services Ltd.

Maurin M, Raoult D (1993). Antimicrobial susceptibility of *Rochalimaea quintana*, *Rochalimaea vinsonii*, and the newly recognized *Rochalimaea henselae*. *J Antimicrob Chemother* **32**: 587.

McCracken GH Jr (1983). Pharmacokinetic and bacteriological correlations between antimicrobial therapy of experimental meningitis in rabbits and meningitis in humans: a review. *J Antimicrob Chemother* **12** (Suppl D): 97.

McCracken GH Jr (1984). Management of bacterial meningitis Current status and future prospects. *Amer J Med* **76** (Suppl): 215.

McCracken GH Jr, Nelson JD, Grimm L (1982). Pharmacokinetics and bacteriological efficacy of cefoperazone, cefuroxime, ceftriaxone, and moxalactam in experimental *Streptococcus pneumoniae* and *Haemophilus influenzae* meningitis. *Antimicrob Ag Chemother* **21**: 262.

McCracken GH Jr, Siegel JD, Threlkeld N, Thomas M (1983). Ceftriaxone pharmacokinetics in newborn infants. *Antimicrob Ag Chemother* **23**: 341.

McCracken GH Jr, Nelson JD, Kaplan SL *et al.* (1987). Consensus report: antimicrobial therapy for bacterial meningitis in infants and children. *Pediatr Infect Dis J* **6**: 501.

McNeil MM, Brown JM, Jarvis WR, Ajello L (1990). Comparison of species distribution and antimicrobial susceptibility of aerobic Actinomycetes from clinical specimens. *Rev Infect Dis* **12**: 778.

Merianos A, Gilles M, Chuah J (1994). Ceftriaxone in the treatment of chronic donovanosis in Central Australia. *Genitourin Med* **70**: 84.

Merino D, Saavedra J, Pujol E *et al.* (1994). *Haemophilus aprophilus* as a rare cause of arthritis. *Clin Infect Dis* **19**: 320.

Mermel LA, Spiegel CA (1992). Nosocomial sepsis due to *Serratia odorifera* biovar 1. *Clin Infect Dis* **14**: 208.

Merle-Melet M, Seta N, Farinotti R, Carbon C (1989). Reduction in biliary excretion of ceftriaxone by diclofenac in rabbits. *Antimicrob Ag Chemother* **33**: 1506.

Merle-Melet M, Bresler L, Lokiec F *et al.* (1992). Effects of diclofenac on ceftriaxone pharmacokinetics in humans. *Antimicrob Ag Chemother* **36**: 2331.

Moody KD, Adams RL, Barthold SW (1994). Effectiveness of antimicrobial treatment against *Borrelia burgdorferi* infection in mice. *Antimicrob Ag Chemother* **38**: 1567.

Meyers BR, Srulevitch ES, Jacobson J, Hirschman SZ (1983). Crossover study of the pharmacokinetics of ceftriaxone administered intravenously or intramuscularly to healthy volunteers. *Antimicrob Ag Chemother* **24**: 812.

Moosa A, Rubidge CJ (1989). Once daily cefriaxone vs chloramphenicol for treatment of typhoid fever in children. *Pediatr Infect Dis J* **8**: 696.

Morgan JR, Paull A, O'Sullivan M, Williams BD (1985). The penetration of ceftriaxone into synovial fluid of the inflamed joint. *J Antimicrob Chemother* **16**: 367.

Moskovitz BL (1984). Clinical adverse effects during ceftriaxone therapy. *Amer J Med* **77** (4c): 84.

Motley M, Sarafian SK, Knapp JS *et al.* (1992). Correlation between *in vitro* antimicrobial susceptibilities and beta-lactamase plasmid contents of isolates of *Haemophilus ducreyi* from the United States. *Antimicrob Ag Chemother* **36**: 1639.

Mustafa MM, Ramilo O, Mertsola J *et al.* (1989). Modulation of inflammation and cachectin activity in relation to treatment of experimental *Haemophilus influenzae* type b meningitis. *J Infect Dis* **160**: 818.

Muytjens HL, Van der Ros-van de Repe J (1982). Comparative activities of 13 beta-lactam antibiotics. *Antimicrob Ag Chemother* **21**: 925.

Nahass RG, Cook S, Weinstein MP (1989). Vertebral osteomyelitis due to *Haemophilus aprophilus*: treatment with ceftriaxone. *J Infect Dis* **159**: 811.

Nath SK, Foster GA, Mandell LA, Rotstein C (1994). Antimicrobial activity of ceftriaxone versus cefotaxime: negative effect of serum albumin binding of ceftriaxone. *J Antimicrob Chemother* **33**: 1239.

Nathoo KJ, Mason PR, Gwanzura L *et al.* (1993). Severe *Klebsiella* infection as a cause of mortality in neonates in Harare, Zimbabwe: evidence from postmortem blood cultures. *Pediatr Infect Dis J* **12**: 840.

Nau R, Prange HW, Muth P *et al.* (1993). Passage of cefotaxime and ceftriaxone into cerebrospinal fluid of patients with uninflamed meninges. *Antimicrob Ag Chemother* **37**: 1518.

Neal TJ, O'Donoghue MAT, Ridgway EJ, Allen KD (1992). *In-vitro* activity of ten antimicrobial agents against penicillin-resistant *Streptococcus pneumoniae*. *J Antimicrob Chemother* **30**: 39.

Nelson JD (1983). A primer for pediatricians on new cephalosporin antibiotics. *Amer J Dis Child* **137**: 1041.

Neu HC, Meropol NJ, Fu KP (1981). Antibacterial activity of ceftriaxone (RO 13–9904)., a beta-lactamase-stable cephalosporin. *Antimicrob Ag Chemother* **19**: 414.

Ng WS, Chau PY, Ling J *et al.* (1983). Penicillinase-producing *Neisseria gonorrhoeae* isolates from different localities in South East Asia Susceptibility to 15 antibiotics. *Brit J Vener Dis* **59**: 232.

Nilsson-Ehle I, Nord CE, Ursing B (1985). Ceftriaxone: pharmacokinetics and effect on the intestinal microflora in patients with acute bacterial infections. *Scand J Infect Dis* **17**: 77.

Noel GJ, Teele DW (1986). *In vitro* activities of selected new and long-acting cephalosporins against *Pasteurella multocida*. *Antimicrob Ag Chemother* **29**: 344.

Oksi J, Mertsola J, Reunanen M *et al.* (1994). Subacute multiple-site osteomyelitis caused by *Borrelia burgdorferi*. *Clin Infect Dis* **19**: 891.

Palenque E, Otero JR, Noriega AR (1986). *In vitro* susceptibility of *Brucella melitensis* to new cephalosporins crossing the blood-brain barrier. *Antimicrob Ag Chemother* **29**: 182.

Panikabutra K, Ariyarit C, Chitwarakorn A *et al.* (1985). Randomised comparative study of ceftriaxone and spectinomycin in gonorrhoea. *Genitourin Med* **61**: 106.

Paris MM, Hickey SM, Uscher MI *et al.* (1994). Effect of dexamethasone on therapy of experimental penicillin- and cephalosporin- resistant pneumococcal meningitis. *Antimicrob Ag Chemother* **38**: 1320.

Patel IH, Kaplan SA (1984). Pharmacokinetics profile of ceftriaxone in man. *Amer J Med* **77** (4c): 17.

Patel IH, Chen S, Parsonnett M *et al.* (1981). Pharmacokinetics of ceftriaxone in humans. *Antimicrob Ag Chemother* **20**: 634.

Patel IH, Weinfeld RE, Konikoff J, Parsonnet M (1982). Pharmacokinetics and tolerance of ceftriaxone in humans after single-dose intramuscular administration in water and lidocaine diluents. *Antimicrob Ag Chemother* **21**: 957.

Patel IH, Sugihara JG, Weinfeld RE *et al.* (1984). Ceftriaxone pharmacokinetics in patients with various degrees of renal impairment. *Antimicrob Ag Chemother* **25**: 438.

Paull A, Morgan JR (1986). Emergence of ceftriaxone-resistant strains of *Pseudomonas aeruginosa* in cystic fibrosis patients. *J Antimicrob Chemother* **18**: 635.

Peltola H, Anttila M, Renkonen O-V and The Finnish Study Group (1989). Randomised comparison of chloramphenicol, ampicillin, cefotaxime and ceftriaxone for childhood bacterial meningitis. *Lancet* **i**: 1281.

Pollock AA, Tee PE, Patel IH *et al.* (1982). Pharmacokinetic characteristics of intravenous ceftriaxone in normal adults. *Antimicrob Ag Chemother* **22**: 816.

Pollock HM, Holt J, Murray C (1983). Comparison of susceptibilities of anaerobic bacteria to cefmenoxime, ceftriaxone and other antimicrobial compounds. *Antimicrob Ag Chemother* **23**: 780.

Reed RP, Klugman KP (1994). Neonatal typhoid fever. *Pediatr Infect Dis J* **13**: 774.

Rice RJ, Knapp JS (1994). Antimicrobial susceptibilities of *Neisseria gonorrhoeae* strains representing five distinct resistance phenotypes. *Antimicrob Ag Chemother* **38**: 155.

Rodriguez C, Olcoz MT, Izquierdo G, Moreno S (1990). Endocarditis due to ampicillin-resistant nontyphoid salmonella: cure with a third-generation cephalosporin. *Rev Infect Dis* **12**: 817.

Rolfe RD, Finegold SM (1982). Comparative *in vitro* activity of ceftriaxone against anaerobic bacteria. *Antimicrob Ag Chemother* **22**: 338.

Rothwell DL, Bremner DA, Taylor KM (1983). Treatment of complicated urinary tract infections with the long acting cephalosporin, ceftraixone. *N Z Med J* **96**: 392.

Russo TA, Cook S, Gorbach SL (1988). Intramuscular ceftriaxone in home parenteral therapy. *Antimicrob Ag Chemother* **32**: 1439.

Sakata Y, McCracken GH Jr, Thomas ML, Olsen KD (1984). Pharmacokinetics and therapeutic efficacy of imipenem, ceftazidime, and ceftriaxone in experimental meningitis due to an ampicillin- and chloramphenicol-resistant strain of *Haemophilus influenzae* type b. *Antimicrob Ag Chemother* **25**: 29.

Salvador P, Smith RG, Weinfeld RE *et al.* (1983). Clinical pharmacology of ceftriaxone in patients with neoplastic disease. *Antimicrob Ag Chemother* **23**: 583.

Samonis G, Gikas A, Anaissie EJ *et al.* (1993). Prospective evaluation of effects of braod-spectrum antibiotics on gastrointestinal yeast colonization in humans. *Antimicrob Ag Chemother* **37**: 51.

Sanders CC, Sanders WE Jr (1983). Emergence of resistance during therapy with the newer beta-lactam antibiotics: role of inducible beta-lactamases and implications for the future. *Rev Infect Dis* **5**: 639.

Schaad UB, Stoeckel K (1982). Single-dose pharmacokinetics of ceftriaxone in infants and young children. *Antimicrob Ag Chemother* **21**: 248.

Schaad UB, McCracken GH Jr, Loock CA, Thomas ML (1981). Pharmacokinetics and bacteriologic efficacy of moxalactam, cefotaxime, cefoperazone, and rocephin in experimental bacterial meningitis. *J Infect Dis* **143**: 156.

Schaad UB, Tschappeler H, Lentze MJ (1986). Transient formation of precipitations in the gallbladder associated with ceftriaxone therapy. *Pediatr Infect Dis* **5**: 708.

Schaad UB, Suter S, Gianella-Borradori A *et al.* (1990). A comparison of ceftriaxone and cefuroxime for the treatment of bacterial meningitis in children. *New Engl J Med* **322**: 141.

Schaad UB, Kaplan SL, McCracken GHJr (1995). Steroid therapy for bacterial meningitis. *Clin Infect Dis* **20**: 685.

Scheck DN, Hook EW (1994). Neurosyphilis. *Inf Dis Clin N Amer* **8**: 769.

Scheld WM, Rocha H, Sande MA, Bryan JP (1984). Rationale for clinical trials evaluating ceftriaxone in the therapy of bacterial meningitis. *Amer J Med* **17** (4c): 42.

Schmid GP (1990). Treatment of chancroid, 1989. *Rev Infect Dis* **12** (Suppl 6): 580.

Schmidt ME, Smith MA, Levy CS (1993). Endophthalmitis caused by unusual Gram-negative bacilli: three case reports and review. *Clin Infect Dis* **17**: 686.

Schwartz B, Al Tobaiqi A, Al-Ruwais A *et al.* (1988). Comparative efficacy of ceftriaxone and rifampicin in eradicating pharyngeal carriage of Group A *Neisseria meningitidis*. *Lancet* **i**: 1239.

Schwebke JR, Whittington W, Rice RJ *et al.* (1995). Trends in susceptibility of *Neisseria gonorrhoeae* to ceftriaxone from 1985 through 1991. *Antimicrob Ag Chemother* **39**: 917.

Scribner RK, Marks MI, Weber A, Pai CH (1982). *Yersinia enterocolitica*: comparative *in vitro* activities of seven new beta-lactam antibiotics. *Antimicrob Ag Chemother* **22**: 140.

Shaefer CF, Trincher RC, Rissing JP (1983). Melioidosis: recrudescence with a strain resistant to multiple antimicrobials. *Amer Rev Respir Dis* **128**: 173.

Shannon K, King A, Warren C, Phillips I (1980). *In vitro* antibacterial activity and susceptibility of the cephalosporin RO 13–9904 to beta-lactamases. *Antimicrob Ag Chemother* **18**: 292.

Sherman JW, Conte JE Jr (1987). Ceftriaxone treatment of multidrug-resistant Salmonella osteomyelitis. *Amer J Med* **83**: 137.

Skoutelis A, Petrochilos J, Bassaris H (1994). Successful treatment of thoracic actinomycosis with ceftriaxone. *Clin Infect Dis* **19**: 161.

Smith CR, Petty BG, Hendrix CW *et al.* (1989). Ceftriaxone compared with cefotaxime for serious bacterial infections. *J Infect Dis* **160**: 442.

Smith MD, Duong NM, Hoa NTT *et al.* (1994). Comparison of ofloxacin and ceftriaxone for short-course treatment of enteric fever. *Antimicrob Ag Chemother* **38**: 1716.

Sng EH, Lim AL, Yeo KL (1984). Susceptibility to antimicrobials of *Neisseria gonorrhoeae* isolated in Singapore: implications on the need for more effective treatment regimens and control strategies. *Brit J Vener Dis* **60**: 374.

Soe GB, Overturf GD (1987). Treatment of typhoid fever and other systemic salmonelloses with cefotaxime, ceftriaxone, cefoperazone and other newer cephalosporins. *Rev Infect Dis* **9**: 719.

Sorbello AF, O'Donnell J, Kaiser-Smith J *et al.* (1994). Infective endocarditis due to *Pasteurella dagmatis*: case report and review. *Clin Infect Dis* **18**: 336.

Spanish Ceftriaxone Study Group (1989). Ceftriaxone monotherapy for severe bacteremic infections. *Chemotherapy* **35** (Suppl 2): 27.

Spector R (1987). Ceftriaxone transport through the blood-brain barrier. *J Infect Dis* **156**: 209.

Stamboulian D, Bonvehi P, Arevalo C *et al.* (1991). Antibiotic management of outpatients with endocarditis due to penicillin-susceptible streptococci. *Rev Infect Dis* **13** (Suppl 2): 160.

Steele RW, Bradsher RW (1983a). Comparison of ceftriaxone with standard therapy for bacterial meningitis. *J Pediatr* **103**: 138.

Steele RW, Bradsher RW (1983b). Ceftriaxone for the treatment of serious infections. *Amer J Dis Child* **137**: 1044.

Steele RW, Eyre LB, Bradsher RW *et al.* (1983). Pharmacokinetics of ceftriaxone in pediatric patients with meningitis. *Antimicrob Ag Chemother* **23**: 191.

Steib A, Jacoberger B, Von Bandel M *et al.* (1993). Concentrations in plasma and tissue penetrations of ceftriaxone and ornidazole during liver transplantation. *Antimicrob Ag Chemother* **37**: 1873.

Sun H, Chow MSS, Maderazo EG (1991). Characteristics of ceftriaxone binding to immunoglobulin G and potential clinical significance. *Antimicrob Ag Chemother* **35**: 2232.

Tan TQ, Schutze GE, Mason EOJr, Kaplan SL (1994). Antibiotic therapy and acute outcome of meningitis due to *Streptococcus pneumoniae* considered intermediately susceptible to broad-spectrum cephalosporins. *Antimicrob Ag Chemother* **38**: 918.

Tantawichien T, Tungsanga K, Swasdikul D (1994). Reversible severe neutropenia after ceftriaxone. *Scand J Infect Dis* **26**: 109.

Täuber MG, Doroshow CA, Hackbarth CJ *et al.* (1984). Antibacterial activity of beta-lactam antibiotics in experimental meningitis due to *Streptococcus pneumoniae*. *J Infect Dis* **149**: 568.

Tawara S, Matsumoto S, Kamimura T, Goto S (1992). Effect of protein binding in serum on therapeutic efficacy of cephem antibiotics. *Antimicrob Ag Chemother* **36**: 17.

Taylor DN, Pitarangsi C, Echeverria P *et al.* (1985). Comparative study of ceftriaxone and trimethoprim-sulfamethoxazole for the treatment of chancroid in Thailand. *J Infect Dis* **152**: 1002.

The International Antimicrobial Therapy Cooperative Group of the European Organization for Research and Treatment of Cancer (1993). Efficacy and toxicity of single daily doses of amikacin and ceftriaxone versus multiple daily doses of amikacin and ceftazidime for infection in patients with cancer and granulocytopenia. *Ann Intern Med* **119**: 584.

Ti T-Y, Monteiro EH, Lam S, Lee H-S (1985). Ceftriaxone therapy in bacteremic typhoid fever. *Antimicrob Ag Chemother* **28**: 540.

Torres H, Raoult D (1993). *In vitro* activities of ceftriaxone and fusidic acid against 13 isolates of *Coxiella burnetii*, determined using the shell vial assay. *Antimicrob Ag Chemother* **37**: 491.

Tunkel AR, Wispelwey B, Scheld WM (1990). Bacterial meningitis: recent advances in pathophysiology and treatment. *Ann Intern Med* **112**: 610.

Tyndall M, Malisa M, Plummer FA *et al.* (1993). Ceftriaxone no longer predictably cures chancroid in Kenya. *J Infect Dis* **167**: 469.

Uriz S, Pineda V, Grau M *et al.* (1991). *Neisseria meningitidis* with reduced sensitivity to penicillin: observations in 10 children. *Scand J Infect Dis* **23**: 171.

Verbist L, Verhaegen J (1981). *In vitro* activity of RO 13–9904, a new beta-lactamase-stable cephalosporin. *Antimicrob Ag Chemother* **19**: 222.

Wahlberg P, Grunlund H, Nyman D *et al.* (1994). Treatment of late Lyme borreliosis. *J Infect* **29**: 255.

Wall RA (1988). The chemoprophylaxis of meningococcal infection. *J Antimicrob Chemother* **21**: 698.

Wallace RJ Jr, Steele LC, Sumter G, Smith JM (1988). Antimicrobial susceptibility patterns of *Nocardia asteroides*. *Antimicrob Ag Chemother* **32**: 1776.

Wallace MR, Yousif AA, Mahroos GA *et al.* (1993). Ciprofloxacin versus ceftriaxone in the treatment of multiresistant typhoid fever. *Eur J Clin Microbiol Infect Dis* **12**: 907.

Watanakunakorn C (1983). *In vitro* activity of ceftriaxone alone and in combination with gentamicin, tobramycin and amikacin against *Pseudomonas aeruginosa*. *Antimicrob Ag Chemother* **24**: 305.

Weber K, Pfister H-W (1994). Clinical management of Lyme borreliosis. *Lancet* **343**: 1017.

Welling GW, Holtrop A, Slootmaker-van der Meulen C *et al.* (1992). Inactivation of ceftriaxone by faecal enzyme preparations during ceftriaxone treatment. *J Antimicrob Chemother* **30**: 234.

Westphal J-F, Jehl F, Vetter D (1994). Pharmacological, toxicologic, an microbiological considerations in the choice of initial antibiotic therapy for serious infections in patients with cirrhosis of the liver. *Clin Infect Dis* **18**: 324.

Wise R, Andrews JM (1983). A comparison of the pharmacokinetics and tissue penetratin of ceftriaxone, moxalactam and cefotaxime. *Eur J Clin Microbiol* **2**: 505.

Zajdowicz TR, Sanches PL, Berg SW *et al.* (1983). Comparison of ceftriaxone with cefoxitin in the treatment of penicillin-resistant gonococcal urethritis. *Brit J Vener Dis* **59**: 176.

Zenker PN, Rolfs RT(1990). Treatment of syphilis. *Rev Infect Dis* **12** (Suppl 6): 590.

Ceftazidime

Description

Ceftazidime, another third-generation cephalosporin, derived from cephalosporin C (p. 251), was developed by Glaxo Laboratories (O'Callaghan *et al.*, 1980). Like other cephalosporins of this group, it is resistant to the usual beta-lactamases of most Gram-negative bacteria, and it is active against most of these, including *Pseudomonas aeruginosa* (Verbist and Verhaegen, 1981). It is a parenteral antibiotic and clinically it is used as the monosodium salt which is highly soluble in water.

Sensitive Organisms

1 Pseudomonas aeruginosa

High degree of activity against this organism is one of the most important properties of ceftazidime. It is more active against *Ps. aeruginosa* than other third-generation cephalosporins such as cefoperazone (p. 324) (Table I.28) (Verbist and Verhaegen, 1981; Harper, 1981; Alford, 1983; Chamberland *et al.*, 1992). Most aminoglycoside-resistant strains are usually ceftazidime-sensitive (Bassey *et al.*, 1984; Wu *et al.*, 1984).

Ceftazidime-resistant variants of *Ps. aeruginosa* can be selected *in vitro* by exposing the organisms to various concentrations of ceftazidime in agar (Piddock and Traynor, 1991). Such strains can also arise when difficult infections, such as *Ps. aeruginosa* endocarditis, are treated by ceftazidime in animals (Bayer *et al.*, 1987a; 1988a; Fantin *et al.*, 1994), and they can also arise during treatment of *Ps. aeruginosa* infections with ceftazidime in humans (Maslow *et al.*, 1983; Bosso *et al.*, 1989; Richards *et al.*, 1989). The main mechanism of resistance appears to be increased production of chromosomally mediated type 1 beta-lactamase (p. 322). Increase of this enzyme may arise due to a chromosomal mutation or more commonly by enzyme induction, and many beta-lactam antibiotics can act as inducers. When this enzyme is overproduced it can slowly inactivate ceftazidime as well as most other beta-lactam antibiotics with the exception of imipenem (p. 229). In cystic fibrosis patients' serum and sputum antibodies against this chromosomal beta-lactamase can be detected. These antibodies are specific markers for resistance development of *Ps. aeruginosa* to ceftazidime and other beta-lactams (Ciofu *et al.*, 1995). Decreased outer membrane permeability can also play some part in the ceftazidime resistance of *Ps. aeruginosa* (Bayer *et al.*, 1987a,b; Giwercman *et al.*, 1990, 1992). When ceftazidime is used widely in any hospital or unit, ceftazidime-resistant strains of *Ps. aeruginosa* (and some other Gram-negative bacteria such as *Enterobacter* spp.) increase in frequency. Once restrictions are placed on the use of ceftazidime, susceptibility of *Ps. aeruginosa* to ceftazidime partially recovers (Sanders and Sanders, 1988; Jones, 1992). In a survey of 24 hospitals in the UK in 1993, 9.6% of *Ps. aeruginosa* strains were ceftazidime-resistant (Chen *et al.*, 1995).

More recently plasmid-mediated extended-spectrum beta-lactamases have appeared which can hydrolyze third-generation cephalosporins (p. 323). They have been more common in some Enterobacteriaceae, such as *Klebsiella* spp. (p. 323). However, Watanabe *et al.* (1991) described a *Ps. aeruginosa* isolate, which contained a plasmid-mediated beta-lactamase which conferred resistance not only to ceftazidime and most other cephalosporins and penicillins, but also to imipenem (p. 230) and meropenem. Nordmann *et al.* (1993) described a novel extended-spectrum beta-lactamase in a clinical isolate of *Ps. aeruginosa*, which hydrolyzed ceftazidime, most penicillins and cephalosporins, but not cephamycins and imipenem. This enzyme was inhibited by clavulanic acid. Unlike other extended-spectrum beta-lactamases, which are plasmid-mediated (p. 323), this beta-lactamase appeared to be chromosomally encoded.

2 Enterobacteriaceae

All of these, including *E. coli*, the *Klebsiella* and *Enterobacter* spp., *Pr. mirabilis*, *Pr. vulgaris*, *Morganella morganii* and the *Citrobacter, Providencia, Salmonella, Shigella Serratia, Hafnia* and *Yersinia* spp. are normally ceftazidime-sensitive (Verbist and Verhaegen, 1981; Goossens *et al.*, 1982; Hornstein *et al.*, 1985; Dornbusch *et al.*, 1988; Martin *et al.*, 1989; Mehtar *et al.*, 1990).

Some of the Enterobacteriaceae, such as *Enterobacter* spp., *Citrobacter* spp., *Proteus vulgaris*, *Providencia* spp., *Morganella morganii*, *Hafnia* and *Serratia* spp., harbor low levels of chromosomally mediated beta-lactamases. When the production of these enzymes is markedly increased due to enzyme induction or chromosomal mutation, then these enzymes can hydrolyze ceftazidime and the organisms become resistant to the drug as well as to other third-generation cephalosporins, such as cefotaxime (p. 322). The bacteria with this type of beta-lactam resistance can become widespread in a hospital or a special unit if ceftazidime is widely used. Partial return to ceftazidime sensitivity may occur when the use of ceftazidime is restricted. This type of resistance often arises *in vivo* during ceftazidime treatment of patients (Quinn *et al.*, 1987; Sanders and Sanders, 1988; Johnson and Ramphal, 1990a; Piddock *et al.*, 1990; Jones, 1992; Thomson *et al.*, 1993).

A few strains of *Escherichia coli* have been found which were resistant to ceftazidime, but not to other third-generation cephalosporins. Altered outer membrane proteins appeared to be the resistance mechanism, but in one strain an unusual chromosomally mediated beta-lactamase was also detected, which appeared to contribute to the strains resistance to ceftazidime (Bakken *et al.*, 1987; Weber *et al.*, 1990).

The plasmid-mediated extended-spectrum beta-lactamases, which can hydrolyze cefotaxime (p. 323) and other third-generation cephalosporins, including ceftazidime, were first detected in the mid-1980s in Europe, but now they have spread to many countries, including the UK and USA (p. 323). Initially they were mainly found in *Klebsiella pneumoniae* and *E. coli*, but they soon spread to some other Enterobacteriaceae. Some of these enzymes hydrolyze only third-generation cephalosporins, but not cephamycins and are inhibited by beta-lactamase-inhibitors. Others hydrolyze cephamycins as well and are not inhibited by beta-lactamase inhibitors (p. 193). There have been numerous reports describing ceftazidime-resistant strains of *Kl. pneumoniae* and *E. coli* in which the resistance was mediated by plasmid encoded extended-spectrum beta-lactamases. The enzymes described varied in different reports; some largely hydrolyzed ceftazidime, but others affected other third-generation cephalosporins as well. If cefotaxime only is used for sensitivity testing of *Kl. pneumoniae* and other Gram-negative bacilli, ceftazidime resistance can be overlooked. For instance, an extended-spectrum beta-lactamase was described in *Salmonella* spp. by Morosini *et al.* (1995). This organism showed high-level resistance to ceftazidime and aztreonam but relatively low-level resistance to cefotaxime and ceftriaxone. Some reports described the isolation of one or a few resistant strains, but others reported hospital outbreaks by ceftazidime-resistant *Kl. pneumoniae* or *E. coli* (Chanal *et al.*, 1988; Petit *et al.*, 1988; Peduzzi *et al.*, 1989; Quinn *et al.*, 1989; Sirot *et al.*, 1989; Vuye *et al.*, 1989; Smith *et al.*, 1990; Thomson *et al.*, 1991; Naumovski *et al.*, 1992; Rasmussen *et al.*, 1993; Bradford *et al.*, 1994; Burwen *et al.*, 1994; Hibbert-Rogers *et al.*, 1994; Urban *et al.*, 1994).

Extended spectrum beta-lactamases have also been detected in ceftazidime-resistant strains of other Enterobacteriaceae, such as *Kl. oxytoca* (Heritage *et al.*, 1992), *Enterobacter* spp. (Drabu *et al.*, 1989; Rice *et al.*, 1990), *Citrobacter freundii* (Gutmann *et al.*, 1988) and *Serratia marcescens* (Payne *et al.*, 1991).

3 Other aerobic Gram-negative bacteria

Neisseria meningititis, N. gonorrhoeae, Haemophilus influenzae, H. parainfluenzae, H. ducreyi and *Moraxella catarrhalis*, including beta-lactamase producers of these organisms, are sensitive to ceftazidime (Harper, 1981; Knothe and Dette, 1981; Coovadia and Ramsaroop, 1984; Alvarez *et al.*, 1985). *Pasteurella multocida* and *Legionella pneumophila* are also usually sensitive (Harper, 1981). *Campylobacter jejuni* (MIC 6.25 µg per ml) is only moderately sensitive (Van der Auwera and Scorneaux, 1985). *Aeromonas* spp. may be ceftazidime-sensitive, but some strains possess inducible chromosomally mediated beta-lactamases and may be ceftazidime-resistant (Bakken *et al.*, 1988). *Acinetobacter baumannii* may be ceftazidime-sensitive, but many strains are moderately or highly resistant. Altered PBPs, decreased outer membrane permeability and induced chromosomally mediated beta-lactamases all seem to play a part in this resistance (Obara and Nakae, 1991; Sato and Nakae, 1991; Anstey *et al.*, 1992). The rare human pathogens, *Chryseamonas luteola* and *Flavimonas oryxihabitans* are usually sensitive to ceftazidime (Kostman *et al.*, 1991). *Vibrio vulnificus*, which can cause a severe gastrointestinal infection or septicemia, is usually ceftazidime-sensitive (Chuang *et al.*, 1992).

Burkholderia (previously *Pseudomonas*) *pseudomallei* is usually ceftazidime-sensitive, but imipenem (p. 230) is even more active against this organism (Puthucheary and Parasakthi, 1987; McEniry *et al.*, 1988; Dance *et al.*, 1989; Sookpranee *et al.*, 1991). This organism usually produces a weekly inducible chromosomal beta-lactamase which hydrolyzes cefuroxime, cefoperazone and cefotaxime, but not ceftazidime (Livermore *et al.*, 1987). Others have detected a different beta-lactamase in a strain of *B. pseudomallei*, which hydrolyzed ceftazidime, but not other cephalosporins. This strain was isolated from a patient who was treated by ceftazidime (Godfrey *et al.*, 1991). With increased use of ceftazidime for the treatment of this disease, some resistant strains have also been reported by others (Dance *et al.*, 1991). In chronic melioidosis which is very refractory to antibiotic treatment, *B. pseudomallei* often grows in microcolonies and biofilms. Vorachit *et al.* (1993) demonstrated *in vitro* that this organism's biofilm cells were very resistant to ceftazidime, needing a concentration some 200 times higher than their usual MICs for inhibition. This resistance of *B. pseudomallei* biofilms to ceftazidime may explain the lack of success with antibiotics in the treatment of chronic melioidosis (p. 379). *Burkholderia* (previously *Pseudomonas*) *cepacia* may be ceftazidime-sensitive, but isolates from cystic fibrosis patients are often resistant. In some of these isolates altered outer membrane permeability appears to be the main resistance mechanism (Aronoff, 1988; Kumar *et al.*, 1992; Simpson *et al.*, 1994). *Stenotrophomonas maltophilia* is usually ceftazidime-resistant (Davies *et al.*, 1983). However, Victor *et al.* (1994) studied 14 episodes of *S. maltophilia* bacteremia in immunocompromised patients and found that 50% of the isolates were ceftazidime-sensitive.

Organism	MICs (µg per ml)
Gram-positive bacteria	
Streptococci, Groups A, C and G	0.25
Streptococci, Group B	0.5
Streptococcus viridans	4.0
Streptococcus pneumoniae	2.0
Enterococcus faecalis	> 64.0
Staphylococcus aureus	8.0
Staphylococcus epidermidis	32.0
Clostridium spp.	> 64.0
Gram-negative bacteria	
Escherichia coli	0.25
Klebsiella pneumoniae	1.0
Enterobacter spp.	0.25
Citrobacter spp.	4.0
Proteus spp.	0.125
Providencia spp.	1.0
Serratia spp.	1.0
Salmonella spp.	0.25
Shigella spp.	0.25
Yersinia enterocolitica	1.0
Neisseria gonorrhoeae	0.06
Haemophilus influenzae	0.25
Acinetobacter spp.	8.0
Pseudomonas aeruginosa	4.0
Burkholderia pseudomallei	4.0
Bacteroides fragilis	64.0

Table I.28
Compiled from data published by Bint *et al.* (1981), Clarke and Zemcov (1981), Jones *et al.* (1981), Neu (1981), Phillips *et al.* (1981) and Dance *et al.* (1989)

4 Anaerobic Gram-negative bacteria

Some of these such as *Fusobacterium* and *Veilonella* spp. are usually ceftazidime-sensitive, but most other anaerobes, especially those of the *Bacteroides fragilis* group are resistant (Chow and Bartlett, 1981; Harper, 1981; Aldridge *et al.*, 1984).

5 Gram-positive bacteria

Streptococcus pyogenes, Group B streptococci, *Strep. viridans* and *Strep. bovis* are sensitive (Neu, 1981). Penicillin G-sensitive pneumococci are less susceptible to ceftazidime (MIC 2 μg per ml) than to penicillin G (p. 5), cefotaxime (p. 320) and ceftriaxone (p. 352). Strains with intermediate and high-level penicillin G-resistance are also much less sensitive to ceftazidime than to penicillin G, cefotaxime and ceftriaxone, the MICs of both these strains to ceftazidime being 16 μg per ml (Spangler *et al.*, 1994). *Staphylococcus aureus* and coagulase-negative staphylococci, including beta-lactamase-producing strains, but not methicillin-resistant strains, are also only moderately susceptible (Table I.28). The activity of other cephalosporins such as cephalothin (p. 251) or cefotaxime (p. 319) is greater against these organisms. *Enterococcus faecalis* and other enterococci are resistant, and so is also *Listeria monocytogenes* (Neu, 1981).

Anaerobic streptococci such as the *Peptococcus* and *Peptostreptococcus* spp. are usually ceftazidime-sensitive. *Clostridium perfringens* is moderately susceptible, but other *Clostridium* spp., including *Cl. difficile*, are resistant. *Lactobacillus* spp. is also usually ceftazidime-resistant (Chow and Bartlett, 1991).

6 Minimum inhibitory concentrations

The MICs of ceftazidime against some selected bacterial species are shown in Table I.28.

Mode of Administration and Dosage

Ceftazidime is not absorbed after oral administration, and it is given by either the i.m., or, more commonly, i.v. route.

1 Adults

The dosage can be varied widely, according to the nature and severity of the infection. For the treatment of urinary tract infections, low dosages such as 0.5 or 1.0 g i.m. or i.v. 12-hourly may suffice (Gentry *et al.*, 1983). For moderately severe systemic infections the drug has been given in dosages of either 3 g per day (1 g 8-hourly) or 4 g per day (2 g 12-hourly). For severe infections, such as septicemia, a common dosage is 6 g per day (2 g 8-hourly) (Scully and Neu, 1984; Cone *et al.*, 1985; Engle *et al.*, 1985; Pizzo *et al.*, 1986; Verhagen *et al.*, 1987; Cade *et al.*, 1993). Intravenously each dose can be given as a bolus, but more commonly it is diluted in 30–50 ml of intravenous fluid and administered as a 30-min infusion, similar to penicillin G (p. 20).

There is some evidence from studies in *in vitro* pharmacokinetic models that continuous infusion of ceftazidime, with a continuous serum level higher than four times the MIC of the organism, may be more effective than intermittent administration for the treatment of *Ps. aeruginosa* infections (Mouton and den Hollander, 1994).

2 Children

For moderate infections the recommended dosage is 100 mg per kg per day, administered in three divided doses, but for severe infections such as septicemia or bacterial meningitis a dosage of 150 mg per kg per day is used, again given in three divided doses (Rodriguez *et al.*, 1985; Hatch *et al.*, 1986; Granowetter *et al.*, 1988; Saha *et al.*, 1993).

3 Newborn babies

The serum half-life of ceftazidime is prolonged in newborn babies and during the first 2 weeks of life the recommended dosage is 50 mg per kg per day, given in two divided doses. Thereafter ceftazidime clearance rapidly increases with increase in postnatal age, after 2 weeks of age the dosage of the drug may need to be increased, and after 4 weeks of age the dosage recommended for children is appropriate (Mulhall and de Louvois, 1985).

4 Patients over 65 years of age

The renal clearance of ceftazidime is somewhat reduced in these subjects, but some authors consider that the changes are relatively minor, and they do not recommend a dosage reduction of ceftazidime in these patients (Le Bel et al., 1985; Deeter et al., 1990). Others reported that most patients in this age group had estimated creatinine clearances of less than 50 ml per min, and recommended that ceftazidime dosage of 1.0 g 12-hourly was usually satisfactory even for patients with severe infections (Jonsson and Walder, 1992; Vlasses et al., 1993).

5 Patients with renal failure

In these patients dosage reduction is necessary because the elimination rate of ceftazidime is considerably decreased. Höffler et al. (1983) recommended dosage schedules for patients with varying degree of renal failure (Table I.29). Appropriate dosage reductions are tabulated for regimens of either 3, 4 or 6 g per 24 h in adults with normal renal function. Individual doses are given in grams (g) and the intervals between doses in hours (h). All doses given are related to a body weight of 70 kg.

Table I.29
After Höffler et al. (1983), with permission

Serum creatinine (mg %)	Glomerular filtration rate (ml per min)	Percentage of normal dose	Dosage 1 (3g per 24h)		Dosage 2 (4g per 24h)		Dosage 3 (6g per 24h)	
			(g)	(h)	(g)	(h)	(g)	(h)
0.8	120	100	1	8	2	12	2	8
2.0	45	50	1	12	1	12	1.5	12
3.5	18	20	0.5	24	0.5	12	1.5	24
6.0	8	12.5	0.5	24	0.5	24	1	24
15.5	2	10	0.5[a]	24	0.5[a]	24	0.5[a]	24
–	0.5	7	0.25[a]	24	0.25[a]	24	0.5[a]	24

[a] These were based on calculations from patients dialyzed three times per week, during which ceftazidime was removed. It was considered that the lower daily doses of 0.25 g could be rounded up to 0.5 g without risk of toxicity.

The disposition of ceftazidime in surgical patients is dependent on creatinine clearance and is not significantly altered by surgery or acute infectious processes (Heim-Duthoy et al., 1988). Ackerman et al. (1984) demonstrated a good correlation between creatinine clearance and ceftazidime clearance in 11 patients with creatinine clearance values of 6–113 ml per min. Whilst twice-daily doses are commonly used in patients with impaired renal function, these authors estimated that daily doses of 1.0 g delivered i.v. over 30 min would provide mean peak and trough concentrations of 55.7 and 5.2 μg per ml, respectively, in patients with a creatinine clearance below 40 ml per min.

In infected patients undergoing peritoneal dialysis, ceftazidime may be given by either the i.v. or intraperitoneal route. After a 1.0-g i.v. bolus dose, mean serum levels at 0.25, 2 and 12 h after the start of peritoneal dialysis were 50.6, 35.6 and 22.7 μg per ml, respectively. The mean peak level in peritoneal fluid was 13.2 μg per ml, approximately 3 h after the start of dialysis. When 1.0 g was given via an intraperitoneal catheter, mean serum levels at 0.25, 2 and 8 h were 14.2, 40.0 and 32.5 μg per ml, respectively. In three patients given 200 mg of ceftazidime in 2 liter dialysis treatments for each of 12 cycles, mean serum levels increased from 1.3 μg per ml at 1 h to 25.3 μg per ml at 12 h (Tourkantonis and Nicolaidis, 1983). From these results, a dose of 0.5 g every 24 h by catheter with an extra 0.5 g at the end of peritoneal dialysis was recommended for such patients.

Hemofiltration in which substances and body fluid are transported across a membrane by transmembrane pressure alone, is frequently used in the intensive care situation. In six patients with renal insufficiency and mild infections a single dose of 0.5 g ceftazidime given after hemofiltration into the extracorporeal circulation was sufficient for up to 48 h (Gravert et al., 1983). In another study ceftazidime was given to critically ill patients with septic multiorgan failure during intermittent hemofiltration. A 1 g i.v. dose of ceftazidime was given 2 h before the beginning of hemofiltration, and this established a safe, effective and non-toxic drug level during the hemofiltration period. It was more difficult to estimate the ceftazidime requirements during the interhemofiltration periods, as there were large variations between individual patients. A 0.5 g i.v. dose of ceftazidime may be appropriate after the first hemofiltration. The authors suggested that ceftazidime serum level monitoring was necessary to determine further ceftazidime dosage (Kinowski et al., 1993).

When ceftazidime was given together with tobramycin to patients with renal failure, there was a slight further decrease in ceftazidime elimination, but no further alteration in dosing was necessary (Aronoff et al., 1990).

6 Patients with liver disease

Ceftazidime can be administered without accumulation or toxicity to patients with chronic liver disease. Dosage adjustment is not necessary provided that the renal function is normal (Pasko et al., 1985; El Touny et al., 1991).

7 Patients with cystic fibrosis

These patients often need increased doses, but with ceftazidime the best results are achieved if the otherwise maximal dose of 150 mg per kg per day (up to maximum of 6 g per day) is administered i.v. in three divided doses (Padoan et al., 1987; Reed et al., 1987).

Serum Levels in Relation to Dosage

1 Intravenous administration

Mean serum levels after ceftazidime was given to six male volunteers by 5 min i.v. infusions are shown in Table I.30. The serum half-life of the drug was approximately 2 h.

Infusions of 2 g over 15 min given every 8 h to febrile cancer patients, provided serum levels which remained above the MICs for 90% of bacterial pathogens frequently recovered from the blood of such patients throughout the dosing interval. There was a poor relationship between estimated creatinine clearance and ceftazidime clearance in this study (Drusano et al., 1985). If vancomycin was administered i.v. together with ceftazidime, the serum levels of ceftazidime were unchanged (Boeckh et al., 1988).

2 Intramuscular administration

Patients with exacerbations of chronic bronchitis were given 1.0- or 2.0-g i.m. injections of ceftazidime. Peak serum levels, reached 30–60 min post-injection, measured 34.4 and 37.8 μg per ml, respectively for these two doses (Davies et al., 1983).

3 Neonates

Ceftazidime administered to premature neonates either i.v. as a 1–2 min bolus injection or i.m. at a dosage of 25 mg per kg every 12 h, produced peak serum concentrations at 15 min and 1.5 h of 77 and 56 μg per ml, respectively (Mulhall and de Louvois, 1985).

4 Cystic fibrosis patients

Mean serum concentrations 15 min after the first and eighth i.v. dose of 35 mg per kg of ceftazidime given every 8 h to six children with this disease (age range 5–14 years) were 97 and 110 μg per ml, respectively (Turner et al., 1984).

Table I.30
After Lüthy et al. (1981), with permission

Dose (g)	Mean serum level (μg per ml) at			
	10 min	6 h	8 h	12 h
0.5	49.9	2.1	1.0	0.3
1.0	107.0	4.4	2.1	0.5
1.0 + probenecid	98.9	4.2	2.1	0.5
2.0	181.0	6.6	3.8	1.1

Excretion

1 Urine

The major route of excretion of ceftazidime is via the kidneys. After i.v. injections of 0.5 and 1.0 g urinary levels of the drug remained as high as 120.9 and 502.8 µg per ml, respectively, 4–6 h later. Urinary recovery rates during 24 h were 90.3% and 88.7% respectively. As concomitant administration of probenecid did not alter either serum levels or urinary recovery, the mechanism of renal excretion was considered to be mainly by glomerular filtration. No active metabolites were detected in urine (Saito, 1983).

2 Bile

A small amount of ceftazidime is excreted via the bile. If the biliary tract is unobstructed, after a 2-g i.v. dose, the 12 h biliary recovery in one study was 0.21% of the dose. The respective ceftazidime concentrations in choledochal and gallbladder bile sampled perioperatively in ten patients 1 h after ceftazidime 2 g i.v. were 78.3 and 17.9 µg per ml (Brogard et al., 1987).

Distribution of the Drug in Body

The serum protein binding of ceftazidime is only 17% (O'Callaghan et al., 1980; Mulhall and de Louvois, 1985). The effect of protein binding on antibiotic efficacy is controversial. Some authors support the concept that only the unbound drug is microbiologically active (Lam et al., 1988), but many disagree with this (p. 95).

1 Extravascular fluid

Levels in induced blister fluid obtained after 1.0 g was given i.v. to volunteers reached a mean peak concentration of 44.7 µg per ml 1 h after injection, and the drug was still detectable at 8 h (Ryan et al., 1982).

2 Ascitic and peritoneal fluid

After ceftazidime was given as a 1-g i.v. bolus dose over 2 min to patients with ascites, normal renal function and serum albumin levels between 2.8 and 3.3 g per 100 ml, it rapidly diffused into the peritoneal space and concentrations greater than 10 µg per ml persisted for at least 6 h (Benoni et al., 1984). The drug penetrated well into normal peritoneal fluid of patients undergoing elective abdominal surgery, where a concentration approximately two-thirds of the concomitant serum level was attained (Corbett et al., 1985).

3 Pleural fluid

The drug penetrated into large pleural effusions of patients with bronchogenic carcinoma, where levels of 17 and 28 µg per ml were obtained 1 and 4 h, respectively after a 2-g i.v. bolus dose (Walstad et al., 1983).

4 Cerebrospinal fluid and brain

A patient with bacterial meningitis and normal renal function who was given 1.0 g ceftazidime i.v. three times daily had a serum level of 56 µg per ml 1 h after a dose and a CSF level of 2.4 µg per ml 2 h after the dose (Abbas et al., 1983). In 14 patients with normal meninges, given a 2-g i.v. bolus, CSF concentrations were less than 1 µg per ml. In five patients with meningitis given the same dose, CSF levels were 18, 17, 16, 1 and 0.8 µg per ml 30–60 min after treatment, although the CSF findings in these five patients were practically identical (Walstad et al., 1983). In a similar study, after 2-g or 3-g i.v. doses which produced similar serum concentrations, CSF levels were substantially lower in patients without meningitis (mean 0.8 µg per ml) than in those with meningitis (mean 22.6 µg per ml). In the patients with meningitis, trough CSF ceftazidime levels 6–7 h post-infusion ranged from 10.5 to 36.7 µg per ml. There was no correlation between CSF penetration and either the degree of CSF pleocytosis or protein concentration (Fong and Tomkins, 1984).

The penetration of ceftazidime into intracranial abscesses were investigated in nine patients who were receiving i.v. ceftazidime in dosages ranging from 0.5 g to 2 g 8-hourly. Concentrations of ceftazidime varying between 2.7 and 27.0 µg per ml were detected in the pus of the abscesses (Green et al., 1989).

5 Breast milk

In 11 puerperal women given ceftazidime 2 g i.v. every 8 h for 5 days for endometritis, the mean trough and peak breast milk levels were 3.8 and 5.2 µg per ml, respectively (Blanco et al., 1983).

6 Respiratory secretions

Sputum concentrations measured after 1- and 2-g i.m. doses peaked at 3 and 5 h with values of 3 and 3.5 µg per ml (Davies *et al.*, 1983). Five adult intubated intensive-care patients were given either 1, 2 or 3 g ceftazidime i.v. Ceftazidime appeared rapidly in bronchial secretions reaching mean maximal concentrations of 2.2, 4.81 and 5.69 µg per ml respectively in the first sampling period (0–2 h) (Langer *et al.*, 1991). In six children with cystic fibrosis, mean sputum concentrations of 2.7 and 2.6 µg per ml, respectively, were found after the first and eighth dose of 35 mg per kg of ceftazidime (Turner *et al.*, 1984). Assael *et al.* (1983) gave 50 mg per kg doses to such patients (average age 14.2 years). Sputum levels obtained at 2 h (4.13 µg per ml) exceeded the MICs for 50% of *Ps. aeruginosa* isolates from these patients, but the MIC for 90% of the isolates was never reached. In another study of 14 patients with cystic fibrosis given a similar dose, the maximum sputum concentration usually obtained 1 h after the infusion, ranged from 0.7 to 9.8 µg per ml (Strandvik *et al.*, 1983).

7 Heart valves and vegetations

In an animal study rabbits with combined tricuspid and aortic endocarditis due to *Ps. aeruginosa* received single i.v. doses of ceftazidime (50 mg per kg). The antibiotic penetrated much better into tricuspid than aortic valve vegetations and the times above the MBCs for tricuspid vegetations were significantly longer than those achieved within aortic vegetations (Bayer *et al.*, 1988b). Humans undergoing open-heart surgery, were given an i.v. bolus injection of 2 g ceftazidime over 5 min. Ceftazidime concentrations in cardiac valvular tissue were 37.4 µg per g soon after administration of the antibiotic, and this declined to 6.3 µg per g within 10 h (Frank *et al.*, 1987).

8 Prostate

After a 2-g i.v. dose, prostatic tissue taken at about 1.0, 1.5, 4.0 and 6.9 h after dosing had levels of 10.1, 6.0, 3.6, and 2.5 µg per g, respectively of ceftazidime and were roughly 14% of mean concurrent serum levels (Abbas *et al.*, 1985).

9 Uterus and fallopian tubes

When a bolus i.v. injection of 2 g ceftazidime was given over 5 min at varying times before hysterectomy, peak tissue concentrations were reached 1–2 h later and were approximately 19 µg per ml for myometrium, endometrium and salpinges. They remained above 8 µg per ml for at least 5 h (Daschner *et al.*, 1983).

10 Eye

In a study a dose of 50 mg per kg of ceftazidime was given to rabbits who had acute endophthalmitis in one eye and whose other eye was normal. The mean penetration of the drug into aqueous humor in the eyes with and without endophthalmitis was 64 and 10%, respectively. In the vitreous body the corresponding penetration was 5 and 1% (Walstad *et al.*, 1987).

11 Skin, fat and muscle

Tissue samples were obtained from 39 patients given 2 g of ceftazidime i.v. 12-hourly for 48 h as chemoprophylaxis for cardiac surgery. Mean ceftazidime tissue levels per g 100–130 min after a dose were 20 µg for bone, 7.1 µg for skin, 9.2 µg for fat, 12.7 µg for heart muscle and 9.4 µg for skeletal muscle. Mean serum levels at 1.5, 4, and 12 h were 70, 27 and 5.5 µg per ml, respectively (Adam *et al.*, 1983).

12 Bone

In one study patients undergoing hip arthroplasty received ceftazidime 1 g i.v. at the time of induction of anesthesia, followed by two doses of 0.5 g, given i.m. 6 and 12 h later. The mean bone ceftazidime concentration showed a general rise towards a maximum of approximately 20 µg per g when the interval between antibiotic injection and removal of bone sample was 35–40 min (Leigh *et al.*, 1985).

Mode of Action

Ceftazidime acts on the bacterial cell wall in a manner similar to penicillin G (p. 25). Like other newer antipseudomonal cephalosporins, the drug shows an initial affinity for penicillin-binding protein PBP3 (p. 334), followed by PBP1a. This is reflected in morphological changes observed in bacteria treated with ceftazidime (Harper, 1981; Elliott and Greenwood, 1984; Ullmann and Hammer-Uschtrin, 1984).

Toxicity

Similar to other cephalosporins such as cephalothin (p. 256) and cefotaxime (p. 256), ceftazidime is a drug with low toxicity. Hypersensitivity manifestations such as rashes, usually mild, have occurred in some 2% of patients treated (Foord, 1983). The drug sometimes may be cross-allergenic with the penicillins. Eosinophilia, positive Coombs' test without hemolysis and mild, reversible elevations in liver enzymes have also been associated with ceftazidime treatment (Clumeck et al., 1983; Lundbergh et al., 1983; Mastella et al., 1983; Van Dalen et al., 1983).

As with all beta-lactam antibiotics (p. 33) leukopenia may occur. It developed in two patients described by Eron et al. (1983) and Pettersson et al. (1983) reported one case in which granulocytopenia persisted for 4 months. It is not known whether ceftazidime or other beta-lactam antibiotics prolong the period of neutropenia when used for treatment of infections in neutropenic cancer patients. In one study the use of two beta-lactam agents (e.g. ceftazidime plus piperacillin) in these patients, rather than one, did not appear to prolong neutropenia (Kibbler et al., 1989a). Nephrotoxicity has been uncommon. In an investigation of this complication in rats, ceftazidime appeared to be no more nephrotoxic than cefazolin (p. 286) (Luft et al., 1984). Ceftazidime does not interfere with the functions of human macrophages. On the contrary, at half the MIC, the antibiotic caused macrophages to ingest and kill Staph. aureus and Ps. aeruginosa at a higher rate than did macrophages without the drug (Cuffini et al., 1987).

Ceftazidime given i.v. has some effect on fecal flora. When the drug was given alone or combined with gentamicin or tobramycin, there were no major changes in fecal anaerobic bacteria. Enterobacteriaceae were usually eliminated. In some patients there was overgrowth of enterococci and yeasts and sometimes also Cl. difficile (Sakata et al., 1986; Meijer-Severs and Joshi, 1989; Murdoch et al., 1990). Although Cl. difficile was isolated from the stools of 27% of a group of premature babies receiving the drug, this percentage was not much greater than that found in healthy babies not receiving antibiotics. There was no increase in the frequency of necrotizing enterocolitis above that normally found in this population (Mulhall and de Louvois, 1985).

Clinical Uses of the Drug

1 Initial therapy for febrile neutropenic cancer patients

There is no uniform agreement which antibiotic or antibiotic combination is the best initial treatment for these patients. Because ceftazidime is active against most aerobic Gram-negative bacilli, including Ps. aeruginosa, many authors have used ceftazidime monotherapy initially with success (De Pauw et al., 1985; Pizzo et al., 1986; Verhagen et al., 1987; Granowetter et al., 1988; Novakova et al., 1990; 1991; Samuelsson et al., 1992; De Pauw et al., 1994). However, in patients whose fever persists, or where there is bacteriological confirmation of infection with an organism resistant to ceftazidime, the chemotherapy has to be changed appropriately. More recently infections by methicillin-resistant Staph. aureus, or Staph. epidermidis as well as other Gram-positive organisms such as Strep. viridans have become more common in these patients. If in any hospital Gram-positive organisms are commonly isolated in this setting, initial therapy should be a ceftazidime/vancomycin combination (Hughes et al., 1990; Armstrong, 1991; Sanders et al., 1991; Pizzo, 1993; Bochud et al., 1994). The other beta-lactam antibiotic suitable for monotherapy is imipenem (p. 236), and one study suggested that imipenem was slightly superior for this purpose (Liang et al., 1990).

It is controversial whether one of the aminoglycosides should be added routinely to ceftazidime for the treatment of these patients (Bodey, 1993). Certainly regimens such as ceftazidime/amikacin have been satisfactory (Viscoli et al., 1991), but there is no proof that the addition of amikacin is necessary on a routine basis. There is some evidence that in high-risk patients, who are profoundly and persistently neutropenic, the response rate may be better if two antibiotics are used (e.g. ceftazidime plus amikacin) to both of which the Gram-negative bacillus causing bacteremia is sensitive (Wade, 1989). A double beta-lactam combination such as ceftazidime plus piperacillin has also been satisfactory as initial therapy (Kibbler et al., 1989b). But when Anaissie et al. (1988) compared ceftazidime plus vancomycin with ceftazidime, piperacillin and vancomycin, the conclusion was that ceftazidime plus vancomycin provided adequate initial therapy and that the further addition of piperacillin did not improve the results.

Chemotherapy in these patients should be continued until the resolution of neutropenia and fever. If after 7 days no bacteriological diagnosis for the fever is made, and if the fever and neutropenia continue, a fungal infection is likely and empirical treatment for this with an antifungal agent such as amphotericin B (p. 1245) should be started (Hughes *et al.*, 1990; Pizzo, 1993). The use of granulocyte colony-stimulating factor along with chemotherapy for certain cancers may reduce the incidence of fever with neutropenia and culture confirmed infections in these patients (Crawford *et al.*, 1994).

In recent years outpatient management of patients with fever and low-risk neutropenia has been tried with success. Regimens used have included oral clindamycin plus ciprofloxacin or ofloxacin alone 400 mg orally 12-hourly (Anaissie and Vadhan-Ray, 1995; Malik *et al.*, 1995).

2 Pseudomonas aeruginosa meningitis

Ceftazidime is effective in *H. influenzae* meningitis in children (Hatch *et al.*, 1986), but for this either cefotaxime (p. 336) or ceftriaxone (p. 359) are preferred. The same is true for bacterial meningitis caused by *E. coli* and other Enterobacteriaceae (Elliott *et al.*, 1986). For *Ps. aeruginosa* meningitis ceftazidime is probably the drug of choice, but it does not always succeed. Probably an aminoglycoside should be added, but as this penetrates poorly into the CSF, parenteral ceftazidime plus intraventricular aminoglycoside may be necessary (Fong and Tomkins, 1985; Williams and Foord, 1985; Korvick and Yu, 1991; Saha *et al.*, 1993). Ciprofloxacin (p. 1027) may also be useful for the treatment of *Ps. aeruginosa* meningitis.

3 Pseudomonas aeruginosa endocarditis

Ticarcillin plus tobramycin has been regarded as optimal therapy (p. 156). Whether ceftazidime may have advantages over ticarcillin is uncertain (Korvick and Yu, 1991). One animal study showed that ceftazidime plus amikacin, given at high doses and short intervals could have a place in the therapy of patients with left-sided endocarditis caused by *Ps. aeruginosa* (Pefanis *et al.*, 1993). *In vivo* resistance of *Ps. aeruginosa* to ceftazidime may arise during the treatment of *Ps. aeruginosa* endocarditis (Bayer *et al.*, 1987a).

4 Other serious Ps. aeruginosa infections such as septicemia, pneumonia, osteomyelitis and pyelonephritis

Ceftazidime has been used with some success for all of these conditions. Often an aminoglycoside has been used as well. Other beta-lactam agents are available for these infections such as ticarcillin (p. 156) or piperacillin (p. 174) and it is not determined which is the optimal therapy (Cox, 1983; Young, 1985; Bragman *et al.*, 1986; Bach and Cocchetto, 1987; Mandell *et al.*, 1987; Korvick and Yu, 1991; Cade *et al.*, 1993). Severe *Ps. aeruginosa* sinusitis in HIV-infected patients has been successfully treated by ceftazidime/gentamicin combination (O'Donnell *et al.*, 1993). In AIDS patients *Ps. aeruginosa* septicemia responded better if ceftazidime was combined with an aminoglycoside such as gentamicin (Mendelson *et al.*, 1994). For serious *Ps. aeruginosa* infections the dosage of ceftazidime given should be adequate. In one burns unit *Ps. aeruginosa* infections appeared when ceftazidime was given in a dose of 3 g daily. The outbreak was controlled by increasing the daily ceftazidime dosage to 6 g and by reinforcement of isolation precautions (Richard *et al.*, 1994).

5 Pseudomonas aeruginosa infections in patients with cystic fibrosis

These infections are difficult to treat, but some success has been obtained in the treatment of bronchopulmonary infections by using either i.v. ceftazidime alone or combining it with an aminoglycoside such as tobramycin (Pedersen *et al.*, 1986; Padoan *et al.*, 1987). Ceftazidime-resistant strains of *Ps. aeruginosa*, usually due to induced chromosomal beta-lactamases (p. 322), often arise during therapy (Schryvers *et al.*, 1987). The long-term administration of ceftazidime to patients chronically colonized with *Ps. aeruginosa* is usually associated with the development of ceftazidime resistance (Mouton *et al.*, 1993).

Ceftazidime may be the best antibiotic to treat *Burkholderia (Pseudomonas) cepacia* infections in cystic fibrosis patients, but these infections are very difficult to treat (Thomassen *et al.*, 1986).

6 Melioidosis

White *et al.* (1989) first conducted an open randomized trial to compare ceftazidime alone (120 mg per kg per day) with conventional therapy, which was chloramphenicol (100 mg per kg per day) plus doxycycline (4 mg per kg per day) plus trimethoprim (10 mg per kg per day) and sulfamethoxazole (50 mg per kg per day), in the treatment of severe melioidosis. In the ceftazidime-treated group 37% of patients died, whilst with the conventional therapy 74% of patients died. Ceftazidime treatment lowered the mortality by 50% and the authors recommended that the drug now should be the treatment of choice for melioidosis. In another trial Sookpranee *et al.* (1992) compared ceftazidime plus co-trimoxazole with the conventional therapy of chloramphenicol, doxycycline and co-trimoxazole in the treatment of patients with severe melioidosis. Ceftazidime plus co-trimoxazole was superior and the authors recommended this combination as the treatment of choice. In another trial i.v. ceftazidime was superior to i.v. amoxycillin/clavulanic acid (Suputtamongkol *et al.*, 1994). Ceftazidime alone is also effective treatment for *Burkholderia pseudomallei* liver abscess (Vatcharapreechasakul *et al.*, 1992). Initial parenteral treatment with ceftazidime is effective in acute melioidosis, but following the i.v. treatment the patients often need prolonged oral chemotherapy with either co-amoxiclav or combination regimen of chloramphenicol, doxycycline and co-trimoxazole. The optimum choice and duration of oral antibiotic treatment to prevent a relapse has not been determined (Chaowagul *et al.*, 1993). Corneal ulcers caused by *B. pseudomallei* can also be cured by topical and/or parenteral ceftazidime followed by oral co-amoxiclav to complete a total of 8 weeks course (Siripanthong *et al.*, 1991).

7 Malignant otitis externa

This usually occurs in elderly diabetics, but may also occur in HIV-infected patients. It is an invasive, potentially devastating infection of the external ear canal and is nearly always caused by *Ps. aeruginosa*. Monotherapy with ceftazidime may be the treatment of choice (Johnson and Ramphal, 1990b; McElroy and Marks, 1991).

8 Other infections caused by Gram-negative bacilli

Ceftazidime can be used to treat infections caused by Enterobacteriaceae, but cefotaxime (p. 338) or ceftriaxone (p. 360) are usually preferred. It is reasonable to use ceftazidime to treat a condition such as nosocomial pneumonia in an intensive-care unit patient, where the bacterial aetiology can not be immediately determined and where *Ps. aeruginosa* may be involved. Ceftazidime plus an aminoglycoside may be used in severe *Vibrio vulnificus* infections although the organism is also sensitive to cefotaxime and ceftriaxone (Chuang *et al.*, 1992).

References

Abbas AMA, Taylor MC, Newby D *et al.* (1983). Ceftazidime: a new approach in the treatment of moderate and serious infections. *J Antimicrob Chemother* **12** (Suppl A): 147.

Abbas AMA, Taylor MC, Da Silva C *et al.* (1985). Penetration of ceftazidime into the human prostate gland following intravenous injection. *J Antimicrob Chemother* **15**: 119.

Ackerman BH, Ross J, Tofte RW, Rotschafer JC (1984). Effect of decreased renal function on the pharmacokinetics of ceftazidime. *Antimicrob Ag Chemother* **25**: 785.

Adam D, Reichart B, Williams KJ (1983). Penetration of ceftazidime into human tissue in patients undergoing cardiac surgery. *J Antimicrob Chemother* **12** (Suppl A): 269.

Aldridge KE, Sanders CV, Janney A *et al.* (1984). Comparison of the activities of penicillin G and new beta-lactam antibiotics against clinical isolates of *Bacteroides* species. *Antimicrob Ag Chemother* **26**: 410.

Alford RH (1983). Comparison of ceftazidime and N-formimidoyl thienamycin against gentamicin-sensitive and resistant *Pseudomonas aeruginosa*. *J Antimicrob Chemother* **11**: 599.

Alvarez S, Jones M, Holtsclaw-Berk S *et al.* (1985). *In vitro* susceptibilities and beta-lactamase production of 53 clinical isolates of *Branhamella catarrhalis*. *Antimicrob Ag Chemother* **27**: 646.

Anaissie EJ, Vadhan-Ray S (1995). Is it time to redefine the management of febrile neutropenia in cancer patients? *Amer J Med* **98**: 221.

Anaissie EJ, Fainstein V, Bodey GP *et al.* (1988). Randomized trial of beta-lactam regimens in febrile neutropenic cancer patients. *Amer J Med* **84**: 581.

Anstey NM, Currie BJ, Withnall KM (1992). Community-acquired *Acinetobacter* pneumonia in the Northern Territory of Australia. *Clin Infect Dis* **14**: 83.

Armstrong D (1991). Empiric therapy for the immunocompromised host. *Rev Infect Dis* **13** (Suppl 9): 763.

Aronoff GR, Brier RA, Sloan RS, Brier ME (1990). Interactions of ceftazidime and tobramycin in patients with normal and impaired renal function. *Antimicrob Ag Chemother* **34**: 1139.

Aronoff SC (1988). Outer membrane permeability in *Pseudomonas cepacia*: diminished porin content in a beta-lactam-resistant mutant and in resistant cystic fibrosis isolates. *Antimicrob Ag Chemother* **32**: 1636.

Assael BM, Boccazzi A, Caccamo ML *et al.* (1983). Clinical pharmacology of ceftazidime in patients. *J Antimicrob Chemother* **12** (Suppl A): 341.

Bach MC, Cocchetto DM (1987). Ceftazidime as single-agent therapy for Gram-negative aerobic bacillary osteomyelitis. *Antimicrob Ag Chemother* **31**: 1605.

Bakken JS, Sanders CC, Thomson KS (1987). Selective ceftazidime resistance in *Escherichia coli*: association with changes in outer membrane protein. *J Infect Dis* **155**: 1220.

Bakken JS, Sanders CC, Clark RB, Hori M (1988). Beta lactam resistance in Aeromonas spp caused by inducible beta-lactamases active against penicillins, cephalosporins, and carbapenems. *Antimicrob Ag Chemother* **32**: 1314.

Bassey CM, Baltch AL, Smith RP *et al.* (1984). Comparative *in vitro* activities of enoxacin (CI-919, AT-2266). and eleven antipseudomonal agents against aminoglycoside-susceptible and -resistant *Pseudomonas aeruginosa* strains. *Antimicrob Ag Chemother* **26**: 417.

Bayer AS, Peters J, Parr TR Jr *et al.* (1987a). Role of beta-lactamase in *in vivo* development of ceftazidime resistance in experimental *Pseudomonas aeruginosa* endocarditis. *Antimicrob Ag Chemother* **31**: 253.

Bayer AS, Selecky M, Babel K *et al.* (1987b). Bactericidal interactions of a beta-lactam and beta-lactamase inhibitors in experimental *Pseudomo-*

nas aeruginosa endocarditis caused by a constitutive overproducer of type Id beta-lactamase. *Antimicrob Ag Chemother* **31**: 1750.

Bayer AS, Hirano L, Yih J (1988a). Development of beta-lactam resistance and increased quinolone MICs during therapy of experimental *Pseudomonas aeruginosa* endocarditis. *Antimicrob Ag Chemother* **32**: 231.

Bayer AS, Crowell DJ, Yih J *et al.* (1988b). Comparative pharmacokinetics and pharmacodynamics of amikacin and ceftazidime in tricuspid and aortic vegetations in experimental *Pseudomonas endocarditis*. *J Infect Dis* **158**: 355.

Benoni G, Arosio MG, Raimondi E *et al.* (1984). Distribution of ceftazidime in ascitic fluid. *Antimicrob Ag Chemother* **25**: 760.

Bint AJ, Yeoman P, Kilburn R *et al.* (1981). The *in vitro* activity of ceftazidime compared with that of other cephalosporins. *J Antimicrob Chemother* **8** (Suppl B): 47.

Blanco JD, Jorgensen JH, Castaneda YS, Crawford SA (1983). Ceftazidime levels in human breast milk. *Antimicrob Ag Chemother* **23**: 479.

Bochud P-Y, Calandra T, Francioli P (1994). Bacteremia due to viridans streptococci in neutropenic patients: a review. *Amer J Med* **97**: 256.

Bodey GP (1993). Empirical antibiotic therapy for fever in neutropenic patients. *Clin Infect Dis* **17** (Suppl 2): 378.

Boeckh M, Lode H, Borner K *et al.* (1988). Pharmacokinetics and serum bactericidal activity of vancomycin alone and in combination with ceftazidime in healthy volunteers. *Antimicrob Ag Chemother* **32**: 92.

Bosso JA, Allen JE, Matsen JM (1989). Changing susceptibility of *Pseudomonas aeruginosa* isolates from cystic fibrosis patients with the clinical use of newer antibiotics. *Antimicrob Ag Chemother* **33**: 526.

Bradford PA, Cherubin CE, Idemyor V *et al.* (1994). Multiply resistant *Klebsiella pneumoniae* strains from two Chicago hospitals: identification of the extended-spectrum TEM-12 and TEM-10 ceftazidime-hydrolysing beta-lactamases in a single isolate. *Antimicrob Ag Chemother* **38**: 761.

Bragman S, Sage R, Booth L, Noone P (1986). Ceftazidime in the treatment of serious *Pseudomonas aeruginosa* sepsis. *Scand J Infect Dis* **18**: 425.

Brogard JM, Jehl F, Paris-Bockel D *et al.* (1987). Biliary elimination of ceftazidime. *J Antimicrob Chemother* **19**: 671.

Burwen DR, Banerjee SN, Gaynes RP *et al.* (1994). Ceftazidime resistance among selected nosocomial Gram-negative bacilli in the United States. *J Infect Dis* **170**: 1622.

Cade JF, Presneill J, Sinickas V, Hellyar A (1993). The optimal dosage of ceftazidime for severe lower respiratory tract infections. *J Antimicrob Chemother* **32**: 611.

Chamberland S, L'Ecuyer J, Lessard C *et al.* (1992). Antibiotic susceptibility profiles of 941 Gram-negative bacteria isolated from septicemic patients throughout Canada. *Clin Infect Dis* **15**: 615.

Chanal CM, Sirot DL, Labia R *et al.* (1988). Comparative study of a novel plasmid-mediated beta-lactamase, CAZ-2, and the CTX-1 and CAZ-1 enzymes conferring resistance to broad-spectrum cephalosporins. *Antimicrob Ag Chemother* **32**: 1660.

Chaowagul W, Suputtamongkob Y, Dance DAB *et al.* (1993). Relapse of melioidosis: incidence and risk factors. *J Infect Dis* **168**: 1181.

Chen HY, Yuan M, Ibrahim-Elmagboul IB, Livermore DM (1995). National survey of susceptibility to antimicrobials amongst clinical isolates of *Pseudomonas aeruginosa*. *J Antimicrob Chemother* **35**: 521.

Chow AW, Bartlett KH (1981). Comparative *in vitro* activity of ceftazidime (GR-20263) and other beta-lactamase stable cephalosporins against anaerobic bacteria. *J Antimicrob Chemother* **8**: 91.

Chuang Y-C, Yuan C-Y, Liu C-Y *et al.* (1992). *Vibrio vulnificus* infection in Taiwan: report of 28 cases and review of clinical manifestations and treatment. *Clin Infect Dis* **15**: 271.

Ciofu O, Giwercman B, Walter-Rasmussen J *et al.* (1995). Antibodies against *Pseudomonas aeruginosa* chromosomal beta-lactamase in patients with cystic fibrosis are markers of the development of resistance of *P. aeruginosa* to beta-lactams. *J Antimicrob Chemother* **35**: 295.

Clarke AM, Zemcov SJV (1981). *In vitro* activity of ceftazidime compared with other beta-lactam antibiotics. *J Antimicrob Chemother* **8** (Suppl B): 57.

Clumeck N, Gordts B, Dab I *et al.* (1983). Ceftazidime as a single agent in the treatment of severe *Pseudomonas aeruginosa* infections. *J Antimicrob Chemother* **12** (Suppl A): 207.

Cone LA, Woodard DR, Stoltzman DS, Byrd RG (1985). Ceftazidime versus tobramycin-ticarcillin in the treatment of pneumonia and bacteremia. *Antimicrob Ag Chemother* **28**: 33.

Coovadia YM, Ramsaroop U (1984). *In vitro* antimicrobial susceptibilities of penicillinase-producing and non-penicillinase-producing strains of *N gonorrhoeae* isolated in Durban, South Africa. *Antimicrob Ag Chemother* **26**: 770.

Corbett CRR, McFarland RJ, Spender GR, Ryan DM (1985). The penetration of ceftazidime into peritoneal fluid in patients undergoing elective abdominal surgery. *J Antimicrob Chemother* **16**: 261.

Cox CE (1983). A comparison of ceftazidime and tobramycin in the treatment of complicated urinary tract infections. *J Antimicrob Chemother* **12** (Suppl A): 47.

Crawford J, Ozer H, Stoller R *et al.* (1994). Reduction by granulocyte colony-stimulating factor of fever and neutropenia induced by chemotherapy in patients with small-cell lung cancer. *Clin Infect Dis* **18** (Suppl 2): 189.

Cuffini AM, Carlone NA, Xerri L, Pizzoglio MF (1987). Synergy of ceftazidime and human macrophages on phagocytosis and killing of *Staphylococcus aureus* and *Pseudomonas aeruginosa*. *J Antimicrob Chemother* **20**: 261.

Dance DAB, Wuthiekanun V, Chaowagul W, White NJ (1989). The antimicrobial susceptibility of *Pseudomonas pseudomallei*. Emergence of resistance *in vitro* and during treatment. *J Antimicrob Chemother* **24**: 295.

Dance DAB, Wuthiekanun V, Chaowagul W *et al.* (1991). Development of resistance to ceftazidime and co-amoxiclav in *Pseudomonas pseudomallei*. *J Antimicrob Chemother* **28**: 321.

Daschner FD, Petersen EE, Just H-M, Hillemanns HG (1983). Penetration of ceftazidime into serum, myometrium, endometrium, salpinges and subcutaneous tissue. *J Antimicrob Chemother* **12** (Suppl A): 247.

Davies BI, Maesen FPV, van Noord JA (1983). Treatment of chronic and recurrent respiratory infection with intramuscular ceftazidime. *J Antimicrob Chemother* **12** (Suppl A): 1.

Deeter RG, Weinstein MP, Swanson KA *et al.* (1990). Crossover assessment of serum bactericidal activity and pharmacokinetics of five broad spectrum cephalosporins in the elderly. *Antimicrob Ag Chemother* **34**: 1007.

De Pauw B, Williams K, De Neeff J *et al.* (1985). A randomized prospective study of ceftazidime versus ceftazidime plus flucloxacillin in the empiric treatment of febrile episodes in severely neutropenic patients. *Antimicrob Ag Chemother* **28**: 824.

De Pauw BE, Deresinski SC, Feld R *et al.* (1994). Ceftazidime compared with piperacillin and tobramycin for the empiric treatment of fever in neutropenic patients with cancer. A multicenter randomized trial. *Ann Intern Med* **120**: 834.

Dornbusch K, Bengtsson S, Brorson JE *et al.* (1988). Susceptibility to beta-lactam antibiotics and gentamicin of Gram-negative bacilli isolated from hospitalized patients: a Swedish multicenter study. *Scand J Infect Dis* **20**: 641.

Drabu YJ, Blakemore PH, Cox DM, McLaren A (1989). Plasmid-mediated ceftazidime resistance. *J Antimicrob Chemother* **23**: 287.

Drusano GL, Joshi J, Forrest A *et al.* (1985). Pharmacokinetics of ceftazidime, alone or in combination with piperacillin or tobramycin in the sera of cancer patients. *Antimicrob Ag Chemother* **27**: 605.

Elliott TSJ, Greenwood D (1984). The morphological response of *Pseudomonas aeruginosa* to aztreonam, cefoperazone, ceftazidime and N-formimidoyl thienamycin. *J Med Microbiol* **17**: 159.

Elliott TSJ, Ispahani P, Cowlishaw WA (1986). Gram-negative bacillary meningitis in neonates: a glimmer of therapeutic success. *J Antimicrob Chemother* **17**: 245.

El Touny M, El Guinaidy MA, El Barry MA *et al.* (1991). Pharmacokinetics of ceftazidime in patients with liver cirrhosis and ascites. *J Antimicrob Chemother* **28**: 95.

Engle JC, Lifland PW, Schleupner CJ (1985). Comparison of ceftazidime with cefamandole for therapy of community-acquired pneumonia. *Antimicrob Ag Chemother* **28**: 146.

Eron LJ, Park CH, Hixon DL et al. (1983). Ceftazidime in patients with *Pseudomonas* infections. *J Antimicrob Chemother* **12** (Suppl A): 161.

Fantin B, Farinotti R, Thabout A, Carbon C (1994). Conditions for the emergence of resistance to cefpirome and ceftazidime in experimental endocarditis due to *Pseudomonas aeruginosa*. *J Antimicrob Chemother* **33**: 563.

Fong IW, Tomkins KB (1984). Penetration of ceftazidime into the cerebrospinal fluid of patients with and without evidence of meningeal inflammation. *Antimicrob Ag Chemother* **26**: 115.

Fong IW, Tomkins KB (1985). Review of *Pseudomonas aeruginosa* meningitis with special emphasis on treatment with ceftazidime. *Rev Infect Dis* **7**: 604.

Foord RD (1983). Ceftazidime: aspects of efficacy and tolerance. *J Antimicrob Chemother* **12** (Suppl A): 399.

Frank U, Kappstein I, Schmidt-Eisenlohr E et al. (1987). Penetration of ceftazidime into heart valves and subcutaneous and muscle tissue of patients undergoing open-heart surgery. *Antimicrob Ag Chemother* **31**: 813.

Gentry LO, Douthit MB, Childs SJ, Madsen PO (1983). A random comparative trial of 025, 05 and 10g ceftazidime twice daily in urinary tract infection. *J Antimicrob Chemother* **12** (Suppl A): 53.

Giwercman B, Lambert PA, Rosdahl VT et al. (1990). Rapid emergence of resistance in *Pseudomonas aeruginosa* in cystic fibrosis patients due to *in-vivo* selection of stable partly derepressed beta-lactamase producing strains. *J Antimicrob Chemother* **26**: 247.

Giwercman B, Meyer C, Lambert PA et al. (1992). High-level beta-lactamase activity in sputum samples from cystic fibrosis patients during antipseudomonal treatment. *Antimicrob Ag Chemother* **36**: 71.

Godfrey AJ, Wong S, Dance DAB et al. (1991). *Pseudomonas pseudomallei* resistance to beta-lactam antibiotics due to alterations in the chromosomally encoded beta-lactamase. *Antimicrob Ag Chemother* **35**: 1635.

Goossens H, Vanhoof R, Grados O et al. (1982). Ceftazidime activity on multi-resistant *Salmonella*. *Lancet* **ii**: 769.

Granowetter L, Wells H, Lange BJ (1988). Ceftazidime with or without vancomycin vs cephalothin, carbenicillin and gentamicin as the initial therapy of febrile neutropenic pediatric cancer patient. *Pediatr Infect Dis J* **7**: 165.

Gravert C, Schulz E, Sack K (1983). Ceftazidime in intensive care medicine and hemofiltration. *J Antimicrob Chemother* **12** (Suppl A): 177.

Green HT, O'Donoghue AT, Shaw MDM, Dowling C (1989). Penetration of ceftazidime into intracranial abscess. *J Antimicrob Chemother* **24**: 431.

Gutmann L, Kitzis MD, Billot-Klein D et al. (1988). Plasmid-mediated beta-lactamase (TEM-7). involved in resistance to ceftazidime and aztreonam. *Rev Infect Dis* **10**: 860.

Harper PB (1981). The *in-vitro* properties of ceftazidime. *J Antimicrob Chemother* **8** (Suppl B): 5.

Hatch D, Overturf GD, Kovacs A et al. (1986). Treatment of bacterial meningitis with ceftazidime. *Pediatr Infect Dis* **5**: 416.

Heim-Duthoy KL, Bubrick MP, Cocchetto DM, Matzke GR(1988). Disposition of ceftazidime in surgical patients with intra-abdominal infection. *Antimicrob Ag Chemother* **32**: 1845.

Heritage J, Hawkey PM, Todd N, Lewis IJ (1992). Transposition of the gene encoding a TEM-12 extended-spectrum beta-lactamase. *Antimicrob Ag Chemother* **36**: 1981.

Hibbert-Rogers LCF, Heritage J, Todd N, Hawkey PM (1994). Convergent evolution of TEM-26, a beta-lactamase with extended-spectrum activity. *J Antimicrob Chemother* **33**: 707.

Höffler D, Koeppe P, Williams KJ (1983). The pharmacokinetics of ceftazidime in normal and impaired renal function. *J Antimicrob Chemother* **12** (Suppl A): 241.

Hoogkamp-Korstanje JAA, Van Erpecum KJ, Jan Kamp H (1985). Ceftazidime in serious hospital-acquired infections. *J Antimicrob Chemother* **15**: 743.

Hornstein MJ, Jupeau AM, Scavizzi MR et al. (1985). *In vitro* susceptibilities of 126 clinical isolates of *Yersinia enterocolitica* to 21 beta-lactam antibiotics. *Antimicrob Ag Chemother* **27**: 806.

Hughes WT, Armstrong D, Bodey GP et al. (1990). Guidelines for the use of antimicrobial agents in neutropenic patients with unexplained fever. *J Infect Dis* **161**: 381.

Johnson MP, Ramphal R (1990a). Beta-lactam-resistant *Enterobacter bacteremia* in febrile neutropenic patients receiving monotherapy. *J Infect Dis* **162**: 981.

Johnson MP, Ramphal R (1990b). Malignant external otitis: report on therapy with ceftazidime and review of therapy and prognosis. *Rev Infect Dis* **12**: 173.

Jones RN (1992). The current and future impact of antimicrobial resistance among nosocomial bacterial pathogens. *Diagn Microbiol Infect Dis* **15**: 3S.

Jones RN, Barry AL, Thornsberry C et al. (1981). Ceftazidime, a *Pseudomonas*-active cephalosporin: *in vitro* antimicrobial activity evaluation including recommendations for disc diffusion susceptibility tests. *J Antimicrob Chemother* **8** (Suppl B): 187.

Jonsson M, Walder M (1992). Pharmacokinetics of ceftazidime in acutely ill hospitalised elderly patients. *Eur J Clin Microbiol Infect Dis* **11**: 15.

Kibbler CC, Prentice HG, Sage RJ et al. (1989a). Do double-beta-lactam combinations prolong neutropenia in patients undergoing chemotherapy or bone marrow transplantation for hematological disease. *Antimicrob Ag Chemother* **33**: 503.

Kibbler CC, Prentice HG, Sage RJ et al. (1989b). A comparison of double-beta-lactam combinations with netilmicin/ureidopenicillin regimens in the empirical therapy of febrile neutropenic patients. *J Antimicrob Chemother* **23**: 759.

Kinowski J-M, de la Coussaye J-E, Bressolle F et al. (1993). Multiple-dose pharmacokinetics of amikacin and ceftazidime in critically ill patients with septic multiple-organ failure during intermittent hemofiltration. *Antimicrob Ag Chemother* **37**: 464.

Knothe H, Dette GA (1981). The *in-vitro* activity of ceftazidime against clinically important pathogens. *J Antimicrob Chemother* **8** (Suppl B): 33.

Korvick JA, Yu VL (1991). Antimicrobial agent therapy for *Psudomonas aeruginosa*. *Antimicrob Ag Chemother* **35**: 2167.

Kostman JR, Solomon F, Fekete T (1991). Infections with *Chryseomonas luteola* (CDC group Ve-1) and *Flavimonas oryzihabitans* (CDC group Ve-2) in neurosurgical patients. *Rev Infect Dis* **13**: 233.

Kumar A, Hay MB, Maier GA, Dyke JW (1992). Post-antibiotic effect of ceftazidime, ciprofloxacin, imipenem, piperacillin and tobramycin for *Pseudomonas cepacia*. *J Antimicrob Chemother* **30**: 597.

Lam YWF, Duroux MH, Gambertoglio JG et al. (1988). Effect of protein binding on serum bactericidal activities of ceftazidime and cefoperazone in healthy volunteers. *Antimicrob Ag Chemother* **32**: 298.

Langer M, Cantoni P, Bellosta C, Boccazzi A (1991). Penetration of ceftazidime into bronchial secretions in critically ill patients. *J Antimicrob Chemother* **28**: 925.

Le Bel M, Barbeau G, Vallee F, Bergeron MG (1985). Pharmacokinetics of ceftazidime in elderly volunteers. *Antimicrob Ag Chemother* **28**: 713.

Leigh DA, Griggs J, Tighe CM et al. (1985). Pharmacokinetic study of ceftazidime in bone and serum of patients undergoing hip and knee arthroplasty. *J Antimicrob Chemother* **16**: 637.

Liang R, Yung R, Chiu E et al. (1990). Ceftazidime versus imipenem-cilastatin as initial monotherapy for febrile neutropenic patients. *Antimicrob Ag Chemother* **34**: 1336.

Livermore DM, Chau PY, Wong AIW, Leung YK (1987). Beta-lactamase of *Pseudomonas pseudomallei* and its contribution to antibiotic resistance. *J Antimicrob Chemother* **20**: 313.

Luft FC, Visscher DW, Nierste DM et al. (1984). Ceftazidime nephrotoxicity in rats. *Antimicrob Ag Chemother* **25**: 513.

Lundbergh P, Jarstrand C, Morfeldt-Manson L, Weiland O (1983). Ceftazidime in septicemia. *J Antimicrob Chemother* **12** (Suppl A): 199.

Lüthy R, Blaser J, Bonetti A et al. (1981). Human pharmacokinetics of ceftazidime in comparison to moxalactam and cefotaxime – abstract. *J Antimicrob Chemother* **8** (Suppl B): 273.

Malik IA, Khan WA, Karim M et al. (1995). Feasibility of outpatient management of fever in cancer patients with low-risk neutropenia: results of a prospective randomized trial. *Amer J Med* **98**: 224.

Mandell LA, Nicolle LE, Ronald AR (1987). A prospective randomized trial of ceftazidime versus cefazolin/tobramycin in the treatment of hospitalized patients with pneumonia. *J Antimcirob Chemother* **20**: 95.

Martin MA, Pfaller MA, Rojas PB (1989). *In vitro* susceptibility of nosocomial Gram-negative bloodstream pathogens to quinolones and other antibiotics – a statistical approach. *J Antimicrob Chemother* **23**: 353.

Maslow MJ, Rosenberg A, Pollock AA *et al.* (1983). Ceftazidime therapy of infections caused by Enterobacteriaceae and *Pseudomonas aeruginosa. J Antimicrob Chemother* **12** (Suppl A): 213.

Mastella G, Agostini M, Barlocco G *et al.* (1983). Alternative antibiotics for the treatment of pseudomonas infections in cystic fibrosis. *J Antimicrob Chemother* **12** (Suppl A): 297.

McElroy EAJr, Marks GL (1991). Fatal necrotizing otitis externa in a patient with AIDS. *Rev Infect Dis* **13**: 1246.

McEniry DW, Gillespie SH, Felmingham D (1988). Susceptibility of *Pseudomonas pseudomallei* to new beta-lactam and aminoglycoside antibiotics. *J Antimicrob Chemother* **21**: 171.

Mehtar S, Drabu YJ, Blackmore PH (1990). The *in-vitro* activity of piperacillin/tazobactam, ciprofloxacin, ceftazidime and imipenem against multiple resistant Gram-negative bacteria. *J Antimicrob Chemother* **25**: 915.

Meijer-Severs GJ, Joshi JH (1989). The effect of new broad-spectrum antibiotics on faecal flora of cancer patients. *J Antimicrob Chemother* **24**: 605.

Mendelson MH, Gurtman A, Szabo S *et al.* (1994). *Pseudomonas aeruginosa* bacteremia in patients with AIDS. *Clin Infect Dis* **18**: 886.

Morosini MI, Canton R, Martinez-Beltran J *et al.* (1995). New extended spectrum TEM-type beta-lactamase from *Salmonella enterica* subsp. *enterica* isolated in a nosocomial outbreak. *Antimicrob Ag Chemother* **39**: 458.

Mouton JW, den Hollander JG (1994). Killing of *Ps aeruginosa* during continuous and intermittent infusion of ceftazidime in an *in vitro* pharmacokinetic model. *Antimicrob Ag Chemother* **38**: 931.

Mouton JW, den Hollander JG, Horrevorts AM (1993). Emergence of antibiotic resistance among *Pseudomonas aeruginosa* isolates from paients with cystic fibrosis. *J Antimicrob Chemother* **31**: 919.

Mulhall A, de Louvois J (1985). The pharmacokinetics and safety of ceftazidime in the neonate. *J Antimicrob Chemother* **15**: 97.

Murdoch DA, Gibbs S, Price CGA *et al.* (1990). Effect of ceftazidime and gentamicin on the oropharyngeal and faecal flora of patients with haematological malignancies. *J Antimicrob Chemother* **26**: 419.

Naumovski L, Quinn JP, Miyashiro D *et al.* (1992). Outbreak of ceftazidime resistance due to a novel extended-spectrum beta-lactamase in isolates from cancer patients. *Antimicrob Ag Chemother* **36**: 1991.

Neu HC (1981). *In vitro* activity of ceftazidime, a beta-lactamase stable cephalosporin. *J Antimicrob Chemother* **8** (Suppl B): 131.

Nordmann P, Ronco E, Naas T *et al.* (1993). Characterization of a novel extended spectrum beta-lactamase from *Pseudomonas aeruginosa. Antimicrob Ag Chemother* **37**: 962.

Novakova I, Donnelly P, De Pauw B (1990). Amikacin plus piperacillin versus ceftazidime as initial therapy in granulocytopenic patients with presumed bacteremia. *Scand J Infect Dis* **22**: 705.

Novakova I, Donnelly JP, De Pauw B (1991). Ceftazidime as monotherapy or combined with teicoplanin for initial empiric treatment of presumed bacteremia in febrile granulocytopenic patients. *Antimicrob Ag Chemother* **35**: 672.

O'Callaghan CH, Acred P, Harper PB *et al.* (1980). GR 20263, a new broad-spectrum cephalosporin with antipseudomonal activity. *Antimicrob Ag Chemother* **17**: 876.

O'Donnell JG, Sorbello AF, Condoluci DV, Barnish MJ (1993). Sinusitis due to *Pseudomonas aeruginosa* in patients with human immunodeficiency virus infection. *Clin Infect Dis* **16**: 404.

Obara M, Nakae T (1991). Mechanisms of resistance to beta-lactam antibiotics in *Acinetobacter calcoaceticus. J Antimicrob Chemother* **28**: 791.

Padoan R, Cambisano W, Costantini D *et al.* (1987). Ceftazidime

monotherapy vs combined therapy in *Pseudomonas* pulmonary infections in cystic fibrosis. *Pediatr Infect Dis J* **6**: 648.

Pasko MT, Beam TR, Spooner JA, Camera DS (1985). Safety and pharmacokinetics of ceftazidime in patients with chronic hepatic dysfunction. *J Antimicrob Chemother* **15**: 365.

Payne DJ, Marriott MS, Amyes SGB (1991). Plasmid mediated ceftazidime resistance identified in a strain of *Serratia marcescens* isolated in Belgium. *J Antimicrob Chemother* **27**: 689.

Pedersen SS, Pressler T, Pedersen M *et al.* (1986). Immediate and prolonged clinical efficacy of ceftazidime versus ceftazidime plus tobramycin in chronic *Pseudomonas aeruginosa* infection in cystic fibrosis. *Scand J Infect Dis* **18**: 133.

Peduzzi J, Barthelemy M, Tiwari K *et al.* (1989). Structural features related to hydrolytic activity against ceftazidime of plasmid-mediated SHV-type CAZ-5 beta-lactamase. *Antimicrob Ag Chemother* **33**: 2160.

Pefanis A, Giamarellou H, Karayiannakos P, Donta I (1993). Efficacy of ceftazidime and aztreonam alone or in combination with amikacin in experimental left-sided *Pseudomonas aeruginosa* endocarditis. *Antimicrob Ag Chemother* **37**: 308.

Petit A, Sirot DL, Chanal CM *et al.* (1988). Novel plasmid-mediated beta-lactamase in clinical isolates of *Klebsiella pneumoniae* more resistant to ceftazidime than to other broad-spectrum cephalosporins. *Antimicrob Ag Chemother* **32**: 626.

Pettersson T, Storgards E, Ahnvonen P (1983). Treatment of lower respiratory tract infections with ceftazidime. *J Antimicrob Chemother* **12** (Suppl A): 31.

Phillips I, Warren C, Shannon K, King A (1981). Ceftazidime: *in vitro* antibacterial activity and susceptibility to beta-lactamases compared with that of cefotaxime, moxalactam and other beta-lactam antibiotics. *J Antimicrob Chemother* **8** (Suppl B): 23.

Piddock LJV, Traynor EA (1991). Beta-lactamase expression and outer membrane protein changes in cefpirome-resistant and ceftazidime-resistant Gram-negative bacteria. *J Antimicrob Chemother* **28**: 209.

Piddock LJV, Traynor EA, Wise R (1990). A comparison of the mechanisms of decreased susceptibility of aztreonam-resistant and ceftazidime-resistant Enterobacteriaceae. *J Antimicrob Chemother* **26**: 749.

Pizzo PA (1993). Management of fever in patients with cancer and treatment-induced neutropenia. *New Engl J Med* **328**: 1323.

Pizzo PA, Hathorn JW, Hiemenz J *et al.* (1986). A randomized trial comparing ceftazidime alone with combination antibiotic therapy in cancer patients with fever and neutropenia. *New Engl J Med* **315**: 552.

Puthucheary SD, Parasakthi N (1987). Antimicrobial susceptibility of *Pseudomonas pseudomallei. J Antimicrob Chemother* **20**: 921.

Quinn JP, Di Vincenzo CA, Foster J (1987). Emergence of resistance to ceftazidime during therapy for *Enterobacter cloacae* infections. *J Infect Dis* **155**: 942.

Quinn JP, Miyashiro D, Sahm D *et al.* (1989). Novel plasmid-mediated beta-lactamase (TEM-10). conferring selective resistance to ceftazidime and aztreonam in clinical isolates of *Klebsiella pneumoniae. Antimicrob Ag Chemother* **33**: 1451.

Rasmussen BA, Bradford PA, Quinn JP *et al.* (1993). Genetically diverse ceftazidime-resistant isolates from a single center: biochemical and genetic characterization of TEM-10 beta-lactamases encoded by different nucleotide sequences. *Antimicrob Ag Chemother* **37**: 1989.

Reed MD, Stern RC, O'Brien CA *et al.* (1987). Randomized double-blind evaluation of ceftazidime dose ranging in hospitalized patients with cystic fibrosis. *Antimicrob Ag Chemother* **31**: 698.

Rice LB, Willey SH, Papanicolaou GA *et al.* (1990). Outbreak of ceftazidime resistance caused by extended-spectrum beta-lactamases at a Massachusetts chronic-care facility. *Antimicrob Ag Chemother* **34**: 2193.

Richard P, Le Floch R, Chamoux C *et al.* (1994). *Pseudomonas aeruginosa* outbreak in a burn unit: role of antimicrobials in the emergence of multiply resistant strains. *J Infect Dis* **170**: 377.

Richards S, Iliadis A, Nichols WW (1989). Beta-lactamase levels and inducibility in sequential isolates of *Pseudomonas aeruginosa* from a patient undergoing ceftazidime therapy. *J Antimicrob Chemother* **23**: 795.

Rodriguez WJ, Khan WN, Gold B *et al.* (1985). Ceftazidime in the treatment of meningitis in infants and children over one month of age. *Amer J Med* **79** (2A): 52.

Ryan DM, Hodges B, Spencer GR, Harding SM (1982). Simultaneous comparison of three methods of assessing ceftazidime penetration into extravascular fluid. *Antimicrob Ag Chemother* **22**: 995.

Saha V, Stansfield R, Masterton R, Eden T (1993). The treatment of *Pseudomonas aeruginosa* meningitis-old regime or newer drugs? *Scand J Infect Dis* **25**: 81.

Saito A (1983). Studies on absorption, distribution, metabolism and excretion of ceftazidime in Japan. *J Antimicrob Chemother* **12** (Suppl A): 255.

Sakata H, Fujita K, Yoshioka H (1986). The effect of antimicrobial agents on fecal flora of children. *Antimicrob Ag Chemother* **29**: 225.

Samuelsson J, Lönnqvist B, Palmblad J (1992). Ceftazidime as initial therapy in febrile patients with acute leukemia during induction chemotherapy. *Scand J Infect Dis* **24**: 89.

Sanders WEJr, Sanders CC (1988). Inducible beta-lactamases: clinical and epidemiologic implications for use of newer cephalosporins. *Rev Infect Dis* **10**: 830.

Sanders JW, Powe NR, Moore RD (1991). Ceftazidime monotherapy for empiric treatment of febrile neutropenic patients: a metaanalysis. *J Infect Dis* **164**: 907.

Sato K, Nakae T (1991). Outer membrane permeability of *Acinetobacter calcoaceticus* and its implication in antibiotic resistance. *J Antimicrob Chemother* **28**: 35.

Schryvers AB, Ogunariwo J, Chamberland S *et al.* (1987). Mechanism of *Pseudomonas aeruginosa* persistence during treatment with broad-spectrum cephalosporins of lung infections in patients with cystic fibrosis. *Antimicrob Ag Chemother* **31**: 1438.

Scully BE, Neu HC (1984). Clinical efficacy of ceftazidime. Treatment of serious infections due to multiresistant *Pseudomonas* and other Gram-negative bacteria. *Arch Intern Med* **144**: 57.

Simpson IN, Finlay J, Winstanley DJ *et al.* (1994). Multi-resistance isolates possessing characteristics of both *Burkholderia (Pseudomonas) cepacia* and *Burkholderia gladioli* from patients with cystic fibrosis. *J Antimicrob Chemother* **34**: 353.

Siripanthong S, Teerapantuwat S, Prugsanusak W *et al.* (1991). Corneal ulcer caused by *Pseudomonas pseudomallei*: report of three cases. *Rev Infect Dis* **13**: 335.

Sirot D, Chanal C, Labia R *et al.* (1989). Comparative study of five plasmid-mediated ceftazidimases isolated in *Klebsiella pneumoniae*. *J Antimicrob Chemother* **24**: 509.

Smith CE, Tillman BS, Howell AW *et al.* (1990). Failure of ceftazidime amikacin therapy for bacteremia and meningitis due to *Klebsiella pneumoniae* producing an extended-spectrum beta-lactamase. *Antimicrob Ag Chemother* **34**: 1290.

Sookpranee T, Sookpranee M, Mellencamp MA, Preheim LC (1991). *Pseudomonas pseudomallei*, a common pathogen in Thailand that is resistant to the bactericidal effects of many antibiotics. *Antimicrob Ag Chemother* **35**: 484.

Sookpranee M, Boonma P, Susaengrat W *et al.* (1992). Multicenter prospective randomized trial comparing ceftazidime plus co-trimoxazole with chloramphenicol plus doxycycline and co-trimoxazole for treatment of severe melioidosis. *Antimicrob Ag Chemother* **36**: 158.

Spangler SK, Jacobs MR, Appelbaum PC (1994). Susceptibilities of 177 penicillin-susceptible and-resistant pneumococci to FK037, cefpirome, cefepime, ceftriaxone, cefotaxime, ceftazidime, imipenem, biapenem, meropenem and vancomycin. *Antimicrob Ag Chemother* **38**: 898.

Strandvik B, Malmborg AS, Alfredson H, Ericsson A (1983). Clinical results and pharmacokinetics of ceftazidime treatment in patients with cystic fibrosis. *J Antimicrob Chemother* **12** (Suppl A): 283.

Suputtamongkol Y, Raychanuwong A, Chaowagul W *et al.* (1994). Ceftazidime vs. amoxicillin/clavulanate in the treatment of severe melioidosis. *Clin Infect Dis* **19**: 846.

Thomassen MJ, Demko CA, Doershuk CF *et al.* (1986). *Pseudomonas cepacia*: decrease in colonization in patients with cystic fibrosis. *Am Rev Respir Dis* **134**: 669.

Thomson KS, Sanders CC, Washington JAII (1991). High-level resistance to cefotaxime and ceftazidime in *Klebsiella pneumoniae* isolates from Cleveland, Ohio. *Antimicrob Ag Chemother* **35**: 1001.

Thomson KS, Sanders CC, Washington JAII (1993). Ceftazidime resistance in *Hafnia alvei*. *Antimicrob Ag Chemother* **37**: 1375.

Tourkantonis A, Nicolaidis P (1983). Pharmacokinetics of ceftazidime in patients undergoing peritoneal dialysis. *J Antimicrob Chemother* **12** (Suppl A): 263.

Turner A, Pedler SJ, Carswell F *et al.* (1984). Sputum and serum concentrations of ceftazidime in patients with cystic fibrosis. *J Antimicrob Chemother* **14**: 521.

Ullmann U, Hammer-Uschtrin U (1984). Influence of cefmenoxime, ceftriaxone, latamoxef and ceftazidime on the lysis of *Klebsiella pneumoniae*: a light and electron microscopic study. *Amer J Med* **77** (6A): 21.

Urban C, Meyer KS, Mariano N *et al.* (1994). Identification of TEM-26 beta-lactamase responsible for a major outbreak of ceftazidime-resistant *Klebsiella pneumoniae*. *Antimicrob Ag Chemother* **38**: 392.

Van Dalen R, Muytjens HL, Gimbrere JSF (1983). Ceftazidime treatment in intensive care patients. *J Antimicrob Chemother* **12** (Suppl A): 189.

Van der Auwera P, Scorneaux B (1985). *In vitro* susceptibility of *Campylobacter jejuni* to 27 antimicrobial agents and various combinations of beta-lactams with clavulanic acid or sulbactam. *Antimicrob Ag Chemother* **28**: 37.

Vatcharapreechasakul T, Suputtamongkol Y, Dance DAB *et al.* (1992). *Pseudomonas pseudomallei* liver abscesses: a clinical, laboratory, and ultrasonographic study. *Clin Infect Dis* **14**: 412.

Verbist L, Verhaegen J (1981). Ceftazidime: comparative *in vitro* study. *J Antimicrob Chemother* **8** (Suppl B): 67.

Verhagen CS, De Pauw B, De Witte T *et al.* (1987). Randomized prospective study of ceftazidime versus ceftazidime plus cephalothin in empiric treatment of febrile episodes in severely neutropenic patients. *Antimicrob Ag Chemother* **31**: 191.

Victor MA, Arpi M, Bruun B *et al.* (1994). *Xanthomonas maltophilia* bacteremia in immunocompromised hematological patients. *Scand J Infect Dis* **26**: 163.

Viscoli C, Moroni C, Boni L *et al.* (1991). Ceftazidime plus amikacin versus ceftazidime plus vancomycin as empiric therapy in febrile neutropenic children with cancer. *Rev Infect Dis* **13**: 397.

Vlasses PH, Bastion WA, Behal R, Sirgo MA (1993). Ceftazidime dosing in the elderly: economic implications. *Ann Pharmacother* **27**: 967.

Vorachit M, Lam K, Jayanetra P, Costerton JW (1993). Resistance of *Pseudomonas pseudomallei* growing as a biofilm on silastic discs to ceftazidime and co-trimoxazole. *Antimicrob Ag Chemother* **37**: 2000.

Vuye A, Verschraegen G, Claeys G (1989). Plasmid-mediated beta-lactamases in clinical isolates of *Klebsiella pneumoniae* and *Escherichia coli* resistant to ceftazidime. *Antimicrob Ag Chemother* **33**: 757.

Wade JC (1989). Antibiotic therapy for the febrile granulocytopenic cancer patient: Combination therapy vs monotherapy. *Rev Infect Dis* **11** (Suppl 7): 1572.

Walstad RA, Hellum KB, Blika S *et al.* (1983). Pharmacokinetics and tissue penetration of ceftazidime: studies on lymph, aqueous humour, skin blister, cerebrospinal and pleural fluid. *J Antimicrob Chemother* **12** (Suppl A): 275.

Walstad RA, Blika S, Thurmann-Nielsen E, Halvorsen TB (1987). The penetration of ceftazidime into the inflamed rabbit eye. *Scand J Infect Dis* **19**: 131.

Watanabe M, Iyobe S, Inoue M, Mitsuhashi S (1991). Transferable imipenem resistance in *Pseudomonas aeruginosa*. *Antimicrob Ag Chemother* **35**: 147.

Weber DA, Sanders CC, Bakken JS, Quinn JP (1990). A novel chromosomal TEM derivative and alterations in outer membrane proteins together mediate selective ceftazidime resistance in *Escherichia coli*. *J Infect Dis* **162**: 460.

White NJ, Dance DAB, Chaowagul W *et al.* (1989). Halving mortality of severe melioidosis by ceftazidime. *Lancet* **ii**: 697.

Williams KJ, Foord RD (1985). Ceftazidime for *Pseudomonas* meningitis. *Lancet* **i**: 464.

Wu DH, Baltch AL, Smith RP (1984). *In vitro* comparison of *Pseudomonas aeruginosa* isolates with various susceptibilities to aminoglycosides and ten beta-lactam antibiotics. *Antimicrob Ag Chemother* **25**: 488.

Young LS (1985). Ceftazidime in the treatment of nosocomial sepsis. *Amer J Med* **79** (2A): 89.

Aztreonam

Description

Aztreonam belongs to a new class of beta-lactam antibiotics (p. 3), known as monobactams. Unlike penicillins and cephalosporins they only have the beta-lactam ring, and the thiazolidine ring, characteristic of penicillins, or the dihydrothiazide ring, characteristic of cephalosporins, is missing. In monobactams, a sulphonate group replaces the second ring. Monobactams are synthesized by bacteria. Aztreonam (3 aminothiazole-oxime, 4 alpha methyl 1 monobactamic acid) is a synthetic member of this group, developed at the Squibb Institute for Medical Research. The antibacterial spectrum of this drug is not as wide as that of the third-generation cephalosporins (p. 319) and it somewhat resembles that of the aminoglycosides (Sykes *et al.*, 1981; Sykes and Bonner, 1985).

Sensitive Organisms

Only Gram-negative aerobic bacteria are sensitive to aztreonam. The drug is quite active against the Enterobacteriaceae such as *Escherichia coli*, *Proteus mirabilis*, other *Proteus* spp. and the *Klebsiella*, *Enterobacter*, *Serratia*, *Providencia*, *Citrobacter*, *Salmonella*, *Shigella*, *Edwardsiella* and *Yersinia* spp. and *Morganella morganii* (Sykes *et al.*, 1981; Jacobus *et al.*, 1982; Barry *et al.*, 1985; Tunkel and Scheld, 1990). *Neisseria gonorrhoeae* and *Haemophilus influenzae*, including beta-lactamase producers are also quite sensitive (Barry *et al.*, 1985). However, *H. influenzae* strains which do not produce beta-lactamase, but have MICs for ampicillin of 4 μg per ml or higher (intrinsic resistance), also have increased MICs for aztreonam (MICs 1 μg per ml instead of 0.12 as for ampicillin-sensitive strains) (Powell and Williams, 1987). *Neisseria meningitidis* is aztreonam-sensitive (Barry *et al.*, 1985), but *Campylobacter jejuni* is resistant (Goossens *et al.*, 1985).

Pseudomonas aeruginosa (usual MIC 8 μg per ml) is aztreonam-susceptible but ceftazidime (p. 369) is usually twice as active. Aztreonam is also commonly effective against gentamicin- or carbenicillin-resistant *Ps. aeruginosa* isolates (Fainstein *et al.*, 1982; Barry *et al.*, 1985; Ng *et al.*, 1985; Tunkel and Scheld, 1990). However, in one study 10 of 43 strains of *Ps. aeruginosa* isolated from cystic fibrosis patients were resistant to aztreonam, although the drug had never been used in that population (Gordts *et al.*, 1984). With *Ps. aeruginosa* strains isolated from cystic fibrosis patients, 56.4% exhibited *in vitro* aztreonam/tobramycin synergism, and 49.3% aztreonam/gentamicin synergism (Bosso *et al.*, 1987). *Aeromonas* spp. are aztreonam-sensitive (Morita *et al.*, 1994). *Burkholderia* (*Pseudomonas*) *cepacia* and *Ps. stutzeri* are usually sensitive, but the *Acinetobacter* spp., *Ps. diminuta*, *Ps. putida*, *Stenotrophomonas maltophilia* and *Flavobacterium* spp. are aztreonam-resistant (Jacobus *et al.*, 1982; Strandberg *et al.*, 1983; Tunkel and Scheld, 1990).

Gram-negative anaerobic bacteria and all Gram-positive bacteria are aztreonam-resistant (Jacobus *et al.*, 1982; Barry *et al.*, 1985).

Aztreonam is stable to the common plasmid-mediated enzymes of Gram-negative bacteria such as TEM (Sykes and Bonner, 1985). Compared with the third-generation cephalosporins, such as cefotaxime (p. 322), *in vivo* development of resistance due to the inducible chromosomally mediated beta-lactamases in organisms such as *Enterobacter*, *Citrobacter* and *Providencia* spp., *Pr. vulgaris*, *Serratia marcescens* and *Ps. aeruginosa*, has been uncommon during aztreonam therapy. This appears to be because, compared with drugs like cefoxitin (p. 295) and cefotaxime (p. 322), aztreonam is a poor enzyme inducer. Occasionally high level production of these enzymes can arise spontaneously because of chromosomal mutation. In this case, the organisms involved show aztreonam-resistance (Sykes and Bonner, 1985; Tunkel and

Organism	MIC (µg per ml)
Gram-negative bacteria	
Escherichia coli	<0.1–1.0
Klebsiella spp.	<0.1–>100.0
Enterobacter cloacae	<0.1–64.0
Enterobacter aerogenes	0.1–50.0
Serratia marcescens	0.1–6.3
Proteus mirabilis	<0.1–0.1
Proteus vulgaris	<0.1–0.1
Morganella morganii	<0.1–1.6
Providencia stuartii	<0.1–0.1
Shigella spp.	<0.1–12.5
Salmonella typhi	0.097–0.39
Salmonella spp.	0.1–1.0
Citrobacter freundii	<0.1–50.0
Yersinia enterocolitica	<0.097–3.12
Pseudomonas aeruginosa	0.195–50.0
Haemophilus influenzae	<0.1–0.2
Neisseria gonorrhoeae	<0.1–0.4
Bacteroides fragilis	>100.0

Table I.31
Compiled from data published by Fainstein *et al.* (1982), Jacobus *et al.* (1982), Scribner *et al.* (1982), Sykes *et al.* (1982), Goossens *et al.* (1984; 1985), Gordts *et al.* (1984)

Scheld, 1990). Resistant mutants of *Enterobacter cloacae*, *Citrobacter freundii*, *S. marcescens*, *Morganella morganii* and *Providencia stuartii*, have been selected *in vitro*, when they were exposed to low concentrations of aztreonam. The mechanism of the resistance was increased production of chromosomally mediated beta-lactamases (Piddock *et al.*, 1990).

The plasmid-mediated extended-spectrum beta-lactamases hydrolyze aztreonam just as they inactivate the third-generation cephalosporins (p. 323). They have been mainly found in *Klebsiella* spp. and *E. coli*, but sometimes also in other Enterobacteriaceae such as *Citrobacter* spp. Strains harboring these beta-lactamases are aztreonam-resistant (Gutmann *et al.*, 1988; Philippon *et al.*, 1989; Jacoby and Carreras, 1990; Wu *et al.*, 1991).

Table I.31 shows the MICs of aztreonam against some selected bacterial species.

Mode of Administration and Dosage

Aztreonam is poorly absorbed after oral administration, peak serum levels of only 0.1–0.2 µg per ml being obtained 2 h after 0.5 oral doses (Swabb *et al.*, 1983b). The drug is usually administered by the parenteral route.

1 Adults

For moderate infections doses of 1–2 g every 8–12 h given i.m. or i.v. may be sufficient (Clergeot *et al.*, 1989). For seriously ill patients such as those with septicemia or meningitis doses of 2 g 8-hourly or 6-hourly have been used i.v. (De Maria *et al.*, 1989; Farid *et al.*, 1990; Lentnek and Williams, 1991; Gotuzzo *et al.*, 1994). The drug is administered i.v. in a similar manner to penicillin G (p. 20).

2 Children

For moderate infections a dosage of 30 mg per kg, given i.v. every 6–8 h is sufficient. For severe infections a dosage of 50 mg per kg, administered 6- or 8- hourly is recommended (Stutman *et al.*, 1984; Girgis *et al.*, 1988; Stutman, 1991).

3 Newborn and premature infants

A dose of 30 mg per kg and a dosage interval of 8–12 h is recommended for the treatment of premature infants (Cuzzolin *et al.*, 1991). For low birth weight infants during their first week of life the same dosage of aztreonam is appropriate. Other infants can be treated by aztreonam

90–125 mg per kg per day, administered in two or three divided doses. Children older than 4–6 weeks can be given the same doses as recommended for children (see above) (Stutman *et al.*, 1984; Likitnukul *et al.*, 1987; Sklavunu-Tsurutsoglu *et al.*, 1991).

4 Patients with renal failure

These patients require dosage modification. Renal clearance of the drug correlates closely with the creatinine clearance, which can be estimated from the patient's serum creatinine, age and sex. Mihindu *et al.* (1983) studied non-infected volunteers with various degrees of renal failure, and found that the elimination half-life of aztreonam increased from about 2 h in normal subjects to 6 h in anephric patients. They recommended that for patients with creatinine clearances of 60 ml per min, 30 ml per min and anephric patients, the drug should be given at the usual intervals, but the normal dose should be reduced to 75%, 50% and 25%, respectively. Mattie and Matze-van der Lans (1986) studied patients with severe Gram-negative infections, who had varying degrees of renal failure. In these patients the plasma half-life of aztreonam was prolonged to 9 h and 40 min in patients with markedly impaired renal function. These authors recommended that in patients with creatinine clearance >50 ml per min, the usual dose can be given 8-hourly. At a clearance of between 30 and 50 ml per min, the usual dose should be given 12-hourly. For patients with a creatinine clearance between 0 and 30 ml per min, they suggested a normal loading dose followed by a maintenance dose between 40 and 80% of the loading dose every 12 h. Serum aztreonam clearance may improve during therapy, probably reflecting improved renal function (Janicke *et al.*, 1985).

About 38% of the dose of aztreonam is removed during a 4 h hemodialysis and during dialysis the drugs half-life is only 2.7 h. It is recommended that half of the maintenance dose be administered after each hemodialysis session (Tunkel and Scheld, 1990).

Intraperitoneal aztreonam can be used to treat peritonitis in patients who are undergoing continuous ambulatory peritoneal dialysis. It is often used together with vancomycin which provides cover for Gram-positive organisms. Brown *et al.* (1990) added 3 g aztreonam to the first exchange in each 24 h period plus vancomycin 0.5 g on the first day and 250 mg on each subsequent days for a total of 10 days. This produced satisfactory serum and peritoneal concentrations of both drugs and a good clinical outcome. Dratwa *et al.* (1991), after initial combination therapy, used intraperitoneal aztreonam alone for the treatment of peritonitis caused by Gram-negative organisms. These authors added 0.5 g of aztreonam per liter in the first dialysate bag and 250 mg per liter in all subsequent bags. Again the serum and dialysate aztreonam levels were satisfactory and most patients recovered.

5 Patients with liver disease

Those with primary biliary cirrhosis and alcoholic cirrhosis have prolonged elimination half-lives (2.2 and 3.2 h, respectively) compared with normal subjects (1.9 h). Renal and non-renal clearances were reduced in patients with alcoholic cirrhosis. If long-term therapy with high doses is given, some dosage reduction is warranted in these patients (MacLeod *et al.*, 1984; El Touny *et al.*, 1992).

6 Patients with severe burns

In these patients the volume of distribution of aztreonam is increased, but the drug's clearance is not affected and it remains strongly associated with creatinine clearance. Larger aztreonam doses in these patients may be necessary (Friedrich *et al.*, 1991).

Serum Levels in Relation to Dosage

When i.m. doses of 1.0 g and 2.0 g were given to normal volunteers, serum levels at 1 h were 22.0 and 46.0 and at 4 h 8.9 and 18.4 μg per ml, respectively (Swabb, 1985). Normal subjects given 3-min i.v. infusions of 0.5, 1.0 and 2.0 g of aztreonam, had mean peak serum levels of 58, 125 and 242 μg per ml, respectively, 5 min after the infusion; 1 h after infusion these levels had fallen to 11.8, 23.3 and 48.6 μg per ml, respectively (Swabb *et al.*, 1981). Serum concentrations at 30 min in nine patients after a single 2.0 g i.v. dose, delivered over 5 min, ranged from 40 to 120 (mean 80.1) μg per ml (Bechard *et al.*, 1985). Scully *et al.* (1983) gave healthy volunteers doses of 0.5 g, 1.0 g and 2.0 g by 30 min infusions. Peak serum levels at the end of the infusions were 65.5, 164 and 255 μg per ml, respectively. Serum levels after a 1.0-g dose exceeded the MIC for 90% of the Enterobacteriaceae by 4- to 8-fold for 8 h and exceeded the MIC for *Ps. aeruginosa* for 4 h. In volunteers given 0.5 g or 1.0 g i.v. by 2 min infusion every 8 h, mean peak levels were 39 and 99 μg per ml, respectively, 10 min after the dose, and mean trough levels immediately prior to the next dose were 1.0 and 2.5 μg per ml, respectively. When these volunteers were given the same doses by the i.m. route every 8 h, mean peak serum levels of 18 and 36 μg per ml were reached in 60 min, and mean trough levels were 1.8 and 3.8 μg per ml, respectively (Swabb *et al.*, 1983a).

Excretion

1 Urine

The main method of elimination of aztreonam is via the kidneys and about 68% of an administered dose is excreted unchanged in the urine (Swabb *et al.*, 1982). Approximately equal amounts of serum aztreonam unbound to protein are cleared by renal tubular secretion and glomerular filtration. Probenecid (p. 24) reduced renal tubular secretion by about 50%, but it only slightly increased the steady-state serum concentration and elimination half-life of aztreonam (Swabb, 1985).

2 Bile

Levels of the drug reached in bile obtained by T-tube drainage after cholecystectomy peaked at about 40 μg per ml (range 9.7–88.2) 2.4 h after a single i.v. 1.0-g dose. Peak biliary levels 70% lower were found in other patients who had received the same dose, but who had biliary obstruction recently relieved by external drainage. This suggested that the secretory capacity of the liver had not fully recovered after biliary decompression (Martinez *et al.*, 1984).

3 Feces

Only 1% of an administered dose of the drug is found unchanged in the feces; presumably this is derived from biliary secretion.

4 Inactivation in body

Aztreonam is not extensively metabolized. Its major metabolite in humans (designated SQ26,992), results from hydrolytic opening of the beta-lactam ring. The site of its formation is unknown. It is eliminated at a much slower rate than the parent compound (Swabb *et al.*, 1983c) and appears to be devoid of any significant antimicrobial activity (Kripalani *et al.*, 1984).

Distribution of the Drug in Body

In animals with non-inflamed meninges, the CSF aztreonam levels are low (1–3 μg per ml) after its administration i.v., but in animals with induced *Ps. aeruginosa* meningitis, they ranged from 10.2 to 14.6 μg per ml (Strausbaugh *et al.*, 1986). Concentrations in the CSF of children with inflamed meninges following a single i.v. dose of 30 mg per kg, averaged 17.3% of the serum concentration; CSF aztreonam concentrations ranged from 2.1 to 20.8 μg per ml and penetration decreased as the inflammation lessened (Stutman *et al.*, 1984). In adults 2–8 h after a single 2-g i.v. dose, a mean CSF concentration of 7.2 μg per ml was attained in five patients with either bacterial, cryptococcal or carcinomatous meningitis (Greenman *et al.*, 1985). In another study in patients with bacterial meningitis, three aztreonam doses of 30 mg per kg were given i.v. at 8 h intervals, first between days 2 and 4 and again between days 11 and 20, after onset of meningitis. The concentrations of aztreonam in the CSF ranged from 3.5 to 62 μg per ml, depending on the sampling time and the time elapsed since the onset of the disease (Modai *et al.*, 1986).

Mean levels measured in bronchial secretions of nine intubated patients after a 5 min 2.0-g infusion of aztreonam, were highest at 4 h after the infusion; 2, 4 and 8 h after the dosing the levels were 0.04–14.1, 2.1–10.7 and 0.5–4.5 μg per ml, respectively (Bechard *et al.*, 1985). In another study in similar patients, after a 2-g i.v. dose, maximum concentrations in bronchial secretions were reached in 2 h, and they ranged from 4.8 to 18.7 μg per ml (Boccazzi *et al.*, 1989). Tissue concentrations measured in severely diseased human kidneys (mean 77 μg per g) were similar to concurrent serum levels (Watson *et al.*, 1984). The mean level in prostatic tissue obtained by transurethral resection was 7.8 μg per g, 50–180 min after a single 1-g i.m. aztreonam dose. This was about 25% of the concurrent serum level, but was still higher than the MICs of most Enterobacteriaceae implicated in chronic prostatitis (Madsen *et al.*, 1984). The drug rapidly penetrated induced blister fluid in normal volunteers; 1 h after infusion of 1 g the concentration was approximately 50% of the serum level and at 1.8 h a mean maximum level of 25.4 μg per ml was attained (Wise *et al.*, 1982). In ascitic fluid a concentration of 6.2 μg per ml was reached 4 h after an i.v. dose of 1 g (El Touny *et al.*, 1992).

Eighteen patients, who required joint replacement, were given a single 2-g i.v. dose of aztreonam preoperatively. The mean drug concentration in the synovial fluid was 83.0 μg per ml and in cancellous bone 16.0 μg per g (MacLeod *et al.*, 1986). After a 2-g i.v. aztreonam dose, the tissue concentrations 1–2 h after the dose were 5.3, 9.2 and 65.4 μg per g in fat, muscle and liver, respectively (Condon *et al.*, 1986). In animals aztreonam penetrated well into intra-abdominal abscesses (Youngs *et al.*, 1989). In rats aztreonam was secreted in breast milk (Singhvi *et al.*, 1984), and in rabbits, subconjunctival injections of the drug resulted in good levels in the vitreous humor (Barza and McCue, 1983). Fifteen patients awaiting cataract extraction were given a 2 g i.v. bolus injection of aztreonam. The mean aztreonam concentrations in the aqueous humor, 1, 2 and 4 h after the injection were 1.22, 1.46 and 2.2 μg per ml, respectively (Haroche *et al.*, 1986).

Protein binding of aztreonam has been reported variously as between 30% and 50% (Jacobus *et al.*, 1982; Swabb, 1985).

Mode of Action

The intrinsic activity of monobactams against bacteria is determined by their binding to particular penicillin-binding proteins (PBPs) (p. 27) and this is in turn determined by the nature of the substituents on their beta-lactam nucleus (Georgopapadakou *et al.*, 1983). Aztreonam, similar to the cephalosporins (p. 334), specifically affects septum formation in *E. coli* (and most likely other aerobic Gram-negative bacteria) and it produces filamentous forms of bacteria (p. 27) (Georgopapadakou *et al.*, 1982). This appears to be due to the high affinity of aztreonam for PBP 3 of Gram-negative bacteria and this may be sufficient to cause cell death. The drug is bactericidal (Shah *et al.*, 1981). Aztreonam is highly resistant to enzymatic hydrolysis by beta-lactamases because it has poor substrate affinity for these enzymes (Sykes *et al.*, 1982). It binds tightly as a competitive substrate to P99 cephalosporinase from *E. cloacae*, strongly inhibiting that enzyme as well (Bush *et al.*, 1982).

Toxicity

1 Hypersensitivity reactions

Aztreonam is a monocyclic beta-lactam antibiotic. Studies in humans as well as animals have demonstrated only a low level of immunologic cross-reactivity between aztreonam and IgG antibodies to penicillin G and cephalothin (Adkinson *et al.*, 1984, 1985). Cross-reactivity with penicillins and cephalosporins seems to be rare. When skin tests were performed on 41 penicillin-allergic subjects with positive reactions for IgE antibody to penicillin (p. 30) there was no cross-reactivity with aztreonam reagents (Saxon *et al.*, 1984). In a retrospective clinical study of hypersensitivity reactions to aztreonam and other beta-lactam antibiotics in cystic fibrosis patients receiving multiple treatment courses 50.9% of patients receiving piperacillin, 13% of patients receiving ceftazidime, but only 6.5% of patients receiving aztreonam, developed reactions (Koch *et al.*, 1991). In two prospective studies 15 and 18 cystic fibrosis patients who had previously experienced severe penicillin or cephalosporin allergic reactions, and whose allergy was confirmed by skin tests, were treated by aztreonam. They had negative aztreonam skin tests. In the first study 13 patients tolerated aztreonam well, but two developed drug fever. In the second study all 18 patients tolerated aztreonam. However, two of these patients had anaphylaxis on re-exposure to aztreonam (Jensen *et al.*, 1991; Moss *et al.*, 1991). Therefore despite the reduced immunogenicity and cross-reactivity, aztreonam should be administered with caution to patients who are allergic to other beta-lactam antibiotics.

2 Other side-effects

The safety profile of aztreonam in clinical trials has been analyzed by Newman *et al.* (1985). Of 2388 patients who received multiple doses, 163 (6.8%) experienced 172 adverse effects. The most common were local reactions at the injection site, rash, diarrhea, nausea and/or vomiting, and slight elevations of SGOT and SGPT levels. Treatment was discontinued in 51 (2.1%) of the 2388 patients. Aztreonam does not aggravate pre-existing renal damage in elderly patients with diminished renal function, provided that the dose is appropriately reduced (Sattler *et al.*, 1985). In non-neutropenic patients believed to be at increased risk for renal dysfunction, aztreonam is a less toxic alternative to aminoglycoside therapy for aerobic Gram-negative infections (Moore *et al.*, 1992). Aztreonam does not interfere with platelet function and coagulation in humans (Tartaglione *et al.*, 1986). The drug does not interfere with human polymorphonuclear leucocyte function; brief exposure of *E. coli* and other bacteria to aztreonam actually enhanced phagocytosis (Pruul *et al.*, 1988).

The fecal flora is changed by aztreonam treatment. The counts of Gram-negative aerobic bacilli decrease, streptococci increase, but anaerobes show no change (Sakata *et al.*, 1990). Some of the aztreonam in the large bowel is inactivated by fecal enzymes (Welling and Groen, 1989).

Clinical Uses of the Drug

1 Gram negative organism septicemia

All but two of 20 patients with Gram-negative aerobic rod septicemia treated with 2 g of aztreonam i.v. 6-hourly by Greenberg *et al.* (1984) were cured. Scully and Neu (1985) treated 87 patients with aztreonam, most of whom had severe infections caused by aerobic Gram-negative rods. Eleven had bacteremia and 10 of these were cured, including four due to *Ps. aeruginosa*. Aztreonam alone is at least as effective as one of the aminoglycosides for the treatment of proven aerobic Gram-negative organism septicemias; aminoglycosides have the disadvantage of nephrotoxicity, but aztreonam therapy often leads to superinfections, mainly by *E. faecalis* (Gudiol *et al.*, 1986; Pierard *et al.*, 1986; Smith *et al.*, 1988; De Maria *et al.*, 1989). In one study aztreonam appeared equally as effective as ceftazidime (p. 379) for the treatment of septicemias due to Gram-negative rods but there were no *Ps. aeruginosa* infections in this trial (Lagast *et al.*, 1986).

2 Initial therapy for neutropenic patients with fever

Aztreonam combined with flucloxacillin has been used for these patients, but this was somewhat unsatisfactory as flucloxacillin did not provide cover for methicillin-resistant staphylococci (Heney *et al.*, 1991). Aztreonam plus vancomycin was satisfactory for these patients, and the addition of a third drug, amikacin, did not improve the results (Jones *et al.*, 1985; 1986).

3 Bacterial meningitis

Aztreonam is quite effective for the treatment of *H. influenzae* meningitis (Girgis *et al.*, 1988), but for this cefotaxime (p. 336) or cefriaxone (p. 359) are preferred. In animals aztreonam was as effective as imipenem, ceftazidime and mezlocillin for the treatment of *E. coli* meningitis (McCracken *et al.*, 1985). In one study 16 patients with meningitis due to Enterobacteriaceae and six due to *Pseudomonas* spp. were treated by aztreonam, and the results obtained were satisfactory (Lentnek and Williams, 1991).

4 Severe neonatal sepsis

Here ampicillin/aztreonam combination has proved to be about as effective as the traditional ampicillin/amikacin regimen (Lebel and McCracken, 1988; Stutman, 1991).

5 Respiratory tract infections

Giamarellou *et al.* (1984) reported the successful use of aztreonam for the treatment of a patient with lung infection due to *E. cloacae*, associated with the adult respiratory distress syndrome. Thirteen of 19 patients with Gram-negative bacterial pneumonia treated with aztreonam by Greenberg *et al.* (1984) were cured. Aztreonam may be a useful alternative to aminoglycosides for these infections (Neu, 1985, 1987), but Schiff and Pennington (1984) found tobramycin to be more effective than aztreonam, piperacillin or azlocillin for experimental *Ps. aeruginosa* pneumonia. Davies *et al.* (1985) used aztreonam in 36 patients with acute exacerbations of chronic bronchitis due to Gram-negative pathogens, such as *H. influenzae*, *Moraxella catarrhalis* and *Ps. aeruginosa*. Results of treatment were poor in many patients mainly because aztreonam-resistant *Strep. pneumoniae* strains emerged. By contrast, Nolen *et al.* (1985) found aztreonam to be effective in 35 patients with lower respiratory tract infections caused by Gram-negative bacilli, but clindamycin was given concomitantly until the pathogen was identified and the presence of Gram-positive bacteria was ruled out.

6 Pulmonary infections in patients with cystic fibrosis

Aztreonam is quite effective for these infections if they are caused by susceptible pathogens, such as *Ps. aeruginosa* (Scully *et al.*, 1985; Bosso and Black, 1988; Lebel and McCracken, 1988; Salh *et al.*, 1992).

7 Urinary tract infections

Greenberg *et al.* (1984) reported that aztreonam cured 45 of 67 patients with pyelonephritis. Seven patients developed enterococcal bladder superinfections. Relapse occurred in ten patients 4 weeks after ceasing therapy; two of these were young women without obvious predisposing factors. In a comparative study with gentamicin, 23 of 35 patients treated with aztreonam were cured compared with 9 of 17 treated with gentamicin. Relapses and reinfections occurred in each group. Fourteen of the aztreonam group but only one of the gentamicin group became colonized with Group D streptococci (Sattler *et al.*, 1984). Another 39 patients with urinary tract infections (12 with concomitant bacteremia) were treated by aztreonam; results of treatment were satisfactory, but several patients developed colonization or superinfection by *Candida* spp., *E. faecalis* or *Staph. aureus* (Romero-Vivas *et al.*, 1985). In another trial aztreonam was about as effective as cefotaxime (p. 338) for the treatment of complicated urinary tract infections (Naber *et al.*, 1986).

8 Typhoid fever and other Salmonella infections

Aztreonam is effective in the treatment of systemic *Salmonella* infections in experimental animals (Bonina *et al.*, 1990). Farid *et al.* (1990) cured four typhoid fever patients with aztreonam. In a randomized trial in children aztreonam appeared about as effective as chloramphenicol for typhoid (Tanaka-Kido *et al.*, 1990). However, in a controlled trial in adults aztreonam was inferior to chloramphenicol with regard to clinical effectiveness and time of defervescence, but it was more effective in the elimination of the infecting *Salmonella* organisms from the bloodstream (Gotuzzo *et al.*, 1994). Using 2 g aztreonam i.v. 6-hourly for 16 days Righter and Vaughan-Neil (1984) eradicated *Salm. hadar* carriage in an elderly female in whom previous courses of oral co-trimoxazole and ampicillin had failed.

9 Bacterial gastroenteritis

Aztreonam, despite its poor absorption after oral administration, appears effective when given orally in a dose of 100 mg three times daily for 5 days in patients with bacterial diarrhea. When given to Americans, who were temporarily living in Mexico, aztreonam reduced the average duration of diarrhea, compared with the placebo, by an average of 40 h. Pathogen eradication occurred in 95% of those receiving aztreonam and in 70% of those receiving placebo. The bacterial pathogens encountered in this study included enterotoxigenic *E. coli*, *Shigella* spp., *Salmonella* spp., *Yersinia enterocolitica*, *Vibrio* spp., *Aeromonas* spp. and *Plesiomonas shigelloides* (Du Pont *et al.*, 1992).

10 Osteomyelitis

In an experimental rabbit model of osteomyelitis due to *Ps. aeruginosa*, aztreonam given for 4 weeks, failed to eradicate the organism (Norden and Budinsky, 1988). Seven patients, in three of whom recent treatment with aminoglycosides had failed despite sensitivity of the organisms involved, were treated for 6 weeks with 1–2 g of aztreonam i.m. or i.v. every 8 h. All patients had a clinical response within 1 week. When reviewed 10 months later, four patients (two with infections due to *Ps. aeruginosa*, one due to *Citrobacter freundii* and the other due to *Pr. mirabilis*) were considered clinically and bacteriologically cured (Giamarellou *et al.*, 1984). Aztreonam was used successfully in 11 patients with osteomyelitis and six with septic arthritis caused by Gram-negative bacilli. Duration of treatment ranged from 14 to 55 days and the period of follow up was 4–18 months (Simons and Lee, 1985). In another study Conrad *et al.* (1991) treated ten patients with septic arthritis and 18 with osteomyelitis, all due to *Ps. aeruginosa*. Most patients were cured.

11 Selective reduction of bowel flora

The poor oral absorption of aztreonam (<1%) and its good activity against aerobic Gram-negative bacteria and not anaerobes, suggests that it may be useful for this purpose (p. 881). In ten volunteers elimination of Gram-negative aerobes was achieved by using either 300 mg or 1500 mg daily doses of oral aztreonam after an average of 4.4 and 3.0 days, respectively. Treatment was continued for 5 days. Fecal counts of enterococci tended to show marked increases with the higher dose regimen towards the end of the 5-day treatment period. Yeast counts also rose but not to an important degree. Anaerobic bacterial counts were unaffected (de Vries-Hospers *et al.*, 1984).

12 Malignant otitis externa

This is a rare condition with a predilection for elderly diabetics (p. 379). *Pseudomonas aeruginosa* invades the soft tissues of the canal and then the bones of the skull become involved.

Cranial nerve palsies and meningitis may follow. Surgical dèbridement may be necessary. Giamarellou *et al.* (1984) used aztreonam in a patient in whom several courses of aminoglycosides had previously been unsuccessful. The patient received 6 g daily for 6 weeks and when assessed at 10 months he was considered to be cured.

13 Gonorrhea

A single i.m. injection of 1 g aztreonam is satisfactory therapy for uncomplicated urethral gonorrhea in men and is probably effective for endocervical and rectal infection as well (Gottlieb and Mills, 1985). This regimen also cures gonorrhea in males and females caused by beta-lactamase-producing strains (Miller *et al.*, 1983; Evans *et al.*, 1986; Mohanty *et al.*, 1988).

14 Chemoprophylaxis in surgery

Aztreonam/metronidazole proved to be unsatisfactory prophylaxis in elective colorectal surgery, as sepsis due to Gram-positive organisms, particularly *Staph. aureus*, occurred (Morris *et al.*, 1990), but clindamycin plus aztreonam was effective for this purpose, and the results obtained were similar to those with clindamycin/gentamicin (Rodolico *et al.*, 1991). Clindamycin/aztreonam was also satisfactory as prophylaxis in gynecologic surgery and the results obtained were similar to those with clindamycin/cefotaxime (Mangioni *et al.*, 1991). One of the first- or second-generation cephalosporins, however, are effective and preferable for prophylaxis in this situation (p. 287).

References

Adkinson NF Jr, Swabb EA, Sugerman AA (1984). Immunology of the monobactom aztreonam. *Antimicrob Ag Chemother* **25**: 93.

Adkinson NF Jr, Saxon A, Spence MR, Swabb EA (1985). Cross allergenicity and immunogenicity of aztreonam. *Rev Infect Dis* **7** (Suppl 4): 613.

Barry AL, Thornsberry C, Jones RN, Gavan TL (1985). Aztreonam: antibacterial activity, beta-lactamase stability, and interpretive standards and quality control guidelines for disk-diffusion susceptibility tests. *Rev Infect Dis* **7** (Suppl 4): 594.

Barza M, McCue M (1983). Pharmacokinetics of aztreonam in rabbit eyes. *Antimicrob Ag Chemother* **24**: 468.

Bechard DL, Hawkins SS, Dhruv R, Friedhoff LT (1985). Penetration of aztreonam into human bronchial secretions. *Antimicrob Ag Chemother* **27**: 263.

Boccazzi A, Langer M, Mandelli M *et al.* (1989). The pharmacokinetics of aztreonam and penetration into the bronchial secretions of critically ill patients. *J Antimicrob Chemother* **23**: 401.

Bonina L, Carbone M, Matera G *et al.* (1990). Beta-lactam antibiotics (aztreonam, ampicillin, cefazolin and ceftazidime). in the control and eradication of *Salmonella typhimurium* in naturally resistant and susceptible mice. *J Antimicrob Chemother* **25**: 813.

Bosso JA, Black PG (1988). Controlled trial of aztreonam vs tobramycin and azlocillin for acute pulmonary exacerbations of cystic fibrosis. *Pediatr Infect Dis J* **7**: 171.

Bosso JA, Saxon BA, Matsen JM (1987). *In vitro* activity of aztreonam combined with tobramycin and gentamicin against clinical isolates of *Pseudomonas aeruginosa* and *Pseudomonas cepacia* from patients with cystic fibrosis. *Antimicrob Ag Chemother* **31**: 1403.

Brown J, Altmann P, Cunningham J *et al.* (1990). Pharmacokinetics of once daily intra-peritoneal aztreonam and vancomycin in the treatment of CAPD peritonitis. *J Antimicrob Chemother* **25**: 141.

Bush K, Freudenberger JS, Sykes RB (1982). Interaction of aztreonam and related monobactams with beta-lactamases from Gram-negative bacteria. *Antimicrob Ag Chemother* **22**: 414.

Clergeot A, Steru D, Rosset M-A, Carbon C (1989). Efficacy and safety of low dose aztreonam in the treatment of moderate to severe Gram-negative bacterial infections. *J Antimicrob Chemother* **23**: 753.

Condon RE, Friedhoff LT, Edmiston CE, Levinson B (1986). Aztreonam concentration in abdominal tissues and bile. *Antimicrob Ag Chemother* **29**: 1101.

Conrad DA, Williams RR, Couchman TL, Lentneck AL (1991). Efficacy of aztreonam in the treatment of skeletal infections due to *Pseudomonas aeruginosa*. *Rev Infect Dis* **13** (Suppl 7): 634.

Cuzzolin L, Fanos V, Zambreri D *et al.* (1991). Pharmacokinetics and renal tolerance of aztreonam in premature infants. *Antimicrob Ag Chemother* **35**: 1726.

Davies BI, Maesen FPV, Teengs JP (1985). Aztreonam in patients with acute purulent exacerbations of chronic bronchitis: failure to prevent emergence of pneumococcal infections. *J Antimicrob Chemother* **15**: 375.

De Maria AJr, Treadwell TL, Saunders CA *et al.* (1989). Randomized clinical trial of aztreonam and aminoglycoside antibiotics in the treatment of serious infections caused by Gram-negative bacilli. *Antimicrob Ag Chemother* **33**: 1137.

de Vries-Hospers HG, Welling GW, Swabb EA, van der Waaij D (1984). Selective decontamination of the digestive tract with aztreonam: a study of 10 healthy volunteers. *J Infect Dis* **150**: 636.

Dratwa M, Glupczynski Y, Lameire N *et al.* (1991). Treatment of Gram-negative peritonitis with aztreonam in patients undergoing continuous ambulatory peritoneal dialysis. *Rev Infect Dis* **13** (Suppl 7): 645.

Du Pont HL, Ericsson CD, Mathewson JJ *et al.* (1992). Oral aztreonam, a poorly absorbed yet effective therapy for bacterial diarrhea in US travelers to Mexico. *JAMA* **267**: 1932.

El Touny M, El Guinaidy M, Barry MA *et al.* (1992). Pharmacokinetics of aztreonam in patients with liver cirrhosis, and ascites. *J Antimicrob Chemother* **30**: 387.

Evans DTP, Crooks AJR, Jones C *et al.* (1986). Treatment of uncomplicated gonorrhoea with single dose aztreonam. *Genitourin Med* **62**: 318.

Fainstein V, Weaver S, Bodey GP (1982). Comparative *in vitro* study of SQ 26776. *Antimicrob Ag Chemother* **21**: 294.

Farid Z, Girgis NI, Kamal M *et al.* (1990). Successful aztreonam treatment of acute typhoid fever after chloramphenicol failure. *Scand J Infect Dis* **22**: 505.

Friedrich LV, White RL, Kays MB *et al.* (1991). Aztreonam pharmacokinetics in burn patients. *Antimicrob Ag Chemother* **35**: 57.

Georgopapadakou NH, Smith SA, Sykes RB (1982). Mode of action of aztreonam. *Antimicrob Ag Chemother* **21**: 950.

Georgopapadakou NH, Smith SA, Cimarusti CM, Sykes RB (1983). Binding of monobactams to penicillin-binding proteins of *Escherichia coli* and *Staphylococcus aureus*: relation to antibacterial activity. *Antimicrob Ag Chemother* **23**: 98.

Giamarellou H, Galanakis N, Douzinas E (1984). Evaluation of aztreonam in difficult to treat infections with prolonged post-treatment follow-up. *Antimicrob Ag Chemother* **26**: 245.

Girgis NI, Abu El Ella AH, Farid Z et al. (1988). Parenteral aztreonam in the treatment of *Haemophilus influenzae* type b meningitis in Egyptian children. *Scand J Infect Dis* **20**: 111.

Goossens H, Vanhoof R, De Mol P et al. (1984). *In-vitro* susceptibility of salmonellae to antimicrobial agents. *J Antimicrob Chemother* **13**: 559.

Goossens H, De Mol P, Coignau H et al. (1985). Comparative *in vitro* activities of aztreonam, ciprofloxacin, norfloxacin, ofloxacin, HR 810 (a new cephalosporin), RU 28965 (a new macrolide), and other agents against enteropathogens. *Antimicrob Ag Chemother* **27**: 388.

Gordts B, Vandenboore C, Van der Auwera P, Butzler JP (1984). Comparison between the *in-vitro* activity of new agents on *Pseudomonas aeruginosa* isolates from cystic fibrosis patients and other chronic infections. *J Antimicrob Chemother* **14**: 25.

Gottlieb A, Mills J (1985). Effectiveness of aztreonam for the treatment of gonorrhea. *Antimicrob Ag Chemother* **27**: 270.

Gotuzzo E, Echevarria J, Carrillo C et al. (1994). Randomized comparison of aztreonam and chloramphenicol in treatment of typhoid fever. *Antimicrob Ag Chemother* **38**: 558.

Greenberg RN, Reilly PM, Luppen KL et al. (1984). Treatment of serious Gram-negative infections with aztreonam. *J Infect Dis* **150**: 623.

Greenman RL, Arcey SM, Dickinson GM et al. (1985). Penetration of aztreonam into cerebrospinal fluid in the presence of meingeal inflammation. *J Antimicrob Chemother* **15**: 637.

Gudiol F, Pallares R, Ariza X et al. (1986). Comparative clinical evaluation of aztreonam versus aminoglycosides in Gram-negative septicaemia. *J Antimicrob Chemother* **17**: 661.

Gutmann L, Kitzis MD, Billot-Klein D et al. (1988). Plasmid-mediated beta-lactamase (TEM-7) involved in resistance to ceftazidime and aztreonam. *Rev Infect Dis* **10**: 860.

Haroche G, Salvanet A, Lafaix Ch et al. (1986). Pharmacokinetics of aztreonam in the aqueous humour. *J Antimicrob Chemother* **18**: 195.

Heney D, Lewis IJ, Ghoneim ATM et al. (1991). Aztreonam therapy in children with febrile neutropenia: a randomized trial of aztreonam plus flucloxacillin versus piperacillin plus gentamicin. *J Antimicrob Chemother* **28**: 117.

Jacobus NV, Ferreira MC, Barza M (1982). *In vitro* activity of aztreonam, a monobactam antibiotic. *Antimicrob Ag Chemother* **22**: 832.

Jacoby GA, Carreras I (1990). Activities of beta-lactam antibiotics against *Escherichia coli* strains producing extended-spectrum beta-lactamases. *Antimicrob Ag Chemother* **34**: 858.

Janicke DM, Cafarell RF, Parker SW et al. (1985). Pharmacokinetics of aztreonam in patients with Gram-negative infections. *Antimicrob Ag Chemother* **27**: 16.

Jensen T, Pedersen SS, Høiby N, Koch C (1991). Safety of aztreonam in patients with cystic fibrosis and allergy to beta-lactam antibiotics. *Rev Infect Dis* **13** (Suppl 7): 594.

Jones P, Rolston K, Fainstein V et al. (1985). Aztreonam plus vancomycin (plus amikacin). vs moxalactam plus ticarcillin for the empiric treatment of febrile episodes in neutropenic cancer patients. *Rev Infect Dis* **7** (Suppl 4): 741.

Jones PG, Rolston KVI, Fainstein V et al. (1986). Aztreonam therapy in neutropenic patients with cancer. *Amer J Med* **81**: 243.

Koch C, Hjelt K, Pedersen SS et al. (1991). Retrospective clinical study of hypersensitivity reactions to aztreonam and six other beta-lactam antibiotics in cystic fibrosis patients receiving multiple treatment courses. *Rev Infect Dis* **13** (Suppl 7): 608.

Kripalani KJ, Singhvi SM, Weinstein SH et al. (1984). Disposition of (14 C). aztreonam in rats, dogs and monkeys. *Antimicrob Ag Chemother* **26**: 119.

Lagast H, Klastersky J, Kains JP et al. (1986). Empiric antimicrobial therapy with aztreonam or ceftazidime in Gram-negative septicemia. *Amer J Med* **80** (5c): 79.

Lebel MH, McCracken GH Jr (1988). Aztreonam: review of the clinical experience and potential uses in pediatrics. *Pediatr Infect Dis J* **7**: 331.

Lentnek AL, Williams RR (1991). Aztreonam in the treatment of Gram-negative bacterial meningitis. *Rev Infect Dis* **13** (Suppl 7): 586.

Likitnukul S, McCracken GH Jr, Threlkeld N et al. (1987). Pharmacokinetics and plasma bactericidal activity of aztreonam in low-birth-weight infants. *Antimicrob Ag Chemother* **31**: 81.

MacLeod CM, Bartley EA, Payne JA (1984). Effects of cirrhosis on kinetics of aztreonam. *Antimicrob Ag Chemother* **26**: 493.

MacLeod CM, Bartley EA, Galante JO et al. (1986). Aztreonam penetration into synovial fluid and bone. *Antimicrob Ag Chemother* **29**: 710.

Madsen PO, Dhruv R, Friedhoff LT (1984). Aztreonam concentrations in human prostatic tissue. *Antimicrob Ag Chemother* **26**: 20.

Mangioni C, Bianchi L, Bolis PF et al. (1991). Multicenter trial of prophylaxis with clindamycin plus aztreonam or cefotaxime in gynecologic surgery. *Rev Infect Dis* **13** (Suppl 7): 621.

Martinez OV, Levi JU, Devlin RG (1984). Biliary excretion of aztreonam in patients with biliary tract disease. *Antimicrob Ag Chemother* **25**: 358.

Mattie H, Matze-van der Lans A (1986). Pharmacokinetics of aztreonam in infected patients. *J Antimicrob Chemother* **17**: 215.

McCracken GH Jr, Sakata Y, Olsen KD (1985). Aztreonam therapy in experimental meningitis due to *Haemophilus influenzae* type b and *Escherichia coli* K 1. *Antimicrob Ag Chemother* **27**: 655.

Mihindu JCL, Scheld WM, Bolton ND et al. (1983). Pharmacokinetics of aztreonam in patients with various degrees of renal dysfunction. *Antimicrob Ag Chemother* **24**: 252.

Miller LK, Sanchez PL, Berg SW et al. (1983). Effectiveness of aztreonam, a new monobactam antibiotics, against penicillin-resistant gonococci. *J Infect Dis* **148**: 612.

Modai J, Vittecoq D, Decazes JM et al. (1986). Penetration of aztreonam into cerebrospinal fluid of patients with bacterial meningitis. *Antimicrob Ag Chemother* **29**: 281.

Mohanty KC, Fimls RD, Strachan RG (1988). A comparative study of aztreonam and procaine penicillin/probenecid in the treatment of uncomplicated gonorrhoea. *Scand J Infect Dis* **20**: 33.

Moore RD, Lerner SA, Levine DP (1992). Nephrotoxicity and ototoxicity of aztreonam versus aminoglycoside therapy in seriously ill nonneutropenic patients. *J Infect Dis* **165**: 683.

Morita K, Watanabe N, Kurata S, Kanamori M (1994). Beta-lactam resistance of motile *Aeromonas* isolates from clinical and environmental sources. *Antimicrob Ag Chemother* **38**: 353.

Morris DL, Wilson SR, Pain J et al. (1990). A comparison of aztreonam/metronidazole and cefotaxime/metronidazole in elective colorectal surgery: antimicrobial prophylaxis must include Gram-positive cover. *J Antimicrob Chemother* **25**: 673.

Moss RB, McClelland E, Williams RR et al. (1991). Evaluation of the immunologic cross-reactivity of aztreonam in patients with cystic fibrosis who are allergic to penicillin and/or cephalosporin antibiotics. *Rev Infect Dis* **13** (Suppl 7): 598.

Naber KG, Dette GA, Kees F et al. (1986). Pharmacokinetics, *in vitro* activity, therapeutic efficacy and clinical safety of aztreonam vs. cefotaxime in the treatment of complicated urinary tract infections. *J Antimicrob Chemother* **17**: 517.

Neu HC (1985). Current state of infectious diseases – potential areas of directed therapy with aztreonam. *Amer J Med* **78** (2A): 77.

Neu HC (1987). New antibiotics: areas of appropriate use. *J Infect Dis* **155**: 403.

Newman TJ, Dreslinski GR, Tadros SS (1985). Safety profile of aztreonam in clinical trials. *Rev Infect Dis* **7** (Suppl 4): 648.

Ng WWS, Chau PY, Leung YK, Livermore DM (1985). *In vitro* activities of Ro 17–2301 and aztreonam compared with those of other new beta-lactam antibiotics against isolates of *Pseudomonas aeruginosa*. *Antimicrob Ag Chemother* **27**: 872.

Nolen TM, Phillips HL, Hall HJ (1985). Comparison of aztreonam and tobramycin in the treatment of lower respiratory tract infections caused by Gram-negative bacilli. *Rev Infect Dis* **7** (Suppl 4): 666.

Norden CW, Budinsky A (1988). Aztreonam therapy for experimental osteomyelitis caused by *Pseudomonas aeruginosa*. *J Infect Dis* **158**: 660.

Philippon A, Labia R, Jacoby G (1989). Extended-spectrum beta-lactamases. *Antimicrob Ag Chemother* **33**: 1131.

Piddock LJV, Traynor EA, Wise R (1990). A comparison of the mechanisms of decreased susceptibility of aztreonam-resistant and ceftazidime-resistant Enterobacteriaceae. *J Antimicrob Chemother* **26**: 749.

Pierard D, Boelaert J, Van Landuyt HW *et al.* (1986). Aztreonam treatment of Gram-negative septicemia. *Antimicrob Ag Chemother* **29**: 359.

Powell M, Williams JD (1987). *In vitro* activities of aztreonam, imipenem and amoxycillin-clavulanate against ampicillin-resistant *Haemophilus influenzae*. *Antimicrob Ag Chemother* **31**: 1871.

Pruul H, Lewis G, McDonald PJ (1988). Enhanced susceptibility of Gram-negative bacteria to phagocytic killing by human polymorphonuclear leucocytes after brief exposure to aztreonam. *J Antimicrob Chemother* **22**: 675.

Righter J, Vaughan-Neil EF (1984). Treatment of *Salmonella* carrier with aztreonam. *J Antimicrob Chemother* **13**: 403.

Rodolico G, Puleo S, Blandino G *et al.* (1991). Colorectal surgery: short term prophylaxis with clindamycin plus aztreonam or gentamicin. *Rev Infect Dis* **13** (Suppl 7): 612.

Romero-Vivas J, Rodriguez-Creixems M, Bouza E *et al.* (1985). Evaluation of aztreonam in the treatment of severe bacterial infections. *Antimicrob Ag Chemother* **28**: 222.

Sakata H, Kakehashi H, Fujita K, Yoshioka H (1990). Effects of aztreonam on fecal flora and on vitamin K metabolism. *Antimicrob Ag Chemother* **34**: 1045.

Salh B, Bilton D, Dodd M *et al.* (1992). A comparison of aztreonam and ceftazidime in the treatment of respiratory infections in adults with cystic fibrosis. *Scand J Infect Dis* **24**: 215.

Sattler FR, Moyer JE, Schramm M *et al.* (1984). Aztreonam compared with gentamicin for treatment of serious urinary tract infection. *Lancet* **i**: 1315.

Sattler FR, Schramm M, Swabb EA (1985). Safety of aztreonam and SQ 26,992 in elderly patients with renal insufficiency. *Rev Infect Dis* **7** (Suppl 4): 622.

Saxon A, Hassner A, Swabb EA *et al.* (1984). Lack of cross-reactivity between aztreonam, a monobactam antibiotic, and penicillin in penicillin-allergic subjects. *J Infect Dis* **149**: 16.

Schiff JB, Pennington JE (1984). Comparative efficacies of piperacillin, azlocillin, ticarcillin, aztreonam and tobramycin against experimental *Pseudomonas aeruginosa* pneumonia. *Antimicrob Ag Chemother* **25**: 49.

Scribner RK, Marks MI, Weber A, Pai CH (1982). *Yersinia enterocolitica*: comparative *in vitro* activities of seven new beta-lactam antibiotics. *Antimicrob Ag Chemother* **22**: 140.

Scully BE, Neu HC (1985). Use of aztreonam in the treatment of serious infections due to multiresistant Gram-negative organisms, including *Pseudomonas aeruginosa*. *Amer J Med* **78** (2A): 251.

Scully BE, Swabb EA, Neu HC (1983). Pharmacology of aztreonam after intravenous infusion. *Antimicrob Ag Chemother* **24**: 18.

Scully BE, Ores CN, Prince AS, Neu HC (1985). Treatment of lower respiratory tract infections due to *Pseudomonas aeruginosa* in patients with cystic fibrosis. *Rev Infect Dis* **7** (Suppl 4): 669.

Shah PM, Losert-Bruggner B, Stille W (1981). Bactericidal activity of SQ 26776. *J Antimicrob Chemother* **8** (Suppl E): 77.

Simons WJ, Lee TJ (1985). Aztreonam in the treatment of bone and joint infections caused by Gram-negative bacilli. *Rev Infect Dis* **7** (Suppl 4): 783.

Singhvi SM, Ita CE, Shaw JM *et al.* (1984). Distribution of aztreonam into fetuses and milk of rats. *Antimicrob Ag Chemother* **26**: 132.

Sklavunu-Tsurutsoglu S, Gatzola-Karaveli M, Hatziioannidis K, Tsurutsoglu G (1991). Efficacy of aztreonam in the treatment of neonatal sepsis. *Rev Infect Dis* **13** (Suppl 7): 591.

Smith G, Bunney RG, Farrell ID, Wood MJ (1988). The use of aztreonam in serious Gram-negative infections. *J Antimicrob Chemother* **21**: 233.

Strandberg DA, Jorgensen JH, Drutz DJ (1983). Activities of aztreonam and new cephalosporins against infrequently isolated Gram-negative bacilli. *Antimicrob Ag Chemother* **24**: 282.

Strausbaugh LJ, Bodem CR, Laun PR (1986). Penetration of aztreonam into cerebrospinal fluid and brain of noninfected rabbits and rabbits with experimental meningitis caused by *Pseudomonas aeruginosa*. *Antimicrob Ag Chemother* **30**: 701.

Stutman HR (1991). Clinical experience with aztreonam for treatment of infections in children. *Rev Infect Dis* **13** (Suppl 7): 582.

Stutman HR, Marks MI, Swabb EA (1984). Single-dose pharmacokinetics of aztreonam in pediatric patients. *Antimicrob Ag Chemother* **26**: 196.

Swabb EA (1985). Review of the clinical pharmacology of the monobactam antibiotic aztreonam. *Amer J Med* **78** (2A): 11.

Swabb EA, Leitz MA, Pilkiewicz FG, Sugerman AA (1981). Pharmacokinetics of the monobactam SQ 26,776 after single intravenous doses in healthy subjects. *J Antimicrob Chemother* **8** (Suppl E): 131.

Swabb EA, Sugerman AA, Platt TB *et al.* (1982). Single-dose pharmacokinetics of the monobactam aztreonam (SQ 26,776). in healthy subjects. *Antimicrob Ag Chemother* **21**: 944.

Swabb EA, Sugerman AA, McKinstry DN (1983a). Multiple dose pharmacokinetics of the monobactam aztreonam (SQ 26,776). in healthy subjects. *Antimicrob Ag Chemother* **23**: 125.

Swabb EA, Sugerman AA, Stern M (1983b). Oral bioavailability of the monobactam aztreonam (SQ 26,776). in healthy subjects. *Antimicrob Ag Chemother* **23**: 548.

Swabb EA, Singhvi SM, Leitz MA *et al.* (1983c). Metabolism and pharmacokinetics of aztreonam in healthy subjects. *Antimicrob Ag Chemother* **24**: 394.

Sykes RB, Bonner DP (1985). Discovery and development of the monobactams. *Rev Infect Dis* **7** (Suppl 4): 579.

Sykes RB, Bonner DP, Bush K *et al.* (1981). Monobactams-monocylic beta-lactam antibiotics produced by bacteria. *J Antimicrob Chemother* **8** (Suppl E): 1.

Sykes RB, Bonner DP, Bush K, Georgopapadakou NH (1982). Aztreonam (Sq 26,776). a synthetic monobactam specifically active against aerobic Gram-negative bacteria. *Antimicrob Ag Chemother* **21**: 85.

Tanaka-Kido J, Ortega L, Santos JI (1990). Comparative efficacies of aztreonam and chloramphenicol in children with typhoid fever. *Pediatr Infect Dis J* **9**: 44.

Tartaglione TA, Duma RJ, Qureshi GD (1986). *In vitro* and *in vivo* studies of the effect of aztreonam on platelet function and coagulation in normal volunteers. *Antimicrob Ag Chemother* **30**: 73.

Tunkel AR, Scheld WM (1990). Aztreonam. *Infect Control Hosp Epidemiol* **11**: 486.

Watson AJS, Stout RL, Whelton A (1984). The intrarenal distribution of aztreonam in healthy and diseased kidneys: clinical therapeutic implications. *J Infect Dis* **150**: 623.

Welling GW, Groen G (1989). Inactivation of aztreonam by faecal supernatants of healthy volunteers as determined by HPLC. *J Antimicrob Chemother* **24**: 805.

Wise R, Dyas A, Hegarty A, Andrews JM (1982). Pharmacokinetics and tissue penetration of aztreonam. *Antimicrob Ag Chemother* **22**: 969.

Wu SW, Dornbusch K, Göransson E *et al.* (1991). Characterization of *Klebsiella oxytoca* septicaemia isolates resistant to aztreonam and cefuroxime. *J Antimicrob Chemother* **28**: 389.

Youngs DJ, Burdon DW, Keighley MRB (1989). The penetration of aztreonam, a monobactam antibiotic, into intra-abdominal abscesses. *J Antimicrob Chemother* **24**: 425.

Cefotetan

Description

Cefotetan disodium is a semisynthetic parenteral cephamycin, which has a 7 alpha methoxy group, similar to cefoxitin (Komiya *et al.*, 1981; Ayers *et al.*, 1982). Unlike cefoxitin, cefotetan has an N-methylthiotetrazole side-chain (Cohen *et al.*, 1987).

Cefotetan possesses a high degree of resistance to both plasmid-mediated and chromosomally determined beta-lactamases (p. 192) produced by Gram-negative bacteria (Phillips *et al.*, 1983). It is some 4- to 8-fold more active than cefoxitin against the Enterobacteriaceae such as *Escherichia coli*, and the *Klebsiella, Proteus, Providencia, Serratia, Salmonella* and *Shigella* spp. Cefotetan inhibits many *Enterobacter* and *Citrobacter* spp. strains which are cefoxitin-resistant. The drug is nearly as active against all of these bacteria as the third-generation cephalosporins, but, for instance, compared with cefotaxime (p. 320), it is still some 2- to 4-fold less potent against most strains (Chattopadhyay and Teli, 1982; Wise *et al.*, 1982; Dette *et al.*, 1983; Phillips *et al.*, 1983; Neu, 1986). The drug is active against *Haemophilus influenzae* and *Neisseria gonorrhoeae*, including strains of both which produce beta-lactamase. It has poor activity against *Acinetobacter* spp. *Pseudomonas aeruginosa* is cefotetan-resistant. Most other *Pseudomonas* spp. and *Stenotrophomonas maltophilia* are also resistant (Ayers *et al.*, 1982; Phillips *et al.*, 1983).

Most plasmid-mediated extended-spectrum beta-lactamases (p. 323), which occur most frequently in *Klebsiella* spp. and *E. coli*, do not hydrolyze the cephamycins with the 7 alpha methoxy groups such as cefoxitin or cefotetan. More recently, however, other types of plasmid-mediated extended-spectrum beta-lactamases have appeared in some Enterobacteriaceae, which can hydrolyze cefoxitin and cefotetan (Jacoby and Archer, 1991) (p. 323). Some authors have reported that cefotetan was usually some 8-fold less active than cefoxitin against *Bacteroides fragilis* and other Gram-negative anaerobes of the *B. fragilis* group (p. 295), such as *B. distasonis, B. ovatus* and *B. thetaiotaomicron* (Wise *et al.*, 1982; Clarke and Zemcov, 1983, Moosdeen *et al.*, 1983). Others have reported that these two drugs had comparable activity against *B. fragilis*, but cefotetan was less potent than cefoxitin against other members of the *B. fragilis* group (Werner, 1983; Watt and Brown, 1985; O'Keefe *et al.*, 1987; Wexler and Finegold, 1988). Cefotetan is also slightly less active than cefoxitin against *Prevotella* (*Bacteroides*) spp. such as P. disiens, but it is slightly more active against Fusobacterium spp. (Ohm Smith and Sweet, 1987; Appelbaum *et al.*, 1991). Cefoxitin-resistant Gram-negative anaerobes are usually also cefotetan-resistant (Andrew and Greenwood, 1987; Aldridge and Stratton, 1991).

Anaerobic Gram-positive cocci and the *Clostridium* spp. are cefotetan-sensitive, including *Cl. difficile* (Watt and Brown, 1985; Ohm-Smith and Sweet, 1987; Wexler and Finegold, 1988).

Cefotetan is less active than cefoxitin (p. 293) against aerobic Gram-positive bacteria such as *Staphylococcus aureus* and the streptococci. Methicillin-resistant *Staph. aureus* strains and *Enterococcus faecalis* are resistant (Ayers *et al.*, 1982; Wise *et al.*, 1982; Clarke and Zemcov, 1983).

The main difference between cefotetan and cefoxitin is that the former has a more prolonged serum elimination half-life (approximately 3.5 h), so that it can be administered i.m. or i.v. at 12-hourly intervals (Carver *et al.*, 1989). For the treatment of urinary tract infections or mild systemic infections, an adult dosage of 1 g 12-hourly may suffice, but for moderate and severe systemic infections a dosage of 2 g, 12-hourly is commonly used (Nakagawa *et al.*, 1982; Cox *et al.*, 1983; Nolen *et al.*, 1983). A dosage of 3 g 12-hourly should not be exceeded. In patients with renal failure dosage should be reduced and serum levels monitored (Ohkawa *et al.*, 1983). A dosage schedule for patients with various degrees of renal failure has been suggested. If the creatinine clearance (in ml per min per 1.73 m^2) is 30 or greater, the cefotetan dosage can be 1–2 g 12-hourly. If this clearance is 10–30, 1–2 g should be administered every 24 h and if the clearance is less than 10, the dosage recommended is 1 or 2 g every 48 h. A loading dose of 1 or 2 g should always be administered initially (Smith *et al.*, 1986). In patients treated by hemodialysis a quarter of the normal dose should be given on days without dialysis, but half of the normal dose is recommended after each dialysis. Little cefotetan is removed by peritoneal dialysis (Browning *et al.*, 1986).

In patients with normal renal function some 80% of the administered dose of cefotetan is excreted in the urine as the active unchanged drug (Ohkawa *et al.*, 1983). A small proportion is eliminated via the bile. In patients with non-obstructed bile ducts, biliary cefotetan concentrations usually exceed simultaneous serum levels (Owen *et al.*, 1983).

Some side-effects of cefotetan are about the same as those of the cephalosporins and cefoxitin (p. 306). Hypersensitivity reactions and gastrointestinal symptoms, such as diarrhea, have been reported (Cox *et al.*, 1983; Trollfors *et al.*, 1986). In common with cefamandole (p. 306) and cefoperazone (p. 335), cefotetan has a N-methylthiotetrazole side-chain (p. 350). In the cephalosporins this side-chain has been associated with prolongation of the prothrombin time (p. 350) and the disulfiram reaction. There is, therefore, a risk of hypoprothrombinemia if cefotetan is given to patients with pre-existing impaired coagulation or to others receiving anticoagulant therapy (Trollfors *et al.*, 1986; Cohen *et al.*, 1987; Sieradzan *et al.*, 1988; Wurtz and Sande, 1989). In situations associated with vitamin K$_1$ deficiency, prophylactic vitamin K$_1$ should be administered. Patients receiving cefotetan therapy are also at risk to develop disulfiram-type reaction if they ingest alcohol (Kline *et al.*, 1987). One patient treated by cefotetan developed an immune hemolytic anemia, similar to that produced by ceftriaxone (p. 358) (Chenoweth *et al.*, 1992).

The clinical role of cefotetan is similar to that of cefoxitin (p. 308). Because of its more convenient 12-hourly dosage regimen, cefotetan may be preferred to cefoxitin. Cefotetan is about as effective as cefoxitin for treatment of urinary tract infections (Cox *et al.*, 1983). It may not be quite as effective as cefoxitin in intra-abdominal infections because of its inferior antibacterial activity against anaerobes of *B. fragilis* group (p. 395). However, many clinical studies have shown that the two drugs are of about equal efficacy for this indication (Ward and Richards, 1989). It is accepted that cefotetan, similar to cefoxitin (p. 309), can be used as single-drug prophylaxis in patients undergoing colorectal surgery. A 2-g dose is usually given i.v. just before the operation and an additional dose of 1 g administered i.v. before closure of the abdomen (Martin *et al.*, 1992; Dellinger *et al.*, 1994).

In one study of perioperative prophylaxis in patients undergoing emergency abdominal surgery, cefotetan 2 g 12-hourly i.v. for three doses was compared with a gentamicin/tinidazole regimen. Of the anaerobes isolated at operation 13% were cefotetan-resistant. In addition, anaerobes, predominantly *B. fragilis*, were isolated from six of 14 infected wounds following cefotetan prophylaxis. Therefore cefotetan alone may not be adequate for patients undergoing emergency colorectal procedures, and if the drug is used, it should be combined with one of the nitroimidazoles (p. 949) (Tanner *et al.*, 1986). Prophylaxis with single i.v. doses of either 1 g cefotetan or 1 g cefazolin have been compared in patients undergoing elective upper gastrointestinal surgery (Leaper *et al.*, 1986) and elective cholecystectomy (Drumm *et al.*, 1985). In the former group there were significantly fewer postoperative infections in cefotetan-treated patients, but in the second group there was no difference between the two drug regimens. A single 1-g i.v. dose of cefotetan was superior to the same dose of cefazolin for prophylaxis in women undergoing elective total abdominal hysterectomy (Hemsell *et al.*, 1995).

One comparative study showed that cefotetan in a dose of 2 g i.v. once-daily was equally as effective as cefoxitin 1–2 g i.v. 8-hourly for the treatment of infections of skin and superficial soft tissue. The organisms isolated from these patients included *Staph. aureus*, *Streptococcus* spp., *E. coli*, *Proteus mirabilis*, *B. fragilis*, other *Bacteroides* spp. and *Peptococcus* and *Peptostreptococcus* spp. (Geckler *et al.*, 1988). Also cefotetan 2 g i.v. 12-hourly plus doxycycline 100 mg i.v. 12-hourly was comparable with cefoxitin 2 g i.v. 6-hourly plus doxycycline 100 mg i.v. 12-hourly in the inpatient treatment of acute salpingitis (Walker *et al.*, 1991).

References

Aldridge KE, Stratton CW (1991). Bactericidal activity of ceftizoxime, cefotetan, and clindamycin against cefoxitin-resistant strains of *Bacteroides fragilis* group. *J Antimicrob Chemother* **28**: 701.

Andrew JH, Greenwood D (1987). Susceptibility of cefotetan and Sch 34343 to beta-lactamases produced by strains of *Bacteroides* that hydrolyze cefoxitin and imipenem. *J Antimicrob Chemother* **19**: 591.

Appelbaum PC, Spangler SK, Jacobs MR (1991). Susceptibilities of 394 *Bacteroides fragilis*, non-*B fragilis* group *Bacteroides* species, and *Fusobacterium* species to newer antimicrobial agents. *Antimicrob Ag Chemother* **35**: 1214.

Ayers LW, Jones RN, Barry AL *et al.* (1982). Cefotetan, a new cephamycin: comparison of *in vitro* antimicrobial activity with other cephems, beta-lactamase stability, and preliminary recommendations for disc diffusion testing. *Antimicrob Ag Chemother* **22**: 859.

Browning MJ, Holt HA, White LO *et al.* (1986). Pharmacokinetics of cefotetan in patients with end-stage renal failure on maintenance dialysis. *J Antimicrob Chemother* **18**: 103.

Carver PL, Nightingale CH, Quintiliani R (1989). Pharmacokinetics and pharmacodynamics of total and unbound cefoxitin and cefotetan in healthy volunteers. *J Antimicrob Chemother* **23**: 99.

Chattopadhyay B, Teli JC (1982). Comparison of *in-vitro* activity of cefotetan (ICI 156834)., a new cephamycin derivative with that of cefoxitin. *J Antimicrob Chemother* **10**: 151.

Chenoweth CE, Judd WJ, Steiner EA, Kauffman CA (1992). Cefotetan-induced immune hemolytic anemia. *Clin Infect Dis* **15**: 863.

Clarke AM, Zemcov SJV (1983). Antibacterial activity of the cephamycin cefotetan: an *in vitro* comparison with other beta-lactam antibiotics. *J Antimicrob Chemother* **11** (Suppl A): 67.

Cohen H, Mackie IJ, Walshe K *et al.* (1987). The effects of cefotetan disodium on haemostasis. *J Hosp Infect* **10**: 51.

Cox CE, Childs SJ, Wells WG *et al.* (1983). Preliminary report on a comparative trial of cefotetan and cefoxitin in the treatment of urinary tract infections. *J Antimicrob Chemother* **11** (Suppl A): 227.

Dellinger EP, Gross PA, Barrett TL *et al.* (1994). Quality standards for antimicrobial prophylaxis in surgical procedures. *Clin Infect Dis* **18**: 422.

Dette GA, Knothe H, Henckel S (1983). Cefotetan: antimicrobial activity *in vitro* compared with that of cefotaxime. *J Antimicrob Chemother* **11** (Suppl A): 11.

Drumm J, Donovan IA, Wise R (1985). A comparison of cefotetan and cephazolin for prophylaxis against wound infection after elective cholecystectomy. *J Hosp Infect* **6**: 277.

Geckler RW, Eng RHK, Fabian TC *et al.* (1988). A multicenter comparative study of cefotetan once daily and cefoxitin thrice daily for the treatment of infections of the skin and superficial soft tissue. *Am J Surg* **155** (5A): 91.

Hemsell DL, Johnson ER, Hemsell PG *et al.* (1995). Cefazolin is inferior to cefotetan as single-dose prophylaxis for women undergoing elective total abdominal hysterectomy. *Clin Infect Dis* **20**: 677.

Jacoby GA, Archer GL (1991). New mechanisms of bacterial resistance to antimicrobial agents. *New Engl J Med* **324**: 601.

Kline SS, Mauro VG, Forney RB *et al.* (1987). Cefotetan-induced disulfiram-type reactions and hypoprothrombinemia. *Antimicrob Ag Chemother* **31**: 1328.

Komiya M, Kijuchi Y, Tachibana A, Yano K (1981). Pharmacokinetics of new broad-spectrum cephamycin, YM09330, parenterally administered to various experimental animals. *Antimicrob Ag Chemother* **20**: 176.

Leaper DJ, Cooper MJ, Turner A (1986). A comparative trial between cefotetan and cephazolin for wound sepsis prophylaxis during elective upper gastrointestinal surgery with an investigation of cefotetan penetration into the obstructed biliary tree. *J Hosp Infect* **7**: 269.

Martin C, Portet C, Lambert D *et al.* (1992). Pharmacokinetics and tissue penetration of single-dose cefotetan used for antimicrobial prophylaxis in patients undergoing colorectal surgery. *Antimicrob Ag Chemother* **36**: 1115.

Moosdeen F, Maskel J, Philpott-Howard J, Williams JD (1983). Cefotetan activity against Gram-negative aerobes and anaerobes. *J Antimicrob Chemother* **11** (Suppl A): 59.

Nakagawa K, Koyama M, Tachibana A *et al.* (1982). Pharmacokinetics of cefotetan (YM09330). in humans. *Antimicrob Ag Chemother* **22**: 935.

Neu HC (1986). Beta-lactam antibiotics: structural relationships affecting *in vitro* activity and pharmacologic properties. *Rev Infect Dis* **8** (Suppl 3): 237.

Nolen TM, Phillips HL, Hall HJ (1983). Clinical evaluation of cefotetan in the treatment of lower respiratory tract infections. *J Antimicrob Chemother* **11** (Suppl A): 233.

Ohkawa M, Hirano S, Tokunaga S *et al.* (1983). Pharmacokinetics of cefotetan in normal subjects and patients with impaired renal function. *Antimicrob Ag Chemother* **23**: 31.

Ohm-Smith MJ, Sweet RL (1987). *In vitro* activity of cefmetazole, cefotetan, amoxicillin-clavulanic acid, and other antimicrobial agents against anaerobic bacteria from endometrial cultures of women with pelvic infections. *Antimicrob Ag Chemother* **31**: 1434.

O'Keefe JP, Venezio FR, Divincenzo CA, Shatzer KL (1987). Activity of newer beta-lactam agents against clinical isolates of *Bacteroides fragilis* and other *Bacteroides* species. *Antimicrob Ag Chemother* **31**: 2002.

Owen AWMC, Manson J McK, Yates RA *et al.* (1983). The pharmacokinetics of cefotetan excretion in the unobstructed biliary tree. *J Antimicrob Chemother* **11** (Suppl A): 217.

Phillips I, King A, Shannon K, Warren C (1983). Cefotetan: *in-vitro* antibacterial activity and susceptibility to beta-lactamases. *J Antimicrob Chemother* **11** (Suppl A): 1.

Sieradzan RR, Bottner WA, Fasco MJ, Bertino JS Jr (1988). Comparative effects of cefoxitin and cefotetan on vitamin K metabolism. *Antimicrob Ag Chemother* **32**: 1446.

Smith BR, Le Frock JL, Thyrum PT *et al.* (1986). Cefotetan pharmacokinetics in volunteers with various degrees of renal function. *Antimicrob Ag Chemother* **29**: 887.

Tanner AG, Thom BT, Strachan CJL (1986). Cefotetan compared with gentamicin and tinidazole in acute abdominal surgery. *J Hosp Infect* **7**: 49.

Trollfors B, Norrby R, Bergmark J *et al.* (1986). Comparative toxicity of gentamicin and cefotetan. *Scand J Infect Dis* **18**: 139.

Walker CK, Landers DV, Ohm-Smith MJ *et al.* (1991). Comparison of cefotetan plus doxycycline with cefoxitin plus doxycycline in the inpatient treatment of acute salpingitis. *Sex Transm Dis* **18**: 119.

Ward A, Richards DM (1989). Cefotetan A review of its antibacterial activity, pharmacokinetic properties and therapeutic use. *Drugs*. ADIS Press Limited. This version updated in May 1989 from the published version which appeared in *Drugs* **30**: 382.

Watt B, Brown FV (1985). The comparative *in-vitro* activity of cefotetan against anaerobic bacteria. *J Antimicrob Chemother* **15**: 671.

Werner H (1983). Inhibitory activity of cefotetan and other beta-lactams against anaerobes. *J Antimicrob Chemother* **11** (Suppl A): 107.

Wexler HM, Finegold SM (1988). *In vitro* activity of cefotetan compared with that of other antibacterial agents against anaerobic bacteria. *Antimicrob Ag Chemother* **32**: 601.

Wise R, Andrews JM, Hancock J (1982). *In vitro* activity of cefotetan, a new cephamycin derivative, compared with that of other beta-lactam compounds. *Antimicrob Ag Chemother* **21**: 486.

Wurtz RM, Sande MA (1989). Cefotetan and coagulopathy. *J Infect Dis* **160**: 555.

Cefpirome

Description

Cefpirome is a parenterally administered, beta-lactamase stable cephalosporin, which has been described as an extended spectrum or fourth-generation cephalosporin. Against all species of Enterobacteriaceae it is slightly more active than cefotaxime (p. 320) (Jones *et al.*, 1984; Wise *et al.*, 1985). Also, compared with the third-generation cephalosporins, it has enhanced activity against Gram-positive bacteria (Chandrasekar *et al.*, 1985; Thornsberry, 1985).

Sensitive Organisms

1 Gram-positive bacteria

Most Gram-positive bacteria are cefpirome-sensitive. These include *Staphylococcus aureus* and coagulase-negative staphylococci, including penicillin G-resistant strains. Some authors have found methicillin-resistant strains marginally sensitive (MICs 8–32 μg per ml), but others have reported them to be resistant (MIC 128 μg per ml). The drug is also highly active against *Streptococcus pyogenes*, *Strep. pneumoniae*, Group B streptococci, *Strep. bovis* and *Strep. viridans*. *Enterococcus faecalis* (MIC 16 μg per ml) is more sensitive to cefpirome than to most other cephalosporins. The clinical significance of this is not known (Jones *et al.*, 1984; Chandrasekar *et al.*, 1985; Thornsberry, 1985; Wise *et al.*, 1985; Eng *et al.*, 1989; Cheng *et al.*, 1993). The MICs of cefpirome for pneumococcal strains with intermediate penicillin G-resistance (0.1–1 μg per ml) and high level penicillin G resistance (1–2 μg per ml) are lower than the MICs of penicillin G for these strains (Spangler *et al.*, 1994; Yoshida *et al.*, 1995). *Nocardia asteroides* is moderately sensitive, MICs being 8 μg per ml for 80% of strains tested (Gombert *et al.*, 1987).

Some authors reported most of the Gram-positive anaerobes, such as the *Peptococcus*, *Clostridium* and *Lactobacillus* spp., to be moderately sensitive, but *Cl. difficile* moderately resistant, most strains needing 16 μg per ml of cefpirome for inhibition (Jones and Gerlach, 1985). However, Cheng *et al.* (1993) tested 12 *Clostridium* spp. strains and six *Peptostreptococcus* spp. strains and found them to be cefpirome-resistant.

2 Gram-negative aerobic bacteria

All species of Enterobacteriaceae such as *E. coli*, the *Klebsiella*, *Enterobacter*, *Proteus*, *Providencia*, *Citrobacter*, *Salmonella*, *Shigella* and *Serratia* spp. and *Morganella morganii* are cefpirome-sensitive; the potency of this drug being about the same as cefotaxime (p. 320) against these bacteria (Jones *et al.*, 1984; Clarke *et al.*, 1985; Wise *et al.*, 1985; Reeves *et al.*, 1993).

Chromosomally mediated beta lactamases, which can be derepressed or induced in species such as *Enterobacter*, *Providencia*, *Citrobacter*, *Proteus vulgaris* and *Morganella morganii*, have much lower affinity for cefpirome than for the third-generation cephalosporins. Strains of these bacteria which hyperproduce these enzymes, in general remain cefpirome-sensitive, but the MICs are slightly raised. It may be that cefpirome will be therapeutically useful for infections caused by these bacteria, even when the enzymes are induced. Cefpirome is also a weak enzyme inducer and therefore it is less likely, compared with the third-generation cephalosporins, that such mutants would be selected during cefpirome therapy (Kobayashi *et al.*, 1986; Satake *et al.*, 1989; Hancock and Bellido, 1992; Reeves *et al.*, 1993). In two studies ceftazidime-resistant

Enterobacteriaceae, including *Enterobacter* spp., were often still sensitive to cefpirome (Spencer *et al.*, 1993; Sader and Jones, 1994). Cefpirome also penetrates the porin channels of most Enterobacteriaceae better than third-generation cephalosporins (Bellido *et al.*, 1991a,b; Hancock and Bellido, 1992; Cheng *et al.*, 1993). The drug also exhibits high-affinity to *E. coli* PBP3 (Pucci *et al.*, 1991). One study showed that *in vitro* both ceftazidime- (p. 369) and cefpirome-selected mutants of *Enterobacter cloacae* expressing derepressed beta-lactamase, but it was much easier to select ceftazidime-resistant than cefpirome-resistant mutants (Piddock and Taynor, 1991).

The extended-spectrum beta-lactamases (p. 323) are likely to affect cefpirome. One plasmid-mediated, extended-spectrum beta-lactamase, produced by a strain of *E. coli*, made the strain with an MIC of 8 μg per ml, moderately cefpirome-resistant (Jacoby and Carreras, 1990).

Both *Haemophilus influenzae* and *Neiseeria gonorrhoeae* are highly cefpirome susceptible, irrespective of beta-lactamase production. Most *Acinetobacter* spp. strains are inhibited by 8 μg per ml (Clarke *et al.*, 1985; Wise *et al.*, 1985; Rolston and Bodey, 1986; Verbist *et al.*, 1993). *Pseudomonas aeruginosa* with an MIC of 8 μg per ml is cefpirome-sensitive, but ceftazidime (MIC 4 μg per ml) is slightly more active. Usually *Ps. aeruginosa* strains which have induced or derepressed chromosomally mediated beta-lactamases, remain cefpirome-sensitive (Cabezudo *et al.*, 1989; Cheng *et al.*, 1993; Reeves *et al.*, 1993; Verbist *et al.*, 1993), but this depends on the degree of derepression. Strains with partial derepression are cefpirome-sensitive, but strains with total derepression are moderately resistant (MIC 16–32 μg per ml) (Gargalianos *et al.*, 1988). Also Watanabe *et al.* (1992) found that most ceftazidime-resistant strains were also cefpirome-resistant. Also *Ps. aeruginosa* isolates resistant to an aminoglycoside, were significantly more resistant to cefpirome (Raizes and Cantey, 1988). Cefpirome/tobramycin *in vitro* was synergistic against 32% of *Ps. aeruginosa* isolates (Chin and Neu, 1989).

The *Moraxella* spp., *Aeromonas* spp., *Campylobacter* spp., *Ps. fluorescens* and *Ps. putida* are cefpirome-sensitive. *Burkholderia* (*Pseudomonas*) *cepacia*, *Ps. stutzeri* and *Stenotrophomonas maltophilia* are resistant (Goossens *et al.*, 1985; Van der Auwera and Scorneaux, 1985; Appelbaum *et al.*, 1986; Cheng *et al.*, 1993; Reeves *et al.*, 1993).

3 Gram-negative anaerobic bacteria

Cefpirome has about the same activity as cefotaxime (p. 321) against Gram-negative anaerobes; it only inhibits some 50% of strains of the *Bacteroides fragilis* group at a concentration of <16 μg per ml. The *Prevotella* spp. and *Fusobacterium* spp. are more sensitive (Jones and Gerlach, 1985; Pascual *et al.*, 1987).

Mode of Administration and Dosage

1 Adults

Cefpirome is not absorbed after oral administration, therefore it has to be given either by the i.m. or i.v. routes. After a 1 g i.v. dose the drug has a half-life of approximately 2 h, and the serum has adequate bactericidal concentration against all cefpirome-sensitive organisms for 8 h after this dose (Paradis *et al.*, 1992). Cefpirome has been given to patients in clinical trials either i.m. or i.v. in dosages of 0.5 g, 1 g or 2 g i.m. or i.v. 12-hourly. Intravenously the drug has been usually given by a short, 30- to 60-min i.v. infusion, similar to penicillin G (p. 20) (Carbon *et al.*, 1992; Meyer *et al.*, 1992; Craig, 1993; Norrby and Geddes, 1993). The 0.5 or 1 g 12-hourly dosage is adequate for the treatment of urinary tract infections or systemic infections due to highly susceptible organisms. For systemic infections due to organisms such as *Ps. aeruginosa*, the dosage of 2 g i.v. 12-hourly is advocated (Wilcox *et al.*, 1991).

2 Patients with renal failure

Cefpirome is mainly eliminated from the body via the kidneys (p. 400) therefore the dosage should be reduced in these patients. If the glomerular filtration rate (GFR) is 20–50 ml per min, 50% of the usual dosage should be given. If the GFR is below 20 ml per min, 25% of the usual daily dosage is recommended. If the patient is treated by hemodialysis, a supplementary dose after each session is needed (Lameire *et al.*, 1989; Wilcox *et al.*, 1991).

Serum Levels in Relation to Dosage

1. After an i.m. dose of cefpirome of 1 g, the maximum average serum level is 23.2 µg per ml and this is reached 1.9 h after the injection. The serum level thereafter falls and is less than 1 µg per ml at 12 h. Doubling the dose, doubles the serum level, but does not significantly prolong the serum level beyond 12 h. The terminal half-life of cefpirome after an i.m. dose is 2 h (Meyer *et al.*, 1992).

2. After a slow 1 h 1 g cefpirome i.v. infusion the peak level straight after the infusion is approximately 60 µg per ml, and if a 2-g dose is administered similarly, the peak level is doubled (119 µg per ml). Thereafter the serum level falls, the average half-life is again 2 h and the level approaches 1 µg per ml in 12 h. There is no accumulation of cefpirome after multiple 12-hourly doses (Craig, 1993).

Excretion

Cefpirome is eliminated in the urine by glomerular filtration. Most studies have shown that the urinary recovery at 24–48 h ranges from 66 to 100%. Using very sensitive assays, 96% of the administered dose can be recovered from the urine. The drug is not metabolized in the body to any appreciable extent (Meyer *et al.*, 1992; Craig, 1993). Some 4% may be eliminated in the feces, presumably because of biliary excretion.

Distribution of the Drug in Body

Cefpirome is only 10% serum protein bound (Wilcox *et al.*, 1991). It penetrates into the CSF to some extent in patients with normal meninges. After a single 2-g i.v. dose was given to 20 patients scheduled for myelogram, the mean CSF concentrations were 0.5, 0.57, 0.76 and 0.83 µg per ml at 1–2 h, 2–4 h, 4–6 h and 6–8.3 h post-dose, respectively (Nix *et al.*, 1992). In another study a 2-g i.v. cefpirome dose was given to 25 patients, who were treated by other antibiotics for bacterial meningitis. The cefpirome was given on days 2 and 3 after the onset of therapy. The mean concentrations of cefpirome in CSF ranged from 2.26 to 4.17 µg per ml. Samples of CSF were obtained at 2, 4, 8 or 12 h after the infusion of cefpirome (Wolff *et al.*, 1992). In an animal study of induced *H. influenzae* type b and *E. coli* meningitis, high CSF levels of cefpirome were found (Jafari *et al.*, 1991).

After a 1-g i.v. dose of cefpirome, the peak serum concentration was 34.5 µg per ml and the concentration in the bronchial mucosa at that time was 19.3 µg per g and that in the epithelial lining fluid 7.2 µg per ml (Baldwin *et al.*, 1991). After a 1-g i.v. dose, the drug penetrated rapidly into inflammatory fluid with a mean peak concentration of 39.2 µg per ml (Kavi *et al.*, 1988).

Toxicity

Relatively few adverse reactions have been attributed to cefpirome and the side-effects reported are similar to those which occur with other cephalosporins. Allergic reactions, neutropenia, increase in liver enzymes such as SGPT and alkaline phosphatase, increase in serum creatinine, drug fever, disturbed taste sensation and *Cl. difficile* diarrhea have been reported in a small number of patients (Norrby *et al.*, 1988; Carbon *et al.*, 1992; Norrby 1993). Cefpirome exhibits only very mild effects on fecal flora (Knothe *et al.*, 1992).

Cefpirome does not interfere with the function of polymorphonuclear leucocytes, but it shows a positive effect on phagocytosis (Moran *et al.*, 1994). Cefpirome in the serum can interfere with serum creatinine estimation by the Jaffe method. Falsely high serum creatinine levels will result, but blood urea readings are unaffected. In patients receiving cefpirome, especially those with impaired renal function, estimation of creatinine must be made by specific methods such as the enzymatic method or high-powered liquid chromatography HPLC (Kulkarni *et al.*, 1991).

Clinical Uses of the Drug

In an animal study Valdes *et al.* (1990) demonstrated that cefpirome was effective therapy in leukopenic mice with *Ps. aeruginosa* infection. Addition of gentamicin or rifampicin did not improve the results.

In clinical trials, patients with complicated urinary tract infections have responded to cefpirome at least as well as to ceftazidime (Norrby *et al.*, 1988; Study Group, 1992; Norrby,

1993). Patients with community acquired or nosocomial pneumonia, those with skin and soft tissue infections and those with septicemia (usually due to Gram-negative organisms), also have responded well and the results have been about the same as obtained with ceftriaxone or ceftazidime regimens (Norrby *et al.*, 1988; Carbon *et al.*, 1992; Norrby, 1993; Norrby and Geddes, 1993). The exact role in chemotherapy for this cephalosporin is yet to be determined.

References

Appelbaum PC, Spangler SK, Sollenberger L (1986). Susceptibility of non-fermentative Gram-negative bacteria to ciprofloxacin, norfloxacin, amifloxacin, pefloxacin and cefpirome. *J Antimicrob Chemother* **18**: 675.

Baldwin DR, Maxwell SRJ, Honeybourne D *et al.* (1991). The penetration of cefpirome into the potential sites of pulmonary infection. *J Antimicrob Chemother* **28**: 79.

Bellido F, Pechere J-C, Hancock REW (1991a). Novel method for measurement of outer membrane permeability to new beta-lactams in intact *Enterobacter cloacae* cells. *Antimicrob Ag Chemother* **35**: 68.

Bellido F, Pechere J-C, Hancock REW (1991b). Reevaluation of the factors involved in the efficacy of new beta-lactams against *Enterobacter cloacae*. *Antimicrob Ag Chemother* **35**: 73.

Cabezudo I, Pfaller M, Bale M, Wenzel R (1989). *In vitro* comparison of cefpirome and four other beta-lactam antibiotics alone and in combination with tobramycin against clinical isolates of *Pseudomonas aeruginosa*. *Diagn Microbiol Infect Dis* **12**: 337.

Carbon C and Cefpirome Study Group (1992). Prospective randomized phase II study of intravenous cefpirome 1 g or 2 g b.d. in the treatment of hospitalized patients with different infections. *J Antimicrob Chemother* **29** (Suppl A): 87.

Chandrasekar PH, Price S, Levine DP (1985). *In-vitro* evaluation of cefpirome (HR 810), teicoplanin and four other antimicrobials against enterococci. *J Antimicrob Chemother* **16**: 179.

Cheng AFB, Ling TKW, Lam AW *et al.* (1993). The antimicrobial activity and beta-lactamase stability of cefpirome, a new fourth-generation cephalosporin in comparison with other agents. *J Antimicrob Chemother* **31**: 699.

Chin N-X, Neu HC (1989). Synergy of new C-3 substituted cephalosporins and tobramycin against *Pseudomonas aeruginosa* and *Pseudomonas cepacia*. *Diagn Microbiol Infect Dis* **12**: 343.

Clarke AM, Zemcov SJV, Wright JM (1985). HR 810 and BMY-28142, two new cephalosporins with broad-spectrum activity: an *in-vitro* comparison with other beta-lactam antibiotics. *J Antimicrob Chemother* **15**: 305.

Craig WA (1993). The pharmacokinetics of cefpirome-rationale for a twelve-hour dosing regimen. *Scand J Infect Dis* (Suppl 91): 33.

Eng RHK, Cherubin CE, Smith SM *et al.* (1989). *In-vitro* and *in-vivo* activity of cefpirome (HR 810). against methicillin susceptible and-resistant *Staphylococcus aureus* and *Streptococcus faecalis*. *J Antimicrob Chemother* **23**: 373.

Gargaliamos P, Oppenheim BA, Skepastianos P *et al.* (1988). Activity of cefpirome (HR 810). against *Pseudomonas aeruginosa* strains with characterised resistance mechanisms to beta lactam antibiotics. *J Antimicrob Chemother* **22**: 841.

Gombert ME, Aulicino TM, DuBouchet L, Berkowitz LR (1987). Susceptibility of *Nocardia asteroides* to new quinolones and beta lactams. *Antimicrob Ag Chemother* **31**: 2013.

Goossens H, De Mol P, Coignau H *et al.* (1985). Comparative *in vitro* activities of aztreonam, ciprofloxacin, norfloxacin, ofloxacin, HR 810 (a new cephalosporin), RU 28965 (a new macrolide), and other agents against enteropathogens. *Antimicrob Ag Chemother* **27**: 388.

Hancock REW, Bellido F (1992). Factors involved in the enhanced efficacy against Gram-negative bacteria of fourth generation cephalosporins. *J Antimicrob Chemother* **29** (Suppl A): 1.

Jacoby GA, Carreras I (1990). Activities of beta-lactam antibiotics against *Escherichia coli* strains producing extended-spectrum beta-lactamases. *Antimicrob Ag Chemother* **34**: 858.

Jafari HS, Saez-Llorens X, Ramilo O *et al.* (1991). Pharmacokinetics and antibacterial efficacy of cefpirome (HR 810) in experimental *Escherichia coli* and *Haemophilus influenzae* type b meningitis. *Antimicrob Ag Chemother* **35**: 220.

Jones RN, Gerlach EH (1985). Antimicrobial activity of HR 810 against 419 strict anaerobic bacteria. *Antimicrob Ag Chemother* **27**: 413.

Jones RN, Thornsberry C, Barry AL (1984). *In vitro* evaluation of HR 810, a new wide-spectrum aminothiazolyl alpha-methoxyimino cephalosporin. *Antimicrob Ag Chemother* **25**: 710.

Kavi J, Andrews JM, Ashby JP *et al.* (1988). Pharmacokinetics and tissue penetration of cefpirome, a new cephalosporin. *J Antimicrob Chemother* **22**: 911.

Knothe H, Schäfer V, Sammann A *et al.* (1992). Influence of cefpirome on pharyngeal and faecal flora after single and multiple intravenous administrations of cefpirome to healthy volunteers. *J Antimicrob Chemother* **29** (Suppl A): 81.

Kobayashi S, Arai S, Hayashi S, Fujimoto K (1986). Beta-lactamase stability of cefpirome (HR 810), a new cephalosporin with a broad antimicrobial spectrum. *Antimicrob Ag Chemother* **30**: 713.

Kulkarni S, Wilson APR, Grüneberg RN *et al.* (1991). Interference of cefpirome with the measurement of plasma creatinine. *J Antimicrob Chemother* **28**: 617.

Lameire NH, Rosenkranz B, Malerczyk V (1989). Influence of renal functional impairment and hemodialysis on the pharmacokinetics of cefpirome In *Program and Abstracts of the 29th Interscience Conference on Antimicrobial Agents and Chemotherapy, Houston, TX, 1989.* (Abst. 1218, p. 308). Washington, DC: American Society for Microbiology.

Meyer BH, Muller FO, Luus HG *et al.* (1992). Safety, tolerance and pharmacokinetics of cefpirome administered intramuscularly to healthy subjects. *J Antimicrob Chemother* **29** (Suppl A): 63.

Moran FJ, Puente LF, Perez-Giraldo C *et al.* (1994). Effects of cefpirome in comparison with cefuroxime against human polymorphonuclear leucocytes *in vitro*. *J Antimicrob Chemother* **33**: 57.

Nix DE, Wilton JH, Velasquez N *et al.* (1992). Cerebrospinal fluid penetration of cefpirome in patients with non-inflamed meninges. *J Antimicrob Chemother* **29** (Suppl A): 51.

Norrby SR (1993). Cefpirome: efficacy in the treatment of urinary and respiratory tract infections and safety profile. *Scand J Infect Dis* (Suppl 91): 41.

Norrby SR, Geddes AM (1993). Efficacy of cefpirome in the treatment of septicaemia. *Scand J Infect Dis* (Suppl 91): 51.

Norrby SR, Dotevall L, Eriksson M *et al.* (1988). Efficacy and safety of cefpirome (HR 810). *J Antimicrob Chemother* **22**: 541.

Paradis D, Vallee F, Allard S *et al.* (1992). Comparative study of pharmacokinetics and serum bactericidal activities of cefpirome, ceftazidime, ceftriaxone, imipenem, and ciprofloxacin. *Antimicrob Ag Chemother* **36**: 2085.

Pascual A, Borobio V, Garcia-Iglesias MC, Perea EJ (1987). Comparative *in vitro* activity of cefodizime, cefpirome, carumonam and RU 28965 with other antimicrobials against anaerobes. *J Antimicrob Chemother* **19**: 701.

Piddock LJV, Traynor EA (1991). Beta-lactamase expression and outer membrane protein changes in cefpirome-resistant and ceftazidime-resistant Gram-negative bacteria. *J Antimicrob Chemother* **28**: 209.

Pucci MJ, Boice-Sowek J, Kessler RE, Dougherty TJ (1991). Comparison of cefepime, cefpirome, and cefaclidine binding affinities for penicillin-binding proteins in Escherichia coli K-12 and *Pseudomonas aeruginosa* SC 8329. *Antimicrob Ag Chemother* **35**: 2312.

Raizes EG, Cantey JR (1988). *In-vitro* activity of cefpirome compared with that of other agents. *J Antimicrob Chemother* **21**: 177.

Reeves DS, Bywater MJ, Holt HA (1993). The activity of cefpirome and ten other antibacterial agents against 2858 clinical isolates collected from 20 centres. *J Antimicrob Chemother* **31**: 345.

Rolston KVI, Bodey GP (1986). *In vitro* susceptibility of *Acinetobacter* species to various antimicrobial agents. *Antimicrob Ag Chemother* **30**: 769.

Sader HS, Jones RN (1994). *In vitro* antimicrobial activity of cefpirome against ceftazidime-resistant isolates from two multicenter studies. *Eur J Clin Microbiol Infect Dis* **13**: 675.

Satake S, Hiraoka M, Mitsuhashi S (1989). Interaction of cefpirome and a cephalosporinase from *Citrobacter freundii* G N 7391. *Antimicrob Ag Chemother* **33**: 398.

Spangler SK, Jacobs MR, Appelbaum PC (1994). Susceptibilities of 177 penicillin-susceptible and -resistant pneumococci to FK 037, cefpirome, cefepime, ceftriaxone, cefotaxime, ceftazidime, imipenem, biapenem, meropenem, and vancomycin. *Antimicrob Ag Chemother* **38**: 898.

Spencer RC, for the International Study Group (1993). Cross-susceptibility of cefpirome and four other beta-lactams against isolates from haematology/oncology and intensive care units. *Scand J Infect Dis* (Suppl 91): 25.

Study Group (1992). Cefpirome versus ceftazidime in the treatment of urinary tract infections. *J Antimicrob Chemother* **29** (Suppl A): 95.

Thornsberry C (1985). Review of *in vitro* activity of third-generation cephalosporins and other newer beta-lactam antibiotics against clinically important bacteria. *Amer J Med* **79** (Suppl 2A): 14.

Valdes JM, Baltch AL, Smith RP *et al.* (1990). Comparative therapy with cefpirome alone and in combination with rifampin and/or gentamicin against a disseminated *Pseudomonas aeruginosa* infection in leukopenic mice. *J Infect Dis* **162**: 1112.

Van der Auwera P, Scorneaux B (1985). *In vitro* susceptibility of *Campylobacter jejuni* to 27 antimicrobial agents and various combinations of beta-lactams with clavulanic acid or sulbactam. *Antimicrob Ag Chemother* **28**: 37.

Verbist L, for the International Study Group (1993). Epidemiology and sensitivity of 8625 ICU and hematology/oncology bacterial isolates in Europe. *Scand J Infect Dis* (Suppl 91): 14.

Watanabe N, Hiruma R, Katsu K (1992). Comparative *in-vitro* activities of newer cephalosporins cefclidin, cefepime, and cefpirome against ceftazidime- or imipenem-resistant *Pseudomonas aeruginosa*. *J Antimicrob Chemother* **30**: 633.

Wilcox MH, Pithie A, Smith G *et al.* (1991). Relationship between cefpirome clearance, serum creatinine, weight and age in patients treated for infection. *J Antimicrob Chemother* **28**: 291.

Wise R, Andrews JM, Cross C, Piddock LJV (1985). The antimicrobial activity of cefpirome, a new cephalosporin. *J Antimicrob Chemother* **15**: 449.

Wolff M, Chavanet P, Kazmierczak A *et al.* (1992). Diffusion of cefpirome into the cerebrospinal fluid of patients with purulent meningitis. *J Antimicrob Chemother* **29** (Suppl A): 59.

Yoshida R, Kaku M, Kohno S *et al.* (1995). Trends in antimicrobial resistance of *Streptococcus pneumoniae* in Japan. *Antimicrob Ag Chemother* **39**: 1196.

Cefepime

Description

Similar to cefpirome (p. 398), cefepime is referred to as an extended spectrum or fourth-generation parenteral cephalosporin. It has a wider spectrum and greater potency than the third-generation cephalosporins. In particular derepression of chromosomal beta-lactamases of Gram-negative bacilli has less effect on the *in vitro* activity of cefepime than that on third-generation cephalosporins (Neu *et al.*, 1986; Phelps *et al.*, 1986; Sanders, 1993).

Sensitive Organisms

1 Gram-positive bacteria

Against these bacteria cefepime has about the same potency as cefotaxime (p. 319), but it exceeds that of ceftazidime (p. 372). However, compared with cefpirome (p. 398), cefepime is slightly less active. Organisms such as *Staphylococcus aureus*, coagulase-negative staphylococci (including beta-lactamase producers of both), *Streptococcus pyogenes*, *Strep. pneumoniae*, *Strep. viridans*, *Strep. bovis* and Group B, C, and G streptococci are quite sensitive. Methicillin-resistant staphylococci and *Enterococcus faecalis* are resistant. *Listeria monocytogenes* (MIC 16–30 µg per ml) is moderately resistant. The anaerobic Gram-positive cocci and *Clostridium* spp. are cefepime-sensitive but *Cl. difficile* is resistant (Conrad *et al.*, 1985; Fuchs *et al.*, 1985; Jones *et al.*, 1985; Neu *et al.*, 1986; Duval *et al.*, 1993; Thornsberry *et al.*, 1993). The MICs of cefepime for pneumococci relatively or highly resistant to penicillin G (p. 5) are lower than the MICs of penicillin G. The MICs of cefepime for these strains are comparable with those of cefotaxime (p. 320) and ceftriaxone (p. 352). In one study 29 of 33 penicillin G-resistant and 84 of 85 relatively penicillin G-resistant isolates were susceptible to cefepime at concentrations of ≥1.0 µg per ml (Yee *et al.*, 1993).

2 Gram-negative aerobic bacteria

The Enterobacteriaceae, such as *Escherichia coli*, the *Klebsiella*, *Enterobacter*, *Proteus*, *Providencia*, *Citrobacter*, *Hafnia*, *Edwardsiella*, *Salmonella*, *Shigella* and *Yersinia* spp. and *Serratia marcescens* and *Morganella morganii* are cefepime-sensitive (Khan *et al.*, 1984; Fuchs *et al.*, 1985; Neu *et al.*, 1986; Thornsberry *et al.*, 1993). Against organisms, such as *E. coli*, *Klebsiella* spp. and *Proteus mirabilis*, which do not possess chromosomally mediated beta-lactamases, the activity of cefepime is about the same as that of cefotaxime and cefpirome and usually superior to that of ceftazidime (Van Ogtrop *et al.*, 1990; Mattie *et al.*, 1992; Sanders, 1993), but bacteria which possess inducible beta-lactamases, such as *Pr. vulgaris*, the *Enterobacter*, *Providencia*, *Citrobacter* and *Hafnia* spp., *S. marcescens* and *Morganella morganii*, are more susceptible to cefepime (and cefpirome) than to third-generation cephalosporins. These bacteria also usually remain cefepime-sensitive when their enzymes are induced or derepressed (Jacoby and Sutton, 1985; Phelps *et al.*, 1986; Rolston *et al.*, 1986; Hiraoka *et al.*, 1988; Chong *et al.*, 1993; Ehrhardt and Sanders, 1993; Thornsberry *et al.*, 1993). Cefotaxime- and ceftazidime-resistant Enterobacteriaceae, and also those which are resistant to aminoglycosides, are usually cefepime-sensitive (Fung-Tomc *et al.*, 1989, 1991).

Several factors make derepressed mutants of Enterobacteriaceae, which harbor inducible chromosomally mediated beta-lactamases, still usually cefepime-sensitive. First of all cefepime has a much lower affinity for these enzymes than the third-generation cephalosporins. It is also a poor inducer of these beta-lactamases. The cefepime molecule penetrates the outer cell membrane of Gram-negative organisms more rapidly. It also has good affinity for both PBP2 and 3 of *E. coli* (Nikaido *et al.*, 1990; Bellido *et al.*, 1991ab; Pucci *et al.*, 1991; Chen and Livermore, 1993; Grassi and Grassi, 1993). Nevertheless, fully derepressed mutants of these Enterobacteriaceae often have slightly elevated MICs for cefepime (Chen and Livermore, 1993; Sanders, 1993). Cefepime-resistant strains of some of these Enterobacteriaceae can be selected *in vitro* (Piddock and Griggs, 1991) and *in vivo* in animal models with *Enterobacter cloacae* infections (Pechere and Vladoianu, 1992). Some extended-spectrum plasmid-mediated beta-lactamases (p. 323) can probably hydrolyze cefepime. These enzymes are most frequently found in *Kl. pneumoniae* and *E. coli*. One *E. coli* strain, producing such an enzyme was moderately cefepime-resistant (MIC 8 µg per ml or less) (Jacoby and Carreras, 1990).

Haemophilus influenzae, Neisseria gonorrhoeae and *N. meningitidis* are cefepime-sensitive irrespective of beta-lactamase production (MICs <0.25 µg per ml), but *H. influenzae* strains with intrinsic resistance to ampicillin (p. 114) are some 8- to 64-fold less susceptible to cefepime than sensitive strains. *Gardnerella vaginalis* is also quite susceptible. *Bordetella pertussis, Brucella* spp., *Campylobacter* spp. and *Moraxella catarrhalis* are slightly less sensitive (MICs 0.25–2 µg per ml). *Aeromonas* and *Acinetobacter* spp. are also susceptible (Bodey *et al.*, 1985; Conrad *et al.*, 1985; Fuchs *et al.*, 1985; Neu *et al.*, 1986; Duval *et al.*, 1993; Sanders, 1993).

Cefepime is approximately half as active against *Pseudomonas aeruginosa* (MIC 8 µg per ml) compared with ceftazidime (p. 369) (Fuchs *et al.*, 1985; Neu *et al.*, 1986; Duval *et al.*, 1993; Thornsberry *et al.*, 1993). Most isolates of *Ps. aeruginosa* from patients with cystic fibrosis are cefepime-sensitive and in 26% of these strains cefepime/tobramycin synergism could be demonstrated *in vitro* (Bosso *et al.*, 1991). Strains of *Ps. aeruginosa* producing chromosomal beta-lactamases may be cefepime-sensitive (Fung-Tomc *et al.*, 1988), but when these strains produce high levels of chromosomal beta-lactamase because of induction or complete derepression, they are cefepime-resistant. Then there also is complete cross-resistance between ceftazidime and cefepime (Watanabe *et al.*, 1992). Cefepime bounds poorly to PBP2 of *Ps. aeruginosa*, but shows good binding to PBP3 (Pucci *et al.*, 1991). In general *Ps. aeruginosa* also has a lower outer membrane permeability compared with most of the Enterobacteriaceae (Hancock and Bellido, 1992). Cefepime is usually active against aminoglycoside-resistant *Ps. aeruginosa* strains (Tsuji *et al.*, 1985; Neu *et al.*, 1986).

The activity of cefepime against other *Pseudomonas* spp. is variable; *Ps. putida, Ps. stutzeri* and *Ps. fluorescens* are moderately susceptible, but *Burkholderia (Pseudomonas) cepacia, Ps. acidovorans* and *Stenotrophomonas maltophilia* are usually resistant (Conrad *et al.*, 1985; Neu *et al.*, 1986; Bosso *et al.*, 1991; Thornsberry *et al.*, 1993).

3 Gram-negative anaerobic bacteria

Prevotella melaninogenica is moderately susceptible, but the activity of cefepime is poor against other Gram-negative anaerobes such as *B. fragilis, B. bivius, B. thetaiotamicron* and *B. vulgatus* (Jones *et al.*, 1985; Neu *et al.*, 1986; Duval *et al.*, 1993).

4 Other bacteria

Cefepime is moderately active against bacteria of the *Mycobacterium avium* complex (MIC 8–16 µg per ml) (Cynamon *et al.*, 1987).

Mode of Administration and Dosage

Cefepime is not absorbed after oral administration, and it is usually administered by the i.v. route.

1 Adults

For moderately severe infections such as pneumonia or pyelonephritis a dosage of 1 g i.v. 12-hourly has been used (Oster *et al.*, 1990; Edelstein *et al.*, 1991; Giamarellou, 1993). Each dose is usually diluted in 30 ml of i.v. fluid and this is then administered as a 30-min infusion, similar to penicillin G (p. 20). For more severe infections such as complicated urinary tract infections due to *Ps. aeruginosa*, patients with Gram-negative bone infections and septicemia a dosage of 2 g i.v. 12-hourly appears appropriate (Gentry and Rodriguez-Gomez, 1991; Mouton *et al.*, 1993). When cefepime was used as monotherapy for treatment of fever in granulocytopenic cancer patients, a dosage as high as 2 g 8-hourly was employed (Eggimann *et al.*, 1993).

2 Patients older than 65 years

The normal cefepime terminal half-life of 2 h is prolonged to about 3 h in elderly patients, but the magnitude of age-related changes in the pharmacokinetics of cefepime is not significant enough to recommend dosage adjustment in these patients with renal function normal for their age (Barbhaiya et al., 1992b).

3 Patients with renal failure

A dosage reduction for these patients is necessary. If there is some renal functional impairment, but creatinine clearance is still >30 ml per min, a dosage of 1 g 12-hourly is recommended. If creatinine clearance is 10–30 ml per min the dosage is 0.5 g once every 24 h, but if creatinine clearance is <10 ml per min, the suggested dosage is 250 mg once every 24 h. If patients are treated by hemodialysis a supplementary dose of 250 mg is recommended after each hemodialysis (Cronqvist et al., 1992). In patients undergoing continuous ambulatory peritoneal dialysis, a cefepime dosage of 1 or 2 g i.v. every 48 h would maintain the antibiotic levels in plasma and peritoneal fluid above the MICs of susceptible bacteria (Barbhaiya et al., 1992d).

4 Patients with cystic fibrosis

The elimination half-life of cefepime in these patients is 11% shorter than in other patients, but the difference in pharmacokinetics is minor and from this point of view no change in dosage is recommended. However, in these patients respiratory infections due to *Ps. aeruginosa* are usually treated. The MICs of *Ps. aeruginosa* strains in these patients are usually 16 μg per ml. To maintain trough serum levels above this MIC, a dosage of 2 g 6-hourly is recommended (Huls et al., 1993).

Serum Levels in Relation to Dosage

Single doses of cefepime of 250 mg, 0.5 g, 1 g and 2 g were given to normal adults by a 30-min infusion. The mean peak serum levels straight after the infusion were 17.9, 31.9, 61.1 and 126 μg per ml, respectively. Doubling the dose resulted in approximately double the peak serum level. The levels of cefepime in plasma declined with a terminal elimination half-life of about 2 h at each dose level. Total clearance for all doses ranged between 122 and 136 ml per min. The cefepime serum level approached 1 μg per ml 8–12 h after administration. When each of the four above doses were given 8-hourly, there was no drug accumulation in the body (Barbhaiya et al., 1990, 1992a; Van der Auwera and Santella, 1993). When cefepime was administered together with amikacin, the pharmacokinetic parameters of both drugs remained unchanged (Barbhaiya et al., 1992c). The pharmacokinetics of cefepime in patients with infections is about the same as in healthy volunteers (Kovarik et al., 1990).

Excretion

1 Urine

Cefepime is mainly eliminated via the kidney as the unchanged active drug by glomerular filtration. Urinary recovery of intact cefepime is about 82% of the administered dose. Cefepime concentrations in urine after administration of the low dose of 250 mg i.v. were approximately 190 μg per ml during the first 2 h, and this concentration was about 90 μg per ml at 8 h (Barbhaiya et al., 1990, 1992a).

2 Inactivation in body

A small amount of the administered dose of cefepime is converted in the body to an inactive non-toxic metabolite N-methyl pyrrolidine N oxide (Van der Auwera and Santella, 1993).

Distribution of the Drug in Body

Cefepime is about 16% serum protein bound (Van der Auwera and Santella, 1993). In bacterial meningitis in animals, the average CSF cefepime level was 9.6 μg per ml which was about 16% of the simultaneous serum level (Kim and Bayer, 1985; Täuber et al., 1985). Non-infected newborn rats who had a peak serum level of cefepime of 43 μg per ml, achieved peak cefepime levels in the CSF and brain tissue of 9.5 μg per ml and 2.2 μg per g, respectively (Tsai et al., 1990).

Cefepime penetrated well into human suction-induced blister fluid (Kalman et al., 1992). In patients undergoing diagnostic bronchoscopy, after a single 2-g dose of cefepime, the mean bronchial mucosal concentration of the drug was 24.1 μg per g and the mean serum concentration was 40.4 μg per ml. The mean percentage penetration was 59.8% (Chadha et al., 1990). In one study 30 patients underwent elective prostatectomy. Five patients were each given cefepime 2 g i.v. 1, 3, 6, 9, 12 and 18 h preoperatively. The mean percentage penetration into prostatic tissue at 1 h was 51%, at 3 h 42%, at 6 h 43%, at 9 h 76%, at 12 h 79% and at 18 h 138%. The half-life of cefepime in prostatic tissue (2.8 h) was longer than that in serum (Arkell *et al.*, 1992). One animal study showed that cefepime concentration in tissues of paralyzed limbs were the same as in non-paralyzed limbs (Darouiche *et al.*, 1989).

Toxicity

Toxic effects appear to be infrequent and similar to those observed with other cephalosporins such as ceftazidime (p. 377). Phlebitis due to i.v. administration has been fairly frequently seen. Skin rashes, nausea, diarrhea, transient elevations of SGOT and SGPT and headache have been observed in a small number of patients. One patient had *Cl. difficile* in the stool and diarrhea (Oster *et al.*, 1990; Edelstein *et al.*, 1991; Eggimann *et al.*, 1993; Mouton *et al.*, 1993; Kieft *et al.*, 1994). Cefepime does change the fecal flora; during administration of the drug there was a decrease in the number of *E. coli* and bifidobacteria in feces, whereas *Bacteroides* spp. and *Clostridium*, including *Cl. difficile* showed a slight increase (Bächer *et al.*, 1992).

Clinical Uses of the Drug

1 Monotherapy for empirical treatment of fever in granulocytopenic cancer patients

In one pilot study, cefepime in a dose of 2 g i.v. 8-hourly was given to 91 evaluable patients with such fever. Overall response rates were 86% for Gram-negative infections, and 44% for Gram-positive infections. Twenty-six patients (29%) did not respond to cefepime monotherapy, and 23 of these responded after the addition of other antibiotics (Eggimann *et al.*, 1993). These results are approximately the same as previously obtained with ceftazidime monotherapy (p. 377).

2 Serious bacterial infections such as septicemia caused by Enterobacteriaceae, Ps. aeruginosa and Gram-positive bacteria such as Strep. pneumoniae and Staph. aureus

Cefepime in a dose of 2 g i.v. 12-hourly has been quite effective for the treatment of such severe infections, which normally occur in the hospital setting. In comparative studies the results of treatment have been about the same as those with ceftazidime (Hoepelman *et al.*, 1993; Mouton *et al.*, 1993; Kieft *et al.*, 1994; Schrank *et al.*, 1995).

3 Pneumonia

This disease, caused by *H. influenzae* or *Strep. pneumoniae* has responded satisfactorily to cefepime 1 g i.v. 12-hourly in clinical trials (Oster *et al.*, 1990; Edelstein *et al.*, 1991). Severe nosocomial pneumonia in intensive care units was successfully treated by cefepime 2 g i.v. 12-hourly plus amikacin 7.5 mg per kg 12-hourly. The main pathogens here were *Staph. aureus*, *Ps. aeruginosa* and *Klebsiella*, *Enterobacter* and *Serratia* spp. (Gouin *et al.*, 1993).

4 Osteomyelitis

In an animal study, cefepime administered for 4 weeks to rabbits with chronic experimental osteomyelitis due to *Staph. aureus* sterilized the bones of 53% of treated animals. This agent appeared as effective as other cephalosporins and penicillinase-resistant penicillins, but not as effective as clindamycin (Norden and Gill, 1990). In one clinical study 23 patients with osteomyelitis, mainly due to *Staph. aureus*, were treated with cefepime 2 g i.v. 12-hourly. Twenty were cured, but treatment failed in three (Jauregui *et al.*, 1993).

5 Other infections

Results comparable with those with ceftazidime have been obtained with the use of cefepime in complicated urinary tract infections and in skin and surgical wound infections (Oster *et al.*, 1990; Gentry and Rodriguez-Gomez, 1991). In children aged 2 months to 15 years, cefepime had equal efficacy and safety as cefotaxime for the treatment of bacterial meningitis (Sáez-Llorens *et al.*, 1995).

References

Arkell D, Ashrap M, Andrews JM, Wise R (1992). An evaluation of the penetration of cefepime into prostate tissue in patients undergoing elective prostatectomy. *J Antimicrob Chemother* **29**: 473.

Bächer K, Schaeffer M, Lode H *et al.* (1992). Multiple dose pharmacokinetics, safety, and effects on faecal microflora, of cefepime in healthy volunteers. *J Antimicrob Chemother* **30**: 365.

Barbhaiya RH, Forgue ST, Gleason CR *et al.* (1990). Safety, tolerance, and pharmacokinetic evaluation of cefepime after administration of single intravenous dose. *Antimicrob Ag Chemother* **34**: 1118.

Barbhaiya RH, Forgue ST, Gleason CR *et al.* (1992a). Pharmacokinetics of cefepime after single and multiple intravenous administrations in healthy subjects. *Antimicrob Ag Chemother* **36**: 552.

Barbhaiya RH, Knupp CA, Pittman KA (1992b). Effects of age and gender on pharmacokinetics of cefepime. *Antimicrob Ag Chemother* **36**: 1181.

Barbhaiya RH, Knupp CA, Pfeffer M, Pittman KA (1992c). Lack of pharmacokinetic interaction between cefepime and amikacin in humans. *Antimicrob Ag Chemother* **36**: 1382.

Barbhaiya RH, Knupp CA, Pfeffer M *et al.* (1992d). Pharmacokinetics of cefepime in patients undergoing continuous ambulatory peritoneal dialysis. *Antimicrob Ag Chemother* **36**: 1387.

Bellido F, Pechere J-C, Hancock REW (1991a). Novel method for measurement of outer membrane permeability to new beta-lactams in intact *Enterobacter cloacae* cells. *Antimicrob Ag Chemother* **35**: 68.

Bellido F, Pechere J-C, Hancock REW (1991b). Reevaluation of the factors involved in the efficacy of new beta-lactams against *Enterobacter cloacae*. *Antimicrob Ag Chemother* **35**: 73.

Bodey GP, Ho DH, Le Blanc B (1985). *In vitro* studies of BMY-28142, a new broad-spectrum cephalosporin. *Antimicrob Ag Chemother* **27**: 265.

Bosso JA, Saxon BA, Matsen JM (1991). Comparative activity of cefepime, alone and in combination, against clinical isolates of *Pseudomonas aeruginosa* and *Pseudomonas cepacia* from cystic fibrosis patients. *Antimicrob Ag Chemother* **35**: 783.

Chadha D, Wise R, Baldwin DR *et al.* (1990). Cefepime concentrations in bronchial mucosa and serum following a single 2 gram intravenous dose. *J Antimicrob Chemother* **25**: 959.

Chen HY, Livermore DM (1993). Effects of beta-lactamase inducibility and derepression on the activity of cefepime and cefpirome against Gram-negative bacteria. *J Antimicrob Chemother* **32**: 651.

Chong Y, Lee K, Kwon OH (1993). *In-vitro* activities of cefepime against *Enterobacter cloacae*, *Serratia marcescens*, *Pseudomonas aeruginosa* and other aerobic Gram-negative bacilli. *J Antimicrob Chemother* **32** (Suppl B): 21.

Conrad DA, Scribner RK, Weber AH, Marks MI (1985). *In vitro* activity of BMY-28142 against pediatric pathogens, including isolates from cystic fibrosis sputum. *Antimicrob Ag Chemother* **28**: 58.

Cronqvist J, Nilsson-Ehle I, Oqvist B, Norrby SR (1992). Pharmacokinetics of cefepime dihydrochloride arginine in subjects with renal impairment. *Antimicrob Ag Chemother* **36**: 2676.

Cynamon MH, Palmer GS, Sorg TB (1987). Comparative *in vitro* activities of ampicillin, BMY 28142, and imipenem against *Mycobacterium avium* complex. *Diagn Microbiol Infect Dis* **6**: 151.

Darouiche R, Musher D, Hamill R *et al.* (1989). Cephalosporin penetration into soft tissue of paralysed limbs. *Antimicrob Ag Chemother* **33**: 1326.

Duval J, Soussy CJ, Acar JF *et al.* (1993). *In vitro* antibacterial activity of cefepime: a multicentre study. *J Antimicrob Chemother* **32** (Suppl B): 55.

Edelstein H, Chirurgi V, Oster S *et al.* (1991). A randomized trial of cefepime (BMY-28142). and ceftazidime for the treatment of pneumonia. *J Antimicrob Chemother* **28**: 569.

Eggimann P, Glauser MP, Aoun M *et al.* (1993). Cefepime monotherapy for the empirical treatment of fever in granulocytopenic cancer patients. *J Antimicrob Chemother* **32** (Suppl B): 151.

Ehrhardt AF, Sanders CC (1993). Beta-lactam resistance among *Enterobacter* species. *Antimicrob Chemother* **32** (Suppl B): 1.

Fuchs PC, Jones RN, Barry AL, Thornsberry C (1985). Evaluation of the *in vitro* activity of BMY-28142, a new broad-spectrum cephalosporin. *Antimicrob Ag Chemother* **27**: 679.

Fung-Tomc J, Huczko E, Pearce M, Kessler RE (1988). Frequency of *in vitro* resistance of *Pseudomonas aeruginosa* to cefepime, ceftazidime, and cefotaxime. *Antimicrob Ag Chemother* **32**: 1443.

Fung-Tomc J, Dougherty TJ, De Orio FJ *et al.* (1989). Activity of cefepime against ceftazidime- and cefotaxime-resistant Gram-negative bacteria and its relationship to beta-lactamase levels. *Antimicrob Ag Chemother* **33**: 498.

Fung-Tomc J, Huczko E, Kolek B *et al.* (1991). *In vitro* activities of cefepime alone and with amikacin against aminoglycoside-resistant Gram-negative bacteria. *Antimicrob Ag Chemother* **35**: 2652.

Gentry LO, Rodriguez-Gomez G (1991). Randomized comparison of cefepime and ceftazidime for treatment of skin, surgical wound, and complicated urinary tract infections in hospitalized subjects. *Antimicrob Ag Chemother* **35**: 2371.

Giamarellou H (1993). Low dosage cefepime as treatment for serious bacterial infections. *J Antimicrob Chemother* **32** (Suppl B): 123.

Gouin F, Papazian L, Martin C *et al.* (1993). A non-comparative study of the efficacy and tolerance of cefepime in combination with amikacin in the treatment of severe infections in patients in intensive care. *J Antimicrob Chemother* **32** (Suppl B): 205.

Grassi GG, Grassi C (1993). Cefepime: overview of activity *in vitro* and *in vivo*. *J Antimicrob Chemother* **32** (Suppl B): 87.

Hancock REW, Bellido F (1992). Factors involved in the enhanced efficacy against Gram-negative bacteria of fourth generation cephalosporins. *J Antimicrob Chemother* **29** (Suppl A): 1.

Hiraoka M, Inoue M, Mitsuhashi S (1988). Hydrolytic rate at low drug concentrations as a limiting factor in resistance to newer cephalosporins. *Rev Infect Dis* **10**: 746.

Hoepelman AIM, Kieft H, Aoun M *et al.* (1993). International comparative study of cefepime and ceftazidime in the treatment of serious bacterial infections. *J Antimicrob Chemother* **32** (Suppl B): 175.

Huls CE, Prince RA, Sailheimer DK, Bosso JA (1993). Pharmacokinetics of cefepime in cystic fibrosis patients. *Antimicrob Ag Chemother* **37**: 1414.

Jacoby GA, Carreras I (1990). Activities of beta-lactam antibiotics against *Escherichia coli* strains producing extended-spectrum beta-lactamases. *Antimicrob Ag Chemother* **34**: 858.

Jacoby GA, Sutton L (1985). Beta-lactamases and beta-lactam resistance in *Escherichia coli*. *Antimicrob Ag Chemother* **28**: 703.

Jauregui L, Matzke D, Scott M *et al.* (1993). Cefepime as treatment for osteomyelitis and other severe bacterial infections. *J Antimicrob Chemother* **32** (Suppl B): 141.

Jones RN, Barry AL, Packer RR (1985). BMY-28142, cefbuperazone (T-1982)., and Sch 34343 Antimicrobial activity against 94 anaerobes compared to seven other antimicrobial agents. *Diagn Microbiol Infect Dis* **3**: 263.

Kalman D, Barriere SL, Johnson BL Jr (1992). Pharmacokinetic disposition and bactericidal activities of cefepime, ceftazidime, and cefoperazone in serum and blister fluid. *Antimicrob Ag Chemother* **36**: 453.

Kessler RE, Bies M, Buck RE *et al.* (1985). Comparison of a new cephalosporin, BMY-28142, with other broad spectrum beta-lactam antibiotics. *Antimicrob AG Chemother* **27**: 207.

Khan NJ, Bihl JA, Schell RF *et al.* (1984). Antimicrobial activities of BMY-28142, cefbuperazone and cefpiramide compared with those of other cephalosporins. *Antimicrob Ag Chemother* **26**: 585.

Kieft H, Hoepelman AIM, Rozenberg-Arska M *et al.* (1994). Cefepime compared with ceftazidime as initial therapy for serious bacterial infections and sepsis syndrome. *Antimicrob Ag Chemother* **38**: 415.

Kim KS, Bayer AS (1985). Efficacy of BMY-28142 in experimental bacteremia and meningitis caused by *Escherichia coli* and Group B streptococci. *Antimicrob Ag Chemother* **28**: 51.

Kovarik JM, Ter Maaten JC, Rademaker CMA *et al.* (1990). Pharmacokinetics of cefepime in patients with respiratory tract infections. *Antimicrob Ag Chemother* **34**: 1885.

Mattie H, Razab Sekh BA, Van Ogtrop ML, Van Strijen E (1992). Comparison of antibacterial effects of cefepime and ceftazidime against *Escherichia coli in vitro* and *in vivo*. *Antimicrob Ag Chemother* **36**: 2439.

Mouton Y, Chidiac C, Humbert G *et al.* (1993). A non-comparative, multicentre study of cefepime in the treatment of serious bacterial infections. *J Antimicrob Chemother* **32** (Suppl B).: 133.

Neu HC, Chin N-X, Jules K, Labthavikul P (1986). The activity of BMY-28142, a new broad spectrum beta-lactamase stable cephalosporin. *J Antimicrob Chemother* **17**: 441.

Nikaido H, Liu W, Rosenberg EY (1990). Outer membrane permeability and beta-lactamase stability of dipolar ionic cephalosporins containing methoxyimino substituents. *Antimicrob Ag Chemother* **34**: 337.

Norden CW, Gill EA (1990). Cefepime for treatment of experimental chronic osteomyelitis due to *Staphylococcus aureus*. *J Infect Dis* **162**: 1218.

Oster S, Edelstein H, Cassano K, McCabe R (1990). Open trial of cefepime (BMY 28142) for infections in hospitalized patients. *Antimicrob Ag Chemother* **34**: 954.

Pechere J-C, Vladoianu IR (1992). Development of resistance during ceftazidime and cefepime therapy in a murine peritonitis model. *J Antimicrob Chemother* **29**: 563.

Phelps DJ, Carlton DD, Farrell CA, Kessler RE (1986). Affinity of cephalosporins for beta-lactamases as a factor in antibacterial efficacy. *Antimicrob Ag Chemother* **29**: 845.

Piddock LJV, Griggs DJ (1991). Selection and characterization of cefepime-resistant Gram-negative bacteria. *J Antimicrob Chemother* **28**: 669.

Pucci MJ, Boice-Sowek J, Kessler RE, Dougherty TJ (1991). Comparison of cefepime, cefpirome, and cefaclidine binding affinities for penicillin-binding proteins in *Escherichia coli* K-12 and *Pseudomonas aeruginosa* SC8329. *Antimicrob Ag Chemother* **35**: 2312.

Rolston KVI, Alvarez ME, Hsu K-C, Bodey GP (1986). In-vitro activity of cefpirome (HR-810)., WIN-49375, BMY-28142 and other antibiotics against nosocomially important isolates from cancer patients. *J Antimicrob Chemother* **17**: 453.

Sáez-Llorens X, Castaño E, Garcia R *et al.* (1995). Prospective randomized comparison of cefepime and cefotaxime for treatment of bacterial meningitis in infants and children. *Antimicrob Ag Chemother* **39**: 937.

Sanders CC (1993). Cefepime: the next generation? *Clin Infect Dis* **17**: 369.

Schrank JHJr, Kelly JW, McAllister CK (1995). Randomized comparison of cefepime and ceftazidime for treatment of hospitalized patients with Gram-negative bacteremia. *Clin Infect Dis* **20**: 56.

Steele JCH Jr, Edwards BH, Rissing JP (1985). In-vitro activity of BMY-28142, a new aminothiazolyl cephalosporin. *J Antimicrob Chemother* **16**: 463.

Täuber MG, Hackbarth CJ, Scott KG *et al.* (1985). New cephalosporins cefotaxime, cefpimizole, BMY 28142, and HR 810 in experimental pneumococcal meningitis in rabbits. *Antimicrob Ag Chemother* **27**: 340.

Thornsberry C, Brown SD, Yee YC *et al.* (1993). *In vitro* activity of cefepime and other antimicrobials: survey of European isolates. *J Antimicrob Chemother* **32** (Suppl B): 31.

Tsai YH, Bies M, Leitner F, Kessler RE (1990). Therapeutic studies of cefepime (BMY 28142) in murine meningitis and pharmacokinetics in neonatal rats. *Antimicrob Ag Chemother* **34**: 733.

Tsuji A, Maniatis A, Bertram MA, Young LS (1985). *In vitro* activity of BMY-28142 in comparison with those of other beta-lactam antimicrobial agents. *Antimicrob Ag Chemother* **27**: 515.

Van der Auwera P, Santella PJ (1993). Pharmacokinetics of cefepime: a review. *J Antimicrob Chemother* **32** (Suppl B): 103.

Van Ogtrop ML, Mattie H, Guiot HFL *et al.* (1990). Comparative study of the effects of four cephalosporins against *Escherichia coli in vitro* and *in vivo*. *Antimicrob Ag Chemother* **34**: 1932.

Watanabe N, Hiruma R, Katsu K (1992). Comparative *in-vitro* activities of newer cephalosporins cefclidin, cefepime and cefpirome against ceftazidime- or imipenem-resistant *Pseudomonas aeruginosa*. *J Antimicrob Chemother* **30**: 633.

Yee YC, Thornsberry C, Brown SD *et al.* (1993). A comparative study of the *in-vitro* activity of cefepime and other antimicrobial agents against penicillin-susceptible and penicillin-resistant Streptococcus pneumoniae. *J Antimicrob Chemother* **32** (Suppl B): 13.

Cefixime

Description

Cefixime is an orally administered cephalosporin with a wider antimicrobial spectrum than earlier oral cephalosporins, such as cephalexin (p. 263) and cefaclor (p. 273). It is referred to as a third-generation oral cephalosporin, but its spectrum of activity is not quite as wide as that of parenteral third-generation cephalosporins such as cefotaxime (p. 319) (The Medical Letter, 1989).

Sensitive Organisms

1 Gram-positive bacteria

Cefixime has good activity against Groups A and B hemolytic streptococci and *Streptococcus pneumoniae*, but *Staphylococcus aureus*, coagulase negative staphylococci, *Enterococcus faecalis* and other enterococci are resistant. *Listeria monocytogenes* and Gram-positive anaerobes such as *Peptostreptococcus* and *Clostridium* spp. are also cefixime-resistant (Stone *et al.*, 1989; Lehtonen and Huovinen, 1993; Sader *et al.*, 1993). Penicillin G-resistant pneumococci also have increased MICs to cefixime (Barry *et al.*, 1994).

2 Gram-negative bacteria

Neisseria gonorrhoeae and *Haemophilus influenzae* are cefixime-sensitive irrespective of beta-lactamase production. However, the MICs of cefixime are considerably higher against ampicillin-resistant *H. influenzae* strains which do not produce beta-lactamase, than MICs of ampicillin-sensitive strains and those that produce beta-lactamase (Table I.32). *Haemophilus parainfluenzae* is also sensitive (Mendelman *et al.*, 1989; Mortensen and Himes, 1990; Nash *et al.*, 1991; Sader *et al.*, 1993). Both *Bordetella pertussis* and *B. parapertussis* are moderately cefixime-resistant (Hoppe and Müller, 1990). The majority of *Moraxella catarrhalis* isolates now produce one of two different beta-lactamases, referred to as BRO-1 and BRO-2. The majority of strains produce BRO-1 enzyme. Cefixime is more active against isolates which produce BRO-2 enzyme (MIC 0.063) compared with those that produce BRO-1 (MIC 0.25 µg per ml) (Nash *et al.*, 1991; Fung *et al.*, 1994).

Among the Enterobacteriaceae, *Escherichia coli*, the *Klebsiella*, *Proteus* and *Providencia* spp. are usually cefixime-sensitive. Most strains of *Serratia marcescens* are also sensitive. *Citrobacter diversus* is usually sensitive but *Citrobacter freundii* is resistant. Most strains of *Enterobacter* spp. and *Morganella morganii* are resistant. Cefixime is not a good inducer of chromosomally mediated beta-lactamases (Class 1 beta-lactamases) of the Enterobacteriaceae which produce these enzymes (p. 322). Yet this resistance mechanism probably explains the insensitivity of *Enterobacter* spp. and *Morganella morganii* to this drug (Sanders, 1989; Stone *et al.*, 1989; MacGowan *et al.*, 1992; Sader *et al.*, 1993). If one of the Enterobacteriaceae, such as *Klebsiella pneumoniae*, harbors extended-spectrum beta-lactamase (p. 323), it is usually cefixime-resistant (Kitzis *et al.*, 1990).

Pasteurella multocida is cefixime-sensitive (Avril *et al.*, 1991), as is *Helicobacter pylori* (Ikeda *et al.*, 1990). *Acinetobacter* spp., *Ps. aeruginosa*, other *Pseudomonas* spp. and *Stenotrophomonas maltophilia* are resistant (Stone *et al.*, 1989; Sader *et al.*, 1993). The activity of cefixime against Gram-negative anaerobes such as *Bacteroides fragilis* is poor (Table I.32) (Stone *et al.*, 1989; Sader *et al.*, 1993).

Organism	MICs (μg per ml)
Gram-positive bacteria	
Streptococcus pneumoniae	0.12
Staphylococcus aureus	>128.0
Gram-negative bacteria	
Neisseria gonorrhoeae	0.008
Haemophilus influenzae, ampicillin-sensitive	0.04
Haemophilus influenzae, beta-lactamase producer	0.04
Haemophilus influenzae, intrinsically ampicillin-resistant	0.96
Escherichia coli	1.0
Klebsiella spp.	0.12
Enterobacter spp.	>128.0
Proteus mirabilis	0.06
Serratia marcescens	4.0
Pseudomonas aeruginosa	>16.0
Bacteroides fragilis	>4.0

Table I.32
Compiled from data published by Mendelman *et al.* (1989), Stone *et al.* (1989) and Sader *et al.* (1993)

3 Other organisms

Borrelia burgdorferi is moderately cefixime-sensitive (MIC 0.8 μg per ml), but against this spirochete ceftriaxone (p. 353) is more active (MIC 0.02 μg per ml) (Agger *et al.*, 1992).

4 Minimum inhibitory concentrations

The MICs of cefixime against some selected bacterial species are shown in Table I.32.

Mode of Administration and Dosage

The usual adult dosage of cefixime is 400 mg orally once-daily (Kiani *et al.*, 1988; Verghese *et al.*, 1990; Raz *et al.*, 1994). For treatment of uncomplicated gonorrhea the oral administration of a single-dose cefixime of 400 mg is recommended (Portilla *et al.*, 1992; CDC, 1993). The dosage in children is 8 mg per kg per day, administered in one daily dose (Piippo *et al.*, 1991; Rodriguez *et al.*, 1993).

Serum Levels in Relation to Dosage

Cefixime is partially absorbed after oral administration. After a 400-mg oral cefixime dose to adults, a maximal serum level from 2.76 to 4.5 μg per ml is reached 3–4 h after administration. Thereafter the serum level falls with a terminal half-life of 3.7 h. The serum level is still about 1 μg per ml in 12 h, but approaches zero in 24 h. Multiple-dose administration of 400 mg cefixime once every 24 h does not lead to any drug accumulation in the serum. By 12 h the mean quantity of cefixime absorbed is about 31% (Healy *et al.*, 1989; Duverne *et al.*, 1992; Fassbender *et al.*, 1993). If antacids containing aluminum and magnesium are administered 2 h before cefixime dose, together with cefixime or 2 h after, the serum levels of cefixime appear slightly increased, but the difference is not significant (Healy *et al.*, 1989).

Intestinal absorption of cefixime in the rat occurs by an active mechanism involving a pH-dependent dipeptide transporter similar to that of amoxycillin (p. 173). The same mechanism probably operates in humans, because if this is the case the drug's absorption should be enhanced by a calcium channel blocker such as nifedipine. Duverne *et al.* (1992) demonstrated that co-administration of nifedipine considerably enhanced the absorption of cefixime in humans. The absolute bioavailability of cefixime alone was 31%, compared with 53% in the presence of nifedipine.

Excretion

1 Urine

About 21.2% of the administered dose of cefixime is excreted via the kidney as the active drug (Fassbender *et al.*, 1993). After a single oral dose of 400 mg, maximal urinary concentrations averaged 216.6 µg per ml and these were reached in urine during the 2–4 h or 4–6 h period after dosing. Minimum urinary concentrations occurred during the 12–24 h collection interval and averaged 19 µg per ml (Healy *et al.*, 1989).

2 Bile

A considerable amount of active cefixime is eliminated via the bile. In patients with T-tube drainage after cholecystectomy about 5% of the administered dose of cefixime was eliminated this way. In these patients following a single 200-mg dose of cefixime, the average peak concentration of cefixime in bile reached 56.9 µg per ml. A concentration of approximately 4.3 µg per ml was still present 20 h after dosing (Westphal *et al.*, 1993).

3 Inactivation in body

Some cefixime may be metabolized in the body, but no metabolites have been identified (Fassbender *et al.*, 1993).

Distribution of the Drug in Body

This has been little studied. The mean concentration of cefixime was 25 µg per g in gallbladder tissue 13–17 h after a 400-mg dose. Concentrations ranged from 0.53 to 0.74 µg per g in tonsillar tissue 5 h after a 4 mg per kg dose. Cefixime is about 70% serum protein bound (Fassbender *et al.*, 1993).

Toxicity

Some patients treated with cefixime have developed rashes (Kiani *et al.*, 1988; Rodruguez *et al.*, 1993). Gastrointestinal symptoms such as nausea, vomiting and in particular diarrhea appear to be the main adverse effects from cefixime. In some patients the diarrhea was severe and one patient had moderate diarrhea with *Cl. difficile* in stools (Kiani *et al.*, 1988; Verghese *et al.*, 1990; Piippo *et al.*, 1991). In one study cefixime 200 mg twice-daily for 7 days was given to ten volunteers. There was marked decrease in streptococci and *E. coli* in the intestinal flora and an increase in enterococci. In the anaerobic microflora the numbers of cocci, clostridia and bacteroides were suppressed. *Clostridium difficile* was isolated in five subjects, but cytotoxin was only detected in one. Slightly soft stools were noted by seven subjects, and one had abdominal pain and diarrhea (Nord *et al.*, 1988). In another volunteer trial 400 mg of oral cefixime daily was given to six subjects for 10 days. In five of six cefixime-treated volunteers *Cl. difficile* was detected. The strains of *Cl. difficile* differed from one volunteer to another, but they were all resistant to cefixime. Antibiotic activity was found in the feces of four volunteers. A few of them had loose stools. This did not correlate with the presence of *Cl. difficile*, but there was correlation between passage of loose stools and fecal antibiotic activity (Chachaty *et al.*, 1992). These findings were confirmed in a later study using 51 volunteers (Chachaty *et al.*, 1993).

There is one report where three children developed abdominal pain and diarrhea in association with cefixime therapy. Two of the patients had blood and mucus in stools and one had watery diarrhea. In all three *Cl. difficile* toxin was detected. Two of them were sigmoidoscoped; both showed erythema and edema of the rectosigmoid mucosa, and in one pseudomembranes were present. All recovered with oral vancomycin therapy (Gremse *et al.*, 1994).

Clinical Uses of the Drug

1 Respiratory tract infections

Cefixime has been used to treat infections such as bacterial bronchitis, pharyngitis and tonsillitis. The results of treatment were good, but not superior to those obtained with oral amoxycillin (Kiani *et al.*, 1988). In another trial 86 patients with acute bacterial exacerbations of chronic bronchitis were randomized to receive either a single 400-mg daily dose of cefixime or 250 mg cephalexin orally four times a day. A total of 70.8% of the cefixime group and 50% of the cephalexin group were clinically cured. However, when the categories of cured and improved were combined, no significant difference was noted between treatment groups (Verghese *et al.*, 1990).

2 Otitis media

Cefixime in a dose of 8 mg per kg per day for 7–10 days has been confirmed as a quite effective treatment for this disease in children, but in two studies its efficacy was about the same as that of cefaclor 40 mg per kg per day, given in three divided doses (Piippo *et al.*, 1991; Rodriguez *et al.*, 1993).

3 Sequential treatment after initial i.v. chemotherapy by parenteral cephalosporins for severe infections

Oral cefixime therapy may be feasible for severe infections such as nosocomial pneumonia, complicated urinary tract infections etc, after initial satisfactory response has been obtained with drugs like i.v. cefotaxime (p. 338) or ceftriaxone (p. 360). Well designed clinical studies are necessary to prove the effectiveness of sequential therapy with oral cephalosporins for serious infections in hospitalized patients (Janknegt and van der Meer, 1994).

4 Urinary tract infections

In one randomized study cefixime 400 mg daily and ofloxacin 200 mg 12-hourly, both given for 3 days, were equally effective in the treatment of uncomplicated urinary tract infections in women (Raz *et al.*, 1994).

5 Gonorrhea

Single-dose cefixime 200 mg or 800 mg have been used successfully for the treatment of uncomplicated gonorrhea (Dunnett and Moyer, 1992; Verdon *et al.*, 1993). It is now accepted that a 400-mg single dose is the best (Portilla *et al.*, 1992), and this is now recommended by Centers of Disease Control as an alternative for i.m. ceftriaxone (p. 361) for the treatment of uncomplicated gonorrhea (CDC, 1993). Cefixime is not effective for coexistent *Chlamydia trachomatis* and *Ureaplasma urealyticum* infections (Megran *et al.*, 1990).

6 Typhoid fever

In a clinical trial in typhoid fever in children, oral cefixime 5 mg per kg 12-hourly for 14 days, appeared equally as effective as i.v. ceftriaxone (p. 360) (Bhutta *et al.*, 1994).

References

Agger WA, Callister SM, Jobe DA (1992). *In vitro* susceptibilities of *Borrelia burgdorferi* to five oral cephalosporins and ceftriaxone. *Antimicrob Ag Chemother* **36**: 1788.

Avril JL, Mesnard R, Donnio P-Y (1991). *In-vitro* activities of penicillin, amoxycillin and certain cephalosporins, including cefpodoxime, against human isolates of *Pasteurella multocida*. *J Antimicrob Chemother* **28**: 483.

Barry AL, Pfaller MA, Fuchs PC, Packer RR (1994). *In vitro* activities of 12 orally administered antimicrobial agents against four species of bacterial respiratory pathogens from US medical centers in 1992 and 1993. *Antimicrob Ag Chemother* **38**: 2419.

Bhutta ZA, Khan IA, Molla AM (1994). Therapy of multidrug-resistant typhoid fever with oral cefixime vs. intravenous ceftriaxone. *Pediatr Infect Dis J* **13**: 990.

CDC (Centers for Disease Control) (1993). Sexually transmitted diseases treatment guidelines. *MMWR* **42** (No RR-14): 56.

Chachaty E, Depitre C, Mario N *et al.* (1992). Presence of *Clostridium difficile* and antibiotic and beta-lactamase activities in feces of volunteers treated with oral cefixime, oral cefpodoxime proxetil, or placebo. *Antimicrob Ag Chemother* **36**: 2009.

Chachaty E, Bourneix C, Renard S *et al.* (1993). Shedding of *Clostridium difficile*, fecal beta-lactamase activity, and gastrointestinal symptoms in 51 volunteers treated with oral cefixime. *Antimicrob Ag Chemother* **37**: 1432.

Dunnett DM, Moyer MA (1992). Cefixime in the treatment of uncomplicated gonorrhea. *Sex Transm Dis* **19**: 92.

Duverne C, Bouten A, Deslandes A *et al.* (1992). Modification of cefixime bioavailability by nifedipine in humans: involvement of the dipeptide carrier system. *Antimicrob Ag Chemother* **36**: 2462.

Fassbender M, Lode H, Schabert T *et al.* (1993). Pharmacokinetics of new oral cephalosporins, including a new carbacephem. *Clin Infect Dis* **16**: 646.

Fung C-P, Yeo S-F, Livermore DM (1994). Susceptibility of *Moraxella catarrhalis* isolates to beta-lactam antibiotics in relation to beta-lactamase pattern. *J Antimicrob Chemother* **33**: 215.

Gremse DA, Dean PC, Farquhar DS (1994). Cefixime and antibiotic-associated colitis. *Pediatr Infect Dis J* **13**: 331.

Healy DP, Sahai JV, Sterling LP, Racht EM (1989). Influence of an antacid containing aluminium and magnesium on the pharmacokinetics of cefixime. *Antimicrob Ag Chemother* **33**: 1994.

Hoppe JE, Müller J (1990). *In vitro* susceptibilities of *Bordetella pertussis* and *Bordetella parapertussis* to six new oral cephalosporins. *Antimicrob Ag Chemother* **34**: 1442.

Ikeda F, Yokota Y, Mine Y, Tatsuta M (1990). Activity of cefixime against *Helicobacter pylori* and affinities for the penicillin-binding proteins. *Antimicrob Ag Chemother* **34**: 2426.

Janknegt R, van der Meer JWM (1994). Sequential therapy with intravenous and oral cephalosporins. *J Antimicrob Chemother* **33**: 169.

Kiani R, Johnson D, Nelson B (1988). Comparative, multicenter studies of cefixime and amoxicillin in the treatment of respiratory tract infections. *Amer J Med* **85** (Suppl 3A): 6.

Kitzis M-D, Liassine N, Ferrè B et al. (1990). *In vitro* activities of 15 oral beta-lactams against *Klebsiella pneumoniae* harboring new extended-spectrum beta-lactamases. *Antimicrob Ag Chemother* **34**: 1783.

Lehtonen L, Huovinen P (1993). Susceptibility of respiratory tract pathogens in Finland to cefixime and nine other antimicrobial agents. *Scand J Infect Dis* **25**: 373.

MacGowan AP, Holt HA, Bedford KA, Reeves DS (1992). The activity of cefixime against 715 urinary isolates of Enterobacteriaceae isolated from general practice and out-patients in twenty centres across the British Isles. *J Antimicrob Chemother* **30**: 554.

Megran DW, Lefebvre K, Willetts V, Bowie WR (1990). Single-dose oral cefixime versus amoxicillin plus probenecid for the treatment of uncomplicated gonorrhea in men. *Antimicrob Ag Chemother* **34**: 355.

Mendelman PM, Henritzy LL, Chaffin DO et al. (1989). *In vitro* activities and targets of three cephem antibiotics against Haemophilus influenzae. *Antimicrob Ag Chemother* **33**: 1878.

Mortensen JE, Himes SL (1990). Comparative *in vitro* activity of cefixime against *Haemophilus influenzae* isolates, including ampicillin-resistant, non-beta-lactamase-producing isolates from pediatric patients. *Antimicrob Ag Chemother* **34**: 1456.

Nash DR, Flanagan C, Steele LC, Wallace RJ Jr (1991). Comparison of the activity of cefixime and activities of other oral antibiotics against adult clinical isolates of *Moraxella* (*Branhamella*) *catarrhalis* containing BRO-1 and BRO-2 and *Haemophilus influenzae*. *Antimicrob Ag Chemother* **35**: 192.

Nord CE, Movin G, Stalberg D (1988). Impact of cefixime on the normal intestinal microflora. *Scand J Infect Dis* **20**: 547.

Piippo T, Stefansson S, Pitkäjärvi T, Lundberg C (1991). Double-blind comparison of cefixime and cefaclor in the treatment of acute otitis media in children. *Scand J Infect Dis* **23**: 459.

Portilla I, Lutz B, Montalvo M, Mogabgab WJ (1992). Oral cefixime versus intramuscular ceftriaxone in patients with uncomplicated gonococcal infections. *Sex Transm Dis* **19**: 94.

Raz R, Rottensterich E, Leshem Y, Tabenkin H (1994). Double-blind study comparing 3-day regimens of cefixime and ofloxacin in treatment of uncomplicated urinary tract infections in women. *Antimicrob Ag Chemother* **38**: 1176.

Rodriguez WJ, Khan W, Sait T et al. (1993). Cefixime vs cefaclor in the treatment of acute otitis media in children: a randomized, comparative study. *Pediatr Infect Dis J* **12**: 70.

Sader HS, Jones RN, Washington JA et al. (1993). *In vitro* activity of cefpodoxime compared with other oral cephalosporins tested against 5556 recent clinical isolates from five medical centers. *Diagn Microbiol Infect Dis* **17**: 143.

Sanders CC (1989). Beta-lactamase stability and *in vitro* activity of oral cephalosporins against strains possessing well-characterized mechanisms of resistance. *Antimicrob Ag Chemother* **33**: 1313.

Stone JW, Linong G, Andrews JM, Wise R (1989). Cefixime, *in-vitro* activity, pharmacokinetics and tissue penetration. *J Antimicrob Chemother* **23**: 221.

The Medical Letter (1989). Cefixime – a new oral cephalosporin. *The Medical Letter* **31**: 73.

Verdon MS, Douglas JM Jr, Wiggins SD, Handsfield HH (1993). Treatment of uncomplicated gonorrhea with single doses of 200 mg cefixime. *Sex Transm Dis* **20**: 290.

Verghese A, Roberson D, Kalbfleisch JH, Sarubbi F (1990). Randomized comparative study of cefixime versus cephalexin in acute bacterial exacerbations of chronic bronchitis. *Antimicrob Ag Chemother* **34**: 1041.

Westphal JF, Jehl F, Schloegel M et al. (1993). Biliary excretion of cefixime: assessment in patients provided with T-tube drainage. *Antimicrob Ag Chemother* **37**: 1488.

Cefprozil (BMY 28100)

Description

Similar to cefixime (p. 409), cefprozil is an oral third-generation cephalosporin. Its spectrum of activity is wider than that of cephalexin (p. 263) and also slightly wider than that of cefaclor (p. 273). Especially against Gram-negative bacteria its activity is not as wide as that of parenteral third-generation cephalosporins, such as cefotaxime (p. 319) (Chin and Neu, 1987; Eliopoulos *et al.*, 1987).

Sensitive Organisms

1 Gram-positive bacteria

Cefprozil is active against *Staphylococcus aureus*, including beta-lactamase-producing strains, but not methicillin-resistant strains. *Staphylococcus epidermidis* and *Staph. saprophyticus* are also usually sensitive (except methicillin-resistant strains), but *Staph. haemolyticus* and *Staph. hominis* are resistant. *Streptococcus pyogenes* and Groups B, C, F and G streptococci are sensitive. *Streptococcus pneumoniae* is quite sensitive and penicillin G-resistant strains (p. 5) with cefprozil MIC of $4\,\mu$g per ml may be more susceptible to this drug than to penicillin G. *Streptococcus viridans* is sensitive, but strains with high-level penicillin G-resistance are also cefprozil-resistant (MIC $32\,\mu$g per ml) (Table I.33). *Streptococcus bovis* is sensitive but *Enterococcus faecalis* (MIC $16\,\mu$g per ml) is only moderately sensitive and *E. faecium* (MIC $32–64\,\mu$g per ml) is resistant (Table I.33). *Listeria monocytogenes* is sensitive, but *Corynebacterium jeikeium* is resistant. Among Gram-positive anaerobes, the *Peptostreptococci* and *Clostridium* spp. are sensitive. *Clostridium difficile* with an MIC of $4–8\,\mu$g per ml is also moderately sensitive, but the clinical significance of this is not known (Chin and Neu, 1987; Eliopoulos *et al.*, 1987; Kayser, 1987; Leitner *et al.*, 1987; Mazzulli *et al.*, 1990; Thornsberry, 1992; Barry *et al.*, 1994).

2 Gram-negative bacteria

Neisseria meningitidis, N. gonorrhoeae, Haemophilus influenzae and *Moraxella catarrhalis* are usually cefprozil-sensitive, irrespective of beta-lactamase production. Among the Enterobacteriaceae *Escherichia coli, Proteus mirabilis, Citrobacter diversus* and most *Salmonella, Shigella* and *Klebsiella* spp. are sensitive. But *Pr. vulgaris, Citrobacter freundii, Morganella morganii, Serratia marcescens, Yersinia enterocolitica* and the *Providencia* and *Enterobacter* spp. are cefprozil-resistant (Table I.33). The *Acinetobacter* spp., *Ps. aeruginosa*, other *Pseudomonas* spp. and *Stenotrophomonas maltophilia* are resistant. Among Gram-negative anaerobes the *Prevotella* (previously *Bacteroides*) spp. such as *P. melaninogenica* and *Fusobacterium* spp. may be sensitive, but other *Bacteroides* spp., and in particular *B. fragilis*, are resistant (Chin and Neu, 1987; Eliopoulos *et al.*, 1987; Leitner *et al.*, 1987; Scribner *et al.*, 1987; Arguedas *et al.*, 1991; Thornsberry, 1992; Goldstein *et al.*, 1995).

3 Minimum inhibitory concentrations

The MICs of cefprozil for some selected bacterial species are shown in Table I.33.

Organism	MICs (μg per ml)
Gram-positive bacteria	
Staphylococcus aureus (methicillin-sensitive)	1.0
Staphylococcus epidermidis (methicillin-sensitive)	8.0
Streptococcus pneumoniae	0.06
Streptococcus pyogenes	0.06
Streptococcus viridans (penicillin G-sensitive)	0.125
Streptococcus viridans (penicillin G-resistant)	32.0
Enterococcus faecalis	16.0
Enterococcus faecium	64.0
Listeria monocytogenes	4.0
Clostridium difficile	4.0
Gram-negative bacteria	
Neisseria gonorrhoeae	8.0
Haemophilus influenzae	2.0
Moraxella catarrhalis	2.0
Escherichia coli	8.0
Klebsiella pneumoniae	0.25–>64.0
Proteus mirabilis	1.0
Citrobacter diversus	2.0
Enterobacter spp.	>128.0
Pseudomonas aeruginosa	>128.0
Bacteroides fragilis	>128.0

Table I.33
Compiled from data published by Chin and Neu (1987), Eliopoulos *et al.* (1987) and Leitner *et al.* (1987)

Mode of Administration and Dosage

1 Adults

Cefprozil is administered orally either once- or twice-daily. For milder infections such as uncomplicated urinary tract infections or acute Group A beta-hemolytic streptococcal pharyngitis a dosage of 0.5 g once-daily is sufficient (Christenson *et al.*, 1991a,b; McCarty and Renteria, 1992). In more severe infections such as lower respiratory tract infections a dosage of 0.5 g 12-hourly is recommended (Pelletier, 1992).

2 Children

Depending on the nature and severity of infection, cefprozil has been given to children in dosages of 15, 20 or 30 mg per kg per day. The larger dosages have been usually administered orally in two divided doses (Saez-Llorens *et al.*, 1990; Stutman and Arguedas, 1992; Milatovic *et al.*, 1993).

3 Patients with renal failure

In patients with creatinine clearance of <30 ml per min, the dosage of cefprozil should be reduced by 50%. The drug is effectively removed by hemodialysis, and so a supplemental dose of 50% of the maintenance dose should be given following the dialysis procedure (Barriere, 1992).

Serum Levels in Relation to Dosage

After oral administration cefprozil is rapidly absorbed, reaching maximum serum level 1–2 h after administration. After a 0.5 mg oral dose to adults this peak is about 9.3 μg per ml. Doubling the dose nearly doubles the peak serum concentration. After the peak, the serum level falls with a terminal half-life of 1.2 h and by 8 h the serum level is less than 1 μg per ml (Nye *et al.*, 1990; Barbhaiya *et al.*, 1990a). Approximately 94% of the orally administered dose is absorbed

(Barriere, 1992). There is no accumulation of the drug in serum if multiple 0.5 g doses are administered 8- or 12-hourly (Barbhaiya *et al.*, 1990 b; Lode *et al.*, 1992). The presence of food in stomach (Babhaiya *et al.*, 1990c) and the co-administration of antacids (Shyu *et al.*, 1992) do not interfere with the absorption of cefprozil.

In children after the administration of 15 mg per kg and 30 mg per kg single doses, peak concentrations of 11.6 and 15.93 μg per ml, respectively, occurred 1 h after the dose. The respective mean half-lives of cefprozil were 1.77 and 2.14 h (Saez-Llorens *et al.*, 1990). This shows that cefprozil is excreted somewhat more slowly in children than in adults.

Excretion

1 Urine

Most of the absorbed cefprozil is eliminated via the kidney. Overall about 61% of the administered dose is excreted in the urine as the active unchanged drug. The renal clearance is about 200 ml per min. This suggests that cefprozil is excreted by both glomerular filtration and tubular secretion. Mean concentrations of the drug in urine are highest during the first 4 h after the dose and range from 175 to 658 μg per ml following doses of 250 mg and 1 g, respectively (Barbhaiya *et al.*, 1990a,b; Barriere, 1992; Lode *et al.*, 1992).

2 Bile and inactivation in body

More cefprozil is absorbed (94% of dose) (see above) than is excreted in the urine (61% of dose), but it is not known what happens in the body to the fraction not excreted in urine. In patients who have hepatic disease, the kinetic disposition of cefprozil was only minimally altered. The kidney has the primary role in elimination of this drug (Barriere, 1992). No metabolites have been detected in urine (Lode *et al.*, 1992).

Distribution of the Drug in Body

Cefprozil is about 42% serum protein bound (Fassbender *et al.*, 1993). It has been found to penetrate well into skin blister fluid, the mean concentration reached there after an oral dose of 0.5 g was 5.8 μg per ml. The skin blister fluid concentration has been found to decline more slowly than that in plasma (Barbhaiya *et al.*, 1990d). Less than 0.3% of a cefprozil dose has been recovered from the breast milk in the 24 h period after administration (Barriere, 1992). Cefprozil penetrates well into tonsillar and adenoidal tissue. In patients undergoing tonsillectomy and/or adenoidectomy, the median ratios of cefprozil concentration in tonsillar tissue to that of plasma were 0.37 and 0.47 for patients receiving 7.5 mg or 20 mg per kg single doses of cefprozil, respectively. The corresponding median ratios for adenoidal tissue were 0.46 and 0.82, respectively (Shyu *et al.*, 1993).

Toxicity

Adverse effects have been uncommon and similar to those observed with other oral cephalosporins. Rash and urticaria have been occasionally seen. Vomiting and diarrhea have been reported, but diarrhea with cefprozil has been less common than with cefixime (p. 411), which is less completely absorbed. Cefprozil also only causes a minimal disturbance of the normal fecal flora such as slight decrease in enterobacteria and a slight increase in enterococci and *Bacteroides* spp. A few patients have shown slight and reversible increase in liver enzymes (Lode *et al.*, 1992; Wilber *et al.*, 1992). Leukopenia also has been reported (Christenson *et al.*, 1991a).

Clinical Uses of the Drug

1 Group A beta hemolytic streptococcal pharyngitis

Good results have been obtained in this disease using cefprozil 0.5 g daily for adults for 10 days (Christenson *et al.*, 1991a). In a study in children cefprozil, in a dose of 7.5 mg per kg body weight twice a day, was given for 10 days and a control group received oral penicillin V (p. 74). The clinical responses in patients treated with cefprozil were significantly better than those in patients who received penicillin V (95.3 versus 88.1%). Eradication of the original serotype of Group A streptococci was achieved in 91.3% of patients treated with cefprozil, and 87.4% of patients treated with penicillin V; the difference here was not statistically significant. Beta-lactamase-producing *Staph. aureus* was more frequently isolated from the throat flora during penicillin V therapy (Milatovic *et al.*, 1993). Cefprozil has also been superior to cefaclor in the treatment of this disease (McCarty and Renteria, 1992).

Despite these superior results with cefprozil, largely due to the fact that penicillin V is much cheaper, the latter at present still remains the drug of choice for the treatment of this disease. There is evidence that many patients with penicillin V 'bacteriological failures' are actually patients with viral pharyngitis and a streptococcal carrier state. The eradication of carrier state is not important unless there is a rheumatic fever outbreak. A carrier does not develop rheumatic fever. It is possible that oral cephalosporins such as cefprozil may be more effective than penicillin V in eradicating the carrier state. The use of cefprozil perhaps could be justified during a rheumatic fever outbreak. In addition, drugs like cefprozil or clindamycin (p. 597) are more effective for patients who relapse clinically after penicillin treatment. In the pharynx there may be beta-lactamase-producing organisms such as *Staph. aureus* or anaerobes, which do not cause disease, but produce beta-lactamases, which inactivate penicillin, but not drugs like cefprozil or clindamycin. This may explain the superiority of these drugs in the treatment of streptococcal pharyngitis in some cases, but this is still controversial (Peter, 1992).

2 Otitis media

In randomized trials cefprozil has been compared with co-amoxiclav, cefaclor and cefixime for the treatment of this disease. The rate of clinical cure or improvement was similar with all these drugs. However, diarrhea with cefprozil was less common than with cefixime or co-amoxiclav (Stutman and Arguedas, 1992; Gehanno *et al.*, 1994). For routine empirical treatment of uncomplicated acute otitis media, amoxycillin (p. 140) is still the drug of choice, but persistence of signs and symptoms of infection during therapy calls for a change to an antibiotic effective against beta-lactamase-producing bacteria. Then drugs such as co-trimoxazole (p. 864), co-amoxiclav (p. 201) or one of the oral cephalosporins such as cefprozil can be selected (Bluestone, 1992).

3 Lower respiratory tract infections

In the treatment of bronchitis and acute exacerbation of chronic bronchitis, cefprozil 0.5 g 12-hourly has been compared with standard regimens of cefaclor (p. 278), cefuroxime axetil (p. 311) and co-amoxiclav (p. 201). The clinical efficacy of cefprozil was superior to that of cefuroxime axetil, but equal to those of cefaclor and co-amoxiclav. There was less diarrhea in cefprozil-treated patients compared with those treated with co-amoxiclav. The value of cefprozil in the treatment of pneumonia has yet to be established (Pelletier, 1992).

4 Acute uncomplicated urinary tract infections

Cefprozil in a dose of 0.5 g daily, given for 10 days, has efficacy comparable with cefaclor 250 mg, given three times daily, for the same period (Christenson, 1991b; Iravani, 1991).

5 Skin and skin-structure infections

For these infections, caused mainly by streptococci and *Staph. aureus*, cefprozil in a dose of 0.5 g once-daily has about the same efficacy as 250 mg of cefaclor administered three times daily or 400 mg of erythromycin administered four times daily (Nolen, 1992).

References

Arguedas AG, Arrieta AC, Stutman HR *et al.* (1991). *In-vitro* activity of cefprozil (BMY 28100). and loracarbef (LY 163892). against pathogens obtained from middle ear fluid. *J Antimicrob Chemother* **27**: 311.

Barbhaiya RH, Gleason CR, Shyu WC *et al.* (1990a). Phase I study of single-dose BMY-28100, a new oral cephalosporin. *Antimicrob Ag Chemother* **34**: 202.

Barbhaiya RH, Shukla UA, Gleason CR *et al.* (1990b). Phase I study of multiple-dose cefprozil and comparison with cefaclor. *Antimicrob Ag Chemother* **34**: 1198.

Barbhaiya RH, Shukla UA, Gleason CR *et al.* (1990c). Comparison of the effects of food on the pharmacokinetics of cefprozil and cefaclor. *Antimicrob Ag Chemother* **34**: 1210.

Barbhaiya RH, Shukla UA, Gleason CR *et al.* (1990d). Comparison of cefprozil and cefaclor pharmacokinetics and tissue penetration. *Antimicrob Ag Chemother* **34**: 1204.

Barriere SL (1992). Pharmacology and pharmacokinetics of cefprozil. *Clin Infect Dis* **14** (Suppl 2): 184.

Barry AL, Pfaller MA, Fuchs PC, Packer RR (1994). *In vitro* activities of 12 orally administered antimicrobial agents against four species of bacterial respiratory pathogens from US medical centers in 1992 and 1993. *Antimicrob Ag Chemother* **38**: 2419.

Bluestone CD (1992). Current therapy for otitis media and criteria for evaluation of new antimicrobial agents. *Clin Infect Dis* **14** (Suppl 2): 197.

Chin N-X, Neu HC (1987). Comparative antibacterial activity of a new oral cephalosporin, BMY- 28100. *Antimicrob Ag Chemother* **31**: 480.

Christenson JC, Swenson E, Gooch WM III, Herrod JN (1991a). Comparative efficacy and safety of cefprozil (BMY-28100). and cefaclor in the treatment of acute Group A beta-hemolytic streptococcal pharyngitis. *Antimicrob Ag Chemother* **35**: 1127.

Christenson JC, Gooch WM, Herrod JN, Swenson E (1991b). Comparative efficacy and safety of cefprozil and cefaclor in the treatment of acute uncomplicated urinary tract infections. *J Antimicrob Chemother* **28**: 581.

Eliopoulos GM, Reiszner E, Wennersten C, Moellering RC Jr (1987). *In vitro* activity of BMY-28100, a new oral cephalosporin. *Antimicrob Ag Chemother* **31**: 653.

Fassbender M, Lode H, Schaberg T *et al.* (1993). Pharmacokinetics of new oral cephalosporins, including a new carbacephem. *Clin Infect Dis* **16**: 646.

Gehanno P, Berche P, Boucot I *et al.* (1994). Comparative efficacy and safety of cefprozil and amoxycillin/clavulanate in the treatment of acute otitis media in children. *J Antimicrob Chemother* **33**: 1209.

Goldstein EJC, Nesbit CA, Citron DM (1995). Comparative *in vitro* activities of azithromycin, Bay y 3118, levofloxacin, sparfloxacin and 11 other oral antimicrobial agents against 194 aerobic and anaerobic bite wound isolates. *Antimicrob Ag Chemother* **39**: 1097.

Iravani A (1991). Comparison of cefprozil and cefaclor for treatment of acute urinary tract infections in women. *Antimicrob Ag Chemother* **35**: 1940.

Kayser FH (1987). Comparative antibacterial activity of the new oral cephalosporin BMY-28100. *Eur J Clin Microbiol* **6**: 309.

Leitner F, Pursiano TA, Buck RE *et al.* (1987). BMY 28100, a new oral cephalosporin. *Antimicrob Ag Chemother* **31**: 238.

Lode H, Müller C, Borner K *et al.* (1992). Multiple-dose pharmacokinetics of cefprozil and its impact on intestinal flora of volunteers. *Antimicrob Ag Chemother* **36**: 144.

Mazzulli T, Simor AE, Jaeger R *et al.* (1990). Comparative *in vitro* activities of several new fluoroquinolones and beta-lactam antimicrobial agents against community isolates of *Streptococcus pneumoniae*. *Antimicrob Ag Chemother* **34**: 467.

McCarty JM, Renteria A (1992). Treatment of pharyngitis and tonsillitis with cefprozil: review of three multicenter trials. *Clin Infect Dis* **14** (Suppl 2): 224.

Milatovic D, Adam D, Hamilton H, Materman E (1993). Cefprozil versus penicillin V in treatment of streptococcal tonsillopharyngitis. *Antimicrob Ag Chemother* **37**: 1620.

Nolen TM (1992). Clinical trials of cefprozil for treatment of skin and skin-structure infections: review. *Clin Infect Dis* **14** (Suppl 2): 255.

Nye K, O'Neill P, Andrews JM, Wise R (1990). Pharmacokinetics and tissue penetration of cefprozil. *J Antimicrob Chemother* **25**: 831.

Pelletier LL Jr (1992). Review of the experience with cefprozil for the treatment of lower respiratory tract infections. *Clin Infect Dis* **14** (Suppl 2): 238.

Peter G (1992). Streptococcal pharyngitis: current therapy and criteria for evaluation of new agents. *Clin Infect Dis* **14** (Suppl 2): 218.

Saez-Llorens X, Shyu WC, Shelton S *et al.* (1990). Pharmacokinetics of cefprozil in infants and children. *Antimicrob Ag Chemother* **34**: 2152.

Scribner RK, Marks MI, Finkhouse BD (1987). *In vitro* activity of BMY-28100 against common isolates from pediatric infections. *Antimicrob Ag Chemother* **31**: 630.

Shyu WC, Wilber RB, Pittman KA, Barbhaiya RH (1992). Effect of antacid on the bioavailability of cefprozil. *Antimicrob Ag Chemother* **36**: 962.

Shyu WC, Reilly J, Campbell DA *et al.* (1993). Penetration of cefprozil into tonsillar and adenoidal tissues. *Antimicrob Ag Chemother* **37**: 1180.

Stutman HR, Arguedas AG (1992). Comparison of cefprozil with other antibiotic regimens in the treatment of children with acute otitis media. *Clin Infect Dis* **14** (Suppl 2): 204.

Thornsberry C (1992). Review of the *in vitro* antibacterial activity of cefprozil, a new oral cephalosporin. *Clin Infect Dis* **14** (Suppl 2): 189.

Wilber RB, Doyle CA, Durham SJ *et al.* (1992). Safety profile of cefprozil. *Clin Infect Dis* **14** (Suppl 2): 264.

Ceftibuten

Description

Ceftibuten is another third-generation oral cephalosporin, similar to cefixime (p. 409) and cefprozil (p. 414). It has good activity against aerobic Gram-negative bacilli and it is stable to the common plasmid-mediated beta-lactamases (Jones and Barry, 1988; Bragman and Casewell, 1990).

Sensitive Organisms

1 Gram-positive bacteria

Groups A, C and G streptococci are ceftibuten-sensitive, but Group B hemolytic streptococci are usually resistant. *Streptococcus pneumoniae* is susceptible, except that strains with intermediate or high-level penicillin G resistance are ceftibuten-resistant. *Enterococcus faecalis* and other enterococci are resistant. *Staphylococcus aureus*, coagulase-negative staphylococci, *Strep. viridans* and *Strep. bovis* are also resistant as are *Corynebacterium jeikeium*, *Listeria monocytogenes* and Gram-positive anaerobes such as *Peptococcus* and *Peptostreptococcus* spp. and *Clostridium* (Jones and Barry, 1988; Jones, 1993; Neu, 1993).

2 Gram-negative bacteria

Ceftibuten is active against *Neisseria meningitidis*, *N. gonorrhoeae*, *Haemophilus influenzae* and *Moraxella catarrhalis*, irrespective of beta-lactamase production. Most Enterobacteriaceae, such as *Escherichia coli*, the *Klebsiella*, *Proteus*, *Providencia*, *Salmonella* and *Shigella* spp., *Morganella morganii*, *Yersinia enterocolitica* and *Citrobacter diversus* are susceptible. *Citrobacter freundii*, *Serratia marcescens* and the *Enterobacter* spp. are usually resistant. Among other Gram-negative bacteria *Aeromonas* and *Brucella* spp. are sensitive, but most strains of *Acinetobacter* spp. are resistant. *Helicobacter pylori* is sensitive, *Campylobacter jejuni* is only moderately so but *Ps. aeruginosa*, other *Pseudomonas* spp. and *Stenotrophomonas maltophilia* are resistant. *Bacteroides fragilis* and other Gram-negative anaerobes are ceftibuten-resistant (Jones and Barry, 1988; Shawar *et al.*, 1989; Bragman and Casewell, 1990; Wise *et al.*, 1990b; Jones, 1993; Neu, 1993).

Ceftibuten is not hydrolyzed by some extended-spectrum beta-lactamases. Strains of *Klebsiella pneumoniae* which had acquired plasmid-mediated extended-spectrum beta-lactamases and which were resistant to ceftazidime and other third-generation cephalosporins, were generally ceftibuten-sensitive (Kitzis *et al.*, 1990; Jones, 1993). *In vitro* synergism between ceftibuten and aminoglycosides could usually be demonstrated against *E. coli* and *Kl. pneumoniae*, but not against the strains of *Kl. pneumoniae* which produced extended-spectrum beta-lactamases. Combination of ceftibuten and ciprofloxacin showed neither synergy nor antagonism (Guèrillot *et al.*, 1993).

3 Minimum inhibitory concentrations

The MICs of ceftibuten against some selected bacterial species are shown in Table I.34.

Organism	MIC (μg per ml)
Gram-positive bacteria	
Streptococcus pyogenes	0.5
Streptococcus Group B	32.0
Streptococcus Group G	1.0
Streptococcus pneumoniae (penicillin G-sensitive)	8.0
Streptococcus pneumoniae (penicillin G-resistant)	>32.0
Staphylococcus aureus	Resistant
Gram-negative bacteria	
Haemophilus influenzae	≤0.06
Moraxella catarrhalis	4.0
Neisseria gonorrhoeae	0.03
Escherichia coli	0.25
Kllebsiella pneumoniae	0.25
Proteus mirabilis	≤0.06
Citrobacter diversus	≤0.06
Citrobacter freundii	>32.0
Enterobacter aerogenes	>32.0
Morganella morganii	8.0
Serratia marcescens	32.0
Campylobacter jejuni	16.0
Pseudomonas aeruginosa	>32.0
Bacteroides fragilis	>32.0

Table I.34
Compiled from data published by Jones and Barry (1988), Shawar *et al.* (1989) and Neu (1993)

Mode of Administration and Dosage

Ceftibuten is administered orally. The daily adult dosage is 400 mg which is usually given as a single daily dose, but a dosage of 200 mg 12-hourly can also be used (Chirurgi *et al.*, 1991; Neu, 1993). The postantibiotic effect of ceftibuten for *Strep. pyogenes* was 2.7–>10 h, for *Strep. pneumoniae* 1.1–3.4 h, for *H. influenzae* 1–1.1 h and for *M. catarrhalis* 1.5–1.8 h. This suggests that ceftibuten can be administered once-daily (Chin *et al.*, 1993).

In children the dosage is 9 mg per kg once-daily (Barr *et al.*, 1993; Pichichero *et al.*, 1993).

In patients with renal failure the ceftibuten dose only needs to be reduced if the creatinine clearance falls below 49 ml per min. In patients with a creatinine clearance of 30–49 ml per min, ceftibuten should be given in a dosage of 200 mg daily. In those with creatinine clearance of 5–29 ml per min, the dosage should be 100 mg daily. In patients with creatinine clearance of <5 ml per min and who are treated by thrice-weekly hemodialysis, 300 mg of ceftibuten should be given three times weekly i.e. once after each hemodialysis (Kelloway *et al.*, 1991).

Serum Levels in Relation to Dosage

Ceftibuten is administered orally as the microbiologically active *cis* isomer. It is well absorbed from the gastrointestinal tract. About 94% of the administered dose is absorbed. Following oral administration, the metabolite ceftibuten *trans* isomer, with antibacterial activity of about one-eighth that of *cis* isomer, is detected in plasma and accounts for 7–10% of the dose recovered from urine of healthy subjects with normal renal function. Most of ceftibuten circulates in the plasma as the active *cis* isomer. After a 200 mg oral ceftibuten dose to adults, a mean peak serum level of 10.9 μg per ml was obtained 1.8 h after administration. The mean elimination half-life from plasma was 2.5 h. The serum level was still approximately 1 μg per ml 12 h after administration. There was no accumulation of ceftibuten in serum after multiple doses of 200 mg 12-hourly. Food in the stomach slightly delayed and reduced the maximal serum level, but the overall bioavailability was not affected (Wise *et al.*, 1990a; Kelloway *et al.*, 1991; Lin *et al.*,

1995a). Doubling the dose to 400 mg, approximately doubled the serum concentrations (Lin *et al.*, 1995b).

In children, after the administration of a 9 mg per kg dose, the peak serum level was 12–16 μg per ml, attained about 2 h after administration. The mean elimination half-life was 2h and at 12 h the serum level was down to about 1 μg per ml. Food in the stomach slightly affected the rate and extent of absorption of the drug which was administered as a suspension (Kearns *et al.*, 1991; Barr *et al.*, 1993).

Excretion

1 Urine

In healthy volunteers, about 94% of an administered dose of ceftibuten is excreted in urine as either the unchanged active *cis* isomer or as the metabolite *trans* isomer. The *trans* isomer accounts for only 7–10% of the dose recovered in the urine in healthy volunteers. In adults practically all the administered dose of ceftibuten is eliminated via the kidney (Wise *et al.*, 1990a; Kelloway *et al.*, 1991). It is possible that in children younger than 5 years there is some non-renal elimination of ceftibuten, but the data are not conclusive (Kearns *et al.*, 1991; Barr *et al.*, 1993).

Distribution of the Drug in Body

Ceftibuten penetrates rapidly and well into inflammatory exudates (Wise *et al.*, 1990a). It also penetrates into the middle ear fluid in children with acute otitis media; within 4 h concentrations in middle ear fluid were similar to those in plasma (Barr *et al.*, 1993). Ceftibuten is 63% serum protein bound (Fassbender *et al.*, 1993).

Toxicity

Reported toxic reactions have been mild and similar to those seen with other cephalosporins. Eosinophilia, elevated serum transaminase, mild nausea and diarrhea have been the main adverse effects (Chirurgi *et al.*, 1991; Pichichero *et al.*, 1993).

Clinical Uses of the Drug

1 Group A hemolytic streptococcal pharyngitis

Similar to cefprozil (p. 416), ceftibuten in one clinical trial was found to be superior to penicillin V in the treatment of streptococcal pharyngitis. Both clinical improvement and eradication of streptococci from the pharynx were more satisfactory in the ceftibuten-treated children (Pichichero *et al.*, 1993). The use of third-generation oral cephalosporins for the treatment of this disease is discussed on p. 417.

2 Bronchitis

In one relatively small study ceftibuten appeared as safe and as effective as cefaclor (p. 278) for the treatment of this disease (Chirurgi *et al.*, 1991).

References

Barr WH, Affrime M, Lin C-C, Batra V (1993). Pharmacokinetics of ceftibuten in children. *Pediatr Infect Dis J* **12**: S55.

Bragman SGL, Casewell MW (1990). The *in-vitro* activity of ceftibuten against 475 clinical isolates of Gram-negative bacilli, compared with cefuroxime and cefadroxil. *J Antimicrob Chemother* **25**: 221.

Chin NX, Huang HB, Neu HC (1993). Postantibiotic effect of ceftibuten on respiratory pathogens. *Pediatr Infect Dis J* **12**: S45.

Chirurgi VA, Edelstein H, Oster SE *et al.* (1991). Ceftibuten versus cefaclor for the treatment of bronchitis. *J Antimicrob Chemother* **28**: 577.

Fassbender M, Lode H, Schaberg T *et al.* (1993). Pharmacokinetics of new oral cephalosporins, including a new carbacephem. *Clin Infect Dis* **16**: 646.

Guèrillot F, Carret G, Flandrois JP (1993). A statistical evaluation of the bactericidal effects of ceftibuten in combination with aminoglycosides and ciprofloxacin. *J Antimicrob Chemother* **32**: 685.

Jones RN (1993). Ceftibuten: a review of antimicrobial activity, spectrum and other microbiological features. *Pediatr Infect Dis J* **12**: S37.

Jones RN, Barry AL (1988). Antimicrobial activity, spectrum, and recommendations for disk diffusion susceptibility testing of ceftibuten (7432-S; SCH 39720), a new orally administered cephalosporin. *Antimicrob Ag Chemother* **32**: 1576.

Kearns GL, Reed MD, Jacobs RF *et al.* (1991). Single-dose pharmacokinetics of ceftibuten (SCH 39720) in infants and children. *Antimicrob Ag Chemother* **35**: 2078.

Kelloway JS, Awni WM, Lin CC *et al* (1991). Pharmacokinetics of ceftibuten-*cis* and its trans metabolite in healthy volunteers and in patients with chronic renal insufficiency. *Antimicrob Ag Chemother* **35**: 2267.

Kitzis M-D, Liassine N, Ferrè B *et al.* (1990). *In vitro* activities of 15 oral beta-lactams against *Klebsiella pneumoniae* harboring new extended-spectrum beta-lactamases. *Antimicrob Ag Chemother* **34**: 1783.

Lin C, Radwanski E, Afrime M, Cayen MN (1995a). Multiple-dose pharmacokinetics of ceftibuten in healthy volunteers. *Antimicrob Ag Chemother* **39**: 356.

Lin C, Lim J, Radwanski E *et al.* (1995b). Pharmacokinetics and dose proportionality of ceftibuten in men. *Antimicrob Ag Chemother* **39**: 359.

Neu HC (1993). Ceftibuten: minimal inhibitory concentrations, post-antibiotic effect, beta-lactamase stability – a rationale for dosing programs. *Pediatr Infect Dis J* **12**: S49.

Pichichero ME, McLinn SE, Gooch WM III *et al.* (1993). Ceftibuten vs. penicillin V in Group A beta-hemolytic streptococcal pharyngitis. *Pediatr Infect Dis J* **12**: S64.

Shawar R, LaRocco M, Cleary TG (1989). Comparative *in vitro* activity of ceftibuten (Sch 39720) against bacterial enteropathogens. *Antimicrob Ag Chemother* **33**: 781.

Wise R, Nye K, O'Neill P *et al.* (1990a). Pharmacokinetics and tissue penetration of ceftibuten. *Antimicrob Ag Chemother* **34**: 1053.

Wise R, Andrews JM, Ashby JP, Thornber D (1990b). Ceftibuten – *in vitro* activity against respiratory pathogens, beta-lactamase stability and mechanism of action. *J Antimicrob Chemother* **26**: 209.

Cefpodoxime

Description

Cefpodoxime is another oral third-generation cephalosporin, which has good stability to beta-lactamases and activity against Gram-negative and some Gram-positive bacteria. It is not absorbed from the gastrointestinal tract as such; therefore the carboxy group on the cephem nucleus of cefpodoxime has been esterified to produce the oral prodrug, antibacterially inactive cefpodoxime proxetil. This ester is about 50% absorbed; thereafter it is de-esterified in the intestinal mucosa and the active drug cefpodoxime is released into the blood (Borin *et al.*, 1990; Sader *et al.*, 1993).

Sensitive Organism

1 Gram-positive bacteria

The hemolytic streptococci of Groups A, B, C, G and F are cefpodoxime-sensitive. Penicillin-sensitive strains of *Streptococcus pneumoniae* are also susceptible, but strains of pneumococci with any degree of penicillin G resistance have higher MICs for cefpodoxime than those for penicillin G-sensitive strains (Table I.35). *Staphylococcus aureus* and coagulase-negative staphylococci, irrespective of beta-lactamase production are susceptible, but methicillin-resistant strains are not. *Enterococcus faecalis* and other enterococci are cefpodoxime-resistant (Fass and Helsel, 1988; Jones and Barry, 1988; Spangler *et al.*, 1993; Sader *et al.*, 1993). *Streptococcus viridans*, *Pasteurella multocida* and the anaerobic cocci and *Clostridium* spp., including *Cl. difficile* are sometimes susceptible (Wise *et al.*, 1990; Avril *et al.*, 1991; Sader *et al.*, 1993).

2 Gram-negative bacteria

Neisseria meningitidis, *N. gonorrhoeae* and *Haemophilus influenzae* are cefpodoxime-sensitive, irrespective of beta-lactamase production (Jones and Barry, 1988; Li-Puma *et al.*, 1990; Fekete *et al.*, 1991; Valentini *et al.*, 1994). The same is true for *Moraxella catarrhalis* (Sarubbi *et al.*, 1989), but the MICs for ampicillin-resistant non-beta-lactamase producing *H. influenzae* strains are somewhat elevated (Table I.35). *Bordetella pertussis* and *B. parapertussis* are moderately resistant (Hoppe and Müller, 1990). The Enterobacteriaceae such as *Escherichia coli*, the *Klebsiella*, *Salmonella* and *Shigella* spp., *Citrobacter diversus*, *Proteus mirabilis*, *Pr. vulgaris*, *Providencia rettgeri* and *Providencia stuartii* are usually cefpodoxime-sensitive. *Enterobacter* spp., *Citrobacter freundii*, *Serratia marcescens*, *Morganella morganii* and *Yersinia enterocolitica* are usually resistant (Fass and Helsel, 1988; Jones and Barry, 1988; Wise *et al.*, 1990; Sader *et al.*, 1993; Valentini *et al.*, 1994).

Among other aerobic Gram-negative bacteria the Aeromonas spp. and *Acinetobacter* spp. are usually resistant, as is *Campylobacter jejuni*. *Pseudomonas aeruginosa*, other *Pseudomonas* spp. and *Stenotrophomonas maltophilia* are always resistant (Fass and Helsel, 1988; Sader *et al.*, 1993; Valentini *et al.*, 1994).

The Gram-negative anaerobes such as *Bacteroides fragilis* are cefpodoxime-resistant (Wise *et al.*, 1990; Sader *et al.*, 1993). The anaerobic Gram-negative coccobacillus, *Actinobacillus actinomycetemcomitans*, which causes peridontal disease, is cefpodoxime-sensitive. The drug also appeared to enhance the action of neutrophils against this organism (Baker *et al.*, 1995).

3 Minimum inhibitory concentrations

The MICs of cefpodoxime against some selective bacterial species are shown in Table I.35.

Organism	MICs (μg per ml)
Gram-positive bacteria	
Staphylococcus aureus	4.0
Streptococcus pyogenes	0.015
Streptococcus pneumoniae:	
penicillin G-sensitive	0.25
intermediate resistance	4.0
penicillin G-resistant	4.0
Gram-negative bacteria	
Neisseria gonorrhoeae	0.06
Haemophilus influenzae:	
ampicillin-sensitive	0.12
beta-lactamase producer	0.25
intrinsically ampicillin-resistant	1.0
Moraxella catarrhalis	1.0
Escherichia coli	1.0
Klebsiella pneumoniae	1.0
Citrobacter diversus	0.25
Citrobacter freundii	>16.0
Enterobacter aerogenes	>16.0
Proteus mirabilis	0.06
Pseudomonas aeruginosa	2.0–>16.0
Bacteroides fragilis	8.0–>128.0

Table I.35
Compiled from data published by Fass and Helsel (1988), Jones and Barry (1988), Dabernat *et al.* (1990), Wise *et al.* (1990), Sader *et al.* (1993) and Spangler *et al.* (1993)

Mode of Administration and Dosage

The dosage of cefpodoxime proxetil is expressed in milligrams of active cefpodoxime. A dosage of 100 mg 12-hourly is sufficient for relatively mild infections caused by highly susceptible organisms such as streptococcal pharyngitis and acute bronchitis. A dosage of 200 mg 12-hourly is recommended for the treatment of more severe infections such as bacterial pneumonia or acute exacerbations of chronic bronchitis (Periti *et al.*, 1990; Safran, 1990; Portier *et al.*, 1994).

In patients with renal failure, a dosage reduction is appropriate if the creatinine clearance is below 50 ml per min. Patients with a creatinine clearance between 30 and 49 ml per min should be given a cefpodoxime proxetil dosage of 200 mg every 12–24 h and for those with creatinine clearance between 5–29 ml per min, a dosage of 200 mg every 24 h is sufficient (St Peter *et al.*, 1992). Hemodialysis removes nearly 25% of the administered dose and therefore a supplemental dose after this procedure is needed. Peritoneal dialysis only has a minimal effect on cefpodoxime clearance, so in renal failure patients, treated by continuous ambulatory peritoneal dialysis, supplemental doses are not necessary. A single 200-mg daily dose is sufficient for these (Johnson *et al.*, 1993).

Serum Levels in Relation to Dosage

After a single 200-mg dose of oral cefpodoxime proxetil, a mean peak serum level of 2.18 μg per ml of cefpodoxime is reached in about 3 h. The serum level thereafter falls and it is less than 0.5 μg per ml in 12 h. The elimination half-life is 2.7 h. If 400 mg cefpodoxime proxetil is administered the serum levels are approximately doubled. Cefpodoxime does not accumulate in serum if 200-mg or 400-mg doses are given every 12 h. Altogether approximately 50% of the administered dose of cefpodoxime proxetil is absorbed after oral administration and released into the circulation as active cefpodoxime (Borin *et al.*, 1990; O'Neill *et al.*, 1990; Tremblay *et al.*, 1990).

Cefpodoxime proxetil is slightly better absorbed if it is given together with food (Wise, 1990; Borin and Forbes, 1995). Optimal absorption of cefpodoxime requires low gastric pH. Therefore the co-administration of antacids and H_2 receptor antagonists significantly reduce the absorption of this drug (Saathoff *et al.*, 1992).

Excretion

Cefpodoxime excretion is predominantly renal. Approximately 80% of the absorbed dose is excreted in urine as the active drug (Tremblay *et al.*, 1990). The mean 8–12 h urine concentration following 200 mg of cefpodoxime was 19.8 μg per ml and from 12–24 h, 3.9 μg per ml (Wise, 1990). The drug is excreted by both glomerular filtration and tubular secretion. Probenecid delays tubular secretion resulting in higher serum levels (St Peter *et al.*, 1992).

A small amount of absorbed cefpodoxime undergoes biotransformation in humans (Johnson *et al.*, 1993).

Distribution of the Drug in Body

Cefpodoxime is approximately 40% serum protein bound (Fassbender *et al.*, 1993). The drug has penetrated into blister fluid reaching concentrations there which were 67–103% of the serum levels at the time (Borin *et al.*, 1990; O'Neill *et al.*, 1990). The mean penetration of cefpodoxime in bronchial mucosal fluid was recorded as 54% (Baldwin *et al.*, 1992). The mean concentrations of this drug in lung tissue were recorded as 0.63, 0.52 and 0.19 μg per g at 3, 6 and 12 h after administration of a 200-mg cefpodoxime proxetil dose, respectively (Couraud *et al.*, 1990). In another study the ratios between concentrations in lung parenchyma and simultaneous concentrations in plasma were 84.7 and 51.2% at 3 and 6 h, respectively, after administration of 200 mg oral cefpodoxime proxetil (Muller-Serieys *et al.*, 1992). In pleural effusions in patients who received a single 200-mg dose, the concentrations were 0.62, 1.84 and 0.78 μg per ml at 3, 6 or 12 h after the dose, respectively (Dumont *et al.*, 1990). In tonsillar tissue after a dose of 100 mg of cefpodoxime proxetil, the concentrations after 4 and 7 h were 0.24 and 0.09 μg per g, respectively, this being approximately 23% of plasma concentrations (Gehanno *et al.*, 1990a).

Toxicity

Similar to other cephalosporins, cefpodoxime proxetil is a drug with low toxicity. Skin eruptions and pruritus have occurred in a few patients. Neutropenia, eosinophilia and mildly abnormal liver function tests have also been noted infrequently. Nausea, vomiting, soft stools and diarrhea have been slightly more frequent. During clinical trials up until 1990, no pseudomembranous colitis had been observed (Safran, 1990). In one trial six healthy adult volunteers were given 400 mg of oral cefpodoxime proxetil daily for 10 days. Before treatment no volunteers had *Cl. difficile* in stools, but during treatment *Cl. difficile* was detected in the stools of all volunteers. These strains were cefpodoxime-resistant. Intestinal side-effects were limited to modification of stool consistency. There was no association between the passage of loose stools and carriage of toxigenic or non-toxigenic strains of *Cl. difficile*. However, there was a significant correlation between the passage of loose stools and the presence of fecal antibiotic activity (Chachaty *et al.*, 1992). In another study with healthy volunteers overgrowth of enterococci and yeasts were noted during administration of cefpodoxime proxetil (Edlund *et al.*, 1994).

Clinical Uses of the Drug

1 Group A hemolytic streptococcal pharyngitis

A total of 220 adults and children over 10 yeas of age with this disease were randomized to receive either cefpodoxime proxetil 100 mg 12-hourly for 5 days or penicillin V 600 mg 8-hourly orally for 10 days. Clinical and bacteriological cure was high (over 90%) in both groups, but the advantage of cefpodoxime appeared to be the shorter course of treatment (Portier *et al.*, 1994). The possible role of the oral third-generation cephalosporins in the treatment of streptococcal pharyngitis is discussed on p. 417.

2 Respiratory tract infections

For the treatment of bacterial sinusitis, cefpodoxime (84% clinical cure) was found to be superior to cefaclor (68% clinical cure) (Gehanno *et al.*, 1990b). In patients with bronchopneumonia cefpodoxime proxetil 200 mg 12-hourly orally was equally as effective as i.m. ceftriaxone 1 g daily, both given for a 10-day period (Zuck *et al.*, 1990). In patients with exacerbations of chronic bronchitis cefpodoxime proxetil was effective and the results of treatment were similar to those obtained with co-amoxiclav (p. 200) (Periti *et al.*, 1990).

3 Otitis media

In one clinical study cefpodoxime was found to be superior to amoxycillin/clavulanic acid for the treatment of otitis media in children (Gehanno *et al.*, 1994).

4 Gonorrhea

In uncomplicated disease in males a single oral dose of cefpodoxime proxetil 100 mg or even 50 mg was curative (Novak *et al.*, 1992).

References

Avril JL, Mesnard R, Donnio P-Y (1991). *In-vitro* activities of penicillin, amoxycillin and certain cephalosporins, including cefpodoxime, against human isolates of *Pasteurella multocida*. *J Antimicrob Chemother* **28**: 473.

Baker PJ Busby WF, Wilson ME (1995). Subinhibitory concentrations of cefpodoxime alter membrane protein expression of *Actinobacillus actinomycetemcomitans* and enhance its susceptibility to killing by neutrophils. *Antimicrob Ag Chemother* **39**: 406.

Baldwin DR, Wise R, Andrews JM, Honeybourne D (1992). Concentrations of cefpodoxime in serum and bronchial mucosal biopsies. *J Antimicrob Chemother* **30**: 67.

Borin MT, Forbes KK (1995). Effect of food on absorption of cefpodoxime proxetil oral suspension in adults. *Antimicrob Ag Chemother* **39**: 273.

Borin MT, Hughes GS, Spillers CR, Patel RK (1990). Pharmacokinetics of cefpodoxime in plasma and skin blister fluid following oral dosing of cefpodoxime proxetil. *Antimicrob Ag Chemother* **34**: 1094.

Chachaty E, Depitre C, Mario N et al. (1992). Presence of *Clostridium difficile* and antibiotic and beta-lactamase activities in feces of volunteers treated with oral cefixime, and cefpodoxime proxetil, or placebo. *Antimicrob Ag Chemother* **36**: 2009.

Couraud L, Andrews JM, Lecoeur H et al. (1990). Concentrations of cefpodoxime in plasma and lung tissue after a single oral dose of cefpodoxime proxetil. *J Antimicrob Chemother* **26** (Suppl E): 35.

Dabernat H, Avril JL, Boussougant Y (1990). *In-vitro* activity of cefpodoxime against pathogens responsible for community-acquired respiratory tract infections. *J Antimicrob Chemother* **26** (Suppl E): 1.

Dumont R, Guetat F, Andrews JM et al. (1990). Concentrations of cefpodoxime in plasma and pleural fluid after a single oral dose of cefpodoxime proxetil. *J Antimicrob Chemother* **26** (Suppl E): 41.

Edlund C, Stark C, Nord CE(1994). The relationship between an increase in beta-lactamase activity after oral administration of three new cephalosporins and protection against intestinal ecological disturbances. *J Antimicrob Chemother* **34**: 127.

Fass RJ, Helsel VL(1988). *In vitro* activity of U-76252 (CS-807), a new oral cephalosporin. *Antimicrob Ag Chemother* **32**: 1082.

Fassbender M, Lode H, Schaberg T et al. (1993). Pharmacokinetics of new oral cephalosporins, including a new carbacephem. *Clin Infect Dis* **16**: 646.

Fekete T, Woodwell J, Cundy KR (1991). Susceptibility of *Neisseria gonorrhoeae* to cefpodoxime: determination of MICs and disk diffusion zone diameters. *Antimicrob Ag Chemother* **35**: 497.

Gehanno P, Andrews JM, Ichou F et al. (1990a). Concentrations of cefpodoxime in plasma and tonsillar tissue after a single oral dose of cefpodoxime proxetil. *J Antimicrob Chemother* **26** (Suppl E): 47.

Gehanno P, Depondt J, Barry B et al. (1990b). Comparison of cefpodoxime proxetil with cefaclor in the treatment of sinusitis. *J Antimicrob Chemother* **26** (Suppl E): 87.

Gehanno P, Barry B, Bobin S, Safran C (1994). Twice daily cefpodoxime proxetil compared with thrice daily amoxicillin/clavulanic acid for treatment of acute otitis media in children. *Scand J Infect Dis* **26**: 577.

Hoppe JE, Müller J (1990). *In vitro* susceptibilities of *Bordetella pertussis* and *Bordetella parapertussis* to six new oral cephalosporins. *Antimicrob Ag Chemother* **34**: 1442.

Johnson CA, Ateshkadi A, Zimmerman SW et al. (1993). Pharmacokinetics and *ex vivo* susceptibility of cefpodoxime proxetil in patients receiving continuous ambulatory peritoneal dialysis. *Antimicrob Ag Chemother* **37**: 2650.

Jones RN, Barry AL (1988). Antimicrobial activity and disk diffusion susceptibility testing of U-76,253A (R-3746), the active metabolite of the new cephalosporin ester, U-76,252 (CS-807). *Antimicrob Ag Chemother* **32**: 443.

Li Puma JJ, Daley B, Stull TL (1990). *In-vitro* activities of trospectomycin, cefpodoxime, and second-generation cephalosporins against *Haemophilus influenzae* type b. *J Antimicrob Chemother* **25**: 535.

Muller-Serieys C, Bancal C, Dombret MC et al. (1992). Penetration of cefpodoxime proxetil in lung parenchyma and epithelial lining fluid of noninfected patients. *Antimicrob Ag Chemother* **36**: 2099.

Novak E, Paxton LM, Tubbs HJ et al. (1992). Orally administered cefpodoxime proxetil for treatment of uncomplicated gonococcal urethritis in males: a dose-response study. *Antimicrob Ag Chemother* **36**: 1764.

O'Neill P, Nye K, Douce G et al. (1990). Pharmacokinetics and inflammatory fluid penetration of cefpodoxime proxetil in volunteers. *Antimicrob Ag Chemother* **34**: 232.

Periti P, Novelli A, Schildwachter G et al. (1990). Efficiency and tolerance of cefpodoxime proxetil compared with co-amoxiclav in the treatment of exacerbation of chronic bronchitis. *J Antimicrob Chemother* **26** (Suppl E): 63.

Portier H, Chavanet P, Waldner-Combernoux A et al. (1994). Five versus ten days treatment of streptococcal pharyngotonsillitis: a randomized controlled trial comparing cefpodoxime proxetil and phenoxymethyl penicillin. *Scand J Infect Dis* **26**: 59.

Saathoff N, Lode H, Neider K et al. (1992). Pharmacokinetics of cefpodoxime proxetil and interactions with an antacid and an H$_2$ receptor antagonist. *Antimicrob Ag Chemother* **36**: 796.

Sader HS, Jones RN, Washington JA et al. (1993). *In vitro* activity of cefpodoxime compared with other oral cephalosporins tested against 5556 recent clinical isolates from five medical centers. *Diagn Microbiol Infect Dis* **17**: 143.

Safran C (1990). Cefpodoxime proxetil: dosage, efficacy and tolerance in adults suffering from respiratory tract infections. *J Antimicrob Chemother* **26** (Suppl E): 93.

Sarubbi FA, Verghese A, Caggiano C et al. (1989). *In vitro* activity of cefpodoxime proxetil (U-76,252; CS-807). against clinical isolates of *Branhamella catarrhalis*. *Antimicrob Ag Chemother* **33**: 113.

Spangler SK, Jacobs MR, Pankuch GA, Appelbaum PC (1993). Susceptibility of 170 penicillin-susceptible and penicillin-resistant pneumococci to six oral cephalosporins, four quinolones, desacetylcefotaxime, Ro 23–9424 and RP 67829. *J Antimicrob Chemother* **31**: 273.

St Peter JV, Borin MT, Hughes GS et al. (1992). Disposition of cefpodoxime proxetil in healthy volunteers and patients with impaired renal function. *Antimicrob Ag Chemother* **36**: 126.

Tremblay D, Dupront A, Ho C *et al.* (1990). Pharmacokinetics of cefpodoxime in young and elderly volunteers after single doses. *J Antimicrob Chemother* **26** (Suppl E): 21.

Valentini S, Coratza G, Rossolini GM *et al.* (1994). *In-vitro* evaluation of cefpodoxime. *J Antimicrob Chemother* **33**: 495.

Wise R (1990). The pharmacokinetics of the oral cephalosporins – a review. *J Antimicrob Chemother* **26** (Suppl E): 13.

Wise R, Andrews JM, Ashby JP, Thornber D (1990). The *in-vitro* activity of cefpodoxime: a comparison with other oral cephalosporins. *J Antimicrob Chemother* **25**: 541.

Zuck P, Rio Y, Ichou F (1990). Efficacy and tolerance of cefpodoxime proxetil compared with ceftriaxone in vulnerable patients with bronchopneumonia. *J Antimicrob Chemother* **26** (Suppl E): 71.

Streptomycin

Description

Streptomycin was isolated from *Streptomyces griseus* in 1944 by Schatz, Bugie and Waksman. It belongs to a group of antibiotics known as the aminoglycosides or aminohexoses, which are basic compounds containing amino sugars. They also have an aminocyclitol structure and are more correctly called aminoglycoside aminocyclitols (Moellering, 1983). Many streptomycin salts can be prepared, but the sulfate, being the least painful and irritative on i.m. injection, is used clinically.

Sensitive Organisms

1 Mycobacteria

Streptomycin is particularly active against both human and bovine strains of *Mycobacterium tuberculosis*. Some strains of *M. kansasii* (Harris *et al.*, 1975; Pezzia *et al.*, 1981) and *M. marinum* (Wallace and Wiss, 1981) may be streptomycin-sensitive, but in general these and the other 'atypical' mycobacteria are streptomycin-resistant (Kuze *et al.*, 1981) (p. 1211). Although *M. ulcerans* is usually sensitive to streptomycin *in vitro*, infection due to this organism does not usually respond to treatment with any chemotherapeutic agents (p. 1212). Chiodini *et al.* (1984) isolated three strains of unclassified *Mycobacterium* spp. from patients with Crohn's disease, which were streptomycin-sensitive. Streptomycin has only a low bactericidal activity against the *Mycobacterium avium* complex (Heifets and Lindholm-Levy, 1989). In experimental animals, the therapeutic activity of streptomycin against infections by these mycobacteria is improved if liposome-encapsulated streptomycin is used (Ashtekar *et al.*, 1991; Gangadharam *et al.*, 1991; 1995; Majumdar *et al.*, 1992). In animals, combined streptomycin/clofazimine therapy is also more effective than streptomycin alone for treatment of infections by these organisms (Gangadharam and Parikh, 1992).

Streptomycin, used in high doses (150 mg per kg body weight) is effective for *M. leprae* infection in the mouse foot-pad. There is no evidence that streptomycin and other aminoglycosides are useful in the treatment of human leprosy (Gelber *et al.*, 1984).

2 Gram-negative bacteria

Streptomycin is active against a large number of Gram-negative bacteria such as *Escherichia coli*, the *Enterobacter*, *Klebsiella*, *Proteus*, *Providencia*, *Serratia*, *Citrobacter*, *Salmonella*, *Shigella* and *Brucella* spp., *Neisseria meningitidis*, *N. gonorrhoeae*, *Haemophilus influenzae*, *H. ducreyi*, *Pasteurella multocida*, *Francisella tularensis*, *Campylobacter* and *Yersinia* spp., such as *Y. pestis*, *Y. pseudotuberculosis* and *Y. enterocolitica*. Some strains of *Pseudomonas aeruginosa* and *Stenotrophomonas maltophilia* are also sensitive (Moellering, 1983; Sanson-Le Pors *et al.*, 1985; Bosch *et al.*, 1986). The anaerobes, such as *Bacteroides fragilis*, are streptomycin-resistant (Kislak, 1972; Schlessinger, 1988) (p. 432).

3 Gram-positive bacteria

Some strains of *Staphylococcus aureus* are sensitive. Resistance of this organism to streptomycin is plasmid-mediated, but a transposon can also be involved (Udo and Grubb, 1991). Most other Gram-positive cocci and bacilli are resistant. Groups A, B and G streptococci, viridans streptococci and non-enterococcal Group D streptococci, such as *Streptococcus bovis*, are usually relatively resistant to streptomycin (MICs 5.0–250 μg per ml). This is referred to as low-level resistance, and organisms with this resistance are killed synergistically by penicillin G/streptomycin combination. This synergism probably occurs because penicillin G has a direct effect on the membrane potential (p. 432), leading to stimulation of streptomycin uptake (Yee *et al.*, 1986). Some strains of all these streptococci can exhibit high-level streptomycin-resistance (MICs >2000 µg per ml). These strains are not killed synergistically by a penicillin G and streptomycin combination, but they usually are by a penicillin/gentamicin combination (Horodniceanu *et al.*, 1982; Farber *et al.*, 1983; Enzler *et al.*, 1987; Farber and Yee, 1987).

Enterococcus faecalis is always resistant to concentrations of streptomycin which can be attained *in vivo*, but penicillin G and streptomycin act synergistically against some strains *in vitro* and *in vivo* (Matsumoto *et al.*, 1980). Strains of *E. faecalis* unaffected by this combination are highly streptomycin-resistant (MICs ≥2,000 µg per ml). In contrast, strains against which the two drugs act synergistically, require only 250 µg per ml or less of streptomycin alone for inhibition (Ruhen and Darrell, 1973; Eliopoulos *et al.*, 1984). In clinical isolates collected in the UK in 1975, 23% of *E. faecalis* strains had a high-level resistance to streptomycin. These strains usually had a low level of resistance to gentamicin, tobramycin and amikacin; each of these aminoglycosides when combined with penicillin G or amoxycillin showed synergism against the organisms (Basker *et al.*, 1977). Of 203 strains of *E. faecalis* isolated at the Massachusetts General Hospital during the period 1973–1976, depending on the source of the isolate, 36–54% had high-level resistance to streptomycin, 16–49% to kanamycin and 0.14% to amikacin. A combination of penicillin G and amikacin failed to show synergism against a number of strains (Calderwood *et al.*, 1977), but penicillin G plus gentamicin or tobramycin were synergistic against all strains tested. Combinations of penicillin G and sisomicin (Calderwood *et al.*, 1977; Gutschik *et al.*, 1977) or penicillin G and netilmicin (Sanders, 1977) were also synergistic against *E. faecalis* strains highly resistant to streptomycin. Despite extensive use of gentamicin, it was only in 1983 that *E. faecalis* strains with 'high-level' gentamicin and other aminoglycoside resistance were reported. With these strains it appeared initially that penicillin G/aminoglycoside synergism could not be obtained with any of the available aminoglycosides. However, it was later reported that, presumably because streptomycin had been used very little for the treatment of *E. faecalis* endocarditis in recent years, some 20% of strains exhibiting high-level gentamicin-resistance did not show high-level resistance to streptomycin. With such strains penicillin G/streptomycin could be used to treat *E. faecalis* endocarditis successfully (Wurtz *et al.*, 1991; Watanakunakorn, 1992).

The number of strains of 'streptomycin-susceptible' *E. faecalis* affected synergistically by antibiotic combinations containing either 20 or 10 µg per ml of streptomycin, is similar, but the magnitude of killing is greater with combinations containing 20 µg per ml of streptomycin (Matsumoto *et al.*, 1980). Based on these *in vitro* data, streptomycin dosages designed to achieve a peak serum concentration of 20 µg per ml appear to be preferable to lower dosages when *E. faecalis* endocarditis is treated by penicillin G/streptomycin. High-level streptomycin-resistance in clinical enterococcal isolates is either due to the production of streptomycin-modifying enzymes or a ribosomal resistance to the drug (p. 432) (Eliopoulos *et al.*, 1984).

Vancomycin and streptomycin in combination are synergistic against some strains of *E. faecalis* (Westenfelder *et al.*, 1973; Kaye, 1982).

Some of the Actinomycetes (p. 435), such as *Streptomyces somaliensis* and *Actinomadura madurae*, may be sensitive to streptomycin (Mahgoub, 1976; Tight and Bartlett, 1981).

4 Acquired resistance

Practically all of the bacteria usually sensitive to streptomycin, including *M. tuberculosis*, can readily become resistant. Patients who have not received previous treatment, but who have tubercle bacilli resistant to streptomycin or other antituberculosis drugs, are described as having primary drug-resistance. This is relatively rare in countries such as the UK, North America and Australia. Studies in Massachusetts in 1972 and 1975/76 showed prevalence of primary resistance to streptomycin of 1.65 and 2.05%, respectively (Stottmeier and Burkes, 1974; Stottmeier and Baker, 1977). In the early 1980s in the USA primary drug-resistance of *M. tuberculosis* to streptomycin (3.8%) and other antituberculosis drugs did not appear to be increasing (CDC, 1983) (p. 1180).

Primary drug-resistance to streptomycin and other antituberculosis drugs was higher in developing countries such as South-East Asia, Africa, the Philippines and Latin America (Dutt and Stead, 1982). Acquired (secondary) drug-resistance in tuberculosis occurs as a result of previous chemotherapy (p. 1180).

As streptomycin has been used less than other antituberculosis drugs in recent years, the outbreaks in New York, USA and elsewhere of multidrug-resistant tuberculosis, has shown *M.*

tuberculosis strains resistant to drugs such as isoniazid and rifampicin, and less so to streptomycin, but streptomycin-resistant strains have also been encountered (Bloch *et al.*, 1994) (p. 1181).

Transposons and plasmids have not been found in streptomycin-resistant strains of *M. tuberculosis*. The resistance appears to be due to a mutation in the gene which encodes ribosomal protein, but a permeability barrier may also be responsible (Honoré and Cole, 1994; Meier *et al.*, 1994).

Streptomycin-resistant Gram-negative bacilli have been common for many years. Sabath (1969) reported that 50% of *E. coli*, and 73% of *Klebsiella*, 58% of *Enterobacter* and 44% of *Proteus* spp. isolated in a Boston hospital during 1967 were resistant to streptomycin. In London from 1967 to 1969, more than half of the *Shigella sonnei* strains isolated were resistant to this drug (Davies *et al.*, 1970). In the 1940s and 1950s streptomycin was found to be a poor drug for therapy of urinary tract infections due to aerobic Gram-negative bacteria, because resistant strains emerged during therapy and led to recurrences (Sugarman and Pesanti, 1980).

Because of this, in the 1960s kanamycin and then gentamicin replaced streptomycin for the treatment of infections caused by Enterobacteriaceae. A consequence of the curtailed use of streptomycin has been the apparent subsequent increase in susceptibility to streptomycin among many species of Gram-negative bacilli. A more recent survey in one Boston hospital showed that only 36% of *E. coli*, 19% of *Klebsiella pneumoniae*, 7% of *Enterobacter aerogenes*, 13% of *Proteus mirabilis* and 47% of *Pr. rettgeri* were streptomycin-resistant (Moellering, 1983).

Haemophilus ducreyi resistant to streptomycin and kanamycin has been reported. Resistance was mediated by a plasmid which coded for the production of two aminoglycoside modifying phosphotransferases (p. 454) (Sanson-Le Pors *et al.*, 1985).

There is partial cross-resistance between streptomycin, kanamycin and neomycin. Strains of *M. tuberculosis* and other bacteria resistant to kanamycin, amikacin or neomycin, are nearly always resistant to streptomycin, but the reverse is not always true and streptomycin-resistant bacteria are frequently still sensitive to the other three drugs. Streptomycin-resistant strains of *M. tuberculosis* are usually sensitive to capreomycin (p. 1231).

5 Minimum inhibitory concentrations

The MICs of sensitive strains of *Staph. aureus* and Gram-negative bacteria are usually in the range of 1–8 µg per ml. Organisms with an MIC greater than 16 µg per ml are resistant. The usual MIC of streptomycin for *M. tuberculosis* is 8 µg per ml.

Mode of Administration and Dosage

1 Adults

Streptomycin is not absorbed from the gastrointestinal tract, and it is usually given by the i.m. route, but it can be given i.v. in the same dosage, in which case each dose is usually administered as a 30 min i.v. infusion (Morris and Cooper, 1994). The usual adult dosage is 1.0 g daily (15 mg per kg per day), given either as one daily dose or in two divided doses. For serious infections, such as miliary tuberculosis, this dose can be doubled for short periods, preferably for no longer than 1 week. Doses higher than 2 g daily should never be given. In patients over the age of 40 years, if prolonged treatment is indicated as for tuberculosis, a lower dosage, such as 0.75 g or even 0.5 g daily, is recommended to avoid toxicity, even if the patient's renal function appears normal.

2 Children

In these the i.m. or i.v. dosage is 20–40 mg per kg body weight per day, given once-daily or in two divided doses. For short-term treatment of serious infections the higher dosage may be used, but for long-term treatment of tuberculosis the lower dosage is advisable.

3 Newborn infants

The dosage in these patients should be lower and 10–20 mg per kg body weight per day is recommended (Yaffe and Back, 1966). A streptomycin dosage of 7.5 mg per kg given every 12 h is satisfactory for most infants (Herngren *et al.* 1977). Preterm infants 1–3 days old excrete approximately 30% of the administered dose within 12 h, compared with approximately 70% excretion by older children and adults (McCracken and Nelson, 1983).

4 Patients with renal failure

Streptomycin accumulates in these patients, so a modified dosage depending on streptomycin serum levels is necessary. A peak serum level of 40–50 μg per ml attained 1 h after i.m. injection, should not be exceeded. Persistent levels over 20 μg per ml are undesirable and levels estimated 24 h after injection should not exceed 3 μg per ml (Commonwealth Dept, 1977). The streptomycin half-life in patients with normal renal function is 2.4–2.7 h, but in patients with severe oliguria or anuria, this may be prolonged to 50–100 h. These patients may be treated by using a loading dose of 1 g, followed by half this dose every 3–4 days. Patients who have a creatinine clearance value of less than 10 ml per min, should be treated in the same way as anuric patients. Uremic patients whose creatinine clearance is in excess of 10 ml per min excrete the drug more rapidly. For these a loading dose of 1 g, followed by half this dose every 1 or 2 days is usually satisfactory (Kunin, 1967).

Streptomycin is removed slowly from the body by hemodialysis, and this is the treatment of choice for acute streptomycin poisoning (Edwards and Whyte, 1959). A safe effective dosage for patients undergoing hemodialysis is 10 mg per kg, every 5–7 days (Usuda and Sekine, 1978).

5 Intrathecal administration

This was once used in a daily adult dosage of 25–50 mg to treat tuberculous meningitis. Meningeal irritation occurred in a number of patients, and nowadays administration of streptomycin by this route is not recommended (p. 1201).

Serum Levels in Relation to Dosage

Streptomycin is rapidly absorbed after i.m. administration, and the peak serum level is reached within 1 h (Fig. I.20). Doubling the dose doubles the serum concentration. A measurable level is usually maintained for approximately 12 h following a 0.5 g dose in an adult, and for up to 24 h after a 1.0 g dose.

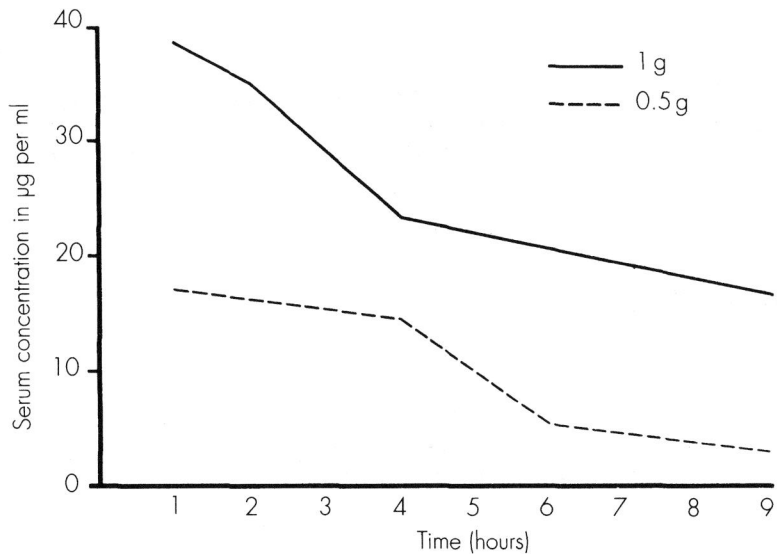

Fig. I.20.
Serum levels of streptomycin after i.m. administration of 0.5 and 1.0 g doses. (Redrawn after Welch, 1954, with permission.)

Excretion

1 Urine

Streptomycin is rapidly excreted by glomerular filtration. In patients with normal renal function, most excretion occurs during the first 12 h after i.m. injection, but the amount may vary from 40 to 90% of the administered dose in different individuals (Adcock and Hettig, 1946; Buggs *et al.*, 1946). High concentrations of the active drug are attained in urine, e.g. 200–400 μg per ml after an i.m. dose of 0.5 g.

2 Bile

Small amounts of streptomycin, probably only 1% of the total dose, are excreted unchanged in the bile. Streptomycin concentrations in bile of 10–20 μg per ml have been recorded after the administration of the usual doses.

3 Inactivation in body

From 10 to 30% of parenterally administered streptomycin does not appear to be excreted, and is presumably inactivated in the body but no streptomycin metabolites have been identified.

Distribution of the Drug in Body

Streptomycin diffuses rapidly into body fluids and tissues. It enters ascitic and pleural fluids. After a single i.m. injection the concentration in these is initially much lower than that in the serum, but some 4 to 6 h later, as the serum level falls, the level in the aberrant fluid may equal that found in the serum at the time (Adcock and Hettig, 1946). Streptomycin penetrates well the walls of tuberculous abscesses and achieves adequate levels even in caseous tissues (Fellander et al., 1952).

Streptomycin does not enter the CSF unless the meninges are inflamed. The CSF streptomycin concentration is usually much lower than the serum level even in patients with acute meningitis (Buggs et al., 1946). The drug crosses the placenta and simultaneous fetal blood levels are usually at least 50% of maternal serum concentrations (Conway and Birt, 1965). Streptomycin enters polymorphs and kills phagocytosed bacteria, but its activity against these is less than that observed against extracellular bacteria (Utili et al., 1991).

Streptomycin is approximately 34% serum protein bound (Gordon et al., 1972).

Mode of Action

The mode of action of streptomycin and other aminoglycosides on bacteria has been extensively studied and the processes involved are very complicated. A full review of the extensive literature available is beyond the scope of this book. The following informative reviews should be consulted: Hancock (1981a,b), David (1982), Moellering (1983), Davis (1987), Taber et al. (1987) and Nichols (1989).

Streptomycin and other aminoglycoside antibiotics interfere with bacterial protein synthesis (p. 561). This action of streptomycin is dependent on its ability to bind to a particular protein or proteins of the 30 S subunit of bacterial ribosomes. As with some other aminoglycoside antibiotics (neomycin, kanamycin and gentamicin), this binding of streptomycin to the subunit results in a misreading (or miscoding) of m-RNA codons. Consequently, wrong amino acids are incorporated into growing peptide chains and faulty bacterial proteins are produced. The resultant alteration in the protein molecule may be small and it does not necessarily affect all bacterial proteins. Therefore, this effect alone may not be lethal to bacteria, yet streptomycin and other aminoglycosides are rapidly bactericidal. Numerous hypotheses have been put forward over the years to explain this. The most likely explanation seems to be that streptomycin also leads to the production of abnormal membrane proteins of the bacterial cell, which cause alterations in membrane permeability, and this plays an essential role in the bactericidal action of aminoglycosides (Bryan and Kwan, 1983; Davis, 1987, 1988; Wyka and St John, 1990).

Bryan and Van den Elzen (1977) investigated the processes by which streptomycin (and gentamicin) are taken up by bacteria. They postulated that these antibiotics initially associate with the cell wall and external surface of the cytoplasmic membrane on an electrostatic basis which is energy-independent. The next phase is energy-dependent and involves binding of the antibiotics to membranous structures and respiratory quinones to form complexes, for their transport into the cell. There is a good correlation between susceptibility of bacteria to aminoglycosides and their possession of respiratory quinones. For instance, quinones are not present in obligate anaerobes such as the clostridia, which are resistant to aminoglycosides. The third phase is also energy-dependent, and involves membrane-bound aminoglycoside becoming bound to higher-affinity binding sites on membrane-associated ribosomes, which carry out protein synthesis. This results in a more rapid transport of the drugs into the cell. This hypothesis suggests that uptake of aminoglycosides is dependent on energy derived from aerobic metabolism (Saunders and Saunders, 1977).

Bacterial resistance to streptomycin may be due to aminoglycoside modifying enzymes, which are usually plasmid-mediated (p. 453) (Shannon and Phillips, 1982; Pinto-Alphandary et al., 1990), or due to genetic mutation causing a change in a particular protein of the 30 S ribosome subunit. This mutation results in decreased ribosomal binding of streptomycin (Hancock, 1981a; Perkins et al., 1992). A third resistance mechanism is alteration in bacterial cell permeability. Streptomycin and other aminoglycosides are inactive under anaerobic conditions because intracellular transport of these agents is markedly impaired in the absence of oxygen (see above). Thus all anaerobes are resistant to aminoglycosides, even though they contain ribosomes that are susceptible to these drugs in vitro (Davies, 1983; Moellering, 1983). Some strains of Ps. aeruginosa and other Gram-negative bacilli do not possess inactivating enzymes or ribosomal mutations, yet they are resistant to streptomycin and other aminoglycosides. In a proportion of these resistance is due to a permeability barrier at the cell wall, and in some *Ps. aeruginosa* strains a 'low-level' aminoglycoside-resistance is associated with a change in the structure of the lipopolysaccharide in their cell walls (Bryan *et al.*, 1984).

Mutant strains may occur which are streptomycin-dependent, i.e. the ribosomes of such bacteria require streptomycin for 'normal' protein synthesis (Hancock, 1981a). A mutation in 16 SrRNA appears to be associated with streptomycin dependence in *M. tuberculosis* (Honoré *et al.*, 1995).

Toxicity

1 Ototoxicity

This is the most serious toxic effect of streptomycin, usually resulting in vestibular disturbance with vertigo, but deafness can also occur (Cawthorne and Ranger, 1957; Assael *et al.*, 1982). The risk of vestibular disturbance is related to total dosage, and also to excessively high serum levels maintained for short periods. Peak serum levels of 40 μg per ml should probably not be exceeded, and persistent levels greater than 20 μg per ml should be avoided. In patients aged more than 40 years, the risk of damage is higher despite apparently normal renal function. In addition, patients in this age group cannot compensate for vestibular damage as well as younger people. There appears to be considerable individual variation in susceptibility to ototoxicity.

Concomitant administration of a loop-inhibiting diuretic, such as frusemide or ethacrynic acid, potentiate ototoxicity due to streptomycin and other aminoglycosides (p. 466). Animal studies also suggest that loud noise may aggravate aminoglycoside ototoxicity, and it seems prudent to minimize the exposure to noise of patients receiving these antibiotics (Brummett, 1983).

If streptomycin is given in the usual dosage for prolonged periods during pregnancy, the fetus may suffer ear damage, but severe effects appear to be uncommon. Robinson and Cambon (1964) reported two cases of congenital hearing loss, that were probably caused by streptomycin administered to mothers during pregnancy. Conway and Birt (1965) examined 17 children aged 6–13 years, whose mothers had received streptomycin during pregnancy. None of these children had any obvious disability, but detailed examination revealed minor abnormalities of VIIIth nerve function in eight; abnormalities in caloric tests were present in six and in the audiograms in four. Such children may be more liable to ototoxicity if they receive streptomycin or related drugs subsequently.

2 Nephrotoxicity

In animals streptomycin is the least nephrotoxic of the aminoglycoside antibiotics (p. 445) and human nephrotoxicity is rare (Appell and Neu, 1977; Luft *et al.*, 1983). Monitoring of renal function in ill patients is advisable to detect deterioration due to any cause because this may lead to accumulation of the drug and ototoxicity.

3 Hypersensitivity

The most common manifestations are rash and fever. The rash is usually morbilliform or urticarial, but occasionally severe or even fatal exfoliative dermatitis may develop. Stevens-Johnson syndrome (p. 816) caused by streptomycin has been reported (Sarkar *et al.*, 1982). Other features include joint pains, lymphadenopathy or possibly hepatitis (Thompson, 1969). Anaphylaxis is rare. In most patients allergic manifestations subside when streptomycin is stopped, but treatment with corticosteroids may be required for severe reactions. Desensitization to streptomycin can be attempted. Nowadays as more first-line antituberculosis drugs are available (p. 1211) one of these is usually substituted for streptomycin if it causes hypersensitivity, but if a multidrug-resistant *M. tuberculosis* strain (p. 1181) is involved, which is streptomycin-sensitive, desensitization may be necessary.

4 Neurotoxicity

Streptomycin and other aminoglycosides (p. 537) can interfere with neuromuscular transmission and thereby cause postoperative respiratory depression, a drug-induced myasthenic syndrome or unmasking or aggravation of myasthenia gravis. Aminoglycosides cause a combined presynaptic and postsynaptic block which results from interference with calcium ion fluxes at the nerve terminal (Argov and Mastaglia, 1979). In the past, sometimes large amounts of streptomycin (up to 5 g in adults) were introduced into the peritoneal cavity during surgery. This was often well absorbed from the inflamed peritoneum causing neuromuscular blockade (McQuillen *et al.*, 1968). Neuromuscular blockade in these patients was enhanced by prior use of muscle relaxants and other anesthetic agents, but antagonized by calcium and neostigmine. Streptomycin is no longer used intraperitoneally.

Some patients develop circumoral paresthesiae, and others rarely develop a temporary lack of mental concentration after streptomycin injections.

5 Hematological side-effects

Agranulocytosis and aplastic anemia have been reported rarely following streptomycin therapy. A bleeding disorder due to the development of a transient Factor V inhibitor, possibly related to streptomycin treatment has been described (Feinstein *et al.*, 1973).

6 Drug interactions

Heparin inhibits the activity of aminoglycosides and specimens for aminoglycoside measurement should not be collected in heparinized tubes. When heparin is used clinically as an anticoagulant, the amount in the blood does not reach levels that affect the aminoglycoside activity (Nilsson *et al.*, 1981).

Clinical Uses of the Drug

1 Tuberculosis

Streptomycin is still one of the standard first-line drugs for this disease and it is used initially in combination with two or sometimes three other first-line drugs. In such regimens isoniazid (p. 1194) is always included, usually with rifampicin, and sometimes pyrazinamide or ethambutol. Nowadays streptomycin is not commonly included in the initial regimens; in most situations, isoniazid in combination with two of the above oral drugs may be used satisfactorily (p. 1194). Some authors prefer to use streptomycin in combination with isoniazid and rifampicin for the initial treatment of tuberculous meningitis (Doganay *et al.*, 1989).

Streptomycin in a dose of 1.0 g two or three times weekly is also suitable for the fully supervised intermittent chemotherapy of pulmonary tuberculosis (p. 1195). The drug is often included in the initial phase of treatment in the short-course chemotherapy of pulmonary tuberculosis (p. 1195).

Streptomycin is not suitable for initial treatment of tuberculosis in areas where multidrug-resistant tuberculosis is prevalent, because many *M. tuberculosis* strains resistant to isoniazid and rifampicin are also streptomycin-resistant (Frieden *et al.*, 1993). Streptomycin may be useful in combination with other drugs, if the strain is confirmed to be streptomycin-sensitive (p. 1199).

2 Mycobacterium avium-complex infections

Animal experiments have demonstrated that liposome-encapsulated streptomycin or other aminoglycosides such as gentamicin (p. 476) or amikacin (p. 516) may be effective for the treatment of these infections (Düzgünes *et al.*, 1991).

3 Brucellosis

The best treatment for this disease has been oral tetracycline (p. 741) plus i.m. streptomycin (1 g daily), with both drugs being given for 2–3 weeks and the tetracycline continued for 4–6 additional weeks (Young, 1983). Other forms of therapy for this disease are now available. Co-trimoxazole (p. 871) alone is not as effective whereas a rifampicin/doxycycline combination (Ariza *et al.*, 1992) and co-trimoxazole/rifampicin combination (Khuri-Bulos *et al.*, 1993) are about as effective as tetracycline/streptomycin. The quinolones such as ciprofloxacin (p. 1031) and ofloxacin (p. 1126) have also been used for the treatment of brucellosis. *In vitro* studies suggest that kanamycin or gentamicin combined with tetracycline may be more effective than the classical streptomycin/tetracycline regimen (Robertson *et al.*, 1973). A few patients have been treated successfully using a gentamicin/tetracycline regimen (p. 476).

Animal studies indicate that aminoglycosides encapsulated in multilamellar liposomes are more effective than free aminoglycosides for the treatment of intracellular infections such as brucellosis (Fountain *et al.*, 1985). Liposomes are synthetic phospholipid bilayer vesicles. They are non-toxic and biodegradable and can protect the entrapped drugs from enzymatic attack until they reach the target cells. In another animal experiment, salmonellosis, a disease typically caused by intracellular bacteria, was treated successfully by streptomycin delivered in a liposome-entrapped form (Tadakuma *et al.*, 1985).

4 Bacterial endocarditis

Streptomycin combined with either penicillin G or ampicillin, was considered for many years as the treatment of choice for *E. faecalis* endocarditis (p. 42). Penicillin G and streptomycin did not show synergism *in vitro* against every strain of *E. faecalis* (p. 42), whereas a penicillin G/gentamicin combination was synergistic against nearly all strains (p. 42). For this reason, the latter combination was commonly used for the treatment of this disease. Gentamicin in a low dose of 3 mg per kg per day is no more nephrotoxic than streptomycin, and when used in this dose with penicillin G, it is satisfactory for the treatment of *E. faecalis* endocarditis (Wilson *et al.*, 1984) (p. 42). A vancomycin/streptomycin combination (p. 778) may be used for the treatment of *E. faecalis* endocarditis, if the penicillins are contraindicated (Westenfelder *et al.*, 1973).

Now when *E. faecalis* strains with high-level gentamicin-resistance have emerged (p. 455) penicillin G/gentamicin therapy is ineffective for the treatment of *E. faecalis* endocarditis caused by such strains. But some 20% of these strains show only low-level streptomycin-resistance, and if this is the case the combination of penicillin G/streptomycin is effective for this disease (Henry *et al.*, 1986; Bhattacharya and Warren, 1993).

Several antibiotic regimens are effective for the treatment of *Strep. viridans* endocarditis. In one a penicillin G/streptomycin combination is used for only 2 weeks, and in another this combination treatment is followed by 2 more weeks of penicillin G alone. Alternatively penicillin G alone can be used for 4–6 weeks (p. 41). All these regimens are effective clinically (p. 41) (Tuazon *et al.*, 1986). Penicillin G and streptomycin are synergistic against most penicillin G-sensitive *Strep. viridans* strains both *in vitro* and in animal endocarditis (Sande and Irvin, 1974).

5 Plaque and tularemia

Streptomycin has been the preferred drug for the treatment of plaque. It should be given i.m. in a dosage of 30 mg per kg per day in two divided doses for 10 days. Tetracycline (p. 744) is a suitable alternative and oral chloramphenicol and i.m. gentamicin are also effective (Butler, 1994; CDC, 1994). Studies in animals have shown that ceftriaxone and ofloxacin are equally effective (Bonacorsi *et al.*, 1994). For the treatment of tularemia, streptomycin or gentamicin (p. 475) are the drugs of choice (Capellan and Fong, 1993), but one of the tetracyclines (p. 744) are also effective and limited data suggest that fluoroquinolones, such as ciprofloxacin, may also prove useful (Risi and Pombo, 1995).

6 Venereal diseases

Streptomycin may be effective for the treatment of chancroid and granuloma inguinale but not for lymphogranuloma venereum (Willcox, 1977). Tetracyclines are the preferred drugs for the two latter infections, but due to the occurrence of resistant *H. ducreyi* strains, other drugs are required for chancroid (p. 744). Because of the high prevalence of streptomycin-resistant gonococcal strains present in many parts of the world (Report, 1978), streptomycin is not recommended for the treatment of gonorrhea. Streptomycin is effective for non-specific urethritis caused by *Ureaplasma urealyticum* but not for that caused by *Chlamydia trachomatis* (p. 746).

7 Mycetoma

This infection is caused either by actinomycetes (actinomycetoma) or fungi (eumycetoma), but usually only those caused by actinomycetes respond to chemotherapy (Annotation, 1977). The actinomycetes include *Nocardia asteroides*, *N. brasiliensis*, *Actinomadura madurea*, *Streptomyces somaliensis*, *Actinomadura pelletierii* and *Actinomyces israelii*. Mahgoub (1976) treated 144 patients with a mycetoma caused by one of the actinomycetes (*S. somaliensis*, *A. pelletierii*, *A. madurae* and *N. brasiliensis*) with various drug regimens. He obtained a 63.2% cure rate and another 21.5% of patients showed clinical improvement; the most effective treatments were dapsone plus streptomycin or co-trimoxazole plus streptomycin; sulfadoxine-pyrimethamine plus streptomycin, and rifampicin plus streptomycin also gave good results.

References

Adcock JD, Hettig RA (1946). Absorption, distribution and excretion of streptomycin. *Arch Intern Med* 77: 179.

Annotation (1977). Treatment of mycetoma. *Lancet* ii: 23.

Appel GB, Neu HC (1977). The nephrotoxicity of antimicrobial agents (second of three parts). *New Engl J Med* 296: 722.

Ariza J, Gudiol F, Pallares R *et al.* (1992). Treatment of human brucellosis with doxycycline plus rifampin or doxycycline plus streptomycin. *Ann Intern Med* 117: 25.

Argov Z, Mastaglia FL (1979). Disorders of neuromuscular transmission caused by drugs. *New Engl J Med* 301: 403.

Assael BM, Parini R, Rusconi F (1982). Ototoxicity of aminoglycoside antibiotics in infants and children. *Ped Infect Dis* 1: 357.

Ashtekar D, Düzgünes N, Gangadharam PRJ (1991). Activity of free and liposome encapsulated streptomycin against *Mycobacterium avium* complex (MAC) inside peritoneal macrophages. *J Antimicrob Chemother* 28: 615.

Basker MJ, Slocombe B, Sutherland R (1977). Aminoglycoside-resistant enterococci. *J Clin Path* 30: 375.

Bhattacharya M, Warren JR (1993). Treatment of infections due to enterococci with high-level gentamicin resistance and streptomycin susceptibility. *Clin Infect Dis* 16: 330.

Bloch AB, Cauthen GM, Onorato IM *et al.* (1994). Nationwide survey of drug-resistant tuberculosis in the United States. *JAMA* 271: 665.

Bonacorsi SP, Scavizzi MR, Guiyoule A *et al.* (1994). Assessment of a fluoroquinolone, three beta-lactams, two aminoglycosides, and a cycline in the treatment of murine *Yersinia pestis* infection. *Antimicrob Ag Chemother* 38: 481.

Bosch J, Liñares J, Lopez de Goicoechea MJ *et al.* (1986). *In vitro* activity of ciprofloxacin, ceftriaxone and five other antimicrobial agents against 95 strains of *Brucella melitensis*. *J Antimicrob Chemother* 17: 459.

Brummett RE (1983). Animal models of aminoglycoside antibiotic ototoxicity. *Rev Infect Dis* 5 (Suppl 2): 294.

Bryan LE, Kwan S (1983). Roles of ribosomal binding, membrane potential, and electron transport in bacterial uptake of streptomycin and gentamicin. *Antimicrob Ag Chemother* 23: 835.

Bryan LE, Van Den Elzen HM (1977). Effects of membrane-energy mutations and cations on streptomycin and gentamicin accumulation by bacteria: a model for entry of streptomycin in susceptible and resistant bacteria. *Antimicrob Ag Chemother* 12: 163.

Bryan LE, O'Hara K, Wong S (1984). Lipopolysaccharide changes in impermeability-type aminoglycoside resistance in *Pseudomonas aeruginosa*. *Antimicrob Ag Chemother* 26: 250.

Buggs CW, Pilling MA, Bronstein B, Hirshfield JW (1946). The absorption, distribution, and excretion of streptomycin in man. *J Clin Invest* 25: 94.

Butler T (1994). *Yersinia* infections: centennial of the discovery of the plague bacillus. *Clin Infect Dis* 19: 655.

Calderwood SA, Wennersten C, Moellering RC Jr *et al.* (1977). Resistance to six aminoglycosidic aminocyclitol antibiotics among enterococci: prevalence, evolution, and relationship to synergism with penicillin. *Antimicrob Ag Chemother* 12: 401.

Capellan J, Fong IW (1993). Tularemia from a cat bite: case report and review of feline-associated tularemia. *Clin Infect Dis* 16: 472.

Cawthorne T, Ranger D (1957). Toxic effect of streptomycin upon balance and hearing. *Brit Med J* 1: 1444.

CDC (Centers for Disease Control) (1983). Primary resistance to anti-tuberculosis drugs – United States. *MMWR* 32: 521.

CDC (Centers for Disease Control) (1994). Human plague – India, 1994. *MMWR* 43: 689.

Chiodini RJ, Van Kruiningen HJ, Thayer WR *et al.* (1984). *In vitro* antimicrobial susceptibility of *Mycobacterium* sp. isolated from patients with Crohn's disease. *Antimicrob Ag Chemother* 26: 930.

Commonwealth Department of Health Australia (1977). *Treatment of Tuberculosis with Particular Reference to Chemotherapy* 4th edn. Canberra: Australian Government Publishing Service.

Conway N, Birt BD (1965). Streptomycin in pregnancy: effect on the foetal ear. *Brit Med J* 2: 260.

Davies JE (1983). Resistance to aminoglycosides: mechanisms and frequency. *Rev Infect Dis* 5 (Suppl 2): 261.

Davies JR, Farrant WN, Uttley AHC (1970). Antibiotic resistance of *Shigella sonnei*. *Lancet* ii: 1157.

Davis BD (1982). Bactericidal synergism between beta-lactams and aminoglycosides: mechanism and possible therapeutic implications. *Rev Infect Dis* 4: 237.

Davis BD (1987). Mechanism of bactericidal action of aminoglycosides. *Microbiol Rev* 51: 341.

Davis BD (1988). The lethal action of aminoglycosides. *J Antimicrob Chemother* 22: 1.

Doganay M, Bakir M, Dökmetas I (1989). Treatment of tuberculous meningitis in adults with a combination of isoniazid, rifampicin and streptomycin: a prospective study. *Scand J Infect Dis* 21: 81.

Düsgünes N, Ashtekar DR, Flasher DL *et al.* (1991). Treatment of *Mycobacterium avium* intracellulare complex infection in beige mice with free and liposome-encapsulated streptomycin: role of liposome type and duration of treatment. *J Infect Dis* 164: 143.

Dutt AK, Stead WW (1982). Present chemotherapy for tuberculosis. *J Infect Dis* 146: 698.

Edwards KDG, Whyte HM (1959). Streptomycin poisoning in renal failure: an indication for treatment with an artificial kidney. *Brit Med J* 1: 752.

Eliopoulos GM, Farber BF, Murray BE *et al.* (1984). Ribosomal resistance of clinical enterococcal isolates to streptomycin. *Antimicrob Ag Chemother* 25: 398.

Enzler MJ, Rouse MS, Henry NK *et al.* (1987). *In vitro* and *in vivo* studies of streptomycin-resistant, penicillin-susceptible streptococci from patients with infective endocarditis. *J Infect Dis* 155: 954.

Farber BF, Yee Y (1987). High-level aminoglycoside resistance mediated by aminoglycoside-modifying enzymes among viridans streptococci: implications for the therapy for endocarditis. *J Infect Dis* 155: 948.

Farber BF, Eliopoulos GM, Ward JI *et al.* (1983). Resistance to penicillin-streptomycin synergy among clinical isolates of viridans streptococci. *Antimicrob Ag Chemother* 24: 871.

Feinstein DI, Rapaport SI, Chong MMY (1973). Factor V inhibitor: report of a case, with comments on a possible effect of streptomycin. *Ann Intern Med* 78: 385.

Fellander M, Hiertonn T, Wallmark G (1952). Studies on the concentration of streptomycin in the treatment of bone and joint tuberculosis. *Acta Tuberculosea Scand* 27: 176.

Fountain MW, Weiss SJ, Fountain AG *et al.* (1985). Treatment of *Brucella canis* and *Brucella abortus in vitro* and *in vivo* by stable plurilamellar vesicle-encapsulated aminoglycosides. *J Infect Dis* 152: 529.

Frieden TR, Sterling T, Pablos-Meudez A *et al.* (1993). The emergence of drug-resistant tuberculosis in New York City. *New Engl J Med* 328: 521.

Gangadharam PRJ, Parikh K (1992). *In-vivo* activity of streptomycin and clofazimine against established infections of *Mycobacterium avium* complex in beige mice. *J Antimicrob Chemother* 30: 833.

Gangadharam PRJ, Ashtekar DR, Ghori N *et al.* (1991). Chemotherapeutic potential of free and liposome encapsulated streptomycin against experimental *Mycobacterium avium* complex infections in beige mice. *J Antimicrob Chemother* 28: 425.

Gangadharam PRJ, Ashtekar DR, Flasher DL, Düzgünes N (1995). Therapy of *Mycobacterium avium* complex infections in beige mice with streptomycin encapsulated in sterically stabilized liposomes. *Antimicrob Ag Chemother* 39: 725.

Gelber RH, Henika PR, Gibson JB (1984). The bactericidal activity of various aminoglycoside antibiotics against *Mycobacterium leprae* in mice. *Lepr Rev* 55: 341.

Gordon RC, Regamey C, Kirby WMM (1972). Serum protein binding of the aminoglycoside antibiotics. *Antimicrob Ag Chemother* 2: 214.

Gutschik E, Jepsen OB, Mortensen I (1977). Effect of combinations of penicillin and aminoglycosides on *Streptococcus faecalis*: a comparative study of seven aminoglycoside antibiotics. *J Infect Dis* **135**: 832.

Hancock REW (1981a). Aminoglycoside uptake and mode of action – with special reference to streptomycin and gentamicni. 1. Antagonists and mutants. *J Antimicrob Chemother* **8**: 249.

Hancock REW (1981b). Aminoglycoside uptake and mode of action – with special reference to streptomycin and gentamicin. II. Effects of aminoglycosides on cells. *J Antimicrob Chemother* **8**: 429.

Harris GD, Johanson WG Jr, Nicholson DP (1975). Response to chemotherapy of pulmonary infection due to *Mycobacterium kansasii*. *Amer Rev Resp Dis* **112**: 31.

Heifets L, Lindholm-Levy P (1989). Comparison of bactericidal activities of streptomycin, amikacin, kanamycin and capreomycin against *Mycobacterium avium* and *M tuberculosis*. *Antimicrob Ag Chemother* **33**: 1298.

Henry NK, Wilson WR, Geraci JE (1986). Treatment of streptomycin-susceptible enterococcal experimental endocarditis with combinations of penicillin and low- or high-dose streptomycin. *Antimicrob Ag Chemother* **30**: 725.

Herngren L Boréus LO, Jalling B, Lagercrantz R (1977). Pharmacokinetic aspects of streptomycin treatment of neonatal septicaemia. *Scand J Infect Dis* **9**: 301.

Honoré N, Cole ST (1994). Streptomycin resistance in mycobacteria. *Antimicrob Ag Chemother* **38**: 238.

Honoré N, Marchal G, Cole ST (1995). Novel mutation in 16S r RNA associated with streptomycin dependence in *Mycobacterium tuberculosis*. *Antimicrob Ag Chemother* **39**: 769.

Horodniceanu T, Buu-Hoï A, Delbox F, Bieth G (1982). High-level aminoglycoside resistance in Group A, B, G, D (*Streptococcus bovis*), and viridans streptococci. *Antimicrob Ag Chemother* **21**: 176.

Kaye D (1982). Enterococci Biologic and epidemiologic characteristics and *in vitro* susceptibility. *Arch Intern Med* **142**: 2006.

Khuri-Bulos NA, Daoud AH, Azab SM (1993). Treatment of childhood brucellosis: results of a prospective trial on 113 children. *Pediatr Infect Dis J* **12**: 377.

Kislak Jw (1972). The susceptibility of *Bacteroides fragilis* to 24 antibiotics. *J Infect Dis* **125**: 295.

Kunin CM (1967). A guide to use of antibiotics in patients with renal disease. *Ann Intern Med* **67**: 151.

Kuze F, Kurasawa T, Bando K *et al.* (1981). *In vitro* and *in vivo* susceptibility of atypical mycobacteria to various drugs. *Rev Infect Dis* **3**: 885.

Luft FC, Bennett WH, Gilbert DN (1983). Experimental aminoglycoside nephrotoxicity: accomplishments and future potential. *Rev Infect Dis* **5** (Suppl 2): 268.

Mahgoub EL (1976). Medical management of mycetoma. *Bull Wld Hlth Org* **54**: 303.

Majumdar S, Flasher D, Friend DS *et al.* (1992). Efficacies of liposome-encapsulated streptomycin and ciprofloxacin against *Mycobacterium avium-M intracellulare* complex infections in human peripheral blood monocyte/macrophages. *Antimicrob Ag Chemother* **36**: 2808.

Matsumoto JY, Wilson WR, Wright AJ *et al.* (1980). Synergy of penicillin and decreasing concentrations of aminoglycosides against enterococci from patients with infective endocarditis. *Antimicrob Ag Chemother* **18**: 944.

McCracken GH Jr, Nelson JD (1983). *Antimicrobial Therapy for Newborns* 2nd edn p. 49. New York: Grune & Stratton.

McQuillen MP, Cantor HE, O'Rourke JR (1968). Myasthenic syndrome associated with antibiotics. *Arch Neurol* **18**: 402.

Meier A, Kirschner P, Bange F-C *et al.* (1994). Genetic alterations in streptomycin-resistant *Mycobacterium tuberculosis*: mapping of mutations conferring resistance. *Antimicrob Ag Chemother* **38**: 228.

Moellering RC Jr (1983). *In vitro* antibacterial activity of the aminoglycoside antibiotics. *Rev Infect Dis* **5** (Suppl 2): 212.

Morris JT, Cooper RH (1994). Intravenous streptomycin: a useful route of administration. *Clin Infect Dis* **19**: 1150.

Nichols WW (1989). The enigma of streptomycin transport. *J Antimicrob Chemother* **23**: 673.

Nilsson L, Maller R, Ånsêhn S (1981). Inhibition of aminoglycoside activity by heparin. *Antimicrob Ag Chemother* **20**: 155.

Perkins BA, Hamill RJ, Musher DM, O'Hara C (1992). *In vitro* activities of streptomycin and 11 oral antimicrobial agents against clinical isolates of *Klebsiella rhinoscleromatis*. *Antimicrob Ag Chemother* **36**: 1785.

Pezzia W, Raleigh JW, Bailey MC *et al.* (1981). Treatment of pulmonary disease due to *Mycobacterium kansasii*: recent experience with rifampin. *Rev Infect Dis* **3**: 1035.

Pinto-Alphandary H, Mabilat C, Courvalin P (1990). Emergence of aminoglycoside resistance genes aadA and aadE in the genus *Campylobacter*. *Antimicrob Ag Chemother* **34**: 1294.

Report of a WHO Scientific Group (1978). *Neisseria gonorrhoeae* and gonococcal infections. *Wld Hlth Org Techn Rep Ser* No. 616.

Risi GF, Pombo DJ (1995). Relapse of tularemia after aminoglycoside therapy: case report and discussion of therapeutic options. *Clin Infect Dis* **20**: 174.

Robertson L, Farrell ID, Hinchliffe PM (1973). The sensitivity of *Brucella abortus* to chemotherapeutic agents. *J Med Microbiol* **6**: 549.

Robinson GC, Cambon KG (1964). Hearing loss in infants of tuberculous mothers treated with streptomycin during pregnancy. *New Engl J Med* **271**: 949.

Ruhen RW, Darrell JH (1973). Antibiotic synergism against Group D streptococci in the treatment of endocarditis. *Med J Aust* **2**: 114.

Sabath LD (1969). Current concepts: drug resistance of bacteria. *New Engl J Med* **280**: 91.

Sande MA, Irvin RG (1974). Penicillin-aminoglycoside synergy in experimental *Streptococcus viridans* endocarditis. *J Infect Dis* **129**: 572.

Sanders CC (1977). Synergy of penicillin-netilmicin combinations against enterococci including strains highly resistant to streptomycin or kanamycin. *Antimicrob Ag Chemother* **12**: 195.

Sanson-Le Pors M-J, Casin IM, Collatz E (1985). Plasmid-mediated aminoglycoside phosphotransferases in *Haemophilus ducreyi*. *Antimicrob Ag Chemother* **28**: 315.

Sarkar SK, Purohit SD, Sharma TN *et al.* (1982). Stevens-Johnson syndrome caused by streptomycin. *Tubercle* **63**: 137.

Saunders JR, Saunders VA (1977). Energetics and antibiotic uptake. *Nature* **270**: 475.

Schatz A, Bugie E, Waksman SA (1944). Streptomycin, a substance exhibiting antibiotic activity against Gram-positive and Gram-negative bacteria. *Proc Soc Exper Biol Med* **55**: 66.

Schlessinger D (1988). Failure of aminoglycoside antibiotics to kill anaerobic, low-pH, and resistant cultures. *Clin Microbiol Rev* **1**: 54.

Shannon K, Phillips I (1982). Mechanisms of resistance to aminoglycosides in clinical isolates. *J Antimicrob Chemother* **9**: 91.

Stottmeier KD, Baker S (1977). Primary drug-resistant tuberculosis in Massachusetts, 1975/6. *New Engl J Med* **296**: 823.

Stottmeier KD, Burkes J (1974). Primary drug-resistant *Mycobacterium tuberculosis* isolated in Massachusetts in 1972. *J Infect Dis* **130**: 293.

Sugarman B, Pesanti E (1980). Treatment failures secondary to *in vivo* development of drug resistance by microorganism. *Rev Infect Dis* **2**: 153.

Taber HW, Mueller JP, Miller PF, Arrow AS (1987). Bacterial uptake of aminoglycoside antibiotics. *Microbiol Rev* **51**: 439.

Tadakuma T, Ikewaki N, Yasuda T *et al.* (1985). Treatment of experimental salmonellosis in mice with streptomycin entrapped in liposomes. *Antimicrob Ag Chemother* **28**: 28.

Thompson JE (1969). The management of hypersensitivity reactions to antituberculosis drugs. *Med J Aust* **2**: 1058.

Tight RR, Bartlett MS (1981). Actinomycetoma in the United States. *Rev Infect Dis* **3**: 1139.

Tuazon CU, Gill V, Gill F (1986). Streptococcal endocarditis: single vs combination antibiotic therapy and the role of various species. *Rev Infect Dis* **8**: 54.

Udo EE, Grubb WB (1991). Transposition of genes encoding kanamycin, neomycin and streptomycin resistance in *Staphylococcus aureus*. *J Antimicrob Chemother* **27**: 713.

Usuda Y, Sekine O (1978). Chemotherapy of tuberculosis in patients on dialysis. In *Current Chemotherapy: Proceedings of the 10th International Congress of Chemotherapy, Zurich/Switzerland, 1977* (Siegenthaler W, Lüthy R, eds), p. 241. Washington DC: American Society for Microbiology.

Utili R, Adinolfi LE, Dilillo M *et al.* (1991). Activity of aminoglycosides against phagocytosed bacteria. *J Antimicrob Chemother* **28**: 897.

Wallace RJ Jr, Wiss K (1981). Susceptibility of *Mycobacterium marinum* to tetracyclines and aminoglycosides. *Antimicrob Ag Chemother* **20**: 610.

Watanakunakorn C (1992). Rapid increase in the prevalence of high-level aminoglycoside resistance among enterococci isolated from blood cultures during 1989–1991. *J Antimicrob Chemother* **30**: 289.

Welch H (1954). *Principles and Practice of Antibiotic Therapy*, p. 103. New York: Medical Encyclopedia Inc.

Westenfelder GO, Paterson PY, Reisberg BE, Carlson GM (1973). Vancomycin-streptomycin synergism in enterococcal endocarditis. *JAMA* **223**: 37.

Willcox RR (1977). How suitable are available pharmaceuticals for the treatment of sexually transmitted diseases? (2). Conditions presenting as sores or tumours. *Brit J Vener Dis* **53**: 340.

Wilson WR, Wilkowske CJ, Wright AJ *et al.* (1984). Treatment of streptomycin-susceptible and streptomycin-resistant enterococcal endocarditis. *Ann Intern Med* **100**: 816.

Wurtz R, Sahm D, Flaherty J (1991). Gentamicin-resistant, streptomycin-susceptible *Enterococcus* (*Streptococcus*) *faecalis* bacteremia. *J Infect Dis* **163**: 1393.

Wyka MA, StJohn AC (1990). Effect of production of abnormal proteins on the rate of killing of *Escherichia coli* by streptomycin. *Antimicrob Ag Chemother* **34**: 534.

Yaffe SJ, Back N (1966). Pediatric pharmacology. *Postgrad Med* **40**: 193.

Yee Y, Farber B, Mates S (1986). Mechanism of penicillin-streptomycin synergy for clinical isolates of viridans streptococci. *J Infect Dis* **154**: 531.

Young EJ (1983). Human brucellosis. *Rev Infect Dis* **5**: 821.

Kanamycin

Description

Kanamycin was isolated in Japan from *Streptomyces kanamyceticus* (Umezawa *et al.*, 1957). The drug is an aminoglycoside, chemically similar to streptomycin (p. 428). Clinically it is used as a sulfate. Kanamycin is now only rarely used; its main place nowadays is for the treatment of tuberculosis caused by multidrug-resistant *Myobacterium tuberculosis* strains (Iseman, 1993).

Sensitive Organisms

1 Gram-negative aerobic bacteria

Kanamycin is active against most of the Enterobacteriaceae such as *Escherichia coli*, the *Enterobacter*, *Klebsiella*, *Proteus*, *Salmonella*, *Shigella*, *Providencia*, *Serratia*, *Citrobacter*, *Hafnia*, *Edwardsiella* and *Arizona* spp. *Yersinia pestis* (Butler *et al.*, 1974), *Y. enterocolitica* (Hammerberg *et al.*, 1977) and *Y. pseudotuberculosis* (Brodie *et al.*, 1973) are also kanamycin-sensitive. Resistance to kanamycin of Enterobacteriaceae, which are normal inhabitants of the human bowel, first became a significant problem about 10 years after its discovery (Sabath, 1969; Roe and Lowbury, 1972; Terman *et al.*, 1972). Resistant Enterobacteriaceae at that time were more frequent in hospital-acquired infections (Dans *et al.*, 1970; Baker *et al.*, 1974).

During the 1970s and early 1980s, presumably because kanamycin was largely replaced by gentamicin (p. 450) in many hospitals, kanamycin-resistant strains were no longer increasing and their prevalence actually decreased in many areas. In seven North American nurseries, the percentage of *E. coli* strains resistant to kanamycin isolated from neonates, decreased from a high of 71% in 1971 to 12% in 1974; this coincided with the substitution of gentamicin for kanamycin for the treatment of neonatal infections (Howard and McCracken, 1975). In a survey in a London hospital, only about 10% of all Enterobacteriaceae isolates were kanamycin-resistant (Phillips *et al.*, 1977). In one Boston hospital only 15% of *E. coli*, 16% of *Klebsiella pneumoniae*, 4% of *Enterobacter aerogenes*, 9% of *Proteus mirabilis*, and 12% of *Providencia stuartii* strains were kanamycin-resistant (Moellering, 1983). Kanamycin resistance of Enterobacteriaceae is most commonly due to plasmid-mediated production of a series of aminoglycoside-modifying enzymes (p. 453). Three major types of enzymes catalyze the modification of aminoglycosides; these act by acetylation of an amino group or phosphorylation or adenylylation of a hydroxy group. A number of subtypes of these acetyltransferases, phosphotransferases, and adenylyltransferases exist. In the bacterial cell these enzymes may be located in the periplasmic space (p. 454) or bound to the cytoplasmic membrane. Kanamycin and other aminoglycosides that are acetylated, phosphorylated or adenylylated do not bind well to ribosomes, and hence their uptake is poor or does not occur and the result is resistance. Aminoglycosides vary in their ability to resist enzymatic modification and of those in clinical use, amikacin (p. 505) is the most resistant. A second mechanism of bacterial resistance to kanamycin and other aminoglycosides results from alterations in bacterial permeability to these drugs (p. 453). Mutational resistance due to a change of the 30 S subunit of the ribosome (p. 452) can lead to streptomycin-resistant Gram-negative bacilli, but such ribosomal resistance to other aminoglycosides does not occur in clinical isolates (Foster, 1983; Moellering, 1983; Neu, 1984).

Among other Gram-negative bacteria, the *Neisseria* spp. (*meningococci* and *gonococci*), *Haemophilus influenzae*, *H. ducreyi*, and the *Brucella* spp. are usually kanamycin-sensitive, but *Pseudomonas aeruginosa* is resistant (Finegold, 1959). Some gonococcal strains are resistant to kanamycin, but beta-lactamase-producing strains (p. 15) are usually susceptible. Gonococcal strains which do not produce beta-lactamase but which are intrinsically resistant to penicillin G (p. 14) are usually moderately or highly kanamycin-resistant (Cohen *et al.*, 1983; Fransen *et al.*, 1984). Strains of *H. ducreyi* resistant to streptomycin and kanamycin have been reported. These strains produce plasmid-mediated aminoglycoside modifying enzymes (Sanson-Le Pors *et al.*, 1985).

Acinetobacter spp. is usually sensitive to kanamycin, but resistant strains occur. *Legionella pneumophila* is sensitive to kanamycin in vitro (MIC 0.5–2.0 μg per ml) (Thornsberry *et al.*, 1978). *Campylobacter jejuni* is sensitive to the aminoglycosides, including kanamycin (MIC 0.25–4.0 μg per ml) (p. 452) (Michel *et al.*, 1983). Resistant strains of *Campylobacter jejuni* have been detected; the resistance in these strains are due to plasmids which usually code for the production of kanamycin phosphotransferase. The resistance gene can also translocate between plasmid and chromosomal DNA (Kotarski *et al.*, 1986; Tenover and Elvrum, 1988; Tenover *et al.*, 1992).

2 Gram-negative anaerobic bacteria

Most of these are kanamycin-resistant. The drug has moderate activity against some strains of *Fusobacterium* spp. and *Prevotella* (*Bacteroides*) *melaninogenica*, but all others and in particular *Bacteroides fragilis* are resistant (Martin *et al.*, 1972).

3 Gram-positive bacteria

Staphylococcus aureus (irrespective of beta-lactamase production) and *Staph. epidermidis* are kanamycin-sensitive, but all other Gram-positive bacteria, such as *Streptococcus pyogenes*, *Strep. pneumoniae*, *Strep. viridans*, *Enterococcus faecalis* and the *Nocardia*, *Actinomyces* and *Clostridium* spp., are resistant. Kanamycin-resistant staphylococci, which were nearly always also neomycin-resistant (p. 533), were detected in some hospitals in the 1960s (Barber and Waterworth, 1966), and resistance to both of these drugs was mediated by a plasmid (Stiffler *et al.*, 1974). Nowadays, *Staph. aureus* and *Staph. epidermidis* strains with multiple resistance to several aminoglycosides, such as kanamycin, gentamicin and tobramycin, are more common. These staphylococcal strains contain aminoglycoside-modifying enzymes; the production of these may be chromosomally mediated (Kayser *et al.*, 1981), but in most resistant strains they are mediated by transferable plasmids (Archer and Johnston, 1983). Methicillin-resistant *Staph. aureus* which caused widespread outbreaks of nosocomial sepsis in the early 1980s in the USA, UK and Australia, were also resistant to most aminoglycosides (p. 80).

Usually *E. faecalis* is resistant to kanamycin concentrations which are attained in the serum with ordinary doses. The combination of penicillin G and kanamycin, similar to penicillin G/streptomycin (p. 429), often acts synergistically against this organism. A penicillin G/kanamycin combination is synergistic against occasional *E. faecalis* strains for which penicillin G/streptomycin is not synergistic. Kanamycin instead of streptomycin, combined with penicillin G was more effective for treatment of endocarditis caused by such *E. faecalis* strains (Garrod and Waterworth, 1962). These strains are uncommon, because most of those which show high-level resistance to streptomycin (p. 429), also show similar resistance to kanamycin (MIC >2000 μg per ml).

Similar to streptomycin (p. 428), Groups A, B and G streptococci, viridans streptococci and non-enterococcal Group D streptococci, are usually relatively resistant to kanamycin (MICs 5.0–250 μg per ml). These organisms with this low-level resistance are usually killed synergistically by a penicillin G/kanamycin combination. Some strains of all these streptococci may exhibit high-level kanamycin resistance (MICs >2000 μg per ml). These strains are not killed synergistically by a penicillin G and kanamycin combination, whereas they are by a penicillin G/gentamicin combination (Horodniceanu *et al.*, 1982).

Nocardia asteroides is usually kanamycin-resistant. Wallace *et al.* (1983) found only 31% of strains tested to be susceptible. *Nocardia brasiliensis* was nearly always resistant. By contrast, *N. caviae* was usually sensitive, with 75% of the strains being susceptible.

4 Mycobacteria

Mycobacterium tuberculosis is kanamycin-sensitive, but resistant strains can emerge. Multidrug-resistant strains of *M. tuberculosis*, which may be resistant to isoniazid, rifampicin, pyrazinamide, ethambutol and streptomycin, are usually kanamycin-sensitive (Frieden *et al.*, 1993; Bloch *et al.*, 1994) (p. 1200).

Among the 'atypical mycobacteria', *M. kansasii* (Kuze *et al.*, 1981), *M. marinum* (Sanders and Wolinsky, 1980; Wallace and Wiss, 1981) and *M. chelonae* (Becker *et al.*, 1980) are usually kanamycin-sensitive. Usually *M. fortuitum* is also susceptible, but some strains are resistant and

Organism	MIC (μg per ml)
Gram-positive bacteria	
Staphylococcus aureus	0.5–2.0
Streptococcus pyogenes	64.0–256.0
Enterococcus faecalis	8.0–32.0
Gram-negative bacteria	
Escherichia coli	2.0–8.0
Klebsiella aerogenes	1.0–4.0
Proteus mirabilis	2.0–8.0
Proteus vulgaris	2.0–8.0
Morganella morganii	2.0–8.0
Providencia rettgeri	2.0–4.0
Salmonella spp.	1.0–4.0
Pseudomonas aeruginosa	8.0–128.0

Table I.36
After Barber and Waterworth (1966)

this is mediated by plasmids coding for aminoglycoside-modifying enzymes (Hull *et al.*, 1984). Other 'atypical mycobacteria', such as the *M. avium* complex, are kanamycin-resistant (Davidson *et al.*, 1981; Zimmer *et al.*, 1982). An unclassified *Mycobacterium* spp. which was isolated from three patients with Crohn's disease, was kanamycin-sensitive (Chiodini *et al.*, 1984).

Kanamycin is bactericidal to *M. leprae* infection in the mouse foot-pad, provided a high daily dose of 100 mg per kg body weight is used. The practicality and usefulness of kanamycin and other aminoglycosides in the treatment of human leprosy has not been established (Gelber *et al.*, 1984).

5 Other organisms

Treponema pallidum, leptospirae, mycoplasmas, chlamydia and fungi are kanamycin-resistant.

6 Minimum inhibitory concentrations

Table I.36 shows the MICs of kanamycin against some selected bacterial species.

Mode of Administration and Dosage

1 Parenteral administration

Kanamycin is poorly absorbed from the gastrointestinal tract, and it is administered by the i.m. or i.v. route. The adult dosage is 15 mg per kg body weight per day, most commonly administered in two divided doses, but similar to amikacin (p. 507) it can be given as a single daily dose. A common dosage for adults is 0.5 g 12-hourly or 1.0 g once every 24 h. Occasionally this dosage may be increased to 0.5 g 8-hourly for severe infections, but only for short periods. Usually adult dosages higher than 1.0 g per day are unnecessary even for very severe infections, and kanamycin should not be used for periods longer than 14 days (Murdoch *et al.*, 1962).

Hieber and Nelson (1976) and Hieber *et al.* (1980) demonstrated that the usual dosage of 15 mg per kg per day fails to produce therapeutic serum concentrations in many children aged 2 months to 12 years. Accordingly, it was recommended that the daily kanamycin dosage for this age group should be increased to 30 mg per kg, given in three divided doses.

The drug may be administered i.v. using the same dosage as used for i.m. therapy. The best method is to dissolve each dose in 20–50 ml of i.v. solution in a pediatric buretrol or a secondary i.v. bottle, for infusion over 20 to 30 min. Kanamycin doses well diluted, can also be given by intermittent injection into the i.v. tubing (McCracken *et al.*, 1977). Kanamycin administration by continuous i.v. infusion is not generally advocated. The drug is incompatible with many additives to i.v. fluids. Nevertheless, it is stable for at least 12 h in all commonly used glucose-saline i.v. fluids (Wyatt *et al.*, 1972), so that under special circumstances it may be added to i.v. bottles and administered by continuous infusion.

2 Patients with renal failure

These require a modified dosage. A loading dose of 0.5–1.0 g can be safely administered i.m. or i.v. to any uremic patient. The peak serum kanamycin concentration attained after the first dose is higher in patients with renal failure (Mawer *et al.*, 1972a). With a single dose there is usually no danger of toxicity, and the first dose often has to be given before the patient's renal function is known. Thereafter, the frequency with which the standard 0.5 g dose can be repeated, depends on the severity of the renal failure (Kunin, 1966).

There is an approximate linear relationship between the serum kanamycin half-life and the serum creatinine concentration (Cutler and Orme, 1969). Kanamycin in a dose of 0.5 g given every third half-life results in therapeutic non-toxic levels in patients with renal failure. The serum half-life in hours, is approximately equal to the patient's serum creatinine in mg % multiplied by 4. (For conversion of creatinine values from SI units to mg %, see p. 460).

Table I.37 exemplifies the use of this formula. This calculation may be simplified further; the interval between kanamycin doses is obtained by multiplying the serum creatinine (in mg %) by 12, which is the usual period in hours between doses for patients with normal renal function (McCloskey and Becker, 1971). Alternatively, the time intervals between doses may be left unchanged, but individual doses suitably reduced; the maintenance dose can be calculated by dividing the ordinary dose by the patient's creatinine in mg %. Methods using a combination of individual dose reduction and extension of the intervals between doses, are also useful (Healy *et al.*, 1973). Computer-assisted prescribing of kanamycin has been used for patients with renal failure and a nomogram for kanamycin dosage has been published (Mawer *et al.*, 1972a,b). With these methods, which aim for more precision, the loading dose, maintenance dose and intervals between doses, are all altered in an attempt to maintain serum kanamycin levels within the range of 10–30 µg per ml, for 2 h after each dose.

All these dosage schedules are useful guides, but when possible dosage should be governed by serum kanamycin estimations (Reeves, 1977). In many patients renal function varies from day to day, and often improves when infection is controlled. Suitable times to collect blood for kanamycin assays are 1 h after an i.m. dose or 30 min after an i.v. dose and then just before the next dose. The first or peak level should not exceed 30 µg per ml and the second or trough level should approach zero and should not exceed 10 µg per ml (see amikacin p. 508).

Kanamycin is removed from the body by hemodialysis. In anephric patients undergoing this procedure, the kanamycin half-life is approximately 4.9 h. During a 6–8 h hemodialysis some 50% of kanamycin is removed from the body, while about 70–80% of the drug is removed during a 12 h dialysis (Danish *et al.*, 1974). Therapeutic non-toxic levels of kanamycin will usually be maintained in anephric patients managed by twice-weekly hemodialysis, if a dose of 7 mg per kg is given after each dialysis. Hemodialysis is the best way to treat kanamycin overdosage.

This drug is also removed by peritoneal dialysis. In anuric patients treated by peritoneal dialysis (2 liter exchanges every 2.5 h), after a dose of 0.5 g kanamycin i.m., serum levels decrease promptly during the first 6–12 h and the half-life of the drug during this time is approximately 5 h, a figure similar to the normal one. As dialysis continues, removal of the drug

Renal function	Kanamycin half-life	Frequency of administration of adult dose of 0.5 g
Normal	4 h	4 × 3 = 12-hourly
Renal failure with serum creatinine of 6 mg %	6 × 4 = 24 h	24 × 3 = 72-hourly

Serum kanamycin half-life in hours = serum creatinine in mg % × 4.
The dose of kanamycin should be administered once every third half-life of the drug.

Table I.37

is slower and the half-life is prolonged to 48 h. The average rate of removal of kanamycin is 4.4 mg per h during peritoneal dialysis (about 100 mg per day). This suggests that a daily dose of 250 mg during peritoneal dialysis would suffice for anuric patients (Greenberg and Sanford, 1967).

A significant amount of kanamycin is absorbed if the drug is added to peritoneal dialysis fluid. If 0.5 g of kanamycin is introduced into the peritoneal cavity, serum levels are reached which are approximately 30% of those obtained with the same i.m. dose (Sanford, 1966). More commonly 20 mg of the drug is added to each liter of peritoneal dialysis fluid (concentration 20 µg per ml) to prevent or treat intraperitoneal infections (Atkins et al., 1973). In such patients, who are not receiving kanamycin by other routes, after 16 h of dialysis the serum kanamycin concentration stabilizes at approximately 45% of the dialysis inflow level.

3 Patients aged more than 50 years

Compared with younger adults the half-life of kanamycin and many other drugs may be prolonged or even doubled in these older patients, despite normal serum creatinine levels. For this reason, dosage may require suitable reduction in this age group (Hansen et al., 1970).

4 Newborn and premature infants

Many of these infants, similar to children (p. 441), need a higher kanamycin dosage than adults. In infants who weigh more than 2000 g at birth, peak serum levels of kanamycin after i.m. doses of 7.5 mg per kg, are below the desired therapeutic range of 15–25 µg per ml. The same also applies to all babies aged more than 7 days (Howard and McCracken, 1975). It is recommended that babies whose birth weight is less than 2000 g should receive 7.5 mg per kg i.m. every 12 h, until 7 days of age, and thereafter 10 mg per kg every 12 h. Infants weighing more than 2000 g at birth should receive 10 mg per kg i.m. every 12 h until 7 days of age, and thereafter 10 mg per kg every 8 h (McCracken and Threlkeld, 1976; McCracken and Nelson, 1983).

Kanamycin can be safely administered to neonates by the i.v. route, provided that each dose is dissolved in a suitable volume of i.v. fluid and then given as a constant infusion over 20–30 min. When administered this way the resultant serum levels are similar to those after i.m. administration. The i.v. kanamycin dosage for infants is the same as that recommended for i.m. use (McCracken and Nelson, 1983).

5 Pregnant patients

These patients have lower serum levels after usual therapeutic doses (p. 444). Monitoring of maternal serum levels throughout therapy is recommended not only to minimize fetal exposure to excessive drug levels, but also to ensure the optimal outcome of treatment through the avoidance of subtherapeutic levels in the mother (Chow and Jewesson, 1985).

6 Intrathecal administration

This is usually unnecessary for the treatment of meningitis. However, in infants who have associated anatomical abnormalities such as meningomyeloceles or who have shunts inserted because of hydrocephalus, intrathecal and intraventricular kanamycin has been used in addition to systemic treatment. Intrathecal doses of kanamycin used for infants have ranged from 5 to 25 mg daily (Lorber, 1967).

7 Oral administration

Kanamycin can be used orally in liver failure (p. 447) in a dosage of 4–8 g per day (1–2 g 6-hourly). Some of this is absorbed, and in patients with impaired renal function, after several days treatment serum levels can approach those usually attained after parenteral administration.

Serum Levels in Relation to Dosage

After i.m. injection, kanamycin can be detected in the serum in 15–30 min, and a peak level is reached in about 1 h. At 2 h the level is somewhat lower and thereafter, it falls rapidly; the half-life in serum being about 4 h (Fig. I.21). The levels are usually low 6–8 h after injection and negligible at 12 h. The drug does not accumulate with repeated doses of 0.5 g given 12-hourly to adults, unless the patient has impaired renal function. The serum half-life of kanamycin in severely uremic patients may be prolonged to 70–80 h.

Following a 30-min i.v. infusion of kanamycin to adults, serum levels as high as 34–48 µg per ml are attained immediately after the infusion. Then a short (0.5 h) distribution phase occurs, during which serum levels fall to 20–30 µg per ml, a value similar to the peak level attained after

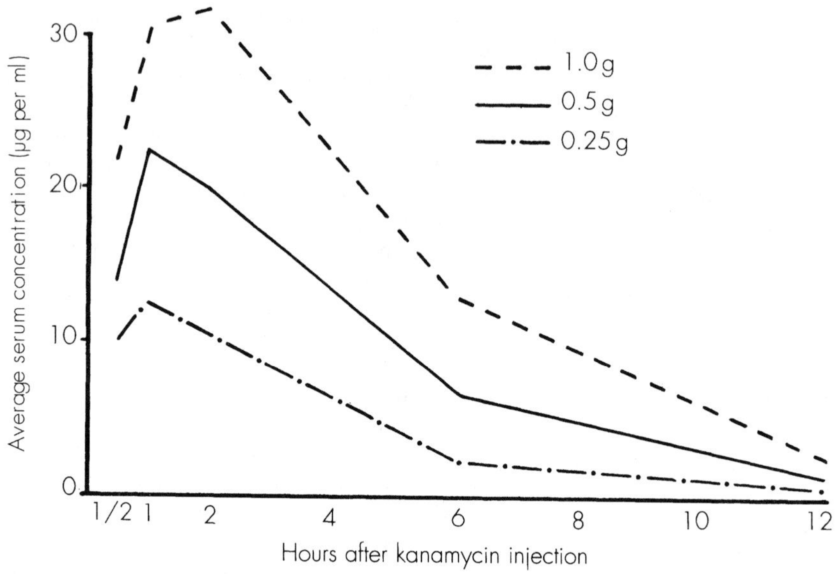

Fig. I.21.
Average serum concentration following single i.m. injections of kanamycin at three dose levels: 0.25, 0.5 and 1.0 g. (Redrawn after Welch *et al.*, 1958, with permission.)

i.m. dosing. Thereafter, the serum level declines in a similar manner to that after i.m. administration (see amikacin, p. 508).

Serum concentrations of kanamycin are consistently lower in pregnant than in non-pregnant patients; this is due to both an increase in the distribution volume and the glomerular filtration rate (Chow and Jewesson, 1985).

Excretion

1 Urine

Most i.m. administered kanamycin (50–80%) is excreted in the urine in an active unchanged form and this mainly occurs in the first 6 h. High concentrations of the active drug are attained in urine and with normal doses these are in the range 100–600 μg per ml (Welch *et al.*, 1958, Kunin, 1966). The mechanism for renal excretion of kanamycin is glomerular filtration. Probenecid does not delay kanamycin excretion (Berger *et al.*, 1959). Kanamycin clearance is slightly less than simultaneously determined creatinine clearance, indicating that some of the antibiotic undergoes tubular reabsorption after glomerular filtration (see amikacin, p. 511). Boger and Gavin (1959) found that the clearance rate in an adult patient was about 80% of simultaneous creatinine clearance, but Berger *et al.* (1959) reported that kanamycin was cleared at a somewhat higher rate in children.

2 Bile

After i.m. administration only about 1% of the dose is excreted in the bile. Biliary concentrations are similar to those obtained in sera, but the peak is not reached until 6 h after injection (Hansbrough *et al.*, 1981).

3 Inactivation in body

This probably does occur to a minor extent, but the fate of the small fraction of kanamycin that cannot be recovered in the free form in urine and bile is unknown (Kunin, 1966).

Distribution of the Drug in Body

Kanamycin diffuses into pleural and ascitic fluids, where it may reach concentrations similar to those obtained in serum at the time (Finegold, 1959). Only traces of kanamycin can be detected in the CSF of patients with uninflamed meninges, in saliva (Boger and Gavin, 1959), and in bronchial secretions (Finegold, 1959). After usual kanamycin doses, drug levels in the gall bladder wall range from 8.0 to 14.0 μg per g. The presence of an obstructed cystic duct does not preclude the entry of kanamycin into gallbladder bile; this may reflect passage of the drug through the gallbladder wall rather than accumulation via bile secretion (Hansbrough *et al.*, 1981). The drug is transferred across the placenta and fetal serum levels are 30–50% of those in the mother. Small amounts of kanamycin are excreted in the breast milk, where a concentration of 2.0 μg per ml is reached after usual therapeutic doses (Chow and Jewesson, 1985). In animals, kanamycin accumulates in the renal cortex, probably intracellularly (Luft and Kleit, 1974).

The drug's serum protein binding, if any, is low (Gordon et al., 1972).

Mode of Action

The mode of action of kanamycin and other aminoglycosides on bacteria is similar to that of streptomycin (p. 432).

Toxicity

1 Ototoxicity

This is the most important toxic effect of kanamycin, causing deafness through irreversible cochlear damage. Vestibular function may also be affected but this is less common than with streptomycin (Finegold, 1959, 1966). Several factors predispose to ototoxicity such as pre-existing renal impairment and high kanamycin serum levels. In animals, the magnitude of ototoxicity resulting from kanamycin appears to be related to the total daily dose and not the dosing schedule (Davis et al., 1984). Other factors which contribute to ototoxicity include prolonged use of the drug, increasing age of the patient, pre-existing hearing loss and possibly also previous treatment with ototoxic drugs.

Kanamycin is potentially more toxic for cochlear function than streptomycin, but less so than neomycin (Frost et al., 1959). 'Acute ototoxicity' most commonly occurs when there are sustained kanamycin serum levels higher than 30 μg per ml. 'Chronic ototoxicity' may occur when a large total dose is administered over a long period, even if the daily dose is small. For this reason, if possible, the total adult dose for a course of treatment should not exceed 14 g. Children with normal renal function usually tolerate treatment well if the total dose administered does not exceed 500 mg per kg (Yow, 1966). Ototoxicity was frequent (6–39% in different series), when kanamycin was used for prolonged periods in pulmonary tuberculosis (Kass, 1966). By contrast, a survey in Boston showed that only four (1.6%) of 243 medical inpatients receiving kanamycin developed deafness (A Cooperative Study, 1973). Kanamycin-treated patients should be questioned daily for tinnitus and for a sensation of 'pressure or fullness in the ears', which indicate that the drug should be stopped. Serial weekly audiograms should be performed, where feasible, during therapy (Finegold, 1966).

The use of other ototoxic drugs together with kanamycin are to be avoided, whenever possible. Sudden deafness may occur in association with the i.v. use of the diuretic, ethacrynic acid (A Cooperative Study, 1973). In some of these patients aminoglycosides, such as kanamycin and or gentamicin, had been used concurrently, so their combination with this diuretic may be more liable to cause ototoxicity (Meriwether et al., 1971). In animals, ototoxicity of kanamycin and other aminoglycosides is augmented by concomitant administration of loop-inhibiting diuretics such as frusemide and ethacrynic acid. Ototoxicity is also aggravated if animals are exposed to loud sounds while receiving kanamycin (Brummett, 1983).

Kanamycin ototoxicity appears to be rare in newborn and premature infants. Many children given kanamycin in the recommended dosage in infancy, have had audiometric, vestibular and psychometric evaluations performed when they were aged 4 years. No significant hearing loss or vestibular dysfunction was identified in these patients compared with controls who had never received the drug (Finitzo-Hieber et al., 1979). Also, in spite of the widespread use of kanamycin, very few cases of neonatal ototoxicity have been recorded following short-term maternal administration of the drug during late pregnancy (Chow and Jewesson, 1985).

2 Nephrotoxicity

Similar to other aminoglycosides, such as neomycin (p. 536) and gentamicin (p. 467), kanamycin may cause renal damage. Kanamycin is not as nephrotoxic as neomycin, but it is more toxic than streptomycin, which is the least nephrotoxic aminoglycoside (Appel and Neu, 1977). Although kanamycin is only excreted by glomerular filtration and not by tubular secretion (p. 444), it accumulates in renal cortical tissue (Buss et al., 1984), and can cause changes in the proximal tubules that range from cloudy swelling to acute necrosis. Mild renal toxicity with the appearance of casts, red and white cells and protein in the urine is relatively common. Increasing azotemia is infrequent, except perhaps in older patients. Oliguric renal failure with features of acute tubular necrosis may occasionally develop. Recovery from these more severe nephrotoxic effects is usually slow and may only be partial (Appel and Neu, 1977; Bennett et al., 1977). Early recognition of kanamycin nephrotoxicity is also important because it may predispose patients to ototoxicity (Finegold 1959, 1966).

Animal studies with other aminoglycosides such as gentamicin, tobramycin and netilmicin, indicate that antibiotic – induced nephrotoxicity can be minimized if the total daily dose of the drug is administered as a single daily injection (Bennett *et al.*, 1979; Davis *et al.*, 1984). This does not apply to ototoxicity (p. 458).

3 Neuromuscular blockade

Similar to streptomycin (p. 433) and neomycin (p. 537), kanamycin can cause paralysis which may affect respiration, especially if a large dose is introduced intraperitoneally in an anesthetized patient (Finegold, 1966). The drug may cause postoperative respiratory depression when administered before or during operations, a myasthenic syndrome unrelated to an operation or transient deterioration in patients with myasthenia gravis (Argov and Mastaglia, 1979).

4 Other neurotoxicity

Many other infrequent neurotoxic side-effects have been attributed to kanamycin. These include circumoral and other paresthesiae, headaches, restlessness, nervousness, tachycardia, blurring of vision, and an acute brain syndrome with hysterical features (Finegold, 1966; Snavely and Hodges, 1984).

5 Hypersensitivity

Pruritus, rash, drug fever and even anaphylaxis have been reported, but these are rare (Finegold, 1966). Eosinophilia without clinical manifestations is more common.

6 Side-effects after oral administration

Vomiting and diarrhea can result. The severe but rare complication of staphylococcal enterocolitis may occur as with neomycin (p. 537). Prolonged oral kanamycin administration can induce malabsorption with steatorrhea, but neomycin (p. 537) appears to be more potent in this regard (Faloon *et al.*, 1966).

7 Drug interactions

All aminoglycosides are partially inactivated by high concentrations of any of the penicillins both *in vitro* and *in vivo*. This effect has been more extensively studied with gentamicin (p. 471), tobramycin (p. 157) and amikacin (p. 157), because they have been often used together with high doses of anti-pseudomonal penicillins such as carbenicillin (p. 155) or ticarcillin (p. 157). *In vitro*, the penicillins inactivate kanamycin to about the same degree as gentamicin and tobramycin but this occurs less readily with amikacin (Farchione, 1981). Studies with gentamicin (p. 471) and amikacin have shown that heparin reversibly inhibits aminoglycoside activity in a dose-dependent way. This may also apply to kanamycin. Specimens for aminoglycoside measurements should not be obtained in heparinized tubes. When heparin is used clinically as an anticoagulant, its serum level is not high enough to affect aminoglycoside activity (Nilsson *et al.*, 1981).

Clinical Uses of the Drug

1 Septicemia due to Gram-negative enteric bacilli

These septicemias are usually associated with some predisposing disease state such as pyelonephritis, cholangitis, agranulocytosis, immunosuppression or they may be associated with operative procedures. Prior to the advent of gentamicin (p. 471) and the third-generation cephalosporins such as cefotaxime (p. 338) and at the time when kanamycin-resistant Gram-negative bacilli were still rare, kanamycin was regarded as the antibiotic of first choice for the treatment of these infections (Murdoch *et al.*, 1962). Nowadays the drug is no longer used for these diseases.

2 Tuberculosis

Kanamycin has never been regarded as a first-line drug for the treatment of this disease, but in the past it was sometimes used as a reserve drug for treatment of patients whose *M. tuberculosis* had become resistant to the first line drugs. Nowadays, when multidrug-resistant tuberculosis has arisen in New York, USA and elsewhere, kanamycin is again used, often in combination with ofloxacin or ciprofloxacin, cycloserine, ethionamide or other drugs (Iseman, 1993). The management of multidrug-resistant tuberculosis is described in the chapter on isoniazid (p. 1200).

3 Bowel sterilization

Oral kanamycin is sometimes preferred to neomycin (p. 539) for bowel sterilization in patients with liver failure, especially if they also have renal failure (Kunin, 1966). Both of these drugs are slightly absorbed from the gastrointestinal tract, but kanamycin has a lower ototoxic and nephrotoxic potential. Kanamycin is also less liable to cause changes in the intestinal mucosa and malabsorption (Faloon et al., 1966).

4 Gonorrhea

Kanamycin has been used as an alternative to penicillin G (p. 45) for the treatment of this disease. Satisfactory results in acute uncomplicated gonorrhea, including cases caused by beta-lactamase producing gonococci, have been obtained using single 2.0 g i.m. doses (Report, 1978; Hira et al., 1985). However, other drugs such as ceftriaxone (p. 361), cefixime (p. 412), ciprofloxacin (p. 1022) and ofloxacin (p. 1122) are now preferred. Gonococcal ophthalmia neonatorum caused by beta-lactamase producing strains has been treated by single-dose i.m. kanamycin regimens. Fransen et al. (1984) found that single i.m. doses of 75 or 150 mg kanamycin were only effective when combined with gentamicin eye ointment for 3 days, but Latif et al. (1988) obtained good results by single i.m. doses of 100 mg kanamycin and hourly ocular irrigation with saline. Other drugs such as ceftriaxone (p. 361) are now preferred for this infection. Kanamycin is currently no longer recommended for gonorrhea by the Centers for Disease Control in the USA (Moran and Levine, 1995).

5 Necrotizing enterocolitis

This is a disease predominantly affecting infants of low birth weight who have received intensive care treatment. It is characterized by abdominal distension, ileus, passage of blood in stools, intestinal perforation, septic shock and a high mortality (20–40%). Prophylaxis with oral kanamycin or gentamicin (p. 475) may lower the frequency of the disease or have no appreciable effect. The acutely ill neonate requires immediate treatment. Antibiotics appropriate for the known sensitivities of the nursery patients' enteric flora should be used e.g. ticarcillin or clindamycin and an aminoglycoside such as kanamycin or gentamicin. Although necrotizing enterocolitis may be the final outcome from multiple etiological agents or adverse events, epidemiological observations support an important role for bacteria or their toxins. Specific organisms thought to be associated with this disease include E. coli, Klebsiella and Enterobacter spp., Ps. aeruginosa, Salmonella spp., Clostridium perfringens and Cl. difficile. Coronavirus, rotavirus, and enteroviruses have also been implicated (Egan et al., 1976; 1977; Kliegman and Fanaroff, 1984; Lawrence, 1986). Vancomycin has been used when Cl. difficile was implicated (p. 779).

References

A Cooperative Study (1973). Drug-induced deafness. *JAMA* **224**: 515.

Appel GB, Neu HC (1977). The nephrotoxicity of antimicrobial agents (second of three parts). *New Engl J Med* **296**: 722.

Archer GL, Johnston JL (1983). Self-transmissible plasmids in staphylococci that encode resistance to aminoglycosides. *Antimicrob Ag Chemother* **24**: 70.

Argov Z, Mastaglia FL (1979). Disorders of neuromuscular transmission caused by drugs. *New Engl J Med* **301**: 409.

Atkins RC, Mion C, Despaux E et al. (1973). Peritoneal transfer of kanamycin and its use in peritoneal dialysis. *Kidney Int* **3**: 391.

Baker CJ, Barrett FF, Clark DJ (1974). Incidence of kanamycin resistance among *Escherichia coli* isolates from neonates. *J Pediatr* **84**: 126.

Barber M, Waterworth PM (1966). Activity of gentamicin against *Pseudomonas* and hospital staphylococci. *Brit Med J* **1**: 203.

Becker GJ, Walker RG, Dziukas LJ et al. (1980). Renal infection with *Mycobacterium chelonei*. *Aust NZ J Med* **10**: 44.

Bennett WM, Plamp C, Porter GA (1977). Drug-related syndromes in clinical nephrology. *Ann Intern Med* **87**: 582.

Bennett WM, Plamp CE, Gilbert DN et al. (1979). The influence of dosage regimen on experimental gentamicin nephrotoxicity: dissociation of peak serum levels from renal failure. *J Infect Dis* **140**: 576.

Berger SH, Bergstrom WH, Wehrle PF (1959). Renal clearance of kanamycin in children. *Antibiotic Annual 1958–1959*: 684.

Bloch AB, Cauthen GM, Onorato IM et al. (1994). Nationwide survey of drug-resistant tuberculosis in the United States. *JAMA* **271**: 665.

Boger WP, Gavin JJ (1959). Kanamycin: its cerebrospinal fluid diffusion, renal clearance, and comparison with streptomycin. *Antibiotic Annual 1958–1959*: 677.

Brodie MJ, Boot PA, Girdwood RWA (1973). Severe *Yersinia pseudotuberculosis* infection diagnosed at laparoscopy. *Brit Med J* **4**: 88.

Brummett RE (1983). Animal models of aminoglycoside antibiotic ototoxicity. *Rev Infect Dis* **5** (Suppl 2): 294.

Buss WC, Piatt MK, Kauten R (1984). Inhibition of mammalian microsomal protein synthesis by aminoglycoside antibiotics. *J Antimicrob Chemother* **14**: 231.

Butler T, Bell WR, Linh NN *et al.* (1974). Yersinia pestis infection in Vietnam. I. Clinical and hematological aspects. *J Infect Dis* (May Suppl) **129**: 78.

Chiodini RJ, Van Kruiningen HJ, Thayer WR *et al.* (1984). *In vitro* antimicrobial susceptibility of *Mycobacterium* sp. isolated from patients with Crohn's disease. *Antimicrob Ag Chemother* **26**: 930.

Chow AW, Jewesson PJ (1985). Pharmacokinetics and safety of antimicrobial agents during pregnancy. *Rev Infect Dis* **7**: 287.

Cohen MS, Cooney MH, Blackman E, Sparling PF (1983). *In vitro* antimicrobial susceptibility of penicillinase-producing and intrinsically resistant Neisseria gonorrhoeae strains. *Antimicrob Ag Chemother* **24**: 597.

Cutler RE, Orme BM (1969). Correlation of serum creatinine concentration and kanamycin half-life. Therapeutic implications. *JAMA* **209**: 539.

Danish M, Schultz R, Jusko WJ (1974). Pharmacokinetics of gentamicin and kanamycin during hemodialysis. *Antimicrob Ag Chemother* **6**: 841.

Dans PE, Barrett FF, Casey JI, Finland M (1970). *Klebsiella-Enterobacter* at Boston City Hospital, 1967. *Arch Intern Med* **125**: 94.

Davidson PT, Khanijo V, Goble M, Moulding TS (1981). Treatment of disease due to *Mycobacterium intracellulare*. *Rev Infect Dis* **3**: 1052.

Davis RR, Brummett RE, Bendrick TW, Himes DL (1984). Dissociation of maximum concentration of kanamycin in plasma and perilymph from ototoxic effect. *J Antimicrob Chemother* **14**: 291.

Egan EA, Mantilla G, Nelson RM, Eitzman DV (1976). A prospective controlled trial of oral kanamycin in the prevention of neonatal necrotizing enterocolitis. *J Pediatr* **89**: 467.

Egan EA, Nelson RM, Mantilla G, Eitzman DV (1977). Additional experience with routine use of oral kanamycin prophylaxis for necrotizing enterocolitis in infants under 1500 grams. *J Pediatr* **90**: 331.

Faloon WW, Paes IC, Woolfolk D *et al.* (1966). Effect of neomycin and kanamycin upon intestinal absorption. *Ann NY Acad Sci* **132**: 879.

Farchione LA (1981). Inactivation of aminoglycosides by penicillins. *J Antimicrob Chemother* **8** (Suppl A): 27.

Finegold SM (1959). Kanamycin. *Arch Intern Med* **104**: 15.

Finegold SM (1966). Toxicity of kanamycin in adults. *Ann NY Acad Sci* **132**: 942.

Finitzo-Hieber T, McCracken GH Jr, Roeser RJ *et al.* (1979). Ototoxicity in neonates treated with gentamicin and kanamycin: results of a four-year controlled follow-up study. *Pediatrics* **63**: 443.

Foster TJ (1983). Plasmid-determined resistance to antimicrobial drugs and toxic metal ions in bacteria. *Microbiol Rev* **47**: 361.

Fransen L, Nsanze H, D'Costa L *et al.* (1984). Single-dose kanamycin therapy of gonococcal ophthalmia neonatorum. *Lancet* **ii**: 1234.

Frieden TR, Sterling T, Pablos-Mendez A *et al.* (1993). The emergence of drug-resistant tuberculosis in New York City. *New Engl J Med* **328**: 521.

Frost JO, Daly JF, Hawkins JE Jr (1959). The ototoxicity of kanamycin in man. *Antibiotic Annual 1958–1959*: 700.

Garrod LP, Waterworth PM (1962). Methods of testing combined antibiotic bactericidal action and the significance of the results. *J Clin Path* **15**: 328.

Gelber RH, Henika PR, Gibson JB (1984). The bactericidal activity of various aminoglycoside antibiotics against *Mycobacterium leprae* in mice. *Lepr Rev* **55**: 341.

Gordon RC, Regamey C, Kirby WMM (1972). Serum protein binding of the aminoglycoside antibiotics. *Antimicrob Ag Chemother* **2**: 214.

Greenberg PA, Sanford JP (1967). Removal and absorption of antibiotics in patients with renal failure undergoing peritoneal dialysis. *Ann Intern Med* **66**: 465.

Hammerberg S, Sorger S, Marks MI (1977). Antimicrobial susceptibilities of *Yersinia enterocolitica* Biotype 4, Serotype 0: 3. *Antimicrob Ag Chemother* **11**: 566.

Hansbrough JF, Clark JE, Reimer LG (1981). Concentrations of kanamycin and amikacin in human gallbladder bile and wall. *Antimicrob Ag Chemother* **20**: 515.

Hansen JM, Kampmann J, Laursen H (1970). Renal excretion of drugs in the elderly. *Lancet* **i**: 1170.

Healy JK, Drum PJ, Elliott AJ (1973). Kanamycin dosage in renal failure. *Aust NZ J Med* **3**: 474.

Hieber JP, Nelson JD (1976). Re-evaluation of kanamycin dosage in infants and children. *Antimicrob Ag Chemother* **9**: 899.

Hieber JP, Kusmiesz H, Nelson JD (1980). Kanamycin in children: pharmacology and lack of toxicity of an increased dosage regimen. *J Pediatr* **96**: 1089.

Hira SK, Attili VR, Kamanga J *et al.* (1985). Efficacy of gentamicin and kanamycin in the treatment of uncomplicated gonococcal urethritis in Zambia. *Sex Trans Dis* **12**: 52.

Horodniceanu T, Buu-Hoi A, Delbox F, Bieth G (1982). High-level aminoglycoside resistance in Groups A, B, G, D (*Streptococcus bovis*), and viridans streptococci. *Antimicrob Ag Chemother* **21**: 176.

Howard JB, McCracken GH Jr (1975). Reappraisal of kanamycin usage in neonates. *J Pediatr* **86**: 949.

Hull SI, Wallace RJ Jr, Bobey DG *et al.* (1984). Presence of aminoglycoside acetyltransferase and plasmids in *Mycobacterium fortuitum*. *Amer Rev Respir Dis* **129**: 614.

Iseman MD (1993). Treatment of multidrug-resistant tuberculosis. *New Engl J Med* **329**: 784.

Kass I (1966). Kanamycin in the therapy of pulmonary tuberculosis in the United States. *Ann NY Acad Sci* **132**: 892.

Kayser FH, Homberger F, Devaud M (1981). Aminocyclitol-modifying enzymes specified by chromosomal genes in *Staphylococcus aureus*. *Antimicrob Ag Chemother* **19**: 766.

Kliegman RM, Fanaroff AA (1984). Necrotizing enterocolitis. *New Engl J Med* **310**: 1093.

Kotarski SF, Merriwether TL, Thalcevic GT, Gemski P (1986). Genetic studies of kanamycin resistance in *Campylobacter jejuni*. *Antimicrob Ag Chemother* **30**: 225.

Kunin CM (1966). Absorption, distribution, excretion and fate of kanamycin. *Ann NY Acad Sci* **132**: 811.

Kuze F, Kurasawa T, Bando K *et al.* (1981). *In vitro* and *in vivo* susceptibility of atypical mycobacteria to various drugs. *Rev Infect Dis* **3**: 885.

Latif A, Mason P, Marowa E *et al.* (1988). Management of gonococcal ophthalmia neonatorum with single-dose kanamycin and ocular irrigation with saline. *Sex Transm Dis* **15**: 108.

Lawrence G (1986). Necrotizing enteritis and *Clostridium perfringens*. *J Infect Dis* **153**: 803.

Lorber J (1967). Intrathecal and intraventricular kanamycin in the treatment of meningitis and ventriculitis in infants. *Postgrad Med J* (May Suppl), p. 52.

Luft FC, Kleit SA (1974). Renal parenchymal accumulation of aminoglycoside antibiotics in rats. *J Infect Dis* **130**: 656.

Martin WJ, Gardner M, Washington JA II (1972). *In vitro* antimicrobial susceptibility of anaerobic bacteria isolated from clinical specimens. *Antimicrob Ag Chemother* **1**: 148.

Mawer GE, Knowles BR, Lucas SB *et al.* (1972a). Computer-assisted prescribing of kanamycin for patients with renal insufficiency. *Lancet* **i**: 12.

Mawer GE, Lucas SB, McGough JG (1972b). Nomogram for kanamycin dosage. *Lancet* **ii**: 45.

McCloskey RV, Becker GG (1971). Evaluation of the Cutler-Orme method for administration of kanamycin during renal failure. *Antimicrob Ag Chemother* **1970**: 161.

McCracken GH Jr, Nelson JD (1983). *Antimicrobial Therapy for Newborns* 2nd edn, p. 49. New York: Grune & Stratton.

McCracken GH Jr, Threlkeld N (1976). Kanamycin dosage in newborn infants. *J Pediatr* **89**: 313.

McCracken GH Jr, Threlkeld N, Thomas ML (1977). Intravenous administration of kanamycin and gentamicin in newborn infants. *Pediatrics* **60**: 463.

Meriwether WD, Mangi RJ, Serpick AA (1971). Deafness following standard intravenous dose of ethacrynic acid. *JAMA* **216**: 795.

Michel J, Rogol M, Dickman D (1983). Susceptibility of clinical isolates of *Campylobacter jejuni* to sixteen antimicrobial agents. *Antimicrob Ag Chemother* **23**: 796.

Moellering RC Jr (1983). *In vitro* antibacterial activity of the aminoglycoside antibiotics. *Rev Infect Dis* **5** (Suppl 2): 212.

Moran JS, Levine WC (1995). Drugs of choice for the treatment of uncomplicated gonococcal infections. *Clin Infect Dis* **20** (Suppl 1): 47.

Murdoch JMcC, Geddes AM, Syme J (1962). Studies with kanamycin sulphate. *Lancet* **i**: 457.

Neu HC (1984). Changing mechanisms of bacterial resistance. *Amer J Med* **76**: 11.

Nilsson L, Maller R, Ånsêhn S (1981). Inhibition of aminoglycoside activity by heparin. *Antimicrob Ag Chemother* **20**: 155.

Phillips I, Eykyn S, King BA *et al.* (1977). The *in vitro* antibacterial activity of nine aminoglycosides and spectinomycin on clinical isolates of common Gram-negative bacteria. *J Antimicrob Chemother* **3**: 403.

Reeves DS (1977). Prescription of aminoglycosides by nomogram. *J Antimicrob Chemother* **3**: 533.

Report of a WHO Scientific Group (1978). *Neisseria gonorrhoeae* and gonococcal infections. *Wld Hlth Org Techn Rep Ser* No. 616: 96.

Roe E, Lowbury EJL (1972). Changes in antibiotic sensitivity patterns of Gram-negative bacilli in burns. *J Clin Path* **25**: 176.

Sabath LD (1969). Current concepts: drug resistance of bacteria. *New Engl J Med* **280**: 91.

Sanders WJ, Wolinsky E (1980). *In vitro* susceptibility of *Mycobacterium marinum* to eight antimicrobial agents. *Antimicrob Ag Chemother* **18**: 529.

Sanford J (1966). Panel discussion: toxicity of kanamycin in adults. *Ann NY Acad Sci* **132**: 970.

Sanson-Le Pors M-J, Casin IM, Collatz E (1985). Plasmid-mediated aminoglycoside phosphotransferases in *Haemophilus ducreyi*. *Antimicrob Ag Chemother* **28**: 315.

Snavely SR, Hodges GR (1984). The neurotoxicity of antibacterial agents. *Ann Intern Med* **101**: 92.

Stiffler PW, Sweeney HM, Schneider M, Cohen S (1974). Isolation and characterization of a kanamycin resistant plasmid from *Staphylococcus aureus*. *Antimicrob Ag Chemother* **6**: 516.

Tenover FC, Elvrum PM (1988). Detection of two different kanamycin resistance genes in naturally occurring isolates of *Campylobacter jejuni* and *Campylobacter coli*. *Antimicrob Ag Chemother* **32**: 1170.

Tenover FC, Fennell CL, Lee L, Le Blanc DJ (1992). Characterisation of two plasmids from *Campylobacter jejuni* isolates that carry the aph A-7 kanamycin resistance determinant. *Antimicrob Ag Chemother* **36**: 712.

Terman JW, Alford RH, Bryant RE (1972). Hospital-acquired *Klebsiella* bacteremia. *Amer J Med Sci* **264**: 191.

Thornsberry C, Baker CN, Kirven LA (1978). *In vitro* activity of antimicrobial agents on Legionnaires' disease bacterium. *Antimicrob Ag Chemother* **13**: 78.

Umezawa H, Ueda M, Maeda K *et al.* (1957). Production and isolation of a new antibiotic, kanamycin. *J Antibiot Japan* Ser A **10**: 181.

Wallace RJ Jr, Wiss K (1981). Susceptibility of *Mycobacterium marinum* to tetracyclines and aminoglycosides. *Antimicrob Ag Chemother* **20**: 610.

Wallace RJ Jr, Wiss K, Curvey R *et al.* (1983). Differences among *Nocardia* spp in susceptibility to aminoglycosides and beta-lactam antibiotics and their potential use in taxonomy. *Antimicrob Ag Chemother* **23**: 19.

Welch H, Wright WW, Weinstein HI, Ataffa AW (1958). *In vitro* and pharmacological studies with kanamycin. *Ann NY Acad Sci* **76**: 66.

Wyatt RG, Okamoto GA, Feigin RD (1972). Stability of antibiotics in parenteral solutions. *Pediatrics* **49**: 22.

Yow M (1966). Kanamycin in pediatric practice with special reference observations on ototoxicity. *Ann NY Acad Sci* **132**: 1037.

Zimmer BL, De Young DR, Roberts GD (1982). *In vitro* synergistic activity of ethambutol, isoniazid, kanamycin, rifampin, and streptomycin against *Mycobacterium avium-intracellulare* complex. *Antimicrob Ag Chemother* **22**: 148.

Gentamicin

Description

Gentamicin is produced by a species of bacteria of the genus *Micromonospora* and was discovered in the Schering Research Laboratories (Weinstein *et al.*, 1964). It is structurally related to the other aminoglycosides, streptomycin, kanamycin, neomycin, amikacin, tobramycin, sisomicin and netilmicin. Gentamicin is used clinically as the sulfate salt.

For about a decade after its discovery gentamicin was usually the preferred drug for the treatment of severe infections caused by Gram-negative aerobic bacteria, particularly in hospitals. Since the mid-1970s, its usefulness has decreased in some areas by the emergence of bacterial resistance. Alternative effective drugs have also become available such as the third-generation cephalosporins (p.338) and the new quinolones (p.981).

Sensitive Organisms

1 Gram-negative aerobic bacteria

Gentamicin is active against nearly all of the Enterobacteriaceae, such as *Escherichia coli*, the *Enterobacter*, *Klebsiella*, *Proteus*, *Salmonella*, *Shigella*, *Providencia*, *Serratia*, *Citrobacter*, *Hafnia*, *Edwardsiella* and *Arizona* spp. (Weinstein *et al.*, 1964; Jao and Jackson, 1964; Panwalker *et al.*, 1980; John *et al.*, 1982; Guimaraes *et al.*, 1985). An exception is *Providencia stuartii*, which unlike other *Providencia* spp. sometimes needs high gentamicin concentrations for inhibition (MICs <0.5->32.0 µg per ml) (Penner and Preston, 1980; Penner *et al.*, 1982). *Yersinia pestis*, *Y. pseudotuberculosis*, *Y. enterocolitica*, *Yersinia*-like organisms and atypical strains of *Yersinia* are also usually gentamicin-sensitive (Butler *et al.*, 1974; Hammerberg *et al.*, 1977; Soriano and Vega, 1982; Pham *et al.*, 1991).

For a period after its introduction, gentamicin-resistant strains of even those Enterobacteriaceae which are normal inhabitants of the human bowel, were uncommon (Sabath, 1969). This contrasted with the high prevalence of kanamycin-resistant organisms at the time (p.439). Since then gentamicin has been extensively used and the prevalence of Enterobacteriaceae resistant to it has gradually increased in many hospitals or special hospital areas, such as burns, intensive care units and long-term care facilities (Roe and Lowbury, 1972; Moellering, 1983; John and Ribner, 1991).

Hospital infections and outbreaks caused by gentamicin-resistant *Klebsiella* spp. became especially prevalent (Richmond *et al.*, 1975; Casewell *et al.*, 1977; Forbes *et al.*, 1977; Gerding *et al.*, 1979; Ackerman *et al.*, 1983; Alford and Hall, 1987). The frequency of such strains often declined rapidly when the use of gentamicin was restricted in a hospital, and increased again several months after restrictions were removed (Noriega *et al.*, 1975). Similarly, in hospitals where amikacin (p.515) was used as the principal aminoglycoside, the prevalence of gentamicin-resistant *Klebsiella* spp. and other resistant Gram-negative aerobic bacilli usually decreased (Ristuccia and Cunha, 1982; Aronsson *et al.*, 1991; Gerding *et al.*, 1991).

Resistant strains of *Serratia marcescens* have been relatively uncommon in the UK (Phillips *et al.*, 1977; Knight and Casewell, 1981), but they have been a problem in several North American Hospitals (Meyer *et al.*, 1976; Schaberg *et al.*, 1976; John and McNeil, 1981; Rutala *et al.*, 1981; Alford and Hall, 1987). In one patient with *S. marcescens* bacteremia and pneumonia, treated by a cefazolin/gentamicin combination, multiple resistance to aminoglycosides and beta-lactams emerged during therapy (Sanders and Watanakunakorn, 1986).

Gentamicin-resistant strains of other Enterobacteriaceae, particularly those which are normal inhabitants of human bowel, have been isolated from hospital patients. Reports include resistant *E. coli* (Drasar *et al.*, 1976; Ike *et al.*, 1981; Bengtsson *et al.*, 1986; Chaslus-Dancla *et al.*, 1986), *Enterobacter* spp. (Drasar *et al.*, 1976; Phillips *et al.*, 1977; John *et al.*, 1982); *Proteus* spp. (Shafi and Datta, 1975; Drasar *et al.*, 1976), *Providencia* spp. (Drasar *et al.*, 1976; Shlaes *et al.*, 1983) and *Citrobacter* spp. (Richmond *et al.*, 1975; Drasar *et al.*, 1976). During an investigation of an outbreak of calf salmonellosis, gentamicin-resistant *Salmonella typhimurium* strains were found, which were also resistant to ampicillin, chloramphenicol, kanamycin, streptomycin, tetracycline and trimethoprim. Intestinal *E. coli* strains from 11 of 24 animals sampled showed the same multiple antibiotic-resistance pattern (Chaslus-Dancla *et al.*, 1986).

Nowadays the third-generation cephalosporins such as cefotaxime (p.319) have replaced gentamicin for many indications and when gentamicin is used it is usually combined with a beta-lactam agent. Overall gentamicin-resistant Enterobacteriaceae have become again less common in hospitals. Most Enterobacteriaceae were sensitive to gentamicin in one large USA hospital (Gerding *et al.*, 1991), in Canada (Chamberland *et al.*, 1992) and in Central and Northern Europe; in Southern Europe the resistance levels were somewhat higher (Dornbusch *et al.*, 1990). All but one of 176 *Proteus mirabilis* strains isolated from blood cultures in one USA hospital during 1980–1992, were gentamicin-sensitive (Watanakunakorn and Perni, 1994).

Gentamicin-resistant strains of *E. coli*, produced *in vitro* by passage in a gentamicin-containing medium, show complete cross-resistance with streptomycin, neomycin, kanamycin and tobramycin. In contrast, naturally occurring gentamicin-resistant strains are not necessarily resistant to the three older drugs, but are usually resistant to tobramycin (p.489) (Houang and Greenwood, 1977). Many strains of Enterobacteriaceae which are resistant to gentamicin, are sensitive to either amikacin (p.504) or netilmicin (p.523), but they are usually resistant to tobramycin (p.489) and sisomicin (p.522).

Pseudomonas aeruginosa is quite sensitive and activity against this organism is one of the important features of gentamicin. Resistant strains have been noted in many hospitals since the advent of this drug. With its increased clinical use both parenterally and topically, the prevalence of such strains has gradually increased. Nevertheless, in most hospitals gentamicin-resistant *Ps. aeruginosa* isolates were still relatively uncommon in the 1970s (Duncan, 1974; Dean *et al.*, 1977). The incidence of gentamicin-resistance in *Ps. aeruginosa* strains isolated from patients in a large Canadian hospital was followed for 11 years after 1968. For the first 5 years the proportion of resistant strains was about 5%, but then it gradually rose to 9% (Duncan *et al.*, 1981). Outbreaks of infections or colonizations of patients by gentamicin-resistant *Ps. aeruginosa* have occurred in special hospital areas (or sometimes throughout a hospital), usually following the widespread use of this drug. Examples are outbreaks in a burns unit (Bridges *et al.*, 1979), in a surgical ward (Falkiner *et al.*, 1977), in an intensive care unit (Olson *et al.*, 1985) and in a cancer research center (Greene *et al.*, 1973). In the USA, a 12-month survey in 1974–1975 at one hospital showed that 19.1% of *Ps. aeruginosa* isolates were gentamicin-resistant (Meyer *et al.*, 1976), and in another hospital the percentage of resistant isolates increased from 13.9 in 1969 to 38.9 in 1972 (Maliwan *et al.*, 1975). In one USA hospital gentamicin-resistant *Ps. aeruginosa* strains first appeared in 1973, and then their frequency varied up till 1977, comprising 0–3% of isolates (Rubens *et al.*, 1981). In special hospital areas where the emergence and spread of gentamicin-resistant *Ps. aeruginosa* was related to excessive use of both parenteral and topical gentamicin, the percentage of resistant strains decreased when the clinical use of the drug was restricted (Holder, 1976; Roberts and Douglas, 1978). More recent surveys indicate that in general gentamicin-resistant *Ps. aeruginosa* strains are more common in hospitals than resistant Enterobacteriaceae (Alford and Hall, 1987; Nilsson *et al.*, 1987; Chamberland *et al.*, 1992).

Similar to gentamicin-resistant Enterobacteriaceae (p.450), gentamicin-resistant *Ps. aeruginosa* strains are often sensitive to amikacin (p.505) and may be sometimes sensitive to netilmicin (p.523). Unlike the Enterobacteriaceae, a proportion of these strains have remained sensitive to tobramycin (p.489) (Meyer *et al.*, 1976; Kauffman *et al.*, 1978).

Burkholderia (previously *Pseudomonas*) *cepacia*, *Ps. multivorans*, *Ps. putida*, *Ps. fluorescens* and *Stenotrophomonas maltophilia* are usually gentamicin-resistant. *Pseudomonas stutzeri* and *Ps. putrefaciens* may be gentamicin-sensitive, but resistant strains occur (Uwaydah and Taqi-Eddin, 1976; Phillips *et al.*, 1977; Moody and Young, 1979; Kim *et al.*, 1989). Usually *Ps. paucimobilis* is sensitive (Reina *et al.*, 1991).

Among other Gram-negative bacteria, the *Neisseria* spp. (meningococci and gonococci) are only moderately sensitive to gentamicin, the degree varying with individual strains. *Haemophilus influenzae* is also only moderately sensitive. The *Brucella* and *Moraxella* spp., *Pasteurella multocida* (Waitz and Weinstein, 1969) and *Francisella tularensis* (Alford *et al.*, 1972), are usually susceptible. *Acinetobacter* spp. is also usually gentamicin-sensitive (Obana *et al.*, 1985; Anstey *et al.*, 1992; Tilley and Roberts, 1994). In one outbreak of infections and colonizations in an intensive care unit in France, the *Acinetobacter baumanii* strain had become resistant to all cephalosporins, quinolones and aminoglycosides, including gentamicin. The strain was sensitive to colistin and imipenem (Lortholary *et al.*, 1995). Imipenem-resistance of this organism has also been described (p.229). *Aeromonas* spp. are also usually gentamicin-sensitive (Harris *et al.*, 1985) but the *Alcaligenes* spp. are commonly resistant to gentamicin and other aminoglycosides (Uwaydah and Taqi-Eddin, 1976). The *Flavobacterium* spp., which may be sensitive to rifampicin (p.677), erythromycin (p.609) and vancomycin (p.767), are always resistant to aminoglycosides including gentamicin (Drasar *et al.*, 1976; Lee *et al.*, 1977).

Legionella pneumophilia is sensitive to gentamicin (MIC 0.12–0.5 μg per ml) (Thornsberry *et al.*, 1978; Gibson and Fitzgeorge, 1983). The drug administered prophylactically or up to 48 h after infection, can prevent the death of embryonated eggs infected with this organism (Lewis *et al.*, 1978), but it does not prevent the death of infected guinea pigs (Fraser *et al.*, 1978). Gentamicin is also ineffective for the treatment of legionellosis in humans. *Legionella pneumophila* replicates intracellularly in human monocytes, and it is possible that testing antimicrobial susceptibility in human monocytes may correlate better with *in vivo* efficacy of antibiotics for legionellosis (Bacheson *et al.*, 1981). *Legionella micdadei*, similarly is gentamicin-sensitive *in vitro*, but the drug is ineffective for treatment of human infections caused by this organism (Dowling *et al.*, 1982). *Campylobacter jejuni* is sensitive to gentamicin and also to other aminoglycosides, such as kanamycin (p.440) and amikacin (p.504) (Ahonkhai *et al.*, 1981; Michel *et al.*, 1983). The drug is also quite active against *Campylobacter fetus*, an organism associated with septicemia and endocarditis in immunocompromised hosts (Chow *et al.*, 1978; Goossens *et al.*, 1989). *Helicobacter pylori* is gentamicin-sensitive (McNuity *et al.*, 1985; Goodwin *et al.*, 1986). The aerotolerant *Campylobacter* spp. such as *C. cryaerophila* and *C. butzleri* are usually gentamicin-sensitive (Kiehlbauch *et al.*, 1992). So is also *Helicobacter cinaedi*, which can cause bacteremia and cellulitis in immunocompromised patients (Kiehlbauch *et al.*, 1994; Burman *et al.*, 1995).

2 Gram-negative anaerobic bacteria

All these, such as *Fusobacterium* spp., *Prevotella* (*Bacteroides*) *melaninogenica*, *Bacteroides fragilis* and other *Bacteroides* spp. are gentamicin-resistant (Brook *et al.*, 1984). Their mechanism of resistance is described on p.453. Gentamicin, combined with either penicillin G, clindamycin or metronidazole may significantly reduce the MICs of the latter three drugs against some strains of *P. melaninogenica* (Brook *et al.*, 1984). Gentamicin does not interfere with the *in vitro* activity of clindamycin or chloramphenicol against *B. fragilis* (Klastersky and Husson, 1977). Gentamicin plus clindamycin or metronidazole may act synergistically against some *B. fragilis* strains (Okubadejo and Allen, 1975; Brook *et al.*, 1984). This may be due to increased transport of gentamicin into the cells of anaerobic bacteria in the presence of other antimicrobials (p.589). Chloramphenicol may interfere with the action of gentamicin on aerobic Gram-negative bacilli, such as *E. coli*, but this antagonism, although observed *in vitro*, probably is of little significance *in vivo* (p.549).

3 Mechanisms of resistance of Gram-negative bacteria to gentamicin

There are three known mechanisms by which Gram-negative bacteria develop resistance to gentamicin and other aminoglycosides.

a Ribosomal mutation This causes an alteration at the site of aminoglycoside attachment to the ribosome thereby interfering with the drug's ability to bind to the ribosome (p.432). Gram-negative bacteria readily develop high-level resistance to streptomycin by this mechanism (p.432), because this drug appears to bind to a single site on the 30S subunit of the ribosome. Other aminoglycosides, such as kanamycin, gentamicin, tobramycin and amikacin, appear to bind to multiple sites on both ribosomal subunits, and high-level ribosomal resistance to these drugs is rare and cannot be selected *in vitro* by a single mutational step. Low level gentamicin-resistance due to changes in ribosomal proteins has been reported, and stepwise high-level resistance may develop if an organism is exposed *in vitro* to progressively higher concentrations of the drug. These mutants are avirulent and revert rapidly to sensitivity when grown in the absence of gentamicin (Shannon and Phillips, 1982; Foster, 1983; Moellering, 1983).

b Decreased cell permeability   Uptake of gentamicin and other aminoglycosides in sensitive strains of Gram-negative bacteria occurs in three stages (Bryan and Van den Elzen, 1977; Foster, 1983; Neu, 1984a; Taber *et al.*, 1987). These antibiotics initially associate with the cell wall and then pass passively through outer membrane pores. The next phase is energy-dependent and involves binding of the antibiotics to membranous structures and respiratory quinones (p.432) to form complexes for their transport into cell. The third phase is also energy-dependent and involves membrane-bound aminoglycoside becoming bound to ribosomes. Uptake of aminoglycosides is dependent on energy derived from aerobic metabolism. All anaerobic bacteria are aminoglycoside-resistant because intracellular transport of these agents is markedly impaired in the absence of oxygen. These bacteria are resistant, even though they contain ribosomes which are susceptible to aminoglycosides (Bryan *et al.*, 1979; Moellering, 1983). Failure of intracellular transport is also closely linked with the third mechanism of resistance, enzymatic modification (see below). Aminoglycosides which are modified by acetylation etc. appear to be unable to react with ribosomes and inhibit protein synthesis, and they only exhibit the first two phases of transport into the bacterial cell (Foster, 1983; Neu, 1984a; Taber *et al.*, 1987).

Some strains of *Ps. aeruginosa* and other Gram-negative bacilli do not possess inactivating enzymes or ribosomal mutations, yet they are resistant to gentamicin and other aminoglycosides. In some of these resistance is due to a transport defect. These mutants may have changes in cytochromes, respiratory quinones or a reduction of the synthesis of components of the electron transport chain (Bryan and Kwan, 1981). This type of resistance leads to generalized cross-resistance to all aminoglycosides, although the level of resistance may be low (Davies, 1983). It probably occurs by a chromosomal mutation affecting the gene for aminoglycoside transport (Hardy *et al.*, 1980). In other bacterial strains resistance may be due to a permeability barrier at the cell wall; in some *Ps. aeruginosa* strains a low level aminoglycoside-resistance is associated with a change in the structure of the lipopolysaccharide in their cell walls (Bryan *et al.*, 1984; Shearer and Legakis, 1985; Bryan, 1988; Young *et al.*, 1992; Kadurugamuwa *et al.*, 1993). *Burkholderia cepacia* does not appear to utilize the self-promoted pathway for gentamicin uptake and its outer membrane is arranged in a way that protects cation binding sites on the lipopolysacharide layer in cell wall (Moore and Hancock, 1986).

c Aminoglycoside modifying enzymes   High-level resistance of Enterobacteriaceae and *Ps. aeruginosa* most commonly occurs due to the acquisition of plasmids, (p.549) which code for the production of enzymes, modifying gentamicin by either acetylation, adenylylation or phosphorylation (Bryan *et al.*, 1974; Shannon *et al.*, 1978; Shaw *et al.*, 1993). These plasmids have been implicated in many hospital outbreaks of infections caused by resistant aerobic Gram-negative bacteria, in which gentamicin-resistance is often associated with resistance to other antibiotics (Richmond *et al.*, 1975; Davey and Pittard, 1977; John and McNeill, 1981; Takahashi and Nagano, 1985; Lee *et al.*, 1986; Lovering *et al.*, 1988). Some authors have found that simultaneous emergence of resistance to beta-lactams and aminoglycosides is rare (Stratton *et al.*, 1987). But *Acinetobacter baumannii* strains have been described resistant to third-generation cephalosporins because of beta-lactamase production, resistant to gentamicin because of production of aminoglycoside-modifying enzymes and resistant to chloramphenicol because of chloramphenicol acetyltransferase (p.549) (Vila *et al.*, 1993). Clinical isolates of Enterobacteriaceae which harbor extended-spectrum beta-lactamases (p.323) may be gentamicin-resistant (Fernandez-Rodriguez *et al.*, 1992) or amikacin-resistant (Mainardi *et al.*, 1994) because they also produce aminoglycoside-modifying enzymes.

Plasmids coding for resistance to gentamicin, other aminoglycosides and many other antibiotics, vary greatly in size and in the types of antibiotic-resistance genes they possess. Plasmids may be conjugative or non-conjugative in type (p.549) (Rubens *et al.*, 1981; Takahashi and Nagano, 1985; Mayer *et al.*, 1986). Aminoglycoside-resistance genes have also been found in DNA sequences or transposons, which can be translocated not only from one plasmid to another in a bacterial cell, but also between plasmids and bacterial chromosomes or bacteriophage genomes (Rubens *et al.*, 1981; Davies, 1983; Neu, 1984b; Mucha and Farrand, 1986; Coleman *et al.*, 1994). This was exemplified by a study of resistance to gentamicin between 1973 and 1977 by Rubens *et al.* (1981). In strains of *S. marcescens* isolated early in a hospital outbreak, gentamicin-resistance was mediated by a common 9.8-megadalton non-conjugative plasmid. A 100-megadalton conjugative plasmid, which conferred resistance to other antibiotics, coexisted with the small gentamicin plasmid in resistant *Serratia* spp. strains. Transposition between the 100- and 9.8-megadalton plasmid in this species resulted in the formation of a 105-megadalton conjugative plasmid which mediated gentamicin-resistance. The genes conferring resistance to gentamicin were located on a transposable DNA sequence (transposon) of 6.2-megadalton molecular weight, which had originally comprised part of the 9.8-megadalton plasmid but had now been transposed to the 100-megadalton plasmid.

At the molecular level, resistance to gentamicin and other aminoglycosides is determined by a group of relatively small genes, which may be located on the chromosome, plasmids, transposons and possibly bacteriophages (Davies, 1983; Lupski, 1987; Shaw et al., 1991; Coleman et al., 1994). Different genes code for the production of different aminoglycoside-modifying enzymes. These genes and their corresponding enzymes have been studied by DNA probe technology. This has been helpful in monitoring the spread of particular resistance genes within a hospital and in delineating the number of genes involved in hospital outbreaks. The technique is also useful in defining the modes of transmission of resistant organisms and may be important in epidemiological studies of antimicrobial resistance (Tenover et al., 1984; Groot Obbink et al., 1985; Young et al., 1985; Tenover, 1986; Barg, 1988; Tenover et al., 1989; Ho and Ng, 1993). The polymerase chain reaction has also been used to identify genes encoding aminoglycoside-modifying enzymes (Vanhoof et al., 1992).

Aminoglycoside-resistance genes code for the production of enzymes which modify these drugs by either acetylation, adenylylation or phosphorylation (Foster, 1983; Moellering, 1983; Neu, 1984a,b; Lovering et al., 1986; Shaw et al., 1993). These enzymes, unlike beta-lactamases (p.26), are not secreted extracellularly and thereby have no effect on the drug outside the cell. They may be located in the periplasmic space (p.26) or in the cytoplasm. Aminoglycosides modified by these enzymes cannot bind to ribosomes (p.432).

There are at least four acetyltransferases which modify aminoglycosides by acetylation, which are designated AAC-1; AAC-2', AAC-3 and AAC-6'. The enzymes AAC-3 and AAC-6' are each further subdivided into several types. These enzymes are found in various Gram-negative bacilli, but AAC-6' is also produced by enterococci. Gentamicin can be modified by AAC-2' and by some types of AAC-3 and AAC-6' enzymes, but amikacin is only affected by the AAC-6' group.

Adenylylation may be caused by at least five adenylyltransferases, designated ANT-2'', ANT-3'', ANT-4', ANT-6 and ANT-9. ANT-4' is further subdivided in two types. ANT-2'' can modify gentamicin, and ANT-4' can modify amikacin.

There are at least ten phosphotransferases, designated APH-3'-I, APH-3'-II, APH-3'-III, APH-3'-IV, APH-3'-V, APH-3'-VI, APH-3'-VII, APH-3''-I, APH-6-I and APH-4-I. Most of these can be elaborated by various Gram-negative bacilli. APH-3'-II and APH-3'-VI can modify gentamicin, but amikacin is only modified by APH-3'-VI.

In summary, gentamicin is susceptible to modification by at least nine enzymes elaborated by Gram-negative bacilli, but amikacin (p.505) is only affected by three of them (Shaw et al., 1989; 1993; Barg and Cooper, 1990; Pitt et al., 1990; Vliegenthart et al., 1991; Rather et al., 1993).

4 Gram-positive bacteria

All strains of Staph. aureus were initially highly sensitive to gentamicin (Barber and Waterworth, 1966; Hoeprich, 1969; Jordan and Hoeprich, 1977). By the mid-1970s, almost a decade after the introduction of gentamicin, reports of outbreaks of infections in hospitals caused by gentamicin-resistant strains of Staph. aureus, appeared (Speller et al., 1976; Wyatt et al., 1977; Lewis and Altemeier, 1978; McGowan et al., 1979). These strains were often resistant to many other antibiotics such as penicillin G, tetracyclines, streptomycin, neomycin, kanamycin, tobramycin, erythromycin and clindamycin. In some of these outbreaks there was evidence that prior excessive use of gentamicin, particularly topically, was a factor.

Shanson et al. (1976) first reported nosocomial infection with Staphylococcus aureus strains resistant to gentamicin and methicillin, as well as to other antibiotics. In the late 1970s and early 1980s there were large hospital outbreaks in the USA, Australia and UK caused by methicillin-resistant Staph. aureus strains which were co-resistant to gentamicin and to most other antibiotics then available, except vancomycin, rifampicin and sodium fusidate (p.80) (Dowd et al., 1983; Gillespie et al., 1984; Townsend et al., 1984).

Resistance of Staph. aureus to gentamicin is mediated by plasmids (p.549), which code for the production of gentamicin-modifying enzymes. Three enzymes are mainly involved in gentamicin modification, 4'-adenylyltransferase (ANT-4'), 3' phosphotransferase (APH-3'‾III) and the bifunctional enzyme 6' acetyltransferase (AAC-6')/2'' phosphotransferase (APH-2'') (Storrs et al., 1988; Hodel-Christian and Murray, 1991; Shaw et al., 1993; Archer and Climo, 1994; Vanhoof et al., 1994).

Gentamicin-resistance genes are usually located on conjugative or non-conjugative plasmids (Schaberg et al., 1985; Byrne et al., 1990), but some can also be located on the chromosome (Storrs et al., 1988; Jordens and Hall, 1989). As in the case of Gram-negative bacilli (p.453), transfer of transposons from the chromosome into plasmids, from one plasmid to another, and a stable integration of an entire plasmid into the chromosome, may occur (Dowd *et al.*, 1983; Townsend *et al.*, 1983; Witte and Dünnhaupt, 1984; Thomas and Archer, 1989; Archer and Scott, 1991; Hodel-Christian and Murray, 1991). In addition, high-level mutational resistance of *Staph. aureus* to gentamicin and all other aminoglycosides, has probably emerged during gentamicin therapy, possibly due to a chromosomal mutation (Heritage *et al.*, 1986).

In some *Staph. aureus* strains, similar to Gram-negative bacilli (p.453), the resistance mechanism is probably decreased intracellular uptake of gentamicin or abnormal intracellular transport of the drug. Such resistance probably arises from a chromosomal mutation. These organisms exhibit a broad spectrum of resistance that applies to all clinically useful aminoglycosides, including amikacin (Miller *et al.*, 1980; Moellering, 1983).

If gentamicin MICs against *Staph. aureus* strains are estimated under anaerobic conditions, they are some 10-fold greater than those determined aerobically. This may be of clinical significance as some *Staph. aureus* infections, such as osteomyelitis and some deep-seated abscesses, are essentially anaerobic (Harrell and Evans, 1978; Mates *et al.*, 1983).

Staphylococcus epidermidis, including penicillin G- and methicillin-resistant strains were initially gentamicin-sensitive (Laverdiere *et al.*, 1978). Now the position is rather similar to that of *Staph. aureus*, in that plasmid-mediated gentamicin-resistance among *Staph. epidermidis* strains is common in hospitals. These strains are often resistant to multiple antibiotics, including methicillin (p.81). Plasmids may be transferred from *Staph. epidermidis* to *Staph. aureus* and *vice versa* (Jaffe *et al.*, 1980, 1982; Archer and Johnston, 1983; Archer *et al.*, 1985; Archer and Scott, 1991).

In contrast to *Staph. epidermidis*, most strains of *Staph. saprophyticus* are still gentamicin-sensitive (Bourgault and Gauvreau, 1983). Other Gram-positive cocci, such as *Streptococcus pyogenes*, Group B streptococci, *Strep. pneumoniae*, and the alpha-hemolytic streptococci (*Strep. viridans*), have only a low degree of sensitivity to gentamicin. These organisms usually do not exhibit high-level gentamicin-resistance and so penicillin G (or ampicillin), combined with gentamicin acts synergistically against Group A and B streptococci (Schauf *et al.*, 1976; Baker *et al.*, 1981). Similar to streptomycin (p.429), gentamicin combined with penicillin G acts synergistically against most *Strep. viridans* strains (Sande and Irvin, 1974). However, against penicillin G-sensitive and -resistant strains of pneumococci, gentamicin only mildly enhances the bactericidal activity of penicillin G and cefotaxime (Gross *et al.*, 1995).

Plasmid or chromosomally mediated high-level gentamicin-resistance has been described in some strains of Group B streptococci (Buu-Hoï *et al.*, 1990; Kaufhold *et al.*, 1992) and chromosomally mediated high-level gentamicin-resistance in *Strep. mitis* (Kaufhold and Potgieter, 1993). For these strains penicillin G (or ampicillin) plus gentamicin does not exhibit synergism. With *Strep. pyogenes* high-level streptomycin- and kanamycin-resistance has been detected but no high-level gentamicin-resistance (Van Asselt *et al.*, 1992).

Enterococcus faecalis is moderately resistant (MIC 5.0–125.0 µg per ml) but in studies gentamicin combined with penicillin G (or ampicillin) was usually synergistic against this organism. This applied to the majority of *E. faecalis* strains, whereas penicillin G/streptomycin (p.429) and penicillin G/kanamycin (p.440) combinations were not found to be synergistic against a large proportion of strains (Ruhen and Darrell, 1973; Calderwood *et al.*, 1977). *in vitro* observations and animal studies have suggested that a peak serum gentamicin concentration of 3.0 µg per ml may be sufficient to obtain optimal penicillin G/gentamicin synergism for the treatment of *E. faecalis* endocarditis (Matsumoto *et al.*, 1980; Carrizosa and Levison, 1981). Penicillin G/gentamicin synergism could not be demonstrated against a small number of *E. faecalis* strains, but these were killed synergistically by penicillin G/tobramycin. Such strains have been of the 'small-colony variant' type and not highly resistant to gentamicin alone. Their resistance appeared to be related to a specific defect in the intracellular uptake of gentamicin (but not tobramycin) in the presence of penicillin G (Moellering *et al.*, 1980; Eliopoulos and Moellering, 1982). A penicillin G/tobramycin combination did not exhibit synergism against *Strep. faecium* (p.42).

In the 1980s the situation changed because strains of *E. faecalis* appeared which had high-level resistance (MICs higher than 2000 µg per ml) to gentamicin (Horodniceanu *et al.*, 1979; Mederski-Samoray and Murray 1983; Murray *et al.*, 1983). The MIC of gentamicin of these strains was >2000 µg per ml, which is much higher than MICs of those with only low-level resistance (see above) (Zervos *et al.*, 1986b). A combination of penicillin G (or ampicilin) plus gentamicin is not synergistic against *E. faecalis* strains with high-level resistance to gentamicin (Patterson and Zervos, 1990; Leclercq *et al.*, 1992). High-level resistance to gentamicin in such strains is mediated by the production of an aminoglycoside-modifying enzyme with both 6'acetyltransferase (AAC-6') and 2'' phosphotransferase (APH-2'') activities (p.454) (Patterson and Zervos, 1990; Woodford *et al.*, 1992). The same enzymes modify all other aminoglycosides except streptomycin, so *E. faecalis* strains with high-level gentamicin-resistance always have high-level resistance (and lack of synergism with penicillin G) to tobramycin, kanamycin, amikacin, netilmicin and sisomicin. High-level streptomycin-resistance is due to an enzyme that appears to adenylylate the 6-hydroxy position of the drug. However, only some 10–20% of *E. faecalis*, with high-level gentamicin-resistance, exhibit low-level streptomycin-resistance and penicillin G/streptomycin synergism (p.429). This percentage, however, varies greatly between different institutions and it may be as low as 0% or as high as 49% (Herman and Gerding, 1991a,b; Murray, 1991; Noskin *et al.*, 1991; Thal *et al.*, 1993).

In recent years *E. faecalis* strains with high-level gentamicin-resistance have become quite prevalent in US hospitals. Whilst in some institutions they still may be absent, in others their prevalence exceeds 50% (Hoffmann and Moellering, 1987; Zervos *et al.*, 1987; Weems *et al.*, 1989; Patterson and Zervos, 1990; Watanakunakorn, 1992; Antalek *et al.*, 1995). Such strains have been also detected in other countries including Canada (Bryce *et al.*, 1991), UK (Smyth and Holliman, 1988; Smyth *et al.*, 1989; Gray *et al.*, 1991; Guiney and Urwin, 1993), Argentina (Murray *et al.*, 1992), Thailand (Murray *et al.*, 1983), Italy and Chile (Hodel-Christian and Murray, 1992), Africa and Japan (Patterson and Zervos, 1990), and in Singapore (Chiew *et al.*, 1993). In one study in the USA, enterococci with high-level gentamicin-resistance were not detected in feces of healthy volunteers, but they were present in feces of 15% of hospitalized individuals (Coque *et al.*, 1995).

The high-level gentamicin-resistance of *E. faecalis* is plasmid-mediated which codes for the production of the specific aminoglycoside modifying enzymes involved (p.455). The plasmid is transferable by conjugation from a resistant to a susceptible strain. Gentamicin-resistance plasmids of *E. faecalis* from diverse geographic areas are heterogeneous, and a variety of conjugative and non-conjugative plasmids are involved (Zervos *et al.*, 1986a; Patterson *et al.*, 1988a; Patterson and Zervos, 1990; Hodel-Christian and Murray, 1992). A transposon can also mediate high-level gentamicin-resistance (Hodel Christian and Murray, 1990, 1991, 1992; Rice *et al.*, 1995). The gentamicin-resistance gene can also be located in the chromosome and from there it can be transposed into various plasmids via transposons (Thal *et al.*, 1994).

Most beta-lactamase producing *E. faecalis* strains (p.10) also show high-level gentamicin-resistance (Ingerman *et al.*, 1987; Markowitz *et al.*, 1991). The beta-lactamase genes and gentamicin-resistance genes in these strains appeared to be integrated into the bacterial chromosome. The co-transmissibility of these resistance determinants makes it likely that they are incorporated into a multiresistance transposable genetic element (Rice *et al.*, 1991a).

A combination of gentamicin with vancomycin is synergistic against *E. faecalis* (p.764) (Chen, 1986), except, as with penicillin G, if a strain with high-level gentamicin-resistance is involved.

Enterococcus faecium usually exhibits low-level gentamicin-resistance, similar to *E. faecalis*. These strains are killed synergistically by penicillin G/gentamicin, but not by combinations of penicillin G and most other aminoglycosides. Penicillin G/streptomycin and penicillin G/amikacin are only synergistic against those strains which are not highly resistant to streptomycin and kanamycin, respectively. Combinations of penicillin G with kanamycin, tobramycin, sisomicin or netilmicin fail to produce synergism against any *E. faecium* strains (Moellering *et al.*, 1979). Genes coding for high-level gentamicin-resistance in *E. faecalis* can be transferred to *E. faecium in vitro*, and *in vivo*. Such *E. faecium* strains exhibit high-level gentamicin-resistance and are unaffected by penicillin G/gentamicin synergism (Chen and Williams, 1985; Eliopoulos *et al.*, 1988; Woodford *et al.*, 1992). High-level gentamicin-resistant strains of *E. faecium* may be becoming more common (Noskin *et al.*, 1995). Handwerger *et al.* (1993) described a nosocomial outbreak due to a single strain of such *E. faecium*, involving nine patients in a USA hospital. In addition this strain was highly resistant to penicillin G and vancomycin. Woodford *et al.* (1993) found that the plasmid profiles from high-level gentamicin-resistant *E. faecium* strains were similar in isolates from Europe, Singapore and Australia suggesting a single origin for these strains. But the plasmid from one such *E. faecium* strain isolated in USA showed little homology with the other plasmids studied.

Genes homologous to the *E. faecalis* high-level gentamicin-resistance gene can also be demonstrated in three additional enterococcal spp, *E. avium*, *E. gallinarium* and *E. raffinosus*. Transfer of these resistance determinants between and among various species can occur, but there is some heterogeneity between the resistance genes in the various species (Grayson *et al.*, 1991; Sahm and Gilmore, 1994).

Listeria monocytogenes is moderately sensitive to gentamicin (MIC 0.25–1.0 μg per ml) (Prichard *et al.*, 1983; Larsson *et al.*, 1985). As with *E. faecalis*, a penicillin G/gentamicin or an

Organism	MIC (μg per ml)
Gram-positive bacteria	
Staphylococcus aureus	0.12–1.0
Streptococcus pyogenes	16.0
Streptococcus pneumoniae	16.0–32.0
Enterococcus faecalis	6.25–200.0
Listeria monocytogenes	0.25–1.0
Gram-negative bacteria	
Escherichia coli	1.0–4.0
Klebsiella aerogenes	1.0–2.0
Klebsiella (other spp.)	0.06–1.0
Proteus mirabilis	2.0–8.0
Proteus vulgaris	1.0–4.0
Morganella morganii	1.0–4.0
Providencia rettgeri	<0.5–4.0
Providencia alcalifaciens	2.0–4.0
Providencia stuartii	8.0–>32.0
Salmonella spp.	0.25–1.0
Pseudomonas aeruginosa	1.0–8.0

Table I.38
Compiled from data published by Barber and Waterworth (1966), Penner and Preston (1980), Tofte *et al.* (1984) and Larsson *et al.* (1985)

ampicillin/gentamicin combination acts synergistically against this organism (p.12) (Azimi *et al.*, 1979; MacGowan *et al.*, 1990). The *Bacillus* and *Corynebacterium* spp. are sensitive to a degree (Waitz and Weinstein, 1969). *Bacillus cereus* is moderately sensitive (MIC 2.0 μg per ml) and both clindamycin or vancomycin may act synergistically with gentamicin against this organism (Gigantelli *et al.*, 1991). Most *Nocardia asteroides* strains are gentamicin-resistant, but *N. brasiliensis* and *N. caviae* are usually sensitive (Bach *et al.*, 1973; Wallace *et al.*, 1983). Anaerobic Gram-positive bacilli, such as *Clostridium perfringens* and *Cl. difficile*, are gentamicin-resistant (Brook and Walker, 1985).

5 Mycobacteria

Gentamicin has no activity against *Mycobacterium tuberculosis* at clinically attainable concentrations, most strains having an MIC of 64 μg per ml or higher. It also has no activity against other mycobacteria (Gangadharam and Candler, 1977; Wallace and Wiss, 1981). Administration of gentamicin is unlikely to impede the bacteriological diagnosis of tuberculosis. It is also inactive against *M. leprae* (Gelber *et al.*, 1984).

6 Other organisms

Mycoplasma pneumoniae and *M. hominis* are sensitive to gentamicin. Yeasts, other fungi and *Entamoeba histolytica* are resistant (Waitz and Weinstein, 1969).

7 Minimum inhibitory concentrations

Table I.38 shows the MICs of gentamicin against some selected bacterial species.

Mode of Administration and Dosage

1 Once-daily administration to adults

The dose of gentamicin usually recommended for this is 4.0–5.0 mg per kg i.m. or i.v. once-daily. Intravenously the drug has usually been given as a 30-min infusion (Prins *et al.*, 1993; Ellis-Pegler *et al.*, 1994). There are several reasons for once-daily administration of gentamicin and other aminoglycosides. First of all bacterial killing with aminoglycosides is enhanced by the high peak drug level attained by this method which achieves a relatively short lived high serum level/MIC ratio. The area under the serum concentration time curve is less important (Moore et al., 1987; Jackson et al., 1990; Drusano, 1991; Bastone et al., 1993). With aminoglycosides this high serum level need not be prolonged because these drugs have a significant post-antibiotic effect against most sensitive bacteria. The post-antibiotic effect is the recovery period or persistent suppression of bacterial growth following a short (1- or 2 h) antimicrobial exposure (Karlowsky et al., 1994a). Initial high antibiotic concentration and increased time of exposure prolong the post-antibiotic effect, and so after one large daily gentamicin dose the post-antibiotic effect can be as long as 5–10 h (Vogelman et al., 1988; Isaksson et al., 1988, 1993; Fantin et al., 1990; MacKenzie and Gould, 1993; Karlowsky et al., 1994b).

There is also evidence that the administration of subsequent aminoglycoside doses, while there is still detectable aminoglycoside present, may inhibit their bacterial killing capacity. This phenomenon is called 'adaptive resistance after first exposure'. Bacteria may become very resistant for several hours before gradual return of their full sensitivity. The mechanism for adaptive resistance is thought to be downregulation of aminoglycoside uptake during the period of accelerated energy dependent drug transport (Daikos et al., 1990; Barclay et al., 1992).

The once-daily administration of gentamicin and other aminoglycosides has several advantages. The dosage calculation is easy; there is a guaranteed peak serum concentration in the therapeutic range, and fewer assays are required. As gentamicin nowadays is nearly always used together with a beta-lactam agent, breakthrough infections are unlikely to occur (Parker and Davey, 1993). The trough gentamicin serum levels need only be measured and these should be undetectable or at least less than 1 μg per ml (Parker and Davey, 1993; MacGowan and Reeves, 1994), but as with netilmicin (p.525), a serum level performed 8 h after administration may be informative. At this time the level should be in the range of 1.5–6 μg per ml. If the serum concentration at this time is lower than 1.5 μg per ml, the daily gentamicin dose may be too low. If the level is higher than 6 μg per ml, the patient may be at risk of toxicity.

Once-daily aminoglycoside administration has been studied in several comparative studies with conventional 8-hourly administration. Clinical efficacy has been about the same. A few studies have shown less ototoxicity with once-daily administration, but in most there was no difference with the two methods. The once-daily dosing of gentamicin and other aminoglycosides resulted in a decreased renal uptake of these agents, and this may have led to less nephrotoxicity. Initially studies were lacking in neutropenic patients, but now there is evidence that once-daily gentamicin can be used in these together with the appropriate beta-lactam antibiotic. Most of the studies have been performed in adults only (Nordström et al., 1990; Gilbert, 1991; Parker and Davey, 1993; Prins et al., 1993; Ellis-Pegler et al., 1994). Once-daily gentamicin plus penicillin is satisfactory for Strep. viridans endocarditis (Brandt et al., 1996), but for enterococcal endocarditis 1 mg per kg 8-hourly is preferable.

In most trials gentamicin has been given once-daily in a dosage of 4–5 mg per kg per day. Nicolau et al. (1995) administered a gentamicin dosage of 7 mg per kg i.v. every 24 h to patients with estimated creatinine clearance of ≥60 ml per min. The same dose was given once every 36 h to those with creatinine clearance of 59–40 ml per min and once every 48 h to those with creatinine clearance of 39–20 ml per min. These authors treated more severe infections by this higher dosage regimen. As expected a few patients developed ototoxicity or nephrotoxicity, but overall these side-effects were infrequent. The results of treatment were good. Serum level monitoring was performed anywhere between 6–14 h after the dose. If at 6 h the serum level was higher than 7.5 μg per ml, the dosing interval had to be extended or the individual dose reduced. At 14 h the gentamicin level was expected to be nearly zero. At 8 h the highest safe level was some 6 μg per ml and at 10 h this was approximately 5 μg per ml.

It appears that the administration of a single 7 mg per kg daily gentamicin dose is suitable when this drug alone is used to treat serious infections. The usual 4–5 mg per kg daily dose is probably sufficient when gentamicin is used together with a beta-lactam antibiotic.

2 Traditional 8-hourly administration

Some clinicians may still prefer to administer gentamicin this way. It may be the best method in a developing country, where a suitable beta-lactam antibiotic may not be available, and gentamicin may have to be used singly to treat a severe infection caused by a Gram-negative rod. The 8-hourly administration has been traditional, but the daily gentamicin dose can also be given in two divided doses.

A commonly recommended adult dosage was 80 mg 8-hourly or 4.5 mg per kg body weight per day, given i.m. or i.v. in three divided doses (Darrell and Waterworth, 1967; Gingell and

Waterworth, 1968). This dosage usually produced mean peak serum levels of 4–6 μg per ml in most adults (Siber *et al.*, 1975).

For seriously ill patients a larger dosage may be needed to obtain higher peak serum levels and a satisfactory clinical outcome. As there is only a narrow safety margin between therapeutically effective and toxic serum levels, near toxic doses are often required for the successful treatment of such patients. In these circumstances, it is preferable to calculate each patient's dosage according to body weight, rather than rely on a single 'standard' adult dosage. During the first day of treatment of critically ill patients, a dosage ranging from 5 mg per kg body weight per day (Noone *et al.*, 1974) to 7–8 mg per kg per day (Riff and Jackson, 1971), or even higher (Zaske *et al.*, 1982), given in three divided doses, has been used. Subsequent gentamicin dosage is then determined according to results of serum level estimation (see below), a gentamicin dosage nomogram (p.461), or both. After the first day of therapy the dosage can often be reduced.

The maintenance dosage will vary in different patients because there is wide interpatient variation in gentamicin elimination. Well known patient variables include renal function (p.460) and age (p.461). In adults there is often a significant inverse correlation between peak serum levels of gentamicin and hematocrit values (Barza *et al.*, 1975). Serum levels may also be lower in febrile compared with non-febrile patients (Pennington *et al.*, 1975). Narcotic drug abusers appear to eliminate or possibly inactivate gentamicin more rapidly, and therefore low therapeutically inadequate serum levels may result if the usual dosage is given (King *et al.*, 1985). Similar to many other antibiotics, such as penicillin G (p.24), serum gentamicin levels are consistently lower in pregnant than in non-pregnant patients (Chow and Jewesson, 1985). Overweight patients need less gentamicin per kg of body weight and conversely underweight ones need more, mainly because the volume of distribution of the drug is higher in the latter group (Traynor *et al.*, 1995). If the drug is used in high dosage for serious infections, serum level estimations are necessary in all patients, including those with normal renal function (Follath *et al.*, 1981; Zaske *et al.*, 1982).

In patients with Gram-negative septicemia, increased mortality has been correlated with early inadequate gentamicin serum levels (Moore *et al.*, 1984; Drusano, 1988). Dosage should be adjusted to produce peak serum levels of about 6–10 μg per ml, which occur about 1 h after i.m. injection, and after the rapid distribution phase after an i.v. administration. A common method used for i.v. administration is to dilute each 8-hourly dose in 30–50 ml of i.v. fluid (or smaller volume for children) for infusion over 20–30 min. With this method the rapid distribution phase is completed 30 min after the conclusion of a 30-min infusion (Siber *et al.*, 1979; Ristuccia and Cunha, 1982). Infusion of a gentamicin dose over 20–30 min is the recommended method of i.v. administration to neonates (McCracken *et al.*, 1977; McCracken and Nelson, 1983). In adults and older children the undiluted 8-hourly dose of gentamicin can be injected directly into the i.v. tubing over 2–3 min (Mendelson *et al.*, 1976). If this is done, the rapid distribution phase of the drug is completed in 60 min.

Serum levels just before the next dose (trough levels) should not exceed 1.5–2.0 μg per ml (McGhie *et al.*, 1974). In some patients the commonly used adult dosage of 80 mg 8-hourly may produce toxic serum levels (see above), but in others this may be insufficient. A proportion of adults require a maintenance dosage of 120 mg or even 160 mg every 8 h (up to 7 mg per kg per day), to achieve adequate serum levels and a satisfactory therapeutic result.

The administration of gentamicin by a continued i.v. infusion in the ordinary doses is not advocated, as low serum levels may result (Powell *et al.*, 1983).

3 Parenteral administration to children

As with kanamycin (p.441), children need relatively higher doses of gentamicin than adults to achieve similar serum levels. For children less than 5 years of age, a dosage of 7.5 mg per kg body weight per day is recommended, while for those aged 5–10 years, a dosage of 6 mg per kg per day is appropriate, both given in three divided doses. These regimens produce serum levels similar to those attained in adults with the commonly used dosage of 4.5 mg per kg per day (p.485). Therefore, in some children with severe infections, higher dosages than these may be needed, particularly for initiation of therapy (Echeverria *et al.*, 1975; Siber *et al.*, 1975). In a study involving relatively small numbers of children, gentamicin in a dosage of 4.5 mg per kg per day, given once-daily, appeared equally as safe and effective as the same daily dose, administered in three divided doses (Elhanan *et al.*, 1995).

4 Newborn and premature infants

The serum gentamicin half-life is prolonged in babies during the first week of life. Such patients should only be given 5 mg per kg per day, administered in two divided doses; all other infants may be given 7.5 mg per kg per day in three divided doses, the dosage recommended for older children (Nelson and McCracken, 1972; Ingham and Emslie, 1972; McCracken and Nelson, 1983). Like in adults (p.459), there is a considerable variation in the serum levels attained with these dosages in individual infants, and serum gentamicin levels should be monitored (Leff *et al.*, 1984; de Louvois, 1987). In one study in full-term neonates a once-daily administration of gentamicin in a dosage of 3.5–4 mg per kg of body weight, infused i.v. over 30 min, was found to be safe and effective (Skopnik and Heimann, 1995).

Smaller doses than those above have been recommended by Szefler *et al.* (1980) and by Edwards *et al.* (1986) for pre-term babies during the first week of life. For those of gestational age of 28 weeks or less, they recommended a dosage of 2.5 mg per kg, once every 24h, and for those of gestational age of 29–35 weeks, 2.5 mg per kg every 18 h. A dosing interval of 24 h was also recommended for infants weighing less than 1500 g and 18 h interval for those weighing between 1500 and 3250 g (Keyes *et al.*, 1989).

5 Patients with renal failure

These patients require a modified dosage schedule. A number of dosage recommendations for patients with renal failure are available. A simple method is to assume that, as with kanamycin (p.442), there is a linear relationship between the gentamicin half-life and the patient's serum creatinine concentration. The gentamicin half-life (measured in hours) is roughly equal to the serum creatinine concentration (mg %)* multiplied by 4.

In patients with renal failure the usual gentamicin dose of 80 to 120 mg (2.5 mg per kg in children) may be administered i.m. or i.v. once every two calculated half-lives. For example an adult with a normal creatinine of 1.0 mg % may be given 80 mg every $(1 \times 4 \times 2) = 8$ hours, whilst a patient with severe renal failure (creatinine 10 mg %) should be given this dose once every $(10 \times 4 \times 2) = 80$ hours (McHenry *et al.*, 1971). A simplification of this is to calculate the period in hours between doses by multiplying the patient's serum creatinine (mg %) by 8 (Goodman *et al.*, 1975). This method has the disadvantage that there may be a prolonged period during which gentamicin serum levels are non-therapeutic, prior to the next dose.

An alternative is to reduce the individual doses of the drug which are administered at constant intervals (Cutler *et al.*, 1972). A loading dose of 1.5–2.5 mg per kg is given, but the subsequent 8-hourly dose is calculated by dividing the loading dose by the patient's serum creatinine in mg %. Regular administration in this way to patients with impaired renal function results in an almost steady-state therapy. This method aims to produce serum gentamicin levels which continuously approximate or slightly exceed the MICs of gentamicin for many aerobic Gram-negative bacilli (Goodman *et al.*, 1975).

However, the gentamicin half-life often correlates poorly with serum creatinine (Kaye *et al.*, 1974; Barza *et al.*, 1975), and it correlates better with creatinine clearance in ml per min (Cronberg, 1994). An initial loading dose of gentamicin (4.5 mg per kg for single-daily dose therapy and 2.5 mg per kg for traditional 8-hourly administration) can be given to any patient with renal failure. Thereafter maintenance doses should be given at the usual dosage intervals, as with amikacin (p.509). The maintenance dose is obtained by dividing the value of the observed creatinine clearance in ml per min by the value of the normal creatinine clearance in ml per min, and then multiplying this result by the value of normal individual dose in mg. The creatinine clearance of a patient can be obtained from the following formula:

$$\text{Creatinine clearance (ml per min)} = \frac{(140 - \text{age in years}) \times \text{weight in kg}}{\text{creatinine in mg } \% \times 72}$$

For females the factor in the divisor is 85 and not 72.

If SI units are used, the formula is:

$$\text{Creatinine clearance (ml per min)} = \frac{(140 - \text{age in years}) \times \text{weight in kg}}{\text{creatinine in micromol } (\mu\text{mol}) \text{ per liter} \times 0.81}$$

For females the factor in the divisor is 0.85 and not 0.81.

As in the case of kanamycin, nomograms for gentamicin dosage have been published (Chan *et al.*, 1972; Mawer *et al.*, 1974; Bryan and Stone, 1977). These provide loading and maintenance

---

* The serum creatinine in mg % may be calculated by multiplying the creatinine value in mmol/liter (SI units) by a factor of 12. For instance, a serum creatinine of 0.1 mmol/liter equals 1.2 mg % and a serum creatinine of 1.0 mg % equals 0.088 mmol/liter.

doses and intervals between doses and are designed to produce peak serum gentamicin concentrations of 5–10 μg per ml and trough concentrations of 2–3 μg per ml (Aronoff and Luft, 1979). Calculations by a nomogram are more accurate than the other methods described, particularly when large gentamicin dosage is needed for severe infections.

Nevertheless, all of these methods of calculating dosage, including nomograms, are at the best only useful approximations, so that whenever possible maintenance doses of gentamicin should be governed by serum level estimations (Follath et al., 1981; Bennett et al., 1983; Matzke et al., 1983). Gentamicin serum levels can be estimated within 4 h by many methods (Follath et al., 1981; Ratcliff et al., 1981).

Gentamicin is removed from the body by hemodialysis, and its half-life in anephric patients of approximately 50 h, is reduced to abut 10 h during dialysis (Halpren et al., 1976). Patients receiving regular hemodialysis two or three times a week can usually be treated satisfactorily by a dosage of 1.5–2.0 mg per kg body weight, given at end of each 8-h dialysis (Curtis et al., 1967). This regimen results in therapeutic serum levels during most of a 48 h interdialysis period, but they are in an ineffective range for the duration of the next hemodialysis (Halpren et al., 1976). For this reason, these authors suggested that after an initial post-dialysis dose of 1.5–2.0 mg per kg, patients undergoing dialysis every 48 h should be given 50% of the initial dose immediately preceding, and again following each dialysis. This schedule avoids both ineffective concentrations during dialysis, and potentially toxic peak concentrations after dialysis. If 6 h dialyses are used twice or thrice a week, it is suggested that a loading dose of 1.5–2.0 mg per kg be given after the first dialysis, but thereafter only 75% of this dose after each subsequent dialysis (Danish et al., 1974). Since these studies were concluded, several other artificial kidneys have become available which vary markedly with respect to their gentamicin elimination and clearance characteristics (Matzke et al., 1984). Therefore, gentamicin serum level monitoring is essential.

Peritoneal dialysis also removes gentamicin, but the rate of clearance varies according to the degree of peritoneal inflammation (Smithivas et al., 1971). A single daily dose of 1.5–2.0 mg per kg of i.m. gentamicin may result in therapeutic non-toxic serum levels in uremic patients undergoing peritoneal dialysis, but this should be confirmed by serum level estimations. Gentamicin may also be added to peritoneal dialysis fluid in a concentration of 5–10 mg per liter. If this is used to treat peritonitis, results are improved if parenteral gentamicin is also administered (Smithivas et al., 1971; Hyams et al., 1971; Pancorbo and Comty, 1981).

6 Patients older than 60 years

These patients may have a reduced creatinine clearance and thus reduced gentamicin clearance despite normal serum creatinine values. Dosages may have to be reduced in these patients and serum gentamicin levels monitored (Ljungberg and Nilsson-Ehle, 1987).

7 Patients with cystic fibrosis

In patients with mild cystic fibrosis, standard doses of gentamicin result in safe and therapeutically adequate serum levels, and increased dosage is not necessary. In patients with more severe cystic fibrosis, similar to some penicillins (p.82), lower serum levels are attained with usual gentamicin doses. Such patients have a significantly larger apparent volume of distribution of gentamicin and also an increased plasma clearance of the drug, which does not show the expected correlation with creatinine clearance. These patients need higher gentamicin dosage, but because there is much individual variation, a generalized approach to gentamicin dosing is not feasible. Therapy should be individualized for each patient which is only possible with serum level monitoring (Kearns et al., 1982; MacDonald et al., 1983). Nevertheless, Hendeles et al. (1987) recommended an initial gentamicin dosage of 3 mg per kg administered every 6 h in children and every 8 h for adults.

8 Patients with hematological malignancies

Some authors have produced evidence that patients with leukemia and other hematological malignancies have an increased clearance of gentamicin and other aminoglycosides, necessitating somewhat increased dosages when infections are treated in these patients (Zeitany et al., 1990; Bertino et al., 1991), but the findings in these studies are disputed by Inciardi and Batra (1993).

9 Exchange transfusion

This procedure is sometimes advocated as adjuvant therapy for treatment of neonatal septicemia. Kliegman et al. (1980) found that a double-volume exchange transfusion decreased serum gentamicin levels in the immediate post-exchange period and suggested that dosage during this period should be adjusted according to serum levels. Other authors considered that exchange transfusion did not significantly alter the elimination of gentamicin. This procedure only modified the elimination of drugs with relatively small distribution volumes and with endogenous clearance rates that were slow relative to the blood flow rates of exchange transfusion (Green, 1981).

10 Intrathecal and intraventricular administration

Gentamicin was administered by these routes for the treatment of meningitis due to Gram-negative bacilli (Newman and Holt, 1971; Moellering and Fischer, 1972). The dosage for newborn babies was 1.0–2.5 mg daily (Nelson and McCracken 1972; Lee et al., 1977; McCracken et al., 1980). For adults the dosage was 5–10 mg daily (Rahal, 1972; Kaiser and McGee, 1975), although doses as high as 20 mg daily have been used safely (Smilack and McCloskey, 1972).

The role of intrathecal gentamicin in conjunction with parenteral treatment, for neonatal meningitis or meningitis caused by Gram-negative enteric bacilli in other age groups, was controversial (Swartz, 1981). In one comparative trial, 117 infants with meningitis due to Gram-negative enteric organisms were treated by either ampicillin plus gentamicin given parenterally, or by the same parenteral drugs plus intrathecal gentamicin; there was no additional benefit from intrathecal therapy (McCracken and Mize, 1976). Gentamicin administration into the lumbar intrathecal space resulted in adequate drug concentrations in lumbar CSF, but not in ventricular CSF. Gentamicin administered into the cerebral ventricles produced adequate concentrations in both the ventricles and lumbar CSF (Kaiser and McGee, 1975). Intraventricular administration of gentamicin (or other antibiotics) may therefore be preferable to the intrathecal route. The USA Neonatal Meningitis Cooperative Study Group carried out a trial on the use of intraventricular gentamicin in the treatment of meningitis with ventriculitis in 52 infants. There was a higher death rate among infants who received daily intraventricular gentamicin (2.5 mg) plus systemic treatment (42.9%) than in those who received systemic antibiotics alone (12.5%) (McCracken et al., 1980; McCracken and Mize, 1980). Gentamicin was usually delivered by repeated percutaneous intraventricular injections, and porencephaly developed in needle-track sites of several infants. More encouraging results were reported in neonatal meningitis when amikacin was injected into the ventricles via a Rickman reservoir (p.510). Intraventricular administration of gentamicin by any method is not without problems and risks, and it should not be used routinely for meningitis caused by Gram-negative bacilli, but it should be reserved for problem patients, not responding or not likely to respond to parenteral therapy alone (Kaiser and McGee, 1975; Kourtopoulos and Holm, 1976; Olson et al., 1977; Pickering et al., 1978). With the availability of third-generation cephalosporins, such as cefotaxime (p.336) and ceftriaxone (p.359) which penetrate well into the CSF, the need for intraventricular gentamicin should be infrequent.

11 Intratracheal gentamicin

This drug is sometimes instilled directly into the trachea either via an endotracheal tube or tracheostomy in patients with severe pneumonia. If 40 mg of gentamicin is instilled in trachea 4-hourly, some of this is absorbed. However, serum levels in one study did not rise above 1.0 μg per ml, provided the renal function was normal, and the authors recommended that if an i.v. aminoglycoside is also given to such patients, its dosage need not be modified (Crosby et al., 1987).

12 Gentamicin dosage in patients with various disease states

In patients with severe trauma the volume of distribution of gentamicin is usually increased and larger doses may be needed, but there is a large interpatient variation. A loading dose of 3 mg per kg of gentamicin is suggested, but serum level monitoring is needed to determine further dosing (Townsend et al., 1989). Similarly, in other critically ill intensive care patients, both adults (Hassan and Ober, 1987) and children (Kraus et al., 1993) the volume of distribution of gentamicin is increased and similar higher initial doses are needed. For children an initial dosage of 9 mg pr kg per day, given in three divided doses, is suggested. Serum level monitoring is again necessary to determine further dosing.

In patients with severe burns, the elimination half-life of gentamicin is usually decreased. Volume of distribution may be increased or unchanged. It is hard to give a dosage recommendation for these and so dosage has to be individualized and serum levels monitored (Boucher et al., 1992). The gentamicin pharmacokinetics and dosage requirements of febrile neutropenic patients do not differ from those of other patients (Bianco et al., 1989).

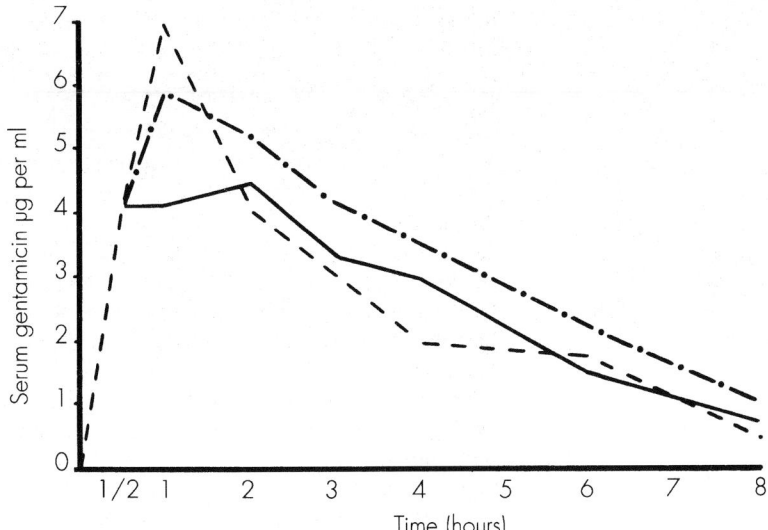

Fig. I.22.
Serum gentamicin levels in three cases with normal renal function after 80 mg i.m. (Redrawn after Gingell and Waterworth, 1968, with permission from the BMJ Publishing Group.)

Serum Levels in Relation to Dosage

The mean peak serum level of gentamicin, after i.m. injection of 80 mg in an adult is 7.0 μg per ml (range 4.2–12.0 μg per ml). This level is attained in 0.5–2.0 h after the injection (Gingell and Waterworth, 1968). Doubling the dose results in approximately twice the serum concentrations (Jao and Jackson, 1964). The serum half-life of the drug in patients with normal renal function is approximately 4 h, and 8 h after injection the serum level falls to about 1.0 μg per ml (Fig. I.22). The serum half-life in patients with severe renal failure may be prolonged to 40–50 h.

In neonates and young children, serum levels similar to those shown in Fig. I.22 are attained after administration of 2.5 mg per kg of gentamicin i.m. (McCracken, 1972; Nelson and McCracken, 1972).

Intravenous gentamicin produces serum levels comparable with those obtained after i.m. injection, provided that the dose is infused over 20–30 min and the peak level is estimated in a serum sample collected 30–60 min after the end of the infusion (McCracken *et al.*, 1977; Dyas *et al.*, 1983). After an i.v. injection given over 2–3 min, the serum half-life of the drug is also similar to that after i.m. administration, but the immediate 'peak' serum level is variable. In some patients this peak transiently exceeds 12.5 μg per ml, and in others levels measured 5–10 min after the injection are no higher than those after i.m. administration. Approximately 60 min after the rapid i.v. injection, when the rapid distribution phase of the drug is completed, the serum level approximates to the peak level obtained after the same i.m. dose (Wise *et al.*, 1981; Meunier *et al.*, 1987). This level is commonly regarded as the peak serum level for purposes of serum level monitoring (Follath *et al.*, 1981) (p.459).

The peak serum levels in patients with renal impairment, after a single gentamicin dose are higher than those obtained in normal subjects (Curtis *et al.*, 1967; Riff and Jackson, 1971). In one study, a dose of 1.6 mg per kg body weight was given i.v. to two subjects with normal renal function; serum concentrations of 5 and 7.5 μg per ml, respectively, were detected after 10 min, but in three patients with chronic renal failure, the level at that time was 16 μg per ml (Curtis *et al.*, 1967). Higher peak serum gentamicin levels are expected after the initial dose in patients with renal failure, because this peak is determined not only by the distribution volume, but also by excretion which commences as soon as gentamicin is present in the blood.

MacGowan *et al.* (1994) gave gentamicin once-daily in a dose of 4.5 mg per kg, infused i.v. over 30 min to seven neutropenic adults. Gentamicin serum levels 1, 2, 4, 8 and 24 h after the infusion averaged to 10.9, 7.1, 4.2, 1.8 and 0.16 μg per ml, respectively.

Excretion

1 Urine

Gentamicin is excreted by glomerular filtration almost entirely in the active form (Black *et al.*, 1964). Its renal clearance in normal subjects is about 60 ml per min (Jao and Jackson, 1964). For the first 1 or 2 days of gentamicin therapy, excretion is partly delayed and during this time only about 40% of the administered drug can be recovered from urine. With continued administration, there is equilibration between the serum and body tissues and the daily urinary excretion increases, and after about 1 week nearly all of the daily dose is excreted in the urine. After 2 days treatment with a dose of 2.4 mg per kg per day, the urine concentration is about 40–50 μg per ml (Jao and Jackson, 1964). The urinary gentamicin concentration varies inversely with urine volume and in oliguric patients concentrations as high as 500–1000 μg per ml of urine have been observed (Riff and Jackson, 1971).

2 Bile

A small amount of gentamicin is excreted in bile, but the mean biliary concentration is usually only 30–40% of the mean serum level. Gentamicin is not detected in gallbladder bile in the presence of cystic duct obstruction (Mendelson et al., 1973; Pitt et al., 1973).

Distribution of the Drug in Body

Binding of gentamicin to serum proteins under normal conditions is very low, and estimated values have been in the range 0–25% (Black et al., 1964; Gordon et al., 1972). Serum protein binding of gentamicin and other aminoglycoside antibiotics increases progressively with decreasing concentrations of the divalent cations, calcium and magnesium. In the absence of these cations the drug is approximately 70% protein bound. Therefore, under normal circumstances the binding of aminoglycosides to serum proteins is not pharmacologically important, but significant binding may occur in certain pathological conditions (Ramirez-Ronda et al., 1975).

Very low gentamicin concentrations are attained in the CSF of patients with uninflamed meninges (Riff and Jackson, 1971). In animals with induced bacterial meningitis, lumbar CSF concentration of approximately 4.25 μg per ml is attained after a bolus i.v. dose of 6 mg per kg (Smith et al., 1988). Corticosteroid pretreatment reduces the gentamicin concentration in the CSF, but this has no deleterious effect on the course of treated experimental meningitis (Scheld and Brodeur, 1983). Animal studies have also shown that transient disruption of the blood–brain barrier can be produced by infusion of hyperosmolar solutions such as a 2-molar mannitol into the carotid artery. This procedure results in markedly increased gentamicin concentrations in both CSF and brain tissue. This finding may have clinical relevance as osmotic barrier disruption has been safely performed in humans (Strausbaugh and Brinker, 1983).

Levels in pleural, pericardial and ascitic fluids are usually about 50% of those found in the serum at the time (Riff and Jackson, 1971; Taryle et al., 1981). The drug concentration is higher and may reach 90% of the serum level, in ascitic fluid of patients with bacterial peritonitis (Gerding et al., 1977; Richey and Schleupner, 1981). Gentamicin penetrates well into synovial fluid, even in the absence of bacterial infection, where concentrations consistently exceed 50% of simultaneous serum levels (Dee and Kozin, 1977).

Gentamicin is detectable in bronchial secretions, but concentrations are only 25–50% of simultaneous serum levels (Pennington and Reynolds, 1973; Wong et al., 1975; Pennington, 1981). Gentamicin depends upon a concentration gradient for passive diffusion into bronchial secretions, and it is cleared from these secretions rather rapidly (Pennington and Reynolds, 1975). It crosses the placenta, where the mean peak level in cord serum is 30–40% of that in maternal serum (Yoshioka et al., 1972). Some gentamicin apparently enters or is absorbed onto red cells, and this is released when the serum level falls (Riff and Jackson, 1971). Gentamicin enters human polymorphonuclear leukocytes, where it may reach a concentration of some 80% of the extracellular level of the drug, but unlike some of the lipid soluble antibiotics, such as chloramphenicol (p.561), rifampicin (p.685), clindamycin (p.593) and erythromycin (p.614), gentamicin is not concentrated in leukocytes (Prokesch and Hand, 1982).

Postmortem studies of gentamicin tissue levels in infants who had received the drug during life have shown that the highest concentration was reached in kidney tissue. Adequate tissue concentrations were usually found in lung, heart and skeletal muscle, but the concentrations in brain tissue were usually less than 1.0 μg per g (Phillips and Milner, 1984).

Incomplete recovery of gentamicin from urine during the first few days of therapy (p.463), and the persistence of measurable concentrations in urine of patients with normal renal function for 10 days or more after a final dose, suggest that gentamicin persists in tissues for long periods (Schentag et al., 1977; Schentag and Jusko, 1977; Kahlmeter et al., 1978). Following the final dose of a course of gentamicin, the serum concentration declines in a biphasic fashion; there is an initial rapid decline phase which is similar to that which follows maintenance doses, and then a slow phase, during which low serum concentrations (<0.5 μg per ml) are measurable for 10 or more days. The gentamicin half-life of the second phase, when tissue bound drug is excreted, averages 112 h (Schentag *et al.*, 1977). Trough gentamicin serum levels (p.463) may reflect tissue levels, which in turn may be related to nephrotoxicity (p.467).

Gentamicin undergoes reabsorption from the lumens of the proximal tubules via the brush border and leads to gentamicin deposition in the kidneys (Brion *et al.*, 1984; Beauchamp *et al.*, 1991). Studies in humans (Edwards *et al.*, 1976; Schentag and Jusko, 1977) and in experimental animals (Kornguth and Kunin, 1977), indicate that the kidneys are the major site of gentamicin deposition, accounting for 40% of the total antibiotic in the body. The main site of this deposition is the renal cortex, which contains approximately 85% of the total renal drug (Luft and Kleit, 1974). The same is true for other aminoglycosides, such as kanamycin (p.445), tobramycin (p.495), amikacin (p.512) and netilmicin (p.527), but the less nephrotoxic streptomycin (p.433) is distributed evenly throughout the kidney. In renal cortical tissue, gentamicin levels are often at least 100-fold higher than those in the serum (Schentag and Jusko, 1977). The drug is transported into renal cortical cells by an active process, aerobic phosphorylation (Hsu *et al.*, 1977; Barza *et al.*, 1980). Gentamicin which is generally considered the most nephrotoxic of the above mentioned aminoglycosides (p.469), undergoes the highest degree of tubular reabsorption and reaches the highest concentrations in renal cortical tissue (Contrepois *et al.*, 1985). In animals, frusemide administration alone has no direct effect on renal excretion of gentamicin; also gentamicin levels in the serum and renal tissue are relatively unaffected by changes of fluid infusion. However, frusemide treated animals are highly susceptible to changes in fluid infusion. Glomerular filtration rate and gentamicin elimination is much reduced when fluid intake is low, and this is much improved with increased fluid infusion (Chiu and Long, 1978). In animals in the presence of endotoxin, gentamicin and other aminoglycosides accumulate in the renal cortex to a greater extent (Bergeron and Bergeron, 1986; Tardif *et al.*, 1990).

Gentamicin and other aminoglycosides are also concentrated in the renal medulla and papillae, where the levels are lower than those in the cortex; some drug persists in these tissues for about 25 days after its administration. As bacterial growth is largely limited to the medulla and papillae in pyelonephritis, this accumulation of gentamicin may be important in the therapy of renal infections (Bergeron and Trottier, 1979). In animals with induced *E. faecalis* pyelonephritis, treated by gentamicin for 7 days, there was an increased concentration of gentamicin in the kidneys, compared with animals with no infection. This high level of aminoglycoside in the kidney may be beneficial for the treatment of pyelonephritis, but it may also increase the toxic potential of the drug (Auclair *et al.*, 1988).

In animals, gentamicin is also distributed in heart, liver and muscle tissue, and concentrations in these tissues and the lymph are about the same as in serum (Black *et al.*, 1964; Chisholm *et al.*, 1968). Dan *et al.* (1981) reported that gentamicin concentrations in human interstitial fluid were similar to those in the serum. According to others the interstitial fluid level is lower than that attained in serum, but the drug persists for a longer period of time in this fluid. Nevertheless, after usual gentamicin doses interstitial fluid levels are consistently above the MICs of susceptible organisms (Carbon *et al.*, 1978). With repeated doses gentamicin does not accumulate in tissue fluid (Tan and Salstrom, 1977). Tissue fluid levels are higher during the first 2 h when gentamicin is administered by a 2.5 min i.v. injection than by a 30-min infusion. Beyond 2 h, levels are the same after both of these methods of administration (Kozak *et al.*, 1977).

Gentamicin enters the inner ear fluids of animals, but concentrations reached in perilymph and endolymph are lower than those in the serum. Concentrations of gentamicin in perilymph, although lower, are related to the concentrations present in the blood. The drug appears to enter endolymph very slowly. After cessation of gentamicin administration, the drug leaves these compartments slowly, and in one animal study a concentration of about 1.0 μg per ml persisted for up to 15 days (Tran Ba Huy *et al.*, 1981, 1983). *In vitro*, gentamicin is active against phagocytosed *Staph. aureus* (Van den Broek *et al.*, 1986).

Mode of Action

Gentamicin inhibits bacterial growth by inhibiting protein synthesis, and the main mechanism of its action appears to be similar to that of streptomycin (p.432). The drug is bactericidal *in vitro*, similar to other aminoglycosides (Hahn and Sarre, 1969). Gentamicin also interacts with the cell envelope of *Ps. aeruginosa*; disruption of cell wall occurs in a sequential manner moving from the outer membrane to the inner membrane and may result in lysis of the cell. Gentamicin also appears to displace essential metal cations within the outer membrane. Thereafter, small transient holes are produced which make the outer membrane more permeable to the antibiotic. This membrane effect may contribute to the effects of protein synthesis inhibition during the bacterial killing process (Hancock *et al.*, 1981; Martin and Beveridge, 1986). Gentamicin also inhibits the accumulation of extracellular proteases secreted by *Ps. aeruginosa*, enzymes which contribute to its pathogenicity. This inhibition occurs at gentamicin concentrations lower than those required to inhibit bacterial protein synthesis (Warren *et al.*, 1985).

Gentamicin and other aminoglycosides can produce a decrease in mammalian microsomal protein synthesis at concentrations approximating those accumulated in the renal cortex (p.465) and in perilymph bathing the membranous labyrinth (see below). The ototoxic diuretic, ethacrynic acid (p.445), also has an inhibitory effect on protein synthesis in microsomes isolated from rat brain. Inhibition of mammalian protein synthesis may explain the toxicity of gentamicin (p.467) and other aminoglycosides (Buss *et al.*, 1984, 1985; Buss and Piatt, 1985).

Toxicity

1 Ototoxicity

This is an important side-effect of gentamicin, but in the absence of renal insufficiency it only occurs if high doses are used. The drug can cause both vestibular and cochlear toxicity, but experimentally the vestibular apparatus seems to be at least twice as vulnerable as the cochlea. Huy and Deffrennes (1988) demonstrated in guinea pigs that gentamicin exhibited a 4-fold greater affinity for the vestibule than for the cochlea. Gentamicin and other aminoglycosides penetrate into the perilymph and vestibular and cochlear tissues (p.465) (Dulon *et al.*, 1986). In the vestibular portion of the labyrinth, gentamicin damages the vestibular secretory tissues and the hair cells of the balance receptors. The two areas within the cochlea primarily affected are the hair cells and the stria vascularis (Wersäll *et al.*, 1969; Brummett, 1983). However, in some patients with gentamicin-induced hearing loss, cochlear ganglion cells were damaged, but there was no hair cell loss (Hinojosa and Lerner, 1987). Some patients are hypersusceptible to gentamicin (and other aminoglycoside) ototoxicity. It has been postulated that these patients have a mitochondrial mutation, which is an inherited trait. The mitochondrial ribosomes are implicated as the targets of aminoglycosides that induce hair cell death and deafness (Hutchin and Cortopassi, 1994).

In large-scale retrospective surveys the frequency of gentamicin ototoxicity has been only 2–3% (Jackson and Arcieri, 1971; Kahlmeter and Dahlager, 1984). In contrast, prospective studies of small patient populations have shown a frequency as high as 25% (Meyers, 1970; Fee, 1983; Holm *et al.*, 1983). Vestibular damage rather than deafness is more common with gentamicin and this results in symptoms varying from an acute Meniere's syndrome to slight vertigo or tinnitus. The damage is usually permanent and affected patients remain insecure on ambulation, particularly in the dark, but they can usually compensate for this disability (Jao and Jackson, 1964). Ototoxicity is related to high prolonged serum levels, and in affected patients these have ranged from 8.0 to 16.6 µg per ml (Jao and Jackson, 1964). The transient high peak gentamicin levels, resulting from once-daily gentamicin administration, do not cause ototoxicity (p.458). Delayed ototoxicity occurring 10–14 days after stopping gentamicin has been observed, but is rare except in patients with markedly impaired renal function (Hewitt, 1974).

In contrast to kanamycin (p.445), deafness due to gentamicin has been uncommon. In one retrospective survey of 1327 patients treated with gentamicin, 31 (2.3%) developed ototoxicity (Arcieri *et al.*, 1970). Vestibular impairment was present in 27 patients, eight of whom also had high tone hearing loss, and the remaining four had high tone hearing loss alone. Total deafness due to gentamicin was not observed in this survey, but it has been reported occasionally (Wersäll *et al.*, 1969; A Cooperative Study, 1973). Deafness may be more likely to occur if gentamicin is administered concurrently with i.v. ethacrynic acid (Meriwether *et al.*, 1971; Brummett, 1983; Buss *et al.*, 1985). In animals, concomitant administration of frusemide also potentiates gentamicin-induced cochlear damage (Brummett, 1983). However, when Smith and Lietman (1983) analyzed data from three prospective, controlled clinical studies, they concluded that the use of frusemide was not a major risk factor for the development of aminoglycoside-induced auditory toxicity.

As deafness is a more serious toxic effect than labyrinthine damage, kanamycin and amikacin would appear to be more ototoxic than gentamicin. However, kanamycin and amikacin are easier to use safely, because there is a greater margin between their therapeutically active and toxic serum levels (p.510) (Holm *et al.*, 1983). Animal studies have suggested that tobramycin may be less ototoxic than gentamicin (p.496). In one clinical study tobramycin appeared to cause less vestibular but not cochlear toxicity than gentamicin (Fee, 1983), but in another larger one there was no difference between these two drugs (Smith *et al.*, 1980).

Despite many studies, the incidence of hearing loss from gentamicin and other aminoglycoside therapy is still in doubt. One factor has been the lack of availability of high-frequency testing equipment. Evaluation of higher frequencies detects the ototoxic process before involvement of the frequency range important for verbal communication. Such early identification of auditory damage would allow consideration of treatment alternatives to decrease ototoxic risk (Brummett and Fox, 1989; Mattie et al., 1989; Fausti et al., 1992).

Gentamicin ototoxicity appears to be uncommon in infants and young children. Finitzo-Hieber et al. (1979) followed 116 children for a 4-year period after they had received gentamicin in a dosage of 5–6 mg per kg per day in the neonatal period. No substantial sensorineural hearing loss or vestibular dysfunction was identified. Theoretically, the newborn infant should be more at risk to aminoglycoside ototoxicity. Experimental data indicate that susceptibility of the cochlea to aminoglycoside toxicity is greater during the period of onset of auditory function. Also aminoglycosides are eliminated mainly by glomerular filtration which is poor at birth. Nevertheless, in spite of the widespread use of gentamicin, very few cases of neonatal ototoxicity have been recorded following short-term maternal administration during late pregnancy. There have been at least 17 published studies of auditory evaluations in 1069 infants and children who received gentamicin or other aminoglycoside therapy in the neonatal period. Ototoxicity was said to be present in from 0 to 25% of patients, but there was just as much auditory toxicity in untreated control patients. Despite these results, there is concern that gentamicin and other aminoglycosides may be ototoxic in infants and children. Extensive surveillance and early testing of neonates and children undergoing aminoglycoside treatment as well as prospective comparative studies are required (Assael et al., 1982; Chow and Jewesson, 1985; Nelson and McCracken, 1986).

Similar to neomycin (p.536), gentamicin applied topically to the ear as ear drops, can cause severe inner ear deafness, especially if a perforation of the ear drum is present. For this reason gentamicin ear drops should not be used (Jones, 1978).

2 Nephrotoxicity

Gentamicin is selectively concentrated in renal cortical cells (p.465), and it can cause functional and structural damage to the proximal tubules. With moderate doses there is cloudy swelling of tubules, but at higher doses acute tubular necrosis results (Appel and Neu, 1977; Bennett et al., 1977). Electron microscopic studies of proximal renal tubules in animals show changes within the first 2 days of gentamicin treatment. With continued gentamicin administration, tubular cells lose brush border microvillae, and intracellular organelles undergo swelling. Eventually, the cell becomes necrotic and sloughs into the lumen, leaving a bare basement membrane on which regenerative activity begins (Luft et al., 1983). Similar changes have been observed in human allograft biopsy specimens obtained during gentamicin treatment (Wellwood et al., 1975) and in a premature baby who died of acute renal failure after therapy with gentamicin (Chan and Ng, 1985).

Various proximal tubular enzymes, such as alanine aminopeptidase, may be excreted in the urine during gentamicin treatment. This enzymuria appears to be an early manifestation of gentamicin nephrotoxicity. It precedes the rise of serum creatinine, but it is only of limited value in predicting nephron damage before renal function deteriorates (Beck et al., 1977; Harpur and Davey, 1981; Davey et al., 1983). Vancomycin therapy alone does not result in significant alaninine aminopeptidase excretion, but if both gentamicin and vancomycin are used together, the enzymuria is greater than from gentamicin alone (Ryback et al., 1987). Daily urinary cast counts may be a more rapid means of identifying early tubular damage in critically ill patients given aminoglycosides (Schentag et al., 1979). There are also reports of hypokalemia (Young et al., 1973), renal glycosuria (Ginsburg et al., 1976), hypomagnesemia, hypocalcemia and alkalosis (Appel and Neu, 1977) induced by gentamicin therapy, but their causative role in nephrotoxicity is not clear. Animal studies show that an increased intake of calcium delays and attenuates gentamicin-mediated renal damage because calcium slows the accumulation of the drug in the renal cortex (Bennett et al., 1982). Animals with ligated common bile ducts are more at risk of gentamicin nephrotoxicity, but the effect can be prevented by pretreatment with dietary calcium (Vakil et al., 1989).

Glomerular dysfunction appears to arise subsequent to proximal tubular damage, but the pathogenesis of this is not clear. Glomerular lesions have not been observed in human kidneys (Lietman and Smith, 1983). In animals gentamicin administration results in a decrease in the diameter and density of endothelial finestrae; tobramycin in the same dosage causes only minor alterations in glomerular endothelium (Luft and Evan, 1980).

Gentamicin-induced interstitial nephritis has been described, but is much less common. A 55-year-old man, who developed recurrent acute renal failure apparently due to gentamicin-induced interstitial nephritis was described by Saltissi et al. (1979). Kourilsky et al. (1982)

studied 29 patients with acute interstitial nephritis; in seven of these gentamicin was a possible etiological agent and five of these patients were female. The authors then studied the effect of gentamicin on male and female rats. Interstitial inflammation was greater in female rats even though the renal failure was more severe in male animals.

The most common clinical manifestation of gentamicin nephrotoxicity is a gradual onset over several days of non-oliguric renal failure with proteinuria and rising blood urea and serum creatinine values. This appears dose-related and is usually reversible. The increase in serum creatinine levels usually appears several days after the initiation of gentamicin therapy. Nephrotoxicity varies from clinically trivial effects on the tubules to life-threatening acute tubular necrosis (Appel and Neu, 1977; Lietman and Smith, 1983). Less commonly an acute oliguric renal failure may occur; the oliguric phase lasts about 10 days, and is followed by a diuretic phase and a slow return to 50% or greater of normal renal function (Kahn and Stein, 1972; Hewitt, 1974). Acute severe renal failure may also occur without oliguria (Gary et al., 1976). Russo and Adelman (1980) described a 14-year-old boy who developed a Fanconi syndrome in association with gentamicin therapy. This was evidenced by low serum levels of sodium, potassium, bicarbonate and phosphorus, with corresponding renal losses of these electrolytes plus glucose and urinary enzyme.

Gentamicin nephrotoxicity is likely to be more severe if other aggravating factors, such as hypovolemia and sodium depletion, are present (Bygbjerg and Møller, 1976; Lietman and Smith, 1983). If gentamicin is used together with ticarcillin, there usually would be enough sodium in the 'ticarcillin sodium' preparation to correct any sodium lack (Ohnishi et al., 1989). In animals prolonged endotoxemia enhances the nephrotoxic potential of gentamicin alone and also of that of gentamicin plus vancomycin (Auclair et al., 1990; Ngeleka et al., 1990).

Concomitant administration of frusemide increases gentamicin nephrotoxicity in animals (Adelman et al., 1979). This may not be relevant to humans since frusemide is usually given with due attention to the fluid and salt status of the patient (Lietman and Smith, 1983). In animals cephalosporins appear to protect the kidneys from gentamicin nephrotoxicity (Luft et al., 1976; Bloch et al., 1979). Although some studies in humans have shown that the simultaneous administration of an aminoglycoside with cephalothin is associated with little nephrotoxicity (Brown et al., 1982), most studies have demonstrated potentiation of gentamicin nephrotoxicity by cephalosporins (p.257). Cyclosporine, which itself is a nephrotoxic drug, potentiates gentamicin nephrotoxicity (Sands and Brown, 1989). However, gentamicin, if carefully monitored, can be reasonably safely combined with i.v. cyclosporine in bone marrow transplant recipients (Chandrasekar and Cronin, 1991).

In animals, concomitant administration of hydrocortisone potentiates gentamicin nephrotoxicity (Beauchamp et al., 1986). Hydrocortisone appears to interfere with the postnecrotic cellular regeneration process in the kidney following gentamicin-induced renal damage (Beauchamp and Pettigrew, 1988), but it may also increase the amount of gentamicin accumulation in the kidney (Bergeron et al., 1987). Animal studies have also shown that polyaspartic acid protects them from gentamicin nephrotoxicity despite marked accumulation of aminoglycosides in the kidneys (Gilbert et al., 1989; Swan et al., 1991, 1992, 1993). The clinical significance of this is not known.

In one large study, involving 1489 patients, aminoglycosides, including gentamicin, were administered according to individual pharmacokinetic monitoring. The risk factors identified for aminoglycoside-associated nephrotoxicity were: higher initial steady state trough concentrations, lower initial aminoglycoside clearance, co-administration of amphotericin B, cephalosporins, vancomycin, piperacillin (but not ticarcillin, where the extra sodium might have been protective), and frusemide, longer duration of therapy, pneumonia, rapidly fatal prognosis, leukemia, lower initial calculated creatinine clearance, pre-existing renal or liver disease, protein malnutrition, ascites, pleural effusion, shock, male sex, larger volume of distribution, older age and intensive care patients (Bertino et al., 1993). Another study suggested that gentamicin/vancomycin was more nephrotoxic than gentamicin alone (Goetz and Sayers, 1993).

The frequency of gentamicin renal damage has varied widely in different reports (Lietman and Smith, 1983). For instance, the frequency of nephrotoxicity has varied from 12–14% (Brown et al., 1982; Kahlmeter and Dahlager, 1984), to 26% (Smith et al., 1980) and even to 40% (Feig et al., 1982). Drug-related renal dysfunction developed in 63% of patients with Ps. aeruginosa endocarditis who were treated by high-dose prolonged gentamicin therapy (peak gentamicin serum levels 12–15 μg per ml) (Tablan et al., 1984).

In man nephrotoxicity is related to the gentamicin dose and to the serum levels attained. There is general agreement that serum levels should be monitored. The best time to take the serum sample for 'peak serum level' (p.463) estimation is 1 h after an i.m. injection and 30 min after a 20–30 min i.v. infusion (Ristuccia and Cunha, 1982; Schentag et al., 1982). Some authors prefer to take the serum sample 2 h after an i.m. dose (Trollfors *et al.*, 1980) or 60 min after a 20–30 min i.v. infusion (Smith *et al.*, 1980; Sawyers *et al.*, 1986; Trollfors *et al.*, 1986). Blood for the estimation of trough levels is taken just before the next dose. The optimum therapeutic non-toxic peak concentrations of gentamicin should be between 4.0 and 10.0 μg per ml and trough concentrations 0.5–2.0 μg per ml (Smith *et al.*, 1980; Schentag *et al.*, 1981). With once-daily gentamicin administration, the transient high peak level does not cause toxicity and this need not be monitored (p.458).

With conventional 8-hourly gentamicin administration, there has been controversy as to whether peak or trough serum levels are the best indices for predicting nephrotoxicity.

Although peak drug levels in excess of 12 μg per ml have been associated with an increased frequency of nephrotoxicity (Hewitt, 1974; Tablan *et al.*, 1984; Sawyers *et al.*, 1986), trough levels are probably more useful for predicting accumulation of gentamicin, because they correlate better with early renal impairment (Goodman *et al.*, 1975). Dahlgren *et al.* (1975) monitored gentamicin serum levels in 86 patients, 21 had trough levels over 2.0 μg per ml and in 36% of these the serum creatinine rose. Elevated serum creatinine levels were not observed in patients with trough levels less than 2.0 μg per ml, and peak levels of higher than 10 μg per ml did not correlate with nephrotoxicity. Lietman and Smith (1983) considered that there was no evidence that dosage adjustments on the basis of trough levels leads to less nephrotoxicity. Dose reduction according to trough levels may lead to inadequate peak levels and a poor therapeutic result. These authors disregarded trough levels in terms of dosage adjustment and used them only as a potential early indicator of a falling glomerular filtration rate. Because gentamicin serum levels are unpredictable, it has been customary to monitor both its peaks and troughs (Ristuccia and Cunha, 1982).

Gentamicin should be used cautiously in patients with pre-existing renal disease, and whenever other factors known to impair renal function, such as hypotension or dehydration, are present (Bygbjerg and Møller, 1976). Other authors have also identified some of the risk factors, described by Bertino *et al.* (1993) (p.468) as well as others, and these include duration of gentamicin therapy, the total dose administered and the age of the patient (Sawyers *et al.*, 1986). Gentamicin nephrotoxicity is frequent in patients with liver cirrhosis (Cabrera *et al.*, 1982) and in those with obstructive jaundice (Desai and Tsang, 1988). Contrast media used in radiology have been reported to produce acute renal failure (Bennett *et al.*, 1980) and it is possible that patients receiving gentamicin therapy and contrast media may be more liable to develop renal damage. One animal experiment (Luft *et al.*, 1978) and one clinical study of six patients (Trollfors, 1983) demonstrated that after the development of nephrotoxicity, renal function improved again after some weeks, despite continuing gentamicin administration. These findings require further elucidation.

Most studies have shown that gentamicin has about the same nephrotoxic potential as amikacin (Lietman and Smith, 1983) (p.513), but Holm *et al.* (1983) found that gentamicin was more potent in this respect, and pointed out that it may be easier to use amikacin safely as its serum levels are more predictable after therapeutic doses. After the usual doses of amikacin, serum levels exceed the MICs of susceptible organisms for a longer period than is the case with gentamicin.

It is generally accepted that gentamicin is more nephrotoxic than tobramycin (p.497). Whilst some clinical studies involving a small number of patients failed to disclose any difference between these drugs (Fong *et al.*, 1981; Feig *et al.*, 1982), most prospective randomized studies involving a larger number of patients, showed that gentamicin was more nephrotoxic than tobramycin (Walker and Gentry, 1976; Kahlmeter, 1979; Smith *et al.*, 1980; Schentag *et al.*, 1981). When Tablan *et al.* (1984) used high-dose prolonged aminoglycoside therapy for patients with *Ps. aeruginosa* endocarditis, the frequencies of nephrotoxicity in the gentamicin and tobramycin groups were the same. However, renal damage appeared earlier and at a smaller cumulative dose in patients receiving gentamicin. In animals the relative nephrotoxicities of various aminoglycosides do not correlate with the renal parenchymal accumulation of these agents and may be more dependent on intrinsic toxicity to the renal proximal tubule. While tobramycin accumulates in the renal parenchyma to a lesser degree than gentamicin, this is not true of netilmicin which appears to be even less nephrotoxic than tobramycin (p.527) (Aronoff *et al.*, 1983; Brier *et al.*, 1985).

It is possible that gentamicin administered during pregnancy could lead to potentially serious problems to the fetal kidneys. One animal study showed that this lead to permanent alterations of the glomerular basement membrane of the fetal kidneys, and it was considered possible that these altered glomeruli may be at risk later in life and that they could be the starting point of kidney disease (Smaoui *et al.*, 1993).

3 Neuromuscular blockade

Gentamicin, in common with other aminoglycosides (p.433), can cause this complication. Warner and Sanders (1971) described an adult patient receiving normal doses of gentamicin, who developed respiratory failure 2 days after an operation; renal impairment and a lowered serum calcium may have been contributory. Another patient with Parkinson's disease reported by Holtzman (1976), developed profound weakness after a short course of gentamicin; this recovered after the drug was stopped but recurred on rechallenge. The symptoms in this patient may have been due to a drug interaction with his anti-Parkinsonian medication. That this side-effect of gentamicin has been uncommon is presumably due to the later introduction of the drug when the effects of 'overdosages' of the older aminoglycosides (streptomycin, p. 433; neomycin p. 537) into the peritoneal cavity, were already known.

Gentamicin can unmask or aggravate myasthenia gravis (Argov and Mastaglia, 1979), and potentiate *Clostridium botulinum* toxin, thus producing an exacerbation of clinical botulism (Santos *et al.*, 1981; Schwartz and Eng, 1982).

4 Other neurotoxicity

In rabbits, daily intraventricular gentamicin doses of 0.25 or 0.5 mg per kg were associated with ventriculitis, ventricular dilation, abnormal postural reflexes and ataxia (Hodges *et al.*, 1981). The increased mortality in neonates who received intraventricular gentamicin in the study by McCracken *et al.* (1980) (p.462) might have been related to gentamicin neurotoxicity. Concentrations of gentamicin in the ventricular fluid of the neonates 1–6 h after administration ranged from 10 to 130 μg per ml; these were similar to those found in the cisternal fluid of rabbits in the study described above. Intraventricular gentamicin levels should, therefore, be regularly estimated in patients receiving the drug by this route.

Parenterally administered gentamicin has been associated with psychosis and encephalopathy on rare occasions (Snavely and Hodges, 1984). Two patients developed acute organic brain syndrome, apparently related to gentamicin therapy (Byrd, 1977).

5 Hypersensitivity reactions

Skin rashes due to parenteral gentamicin and skin sensitization due to topical gentamicin occur but are rare (Ristuccia and Cunha, 1982). One case of anaphylaxis, presenting within 1 min of an i.v. gentamicin injection, has been reported (Hall, 1977).

6 Hematological side-effects

A transient leucopenia has been observed occasionally, and one patient developed acute agranulocytosis in association with gentamicin therapy (Chang and Reyes, 1975). *In vitro*, therapeutic concentrations of gentamicin and other aminoglycosides inhibit leucocyte function of migration (Seklecki *et al.*, 1978), chemotaxis (Burgaleta *et al.*, 1982) and candidacidal activity (Ferrari *et al.*, 1980). When gentamicin and other aminoglycosides were administered i.v. to normal volunteers, these drugs did not appear to produce leokocyte dysfunction *in vivo*, as chemotaxis, phagocytosis and killing of *Candida albicans* was unimpaired at 1, 3 and 24 h after aminoglycoside infusion (Venezio and DiVincenzo, 1985).

7 Fetal toxicity

The safety of gentamicin during pregnancy has not been established. The drug crosses the placenta (p.464) but the degree of risk of ototoxicity (p.466) and nephrotoxicity (p.467) to the fetus is not known.

8 Changes in fecal flora

Parenteral gentamicin therapy leads to some changes in fecal flora. Enterococci often increase in the feces as well as gentamicin-resistant *Staph. epidermidis*, and in some patients gentamicin-resistant Gram-negative aerobic bacilli appear (Heritage *et al.*, 1988).

9 Other side-effects

Transient elevations of SGOT levels have occurred, but there has been no other evidence of hepatotoxicity (Klein *et al.*, 1964). Carbohydrate intolerance in term neonates, manifested by greater stool frequency, higher frequency of fecal reducing substances and a greater requirement for dietary manipulation, has been attributed to parenteral antibiotics. Bhatia *et al.* (1986) found these abnormalities in neonates receiving i.v. ampicillin plus gentamicin. This is probably a complication common to many parenteral antibiotics and not specifically to gentamicin. This is another reason against the unwarranted widespread use of antibiotics in newborns (Johnson, 1986).

Some reports suggested that gentamicin interferes with the binding of bilirubin to serum albumin (Kapitulnik *et al.*, 1972). This has not been confirmed by subsequent studies, and gentamicin does not predispose to the development of kernicterus in the human neonate (Wennberg and Rusmussen, 1975; Woods *et al.*, 1976).

Gentamicin and other aminoglycosides are partially inactivated by high concentrations of any of the penicillins both *in vitro* and *in vivo* (p.157). Heparin reversibly inhibits gentamicin activity in a dose-dependent way. Therefore, specimens for gentamicin estimations should not be put in heparinized tubes. When heparin is used clinically as an anticoagulant, its serum level is not high enough to affect the activity of gentamicin (Nilsson *et al.*, 1981).

Clinical Uses of the Drug

1 Septicemia and other severe infections due to aerobic Gram-negative bacilli

Gentamicin is a useful drug for treatment of these infections, and prior to the development of other aminoglycosides, such as tobramycin (p.498) and amikacin (p.514), and the broad-spectrum beta-lactams such as cefotaxime (p.338), ceftriaxone (p.360), ceftazidime (p.377), imipenem (p.236) and other drugs, it was often the only antibiotic available to which organisms causing hospital-acquired infections, were sensitive. Nowadays the situation has changed. Gentamicin-resistant strains of Enterobacteriaceae and *Ps. aeruginosa* are no longer rare in some hospitals, and in this situation amikacin is the preferred aminoglycoside. Many clinicians consider that amikacin should be kept in reserve for the treatment of sepsis due to these resistant organisms. In Australia, where gentamicin-resistance is still uncommon this is the usual practice. In some hospitals in the USA, where gentamicin-resistance was prevalent, amikacin was instituted as a first-line aminoglycoside. During a 1-year surveillance, there was no increase of amikacin-resistance, and resistance levels to gentamicin and tobramycin showed a marked decrease (Price *et al.*, 1981; Betts *et al.*, 1984). The pharmacokinetics of amikacin are probably more predictable (Holm *et al.*, 1983) (p.510) and it has the advantage that, compared with gentamicin, it is only minimally inactivated by high concentrations of the penicillins (p.157). For these reasons some clinicians prefer amikacin to gentamicin, even if gentamicin-resistance is not a problem.

Many bacteriologically confirmed infections caused by aerobic Gram-negative rods, such as meningitis, septicemia, suspected septicemia in neutropenic cancer patients, endocarditis, pneumonia and pyelonephritis are treated increasingly by one of the broad-spectrum beta-lactams (p.377) or by a quinolone (p.1026). An important consideration is whether monotherapy by one of these drugs, such as ceftazidime (p.377) or imipenem (p.236), would be adequate for the immediate empiric therapy of suspected septicemia, particularly in neutropenic patients. Monotherapy with these drugs (pp.236, 377) can certainly be used with success in some patients, but most authors recommend a beta-lactam (e.g. ticarcillin, piperacillin, ceftazidime or imipenem) combination with one of the aminoglycosides, such as gentamicin. Sometimes there may be bactericidal synergy between these antibiotics and the combination may prevent the emergence of resistant bacterial strains (EORTC, 1978; Hathorn and Pizzo, 1986; Jacobs, 1986; Young, 1986; Klastersky, 1989; Hughes *et al.*, 1990). If gentamicin-resistant Gram-negative bacilli are prevalent in any hospital area, another aminoglycoside, usually amikacin (p.514), should be substituted for gentamicin. In areas where methicillin-resistant coagulase-negative staphylococci, *Staph. aureus*, *Corynebacterium* spp. or *Strep. viridans* are frequent causes for septicemia in these patients, vancomycin (p.780) should be included in the initial regimen (Hughes *et al.*, 1990; Gibson *et al.*, 1994). The aminoglycoside in these regimens should be stopped as soon as clinically practicable, especially if there are risk factors for aminoglycoside toxicity (McCormack and Jewesson, 1992). An aminoglycoside alone should not be used for the treatment of suspected or proven Gram-negative rod infections in neutropenic patients, as the results of such treatment are poor, particularly if *Ps. aeruginosa* is the pathogen (Young, 1983; Bodey *et al.*, 1985).

Suspected or confirmed Gram-negative bacterial septicemias in non-neutropenic patients nowadays are also usually treated by a combination of a broad-spectrum beta-lactam (such as cefotaxime etc) plus an aminoglycoside, especially if the infection is severe. For milder infections, a beta-lactam agent alone or an aminoglycoside, such as gentamicin, alone is satisfactory. Gentamicin should be avoided in patients with risk factors for aminoglycoside toxicity (p.466). Korvick *et al.* (1992) reviewed 230 patients with *Klebsiella* spp. septicemia and concluded that for less severely ill patients (immunocompetent, urinary tract portal, mentally alert) monotherapy with either a beta-lactam or an aminoglycoside (to which the organism was susceptible) was satisfactory. On the other hand severely ill patients, who experienced hypotension, benefited from beta-lactam/aminoglycoside combinations. Severe hospital-acquired *Serratia* spp. septicemia would also nowadays be, at least initially, treated by beta-lactam/gentamicin combination (Watanakunakorn, 1989). For severe septicemia caused by *Edwardsiella tarda* the same initial therapy may be appropriate, but as this organism is very sensitive to ciprofloxacin (p.981), perhaps a cefotaxime/ciprofloxacin combination can be used initially (Reinhardt *et al.*, 1985; Janda and Abbott, 1993). Appropriate therapies for *Acinetobacter* pneumonia or septicemia include gentamicin (or another aminoglycoside), an extended-spectrum penicillin (p.165) or imipenem (p.237). For severe infections gentamicin can be combined initially with either the penicillin or imipenem (Anstey *et al.*, 1992; Tilley and Roberts, 1994). Septicemia by the rare Gram-negative pathogen, *Methylobacterium extorquens* in immunocompromised hosts, may respond to gentamicin (Kaye *et al.*, 1992). In an experimental model of Gram-negative endocarditis, Potel *et al.* (1992) predicted that amikacin would be superior to gentamicin or tobramycin for the treatment of this infection.

In intra-abdominal or female genital tract sepsis, mixed infection with both aerobic and anaerobic Gram-negative bacteria may be involved, and gentamicin combined with chloramphenicol (p.569), clindamycin (Bartlett *et al.*, 1977) (p.597) or metronidazole (p.947) are only a few of many suitable treatment regimens. Many regimens, such as cefoxitin alone (p.308) and others are available which do not include an aminoglycoside. In general there is no difference in efficacy between regimens which include or do not contain an aminoglycoside (Ho and Barza, 1987).

For confirmed severe *Ps. aeruginosa* infections, the combination of gentamicin and carbenicillin (or ticarcillin) was used with success (Rodriguez *et al.*, 1970; Bodey *et al.*, 1976). Nowadays several other beta-lactam agents are available to be used together with gentamicin for this purpose, such as piperacillin, ceftazidime etc. It is still uncertain whether these two drug combinations always act synergistically against this organism in patients (p.156). Under certain conditions high ticarcillin concentrations may inactivate gentamicin both *in vitro* and *in vivo* (p.157). In patients with normal renal function, this can be avoided largely if the two antibiotics are not mixed together in i.v. infusion fluids. High sustained concentrations of ticarcillin, which can occur in patients with renal failure, may cause significant gentamicin inactivation; these patients require an increased dosage of gentamicin to compensate for this (p.157). In contrast, if gentamicin is administered together with 5-fluorocytosine, the gentamicin serum level may be increased. This may occur with other aminoglycosides and 5-fluorocytosine and a possible mechanism is competition for renal excretion by the drugs. In this situation gentamicin dosage may need to be decreased and serum levels monitored.

Gentamicin alone, used parenterally, did produce good results in *Ps. aeruginosa* septicemia complicating burns (Stone, 1969). The drug is also useful for the treatment of acute septic arthritis due to Gram-negative bacilli. This form of arthritis commonly occurs in elderly patients with underlying diseases or in patients receiving immunosuppressive drugs (Goldenberg and Cohen, 1976). Nowadays other drugs, such as one of the third-generation cephalosporins may be preferred for these indications. Vertebral osteomyelitis in i.v. drug abusers can be caused by Gram-negative aerobic bacilli including *Ps. aeruginosa*, and gentamicin may be useful as part of the treatment regimen (Sapico and Montgomerie, 1980). In polymicrobial osteomyelitis, Gram-negative aerobic bacteria may be involved in addition to *Staph. aureus*, *E. faecalis* and the anaerobes, and gentamicin may have a place in the treatment combined with other drugs (Pichichero and Friesen, 1982). Infections caused by *Ps. paucimobilis* (Reina *et al.*, 1991) and *Ps. putrefaciens* (Dan *et al.*, 1992) also respond to gentamicin, but some third-generation cephalosporins and quinolones are also effective.

Hospital-acquired pneumonia is commonly caused by Gram-negative aerobic bacilli such as *Ps. aeruginosa*, *E. coli* and *Klebsiella* or *Serratia* spp. (Jonas and Cunha, 1982; Bartlett *et al.*, 1986; McGehee *et al.*, 1988). This disease, and purulent bronchial infections caused by these organisms in patients with chronic lung disease, are difficult to treat. Satisfactory results with gentamicin alone were obtained in a considerable proportion of such patients (Parry *et al.*, 1977), but in general combination therapy with the appropriate beta-lactam, such as ticarcillin (p.156), mezlocillin (p.173) or piperacillin (p.174), is superior (Donowitz and Mandell, 1983). If combined topical (tracheal instillation) and systemic gentamicin is given to patients with pulmonary infection, serum levels should be monitored, because some of the topically administered drug is absorbed (Lake *et al.*, 1975). Activity of gentamicin is reduced in the purulent sputum of patients with cystic fibrosis and bronchiectasis. Apparently some components of the sputum bind a portion of the drug and render it inactive, and in addition the ionic content of the sputum inhibits the drug's activity (Levy *et al.*, 1983).

Gentamicin is a satisfactory drug for the treatment of *Campylobacter jejuni* and *Campylobacter fetus* septicemias in adults (McNulty, 1987; Morrison *et al.*, 1990; Schønheyder *et al.*, 1995). Intraperitoneal gentamicin plus vancomycin is also recommended for the initial treatment of peritonitis in continuous ambulatory peritoneal dialysis patients (Report, 1987).

2 Severe Gram-negative sepsis in children

For neonatal meningitis, ampicillin combined with gentamicin (or amikacin) is still considered to be a satisfactory initial chemotherapy before the organism is identified (p.121), but the empiric selection of antimicrobial agents should also depend on a knowledge of the prevalent nosocomial pathogens in the particular nursery (Baker, 1981). Both ampicillin and gentamicin may be continued parenterally if the causative organism is *E. coli*, *Klebsiella* spp. or another Gram-negative rod. Alternatively monotherapy with i.v. cefotaxime (p.338) or ceftriaxone (p.360) may be used.

Gentamicin has been effective for the treatment of infants and children with other severe Gram-negative rod infections such as septicemia, pyelonephritis, pneumonia, septic arthritis and osteomyelitis (Nunnery and Riley, 1969; Klein *et al.*, 1971; Pittard *et al.*, 1976). Gentamicin (combined with penicillin G or ampicillin) is valuable as initial therapy for newborns with life-threatening bacterial infections (Klein, 1969).

Sepsis in a neonate caused by *Campylobacter fetus* was successfully treated by i.v. ampicillin and gentamicin (Simor *et al.*, 1986). Ten of 11 newborn infants infected during a nosocomial outbreak of *Campylobacter jejuni* meningitis also responded well to the same therapy (Goossens *et al.*, 1986). Chloramphenicol may be effective for *Campylobacter* meningitis, although there are difficulties to use this drug in neonates (p.557) (Simor *et al.*, 1986). It is possible that for non-meningitic *Campylobacter* sepsis, erythromycin (p.618) may be satisfactory. *Yersinia enterocolitica* septicemia in an 8-week-old infant was successfully treated by 10-day course of i.v. gentamicin (St John Sutton *et al.*, 1983). Enterococcal (*E. faecium*) meningitis in a 4-year-old boy failed to respond to ampicillin-chloramphenicol, but cure was obtained when therapy was changed to a synergistic ampicillin/gentamicin combination (Venezio *et al.*, 1984).

3 Urinary tract infections

Gentamicin is effective against most organisms causing urinary tract infections, with the exception of *E. faecalis* (Cox, 1969). The drug is not indicated for most urinary infections which usually respond to safer oral drugs. It is valuable for treatment of infections due to *Ps. aeruginosa*, *Klebsiella* spp. and other Gram-negative bacilli resistant to commonly used drugs, especially if such infections occur in an abnormal urinary tract (Chisholm, 1974). Gentamicin is more effective for urinary tract infections, if the urine is made alkaline. It is approximately 100-fold more active against most strains of Gram-negative bacilli, when tested *in vitro* at a pH of 8.5 than at a pH of 5.0. A concentrated urine has an inhibitory effect on the antibacterial activity of gentamicin, the degree of which depends on the total urine osmolality and also on the presence of individual solutes (Sabath *et al.*, 1970; Papapetropoulou *et al.*, 1983). Relatively small doses of gentamicin are often recommended for the treatment of uncomplicated urinary tract infections, to lessen the risk of toxicity. In this case, alkalinization and dilution of the urine may be important to ensure that optimal conditions for its antibacterial activity are present. Urine alkalinization can be conveniently achieved by concomitant administration of bicarbonate or acetazolamide (Sabath *et al.*, 1970). Gentamicin treatment may fail to eradicate urinary tract infections in patients with renal failure, because their urine may be strongly acid and only relatively low urinary gentamicin concentrations are attained.

For uncomplicated lower urinary tract infection low dosage regimens may be effective; a single daily dose of 160 mg of gentamicin i.m. appears convenient for the treatment of selected adult out-patients (Labovitz *et al.*, 1974). Most patients requiring gentamicin have difficult infections with renal tissue involvement, which are often caused by organisms resistant to many drugs, and these should be treated by gentamicin in full dosage (Chisholm, 1974). Urinary tract infections of infants are often serious and may be accompanied by septicemia, so initial chemotherapy should include a combination, such as amoxycillin plus gentamicin, both drugs being given in full dosage for 10–14 days (Ginsburg and McCracken, 1982).

Gentamicin, because it is stored in renal tissue (p.465), prevents acute retrograde pyelonephritis in experimental animals. The kidneys are protected from infection in the absence of effective levels of gentamicin in urine (Glauser *et al.*, 1979; Bille and Glauser, 1981). Furthermore, intracortical, intramedullary and papillary gentamicin concentrations are higher in animals with induced pyelonephritis than in uninfected controls. Gentamicin administration 12-hourly for 7 or 14 days in animals resulted in continuous levels of the drug in the medulla which persisted above the MICs for *E. coli* for 6 months or more (Bergeron *et al.*, 1982a,b). Persistent high renal tissue levels of gentamicin may be advantageous for the management of human pyelonephritis. Further animal studies have shown that 3 days of gentamicin in combination with either ampicillin, cephalothin or trimethoprim followed by 2 weeks of therapy with a non-aminoglycoside drug, was more effective than either antibiotic alone in pyelonephritis. Such reduction in the duration of gentamicin therapy may diminish its nephrotoxic potential. Controlled trials are necessary to establish whether these findings are applicable to humans (Bergeron, 1985; Bergeron and Marois, 1986).

Gentamicin is often included in chemoprophylaxis before renal transplantation. For example, Tilney *et al.* (1978) at the time of induction of anesthesia used single i.v. doses of 2 g ampicillin, 2 g oxacillin and 1.5 mg per kg body weight of gentamicin. Patients undergoing urological operations often have infected urine and preoperative chemoprophylaxis should be governed by sensitivities of the organism involved. Gentamicin is often suitable and a single preoperative dose of 1.5 mg per kg i.m. or i.v. is given (Cafferkey *et al.*, 1982).

4 Bacterial endocarditis

A combination of penicillin G and gentamicin is the preferred treatment of *E. faecalis* endocarditis (Rice *et al.*, 1991b) (p.42), but *E. faecalis* septicemia without endocarditis may respond to penicillin G or ampicillin alone (Gullberg *et al.*, 1989; Watanakunakorn and Patel, 1993). Strains of *E. faecalis* have now emerged with plasmid-mediated high-level gentamicin resistance (p.42), and with these penicillin G/aminoglycoside synergism cannot be obtained, except that some 10–20% of these strains may exhibit penicillin G/streptomycin synergism (p.429) in which case this latter combination is useful for treatment of *E. faecalis* endocarditis. For other strains with high-level gentamicin-resistance, the optimum treatment of endocarditis is uncertain at present (Herman and Gerding, 1991b). Vancomycin alone has been successful occasionally (Patterson *et al.*, 1988b), but is generally unsatisfactory (p.779). Animal studies indicate that high-dose continuous infusion of ampicillin or high-dose i.v. teicoplanin may have some value (Eliopoulos *et al.*, 1992). Some of the *E. faecalis* strains with high-level gentamicin-resistance produce a hemolysin, and if these strains cause a septicemia without endocarditis, the mortality may still be high (Huycke *et al.*, 1991).

High-level gentamicin-resistant strains of *E. faecium* have now also been reported, and as with *E. faecalis*, there is no known optimal treatment for endocarditis caused by them (Das *et al.*, 1994). Endocarditis due to vancomycin and ampicillin-resistant *E. faecium* is also difficult to treat; animal experiments suggest that the combination of ciprofloxacin, gentamicin and rifampicin may succeed (Whitman *et al.*, 1993). Gentamicin, instead of streptomycin, can also be used in combination with penicillin G to treat *Strep. viridans* endocarditis (p.41).

The role of gentamicin in *Staph. aureus* endocarditis is less certain. The combination of a penicillinase-resistant penicillin with gentamicin usually exhibits *in vitro* synergism against methicillin-sensitive *Staph. aureus* strains (Watanakunakorn and Glotzbecker, 1974). But a multicenter study in the USA, which compared nafcillin (p.105) versus nafcillin/gentamicin therapy for the treatment of *Staph. aureus* endocarditis, revealed that the benefit of the combination was only marginal. There was a more rapid defervescence and blood cultures became sterile more rapidly during the first week; ultimate outcome of the infection was unaffected. It was therefore recommended that gentamicin may be added to the treatment regimen during the first 5–7 days only (p.105). There is also no evidence that a vancomycin/gentamicin combination is superior to vancomycin alone for the treatment of *Staph. aureus* endocarditis caused by methicillin-resistant strains (p.777). However, for the treatment of prosthetic valve endocarditis caused by methicillin-resistant *Staph. epidermidis* strains, it is useful to use vancomycin in combination with both gentamicin and rifampicin (p.778) (Karchmer *et al.*, 1983). In the USA, gentamicin is recommended for the first 2 weeks of therapy only; vancomycin plus rifampicin are then continued for 6–8 weeks. The addition of gentamicin may not improve the clinical outcome, but it prevents the emergence of rifampicin-resistant *Staph. epidermidis* strains during therapy (Rupp and Archer, 1994). With vancomycin plus rifampicin therapy such resistance emerges in some 30% of patients. Gentamicin should not be added to the regimen if the strain is gentamicin-resistant. In this situation it may be reasonable to use vancomycin alone for first 4–5 days and then add rifampicin. This may make emergence of rifampicin-resistant strains less likely, as the population of organisms may be much reduced by vancomyin alone during the first few days. The triple drug combination is also usually synergistic *in vitro* against methicillin-resistant *Staph. epidermidis* strains (Lowy *et al.*, 1983; Yu *et al.*, 1984).

Endocarditis due to Gram-negative bacilli usually occurs in patients with serious underlying diseases or in i.v. drug abusers. Nowadays one of the third-generation cephalosporins, such as cefotaxime, ceftriaxone or ceftazidime, would be the mainstay of treatment, but combination therapy with gentamicin or amikacin may be needed in difficult cases. For *Ps. aeruginosa* endocarditis, a ticarcillin/tobramycin combination is usually preferred (p.156).

Gentamicin 1.5 mg per kg plus cloxacillin 2 g i.v. may be used as chemoprophylaxis before cardiac valve surgery to prevent prosthetic valve endocarditis; a loading dose of each drug is given just before surgery and this is followed by a second dose at the end of cardiopulmonary bypass (Ward *et al.*, 1977). Gentamicin is also recommended for some patients who need endocarditis chemoprophylaxis (p.44).

5 Chemoprophylaxis in abdominal surgery

A single i.m. injection of 80 mg gentamicin, given just before colonic or rectal surgery, is ineffective in prevention of postoperative wound infection, intraperitoneal abscess and fecal fistula formation (Burton *et al.*, 1975). If i.m. or i.v. gentamicin 1.5 mg per kg body weight is combined with either i.v. clindamycin 600 mg, oral tinidazole 2 g, rectal metronidazole 1 g or i.v. metronidazole 500 mg, and both chemotherapeutic agents are given once only just before surgery, there is a significant reduction of postoperative infections after large bowel surgery (p.949). In one controlled study prophylactic i.v metronidazole alone was compared with the combination of metronidazole and gentamicin. There was no difference in mortality and postoperative infections (Morris *et al.*, 1983).

6 Biliary tract infections

Gentamicin, in combination with ampicillin (p.125) or one of the cephalosporins (p.339), is often used to treat acute cholangitis. In seriously ill and particularly elderly patients, drugs such as chloramphenicol (p.569) or clindamycin (p.597) may also be needed to cover the possibility of Gram-negative anaerobic bacterial infection.

7 Necrotizing enterocolitis

Similar to kanamycin (p.447), gentamicin may be useful for the prophylaxis and treatment of this condition. Prophylaxis with oral gentamicin may lower the incidence of this disease (Kliegman and Fanaroff, 1984), but the oral drug is ineffective for treatment (Hansen *et al.*, 1980). The acutely ill neonate needs parenteral antibiotics appropriate for the known sensitivities of the enteric flora in the nursery; combinations such as ticarcillin/gentamicin and clindamycin/gentamicin have been commonly used (Bell *et al.*, 1979; Kliegman and Fanaroff, 1984). Under certain circumstances other antibiotic combinations may be necessary (p.447). In one trial cefotaxime/vancomycin proved superior to ampicillin/gentamicin (Scheifele *et al.*, 1987).

8 Gonorrhea

The uncomplicated disease responds to a single i.m. dose of 280 mg of gentamicin and this dose is non-toxic to adults with normal renal function (Report, 1978). Gentamicin is not currently recommended for the treatment of gonorrhea, but in some areas it may have to be considered for disease produced by beta-lactamase producing gonococci (Hira *et al.*, 1985).

9 Reduction of bowel flora in patients with granulocytopenia

Oral gentamicin in combination with vancomycin has been used with some success to reduce intestinal flora and consequently the frequency of serious infections, such as septicemia, in granulocytopenic patients with leukemia or other malignancies (Hahn *et al.*, 1978). Other antibiotics, including co-trimoxazole have also been used for this purpose (p.881). Other aminoglycosides such as neomycin (p.539) have also been used and oral tobramycin appears to be the best of the aminoglycosides for selective decontamination (Clasener *et al.*, 1987).

10 Other infections

Gentamicin can be given by subconjunctival injection in a dose of 20–40 mg to treat or prevent intra-ocular infections (Mathalone, 1974). The drug is effective in the treatment of tularemia (Mason *et al.*, 1980; Enderlin *et al.*, 1994; Cross *et al.*, 1995), but streptomycin (p.435) is an equally effective alternative (Capellan and Fong, 1993). According to a report from South Africa, in approximately 10% of children with gastroenteritis, severe diarrhea continues and requires therapy for more than 7 days. In this group of children the administration of oral gentamicin plus cholestyramine was beneficial. By some mechanism these drugs improved nitrogen and fat absorption and decreased the stool weight (Hill *et al.*, 1986).

11 Liposome-encapsulated-gentamicin

Animal experiments indicate that gentamicin encapsulated in liposomes can be administered safely by the parenteral route. Liposomes are closed, single or multilamellar vesicles composed of lipids. Gentamicin when encapsulated in liposomes enters cells more readily, and is more effective for the treatment of experimental intracellular infections, such as brucellosis (Morgan and Williams, 1980; Fountain *et al.*, 1985), murine salmonellosis and some Gram-negative extracellular infections such as *Klebsiella* pneumonia (Fierer *et al.*, 1990; Swenson *et al.*, 1990; Karlowsky and Zhanel, 1992).

Liposome-encapsulated-gentamicin is also active against disseminated *Mycobacterium avium* complex infections in animals (Klemens *et al.*, 1990). It also has been tried in AIDS patients with this infection. It was administered as an infusion twice-weekly for 4 weeks in three different dosages – 1.7 mg per kg, 3.4 mg per kg and 5.1 mg per kg of gentamicin per infusion. The MAC colony counts in blood fell by 75% or more in all three groups (Nightingale *et al.*, 1993). The place of gentamicin for the treatment of this infection is uncertain. It should be treated by a regimen of two or preferably three drugs. On present evidence oral clarithromycin (p.648) or azithromycin (p.657) is the preferred first agent and ethambutol (p.1215) is the preferred second drug. The choice for the third agent is between rifampicin (p.692) and rifabutin (p.712), ciprofloxacin (p.1032), amikacin (p.516) or liposome-encapsulated gentamicin (Benson, 1994).

References

A Cooperative Study (1973). Drug-induced deafness. *JAMA* **224**: 515.

Ackerman VP, Groot Obbink DJ, Sivertsen T (1983). Transferable antibiotic resistance in a general hospital: a two year survey. *Aust J Exp Biol Med Sci* **61**: 251.

Adelman RD, Spangler WL, Beasom F *et al.* (1979). Furosemide enhancement of experimental gentamicin nephrotoxicity: comparison of functional and morphological changes with activities of urinary enzymes. *J Infect Dis* **140**: 342.

Ahonkhai VI, Cherubin CE, Sierra F *et al.* (1981). *In vitro* susceptibility of *Campylobacter fetus* subsp. *jejuni* to N-formimidoyl thienamycin, rosaramicin, cefoperazone and other antimicrobial agents. *Antimicrob Ag Chemother* **20**: 850.

Akalin HE, Torun M, Alacam R (1988). Aminoglycoside resistance patterns in Turkey. *Scand J Infect Dis* **20**: 199.

Alford RH, Hall A (1987). Epidemiology of infections caused by gentamicin-resistant Enterobacteriaceae and *Pseudomonas aeruginosa* over 15 years at the Nashville Veterans Administration Medical Center. *Rev Infect Dis* **9**: 1079.

Alford RH, John JT, Bryant RE (1972). Tularemia treated successfully with gentamicin. *Amer Rev Resp Dis* **106**: 265.

Anstey NM, Currie BJ, Withnall KM (1992). Community-acquired *Acinetobacter pneumonia* in the Northern Territory of Australia. *Clin Infect Dis* **14**: 83.

Antalek MD, Mylotte JM, Lesse AJ, Sellick JAJr (1995). Clinical and molecular epidemiology of *Enterococcus faecalis* bacteremia, with special reference to strains with high-level resistance to gentamicin. *Clin Infect Dis* **20**: 103.

Appel GB, Neu HC (1977). The nephrotoxicity of antimicrobial agents (second of three parts). *New Engl J Med* **296**: 722.

Archer GL, Climo MW (1994). Antimicrobial susceptibility of coagulase-negative staphylococci. *Antimicrob Ag Chemother* **38**: 2231.

Archer GL, Johnston JL (1983). Self-transmissible plasmids in staphylococci that encode resistance to aminoglycosides. *Antimicrob Ag Chemother* **24**: 70.

Archer GL, Scott J (1991). Conjugative transfer genes in staphylococcal isolates from the United States. *Antimicrob Ag Chemother* **35**: 2500.

Archer GL, Dietrick DR, Johnston JL (1985). Molecular epidemiology of transmissible gentamicin resistance among coagulase-negative staphylococci in a cardiac surgery unit. *J Infect Dis* **151**: 243.

Arcieri GM, Falco FG, Smith HM, Hobson LB (1970). Clinical research experience with gentamicin: incidence of adverse reactions. *Med J Aust* **1** (Spec Suppl): 30.

Argov Z, Mastaglia FL (1979). Disorders of neuromuscular transmission caused by drugs. *New Engl J Med* **301**: 409.

Aronoff GR, Luft FC (1979). Antimicrobial therapy in patients with impaired renal function. *Dial Transplant* **8**: 14.

Aronoff GR, Pottratz ST, Brier ME *et al.* (1983). Aminoglycoside accumulation kinetics in rat renal parenchyma. *Antimicrob Ag Chemother* **23**: 74.

Aronsson B, Eriksson M, Herin P, Rylander M (1991). Gentamicin-resistant *Klebsiella* spp and *Escherichia coli* in a neonatal intensive care unit. *Scand J Infect Dis* **23**: 195.

Assael BM, Parini R, Rusconi F (1982). Ototoxicity of aminoglycoside antibiotics in infants and children. *Pediatr Infect Dis* **1**: 357.

Auclair P, Lessard C, Bergeron MG (1988). Renal pharmacokinetic changes of gentamicin during enterococcal pyelonephritis. *Antimicrob Ag Chemother* **32**: 736.

Auclair P, Tardif D, Beauchamp D *et al.* (1990). Prolonged endotoxemia enhances the renal injuries induced by gentamicin in rats. *Antimicrob Ag Chemother* **34**: 889.

Azimi PH, Koranyi K, Lindsey KD (1979). *Listeria monocytogenes*. Synergistic effects of ampicillin and gentamicin. *Amer J Clin Path* **72**: 974.

Bach MC, Sabath LD, Finland M (1973). Susceptibility of *Nocardia asteroides* to 45 antimicrobial agents *in vitro*. *Antimicrob Ag Chemother* **3**: 1.

Bacheson MA, Friedman HM, Benson CE (1981). Antimicrobial susceptibility of intracellular *Legionella pneumophila*. *Antimicrob Ag Chemother* **20**: 691.

Baker CJ (1981). Nosocomial septicemia and meningitis in neonates. *Amer J Med* **70**: 638.

Baker CN, Thornsberry C, Facklam RR (1981). Synergism, killing kinetics and antimicrobial susceptibility of Group A and B Streptococci. *Antimicrob Ag Chemother* **19**: 716.

Barber M, Waterworth PM (1966). Activity of gentamicin against *Pseudomonas*, and hospital staphylococci. *Brit Med J* **1**: 203.

Barclay ML, Begg EJ, Chambers ST (1992). Adaptive resistance following single doses of gentamicin in a dynamic *in vitro* model. *Antimicrob Ag Chemother* **36**: 1951.

Barg NL (1988). Construction of a probe for the aminoglycoside

3-V-acetyltransferase gene and detection of the gene among endemic clinical isolates. *Antimicrob Ag Chemother* **32**: 1834.

Barg NL Cooper JF (1990). Endogenous colonization by gentamicin-resistant Gram-negative bacilli elaborating aminoglycoside (3).-5-acetyl-transferase. *Antimicrob Ag Chemother* **34**: 1827.

Bartlett JG, Miao PVW, Gorbach SL (1977). Empiric treatment with clindamycin and gentamicin of suspected sepsis due to anaerobic and aerobic bacteria. *J Infect Dis* **135** (Suppl): 80.

Bartlett JG, O'Keefe P, Tally FP et al. (1986). Bacteriology of hospital-acquired pneumonia. *Arch Intern Med* **146**: 868.

Barza M, Brown RB, Shen D et al. (1975). Predictability of blood levels of gentamicin in man. *J Infect Dis* **132**: 165.

Barza M, Murray T, Hamburger RJ (1980). Uptake of gentamicin by separated, viable renal tubules from rabbits. *J Infect Dis* **141**: 510.

Bastone EB, Li SC, Ioannides-Demos LL et al. (1993). Kill kinetics and regrowth patterns of *Escherichia coli* exposed to gentamicin concentration-time profiles simulating *in vivo* bolus and infusion dosing. *Antimicrob Ag Chemother* **37**: 914.

Beauchamp D, Pettigrew M (1988). Influence of hydrocortisone on gentamicin-induced nephrotoxicity in rats. *Antimicrob Ag Chemother* **32**: 992.

Beauchamp D, Charette F, Auclair P et al. (1986). Effect of hydrocortisone on gentamicin-induced nephrotoxicity. In *Abstracts and Program of the 26th Interscience Conference on Antimicrobial Agents and Chemotherapy, New Orleans* (Abstr. 28). Washington. DC: American Society for Microbiology.

Beauchamp D, Gourde P, Bergeron MG (1991). Subcellular distribution of gentamicin in proximal tubular cells, determined by immunogold labeling. *Antimicrob Ag Chemother* **35**: 2173.

Beck PR, Thomson RB, Chaudhuri AKR (1977). Aminoglycoside antibiotics and renal function: changes in urinary gamma-glutamyl-transferase excretion. *J Clin Path* **30**: 432.

Bell MJ, Shackleford PG, Feigin RD et al. (1979). Alterations in gastrointestinal microflora during antimicrobial therapy for necrotizing enterocelitis. *Pediatrics* **63**: 425.

Bengtsson S, Bernander S, Brorson JE et al. (1986). *In vitro* aminoglycoside resistance of Gram-negative bacilli and staphylococci isolated from blood in Sweden 1980–1984. *Scand J Infect Dis* **18**: 257.

Bennett WM, Plamp C, Porter GA (1977). Drug-related syndromes in clinical nephrology. *Ann Intern Med* **87**: 582.

Bennett WM, Luft F, Porter GA (1980). Pathogenesis of renal failure due to aminoglycosides and contrast media used in roentgenography. *Amer J Med* **69**: 767.

Bennett WM, Elliott WC, Houghton DC et al. (1982). Reduction of experimental gentamicin nephrotoxicity in rats by dietary calcium loading. *Antimicrob Ag Chemother* **22**: 508.

Bennett WM, Aronoff GR, Morrison G et al. (1983). Drug prescribing in renal failure: dosing guidelines for adults. *Amer J Kid Dis* **3**: 155.

Benson CA (1994). Treatment of disseminated disease due to *Mycobacterium avium* complex in patients with AIDS. *Clin Infect Dis* **18**: (Suppl 3): 237.

Bergeron MG (1985). Leading article Theraputic potential of high renal levels of aminoglycosides in pyelonephritis. *J Antimicrob Chemother* **15**: 4.

Bergeron MG, Bergeron Y, (1986). Influence of endotoxin on the intrarenal distribution of gentamicin, netilmicin, tobramycin, amikacin and cephalothin. *Antimicrob Ag Chemother* **29**: 7.

Bergeron MG, Marois Y (1986). Benefit from high intrarenal levels of gentamicin in the treatment of *E coli* pyelonephritis. *Kid Int* **30**: 481.

Bergeron MG, Trottier S (1979). Influence of single or multiple doses of gentamicin and netilmicin on their cortical medullary and papillary distribution. *Antimicrob Ag Chemother* **15**: 635.

Bergeron MG, Bastille A, Lessard C, Gagnon PM (1982a). Significance of intrarenal concentrations of gentamicin for the outcome of experimental pyelonephritis in rats. *J Infect Dis* **146**: 91.

Bergeron MG, Trottier S, Lessard C et al. (1982b). Disturbed intrarenal distribution of gentamicin in experimental pyelonephritis due to *Escherichia coli*. *J Infect Dis* **146**: 436.

Bergeron MG, Bergeron Y, Bauchamp D (1987). Influence of hydrocortisone succinate on intrarenal accumulation of gentamicin in endotoxemic rats. *Antimicrob Ag Chemother* **31**: 1816.

Bertino JS,Jr, Booker LA, Franck P, Rybicki B (1991). Gentamicin pharmacokinetics in patients with malignancies. *Antimicrob Ag Chemother* **35**: 1501.

Bertino JS Jr, Booker LA, Franck PA et al. (1993). Incidence of and significant risk factors for aminoglycoside-associated nephrotoxicity in patients dosed by using individualized pharmacokinetic monitoring. *J Infect Dis* **167**: 173.

Betts RF, Valenti WM, Chapman SW et al. (1984). Five-year surveillance of aminoglycoside usage in a university hospital. *Ann Intern Med* **100**: 219.

Bhatia J, Prihoda AR, Richardson J (1986). Parenteral antibiotics and carbohydrate intolerance in term neonates. *Amer J Dis Child* **140**: 111.

Bianco TM, Dwyer PN, Bertino JSJr (1989). Gentamicin pharmacokinetics, nephrotoxicity, and prediction of mortality in febrile neutropenic patients. *Antimicrob Ag Chemother* **33**: 1890.

Bille J, Glauser MP (1981). Prevention of acute and chronic ascending pyelonephritis in rats by aminoglycoside antibiotics accumulated and persistent in kidneys. *Antimicrob Ag Chemother* **19**: 381.

Black J, Calesnick B, Williams D, Weinstein MJ (1964). Pharmacology of gentamicin, a new broad-spectrum antibiotic. *Antimicrob Ag Chemother* **1963**: 138.

Bloch R, Luft FC, Rankin LI et al. (1979). Protection from gentamicin nephrotoxicity by cephalothin and carbenicillin. *Antimicrob Ag Chemother* **15**: 46.

Bodey GP, Feld R, Burgess MA (1976). Beta-lactum antibiotics alone or in combination with gentamicin for therapy of Gram-negative bacillary infections in neutropenic patients. *Amer J Med Sci* **271**: 179.

Bodey GP, Jadeja L, Elting L (1985). *Pseudomonas* bacteremia. Retrospective analysis of 410 episodes. *Arch Intern Med* **145**: 1621.

Boucher BA, Kuhl DA, Hickerson WL (1992). Pharmacokinetics of systemically administered antibiotics in patients with thermal injury. *Clin Infect Dis* **14**: 458.

Bourgault A-M, Gauvreau L (1983). Antimicrobial susceptibilities of coagulase-negative staphylococci isolated from urinary infections. *Antimicrob Ag Chemother* **23**: 793.

Brandt CM, Warner CB, Rouse MS et al. (1996). Effect of gentamicin dosing interval on efficacy of penicillin or ceftriaxone treatment of experimental endocarditis due to penicillin-susceptible, uftriaxone-tolerant *Viridans* group streptococci. *Antimicrob Ag Chemother* **40**: 2901.

Bridges K, Kidson A, Lowbury EJL, Wilkins MD (1979). Gentamicin and silver-resistant pseudomonas in a burns unit. *Brit Med J* **1**: 446.

Brier ME, Mayer PR, Brier RA et al. (1985). Relationship between rat renal accumulation of gentamicin, tobramycin, and netilmicin and their nephrotoxicities. *Antimicrob Ag Chemother* **27**: 812.

Brion N, Barge J, Godefroy I et al. (1984). Gentamicin, netilmicin, dibekacin and amikacin nephrotoxicity and its relationship to tubular reabsorption in rabbits. *Antimicrob Ag Chemother* **25**: 168.

Brook I, Walker RI (1985). Interaction between penicillin, clindamycin or metronidazole and gentamicin against species of clostridia and anaerobic and facultatively anaerobic Gram-positive cocci. *J Antimicrob Chemother* **15**: 31.

Brook I, Coolbaugh JC, Walker RI, Weiss E (1984). Synergism between penicillin, clindamycin, or metronidazole and gentamicin against species of the *Bacteroides melaninogenicus* and *Bacteroides fragilis* groups. *Antimicrob Ag Chemother* **25**: 71.

Brown AE, Quesada O, Armstrong D (1982). Minimal nephrotoxicity with cephalosporin-aminoglycoside combinations in patients with neoplastic disease. *Antimicrob Ag Chemother* **21**: 592.

Brummett RE (1983). Animal models of aminoglycoside antibiotic ototoxicity. *Rev Infect Dis* **5** (Suppl 2): 294.

Brummett RE, Fox KE (1989). Aminoglycoside-induced hearing loss in humans. *Antimicrob Ag Chemother* **33**: 797.

Bryan CS, Stone WJ (1977). Antimicrobial dosage in renal failure: a unifying nomogram. *Clin Nephrol* **7**: 81.

Bryan LE (1988). General mechanisms of resistance to antibiotics. *J Antimicrob Chemother* **22** (Suppl A): 1.

Bryan LE, Kwan S (1981). Aminoglycoside-resistant mutants of *Pseudomonas aeruginosa* deficient in cytochrome d, nitrite reductase and aerobic transport. *Antimicrob Ag Chemother* **19**: 958.

Bryan LE, Van den Elzen HM (1977). Effects of membrane-energy mutations and cations on streptomycin and gentamicin accumulation by bacteria: a model for entry of streptomycin and gentamicin in susceptible and resistant bacteria. *Antimicrob Ag Chemother* **12**: 163.

Bryan LE, Kowand SK, Van den Elzen HM (1979). Mechanism of aminoglycoside antibiotic resistance in anaerobic bacteria: *Clostridium perfringens* and *Bacteroides fragilis*. *Antimicrob Ag Chemother* **15**: 7.

Bryan LE, O'Hara K, Wong S (1984). Lipopolysaccharide changes in impermeability- type aminoglycoside resistance in *Pseudomonas aeruginosa*. *Antimicrob Ag Chemother* **26**: 250.

Bryce EA, Zemcov SJV, Clarke AM (1991). Species identification and antibiotic resistance patterns of the enterococci. *Eur J Clin Microbiol Infect Dis* **10**: 745.

Burgaleta C, Martinez-Beltrán J, Bouza E (1982). Comparative effects of moxalactam and gentamicin on human polymorphonuclear leukocyte function. *Antimicrob Ag Chemother* **21**: 718.

Burman WJ, Cohn DL, Reves RR, Wilson ML (1995). Multifocal cellulitis and monoarticular arthritis as manifestations of *Helicobacter cinaedi* bacteremia. *Clin Infect Dis* **20**: 564.

Burton RC, Hughes ESR, Cuthbertson AM (1975). Prophylactic use of gentamicin in colonic and rectal surgery. *Med J Aust* **2**: 597.

Buss WC, Piatt MK (1985). Gentamicin administered *in vivo* reduces protein synthesis in microsomes subsequently isolated from rat kidneys but not from rat brains. *J Antimicrob Chemother* **15**: 715.

Buss WC, Piatt MK, Kauten R (1984). Inhibition of mammalian microsomal protein synthesis by aminoglycoside antibiotics. *J Antimicrob Chemother* **14**: 231.

Buss WC, Kauten R, Piatt MK (1985). Inhibitory effects of gentamicin and ethacrynic acid on mammalian microsomal protein synthesis. *J Antimicrob Chemother* **15**: 105.

Butler T, Bell WR, Linh NN *et al.* (1974). *Yersinia pestis* infection in Vietnam. I. Clinical and hematological aspects. *J Infect Dis* (Suppl): **129**: 78.

Buu-Hoi A, Le Bouguenec C, Horaud T (1990). High-level chromasomal gentamicin resistance in *Streptococcus agalactiae* (Group B). *Antimicrob Ag Chemother* **34**: 985.

Bygbjerg IC, Møller R (1976). Gentamicin-induced nephropathy. *Scand J Infect Dis* **8**: 203.

Byrd GJ (1977). Actue organic brain syndrome associated with gentamicin therapy. *JAMA* **238**: 53.

Byrne ME, Gillespie MT, Skurray RA (1990). Molecular analysis of a gentamicin resistance transposonlike element on plasmids isolated from North American *Staphylococcus aureus* strains. *Antimicrob Ag Chemother* **34**: 2106.

Cabrera J, Arroyo V, Ballesta AM *et al.* (1982). Aminoglycoside nephrotoxicity in cirrhosis. *Gastroenterology* **82**: 97.

Cafferkey MT, Falkiner FR, Gillespie WA, Murphy DM (1982). Antibiotics for the prevention of septicaemia in urology. *J Antimicrob Chemother* **9**: 471.

Calderwood SA, Wennersten C, Moellering RC Jr *et al.* (1977). Resistance to six aminoglycosidic aminocyclitol antibiotics among enterococci: prevalence, evolution, and relationship to synergism with penicillin. *Antimicrob Ag Chemother* **12**: 401.

Capellan J, Fong IW (1993). Tularemia from a cat bite: case report and review of feline-associated tularemia. *Clin Infect Dis* **16**: 472.

Carbon C, Contrepois A, Lamotte-Barrillon S (1978). Comparative distribution of gentamicin, tobramycin, sisomicin, netilmicin, and amikacin in interstitial fluid in rabbits. *Antimicrob Ag Chemother* **13**: 368.

Carrizosa J, Levison ME (1981). Minimal concentrations of aminoglycoside

that can synergize with penicillin in enterococcal endocarditis. *Antimicrob Ag Chemother* **20**: 405.

Casewell MW, Dalton MT, Webster M, Phillips I (1977). Gentamicin-resistant *Klebsiella aerogenes* in a urological ward. *Lancet* **ii**: 444.

Chamberland S, L'Ecuyer J, Lessard C *et al.* (1992). Antibiotic susceptibility profiles of 941 Gram-negative bacteria isolated from septicemic patients throughout Canada. *Clin Infect Dis* **15**: 615.

Chan KW, Ng WL (1985). Gentamicin nephropathy in a neonate. *Pathology* **17**: 514.

Chan RA, Benner EJ, Hoeprich PD (1972). Gentamicin therapy in renal failure: a nomogram for dosage. *Ann Intern Med* **76**: 773.

Chandrasekar PH, Cronin SM (1991). Nephrotoxicity in bone marrow transplant recipients receiving aminoglycoside plus cyclosporine or aminoglycoside alone. *J Antimicrob Chemother* **27**: 845.

Chang JC, Reyes B (1975). Agranulocytosis associated with gentamicin. *JAMA* **232**: 1154.

Chaslus-Dancla E, Martel J-L, Carlier C *et al.* (1986). Emergence of aminoglycoside 3-N-acetyltransferase IV in *Escherichia coli* and *Salmonella typhimurium* isolated from animals in France. *Antimicrob Ag Chemother* **29**: 239.

Chen HY (1986). Leading article. Resistance of enterococci to anitbiotic combinations. *J Antimicrob Chemother* **18**: 1.

Chen HY, Williams JD (1985). Transferable resistance and aminoglycoside-modifying enzymes in enterococci. *J Med Microbiol* **20**: 187.

Chiew Y-F, Lim S-W, Kuah B-G, Liew H-Y (1993). Prevalence in Singapore of enterococci with high-level resistance to aminoglycosides and comparison of three methods for their detection. *J Infect* **27**: 125.

Chisholm GD (1974). The use of gentamicin in urinary tract infections with special reference to drug levels in complicated (urological). infections. *Postgrad Med J* **50** (Suppl 7): 23.

Chisholm GD, Calnan JS, Waterworth PM, Reis ND (1968). Distribution of gentamicin in body fluids. *Brit Med J* **2**: 22.

Chiu PJS, Long JF (1978). Effects of hydration on gentamicin excretion and renal accumulation in furosemide-treated rats. *Antimicrob Ag Chemother* **14**: 214.

Chow AW, Jewesson PJ (1985). Pharmacokinetics and safety of antimicrobial agents during pregnancy. *Rev Infect Dis* **7**: 287.

Chow AW, Patten V, Bednorz D (1978). Susceptibility of *Campylobacter fetus* to 22 antimicrobial agents. *Antimicrob Ag Chemother* **13**: 416.

Clasener HAL, Vollaard EJ, Van Saene HKF (1987). Long-term prophylaxis of infection by selective decontamination in leukopenia and in mechanical ventilation. *Rev Infect Dis* **9**: 295.

Coleman K, Athalye M, Clancey A *et al.* (1994). Bacterial resistance mechanisms as therapeutic targets. *J Antimicrob Chemother* **33**: 1091.

Contrepois A, Brion N, Garaud J-J *et al.* (1985). Renal disposition of gentamicin dibekacin, tobramycin, netilmicin, and amikacin in humans. *Antimicrob Ag Chemother* **27**: 520.

Coque TM, Arduino RC, Murray BE (1995). High-level resistance to aminoglycosides: comparison of community and nosocomial fecal isolates of enterococci. *Clin Infect Dis* **20**: 1048.

Cox CE (1969). Gentamicin, a new aminoglycoside antibiotic: clinical and laboratory studies in urinary tract infection. *J Infect Dis* **119**: 486.

Cronberg S (1994). Simplified monitoring of aminoglycosides. *J Antimicrob Chemother* **34**: 819.

Crosby SS, Edwards WAD, Brennan C *et al.* (1987). Systemic absorption of endotracheally administered aminoglycosides in seriously ill patients with pneumonia. *Antimicrob Ag Chemother* **31**: 850.

Cross JT Jr, Schutze GE, Jacobs RF (1995). Treatment of tularemia with gentamicin in pediatric patients. *Pediatr Infect Dis J* **14**: 151.

Curtis JR, McDonald SJ, Weston JH (1967). Parenteral administration of gentamicin in renal failure: patients undergoing intermittent haemodialysis. *Brit Med J* **2**: 537.

Cutler RE, Gyselynck A, Fleet WP, Forrey AW (1972). Correlation of serum creatinine concentration and gentamicin half-life. *JAMA* **29**: 1037.

Dahlgren JG, Anderson ET, Hewitt WL (1975). Gentamicin blood levels: a guide to nephrotoxicity. *Antimicrob Ag Chemother* **8**: 58.

Daikos GL, Jackson GG, Lolans VT, Livermore DM (1990). Adaptive resistance to aminoglycoside antibiotics from first-exposure down regulation. *J Infect Dis* **162**: 414.

Dan M, Halkin H, Rubinstein E (1981). Interstitial fluid concentrations of aminoglycosides. *J Antimicrob Chemother* **7**: 551.

Dan M, Gutman R, Biro A (1992). Peritonitis caused by *Pseudomonas putrefaciens* in patients undergoing continuous ambulatory peritoneal dialysis. *Clin Infect Dis* **14**: 359.

Danish M, Schultz R, Jusko WJ (1974). Pharmacokinetics of gentamicin and kanamycin during hemodialysis. *Antimicrob Ag Chemother* **6**: 841.

Darrell JH, Waterworth PM (1967). Dosage of gentamicin for *Pseudomonas* infections. *Brit Med J* **2**: 535.

Das SS, Anderson JR, Macdonald AA, Somerville KW (1994). Endocarditis due to high level gentamicin resistant *Enterococcus faecium*. *J Infect* **28**: 185.

Davey PG, Geddes AM, Cowley DM (1983). Study of alanine aminopeptidase excretion as a test of gentamicin nephrotoxocity. *J Antimicrob Chemother* **11**: 455.

Davey RB, Pittard J (1977). Plasmids mediating resistance to gentamicin and other antibiotics in Enterobacteriaceae from four hospitals in Melbourne. *Aust J Exper Biol Med Sci* **55**: 299.

Davies JE (1983). Resistance to aminoglycosides: mechanisms and frequency. *Rev Infect Dis* **5** (Suppl 2): 261.

Dean HF, Morgan AF, Asche LV, Holloway BW (1977). Isolates of *Pseudomonas aeruginosa* from Australian hospitals having R-plasmid determined antibiotic resistance. *Med J Aust* **2**: 116.

Dee TH, Kozin F (1977). Gentamicin and tobramycin penetration into synovial fluid. *Antimicrob Ag Chemother* **12**: 548.

de Louvois J (1987). Pharmacokinetics of antibiotics in the newborn. *J Antimicrob Chemother* **20**: 623.

Desai TK, Tsang T-K (1988). Aminoglycoside nephrotoxicity in obstructive jaundice. *Amer J Med* **85**: 47.

Donowitz GR, Mandell GL (1983). Empiric therapy for pneumonia. *Rev Infect Dis* **5** (Suppl 1): 40.

Dornbusch K, Miller GH, Hare RS et al. (1990). Resistance to aminoglycoside antibiotics in Gram-negative bacilli and staphylococci isolated from blood. Report from a European collaborative study. *J Antimicrob Chemother* **26**: 131.

Dowd G, Cafferkey M, Dougan G (1983). Gentamicin and methicillin resistant *Staphylococcus aureus* in Dublin hospitals: molecular studies. *J Med Microbiol* **16**: 129.

Dowling JN, Weyant RS, Pasculle AW (1982). Bacterial activity of antibiotics against *Legionella micdadei* (Pittsburg pneumonia agent). *Antimicrob Ag Chemother* **22**: 272.

Drasar FA, Farrell W, Maskell J, Williams JD (1976). Tobramycin, amikacin, sisomicin, and gentamicin-resistant Gram-negative rods. *Brit Med J* **2**: 1284.

Drusano GL (1988). Role of pharmacokinetics in the outcome of infections. *Antimicrob Ag Chemother* **32**: 289.

Drusano GL (1991). Human pharmacodynamics of beta-lactams, aminoglycosides and their combination. *Scand J Infect Dis* (Suppl 74): 235.

Dulon D, Aran J-M, Zajic G, Schacht J (1986). Comparative uptake of gentamicin, netilmicin, and amikacin in the guinea pig cochlea and vestibule. *Antimicrob Ag Chemother* **30**: 96.

Duncan IBR (1974). Susceptibility of 1500 isolates of *Pseudomonas aeruginosa* to gentamicin, carbenicillin, colistin and polymyxin B. *Antimicrob Ag Chemother* **5**: 9.

Duncan IBR, Rennie RP, Duncan NH (1981). A long-term study of gentamicin-resistant *Pseudomonas aeruginosa* in a general hospital. *J Antimicrob Chemother* **7**: 147.

Dyas A, Wise R, Pijck J et al. (1983). Reproducibility study of the pharmacokinetics of amikacin, gentamicin and tobramycin; a three-way crossover study. *J Antimicrob Chemother* **12**: 371.

Echeverria P, Siber GR, Paisley J et al. (1975). Age-dependent dose response to gentamicin. *J Pediatr* **87**: 805.

Edwards C, Smith CR, Baughman KL et al. (1976). Concentrations of gentamicin and amikacin in human kidneys. *Antimicrob Ag Chemother* **9**: 925.

Edwards C, Low DC, Bissenden JG (1986). Gentamicin dosage for the newborn. *Lancet* **i**: 508.

Elhanan K, Siplovich L, Raz R (1995). Gentamicin once-daily versus thrice-daily in children. *J Antimicrob Chemother* **35**: 327.

Eliopoulos GM, Moellering RC Jr (1982). Antibiotic synergism and antimicrobial combinations in clinical infections. *Rev Infect Dis* **4**: 282.

Eliopoulos GM, Wennersten C, Zighelboim-Daum et al. (1988). High-level resistance to gentamicin in clinical isolates of *Streptococcus (Enterococcus) faecium*. *Antimicrob Ag Chemother* **32**: 1528.

Eliopoulos GM, Thauvin-Eliopoulos C, Moellering RCJr (1992). Contribution of animal models in the search for effective therapy for endocarditis due to enterococci with high-level resistance to gentamicin. *Clin Infect Dis* **15**: 58.

Ellis-Pegler RB, Chambers S, Begg EJ, Barclay ML (1994). Aminoglycoside dosing: time to change. *Aust NZ J Med* **24**: 359.

Enderlin G, Morales L, Jacobs RF, Cross JT (1994). Streptomycin and alternative agents for the treatment of tularemia: review of the literature. *Clin Infect Dis* **19**: 42.

EORTC International Antimicrobial Therapy Project Group (1978). Three antibiotic regiments in the treatment of infection in febrile granulocytopenic patients with cancer. *J Infect Dis* **137**: 14.

Falkiner FR, Keane CT, Dalton M et al. (1977). Cross infection in a surgical ward caused by *Pseudomonas aeruginosa* with transferable resistance to gentamicin and tobramycin. *J Clin Path* **30**: 731.

Fantin B, Ebert S, Leggett J et al. (1990). Factors affecting duration of *in-vivo* postantibiotic effect for aminoglycosides against Gram-negative bacilli. *J Antimicrob Chemother* **27**: 829.

Fausti SA, Henry JA, Schaffer HI et al. (1992). High-frequency audiometric monitoring for early detection of aminoglycoside ototoxicity. *J Infect Dis* **165**: 1026.

Fee WE Jr (1983). Gentamicin and tobramycin: comparison of ototoxicity. *Rev Infect Dis* **5** (Suppl 2): 304.

Feig PU, Mitchell PP, Abrutyn E et al. (1982). Aminoglycoside nephrotoxicity: a double blind prospective randomized study of gentamicin and tobramycin. *J Antimicrob Chemother* **10**: 217.

Fernandez-Rodriguez A, Canton R, Perez-Diaz JC et al. (1992). Aminoglycoside-modifying enzymes in clinical isolates harboring extended-spectrum beta-lactamases. *Antimicrob Ag Chemother* **36**: 2536.

Ferrari FA, Pagani A, Marconi M et al. (1980). Inhibition of candidacidal activity of human neutrophil leukocytes by aminoglycoside antibiotics. *Antimicrob Ag Chemother* **17**: 87.

Fierer J, Hatlen L, Lin J-P et al. (1990). Successful treatment using gentamicin liposomes of Salmonella dublin infections in mice. *Antimicrob Ag Chemother* **34**: 343.

Finitzo-Hieber T, McCracken GH Jr, Roeser RJ et al. (1979). Ototoxicity in neonates treated with gentamicin and kanamycin: results of a four-year controlled follow-up study. *Pediatrics* **63**: 443.

Follath F, Wenk M, Vozeh S (1981). Plasma concentration monitoring of aminoglycosides. *J Antimicrob Chemother* **8** (Suppl A): 37.

Fong IW, Fenton RS, Bird R (1981). Comparative toxicity of gentamicin versus tobramycin: a randomized prospective study. *J Antimicrob Chemother* **7**: 81.

Forbes I, Gray A, Hurse A, Pavillard R (1977). The emergence of gentamicin-resistant *Klebsiellae* in a large general hospital. *Med J Aust* **1**: 14.

Foster TJ (1983). Plasmid-determined resistance to antimicrobial drugs and toxic metal ions in bacteria. *Microbiol Rev* **47**: 361.

Fountain MW, Weiss SJ, Fountain AG et al. (1985). Treatment of *Brucella canis* and *Brucella abortus in vitro* and *in vivo* by stable plurilamellar vesicle-encapsulated aminoglycosides. *J Infect Dis* **152**: 529.

Fraser DW, Wachsmuth IK, Bopp C et al. (1978). Antibiotic treatment of guinea-pigs infected with agent of Legionnaires' disease. *Lancet* **i**: 175.

Gangadharam PRJ, Candler ER (1977). *In vitro* anti-mycobacterial activity of some new aminoglycoside antibiotics. *Tubercle* **58**: 35.

Gary NE, Buzzeo L, Salaki J, Eisinger RP (1976). Gentamicin-associated acute renal failure. *Arch Intern Med* **136**: 1101.

Gelber RH, Henika PR, Gibson JB (1984). The bactericidal activity of various aminoglycoside antibiotics against *Mycobacterium leprae* in mice. *Lepr Rev* **55**: 341.

Gerding DN, Hall WH, Schierl EA (1977). Antibiotic concentrations in ascitic fluid of patients with ascites and bacterial peritonitis. *Ann Intern Med* **86**: 708.

Gerding DN, Buxton AE, Hughes RA *et al.* (1979). Nosocomial multiply resistant *Klebsiella pneumoniae*: epidemiology of an outbreak of apparent index case origin. *Antimicrob Ag Chemother* **15**: 608.

Gerding DN, Larson TA, Hughes RA *et al.* (1991). Aminoglycoside resistance and aminoglycoside usage: ten years experience in one hospital. *Antimicrob Ag Chemother* **35**: 1284.

Gibson DH, Fitzgeorge RB (1983). Persistence in serum and lungs of guinea pigs of erythromycin, gentamicin, chloramphenicol and rifampicin and their *in vitro* activities against *Legionella pneumophila*. *J Antimicrob Chemother* **12**: 235.

Gibson L, MacLeod C, Johnson L *et al.* (1994). Trends in bacterial infections in febrile neutropenic patients: 1986–1992. *Aust NZ J Med* **24**: 374.

Gigantelli JW, Gomez JT, Osato MS (1991). *In vitro* susceptibilities of ocular *Bacillus cereus* isolates to clindamycin, gentamicin, and vancomycin alone or in combination. *Antimicrob Ag Chemother* **35**: 201.

Gilbert DN (1991). Once-daily aminoglycoside therapy. *Antimicrob Ag Chemother* **35**: 399.

Gilbert DN, Wood CA, Kohlhepp SJ (1989). Polyaspartic acid prevents experimental aminoglycoside nephrotoxicity. *J Infect Dis* **159**: 945.

Gillespie MT, May JW, Skurray RA (1984). Antibiotic susceptibilities and plasmid profiles of nosocomial methicillin-resistant *Staphylococcus aureus*; a retrospective study. *J Med Microbiol* **17**: 295.

Gingell JC, Waterworth PM (1968). Dose of gentamicin in patients with normal renal function and renal impairment. *Brit Med J* **2**: 19.

Ginsburg CM, McCracken GH Jr (1982). Urinary tract infections in young infants. *Pediatrics* **69**: 409.

Ginsburg DS, Quintanilla AP, Levin M (1976). Renal glycosuria due to gentamicin in rabbits. *J Infect Dis* **134**: 119.

Glauser MP, Lyons JM, Braude AI (1979). Prevention of pyelonephritis due to *Escherichia coli* in rats with gentamicin store in kidney tissue. *J Infect Dis* **139**: 172.

Goetz MB, Sayers J (1993). Nephrotoxicity of vancomycin and aminoglycoside therapy separately and in combination. *J Antimicrob Chemother* **32**: 325.

Goldenberg DL, Cohen AS (1976). Acute infectious arthritis A review of patients with nongonococcal joint infections (with emphasis on therapy and prognosis). *Amer J Med* **60**: 369.

Goodman EL, Van Gelder J, Holmes R *et al.* (1975). Prospective comparative study of variable dosage and variable frequency regimens for administration of gentamicin. *Antimicrob Ag Chemother* **8**: 434.

Goodwin CS, Blake P, Blincow E (1986). The minimum inhibitory and bactericidal concentrations of antibiotics and anti-ulcer agents against *Campylobacter pyloridis*. *J Antimicrob Chemother* **17**: 309.

Goossens H, Henocque G, Kremp L *et al.* (1986). Nosocomial outbreak of *Campylobacter jejuni* meningitis in newborn infants. *Lancet* **ii**: 146.

Goossens H, Coignau H, Vlaes L, Butzler J-P (1989). *In vitro* evaluation of antibiotic combinations against *Campylobacter fetus*. *J Antimicrob Chemother* **24**: 195.

Gordon RC, Regamey C, Kirby WMM (1972). Serum protein binding of the aminoglycoside antibiotics. *Antimicrob Ag Chemother* **2**: 214.

Gray JW, Stewart D, Pedler SJ (1991). Species identification and antibiotic susceptibility testing of enterococci isolated from hospitalized patients. *Antimicrob Ag Chemother* **35**: 1943.

Grayson ML, Eliopoulos GM, Wennersten CB (1991). Comparison of *Enterococcus raffinosus* with *Enterococcus avium* on the basis of penicillin susceptibility, penicillin-binding protein analysis, and high-level aminoglycoside resistance. *Antimicrob Ag Chemother* **35**: 1408.

Green TP (1981). Gentamicin elimination during exchange transfusion. *J Pediatr* **98**: 507.

Greene WH, Moody M, Schimpff S *et al.* (1973). *Pseudomonas aeruginosa* resistant to carbenicillin and gentamicin. *Ann Intern Med* **79**: 684.

Groot Obbink DJ, Ritchie LJ, Cameron FH *et al.* (1985). Construction of gentamicin resistance gene probe for epidemiological studies. *Antimicrob Ag Chemother* **28**: 96.

Gross ME, Giron KP, Septimus JD *et al.* (1995). Antimicrobial activities of beta-lactam antibiotics and gentamicin against penicillin-susceptible and penicillin-resistant pneumococci. *Antimicrob Ag Chemother* **39**: 1166.

Guimaraes MA, Sage R, Noone P (1985). The comparative activity of aminocyclitol antibiotics against 773 aerobic Gram-negative rods and staphylococci isolated from hospitalized patients. *J Antimicrob Chemother* **16**: 555.

Guiney M, Urwin G (1993). Frequency and antimicrobial susceptibility of clinical isolates of enterococci. *Eur J Clin Microbiol Infect Dis* **12**: 362.

Gullberg RM, Homann SR, Phair JP (1989). Enterococcal bacteremia: analysis of 75 episodes. *Rev Infect Dis* **11**: 74.

Hahn DM, Schimpff SC, Fortner CL *et al.* (1978). Infection in acute leukemia patients receiving oral nonabsorbable antibiotics. *Antimicrob Ag Chemother* **13**: 958,.

Hahn FE, Sarre SG (1969). Mechanism of action of gentamicin. *J Infect Dis* **119**: 364.

Hall FJ (1977). Anaphylaxis after gentamicin. *Lancet* **ii**: 455.

Halpren BA, Azline SG, Coplon NS, Brown DM (1976). Clearance of gentamicin during hemodialysis: comparison of four artificial kidneys. *J Infect Dis* **133**: 627.

Hammerberg S, Sorger S, Marks MI (1977). Antimicrobial susceptibilities of *Yersinia enterocolitica* biotype 4, serotype 0:3. *Antimicrob Ag Chemother* **11**: 566.

Hancock REW, Raffle VJ, Nicas TI (1981). Involvement of the outer membrane in gentamicin and streptomycin uptake and killing in *Pseudomonas aeruginosa*. *Antimicrob Ag Chemother* **19**: 777.

Handwerger S, Raucher B, Altarac D *et al.* (1993). Nosocomial outbreak due to *Enterococcus faecium* highly resistant to vancomycin, penicillin, and gentamicin. *Clin Infect Dis* **16**: 750.

Hansen TN, Ritter DA, Speer ME *et al.* (1980). A randomized, controlled study of oral gentamicin in the treatment of neonatal necrotizing enterocolitis. *J Pediatr* **97**: 836.

Hardy DJ, Legeai RJ, O'Callaghan RJ (1980). *Klebsiella* neonatal infections: mechanism of broadening aminoglycoside resistance. *Antimicrob Ag Chemother* **18**: 542.

Harpur ES, Davey PG (1981). Toxic effects of aminoglycosides. *J Antimicrob Chemother* **7**: 313.

Harrell LJ, Evans JB (1978). Anaerobic resistance of clinical isolates of *Staphylococcus aureus* to aminoglycosides. *Antimicrob Ag Chemother* **14**: 927.

Harris RL, Fainstein V, Elting L *et al.* (1985). Bacteremia caused by *Aeromonas* spp. in hospitalized cancer patients. *Rev Infect Dis* **7**: 314.

Hassan E, Ober JD (1987). Predicted and measured aminoglycoside pharmacokinetic parameters in critically ill patients. *Antimicrob Ag Chemother* **31**: 1855.

Hathorn JW, Pizzo PA (1986). Is there a role for monotherapy with beta-lactam antibiotics in the initial empirical management of febrile neutropenic cancer patients? *J Antimicrob Chemother* **17** (Suppl A): 41.

Hendeles L, Iafrate RP, Stillwell PC, Mangos JA (1987). Individualizing gentamicin dosage in patients with cystic fibrosis: limitations to pharmacokinetic approach. *J Pediatr* **110**: 303.

Heritage J, Settle JAD, Lalani E-NMA, Lacey RW (1986). Probable chromosomal mutation to resistance to all aminoglycosides in *.Staphylococcus aureus* selected by the therapeutic use of gentamicin: a preliminary report. *J Antimicrob Chemother* **17**: 571.

Heritage J, Dyke GW, Johnson D, Lacey RW (1988). Selection of resistance to gentamicin and netilmicin in the faecal flora following prophylaxis for colo-rectal surgery. *J Antimicrob Chemother* **22**: 249.

Herman DJ, Gerding DN (1991a). Antimicrobial resistance among enterococci. *Antimicrob Ag Chemother* **35**: 1.

Herman DJ, Gerding DN (1991b). Screening and treatment of infections caused by resistant enterococci. *Antimicrob Ag Chemother* **35**: 215.

Hewitt WL (1974). Gentamicin: toxicity in perspective. *Postgrad Med J* **50** (Suppl 7): 55.

Hill ID, Mann MD, Househam KC, Bowie MD (1986). Use of oral gentamicin, metronidazole, and cholestyramine in the treatment of severe persistent diarrhoea in infants. *Pediatrics* **77**: 477.

Hinojosa R, Lerner SA (1987). Cochlear neural degeneration without hair cell loss in two patients with aminoglycoside ototoxicity. *J Infect Dis* **156**: 449.

Hira SK, Attili VR, Kamanga J et al. (1985). Efficacy of gentamicin and kanamycin in the treatment of uncomplicated gonococcal urethritis in Zambia. *Sex Trans Dis* **12**: 52.

Ho BSW, Ng MH (1993). Development of a specific probe for the aminoglycoside-(3)-N-acetyltransferase resistance gene. *J Antimicrob Chemother* **31**: 637.

Ho JL, Barza M (1987). Role of aminoglycoside antibiotics in the treatment of intra-abdominal infection. *Antimicrob Ag Chemother* **31**: 485.

Hodel-Christian SL, Murray BE (1990). Mobilization of the gentamicin resistance gene in *Enterococcus faecalis*. *Antimicrob Ag Chemother* **34**: 1278.

Hodel-Christian SL, Murray BE (1991). Characterization of the gentamicin resistace transposon Tn 5281 from *Enterococcus faecalis* and comparison to staphylococcal transposons Tn4001 and Tn4031. *Antimicrob Ag Chemother* **35**: 1147.

Hodel-Christian SL, Murray BE (1992). Comparison of the gentamicin resistance transposon Tn 5281 with regions encoding gentamicin resistance in *Enterococcus faecalis* isolated from diverse geographical locations. *Antimicrob Ag Chemother* **36**: 2259.

Hodges GR, Watanabe I, Singer P et al. (1981). Central nervous system toxicity of intraventricularly administered gentamicin in adult rabbits. *J Infect Dis* **143**: 148.

Hoeprich PD (1969). Gentamicin versus *.Staphylococcus aureus*. *J Infect Dis* **199**: 391.

Hoffmann SA, Moellering RC Jr (1987). The enterococcus: 'putting the bug in our ears'. *Ann Intern Med* **106**: 757.

Holder IA (1976). Gentamicin-resistant *Pseudomonas aeruginosa* in a burns unit. *J Antimicrob Chemother* **2**: 309.

Holm SE, Hill B, Löwestad A et al. (1983). A prospective, randomized study of amikacin and gentamicin in serious infections with focus on efficacy, toxicity and duration of serum levels above the MIC. *J Antimicrob Chemother* **12**: 393.

Holtzman JL (1976). Gentamicin and neuromuscular blockade. *Ann Intern Med* **84**: 55.

Horodniceanu T, Bougueleret L, El-Solh N et al. (1979). High-level, plasmid-borne resistance to gentamicin in *Streptococcus faecalis* subsp zymogenes. *Antimicrob Ag Chemother* **16**: 686.

Houang ET, Greenwood D (1977). Aminoglycoside cross-resistance patterns of gentamicin-resistant bacteria. *J Clin Path* **30**: 738.

Hsu CH, Kurtz TW, Weller JM (1977). *In vitro* uptake of gentamicin by rat renal cortical tissue. *Antimicrob Ag Chemother* **12**: 192.

Hughes WT, Armstrong D, Bodey GP et al. (1990). Guidelines for the use of antimicrobial agents in neutropenic patients with unexplained fever. *J Infect Dis* **161**: 381.

Hutchin T, Cortopassi G (1994). Proposed molecular and cellular mechanism for aminoglycoside ototoxicity. *Antimicrob Ag Chemother* **38**: 2517.

Huy PTB, Deffrennes D (1988). Aminoglycoside binding sites in the inner ears of guinea pigs. *Antimicrob Ag Chemother* **32**: 467.

Huycke MM, Spiegel CA, Gilmore MS (1991). Bacteremia caused by hemolytic, high-level gentamicin-resistant *Enterococcus faecalis*. *Antimicrob Ag Chemother* **35**: 1626.

Hyams PJ, Smithivas T, Matalon R et al. (1977). The use of gentamicin in peritoneal dialysis II Microbiologic and clinical results. *J Infect Dis* **124** (Suppl): 84.

Ike Y, Fujisawa-Kon N, Shimizu S et al. (1981). Identification of R plasmids mediating gentamicin resistance from *Escherichia coli* strains in Japan. *Antimicrob Ag Chemother* **19**: 1070.

Inciardi JF, Batra KK (1993). Nonparametric approach to population pharmacokinetics in oncology patients receiving aminoglycoside therapy. *Antimicrob Ag Chemother* **37**: 1025.

Ingerman M, Pitsakis PG, Rosenberg A et al. (1987). Beta-lactamase production in experimental endocarditis due to aminoglycoside-resistant *Streptococcus faecalis*. *J Infect Dis* **155**: 1226.

Ingham HR, Emslie JAN (1972). Gentamicin dosage. *Brit Med J* **4**: 732.

Isaksson B, Nilsson L, Maller R, Sören L (1988). Postantibiotic effect of aminoglycosides on Gram-negative bacteria evaluated by a new method. *J Antimicrob Chemother* **22**: 23.

Isaksson B, Maller R, Nilsson LE, Nilsson M (1993). Postantibiotic effect of aminoglycosides on staphylococci. *J Antimicrob Chemother* **32**: 215.

Jackson GG, Arcieri G (1971). Ototoxicity of gentamicin in man: a survey and controlled analysis of clinical experience in the United States. *J Infect Dis* **124** (Suppl): 130.

Jackson GG, Lolans VT, Daikos GL (1990). The inductive role of ionic binding in the bactericidal and postexposure effects of aminoglycoside antibiotics with implications for dosing. *J Infect Dis* **162**: 408.

Jacobs RF (1986). Imipenem-cilastatin: the first thienamycin antibiotic. *Pediatr Infect Dis* **5**: 444.

Jaffe HW, Sweeney HM, Nathan C et al. (1980). Identity and interspecific transfer of gentamicin-resistance plasmids in *.Staphylococcus aureus* and *Staphylococcus epidermidis*. *J Infect Dis* **141**: 738.

Jaffe HW, Sweeney HM, Weinstein RA et al. (1982). Structural and phenotypic varieties of gentamicin resistance plasmids in hospital strains of *.Staphylococcus aureus* and coagulase-negative staphylococci. *Antimicrob Ag Chemother* **21**: 773.

Janda JM, Abbott SL (1993). Infections associated with the genus *Edwardsiella*: the role of *Edwardsiella tarda* in human disease. *Clin Infect Dis* **17**: 742.

Jao RL, Jackson GG (1964). Gentamicin sulphate, new antibiotic against Gram-negative bacilli. *JAMA* **189**: 817.

John JF Jr, McNeill WF (1981). Characteristics of *Serratia marcescens* containing a plasmid coding for gentamicin resistance in nosocomial infections. *J Infect Dis* **143**: 810.

John JF Jr, Ribner BS (1991). Antibiotic resistance in long-term care facilities. *Infect Control Hosp Epidemiol* **12**: 245.

John JF Jr, Sharburgh RJ, Bannister ER (1982). *Enterobacter cloacae*: bacteremia, epidemiology and antibiotic resistance. *Rev Infect Dis* **4**: 13.

Johnson JD (1986). Antibiotics and carbohydrate malabsorption in new-borns. *Amer J Dis Child* **140**: 101.

Jonas M, Cunha BA (1982). Bacteremic *Escherichia coli* pneumonia. *Arch Intern Med* **142**: 2157.

Jones RAK (1978). Ototoxicity of gentamicin ear-drops. *Lancet* **i**: 1161.

Jordan GW, Hoeprich PD (1977). Susceptibility of three groups of *.Staphylococcus aureus* to newer antimicrobial agents. *Antimicrob Ag Chemother* **11**: 7.

Jordens JZ, Hall LMC (1989). Chromosomally encoded gentamicin resistance in 'epidemic' methicillin-resistant *Staphylococcus aureus*: detection with a synthetic oligonucleotide probe. *J Antimicrob Chemother* **23**: 327.

Kadurugamuwa JL, Lam JS, Beveridge TJ (1993). Interaction of gentamicin with the A band and B band lipopolysaccharides of *Pseudomonas aeruginosa* and its possible lethal effect. *Antimicrob Ag Chemother* **37**: 715.

Kahlmeter G (1979). Gentamicin and tobramycin Clinical pharmacokinetics and nephrotoxicity. Aspects of assay techniques. *Scand J Infect Dis* (Suppl 18): 7.

Kahlmeter G, Dahlager JI (1984). Aminoglycoside toxicity – a review of clinical studies published between 1975 and 1982. *J Antimicrob Chemother* **13** (Suppl A): 9.

Kahlmeter G, Jonsson S, Kamme C (1978). Longstanding post-therapeutic gentamicin serum and urine concentrations in patients with unimpaired renal function. A pharmacokinetic evaluation. *J Antimicrob Chemother* **4**: 143.

Kahn T, Stein RM (1972). Gentamicin and renal failure. *Lancet* **i**: 498.

Kaiser AB, McGee ZA (1975). Aminoglycoside therapy of Gram-negative bacillary meningitis. *New Engl J Med* **293**: 1215.

Kapitulnik J, Eyal F, Simcha AJ (1972). Gentamicin and bilirubin-binding by plasma. *Lancet* **ii**: 1195.

Karchmer AW, Archer GL, Dismukes WE (1983). *Staphylococcus epidermidis* causing prosthetic valve endocarditis: microbiologic and clinical observations as guides to therapy. *Ann Intern Med* **98**: 447.

Karlowsky JA, Zhanel GG (1992). Concepts on the use of liposomal antimicrobial agents: applications for aminoglycosides. *Clin Infect Dis* **15**: 654.

Karlowsky JA, Zhanel GG, Davidson RJ, Hoban DJ (1994a). Once-daily aminoglycoside dosing assessed by MIC reversion time with *Pseudomonas aeruginosa*. *Antimicrob Ag Chemother* **38**: 1165.

Karlowsky JA, Zhanel GG, Davidson RJ, Hoban DJ (1994b). Postantibiotic effect in *Pseudomonas aeruginosa* following single and multiple aminoglycoside exposures *in vitro*. *J Antimicrob Chemother* **33**: 937.

Kauffman CA, Ramundo NC, Williams SG *et al.* (1978). Surveillance of gentamicin-resistant Gram-negative bacilli in a general hospital. *Antimicrob Ag Chemother* **13**: 918.

Kaufhold A, Potgieter E (1993). Chromosomally mediated high-level gentamicin resistance in *Streptococcus mitis*. *Antimicrob Ag Chemother* **37**: 2740.

Kaufhold A, Podbielski A, Horaud T, Ferrieri P (1992). Identical genes confer high-level resistance to gentamicin upon *Enterococcus faecalis*, *Enterococcus faecium*, and *Streptococcus agalactiae*. *Antimicrob Ag Chemother* **36**: 1215.

Kaye D, Levison ME, Labovitz ED (1974). The unpredictability of serum concentrations of gentamicin: pharmacokinetics of gentamicin in patients with normal and abnormal renal function. *J Infect Dis* **130**: 150.

Kaye KM, Macone A, Kazanjian PH (1992). Catheter infection caused by *Methylobacterium* in immunocompromised hosts: report of three cases and review of the literature. *Clin Infect Dis* **14**: 1010.

Kearns GL, Hilman BC, Wilson JT (1982). Dosing implications of altered gentamicing disposition in patients with cystic fibrosis. *J Pediatr* **100**: 312.

Keyes PS, Johnson CK, Rawlins TD (1989). Predictors of trough serum gentamicin concentrations in neonates. *Am J Dis Child* **143**: 1419.

Kiehlbauch JA, Baker CN, Wachsmuth IK (1992). *In vitro* susceptibilities of aerotolerant *Campylobacter* isolates to 22 antimicrobial agents. *Antimicrob Ag Chemother* **36**: 717.

Kiehlbauch JA, Tauxe RV, Baker CN, Wachsmuth IK (1994). *Helicobacter cinaedi*-associated bacteremia and cellulitis in immunocompromised patients. *Ann Intern Med* **121**: 90.

Kim JH, Cooper RA, Welty-Wolf KE *et al.* (1989). *Pseudomonas putrefaciens* bacteremia. *Rev Infect Dis* **11**: 97.

King CH, Creger RJ, Ellner JJ (1985). Pharmacokinetics of tobramycin and gentamicin in abusers of intravenous drugs. *Antimicrob Ag Chemother* **27**: 285.

Klastersky J (1989). A review of chemoprophylaxis and theapy of bacterial infections in neutropenic patients. *Diagn Microbiol Infect Dis* **12**: 201S.

Klastersky J, Husson M (1977). Bactericidal activity of the combinations of gentamicin with clindamycin or chloramphenicol against species of *Escherichia coli* and *Bacteroides fragilis*. *Antimicrob Ag Chemother* **12**: 135.

Klein JO (1969). Consideration of gentamicin for therapy of neonatal sepsis. *J Infect Dis* **119**: 457.

Klein JO, Eickhoff TC, Finland M (1964). Gentamicin: activity *in vitro* and observations in 26 patients. *Amer J Med Sci* **248**: 528; quoted by Curtis *et al.* (1967).

Klein JO, Herschel M, Therakan RM, Ingall D (1971). Gentamicin in serious neonatal infections: absorption, excretion and clinical results in 25 cases. *J Infect Dis* **124** (Suppl): 224.

Klemens JP, Cynamon MH, Swenson CE, Ginsberg RS (1990). Liposome-encapsulated-gentamicin therapy of *Mycobacterium avium* complex infection in beige mice. *Antimicrob Ag Chemother* **34**: 967.

Kliegman RM, Fanaroff AA (1984). Necrotizing enterocolitis. *New Engl J Med* **310**: 1093.

Kliegman RM, Bertino JS, Fanaroff AA *et al.* (1980). Pharmacokinetics of gentamicin during exchange transfusions in neonates. *J Pediatr* **96**: 927.

Knight S, Casewell M (1981). Dissemination of resistance plasmids among gentamicin-resistant enterobacteria from hospital patients. *Brit Med J* **283**: 755.

Kornguth ML, Kunin CM (1977). Distribution of gentamicin and amikacin in rabbit tissues. *Antimicrob Ag Chemother* **11**: 974.

Korvick JA, Bryan CS, Farber B *et al.* (1992). Prospective observational study of *Klebsiella* bacteremia in 230 patients: outcome for antibiotic combinations versus monotherapy. *Antimicrob Ag Chemother* **36**: 2639.

Kourilsky O, Solez K, Morel-Maroger L *et al.* (1982). The pathology of acute renal failure due to interstitial nephritis in man with comments on the role of interstitial inflammation and sex in gentamicin nephrotoxicity. *Medicine* **61**: 258.

Kourtopoulos H, Holm SE (1976). Intraventricular treatment of *Serratia marcescens* meningitis with gentamicin. *Scand J Infect Dis* **8**: 57.

Kozak AJ, Gerding DN, Peterson LR, Hall WH (1977). Gentamicin intravenous infusion rate: effect on interstitial fluid concentration. *Antimicrob Ag Chemother* **12**: 606.

Kraus DM, Dusik CM, Rodvold KA *et al.* (1993). Bayesian forecasting of gentamicin pharmacokinetics in pediatric intensive care unit patients. *Pediatr Infect Dis J* **12**: 713.

Labovitz E, Levison ME, Kaye D (1974). Single-dose daily gentamicin therapy in urinary tract infection. *Antimicrob Ag Chemother* **6**: 465.

Lake KB, Van Dyke JJ, Rumsfeld JA (1975). Combined topical pulmonary and systemic gentamicin: the question of safety. *Chest* **68**: 62.

Larsson S, Walder MH, Cronberg SN *et al.* (1985). Antimicrobial susceptibilities of *Listeria monocytogenes* strains isolated from 1958 to 1982 in Sweden. *Antimicrob Ag Chemother* **28**: 12.

Laverdiere M, Peterson PK, Verhoef J *et al.* (1978). *In vitro* activity of cephalosporins against methicillin-resistant, coagulase-negative staphylococci. *J Infect Dis* **137**: 245.

Leclercq R, Dutka-Malen S, Brisson-Noël A *et al.* (1992). Resistance of enterococci to aminoglycosides and glycopeptides. *Clin Infect Dis* **15**: 495.

Lee EL, Robinson MJ, Thong ML *et al.* (1977). Intraventricular chemotherapy in neonatal meningitis. *J Pediatr* **91**: 991.

Lee SC, Gerding DN, Cleary PP (1986). Hospital distribution, persistence, and reintroduction of related gentamicin R plasmids. *Antimicrob Ag Chemother* **29**: 654.

Leff RD, Andersen RD, Roberts RJ (1984). Simplified gentamicin dosing in neonates: a time-and cost-efficient approach. *Pediatr Infect Dis* **3**: 208.

Levy J, Smith AL, Kenny MA *et al.* (1983). Bioactivity of gentamicin in purulent sputum from patients with cystic fibrosis or bronchiectasis: comparison with activity in serum. *J Infect Dis* **148**: 1069.

Lewis SA, Altemeier WA (1978). Emergence of clinical isolates of *Staphylococcus aureus* resistant to gentamicin and correlation of resistance with bacteriophage type. *J Infect Dis* **137**: 314.

Lewis VJ, Thacker WL, Shephard CC, McDade JE (1978). *In vivo* susceptibility of the Legionnaires' disease bacterium to 10 antimicrobial agents. *Antimicrob Ag Chemother* **13**: 419.

Lietman PS, Smith CR (1983). Aminoglycoside nephrotoxicity in humans. *Rev Infect Dis* **5** (Suppl 2): 284.

Ljungberg B, Nilsson-Ehle I (1987). Pharmacokinetics of antimicrobial agents in the elderly. *Rev Infect Dis* **9**: 250.

Lortholary O, Fagon JY, Hoi AB *et al.* (1995). Nosocomial acquisition of multiresistant *Acinetobacter baumannii*: risk factors and prognosis. *Clin Infect Dis* **20**: 790.

Lovering AM, White LO, Reeves DS (1986). Identification of individual aminoglycoside-inactivating enzymes in a mixture by HPLC determination of reaction products. *J Antimicrob Chemother* **18**: 139.

Lovering AM, Bywater MJ, Holt HA *et al.* (1988). Resistance of bacterial pathogens to four aminoglycosides and six other antibacterials and prevalence of aminoglycoside modifying enzymes, in 20 UK centres. *J Antimicrob Chemother* **22**: 823.

Lowy FD, Chang DS, Lash PR (1983). Synergy of combinations of vancomycin, gentamicin and rifampin against methicillin-resistant, coagulase-negative staphylococci. *Antimicrob Ag Chemother* **23**: 932.

Luft FC, Evan AP (1980). Comparative effects of tobramycin and gentamicni on glomerular ultrastructure. *J Infect Dis* **142**: 910.

Luft FC, Kleit SA (1974). Renal parenchymal accumulation of aminoglycoside antibiotics in rats. *J Infect Dis* **130**: 656.

Luft FC, Patel V, Yum MN, Kleit SA (1976). Nephrotoxicity of cephalosporin-gentamicin combinations in rats. *Antimicrob Ag Chemother* **9**: 831.

Luft FC, Rankin LI, Sloan RS, Yum MN (1978). Recovery from aminoglycoside nephrotoxicity with continued drug administration. *Antimicrob Ag Chemother* **14**: 284.

Luft FC, Bennett WH, Gilbert DN (1983). Experimental aminoglycoside nephrotoxicity: accomplishments and future potential. *Rev Infect Dis* **5** (Suppl 2): 268.

Lupski JR (1987). Molecular mechanisms for transposition of drug-resistance genes and other movable genetic elements. *Rev Infect Dis* **9**: 357.

MacDonald NE, Anas NG, Peterson RG *et al.* (1983). Renal clearance of gentamicin in cystic fibrosis. *J Pediatr* **103**: 985.

MacGowan AP, Reeves DS (1994). Serum monitoring and practicalities of once-daily aminoglycoside dosing. *J Antimicrob Chemother* **33**: 349.

MacGowan AP, Holt HA, Reeves DS (1990). *In-vitro* synergy testing of nine antimicrobial combinations against *Listeria monocytogenes*. *J Antimicrob Chemother* **25**: 561.

MacGowan AP, Bedford KA, Blundell E *et al.* (1994). The pharmacokinetics of once-daily gentamicin in neutropenic adults with haematological malignancy. *J Antimicrob Chemother* **34**: 809.

MacKenzie FM, Gould IM (1993). The post-antibiotic effect. *J Antimicrob Chemother* **32**: 519.

Mainardi J-L, Zhou XY, Goldstein F *et al.* (1994). Activity of isepamicin and selection of permeability mutants to beta-lactams during aminoglycoside therapy of experimental endocarditis due to *Klebsiella pneumoniae* CF 104 producing an aminoglycoside acetyltransferase 6' modifying enzyme and a TEH-3 beta-lactamase. *J Infect Dis* **169**: 1318.

Maliwan N, Grieble HG, Bird TJ (1975). Hospital *Pseudomonas aeruginosa*: surveillance of resistance to gentamicin and transfer of aminoglycoside R factor. *Antimicrob Ag Chemother* **8**: 415.

Markowitz SM, Wells VD, Williams DS *et al.* (1991). Antimicrobial susceptibility and molecular epidemiology of beta-lactamase-producing, aminoglycoside-resistant isolates of *Enterococcus faecalis*. *Antimicrob Ag Chemother* **35**: 1075.

Martin NL, Beveridge TJ (1986). Gentamicin interaction with *Pseudomonas aeruginosa* cell envelope. *Antimicrob Ag Chemother* **29**: 1079.

Mason WL, Eigelsbach T, Little F, Bates JH (1980). Treatment of tularemia, including pulmonary tularemia with gentamicin. *Amer Rev Respir Dis* **121**: 39.

Mates SM, Patel L, Kaback HR, Miller MH (1983). Membrane potential in anaerobically growing *Staphylococcus aureus* and its relationship to gentamicin uptake. *Antimicrob Ag Chemother* **23**: 526.

Mathalone B (1974). Gentamicin in eye infection. *Postgrad Med J* **50** (Suppl 7): 38.

Matsumoto JY, Wilson WR, Wright AJ *et al.* (1980). Synergy of penicillin and decreasing concentrations of aminoglycosides against enterococci from patients with infective endocarditis. *Antimicrob Ag Chemother* **18**: 944.

Mattie H, Craig WA, Pechère JC (1989). Determinants of efficacy and toxicity of aminoglycosides. *J Antimicrob Chemother* **24**: 281.

Matzke GR, Burkle WS, Cucarotti RL (1983). Gentamicin and tobramycin dosing guidelines: an evaluation. *Drug Intellig Clin Pharm* **17**: 425.

Matzke GR, Halstenson CE, Keane WF (1984). Hemodialysis elimination rates and clearance of gentamicin and tobramycin. *Antimicrob Ag Chemother* **25**: 128.

Mawer GE, Ahmad R, Dobbs SM *et al.* (1974). Prescribing aids for gentamicin. *Brit J Clin Pharmacol* **1**: 45.

Mayer KH, Hopkins JD, Gilleece ES *et al.* (1986). Molecular evolution, species distribution, and clinical consequences of an endemic aminogly-

coside resistance plasmid. *Antimicrob Ag Chemother* **29**: 628.

McCormack JP, Jewesson PJ (1992). A critical reevaluation of the 'therapeutic range' of aminoglycosides. *Clin Infect Dis* **14**: 320.

McCracken GH Jr (1972). Clinical pharmacology of gentamicin in infants 2 to 24 months of age. *Amer J Dis Child* **124**: 884.

McCracken GH Jr, Mize SG (1976). A controlled study of intrathecal antibiotic therapy in Gram-negative enteric meningitis of infancy. *J Pediatr* **89**: 66.

McCracken GH Jr, Mize SG (1980). Intraventricular gentamicin in meningitis. *Lancet* **ii**: 253.

McCracken GH, Nelson JD (1983). *Antimicrobial Therapy for Newborns* 2nd edn, p. 52. New York: Grune & Stratton.

McCracken GH Jr, Threlkeld N, Thomas ML (1977). Intravenous administration of kanamycin and gentamicin in newborn infants. *Pediatrics* **60**: 463.

McCracken GH Jr, Mize SG, Threlkeld N (1980). Intraventricular gentamicin therapy in Gram-negative bacillary meningitis of infancy Report of a second neonatal meningitis Cooperative Study Group. *Lancet* **i**: 787.

McGehee JL, Podnos SD, Pierce AK, Weissler JC (1988). Treatment of pneumonia in patients at risk of infections with Gram-negative bacilli. *AmerJMed* **84**: 597.

McGhie D, Hutchison JGP, Geddes AM (1974). Serum gentamicin. *Lancet* **ii**: 1463.

McGowan JE Jr, Terry PM, Huang T-SR *et al.* (1979). Nosocomial infections with gentamicin-resistant *Staphylococcus aureus*: plasmid analysis as an epidemiologic tool. *J Infect Dis* **140**: 864.

McHenry MC, Gavan TL, Gifford RW Jr *et al.* (1971). Gentamicin dosages for renal insufficiency. *Ann Intern Med* **74**: 192.

McNulty CAM (1987). The treatment of campylobacter infections in man. *J Antimicrob Chemother* **19**: 281.

McNulty CAM, Dent J, Wise R (1985). Susceptibility of clinical isolates of *Campylobacter pyloridis* to 11 antimicrobial agents. *Antimicrob Ag Chemother* **28**: 837.

Mederski-Samoraj BD, Murray BE (1983). High-level resistance to gentamicin in clinical isolates of enterococci. *J Infect Dis* **147**: 751.

Mendelson J, Portnoy J, Sigman H (1973). Pharmacology of gentamicin in the biliary tract of humans. *Antimicrob Ag Chemother* **4**: 538.

Mendelson J, Portnoy J, Dick V, Black M (1976). Safety of the bolus administration of gentamicin. *Antimicrob Ag Chemother* **9**: 633.

Meriwether WF, Mangi RJ, Serpick AA (1971). Deafness following standard intravenous dose of ethacrynic acid. *JAMA* **216**: 795.

Meunier F, Van der Auwera P, Schmitt H *et al.* (1987). Pharmacokinetics of gentamicin after iv infusion or iv bolus. *J Antimicrob Chemother* **19**: 225.

Meyer RD, Lewis RP, Halter J, White M (1976), Gentamicin-resistant *Pseudomonas aeruginosa* and *Serratia marcescens* in a general hospital. *Lancet* **i**: 580.

Meyers RM (1970). Ototoxic effects of gentamicin. *Arch Otolaryngol* **92**: 160.

Michel J, Rogol M, Dickman D (1983). Susceptibility of clinical isolates of *Campylobacter jejuni* to sixteen antimicrobial agents. *Antimicrob Ag Chemother* **23**: 796.

Miller MH, Edberg SC, Mandel LJ *et al.* (1980). Gentamicin uptake in wild-type and aminoglycoside-resistant small-colony mutants of *Staphylococcus aureus*. *Antimicrob Ag Chemother* **18**: 722.

Moellering RC Jr (1983). *In vitro* antibacterial activity of the aminoglycoside antibiotics. *Rev Infect Dis* **5** (Suppl 2): 212.

Moellering RC Jr, Fischer EG (1972). Relationship of intraventricular gentamicin levels to cure of meningitis. *J Pediatr* **81**: 534.

Moellering RC Jr, Korzeniowski OM, Sande M, Wennersten CB (1979). Species-specific resistance to antimicrobial synergism in *Streptococcus faecium* and *Streptococcus faecalis*. *J Infect Dis* **140**: 203.

Moellering RC Jr, Murray BE, Schoenbaum SC *et al.* (1980). A novel mechanism of resistance to penicillin-gentamicin synergism in *Streptococcus faecalis*. *J Infect Dis* **141**: 81.

Moody MR, Young VM (1979). A comparison of antibiograms of 'non-aeruginosa' pseudomonas recovered in two locales. *J Antimicrob Chemother* 5: 143.

Moore RA, Hancock REW (1986). Involvement of outer membrane of *Pseudomonas cepacia* in amingolycoside and polymyxin resistance. *Antimicrob Ag Chemother* 30: 923.

Moore RD, Smith CR, Lietman PS (1984). The association of aminoglycoside plasma levels with mortality in patients with Gram-negative bacteremia. *J Infect Dis* 149: 443.

Moore RD, Lietman PS, Smith CR (1987). Clinical response to aminoglycoside therapy: importance of the ratio of peak concentration to minimal inhibitory concentration. *J Infect Dis* 155: 93.

Morgan JR, Williams KE (1980). Preparation and properties of liposome-associated gentamicin. *Antimicrob Ag Chemother* 17: 544.

Morris DL, Hares MM, Voogt RJ *et al.* (1983). Metronidazole need not be combined with an aminoglycoside when used for prophylaxis in elective colorectal surgery. *J Hosp Infect* 4: 65.

Morrison VA, Lloyd BK, Chia JKS, Tuazon CU (1990). Cardiovascular and bacteremic manifestations of *Campylobacter fetus* infection: case report and review. *Rev Infect Dis* 12: 387.

Mucha DK, Farrand SK (1986). Diversity of determinants encoding carbenicillin, gentamicin, and tobramycin resistance in nosocomial *Pseudomonas aeruginosa. Antimicrob Ag Chemother* 30: 281.

Murray BE (1991). New aspects of antimicrobial resistance and the resulting therapeutic dilemmas. *J Infect Dis* 163: 1185.

Murray BE, Tsao J, Panida J (1983). Enterococci from Bangkok, Thailand, with high-level resistance to currently available aminoglycosides. *Antimicrob Ag Chemother* 23: 799.

Murray BE, Lopardo HA, Rubeglio EA (1992). Intrahospital spread of a single gentamicin-resistant, beta-lactamase-producing strain of *Enterococcus faecalis* in Argentina. *Antimicrob Ag Chemother* 36: 230.

Nelson JD, McCracken GH Jr (1972). Editorial The current status of gentamicin for the neonate and young infant. *Amer J Dis Child* 124: 13.

Nelson JD, McCracken GH Jr (1986). Aminoglycoside toxicity in infants and children. *Ped Infect Dis Newsl* 12: 6.

Neu H (1984a). Current mechanisms of resistance to antimicrobial agents in micro-organisms causing infection in the patient at risk for infection. *Amer J Med* 76 (Suppl): 11.

Neu HC (1984b). Changing mechanisms of bacterial resistance. *Amer J Med* 76: 11.

Newman RL, Holt RJ (1971). Gentamicin in pediatrics. I. Report on intrathecal gentamicin. *J Infect Dis* 124 (Suppl): 254.

Ngeleka M, Beauchamp D, Tardif D *et al.* (1990). Endotoxin increases the nephrotoxic potential for gentamicin and vancomycin plus gentamicin. *J Infect Dis* 161: 721.

Nicolau DP, Freeman CD, Belliveau PP *et al.* (1995). Experience with a once-daily aminoglycoside program administered to 2,184 adult patients. *Antimicrob Ag Chemother* 39: 650.

Nightingale SD, Saletan SL, Swenson CE *et al.* (1993). Liposome-encapsulated gentamicin treatment of *Mycobacterium avium-Mycobacterium intracellulare* complex bacteremia in AIDS patients. *Antimicrob Ag Chemother* 37: 1869.

Nilsson L, Maller R, Ånsêhn S (1981). Inhibition of aminoglycoside activity by heparin. *Antimicrob Ag Chemother* 20: 155.

Nilsson L, Sörèn L, Rådberg G (1987). Frequencies of variants resistant to different aminoglycosides in *Pseudomonas aeruginosa. J Antimicrob Chemother* 20: 255.

Noone P, Parsons TMC, Pattison JR *et al.* (1974). Experience in monitoring gentamicin therapy during treatment of serious Gram-negative sepsis. *Brit Med J* 1: 477.

Nordström L, Ringberg H, Cronberg S *et al.* (1990). Does administration of an aminoglycoside in a single daily dose affect its efficacy and toxicity? *J Antimicrob Chemother* 25: 159.

Noriega ER, Leibowitz RE, Richmond AS *et al.* (1975). Nosocomial infection caused by gentamicin-resistant, streptomycin-sensitive *Klebsiella. J Infect Dis* 131 (Suppl): 45.

Noskin GA, Till M, Patterson BK *et al.* (1991). High-level gentamicin resistance in *Enterococcus faecalis* bacteremia. *J Infect Dis* 164: 1212.

Noskin GA, Peterson LR, Warren JR (1995). *Enterococcus faecium* and *Enterococcus faecalis* bacteremia: acquisition and outcome. *Clin Infect Dis* 20: 296.

Nunnery AW, Riley HD Jr (1969). Gentamicin: clinical and laboratory studies in infants and children. *J Infect Dis* 199: 460.

Obana Y, Nishino T, Tanino T (1985). *In-vitro* and *in-vivo* activities of antimicrobial agents against *Acinetobacter calcoaceticus. J Antimicrob Chemother* 15: 441.

Ohnishi A, Bryant TD, Branch KR *et al.* (1989). Role of sodium in the protective effect of ticarcillin on gentamicin nephrotoxicity in rats. *Antimicrob Ag Chemother* 33: 928.

Okubadejo OA, Allen J (1975). Combined activity of clindamycin and gentamicin on *Bacteroides fragilis* and other bacteria. *J Antimicrob Chemother* 1: 403.

Olson B, Weinstein RA, Nathan C *et al.* (1985). Occult aminoglycoside resistance in *Pseudomonas aeruginosa*: epidemiology and implications for therapy and control. *J Infect Dis* 152: 769.

Olson L, Grotte G, Nordbring F (1977). Successful treatment of *Pseudomonas aeruginosa-ventriculitis* with intraventricular gentamicin in a child with hydrocephalus. *Scand J Infect Dis* 9: 243.

Pancorbo S, Comty C (1981). Pharmacokinetics of gentamicin in patients undergoing continuous ambulatory peritoneal dialysis. *Antimicrob Ag Chemother* 19: 605.

Panwalker AP, Trager GM, Porembski PE (1980). *Klebsiella* species: antimicrobial susceptibilities, bactericidal kinetics, and *in vitro* inactivation of beta-lactam agents. *Antimicrob Ag Chemother* 18: 877.

Papapetropoulou M, Papavassiliou J, Legakis NJ (1983). Effect of the pH and osmolality of urine on the antibacterial activity of gentamicin. *J Antimicrob Chemother* 12: 571.

Parker SE, Davey PG (1993). Practicalities of once-daily aminoglycoside dosing. *J Antimicrob Chemother* 31: 4.

Parry MF, Neu HC, Merlino M *et al.* (1977). Treatment of pulmonary infections in patients with cystic fibrosis: a comparative study of ticarcillin and gentamicin. *J Pediatr* 90: 144.

Patterson JE, Zervos MJ (1990). High-level gentamicin resistance in *Enterococcus*: microbiology, genetic basis, and epidemiology. *Rev Infect Dis* 12: 644.

Patterson JE, Masecar BL, Kauffman CA *et al.* (1988a). Gentamicin resistance plasmids of enterococci from diverse geographical areas are heterogeneous. *J Infect Dis* 158: 212.

Patterson JE, Colodny SM, Zervos MJ (1988b). Serious infection due to beta-lactamase-producing *Streptococcus faecalis* with high-level resistance to gentamicin. *J Infect Dis* 158: 1144.

Penner JL, Preston MA (1980). Differences among *Providencia* species in their *in vitro* susceptibilities to five antibiotics. *Antimicrob Ag Chemother* 18: 868.

Penner JL, Preston MA, Hennessy JN *et al.* (1982). Species differences in susceptibilities of *Proteeae* spp. to six cephalosporins and three aminoglycosides. *Antimicrob Ag Chemother* 22: 218.

Pennington JE (1981). Penetration of antibiotics into respiratory secretions. *Rev Infect Dis* 3: 67.

Pennington JE, Reynolds HY (1973). Concentrations of gentamicin and carbenicillin in bronchial secretions. *J Infect Dis* 128: 63.

Pennington JE, Reynolds HY (1975). Pharmacokinetics of gentamicin sulfate in bronchial secretions. *J Infect Dis* 131: 158.

Pennington JE, Dale DC, Reynolds HY, MacLowry JD (1975). Gentamicin sulfate pharmacokinetics: lower levels of gentamicin in blood during fever. *J Infect Dis* 132: 270.

Pham JN, Bell SM, Lanzarone JYM (1991). Biotype and antibiotic sensitivity of 100 clinical isolates of *Yersinia enterocolitica. J Antimicrob Chemother* 28: 13.

Phillips AMR, Milner RDG (1984). Tissue concentrations of netilmicin and gentamicin in neonates. *J Infect Dis* 149: 474.

Phillips I, Eykyn S, King BA *et al.* (1977). The *in vitro* antibacterial activity of nine aminoglycosides and spectinomycin on clinical isolates of common Gram-negative bacteria. *J Antimicrob Chemother* 3: 403.

Pichichero ME, Friesen HA (1982). Polymicrobial osteomyelitis: report of three cases and review of the literature. *Rev Infect Dis* **4**: 86.

Pickering LK, Ericsson CD, Ruiz-Palacios G *et al.* (1978). Intraventricular and parenteral gentamicin therapy for ventriculitis in children. *Amer J Dis Child* **132**: 480.

Pitt HA, Roberts RB, Johnson WD Jr (1973). Gentamicin levels in the human biliary tract. *J Infect Dis* **127**: 299.

Pitt TL, Livermore DM, Miller G *et al.* (1990). Resistance mechanisms of multiresistant serotype 012 *Pseudomonas aeruginosa* isolated in Europe. *J Antimicrob Chemother* **26**: 319.

Pittard WV III, Thullen JD, Fanaroff AA (1976). Neonatal septic arthritis. *J Pediatr* **88**: 621.

Potel G, Caillon J, Le Gallou F *et al.* (1992). Identification of factors affecting *in vivo* aminoglycoside activity in an experimental model of Gram-negative endocarditis. *Antimicrob Ag Chemother* **36**: 744.

Powell SH, Thompson WL, Luthe MA *et al.* (1983). Once-daily vs continuous aminoglycoside dosing: efficacy and toxicity in animal and clinical studies of gentamicin, netilmicin and tobramycin. *J Infect Dis* **147**: 918.

Price KE, Kresel PA, Farchione LA *et al.* (1981). Epidemiological studies of aminoglycoside resistance in the USA. *J Antimicrob Chemother* **8** (Suppl A): 89.

Prichard MG, Miles HM, Pavillard ER (1983). *Listeria meningitis – in vitro* sensitivities to co-trimoxazole, penicillins and gentamicin. *Aust NZ J Med* **13**: 76.

Prins JM, Büller HR, Kuijper EJ *et al.* (1993). Once versus thrice daily gentamicin in patients with serious infections. *Lancet* **341**: 335.

Prokesch RC, Hand WL (1982). Antibiotic entry into human polymorphonuclear leukocytes. *Antimicrob Ag Chemother* **21**: 373.

Rahal JJ Jr (1972). Treatment of Gram-negative bacillary meningitis in adults. *Ann Intern Med* **77**: 295.

Ramirez-Ronda CH, Holmes RK, Sanford JP (1975). Effects of divalent cations on binding of aminoglycoside antibiotics to human serum proteins and to bacteria. *Antimicrob Ag Chemother* **7**: 239.

Ratcliff RM, Mirelli C, Moran E *et al.* (1981). Comparison of five methods for the assay of serum gentamicin. *Antimicrob Ag Chemother* **19**: 508.

Rather PN, Mann PA, Mierzwa R *et al.* (1993). Analysis of the aac(3).-VIa gene encoding a novel 3-N-acetyl-transferase. *Antimicrob Ag Chemother* **37**: 2074.

Reina J, Bassa A, Llompart I *et al.* (1991). Infections with *Pseudomonas paucimobilis*: report of four cases and review. *Rev Infect Dis* **13**: 1072.

Reinhardt JF, Fowlston S, Jones J, George WL (1985). Comparative *in vitro* activities of selected antimicrobial agents against *Edwardsiella tarda. Antimicrob Ag Chemother* **27**: 966.

Report of a WHO Scientific Group (1978). *Neisseria gonorrhoeae* and gonococcal infections. *Wld Hlth Org Techn Rep Ser* No. 616: 96.

Report of a Working Party of the British Society for Antimicrobial Chemotherapy (1987). Diagnosis and management of peritonitis in continuous ambulatory peritoneal dialysis. *Lancet* **i**: 845.

Rice LB, Eliopoulos GM, Wennersten C *et al.* (1991a). Chromosomally mediated beta-lactamase production and gentamicin resistance in *Enterococcus faecalis. Antimicrob Ag Chemother* **35**: 272.

Rice LB, Calderwood SB, Eliopoulos GM *et al.* (1991b). Enterococcal endocarditis: a comparison of prosthetic and native valve disease. *Rev Infect Dis* **13**: 1.

Rice LB, Carias LL, Marshall SH (1995). Tn 5384, a composite enterococcal mobile element conferring resistance to erythromycin and gentamicin whose ends are directly repeated copies of IS 256. *Antimicrob Ag Chemother* **39**: 1147.

Richey GD, Schleupner CJ (1981). Peritoneal fluid concentrations of gentamicin in patients with spontaneous bacterial peritonitis. *Antimicrob Ag Chemother* **19**: 312.

Richmond AS, Simberkoff MS, Rahal JJ Jr, Schaefler S (1975). R factors in gentamicin-resistant organisms causing hospital infection. *Lancet* **ii**: 1176.

Riff LJ, Jackson GG (1971). Pharmacology of gentamicin in man. *J Infect Dis* **124** (Suppl): 98.

Ristuccia AM, Cunha BA (1982). The aminoglycosides. *Med Clin North Amer* **66**: 303.

Roberts NJ Jr, Douglas RG Jr (1978). Gentamicin use and *Pseudomonas* and *Serratia* resistance: effect of a surgical prophylaxis regimen. *Antimicrob Ag Chemother* **13**: 214.

Rodriguez V, Whitecar JP Jr, Bodey GP (1970). Therapy of infections with the combination of carbenicillin and gentamicin. *Antimicrob Ag Chemother* **1969**: 386.

Roe E, Lowbury EJL (1972). Changes in antibiotic sensitivity patterns of Gram-negative bacilli in burns. *J Clin Path* **25**: 176.

Rubens CE, Farrar WE Jr, McGee ZA, Schaffner W (1981). Evolution of plasmid mediating resistance to multiple antimicrobial agents during a prolonged epidemic of nosocomial infections. *J Infect Dis* **143**: 170.

Ruhen RW, Darrell JH (1973). Antibiotic synergism against group D streptococci in the treatment of endocarditis. *Med J Aust* **2**: 114.

Rupp ME, Archer GL (1994). Coagulase-negative staphylococci: pathogens associated with medical progress. *Clin Infect Dis* **19**: 231.

Russo JC, Adelman RD (1980). Gentamicin-induced Fanconi syndrome. *J Pediatr* **96**: 151.

Rutala WA, Kennedy VA, Loflin HB, Sarubbi FA Jr (1981). *Serratia marcescens* nosocomial infections of the urinary tract associated with urine measuring containers and urinometers. *Amer J Med* **70**: 659.

Ryback MJ, Frankowski JJ, Edwards DJ, Albrecht LM (1987). Alanine aminopeptidase and B$_2$-microglobulin excretion in patients receiving vancomycin and gentamicin. *Antimicrob Ag Chemother* **31**: 1461.

Sabath LD (1969). Current concepts: drug resistance of bacteria. *New Engl J Med* **280**: 91.

Sabath LD, Gerstein DA, Leaf CD, Finland M (1970). Increasing the usefulness of antibiotics: treatment of infections caused by Gram-negative bacilli. *Clin Pharm Ther* **11**: 161.

Sahm DF, Gilmore MS (1994). Transferability and genetic relatedness of high-level gentamicin resistance among enterococci. *Antimicrob Ag Chemother* **38**: 1194.

Saltissi D, Pusey CD, Rainford DJ (1979). Recurrent acute renal failure due to antibiotic-induced interstitial nephritis. *Brit Med J* **1**: 1182.

Sande MA, Irvin RG (1974). Penicillin-aminoglycoside synergy in experimental *Streptococcus viridans* endocarditis. *J Infect Dis* **129**: 572.

Sanders CC, Watanakunakorn C (1986). Emergence of resistance to beta-lactams, aminoglycosides, and quinolones during combination therapy for infection due to *Serratia marcescens. J Infect Dis* **153**: 617.

Sands M, Brown RB (1989). Interactions of cyclosporine with antimicrobial agents. *Rev Infect Dis* **11**: 691.

Santos JI, Swensen P, Glasgow LA (1981). Potentiation of *Clostridium botulinum* toxin by aminoglycoside antibiotics: clinical and laboratory observations. *Pediatrics* **68**: 50.

Sapico FL, Montgomerie JZ (1980). Vertebral osteomyelitis in intravenous drug abusers: report of three cases and review of the literature. *Rev Infect Dis* **2**: 196.

Sawyers CL, Moore RD, Lerner SA, Smith CR (1986). A model for predicting nephrotoxicity in patients treated with aminoglycosides. *J Infect Dis* **153**: 1062.

Schaberg DR, Alford RH, Anderson R *et al.* (1976). An outbreak of nosocomial infection due to multiply resistant *Serratia marcescens*: evidence of interhospital spread. *J Infect Dis* **134**: 181.

Schaberg DR, Power G, Betzold J, Forbes BA (1985). Conjugative R plasmids in antimicrobial resistance of *Staphylococcus aureus* causing nosocomial infections. *J Infect Dis* **152**: 43.

Schauf V, Deveikis A, Riff L, Serota A (1976). Antibiotic-killing kinetics of Group B streptococci. *J Pediatr* **89**: 194.

Scheifele DW, Ginter GL, Olsen E *et al.* (1987). Comparison of two antibiotic regimens for neonatal necrotising enterocolitis. *J Antimicrob Chemother* **20**: 421.

Scheld WM, Brodeur JP (1983). Effect of methylprednisolone on entry of ampicillin and gentamicin into cerebrospinal fluid in experimental pneumococcal and *Escherichia coli* meningitis. *Antimicrob Ag Chemother* **23**: 108.

Schentag JJ, Jusko WJ (1977). Gentamicin persistence in the body. *Lancet* i: 486.

Schentag JJ, Jusko WJ Plaut ME *et al.* (1977). Tissue persistence of gentamicin in man. *JAMA* **238**: 327.

Schentag JJ, Gengo FM, Plaut ME *et al.* (1979). Urinary casts as an indicator of renal tubular damage in patients receiving aminoglycosides. *Antimicrob Ag Chemother* **16**: 468.

Schentag JJ, Plaut ME, Cerra FB (1981). Comparative nephrotoxicity of gentamicin and tobramycin: pharmacokinetic and clinical studies in 201 patients. *Antimicrob Ag Chemother* **19**: 859.

Schentag JJ, Cerra FB, Plaut ME (1982). Clinical and pharmacokinetic characteristics of aminoglycoside nephrotoxicity in 201 critically ill patients. *Antimicrob Ag Chemother* **21**: 721.

Schønheyder HC, Søgaard P, Fredriksen W (1995). A survey of *Campylobacter bacteremia* in three Danish counties, 1989 to 1994. *Scand J Infect Dis* **27**: 145.

Schwartz RH, Eng G (1982). Infant botulism: exacerbation by aminoglycosides. *Amer J Dis Child* **136**: 952.

Seklecki MM, Quintiliani R, Maderazo EG (1978). Aminoglycoside antibiotics moderately impair granulocyte function. *Antimicrob Ag Chemother* **13**: 552.

Shafi MS, Datta N (1975). Infection caused by *Proteus mirabilis* strains with transferable gentamicin-resistance factors. *Lancet* i: 1355.

Shannon KP, Phillips I (1982). Mechanisms of resistance to aminoglycosides in clinical isolates. *J Antimicrob Chemother* **9**: 91.

Shannon KP, Phillips I, King BA (1978). Aminoglycoside resistance among Enterobacteriaceae and *Acinetobacter* species. *J Antimicrob Chemother* **4**: 131.

Shanson DC, Kensit JG, Duke R (1976). Outbreak of hospital infection with a strain of .*Staphylococcus aureus* resistant to gentamicin and methicillin. *Lancet* ii: 1347.

Shaw KJ, Cramer CA, Rizzo M *et al.* (1989). Isolation, characterization, and DNA sequence analysis of an AAC(6').-II gene from *Pseudomonas aeruginosa*. *Antimicrob Ag Chemother* **33**: 2052.

Shaw KJ, Hare RS, Sabatelli FJ *et al.* (1991). Correlation between aminoglycoside resistance profiles and DNA hybridization of clinical isolates. *Antimicrob Ag Chemother* **35**: 2253.

Shaw KJ, Rather PN, Hare RS, Miller GH (1993). Molecular genetics of aminoglycoside genes and familial relationships of the aminoglycoside-modifying enzymes. *Microbiol Rev* **57**: 138.

Shearer BG, Legakis NJ (1985). *Pseudomonas aeruginosa*: evidence for the involvement of lipopolysaccharide in determing outer membrane permeability to carbenicillin and gentamicin. *J Infect Dis* **152**: 351.

Shlaes DM, Currie CA, Rotter G *et al.* (1983). Epidemiology of gentamicin-resistant Gram-negative bacillary colonization in a spinal cord injury unit. *J Clin Microbiol* **18**: 227.

Siber GR, Echeverria P, Smith AL *et al.* (1975). Pharmacokinetics of gentamicin in children and adults. *J Infect Dis* **132**: 637.

Siber GR, Smith AL, Levin MJ (1979). Predictability of peak serum gentamicin concentration with dosage based on body surface area. *J Pediatr* **94**: 135.

Simor AE, Karmali MA, Jadavji T, Roscoe M (1986). Abortion and perinatal sepsis associated with *Campylobacter* infection. *Rev Infect Dis* **8**: 397.

Skopnik H, Heimann G (1995). Once daily aminoglycoside dosing in full term neonates. *Pediatr Infect Dis J* **14**: 71.

Smaoui H, Mallie J-P, Schaeverbeke M *et al.* (1993). Gentamicin administered during gestation alters glomerular basement membrane development. *Antimicrob Ag Chemother* **37**: 1510.

Smilack J, McCloskey RV (1972). Intrathecal gentamicin. *Ann Intern Med* **77**: 1002.

Smith AL, Daum RS, Siber GR *et al.* (1988). Gentamicin penetration into cerebrospinal fluid in experimental *Haemophilus influenzae* meningitis. *Antimicrob Ag Chemother* **32**: 1034.

Smith CR, Lietman PS (1983). Effect of furosemide on aminoglycoside-induced nephrotoxicity and auditory toxicity in humans. *Antimicrob Ag Chemother* **23**: 133.

Smith CR, Lipsky JJ, Laskin OL *et al.* (1980). Double-blind comparison of the nephrotoxicity and auditory toxicity of gentamicin and tobramycin. *New Engl J Med* **302**: 1106.

Smithivas T, Hymans PJ, Matalon R *et al.* (1971). The use of gentamicin in peritoneal dialysis. I. Pharmacologic results. *J Infect Dis* **124** (Suppl): 77.

Smyth EG, Holliman RE (1988). High-level gentamicin resistance in *Strepotococcus faecalis*. *Lancet* i: 1220.

Smyth EG, Stevens PJ, Holliman RE (1989). Prevalence and susceptibility of highly gentamicin resistant *Enterococcus faecalis* in a South London teaching hospital. *J Antimicrob Chemother* **23**: 633.

Snavely SR, Hodges GR (1984). The neurotoxicity of anitbacterial agents. *Ann Intern Med* **101**: 92.

Soriano F, Vega J (1982). The susceptibility of *Yersinia* to eleven antimicrobials. *J Antimicrob Chemother* **10**: 543.

Speller DCE, Raghunath D, Stephens N *et al.* (1976). Epidemic infection by a gentamicin-resistant .*Staphylococcus aureus* in three hospitals. *Lancet* i: 464.

St John Sutton MB, Papadeas V, Pasquariello PS Jr (1983). *Yersinia enterocolitica* septicemia in a normal child. *Amer J Dis Child* **137**: 305.

Stone HH (1969). The diagnosis and treatment of *Pseudomonas sepsis* in major burns. *J Infect Dis* **119**: 504.

Storrs MJ, Courvalin P, Foster TJ (1988). Genetic analysis of gentamicin resistance in methicillin- and gentamicin-resistant strains of *Staphylococcus aureus* isolated in Dublin hospitals. *Antimicrob Ag Chemother* **32**: 1174.

Stratton CW, Weeks LS, Tausk F (1987). Beta-lactamase induction and aminoglycoside susceptibility in *Pseudomonas aeruginosa*. *J Antimicrob Chemother* **19**: 21.

Strausbaugh LJ, Brinker GS (1983). Effect of osmotic blood-brain barrier disruption on gentamicin penetration into the cerebrospinal fluid and brains of normal rabbits. *Antimicrob Ag Chemother* **24**: 147.

Swan SK, Kohlhepp SJ, Kohnen PW *et al.* (1991). Long-term protection of polyaspartic acid in experimental gentamicin nephrotoxicity. *Antimicrob Ag Chemother* **35**: 2591.

Swan SK, Gilbert DN, Kohlhepp SJ *et al.* (1992). Duration of the protective effect of polyaspartic acid on experimental gentamicin nephrotoxicity. *Antimicrob Ag Chemother* **36**: 2556.

Swan SK, Gilbert DN, Kohlhepp SJ *et al.* (1993). Pharmacological limits of the protective effect of polyaspartic acid on experimental gentamicin nephrotoxicity. *Antimicrob Ag Chemother* **37**: 347.

Swartz MN (1981). Editorial. Intraventricular use of aminoglycosides in the treatment of Gram-negative bacillary meningitis: conflicting views. *J Infect Dis* **143**: 293.

Swenson CE, Stewart KA, Hammett JL *et al.* (1990). Pharmacokinetics and *in vivo* activity of liposome-encapsulated gentamicin. *Antimicrob Ag Chemother* **34**: 235.

Szefler SJ, Wynn RJ, Clarke DF *et al.* (1980). Relationship of gentamicin serum concentrations to gestational age in preterm and term neonates. *J Pediatr* **97**: 312.

Taber HW, Mueller JP, Miller PF, Arrow AS (1987). Bacterial uptake of aminoglycoside antibiotics. *Microbiol Rev* **51**: 439.

Tablan OC, Reyes MP, Rintelmann WF, Lerner AM (1984). Renal and auditory toxicity of high-dose, prolonged therapy with gentamicin and tobramycin in *Pseudomonas endocarditis*. *J Infect Dis* **149**: 257.

Takahashi S, Nagano Y (1985). Dissemination of gentamicin-resistant plasmids among strains of Enterobacteriaceae. *J Hosp Infect* **6**: 46.

Tan JS, Salstrom SJ (1977). Levels of carbenicillin, ticarcillin, cephalothin, cefazolin, cefamandole, gentamicin, tobramycin, and amikacin in human serum and interstitial fluid. *Antimicrob Ag Chemother* **11**: 698.

Tardif D, Beauchamp D, Bergeron MG (1990). Influence of endotoxin on the intracortical accumulation kinetics of gentamicin in rats. *Antimicrob Ag Chemother* **34**: 576.

Taryle DA, Good JT Jr, Morgan EJ III *et al.* (1981). Antibiotic concentrations in human parapneumonic effusions. *J Antimicrob Chemother* **7**: 171.

Tenover FC (1986). Studies of antimicrobial resistance genes using DNA probes. *Antimicrob Ag Chemother* **29**: 721.

Tenover FC, Gootz TD, Gordon KP *et al.* (1984). Development of a DNA probe for the structural gene of the 2"-0-adenyltransferase aminoglycoside-modifying enzyme. *J Infect Dis* **150**: 678.

Tenover FC, Phillips KL, Gilbert T *et al.* (1989). Development of a DNA probe from the deoxyribonucleotide sequence of a 3-N-aminoglycoside acetyltransferase [AAC(3).-I] resistance gene. *Antimicrob Ag Chemother* **33**: 551.

Thal LA, Chow JW, Patterson JE *et al.* (1993). Molecular characterization of highly gentamicin-resistant *Enterococcus faecalis* isolates lacking high-level streptomycin resistance. *Antimicrob Ag Chemother* **37**: 134.

Thal LA, Chow JW, Clewell DB, Zervos MJ (1994). Tn 924, a chromosome-borne transposon encoding high-level gentamicin resistance in *Enterococcus faecalis*. *Antimicrob Ag Chemother* **38**: 1152.

Thomas WD Jr, Archer GL (1989). Mobility of gentamicin resistance genes from staphylococci isolated in the United States: identification of Tn 4031, a gentamicin resistance transposon from *Staphylococcus epidermidis*. *Antimicrob Ag Chemother* **33**: 1335.

Thornsberry C, Baker CN, Kirven LA (1978). *In vitro* activity of antimicrobial agents on Legionnaires' disease bacterium. *Antimicrob Ag Chemother* **13**: 78.

Tilley PAG, Roberts FJ (1994). Bacteremia with *Acinetobacter* species: risk factors and prognosis in different clinical settings. *Clin Infect Dis* **18**: 896.

Tilney NL, Strom TB, Vineyard GC, Merrill JP (1978). Factors contributing to the declining mortality rate in renal transplantation. *New Engl J Med* **299**: 1321.

Tofte RW, Solliday J, Crossley KB (1984). Susceptibilities of enterococci to twelve antibiotics. *Antimicrob Ag Chemother* **25**: 532.

Townsend DE, Grubb WB, Ashdown N (1983). Gentamicin resistance in methicillin-resistant *Staphylococcus aureus*. *Pathology* **15**: 169.

Townsend DE, Ashdown N, Greed LC, Grubb WB (1984). Analysis of plasmids mediating gentamicin resistance in methicillin-resistant *Staphylococcus aureus*. *J Antimicrob Chemother* **13**: 347.

Townsend PL, Fink MP, Stein KL, Murphy SG (1989). Aminoglycoside pharmacokinetics: dosage requirements and nephrotoxicity in trauma patients. *Critical Care Medicine* **17**: 154.

Tran Ba Huy P, Manuel C, Meulemans A *et al.* (1981). Pharmacokinetics of gentamicin in perilymph and endolymph of the rat as determined by radioimmunoassay. *J Infect Dis* **143**: 476.

Tran Ba Huy P, Meulemans A, Wassef M *et al.* (1983). Gentamicin persistence in rat endolymph and perilymph after a two-day constant infusion. *Antimicrob Ag Chemother* **23**: 344.

Traynor AM, Nafziger AN, Bertino JS Jr (1995). Aminoglycoside dosing weight correction factors for patients of various body sizes. *Antimicrob Ag Chemother* **39**: 545.

Trollfors B (1983). Gentamicin-associated changes in renal function reversible during continued treatment. *J Antimicrob Chemother* **12**: 285.

Trollfors B, Alestig K, Krantz I, Norrby R (1980). Quantitative nephrotoxicity of gentamicin in nontoxic doses. *J Infect Dis* **141**: 306.

Trollfors B, Norrby R, Bergmark J *et al.* (1986). Comparative toxicity of gentamicin and cefotetan. *Scand J Infect Dis* **18**: 139.

Uwaydah M, Taqi-Eddin A (1976). Susceptibility of non-formentative Gram-negative bacilli to tobramycin. *J Infect Dis* **132** (Suppl): 28.

Vakil N, Abu-Alfa A, Mujais SK (1989). Gentamicin nephrotoxicity in extrahepatic cholestasis: modulation by dietary calcium. *Hepatology* **9**: 519.

Van Asselt GJ, Vliegenthart JS, Petit PLC *et al.* (1992). High-level aminoglycoside resistance among enterococci and group A streptococci. *J Antimicrob Chemother* **30**: 651.

Van den Broek PJ, Buys LFM, Van den Barselaar MT *et al.* (1986). Influence of human monocytes on the antibacterial activity of kanamycin and gentamicin for .*Staphylococcus aureus*. *Antimicrob Ag Chemother* **29**: 1032.

Vanhoof R, Centent J, Van Bossuyt E *et al.* (1992). Identification of the aad B gene coding for the aminoglycoside-2"-0-nucleotidyltransferase, ANT (2"), by means of the polymerase chain reaction. *J Antimicrob Chemother* **29**: 365.

Vanhoof R, Godard C, Content J *et al.* (1994). Detection by polymerase chain reaction of genes encoding aminoglycoside-modifying enzymes in methicillin-resistant *Staphytlococcus aureus* isolates of epidemic phage types. *J Med Microbiol* **41**: 282.

Venezio FR, Di Vincenzo CA (1985). Effects of aminoglycoside antibiotics on polymorphonuclear leukocyte function *in vivo*. *Antimicrob Ag Chemother* **27**: 712.

Venezio FR, Masters D, O'Keefe P (1984). Enterococcal meningitis: failure of treatment with ampicillin and chloramphenicol. *J Infect Dis* **150**: 305.

Vila J, Marcos A, Marco F *et al.* (1993). *In vitro* antimicrobial production of beta-lactamases, aminoglycoside-modifying enzymes, and chloramphenicol acetyltransferase by and susceptibility of clinical isolates of *Acinetobacter baumannii*. *Antimicrob Ag Chemother* **37**: 138.

Vliegenthart JS, Ketelaar-van Gaalen PAG, Van de Klundert JAM (1991). Nucleotide sequence of the aac C3 gene, a gentamicin resistance determinant encoding aminoglycoside- (3).-N-acetyltransferase III expressed in *Pseudomonas aeruginosa* but not in *Escherichia coli*. *Antimicrob Ag Chemother* **35**: 892.

Vogelman B, Gudmundson S, Turnidge J *et al.* (1988). *In vivo* postantibiotic effect in a thigh infection in neutropenic mice. *J Infect Dis* **157**: 287.

Waitz JA, Weinstein MJ (1969). Recent microbiological studies with gentamicin. *J Infect Dis* **119**: 355.

Walker BD, Gentry LO (1976). A randomized comparative study of tobramycin and gentamicin in treatment of acute urinary tract infections. *J Infect Dis* **134** (Suppl): 146.

Wallace RJ Jr, Wiss K (1981). Susceptibility of *Mycobacterium marinum* to tetracyclines and aminoglycosides. *Antimicrob Ag Chemother* **20**: 610.

Wallace RJ Jr, Wiss K, Curvey R *et al.* (1983). Differences among *Nocardia* spp. in susceptibility to aminoglycosides and beta-lactam antibiotics and their potential use in toxonomy. *Antimicrob Ag Chemother* **23**: 19.

Ward C, Jephcott AE, Hardisty CA (1977). Perioperative antibiotic prophlyaxis and prosthetic valve endocarditis. *Postgrad Med J* **53**: 353.

Warner WA, Sanders E (1971). Neuromuscular blockade associated with gentamicin therapy. *JAMA* **215**: 1153.

Warren RL, Baker NR, Johnson J, Stapleton MJ (1985). Selective inhibition of the accumulation of extracellular proteases of *Pseudomonas aeruginosa* by gentamicin and tobramycin. *Antimicrob Ag Chemother* **27**: 468;.

Watanakunakorn C (1989). *Serratia* bacteremia: a review of 44 episodes. *Scand J Infect Dis* **21**: 477.

Watanakunakorn C (1992). Rapid increase in the prevalence of high-level aminoglycoside resistance among enterococci isolated from blood cultures during 1989–1991. *J Antimicrob Chemother* **30**: 289.

Watanakunakorn C, Glotzbecker C (1974). Enhancement of the effects of anti-staphylococcal antibiotics by aminoglycosides. *Antimicrob Ag Chemother* **6**: 802.

Watanakunakorn C, Patel R (1993). Comparison of patients with enterococcal bacteremia due to strains with and without high-level resistance to gentamicin. *Clin Infect Dis* **17**: 74.

Watanakunakorn C, Perni SC (1994). *Proteus* mirabilis bacteremia: a review of 176 cases during 1980–1992. *Scand J Infect Dis* **26**: 361.

Weems JJ Jr, Lowrance JH, Baddour LM, Simpson WA (1989). Molecular epidemiology of nosocomial, multiply aminoglycoside resistant *Enterococcus faecalis*. *J Antimicrob Chemother* **24**: 121.

Weinstein MJ, Luedemann GM, Oden EM, Wagman GH (1964). Gentamicin A new broad-spectrum antibiotic complex. *Antimicrob Ag Chemother* **1963**: 1.

Wellwood JM, Simpson PM, Tighe JR, Thompson AE (1975). Evidence of gentamicin nephrotoxicity in patients with renal allografts. *Brit Med J* **3**: 278.

Wennberg RP, Rasmussen LF (1975). Effects of gentamicin on albumin binding of bilirubin. *J Pediatr* **86**: 611.

Wersäll J, Lundquist PG, Björkroth B (1969). Ototoxicity of gentamicin. *J Infect Dis* **119**: 410.

Whitman MS, Pitsakis PG, Zausner A *et al.* (1993). Antibiotic treatment of experimental endocarditis due to vancomycin- and ampicillin-resistant *Enterococcus faecium. Antimicrob Ag Chemother* **37**: 2069.

Wilson WR (1987). Antimicrobial therapy of streptococcal endocarditis. *J Antimicrob Chemother* **20** (Suppl A): 147.

Wise R, Walker JM, Mitchard M (1981). A comparison of the pharmacokinetics of amikacin and gentamicin. *J Antimicrob Chemother* **8** (Suppl A): 45.

Witte W, Dünnhaupt K (1984). Occurrence of a nonplasmid-located determinant for gentamicin resistance in strains of *Staphylococcus aureus. J Hyg Camb* **93**: 1.

Wong GA, Peirce TH, Goldstein E, Hoeprich PD (1975). Penetration of antimicrobial agents into bronchial secretions. *Amer J Med* **59**: 219.

Woodford N, McNamara E, Smyth E, George RC (1992). High-level resistance to gentamicin in Enterococcus faecium. *J Antimicrob Chemother* **29**: 395.

Woodford N, Morrison D, Cookson B, George RC (1993). Comparison of high-level gentamicin-resistant *Enterococcus faecium* isolates from different continents. *Antimicrob Ag Chemother* **37**: 681.

Woods JT, Bryan LE, Chan G, Schiff D (1976). Gentamicin and albumin-bilirubin binding. *J Pediatr* **89**: 483.

Wyatt TD, Ferguson WP, Wilson TS, McCormick E (1977). Gentamicin-resistant .*Staphylococcus aureus* associated with the use of topical gentamicin. *J Antimicrob Chemother* **3**: 213.

Yoshioka H, Monma T, Matsuda S (1972). Placental transfer of gentamicin. *J Pediatr* **80**: 121.

Young GP, Sullivan J, Hurley T (1973). Hypokalaemia due to gentamicin/cephalexin in leukaemia. *Lancet* **ii**: 855,.

Young LS (1983). Problems in determining the efficacy of aminoglycosides. *Rev Infect Dis* **5** (Suppl 2): 250.

Young LS (1986). Empirical antimicrobial therapy in the neutropenic host. *New Engl J Med* **315**: 580.

Young ML, Bains M, Bell A, Hancock REW (1992). Role of *Pseudomonas aeruginosa* outer membrane protein OprH in polymyxin and gentamicin resistance: isolation of an OprH-deficient mutant by gene replacement techniques. *Antimicrob Ag Chemother* **36**: 2566.

Young SA, Tenover FC, Gootz TD *et al.* (1985). Development of two DNA probes for differentiating the structural genes for subclasses I and II of the aminoglycoside-modifying enzyme 3'-aminoglycoside phosphotransferase. *Antimicrob Ag Chemother* **27**: 739.

Yu VL, Zuravleff JJ, Bornholm J, Archer G (1984). *In-vitro* synergy testing of triple antibiotic combinations against Staphylococcus epidermidis isolates from patients with endocarditis. *J Antimicrob Chemother* **14**: 359.

Zaske DE, Cipolle RJ, Rotschafer JC *et al.* (1982). Gentamicin pharmacokinetics in 1640 patients: method for control of serum concentrations. *Antimicrob Ag Chemother* **21**: 407.

Zeitany RG, El Saghir NS, Santhosh-Kumar CR, Sigmon MA (1990). Increased aminoglycoside dosage requirements in hematologic malignancy. *Antimicrob Ag Chemother* **34**: 702.

Zervos MJ, Mikasell TS, Schaberg DR (1986a). Heterogeneity of plasmids determining high-level resistance to gentamicin in clinical isolates of *Streptococcus faecalis. Antimicrob Ag Chemother* **30**: 78.

Zervos MJ, Dembinski S, Mikesell T, Schaberg DR (1986b). High-level resistance to gentamicin in *Streptococcus faecalis*: risk factors and evidence for exogenous acquisition of infection. *J Infect Dis* **153**: 1075.

Zervos MJ, Kauffman CA, Therasse PM *et al.* (1987). Nosocomial infection by gentamicin-resistant *Streptococcus faecalis. Ann Intern Med* **106**: 687.

Tobramycin

Description

Tobramycin, previously known as nebramycin factor 6, is an aminoglycoside aminocyclitol antibiotic (p.428), which is one of several compounds in an antibiotic complex (nebramycin) produced by *Streptomyces tenebrarius* (Preston and Wick, 1971). It is a similar drug to gentamicin (p.450), but its advantages include greater intrinsic activity against *Pseudomonas aeruginosa*, activity against some gentamicin-resistant *Ps. aeruginosa* strains and lesser nephrotoxicity (p.497).

Sensitive Organisms

The antibacterial spectrum of tobramycin is similar to that of gentamicin (p.450).

1 Gram-negative bacteria

Tobramycin is active against all the Enterobacteriaceae such as *Escherichia coli*, the *Enterobacter*, *Klebsiella*, *Proteus*, *Salmonella*, *Shigella*, *Providencia*, *Serratia*, *Citrobacter*, *Hafnia*, *Edwardsiella*, *Arizona* and *Yersinia* spp. (Waterworth, 1972; Moellering, 1977; Hammerberg *et al.*, 1977). Against some of these bacteria, such as *E. coli*, tobramycin is usually about 2-fold less active and against *Serratia* spp. at least 4-fold less active than gentamicin (Waterworth, 1972; Reynolds *et al.*, 1974; Moellering, 1983; Guimaraes *et al.*, 1985). Similar to gentamicin (p.450), tobramycin is less active against *Providencia stuartii* than other Enterobacteriaceae (Penner *et al.*, 1982).

Enterobacteriaceae exhibit almost complete cross-resistance between tobramycin and gentamicin (Meyer *et al.*, 1976; Houang and McKay-Ferguson, 1976; Seligman, 1978; Moellering, 1983; Bengtsson *et al.*, 1986). Only occasional gentamicin-resistant isolates of this family, such as the *Klebsiella* and *Serratia* spp., may be tobramycin-sensitive (Drasar *et al.*, 1976; Verbist *et al.*, 1978; Bengtsson *et al.*, 1986). Resistance mechanisms of Enterobacteriaceae to tobramycin are the same as with gentamicin (p.452). The most common one is plasmid-mediated production of enzymes which modify tobramycin by either acetylation, adenylylation or phosphorylation (Price *et al.*, 1981; Maes, 1985; Jacoby *et al.*, 1990; Galimand *et al.*, 1993; Shaw *et al.*, 1993). At least seven enzymes can modify tobramycin by acetylation (AAC-3, type II, AAC-3, type III, AAC-3, type IV, AAC-6', type I, AAC-6', type 2, AAC-6'-APH-2'' and AAC-2', type I), three by adenylylation (ANT-2'', type I, ANT-4', type I, and ANT-4', type II) and none by phosphorylation, except the combined enzyme. In addition APH-3', type I can cause low-level tobramycin-resistance in *E. coli* (Menard *et al.* 1993).

Most of these enzymes can be produced by Enterobacteriaceae, but some types of AAC-3 are only produced by *Ps. aeruginosa*. Gentamicin is also susceptible to modification by at least nine of these enzymes (p.454), but amikacin is only susceptible to three of them (p.505).

As with gentamicin (p.450), the prevalence of tobramycin-resistant Enterobacteriaceae in an institution often decreases if the use of the drug is restricted. In one hospital in the USA, the use of gentamicin and tobramycin was restricted after 1980, and they were replaced by amikacin. During the next $4\frac{1}{2}$ years the prevalence of tobramycin-resistant *Serratia* spp. strains decreased from 42.1 to 2.5% (Larson *et al.*, 1986).

An important feature of tobramycin is that *Ps. aeruginosa* is quite sensitive, against which it is about 2- to 4-fold more active than gentamicin (Waterworth, 1972; Wretlind *et al.*, 1974; Perkins *et al.*, 1976; Moellering, 1983; Van der Auwera and Schuyteneer, 1983; Guimaraes *et al.*, 1985). Unlike the Enterobacteriaceae, against *Ps. aeruginosa* cross-resistance between gentamicin and tobramycin is incomplete. In general, strains with only a low level of gentamicin-resistance (MICs 16.0–32.0 μg per ml) are still susceptible to tobramycin concentrations which are attainable *in vivo* (4.0–8.0 μg per ml). This is because of the greater intrinsic activity of tobramycin. Such low-level gentamicin-resistance is usually due to a chromosomally mediated defect of transport of aminoglycosides into the bacterial cell (p.453). These strains are usually also amikacin-resistant (p.506) (Olson *et al.*, 1985). *Pseudomonas aeruginosa* strains with a high degree of gentamicin-resistance (MICs >128.0 μg per ml) are also usually tobramycin-resistant (Kluge *et al.*, 1974; Houang and McKay-Ferguson, 1976; Meyer *et al.*, 1976; Moellering, 1983). The resistance mechanism in most strains of *Ps. aeruginosa* which have high-level gentamicin-resistance is plasmid-mediated production of aminoglycoside-modifying enzymes (p.489). Strains with high-level gentamicin- and tobramycin-resistance are usually amikacin-sensitive (p.504) (Olson *et al.*, 1985). The number of variants resistant to high concentrations of tobramycin is greater in *Ps. aeruginosa* than in *E. coli* (Nilsson *et al.*, 1987).

Some strains of *Ps. aeruginosa* may become tobramycin-resistant because of a different mechanism. These mutants of *Ps. aeruginosa* have impaired ability to transport aminoglycosides due to defects in cytoplasmic transport system that are related to inefficient energy generation (Parr and Bayer, 1988). *Pseudomonas aeruginosa* in sites of chronic infection, such as cystic fibrosis, often form a thick glycocalyx matrix or biofilm around them, which may prevent the accumulation of bactericidal concentrations of the antibiotic at the target (Anwar *et al.*, 1989). Although tobramycin may not be able to eliminate *Ps. aeruginosa* from the bronchi of patients with cystic fibrosis, animal studies have shown that even subinhibitory tobramycin concentrations may suppress *Ps. aeruginosa* exoenzymes, which are damaging to the lung, and thus delay the chronic disease progression (Grimwood *et al.*, 1989). Also mucoid strains of *Ps. aeruginosa*, growing in the presence of sublethal concentrations of aminoglycosides do not produce alginate and may not colonize the epithelial surface. In contrast, bacteria exposed to beta-lactam antibiotics may continue to release extracellular toxins which can damage the tissues (Geers and Baker 1987a,b).

A tobramycin/carbenicillin (p.146) combination shows *in vitro* synergism against many isolates of *Ps. aeruginosa*, but the degree of susceptibility to tobramycin alone cannot be used to predict a synergistic effect (Anderson *et al.*, 1975; Marks *et al.*, 1976). A tobramycin/ticarcillin (p.146) combination is also synergistic *in vitro* against many strains (Comber *et al.*, 1977). Tobramycin combined with one of the other anti-pseudomonal beta-lactams, such as azlocillin (p.164) (Fass, 1982a), piperacillin (p.165) (Fass, 1982b; Lyon *et al.*, 1986), imipenem (p.230) or ceftazidime (p.369), also exhibits *in vitro* synergism against a proportion of *Ps. aeruginosa* strains (Chan and Zabransky, 1987).

Pseudomonas stutzeri may be tobramycin-sensitive, but *Burkholderia (Pseudomonas) cepacia* is usually resistant (Uwaydah and Taqi-Eddin, 1976; Moellering, 1983). The diuretic amiloride is markedly synergistic with tobramycin against *B. cepacia*, and this combination may be potentially useful in the treatment of *B. cepacia* pulmonary infections in children with cystic fibrosis. *Stenotrophomonas maltophilia* is tobramycin-resistant (Cohn *et al.*, 1988).

Among other Gram-negative bacteria, the *Neisseria* spp. (meningococci and gonococci), similar to gentamicin (p.451), are only moderately sensitive to tobramycin. The same also applies to *Haemophilus influenzae* (Moellering, 1983). *Acinetobacter* spp. are usually more sensitive to tobramycin than to gentamicin, but moderately or highly resistant strains occur. The *Alcaligenes* spp. are more commonly resistant (Uwaydah and Taqi-Eddin, 1976). The *Flavobacterium* spp. are always resistant to aminoglycosides including tobramycin (Drasar *et al.*, 1976). *Legionella pneumophila* is sensitive to tobramycin *in vitro* (Thornsberry *et al.*, 1978).

Tobramycin, like gentamicin (p.452), is inactive against *Bacteroides fragilis* and most other anaerobic Gram-negative bacteria (Moellering, 1977; Ristuccia and Cunha, 1982). The explanation for this is the same as in the case of gentamicin (p.453).

2 Gram-positive bacteria

Staphylococcus aureus, including penicillin G- and methicillin-resistant strains may be tobramycin-sensitive (Jordan and Hoeprich, 1977). Gentamicin-resistant *Staph. aureus* strains (p.454), which in the early 1980s became common in hospitals and which were often multiply resistant to many antibiotics including methicillin (p.80), were also always tobramycin-resistant (Vogel *et al.*, 1978; Archer and Johnston, 1983). The resistance mechanisms are the same as with gentamicin (p.454). *Staphylococcus epidermidis* may be sensitive, but many hospital strains are now tobramycin-resistant, as with gentamicin (p.455).

Other Gram-positive cocci, such as *Streptococcus pyogenes*, Group B streptococci, *Strep. pneumoniae* and the alpha-hemolytic streptococci (*Strep. viridans*), have only a low degree of sensitivity or are completely tobramycin-resistant (Britt *et al.*, 1972). The various enterococci,

Organism	MIC (μg per ml)	
	Gentamicin	Tobramycin
Gram-positive bacteria		
Staphylococcus aureus	0.03–0.12	0.12–0.25
Enterococcus faecalis	2.0–4.0	2.0–8.0
Gram-negative bacteria		
Escherichia coli	0.25–1.0	0.25–1.0
Klebsiella spp.	0.06–0.25	0.12–1.0
Serratia marcescens	0.25–0.5	1.0–4.0
Proteus mirabilis	0.25–2.0	1.0–4.0
Providencia rettgeri	<0.5–32.0	<0.5–16.0
Providencia stuartii	<0.5–>32.0	<0.5–>32.0
Pseudomonas aeruginosa	0.25–2.0	0.12–2.0

Table I.39
After Waterworth (1972) and Penner and Preston (1980)

including *Enterococcus faecalis* and *E. faecium* are moderately resistant, being slightly more resistant to tobramycin than to gentamicin (Finland *et al.*, 1976). Similar to gentamicin (p.42), tobramycin acts synergistically with penicillin G against many *E. faecalis* strains (Basker *et al.*, 1977; Calderwood *et al.*, 1977; Gutschik *et al.*, 1977). Some strains of *E. faecalis* are not killed synergistically by a penicillin G/gentamicin combination. These seem to have a specific defect in gentamicin uptake, they are susceptible to a penicillin G/tobramycin combination (p.42) (Moellering *et al.*, 1980; Eliopoulos and Moellering, 1982). Strains of *E. faecalis* with acquired high-level gentamicin-resistance, due to plasmid-mediated aminoglycoside-modifying enzymes, are not killed synergistically by any beta-lactam/aminoglycoside combination, except for a small percentage which are affected by penicillin G/streptomycin-synergism (p.42). There is no synergism between penicillin G and tobramycin against *E. faecium*. However, most strains of *E. faecium* are killed synergistically by a penicillin G/gentamicin combination (p.42). This appears to be because *Strep. faecium* elaborates an enzyme, aminoglycoside-6'-acetyltransferase, which modifies tobramycin but not gentamicin (Eliopoulos and Moellering, 1982).

Similar to gentamicin (p.455), tobramycin only has a low degree of activity against Gram-positive bacilli.

3 Mycobacteria

At clinically attainable concentrations, tobramycin has no activity against *Mycobacterium tuberculosis* or other mycobacteria (Gangadharam and Candler, 1977).

4 Minimum inhibitory concentrations

The MICs of tobramycin, compared with those of gentamicin, against some selected bacterial species, are shown in Table I.39.

Mode of Administration and Dosage

Like gentamicin, tobramycin is not absorbed from the gastrointestinal tract and it is administered either by the i.m. or i.v. routes.

1 Once-daily administration to adults

Similar to gentamicin (p.457), tobramycin can be administered once-daily in a dosage of 4–5 mg per kg body weight i.m. or i.v. as a 30-min infusion (Gilbert, 1991; Potel *et al.*, 1991; Ellis-Pegler *et al.*, 1994). In common with gentamicin, tobramycin has a prolonged post-antibiotic effect (Rescott *et al.*, 1988; Barmada *et al.*, 1993). Hyperoxia prolongs the tobramycin-induced post-antibiotic effect in *Ps. aeruginosa*. This may be clinically relevant when patients with *Ps. aeruginosa* infections are treated with high inspired oxygen tensions (Park *et al.*, 1991).

Initially animal studies suggested that the administration of tobramycin as a single large daily dose i.v. or i.m. may be therapeutically more effective and possibly less toxic than the administration of the same amount of the drug in three divided doses (Kapusnik and Sande, 1986; Herscovici *et al.*, 1988; Wood *et al.*, 1988). However, in neutropenic guinea pigs given tobramycin every 24 h, bacterial regrowth occurred and so tobramycin therapy alone was ineffective. Combined beta-lactam plus once-daily tobramycin was effective, so once-daily tobramycin therapy can be given to neutropenic patients, provided it is given together with a suitable beta-lactam agent (Kapusnik *et al.*, 1988; Ellis-Pegler *et al.*, 1994).

In clinical trials tobramycin was given once-daily either as a 20-min infusion or by continuous infusion over 24 h to 52 patients with cystic fibrosis; large total daily doses of 10–15 mg per kg were used. A mean peak serum level of 32 μg per ml was attained in those who received the drug by 20-min infusion; neither ototoxicity nor nephrotoxicity were observed after 10 days of such therapy (Powell *et al.*, 1983). In another study, tobramycin was given to ten healthy volunteers as a single daily dose of 5.1 mg per kg per day for a period of 9 days. Another ten volunteers received the same total daily dose, but it was given as 1.7 mg per kg every 8 h. Renal side-effects were not observed in either group (Petty *et al.*, 1986).

With once-daily tobramycin in a dosage of 4–5 mg per kg body weight, usually only the trough serum levels need to be monitored, especially if tobramycin is used together with a beta-lactam antibiotic. For severe infections, especially if tobramycin is used alone, a starting dosage of 7 mg per kg (infused i.v. during 30 min) is recommended. Serum levels then can be measured at 1 h and 6–14 h after the start of the infusion, and suitable dosage adjustments made for subsequent daily doses as described by Barclay *et al.* (1995). This is similar to what has been suggested for gentamicin (p.458).

Other authors have found that a 12-hourly tobramycin regimen, in which the total daily dose is given in two equal doses, is satisfactory for the treatment of patients (Lilliestierna *et al.*, 1985).

2 Classical 8-hourly administration to adults

Similar to gentamicin (p.458), the i.m. dosage of tobramycin is the same as the i.v. dosage. For the treatment of mild to moderate infections, tobramycin is usually administered in a dosage of 3.0–4.5 mg per kg body weight per day, given in three divided doses. A common adult dosage is 80 mg every 6 or 8 h (Simon *et al.*, 1973; Kahlmeter, 1979). The dosage can be increased to 5–8 mg per kg per day for serious infections (Lode *et al.*, 1975). Patients with *Ps. aeruginosa* endocarditis need a high dosage of at least 8.0 mg per kg per day (Rybak *et al.*, 1986). As with gentamicin (p.459), there is a wide variation in serum levels attained in different patients, and therefore serum level monitoring is advisable in all seriously ill patients (Follath *et al.*, 1981). Optimally, the peak serum level should be 5–10 μg per ml and the trough level 1–2 μg per ml (Kahlmeter, 1979; Follath *et al.*, 1981). The blood sample for estimation of the peak serum level should be taken 1 h after i.m. dosing. After i.v. administration, the immediate high peak is not measured, but the blood sample for estimation of the peak serum level is taken after the rapid distribution phase is completed (p.463). This is 1 h after administration of a bolus i.v. dose of the drug or 30 min after a 20–30 min i.v. infusion is completed (Ristuccia and Cunha, 1982). In common with gentamicin, the time at which a blood sample was taken for estimation of the peak serum level has varied between investigators. For instance, some have taken the sample 60 min after the completion of a 20–30 min i.v. infusion (Follath *et al.*, 1981; Dyas *et al.*, 1983). Another variable is that sometimes the drug is given by a 60 min, rather than 20- to 30-min infusion (Bauer and Blouin, 1981).

Seriously ill patients should receive a loading dose of at least 2.0 mg per kg of tobramycin (Kahlmeter, 1979). This may not be sufficient for all patients. In one study, 26 consecutive patients with presumed sepsis or septic shock had initial serum levels determined 1 h after completion of a 20-min infusion of tobramycin in a dose of 2.0 mg per kg; 59% of them had levels below the recommended one of at least 5 μg per ml. These peak serum levels might have been higher if they had been estimated 30 min after the infusion. Therefore, it appears that the recommended dosage schedules (1–2 mg per kg 8-hourly) may be too low for patients with severe sepsis. The volume of distribution of the drug in these patients is probably much increased (Summer *et al.*, 1983). Animal studies have shown that low dosage dopamine increases renal clearance of tobramycin (Kirby *et al.*, 1986). It is likely that patients receiving dopamine may need increased tobramycin dosage. Tobramycin elimination is more rapid in i.v. drug abusers and if they are aged less than 35 years they may need a dosage of at least 8 mg per kg per day (King *et al.*, 1985). Similar to gentamicin, pregnant patients need larger doses of tobramycin (p.443).

3 Methods of intravenous administration

Like gentamicin (p.459), tobramycin can be administered intermittently directly into the i.v. tubing over a period of 1–3 min (Dobbs and Mawer, 1976); or even as rapidly as over 15 seconds (Gillett *et al.*, 1976). After such rapid i.v. injections, immediate peak serum concentrations usually exceed 10 μg per ml and sometimes even 20 μg per ml, but they are only transitory. Within 30–60 min serum levels are similar to the peak obtained after an i.m. injection of the same dose; thereafter the half-life of the drug in serum is only slightly shorter than that which occurs with i.m. administration. Transient high serum levels which follow rapid i.v. injections are not associated with any immediate or delayed toxic effects on the VIIIth nerve or the kidney (Dobbs and Mawer, 1976; Gillett *et al.*, 1976). If tobramycin is administered by rapid intermittent i.v. injections, the serum level 1 h after injection should still be about 5 μg per ml, otherwise therapy may be inadequate (Gillett *et al.*, 1976). These authors also found that serum levels were less than 2 μg per ml 6 h after a 1.5 mg per kg i.v. dose. Accordingly, they recommended that tobramycin should be given at intervals of 6 h in a dosage of 6 mg per kg per day, whenever the drug is administered by rapid i.v. injections.

Alternatively, tobramycin, like gentamicin (p.459), may be administered i.v. as an intermittent infusion over 20–30 min, every 8 h (Lode *et al.*, 1975; Setia and Gross, 1976). This is the only method of i.v. administration recommended for neonates (McCracken and Nelson, 1983). Intramuscular administration produces unpredictable serum concentrations in neonates (Bratlid and Fuglesang, 1979). As with gentamicin (p.459), administration of tobramycin by continuous infusion is not advocated (Bodey *et al.*, 1975; Klastersky *et al.*, 1981).

4 Children

In common with gentamicin (p.459), children need a higher dosage. Young children with serious infections should receive at least 7.5 mg per kg per day. A pharmacokinetic evaluation in 50 pediatric patients, showed that therapeutic non-toxic serum levels were only achieved if a high total daily dose of 300 mg per m^2 (approximately 10 mg per kg every 24 h) was given in six divided doses every 4 h. It was recommended that this tobramycin dosage should be given to children and adolescents under 18 years of age (Hoecker *et al.*, 1978) (see also amikacin p.508).

5 Newborn and premature infants

One recommendation is to administer tobramycin in a dosage of 2 mg per kg every 12 h to infants aged 0–7 days, and give the same dose 8-hourly to infants older than 7 days, (McCracken and Nelson, 1983). Premature babies during their first week of life may need a lower tobramycin dosage (Arbeter *et al.*, 1983). Nahata *et al.* (1983, 1984a) suggested the following modifications: for full-term infants during their first week of life 2.5 mg per kg 12-hourly; for those who are less than 34 weeks of gestational age and have a birth weight greater than 1.25 kg, 2.5 mg per kg every 18 h; and babies of the same gestational age who weigh less than 1.25 kg, 3 mg per kg every 24 h. Nevertheless, despite all these recommendations, individual dosage should be adjusted according to tobramycin serum levels. Another problem is that a 2.0 or 2.5 mg per kg individual dose rarely produces therapeutic serum concentrations. Therefore, for seriously ill infants, a higher initial loading dose may be necessary (Marks, 1984). Also the rate and method of i.v. tobramycin administration can markedly influence the amount of drug actually infused and resultant serum concentrations (Nahata *et al.*, 1984b). Nowadays, if tobramycin is given together with a suitable beta-lactam antibiotic, it may not matter if tobramycin serum levels are not high enough.

6 Patients with renal failure

Dosage should be reduced in these patients. This may be accomplished in two ways. Individual tobramycin doses may be left unchanged, but the usual dosage interval of 6–8 h is extended by multiplying it by the value of the patient's serum creatinine measured in mg % (for conversion of serum creatinine from mmol per liter, see gentamicin, p.460). Alternatively, the usual 6–8 h interval between doses may be left unchanged but individual doses reduced by dividing them by the value of the patient's serum creatinine, measured in mg % (Naber *et al.*, 1973; Jaffe *et al.*, 1974; Neu, 1977). These dosage schedules are only rough approximations. The presumed linear relationship between serum creatinine and the tobramycin half-life in the body does not necessarily always hold true, especially at higher creatinine concentrations and particularly with those above 10 mg % (Jaffe *et al.*, 1974). For this reason, tobramycin dosage in patients with impaired renal function should always be governed by regular serum level estimations. Ideally, peak serum levels should be at least 4–5 μg per ml (or for serious infections 5–10 μg per ml), and trough levels should not exceed 2.0 μg per ml (Gillett *et al.*, 1976).

Nomograms developed to assist gentamicin prescribing in these patients (p.461) can also be used for tobramycin. The minimal input data for such nomograms are the patient's age, sex, weight and serum creatinine concentration. The gentamicin nomogram developed by Mawer *et al.* (1974) was used effectively by Tobias *et al.* (1977) to prescribe i.v. tobramycin, particularly when high dosage was required. Tobramycin serum level estimations are still advisable, even if the dosage is prescribed according to a nomogram (p.461).

Tobramycin, like gentamicin (p.461), is removed by hemodialysis; approximately 50% of an administered dose is removed by a 6 h dialysis (Lockwood and Bower, 1973; Jaffe *et al.*, 1974). In anephric patients maintained by regular hemodialysis, the usual single dose of 1.5–2.0 mg per kg, given after each dialysis, will usually maintain therapeutic non-toxic serum levels. Removal of tobramycin by peritoneal dialysis is inefficient, and only about 50% of an administered dose is recovered during 36 h of this procedure (Weinstein *et al.*, 1973; Jaffe *et al.*, 1974). Nevertheless, the tobramycin half-life in anephric patients of 53 h is reduced to 12–16 h when these patients undergo peritoneal dialysis, so that the following dosage schedule is recommended: a loading dose of 2 mg per kg body weight, followed by either the same dose once every 36 h or 1 mg per kg every 12 h (Malacoff *et al.*, 1975).

Tobramycin can be added to peritoneal dialysate to treat *Ps. aeruginosa* peritonitis, a serious complication of continuous ambulatory peritoneal dialysis (Shalit *et al.*, 1985). Usually the drug is added to produce a concentration of 8 μg per ml in each dialysis exchange. Walshe *et al.* (1986) suggested that intermittent intraperitoneal administration with larger doses may be advantageous; higher fluctuating serum levels are attained making parenteral dosing unnecessary; drug administration is simpler and the risk of dialysate contamination is reduced. An intraperitoneal loading dose of 3.0 mg per kg body weight, added to 2 liters of dialysate is recommended; this produces peak tobramycin serum concentrations of 6–8 μg per ml, and after 24 h the serum level is 5 μg per ml and the dialysate concentration is 3.5 μg per ml. An intraperitoneal maintenance dose of 1.2 mg per kg per 2 liters of dialysate once every 24 h is usually sufficient, but this should be governed by serum tobramycin estimations.

7 Patients with cystic fibrosis or burns

As with gentamicin (p.461), these patients need a larger dosage. Some may require one as high as 12 mg per kg body weight per day. There is a large individual variation and dosage should be adjusted according to serum levels. Patients with severe burns may also need a larger dosage as they appear to eliminate the drug more rapidly (McCrae *et al.*, 1976; Setia and Gross, 1976; Levy *et al.*, 1984).

8 Intrathecal and intraventricular administration

In common with gentamicin (p.462), tobramycin can be administered by these routes to adults in single daily doses of 5–10 mg. Intrathecal administration produces adequate antibiotic concentrations in lumbar, but not in ventricular CSF. When it is given into the cerebral ventricles, adequate concentrations are attained in both lumbar and ventricular CSF (Kaiser and McGee, 1975). These methods of administration should be only rarely necessary nowadays.

Serum Levels in Relation to Dosage

After an 80 mg i.m. injection of tobramycin is given to adults, a mean peak serum level of 3.7 μg per ml is attained in 30 min. Six hours later the mean serum level is 0.56 μg per ml, and after 8–12 h the drug is undetectable (Simon *et al.*, 1973). These serum levels are similar to those of gentamicin (p.463). The half-life of tobramycin after i.m. injection is 1.9–2.2 h (Neu, 1977).

If tobramycin is administered i.v. as a 30- to 60-min infusion, the peak serum level attained straight after the infusion and subsequent serum levels, are similar to those obtained after an identical i.m. dose (Lode *et al.*, 1975). When it is given i.v. by rapid injections, transient high peaks are reached soon after the injection, which are proportional to the rate of injection. One hour after rapid i.v. injection the serum level approximates to the peak level after an identical i.m. dose (Gillett *et al.*, 1976). The serum half-life of the drug with this method (1.3–1.5 h) is shorter than that after i.m. administration. Serum levels at 6 h are invariably below 1.0 μg per ml and often below 0.1 μg per ml (Neu, 1977).

When the drug is given by continuous i.v. infusion (6.6 mg per h), the peak serum level is achieved 2.5–3.0 h after commencement of infusion. Thereafter, a steady-state serum concentration which averages 0.94 μg per ml is maintained, and an almost identical result is achieved with gentamicin (Simon et al., 1973) (p.459). If tobramycin is administered by constant infusion at 30 mg per h, a steady-state serum concentration of 3.6–4.5 µg per ml can be attained (Neu, 1977). To achieve steady-state serum levels of at least 3 µg per ml by continuous tobramycin infusion, a total daily dose of 7 mg per kg is needed (Bodey et al., 1975).

With multiple dosing of tobramycin, gradually rising peak and trough serum levels sometimes occur even in patients with stable renal function. This can be probably explained on the basis of a slow tissue uptake and release of the antibiotic (see below). Later in the course of treatment, when the drug has already accumulated in tissues, a given dose is likely to produce a higher serum concentration (Schentag et al., 1978).

Excretion

Tobramycin is excreted by the kidneys in an active unchanged form, producing high urinary concentrations. In patients with normal renal function, 60% of an administered dose is excreted within 6 h (Naber et al., 1973), and 85% within 24 h (Neu, 1977). Excretion is only by glomerular filtration and therefore probenecid has no effect on its elimination (Naber et al., 1973). Like gentamicin (p.465), some of the drug is not excreted and accumulates in the body, particularly in renal cortical tissue (see below). Accumulated tobramycin is slowly excreted by the kidney for 10–20 days after the last dose (Schentag et al., 1978).

In patients with impaired renal function, tobramycin excretion is reduced, but even in those with moderately severe renal failure, urine levels are adequate for the inhibition of tobramycin-sensitive Gram-negative bacilli (Weinstein et al., 1973). The serum half-lives of tobramycin and gentamicin are virtually identical, being 2 h in patients with normal kidneys and 53.4 h in anephric patients (Lockwood and Bower, 1973).

Distribution of the Drug in Body

Binding of tobramycin to serum proteins is very low, and it has been estimated to vary from zero (Gordon et al., 1972) to 25–30% (Naber et al., 1973).

Tobramycin is distributed in human body fluids and tissues in a similar manner to gentamicin (p.464). It diffuses poorly into the CSF of patients with uninflamed meninges, but similar to gentamicin (p.464) in animals rapid infusion of mannitol into the internal carotid artery causes osmotic disruption of the blood–brain barrier, and this enhances penetration of tobramycin into the CSF and the brain tissue (Perkins and Strausbaugh, 1983). Tobramycin levels are low in peritoneal fluid (Weinstein et al., 1973; Gerding et al., 1976), but they usually reach 50% or more of the simultaneous serum level in patients with ascites and bacterial peritonitis (Gerding et al., 1977). The drug penetrates well into synovial fluid even in the absence of bacterial infection, where concentrations consistently exceed 50% of the serum level (Dee and Kozin, 1977).

Tobramycin passes into the bronchial secretions to approximately the same extent as gentamicin (Pennington and Reynolds, 1973). Mean concentrations of tobramycin in bronchial secretions from patients with pneumonia are almost twice those found in normal patients (Alexander et al., 1982). In patients with cystic fibrosis, peak sputum levels exceed the MICs of many Ps. aeruginosa strains, provided that large doses of 5–10 mg per kg per day are used. Tobramycin penetrates the sputum of patients with cystic fibrosis where after a period it accumulates. Although the sputum of these patients antagonizes the antibacterial activity of tobramycin and other aminoglycosides, a 3-week course of i.v. tobramycin combined with an anti-pseudomonal beta-lactam antibiotic may be effective in eradicating Ps. aeruginosa from the sputum of some of these patients (Mendelman et al., 1985). If free tobramycin and tobramycin encapsulated in liposomes is administered to animals intratracheally, the liposome encapsulated drug remains in lungs for a longer period of time (Omri et al., 1994). Other studies have suggested that liposome-encapsulated tobramycin is likely to be more effective than free tobramycin for the treatment of Ps. aeruginosa infections (Poyner et al., 1994). Tobramycin reaches satisfactory concentrations in non-inflamed human interstitial fluid (Tan and Salstrom, 1977). In animals its concentration in interstitial tissue fluid is low compared with that of gentamicin (Chisholm et al., 1973; Carbon et al., 1978).

Tobramycin accumulates in the kidney, where it is selectively concentrated in renal cortical cells (Luft and Kleit, 1974; Bennett et al., 1977), but gentamicin accumulates to a greater extent in this tissue (Whelton et al., 1978; Aronoff et al., 1983). These drugs are only slowly eliminated from renal tissue. Luft and Kleit (1974) found that the half-life of gentamicin in renal tissue was 109 h, whilst that of tobramycin was 74 h. This shorter renal half-life may partly explain the lower renal cortical concentrations of tobramycin compared with gentamicin. Netilmicin also accumulates in renal cortical tissue to a greater extent than tobramycin and it is also more slowly eliminated. Yet the nephrotoxicity (p.528) of these two drugs is about the same. This means that netilmicin is intrinsically less toxic to the kidney, compared with tobramycin (Winslade *et al.*, 1987). In animals with experimental pyelonephritis, tobramycin accumulates to a greater extent in distal renal tubules, than in non-infected kidneys (Bergeron *et al.*, 1987). If tobramycin and vancomycin are given together to experimental animals, vancomycin has no effect on the distribution of tobramycin in the kidneys (Beauchamp *et al.*, 1992). From this it is not clear whether vancomycin would aggravate tobramycin nephrotoxicity (p.775).

The drug crosses the placenta but fetal serum levels are lower than those in the mother. Fetal concentrations were studied in detail by Bernard *et al.* (1977). After administering single 2 mg per kg body weight doses of tobramycin to pregnant women, the drug's half-life in fetal serum was 5.2 h where levels did not exceed 0.58 μg per ml. For the subsequent 34 h the mean placental tissue concentration was 1.4 μg per g. Tobramycin was also detected in amniotic fluid, except in women during their first trimester. Fetal kidney tissue concentrations reached 7.2 μg per g, 34 h after maternal drug administration, higher concentrations in this tissue were obtained when maturation of the fetal kidney was more advanced. Fetal urine concentrations estimated during second trimester ranged from 0.1 to 3.4 μg per ml. Very low tobramycin CSF concentrations (0.1–0.7 μg per ml) were found in fetuses of less than 17 weeks gestation.

Mode of Action

Tobramycin inhibits bacterial growth by inhibiting protein synthesis in a manner similar to that of streptomycin (p.432). Tobramycin-resistant non-typable *H. influenzae* strains isolated from lower respiratory tracts of patients with chronic respiratory tract infections, have altered ribosomes which are less sensitive to misreading of messenger RNA in the presence of tobramycin (Levy *et al.*, 1986). Similar to gentamicin, tobramycin probably also interacts with the cell envelope of some Gram-negative bacilli such as *Ps. aeruginosa* (p.465).

Toxicity

1 Ototoxicity

Tobramycin, like gentamicin (p.466) is prone to cause ototoxicity with high prolonged serum levels of the drug. Wilson and Ramsden (1977) performed electrocochleography on three patients who were receiving tobramycin by rapid i.v. injection. When peak serum tobramycin levels exceeded 8–10 μg per ml, an immediate reduction in cochlear output was observed, which returned to normal as serum levels fell. These patients had no auditory or vestibular symptoms either during or after treatment.

In patients with cystic fibrosis, who are receiving repeated courses of tobramycin, high-frequency audiometry may serve as a useful measure of elevation in pure-tone hearing thresholds that precede noticeable loss of auditory acuity (McRorie *et al.*, 1989). In general, acute and chronic ototoxicity of repeated high-dose tobramycin treatment in cystic fibrosis patients appears to be mild (Pedersen *et al.*, 1987). Also there were no abnormalities in audiometric investigations in ten patients with cystic fibrosis who received one 400 mg nebulized tobramycin dose; the highest serum level recorded at 30 min in one of the patients was 9.9 μg per ml (Mukhopadhyay *et al.*, 1993).

Large-scale retrospective surveys have suggested that the frequency of tobramycin ototoxicity is low. For instance, Neu and Bendush (1976) found ototoxicity in only 21 of 3506 treated patients. In seven of these patients the effects were auditory only, in nine vestibular only and in five both were affected. Subsequent progress of 18 patients was monitored; in 14 side-effects gradually subsided, in three a high frequency audiometric loss persisted and in the rest there was a decrease in hearing. It seemed that pre-existing renal impairment, prior and/or concomitant therapy with other ototoxic drugs, and therapy for 10 days or more with a dose exceeding 3 mg per kg per day, predisposed to ototoxicity. In contrast, smaller prospective studies in which all patients were carefully monitored from beginning of therapy, have shown that ototoxicity was more common; in three such studies this side-effect occurred in 11% (Smith *et al.*, 1980), 12% (Lerner *et al.*, 1983) and as high as 24% of patients (Fee, 1983).

Studies in animals suggest that tobramycin may cause less cochlear and vestibular damage than gentamicin (Brummett *et al.*, 1978; Federspil, 1978; Brummett, 1983). There is insufficient evidence to indicate that this applies to humans (p.466). In one prospective randomized trial involving 187 patients where netilmicin, tobramycin and amikacin were compared, auditory toxicity was detected in 4.4, 10.8 and 23.5% of patients given netilmicin, tobramycin and amikacin, respectively. In this study it was also found that increasing age was the most important predisposing factor for the development of auditory toxicity in patients receiving aminoglycosides (Gatell *et al.*, 1987).

2 Nephrotoxicity

Tobramycin is selectively concentrated in renal cortical cells (p.495) and it produces changes in proximal tubules resembling those produced by gentamicin (p.467). The drug causes renal impairment characterized by excretion of casts, oliguria, proteinuria and a progressive rise in blood urea and serum creatinine values (Appel and Neu, 1977; Lietman and Smith, 1983). Serum creatinine and tobramycin levels should be monitored during therapy. In animals tobramycin accumulates in the kidneys more during the rest period at night and possibly it causes more nephrotoxicity during that time (Lin *et al.*, 1994).

Retrospective surveys have indicated that nephrotoxicity is an infrequent side-effect. In a review of 3506 patients treated by tobramycin, 53 (1.5%) were considered to have developed nephrotoxicity as a result of its use, but its occurrence in another 105 (3%) was of doubtful relation to tobramycin therapy (Bendush and Weber, 1976). Prospective studies of smaller number of patients have usually showed a higher frequency of nephrotoxicity such as 4% (Lerner *et al.*, 1983), 12% (Smith *et al.*, 1980) and 28% (Feig *et al.*, 1982). When Tablan *et al.* (1984) used high tobramycin dosages, aiming to produce peak serum levels of 12–15 μg per ml in patients with *Ps. aeruginosa* endocarditis, nephrotoxicity developed in 44%. Tobramycin-related nephrotoxicity has occurred primarily in patients receiving high doses for prolonged periods. Other predisposing factors may include dehydration and endotoxemia (Bergeron *et al.*, 1986; Joly *et al.*, 1991). In one clinical study there appeared to be no interaction between shock and tobramycin use in causing renal impairment (Ambinder *et al.*, 1985). Tobramycin renal damage may be aggravated by concomitant use of other nephrotoxic drugs. One animal study demonstrated that vancomycin (p.775) potentiated tobramycin nephrotoxicity (Wood *et al.*, 1986). In cancer patients who had recently received high-dose cisplastin (cytotoxic) therapy, tobramycin and other aminoglycosides could be administered safely and they did not significantly increase the risk of renal dysfunction (Cooper *et al.*, 1993). However, similar to gentamicin (p.469), tobramycin nephrotoxicity was more common in patients with obstructive jaundice (Desai and Tsang, 1988).

In common with gentamicin (p.468), a combination of tobramycin with cephalothin may be associated with a higher risk of nephrotoxicity than the use of tobramycin alone (Klastersky *et al.*, 1975; Tobias *et al.*, 1976; Kahlmeter, 1979). With tobramycin (and also gentamicin, p.468) in animals cephalosporins such as cephalothin and ceftriaxone do not potentiate, but actually protect against nephrotoxicity (Barza *et al.*, 1978; Beauchamp *et al.*, 1994). Increased renal toxicity has not been observed when tobramycin was used with either carbenicillin or ticarcillin (p.155) (Klastersky *et al.*, 1975, Appel and Neu, 1977; Neu 1977). One animal study showed that the concomitant administration of ticarcillin probably protected against tobramycin nephrotoxicity (English *et al.*, 1985). As salt depletion aggravates tobramycin nephrotoxicity, the protective effect of ticarcillin may be secondary to the obligatory sodium load associated with the use of this drug (Sabra and Branch, 1990).

In animals gentamicin is more toxic to renal tubules than tobramycin (Whelton *et al.*, 1978; Bennett *et al.*, 1979; Kahlmeter, 1979; Luft *et al.*, 1983). Most prospective, randomized studies have also shown that gentamicin is more nephrotoxic than tobramycin in patients (p.469). However, when Kahlmeter and Dahlager (1984) analyzed results of clinical studies published between 1975 and 1982, involving approximately 10 000 patients treated by aminoglycosides, the average frequencies of nephrotoxicity for gentamicin and tobramycin were 14% and 12.9%, respectively.

3 Other side-effects

Local reactions may occur at the sites of i.m. injections and thrombophlebitis may occur after i.v. administration. Urticaria, eosinophilia or a maculopapular rash have been described but are rare. Elevated SGOT levels have been noted in some patients, but other evidence of hepatotoxicity has not been reported (Bendush and Weber, 1976). Like gentamicin (p.470), tobramycin inhibits various neutrophil functions such as chemotaxis (Sacchi *et al.*, 1981). Psychosis and delirium in one 66-year-old woman was probably caused by tobramycin (McCartney *et al.*, 1982).

Clinical Uses of the Drug

1 Pseudomonas aeruginosa infections

Tobramycin is commonly used in preference to gentamicin for the treatment of confirmed *Ps. aeruginosa* infections, and also for initial emergency treatment of patients with severe infections in whom *Ps. aeruginosa* is a likely pathogen, such as those with neutropenia, burns and cystic fibrosis (Moellering, 1977). In areas where *Ps. aeruginosa* has become a significant cause of septicemia in i.v. narcotic addicts, the combination of tobramycin, ticarcillin and vancomycin has been suggested for initial empiric chemotherapy (Crane *et al.*, 1986). Compared with gentamicin, tobramycin is more active *in vitro* against *Ps. aeruginosa*, and it is also active against a proportion of these organisms which are gentamicin-resistant (p.489). In one animal study tobramycin was more active than gentamicin for the treatment of infections with *Ps. aeruginosa*, when results were analyzed in terms of the therapeutic index (ratio of toxicity to efficacy) (Davis, 1975). In another study these two drugs appeared to be of about the same value for the treatment of induced *Pseudomonas* sepsis in monkeys (Saslaw *et al.*, 1972). There have been few comparative clinical trials in humans of gentamicin and tobramycin for severe *Ps. aeruginosa* infections. In one study the clinical effectiveness of the two drugs appeared about the same (Klastersky *et al.*, 1974).

In experimental *Ps. aeruginosa* infections in animals, such as pneumonia, tobramycin alone has been as effective as a tobramycin/beta-lactam combination (e.g. tobramycin/ticarcillin) (Pennington and Stone, 1979; Schiff and Pennington, 1984). However, a tobramycin/beta-lactam combination was superior to either drug used alone for treatment of *Ps. aeruginosa* pneumonia in neutropenic guinea pigs (Rusnak *et al.*, 1984).

Clinically tobramycin has been used as a single drug with about the same success as gentamicin (p.471) to treat *Ps. aeruginosa* septicemia (Blair *et al.*, 1975), bronchitis and pneumonia (Carmalt *et al.*, 1976) and respiratory infections in children with cystic fibrosis (McCrae *et al.*, 1976). For cystic fibrosis patients, a large well controlled tobramycin dosage is often required to achieve satisfactory serum and sputum concentrations (Li *et al.*, 1991) (p.494). Friis (1979) found that a tobramycin/carbenicillin combination was superior to tobramycin alone for treatment of *Ps. aeruginosa* bronchial infections in such patients. Nowadays most clinicians would recommend the use of combination therapy with an anti-pseudomonal beta-lactam such as ticarcillin (p.156), piperacillin (p.174) or ceftazidime (p.377) plus tobramycin for the treatment of pneumonia and most other serious *Ps. aeruginosa* infections (Korvick and Yu, 1991). In patients with cystic fibrosis, an aerosol administration of 600 mg tobramycin daily as a single drug has been found to be safe and efficaceous short-term treatment (28 days) for endobronchial infections with *Ps. aeruginosa* (Ramsey *et al.*, 1993). In patients with Gram-negative bacterial pneumonia endobronchial administration of 40 mg of tobramycin 8-hourly may be a useful adjunctive therapy to systemically administered antibiotics (Brown *et al.*, 1990).

Likewise tobramycin has been used successfully to treat *Pseudomonas* urinary tract infections (Bennett, 1976; Perkins *et al.*, 1976), soft tissue infections and osteomyelitis (Carmalt *et al.*, 1976; Perkins *et al.*, 1976) and osteochondritis (Jacobs *et al.*, 1989). It has also been of value for wound sepsis, infected burns and peritonitis, where *Ps. aeruginosa* is not infrequently involved in a mixed infection with other organisms (Ishiyama *et al.*, 1976). Serious infections caused by gentamicin-resistant, but tobramycin-sensitive strains of *Ps. aeruginosa* may respond satisfactorily to tobramycin (Moellering *et al.*, 1976).

For initial treatment of severe infections in neutropenic patients with leukemia or cancer, a combination of tobramycin plus an anti-pseudomonal beta-lactam, such as ticarcillin (p.156), piperacillin (p.174) or ceftazidime (p.377) is preferred (Bodey *et al.*, 1985; Korvick and Yu, 1991). A total of 410 episodes of *Ps. aeruginosa* septicemia occurring in patients with cancer were analyzed by Bodey *et al.* (1985). Patients who received an antipseudomonal beta-lactam antibiotic with or without an aminoglycoside had a higher cure rate than patients who received only an aminoglycoside (72% and 71% versus 29%). Therefore tobramycin alone should not be used for the continuation therapy of these patients if *Ps. aeruginosa* proves to be the pathogen.

The preferred combination for the treatment of *Ps. aeruginosa* endocarditis is ticarcillin plus tobramycin (p.156). Large doses of tobramycin are recommended, aiming to obtain peak serum levels of 12–15 μg per ml or even 15–20 μg per ml (Tablan *et al.*, 1984; Rybak *et al.*, 1986; Korvick and Yu, 1991).

2 Infections caused by other Gram-negative bacilli

Urinary tract infections, as well as more serious systemic infections, such as pneumonia, osteomyelitis and septicemia, caused by the Enterobacteriaceae such as *E. coli* and the *Enterobacter*, *Klebsiella* and *Proteus* spp., also respond to tobramycin treatment (Bendush and Weber, 1976; Bennet, 1976; Carmalt *et al.*, 1976).

Most clinicians opt to use the more familiar gentamicin (p.471) rather than tobramycin, for treatment of infections caused by the Enterobacteriaceae. Gentamicin is certainly indicated for *Serratia marcescens* infections, as it is about four-fold more active than tobramycin against this pathogen (p.489). In addition, some strains of *E. coli* and of other Enterobacteriaceae may be about twice as sensitive to gentamicin as tobramycin (p.489). For the treatment of infections caused by Enterobacteriaceae equally sensitive to both of these drugs, tobramycin can be used with success, and some clinicians may prefer it because of its lesser nephrotoxicity (p.497).

References

Alexander MR, Schoell J, Hicklin G *et al.* (1982). Bronchial secretion concentrations of tobramycin. *Amer Rev Respir Dis* **125**: 208.

Ambinder RF, Moore RD, Smith CR *et al.* (1985). Lack of evidence for interaction between tobramycin and shock in their effect on renal function. *Antimicrob Ag Chemother* **27**: 217.

Anderson EL, Gramling PK, Vestal PR, Farrar WE Jr (1975). Susceptibility of *Pseudomonas aeruginosa* to tobramycin or gentamicin alone and combined with carbenicillin. *Antimicrob Ag Chemother* **8**: 300.

Anwar H, Dasgupta M, Lam K, Costerton JW (1989). Tobramycin resistance of mucoid *Pseudomonas aeruginosa* biofilm grown under iron limitation. *J Antimicrob Chemother* **24**: 647.

Appel GB, Neu HC (1977). The nephrotoxicity of antimicrobial agents. (second of three parts) *New Engl J Med* **296**: 722.

Arbeter AM, Saccard CL, Eisner S *et al.* (1983). Tobramycin sulfate elimination in premature infants. *J Pediatr* **103**: 131.

Archer GL, Johnston JL (1983). Self-transmissible plasmids in staphylococci that encode resistance to aminoglycosides. *Antimicrob Ag Chemother* **24**: 70.

Aronoff GR, Pottratz ST, Brier ME *et al.* (1983). Aminoglycoside accumulation kinetics in rat renal parenchyma. *Antimicrob Ag Chemother* **23**: 74.

Barclay ML, Duffull SB, Begg EJ, Buttimore RC (1995). Experience of once-daily aminoglycoside dosing using a target area under the concentration-time curve. *Aust NZ J Med* **25**: 230.

Barmada S, Kohlhepp S, Leggett J *et al.* (1993). Correlation of tobramycin-induced inhibition of protein synthesis with postantibiotic effect in *Escherichia coli*. *Antimicrob Ag Chemother* **37**: 2678.

Barza M, Pinn V, Tanguay P, Murray T (1978). Nephrotoxicity of newer cephalosporins and aminoglycosides alone and in combination in a rat model. *J Antimicrob Chemother* **4** (Suppl A): 59.

Basker MJ, Slocombe B, Sutherland R (1977). Aminoglycoside-resistant enterococci. *J Clin Path* **30**: 375.

Bauer LA, Blouin RA (1981). Influence of age on tobramycin pharmacokinetics in patients with normal renal function. *Antimicrob Ag Chemother* **20**: 587.

Beauchamp D, Gourde P, Simard M, Bergeron MG (1992). Subcellular localization of tobramycin and vancomycin given alone and in combination in proximal tubular cells, determined by immunogold labeling. *Antimicrob Ag Chemother* **36**: 2204.

Beauchamp D, Theriault G, Grenier L *et al.* (1994). Ceftriaxone protects against tobramycin nephrotoxicity. *Antimicrob Ag Chemother* **38**: 750.

Bendush CL, Weber R (1976). Tobramycin sulfate: a summary of worldwide experience from clinical trials. *J Infect Dis* **134** (Suppl): 219.

Bengtsson S, Bernander S, Brorson JE *et al.* (1986). *In vitro* aminoglycoside resistance of Gram-negative bacilli and staphylococci isolated from blood in Sweden 1980–1984. *Scand J Infect Dis* **18**: 257.

Bennett AH (1976). Evaluation of tobramycin in severe urinary tract infections. *J Infect Dis* **134** (Suppl): 156.

Bennett WM, Plamp C, Porter GA (1977). Drug-related syndromes in clinical nephrology. *Ann Intern Med* **87**: 582.

Bennett WM, Plamp CE, Parker RA *et al.* (1979). Renal transport of organic acids and bases in aminoglycoside nephrotoxicity. *Antimicrob Ag Chemother* **16**: 231.

Bergeron MG, Bergeron Y, Marois Y (1986). Autoradiography of tobramycin uptake by the proximal and distal tubules of normal and endotoxin-treated rats. *Antimicrob Ag Chemother* **29**: 1005.

Bergeron MG, Marois Y, Kuehn C, Silverblatt FJ (1987). Autoradiographic study of tobramycin uptake by proximal and distal tubules of normal and pyelonephritic rats. *Antimicrob Ag Chemother* **31**: 1359.

Bernard B, Garcia-Cázares SJ, Ballard CA *et al.* (1977). Tobramycin: maternal-fetal pharmacology. *Antimicrob Ag Chemother* **11**: 688.

Blair DC, Fekety FR Jr, Bruce B *et al.* (1975). Therapy of *Pseudomonas aeruginosa* infections with tobramycin. *Antimicrob Ag Chemother* **8**: 22.

Bodey GP, Chang H-Y, Rodriguez V, Stewart D (1975). Feasibility of administering aminoglycoside antibiotics by continuous intravenous infusion. *Antimicrob Ag Chemother* **8**: 328.

Bodey GP, Jadeja L, Elting L (1985). *Pseudomonas* bacteremia. Retrospective analysis of 410 episodes. *Arch Intern Med* **145**: 1621.

Bratlid D, Fuglesand JE (1979). Clinical pharmacology of tobramycin in infants. *Scand J Infect Dis* **11**: 73.

Britt MR, Garibaldi RA, Wilfert JN, Smith CB (1972). *In vitro* activity of tobramycin and gentamicin. *Antimicrob Ag Chemother* **2**: 236.

Brown RB, Kruse JA, Counts GW *et al.* (1990). Double-blind study of endotracheal tobramycin in the treatment of Gram-negative bacterial pneumonia. *Antimicrob Ag Chemother* **34**: 269.

Brummett RE (1983). Animal models of aminoglycoside antibiotic ototoxicity. *Rev Infect Dis* **5** (Suppl 2): 294.

Brummett RE, Fox KE, Bendrick TW, Himes DL (1978). Ototoxicity of tobramycin, gentamicin, amikacin and sisomicin in the guinea pig. *J Antimicrob Chemother* **4** (Suppl A): 73.

Calderwood SA, Wennersten C, Moellering RC Jr *et al.* (1977). Resistance to six aminoglycosidic aminocyclitol antibiotics among enterococci: prevalence, evolution and relationship to synergism with penicillin. *Antimicrob Ag Chemother* **12**: 401.

Carbon C, Contrepois A, Lamotte-Barrillon S (1978). Comparative distribution of gentamicin, tobramycin, sisomicin, netilmicin and amikacin in interstitial fluid in rabbits. *Antimicrob Ag Chemother* **13**: 368.

Carmalt ED, Cortez LM, Rosenblatt JE (1976). Clinical experience with tobramycin in the treatment of infections due to Gram-negative bacilli. *Amer J Med Sci* **271**: 285.

Chan EL, Zabransky RJ (1987). Determination of synergy by two methods with eight antimicrobial combinations against tobramycin-susceptible and tobramycin-resistant strains of *Pseudomonas*. *Diagn Microbiol Infect Dis* **6**: 157.

Chisholm GD, Waterworth PM, Calnan JS, Garrod LP (1973). Concentration of antibacterial agents in interstitial tissue fluid. *Brit Med J* **1**: 569.

Cohn RC, Jacobs M, Aronoff SC (1988). *In vitro* activity of amiloride combined with tobramycin against pseudomonas isolates from patients with cystic fibrosis. *Antimicrob Ag Chemother* **32**: 395.

Comber KR, Basker MJ, Osborne CD, Sutherland R (1977). Synergy between ticarcillin and tobramycin against *Pseudomonas aeruginosa* and Enterobacteriaceae *in vitro* and *in vivo*. *Antimicrob Ag Chemother* **11**: 956.

Cooper BW, Creger RJ, Soegiarso W *et al.* (1993). Renal dysfunction during high-dose cisplatin therapy and autologous hematopoietic stem cell transplantation: effect of aminoglycoside therapy. *Amer J Med* **94**: 497.

Crane LR, Levine DP, Zervos MJ, Cummings G (1986). Bacteremia in narcotic addicts at the Detroit Medical Center I Microbiology, epidemiology, risk factors, and empiric therapy. *Rev Infect Dis* **8**: 364.

Davis SD (1975). Activity of gentamicin, tobramycin, polymyxin B and colistimethate in mouse protection tests with *Pseudomonas aeruginosa*. *Antimicrob Ag Chemother* **8**: 50.

Dee TH, Kozin F (1977). Gentamicin and tobramycin penetration into synovial fluid. *Antimicrob Ag Chemother* **12**: 548.

Desai TK, Tsang T-K (1988). Aminoglycoside nephrotoxicity in obstructive jaundice. *Amer J Med* **85**: 47.

Dobbs SM, Mawer GE (1976). Intravenous injection of gentamicin and tobramycin without impairment of hearing. *J Infect Dis* **134** (Suppl): 114.

Drasar FA, Farrell W, Maskell J, Williams JD (1976). Tobramycin, amikacin, sisomicin and gentamicin resistant Gram-negative rods. *Brit Med J* **2**: 1284.

Dyas A, Wise R, Pijck J *et al.* (1983). Reproducibility study of the pharmacokinetics of amikacin, gentamicin and tobramycin: a three-way crossover study. *J Antimicrob Chemother* **12**: 371.

Eliopoulos GM, Moellering RC Jr (1982). Antibiotic synergism and antimicrobial combinations in clinical infections. *Rev Infect Dis* **4**: 282.

Ellis-Pegler RB, Chambers S, Begg EJ, Barclay ML (1994). Aminoglycoside dosing: time to change. *Aust NZ J Med* **24**: 359.

English J, Gilbert DN, Kohlhepp S *et al.* (1985). Attenuation of experimental tobramycin nephrotoxicity by ticarcillin. *Antimicrob Ag Chemother* **27**: 897.

Fass RJ (1982a). Comparative *in vitro* activities of beta-lactam-tobramycin combinations against *Pseudomonas aeruginosa* and multidrug-resistant Gram-negative enteric bacilli. *Antimicrob Ag Chemother* **21**: 1003.

Fass RJ (1982b). Comparative *in vitro* activities of azlocillin-cefotaxime and azlocillin-tobramycin combinations against blood and multidrug-resistant bacterial isolates. *Antimicrob Ag Chemother* **22**: 167.

Federspil P (1978). Comparative studies on the ototoxicity of tobramycin and the other aminoglycosides. *Assessment of Aminoglycoside Toxicity*. A Symposium Sponsored by Eli Lilly and Company as a Service to Physicians, p. 69. Bürgenstock, Switzerland, September 24–25, 1977.

Fee WE Jr (1983). Gentamicin and tobramycin: comparison of ototoxicity. *Rev Infect Dis* **5** (Suppl 2): 304.

Feig PU, Mitchell PP, Abrutyn E *et al.* (1982). Aminoglycoside nephrotoxicity: a double blind prospective randomized study of gentamicin and tobramycin. *J Antimicrob Chemother* **10**: 217.

Finland M, Garner C, Wilcox C, Sabath LD (1976). Susceptibility of 'Enterobacteria' to aminoglycoside antibiotics: comparison with tetracyclines, polymyxins, chloramphenicol, and spectinomycin. *J Infect Dis* **134** (Suppl): 57.

Follath F, Wenk M, Vozeh S (1981). Plasma concentration monitoring of aminoglycosides. *J Antimicrob Chemother* **8** (Suppl A): 37.

Friis B (1979). Chemotherapy of chronic infections with mucoid *Pseudomonas aeruginosa* in lower airways of patients with cystic fibrosis. *Scand J Infect Dis* **11**: 211.

Galimand M, Lambert T, Gerbaud G, Courvalin P (1993). Characterization of the aac(6').-Ib gene encoding an aminoglycoside 6'-N-acetyltransferase in *Pseudomonas aeruginosa* BM 2656. *Antimicrob Ag Chemother* **37**: 1456.

Gangadharam PRJ, Candler ER (1977). *In vitro* anti-mycobacterial activity of some new aminoglycoside antibiotics. *Tubercle* **58**: 35.

Gatell JM, Ferran F, Araujo V *et al.* (1987). Univariate and multivariate analyses of risk factors predisposing to auditory toxicity in patients receiving aminoglycosides. *Antimicrob Ag Chemother* **31**: 1383.

Geers TA, Baker NR (1987a). The effect of sublethal concentrations of aminoglycosides on adherence of *Pseudomonas aeruginosa* to hamster tracheal epithelium. *J Antimicrob Chemother* **19**: 561.

Geers TA, Baker NR (1987b). The effect of sublethal levels of antibiotics on the pathogenicity of *Pseudomonas aeruginosa* for tracheal tissue. *J Antimicrob Chemother* **19**: 569.

Gerding DN, Kromhout JP, Sullivan JJ, Hall WH (1976). Antibiotic penetrance of ascitic fluid in dogs. *Antimicrob Ag Chemother* **10**: 580.

Gerding DN, Hall WH, Schierl EA (1977). Antibiotic concentrations in ascitic fluid of patients with ascites and bacterial peritonitis. *Ann Intern Med* **86**: 708.

Gilbert DN (1991). Once-daily aminoglycoside therapy. *Antimicrob Ag Chemother* **35**: 399.

Gillett AP, Falk RH, Andrews J *et al.* (1976). Rapid intravenous injection of tobramycin: suggested dosage schedule and concentrations in serum. *J Infect Dis* **134** (Suppl): 110.

Gordon RC, Regamey C, Kirby WMM (1972). Serum protein binding of the aminoglycoside antibiotics. *Antimicrob Ag Chemother* **2**: 214.

Grimwood K, To M, Rabin HR, Woods DE (1989). Inhibition of *Pseudomonas aeruginosa* exoenzyme expression by subinhibitory antibiotic concentrations. *Antimicrob Ag Chemother* **33**: 41.

Guimaraes MA, Sage R, Noone P (1985). The comparative activity of aminocyclitol antibiotics against 773 aerobic Gram-negative rods and staphylococci isolated from hospitalized patients. *J Antimicrob Chemother* **16**: 555.

Gutschik E, Jepsen OB, Mortensen I (1977). Effect of combinations of penicillin and aminoglycosides on *Streptococcus faecalis*: a comparative study of seven aminoglycoside antibiotics. *J Infect Dis* **135**: 832.

Hammerberg S, Sorger S, Marks MI (1977). Antimicrobial susceptibilities of *Yersinia enterocolitica* Biotype 4, Serotype 0: 3. *Antimicrob Ag Chemother* **11**: 566.

Herscovici L, Grise G, Thauvin C *et al.* (1988). Efficacy and safety of once daily versus intermittent dosing of tobramycin in rabbits with acute pyelonephritis. *Scand J Infect Dis* **20**: 205.

Hoecker JL, Pickering LK, Swaney J *et al.* (1978). Clinical pharmacology of tobramycin in children. *J Infect Dis* **137**: 592.

Houang ET, McKay-Ferguson E (1976). Activities of tobramycin and amikacin against gentamicin-resistant Gram-negative bacilli. *Lancet* **i**: 423.

Ishiyama S, Nakayama I, Iwamoto H *et al.* (1976). Clinical use of tobramycin in patients with surgical infections due to Gram-negative bacilli. *J Infect Dis* **134** (Suppl): 178.

Jacobs RF, McCarthy RE, Elser JM (1989). *Pseudomonas osteochondritis* complicating puncture wounds of the foot in children: a 10-year evaluation. *J Infect Dis* **160**: 657.

Jacoby GA, Blaser MJ, Santanam P *et al.* (1990). Appearance of amikacin and tobramycin resistance due to 4'-aminoglycoside nucleotidyltransferase [ANT(4').-II] in Gram-negative pathogens. *Antimicrob Ag Chemother* **34**: 2381.

Jaffe G, Meyers BR, Hirschman SZ (1974). Pharmacokinetics of tobramycin in patients with stable renal impairment, patients undergoing peritoneal dialysis, and patients on chronic hemodialysis. *Antimicrob Ag Chemother* **5**: 611.

Joly V, Bergeron Y, Bergeron MG, Carbon C (1991). Endotoxin-tobramycin additive toxicity on renal proximal tubular cells in culture. *Antimicrob Ag Chemother* **35**: 351.

Jordan GW, Hoeprich PD (1977). Susceptibility of three groups of *Staphylococcus aureus* to newer antimicrobial agents. *Antimicrob Ag Chemother* **11**: 7.

Kahlmeter G (1979). Gentamicin and tobramycin Clinical pharmacokinetics and nephrotoxicity. Aspects of assay techniques. *Scand J Infect Dis* (Suppl 18): 7.

Kahlmeter G, Dahlager JI (1984). Aminoglycoside toxicity – a review of clinical studies published between 1975 and 1982. *J Antimicrob Chemother* **13** (Suppl A): 9.

Kaiser AB, McGee ZA (1975). Aminoglycoside therapy of Gram-negative bacillary meningitis. *New Engl J Med* **293**: 1215.

Kapusnik JE, Sande MA (1986). Novel approaches for the use of aminoglycosides: the value of experimental models. *J Antimicrob Chemother* **17** (Suppl A): 7.

Kapusnik JE, Hackbarth CJ, Chambers HF *et al* (1988). Single, large, daily dosing versus intermittent dosing of tobramycin for treating experimental *Pseudomonas* pneumonia. *J Infect Dis* **158**: 7.

King CH, Creger RJ, Ellner JJ (1985). Pharmacokinetics of tobramycin and gentamicin in abusers of intravenous drugs. *Antimicrob Ag Chemother* **27**: 285.

Kirby MG, Dasta JF, Armstrong DK (1986). Effect of low-dose dopamine on the pharmacokinetics of tobramycin in dogs. *Antimicrob Ag Chemother* **29**: 168.

Klastersky J, Hensgens C, Henri A, Daneau D (1974). Comparative clinical study of tobramycin and gentamicin. *Antimicrob Ag Chemother* **5**: 133.

Klastersky J Hensgens C, Debusscher L (1975). Empiric therapy for cancer patients: comparative study of ticarcillin-tobramycin, ticarcillin-cephalothin, and cephalothin-tobramycin. *Antimicrob Ag Chemother* **7**: 640.

Klastersky J, Thys JP, Mombelli G (1981). Comparative studies of intermittent and continuous administration of aminoglycosides in the treatment of bronchopulmonary infections due to Gram-negative bacteria. *Rev Infect Dis* **3**: 74.

Kluge RM, Standiford HC, Tatem B *et al.* (1974). Comparative activity of tobramycin, amikacin and gentamicin alone and with carbenicillin against *Pseudomonas aeruginosa. Antimicrob Ag Chemother* **6**: 442.

Korvick JA, Yu VL (1991). Antimicrobial agent therapy for *Pseudomonas aeruginosa. Antimicrob Ag Chemother* **35**: 2167.

Larson TA, Garrett CR, Gerding DN (1986). Frequency of aminoglycoside 6'-N-acetyltransferase among *Serratia* species during increased use of amikacin in the hospital. *Antimicrob Ag Chemother* **30**: 176.

Lerner AM, Reyes MP, Cone LA *et al.* (1983). Randomised, controlled trial of the comparative efficacy, auditory toxicity, and nephrotoxicity of tobramycin and netilmicin. *Lancet* **i**: 1123.

Levy J, Smith AL, Koup JR *et al.* (1984). Disposition of tobramycin in patients with cystic fibrosis: a prospective controlled study. *J Pediatr* **105**: 117.

Levy J, Burns JL, Mendelman PM *et al.* (1986). Effect of tobramycin on protein synthesis in 2-deoxystreptamine aminoglycoside-resistant clinical isolates of *Haemophilus influenzae. Antimicrob Ag Chemother* **29**: 474.

Li SC, Bowes G, Ionnides-Demos LL *et al.* (1991). Dosage adjustment and clinical outcomes of long-term use of high-dose tobramycin in adult cystic fibrosis patients. *J Antimicrob Chemother* **28**: 561.

Lietman PS, Smith CR (1983). Aminoglycoside nephrotoxicity in humans. *Rev Infect Dis* **5** (Suppl 2): 284.

Lilliestierna H, Alestig K, Holm S (1985). Tobramycin therapy – two or three doses per day? *Scand J Infect Dis* **17**: 323.

Lin L, Grenier L, Bergeron Y *et al.* (1994). Temporal changes of pharmacokinetics, nephrotoxicity, and subcellular distribution of tobramycin in rats. *Antimicrob Ag Chemother* **38**: 54.

Lockwood WR, Bower JD (1973). Tobramycin and gentamicin concentrations in the serum of normal and anephric patients. *Antimicrob Ag Chemother* **3**: 125.

Lode H, Kemmerich B, Koeppe P (1975). Comparative clinical pharmacology of gentamicin, sisomicin and tobramycin. *Antimicrob Ag Chemother* **8**: 396.

Luft FC, Kleit SA (1974). Renal parenchymal accumulation of aminoglycoside antibiotics in rats. *J Infect Dis* **130**: 656.

Luft FC, Bennett WH, Gilbert DN (1983). Experimental aminoglycoside nephrotoxicity: accomplishments and future potential. *Rev Infect Dis* **5** (Suppl 2): 268.

Lyon MD, Smith KR, Saag MS *et al.* (1986). *In vitro* activity of piperacillin, ticarcillin, and mezlocillin alone and in combination with aminoglycosides against *Pseudomonas aeruginosa. Antimicrob Ag Chemother* **30**: 25.

Maes P (1985). Evaluation of the resistance mechanisms of gentamicin-resistant Gram-negative bacilli and their susceptibility to tobramycin, netilmicin and amikacin. *J Antimicrob Chemother* **15**: 283.

Malacoff RF, Finkelstein FO, Andriole VT (1975). Effect of peritoneal dialysis on serum levels of tobramycin and clindamycin. *Antimicrob Ag Chemother* **8**: 574.

Marks MI (1984). Pharmacokinetics of tobramycin in neonates. *J Pediatr* **104**: 160.

Marks MI, Hammerberg S, Greenstone G, Silver B (1976). Activity of newer aminoglycosides and carbenicillin alone and in combination against gentamicin-resistant *Pseudomonas aeruginosa. Antimicrob Ag Chemother* **10**: 399.

Mawer GE, Ahmad R, Dobbs SM *et al.* (1974). Prescribing aids for gentamicin. *Brit J Clin Pharmacol* **1**: 45.

McCartney CF, Hatley LH, Kessler JM (1982). Possible tobramycin delirium. *JAMA* **247**: 1319.

McCracken GH Jr, Nelson JD (1983). *Antimicrobial Therapy for Newborns* 2nd edn, p. 57. New York, London: Grune & Stratton.

McCrae WM, Raeburn JA, Hanson EJ (1976). Tobramycin therapy of infections due to *Pseudomonas aeruginosa* in patients with cystic fibrosis: effect of dosage and concentration of antibiotic in sputum. *J Infect Dis* **134** (Suppl): 191.

McRorie TI, Bosso J, Randolph L (1989). Aminoglycoside ototoxicity in cystic fibrosis. *Am J Dis Child* **143**: 1328.

Menard R, Molinas C, Arthur M *et al.* (1993). Overproduction of 3'-aminoglycoside phosphotransferase type I confers resistance to tobramycin in *Escherichia coli. Antimicrob Ag Chemother* **37**: 78.

Mendelman PM, Smith AL, Levy J *et al.* (1985). Aminoglycoside penetration, inactivation and efficacy in cystic fibrosis sputum. *Amer Rev Respir Dis* **132**: 761.

Meyer RD, Lewis RP, Halter J, White M (1976). Gentamicin-resistant *Pseudomonas aeruginosa* and *Serratia marcescens* in a general hospital. *Lancet* **i**: 580.

Moellering RC Jr (1977). Microbiological considerations in the use of tobramycin and related aminoglycosidic aminocyclitol antibiotics. *Med J Aust* **2** (Suppl): 4.

Moellering RC Jr (1983). *In vitro* antibacterial activity of the aminoglycoside antibiotics. *Rev Infect Dis* **5** (Suppl 2): 212.

Moellering RC Jr, Wennersten C, Kunz LJ (1976). Emergence of gentamicin-resistant bacteria: experience with tobramycin therapy of infections due to gentamicin-resistant organisms. *J Infect Dis* **134** (Suppl): 40.

Moellering RC Jr, Murray BE, Schoenbaum SC *et al.* (1980). A novel mechanism of resistance to penicillin-gentamicin synergism in *Streptococcus faecalis. J Infect Dis* **141**: 81.

Mukhopadhyay S, Baer S, Blanshard J *et al.* (1993). Assessment of potential ototoxicity following high-dose nebulized tobramycin in patients with cystic fibrosis. *J Antimicrob Chemother* **31**: 429.

Naber KG, Westenfelder SR, Masden PO (1973). Pharmacokinetics of the aminoglycoside antibiotic tobramycin in humans. *Antimicrob Ag Chemother* **3**: 469.

Nahata MC, Powell DA, Gregoire RP *et al.* (1983). Tobramycin kinetics in newborn infants. *J Pediatr* **103**: 136.

Nahata MC, Powell DA, Durrell DE *et al.* (1984a). Effect of gestational age and birth weight on tobramycin kinetics in newborn infants. *J Antimicrob Chemother* **14**: 59.

Nahata MC, Powell DA, Durrell DB *et al.* (1984b). Effect of infusion methods on tobramycin serum concentrations in newborn infants. *J Pediatr* **104**: 136.

Neu HC (1977). The pharmacology of newer aminoglycosides, with a consideration of the application to clinical situations. *Med J Aust* **2** (Suppl): 13.

Neu HC, Bendush CL (1976). Ototoxicity of tobramycin: a clinical overview. *J Infect Dis* **134** (Suppl): 206.

Nilsson L, Sören L, Rådberg G (1987). Frequencies of variants resistant to diffferent aminoglycosides in *Pseudomonas aeruginosa. J Antimicrob Chemother* **20**: 255.

Olson B, Weinstein RA, Nathan C *et al.* (1985). Occult aminoglycoside resistance in *Pseudomonas aeruginosa*: epidemiology and implications for therapy and control. *J Infect Dis* **152**: 769.

Omri A, Beaulac C, Bouhajib M *et al.* (1994). Pulmonary retention of free and liposome-encapsulated tobramycin after intrathecal administration in uninfected rats and rats infected with *Pseudomonas aeruginosa. Antimicrob Ag Chemother* **38**: 1090.

Park MK, Muhvich KH, Myers RAM, Marzella L (1991). Hyperoxia prolongs the aminoglycoside-induced postantibiotic effect in *Pseudomonas aeruginosa. Antimicrob Ag Chemother* **35**: 691.

Parr TR Jr, Bayer AS (1988). Mechanisms of aminoglycoside resistance in variants of *Pseudomonas aeruginosa* isolated during treatment of experimental endocarditis in rabbits *J Infect Dis* **158**: 1003.

Pedersen SS, Jensen T, Osterhammel D, Osterhammel P (1987). Cumulative and acute toxicity of repeated high-dose tobramycin treatment in cystic fibrosis. *Antimicrob Ag Chemother* **31**: 594.

Penner JL, Preston MA (1980). Differences among *Providencia* species in their *in vitro* susceptibilities to five antibiotics. *Antimicrob Ag Chemother* **18**: 868.

Penner JL, Preston MA, Hennessy JN *et al.* (1982). Species differences in susceptibilities of *Proteeae* spp. to six cephalosporins and three aminoglycosides. *Antimicrob Ag Chemother* **22**: 218.

Pennington JE, Reynolds HY (1973). Tobramycin in bronchial secretions. *Antimicrob Ag Chemother* **4**: 299.

Pennington JE, Stone RM (1979). Comparison of antibiotic regimens for treatment of experimental pneumonia due to *Pseudomonas. J Infect Dis* **140**: 881.

Perkins BA, Strausbaugh LJ (1983). Effect of mannitol infusions into the internal carotid artery on entry of two antibiotics into the cerebrospinal fluid and brains of normal rabbits. *Antimicrob Ag Chemother* **24**: 339.

Perkins RL, Saslaw S, Fass RJ *et al.* (1976). Tobramycin: *in vitro* and clinical evaluation in 30 patients. *Amer J Med Sci* **271**: 297.

Petty BG, Baumgardner JY, Lietman PS (1986). Comparison of renal effects of single vs thrice daily dosing of tobramycin in healthy volunteers. In *Abstracts and Program of the 26th Interscience Conference on Antimicrobial Agents and Chemotherapy, New Orleans* (Abstr. 30). Washington, DC: American Society for Microbiology.

Potel G, Chau NP, Pangon B *et al.* (1991). Single daily dosing of antibiotics: importance of *in vitro* killing rate, serum half-life, and protein binding. *Antimicrob Ag Chemother* **35**: 2085.

Powell SH, Thompson WL, Luthe MA *et al.* (1983). Once-daily vs. continuous aminoglycoside dosing: efficacy and toxicity in animal and clinical studies of gentamicin, netilmicin and tobramycin. *J Infect Dis* **147**: 918.

Poyner EA, Alpar HO, Brown MRW (1994). Preparation, properties and the effects of free and liposomal tobramycin on siderophore production by *Pseudomonas aeruginosa. J Antimicrob Chemother* **34**: 43.

Preston DA, Wick WE (1971). Preclinical assessment of the antibacterial activity of nebramycin factor 6. *Antimicrob Ag Chemother* **1970**: 322.

Price KE, Kresel PA, Farchione LA *et al.* (1981). Epidemiological studies of aminoglycoside resistance in the USA. *J Antimicrob Chemother* **8** (Suppl A): 89.

Ramsey BW, Dorkin HL, Eisenberg JD *et al.* (1993). Efficacy of aerosolized tobramycin in patients with cystic fibrosis. *New Engl J Med* **328**: 1740.

Rescott DL, Nix DE, Holden P, Schentag JJ (1988). Comparison of two methods for determining *in vitro* postantibiotic effects of three antibiotics on *Escherichia coli. Antimicrob Ag Chemother* **32**: 450.

Reynolds AV, Hamilton-Miller JMT, Brumfitt W (1974). Newer aminoglycosides – amikacin and tobramycin: an *in vitro* comparison with kanamycin and gentamicin. *Brit Med J* **3**: 778.

Ristuccia AM, Cunha BA (1982). The aminoglycosides. *Med Clin N Amer* **66**: 303.

Rusnak MG, Drake TA, Hackbarth CJ, Sande MA (1984). Single versus combination antibiotic therapy for pneumonia due to *Pseudomonas aeruginosa* in neutropenic guinea pigs. *J Infect Dis* **149**: 980.

Rybak MJ, Boike SC, Levine DP, Erickson SR (1986). Clinical use and toxicity of high-dose tobramycin in patients with pseudomonal endocarditis. *J Antimicrob Chemother* **17**: 115.

Sabra R, Branch RA (1990). Role of sodium in protection by extended-spectrum penicillins against tobramycin-induced nephrotoxicity. *Antimicrob Ag Chemother* **34**: 1020.

Sacchi F, Marseglia G, Fietta A *et al.* (1981). Effects of aminoglycoside antibiotics on neutrophil chemotaxis. *Antimicrob Ag Chemother* **20**: 258.

Saslaw S, Carlisle HN, Moheimani M (1972). Comparison of tobramycin, gentamicin, colistin, and carbenicillin in *Pseudomonas* sepsis in monkeys. *Antimicrob Ag Chemother* **2**: 164,.

Schentag JJ, Lasezkay G, Cumbo TJ *et al.* (1978). Accumulation pharmacokinetics of tobramycin. *Antimicrob Ag Chemother* **13**: 649.

Schiff JB, Pennington JE (1984). Comparative efficacies of piperacillin, azlocillin, ticarcillin, aztreonam and tobramycin against experimental *Pseudomonas aeruginosa* pneumonia. *Antimicrob Ag Chemother* **25**: 49.

Seligman SJ (1978). Frequency of resistance to kanamycin, tobramycin, netilmicin and amikacin in gentamicin-resistant Gram-negative bacteria. *Antimicrob Ag Chemother* **13**: 70.

Setia U, Gross PA (1976). Administration of tobramycin and gentamicin by the intravenous route every 6 h in patients with normal renal function. *J Infect Dis* **134** (Suppl): 125.

Shalit I, Welch DF, San Joaquin VH, Marks MI (1985). *In vitro* antibacterial activities of antibiotics against *Pseudomonas aeruginosa* in peritoneal dialysis fluid. *Antimicrob Ag Chemother* **27**: 908.

Shaw KJ, Rather PN, Hare RS, Miller GH (1993). Molecular genetics of aminoglycoside resistance genes and familial relationships of the aminoglycoside-modifying enzymes. *Microbiol Rev* **57**: 138.

Simon VK, Mösinger EU, Malerczy V (1973). Pharmacokinetic studies of tobramycin and gentamicin. *Antimicrob Ag Chemother* **3**: 445.

Smith CR, Lipsky JJ, Laskin OL *et al.* (1980). Double-blind comparison of the nephrotoxicity and auditory toxicity of gentamicin and tobramycin. *New Engl J Med* **302**: 1106.

Summer WR, Michael JR, Lipsky JJ (1983). Initial aminoglycoside levels in the critically ill. *Crit Care Med* **11**: 948.

Tablan OC, Reyes MP, Rintelmann WF, Lerner AM (1984). Renal and auditory toxicity of high-dose, prolonged therapy with gentamicin and tobramycin in *Pseudomonas endocarditis. J Infect Dis* **149**: 257.

Tan JS, Salstrom SJ (1977). Levels of carbenicillin, ticarcillin, cephalothin, cefazolin, cefamandole, gentamicin, tobramycin and amikacin in human serum and interstitial fluid. *Antimicrob Ag Chemother* **11**: 698.

Thornsberry C, Baker CN, Kirven LA (1978). *In vitro* activity of antimicrobial agents on Legionnaires' disease bacterium. *Antimicrob Ag Chemother* **13**: 78.

Tobias JS, Whitehouse JM, Wrigley PFM (1976). Severe renal dysfunction after tobramycin/cephalothin therapy. *Lancet* **i**: 425.

Tobias JS, Wrigley PFM, Korde S, Shaw EJ (1977). Nomogram-assisted dosage of tobramycin. *J Antimicrob Chemother* **3**: 305.

Uwaydah M, Taqi-Eddin A (1976). Susceptibility of non-fermentative Gram-negative bacilli to tobramycin. *J Infect Dis* **134** (Suppl): 28.

Van der Auwera P, Schuyteneer F (1983). *In-vitro* susceptibility of *Pseudomonas aeruginosa* to old and new beta-lactam antibiotics and aminoglycosides. *J Antimicrob Chemother* **11**: 511.

Verbist L, Vandepitte J, Vandeven J (1978). Activity of eight aminoglycosides against isolates of *Serratia marcescens* from four hospitals. *J Antimicrob Chemother* **4**: 47.

Vogel L, Nathan C, Sweeney HM *et al.* (1978). Infections due to gentamicin-resistant *Staphylococcus aureus* strain in a nursery for neonatal infants. *Antimicrob Ag Chemother* **13**: 466.

Walshe JJ, Morse GD, Janicke DM, Apicella MA (1986). Crossover pharmacokinetic analysis comparing intravenous and intraperitoneal administration of tobramycin. *J Infect Dis* **153**: 796.

Waterworth PM (1972). The *in vitro* activity of tobramycin compared with that of other aminoglycosides. *J Clin Path* **25**: 979.

Weinstein AJ, Karchmer AW, Moellering RC Jr (1973). Tobramycin concentrations during peritoneal dialysis. *Antimicrob Ag Chemother* **4**: 432.

Whelton A, Carter GG, Craig TJ *et al.* (1978). Comparison of the intrarenal disposition of tobramycin and gentamicin: therapeutic and toxicologic answers. *J Antimicrob Chemother* **4** (Suppl): 13.

Wilson P, Ramsden RT (1977). Immediate effects of tobramycin on human cochlea and correlation with serum tobramycin levels. *Brit Med J* **1**: 259.

Winslade NE, Adelman MH, Evans EJ, Schentag JJ (1987). Single-dose accumulation pharmacokinetics of tobramycin and netilmicin in normal volunteers. *Antimicrob Ag Chemother* **31**: 605.

Wood CA, Kohlhepp SJ, Kohnen PW *et al.* (1986). Vancomycin enhancement of experimental tobramycin nephrotoxicity. *Antimicrob Ag Chemother* **30**: 20.

Wood CA, Norton DR, Kohlhepp SJ *et al.* (1988). The influence of tobramycin dosage regimens on nephrotoxicity, ototoxicity, and anti-bacterial efficacy in a rat model of subcutaneous abscess. *J Infect Dis* **158**: 13.

Wretlind B, Nord CE, Wadström T (1974). *In vitro* sensitivity of isolates of *Pseudomonas aeruginosa* to carbenicillin, gentamicin, tobramycin, and some other antibiotics. *Scand J Infect Dis* **6**: 49.

Amikacin

Description

Amikacin is a semisynthetic aminoglycoside aminocyclitol antibiotic (p.428). It was derived from kanamycin A by acetylation with an S-4-amino-2-hydroxybutyryl (AHB) side-chain at the 1-position of its deoxystreptamine moiety (Kawaguchi, 1976; Pien and Ho, 1981). The drug is almost identical with kanamycin (p.439) in its physical, chemical, pharmacologic and toxicologic properties (Cabana and Taggart, 1973; Hewitt and Young, 1977). However, it has an *in vitro* antibacterial spectrum which is broader than that of kanamycin, gentamicin (p.450) and tobramycin (p.489) (Ries *et al.*, 1973; Meyer, 1981). The presence of the AHB side-chain gives amikacin stability against most of the bacterial plasmid-mediated enzymes, which are responsible for resistance to aminoglycosides (p.453). For this reason, amikacin is active against many gentamicin- and tobramycin-resistant Gram-negative bacilli (Price *et al.*, 1976; Davies and Courvalin, 1977; Gerding and Larson, 1985; Maes, 1985).

Sensitive Organisms

1 Gram-negative bacteria

Amikacin is active against all the Enterobacteriaceae such as *Escherichia coli*, the *Enterobacter*, *Klebsiella*, all *Proteus*, *Salmonella*, *Shigella*, *Providencia*, *Serratia*, *Citrobacter*, *Hafnia*, *Edwardsiella*, *Arizona* and *Yersinia* spp. (Drasar *et al.*, 1976; Kawaguchi, 1976; Hammerberg *et al.*, 1977; Schiffman, 1977; Ball and Gray, 1979; Moellering, 1983; Kwaga and Iversen, 1990).

Pseudomonas aeruginosa is amikacin-sensitive (Davies and Courvalin, 1977; Van der Auwera and Schuyteneer, 1983; Williams *et al.*, 1984). Usually *Ps. stutzeri* and *Ps. fluorescens* are susceptible, but *Burkholderia* (*Pseudomonas*) *cepacia* and *Stenotrophomonas maltophilia* are more commonly resistant (Price *et al.*, 1976; Moellering *et al.*, 1977).

Amikacin, like kanamycin (p.439) is quite active against the *Neisseria* spp. (meningococci and gonococci) and *Haemophilus influenzae* (Phillips *et al.*, 1977). *Pasteurella multocida* is susceptible (Yu and Washington, 1973). *Acinetobacter calcoaceticus* (now referred to as *A. baumanii*), the *Alcaligenes* and *Aeromonas* spp. are usually amikacin-sensitive, but resistant strains occur (Yu and Washington, 1973; Drasar *et al.*, 1976; Phillips *et al.*, 1977; Bergogne Berezin and Joly-Guillou, 1985; Harris *et al.*, 1985). *Acinetobacter* spp. strains can become amikacin-resistant due to chromosomal- or plasmid-mediated production of the aminoglycoside modifying enzymes, 6' aminoglycoside acetyltransferase (AAC-6') or 3'- aminoglycoside phosphotransferase (APH-3') (Lambert *et al.*, 1988; Shaw *et al.*, 1993; Lambert *et al.*, 1994a,b; Ploy *et al.*, 1994). *Flavobacterium* spp. are amikacin-resistant (Drasar *et al.*, 1976). *Legionella pneumophila* is sensitive to amikacin *in vitro* (Thornsberry *et al.*, 1978). Both *Campylobacter jejuni* and *C. fetus* are amikacin-sensitive, similar to gentamicin (p.452).

In common with other aminoglycosides, amikacin is inactive against *Bacteroides fragilis* and most other anaerobic Gram-negative bacteria. The uptake of aminoglycosides by bacteria is an active process requiring oxygen, which cannot occur in anaerobes (p.453) (Moellering, 1977).

2 Gentamicin- and tobramycin-resistant Gram-negative bacteria

The most important feature of amikacin is that it is active against many strains of the Enterobacteriaceae and also a considerable proportion of those of *Ps. aeruginosa*, which have acquired resistance to gentamicin and/or other aminoglycosides. Many early surveys showed that most gentamicin-resistant Enterobacteriaceae (>80%) and a smaller percentage of gentamicin-resistant *Ps. aeruginosa* strains (25–85%) were amikacin-sensitive (Acar *et al.*, 1976; Houang and McKay-Ferguson, 1976; Meyer *et al.*, 1976; Moellering *et al.*, 1977; Seligman, 1978; Price *et al.*, 1981; Gerding and Larson, 1985; Guimaraes *et al.*, 1985; Maes, 1985; Bengtsson *et al.*, 1986).

Resistance of Enterobacteriaceae and *Ps. aeruginosa* to aminoglycosides is usually due to the production of aminoglycoside-modifying enzymes, which act on the antibiotic in the outer layers of the bacterial cell (p.453). These enzymes do not inactivate the antibiotic but inhibit its transport into the cell (p.453). Enzyme modification of aminoglycosides occurs mainly by either acetylation, adenylylation or phosphorylation. Gram-negative bacteria produce many different enzymes, but only three, aminoglycoside 6'-acetyltransferase (AAC-6'), 3'- aminoglycoside phosphotransferase (APH-3') and 4'- aminoglycoside adenylyltransferase (ANT-4') determine resistance to amikacin in clinical isolates (p.454). The genes coding for production of these three enzymes are usually located in plasmids, but they may also reside in the chromosome or on transposons (Sanders and Watanakunakorn, 1986; Tolmasky *et al.*, 1986; 1988; Tolmasky and Crosa, 1987; Champion *et al.*, 1988; Gaynes *et al.*, 1988; Van Nhieu and Collatz, 1988; Jacoby *et al.*, 1990; Hopkins *et al.*, 1991; Lambert *et al.*, 1990, 1993, 1994a). Amikacin's AHB side-chain (p.504) prevents its modification by the majority of plasmid-coded enzymes that determine resistance to other antibiotics. In contrast to amikacin, at least nine enzymes affect gentamicin and ten affect tobramycin (p.489). Greater resistance to enzymes is why many Gram-negative bacilli resistant to gentamicin and other aminoglycosides, are still amikacin-sensitive.

3 Acquired resistance of Gram-negative bacteria

Strains of these bacteria resistant to amikacin were detected in early surveys; some of them might have been naturally occurring and others had acquired resistance. Jauregui *et al.* (1977) in a 10-month survey, detected 37 (0.8%) of 4640 strains of Gram-negative bacilli in one general hospital which were amikacin-resistant. These isolates comprised *Ps. aeruginosa* (6), *Burkholderia* (*Pseudomonas*) *cepacia* (13) other *Pseudomonas* spp. (1) *Serratia marcescens* (6) and other Enterobacteriaceae (11). Moellering *et al.* (1977) surveyed 46 000 isolates of Gram-negative bacilli during a 2-year period in another hospital, and found a small percentage of amikacin-resistant bacteria. The majority of these were *Acinetobacter* and *Flavobacterium* spp. and *S. maltophilia*, but there were also amikacin-resistant strains of *Ps. aeruginosa* and most Enterobacteriaceae.

There have been a number of reports of the emergence of amikacin-resistant organisms during treatment. Over a 2-year period in a burns center Minshew *et al.* (1977) described the appearance of a number of isolates of *E. coli*, *Klebsiella pneumoniae* and *Ps. aeruginosa* with increased resistance to gentamicin, tobramycin and amikacin. In one patient with *Ps. aeruginosa* bronchopneumonia, an amikacin-resistant strain emerged after only 4 days treatment with the drug (Amirak *et al.*, 1977). Amikacin was used to treat 19 patients with gentamicin-resistant *S. marcescens* infections by Craven *et al.* (1977). In four patients with pneumonia or other deep tissue infections, in whom the infection failed to clear promptly, *Serratia* spp. strains became increasingly resistant to amikacin during therapy. In one patient with *Serratia* septicemia, who was treated by ticarcillin/tobramycin and later by cefazolin/gentamicin, the *Serratia* spp. strain became resistant to multiple drugs, including amikacin. The strains showed both alteration of outer membrane proteins and development of AAC-6' activity (p.454) (Sanders and Watanakunakorn, 1986). Increased resistance of Enterobacteriaceae and *Ps. aeruginosa* to amikacin was also reported in neonatal units following increased amikacin usage (Garcia *et al.*, 1989; Friedland *et al.*, 1992).

Because of the above observations, there is an opinion that the use of amikacin should be restricted (p.515), but in some hospitals in the USA, where gentamicin-resistant Gram-negative bacilli had become widespread, amikacin was used as the major unrestricted aminoglycoside for long periods. In some of these hospitals there was no increase of amikacin-resistant strains. In other hospitals the frequency of amikacin-resistant strains increased only marginally over a range of 1.2–1.8% during periods of 1–13 years of usage (Gerding and Larson, 1985; Shulman and Yogev, 1985; Young, 1985; Larson *et al.*, 1986; Powell and Pincus, 1987; Gerding *et al.*, 1991; Muscato *et al.*, 1991; King *et al.*, 1992). This has not been the experience in all hospitals. In one hospital in Chile, during a 9-month period when amikacin was the sole aminoglycoside used clinically, resistance to it was encountered in 42 strains of Enterobacteriaceae. This resistance was mediated by a transferable plasmid, which encoded for the production of 6' aminoglycoside acetyltransferase (AAC-6'), (p.454) (Van Nhieu *et al.*, 1986). In one US hospital the incidence of amikacin-resistance among Gram-negative bacilli increased from 2% to >7% during an 18-month period which coincided with a 3-fold increase in amikacin use. Resistance occurred most frequently amongst strains of *Klebsiella*, *Serratia* and *Pseudomonas* spp., and AAC-6' was detected in some 67% of them. It was concluded that amikacin-resistance is enhanced by its increased usage (Levine *et al.*, 1985).

Instead of modification by enzymes, some bacteria are resistant to amikacin by a different mechanism, presumably due to increase in the permeability barrier to the drug (p.453). This resistance is not plasmid-mediated and not transferable. Such amikacin-resistant Gram-negative bacilli are usually resistant to all other aminoglycosides (p.453) and the resistance is usually of low-level (p.453) (Moellering *et al.*, 1977; Olson *et al.*, 1985; Clark *et al.*, 1988). This resistance is sometimes associated with the acquisition of plasmids which code for the production of one of the phosphotransferases (APH-3') (p.454). With this combination high-level amikacin-resistance in *E. coli* strains may result. These amikacin-resistant strains may emerge not only as a result of exposure to amikacin, but also because of exposure to relatively low levels of gentamicin, the main aminoglycoside used in hospitals where amikacin use is restricted (Perlin and Lerner, 1979; 1986; Bongaerts and Kaptijn, 1981; Woloj *et al.*, 1986).

4 Gram-positive bacteria

Staphylococcus aureus and *Staph. epidermidis*, including penicillin G-resistant strains of both are usually amikacin-sensitive. Methicillin-resistant strains of these organisms may be amikacin-sensitive, but many isolates from hospitals are resistant (p.80) (Guimaraes *et al.*, 1985). Amikacin resistance in staphylococci is usually mediated by plasmids which code for amikacin-modifying enzymes such as 4-adenylyltransferase, 3'-phosphotransferase and 6' acetyltransferase (p.454) (Courvalin and Davies, 1977; Davies and Courvalin, 1977; Neu, 1984; Ubukata *et al.*, 1984). Gentamicin-resistant *Staph. aureus* strains (p.454) may be amikacin-sensitive, but often their MICs for amikacin are 4- to 8-fold higher than those for fully susceptible strains (Vogel *et al.*, 1978).

Other Gram-positive cocci, such as *Streptococcus pyogenes*, *Strep. pneumoniae* and *Enterococcus faecalis*, are amikacin-resistant (Schiffman, 1977; Hewitt and Young, 1977). The combination of penicillin G and amikacin does not act synergistically against many *E. faecalis* strains. If a penicillin G/kanamycin (p.440) combination is not synergistic against a particular *E. faecalis* strain, then this also applies to penicillin G/amikacin (Basker *et al.*, 1977; Calderwood *et al.*, 1977; Gutschik *et al.*, 1977). The absence of synergy by penicillin G/amikacin against *E. faecalis* is due to the production of plasmid-mediated amikacin-modifying enzymes such as 3'-phosphotransferase (Calderwood *et al.*, 1981). Amikacin can actually antagonize the bactericidal effect of penicillin G against *E. faecalis* strains which produce this enzyme (Thauvin *et al.*, 1985).

Nocardia asteroides is amikacin-sensitive, most strains being inhibited by 0.5–1.0 µg per ml (Gutmann *et al.*, 1983; Gombert *et al.*, 1986). Other aerobic *Actinomycetes* such as *N. brasiliensis*, *Actinomadura madurae* and *Streptomyces griseus* are also amikacin sensitive (Boiron and Provost, 1988; McNeil *et al.*, 1990). Gram-positive anaerobic bacilli, such as *Clostridium* and *Actinomyces* spp., are amikacin-resistant, similar to other anaerobes (p.504).

6 Mycobacteria

Mycobacterium tuberculosis is amikacin-sensitive (Gangadharam and Candler, 1977; Sanders *et al.*, 1982; Heifets and Lindholm-Levy, 1989). Approximately 50% of *M. fortuitum* strains and a proportion of those of *M. chelonae* are also susceptible to clinically attainable amikacin concentrations (Dalovisio and Pankey, 1978; Wallace *et al.*, 1979a; Swenson *et al.*, 1982; Ingram *et al.*, 1993). There are three biovariants of *M. fortuitum* and two of *M. chelonae*. These subgroups vary in their susceptibility to amikacin and other antimicrobial agents, so that susceptibility testing is necessary to select appropriate regimens for treatment of infections by these bacteria (Swenson *et al.*, 1985). Usually *M. marinum* is amikacin-sensitive (Sanders and Wolinsky, 1980; Wallace and Wiss, 1981); *M. kansasii* is usually resistant and its MICs are usually higher than 12.8 µg per ml (Sanders *et al.*, 1982).

Mycobacterium avium complex is usually susceptible, most strains having an MIC of 16 µg per ml or lower. The MICs of amikacin for this organism, however, differ according to the laboratory method used. The MBCs are also considerably higher than MICs and they range from 32 to 256 µg per ml (Inderlied *et al.*, 1987; Yajko *et al.*, 1987; Bermudez and Young, 1988; Heifets, 1988; Khardori *et al.*, 1989). Amikacin also appears active against this organism under simulated *in vivo* conditions (Gangadharam *et al.*, 1988a). Liposome-encapsulated amikacin may augment the intracellular killing of *M. avium* complex (Bermudez *et al.*, 1987). *Mycobacterium*

Organism	MIC (µg per ml)
Gram-negative bacteria	
Escherichia coli	1.6–3.1
Klebsiella spp.	1.6–3.1
Enterobacter spp.	1.6–6.3
Serratia marcescens	0.8–3.1
Proteus mirabilis	3.1
Proteus vulgaris	1.6
Morganella morganii	3.1
Providencia rettgeri	1.6
Providencia stuartii	0.8–3.1
Pseudomonas aeruginosa	1.6–12.5
Gram-positive bacteria	
Staphylococcus aureus	0.4–3.1
Streptococcus pyogenes	12.5
Mycobacteria	
Mycobacterium tuberculosis	0.6

Table I.40
After Kawaguchi (1976)

haemophilum, which causes cutaneous lesions in immunosuppressed patients, may be sensitive to amikacin *in vivo*, if it is combined with other antibiotics such as rifampicin and ciprofloxacin (Straus *et al.*, 1994). An unclassified *Mycobacterium* spp. which was isolated from three patients with Crohn's disease, was sensitive to amikacin and kanamycin (Chiodini *et al.*, 1984). Amikacin is bactericidal to *M. leprae* in the mouse foot-pad model, provided that a high daily dose of 100 mg per kg body weight is used. Similar to kanamycin (p.441), amikacin is not useful for the treatment of human leprosy (Gelber *et al.*, 1984).

7 Minimum inhibitory concentrations

The MICs of amikacin against some selected bacterial species are shown in Table I.40. The intrinsic activity of amikacin against kanamycin-sensitive strains is generally equal to, or greater than, that of kanamycin (p.441) (Kawaguchi, 1976). Against gentamicin-sensitive strains, amikacin is 2- to 4-fold less active than gentamicin (p.457) (Bodey and Stewart, 1973; Yu and Washington, 1973). Most Gram-negative bacilli which are resistant to kanamycin, gentamicin and tobramycin, are amikacin-sensitive, but their amikacin MICs may be greater than those of bacteria which are also sensitive to gentamicin and tobramycin (Hewitt and Young, 1977).

Mode of Administration and Dosage

Amikacin is not absorbed from the gastrointestinal tract and it is administered by either the i.m. or i.v. route.

1 Single-daily dose administration

Similar to other aminoglycosides, such as gentamicin (p.457), amikacin can be administered as a single-daily dose. For normal adults the daily dose is 15 mg per kg body weight per day or 1.0 g daily. This can be given i.m. but more commonly i.v. the dose being dissolved in 30–50 ml of i.v. fluid and this then infused in 30 min. In neutropenic patients, however, once-daily administration should only be done if amikacin is combined with an appropriate beta-lactam antibiotic. This may also apply if *Ps. aeruginosa* or *Serratia marcescens* infections are treated. Once-daily amikacin administration may be slightly less nephrotoxic than classical 12-hourly dosing and some investigators have also found it clinically slightly more efficaceous (Maller *et al.*, 1988, 1990, 1993; Garraffo *et al.*, 1990; Beaucaire *et al.*, 1991; Marik *et al.*, 1991a,b; Tulkens, 1991; McGrath *et al.*, 1992; The Int Antimicrob Ther Coop Group, 1993; Ellis-Pegler *et al.*, 1994). A meta-analysis of seven comparative studies showed that there were only very minor differences in efficacy and toxicity between once-daily compared with 12-hourly amikacin administration. The main advantage of once-daily dosing appears to be simplicity of administration (Munckhof *et al.*, 1996). The theoretical justifications for once-daily amikacin administration are the same as those for gentamicin (p.458). Similar to other aminoglycosides (p.458) amikacin has a post-antibiotic effect (Van der Auwera and Klastersky, 1987; Tsui *et al.*, 1993).

The mean peak serum level after once-daily i.v. amikacin infusion of 15 mg per kg over 30 min (blood collected 30 min after the infusion) was 40.9 µg per ml and trough concentration was 1.8 µg per ml (blood collected just before the next infusion) (Maller *et al.*, 1993). As with gentamicin, usually only the trough concentrations need to be monitored.

2 Classical 12-hourly administration to adults

a Intramuscular A common dosage of amikacin, similar to kanamycin (p.441), is 15 mg per kg body weight per day, administered in two divided doses (Gooding *et al.*, 1976; Meyer, 1981). For most adults the dose is approximately 0.5 g every 12 h. For the treatment of serious infections higher doses of 7.5–8.0 mg per kg 8-hourly have been used (Smith *et al.*, 1977; Lau *et al.*, 1977a). As with other aminoglycosides (p.461), serum level monitoring of amikacin is necessary, especially when severe Gram-negative infections are treated. Optimal peak serum levels attained approximately 1 h after i.m. administration) are 20–30 µg per ml and trough levels (concentrations which prevail just prior to the next dose) should not exceed 10 µg per ml (Black *et al.*, 1976; Hewitt and Young, 1977; Follath *et al.*, 1981).

b Intravenous Amikacin can be administered i.v. in the same total daily dosage and at the same intervals, as recommended for the i.m. route. The drug is most commonly given i.v. by dissolving each individual dose in 30–50 ml of i.v. fluid, which is then infused over 30 min via a pediatric buretrol or a secondary i.v. bottle (Lau *et al.*, 1977a; Smith *et al.*, 1977). The serum level just after a 30-min infusion of a standard 7.5 mg per kg dose is usually higher than the peak after the same i.m. dose, but the level 30 min after the completion of the infusion approximates to the peak obtained from i.m. dosing, as at that time the rapid distribution phase is usually completed. For the purposes of serum level monitoring, blood is usually taken 30 min after the completion of the infusion, and the result is regarded as the 'peak' serum level (Lau *et al.*, 1977a; Trenholme *et al.*, 1977).

Similar to other aminoglycosides (p.459), amikacin can also be given by rapid i.v. injections. If individual doses of 0.5 g are given i.v. over a period of 5 min to normal adults, the serum levels during the first hour after injection usually exceed 30 µg per ml, and during the first 15 min they may exceed 50 µg per ml. By 1 h after administration the concentrations approximate the peak serum levels attained after i.m. injections of the same doses. Transiently high serum levels obtained with this method do not appear to be associated with toxicity (Yates *et al.*, 1978; Wise *et al.*, 1981).

3 Children and adolescents

As with kanamycin (p.441) and gentamicin (p.459), younger subjects have a higher glomerular filtration rate of amikacin and therefore excrete more of the drug in proportion to their body weight than adults. Cleary *et al.* (1979) suggested that the optimal initial dosage regimen of amikacin in children is 20 mg per kg daily, administered in divided doses every 6 h. This dosage for children can also be administered as an once-daily dose (Marik *et al.*, 1991a,b). Vogelstein *et al.* (1977) studied 20 patients aged 4–16 years, and found that in many an amikacin dosage as high as 10 mg per kg every 8 h was required to produce satisfactory serum levels. Patients with small weight-to-surface area ratios, such as the young and debilitated, needed 15 mg or occasionally even 20 mg per kg every 8 h. These authors found that dosage based on surface area, rather than body weight, was more satisfactory for these patients. Accordingly, they suggested an amikacin dosage of 420 mg per m^2 administered i.v. every 8 h. This resulted in therapeutic non-toxic serum levels, and there was no accumulation of the drug after four doses.

It seems advisable to use the higher doses either i.m. or i.v. with serum level monitoring, whenever severe infections are treated in children. For milder infections the usual dosage of 7.5 mg per kg 12-hourly may suffice. Many children with moderate or even severe infections have responded to this lower amikacin dosage (Khan *et al.*, 1976; Yow, 1977).

4 Newborn and premature infants

For infants weighing less than 2000 g and who are 0–7 days old, an individual dose of 7.5 mg per kg should be used; for all others the individual dose recommended is 10 mg per kg. The individual dose should be given i.v. (as a 20- to 30-min infusion) every 12 h for infants 0–7 days of age and every 8 h for infants older than 7 days. This equates to a total daily dosage of 15 mg per kg for infants weighing less than 2000 g and 0–7 days of age, 20 mg per kg for infants weighing more than 2000 g and 0–7 days of age and 30 mg per kg for those older than 7 days (Howard and McCracken, 1975; McCracken and Nelson, 1983). For preterm infants, an initial amikacin dose of 10 mg per kg, followed by 7.5 mg per kg 12-hourly may be suitable (Want *et al.*, 1979). Many factors, such as hypoxemia, affect the serum half-life of amikacin in neonates, so that routine monitoring of serum levels is advisable (Myers *et al.*, 1977). Other authors have found that pre-term infants of greater than 30 weeks of postceptional age may need higher dosages such as 9 mg per kg 12-hourly, but there is individual variation, so ongoing serum level monitoring is essential (Kenyon *et al.*, 1990).

5 Patients with renal failure

Dosage should be reduced in a similar manner to kanamycin (p.442), for such patients. The simplest approximate dosage schedule assumes a linear relationship between amikacin's serum half-life and the patient's serum creatinine in mg % (for conversion of creatinine values from SI units, see gentamicin, p.460). Normal individual amikacin doses can be used, but the interval between doses (in hours) is extended to a value which is obtained by multiplying the normal dosage interval (in hours) by the patient's serum creatinine in mg %. Alternatively, the intervals between doses may be left unchanged, but after the initial dose, subsequent maintenance doses are calculated by dividing the usual dose by the patient's creatinine in mg %. These two approaches can also be combined (p.442).

If amikacin dosage is calculated by these methods, frequent monitoring of serum levels are necessary, otherwise considerable errors can occur. This is because the relationship between the drug's half-life and serum creatinine is not always linear (McHenry *et al.*, 1976). Particularly in older patients, the creatinine clearance (and therefore amikacin clearance) is often considerably reduced without a corresponding increase in serum creatinine. These patients may thereby be overdosed with amikacin using the above dosage schedule (Pijck *et al.*, 1976). Calculations are also likely to be quite inaccurate in patients with acute or unstable renal failure (Leroy *et al.*, 1976). There is a better linear relationship between the amikacin serum half-life and the rate of creatinine clearance (McHenry *et al.*, 1976). The formula for estimation of creatinine clearance is given on p.460. This can be used to calculate dosage for patients with renal failure. An initial dose of 7.5 mg per kg body weight is used, and thereafter maintenance doses are given at the usual dosage intervals. The maintenance dose is obtained by dividing the value of the observed creatinine clearance in ml per min by the value of the normal creatinine clearance in ml per min, and then multiplying this result by the value of the calculated normal dose in mg (Schiffman, 1977). A disadvantage of this method is the difficulty in estimating creatinine clearance in acutely ill patients. More accurate dosage schedules can be obtained from nomograms based on creatinine clearance values, as in the case of kanamycin (p.442) (Pijck *et al.*, 1976; Bryan and Stone, 1977). Even with nomogram prescribing in renal failure, several variables remain (see gentamicin, p.461), and serum level monitoring is necessary. For instance, in patients with stable, but impaired renal function, the amikacin half-life in serum increases with increasing duration of therapy, despite a stable creatinine clearance. This is because at the beginning of therapy, the drug accumulates in the tissues, but later when the tissues are saturated, amikacin is only cleared from the central compartment by renal elimination (Blaser *et al.*, 1983).

Amikacin, like kanamycin (p.442), is removed by hemodialysis, and during this procedure its half-life decreases to less than 10% of the pretreatment value. A satisfactory dose for anephric patients undergoing twice-weekly hemodialysis is 5.0–7.5 mg per kg body weight administered i.v. immediately after each dialysis (Regeur *et al.*, 1977). Peritoneal dialysis is less effective in removing amikacin; its serum half-life may be decreased to about 30% of the pretreatment value, but this may vary according to other factors such as peritoneal inflammation (Madhavan *et al.*, 1976; Regeur *et al.*, 1977). Individual dosage adjustment with serum level monitoring is required in patients undergoing peritoneal dialysis. Amikacin can be added to peritoneal dialysis fluid (usually in a concentration of 20–30 μg per ml) to treat bacterial (e.g. *Pseudomonas*) peritonitis associated with chronic ambulatory peritoneal dialysis. Intraperitoneal amikacin alone may be clinically ineffective and supplemental systemic amikacin may be required. In these circumstances serum level monitoring is necessary to avoid toxic serum levels (Shalit *et al.*, 1985). In these patients a single 7.5 mg per kg i.v. dose of amikacin may provide clinically effective concentrations in serum and peritoneal fluid for up to 72 h (Smeltzer *et al.*, 1988).

In renal failure patients treated by hemofiltration, this procedure removes about 60% of the administered amikacin dose. A 7.5 mg per kg dose of amikacin can be given 2 h before the hemofiltration period and half this dose after the first hemofiltration. To determine further dosing serum level monitoring is necessary (Kinowski *et al.*, 1993).

6 Elderly patients

In these, as in normal adults, amikacin can be given as a single-daily dose or the dose divided in two and given 12-hourly. The total daily dosage should be reduced according to the creatinine clearance and in most patients the dosage is likely to be about 11 mg per kg body weight per day (Maller *et al.*, 1990; Vanhaeverbeek *et al.*, 1993).

7 Patients with malignancies

Patients with hematological malignancies and also those with cancer receiving high-dose cancer chemotherapy often have a higher volume of distribution of amikacin and also higher drug clearance. Higher amikacin dosages with serum level monitoring may be necessary in these patients (Kaojarern *et al.*, 1989; Davis *et al.*, 1991).

8 Children with burns

These children also need more amikacin and an initial dosage of 10 mg per kg 6-hourly is recommended. All children studied had increased volumes of distribution of the drug, but these tended to be lower in the older children (Kopcha *et al.*, 1991).

9 Intrathecal and intraventricular administration

Amikacin has been administered intrathecally as an adjunct to systemic therapy to treat meningitis in two adults caused by gentamicin-resistant *Klebsiella* spp. In one patient the daily intrathecal dose was 4 mg (Hamory *et al.*, 1976), and in the other it was 20 mg (Block *et al.*, 1977). Intrathecal therapy was well tolerated and appeared to contribute to the recovery of both patients. As with gentamicin (p.462), the intrathecally administered drug is unlikely to reach the cerebral ventricles. Wright *et al.* (1981) administered amikacin intraventricularly to neonates with Gram-negative rod meningitis. An initial intraventricular instillation of 5 mg of amikacin via a Rickham reservoir was given, and thereafter the dosage was adjusted to maintain the concentration of amikacin in CSF well above the MIC for the infecting organism.

Serum Levels in Relation to Dosage

1 Intramuscular administration

Serum levels of amikacin are very similar to those of kanamycin (p.443). After a 0.5-g dose, a peak serum concentration of about 20 μg per ml is attained approximately 1 h (range 0.75–2.0 h) later. Thereafter, the level falls and is approximately 10 μg per ml at 4 h, 4 μg per ml at 8 h, and it is usually undetectable in serum 12 h after administration. The half-life of amikacin after i.m. injection is approximately 2.3 h (Cabana and Taggart, 1973; Kirby *et al.*, 1976). As with many other antibiotics, serum amikacin levels are lower in pregnant patients (p.443) (Chow and Jewesson, 1985).

2 Intravenous administration

Following a 0.5-g i.v. infusion given over 30 min to adults, serum levels as high as 34–48 μg per ml are attained immediately after the infusion (Schiffman, 1977). After the infusion, a short (0.5 h) distribution phase occurs in most patients, during which serum levels fall to 20–30 μg per ml, a value similar to the peak level attained after i.m. dosing. Thereafter, the serum level declines in a similar manner to that after i.m. administration, and at 12 h very little if any amikacin can be detected in the serum. For purposes of serum level monitoring during therapy, blood for the 'peak' level estimation is usually taken 0.5 h after the cessation of a 30-min infusion, and blood for the 'trough' level is collected shortly before the next infusion (p.442). The serum levels attained after a single 15 mg per kg dose (usually 1.0 g in adults) administered i.v. by the above method are given on p.508. When a 0.5-g dose of amikacin is administered to adults by rapid i.v. injection (over 2–5 min), transient high peaks of up to 60 μg per ml are attained during first 15 min. These rapidly fall to 20–30 μg per ml at 1 h, a value similar to the peak level attained after i.m. administration. Subsequent serum concentrations fall more slowly in a manner similar to the decline, which occurs after i.m. administration (Vogelstein *et al.*, 1977; Walker *et al.*, 1979; Wise *et al.*, 1981).

Excretion

Like kanamycin (p.444), amikacin is eliminated from the body almost entirely by the kidney in an active unchanged form. High concentrations of the active drug are attained in urine. It is excreted entirely by glomerular filtration, but the rate of renal clearance of creatinine is higher than that of either amikacin or kanamycin, indicating that these antibiotics undergo appreciable tubular reabsorption (Kirby *et al.*, 1976). In patients with normal renal function approximately 94% of an administered dose is excreted in the urine within 24 h (Cabana and Taggart, 1973; Kirby *et al.*, 1976). With impaired renal function the half-life of the drug is increased progressively as renal function deteriorates. The normal half-life of 2.3 h may be prolonged to 44 h in patients with minimal renal function and to 86 h in anephric patients (Regeur *et al.*, 1977).

Distribution of the Drug in Body

Serum protein binding of amikacin, like that of kanamycin (p.445), is very low (3.6%) (Kirby *et al.*, 1976). Amikacin does not penetrate into the CSF of patients with normal meninges (Briedis and Robson, 1978), and even in those with bacterial meningitis CSF levels are low when usual parenteral doses are given. Hamory *et al.* (1976) gave an adult patient with *Klebsiella* meningitis, amikacin 7.5 mg per kg i.m. every 12 h; concentrations in the CSF were consistently less than 0.6 μg per ml. Badri *et al.* (1977) found CSF levels in a range of <0.4–3.8 μg per ml in six neonates with bacterial meningitis, who were treated by parenteral amikacin. The findings of Gaillard *et al.* (1995) in older children with bacterial meningitis were similar; the highest average CSF levels of amikacin (2.9 μg per ml) were found in those with low CSF glucose levels. Yogev and Kolling (1981) measured ventricular fluid amikacin levels in ten hydrocephalic children with suspected ventriculitis who were given the drug in a dosage of 7.5 mg per kg 8-hourly. After the fourth or fifth dose, the mean peak ventricular fluid level in five patients with bacterial meningitis was 6.1 μg per ml. In the remaining five patients without bacterial ventriculitis, very low levels (<0.7 μg per ml) of amikacin were detected.

The apparent volume of distribution of amikacin is approximately 23% of body volume or 30% of total body weight, suggesting that it is distributed primarily in extracellular fluids (Cabana and Taggart, 1973; Kirby *et al.*, 1976; Schiffman, 1977). Amikacin diffuses well into normal human interstitial fluid, but concentrations are lower than simultaneous serum levels (Tan and Salstrom, 1977; Lanao *et al.*, 1983). It may also reach adequate concentrations in tissue contiguous with pressure sores in humans with spinal cord injury (Segal *et al.*, 1990). Muscle and fat concentrations were determined in 41 children after i.m. administration of a dose of 7.5 mg per kg body weight (Daschner *et al.*, 1977). After 1.5 h the concentrations peaked in serum (mean 14.9 μg per ml), as well as in muscle (2.2 μg per g) and fat tissue (1.89 μg per g). Thereafter, all these concentrations declined, but they exceeded 1.0 μg per g in muscle and fat for at least 3 and 4 h, respectively. Amikacin crosses the placenta. When a single i.v. injection of 7.5 mg per kg was given to women in labor, amikacin levels of 0.5–6.0 μg per ml were detected in cord blood. After 3 h the babies' serum levels of amikacin were 2- to 10-fold lower than those of the mothers (Mazzei *et al.*, 1976).

Amikacin penetrates relatively poorly into non-infected bronchial secretions. In one study three consecutive i.m. injections (7.5 mg per kg 12-hourly) were given to healthy men. Bronchial secretion concentrations between 1.5 and 2.0 h after the final dose ranged from 2.3 to 8.4 μg per ml. The mean bronchial secretion concentration 7 h after the final dose was less than 1.0 μg per ml (Dull *et al.*, 1979). The drug penetrated better into bronchial secretions of patients with pneumonia, where the concentrations were higher if the drug was given i.v. once-daily rather than in two divided doses (Santré *et al.*, 1995). Amikacin penetrated well into human parapneumonic effusions, where the concentration reached was approximately 80% of the simultaneous serum level (Taryle *et al.*, 1981). Amikacin levels in human bile were lower than those in the serum (approximately 20% of simultaneous serum levels). The concentrations of the drug in gallbladder wall ranged from 4.7 to 34 μg per g after the usual parenteral doses were given (Bermúdez *et al.*, 1981; Hansbrough *et al.*, 1981).

In animals, amikacin penetrated well into the exudate of experimental sterile peritonitis, where its concentrations approximately equated with serum levels at the time (MacGregor, 1977). In other animal studies after repeated injections of the drug, low concentrations (0.4–5.0 μg per g) were detected in most body tissues such as liver, heart, lung and muscle, but not in brain (Kornguth and Kunin, 1977). In animals with induced *Ps. aeruginosa* endocarditis of both tricuspid and aortic valves, amikacin penetrated better into the tricuspid valve vegetations and the time above MBC was also longer in these vegetations (Bayer *et al.*, 1988). After systemic amikacin administration to rabbits the drug reached adequate levels in the aqueous humor of the eye, but chloramphenicol (p.561), a lipophilic compound, gave higher concentrations than amikacin (Mayers *et al.*, 1991).

As with other aminoglycosides (p.465), the major site of antibiotic deposition is the kidney, particularly the renal cortex, where concentrations may exceed 100 μg per g. Reabsorption in the proximal tubule (p.465), the major portion of which is located in the cortex, is mainly responsible for the accumulation of the drug in renal tubular cells (Kornguth and Kunin, 1977; Contrepois *et al.*, 1985). This accumulation appears to be related to nephrotoxicity (p.467). High kidney concentrations were found in five patients who died during therapy with amikacin (Edwards *et al.*, 1976). Concentrations ranged from 365 to 1030 μg per g in the renal cortex and from 270 to 718 μg per g in the medulla. Tissue levels were high in patients with both normal and abnormal renal function.

Mode of Action

This is probably similar to that of other aminoglycosides, such as streptomycin (p.432) and gentamicin (p.465).

Toxicity

1 Ototoxicity

This can occur and, like kanamycin (p.445), amikacin causes predominantly cochlear damage, although vestibular dysfunction can also develop in some patients (Black *et al.*, 1976; Bock *et al.*, 1980; Meyer, 1981). In an analysis of the records of 1548 patients treated with amikacin, high frequency hearing loss occurred in 71 (4.59%), and conversational hearing loss in another eight patients (0.52%). A further ten patients (0.65%) had some vestibular damage, which was usually mild (Lane *et al.*, 1977). In 328 of these patients pre- and post-treatment audiograms could be evaluated. In 11 a hearing loss of 15 decibels or greater occurred at least at one frequency; all of these had received approximately twice as much amikacin as those with audiometric changes. In addition, eight of the 11 patients (72.8%) had received previous aminoglycoside therapy compared with only 34.1% of the 317 patients without cochlear damage. Differences between the mean ages of these groups were not significant.

Some comparative studies, involving relatively small number of patients, suggested that the frequency of amikacin ototoxicity may be similar to that of gentamicin. For instance, Lau *et al.* (1977a) treated 157 leukopenic patients with suspected Gram-negative organism sepsis, randomly by either an amikacin/carbenicillin or a gentamicin/carbenicillin regimen. During 105 courses of amikacin therapy, some hearing loss was documented by pre- and post-treatment audiograms in 21 patients (20%), but only one had clinical hearing loss. Significant audiogram changes were observed following 13 of 96 (13.6%) courses of gentamicin therapy; four of these patients also had tinnitus, but major vestibular symptoms did not occur. Smith *et al.* (1977) also used amikacin or gentamicin randomly to treat 174 patients, 64 of whom were evaluated for auditory toxicity. The frequency of this was similar in both groups, hearing loss developing in 10% of 30 patients receiving gentamicin and in 6% of the 34 receiving amikacin. Two additional patients receiving amikacin noted transient tinnitus. Kahlmeter and Dahlager (1984) surveyed aminoglycoside-induced ototoxicity reported in clinical trials published between 1975 and 1982 which included approximately 10 000 patients. The average frequency of cochlear toxicity was 13.9% for amikacin, 8.3% for gentamicin and 6.1% for tobramycin. The average frequencies of vestibular toxicity for amikacin, gentamicin and tobramycin were similar (3.2 to 3.7%).

In animals amikacin was used in a dosage five times greater than gentamicin, approximately the dosage ratio with which these antibiotics are used clinically. In such studies amikacin selectively produced an impairment of cochlear function, and gentamicin an impairment of vestibular function with also a significant degree of concurrent cochlear damage. The cochlear ototoxicity produced by amikacin was similar in degree and appeared after the same duration of drug administration as the vestibular ototoxicity produced by gentamicin. It appeared that amikacin was selectively toxic to the cochlea at five times the dose of gentamicin which produced both vestibular and cochlear damage (Christensen *et al.*, 1977; Hottendorf, 1977). In animals, amikacin, similar to other aminoglycosides (p.465), penetrated the inner ear fluid compartments and caused hair cell damage. The rate of entry of amikacin into the perilymph space of the inner ear was relatively slow, but it persisted there because of slow elimination (Desjardins-Giasson and Beaubien, 1984). There was no correlation between the concentrations of various aminoglycosides attained in the inner ear and their degree of toxicity (Dulon *et al.*,

1986). Amikacin ototoxicity appeared to be related to the presence of the drug in the perilymph over the total time of amikacin exposure regardless of the level in the perilymph (Beaubien *et al.*, 1991).

As deafness is usually more disabling than vestibular dysfunction, amikacin, like kanamycin (p.445), is potentially more toxic than gentamicin. There are no warning symptoms of early amikacin cochlear toxicity, and performing serial audiograms is often not feasible. Hearing loss caused by amikacin, unlike that due to neomycin (p.536), is usually not progressive once the drug is stopped (Black *et al.*, 1976). Amikacin ototoxicity is usually irreversible, although it ameliorates occasionally (Meyer, 1981). The major risk factors associated with amikacin-induced hearing loss include prolonged duration of therapy (more than 10 days), large total dose (greater than 15 g), increasing age of patient, previous aminoglycoside therapy, elevated serum peak (>30 μg per ml), and trough (>10 μg per ml) concentrations, previous excessive noise exposure and possibly the concomitant use of loop diuretics such as frusemide (Meyer, 1981; Pien and Ho, 1981; Moore *et al.*, 1984; Gatell *et al.*, 1987). Single-daily dose therapy does not appear to be associated with increased ototoxicity (Meunier *et al.*, 1991; Kibbler *et al.*, 1992; The Int Antimicrob Ther Coop Group, 1993).

As with other aminoglycosides (p.445, 467), amikacin ototoxicity has been uncommon in young children (Faden *et al.*, 1982). But Assael *et al.* (1982) believed that it was not possible to draw a general conclusion about the ototoxicity of amikacin and other aminoglycosides in infants and children. More prospective and comparative studies are needed to determine aminoglycoside ototoxicity in these age groups. Finitzo-Hieber *et al.* (1985) used the more reliable method of auditory brain stem response audiometry for detecting hearing impairment in the first months of life. Infants treated by aminoglycosides had conventional audiometric examinations performed when they reached the age of 6 weeks and again when aged 18 months. A total of 150 infants with gestational ages of 27 to 42 weeks were studied; 49 received netilmicin, 50 received amikacin and the others served as controls. The duration of aminoglycoside therapy ranged from 3 to 7 days. Bilateral sensorineural impairment was confirmed in three (2%) of these infants, one given netilmicin, one given amikacin and one was an untreated control. There was a high frequency of transient auditory abnormalities in these infants, who were receiving intensive care. Therefore, it appeared that the risk of developing hearing impairment from a short course amikacin or netilmicin therapy during infancy was small.

2 Nephrotoxicity

Amikacin can cause this side-effect, the clinical features of which are similar to those of gentamicin nephrotoxicity (p.467). In a review 8.7% of 1548 patients treated with amikacin developed changes consistent with impairment of renal function (Lane *et al.*, 1977). These changes were more frequent in patients whose initial serum creatinine values were high, in older patients, in those receiving a larger total dose of amikacin and in those who had also received other nephrotoxic agents, either previously or concurrently. Concomitant administration of frusemide did not appear to be a major risk factor for the development of amikacin-induced nephrotoxicity (Smith and Lietman, 1983).

The nephrotoxic potential of amikacin appears to be about the same as that of gentamicin (Schiffman, 1977). This was demonstrated in three clinical studies (Lau *et al.*, 1977a; Smith *et al.*, 1977; French *et al.*, 1981). But when Kahlmeter and Dahlager (1984) analyzed aminoglycoside nephrotoxicity in approximately 10 000 patients reported in the literature between 1975 and 1982, the average frequencies of nephrotoxicity for gentamicin and amikacin were 14% and 9.4%, respectively. Studies in animals have been somewhat conflicting. Some investigators found that gentamicin and amikacin were about equally nephrotoxic (Hottendorf, 1977; Rankin *et al.*, 1980), whilst others reported gentamicin to be more toxic than amikacin (Hottendof and Gordon, 1980; Brian *et al.*, 1984). Similar to other aminoglycosides (p.469), amikacin may be more nephrotoxic in patients with obstructive jaundice (Desai and Tsang, 1988).

3 Other side-effects

These are infrequent and relatively unimportant. They include hypersensitivity reactions, nausea and vomiting, headache, drug fever, tremor, paresthesiae, arthralgia, eosinophilia, anemia and mild abnormalities in liver function tests (Gooding *et al.*, 1976; Schiffman, 1977). As with other aminoglycosides (p.470), the *in vitro* incubation of aminoglycoside antibiotics with human polymorphonuclear leukocytes induces abnormalities in polymorph function. In contrast, when amikacin or other aminoglycosides are given i.v. to normal volunteers, polymorph function remains normal (Venezio and Di Vencenzo, 1985).

Clinical Uses of the Drug

1 Infections due to aerobic Gram-negative bacilli

Controlled studies indicate that amikacin is equally as effective as gentamicin or tobramycin, for the treatment of serious Gram-negative infections caused by organisms susceptible to all three drugs. Lau *et al.* (1977a) treated 157 leukopenic patients who had fever and evidence of Gram-negative infection, randomly by either an amikacin/carbenicillin or a gentamicin/carbenicillin regimen. The overall clinical response rate was 75% for both groups. Similarly, Smith *et al.* (1977) used amikacin or gentamicin randomly to treat 174 patients with suspected severe Gram-negative infections. Enteric Gram-negative bacilli were subsequently isolated from 71 of these patients, 39 of whom were treated with amikacin and 32 with gentamicin. A favorable response was obtained in 77% of all the patients treated with amikacin and in 78% of those treated with gentamicin. Feld *et al.* (1977) compared amikacin and tobramycin in a randomized study of the treatment of serious infections in 175 cancer patients. An etiological agent was isolated from 74 patients which in 59 (80%) was a Gram-negative bacillus, usually either *Kl. pneumoniae*, *E. coli* or *Ps. aeruginosa*; in these confirmed infections, the response rate was 60% for tobramycin and 64% for amikacin. Salicylates reduce the capsular polysaccharide production in *Kl. pneumoniae* and render this organism more sensitive to all aminoglycosides *in vitro* (Domenico *et al.*, 1990). Salicylates also potentiated amikacin therapy in rodent models of *Kl. pneumoniae* infection. *In vivo* salicylate enhanced phagocytosis rather than antibiotic action. This potentiation of amikacin was abolished in neutropenic animals (Domenico *et al.*, 1993).

Amikacin also has an efficacy comparable with that of tobramycin in the treatment of pulmonary infection due to sensitive strains for *Ps. aeruginosa* in cystic fibrosis patients (Levy *et al.*, 1982). Some amikacin binds to macromolecules in the sputum of cystic fibrosis patients and only the free unbound drug is active against bacteria (Bataillon *et al.*, 1992).

The drug has been compared with gentamicin for the treatment of adults with urinary tract infections. In two randomized studies gentamicin was used in a dosage of 3–4 mg per kg per day, but amikacin was used in a reduced dosage of 9 mg per kg per day (Cox, 1976; Gilbert *et al.*, 1977). Results of treatment using either drug were essentially the same.

Amikacin has been used in many uncontrolled studies to treat various infections caused by gentamicin-sensitive Gram-negative rods. In general it has been about as effective as would be expected from a gentamicin regimen. Mathias *et al.* (1976) treated 42 patients many of whom had pyelonephritis and/or a septicemia. Most patients responded well, but in four with chronic urinary tract infection, *Ps. aeruginosa* isolates acquired amikacin-resistance during therapy. Amikacin has been utilized successfully in Gram-negative bacillary pneumonias (Trenholme *et al.*, 1977), bone and joint Gram-negative infections (Schurman and Wheeler, 1977) and in exacerbations of *Ps. aeruginosa* infections in children and adults with cystic fibrosis (Lau *et al.*, 1977b). In one study amikacin appeared superior to netilmicin (p.529) for the treatment of severe *Ps. aeruginosa* infections (Noone *et al.*, 1989).

Many clinical studies have documented the efficacy of amikacin for the treatment of septicemia and other serious infections caused by gentamicin-resistant aerobic Gram-negative bacilli (Meyer *et al.*, 1975; Tally *et al.*, 1976; Lewis *et al.*, 1977; Tally and Gorbach, 1977; Mosquera *et al.*, 1981). This is the prime indication for amikacin therapy (p.515). It has also been useful for treatment of similar infections in patients with cancer and neutropenia (Valdivieso *et al.*, 1977). Pulmonary infections caused by drug-resistant Gram-negative bacilli usually respond to amikacin (Bartlett, 1977). However, in one trial in which 19 patients with *Serratia* infections were treated, only one of eight patients with pneumonia or other deep tissue infections was cured. In four of the treatment failures *Serratia* spp. strains became increasingly amikacin-resistant during therapy (Craven *et al.*, 1977). Urinary tract infections caused by gentamicin-resistant organisms usually respond well to amikacin (Craven *et al.*, 1977).

Amikacin is valuable for the treatment of serious infections, caused by multiresistant aerobic Gram-negative bacilli, in children of all ages and neonates (Yow, 1977; Shulman and Yogev, 1985). In neonatal meningitis caused by either gentamicin-sensitive or -resistant Gram-negative bacilli, an ampicillin/amikacin combination is equally as effective as cefotaxime used as a single drug (p.337).

For neutropenic cancer patients with presumed infection, empiric emergency chemotherapy is often necessary. Combinations of either amikacin/carbenicillin (Lau *et al.*, 1977a) or amikacin/ticarcillin (Klastersky, 1983) have been used with success. Similarly, amikacin combined with one of the newer beta-lactams, such as mezlocillin, azlocillin, piperacillin, ceftazidime or imipenem also provides an acceptable initial regimen (Young *et al.*, 1981; Young, 1985; Winston *et al.*, 1986). Again, amikacin plus ceftriaxone, each administered once every 24 h, was equally as safe and efficaceous as multiple daily doses of amikacin and ceftazidime for the treatment of these patients (The Internat Antimicrob Ther Coop Group, 1993). Combination therapy is usually worth continuing after isolation of the organism, especially if the two drugs show *in vitro* synergism against it (Klastersky *et al.*, 1976).

A combination of amikacin plus a beta-lactam antibiotic is often valuable for treatment of non-neutropenic patients if a severe infection due to Gram-negative aerobic bacilli is suspected or proven. For instance, ampicillin (or penicillin G) plus amikacin is used for the treatment of severe sepsis, including meningitis, in neonates (Shulman and Yogev, 1985; Moreno *et al.*, 1994). A third-generation cephalosporin, such as cefotaxime, may be combined with amikacin to treat both children or adults with pneumonia caused by Gram-negative bacilli (Karnad *et al.*, 1985). Amikacin plus ticarcillin is probably equally as effective as a tobramycin/ticarcillin combination for the treatment of difficult *Ps. aeruginosa* infections, such as septicemia and endocarditis. If ticarcillin- and tobramycin-resistant *Ps. aeruginosa* strains are encountered, data from animal studies indicate that either an amikacin/ceftazidime or amikacin/imipenem combination may be the best alternative (Bayer *et al.*, 1985; Johnson *et al.*, 1985; Van der Auwera *et al.*, 1986). Aminoglycoside activity is suppressed under conditions of low pH and oxygen tension that are likely to occur in infected tissue, but beta-lactam antibiotics such as cefotaxime, used simultaneously, improve the action of amikacin under these circumstances. This is another reason for using beta-lactam/aminoglycoside combinations when treating severe Gram-negative aerobic bacterial infections (Bryant *et al.*, 1992).

If amikacin is used for emergency treatment of sepsis following large bowel surgery, where infection by both aerobic and anaerobic Gram-negative organisms is possible, it should be combined with either chloramphenicol (p.569). clindamycin (p.597) or metronidazole (p.943) (Dougherty, 1985). Other drugs are also available for anaerobic infections (pp.236, 308, 396).

When amikacin was first introduced for clinical use, it was generally regarded as a 'reserve drug' to be used only for treatment of the serious aerobic Gram-negative bacillary infections described above, if the organism concerned was suspected or proven to be resistant to gentamicin and other aminoglycosides (Hewitt and Young, 1977; Schiffman, 1977). Since then amikacin has been used as the principal aminoglycoside in some hospitals in the USA for several years without the emergence of amikacin-resistance among Gram-negative bacilli (p.505). Therefore, some clinicians consider that there is no need to restrict the use of amikacin (Levin, 1981; Young *et al.*, 1981; Dougherty, 1985; Young, 1985; King *et al.*, 1992). Amikacin has the obvious advantage of being active against most gentamicin- and tobramycin-resistant Gram-negative bacilli. Some also consider that predictable, adequate and non-toxic serum levels are more easily attained with amikacin, compared with gentamicin or tobramycin (p.510) (Levin, 1981; Pien and Ho, 1981). Another advantage of amikacin is that it is the most stable aminoglycoside when used in combination with high doses of the penicillins, such as carbenicillin or ticarcillin (p.157) (Blair *et al.*, 1982; Glew and Pavuk, 1983). However, in some hospitals increased use of amikacin has resulted in emergence of amikacin-resistant Gram-negative bacilli (p.505). It seems prudent to use gentamicin (p.471) for severe infections caused by one of the Enterobacteriaceae and tobramycin (p.497) for *Ps. aeruginosa* infections if the strains involved are sensitive to these drugs. This would restrict amikacin for the treatment of infections caused by strains resistant to other aminoglycosides. In institutions with significant gentamicin- or tobramycin-resistance, amikacin is the aminoglycoside of choice to be included in emergency treatment regimens for suspected severe infections caused by Gram-negative aerobic rods.

2 Nocardia asteroides infections

Amikacin is effective in *N. asteroides* infections in animals (Wallace *et al.*, 1979b; Gombert *et al.*, 1986, 1990). It has been used successfully in human nocardiosis (Yogev *et al.*, 1980; Meier *et al.*, 1986). Co-trimoxazole (p.871) is probably the drug of choice for the treatment of this disease, but amikacin may be a useful therapeutic alternative for patients who develop reactions to sulfonamides or who fail to respond to the usual therapy. One patient with *Nocardia farcinica* infection also responded well to amikacin therapy (Schiff *et al.*, 1993).

3 Mycobacterial infections

Although *M. tuberculosis* is sensitive to amikacin *in vitro*, the drug has no role in the treatment of human tuberculosis, as there is complete cross-resistance between amikacin and kanamycin, and as it has no advantages over kanamycin, (p.446) (Allen *et al.*, 1983). Amikacin has occasionally been used for treatment of multiresistant tuberculosis (p.1199) if kanamycin was not available.

Amikacin, in combination with other drugs, may be clinically useful for the treatment of *M. fortuitum* and *M. chelonae* infections, provided that the strain involved is amikacin-sensitive (p.506). Cutaneous lesions in immunocompetent patients respond well to one or a combination of two drugs, but disseminated infection in immunocompromised patients needs more aggressive therapy with three or more agents. Drugs which may be useful for combination therapy with amikacin include erythromycin (p.621), clarithromycin (p.648), azithromycin, roxithromycin, cefoxitin (p.309), imipenem (p.238) and doxycycline (p.745) (Wallace *et al.*, 1985; Subbarao *et al.*, 1987; Raad *et al.*, 1991; McWhinney *et al.*, 1992; Ingram *et al.*, 1993). Amikacin, either alone or combined with another antibiotic also provides adequate therapy for environmental mycobacterial peritonitis which may be a complication of peritoneal dialysis (Hakim *et al.*, 1993).

Mycobacterium avium complex infections are hard to treat, particularly in patients with AIDS (p.648). Animal studies suggest that amikacin, in combination with other antimycobacterial agents, may be useful for the treatment of these infections (Gangadharam *et al.*, 1988b; Inderlied *et al.*, 1989). In animals liposome-encapsulated amikacin has been more effective for the treatment of disseminated *M. avium* infections (Cynamon *et al.*, 1989; Bermudez *et al.*, 1990). In humans some success has been obtained by using combinations such as amikacin, rifampicin and ethambutol (Baron and Young, 1986; Young *et al.*, 1986; Young, 1988). Other useful agents include rifabutin (p.712) and the newer macrolides such as clarithromycin (p.648) and azithromycin (p.657).

References

Acar JF, Witchitz JL, Goldstein F *et al.* (1976). Susceptibility of aminoglycoside-resistant Gram-negative bacilli to amikacin: delineation of individual resistance patterns. *J Infect Dis* **134** (Suppl): 280.

Allen BW, Mitchison DA, Chan YC *et al.* (1983). Amikacin in the treatment of pulmonary tuberculosis. *Tubercle* **64**: 111.

Amirak ID, Williams RJ, Noone P, Wills M R (1977). Amikacin resistance developing in a patient with *Pseudomonas aeruginosa* bronchopneumonia. *Lancet* **i**: 537.

Assael BM, Parini R, Rusconi F (1982). Ototoxicity of aminoglycoside antibiotics in infants and children. *Pediatr Infect Dis* **1**: 357.

Badri MD, Boysen BE, Chiu TW *et al.* (1977). Amikacin in neonatal infections, evaluation of efficacy and toxicity. *Amer J Med* **62** (Suppl): 172.

Ball P, Gray J (1979). Activity of cefuroxime, cefoxitin and amikacin against *Serratia marcescens*. *J Antimicrob Chemother* **5**: 472.

Baron EJ, Young LS (1986). Amikacin, ethambutol and rifampin for treatment of disseminated *Mycobacterium avium-intracellulare* infections in patients with acquired immune deficiency syndrome. *Diagn Microbiol Infect Dis* **5**: 215.

Bartlett JG (1977). Amikacin treatment of pulmonary infections involving gentamicin-resistant Gram-negative bacilli. *Amer J Med* **62** (Suppl): 151.

Basker MJ, Slocombe B, Sutherland R (1977). Aminoglycoside-resistant enterococci. *J Clin Path* **30**: 375.

Bataillon V, Lhermitte M, Lafitte J-J *et al.* (1992). The binding of amikacin to macromolecules from the sputum of patients suffering from respiratory diseases. *J Antimicrob Chemother* **29**: 499.

Bayer AS, Norman D, Kim KS (1985). Efficacy of amikacin and ceftazidime in experimental aortic valve endocarditis due to *Pseudomonas aeruginosa*. *Antimicrob Ag Chemother* **28**: 781.

Bayer AS, Crowell DJ, Yih J *et al.* (1988). Comparative pharmacokinetics and pharmacodynamics of amikacin and ceftazidime in triscuspid and aortic vegetations in experimental *Pseudomonas endocarditis*. *J Infect Dis* **158**: 355.

Bayer AS, O'Brien T, Norman DC, Nast CC (1989). Oxygen-dependent differences in exopolysacharide production and aminoglycoside inhibitory-bactericidal interactions with *Pseudomonas aeruginosa*–implications for endocarditis. *J Antimicrob Chemother* **23**: 21.

Beaubien AR, Ormsby E, Bayne A *et al.* (1991). Evidence that amikacin ototoxicity is related to total perilymph area under the concentration-time curve regardless of concentration. *Antimicrob Ag Chemother* **35**: 1070.

Beaucaire G, Leroy O, Beuscart C *et al.* (1991). Clinical and bacteriological efficacy, and practical aspects of amikacin given once daily for severe infections. *J Antimicrob Chemother* **27** (Suppl C): 91.

Bengtsson S, Bernarder S, Brorson JE *et al.* (1986). *In vitro* aminoglycoside resistance of Gram-negative bacilli and staphylococci isolated from blood in Sweden 1980–1984. *Scand J Infect Dis* **18**: 257.

Bergogne-Berezin E, Joly-Guillou ML (1985). An underestimated nosocomial pathogen, *Acinetobacter calcoaceticus*. *J Antimicrob Chemother* **16**: 535.

Bermudez LEM, Young LS (1988). Activities of amikacin, roxithromycin, and azithromycin alone or in combination with tumor necrosis factor against *Mycobacterium avium* complex. *Antimicrob Ag Chemother* **32**: 1149.

Bermudez LEM, Wu M, Young LS (1987). Intracellular killing of *Mycobacterium avium* complex by rifapentine and liposome-encapsulated amikacin. *J Infect Dis* **156**: 510.

Bermudez LE, Yau-Young AO, Lin J-P *et al.* (1990). Treatment of disseminated *Mycobacterium avium* complex infection of beige mice with liposome-encapsulated aminoglycosides. *J Infect Dis* **161**: 1262.

Bermudez RH, Lugo A, Ramirez-Ronda CH *et al.* (1981). Amikacin sulfate levels in human serum and bile. *Antimicrob Ag Chemother* **19**: 352.

Black RE, Lau WK, Weinstein RJ *et al.* (1976). Ototoxicity of amikacin. *Antimicrob Ag Chemother* **9**: 956.

Blair DC, Duggan DO, Schroeder ET (1982). Inactivation of amikacin and gentamicin by carbenicillin in patients with end-stage renal failure. *Antimicrob Ag Chemother* **22**: 376.

Blaser J, Rüttimann S, Bhend H, Lüthy R (1983). Increase of amikacin half-life during therapy in patients with renal insufficiency. *Antimicrob Ag Chemother* **23**: 888.

Block CS, Cassel R, Koornhof HJ, Robinson RG (1977). *Klebsiella* meningitis treated with intrathecal amikacin. *Lancet* **i**: 1371.

Bock BV, Edelstein PH, Meyer RD (1980). Prospective comparative study of efficacy and toxicity of netilmicin and amikacin. *Antimicrob Ag Chemother* **17**: 217.

Bodey GP, Stewart D (1973). *In vitro* studies of BB-K8, a new aminoglycoside antibiotic. *Antimicrob Ag Chemother* **4**: 186.

Boiron P, Provost F (1988). *In vitro* susceptibility testing of *Nocardia spp.* and its taxonomic implication. *J Antimicrob Chemother* **22**: 623.

Bongaerts GPA, Kaptijn MP (1981). Aminoglycoside phosphotransferase-II-mediated amikacin resistance in *Escherichia coli*. *Antimicrob Ag Chemother* **20**: 344.

Briedis DJ, Robson HG (1978). Cerebrospinal fluid penetration of amikacin. *Antimicrob Ag Chemother* **13**: 1042.

Brion N, Barge J, Godefroy I *et al.* (1984). Gentamicin, netilmicin, dibekacin and amikacin nephrotoxicity and its relationship to tubular reabsorption in rabbits. *Antimicrob Ag Chemother* **25**: 168.

Bryan CS, Stone WJ (1977). Antimicrobial dosage in renal failure: a unifying nomogram. *Clin Nephrol* **7**: 81.

Bryant RE, Fox K, Oh G, Morthland VH (1992). Beta-lactam enhancement of aminoglycoside activity under conditions of reduced pH and oxygen tension that may exist in infected tissues. *J Infect Dis* **165**: 676.

Cabana BE, Taggart JG (1973). Comparative pharmacokinetics of BB-K8 and kanamycin in dogs and humans. *Antimicrob Ag Chemother* **3**: 478.

Calderwood SA, Wennersten C, Moellering RC Jr *et al.* (1977). Resistance of six aminoglycosidic aminocyclitol antibiotics among enterococci: prevalence, evolution and relationship to synergism with penicillin. *Antimicrob Ag Chemother* **12**: 401.

Calderwood SB, Wennersten C, Moellering RC Jr *et al.* (1981). Resistance of antiobiotic synergism in *Streptococcus faecalis*: further studies with amikacin and with a new amikacin derivative, 4'-deoxy, 6'-N-methylamikacin. *Antimicrob Ag Chemother* **19**: 549.

Champion HM, Bennett PM, Lewis DA, Reeves DS (1988). Cloning and characterization of an AAC (6'). gene from *Serratia marcescens*. *J Antimicrob Chemother* **22**: 587.

Chiodini RJ, Van Kruiningen HJ, Thayer WR *et al.* (1984). *In vitro* antimicrobial susceptibility of *Mycobacterium* sp. isolated from patients with Crohn's disease. *Antimicrob Ag Chemother* **26**: 930.

Chow AW, Jewesson PJ (1985). Pharmacokinetics and safety of antimicrobial agents during pregnancy. *Rev Infect Dis* **7**: 287.

Christensen EF, Reiffenstein JC, Madissoo H (1977). Comparative ototoxicity of amikacin and gentamicin in cats. *Antimicrob Ag Chemother* **12**: 178.

Clark RB, Sandrs CC, Pakiz CB, Hostetter MK (1988). Aminoglycoside resistance among *Pseudomonas aeruginosa* isolates with an unusual disc diffusion antibiogram. *Antimicrob Ag Chemother* **32**: 689.

Cleary TG, Pickering LK, Kramer WG *et al.* (1979). Amikacin pharmacokinetics in pediatric patients with malignancy. *Antimicrob Ag Chemother* **16**: 829.

Contrepois A, Brion N, Garaud J-J *et al.* (1985). Renal disposition of gentamicin, dibekacin, tobramycin, netilmicin, and amikacin in humans. *Antimicrob Ag Chemother* **27**: 520.

Contreras AM, Gamba G, Cortés J *et al.* (1989). Serial trough and peak amikacin levels in plasma as predictors of nephrotoxicity. *Antimicrob Ag Chemother* **33**: 973.

Courvalin P, Davies J (1977). Plasmid mediated aminoglycoside phosphotransferase of broad substrate range that phosphorylates amikacin. *Antimicrob Ag Chemother* **11**: 619.

Cox CE (1976). Amikacin therapy of urinary tract infections. *J Infect Dis* (Suppl) **134**: 362.

Craven PC, Jorgensen JH, Kaspar RL, Drutz DJ (1977). Amikacin therapy of patients with multiply antibiotic-resistant *Serratia marcescens* infections. Development of increasing resistance during therapy. *Amer J Med* **62** (Suppl): 66.

Cynamon MH, Swenson CE, Palmer GS, Ginsberg RS (1989). Liposome-encapsulated-amikacin therapy of *Mycobacterium avium* complex infection in beige mice. *Antimicrob Ag Chemother* **33**: 1179.

Dalovisio JR, Pankey GA (1978). *In vitro* susceptibility of *Mycobacterium fortuitum* and *Mycobacterium chelonei* to amikacin. *J Infect Dis* **137**: 318.

Daschner F, Reiss E, Engert J (1977). Distribution of amikacin in serum, muscle, and fat in children after a single intramuscular injection. *Antimicrob Ag Chemother* **11**: 1081.

Davies J, Courvalin P (1977). Mechanisms of resistance to aminoglycosides. *Amer J Med* **62** (Suppl): 25.

Davis RL, Lehmann D, Stidley CA, Neidhart J (1991). Amikacin pharmacokinetics in patients receiving high-dose cancer chemotherapy. *Antimicrob Ag Chemother* **35**: 944.

Desai TK, Tsang T-K (1988). Aminoglycoside nephrotoxicity in obstructive jaundice. *Amer J Med* **85**: 47.

Desjardins-Giasson S, Beaubien AR (1984). Correlation of amikacin concentrations in perilymph and plasma of continuously infused guinea pigs. *Antimicrob Ag Chemother* **26**: 87.

Domenico P, Hopkins T, Schoch PE, Cunha BA (1990). Potentiation of aminoglycoside inhibition and reduction of capsular polysacharide, production in *Klebsiella pneumoniae* by sodium salicylate. *J Antimicrob Chemother* **25**: 903.

Domenico P, Straus DC, Woods DE, Cunha BA (1993). Salicylate potentiates amikacin therapy in rodent models of *Klebsiella pneumoniae* infection. *J Infect Dis* **168**: 766.

Dougherty SH (1985). Role of amikacin in the management of intra-abdominal sepsis. *Amer J Med* **79** (1A): 28.

Drasar FA, Farrell W, Maskell J, Williams JD (1976). Tobramycin, amikacin, sisomicin and gentamicin-resistant Gram-negative rods. *Brit Med J* **2**: 1284.

Dull WL, Alexander MR, Kasik JE (1979). Bronchial secretion levels of amikacin. *Antimicrob Ag Chemother* **16**: 767.

Dulon D, Aran J-M, Zajic G, Schacht J (1986). Comparative uptake of gentamicin, netilmicin, and amikacin in the guinea pig cochlea and vestibule. *Antimicrob Ag Chemother* **30**: 96.

Edwards CQ, Smith CR, Baughman KL *et al.* (1976). Concentrations of gentamicin and amikacin in human kidneys. *Antimicrob Ag Chemother* **9**: 925.

Ellis-Pegler RB, Chambers S, Begg EJ, Barclay ML (1994). Aminoglycoside dosing: time to change. *Aust NZ JM* **24**: 359.

Faden H, Deshpande G, Grossi M (1982). Renal and auditory toxic effects of amikacin in children with cancer. *Amer J Dis Child* **136**: 223.

Feld R, Valdivieso M, Bodey GP, Rodriguez V (1977). Comparison of amikacin and tobramycin in the treatment of infection in patients with cancer. *J Infect Dis* **135**: 61.

Finitzo-Hieber T, McCracken GH Jr, Brown KC (1985). Prospective controlled evaluation of auditory function in neonates given netilmicin or amikacin. *J Pediatr* **106**: 129.

Follath F, Wenk M, Vozeh S (1981). Plasma concentration monitoring of aminoglycosides. *J Antimicrob Chemother* **8** (Suppl A): 37.

French MA, Cerra FB, Plaut ME, Schentag JJ (1981). Amikacin and gentamicin accumulation pharmacokinetics and nephrotoxicity in critically ill patients. *Antimicrob Ag Chemother* **19**: 147.

Friedland IR, Funk E, Khoosal M, Klugman KP (1992). Increased resistance to amikacin in a neonatal unit following intensive amikacin usage. *Antimicrob Ag Chemother* **36**: 1596.

Gaillard J-L, Silly C, Le Masne A *et al.* (1995). Cerebrospinal fluid penetration of amikacin in children with community-acquired bacterial meningitis. *Antimicrob Ag Chemother* **39**: 253.

Gangadharam PRJ, Candler ER (1977). *In vitro* anti-mycobacterial acitivity of some new aminoglycoside antibiotics. *Tubercle* **58**: 35.

Gangadharam PRJ, Kesavalu L, Rao PNR *et al.* (1988a). Activity of amikacin against *Mycobacterium avium* complex under simulated *in vivo* conditions. *Antimicrob Ag Chemother* **32**: 886.

Gangadharam PRJ, Perumal VK, Podapati NR *et al.* (1988b). *In vivo* activity of amikacin alone or in combination with clofazimine or rifabutin or both against acute experimental *Mycobacterium avium* complex infections in beige mice. *Antimicrob Ag Chemother* **32**: 1400.

Garcia DC, Trevisan AR, Botto L *et al.* (1989). An outbreak of multiply resistant *Pseudomonas aeruginosa* in a neonatal unit: plasmid pattern analysis. *J Hosp Infect* **14**: 99.

Garraffo R, Drugeon HB, Dellamonica P *et al.* (1990). Determination of optimal dosage regimen for amikacin in healthy volunteers by study of pharmacokinetics and bactericidal activity. *Antimicrob Ag Chemother* **34**: 614.

Gatell JM, Ferran F, Araujo V et al. (1987). Univariate and multivariate analyses of risk factors predisposing to auditory toxicity in patients receiving aminoglycosides. Antimicrob Ag Chemother 31: 1383.

Gaynes R, Groisman E, Nelson E et al. (1988). Isolation, characterization, and cloning of plasmid-borne gene encoding a phosphotransferase that confers high-level amikacin resistance in enteric bacilli. Antimicrob Ag Chemother 32: 1379.

Gelber RH, Henika PR, Gibson JB (1984). The bacterial activity of various aminoglycoside antibiotics against Mycobacterium leprae in mice. Lepr Rev 55: 341.

Gerding DN, Larson TA (1985). Aminoglycoside resistance in Gram-negative bacilli during increased amikacin use. Amer J Med 79 (1A): 1.

Gerding DN, Larson TA, Hughes RA et al. (1991). Aminoglycoside resistance and aminoglycoside usage: ten years of experience in one hospital. Antimicrob Ag Chemother 35: 1284.

Gilbert DN, Eubanks N, Jackson J (1977). Comparison of amikacin and gentamicin in the treatment of urinary tract infections. Amer J Med 62 (Suppl): 121.

Glew RH, Pavuk RA (1983). Stability of gentamicin, tobramycin, and amikacin in combination with four beta-lactam antibiotics. Antimicrob Ag Chemother 24: 474.

Gombert ME, Aulicino TM, Du Bouchet L et al. (1986). Therapy of experimental cerebral nocardiosis with imipenem, amikacin, trimethoprim-sulfamethoxazole, and minocycline. Antimicrob Ag Chemother 30: 270.

Gombert ME, Berkowitz LB, Aulicino TM, du Bouchet L (1990). Therapy of pulmonary nocardiosis in immunocompromised mice. Antimicrob Ag Chemother 34: 1766.

Gooding PG, Berman E, Lane AZ, Agre K (1976). A review of results of clinical trials with amikacin. J Infect Dis 134 (Suppl): 441.

Guimares MA, Sgae R, Noone P (1985). The comparative activity of aminocyclito antibiotics against 773 aerobic Gram-negative rods and staphylococci isolated from hospitalized patients. J Antimicrob Chemother 16: 555.

Gutmann L, Goldstein FW, Kitzis MD et al. (1983). Susceptibility of Nocardia asteroides to 46 antibiotics including 22 beta-lactams. Antimicrob Ag Chemother 23: 248.

Gutschik E, Jepsen OB, Mortensen I (1977). Effect of combinations of penicillin and aminoglycosides in Streptococcus faecalis: a comparative study of seven aminoglycoside antibiotics. J Infect Dis 135: 832.

Hakim A, Hisam N, Reuman PD (1993). Environmental Mycobacterial peritonitis complicating peritoneal dialysis: three cases and review. Clin Infect Dis 16: 426.

Hammerberg S, Sorger S, Marks MI (1977). Antimicrobial susceptibilities of Yersinia enterocolitica biotype 4, serotype 0: 3. Antimicrob Ag Chemother 11: 566.

Hamory B, Ignatiadis P, Sande MA (1976). Intrathecal amikacin administration. Use in the treatment of gentamicin-resistant Klebsiella pneumoniae meningitis. JAMA 236: 1973.

Hansborough JF, Clark JE, Reimer LG (1981). Concentrations of kanamycin and amikacin in human gallbladder bile and wall. Antimicrob Ag Chemother 20: 515.

Harris RL, Fainstein V, Elting L et al. (1985). Bacteremia caused by Aeromonas species in hospitalized cancer patients. Rev Infect Dis 7: 314.

Heifets L (1988). MIC as a quantitative measurement of the susceptibility of Mycobacterium avium strains to seven antituberculosis drugs. Antimicrob Ag Chemother 32: 1131.

Heifets L, Lindholm-Levy P (1989). Comparison of bactericidal activities of streptomycin, amikacin, kanamycin, and cepreomycin against Mycobacterium avium and M tuberculosis. Antimicrob Ag Chemother 33: 1298.

Hewitt WL, Young LS (1977). Symposium perspective. Amer J Med 62 (Suppl): 1.

Hopkins JD, Flores A, Del Pilar Pla M et al. (1991). Nosocomial spread of an amikacin resistance gene on both a mobilized, nonconjugative plasmid and a conjugative plasmid. Antimicrob Ag Chemother 35: 1605.

Hottendorf GH (1977). Comparative ototoxicity (cats) and nephrotoxicity (rats) of amikacin and gentamicin. Amer J Med 62 (Suppl): 97.

Hottendorf GH, Gordon LL (1980). Comparative low-dose nephrotoxicities of gentamicin, tobramycin and amikacin. Antimicrob Ag Chemother 18: 176.

Houang ET, McKay-Ferguson E (1976). Activities of tobramycin and amikacin against gentamicin-resistant Gram-negative bacilli. Lancet i: 423.

Howard JB, McCracken GH Jr (1975). Pharmacological evaluation of amikacin in neonates. Antimicrob Ag Chemother 8: 86.

Inderlied CB, Young LS, Yamada JK (1987). Determination of in vitro susceptibility of Mycobacterium avium complex isolates to antimycobacterial agents by various methods. Antimicrob Ag Chemother 31: 1697.

Inderlied CB, Kolonoski PT, Wu M, Young LS (1989). Amikacin, ciprofloxacin and imipenem treatment for disseminated Mycobacterium avium complex infection of beige mice. Antimicrob Ag Chemother 33: 176.

Ingram CW, Tanner DC, Durack DT et al. (1993). Disseminated infection with rapidly growing mycobacteria. Clin Infect Dis 16: 463.

Jacoby GA, Blaser MJ, Santanam P et al. (1990). Appearance of amikacin and tobramycin resistance due to 4'-aminoglycoside nucleotidyltransferase [ANT(4'-II] in Gram-negative pathogens. Antimicrob Ag Chemother 34: 2381.

Jauregui L, Cushing RD, Lerner AM (1977). Gentamicin/amikacin resistant Gram-negative bacilli at Detroit General Hospital, 1975–1976. Amer J Med 62 (Suppl). 39.

Johnson DE, Thompson B, Calia FM (1985). Comparative activities of piperacillin, ceftazidime and amikacin, alone and in all possible combinations, against experimental Pseudomonas aeruginosa infections in neutropenic rats. Antimicrob Ag Chemother 28: 735.

Kahlmeter G, Dahlager JI (1984). Aminoglycosde toxicity – a review of clinical studies published between 1975 and 1982. J Antimicrob Chemother 13 (Suppl A): 9.

Kaojarern S, Maoleekoonpairoj S, Atichartakarn V (1989). Pharmacokinetics of amikacin in hematologic malignancies. Antimicrob Ag Chemother 33: 1406.

Karnad A, Alvarez S, Berk SL (1985). Pneumonia caused by Gram-negative bacilli. Amer J Med 79(1A): 61.

Kawaguchi H (1976). Discovery, chemistry, and activity of amikacin. J Infect Dis 134 (Suppl): 242.

Kenyon CF, Knoppert DC, Lee SK et al. (1990). Amikacin pharmacokinetics and suggested dosage modifications for the preterm infant. Antimicrob Ag Chemother 34: 265.

Khan AJ, Evans HE, Jhaveri R et al. (1976). Amikacin pharmacokinetics in the therapy of childhood urinary tract infections. Pediatrics 58: 873.

Khardori N, Rolston K, Rosenbaum B et al. (1989). Comparative in-vitro activity of twenty antimicrobial agents against clinical isolates of Mycobacterium avium complex. J Antimicrob Chemother 24: 667.

Kibbler CC, McWhinney PHM, Warner P, Prentice HG (1992). Ototoxicity associated with once daily dose of amikacin regimen in febrile neutropenic patients. J Antimicrob Chemother 29: 463.

King JW, White MC, Todd JR, Conrad SA (1992). Alterations in the microbial flora and in the incidence of bacteremia at a University Hospital after adoption of amikacin as the sole formulary aminoglycoside. Clin Infect Dis 14: 908.

Kinowski J-M, de la Coussaye J-E, Bressolle F et al. (1993). Multiple-dose pharmacokinetics of amikacin and ceftazidime in critically ill patients with septic multiple-organ failure during intermittent hemofiltration. Antimicrob Ag Chemother 37: 464.

Kirby WMM, Clarke JT, Libke RD, Regamey C (1976). Clinical pharmacology of amikacin and kanamycin. J Infect Dis 134 (Suppl): 312.

Klastersky J (1983). Empiric treatment of infections in neutropenic patients with cancer. Rev Infect Dis 5 (Suppl 1): 21.

Klastersky J, Hensgens C, Meunier-Carpentier F (1976). Comparative effftectiveness of combinations of amikacin with penicillin G and amikacin with carbenicillin in Gram-negative septicaemia: double-blind clinical trial. *J Infect Dis* **134** (Suppl): 433.

Kopcha RG, Fant WK, Warden GD (1991). Increased dosing requirements for amikacin in burned children. *J Antimicrob Chemother* **28**: 747.

Kornguth ML, Kunin CM (1977). Distribution of gentamicin and amikacin in rabbit tissues. *Antimicrob Ag Chemother* **11**: 974.

Kwaga J, Iversen JO (1990). *In vitro* antimicrobial susceptibilities of *Yersinia enterocolitica* and related species isolated from slaughtered pigs and pork products. *Antimicrob Ag Chemother* **34**: 2423.

Lambert T, Gerbaud G, Courvalin P (1988). Transferable amikacin resistance in *Acinetobacter* spp. due to a new type of 3'-aminoglycoside phosphotransferase. *Antimicrob Ag Chemother* **32**: 15.

Lambert T, Gerbaud G, Bouvet P et al. (1990). Dissemination of amikacin resistance gene aphA6 in *Acinetobacter* spp. *Antimicrob Ag Chemother* **34**: 1244.

Lambert T, Gerbaud G, Galimand M, Courvalin P (1993). Characterization of *Acinetobacter haemolyticus* aac (6').- Ig gene encoding an aminoglycoside 6'-N-acetyltransferase which modifies amikacin. *Antimicrob Ag Chemother* **37**: 2093.

Lambert T, Gerbaud G, Courvalin P (1994a). Characterization of transposon Tn 1528, which confers amikacin resistance by synthesis of aminoglycoside 3'-O-phosphoratransferase type VI. *Antimicrob Ag Chemother* **38**: 702.

Lambert T, Gerbaud G, Courvalin P (1994b). Characterization of the chromosomal aac (6').-Ij gene of *Acinetobacter* sp. 13 and the aac (6').-Ih plasmid gene of *Acinetobacter baumannii*. *Antimicrob Ag Chemother* **38**: 1883.

Lanao JM, Navarro AS, Dominguez-Gil A et al. (1983). Amikacin concentrations in serum and blister fluid in healthy volunteers and in patients with renal impairment. *J Antimicrob Chemother* **12**: 481.

Lane AZ, Wright GE, Blair DC (1977). Ototoxicity and nephrotoxicity of amikacin An overview of Phase II and Phase III experience in the United States. *Amer J Med* **62** (Suppl): 105.

Larson TA, Garrett CR, Gerding DN (1986). Frequency of aminoglycoside 6'-N-acetyltransferase among *Serratia* species during increased use of amikacin in the hospital. *Antimicrob Ag Chemother* **30**: 176.

Lau WK, Young LS, Black RE et al. (1977a). Comparative efficacy and toxicity of amikacin/carbenicillin versus gentamicin/carbenicillin in leukopenic patients. A randomized prospective trial. *Amer J Med* **62** (Suppl): 212.

Lau WK, Young LS, Osher AB, Dooley RR (1977b). Amikacin therapy of exacerbations of *Pseudomonas aeruginosa* infections in patients with cystic fibrosis. *Pediatrics* **60**: 372.

Leroy A, Humbert G, Oksenhendler G, Fillastre JP (1976). Comparative pharmacokinetics of lividomycin, amikacin and sisomicin in normal subjects and in uraemic patients. *J Antimicrob Chemother* **2**: 373.

Levin S (1981). Antibiotics of choice in suspected severe sepsis. *J Antimicrob Chemother* **8** (Suppl A): 133.

Levine JF, Maslow MJ, Leibowitz RE et al. (1985). Amikacin-resistant Gram-negative bacilli: correlation of occurrence with amikacin use. *J Infect Dis* **151**: 295.

Levy J, Baran D, Klastersky J (1982). Comparative study of the anitbacterial activity of amikacin and tobramycin during *Pseudomonas* pulmonary infection in patients with cystic fibrosis. *J Antimicrob Chemother* **10**: 227.

Lewis RP, Meyer RD, Finegold SM (1977). Amikacin therapy of patients with gentamicin-resistant Gram-negative bacillary infection. *Amer J Med* **62** (Suppl): 142.

MacGregor RR (1977). Comparative penetration of amikacin, gentamicin, and penicillin G into exudate fluid in experimental sterile peritonitis. *Antimicrob Ag Chemother* **11**: 110.

Madhavan T, Yaremchuk K, Levin N et al. (1976). Effect of renal failure and dialysis on the serum concentration of the aminoglycoside amikacin. *Antimicrob Ag Chemother* **10**: 464.

Maes P (1985). Evaluation of the resistance mechanisms of gentamicin-resistant Gram-negative bacilli and their susceptibility to tobramycin, netilmicin and amikacin. *J Antimicrob Chemother* **15**: 283.

Maller R, Isaksson B, Nilsson L, Sören L (1988). A study of amikacin given once versus twice daily in serious infections. *J Antimicrob Chemother* **22**: 75.

Maller R, Emanuelsson B-M, Isaksson B, Nilsson L (1990). Amikacin once daily: a new dosing regimen based on drug pharmacokinetics. *Scand J Infect Dis* **22**: 575.

Maller R, Ahrne H, Holmen C et al. (1993). Once- versus twice-daily amikacin regimen: efficacy and safety in systemic Gram-negative infections. *J Antimicrob Chemother* **31**: 939.

Marik PE, Havlik I, Monteagudo FSE, Lipman J (1991a). The pharmacokinetics of amikacin in critically ill adult and paediatric patients: comparison of once- versus twice-daily dosage regimens. *J Antimicrob Chemother* **27** (Suppl C): 81.

Marik PE, Lipman J, Kobilski S, Scribante J (1991b). A prospective randomized study comparing once- versus twice-daily amikacin dosing in critically ill adults and paediatric patients. *J Antimicrob Chemother* **28**: 753.

Mathias RG, Ronald AR, Gurwith MJ et al. (1976). Clinical evaluation of amikacin in treatment of infections due to Gram-negative aerobic bacilli. *J Infect Dis* **134** (Suppl): 394.

Mayers M, Rush D, Madu A et al. (1991). Pharmacokinetics of amikacin and chloramphenicol in the aqueous humor of rabbits. *Antimicrob Ag Chemother* **35**: 1791.

Mazzei T, Paradiso M, Nicoletti I, Periti P (1976). Amikacin in obstetric, gynaecologic, and neonatal infections: laboratory and clinical studies. *J Infect Dis* **134** (Suppl): 374.

McCracken GH Jr, Nelson JD (1983). *Antimicrobial Therapy for Newborns* 2nd edn, p. 59. New York: Grune & Stratton.

McGrath BJ, Bailey EM, Lamp KC, Rybak MJ (1992). Pharmacodynamics of once-daily amikacin in various combinations with cefepime, aztreonam, and ceftazidime against *Pseudomonas aeruginosa* in an *in vitro* infection model. *Antimicrob Ag Chemother* **36**: 2741.

McHenry MC, Wagner JG, Hall PM et al. (1976). Pharmacokinetics of amikacin in patients with impaired renal function. *J Infect Dis* **134** (Suppl): 343.

McNeil MM, Brown JM, Jarvis WR, Ajello L (1990). Comparison of species distribution and antimicrobial susceptibility of aerobic actinomycetes from clinical specimens. *Rev Infect Dis* **12**: 778.

McWhinney PHM, Yates M, Prentice HG et al. (1992). Infection caused by *Mycobacterium chelonae*: a diagnostic and therapeutic problem in the neutropenic patient. *Clin Infect Dis* **14**: 1208.

Meier B, Metzger U, Müller F et al. (1986). Successful treatment of a pancreatic *Nocardia asteroides* abscess with amikacin and surgical drainage. *Antimicrob Ag Chemother* **29**: 150.

Meunier F, Van der Auwera P, Aoun M et al. (1991). Empirical antimicrobial therapy with a single daily dose of ceftriaxone plus amikacin in febrile granulocytopenic patients: a pilot study. *J Antimicrob Chemother* **27** (Suppl C): 129.

Meyer RD (1981). Amikacin. *Ann Intern Med* **95**: 328.

Meyer RD, Lewis RP, Carmalt ED, Finegold SM (1975). Amikacin therapy for serious Gram-negative bacillary infections. *Ann Intern Med* **83**: 790.

Meyer RD, Lewis RP, Halter J, White M (1976). Gentamicin-resistant *Pseudomonas aeruginosa* and *Serratia marcescens* in a general hospital. *Lancet* i: 580.

Minshew BH, Pollock HM, Schoenknecht FD, Sherris JC (1977). Emergence in a burn center of populations of bacteria resistant to gentamicin, tobramycin and amikacin: evidence for the need for changes in zone diameter interpretive standards. *Antimicrob Ag Chemother* **12**: 688.

Moellering RC Jr (1977). Microbiological considerations in the use of tobramycin and related aminoglycosidic aminocyclitol antibiotics. *Med J Aust* **2** (Suppl): 4.

Moellering RC Jr (1983). *In vitro* anitbacterial activity of the aminoglycoside antibiotics. *Rev Infect Dis* **5** (Suppl 2): 212.

Moellering RC Jr, Wennersten C, Kunz LJ, Poitras JW (1977). Resistance to gentamicin, tobramycin and amikacin among clinical isolates of bacteria. *Amer J Med* **62** (Suppl): 30

Moore RD, Smith CR, Lietman PS (1984). Risk factors for the development of auditory toxicity in patients receiving aminoglycosides. *J Infect Dis* **149**: 23.

Moreno MT, Vargas S, Poveda R, Sáez-Llorens X (1994). Neonatal sepsis and meningitis in a developing Latin American country. *Pediatr Infect Dis J* **13**: 516.

Mosquera JM, De Villota ED, De La Serna JL *et al.* (1981). Amikacin treatment of *Serratia* septicemia in critically ill patients. *Crit Care Med* **9**: 633,.

Munckhof WJ, Grayson ML, Turnidge JD (1995). A meta-analysis of studies on the safety and efficacy of aminoglycosides given either once-daily or as divided doses. *J Antimicrob Chemother* **37**: 645.

Muscato JJ, Wilbur DW, Stout JJ, Fahrlender RA (1991). An evaluation of the susceptibility patterns of Gram-negative organisms isolated in cancer centres with aminoglycoside usage. *J Antimicrob Chemother* **27** (Suppl C): 1.

Myers MG, Roberts RJ, Mirhij NJ (1977). Effects of gestational age, birth weight, and hypoxemia on pharmacokinetics of amikacin in serum of infants. *Antimicrob Ag Chemother* **11**: 1027.

Neu HC (1984). Current mechanisms of resistance to antimicrobial agents in micro-organisms causing infection in the patient at risk of infection. *Amer J Med* **11**.

Noone M, Pomeroy L, Sage R, Noone P (1989). Prospective study of amikacin versus netilmicin in the treatment of severe infection in hospitalized patients. *Amer J Med* **86**: 809.

Olson B, Weinstein RA, Nathan C *et al.* (1985). Occult aminoglycoside resistance in *Pseudomonas aeruginosa*: epidemiology and implications for therapy and control. *J Infect Dis* **152**: 769.

Perlin MH, Lerner SA (1979). Amikacin resistance associated with a plasmid borne aminoglycoside phosphotransferase in *Escherichia coli*. *Antimicrob Ag Chemother* **16**: 598.

Perlin MH, Lerner SA (1986). High-level amikacin resistance in *Escherichia coli* due to phosphorylation and impaired aminoglycoside uptake. *Antimicrob Ag Chemother* **29**: 216.

Phillips I, Eykyn S, King BA *et al.* (1977). The *in vitro* antibacterial activity of nine aminoglycosides and spectinomycin on clinical isolates of common Gram-negative bacteria. *J Antimicrob Chemother* **3**: 403.

Pien FD, Ho PWL (1981). Antimicrobial spectrum, pharmacology, adverse effects, and therapeutic use of amikacin sulfate. *Amer J Hosp Pharm* **38**: 981.

Pijck J, Hallynck T, Soep H *et al.* (1976). Pharmacokinetics of amikacin in patients with renal insufficiency: relation to half-life and creatinine clearance. *J Infect Dis* **134** (Suppl): 331.

Ploy M-C, Giamarellou H, Bourlioux P *et al.* (1994). Detection of aac(6').-I genes in amikacin-resistant *Acinetobacter* spp. by PCR. *Antimicrob Ag Chemother* **38**: 2925.

Powell KR, Pincus PH (1987). Five years of experience with the exclusive use of amikacin in a neonatal intensive care unit. *Pediatr Infect Dis J* **6**: 466.

Price KE, De Furia MD, Pursiano TA (1976). Amikacin, an aminoglycoside with marked activity against antibiotic-resistant clinical isolates. *J Infect Dis* **134** (Suppl): 249.

Price KE, Kresel PA, Farchione LA *et al.* (1981). Epidemiological studies of aminoglycoside resistance in the USA. *J Antimicrob Chemother* **8** (Suppl A): 89.

Raad II, Vartivarian S, Khan A, Bodey GP (1991). Catheter-related infections caused by the *Mycobacterium fortuitum* complex: 15 cases and review. *Rev Infect Dis* **13**: 1120.

Rankin LI, Luft FC, Yum MN, Isaacs LL (1980). Comparative nephrotoxicities of dibekacin, amikacin and gentamicin in a rat model. *Antimicrob Ag Chemother* **18**: 983.

Regeur L, Colding H, Jensen H, Kampmann JP (1977). Pharmacokinetics of amikacin during hemodialysis and peritoneal dialysis. *Antimicrob Ag Chemother* **11**: 214.

Ries K, Levison ME, Keye D (1973). *In vitro* evaluation of a new aminoglycoside derivative of kanamycin, a comparison with tobramycin and gentamicin. *Antimicrob Ag Chemother* **3**: 532.

Sanders CC, Watanakunakorn C (1986). Emergence of resistance to beta-lactams, aminoglycosides, and quinolones during combination therapy for infection due to *Serratia marcescens*. *J Infect Dis* **153**: 617.

Sanders WE Jr, Hartwig C, Schneider N *et al.* (1982). Activity of amikacin against mycobacteria *in vitro* and in murine tuberculosis. *Tubercle* **63**: 201.

Sanders WJ, Wolinsky E (1980). *In vitro* susceptibility of *Mycobacterium marinum* to eight antimicrobial agents. *Antimicrob Ag Chemother* **18**: 529.

Santré C, Georges H, Jacquier JM *et al.* (1995). Amikacin levels in bronchial secretions of 10 pneumonia patients with respiratory support treated once daily versus twice daily. *Antimicrob Ag Chemother* **39**: 264.

Schiff TA, McNeil MM, Brown JM (1993). Cutaneous *Nocardia farcinia* infection in a non immunocompromised patient. Case report and review. *Clin Infect Dis* **16**: 756.

Schiffman DO (1977). Evaluation of amikacin sulfate (amikin). A new aminoglycoside antibiotic. *JAMA* **238**: 1547.

Schurman DJ, Wheeler R (1977). Bone and joint Gram-negative infection and amikacin treatment. *Amer J Med* **62** (Suppl): 160.

Segal JL, Brunnemann SR, Eltorai IM (1990). Pharmacokinetics of amikacin in serum and in tissue contiguous with pressure sores in humans with spinal cord injury. *Antimicrob Ag Chemother* **34**: 1422.

Seligman SJ (1978). Frequency of resistance to kanamycin, tobramycin, netilmicin and amikacin in gentamicin-resistant Gram-negative bacteria. *Antimicrob Ag Chemother* **13**: 70.

Shalit I, Welch DF, San Joaquin VH, Marks MI (1985). *In vitro* anitbacterial activities of antibiotics against *Pseudomonas aeruginosa* in peritoneal dialysis fluid. *Antimicrob Ag Chemother* **27**: 908.

Shaw KJ, Rather PN, Hare RS, Miller GH (1993). Molecular genetics of aminoglycoside resistance genes and familial relationships of the aminoglycoside-modifying enzymes. *Microbiol Rev* **57**: 138.

Shulman ST, Yogev R (1985). Treatment of pediatric infections with amikacin as first-line aminoglycoside. *Amer J Med* **79** (1A): 43.

Smeltzer BD, Schwartzman MS, Bertino JSJr (1988). Amikacin pharmacokinetics during continuous ambulatory peritoneal dialysis. *Antimicrob Ag Chemother* **32**: 236.

Smith CR, Lietman PS (1983). Effect of furosemide on aminoglycoside-induced nephrotoxicity and auditory toxicity in humans. *Antimicrob Ag Chemother* **23**: 133.

Smith CR, Baughman KL, Edwards CQ *et al.* (1977). Controlled comparison of amikacin and gentamicin. *New Engl J Med* **296**: 349.

Straus WL, Ostroff SM, Jernigan DB *et al.* (1994). Clinical and epidemiologic characteristics of *Mycobacterium haemophilium*, an emerging pathogen in immunocompromised patients. *Ann Intern Med* **120**: 118.

Subbarao EK, Tarpay MM, Marks MI (1987). Soft tissue infections caused by *Mycobacterium fortuitum* complex following penetrating injury. *Amer J Dis Child* **141**: 1018.

Swenson JM, Thornsberry C, Silcox VA (1982). Rapidly growing mycobacteria: testing of susceptibility to 34 antimicrobial agents by broth microdilution. *Antimicrob Ag Chemother* **22**: 186.

Swenson JM, Wallace RJ Jr, Silcox VA, Thornsberry C (1985). Antimicrobial susceptibility of five subgroups of *Mycobacterium fortuitum* and *Mycobacterium chelonae*. *Antimicrob Ag Chemother* **28**: 807.

The International Antimicrobial Therapy Cooperative Group of the European Organization for Research and Treatment of cancer (1993). Efficacy and toxicity of single daily doses of amikacin and ceftriaxone versus multiple daily doses of amikacin and ceftazidime for infection in patients with cancer and granulocytopenia. *Ann Intern Med* **119**: 584.

Tally FP, Gorbach SL (1977). Review of 152 patients with bacteremias treated with amikacin. *Amer J Med* **62** (Suppl): 137.

Tally FP, Louie TJ, O'Keefe JP *et al.* (1976). Amikacin therapy for severe Gram-negative sepsis: efficacy in infections involving gentamicin-resistant organisms. *J Infect Dis* **134** (Suppl): 428.

Tan JS, Salstrom SJ (1977). Levels of carbenicillin, ticarcillin, cephalothin, cefazolin, cefamandole, gentamicin, tobramycin and amikacin in human serum and interstitial fluid. *Antimicrob Ag Chemother* **11**: 698.

Taryle DA, Good JT Jr, Morgan EJ III *et al.* (1981). Anitbiotic concentrations in human parapneumonic effusions. *J Antimicrob Chemother* **7**: 171.

Thauvin C, Eliopoulos GM, Wennersten C, Moellering RC Jr (1985). Antagonistic effect of penicillin-amikacin combinations against enterococci. *Antimicrob Ag Chemother* **28**: 78.

Thornsberry C, Baker CN, Kirven LA (1978). *In vitro* activity of antimicrobial agents on Legionnaires' disease bacterium. *Antimicrob Ag Chemother* **13**: 78.

Tolmasky ME, Crosa JH (1987). Tn 1331, a novel multiresistance transposon encoding resistance to amikacin and ampicillin in *Klebsiella pneumoniae*. *Antimicrob Ag Chemother* **31**: 1955.

Tolmasky ME, Roberts M, Woloj M, Crosa JH (1986). Molecular cloning of amikacin resistance dterminants from a *Klebsiella pneumoniae* plasmid. *Antimicrob Ag Chemother* **30**: 315.

Tolmasky ME, Chamorro RM, Crosa JH, Marini PM (1988). Transposon-mediated amikacin resistance in *Klebsiella pneumoniae*. *Antimicrob Ag Chemother* **32**: 1416.

Trenholme GM, McKellar PP, Rivera N, Levin S (1977). Amikacin in the treatment of Gram-negative pneumonia. *Amer J Med* **62** (Suppl): 155.

Tsui SYT, Yew WW, Li MSK *et al.* (1993). Postantibiotic effects of amikacin and ofloxacin on *Mycobacterium fortuitum*. *Antimicrob Ag Chemother* **37**: 1001.

Tulkens PM (1991). Pharmacokinetic and toxicological evaluation of a once-daily regimen versus conventional schedules of netilmicin and amikacin. *J Antimicrob Chemother* **27** (Suppl C): 49.

Ubukata K, Yamashita N, Gotoh A, Konno M (1984). Purification and characterization of aminoglycoside-modifying enzymes from *Staphylococcus aureus* and *Staphylococcus epidermidis*. *Antimicrob Ag Chemother* **25**: 754.

Valdivieso M, Keating MJ, Feld R *et al.* (1977). Review of experience with amikacin and other aminoglycoside antibiotics in the treatment of infectious complications in patients with cancer. *Amer J Med* **62** (Suppl): 204.

Van der Auwera P, Klastersky J (1987). Serum bactericidal activity and postantibiotic effect in serum of patients with urinary tract infection receiving high-dose amikacin. *Antimicrob Ag Chemother* **31**: 1061.

Van der Auwera P, Schuyteneer F (1983). *In-vitro* susceptibility of *Pseudomonas aeruginosa* to old and new beta-lactam antibiotics and aminoglycosides. *J Antimicrob Chemother* **11**: 511.

Van der Auwera P, Klastersky J, Lagast H, Husson M (1986). Serum bactericidal activity and killing rate for volunteers receiving imipenem, imipenem plus amikacin, and ceftazidime plus amikacin against *Pseudomonas aeruginosa*. *Antimicrob Ag Chemother* **30**: 122.

Vanhaeverbeek M, Siska G, Herchuelz A (1993). Pharmacokinetics of once-daily amikacin in elderly patients. *J Antimicrob Chemother* **31**: 185.

Van Nhieu GT, Collatz E (1988). Heterogeneity of 6'-N-acetyltransferases of type 4 conferring resistance to amikacin and related aminoglycosides in members of the family Enterobacteriaceae. *Antimicrob Ag Chemother* **32**: 1289.

Van Nhieu GT, Goldstein FW, Pinto ME *et al.* (1986). Transfer of amikacin resistance by closely related plasmids in members of the family Enterobacteriaceae isolated in Chile. *Antimicrob Ag Chemother* **29**: 833.

Venezio FR, Di Vincenzo CA (1985). Effects of aminoglycoside antibiotics on polymorphonuclear leukocyte function *in vivo*. *Antimicrob Ag Chemother* **27**: 712.

Vogel L, Nathan C, Sweeney HM *et al.* (1978). Infections due to gentamicin-resistant *Staphylococcus aureus* strain in a nursery for neonatal infants. *Antimicrob Ag Chemother* **13**: 466.

Vogelstein B, Kowarski AA, Lietman PS (1977). The pharmacokinetics of amikacin in children. *J Pediatr* **91**: 333.

Walker JM, Wise R, Mithcard M (1979). The pharmacokinetics of amikacin and gentamicin in volunteers: a comparison of individual differences. *J Antimicrob Chemother* **5**: 95.

Wallace RJ Jr, Wiss K (1981). Susceptibility of *Mycobacterium marinum* to tetracyclines and aminoglycosides. *Antimicrob Ag Chemother* **20**: 610.

Wallace R J Jr, Dalovisio JR, Pankey GA (1979a). Disc diffusion testing of susceptibility of *Mycobacterium fortuitum* and *Mycobacterium chelonei* to antibacterial agents. *Antimicrob Ag Chemother* **16**: 611.

Wallace RJ Jr, Septimus EJ, Musher DM *et al.* (1979b). Treatment of experimental nocardiosis in mice: comparison of amikacin and sulfonamide. *J Infect Dis* **140**: 244.

Wallace RJ Jr, Swenson JM, Silcox VA, Bullen MG (1985). Treatment of non-pulmonary infections due to *Mycobacterium fortuitum* and *Mycobacterium chelonei* on the basis of *in vitro* susceptibilities. *J Infect Dis* **152**: 500.

Want SV, Jones RAK, Darrell JH (1979). Amikacin dosage in the preterm newborn. *J Antimicrob Chemother* **5**: 527.

Williams RJ, Lindridge MA, Said AA *et al.* (1984). National survey of antibiotic resistance in *Pseudomonas aeruginosa*. *J Antimicrob Chemother* **14**: 9.

Winston DJ, Ho WG, Champlin RE *et al.* (1986). Ureidopenicillins, aztreonam, and thienamycin: efficacy as single-drug therapy of severe infections and potential as components of combined therapy. *J Antimicrob Chemother* **17** (Suppl A): 55.

Wise R, Walker JM, Mitchard M (1981). A comparison of the pharmacokinetics of amikacin and gentamicin. *J Antimicrob Chemother* **8** (Suppl A): 45.

Woloj M, Tolmasky ME, Roberts MC, Crosa JH (1986). Plasmid-encoded amikacin resistance in multiresistant strains of *Klebsiella pneumoniae* isolated from neonates with meningitis. *Antimicrob Ag Chemother* **29**: 315.

Wright PF, Kaiser AB, Bowman CM *et al.* (1981). The pharmacokinetics and efficacy of an aminoglycoside administered into the cerebral ventricles in neonates: implications for further evaluation of this route of therapy in meningitis. *J Infect Dis* **143**: 141.

Yajko DM, Nassos PS, Hadley WK (1987). Broth microdilution testing of susceptibilities to 30 antimicrobial agents of *Mycobacterium avium* strains from patients with acquired immune deficiency syndrome. *Antimicrob Ag Chemother* **31**: 1579.

Yates RA, Mitchard M, Wise R (1978). Disposition studies with amikacin after rapid intravenous and intramuscular administration to human volunteers. *J Antimicrob Chemother* **4**: 335.

Yogev R, Kolling WM (1981). Intraventricular levels of amikacin after intravenous administration. *Antimicrob Ag Chemother* **20**: 583.

Yogev R, Greenslade T, Firlit CF, Lewy P (1980). Successful treatment of *Nocardia asteroides* infection with amikacin. *J Pediatr* **96**: 771.

Young LS (1985). Use of aminoglycosides in immunocompromised patients. *Amer J Med* **79** (1A): 21.

Young LS (1988). *Mycobacterium avium* complex infection. *J Infect Dis* **157**: 863.

Young LS, Meyer-Dudnik DV, Hindler J, Martin WJ (1981). Aminoglycosides in the treatment of bacteraemic infections in the immunocomprised host. *J Antimicrob Chemother* **8** (Suppl A): 121.

Young LS, Inderlied CB, Berlin OG, Gottlieb MS (1986). Mycobacterial infections in AIDS patients, with an emphasis on the *Mycobacterium avium* complex. *Rev Infect Dis* **8**: 1024.

Yow MD (1977). An overview of pediatric experience with amikacin. *Amer J Med* **62** (Suppl): 167.

Yu PKW, Washington JA II (1973). Comparative *in vitro* activity of three aminoglycosidic antibiotics: BB-K8, kanamycin and gentamicin. *Antimicrob Ag Chemother* **4**: 133.

Sisomicin and Netilmicin

Description

1 Sisomicin

This aminoglycoside is produced by *Micromonospora inyoensis* (Crowe and Sanders, 1973). In its antimicrobial spectrum and all other properties, it is very similar to gentamicin (p.450). It is about as effective as gentamicin against all Enterobacteriaceae (Meyers *et al.*, 1975; Drasar *et al.*, 1976; Phillips *et al.*, 1977a). Sisomicin is more active than gentamicin, but not as active as tobramycin (p.489) against *Pseudomonas aeruginosa* (Sanders and Sanders, 1980; Moellering, 1983).

There is almost complete cross-resistance between gentamicin and sisomicin, most gentamicin-resistant Gram-negative bacilli being also sisomicin-resistant (Drasar *et al.*, 1976; Meyer *et al.*, 1976; Verbist *et al.*, 1978). The reason for this is that sisomicin, like gentamicin, is affected by at least eight of the plasmid coded enzymes, which can be produced by Gram-negative bacteria and which modify gentamicin (p.453) (O'Hara *et al.*, 1974; Shaw *et al.*, 1993). On the other hand, sisomicin is active against some organisms which resist gentamicin by non-enzymatic mechanisms (Sanders and Sanders, 1980).

Sisomicin does not offer significant advantages over gentamicin. It has had limited clinical trials, and has been available commercially in Europe, but not in the USA, UK and Australia. The dosage of sisomicin (3–6 mg per kg per day), its methods of administration and pharmacokinetics, are similar to those of gentamicin (p.457) (Pechère *et al.*, 1976; Leroy *et al.*, 1976). The toxicity of these two drugs is also probably about the same (Sanders and Sanders, 1980). Results of treatment of conditions, such as urinary tract infections or Gram-negative organism septicemias, have, in general, been similar to what would be expected from an identical gentamicin regimen (Klastersky *et al.*, 1975).

2 Netilmicin

This is a semisynthetic derivative of sisomicin, which was developed by ethylation of the 1-N position of the deoxystreptamine ring of sisomicin (Rahal *et al.*, 1976; Dhawan *et al.*, 1977). Netilmicin has a similar *in vitro* antibacterial spectrum to that of gentamicin (p.450), but unlike sisomicin, it is active against a proportion of gentamicin-resistant Gram-negative bacilli (Miller *et al.*, 1976). Whilst at least nine of the plasmid-mediated enzymes produced by Gram-negative bacilli affect gentamicin (p.454) and eight affect sisomicin, netilmicin is not affected by all of these enzymes. In general, netilmicin is active against strains of Gram-negative bacilli which modify gentamicin by phosphorylation (APH enzymes) or adenylylation (referred to as either AAD or ANT enzymes). Netilmicin is usually ineffective against bacterial strains, some of which are sensitive to amikacin (p.505), which produce aminoglycoside acetylating (AAC) enzymes (Miller *et al.*, 1976; Guay, 1983; Moellering, 1983; Maes, 1985; Shaw *et al.*, 1993). Therefore, netilmicin is not active against such a wide range of gentamicin-resistant Gram-negative bacilli as amikacin (p.505). Nevertheless, it may be occasionally indicated as an alternative to amikacin, for the treatment of infections caused by gentamicin-resistant but netilmicin-sensitive Gram-negative organisms.

The following details apply to netilmicin only.

Sensitive Organisms

1 Gram-negative bacteria

Netilmicin, like gentamicin (p.450), is active against all the Enterobacteriaceae, such as *Escherichia coli*, the *Enterobacter*, *Klebsiella*, all *Proteus*, *Salmonella*, *Shigella*, *Providencia*, *Serratia*, *Citrobacter*, *Hafnia*, *Edwardsiella*, *Arizona* and *Yersinia* spp. (Eickhoff and Ehret, 1977; Hammerberg *et al.*, 1977; Smith *et al.*, 1977). In general, its activity against gentamicin-susceptible strains of the Enterobacteriaceae, is similar to that of gentamicin. But, gentamicin is more active against *Serratia* spp. (Klastersky *et al.*, 1977; Kantor and Norden, 1977; Habwe and Shadomy, 1979). *Serratia* spp. can also become netilmicin-resistant due to production of an aminoglycoside acetylating enzyme (Hawkey and Constable, 1988).

Pseudomonas aeruginosa is netilmicin-sensitive, but most strains are approximately 2-fold less sensitive than to gentamicin (Brown *et al.*, 1976; Smith *et al.*, 1977; Digranes *et al.*, 1980), and in terms of MICs, 4-fold less active than tobramycin (Moffie *et al.*, 1993). Netilmicin, like gentamicin, is active against the *Neisseria* spp. (meningococci and gonococci) and *Haemophilus influenzae* (Eickhoff and Ehret, 1977). *Acinetobacter* spp. may be netilmicin-sensitive, but resistant strains occur (Meyers and Hirschman, 1977; Phillips *et al.*, 1977b).

In common with other aminoglycosides (p.452), netilmicin is inactive against *Bacteroides fragilis* and other anaerobic Gram-negative bacteria.

2 Gentamicin-resistant Gram-negative bacteria

The main feature of netilmicin is its activity against a percentage of strains of Enterobacteriaceae and also some strains of *Ps. aeruginosa*, with acquired resistance to gentamicin and/or tobramycin (Meyers and Hirschman, 1977; Langstaff *et al.*, 1983; Guimaraes *et al.*, 1985; Bengtsson *et al.*, 1986). Compared with amikacin, netilmicin is not active against as high a percentage of individual species strains, or as wide a range of gentamicin-resistant Gram-negative bacilli (Kantor and Norden, 1977; Seligman, 1978; Guay, 1983). This is due to its greater susceptibility to aminoglycoside-modifying enzymes (p.522).

Gentamicin-resistant strains of *E. coli*, *Proteus mirabilis* and the *Enterobacter*, *Klebsiella*, *Citrobacter* and *Serratia* spp. are usually netilmicin-sensitive, while gentamicin-resistant *Pr. vulgaris*, *Morganella morganii* and *Providencia* spp. are usually resistant to netilmicin (Miller *et al.*, 1976; Dhawan *et al.*, 1977; Verbist *et al.*, 1978; Moellering, 1983). Others have reported that a proportion of gentamicin-resistant strains of *E. coli* and *Serratia marcescens* are also resistant to netilmicin (Fu and Neu, 1976; Meyers and Hirschman, 1977). The majority of gentamicin-resistant *Ps. aeruginosa* strains are also netilmicin-resistant (Fu and Neu, 1976; Marks *et al.*, 1976; Kantor and Norden, 1977), but some investigators have reported a variable proportion of these strains to be netilmicin-sensitive (Dhawan *et al.*, 1977; Meyers and Hirschman, 1977). Strains of *Acinetobacter* spp. which are resistant to gentamicin are usually netilmicin-resistant (Meyers and Hirschman, 1977).

The proportion of gentamicin-resistant Gram-negative bacilli which are netilmicin-sensitive, may vary in different geographical areas. In one study in Belgium 253 gentamicin-resistant Gram-negative bacilli, isolated from clinical material, were tested for sensitivity to tobramycin, netilmicin and amikacin. Amikacin was active against 90% of strains, whereas the activities of netilmicin and tobramycin were the same with only approximately 14% of strains being susceptible. That netilmicin was not superior was explained by local enzyme patterns. In this population of bacteria the acetylating enzyme AAC-3 was predominant, which inactivates gentamicin, tobramycin and netilmicin, but not amikacin (p.505) (Maes, 1985). In a UK hospital 773 clinical isolates from hospital patients were tested for aminoglycoside sensitivity. Gentamicin resistance was found in 21% of strains of *Ps. aeruginosa*, 30% of *Pr. mirabilis* and 29% of other *Proteus* spp. Only about 10% of the isolates of these species were amikacin- and netilmicin-resistant. Differences between amikacin and netilmicin were only marginal, reflecting the relatively low prevalence of acetylating enzyme-producing organisms in this bacterial population (Guimaraes *et al.*, 1985).

3 Gram-positive bacteria

Staphylococcus aureus and *Staph. epidermidis*, including penicillin G-resistant strains are netilmicin-sensitive. Methicillin-resistant strains of these organisms may be netilmicin-sensitive, but in many hospitals, particularly in Australia, these strains are resistant to all aminoglycosides, including netilmicin (p.454). Gentamicin-resistant staphylococci are often susceptible to netilmicin, but netilmicin MICs for these strains may be 4- to 8-fold higher than those for fully susceptible strains. The suitability of netilmicin for treatment of infections caused by these

Organism	MIC (μg per ml)
Gram-negative bacteria (gentamicin-sensitive)	
Escherichia coli	0.2–6.3
Enterobacter spp.	0.2–6.3
Klebsiella spp.	0.2–6.3
Salmonella spp.	0.2–1.6
Serratia marcescens	0.4–50.0
Citrobacter spp.	0.023–0.8
Proteus mirabilis	0.2–25.0
Proteus vulgaris	0.2–12.5
Providencia spp.	0.4–25.0
Pseudomonas aeruginosa	0.2–12.5
Acinetobacter spp.	0.2–25.0
Gram-negative bacteria (gentamicin-resistant)	
Escherichia coli	0.4–12.5
Enterobacter spp.	3.1–12.5
Klebsiella spp.	0.2–6.3
Serratia marcescens	3.1–>100.0
Citrobacter spp.	0.4
Proteus mirabilis	50.0
Proteus vulgaris	3.1–25.0
Pseudomonas aeruginosa	12.5–50.0
Gram-positive bacteria	
Staphylococcus aureus	0.05–0.8
Enterococcus faecalis	3.1–25.0

Table I.41
After Fu and Neu (1976)

staphylococci, therefore depends on the susceptibility of the particular strain (Phillips *et al.*, 1977b; Bengtsson *et al.*, 1986; Davies *et al.*, 1986; McAllister *et al.*, 1987).

Streptococcus pyogenes, *Strep. pneumoniae* and *Enterococcus faecalis* are relatively netilmicin-resistant (Eickhoff and Ehret, 1977). Activity of netilmicin against these organisms is comparable with that of gentamicin (p.455). Similar to penicillin G/gentamicin (p.455) and penicillin G/tobramycin (p.491) combinations, penicillin G and netilmicin act synergistically against a proportion of *E. faecalis* strains *in vitro* (Smith *et al.*, 1977; Sanders, 1977). In one study, netilmicin was at least as effective as gentamicin for bactericidal synergy with penicillin G against *E. faecalis* strains isolated from patients with endocarditis (Shanson *et al.*, 1986). Findings by Rahal and Simberkoff (1986) were somewhat different. They reported that bactericidal synergy occurred with penicillin G with 2- to 4-fold lower netilmicin concentrations than with gentamicin. A penicillin G/netilmicin combination is effective for the treatment of experimental *E. faecalis* endocarditis in animals, caused by both 'streptomycin-susceptible' and 'streptomycin-resistant' (p.429) *E. faecalis* strains (Carrizosa and Kaye, 1978; Korzeniowski *et al.*, 1978). Penicillin G plus netilmicin are not synergistic against *E. faecalis* strains which exhibit 'high-level' gentamicin resistance (p.455). Similar to penicillin G/gentamicin (p.9), penicillin G/netilmicin exhibits bactericidal synergism against penicillin G-tolerant *Strep. viridans* strains (Shanson *et al.*, 1986).

Nocardia asteroides and some other *Nocardia* spp. are netilmicin-sensitive (Martin-Luengo and Valero-Guillen, 1983). All Gram-positive anaerobic bacilli, such as the *Clostridium* spp., are netilmicin-resistant, similar to other aminoglycosides (p.457).

4 Minimum inhibitory concentrations

The MICs of netilmicin against some selected bacterial species are shown in Table I.41.

Mode of Administration and Dosage

1 Once-daily administration

Similar to other aminoglycosides (p.457), netilmicin can be given once-daily i.m. or i.v. The theoretical justifications for this are similar to those of gentamicin (p.458) and other aminoglycosides. Bacterial killing by netilmicin is enhanced by the high peak level, thereafter there is the prolonged post-antibiotic effect, and with more frequent dosing 'adaptive resistance' to netilmicin may develop (Blaser et al., 1985, 1987; Daikos et al., 1991). Netilmicin has been given once-daily i.m. or i.v. in doses of 5–6 mg per kg. If it is given i.v., it is best to dilute the dose in 30–50 ml of i.v. infusion fluid and then to administer this as a short 30-min infusion. Blood for peak serum level estimation is taken 30 min after the conclusion of the infusion and this can be as high as 18–26 μg per ml (Gilbert, 1991).

For treatment of Gram-negative bacteremia, netilmicin, used as single drug, appears equally safe and effective when the total daily dose is administered once-daily, compared with the classical administration of the drug in three divided doses (Sturm, 1989, Gilbert, 1991). For the treatment of Gram-negative pyelonephritis in adults and children netilmicin, 5–6 mg per kg body weight once-daily or 2 mg per kg thrice-daily were again equally efficacious and safe (Van der Auwera et al., 1991; Vigano et al., 1992). For treatment of peritonitis, netilmicin once-daily or thrice-daily, again gave comparable results, but here the netilmicin regimens were combined with metronidazole (Fan et al., 1988; Hollender et al., 1989). For treatment of febrile neutropenic patients, again there was no difference in results with the two netilmicin regimens, but here it was essential to combine netilmicin with a suitable beta-lactam antibiotic (Rozdzinski et al., 1993). *Pseudomonas aeruginosa* infections in cystic fibrosis patients have been treated with a higher once-daily netilmicin dosage of 8 mg per kg (p.461) with success (Smith et al., 1994). With once-daily netilmicin administration one can monitor the peak and trough serum levels. However, Blaser et al. (1994) suggested that adequate information about serum netilmicin concentrations in these patients may be derived from a sample obtained 8 h after administration. Concentrations measured at this time should be in the range of 1.5–6 μg per ml. If the serum concentration at 8 h is lower than this, the netilmicin dosage may be too low, producing too small area under the curve. If the level is higher, the patient may be at risk of toxicity.

The administration of netilmicin once-daily appears about as safe and efficacious as the classical 8-hourly dosing, but the once-daily administration is more convenient (Munckhof et al., 1996).

2 Classical 8-hourly administration to adults

Netilmicin, like gentamicin (p.458), can be administered both i.m. or i.v. in the same dosage. The drug has been used in daily doses of either 3.0, 4.5, 6.0 or 7.5 mg per kg body weight administered in three divided doses at 8-hourly intervals (Klastersky et al., 1977; Panwalker et al., 1978; Kahlmeter, 1980; Aroney et al., 1981). The higher dosages have been used for severely ill patients or for treatment of infections caused by organisms relatively resistant to netilmicin. Solberg et al. (1980) used an adult i.m. dose as high as 200 mg (2.2 to 3.6 mg per kg) netilmicin every 8 h for 10 days to treat patients with severe infections. Others have administered the drug i.v. every 12 h in a dosage of 150 mg (Haverkorn, 1983) or 200 mg (Perera et al., 1982) to treat patients with systemic aerobic Gram-negative rod infections.

Netilmicin can be administered i.v. in the same manner as gentamicin (p.463), either by relatively rapid (3–5 min) injections (Riff and Moreschi, 1977), or by suitably diluting each dose in i.v. fluid for infusion over a 30-min period (Meyers et al., 1977). It may also be feasible to give netilmicin by a constant i.v. infusion using an infusion pump. To maintain constant serum concentrations of 4–6 μg per ml by this method, a higher total daily dose of the drug is needed, which may increase the risk of toxicity (Yap et al., 1977).

3 8-hourly administration to children

A daily dosage of 6 to 7.5 mg per kg body weight is suitable for patients of this age group (Michalsen and Bergan, 1981).

4 Newborn infants

On the basis of pharmacokinetic studies, a dosage of 2.5–3.0 mg per kg administered 12-hourly to infants 0–7 days of age and 8-hourly to those older than 7 days, is recommended. Serum level monitoring is essential when netilmicin is given to these patients (Siegel et al., 1979; McCracken and Nelson, 1983). Small preterm infants may require longer than 12 h intervals between individual 2.5 mg per kg netilmicin doses (Granati et al., 1985).

5 Patients with renal failure

The dose should be adjusted in a similar manner to that of gentamicin (p.460). The mean terminal half-life of netilmicin for subjects with a creatinine clearance value of >70 ml per min is 2.7 h. For those with creatinine clearance values of 25–70 ml per min, 4–25 ml per min and for anephric patients the netilmicin half-lives are approximately 10, 32 and 42 h, respectively. In patients with renal failure, the individual 2.0 mg per kg netilmicin doses, which are usually given 8-hourly, should be administered at longer intervals. These intervals can be calculated by multiplying by 3 the drug's half-life. This is a rough approximation and serum level monitoring and appropriate dosage adjustments are necessary. In anephric patients undergoing chronic hemodialysis, a dose of 2 mg per kg at the end of each dialysis session is usually sufficient (Humbert et al., 1978; Luft et al., 1978).

6 Cystic fibrosis patients

As with other aminoglycosides (p.461), these often need higher dosages. In ten cystic fibrosis patients, Bosso et al. (1985) found that the range of dosages needed to achieve desired peak concentrations in the sera was 7.42–17.02 mg per kg of body weight per day. As there is a large individual variation, routine monitoring of netilmicin concentrations in the sera of these patients is recommended.

Serum Levels in Relation to Dosage

Serum netilmicin levels after both i.m. and i.v. administration resemble those of gentamicin (p.463) (Chung et al., 1980).

1 Intramuscular administration

After an i.m. dose of 1.0 mg per kg body weight to adults, a mean peak serum level of 3.76 μg per ml is reached in 30–40 min. After the peak, the serum level of netilmicin gradually falls with a half-life of 2.0–2.5 h, reaching 1.0 μg per ml at 4 h and usually zero at 8 h (Riff and Moreschi, 1977).

2 Intravenous administration

Serum levels after i.v. administration of 1.0 mg per kg doses of both gentamicin and netilmicin, administered over 3–5 min, have been compared (Riff and Moreschi, 1977). Mean peak serum levels 10 min after the injection were similar for both drugs (5.0 μg per ml), but during the next 30 min (distribution phase) netilmicin serum levels fell more rapidly than those of gentamicin, so that at 40 min the netilmicin level was 2.9 μg per ml whilst that of gentamicin was still 3.6 μg per ml. Netilmicin may be more quickly distributed to a larger extravascular area than gentamicin. From the second hour onwards after the injection (elimination phase), netilmicin and gentamicin had approximately the same half-life of 2 h.

If a 2 mg per kg dose is infused i.v. over 30 min, the mean peak serum level 10 min after the infusion is 16.56 μg per ml. This falls to 12.87, 9.75, 7.89, 3.25, 1.39 and 0.91 μg per ml at 20 min, 40 min, 1 h, 2 h, 6 h and 8 h after the end of the infusion, respectively (Meyers et al., 1977).

Excretion

Like other aminoglycosides, netilmicin is excreted via the kidney by glomerular filtration and it is reabsorbed in the tubules to a limited extent (Chiu et al., 1977). The drug appears in the urine in an unchanged active form, where high urinary concentrations are attained. Approximately 50% of an administered dose is excreted in the urine during the first 6 h (Yap et al., 1977), and 70–80% in the first 24 h (Follath et al., 1978). The urine excretion of netilmicin is almost the same regardless of the route of administration (Riff and Moreschi, 1977).

After i.v. administration of netilmicin, urinary excretion during the first 2 h is slightly less than that after an identical dose of gentamicin. This suggests that the more rapid decline of netilmicin serum levels during the distribution phase (see above) is not due to its more rapid renal excretion, but due to a more rapid extravascular distribution (Riff and Moreschi, 1977).

Distribution of the Drug in Body

In common with other aminoglycosides (p.464), the serum protein binding of netilmicin is low (Welling *et al.*, 1977). The drug appears to be distributed in various body fluids and tissues in a similar manner to gentamicin (p.464). Netilmicin usually does not penetrate into the CSF of patients with uninflamed meninges. In patients who received a single daily dose of 400 mg of the drug i.v., CSF netilmicin concentrations of 0.13–0.45 μg per ml were observed 2–10 h after the end of netilmicin infusion (Nau *et al.*, 1993). In patients with bacterial meningitis after more than one of 8-hourly netilmicin doses, CSF levels ranged from 0.27 to 5.0 μg per ml (Brückner *et al.*, 1983). Netilmicin penetrated into the tissue fluid in much the same way as other aminoglycosides, such as tobramycin (Larson *et al.*, 1983; Blaser *et al.*, 1991).

The drug penetrated into the bronchial secretions in patients with purulent bronchitis, where the concentrations were about 19% of those found in serum (Thys *et al.*, 1979, 1981). When netilmicin in a dosage of 5 mg per kg body weight 12-hourly was given to patients with cystic fibrosis, who had *Ps. aeruginosa* bronchial infections, peak sputum netilmicin concentrations occurred 2–3 h after administration and these averaged 2.6 and 1.5 μg per ml on days 2 and 6 of treatment, respectively (Hjelte *et al.*, 1989).

In animals, netilmicin accumulates in the kidney in the same manner as gentamicin (p.465). The predominant site is the renal cortex, where the concentration is similar to that of gentamicin, but higher than that of tobramycin (Luft *et al.*, 1976; Bowman *et al.*, 1977; Chiu *et al.*, 1977; Luft *et al.*, 1983). Some authors have reported that netilmicin accumulates in the renal cortex of animals to an even greater extend than gentamicin (Brier *et al.*, 1985). The cortical concentrations of netilmicin and other aminoglycosides do not correlate with their degree of nephrotoxicity (p.528) (Parker *et al.*, 1980; Brion *et al.*, 1984; Brier *et al.*, 1985). In patients netilmicin, similar to gentamicin (p.465), accumulates in the body with multiple dosing. This accumulation is probably predominantly in the renal cortical cells (Edwards *et al.*, 1981). In animals netilmicin, like gentamicin (p.465), also accumulates in the renal medulla and the papillae; concentrations in these tissues are lower than in the cortex, but therapeutic levels persist for some 25 days after a 7-day course of the drug (Bergeron and Trottier, 1979).

Mode of Action

This is presumably the same as that of other aminoglycosides, such as streptomycin and gentamicin. Netilmicin and other aminoglycosides also produce a dose-dependent inhibition of amino acid incorporation in microsomes isolated from human liver and rat brain, kidney and liver. This inhibition of microsomal protein synthesis occurs at concentrations that have been shown to accumulate in rodent and human renal cortex and perilymph. This effect may partly explain the toxic effects of these drugs (Buss *et al.*, 1984).

Toxicity

1 Ototoxicity

Characteristic of all aminoglycosides (p.466), netilmicin can cause this complication. Animal studies indicate that netilmicin on a weight for weight basis, is considerably less ototoxic than other aminoglycosides, such as gentamicin and tobramycin (Wersäll, 1984). In animals, netilmicin concentrations in both vestibular and cochlear tissues are slightly lower than those of gentamicin, but their concentrations are about the same in the perilymph. There is no correlation between the concentration of the various aminoglycosides in these tissues and perilymph and their degree of ototoxicity (Dulon *et al.*, 1986).

Clinical studies also indicate that netilmicin-induced ototoxicity has been uncommon and that the drug is probably less toxic to the human inner ear than other aminoglycosides, such as gentamicin, tobramycin and amikacin. Klastersky *et al.* (1977) treated 30 patients with doses of either 4.5, 6.0 or 7.5 mg per kg body weight per day, and ototoxicity was not encountered. Panwalker *et al.* (1978) treated a further 27 patients with netilmicin and studied 21 by serial audiograms. One patient developed unilateral hearing loss, which was partially reversible. They also noted the absence of ototoxicity in two patients in whom very high netilmicin serum levels were maintained for more than a week; in one of these the range of peak serum levels was 15–36 μg per ml, and that of trough levels 10–24 μg per ml. Bergeron *et al.* (1983) treated 28 patients, aged between 17 and 72 years, for an average of 35 days with netilmicin at dosages of 2.4 to 6.9 mg per kg per day. Vestibular toxicity developed in two patients, but there were no audiogram changes.

In a prospective study of 90 adults, Barza *et al.* (1980) compared amikacin and netilmicin ototoxicity. Cochlear toxicity, as measured by a change of audiogram, occurred in four of 14 amikacin recipients and in three of 19 netilmicin recipients. Vestibular toxicity was noted in three of 16 amikacin-treated patients and in one of 15 treated by netilmicin. In another comparative trial 197 patients were treated by either tobramycin or netilmicin, and 55 were evaluated by audiogram. Relatively mild auditory toxicity developed in five of 28 recipients of tobramycin and in two of 27 of those treated by netilmicin (Gatell *et al.*, 1984). In another trial involving 187 patients, auditory toxicity was detected in 4.4, 10.8, and 23.5 % of patients given netilmicin, tobramycin, and amikacin, respectively (Gatell *et al.*, 1987). Also in a study of 118 immunocompromised patients with presumed severe infections, aminoglycoside-associated ototoxicity was less severe and more often reversible with netilmicin than with tobramycin (Bernstein *et al.*, 1986). Either tobramycin/ticarcillin or netilmicin/ticarcillin were used to treat 254 patients with serious Gram-negative bacillary infections by Lerner *et al.* (1983) and 84 tobramycin- and 73 netilmicin-treated patients had serial audiograms. Ototoxicity developed in ten tobramycin-treated patients, but only in two of those who received netilmicin. Kahlmeter and Dahlager (1984) surveyed aminoglycoside-induced ototoxicity in some 10 000 patients described in clinical trials published between 1975 and 1982. The average frequency of cochlear toxicity was 13.9% for amikacin, 8.3% for gentamicin, 6.1% for tobramycin and 2.4% for netilmicin. But in one study involving 89 older adults with serious bacterial infections and pre-existing renal impairment, the ototoxicity due to tobramycin and netilmicin appeared to be about the same (Gorse *et al.*, 1992). Also in a clinical trial where once-daily netilmicin dosage was compared with once-daily gentamicin for treatment of serious infections, there was no difference in ototoxicity between the two groups (Prins *et al.*, 1994).

It appears that netilmicin may be less ototoxic in adults than other aminoglycosides. In a study of infants treated in an intensive care unit, 50 received amikacin and 49 netilmicin for periods of 3–7 days. A third group of 51 healthy untreated neonates were selected as the control group. All these infants were followed up until 18 months of age. Bilateral sensorineural impairment was confirmed in one infant given amikacin, in one given netilmicin and in one untreated infant. As with other aminoglycosides (p.467), the risk in infants developing ototoxicity from a short-course netilmicin therapy appears to be small (Finitzo-Hieber *et al.*, 1985).

2 Nephrotoxicity

This is another characteristic side-effect of aminoglycosides (p.467), shared by netilmicin. In animals netilmicin is less nephrotoxic than gentamicin, but this is not explicable by a difference in the concentrations of these antibiotics in the renal cortex (p.527) (Luft *et al.*, 1976, 1983; Chiu *et al.*, 1977; Luft, 1980). Gentamicin, possibly the most nephrotoxic of the aminoglycosides, is reabsorbed by the renal tubules to a greater extent than the other drugs. In both animals and humans aminoglycoside renal toxicity is probably determined by two major factors, the drug's transport into tubular cells and its intrinsic intracellular toxicity (Brion *et al.*, 1984; Contrepois *et al.*, 1985). In animals, the concomitant administration of non-aminoglycoside antibiotics, such as ampicillin, carbenicillin, methicillin, cefamandole and clindamycin, does not aggravate netilmicin nephrotoxicity (Hagstrom *et al.*, 1978). However, the administration of frusemide enhances the nephrotoxicity of netilmicin in animals, possibly largely due to volume depletion (Adelman *et al.*, 1981). In contrast, diltiazem, a calcium channel blocker, prevents netilmicin-induced renal failure in animals (Lortholary *et al.*, 1993).

Mild reversible nephrotoxicity has been encountered fairly frequently when netilmicin is used clinically. Klastersky *et al.* (1977) noted granular casts in the urine and/or rises in blood urea and serum creatinine values, in seven of ten patients treated by a netilmicin dosage of 7.5 mg per kg body weight per day. These changes were not observed in patients receiving lower dosages. Others also have reported rises in blood urea and serum creatinine, usually reversible, in a small number of patients. Nephrotoxicity appears to be more likely in diabetics and older patients, after prolonged treatment and when a larger total amount of the drug is administered (Panwalker *et al.*, 1978; Trestman *et al.*, 1978; Bergeron *et al.*, 1983; Bhattacharya *et al.*, 1983).

Data from statistically assessable clinical trials, comparing the nephrotoxicity of netilmicin with that of other aminoglycosides, are limited. Lerner *et al.* (1983) treated 254 patients with either tobramycin/ticarcillin or netilmicin/ticarcillin. Drug-related renal dysfunction developed in five (4%) of 114 tobramycin-treated patients whose renal function was monitored and in one (1%) of 116 netilmicin-treated patients. Gatell *et al.* (1984), in a prospective randomized trial, gave tobramycin or netilmicin to 197 patients; 140 of these were evaluated for nephrotoxicity. Renal damage of similar severity developed in seven of 73 (9.6%) recipients of tobramycin and in seven of 67 (10.4%) recipients of netilmicin. Other authors have also found the prevalence of nephrotoxicity to be about the same in netilmicin and tobramycin-treated patients (Bernstein *et al.*, 1986; Gorse *et al.*, 1992). In a trial where once-daily gentamicin was compared with once-daily netilmicin for the treatment of serious infections, the prevalence of nephrotoxicity in the two groups was again about the same (Prins *et al.*, 1994). Kahlmeter and Dahlager (1984) surveyed aminoglycoside nephrotoxicity in approximately 10 000 patients described in clinical trials published between 1975 and 1982. Average frequencies of nephrotoxicity for gentamicin, tobramycin, amikacin and netilmicin were 14%, 12.9%, 9.4% and 8.7%, respectively. It appears that comparative nephrotoxicity is relatively unimportant, compared with clinical and microbiological considerations, when an aminoglycoside is chosen for therapy in a clinical situation (Luft, 1984).

3 Other side-effects

Elevated SGOT values have been noted in some patients. An elevation of serum alkaline phosphatase occurred in 43% of patients treated by Panwalker *et al.* (1978). There was no other evidence of hepatotoxicity. Netilmicin, similar to other aminoglycosides (p.470), can also cause neuromuscular blockade (Paradelis, 1979). Animal studies have suggested that aminoglycosides may have a myocardial depressant effect, and that netilmicin is more potent in this regard than gentamicin or sisomicin (Descotes and Evreux, 1981).

Clinical Uses of the Drug

Netilmicin either alone, or in combination with a beta-lactam antibiotic, such as ticarcillin (p.156), has been used to treat severe infections such as pyelonephritis, biliary tract infections, peritonitis, pleuropulmonary infections and septicemia, caused by gentamicin-sensitive Gram-negative bacilli. Results of treatment have usually been satisfactory and similar to those which would be expected from a similar gentamicin regimen (Klastersky *et al.*, 1977; Panwalker *et al.*, 1978; Snydman *et al.*, 1979; Brandenhoff *et al.*, 1980 Aroney *et al.*, 1981; Perera *et al.*, 1982; Lerner *et al.*, 1983; Lane, 1984; Prins *et al.*, 1994). Most clinicians prefer to use the more familiar and usually cheaper gentamicin for the treatment of these infections, but some may prefer netilmicin because of its probably lesser potential to cause ototoxicity (Jackson, 1984). Netilmicin also appears as effective as amikacin for the treatment of complicated urinary tract infections, caused by Gram-negative bacilli sensitive to both antibiotics (Maigaard *et al.*, 1978). The drug is about as efficaceous clinically as tobramycin, when serious infections due to organisms susceptible to both antibiotics are treated (Bernstein *et al.*, 1986; Gorse *et al.*, 1992).

Edelstein and Meyer (1978) used netilmicin to treat 25 patients with serious Gram-negative bacillary infections, nine of whom had gentamicin-resistant but netilmicin-susceptible pathogens. Previous therapy with gentamicin had been unsuccessful in six, but seven of the nine patients subsequently responded to netilmicin. This drug may have a place in therapeutics on occasions as an alternative to amikacin (p.515), for the treatment of those infections caused by gentamicin-resistant Gram-negative bacilli which remain netilmicin-sensitive.

Netilmicin in combination with vancomycin (p.778) has been used intraperitoneally to treat peritonitis in patients on continuous ambulatory peritoneal dialysis. Prolonged (4–6 h) dwell times for peritoneal fluid administration were used. A loading dose of 1.7 mg per kg netilmicin was added to 2 liters of dialysis fluid. Thereafter, netilmicin in a dosage of 7.5 mg per liter of dialysate was administered 4-hourly during the first day, and then 4.0 mg per liter was given every 6 h. The minimum and maximum netilmicin serum levels achieved were 1.0 and 8.1 μg per ml, respectively (Brauner *et al.*, 1985).

Netilmicin in a single dose of 300 mg i.m. is quite effective for the treatment of gonorrhea, but other drugs are preferred for the treatment of this disease (p.361) (Moran and Levine, 1995).

References

Adelman RD, Spangler WL, Beasom F *et al.* (1981). Frusemide enhancement of netilmicin nephrotoxicity in dogs. *J Antimicrob Chemother* **7**: 431.

Aroney RS, Dalley DN, Levi JA (1981). Treatment of serious systemic infections with netilmicin in combination with other antibiotics. *Med J Aust* **1**: 475.

Barza M, Lauermann MW, Tally FP, Gorbach SL (1980). Prospective, randomized trial of netilmicin and amikacin, with emphasis on eight-nerve toxicity. *Antimicrob Ag Chemother* **17**: 707.

Bengtsson S, Bernander S, Brorson JE *et al.* (1986). *In vitro* aminoglycoside resistance of Gram-negative bacilli and staphylococci isolated from blood in Sweden 1980–1984. *Scand J Infect Dis* **18**: 257.

Bergeron MG, Trottier S (1979). Influence of single or multiple doses of gentamicin and netilmicin on their cortical, medullary and papillary distribution. *Antimicrob Ag Chemother* **15**: 635.

Bergeron MG, Lessard C, Ronald A *et al.* (1983). Three to eight weeks of therapy with netilmicin: toxicity in normal and diabetic patients. *J Antimicrob Chemother* **12**: 245.

Bernstein JM, Gorse GJ, Linzmayer MI *et al.* (1986). Relative efficacy and toxicity of netilmicin and tobramycin in oncology patients. *Arch Intern Med* **146**: 2329.

Bhattacharya BK, Gorringe H, Farr MJ (1983). Netilmicin and nephrotoxicity. *Lancet* **ii**: 216.

Blaser J, Stone BB, Zinner SH (1985). Efficacy of intermittent versus continuous administration of netilmicin in a two-compartment *in vitro* model. *Antimicrob Ag Chemother* **27**: 343.

Blaser J, Stone BB, Groner MC, Zinner SH (1987). Comparative study with enoxacin and netilmicin in a pharmacodynamic model to determine importance of ratio of antibiotic peak concentration to MIC for bactericidal activity and emergence of resistance. *Antimicrob Ag Chemother* **31**: 1054.

Blaser J, Rieder HL, Lüthy R (1991). Interface-area-to-volume ratio of interstitial fluid in humans determined by pharmacokinetic analysis of netilmicin in small and large skin blisters. *Antimicrob Ag Chemother* **35**: 837.

Blaser J, König C, Simmen H-P, Thurnheer U (1994). Monitoring serum concentrations for once-daily netilmicin dosing regimens. *J Antimicrob Chemother* **33**: 341.

Bosso JA, Townsend PL, Herbst JJ, Matsen JM (1985). Pharmacokinetics and dosage requirements of netilmicin in cystic fibrosis patients. *Antimicrob Ag Chemother* **28**: 829.

Bowman RL, Silverblatt FJ, Kaloyanides GJ (1977). Comparison of the nephrotoxicity of netilmicin and gentamicin in rats. *Antimicrob Ag Chemother* **12**: 474.

Brandenhoff P, Stafanger G, Gammelgaard PA *et al.* (1980). Netilmicin therapy of patients with septicaemia and other severe infections. *Scand J Infect Dis* (Suppl 23): 181.

Brauner L, Kahlmeter G, Lindholm T, Simonsen O (1985). Vancomycin and netilmicin as first line treatment of peritonitis in CAPD patients. *J Antimicrob Chemother* **15**: 751.

Brier ME, Mayer PR, Brier RA *et al.* (1985). Relationship between rat renal accumulation of gentamicin, tobramycin, and netilmicin and their nephrotoxicities. *Antimicrob Ag Chemother* **27**: 812.

Brion N, Barge J, Godefroy I *et al.* (1984). Gentamicin, netilmicin, dibekacin and amikacin nephrotoxicity and its relationship to tubular reabsorption in rabbits. *Antimicrob Ag Chemother* **25**: 168.

Brown KN, Benedictson J, Swanby S (1976). *In vitro* comparisons of gentamicin, tobramycin, sisomicin and netilmicin. *Antimicrob Ag Chemother* **10**: 768.

Brückner O, Trautmann M, Kolodziejczyk D *et al.* (1983). Netilmicin in human CSF after parenteral administration in patients with slightly and severely impaired blood CSF barrier. *J Antimicrob Chemother* **11**: 565.

Buss WC, Piatt MK, Kauten R (1984). Inhibition of mammalian microsomal protein synthesis by aminoglycoside antibiotics. *J Antimicrob Chemother* **14**: 231.

Carrizosa J, Kaye D (1978). Penicillin and netilmicin in treatment of experimental enterococcal endocarditis. *Antimicrob Ag Chemother* **13**: 505.

Chiu PJS, Miller GH, Brown AD *et al.* (1977). Renal pharmacology of netilmicin. *Antimicrob Ag Chemother* **11**: 821.

Chung M, Costello R, Symchowicz S (1980). Comparison of netilmicin and gentamicin pharmacokinetics in humans. *Antimicrob Ag Chemother* **17**: 184.

Contrepois A, Brion N, Garaud J-J *et al.* (1985). Renal disposition of gentamicin, dibekacin, tobramycin, netilmicin, and amikacin in humans. *Antimicrob Ag Chemother* **27**: 520.

Crowe CC, Sanders E (1973). Sisomicin: evaluation *in vitro* and comparison with gentamicin and tobramycin. *Antimicrob Ag Chemother* **3**: 24.

Daikos GL, Lolans VT, Jackson GG (1991). First-exposure adaptive resistance to aminoglycoside antibiotics *in vivo* with meaning for optimal clinical use. *Antimicrob Ag Chemother* **35**: 117.

Davies AJ, Clewett J, Jones A, Marshall R (1986). Sensitivity patterns of coagulase-negative staphylococci from neonates. *J Antimicrob Chemother* **17**: 155.

Descotes J, Evreux J Cl (1981). Cardiac depressant effects of some recent aminoglycoside antibiotics. *J Antimicrob Chemother* **7**: 197.

Dhawan V, Marso E, Martin WJ, Young LS (1977). *In vitro* studies with netilmicin compared with amikacin, gentamicin, and tobramycin. *Antimicrob Ag Chemother* **11**: 64.

Digranes A, Dibb WL, Östervold B (1980). The *in vitro* activity of netilmicin against 357 clinical isolates of Enterobacteriaceae, *Pseudomonas aeruginosa* and *Staphylococcus aureus*. *Scand J Infect Dis* (Suppl 23): 30.

Drasar FA, Farrell W, Maskell J, Williams JD (1976). Tobramycin-, amikacin-, sisomicin- and gentamicin- resistant Gram-negative rods. *Brit Med J* **2**: 1284.

Dulon D, Aran J-M, Zajic G, Schacht J (1986). Comparative uptake of gentamicin, netilmicin, and amikacin in the guinea pig cochlea and vestibule. *Antimicrob Ag Chemother* **30**: 96.

Edelstein PH, Meyer RD (1978). Netilmicin therapy of serious Gram-negative bacillary infections. *J Antimicrob Chemother* **4**: 495.

Edwards DJ, Mangione A, Cumbo TJ, Schentag JJ (1981). Predicted tissue accumulation of netilmicin in patients. *Antimicrob Ag Chemother* **20**: 714.

Eickhoff TC, Ehret JM (1977). *In vitro* activity of netilmicin compared with gentamicin, tobramycin, amikacin, and kanamycin. *Antimicrob Ag Chemother* **11**: 791.

Fan ST, Lau WY, Teoh-Chan CH (1988). Once daily administration of netilmicin with thrice daily, both in combination with metronidazole, in gangrenous and perforated appendicitis. *J Antimicrob Chemother* **22**: 69.

Finitzo-Hieber T, McCracken GH Jr, Brown KC (1985). Prospective controlled evaluation of auditory function in neonates given netilmicin or amikacin. *J Pediatr* **106**: 129.

Follath F, Spring P, Wenk M *et al.* (1978). Comparative pharmacokinetics of sisomicin and netilmicin in healthy volunteers. In *Current Chemotherapy: Proceedings of the 10th International Congress of Chemotherapy, Zurich/Switzerland, 1977* (Siegenthaler W, Lüthy R, eds), p. 979. Washington, DC: American Society for Microbiology.

Fu KP, Neu HC (1976). *In vitro* study of netilmicin compared with other aminoglycosides. *Antimicrob Ag Chemother* **10**: 526.

Gatell JM, San Miguel JG, Araujo V *et al.* (1984). Prospective randomized double-blind comparison of nephrotoxicity and auditory toxicity of tobramycin and netilmicin. *Antimicrob Ag Chemother* **26**: 766.

Gatell JM, Ferran F, Araujo V *et al.* (1987). Univariate and multivariate analyses of risk factors predisposing to auditory toxicity in patients receiving aminoglycosides. *Antimicrob Ag Chemother* **31**: 1383.

Gilbert DN (1991). Once-daily aminoglycoside therapy. *Antimicrob Ag Chemother* **35**: 399.

Gorse GJ, Bernstein JM, Cronin RE, Etzell PS (1992). A comparison of netilmicin and tobramycin therapy in patients with renal impairment. *Scand J Infect Dis* **24**: 503.

Granati B, Assael BM, Chung M *et al.* (1985). Clinical pharmacology of netilmicin in preterm and term newborn infants. *J Pediatr* **106**: 664.

Guay DRP (1983). Netilmicin (Netromycin, Schering-Plough). *Drug Intellig Clin Pharm* **17**: 83.

Guimaraes MA, Sage R, Noone P (1985). The comparative activity of aminocyclitol against 773 aerobic Gram-negative rods and staphylococci isolated from hospitalized patients. *J Antimicrob Chemother* **16**: 555.

Habwe V, Shadomy S (1979). Comparative *in vitro* studies with netilmicin, amikacin, gentamicin, sisomicin and tobramycin. *J Antimicrob Chemother* **5**: 73.

Hagstrom GL, Luft FC, Yum MN *et al.* (1978). Nephrotoxicity of netilmicin in combination with non-aminoglycoside antibiotics. *Antimicrob Ag Chemother* **13**: 490.

Hammerberg S, Sorger S, Marks MI (1977). Antimicrobial susceptibilities of *Yersinia enterocolitica* biotype 4, serotype 0:3. *Antimicrob Ag Chemother* **11**: 566.

Haverkorn MJ (1983). Netilmicin 150 mg every 12 hours in systemic infections. *J Antimicrob Chemother* **12**: 209.

Hawkey PM, Constable HK (1988). Selection of netilmicin resistance, associated with incresed 6'aminoglycoside acetyltransferase activity, in *Serratia marcescens. J Antimicrob Chemother* **21**: 535.

Hjelte L, Malmborg A-S, Strandvik B (1989). Serum and sputum concentrations of netilmicin in combination with acylureidopenicillin and cephalosporins in clinical treatment of pulmonary exacerbations in cystic fibrosis. *J Antimicrob Chemother* **23**: 885.

Hollender LF, Bahnini J, DeManzini N *et al.* (1989). A multicentric study of netilmicin once daily versus thrice daily in patients with appendicitis and other intra-abdominal infections. *J Antimicrob Chemother* **23**: 773.

Humbert G, Leroy A, Fillastre JP, Oksenhendler G (1978). Pharmacokinetics of netilmicin in the presence of normal or impaired renal function. *Antimicrob Ag Chemother* **14**: 40.

Jackson GG (1984). The key role of aminoglycosides in antibacterial therapy and prophylaxis. *J Antimicrob Chemother* **13** (Suppl A). 1.

Kahlmeter G (1980). Netilmicin: clinical pharmacokinetics and aspects on dosage schedules. An overview. *Scand J Infect Dis* (Suppl 23): 74.

Kahlmeter G, Dahlager JI (1984). Aminoglycoside toxicity – a review of clinical studies published between 1975 and 1982. *J Antimicrob Chemother* **13** (Suppl A): 9.

Kantor RJ, Norden CW (1977). *In vitro* activity of netilmicin, gentamicin, and amikacin. *Antimicrob Ag Chemother* **11**: 126.

Klastersky J, Hensgens C, Gerard M, Daneau D (1975). Comparison of sisomicin and gentamicin in bacteriuric patients with underlying diseases of the urinary tract. *Antimicrob Ag Chemother* **7**: 742.

Klastersky J, Meunier-Carpentier F, Coppens-Kahan L *et al.* (1977). Clinical and bacteriological evaluation of netilmicin in Gram-negative infections. *Antimicrob Ag Chemother* **12**: 503.

Korzeniowski OM, Wennersten C, Moellering RC Jr, Sande MA (1978). Penicillin-netilmicin synergism against *Streptococcus faecalis. Antimicrob Ag Chemother* **13**: 430.

Lane AZ (1984). Clinical experience with netilmicin. *J Antimicrob Chemother* **13**: (Suppl A): 67.

Langstaff D, Schueler S, Righter J (1983). Netilmicin: *in-vitro* activity compared with that of other aminoglycosides against *Serratia marcescens. J Antimicrob Chemother* **11**: 187.

Larson TA, Gerding DN, Peterson LR (1983). Extravascular penetration of tobramycin and netilmicin in a subcutaneous visking chamber model in rabbits. *Antimicrob Ag Chemother* **24**: 594.

Lerner AM, Reyes MP, Cone LA *et al.* (1983). Randomised, controlled trial of the comparative efficacy, auditory toxicity, and nephrotoxicity of tobramycin and netilmicin. *Lancet* i: 1123.

Leroy A, Humbert G, Oksenhendler G, Fillastre JP (1976). Comparative pharmacokinetics of lividomycin, amikacin and sisomicin in normal subjects and in uraemic patients. *J Antimicrob Chemother* **2**: 373.

Lortholary O, Blanchet F, Nochy D *et al.* (1993). Effects of diltiazem on netilmicin-induced nephrotoxicity in rabbits. *Antimicrob Ag Chemother* **37**: 1790.

Luft FC (1980). The nephrotoxic potential of netilmicin as determined in a rat model. *Scand J Infect Dis* (Suppl 23): 82.

Luft FC (1984). Clinical significance of renal changes engendered by aminoglycosides in man. *J Antimicrob Chemother* **13** (Suppl A): 23.

Luft FC, Yum MN, Kleit SA (1976). Comparative nephrotoxicities of netilmicin and gentamicin in rats. *Antimicrob Ag Chemother* **10**: 845.

Luft FC, Brannon DR, Stropes LL *et al.* (1978). Pharmacokinetics of netilmicin in patients with renal impairment and in patients on dialysis. *Antimicrob Ag Chemother* **14**: 403.

Luft FC, Bennett WH, Gilbert DN (1983). Experimental aminoglycoside nephrotoxicity: accomplishments and future potential. *Rev Infect Dis* **5** (Suppl 2): 268.

Maes P (1985). Evaluation of the resistance mechanism of gentamicin-resistant Gram-negative bacilli and their susceptibility to tobramycin, netilmicin and amikacin. *J Antimicrob Chemother* **15**: 283.

Maigaard S, Frimodt-Möller N, Madsen PO (1978). Comparison of netilmicin and amikacin in treatment of complicated urinary tract infections. *Antimicrob Ag Chemother* **14**: 544.

Marks MI, Hammerberg S, Greenstone G, Silver B (1976). Activity of newer aminoglycosides and carbenicillin, alone and in combination, against gentamicin-resistant *Pseudomonas aeruginosa. Antimicrob Ag Chemother* **10**: 399.

Martin-Luengo F, Valero-Guillen PL (1983). *In vitro* activity of netilmicin against *Nocardia. J Antimicrob Chemother* **12**: 413.

McAllister TA, Mocan H, Murphy AV, Beattie TJ (1987). Antibiotic susceptibility of staphylococci from CAPD peritonitis in children. *J Antimicrob Chemother* **19**: 95.

McCracken GH Jr, Nelson JD (1983). *Antibiotic Therapy for Newborns* 2nd edn, p. 62. New York: Grune & Stratton.

Meyer RD, Kraus LL, Pasiecznik KA (1976). *In vitro* susceptibility of gentamicin-resistant Enterobacteriaceae and *Pseudomonas aeruginosa* to netilmicin and selected aminoglycoside antibiotics. *Antimicrob Ag Chemother* **10**: 677.

Meyers BR, Hirschman SZ (1977). Antimicrobial activity *in vitro* of netilmicin and comparison with sisomicin, gentamicin and tobramycin. *Antimicrob Ag Chemother* **11**: 118.

Meyers BR, Leng B, Hirschman SZ (1975). Comparison of the antibacterial activities of sisomicin and gentamicin against Gram-negative bacteria. *Antimicrob Ag Chemother* **8**: 757.

Meyers BR, Hirschman SZ, Wormser G, Siegel D (1977). Pharmacokinetic study of netilmicin. *Antimicrob Ag Chemother* **12**: 122.

Michalsen H, Bergan T (1981). Pharmacokinetics of netilmicin in children with and without cystic fibrosis. *Antimicrob Ag Chemother* **19**: 1029.

Miller GH, Arcieri G, Weinstein MJ, Waitz JA (1976). Biological activity of netilmicin, a broad-spectrum semisynthetic aminoglycoside antibiotic. *Antimicrob Ag Chemother* **10**: 827.

Moellering RC Jr (1983). *In vitro* antibacterial activity of the aminoglycoside antibiotics. *Rev Infect Dis* **5** (Suppl 2): 212.

Moffie BG, Hoogeterp JJ, Lim T *et al.* (1993). Effectiveness of netilmicin and tobramycin against *Pseudomonas aeruginosa in vitro* and in an experimental tissue infection in mice. *J Antimicrob Chemother* **31**: 403.

Moran JS, Levine WC (1995). Drugs of choice for the treatment of uncomplicated gonococcal infections. *Clin Infect Dis* **20** (Suppl 1): 47.

Munckhof WJ, Grayson ML, Turnidge JD (1996). A meta-analysis of studies on the safety and efficacy of aminoglycosides given either once-daily or as divided doses. *J Antimicrob Chemother* **37**: 645.

Nau R, Scholz P, Sharifi S *et al.* (1993). Netilmicin cerebrospinal fluid concentrations after an intravenous infusion of 400 mg in patients without meningeal inflammation. *J Antimicrob Chemother* **32**: 893.

O'Hara K, Kono M, Mitsuhashi S (1974). Enzymatic inactivation of a new aminoglycoside antibiotic, sisomicin, by resistant strains of *Pseudomonas aeruginosa. Antimicrob Ag Chemother* **5**: 558.

Panwalker AP, Malow JB, Zimelis VM, Jackson GG (1978). Netilmicin: clinical efficacy, tolerance, and toxicity. *Antimicrob Ag Chemother* **13**: 170.

Paradelis AG (1979). Aminoglycoside antibiotics and neuromuscular blockade. *J Antimicrob Chemother* **5**: 737.

Parker RA, Gilbert DN, Houghton DC *et al.* (1980). Comparative nephrotoxicities of high-dose netilmicin and tobramycin in rats. *Antimicrob Ag Chemother* **18**: 346.

Pechère J-C, Pechère M-M, Dugal R (1976). Clinical pharmacokinetics of sisomicin: dosage schedules in renal-impaired patients. *Antimicrob Ag Chemother* **9**: 761.

Perera MR, Amirak ID, Noone P (1982). High-dose netilmicin in patients with life-threatening sepsis. *J Antimicrob Chemother* **9**: 231.

Phillips I, Eykyn S, King BA *et al.* (1977a). The *in vitro* antibacterial activity of nine aminoglycosides and spectinomycin on clinical isolates of common Gram-negative bacteria. *J Antimicrob Chemother* **3**: 403.

Phillips I, Smith A, Shannon K (1977b). Antibacterial activity of netilmicin, a new aminoglycoside antibiotic, compared with that of gentamicin. *Antimicrob Ag Chemother* **11**: 402.

Prins JM, Büller HR, Kuijper Ed J *et al.* (1994). Once-daily gentamicin versus once-daily netilmicin in patients with serious infections – a randomized clinical trial. *J Antimicrob Chemother* **33**: 823.

Rahal JJ, Simberkoff MS (1986). Comparative bactericidal activity of penicillin-netilmicin and penicillin-gentamicin against enterococci. *J Antimicrob Chemother* **17**: 585.

Rahal JJ Jr, Simberkoff MS, Kagan K, Moldover NH (1976). Bactericidal efficacy of Sch 20569 and amikacin against gentamicin-sensitive and resistant organisms. *Antimicrob Ag Chemother* **9**: 595.

Riff LJ, Moreschi G (1977). Netilmicin and gentamicin: comparative pharmacology in humans. *Antimicrob Ag Chemother* **11**: 609.

Rozdzinski E, Kern WV, Reichle A *et al.* (1993). Once-daily versus thrice-daily dosing of netilmicin in combination with beta-lactam antibiotics as empirical therapy for febrile neutropenic patients. *J Antimicrob Chemother* **31**: 585.

Sanders CC (1977). Synergy of penicillin-netilmicin combinations against enterococci including strains highly resistant to streptomycin or kanamycin. *Antimicrob Ag Chemother* **12**: 195.

Sanders WE Jr, Sanders CC (1980). Sisomicin: a review of eight years' experience. *Rev Infect Dis* **2**: 182.

Seligman SJ (1978). Frequency of resistance to kanamycin, tobramycin, netilmicin and amikacin in gentamicin-resistant Gram-negative bacteria. *Antimicrob Ag Chemother* **13**: 70.

Shanson DC, Tadayon M, Bakhtiar M (1986). Bactericidal activity of netilmicin compared with gentamicin and streptomycin, alone and in combination with penicillin, against penicillin tolerant viridans streptococci and enterococci. *J Antimicrob Chemother* **18**: 479.

Shaw KJ, Rather PN, Hare RS, Miller GH (1993). Molecular genetics of aminoglycoside resistance genes and familial relationships of the aminoglycoside-modifying enzymes. *Microbiol Rev* **57**: 135.

Siegel JD, McCracken GH Jr, Thomas ML, Threlkeld N (1979). Pharmacokinetic properties of netilmicin in newborn infants. *Antimicrob Ag Chemother* **15**: 246.

Smith DL, Stableforth DE, Geddes AM (1994). Evaluation of a once-daily netilmicin regimen in the treatment of cystic fibrosis. *J Antimicrob Chemother* **33**: 191.

Smith JA, Morgan JR, Mogyoros M (1977). *In vitro* activity of netilmicin. *Antimicrob Ag Chemother* **11**: 362.

Snydman DR, Tally FP, Landesman SH *et al.* (1979). Netilmicin in Gram-negative bacterial infections. *Antimicrob Ag Chemother* **15**: 50.

Solberg CO, Madsen ST, Digranes A *et al.* (1980). High dose netilmicin therapy: efficacy, tolerance and tissue penetration. *J Antimicrob Chemother* **6**: 133.

Sturm AW (1989). Netilmicin in the treatment of Gram-negative bacteremia: single daily versus multiple daily dosage. *J Infect Dis* **159**: 931.

Thys JP, Mouawad E, Klastersky J (1979). Concentrations of netilmicin in bronchial secretions and serum during intermittent vs continuous infusion: a crossover study in humans. *J Infect Dis* **140**: 634.

Thys JP, Klastersky J, Mombeli G (1981). Peak or sustained antibiotic serum levels for optimal tissue penetration. *J Antimicrob Chemother* **8** (Suppl C): 29.

Trestman I, Parsons J, Santoro J *et al.* (1978). Pharmacology and efficacy of netilmicin. *Antimicrob Ag Chemother* **13**: 382.

Van der Auwera P, Meunier F, Ibrahim S *et al.* (1991). Pharmacodynamic parameters and toxicity of netilmicin (6 milligrams/kilogram/day). given once daily or in three divided doses to cancer patients with urinary tract infection. *Antimicrob Ag Chemother* **35**: 640.

Verbist L, Vandepitte J, Vandeven J (1978). Activity of eight aminoglycosides against isolates of *Serratia marcescens* from four hospitals. *J Antimicrob Chemother* **4**: 47.

Vigano A, Principi N, Brivio L *et al.* (1992). Comparison of 5 milligrams of netilmicin per kilogram of body weight once daily versus 2 milligrams per kilogram thrice daily for treatment of Gram-negative pyelonephritis in children. *Antimicrob Ag Chemother* **36**: 1499.

Welling PG, Baumueller A, Lau CC, Madsen PO (1977). Netilmicin pharmacokinetics after single intravenous doses to elderly male patients. *Antimicrob Ag Chemother* **12**: 328.

Wersäll J (1984). Recent otological evaluation of aminoglycoside antibiotics. *J Antimicrob Chemother* **13** (Suppl A): 31.

Yap B-S, Stewart D, Bodey GP (1977). Clinical pharmacology of netilmicin. *Antimicrob Ag Chemother* **12**: 717.

Neomycin, Framycetin and Paromomycin

Description

These three antibiotics are more toxic, and unlike the aminoglycosides described in the previous chapters, they are not used systemically.

1 Neomycin

First described by Waksman and Lechevalier in 1949, this antibiotic in its marketed form contains two chemically similar components, neomycin B and C.

2 Framycetin

Purification of this drug was carried out by Roussell Laboratories, after it was first described in 1953 by Decaris in France. It is probably identical with neomycin B.

3 Paromomycin

This was isolated from a strain of *Streptomyces rimosus* in 1959.

These aminoglycosides are used clinically as sulfates, which produce stable solutions in water. They are all used much less extensively than in the past.

Sensitive Organisms

1 Gram-negative bacteria

Nearly all the medically important Gram-negative aerobic bacteria are sensitive to these drugs, with the exception of *Pseudomonas aeruginosa*. Anaerobic bacteria, such as *Bacteroides* spp., are resistant. Resistant strains of the usually sensitive organisms such as *Escherichia coli*, *Klebsiella* and *Proteus* spp., are now often encountered in hospitals, and these usually show complete cross-resistance with kanamycin (p.439). Long-term oral administration of neomycin particularly favors emergence of multiresistant plasmid carrying aerobic enteric bacteria. These are usually also resistant to other drugs, such as sulfonamides, tetracyclines, streptomycin, ampicillin and carbenicillin. Such multiresistant bacteria are capable of transferring their resistance to other aerobic enteric bacteria (Valtonen *et al.*, 1977). Neomycin-resistant strains of *Shigella sonnei* (Davies *et al.*, 1970) and the salmonellae (Bissett *et al.*, 1974) have been encountered.

2 Gram-positive bacteria

Staphylococcus aureus and *Staph. epidermidis* are highly sensitive to these drugs, but all streptococci and the Gram-positive bacilli are relatively resistant. Neomycin-resistant strains of *Staph. aureus* were first reported from hospitals in the 1960s (Rountree and Beard, 1965). These staphylococci were also always resistant to framycetin and kanamycin, and the majority were resistant to several other antibiotics including penicillin G, streptomycin, tetracycline and erythromycin. At times they also became resistant to bacitracin (p.542), an antibiotic often used in combination with neomycin in topical applications (Rountree and Beard, 1965). When neomycin-containing topical preparations are used for short-tem control of skin sepsis in conditions such as eczema, the risk of inducing neomycin-resistant strains of *Staph. aureus* is relatively small. If these applications are used for weeks, months or intermittently, staphylococci resistant to neomycin emerge readily. These may be implicated in further attacks of sepsis and they may be difficult to control (Smith *et al.*, 1975). Methicillin-resistant strains of *Staph. aureus* and *Staph. epidermidis*, which became widespread in many hospitals in the late 1970s, were also often resistant to neomycin and other aminoglycosides (p.454).

3 Mycobacteria

Mycobacterium tuberculosis, including multidrug-resistant strains, is sensitive to paromomycin. There is no cross-resistance with streptomycin or any other antimicrobial agent. The MICs of paromomycin for sensitive and multidrug-resistant strains of *M. tuberculosis* range from 0.09 to 1.5 μg per ml. Paromomycin is also active against *M. avium* complex strains, their MICs ranging from 1.56 to 12.5 μg per ml (Kanyok *et al.*, 1994a; Piersimoni *et al.*, 1994). The drug is also active *in vivo* in experimental animals against these mycobacterial infections (Kanyok *et al.*, 1994b).

4 Entamoeba histolytica, Acanthamoebae and Cryptosporidium

Entamoeba histolytica was reported to be sensitive to paromomycin (Courtney *et al.*, 1960), but not to neomycin and framycetin. Both neomycin and paromomycin are active *in vitro* against two species of *Acanthamoeba*, *A. polyphaga* and *A. castellanii*, which can cause eye infections (Nagington and Richards, 1976). Paromomycin in concentrations from 50 to 5000 μg per ml inhibits *Cryptosporidium* infection of a human enterocyte cell line. Concentrations of paromomycin of >1000 μg per ml are achievable in the bowel lumen (Marshall and Flanigan, 1992).

5 Minimum inhibitory concentrations

The MICs of neomycin, framycetin and paromomycin against sensitive organisms are similar to those of kanamycin (Table I.36, p. 441).

Mode of Administration and Dosage

1 Parenteral administration

Neomycin is now never used parenterally. In the past an i.m. adult dosage of 1.0 g or 15 mg per kg body weight per day, given in two to four divided doses was used, but serious toxic effects were common (p.536). Framycetin and paromomycin have not been available for parenteral use in the USA and Australia. However, according to Kanyok *et al.* (1994a), a drug named aminosidine has been used parenterally elsewhere in the world with relatively little toxicity. This drug has now been shown to be identical to paromomycin. It has been given in dosages of 0.5 g i.m. 12-hourly or 1.0 g i.m. daily to adults.

2 Oral administration

These antibiotics are not usually absorbed after oral administration, so they are only used orally to suppress intestinal microbial flora. The usual adult oral dosage of neomycin is 1 g every 6 h (50–100 mg per kg body weight per day for children), but up to 2 g orally every 6 h has also been used. A three-dose regimen of neomycin plus erythromycin (or metronidazole) has been often used as chemoprophylaxis before elective colon operations. Mechanical bowel preparation is performed for 3 days preoperatively and 1.0-g doses of both neomycin and erythromycin are given orally at 19 h, 18 h and 9 h before surgery. This regimen has been used in the USA since 1972 (Gorbach, 1982, 1991).

To suppress bowel flora in patients with hepatic pre-coma or coma, Suh *et al.* (1979) recommended that the optimal neomycin regimen was a dose of 2.0 g given three times on the first day followed by 1.0 g twice-daily.

In the past neomycin dosages of up to 100 mg per kg per day were given to newborn infants and young children to treat gastrointestinal infections. Oral neomycin often induced a malabsorption syndrome in babies (p.537). Treatment of gastrointestinal infections by orally administered neomycin was not effective and neomycin is no longer used for this purpose in any age group (p.538).

The oral dosage of framycetin is 2.0–4.0 g per day in adults or 50 mg per kg body weight for children. Paromomycin has been used orally in a dosage of 1.0–2.0 g daily in adults and 50 mg per kg body weight in children (Bissuel et al., 1994).

3 Intraperitoneal administration

Previously neomycin was instilled into the peritoneal cavity after surgery for the treatment or prevention of peritonitis. A solution of 0.5% neomycin in normal saline was usually used. Intraperitoneal administration of neomycin is no longer advocated (Keighley, 1983), but if such treatment is used, the daily amount instilled in adults should not exceed 1.0 g (or 15 mg per kg body weight in children) and treatment should not be continued longer than 3 days.

4 Bladder irrigation or instillation

For continuous bladder irrigation, a solution containing 40 mg of neomycin per liter was recommended in the past. In addition, even stronger neomycin solutions (e.g. 40–100 ml of a 0.1 or 0.2% solution) were instilled in the bladder for several hours following instrumentation (Clark, 1973). In patients with indwelling catheters, these instillations were performed daily or even more frequently. Solutions containing 1.0% neomycin, 1.0% bacitracin and 0.4% polymyxin B were used in paraplegics for urethral irrigation prior to catheterization (McLeod et al., 1963). It is now accepted that prevention of nosocomial infections of the urinary tract in catheterized patients depends on aseptic catheter care techniques, and neomycin bladder irrigations or instillations are no longer recommended (Haldorson et al., 1978; Turck and Stamm, 1981).

5 Topical administration

Neomycin and framycetin are commonly used topically to treat superficial infections (p.538).

Serum Levels in Relation to Dosage

Serum levels similar to those of kanamycin are attained after i.m. injections of neomycin (Fig. I.21, p.444). After a 0.5 g i.m. dose, a peak serum level of about 20 μg per ml is reached about 1 h later. Although both neomycin and framycetin are generally classed as non-absorbable, some absorption from the gastrointestinal tract does occur. A single oral dose of 4 g neomycin may produce a peak serum level of about 4.0 μg per ml (Kunin et al., 1960). Enema administered neomycin is absorbed to about the same extent (Breen et al., 1972). Prolonged oral administration of these drugs in high dosage may result in toxic blood levels, especially if renal impairment is present. Last and Sherlock (1960) reported neomycin serum level studies in 27 patients with acute and chronic hepatic insufficiency, treated with oral neomycin in a dose rarely exceeding 4 g daily. Detectable serum levels of neomycin were demonstrated in seven patients, which ranged from 0.5 g 40 μg per ml. The development of detectable serum levels correlated with the occurrence of oliguria. Intestinal ulceration did not appear to enhance neomycin absorption (Breen et al., 1972).

These drugs are also absorbed from wounds, the peritoneum, bronchial tree, bladder and even from inflamed skin following cutaneous application (Trimble, 1969; Weinstein et al., 1977). Significant serum levels may result if too large doses are administered at these sites (p.537).

Excretion

If these drugs are present in the serum, excretion is predominantly by the kidneys in a manner similar to kanamycin (p.444), and they may accumulate in the body if there is renal impairment.

Most of orally administered neomycin, framycetin or paromomycin appears in the feces in an active unchanged form.

Distribution of Drugs in Body

Neomycin, administered parenterally, is distributed in the body in a similar fashion to kanamycin (p.444).

Mode of Action

Neomycin, framycetin and paromomycin act on bacteria like other aminoglycosides (p.432).

Toxicity

1 Ototoxicity

Neomycin and framycetin can cause irreversible deafness rather than vestibular dysfunction. This is the principal reason why they are not used parenterally. Neomycin, when first introduced, was given i.m. in doses of 0.5–1.0 g daily and many patients became completely deaf after relatively short courses of 7–15 days (Welch, 1954). Neomycin is considerably more ototoxic than kanamycin (Leading article, 1963). Detection of early ototoxicity usually does not prevent further auditory loss, which often progresses to complete deafness, despite cessation of the drug. Sometimes hearing loss is first noted days or weeks after stopping the drug, and then progressively deteriorates (Kelly *et al.*, 1969; Leading article, 1969).

Sufficient absorption of these drugs may occur after prolonged oral administration (p.535) to cause ototoxicity, especially in the presence of renal impairment. This is most likely to occur in patients with liver failure, who often have associated renal functional impairment, and are treated for prolonged periods with neomycin (A Co-operative Study, 1973). It is advisable to check neomycin serum levels regularly in such patients (Last and Sherlock, 1960). If serum levels higher than 5 or especially 10 µg per ml are detected, the drug should be stopped or the dose reduced.

Ototoxicity can also result from topical neomycin or framycetin therapy. Kelly *et al.* (1969) reported deafness in a patient whose wound was irrigated 4-hourly with 80 ml of a solution containing 0.5% neomycin. The amount of neomycin used for wound irrigation in this patient was 2.4 g daily. Following this report, Trimble (1969) reviewed neomycin-induced deafness, and showed that otoxicity had occurred after use of this drug by all modes of administration – parenteral, aerosol, oral, wound and bowel irrigation and cutaneous application. He also made the observation that, whenever a new neomycin preparation became available, reports of ototoxicity following its use appeared.

Jawetz (1969) pointed out that the absorption of neomycin from a wound or granulating surface, may be comparable with absorption after i.m. injection. Neomycin is not absorbed after application to normal skin or instillation into a normal bladder, but it may be absorbed if the skin or bladder mucosa is inflamed. Weinstein *et al.* (1977) studied ten patients in whom neomycin wound irrigations were used during total hip replacement. A 1.0% neomycin solution was used, and the volume of irrigation solution varied from 500 to 1400 ml in individual patients; it was calculated that these patients received a topical dose ranging from 67 to 203 mg per kg. Although ototoxicity was not observed, systemic absorption and significant neomycin serum levels occurred in all patients.

Neomycin toxicity after topical therapy may be avoided if the total daily amount of the drug administered is calculated, and this is restricted to a safe dose. The dose should not exceed 15 mg per kg per day or 1.0 g daily in adults, for longer than 1–3 days. A lower total daily dose should be used if 'topical therapy' is continued for longer periods.

Animal studies have shown that many antibiotics, such as neomycin, gentamicin, chloramphenicol, tetracycline, erythromycin and polymyxin B, can cause deafness if instilled directly into the intact middle ear. Antibiotic ear drops may therefore be a potential cause of deafness in man, although severe deafness from their use appears to be rare. Nevertheless, in view of their doubtful efficacy and the possibility of ototoxicity, antibiotic ear drops should be avoided where possible, especially in the presence of large perforations and in patients undergoing ear surgery (Annotation, 1976; Brummett, 1983).

Paromomycin may be considerably less ototoxic than neomycin and framycetin and it may be possible to use this drug parenterally to treat mycobacterial infections (Kanyok *et al.*, 1994a). This still needs confirmation.

2 Nephrotoxicity

Neomycin may cause renal damage if administered parentally. In initial trials with i.m. neomycin using daily doses of 0.5–1.0 g, a rising blood urea was observed after 7–15 days of treatment, and in many patients renal damage was severe enough to warrant cessation of the drug (Welch, 1954). By contrast with neomycin ototoxicity, nephrotoxicity is usually reversible. De Beukelaer *et al.* (1971) described a 13-month-old infant who developed acute tubular necrosis and deafness following i.m. neomycin. The nephrotoxicity was reversible, but hearing loss was not. A renal biopsy showed vacuolization of proximal tubular epithelium similar to that observed in animal studies on neomycin nephrotoxicity. Krumlovsky *et al.* (1972) described a 39-year-old woman who developed severe but reversible nephrotoxicity following accidental i.m. administration of neomycin. In this patient the drug was removed by hemodialysis, and this seems to be the treatment of choice for neomycin poisoning.

The danger of renal damage may not be very great when neomycin is used by the oral route. In 27 patients with liver disease treated by oral neomycin, there was no convincing evidence that sufficient quantities of neomycin had been absorbed to cause renal damage (Last and Sherlock, 1960). Nevertheless, such patients should be monitored for declining renal function to avoid toxicity (Appel and Neu, 1977).

Animal studies show that neomycin is the most nephrotoxic of the commonly used aminoglycosides. Parenteral neomycin produces toxic lesions of the proximal renal tubules, which in the rat are manifested by glycosuria, aminoaciduria and proteinuria. These lesions are accompanied by a decrease of enzyme activity in the tubules, but are reversible. Renal toxicity in animals can also be demonstrated after very large oral doses of the drug (Emmerson and Pryse-Davies, 1964; Appel and Neu, 1977).

3 Neuromuscular blockade

Neomycin and framycetin can cause this complication, similar to other aminoglycosides (p.433). In the past when neomycin was often administered intraperitoneally for the treatment of peritonitis, neuromuscular blockade was observed most commonly in children, because the danger of overdosage was greater in this age group. This form of therapy, especially if peritonitis is present, may result in rapid systemic absorption of the drug. Anesthesia and muscle relaxants potentiate neomycin-induced neuromuscular blockade (Emery, 1963). This complication was also observed when neomycin was given by other routes. Ross *et al.* (1963) reported postoperative apnea in a man aged 70 with impaired renal function, who received 6 g oral neomycin prior to operation, a small amount of the drug, probably less than 150 mg, was introduced into the peritoneal cavity during operation. Bush (1962) reported the same effect in a newborn baby, in whom a large area of subcutaneous tissue was sprayed with a neomycin and polymyxin B mixture. This neonate (weight 3.1 kg) probably received a total dose of 166 mg neomycin and 50 000 units of polymyxin B. The polymyxins can also cause neuromuscular blockade (p.672).

4 Gastrointestinal side-effects

Large oral doses of these drugs may cause vomiting or diarrhea. Rubbo *et al.* (1966) found that doses of neomycin as high as 9 g per day used for preoperative chemoprophylaxis, frequently caused these symptoms. Orally administered neomycin, unlike parenteral aminoglycosides, has also been implicated as a cause of antibiotic-associated colitis due to *Clostridium difficile* (Bartlett, 1979). Similar to tetracyclines (p.735), colitis due to *Staph. aureus* overgrowth may also be a rare complication of oral neomycin therapy. It mainly occurred in surgical patients who had received preoperative neomycin as chemoprophylaxis, and the infection appeared to be caused by neomycin-resistant staphylococci (Finegold, 1986). *Staphylococcus aureus*, however, is common in the stools of patients who are receiving broad-spectrum antimicrobial agents and most patients who harbor this organism have no symptoms. It is possible that some cases diagnosed as staphylococcal enterocolitis in the past, were due to *Cl. difficile* (Bartlett, 1979).

Prolonged oral administration of neomycin may also cause atrophic changes in the intestinal mucosa resulting in a malabsorption syndrome (Jacobson and Faloon, 1961). Malabsorption of fat, cholesterol, electrolytes, disaccharides, glucose, xylose, vitamin B_{12} and oral penicillin may result. Neomycin, even in a single dose of 1.0 g, depresses the rate and extent of the absorption of digoxin in man (Lindenbaum *et al.*, 1976).

In infants with *E. coli* gastroenteritis, a mild form of malabsorption was commonly induced by relatively short courses of oral neomycin. Nelson (1971) showed that diarrhea was significantly prolonged, and onset of weight gain was delayed, in infants treated with neomycin for 10 days, compared with infants treated for 3 days.

5 Contact dermatitis

Prolonged application of either neomycin or framycetin to skin lesions may cause sensitization. Kirton and Munro-Ashman (1965) described 70 cases of contact dermatitis due to these drugs. The patients had been treated for lesions such as leg ulcers, otitis externa, blepharitis and eczema. Sensitization was manifested by either an acute exacerbation of the disease or failure to respond to local treatment. In this latter group, the absence of an acute allergic reaction was ascribed to the concomitant use of topical corticosteroids. Patch testing showed that 65 patients were sensitive to neomycin and 50 to framycetin, and in 45 patients there was cross-sensitivity between these two antibiotics. Other studies also suggested that the risk of contact dermatitis was high, especially in eczema of the lower leg and when application is continued for long periods. In contrast, short-term application of neomycin, particularly to children, carried little risk of sensitization (Leading article, 1977).

Clinical Uses of the Drugs

1 Topical treatment of superficial infections

Both neomycin and framycetin have been often used for local treatment of superficial infections due to staphylococci and Gram-negative bacilli. These drugs are best used in combination with other antibiotics to avoid the development of resistant strains. Neomycin is often combined with polymyxin B and bacitracin in various creams, ointments, eye drops, sprays and solutions for topical use. Neomycin is also used in association with various corticosteroids in creams and ointments to treat allergic diseases with secondary bacterial infections.

2 Bacterial intestinal infections

As these antibiotics are only slightly absorbed from the gastrointestinal tract, they were used in the past to treat various bacterial intestinal infections. They are no longer recommended for this purpose.

Orally administered non-absorbable drugs of this group are of no value in gastroenteritis due to enteropathogenic *E. coli* (Emond *et al.*, 1969; Christie, 1973; Ryan *et al.*, 1986). Similarly, antibiotics (absorbable or non-absorbable) are of little or no practical value for the treatment of *Salmonella* gastroenteritis. They do not shorten the clinical illness, and may prolong the *Salmonella* carrier state. This was confirmed in a controlled trial with neomycin (Joint Project, 1970). In patients with severe *Salmonella* gastroenteritis in whom septicemia is suspected or confirmed, treatment with either chloramphenicol (p.568), amoxycillin (p.141), co-trimoxazole (p.867) or ciprofloxacin (p.1016) is indicated.

Neomycin and related drugs do not benefit mild to moderate cases of *Shigella sonnei* dysentery. Severe *Shigella* dysentery with marked systemic symptoms, which occurs more frequently with *Sh. flexneri and Sh. dysenteriae* type 1 infections, may require chemotherapy, but absorbable antibiotics such as ampicillin (p.122), co-trimoxazole (p.868) or ciprofloxacin (p.1016) are indicated.

3 Parasitic infections

Oral paromomycin was found to be effective in amebic dysentery, but it had no effect on hepatic amebiasis (Courtney *et al.*, 1960). As metronidazole (p.951) is the best drug for all forms of amebiasis, paromomycin now has little place in the treatment of this disease. Paromomycin may be used for mild to moderate cases of amebic dysentery during pregnancy, when metronidazole may be contraindicated. However, for severe cases it is still advisable to use metronidazole, at least initially (McAuley and Juranek, 1992).

Paromomycin has been used for the treatment of *Taenia saginata, T. solium, Hymenolepsis nana* and *Diphyllobothrium latum* intestinal infestations. Tanowitz and Wittner (1973) used a single 4 g dose of the drug successfully to treat five patients with *Diphyllobothrium latum* infection. Niclosamide ('Yomesan'), is a better choice for these infections. In animals, topical treatment with 15% paromomycin sulfate, 12%, methylbenzethonium, 12% benzethonium chloride and 12% cetalkonium chloride, all incorporated in white soft paraffin, was effective for the treatment of cutaneous leishmaniasis (El-On *et al.*, 1984).

Amebic keratitis may be treated by topical neomycin or paromomycin in combination with other drugs, but the results of treatment are often disappointing. These drugs also, if used for prolonged periods, have ocular toxic effects (Osato *et al.*, 1991).

Cryptosporidium parvum is a protozoan parasite that is a common cause of diarrhea worldwide. In normal hosts cryptosporidiosis typically presents with watery diarrhea that resolves spontaneously, but in HIV-infected patients with profound immunosuppression, cryptosporidiosis causes prolonged diarrhea and wasting (White *et al.*, 1994). In dexamethasone-treated rats, paromomycin could not eradicate cryptosporidiosis, but a decrease in the intensity of ileal parasitism was achieved (Verdon *et al.*, 1994). In another animal study paromomycin reduced the severity of ileal infections; however the drug was ineffective against cecal and biliary tract cryptosporidiosis (Regh, 1994). Clinically in AIDS patients paromomycin has been used orally in doses of 250 mg 6-hourly, 0.5 g 6-hourly or 1.0 g 12-hourly. Usually 2 weeks of paromomycin treatment results in improvement. A decrease in frequency of diarrheal episodes and stablization of body weight usually occurs. *Cryptosporidium* oocyst excretion also decreases, but the parasite is only occasionally eliminated from the bowel. Following paromomycin treatment, relapses are common. The optimum duration of treatment is not yet clear. Continuous maintenance therapy may be needed to prevent relapses (Fichtenbaum *et al.*, 1993; Wallace *et al.*, 1993; Bissuel *et al.*, 1994; White *et al.*, 1994). Animal studies suggest that higher paromomycin doses may be more effective, but these may not be tolerated by patients (Tzipori *et al.*, 1995; White *et al.*, 1995).

4 Preoperative chemoprophylaxis in large bowel surgery

Both oral neomycin and framycetin were often used in the past to suppress the normal flora of the large bowel prior to surgery. This was of doubtful efficacy and neomycin or framycetin, used alone, are now no longer recommended for this purpose. The combination regimen of oral neomycin plus erythromycin (p.534) is still used in the USA prior to elective operations on the colon. The use of non-absorbable antibiotics encourages the emergence of resistant organisms in the bowel (Finegold, 1986). Emergence of resistant organisms may result in bowel superinfections and diseases such as *Cl. difficile* or staphylococcal colitis (p.537).

Postoperative infections are best prevented in high-risk patients by the use of other more appropriate antibiotics. These must be present in high concentrations in the tissues before bacterial contamination occurs, and this implies their i.v. or i.m. use just before or at the beginning of an operation (Keighley, 1983) (p.949).

5 Hepatic failure

Oral neomycin is commonly used for suppression of intestinal flora in this condition (Suh *et al.*, 1979) but framycetin or kanamycin can also be used for this purpose.

6 Reduction of bowel flora in patients with granulocytopenia

Oral neomycin or framycetin, usually in combination with other non-absorbable antibiotics, has been used to suppress intestinal aerobic bacteria in leukemic patients during neutropenic episodes. This has met with some success in reducing the frequency of septicemia, other infections and pyrexial episodes, because most of the causative organisms in such patients arise from the bowel (Keating and Penington, 1973; Storring *et al.*, 1977; Clasener *et al.*, 1987). Many aerobic Gram-negative bacilli in hospitals may now be neomycin-resistant, and drugs such as oral gentamicin (p.435) or co-trimoxazole (p.881) are often preferred.

Anaerobes have an inhibitory effect on the growth of aerobic microorganisms in the bowel. This effect is referred to as colonization resistance (Guiot *et al.*, 1981; Clasener *et al.*, 1987). Furthermore, anaerobes do not cause serious infections in neutropenic patients. Therefore, a combination of antibiotics with activity against Gram-negative aerobes and fungi, but not against anaerobes should be chosen for administration to these patients. The use of such antibiotic regimens has been referred to as selective antimicrobial modulation or selective decontamination of human microbial flora. Oral antibiotic regimens, such as the combination of neomycin, polymyxin B, amphotericin B and nalidixic acid (Guiot *et al.*, 1981; 1983), oral vancomycin, gentamicin plus nystatin or co-trimoxazole alone (p.881) have been used for this purpose. There is no generally accepted ideal regimen. Emergence of drug resistance and drug reactions are common problems. The use of these regimens has prolonged infection-free intervals in individual patients, but there is no evidence that a specific prophylactic regimen is associated with more prolonged overall survival (Young, 1983).

Neomycin is very active against sensitive Gram-negative aerobes in the bowel (Arabi *et al.*, 1979) and high concentrations of the drug are reached in the colon after oral administration. Yet a neomycin dosage of at least 250 mg orally 6-hourly is required for selective decontamination of the bowel (Guiot *et al.*, 1983). This seems to be because some neomycin (and other antibiotics) is biologically inactivated by intestinal contents (Veringa and Van der Waaij, 1984). In addition, drugs such as neomycin and polymyxin B may be approximately 90% bound to solid parts of feces in the intestinal lumen, and only the free unbound antibiotic is antibacterially active (Hazenberg *et al.*, 1986).

7 Bladder infections

Neomycin solutions were often instilled into the bladder for prophylactic purposes after cystoscopy and other procedures. Such solutions were also used for bladder washouts to treat or prevent infections in patients with continuous catheter drainage. The use of neomycin for these purposes is no longer recommended (Haldorson *et al.*, 1978).

8 Hypercholesterolemia

Long-term administration of oral neomycin in a dose of 1.5 g daily has a serum cholesterol-lowering effect. This appears to be primarily due to inhibition of intestinal absorption of cholesterol, resulting in enhanced elimination of cholesterol as neutral sterols in the feces (Miettinen and Toivonen, 1975). This long-term neomycin treatment, however, has a profound effect on the aerobic intestinal flora (p.537), and neomycin is not used for this purpose.

References

A Cooperative Study (1973). Drug-induced deafness. *JAMA* **224**: 515.

Annotation (1976). Ear-drops. *Lancet* **i**: 896.

Appel GB, Neu HC (1977). The nephrotoxicity of antimicrobial agents (second of three parts). *New Engl J Med* **296**: 722.

Arabi Y, Dimock F, Burdon DW *et al.* (1979). Influence of neomycin and metronidazole on colonic microflora of volunteers. *J Antimicrob Chemother* **5**: 531.

Bartlett JG (1979). Antibiotic-associated pseudomembranous colitis. *Rev Infect Dis* **1**: 530.

Bissett ML, Abbott SL, Wood RM (1974). Antimicrobial resistance and R factors in *Salmonella* isolated in California (1971–1972). *Antimicrob Ag Chemother* **5**: 161.

Bissuel F, Cotte L, Rabodonirina M *et al.* (1994). Paramomycin: an effective treatment for cryptosporidial diarrhea in patients with AIDS. *Clin Infect Dis* **18**: 447.

Breen KJ, Bryant RE, Levinson JD, Schenker S (1972). Neomycin absorption in man. *Ann Intern Med* **76**: 211.

Brummett RE (1983). Animal models of aminoglycoside antibiotic ototoxicity. *Rev Infect Dis* **5** (Suppl 2): 294.

Bush GH (1962). Antibiotic paralysis. *Brit Med J* **2**: 1062.

Christie AB (1973). Treatment of gastrointestinal infections: a clinician's viewpoint. In *Current Antibiotic Therapy* (Geddes AM, Williams JD, eds), p. 183. Edinburgh, London: Churchill Livingstone.

Clark LW (1973). Neomycin in the prevention of postcatheterization bacteriuria. *Med J Aust* **1**: 1034.

Clasener HAL, Vollaard EJ, Van Saene HKF (1987). Long-term prophylaxis of infection by selective decontamination in leukopenia and in mechanical ventilation. *Rev Infect Dis* **9**: 295.

Courtney KO, Thompson PE, Hodgkinson R, Fitzsimmons JR (1960). Paromomycin as a therapeutic substance for intestinal amebiasis and bacterial enteritis. *Antibiotics Annual 1959–1960*: 304.

Davies JR, Farrant WN, Uttley AHC (1970). Antibiotic resistance of *Shigella* sonnei. *Lancet* **ii**: 1157.

De Beukelaer MM, Travis LB, Dodge WF, Guerra FA (1971). Deafness and acute tubular necrosis following parenteral administration of neomycin. *Amer J Dis Child* **121**: 250.

El-On J, Jacobs GP, Witztum E, Greenblatt CL (1984). Development of topical treatment for cutaneous leishmaniasis caused by *Leishmania major* in experimental animals. *Antimicrob Ag Chemother* **26**: 745.

Emery ERJ (1963). Neuromuscular blocking properties of antibiotics as a cause of postoperative apnoea. *Anaesthesia* **18**: 57.

Emmerson BT, Pryse-Davies J (1964). Studies on the nephrotoxic effect of neomycin. *Aust Ann Med* **13**: 149.

Emond RTD, Gray JA, Smith H, Young SEJ (1969). Antibiotics in acute gastroenteritis. *Lancet* **i**: 1312.

Fichtenbaum CJ, Ritchie DJ, Powderly WG (1993). Use of paromomycin for treatment of cryptosporidiosis in patients with AIDS. *Clin Infect Dis* **16**: 298.

Finegold SM (1986). Intestinal microbial changes and disease as a result of antimicrobial use. *Pediat Infect Dis* **5** (Suppl): 88.

Gorbach SL (1982). Prophylactic antibiotics-indications in surgical patients. *Scand J Infect Dis* (Suppl 36): 134.

Gorbach SL (1991). Antimicrobial prophylaxis for appendecectomy and colorectal surgery. *Rev Infect Dis* **13** (Suppl 10): 815.

Guiot HFL, Van der Meer JWM, Van Furth R (1981). Selective antimicrobial modulation of human microbial flora: infection prevention in patients with decreased host defense mechanisms by selective elimination of potentially pathogenic bacteria. *J Infect Dis* **143**: 644.

Guiot HFL, Van den Broek PJ, Van der Meer JWM, Van Furth R (1983). Selective antimicrobial modulation of the intestinal flora of patients with acute nonlymphocytic leukemia: a double blind placebo-controlled study. *J Infect Dis* **147**: 615.

Haldorson AM, Keys TF, Maker MD, Opitz JL (1978). Nonvalue of neomycin instillation after intermittent urinary catheterization. *Antimicrob Ag Chemother* **14**: 368.

Hazenberg MP, Pennock-Schröder AM, Van de Merwe JP (1986). Reversible binding of polymyxin B and neomycin to the solid part of faeces. *J Antimicrob Chemother* **17**: 333.

Jacobson ED, Faloon WW (1961). Malabsorptive effects of neomycin in commonly used doses. *JAMA* **175**: 187.

Jawetz E (1969). Neomycin ototoxicity: dossier and doses. *New Engl J Med* **281**: 219.

Joint Project by Members of the Association for the Study of Infectious Disease (1970). Effect of neomycin in the non-invasive *Salmonella* infections of the gastrointestinal tract. *Lancet* **ii**: 1159.

Kanyok TP, Reddy MV, Chinnaswamy J *et al.* (1994a). Activity of aminosidine (paromomycin). for *Mycobacterium tuberculosis* and *Mycobacterium avium*. *J Antimicrob Chemother* **33**: 323.

Kanyok TP, Reddy MV, Chinnaswamy J *et al.* (1994b). *In vivo* activity of paromomycin against susceptible and multidrug-resistant *Mycobacterium tuberculosis* and *M avium* complex strains. *Antimicrob Ag Chemother* **38**: 170.

Keating MJ, Penington DG (1973). Prophylaxis against septicaemia in acute leukaemia: the use of oral framycetin. *Med J Aust* **2**: 213.

Keighley MRB (1983). Perioperative antibiotics. *Brit Med J* **286**: 1844.

Kelly DR, Nilo ER, Berggren RB (1969). Deafness after topical neomycin wound irrigation. *New Engl J Med* **280**: 1338.

Kirton V, Munro-Ashman D (1965). Contact dermatitis from neomycin and framycetin. *Lancet* **i**: 138.

Krumlovsky FA, Emmerman J, Parker RH *et al.* (1972). Dialysis in treatment of neomycin overdosage. *Ann Intern Med* **76**: 443.

Kunin CM, Chalmers TC, Leevy CM *et al.* (1960). Absorption of orally administered neomycin and kanamycin. *New Engl J Med* **262**: 380.

Last PM, Sherlock S (1960). Systemic absorption of orally administered neomycin in liver disease. *New Engl J Med* **262**: 385.

Leading Article (1963). Antibiotic ototoxicity. *Brit Med J* **2**: 68.

Leading Article (1969). Deafness after topical neomycin. *Brit Med J* **4**: 181.

Leading Article (1977). Steroid-antibiotic combinations. *Brit Med J* **1**: 1303.

Lindenbaum J, Maulitz RM, Butler VP Jr (1976). Inhibition of digoxin absorption by neomycin. *Gastroenterology* **71**: 399.

Marshall RJ, Flanigan TP (1992). Paromomycin inhibits *Cryptosporidium* infection of a human enterocyte cell line. *J Infect Dis* **165**: 772.

McAuley JB, Juranek DD (1992). Paromomycin in the treatment of mild-to-moderate intestinal amebiasis. *Clin Infect Dis* **15**: 551.

McLeod JW, Mason JM, Pilley A (1963). Prophylactic control of infection of the urinary tract consequent on catheterization. *Lancet* **i**: 292.

Miettinen TA, Toivonen I (1975). Treatment of severe and mild hypercholesterolaemia with probucol and neomycin. *Postgrad Med J* **51** (Suppl): 71.

Nagington J, Richards JE (1976). Chemotherapeutic compounds and *Acanthamoebae* from eye infections. *J Clin Path* **29**: 648.

Nelson JD (1971). Duration of neomycin therapy for enteropathogenic *Escherichia coli* diarrhoeal disease: a comparative study of 113 cases. *Pediatrics* **48**: 248.

Osato MS, Robinson NM, Wilhelmus KR, Jones DB (1991). *In vitro* evaluation of antimicrobial compounds for cysticidal activity against Acanthamoeba. *Rev Infect Dis* **13** (Suppl 5): 431.

Piersimoni C, Bornigia S, De Sio G, Scalise G (1994). Bacterostatic and bactericidal activities of paromomycin against *Mycobacterium avium* complex isolates. *J Antimicrob Chemother* **34**: 421.

Rehg JE (1994). A comparison of anticryptosporidial activity of paromomycin with that of other aminoglycosides and azithromycin in immunosuppressed rats. *J Infect Dis* **170**: 934.

Ross EDT, Settle JAD, Telfer ABM (1963). Oral neomycin: a possible anaesthetic hazard. *Brit Med J* **2**: 1109.

Rountree PM, Beard MA (1965). The spread of neomycin-resistant staphylococci in a hospital. *Med J Aust* **1**: 498.

Rubbo SD, Hughes ESR, Blainey B, Russell IS (1966). Role of preoperative chemoprophylaxis in bowel surgery. *Antimicrob Agents Chemother* **1965**: 649.

Ryan CA, Tauxe RV, Hosek GW *et al.* (1986). *Escherichia coli* 0157:H7 diarrhoea in a nursing home: clinical, epidemiological, and pathological findings. *J Infect Dis* **154**: 631.

Smith RJ, Alder VG, Warin RP (1975). Pyogenic cocci in infantile eczema throughout one year. *Brit Med J* **3**: 199.

Storring RA, McElwain TJ, Jameson B, Wiltshaw E (1977). Oral non-absorbed antibiotics prevent infection in acute non-lymphoblastic leukaemia. *Lancet* **ii**: 837.

Suh B, Stephens JL, Kunin CM (1979). Oral neomycin dosage schedules for suppression of ammonia production by bowel flora. *Antimicrob Ag Chemother* **16**: 519.

Tanowitz HB, Wittner M (1973). Paromomycin in the treatment of *Diphylobothrium latum* infections. *J Trop Med* **76**: 151.

Trimble GX (1969). Neomycin ototoxicity: dossier and doses. *New Engl J Med* **281**: 219.

Turck M, Stamm W (1981). Nosocomial infection of the urinary tract. *Amer J Med* **70**: 655,.

Tzipori S, Griffiths J, Theodes C (1995). Paromomycin treatment against cryptosporidiosis in patients with AIDS. *J Infect Dis* **171**: 1069.

Valtonen MV, Suomalainen RJ, Ylikahri RH, Valtonen VV (1977). Selection of multiresistant coliforms by long-term treatment of hypercholesterolaemia with neomycin. *Brit Med J* **1**: 683.

Verdon R, Polianski J, Gaudebout C *et al.* (1994). Evaluation of curative anticryptosporidial activity of paromomycin in a dexamethasone-treated rat model. *Antimicrob Ag Chemother* **38**: 1681.

Veringa EM, Van der Waaij D (1984). Biological inactivation by faeces of antimicrobial drugs applicable in selective decontamination of the digestive tract. *J Antimicrob Chemother* **14**: 605.

Waksman SA, Lechevalier HA (1949). Neomycin, a new antibiotic active against streptomycin-resistant bacteria, including tuberculosis organisms. *Science* **109**: 305; quoted by Welch (1954).

Wallace MR, Nguyen M-T, Newton JAJr (1993). Use of paromomycin for the treatment of cryptosporidiosis in patients with AIDS. *Clin Infect Dis* **17**: 1070.

Weinstein AJ, McHenry M, Gavan TL (1977). Systemic absorption of neomycin irrigating solution. *JAMA* **238**: 152.

Welch H (1954). *Principles and Practice of Antibiotic Therapy* p. 158. New York: Medical Encyclopedia Inc.

White AC Jr, Chappell CL, Hayat CS *et al.* (1994). Paramomycin for cryptosporidiosis in AIDS: a prospective, double-blind trial. *J Infect Dis* **170**: 419.

White AC Jr, Goodgame RW, Chappell CL (1995). Paromomycin treatment against cryptosporidiosis in patients with AIDS. *J Infect Dis* **171**: 1071.

Young LS (1983). Antimicrobial prophylaxis against infection in neutropenic patients. *J Infect Dis* **147**: 611.

Bacitracin and Gramicidin

Description

Similar to the polymyxins (p. 667), these are peptide antibiotics which are composed of peptide-linked amino acids.

1 Bacitracin

This was isolated from a strain of *Bacillus* spp. (Johnson *et al.*, 1945), which was originally classified as *Bacillus subtilis*, but now it is known as *B. licheniformis* (Katz and Demain, 1977). From the time of its discovery until about 1960, bacitracin was used systemically, mainly for the treatment of severe staphylococcal infections (Jawetz, 1968). Because of its toxicity and the availability of other antibiotics, it is now mainly restricted to topical use. For this reason, descriptions of its pharmacokinetics and detailed toxicology are not included.

2 Gramicidin

In 1939 an antibiotic named tyrothricin was isolated from *Bacillus brevis* by Dubos. Later it was shown that tyrothricin consisted of two antibiotics, gramicidin and tyrocidine. Gramicidin was the more active drug of the two, but it was too toxic to be used systemically. It is now used in a number of topical preparations.

Sensitive Organisms

Bacitracin is highly active against most Gram-positive bacteria, particularly *Staphylococcus aureus* and *Streptococcus pyogenes*. Group C and G beta-hemolytic streptococci are usually less susceptible and Group B streptococci are usually resistant (Baker *et al.*, 1976; Finland *et al.*, 1976). *Clostridium difficile* is usually sensitive and the majority of strains are synergistically inhibited by the combination of bacitracin and rifampicin (Bacon *et al.*, 1991). Pathogenic *Neisseria* (meningococci and gonococci) are also sensitive, but Gram-negative bacilli are resistant.

Acquired bacterial resistance to bacitracin is unusual, but resistant *Staph. aureus* strains have been occasionally detected. In one hospital, where topical preparations containing both bacitracin and neomycin were commonly used, staphylococci resistant to both of these drugs were encountered (Rountree and Beard, 1965).

Gramicidin is also highly active against Gram-positive bacteria, but the *Neisseria* spp. are relatively resistant and Gram-negative bacilli are completely resistant.

Mode of Action

Bacitracin interferes with bacterial cell wall synthesis. It is a specific inhibitor of the dephosphorylation of a lipid pyrophosphate, a reaction which occurs during the second stage of bacterial cell wall synthesis (Strominger, 1973).

Bacitracin probably also damages the bacterial cytoplasmic membrane, and unlike the penicillins (p. 28), it is active against protoplasts. Gramicidin acts on bacteria by altering the function of their cytoplasmic membrane (Carter and McCarthy, 1966). It may also be a potent and specific inhibitor of the transcription reaction and inhibit the binding of DNA-dependent RNA polymerase (transcriptase) to DNA (Dancer, 1977) (p. 561).

Toxicity

Nephrotoxicity is the main toxic effect of bacitracin, if it is administered systemically, but it seldom causes side-effects when it is used topically. The renal toxicity of this drug may be largely due to the fact that it causes renal vasoconstriction (Drapeau *et al.*, 1992). Serum levels comparable with those obtained after parenteral administration can result if bacitracin is used for mediastinal irrigation or intraperitoneal lavage, so that its use by these routes should be avoided (Westerman, 1983). Applied locally to skin or mucous membranes the drug is non-irritating and allergic sensitization is rare.

Gramicidin also has virtually no side-effects when used topically.

Clinical Uses of the Drugs

1 Topical use

Bacitracin was commonly used in various topical antibiotic applications such as creams, ointments, antibiotic sprays and powders and also in solutions for wound irrigation or bladder instillation, etc. Most commonly it was combined with both neomycin and polymyxin B, providing an effective 'cover' for all bacterial species (pp.538, 674).

Gramicidin is also used in topical preparations such as eye and ear drops, creams and ointments, and like bacitracin, it is often combined with neomycin and polymyxin B.

Nowadays for the treatment of impetigo, antiseptics such as chlorhexidine or povidone-iodine are preferred. In general antibiotics, except for mupirocin (p. 544) are avoided for the treatment of this disease. However, antiseptics and mupirocin eradicated coagulase-negative staphylococci from the skin surface and from the underlying stratum corneum, but repopulation with the organisms of stratum corneum soon resulted. By contrast neomycin, bacitracin and polymyxin B ointment not only eradicated organisms from both sites, but also prevented repopulation of the stratum corneum by coagulase-negative staphylococci. These findings may have clinical relevance, for prevention of infections when catheters are introduced via the skin (Hendley and Ashe, 1991).

2 Pseudomembranous colitis

In addition to vancomycin (p. 779) and metronidazole (p. 949), bacitracin is another drug which has been used to treat antibiotic-associated colitis. It has been effective for this purpose in an oral dosage of 25 000 units four times daily. Further data are required before the place of bacitracin can be defined as published evidence on bacitracin for the treatment of this disease is limited and some strains of *Cl. difficile* are highly resistant to this drug (Bartlett, 1992).

References

Bacon AE, McGrath S, Fekety R, Holloway WJ (1991). *In vitro* synergy studies with *Clostridium difficile*. Antimicrob Ag Chemother **35**: 582.

Baker CJ, Webb BJ, Barrett FF (1976). Antimicrobial susceptibility of Group B streptococci isolated from a variety of clinical sources. *Antimicrob Ag Chemother* **10**: 128.

Bartlett JG (1992). *Clostridium difficile*-associated diarrhea and colitis. In: *Infectious Diseases* (Gorbach SL, Bartlett JG, Blacklow NR, eds) p. 162. Philadelphia, London: WB Saunders Co.

Carter W, McCarthy KS (1966). Molecular mechanisms of antibiotic action. *Ann Intern Med* **64**: 1087.

Dancer BN (1977). Antibiotics and bacterial sporulation. *Nature* **267**: 485.

Drapeau G, Petitclerc E, Toulouse A, Marceau F (1992). Dissociation of the antimicrobial activity of bacitracin USP from its renovascular effects. *Antimicrob Ag Chemother* **36**: 955.

Finland M, Garner C, Wilcox C, Sabath LD (1976). Susceptibility of beta-hemolytic streptococci to 65 antibacterial agents. *Antimicrob Ag Chemother* **9**: 11.

Hendley JO, Ashe KM (1991). Effect of topical antimicrobial treatment on aerobic bacteria in the stratum corneum of human skin. *Antimicrob Ag Chemother* **35**: 627.

Jawetz E (1968). Polymyxins, colistin, bacitracin, ristocetin, and vancomycin. *Pediatr Clin N Amer* **15**: 85.

Johnson BA, Anker H, Meleney FL (1945). Bacitracin: a new antibiotic produced by a member of the B subtilis group. *Science* **102**: 376.

Katz E, Demain AL (1977). The peptide antibiotics of bacillus: chemistry, bio-genesis, and possible functions. *Bacteriol Rev* **41**: 449.

Rountree PM, Beard MA (1965). The spread of neomycin-resistant staphylococci in a hospital. *Med J Aust* **1**: 498.

Strominger JL (1973). The actions of penicillin and other antibiotics on bacterial cell wall synthesis. *Hopkins Med J* **133**: 63.

Westerman EL (1983). Toxicity of mediastinal irrigation with bacitracin. *JAMA* **250**: 899.

Mupirocin

Description

Antibacterial activity of *Pseudomonas fluorescens* was first recorded in 1887 (Baader and Garre, 1887), but it was not until 1971 that Fuller *et al.* isolated the major metabolite which accounted for most of this activity. Formerly called pseudomonic acid A, this substance now has the name of mupirocin. Structurally different to other antibiotics, it contains the biogenetically unique 9-hydroxy-nonanoic acid moiety (Chain and Mellows, 1977; Alexander *et al.*, 1978). Mupirocin is useful for the topical treatment of superficial infections, particularly those due to staphylococci. For treatment of skin infections such as impetigo, mupirocin is available as 2% ointment in polyethylene glycol base. However, this base is irritant to mucous membranes, open wounds or burns. For treatment of these areas, another formulation of the agent, 2% calcium mupirocin in a white soft-paraffin base has been developed. This is suitable for the application to the nasal mucosa (Casewell and Hill, 1987; Doebbeling *et al.*, 1993).

Sensitive Organisms

Mupirocin is quite active against a wide range of Gram-positive and some Gram-negative bacteria (Sutherland *et al.*, 1985). It is active against *Staphylococcus aureus* (mode MIC 0.12 μg per ml) including beta-lactamase producing, methicillin-resistant and multiply antibiotic-resistant strains (Casewell and Hill, 1985). It is equally active against coagulase-negative staphylococci, such as *Staph. epidermidis*, *Staph. saphrophyticus*, *Staph. hominis* and *Staph. haemolyticus.* Beta-hemolytic streptococci of groups A, B, C and G, viridans streptococci and *Streptococcus pneumoniae* are susceptible to 0.12–0.5 μg per ml of mupirocin, but the group D enterococci, *Enterococcus faecalis* and *E. faecium*, and the non-enterococcal *Strep. bovis* are more resistant (MICs 32–64 μg per ml). For *Erysipelothrix rhusiopathiae* and *Listeria monocytogenes* the MIC is 8.0 μg per ml. *Corynebacterium* spp. and the anaerobic Gram-positive bacteria, such as *Peptococcus*, *Peptostreptococcus*, *Clostridium* spp. and *Propionibacterium acnes* are resistant. Of the Gram-negative bacteria, *Haemophilus influenzae*, *Neisseria gonorrhoeae*, *N. meningitidis*, *Moraxella catarrhalis*, *Bordetella pertussis* and *Pasteurella multocida* are quite sensitive (MICs 0.02–0.25 μg per ml). Other Gram-negative organisms, such as *Escherichia coli*, *Klebsiella pneumoniae*, *Enterobacter* and *Proteus* spp. (MICs 64–128 μg per ml), *Morganella morganii*, *Pseudomonas aeruginosa*, *Serratia marcescens* and *Bacteroides fragilis* (MICs >1600 μg per ml), are resistant. *Chlamydia trachomatis* and fungi, such as *Candida albicans*, *Pityrosporum ovale*, *Aspergillus fumigatus* and *Trichophyton mentagrophytes*, are resistant. There is no cross-resistance between mupirocin and any of the major groups of antibiotics. Resistant strains of *Staph. aureus* can be selected by culture *in vitro* in the presence of mupirocin but their frequency is low. The drug is more active in acid medium, it is highly protein bound (95%) and its MBCs against *Staph. aureus* are 8- to 32-fold higher than its MICs (Sutherland *et al.*, 1985; Casewell and Hill, 1987; Aldridge, 1992; Maple *et al.*, 1992).

Absorption and Inactivation

Although mupirocin is well absorbed after oral and parenteral administration, its serum concentrations are short-lived because of extensive degradation to an antibacterially inactive metabolite, monic acid (Sutherland *et al.*, 1985). Therefore, it is only useful clinically when used topically.

Mode of Action and Acquired Resistance

Mupirocin acts on bacteria by binding reversibly to the isoleucyl-t RNA synthetase (Hughes and Mellows, 1980) which prevents isoleucine incorporation and this inhibits protein synthesis (Hughes and Mellows, 1978). Resistance to mupirocin involves restricted access to the binding site on isoleucyl-t RNA synthetase (Capobianco et al., 1989). Resistant strains of Staph. aureus do not modify or degrade the antibiotic. The resistance determinants are located on plasmids (Farmer et al., 1992).

Mupirocin-resistance in staphylococci can be either low-level (MICs 32–64 µg per ml) or high-level (MICs >1024 µg per ml or even > 5000 µg per ml. In strains with low-level resistance a different chromosomally encoded isoleucyl-t RNA synthetase has been detected. This enzyme was inhibited less by mupirocin than the enzyme from fully susceptible strains. The determinants of the high-level mupirocin-resistance reside on large conjugative plasmids or transposons. These resistance determinants can be transferred from Staph. aureus to coagulase-negative staphylococci. These highly resistant strains appear to possess another isoleucyl-t RNA synthetase which is completely mupirocin-resistant (Cookson, 1990; Gilbart et al., 1993; Janssen et al., 1993; Hodgson et al., 1994; Morton et al., 1995). Mupirocin-resistance has been detected in methicillin-resistant staphylococci and also in borderline oxacillin-resistant Staph. aureus (Layton and Patterson, 1994). Low-level mupirocin-resistance is of questionable clinical significance, but high-level resistance is associated with therapeutic failures (Smith and Kennedy, 1988).

Mupirocin-resistance is more likely to arise if it is used for prolonged periods in facilities with endemic MRSA colonizations. Resistance is much less likely if the drug is used short-term in outbreak situations (p. 546) (Kauffman et al., 1993). Resistance to mupirocin is also more likely to develop if it is used in patients with indwelling foreign bodies such as nasal feeding tubes, tracheostomies and nasotracheal tubes. Also in large decubitus ulcers staphylococci may not be eradicated and mupirocin-resistant strains are likely to develop (Neu, 1990).

Toxicity

No adverse reactions have been associated with topical treatment except for soreness and itching around the nose, which may have been due to the ointment containing polyethylene glycol, which is now not recommended for intranasal use (Casewell and Hill, 1986).

Clinical Uses of the Drug

1 Eradication of nasal carrier state of Staph. aureus

In a controlled trial involving 32 healthy volunteers, Casewell and Hill (1986) showed that 2% mupirocin ointment applied four times daily for 5 days, eliminated nasal carriage of Staph. aureus within 2 days; 2 weeks after the course Staph. aureus could not be detected. Eventually 14 subjects resumed carriage, ten with a different phage type and four with their pretreatment strains. Leigh and Joy (1993) compared mupirocin nasal ointment and chlorhexidine neomycin 'Naseptin' cream, both given for 7 days for removing nasal carriage of Staph. aureus. There was a better response to mupirocin, which also had a prolonged effect in preventing recolonization. During a hospital outbreak of methicillin-resistant Staph. aureus (MRSA), involving more than 200 patients, 40 patients and 32 hospital staff who were nasal carriers of MRSA, received topical application of 2% mupirocin ointment. Nasal carriage was eliminated in all patients and staff, usually within the first 48h of treatment (Hill et al., 1988). Six clinical trials in six institutions with mupirocin ointment for the elimination of nasal Staph. aureus carrier state in the USA were analyzed by Doebbeling et al. (1993). The data demonstrated that calcium mupirocin ointment, administered intranasally for 5 days was safe and effective in eliminating stable nasal carriage of Staph. aureus. The experience of Reagan et al. (1991) and Fernandez et al. (1995) with healthy health-care workers, who were nasal carriers of Staph. aureus, was similar. In one nursing home 39 patients (38.2%) were colonized, 18 with methicillin-sensitive Staph. aureus strains and 21 with MRSA. These patients were treated with mupirocin ointment applied to anterior nares twice-daily for 7 days. After treatment colonization persisted in three patients. At 2 months follow-up, 11 patients became transiently recolonized and three became permanently recolonized with Staph. aureus (Cederna et al., 1990).

In another study the long-term effect of a single 5-day application of intranasal mupirocin calcium ointment was investigated in 68 healthy volunteers who had stable Staph. aureus carriage. Half of them received mupirocin and the other half placebo. At 6 months nasal carriage was still present in 48% in the treatment group versus 72% in controls; at 1 year nasal carriage was 53% versus 76% in these two groups, respectively. About half of treated subjects were recolonized with a new strain at 1 year, and the other half reisolated the original strain (Doebbeling *et al.*, 1994). In a long-term care facility, Kauffman *et al.* (1993) found that mupirocin ointment used short-term, was effective at decreasing colonization with MRSA. However, long-term use of the ointment selected mupirocin-resistant MRSA strains. In a 26-bed spinal cord injury unit, where some patients not only had MRSA nasal colonization but also infected decubitus ulcers, the combination of a 2-week course of oral minocycline and rifampicin plus a 5-day course of intranasal mupirocin, successfully eliminated MRSA from most patients (Dorouiche *et al.*, 1991). In another study topical mupirocin ointment was equally effective to oral co-trimoxazole plus topical fusidic acid for the eradication of nasal carriage of MRSA (Parras *et al.*, 1995).

2 Impetigo

For treatment of this disease 2% mupirocin in polyethylene glycol base, applied topically three times daily for 8 days has been compared with treatment by oral erythromycin. Results of treatment were about the same, but erythromycin occasionally caused mild diarrhea (Goldfarb *et al.*, 1988; Britton *et al.*, 1990). If patients are infected with erythromycin-resistant *Staph. aureus* strains (p. 607), then mupirocin treatment is superior (Dagan and Bar David, 1992).

3 Burn wounds infected by Staph. aureus

Mupirocin ointment, applied to burn wounds twice-daily has been effective in eliminating MRSA from them. It has only been used in burn wounds involving less than 20% of the total body surface area (Rode *et al.*, 1988, 1989).

References

Aldridge KE (1992). *In vitro* antistaphylococcal activities of two investigative fluoroquinolones, CI-960 and WIN 57273, comparded with those of ciprofloxacin, mupirocin (pseudomonic acid),and peptide-class antimicrobial agents. *Antimicrob Ag Chemother* **36**: 851.

Alexander RG, Clayton JP, Luk K *et al.* (1978). The chemistry of pseudomonic acid 1: the absolute configuration of pseudomonic acid. *J Chem Soc Perkin* **1**: 294, quoted by Casewell and Hill (1985).

Baader A, Garre C (1887). Ueber Antagonisten under den Bacterien. *Correspondenz-Blatt fur Schweizer Aerzte* **13**: 385, quoted by Casewell and Hill (1985).

Britton JW, Fajardo JE, Krafte-Jacobs B (1990). Comparison of mupirocin and erythromycin in the treatment of impetigo. *J Pediatrics* **117**: 827.

Capobianco JO, Doran CC, Goldman RC (1989). Mechanism of mupirocin transport into sensitive and resistant bacteria. *Antimicrob Ag Chemother* **33**: 156.

Casewell MW, Hill RLR (1985). *In-vitro* activity of mupirocin ('pseudomonic acid'). against clinical isolates of *Staphylococcus aureus*. *J Antimicrob Chemother* **15**: 523.

Casewell MW, Hill RLR (1986). Elimination of nasal carriage of *Staphylococcus aureus* with mupirocin ('pseudomonic acid'). – a controlled trial. *J Antimicrob Chemother* **17**: 365.

Casewell MW, Hill RLR (1987). Mupirocin ('pseudomonic acid'). – a promising new topical antimicrobial agent. *J Antimicrob Chemother* **19**: 1.

Cederna JE, Terpenning MS, Ensberg M *et al.* (1990). *Staphylococcus aureus* nasal colonization in a nursing home: eradication with mupirocin. *Infect Control Hosp Epidemiol* **11**: 13.

Chain EB, Mellows G (1977). The structure of pseudomonic acid A, a novel antibiotic produced by *Pseudomonas fluorescens*. *J Chem Soc Perkin* **1**: 294, quoted by Casewell and Hill (1985).

Cookson BD (1990). Mupirocin resistance in staphylococci. *J Antimicrob Chemother* **25**: 497.

Dagan R, Bar-David Y (1992). Double-blind study comparing erythromycin and mupirocin for treatment of impetigo in children: implications of a high prevalence of erythromycin-resistant *Staphylococcus aureus* strains. *Antimicrob Ag Chemother* **36**: 287.

Darouiche R, Wright C, Hamill R *et al.* (1991). Eradication of colonization by methicillin-resistant *Staphylococcus aureus* by using oral minocy-cline-rifampin and topical mupirocin. *Antimicrob Ag Chemother* **35**: 1612.

Doebbeling BN, Breneman DL, Neu HC *et al.* (1993). Elimination of *Staphylococcus aureus* nasal carriage in health care workers: analysis of six clinical trials with calcium mupirocin ointment. *Clin Infect Dis* **17**: 466.

Doebbeling BN, Reagan DR, Pfaller MA *et al.* (1994). Long-term efficacy of intranasal mupirocin ointment A prospective cohort study of *Staphylococcus aureus* carriage. *Arch Intern Med* **154**: 1505.

Farmer TH, Gilbart J, Elson SW (1992). Biochemical basis of mupirocin resistance in strains of *Staphylococcus aureus*. *J Antimicrob Chemother* **30**: 587.

Fernandez C, Gaspar C, Torrelas A *et al.* (1995). A double-blind, randomized, placebo-controlled clinical trial to evaluate the safety and efficacy of mupirocin calcium ointment for eliminating nasal carriage of *Staphylococcus aureus* among hospital personnel. *J Antimicrob Chemother* **35**: 399.

Fuller AT, Mellows G, Woodford M *et al.* (1971). Pseudomonic acid: an antibiotic produced by *Pseudomonas fluorescens*. *Nature* **243**: 416.

Gilbart J, Perry CR, Slocombe B (1993). High-level mupirocin resistance in *Staphylococcus aureus*: evidence for two distinct isoleucyl-tRNA synthetases. *Antimicrob Ag Chemother* **37**: 32.

Goldfarb J, Crenshaw D, O'Horo J *et al.* (1988). Randomized clinical trial of topical mupirocin versus oral erythromycin for impetigo. *Antimicrob Ag Chemother* **32**: 1780.

Hill RLR, Duckworth GJ, Casewell MW (1988). Elimination of nasal carriage of methicillin-resistant *Staphyloccus aureus* with mupirocin during a hospital outbreak. *J Antimicrob Chemother* **22**: 377.

Hodgson JE, Curnock SP, Dyke KGH *et al.* (1994). Molecular characterization of the gene encoding high-level mupirocin resistance in

Staphylococcus aureus J2870. *Antimicrob Ag Chemother* **38**: 1205.

Hughes J, Mellows G (1978). On the mode of action of pseudomonic acid: inhibition of protein synthesis in *Staphylococcus aureus*. *J Antibiot* **31**: 330.

Hughes J, Mellows G (1980). Interaction of pseudomonic acid A with *Escherichia coli* B isoleucyl-t-RNA synthetase. *Biochem J* **191**: 209.

Janssen DA, Zarins LT, Schaberg DR *et al.* (1993). Detection and characterization of mupirocin resistance in *Staphylococcus aureus*. *Antimicrob Ag Chemother* **37**: 2003.

Kauffman CA, Terpenning MS, He X *et al.* (1993). Attempts to eradicate methicillin-resistant *Staphylococcus aureus* from a long-term-care facility with the use of mupirocin ointment. *Amer J Med* **94**: 371.

Layton MC, Patterson JE (1994). Mupirocin resistance among consecutive isolates of oxacillin-resistant and boarderline oxacillin-resistant *Staphylococcus aureus* at a university hospital. *Antimicrob Ag Chemother* **38**: 1664.

Leigh DA, Joy G (1993). Treatment of familial staphylococcal infection – comparison of mupirocin nasal ointment and chlorhexidine/neomycin (Naseptin). cream in eradication of nasal carriage. *J Antimicrob Chemother* **31**: 909.

Maple PAC, Hamilton-Miller JMT, Brumfitt W (1992). Comparison of the *in-vitro* activities of the topical antimicrobials azelaic acid, nitrofurazone, silver sulphadiazine and mupirocin against methicillin-resistant *Staphylococcus aureus*. *J Antimicrob Chemother* **29**: 661.

Morton TM, Johnston JL, Patterson J, Archer GL (1995). Characterization of conjugative staphylococcal mupirocin resistance plasmid. *Antimicrob Ag Chemother* **39**: 1272.

Neu HC (1990). The use of mupirocin in controlling methicillin-resistant *Staphylococcus aureus*. *Infect Control Hosp Epidemiol* **11**: 11.

Parras F, Guerrero M del C, Bouza E *et al.* (1995). Comparative study of mupirocin and oral co-trimoxazole plus topical fusidic acid in eradication of nasal carriage of methicillin-resistant *Staphylococcus aureus*. *Antimicrob Ag Chemother* **39**: 175.

Reagan DR, Doebbeling BN, Pfaller MA *et al.* (1991). Elimination of coincident *Staphylococcus aureus* nasal and hand carriage with intranasal application of mupirocin calcium ointment. *Ann Intern Med* **114**: 101.

Rode H, De Wet PM, Millar AJW, Cywes S (1988). Bactericidal efficacy of mupirocin in multi-antibiotic resistant *Staphylococcus aureus* burn wound infection. *J Antimicrob Chemother* **21**: 589.

Rode H, Hanslo D, de Wet PH *et al.* (1989). Efficacy of mupirocin in methicillin-resistant *Staphylococcus aureus* burn wound infection. *Antimicrob Ag Chemother* **33**: 1358.

Smith GE, Kennedy CTC (1988). *Staphylococcus aureus* resistant to mupirocin. *J Antimicrob Chemother* **21**: 141.

Sutherland R, Boon RJ, Griffin KE *et al.* (1985). Antibacterial activity of mupirocin (pseudomonic acid), a new antibiotic for topical use. *Antimicrob Ag Chemother* **27**: 495.

Chloramphenicol and Thiamphenicol

Description

1 Chloramphenicol

Originally isolated from *Streptomyces venezuelae* (Ehrlich *et al.*, 1947), this was the first broad-spectrum antibiotic discovered. It has a benzene ring in its structure and has the chemical formula of D(-)-threo-p-nitrophenyl-2-dichloracetamido-1, 3-propanediol (Woodward and Wisseman, 1958). The chemical structure of chloramphenicol and a method for its synethetization were elucidated by Parke Davis Laboratories.

2 Thiamphenicol

This is an analog of chloramphenicol, in which the p-nitro group on the benzene ring is replaced by a methyl-sulphonyl group. It is more soluble and also more stable in solution than chloramphenicol. Unlike chloramphenicol (p. 560), thiamphenicol is not conjugated with glucuronic acid in the liver to any extent, and in patients with normal renal function most of an administered dose is excreted in the urine in an active unchanged form. High urine levels of active thiamphenicol are attained (Tacquet *et al.*, 1974; Furman *et al.*, 1976). In patients with renal failure thiamphenicol dosage, unlike that of chloramphenicol (p. 557), should be appropriately reduced (Dettli and Spring, 1974). The daily dose of thiamphenicol for patients with advanced renal failure is approximately 0.75 g, instead of the usual one of 3.0 g (Tacquet *et al.*, 1974).

The antimicrobial spectrum of thiamphenicol is similar to that of chloramphenicol. Overall, chloramphenicol is more active, being so against many enterobacteria, *Staphylococcus aureus*, *Enterococcus faecalis* and *Streptococcus pneumoniae* (Neu and Fu, 1980; Glupczynski *et al.*, 1983; Marca *et al.*, 1984). Chloramphenicol and thiamphenicol are equally active against *Neisseria gonorrhoeae*, including beta-lactamase-producing strains (Duck *et al.*, 1978). In therapeutic doses thiamphenicol, like chloramphenicol, causes hemopoietic toxicity (p. 565). Early bone marrow suppression mainly involving erythropoiesis is more severe with thiamphenicol than with chloramphenicol. However, thiamphenicol-induced bone marrow damage, even if severe, is said to be always reversible. Also thiamphenicol apparently has not been implicated as a cause of fatal bone marrow aplasia among 69 million treated patients (Francheschinis, 1981). Thiamphenicol has been widely used in Europe and Japan, especially for the treatment of respiratory infections. The drug has been used successfully to treat gonorrhea (single oral dose of 2.5 g) and for chancroid, single oral dose of 2.5 g followed by 1.25 g in a week if the lesion is not healed (Latif, 1982; Latif *et al.*, 1982, 1986). When used as a single oral 2.5-g dose for gonorrhea, thiamphenicol was ineffective in eliminating co-existent *Chlamydia trachomatis* from patients (Perroud and Miedzybrodzka, 1978). In a study in the Philippines, a single oral dose of 2.5 g thiamphenicol was equally as effective as single-dose treatment with procaine penicillin G plus probenecid for gonorrhea due to non-beta-lactamase-producing strains, and equally as effective as single-dose treatment with spectinomycin or cefuroxime for disease due to beta-lactamase-producers (Tupasi *et al.*, 1982, 1983). Thiamphenicol is not available in the USA and Australia.

The following data only apply to chloramphenicol.

Sensitive Organisms

Chloramphenicol has a wide range of activity.

1 Gram-negative aerobic bacteria

The Enterobacteriaceae are normally sensitive to chloramphenicol, *Escherichia coli* and the *Enterobacter*, *Klebsiella*, *Proteus*, *Serratia*, *Citrobacter*, *Providencia*, *Hafnia*, *Edwardsiella* and *Arizona* spp. are usually susceptible. *Yersinia pestis* (Butler *et al.*, 1974) and *Y. enterocolitica* (Preston *et al.*, 1994) are also usually chloramphenicol-sensitive.

The prevalence of chloramphenicol-resistant variants of these organisms has slowly increased over the years, but acute infections due to resistant strains are still uncommon unless hospital acquired. During a 2-month survey in a Boston hospital in 1967, Sabath (1969) found that 15% of *E. coli* and 55% of *Klebsiella*, 47% of *Enterobacter*, 28% of *Proteus* and 60% of *Serratia* spp. strains isolated were chloramphenicol-resistant. Other surveys indicated that approximately 80% of clinical isolates of *Serratia marcescens* were chloramphenicol-sensitive (Cooksey *et al.*, 1975; Mills and Drew, 1976). However, in some nosocomial infections due to this organism, the epidemic strain has at times been resistant to chloramphenicol, and also to other antibiotics such as ampicillin, carbenicillin, tetracycline, streptomycin, kanamycin and gentamicin (Schaberg *et al.*, 1977). Such multidrug-resistance is often plasmid-mediated (see below), and it can be transferred in the urine or elsewhere from a multidrug-resistant *S. marcescens* strain to other Enterobacteriaceae such as *E. coli* (Schaberg *et al.*, 1977). The clinical use of chloramphenicol is a major factor in selecting chloramphenicol-resistant strains. For example, the routine use of chloramphenicol for treating neonatal sepsis resulted in the emergence of chloramphenicol-resistance in up to 50% of enterobacteria (*E. coli* or *Klebsiella*) in one neonatal intensive care unit (Prober *et al.*, 1983). Of enteropathogenic *E. coli* strains collected in the UK during 1980 and 1981, 29% were resistant to chloramphenicol and all of these were resistant to other antibiotics (Gross *et al.*, 1982). Chloramphenicol-resistant Enterobacteriaceae are also common in developing countries. In one study in Nigeria, some 80% of *E. coli*, and *Klebsiella* and *Proteus* spp., isolated from hospitalized patients, were chloramphenicol-resistant (Montefiore *et al.*, 1989).

Chloramphenicol-resistant bacterial strains, which possess plasmid-mediated resistance, produce an enzyme, acetyltransferase, which inactivates the drug (Coleman *et al.*, 1994). Some chloramphenicol-resistant strains of *E. coli* do not produce acetyltransferase. These *E. coli* cells possess an active efflux system which results in removal of chloramphenicol from the periplasmic space. The genes for this type of resistance probably reside in bacterial chromosomes (McMurry *et al.*, 1994).

The combination of chloramphenicol and gentamicin may exhibit some antagonism against Enterobacteriaceae such as *E. coli* and *Klebsiella* spp. (D'Alessandri *et al.*, 1976). Chloramphenicol appears to suppress the rapid bactericidal activity of gentamicin against these organisms (Klastersky and Husson, 1977). Other *in vitro* studies showed that chloramphenicol antagonized the bactericidal effect of gentamicin and of ampicillin plus gentamicin against *E. coli* (Paisley and Washington, 1979). The drug also shows antagonism *in vitro* to cefotaxime and ceftriaxone, and to a lesser extent to aztreonam and imipenem (Brown and Alford, 1984; Asmar *et al.*, 1988).

Salmonella typhi, other salmonellae and the shigellae are usually chloramphenicol-sensitive, but over the years some changes in the sensitivities of these organisms have occurred. Chloramphenicol-resistant shigellae were first observed in Japan (Suzuki *et al.*, 1956), and it was soon established that this resistance may be transferred from *E. coli* to shigellae. Such transfer was demonstrated *in vitro*, in laboratory animals and in human volunteers. Bacterial resistance to antibiotics acquired by this method is termed transferable drug resistance.

The transfer of resistance to an antibiotic (or to multiple antibiotics) from one bacterial species to another occurs during bacterial conjugation and is controlled by plasmids (Buu-Hoi *et al.*, 1986; Couturier *et al.*, 1988). Conjugation is the process which occurs when bacterial cells come in contact, and genetic material is passed from one organism to another. Plasmids are extra chromosomal genetic elements which are capable of independent replication and are stably inherited. Certain plasmids called 'resistance plasmids' (R plasmids) carry genetic information for resistance to antibiotics and/or other antibacterial drugs. Other plasmids which bring about the transfer of DNA by conjugation are called conjugative plasmids; these were previously called infectious or transmissible plasmids. Many R plasmids are also conjugative plasmids, so that they have the additional ability to transfer their genetic information for antibiotic-resistance by conjugation. Other R plasmids must be associated with conjugative plasmids before transfer of resistance from one organism to another can occur.

Transferable drug resistance mediated by plasmids occurs amongst the Enterobacteriaceae, and many other organisms such as *Pseudomonas aeruginosa* (p. 453), *Vibrio cholerae* (p. 724).

Haemophilus influenzae (p. 113), and beta-lactamase-producing *N. gonorrhoeae* (p. 115). DNA sequences carrying resistance genes can be transposed from one plasmid to another, or from plasmid to bacterial chromosome or to bacteriophage or *vice versa* (Datta, 1977). The specific lengths of DNA involved in such transpositions have been termed transposons (Grinsted, 1986; Lupski, 1987). The specific beta-lactamase (TEM enzyme) which confers resistance to the penicillins is plasmid-mediated. The genetic material conferring this quality on the organism has been transferred by means of transposons from plasmids of enterobacteria to plasmids in *N. gonorrhoeae* and *H. influenzae* (Datta, 1977). In this way ampicillin-resistant strains of *H. influenzae* (p. 113) and penicillin-resistant strains of *N. gonorrhoeae* (p. 15), have emerged.

For many years, R plasmid-mediated chloramphenicol-resistant shigellae were common in Japan and later appeared in other countries. During three large early surveys of *Shigella* spp. isolated from patients in North America, chloramphenicol-resistant variants were either not detected or were very rare (Farrar and Eidson, 1971; Ross *et al.*, 1972; Neu *et al.*, 1975a). In Sweden, Urban (1972) found that 18% of 94 *Sh. flexneri* and *Sh. sonnei* strains during 1970 were resistant to chloramphenicol. During 1959 and 1970 a major epidemic of bacillary dysentery due to *Sh. dysenteriae* type 1 (*Shiga bacillus*) occurred in Central America and this spread to Mexico in 1971. The *Shigella* strain involved possessed plasmid-mediated resistance to chloramphenicol, tetracycline, streptomycin and sulfonamides (Thorne and Farrar, 1973; Balows, 1977). This pattern of resistance was similar to that found in the strain of *Salm. typhi*, which caused an extensive outbreak of typhoid fever in Mexico during 1972 (see below). Surprisingly, the plasmids from the epidemic strains of *Sh. dysenteriae* type 1 and those from *Salm. typhi* belonged to different compatibility groups, demonstrating that although these two epidemic organisms had similar antibiotic resistance patterns, their resistance was mediated by two unrelated plasmids (Thorne and Farrar, 1974). During this dysentery epidemic, a small number of strains of *Sh. dysenteriae* type 1 were isolated from patients which were additionally resistant to ampicillin (p. 111). This ampicillin-resistance was due to a separate plasmid. These strains with dual-plasmid resistance never became widespread in Central America. Only a very few 'imported' cases of *Shigella* dysentery were reported in the USA during the outbreak in Central America and Mexico (Balows, 1977). Chloramphenicol-resistance was frequent amongst *Shigella* isolates in Lebanon (Uwaydah and Osseiran, 1981). In the UK, the percentage of *Shigella* spp. strains isolated which were resistant to chloramphenicol rose from 2.6 in 1974 to 52.1 in 1983 (Gross *et al.*, 1984). In Bangladesh and India most strains of *Sh. dysenteriae* were resistant to chloramphenicol, streptomycin, tetracycline and co-trimoxazole, resistance being plasmid-mediated (Farrar, 1985; Panigrahi *et al.*, 1987). In many other developing countries *Shigella dysenteriae* type 1 strains were resistant to chloramphenicol, ampicillin, nalidixic acid, tetracycline and co-trimoxazole e.g. in Burundi, Africa (Ries *et al.*, 1994). In Cordoba, Argentina, most *Shigella* spp. strains were resistant to the same antibiotics (Brito-Alayon *et al.*, 1994). In North eastern Brazil during the period 1988 to 1993 most *Shigella* spp. strains were multiply-resistant to ampicillin, co-trimoxazole, streptomycin, tetracycline and chloramphenicol (Lima *et al.*, 1995).

Chloramphenicol-resistance mediated by plasmids can also be transferred from *E. coli* to salmonellae (Smith, 1973). Resistant strains of these organisms, including *Salm. typhi*, had been occasionally detected in the past (Oles and Stanio-Pyrkosz, 1964; Gill and Hook, 1966). Emergence of chloramphenicol-resistant *Salm. typhi* during treatment was first detected in Britain (Colquhoun and Weetch, 1950). Large surveys indicated that such strains were very rare (Winshell *et al.*, 1970). Later in a study in California a higher prevalence of chloramphenicol-resistant salmonellae was detected. Of *Salm. typhi* strains 16% were resistant, but only 4% or less of strains of other species were resistant, with most species being only 1% or less resistant (Bissett *et al.*, 1974). Some of the resistant *Salm. typhi* isolates detected in this survey were obtained from imported typhoid cases during the 1972 epidemic in Mexico.

From February 1972 until June 1973, an epidemic of typhoid fever involving over 10 000 cases, occurred in Mexico. The *Salm. typhi* strain concerned possessed plasmid-mediated resistance to chloramphenicol as well as resistance to tetracycline, streptomycin and sulfonamides (Vasquez *et al.*, 1972; Olarte and Galindo, 1973), which was mediated by a single plasmid (Balows, 1977). The MIC of chloramphenicol for this strain was as high as 150 µg per ml, compared with 0.75–5.0 µg per ml for sensitive strains (WHO, 1974a; Anderson, 1975). During this epidemic a few *Salm. typhi* strains were isolated from patients, which were additionally resistant to ampicillin (p. 110). Ampicillin-resistance was mediated by a separate plasmid (Balows, 1977). Fortunately, strains with this dual resistance did not spread to any extent, and the vast majority of chloramphenicol-resistant organisms remained ampicillin-sensitive (Overturf *et al.*, 1973; Datta and Olarte, 1974). After the epidemic in Mexico abated in

1973, typhoid remained endemic in the area, but surprisingly the previously resistant *Salm. typhi* strains were replaced by chloramphenicol-sensitive ones (Balows, 1977).

During the typhoid fever epidemic in Mexico, eight cases of typhoid fever due to the Mexican epidemic strain were reported in the USA, and most of the patients concerned had recently travelled in Mexico. Associated with the Mexican epidemic, a smaller number of imported cases of typhoid were also detected in other countries such as UK (Anderson and Smith, 1972), Switzerland and Canada (Balows, 1977). Some 15–20 years ago plasmid-mediated chloramphenicol-resistant *Salm. typhi* strains were detected in countries such as South Vietnam (Butler *et al.*, 1973; Brown *et al.*, 1975), Thailand (Lampe and Mansuwan, 1973), India (WHO, 1974b), Indonesia (Sanborn *et al.*, 1975; Ling and Chau, 1984) and Bangladesh (Huo and Samadi, 1982). Although precise data were not available, it appeared likely that typhoid fever due to chloramphenicol-resistant *Salm. typhi* strains was already prevalent in South-East Asia, and that this prevalence was increasing (Anderson, 1975). In India, occasional strains of *Salm. typhi* resistant to chloramphenicol and even ampicillin have been isolated since 1962, but since 1972 multiple antibiotic-resistant strains of *Salm. typhi* and of other salmonellae have been encountered increasingly. The *Salm. typhi* strains were uniformly resistant to chloramphenicol, streptomycin, sulfonamides and tetracycline; whilst the non-*typhi* salmonellae were commonly resistant to ampicillin as well; transmissible plasmids were demonstrated in all of these strains (Sharma *et al.*, 1979). Of 241 strains of *Salm. typhi* isolated in Peru during 1981–1983, 72 (29.9%) were resistant to chloramphenicol; this was plasmid-mediated and four different resistance patterns were described; chloramphenicol- (and tetracycline) resistance was associated with sulfonamide-resistance in 71 strains, ampicillin-resistance in 15, and trimethoprim-resistance in 34. These resistant strains were sensitive to ceftriaxone, aztreonam, imipenem, ampicillin/clavulanic acid and to the quinolones, norfloxacin and ciprofloxacin. Strains of *Salm. typhi* resistant to chloramphenicol, ampicillin, sulfonamides and trimethoprim were isolated in Japan and France (Goldstein *et al.*, 1986). Acquired resistance of *Salm. typhi* to chloramphenicol can also occur during treatment by the acquisition of the resistance gene(s) (plasmid or transposon) from other intestinal organisms. Datta *et al.* (1981) described *in vivo* acquired resistance of a strain to chloramphenicol and co-trimoxazole. Threlfall *et al.* (1982) reported another strain in which acquired resistance to chloramphenicol and ampicillin occurred during treatment. More recently Schwalbe *et al.* (1990) reported the recovery of *Salm. typhi* which acquired resistance to chloramphenicol, ampicillin, co-trimoxazole and gentamicin subsequent to multiple antibiotic therapy. Isolates of *E. coli* and *Klebsiella pneumoniae* were recovered from the same stool samples and these displayed identical resistance patterns.

Initial surveys in the USA indicated that *Salm. typhi* strains resistant to chloramphenicol were rare. Chloramphenicol-resistant isolates of other salmonellae were also uncommon; the frequency of such strains was only approximately one per 1000 of *Salmonella* isolates (Neu *et al.*, 1975b; Cherubin *et al.*, 1977). In 1967 there were no chloramphenicol-resistant non-typhoid salmonellae detected in isolates sent to the CDC in the USA, whereas six isolates (0.8%) were resistant in 1975. These strains were usually resistant to multiple antibiotics including ampicillin (Ryder *et al.*, 1980). Of 209 strains of *Salm. typhi* isolated in the USA in 1975 and 1976, 95% were sensitive to ampicillin and chloramphenicol (Ryder and Blake, 1979). The proportion of imported cases of typhoid fever in the USA was gradually rising. They constituted only 33% of the total during 1967–1972, but the proportion of imported cases rose to 69% in 1984. The major sources of the 1975–1984 cases were Mexico (39%) and India (14%). Antimicrobial resistance was still only a minor problem (Ryan *et al.*, 1989). In 1985 an outbreak of salmonellosis occurred in California. The organism, *Salm. newport*, was resistant to chloramphenicol and its source was traced through hamburgers to dairy farms (Spika *et al.*, 1987). Non-typhoid salmonellosis is commonly believed to be a zoonosis and therefore antibiotic resistance is presumed in most cases to be first acquired by the animal host (Leading article, 1982) (p. 110).

Salmonella typhimurium strains with resistance to both chloramphenicol and ampicillin were noted in Canada. From January 1973 to July 1975, 12% (6 of 51) of infections due to this organism at the Hospital for Sick Children in Toronto were caused by such resistant strains (Grant *et al.*, 1976). Chloramphenicol-resistant strains of *Salm. typhi* and other salmonellae were more common in certain European countries such as Holland and France than in the USA (Cherubin *et al.*, 1977). Since 1977 two types of *Salm. typhimurium* with plasmid-mediated multiple antibiotic-resistance (including to chloramphenicol) were involved in bovine and human infections in the UK (Threlfall *et al.*, 1978).

Plasmid-encoded multiresistant (usually to ampicillin, chloramphenicol, kanamycin, streptomycin, sulfonamides, tetracycline, gentamicin and trimethoprim) *Salm. typhimurium* strains have caused outbreaks of enteritis and systemic disease in India and Saudi Arabia but these did not appear to be water or food-borne (Rowe *et al.*, 1980; Rangnekar *et al.*, 1983). More recently in Pakistan 20% of cases of typhoid fever were caused by strains of *Salm. typhi* resistant to ampicillin, chloramphenicol and co-trimoxazole (Bhutta *et al.*, 1991). Multiresistant *Salm. typhi* has also been reported from India (Jesudasan and John, 1990) and from Bangladesh (Albert *et al.*, 1991). In 1979 a nosocomial outbreak of *Salm. typhimurium* began in Durban, South Africa which was particularly severe in a pediatric surgical ward; over a 2-year period 488 patients were infected. The strain was resistant to chloramphenicol, ampicillin, streptomycin, spectinomycin, sulfona-mides, trimethoprim and nalidixic acid; resistances to drugs other than nalidixic acid were specified by plasmids (Robins-Browne *et al.*, 1983). Resistance to chloramphenicol of salmonella isolated in Rome in 1977–78 was common; this was particularly so of strains of *Salm. wien* which usually showed multiple antibiotic-resistance (Falbo *et al.*, 1982). It is known that *Salm. wien*, resistant to many antibiotics including chloramphenicol, has been the cause of many outbreaks of nosocomial infection in Europe (Cherubin, 1981). In one Spanish hospital from 1988 to 1991 the overall rates of non-*Salm. typhi Salmonella* spp. resistance to ampicillin, chloramphenicol, and co-trimoxazole were 32, 11 and 2%, respectively (Muñoz *et al.*, 1993). Chloramphenicol-resistant salmonellae were reported to be relatively uncommon in Japan (Tanaka *et al.*, 1976) and Korea (Chun *et al.*, 1977). In Hong Kong *Salm. typhi* strains resistant to chloramphenicol were rare, but among other salmonellae 23% were resistant to chloramphenicol (Ling *et al.*, 1991). In recent years the prevalence of chloramphenicol-resistant *Salm. typhi* strains have been increasing in Oman (Elshafie and Rafay, 1992). A chloramphenicol-resistant *Salm. typhi* strain has been reported from Chile which carried no plasmid and had no chloramphenicol acetyltransferase activity. This isolate appeared to lack the main porin protein which usually serves as porin for entry of chloramphenicol in the bacterial cell wall (Toro *et al.*, 1990).

Most other Gram-negative bacteria are sensitive to chloramphenicol. The *Neisseria* (meningococci and gonococci) are very sensitive. Strains of meningococci resistant to chloramphenicol have been reported, but are rare (Report, 1976). Gonococci, including beta-lactamase-producing strains (p. 115) are nearly always chloramphenicol-sensitive (Report, 1978). *Haemophilus influenzae* (Williams and Andrews, 1974; Righter and Luchsinger, 1988) and *H. parainfluenzae* (Mayo and McCarthy, 1977) are very sensitive. In tests of bactericidal action against *H. influenzae* type b strains, chloramphenicol is more rapidly effective than ampicillin (p. 112) (Turk, 1977). Feldman (1978) found that chloramphenicol and ampicillin acted synergistically against a proportion of both ampicillin-sensitive and -resistant *H. influenzae* strains, but others using different methodology showed that chloramphenicol could inhibit the bactericidal activity of ampicillin against this organism (Rocco and Overturf, 1982). Neither synergy nor antagonism was detected using chloramphenicol plus rifampicin against *H. influenzae* (Jadavji *et al.*, 1984).

Chloramphenicol-resistant isolates of *Haemophilus* spp. have been detected. Cavanagh *et al.* (1975) isolated a resistant strain of *H. parainfluenzae* from the pharynx of a patient in the UK. Chloramphenicol-resistant non-typable strains of *H. influenzae* were isolated from the throat of a 4-year-old girl in Holland (Manten *et al.*, 1976) and from the blood of a woman with agammaglobulinemia in the USA (CDC, 1976). Strains of *H. influenzae* type b resistant to chloramphenicol, but sensitive to ampicillin have been isolated in the USA (Barrett *et al.*, 1972) and the UK from the CSF of children with meningitis, one of whom failed to respond to chloramphenicol therapy (Kinmonth *et al.*, 1978). A chloramphenicol-resistant but ampicillin-sensitive strain of *H. influenzae* type b (Peel *et al.*, 1979) and another with the same sensitivity pattern (Richardson *et al.*, 1979) were isolated from Indo-Chinese refugees who were recent arrivals in Australia. Strains of *H. influenzae* type b resistant to chloramphenicol and ampicillin were isolated in the USA (Uchiyama *et al.*, 1980; Mendelman *et al.*, 1984; Doern *et al.*, 1988; Givner *et al.*, 1989; George *et al.*, 1991; Jorgensen, 1992), the UK (Garvey and McMullin, 1983; Howard and Williams, 1988; Powell and Price, 1990; Dimopoulou *et al.*, 1992), Australia (Moore *et al.*, 1985; Hansman, 1985; Wild *et al.*, 1986; Collignon *et al.*, 1992), Spain (Catry and Vaz Pato, 1983), and Dominican Republic (CDC, 1984). Most of these strains were isolated from patients with serious infections such as meningitis or bacteremia. Simasathien *et al.* (1980) described three children from an orphanage in Bangkok who died of meningitis caused by *H. influenzae* type b which was resistant to chloramphenicol and ampicillin. In contrast a study in Pakistan showed that 47.5% of *H. influenzae* strains were resistant to co-trimoxazole, 5.1% to ampicillin, but none to chloramphenicol (Mastro *et al.*, 1993). In a report from Gambia, West Africa 1.8% of *H. influenzae* strains were chloramphenicol-resistant, but none were resistant to ampicillin (Bijlmer *et al.*, 1994).

Non-encapsulated *H. influenzae* strains which were resistant to chloramphenicol and ampicillin have also been detected in the UK (Heymann *et al.*, 1981; Sills *et al.*, 1983). Most of these chloramphenicol-resistant *Haemophilus* spp. isolates were also tetracycline-resistant. Resistance to chloramphenicol was mediated by a plasmid which coded for the production of an enzyme, chloramphenicol acetyltransferase, which inactivated the drug (Van Klingeren *et al.*, 1977; Shaw *et al.*, 1978; Doern *et al.*, 1988). Multiple antibiotic-resistance of a non-encapsulated strain of *H. influenzae* was transmissible easily to *E. coli* (Rotimi and Turk, 1981). Burns *et al.* (1985) showed that some chloramphenicol-resistant non-encapsulated *H. influenzae* strains did not produce chloramphenicol acetyltransferase and resistance appeared to be due to a chromosomally mediated relative permeability barrier caused by the loss of a porin protein of the outer membrane (p. 26). Mendelman *et al.* (1984) also reported similar isolates of *H. influenzae*. Chloramphenicol accumulation by *H. influenzae* normally occurs by energy-dependent transport (Burns and Smith, 1987).

Overall, chloramphenicol-resistant *Haemophilus* spp. strains remain relatively rare, at least in developed countries. Data are not available for many developing countries. In the USA, all of 150 *Haemophilus* isolates (mainly *H. influenzae* and *H. parainfluenzae*) from patients with chronic bronchitis were chloramphenicol-sensitive (Kauffman *et al.*, 1979); of 409 *H. influenzae* strains isolated from healthy children only one non-typable strain was resistant to chloramphenicol and tetracycline (Lerman *et al.*, 1979); of clinical isolates of *H. influenzae* tested by Simon *et al.* (1980) only one was chloramphenicol-resistant and there were none amongst the 94 tested by Granato *et al.* (1983). The resistance of *H. influenzae* type b strains in the USA is less than 1% (CDC, 1984; Jorgensen, 1992). Surveys in the UK have given similar results. In 1977 and 1981 the prevalence of chloramphenicol plus tetracycline-resistance amongst *H. influenzae* strains rose from 0.25% to 1.03% (Howard *et al.*, 1978; Philpott-Howard and Williams, 1982). Mehtar and Aminiafshar (1983) found about 2% of *H. influenzae* and *H. parainfluenzae* strains to be chloramphenicol-resistant in London. In early 1991, only 0.8% of *H. influenzae* were chloramphenicol-resistant in Scotland (Powell *et al.*, 1992). Of 169 blood and CSF isolates of *H. influenzae* collected in Canada from 1976 to 1983, none were chloramphenicol-resistant (Bannatyne *et al.*, 1985), but a 0.04% chloramphenicol-resistance has been reported from Canada since then (Jorgensen, 1992). All strains of *H. influenzae* tested in Sweden were sensitive (Forsgren and Walder, 1982). In West Germany of 523 clinical isolates of *H. influenzae* and *H. parainfluenzae*, seven were chloramphenicol-resistant (Braveny and Machka, 1980). The picture is quite different in Spain. In the period 1981 to 1983, of 225 *H. influenzae* strains isolated from pediatric patients, 52.2% were resistant to chloramphenicol; this resistance was often associated with resistance to ampicillin, tetracycline and co-trimoxazole (Campos *et al.*, 1984, 1987). However, in Cape Town, South Africa 95% of strains tested were still chloramphenicol-sensitive (Hussey *et al.*, 1994).

Usually *H. ducreyi* is chloramphenicol-sensitive (Hammond *et al.*, 1978), but resistant strains have been isolated in South-East Asia; the USA and France (Sanson-LePors *et al.*, 1983; Roberts *et al.*, 1985). The latter authors found that although chloramphenicol-resistant strains of both *H. ducreyi* and *H. parainfluenzae* produced chloramphenicol acetyltransferases, resistance determinants were located on conjugative plasmids in *H. ducreyi* but were chromosomally located in *H. parainfluenzae*.

The *Brucella* spp., *Bordetella pertussis* and *Pasteurella multocida* are chloramphenicol-susceptible. The same is true for *Vibrio parahaemolyticus* (Joseph *et al.*, 1978). Also *V. cholerae* is sensitive, but rare resistant strains have been detected (p. 724). Strains of *V. cholerae* biotype El Tor isolated in an epidemic in Tanzania were resistant to multiple antibiotics including chloramphenicol and tetracycline (Mhalu *et al.*, 1979) and resistance was transferable by a plasmid (Towner *et al.*, 1979). Strains of *V. cholerae* non-O-group 1 which caused gastroenteritis in the USA were susceptible to chloramphenicol and tetracycline (Morris *et al.*, 1981). Also the more recently reported multiresistant *V. cholerae* O1 El Tor in Argentina remained susceptible to chloramphenicol (Rossi *et al.*, 1993). The *Moraxella* spp. are chloramphenicol-sensitive (De Leys and Juni, 1977). *Burkholderia (Pseudomonas) pseudomallei* with a median MIC of 6.4 µg per ml is only sensitive to a degree (Eickhoff *et al.*, 1970; Howe *et al.*, 1971; Calabi, 1973). The cidal action of ceftazidime (p. 371) against this organism is antagonized by chloramphenicol *in vitro* (Dance *et al.*, 1989). *Pseudomonas aeruginosa* is always completely resistant. This now appears mainly due to an active efflux pump which removes chloramphenicol from the bacterial cell, rather than due to a permeability barrier (Li *et al.*, 1994). *Burkholderia (Pseudomonas) cepacia* is also resistant (Burns *et al.*, 1989). *Campylobacter jejuni* is sensitive to chloramphenicol but a few resistant strains occur (Vanhoof *et al.*, 1978; Ringertz *et al.*, 1981; Michel *et al.*, 1983). *Helicobacter pylori* is also sensitive (Goodwin *et al.*, 1986). Most strains of *Aeromonas* spp. are susceptible (Gray, 1984; Janda *et al.*, 1994). *Flavobacteria* are resistant (Aber *et al.*, 1978).

Legionella pneumophila (MIC 0.5 µg per ml) is sensitive to chloramphenicol *in vitro* (Thornsberry *et al.*, 1978; Saravolatz *et al.*, 1980), and the drug also prevents death of infected embryonated eggs (Lewis *et al.*, 1978). Other Legionellaceae, such as *L. micdadei*, *L. bozemanii*, *L. gormanii*, and *L. dumoffii*, are sensitive to chloramphenicol *in vitro* (Pasculle *et al.*, 1981). However, chloramphenicol is not as active as erythromycin (p. 609) and especially rifampicin (p. 677) against *L. pneumophila in vivo*; in one experiment chloramphenicol, unlike these other two drugs, did not prevent the death of guinea pigs infected intraperitoneally (Fraser *et al.*, 1978). Chloramphenicol penetrates the lungs of guinea pigs to a lesser extent than rifampicin and erythromycin (Gibson and Fitzgeorge, 1983). Chloramphenicol is also not effective for the treatment of experimental *L. micdadei* infection in guinea pigs (Pasculle *et al.*, 1985).

2 Gram-negative anaerobic bacteria

Chloramphenicol is one of the most active chemotherapeutic agents against these bacteria. Most bacteria of the *Bacteroides fragilis* group are susceptible (Kirby *et al.*, 1980; Snydman *et al.*, 1980; Cuchural *et al.*, 1981; Hill and Ayers, 1985). In particular, *B. fragilis* is nearly always so. In surveys of the bacteria of the *B. fragilis* group in the USA (Cuchural *et al.*, 1988; Appleman *et al.*, 1991; Citron *et al.*, 1995), in Canada (Bourgault *et al.*, 1992), in the UK (Fox and Phillips, 1987), in France (Patey *et al.*, 1994) and in Korea (Lee *et al.*, 1992), no chloramphenicol-resistant strains were detected. Plasmids which code for chloramphenicol-resistance have been detected in strains of *B. ochraceus* (Guiney and Davis, 1978) and *B. uniformis* (Martínez-Suárez *et al.*, 1985; Wexler and Finegold, 1987). Britz and Wilkinson (1978) described a resistant strain of *B. fragilis* due to the production of a chloramphenicol acetyltransferase which was constitutively produced.

The *Prevotella*, *Fusobacterium* and *Veillonella* spp. are usually quite susceptible (Sutter and Finegold, 1976; George *et al.*, 1981). When a gentamicin/chloramphenicol combination is used clinically to treat suspected mixed aerobic and anaerobic intra-abdominal infections (p. 569), gentamicin does not interfere with the activity of chloramphenicol against *B. fragilis* (Klastersky and Husson, 1977). The uncommonly encountered, motile, anaerobic Gram-negative bacilli such as *Butyrivibrio*, *Succinivibrio*, *Anaerovibrio*, *Wolinella*, *Desulfovibrio*, *Selenomonas* and *Anaerobiospirillum* spp. are nearly always chloramphenicol-sensitive (Johnson and Finegold, 1987).

3 Gram-positive cocci

Staphylococcus aureus (including beta-lactamase-producing strains), *Staph. epidermidis*, *Strep. pyogenes*, *Strep. pneumoniae*, alpha hemolytica streptococci (*Strep. viridans*) and *E. faecalis*, are usually sensitive. Group B streptococci are nearly always chloramphenicol-sensitive; some authors have found 1.0–2.0% of isolates to be resistant (Anthony and Concepcion, 1975; Baker *et al.*, 1976). Resistant strains of *Staph. aureus* (Sabath, 1969), *Staph. epidermidis* (Bentley *et al.*, 1970) and *Staph. haemolyticus* (Schwartz and Cardoso, 1991a) occur, but in contrast to the tetracyclines (p. 720), chloramphenicol-resistance is less common. In particular resistant strains of 'community staphylococci' have been relatively uncommon (Bennet and Kucers, 1970; Hassam *et al.*, 1978). Methicillin-resistant strains of *Staph. aureus* have usually been resistant to chloramphenicol, but some strains may now be sensitive in developed countries, as the drug has been used very little in recent years. The resistance of staphylococci to the drug is plasmid-mediated, which codes for the production of chloramphenicol acetyltransferase (Schwarz and Cardoso, 1991b).

Chloramphenicol-resistant *Strep. pyogenes* strains have become common in Japan (Nakae *et al.*, 1977), but they appear to be rare elsewhere (Bourbeau and Campos, 1982). Pneumococci resistant to chloramphenicol are still generally rare (Perlino and Lichtenberger, 1984), but they have been detected in Poland, France, Britain, West Africa, Australia and the USA (Hansman, 1978; Howard *et al.*, 1978; Dang-Van *et al.*, 1978; Istre *et al.*, 1983). Most of these resistant strains produce a plasmid-mediated chloramphenicol acetyltransferase, which inactivates the drug (Dang-Van *et al.*, 1978). In South Africa pneumococci which were resistant to multiple antibiotics, including penicillin G and chloramphenicol, were detected and they were associated with serious infections (CDC, 1977; Oppenheim *et al.*, 1986; Klugman and Koornhof, 1988). During 1983–1984, a cluster of nine strains of *Strep. pneumoniae* isolated from patients in New York were found to be resistant to penicillin G, other beta-lactam antibiotics, chloramphenicol, tetracycline and co-trimoxazole; they were sensitive to erythromycin, clindamycin, vancomycin and rifampicin (Simberkoff *et al.*, 1986). Pneumococci resistant to penicillin G, chloramphenicol and frequently to other antibiotics have been common in Spain (p. 5) and they are also increasing in prevalence in other countries, such as Pakistan (Mastro *et al.*, 1993) and Korea (Lee *et al.*, 1995).

Chloramphenicol-resistant *E. faecalis* strains are not uncommon, and most of these variants show resistance to two or more antimicrobial agents. This resistance also appears to be plasmid-mediated; one plasmid was identified in *E. faecalis*, which coded for resistance to chloramphenicol and erythromycin and also for high-level resistance to streptomycin and lincomycin (Marder and Kayser, 1977). The biochemical mechanism of chloramphenicol-resistance in *E. faecalis* is inactivation of the drug by the enzyme, chloramphenicol acetyltransferase (Courvalin *et al.*, 1978; Trieu-Cuot *et al.*, 1993). Enterococcal-resistance genes can be located on the bacterial chromosome or transposons (Pepper *et al.*, 1987). Tofte *et al.* (1984) tested the susceptibility of 347 strains of *E. faecalis* (and its subspecies) and found them to be moderately resistant to chloramphenicol (MIC 12.5–25.0 μg per ml). However, in one study in USA, where chloramphenicol has been used very little in hospitals in recent years, 14 strains of *E. faecium*, which were resistant to penicillin G and vancomycin, were all chloramphenicol-sensitive (Norris *et al.*, 1995).

Anaerobic Gram-positive cocci, such as the *Peptococcus* and *Peptostreptococcus* spp. and the anaerobic streptococci, are all susceptible to chloramphenicol (Sutter and Finegold, 1976; Ohm-Smith *et al.*, 1982).

4 Gram-positive bacilli

Corynebacterium diphtheriae, *Listeria monocytogenes* and *Bacillus anthracis* are nearly always sensitive. *C. jeikeium* is usually resistant to chloramphenicol (Gill *et al.*, 1981). The *Nocardia* spp. are chloramphenicol-resistant (Gutman *et al.*, 1983). *Rhodococcus equi* is usually sensitive (Harvey and Sunstrum, 1991; Sirera *et al.*, 1991).

Among the anaerobic Gram-positive bacilli *Clostridium tetani*, *Cl. perfringens*, most other *Clostridium* spp. and the *Actinomyces*, *Lactobacillus*, *Eubacterium*, *Bifidobacterium* and *Propionibacterium* spp. are chloramphenicol-sensitive (Sutter and Finegold, 1976; Schwartzman *et al.*, 1977; Rood *et al.*, 1978; Denys *et al.*, 1983; Pollock *et al.*, 1983). Chloramphenicol-resistant strains of *Cl. perfringens* have been isolated and the resistance is plasmid-mediated (Rood *et al.*, 1989; Bannam and Rood, 1991). *Clostridium difficile* may be chloramphenicol-sensitive, but many strains, particularly those of serogroup C, are resistant (Delmee and Avesani, 1988; Wren *et al.*, 1988).

5 Other organisms

Treponema pallidum, leptospirae and mycoplasmas are chloramphenicol-sensitive. Mycobacteria, fungi and protozoa are resistant. Chloramphenicol is active against the rickettsiae which cause the various typhus fevers and Rocky Mountain spotted fever (Wisseman *et al.*, 1974). The action of chloramphenicol is rickettsiastatic against *Rickettsia rickettsii*, so that treatment for at least 6 days is necessary until an effective immune response is mounted in Rocky Mountain spotted fever (Wisseman and Ordonez, 1986). *Coxiella burnetii*, the agent causing Q fever, is also sensitive, as are the *Chlamydia*, a genus which includes the causative agents of pneumonia, psittacosis, lymphogranuloma venereum, trachoma and inclusion body conjunctivitis (p. 746).

6 Minimum inhibitory concentrations

The MICs of chloramphenicol against some selected bacterial species are shown in Table I.42. Organisms with an MIC of 16 μg per ml can be considered to be susceptible to chloramphenicol. This is also called the 'breakpoint' i.e. a concentration of an antimicrobial agent which can be achieved in blood with optimal therapy (Kirby *et al.*, 1980).

Mode of Administration and Dosage

Chloramphenicol can be administered orally, i.m. or i.v. Oral administration is satisfactory for many conditions, but for severely ill patients, initial administration by one of the parenteral routes is preferable, because absorption of the oral drug may be poor.

There are no generally accepted optimal therapeutic non-toxic serum levels; peak levels ranging from 15 to 25 (Kauffman *et al.*, 1981b; Yogev *et al.*, 1981), 30 μg per ml (Mulhall *et al.*, 1983c) or 35 μg per ml (Smith and Weber, 1983) have been suggested for children. Because of the erratic peak serum levels which occur following i.v. administration of the succinate to infants and children (p. 558), Lietman (1981) suggested that dosage could be adjusted to achieve reasonable trough serum levels – these should be kept as high as the MIC of the offending organism (at least 5 μg per ml if this is unknown) and below 10 μg per ml. In most patients this would result in peak serum values below 20 μg per ml and transient bone-marrow suppression (p. 565) would be avoided.

Organism	MIC range (μg per ml)	MIC of most strains strains less than:
Gram-positive bacteria		
Staphylococcus aureus	1.0–5.0	12.5
Staphylococcus epidermidis	1.0–6.25	2.5
Streptococcus pyogenes	0.3–6.0	3.0
Streptococcus pneumoniae	0.06–12.5	2.5
Streptococcus viridans	0.6–2.5	1.0
Bacillus anthracis	0.75–5.0	3.0
Clostridium perfringens	2.0–4.0	4.0
Actinomyces spp.	0.5–8.90	2.0
Gram-negative bacteria		
Escherichia coli	3.0–50.0	6.0
Enterobacter spp.	0.5–64.0	12.0
Klebsiella pneumoniae	0.5–25.0	3.1
Serratia marcescens	2.5–5.0	2.5
Proteus vulgaris	0.12–>250.0	15.0
Salmonella typhi	0.75–5.0	1.56
Shigella sonnei	2.5–6.0	5.0
Neisseria gonorrhoeae	0.078–6.3	1.0
Neisseria gonorrhoeae (beta-lactamase producing)	0.5–8.0	2.0
Neisseria meningitidis	0.78–6.25	1.5
Haemophilus influenzae	0.2–3.5	2.0
Bordetella pertussis	0.2–12.5	1.0
Pseudomonas aeruginosa	8.0–1000.0	Resistant
Bacteroides fragilis	0.5–16.0	8.0
Other *Bacteroides* spp.	0.1–16.0	2.0
Fusobacterium spp.	0.5–2.0	1.0

Table I.42
Compiled from data published by Welch (1954), Sutter and Finegold (1976) and Report (1978)

1 Oral administration

The recommended dosage for adults and children is 50 mg per kg body weight per day, given in equally divided doses every 6 h. The manufacturers have stated that a daily dose of 100 mg per kg can be used for short periods if there is need to produce high serum levels. The dosage for adults should not exceed 4 g per day.

The oral administration of unaltered chloramphenicol is difficult in young children, because they cannot swallow capsules, and chloramphenicol elixir is exceedingly bitter. The tasteless compound, chloramphenicol palmitate, is used for children. This substance has no antibacterial activity, and must be hydrolyzed by enzymes in the gut before absorption of liberated active chloramphenicol can occur. Initial preparation of this compound did not produce adequate serum levels after oral administration, but subsequently particle size was controlled to produce satisfactory blood levels.

Pharmacological studies have shown that the palmitate suspension produces good serum levels in children. In infants, serum levels obtained after oral administration are more predictable than those obtained after the succinate ester is given i.v. (p. 559). Kauffman *et al.* (1981b) (p. 558) recommended a dose of 75 mg per kg per day as a starting one for most infants beyond the newborn period; subsequent dosage should be adjusted according to serum levels obtained. Tuomanen *et al.* (1981) found that a dose of 75 mg per kg per day of the palmitate was effective for children with *H. influenzae* meningitis, and was less likely than higher doses to cause neutropenia.

2 Parenteral administration

The ester, chloramphenicol sodium succinate, is used for this purpose. It is a highly water soluble preparation which can be easily administered by either the i.m. or i.v. route. This ester has no antibacterial activity, but after administration it is converted to active chloramphenicol (p. 558). For i.m. administration the contents of a 1.2-g vial may be dissolved in as little as 2.0 ml of 'water for injection', resulting in a 40% solution. For intermittent i.v. injections, it is recommended that a more dilute 10% solution be used, and the dose slowly injected into a vein or drip tubing over 1 min. Rapid i.v. injection of a more concentrated solution is not dangerous, but the patient may experience an intensely bitter taste lasting a few minutes, and concentrated solutions may also cause thrombophlebitis. Commonly the diluted succinate is placed in a buretrol for intermittent i.v. infusion. The duration of the infusion is an important factor in determining the percentage of the succinate which is actually delivered to the patient. To make valid comparisons of chloramphenicol serum levels, the rate of infusion from the buretrol should be standardized. For adults, the contents of the buretrol are commonly infused over a period of 30 min. McCracken and Nelson (1983) recommended a 15- to 30-min infusion period for neonates. Lower peak serum chloramphenicol levels are obtained when the drug is administered via a buretrol than when it is given directly into the i.v. tubing.

Chloramphenicol succinate ester is stable in all commonly used i.v. fluids, so it can be added to i.v. bottles for continuous infusion, but incompatibility may occur in the presence of other i.v. additives. It is recommended that the dose of i.v. or i.m. chloramphenicol sodium succinate should be identical to oral chloramphenicol dosage. Nevertheless, resultant serum levels after administration of the succinate i.v. to infants and children are highly variable (p. 559) so that regular serum level monitoring, particularly of infants, is warranted.

3 Newborn and premature infants

The manufacturers (1995) recommended a dosage of 25 mg per kg per day given in four divided doses at 6 h intervals for newborn infants and for those in whom immature renal and/or hepatic function was suspected; full term infants older than 2 weeks can receive 50 mg per kg per day given in four divided doses at 6 h intervals, but pharmacokinetic studies (p. 558) have shown that the absorption of the palmitate suspension is unreliable in neonates and it should not be used. Serum levels following the i.v. administration of chloramphenicol succinate to neonates are variable and not predictable, so that serum level monitoring every 48 h to enable suitable dosage adjustment is recommended (p. 559). A therapeutic non-toxic serum level range of 15–25 μg per ml has been recommended (p. 559). Rajchgot et al. (1982) studied serum levels in premature neonates (p. 559) and as a result they suggested that such patients should receive an initial loading dose of 20 mg per kg. Black et al. (1978) treated one neonate with bacterial meningitis using i.v. chloramphenicol, which was commenced on the 5th day of life and continued for 3 weeks. Serum level monitoring showed that in order to maintain serum levels in the therapeutic range of 10–20 μg per ml, the daily chloramphenicol dose had to be progressively increased from 20 to 95 mg per kg with increasing age of the infant.

4 Patients with renal failure

Active chloramphenicol does not accumulate in these patients, and the drug may be administered in the usually recommended doses (Kunin, 1967). The drug may be more toxic to the bone marrow of uremic patients, probably because of pre-existing bone marrow depression often associated with renal failure. Inactive chloramphenicol metabolites accumulate in the serum of patients with renal failure (p. 560) but these have not been associated with toxicity (Smith and Weber, 1983). In using chloramphenicol to treat a severe infection in such patients, this increased risk of toxicity cannot be avoided, because dosage reduction results in inadequate serum levels of the active drug. Peritoneal dialysis does not alter the serum half-life of active chloramphenicol (Greenberg and Sanford, 1967). Slaughter et al. (1980) studied two patients with renal failure and hepatic dysfunction; increased clearance of chloramphenicol occurred during hemodialysis. They considered that the normal maintenance dose of the drug should be administered after dialysis to avoid possible increased clearance.

5 Patients with liver disease

In patients with liver dysfunction the total body clearance of chloramphenicol is reduced (Koup et al., 1979a). This is to be expected because the drug is metabolized in the liver (p. 560). If chloramphenicol is used in patients with liver disease, serum levels should be monitored and dosage reduced as appropriate.

Serum Levels in Relation to Dosage

With the use of more specific methods for drug assay, there is now a better understanding of the pharmacology of chloramphenicol and of its prodrugs (palmitate and succinate).

1 Oral administration

Chloramphenicol, administered orally in capsules, is rapidly and completely absorbed from the intestinal tract, and has somewhat greater bioavailability than orally administered palmitate (see below) (Smith and Weber, 1983). The peak serum level occurs about 2 h after dosing; after a 1-g dose in adults it is approximately 10–13 µg per ml (DuPont *et al.*, 1970). Doubling the usual oral dose, doubles the serum concentrations attained. The half-life of active chloramphenicol in serum is 1.6–3.3 h (Kunin *et al.*, 1959), but therapeutic levels may still be detected 6–8 h after the dose.

The biologically inactive palmitate ester is not absorbed as such, but it is hydrolyzed (presumably by pancreatic enzymes) in the upper intestinal tract to free chloramphenicol which is well absorbed. Incomplete hydrolysis or metabolism before it reaches the systemic circulation, may be factors in causing the lower bioavailability of the palmitate compared with free chloramphenicol (Smith and Weber, 1983). Nevertheless, chloramphenicol palmitate is more bioavailable than i.v. administered chloramphenicol succinate (see below) in infants in children (Kauffman *et al.*, 1981b; Yogev *et al.*, 1981). A men peak serum level of 19.3 µg per ml was reached 2–3 h after ingestion of an oral dose of 25 mg per kg palmitate in children aged up to 12 years (Pickering *et al.*, 1980). This was slightly lower than the mean peak level of 28.2 µg per ml which occurred 2–3 h after infusion of the same dose of the succinate ester; thereafter serum levels resulting from oral and i.v. administration were similar and at 6 h many levels were still in excess of 12 µg per ml. Yogev *et al.* (1981) gave the same dose orally (palmitate) and i.v. (succinate infused over 30 min) to infants aged 5–23 months with *H. influenzae* meningitis. Mean peak serum levels were 18.5 (after 2–3 h) and 15.0 µg per ml (after 45 min) following oral and i.v. administration, respectively. The mean serum half-life of the drug was longer after oral (6–5 h) than after i.v. (4.0 h) administration. In addition, with repeated oral doses there was an increase in the drug's half-life so that sometimes it accumulated producing peak serum levels in excess of 30 µg per ml. Kauffman *et al.* (1981b) gave chloramphenicol palmitate to children aged 2 months to 14 years; their studies showed that a dose of 60–75 mg per kg per day (given in divided doses every 6 h) usually resulted in serum levels of 15–25 µg per ml, whereas higher doses resulted in concentrations greater than 25 µg per ml in more than half their patients. They recommended a starting dose of 75 mg per kg per day for patients beyond the newborn period. Ekblad *et al.* (1985) also showed that oral chloramphenicol produced good serum levels in infants and children (p. 556).

Serum levels resulting from oral administration of chloramphenicol palmitate are not as predictable in neonates. In a study of seven neonates (four preterm, three term), the bioavailability of palmitate (given via a gastric tube) was lower than that after i.v. administered succinate – in the three preterm neonates (<40 weeks post-conceptional age) the dosage of palmitate required to maintain adequate serum levels was twice that of the succinate dose given i.v. Maximum serum levels were 5.5–23.1 µg per ml after a 50 mg per kg per day dosage of palmitate and occurred at or after 4 h. Furthermore, in all but two of the seven neonates, the serum concentrations failed to decline over 6 h. The investigators (Shankaran and Kauffman, 1984) considered that the variable serum levels after palmitate in neonates were probably related to prolonged and erratic absorption, due to delayed gastric emptying or decreased hydrolysis of the palmitate ester. Similar findings and explanations were given by Weiss *et al.* (1960) in an earlier report. In a larger study involving 90 babies (<1 year of age), including 64 neonates, Mulhall *et al.* (1983a) also found that oral administration in neonates resulted in lower steady state serum levels than those following i.v. administration.

2 Intravenous administration

Results of pharmacological studies using the prodrug chloramphenicol succinate i.v. have been variable. Data from many early studies are not relevant because methods used for drug quantitation measured total aromatic nitro-compounds (conjugated and unconjugated chloramphenicol and metabolites) and were not specific for free chloramphenicol or its succinate. It was, therefore, some time before it was recognized that there was appreciable urinary excretion of chloramphenicol succinate (see below), which reduced its bioavailability. Chloramphenicol succinate has no antibacterial activity as such, and after parenteral administration it is hydrolyzed in the liver to produce free active chloramphenicol. This rate of hydrolysis is highly variable in different individuals and unhydrolyzed succinate can be excreted unchanged in the urine, the extent of which is also quite variable in different individuals. Pharmacokinetics are further complicated by the metabolism of free chloramphenicol to chloramphenicol glucuronide in the liver (see below). Therefore, serum levels of chloramphenicol after i.v. administration of succinate depend on the rate of hydrolysis of chloramphenicol succinate, the rate of excretion of chloramphenicol succinate and the rate of glucuronidization of chloramphenicol to biological inactive chloramphenicol glucuronide (Lietman, 1981). The renal excretion of chloramphenicol succinate and consequent loss of available chloramphenicol explains why the orally administered chloramphenicol palmitate has greater bioavailability. Variable metabolism and variable excretion of the succinate are the reasons for the lack of correlation between the dose of i.v. succinate and resultant serum levels, and the varied results obtained in different studies a number of which are now summarized.

Friedman et al. (1979) gave chloramphenicol succinate to 54 infants and children (aged 1 day to 11 years) in dosages of 12.5–100 mg per kg per day usually in four divided doses by i.v. infusions over periods varying from 5 min to 2 h; the half-life of the drug at all ages had a wide range (0.87–17.8 h). Sack et al. (1980) gave similar i.v. dosages of the succinate in four divided doses to 17 children (aged 1 month to 6 years) by 60 min infusions. They also found wide variability of serum half-lives (range, 2.1–8.3 h) and of body clearances of the drug which was not accounted for by renal or liver disease; serum chloramphenicol succinate concentrations 1 h after infusion were low (mean, 2.8 μg per ml). Ekblad et al. (1985) reported the use of various chloramphenicol preparations in 52 children aged 3 months to 14 years. When the succinate was given in a dosage of 150 mg per kg per day in four divided doses (infusion times 30 min), the mean peak serum level was 33.5 μg per ml; when it was given in a dosage of 100 mg per kg per day the mean peak serum level was 24.7 μg per ml; and almost identical levels were obtained when the same dose was given as oral chloramphenicol in capsules or as chloramphenicol palmitate.

In studies on low birth weight infants, Glazer et al. (1980) found that chloramphenicol serum levels were highly variable and not predictable. Doses of 15–50 mg per kg per day were given in one to three divided doses by 15-min infusion. Peak serum levels (measured in blood samples taken 0.5–2.0 h after infusion) were 11.2–36.2 and 10.0–36.2 μg per ml for infants aged 1–8 days (13) and 11 days to 8 weeks (5), respectively. The serum half-life in the group of older infants was 5.5–15.7 h, whereas for the younger group it was 10.0–36.0 h and in some there was no decline in serum levels over the dosing period and possibly accumulation with serial dosing. Kauffman et al. (1981a) also showed that serum half-lives of chloramphenicol were inversely related to age and that the succinate persisted in serum up to 6 h after a dose and comprised a larger fraction of total chloramphenicol in infants under 1 month of age than in older infants and children. Mulhall et al. (1983a) studied pharmacokinetics of chloramphenicol administered i.v. and orally to 90 babies (less than one year of age, including 64 neonates). Dosages used were: 25 mg per kg per day for premature babies and term babies less than 7 days old; 37.5–50.0 mg per kg per day for neonates aged 7–28 days; and for infants 50–100 mg per kg per day. After i.v. administration serum concentrations were related to dosage in neonates but not in infants. Clearance of chloramphenicol was related to postnatal age in infants and gestational age in neonates; concomitant penicillin therapy also reduced clearance. In some babies peak serum levels greater than 25 μg per ml occurred whilst in others they were less than 10 μg per ml when the above dosages were given. Erratic chloramphenicol serum levels in these babies was ascribed to possible defective liver metabolism of the drug and immature renal function. The authors recommended that whenever chloramphenicol is administered to babies, serum levels should be monitored every 48 h, and that dosage should be adjusted to keep peak serum levels at 20–30 μg per ml, and trough serum levels below 15 μg per ml. Rajchgot et al. (1982) gave 39 courses of i.v. chloramphenicol succinate over a 30-min period by infusion pump to 35 neonates; 13 premature neonates received an initial dose of 12.5 mg per kg and 26 received a loading dose of 20 mg per kg. Neonates receiving the former dose did not achieve serum concentrations >10 μg per ml (mean peak level 8.8 μg per ml), whereas after a 20 mg per kg dose all neonates had concentrations >10 μg per ml (mean peak level, 15.9 μg per ml). Chloramphenicol levels peaked at 4 h in neonates ≥2 days postnatal age and at 2 h in neonates 3–55 days postnatal age. Chloramphenicol succinate serum levels were higher in younger than in older neonates at both 2 and 4 h after the dose, possibly due to slower hydrolysis in the liver or a prolonged distribution phase.

There are a limited number of pharmacokinetic studies of the use of chloramphenicol succinate given i.v. to adults. The serum half-life in adults is about 1.2 h and renal clearance of the succinate is less in adults than in children (Smith and Weber, 1983). In one study, in typhoid fever patients, with equivalent doses of chloramphenicol the serum concentrations of patients treated i.v. were significantly lower than those of patients on oral therapy (Ti et al., 1990).

3 Intramuscular administration

DuPont *et al.* (1970) found that after i.m. administration, serum levels of active chloramphenicol were about 50% lower than those achieved after identical oral doses; approximately one-third of the i.m. administered drug was present in serum in the form of antimicrobially inactive unhydrolyzed ester, and the serum concentration of active chloramphenicol did not rise with continued i.m. administration. These authors also observed that patients with induced typhoid fever responded more rapidly to oral chloramphenicol in a dosage of 1 g 8-hourly, than to an identical i.m. dosage of chloramphenicol succinate. Accordingly, they recommended that higher than the recommended dosage of the succinate for i.v. administration, should be used when it is given i.m., but as pointed out by Shann *et al.* (1985), although chloramphenicol serum levels are higher after oral administration than after i.m. administration of succinate, it should not be concluded that i.v. is superior to i.m. administration. Moreover, Glazko *et al.* (1977) found that the bioavailability was the same when chloramphenicol succinate was administered i.m. or i.v. to adults. It has been our experience and that of others (Barrett *et al.*, 1972), that i.m. chloramphenicol sodium succinate, administered in the usually recommended doses, gives good results in severe infections such as *H. influenzae* meningitis.

Shann *et al.* (1985) reported the results of studies in which chloramphenicol succinate was given to 57 children by the i.m. route and to 13 others i.v. Their ages ranged from 28 days to less than 6 years. The same dosage of 25 mg per kg every 6 h was used by both routes. After i.m. administration the peak serum level (specimen taken 1 h after administration) was 19.5 μg per ml after the first dose and 31.4 μg per ml after two or more doses; the lowest peak level after i.m. administration was 13 μg per ml. After the drug was given i.v. (bolus injection over about 1 min), the mean peak serum level (specimen taken 1 h later) was 19.4 μg per ml after the first dose and 28.2 μg per ml after two or more doses. After 6 h following the first i.m. or i.v. dose, mean serum levels were in excess of 10 μg per ml; and with repeated doses mean serum levels at 5 h were greater than 15 μg per ml after administration of the drug by either route. The area under the curve was not significantly different after i.m. or i.v. administration.

Excretion

1 Urine

About 90% of administered chloramphenicol is excreted in urine, but only 5–10% is in the unchanged active form. Chloramphenicol is rapidly conjugated with glucuronic acid in the healthy human liver, and the conjugates are antibacterially inactive. Active chloramphenicol is excreted only by glomeruli, but the inactive derivatives are also eliminated by tubular secretion (Weiss *et al.*, 1960). Although most administered chloramphenicol is excreted in the form of inactive metabolites, urine concentrations of the active drug are still sufficiently high to be effective for treatment of urinary infections. Urine levels exceeding 200 μg per ml of the active drug have been found following a single oral dose of 1.5 g (Glazko *et al.*, 1949). However, much less active chloramphenicol is excreted in the urine of patients with renal failure, and some of these patients may have no antibacterial effect in the urine (Lindberg *et al.*, 1966).

As most active chloramphenicol disappears from the body primarily by conversion in liver, the active drug does not accumulate in the serum of anuric patients (Kunin *et al.*, 1959; Greenberg and Sanford, 1967). Inactive chloramphenicol metabolites, which are probably not toxic, do accumulate in the serum of such patients.

After i.v. administration of chloramphenicol succinate a variable amount (6–73%) of this unchanged ester is excreted by the kidneys (Lietman, 1981). Immaturity of renal excretory mechanisms is probably one factor causing the unpredictability of serum levels in neonates after the oral administration of chloramphenicol palmitate and after the i.v. administration of chloramphenicol succinate (pp. 558, 559).

2 Inactivation in body

Chloramphenicol is metabolized in the liver and the major metabolite is chloramphenicol glucuronide (see above). Minor metabolites, some of which have little antibacterial activity, have been detected in humans (Smith and Weber, 1983). Further work has shown that chloramphenicol is metabolized by a number of pathways to produce oxidized, reduced and conjugated metabolites that can be detected in the serum by modern methods. These metabolites are probably not involved in the drug's toxicity (Holt *et al.*, 1995). Immaturity of hepatic metabolizing mechanisms are probably a factor causing unpredictable pharmacokinetic results in neonates after palmitate and succinate administration. Interference with metabolism is also the probable reason for the accumulation of chloramphenicol in patients with liver dysfunction (p. 557).

3 Bile

Only small amounts of chloramphenicol (2–3% of the administered dose) are excreted in bile, mostly in the inactive form. The concentration of active chloramphenicol in bile is usually lower than that in the serum at the time (Woodward and Wisseman, 1958).

4 Feces

About 1% of an orally administered dose of chloramphenicol is excreted in the feces, mainly in the inactive form. It probably reaches the intestinal tract via the bile.

Distribution of the Drug in Body

Chloramphenicol has high lipid solubility and diffuses into many body tissues and readily penetrates into pleural and ascitic fluids, and also crosses the placenta (Woodward and Wisseman, 1958). Concentrations of the drug in the ascitic fluid of patients with bacterial peritonitis usually exceed half of the serum level at the time (Gerding *et al.*, 1977). Also unlike many other antibiotics, it penetrates well into all parts of the eye (Mayers *et al.*, 1991), and into the CSF even in the absence of meningitis. The CSF concentration may be 50% or more of that found in the serum of patients with normal meninges, a higher proportion than that attained with any other antibiotic. There have been many reports confirming that CSF levels of the order of 65% of the simultaneous serum level are obtained in patients with and without meningitis (Dunkle, 1978; Friedman *et al.*, 1979; Pickering *et al.*, 1980; Yogev *et al.*, 1981; Mulhall *et al.*, 1983a). Salivary levels of chloramphenicol are related to serum levels, but there is considerable variability (Koup *et al.*, 1979b). *In vitro*, chloramphenicol is concentrated in polymorphonuclear leucocytes (Prokesch and Hand, 1982; Jacobs and Wilson, 1983), in nucleated human polymorphonucler leukocytes (PMN cytoplasts) (Hand and King-Thomson, 1990) and the alveolar macrophages obtained from smokers (Hand *et al.*, 1985). If chloramphenicol succinate is used for local treatment of wounds, it is hydrolyzed to the active drug in the wound fluid (Nilsson-Ehle and Hedström, 1987).

Serum protein binding of chloramphenicol is about 44% (Koup *et al.*, 1979b).

Mode of Action

Chloramphenicol is a potent inhibitor of bacterial protein synthesis (Goldberg, 1965). It is of some clinical importance to understand the mechanism of action of chloramphenicol and also that of the other antibiotics which interfere with bacterial protein synthesis. For this reason, the following description of bacterial protein synthesis is included.

The basic mechanisms involved in the synthesis of bacterial and human proteins are similar. Fortunately, there are sufficient differences between their metabolic processes to allow certain antibiotics to be selectively toxic to bacteria.

Deoxyribonucleic acid (DNA), contained in the nucleus, has the genetic control of the synthesis of all specific cellular proteins including enzymes. For this purpose DNA directs the formation of three types of ribonucleic acid (RNA).

a   Messenger RNA (m-RNA)   The genetic code of DNA for the specific organism is copied onto m-RNA, the process being catalyzed by a polymerase called DNA-dependent RNA polymerase (transcriptase). This 'transcription' of information onto m-RNA, determines the amino acid sequence of the proteins to be synthesized. Messenger RNA is an elongated strand consisting of many segments or codons, each of which is specific for a particular amino acid. This RNA migrates out into the cytoplasm, where in association with small organelles, the ribosomes, it acts as a template to direct synthesis of specific cellular proteins ('translation' of genetic message).

b   Transfer RNA (t-RNA)   This RNA acts as a carrier to transport amino acids to the proper site on the template of m-RNA. For each amino acid to be incorporated into a protein molecule, there is a specific t-RNA molecule. The specific part of t-RNA for the amino acid carried is called the anticodon, and this is complementary to the codon on m-RNA for that particular amino acid.

c   Ribosome RNA (r-RNA)   Ribosomes consist of this particular ribonucleic acid and various proteins. The ribosome can be considered as the 'work-bench' upon which various amino acids are joined in a predetermined arrangement to produce the polypeptide chains of the many proteins required for cell metabolism (Nomura, 1969). Ribosomes from bacteria can be distinguished from those of mammalian cells on the basis of their sedimentation coefficients (S values). Broadly speaking, bacteria contain 70 S ribosomes and mammalian cells 80 S ribosomes, and this distinction is useful in the context of antibiotic action, because many antibiotics selectively act against 70 S ribosomes. However, some 70 S ribosomes are also found in mammalian mitochondria.

The first step in protein synthesis is activation of amino acids, which is carried out by activating enzymes specific for each amino acid, known as aminoacyl-RNA synthetases. These activated amino acid molecules are then attached to the specific t-RNA molecules which are coded for this purpose. This process is catalyzed by specific enzymes known as aminoacyl-t-RNA synthetases. The resultant aminoacyl-t-RNA molecules then migrate to the ribosome-m-RNA complex for the synthesis of amino acid chains as specified by the m-RNA template.

The process by which polypeptide chains are manufactured from amino acids at the ribosomes is complicated. Bacterial 70 S ribosomes consist of two unequal portions, a larger '50 S' subunit and a smaller '30 S' subunit. Certain 'initiation factors' appear to be necessary for the commencement of polypeptide chain synthesis at the ribosomes. As a result it seems that m-RNA initially binds to the 30 S subunit and sequentially t-RNA and then the 50 S subunit to form the complete 70 S 'initiation complex' or active ribosome, necessary for protein synthesis.

The two parts of the aggregated or active ribosome particle have different functions. Messenger RNA is bound to the 30 S portion of the ribosome, whilst the 50 S subunit is a site for attachment of amino acids and a site for holding the growing peptide chains. These sites, known respectively as the acceptor (A) site and the peptidyl donor (P) site, are in close proximity to each other, and each site is also in juxtaposition to one m-RNA codon. The next step is the binding of individual aminoacyl-t-RNA molecules to each A site on the ribosome as directed by the m-RNA codon in juxtaposition. This binding process is catalyzed by a complex enzyme, called transfer factor T.

Growth of peptide chains is achieved by the transfer and binding of a peptide chain from a nearby P site, onto the amino acid at the A site. This results in the release of the deacylated or old t-RNA which has lost its peptide chain at the P site. The aminoacyl-t-RNA complex at the former A site then becomes the carrier of the newly elongated peptide chain. This process called 'transpeptidation' is catalyzed by an enzyme, peptidyl transferase, which is part of the 50 S subunit of the ribosome.

To enable further growth of the peptide chain, the newly elongated peptide chain is then moved into a donor or P site, by a process called translocation. This involves the movement of the ribosome along the strand of RNA, resulting in the m-RNA codon for the next amino acid to be incorporated, to be brought into juxtaposition to the donor site, as the new acceptor site. Translocation is catalyzed by a translocase enzyme called G factor.

Protein synthesis occurs at the various ribosome-m-RNA complexes, and this enables multiple proteins to be synthesized at the same time. Other proteins are involved in the release of the completed polypeptide chains from the ribosome complexes.

Most of these steps in bacterial protein synthesis may be attacked by antibiotics with consequent disruption of cell metabolism.

The inhibitory action of chloramphenicol on bacterial protein synthesis is dependent on its ability to bind to a protein of the 50 S subunit of the ribosome. This protein is an essential component of peptidyl transferase which is involved in the transpeptidation reaction which occurs at the ribosomal acceptor site (Gale *et al.*, 1972; Vince *et al.*, 1975; Harvey and Koch, 1980). In bacterial cells, which have been exposed to chloramphenicol for a short time, protein synthesis may resume when the drug is withdrawn. Peptide chains, whose synthesis was interrupted by chloramphenicol, can again be completed when the drug is removed. This explains the bacteriostatic rather than bactericidal action which this drug has against certain bacteria (Green *et al.*, 1975). With more prolonged exposure, chloramphenicol has additional effects on bacteria resulting in excretion of cellular macromolecules, lysis of cells and degradation of ribosomes; these effects eventually lead to cell death. This bactericidal effect is dependent on the growth phase of the bacterial cells. Actively dividing cells rapidly lose viability, but resting or slowly dividing cells remain viable for long periods (Bacchus and Javor, 1975; Gupta, 1975).

Chloramphenicol resistance is most frequently due to the production of an enzyme chloramphenicol acetyltransferase which acetylates and inactivates the drug and which is usually plasmid encoded. Various chloramphenicol acetyltransferases have been found in many Gram-negative and Gram-positive bacteria. Some of these enzymes are produced constitutively, others are inducible (Foster, 1983; Neu, 1984). Some Gram-negative bacteria which are chloramphenicol-resistant do not express chloramphenicol acetyltransferase, and resistance seems to be due to a permeability barrier at the cytoplasmic membrane (p. 26) (Foster, 1983). Transposons (p. 550) have been detected in strains of *Ps. aeruginosa* and *E. coli* which encode resistance due to alterations in the cells outer membrane permeability (Burns *et al.*, 1989). A similar mechanism of resistance has been described with *H. influenzae* (p. 553).

It was suggested that the hemopoietic toxicity of chloramphenicol occurs because the drug inhibits human cell protein synthesis (Weisbeger *et al.*, 1969). Immature or proliferating erythrocytes are much more susceptible to chloramphenicol than other mammalian cells. Furthermore, the anamnestic antibody response to tetanus toxoid can be suppressed by chloramphenicol, suggesting that it may inhibit protein synthesis (Daniel *et al.*, 1965). This inhibitory effect has been shown experimentally in tissue cultures of lymph node fragments (Ambrose and Coons, 1963).

The mechanism by which chloramphenicol inhibits protein synthesis in mammalian cells is probably different from that operating in bacteria. It is generally accepted that chloramphenicol does not inhibit ribosomal protein synthesis in mammals (Beard and Weisberger, 1972; Yunis, 1974). Mammalian cells contain 80 S ribosomes, and the protein synthesis in these, unlike that in bacterial 70 S ribosomes, appears to be unaffected by chloramphenicol. In human and other mammalian cells the mitochondria (which contain 70 S particles) are also capable of independent protein synthesis. Martelo *et al.* (1969) demonstrated that therapeutic concentrations of chloramphenicol inhibited protein synthesis by human and rabbit bone marrow mitochondria. Furthermore, Yunis *et al.* (1970) observed mitochondrial damage by electron microscopy in bone marrow cells obtained from patients treated with chloramphenicol. However, there is also some evidence suggesting that chloramphenicol only acts on human mitochondria in experimental situations, as normally mitochondria are impermeable to this drug (Gale *et al.*, 1972). Nevertheless, the effect of chloramphenicol on mitochondria appears to be the explanation of the dose-related hemopoietic toxicity of the drug (p. 565), but the pathogenesis of the rare aplastic anemia (see below) remains unknown.

Chloramphenicol is usually classed as a 'bacteriostatic' agent, because *in vitro* this drug usually arrests the multiplication of bacteria, but does not reduce the number of living organisms. However, chloramphenicol in high concentrations may be 'cidal' to some organisms, and it is even 'cidal' in clinically achievable concentrations against *H. influenzae*, *Strep. pneumoniae* and *N. meningitidis* (Rahal and Simberkof, 1979). These authors ascribe the success of chloramphenicol for the treatment of meningitis due to these bacteria, to this action. Chloramphenicol at similar concentrations is bacteriostatic for Enterobacteriaceae, which may be why it is not so effective in meningitis due to these bacilli. The distinction between so called 'bactericidal' and 'bacteriostatic' agents is only relative, and many other factors influence the action of antibiotics on bacteria *in vivo*.

From a practical point of view it is wrong to assume that a 'bactericidal' drug will always be clinically superior to a 'bacteriostatic' one. For example, chloramphenicol is more effective than some other drugs with a 'bactericidal action' in the treatment of typhoid fever. Even then, in some *in vitro* tests chloramphenicol may be bactericidal against *Salm. typhi* (Preblud *et al.*, 1984). One situation in which bactericidal drugs appear to be superior is in the treatment of bacterial endocarditis, an infection of a relatively avascular tissue.

Toxicity

1 Bone marrow depression

This is the most important toxic effect of chloramphenicol (Yunis and Bloomberg, 1964). Two forms of bone marrow depression occur:

a Aplastic anemia This is a rare complication, but has a high mortality. Initially its frequency was variously estimated as 1 in 500 to 1 in 100 000 of treated patients (Willcox, 1967). A survey in California showed that the calculated risk of dying from aplastic anemia was 1 in 21 671 after an average adult course of 7.5 g of the drug. This chloramphenicol-associated fatal aplastic anemia was 13-fold more common than aplastic anemia in the population not treated by chloramphenicol. Fatal aplastic anemia was estimated to occur with a frequency of 1 in 24 500 to 1 in 40 800 courses of treatment with chloramphenicol (Wallerstein *et al.*, 1969; Wallerstein, 1969). Between 1965 and 1971 inclusive, 31 cases of aplastic anemia following exposure to chloramphenicol were observed in Hamburg and surrounding districts. The frequency was estimated at 1 in 11 500 and the death rate as 1 in 18 500 (Hausmann and Skrandies, 1974). In Sweden during a 6-year period 1966–1971, seven patients with chloramphenicol-induced aplastic anemia were reported, and six of them died. In this study the risk of developing aplastic anemia after a course of chloramphenicol was calculated to be 1 in 19 000 (Böttiger, 1974). It is apparent that the estimated risks of aplastic anemia from chloramphenicol in these surveys from different countries are in accord.

Bone marrow aplasia due to chloramphenicol usually results in aplastic anemia with pancytopenia, and other forms, such as erythroid hypoplasia, selective leucopenia or thrombocytopenia are less common. The mortality in aplastic anemia with pancytopenia has been in excess of 50% (Davis and Rubin 1972). Some recoveries have occurred after prolonged periods of bone marrow aplasia and nowadays the death of some patients can be prevented by bone marrow transplantation (Storb et al., 1980). This blood dyscrasia may develop during the first 1 or 2 weeks of chloramphenicol treatment, but in the majority of patients the disorder only becomes evident after a latent period of weeks or months. It has been difficult to correlate amounts of the drug administered and the frequency of aplastic anemia (Best, 1967).

Holt (1967) noted that there had been no recorded cases of marrow aplasia following the administration of the drug by parenteral routes alone. The view that aplastic anemia was virtually exclusively associated with the oral administration of chloramphenicol was held for some time (Gleckman, 1975). There is accumulating evidence which implicates chloramphenicol administered parenterally and probably chloramphenicol administered topically to the eye, as causes of aplastic anemia.

In the period 1967–1975, Pickering et al. (1980) state that the manufacturers were aware of five cases of aplastic anemia attributed to parenterally administered chloramphenicol which had been reported in the medical literature. Daum et al. (1979) described a patient who developed fatal aplastic anemia which was diagnosed after 12 days' treatment with i.v. chloramphenicol succinate during which hematological changes suggested dose-related hemopoietic toxicity (see below). Plaut and Best (1982) related two other cases of aplastic anemia following i.v. use of the drug. They also recorded additional information on a previous review of chloramphenicol-associated blood dyscrasias (Best, 1967), i.e. the route of administration among 149 cases was oral in 83%, parenteral in 14% and rectal in 3%. Wallerstein et al. (1969) found that of ten cases of aplastic anemia, eight patients had received chloramphenicol orally and two had received the drug orally and i.m. Feder et al. (1981) in a review mention several other reported cases of aplastic anemia associated with parenterally administered chloramphenicol. A possible role of parenterally administered chloramphenicol as a cause of aplastic anemia has been difficult to establish statistically; more patients have received the drug orally than parenterally; the number of patients who have received the drug parenterally is unknown; and aplastic anemia is rare (Lietman, 1981; Yogev et al., 1981). In a review West et al. (1988) stated that they were aware of ten cases of fatal aplastic anemia complicating therapy with parenteral chloramphenicol. In two patients who also received i.v. cimetidine, the aplastic anemia supervened rapidly and these patients soon died.

There have been a number of anecdotal reports of an association of chloramphenicol applied topically to the eye (eye drops and ointments) and the development of aplastic anemia (Rosenthal and Blackman, 1965; Davidson, 1974; Carpenter, 1975; Abrams et al., 1980; Fraunfelder et al., 1982; Fraunfelder and Bagby, 1983). There are several possible routes by which chloramphenicol can enter the body after topical application to the eye – by absorption through the nasal mucosa after passing through the nasolacrimal ducts, by absorption into the aqueous humor which occurs readily (Fraunfelder et al., 1982) or possibly by absorption from the gut after swallowing tears which contain the drug (Carpenter, 1975). In many of the cases ascribed to ophthalmic administration, topical administration was continued for many months, but this, like bone marrow aplasia after parenteral administration of chloramphenicol is not a prerequisite since this complication is idiosyncratic. It can be argued that it has not been proven that the ophthalmic preparation of chloramphenicol is a cause of aplastic anemia; the occurrences may be coincidental or other drugs known or unknown may have been the causative agents. But administration of chloramphenicol topically to the eye, sometimes months previously, may be overlooked by the patient and the attending physician in cases of aplastic anemia. Also, as Fraunfelder and Bagby (1982) point out, the confirmation of a definite relationship between ophthalmic chloramphenicol and aplastic anemia would require a great number of patient observations. Until and if, this association is confirmed, it seems prudent to avoid topical chloramphenicol in patients with a previous history or family history of drug-related hemopoietic toxicity and its long-term use (Fraunfelder et al., 1982).

A report of aplastic anemia in identical twins given chloramphenicol is of interest (Nagao and Mauer, 1969). In an attempt to explain this occurrence, Dameshek (1969) postulated that there may be a genetically determined defect in the bone marrow cells of some individuals, rendering them particularly susceptible to chloramphenicol bone marrow aplasia.

There is some confusion over the association of liver diseases, aplastic anemia and chloramphenicol administration. Hodgkinson (1973) described five patients who developed aplastic anemia after receiving chloramphenicol during the pre-icteric phase of hepatitis, presumed of viral etiology. Viral hepatitis *per se* has been regarded as an important cause of aplastic anemia, and it was thought that chloramphenicol and the hepatitis virus(es) may have an additive toxic effect on the bone marrow, but if a hepatitis virus is a cause of aplastic anemia it is not hepatitis A or hepatitis B (Bennett and Lucas, 1979; Bannister *et al.*, 1983). Nevertheless, there are numerous reports of an association of liver damage with aplastic anemia and chloramphenicol administration (oral and i.v.); usually chloramphenicol administration precedes the hepatitis and pancytopenia (Bennett and Lucas, 1979; Casale *et al.*, 1982). The etiology of this syndrome which is usually fatal is not clear and there is no evidence to indicate that the liver damage is caused by a hepatitis virus, or, for that matter, by chloramphenicol. If abnormalities of liver function appear during chloramphenicol administration, the drug should be discontinued because in patients with this syndrome, liver function tests became abnormal prior to or concomitant with hemopoietic toxicity (Casale *et al.*, 1982).

b   Hemopoietic toxicity   Side-effects grouped under this heading are much more common than aplastic anemia and they appear to be dose -related and reversible. There is some evidence from animal experiments that chloramphenicol suppresses the activity of ferrochelatase, an enzyme which normally catalyses hemoglobin synthesis within the mitochondria of bone marrow erythroid cells (Manyan *et al.*, 1972). Chloramphenicol in concentrations which are achieved in serum during therapy, also inhibits bone marrow colony formation *in vitro* (Howell *et al.*, 1975). A number of studies in humans (Scott *et al.*, 1965; Hughes, 1968; 1973) indicate that the administration of large doses of chloramphenicol for several weeks is sometimes associated with:

1   Reduced iron utilization for hemoglobin synthesis as indicated by rising serum iron levels.

2   Vacuolation of erythroblasts, or a progressive increase in the marrow myeloid-erythroid ratio, a low reticulocyte count and falling hemoglobin, suggesting interference with the production and maturation of erythroid cells. The use of phenylalanine reduces this vacuolation of the erythroblasts (Ingall *et al.*, 1965), but there is no evidence that this amino acid is useful for the treatment of patients with aplastic anemia.

3   Thrombocytopenia and leucopenia with vacuolation of marrow granulocyte precursors.

These changes occurred regularly when the serum levels of active chloramphenicol were 25 μg per ml or greater, suggesting that these toxic effects are a pharmacological property of the drug (Scott *et al.*, 1965) (see also Mode of Action, p.563). Similar changes occurred more rapidly in patients with hepatic diseases, especially in those with jaundice or ascites, who developed high active chloramphenicol serum levels more rapidly. Such side-effects are usually reversible after cessation of the drug; the serum iron falls abruptly, reticulocytosis appears and the bone marrow and the peripheral blood returns to normal within a few days. In some cases erythropoietic recovery may occur even if chloramphenicol is continued (Hughes, 1973). This is more likely if the reticulocyte count exceeds 0.5% and if the myeloid-erythroid ratio is less than 10:1. However, in other patients, especially if neutropenia and thrombocytopenia have already developed, more severe bone marrow depression may occur if the drug is continued (Hughes, 1973). It therefore seems that a different mechanism is responsible for the development of the rare and irreversible aplastic anemia.

2 Other hemopoietic side-effects

Chloramphenicol prevents the expected reticulocyte response in patients with pernicious anemia treated by vitamin B_{12}. Similarly, it prevents the expected response to iron in patients with iron deficiency anemia. These phenomena are probably explicable in terms of the known mode of action of chloramphenicol on rapidly multiplying cells (Weisberger *et al.*, 1969). Hemolytic anemia developed in three patients with glucose-6-phosphate dehydrogenase deficiency who were treated by chloramphenicol for typhoid fever (McCaffrey *et al.*, 1971). The drug only caused a mild hemolytic reaction in two of these patients when, free from the infection, they were studied 1 year later. Paradoxically, Adams and Pearson (1983) described a boy with chronic neutropenia, in whom chloramphenicol stimulated neutrophil maturation and release; the drug was used for this purpose for more than 12 months. *In vitro*, chloramphenicol in therapeutic concentrations, markedly depresses leukocyte migration (Forsgren and Schmeling, 1977) and may suppress antigen-induced lymphocyte blastogenesis (DaMert and Sohnle, 1979); in high concentrations such as 200 μg per ml it also impairs phagocytosis (Melby and Midtvedt, 1977). The clinical significance of these observations is not clear.

Shu *et al.* (1987) conducted a population-based case-control interview study of 309 childhood leukemia cases and 618 age- and sex-matched controls and this showed a significant relation between previous use of chloramphenicol and risk of both acute lymphocytic leukemia and acute non-lymphocytic leukemia. This association may have non-causal explanations, but further investigations are warranted.

3 Gray (baby) syndrome

This is a type of circulatory collapse which can occur in premature and newborn infants and is associated with excessively high serum levels of chloramphenicol (Sutherland, 1959). In a trial reported by Burns *et al.* (1959), chloramphenicol was given to 61 premature infants in high doses ranging from 100 to 165 mg per kg daily. Approximately 60% of these infants died. Features were abdominal distension, vomiting, pallor, cyanosis and circulatory collapse, which usually resulted in death. The gray baby syndrome is characterized by an onset 2–9 days after treatment is begun, hypotonia, lethargy, ashen-gray colour, tachypnea or apnea, unresponsiveness, distension, peripheral hypoperfusion, hypotension, hypothermia and acidosis. The mortality is often over 50% and surviving babies usually gradually recover 24–36 h after chloramphenicol is stopped. The term 'gray' syndrome was coined from the appearance of these babies. A potentially reversible alteration of myocardial function is part of the syndrome (Biancaniello *et al.*, 1981; Fripp *et al.*, 1983) and may be due to a direct action of chloramphenicol on myocardial function rather than due to inhibition of mitochondrial function (p. 563) (Werner *et al.*, 1985); this also accounts for cardiovascular collapse which has occurred within hours of a single large dose (Sutherland, 1959). The occurrence of this syndrome particularly in neonates is probably related to immaturity of the liver resulting in decreased glucuronidization of chloramphenicol and reduced renal excretion of both free chloramphenicol and its succinate ester (p. 560). As chloramphenicol readily crosses the placenta, it should be used with caution in late pregnancy or during labor, because of the risk, albeit low, of this toxic effect in the newborn. The use of chloramphenicol may also be best avoided during lactation, as the drug is excreted in human milk.

A similar syndrome can occur in older children ('gray toddler syndrome') and adults who have received accidental chloramphenicol overdosage. Thompson *et al.* (1975) described three patients. One, a 70-year-old woman who received one 20-g dose, died 11 h later. The second patient was a 26-year-old woman who received an initial 1.0-g dose followed in 7 and 12 h by two 10-g doses. She developed severe shock, cyanosis and coma 5 h after the last dose, but she responded slowly to fluids and dopamine and made a full recovery. The serum active chloramphenicol level 5.5 h after her last dose was 201 μg per ml. The third patient was a 4½-month-old infant, who following chloramphenicol overdosage became unresponsive with hypothermia and abdominal distension. The serum chloramphenicol level was 174 μg per ml. The infant recovered after an exchange transfusion and other measures.

In more recent times, the gray syndrome in babies also usually has been due to accidental overdosage with chloramphenicol (Kessler *et al.*, 1980; Mauer *et al.*, 1980; Stevens *et al.*, 1981, Freundlich *et al.*, 1983). In these reports of infants with toxicity, serum chloramphenicol levels ranged from 98 to 180 μg per ml; but the gray syndrome has been reported with a serum level as low as 40 μg per ml (Glazer *et al.*, 1980). Even when a reduced dosage of i.v. chloramphenicol succinate is used in infants, resultant serum levels are erratic and dosage should be monitored according to serum levels to avoid toxicity (p. 557).

Surprisingly, sometimes high serum chloramphenicol levels may occur without signs of toxicity. For instance, Stevens *et al.* (1981) reported a 10-week-old boy who received an accidental overdosage of chloramphenicol and whose serum level reached 130 μg per ml and then declined to 0 over the next 40 h without clinical evidence of toxicity. Mulhall *et al.* (1983b) reviewed toxicity in 64 neonates given chloramphenicol; ten exhibited clinical features attributed to toxicity (five gray syndrome, four hematological toxicity, one was described as being very gray). Of those with toxicity, one received an accidental overdose and nine received the prescribed dose, although in six this was greater than that recommended. Peak serum concentrations in these ten babies ranged from 28 to 180 μg per ml and trough levels from 19 to 47 μg per ml. In 27 neonates serum chloramphenicol levels above the therapeutic range were observed (two had received a 10-fold overdose) without signs of toxicity; in seven of these it was in excess of 50 μg per ml. Toxicity was not related to the duration of the high serum level but seemed to be more common in infants aged less than 9 days. Mulhall *et al.* (1983b) considered that chloramphenicol could be used safely in neonates if serum concentrations are maintained in the range of 15–25 μg per ml.

It can be inferred from the foregoing that infants with high serum chloramphenicol levels and no clinical abnormalities can be safely observed after discontinuation of the drug. Associated liver dysfunction may be an increased risk factor in such infants (Stevens *et al.*, 1981). Chloramphenicol intoxication in infants with the features of the gray syndrome has been treated by exchange transfusion with variable results (Kessler *et al.*, 1980; Stevens *et al.*, 1981) and more successfully by using charcoal-column hemoperfusion (Mauer *et al.*, 1980; Freundlich *et al.*, 1983).

4 Optic neuritis

This complication has been described in a small number of patients treated with chloramphenicol, and sometimes this resulted in optic atrophy and blindness (Cocke *et al.*, 1966; Snaveley and Hodges, 1984). Most of these patients were children with cystic fibrosis receiving prolonged chloramphenicol treatment for pulmonary infection. Blindness may occur without recognizable fundal changes. Vision may partly return after cessation of the drug, but this is not invariable. Large doses of B group vitamins have been used to treat this condition. This complication is an additional reason to avoid prolonged courses of chloramphenicol. Peripheral neuritis has been described in association with optic neuritis (Ramilo *et al.*, 1988). Other neurotoxic symptoms, such as headache, depression, ophthalmoplegia, mental confusion and delirium have been occasionally attributed to chloramphenicol.

5 Gastrointestinal side-effects

Nausea, vomiting and diarrhea occasionally occur, but these are much less common than with the tetracyclines. Pseudomembranous colitis (p. 594) may occur, but this complication is rare. Glossitis and stomatitis, sometimes associated with thrush, may also be encountered.

6 Hypersensitivity reactions

These are very rare, but contact dermatitis, rashes, drug fever, and even occasional instances of anaphylaxis and angioneurotic edema have been reported. Jarisch-Herxheimer reactions have been described in patients treated for syphilis (Welch, 1954), and also during therapy for typhoid fever. Cahill (1962) reported a patient who developed a severe hemorrhagic reaction associated with chloramphenicol. There was no evidence of bone marrow depression, or coagulation defects, and bleeding appeared to be due to a capillary defect presumably due to hypersensitivity.

7 Bleeding due to increase of prothrombin time

This may occur as a result of prolonged oral administration of the drug. Decreased vitamin K synthesis results from a reduction of intestinal bacteria, and this defect can be rapidly corrected by the administration of parenteral vitamin K (Cahill, 1962).

8 Ototoxicity

Hearing loss has been noted in a few children with *H. influenzae* meningitis, who have been treated by chloramphenicol. This was almost certainly a sequel to their meningitis and not a drug toxicity (Svenungsson *et al.*, 1976). Studies in animals have shown that chloramphenicol ear drops can cause deafness, especially if the drops have a higher concentration than 5% and if they are instilled in the middle ear cavity (Morizono and Johnstone, 1975). Chloramphenicol ear drops are seldom indicated, especially in the presence of large perforations (see also neomycin, p.536).

9 Drug interactions

Chloramphenicol inhibits the activity of certain liver enzymes, and it interferes with the biotransformation of tolbutamide, diphenylhydantoin (phenytoin), and dicoumarol. Toxicity due to these three drugs may occur if they are administered in usual doses to a patient who is also receiving chloramphenicol (Christensen and Skovsted, 1969; Rose *et al.*, 1977). Moreover, concurrent administration of phenytoin and chloramphenicol succinate may result in elevated serum chloramphenicol levels into the potentially toxic range. In 17 children treated by i.v. chloramphenicol succinate alone (25 mg per kg per dose given over 10–15 min), mean peak and trough serum chloramphenicol levels were 25.3 and 13.4 µg per ml, respectively; in six others receiving phenytoin as well, the mean peak serum level was 41.7 µg per ml. It was thought that phenytoin interacts with chloramphenicol causing phenytoin toxicity and elevated chloramphenicol serum levels by competition for binding sites rather than by induction of hepatic enzymes (Krasinski *et al.*, 1982). Observations in one patient suggested that phenytoin and phenobarbitone may lower serum chloramphenicol levels (Powell *et al.*, 1981). In the study by Krasinski *et al.* (1982), concurrent administration of phenobarbital in six children resulted in lower mean serum peak and trough levels of 16.6 and 7.5 μg per ml, respectively. One study in adults indicated that paracetamol (acetaminophen) decreased chloramphenicol clearance from the body (Buchanan and Moodley, 1979), but a study in children failed to confirm this (Kearns *et al.*, 1985). Concomitant administration of rifampicin may lower chloramphenicol serum levels (p. 693).

Clinical Uses of the Drug

1 Salmonella infections

Chloramphenicol remains an excellent drug for treatment of typhoid and paratyphoid fever, but ampicillin (p. 121), amoxycillin (p. 141) and co-trimoxazole (p. 867) are also effective (Herzog, 1976; Butler *et al.*, 1977). In developed countries the more expensive, but effective drugs such as ciprofloxacin (p. 1016) or ceftriaxone (p. 360) can also be used for this disease, but it would be preferable to use these only if the *Salm. typhi* strain is resistant to the above three cheaper drugs. It is reasonable to use ciprofloxacin or ceftriaxone initially for patients with suspected typhoid acquired in South-East Asia or other areas where resistant typhoid bacilli are known to exist. Typhoid fever is usually treated by chloramphenicol for a period of 2 weeks (Hoffman *et al.*, 1975; Snyder *et al.*, 1976). A study by Hoffman *et al.* (1984) showed that if high doses of dexamethasone are used with chloramphenicol for patients who are delirious, obtunded, stuporous, comatose, or in shock, case fatality is reduced.

Chloramphenicol is not indicated in uncomplicated salmonella gastroenteritis (Nelson, 1981). Treatment is warranted in severe cases, especially if a septicemia is present. In abdominal aortitis chloramphenicol has not been very effective, and one of the bactericidal drugs are more satisfactory (Ljungberg and Braconier, 1986). Treatment is usually also necessary in some immunocompromised patients, such as those with HIV infection, but drugs other than chloramphenicol are also often preferred for these (Sperber and Schleupner, 1987). Chloramphenicol, however, is still probably the best antibiotic for treatment of *Salmonella* meningitis (Davis, 1981). Septicemias due to salmonellae, such as *Salm. chlorae-suis* and *Salm. typhimurium*, do not respond as well and predicably as typhoid fever, but chloramphenicol is still one of the best antibiotics available for their treatment. Chloramphenicol is of no value for the eradication of the *Salmonella* carrier state, and this applies both to persistent typhoid carriers and the usually short-lived carrier state due to other *Salmonella* spp. In addition, treatment of patients with acute *Salmonella* gastroenteritis with chloramphenicol usually prolongs the period of excretion of salmonellae after clinical recovery (Aserkoff and Bennett, 1969).

2 Shigella infections

For the vast majority of cases of *Shigella* dysentery, chloramphenicol is not indicated, but it is a valuable drug for the rare severe case with extensive tissue involvement or associated septicemia (Duncan *et al.*, 1981). If antibiotics are indicated in shigellosis, either ampicillin (p. 122) or co-trimoxazole (p. 868) are usually used. These two drugs are also effective alternatives for severe cases if chloramphenicol-resistant *Shigella* spp. strains (p. 550) are involved.

3 Rickettsial diseases

Chloramphenicol is effective for treatment of epidemic typhus fever, scrub typhus, murine typhus, Rocky Mountain spotted fever and Mediterranean spotted fever (Snyder and Woodward, 1970; Breitschwerdt *et al.*, 1991; Raoult and Drancourt, 1991). The tetracyclines are equally effective (p. 748), and are usually used in moderate cases, because they are potentially less toxic. Chloramphenicol is preferable for very ill patients, because parenteral forms of the tetracyclines are not as satisfactory and also most tetracyclines cannot be used in the presence of renal failure (p. 728). Chloramphenicol is also preferred in pregnant patients (Walker, 1995).

4 Bacterial meningitis

Penicillin G and chloramphenicol has been a very useful combination for the initial treatment of this disease in children, before the causative organism was identified (Lindberg *et al.*, 1977). Chloramphenicol alone is very effective for the treatment of meningitis due to *H. influenzae* type b (Feigin *et al.*, 1976; Sangster *et al.*, 1982). Orally administered chloramphenicol palmitate is just as effective as i.v. administered succinate for the treatment of *H. influenzae* meningitis (Shann and Germer, 1981; Tuomanen *et al.*, 1981). Since the widespread occurrence of strains of *H. influenzae* resistant to ampicillin (p. 112), chloramphenicol became the preferred drug for serious infections due to this organism. Many clinicians, particularly in North America, gave both ampicillin and chloramphenicol, until the results of antibiotic sensitivity tests on the strain involved, were available (Enzenauer and Bass, 1983; McCabe, 1983). Fortunately, strains of *H. influenzae* resistant to both ampicillin and chloramphenicol are still rare (p. 552). Nowadays, however, most clinicians in developed countries would use one of the third-generation cephalosporins, such as cefotaxime (p. 336) or ceftriaxone (p. 359) for both the initial and continuation treatment of *H. influenzae* meningitis (The Research Committee, 1995).

Chloramphenicol is also effective for rarer types of meningitis, such as that due to *Staph. aureus*. It is also an effective alternative drug for meningococcal and pneumococcal meningitis in penicillin-allergic patients (Gleckman, 1975). Chloramphenicol is a good alternative drug to penicillin G for treatment of meningococcal meningitis (Whittle *et al.*, 1973; Halstensen *et al.*, 1987), but the third-generation cephalosporins are also very effective (pp. 336, 359). Mulhall *et al.* (1983c) reported comparatively good results using chloramphenicol for the treatment of neonatal meningitis, but many of their patients also received additional antibiotics. Others have found that results after using chloramphenicol for Gram-negative bacillary meningitis in neonates and adults, are disappointing (Cherubin *et al.*, 1982). This is possibly due to the lack of bactericidal action against Enterobacteriaceae at the concentrations achieved in CSF (p. 563). Third-generation cephalosporins, such as cefotaxime (p. 337) or ceftriaxone (p. 359), give better results in Gram-negative meningitis. Chloramphenicol may have a place in mixed bacterial meningitis, but initially combination therapy such as cefotaxime/chloramphenicol or cefotaxime/metronidazole would be preferred (Downs *et al.*, 1987). For *B. fragilis* meningitis metronidazole appears preferable to chloramphenicol (Feder, 1987). Several cases of *Campylobacter* meningitis have been successfully treated with chloramphenicol (Norrby *et al.*, 1980; Thomas *et al.*, 1980; McNulty, 1987). Chloramphenicol plus an aminoglycoside has been curative in a few patients with *L. monocytogenes* meningitis (Bouvet *et al.*, 1982). In one patient with Whipple's disease in whom meningoencephalitis developed when penicillin G treatment was withdrawn (p. 51), the infection was controlled by long-term chloramphenicol therapy (Feldman *et al.*, 1980).

5 Haemophilus influenzae infections

Apart from meningitis *H. influenzae* type b may cause other severe infections, particularly in children, such as epiglottitis, osteomyelitis, cellulitis and pneumonia, all of which are usually associated with septicemia. Chloramphenicol is very effective for these diseases and it is the preferred drug in the developing countries if the strain involved is resistant to ampicillin (Faden, 1979; Ginsburg *et al.*, 1979; Hirschmann and Everett, 1979). In the developed countries one of the third-generation cephalosporins such as cefotaxime (p. 338) or ceftriaxone (p. 360) are now usually used for these indications.

6 Cerebral abscess

Penicillin G combined with chloramphenicol is a time-honoured combination for this infection (Schliamser *et al.*, 1988), but a penicillin G/metronidazole combination is gaining in popularity (p. 948). In post-traumatic abscesses and in spinal extradural abscesses, *Staph. aureus* is the predominant organism. These would also usually respond to chloramphenicol, but if the bacterial etiology is known, a specific anti-staphylococcal agent, such as cloxacillin (p. 97), can be used.

7 Staphylococcal infections

Chloramphenicol is effective for many life-threatening *Staph. aureus* infections, but its use has been largely supplanted by the penicillinase-resistant penicillins (p. 97).

8 Gram-negative anaerobic bacterial infections

Gram-negative anaerobes, particularly *B. fragilis*, are causative agents of a wide range of major infections in man (pp. 946).

Many mixed aerobic/anaerobic infections such as peritonitis, need appropriate surgical treatment, but antibiotics are often also essential. Chloramphenicol, metronidazole (p. 947), clindamycin (p. 597), cefoxitin (p. 306), cefotetan (p. 396), imipenem (p. 236), ticarcillin (p. 157), ticarcillin/clavulanic acid, ampicillin/sulbactam (p. 214) and piperacillin/tazobactam (p. 224) are all effective drugs for the treatment of anaerobic infections. In trials comparing these drugs (metronidazole and clindamycin would be combined with an aminoglycoside) for the treatment of intra-abdominal or female genital tract infections, no one combination has proved superior (p. 947) (Finegold and Wexler, 1988).

9 Gram-negative aerobic enteric bacterial infections

Chloramphenicol is effective in many severe infections due to these organisms, except those due to *Ps. aeruginosa*. It should never be used for uncomplicated urinary tract infections, which respond to safer drugs. For the treatment of severe infections caused by aerobic Gram-negative enteric bacteria, aminoglycosides, such as kanamycin (p. 446) or gentamicin (p. 471), or a third-generation cephalosporin, are usually preferred. The drug may be used for *Aeromonas* spp. septicemia, but other drugs such as ceftriaxone or ciprofloxacin (p. 1019) are also suitable (Janda *et al.*, 1994).

10 Melioidosis

This disease, caused by *Burkholderia (Pseudomonas) pseudomallei*, may be subacute or chronic, but sometimes presents as an acute septicemia, often with pulmonary involvement, and has a high mortality. Opinion on the ideal type of chemotherapy for this disease was not uniform. For severe cases, some authors favored the use of large doses of chloramphenicol (sometimes as much as 3 g every 6 h for adults) combined with novobiocin and kanamycin (Sheehy *et al.*, 1967; Weber *et al.*, 1969). Others preferred tetracycline, either alone or in combination with novobiocin (Howe *et al.*, 1971; Calabi, 1973). Co-trimoxazole was also of value (p. 873). Tetracyclines (p. 743) either alone or in combination with chloramphenicol were most commonly used for the treatment of this disease (Everett and Nelson, 1975). Nowadays ceftazidime (p. 378) perhaps combined with co-trimoxazole is regarded as the best treatment for severe systemic melioidosis (Sookpranee *et al.*, 1992; Vatcharapreechasakul *et al.*, 1992; Chaowagul *et al.*, 1993).

11 Bacterial eye infections

Chloramphenicol penetrates into both the aqueous and vitreous humors after systemic administration, and is therefore useful for the treatment of intraocular infections. It also penetrates into the aqueous humor after topical application to eye (Hodgman, 1961). Both clindamycin and chloramphenicol, each of which have good intraocular penetration, have been used to treat *Bacillus cereus panophthalmitis*, which occurs particularly in drug abusers; eye enucleation, however, is usually necessary because of the fulminating nature of the infection (Shamsuddin *et al.*, 1982).

12 Chlamydial eye infections

Topically administered chloramphenicol is ineffective for the treatment of trachoma (p. 746). Also such treatment only suppresses infection in chlamydial ophthalmia neonatorum, so that treatment with erythromycin is recommended (p. 619).

13 Venereal diseases

Romanowski *et al.* (1983) reported the successful treatment of a penicillin-allergic patient with neurosyphilis by chloramphenicol. Penicillin G (p. 47) is the usual recommended treatment for this disease and the alternate drug for penicillin-allergic patients is tetracycline (p. 747).

14 Louse-borne relapsing fever

This responds to single-dose oral treatment with chloramphenicol (p. 748).

15 Rhodococcus equi infections

Chloramphenicol is suitable to treat these infections in patients with or without HIV infections, although alternatives such as erythromycin plus rifampicin (p. 620), ciprofloxacin and vancomycin (p. 782) are also available (Harvey and Sunstrum, 1991; Sirera *et al.*, 1991).

16 Enterococcal infections

Enterococci, particularly *E. faecium* in the USA, have recently become resistant to multiple antibiotics, including penicillin G, ampicillin and vancomyin (p. 765). Some of these may be chloramphenicol-sensitive and the drug has proved to be effective in the treatment of infections such as *E. faecium* bacteremia (Norris *et al.*, 1995). It is unlikely to be effective for enterococcal endocarditis.

References

Aber RC, Wennersten C, Moellering RC Jr (1978). Antimicrobial susceptibility of flavobacteria. *Antimicrob Ag Chemother* **14**: 483.

Abrams SM, Degnan TJ, Viniguerra V (1980). Marrow aplasia following topical application of chloramphenicol eye ointment. *Arch Intern Med* **140**: 576.

Adams GR, Pearson HA (1983). Chloramphenicol-responsive chronic neutropenia. *New Engl J Med* **309**: 1039.

Albert MJ, Haider K, Nahar S *et al.* (1991). Multiresistant *Salmonella typhi* in Bangladesh. *J Antimicrob Chemother* **27**: 554.

Ambrose CT, Coons AH (1963). Studies on antibody production: VIII. The inhibitory effect of chloramphenicol on the synthesis of antibody in tissue culture. *J Exp Med* **117**: 1075; quoted by Weisberger *et al.* (1969).

Anderson ES (1975). The problem and implications of chloramphenicol resistance in the typhoid bacillus. *J Hyg Camb* **74**: 289.

Anderson ES, Smith HR (1972). Chloramphenicol resistance in the typhoid bacillus. *Brit Med J* **3**: 329.

Anthony BF, Concepcion NF (1975). Group B streptococcus in a general hospital. *J Infect Dis* **132**: 561.

Appleman MD, Heseltine PNR, Cherubin CE (1991). Epidemiology, antimicrobial susceptibility, pathogenicity, and significance of *Bacteroides fragilis* group organisms isolated at Los Angeles County – University of Southern California Medical Center. *Rev Infect Dis* **13**: 12.

Aserkoff B, Bennett JV (1969). Effect of antibiotic therapy in acute salmonellosis on the fecal excretion of salmonellae. *New Engl J Med* **281**: 636.

Asmar BI, Prainito M, Dajani AS (1988). Antagonistic effect of chloramphenicol in combination with cefotaxime or ceftriaxone. *Antimicrob Ag Chemother* **32**: 1375.

Bacchus AN, Javor GT (1975). Stability of *Escherichia coli* membrane proteins during chloramphenicol treatment. *Antimicrob Ag Chemother* **8**: 387.

Baine WB, Farmer JJ III, Gangarosa EJ *et al.* (1977). Typhoid fever in the United States associated with the 1972–1973 epidemic in Mexico. *J Infect Dis* **135**: 649.

Baker CJ, Webb BJ, Barrett FF (1976). Antimicrobial susceptibility of Group B streptococci isolated from a variety of clinical sources. *Antimicrob Ag Chemother* **10**: 128.

Balows A (1977). An overview of recent experiences with plasmid-mediated antibiotic resistance or induced virulence in bacterial diseases. *J Antimicrob Chemother* **3** (Suppl C): 3.

Bannam TL, Rood JI (1991). Relationship between the *Clostridium perfringens* catQ gene product and chloramphenicol acetyltransferases from other bacteria. *Antimicrob Ag Chemother* **35**: 471.

Bannatyne RM, Toma S, Cheung R, Hodge D (1985). Antibiotic susceptibility of blood and cerebrospinal fluid isolates of *Haemophilus influenzae*. *J Antimicrob Chemother* **15**: 187.

Bannister P Miloszewski K, Barnard D, Losowsky MS (1983). Fatal marrow aplasia associated with non-A, non-B hepatitis. *Brit Med J* **286**: 1314.

Barrett FF, Taber LH, Morris CR *et al.* (1972). A 12 year review of the antibiotic management of *Hemophilus influenzae* meningitis. *J Pediatr* **81**: 370.

Beard NS Jr, Weisberger AS (1972). Protein synthesis by reticulocyte ribosomes IV. Factors involved in formation of the mRNA-sRNA-ribosome complex and the absence of inhibition by chloramphenicol. *Amer J Med Sci* **263**: 215.

Bennett N McK, Kucers A (1970). Staphylococcal and Gram-negative septicaemia. *Aspects of Infection. Proc Symp Auckland, Sydney and Melbourne*, p. 123. Melbourne, Australia: Mercedes Publishing Services.

Bennett N McK, Lucas CR (1979). Does viral hepatitis cause aplastic anaemia? *Aust NZ J Med* **9**: 667.

Bentley DW, Hahn JJ, Lepper MH (1970). Transmission of chloramphenicol-resistant *Staphylococcus epidermidis*: epidemiologic and laboratory studies. *J Infect Dis* **122**: 365.

Best WR (1967). Chloramphenicol-associated blood dyscrasias. *JAMA* **201**: 181.

Betriu C, Campos E, Cabronero C *et al.* (1990). Susceptibilities of species of the *Bacteroides fragilis* group to 10 antimicrobial agents. *Antimicrob Ag Chemother* **34**: 671.

Bhutta ZA, Naqvi SH, Razzaq RA, Farooqui BJ (1991). Multidrug-resistant typhoid in children: presentation and clinical features. *Rev Infect Dis* **13**: 832.

Biancaniello T, Meyer RA, Kaplan S (1981). Chloramphenicol and cardiotoxicity. *J Pediatr* **98**: 828.

Bijlmer HA, Van Alphen L, Greenwood BM *et al.* (1994). Antibiotic susceptibility of invasive and non-invasive isolates of *Haemophilus influenzae* from the Gambia, West Africa. *J Antimicrob Chemother* **34**: 275.

Bissett ML, Abbott SL, Wood RM (1974). Antimicrobial resistance and R factors in salmonella isolated in California (1971–1972). *Antimicrob Ag Chemother* **5**: 161.

Black SB, Levine P, Shinefield HR (1978). The necessity for monitoring chloramphenicol levels when treating neonatal meningitis. *J Pediatr* **92**: 235.

Böttiger LE (1974). Drug-induced aplastic anaemia in Sweden with special reference to chloramphenicol. *Postgrad Med J* **50** (Suppl 5): 127.

Bourbeau PM, Campos JM (1982). Current antibiotic susceptibility of group A B-hemolytic streptococci. *J Infect Dis* **145**: 916.

Bourgault A-M, Lamothe F, Hoban DJ *et al.* (1992). Survey of *Bacteroides fragilis* group susceptibility patterns in Canada. *Antimicrob Ag Chemother* **36**: 343.

Bouvet E, Suter F, Gibert C *et al.* (1982). Severe meningitis due to *Listeria monocytogenes*. A review of 40 cases in adults. *Scand J Infect Dis* **14**: 267.

Braveny I, Machka K (1980). Multiply resistant *Haemophilus influenzae* and *para-influenzae* in West Germany. *Lancet* **ii**: 752.

Breitschwerdt EB, Davidson MG, Aucoin DP *et al.* (1991). Efficacy of chloramphenicol, enrofloxacin, and tetracycline for treatment of experimental Rocky Mountain spotted fever in dogs. *Antimicrob Ag Chemother* **35**: 2375.

Brito-Alayon NE, Blando AM, Monzon-Moreno C (1994). Antibiotic resistance patterns and plasmid profiles for *Shigella* spp isolated in Cordoba, Argentina. *J Antimicrob Chemother* **34**: 253.

Britz ML, Wilkinson RG (1978). Chloramphenicol acetyltransferase of *Bacteroides fragilis*. *Antimicrob Ag Chemother* **14**: 105.

Brown JD, Mo DH, Rhoades ER (1975). Chloramphenicol-resistant *Salmonella typhi* in Saigon. *JAMA* **231**: 162.

Brown TH, Alford RH (1984). Antagonism by chloramphenicol of broad spectrum beta-lactam antibiotics against *Klebsiella pneumonia*. *Antimicrob Ag Chemother* **25**: 405.

Buchanan N, Houdley GP (1979). Interaction between chloramphenicol and paracetamol. *Brit Med J* **2**: 307.

Burns JL, Smith AL (1987). Chloramphenicol accumulation by *Haemophilus influenzae*. *Antimicrob Ag Chemother* **31**: 686.

Burns JL, Mendelman PM, Levy J *et al.* (1985). A permeability barrier as a mechanism of chloramphenicol resistance in *Haemophilus influenzae*. *Antimicrob Ag Chemother* **27**: 46.

Burns JL, Hedin LA, Lien DM (1989). Chloramphenicol resistance in *Pseudomonas cepacia* because of decreased permeability. *Antimicrob Ag Chemother* **33**: 136.

Burns LE, Hodgman JE, Cass AB (1959). Fatal circulatory collapse in premature infants receiving chloramphenicol. *New Engl J Med* **261**: 1318.

Butler T, Linh NN, Arnold K, Pollack M (1973). Chloramphenicol-resistant typhoid fever in Vietnam associated with R-factor. *Lancet* **2**: 983.

Butler T, Bell WR, Linh NN *et al.* (1974). *Yersinia pestis* infection in Vietnam. I. Clinical and hematologic aspects. *J Infect Dis* **129** (Suppl): 78.

Butler T, Linh NN, Arnold K et al. (1977). Therapy of antimicrobial-resistant typhoid fever. Antimicrob Ag Chemother 11: 645.

Buu-Hoi A, Goldstein FW, Acar JF (1986). R-factors in Gram-positive and Gram-negative aerobic bacteria selected by antimicrobial therapy. Scand J Infect Dis (Suppl 49): 46.

Cahill KM (1962). Chloramphenicol hypersensitivity. A severe haemorrhagic reaction. Lancet ii: 277.

Calibi O (1973). Bactericidal synergism of novobiocin and tetracycline against Pseudomonas pseudomallei. J Med Microbiol 6: 293.

Campos J, Garcia-Tornel S, Sanfeliu I (1984). Susceptibility studies of multiply resistant Haemophilus influenzae isolated from pediatric patients and contacts. Antimicrob Ag Chemother 25: 706.

Campos J, Garcia-Tornel S, Musser JM et al. (1987). Molecular epidemiology of multiply-resistant Haemophilus influenzae type b in day care centers. J Infect Dis 156: 483.

Campos J, Chanyangam M, de Groot R et al. (1989). Genetic relatedness of antibiotic resistance determinants in multiply resistant Haemophilus influenzae. J Infect Dis 160: 810.

Carpenter G (1975). Chloramphenicol eye-drops and marrow aplasia. Lancet ii: 326.

Casale TB, Macher AM, Fauci AS (1982). Complete hematologic and hepatic recovery in a patient with chloramphenicol hepatitis-pancytopenia syndrome. J Pediatr 101: 1025.

Catry MA, Vaz Pato MV (1983). Haemophilus influenzae type b resistant to ampicillin and chloramphenicol. Brit Med J 287: 1471.

Cavanagh P, Morris CA, Mitchell NJ (1975). Chloramphenicol resistance in Haemophilus species. Lancet i: 696.

CDC (Center for Disease Control) (1977). Multiple-antibiotic resistance of pneumococci – South Africa. MMWR 26: 285.

CDC (Center for Disease Control) (1984). Ampicillin and chloramphenicol resistance in systemic Haemophilus influenzae disease. MMWR 33: 35.

Chaowagul W, Suputtamongkol Y, Dance DAB et al. (1993). Relapse in melioidosis: incidence and risk factors. J Infect Dis 168: 1181.

Cherubin CE (1981). Antibiotic resistance of Salmonella in Europe and the United States. Rev Infect Dis 3: 1105.

Cherubin CE, Neu HC, Rahal JJ, Sabath LD (1977). Emergence of resistance to chloramphenicol in Salmonella. J Infect Dis 135: 807.

Cherubin CE, Corrado ML, Nair SR et al. (1982). Treatment of Gram-negative bacillary meningitis: role of the new cephalosporin antibiotics. Rev Infect Dis 4 (Suppl): 453.

Christensen LK, Skovsted L (1969). Inhibition of drug metabolism by chloramphenicol. Lancet ii: 1397.

Chun D, Seol SY, Cho DT, Tak R (1977). Drug resistance and R plasmids in Salmonella typhi isolated in Korea. Antimicrob Ag Chemother 11: 209.

Citron DM, Goldstein EJC, Kenner MA et al. (1995). Activity of ampicillin/sulbactam, ticarcillin/clavulanate, clarithromycin, and eleven other antimicrobial agents against anaerobic bacteria isolated from infections in children. Clin Infect Dis 20 (Suppl 2): 356.

Cocke JG Jr, Brown RE, Geppert LJ (1966). Optic neuritis with prolonged use of chloramphenicol. J Pediatr 68: 27.

Coleman K, Athalye M, Clancey A et al. (1994). Bacterial resistance mechanisms as therapeutic targets. J Antimicrob Chemother 33: 1091.

Collignon PJ, Bell JM, MacInnes SJ et al. (1992). A national collaborative study of resistance to antimicrobial agents in Haemophilus influenzae in Australian hospitals. J Antimicrob Chemother 30: 153.

Colquhoun J, Weetch RS (1950). Resistance to chloramphenicol developing during treatment of typhoid fever. Lancet ii: 621.

Cooksey RC, Bannister ER, Farrar WE Jr (1975). Antibiotic resistance patterns of clinical isolates of Serratia marcescens. Antimicrob Ag Chemother 7: 396.

Cooper JA, Lietman PS (1977). Chloramphenicol in Haemophilus endocarditis. Lancet ii: 871.

Couturier M, Bex F, Bergquist PL, Maas WK (1988). Identification and classification of bacterial plasmids. Microbiol Rev 52: 375.

Courvalin PM, Shaw WV, Jacob AE (1978). Plasmid-mediated mechanisms of resistance to aminoglycoside-aminocyclitol antibiotics and to chloramphenicol in Group D streptococci. Antimicrob Ag Chemother 13: 716.

Cuchural G, Jacobus N, Gorbach SL, Tally FP (1981). A survey of Bacteroides susceptibility in the United States. J Antimicrob Chemother 8 (Suppl D): 27.

Cuchural GJ Jr, Tally FP, Jacobus NV et al. (1988). Susceptibility of the Bacteroides fragilis Group in the United States: analysis by site of isolation. Antimicrob Ag Chemother 32: 717.

D'Alessandri RM, McNeely DJ, Kluge RM (1976). Antibiotic synergy and antagonism against clinical isolates of Klebsiella species. Antimicrob Ag Chemother 10: 889.

DaMert GJ, Sohnle PG (1979). Effect of chloramphenicol on in vitro function of lymphocytes. J Infect Dis 139: 220.

Dameshek W (1969). Chloramphenicol aplastic anaemia in identical twins – a clue to pathogenesis. New Engl J Med 281: 42.

Dance DAB, Wuthiekanun V, Chaowagul W, White NJ (1989). Interactions in vitro between agents used to treat melioidosis. J Antimicrob Chemother 24: 311.

Dang-Van A, Tiraby G, Acar JF et al. (1978). Chloramphenicol resistance in Streptococcus pneumoniae: enzymatic acetylation and possible plasmid linkage. Antimicrob Ag Chemother 13: 577.

Daniel TM, Suhrland LG, Weisberger AS (1965). Suppression of the anamnestic response to tetanus toxoid in man by chloramphenicol. New Engl J Med 273: 367.

Datta N (1977). Classification of plasmids as an aid to understanding their epidemiology and evolution. J Antimicrob Chemother 3 (Suppl C): 19.

Datta N, Olarte J (1974). R factors in strains of Salmonella typhi and Shigella dysenteriae 1 isolated during epidemics in Mexico: Classification by compatibility. Antimicrob Ag Chemother 5: 310.

Datta N, Richards H, Datta C (1981). Salmonella typhi in vivo acquires resistance to both chloramphenicol and co-trimoxazole. Lancet i: 1181.

Daum RS, Cohen DL, Smith AL (1979). Fatal aplastic anaemia following apparent 'dose-related' chloramphenicol toxicity. J Pediatr 94: 403.

Davidson SI (1974). Systemic effects of eye-drops. Trans Ophthal Soc UK 94: 487.

Davis RC (1981). Salmonella sepsis in infancy. Amer J Dis Child 135: 1096.

Davis S, Rubin AD (1972). Treatment and prognosis in aplastic anaemia. Lancet i: 871.

DeLeys RJ, Juni E (1977). Unusual effects of penicillin G and chloramphenicol on the growth of Moraxella osloensis. Antimicrob Ag Chemother 12: 573.

Delmee M, Avesani V (1988). Correlation between serogroup and susceptibility to chloramphenicol, clindamycin, erythromycin, rifampicin and tetracycline among 308 isolates of Clostridium difficile. J Antimicrob Chemother 22: 325.

Denys GA, Jerris RC, Swenson JM, Thornsberry C (1983). Susceptibility of Propionibacterium acnes clinical isolates to 22 antimicrobial agents. Antimicrob Ag Chemother 23: 335.

Dettli L, Spring P (1974). The dosage regimen of thiamphenicol in patients with kidney disease. Postgrad Med J 50 (Suppl 5): 32.

Dimopoulou ID, Kraak WAG, Anderson EC et al. (1992). Molecular epidemiology of unrelated clusters of multiresistant strains of Haemophilus influenzae. J Infect Dis 165: 1069.

Doern GV, Jorgensen JH, Thornsberry C et al. (1988). National collaborative study of the prevalence of antimicrobial resistance among clinical isolates of Haemophilus influenzae. Antimicrob Ag Chemother 32: 180.

Downs NJ, Hodges GR, Taylor SA (1987). Mixed bacterial meningitis. Rev Infect Dis 9: 693.

Duck PD, Dillon JR, Eidus L (1978). Effects of thiamphenicol and chloramphenicol in inhibiting Neisseria gonorrhoeae isolates. Antimicrob Ag Chemother 14: 788.

Duncan B, Fulginiti VA, Sieber OF Jr, Ryan KJ (1981). Shigella sepsis. Amer J Dis Child 135: 151.

Dunkle LM (1978). Central nervous system chloramphenicol concentration in premature infants. Antimicrob Ag Chemother 13: 427.

DuPont HL, Hornick RB, Weiss CF et al. (1970). Evaluation of chloramphenicol acid succinate therapy of induced typhoid fever and Rocky Mountain spotted fever. New Engl J Med 282: 53.

Ehrlich J, Bartz QR, Smith RM et al. (1974). Chloromycetin, a new antibiotic from a soil antimonycete. Science 106: 417; quoted by Welch (1954).

Eickhoff TC, Bennett JV, Hayes PS, Feely J (1970). Pseudomonas pseudomallei: susceptibility to chemotherapeutic agents. J Infect Dis 121: 95.

Ekblad H, Ruuskanen O, Lindberg R, Iisalo E (1985). The monitoring of serum chloramphenicol levels in children with severe infections. J Antimicrob Chemother 15: 489.

Elshafie SS, Rafay AM (1992). Chloramphenicol-resistant typhoid fever: an emerging problem in Oman. Scand J Infect Dis 24: 819.

Enzenauer RW, Bass JW (1983). Initial antibiotic treatment of purulent meningitis in infants 1 to 2 months of age. Amer J Dis Child 137: 1055.

Everett ED, Nelson RA (1975). Pulmonary melioidosis. Observations in thirty-nine cases. Amer Rev Resp Dis 112: 331.

Faden HS (1979). Treatment of Haemophilus influenzae type B epiglottitis. Pediatrics 63: 402.

Falbo V, Caprioli A, Mondello F et al. (1982). Antimicrobial resistance among salmonella isolates from hospitals in Rome. J Hyg Camb 88: 275.

Farrar WE (1985). Antibiotic resistance in developing countries. J Infect Dis 152: 1103.

Farrar WE Jr, Eidson M (1971). Antibiotic resistance in Shigella mediated by R factors. J Infect Dis 123: 477.

Feder HM Jr (1987). Bacteroides fragilis meningitis. Rev Infect Dis 9: 783.

Feder HM Jr, Osier C, Maderazo EG (1981). Chloramphenicol: a review of its use in clinical practice. Rev Infect Dis 3: 479.

Feigin RD, Stechenberg BW, Chang MJ et al. (1976). Prospective evaluation of treatment of Hemophilus influenzae meningitis. J Pediatr 88: 542.

Feldman M, Hendler RS, Morrison EB (1980). Acute meningoencephalitis after withdrawal of antibiotics in Whipple's disease. Ann Intern Med 93: 709.

Feldman WE (1978). Effect of ampicillin and chloramphenicol against Haemophilus influenzae. Pediatrics 61: 406.

Feldman WE, Zweighaft T (1979). Effect of ampicillin and chloramphenicol against Streptococcus pneumoniae and Neisseria meningitidis. Antimicrob Ag Chemother 15: 240.

Ferrari V, Della Bella D (1974). Comparison of chloramphenicol and thiamphenicol metabolism. Postgrad Med J 50 (Suppl 5): 17.

Finegold SM, Wexler HM (1988). Theapeutic implications of bacteriologic findings in mixed aerobic-anaerobic infections. Antimicrob Ag Chemother 32: 611.

Forsgren A, Schmeling D (1977). Effect of antibiotics on chemotaxis of human leukocytes. Antimicrob Ag Chemother 11: 580.

Forsgren A, Walder M (1982). Haemophilus influenzae, pneumococci, Group A streptococci and Staphylococcus aureus: sensitivity of outpatient strains to commonly prescribed antibiotics. Scand J Infect Dis 14: 39.

Foster TJ (1983). Plasmid-determined resistance to antimicrobial drugs and toxic metal ions in bacteria. Microbiol Rev 47: 361.

Fox AR, Phillips I (1987). The antibiotic sensitivity of Bacteroides fragilis group in the United Kingdom. J Antimicrob Chemother 20: 477.

Franceschinis R (1981). Drug utilization data for chloramphenicol and thiamphenicol in recent years. In Safety Related to Chloramphenicol and Thiamphenicol Therapy (Najean Y, Tognoni G, Yunis AA, eds), pp 81–9 New York: Raven Press, quoted by Glupczynski et al., 1983.

Fraser DW, Wachsmuth IK, Bopp C et al. (1978). Antibiotic treatment of guinea-pigs infected with agent of Legionnaires' disease. Lancet i: 175.

Fraunfelder FT, Bagby GG (1982). Fatal aplastic anaemia. JAMA 247: 2499.

Fraunfelder FT, Bagby GC Jr (1983). Ocular chloramphenicol and aplastic anemia. New Engl J Med 308: 1536.

Fraunfelder FT, Bagby GC Jr, Kelly DJ (1982). Fatal aplastic anemia following topical administration of ophthalmic chloramphenicol. Amer J Ophthalmol 93: 356.

Freundlich M, Cynamon H, Tamer A et al. (1983). Management of chloramphenicol intoxication in infancy by charcoal hemoperfusion. J Pediatr 103: 485.

Friedman CA, Lovejoy FC, Smith AL (1979). Chloramphenicol disposition in infants and children. J Pediatr 95: 1071.

Fripp RR, Carter MC, Werner CJ et al. (1983). Cardiac function and acute chloramphenicol toxicity. J Pediatr 103: 487.

Furman KI, Koornhof HJ, Kilroe-Smith TA et al. (1976). Peritoneal transfer of thiamphenicol during peritoneal dialysis. Antimicrob Ag Chemother 9: 557.

Gale EF, Cundliffe E, Reynolds PE et al. (1972). The Molecular Basis of Antibiotic Action, p. 332. New York: John Wiley & Sons.

Garvey RJP, McMullin GP (1983). Meningitis due to beta lactamase producing type b Haemophilus influenzae resistant to chloramphenicol. Brit Med J 287: 1183.

George MJ, Kitch B, Henderson FW, Gilligan PH (1991). In vitro activity of orally administered antimicrobial agents against Haemophilus influenzae recovered from children monitored longitudinally in a group day-care center. Antimicrob Ag Chemother 35: 1960.

George WL, Kirby BD, Sutter VL et al. (1981). Gram-negative anaerobic bacilli; their role in infection and patterns of susceptibility to antimicrobial agents. II. Little known Fusobacterium species and miscellaneous genera. Rev Infect Dis 3: 599.

Gerding DN, Hall WH, Schierl EA (1977). Antibiotic concentrations in ascitic fluid of patients with ascites and bacterial peritonitis. Ann Intern Med 86: 708.

Gibson DH, Fitzgeorge RB (1983). Persistence in serum and lungs of guinea pigs of erythromycin, gentamicin, chloramphenicol and rifampicin and their in vitro activities against Legionella pneumophila. J Antimicrob Chemother 12: 235.

Gill FA, Hook EW (1966). Salmonella strains with transferable antimicrobial resistance. JAMA 198: 1267.

Gill VJ, Manning C, Lamson M et al. (1981). Antibiotic-resistant group JK bacteria in hospitals. J Clin Microbiol 13: 472.

Ginsburg CM, Howard JB, Nelson JD (1979). Report of 65 cases of Haemophilus influenzae b pneumonia. Paediatrics 64: 283.

Givner LB, Abramson JS, Wasilauskas B (1989). Meningitis due to Haemophilus influenzae type b resistant to ampicillin and chloramphenicol. Rev Infect Dis 11: 329.

Glazer JP, Danish MA, Plotkin SA, Jaffe SJ (1980). Disposition of chloramphenicol in low birth weight infants. Paediatrics 66: 573.

Glazko AJ, Wolf LM, Dill WA, Bratton AC Jr (1949). Biochemical studies on chloramphenicol (chloromycetin). II. Tissue distribution and excretion studies. J Pharmacol Exper Ther 96: 445; quoted by Woodward and Wisseman (1958).

Glazko AJ, Dill WA, Kinkel AW et al. (1977). Absorption and excretion of parenteral doses of chloramphenicol sodium succinate in comparison with peroral doses of chloramphenicol. Clin Pharmacol Ther 21: 104.

Gleckman RA (1975). Warning – chloramphenicol may be good for your health. Arch Intern Med 135: 1125.

Glupczynski Y, Yourassowsky E, Van der Linden MP, Crokaert F (1983). Susceptibility of Streptococcus pneumoniae to chloramphenicol and thiamphenicol. J Antimicrob Chemother 11: 488.

Goldberg IH (1965). Mode of action of antibiotics II Drugs affecting nucleic acid and protein synthesis. Amer J Med 39: 722.

Goldstein FW, Chumpiatz JC, Guevara JM et al. (1986). Plasmid-mediated resistance to multiple antibiotics in Salmonella typhi. J Infect Dis 153: 261.

Goodwin CS, Blake P, Blincow E (1986). The minimum inhibitory and bactericidal concentrations of antibiotics and anti-ulcer agents against Campylobacter pyloridis. J Antimicrob Chemother 17: 309.

Gould T, Roberts RJ (1979). Therapeutic problems arising from the use of the intravenous route for drug administration. J Pediatr 95: 465.

Granato PA, Jurek EA, Weiner LB (1983). Biotypes of Haemophilus influenzae: relationship to clinical source of isolation, serotype and antibiotic susceptibility. Amer J Clin Path 79: 73.

Grant RB, Bannatyne RM, Shapley AJ (1976). Resistance to chloramphenicol and ampicillin of *Salmonella typhimurium* in Ontario, Canada. *J Infect Dis* **134**: 354.

Gray SJ (1984). *Aeromonas hydrophila* in livestock: incidence, biochemical characteristics and antibiotic susceptibility. *J Hyg Camb* **92**: 365.

Green CE, Cameron HJ, Julian GR (1975). Recovery of polysome function of T4-infected *Escherichia coli* after brief treatment with chloramphenicol and rifampin. *Antimicrob Ag Chemother* **7**: 549.

Greenberg PA, Sanford JP (1967). Removal and absorption of antibiotics in patients with renal failure undergoing peritoneal dialysis. *Ann Intern Med* **66**: 465.

Grinsted J (1986). Evolution of transposable elements. *J Antimicrob Chemother* **18** (Suppl C): 77.

Gross RJ, Ward LR, Threlfall EJ et al. (1982). Drug resistance among infantile enteropathogenic *Escherichia coli* strains isolated in the United Kingdom. *Brit Med J* **285**: 472.

Gross RJ, Threlfall EJ, Ward LR, Rowe B (1984). Drug resistance in *Shigella dysenteriae*, *S. flexneri* and *S. boydii* in England and Wales: increasing incidence of resistance to trimethoprim. *Brit Med J* **288**: 784.

Guiney DG Jr, Davis CE (1978). Identification of a conjugative R plasmid in *Bacteroides ochraceus* capable of transfer to *Escherichia coli*. *Nature* **274**: 181.

Gupta RS (1975). Killing and lysis of *Escherichia coli* in the presence of chloramphenicol: relation to cellular magnesium. *Antimicrob Ag Chemother* **7**: 748.

Gutmann L, Goldstein FW, Kitzis MD et al. (1983). Susceptibility of *Nocardia asteroides* to 46 antibiotics, including 22 β-lactams. *Antimicrob Ag Chemother* **23**: 248.

Halstensen A, Vollset SE, Haneberg B et al. (1987). Antimicrobial therapy and case fatality in meningococcal disease. *Scand J Infect Dis* **19**: 403.

Hammond GW, Lian CJ, Wilt JC, Ronald AR (1978). Antimicrobial susceptibility of *Haemophilus ducreyi*. *Antimicrob Ag Chemother* **13**: 608.

Hand WL, King-Thompson NL (1990). Uptake of antibiotics by human polymorphonuclear leukocyte cytoplasts. *Antimicrob Ag Chemother* **34**: 1189.

Hand WL, Boozer RM, King-Thompson NL (1985). Antibiotic uptake by alveolar macrophages of smokers. *Antimicrob Ag Chemother* **27**: 42.

Hansman D (1978). Chloramphenicol-resistant pneumococci in West Africa. *Lancet* **i**: 1102.

Hansman D (1985). Multiple drug resistance in *Haemophilus influenzae* type b. *Med J Aust* **142**: 536.

Harvey RJ, Koch AL (1980). How partially inhibitory concentrations of chloramphenicol affect the growth of *Escherichia coli*. *Antimicrob Ag Chemother* **18**: 323.

Harvey RL, Sunstrum JC (1991). *Rhodococcus equi* infection in patients with and without human immunodeficiency virus infection. *Rev Infect Dis* **13**: 139.

Hassam ZA, Shaw EJ, Shooter RA, Caro DB (1978). Changes in antibiotic sensitivity in strains of *Staphylococcus aureus*, 1952–78. *Brit Med J* **2**: 536.

Hausmann K, Skrandies G (1974). Aplastic anaemia following chloramphenicol therapy in Hamburg and surrounding districts. *Postgrad Med J* **50** (Suppl 5): 131.

Herzog CH (1976). Drug treatment of typhoid fever. *Brit Med J* **2**: 941.

Heymann CS, Turk DC, Rotimi VO (1981). Multiple antibiotic resistance in *Haemophilus influenzae*. *Lancet* **i**: 553.

Hill GB, Ayers OM (1985). Antimicrobial susceptibilities of anaerobic bacteria isolated from female genital tract infections. *Antimicrob Ag Chemother* **27**: 324.

Hirschmann JV, Everett ED (1979). *Haemophilus influenzae* infections in adults: report of nine cases and a review of the literature. *Medicine* **58**: 80.

Hodgkinson R (1973). The chloramphenicol-hepatitis-aplastic anaemia syndrome. *Med J Aust* **1**: 939.

Hodgman JE (1961). Chloramphenicol. *Pediatr Clin N Amer* **8**: 1027.

Hoffman SL, Punjabi NH, Kumala S et al. (1984). Reduction of mortality in chloramphenicol-treated severe typhoid fever by high-dose dexamethasone. *New Engl J Med* **310**: 82.

Hoffman TA, Ruiz CJ, Counts GW et al. (1975). Waterborne typhoid fever in Dade County, Florida – clinical and therapeutic evaluation of 105 bacteremic patients. *Amer J Med* **59**: 481.

Holt DE, Hurley R, Harvey D (1995). A reappraisal of chloramphenicol metabolism: detection and quantification of metabolites in sera of children. *J Antimicrob Chemother* **35**: 115.

Holt R (1967). The bacterial degradation of chloramphenicol. *Lancet* **i**: 1259.

Howard AJ, Williams HM (1988). The prevalence of antibiotic resistance in *Haemophilus influenzae* in Wales. *J Antimicrob Chemother* **21**: 251.

Howard AJ, Hince CJ, Williams JD (1978). Antibiotic resistance in *Streptococcus pneumoniae* and *Haemophilus influenzae*. Report of a study group on bacterial resistance. *Brit Med J* **1**: 1657.

Howe C, Sampath A, Spotnitz M (1971). The *Psuedomallei* group: a review. *J Infect Dis* **124**: 598.

Howell A, Andrews TM, Watts RWE (1975). Bone-marrow cells resistant to chloramphenicol in chloramphenicol-induced aplastic anaemia. *Lancet* **i**: 65.

Hughes DWO'G (1968). Studies on chloramphenicol: 1. Assessment of haemopoietic toxicity. *Med J Aust* **2**: 436.

Hughes DWO'G (1973). Studies on chloramphenicol. II. Possible determinants and progress of haemopoietic toxicity during chloramphenicol therapy. *Med J Aust* **2**: 1142.

Huo MI, Samadi AR (1982). Chloramphenicol-resistant *Salmonella typhi* Vi phage type A isolated from a patient in Bangladesh. *Lancet* **i**: 1125.

Hussey G, Hitchcock J, Hanslo D et al. (1994). Serotypes and antimicrobial susceptibility of *Haemophilus influenzae*. *J Antimicrob Chemother* **34**: 1031.

Ingall D, Sherman JD, Cockburn F, Klein R (1965). Amelioration by ingestion of phenylalanine of toxic effects of chloramphenicol on bone marrow. *New Engl J Med* **272**: 180.

Istre GR, Humphreys JT, Albrecht KD et al. (1983). Chloramphenicol and penicillin resistance in pneumococci isolated from blood and cerebrospinal fluid: a prevalence study in metropolitan Denver. *J Clin Microbiol* **17**: 472.

Jacobs RF, Wilson CB (1983). Intracellular penetration and antimicrobial activity of antibiotics. *J Antimicrob Chemother* **12** (Suppl C): 13.

Jadavji T, Prober CG, Cheung R (1984). *In vitro* interactions between rifampin and ampicillin or chloramphenicol against *Haemophilus influenzae*. *Antimicrob Ag Chemother* **26**: 91.

Janda JM, Guthertz LS, Kokka RP, Shimada T (1994). *Aeromonas* spp in septicemia: laboratory characteristics and clinical observations. *Clin Infect Dis* **19**: 77.

Jesudasan MJ, John TJ (1990). Multiresistant *Salmonella typhi* in India. *Lancet* **336**: 252.

Johnson CC, Finegold SM (1987). Uncommonly encountered, motile, anaerobic Gram-negative bacilli associated with infection. *Rev Infect Dis* **9**: 1150.

Jorgensen JH (1992). Update on mechanisms and prevalence of antimicrobial resistance in *Haemophilus influenzae*. *Clin Infect Dis* **14**: 1119.

Joseph SW, DeBell RM, Brown WP (1978). *In vitro* response to chloramphenicol, tetracycline, ampicillin, gentamicin, and beta-lactamase production by halophilic *Vibrios* from human and environmental sources. *Antimicrob Ag Chemother* **13**: 244.

Kauffman CA, Bergman AG, Hertz CS (1979). Antimicrobial resistance of *Haemophilus* species in patients with chronic bronchitis. *Amer Rev Respir Dis* **120**: 1382.

Kauffman RE, Miceli JN, Strebel L et al. (1981a). Pharmacokinetics of chloramphenicol and chloramphenicol succinate in infants and children. *J Pediatr* **98**: 315.

Kauffman RE, Thirumoorthi MC, Buckley JA et al. (1981b). Relative bioavailability of intravenous chloramphenicol succinate and oral chloramphenicol palmitate in infants and children. *J Pediatr* **99**: 963.

Kearns GL, Bocchini JA Jr, Brown RD *et al.* (1985). Absence of pharmacokinetic interaction between chloramphenicol and acetaminophen in children. *J Pediatr* **107**: 134.

Kessler DL, Smith AL, Woodrum DE (1980). Chloramphenicol toxicity in a neonate treated with exchange transfusion. *J Pediatr* **96**: 140.

Kinmonth AL, Storrs CN, Mitchell RG (1978). Meningitis due to chloramphenicol-resistant *Haemophilus influenzae* type b. *Brit Med J* **1**: 694.

Kirby BD, George WL, Sutter VL *et al.* (1980). Gram-negative anaerobic bacilli: their role in infection and patterns of susceptibility to antimicrobial agents I Little-known *Bacteroides* species. *Rev Infect Dis* **2**: 914.

Klastersky J, Husson M (1977). Bactericidal activity of the combination of gentamicin with clindamycin or chloramphenicol against species of *Escherichia coli* and *Bacteroides fragilis*. *Antimicrob Ag Chemother* **12**: 135.

Klugman KP, Koornhof HJ (1988). Drug resistance patterns and serogroups or serotypes of pneumococcal isolates, from cerebrospinal fluid or blood, 1979–1986. *J Infect Dis* **158**: 956.

Koup JR, Lau AH, Brodsky B, Slaughter RL (1979a). Chloramphenicol pharmacokinetics in hospitalized patients. *Antimicrob Ag Chemother* **15**: 651.

Koup JR, Lau AH, Brodsky B, Slaughter RL (1979b). Relationship between serum and saliva chloramphenicol concentrations. *Antimicrob Ag Chemother* **15**: 658.

Krasinski K, Kusmiesz H, Nelson JD (1982). Pharmacologic interactions among chloramphenicol, phenytoin and phenobarbital. *Pediatr Infect Dis* **1**: 232.

Kunin CM (1967). A guide to use of antibiotics in patients with renal disease. *Ann Intern Med* **67**: 151.

Kunin CM, Glazko AJ, Finland M (1959). Persistence of antibiotics in blood of patients with acute renal failure. II. Chloramphenicol and its metabolic products in the blood of patients with severe renal disease or hepatic cirrhosis. *J Clin Invest* **38**: 1498; quoted by Hodgman (1961).

Lampe RM, Mansuwan P (1973). Chloramphenicol-resistant *Salmonella typhosa*. *New Engl J Med* **289**: 1203.

Latif AS (1982). Thiamphenicol in the treatment of chancroid in men. *Brit J Vener Dis* **58**: 54.

Latif AS, Lencioni R, Crocchiolo P, Esposito R (1982). Single-dose thiamphenicol for chancroid. *Lancet* **ii**: 1225.

Latif AS, Marowa E, Mason PR *et al.* (1986). Treatment of infection due to penicillinase-producing *Neisseria gonorrhoeae* with oral thiamphenicol and with oral lymecycline. *Sex Transm Dis* **13**: 156.

Leading Article (1982). Drug resistance in salmonellas. *Lancet* **i**: 1391.

Lee H-J, Park J-Y, Jang S-H *et al.* (1995). HIgh incidence of resistance to multiple antimicrobials in clinical isolates of *Streptococcus pneumoniae* from a University Hospital in Korea. *Clin Infect Dis* **20**: 826.

Lee K, Jang IH, Kim YJ, Chong Y (1992). *In vitro* susceptibilities of the *Bacteroides fragilis* group to 14 antimicrobial agents in Korea. *Antimicrob Ag Chemother* **36**: 195.

Leelarasamee A, Bovernkitti S (1989). Melioidosis: review and update. *Rev Infect Dis* **11**: 413.

Lerman SJ, Kucera JC, Brunken JM (1979). Nasopharyngeal carriage of antibiotic-resistant *Haemophilus influenzae* in healthy children. *Pediatrics* **64**: 287.

Lewis VJ, Thacker WL, Shepard CC, McDade JE (1978). *In vivo* susceptibility of the Legionnaires' disease bacterium to ten antimicrobial agents. *Antimicrob Ag Chemother* **13**: 419.

Li X-Z, Livermore DM, Nikaido H (1994). Role of efflux pump(s). in intrinsic resistance of *Pseudomonas aeruginosa*: resistance to tetracycline, chloramphenicol, and norfloxacin. *Antimicrob Ag Chemother* **38**: 1732.

Lietman PS (1981). Editorial Oral chloramphenicol therapy. *J Pediatr* **99**: 905.

Lima AAM, Lima NL, Pinho MCN *et al.* (1995). High frequency of strains multiply resistant to ampicillin, trimethoprim-sulfamethoxazole, strepto-

mycin, chloramphenicol and tetracycline isolated from patients with shigellosis in Northeastern Brazil during the period 1988 to 1993. *Antimicrob Ag Chemother* **39**: 256.

Lindberg AA, Nilsson L. H, Bucht H, Kallings LO (1966). Concentration of chloramphenicol in the urine and blood in relation to renal function. *Brit Med J* **2**: 724.

Lindberg J, Rosenhall U, Nylen O, Ringner A (1977). Long-term outcome of *Hemophilus influenzae* meningitis related to antibiotic treatment. *Pediatrics* **60**: 1.

Ling J, Chau PY (1984). Plasmids mediating resistance to chloramphenicol, trimethoprim and ampicillin in *Salmonella typhi* strains isolated in Southeast asian region. *J Infect Dis* **149**: 652.

Ling JM, Zhou G-M, Woo THS, French GL (1991). Antibiotic susceptibilities and beta-lactamase production of Hong Kong isolates of gastroenteric salmonellae and *Salmonella typhi*. *J Antimicrob Chemother* **28**: 877.

Ljungberg B, Braconier JH (1986). Abdominal aortitis and infected aneurysms due to *Salmonella*. *Scand J Infect Dis* **18**: 401.

Lupski JR (1987). Molecular mechanisms for transposition of drug-resistance genes and other movable genetic elements. *Rev Infect Dis* **9**: 357.

Manten A, van Klingeren B, Dessens-Kroon M (1976). Chloramphenicol resistance in *Haemophilus influenzae*. *Lancet* **i**: 702.

Manyan DR, Arimura GK, Yunis AA (1972). Chloramphenicol-induced erythroid suppression and bone marrow ferrochelatase activity in dogs. *J Lab Clin Med* **79**: 137.

Marca G, Mattina R, Dubini F, Cocuzza G (1984). *In-vitro* antibacterial activity of Sch 25393, a fluorinated analogue of thiamphenicol. *J Antimicrob Chemother* **13**: 423.

Marder HP, Kayser FH (1977). Transferable plasmids mediating multiple-antibiotic resistance in *Streptococcus faecalis* subsp. *liquefaciens*. *Antimicrob Ag Chemother* **12**: 261.

Martelo OJ, Manyan DR, Smith US, Yunis AA (1969). Chloramphenicol and bone marrow mitochondria. *J Lab Clin Med* **74**: 927.

Martinez-Suárez JV, Baquero F, Reig M, Pérez-Diaz JC (1985). Transferable plasmid-linked chloramphenicol acetyltransferase conferring high-level resistance in Bacteroides uniformis. *Antimicrob Ag Chemother* **28**: 113.

Mastro TD, Nomani NK, Ishaq Z *et al.* (1993). Use of nasopharyngeal isolates of *Streptococcus pneumoniae* and *Haemophilus influenzae* from children in Pakistan for surveillance for antimicrobial resistance. *Pediatr Infect Dis J* **12**: 824.

Mauer SM, Chavers BM, Kjellstrand CM (1980). Treatment of an infant with severe chloramphenicol intoxication using charcoal-column hemoperfusion. *J Pediatr* **96**: 136.

Mayers M, Rush D, Madu A *et al.* (1991). Pharmacokinetics of amikacin and chloramphenicol in the aqueous humor of rabbits. *Antimicrob Ag Chemother* **35**: 1791.

Mayo JB, McCarthy LR (1977). Antimicrobial susceptibility of *Haemophilus parainfluenzae*. *Antimicrob Ag Chemother* **11**: 844.

McCabe WR (1983). Empiric therapy for bacterial meningitis. *Rev Infect Dis* **5** (Suppl): 74.

McCaffrey RP, Halsted CH, Wahab MFA, Robertson RP (1971). Chloramphenicol-induced hemolysis in caucasian glucose-6-phosphate dehydrogenase deficiency. *Ann Intern Med* **74**: 722.

McCracken GH Jr, Nelson JD (1983). *Antimicrobial Therapy for Newborns*, p. 68. New York: Grune & Stratton.

McMurry LM George AM, Levy SB (1994). Active efflux of chloramphenicol in susceptible *Escherichia coli* strains and in multiple-antibiotic-resistant (Mar). mutants. *Antimicrob Ag Chemother* **38**: 542.

McNulty CAM (1987). The treatment of campylobacter infections in man. *J Antimicrob Chemother* **19**: 281.

Mehtar S, Aminiafshar S (1983). Antibiotic resistance amongst various types of *Haemophilus* species. *J Antimicrob Chemother* **12**: 565.

Melby K, Midvedt T (1977). The effect of eight antibacterial agents on the phagocytosis of 32P-labelled *Escherichia coli* by rat polymorphonuclear cells. *Scand J Infect Dis* **9**: 9.

Mendelman PM, Doroshow CA, Gandy SL *et al.* (1984). Plasmid-mediated resistance in multiply resistant *Haemophilus influenzae* typb b causing meningitis: molecular characterization of one strain and review of the literature. *J Infect Dis* **150**: 30.

Mhalu FS, Mmari PW, Ijumba J (1979). Rapid emergence of *El Tor Vibrio* cholerae resistant to antimicrobial agents during first six months of fourth cholera epidemic in Tanzania. *Lancet* **i**: 345.

Michel J, Rogol M, Dickman D (1983). Susceptibility of clinical isolates of *Campylobacter jejuni* to sixteen antimicrobial agents. *Antimicrob Ag Chemother* **23**: 796.

Mills J, Drew D (1976). *Serratia marcescens* endocarditis: a regional illness associated with intravenous drug abuse. *Ann Intern Med* **84**: 29.

Montefiore D, Rotimi JO, Adeyemi-Doro FAB (1989). The problem of bacterial resistance to antibiotics among strains isolated from hospital patients in Lagos and Ibadan, Nigeria. *J Antimicrob Chemother* **23**: 641.

Moore A, Summerford M, Jarvinen A, Hansman D (1985). Multiply resistant *Haemophilus influenzae* type b and bacteraemia. *Med J Aust* **142**: 78.

Morizono T, Johnstone BM (1975). Ototoxicity of chloramphenicol ear drops with propylene glycol as solvent. *Med J Aust* **2**: 634.

Morris JG Jr, Wilson R, Davis BR *et al.* (1981). Non-O-Group 1 *Vibrio cholerae* gastroenteritis in the United States. Clinical, epidemiologic, and laboratory characteristics of sporadic cases. *Ann Intern Med* **94**: 656.

Mulhall A, De Louvois J, Hurley R (1983a). The pharmacokinetics of chloramphenicol in the neonate and young infant. *J Antimicrob Chemother* **12**: 629.

Mulhall A, De Louvois J, Hurley R (1983b). Chloramphenicol toxicity in neonates: its incidence and prevention. *Brit Med J* **287**: 1424.

Mulhall A, De Louvois J, Hurley R (1983c). Efficacy of chloramphenicol in the treatment of neonatal and infantile meningitis: a study of 70 cases. *Lancet* **ii**: 284.

Muñoz P, Diaz MD, Rodriguez-Créixems M *et al.* (1993). Antimicrobial resistance of *Salmonella* isolates in a Spanish hospital. *Antimicrob Ag Chemother* **37**: 1200.

Nagao T, Mauer AM (1969). Concordance for drug-induced aplastic anaemia in identical twins. *New Engl J Med* **281**: 7.

Nakae M, Murai T, Kaneko Y, Mitsuhashi S (1977). Drug-resistance in *Streptococcus pyogenes* isolated in Japan (1974–1975). *Antimicrob Ag Chemother* **12**: 427.

Nelson JD (1981). Antibiotic therapy for salmonella syndromes. *Amer J Dis Child* **135**: 1093.

Neu H (1984). Current mechanisms of resistance to antimicrobial agents in micro-organisms causing infection in the patient at risk. *Amer J Med* **76**: 11.

Neu HC, Fu KP (1980). *In vitro* activity of chloramphenicol and thiamphenicol analogs. *Antimicrob Ag Chemother* **18**: 311.

Neu HC, Cherubin CE, Longo ED, Winter J (1975a). Antimicrobial resistance of shigella isolated in New York City in 1973. *Antimicrob Ag Chemother* **7**: 833.

Neu HC, Cherubin CE, Longo ED *et al.* (1975b). Antimicrobial resistance and R-factor transfer among isolates of *Salmonella* in the Northeastern United States: a comparison of human and animal isolates. *J Infect Dis* **132**: 617.

Nilsson-Ehle I, Hedström SA (1987). Hydrolysis of chloramphenicol succinate in local treatment of soft tissue infections. *J Antimicrob Chemother* **19**: 138.

Nomura M (1969). Ribosomes. *Scient Amer* **221**: 28.

Norrby R, McCloskey RV, Zackrisson G, Falsen E (1980). Meningitis caused by *Campylobacter fetus* spp. *jejuni*. *Brit Med J* **280**: 1164.

Norris AH, Reilly JP, Edelstein PH *et al.* (1995). Chloramphenicol for the treatment of vancomycin-resistant enterococcal infections. *Clin Infect Dis* **20**: 1137.

Ohm-Smith MJ, Hadley WK, Sweet RL (1982). *In vitro* activity of new beta-lactam antibiotics and other antimicrobial drugs against anaerobic isolates from obstetric and gynaecological infection. *Antimicrob Ag Chemother* **22**: 711.

Olarte J, Galindo E (1973). *Salmonella typhi* resistant to chloramphenicol, ampicillin and other antimicrobial agents: strains isolated during an extensive typhoid fever epidemic in Mexico. *Antimicrob Ag Chemother* **4**: 597.

Oles A, Stanio-Pyrkosz B (1964). Chloromycetin resistance of *Salmonella typhi* strains isolated from carriers and cases of typhoid fever. *J Hyg Epid Microb Immunol* **8**: 169.

Oppenheim B, Koornhof HJ, Austrian R (1986). Antibiotic-resistant pneumococcal disease in children at Baragwanath Hospital, Johannesburg. *Pediatr Infect Dis* **5**: 520.

Overturf G, Marton KI, Mathies AW Jr (1973). Antibiotic resistance in typhoid fever. *New Engl J Med* **289**: 463.

Paisley JW, Washington JA II (1979). Susceptibility of *Escherichia coli* K1 to four combinations of antimicrobial agents potentially useful for treatment of neonatal meningitis. *J Infect Dis* **140**: 183.

Panigrahi D, Agarwal KC, Verma AD, Dubey ML (1987). Incidence of shigellosis and multi-drug resistant shigellae: a 10 year study. *J Trop Med Hyg* **90**: 25.

Pasculle AW, Dowling JN, Weyant RS *et al.* (1981). Susceptibility of Pittsburg pneumonia agent (*Legionella micdadei*). and other newly recognized members of the genus *Legionella* to nineteen antimicrobial agents. *Antimicrob Ag Chemother* **20**: 793.

Pasculle AW, Dowling JN, Frola FN *et al.* (1985). Antimicrobial therapy of experimental *Legionella micdadei* pneumonia in guinea pigs. *Antimicrob Ag Chemother* **28**: 730.

Patey O, Varon E, Prazuck T *et al.* (1994). Multicentre survey in France of the antimicrobial susceptibilities of 416 blood culture isolates of the *Bacteroides fragilis* group. *J Antimicrob Chemother* **33**: 1029.

Peel MM, Tibbits DR, Forsyth JRL (1979). Chloramphenicol-resistant *Haemophilus influenzae*. *Med J Aust* **1**: 130.

Pepper K, Horaud T, Le Bouguenec C, De Caspedes G (1987). Location of antibiotic resistance markers in clinical isolates of *Enterococcus faecalis* with similar antibiotypes. *Antimicrob Ag Chemother* **31**: 1394.

Perlino CA, Lichtenberger CJ (1984). Antibiotic susceptibility and serotype distribution of *Streptococcus pneumoniae*. *Amer Rev Respir Dis* **129**: 1018.

Perroud HM, Miedzybrodzka K (1978). Chlamydial infection of the urethra in men. *Brit J Vener Dis* **54**: 45.

Philpott-Howard J, Williams JD (1982). Increase in antibiotic resistance in *Haemophilus influenzae* in the United Kingdom since 1977: report of study group. *Brit Med J* **284**: 1597.

Pickering LK, Hoecker JL, Kramer WG *et al.* (1980). Clinical pharmacology of two chloramphenicol preparations in children: sodium succinate (IV). and palmitate (oral). esters. *J Pediatr* **96**: 757.

Plaut ME, Best WR (1982). Aplastic anemia after parental chloramphenicol: warning renewed. *New Engl J Med* **306**: 1486.

Pollock HM, Holt J, Murray C (1983). Comparison of susceptibilities of anaerobic bacteria to cefmenoxime, ceftriaxone and other antimicrobial compounds. *Antimicrob Ag Chemother* **23**: 780.

Powell DA, Nahata MC, Durrell DC *et al.* (1981). Interactions among chloramphenicol, phenytoin, and phenobarbital in a pediatric patient. *J Pediatrics* **98**: 1001.

Powell M, Price EH (1990). Invasive infections due to *Haemophilus influenzae* type b resistant to ampicillin and chloramphenicol. *J Antimicrob Chemother* **26**: 149.

Powell M, Fah YS, Seymour A *et al.* (1992). Antimicrobial resistance in *Haemophilus influenzae* from England and Scotland in 1991. *J Antimicrob Chemother* **29**: 547.

Preblud SR, Gill CJ, Campos JM (1984). Bactericidal activities of chloramphenicol and eleven other antibiotics against *Salmonella* spp. *Antimicrob Ag Chemother* **25**: 327.

Preston MA, Brown S, Borczyk AA *et al.* (1994). Antimicrobial susceptibility of pathogenic Yersinia enterocolitica isolated in Canada from 1972 to 1990. *Antimicrob Ag Chemother* **38**: 2121.

Prober CG, Rajchgot P, Bannatyne RM *et al.* (1983). Impact of chloramphenicol use on bacterial resistance in a neonatal intensive care unit. *Lancet* **ii**: 158.

Prokesch RC, Hand WL (1982). Antibiotic entry into human polymorphonuclear leukocytes. *Antimicrob Ag Chemother* **21**: 373.

Rahal JJ Jr, Simberkoff MS (1979). Bactericidal and bacteriostatic action of chloramphenicol against meningeal pathogens. *Antimicrob Ag Chemother* **16**: 13.

Rajchgot P, Prober CG, Soldin S et al. (1982). Initiation of chloramphenicol therapy in the newborn infant. *J Pediatr* **101**: 1018.

Ramilo O, Kinane BT, McCracken GHJr (1988). Chloramphenicol neurotoxicity. *Pediatr Infect Dis J* **7**: 358.

Rangnekar VM, Banker DD, Jhala HI (1983). Antimicrobial resistance and incompatibility groups of R plasmids in *Salmonella typhimurium* isolated from human sources in Bombay from 1978 to 1980. *Antimicrob Ag Chemother* **23**: 54.

Raoult D, Drancourt M (1991). Antimicrobial therapy of Rickettsial diseases. *Antimicrob Ag Chemother* **35**: 2457.

Report of a WHO Study Group (1976). Cerebrospinal meningitis control. *Wld Hlth Org Techn Rep Ser* No. **588**, p. 21.

Report of a WHO Scientific Group (1978). *Neisseria gonorrhoeae* and gonococcal infections. *Wld Hlth Org Techn Rep Ser* No. **616**, p. 130.

Richardson CJL, Hume D, Masters PL (1979). Chloramphenicol-resistant *Haemophilus influenzae*. *Med J Aust* **2**: 429.

Ries AA, Wells JG, Olivola D et al. (1994). Epidemic *Shigella* dysenteriae type 1 in Burundi: panresistance and implications for prevention. *J Infect Dis* **169**: 1035.

Righter J, Luchsinger I (1988). *Haemophilus influenzae* from four laboratories in one Canadian City. *J Antimicrob Chemother* **22**: 333.

Ringertz S, Rockhill RC, Ringertz O, Sutomo A (1981). Susceptibility of *Campylobacter fetus* subsp. *jejuni*, isolated from patients in Jakarta, Indonesia, to ten antimicrobial agents. *J Antimicrob Chemother* **8**: 333.

Roberts MC, Actis LA, Crosa JH (1985). Molecular characterization of chloramphenicol-resistant *Haemophilus parainfluenzae* and *Haemophilus ducreyi*. *Antimicrob Ag Chemother* **28**: 176.

Robins-Browne RM, Rowe B, Ramsaroop R et al. (1983). A hospital outbreak of multiresistant *Salmonella typhimurium* belonging to phage type 193. *J Infect Dis* **147**: 210.

Rocco V, Overturf G (1982). Chloramphenicol inhibition of the bactericidal effect of ampicillin against *Haemophilus influenzae*. *Antimicrob Ag Chemother* **21**: 349.

Romanowski B, Starreveld E, Jarema AJ (1983). Treatment of neurosyphilis with chloramphenicol. A case report. *Brit J Vener Dis* **59**: 225.

Rood JI, Maher EA, Somers EB et al. (1978). Isolation and characterization of multiply antibiotic-resistant *Clostridium perfringens* strains from porcine feces. *Antimicrob Ag Chemother* **13**: 871.

Rood JI, Jefferson S, Bannam TL et al. (1989). Hybridization analysis of three chloramphenicol resistance determinants from *Clostridium perfringens* and *Clostridium difficile*. *Antimicrob Ag Chemother* **33**: 1569.

Rose JQ, Choi HK, Schentag JJ et al. (1977). Intoxication caused by interaction of chloramphenicol and phenytoin. *JAMA* **237**: 2630.

Rosenthal RI, Blackman A (1965). Bone-marrow hypoplasia following use of chloramphenicol eye drops. *JAMA* **191**: 136.

Ross S, Controni G, Khan W (1972). Resistance of shigellae to ampicillin and other antibiotics. *JAMA* **221**: 45.

Rossi A, Galas M, Binztein N et al. (1993). Unusual multiresistant *Vibrio cholerae* O1 El Tor in Argentina. *Lancet* **342**: 1172.

Rotimi JO, Turk DC (1981). Transferable multiple antibiotic resistance in *Haemophilus influenzae*. *J Antimicrob Chemother* **8**: 187.

Rowe B, Frost JA, Threlfall EJ, Ward LR (1980). Spread of a multiresistant clone of *Salmonella typhimurium* phage type 66/122 in South-East Asia and the Middle East. *Lancet* **i**: 1070.

Ryan CA, Hargrett-Bean NT, Blake PA (1989). *Salmonella typhi* infections in the United States, 1975–1984: increasing role of foreign travel. *Rev Infect Dis* **11**: 1.

Ryder RW, Blake PA (1979). Typhoid fever in the United States, 1975 and 1976. *J Infect Dis* **139**: 124.

Ryder RW, Blake PA, Murlin AC et al. (1980). Increase in antibiotic resistance among isolates of *Salmonella* in the United States. *J Infect Dis* **142**: 485.

Sabath LD (1969). Current concepts: drug resistance of bacteria. *New Engl J Med* **280**: 91.

Sack CM, Koup JR, Smith AL (1980). Chloramphenicol pharmacokinetics in infants and young children. *Pediatrics* **66**: 579.

Sanborn WR, Lesmana M, Dennis DT et al. (1975). Antibiotic-resistant typhoid in Indonesia. *Lancet* **2**: 408.

Sangster G, Murdoch JMcC, Gray JA (1982). Bacterial meningitis 1940–79. *J Infect* **5**: 245.

Sanson-Le Pors MJ, Casin I, Ortenberg M, Perol Y (1983). *In vitro* susceptibility of thirty strains of *Haemophilus ducreyi* to several antibiotics including six cephalosporins. *J Antimicrob Chemother* **11**: 271.

Saravolatz LD, Pohlod DJ, Quinn EL (1980). Antimicrobial susceptibility of *Legionella pneumophila* serogroups I-IV. *Scand J Infect Dis* **12**: 215.

Schaberg DR, Highsmith AK, Wachsmuth IK (1977). Resistance plasmid transfer of *Serratia marcescens* in urine. *Antimicrob Ag Chemother* **11**: 449.

Schliamser SE, Bächman K, Norrby SR (1988). Intracranial abscesses in adults: an analysis of 54 consecutive cases. *Scand J Infect Dis* **20**: 1.

Schwalbe RS, Hoge CW, Morris JGJr et al. (1990). *In vivo* selection for transmissible drug resistance in *Salmonella typhi* during antimicrobial therapy. *Antimicrob Ag Chemother* **34**: 161.

Schwartzman JD, Reller LB, Wang W-L (1977). Susceptibility of *Clostridium perfringens* isolated from human infections to twenty antibiotics. *Antimicrob Ag Chemother* **11**: 695.

Schwarz S, Cardoso M (1991a). Molecular cloning, purification, and properties of a plasmid-encoded chloramphenicol acetyltransferase from *Staphylococcus haemolyticus*. *Antimicrob Ag Chemother* **35**: 1277.

Schwarz S, Cordoso M (1991b). Nucleotide sequence and phylogeny of a chloramphenicol acetyltransferase encoded by the plasmid p SCS7 from *Staphylococcus aureus*. *Antimicrob Ag Chemother* **35**: 1551.

Scott JL, Finegold SM, Belkin GA, Lawrence JS (1965). A controlled double-blind study of the hematologic toxicity of chloramphenicol. *New Engl J Med* **272**: 1137.

Shamsuddin D, Tuazon CU, Levy C, Curtin J (1982). *Bacillus cereus* panophthalmitis: source of the organism. *Rev Infect Dis* **4**: 97.

Shankaran S, Kauffman RE (1984). Use of chloramphenicol palmitate in neonates. *J Pediatr* **105**: 113.

Shann F, Germer S (1981). Treatment of bacterial meningitis in children without intravenous fluids. *Med J Aust* **1**: 577.

Shann F, Linnemann V, Mackenzie A et al. (1985). Absorption of chloramphenicol sodium succinate after intramuscular administration in children. *New Engl J Med* **313**: 410.

Sharma KB, Bhat MB, Pasricha A, Vaze S (1979). Multiple antibiotic resistance among salmonellae in India. *J Antimicrob Chemother* **5**: 15.

Shaw RG, McLean JA (1957). Chloramphenicol and aplastic aneamia. *Med J Aust* **1**: 352.

Shaw WV, Bouanchaud DH, Goldstein FW (1978). Mechanism of transferable resistance to chloramphenicol in *Haemophilus parainfluenzae*. *Antimicrob Ag Chemother* **13**: 326.

Sheehy TW, Deller JJ Jr, Weber DR (1967). Melioidosis. *Ann Intern Med* **67**: 897.

Shu XO, Gao YT, Linet MS et al. (1987). Chloramphenicol use and childhood leukaemia in Shanghai. *Lancet* **ii**: 934.

Sills JA, McMahon P, Hall E, Fitzgerald T (1983). *Haemophilus influenzae* type b resistant to chloramphenicol and ampicillin. *Brit Med J* **286**: 722.

Simasathien S, Duangmani C, Echeverria P (1980). *Haemophilus influenzae* type b resistant to ampicillin and chloramphenicol in an orphanage in Thailand. *Lancet* **ii**: 1214.

Simberkoff MS, Lukaszewski M, Cross A (1986). Antibiotic-resistant isolates of *Streptococcus pneumoniae* from clinical specimens: a cluster of serotype 19A organisms in Brooklyn, New York. *J Infect Dis* **153**: 78.

Simon HB, Southwick FS, Moellering RC Jr, Sherman E (1980). *Hemophilus influenzae* in hospitalized adults: current perspectives. *Amer J Med* **69**: 219.

Sirera G, Romeu J, Clotet B et al. (1991). Relapsing systemic infection due to *Rhodococcus equi* in a drug abuser seropositive for human immunodeficiency virus. *Rev Infect Dis* **13**: 509.

Slaughter RL, Cerra FB, Koup JR (1980). Effect of hemodialysis on total body clearance of chloramphenicol. *Amer J Hosp Pharm* **37**: 1083.

Smith A, Weber A (1983). Pharmacology of chloramphenicol. *Pediatr Clin North Amer* **30**: 209.

Smith HW (1973). Chloramphenicol resistance in *Escherichia coli. J Med Microbiol* **6**: 347.

Snaveley SR, Hodges GR (1984). The neurotoxicity of antibacterial agents. *Ann Intern Med* **101**: 92.

Snyder MJ, Woodward TE (1970). The clinical use of chloramphenicol. *Med Clin N Amer* **54**: 1187.

Snyder MJ, Perroni J, Gonzalez O *et al.* (1976). Comparative efficacy of chloramphenicol, ampicillin and co-trimoxazole in the treatment of typhoid fever. *Lancet* **2**: 1155.

Snydman DR, Tally FP, Knuppel R *et al.* (1980). *Bacteroides bivius* and *Bacteroides disiens* in obstetrical patients: clinical findings and antimicrobial susceptibilities. *J Antimicrob Chemother* **6**: 519.

Sookpranee M, Boonma P, Susaengrat W *et al.* (1992). Multicenter prospective randomized trial comparing ceftazidime plus co-trimoxazole with chloramphenicol plus doxycycline and co-trimoxazole for treatment of severe melioidosis. *Antimicrob Ag Chemother* **36**: 158.

Sperber SJ,Schleupner CJ (1987). Salmonellosis during infection with human immunodeficiency virus. *Rev Infect Dis* **9**: 925.

Spika JS, Waterman SH, Hoo GWS *et al.* (1987). Chloramphenicol-resistant *Salmonella* newport traced through hamburger to dairy farms. *New Engl J Med* **316**: 565.

Stevens DC, Kleiman MB, Leitman PS, Schreiner RL (1981). Exchange transfusion in acute chloramphenicol toxicity. *J Pediatr* **99**: 651.

Storb R, Thomas ED, Buckner CD (1980). Marrow transplantation in thirty 'untransfused' patients with severe aplastic anemia. *Ann Intern Med* **92**: 30.

Sutherland JM (1959). Fatal cardiovascular collapse of infants receiving large amounts of chloramphenicol. *Amer J Dis Child* **97**: 761.

Sutter VL, Finegold SM (1976). Susceptibility of anaerobic bacteria to 23 antimicrobial agents. *Antimicrob Ag Chemother* **10**: 736.

Suzuki SA, Nakazawa S, Ushioda T (1956). Yearly changes of drug resistance of *Shigella* strains isolated in Kyoto for five years from 1951. *Chemotherapy* **4**: 336; quoted by Farrar and Eidson (1971).

Svenungsson B, Bengtsson E, Fluur E, Siegborn J (1976). Hearing loss as a sequel to chloramphenicol and ampicillin treatment of *Haemophilus influenzae* meningitis. *Scand J Infect Dis* **8**: 175.

Tacquet A, Devulder B, Cuvelier D, Legros J (1974). Pharmacokinetic aspects of thiamphenicol in subjects with normal renal function and in patients with chronic renal insufficiency, with or without haemodialysis. *Postgrad Med J* **50** (Suppl 5): 36.

Tanaka T, Ikemura K, Tsunoda M *et al.* (1976). Drug resistance and distribution of R factors in *Salmonella* strains. *Antimicrob Ag Chemother* **9**: 61.

The Research Committee of BSSI (1995). Bacterial meningitis: causes for concern *J Infect* **30**: 89.

Thomas K, Chan KN, Ribeiro CD (1980). *Campylobacter* jejuni/coli meningitis in a neonate. *Brit Med J* **280**: 1301.

Thompson WL, Anderson SE Jr, Lipsky JJ, Lietman PS (1975). Overdoses of chloramphenicol. *JAMA* **234**: 149.

Thorne GM, Farrar WE Jr (1973). Genetic properties of R factors associated with epidemic strains of *Shigella dysenteriae* type 1 from Central America and *Salmonella typhi* from Mexico. *J Infect Dis* **128**: 132.

Thorne GM, Farrar WE Jr (1974). Superinfection compatibility of R factors in *Shigella dysenteriae* type 1 from Central America and *Salmonella typhi* from Mexico. *J Infect Dis* **130**: 284.

Thornsberry C, Baker CN, Kirven LA (1978). *In vitro* activity of antimicrobial agents on Legionnaires' disease bacterium. *Antimicrob Ag Chemother* **13**: 78.

Threlfall EJ, Ward LR, Rowe B (1978). Spread of multiresistant strains of *Salmonella typhimurium* phage types 204 and 193 in Britain. *Brit Med J* **1**: 997.

Threlfall EJ, Ward LR, Rowe B, Robins-Browne R (1982). Acquisition of resistance by *Salmonella typhi in vivo*: the importance of plasmid characterisation. *Lancet* **i**: 740.

Ti T-Y, Monteiro EH, Lam S, Lee H-S (1990). Chloramphenicol concentrations in sera of patients with typhoid fever being treated with oral or intravenous preparation. *Antimicrob Ag Chemother* **34**: 1809.

Tofte RW, Solliday J, Crossley KB (1984). Susceptibilities of enterococci to twelve antibiotics. *Antimicrob Ag Chemother* **25**: 532.

Toro CS, Lobos SR, Calderon I *et al* (1990). Clinical isolate of a porinless *Salmonella typhi* resistant to high levels of chloramphenicol. *Antimicrob Ag Chemother* **34**: 1715.

Towner KJ, Pearson NJ, O'Grady F (1979). Resistant *Vibrio cholerae* El Tor in Tanzania. *Lancet* **ii**: 147.

Trieu-Cuot P, de Cespédìs G, Bentorcha F *et al.* (1993). Study of heterogenoity of chloramphenicol acetyltransferase (CAT) genes in streptococci and enterococci by polymerase chain reaction: characterization of new CAT determinant. *Antimicrob Ag Chemother* **37**: 2593.

Tuomanen EI, Powell KR, Marks MI *et al.* (1981). Oral chloramphenicol in the treatment of *Haemophilus influenzae* meningitis. *J Pediatr* **99**: 968.

Tupasi TE, Crisologo LB, Torres CA, Calubiran OV (1982). Comparison of spectinomycin, cefuroxime, thiamphenicol and penicillin G in the treatment of uncomplicated gonococcal infections in women. *J Infect Dis* **145**: 583.

Tupasi TE, Crisologo LB, Torres CA *et al.* (1983). Cefuroxime, thiamphenicol, spectinomycin, and penicillin G in uncomplicated infections due to penicillinase-producing strains of *Neisseria gonorrhoeae. Brit J Vener Dis* **59**: 172.

Turk DC (1977). A comparison of chloramphenicol and ampicillin as bacterial agents for *Haemophilus influenzae* type b. *J Med Microbiol* **10**: 127.

Uchiyama N, Greene GR, Kitts DB, Thrupp LD (1980). Meningitis due to *Haemophilus influenzae* type b resistant to ampicillin and chloramphenicol. *J Pediatr* **97**: 421.

Urban T (1972). Transferable multiple drug resistance of *Shigella* strains isolated in Sweden. *Scand J Infect Dis* **4**: 221.

Uwaydah M, Osseiran M (1981). Susceptibility of recent *Shigella* isolates to mecillinam, ampicillin, tetracycline, chloramphenicol and cotrimoxazole. *J Antimicrob Chemother* **7**: 619.

Van Klingeren B, Van Embden JDA, Dessens-Kroon M (1977). Plasmid-mediated chloramphenicol resistance in *Haemophilus influenzae. Antimicrob Ag Chemother* **11**: 383.

Vanhoof R, Vanderlinden MP, Dierickx R *et al.* (1978). Susceptibility of *Campylobacter fetus* subsp. *jejuni* to twenty-nine antimicrobial agents. *Antimicrob Ag Chemother* **14**: 553.

Vatcharapreechasakul T, Suputtamongkol Y, Dance DAB *et al.* (1992). *Pseudomonas pseudomallei* liver abscesses: a clinical laboratory and ultrasonographic study. *Clin Infect Dis* **14**: 412.

Vazquez J, Calderon E, Rodriguez RS (1972). Chloramphenicol-resistance strains of *Salmonella typhosa. New Engl J Med* **286**: 1220.

Vince R, Almquist RG, Ritter CL, Daluge S (1975). Chloramphenicol binding site with analogues of chloramphenicol and puromycin. *Antimicrob Ag Chemother* **8**: 439.

Walker DH (1995). Rocky Mountain Spotted Fever: a seasonal alert. *Clin Infect Dis* **20**: 1111.

Wallerstein RO (1969). Chloramphenicol toxicity. *Lancet* **ii**: 695.

Wallerstein RO, Conduit PK, Kasper CK *et al.* (1969). Statewide study of chloramphenicol therapy and fatal aplastic anemia. *JAMA* **208**: 2045.

Weber DR, Douglas LE, Brundage WG, Stallkamp TC (1969). Acute varieties of melioidosis occurring in US soldiers in Vietnam. *Amer J Med* **46**: 234.

Weisberger AS, Wessler S, Avioli LV (1969). Mechanisms of action of chloramphenicol. *JAMA* **209**: 97.

Weiss CF, Glazko AJ, Weston JK (1960). Chloramphenicol in the newborn infant: a physiologic explanation of its toxicity when given in excessive doses. *New Engl J Med* **262**: 787.

Welch H (1954). *Principles and Practice of Antibiotic Therapy*, p. 205. New York: Medical Encyclopedia Inc.

Werner JC, Whitman V, Schuler HG *et al.* (1985). Acute myocardial effects of chloramphenicol in newborn pigs: a possible insight into the gray baby syndrome. *J Infect Dis* **152**: 344.

West BC, De Vault GAJr, Clement JC, Williams DM (1988). Aplastic anemia associated with parenteral chloramphenicol: review of 10 cases, including the second case of possible increased risk with cimetidine. *Rev Infect Dis* **10**: 1048.

Wexler HM, Finegold SM (1987). Antimicrobial resistance in *Bacteroides*. *J Antimicrob Chemother* **19**: 143.

Whittle HC, Davidson NMcD, Greenwood BM *et al.* (1973). Trial of chloramphenicol for meningitis in Northern Savanna of Africa. *Brit Med J* **3**: 379.

WHO (1974a). Transferable drug resistance in *Salmonella* in South and Central America. *WHO Wkly Epidem Rec* **49**: 65.

WHO (1974b). *Salmonella* surveillance Group H resistance factors in Southern Asia. *WHO Wkly Epidem Rec* **49**: 245.

WHO (1974c). *Salmonella* surveillance. Chloramphenicol-resistant *Salmonella typhi* in Viet-Nam (Rep. of) and Thailand. *WHO Wkly Epidem Rec* **49**: 295.

Wild BE, Pearman JW, Richardson CJL *et al.* (1986). Multiply-antibiotic-resistant *Haemophilus influenzae* type b meningitis in Western Australia. *Med J Aust* **144**: 666.

Willcox PHA (1967). Chloramphenicol. *Brit Med J* **2**: 443.

Williams JD, Andrews J (1974). Sensitivity of *Haemophilus influenzae* to antibiotics. *Brit Med J* **1**: 134.

Winshell EB, Cherubin C, Winter J, Neu HC (1970). Antibiotic resistance of *Salmonella* in the Eastern United States. *Antimicrob Ag Chemother* – **1969**: 86.

Wisseman CL Jr, Ordonez SV (1986). Action of antibiotics on *Rickettsia rickettsii*. *J Infect Dis* **153**: 626.

Wisseman CL Jr, Waddell AD, Walsh WT (1974). *In vitro* studies of the action of antibiotics on *Rickettsia prowazeki* by two basic methods of cell culture. *J Infect Dis* **130**: 564.

Woodward TE, Wisseman CL Jr (1958). *Chloromycetin* (*Chloramphenicol*). New York: Medical Encyclopedia Inc.

Wren BW, Mullany P, Clayton C, Tabaqchali S (1988). Molecular cloning and genetic analysis of a chloramphenicol acetyltransferase determinant from *Clostridium difficile*. *Antimicrob Ag Chemother* **32**: 1213.

Yogev R, Kolling WM, Williams T (1981). Pharmacokinetic comparison of intravenous and oral chloramphenicol in patients with *Haemophilus influenzae* meningitis. *Pediatrics* **67**: 656.

Yunis AA (1974). Concluding remarks International symposium on chloramphenicol-thiamphenicol. *Postgrad Med J* **50** (Suppl5): 149.

Yunis AA, Bloomberg GR (1964). Chloramphenicol toxicity: clinical features and pathogenesis. *Progr Hemat* **4**: 138.

Yunis AA, Smith US, Restrepo A (1970). Reversible bone marrow suppression from chloramphenicol: a consequence of mitochondrial injury. *Arch Intern Med* **126**: 272.

Fusidate Sodium

Description

Fusidic acid, obtained from the fungus *Fusidium coccineum*, has a steroid structure and is chemically related to cephalosporin P, which is one of the antibiotics formed by the mould *Cephalosporium acremonium*. The sodium salt of fusidic acid (sodium fusidate) is used clinically. This antibiotic was developed by Leo Laboratories in Copenhagen.

A number of derivatives of fusidic acid have been prepared, but their antibacterial activity is low compared with sodium fusidate (Godtfredsen et al., 1966).

Sensitive Organisms

1 Gram-positive bacteria

The most significant feature of fusidate sodium is its high degree of activity against *Staphylococcus aureus*, including beta-lactamase producing strains. Resistant strains of *Staph. aureus* can be readily produced by growing the organism in the presence of increasing concentrations of fusidate sodium (Godtfredsen et al., 1962; Hilson, 1962). The development of resistance during treatment, whilst uncommon (Taylor and Bloor, 1962; Rao et al., 1972), has occurred (Amirak et al., 1981). Another important feature about this drug is that it is active against many strains of methicillin-resistant *Staph. aureus* (Garrod, 1968; Hoeprich et al., 1970; Verbist, 1990); reports of fusidic acid resistance in such organisms are, however, increasing (Moorhouse et al., 1985). Also, in 16 of 18 strains tested by Foldes et al. (1983) their MBCs were 4-fold higher than their MICs for fusidate sodium. Usually *Staph. epidermidis*, including methicillin-resistant strains, is also sensitive to fusidate sodium.

Compared with staphylococci, all other aerobic Gram-positive cocci are much less susceptible to fusidate sodium. Enterococcal strains studied by Traub et al. (1986) were inhibited but the drug was not bactericidal. The strains of *Streptococcus pneumoniae* resistant to multiple antibiotics, which were isolated in South Africa in 1977, were only partially resistant (MIC 2 μg per ml) to fusidate sodium (CDC, 1977). Gram-positive anaerobic cocci such as the *Peptococcus* and *Peptostreptococcus* spp. are sensitive. The same is true for Gram-positive bacteria, aerobic and anaerobic, such as *Corynebacterium diphtheriae*, other corynebacteria, *Clostridium tetani*, *Cl. perfringens*, other *Clostridium* spp., including *Cl. difficile* (Verbist, 1990). However, Aronsson et al. (1994) found that *Cl. difficile* was not always very sensitive and that its MICs ranged from 0.5 to 64 μg per ml.

2 Gram-negative bacteria

Gram-negative aerobic bacteria, with the exception of *Neisseria* spp. and *Legionella pneumophila* are sodium fusidate-resistant, but *Bacteroides fragilis*, other members of the *B. fragilis* group and *Prevotella meloninogenica* are usually sensitive. The *Fusobacteria* are resistant (Stirling and Goodwin, 1977; Verbist, 1990).

3 Other organisms

Fusidate sodium has some action against *Mycobacterium tuberculosis*, but this is of no clinical importance (Verbist, 1990). However, the drug is highly active against extracellular and intracellular *M. leprae* (Franzblau et al., 1992). Fusidate sodium has some activity against *Coxiella burnetii* (Torres and Raoult, 1993). The drug inhibited 80–90% of growth of *Plasmodium falciparum* strains in an *in vitro* culture system at levels of 50 μg per ml (Black et al., 1985).

Organisms	Concentrations required for inhibition of 50% of strains
Gram-positive bacteria	
Staphylococcus aureus	0.066
Staphylococcus aureus (beta-lactamase producer)	0.059
Staphylococcus aureus (methicillin-resistant)	0.19
Staphylococcus epidermidis	0.25
Staphylococcus saprophyticus	2.0
Streptococcus pyogenes	6.8
Streptococcus pneumoniae	8.6
Enterococcus faecalis	4.0
Corynebacterium diphtheriae	0.0044
Clostridium tetani	0.016
Gram-negative bacteria	
Escherichia coli	>100.0
Klebsiella pneumoniae	35.0
Neisseria meningitidis	0.56
Bacteroides fragilis	2.0

Table I.43
Compiled from data published by Godtfredsen *et al.* (1962), Richardson and Marples (1980), Guenthner and Wenzel (1984) and Verbist (1990)

4 Minimum inhibitory concentrations

Table I.43 shows the MICs of fusidate sodium against some selected bacterial species. Staphylococci are almost 100-fold more sensitive than most streptococcal species.

Mode of Administration and Dosage

1 Oral administration

Fusidate sodium is usually administered by the oral route. The usual adult dosage is 0.5 g 8-hourly, but for severe infections this dose can be doubled. The recommended dosages for children are up to 1 year of age, 50 mg per kg body weight per day, given in three divided doses; 1–5 years, 250 mg three times daily; 6–12 years 0.5 g three times daily. To reduce dyspepsia it may be taken with meals. Initially sodium fusidate for adults was available in enteric-coated tablets, but now new film-coated tablets are available. Absorption of the drug from the new film-coated tablets is nearly complete, and the serum levels attained are about the same as those attained after i.v. administration (MacGowan *et al.*, 1989; Taburet *et al.*, 1990).

2 Intravenous administration

Previously a special preparation diethanolamine fusidate was available for i.v. administration. This preparation often caused venospasm and thrombosis (Webb *et al.*, 1968). Now a new i.v. preparation of sodium fusidate is available, which also often causes thrombophlebitis, but apparently this problem is not so severe as with the earlier preparation (Portier, 1990). The adult dose of sodium fusidate is 500 mg i.v. 8-hourly. Each dose should be dissolved in 50 ml of sterile buffer, then diluted further in 200–250 ml of normal saline and this should be infused i.v. over 2 h or even longer. The dosage for children is 20 mg per kg body weight daily, administered in three divided doses. Each dose again should be infused slowly (Eykyn, 1990; Portier, 1990; Taburet *et al.*, 1990).

3 Patients with renal failure

Fusidate sodium can be administrated in the usual doses to these patients.

4 Patients with intrahepatic cholestasis

These patients usually have a lower serum albumin. This results in higher serum levels of free unbound fusidate sodium and so there is an increased distribution of the drug in tissues and increased hepatic metabolism. However, the higher bilirubinemia in these patients results in competition with sodium fusidate for the limited glucuronidation mechanism. This compensates for the increased elimination of the drug because of low serum albumin. It therefore appears that sodium fusidate can be administered in the usual doses even to patients with high bilirubinemia. This may not apply to patients with acute liver disease and severe hepatic impairment (Peter et al., 1993).

Serum Levels in Relation to Dosage

After a single oral dose of 0.5 g of the old enteric-coated tablets, the peak serum level was usually achieved in 2 h and it was about 27 μg per ml. The level then gradually fell, and detectable amounts were still present after 24 h (Godtfredsen et al., 1962). These authors also showed that there was considerable individual variation in the amount of the drug absorbed from the alimentary tract. At 1 h the lowest level recorded was 0.7 μg per ml, and the highest 35 μg per ml, and although peak levels at 2 h were more uniform, they still ranged from 14 to 38 μg per ml. With a dosage of 0.5 g 8-hourly, the drug steadily accumulated in the body. After 96 h of such a regimen, a mean serum level of 71 μg per ml was obtained, but some individuals showed serum levels just over 100 μg per ml (Godtfredsen et al., 1962). With a lower dosage of 0.5 g every 12 h, there was usually no accumulation, and the serum concentration soon stabilized at about 20 μg per ml. Stirling and Goodwin (1977) gave two volunteers two oral doses of 1 g at an interval of 6 h, and serum concentrations of 54 and 59 μg per ml, respectively, were obtained.

After a single 500-mg oral dose of the film coated sodium fusidate tablets given to adults, a peak serum level of about 33 μg per ml was attained in 2 h; thereafter the serum level fell with a mean half-life of 16 h. Doubling the doses resulted in double the serum concentration. Food significantly reduced the maximum serum level, but it did not affect the total amount of drug absorbed (MacGowan et al., 1989; Taburet et al., 1990).

After a single i.v. infusion of 500 mg sodium fusidate over 2 h, the peak serum level just after the infusion was 52 μg per ml; if this dose is given i.v. 8-hourly for 3 days, the peak serum level after the last infusion is approximately 123 μg per ml. Thus there is some accumulation of the drug in body with repeated infusions (Taburet et al., 1990).

Excretion

1 Urine

Very little active fusidate sodium is excreted by the kidneys, and only about 1% of the administered dose can be recovered from the urine. After 4 days treatment with standard doses, the urine only contains 0.8 μg per ml or less of the active drug (Godtfredsen et al., 1962).

2 Bile

Some fusidate sodium is excreted and concentrated in bile. A fraction of the administered dose can be recovered in active form from the feces; some of this may be non-absorbed drug, and some presumably due to biliary excretion.

3 Inactivation in body

The total amount of detectable drug excreted in the urine, feces and bile does not account for all of the administered dose. A major proportion of the drug is converted to metabolites in the liver, some of which have weak antibiotic activity (Reeves, 1987).

Distribution of the Drug in Body

Fusidate sodium is well distributed throughout the body. It has been demonstrated in samples of subcutaneous fat, kidney, muscle and prostate taken from patients undergoing surgery a few hours after its administration. Bergeron et al. (1985) found levels in atrial appendages of approximately 11 μg per g of tissue 1 h after a 2-h i.v infusion of 580 mg of diethanolamine fusidate with a resultant mean tissue:serum ratio of 0.33. It also passes through the placenta and can be found in fetal tissue. Very little of the drug is detectable in the CSF of patients with normal meninges. Fusidate sodium is effective even in the presence of large collections of pus, possibly because of its ability to penetrate well into purulent collections (Crosbie, 1963). It also penetrates well into pus of a cerebral abscess (De Louvois et al., 1977), and into the synovial fluid of inflamed joints (Sattar et al., 1983).

In vitro studies suggest that fusidate sodium is very highly protein bound; one study showed that the binding was as high as 97.2% (Rolinson and Sutherland, 1965). The *in vitro* activity of the drug is reduced 64-fold in the presence of 50% serum (Barber and Waterworth, 1962). Despite this very high degree of serum protein binding, the drug is quite effective clinically. This can be partly explained by the wide margin between its MIC for staphylococci and the serum levels achieved after usual doses. The clinical significance of protein binding of antibiotics is discussed on p 95.

Mode of Action

Fusidate sodium is related chemically to cephalosporin P, but the cephalosporin antibiotics (pp.251) are derived from cephalosporin C. In contrast to the cephalosporins, which inhibit bacterial cell wall synthesis, fusidate sodium inhibits bacterial protein synthesis (Harvey *et al.*, 1966), by interfering with the 'G' factor (p. 562) involved in translocation, and possibly by other mechanisms (Tanaka *et al.*, 1968). Mutants resistant to fusidate sodium have an altered 'G' factor (Tanaka *et al.*, 1971). This different mode of action probably explains the lack of cross-resistance between fusidate sodium and the penicillinase-resistant penicillins and cephalosporins. For this reason, methicillin-resistant staphylococci are usually sensitive to fusidate sodium. Inhibition of protein synthesis results in less Protein A on the surface of *Staph. aureus*, rendering the organism more susceptible to phagocytosis (Gemmell and O'Dowd, 1983). Gram-negative bacilli were thought to be fusidate sodium-resistant, probably because the drug could not penetrate their cell walls; fusidate sodium inhibits the protein synthesis of *E. coli* in cell free systems. Bennett and Shaw (1983) showed that one type of plasmid-associated fusidate sodium-resistance in *E. coli* involves binding of the drug to type I chloramphenicol acetyltransferase (p. 562) with consequent 'sequestering' of the drug, and prevention of its attachment to the translational elongation factor G (see above) (Proctor *et al.*, 1983). Results of *in vitro* tests with fusidate sodium illustrate that the distinction between the 'bactericidal' and 'bacteriostatic' drugs is only relative. Some investigators have reported that this drug is mainly bacteriostatic (Hilson, 1962), whereas others have found it bactericidal (Newman *et al.*, 1962). These differing results seem to depend on such factors as the concentration of the drug used, the inoculum size and the sensitivity of the particular *Staph. aureus* strain (p. 580).

Toxicity

In general, fusidate sodium can be regarded as a non-toxic antibiotic. When administered orally, only mild upper gastrointestinal discomfort and diarrhea have been noted. Investigations have failed to show any evidence of renal or hemopoietic toxicity. There is a risk of thrombophlebitis after i.v. administration into a peripheral vein for more than 24 h (Iwarson *et al.*, 1981), but this appears to be less with the newer sodium fusidate i.v. preparation. No severe allergic reactions have been observed, but occasional mild rashes have been reported. The drug appears to be safe in penicillin-allergic patients. Allergic contact dermatitis has been reported after topical fusidate sodium use. In one case this was attributed to formaldehyde in the ointment (Andersen *et al.*, 1983). In chronic infections fusidate sodium has been given for several months without obvious toxic effects (Crosbie, 1963; Dodson, 1963).

It is not known whether fusidate sodium accumulates in the presence of liver disease and therefore it should be used cautiously in patients with impaired liver function. It seems safe in patients with cholestasis (p. 582). Used i.v. the drug does appear to impair liver function. In a group of patients with staphylococcal septicemia treated with i.v. fusidate sodium or other antibiotics, the rates of development of jaundice in these two groups were 34% and 2%, respectively. Of the jaundiced patients, 48% received the old fusidate sodium i.v. compared with 13% by mouth; jaundice appeared within 48 h of commencing this drug in 93%; it was associated with deepening of jaundice in 68% of those with pre-existing jaundice (Humble *et al.*, 1980). When fusidate sodium was stopped, serum bilirubin values fell to normal within 4 days in those who were anicteric before treatment. In six of 32 patients receiving the drug i.v. liver function tests suggested a cholestatic picture; in the remainder, the mechanism of production of jaundice was unknown (Humble *et al.*, 1980; McAreavey and Redding, 1983). The new i.v. sodium fusidate preparation can also cause jaundice; whether it does so less frequently is not yet clear. Some 6% of patients receiving the new film-coated sodium fusidate tablets also have developed jaundice (Eykyn, 1990; Portier, 1990).

Because of its steroid structure it was thought that this drug may possibly have some metabolic effects, unrelated to its antibacterial activity. Wynn (1965) showed that no significant metabolic changes were associated with fusidate sodium administration. It had a mild protein catabolic effect, it lowered urinary calcium excretion, and also caused mild temporary impairment of bromsulphthalein excretion by the liver. It is conceivable that the latter finding may have some relation to the ability of the drug to impair liver function. Human leucocytes incubated with fusidate sodium show markedly depressed migration (Forsgren and Schmeling, 1977). The clinical significance of this observation is unknown. The drug is strongly bound to human albumin (p. 583) and competes with bilirubin for binding sites. It should, therefore, be administered with caution to newborn infants, particularly if premature, icteric or acidotic, in order to avoid the risk of bilirubin encephalopathy induced by displacement of bilirubin from the carrier protein (Brodersen, 1985).

Clinical Uses of the Drug

1 Staphylococcal infections

Treatment of these infections is the main indication for fusidate sodium. It has been used for furunculosis, abscesses, infected wounds or burns, osteomyelitis, pneumonia, septicemia and endocarditis. Most clinical studies show that the results of treatment of these diseases have been good (Crosbie, 1963; Jensen and Lassen, 1964; Matsaniotis et al., 1967; Coombs and Menday, 1985). The introduction of the older parenteral form of fusidic acid in 1969 and later the i.v. sodium fusidate, overcame its previous disadvantage of only being an oral drug. Fusidate sodium given i.v. has been used successfully to treat severe staphylococcal infections (Eykyn, 1990; Portier, 1990). Resistant Staph. aureus strains, which emerge very easily in vitro (p. 580) have appeared in vivo during the treatment of burns (Lowbury et al., 1962), but this has not been a common problem during treatment of other infections. Fusidate sodium has been used alone or in combination with another anti-staphylococcal drug such as cloxacillin for the prolonged treatment of staphylococcal pulmonary infections complicating cystic fibrosis without the emergence of drug-resistance (Norman, 1967; Jensen et al., 1990). Combinations of fusidate sodium and oxacillin or dicloxacillin have also been employed with success to treat Staph. aureus infections in cystic fibrosis patients (Szaff and Høiby, 1982). It is recommended that fusidate sodium should be combined with another antistaphylococcal agent, particularly for treatment of infections due to methicillin-resistant staphylococci (Jensen, 1968; Jensen and Lasen, 1969). Such combinations do not act synergistically, but may prevent the emergence of further drug resistance (Drugeon et al., 1994). This applies to combinations of rifampicin/ fusidate sodium (p. 695) and novobiocin/fusidate sodium (p. 666). Antagonism between fusidate sodium and penicillin G (or one of the semisynthetic penicillins such as methicillin) can be readily demonstrated in vitro with many staphylococcal strains (O'Grady and Greenwood, 1973). Hudson (1985) reported a child with staphylococcal endocarditis who failed to improve with treatment by a combination of fusidate sodium and flucloxacillin, when reasonable bactericidal serum titers were achieved. Clinical improvement occurred only when fusidate sodium was ceased and flucloxacillin was continued alone. In contrast, four infants with staphylococcal neonatal osteomyelitis failed to improve with cloxacillin, surgery and gentamicin treatment and control was only achieved when fusidate sodium was added to the regimen (Bergdahl et al., 1981). Forty-five patients with acute hematogenous osteomyelitis were treated with i.v. cloxacillin and fusidate sodium i.v. for 3 weeks and then orally for another 6 weeks. Only seven patients required operation in addition to this antibiotic therapy (O'Brien et al., 1982). The experience of Coombs (1990) who used fusidate sodium plus flucloxacillin for the treatment of staphylococcal osteomyelitis, was similar. One animal study with induced MRSA endocarditis showed that vancomycin alone was effective and that vancomycin plus sodium fusidate was no better. Fusidate sodium alone was not effective and resistant strains to this drug emerged during therapy (Fantin et al., 1993).

Fusidate sodium is an effective anti-staphylococcal agent but it is not recommended for initial treatment of severe staphylococcal infections. Other drugs such as the penicillinase-resistant penicillins (pp. 97, 105), or cephalothin (p. 258) are preferred. Fusidate sodium may be useful for continuation oral therapy after the acute phase of the illness has responded, but it is mainly a reserve drug for the treatment of infections due to methicillin-resistant strains. Here it is best to combine it with another drug, such as rifampicin (p. 695).

Topical fusidate sodium has been used to treat superficial staphylococcal soft tissue infections (Pakrooh, 1978) and to eradicate the staphylococcal nasal carrier state (Newman et al., 1962). Mackechnie-Jarvis (1985) successfully treated a number of patients with Staph. aureus infections surrounding intramedullary nails with fusidate sodium irrigations; he found this technique enabled him to leave the nail in situ till the fracture had healed. Topical use of the drug is no longer recommended because it encourages the emergence of resistant strains, and thereby compromises its value for the treatment of systemic infections due to methicillin-resistant organisms.

2 Other infections

A combination of rifampicin and fusidate sodium was used to eradicate multiply-resistant strains of *Strep. pneumoniae* in South Africa (p. 5). Oral fusidate sodium in a high dose of 15 mg per kg (up to a maximum of 1.0 g) every 8 h was used to treat five patients successfully with *B. fragilis* infections (Stirling and Goodwin, 1977). Cronberg *et al.* (1984) showed that 0.5 g of fusidate sodium daily appeared to be as effective as vancomycin (p. 779) or metronidazole (p. 949) for the treatment of *Cl. difficile*-induced colitis. A renal transplant patient with a lung abscess from which *L. pneumophila* was grown, failed to respond to erythromycin therapy, but was cured when fusidate sodium was added to the regimen; the MIC of sodium fusidate for the organism was 0.5 µg per ml (Friis-Møller *et al.*, 1985). Sodium fusidate as a single drug was assessed in nine lepromatous leprosy patients. All patients showed clinical improvement; it appeared to be a weakly bactericidal antileprosy agent, which may have a role in multidrug treatment of leprosy (Franzblau *et al.*, 1994).

References

Amirak ID, Li AK, Williams RJ, Noone P (1981). A fatal infection caused by methicillin-resistant *Staphylococcus aureus* acquiring resistance to gentamicin and fusidic acid during therapy. *J Infect* **3**: 50.

Andersen KE, Bundgaard H, Johansen M (1983). Allergic contact dermatitis from formaldehyde in Fucidin ointment. *Contact Dermat* **9**: 78.

Aronsson B, Möllby R, Nord CE (1994). Diagnosis and epidemiology of *Clostridium difficile* enterocolitis in Sweden. *J Antimicrob Chemother* **14** (Suppl D): 85.

Barber M, Waterworth P (1962). Antibacterial activity *in vitro* of fucidin. *Lancet* **i**: 931.

Bennett AD, Shaw WV (1983). Resistance to fusidic acid in *Escherichia coli* mediated by the Type 1 variant of chloramphenicol acetyltransferase. A plasmid-encoded mechanism involving antibiotic binding. *Biochem J* **215**: 29.

Bergdahl S, Elinder G, Eriksson M (1981). Treatment of neonatal osteomyelitis with cloxacillin in combination with fusidic acid. *Scand J Infect Dis* **13**: 281.

Bergeron MG, Desaulniers D, Lessard C *et al.* (1985). Concentrations of fusidic acid, cloxacillin, and cefamandole in sera and atrial appendages of patients undergoing cardiac surgery. *Antimicrob Ag Chemother* **27**: 928.

Black FT, Wildfang IL, Borgbjerg K (1985). Activity of fusidic acid against *Plasmodium falciparum in vitro*. *Lancet* **i**: 578.

Brodersen R (1985). Fusidic acid binding to serum albumin and interaction with binding of bilirubin. *Acta Paediatr Scand* **74**: 874.

CDC (Center for Disease Control) (1977). Multiple-antibiotic resistance of pneumococci – South Africa. *MMWR* **26**: 285.

Coombs RRH (1990). Fusidic acid in staphylococcal bone and joint infection. *J Antimicrob Chemother* **25** (Suppl B): 53.

Coombs RR, Menday AP (1985). Fusidic acid in orthopedic infections due to coagulase-negative staphylococci. *Curr Med Res Opin* **9**: 587.

Cronberg S, Castor B, Thoren A (1984). Fusidic acid for the treatment of antibiotic-associated colitis induced by *Clostridium difficile*. *Infections* **12**: 276.

Crosbie RB (1963). Treatment of staphylococcal infections with 'fucidin'. *Brit Med J* **1**: 788.

De Louvois J, Gortvai P, Hurley R (1977). Antibiotic treatment of abscesses of central nervous systems. *Brit Med J* **2**: 985.

Dodson B (1963). Fusidic acid in the management of phage-type 80 staphylococcal infection. *Lancet* **ii**: 659.

Drugeon HB, Caillon J, Juvin ME (1994). *In vitro* antibacterial activity of fusidic acid alone and in combination with other antibiotics against methicillin-sensitive and -resistant *Staphylococcus aureus*. *J Antimicrob Chemother* **34**: 899.

Eykyn SJ (1990). Staphylococcal bacteraemia and endocarditis and fusidic acid. *J Antimicrob Chemother* **25** (Suppl B): 33.

Fantin B, Leclereq R, Duval J, Carbon C (1993). Fusidic acid alone or in combination with vancomycin for therapy of experimental endocarditis due to methicillin-resistant *Staphylococcus aureus*. *Antimicrob Ag Chemother* **37**: 2466.

Foldes M, Munro R, Sorrell TC *et al.* (1983). *In vitro* effects of vancomycin, rifampicin and fusidic acid, alone and in combination, against methicillin-resistant *Staphylococcus aureus*. *J Antimicrob Chemother* **11**: 21.

Forsgren A, Schmeling D (1977). Effect of antibiotics on chemotaxis of human leukocytes. *Antimicrob Ag Chemother* **11**: 580.

Franzblau SG, Biswas AN, Harris EB (1992). Fusidic acid is highly active against extracellular and intracellular *Mycobacterium leprae*. *Antimicrob Ag Chemother* **36**: 92.

Franzblau SG, Chan GP, Garcia-Ignacio BG *et al.* (1994). Clinical trial of fusidic acid for lepromatous leprosy. *Antimicrob Ag Chemother* **38**: 1651.

Friis-Møller A, Rechnitzer C, Nielsen L, Madsen S (1985). Treatment of *Legionella* lung abscess in a renal transplant recipient with erythromycin and fusidic acid. *Eur J Clin Microbiol* **4**: 513.

Garrod LP (1968). Methicillin-resistant staphylococci. *Lancet* **ii**: 871.

Gemmell CG, O'Dowd A (1983). Regulation of Protein A synthesis in *Staphylococcus aureus* by certain antibiotics: its effect on phagocytosis by leukocytes. *J Antimicrob Chemother* **12**: 587.

Godtfredsen WO, Roholt K, Tybring L (1962). Fucidin: a new orally active antibiotic. *Lancet* **i**: 928.

Godtfredsen WO, Albrethsen C, Daehne WV *et al.* (1966). Transformations of fusidic acid and the relationship between structure and antibacterial activity. *Antimicrob Ag Chemother* **1965**: 132.

Guenthner SH, Wenzel RP (1984). *In vitro* activities of teichomycin, fusidic acid, flucloxacillin, fosfomycin, and vancomycin against methicillin-resistant *Staphylococcus aureus*. *Antimicrob Ag Chemother* **26**: 268.

Harvey CL, Knights SG, Sih CJ (1966). On the mode of action of fusidic acid. *Biochemistry* **5**: 3320.

Hilson GRF (1962). *In vitro* studies of a new antibiotic (Fucidin). *Lancet* **i**: 932.

Hoeprich PD, Benner EJ, Kayser FH (1970). Susceptibility of methicillin resistant *Staphylococcus aureus* to 12 antimicrobial agents. *Antimicrob Ag Chemother* **1969**: 104.

Hudson SJ (1985). Treatment of bacterial endocarditis. *Lancet* **i**: 1249.

Humble MW, Eykyn S, Phillips I (1980). Staphylococcal bacteremia, fusidic acid and jaundice. *Brit Med J* **280**: 1495.

Iwarson S, Fasth S, Olaison L, Hulten L (1981). Adverse reactions to intravenous administration of fusidic acid. *Scand J Infect Dis* **13**: 65.

Jensen K (1968). Methicillin-resistant staphylococci. *Lancet* **ii**: 1078.

Jensen K, Lassen HCA (1964). Fulminating staphylococcal infections treated with fucidin and penicillin or semisynthetic penicillin. *Ann Intern Med* **60**: 790.

Jensen K, Lassen HCA (1969). Combined treatment with antibacterial chemotherapeutical agents in staphylococcal infections. *Quart J Med New Ser 38* **149**: 91.

Jensen T, Lanng S, Faber M *et al.* (1990). Clinical experiences with fusidic acid in cystic fibrosis patients. *J Antimicrob Chemother* **25** (Suppl B): 45.

Lowbury EJL, Cason JS, Jackson D *et al.* (1962). Fucidin for staphylococcal infection of burns. *Lancet* **ii**: 478.

MacGowan AP, Greig MA, Andrews JM *et al.* (1989). Pharmacokinetics and tolerance of a new film-coated tablet of sodium fusidate administered as a single oral dose to healthy volunteers. *J Antimicrob Chemother* **23**: 409.

Mackechnie-Jarvis AC (1985). Simple wound irrigation system to treat staphylococcal infection of intramedullary nails. *Lancet* **i**: 1035.

McAreavey D, Redding PJ (1983). Staphylococcal septicemia complicated by probable cloxacillin neurotoxicity and by jaundice induced by fusidic acid. *Scot Med J* **28**: 179.

Moorhouse EC, Mulvihill TE, Jones L *et al.* (1985). The *in vitro* activity of some antimicrobial agents against methicillin-resistant *Staphylococcus aureus*. *J Antimicrob Chemother* **15**: 291.

Newman RL, Bhat KM, Hackney R *et al.* (1962). Fusidic acid; laboratory and clinical assessment. *Brit Med J* **2**: 1645.

Norman AP (1967). Fusidic acid in cystic fibrosis. *Lancet* **ii**: 516.

O'Brien T, McManus F, MacAuley PH, Ennis JT (1982). Acute haematogenous osteomyelitis. *J Bone Jt Surg* **64**: 450.

O'Grady F, Greenwood D (1973). Interactions between fusidic acid and penicillins. *J Med Microbiol* **6**: 441.

Pakrooh H (1978). A comparison of sodium fusidate ointment ('Fucidin'). alone versus oral antibiotic therapy in soft tissue infections. *Curr Med Res Opin* **5**: 289.

Peter J-D, Jehl F, Pottecher T *et al.* (1993). Pharmacokinetics of intravenous fusidic acid in patients with cholestasis. *Antimicrob Ag Chemother* **37**: 501.

Portier H (1990). A multicentre, open, clinical trial of a new intravenous formulation of fusidic acid in severe staphylococcal infections. *J Antimicrob Chemother* **25** (Suppl B): 39.

Proctor GN, McKell J, Rownd RH (1983). Chloramphenicol acetyltransferase may confer resistance to fusidic acid by sequestering the drug. *J Bacteriol* **155**: 937.

Rao R, Webster ABD, Sunderland DR *et al.* (1972). Cloxacillin and sodium fusidate in management of shunt infections. *Brit Med J* **3**: 618.

Reeves DS (1987). The pharmacokinetics of fusidic acid. *J Antimicrob Chemother* **20**: 467.

Richardson JF, Marples RR (1980). Differences in antibiotic susceptibility between *Staphylococcus epidermidis* and *Staphylococcus saprophyticus*. *J Antimicrob Chemother* **6**: 499.

Rolinson GN, Sutherland R (1965). The binding of antibiotics to serum proteins. *Brit J Pharmacol* **25**: 638.

Sanford MD, Widmer AF, Bale MJ *et al.* (1994). Efficient detection and long-term persistence of the carriage of methicillin-resistant *Staphylococcus aureus*. *Clin Infect Dis* **19**: 1123.

Sattar MA, Barrett SP, Cawley MI (1983). Concentrations of some antibiotics in synovial fluid after oral administrations, with special reference to antistaphylococcal activity. *Ann Rheum Dis* **42**: 67.

Stirling J, Goodwin S (1977). Susceptibility of *Bacteroides fragilis* to fusidic acid. *J Antimicrob Chemother* **3**: 522.

Szaff M, Høiby N (1982). Antibiotic treatment of *Staphylococcus aureus* infection in cystic fibrosis. *Acta Paediatr Scand* **71**: 821.

Taburet AM, Guibert J, Kitzis MD *et al.* (1990). Pharmacokinetics of sodium fusidate after single and repeated infusions and oral administration of new formulation. *J Antimicrob Chemother* **25** (Suppl B): 23.

Tanaka N, Kinoshita T, Masukawa H (1968). Mechanism of protein synthesis inhibition by fusidic acid and related antibiotics. *Biochem Biophys Res Commun* **30**: 278.

Tanaka N, Kawano G, Kinoshita T (1971). Chromosomal location of a fusidic acid resistant marker in *Escherichia coli. Biochem Biophys Res Commun* **42**: 564.

Taylor G, Bloor K (1962). Antistaphylococcal activity of fucidin. *Lancet* **i**: 935.

Torres H, Raoult D (1993). *In vitro* activities of ceftriaxone and fusidic acid against 13 isolates of *Coxiella burnetii*, determined using the shell vial assay. *Antimicrob Ag Chemother* **37**: 491.

Traub WH, Spohr M, Bauer D (1986). *Streptococcus fecalis: in vitro* susceptibility to antimicrobial drugs, single and combined, with and without defibrinated human blood. *Chemotherapy* **32**: 270.

Verbist L (1990). The antimicrobial activity of fusidic acid. *J Antimicrob Chemother* **25** (Suppl B): 1.

Webb J, Wilson HG, Rao A (1968). Staphylococcal endocarditis treated by intravenous administration of fusidic acid and penicillin. *Med J Aust* **1**: 131.

Wynn V (1965). Metabolic effects of the steroid antibiotic fusudic acid. *Brit Med J* **1**: 1400.

Lincomycin and Clindamycin

Description

Lincomycin was isolated from a strain of *Streptomyces lincolnensis* in the Upjohn Research Laboratories (Lewis *et al.*, 1963). The drug is not chemically related to erythromycin, but there are certain similarities between lincomycin and the antibiotics of the macrolide group. Many chemical modifications of the lincomycin molecule have been developed (lincosamides) in an attempt to produce an improved antibiotic. Of these, clindamycin (7-chloro-7-deoxylincomycin), was the most promising (Magerlein *et al.*, 1967) and this drug is clinically superior to lincomycin. Initially in North America the generic name of clinimycin was adopted for this compound, but now the name clindamycin is used universally. The information below will only apply to clindamycin.

Sensitive Organisms

The antibacterial spectrum of clindamycin is rather similar to that of erythromycin, with some important differences.

1 Gram-positive aerobic bacteria

Clindamycin is active against most of these bacteria. *Staphylococcus aureus* (including beta-lactamase-producing strains), coagulase-negative staphylococci, *Streptococcus pyogenes*, Groups B, C and G streptococci, *Strep. pneumoniae*, *Strep. viridans* and *Strep. bovis* are usually susceptible. Unlike erythromycin, this drug is inactive against *Enterococcus faecalis*. Of the other enterococci, *E. faecium* is resistant but *E. durans* is sensitive (Karchmer *et al.*, 1975). *Corynebacterium diphtheriae* is highly sensitive to clindamycin (Zamiri and McEntegart 1972). *Bacillus anthracis*, *B. cereus* and the *Nocardia* spp. are sensitive (Keusch and Present, 1976; Gigantelli *et al.*, 1991).

In clinical practice sensitivity testing is still commonly not performed on the usually clindamycin-sensitive streptococci, but resistant strains have been detected amongst all these species. *Streptococcus pyogenes* resistant to clindamycin has been reported (Kohn and Evans, 1970; Drapkin *et al.*, 1976; Jenssen *et al.*, 1987). Similarly some strains of Group B streptococci are clindamycin-resistant (Jenssen *et al.*, 1987). Strains of *Strep. pneumoniae* resistant to clindamycin (and erythromycin) have been detected (Champion *et al.*, 1978; Liñares *et al.*, 1983). The penicillin G-resistant pneumococci, isolated in South Africa during 1977 (p. 5), were also resistant to clindamycin (CDC, 1977). Multiply-resistant pneumococci, susceptible to beta-lactam antibiotics, but resistant to erythromycin, clindamycin, co-trimoxazole and tetracycline were also reported from South Africa (Klugman *et al.*, 1986). In many areas of the world, such as South Africa and Spain (p. 5), penicillin G-resistant pneumococci are now also clindamycin-resistant, but in most areas in the USA they are still clindamycin-sensitive (Nelson *et al.*, 1994). Strains of the *viridans* group of streptococci, resistant to clindamycin (usually also to erythromycin) have been isolated from the mouth sockets of recently removed teeth and blood of patients receiving these drugs (Phillips *et al.*, 1976).

Staphylococci resistant to clindamycin are more common, and sensitivity testing is always indicated in clinical practice. As with erythromycin (p. 607), staphylococci resistant to clindamycin can be easily produced *in vitro*, and may occasionally emerge during treatment *in vivo*. Methicillin-resistant strains of *Staph. aureus* (p. 80) are now often resistant to clindamycin (Reeves *et al.*, 1991).

Most clindamycin-resistant Gram-positive bacteria are also resistant to erythromycin and other macrolides and type-B streptogramins. This is known as MLS-resistance. These MLS antibiotics share a common or overlapping binding site in the ribosome. A ribosomal mutation makes the ribosome insensitive to all these antibiotics. Expression of MLS-resistance in Gram-positive cocci may be constitutive or inducible. When expression is constitutive, the strains are resistant to all macrolides, all lincosomides (including clindamycin) and streptogramin B-type antibiotics. When expression is inducible, the strains are resistant to erythromycin, roxithromycin, oleandomycin and azithromycin only (Weisblum, 1995). Clindamycin remains active. This dissociated resistance is due to differences in the inducing abilities of the various MLS antibiotics. *Staphylococcus aureus* and other staphylococci can also owe their resistance to clindamycin due to enzymatic inactivation of the drug; the enzyme production is specified by small non-conjugative plasmids. The third resistance mechanism to clindamycin involves active efflux of the antibiotic from the periplasmic space (p. 26). This mainly occurs in Gram-negative bacteria (Courvalin *et al.*, 1985; Arthur *et al.*, 1987; Jenssen *et al.*, 1987; Quiros *et al.*, 1988; Leclercq and Courvalin, 1991a,b). In the laboratory clindamycin resistance of staphylococci can be overlooked if the test is done by clindamycin; testing with lincomycin is more reliable (Leclercq *et al.*, 1987).

In previous studies with lincomycin, which may also apply to clindamycin, it was shown that if erythromycin-resistant and erythromycin-sensitive *Staph. aureus* strains were passaged in the presence of lincomycin, the erythromycin-resistant strains rapidly became lincomycin-resistant, whereas the erythromycin-sensitive ones slowly developed a lesser degree of lincomycin-resistance (Duncan, 1968; McGehee *et al.*, 1969). Lincomycin also exhibited the 'dissociated type of resistance' (p. 607) characteristic of the macrolides, i.e. strains of *Staph. aureus.* resistant to erythromycin but sensitive to lincomycin were found to be lincomycin-resistant, if tested in the presence of erythromycin (Barber and Waterworth, 1964). These phenomena can be explained by the mode of action of lincomycin, clindamycin and the macrolides (p. 614). It was then advised that lincomycin should not be selected for the treatment of infections due to *Staph. aureus* strains which are erythromycin-resistant but sensitive to lincomycin because lincomycin-resistance may develop *in vivo* (Duncan, 1968). The same almost certainly applies to clindamycin.

2 Gram-positive anaerobic bacteria

Clostridium tetani and *Cl. perfringens* are sensitive; so is *Cl. septicum* (Gabay *et al.*, 1981). However, some *Cl. perfringens* strains and strains of less common human pathogens, such as *Cl. sporogenes*, *Cl. tertium*, *Cl. bifermentans*, *Cl. novyi*, *Cl. ramosum* and *Cl. sordelli*, may be clindamycin-resistant (Wilkins and Thiel, 1973; Staneck and Washington, 1974; Dornbusch *et al.*, 1975; Sutter and Finegold, 1976). Amongst the other anaerobic Gram-positive organisms, the *Peptococcus, Peptostreptococcus, Eubacterium, Propionibacterium, Bifidobacterium* and *Lactobacillus* spp. are usually sensitive (Sutter and Finegold, 1976; Denys *et al.*, 1983). *Peptostreptococcus* spp. strains, resistant to clindamycin, have been reported (Reig *et al.*, 1982b). Bayer *et al.* (1978) showed that whilst 98% of 40 strains of *Lactobacillus* spp. were inhibited by 5 μg per ml of clindamycin or less, such levels were only bactericidal for less than one-fifth of these strains. The same phenomenon was found to exist with penicillin G, only one-quarter of the strains having an MBC within achievable serum concentrations. A synergistic combination such as a penicillin G and an aminoglycoside (p. 13) may therefore be necessary to achieve a cure in some infections caused by lactobacilli. Most strains of *Actinomyces israelii* are sensitive to clindamycin (Sutter and Finegold, 1976; Holmberg *et al.*, 1977). Similarly *Bifodobacterium* and *Eubacterium* spp. or usually clindamycin-sensitive (Brook and Frazier, 1993). *Clostridium difficile* may be clindamycin-sensitive or -resistant and the proportion of sensitive strains has varied from 10% to 90% in different studies (Levett, 1988). During outbreaks of diarrhea associated with *Cl. difficile*, the strains are usually clindamycin-resistant and they contain a plasmid, probably located on the chromosome. This codes for transferable macrolide-lincosamide-streptogramin B (MLS) resistance (p. 587). This resistance can be transferred from *Cl. difficile* to *Staph. aureus* (Hächler *et al.*, 1987; Clabots *et al.*, 1988). In one study almost all of 161 isolates of *Cl. difficile* of serogroups A, F, G, H and X were susceptible to clindamycin and other antibiotics, but 32 toxigenic isolates of serogroup C were clindamycin-resistant (Delmèe and Avesani, 1988).

3 Gram-negative aerobic bacteria

Practically all the aerobic Gram-negative bacteria are resistant to clindamycin. A difference between this drug and erythromycin is that bacteria, such as *Neisseria meningitidis, N. gonorrhoeae* and *Haemophilus influenzae* which are characteristically sensitive to erythromycin are clindamycin-resistant (McGehee *et al.*, 1968; Klainer, 1987). Some authors have found that clindamycin is more active against *H. influenzae* than lincomycin *in vitro* (Geddes *et al.*, 1970), but clinical results have usually been disappointing. *Campylobacter jejuni* is sensitive to clindamycin (Michel *et al.*, 1983), but as with erythromycin (p. 609), *Campylobacter coli* is much more resistant with 90% of strains requiring 128 μg per ml for inhibition compared with a value of 8 μg per ml for *Campylobacter jejuni* (Elharrif *et al.*, 1985). *Capnocytophaga canimorosus* (DF-2), a slowly growing Gram-negative bacillus, which is associated with bacteremic illness and dog bites or other animal exposure, particularly in the immunocompromized, is clindamycin-sensitive (Findling *et al.*, 1980). The *Flavobacteria* may be clindamycin-sensitive (Sheridan *et al.*, 1993). Of 21 different antibiotics, tested by McCarthy *et al.* (1979), erythromycin and clindamycin had the greatest inhibitory effect on *Gardnerella vaginalis*, a microaerophilic organism (p. 947).

4 Gram-negative anaerobic bacteria

An important property of clindamycin is that it has good activity against the *Bacteroides fragilis* group of anaerobic bacteria. Early studies showed that most strains of these bacteria were inhibited by 2 μg per ml or less of clindamycin (Kislak, 1972; Bodner *et al.*, 1972; Sutter *et al.*, 1973; Zabransky *et al.*, 1973). Gradually over the years a proportion of these bacteria have become clindamycin-resistant. In general *B. fragilis* has remained more sensitive to clindamycin than other members of the *B. fragilis* group (p. 295), such as *B. thetaiotaomicron*, *B. ovatus*, and *B. vulgatus* and *B. distasonis* (Fox and Phillips, 1987; Betriu *et al.*, 1990; Appleman *et al.*, 1991; Tanaka-Bandoh *et al.*, 1995). In one survey in the USA only 5% of isolates of bacteria of the *B. fragilis* group were clindamycin-resistant (Cuchural *et al.*, 1988). In another survey in Los Angeles resistance to clindamycin ranged from 8% to 22% among species and was most common among isolates of *B. distasonis* and *B. thetaiotaomicron* (Appleman *et al.*, 1991). In a study in Detroit, clindamycin-resistance was detected in 38% of the *B. fragilis* group, which was a marked increase from the 4% detected 10 years ago at the same institution (Brown, 1988). In an early survey in UK, clindamycin-resistance was uncommon; only 1% of *B. fragilis* strains and 10% of other *B. fragilis* isolates were resistant (Fox and Phillips, 1987). In a more recent Canadian study 7.3% of *B. fragilis* strains and 9.4% of non-*B. fragilis* strains were clindamycin-resistant (Turgeon *et al.*, 1994). Similarly in France resistance among the *B. fragilis* strains was lower (9.5%) than among the other species of *B. fragilis* group (20.3%), the highest incidence of resistance (23%) was recorded for *B. distasonis* strains (Patey *et al.*, 1994). Resistance patterns of these bacteria to clindamycin may vary widely between various countries and also between institutions in the same city (Bawdon *et al.*, 1979). In one children's hospital in the USA, where clindamycin had been extensively used to treat intra-abdominal infections, 62% of *B. fragilis* group isolates and 13% of *B. fragilis* strains were clindamycin-resistant (Citron *et al.*, 1995). One *B. fragilis* strain has been reported, which was resistant to metronidazole, imipenem and co-amoxiclav, but this was clindamycin-sensitive (Turner *et al.*, 1995).

Clindamycin is quite active against other Gram-negative anaerobes such as *Prevotella disiens* and *Prevotella melaninogenica* and the *Fusobacterium* spp. (Sutter and Finegold, 1976; Sutter, 1977; Leigh, 1981). *Bacteroides gracilis*, which normally resides in the oral cavity, may be clindamycin-sensitive, but some strains are resistant (Lee *et al.*, 1993).

In addition to the above commonly encountered Gram-negative anaerobic bacteria there is also a group of motile Gram-negative anaerobic bacilli which belong to genera such as *Butyrivibrio*, *Succinimonas*, *Anaerovibrio* and other genera. Some, but not all of these bacteria are sensitive to clindamycin (Johnson and Finegold, 1987).

The mechanism of *Bacteroides* spp. resistance to clindamycin is usually due to a change in the target ribosome which leads to erythromycin, clindamycin and streptogramin B-resistance, similar to the mechanism in Gram-positive bacteria (p. 587) (Fletcher and Macrina, 1991; Jimenez-Diaz *et al.*, 1992; Reig *et al.*, 1992a). The resistance gene in *Bacteroides* spp. can be located in plasmids or on the chromosome; it can be transferred between species by a plasmid or transposon (Privitera *et al.*, 1979, 1981; Tally and Malamy, 1986; Halula and Macrina, 1990).

Because there are clinical indications to combine clindamycin with an aminoglycoside, the interactions of these drugs against Gram-negative bacteria have been studied *in vitro*. Fass *et al.* (1974) did not detect antagonism between clindamycin and gentamicin, but found synergism with some strains of Enterobacteriaceae (a number being resistant to both drugs) and *Pseudomonas aeruginosa*. Leng *et al.* (1975) used combinations of either clindamycin or erythromycin with gentamicin or colistin against Enterobacteriaceae and *Ps. aeruginosa* and also demonstrated synergism and no antagonism. Klastersky and Husson (1977) demonstrated that gentamicin did not interfere with activity of clindamycin against *B. fragilis*, and that clindamycin did not influence the activity of gentamicin against *Escherichia coli*.

Organism	MIC (μg per ml)	
	Range	Median
Gram-positive bacteria		
Staphylococcus aureus	0.04–0.8	0.1
Streptococcus pyogenes	0.02–0.1	0.04
Streptococcus pneumoniae	<0.002–0.04	0.01
Streptococcus viridans	0.005–0.04	0.02
Enterococcus faecalis	12.5–>100.0	100.0
Gram-negative bacteria		
Escherichia coli	>100.0	>100.0
Neisseria meningitidis	6.3–25.0	12.5
Haemophilus influenzae	6.3–50.0	12.5
Bacteroides fragilis	<0.25–>256.0	4.0[a]

[a] MIC for 90% of strains

Table I.44
After McGehee *et al.* (1968), Tally *et al.* (1985)

5 Other organisms

The mycoplasma and *Ureaplasma urealyticum* are clindamycin-resistant (McGehee *et al.*, 1968). Clindamycin alone has some activity against *Chlamydia trachomatis* (MICs 0.25–2.0 μg per ml) (p. 598) Rice *et al.*, 1995). Furthermore the drug is synergistic with an aminoglycoside such as gentamicin, and the combination may be useful clinically (Pearlman *et al.*, 1990). *Coxiella burnetii* is apparently sensitive (Geddes, 1983). The leptospirae appear to be susceptible to lincomycin (and probably also to clindamycin) when tested in experimental animals (Lewis *et al.*, 1963). Clindamycin is much less active than erythromycin or penicillin G for the treatment of established syphilitic lesions on rabbits (Brause *et al.*, 1976).

The true fungi and *Mycobacterium tuberculosis* are clindamycin-resistant. But clindamycin shows some activity against *M. leprae* (Franzblau, 1991). The combination of clindamycin and primaquine is effective in both *in vitro* and *in vivo* models of *Pneumocystis carinii* infection (Queener *et al.*, 1988; Smith, 1991). Clindamycin is effective in animals infected with chloroquine-resistant and -sensitive *Plasmodium falciparum* (Powers and Jacobs, 1972). It is also effective against *Pl. vivax*, but not against the exo-erythrocytic parasites (Keusch and Present, 1976). Clindamycin is effective in experimental toxoplasmosis in mice (Araujo and Remington, 1974). In cultured mammalian cells clindamycin reduces the level of replication of *Toxoplasma gondii*, it affects the protein synthesis of free parasites and it also impairs the ability of the parasite to infect host cells. Mutants of *T. gondii*, resistant to clindamycin, can be selected and these usually show cross-resistance to spiromycin (p. 630) and azithromycin (p. 654) (Pfefferkorn *et al.*, 1992; Blais *et al.*, 1993 Pfefferkorn and Borotz, 1994; Fichera *et al.*, 1995).

6 Minimum inhibitory concentrations

The *in vitro* activity of clindamycin is not affected by variations in the size of the inoculum (Meyers and Kaplan, 1969), and in contrast to erythromycin, clindamycin does not become less active when the pH is lowered by the addition of carbon dioxide to the system (Kislak, 1972). The MICs of clindamycin for some selected bacterial species are shown in Table I.44.

Mode of Administration and Dosage

1 Oral administration

The hydrochloride salt of clindamycin is used orally. A dosage of 150 mg every 6 h is recommended for adults, but this may be increased to 300 mg or 450 mg 6-hourly for the treatment of serious infections. Two dosage ranges are recommended for children depending on the severity of the infection, 8–16 mg or 16–20 mg per kg body weight per day, each given in three or four divided doses. Clindamycin is not recommended for infants aged less than 1 month. The ester clindamycin palmitate hydrochloride is available as a suspension for administration to children and elderly patients who are unable to swallow capsules. This is a water soluble compound which is hydrolyzed *in vivo* to the active base. The dosage of this preparation is similar to that of clindamycin hydrochloride.

2 Parenteral administration

Clindamycin is poorly soluble in solutions at neutral pH and it is too irritating for parenteral use so that an ester, clindamycin-2-phosphate, is used for i.m. and i.v. administration. The i.m. dosage for adults is 0.6–2.4 g per day, depending on the severity of the infection, given in two to four divided doses. For i.v. infusion clindamycin phosphate must be diluted at least one part to 25 parts of infusion solution, and depending on the volume, this is infused over a period of 20–45 min. For example, a 600-mg dose (available in 4 ml) should be diluted to 100 ml and infused over a minimum period of 20 min. The administration of more than 1.2 g i.v. in a single hour infusion is not recommended. The adult i.v. dose is 0.9–2.7 g per day, depending on the severity of the infection, given in two to four divided doses. Buchwald *et al.* (1989) compared the adult dosage for serious infections of 600 mg 6-hourly with 600 mg 8-hourly. Both dosages were equal in efficacy, but the patients who received the 6-hourly regimen had more side-effects. It was concluded that 600 mg 8-hourly is the optimal dosage for patients with serious infections. The administration of clindamycin phosphate i.v. at 12-hourly intervals has been investigated. Plaisance *et al.* (1989), after a pharmacokinetic study, concluded that i.v. clindamycin in a dosage of 1.2 g 12-hourly would probably be unsatisfactory, but Flaherty *et al.* (1988) thought that such regimen would probably be suitable and that it may represent an alternative dosing strategy for clindamycin.

For children over 1 month old a dosage of 15–40 mg per kg body weight per day, depending on the severity of the infection, is given in two to four divided doses. Others have suggested that infants at term, and also those older than 4 weeks or weighing more than 3.5 kg should receive 20 mg per kg per day in four divided doses. For premature neonates, a schedule of 5 mg per kg every 8 h has been recommended (Bell *et al.*, 1984).

3 Patients with renal failure

Although some clindamycin is excreted in urine, its main excretion pathway is probably by the liver (p. 593). The clindamycin half-life (normally about 3 h) is not appreciably altered in patients with only moderate renal functional impairment (Eastwood and Gower, 1974; Malacof *et al.*, 1975; Peddie *et al.*, 1975; Keusch and Present, 1976). For patients with mild to moderate renal failure, no dosage adjustments of clindamycin are necessary (Eastwood and Gower, 1974; Peddie *et al.*, 1975). In functionally anephric patients, Malacoff *et al.* (1975) found that the peak serum levels were about 2-fold greater than those expected in normal patients after the same parenteral dosage. They therefore recommended that half the normal dose should be used in such patients. Clindamycin is not significantly removed by hemodialysis (Eastwood and Gower, 1974; Peddie *et al.*, 1975) or by peritoneal dialysis (Malacoff *et al.*, 1975).

4 Patients with liver disease

Some studies have indicated that the clindamycin half-life might be prolonged up to 5-fold in patients with severe liver disease (Brandl *et al.*, 1972; Keusch and Present, 1976), but Hinthorn *et al.* (1976) only found a 39% increase in patients with cirrhosis. Williams *et al.* (1975) studying patients with moderate to severe hepatic dysfunction detected serum levels which were nearly 3-fold higher than those found in patients with normal liver function. There was also an association between the serum levels after 5 h and the degree of elevation of the SGOT. Eng *et al.* (1981) were unable to confirm the latter relationship; they found that there was a direct correlation between the serum half-life and the indirect bilirubin level, provided there were no factors contributing to increased production of bilirubin and there was no extra hepatic obstruction. These results indicate that clindamycin serum levels should be monitored in patients with liver disease, because sometimes appropriate dosage reduction may be necessary.

Serum Levels in Relation to Dosage

1 Oral administration

Clindamycin is well absorbed from the gastrointestinal tract, and peak serum levels occur 1–2 h after administration. Following a single 150-mg oral dose to adults, peak serum levels are in the range 2.5–3.0 μg per ml (Peddie *et al.*, 1975). Peak levels after oral doses of 300 and 600 mg are about 4 and 8 μg per ml, respectively (Keusch and Present, 1976) (Fig. I.23). Furthermore, the presence of food in the stomach does not significantly impair the absorption of clindamycin (McGehee *et al.*, 1968; Wagner *et al.*, 1968). Higher serum levels occur when clindamycin is

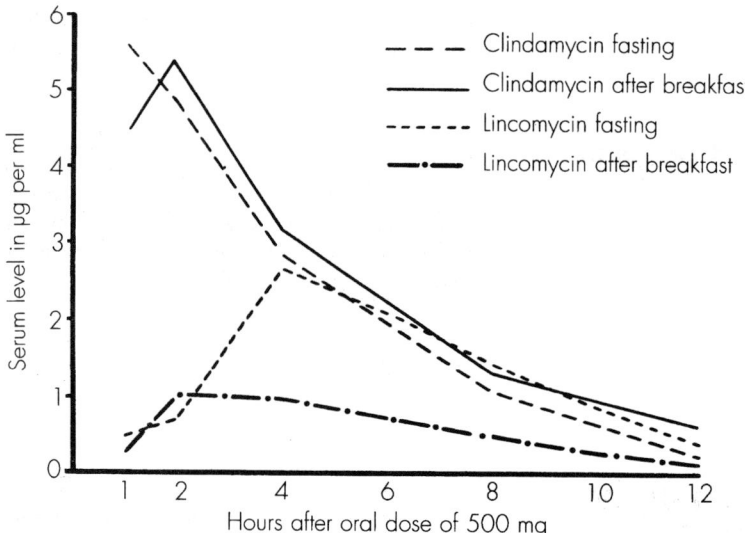

Fig. I.23.
Effect of food on serum concentrations
of lincomycin and clindamycin after oral
administration. (Redrawn after
McGehee *et al.*, 1968, with permission.)

given orally to patients with celiac disease, jejunal diverticulosis and Crohn's disease (Keusch and Present, 1976). Also in AIDS patients the bioavailability of orally administered clindamycin is some 1.5-fold higher than in normal patients (Gatti *et al.*, 1993). The ester, clindamycin palmitate hydrochloride, is also well absorbed from the gastrointestinal tract, and serum levels attained with this compound are nearly the same as those with clindamycin capsules (Campbell *et al.*, 1973).

2 Parenteral administration

Satisfactory serum levels are attained with i.m. or i.v. administration of clindamycin-2-phosphate. Following a 300-mg i.m. dose a mean peak level of 4.9 µg per ml is attained at 2.5 h and this falls to 2.8 µg per ml 8 h after administration. Diabetic patients tend to have lower serum clindamycin levels after i.m. administration (Fass and Saslaw, 1972); a similar phenomenon occurs with penicillin G (p. 22). The i.v. infusion of 300 mg over a 30-min period results in a mean peak serum level of 14.7 µg per ml, which falls to 4.9 µg per ml at 2–4 h, and to 3.9 µg per ml 8 h after the infusion (Fass and Saslaw, 1972). Serum levels varying from 2.6 to 26.0 µg per ml after a 300-mg dose, and from 6 to 29.0 µg per ml after a 600-mg dose, both given by infusions over a period of 30–40 min, were detected in patients treated by Hugo *et al.* (1977). Doses of 5 mg per kg given three or four times daily as 30-min i.v. infusions to neonates (premature and term) less than 28 days old resulted in mean peak serum levels of 10.92 and 10.45 µg per ml, respectively; similar doses in infants between 4 weeks and 1 year resulted in a mean peak serum level of 12.69 µg per ml (Bell *et al.*, 1984).

Excretion

1 Urine

Some clindamycin is excreted in urine (Brown *et al.*, 1975). After a single oral dose of this drug administered either fasting or after food, 13% of the administered dose can be recovered from the urine in the active form within 24 h (McGehee *et al.*, 1968). In contrast, in severe renal disease, less than 1% of the active drug may be detected in the urine in 24 h (Peddie *et al.*, 1975). Williams *et al.* (1975) found an increased urinary excretion after i.v. clindamycin in patients with severe hepatic dysfunction, suggesting that the kidneys may have some compensatory excretory ability in patients with liver disease. In those with normal renal function, high urinary concentrations of clindamycin are obtained with the usual doses. The urinary activity is due to a mixture of the unchanged drug and the presence of active metabolites (see below).

With parenteral clindamycin administered to adults every 8 h, 8% of an i.m. dose and 28% of an i.v. dose are recovered from the urine during the 8 h after each injection or infusion (Fass and Saslaw, 1972). In premature and term infants less than 4 weeks old 14–16% of an i.v. dose is recoverable in the urine and this increases to 22.8% for infants between 1 and 12 months of age (Bell *et al.*, 1984). The renal excretion of clindamycin is important clinically, because in the presence of severe renal impairment, dosage reduction of this drug is necessary (p. 591).

2 Bile

Clindamycin appears to be extensively eliminated by hepatic mechanisms. Biliary levels of 48 and 55 µg per ml of clindamycin have been detected in two patients receiving an i.v. dosage of 600 mg every 6 h (Williams *et al.*, 1975).

3 Inactivation in body

The excretion of clindamycin in urine and bile does not account for all of the administered dose, and a substantial proportion of the drug appears to be inactivated in the body, presumably mainly in the liver. Active metabolites (N-demethyl clindamycin and clindamycin sulfoxide) and inactive metabolites are excreted in urine. Clindamycin is metabolized at an increased rate in children (Leading article, 1975).

4 Feces

After a single oral dose of clindamycin, less than 5% of the active drug is excreted in the feces (Keusch and Present, 1976).

Distribution of the Drug in Body

Clindamycin is well distributed in the body. Concentrations in saliva are similar to those in serum (Keusch and Present, 1976), and in gingival crevicular fluid they remained in excess of MICs for regional flora for more than 6 h (Walker *et al.*, 1981). Satisfactory levels were reached in the sputum of patients with purulent chest infections (Raeburn and Devine, 1971). In their review, Keusch and Present (1976) considered that penetration of clindamycin into the central nervous system and the eye was poor. However, Shamsuddin *et al.* (1982) reported successful treatment of *Bacillus cereus* panophthalmitis with clindamycin, and earlier work with rabbits demonstrated that good levels could be achieved in ocular tissues (Tabbara and O'Connor, 1975).

High biliary concentrations of clindamycin occur (see above) after i.v. clindamycin phosphate, and these may be two to three times higher than the serum levels (Brown *et al.*, 1976). However, in the presence of obstruction of the common bile duct, no drug could be detected in the bile, and there was reduced clindamycin in the gallbladder wall, but concentrations were a little higher in the liver than in patients with no obstruction. Clindamycin penetrated well into the ascitic fluid of patients with bacterial peritonitis (Gerding *et al.*, 1977). It also penetrated well into the base of decubitus ulcers, 80% of tissue samples having levels higher than 2.5 µg per g after an i.v. infusion of 600 mg over 10 min (Berger *et al.*, 1978). Clindamycin also penetrated well in the infected tissue in diabetics with infected feet (Duckworth *et al.*, 1993). After i.v. administration of clindamycin phosphate, the concentration of clindamycin in fundal mucosa and gastric juice was 1.5 to 2-fold higher than the serum concentrations. The accumulation in the stomach of the drug occurred against a concentration gradient, suggesting that an active process was involved (Hextall *et al.*, 1994). The findings in an animal study were similar (Westblom *et al.*, 1990).

Following the administration of six doses of 600 mg of clindamycin every 8 h to patients undergoing colorectal surgery, levels in feces rose steadily to greater than 200 µg per g on day 5; measurable effects on the colonic microflora were present 24 h after the first dose. Mean mucosal tissue level was 10.3 µg per g at less than 1 h (Kager *et al.*, 1981). Clindamycin crosses the placenta (Philipson *et al.*, 1973). Some clindamycin is also found in breast milk (Chow and Jewesson, 1985). The drug penetrates well into bone (Dornbusch *et al.*, 1977; Summersgill *et al.*, 1982). There is a marked uptake of clindamycin by the alveolar macrophages of smokers (compared with non-smokers) to attain an antibiotic concentration more than 50 times that of the extracellular fluid (Hand *et al.*, 1985).

Clindamycin promotes *in vitro* phagocytosis and killing of *E. coli* by polymorphonuclear leukocytes (Bassaris *et al.*, 1984, 1987). Others have shown that the drug increases the opsonization, complement fixation and phagocytosis of other bacteria (Howard and Soucy, 1983; Milatovic *et al.*, 1983; Gemmell, 1984). Intracellular killing by neutrophils of a clindamycin-resistant strain of *Staph. aureus* was, however, modestly increased when the patient was treated with this drug; one possibility for this apparent synergy with intracellular killing mechanism would be the increase in the intracellular concentration of clindamycin (Faden *et al.*, 1985). Jacobs and Wilson (1983) are among many who have shown an increased uptake by neutrophils of clindamycin (and chloramphenicol and trimethoprim) compared with penicillin G, and a relationship between this phenomenon and increased intracellular killing of *H. influenzae* and *Staph. aureus*. Anderson *et al.* (1986) suggested that it was the interaction between the intracellular killing systems and the antibiotic within the phagocytes which resulted in the beneficial bacteriostatic effect of clindamycin against intracellular *Staph. aureus*. However, other authors have shown that clindamycin, which is markedly concentrated in human polymorphonuclear leukocytes, exhibits poor activity against intraphagocytic *Staph. aureus* and other bacteria, such as *Actinobacillus actinomycetemcomitans*, *Eikenella corrodens* and *Capnocytophaga ochracea*, the latter three species being bacteria which cause peridontal disease (Hand and King-Thompson, 1986; Baker and Wilson, 1988; Hand *et al.*, 1990).

Clindamycin is about 60% bound to serum proteins (Eastwood and Gower, 1974).

Mode of Action

Clindamycin inhibits bacterial protein synthesis and acts specifically on the 50S subunit (p. 562) of the bacterial ribosome, most likely by affecting the process of peptide chain initiation (p. 562) (Reusser, 1975). It may also stimulate dissociation of peptidyl-tRNA from ribosomes (Menninger and Coleman, 1993). *Escherichia coli* exposed to subminimal inhibitory concentrations of clindamycin shows less adherence to buccal mucosal cells, and this may be a consequence of this suppression of protein synthesis (Bassaris *et al.*, 1984).

Presumably it is suppression of protein synthesis which also enabled Sanders *et al.* (1983) to show that clindamycin is an effective *in vitro* inhibitor of the derepression of bacterial beta-lactamases which would otherwise have been produced by certain non-fastidious Gram-negative bacilli exposed to various beta-lactam antibiotics (p. 322). Similarly, Schlievert and Kelly (1984) showed inhibition of toxin production in toxic shock syndrome-producing strains of *Staph. aureus* (p. 98) by levels of clindamycin which do not inhibit bacterial growth.

Toxicity

1 Gastrointestinal side-effects

Clindamycin administration results in changes in intestinal microflora. Numbers of enterococcal spp. increase and all anaerobes decrease (Nord and Heimdahl, 1986). Oral or parenteral administration of clindamycin may cause nausea, vomiting, abdominal cramps and diarrhea. A metallic taste in the mouth may follow i.v. administration of clindamycin. Esophageal ulceration due to temporary lodgement of a clindamycin capsule in the lower esophagus has been reported (Sutton and Gosnold, 1977). The mechanism of mucosal damage in this case was similar to that which occurs with the tetracyclines (p. 734).

2 Pseudomembranous colitis

It was first observed that lincomycin-induced diarrhea may occasionally be severe, simulate acute ulcerative colitis, and persist for 1 or 2 weeks after the drug is stopped (Kaplan and Weinstein, 1968). Subsequently, there were numerous reports on the occurrence of pseudomembranous colitis following oral or parenteral lincomycin administration (Benner and Tellman, 1970; Scott *et al.*, 1973; Le Frock *et al.*, 1975; Gibson *et al.*, 1975; Clark *et al.*, 1976; Munk *et al.*, 1976). Despite the early emphasis on pseudomembranous colitis, it was soon recognized that this was the severe end of a spectrum of disease in which the most common clinical presentation was a self-limiting diarrhea (Bartlett, 1985, 1990, 1992, 1994). Most patients improve spontaneously when the implicated antibiotic is discontinued (Young *et al.*, 1985; Kelly *et al.*, 1994). Severe diarrhea and pseudomembranous colitis have also occurred in association with oral or parenteral clindamycin therapy (Cohen *et al.*, 1973; Tedesco *et al.*, 1974; Dallos, 1975; Gibson *et al.*, 1975; Le Frock *et al.*, 1975; Friedman *et al.*, 1976; Lemos *et al.*, 1976; Gurwith *et al.*, 1977; Lusk *et al.*, 1977; Neu *et al.*, 1977; Robertson *et al.*, 1977; Swartzberg *et al.*, 1977;). In early retrospective and prospective studies the frequency of clindamycin-associated diarrhea varied from 0.3 to 21% and for pseudomembranous colitis from 1.9 to 10%. In many early reports there appeared to be a geographical clustering of cases (Kabins and Spira, 1975), a greater frequency in older age groups and in patients who had undergone abdominal surgery (Clark *et al.*, 1976; Kappas *et al.*, 1978). In most instances, clindamycin diarrhea and colitis were more common after oral than parenteral therapy but were not related to the duration of therapy.

Symptoms of colitis associated with clindamycin may be mild and may resolve without any specific treatment. If pseudomembranous colitis is present the diarrhea is frequently profuse and watery, but rectal bleeding is uncommon. It may be associated with cramping abdominal pain. A neutrophil leucocytosis is common. The disease may be complicated by dehydration, hypotension and hypoalbuminemia, toxic megacolon, colonic perforation and fatalities have also occurred (Fekety and Shah, 1993; Kelly *et al.*, 1994). In patients who had a laparotomy, a baggy dilated colon associated with ascites was found (Wells, 1974). Sigmoidoscopy, proctoscopy or colonoscopy may only reveal a non-specific colitis with a red edematous and friable mucosa (Gibson *et al.*, 1975), but the diagnostic feature of pseudomembranous colitis, white-yellow raised plaques of variable size are usually visible. These plaques can sometimes be felt on digital examination. They consist of fibrin, mucus, epithelial debris and polymorphs. Underlying dilated mucous glands are often present in the mucosa. The plaques may slough, and ulcerate into the muscle coat. Price and Davies (1977) considered that the earliest pathological lesion was focal epithelial necrosis or irregularity with polymorphs, and an eosinophilic exudate in the lamina propria. Barium studies showed widening and distortion of haustral folds, irregularities, ulceration, thumb-printing and a cobble-stone appearance (Le Frock et al., 1975; Bartlett, 1992). Recovery usually occurred within three weeks of stopping the drug but prolonged diarrhea and relapses were also reported (Lambert, 1975; Swartzberg et al., 1977). Early treatment was symptomatic; i.v. fluid therapy in severe cases and some patients underwent subtotal colectomy (Boyd and Denbesten, 1976). Corticosteroids were of no value.

Pseudomembranous colitis is not a new disease and it had been described in the pre-antibiotic era (Keusch and Present, 1976; Gorbach and Bartlett, 1977). It was often associated with colonic obstruction (especially due to carcinoma) or as a sequel to abdominal surgery. It has long been recognized that antibiotics may be associated with the development of pseudomembranous colitis (Reiner et al., 1952; Goulston and McGovern, 1965). Pseudomembranous colitis has been described after the use of almost all antibiotics except vancomycin. Apart from clindamycin, the most commonly implicated drugs have been ampicillin, amoxycillin and the cephalosporins (Bartlett, 1992). That an identical clinical picture could be caused by a variety of antibiotics and perhaps by physiological alterations in the bowel, indicated a common etiological factor in this disease. Clustering of cases suggested the possibility of an infective agent.

A variety of possibilities were considered for the etiology of pseudomembranous colitis until Larson et al. (1977) detected a cytopathogenic toxin in the feces of patients with the disease. At first this heat-labile toxin was thought to be elaborated from Clostridium sordelli (Rifkin et al., 1977; Larson and Price, 1977), but it was later shown to be produced by Cl. difficile (Bartlett et al., 1978; Burdon and George, 1978; George et al., 1978a,b). Following this description of Cl. difficile as an enteric pathogen capable of causing disease mainly in the presence of antibiotic exposure, swift progress followed. Within 2 years a good diagnostic assay of the toxin was developed, the clinical and pathological spectrum of the disease was described and the risk factors and the characterization of two toxins (A and B) to account for the pathophysiologic events were defined. The toxins may also be involved in the etiology of non-antibiotic pseudomembranous colitis (Gerding, 1989; Kelly et al., 1994). Clostridium difficile appears to be commonly present as a normal inhabitant of the gut but this may vary geographically, accounting for differences in the reported frequency of pseudomembranous colitis. In hospitals and nursing homes, Cl. difficile spores exist as environmental pathogens, and patients in these institutions receive antibiotics and become colonized by Cl. difficile. This accounts for the outbreaks of pseudomembranous colitis which have occurred in hospitals and long-term care institutions. Increased age and more severe underlying illness were associated more commonly with Cl. difficile carriage and diarrhea (McFarland et al., 1990; Simor et al., 1993; Samore et al., 1994b). In hospitals the patients infected should be nursed with routine enteric precautions (Bartlett, 1992). But high incidence of nosocomial Cl. difficile diarrhea does not necessarily indicate a clonal epidemic as often a diversity of Cl. difficile strains are involved (Samore et al., 1994a).

In addition to the antibiotics, Cl. difficile colitis has also been caused by antineoplastic chemotherapy. These chemotherapeutic agents can alter the normal bowel flora, cause intestinal inflammatory changes, which potentiate both the growth of Cl. difficile and it production of toxin (Anand and Glatt, 1993).

There are several biotypes of Cl. difficile some of which are non-toxigenic. Normally the growth of Cl. difficile is limited by other intestinal bacteria and insignificant amounts of the toxins are produced. Following the administration of antibiotics (or possibly after altered bowel physiology), the organism multiplies and produces larger amounts of the toxins. The exact mechanisms of action of these toxins on the bowel wall is still not fully understood. Often Cl. difficile is resistant to penicillins, cephalosporins, aminoglycosides, clindamycin, tetracycline and erythromycin (George et al., 1978a). Only a percentage of strains may be resistant to clindamycin (Larson et al., 1978). The survival of this organism in the gut at the expense of other intestinal organisms explains the occurrence of pseudomembranous colitis after the use of antibiotics. The main method used nowadays for the diagnosis of Cl. difficile colitis is the demonstration of Cl. difficile toxins in the stools. This is done by a tissue culture assay (Bartlett, 1994; Kelly et al., 1994).

Clostridium difficile may be sensitive to metronidazole, sulfonamides, vancomycin (George et al., 1978a), bacitracin (Chang et al., 1980) and fusidic acid (Cronberg et al., 1984). Most of these drugs have now been used to treat patients with pseudomembranous colitis who did not improve after ceasing antibiotics (Keighley *et al.*, 1978; Tedesco *et al.*, 1978; Cherry *et al.*, 1982; Teasley *et al.*, 1983; Bartlett, 1984; Cronberg *et al.*, 1984; Young *et al.*, 1985). Vancomycin is the preferred treatment for patients who are seriously ill (p. 779). For those less seriously ill, oral metronidazole (p. 949) is usually recommended (Gerding, 1989; Fekety and Shah, 1993; Bartlett, 1994). Replacing the colonic flora has been suggested, and successfully employed, using either lactobacilli or other preparations (Fekety and Shah, 1993).

The problem of relapse after treatment with vancomycin (p. 780) was first reported by George *et al.* (1979) but has been subsequently reported to occur at a frequency ranging between 5 and 55% (Bartlett, 1985). It appears that the phenomenon may be attributable to a failure to eradicate the organism, perhaps associated with its ability to sporulate under adverse conditions. Relapses are unpredictable but may occur more frequently in the elderly and those who have undergone abdominal surgery (Young *et al.*, 1986). Relapses may respond to a second or third course of the same antibiotic as before, or one of the alternative therapies (Schwan *et al.*, 1984; Bartlett, 1985). Toxin A produced by *Cl. difficile*, binds to epithelial cells within the intestine which results in destruction of these cells. This destruction is the crucial step leading to development of diarrhea and thereafter the potent cytotoxin B can gain access to underlying tissues and cause further damage. Various synthetic oligosaccharides bind to toxin A. They have been shown to neutralize toxin A from stool samples, and they could serve as a potential therapy for *Cl. difficile*-associated diarrhea (Heerze *et al.*, 1994).

3 Hypersensitivity reactions

Rashes may occur with clindamycin (Levison *et al.*, 1974), and in one study they occurred with a surprisingly high frequency of 10% (Geddes *et al.*, 1970). Drug fever and eosinophilia may occur with clindamycin and one case of Stevens-Johnson syndrome has been attributed to it (Fulghum and Catalano, 1973). Clindamycin is not cross-allergenic with the penicillins, and may be safely used in penicillin-allergic patients.

4 Hepatotoxicity

Minor abnormalities of liver function tests, such as an elevated SGOT level, have been observed in patients receiving clindamycin (Fass and Saslaw, 1972; Levison *et al.*, 1974; Williams *et al.*, 1975). Rarely, jaundice has been associated with clindamycin therapy (Elmore *et al.*, 1974; Levison *et al.*, 1974). Clindamycin has been given parenterally to patients with liver disease without causing aggravation (Williams *et al.*, 1975; Hinthorn *et al.*, 1976). Elevations of SGOT levels occurring with i.m. clindamycin may not be due to hepatotoxicity but to injection-produced muscle damage (Fass and Saslaw, 1972). In addition, McGehee *et al.* (1968) showed that some of the apparently elevated SGOT levels observed in patients receiving clindamycin were due to interference with the colorimetric method of estimating SGOT, by the drugs or their metabolites. If the SGOT was measured by a specific enzymatic method, no elevations could be detected. Similar observations have been made in patients receiving erythromycin estolate.

5 Side-effects from parenteral clindamycin

Clindamycin administered i.v. by the recommended method is quite safe, but with high doses phlebitis can be a problem. Clindamycin given i.m. is usually well tolerated and injections are relatively painless.

6 Miscellaneous side-effects

Neutropenia has been occasionally noted in patients receiving clindamycin. The safety of clindamycin in pregnancy has not been established, but to date there is no evidence that it is harmful.

Clinical Uses of the Drug

1 Staphylococcal infections

Clindamycin is effective even in severe staphylococcal infections, but it is not regarded as the drug of first choice (Geddes *et al.*, 1970; Fass and Saslaw, 1972). Many authors consider that the drug is particularly effective for staphylococcal osteomyelitis and septic arthritis (Kosmidis *et al.*, 1973; Finch *et al.*, 1975; Rodriguez *et al.*, 1977; Geddes *et al.*, 1977). Staphylococcal infections in patients with cystic fibrosis were successfully treated with clindamycin: clearing was obtained more frequently in those with mild or moderate pulmonary disease (Shapera *et al.*, 1981). Clindamycin has been used to treat staphylococcal endocarditis with some success but several failures have been described due to the development of *in vivo* resistance (Burch *et al.*, 1976; Watanakunakorn, 1976; Cherubin and Nair, 1978; Scheld *et al.*, 1982).

Staphylococcus epidermidis infections can also be treated by clindamycin, provided that the strain is clindamycin-sensitive. Furthermore, studies in an *in vitro* model have shown that subinhibitory concentrations of clindamycin may have a role in the prevention of microbial adherence to vascular catheters (Khardori *et al.*, 1991).

2 Streptococcal and pneumococcal infections

Clindamycin may be indicated occasionally in these infections for patients allergic to penicillin G and the cephalosporins. Oral clindamycin 75 mg two or three times daily may be substituted for oral penicillin V for prophylaxis against rheumatic fever (Massell, 1979). Clindamycin has been used successfully for the treatment of *Strep. pyogenes* throat and skin infections and pneumococcal pneumonia (Geddes *et al.*, 1970; Newel, 1970; Lines *et al.*, 1973; Breese *et al.*, 1974, Dillon and Derrick, 1975). Clindamycin usually cures clinically and bacteriologically streptococcal pharyngitis, if there has been a clinical or bacteriological failure after 10 days of penicillin V treatment. The explanation may be that this treatment selects beta-lactamase-producing bacterial species in the throat, which leads to treatment failure due to inactivation of the penicillin V (Orrling *et al.*, 1994; Nord, 1995). Clindamycin, compared with penicillin G, also more effectively reduces the frequency of encapsulation of *Strep. pyogenes*, the latter being a known virulence factor of this organism (Brook *et al.*, 1995).

In experimental streptococcal myositis, clindamycin has demonstrated a superior efficacy to penicillin G (Stevens *et al.*, 1988). Poor results in cases of severe *Strep. pyogenes* myositis in humans have been reported with penicillin G treatment (Stevens, 1994). The same may be true for Group A streptococcal necrotizing fasciitis, and some authors prefer clindamycin to penicillin G (p. 35) for the treatment of this disease (Brogan *et al.*, 1995). It is possible that large doses of i.v. clindamycin may sometimes succeed in treatment of pneumococcal meningitis caused by strains with some degree of penicillin G-resistance, but this would only be the case if the strain is clindamycin-sensitive (p. 587). A few cases of pneumococcal endocarditis have been successfully treated with i.v. clindamycin (Keane and Rose, 1973). *Streptococcus viridans* endocarditis also responds to parenteral clindamycin (Freeman and Roberts, 1976).

Clindamycin also appears useful for the treatment of chronic suppurative ear infections, mainly because both aerobic and anaerobic bacteria are usually involved (Cooke and Raghuvaran, 1974; Brook, 1994).

3 Diphtheria

A 7-day course of oral clindamycin (or erythromycin) was just as effective as a single injection of benzathine penicillin G in eradicating *C. diphtheriae* from the nasopharynx of asymptomatic carriers (McCloskey *et al.*, 1974).

4 Clostridium perfringens infections

Studies in experimental animals have shown that clindamycin is superior to penicillin G (p. 49) for the treatment of this disease (Stevens *et al.*, 1987a,b, 1993). This may be because in addition to its antibacterial properties, clindamycin is a potent suppressor of bacterial toxin synthesis and it also has immunomodulatory effects (Stevens *et al.*, 1995).

5 Actinomycosis

This disease has been successfully treated with prolonged clindamycin therapy. It may be the most satisfactory alternative to penicillin G in penicillin allergic patients (Fass and Saslaw, 1972; Rose and Rytel, 1972).

6 Gram-negative anaerobic bacterial infections

In clinical practice mixed aerobic/anaerobic infections occur most frequently. In aspiration pneumonia and lung abscess Gram-positive aerobes such as *Staph. aureus* and *Strep. pyogenes* are involved, as well as Gram-positive anaerobes (*Peptococcus* spp.) and Gram-negative anaerobes such as *Prevotella melaninogenica* and *Fusobacterium* spp. In the past penicillin G (p. 38) was considered as the drug of choice for these infections, but many of the Gram-negative anaerobes involved now produce beta-lactamases and penicillin G plus clindamycin or clindamycin alone now is a much better treatment option (Brook, 1979; Levison *et al.*, 1983; Finegold and Wexler, 1988; Lode, 1988, Tally, 1988; Bartlett, 1993).

In intra-abdominal infections the pathogens involved are *B. fragilis*, other members of the *B. fragilis* group and Gram-negative aerobes such as the Enterobacteriaceae. A combination of clindamycin and an aminoglycoside such as gentamicin, is effective for these infections (Bartlett *et al.*, 1977; Heseltine *et al.*, 1983; Nichols, 1983; Tally, 1988; Nichols and Smith, 1993; McClean *et al.*, 1994). However, nowadays many alternatives are available such as metronidazole/gentamicin (p. 947), chloramphenicol/gentamicin (p. 569), cefoxitin (p. 308), cefotetan (p. 396), ceftizoxime (p. 340), imipenem/cilastatin (p. 236), ticarcillin/clavulanic acid (p. 202), ampicillin/sulbactam (p. 214) and piperacillin/tazobactam (p. 224). If in a given area clindamycin-resistant strains of *B. fragilis* are encountered, it is best to select one of the alternatives and not clindamycin/gentamicin (McClean *et al.*, 1994). One patient recovered from intra-abdominal infection and empyema with clindamycin/gentamicin, when the *B. fragilis* strain involved was resistant to metronidazole, co-amoxiclav and imipenem, but sensitive to clindamycin (Turner *et al.*, 1995).

Clindamycin is also useful for *B. fragilis* septicemia (Bartlett *et al.*, 1972; Douglas and Kislak, 1973; Mitchell and Simpson, 1973; Fry *et al.*, 1979) and septic arthritis (Rosenkranz *et al.*, 1990). Clindamycin/gentamicin, despite its inferior activity against *Chlamydia trachomatis*, is as satisfactory treatment for pelvic inflammatory disease as cefoxitin/doxycycline (p. 45) (Peterson *et al.*, 1990). Clindamycin, often combined with another drug is also useful in other mixed aerobic/anaerobic infections, such as sepsis associated with decubitus ulcers (Chow *et al.*, 1977), foot infections in diabetics, chronic sinusitis, space infections in neck, Ludwigs angina, peridontal abscess, suppurative cholangitis, liver abscess, septic abortion and osteomyelitis (Bamberger *et al.*, 1987; Tally, 1988; Nord, 1995).

7 Capnocytophaga canimorosus (DF-2) septicemia

Clindamycin has been used successfully to treat the fulminant septicemia that may follow a dog bite causing infection with this organism in splenectomized patients (Kalb *et al.*, 1985).

8 Acne

Some authors have found clindamycin, in a small dose of 150 mg daily, beneficial for this condition (Leading article, 1973). Other have used clindamycin topically as a 1% lotion with apparently good effect (Adams *et al.*, 1981) and in another study, twice-daily topical applications of 1% clindamycin phosphate were more successful in reducing inflammation in this condition than oral tetracycline 500 mg twice-daily (Braathen, 1985).

9 Q-fever endocarditis

Clindamycin has been sometimes added to a tetracycline for the treatment of this disease (p. 749).

10 Toxoplasmic encephalitis in patients with the acquired immunodeficiency syndrome

Clindamycin in a dosage of 600 mg four times daily plus pyrimethamine 75 mg once-daily is an acceptable alternative to sulfadiazine/pyrimethamine for the treatment of this disease. Initial studies in animal models suggested that clindamycin may have a role in the treatment of toxoplasmosis (Hofflin and Remington, 1987; Piketty *et al.*, 1990; Filice and Pomeroy, 1991). Subsequent clinical studies have confirmed that approximately 70% of AIDS patients with this disease respond to clindamycin/pyrimethamine therapy. Patients who have early neurologic deterioration despite this treatment or who do not improve neurologically after 10–14 days should be considered candidates for brain biopsy (Leport *et al.*, 1989; Dannemann *et al.*, 1991; Foppa *et al.*, 1991; Katlama, 1991; Ruf and Pohle, 1991; Luft and Remington, 1992; Luft *et al.*, 1993).

11 Pneumocystis carinii pneumonia

The combination of clindamycin and primaquine is effective for the treatment of *Pneumocystis carinii* pneumonia in AIDS patients. This combination has been usually only given to patients with mild to moderate pneumonia. The value of this treatment has mainly been established in open trials, but in a few comparative studies for mild to moderate *P. carinii* pneumonia it has been as effective as standard treatment with co-trimoxazole (p. 874). Rash has been the most commonly observed adverse effect, but this usually resolved despite continued therapy. Some 5–10% of patients developed diarrhea and leukopenia. Methemoglobinemia was common with doses of 30 mg of primaquine a day, but it did not exceed 20%, did not cause significant symptoms and did not necessitate discontinuation of treatment. Primaquine cannot be used in patients who have glucose-6-phosphate dehydrogenase deficiency. The clindamycin/primaquine treatment should usually be administered for over 3 weeks. The recommended dosage is primaquine 15–30 mg daily and clindamycin 600 mg 8-hourly or 600 mg 6-hourly. Clindamycin can be given i.v. initially, but for many patients this is unnecessary. Such clindamycin/primaquine therapy has proven to be well tolerated and effective for mild to moderate cases of *P. carinii* pneumonia (Toma *et al.*, 1989, 1993; Black *et al.*, 1991, 1994; Ruf *et al.*, 1991; Noskin *et al.*, 1992; Vildé and Remington, 1992).

12 Malaria

Clindamycin is effective treatment for *Pl. falciparum* malaria, but it produces a rather slow response. In endemic areas it has been used with some success for the treatment of uncomplicated falciparum malaria, either as a single drug or in combination with quinine. For semi-immune patients it has also been used in combination with doxycycline. Clindamycin should not be prescribed for non-immune patients and it also is not suitable for treatment of severe complicated falciparum malaria (Kremsner *et al.*, 1988, 1989; Kremsner, 1990). But in one clinical trial of severe falciparum malaria in children a 4-day regimen of quinine plus clindamycin proved to be slightly superior to standard 7-day quinine regimen (Kremsner *et al.*, 1995).

References

Adams SJ, Cooke EM, Cunliffe WJ (1981). The use of oral and topical antibiotics in acne. *J Antimicrob Chemother* 7 (SupplA): 75.

Anand A, Glatt AE (1993). *Clostridium difficile* infection associated with antineoplastic chemotherapy: a review. *Clin Infect Dis* 17: 109.

Anderson R, Joone G, Van Rensburg CEJ (1986). An *in vitro* investigation of the intracellular bioactivity of amoxicillin, clindamycin and erythromycin for *Staphylococcus aureus*. *J Infect Dis* 153: 593.

Appleman MD, Heseltine PNR, Cherubin CE (1991). Epidemiology, antimicrobial susceptibility, pathogenicity, and significance of *Bacterioides fragilis* group organisms isolated at Los Angeles County – University of Southern California Medical Center. *Rev Infect Dis* 13: 12.

Araujo FG, Remington JS (1974). Effect of clindamycin on acute and chronic toxoplasmosis in mice. *Antimicrob Ag Chemother* 5: 647.

Arthur M, Brisson-Noel A, Courvalin P (1987). Origin and evolution of genes specifying resistance to macrolide, lincosamide and streptogramin antibiotics: data and hypotheses. *J Antimicrob Chemother* 20: 783.

Baker PJ, Wilson ME (1988). Effect of clindamycin on neutrophil killing of Gram-negative periodontal bacteria. *Antimicrob Ag Chemother* 32: 1521.

Bamberger DM, Daus GP, Gerding DN (1987). Osteomyelitis in the feet of diabetic patients. Long-term results, prognostic factors, and the role of antimicrobial and surgical therapy. *Amer J Med* 83: 653.

Barber M, Waterworth PM (1964). Antibacterial activity of lincomycin and pristinamycin: a comparison with erythromycin. *Brit Med J* 2: 603.

Bartlett JG (1984). Treatment of antibiotic-associated pseudomembranous colitis. *Rev Infect Dis* 6 (Suppl): 235.

Bartlett JG (1985). Treatment of *Clostridium difficile* colitis. *Gastroenterology* 89: 1192.

Bartlett JG (1990). *Clostridium difficile*: clinical considerations. *Rev Infect Dis* 12 (Suppl 2): 243.

Bartlett JG (1992). Antibiotic-associated diarrhea. *Clin Infect Dis* 15: 573.

Bartlett JG (1993). Anaerobic bacterial infections of the lung and pleural space. *Clin Infect Dis* 16 (Suppl 4): 248.

Bartlett JG (1994). *Clostridium difficile*: history of its role as an enteric pathogen and the current state of knowledge about the organism. *Clin Infect Dis* 18 (Suppl 4): 265.

Bartlett JG, Sutter VL, Finegold SM (1972). Treatment of anaerobic infection with lincomycin and clindamycin. *New Engl J Med* 287: 1066.

Bartlett JG, Miao PVW, Gorbach SL (1977). Empiric treatment with clindamycin and gentamicin of suspected sepsis due to anaerobic and aerobic bacteria. *J Infect Dis* 135 (Suppl): 80.

Bartlett JG, Chang TW, Onderdonk AB (1978). Will the real *Clostridium* species responsible for antibiotic-associated colitis please step forward. *Lancet* i: 338.

Bassaris HP, Lianou PE, Papavassiliou JT (1984). Interactions of subminimal inhibitory concentrations of clindamycin and *Escherichia coli*: effects on adhesion and polymorphonuclear leukocyte function. *J Antimicrob Chemother* 13: 361.

Bassaris HP, Lianou PE, Skoutelis A Th, Papavassiliou J Th (1987). *In vivo* efffects of clindamycin on polymorphonuclear leucocyte phagocytosis and killing of Gram-negative organisms. *J Antimicrob Chemother* 19: 467.

Bawdon RE, Rozmiej E, Palchaudhuri S, Krakowiak J (1979). Variability of the susceptibility pattern of *Bacteroides fragilis* in four Detroit area hospitals. *Antimicrob Ag Chemother* 16: 664.

Bayer AS, Chow AW, Concepcion N, Guze LB (1978). Susceptibility of 40 lactobacilli to six antimicrobial agents with broad Gram-positive anaerobic spectra. *Antimicrob Ag Chemother* 14: 720.

Bell MJ, Shackelford P, Smith R, Schredder K (1984). Pharmacokinetics of clindamycin phosphate in the first year of life. *J Pediatrics* 105: 482.

Benner EJ, Tellman WH (1970). Pseudomembranous colitis as a sequel to oral lincomycin therapy. *Amer J Gastroent* 54: 55.

Berger SA, Barza M, Haher J et al. (1978). Penetration of clindamycin into decubitus ulcers. *Antimicrob Ag Chemother* 14: 498.

Betriu C, Campos E, Cabronero C et al. (1990). Susceptibilities of species of the *Bacteroides fragilis* group to 10 antimicrobial agents. *Antimicrob Ag Chemother* 34: 671.

Black JR, Feinberg J, Murphy RL et al. (1991). Clindamycin and primaquine as primary treatment for mild and moderately severe *Pneumocystis carinii* pneumonia in patients with AIDS. *Eur J Clin Microbiol Infect Dis* 10: 204.

Black JR, Feinberg J, Murphy RL et al. (1994). Clindamycin and primaquine therapy for mild- to-moderate episodes of *Pneumocystis carinii* pneumonia in patients with AIDS: AIDS clinical trials group 044. *Clin Infect Dis* 18: 905.

Blais J, Tardif C, Chamberland S (1993). Effect of clindamycin on intracellular replication, protein synthesis, and infectivity of *Toxoplasma gondii*. *Antimicrob Ag Chemother* 37: 2571.

Bodner SJ, Koenig MG, Treanor LL, Goodman JS (1972). Antibiotic susceptibility testing of *Bacteroides. Antimicrob Ag Chemother* **2**: 57.

Bowden TA Jr, Mansberger AR Jr, Lykins LE (1981). Pseudomembranous enterocolitis mechanism of restoring floral homeostatis. *Amer Surg* **47**: 178.

Boyd WC, Denbesten L (1976). Subtotal colectomy for refractory *Pseudomembranous* enterocolitis. *JAMA* **235**: 181.

Braathen LR (1985). Topical clindamycin versus oral tetracycline and placebo in acne vulgaris. *Scand J Infect Dis* (Suppl 43): 71.

Brandl RC, Arkenau C, Simon C et al. (1972). Zur Pharmakokinetik von Clindamycin bei gestörter Leber-und Nierenfunktion. *Dtsch Med Wöckenschr* **97**: 1057.

Brause BD, Borges JS, Roberts RB (1976). Relative efficacy of clindamycin erythromycin and penicillin in treatment of *Treponema pallidum* in skin syphilomas of rabbits. *J Infect Dis* **134**: 93.

Breese BB, Disney FA, Talpey W et al. (1974). Streptococcal infections in children Comparison of the therapeutic effectiveness of erythromycin administered twice daily with erythromycin, penicillin phenoxymethyl, and clindamycin administered three times daily. *Amer J Dis Child* **128**: 457.

Brogan TV, Nizet V, Waldhausen JHT et al. (1995). Group A streptococcal necrotizing fasciitis complicating primary varicella: a series of fourteen patients. *Pediatr Infect Dis J* **14**: 588.

Brook I (1979). Clindamycin in treatment of aspiration pneumonia in children. *Antimicrob Ag Chemother* **15**: 342.

Brook I (1994). Management of chronic suppurative otitis media: superiority of therapy effective against anaerobic bacteria. *Pediatr Infect Dis J* **13**: 188.

Brook I, Frazier EH (1993). Significant recovery of nonsporulating anaerobic rods from clinical specimens. *Clin Infect Dis* **16**: 476.

Brook I, Gober AE, Leyva F (1995). *In vitro* and *in vivo* effects of penicillin and clindamycin on expression of Group A beta-hemolytic streptococcal capsule. *Antimicrob Ag Chemother* **39**: 1565.

Brown RB, Barza M, Brusch JL et al. (1975). Pharmacokinetics of lincomycin and clindamycin phosphate in a canine model. *J Infect Dis* **131**: 252.

Brown RB, Martyak SM, Barza M et al. (1976). Penetration of clindamycin phosphate into the abnormal human biliary tract. *Ann Intern Med* **84**: 168.

Brown WJ (1988). National committee for clinical laboratory standards agar dilution susceptibility testing of anaerobic Gram-negative bacteria. *Antimicrob Ag Chemother* **32**: 385.

Buchwald D, Soumerae SB, Vandevanter N et al. (1989). Effect of hospitalwide change in clindamycin dosing schedule on clinical outcome. *Rev Infect Dis* **11**: 619.

Burch KH, Quinn EL, Cox F et al. (1976). Intramuscular clindamycin for therapy of infective endocarditis. Report of 23 cases and review of the literature. *Amer J Cardiol* **38**: 929.

Burdon DW, George RH (1978). Pseudomembranous colitis. *Lancet* **i**: 444.

Campbell IW, Hossack DJN, Munro JF (1973). Absorption and urinary excretion of clindamycin palmitate in the elderly. *Curr Med Res Opin* **1**: 369.

CDC (Center for Disease Control) (1977). Multiple-antibiotic resistance of pneumococci-South Africa. *MMWR* **26**: 285.

Champion LAA, Wald ER, Luddy RE, Schwartz AD (1978). *Streptococcus pneumoniae* resistant to erythromycin and clindamycin. *J Pediatr* **92**: 505.

Chang T-W, Gorbach SL, Bartlett JG, Saginur R (1980). Bacitracin treatment of antibiotic associated colitis and diarrhea caused by *Clostridium difficile* toxin. *Gastroenterology* **78**: 1584.

Cherry RD, Portnoy D, Jabbari M et al. (1982). Metronidazole: an alternate therapy for antibiotic-associated colitis. *Gastroenterology* **82**: 849.

Cherubin CE, Nair SR (1978). Clindamycin in infective endocarditis. *JAMA* **239**: 626.

Chow AW, Galpin JE, Guze LB (1977). Clindamycin for treatment of sepsis caused by decubitus ulcers. *J Infect Dis* **135** (Suppl): 65.

Chow AW, Jewesson PJ (1985). Pharmacokinetics and safety of antimicrobial agents during pregnancy. *Rev Infect Dis* **7**: 287.

Citron DM, Goldstein EJC, Kenner MA et al. (1995). Activity of ampicillin/sulbactam, ticarcillin/clavulanate, clarithromycin and eleven other antimicrobial agents against anaerobic bacteria isolated from infections in children. *Clin Infect Dis* **20** (Suppl 2): 356.

Clabots CR, Peterson LR, Gerding DN (1988). Characterization of a nosocomial *Clostridium difficile* outbreak by using plasmid profile typing and clindamycin susceptibility testing. *J Infect Dis* **158**: 731.

Clark CE, Thompson H, McLeisch AR et al. (1976). Pseudomembranous colitis following prophylactic antibiotics in bowel surgery. *J Antimicrob Chemother* **2**: 167.

Cohen LE, McNeill CJ, Wells RF (1973). Clindamycin-associated colitis. *JAMA* **223**: 1379.

Cooke ETM, Raghuvaran G (1974). Clindamycin in conjunction with surgery of the chronic suppurative ear. *Brit J Clin Pract* **28**: 57.

Courvalin P, Ounissi H, Arthur M (1985). Multiplicity of macrolide-lincosamide-streptogramin antibiotic resistance determinants. *J Antimicrob Chemother* **16** (Suppl A): 91.

Cronberg S, Castor B, Thoren A (1984). Fusidic acid for the treatment of antibiotic-associated colitis induced by *Clostridium difficile. Infection* **12**: 276.

Cuchural GJ Jr, Tally FP, Jacobus NV et al. (1988). Susceptibility of the *Bacteroides fragilis* Group in the United States: analysis by site of isolation. *Antimicrob Ag Chemother* **32**: 717.

Dall L, Keilhofner M, Herndon B et al. (1990). Clindamycin effect on glycocalyx production in experimental viridans streptococcal endocarditis. *J Infect Dis* **161**: 1221.

Dallos V (1975). Clindamycin – a retrospective study of its side-effects. *J Antimicrob Chemother* **1**: 411.

Dannemann BR, McCutchan JA, Israelski DM et al. (1991). Treatment of acute toxoplasmosis with intravenous clindamycin. *Eur J Clin Microbiol Infect Dis* **10**: 193.

Delmée M, Avesani V (1988). Correlation between serogroup and susceptibility to chloramphenicol, clindamycin, erythromycin, rifampicin and tetracycline among 308 isolates of *Clostridium difficile. J Antimicrob Chemother* **22**: 325.

Denys GA, Jerris RC, Swenson JM, Thornsberry C (1983). Susceptibility of *Propionibacterium acnes* clinical isolates of 22 antimicrobial agents. *Antimicrob Ag Chemother* **23**: 335.

Dillon HC, Derrick CW (1975). Clinical experience with clindamycin hydrochloride 1 Treatment of streptococcal and mixed streptococcal-staphylococcal skin infection. *Pediatrics* **55**: 205.

Dornbusch K, Nord C-E, Dahlbäck A (1975). Antibiotic susceptibility of *Clostridium* species isolated from human infections. *Scand J Infect Dis* **7**: 127.

Dornbusch K, Carlström A, Hugo H, Lidström A (1977). Antibacterial activity of clindamycin and lincomycin in human bone. *Antimicrob Chemother* **3**: 153.

Douglas RL, Kislak JW (1973). Treatment of *Bacteroides fragilis* bacteremia with clindamycin. *J Infect Dis* **128**: 569.

Drapkin MS, Karchmer AW, Moellering RC Jr (1976). Bacteremic infections due to clindamycin-resistant streptococci. *JAMA* **236**: 263.

Duckworth C, Fisher JF, Carter SA et al. (1993). Tissue penetration of clindamycin in diabetic foot infections. *J Antimicrob Chemother* **31**: 581.

Duncan IBR (1968). Development of lincomycin resistance by staphylococci. *Antimicrob Ag Chemother* **1967**: 723.

Eastwood JB, Gower PE (1974). A study of the pharmacokinetics of clindamycin in normal subjects and patients with chronic renal failure. *Postgrad Med J* **50**: 710.

Elharrif Z, Megraud F, Marchand A-M (1985). Susceptibility of *Campylobacter jejuni* and *Campylobacter coli* to macrolides and related compounds. *Antimicrob Ag Chemother* **28**: 695.

Elmore M, Rissing JP, Rink L, Brooks GF (1974). Clindamycin-associated hepatotoxicity. *Amer J Med* **57**: 627.

Eng RHK, Gorski S, Person A et al. (1981). Clindamycin elimination in patients with liver disease. *J Antimicrob Chemother* **8**: 277.

Faden H, Hong JJ, Ogra PL (1985). *In vivo* effects of clindamycin on neutrophil function. *J Antimicrob Chemother* **16**: 649.

Fass RJ, Saslaw S (1972). Clindamycin: clinical and laboratory evaluation of parenteral therapy. *Amer J Med Sci* **263**: 369.

Fass RJ, Rotilie CA, Prior RB (1974). Interaction of clindamycin and gentamicin *in vitro*. *Antimicrob Ag Chemother* **6**: 582.

Feigin RD, Pickering LK, Anderson D *et al.* (1975). Clindamycin treatment of osteomyelitis and septic arthritis in children. *Pediatrics* **55**: 213.

Fekety R, Shah AB (1993). Diagnosis and treatment of *Clostridium difficile* colitis. *JAMA* **269**: 71.

Fichera ME, Bhopale MK, Roos DS (1995). *In vitro* assays elucidate peculiar kinetics of clindamycin action against *Toxoplasma gondii*. *Antimicrob Ag Chemother* **39**: 1530.

Filice GA, Pomeroy C (1991). Effect of clindamycin on pneumonia from reactivation of *Toxoplasma gondii* infection in mice. *Antimicrob Ag Chemother* **35**: 780.

Finch RG, Phillips I, Geddes AM (1975). A clinical, microbiological and toxicological assessment of clindamycin phosphate. *J Antimicrob Chemother* **1**: 297.

Findling JW, Pholman GP, Rose HD (1980). Fulminant Gram-negative bacillemia (DF-2). following a dog bite in an asplenic woman. *Amer J Med* **68**: 154.

Finegold SM, Wexler HM (1988). Therapeutic implications of bacteriologic findings in mixed aerobic-anaerobic infections. *Antimicrob Ag Chemother* **32**: 611.

Flaherty JF, Rodondi LC, Guglielmo BJ *et al.* (1988). Comparative pharmacokinetics and serum inhibitory activity of clindamycin in different dosing regimens. *Antimicrob Ag Chemother* **32**: 1825.

Fletcher HM, Macrina FL (1991). Molecular survey of clindamycin and tetracycline resistance determinants in *Bacteroides* spp. *Antimicrob Ag Chemother* **35**: 2415.

Foppa CU, Bini T, Gregis G *et al.* (1991). A retrospective study of primary and maintenance therapy of toxoplasmic encephalitis with oral clindamycin and pyrimethamine. *Eur J Clin Microbiol Infect Dis* **10**: 187.

Fox AR, Phillips I (1987). The antibiotic sensitivity of *Bacteroides fragilis* group in the United Kingdom. *J Antimicrob Chemother* **20**: 477.

Franzblau SG (1991). *In vitro* activities of aminoglycosides, lincosamides, and rifamycins against *Mycobacterium leprae*. *Antimicrob Ag Chemother* **35**: 1232.

Freeman R, Roberts DW (1976). A case of subacute bacterial endocarditis treated with parenteral clindamycin (clindamycin-2-phosphate). *Postgrad Med J* **52**: 595.

Friedman GD, Gérard MJ, Ury HK (1976). Clindamycin and diarrhea. *JAMA* **236**: 2498.

Fry DE, Garrison RN Polk HC Jr (1979). Clinical implications in *Bacteroides bacteremia*. *Surg Gynecol Obstet* **149**: 189.

Fulghum DD, Catalano PM (1973). Stevens-Johnson syndrome from clindamycin. A case report. *JAMA* **223**: 318.

Gabay EL, Rolfe RD, Finegold SM (1981). Susceptibility of *Clostridium septicum* to 23 antimicrobial agents. *Antimicrob Ag Chemother* **20**: 852.

Gatti G, Flaherty J, Bubp J *et al.* (1993). Comparative study of bioavailabilities and pharmacokinetics of clindamycin in healthy volunteers and patients with AIDS. *Antimicrob Ag Chemother* **37**: 1137.

Geddes AM (1983). Leading article. Q Fever. *Brit Med J* **287**: 927.

Geddes AM, Bridgwater FAJ, Williams DN *et al.* (1970). Clinical and bacteriological studies with clindamycin. *Brit Med J* **2**: 703.

Geddes AM, Dwyer NStJ, Ball AP, Amos RS (1977). Clindamycin in bone and joint infections. *J Antimicrob Chemother* **3**: 501.

Gemmell CG (1984). Clindamycin and its action on the susceptibility of pathogenic bacteria to phagocytosis. *Scand J Infect Dis* (Suppl 43): 17.

George RH, Symonds JM, Dimock F *et al.* (1978a). Identification of *Clostridium difficile* as a cause of pseudomembranous colitis. *Brit Med J* **1**: 695.

George WL, Sutter VL, Goldstein EJC *et al.* (1978b). Aetiology of antimicrobial-agent-associated colitis. *Lancet* **i**: 802.

George WL, Sutter VL, Citron D, Finegold SM (1979). Selective and differential medium for isolation of *Clostridium difficile*. *J Clin Microbiol* **9**: 214.

Gerding DN (1989). Disease associated with *Clostridium difficile* infection. *Ann Intern Med* **110**: 255.

Gerding DN, Hall WH, Schierl EA (1977). Antibiotic concentrations in ascitic fluid of patients with ascites and bacterial peritonitis. *Ann Intern Med* **86**: 708.

Gibson GE, Rowland R, Hecker R (1975). Diarrhoea and colitis associated with antibiotic treatment.. *Aust NZ J Med* **5**: 340.

Gigantelli JW, Gomez JT, Orato MS (1991). *In vitro* susceptibilities of ocular *Bacillus cereus* isolates to clindamycin, gentamicin, and vancomycin alone or in combination. *Antimicrob Ag Chemother* **35**: 201.

Gorbach SL, Bartlett JG (1977). Pseudomembranous enterocolitis; a review of its diverse forms. *J Infect Dis* **135** (Suppl): 89.

Goulston SJM, McGovern VJ (1965). Pseudomembranous colitis. *Gut* **6**: 207.

Gurwith MJ, Rabin HR, Love K and the Cooperative Antibiotic Diarrhea Study Group (1977). Diarrhea associated with clindamycin and ampicillin therapy: preliminary results of a cooperative study. *J Infect Dis* **135** (Suppl): 104.

Hächler H, Berger-Bächi B, Kayser FH (1987). Genetic characterization of a *Clostridium difficile* erythromycin-clindamycin resistance determinant that is transferable to *Staphylococcus aureus*. *Antimicrob Ag Chemother* **31**: 1039.

Halula M, Macrina FL (1990). Tn 5030: a conjugative transposon conferring clindamycin resistance in *Bacteroides* species. *Rev Infect Dis* **12** (Suppl 2): 235.

Hand WL, King-Thompson NL (1986). Contrasts between phagocyte antibiotic uptake and subsequent intracellular bactericidal activity. *Antimicrob Ag Chemother* **29**: 135.

Hand WL, Boozer RM, King-Thompson NL (1985). Antibiotic uptake by alveolar macrophages of smokers. *Antimicrob Ag Chemother* **27**: 42.

Hand WL, Hand DL, King-Thompson NL (1990). Antibiotic inhibition of the respiratory burst response in human polymorphonuclear leukocytes. *Antimicrob Ag Chemother* **34**: 863.

Heerze LD, Kelm MA, Talbot JA, Armstrong GD (1994). Oligosaccharide sequences attached to an inert support (SYNSORB. as potential therapy for antibiotic-associated diarrhea and pseudomembranous colitis. *J Infect Dis* **169**: 1291.

Heseltine PNR, Yellin AE, Appleman MD *et al.* (1983). Perforated and gangrenous appendicitis: an analysis of antibiotic failures. *J Infect Dis* **148**: 322.

Hextall A, Radley S, Andrews JM *et al.* (1994). Mucosal concentration and excretion of clindamycin by the human stomach. *J Antimicrob Chemother* **33**: 595.

Hinthorn DR, Baker LH, Romig DA *et al.* (1976). Use of clindamycin in patients with liver disease. *Antimicrob Ag Chemother* **9**: 498.

Hofflin JM, Remington JS (1987). Clindamycin in a murine model of toxoplasmic encephalitis. *Antimicrob Ag Chemother* **31**: 492.

Holmberg K, Nord CE, Dornbusch K (1977). Antimicrobial *in vitro* susceptibility of *Actinomyces israelii* and *Arachnia propionica*. *Scand J Infect Dis* **9**: 40.

Howard RJ, Soucy DM (1983). Potentiation of phagocytosis of *Bacteroides fragilis* following incubation with clindamycin. *J Antimicrob Chemother* **12** (Suppl C): 63.

Hugo H, Dornbusch K, Sterner G (1977). Studies of the clinical efficacy, serum levels and side effects of clindamycin phosphate administered intravenously. *Scand J Infect Dis* **9**: 221.

Jacobs RF, Wilson CB (1983). Intracellular penetration and antimicrobial activity of antibiotics. *J Antimicrob Chemother* **12** (Suppl C): 13.

Jenssen WD, Thakker-Varia S, Dubin DT, Weinstein MP (1987). Prevalence of macrolides-lincosamides-streptogramin B resistance and erm gene classes among clinical strains of staphylococci and streptococci. *Antimicrob Ag Chemother* **31**: 883.

Jimenez-Diaz A, Reig M, Baquero F, Ballesta JPG (1992). Antibiotic sensitivity of ribosomes from wild-type and clindamycin-resistant

Bacteroides vulgatus strains. *J Antimicrob Chemother* **30**: 295.

Johnson CC, Finegold SM (1987). Uncommonly encountered, motile, anaerobic Gram-negative bacilli associated with infection. *Rev Infect Dis* **9**: 1150.

Kabins SA, Spira TJ (1975). Outbreak of clindamycin-associated colitis. *Ann Intern Med* **83**: 830.

Kager L, Liljequist L, Malmborg AS, Nord CE (1981). Effect of clindamycin prophylaxis on the colonic microflora in patients undergoing colorectal surgery. *Antimicrob Ag Chemother* **20**: 736.

Kalb R, Kaplan MH, Tenebaum MJ *et al.* (1985). Cutaneous infections at dog bite wounds associated with fulminant DF-2 septicemia. *Amer J Med* **78**: 687.

Kaplan E, Weinstein L (1968). Lincomycin. *Pediatr Clin N Amer* **15**: 131.

Kappas A, Shinagawa N, Arabi Y *et al.* (1978). Diagnosis of pseudomembranous colitis. *Brit Med J* **1**: 675.

Karchmer AW, Moellering RC Jr, Watson BK (1975). Susceptibility of various serogroups of streptococci to clindamycin and lincomycin. *Antimicrob Ag Chemother* **7**: 164.

Katlama C (1991). Evaluation of the efficacy and safety of clindamycin plus pyrimethamine for induction and maintenance therapy of toxoplasmic encephalitis in AIDS. *Eur J Clin Microbiol Infect Dis* **10**: 189.

Keane JT, Rose HD (1973). Pneumococcal endocarditis treated with clindamycin. *JAMA* **226**: 1120.

Keighley MRB, Burdon DW, Arabi Y *et al.* (1978). Randomized controlled trial of vancomycin for pseudomembranous colitis and postoperative diarrhea. *Brit Med J* **12**: 1667.

Kelly CP, Pothoulakis C, La Mont JT (1994). *Clostridium difficile* colitis. *New Engl J Med* **330**: 257.

Keusch GT, Present DH (1976). Summary of a workshop on clindamycin colitis. *J Infect Dis* **133**: 578.

Khardori N, Wong E, Nguyen H *et al.* (1991). Effect of subinhibitory concentrations of clindamycin and trospectomycin on the adherence of *Staphylococcus epidermidis* in an *in vitro* model of vascular catheter colonization. *J Infect Dis* **164**: 108.

Kislak JW (1972). The susceptibility of *Bacteroides fragilis* to 24 antibiotics. *J Infect Dis* **125**: 295.

Klainer AS (1987). Clindamycin. *Med Clin N Amer* **71**: 1169.

Klastersky J, Husson M (1977). Bactericidal activity of the combination of gentamicin with clindamycin or chloramphenicol against species of *Escherichia coli* and *Bacteroides fragilis*. *Antimicrob Ag Chemother* **12**: 135.

Klugman K, Koornhof HJ, Kuhnie V *et al.* (1986). Meningitis and pneumonia due to novel multiply resistant pneumococci. *Brit Med J* **292**: 730.

Kohn J, Evans AJ (1970). Group A streptococci resistant to clindamycin. *Brit Med J* **2**: 423.

Kosimidis JC, Corbett V, Cole AJL *et al.* (1973). The treatment of paediatric infections with the lincomycins. *Brit J Clin Pract* **27**: 315.

Kremsner PG (1990). Clindamycin in malaria treatment. *J Antimicrob Chemother* **25**: 9.

Kremsner PG, Zotter GM, Feldmeier H *et al.* (1988). A comparative trial of three regimens for treating uncomplicated *Falciparum* malaria in Acre, Brazil. *J Infect Dis* **158**: 1368.

Kremsner PG, Zotter GM, Feldmeier H *et al.* (1989). Clindamycin treatment of *Falciparum* malaria in Brazil. *J Antimicrob Chemother* **23**: 275.

Kremsner PG, Radloff P, Metzger W *et al.* (1995). Quinine plus clindamycin improves chemotherapy of severe malaria in children. *Antimicrob Ag Chemother* **39**: 1603.

Lambert HP (1975). Unwanted effects of antibiotics: some recent additions. *J Antimicrob Chemother* **1**: 2.

Larson HE, Price AB (1977). Pseudomembranous colitis: presence of clostridial toxin. *Lancet* **ii**: 1312.

Larson HE, Parry JV, Price AB *et al.* (1977). Undescribed toxin in pseudomembranous colitis. *Brit Med J* **1**: 1246.

Larson HE, Price AB, Honour P, Borriello SP (1978). *Clostridium difficile* and the aetiology of pseudomembranous colitis. *Lancet* **i**: 1063.

Leading Article (1973). Antibiotics in acne vulgaris. *Brit Med J* **1**: 65.

Leading Article (1975). Drug metabolism and increasing age. *Brit Med J* **2**: 581.

Le Frock JL, Klainer AS, Chen S *et al.* (1975). The spectrum of colitis associated with lincomycin and clindamycin therapy. *J Infect Dis* **131** (Suppl): 108.

Leclercq R, Courvalin P (1991a). Bacterial resistance to macrolide, lincosamide, and streptogramin antibiotics by target modification. *Antimicrob Ag Chemother* **35**: 1267.

Leclercq R, Courvalin P (1991b). Intrinsic and unusual resistance to macrolide, lincosamide, and stroptogramin antibiotics in bacteria. *Antimicrob Ag Chemother* **35**: 1273.

Leclercq R, Brisson-Noel A, Duval J, Courvalin P (1987). Phenotypic expression and genetic heterogeneity of lincosamide inactivation in *Staphylococcus* spp. *Antimicrob Ag Chemother* **31**: 1887.

Lee D, Goldstein EJC, Citron DM, Ross S (1993). Empyema due to *Bacteroides gracilis*: case report and *in vitro* susceptibilities to eight antimicrobial agents. *Clin Infect Dis* **16** (Suppl 4): 263.

Leigh DA (1981). Antibacterial activity and pharmacokinetics of clindamycin. *J Antimicrob Chemother* **7** (Suppl A): 3.

Lemos LB, Baba N, De Araujo OJ (1976). Clindamycin-induced pseudomembranous colitis. *Amer J Clin Path* **65**: 455.

Leng B, Meyers BR, Hirschman SZ, Keusch GT (1975). Susceptibility of Gram-negative bacteria to combinations of antimicrobial agents *in vitro*. *Antimicrob Ag Chemother* **8**: 164.

Leport C, Bastuji-Garin S, Perronne C *et al.* (1989). An open study of the pyrimethamine-clindamycin combination in AIDS patients with brain toxoplasmosis. *J Infect Dis* **160**: 557.

Levett PN (1988). Antimicrobial susceptibility of *Clostridium difficile* determined by disc diffusion and breakpoint methods. *J Antimicrob Chemother* **22**: 167.

Levison ME, Bran JL, Ries K (1974). Treatment of anaerobic bacterial infections with clindamycin 2 phosphate. *Antimicrob Ag Chemother* **5**: 276.

Levison ME, Mansura CT, Lorber B *et al.* (1983). Clindamycin compared with penicillin for the treatment of anaerobic lung abscess. *Ann Intern Med* **98**: 466.

Lewis C, Clapp HW, Grady JE (1963). *In vitro* and *in vivo* evaluation of lincomycin, a new antibiotic. *Antimicrob Ag Chemother* **1962**: 570.

Liñares J, Garau J, Dominguez C, Perez JL (1983). Antibiotic resistance and serotypes of *Streptococcus pneumoniae* from patients with community-acquired pneumococcal disease. *Antimicrob Ag Chemother* **23**: 545.

Lines DR, Vimpani GV, Pearson CC (1973). The use of 7–chloro-lincomycin in the treatment of childhood respiratory disease. *Med J Aust* **1**: 439.

Lode H (1988). Microbiological and clinical aspects of aspiration pneumonia. *J Antimicrob Chemother* **21** (Suppl C): 83.

Luft BJ, Remington JS (1992). Toxoplasmic encephalitis in AIDS. *Clin Infect Dis* **15**: 211.

Luft BJ, Hafner R, Korzun AH *et al.* (1993). Toxoplasmic encephalitis in patients with the acquired immunodeficiency syndrome. *New Engl J Med* **329**: 995.

Lusk RH, Fekety FR Jr, Silva J Jr *et al.* (1977). Gastrointestinal side effects of clindamycin and ampicillin therapy. *J Infect Dis* **135** (Suppl): 111.

Magerlein BJ, Birkenmeyer RD, Kagam F (1967). Chemical modification of lincomycin. *Antimicrob Ag Chemother* **1966**: 727.

Malacoff RF, Finkelstein FO, Andriole VT (1975). Effect of peritoneal dialysis on serum levels of tobramycin and lincomycin. *Antimicrob Ag Chemother* **8**: 574.

Massell BF (1979). Prophylaxis of streptococcal infections and rheumatic fever. A comparison of orally-administered clindamycin and penicillin. *JAMA* **241**: 1589.

McCarthy LR, Mickelson PA, Smith EG (1979). Antibiotic susceptibility of *Haemophilus vaginale* (*Corynebacterium vaginale*). to 21 antibiotics. *Antimicrob Ag Chemother* **16**: 186.

McClean KL, Sheehan GJ, Harding GKM (1994). Intraabdominal infection: a review. *Clin Infect Dis* **19**: 100.

McCloskey RV, Green MJ, Eller J, Smilack J (1974). Treatment of diphtheria carriers: benzathine penicillin, erythromycin, and clindamycin. *Ann Intern Med* **81**: 788.

McFarland LV, Suravicz CM, Stamm WE (1990). Risk factors for *Clostridium difficile* carriage and *C difficile*-associated diarrhea in a cohort of hospitalized patients. *J Antimicrob Chemother* **162**: 678.

McGehee RF Jr, Smith CB, Wilcox C, Finland M (1968). Comparative studies of antibacterial activity *in vitro* and absorption and excretion of lincomycin and clindamycin. *Amer J Med Sci* **256**: 279.

McGehee RF Jr, Barrett FF, Finland M (1969). Resistance of *Staphylococcus aureus* to lincomycin, clinimycin and erythromycin. *Antimicrob Ag Chemother* **1968**: 392.

Menninger JR, Coleman RA (1993). Lincosamide antibiotics stimulate dissociation of peptidyl-tRNA from ribosomes. *Antimicrob Ag Chemother* **37**: 2027.

Meyers BR, Kaplan KWS (1969). Microbiological and pharmacological behaviour of 7-chloro-lincomycin. *Appl Microbiol* **17**: 653.

Michel J, Rogol M, Dickman D (1983). Susceptibility of clinical isolates of *Campylobacter jejuni* to sixteen antimicrobial agents. *Antimicrob Ag Chemother* **23**: 796.

Milatovic D, Braveny I, Verhoef J (1983). Clindamycin enhances opsonization of *Staphylococcus aureus*. *Antimicrob Ag Chemother* **24**: 413.

Mitchell AAB, Simpson RG (1973). Bacteroides septicaemia. *Curr Med Res Opin* **1**: 385.

Munk JF, Collopy BT, Connell JL et al. (1976). Lincomycin-clindamycin-associated pseudomembranous colitis. *Med J Aust* **2**: 95.

Nelson CT, Mason EO Jr, Kaplan SL (1994). Activity of oral antibiotics in middle ear and sinus infections caused by penicillin-resistant *Streptococcus pneumoniae*: implications for treatment. *Pediatr Infect Dis J* **13**: 585.

Neu HC, Prince A, Neu CO, Garvey GJ (1977). Incidence of diarrhea and colitis assocaited with clindamycin therapy. *J Infect Dis* **35** (Suppl): 120.

Newell AC (1970). Clinical trial of a new antibiotic. *Med J Aust* **2**: 321.

Nichols RL (1983). Empiric antibiotic therapy for intra-abdominal infections. *Rev Infect Dis* **5** (Suppl): 90.

Nichols RL, Smith JW (1993). Wound and intraabdominal infections: microbiological considerations and approaches to treatment. *Clin Infect Dis* **16** (Suppl 4): 266.

Nord CE (1995). The role of anaerobic bacteria in recurrent episodes of sinusitis and tonsillitis. *Clin Infect Dis* **20**: 1512.

Nord CE, Haeimdahl A (1986). Impact of orally administered antimicrobial agents on human oropharyngeal and colonic microflora. *J Antimicrob Chemother* **18** (Suppl C): 159.

Noskin GA, Murphy RL, Black JR, Phair JP (1992). Salvage therapy with clindamycin/primaquine for *Pneumocystis carinii* pneumonia. *Clin Infect Dis* **14**: 183.

Orrling A, Stjernquist-Desatnik A, Schalén C, Kamme C (1994). Clindamycin in persisting streptococcal pharyngotonsillitis after penicillin treatment. *Scand J Infect Dis* **26**: 535.

Patey O, Varon E, Prazuck T et al. (1994). Multicentre survey in France of the antimicrobial susceptibilities of 416 blood culture isolates of the *Bacteroides fragilis* group. *J Antimicrob Chemother* **33**: 1029.

Pearlman MD, Faro S, Riddle GD, Tortolero G (1990). *In vitro* synergy of clindamycin and aminoglycosides against *Chlamydia trachomatis*. *Antimicrob Ag Chemother* **34**: 1399.

Peddie BA, Dann E, Bailey RR (1975). The effect of impairment of renal function and dialysis on the serum and urine levels of clindamycin. *Aust NZ J Med* **5**: 198.

Peterson HB, Galaid EI, Zanilman JM (1990). Pelvic inflammatory disease: review of treatment options. *Rev Infect Dis* **12** (Suppl 6): 656.

Pfefferkorn ER, Borotz SE(1994). Comparison of mutants of *Toxoplasma gondii* selected for resistance to azithromycin, spiramycin, or clindamycin. *Antimicrob Ag Chemother* **38**: 31.

Pfefferkorn ER, Nothnagel RF, Borotz SE (1992). Parasiticidal effect of clindamycin on *Toxoplasma gondii* grown in cultured cells and selection of a drug-resistant mutant. *Antimicrob Ag Chemother* **36**: 1091.

Philipson A, Sabath LD, Charles D (1973). Transplacental passage of erythromycin and clindamycin. *New Engl J Med* **288**: 1219.

Phillips I, Warren C, Harrison JM et al. (1976). Antibiotic susceptibility of streptococci from the mouth and blood of patients treated with penicillin or lincomycin and clindamycin. *J Med Microbiol* **9**: 393.

Piketty C, Derouin F, Rouveix B, Pocidalo J-J (1990). *In vivo* assessment of antimicrobial agents against *Toxoplasma gondii* by quantification of parasites in the blood, lungs and brain of infected mice. *Antimicrob Ag Chemother* **34**: 1467.

Plaisance KI, Drusano GL, Forrest A et al. (1989). Pharmacokinetic evaluation of two dosage regimens of clindamycin phosphate. *Antimicrob Ag Chemother* **33**: 618.

Powers KG, Jacobs RL (1972). Activity of two chlorinated lincomycin analogues against chloroquine-resistant falciparum malaria in owl monkeys. *Antimicrob Ag Chemother* **1**: 49.

Price AB, Davies DR (1977). Pseudomembranous colitis. *J Clin Path* **30**: 1.

Privitera G, Dublanchet A, Sebald M (1979). Transfer of multiple antibiotic resistance between subspecies of *Bacteroides fragilis*. *J Infect Dis* **139**: 97.

Privitera G, Fayolle F, Sebald M (1981). Resistance to tetracycline, erythromycin and clindamycin in the *Bacteroides fragilis* group: inducible versus constitutive tetracycline resistance. *Antimicrob Ag Chemother* **20**: 314.

Queener SF, Bartlett MS, Richardson JD et al. (1988). Activity of clindamycin with primaquine against *Pneumocystis carinii in vitro* and *in vivo*. *Antimicrob Ag Chemother* **32**: 807.

Quiros LM, Fidalgo S, Mendez FJ et al. (1988). Novel mechanisms of resistance to lincosamides in *Staphylococcus* and *Arthrobacter* spp. *Antimicrob Ag Chemother* **32**: 420.

Raeburn JA, Devine JD (1971). Clindamycin levels in sputum in a patient with purulent chest disease due to cystic fibrosis. *Postgrad Med J* **47**: 366.

Reeves DS, Holt HA, Phillips I et al. (1991). Activity of clindamycin against *Staphylococcus aureus* and *Staphylococcus epidermidis* from four UK centres. *J Antimicrob Chemother* **27**: 469.

Reig M, Fernandez MC, Ballesta JPG, Baquero F (1992a). Inducible expression of ribosomal clindamycin resistance in *Bacterioides vulgatus*. *Antimicrob Ag Chemother* **36**: 639.

Reig M, Moreno A, Baquero F (1992b). Resistance of *Peptostreptococcus* spp. to macrolides and lincosamides: inducible and constitutive phenotypes. *Antimicrob Ag Chemother* **36**: 662.

Reiner L, Schlesinger MJ, Miller GM (1952). Pseudomembranous colitis following aureomycin and chloramphenicol. *Arch Path* **54**: 39.

Reusser F (1975). Effect of lincomycin and clindamycin on peptide chain initiation. *Antimicrob Ag Chemother* **7**: 32.

Rice RJ, Bhullar V, Mitchell SH et al. (1995). Susceptibilies of *Chlamydia trachomatis* isolates causing uncomplicated female genital tract infections and pelvic inflammatory disease. *Antimicrob Ag Chemother* **39**: 760.

Rifkin GD, Fekety FR, Silva J Jr (1977). Antibiotic-induced colitis Implication of a toxin neutralised by *Clostridium sordellii* antitoxin. *Lancet* **ii**: 1103.

Robertson MB, Breen KJ, Desmond PV et al. (1977). Incidence of antibiotic-related diarrhoea and pseudomembranous colitis. A prospective study of lincomycin, clindamycin and ampicillin. *Med J Aust* **1**: 243.

Rodriguez W, Ross S, Khan W et al. (1977). Clindamycin in the treatment of osteomyelitis in children. A report of 29 cases. *Amer J Dis Child* **131**: 1088.

Rose HD, Rytel MW (1972). Actinomycosis treated with clindamycin. *JAMA* **221**: 1052.

Rosenkranz P, Lederman MM, Gopalakrishna KV, Ellner JJ (1990). Septic arthritis caused by *Bacteroides fragilis*. *Rev Infect Dis* **12**: 20.

Ruf B, Pohle HD (1991). Role of clindamycin in the treatment of acute toxoplasmosis of the central nervous system. *Eur J Clin Microbiol Infect Dis* **10**: 183.

Ruf B, Rohde I, Pohle HD (1991). Efficacy of clindamycin/primaquine versus trimethoprim/sulfamethoxazole in primary treatment of *Pneumocystis carinii* pneumonia. *Eur J Clin Microbiol Infect Dis* **10**: 207.

Samore MH, Bettin KM, De Girolami PC *et al.* (1994a). Wide diversity of *Clostridium difficile* types at a tertiary referral hospital. *J Infect Dis* **170**: 615.

Samore MH, De Girolami PC, Tlucko A *et al.* (1994b). *Clostridium difficile* colonization and diarrhea at a tertiary care hospital. *Clin Infect Dis* **18**: 181.

Sanders CC, Sanders WE Jr, Goering RV (1983). Effects of clindamycin on derepression of beta-lactamases in Gram-negative bacteria. *J Antimicrob Chemother* **12** (Suppl C): 97.

Scheld WM, Johnson ML, Gerhardt EB, Sande MA (1982). Clindamycin therapy of experimental *Staphylococcus aureus* endocarditis. *Antimicrob Ag Chemother* **21**: 646.

Schlievert PM, Kelly JA (1984). Clindamycin-induced suppression of toxic-shock syndrome-associated exotoxin production. *J Infect Dis* **149**: 471.

Schwan A, Sjölin S, Troffestam U, Aronsson B (1984). Relapsing *Clostridium difficile* enterocolitis by rectal infusion of normal feces. *Scand J Infect Dis* **16**: 211.

Scott AJ, Nicholson GI, Kerr AR (1973). Lincomycin as a cause of pseudomembranous colitis. *Lancet* ii: 1232.

Shamsuddin D, Tuazon CU, Levy C, Curtin J (1982). *Bacillus cereus* panophthalmitis: source of the organism. *Rev Infect Dis* **4**: 97.

Shapera RM, Warwick WJ, Matsen JM (1981). Clindamycin therapy of staphylococcal pulmonary infections in patients with cystic fibrosis. *J Pediatrics* **99**: 647.

Sheridan RL, Ryan CM, Pasternack MS *et al.* (1993). Flavobacterial sepsis in massively burned pediatric patients. *Clin Infect Dis* **17**: 185.

Simor AE, Yake SL, Tsimidis K (1993). Infection due to *Clostridium difficile* among elderly residents of a long-term care facility. *Clin Infect Dis* **17**: 672.

Smith JW (1991). Studies of the susceptibility of *Pneumocystis carinii* to clindamycin/primaquine in rats. *Eur J Clin Microbiol Infect Dis* **10**: 201.

Staneck JL, Washington JAII (1974). Antimicrobial susceptibilities of anaerobic bacteria: recent clinical isolates. *Antimicrob Ag Chemother* **6**: 311.

Stevens DL (1994). Invasive group A streptococcal infections: the past, present and future. *Pediatr Infect Dis J* **13**: 561.

Stevens DL, Maier KA, Mitten JE (1987a). Effect of antibiotics on toxin production and viability of *Clostridium perfringens*. *Antimicrob Ag Chemother* **31**: 213.

Stevens DL, Laine BM, Mitten JE (1987b). Comparison of single and combination antimicrobial agents for prevention of experimental gas gangrene caused by *Clostridium perfringens*. *Antimicrob Ag Chemother* **31**: 312.

Stevens DL, Gibbons AE, Bergstrom R, Winn J (1988). The Eagle effect revisited: efficacy of clindamycin, erythromycin, and penicillin in the treatment of streptococcal mycositis. *J Infect Dis* **158**: 23.

Stevens DL, Bryant AE, Adams K, Mader JT (1993). Evaluation of therapy with hyperbaric oxygen for experimental infection with *Clostridium perfringens*. *Clin Infect Dis* **17**: 231.

Stevens DL, Bryant AE, Hackett SP (1995). Antibiotic effects on bacterial viability, toxin production, and host response. *Clin Infect Dis* **20** (Suppl 2): 154.

Summersgill JT, Schupp LG, Raff MJ (1982). Comparative penetration of metronidazole, clindamycin, chloramphenicol, cefoxitin, ticarcillin, and moxalactam into bone. *Antimicrob Ag Chemother* **21**: 601.

Sutter VL (1977). *In vitro* susceptibility of anaerobes: comparison of clindamycin and other antimicrobial agents. *J Infect Dis* **135** (Suppl): 7.

Sutter VL, Finegold SM (1976). Susceptibility of anaerobic bacteria to 23 antimicrobial agents. *Antimicrob Ag Chemother* **10**: 736.

Sutter VL, Kwok Y-Y, Finegold SM (1973). Susceptibility of *Bacteroides fragilis* to six antibiotics determined by standardized antimicrobial disc susceptibility testing. *Antimicrob Ag Chemother* **3**: 188.

Sutton DR, Gosnold JK (1977). Oesophageal ulceration due to clindamycin. *Brit Med J* **1**: 1598.

Swartzberg JE, Maresca RM, Remington JS (1977). Clinical study of gastrointestinal complications associated with clindamycin therapy. *J Infect Dis* **135** (Suppl): 99.

Tabbara KF, O'Connor GR (1975). Ocular tissue absorption of clindamycin phosphate. *Arch Ophthal* **93**: 1183.

Tally FP (1983). Susceptibility of the *Bacteroides fragilis* group in the United States in 1981. *Antimicrob Ag Chemother* **23**: 536.

Tally FP (1988). Factors affecting the choice of antibiotics in mixed infections. *J Antimicrob Chemother* **22** (Suppl A): 87.

Tally FP, Malamy MH (1986). Resistance factors in anaerobic bacteria. *Scand J Infect Dis* (Suppl 49): 56.

Tally FP, Cuchural GJ Jr, Jacobus NV *et al.* (1985). Nationwide study of the susceptibility of the *Bacteroides fragilis* group in the United States. *Antimicrob Ag Chemother* **28**: 675.

Tanaka-Bandoh K, Kato N, Watanabe K, Ueno K (1995). Antibiotic susceptibility profiles of *Bacteroides fragilis* and *Bacteroides thetaiotaomicron* in Japan from 1990 to 1992. *Clin Infect Dis* **20** (Suppl 2): 352.

Teasley DG, Olson MM, Gebhard RL *et al.* (1983). Prospective randomized trial of metronidazole versus vancomycin for *Clostridium difficile*-associated diarrhea and colitis. *Lancet* i: 1043.

Tedesco FJ (1982). Treatment of recurrent antibiotic-associated pseudomembranous colitis. *Amer J Gastroenterol* **77**: 220.

Tedesco FJ, Barton RW, Alpers DH (1974). Clindamycin-associated colitis A prospective study. *Ann Intern Med* **81**: 429.

Tedesco F, Gurwith M, Markham R *et al.* (1978). Oral vancomycin for antibiotic-associated pseudomembranous colitis. *Lancet* ii: 226.

Toma E, Fournier S, Poisson M *et al.* (1989). Clindamycin and primaquine for *Pneumocystis carinii* pneumonia. *Lancet* i: 1046.

Toma E, Fournier S, Dumont M *et al.* (1993). Clindamycin/primaquine versus trimethoprim-sulfamethoxazole as primary therapy for *Pneumocystis carinii* pneumonia in AIDS: a randomized, double-blind pilot trial. *Clin Infect Dis* **17**: 178.

Turgeon P, Turgeon V, Gordeau M *et al.* (1994). Longitudinal study of susceptibilities of species of the *Bacteroides fragilis* group to five antimicrobial agents in three medical centers. *Antimicrob Ag Chemother* **38**: 2276.

Turner P, Edwards R, Weston V *et al.* (1995). Simultaneous resistance to metronidazole, co-amoxiclav, and imipenem in clinical isolate of *Bacteroides fragilis*. *Lancet* **345**: 1275.

Vildé J-L, Remington JS (1992). Role of clindamycin with or without another agent for pneumocystosis in patients with AIDS. *J Infect Dis* **166**: 694.

Wagner JG, Novak E, Patel NC *et al.* (1968). Absorption, excretion and half-life of clinimycin in normal adult males. *Amer J Med Sci* **256**: 25.

Walker CB, Gordon JM, Cornwall HA *et al.* (1981). Gingival crevicular fluid levels of clindamycin compared with its minimal inhibitory concentrations for periodontal bacteria. *Antimicrob Ag Chemother* **19**: 867.

Watanakunakorn C (1976). Clindamycin therapy of *Staphylococcus aureus* endocarditis Clinical relapse and development of resistance to clindamycin, lincomycin and erythromycin. *Amer J Med* **60**: 419.

Weisblum B (1995). Insights into erythromycin action from studies of its activity as inducer of resistance. *Antimicrob Ag Chemother* **39**: 793.

Wells RF (1974). Editorial. Clindamycin-associated colitis. *Ann Intern Med* **81**: 547.

Westblom TU, Duriex DE, Madan E, Belshe RB (1990). Guinea pig model for antibiotic transport across gastric mucosa: inhibitory tissue concentrations of clindamycin against *Helicobacter pylori* (*Campylobacter pylori*). following two separate dose regimens. *Antimicrob Ag Chemother* **34**: 25.

Wilkins TD, Thiel T (1973). Resistance of some species of *Clostridium* to clindamycin. *Antimicrob Ag Chemother* **3**: 136.

Williams DN, Crossley K, Hoffman C, Sabath LD (1975). Parenteral clindamycin phosphate: pharmacology with normal and abnormal liver function and effect on nasal staphylococci. *Antimicrob Ag Chemother* **7**: 153.

Young GP, Ward PB, Bayley N *et al.* (1985). Antibiotic associated-colitis due to *Clostridium difficile*: double blind comparison of vancomycin with bacitracin. *Gastroenterology* **89**: 1038.

Young GP, Bayley N, Ward P *et al.* (1986). Antibiotic associated colitis caused by *Clostridium difficile*: relapse and risk factors. *Med J Aust* **144**: 303.

Zabransky RJ, Johnston JA, Hauser KJ (1973). Bacteriostatic and bactericidal activities of various antibiotics against *Bacteroides fragilis*. *Antimicrob Ag Chemother* **3**: 152.

Zamiri I, McEntegart MG (1972). The sensitivity of diphtheria bacilli to eight antibiotics. *J Clin Path* **25**: 716.

Erythromycin

Description

Erythromycin was isolated from a strain of *Streptomyces erythreus* (McGuire *et al.*, 1952) and it belongs to a group of antibiotics known as the 'macrolides' which have in common a macrocyclic lactone ring. Erythromycin has a 14-membered lactone ring. These antibiotics are all weak bases, only slightly soluble in water. There are many antibiotics in this group, but of the older derivatives, apart from erythromycin, only spiramycin, josamycin and rosaramicin (p. 629) are still being used clinically. More recently newer macrolides, such as roxithromycin (p. 637), clarithromycin (p. 643) and azithromycin (p. 653) have been developed. These, compared with erythromycin, have new clinical uses.

Erythromycin base is very bitter, insoluble in water and inactivated by acid. To prevent inactivation by gastric secretions, erythromycin base has been manufactured in various acid resistant forms, such as enteric-coated tablets and granules. Depending on the preparation, these acid-resistant forms are better absorbed and produce more consistent serum levels. Their absorption is still influenced by food and therefore they should be given at least 1 h prior to meals. Various erythromycin salts and esters subsequently became available for clinical use, which are more acid-resistant. Four of these have been used clinically.

1 Erythromycin stearate (a salt).

2 Erythromycin ethyl succinate (an ester).
These two preparations are still susceptible to acid inactivation. Despite the fact that they are marketed with a buffering agent or as film-coated or enteric-coated tablets, they should be administered at least 1 h before a meal.

3 Propinyl erythromycin ester lauryl sulfate (erythromycin estolate) (the salt of an ester).

4 Stearate salt of 2'-acetyl ester of erythromycin (erythromycin ascitrate) (Tuominen *et al.*, 1988).

These last two formulations are more resistant to inactivation by gastric acid and they can be administered in the fasting state or after food. Erythromycin is widely used as an alternative to the beta-lactam agents for the treatment and prevention of infections caused by Gram-positive organisms, *Campylobacter* and *Legionella* infections, and of infections caused by non-bacterial agents such as *Chlamydia* and *Mycoplasma* spp.

Sensitive Organisms

1 Gram-positive aerobic bacteria

Erythromycin is normally highly active against organisms such as *Streptococcus pyogenes*, Groups B, C, and G streptococci, *Strep. pneumoniae*, *Strep. viridans*, *Strep. bovis*, *Staph. aureus* (including beta-lactamase-producing strains) and coagulase-negative staphylococci. *Enterococcus faecalis* is somewhat less susceptible (Table I.45). Nutritionally variant strains of streptococci are usually sensitive. The MIC and MBC of erythromycin for 90% of these organisms in one series were 0.13 and 2.0 μg per ml, respectively (Gephart and Washington, 1982).

All of these normally sensitive streptococci can develop erythromycin-resistance. Strains of *Strep. pyogenes* resistant to erythromycin were first reported in 1968 (Dixon, 1968; Sanders *et al.*, 1968). The frequency of these resistant strains of *Strep. pyogenes* has increased in various areas since that time. In northern Canada in 1972, 1.3% were resistant to erythromycin (Dixon and Lipinski, 1972) and in the USA in 1982 3% of the isolates were resistant (Bourbeau and Campos, 1982). In a later study in the USA 4% of *Strep. pyogenes* strains were erythromycin-resistant (Coonan and Kaplan, 1994), in Western Australia the percentage of resistant strains was 17.6% (Stingemore *et al.*, 1989), in Sweden 5.9% (Zackrisson *et al.*, 1988) and in Finland in certain areas of the country it rose to 29–54% (Seppälä *et al.*, 1993). In Japan the resistance rates were some 22% in 1981 and 1982, but these have decreased markedly in recent years because of lesser erythromycin use (Fujita *et al.*, 1994). Also during 1971 and 1972 in northern Canada, 0.6% of Group B, 1–2% of Group C and 1.3% of Group G streptococci were resistant to erythromycin (Dixon and Lipinski, 1974). Of 707 clinical isolates of Group B streptococci from one hospital in California, 1–2% were resistant to erythromycin or clindamycin, but cross-resistance between these two antibiotics was not absolute (Anthony and Concepcion, 1975).

Initially strains of *Strep. pneumoniae* resistant to erythromycin were rare (Kislak *et al.*, 1965; Champion *et al.*, 1978, Casal, 1982; Liñares *et al.*, 1983). The multiple antibiotic-resistant strains of pneumococci isolated in South Africa during 1977 (p. 5) were resistant to erythromycin (CDC, 1977c). Later in Spain of a total of 163 *Strep. pneumoniae* isolates, 42.5% were penicillin G-resistant and 10.8% erythromycin-resistant (García-Leoni *et al.*, 1992). In another study in Spain overall 16 of 78 isolates (20.5%) were resistant to erythromycin, and this resistance was found in 2.5%, 33.3% and 45% of penicillin-sensitive, intermediately penicillin-resistant and penicillin-resistant strains, respectively (Soriano and Fernández-Roblas, 1993). During 1979–1987, only 0.3% of pneumococcal strains in the USA were erythromycin-resistant, but later in one area of that country 5% of strains were resistant (Lonks and Medeiros, 1993). In a study in Korea 70% of *Strep. pneumoniae* isolates showed penicillin G-resistance; 52% of these were also erythromycin-resistant (Lee *et al.*, 1995). Strains with combined penicillin G and erythromycin resistance have also been detected in a day-care center in the USA (Barnes *et al.*, 1995).

Resistant strains of *Strep. viridans* have also been reported (Sprunt *et al.*, 1970; Yagi *et al.*, 1978).

Most staphylococci are still erythromycin-sensitive (Hassam *et al.*, 1978), but resistant strains have been encountered with increasing frequency, particularly in hospitals and newborn nurseries (Fidalgo *et al.*, 1988; Hedberg *et al.*, 1990; Back *et al.*, 1993). Methicillin-resistant staphylococci now are also usually erythromycin-resistant (p. 77). When erythromycin use in a community or hospital area is reduced, the percentage of resistant strains often decreases. For instance, Lilly and Lowbury (1978) noted a fall in the proportion of erythromycin-resistant *Staph. aureus* strains isolated after cessation of 'routine' prophylaxis with erythromycin in a burns unit. With staphylococci there is some cross-resistance between all the macrolides, and also, to some extent, between them and chemically unrelated clindamycin (p. 588). Most staphylococcal strains resistant to clindamycin and spiramycin are also resistant to erythromycin, but erythromycin-resistant strains are not always resistant to spiramycin and clindamycin. A characteristic feature of the macrolide antibiotics is the 'dissociated type of resistance', which was first described by Garrod (1957). This phenomenon also occurs with clindamycin (p. 588).

Enterococcus faecalis also easily acquires erythromycin-resistance. In 1976 in Zürich, up to 30% of *E. faecalis* strains were resistant (Marder and Kayser, 1977). An even greater level of resistance among urinary isolates of enterococci in the USA was demonstrated by Tofte *et al.* (1984). Erythromycin-resistant enterococci in the USA have been also isolated from pigs and chickens and some of them are also resistant to other antibiotics such as tetracycline and chloramphenicol (Rollins *et al.*, 1985; Pepper *et al.*, 1987).

Bacillus anthracis and *Listeria monocytogenes* are erythromycin-sensitive (Wiggins *et al.*, 1978). However, at 48 h incubation, erythromycin is bacteriostatic while penicillin G would kill most of the *L. monocytogenes* strains tested. Because erythromycin and penicillin are antagonistic *in vitro*, the combination is not recommended for the treatment of *L. monocytogenes* infections (Winslow *et al.*, 1983). Similar antagonism has been demonstrated between erythromycin and gentamicin (Penn *et al.*, 1982). *Corynebacterium diphtheriae* is very susceptible (Zamiri and McEntegart, 1972), but resistant strains have been detected occasionally (Jellard and Lipinski, 1973; Coyle *et al.*, 1979). The toxigenic strains of *C. diphtheriae* isolated recently in northwestern Russia and surrounding countries are erythromycin-sensitive (Maple *et al.*, 1994). The *Nocardia* are variable in their susceptibility. Bach *et al.* (1973) found that erythromycin in a concentration of 0.8 µg per ml inhibited 40% of *N. asteroides* strains tested, but MICs for most of the others were greater than 100 µg per ml. The resistant *N. asteroides* strains inactivate erythromycin by either phosphorylation or glycosylation (Yazawa *et al.*, 1994). *Rhodococcus equi* is erythromycin-sensitive (Decré *et al.*, 1991; Verville *et al.*, 1994).

The resistance mechanisms of Gram-positive bacteria to erythromycin are similar to those for clindamycin (p. 587). The most prevalent mechanism is target site modification, which involves dimethylation of adenine in 23 rRNA. This leads to reduced binding of macrolide, lincosamide and streptogramin B antibiotics to their shared 50S rRNA target site (MLS type of resistance) (Arthur et al., 1987b; Jenssen et al., 1987; Eady et al., 1990; Leclercq and Courvalin, 1991a; Weisblum, 1995). The genes determining this type of resistance are located on either chromosomes, plasmids or transposons. In *Staphylococcus aureus* the genes encoding this resistance have been designated as erm A, erm B, and erm C (Westh et al., 1995). The second known resistance mechanism involves active efflux of the antibiotic from the periplasmic space, which is also genetically determined (Leclercq and Courvalin, 1991b; Eady et al., 1993). The third mechanism is enzymatic inactivation of erythromycin which may be plasmid-mediated (Leclercq and Courvalin, 1991b; Yazawa et al., 1994).

2 Gram-positive anaerobic bacteria

Erythromycin has a wide range of activity against Gram-positive anaerobic bacteria. It is active against *Eubacterium*, *Propionibacterium*, *Bifidobacterium*, *Lactobacillus* and *Peptostreptococcus* spp., and also against most strains of *Peptococcus* spp. (Sutter and Finegold, 1976). *Actinomyces israeli* (the causative agent of human actinomycosis) is also sensitive (Sutter and Finegold, 1976; Holmberg et al., 1977). *Clostridium tetani* and *Cl. perfringens* are also usually susceptible (Brazier et al., 1985). Some strains of *Cl. perfringens* are resistant; the resistance is determined by a gene which codes for the most common resistance mechanism for erythromycin-target site modification (see above) (Berryman et al., 1994). In one study 308 *Cl. difficile* isolates were tested for erythromycin sensitivity. Almost all of the 161 isolates of serogroups A, F, G, H and X were erythromycin-sensitive, but most of 32 toxigenic isolates of serogroup C were resistant. Other serogroups showed variable patterns (Delmée and Avesani, 1988). The main resistance mechanism for *Cl. difficile* is again target site modification (Hächler et al., 1987; Berryman and Rood, 1989).

3 Gram-negative bacteria

Erythromycin is active against *Neisseria meningitidis*. *Haemophilus influenzae*, including ampicillin-resistant strains, is only moderately susceptible (Table I.45) (Righter and Luchsinger, 1988). *Bordetella pertussis* is sensitive and there was no change in its sensitivity to erythromycin in isolates collected between 1969 and 1981 (Bannatyne and Cheung, 1982, but recently, a strain of erythromycin-resistant *B. pertussis* was isolated in *Arizona*, USA from a child suffering from *pertussis* (Leads from the MMWR, 1995). Susceptibility of *H. ducreyi* to antibiotics varies geographically. Bilgeri et al. (1982) reported 90% of 103 isolates of *H. ducreyi* as having an erythromycin MIC equal to or less than 0.03 μg per ml. Erythromycin and clindamycin were the most active antibiotics against 56 strains of *Gardnerella vaginalis*, all strains being inhibited by 0.06 μg per ml or less (McCarthy et al., 1979).

Neisseria gonorrhoeae is sensitive, but strains with diminished sensitivity or which are completely resistant occur. In clinical isolates of *N. gonorrhoeae* there is usually a correlation between the degree of sensitivity with penicillin G, tetracycline, erythromycin and chloramphenicol (Report, 1978). Some 35% of beta-lactamase-producing strains isolated in the USA and East Asia were resistant to erythromycin in a concentration of 1.0 μg per ml (CDC, 1978). Ng et al. (1983) examined strains of *N. gonorrhoeae* from various South-East Asian countries and found that 80% of the beta-lactamase-producing strains and 75% of the non-beta-lactamase-producers had MICs equal or greater than 2 μg per ml. *Moraxella catarrhalis* is usually very sensitive to erythromycin (Brorson et al., 1981), but Brown et al. (1989), who studied 457 strains of this organism, found that 16 of the isolates were only moderately sensitive and the MIC of one isolate was >8 μg per ml. Some strains of *Brucella* spp. are sensitive to erythromycin (Abbott Laboratories, 1966).

Escherichia coli, the *Enterobacter*, *Klebsiella*, *Proteus*, *Salmonella* and *Shigella* spp. and *Ps. aeruginosa* are erythromycin-resistant. *Escherichia coli* and other Enterobacteriaceae are resistant because they have a modified target site (MLS resistance, see above) or because they produce a plasmid-mediated erythromycin esterase which inactivates the drug (Arthur and Courvalin, 1986; Arthur et al., 1987b). Antibacterial activity of erythromycin against Gram-negative bacilli is influenced by pH and it increases markedly as the pH rises to 8.5. Most *E. coli* and *Klebsiella* spp. strains can be inhibited by erythromycin concentrations attained in urine with ordinary therapeutic doses, provided the urine is made alkaline (Sabath et al., 1968).

Campylobacter jejuni is usually sensitive to erythromycin. Early studies showed that some 90% of isolates were inhibited by less than 1.0 μg per ml (Vanhoof et al., 1980; Karmali et al.,

1981). Similarly, of 28 strains of *C. jejuni* isolates in Jakarta, Indonesia, 90% were sensitive to 0.5 µg per ml or less of erythromycin (Ringertz *et al.*, 1981). In more recent years *C. jejuni* strains resistant to erythromycin were still uncommon in Sweden (Sjögren *et al.*, 1992) and Spain (Reina *et al.*, 1994; Sánchez *et al.*, 1994), but in Thailand 53% of orphanage-acquired strains and 11% of community-acquired *C. jejuni* strains were erythromycin-resistant (Taylor *et al.*, 1987). *Campylobacter coli* (Secker, 1983; Taylor *et al.*, 1987; Reina *et al.*, 1994) and *C. fetus* (Chow *et al.*, 1978) are usually moderately or completely erythromycin-resistant. *Helicobacter pylori* is sensitive to erythromycin (McNulty *et al.*, 1985), but strains with increased MICs can be selected *in vitro* in the presence of the antibiotic (Haas *et al.*, 1990). The resistance of *Campylobacter* spp. to erythromycin appears to be chromosomally determined which codes for a change in a ribosomal protein (Taylor and Courvalin, 1988; Yan and Taylor, 1991).

Early *in vitro* and animal studies on *Legionella pneumophila* indicated that erythromycin might be effective against this organism (CDC, 1977a,b). Subsequent *in vitro* (Thornsberry *et al.*, 1978; Edelstein and Meyer, 1980; Moffie and Mouton, 1988) and *in vivo* studies in guinea pigs (Fraser *et al.*, 1978) and embryonated eggs (Lewis *et al.*, 1978) have confirmed that erythromycin is one of the most active drugs against this organism. This agent is also active against *L. pneumophila* within human monocyte-derived macrophages (Vildé *et al.*, 1986). Methylprednisolone does not diminish the intracellular activity of erythromycin on *L. pneumophila* (Higa *et al.*, 1993). Other members of this genus, *L. micdadei* (the Pittsburg pneumonia agent), *L. bozemanii*, *L. gormanii*, *L. dumoffii*, *L. longbeachae*, and *L. anisa* are also sensitive to erythromycin (Pasculle *et al.*, 1981; Dowling *et al.*, 1982; Fallon and Stack, 1990; Nimmo and Bull, 1995). Strains of *L. pneumophila* and *L. micdadei* have been produced after passage *in vitro* in a medium containing erythromycin, which were resistant to erythromycin and cross-resistant to rosaramicin (p. 630) (Dowling *et al.*, 1985). *Flavobacterium* spp. may also be sensitive to erythromycin (Lee *et al.*, 1977). *Bartonella* (formerly *Rochalimaea*) *quintana* and *Bartonella henselae*, the agents which cause bacillary angiomatosis and bacillary peliosis in AIDS patients, are erythromycin-sensitive (Koehler and Tappero, 1993; Maurin and Raoult, 1993; Regnery and Tappero, 1995). *Pasteurella multocida* is resistant (Goldstein *et al.*, 1988).

Erythromycin has a variable activity against anaerobic Gram-negative bacteria. Most strains of *Bacteroides* spp. can be inhibited by moderately high erythromycin concentrations, but such high levels are only attained in the serum after parenteral administration (Zabransky *et al.*, 1973; Gorbach and Bartlett, 1974). Sutter and Finegold (1976) studied susceptibility of anaerobic organisms to erythromycin. Although all strains of *Prevotella melaninogenica* and some *Bacteroides* spp. were susceptible to 1.0 µg per ml, *B. fragilis* and the *Fusobacterium* spp. were usually resistant. Harvey *et al.* (1981) found that a concentration of erythromycin of 6 µg per ml was usually required to inhibit more than 90% of *B. fragilis*, other *Bacteroides* spp. and *Fusobacterium* spp.

4 Spirochetes

Treponema pallidum is erythromycin-sensitive (Brause *et al.*, 1976; Norris and Edmondson, 1988), although strains which exhibit high-level erythromycin resistance have been detected (Stamm *et al.*, 1988). Erythromycin exhibits only a relatively low degree of activity against *Borrelia burgdorferi* (Johnson *et al.*, 1987).

5 Rickettsiae

In vitro activity of erythromycin against *Rickettsia prowazeki* has been demonstrated in cell culture, but the rate of killing of rickettsiae was slow (Wisseman *et al.*, 1974). *Rickettsia rickettsii* and *R. conorii* are erythromycin-resistant (Raoult *et al.*, 1988).

6 Chlamydiae

With *Chlamydia trachomatis*, cell culture and clinical studies have indicated that tetracycline (p. 726) and erythromycin are the most effective antibiotics against this organism (Kuo *et al.*, 1977; Lee *et al.*, 1978; Schachter *et al.*, 1986). A few strains of *C. trachomatis* have been shown to be relatively resistant to erythromycin (Mourad *et al.*, 1980). *Chlamydia pneumoniae* is also erythromycin-sensitive, but chlarithromycin (p. 645) is some 8-fold more active *in vitro* (Chirgwin *et al.*, 1989; Fenelon *et al.*, 1990; Hammerschlag, 1994; Roblin *et al.*, 1994).

7 Mycoplasmas

Mycoplasma pneumoniae is very susceptible to erythromycin (Jao and Finland, 1967). Erythromycin-resistant *M. pneumoniae* variants can be obtained *in vitro* by serial subculture of the organism in the presence of the drug. Such erythromycin-resistance is usually accompanied

Organism	MIC (µg per ml)
Gram-positive bacteria	
Staphylococcus aureus	0.5
Streptococcus pyogenes	0.04
Streptococcus pneumoniae	0.10
Streptococcus viridans	0.5
Enterococcus faecalis	1.5
Listeria monocytogenes	0.16
Clostridium tetani	0.09
Gram-negative bacteria	
Neisseria gonorrhoeae	0.94
Haemophilus influenzae	2.5
Bordetella pertussis	1.56
Legionella pneumophila	0.25
Fusobacterium spp.	19.0
Miscellaneous	
Mycoplasma pneumoniae	0.0125

Table I.45
After Abbott Laboratories (1966)
Edelstein and Meyer (1980) and Baker
et al. (1983)

by resistance to other macrolides (Niitu *et al.*, 1974). In one report a strain of *M. pneumoniae* acquired resistance to erythromycin during treatment (Niitu *et al.*, 1970). Erythromycin is also active against *M. genitalium* (Renaudin *et al.*, 1992), but not against *M. hominis* (Csonka and Spitzer, 1969).

8 Ureaplasma urealyticum

Ureaplasma urealyticum is sensitive to erythromycin, but some strains with intermediate or complete resistance occur (Spaepen *et al.*, 1976; Waites *et al.*, 1992). Tetracycline-resistant strains of *U. urealyticum* may sometimes be sensitive to erythromycin (Ford and Smith, 1974).

9 Mycobacteria

Mycobacterium tuberculosis is resistant to erythromycin, but some atypical mycobacteria are erythromycin-sensitive particularly *M. chelonae* (Molavi and Weinstein, 1971). *Mycobacterium avium* is sensitive, but to a lower degree (Swenson *et al.*, 1982).

10 Minimum inhibitory concentrations

The MICs of erythromycin against some selected bacterial species are shown in Table I.45.

Mode of Administration and Dosage

1 Oral administration

Erythromycin is usually administered by the oral route. The dosage is 30–50 mg per kg per day given in three or four divided doses. Erythromycin estolate and erythromycin ethylsuccinate have also been given in a dose of 30 mg per kg per day in two divided doses (Ginsburg *et al.*, 1982).

2 Intramuscular administration

Erythromycin can be administered i.m. in the form of erythromycin ethyl succinate. The adult dosage is 100–200 mg 8-hourly, but these injections are large and painful, so that this route of administration is rarely used.

3 Intravenous administration

The drug, as erythromycin lactobionate, can be used i.v. for treatment of severe infections. The dosage is 300–500 mg 6-hourly for adults and 30–50 mg per kg per day for children (given in four divided doses). Adult doses as high as 4–6 g daily have been given without toxic effects. The drug should be given i.v. by intermittent or continuous i.v. infusions. For intermittent administration each dose should be dissolved in 100–200 ml of infusion fluid and this should be infused relatively slowly (see below). The severity of venous irritation, which ranges from localized discomfort to thrombophlebitis is minimized by slower infusions. Too rapid i.v. infusion has also been associated with a high frequency of side-effects such as abdominal cramps, nausea, vomiting, pancreatitis and hepatic failure (Marlin et al., 1983; Putzi et al., 1983; Farrar et al., 1993). Ventricular arrhythmias can also occur, which appear to be more likely with rapid infusions (p. 615) (Schoenenberger et al., 1990). Being compatible with commonly used i.v. fluids, the drug can be added to i.v. drip bottles and administered by continuous infusion, but possible incompatible additives should be avoided. The manufacturers currently recommend continuous infusion but they state that if intermittent administration is necessary, each 6-hourly dose should be infused in 20–60 min. The 20-min infusion seems too fast, in view of the cardiac arrythmias reported (p. 615). Definite recommendations at this time are not available, but it seems to us that if the 6-hourly dose is 500 mg, it should be infused in 0.5–1.0 h. If the 6-hourly dose is 1.0 g, it probably should not be infused faster than in 1–2 h.

4 Patients with renal failure

The normal serum half-life of erythromycin of 1.4 h is only prolonged to 4.8–5.8 h in anuric patients, so that only minor, if any, dosage reduction of erythromycin is necessary in patients with severe renal failure (Kunin, 1967).

5 Patients with liver disease

Erythromycin may accumulate in patients with severe liver disease. If large doses are administered to such patients, serum level monitoring and dosage reduction may be necessary.

6 Newborn and premature infants

The oral dosage recommended for older children may be safely used in this age group. Burns and Hodgman (1963) administered 40 mg per kg per day of erythromycin estolate in four divided doses to 26 premature infants. Satisfactory serum levels, no evidence of accumulation and no toxic effects were observed. Erythromycin lactobionate i.v. should be administered to these patients in a dosage of 40 mg per kg per day in four divided doses, and each dose should be infused no faster than over 60 min (Gouyon et al., 1994; Waites et al., 1994).

7 Pregnant patients

Because of its propensity to cause hepatotoxicity (p. 615), erythromycin estolate should not be used in such patients. Other erythromycin preparations are safe in pregnancy.

8 Topical use

Erythromycin preparations of varying concentrations as ointments, lotions and gels have been employed in the treatment of acne vulgaris (Chalker et al., 1983; Lesher et al., 1985).

Serum Levels in Relation to Dosage

1 Erythromycin base

This is destroyed by acid in the stomach, so that tablets are manufactured with an acid-resistant coating, which subsequently dissolve in duodenum.

2 Erythromycin stearate

It is less readily destroyed in the stomach and dissociates in the duodenum liberating active erythromycin, which is absorbed. Peak serum levels after oral administration of erythromycin

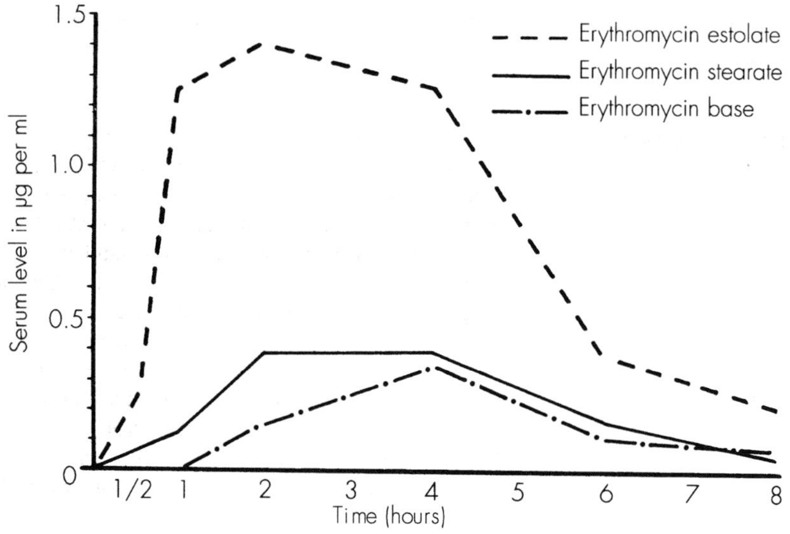

Fig. I.24.
Average serum concentrations in adults after oral administration of 250 mg erythromycin base, stearate and estolate. (Redrawn after Griffith and Black, 1962, with permission.)

base and stearate appear approximately the same, except that the absorption of the base may be slightly more delayed (Fig. I.24). Triggs and Ashley (1978) showed in volunteers that although mean serum levels were low after a single dose of erythromycin stearate, these were considerably higher after repeated doses. Doubling the dose of these compounds approximately doubles the serum concentrations. Food in stomach diminishes the absorption of both base and stearate (Disanto and Chodos, 1981). Furthermore, there is marked individual variation in the serum levels achieved after the administration of all forms of oral erythromycin (Griffith and Black, 1964; Lake and Bell, 1969).

3 Erythromycin estolate

Unlike the base and the stearate, it is acid-stable and absorbed from the gastrointestinal tract more completely. It is absorbed mainly as ester, of which about 41% is hydrolyzed in serum to active erythromycin (Croteau *et al.*, 1988). Figure I.24 shows the total free erythromycin plus inactive erythromycin estolate circulating in serum after erythromycin estolate administration, but the serum level of active erythromycin is still higher than the level after administration of the base or stearate.

4 Erythromycin ethylsuccinate

This is another ester which is well absorbed from the gastrointestinal tract. Absorption is delayed by food, however, and the highest and earliest peak serum levels after an 800 mg dose (2.23 μg per ml) occur under fasting conditions (Thompson *et al.*, 1980). After absorption about 69% of this ester is hydrolyzed to active erythromycin, but the estolate ester is still considered to have an advantage in pharmacokinetics as it has a longer half-life (5.47 versus 2.72 h) and a larger area-under-the-curve (Croteau *et al.*, 1988). In another study Bérubé *et al.* (1988) also found that after single doses of erythromycin estolate (500 mg) and erythromycin ethylsuccinate (600 mg), the bactericidal titers at 2 and 8 h against *Strep. pyogenes* and *Strep. pneumoniae* were significantly higher with erythromycin estolate than with ethylsuccinate ester.

Eriksson *et al.* (1981) reported a decreased absorption of erythromycin suspension (both stearate and ethyl succinate) in infants less than 1 month old, and the stearate suspension was also poorly absorbed in infants 1–6 months old. In a pharmacokinetic study of infants under 4 months of age comparing the estolate and ethylsuccinate esters, no differences were found between peak serum concentrations or the time taken to reach them, but the elimination half-life of the estolate was longer (Patamasucon *et al.*, 1981).

5 Erythromycin ascitrate

This ester is well absorbed after oral administration, provided it is given in a tablet with acid resistant coating. The total serum level reached is about 3.9-fold higher than that after the same dose of erythromycin base with acid resistant coating (Fig. I.24). In plasma, however, only about one-third of erythromycin ascitrate is hydrolyzed to active erythromycin. The absorption of this ester in some patients may be impaired by food. Concomitant administration of cimetidine does not affect the serum levels attained after erythromycin ascitrate (Männistö *et al.*, 1988; Tuominen *et al.*, 1988).

6 Parenteral erythromycin

Satisfactory serum levels are achieved after parenteral erythromycin administration. After an i.m. injection of 100 mg of erythromycin ethyl succinate in adults, the mean peak level after 1 h is 0.64 μg per ml; this level is maintained for nearly 6 h and measurable serum concentrations persist for at least 12 h (Metzger *et al.*, 1959). Following a single i.v. injection of 200 mg of erythromycin lactobionate, the mean serum level in adults is 3.0 μg per ml 1 h after injection and detectable levels persist for at least 6 h (Abbott Laboratories, 1966). If erythromycin lactobionate is given by continuous infusion at a rate of 1.0 g every 12 h, serum levels of about 4–6 μg per ml are maintained from 8 h onwards (Neaverson, 1976). Peak concentrations attained after 1 h intermittent i.v. erythromycin infusions in the usual doses (p. 611) are usually some 4- to 10-fold greater than those attained after oral erythromycin (Farrar *et al.*, 1993). When erythromycin lactobionate was given to preterm neonates i.v. in dosages of either 25 or 40 mg per kg per day in four divided doses 6-hourly (each dose infused over 60 min), the peak serum levels varied from 3.05 to 3.69 and 1.92 to 2.9 μg per ml for the 40- and 25-mg per kg per day dosage groups, respectively (Waites *et al.*, 1994).

7 Patients with liver disease

When 500 mg of erythromycin base was given to patients with alcoholic liver disease and to normal subjects after a 12 h fast, in the former the normally delayed absorption (lag time) was shorter (2 versus 3 h), an earlier peak was obtained (4.6 versus 6.3 h) and higher peak concentrations were observed (2.04 versus 1.5 μg per ml). A slower elimination time also occurred in patients with liver disease, so that some adjustment of the dose may be required in such patients (p. 611) (Kroboth *et al.*, 1982).

Excretion

1 Urine

Erythromycin is partly excreted in urine, and only about 2.5% of an orally administered dose and 15% of a parenterally administered dose is recoverable from the urine in the active form (Abbott Laboratories, 1966). Urinary concentrations of the active drug are usually low and variable. As renal excretion is not the main method of erythromycin elimination from the body, there is no significant accumulation of the drug in uremic patients.

2 Bile

A considerable proportion of erythromycin is excreted in the bile, where high levels of the active drug are attained. Some erythromycin excreted in this way is reabsorbed from the intestine.

3 Inactivation in body

A large proportion of administered erythromycin cannot be accounted for by combined renal and biliary excretion, and so a considerable amount appears to be inactivated in the body, probably in the liver (Osono and Umezawa, 1985).

Distribution of the Drug in Body

Erythromycin is widely distributed in tissues, and is concentrated in the liver and spleen. It persists in the tissues for longer periods than in the serum. The related macrolide antibiotic, spiramycin (p. 631) and some newer macrolides (p. 656) produce even higher and better sustained tissue concentrations than erythromycin.

Adequate concentrations of erythromycin are found in pleural and ascitic fluids. The drug reaches high levels in tear fluid in infants with purulent conjunctivitis (Sandström and Ringertz, 1988). It enters middle-ear exudates in sufficient concentration to inhibit the highly sensitive organisms *Strep. pyogenes* and *Strep. pneumoniae*, but not necessarily all strains of *H. influenzae* (Bass *et al.*, 1971). Adequate levels of erythromycin are found in tonsils after oral administration, the levels being higher after the estolate suspension than after ethylsuccinate suspension (Ginsburg *et al.*, 1976). The tonsillar concentrations are also adequate after oral erythromycin ascitrate administration and more of this ester is hydrolyzed to active erythromycin in the tonsillar tissue than in the serum (Gordin *et al.*, 1988a). In patients with lobar pneumonia treated with i.v. erythromycin lactobionate, effective concentrations were reached in the infected and uninfected lung tissue within 10 min and maintained for at least 1 h (Wollmer *et al.*, 1982). Thiopronine, a mucolytic agent, elevated concentrations of erythromycin in rat lung by 36 and 26% at 1.5 and 3.0 h, respectively (Coppi and Alberti, 1984). Mean sputum levels of 2.6 μg per ml have been recorded when erythromycin lactobionate was given by infusion in a dose of 1 g every 12 h (Neaverson, 1976). However, after 500 mg erythromycin stearate was given orally every 8 h for 7 days, sputum levels in 24 h collections did not exceed 1.0 μg per ml in five of six patients (Clarke *et al.*, 1980). After an oral dose of 500 mg erythromycin ethylsuccinate or stearate, the gastric mucosal concentration was higher than the MIC of *H. pylori* (McNulty *et al.*, 1988).

Erythromycin does not enter the CSF in the absence of meningitis, but as with many antibiotics, the drug may be detectable in the CSF when the meninges are inflamed (Griffith and Black, 1970). Peak concentrations in lymph after oral therapy were 24% of the peak serum concentrations and the mean lymph: serum concentration ratio was 0.35 (Bergan *et al.*, 1982). After i.v. administration of erythromycin lactobionate, the concentrations in normal cancelous bone were approximately 30% of concomitant serum levels (Rosdahl *et al.*, 1979). Erythromycin crosses the placenta, but serum concentrations attained in the infant are considerably lower and less predictable than those in the mother (South *et al.*, 1964; Philipson *et al.*, 1973). Erythromycin is only 18% protein bound (Kunin, 1967).

Erythromycin is concentrated in human polymorphonuclear leukocytes some 10–20 times the concentration in extracellular fluid (Prokesch and Hand, 1982; Ishiguro *et al.*, 1989). Phagocytosis by neutrophils appears to be unaffected by erythromycin (Naess and Solberg, 1988), but erythromycin may stimulate neutrophil migration (Anderson, 1989). In alveolar macrophages from smokers and non-smokers, the uptake of erythromycin was lower in the cells derived from the latter group (Hand *et al.*, 1985).

Mode of Action

Erythromycin interferes with bacterial protein synthesis at the ribosomes. This drug, similar to other macrolide antibiotics, becomes bound to the 50 S subunit of the ribosome (Goldman *et al.*, 1990). Chloramphenicol (p. 561) and clindamycin (p. 594) also become attached to this site. The exact stage of bacterial protein synthesis affected by erythromycin is not known with certainty but it was suggested that it may interfere with the 'translocation reaction' (p. 562) which is catalyzed by an enzyme, translocase (Cundliffe and McQuillen, 1967). During this reaction the growing peptide chain with its t-RNA moves from the 'acceptor site' to the 'donor site' on the ribosome. Erythromycin probably binds to the donor site, and by competing for this site of attachment, prevents translocation of the peptide chain from the acceptor to the donor site (Oleinick and Corcoran, 1969). More recently it has been suggested that erythromycin stimulates dissociation of peptidyl-tRNA from the ribosomes during the elongation phase, leading to inhibition of protein synthesis (Mazzei *et al.*, 1993).

It is possible that one reason why Gram-negative bacilli are resistant to erythromycin is because it cannot penetrate their cell walls. Stable L-forms of *Pr. mirabilis*, which have no cell walls, are very susceptible to erythromycin (Guze and Kalmanson, 1964; Gutman *et al.*, 1967).

Erythromycin has been shown to produce other effects in addition to its direct antimicrobial activity. It appears to act as immunomodulator or bacterial virulence suppressing agent, especially against *Ps. aeruginosa* infections (Hirakata *et al.*, 1992; Ras *et al.*, 1992).

Toxicity

1 Gastrointestinal side-effects

Symptoms such as nausea, vomiting and diarrhea are fairly frequently encountered with oral erythromycin, but these are only occasionally severe. Erythromycin stimulates the gastro-intestinal motor activity of dogs. This may explain some of these side-effects, particularly when associated with i.v. administration of the drug; some of the effect can be blocked with atropine sulfate (Itoh *et al.*, 1984). Also in human volunteers both oral and i.v. erythromycin increased the amplitude and frequency of gastric contractions. Some of the volunteers felt nauseated and a few vomited (Williams and Sefton, 1993; Williams, 1995). Pseudomembranous colitis (p. 594) has been reported in conjunction with the use of this antibiotic (Ganz *et al.*, 1979).

2 Hepatotoxicity

Initially this was thought to occur after administration of erythromycin estolate, but not after other erythromycin preparations (Masel, 1962; Sherlock 1968). It was postulated that the propionyl ester linkage at the 2' position conferred this property on the estolate and that there was no cross-sensitivity with other erythromycin preparations (Tolman et al., 1974). Jaundice usually occurs about 10–12 days after starting treatment, but it may occur within 1 or 2 days in patients who had previously experienced the drug (Robinson, 1961; Gilbert, 1962). Some patients may experience severe abdominal pain, which may lead to an erroneous diagnosis of cholelithiasis (Oliver et al., 1973). Other symptoms include fever and pruritus and a rash may occasionally occur. Jaundice may be clinical or subclinical and hepatic enlargement is usually present. Eosinophilia is common, liver function tests usually indicate cholestasis and the jaundice is probably due to 'hypersensitivity cholestasis'. Liver histology usually reveals a picture of intrahepatic cholestasis.

The jaundice and other symptoms usually subside when the drug is stopped, but occasionally jaundice may persist for weeks, and in one case reported by Brown (1963) it persisted for about 3 months. There have been no deaths associated with erythromycin jaundice, and the subsequent development of chronic liver disease has not been reported. The exact frequency of this complication was not known. It is possible that this complication may be more frequent during pregnancy (McCormack et al., 1977).

It now appears that similar cholestatic jaundice can arise after other erythromycin preparations and that it may not be more common with the estolate than with the others. Inman and Rawson (1983) reported three cases of similar jaundice associated with erythromycin stearate. Carson et al. (1993) estimated that annually in the USA 66 cases of acute symptomatic liver disease, resulting in hospitalization, were caused by erythromycin. None of these patients had taken erythromycin estolate, but this study demonstrated that jaundice occurred after erythromycin ethylsuccinate and erythromycin stearate. Derby et al. (1993) studied a total of 366 064 patients who had received one or more prescriptions of erythromycin. They estimated that the risk of cholestatic jaundice associated with erythromycin was approximately 3.6 per 100 000 users. It did not appear that erythromycin estolate caused jaundice more frequently than other erythromycin preparations, although only 3 036 patients received the estolate. Lehtonen et al. (1991) administered erythromycin ascitrate to 1549 patients. Only three patients (0.2%) developed hepatic damage attributable to the drug.

3 Skin rashes

These may occur as a single manifestation, but are rare. The risk of erythromycin hypersensitivity appears to be higher in patients allergic to other antibiotics, such as the penicillins (Boguniewicz and Leung, 1995).

4 Ototoxicity

Tinnitus and transient deafness have been described in a small number of patients, mainly in association with the i.v. administration of erythromycin lactobionate (Minz et al., 1973; Quinnan and McCabe, 1978; Snavely and Hodges, 1984), but also after oral administration (Eckman et al., 1975; Van Marion et al., 1978). In a number of these patients, renal failure and/or liver damage may have predisposed to high serum levels of erythromycin (Quinnan and McCabe, 1978; Van Marion et al., 1978; Umstead and Neumann, 1986). In one patient symptoms were noted only after three 1.0-g doses of i.v. erythromycin lactobionate (Miller, 1982). In most patients erythromycin-induced ototoxicity has been a reversible event which occurred with high doses, such as 1 g i.v. 6-hourly, or in patients with hepatic or renal abnormalities (Brummett and Fox, 1989).

5 Cardiac toxicity

Schoenenberger et al. (1990) described a 61-year-old woman with pneumonia who was treated with erythromycin lactobionate i.v. 1.0 g 8-hourly (each dose infused over 90 min). During the fifth infusion she developed prolongation of the Q-T interval, multiple ventricular extrasystoles, and an episode of non-sustained torsades de pointes occurred. These abnormalities subsided after the erythromycin infusion, but recurred with subsequent infusions. After the tenth infusion, erythromycin was stopped and there were no further cardiac abnormalities. Dan and Feigl (1993) reported a 17-year-old girl who was treated with erythromycin lactobionate 600 mg i.v. 6-hourly for pneumonia. During the second infusion she developed extreme weakness and hypotension. Erythromycin infusion was stopped and she improved with fluids, hydrocortisone and dopamine. A dose of 500 mg oral erythromycin was administered 16 h later and similar hypotension recurred 1½ h after the dose. Brandriss et al. (1994) reported a 35-year-old woman who was treated with i.v. erythromycin (1 g 6-hourly) for pneumonia. From the fifth day of treatment she developed intermittent ventricular bigemy and short episodes of ventricular tachycardia. Initially erythromycin therapy was not suspected as the cause and the episodes of ventricular tachycardia responded to lidocaine; however, later it was obvious that some episodes of cardiac arrythmia started soon after commencement of erythromycin infusion. On day 10, erythromycin was stopped and no further cardiac abnormalities occurred. These authors also reviewed 11 other cases published in English literature. Most of them had some underlying cardiac abnormality. Nine received i.v. erythromycin. Ten patients developed polymorphic ventricular tachycardia characteristic of torsades de pointes; these abnormalities occurred during or after erythromycin infusion. Four adult patients have been reported to the Australian Drug Reactions Advisory Committee, who developed serious cardiac arrythmias whilst receiving intermittent i.v. infusions of erythromycin lactobionate; two of them died (ADRAC, 1995).

Premature infants are now more commonly treated with i.v. erythromycin, mainly for *Ureaplasma urealyticum* infections. Farrar *et al.* (1993) reported two infants treated with i.v. erythromycin. One received 20 mg per kg per day in two divided doses and the other 26 mg per kg per day in four divided doses. Each dose was infused in 30 min. Both developed bradycardia and shock during the first infusion. Both were resuscitated, but one of them died later from pulmonary complications. Gouyon *et al.* (1994) described two infants who were treated by 20–25 mg per kg of i.v. erythromycin, 12-hourly, and each dose was infused over 30 min (total dose 40–50 mg per kg per day). Both infants developed severe cardiac abnormalities; one of them had a lethal ventricular tachycardia. Both infants died. Waites *et al.* (1993) and Sims *et al.* (1994) consider that i.v. erythromycin lactobionate may be safe in infants in doses of 25–40 mg per kg per day, provided that it is administered in four divided doses and provided that each dose is not infused faster than over 60 min. However, it seems that further evaluation of the pharmacokinetics and safety of i.v. erythromycin in the neonatal population is necessary.

Terfenadine, a non-sedating histamine H_1-antagonist accumulates in the serum if it is used together with oral erythromycin. Terfanadine then is associated with altered cardiac repolarization. The concomitant use of erythromycin and terfenadine is contraindicated (Honig *et al.*, 1994).

6 Drug interactions

Two review articles have concluded that there is sufficient data to suggest that erythromycin can, in some individuals, inhibit the elimination of methylprednisolone, theophylline, carbamazepine and warfarin (Descotes *et al.*, 1985; Ludden, 1985). This has been more closely studied for some of these drugs such as carbamazepine (Wroblewski *et al.*, 1986). The mean change in drug clearance was about 20–25% in most cases, with some patients having a much larger change than others. The type of erythromycin used may also be important. Concomitant erythromycin administration may cause elevation of cyclosporine serum levels by interfering with its metabolism in liver. This can lead to acute reversible impairment of renal function (Martell *et al.*, 1986; Ben-Ari *et al.*, 1988).

7 Changes in bowel flora

Oral erythromycin administration decreased both aerobic and anaerobic bacteria in the colon. New colonizing *Clostridium* spp., in some cases including *Cl. difficile*, enterobacteria and fungi appeared in the colon (Nord and Heimdahl, 1986; Kaukoranta-Tolvanen *et al.*, 1989).

8 Miscellaneous side-effects

Interstitial nephritis and acute renal failure has been reported after oral erythromycin (Rosenfeld *et al.*, 1983). An episode of erythromycin-induced hemolytic anemia has been described by Wong *et al.* (1981). Reversible selective Factor X deficiency and acute liver failure have been reported in a patient with chest infection treated with erythromycin base (Hosker and Jewell, 1983).

Clinical Uses of the Drug

1 Streptococcal and pneumococcal infections

Erythromycin is an effective alternative to penicillin G for the treatment of many of these infections in penicillin-allergic patients. Streptococcal tonsillitis, scarlet fever and erysipelas can be successfully treated by erythromycin. Erythromycin base or estolate given twice-daily is just as effective for streptococcal tonsillitis as when given 6- or 8-hourly provided that the same total daily dose is used (Breese *et al.*, 1974; Ginsburg and Eichenwald, 1976; Hovi *et al.*, 1987). In one study erythromycin estolate in a dose of 15 mg per kg 12-hourly proved to be superior to erythromycin ethylsuccinate, given in the same dosage (Ginsburg *et al.*, 1982). In another study erythromycin ethylsuccinate given at 50 mg per kg per day in two doses produced a high frequency of gastrointestinal symptoms and a greater bacteriologic failure rate in treating *Strep. pyogenes* pharyngitis than twice-daily estolate (30 mg per kg per day), each drug being given for 10 days (Ginsburg *et al.*, 1984).

Large doses of erythromycin i.v. were used in the past for *Strep. viridans* endocarditis in penicillin-allergic patients, but now cephalothin (p. 258) or ceftriaxone (p. 362) are preferred. It also has been used under the same circumstances for *E. faecalis* endocarditis, but vancomycin plus gentamicin (p. 778) is now preferred.

Erythromycin is also an effective alternative to penicillin G for the treatment of pneumococcal pneumonia. It is effective for severe infections, such as pneumococcal meningitis, if it is used in large doses (4–6 g daily) i.v., but chloramphenicol (p. 569), cefotaxime (p. 336) or ceftriaxone (p. 359) are preferable for this disease if penicillin G is contraindicated.

2 Chemoprophylaxis

For endocarditis chemoprophylaxis oral erythromycin stearate 1.0 g orally 2 h before the dental procedure and 0.5 g 6 h later is recommended for standard risk penicillin-allergic patients (p. 44). This erythromycin regimen is also suitable for standard risk patients who have been taking long-term penicillin prophylaxis for rheumatic fever (p. 44). Erythromycin may cause some gastrointestinal side-effects in these patients (Sefton *et al.*, 1990).

Erythromycin is the most suitable alternative to penicillin for prophylaxis against rheumatic fever (Ginsburg and Eichenwald, 1976). Suitable dosage is a single daily dose of 200 mg for children and adults weighing more than 36 kg and 100 mg for those of lower weight. This chemoprophylaxis has been used continuously for over 4 years without side-effects or the development of resistant strains of *Strep. pyogenes*. Erythromycin-resistant strains of *Strep. viridans* often appear in the pharynx of patients receiving long-term erythromycin prophylaxis. In ten volunteers given three 1.0-g doses of erythromycin stearate, erythromycin-resistant strains of *Strep. viridans* persisted in eight of the ten subjects at 23 weeks and were still present in five of eight subjects examined at 43 weeks (Harrison *et al.*, 1985). In such patients with rheumatic heart disease receiving long-tem erythromycin, who require temporary protection against endocarditis at the time of dental procedures, etc., prophylaxis by an unrelated antibiotic, such as one of the cephalosporins, is indicated. Clindamycin is not suitable for this purpose, as erythromycin-resistant *Strep. viridans* strains are also often clindamycin-resistant (Sprunt *et al.*, 1970).

In military recruits benzathine penicillin is usually used to prevent *Strep. pyogenes* epidemics (p. 51). Fujikawa *et al.* (1992) showed that low-dose oral erythromycin (250 mg twice-daily) was also suitable for this purpose and it can be recommended for penicillin-allergic recruits. Oral antibiotic prophylaxis with cotrimoxazole and erythromycin reduced the incidence of fever and infection in some granulocytopenic patients, but the benefit was limited, and restricted to those with good compliance (Pizzo *et al.*, 1983) (p. 882).

3 Respiratory tract infections

Pneumococci and *H. influenzae* are the common pathogens in bacterial bronchitis and erythromycin is one of several effective drugs for the treatment of acute infections (Gordin *et al.*, 1988b; Söderström *et al.*, 1991). Erythromycin is also useful for the treatment of otitis media caused by pneumococci or *Strep. pyogenes*, but it is of doubtful efficacy if this infection is caused by *H. influenzae* (Ginsburg and Eichenwald, 1976). The combination of erythromycin with sulfisoxazole (p. 821) is a more satisfactory treatment for *H. influenzae* otitis media than erythromycin alone (Bergeron *et al.*, 1987; Berman, 1995). Some failures of erythromycin therapy in otitis media may be due to erythromycin-resistant *Strep. pneumoniae* strains (p. 607) (Tarpay *et al.*, 1982). Amoxicillin is usually the preferred drug for otitis media (p. 140). *Streptococcus pyogenes* and pneumococcal sinusitis also responds well to erythromycin, but that due to *H. influenzae* may not do so (Kalm *et al.*, 1975). Respiratory tract infections due to *Moraxella catarrhalis* usually respond well to erythromycin (Darelid *et al.*, 1993).

4 Staphylococcal infections

Severe *Staph. aureus* infections, such as septicemia may be successfully treated by large doses of i.v. erythromycin if the organism is susceptible (Shoemaker and Yow, 1954), but other drugs are preferred. Prolonged chemotherapy is often necessary for patients with severe disseminated staphylococcal infections, particularly those with extensive osteomyelitis (Bennett and Kucers, 1970), and oral erythromycin may be suitable for the extended treatment, though alternatives such as penicillinase-resistant penicillins are available. Oral erythromycin may be useful for treatment of staphylococcal diseases such as boils, carbuncles and wound infections. An oral dose of 1.0 g daily given for 7 days was effective in eradicating staphylococci from healthy nasal carriers (Wilson et al., 1977).

5 Legionella infections

Erythromycin remains the drug of choice for Legionella pneumonia. Other drugs such as rifampicin, spiramycin, ciprofloxacin, pefloxacin, tetracyclines and possibly cotrimoxazole also have some effect but no controlled trials have been performed. Retrospective reviews favor the use of erythromycin. Mild infections may be treated by oral erythromycin, but moderately severe cases should be treated by i.v. erythromycin 0.5 g 6-hourly and more severe cases by i.v. erythromycin 1.0 g 6-hourly. The high dosage i.v. should always be given to patients with immunosuppression. A combination of i.v. erythromycin plus rifampicin (1 200 mg daily) is recommended for very ill patients and for those not responding to erythromycin (Meyer, 1983; Fraser et al., 1978; Muder et al., 1989; Nguyen et al., 1991; Edelstein, 1993). Legionella infections may occur in renal transplant patients. Intravenous erythromycin is again the treatment of choice, and rifampicin should be added if there is no response. Both erythromycin and rifampicin have important and opposite effects on cyclosporine metabolism, which may result, respectively, in increased cyclosporine toxicity or graft loss (p. 690). Patients who must continue cyclosporine will, therefore, require frequent monitoring of cyclosporine levels (Ampel and Wing, 1990). Alternatively the Legionella infection in these patients may be treated with one of the fluoroquinolones (p. 1024) (Edelstein, 1993). AIDS patients may develop Legionella pneumonia, but this has not occurred in patients receiving prophylactic cotrimoxazole. Some of these patients have responded to high-dose cotrimoxazole, but once the correct diagnosis is made, high dose i.v. erythromycin is preferable (Edelstein, 1993; Blatt et al., 1994).

Some 20% of patients with Legionella pneumonia are septicemic and they may develop extrapulmonary lesions. Lesions such as Legionella peritonitis, bowel abscess, colitis and cellulitis have been described. Bowel lesions may develop due to ingestion of the bacteria, rather than due to septicemia. Treatment of choice again is erythromycin (Edelstein, 1993; Waldor et al., 1993). A patient with prosthetic valve endocarditis caused by L. pneumophila was reported to be improving after valve surgery and 2 months therapy with i.v. erythromycin (4.0 g per day) and rifampicin 600 mg per day orally. It was planned to give 6 months therapy (McCabe et al., 1984).

Legionella micdadei also causes pneumonia, but this occurs mainly as a nosocomial infection in immunocompromised hosts, such as renal transplant and bone-marrow transplant patients, patients receiving steroids and those who are hospitalized for prolonged periods (Schwebke et al., 1990). However, waterborne outbreaks have also occurred in the community (Goldberg et al., 1989). For L. micdadei pneumonia erythromycin again is the drug of choice (Wing et al., 1981; Schwebke et al., 1990). In cases of apparent failure of therapy with erythromycin, cotrimoxazole may be beneficial (Rudin et al., 1984).

6 Campylobacter infections

In Campylobacter enteritis, if erythromycin is given early, there may be some lessening of pain and the post-infection carrier state is shortened. However, therapy by this drug does not reduce the duration or severity of diarrhea and other symptoms. The disease is usually short-lived and self-limiting and no chemotherapy is necessary, unless the eradication of organisms from stools is important. If erythromycin is used, a dose of oral erythromycin 0.5 g 6-hourly is sufficient (Pai et al., 1983; Mandal et al., 1984; Williams et al., 1989). For Campylobacter jejuni septicemia, gentamicin (p. 473) is the preferred drug (McNulty, 1987). In contrast, in immunosuppressed patients such as those with HIV infection, Campylobacter jejuni enteritis can be prolonged and severe, necessitating prolonged erythromycin therapy. In some of these patients so treated, erythromycin-resistant C. jejuni may develop in vivo during treatment (Perlman et al., 1988).

In a series of patients with Campylobacter fetus bacteremia, relapse of one patient after therapy with erythromycin, and progress in vertebral osteomyelitis in another during treatment, suggested that erythromycin alone may not be suitable therapy (Francioli et al., 1985). Erythromycin has not proved to be successful in eradication of Helicobacter pylori from stomach (McNulty et al., 1986; McNulty, 1987). Combination of bismuth subcitrate, tetracycline and metronidazole is effective for this purpose (p. 743).

7 Bartonella (formerly Rochalimaea) infections

Bacteria of this genus cause cat scratch disease, trench fever and two newly recognized clinical syndromes in HIV-infected patients – bacillary angiomatosis and bacillary peliosis. In bacillary angiomatosis there are localized vascular proliferative lesions in skin and extracutaneous organs and in bacillary peliosis there are changes in the hepatic or splenic parenchyma. In addition, in these patients bacteremia may occur, and lesions may develop in other parts of the body. There are three main species of this genus, *Bartonella quintana*, *B. henselae* and *B. elizabethae*. In World War I *B. quintana* caused trench fever and this was probably louse-borne; *B. henselae* is carried by cats and it causes cat-scratch disease. All three species can cause the severe syndromes occurring in HIV-infected patients. Additionally, *B. quintana* bacteremia has been described in patients with chronic alcoholism (Spach *et al.*, 1995a) and endocarditis due to this organism has been reported in homeless men (Drancourt *et al.*, 1995; Spach *et al.*, 1995b).

Antimicrobial treatment of severe infections in AIDS patients due to these bacteria has never been systematically studied, but erythromycin has been most often used with success. For mild disease oral erythromycin may be used but for severe infections the drug should be given i.v. Doxycycline has also been used with success in some patients (p. 744). Therapy should usually be continued for 4–6 weeks (Schwartzman, 1992; Koehler and Tappero, 1993; Koehler *et al.*, 1994; Tompkins, 1994; McGregor and Sorrell, 1995).

8 Mycoplasma infections

Pneumonia due to *M. pneumoniae* responds well to erythromycin and the tetracyclines (p. 745). Although treatment by either of these drugs reduces the length of illness, mycoplasmas may often persist in respiratory tract secretions both during and after therapy. Prolonged treatment for 2–3 weeks is often needed (Shames *et al.*, 1970; Wenzel *et al.*, 1976; Martin and Bates, 1991). Mycoplasma hominis has been implicated in pelvic inflammatory disease, postabortal and postpartum fever. Infections caused by this *Mycoplasma* spp. do not respond to erythromycin, but the tetracyclines are effective (p. 745) (Plummer *et al.*, 1987).

9 Chlamydia infections

Non-gonococcal urethritis caused by *Chlamydia trachomatis* usually responds to a 7-day course of oral erythromycin, although a tetracycline such as doxycycline is probably more effective (Scheibel *et al.*, 1982; CDC, 1993). Newer agents such as azithromycin (p. 658) and ofloxacin (p. 1122) are also effective for this infection. Erythromycin is the drug of choice for infections in pregnant women, nursing mothers, infants and children (Toomey and Barnes, 1990). A 7-day course is usually sufficient but persistent or recurrent cases should receive 3 weeks of the drug (Hooton *et al.*, 1990). In settings in which the prevalence of *Chlamydia* infection is high, a routine screening program of pregnant women for cervical *C. trachomatis*, followed by treatment of those infected, would usually prevent *C. trachomatis* infection in their infants (Schachter *et al.*, 1986). Also *C. trachomatis* causes pneumonia in infants 3 weeks to 4 months of age. It usually has no fever and paroxysmal cough (with no whoop) is characteristic. Apneic attacks may occur. The recommended treatment is erythromycin 50 mg per kg per day orally in four divided doses for 2 weeks (Braithwaite *et al.*, 1983; CDC, 1993). In infants less than 30 days old *C. trachomatis* also caused ophthalmia neonatorum and infections of oropharynx, urogenital tract and rectum. These all should be treated by erythromycin 50 mg per kg per day orally, given in four divided doses, for 10–14 days (CDC, 1993). The addition of topical treatment for ophthalmia seems unnecessary, but the results of treatment of this condition are not uniformly satisfactory (Oriel, 1984). It also appears unrewarding to use erythromycin ointment or silver nitrate solution prophylactically to prevent chlamydial ophthalmia neonatorum in infants whose mothers have cervical *C. trachomatis* infection (Bell *et al.*, 1987). Oral erythromycin has been used as treatment for trachoma, but it is only marginally more effective than topical erythromycin or topical tetracycline (p. 746) (Dawson and Schachter, 1985).

Pneumonia in older children and adults caused by *C. pneumoniae* can be treated by erythromycin 0.5 g 6-hourly for 2–3 weeks. Treatment by doxycycline (p. 747) or azithromycin (p. 658) gives equally satisfactory results (Grayston *et al.*, 1990; Ekman *et al.*, 1993; Hammerschlag, 1994).

It has been stated that one of the tetracyclines are the only drugs effective for psittacosis (caused by *C. psittaci*) (p. 746), but Hammers-Berggren *et al.* (1991) found erythromycin also satisfactory.

10 Ureaplasma urealyticum infections

For non-gonococcal urethritis due to this organism, doxycycline is the drug of choice (p. 742), but erythromycin is also effective and is suitable for pregnant women (CDC, 1993). *Ureaplasma urealyticum* may also cause postpartum infections, which can be treated by doxycycline or erythromycin (Plummer *et al.*, 1987). This organism also caused neonatal bacteremia, pneumonia or meningitis. Severe cases should be treated by i.v. erythromycin (dosage, p. 611) (Waites *et al.*, 1992, 1993). For meningitis it is probably wise to use both erythromycin and chloramphenicol initially, pending results of sensitivity testing (Stahelin-Massik *et al.*, 1994).

11 Pertussis

Erythromycin may prevent whooping cough in exposed susceptible individuals, and may also attenuate the illness if given early in the course of the disease (Linnemann *et al.*, 1975; Altemeier and Ayoub, 1977; Bergquist *et al.*, 1987). Mothers with pertussis can safely nurse their infants if both receive erythromycin (Granström *et al.*, 1987). In one pertussis outbreak in a facility for developmentally disabled, erythromycin prophylaxis was effective in exposed patients. Carbamazepine toxicity occurred in seven (19%) of 37 residents when this drug was administered together with erythromycin (Steketee *et al.*, 1988).

Once the paroxysmal stage is reached, erythromycin, like other antibiotics, does not influence the natural course of the illness. It may be useful in preventing secondary bacterial infection and it also eliminates pertussis organisms from the nasopharynx, possibly rendering the patients non-infectious and reducing the number of secondary cases (Bass *et al.*, 1969; Nelson, 1969; Bergquist *et al.*, 1987). It appears worthwhile using erythromycin in pertussis in children younger than 6 months, diagnosed early, and for older children if they are seriously ill or diagnosed during the first week or so of their symptoms. Bass (1985) considered that erythromycin estolate in a dosage of 50 mg per kg per day for 14 days was preferable to treat pertussis because of the higher serum levels attained (p. 612). In one child infected with an erythromycin-resistant strain of *Bordetella pertussis*, the clinical course worsened during erythromycin therapy and nasopharyngeal cultures remained positive for this organism (Lewis *et al.*, 1995).

12 Diphtheria

Erythromycin is active against *C. diphtheriae*, but the administration of specific diphtheria antitoxin is essential for treatment of the disease itself, but a course of erythromycin (or penicillin G or V) for 7–14 days should also be given so that the organism will be eradicated, toxin production terminated, and the likelihood of transmission decreased (Farizo *et al.*, 1993; Wilson, 1995). Erythromycin is effective in eliminating *C. diphtheriae* from carriers (Ginsburg and Eichenwald, 1976). Miller *et al.* (1974), however, found a 21% relapse rate 2 weeks after a 6-day course of erythromycin, but this may have been due to reinfection. Erythromycin for 7 days or an injection of benzathine penicillin has been recommended for unimmunized household contacts of diphtheria (CDC, 1985).

13 Rhodococcus equi infections

This organism can cause pneumonia in normal individuals, but more commonly it causes a destructive cavitating pneumonia in patients with immune system dysfunction, especially in patients with AIDS. Several antibiotics are effective against this organism such as erythromycin, rifampicin, ciprofloxacin, aminoglycosides and vancomycin. So far erythromycin combined with rifampicin has been most commonly used for treatment, which may have to be prolonged (Harvey and Sunstrum, 1991; Gillet-Juvin *et al.*, 1994; Verville *et al.*, 1994).

14 Gas gangrene

Erythromycin in large doses i.v. is an effective alternative to penicillin G for the treatment of this disease in penicillin-allergic patients. Occasionally strains of *Cl. perfringens* may be resistant to erythromycin. In such cases clindamycin, chloramphenicol or metronidazole can be used (pp. 555, 597, 949).

15 Actinomycosis

Erythromycin or one of the tetracyclines may be the best alternatives to penicillin G for the treatment of this disease in penicillin-allergic patients (Holmberg *et al.*, 1977).

16 Chancroid

Erythromycin 500 mg orally four times daily for 7 days is one of several effective therapies for chancroid. Ceftriaxone (p. 362) or azithromycin (p. 658) are the others most commonly recommended (Dangor *et al.*, 1990; Schmid, 1990; CDC, 1993). Chancroid is harder to cure in HIV-positive patients; the above dose of erythromycin is usually sufficient, but a lower dose such as 250 mg 8-hourly for 7 days may be inadequate (Behets *et al.*, 1995).

17 Relapsing fever

A single oral dose of 0.5 g erythromycin (or tetracycline) is considered optimal therapy for louse-borne relapsing fever due to *Borrelia recurrentis* (p. 748). Erythromycin rather than tetracycline should be used in pregnant patients and children. Both drug regimens produce the Jarisch–Herxheimer reaction, but the associated hypotension can be minimized by i.v. fluids.

18 Flavobacterium meningosepticum meningitis

This rare form of meningitis usually occurs in children. In addition to i.v. erythromycin, intraventricular and intrathecal drug has been used in 1.0- or 10-mg doses without evidence of toxicity (Maderazo *et al.*, 1974). Treatment failure has been reported in an adult, because of development of resistance to erythromycin during therapy. Rifampicin may be a suitable alternative (Rios *et al.*, 1978) (p. 700).

19 Mycobacterial infections

Mycobacterium chelonae chest infection was successfully treated with 2.0 g oral erythromycin daily in one patient (Irwin *et al.*, 1982). Erythromycin has also been combined with various other drugs, such as cefoxitin (p. 309) and amikacin (p. 516) for the treatment of *M. chelonae* and *M. fortuitum* infections. Erythromycin demonstrated no advantage over isoniazid in a controlled trial of treatment of adverse reactions to bacille Calmette-Guérin (BCG) vaccination (Hanley *et al.*, 1985) (p. 1203). Caglayan *et al.* (1987) could not demonstrate any superiority of erythromycin over placebo for the treatment of regional lymphadenitis and abscesses which followed BCG vaccinations. But Murphy *et al.* (1989) reported two patients in whom post-BCG vaccination abscesses appeared to heal with erythromycin therapy.

20 Q fever

Five patients with Q fever pneumonia all showed reduction or resolution of fever within 48 h of commencing treatment with i.v. erythromycin in a dosage of 500 mg 6-hourly (D'Angelo and Hetherington, 1979). Pérez-del-Molino *et al.* (1991) had similar experience with both i.v. and oral erythromycin.

21 Acne

Erythromycin has been used for this disease on the same basis as the tetracyclines (p. 749) (Ginsburg and Eichenwald, 1976). The drug in various suitable vehicles has also been used topically (Stoughton, 1979; Eady *et al.*, 1982).

22 Syphilis

Erythromycin in a dosage of 2 g daily for 10–15 days has been used to treat primary or secondary syphilis in penicillin-allergic pregnant women. The disease in the mother is usually cured, but placental transfer of the drug is inconsistent and the fetus may remain infected (Rolfs, 1995). If possible, desensitization to penicillin G, is preferable (p. 47).

References

Abbott Laboratories (1966). *Erythromycin A Review of Its Properties and Clinical Status*. North Chicago, Illinois: Abbott Laboratories, Scientific Division.

ADRAC (1995). Serious arrhythmias with intravenous erythromycin. *Austral Adverse Drug React Bull* **14**, No 1: 2.

Altemeier WAIII, Ayoub EM (1977). Erythromycin prophylaxis for pertussis. *Pediatrics* **59**: 623.

Ampel NM, Wing EJ (1990). *Legionella* infection in transplant patients. *Semin Resp Infect* **5**: 30.

Anderson R (1989). Erythromycin and roxithromycin potentiate human neutrophil locomotion *in vitro* by inhibition of leukoattractant-activated superoxide generation and autooxidation. *J Infect Dis* **159**: 966.

Anthony BF, Concepcion NF (1975). Group B streptococcus in a general hospital. *J Infect Dis* **132**: 561.

Arthur M, Courvalin P (1986). Contribution of two different mechanisms to erythromycin resistance in *Escherichia coli*. *Antimicrob Ag Chemother* **30**: 694.

Arthur M, Andremont A, Courvalin P (1987a). Distribution of erythromycin esterase and rRNA methylase genes in members of the family Enterobacteriaceae highly resistant to erythromycin. *Antimicrob Ag Chemother* **31**: 404.

Arthur M, Brisson-Nšel A, Courvalin P (1987b). Origin and evolution of genes specifying resistance to macrolide, lincosamide and streptogramin antibiotics: data and hypotheses. *J Antimicrob Chemother* **20**: 783.

Bach MC, Sabath LD, Finland M (1973). Susceptibility of *Nocardia asteroides* to 45 antimicrobial agents *in vitro*. *Antimicrob Ag Chemother* **3**: 1.

Back NA, Linnemann CCJr, Pfaller MA *et al.* (1993). Recurrent epidemics caused by a single strain of erythromycin-resistant *Staphylococcus aureus*. The importance of molecular epidemiology. *JAMA* **270**: 1329.

Baker PJ, Slots J, Genco RJ, Evans RT (1983). Minimal inhibitory concentrations of various antimicrobial agents for human oral anaerobic bacteria. *Antimicrob Ag Chemother* **24**: 420.

Bannatyne RM, Cheung R (1982). Antimicrobial susceptibility of *Bordetella pertussis* strains isolated from 1960 to 1981. *Antimicrob Ag Chemother* **21**: 666.

Barnes DM, Whittier S, Gilligan PH *et al.* (1995). Transmission of multidrug-resistant serotype 23F *Streptococcus pneumoniae* in group day care: evidence suggesting capsular transformation of the resistant strain *in vivo*. *J Infect Dis* **171**: 890.

Bass JW (1985). Pertussis: current status of prevention and treatment. *Ped Infect Dis* **4**: 614.

Bass JW, Klenk EL, Kotheimer JB *et al.* (1969). Antimicrobial treatment of pertussis. *J Pediatr* **75**: 768.

Bass JW, Steele RW, Wiebe RA, Dierdorff EP (1971). Erythromycin concentrations in middle ear exudates. *Pediatrics* **48**: 417.

Behets FM-T, Liomba G, Lule G *et al.* (1995). Sexually transmitted diseases and human immunodeficiency virus control in Malawi: a field study of genital ulcer disease. *J Infect Dis* **171**: 451.

Bell TA, Sandstršm KI, Gravett MG, *et al.*, (1987). Comparison of ophthalmic silver nitrate solution and erythromycin ointment for prevention of naturally acquired *Chlamydia trachomatis*. *Sex Trans Dis* **14**: 195.

Ben-Ari J, Eisenstein B, Davidovits M *et al.* (1988). Effect of erythromycin on blood cyclosporine concentrations in kidney transplant patients. *JPediatrics* **112**: 992.

Bennett NMcK, Kucers A (1970). Staphylococcal and Gram-negative septicaemia. *Aspects of Infection. Proc Symp Auckland, Sydney and Melbourne*, p. 123. Melbourne, Australia: Mercedes Publishing Services.

Bergan T, Engeset A, Olszewski W *et al.* (1982). Penetration of erythromycin into human peripheral lymph. *J Antimicrob Chemother* **10**: 319.

Bergeron MG, Ahronheim G, Richard JE *et al.* (1987). Comparative efficacies of erythromycin-sulfisoxazole and cefaclor in acute otitis media: a double blind randomized trial. *Pediatr Infect Dis J* **6**: 654.

Bergquist S-O, Bernander S, Dahnsjö H, Sundelfö B (1987). Erythromycin in the treatment of pertussis: a study of bacteriologic and clinical effects. *Pediatr Infect Dis J* **6**: 458.

Berman S (1995). Otitis media in children. *New Engl J Med* **332**: 1560.

Berryman DI, Rood JI (1989). Cloning and hybridization analysis of ermP, a macrolide-lincosamide-streptogramin B resistance determinant from *Clostridium perfringens*. *Antimicrob Ag Chemother* **33**: 1346.

Berryman DI, Lyristis M, Rood JI (1994). Cloning and sequence analysis of erm Q, the predominant macrolide-lincosamide-streptogramin B resistance gene in *Clostridium perfringens*. *Antimicrob Ag Chemother* **38**: 1041.

Berubé D, Kirouac D, Croteau D *et al.* (1988). Plasma bactericidal activity after administration of erythromycin estolate and erythromycin ethylsuccinate to healthy volunteers. *Antimicrob Ag Chemother* **32**: 1227.

Bilgeri YR, Ballard RC, Duncan MO *et al.* (1982). Antimicrobial susceptibility of 103 strains of *Haemophilus ducreyi* isolated in Johannesburg. *Antimicrob Ag Chemother* **22**: 686.

Blatt SP, Dolan MJ, Hendrix CW, Melcher GP (1994). Legionaires disease in human immunodeficiency virus-infected patients: eight cases and review. *Clin Infect Dis* **18**: 227.

Boguniewicz M, Leung DYM (1995). Hypersensitivity reactions to antibiotics commonly used in children. *Pediatr Infect Dis J* **14**: 221.

Bourbeau P, Campos JM (1982). Current antibiotic susceptibility of Group A beta-hemolytic streptococci. *J Infect Dis* **145**: 916.

Braithwaite J, Davidson F, Lambert HP, Williams M (1983). Infant chlamydial pneumonia. *Brit Med J* **286**: 1394.

Brandriss MW, Richardson WS, Barold SS (1994). Erythromycin-induced QT prolongation and polymorphic ventricular tachycardia (torsades de pointes): case report and review. *Clin Infect Dis* **18**: 995.

Brause BD, Borges JS, Roberts RB (1976). Relative efficacy of clindamycin, erythromycin and penicillin in treatment of *Treponema pallidum* in skin syphilomas of rabbits. *J Infect Dis* **134**: 93.

Brazier JS, Levett PN, Stannard AJ *et al.* (1985). Antibiotic susceptibility of clinical isolates of *Clostridia*. *J Antimicrob Chemother* **15**: 181.

Breese BB, Disney FA, Talpey W *et al.* (1974). Streptococcal infections in children Comparison of the therapeutic effectiveness of erythromycin administered twice daily with erythromycin, penicillin phenoxymethyl, and clindamycin administered three times daily. *Amer J Dis Child* **128**: 457.

Brorson J-E, Martinell J, Wilske H (1981). *Branhamella catarrhalis*: antibiotic susceptibility and beta-lactamase production. *J Antimicrob Chemother* **7**: 208.

Brown AR (1963). Two cases of untoward reaction after 'Ilosone'. *Brit Med J* **2**: 913.

Brown BA, Wallace RJJr, Flanagan CW *et al.* (1989). Tetracycline and erythromycin resistance among clinical isolates of *Branhamella catarrhalis*. *Antimicrob Ag Chemother* **33**: 1631.

Brummett RE, Fox KE (1989). Vancomycin and erythromycin-induced hearing loss in humans. *Antimicrob Ag Chemother* **33**: 791.

Burns L, Hodgman J (1963). Studies of prematures, given erythromycin estolate. *Amer J Dis Child* **106**: 280.

Caglayan S, Yegin O, Kayran K *et al.* (1987). Is medical therapy effective for regional lymphadenitis following BCC vaccination. *Amer J Dis Child* **141**: 1213.

Carson JL, Strom BL, Duff A *et al.* (1993). Acute liver disease associated with erythromycins, sulfonamides, and tetracyclines. *Ann Intern Med* **119**: 576.

Casal J (1982). Antimicrobial susceptibility of *Streptococcus pneumoniae*: serotype distribution of penicillin-resistant strains in Spain. *Antimicrob Ag Chemother* **22**: 222.

CDC (Center for Disease Control) (1977a). Follow-up on Legionnaires' disease. *MMWR* **26**: 111.

CDC (Center for Disease Control) (1977b). Follow-up on Legionnaires' disease – Pennsylvania. *MMWR* **26**: 152.

CDC (Center for Disease Control) (1977c). Multiple-antibiotic resistance of pneumococci – South Africa. *MMWR* **26**: 285.

CDC (Center for Disease Control) (1978). Penicillinase-(beta-lactamase-). producing *Neisseria gonorrhoeae* worldwide. *MMWR* **27**: 10.

CDC (Centers for Disease Control) (1985). ACIP, diphtheria, tetanus and pertussis Guidelines for vaccine prophylaxis and other preventive measures. *MMWR* **34**: 405.

CDC (Centers for Disease Control) (1993). Sexually transmitted diseases treatment guidelines. *MMWR* **42** (No RR-14): 20, 47.

Chalker DK, Shalita A, Smith JG Jr, Swann RW (1983). A double-blind study of the effectiveness of a 3% erythromycin and 5% benzoyl peroxide combination in the treatment of acne vulgaris. *J Amer Acad Dermatol* **9**: 933.

Champion LAA, Wald ER, Luddy RE, Schwartz AD (1978). *Streptococcus pneumoniae* resistant to erythromycin and clindamycin. *J Pediatr* **92**: 505.

Chirgwin K, Roblin PM, Hammerschlag MR (1989). *In vitro* susceptibilities of *Chlamydia pneumoniae* (*Chlamydia* sp. strain TWAR). *Antimicrob Ag Chemother* **33**: 1634.

Chow AW, Patten V, Bednorz D (1978). Susceptibility of *Campylobacter fetus* to twenty-two antimicrobial agents. *Antimicrob Ag Chemother* **13**: 416.

Clarke CW, May CS, Robinson W, Hampshire P(1980). A new formulation of erythromycin stearate: blood and sputum levels in patients with chronic lower respiratory tract infection. *J Antimicrob Chemother* **6**: 389.

Coonan KM, Kaplan EL (1994). *In vitro* susceptibility of recent North

American Group A streptococcal isolates to eleven oral antibiotics. *Pediatr Infect Dis J* **13**: 630.

Coppi G, Alberti D (1984). Thiopronine and lung levels of erythromycin. *J Antimicrob Chemother* **14**: 307.

Coyle MB, Minshew BH, Bland JA, Hsu PC (1979). Erythromycin and clindamycin resistance in *Corynebacterium diphtheriae* from skin lesions. *Antimicrob Ag Chemother* **16**: 525.

Croteau D, Bergeron MG, Le Bel M (1988). Pharmacokinetic advantages of erythromycin estolate over ethylsuccinate as determined by high-pressure liquid chromatography. *Antimicrob Ag Chemother* **32**: 561.

Csonka GW, Spitzer RJ (1969). Lincomycin, non-gonococcal urethritis, and mycoplasmata. *Brit J Vener Dis* **45**: 52.

Cundliffe E, McQuillen K (1967). Bacterial protein synthesis: the effect of antibiotics. *J Mol Biol* **30**: 137.

D'Angelo LJ, Hetherington R (1979). Q fever treated with erythromycin. *Brit Med J* **2**: 305.

Dan M, Feigl D (1993). Erythromycin-associated hypotension. *Pediatr Infect Dis J* **12**: 692.

Dangor Y, Ballard RC, Miller SD, Koornhof HJ (1990). Treatment of chancroid. *Antimicrob Ag Chemother* **34**: 1308.

Darelid J, Lšfgren S, Malmvall B-E (1993). Erythromycin treatment is beneficial for longstanding *Moraxella catarrhalis* associated cough in children. *Scand J Infect Dis* **25**: 323.

Dawson CR, Schachter J (1985). Strategies for treatment and control of blinding trachoma: cost-effectiveness of topical and systemic antibiotics. *Rev Infect Dis* **7**: 768.

Decré, Buré A, Pangon B *et al.* (1991). *In vitro* susceptibility of *Rhodococcus equi* to 27 antibiotics. *J Antimicrob Chemother* **28**: 311.

Delmée M, Avesani V (1988). Correlation between serogroup and susceptibility to chloramphenicol, clindamycin, erythromycin, rifampicin and tetracycline among 308 isolates of *Clostridium difficile*. *J Antimicrob Chemother* **22**: 325.

Derby LE, Jick H, Henry DA, Dean AD (1993). Erythromycin-associated cholestatic hepatitis. *Med J Aust* **158**: 600.

Descotes J, Andre P, Evreux JC (1985). Pharmacokinetic drug interactions with macrolide antibiotics. *J Antimicrob Chemother* **15**: 659.

Disanto AR, Chodos DJ (1981). Influence of study design in assessing food effects on absorption of erythromycin base and erythromycin stearate. *Antimicrob Ag Chemother* **20**: 190.

Dixon JMS (1968). Group A streptococcus resistant to erythromycin and lincomycin. *Can Med Assoc J* **9**: 1093.

Dixon JMS, Lipinski AE (1972). Resistance of Group A beta-hemolytic streptococci to lincomycin and erythromycin. *Antimicrob Ag Chemother* **1**: 333.

Dixon JMS, Lipinski AE (1974). Infections with beta-hemolytic streptococcus resistant to lincomycin and erythromycin and observations on zonal-pattern resistance to lincomycin. *J Infect Dis* **130**: 351.

Dowling JN, Weyant RS, Pasculle AW (1982). Bactericidal activity of antibiotics against *Legionella micdadei* (Pittsburg pneumonia agent). *Antimicrob Ag Chemother* **22**: 272.

Dowlng JN, McDevitt DA, Pasculle AW (1985). Isolation and preliminary characterization of erythromycin-resistant variants of *Legionella micdadei* and *Legionella pneumophila*. *Antimicrob Ag Chemother* **27**: 272.

Drancourt M, Mainardi JL, Brouqui P *et al.* (1995). *Bartonella (Rochalimae) quintana* endocarditis in three homeless men. *New Engl J Med* **332**: 419.

Eady EA, Holland KT, Cunliffe WJ *et al.* (1982). The use of antibiotics in acne therapy: oral or topical administration. *J Antimicrob Chemother* **10**: 89.

Eady EA, Ross JI, Cove JH (1990). Multiple mechanisms of erythromycin resistance. *J Antimicrob Chemother* **26**: 461.

Eady EA, Ross JI, Tipper JL *et al.* (1993). Distribution of genes encoding erythromycin ribosomal methylases and an erythromycin efflux pump in epidemiologically distinct groups of staphylococci. *J Antimicrob Chemother* **31**: 211.

Eckman MR, Johnson T, Riess R (1975). Partial deafness after erythromycin. *New Engl J Med* **292**: 649.

Edelstein PH (1993). Legionnaires disease. *Clin Infect Dis* **16**: 741.

Edelstein PH, Meyer RD (1980). Susceptibility of *Legionella pneumophila* to twenty antimicrobial agents. *Antimicrob Ag Chemother* **18**: 403.

Ekman M-R, Grayston JT, Visakorpi R *et al.* (1993). An epidemic of infections due to *Chlamydia pneumoniae* in military conscripts. *Clin Infect Dis* **17**: 420.

Eriksson M, Bolme P, Blennow M (1981). Absorption of erythromycin from pediatric suspension in infants and children. *Scand J Infect Dis* **13**: 211.

Fallon RJ, Stack BHR (1990). Legionaires' disease due to *Legionella anisa*. *J Infect* **20**: 227.

Farízo KM, Strebel PM, Chen RT *et al.* (1993). Fatal respiratory disease due to *Corynebacterium diphtheriae*: case report and review of guidelines for management, investigation, and control. *Clin Infect Dis* **16**: 59.

Farrar HC, Walsh-Sukys MC, Kyllonen K, Blumber JL (1993). Cardiac toxicity associated with intravenous erythromycin lactobionate: two case reports and a review of the literature. *Pediatr Infect Dis J* **12**: 688.

Fenelon LE, Mumtaz G, Ridgway GL (1990). The *in vitro* antibiotic susceptibility of *Chlamydia pneumoniae*. *J Antimicrob Chemother* **26**: 763.

Fidalgo S, Mendez FJ, Hardisson C, Salas JA (1988). Epidemiology of macrolide and lincosamide resistance in species of staphylococci in a general hospital. *J Hosp Inf* **11**: 36.

Ford DK, Smith JR (1974). Non-specific urethritis associated with a tetracycline-resistant T-mycoplasma. *Brit J Vener Dis* **50**: 373.

Francioli P, Herzstein J, Grob JP, *et al.* (1985). *Campylobacter fetus* subspecies *fetus* bacteremia. *Arch Intern Med* **145**: 289.

Fraser DW, Wachsmuth IK, Bopp C *et al.* (1978). Antibiotic treatment of guinea-pigs infected with agent of Legionnaires' disease. *Lancet* **i**: 175.

Fujikawa J, Struewing JP, Hyams KC *et al.* (1992). Oral erythromycin prophylaxis against *Streptococcus pyogenes* infection in penicillin-allergic military recruits: a randomized clinical trial. *J Infect Dis* **166**: 162.

Fujita K, Morono K, Yoshikawa M, Murai T (1994). Decline in erythromycin resistance of Group A streptococci in Japan. *Pediatr Infect Dis J* **13**: 1075.

Ganz NM, Dickerson J, Bartlett JG (1979). Pseudomembranous colitis associated with erythromycin. *Ann Intern Med* **91**: 866.

García-Leoni ME, Cercanado E, Rodeño P *et al.* (1992). Susceptibility of *Streptococcus pneumoniae* to penicillin: a prospective microbiological and clinical study. *Clin Infect Dis* **14**: 427.

Garrod LP (1957). The erythromycin group of antibiotics. *Brit Med J* **2**: 57.

Gephart JF, Washington JAII (1982). Antimicrobial susceptibilities of nutritionally variant streptococci. *J Infect Dis* **146**: 536.

Gilbert FI (1962). Cholestatic hepatitis caused by esters of erythromycin and oleandomycin. *JAMA* **182**: 1048.

Gillet-Juvin K, Stern M, Israël-Biet D *et al.* (1994). A highly unusual combination of pulmonary pathogens in an HIV infected patient. *Scand J Infect Dis* **26**: 215.

Ginsburg CH, Eichenwald HF (1976). Erythromycin: a review of its uses in pediatric practice. *J Pediatr* **89**: 872.

Ginsburg CH, McCracken GHJr, Culbertson MCJr (1976). Concentrations of erythromycin in serum and tonsil: comparison of the estolate and ethyl succinate suspensions. *J Pediatr* **89**: 1011.

Ginsburg CH, McCracken GHJr, Crow SD *et al.* (1984). Erythromycin therapy for Group A streptococcal pharyngitis. *Amer J Dis Child* **138**: 536.

Ginsburg CM, McCracken GH Jr, Steinberg JB *et al.* (1982). Management of Group A streptococcal pharyngitis: a randomized controlled study of twice-daily erythromycin ethylsuccinate versus erythromycin estolate. *Pediatr Infect Dis* **1**: 384.

Goldberg DJ, Wrench JG, Collier PW *et al.* (1989). Lochgoilhead fever: outbreak of non-pneumonic legionellosis due to *Legionella micdadei*. *Lancet* **i**: 316.

Goldman RC, Fesik SW, Doran CC (1990). Role of protonated and neutral forms of macrolides in binding to ribosomes from Gram-positive and Gram-negative bacteria. *Antimicrob Ag Chemother* **34**: 426.

Goldstein EJC, Citron DM, Richwald GA (1988). Lack of *in vitro* efficacy of oral forms of certain cephalosporins, erythromycin and oxacillin against *Pasteurella multocida*. *Antimicrob Ag Chemother* **32**: 213.

Gorbach SL, Bartlett JG (1974). Anaerobic infections (third of three parts). *New Engl J Med* **290**: 1289.

Gordin A, Männistö PT, Antikainen R *et al.* (1988a). Concentrations of erythromycin, 2^1 – acetyl erythromycin, and their anhydro forms in plasma and tonsillar tissue after repeated dosage of erythromycin stearate and erythromycin acistrate. *Antimicrob Ag Chemother* **32**: 1019.

Gordin A, Kalima S, Hulmi S *et al.* (1988b). Comparison of erythromycin ascitrate and enterocoated erythromycin base in acute respiratory infections. *J Antimicrob Chemother* **21** (Suppl D): 85.

Gouyon JB, Benoit A, Bétremieux P *et al.* (1994). Cardiac toxicity of intravenous erythromycin lactobionate in preterm infants. *Pediatr Infect Dis J* **13**: 840.

Granström G, Sterner G, Nord CE, Granström M (1987). Use of erythromycin to prevent pertussis in newborns of mothers with pertussis. *J Infect Dis* **155**: 1210.

Grayston JT, Campbell LA, Kuo C-C *et al.* (1990). A new respiratory tract pathogen: *Chlamydia pneumoniae* strain TWAR. *J Infect Dis* **161**: 618.

Griffith RS, Black HR (1962). A comparison of blood levels after oral administration of erythromycin and erythromycin estolate. *Antibiot Chemother* **12**: 398.

Griffith RS, Black HR (1964). Comparison of the blood levels obtained after single and multiple doses of erythromycin estolate and erythromycin stearate. *Amer J Med Sci* **247**: 69.

Griffith RS, Black HR (1970). Erythromycin. *Med Clin N Amer* **54**: 1199.

Gutman L, Schaller J, Wedgwood RJ (1967). Bacterial L-forms in relapsing urinary-tract infection. *Lancet* **i**: 464.

Guze LB, Kalmanson GM (1964). Action of erythromycin on 'protoplasts *in vivo*'. *Science* **146**: 1558.

Haas CE, Nix DE, Schentag JJ (1990). *In vitro* selection of resistant *Helicobacter pylori*. *Antimicrob Ag Chemother* **34**: 1637.

Hächler H, Berger-Bächi B, Kayser FH (1987). Genetic characterization of a *Clostridium difficile* erythromycin-clindamycin resistance determinant that is transferable to *Staphylococcus aureus*. *Antimicrob Ag Chemother* **31**: 1039.

Hammers-Berggren S, Granath F, Julander I, Kalin M (1991). Erythromycin for treatment of ornithosis. *Scand J Infect Dis* **23**: 159.

Hammerschlag MR (1994). Antimicrobial susceptibility and therapy of infections caused by *Chlamydia pneumoniae*. *Antimicrob Ag Chemother* **38**: 1873.

Hand WL, Boozer RM, King-Thompson NL (1985). Antibiotic uptake by alveolar macrophages of smokers. *Antimicrob Ag Chemother* **27**: 42.

Hanley SP, Guml J, Macforlave JT (1985). Comparison of erythromycin and isoniazid in treatment of adverse reactions to BCG vaccinations. *Brit Med J* **290**: 970.

Harrison GAJ, Stross WP, Rubin MP *et al.* (1985). Resistance in oral streptococci after repeated three-dose erythromycin prophylaxis. *J Antimicrob Chemother* **15**: 471.

Harvey KJ, Miles H, Hurse A, Carson M (1981). *In-vitro* activity of erythromycin against anaerobic microorganisms. *Med J Aust* **1**: 474.

Harvey RL, Sunstrum JC (1991). *Rhodococcus equi* infection in patients with and without human immunodeficiency virus infection. *Rev Infect Dis* **13**: 139.

Hassam ZA, Shaw EJ, Shooter RA (1978). Changes in antibiotic sensitivity in strains of *Staphylococcus aureus*, 1952–78. *Brit Med J* **2**: 536.

Hedberg K, Ristinen TL, Soler JT *et al.* (1990). Outbreak of erythromycin-resistant staphylococcal conjunctivitis in a newborn nursery. *Pediatr Infect Dis J* **9**: 268.

Higa F, Saito A, Inadome J *et al.* (1993). Influence of methylprednisolone on the intracellular antimicrobial activity of erythromycin and clindamycin against *Legionella pneumophila*. *J Antimicrob Chemother* **31**: 901.

Hirakata Y, Kaku M, Mizukane R *et al.* (1992). Potential effect of erythromycin on host defense systems and virulence of *Pseudomonas aeruginosa*. *Antimicrob Ag Chemother* **36**: 1922.

Holmberg K, Nord C-E, Dornbusch K (1977). Antimicrobial *in vitro* susceptibility of *Actinomyces israelii* and *Arachnia propionica*. *Scand J Infect Dis* **9**: 40.

Honig PK, Wortham DC, Zamani K, Cantilena LR (1994). Comparison of the effect of the macrolide antibiotics erythromycin, clarithromycin and azithromycin on terfenadine steady-state pharmacokinetics and electrocardiographic parameters. *Drug Invest* **7**: 148.

Hooton TM, Wong ES, Barnes RC *et al.* (1990). Erythromycin for persistent or recurrent nongonococcal urethritis. *Ann Intern Med* **113**: 21.

Hosker JP, Jewell DP (1983). Transient, selective Factor X deficiency and acute liver failure following a chest infection treated with erythromycin BP. *Postgrad Med J* **59**: 514.

Hovi T, Svahn T, Valtonen V (1987). Twice-a-day regimen of erythromycin base is effective in the treatment of acute streptococcal tonsillitis. *Scand J Infect Dis* **19**: 661.

Inman WHW, Rawson NSB (1983). Erythromycin estolate and jaundice. *Brit Med J* **286**: 1954.

Irwin RS, Pratter MR, Corwin RW *et al.* (1982). Pulmonary infection with *Mycobacterium chelonei*: successful treatment with one drug based on disk diffusion susceptibility data. *J Infect Dis* **145**: 772.

Ishiguro M, Koga H, Kohno S *et al.* (1989). Penetration of macrolides into human polymorphonuclear leucocytes. *J Antimicrob Chemother* **24**: 719.

Itoh Z, Suzuki T, Nakaya M *et al.* (1984). Gastrointestinal motor-stimulating activity of macrolide antibiotics and analysis of their side-effects on the canine gut. *Antimicrob Ag Chemother* **26**: 863.

Jao RL, Finland M (1967). Susceptibility of *Mycoplasma pneumoniae* to 21 antibiotics *in vitro*. *Amer J Med Sci* **253**: 639.

Jellard CH, Lipinski AE (1973). *Corynebacterium diphtheriae* resistant to erythromycin and lincomycin. *Lancet* **i**: 156.

Jenssen WD, Thakker-Varia S, Dubin OT, Weinstein MP (1987). Prevalence of macrolides-lincosamides-streptogramin B resistance and erm gene classes among clinical strains of staphylococci and streptococci. *Antimicrob Ag Chemother* **31**: 883.

Johnson, RC, Kodner C, Russell M (1987). *In vitro* and *in vivo* susceptibility of the Lyme disease spirochete *Borrelia burgdorferi* to four antimicrobial agents. *Antimicrob Ag Chemother* **31**: 164.

Kalm O, Kamme C, Bergström B *et al.* (1975). Erythromycin stearate in acute maxillary sinusitis. *Scand J Infect Dis* **7**: 209.

Karmali MA, DeGrandis S, Fleming PC (1981). Antimicrobial susceptibility of *Campylobacter jejuni* with special reference patterns of Canadian isolates. *Antimicrob Ag Chemother* **19**: 593.

Kaukoranta-Tolvanen S-S, Renkonen O-V, Gordin A *et al.* (1989). Effect of erythromycin ascitrate and erythromycin stearate on human colonic microflora. *Scand J Infect Dis* **21**: 717.

Kislak JW, Razavi LMB, Daly AK, Finland M (1965). Susceptibility of pneumococci to nine antibiotics. *Amer J Med Sci* **250**: 261.

Koehler JE, Tappero JW (1993). Bacillary angiomatosis and bacillary peliosis in patients infected with Human Immunodeficiency Virus. *Clin Infect Dis* **17**: 612.

Koehler JE, Glaser CA, Tappero JW (1994). *Rochalimaea henselae* infection A new zoonosis with the domestic cat as reservoir. *JAMA* **271**: 531.

Kroboth PD, Brown A, Lyon JA *et al.* (1982). Pharmacokinetics of single-dose erythromycin in normal and alcoholic liver disease subjects. *Antimicrob Ag Chemother* **21**: 135.

Kunin CM (1967). A guide to use of antibiotics in patients with renal disease. *Ann Intern Med* **67**: 151.

Kuo C-C, Wang S-P, Grayston JT (1977). Antimicrobial activity of several antibiotics and a sulfonamide against *Chlamydia trachomatis* organisms in cell culture. *Antimicrob Ag Chemother* **12**: 80.

Lake B, Bell SM (1969). Variations in absorption of erythromycin. *Med J Aust* **1**: 449.

Lambert H (1979). Antimicrobial drugs in the treatment and prevention of pertussis. *J Antimicrob Chemother* **5**: 329.

Leads from the Morbidity and Mortality Weekly Report Atlanta Ga (1995). Erythromycin-resistant *Bordetella pertussis*-Yuma County, Arizona, May–October 1994. *JAMA* **273**: 131.

Leclercq R, Courvalin P (1991a). Bacterial resistance to macrolide, lincosamide, and streptogramin antibiotics by target modification. *Antimicrob Ag Chemother* **35**: 1267.

Leclercq R, Courvalin P (1991b). Intrinsic and unusual resistance to macrolide, lincosamide, and streptogramin antibiotics in bacteria. *Antimicrob Ag Chemother* **35**: 1273.

Lee CK, Bowie WR, Alexander ER (1978). *In vitro* assays of the efficacy of antimicrobial agents in controlling *Chlamydia trachomatis* propogation. *Antimicrob Ag Chemother* **13**: 441.

Lee EL, Robinson MJ, Thong ML *et al.* (1977). Intraventricular chemotherapy in neonatal meningitis. *J Pediatr* **91**: 991.

Lee HJ, Park J-Y, Jang S-H *et al.* (1995). High incidence of resistance to multiple antimicrobials in clinical isolates of *Streptococcus pneumoniae* from a University Hospital in Korea. *Clin Infect Dis* **20**: 826.

Lehtonen L, Lankinen KS, Wikberg R *et al.* (1991). Hepatic safety of erythromycin ascitrate in 1549 patients with respiratory tract and skin infections. *J Antimicrob Chemother* **27**: 233.

Lesher JL Jr, Chalker DK, Smith JG Jr *et al.* (1985). An evaluation of a 2% erythromycin ointment in the topical therapy of acne vulgaris. *J Amer Acad Dermatol* **12**: 526.

Lewis K, Saubolle MA, Tenover FC *et al.* (1995). Pertussis caused by an erythromycin-resistant strain of *Bordetella pertussis*. *Pediatr Infect Dis J* **14**: 388.

Lewis VJ, Thacker WL, Shepard CC, McDade JE (1978). *In vivo* susceptibility of the Legionnaires' disease bacterium to ten anti-microbial agents. *Antimicrob Ag Chemother* **13**: 419.

Lilly HA, Lowbury EJL (1978). Antibiotic resistance of *Staphylococcus aureus* in a burns unit after stopping routine prophylaxis with erythromycin. *J Antimicrob Chemother* **4**: 545.

Liñares J, Garau J, Dominguez C, Perez JL (1983). Antibiotic resistance and serotypes of *Streptococcus pneumoniae* from patients with community-acquired pneumococcal disease. *Antimicrob Ag Chemother* **23**: 545.

Linnemann CC Jr, Ramundo N, Perlstein PH *et al.* (1975). Use of pertussis vaccine in an epidemic involving hospital staff. *Lancet* **ii**: 540.

Lonks JR, Medeiros AA (1993). High rate of erythromycin and clarithromycin resistance among *Streptococcus pneumoniae* isolates from blood cultures from Providence, RI. *Antimicrob Ag Chemother* **37**: 1742.

Ludden TM (1985). Pharmacokinetic interactions of the macrolide antibiotics. *Clin Pharmacokinet* **10**: 63.

Männistö PT, Taskinen J, Ottoila P *et al.* (1988). Fate of single oral doses of erythromycin ascitrate, erythromycin stearate, and pelleted erythromycin base analysed by mass-spectrometry in plasma of healthy human volunteers. *J Antimicrob Chemother* **21** (Suppl D): 33.

Maderazo EG, Bassaris HP, Quintiliani R (1974). *Flavobacterium meningosepticum* meningitis in a newborn infant. Treatment with intraventricular erythromycin. *J Pediatr* **85**: 675.

Malmborg A-S (1979). Effect of food on absorption of erythromycin. A study of two derivatives, the stearate and the base. *J Antimicrob Chemother* **5**: 591.

Mandal BK, Ellis ME, Dunbar EM, Whale K (1984). Double-blind placebo-controlled trial of erythromycin in the treatment of clinical *Campylobacter* infections. *J Antimicrob Chemother* **13**: 619.

Maple PAC, Efstratiou A, Tseneva G *et al.* (1994). The *in vitro* susceptibilities of toxigenic strains of *Corynebacterium diphtheriae* isolated in northwestern Russia and surrounding areas to ten antibiotics. *J Antimicrob Chemother* **34**: 1037.

Marder HP, Kayser FH (1977). Transferable plasmids mediating multiple-antibiotic resistance in *Streptococcus faecalis* subsp liquefaciens. *Antimicrob Ag Chemother* **12**: 261.

Marlin GE, Thompson PJ, Jenkins CR *et al.* (1983). Study of serum levels, venous irritation, and gastrointestinal side-effects with intravenous erythromycin lactobionate in patients with bronchopulmonary infection. *Hum Toxicol* **2**: 593.

Martell R, Heinrichs D, Stiller CR *et al.* (1986). The effects of erythromycin in patients treated with cyclosporine. *Ann Intern Med* **104**: 660.

Martin RE, Bates JH (1991). Atypical pneumonia. *Inf Dis Clin N Amer* **5**: 585.

Masel MA (1962). Erythromycin hepato-sensitivity: a preliminary report of two cases. *Med J Aust* **1**: 560.

Maurin M, Raoult D (1993). Antimicrobial susceptibility of *Rochalimaea quintana, Rochalimaea vinsonii*, and the newly recognized *Rochalimaea henselae*. *J Antimicrob Chemother* **32**: 587.

Mazzei T, Mini E, Novelli A, Periti P (1993). Chemistry and mode of action of macrolides. *J Antimicrob Chemother* **31** (Suppl C): 1.

McCabe RE, Baldwin JC, McGregor CA *et al.* (1984). Prosthetic valve endocarditis caused by *Legionella pneumophila*. *Ann Intern Med* **100**: 525.

McCarthy LR, Mickelson PA, Smith EG (1979). Antibiotic susceptibility of *Haemophilus vaginalis* (*Corynebacterium vaginale*). to 21 antibiotics. *Antimicrob Ag Chemother* **16**: 186.

McCormack WM, George H, Donner A *et al.* (1977). Hepatotoxicity of erythromycin estolate during pregnancy. *Antimicrob Ag Chemother* **12**: 630.

McGregor AR, Sorrell TC (1995). Infectious diseases. *Med J Aust* **162**: 104.

McGuire JM, Bunch RL, Anderson RC *et al.* (1952). 'Ilotycin', a new antibiotic. *Antibiot Chemother* **2**: 281; quoted by Abbott Laboratories (1966).

McNulty CAM (1987). The treatment of *Campylobacter* infections in man. *J Antimicrob Chemother* **19**: 281.

McNulty CAM, Dent J, Wise R (1985). Susceptibility of clinical isolates of *Campylobacter pyloridis* to 11 antimicrobial agents. *Antimicrob Ag Chemother* **28**: 837.

McNulty CAM, Gearty JC, Crump B *et al.* (1986). *Campylobacter pyloridis* and associated gastritis: investigator blind, placebo controlled trial of bismuth salicylate and erythromycin ethylsuccinate. *Brit Med J* **293**: 645.

McNulty CAM, Dent JC, Ford GA, Wilkinson SP (1988). Inhibitory antimicrobial concentrations against *Campylobacter pylori* in gastroc mucosa. *J Antimicrob Chemother* **22**: 729.

Metzger WI, Jenkins CJJr, Harris CJ *et al.* (1959). Laboratory and clinical studies of intramuscular erythromycin. *Antibiot Annual 1958–1959*: 383.

Meyer RD (1983). *Legionella* infections: a review of five years of research. *Rev Infect Dis* **5**: 258.

Miller LW, Bickham S, Jones WL *et al.* (1974). Diphtheria carriers and the effect of erythromycin therapy. *Antimicrob Ag Chemother* **6**: 166.

Miller SM (1982). Erythromycin toxicity. *Med J Aust* **2**: 242.

Mintz U, Amir J, Pinkhas J, de Vries A (1973). Transient perceptive deafness due to erythromycin lactobionate. *JAMA* **225**: 1122.

Moffie BG, Mouton RP (1988). Sensitivity and resistance of *Legionella pneumophila* to some antibiotics and combination of antibiotics. *J Antimicrob Chemother* **22**: 457.

Molavi A, Weinstein L (1971). *In vitro* activity of erythromycin against atypical mycobacteria. *J Infect Dis* **123**: 216.

Mourad A, Sweet RL, Sugg N, Schachter J (1980). Relative resistance to erythromycin in *Chlamydia trachomatis*. *Antimicrob Ag Chemother* **18**: 696.

Muder RR, Yu VL, Fang G-D (1989). Community-acquired Legionnaires' disease. *Semin Resp Infect* **4**: 32.

Murphy PM, Mayers DL, Brock NF, Wagner KF (1989). Cure of Bacille Calmette-Guérin vaccination abscesses with erythromycin. *Rev Infect Dis* **11**: 335.

Naess A, Solberg CO (1988). Effects of two macrolide antibiotics on human leukocyte membrane receptors and functions. *APMIS* **96**: 503.

Neaverson MA (1976). Intravenous administration of erythromycin; serum, sputum and urine levels. *Curr Med Res Opin* **4**: 359.

Nelson JD (1969). Antibiotic treatment of pertussis. *Pediatrics* **44**: 474.

Ng WS, Chau PY, Ling J *et al.* (1983). Penicillinase-producing *Neisseria gonorrhoeae* isolates from different localities in South East Asia. Susceptibility to 15 antibiotics. *Brit J Vener Dis* **59**: 232.

Nguyen MH, Stout JE, Yu VL (1991). Legionellosis. *Inf Dis Clin N Amer* **5**: 561.

Niitu Y, Hasegawa S, Suetake T *et al.* (1970). Resistance of *Mycoplasma pneumoniae* to erythromycin and other antibiotics. *J Pediatr* **76**: 438.

Niitu Y, Hasegawa S, Kibota H (1974). *In vitro* development of resistance to erythromycin, other macrolide antibiotics, and lincomycin in *Mycoplasma pneumoniae*. *Antimicrob Ag Chemother* **5**: 513.

Nimmo GR, Bull JZ (1995). Comparative susceptibility of *Legionella pneumophila* and *Legionella longbeachae* to 12 antimicrobial agents. *J Antimicrob Chemother* **36**: 219.

Nord CE, Heimdahl A (1986). Impact of orally administered antimicrobial agents on human oropharyngeal and colonic microflora. *J Antimicrob Chemother* **18** (Suppl C): 159.

Norris SJ, Edmondson DG (1988). *In vitro* culture system to determine MICs and MBCs of antimicrobial agents against *Treponema pallidum* subsp *pallidum* (Nichols strain). *Antimicrob Ag Chemother* **32**: 68.

Oleinick NL, Corcoran JW (1969). Two types of binding of erythromycin to ribosomes from antibiotic-sensitive and -resistant *Bacillus subtilis* 168. *J Biol Chem* **244**: 727.

Oliver LE, Iser JH, Stening GF, Smallwood RA (1973). 'Biliary colic' and ilosone. *Med J Aust* **1**: 1148.

Oriel JD (1984). Ophthalmia neonatorum: relative efficacy of current prophylactic practices and treatment. *J Antimicrob Chemother* **14**: 209.

Osono T, Umezawa H (1985). Pharmacokinetics of macrolides, licosamides and streptogramins. *J Antimicrob Chemother* **16** (Suppl A): 151.

Pai CH, Gillis F, Tuomanen E, Marks MI (1983). Erythromycin in treatment of *Campylobacter* enteritis in children. *Amer J Dis Child* **137**: 286.

Pasculle AW, Dowling JN, Frola FN *et al.* (1981). Susceptibility of Pittsburg pneumonia agent (*Legionella micdadei*). and other newly recognized members of the genus *Legionella* to nineteen antimicrobial agents. *Antimicrob Ag Chemother* **20**: 793.

Patamasucon P, Kaojarer S, Kusmiez H, Nelson JD (1981). Pharmacokinetics of erythromycin ethylsuccinate and estolate in infants under 4 months of age. *Antimicrob Ag Chemother* **19**: 736.

Penn RL, Ward TT, Steigbigel RT (1982). Effect of erythromycin in combination with penicillin, ampicillin or gentamicin on the growth of *Listeria monocytogenes*. *Antimicrob Ag Chemother* **22**: 289.

Pepper K, Horaud T, Le Bouguénec C, De Caspédès G (1987). Location of antibiotic resistance markers in clinical isolates of *Enterococcus faecalis* with similar antibiotics. *Antimicrob Ag Chemother* **31**: 1394.

Pérez-del-Molino A, Aguado JM, Riancho JA *et al.* (1991). Erythromycin and the treatment of *Coxiella burnetii* pneumonia. *J Antimicrob Chemother* **28**: 455.

Perlman DM, Ampel NM, Schifman RB, *et al.* (1988). Persistent *Campylobacter jejuni* infections in patients infected with human immunodeficiency virus (HIV). *Ann Intern Med* **108**: 540.

Philipson A, Sabath LD, Charles D (1973). Transplacental passage of erythromycin and clindamycin. *New Engl J Med* **288**: 1219.

Pizzo PA, Robichaud KJ, Edwards BK *et al.* (1983). Oral antibiotic prophylaxis in patients with cancer: a double-blind randomized placebo-controlled trial. *J Pediatr* **102**: 125.

Plummer DC, Garland SM, Gilbert GL (1987). Bacteraemia and pelvic infection in women due to *Ureaplasma urealyticum* and *Mycoplasma hominis*. *Med J Aust* **146**: 135.

Prokesch RC, Hand WL (1982). Antibiotic entry into human polymorphonuclear leukocytes. *Antimicrob Ag Chemother* **21**: 373.

Putzi R, Blaser J, Luthy R *et al.* (1983). Side-effects due to the intravenous infusion of lactobionate. *Infection* **11**: 161.

Quinnan GVJr, McCabe WR (1978). Ototoxicity of erythromycin. *Lancet* **i**: 1160.

Raoult D, Roussellier P, Tamalet J (1988). *In vitro* evaluation of josamycin, spiramycin, and erythromycin against *Rickettsia rickettsii* and *R. conorii*. *Antimicrob Ag Chemother* **32**: 255.

Ras GJ, Anderson R, Taylor GW *et al.* (1992). Clindamycin, erythromycin, and roxithromycin inhibit the proinflammatory interactions of *Pseudomonas aeruginosa* pigments with human neutrophils *in vitro*. *Antimicrob Ag Chemother* **36**: 1236.

Regnery R, Tappero J (1995). Unraveling mysteries associated with cat-scratch disease, bacillary angiomatosis, and related syndromes. *Emerging Infect Dis* **1**: 16.

Reina J, Ros MJ, Serra A (1994). Susceptibilities to 10 antimicrobial agents of 1220 *Campylobacter* strains isolated from 1987 to 1993 from feces of pediatric patients. *Antimicrob Ag Chemother* **38**: 2917.

Renaudin H, Tully JG, Bebear C (1992). *In vitro* susceptibilities of *Mycoplasma genitalium* to antibiotics. *Antimicrob Ag Chemother* **36**: 870.

Report of a WHO Scientific Group (1978). *Neisseria gonorrhoeae* and gonococcal infections. *Wld Hlth Org Rep Ser* No. 616, p. 99.

Righter J, Luchsinger I (1988). *Haemophilus influenzae* from four laboratories in one Canadian City. *J Antimicrob Chemother* **22**: 333.

Ringertz S, Rockhill RC, Ringertz O, Sutomo A (1981). Susceptibility of *Campylobacter fetus* subsp. *jejuni*, isolated from patients in Jakarta, Indonesia, to ten antimicrobial agents. *J Antimicrob Chemother* **8**: 333.

Rios I, Klimek JJ, Maderazzo E, Quintiliani R (1978). *Flavobacterium meningosepticum* meningitis: report of selected aspects. *Antimicrob Ag Chemother* **14**: 444.

Robinson MM (1961). Antibiotics increase incidence of hepatitis. *JAMA* **178**: 89.

Roblin PM, Montalban G, Hammerschlag MR (1994). Susceptibilities to clarithromycin and erythromycin of isolates of *Chlamydia pneumoniae* from children with pneumonia. *Antimicrob Ag Chemother* **38**: 1588.

Rolfs RT (1995). Treatment of syphilis. *Clin Infect Dis* **20** (Suppl 1): 23.

Rollins LD, Lee LN, LeBlanc DJ (1985). Evidence for a disseminated erythromycin resistance determinant mediated by Tn917–like sequences among Group D streptococci isolated from pigs, chickens and humans. *Antimicrob Ag Chemother* **27**: 439.

Rosdahl VT, Sørensen TS, Colding H (1979). Determination of antibiotic concentrations in bone. *J Antimicrob Chemother* **5**: 275.

Rosenfeld J, Gura J, Boner G *et al.* (1983). Interstitial nephritis with acute renal failure after erythromycin. *Brit Med J* **286**: 938.

Rudin JE, Evans TL, Wing EJ (1984). Failure of erythromycin in treatment of *Legionella micdadei* pneumonia. *Amer J Med* **76**: 318.

Sánchez R, Fernández-Baca V, Diaz MD *et al.* (1994). Evolution of susceptibilities of *Campylobacter* spp. to quinolones and macrolides. *Antimicrob Ag Chemother* **38**: 1879.

Sabath LD, Gerstein DA, Loder PB, Finland M (1968). Excretion of erythromycin and its enhanced activity in urine against Gram-negative bacilli with alkalinization. *J Lab Clin Med* **72**: 916.

Sanders E, Foster MT, Scott D (1968). Group A beta-haemolytic streptococci resistant to erythromycin and lincomycin. *New Engl J Med* **278**: 538.

Sandström I, Ringertz O (1988). Levels of erythromycin in tear fluid and serum in infants with conjunctivitis. *Scand J Infect Dis* **20**: 429.

Schachter J, Sweet RL, Grossman M *et al.* (1986). Experience with the routine use of erythromycin for chlamydial infections in pregnancy. *New Engl J Med* **314**: 276.

Scheibel JH, Kristensen JK, Hentzer B *et al.* (1982). Treatment of chlamydial urethritis in men and *Chlamydia trachomatis*-positive female partners: comparison of erythromycin and tetracycline in treatment courses of one week. *Sex Transm Dis* **9**: 128.

Schmid GP (1990). Treatment of chancroid. *Rev Infect Dis* **12** (Suppl 6): 580.

Schoenenberger RA, Haefeli WE, Weiss P, Ritz RF (1990). Association of intravenous erythromycin and potentially fatal ventricular tachycardia with QT prolongation (torsades de pointes). *Brit Med J* **300**: 1375.

Schwartzman WA (1992). Infections due to Rochalimaea: the expanding clinical spectrum. *Clin Infect Dis* **15**: 893.

Schwebke JR, Hackman R, Bowden R (1990). Pneumonia due to *Legionella micdadei* in bone marrow transplant recipients. *Rev Infect Dis* **12**: 824.

Secker DA (1983). Erythromycin resistance only found in *Campylobacter coli*. *J Antimicrob Chemother* **12**: 414.

Sefton AM, Maskell JP, Kerawalla C *et al.* (1990). Comparative efficacy and tolerance of erythromycin and josamycin in the prevention of bacteraemia following dental extraction. *J Antimicrob Chemother* **25**: 975.

Seppölö H, Nissinen A, Yu Q, Huovinen P (1993). Three different phenotypes of erythromycin-resistant *Streptococcus pyogenes* in Finland. *J Antimicrob Chemother* **32**: 885.

Shames JM, George RB, Holliday WB *et al.* (1970). Comparison of antibiotics in the treatment of *Mycoplasma pneumonia*. *Arch Intern Med* **125**: 680.

Sherlock S (1968). Drugs and the liver. *Brit Med J* **1**: 227.

Shoemaker EH, Yow EM (1954). Clinical evaluation of erythromycin. *Arch Intern Med* **93**: 397.

Sims PJ Waites KB, Crouse DT (1994). Erythromycin lactobionate toxicity in preterm neonates. *Pediatr Infect Dis J* **13**: 164.

Sjögren E, Kaijser B, Werner M (1992). Antimicrobial susceptibilities of *Campylobacter jejuni* and *Campylobacter coli* isolated in Sweden: a 10-year follow-up report. *Antimicrob Ag Chemother* **36**: 2847.

Snavely SR, Hodges GR (1984). The neurotoxicity of antibacterial agents. *Ann Intern Med* **101**: 92.

Söderström M, Blomberg J, Christensen P, Hovelius B (1991). Erythromycin and phenoxymethylpenicillin (penicillin V). in the treatment of respiratory tract infections as related to microbiological findings and serum C-reactive protein. *Scand J Infect Dis* **23**: 347.

Soriano F, Fernández-Roblas R (1993). High rates of erythromycin-resistant *Streptococcus pneumoniae* among penicillin-resistant strains. *J Antimicrob Chemother* **31**: 440.

South MA, Short DH, Knox JM (1964). Failure of erythromycin estolate therapy in *in utero* syphilis. *JAMA* **190**: 70.

Spach DH, Kanter AS, Dougherty MJ *et al.* (1995a). *Bartonella (Rochalimaea). quintana* bacteremia in inner city patients with chronic alcoholism. *New Engl J Med* **332**: 424.

Spach DH, Kanter AS, Daniels NA *et al.* (1995b). *Bartonella (Rochalimaea).* species as a cause of apparent culture negative endocarditis. *Clin Infect Dis* **20**: 1044.

Spaepen MS, Kundsin RB, Horne HW (1976). Tetracycline-resistant T-mycoplasmas (*Ureaplasma urealyticum*). from patients with a history of reproductive failure. *Antimicrob Ag Chemother* **9**: 1012.

Spika JS, Facklam RR, Plikaytis BD *et al.* (1991). Antimicrobial resistance of *Streptococcus pneumoniae* in the United States 1979–1987. *J Infect Dis* **163**: 1273.

Sprunt K, Leidy G, Redman W (1970). Cross-resistance between lincomycin and erythromycin in viridans streptococci. *Pediatrics* **46**: 84.

Stahelin-Massik J, Levy F, Friderich P, Schaad UB (1994). Meningitis caused by *Ureaplasma urealyticum* in a full term neonate. *Pediatr Infect Dis J* **13**: 419.

Stamm LV, Stapleton JT, Bassford PJ Jr, (1988). *In vitro* assay to demonstrate high-level erythromycin resistance of a clinical isolate of *Trepanema pallidum*. *Antimicrob Ag Chemother* **32**: 164.

Steketee RW, Wassilak SGF, Adkins WN *et al.* (1988). Evidence of a high attack rate and efficacy of erythromycin prophylaxis in a pertussis outbreak in a facility for the developmentally disabled. *J Infect Dis* **157**: 434.

Stingemore N, Francis GRJ, Toohey M, McGechie DB (1989). The emergence of erythromycin resistance in *Streptococcus pyogenes* in Freemantle, Western Australia. *Med J Aust* **150**: 626.

Stoughton RB (1979). Topical antibiotics for acne vulgaris. Current usage. *Arch Dermatol* **115**: 486.

Sutter VL, Finegold SM (1976). Susceptibility of anaerobic bacteria to 23 antimicrobial agents. *Antimicrob Ag Chemother* **10**: 736.

Swenson JM, Thornsberry C, Silcox VA (1982). Rapidly growing mycobacteria: testing of susceptibility to 34 antimicrobial agents by broth microdilution. *Antimicrob Ag Chemother* **22**: 186.

Tarpay MM, Welch DF, Salari H, Marks MI (1982). *In vitro* activity of antibiotics commonly used in the treatment of otitis media against *Streptococcus pneumoniae* isolates with different susceptibilities to penicillin. *Antimicrob Ag Chemother* **22**: 145.

Taylor DE, Courvalin P (1988). Mechanisms of antibiotic resistance in *Campylobacter* species. *Antimicrob Ag Chemother* **32**: 1107.

Taylor DN, Blaser MJ, Echeverria P *et al.* (1987). Erythromycin-resistant *Campylobacter* infections in Thailand. *Antimicrob Ag Chemother* **31**: 438.

Thompson PJ, Burgess KR, Marlin GE (1980). Influence of food absorption of erythromycin ethyl succinate. *Antimicrob Ag Chemother* **18**: 829.

Thornsberry C, Baker CN, Kirven LA (1978). *In vitro* activity of antimicrobial agents on Legionnaires' disease bacterium. *Antimicrob Ag Chemother* **13**: 78.

Tofte RW, Solliday J, Crossley KB (1984). Susceptibilities of enterococci to twelve antibiotics. *Antimicrob Ag Chemother* **25**: 532.

Tolman KG, Sannella JJ, Freston JW (1974). Chemical structure of erythromycin and hepatotoxicity. *Ann Intern Med* **81**: 58.

Tompkins LS (1994). Rochalimaea infections Are they zoonoses? *JAMA* **271**: 553.

Toomey KE, Barnes RC (1990). Treatment of *Chlamydia trachomatis* genital infection. *Rev Infect Dis* **12** (Suppl 6): 645.

Triggs EJ, Ashley JJ (1978). Oral administration of erythromycin stearate: effect of dosage form of plasma levels. *Med J Aust* **2**: 121.

Tuominen RK, Männistö PT, Pohto P *et al.* (1988). Absorption of erythromycin acistrate and erythromycin base in the fasting and non-fasting state. *J Antimicrob Chemother* **21** (Suppl D): 45.

Umstead GS, Neumann KH (1986). Erythromycin ototoxicity and acute psychotic reaction in cancer patients with hepatic dysfunction. *Arch Intern Med* **146**: 897.

Vanhoof R, Gordts B, Dierickx R *et al.* (1980). Susceptibility of *Campylobacter fetus* subsp. *jejuni* to 25 antimicrobial agents. *Antimicrob Ag Chemother* **14**: 533.

Van Marion WF, Van der Meer JWM, Kalff MW, Schicht SM (1978). Ototoxicity of erythromycin. *Lancet* **ii**: 214.

Verville TD, Huycke MM, Greenfield RA *et al.* (1994). *Rhodococcus equi* infections of humans. *Medicine* **73**: 119.

Vildé JL, Dournon E, Rajagopalan P (1986). Inhibition of *Legionella pneumophila* multiplication within human macrophages by antimicrobial agents. *Antimicrob Ag Chemother* **30**: 743.

Waites KB, Crouse DT, Cassell GH (1992). Antibiotic susceptibilities and therapeutic options for Ureaplasma urealyticum infections in neonates. *Pediatr Infect Dis J* **11**: 23.

Waites KB, Crouse DT, Cassell GH (1993). Therapeutic concentrations for *Ureaplasma urealyticum* infections in neonates. *Clin Infect Dis* **17** (Suppl 1): 208.

Waites KB, Sims PJ, Crouse DT *et al.* (1994). Serum concentrations of erythromycin after intravenous infusion in preterm neonates treated for *Ureaplasma urealyticum* infection. *Pediatr Infect Dis J* **13**: 287.

Waldor MK, Wilson B, Swartz M (1993). Cellulitis caused by *Legionella pneumophila*. *Clin Infect Dis* **16**: 51.

Weisblum B (1995). Erythromycin resistance by ribosome modification. *Antimicrob Ag Chemother* **39**: 577.

Wenzel RP, Hendley JO, Dodd WK, Gwaltney JMJr (1976). Comparison of josamycin and erythromycin in the therapy of *Mycoplasma pneumoniae* pneumonia. *Antimicrob Ag Chemother* **10**: 899.

Westh H, Hougaard DM, Vuust J, Rosdahl VT (1995). Prevalence of erm gene classes in erythromycin-resistant *Staphylococcus aureus* strains isolated between 1959 and 1988. *Antimicrob Ag Chemother* **39**: 369.

Wiggins GL, Albritton WL, Feeley JC (1978). Antibiotic susceptibility of clinical isolates of *Listeria monocytogenes*. *Antimicrob Ag Chemother* **13**: 854.

Williams D, Schorling J, Barrett LJ *et al.* (1989). Early treatment of *Campylobacter jejuni* enteritis. *Antimicrob Ag Chemother* **33**: 248.

Williams JD (1995). Selective toxicity and concordant pharmacodynamics of antibiotics and other drugs. *J Antimicrob Chemother* **35**: 721.

Williams JD, Sefton AM (1993). Comparison of macrolide antibiotics. *J Antimicrob Chemother* **31** (Suppl C): 11.

Wilson SZ, Martin RR, Putman M (1977). *In vitro* effects of josamycin, erythromycin, and placebo therapy on nasal carriage of *Staphylococcus aureus*. *Antimicrob Ag Chemother* **11**: 407.

Wilson APR (1995). Treatment of infection caused by toxigenic and non-toxigenic strains of *Corynebacterium diphtheriae*. *J Antimicrob Chemother* **35**: 717.

Wing EJ, Schafer FJ, Pasculle AW (1981). Successful treatment of *Legionella micdadei* (Pittsburgh pneumonia agent). pneumonia with erythromycin. *Amer J Med* **71**: 386.

Winslow DL, Damme J, Dieckman E (1983). Delayed bactericidal activity of beta-lactam antibiotics against *Listeria monocytogenes*: antagonism of chloramphenicol and rifampin. *Antimicrob Ag Chemother* **23**: 555.

Wisseman CLJr, Waddell AD, Walsh WT (1974). *In vitro* studies of the action of antibiotics on *Rickettsia prowazeki* by two methods of cell culture. *J Infect Dis* **130**: 564.

Wollmer P, Pride NB, Rhodes CG *et al.* (1982). Measurement of pulmonary erythromycin concentration in patients with lobar pneumonia by means of positron tomography. *Lancet* **ii**: 1361.

Wong KY, Boose GM, Issitt CH *et al.* (1981). Erythromycin-induced hemolytic anaemia. *J Pediatr* **98**: 647.

Wroblewski BA, Singer WD, Whyte J (1986). Carbamazepine-erythromycin interaction. Case studies and clinical significance. *JAMA* **255**: 1165.

Yagi Y, McLellan TS, Frez WA, Clewell DB (1978). Characterization of a small plasmid determining resistance of erythromycin, lincomycin, and vernamycin B in a strain of *Streptococcus sanguis* isolated from dental plaque. *Antimicrob Ag Chemother* **13**: 884.

Yan W, Taylor DE (1991). Characterization of erythromycin resistance in *Campylobacter jejuni* and *Campylobacter coli*. *Antimicrob Ag Chemother* **35**: 1989.

Yazawa K, Mikami Y, Sakamoto T *et al.* (1994). Inactivation of the macrolide antibiotics erythromycin, midecamycin, and rokitamycin by pathogenic *Nocardia* species. *Antimicrob Ag Chemother* **38**: 2197.

Zabransky RJ, Johnston JA, Hauser KJ (1973). Bacteriostatic and bactericidal activities of various antibiotics against *Bacteroides fragilis*. *Antimicrob Ag Chemother* **3**: 152.

Zackrisson G, Lind L, Roos K, Larsson P (1988). Erythromycin-resistant beta-hemolytic streptococci Group A in Göteborg, Sweden. *Scand J Infect Dis* **20**: 419.

Zamiri I, McEntegart MG (1972). The sensitivity of diphtheria bacilli to eight antibiotics. *J Clin Path* **25**: 716.

Spiramycin, Josamycin and Rosaramicin

Description

Like erythromycin, these three antibiotics belong to the macrolide group (p. 606).

1 Spiramycin

Spiramycin was isolated by Pinnert-Sindico *et al.* (1955) from a strain of *Streptomyces ambofaciens* in France. The antibiotic has been used extensively in that country, but experience with it in Britain, North America and Australia has been limited.

2 Josamycin

Josamycin was produced from *Streptomyces narbonensis* var. *josamyceticus* (Osono *et al.*, 1967; Nitta *et al.*, 1967).

3 Rosaramicin

Rosaramicin a somewhat newer macrolide, was produced by *Micromonospora rosaria*, and was formerly called rosamicin (Wagman *et al.*, 1972; Waitz *et al.*, 1972).

Sensitive Organisms

The antibacterial spectrum of these three drugs is similar to that of erythromycin (p. 606), and the most active of the three seems to be rosaramicin.

1 Gram-positive bacteria

These drugs are active against bacteria such as *Staphylococcus aureus* (including beta-lactamase producing strains), coagulase-negative staphylococci, *Streptococcus pyogenes*, *Strep. pneumoniae* and most strains of *Enterococcus faecalis*. While some authors have shown that josamycin has similar activity to erythromycin against *Staph. aureus* (Strausbaugh *et al.*, 1976a; Westerman *et al.*, 1976), others have found the activity of the drug to be inferior to that of erythromycin and rosaramicin (Shadomy *et al.*, 1976). Resistance of *Staph. aureus* to spiramycin is mainly due to the same mechanism which operates with clindamycin and erythromycin (MLS-resistance) (p. 587). Spiramycin-resistant strains are always erythromycin-resistant, but some erythromycin-resistant strains may be spiramycin-sensitive (Chabbert, 1988). Resistance of *Staph. aureus* to rosaramicin is usually also of the MLS type and appears to be mainly constitutive (p. 588). No cultures tested by Lacey (1981) showed inducible resistance to rosaramicin. Erythromycin is more active against Group A streptococci than rosaramicin (Saroglou and Bisno, 1978), and rosaramicin is also inferior to many other agents in its inhibition of *E. faecalis* (Tofte *et al.*, 1984). *Corynebacterium diphtheriae* and *Bacillus anthracis* are sensitive to spiramycin and rosaramicin.

Of the Gram-positive anaerobes, the *Peptococcus*, *Peptostreptococcus*, *Propionibacterium* and *Eubacterium* spp. are sensitive to josamycin, but *Clostridium* spp. strains may be resistant (Long *et al.*, 1976). Rosaramicin is also active against anaerobes (Sutter and Finegold, 1976). For Gram-positive anaerobes it is much more active than erythromycin against *Peptococcus* spp., but of about equal activity against the others, such as *Peptostreptococcus*, *Eubacterium*, *Propionibacterium*, *Actinomyces* and *Lactobacillus* spp. *Clostridium tetani* and *Cl. perfringens* are sensitive to spiramycin and rosaramicin.

2 Gram-negative bacteria

While *Neisseria meningitidis* is generally sensitive to these antibiotics, approximately half of 80 strains of *N. gonorrhoeae* (none of them produced beta-lactamase) isolated in Brussels in 1978 were resistant to spiramycin (Gordts *et al.*, 1982), as were about one-third of 517 Canadian strains, again none producing beta-lactamase, isolated in 1973–74; two-thirds of a smaller number of penicillinase-producing strains were spiramycin-resistant (Dillon *et al.*, 1978), but 50% of 100 gonococcal isolates from South Africa were susceptible to 0.02 μg per ml or less of rosaramicin (Liebowitz *et al.*, 1982). Rosaramicin is more active than penicillin G, erythromycin and tetracycline against *N. gonorrhoeae*; this activity also encompasses beta-lactamase-producing strains (Sanders and Sanders, 1977).

Neisseria meningitidis and *Bordetella pertussis* are sensitive to spiramycin and josamycin. While spiromycin is not very active against *Haemophilus influenzae*, the *in vitro* activity of rosaramicin is greater than that of chloramphenicol, ampicillin or erythromycin (Sanders and Sanders, 1977). All 23 strains of *H. ducreyi* tested by Feltham *et al.* (1979) were inhibited by 0.06 μg per ml or less of rosaramicin. *Campylobacter* spp. are readily inhibited by these three antibiotics, but some variation in sensitivity between subspecies occurs, which may assist laboratory differentiation (Ahonkai *et al.*, 1981; Wang *et al.*, 1984). For instance, *Campylobacteria jejuni* was somewhat more sensitive than *C. coli* to both spiramycin and josamycin, and human strains of *C. coli* were more susceptible to these two drugs than *C. coli* strains isolated from swine (Elharrif *et al.*, 1985). *Legionella* spp. were very susceptible to rosaramicin, the mean MIC of 33 strains was only one-fifth of the corresponding MIC of erythromycin (Edelstein *et al.*, 1982). Josamycin has therapeutic efficacy in experimental *Legionella pneumophila* pneumonia in guinea-pigs (Saito *et al.*, 1985). Spiramycin is also active against *L. pneumophila* and *Moraxella catarrhalis* (Chabbert, 1988).

While 60% of *Fusobacterium* spp. tested by Long *et al.* (1976) were resistant to a concentration of 2.0 μg per ml of josamycin, it is more active against *Bacteroides fragilis* than spiramycin (Strausbaugh *et al.*, 1976a). Rosaramicin is generally more active than erythromycin against Gram-negative anaerobes such as the *Bacteroides* and *Fusobacterium* spp. All strains of *Bacteroides fragilis* tested by Sutter and Finegold (1976) were inhibited by concentrations of rosaramicin of 4 μg per ml or less.

3 Other organisms

Mycoplasmas are sensitive to all three antibiotics, as is *Ureaplasma urealyticum* (Robertson *et al.*, 1981; Chabbert, 1988). *Chlamydia trachomatis* is sensitive to rosaramicin and spiramycin; spiramycin also has some activity against *C. psittaci* (Orfila *et al.*, 1988). *Rickettsia rickettsii* and *R. conorii* are sensitive to josamycin, but not to spiramycin (Raoult *et al.*, 1988). *Cryptosporidium* spp. appears somewhat sensitive to spiramycin *in vivo*; its sensitivity to antibiotics cannot be tested *in vitro* (Fayer and Ungar, 1986; Soave and Armstrong, 1986; Moskovitz *et al.*, 1988). Spiramycin also has some activity against *Toxoplasma gondii* in tissue

Organism	MIC (μg per ml)	
	Spiramycin	Rosaramicin
Gram-positive organisms		
Staphylococcus aureus	0.3–25.0	0.5–2.0
Streptococcus pyogenes	0.25–1.0	0.12–0.5
Streptococcus pneumoniae	0.2–1.2	0.12–0.25
Enterococcus faecalis	1.0–5.0	0.5–4.0
Clostridium perfringens	2.0–8.0	0.5–1.0
Gram-negative bacteria		
Neisseria meningitidis	0.3–3.0	0.06–0.5
Haemophilus influenzae	16.0–32.0	0.5–2.0
Campylobacter spp.	0.5–>32.0	–
Bacteroides fragilis	4.0–16.0	1.0–2.0

Table I.46

Compiled from data published by Smith *et al.* (1981), Kernbaum (1982) and Elharrif *et al.* (1985)

culture and in mouse models of infection (Chang and Pechére, 1988a,b; Derouin and Chastang, 1988; Wong and Remington, 1994).

4 Minimum inhibitory concentrations

The MICs of spiramycin and rosaramicin against some selected bacterial species are shown in Table I.46.

Mode of Administration and Dosage

Spiramycin and josamycin were administered only by the oral route, but now an i.v. preparation of spiramycin is available (Mayaud et al., 1988). Rosaramicin may be given orally or i.v. The usual dosage of spiramycin is 2–3 g orally per day, given in two to four divided doses; this may be increased to 4 g daily in severe infections. Intravenously spiramycin is usually given in a dosage of 1.0 g 8-hourly (Mayaud et al., 1988). The spiramycin dosage for children is 50–100 mg per kg daily given in two to four divided doses. The simultaneous administration of food does not affect its bioavailability. The oral josamycin dosage is similar (Wenzel et al., 1976). Rosaramicin has been administered in a dosage of 250 mg orally four times daily (Brunham et al., 1982).

Serum Levels in Relation to Dosage

Serum levels of spiramycin during continuous oral administration of 3 g per day in adults ranged from 1.6 μg to 2.8 μg per ml (Chabbert, 1955). Hudson et al. (1956) administered oral spiramycin to 26 adults with a loading dose of 2 g followed by 1 g every 6 h. Serum levels taken 2, 4 and 6 h after each dose ranged from 1.0 to 6.7 μg per ml. After the patients had received 11 doses, the lowest serum level detected was 2 μg per ml, indicating that some accumulation had occurred after treatment for 3 days. According to MacFarlane et al. (1968), serum and tissue spiramycin concentrations are maximal after treatment for 7 days.

Pharmacological studies indicate that after oral administration, josamycin behaves similarly to erythromycin (Strausbaugh et al., 1976b). Compared with erythromycin, there was a tendency for josamycin to accumulate over the first 48 h, resulting in higher peak and trough levels.

After a 1-h i.v. infusion of 0.5 g of rosaramicin in a volume of 200 ml, a peak serum level of over 3.0 μg per ml was obtained in 12 healthy males and this level declined to between 0.1 and 0.2 μg per ml over the next 12 h (Lin et al., 1984). Peak serum levels of 0.3–0.5 μg per ml were obtained 1.5–2 h after oral administration of 0.5 g of the drug (as tablet or oral solution) to the same subjects.

Excretion

1 Spiramycin

Only 5–15% of an orally administered dose can be recovered from the urine, but there is significant biliary excretion with bile levels being 15- to 40-fold higher than those found in sera. Inactivation of the drug in the body accounts for most of the ingested dose, but the process is apparently slower than with erythromycin. The biologic half-life is reported to be between 4–8 h.

2 Josamycin

This is metabolized in the liver and excreted in the bile in an inactive form (Mitsuhashi, 1971). Less than 20% of the drug is excreted in the urine in the active form, but high urinary concentrations are obtained.

3 Rosaramicin

Extensive biliary excretion of both active and metabolized drug is also thought to be responsible for the appearance of 87% of an administered dose of rosaramicin in the feces. Extensive metabolism of the drug occurs. Unchanged rosaramicin accounted for only 7–9% of the drug excreted in urine (Lin et al., 1984).

Distribution of the Drugs in Body

High concentrations of spiramycin appear to persist in various organs for prolonged periods. The drug is secreted in saliva in which its peak concentrations are 1.3 to 4.8 times higher than those in serum (Kamme et al., 1978). Spiramycin quickly penetrates bronchial secretions; 3 h after dosing; its concentration in these secretions is equal to the serum level and this does not vary with the severity of bronchial inflammation. Tissue concentrations of spiramycin may still be high when the serum spiramycin has fallen to a low level; e.g. 12 h after a dose of 2 g per day for 16 days, levels of 21 and 27 μg per ml were obtained in prostate and muscle, respectively (MacFarlane *et al.*, 1968). However, spiramycin diffuses poorly in large collections of tissue fluid (Davey *et al.*, 1987). Spiramycin virtually does not enter the CSF, even in patients with meningitis. The transplacental passage and distribution of spiramycin in the tissues in the fetus has been studied in rhesus monkeys. The fetal–maternal serum level ratio was 0.27 to 0.58; the higher fetal–maternal serum ratios occurred when larger doses of the drug were given i.v. rather than orally. It appeared that spiramycin accumulated in the soft tissue, especially in the liver and spleen, of both the mother and the fetus. The concentration in placental tissue was about 10- 20-fold higher than the level in fetal serum. Its concentration in the amniotic fluid was about 5-fold higher than the level in fetal serum (Schoondermark-Van de Ven *et al.*, 1994a).

Strausbaugh *et al.* (1976b) showed that josamycin penetrated well into saliva sweat and tears. The drug was concentrated up to 20-fold in phagocytic cells compared with serum (Labro and Babin-Chevaye, 1989).

Rosaramicin is concentrated in human prostatic tissue and, therefore, it has been suggested that it may be useful for the treatment of bacterial prostatitis (Baumueller *et al.*, 1977). After a single 250-mg dose was given to ten lactating mothers, only 0.0025% of the dose was recoverable from breast milk over the first 10 h. Drug-induced toxicity in an infant via breast milk is, therefore, unlikely (Stoehr *et al.*, 1985).

Mode of Action

The mode of action of all macrolide antibiotics on bacteria is similar (see erythromycin, p. 614).

Toxicity

1 Spiramycin

Gastrointestinal side-effects (nausea, vomiting, dry mouth and abdominal pain, (particularly if high doses were used), and occasional skin rashes; including a report of a patient developing urticaria, have occurred. Asthma has been reported following occupational exposure to spiramycin in the pharmaceutical industry (Davies and Pepys, 1975; Moscato *et al.*, 1984). Contact dermatitis has been described in several veterinary surgeons (Hjorth and Roed-Petersen, 1980). There is a report of atypical antibiotic-associated colitis associated with spiramycin therapy (Di Febo *et al.*, 1982) and Biermann *et al.* (1988) reported a case of pseudomembranous colitis caused by spiramycin. With oral spiramycin therapy, resistant Enterobacteriaceae, increase in the fecal flora (Andremont *et al.*, 1991). Spiramycin has not been implicated as causing significant drug interactions by interfering with other drug hepatic metabolism (Ludden, 1985). The 14-membered lactone ring macrolide antibiotics, such as erythromycin, often cause drug interactions (p. 616). Spiramycin is a 16-membered lactone ring macrolide, and its use is not associated with drug interactions (Descotes *et al.*, 1985; Mayaud *et al.*, 1988).

2 Josamycin

Josamycin has generally only been associated with mild gastrointestinal side-effects (Mitsuhashi, 1971). Unlike erythromycin (p. 616), it does not inhibit the clearance of theophylline and is also not involved in other drug reactions, so it might be preferred when a macrolide is needed in association with theophylline and some other drugs (Pessayre, 1983; Descotes *et al.*, 1985).

3 Rosaramicin

This has been reported to be associated with elevated serum alanine aminotransferase levels in four of 18 women receiving the drug for chlamydial infection of the cervix (Robson *et al.*, 1983). Gastrointestinal side-effects have been frequently observed in treatment trials. They occurred when usual doses were employed and appeared to be more frequent than those associated with erythromycin.

Clinical Uses of the Drugs

1 Spiramycin

This has been used for indications similar to those for oral erythromycin (p. 616). It has been used as an alternative to penicillin G for streptococcal and pneumococcal infections, and also for treatment of staphylococcal infections. Despite the inferior antibacterial activity of spiramycin, compared with erythromycin, clinicians mainly in France have obtained good results with spiramycin in all these infections (Kernbaum, 1982; De Cock and Poels, 1988; Modai, 1988). This may be explained by the special pharmacological behavior of this drug (p. 631). In one uncontrolled trial i.v. spiramycin in a dosage of 1.0 g 8-hourly appeared to be about equal in efficacy to i.v. erythromycin for the treatment of *Legionella pneumonia* (Mayaud *et al.*, 1988). Spiramycin given as nine doses (a 2-g loading dose followed by 1 g 12-hourly for 4 days) to 59 healthy adult nasopharyngeal carriers of meningococci resulted in a reduction in carriage of 85 and 59% respectively, on the 2nd and 12th post-treatment days. It was concluded that spiramycin may be an effective alternative to rifampicin (p. 697) for the chemoprophylaxis of secondary meningococcal disease (Engelen *et al.*, 1981).

Hyperendemic trachoma in children was treated for 6 weeks with topical ointment containing 1% rifampicin, oxytetracycline or spiramycin. Similar cure rates were obtained, but re-culture 7 months later revealed a 27% positive culture rate for the spiramycin treated group, while the rate for the other groups was less than 2% (Darougar *et al.*, 1980). In one trial spiramycin appeared to be a satisfactory treatment for non-gonococcal urethritis in men, mainly caused by *C. trachomatis* (Segev *et al.*, 1988). In another comparative study spiramycin in a dosage of 1.0 g twice-daily for 14 days was equally as effective as doxycycline 100 mg twice-daily for 14 days for the treatment of *C. trachomatis* genital infections in both men and women (Dylewski *et al.*, 1993).

Spiramycin is recommended for the treatment of toxoplasmosis during the first trimester of pregnancy, when pyrimethamine is contraindicated (p. 913). In one prospective study of 375 pregnant women with high initial toxoplasma antibody titers or seroconversion during pregnancy, spiramycin treatment reduced the frequency of fetal toxoplasma infections (Desmonts and Couvreur, 1974). However, from this study it also appeared that spiramycin did not influence the course of established fetal toxoplasmosis. Pregnant women in first trimester should be treated by 3 g spiramycin per day in divided doses. Compared with the level in maternal serum, the concentration of spiramycin in cord serum is only half as high (p. 632). The spiramycin levels in fetal blood may be insufficient for the treatment of fetus *in utero*. In the second and third trimesters of pregnancy the more effective pyrimethamine/sulfadiazine should be used (p. 913).

In HIV-infected patients, chronic (latent) *Toxiplasma gondii* infection may reactivate and the result can be life-threatening disease in the woman and transmission of *T. gondii*, HIV or both to the fetus. These women may also acquire acute toxoplasmosis during pregnancy. It is recommended that they should be treated by spiramycin 3 g per day during the first trimester of pregnancy, but it is unlikely that spiramycin will prevent the development of toxoplasmic encephalitis in either mother or fetus. Treatment with pyrimethamine/sulfadiazine should be considered from the 17th week of gestation (Wong and Remington, 1994). The effectiveness of spiramycin for the treatment of rhesus monkey fetuses congenitally infected with *T. gondii* has been studied. The monkeys were infected at day 90 of pregnancy. Treatment with spiramycin was started as soon as fetal infection was proven and was continued until birth. Concentration of spiramycin in neonatal tissue was 5- to 28-fold higher than the corresponding concentration in neonatal serum. But no spiramycin was found in the fetal brains. It appeared that early treatment with spiramycin may prevent transmission of infection to the fetus but most probably cannot cure an existing brain infection in the fetus (Schoondermark-Van de Ven *et al.*, 1994b).

Spiramycin has been tried in *Cryptosporidium* diarrhea. A controlled study in young children with this disease showed that spiramycin 75 mg per kg per day in two divided doses for 5 days was no better than placebo (Wittenberg *et al.*, 1989). In older children and young normal adults *Cryptosporidium* diarrhea is an acute self-limiting illness which requires no chemotherapy (Hart *et al.*, 1984). However, this parasite causes prolonged debilitating diarrhea and even death in HIV-infected patients (CDC, 1984). There is no satisfactory treatment for this. Spiramycin has resulted in some improvement in symptoms in a few patients, but similar to paromomycin (p. 538), it does not cure the disease (Portnoy *et al.*, 1984; Soave and Armstrong, 1986). *Cryptosporidium* diarrhea has also occurred in patients with hematological malignancies; this resolved without treatment in some patients and spiramycin therapy was of no value (Gentile *et al.*, 1991). In one bone marrow transplantation unit there was an outbreak of *Cryptosporidium* diarrhea. Four patients were treated with spiramycin 3 g per day and three of the four patients recovered from diarrhea and stopped excreting *Cryptosporidium* oocysts during therapy. However, simultaneous marrow engraftment may have contributed to their recovery (Martino *et al.*, 1988). *Cryptosporidium* can also infect other body tissues in immunodeficient patients; one 17-year-old boy with congenital hypogammaglobulinemia developed *Cryptosporidium* sinusitis (Davis and Heyman, 1988) and in one bone-marrow transplant patient pulmonary cryptosporidiosis occurred (Kibbler *et al.*, 1987). In the first patient symptoms resolved after spiramycin therapy, and in the second spiramycin appeared to eradicate *Cryptosporidium* from the lungs, but the patient died from cytomegalovirus (CMV) pneumonitis.

2 Josamycin

Josamycin propionate, a tasteless derivative suitable for use in a pediatric suspension, appeared to be highly effective in an open trial for the infections in a pediatric practice. Side-effects were few. However, the infections were mainly diagnosed on clinical grounds (Privitera *et al.*, 1984). In one controlled study, josamycin and erythromycin, both given in an oral dose of 2.0 g daily in four divided doses, were equally effective in adults with mycoplasma pneumonia (Wenzel *et al.*, 1976). Similarly, josamycin and erythromycin were equally effective in reducing the carrier rates of *Staph. aureus* (Wilson *et al.*, 1977). A 5-day treatment with josamycin was satisfactory for non-severe community-acquired pneumonia (Mensa *et al.*, 1993). A 5-day josamycin regimen was as effective as 1-day doxycycline treatment for Mediterranean spotted fever, a tick-borne rickettsiosis caused by *Rickettsia conorii* (p. 748) (Bella *et al.*, 1990).

3 Rosaramicin

This drug in a dose of 1 g daily and erythromycin stearate 2 g daily were equally effective when given for 7 days to women with *C. trachomatis* cervicitis. Cultures obtained 11 and 32 days later were negative in all except one erythromycin-treated patient (Robson *et al.*, 1983). A similar result was obtained in another controlled trial in which tetracycline 2 g daily and rosaramicin 250 mg four times daily, each for 7 days, were compared (Brunham *et al.*, 1982). Rosaramicin, while equally effective, produced a higher rate of gastrointestinal side-effects in this trial. Non-gonococcal urethritis in men was treated in two controlled trials with either rosaramicin or tetracycline, each given in a dosage of 1 g per day for 7 days, with equivalent good results. Again gastrointestinal side-effects were more common in the rosaramicin treated group (Juvakoski *et al.*, 1981; Darne *et al.*, 1982). A high (28%) prevalence of gastrointestinal side-effects was also recorded when two regimens of rosaramicin (2 g and 1.5 g daily for 4 days) were compared in the treatment of gonococcal urethritis in males. After treatment 39 of 40 patients were asymptomatic and had negative cultures (Dacso *et al.*, 1980).

A comparative study of erythromycin base 500 mg and rosaramicin 250 mg, each four times daily for 10 days in the treatment of genital ulcers due to *Haemophilus ducreyi* in Kenyan men, resulted in similar healing times of from 5 days to 2 weeks and no treatment failures in either group (Plummer *et al.*, 1983).

References

Ahonkai VI, Cherubin CE, Sierra MF *et al.* (1981). *In vitro* susceptibility of *Campylobacter fetus* subsp. *jejuni* to N-formimidoyl thienamycin, rosaramicin, cefoperazone, and other antimicrobial agents. *Antimicrob Ag Chemother* **20**: 850.

Andremont A, Trancréde C, Desnottes J-F (1991). Effect of spiramycin on the faecal and oral bacteria in human volunteers. *J Antimicrob Chemother* **27**: 355.

Baumueller A, Hoyme U, Madsen PO (1977). Rosamicin – a new drug for the treatment of bacterial prostatitis. *Antimicrob Ag Chemother* **12**: 240.

Bella F, Font B, Uriz S *et al.* (1990). Randomized trial of doxycycline versus josamycin for Mediterranean spotted fever. *Antimicrob Ag Chemother* **34**: 937.

Biermann C, Loken A, Riise R (1988). Comparison of spiramycin and

doxycycline in the treatment of lower respiratory infections in general practice. *J Antimicrob Chemother* **22** (Suppl B): 155.

Brunham RC, Kuo CC, Stevens CE, Holmes KK (1982). Therapy of cervical chlamydial infection. *Ann Intern Med* **97**: 216.

CDC (Centers for Disease Control) (1984). Update: treatment of cryptosporidiosis in patients with the acquired immune deficiency syndrome (AIDS).. *MMWR* **33**: 117.

Chabbert Y (1955). *In vitro* studies with spiramycin. *Ann Inst Pasteur* **89**: 434.

Chabbert YA (1988). Early studies on *in-vitro* and experimental activity of spiramycin: a review. *J Antimicrob Chemother* **22** (Suppl B): 1.

Chang HR, Pechère J-CF (1988a). Activity of spiramycin against *Toxoplasma gondii in vitro*, in experimental infections and in human infections. *J Antimicrob Chemother* **22** (Suppl B): 87.

Chang HR, Pechère J-CF (1988b). *In vitro* effects of four macrolides (roxithromycin, spiramycin, azithromycin (CP-62,993). and A-56268 on *Toxoplasma gondii*. *Antimicrob Ag Chemother* **32**: 524.

Dacso C, Greenberg S, Martin RR (1980). Rosaramicin treatment of gonococcal urethritis in men. *Sex Transm Dis* **7**: 133.

Darne JF, Ridgway GL, Oriel JD (1982). Rosaramicin and tetracycline in the treatment of non-gonococcal urethritis. A comparison of clinical and microbiological results. *Brit J Vener Dis* **58**: 117.

Darougar S, Jones BR, Viswalingam N *et al.* (1980). Topical therapy of hyperendemic trachoma with rifamicin, oxytetracycline or spiramycin eye ointments. *Br J Ophthalmol* **64**: 37.

Davey PG, Jacobus NV, Tally FP (1987). Comparative efficacy of clindamycin, erythromycin and spiramycin against *Staphylococcus aureus* in the rat croton oil pouch model. *J Antimicrob Chemother* **20**: 705.

Davies RJ, Pepys J (1975). Asthma due to inhaled chemical agents – the macrolide antibiotic spiramycin. *Clin Allergy* **5**: 99.

Davis JJ, Heyman MB (1988). Cryptosporidosis and sinusitis in an immunodeficient adolescent. *J Infect Dis* **158**: 649.

De Cock L, Poels R (1988). Comparison of spiramycin with erythromycin for lower respiratory tract infections. *J Antimicrob Chemother* **22** (Suppl B): 159.

Derouin F, Chastang C (1988). Enzyme immunoassay to assess efffect of antimicrobial agents on *Toxoplasma gondii* in tissue culture. *Antimicrob Ag Chemother* **32**: 303.

Descotes J, André P, Evreux JC (1985). Pharmacokinetic drug interactions with macrolide antibiotics. *J Antimicrob Chemother* **15**: 659.

Desmonts G, Couvreur J (1974). Congenital toxoplasmosis. A prospective study of 378 pregnancies. *New Engl J Med* **290**: 1110.

Di Febo G, Milazzo G, Gizzi G *et al.* (1982). Antibiotic-associated colitis: always pseudomembranous? *Endoscopy* **14**: 128.

Dillon JR, Duck PD, Eidus L (1978). A comparison of the *in vitro* activity of rosamicin, erythromycin, spiramycin, penicillin and tetracycline against *N gonorrhoeae* including beta-lactamase producing isolates. *J Antimicrob Chemother* **4**: 477.

Dylewski J, Clecner B, Dubois J *et al.* (1993). Comparison of spiramycin and doxycycline for treatment of *Chlamydia trachomatis* genital infections. *Antimicrob Ag Chemother* **37**: 1373.

Edelstein PH, Pasiecznik KA, Yasui VK, Meyer RD (1982). Susceptibility of *Legionella* spp. to mycinamicin I and II and other macrolide antibiotics: effects of media composition and origin of organisms. *Antimicrob Ag Chemother* **22**: 90.

Elharrif Z, Megraud F, Marchand A-M (1985). Susceptibility of *Campylobacter jejuni* and *Campylobacter coli* to macrolides and related compounds. *Antimicrob Ag Chemother* **28**: 695.

Engelen F, Vandepitte J, Verbist L, DeMaeyer-Cleempoel S (1981). Effect of spiramycin on the nasopharyngeal carriage of *Neisseria meningitidis*. *Chemotherapy* **27**: 325.

Fayer R, Ungar BLP (1986). *Cryptosporidium* spp. and cryptosporidiosis. *Microbiol Rev* **50**: 458.

Feltham S, Ronald AR, Albritton WL (1979). A comparison of the *in vitro* activity of rosaramicin, erythromycin, clindamycin, metronidazole and ornidazole against *H. ducreyi* including beta-lactamase producing strains. *J Antimicrob Chemother* **5**: 731.

Gentile G, Venditti M, Micozzi A *et al.* (1991). Cryptosporidiosis in patients with hematologic malignancies. *Rev Infect Dis* **13**: 842.

Gordts B, Vanhoof R, Hubrechts JM *et al.* (1982). *In vitro* activity of 21 antimicrobial agents against *Neisseria gonorrhoeae* in Brussels. *Brit J Vener Dis* **58**: 23.

Hart CA, Baxby D, Blundell M (1984). Gastroenteritis due to *Cryptosporidium*: a prospective survey in a children's hospital. *J Infect* **9**: 264.

Hjorth N, Roed-Petersen J (1980). Allergic contact dermatitis in veterinary surgeons. *Contact Dermat* **6**: 27.

Hudson DG, Yoshihara GM, Kirby WMM (1956). Spiramycin, clinical and laboratory studies. *Arch Intern Med* **97**: 57.

Juvakoski T, Allgulander C, Lassus A (1981). Rosaramicin and tetracycline treatment in *Chlamydia trachomatis*-positive and -negative non-gonococcal urethritis. *Sex Transm Dis* **8**: 12.

Kamme C, Kahlmeter G, Melander A (1978). Evaluation of spiramycin as a therapeutic agent for elimination of nasopharyngeal pathogens. *Scand J Infect Dis* **10**: 135.

Kernbaum S (1982). Spiramycin therapeutic use in man. *Semaine des Hopitaux* **58**: 289.

Kibbler CC, Smith A, Hamilton-Dutoit SJ *et al.* (1987). Pulmonary cryptosporidiosis occurring in a bone marrow transplant patient. *Scand J Infect Dis* **19**: 581.

Labro MT, Babin-Chevaye C (1989). Synergistic interaction of josamycin with human neutrophils bactericidal function *in vitro*. *J Antimicrob Chemother* **24**: 731.

Lacey RW (1981). *In vitro* evaluation of rosaramicin. *J Antimicrob Chemother* **7**: 293.

Liebowitz LD, Ballard RC, Koornhof HJ (1982). *In vitro* susceptibility and cross-resistance of South African isolates of *Neisseria gonorrhoeae* to 14 antimicrobial agents. *Antimicrob Ag Chemother* **22**: 598.

Lin C-C, Chung M, Gural R *et al.* (1984). Pharmacokinetics of rosaramicin in humans. *Antimicrob Ag Chemother* **26**: 522.

Long SS, Mueller S, Swenson RM (1976). *In vitro* susceptibilities of anaerobic bacteria to josamycin. *Antimicrob Ag Chemother* **9**: 859.

Ludden TM (1985). Pharmacokinetic interactions of the macrolide antibiotics. *Clin Pharmacokinet* **10**: 63.

MacFarlane J, Mitchell A, Walsh J, Roverbson J (1968). Spiramycin in the prevention of postoperative staphylococcal infection. *Lancet* **i**: 1.

Martino P, Gentile G, Caprioli A *et al.* (1988). Hospital-acquired cryptosporidiosis in a bone marrow transplantation unit. *J Infect Dis* **158**: 647.

Mayaud C, Dournon E, Montagne V *et al.* (1988). Efficacy of intravenous spiramycin in the treatment of severe Legionnaires disease. *J Antimicrob Chemother* **22** (Suppl B): 179.

Mensa J, Trilla A, Moreno A *et al.* (1993). Five-day treatment of non-severe, community-acquired pneumonia with josamycin. *J Antimicrob Chemother* **31**: 749.

Mitsuhashi S (ed). (1971). *Drug Action and Drug Resistance in Bacteria*. Tokyo: University Park Press.

Modai J (1988). The clinical use of macrolides. *J Antimicrob Chemother* **22** (Suppl B): 145.

Moscato G, Naldi N, Candura F (1984). Bronchial asthma due to spiramycin and adipic acid. *Clin Allergy* **14**: 355.

Moskovitz BL, Stanton TL, Kusmierek JJE (1988). Spiramycin therapy for cryptosporidial diarrhoea in immunocompromised patients. *J Antimicrob Chemother* **22** (Suppl B): 189.

Nitta K, Yano K, Miyamoto F *et al.* (1967). A new antibiotic, josamycin. II. Biological studies. *J Antibiot* (Tokyo) **20**: 181.

Orfila J, Haider F, Thomas D (1988). Activity of spiramycin against chlamydia, *in vitro* and *in vivo*. *J Antimicrob Chemother* **22** (Suppl B): 73.

Osono T, Oka Y, Watanabe S *et al.* (1967). A new antibiotic, josamycin. I. Isolation and physicochemical characteristics. *J Antibiot* (Tokyo) **20**: 174.

Pessayre D (1983). Effects of macrolide antibiotics on drug metabolism in rats and humans. *Int J Clin Pharmacol Res* **13**: 449.

Pinnert-Sindico S, Ninet L, Preud'Homme J, Cosar C (1955). A new antibiotic: spiramycin. *Antibiotics Annual, 1954–55*:724–727..

Plummer FA, D'Costa LJ, Nsanze H *et al.* (1983). Antimicrobial therapy of chancroid: effectiveness of erythromycin. *J Infect Dis* **148**: 726.

Portnoy D, Whiteside ME, Buckley EIII, Macleod CL (1984). Treatment of intestinal cryptosporidiosis with spiramycin. *Ann Intern Med* **101**: 202.

Privitera G, Bonino S, Del Mastro S (1984). Clinical multicentre trial with josamycin propionate in pediatric patients. *Int J Clin Pharmacol Res* **4**: 201.

Raoult D, Roussellier P, Tamalet J (1988). *In vitro* evaluation of josamycin, spiramycin, and erythromycin against *Rickettsia rickettsii* and *R. conorii*. *Antimicrob Ag Chemother* **32**: 255.

Robertson JA, Coppola JE, Heisler OR (1981). Standardized method for determining antimicrobial susceptibility of strains of *Ureaplasma urealy-*

ticum and their response to tetracycline, erythromycin and rosaramicin. *Antimicrob Ag Chemother* **20**: 53.

Robson HG, Shah PP, Lalonde RG *et al.* (1983). Comparison of rosaramicin and erythromycin stearate for treatment of cervical infection with *Chlamydia trachomatis. Sex Transm Dis* **10**: 130.

Saito A, Sawatari K, Fukuda Y *et al.* (1985). Susceptibility of *Legionella pneumophila* to ofloxacin *in vitro* and in experimental Legionella pneumonia in guinea pigs. *Antimicrob Ag Chemother* **28**: 15.

Sanders CC, Sanders WEJr (1977). *In vitro* activity of rosamicin against *Neisseria* and *Haemophilus*, including penicillinase-producing strains. *Antimicrob Ag Chemother* **12**: 293.

Saroglou G, Bisno AL (1978). Susceptibility of skin and throat strains of Group A streptococci to rosamicin and erythromycin. *Antimicrob Ag Chemother* **13**: 701.

Schoondermark-Van de Ven E, Galama J, Camps W *et al.* (1994a). Pharmacokinetics of spiramycin in the rhesus monkey: transplacental passage and distribution in tissue in the fetus. *Antimicrob Ag Chemother* **38**: 1922.

Schoondermark-Van de Ven E, Melchers W, Camps W *et al.* (1994b). Effectiveness of spiramycin for treatment of congenital *Toxoplasma gondii* infection in rhesus monkeys. *Antimicrob Ag Chemother* **38**: 1930.

Segev S, Samra Z, Eliav E *et al.* (1988). The efficacy and safety of spiramycin in the treatment of nongonococcal urethritis in men. *J Antimicrob Chemother* **22** (Suppl B): 183.

Shadomy S, Tipple M, Paxton L (1976). Josamycin and rosamicin: *in vitro* comparisons with erythromycin and clindamycin. *Antimicrob Ag Chemother* **10**: 773.

Smith JA, Skidmore AG, Salit IE (1981). Rosaramicin: *in vitro* activity against common bacterial isolates. *J Antimicrob Chemother* **7**: 505.

Soave R, Armstrong D (1986). Cryptosporidium and cryptosporidosis. *Rev Infect Dis* **8**: 1012.

Stoehr GP, Juhl RP, Veals J *et al.* (1985). The excretion of rosaramicin in breast milk. *J Clin Pharmacol* **25**: 89.

Strausbaugh LJ, Dilworth JA, Gwaltney JMJr, Sande MA (1976a). *In vitro* susceptibility studies with josamycin and erythromycin. *Antimicrob Ag Chemother* **9**: 546.

Strausbaugh LJ, Bolton WK, Dilworth JA *et al.* (1976b). Comparative pharmacology of josamycin and erythromycin stearate. *Antimicrob Ag Chemother* **10**: 450.

Sutter VL, Finegold SM (1976). Rosamicin: *in vitro* activity against anaerobes and comparison with erythromycin. *Antimicrob Ag Chemother* **9**: 350.

Tofte RW, Solliday JA, Crossley KB (1984). Susceptibilities of enterococci to twelve antibiotics. *Antimicrob Ag Chemother* **25**: 532.

Wagman GH, Waitz JA, Marquez J *et al.* (1972). A new micromonospora-produced macrolide antibiotic, rosamicin. *J Antibiot* (Tokyo) **25**: 641.

Waitz JA, Drube CG, Moss ELJr, Weinstein MJ (1972). Biological studies with rosamicin, a new micromonospora-produced macrolide antibiotic. *J Antibiot* (Tokyo) **25**: 647.

Wang WL, Reller LB, Blaser MJ (1984). Comparison of antimicrobial sensitivity patterns of *Campylobacter jejuni* and *Campylobacter coli. Antimicrob Ag Chemother* **26**: 351.

Wenzel RP, Hendley JO, Dodd WK, Gwaltney JMJr (1976). Comparison of josamycin and erythromycin in the therapy of *Mycoplasma pneumoniae* pneumonia. *Antimicrob Ag Chemother* **10**: 899.

Westerman EL, Williams TWJr, Moreland N (1976). *In vitro* activity of josamycin against aerobic Gram-positive cocci and anaerobes. *Antimicrob Ag Chemother* **9**: 988.

Wilson SZ, Martin RP, Putman M (1977). *In vivo* effects of josamycin, erythromycin, and placebo therapy on nasal carriage of *Staphylococcus aureus. Antimicrob Ag Chemother* **11**: 407.

Wittenberg DF, Miller NM, Van den Ende J (1989). Spiramycin is not efffective in treating *Cryptosporidium diarrhea* in infants: results of a double-blind randomized trial. *J Infect Dis* **159**: 131.

Wong S-Y, Remington JS (1994). Toxoplasmosis in pregnancy. *Clin Infect Dis* **18**: 853.

Roxithromycin

Description

Roxithromycin is a new macrolide antibiotic; it is a chemical modification of erythromycin and it contains a 14-membered macrolide lactone ring (Kirst and Sides, 1989a). Its *in vitro* antibacterial activity is similar to erythromycin and against most erythromycin-sensitive organisms it has a similar or slightly lower activity (Pechère and Auckenthaler, 1987; Barry *et al.*, 1988). The main difference between erythromycin and roxithromycin is in pharmacokinetics; the latter produces higher serum levels and is also more slowly excreted, so that an oral dosage of 150 mg 12-hourly or 300 mg once-daily is appropriate (Nilsen, 1987; Puri and Lassman, 1987).

Sensitive Organisms

1 Gram-positive bacteria

Gram-positive cocci such as *Staphylococcus aureus*, coagulase negative staphylococci, *Streptococcus pyogenes*, Groups B, C and G streptococci, *Strep. pneumoniae*, *Strep. bovis*, *Strep. viridans* and *Enterococcus faecalis* are about as sensitive to roxithromycin than to erythromycin. Some authors have found that erythromycin is slightly more active against these pathogens than roxithromycin. There is complete cross-resistance between these drugs; erythromycin-resistant organisms are also roxithromycin-resistant (Barlam and Neu, 1984; Pechère and Auckenthaler, 1987; Barry *et al.*, 1988). Gram-positive bacilli such as *Listeria monocytogenes*, are slightly less sensitive to roxithromycin than to erythromycin (Barlam and Neu, 1984). *Nocardia asteroides* is resistant (Pechère and Auckenthaler, 1987). Among the Gram-positive anaerobic cocci, the *Peptococcus* and *Peptostreptococcus* spp. are usually roxithromycin-sensitive. *Clostridium perfringens* is usually sensitive but slightly less so than to erythromycin. Some *Cl. difficile* strains are sensitive, but others are completely resistant (Dubreuil, 1987).

2 Gram-negative bacteria

Neisseria meningitidis and *N. gonorrhoeae* are usually roxithromycin-sensitive, but erythromycin-resistant strains are also roxithromycin-resistant. *Haemophilus influenzae*, *Bordetella pertussis* and *Moraxella catarrhalis* are sensitive, but some 2- to 4-fold less so than to erythromycin. *Legionella pneumophila* and *L. micdadei* are as sensitive to roxithromycin as they are to erythromycin. The same is true for *Haemophilus ducreyi*. *Campylobacter* spp. are slightly less sensitive to roxithromycin, compared with erythromycin. *Gardnerella vaginalis* is sensitive. Similar to erythromycin, roxithromycin has no activity against the Enterobacteriaceae, *Acinetobacter* spp. and *Pseudomonas aeruginosa*. Of the Gram-negative anaerobes, only some 50% of the bacteria of the *B. fragilis* group are roxithromycin-sensitive. Other *Bacteroides* spp. are more susceptible, but most Fusobacteria are resistant (Jones *et al.*, 1983; Barlam and Neu, 1984; Dubreuil, 1987; Ridgway, 1987; Barry *et al.*, 1988; Hardy *et al.*, 1988, Kirst and Sides, 1989a; Liebers *et al.*, 1989; Kitsukawa *et al.*, 1991; Vaara, 1993).

3 Other organisms

Chlamydia trachomatis, *C. psittaci*, *Ureaplasma urealyticum*, *Mycoplasma pneumoniae* and *M. hominis* are sensitive to roxithromycin as they are to erythromycin (Pechère and Auckenthaler, 1987; Ridgway, 1987). Roxithromycin appears effective in experimental *Treponema pallidum* infections in rabbits (Lukehart and Baker-Zander, 1987). *Rickettsia rickettsii* and *R. conorii* are

Organism	MIC (μg per ml)	
	Erythromycin	Roxithromycin
Gram-positive organisms		
Staphylococcus aureus	0.8	0.8
Streptococcus pyogenes	0.8	1.6
Streptococcus Group B	0.4	0.8
Streptococcus pneumoniae	<0.1	0.2
Enterococcus faecalis	1.6	6.3
Listeria monocytogenes	0.5	1.0
Gram-negative bacteria		
Haemophilus influenzae	4.0	8.0
Moraxella catarrhalis	0.25	1.0
Campylobacter jejuni	1.0	4.0
Legionella pneumophila	2.0	0.5
Bordetella pertussis	0.03	0.25

Table I.47
Compiled from data published by Barlam and Neu (1984), *Barry et al.* (1988) and Hardy *et al.* (1988)

susceptible to roxithromycin (Drancourt and Raoult, 1989). Roxithromycin has significant *in vitro* activity against a variety of atypical mycobacteria such as *Mycobacterium scrofulaceum, M. szulgai, M. malmoense, M. xenopi, M. marinum, M. kansasii, M. chelonae* and *M. fortuitum*. It is also active against the *M. avium* complex *in vitro* and in mice *in vivo*. Against this organism the activity of roxithromycin is enhanced if it is used together with ethambutol (p. 1211) and a third drug such as rifampicin, amikacin, ofloxacin, or rifabutin (Bermudez and Young, 1988; Rastogi *et al.*, 1993, 1994, 1995a; Struillou *et al.*, 1995). However, *M. tuberculosis* is roxithromycin-resistant (Rastogi *et al.*, 1995b).

Roxithromycin is active against *M. leprae* infections in mouse footpads, but clarithromycin (p. 645) shows superior activity (Franzblau and Hastings, 1988; Gelber *et al.*, 1991). *Toxoplasma gondii* infections in mice were successfully treated by roxithromycin, but the drug often did not eradicate the organisms from the brain (Chang and Pechère, 1987). Also *in vitro* studies showed that roxithromycin had activity against this parasite, but high concentrations of the drug were needed to have a killing effect on *T. gondii* (Chang and Pechère, 1988). In a murine model of toxoplasmic encephalitis roxithromycin was synergistic with gamma interferon (Hofflin and Remington, 1987). In animal studies roxithromycin alone was also relatively ineffective for toxoplasmosis, but its efficacy was improved if it was combined with either sulfadiazine or pyrimethamine (Romand *et al.*, 1995).

4 Minimum inhibitory concentrations

The MICs of roxithromycin, compared with those of erythromycin for some selected bacterial species are shown in Table I.47.

Mode of Administration and Dosage

Roxithromycin can only be administered by the oral route.

1 Adults

The usual dosage of roxithromycin is 300 mg orally daily. Commonly 150 mg 12-hourly is given (Puri and Lassman, 1987; Paulsen *et al.*, 1992; Cooper *et al.*, 1994).

2 Children

The dosage for these is 2.5–5 mg per kg, administered 12-hourly (Kafetzis and Blanc, 1987; Stenberg and Mårdh, 1991).

3 Patients with renal failure

The terminal elimination half-life of the drug in one study was significantly prolonged in patients with severe renal failure (15.5 h) compared with that in patients with normal renal function (7.9 h). It was suggested that in patients with severe renal failure the dosage interval between individual roxithromycin doses should be doubled (Halstenson et al., 1990). Very little roxithromycin is eliminated by continuous ambulatory peritoneal dialysis (Lam et al., 1995).

4 Patients with liver disease

In patients with alcoholic cirrhosis, the increase in renal clearance of roxithromycin offsets the reduction of hepatic clearance, and no dosage modification is necessary in most patients (Periti and Mazzei, 1987).

Serum Levels in Relation to Dosage

When 150 mg of roxithromycin was given to normal adults every 12 h for 3 days, the mean peak levels (attained 1.5 h after the dose) increased from 4.4 μg per ml on day 1 to 5.9 μg per ml on day 2 and 7.4 μg per ml on day 3 (Wise et al., 1987). Steady-state serum levels were usually reached by day 4. The minimum plasma concentrations of roxithromycin at steady-state (days 4–11) ranged from 3.22 to 3.69 μg per ml. The maximal serum level during this time was about 9.3 μg per ml. The drug is eliminated with a half-life of about 10 h. Doubling the dose increases, but does not double the peak serum level. The absorption of roxithromycin is not impaired by concomitant administration of milk or food (Puri and Lassman, 1987; Kirst and Sides, 1989b).

Excretion

1 Urine

Only about 10% of the administered dose of roxithromycin is excreted in urine in the active unchanged form, but small amounts of three metabolites are also excreted via the kidney (Puri and Lassman, 1987; Wise et al., 1987).

2 Pulmonary

Some 10–20% of the administered dose is eliminated in expired air (Puri and Lassman, 1987; Wise et al., 1987).

3 Feces

Some 54% of an administered dose of roxithromycin is eliminated in the feces; some of this is excreted via the bile and some represents unabsorbed drug. Roxithromycin is not extensively metabolized in the liver, but about 30% of the drug eliminated in the feces consists of inactive metabolites (Periti and Mazzei, 1987; Puri and Lassman, 1987).

Distribution of the Drug in Body

Roxithromycin penetrates well into blister fluid; in one study the mean percent penetration was 85% (Wise et al., 1987). After oral dosing a very high concentration was achieved in pulmonary, prostatic, tonsillar and skin tissue and in epidydimis. However, roxithromycin was not detected in the CSF of subjects with non-inflamed meninges (Chastre et al., 1987; Puri and Lassman, 1987; Campa et al., 1990; Costa et al., 1992). Less than 0.05% of a single 300-mg dose is excreted in the breast milk of lactating women (Puri and Lassman, 1987). Roxithromycin is concentrated in human monocytes (Hand and King-Thompson, 1989). The drug is also concentrated in neutrophils and macrophages (Labro et al., 1989) and it stimulates human neutrophil migration in vitro (Anderson, 1989).

The drug is 86–91% serum protein bound when serum concentration is 10 μg per ml (Wise et al., 1987). The free serum fraction of roxithromycin increases with increasing serum levels (Puri and Lassman, 1987).

Mode of Action

This is similar for all macrolide antibiotics (see erythromycin, p. 614). Similar to erythromycin, roxithromycin appears to have actions in body other than just antibacterial activity. It may prevent tissue damage in Ps. aeruginosa infections (Ras et al., 1992). Animal experiments suggest that after prolonged treatment roxithromycin may not only enhance the host defence system through increased cytokine synthesis by host cells, but also exhibit an anti-inflammatory activity (Kita et al., 1993).

Toxicity

Roxithromycin therapy has caused vomiting in a few children (Kafetzis and Blanc, 1987). In adults the gastrointestinal tolerance of roxithromycin compares favorably with that of doxycycline and erythromycin ethylsuccinate. Mild abnormalities of liver function tests have been noted in 1.9% of treated patients. Other side-effects such as allergic rashes or *Candida* overgrowth have been rare (Blanc *et al.*, 1987; Peterslund *et al.*, 1989; Paulsen *et al.*, 1992).

Although roxithromycin is a 14-membered lactone ring macrolide, it has been reported that, unlike erythromycin (p. 616), it does not interfere with the metabolism of theophylline and carbamazepine (Saint-Salvi *et al.*, 1987). The effect of roxithromycin on the human fecal flora is relatively weak. The main effect is a decrease in Enterobacteriaceae (Pecquet *et al.*, 1991).

Clinical Uses of the Drug

1 Community-acquired respiratory infections

Roxithromycin has been effective in the treatment of sinusitis, otitis media, bronchitis and pneumonia, caused by pathogens such as *Strep. pyogenes*, *Strep. pneumoniae*, *H. influenzae*, *M. catarrhalis*, *Mycoplasma pneumoniae* and *Chlamydia psittaci*. It has performed quite well in proven *H. influenzae* bronchitis and pneumonia and it appears that the relatively low *in vitro* activity against this organism is well compensated by the higher serum and tissue levels of roxithromycin, compared with erythromycin (Gentry, 1987; Kirst and Sides, 1989b; Peterslund *et al.*, 1989; Paulsen *et al.*, 1992; Cooper *et al.*, 1994). However, roxithromycin is not as good as erythromycin for streptococcal pharyngitis (Melcher *et al.*, 1988).

2 Chlamydia trachomatis and Ureaplasma urealyticum infections

In animal experiments roxithromycin was effective for treatment of *C. trachomatis* salpingitis, but fertility was not always preserved (Zana *et al.*, 1991). In treatment of non-gonococcal urethritis in males, roxithromycin in a dosage of 150 mg 12-hourly eradicated 97% of *C. trachomatis* infections, 88% of *Ureaplasma urealyticum* and 73% of those due to *M. homini* (Lassus and Seppala, 1987). Chlamydial conjunctivitis in newborns and adults has also been treated with some success with oral roxithromycin (Stenberg and Mårdh, 1991).

3 Legionella pneumonia

Roxithromycin was effective for the treatment of induced Legionnaires' disease in guinea pigs (Fitzgeorge and Featherstone, 1989).

4 Chemoprophylaxis in neutropenic patients

In a prospective, randomized, open trial, the efficacy of oral roxithromycin (150 mg 12-hourly) as additional chemoprophylaxis to ofloxacin was evaluated in 131 adult patients with acute leukemia or bone marrow transplant recipients. In comparison with patients given ofloxacin alone, fewer patients receiving both drugs developed bacteremia caused by *Strep. viridans*. The authors considered that routine use of roxithromycin prophylaxis was not justified, but that it may be valuable in areas where there is a high risk of streptococcal infections (Kern *et al.*, 1994). Other authors have also used a quinolone such as ciprofloxacin plus roxithromycin as chemoprophylaxis in neutropenic patients with some success (Verhoef, 1993).

5 Prophylaxis against experimental pneumocystosis and toxoplasmosis

In one study corticosteroid-treated rats naturally infected by *Pneumocystis carinii* were challenged with a strain of *T. gondii*. In rats that received co-trimoxazole or pyramethamine plus dapsone, *T. gondii* was eradicated and *P. carinii* pneumonia prevented. In contrast, roxithromycin provided significant protection only against *T. gondii* infection (Brun-Pascaud *et al.*, 1994).

6 Isospora belli infection

This infection is normally self-limiting but it causes a chronic debilitating diarrhea in HIV-positive immunodeficient patients. This infection is usually treated by co-trimoxazole (p. 870), but Musey *et al.* (1988) treated one AIDS patient with this infection using roxithromycin 2.5 mg per kg 12-hourly. He had previously failed to respond to co-trimoxazole. This patient responded well to roxithromycin and stool cultures after treatment were negative.

References

Anderson R (1989). Erythromycin and roxithromycin potentiate human neutrophil locomotion *in vitro* by inhibition of leukoattractant-activated superoxide generation and autooxidation. *J Infect Dis* **159**: 966.

Barlam T, Neu HC (1984). *In vitro* comparison of the activity of RU 28965, a new macrolide, with that of erythromycin against aerobic and anaerobic bacteria. *Antimicrob Ag Chemother* **25**: 529.

Barry AL, Jones RN, Thornsberry C (1988). *In vitro* activities of azithromycin (CP 62,993). clarithromycin (A-56268; TE-031). erythromycin, roxithromycin and clindamycin. *Antimicrob Ag Chemother* **32**: 752.

Bermudez LEM, Young LS (1988). Activities of amikacin, roxithromycin, and azithromycin alone or in combination with tumor necrosis factor against *Mycobacterium avium* complex. *Antimicrob Ag Chemother* **32**: 1149.

Blanc F, D'Enfert J, Fiessinger S *et al.* (1987). An evaluation of tolerance of roxithromycin in adults. *J Antimicrob Chemother* **20** (Suppl B): 179.

Brun-Pascaud M, Chau F, Simonpoli A-M *et al.* (1994). Experimental evaluation of combined prophylaxis against murine pneumocystosis and toxoplasmosis. *J Infect Dis* **170**: 653.

Campa M, Zolfino I, Senesi S *et al.* (1990). The penetration of roxithromycin into human skin. *J Antimicrob Chemother* **26**: 87.

Chang HR, Pechère J-CF (1987). Effect of roxithromycin on acute toxoplasmosis in mice. *Antimicrob Ag Chemother* **31**: 1147.

Chang HR, Pechère J-CF (1988). *In vitro* effects of four macrolides (roxithromycin, spiramycin, azithromycin (CP-62,993). and A-56268 on *Toxoplasma gondii*. *Antimicrob Ag Chemother* **32**: 524.

Chastre J, Brun P, Fourtillan JB *et al.* (1987). Pulmonary disposition of roxithromycin (RU 28965). a new macrolide antibiotic. *Antimicrob Ag Chemother* **31**: 1312.

Cooper BC, Mullins PR, Jones MR, Lang SDR (1994). Clinical efficacy of roxithromycin in the treatment of adults with upper and lower respiratory tract infection due to *Haemophilus influenzae*. A meta-analysis of 12 clinical studies. *Drug Invest* **7**: 299.

Costa P, d'Arramon FD, Gouby A *et al.* (1992). Disposition of roxithromycin in the epididymis after repeated oral administration. *J Antimicrob Chemother* **30**: 197.

Drancourt M, Raoult D (1989). *In vitro* susceptibilities of *Rickettsia rickettsii* and *Rickettsia conorii* to roxithromycin and pristinamycin. *Antimicrob Ag Chemother* **33**: 2146.

Dubreuil L (1987). *In-vitro* comparison of roxithromycin and erythromycin against 900 anaerobic bacterial strains. *J Antimicrob Chemother* **20** (Suppl B): 13.

Fitzgeorge RB, Featherstone ASR (1989). Roxithromycin therapy in experimental airborne Legionnaires' disease. *J Antimicrob Chemother* **23**: 462.

Franzblau SG, Hastings RC (1988). *In vitro* and *in vivo* activities of macrolides against *Mycobacterium leprae*. *Antimicrob Ag Chemother* **32**: 1758.

Gelber RH, Siu P, Tsang M, Murray LP (1991). Activities of various macrolide antibiotics against *Mycobacterium leprae* infection in mice. *Antimicrob Ag Chemother* **35**: 760.

Gentry LO (1987). Roxithromycin, a new macrolide antibiotic, in the treatment of infections in the lower respiratory tract: an overview. *J Antimicrob Chemother* **20** (Suppl B): 145.

Halstenson CE, Opsahl JA, Schwenk MH *et al.* (1990). Disposition of roxithromycin in patients with normal and severely impaired renal function. *Antimicrob Ag Chemother* **34**: 385.

Hand WL, King-Thompson NL (1989). The entry of antibiotics into human monocytes. *J Antimicrob Chemother* **23**: 681.

Hardy DJ, Hensey DM, Bejer JM *et al.* (1988). Comparative *in vitro* activities of new 14-, 15-, and 16-membered macrolides. *Antimicrob Ag Chemother* **32**: 1710.

Hofflin JM, Remington JS (1987). *In vivo* synergism of roxithromycin (RU 965). and interferon against *Toxoplasma gondii*. *Antimicrob Ag Chemother* **31**: 346.

Jones RN, Barry AL, Thornsberry C (1983). *In vitro* evaluation of three new macrolide antimicrobial agents, RU 28965, RU 29065, and RU 29702, and comparisons with other orally administered drugs. *Antimicrob Ag Chemother* **24**: 209.

Kafetzis DA, Blanc F (1987). Efficacy and safety of roxithromycin in treating paediatric patients. A European multicentre study. *J Antimicrob Chemother* **20** (Suppl B): 171.

Kern WV, Hay B, Kern P *et al.* (1994). A randomized trial of roxithromycin in patients with acute leukemia and bone marrow transplant recipients receiving fluoroquinolone prophylaxis. *Antimicrob Ag Chemother* **38**: 465.

Kirst HA, Sides GD (1989a). New direction for macrolide antibiotics: structural modifications and *in vitro* activity. *Antimicrob Ag Chemother* **33**: 1413.

Kirst HA, Sides GD (1989b). New directions for macrolide antibiotics: pharmacokinetics and clinical efficacy. *Antimicrob Ag Chemother* **33**: 1419.

Kita E, Sawaki M, Mikasa K *et al.* (1993). Alterations of host response by a long-term treatment of roxithromycin. *J Antimicrob Chemother* **32**: 285.

Kitsukawa K, Hara J, Saito A (1991). Inhibition of *Legionella pneumophila* in guinea pig peritoneal macrophages by new quinolone, macrolide and other antimicrobial agents. *J Antimicrob Chemother* **27**: 343.

Labro MT, El Benna J, Babin-Chevaye C (1989). Comparison of the *in-vitro* effect of several macrolides on the oxidative burst of human neutrophils. *J Antimicrob Chemother* **24**: 561.

Lam YWF, Flaherty JF, Yumena L *et al.* (1995). Roxithromycin disposition in patients on continuous ambulatory peritoneal dialysis. *J Antimicrob Chemother* **36**: 157.

Lassus A, Seppala A (1987). Roxithromycin in nongonococcal urethritis. *J Antimicrob Chemother* **20** (Suppl B): 157.

Liebers DM, Baltch AL, Smith RP *et al.* (1989). Susceptibility of *Legionella pneumophila* to eight antimicrobial agents including four macrolides under different assay conditions. *J Antimicrob Chemother* **23**: 37.

Lukehart SA, Baker-Zander SA (1987). Roxithromycin (RU 965).: effective therapy for experimental syphilis infection in rabbits. *Antimicrob Ag Chemother* **31**: 187.

Melcher GP, Hadfield TL, Gaines JK, Winn RE (1988). Comparative efficacy and toxicity of roxithromycin and erythromycin ethylsuccinate in the treatment of streptococcal pharyngitis in adults. *J Antimicrob Chemother* **22**: 549.

Musey KL, Chidiac C, Beaucaire G *et al.* (1988). Effectiveness of roxithromycin for treating *Isospora belli* infection. *J Infect Dis* **158**: 646.

Nilsen OG (1987). Comparative pharmacokinetics of macrolides. *J Antimicrob Chemother* **20** (Suppl B): 81.

Paulsen O, Christensson BA, Hebelka M *et al.* (1992). Efficacy and tolerance of roxithromycin in comparison with erythromycin stearate in patients with lower respiratory tract infections. *Scand J Infect Dis* **24**: 219.

Pechère J-C, Auckenthaler R (1987). *In-vitro* activity of roxithromycin against respiratory and skin pathogens. *J Antimicrob Chemother* **20** (SupplB): 1.

Pecquet S, Chachaty E, Tancréde C, Andremont A (1991). Effects of roxithromycin on fecal bacteria in human volunteers and resistance to colonization in gnotobiotic mice. *Antimicrob Ag Chemother* **35**: 548.

Periti P, Mazzei T (1987). Pharmacokinetics of roxithromycin in renal and hepatic failure and drug interactions. *J Antimicrob Chemother* **20** (Suppl B): 107.

Peterslund NA, Hönninen P, Schreiner A *et al.* (1989). Roxithromycin in the treatment of pneumonia. *J Antimicrob Chemother* **23**: 737.

Puri SK, Lassman HB (1987). Roxithromycin: a pharmacokinetic review of a macrolide. *J Antimicrob Chemother* **20** (Suppl B): 89.

Ras GJ, Anderson R, Taylor GW *et al.* (1992). Clindamycin, erythromycin, and roxithromycin inhibit the proinflammatory interactions of *Pseudomo-*

nas aeruginosa pigments with human neutrophils *in vitro*. *Antimicrob Ag Chemother* **36**: 1236.

Rastogi N, Goh KS, Bryskier A (1993). *In vitro* activity of roxithromycin against 16 species of atypical mycobacteria and effect of pH on its radiometric MICs. *Antimicrob Ag Chemother* **37**: 1560.

Rastogi N, Goh KS, Bryskier A (1994). Activities of roxithromycin used alone and in combination with ethambutol, rifampin, amikacin, ofloxacin and clofazimine against *Mycobacterium avium* complex. *Antimicrob Ag Chemother* **38**: 1433.

Rastogi N, Labrousse V, Bryskier A (1995a). Intracellular activities of roxithromycin used alone and in association with other drugs against *Mycobacterium avium* complex in human macrophages. *Antimicrob Ag Chemother* **39**: 976.

Rastogi N, Goh KS, Ruiz P, Casal M (1995b). *In vitro* activity of roxithromycin against the *Mycobacterium tuberculosis* complex. *Antimicrob Ag Chemother* **39**: 1162.

Ridgway GL (1987). A review of the *in-vitro* activity of roxithromycin against genital pathogens. *J Antimicrob Chemother* **20** (Suppl B): 7.

Romand S, Bryskier A, Moutot M, Derouin F (1995). *In-vitro* and *in-vivo* activities of roxithromycin in combination with pyrimethamine or sulphadiazine against *Toxoplasma gondii*. *J Antimicrob Chemother* **35**: 821.

Saint-Salvi B, Tremblay D, Surjus A, Lefebvre MA (1987). A study of the interaction of roxithromycin with theophylline and carbamazepine. *J Antimicrob Chemother* **20** (Suppl B): 121.

Stenberg K, Mårdh P-A (1991). Treatment of chlamydial conjunctivitis in newborns and adults with erythromycin and roxithromycin. *J Antimicrob Chemother* **28**: 301.

Struillou L, Cohen Y, Lounis N *et al.* (1995). Activities of roxithromycin against *Mycobacterium avium* infections in human macrophages and C57BL/6 mice. *Antimicrob Ag Chemother* **39**: 878.

Vaara M (1993). Outer membrane permeability barrier to azithromycin, clarithromycin, and roxithromycin in Gram-negative enteric bacteria. *Antimicrob Ag Chemother* **37**: 354.

Verhoef J (1993). Prevention of infections in the neutropenic patients. *Clin Infect Dis* **17** (Suppl 2): 359.

Wise R, Kirkpatrick B, Ashby J, Andrews JM (1987). Pharmacokinetics and tissue penetration of roxithromycin after multiple dosing. *Antimicrob Ag Chemother* **31**: 1051.

Zana J, Muffat-Joly M, Thomas D *et al.* (1991). Roxithromycin treatment of mouse chlamydial salpingitis and protective effect on fertility. *Antimicrob Ag Chemother* **35**: 430.

Clarithromycin

Description

Clarithromycin (6–0-methyl erythromycin) is a new 14-membered macrolide, chemically related to erythromycin (Vallée *et al.*, 1991). Its *in vitro* activity against most aerobic microorganisms is equal to or twice that of erythromycin, except for *Haemophilus influenzae* for which it is half as active (Fernandes *et al.*, 1986; Hardy *et al.*, 1988a).

In man, clarithromycin has four metabolites, the most important of which is 14-hydroxy clarithromycin which is twice as active as the parent compound against *H. influenzae*. Furthermore, clarithromycin and its metabolite act synergistically against *H. influenzae*, so that the activity of the combination is further enhanced (Hardy *et al.*, 1990; Dabernat *et al.*, 1991).

Clarithromycin has proved clinically useful for infections similar to those for which erythromycin (p. 616) is used, but it is superior to erythromycin pharmacologically (Neu, 1991). In addition it has proved to be an active agent for treatment of *Mycobacterium avium* complex infection in AIDS patients (Lane *et al.*, 1994).

Sensitive Organisms

1 Gram-positive bacteria

Staphylococcus aureus, including beta-lactamase-producing strains, are sensitive to clarithromycin and its 14-hydroxy metabolite, but methicillin-resistant strains are usually resistant. The same is true for coagulase-negative staphylococci. Group A hemolytic streptococci, and streptococci of Groups B, C and G are similarly sensitive to both. *Streptococcus pneumoniae* and *Strep. viridans* are also susceptible. Similar to erythromycin (p. 606) *Enterococcus faecalis* is less sensitive to clarithromycin. In general most of these organisms are about twice as sensitive to clarithromycin as to erythromycin, and they are about equally sensitive to the metabolite and erythromycin (Barry *et al.*, 1987; Benson *et al.*, 1987; Eliopoulos *et al.*, 1987; Floyd-Reising *et al.*, 1987; Neu, 1991; Goldstein and Citron, 1993; Hardy, 1993). These bacteria can become resistant to clarithromycin and erythromycin and the most common mechanism is methylase production (which can be constitutive or induced), which is responsible for methylating the ribosome binding site of macrolides, lincosamides and streptogramin B (MLS resistance) (p. 587). Therefore there is usually complete cross-resistance between clarithromycin and erythromycin (Fernandes *et al.*, 1989a, Fass, 1993). In two studies in the USA 5% of *Strep. pneumoniae* isolates were clarithromycin-resistant (Lonks and Medeiros, 1993; Barry *et al.*, 1994). In the latter survey only 71% of 58 penicillin G-resistant *Strep. pneumoniae* isolates were erythromycin- and clarithromycin-susceptible. *Stomatococcus mucilaginosus* and the *Micrococcus* spp. are more sensitive to clarithromycin, compared with erythromycin (Von Eiff *et al.*, 1995).

Clarithromycin is also active against *Listeria* monocytogenes and *Corynebacterium* spp. *Corynebacterium jeikeium* is resistant (Benson *et al.*, 1987; Hardy *et al.*, 1988a; Bauer and Hof, 1992; Goldstein and Citron, 1993).

The anaerobic Gram-positive cocci such as *Peptostreptococcus* spp. are usually moderately clarithromycin-sensitive. The same is true for *Clostridium* spp. and *Propionibacterium acnes* (Fernandes *et al.*, 1986; Fass, 1993; Goldstein and Citron, 1993).

2 Gram-negative bacteria

Neisseria meningitidis and *N. gonorrhoeae* (unless erythromycin-resistant) are clarithromycin-sensitive (Barry *et al.*, 1987; Eliopoulos *et al.*, 1987). The same is true for *Bordetella pertussis* and *B. parapertussis* (Hardy, 1993). *Haemophilus influenzae* is only moderately sensitive to clarithromycin (MICs 2–8 μg per ml), but its metabolite 14-hydroxy-clarithromycin is more active against this pathogen (MICs 1–4 μg per ml), The combination of the drug with its metabolite is bactericidal and synergistic against *H. influenzae*. This has been confirmed in a mouse model of *H. influenzae* infection and in human volunteers (Dabernat *et al.*, 1991; Jorgensen *et al.*, 1991; Walker *et al.*, 1994). Also *H. parainfluenzae* is moderately sensitive (Benson *et al.*, 1987), but *H. ducreyi* is very sensitive (MICs 0.002–0.06 μg per ml) (Dangor *et al.*, 1988).

Clarithromycin is also active against *Moraxella catarrhalis*, *Pasteurella multocida* and *Campylobacter jejuni* (Eliopoulos *et al.*, 1987; Endtz *et al.*, 1993; Fass, 1993). One report described the *in vivo* development of clarithromycin-resistance in a strain of *C. jejuni* during treatment with this drug of an AIDS patient with *C. jejuni* diarrhea (Funke *et al.*, 1994). Most strains of *C. coli* and *C. fetus* are also sensitive (Sánchez *et al.*, 1994). Clarithromycin is quite active against *Helicobacter pylori in vitro* (Hardy *et al.*, 1988b). *Legionella pneumophila* is more sensitive to clarithromycin, compared with erythromycin (Eliopoulos *et al.*, 1987; Liebers *et al.*, 1988; Reda *et al.*, 1994). The inhibitory activity of clarithromycin against Legionella spp. is enhanced by its 14-hydroxy metabolite, and the drug and its metabolite are also active against other *Legionella* spp., such as *L. bozemanii*, *L. dumoffii*, *L. gormanii*, *L. jordanis*, *L. longbeachae* and *L. micdadei* (Jones *et al.*, 1990). *Vibrio* spp. are also moderately sensitive to clarithromycin (Benson *et al.*, 1987; Yamamoto *et al.*, 1995).

The Enterobacteriaceae and *Pseudomonas aeruginosa* are clarithromycin-resistant (Benson *et al.*, 1987; Chin *et al.*, 1987).

Some Gram-negative anaerobes such as *Prevotella melaninogenica* may be moderately clarithromycin-sensitive, but *Bacteroides fragilis*, other members of the *B. fragilis* group and *Fusobacterium* spp. are usually resistant (Chin *et al.*, 1987; Hardy *et al.*, 1988a; Fass, 1993; Spangler *et al.*, 1994, 1995).

3 Mycobacteria

Clarithromycin has some activity against *M. tuberculosis* (MIC 1.3–10 μg per ml); it is more active than erythromycin, but less active than fluoroquinolones such as ciprofloxacin (p. 985) (Gorzynski *et al.*, 1989). One study showed that strains of *M. tuberculosis* resistant to isoniazid, rifampicin or ethambutol became sensitive to these drugs if their sensitivity was tested in the presence of clarithromycin in a concentration of 2.0 μg per ml plus its metabolite 14-hydroxy-clarithromycin in a concentration of 0.5 μg per ml. The clinical significance of this is not yet known (Cavalieri *et al.*, 1995).

Clarithromycin is more active against *M. paratuberculosis* (MIC 0.25 μg per ml) (Rastogi *et al.*, 1992). The drug is quite active against *M. fortuitum*, *M. chelonae* and *M. chelonae*-like organisms (Brown *et al.*, 1992a); *M. marinum* is also sensitive (Forsgren, 1993). The slowly growing mycobacteria such as *M. gordonae*, *M. scrofulaceum*, *M. szelgai* and *M. kansasii* are also susceptible. Also *M. haemophilum* is sensitive, but *M. simiae* is relatively resistant (Biehle and Cavalieri, 1992; Brown *et al.*, 1992b; Bernard *et al.*, 1993; Valero *et al.*, 1994; Sanders *et al.*, 1995).

Of special interest is the activity of clarithromycin against the *Mycobacterium avium* complex both *in vitro* and *in vivo* . The usual MIC has been accepted as 4 μg per ml, but depending on the method used, lower and higher MICs have been reported by various authors. When clarithromycin was combined with either ethambutol, rifampicin or both, the combinations showed increased bactericidal activity against this organism (Fernandes *et al.*, 1989b; Naik and Ruck, 1989; Rastogi and Labrousse, 1991; Truffot-Pernot *et al.*, 1991; Heifets *et al.*, 1992; Gevaudan *et al.*, 1993; Rastogi *et al.*, 1995).

Clarithromycin was also active against *M. avium* growing inside macrophages obtained from mice and also against this organism growing inside alveolar macrophages obtained from HIV-infected humans. The clarithromycin metabolite, 14-OH clarithromycin was also active against this organism growing inside macrophages (Perronne *et al.*, 1990; Cohen *et al.*, 1992; Yajko *et al.*, 1992; Mor and Heifets, 1993a,b; Mor *et al.*, 1994). Liposome encapsulated clarithromycin appeared more active against *M. avium* growing in human macrophages (Onyeji *et al.*, 1994). Clarithromycin was also effective *in vivo* in mice models infected with *M. avium*. The addition of amikacin prevented the emergence of clarithromycin-resistant mutants and rifabutin (p. 709), a new rifamycin KRM 1648 , or ethambutol (p. 1211) were synergistic with clarithromycin in the mouse model (Klemens *et al.*, 1992; Bermudez *et al.*, 1994; Cynamon *et al.*, 1994; Ji *et al.*, 1994;

Furney *et al.*, 1995; Lounis *et al.*, 1995). Also in AIDS patients treated by clarithromycin alone for *M. avium* bacteremia, blood cultures became negative in 6 weeks (Dautzenberg *et al.*, 1991; Heifets *et al.*, 1993; Lane *et al.*, 1994). However, if clarithromycin was used alone in humans for longer periods, the *M. avium* strains became clarithromycin-resistant and they showed cross-resistance to azithromycin (Heifets *et al.*, 1993), other macrolides and related drugs such as clindamycin and streptogramins (Doucet-Populaire *et al.*, 1995). The same thing happened if *M. avium* infected mice were treated for prolonged periods with clarithromycin monotherapy (Ji *et al.*, 1992). The resistance mechanism is of the MLS type which also operates in Gram-positive bacteria (p. 587) (Meier *et al.*, 1994). Therefore, although clarithromycin is a useful drug for treatment of *M. avium* infections in AIDS patients (p. 648), it cannot be used alone, but should be combined with at least two other effective drugs.

Clarithromycin is also rapidly bactericidal against *Mycobacterium leprae* growing in mouse foot pads (Gelber *et al.*, 1991) and in humans with lepromatous leprosy (Ji *et al.*, 1993).

4 Other organisms

Clarithromycin is active, and more so than erythromycin, against *Chlamydia trachomatis* (Segreti *et al.*, 1987). *Chlamydia pneumoniae* is also susceptible (Chirgwin *et al.*, 1989; Hammerschlag, 1994; Roblin *et al.*, 1994). Clarithromycin is effective against *Mycoplasma pneumoniae*, but not *M. hominis*. *Ureaplasma urealyticum* is also usually sensitive but resistant strains occur (Waites *et al.*, 1988). The drug is effective in treating active *Treponema pallidum* infections in hamsters (Alder *et al.*, 1993a). Clarithromycin and its metabolite had a superior antimicrobial activity compared with doxycycline (p. 726) against *Borrelia burgdorferi* (Levin *et al.*, 1993). Clarithromycin is active *in vitro* against *Rickettsia rickettsii*, *R. conorii*, *R. israeli* and *Coxiella burnetii* (Maurin and Raoult, 1993).

Clarithromycin has some *in vivo* activity against *T. gondii* infections in mice (Chang *et al.*, 1988) and this activity is improved if clarithromycin is combined with minocycline (Araujo *et al.*, 1992; Derouin *et al.*, 1992).

5 Minimum inhibitory concentrations

The MICs of clarithromycin, compared with those of erythromycin, are shown in Table I.48.

Organism	MIC (µg per ml)	
	Erythromycin	Clarithromycin
Gram-positive bacteria		
Staphylococcus aureus	0.5	0.25
Streptococcus pneumoniae	0.12	0.06
Streptococcus pyogenes	0.25	0.12
Listeria monocytogenes	0.25	0.5
Gram-negative bacteria		
Haemophilus influenzae	2.0–4.0	2.0–8.0
Moraxella catarrhalis	0.5	0.25
Legionella pneumophila	1.0	0.25
Campylobacter jejuni	2.0	8.0
Other organisms		
Chlamydia trachomatis	0.06	0.008
Chlamydia pneumoniae	0.08–0.1	0.015–0.03
Coxiella burnetii	0.5	0.5
Rickettsia rickettsii	8.0	2.0

Table I.48
Compiled from data published by Fernandes *et al.* (1986), Barry *et al.* (1987), Benson *et al.* (1987), Segreti *et al.* (1987), Maurin and Raoult (1993) and Hammerschlag (1994)

Mode of Administration and Dosage

1 Adults

The usual dosage of clarithromycin, used for milder infections such as those of the respiratory tract is 250 mg orally 12-hourly (Bachand, 1991; Wettengel *et al.*, 1993). For infections due to atypical mycobacteria such as *M. chelonae* an adult dose of 500 mg 12-hourly is usual (Zahid *et al.*, 1994). For treatment of *Mycobacterium avium* complex infections in AIDS patients, when clarithromycin was used as a single drug in clinical trials, a dose of 1.0 g 12-hourly was often used, but 500 mg 12-hourly is sufficient when clarithromycin is used as one of the drugs in a three- or four-drug regimen for the treatment of this disease (Benson and Ellner, 1993; Benson, 1994). As the concomitant administration of rifampicin or rifabutin reduces the serum levels of clarithromycin (see below), the dose of the latter may need to be increased when these drugs are used together, but such increase of the dosage of clarithromycin is often poorly tolerated (p. 647).

2 Children

The usual dose, used for respiratory tract infections, is 7.5 mg per kg twice-daily (Still *et al.*, 1993; Hammerschlag, 1994).

3 Patients with renal failure and liver disease

A dose reduction of clarithromycin is recommended for patients with creatinine clearance rates of <30 ml per min. Dosage adjustment is not necessary for patients with impaired hepatic function (Rodvold and Piscitelli, 1993).

Serum Levels in Relation to Dosage

Clarithromycin is acid-stable and is well absorbed after oral administration. After absorption approximately half of the absorbed dose is converted in the body to active metabolite 14-hydroxy-clarithromycin. After single doses of 250 mg and 500 mg, the peak serum levels are 0.78 µg per ml and 2.12 µg per ml, respectively, and these levels are attained in 2–3 h. The peak serum level of the active metabolite is 0.65 µg per ml after a clarithromycin dose of 250 mg and 1.0 µg per ml after a dose of 500 mg. For investigational use i.v. clarithromycin lactobionate is available. When this compound in a dose of 250 mg is given i.v. over 45 min, a maximum serum concentration of clarithromycin, attained immediately after the infusion is 2.78 µg per ml and the peak metabolite level is only 0.45 µg per ml, attained in 2 h. The half-life after oral clarithromycin with a 250-mg oral dose is 2.7 h and that of the metabolite is 4.9 h. The half-life after i.v. clarithromycin in the same dose is 2.8 h and that of the metabolite 5.1 h. The areas-under-the-curve of clarithromycin plus metabolite after oral and i.v. administration are approximately the same and the fraction of the oral drug absorbed is about 89%. The presence of food in stomach increases the bioavailability of the drug. The pharmacokinetics of clarithromycin is not linear and the peak serum level of the drug itself increases to more than double after doubling the dose. This is due to saturation of the metabolic pathway for the production of the metabolite (Chu *et al.*, 1992a,b; Rodvold and Piscitelli, 1993). There is some accumulation of clarithromycin in the serum with repeated doses of 250 mg 12-hourly, but steady-state is reached after the fifth dose and the peak serum concentration of the drug itself then is approximately 1.0 µg per ml (Guay and Craft, 1993). Concomitant administration of rifabutin significantly reduces clarithromycin serum levels due to hepatic enzyme induction. This effect is even more marked with rifampicin (Havlir, 1994; Wallace *et al.*, 1995). Conversely, clarithromycin increases rifabutin serum levels (p. 710). Clarithromycin does not alter the bioavailability of zidovudine, provided it is given 2 h before or after the administration of the latter (Vance *et al.*, 1995).

In children, after a 7.5 mg per kg dose of clarithromycin suspension the peak serum level, attained in 3 h was approximately 4.0 µg per ml. The peak level of the metabolite, attained in 4 h was approximately 1.0 µg per ml. Food did not influence the absorption and there was no accumulation of the drug after multiple doses (Gan *et al.*, 1992; Guay and Craft, 1993).

Excretion

Clarithromycin is metabolized in the liver and several metabolites are formed, but 14-hydroxyclarithromycin is the only microbiologically active metabolite, and it is also the only metabolite found in plasma in high concentrations. Approximately 20–30% of an oral dose is excreted in urine as active clarithromycin and another 10–15% is recoverable in urine as the active metabolite (Chu *et al.*, 1992 b; Rodvold and Piscitelli, 1993).

Distribution of the Drug in Body

Clarithromycin is well distributed in many body fluids and tissues. Patients receiving the drug in a dosage of 250 mg orally 12-hourly reached peak tissue levels 4 h after administration and the mean peak concentrations in nasal mucosa and in tonsil were 8.32 and 6.47 μg per g, respectively (Fraschini *et al.*, 1991). Patients who were to undergo lung resection were given clarithromycin 500 mg orally every 12 h for a minimum of five doses and lung resection was performed approximately 4 h after the final dose. The concentrations of the drug and its 14-hydroxymetabolite in the lung tissue at this time averaged 54.3 and 5.12 μg per g, respectively, with a mean calculated ratio of concentrations of the parent to metabolite being 11.3 in lung tissue and 2.4 in plasma (Fish *et al.*, 1994). The drug is also concentrated in epithelial lining fluid and in alveolar cells (Conte *et al.*, 1995). Patients with infective exacerbations of chronic bronchiectasis, were given a single 250-mg clarithromycin dose orally. Maximum sputum concentrations were 0.52 μg per ml of clarithromycin 5 h after the dose and 0.3 μg per ml of the metabolite 6.5 h after the dose (Tsang *et al.*, 1994). Clarithromycin suspension was given in a dosage of 7.5 mg per kg 12-hourly for 7 days to children with otitis media. The fifth dose was given 2.5 h before aspiration of middle ear effusion. In the middle ear effusions mean concentrations of clarithromycin (2.5 μg per ml) and metabolite (1.3 μg per ml) were higher than the serum concentrations (1.7 and 0.8 μg per ml, respectively) (Guay and Craft, 1993; Sundberg and Cederberg, 1994).

Clarithromycin is approximately 70% bound to serum proteins (Chu *et al.*, 1992 a).

Mode of Action

This is similar to all macrolide antibiotics (see erythromycin, p. 614). In addition to its antibacterial activity, clarithromycin, similar to erythromycin acts as an immunomodulator. Combined treatment with this macrolide and the immunosuppressant such as cyclosporin A results in increased inhibition of T-cell proliferation (Morikawa *et al.*, 1994). Clarithromycin also eradicates the glycocalyx matrix produced by *Ps. aeruginosa* and *Staph. epidermidis*. This clarithromycin effect is not related to its antibacterial activity, but this action makes the relevant antibiotics more potent *in vivo* against these pathogens (Yasuda *et al.*, 1993, 1994).

Toxicity

Clarithromycin can cause gastrointestinal disturbances. They appear to be more common than with penicillin V (Still *et al.*, 1993), but this side-effect has been less common with clarithromycin than with amoxycillin/clavulanic acid (McCarthy *et al.*, 1993) and also less common than with erythromycin (Anderson *et al.*, 1991). When high-dose oral clarithromycin (1 g 12-hourly) was used to treat chronic mycobacterial infections in elderly patients, all patients developed symptoms such as bitter taste, nausea, vomiting and central nervous system disturbances. Elevated liver enzymes developed in 38%. A dosage reduction to 500 mg 12-hourly was better tolerated by most patients (Wallace *et al.*, 1993). Clarithromycin alters the intestinal microflora; streptococci and enterobacteria decrease. Anaerobic bacteria also decrease, but there is usually no overgrowth with resistant organisms (Brismar *et al.*, 1991). In one patient treated with clarithromycin, pseudomembranous colitis occurred, which responded to vancomycin (Braegger and Nadal, 1994).

Other side-effects with clarithromycin appear uncommon. Some patients have reported depression (Anderson *et al.*, 1991). One AIDS patient who was treated for *M. avium* infection with clarithromycin 1 g 12-hourly plus ciprofloxacin developed corneal opacities, which improved when clarithromycin was stopped (Dorrell *et al.*, 1994). In another AIDS patient, who was receiving several drugs, the development of thrombocytopenia appeared to be temporally related to clarithromycin therapy (Price and Tuazon, 1992). Thrombocytopenic purpura also developed in one patient who was treated with clarithromycin for pneumonia (Oteo *et al.*, 1994). In a few patients transient elevations of liver enzymes such as serum alanine aminotransferase, serum aspartate aminotransferase and alkaline phosphatase have been noted during clarithromycin therapy (Poirier, 1991; Brown *et al.*, 1995). Two AIDS patients who were treated with clarithromycin developed reversible psychosis. This recurred when the drug was resumed (Nightingale *et al.*, 1995). Acute uveitis may develop if clarithromycin is used together with rifabutin, but this appears to be due to elevated serum levels of the latter (p. 711).

Clarithromycin, similar to erythromycin (p. 616), significantly affects the pharmacokinetics of terfenadine, a non-sedating antihistamine. Terfenadine serum levels are elevated, which can result in cardiac toxicity. These two drugs should not be used together (Honig *et al.*, 1994). It is not yet clear whether clarithromycin shows drug interactions with the other drugs which interact with erythromycin, such as theophylline, carbamazepine, digitalis glycosides, analgesics and anti-asthmatic medications (p. 616) (Craft and Siepman, 1993).

Clinical Uses of the Drug

1 Mycobacterium avium complex bacteremia in AIDS patients

Clarithromycin (or azithromycin, p. 657) are now prime drugs for treatment of this disease. They should not be used as single drugs, as resistance of *M. avium* develops *in vivo*, but one of them is now usually preferred as the first choice for the treatment regimen. For clarithromycin, a dosage of 500 mg orally 12-hourly is usually sufficient. The regimen should also usually contain ethambutol in an oral dosage of 15 mg per kg per day (p. 1215). Sometimes three or even four drugs are used and the available drugs for the third and fourth drug are rifabutin 300 mg orally daily (p. 712), ciprofloxacin 750 mg orally 12-hourly (p. 1032), and amikacin 7.5 mg per kg i.m. or i.v. 12-hourly. Therapy should be continued for life, but for long-term treatment two oral drugs are selected, such as clarithromycin plus ciprofloxacin (De Lalla *et al.*, 1992; Benson and Ellner, 1993; Benson, 1994; Lane *et al.*, 1994). Animal experiments suggest that the granulocyte colony-stimulating factor may potentiate the activity of clarithromycin against *M. avium* (Lazard *et al.*, 1993). Rifabutin 300 mg daily (p. 711) is currently recommended for prevention of *M. avium* complex bacteremia in AIDS patients (Gordin and Masur, 1994), but clarithromycin in a dosage of 500 mg 12-hourly is currently being evaluated for this indication. Preliminary results showed that the drug is quite effective for this purpose, but when *M. avium* was isolated from patients receiving clarithromycin, a high percentage of the isolates were clarithromycin-resistant (Ostroff *et al.*, 1995).

Similar regimens to the above, which include clarithromycin, are also useful for the treatment of *M. avium* complex pulmonary disease in AIDS patients (Kalayjian *et al.*, 1995).

2 Other Mycobacterial infections

Clinical disease due to *M. chelonae* usually presents with skin and soft tissue infection, abscesses or osteomyelitis (Wallace *et al.*, 1992; Ingram *et al.*, 1993; Zahid *et al.*, 1994). Clarithromycin in a dosage of 500 mg 12-hourly has been useful for the treatment *M. chelonae* and *M. fortuitum* infections. It can be used as monotherapy or combined with ciprofloxacin. Most patients should be treated for at least 6 weeks after clinical resolution of the primary infection. Prolonged therapy for months to years may be required in severely compromised patients. In one 60-year-old heart transplant patient with disseminated *M. chelonae* infection, monotherapy with clarithromycin failed because of the rapid development of resistance to the drug (Tebas *et al.*, 1995). The authors suggested that two drugs should be used in treatment and either ciprofloxacin, tobramycin or imipenem can be combined with clarithromycin. In normal hosts, *M. marinum* causes cutaneous infections (swimming pool granuloma) but severe dermatological disease may occur in HIV-infected patients. Severe disease in an AIDS patient responded to clarithromycin 1 g 12-hourly (Bonnet *et al.*, 1994). The drug is not currently used for treatment of tuberculosis, but it may gain a place in a multidrug regimen for the treatment of multidrug-resistant *M. tuberculosis* infections (p. 1119). Clarithromycin in combination with ethambutol and ciprofloxacin may be useful for *M. genavense* infections in AIDS patients (Berman *et al.*, 1994; Matsiota-Bernard *et al.*, 1995).

3 Leprosy

In a clinical trial clarithromycin was given to nine previously untreated lepromatous leprosy patients. Patients received two 1500-mg doses on the first day, followed by 7 days of no treatment, in order to evaluate the efficacy of intermittent therapy. Thereafter they received 1000 mg daily for 2 weeks followed by 500 mg daily for 9 weeks. Within 3 weeks, biopsy-derived *M. leprae* specimens were non-infectious for mice and significant clinical improvement was evident after 4 weeks of treatment. Clarithromycin appeared rapidly bactericidal for *M. leprae* in humans (Chan *et al.*, 1994).

4 Toxoplasma encephalitis in AIDS patients

In one uncontrolled clinical trial clarithromycin 2 g daily plus pyrimethamine 75 mg daily for 6 weeks appeared about equally effective to the conventional therapy of sulfadiazine plus pyrimethamine (p. 823) for therapy of acute *Toxoplasma* encephalitis in patients with AIDS (Fernandez-Martin *et al.*, 1991).

5 Rhodococcus equi pneumonia in AIDS patients

In one AIDS patient clarithromycin (500 mg 8-hourly) plus minocycline eradicated this infection which had previously responded poorly to other antibiotics (Pialoux *et al.*, 1993).

6 Lyme disease

Studies in animals suggest that clarithromycin may be useful for the treatment of Lyme disease (Alder *et al.*, 1993b) and a pilot study on early Lyme disease in humans showed that the drug in a dosage of 500 mg twice-daily for 21 days was effective (Dattwyler *et al.*, 1996).

7 Community-acquired respiratory infections

All of these respond to older and cheaper drugs, but clarithromycin is also effective for most of them. In *Strep. pyogenes* pharyngitis clarithromycin is clinically similar to oral penicillin V, but it eradicated the organism from the pharynx more efficiently than penicillin (Still *et al.*, 1993). Clarithromycin is about as effective as amoxycillin for the treatment of otitis media (Pukander *et al.*, 1993). Community-acquired bronchitis or pneumonia, caused by *Strep. pneumoniae*, *H. influenzae*, *M. catarrhalis*, *M. pneumoniae* and *Chlamydia pneumoniae* respond quite satisfactorily to clarithromycin in an adult dosage of 250 mg 12-hourly (Aldons, 1991; Anderson *et al.*, 1991; Bachand, 1991; Grayston, 1992, 1994; Wettengel *et al.*, 1993; Hammerschlag, 1994). *Mycoplasma pneumoniae* and *C. pneumoniae* infections in children respond satisfactorily to the drug in a dosage of 7.5 mg per kg, given twice-daily (Block *et al.*, 1995). One animal study showed that clarithromycin may be a promising drug for treatment of *Legionella pneumophila* pneumonia (Kohno *et al.* 1989).

8 Helicobacter pylori infections

Combined treatment with clarithromycin and omeprazole eradicated *H. pylori* from some 87% of patients. Omeprazole increased concentrations of clarithromycin in gastric tissue and mucus and this may be one of the explanations for the success of this regimen (Gustavson *et al.*, 1995). Over 95% of pre-treatment strains of *H. pylori* are clarithromycin-sensitive (Xia *et al.*, 1996). This contrasts with metranidazole to which a high percentage of such strains may be resistant (p. 937).

9 Pneumocystis carinii pneumonia

Animal studies suggest that the combination of clarithromycin plus sulfamethoxazole may be effective for *P. carinii* pneumonia (Alder *et al.*, 1994).

References

Alder J, Jarvis K, Mitten M *et al.* (1993a). Clarithromycin therapy of experimental *Treponema pallidum* infections in hamsters. *Antimicrob Ag Chemother* **37**: 864.

Alder J, Mitten M, Jarvis K *et al.* (1993b). Efficacy of clarithromycin for treatment of experimental Lyme disease *in vivo*. *Antimicrob Ag Chemother* **37**: 1329.

Alder J, Mitten M, Shipkowitz N *et al.* (1994). Treatment of experimental *Pneumocystis carinii* infection by combination of clarithromycin and sulphamethoxazole. *J Antimicrob Chemother* **33**: 253.

Aldons PM (1991). A comparison of clarithromycin with ampicillin in the treatment of outpatients with acute bacterial exacerbation of chronic bronchitis. *J Antimicrob Chemother* **27** (Suppl A): 101.

Anderson G, Esmonde TS, Coles S *et al.* (1991). A comparative safety and efficacy study of clarithromycin and erythromycin stearate in community-acquired pneumonia. *J Antimicrob Chemother* **27** (Suppl A): 117.

Araujo FG, Prokocimer P, Lin T, Remington JS (1992). Activity of clarithromycin alone or in combination with other drugs for treatment of murine toxoplasmosis. *Antimicrob Ag Chemother* **36**: 2454.

Bachand RJJr (1991). Comparative study of clarithromycin and ampicillin in the treatment of patients with acute bacterial exacerbations of chronic bronchitis. *J Antimicrob Chemother* **27** (Suppl A): 91.

Barry AL, Thornsberry C, Jones RN (1987). *In vitro* activity of new macrolide, A-56268, compared with that of roxithrommycin, erythromycin and clindamycin. *Antimicrob Ag Chemother* **31**: 343.

Barry AL, Pfaller MA, Fuchs PC, Packer RR (1994). *In vitro* activities of 12 orally administered antimicrobial agents against four species of bacterial respiratory pathogens from US medical centers in 1992 and 1993. *Antimicrob Ag Chemother* **38**: 2419.

Bauer J, Hof H (1992). Activity of clarithromycin against murine listeriosis. *J Antimicrob Chemother* **29**: 435.

Benson CA (1994). Treatment of disseminated disease due to the *Mycobacterium avium* complex in patients with AIDS. *Clin Infect Dis* **18** (Suppl 3): 237.

Benson CA, Ellner JJ (1993). Mycobacterium avium complex infection and AIDS: advances in theory and practice. *Clin Infect Dis* **17**: 7.

Benson CA, Segreti J, Beaudette FE *et al.* (1987). *In vitro* activity of A-56268 (TE-031), a new macrolide, compared with that of erythromycin and clindamycin against selected Gram-positive and Gram-negative organisms. *Antimicrob Ag Chemother* **31**: 328.

Berman SM, Kim RC, Haghighat D *et al.* (1994). Mycobacterium genavense infection presenting as a solitary brain mass in a patient with AIDS: case report and review. *Clin Infect Dis* **19**: 1152.

Bermudez LE, Kolonoski P, Young LS, Inderlied CB (1994). Activity of KRM 1648 alone or in combination with ethambutol or clarithromycin against *Mycobacterium avium* in beige mouse model of disseminated infection. *Antimicrob Ag Chemother* **38**: 1844.

Bernard EM, Edwards FF, Kiehn TE *et al.* (1993). Activities of antimicrobial agents against clinical isolates of *Mycobacterium haemophilum*. *Antimicrob Ag Chemother* **37**: 2323.

Biehle J, Cavalieri SJ (1992). *In vitro* susceptibility of *Mycobacterium kansasii* to clarithromycin. *Antimicrob Ag Chemother* **36**: 2039.

Block S, Hedrick J, Hammerschlag MR *et al.* (1995). *Mycoplasma pneumoniae* and *Chlamydia pneumoniae* in pediatric community-acquired pneumonia: comparative efficacy and safety of clarithromycin vs erythromycin ethylsuccinate. *Pediatr Infect Dis J* **14**: 471.

Bonnet E, Debat-Zoguerch D, Petit N *et al.* (1994). Clarithromycin: a potent agent against infections due to *Mycobacterium marinum*. *Clin Infect Dis* **18**: 664.

Braegger CP, Nadal D (1994). Clarithromycin and pseudomembranous enterocolitis. *Lancet* **343**: 241.

Brismar B, Edlund C, Nord CE (1991). Comparative effects of clarithromycin and erythromycin on the normal intestinal microflora. *Scand J Infect Dis* **23**: 635.

Brown BA, Wallace RJJr, Onyi GO *et al.* (1992a). Activities of four macrolides, including clarithromycin, against *Mycobacterium fortuitum*, *Mycobacterium chelonae*, and *M. chelonae*-like organisms. *Antimicrob Ag Chemother* **36**: 180.

Brown BA, Wallace RJJr, Onyi GO (1992b). Activities of clarithromycin against eight slowly growing species of nontuberculous mycobacteria, determined by using a broth microdilution MIC system. *Antimicrob Ag Chemother* **36**: 1987.

Brown BA, Wallace RJJr, Griffith DE, Girard W (1995). Clarithromycin-induced hepatotoxicity. *Clin Infect Dis* **20**: 1073.

Cavalieri SJ, Biehle JR, Sanders WEJr (1995). Synergistic activities of clarithromycin and antituberculous drugs against multidrug-resistant *Mycobacterium tuberculosis*. *Antimicrob Ag Chemother* **39**: 1542.

Chan GP, Garcia-Ignacio BY, Chavez VE *et al.* (1994). Clinical trial of clarithromycin for lepromatous leprosy. *Antimicrob Ag Chemother* **38**: 515.

Chang HR, Rudareanu FC, Pechère J-C (1988). Activity of A-56268 (TE-031), a new macrolide, against *Toxoplasma gondii* in mice. *J Antimicrob Chemother* **22**: 359.

Chin N-X, Neu NM, Labthavikul P *et al.* (1987). Activity of A-56268 compared with that of erythromycin and other oral agents against aerobic and anaerobic bacteria. *Antimicrob Ag Chemother* **31**: 463.

Chirgwin K, Roblin PM, Hammerschlag MR (1989). *In vitro* susceptibilities of *Chlamydia pneumoniae* (Chlamydia sp. strain TWAR). *Antimicrob Ag Chemother* **33**: 1634.

Chu S-Y, Deaton R, Cavanaugh J (1992a). Absolute bioavailability of clarithromycin after oral administration in humans. *Antimicrob Ag Chemother* **36**: 1147.

Chu S-Y, Sennello LT, Bunnell ST *et al.* (1992b). Pharmacokinetics of clarithromycin, a new macrolide, after single ascending oral doses. *Antimicrob Ag Chemother* **36**: 2447.

Cohen Y, Perronne C, Truffot-Pernot C *et al.* (1992). Activities of WIN-57273, minocycline, clarithromycin, and 14-hydroxy-clarithromycin against *Mycobacterium avium* complex in human macrophages. *Antimicrob Ag Chemother* **36**: 2104.

Conte JE Jr, Golden JA, Duncan S *et al.* (1995). Intrapulmonary pharmacokinetics of clarithromycin and of erythromycin. *Antimicrob Ag Chemother* **39**: 334.

Craft JC, Siepman N (1993). Overview of safety profile of clarithromycin suspension in pediatric patients. *Pediatr Infect Dis J* **12** (Suppl 3): 142.

Cynamon MH, Klemens SP, Grossi MA (1994). Comparative activities of azithromycin and clarithromycin against *Mycobacterium avium* infection in beige mice. *Antimicrob Ag Chemother* **38**: 1452.

Dabernat H, Delmas C, Seguy M *et al.* (1991). The activity of clarithromycin and its 14-hydroxy metabolite against *Haemophilus influenzae*, determined by *in-vitro* and serum bactericidal tests. *J Antimicrob Chemother* **27** (Suppl A): 19.

Dangor Y, Miller SD, Exposto F da L, Koornhof HJ (1988). Antimicrobial susceptibilities of Southern African isolates of *Haemophilus ducreyi*. *Antimicrob Ag Chemother* **32**: 1458.

Dattwyler RJ, Grunwaldt E, Luft BJ (1996). Clarithromycin in treatment of early Lyme disease: a pilot study. *Antimicrob Ag Chemother* **40**: 468.

Dautzenberg B, Truffot C, Legris S *et al.* (1991). Activity of clarithromycin against *Mycobacterium avium* infection in patients with the acquired immune deficiency syndrome: a controlled clinical trial. *Am Rev Respir Dis* **144**: 564.

De Lalla F, Maserati R, Scarpellini P *et al.* (1992). Clarithromycin-ciprofloxacin-amikacin for therapy of *Mycobacterium avium-Mycobacterium intracellulare* bacteremia in patients with AIDS. *Antimicrob Ag Chemother* **36**: 1567.

Derouin F, Caroff B, Chau F *et al.* (1992). Synergistic activity of clarithromycin and minocycline in an animal model of acute experimental toxoplasmosis. *Antimicrob Ag Chemother* **36**: 2852.

Dorrell L, Ellerton C, Cottrell DG, Snow MH (1994). Toxicity of clarithromycin in the treatment of *Mycobacterium avium* complex infection in a patient with AIDS. *J Antimicrob Chemother* **34**: 605.

Doucet-Populaire F, Truffot-Pernot C, Grosset J, Jarlier V (1995). Acquired resistance in *Mycobacterium avium* complex strains isolated from AIDS patients and beige mice during treatment with clarithromycin. *J Antimicrob Chemother* **36**: 129.

Eliopoulos GM, Reiszner E, Ferraro MJ, Moellering RC (1987). Comparative *in-vitro* activity of A-56268 (TE-031), a new macrolide antibiotic. *J Antimicrob Chemother* **20**: 671.

Endtz HP, Broeren M, Mouton RP (1993). *In vitro* susceptibility of quinolone-resistant *Campylobacter jejuni* to new macrolide antibiotics. *Eur J Clin Microbiol Infect Dis* **12**: 48.

Fass RJ (1993). Erythromycin, clarithromycin, and azithromycin: use of frequency distribution curves, scattergrams, and regression analyses to compare *in vitro* activities and describe cross-resistance. *Antimicrob Ag Chemother* **37**: 2080.

Fernandes PB, Bailer R, Swanson R *et al.* (1986). *In vitro* and *in vivo* evaluation of A-56268 (TE-031), a new macrolide. *Antimicrob Ag Chemother* **30**: 865.

Fernandes PG, Baker WR, Freiberg LA *et al.* (1989a). New macrolides active against *Streptococcus pyogenes* with inducible or constitutive type of macrolide-lincosamide-streptogramin B resistance. *Antimicrob Ag Chemother* **33**: 78.

Fernandes PG, Hardy DJ, McDaniel D *et al.* (1989b). *In vitro* and *in vivo* activities of clarithromycin against *Mycobacterium avium*. *Antimicrob Ag Chemother* **33**: 1531.

Fernandez-Martin J, Leport C, Morlat P *et al.* (1991). Pyrimethamine-clarithromycin combination for therapy of acute toxoplasma encephalitis in patients with AIDS. *Antimicrob Ag Chemother* **35**: 2049.

Fish DN, Godfried MH, Danziger LH, Rodvold KA (1994). Penetration of clarithromycin into lung tissues from patients undergoing lung resection. *Antimicrob Ag Chemother* **38**: 876.

Floyd-Reising S, Hindler JA, Young LS (1987). *In vitro* activity of A-56268 (TE-031), a new macrolide antibiotic, compared with that of erythromycin and other antimicrobial agents. *Antimicrob Ag Chemother* **31**: 640.

Forsgren A (1993). Antibiotic susceptibility of *Mycobacterium marinum*. *Scand J Infect Dis* **25**: 779.

Fraschini F, Scaglione F, Pintucci G *et al.* (1991). The diffusion of clarithromycin and roxithromycin into nasal mucosa, tonsil and lung in humans. *J Antimicrob Chemother* **27** (Suppl A): 61.

Funke G, Baumann R, Penner JL, Altwegg M (1994). Development of resistance to macrolide antibiotics in an AIDS patient treated with clarithromycin for *Campylobacter jejuni* diarrhea. *Eur J Clin Microbiol Infect Dis* **13**: 612.

Furney SK, Skinner PS, Farrer J, Orme IM (1995). Activities of rifabutin, clarithromycin, and ethambutol against two virulent strains of *Mycobacterium avium* in a mouse model. *Antimicrob Ag Chemother* **39**: 786.

Gan VN, Chu S-Y, Kusmiesz HT, Craft JC (1992). Pharmacokinetics of clarithromycin suspension in infants and children. *Antimicrob Ag Chemother* **36**: 2478.

Gelber RH, Siu P, Tsang M, Murray LP (1991). Activities of various macrolide antibiotics against *Mycobacterium leprae* infection in mice. *Antimicrob Ag Chemother* **35**: 760.

Gevaudan MJ, Bollet C, Mallet MN, de Micco P (1993). *In-vitro* evaluation of clarithromycin, temafloxacin, and ethambutol in combination against *Mycobacterium avium* complex. *J Antimicrob Chemother* **31**: 725.

Goldstein EJC, Citron DM (1993). Comparative susceptibilities of 173 aerobic and anaerobic bite wound isolates to sparfloxacin, temafloxacin, clarithromycin, and older agents. *Antimicrob Ag Chemother* **37**: 1150.

Gordin F, Masur H (1994). Prophylaxis of *Mycobacterium avium* complex bacteremia in patients with AIDS. *Clin Infect Dis* **18** (Suppl 3): 223.

Gorzynski EA, Gutman SI, Allen W (1989). Comparative antimycobacterial activities of difloxacin, temofloxacin, enoxacin, pefloxacin, reference fluoroquinolones, and new macrolide, clarithromycin. *Antimicrob Ag Chemother* **33**: 591.

Grayston JT (1992). Infections caused by *Chlamydia pneumoniae* strain TWAR. *Clin Infect Dis* **15**: 757.

Grayston JT (1994). Chlamydia pneumoniae (TWAR). Infections in children. *Pediatr Infect Dis J* **13**: 675.

Guay DRP, Craft JC (1993). Overview of the pharmacology of clarithromycin suspension in children and a comparison with that in adults. *Pediatr Infect Dis J* **12** (Suppl 3): 106.

Gustavson LE, Kaiser JF, Edmonds AL *et al.* (1995). Effect of omeprazole on concentrations of clarithromycin in plasma and gastric tissue at steady state. *Antimicrob Ag Chemother* **39**: 2078.

Hammerschlag MR (1994). Antimicrobial susceptibility and therapy of infections caused by *Chlamydia* pneumoniae. *Antimicrob Ag Chemother* **38**: 1873.

Hardy DJ (1993). Extent and spectrum of the antimicrobial activity of clarithromycin. *Pediatr Infect Dis J* **12** (Suppl 3): 99.

Hardy DJ, Hensey DM, Bejer JM *et al.* (1988a). Comparative *in vitro* activities of new 14-, 15-, and 16-membered macrolides. *Antimicrob Ag Chemother* **32**: 1710.

Hardy DJ, Hanson CW, Hensey DM *et al.* (1988b). Susceptibility of *Campylobacter pylori* to macrolides and fluoroquinolones. *J Antimicrob Chemother* **22**: 631.

Hardy DJ, Swanson RN, Rode RA *et al.* (1990). Enhancement of the *in vitro* and *in vivo* activities of clarithromycin against *Haemophilus influenzae* by 14-hydroxy-clarithromycin, its major metabolite in humans. *Antimicrob Ag Chemother* **34**: 1407.

Havlir DV (1994). *Mycobacterium avium* complex: advances in therapy. *Eur J Clin Microbiol Infect Dis* **13**: 915.

Heifets LB, Lindholm-Levy PJ, Comstock RD (1992). Bacteriostatic and bactericidal activities of gentamicin alone and in combination with clarithromycin against *Mycobacterium avium*. *Antimicrob Ag Chemother* **36**: 1695.

Heifets LB, Mor N, Vanderkolk J (1993). *Mycobacterium avium* strains resistant to clarithromycin and azithromycin. *Antimicrob Ag Chemother* **37**: 2364.

Honig PK, Wortham DC, Zamani K, Cantilena LR (1994). Comparison of the effect of the macrolide antibiotics erythromycin, clarithromycin and azithromycin on terfenadine steady-state pharmacokinetics and electrocardiographic parameters. *Drug Invest* **7**: 148.

Ingram CW, Tanner DC, Durack DT *et al.* (1993). Disseminated infection with rapidly growing mycobacteria. *Clin Infect Dis* **16**: 463.

Ji B, Lounis N, Truffot-Pernot C, Grosset J (1992). Selection of resistant mutants of *Mycobacterium avium* in beige mice by clarithromycin monotherapy. *Antimicrob Ag Chemother* **36**: 2839.

Ji B, Jamet P, Perani EG *et al.* (1993). Powerful bactericidal activities of clarithromycin and minocycline against *Mycobacterium leprae* in lepromatous leprosy. *J Infect Dis* **168**: 188.

Ji B, Lounis N, Truffot-Pernot C, Grosset J (1994). Effectiveness of various antimicrobial agents against *Mycobacterium avium* complex in beige mouse model. *Antimicrob Ag Chemother* **38**: 2521.

Jones RN, Erwin ME, Barrett MS (1990). *In vitro* activity of clarithromycin (TE-031, A-67268). and 140H-clarithromycin alone and in combination against *Legionella* species. *Eur J Clin Microbiol Infect Dis* **9**: 846.

Jorgensen JH, Maher LA, Howell AW(1991). Activity of clarithromycin and its principal human metabolite against *Haemophilus influenzae*. *Antimicrob Ag Chemother* **35**: 1524.

Kalayjian RC, Toossi Z, Tomashefski JF Jr *et al.* (1995). Pulmonary disease due to infection by *Mycobacterium avium* complex in patients with AIDS. *Clin Infect Dis* **20**: 1186.

Klemens SP, De Stefano MS, Cynamon MH (1992). Activity of clarithromycin against *Mycobacterium avium* complex infection in beige mice. *Antimicrob Ag Chemother* **36**: 2413.

Kohno S, Koga H, Yamaguchi K *et al.* (1989). A new macrolide, TE-031(A-56268), in treatment of experimental Legionaires' disease. *J Antimicrob Chemother* **24**: 397.

Lane HC, Laughon BE, Falloon J *et al.* (1994). Recent advances in the management of AIDS-related opportunistic infections. *Ann Intern Med* **120**: 945.

Lazard T, Perronne C, Cohen Y *et al.* (1993). Efficacy of granulocyte colony-stimulating factor and RU-40555 in combination with clarithromycin against *Mycobacterium avium* complex infection in C57BL/6 mice. *Antimicrob Ag Chemother* **37**: 692.

Levin JM, Nelson JA, Segreti J *et al.* (1993). *In vitro* susceptibility of *Borrelia burgdorferi* to 11 antimicrobial agents. *Antimicrob Ag Chemother* **37**: 1444.

Liebers DM, Baltch AL, Smith RP *et al.* (1988). Comparative *in vitro* activities of A-56268 (TE-031). and erythromycin against 306 clinical isolates. *J Antimicrob Chemother* **21**: 565.

Lonks JR, Medeiros AA (1993). High rate of erythromycin and clarithromycin resistance among *Streptococcus pneumoniae* isolates from blood cultures from Providence, RI. *Antimicrob Ag Chemother* **37**: 1742.

Lounis N, Ji B, Truffot-Pernot C, Grosset J (1995). Selection of clarithromycin-resistant *Mycobacterium avium* complex during combined therapy using the beige mouse model. *Antimicrob Ag Chemother* **39**: 608.

Matsiota-Bernard P, Thierry D, De Truchis P *et al.* (1995). *Mycobacterium genavense* infection in a patient with AIDS who was successfully treated with clarithromycin. *Clin Infect Dis* **20**: 1565.

Maurin M, Raoult D (1993). *In vitro* susceptibilities of spotted fever group Rickettsiae and *Coxiella burnetii* to clarithromycin. *Antimicrob Ag Chemother* **37**: 2633.

McCarthy JM, Phillips A, Wiisanen R (1993). Comparative safety and efficacy of clarithromycin and amoxillin/clavulanate in the treatment of acute otitis media in children. *Pediatr Infect Dis J* **12** (Suppl 3): 122.

Meier A, Kirschner P, Spinger B *et al.* (1994). Identification of mutations in 23S rRNA gene of clarithromycin-resistant *Mycobacterium intracellulare*. *Antimicrob Ag Chemother* **38**: 381.

Mor N, Heifets L (1993a). MICs and MBCs of clarithromycin against *Mycobacterium avium* within human macrophages. *Antimicrob Ag Chemother* **37**: 111.

Mor N, Heifets L (1993b). Inhibition of intracellular growth of *Mycobacterium avium* by one pulsed exposure of infected macrophages to clarithromycin. *Antimicrob Ag Chemother* **37**: 1380.

Mor N, Vanderkolk J, Mezo N, Heifets L (1994). Effects of clarithromycin and rifabutin alone and in combination on intracellular and extracellular replication of *Mycobacterium avium*. *Antimicrob Ag Chemother* **38**: 2738.

Morikawa K, Oseko F, Morikawa S, Iwamoto K (1994). Immunomodulatory effects of three macrolides, midecamycin acetate, josamycin, and clarithromycin, on human T-lymphocyte function *in vitro*. *Antimicrob Ag Chemother* **38**: 2643.

Naik S, Ruck R (1989). *In vitro* activities of several new macrolide antibiotics against *Mycobacterium avium* complex. *Antimicrob Ag Chemother* **33**: 1614.

Neu HC (1991). The development of macrolides: clarithromycin in perspective. *J Antimicrob Chemother* **27** (Suppl A): 1.

Nightingale SD, Koster FT, Mertz GJ, Loss SD (1995). Clarithromycin-induced mania in two patients with AIDS. *Clin Infect Dis* **20**: 1564.

Onyeji CO, Nightingale CH, Nicolau DP, Quintiliani R (1994). Efficacies of liposome-encapsulated clarithromycin and ofloxacin against *Mycobacterium avium-M. intracellulare* complex in human macrophages. *Antimicrob Ag Chemother* **38**: 523.

Ostroff SM, Spiegel RA, Feinberg J *et al.* (1995). Preventing disseminated

Mycobacterium avium complex disease in patients infected with human immunodeficiency virus. *Clin Infect Dis* **21** (Suppl 1): 72.

Oteo JA, Gómez-Cadiñanos A, Rosel L, Casas JM (1994). Clarithromycin-induced thrombocytopenic purpura. *Clin Infect Dis* **19**: 1170.

Perronne C, Gikas A, Truffot-Pernot C *et al.* (1990). Activities of clarithromycin, sulfisoxazole, and rifabutin against *Mycobacterium avium* complex multiplication within human macrofages. *Antimicrob Ag Chemother* **34**: 1508.

Pialoux G, Goldstein F, Dupont B *et al.* (1993). Combination antibiotic treatment with clarithromycin for human immunodeficiency virus-associated *Rhodococcus equi* infection. *Clin Infect Dis* **17**: 513.

Poirier R (1991). Comparative study of clarithromycin and roxithromycin in the treatment of community-acquired pneumonia. *J Antimicrob Chemother* **27** (Suppl A): 109.

Price TA, Tuazon CU (1992). Clarithromycin-induced thrombocytopenia. *Clin Infect Dis* **15**: 563.

Pukander JS, Jero JP, Kaprio EA, Sorri MJ (1993). Clarithromycin versus amoxicillin suspensions in the treatment of pediatric patients with acute otitis media. *Pediatr Infect Dis J* **12** (Suppl 3): 118.

Rastogi N, Labrousse V (1991). Extracellular and intracellular activities of clarithromycin used alone and in association with ethambutol and rifampin against *Mycobacterium avium* complex. *Antimicrob Ag Chemother* **35**: 462.

Rastogi N, Goh KS, Labrousse V (1992). Activity of clarithromycin compared with those of other drugs against *Mycobacterium paratuberculosis* and further enhancement of its extracellular and intracellular activities by ethambutol. *Antimicrob Ag Chemother* **36**: 2843.

Rastogi N, Bauriaud R-M, Bourgoin A *et al.* (1995). French multicenter study involving eight test sites for radiometric determination of activities of 10 antimicrobial agents against *Mycobacterium avium* complex. *Antimicrob Ag Chemother* **39**: 638.

Reda C, Quaresima T, Pastoris MC (1994). *In vitro* activity of six intracellular antibiotics against *Legionella pneumophila* strains of human and environmental origin. *J Antimicrob Chemother* **33**: 757.

Roblin PM, Montalban G, Hammerschlag MR (1994). Susceptibilities to clarithromycin and erythromycin of isolates of *Chlamydia pneumoniae* from children with pneumonia. *Antimicrob Ag Chemother* **38**: 1588.

Rodvold KA, Piscitelli SC (1993). New oral macrolide and fluoroquinolone antibiotics: an overview of pharmacokinetics, interactions, and safety. *Clin Infect Dis* **17** (Suppl 1): 192.

Sánchez R, Fernández-Baca V, Diaz MD *et al.* (1994). Evolution of susceptibilities of *Campylobacter* spp to quinolones and macrolides. *Antimicrob Ag Chemother* **38**: 1879.

Sanders JW, Walsh AD, Snider RL, Sahn EE (1995). Disseminated *Mycobacterium scrofulosum* infection: a potentially treatable complication of AIDS. *Clin Infect Dis* **20**: 549.

Segreti J, Kessler HA, Kapell KS, Trenholme GM (1987). *In vitro* activity of A-56268 (TE-031). and four other antimicrobial agents against *Chlamydia trachomatis*. *Antimicrob Ag Chemother* **31**: 100.

Spangler SK, Jacobs MR, Appelbaum PC (1994). Effect of CO_2 on susceptabilities of anaerobes to erythromycin, azithromycin, clarithromycin and roxithromycin. *Antimicrob Ag Chemother* **38**: 211.

Spangler SK, Jacobs MR, Appelbaum PC (1995). Susceptibilities of 201 anaerobes to erythromycin, azithromycin, clarithromycin, and roxithromycin by oxyrase agar dilution and E test methodologies. *J Clin Microbiol* **33**: 1366.

Still JG, Hubbard WC, Poole JM *et al.* (1993). Comparison of clarithromycin and penicillin VK suspensions in the treatment of children with streptococcal pharyngitis and review of currently available alternative antibiotic therapies. *Pediatr Infect Dis J* **12** (Suppl 3): 134.

Sundberg L, Cederberg Å (1994). Penetration of clarithromycin and its 14-hydroxy metabolite into middle ear effusion in children with secretory otitis media. *J Antimicrob Chemother* **33**: 299.

Tebas P, Sultan F, Wallace RJ Jr, Fraser V (1995). Rapid development of resistance to clarithromycin following monotherapy for disseminated

Mycobacterium chelonae infection in a heart transplant patient. *Clin Infect Dis* **20**: 443.

Truffot-Pernot C, Ji B, Grosset J (1991). Effect of pH on the *in vitro* potency of clarithromycin against *Mycobacterium avium* complex. *Antimicrob Ag Chemother* **35**: 1677.

Tsang KWT, Roberts P, Read RC *et al.* (1994). The concentrations of clarithromycin and its 14-hydroxy metabolite in sputum of patients with bronchiectasis following single dose oral administration. *J Antimicrob Chemother* **33**: 289.

Valero G, Moreno F, Graybill JR (1994). Activities of clarithromycin, ofloxacin, and clarithromycin plus ethambutol against *Mycobacterium simiae* in murine model of disseminated infection. *Antimicrob Ag Chemother* **38**: 2676.

Vallée E, Azoulay-Dupuis E, Swanson R *et al.* (1991). Individual and combined activities of clarithromycin and its 14-hydroxy metabolite in murine model of *Haemophilus influenzae* infection. *J Antimicrob Chemother* **27** (Suppl A): 31.

Vance E, Watson-Bitar M, Gustavson L, Kazanjian P (1995). Pharmacokinetics of clarithromycin and zidovudine in patients with AIDS. *Clin Infect Dis* **39**: 1355.

Von Eiff C, Hermann M, Peters G (1995). Antimicrobial susceptibilities of *Stomatococcus mucilaginosus* and of *Micrococcus* spp. *Antimicrob Ag Chemother* **39**: 268.

Waites KB, Cassell GH, Canupp KC, Fernandes PB (1988). *In vitro* susceptibilities of mycoplasmas and ureaplasmas to new macrolides and aryl-fluoroquinolones. *Antimicrob Ag Chemother* **32**: 1500.

Walker KJ, Larsson AJ, Zabinski RA, Rotschafer JC (1994). Evaluation of antimicrobial activities of clarithromycin and 14-hydroxyclarithromycin against three strains of *Haemophilus influenzae* by using an *in vitro* pharmacodynamic model. *Antimicrob Ag Chemother* **38**: 2003.

Wallace RJ Jr, Brown BA, Onyi GO (1992). Skin, soft tissue, and bone infections due to *Mycobacterium chelonae* chelonae: importance of prior corticosteroid therapy, frequency of disseminated infections, and resistance to oral antimicrobials other than clarithromycin. *J Infect Dis* **166**: 405.

Wallace RJ Jr, Brown BA, Griffith DE (1993). Drug intolerance to high-dose clarithromycin among elderly patients. *Diagn Microbiol Infect Dis* **16**: 215.

Wallace RJ Jr, Brown BA, Griffith DE (1995). Reduced serum levels of clarithromycin in patients treated with multidrug regimens including rifampin or rifabutin for *Mycobacterium avium–M. intracellulare* infection. *J Infect Dis* **171**: 747.

Wettengel R, Vetter N, Waardenburg FA (1993). Clarithromycin versus cefaclor for the treatment of mild-to-moderate acute bacterial bronchitis. *J Antimicrob Chemother* **31**: 963.

Xia H-X, Buckley M, Keane CT, O'Morain CA (1996). Clarithromycin resistance in *Helicobacter pylori*: prevalence in untreated dyspeptic patients and stability *in vitro*. *J Antimicrob Chemother* **37**: 473.

Yajko DM, Nassos PS, Sanders CA *et al.* (1992). Comparison of the intracellular activities of clarithromycin and erythromycin against *Mycobacterium avium* complex strains in J774 cells and in alveolar macrophages from human immunodeficiency virus type 1-infected individuals. *Antimicrob Ag Chemother* **36**: 1163.

Yamamoto T, Nair GB, Albert MJ (1995). Survey of *in vitro* susceptibilities of *Vibrio cholerae* 01 and 0139 to antimicrobial agents. *Antimicrob Ag Chemother* **39**: 241.

Yasuda H, Ajiki Y, Koga T *et al.* (1993). Interaction between biofilms formed by *Pseudomonas aeruginosa* and clarithromycin. *Antimicrob Ag Chemother* **37**: 1749.

Yasuda H, Ajiki Y, Koga T, Yokota T (1994). Intraction between clarithromycin and biofilms formed by *Staphylococcus epidermidis*. *Antimicrob Ag Chemother* **38**: 138.

Zahid MA, Klotz SA, Goldstein E, Bartholomew W (1994). *Mycobacterium chelonae* (*M. chelonae* subspecies chelonae): report of a patient with a sporotrichoid presentation who was successfully treated with clarithromycin and ciprofloxacin. *Clin Infect Dis* **18**: 999.

Azithromycin

Description

Azithromycin is a new macrolide antibiotic, differing structurally from erythromycin (p. 606) in the possession of a unique 15-membered macrolide ring and bearing a methyl substituted nitrogen at position 9a. It is the first of a novel subclass of macrolides referred to as azalides. Azithromycin has greater *in vitro* activity than erythromycin against some Gram-negative bacteria and improved pharmacokinetics (Dunkin *et al.*, 1988; Maskell *et al.*, 1990). The drug also shows activity against non-tuberculous mycobacteria, including *Mycobacterium avium* complex (Cynamon and Klemens, 1992; Klemens and Cynamon, 1994a) and some parasites, such as *Toxoplasma gondii* (Huskinson-Mark *et al.*, 1991).

Sensitive Bacteria

1 Gram-positive bacteria

Similar to erythromycin (p. 606), azithromycin is active against erythromycin-sensitive strains of *Streptococcus pyogenes*, Groups B, C and G streptococci, *Strep. pneumoniae*, *Strep. viridans*, *Strep. bovis*, *Staphylococcus aureus*, coagulase-negative staphylococci, *Enterococcus faecalis* and *E. faecium*. *Listeria monocytogenes* is also moderately susceptible. Some authors have found the activity of azithromycin against these organisms to be about the same as that of erythromycin, but most have reported azithromycin to be some 4- to 8-fold less active. There is complete cross-resistance between erythromycin and azithromycin for all of these bacteria (Retsema *et al.*, 1987; Barry *et al.*, 1988; Dunkin *et al.*, 1988; Maskell *et al.*, 1990; Williams *et al.*, 1992; Barry and Fuchs, 1995). Most *Strep. pyogenes* isolates in southern Taiwan are now azithromycin- and erythromycin-resistant (Hsueh *et al.*, 1995).

Gram-positive anaerobic cocci such as the *Peptostreptococcus* spp. are also azithromycin-sensitive. The same is true for Gram-positive anaerobic rods such as the *Clostridium*, *Actinomyces*, *Propionibacterium*, *Eubacterium* and *Lactobacillus* spp. (Barry *et al.*, 1988; Maskell *et al.*, 1990; Williams *et al.*, 1992).

2 Gram-negative bacteria

Azithromycin is more active against *Neisseria meningitidis* and *N. gonorrhoeae* than erythromycin (Barry *et al.*, 1988; Slaney *et al.*, 1990). *Haemophilus influenzae* and *Moraxella catarrhalis* are some 4-fold more sensitive to azithromycin than to erythromycin (Barry *et al.*, 1988; Maskell *et al.*, 1990; Barry and Fuchs, 1995). Azithromycin also has a rapid bactericidal effect on *H. influenzae* (Goldstein *et al.*, 1990). *Haemophilus ducreyi* is also more susceptible to azithromycin than erythromycin (Slaney *et al.*, 1990; Motley *et al.*, 1992). Azithromycin is about as active as erythromycin against *Legionella pneumophila* and *L. micdadei in vitro*, but the new drug appears to be more active against these pathogens intracellularly (Edelstein and Edelstein, 1991; Donowitz and Earnhardt, 1993). *Campylobacter jejuni* and *C. coli* are about as sensitive to azithromycin as they are to erythromycin and erythromycin-resistant strains are also azithromycin-resistant (Taylor and Chang, 1991; Rautelin *et al.*, 1993). Quinolone-resistant strains of *C. jejuni* are usually azithromycin-sensitive (Endtz *et al.*, 1993).

The *Brucella* spp. with MICs of 0.5–2.0 μg per ml are moderately azithromycin-sensitive (Landinez *et al.*, 1992; Garcia-Rodriguez *et al.*, 1993). *Vibrio cholerae*, both biotype *El Tor* 01 and the classical biotype 01 are highly sensitive to azithromycin. The same is true for the new *V. cholerae* 0139 Bengal strain (Yamamoto *et al.*, 1995). This new *V. cholerae* 0139 strain was sensitive to tetracycline (p. 722), but resistant to co-trimoxazole and furazolidone (Waldor and Mekalanos, 1994). Azithromycin also shows some activity against other Gram-negative bacteria such as the *Bartonella* (*Rochalimaea*) spp., *Cardiobacterium hominis* and the *Pasteurella*, *Aeromonas* and *Acinetobacter* spp, but *Ps. aeruginosa* is completely resistant (Retsema *et al.*, 1987; Kitzis *et al.*, 1990; Guerra *et al.*, 1993; Goldstein *et al.*, 1995).

Unlike erythromycin (p. 608), azithromycin is active against some of the Enterobacteriaceae, particularly the enteropathogens such as enteropathogenic *Escherichia coli* and the *Shigella* and *Salmonella* spp. Azithromycin is particularly effective against these pathogens intracellularly (Retsema *et al.*, 1987; Gordillo *et al.*, 1993; Rakita *et al.*, 1994). It also has some activity against other *E. coli* strains, *Yersinia enterocolitica*, and *Citrobacter diversus*. *Klebsiella* and *Enterobacter* spp. and *Citrobacter freundii* are more resistant and the *Proteus* and *Serratia* spp. and *Yersinia pestis* are completely resistant ((Retsema *et al.*, 1987; Smith *et al.*, 1995).

Among the Gram-negative anaerobic bacteria, the *Prevotella* spp. such as *P. melaninogenica*, *P. oralis*, *P. intermedia* and *P. disiens* are azithromycin-sensitive. The same is true of *Fusobacterium* spp. *Actinobacillus actinomycetemcomitans* and *Eikenella corrodens* are also sensitive. *Veillonela* spp., *Bacteroides fragilis* and other members of the *B. fragilis* group are moderately resistant (Barry *et al.*, 1988; Kitzis *et al.*, 1990; Pajukanta *et al.*, 1992; Williams *et al.*, 1992; Goldstein *et al.*, 1995).

The explanation why azithromycin is more active than erythromycin against Gram-negative bacteria is probably because of the former's better penetration across the bacterial permeability barriers. It is unlikely that azithromycin passes more easily through the usual porins in the outer membrane (p. 26), but azithromycin has an extra positive charge created by the presence of a methyl-substituted nitrogen in the 15-membered macrolide ring (p. 653). This may allow it to have a better access to the self-promoted uptake pathway through the bacterial cell wall (Farmer *et al.*, 1992; Pruul and McDonald, 1992).

3 Mycobacteria

Azithromycin is active against *Mycobacterium avium* complex. Its activity has been assessed in *in vitro* cultures of human macrophages infected by *Mycobacterium avium* and also in *in vivo* models of infected beige mice or immunosuppressed rats. Some studies have shown azithromycin to be somewhat less active than clarithromycin (p. 644) but others have found the two drugs to be of about equal activity (Bermudez and Young, 1988; Perronne *et al.*, 1991; Cynamon and Klemens, 1992; Brown *et al.*, 1993; Klemens and Cynamon, 1994b). Azithromycin encapsulated in stable liposomes appears superior to the non-encapsulated drug in inhibition of *M. avium* growth within cultured macrophages (Oh *et al.*, 1995).

Against some other non-tuberculous mycobacteria, such as *M. kansasii*, *M. xenopi*, *M. simiae* and *M. malmoense*, azithromycin has good and comparable activity with clarithromycin (Klemens and Cynamon, 1994a).

4 Other organisms

Mycoplasma pneumoniae is highly sensitive to azithromycin (Ishida *et al.*, 1994). Both *Chlamydia trachomatis* and *Chlamydia pneumoniae* have been extensively studied *in vitro* and in experimental animals, and all authors have found them azithromycin-sensitive. *Chlamydia psittaci* is also susceptible (Walsh *et al.*, 1987; Engel, 1992; Hammerschlag *et al.*, 1992; Welsh *et al.*, 1992; Agacfidan *et al.*, 1993; Niki *et al.*, 1994; Malinverni *et al.*, 1995). Results of clinical studies indicate that the drug is also effective against *Ureaplasma urealyticum* (Steingrimsson *et al.*, 1990, 1994). Azithromycin is active against *Treponema pallidum* infection in a rabbit model (Lukehart *et al.*, 1990). *Borrelia burgdorferi* is also sensitive, both *in vitro* and in experimental animals (Johnson *et al.*, 1990).

Several *in vitro* microassays have been developed to study the efficacy of antimicrobial agents against *Toxoplasma gondii*. Results with these *in vitro* methods plus studies in animals have demonstrated that azithromycin has potent activity against this parasite and that it is more active than erythromycin or spiramycin (Araujo *et al.*, 1988; Chamberland *et al.*, 1991; Huskinson-Mark *et al.*, 1991; Dumas *et al.*, 1994). Azithromycin inhibits *T. gondii* protein synthesis (Blais *et al.*, 1993). Azithromycin plus pyrimethamine (p. 906) in one *in vitro* study only showed an additive effect on this parasite and true synergism was not demonstrated (Cantin and Chamberland, 1993). However, in an animal study Derouin *et al.* (1992) observed marked synergism with azithromycin/pyrimethamine and azithromycin/sulfadiazine against *T. gondii*. Mutants resistant to azithromycin, spiramycin and clindamycin can be selected in the *in vitro* cultures of this parasite (Pfefferkorn and Borotz, 1994).

	MIC (μg per ml)	
Organisms	Azithromycin	Erythromycin
Gram-positive bacteria		
Staphylococcus aureus	2.0	0.5
Streptococcus pneumoniae	2.0	0.12
Enterococcus spp.	16.0	4.0
Gram-negative bacteria		
Neisseria gonorrhoeae	0.25	1.0
Haemophilus influenzae	4.0	16.0
Moraxella catarrhalis	0.12	0.5
Legionella spp.	2.0	1.0
Campylobacter spp.	0.5	2.0
Salmonella enteritidis	2.0	64.0
Shigella flexneri	1.0	16.0
Bacteroides fragilis	>16.0	>16.0
Prevotella melaninogenica	0.5	4.0
Chlamydia spp.		
Chlamydia trachomatis	0.125	0.5
Chlamydia pneumoniae	0.125	0.25

Table I.49
Compiled from data published by Retsema *et al.* (1987), Barry *et al.* (1988), Williams *et al.* (1992) and Niki *et al.* (1994)

Rehg (1991) demonstrated that azithromycin had some activity against *Cryptosporidium parvum* in immunosuppressed animals. It was more effective than spiramycin. In the same animals azithromycin was more effective than paramomycin (p. 534) against *Cryptosporidium* infection involving the ileum, cecum or biliary tract (Rehg, 1994). Azithromycin also has some activity against malaria parasites (Gingras and Jensen, 1993; Andersen *et al.*, 1994).

5 Minimum inhibitory concentrations

The MICs of azithromycin against some selected bacterial and chlamydial spp. are shown in Table I.49. Those of erythromycin are included for comparison.

Mode of Administration and Dosage

Azithromycin is administered by the oral route. The adult dose for mild to moderate illnesses, such as various respiratory tract infections, is 500 mg once-daily on the first day and 250 mg once-daily for the next 4 days. Alternatively 500 mg once-daily for only 3 days can be given (Foulds *et al.*, 1990; Bradbury, 1993; Foulds and Johnson, 1993). The dosage for children is 10 mg per kg as a single dose on day 1 of treatment followed by 5 mg per kg once-daily for the next 4 days. Alternatively 10 mg per kg, once-daily can be given for 3 days only (Hamill 1993; Nahata *et al.*, 1993, 1995; Schaad, 1993). Because of the high and persistent tissue concentrations these short courses of azithromycin are approximately equivalent to 10-day courses of oral erythromycin and other oral agents such as co-amoxiclav (p. 200) (Klein, 1994).

When azithromycin is included in a regimen to treat *M. avium* complex bacteremia in AIDS patients, the dosage recommended is 500 mg once-daily for long periods in adults and 10–20 mg per kg per day in children (Masur *et al.*, 1993; Benson, 1994). The dosage of azithromycin (combined with pyrimethamine, p. 907), used in trials for treatment of acute toxoplasmic encephalitis in AIDS patients has also been 500 mg daily for 4 weeks (Saba *et al.*, 1993).

As only some 4.5–6% of an administered dose of azithromycin is excreted in the urine as the active drug (Cooper *et al.*, 1990; Foulds *et al.*, 1990), dosage modification of the drug is not necessary in patients with renal failure. The elimination half-life of azithromycin is somewhat longer in patients with liver disease than in normal subjects, but in patients with mild to moderate liver cirrhosis its dosage need not be modified when only short courses (3–5 days) are given (Mazzei *et al.*, 1993).

Serum Levels in Relation to Dosage

After a single 500 mg oral dose of azithromycin a mean peak serum level of 0.4 μg per ml was reached in 2–4 h. The serum level thereafter declined to 0.1 μg per ml at 6 h and 0.04 μg per ml at 12 h. This initial rather rapid fall of serum levels was not due to the drug's elimination, but due to extensive uptake of azithromycin in the tissues. The half-life of the drug during this time was only 2.8 h. When a 3-day regimen of the drug was given (500 mg daily), the peak serum level after the last dose was 0.42 μg per ml. With a 5-day regimen (500 mg on first day and 250 mg daily for the next 4 days), the peak serum level after the last dose decreased to 0.18 μg per ml. After the last dose of both regimens, the elimination of azithromycin from plasma followed a polybasic pattern. The average half-life estimated from peak time to 8 h after administration was 2.4 h with the 3-day regimen an 2.2 h with the 5-day regimen. This again was mainly due to rapid uptake of the drug by tissues. During 8–48 h after the last dose the average apparent half-lives were 27.9 h (3-day regimen) and 35.8 h (5-day regimen). This second slow decline of the serum levels was probably largely because of elimination of the drug from the body. About 40% of an administered oral dose of azithromycin is absorbed (Cooper *et al.*, 1990; Foulds *et al.*, 1990; Wildfeuer *et al.*, 1993). The serum levels in children are similar to those in adults if they are given a single dose of azithromycin 10 mg per kg on day 1 and 5 mg per kg daily for the next 4 days (Nahata *et al.*, 1993).

Excretion

1 Urine

Only 4–6% of an orally administered dose of azithromycin is excreted via the kidney as the active drug (Cooper *et al.*, 1990; Wildfeuer *et al.*, 1993).

2 Bile and inactivation in body

Part of the absorbed dose of the drug may be eliminated via the bile, but most of it is presumably metabolized by the liver.

3 Distribution of the Drug in Body

The most important property of azithromycin is that it is very widely distributed in body fluids and tissues and most tissue levels are much higher than serum levels. In animals in some tissues the levels of the drug were 100-fold higher than those in the serum. Concentrations were particularly high in spleen, liver, kidneys, lung, lymph nodes and tonsils, but they were some 10-fold lower in muscle and fat. Azithromycin tissue levels were 20-fold higher in eye than those in serum, but only 1.2-fold higher in the brain (Shepard and Falkner, 1990). In animals with induced infections due to *Strep. pyogenes*, *Strep. pneumoniae*, Group B. streptococci, *H. influenzae* and *Legionella pneumophila* the drug was very effective and this correlated with its high tissue levels in the infected organs (Girard *et al.*, 1987; Tissi *et al.*, 1995). But in experimental *Staph. aureus* osteomyelitis, azithromycin was less effective than rifampicin or clindamycin, despite the fact that the peak azithromycin concentration in bone was more than 30 times higher than levels in the serum (O'Reilly *et al.*, 1992).

Azithromycin is highly concentrated in polymorphonuclear leukocytes (Bonnet and Van der Auwera, 1992). There is evidence from animal and human volunteer studies that neutrophils migrate to sites of infection and may release the drug in the infected environment. This may further increase its concentration in infected tissues (Gladue *et al.*, 1989; Frank *et al.*, 1992; Vallee *et al.*, 1992; Veber *et al.*, 1993; Freeman *et al.*, 1994; Mandell, 1994). Despite the high concentrations of azithromycin in granulocytes, paradoxically Meyer *et al.* (1993) could not demonstrate enhanced killing of *Staph. aureus* ingested by neutrophils. However, there was an enhanced killing of *Staph. aureus* within human monocytes which also have high intracellular concentrations of the drug.

Azithromycin is also concentrated in macrophages and the concentration of the drug in these cells was further enhanced in experimental animals infected by *L. pneumophila*, when the macrophages had ingested intracellular organisms (Stamler *et al.*, 1994). The same is true of macrophages which contain *M. avium* and the azithromycin concentration in these cells was further enhanced if they were stimulated by tumor necrosis factor or recombinant human gamma interferon (Bermudez *et al.*, 1991). Azithromycin is also concentrated in *T. gondii* infected macrophages (Blais *et al.*, 1994; Schwab *et al.*, 1994). This may explain why azithromycin has some effect in cerebral toxoplasmosis. In addition, Dumas *et al.* (1994) found that in animals with induced cerebral toxoplasmosis, the concentrations of azithromycin in the brains ranged from 0.7 to 2.3 μg per g, which is higher than the usual serum levels. The normal brain is the only tissue in which azithromycin levels are only about the same as those in the serum (p. 656).

The drug is also concentrated in human skin fibroblasts (Gladue and Snider, 1990) and in human endometrial epithelial cells, but when the latter were infected by *C. trachomatis*, the concentration of azithromycin in them remained much the same (Raulston, 1994). In women with cervical chlamydial infection, after a single oral 1-g dose of the drug, the azithromycin concentrations in cervical mucus on day 7 and day 14 after this dose were still higher than the MIC of *C. trachomatis* (Worm and Østerlind, 1995).

The serum protein binding of azithromycin varies with its concentration in the serum. At concentrations of 0.02 and 0.05 μg per ml, the protein binding was approximately 50%. The binding declined to 23% at 0.1 μg per ml, 18% at 0.3 μg per ml, 12% at 0.5 μg per ml and 7.5% at 1.0 μg per ml (Foulds *et al.*, 1990).

Mode of Action

The mode of action of azithromycin on bacteria is similar to that of other macrolides (p. 614). It also inhibits *T. gondii* protein synthesis (Blais *et al.*, 1993). Similar to other macrolides, azithromycin appears to have actions in body other than just antibacterial activity. It may prevent tissue damage in body caused by *Ps. aeruginosa* and in this respect it appears more potent than other macrolides (p. 614) (Molinari *et al.*, 1993).

Toxicity

Azithromycin appears to be a safe drug and mild gastrointestinal symptoms have been the main side-effect. Skin rashes have been rarely seen. Similarly, headache or dizziness have been occasionally noted. The drug has had no consistent effect on laboratory safety tests (Hopkins, 1991, 1993; Hopkins and Williams, 1995). The principal side-effect in AIDS patients has also been loose stools or diarrhea, usually not necessitating cessation of treatment (Young *et al.*, 1991). In addition abnormal liver function tests and reversible hearing loss has been reported when azithromycin in a dose of 500 mg daily has been used in AIDS patients long-term (Saba *et al.*, 1993; Wallace *et al.*, 1994a).

Unlike erythromycin (p. 616), azithromycin does not inhibit the metabolism of other drugs by the liver (Amacher *et al.*, 1991). It has no effect on serum zidovudine levels in AIDS patients (Chave *et al.*, 1992). It also has no effect on terfenadine pharmacokinetics or cardiac pharmacodynamics (Honig *et al.*, 1994).

Clinical Uses of the Drug

1 Mycobacterium avium complex infection in AIDS patients

In an uncontrolled phase I trial azithromycin was given at a dose of 500 mg per day to patients with AIDS and *M. avium* bacteremia for variable lengths of time. Quantitative blood levels of *M. avium* decreased for patients who had 5, 20 or 30 days of azithromycin therapy. Most patients treated for 2 days or more reported resolution of fever and night sweats, but other symptoms such as fatigue continued (Young *et al.*, 1991). For treatment of this condition a regimen of two, three or four drugs should be used. Although there is less clinical experience so far with azithromycin than with clarithromycin, it is recommended that azithromycin can be a suitable alternative to clarithromycin as the number one drug for the treatment regimen. The second, third or possibly fourth drugs should be the same as when clarithromycin is used as the first drug (p. 648) (Masur *et al.*, 1993; Benson, 1994). Once-weekly dosage of 1200 mg azithromycin is also effective for prophylaxis against disseminated *M. avium* complex disease in AIDS patients (Havlir *et al.*, 1996).

2 Toxoplasmic encephalitis in AIDS patients

Azithromycin, used as a single drug is not effective for this condition (Luft and Remington, 1992; Lane *et al.*, 1994). However, azithromycin combined with pyrimethamine may be more effective. In an uncontrolled study 14 AIDS patients who had toxoplasmic encephalitis were treated by 500 mg of azithromycin daily plus pyrimethamine 75 mg daily for 4 weeks; eight of them were evaluable for clinical response and five responded favorably (Saba *et al.*, 1993).

3 Salmonella infections

In animal studies azithromycin was as effective as ciprofloxacin for *Salmonella typhimurium* infections (Butler and Girard, 1993). However, in three of four patients with typhoid fever there was no clinical response by the 4th and 5th days, when azithromycin was used in a dosage of 1 g on day 1 and then 500 mg daily. Probably the low serum levels of azithromycin (p. 656) were inadequate to clear the *Salm. typhi* bacteremia (Wallace *et al.*, 1994b).

4 Syphilis

In a pilot study, azithromycin in a dose of 500 mg daily for 10 days was effective for primary or secondary syphilis in 11 of 13 HIV-negative patients. Further trials and assessment of other dosage regimens are indicated (Verdon *et al.*, 1994).

5 Bacillary angiomatosis

One AIDS patient with this disease responded rapidly to a 14-day course of azithromycin 1 g daily (Guerra *et al.*, 1993). This disease, caused by *Bartonella* (*Rochalimaea*) spp. is known to respond well to erythromycin therapy (p. 619).

6 Malaria chemoprophylaxis

In a human volunteer study four subjects received 500 mg of azithromycin orally on day 1, followed by 250 mg daily for 7 further days. They were infected by a chloroquine-resistant strain of *Pl. falciparum* on the 3rd day. Three of the four subjects were protected compared with none of 15 controls. The volunteer not protected had low serum levels of the drug, probably because of poor absorption (Kuschner *et al.*, 1994).

In another human volunteer study two cohorts of ten volunteers were used. For cohort 1, azithromycin 500 mg on first day and then 250 mg daily were given for 14 days before challenge with *P. falciparium*-infected mosquitos and the drug was continued for 7 days after the challenge. In this group, only four of the ten volunteers did not develop parasitemia. However, in cohort 2 (ten volunteers) azithromycin again in the same dosage was started 14 days before the challenge, but continued for 28 days after the challenge. None of these volunteers developed parasitemia. It was concluded that azithromycin may be as effective as mefloquine or doxycycline as a prophylactic agent for malaria (Anderson *et al.*, 1995).

7 Gonorrhea

A single-dose of azithromycin 2 g orally cures uncomplicated gonorrhea, but this high dose causes gastrointestinal symptoms and other drugs are preferred to treat this disease (pp. 361, 412) (Moran and Levine, 1995).

8 Non-gonococcal urethritis and trachoma

A single 1-g dose of azithromycin has comparable efficacy to a 7-day course of doxycycline 100 mg 12-hourly in both men and women with genital *Chlamydia trachomatis* infection. This disease caused by *Ureaplasma urealyticum* in men also responds to this single-dose azithromycin (Steingrimson *et al.*, 1994; Stamm *et al.*, 1995; Weber and Johnson, 1995). An advantage of azithromycin is that it allows directly administered single-dose therapy (Magid *et al.*, 1996).

Azithromycin is also a new promising drug for treatment of trachoma (Thylefors, 1966).

9 Chancroid

A single 1-g oral dose of azithromycin is as effective as a 250-mg i.m. dose of ceftriaxone (p. 362) for the treatment of this disease (Martin *et al.*, 1995).

10 Community-acquired respiratory tract infections

A shorter (3–5 day course) of azithromycin is as effective as a 5–10 day course of erythromycin and other older antibiotics such as amoxycillin, co-amoxiclav, cefaclor and others in most of these infections. However, the older antibiotics are cheaper and at this time are preferred to azithromycin. Azithromycin is quite effective for streptococcal pharyngitis (Hamill, 1993; Klein, 1994), otitis media (Schaad, 1993; Neu, 1995), acute bronchitis and acute exacerbation of chronic bronchitis (Mertens *et al.*, 1992; Hoepelman *et al.*, 1993). Community-acquired bacterial pneumonia also usually responds well to azithromycin (Kinasewitz and Wood, 1991; Myburgh *et al.*, 1993), as does pneumonia caused by *Mycoplasma pneumoniae* (Bébéar *et al.*, 1993;

Schönwald *et al.*, 1994) and that caused by *Chlamydia pneumoniae* (Grayston, 1994; Hammerschlag, 1994). Chronic pharyngitis caused by *C. pneumoniae* may respond to a more prolonged azithromycin therapy (Falck *et al.*, 1995). In one study azithromycin, administered orally in a dose of 500 mg on the 1st day and 250 mg daily for further 4 days, or 500 mg once-daily for 3 days, proved to be effective therapy in 16 patients with community-acquired pneumonia caused by *Legionella pneumophila* (Kuzman *et al.*, 1995).

11 Campylobacter enteritis

Azithromycin in a dosage of 500 mg daily for 3 days was used with success in Thailand for this disease, where ciprofloxacin-resistant *Campylobacter* spp. strains were common (Kuschner *et al.*, 1995). However, another study in US troops deployed in Hat Yai in southern Thailand showed that 31% of *Campylobacter* spp. strains from patients with diarrhea were also azithromycin-resistant (Murphy *et al.*, 1996).

12 Lyme disease

In a progressive randomized study involving a total of 64 patients with erythema migrans, azithromycin in a dosage of 250 mg twice-daily for 2 days, followed by 250 mg once-daily for 8 days appeared to be of about the same efficacy as a 14-day course of either oral phenoxymethylpenicillin or oral doxycycline (Strle *et al.*, 1992). In another trial involving 246 adult patients with erthema migrans, azithromycin in a dosage of 500 mg once-daily for 7 days was compared with amoxycillin 500 mg three times daily for 20 days. Amoxycillin was definitely more effective than azithromycin in completely resolving the acute manifestations of the disease and preventing relapse within 180 days of infection (Luft *et al.*, 1996).

References

Agacfidan A, Moncada J, Schachter J (1993). *In vitro* activity of azithromycin (CP-62,993). against *Chlamydia trachomatis* and *Chlamydia pneumoniae*. *Antimicrob Ag Chemother* **37**: 1746.

Amacher DE, Schomaker SJ, Retsema JA (1991). Comparison of the effects of the new azalide antibiotic, azithromycin, and erythromycin estolate on rat liver cytochrome P-450. *Antimicrob Ag Chemother* **35**: 1186.

Andersen SL, Ager AL, McGreevy P *et al.* (1994). Efficacy of azithromycin as a causal prophylactic agent against murine malaria. *Antimicrob Ag Chemother* **38**: 1862.

Anderson SL, Berman J, Kuschner R *et al.* (1995). Prophylaxis of *Plasmodium falciparum* malaria with azithromycin administered to volunteers. *Ann Intern Med* **123**: 771.

Araujo FG, Guptill DR, Remington JS (1988). Azithromycin, a macrolide antibiotic with potent activity against *Toxoplasma gondii*. *Antimicrob Ag Chemother* **32**: 755.

Barry AL, Fuchs PC (1995). *In vitro* activities of a streptogramin (RP59500), three macrolides, and an azalide against four respiratory tract pathogens. *Antimicrob Ag Chemother* **39**: 238.

Barry AL, Jones RN, Thornsberry C (1988). *In vitro* activities of azithromycin (CP 62,493), clarithromycin (A-56268; TE-031), erythromycin, roxithromycin and clindamycin. *Antimicrob Ag Chemother* **32**: 752.

Bébéar C, Dupon M, Renaudin H, de Barbeyrac B (1993). Potential improvements in therapeutic options for Mycoplasmal respiratory infections. *Clin Infect Dis* **17** (Suppl 1): 202.

Benson CA (1994). Treatment of disseminated disease due to the *Mycobacterium avium* complex in patients with AIDS. *Clin Infect Dis* **18** (Suppl 3): 237.

Bermudez LEM, Young LS (1988). Activities of amikacin, roxithromycin, and azithromycin alone or in combination with tumor necrosis factor against *Mycobacterium avium* complex. *Antimicrob Ag Chemother* **32**: 1149.

Bermudez LE, Inderlied C, Young LS (1991). Stimulation with cytokines enhances penetration of azithromycin into human macrophages. *Antimicrob Ag Chemother* **35**: 2625.

Blais J, Garneau V, Chamberland S (1993). Inhibition of *Toxoplasma gondii* protein synthesis by azythromycin. *Antimicrob Ag Chemother* **37**: 1701.

Blais J, Beauchamp D, Chamberland S (1994). Azithromycin uptake and intracellular accumulation by *Toxoplasma gondii*-infected macrophages. *J Antimicrob Chemother* **34**: 371.

Bonnet M, Van der Auwera P (1992). *In vitro* and *in vivo* intraleukocytic accumulation of azithromycin (CP-62,993). and its influence on *ex vivo* leukocyte chemiluminescence. *Antimicrob Ag Chemother* **36**: 1302.

Bradbury F (1993). Comparison of azithromycin versus clarithromycin in the treatment of patients with lower respiratory tract infections. *J Antimicrob Chemother* **31** (Suppl E): 153.

Brown ST, Edwards FF, Bernard EM *et al.* (1993). Azithromycin, rifabutin, and rifapentine for treatment and prophylaxis of *Mycobacterium avium* complex in rats treated with cyclosporine. *Antimicrob Ag Chemother* **37**: 398.

Butler T, Girard AE (1993). Comparative efficacies of azithromycin and ciprofloxacin against experimental *Salmonella typhimurium* infection in mice. *J Antimicrob Chemother* **31**: 313.

Cantin L, Chamberland S (1993). *In vitro* evaluation of the activities of azithromycin alone and combined with pyrimethamine against *Toxoplasma gondii*. *Antimicrob Ag Chemother* **37**: 1993.

Chamberland S, Kirst HA, Current WL (1991). Comparative activity of macrolides against *Toxoplasma gondii* demonstrating utility of an *in vitro* microassay. *Antimicrob Ag Chemother* **35**: 903.

Chave J-P, Munafo A, Chatton J-Y *et al.* (1992). Once-a-week azithromycin in AIDS patients: tolerability, kinetics, and effects on zidovudine disposition. *Antimicrob Ag Chemother* **36**: 1013.

Cooper MA, Nye K, Andrews JM, Wise R (1990). The pharmacokinetics and inflammatory fluid penetration of orally administered azithromycin. *J Antimicrob Chemother* **26**: 533.

Cynamon MH, Klemens SP (1992). Activity of azithromycin against *Mycobacterium avium* infections in beige mice. *Antimicrob Ag Chemother* **36**: 1611.

Derouin F, Almadany R, Chau F et al. (1992). Synergistic activity of azithromycin and pyrimethamine or sulfadiazine in acute experimental toxoplasmosis. *Antimicrob Ag Chemother* **36**: 997.

Donowitz GR, Earnhardt KI (1993). Azithromycin inhibition of intracellular *Legionella micdadei*. *Antimicrob Ag Chemother* **37**: 2261.

Dumas J-L, Chang R, Mermillod B et al. (1994). Evaluation of the efficacy of prolonged administration of azithromycin in a murine model of chronic toxoplasmosis. *J Antimicrob Chemother* **34**: 111.

Dunkin KT, Jones S, Howard AJ (1988). The in vitro activity of CP-62,993 against *Haemophilus influenzae*, *Branhamella catarrhalis*, staphylococci and streptococci. *J Antimicrob Chemother* **21**: 405.

Edelstein PH, Edelstein MAC (1991). *In vitro* activity of azithromycin against clinical isolates of *Legionella* species. *Antimicrob Ag Chemother* **35**: 180.

Endtz HP, Broeren M, Muton RP (1993). *In vitro* susceptibility of quinolone-resistant *Campylobacter jejuni* to new macrolide antibiotics. *Eur J Clin Microbiol Infect Dis* **12**: 48.

Engel JN (1992). Azithromycin-induced block of elementary body formation in *Chlamydia trachomatis*. *Antimicrob Ag Chemother* **36**: 2304.

Falck G, Heyman L, Gnarpe J, Gnarpe H (1995). *Chlamydia pneumoniae* and chronic pharyngitis. *Scand J Infect Dis* **27**: 179.

Farmer S, Li Z, Hancock REW (1992). Influence of outer membrane mutations on susceptibility of *Escherichia coli* to the dibasic macrolide azithromycin. *J Antimicrob Chemother* **29**: 27.

Foulds G, Johnson RB (1993). Selection of dose regimens of azithromycin. *J Antimicrob Chemother* **31** (Suppl E): 39.

Foulds G, Shepard RM, Johnson RB (1990). The pharmacokinetics of azithromycin in human serum and tissues. *J Antimicrob Chemother* **25** (Suppl A): 73.

Frank MO, Sullivan GW, Carper HT, Mandell GL (1992). *In vitro* demonstration of transport and delivery of antibiotics by polymorphonuclear leukocytes. *Antimicrob Ag Chemother* **36**: 2584.

Freeman CD, Nightingale CH, Nicolau DP et al. (1994). Intracellular and extracellular penetration of azithromycin into inflammatory and non-inflammatory blister fluid. *Antimicrob Ag Chemother* **38**: 2449.

Garcia-Rodriguez JA, Bellido JLM, Fresnadillo MJ, Trujillano I (1993). *In vitro* activities of new macrolides and rifapentine against Brucella spp. *Antimicrob Ag Chemother* **37**: 911.

Gingras BA, Jensen JB (1993). Antimalarial activity of azithromycin and erythromycin against *Plasmodium berghei*. *Am J Trop Med Hyg* **49**: 101.

Girard AE, Girard D, English AR et al. (1987). Pharmacokinetic and in vivo studies with azithromycin (CP-62,993), a new macrolide with an extended half-life and excellent tissue distribution. *Antimicrob Ag Chemother* **31**: 1948.

Gladue RP, Snider ME (1990). Intracellular accumulation of azithromycin by cultured human fibroblasts. *Antimicrob Ag Chemother* **34**: 1056.

Gladue RP, Bright GM, Isaacson RE, Newborg MF (1989). *In vitro* and *in vivo* uptake of azithromycin (CP-62,993) by phagocytic cells: possible mechanism of delivery and release at sites of infection. *Antimicrob Ag Chemother* **33**: 277.

Goldstein EJC, Nesbit CA, Citron DM (1995). Comparative *in vitro* activities of azithromycin, Bay Y 3118, levofloxacin, sparfloxacin, and 11 other oral antimicrobial agents against 194 aerobic and anaerobic bite wound isolates. *Antimicrob Ag Chemother* **39**: 1097.

Goldstein FW, Emirian MF, Coutrot A, Acar JF (1990). Bacteriostatic and bactericidal activity of azithromycin against *Haemophilus influenzae*. *J Antimicrob Chemother* **25** (Suppl A): 25.

Gordillo ME, Singh KV, Murray BE (1993). *In vitro* activity of azithromycin against bacterial enteric pathogens. *Antimicrob Ag Chemother* **37**: 1203.

Grayston JT (1994). *Chlamydia pneumoniae* (TWAR) infection in children. *Pediatr Infect Dis J* **13**: 675.

Guerra LG, Neira CJ, Boman D et al. (1993). Rapid response of AIDS-related bacillary angiomatosis to azithromycin. *Clin Infect Dis* **17**: 264.

Hamill J (1993). Multicentre evaluation of azithromycin and penicillin V in the treatment of acute streptococcal pharyngitis and tonsillitis in children. *J Antimicrob Chemother* **31** (Suppl E): 89.

Hammerschlag MR (1994). Antimicrobial susceptibility and therapy of infections caused by *Chlamydia pneumoniae*. *Antimicrob Ag Chemother* **38**: 1873.

Hammerschlag MR, Qumei KK, Roblin PM (1992). *In vitro* activities of azithromycin, clarithromycin, L-ofloxacin and other antibiotics against *Chlamydia pneumoniae*. *Antimicrob Ag Chemother* **36**: 1573.

Havlir DV, Dube MP, Sattler FR et al. (1996). Prophylaxis against disseminated *Mycobacterium avium* complex with weekly azithromycin, daily rifabutin or both. *New Engl J Med* **335**: 392.

Hoepelman AIM, Sips AP, Van Helmond JLM et al. (1993). A single-blind comparison of three-day azithromycin and ten-day co-amoxiclav treatment of acute lower respiratory tract infections. *J Antimicrob Chemother* **31** (Suppl E): 147.

Honig PK, Wortham DC, Zamani K, Cantilena LR (1994). Comparison of the effect of the macrolide antibiotics erythromycin, clarithromycin and azithromycin on terfenadine steady-state pharmacokinetics and electro-cardiographic parameters. *Drug Invest* **7**: 148.

Hopkins S (1991). Clinical toleration and safety of azithromycin. *Amer J Med* **91** (Suppl 3A): 40.

Hopkins S (1993). Clinical safety and tolerance of azithromycin in children. *J Antimicrob Chemother* **31** (Suppl E): 111.

Hopkins SJ, Williams D (1995). Clinical tolerability and safety of azithromycin in children. *Pediatr Infect Dis J* **14**: S67.

Hsueh P-R, Chen H-M, Huang H-A, Wu J-J (1995). Decreased activity of erythromycin against *Streptococcus pyogenes* in Taiwan. *Antimicrob Ag Chemother* **39**: 2239.

Huskinson-Mark J, Araujo FG, Remington JS (1991). Evaluation of the effect of drugs on the cyst form of *Toxoplasma gondii*. *J Infect Dis* **164**: 170.

Ishida K, Kaku M, Irifune K et al. (1994). *In vitro* and in vivo activities of macrolides against *Mycoplasma pneumoniae*. *Antimicrob Ag Chemother* **38**: 790.

Johnson RC, Kodner C, Russell M, Girard D (1990). *In-vitro* and *in-vivo* susceptibility of *Borrelia burgdorferi* to azithromycin. *J Antimicrob Chemother* **25**: (Suppl A): 33.

Kinasewitz G, Wood RG (1991). Azithromycin versus cefaclor in the treatment of acute bacterial pneumonia. *Eur J Clin Microbiol Infect Dis* **10**: 872.

Kitzis MD, Goldstein FW, Miegi M, Acar JF (1990). *In vitro* activity of azithromycin against various Gram-negative bacilli and anaerobic bacteria. *J Antimicrob Chemother* **25** (Suppl A): 15.

Klein JO (1994). Management of streptococcal pharyngitis. *Pediatr Infect Dis J* **13**: 572.

Klemens SP, Cynamon MH (1994a). Activities of azithromycin and clarithromycin against non-tuberculous *Mycobacteria* in beige mice. *Antimicrob Ag Chemother* **38**: 1455.

Klemens SP, Cynamon MH (1994b). Intermittent azithromycin for treatment of *Mycobacterium avium* infection in beige mice. *Antimicrob Ag Chemother* **38**: 1721.

Kuschner RA, Heppner DG, Andersen SL et al. (1994). Azithromycin prophylaxis against a chloroquine-resistant strain of *Plasmodium falciparum*. *Lancet* **343**: 1394.

Kuschner RA, Trofa AF, Thomas RJ et al. (1995). Use of azithromycin for the treatment of *Campylobacter enteritis* in travellers to Thailand, an area where ciprofloxacin resistance is prevalent. *Clin Infect Dis* **21**: 536.

Kuzman I, Soldo I, Schönwald S, Čulig J (1995). Azithromycin for treatment of community acquired pneumonia caused by *Legionella pneumophila*: a retrospective study. *Scand J Infect Dis* **27**: 503.

Landinez R, Liñares J, Loza E et al. (1992). *In vitro* activity of azithromycin and tetracycline against 358 clinical isolates of *Brucella melitensis*. *Eur J Clin Microbiol Infect Dis* **11**: 265.

Lane HC, Laughon BE, Falloon J (1994). Recent advances in the management of AIDS-related opportunistic infections. *Ann Intern Med* **120**: 945.

Luft BJ, Remington JS (1992). Toxoplasmic encephalitis in AIDS. *Clin Infect Dis* **15**: 211.

Luft BJ, Dattwyler RJ, Johnson RC *et al.* (1996). Azithromycin compared with amoxicillin in the treatment of erythema migrans. A double-blind, randomized, controlled trial. *Ann Intern Med* **124**: 785.

Lukehart SA, Fohn MJ, Baker-Zander SA (1990). Efficacy of azithromycin for therapy of active syphilis in the rabbit model. *J Antimicrob Chemother* **25** (Suppl A): 91.

Magid D, Douglas JMJr, Schwartz JS (1996). Doxycycline compared with azithromycin for treating women with genital *Chlamydia trachomatis* infections: an incremental cost-effective analysis. *Ann Intern Med* **124**: 389.

Malinverni R, Kuo C-C, Campbell LA *et al.* (1995). Effects of two antibiotic regimens on course and persistence of experimental *Chlamydia pneumoniae* TWAR pneumonitis. *Antimicrob Ag Chemother* **39**: 45.

Mandell GL (1994). Delivery of antibiotics by phagocytes. *Clin Infect Dis* **19**: 922.

Martin DH, Sargent SJ, Wendel GDJr *et al.* (1995). Comparison of azithromycin and ceftriaxone for the treatment of chancroid. *Clin Infect Dis* **21**: 409.

Maskell JP, Sefton AM, Williams JD (1990). Comparative *in-vitro* activity of azithromycin and erythromycin against Gram-positive cocci, *Haemophilus influenzae* and anaerobes. *J Antimicrob Chemother* **25** (Suppl A): 19.

Masur H and the Public Health Service Task Force on Prophylaxis and Therapy for *Mycobacterium avium* complex (1993). Recommendations on prophylaxis and therapy for disseminated *Mycobacterium avium* complex disease in patients infected with the human immunodeficiency virus. *New Engl J Med* **329**: 898.

Mazzei T, Surrenti C, Novelli A *et al.* (1993). Pharmacokinetics of azithromycin in patients with impaired hepatic function. *J Antimicrob Chemother* **31** (Suppl E): 57.

Mertens JCC, Van Berneveld PWC, Asin HRG *et al.* (1992). Double-blind randomized study comparing the efficacies and safeties of a short (3-day). course of azithromycin and a 5-day course of amoxicillin in patients with acute exacerbations of chronic bronchitis. *Antimicrob Ag Chemother* **36**: 1456.

Meyer AP, Bril-Bazuin C, Mattie H, Van den Broek PJ (1993). Uptake of azithromycin by human monocytes and enhanced intracellular antibacterial activity against *Staphylococcus aureus*. *Antimicrob Ag Chemother* **37**: 2318.

Molinari G, Guzmán CA, Pesce A, Schito GC (1993). Inhibition of *Pseudomonas aeruginosa* virulence factors by subinhibitory concentrations of azithromycin and other macrolide antibiotics. *J Antimicrob Chemother* **31**: 681.

Moran JS, Levine WC (1995). Drugs of choice for the treatment of uncomplicated gonococcal infections. *Clin Infect Dis* **20** (Suppl 1): 47.

Motley M, Sarafian SK, Knapp JS *et al.* (1992). Correlation between *in vitro* antimicrobial susceptibilities and beta-lactamase plasmid contents of isolates of *Haemophilus ducreyi* from the United States. *Antimicrob Ag Chemother* **36**: 1639.

Murphy GS, Echeverria P, Jackson LR *et al.* (1996). Ciprofloxacin- and azithromycin- resistant *Campylobacter* causing travelers' diarrhea in US troops deployed to Thailand in1994. *Clin Infect Dis* **22**: 868.

Myburgh J, Nagel GJ, Petschel E (1993). The efficacy and tolerance of a three-day course of azithromycin in the treatment of community-acquired pneumonia. *J Antimicrob Chemother* **31** (Suppl E): 163.

Nahata MC, Koranyi KI, Gadgil SD *et al.* (1993). Pharmacokinetics of azithromycin in pediatric patients after oral administration of multiple doses of suspension. *Antimicrob Ag Chemother* **37**: 314.

Nahata MC, Koranyi KI, Luke DR, Foulds G (1995). Pharmacokinetics of azithromycin in pediatric patients with acute otitis media. *Antimicrob Ag Chemother* **39**: 1875.

Neu HC (1995). Otitis media: antibiotic resistance of causative pathogens and treatment alternatives. *Pediatr Infect Dis J* **14**: S51.

Niki Y, Kumura M, Miyashita N, Soejima R (1994). *In vitro* and *in vivo* activities of azithromycin, a new azalide antibiotic, against *Chlamydia*. *Antimicrob Ag Chemother* **38**: 2296.

Oh Y-K, Nix DE, Straubinger RM (1995). Formulation and efficacy of liposome-encapsulated antibiotics for therapy of intracellular *Mycobacterium avium* infection. *Antimicrob Ag Chemother* **39**: 2104.

O'Reilly T, Kunz S, Sande E *et al.* (1992). Relationship between antibiotic concentration in bone and efficacy of treatment of staphylococcal osteomyelitis in rats: azithromycin compared with clindamycin and rifampin. *Antimicrob Ag Chemother* **36**: 2693.

Pajukanta R, Asikainen S, Saarela M *et al.* (1992). *In vitro* activity of azithromycin compared with that of erythromycin against *Actinobacillus actinomycetemcomitans*. *Antimicrob Ag Chemother* **36**: 1241.

Perronne C, Gikas A, Truffot-Pernot C *et al.* (1991). Activities of sparfloxacin, azithromycin, temafloxacin, and rifapentine compared with that of clarithromycin against multiplication of *Mycobacterium avium* complex within human macrophages. *Antimicrob Ag Chemother* **35**: 1356.

Pfefferkorn, ER, Borotz SE (1994). Comparison of mutants of *Toxoplasma gondii* selected for resistance to azithromycin, spiramycin, or clindamycin. *Antimicrob Ag Chemother* **38**: 31.

Pruul H, McDonald PJ (1992). Potentiation of azithromycin activity against *Escherichia coli* by human serum ultrafiltrate. *J Antimicrob Chemother* **30**: 497.

Rakita RM, Jacquez-Palaz K, Murray BE (1994). Intracellular activity of azithromycin against bacterial enteric pathogens. *Antimicrob Ag Chemother* **38**: 1915.

Raulston JE (1994). Pharmacokinetics of azithromycin and erythromycin in human endometrial epithelial cells and in cells infected with *Chlamydia trachomatis*. *J Antimicrob Chemother* **34**: 765.

Rautelin H, Renkonen O-V, Kosunen TU (1993). Azithromycin resistance in *Campylobacter jejuni* and *Campylobacter coli*. *Eur J Clin Microbiol Infect Dis* **12**: 864.

Rehg JE (1991). Activity of azithromycin against *Cryptosporidia* in immunosuppressed rats. *J Infect Dis* **163**: 1293.

Rehg JE (1994). A comparison of anticryptosporidial activity of paromomycin with that of other aminoglycosides and azithromycin in immunosuppressed rats. *J Infect Dis* **170**: 934.

Retsema J, Girard A, Schelkly W *et al.* (1987). Spectrum and mode of action of azithromycin (CP-62,993), a new 15-membered-ring macrolide with improved potency against Gram-negative organisms. *Antimicrob Ag Chemother* **31**: 1939.

Saba J, Morlat P, Raffi F *et al.* (1993). Pyrimethamine plus azithromycin for treatment of acute toxoplasmic encephalitis in patients with AIDS. *Eur J Clin Microbiol Infect Dis* **12**: 853.

Schaad UB (1993). Multicentre evaluation of azithromycin in comparison with co-amoxiclav for the treatment of acute otitis media in children. *J Antimicrob Chemother* **31** (Suppl E): 81.

Schönwald S, Baršic B, Klinar I, Gunjača M (1994). Three-day azithromycin compared with ten-day roxithromycin treatment of atypical pneumonia. *Scand J Infect Dis* **26**: 706.

Schwab JC, Cao Y, Slowik MR , Joiner KA (1994). Localization of azithromycin in *Toxoplasma gondii*-infected cells. *Antimicrob Ag Chemother* **38**: 1620.

Shepard RM, Falkner FC (1990). Pharmacokinetics of azithromycin in rats and dogs. *J Antimicrob Chemother* **25** (Suppl A): 49.

Slaney L, Chubb H, Ronald A, Brunham R (1990). *In vitro* activity of azithromycin, erythromycin, ciprofloxacin and norfloxacin against *Neisseria gonorrhoeae*, *Haemophilus ducreyi* and *Chlamydia trachomatis*. *J Antimicrob Chemother* **25** (Suppl A): 1.

Smith MD, Vinh DX, Hoa NTT *et al.* (1995). *In vitro* antimicrobial susceptibilities of strains of *Yersinia pestis*. *Antimicrob Ag Chemother* **39**: 2153.

Stamler DA, Edelstein MAC, Edelstein PH (1994). Azithromycin pharmacokinetics and intracellular concentrations in *Legionella pneumophila*-infected and uninfected guinea pigs and their alveolar macrophages. *Antimicrob Ag Chemother* **38**: 217.

Stamm WE, Hicks CB, Martin DH *et al.* (1995). Azithromycin for empirical treatment of the nongonococcal urethritis syndrome in men. A randomized double-blind study. *JAMA* **274**: 545.

Steingrimsson O, Olafsson JH, Thorarinsson H *et al.* (1990). Azithromycin in the treatment of sexually transmitted disease. *J Antimicrob Chemother* **25** (Suppl A): 109.

Steingrimsson O, Ólafsson JH, Thorarinsson H *et al.* (1994). Single dose azithromycin treatment of gonorrhea and infections caused by *C. trachomatis* and *U. urealyticum* in men. *Sex Transm Dis* **21**: 43.

Strle, F, Ruzic E, Cimperman J (1992). Erythema migrans: comparison of treatment with azithromycin, doxycycline and phenoxymethylpenicillin. *J Antimicrob Chemother* **30**: 543.

Taylor DE, Chang N (1991). *In vitro* susceptibilities of *Campylobacter jejuni* and *Campylobacter coli* to azithromycin and erythromycin. *Antimicrob Ag Chemother* **35**: 1917.

Thylefors B (1996). Azithromycin: a new opportunity for control of trachoma. *WHO Drug Information* **10**: 132.

Tissi L, von Hunolstein C, Mosci P *et al.* (1995). *In vivo* efficacy of azithromycin in treatment of systemic infection and septic arthritis induced by type IV Group B streptococcus strains in mice: comparative study with erythromycin and penicillin G. *Antimicrob Ag Chemother* **39**: 1938.

Vallee E, Azoulay-Dupuis E, Pocidalo J-J, Bergogne-Berezin E (1992). Activity and local delivery of azithromycin in a mouse model of *Haemophilus influenzae* lung infection. *Antimicrob Ag Chemother* **36**: 1412.

Veber B, Vallee E, Desmonts JM *et al.* (1993). Correlation between macrolide lung pharmacokinetics and therapeutic efficacy in a mouse model of pneumococcal pneumonia. *J Antimicrob Chemother* **32**: 473.

Verdon MS, Handsfield HH, Johnson RB (1994). Pilot study of azithromycin for treatment of primary and secondary syphilis. *Clin Infect Dis* **19**: 486.

Waldor MK, Mekalanos JJ (1994). Emergence of new cholera pandemic: molecular analysis of virulance determinants in *Vibrio cholerae* 0139 and

development of a live vaccine prototype *J Infect Dis* **170**: 278.

Wallace MR, Miller LK, Nguyen M-T, Shields AR (1994a). Ototoxicity with azithromycin. *Lancet* **343**: 241.

Wallace MR, Yousif AA, Habib NF, Tribble DR (1994b). Azithromycin and typhoid. *Lancet* **343**: 1497.

Walsh M, Kappus EW, Quinn TC (1987). *In vitro* evaluation of CP-62,993, erythromycin, clindamycin, and tetracycline against *Chlamydia trachomatis*. *Antimicrob Ag Chemother* **31**: 811.

Weber JT, Johnson RE (1995). New treatments for *Chlamydia trachomatis* genital infection. *Clin Infect Dis* **20** (Suppl 1): 66.

Welsh LE, Gaydos CA, Quinn TC (1992). *In vitro* evaluation of activities of azithromycin, erythromycin and tetracycline against *Chlamydia trachomatis* and *Chlamydia pneumoniae*. *Antimicrob Ag Chemother* **36**: 291.

Wildfeuer A, Laufen H, Leitold M, Zimmermann T (1993). Comparison of pharmacokinetics of three-day and five-day regimens of azithromycin in plasma and urine. *J Antimicrob Chemother* **31** (Suppl E): 51.

Williams JD, Maskell JP, Shain H *et al.* (1992). Comparative *in-vitro* activity of azithromycin, macrolides (erythromycin, clarithromycin and spiramycin). and streptogramin RP 59500 against oral organisms. *J Antimicrob Chemother* **30**: 27.

Worm A-M, Østerlind A (1995). Azithromycin levels in cervical mucus and plasma after a single 1.0 g oral dose for chlamydial cervicitis. *Genitourin Med* **71**: 244.

Yamamoto T, Nair GB, Albert MJ *et al.* (1995). Survey of *in vitro* susceptibilities of *Vibrio cholerae* 01 and 0139 to antimicrobial agents. *Antimicrob Ag Chemother* **39**: 241.

Young LS, Wiviott L, Wu M *et al.* (1991). Azithromycin for treatment of *Mycobacterium avium–intracellulare* complex infection in patients with AIDS. *Lancet* **338**: 1107.

Novobiocin

Description

Novobiocin was isolated from *Streptomyces niveus* in the Upjohn Research Laboratories and initially was given the generic name of 'Streptonivicin' (Smith *et al.*, 1956). It was also isolated almost simultaneously in other laboratories, and was given several other names. Novobiocin is no longer available commercially in most countries and is only seldom used. A short chapter on novobiocin is included in this book because of recent evidence that it is effective *in vitro* (French *et al.*, 1993) and *in vivo* (Quale *et al.*, 1994) against multiresistant strains of *Enterococcus faecium*.

Sensitive Organisms

1 Gram-positive cocci

Novobiocin is active against some of these bacteria, such as *Staphylococcus aureus* (including beta-lactamase-producing strains) and the pneumococcus. Its MIC against strains of methicillin-resistant *Staph. aureus* is ≤0.25 μg per ml (Walsh *et al.*, 1985), and against such strains when combined with rifampicin it shows neither synergy nor antagonism, but emergence of resistance to either agent seems prevented (Walsh *et al.*, 1986). *Streptococcus pyogenes* is much less sensitive and *Strep. viridans* strains vary in their sensitivity. *Enterococcus faecalis* is usually moderately resistant, but *E. faecium*, including multiresistant strains is sensitive (French *et al.*, 1993) (Table I.50).

2 Gram-positive bacilli

Gram-positive bacilli, such as *Bacillus anthracis*, *Clostridium tetani*, *Cl. perfringens* and *Corynebacterium diphtheriae*, are novobiocin-sensitive.

3 Gram-negative bacteria

Some of these, such as *Haemophilus influenzae* and the pathogenic *Neisseria* spp. are sensitive. *Proteus vulgaris* may be sensitive to moderate novobiocin concentrations, but other *Proteus* spp. are resistant. Other Gram-negative bacilli, such as *Escherichia coli*, *Enterobacter* and *Klebsiella* spp., salmonellae, shigellae and *Pseudomonas aeruginosa*, are novobiocin-resistant. Novobiocin alone may inhibit *Burkholderia (Pseudomonas) pseudomallei*, but only in concentrations that can be attained with very high systemic doses. However, *in vitro*, concentrations as low as 0.2 μg per ml, if combined with tetracycline, exert a bactericidal synergistic effect against this organism (Calabi, 1973).

4 Acquired resistance

Staphylococcus aureus and many other bacteria, usually sensitive to this drug readily acquire resistance following repeated subculturing *in vitro* in the presence of the antibiotic (Finland and Nichols, 1957).

5 Minimum inhibitory concentrations

Usual MICs of novobiocin against some selected bacteria are shown in Table I.50.

Organism	MIC (μg per ml)
Staphylococcus aureus	0.12–1.0
Streptococcus pyogenes	0.5–4.0
Streptococcus pneumoniae	0.5
Enterococcus faecalis	8.0–16.0
Enterococcus faecium	0.5–1.0
Clostridium perfringens	1.0
Neisseria gonorrhoeae	1.0–4.0
Haemophilus influenzae	1.0

Table I.50
Compiled from data published by *Today's Drugs* (1963) and French *et al.* (1993)

Mode of Administration and Dosage

1 Oral administration

Novobiocin is most commonly administered by the oral route. The usual adult dosage is 2 g per day, administered in four divided doses, and for children 30 mg per kg body weight per day, in four divided doses. The drug should not be administered to infants under 1 month old, because it may cause hyperbilirubinemia (p. 665). The dose of novobiocin may be varied. Smaller doses have been used to treat mild infections, and larger doses (4 g per day in adults and up to 100 mg per kg per day in children) for serious infections (Finland and Nichols, 1957).

2 Parenteral administration

Novobiocin may be given by i.m. injection, and the usual adult dose is 0.5 g 8-hourly. These injections are painful, and solutions of novobiocin are incompatible with procaine.

The drug can also be given i.v. If it is to be administered by continuous i.v. infusion, a 0.5-g dose should be dissolved in 5 ml of diluent, and then added to 500 ml isotonic saline for infusion in 6–8 h. Novobiocin is incompatible with 5% dextrose. Novobiocin can also be administered by intermittent i.v. injections, and, for this purpose, a 0.5-g dose should be diluted in at least 30 ml, before injection slowly into the drip tubing over a period of 5–10 min.

3 Patients with renal failure

Dosage modification is not necessary for patients with renal failure (Kunin, 1967).

4 Patients with liver disease

Novobiocin is best avoided in patients with liver disease, but if it is used, serum level monitoring and dose reduction may be necessary, because novobiocin is mainly excreted via the bile (p. 665).

Serum Levels in Relation to Dosage

Novobiocin is well absorbed from the alimentary tract. After a single oral dose of 0.5-g to adults, a peak serum level of 10–20 μg per ml is attained in 1–4 h. Thereafter, these levels fall slowly, but therapeutically effective levels may persist for 24 h or longer (Wright *et al.*, 1956). Doubling the dose doubles the serum concentrations. If a dose of 0.5 g is administered orally every 6 h, there is often some accumulation, and after four doses the peak serum level may reach 100 μg per ml (Martin *et al.*, 1955). When an oral dose of 0.5 g novobiocin was given orally twice-daily to adult volunteers for 27 doses, the mean serum concentration prior to dose 27 was 21.6 μg per ml; this rose to a mean peak serum level of 55.5 μg per ml 2 h after the dose. When oral rifampicin (300 mg 12-hourly) was given concomitantly, the comparative values before and after the 27th dose were 6.9 and 49.2 μg per ml, respectively. Similarly, novobiocin levels were lower when rifampicin was co-administered than when novobiocin was given alone at 8 h (7.9 versus 21.6 μg per ml) and at 12 h after the 27th dose (3.0 versus 16.0 μg per ml). The half-life of novobiocin (5.85 h) was reduced to 2.66 h when administered in combination with rifampicin. These changes were due to a change in novobiocin clearance rather than a change in its absorption (Drusano *et al.*, 1986).

Excretion

1 Urine

Only about 3% of administered novobiocin is excreted via the kidney, and urine concentrations of the active drug are usually lower than serum concentrations (Martin *et al.*, 1955).

2 Bile

Novobiocin is mainly excreted in the bile in which its concentration is usually high. The effect of rifampicin on serum levels of novobiocin (see above) suggests that rifampicin may induce hepatic metabolism of novobiocin or alternatively compete with the same protein binding site (Drusano *et al.*, 1986).

Distribution of the Drug in Body

Novobiocin slowly diffuses into most body tissues, but only small amounts penetrate into the CSF when the meninges are uninflamed, and concentrations in pleural and ascitic fluids are usually lower than simultaneous serum levels. Of the tissues studied, the liver and large intestine had the highest novobiocin content (Taylor *et al.*, 1956).

Novobiocin is one of the antibiotics which is most highly bound to serum proteins. Over 90% of the drug is reversibly bound to serum albumin, and some investigators have estimated its serum binding to be as high as 99.2% (Rolinson and Sutherland, 1965). *In vitro* its antibacterial activity is markedly decreased in the presence of 10% serum. Nevertheless, the drug is therapeutically effective (Leading article, 1966). This may be partly because the serum levels of novobiocin are usually quite high in relation to the MICs of highly susceptible organisms. The peak serum level of 'free novobiocin' after an oral dose of 0.5 g is 0.28 µg per ml (the total level being 35 µg per ml), which still exceeds the MIC (0.20 µg per ml) of a highly sensitive *Staph. aureus* (Rolinson, 1967). The significance of antibiotic serum binding is discussed on p. 95.

Mode of Action

Novobiocin inhibits DNA and bacterial protein synthesis by binding to DNA topoisomerase 11 (gyrase) an enzyme which is associated with the supercoiling of DNA (p. 971).

Toxicity

1 Gastrointestinal side-effects

Symptoms such as nausea, abdominal pain and diarrhea are fairly common with oral novobiocin therapy, but are usually not severe enough to necessitate cessation of treatment.

2 Hypersensitivity reactions

Erythematous or urticarial rashes are quite common, and may occur in 10–15% of patients if treatment is continued for 1 week or longer. Drug fever may also occur. More serious allergic manifestations, such as Stevens-Johnson syndrome, have also been encountered (Martin and Wellman, 1967). Hemorrhagic cutaneous lesions have been described, possibly due to a coumarin-like effect of the drug. Rarely allergic pneumonitis or myocarditis may occur (Riley, 1970).

3 Hematological changes

Eosinophilia is common, and usually occurs in association with hypersensitivity reactions. Rarely anemia, leucopenia, agranulocytosis, thrombocytopenia and pancytopenia have been reported (Martin and Wellman, 1967). Montgomery (1963) reported hemolytic anemia with positive direct and indirect Coombs' tests in a 6-year-old girl in association with novobiocin administration.

4 Interference with liver function

Yellow discoloration of sclerae, commonly seen in patients treated by novobiocin, is usually due to transient deposition of a harmless pigment derivative of the drug. However, in young children novobiocin may interfere with bilirubin conjugation, resulting in hyperbilirubinemia. This is particularly likely in newborns, in whom the enzyme systems for bilirubin conjugation are immature (Sutherland and Keller, 1961). For this reason, novobiocin is contraindicated in infants less than 1 month old.

The serum bilirubin should be estimated if scleral discoloration appears in older children or adults. A normal bilirubin indicates that the yellow color is due to novobiocin metabolites, and the drug need not be discontinued (Martin and Wellman, 1967).

Clinical Uses of the Drug

1 Staphylococcal infections

Novobiocin formerly had a role in the treatment of these infections. With the advent of the penicillinase-resistant penicillins and other anti-staphylococcal agents, novobiocin is no longer used for this indication, except perhaps as a adjunct to other drugs, for the treatment of methicillin-resistant staphylococcal infections. For instance, novobiocin/sodium fusidate and novobiocin/rifampicin combinations have been used successfully to treat staphylococcal infections of this nature (Jensen, 1968). These combinations have only been used to prevent the emergence of further drug-resistance among such strains, and there is no evidence that they act synergistically.

2 Multiresistant Enterococcus faecium infections

In an animal study Quale *et al.* (1994) found the combination of novobiocin plus ciprofloxacin effective for endocarditis caused by strains of *E. faecium* resistant to ampicillin, vancomycin and aminoglycosides. Further studies using this combination for infections due to multidrug-resistant strains of *E. faecium* are warranted.

References

Calibi O (1973). Bactericidal synergism of novobiocin and tetracycline against *Pseudomonas pseudomallei. J Med Microbiol* **6**: 293.

Drusano GL, Townsend RJ, Walsh TJ *et al.* (1986). Steady-state serum pharmacokinetics of novobiocin and rifampin alone and in combination. *Antimicrob Ag Chemother* **30**: 42.

Finland M, Nichols RL (1957). Novobiocin. *Practitioner* **179**: 84.

French P, Venuti E, Fraimow HS (1993). *In vitro* activity of novobiocin against multiresistant strains of *Enterococcus faecium. Antimicrob Ag Chemother* **37**: 2736.

Jensen K (1968). Methicillin-resistant staphylococci. *Lancet* **ii**: 1078.

Kunin CM (1967). A guide to use of antibiotics in patients with renal disease. *Ann Intern Med* **67**: 151.

Leading Article (1966). Serum binding of antibiotics. *Brit Med J* **1**: 1059.

Martin WJ, Wellman WE (1967). Clinically useful antimicrobial agents. *Postgrad Med* **42**: 350.

Martin WJ, Heilman FR, Nichols DR *et al.* (1955). Streptonivicin (albamycin): a new antibiotic; preliminary report. *Proc Mayo Clin* **30**: 540.

Montgomery JR (1963). Haemolytic reaction after novobiocin therapy. *New Engl J Med* **269**: 966.

Quale JM, Landman D, Mobarakai N (1994). Treatment of experimental endocarditis due to multidrug resistant *Enterococcus faecium* with ciprofloxacin and novobiocin. *J Antimicrob Chemother* **34**: 797.

Riley HD (1970). Vancomycin and novobiocin. *Med Clin N Amer* **54**: 1277.

Rolinson GN (1967). The significance of protein binding of antibiotics *in vitro* and *in vivo*. In *Recent Advances in Medical Microbiology* (Waterson AP, ed.), p. 254. Edinburgh: J & A Churchill.

Rolinson GN, Sutherland R (1965). The binding of antibiotics to serum proteins. *Brit J Pharmacol* **25**: 638.

Smith CG, Dietz A, Sokolski WT, Savage GM (1956). Streptonivicin, a new antibiotic. I. Discovery and biologic studies. *Antibiot Chemother* **6**: 135.

Sutherland JM, Keller WH (1961). Novobiocin and neonatal hyper-bilirubinemia. *Amer J Dis Child* **101**: 447.

Taylor RM, Miller WL, Van der Brook MJ (1956). Streptonivicin, a new antibiotic. V. Absorption, distribution and excretion. *Antibiot Chemother* **6**: 162.

Today's Drugs (1963). Alternatives to penicillin. *Brit Med J* **1**: 1213.

Walsh TJ, Hansen SL, Tatem BA *et al.* (1985). Activity of novobiocin against melthicillin-resistant *Staphylococcus aureus. J Antimicrob Chemother* **15**: 435.

Walsh TJ, Auger F, Tatem BA *et al.* (1986). Novobiocin and rifampicin in combination against methicillin-resistant *Staphylococcus aureus*; an *in-vitro* comparison with vancomycin plus rifampicin. *J Antimicrob Chemother* **17**: 75.

Wright WW, Putnam LE, Welch H (1956). Novobiocin: serum concentrations and urinary excretion following oral administration in man. *Antibiot Med* **2**: 311.

Polymyxins

Description

The polymyxins are a group of antibiotics, which were first isolated in 1947 from a spore-bearing soil bacillus (*Bacillus polymyxa*). It was soon shown that a number of chemically different polymyxins, named A, B, C, D and E could be obtained from different strains of this bacillus. These compounds, like bacitracin (p. 542), have a polypeptide structure.

Initially only polymyxin B in the form of its sulfate was commercially available. Polymyxin B was not available commercially in a pure form, and its activity and dosage were usually measured in units. One mg of pure polymyxin B is equivalent to 10 000 units, and commercial preparations contained not less than 6000 units per ml.

Colistin, which became available for clinical use in 1959, had been isolated in 1949 in Japan from *Bacillus polymyxa* var. *colistinus*. Initially it was thought to be a new antibiotic, but was soon shown to be identical with polymyxin E (Wilkinson, 1963). However, the drug was supplied in a new form as the sulfomethyl derivative (methane sulfonate) of polymyxin E, also known as colistimethate sodium. When polymyxin E (colistin) was marketed, a new unit was adopted, which was one-third the value of that used for polymyxin B. One mg of pure polymyxin E (colistin) was equivalent to 30 000 units.

The other polymyxins (A, C and D) are too toxic for clinical use.

Colistin methane sulfonate, when introduced, was represented as a better drug than polymyxin B sulfate on the grounds of reduced toxicity. The methane sulfonates of both of these drugs are indeed less toxic, but they have an inferior antibacterial activity than the sulfates. Eickhoff and Finland (1965) showed that the sulfates had about eight times more activity than the methane sulfonates against *Ps. aeruginosa*. Nord and Hoeprich (1964) showed that polymyxin E (colistin) sulfate was less toxic to white mice than polymyxin B sulfate, and that the methane sulfonates of both drugs were even less toxic. The activity of these four derivatives against *Pseudomonas aeruginosa* was found to be directly related to their toxicity, and so an equally toxic dose of each achieves about the same antibacterial effect.

Both polymyxin B and E were available either as the sulfate or methane sulfonate for parenteral administration and other uses. At this time these drugs are not used clinically, as the aminoglycosides and some broad-spectrum beta-lactam agents are more effective against *Ps. aeruginosa* and other Gram-negative bacteria, and they are also less toxic than the polymyxins.

Sensitive Organisms

All of the polymyxins have a similar antibacterial spectrum, but there are quantitative differences in their activity.

1 Gram-negative enteric bacilli

The polymyxins are highly active against most of the important Gram-negative bacteria which are normally inhabitants of the human bowel. *Escherichia coli*, *Enterobacter* and *Klebsiella* spp. and also *Ps. aeruginosa* are highly susceptible, but all *Proteus* spp. are resistant (Schwartz *et al.*, 1960; Taylor and Alison, 1962). *Serratia marcescens* is also usually resistant (Greenfield and Feingold, 1970) and *Bacteroides fragilis* is invariably resistant (Kislak, 1972). The *Prevotella* and *Fusobacterium* spp. are more sensitive (Hamilton-Miller, 1975).

| | MIC (μg per ml) | |
Organism	Polymyxin B sulfate	Colistin methane sulfonate
Escherichia coli	0.02–11.1	0.04–3.7
Enterobacter spp.	0.02–11.1	0.41–33.3
Klebsiella pneumoniae	0.02–0.41	0.01–3.7
Serratia marcescens	11.1	11.1
Proteus spp.	100.0	100.0
Salmonella typhi	0.02	0.14
Shigella sonnei	0.02	0.14
Pseudomonas aeruginosa	0.02–3.7	1.2–33.3

Table I.51
Condensed from Schwartz *et al.* (1960)

2 Other Gram-negative bacteria

The polymyxins are active against *Haemophilus influenzae*, *Bordetella pertussis*, the salmonellae and shigellae. The pathogenic *Neisseria* spp. (meningococci and gonococci), and the *Brucella* spp. are resistant (Schwartz *et al.*, 1960). Classical *Vibrio cholerae* 01 is sensitive to the polymyxins, but the *El Tor* biotype is resistant. The new *V. cholerae* 0139 Bengal strain, similar to *El Tor* vibrios is polymyxin B-resistant. Sensitivity to polymyxin is one of the laboratory tests which can be used to distinguish these *V. cholerae* strains (Mukerjee 1964; Cholera Working Group, 1993; Yamamoto *et al.*, 1995). *Acinetobacter* spp. is sensitive (Kuck, 1976), and so is *Legionella pneumophila* (Thornsberry *et al.*, 1978). *Burkholderia* (*Pseudomonas*) *cepacia* is polymyxin-resistant (Moore and Hancock, 1986).

3 Gram-positive bacteria

These are all resistant to the polymyxins.

4 Acquired resistance

An important property of the polymyxins is that the bacteria usually sensitive to these drugs do not readily acquire resistance. Occasionally resistant *Ps. aeruginosa* strains were encountered and these showed complete cross-resistance between polymyxin B and colistin. Some *Ps. aeruginosa* strains, while developing resistance to polymyxins, had increased sensitivity to antibiotics, such as chloramphenicol and in particular tetracycline, to which these organisms are normally resistant (Brown *et al.*, 1972). The clinical significance of this observation is not clear.

5 Minimum inhibitory concentrations

The MICs of polymyxin B sulfate and colistin methane sulfonate against some bacterial species are shown in Table I.51. Polymyxin B is more active, particularly against *Ps. aeruginosa*.

Mode of Administration and Dosage

The polymyxins are not absorbed from the gastrointestinal tract, and they are administered i.m. or i.v. for treatment of systemic infections.

1 Polymyxin B sulfate

The usual i.m. dosage for adults and children older than 2 years is 25 000–30 000 units (2.5–3.0 mg) per kg body weight per day, given in four to six divided doses. A dosage of up to 40 000 units per kg daily has been recommended for infants with normal renal function. A total daily dose of 2 000 000 units should not be exceeded. Intramuscular injections are quite painful, but this can be circumvented by adding procaine when preparing the drug for i.m. injections.

Polymyxin B sulfate can be given i.v. in a dosage of 15 000–25 000 units per kg per day for adults and children older than 2 years; infants with normal renal function can be given up to 40 000 units per kg daily. The contents of a vial (500 000 units) are dissolved in 300–500 ml of 5% dextrose and the drug is infused usually over a period of 60–90 min. Rapid i.v. injections should be avoided, because of the risk of neuromuscular blockade (p. 672). The recommended dose should be added to at least 100 ml of fluid and infused over a period of not less 20–30 min. The daily dose can be given in two to four divided doses.

2 Colistin (polymyxin E) methane sulfonate

The usual i.m. dosage of this drug is 2.5–5.0 mg per kg per day, given in two or four divided doses. For severe infections the higher dose of 5.0 mg per kg per day should be used. The dosage of 2.5–5.0 mg per kg body weight per day is also safe for newborn infants (Lawson and Hewstone, 1964). Unlike most other antibiotics which are excreted from the body in the urine, colistin does not have a prolonged half-life in premature babies (Axline *et al.*, 1967; Weinstein and Dalton, 1968).

Colistin methane sulfonate is given i.v. in the same dosage as used by the i.m. route, 2.5–5.0 mg per kg body weight per day, given in two divided doses. Baines and Rifkind (1964) administered a dose of 2.0–2.5 mg per kg every 12 h by dissolving the dose in 100 ml of 5% glucose which was then infused over 20–30 min. Cox and Harrison (1971) gave the drug i.v. in two stages. Half the daily dose (1.25–2.5 mg per kg) was given by rapid i.v. injection over 2–3 min, and the other half was administered as a slow infusion, lasting 20 h or longer, commencing 2 h after the loading dose. The rate of drug administration during this infusion was 5–6 mg per h. Some patients experienced parasthesiae, but no other adverse effects were noted. The manufacturers recommended that for direct intermittent i.v. administration, half of the total daily dose should be injected over 3–5 min every 12 h. Alternatively, half of the total daily dose can be administered in this way as a loading dose and then 1–2 h later the remainder of the total daily dose can be given by i.v. infusion at a rate of 5–6 mg per h in patients with normal renal function.

3 Patients with renal failure

The polymyxins accumulate in these patients, so a modified dosage schedule with serum level monitoring is necessary (MacKay and Kaye, 1964).

One method of administration of these drugs to patients with renal failure is to use the usual recommended dose, but to adjust the intervals between doses according to the degree of renal functional impairment. In anuric patients in whom the serum half-life of polymyxin B or colistin methane sulfonate is 2–3 days, the interval between these doses, given either i.m. or i.v., should be 3–4 days (Kunin, 1967). Curtis and Eastwood (1968) suggested that colistin methane sulfonate in a dosage of 2–3 mg per kg body weight, given i.v. once every 3 days is suitable for patients with severe renal failure. A corresponding dosage of polymyxin B sulfate for this purpose is about 1.0 mg per kg body weight every 3 days. Curtis and Eastwood (1968) found that small, but significant amounts of colistin methane sulfonate were removed by hemodialysis, and recommended that a dose of 2–3 mg per kg body weight of the drug given at the end of each dialysis was suitable for patients undergoing twice-weekly hemodialysis. In contrast, Goodwin and Friedman (1968) found that measurable quantities of the drug were not removed by hemodialysis. The clearance of colistin methane sulfonate during peritoneal dialysis is insignificant, and there is no need to increase its dosage in patients undergoing this procedure (Greenberg and Sanford, 1967; Curtis and Eastwood, 1968; Goodwin and Friedman, 1968). A dosage schedule of colistin methane sulfonate for patients with renal impairment was recommended by Goodwin and Friedman (1968), which differs somewhat from those of Kunin (1967) and Curtis and Eastwood (1968). Smaller doses at shorter intervals were used to avoid periods during which non-therapeutic serum levels may occur. They recommended the following dosage schedule for colistin methane sulfonate, assuming that the usual daily dose is 2.5 mg per kg per day (150 mg daily or 75 mg 12-hourly for adults).

a Patients with moderate renal impairment (creatinine clearance exceeding 20 ml per min) *Dose*: 75–100% of the daily dose given in two divided doses every 12 h. The duration of serum levels in these patients was almost the same as in subjects with normal renal function.

b Patients with severe renal failure (creatinine clearance 5–20 ml per min) *Dose*: 50% of the daily dose given in two divided doses every 12 h.

c Patients with negligible renal function (creatinine clearance less than 5 ml per min) *Dose*: 30% of the daily dose given in two divided doses every 12–18 h.

The higher recommended daily dose of 5 mg per kg per day of colistin methane sulfonate should be used cautiously in the above schedule, because toxic blood levels may result in some patients with renal failure. Goodwin and Friedman (1968) did not study polymyxin B sulfate but their dosage schedule can probably be applied to this drug (Kunin, 1968), assuming that the usual daily dose is 1.5–2.5 mg per kg. Nevertheless, such dosage schedules are only an approximate guide and regular serum level monitoring is necessary in all patients with renal failure. In addition, the polymyxins are bound to various tissues, where they may persist when serum levels are already low.

4 Aerosol administration

Polymyxin B may be used as inhalation therapy for *Ps. aeruginosa* bronchial infections, but this is usually not very effective (p. 673). The total daily aerosol dose of polymyxin B should not exceed the daily dose recommended for parenteral use. The drug is a bronchial irritant and concentrations higher than 10 mg per ml should not be used for inhalation (Marschke and Sarauw, 1971). Colistin inhalations, one million units dissolved in 3 ml of sterile water, administered twice-daily, have also been given to cystic fibrosis patients with chronic *Ps. aeruginosa* lung infections (Jensen *et al.*, 1987).

Serum Levels in Relation to Dosage

After a single i.m. injection of 50 mg polymyxin B sulfate to adults, the peak serum level is reached after about 2 h. The peak serum level is subject to considerable individual variation, and it may be as high as 8 µg per ml or as low as 1–2 µg per ml. The serum level thereafter declines slowly, and detectable levels are usually present for about 8–12 h. The half-life of polymyxin B sulfate in serum is about 6 h (Kunin, 1967). Some accumulation of the drug usually occurs, and peak levels in patients given 2.5 mg per kg per day for over a week may reach 15 µg per ml.

After a single i.m. injection of colistin methane sulfonate in a dose of 2.5 mg per kg body weight to children (about 150 mg for adults), a peak serum level of 5–7 µg per ml occurs in 1–2 h and detectable levels persist for 8–12 h (Fig. I.25). The serum half-life of this drug is only 1.6–2.7 h (Kunin, 1967).

As with polymyxin B sulfate, repeated administration yields higher serum levels. McMillan *et al.* (1962) measured serum levels in adult patients receiving 120 mg of colistin methane sulfonate i.m. at 8-hourly intervals. They found that a maximum level of 11–12 µg per ml, achieved 2–3 h after the injection, was maintained for 5–6 h and then fell progressively.

If colistin methane sulfonate is administered i.v. using an initial rapid injection, followed by a slow infusion (p. 669), relatively constant serum levels of 5–6 µg per ml are maintained in most patients (Cox and Harrison, 1971).

Fig. I.25.
Average serum levels of colistin methane sulfonate after a single intramuscular dose of 2.5 mg per kg body weight in children. (Redrawn after Ross *et al.*, 1960.)

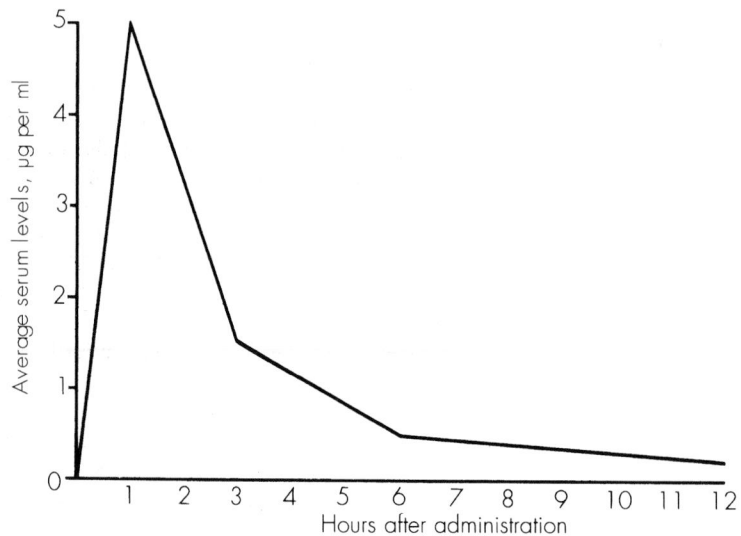

Excretion

1 Urine

The polymyxins are mainly excreted by the kidney, but there is a time lag in the excretion of the sulfates after the initial dose. Only about 0.1% of polymyxin B sulfate is recovered from urine during the first 12 h after injection, thereafter urinary excretion increases and with continuing administration in the usual dosage, the urinary concentration varies from 20 to 100 μg per ml. Overall, about 60% of the injected dose of polymyxin B sulfate can be recovered from the urine (Hoeprich, 1970).

The methane sulfonate derivatives are more rapidly excreted via the kidney. About 40% of colistin methane sulfonate is excreted in the urine in the first 8 h following injection. The urine levels of colistin (and polymyxin B sulfate) vary according to fluid intake. Urinary colistin concentrations may reach more than 200 μg per ml after usual therapeutic doses, but when fluid intake is high, values of only 20 μg per ml or less may occur (McMillan et al., 1962).

The polymyxins accumulate in patients with impaired renal function.

2 Inactivation in body

The polymyxins are not excreted in bile. The fraction of the administered dose not recoverable from the urine is probably slowly inactivated in the body, possibly by normal tissues (Kunin and Edmondson, 1968). The serum half-life of the polymyxins in anuric patients is usually 2–3 days (Kunin, 1967), but Goodwin and Friedman (1968) showed that it may be considerably shorter in some patients with virtually no renal function. This suggests that there is considerable variation in the rate of inactivation of polymyxins by the 'non-renal mechanisms'.

Distribution of the Drugs in Body

Although reports conflict on the degree of dialysability of the polymyxins by hemodialysis (Curtis and Eastwood, 1968; Goodwin and Friedman, 1968), all authors agree that these drugs dialyze poorly by any method. This is probably due to the large molecular size of the polymyxins, rather than their protein binding (Kunin, 1967). For this reason, the polymyxins do not appear to diffuse well into pleural or joint cavities or infective foci in general, but quantitative date are not available. These drugs also do not diffuse readily into normal CSF (Wynne and Cooke, 1966).

Animal studies show that the polymyxins become bound to and persist in various body tissues such as the liver, kidney, brain, heart, muscle and lung (Kunin and Bugg, 1971). The drugs persist in these tissues for up to 72 h after single injections and for up to 5 days after a course of injections. Comparatively more colistin methane sulfonate than polymyxin B sulfate is localized in the kidney, lung and liver, but much higher levels of polymyxin B sulfate than colistin methane sulfonate are found in the brain. The clinical significance of these observations is uncertain.

According to Kunin (1967), the degree of the protein binding of the polymyxins is low.

Mode of Action

The polymyxins are bactericidal to Gram-negative bacteria because they interfere with the structure and function of their outer and cytoplasmic membranes (p. 26). These membranes have specific transport systems, which determine the permeability characteristics of the cell. Damage to this osmotic barrier leads to leakage of intracellular components. The structure of the polymyxins allows them to interact with the lipopolysaccharides and phospholipids of the outer membrane; they also interact electrostatically with the outer membrane by competitively displacing divalent cations (calcium and magnesium) from the negatively charged phosphate groups of membrane lipids (Dixon and Chopra, 1986). Resistance of Ps. aeruginosa to polymyxin seems to occur by means of a variety of structural and chemical changes in the outer membrane of the bacteria (Moore et al., 1984; Shand et al., 1988; Conrad and Galanos, 1989; Young et al., 1992).

Polymyxin B, apart from its antibacterial activity, has been shown to have another property in animal studies. It appears to moderate experimental shock, when animals are injected with endotoxins from Gram-negative bacteria such as E. coli. It had no effect when endotoxins from meningococci were used. A derivative of polymyxin B, polymyxin B nonapeptide, which is not antibacterial, and is less toxic than polymyxin B, also has anti-endotoxin activity, similar to that of polymyxin B (Flynn et al., 1987; Danner et al., 1989; Baldwin et al., 1991). Clinical studies with this have not been pursued.

Toxicity

The polymyxins, even when administered in the recommended doses, frequently cause side-effects. For instance, in a study of 288 patients treated by colistin methane sulfonate (sodium colistimethate), untoward effects were observed in 25.1% (Koch-Weser *et al.*, 1970).

1 Nephrotoxicity

This is the most serious toxic effect of the polymyxins. Polymyxin B compounds are more nephrotoxic than colistin (polymyxin E) compounds, and the sulfate derivatives of both these drugs are more toxic than their corresponding methane sulfonates. The antibacterial activity of these compounds is proportional to their toxicity, so that for a certain degree of antibacterial effect, the toxicity is the same whichever preparation is used (p. 667). Patients with pre-existing renal impairment can be treated by polymyxins if a modified dosage is used, and renal function sometimes improves as the infection is controlled by polymyxin therapy.

Nephrotoxicity, occurring in 20.2% of patients, was the most common side-effect observed by Koch-Weser *et al.* (1970). Proteinuria, hematuria and casts in the urine may occur, but rising blood urea and serum creatinine values are the most invariable features. These usually occur within the first 4 days of therapy. Acute tubular necrosis may result and this may not be preceded by progressive renal functional impairment. Renal impairment may sometimes continue to progress for 1 or 2 weeks after the drug has been stopped. Koch-Weser *et al.* (1970) also observed that, after excluding patients in whom dosage had not been appropriately reduced, the frequency of nephrotoxicity in patients with normal and in those with pre-existing renal impairment was the same. The simultaneous administration of cephalothin (p. 257) was associated with a higher frequency of nephrotoxicity. The majority of the patients developing renal impairment had received sodium colistimethate in the recommended doses. However, nephrotoxicity was more common in heavier patients, probably because a dose according to body weight tends to produce overdosage in such individuals, and surface area would correlate better with glomerular filtration rate and blood volume. In doses of 3 mg (30 000 units) per kg per day, polymyxin B may cause nephrotoxicity in patients with normal renal function, but lower doses may cause renal damage in patients with pre-existing renal impairment (Appel and Neu, 1977).

The use of polymyxins in doses higher than those recommended is dangerous and potentially fatal; this may result in oliguric renal failure due to acute tubular necrosis. Price and Graham (1970) reported 14 patients with refractory *Klebsiella* spp. infections treated by colistin in doses about six times higher than usually recommended, who all developed acute renal failure. This complication has also occurred in children who have received accidental colistin overdosages (Ryan *et al.*, 1969; Brown *et al.*, 1970). One child aged 10 months, who had accidentally received 250 mg colistin i.m. (approximately 38.5 mg per kg), had a serum colistin level of 320 μg per ml a few hours later. This child subsequently developed oliguric renal failure, but eventually recovered. Peritoneal dialysis did not remove colistin from this patient, but exchange transfusion appeared to be effective (Brown *et al.*, 1970).

2 Neurotoxicity

The polymyxins can cause giddiness, disturbances of sensation, such as numbness and paresthesiae mainly affecting the face, nausea and vomiting, muscle weakness and peripheral neuropathy (Koch-Weser *et al.*, 1970). These usually occur within the first 4 days of treatment and disappear when the drug is stopped. More severe neurotoxic disturbances such as mental confusion, coma, psychosis, convulsions or ataxia may also occur. These may be more frequent in patients receiving large doses or in those with renal functional impairment (Wolinsky and Hines, 1962).

Another serious neurotoxic effect is reversible neuromuscular blockade, which may result in respiratory paralysis (Perkins, 1964; Lindesmith *et al.*, 1968). This may appear quickly and be without premonitory minor side-effects of neurotoxicity (Koch-Weser *et al.*, 1970). The occurrence of paralysis due to polymyxins and other antibiotics was reviewed by McQuillen *et al.* (1968). Neuromuscular blockade was related to the dose of the antibiotic given, but this was not the only factor. In most reported cases paralysis occurred postoperatively, and there were usually other potentiating factors such as ether anesthesia, sedatives, neuromuscular blocking agents, hypocalcemia, renal disease, hypoxia and chronic debilitating illnesses.

Polymyxin-induced neuromuscular blockade differs from that induced by the aminoglycosides (Lindesmith *et al.*, 1968). Neomycin, kanamycin and streptomycin apparently produce a competitive blockade (p. 537), which may be reversed by neostigmine, but the polymyxins cause a non-competitive blockade which is never reversed by neostigmine. Respiratory paralysis due to the polymyxins must be treated by artificial ventilation, and calcium administration may be helpful in some cases. Neuromuscular blockade usually improves within 24 h after the antibiotic is stopped.

It has been suggested that the polymyxins are particularly suitable for treatment of *Ps. aeruginosa* infections in anephric patients, because nephrotoxicity is not a consideration (Curtis and Eastwood, 1968), but neurotoxicity can be a serious hazard in chronically anemic patients because their nervous system appears to be more susceptible to polymyxin toxicity than that of patients with either acute renal failure or normal renal function (Richet *et al.*, 1970).

Experiments in animals indicate that ear drops containing various antibiotics including polymyxins may be ototoxic and cause deafness. In view of this and the doubt about the efficacy of such treatment, the use of antibiotic ear drops has been discouraged, especially in the presence of large perforations, where ear surgery has been performed, or for preoperative prophylaxis (Annotation, 1976).

3 Hypersensitivity reactions

Rashes, pruritus and drug fever have been observed with polymyxin therapy (Hoeprich, 1970; Koch-Weser *et al.*, 1970). Two patients were reported who developed bronchospasm as a result of aerosol therapy with the usual doses of polymyxin B. This may have been due to an allergic reaction or bronchial irritation (Marschke and Sarauw, 1971). One patient with aplastic anemia and polymyxin allergy was reported by Lakin *et al.* (1975). After immunosuppression and receipt of a bone-marrow graft, and whilst lacking T cell activity, he developed a rash and fever attributed to intranasal polymyxin B which was associated with specific IgE antibody. These authors considered that there could be an increased frequency of type 1 hypersensitivity in immunosuppressed patients because the normal suppressor effect of T cell on B cell-mediated IgE synthesis may be absent.

4 Leukopenia and hepatotoxicity

On rare occasions leukopenia and hepatotoxicity have been observed during colistin therapy but a definite causal relationship has not been established.

Clinical Uses of the Drugs

1 Pseudomonas aeruginosa infections

In the past polymyxins were often used for the treatment of *Ps. aeruginosa* infections such as septicemia, meningitis, pneumonia and wound, burn and urinary tract infections. Nowadays, one of the aminoglycosides such as gentamicin (p. 471), tobramycin (p. 493) or amikacin (p. 514) or a beta-lactam agent such as ticarcillin (p. 156), piperacillin (p. 174) or ceftazidime (p. 377), either singly or in combination, are preferred for these infections.

Usually *Ps. aeruginosa* septicemia occurs in patients with severe associated diseases; nevertheless, some success was obtained by the use of the polymyxins in this disease (Murdoch, 1964). *Pseudomonas* has also been eliminated from infected burns by using one of the polymyxins both parenterally and locally. The treatment of chronic purulent *Ps. aeruginosa* bronchial infections by these drugs was unsatisfactory (Pines *et al.*, 1967), though occasional successes were reported (Lieberson *et al.*, 1969). In addition, in one study in which polymyxin B was administered by aerosol to critically ill patients in an attempt to prevent *Ps. aeruginosa* pneumonia, results were unfavorable. A number of these patients developed pneumonia due to organisms which were polymyxin-resistant and which were uncommon pathogens, such as *Stenotrophomonas maltophilia*, *Burkholderia* (*Pseudomonas*) *cepacia*, *Flavobacterium* and *Serratia* spp. and *Entococcus faecalis* (Feeley *et al.*, 1975).

Ps. aeruginosa urinary tract infections were also treated, with reasonably satisfactory results (Edgar and Dickinson, 1962). It was suggested that colistin methane sulfonate may be superior to polymyxin B sulfate for the treatment of these infections, because high urinary concentrations are more rapidly attained after administration (Goodwin, 1970). However, the urine levels of polymyxin B sulfate also become adequate after a lag period of approximately 12 h and remain high with continuing treatment (p. 671).

Because of the availability of effective and less toxic drugs, the polymyxins have now been relegated to the position of reserve drugs for the parenteral treatment of *Ps. aeruginosa* infections.

2 Infections due to other Gram-negative bacilli

The polymyxins were not the drugs of choice for septicemia, meningitis, pyelonephritis, etc., caused by organisms such as *E. coli* and *Klebsiella* spp., but they were used when these bacteria had become resistant to commonly used antibiotics. Colley and Frankel (1963) used colistin methane sulfonate with moderate success in 18 male paraplegic patients, who had chronic *Klebsiella aerogenes* infections of the urinary tract.

3 Topical antibiotic therapy

Polymyxin B sulfate was combined with the two other commonly used topical antibiotics, neomycin and bacitracin, because the latter two are ineffective against *Ps. aeruginosa*. These three antibiotics have been marketed in various creams, ointments, eye and ear drops, sprays, solutions for wound irrigation and bladder instillation, etc. (pp. 538, 543). Polymyxin B sulfate is particularly suitable for topical therapy, because development of bacterial resistance to this drug is uncommon. Toxicity is not a problem with topical therapy, and therefore the polymyxin with the greatest therapeutic activity, polymyxin B sulfate is always selected for this purpose.

4 Reduction of bowel flora in patients with leukemia

Polymyxins are one of several drugs which when given orally, produce 'selective decontamination' of the gut flora (p. 881) and they have been used in combination with other antibiotics to reduce bacterial infections in granulocytopenic patients (p. 539). A daily dose of 400–800 mg polymyxin B was recommended for this purpose. The reason for this relatively high dose is because polymyxin B is bound to solid part of feces. Reversible binding of polymyxin to feces allows a free antibiotic concentration which is low enough to spare insensitive obligate anaerobic flora but high enough to eliminate the sensitive, aerobic Gram-negative rods (Hazenberg, 1986; Alcock and Ledingham, 1988).

Reference

Alcock SR, Ledingham I McA (1988). Selective decontamination of the digestive tract and prevention of infection in intensive care units. *J Antimicrob Chemother* **22**: 97.

Annotation (1976). Ear drops. *Lancet* i: 896.

Appel GB, Neu HC (1977). The nephrotoxicity of antimicrobial agents (second of three parts). *New Engl J Med* **296**: 722.

Axline SG, Yaffe SJ, Simon HJ (1967). Clinical pharmacology of antimicrobials in premature infants: II. Ampicillin, methicillin, oxacillin, neomycin, and colistin. *Pediatrics* **39**: 97.

Baines RD, Rifkind D (1964). Intravenous administration of sodium colistimethate. *JAMA* **190**: 278.

Baldwin G, Alpert G, Caputo GL *et al.* (1991). Effect of polymyxin B on experimental shock from meningococcal and *Escherichia coli* endotoxins. *J Infect Dis* **164**: 542.

Brown JM, Dorman DC, Roy LP (1970). Acute renal failure due to overdosage of colistin. *Med J Aust* **2**: 923.

Brown MRW, Fenton EM, Watkins WM (1972). Tetracycline-sensitive/polymyxin-resistant *Pseudomonas aeruginosa*. *Lancet* ii: 86.

Cholera Working Group, International Centre for Diarrhoeal Diseases Research, Bangladesh (1993). Large epidemic of cholera-like disease in Bangladesh caused by *Vibrio cholerae* 0139 synonym Bengal. *Lancet* **342**: 387.

Colley EW, Frankel HL (1963). 'Colomycin' treatment of *Klebsiella aerogenes* infection of urinary tract in paraplegia. *Brit Med J* **2**: 790.

Conrad RS, Galanos C (1989). Fatty acid alterations and polymyxin B binding by lipopolysacharides from *Pseudomonas aeruginosa* adapted to polymyxin B resistance. *Antimicrob Ag Chemother* **33**: 1724.

Cox CE, Harrison LH (1971). Intravenous sodium colistimethate therapy of urinary tract infections: pharmacological and bacteriological studies. *Antimicrob Ag Chemother* **1970**: 296.

Curtis JR, Eastwood JB (1968). Colistin sulphomethate sodium administration in the presence of severe renal failure and during haemodialysis and peritoneal dialysis. *Brit Med J* **1**: 484.

Danner RL, Joiner KA, Rubin M *et al.* (1989). Purification, toxicity, and antiendotoxin activity of polymyxin B nonapeptide. *Antimicrob Ag Chemother* **33**: 1428.

Dixon RA, Chopra I (1986). Leakage of periplasmic proteins from *Escherichia coli* mediated by polymyxin B nonapeptide. *Antimicrob Ag Chemother* **29**: 781.

Edgar WM, Dickinson KM (1962). A trial of colistin methane sulphonate in urinary infection with *Pseudomonas pyocyanea*. *Lancet* ii: 739.

Eickhoff TC, Finland M (1965). Polymyxin B and colistin: *in vitro* activity against *Pseudomonas aeruginosa*. *Amer J Med Sci* **249**: 172.

Feeley TW, Du Moulin GC, Hedley-Whyte J *et al.* (1975). Aerosol polymyxin and pneumonia in seriously ill patients. *New Engl J Med* **293**: 471.

Flynn PM, Shenep JL, Stokes DC *et al.* (1987). Polymyxin B moderates acidosis and hypotension in established Gram-negative septicemia. *J Infect Dis* **156**: 706.

Goodwin NJ (1970). Colistin and sodium colistimethate. *Med Clin N Amer* **54**: 1267.

Goodwin NJ, Friedman EA (1968). The effects of renal impairment, peritoneal dialysis, and hemodialysis on serum sodium colistimethate levels. *Ann Intern Med* **68**: 984.

Greenberg PA, Sanford JP (1967). Removal and absorption of antibiotics in patients with renal failure undergoing peritoneal dialysis. *Ann Intern Med* **66**: 465.

Greenfield S, Feingold DS (1970). The synergistic action of the sulfonamides and the polymyxins against *Serratia marcescens*. *J Infect Dis* **121**: 555.

Hamilton-Miller JMT (1975). Antimicrobial agents acting against anaerobes. *J Antimicrob Chemother* **1**: 273.

Hazenberg MP, Pennock-Schröder AM, Van de Merwe JP (1986). Reversible binding of polymyxin B and neomycin to the solid part of faeces. *J Antimicrob Chemother* **17**: 333.

Hoeprich PD (1970). The polymyxins. *Med Clin N Amer* **54**: 1257.

Jensen T, Pedersen SS, Garne S et al. (1987). Colistin inhalational therapy in cystic fibrosis patients with chronic *Pseudomonas aeruginosa* lung infection. *J Antimicrob Chefmother* **19**: 831.

Kislak JW (1972). The susceptibility of *Bacteroides fragilis* to 24 antibiotics. *J Infect Dis* **125**: 295.

Koch-Weser J, Sidel VW, Federman EB et al. (1970). Adverse effects of sodium colistimethate. Manifestations and specific reaction rates during 317 courses of therapy. *Ann Intern Med* **72**: 857.

Kuck NA (1976). *In vitro* and *in vivo* activities of minocycline and other antibiotics against *Acinetobacter* (Herellea-Mima). *Antimicrob Ag Chemother* **9**: 493.

Kunin CM (1967). A guide to use of antibiotics in patients with renal disease. *Ann Intern Med* **67**: 151.

Kunin CM (1968). More on antimicrobials in renal failure. *Ann Intern Med* **69**: 397.

Kunin CM, Bugg A (1971). Binding of polymyxin antibiotics to tissues: the major determinant of distribution and persistence in the body. *J Infect Dis* **124**: 394.

Kunin CM, Edmondson WP (1968). Inhibition of antibiotics in bacteriologic agar. *Proc Soc Exp Biol (NY)* **129**: 118.

Lakin JD, Strong DM, Sell KW (1975). Polymyxin B reactions, IgE antibody, and T-cell deficiency. *Ann Intern Med* **83**: 204.

Lawson JS, Hewstone AS (1964). Toxic effects of colistin methane sulphonate in the new-born. *Med J Aust* **1**: 917.

Lieberson AD, Winter LW, Behnke RH, Martin RR (1969). Extensive *Pseudomonal pneumonia* ultimately responding to polymyxin therapy. *Amer Rev Resp Dis* **100**: 558.

Lindesmith LA, Baines RDJr, Bigelow DB, Petty TL (1968). Reversible respiratory paralysis associated with polymyxin therapy. *Ann Intern Med* **68**: 318.

MacKay D, Kaye D (1964). Serum concentrations of colistin in patients with normal and impaired renal function. *New Engl J Med* **270**: 394.

Marschke G, Sarauw A (1971). Polymyxin inhalation therapeutic hazard. *Ann Intern Med* **74**: 144.

McMillan M, Price TML, MacLaren DM, Scott GW (1962). *Pseudomonas pyocyanea* infection treated with colistin methane sulphonate. *Lancet* **ii**: 737.

McQuillen MP, Cantor HE, O'Rourke JR (1968). Myasthenic syndrome associated with antibiotics. *Arch Neurol* **18**: 402.

Moore RA, Hancock REW (1986). Involvement of outer membrane of *Pseudomonas cepacia* in aminoglycoside and polymyxin resistance. *Antimicrob Ag Chemfother* **30**: 923.

Moore RA, Chan L, Hancock REW (1984). Evidence for two distinct mechanisms of resistance to polymyxin B in *Pseudomonas aeruginosa*. *Antimicrob Ag Chemother* **26**: 539.

Mukerjee S (1964). Cholera El Tor in Calcutta. *Brit Med J* **2**: 546.

Murdoch J McC (1964). The treatment of severe *Pseudomonas pyocyanea* infections with colistin. *Proc Third Int Cong Chemother Stuttgart*, p. 319.

Nord NM, Hoeprich PD (1964). Polymyxin B and colistin, a critical comparison. *New Engl J Med* **270**: 1030.

Perkins RL (1964). Apnea with intramuscular colistin therapy. *JAMA* **190**: 421.

Pines A, Raafat H, Plucinski K (1967). Gentamicin and colistin in chronic purulent bronchial infections. *Brit Med J* **2**: 543.

Price DJE, Graham DI (1970). Effects of large doses of colistin sulphomethate sodium on renal function. *Brit Med J* **4**: 525.

Richet G, Lopez de Novales E, Verroust P (1970). Drug intoxication and neurological episodes in chronic renal failure. *Brit Med J* **2**: 394.

Ross P, Puig JR, Zaremba EA (1960). Colistin: some preliminary laboratory and clinical observations in specific gastroenteritis in infants and children. *Antibiot Annual 1959–1960*: 89.

Ryan KJ, Schainuck LI, Hickman RO, Striker GE (1969). Colistimethate toxicity Report of a fatal case in a previously healthy child. *JAMA* **207**: 2099.

Schwartz BS, Warren MR, Barkley FA, Landis L (1960). Microbiological and pharmacological studies of colistin sulfate and sodium colistinmethanesulfonate. *Antibiot Annual -1959–1969*: 41.

Shand GH, Anwar H, Brown MRW (1988). Outer membrane proteins of polymyxin-resistant *Pseudomonas aeruginosa*: effect of magnesium depletion. *J Antimicrob Chemother* **22**: 811.

Taylor G, Allison H (1962). 'Colomycin' – laboratory and clinical investigations. *Brit Med J* **2**: 161.

Thornsberry C, Baker CN, Kirven LA (1978). *In vitro* activity of antimicrobial agents on Legionnaires' disease bacterium. *Antimicrob Ag Chemother* **13**: 78.

Weinstein L, Dalton AC (1968). Host determinants of response to antimicrobial agents. *New Engl J Med* **279**: 467.

Wilkinson S (1963). Identity of colistin and polymyxin E. *Lancet* **i**: 922.

Wolinsky E, Hines JD (1962). Neurotoxic and nephrotoxic effects of colistin in patients with renal disease. *New Engl J Med* **266**: 759.

Wynne JM, Cooke EM (1966). Passage of chloramphenicol and sodium colistimethate into the cerebrospinal fluid; studies of hydrocephalic children. *Amer J Dis Child* **112**: 422.

Yamamoto T, Nair GB, Albert MJ et al. (1995). Survey of *in vitro* susceptibilities of *Vibrio cholerae* 01 and 0139 to antimicrobial agents. *Antimicrob Ag Chemother* **39**: 241.

Young ML, Bains M, Bell A, Hancock REW (1992). Role of *Pseudomonas aeruginosa* outer membrane protein OprH in polymyxin and gentamicin resistance: isolation of an OprH-deficient mutant by gene replacement techniques. *Antimicrob Ag Chemother* **36**: 2566.

Rifampicin (Rifampin)

Description

In 1957 a new class of antibiotics called rifamycins was recognized at Lepetit laboratories in Italy (Sensi, 1983). These antibiotics were isolated from a microorganism *Nocardia mediterranei*. Chemical modifications to one of the original compounds, designated rifamycin B, resulted in others with increased antibacterial activity. Two of these were introduced for clinical use in some countries, rifamycin SV in 1963 and rifamycin B diethylamide or rifamide in 1965; both were active against *Mycobacterium tuberculosis* and various other bacteria but they were excreted rather quickly by the liver and required parenteral administration. Further chemical modifications of rifamycin were made with the aim of producing a drug which was absorbed after oral administration, had a more prolonged antibacterial level in the blood, and a greater activity against mycobacteria and other bacteria. Rifampicin or rifampin was synthesized in 1965 and introduced for clinical use in 1968. The name rifampin is used in the USA whilst the drug is called rifampicin in Europe and Australia. Rifampicin has the chemical formula of 3–4 (4-methylpiperazinyl-iminomethylidene)-rifamycin SV (Sensi *et al.*, 1967).

Rifampicin is a most valuable drug for the treatment of tuberculosis, leprosy and an expanding range of other infections. Other derivatives of rifampicin may prove to be useful for treatment of tuberculosis and other mycobacterial disease. The main one of these at present is rifabutin, which is recommended for the chemoprophylaxis of *Mycobacterium avium* complex infections in AIDS patients (p. 771).

The following details only apply to rifampicin.

Sensitive Organisms

1 Gram-positive bacteria

Rifampicin is highly active against *Staphylococcus aureus* and coagulase-negative staphylococci such as *Staph. epidermidis*, *Staph. saprophyticus*, *Staph. haemolyticus*, *Staph. hominis*, *Staph. lugdunensis*, *Staph. schleiferi* and *Staph. warneri*. Beta-lactamase-producing strains and methicillin-resistant strains of these bacteria are also usually rifampicin-sensitive. Rifampicin-resistant mutants of these staphylococci easily arise *in vitro* and *in vivo* in the presence of rifampicin as a single drug. The emergence of *in vivo* rifampicin-resistance, particularly of methicillin-resistant strains, can be usually, but not invariably, prevented by the use of antibiotic combinations. Thus combinations such as rifampicin/sodium fusidate, rifampicin/ciprofloxacin and rifampicin/novobiocin have been used with success to treat infections due to methicillin-resistant *Staph. aureus* strains (p. 584). A combination of vancomycin/rifampicin/gentamicin has been useful for treatment of methicillin-resistant *Staph. epidermidis* endocarditis (Archer *et al.*, 1980; Carper *et al.*, 1987; Proctor *et al.*, 1987; Hoogeterp *et al.*, 1988; Tebas *et al.*, 1991; Torre *et al.*, 1992; Archer and Climo, 1994; Kang *et al.*, 1994; Rupp and Archer, 1994).

Streptococcus pyogenes, *Strep. viridans*, Group B streptococci, *Strep. pneumoniae* and anaerobic cocci are also rifampicin-sensitive, but most *Enterococcus faecalis* strains are only moderately susceptible. Strains of *Strep. pneumoniae* detected in South Africa in 1977, which were resistant to penicillin G and many other antibiotics were usually sensitive to rifampicin, but some developed resistance to it (p. 5). Rifampicin-resistant *Strep. pneumoniae* are now more common in some countries, and this may be due to the increase of the prevalence of tuberculosis in the world (p. 1194), for which rifampicin is used (Garcia-Arenzana *et al.*, 1994). *Bacillus anthracis* is sensitive (Sensi *et al.*, 1967; Kunin *et al.*, 1969, Dans *et al.*, 1970). Rifampicin is quite active against *Listeria monocytogenes* (Tuazon *et al.*, 1982; Thornsberry *et al.*, 1983), and it is effective in animal infections with this organism (Scheld, 1983). *Rhodococcus equi* is rifampicin-sensitive (Nordmann *et al.*, 1992; De Marais and Kocka, 1995), but the *Nocardia* are nearly always resistant (Tanzil *et al.*, 1972). *Nocardia brasiliensis* can inactivate rifampicin (Yazawa *et al.*, 1993).

Anaerobic Gram-positive bacilli such as *Clostridium* spp., including *Cl. difficile*, are rifampicin-sensitive (Sensi *et al.*, 1967; Kunin *et al.*, 1969; Bacon *et al.*, 1991). In animals rifampicin, clindamycin or tetracycline are more effacious than penicillin G for the treatment of fulminant gas gangrene caused by *Cl. perfringens*. Toxin suppression and rapid bacterial killing may explain this superiority (Stevens *et al.*, 1987).

2 Gram-negative bacteria

Meningococci are highly sensitive to rifampicin. A small percentage now are rifampicin-resistant because of the widespread use of the drug for the prevention of secondary cases among contacts of patients with invasive meningococcal disease (p. 697). Severe meningococcal disease due to rifampicin-resistant strains has also been recorded (Yagupsky *et al.*, 1993; Carter *et al.*, 1994). These strains are usually susceptible to penicillin G, and especially so to ceftriaxone (Abadi *et al.*, 1995). *Neisseria gonorrhoeae* is highly sensitive and this includes beta-lactamase-producing strains (p. 15), which are inhibited by a concentration of 2 μg per ml or less (Report, 1978). Gonococcal strains with intrinsic resistance to penicillin G are also often relatively or completely resistant to rifampicin (p. 14). Occasional other strains of gonococci are rifampicin-resistant (Piot *et al.*, 1979). *Haemophilus influenzae*, including ampicillin-resistant strains (p. 112) and ampicillin/chloramphenicol-resistant strains (p. 552) is also usually sensitive (Bannatyne and Cheung, 1978; Simasathien *et al.*, 1980). Resistant mutants of this organism evolve rapidly when cultured in the presence of rifampicin (Mendelman *et al.*, 1982) and *in vivo*, particularly in children who have received rifampicin prophylactically (Murphy *et al.*, 1981; Nicolle *et al.*, 1982a; McCarty *et al.*, 1986; Doern *et al.*, 1988). *Haemophilus ducreyi* is also very susceptible (Hammond *et al.*, 1978) and the MIC for *Bordetella pertussis* is usually ≤2 μg per ml (Zakrisson *et al.*, 1985).

Entrobacteriaceae, such as *Escherichia coli*, the *Enterobacter*, *Klebsiella*, *Proteus*, *Providencia*, *Serratia* and *Citrobacter* spp., are usually resistant, though some strains of *Proteus mirabilis* and *E. coli* may be moderately sensitive (Thornsberry *et al.*, 1983). The salmonellae, shigellae and *Pseudomonas aeruginosa* are resistant. Although *Burkholderia* (*Pseudomonas*) *pseudomallei* is usually resistant *in vitro*, some animal studies suggested that rifampicin was effective against it *in vivo* (Pattamasukon *et al.*, 1975). *Pasteurella multocida* and the majority of anaerobes, such as *Bacteroides* spp., are sensitive (Leigh, 1974). In a mouse model rifampicin was superior to clindamycin and comparable in efficacy to metronidazole in treating *Bacteroides fragilis* infection (Fu *et al.*, 1984). Occasional strains of *B. fragilis* are rifampicin-resistant (Bullock *et al.*, 1981).

Brucella spp. are sensitive and rifampicin is effective for the treatment of experimental brucellosis in animals (Philippon *et al.*, 1977). However, rifampicin-resistance in *B. melitensis* arose *in vivo* in one patient with brucellosis treated with rifampicin plus doxycycline (De Rautlin De La Roy *et al.*, 1986). *Flavobacteria* spp. are sensitive with MICs ≤2 μg per ml (Aber *et al.*, 1978). Rifampicin remains the most active drug against *Legionella pneumophila* with an MIC of usually < 0.03 μg per ml (Lewis *et al.*, 1978; Edelstein and Meyer, 1980; Thornsberry *et al.*, 1978, 1983). Other *Legionella* spp., such as *L. dumoffii*, *L. bozemanii*, *L. micdadei* (Pittsburgh pneumonia agent), *L. gormanii*, *L. longbeachae*, *L. jordanis* and *L. oakridgensis*, are all very sensitive to rifampicin, with *L. longbeachae* and *L. oakridgensis* being slightly more resistant with MICs of 0.25 and 0.12 μg per ml, respectively (Thornsberry *et al.*, 1983). In guinea pigs rifampicin is more effective than erythromycin or gentamicin in eliminating viable *L. pneumophila* from the lungs and also in preventing pulmonary lesions (Gibson *et al.*, 1983). Resistance of *L. pneumophila* does not emerge when the drug is used to treat *Legionella* infections in animals (Edelstein, 1991). Rifampicin also reduces mortality of guinea pigs infected with *L. micdadei* (Pasculle *et al.*, 1985). Rifampicin has almost no activity against *Campylobacter* organisms (Washington *et al.*, 1982), but *Helicobacter pylori* is usually sensitive, as is *H. cinaedi* (Burman *et al.*, 1995). *Francisella tularensis* is usually sensitive and resistant mutants appear to have reduced virulence (Bhatnagar *et al.*, 1994). The *Bartonella* (*Rochalimaea*) spp. are rifampicin-sensitive (MICs 0.25 μg per ml) (Maurin *et al.*, 1995).

3 Mycobacteria

Rifampicin is highly active against *M. tuberculosis* (Clark and Wallace, 1967; Sensi *et al.*, 1967). The rate of spontaneous development of rifampicin-resistant mutants of *M. tuberculosis in vitro* is low (McClatchy *et al.*, 1969). In one trial rifampicin was used alone for 45 days to treat 11 patients with pulmonary tuberculosis; resistant strains were detected in two patients and strains with diminished sensitivity to rifampicin in another four (Baronti and Lukinovich, 1968). Emergence of rifampicin-resistant strains of *M. tuberculosis* during treatment of patients for many years was also not a major problem, but in nearly all trials rifampicin was used together with one or two other antituberculosis drugs. Primary rifampicin-resistance was still only 1.5% in Australia in the year 1991 (Lim, 1995). In the USA primary rifampicin-resistance in tuberculosis initially was also uncommon (Woodley *et al.*, 1972; Hobby *et al.*, 1974). An increasing incidence of rifampicin-resistant strains (reaching 1.96%) was found in Massachusetts in the years 1971 to 1974 mainly amongst patients who had had previous treatment for tuberculosis (acquired or secondary resistance) (Stottmeier, 1976). Primary drug-resistance to antituberculosis drugs was higher in developing countries such as India (Trivedi and Desai, 1988). A higher proportion of strains of *M. tuberculosis* isolated from Indo-Chinese refugees with pulmonary tuberculosis in the USA were resistant to rifampicin; such strains were also always resistant to isoniazid (CDC, 1981b).

Strains of tubercle bacilli isolated from patients in Pakistan which were resistant to rifampicin were also resistant to isoniazid, but many strains which were isoniazid-resistant were susceptible to rifampicin (Siddiqi *et al.*, 1981). Strains acquired in Korea also showed an increased incidence of primary resistance to rifampicin (p. 1180). Rifampicin-resistant strains of *M. africanum* also occur (p. 1180). Strains of *M. tuberculosis* isolated from countries where rifampicin was used widely for both tuberculous and non-tuberculous conditions (Italy, Argentina, Brazil and Spain) did not show a higher incidence of primary resistance than strains from other countries (France, UK and the USA), where the use of rifampicin was largely confined to tuberculosis (Acocella *et al.*, 1977); but during the years 1981–1984 three of 19 strains of *M. tuberculosis* isolated from children in New York, USA had primary rifampicin-resistance (Steiner *et al.*, 1986).

More recently rifampicin-resistant *M. tuberculosis*, often resistant also to isoniazid and other antituberculosis drugs (multidrug-resistant *M. tuberculosis*) became common in the USA (particularly New York City), and also in other countries. Many of the patients who were infected with multidrug-resistant *M. tuberculosis* also had HIV infection. Resistance to rifampicin and other antituberculous drugs developed not only in the strain that caused the initial disease, but also as a result of reinfection with a new strain of *M. tuberculosis* which was drug-resistant (Godfrey-Faussett *et al.*, 1993; Small *et al.*, 1993; Bloch *et al.*, 1994). The problem of multidrug-resistant *M. tuberculosis* is described in more detail in the chapter on isoniazid, p. 1181.

In *M. tuberculosis* a special gene, referred to as *rpo B* gene is associated with rifampicin-resistance. This resistance involves alterations of RNA polymerase. The *rpo B* gene codes for the beta-subunit of the altered RNA polymerase. Substitutions of a limited member of highly conserved amino acids encoded by the *rpo B* gene appears to be the molecular mechanism responsible for 'single-step' high-level resistance to rifampicin in *M. tuberculosis*. These findings have served to develop a strategy to rapidly identify rifampicin-resistant *M. tuberculosis* strains by using the polymerase chain reaction (Telenti *et al.*, 1993; Miller *et al.*, 1994; Williams *et al.*, 1994; Morris *et al.*, 1995). Most strains of *M. tuberculosis* which are rifampicin-resistant are also resistant to other rifamycins, but some are rifabutin-sensitive (p. 709). The type of substitution in the beta subunit of the RNA polymerase in these strains differs from those which are found in strains resistant to both drugs (Bodmer *et al.*, 1995).

Some other mycobacteria may sometimes be sensitive to rifampicin. *Mycobacterium avium* complex may be sensitive, but many strains, especially if they are isolated from AIDS patients, are resistant (Horsburgh *et al.*, 1986; Heifets, 1988). In AIDS patients with *M. avium* complex bacteremia the use of rifampicin as a single drug did not result in a statistically significant reduction of the level of mycobacteremia in 4 weeks (Kemper *et al.*, 1994). But rifampicin potentiated the *in vitro* activity of ethambutol against most strains of this organism (Yajko *et al.*, 1988).

Mycobacterium kansasii may be rifampicin-sensitive (Lillo *et al.*, 1990), but many strains are resistant (Wallace *et al.*, 1994). Usually *M. haemophilum* is sensitive (Kristjansson *et al.*, 1991; Bernard *et al.*, 1993). Also *M. malmoense* is usually rifampicin-sensitive (Zaugg *et al.*, 1993). *Mycobacterium scrofulaceum*, *M. xenopi* and *M. marinum* may be rifampicin-sensitive, but *M. fortuitum*, *M. chelonae*, *M. simiae* and *M. ulcerans* are resistant (Woods and Washington, 1987). Rifampicin-resistant strains of mycobacteria other than *M. tuberculosis* also contain the mutation in the *rpo B* gene, similar to resistant strains of *M. tuberculosis* (Williams *et al.*, 1994). Another resistance mechanism in several fast-growing *Mycobacterium* strains is inactivation of the drug by a process referred to as ribosylation (Dabbs *et al.*, 1995).

Mycobacterium leprae (including strains resistant to sulfones such as dapsone) is also rifampicin-susceptible, the MIC being 0.3 μg per ml when tested against human strains grown in mice. In this test system, it kills bacilli more rapidly than other drugs used for treatment of leprosy, such as the sulfones (Rees *et al.*, 1970; Holmes and Hilson, 1972; Ellard, 1980; WHO, 1994). The high degree of activity of rifampicin against *M. leprae* has now also been confirmed *in vitro* with the BACTEC 460 system (Franzblau, 1991). Rifampicin and dapsone are the two most active antileprosy drugs available. A dose of 600 mg rifampicin produces peak serum level about 30-fold the MIC of *M. leprae*. A 100-mg dose of dapsone only results in weak bactericidal activity, but its peak serum levels exceed the MIC of *M. leprae* (0.003 μg per ml) by about 500-fold (Ellard, 1980). Levy *et al.* (1976) studied the bactericidal effect of rifampicin in human volunteers with untreated multibacillary leprosy by taking repeated skin biopsies for mouse inoculation to determine the rate of killing of *M. leprae*. Organisms were killed equally rapidly by a daily dose of 600 mg or single doses of 1500 or 1200 mg; lower single doses or a daily dose of 300 mg were less effective but, even with these regimens, no viable organisms could be detected within 1–2 weeks, a result which can only be achieved by about 3-months treatment with dapsone. The effect of rifampicin or dapsone treatment on the bacteremia associated with lepromatous leprosy, has also been assessed by testing the ability of organisms taken from the blood to multiply in the mouse footpad. Leprosy bacilli could be detected in the blood by direct smears for at least 12–16 weeks with either form of therapy. However, circulating viable *M. leprae* were only present for up to 6 weeks after initiation of dapsone treatment and for fewer than 4 weeks after starting rifampicin. It was concluded that either dead organisms had continued to circulate or the test system was not sufficiently sensitive to detect viable *M. leprae* (Drutz *et al.*, 1974).

Despite the rapid bactericidal action of rifampicin against *M. leprae*, it should not be concluded that all organisms are rapidly killed and that, therefore, there is no possibility of relapse after a short course of rifampicin. Pattyn *et al.* (1976) detected viable organisms in the nerve of a patient who had taken rifampicin at weekly intervals for 3 months. Viable organisms have also been recovered from nerve and muscle tissue after at least 5 years daily treatment with the drug (Rees, 1975; Rees *et al.*, 1976; Waters *et al.*, 1978).

Collectively these studies indicate that the use of rifampicin results in rapid killing of *M. leprae* which reduces the period of the patient's infectivity. However, prolonged chemotherapy for 2 years is still necessary for patients with multibacillary leprosy (WHO, 1994) (p. 694). In this form persisting *M. leprae* may be responsible for relapse after rifampicin therapy similar to that which may occur after dapsone therapy.

Strains of *M. leprae* resistant to rifampicin have been confirmed by mouse foot-pad studies; these occurred mainly in patients who were receiving rifampicin alone for the treatment of their disease (Jacobson and Hastings, 1976). Similar to rifampicin-resistant *M. tuberculosis* (p. 678) resistant *M. leprae* strains contain a mutant *rpo B* gene. This finding should be of use for the development of a rapid screening procedure, involving the polymerase chain reaction, for monitoring the emergence of rifampicin-resistant *M. leprae* strains (Honore and Cole, 1993).

4 Chlamydia

Rifampicin is active *in vitro* against the agents causing trachoma, non-gonococcal urethritis, lymphogranuloma venereum and psittacosis (Binda *et al.*, 1971), and in this respect some authors have found that it is more active than tetracycline and erythromycin (Blackman *et al.*, 1977; Schachter, 1983). Mutant strains of *Chlamydia trachomatis* resistant to rifampicin can be induced *in vitro* (Keshishyan *et al.*, 1973), but this can be prevented by the addition of subinhibitory amounts of erythromycin or oxytetracycline (Jones *et al.*, 1983). Although rifampicin is also active against *C. psittaci*, it is more active against *C. trachomatis*.

5 Rickettsiae

In vitro studies show that rifampicin is very active against *Rickettsia prowazeki* (MIC 0.008–0.01 μg per ml) and although it is also cidal against this organism at a clinically attainable concentration, the rate of killing is slow (Wisseman *et al.*, 1974). *Coxiella burnetii*, the causative agent of Q fever, is also susceptible (Sawyer *et al.*, 1987; Yeaman *et al.*, 1987).

6 Ehrlichia

The organisms of this genus are sensitive to rifampicin *in vitro* (Brouqui and Raoult, 1990; Dumler and Bakken, 1995).

7 Naegleria

Rifampicin has been reported to have *in vitro* activity against the ameboflagellate *N. fowleri* which causes amebic meningoencephalitis in humans (Thong *et al.*, 1977). A combination of drugs, including rifampicin, may be the best treatment for *N. fowleri* infections (p. 1283).

8 Leishmania

In vitro, at high concentrations, rifampicin has an inhibitory action on these protozoa (Conti and Parenti, 1983). The clinical significance of this is not known.

9 Malaria parasites

One study in humans showed that rifampicin alone in usual therapeutic doses had only partial activity against *P. vivax* infection, and used alone, it was insufficient for cure. It may prove of value in combination antimalarial therapy (Pukrittayakamee *et al.*, 1994).

10 Synergy with other drugs

Many *in vitro* and *in vivo* systems have been designed to test interactions of antibiotic combinations. The outcome of such experiments (synergy, additive effect, indifference or antagonism) on the inhibitory or bactericidal action of antibiotic combinations against a test organism is subject to many experimental variables, some of which cannot always be reproduced. For these reasons, published reports on antibiotic interactions are often conflicting. This is particularly so in the case of rifampicin. Moreover, because experimental conditions can never truly mirror human infection, predictions of the possible clinical efficacy of an antibiotic combination based on experimental data, must be made with caution. Rifampicin, when used in combination with several other chemotherapeutic agents, displays *in vitro* synergy against a wide variety of microorganisms. However, when tested by standard *in vitro* tests for measuring

Organism	MIC (μg per ml)
Gram-positive bacteria	
Staphylococcus aureus	0.02
Staphylococcus epidermidis	0.015
Streptococcus pyogenes	0.099
Streptococcus pneumoniae	0.01
Streptococcus pneumoniae (penicillin G-resistant)	4.0
Streptococcus viridans	0.12
Enterococcus faecalis	4.12
Listeria monocytogenes	0.25
Gram-negative bacteria	
Escherichia coli	5.3
Klebsiella pneumoniae	10.0
Enterobacter spp.	11.3
Proteus mirabilis	3.85
Providencia rettgeri	32.0
Serratia marcescens	64.0
Salmonella typhimurium	7.16
Haemophilus influenzae	1.0
Neisseria gonorrhoeae	0.5
Neisseria meningitidis	0.5
Bacteroides fragilis	0.26
Legionella spp.	≤0.25
Mycobacteria	
Mycobacterium tuberculosis	0.5
Mycobacterium fortuitum	>64.0

Table 1.52
Compiled from data published by Sensi *et al.* (1967), Kerry *et al.* (1975) and Thornsberry *et al.* (1983)

antibiotic interactions (checkerboard techniques, time-kill curves and tests for bactericidal activity in serum), rifampicin in low concentrations produces antagonism or reduces the bactericidal activity of cell wall-active antibiotics such as beta-lactams and vancomycin. Such *in vitro* antagonism neither predicts nor correlates with the action of these combinations *in vivo*; in the body, cell wall-active drugs may act preferentially on rapidly dividing easily accessible organisms and rifampicin may act on slower dividing organisms in less accessible sites (Sande, 1983).

An extensive literature on *in vitro* and *in vivo* synergy of rifampicin with other drugs was summarized in the fourth edition of this book, but it now appears that this has little clinical significance, and so it will not be repeated here. Certainly rifampicin is often used in combination with other drugs, particularly for the treatment of staphylococcal and mycobacterial infections, but the combinations selected are those which prevent the emergence of resistant bacterial strains. *In vitro* synergy results for practical purposes are not used as a basis for the selection of antibiotic combinations used in clinical practice.

11 Minimum inhibitory concentrations

The MICs of rifampicin against some selected bacterial species are shown in Table I.52. Organisms with an MIC of ≤2 µg per ml are regarded as susceptible and those with an MIC of up to 4 µg per ml as moderately sensitive (Thornsberry *et al.*, 1983). Naturally occurring strains of *M. tuberculosis*, both sensitive and resistant to other antituberculosis drugs, are usually inhibited by 0.5 µg per ml or less of rifampicin.

Mode of Administration and Dosage

1 Oral administration

Rifampicin is usually administered orally in a dosage of 10–20 mg per kg per day given in one, two or three divided doses. For elderly patients a smaller dose of 8 mg per kg per day may be given. Recommended doses for the treatment of tuberculosis are 600 mg daily for patients with a weight of 50 kg or more and 450 mg daily for those weighing less than 50 kg. Children should be given 10–20 mg per kg body weight, with a maximum daily dose of 600 mg. The daily amount is usually given in one dose 30 min before breakfast. Although serum levels are slightly lower if the drug is given with food (p. 682), the duration of therapeutically active serum levels is unchanged (Siegler *et al.*, 1974). Nevertheless, failure of a number of patients to respond to short-term chemotherapy of tuberculosis with a rifampicin-based regimen has been attributed to giving rifampicin after breakfast. Therefore, this drug should be given on waking and as long as possible before breakfast (Gill, 1976).

2 Intravenous administration

An i.v. preparation of rifampicin is available. Wake *et al.* (1980) used this to treat one patient in a daily dose of 600 mg for a period of 7 weeks without side-effects attributable to the drug; serum concentrations obtained were comparable with those after oral administration. Kissling *et al.* (1982) reported experience with i.v. rifampicin in 237 patients. The i.v. preparation was used for patients who were unable to swallow, or in whom oral administration was not reliable. It was administered i.v. by rapid injection or infusion in a dosage of 450–600 mg daily for adults (300 mg for children). Most (over 80%) of these patients (the majority had tuberculosis) responded to treatment (rifampicin was always combined with other drugs). The drug was well tolerated when given i.v., with the most common side-effect being thrombophlebitis, which was more frequent if treatment was continued over 30 days. Tan *et al.* (1993) administrated i.v. rifampicin to neonates. A dose of 10 mg per kg per day was used. This was given in two divided doses 12-hourly, and each dose was infused i.v. over 30 min. The drug was well tolerated.

3 Intermittent chemotherapy of tuberculosis

Rifampicin is used in regimens for this type of chemotherapy of tuberculosis (p. 1195). A dosage of 1200 mg twice-weekly is not recommended because of severe side-effects (p. 686). The frequency of side-effects is much lower with a dosage of 900 mg (15 mg per kg) twice-weekly (Citron, 1972; Anastasatu *et al.*, 1973). This and a lower dose of 600 mg, thrice- twice- or once-weekly have been satisfactory for intermittent regimens (p. 1195). Rifampicin in a dose of 600 mg or even 450 mg given on alternate days has also been used. For the treatment of leprosy (p. 694), monthly doses of 600 and 1200 mg have been well tolerated.

4 Patients with renal failure and liver disease

Rifampicin does not accumulate in patients with impaired renal function and for these the usually recommended doses are suitable. Renal clearance of rifampicin is about 12% of the glomerular filtration rate (Acocella, 1983). The drug may accumulate in the presence of liver disease or biliary tract obstruction (p. 683), and so it should be used with caution in patients with chronic alcoholism or known liver disease. The elimination of rifampicin is not affected by hemodialysis or peritoneal dialysis (Binda et al., 1971).

5 Pregnant patients

Because developmental abnormalities have been noted in animals treated with rifampicin, the manufacturers caution against its use in the first trimester of pregnancy. Rifampicin can be used in pregnancy if the appropriate indications are present; its use has not been associated with teratogenic effects (Jentgens, 1975; Stern and Stainton-Ellis, 1977; Bailey et al., 1983). The American Thoracic Society recommends that, where feasible, tuberculosis during pregnancy should be treated by at least two of isoniazid, rifampicin or ethambutol (Bailey et al., 1983).

Serum Levels in Relation to Dosage

Rifampicin is well absorbed from the gastrointestinal tract. Experience with one patient indicated that adequate absorption can occur from the jejunum even in the absence of the ileum (Wake et al., 1980). The peak serum concentration is usually reached 2 h after administration; but this may vary from 1 to 3, or even 4 h, between individuals and also within the same subject (Acocella, 1983). Serum levels are lower if the drug is taken immediately after food (Fig. I.26). A wide range of serum levels have been obtained in different studies, some of which are considerably higher than those depicted in Fig. I.26 (Binda et al., 1971).

There is also a disproportion between peak serum levels (and the area under the curve, and the size of the dose, because larger doses result in greater than proportional peak levels. After 150, 300, 450, 600 and 1200 mg doses, the peak serum levels reached are 2, 4, 6, 10 and >30 µg per ml, respectively. The reason for these disproportional rises is that there is a limit to the rate at which the liver can transport the drug (transport maximum) into the bile (see below); this occurs at a dose of about 300–450 mg. Another effect of this biliary transport maximum is that the peak serum level, half-life and area under the curve are higher when the drug is given as a single daily dose instead of divided doses. The rifampicin serum half-life also seems to increase with dose; it is 2.5, 3 and 5 h for doses of 300, 600 and 900 mg, respectively (Acocella, 1983).

Changes in serum levels occur after continuous administration of rifampicin (Acocella et al., 1971; Acocella and Scotti, 1976). During the first 6 days of treatment, although peak serum levels are unaffected, the levels at 12 h show a decrease. The serum half-life also becomes shorter

Fig. I.26.
Rifampicin serum concentrations in adult humans after a single oral dose of 600 mg on an empty stomach and 600 mg in addition to breakfast. (Redrawn after Verbist and Gyselen, 1968, with permission.)

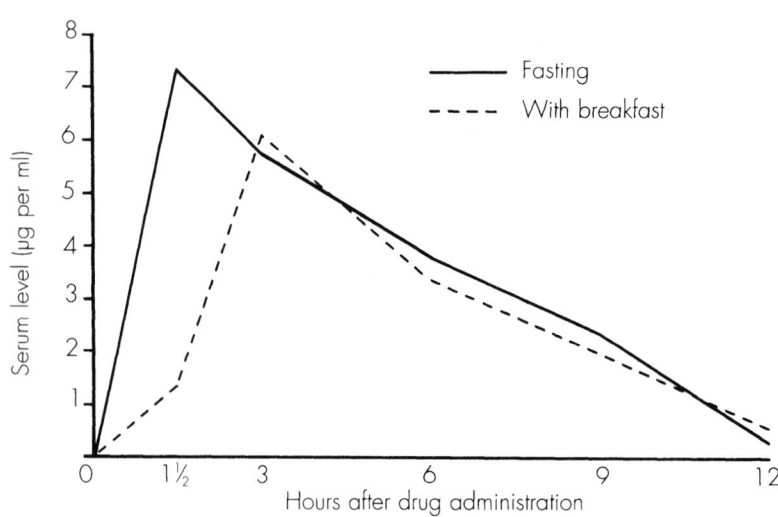

during the first 6 days and this is most evident with daily doses of 900 mg; the half-lives following 600-mg and 900-mg daily doses are then nearly the same (about 2.5–3.0 h). An increased rate of biliary excretion during the first 6 days of treatment occurs, because during this period rifampicin induces enzymes in the liver which increase its own metabolism (p. 689). It appears that in most subjects an equilibrium occurs after 1–2 weeks treatment, and subsequently no more major changes occur (Acocella, 1983).

Pharmacokinetic studies in infants and children (6–58 months old) showed that a mean peak serum level of 9.0–11.5 μg per ml occurs 1 h after a 10 mg per kg body weight oral dose, and the average half-life was 2.9 h (McCracken et al., 1980). When infants were given i.v. rifampicin, 5 mg per kg body weight every 12 h (each dose infused over 30 min), the average peak serum level 30 min after the end of the infusion was 4.02 μg per ml, and the trough level just before the next infusion was 1.11 μg per ml (Tan et al., 1993).

Concomitant administration of certain preparations of para-aminosalicylic acid (PAS) interferes with the absorption of rifampicin from the gastrointestinal tract; this is caused by bentonite an excipient used in PAS granules. If these two drugs are used together, their administration should be separated by an interval of about 8–12 h (Boman et al., 1971). Adequate serum levels also may not be attained if barbiturates are administered concomitantly, presumably as a result of induction of liver enzymes, which metabolize rifampicin (see above) (Council on Drugs, 1972). Archer et al. (1982) found that rifampicin serum levels were lower in patients who were given preoperative opiate and anticholinergic drugs i.m. at the same time; this appeared to be due to decreased gastrointestinal absorption of rifampicin. When ciprofloxacin is administered together with rifampicin, the serum levels of both drugs are not affected (Chandler et al., 1990). When novobiocin is given together with rifampicin, the serum levels of the latter are normal, but novobiocin concentrations in the serum are lowered. This is probably because rifampicin induces hepatic enzymes which metabolize novobiocin, but after the usual doses novobiocin serum levels are still in the therapeutic range (Drusano et al., 1986). In some AIDS patients, who were treated by rifampicin for Mycobacterium avium complex infections or tuberculosis, the serum levels of the drug were low, probably because of impaired absorption (Gordon et al., 1993; Patel et al., 1995). This may lead to failure of chemotherapy and the emergence of rifampicin-resistant M. tuberculosis strains.

Excretion

1 Urine

In general, urinary concentrations and recovery of rifampicin are related to serum levels; the time rifampicin is excreted in the urine is similar to that of its appearance in blood (Acocella, 1983). Murdoch et al. (1969) found that with daily oral doses of 900 mg, 200–400 mg of the active drug could be recovered from urine in the following 24 h. Kunin et al. (1969) showed in five male volunteers given a single dose of 300 mg rifampicin, that 6% of the total dose was excreted in the urine in the active form, and peak urine concentrations of 10–70 μg per ml were obtained within 4–8 h. With small oral doses of 150 mg or less, the drug is nearly all excreted in bile at doses of 300 mg or more the excretory capacity of the liver (see above) is exceeded, rifampicin serum levels rise and the drug appears in the urine (Girling, 1977). Desacetylrifampicin accounts for >50% of all antibacterial activity in the urine on day one of administration, but the percentage is much lower on day 7. Peak urinary concentrations (rifampicin plus desacetylrifampicin) are somewhat lower (200–250 μg per ml) than biliary peaks (300–350 μg per ml) (Acocella, 1983). After single doses of 150–600 mg rifampicin, peak urine levels at 6 h range from 100 to 450 μg per ml. Urine levels and recovery rates of rifampicin decrease with the first few days of treatment due to the increased liver metabolism of the drug (see below) (Acocella, 1978).

2 Bile

After absorption from the intestine, rifampicin is partly metabolized (deacetylated) in the liver by an enzyme induced in the first few days of treatment, to form desacetylrifampicin. This metabolite, which is more water soluble, is then excreted via bile into the intestine where it can be further reabsorbed i.e. an enterohepatic cycle occurs. Unchanged rifampicin excreted in bile is readily reabsorbed from the gut but its deacetylated form is poorly absorbed. Intestinal absorption of rifampicin can increase over time but the ability of the liver to transfer the drug into the bile is limited (transport maximum). When the transport maximum is exceeded then disproportional rises in rifampicin serum concentrations occur (p. 682). Two factors affect the metabolism and transfer of the drug into bile – the functional mass of the liver and its blood flow.

Both of these contribute in varying degrees to high and prolonged serum concentrations of rifampicin, which may occur with liver cirrhosis or chronic viral hepatitis (Acocella, 1983). Increased serum levels may also result in patients with biliary obstruction (Leading article, 1969). Rifampicin levels attained in bile are about 100-fold higher than those in the serum at the time, provided there is no biliary obstruction or impaired liver function (Keberle et al., 1968). Desacetylrifampicin is active antibacterially but less so than the parent drug (Dickinson et al., 1974). In human hepatic bile desacetylrifampicin accounts for 80% of all antibacterial activity; only low levels of this metabolite occur in the blood. In humans, antibacterial activity occurs in the bile 1–2 h after rifampicin administration and reaches a plateau at 4–6 h; this activity is mainly due to desacetylrifampicin; after a 600-mg dose the plateau concentration consists of 300 μg per ml desacetylrifampicin and about 50 μg per ml unmetabolized rifampicin. Desacetylrifampicin is transferred into bile 3-fold faster than rifampicin (Acocella, 1983).

Concomitant administration of probenecid increases serum levels in man probably by depressing hepatic uptake of rifampicin, thereby slowing its deacetylation in the liver and excretion via the bile. Studies by Kenwright and Levi (1973) indicated that the peak serum level could be almost doubled if 2 g probenecid was given orally 30 min before a 300-mg dose of rifampicin. Subsequently, Fallon et al. (1975) confirmed that probenecid increases rifampicin serum levels, but showed that this effect is so uncommon and inconsistent that probenecid has no place as an adjunct to routine rifampicin therapy.

3 Feces

Eventually about 60% of a single dose of the drug is excreted in the feces (Keberle et al., 1968).

4 Inactivation in body

In addition to deacetylation, small amounts of rifampicin may be metabolized in the liver by other mechanisms such as glucuronidation. Some 15–20% of desacetylrifampicin is converted to glucuronide in the liver (Acocella and Conti, 1980).

Distribution of the Drug in Body

Rifampicin penetrates well into most tissues. In man concentrations in the lungs, liver, stomach wall, pleural exudate, ascitic fluid and bone usually exceed simultaneous serum levels (Sensi et al., 1967). Therapeutically active concentrations are attained in tears and saliva (Hoeprich, 1971; McCracken et al., 1980; Cox et al., 1981). After usual therapeutic doses rifampicin levels in nasal secretions exceed the MICs of N. meningitidis and just reach, but do not exceed the MICs of H. influenzae (Darouiche et al., 1990).

A concentration of about 0.5 and 0.73 μg per ml may be reached in normal CSF after usual oral and i.v. doses, respectively. There may be a 4- to 8- fold increase in this concentration if the meninges are inflamed; in patients with tuberculous meningitis therapeutic CSF concentrations can be easily maintained during the first 1–2 months of treatment (Curci et al., 1969; D'Oliveira, 1972; Nau et al., 1992). In another study rifampicin was not detected in the CSF of normal subjects 3 h after a dose of 25 mg per kg, but in patients with tuberculous meningitis significant CSF concentrations were reached in 3 h and maintained for 24 h (Sippel et al., 1974). In animals, rifampicin penetrates into the brain tissue to some extent, but this penetration was mainly into brain cells and little of the drug was found in the cerebral extracellular space (Mindermann et al., 1993). In humans, after a 600-mg oral dose, concentrations of the drug in the aqueous humor of the eye ranged from less than 0.2 to 1.3 μg per ml (Outman et al., 1992). Concentrations which equate with those in the serum, are also attained in human nerve fiber tissue (Guebre-Xabier et al., 1995).

Sputum levels of 1–3 μg per ml occur when fairly large doses of rifampicin are given to patients with chronic bronchitis (Citron and May, 1969). In tuberculous patients, sputum concentrations after daily administration of 900 mg rifampicin, peak at 9 h and may reach 12 μg per ml (Acocella, 1983). Because of its lipid solubility (see below), rifampicin is concentrated in the alveolar macrophages of smokers (Hand et al., 1985). Concentrations of rifampicin equivalent to 65% of simultaneous serum values were detected in cardiac valves (Archer et al., 1982). It also penetrated well into endothelial cells, but bacterial killing by rifampicin within these cells was poor, but when combined with other antibiotics, it potentiated their killing activity against Staph. aureus (Darouiche and Hamill, 1994). Rifampicin appears to diffuse through a Staph. epidermidis biofilm and bactericidal levels of the drug can be attained at the surface of an infected implant (Dunne *et al.*, 1993). It also diffuses well into purulent collections (Suter *et al.*, 1984a) and pancreatic juice (Pederzoli *et al.*, 1985).

Rifampicin crosses the placenta producing clinically significant levels of the drug in the fetus and amniotic fluid (Binda *et al.*, 1971).

Rifampicin has one possibly detrimental effect on phagocytes; it inhibits their chemotactic activity. However, phagocytosis and intracellular killing by granulocytes and monocytes are normal in the presence of rifampicin (Van den Broek, 1989). Also, the drug unlike many other antibiotics, is lipid soluble and it can penetrate the cell membrane and kill intracellular organisms. As it is concentrated in the phagocytes, it may be delivered by these cells to the sites of infection in the body where they migrate (Mandell, 1994). The drug may also be of special value in the treatment of patients whose leucocytes are unable to kill ingested bacteria, e.g. in chronic granulomatous disease (Lobo and Mandell, 1972; Mandell and Vest, 1972), and to eradicate intracellular staphylococci which are present in leukocyte collections (Mandell, 1983; Solberg *et al.*, 1983). At an extracellular concentration of 0.06–5.0 μg per ml rifampicin reduces the number of staphylococci surviving in the polymorphs of patients with chronic granulomatous disease (Höger *et al.*, 1985). Rifampicin also has a unique action against tubercle bacilli in macrophages and closed caseous lesions (p. 1196).

Rifampicin is about 80% bound to serum proteins (Boman, 1973).

Mode of Action

Rifampicin has a specific action of inhibiting bacterial RNA polymerase (p. 561), the enzyme responsible for DNA transcription, by forming a stable drug-enzyme complex (Wehrli, 1983). Hartmann *et al.* (1967), in studies using *E. coli*, first showed that rifampicin inhibits bacterial RNA synthesis by binding to DNA-dependent RNA polymerase. Its mechanism of action on mycobacteria is similar, and rifampicin-resistant strains may possess an altered DNA-dependent RNA polymerase (Konno *et al.*, 1973). Studies by Yamada *et al.* (1985) indicate that this was the case with a rifampicin-resistant strain of *M. tuberculosis*. Mammalian cells also contain RNA polymerase, but rifampicin is selectively toxic to bacteria, because the mammalian cell enzyme is much less sensitive to the drug than its bacterial counterpart (Hartmann *et al.*, 1967; Staehelin *et al.*, 1968). The polymerase in mammalian mitochondria is sensitive to rifampicin, but is probably unaffected by the drug *in vivo* because it appears that intact mitochondria are impermeable to rifampicin (Gadaleta *et al.*, 1970). The RNA polymerase of Gram-negative and Gram-positive bacteria are similarly sensitive to rifampicin but the MICs for Gram-negative bacteria are higher because of reduced penetration of rifampicin through their outer cell membrane (p. 26). The reason for antagonism between rifampicin and antibiotics which act on growing bacteria (p. 27), may be because rifampicin stops bacterial growth (Wehrli, 1983). Rifampicin also inhibits fungal RNA synthesis, provided the drug is used with amphotericin B, which acts on the fungal plasma membrane (p. 1262), thereby increasing cell permeability to rifampicin (Battaner and Kumar, 1974). The antifungal action of rifampicin may not be due to inhibition of fungal RNA polymerase and may be due to inhibition of ribosomal RNA (p. 561) (Medoff, 1983).

Toxicity

In general, rifampicin is a well tolerated drug. Some adverse reactions can occur with either daily or intermittent therapy, whereas others usually only occur when the drug is given intermittently. Serious reactions are uncommon if the recommended dosage schedules for daily and intermittent therapy are followed. Adverse reactions to rifampicin, particularly rash and hepatotoxicity, are more common when tuberculosis is treated in AIDS patients, compared with non-AIDS patients (Chaisson *et al.*, 1987; Small *et al.*, 1991; Van der Ven *et al.*, 1994).

1 Hypersensitivity reactions

Severe generalized hypersensitivity reactions can occur but are rare (Girling, 1977). One of the most common side-effects of rifampicin is the 'cutaneous syndrome'; this may occur in patients receiving daily or intermittent rifampicin therapy and it usually becomes apparent early in the course of treatment. It consists of flushing and/or itching of the skin with or without a rash, involving particularly the face and scalp; redness and watering of the eyes may also occur. Symptoms usually appear 2 to 3 h after a rifampicin dose, are generally self-limiting and only require symptomatic treatment (Girling and Fox, 1971; Aquinas *et al.*, 1972). The frequency of cutaneous reactions varies in different populations, but they may affect up to 5% of patients. If a reaction is persistent or troublesome, desensitization of the patient to rifampicin is necessary (Girling and Hitze, 1979). The procedure for desensitization to antituberculosis drugs is described on p. 1181. On rare occasions an acute shock-like state, probably due to anaphylaxis, has followed rifampicin administration (Nessi *et al.*, 1973; Brook and Pain, 1987). The drug is not cross-allergenic with the penicillins or any other non-related antibiotics.

2 Gastrointestinal side-effects

Anorexia, nausea, abdominal pain, vomiting and diarrhea ('abdominal syndrome') are uncommon side-effects. These symptoms may occur with both daily and intermittent rifampicin therapy and, if unaccompanied by other side-effects, seldom necessitate change in therapy (Girling, 1977). If the patient has been taking rifampicin on an empty stomach (as recommended) these side-effects can be alleviated by taking the drug during or immediately after a meal.

3 Pseudomembranous colitis

This may complicate therapy with many antibiotics; it is usually due to an alteration in bowel flora resulting in the overgrowth of toxin-producing *Cl. difficile* (p. 594). Fournier *et al.* (1980) first reported a patient with pseudomembranous colitis probably due to rifampicin, and Fekety *et al.* (1983) then reviewed reports of six such patients. All had received rifampicin as part of treatment for active tuberculosis; the complication appeared as early as 7 days and as late as 9 months after commencement of rifampicin therapy; *Cl. difficile* was isolated from two patients and one strain tested was toxigenic *in vitro* and resistant to rifampicin; one patient died but the others recovered after discontinuation of chemotherapy or treatment with vancomycin. Usually *Cl. difficile* is very sensitive to rifampicin (MIC <1 μg per ml) (Acocella and Arioli, 1980; Fekety *et al.*, 1983). Experience with hamsters suggest that *Cl. difficile* may become resistant on exposure to rifampicin and then spread to the environment and to contacts (Fekety *et al.*, 1983).

4 Hepatotoxicity

Rifampicin-induced hepatitis is uncommon, occurring in up to 1% of patients (Girling and Hitze, 1979). Rifampicin can often be recommenced in such patients after recovery from hepatitis; but liver function tests should be performed regularly and if abnormalities recur, alternative therapy should be given. Original fears that a rifampicin/isoniazid combination might be markedly more hepatotoxic, have been dispelled with accumulated experience (p. 1190). The rate of hepatotoxicity with this combination in the USA is less than 4%. Many patients receiving rifampicin alone or in combination with other drugs, develop elevations of serum transaminase levels, particularly during the first few weeks of therapy, but most of these are asymptomatic and the transaminase levels return to normal whether rifampicin is stopped or not (Newman *et al.*, 1974; Donald *et al.*, 1987). Baron and Bell (1974) also showed that transient biochemical liver disturbances were common during the early weeks of antituberculosis treatment, irrespective of whether rifampicin was in the regimen, and they did not imply serious toxicity. Interference with bilirubin excretion by rifampicin in the early phase of rifampicin treatment (p. 689) should not be interpreted as hepatoxicity. Rifampicin (with isoniazid) can be safely used in patients with liver disease and in alcoholics, but regular monitoring of liver function tests in such patients is prudent (p. 1190) (Girling, 1977). It may be concluded that mild transient abnormalities of liver function not uncommonly occur in the early weeks of rifampicin treatment, but the risk of overt hepatitis during chemotherapy is small (Girling, 1977). Experience in treating leprosy, suggests that rifampicin may potentiate hepatotoxicity caused by ethionamide or prothionamide (p. 1236). Occasionally acute liver failure, necessitating liver transplantation, has occurred in patients receiving combined rifampicin, isoniazid and pyrazinamide therapy (Mitchell *et al.* (1995).

5 Thrombocytopenia and other hematological changes

Thrombocytopenic purpura, sometimes associated with bleeding, usually occurs with intermittent rifampicin therapy, but it may also occur during daily treatment (Hong Kong/BMRC, 1975).

Blajchman *et al.* (1970) reported a patient in whom severe thrombocytopenia with bleeding occurred during administration and readministration of rifampicin. The thrombocytopenia had an immunological basis, because the patient's serum contained both IgG and IgM antibodies, which could only fix complement to platelets in the presence of rifampicin. These authors also referred to seven similar cases communicated to them, and noted that in all patients thrombocytopenia was associated with high dosage intermittent rifampicin therapy (1200 mg twice-weekly). Poole *et al.* (1971) observed the same complication in three patients under similar circumstances. In view of these reports high intermittent doses of rifampicin should be avoided, and where possible monthly platelet counts should be performed on all patients receiving rifampicin. Thrombocytopenia and other side-effects of intermittent therapy (see below) are much less common when lower rifampicin doses of 900 mg or 600 mg twice-weekly are used (p. 681). All side-effects from intermittent rifampicin therapy are more frequent and severe when either the individual dose or the interval between doses is increased. However, side-effects do not occur when the intervals between doses is as long as 1 month as in the treatment of leprosy (p. 694). These complications may also occur in patients who have been prescribed daily rifampicin, if they do not take the drug regularly and interrupt their medication for several days at a time (Flynn *et al.*, 1974).

Thrombocytopenia usually becomes apparent within 3 h of a dose, and in the absence of further rifampicin, the platelet count returns to normal within 36 h. Fatalities have been recorded due to cerebral hemorrhage when the drug has been continued (Girling, 1977). The occurrence of thrombocytopenia or purpura is a contraindication to the further use of rifampicin. One 75-year-old man who had been treated for 10 days with daily isoniazid, rifampicin and ethambutol, developed rifampicin-induced immune thrombocytopenia. Rifampicin-independent antiplatelet antibodies were implicated in this case (Martinez *et al.*, 1994). Another patient developed bleeding during rifampicin therapy, which was due to circulating inhibitor of factor VIII (Legrand *et al.*, 1987).

Blajchman *et al.* (1970) demonstrated weak serum antibodies against red cells in 19 of 41 patients receiving rifampicin, but these did not appear to be associated with any hematological complications. These rifampicin-dependent antibodies, which bind complement to the surface of red cells, appear to be more common in patients receiving intermittent rifampicin therapy, either in high doses (Poole *et al.*, 1971), or in the lower doses of 600 mg twice-weekly (Poole *et al.*, 1973). However, rifampicin, unlike penicillin G, does not combine firmly with red cells, and hemolytic anemia due to this drug, although reported, appears to be rare (Worlledge 1973a; Girling, 1977). Hemolysis usually becomes evident within 2–3 h after a rifampicin dose and recovery occurs when the drug is stopped. Severe hemolysis with renal failure has been described. Massive hemolysis has been reported in one patient who received rifampicin therapy for nearly a year (Lakshminarayan *et al.*, 1973).

Neutropenia has been detected in a small percentage of patients who have received rifampicin (plus pyrazinamide and isoniazid) for the treatment of tuberculosis (Van Assendelft, 1985).

Human polymorphonuclear leukocytes incubated with rifampicin (or with chloramphenicol, sodium fusidate or tetracyclines) show markedly depressed chemotactic migration (p. 565) (Forsgren and Schmelling, 1977), probably by competing with chemoattractants on leukocytes (Gray *et al.*, 1983). The clinical significance of this observation is not known.

6 Renal failure

Sudden onset of fever and lumbar pain followed by oliguria and then anuria has been described in patients treated with rifampicin (Cordonnier and Muller, 1972; Kleinknecht *et al.*, 1972; Flynn *et al.*, 1974). All of these patients had temporarily discontinued daily rifampicin therapy and symptoms occurred 1–2 h after readministration of the drug. The anuria usually persisted for several days necessitating hemodialysis, but ultimately recovery was complete. Rothwell and Richmond (1974) reported a patient who took rifampicin intermittently of her own accord and who developed acute reversible renal failure in association with moderately severe hepatocellular damage. Renal failure has also occurred when rifampicin administration had been resumed after an interval. In two patients reported by Seufert (1973), acute renal failure was associated with hemolysis, but this did not appear to be the direct cause of the renal damage. Renal failure may also result from shock associated with rifampicin therapy (see above). Pathological changes commonly described with renal failure due to rifampicin have been acute tubular necrosis possibly caused by a period of tubular ischemia (Chan *et al.*, 1975). Studies in other patients have revealed changes of interstitial nephritis (Flynn *et al.*, 1974; Stone *et al.*, 1976; Gabow *et al.*, 1976). An acute interstitial nephritis, similar to that which may be caused by the penicillins (p. 32), has been described as a rare complication of rifampicin; this hypersensitivity reaction is characterized by fever and often by nausea, diarrhea, myalgia, rash, eosinophilia, abnormal liver function tests and renal failure (Nessi *et al.*, 1976). The patient described by Gabow *et al.* (1976) is of interest, because he developed renal failure which was detected by a rising serum creatinine level in the absence of symptoms when rifampicin was readministered after a gap of 36 days; renal biopsy showed interstitial and glomerular changes and antibody deposited about the renal tubules. Permanent renal damage occurred in a 42-year-old woman who resumed rifampicin therapy after a period of 9 months; two renal biopsies showed severe cortical necrosis (Cochran *et al.*, 1975). Some of the pathological changes which have been described, together with the detection of circulating rifampicin-dependent antibodies in high titer in some patients (Chan *et al.*, 1975), suggest that the renal complications of rifampicin have an immunological basis.

Acute renal failure due to rifampicin therapy is uncommon, but is more prone to occur in patients receiving intermittent therapy or those taking the drug irregularly. If the drug is recommenced after an interval, special care should be taken and it may be advisable to reintroduce it in small gradually increasing daily doses (Girling, 1977). If renal failure develops, further use of the drug is contraindicated.

The time of onset of nephrotoxicity after starting rifampicin is unpredictable. Cohn *et al.* (1985) described two cases and found another 83 cases of rifampicin-induced renal insufficiency which had been reported in English and French language journals.

7 Influenza syndrome

This is a collection of symptoms which is common with certain regimens of intermittent rifampicin therapy (Aquinas *et al.*, 1972; Zierski, 1973). The features have been delineated during various clinical trials on patients with tuberculosis (Hong Kong/Brompton Hospital/ BMRC, 1974, 1975; Hong Kong/BMRC, 1974, 1975; Singapore/BMRC, 1975); these have been summarized by Girling (1977).

The 'flu' syndrome is peculiar to intermittent therapy; it consists of fever, headache, malaise and bone pain beginning 1–2 h after a dose of rifampicin and these usually subside spontaneously within 12 h. This syndrome usually does not appear until after 3–6 months of intermittent rifampicin therapy, and it may be accompanied by other side-effects of rifampicin. The frequency of the 'flu' syndrome is much higher both in patients receiving higher doses of the drug (especially 1200 mg or more), and also in patients receiving the drug at weekly intervals compared with others given the same dosage twice-weekly. Some authors have noted that this syndrome is more frequent in females (Eule *et al.*, 1974), and it is more common in men, but not women with increasing age (Hong Kong/BMRC, 1975). Therapy with rifampicin may be continued in most patients, either by using a lower dosage for intermittent therapy or by substituting a daily rifampicin regimen (Girling and Fox, 1971; Aquinas *et al.*, 1972). Attempts to reduce the frequency of this side-effect by adding a small daily supplement of rifampicin to the larger intermittent doses have not been successful enough for practical application (Hong Kong/BMRC, 1974; Singapore/BMRC, 1975). The syndrome appears to be mild and infrequent if rifampicin is given in doses of 600 mg or 450 mg three times weekly or 900 mg, 600 mg or 450 mg twice-weekly or 600 mg once-weekly.

An immunological reaction appears to be involved because many patients with the syndrome develop serum rifampicin-dependent antibodies (Worlledge, 1973b; Hong Kong/Brompton Hospital/BMRC, 1974; Singapore/BMRC, 1975). These antibodies are affected by the rhythm of rifampicin administration. They are rarely detectable with daily administration, possibly because this causes immune tolerance, whereas intermittent therapy favors sensitization. Bassi *et al.* (1976) studied rifampicin antibodies in patients with tuberculosis, 1 day, 1 week, 3 weeks and 8 weeks after discontinuation of daily therapy; the greater number of patients with antibodies was found in the third week. These findings were considered to be more consistent with a hypothesis that continuous rifampicin treatment results in continuous neutralization of antibodies, rather than induction of tolerance. The dose size is also important in determining the presence of antibodies; doses of 450 mg or 600 mg three times-weekly are much less liable to produce antibodies than doses of 900 mg or 600 mg twice- or once-weekly (Girling, 1977). Experience in subsequent trials (Hong Kong/BMRC, 1981, p. 681), where rifampicin was used in a dose of 600 mg three times-weekly, revealed a very low frequency of rifampicin-dependent antibodies and the 'flu' syndrome. There is no evidence from studies in Hong Kong and Singapore that the presence of antibodies to rifampicin affects the therapeutic response to the drug (Hong Kong/ Singapore/BMRC, 1976).

8 Respiratory syndrome

This syndrome is a less common complication of intermittent rifampicin administration (Aquinas *et al.*, 1972; Hong Kong/Brompton Hospital/BMRC, 1974). It consists of dyspnea with or without a wheeze and sometimes a fall in blood pressure and shock. This side-effect is usually managed in a similar manner to the 'flu' syndrome, with which it may be associated and share a common mechanism.

9 Immunosuppression

Rifampicin has been reported to affect both humoral and cell-mediated immunity in animals and man, but results have been inconsistent. For instance, Graber *et al.* (1973) found that rifampicin interfered with the anamnestic response to *Salmonella typhi* vaccine in patients with tuberculosis, but Bassi *et al.* (1975) and Miller (1978), studying similar patients, found no interference with antibody response after administration of killed influenza virus vaccine. Other studies in humans suggested that rifampicin may suppress cell-mediated immunity, as tested for by delayed cutaneous hypersensitivity to purified protein derivative (PPD) of *M. tuberculosis* or by *in vitro* lymphocyte responses. There has been a decreased cutaneous reaction to PPD in some patients treated with rifampicin (Mukerjee *et al.*, 1973). In high concentrations rifampicin suppressed *in vitro* lymphocyte responses to PPD and inhibited the blastic transformation of lymphocytes cultured in the presence of phytohemagglutinin (PHA) (Nilsson, 1971; Grassi and Pozzi, 1972); it also suppressed colony formation by human thymus-derived lymphocytes (Scharre *et al.*, 1981).

Other investigators have found differing results in studies of patients with tuberculosis receiving rifampicin. Ruben *et al.* (1974) noted that suppression of *in vitro* lymphocyte responses to PHA and PPD only occurred in such patients after 12–16 weeks treatment. Gupta *et al.* (1975) demonstrated suppression of T-lymphocyte rosettes in 8 of 18 patients, which usually occurred after a period of 8 weeks; they were also able to demonstrate similar changes in some healthy subjects who had received rifampicin for 2–3 weeks and these changes were reversible after cessation of the drug. Goldstein *et al.* (1976) only found depression of lymphocyte responses to PHA in patients with tuberculosis who had received the drug for 4–24 months and in whom *in vitro* and *in vivo* responses to PPD remained normal. These authors pointed out that the divergent conclusions which have been reached about the immunosuppressive effect of rifampicin can be explained by the diversity of the patients with tuberculosis who have been tested, some of whom may have been anergic due to their disease, and to the variety of test systems used. Humber *et al.* (1980) investigated patients with tuberculosis treated by regimens with and without rifampicin, and tuberculosis contacts receiving either rifampicin or a placebo; rifampicin had no effect on humoral or cellular immunity. In summary, although rifampicin can interfere with lymphocyte function *in vitro*, it is doubtful whether it has any effect on humoral or cellular immunity in patients when used in the usual dosage (Grosset and Leventis, 1983). Certainly there is no evidence that immunosuppressive effects of the drug hinder its effectiveness in the treatment of tuberculosis in man (Gupta *et al.*, 1975). This also applies to the use of rifampicin in leprosy, but in certain forms of this disease immunological reactions may be precipitated as a consequence of the antimicrobial activity of the drug (Anderson, 1983).

10 Fetal abnormalities

These have been observed in rats and mice when large doses of rifampicin were used (Stern and Stainton-Ellis, 1977). Although the manufacturers warn that the drug is contraindicated in pregnancy, particularly during the first trimester because of possible teratogenicity, experience to date indicates that it may be used under appropriate indications (p. 682).

11 Interference with metabolism of other drugs

Rifampicin competes with and thereby decreases the biliary excretion of some substances such as bilirubin, bromsulphalein (BSP) and certain contrast media used in cholecystography (Binda *et al.*, 1971). With bilirubin, at first rifampicin competes with it for excretion so that bilirubin serum levels increase, then probably as a result of enzyme induction (see below), bilirubin glucuronide production and its excretion in bile increases and serum bilirubin levels return to normal. If a BSP retention test is required, it should be performed either before or at least 8–10 h after rifampicin administration(Acocella and Conti, 1980).

Rifampicin induces a gradual proliferation of hepatic cell smooth endoplasmic reticulum in man, which is thought to be a locus for microsomal enzymes responsible for drug metabolism (Jezeguel *et al.*, 1971). Enzymes that deacetylate rifampicin (p. 683) are not located on the smooth endoplasmic reticulum; possibly the stimulation of enzymes at this site which catalyze the conversion of desacetylrifampicin into a glucuronide, is the reason for their increased functional activity after rifampicin administration (Acocella and Conti, 1980). Rifampicin causes enhancement of its own metabolism during the first 6 days of treatment, resulting in lowering of serum levels and half-life values for the drug (p. 683). This also seems to be the main mechanism by which it accelerates the metabolism of a number of other drugs in man. Rifampicin drug interactions have been reviewed by Acocella and Conti (1980) and Baciewicz and Self (1984). A very short-term (2–4 days) administration of rifampicin can induce the oxidative metabolism of other drugs (Borcherding *et al.*, 1992).

The half-life of tolbutamide is shortened in patients with tuberculosis treated by rifampicin (Syvälahti *et al.*, 1974), and diabetic therapy should be adjusted by estimating blood glucose levels. The efficacy of oral contraceptive medication may be impaired, resulting in disturbances of the menstrual cycle and unplanned pregnancy (Skolnick *et al.*, 1976). Induction of liver enzymes by rifampicin causes an increased breakdown of estrogenic hormones (Bolt et al., 1974) and the prognestinic components (Baciewicz and Self, 1984) in oral contraceptive pills. Patients receiving rifampicin treatment are recommended to use contraceptive measures other than oral contraceptive drugs (Acocella and Conti, 1980).

Rifampicin has a pronounced effect on the metabolism of corticosteroids, by increasing catabolism, again presumably by induction of microsomal enzymes (Yamada and Iwai, 1976; Wood, 1987). In three such patients with associated adrenal insufficiency, rifampicin appeared to precipitate acute adrenal crisis (Edwards et al., 1974; Elansary and Earis, 1983); in one of these cases the serum half-life of cortisol was reduced (Edwards et al., 1974). A reduction in circulating corticosteroids by concomitant rifampicin may adversely affect renal transplantation. Buffington et al. (1976) described three patients with renal transplants, who developed progressive loss of renal allograft function during treatment of tuberculosis by rifampicin; this appeared to be due to a decreased glucocorticosteroid effect as a result of increased degradation. Langhoff and Madsen (1983) had a similar patient who was being treated for tuberculosis with rifampicin and isoniazid in whom renal transplant rejection occurred; rapid prednisolone clearance was related to rifampicin therapy; antituberculous treatment was also associated with a fall in blood concentrations of cyclosporine. If rifampicin is required in a renal transplant patient, it may be necessary to double daily doses of corticosteroids. The failure of a child with nephrotic syndrome to respond to corticosteroid treatment was shown to result from a decreased half-life of prednisolone in association with rifampicin therapy (Hendrickse et al., 1979). A study by Powell-Jackson et al. (1983) of six patients with steroid-dependent asthma revealed that the serum half-life and bioavailability of prednisolone was decreased after rifampicin administration, and prednisolone doses had to nearly double to maintain asthma control. In two patients with pulmonary disease usually responsive to corticosteroids, treated by McAllister et al. (1983), presumed steroid response occurred when concomitant treatment with rifampicin was withdrawn. These authors also investigated seven patients who were being treated for pulmonary tuberculosis with rifampicin plus isoniazid and sometimes ethambutol and prednisolone; in five patients it was possible to study them when they were taking prednisolone alone; rifampicin increased serum clearance of prednisolone by 45% and reduced its bioavailability (area under the serum concentration time curve) by 66%. Two patients with giant cell arteritis failed to respond to prednisolone, when rifampicin was also administered (Carrie et al., 1994). Rifampicin does not cause hypothyroidism in normal patients, but this may result in patients with hypothyroidism who are receiving thyroid hormone replacement therapy (Isley, 1987). Experience with another patient has confirmed the observation by Langhoff and Madsen (see above), that concomitant rifampicin administration can reduce serum cyclosporine levels (Daniels et al., 1984).

Rifampicin diminishes the activity of anticoagulants. Studies by O'Reilly (1974, 1975) indicate that rifampicin markedly decreases the effect of warfarin during long-term therapy by enhancing its elimination from plasma, presumably mainly by liver enzyme induction. In patients receiving therapy with both warfarin and rifampicin, an unusually high maintenance dose of warfarin may be required to achieve a therapeutic effect. Romankiewicz and Ehrman (1975) described a patient in whom this effect on warfarin appeared to be maximal 5–7 days after commencing rifampicin therapy, and it persisted for a similar period of time after rifampicin was stopped. There are also reports of rifampicin interfering with the anticoagulant action of other coumarin derivatives, such as phenprocoumon (Baciewicz and Self, 1984).

Symptoms of methadone withdrawal have been described in patients receiving rifampicin which have been attributed to enhanced methadone metabolism in the liver (Kreek et al., 1976; Bending and Skacel, 1977). In the report by Kreek et al. (1976), of 30 patients receiving rifampicin (600–900 mg per day) and also methadone maintenance, symptoms of narcotic withdrawal developed in 21 patients 1–33 days after commencing rifampicin. In pharmacological studies of six of these patients, concomitant administration of rifampicin lowered methadone plasma concentrations and increased the urinary excretion of its major metabolite, consistent with an enhancement of methadone metabolism in the liver. Apparently by inducing its metabolism and perhaps increasing its biliary excretion, rifampicin causes lowering of serum theophylline levels after oral and i.v. administration of aminophylline (Powell-Jackson et al., 1985).

By presumed enzyme induction, concomitant administration of rifampicin can cause a reduction in serum cardiac glycosides (digoxin and digitoxin) levels and be associated with a diminished response of cardiac failure (Acocella and Conti 1980; Novi et al., 1980; Poor et al., 1983; Bussey et al., 1984). It is therefore advisable to estimate serum levels of cardiac glycosides of patients receiving rifampicin. Rifampicin also seems to induce liver enzymes which metabolize quinidine. One patient has been described whose ventricular dysrythmia responded to quinidine but relapsed when rifampicin was added to treat tuberculosis (Acocella and Conti, 1980). In another patient, it seemed that rifampicin increased the metabolism of quinidine thereby reducing its serum concentration; this led to a decline in the serum digoxin concentration, because this in turn is dependent on the serum quinidine concentration (Bussey *et al.*, 1984). Twum-Barima and Carruthers (1981) confirmed in volunteers that 7 days treatment with rifampicin increased the rate of metabolism of quinidine. Induction of quinidine metabolism by rifampicin may increase the production of active metabolites and thereby compensate for the decline in serum quinidine concentration (Bussey *et al.*, 1984). Rifampicin can also increase propanolol metabolism (Herman *et al.*, 1983). Dapsone clearance is enhanced by rifampicin but this does not appear to have any significance in the treatment of leprosy (Acocella and Conti, 1980).

Early studies did not show any interaction between rifampicin and isoniazid (Acocella and Conti, 1980). Mouton *et al.* (1979) showed that isoniazid had an adverse effect on serum rifampicin levels, but this was not considered of clinical importance. But the interactions between these two drugs may be very complex (p. 1187). In addition, the co-administration of rifampicin and pyrazinamide, results in somewhat lower rifampicin serum levels. Pyrazinamide probably affects the hepatic or renal clearance of rifampicin (Fox, 1990; Jain *et al.*, 1993). Interactions between rifampicin and antifungal azole drugs such as ketaconazole, itraconazole and fluconazole are important. Concomitant rifampicin administration reduces the serum levels of ketaconazole and itraconazole and to a lesser extent those of fluconazole. This may lead to failure of antifungal therapy (Doble *et al.*, 1988; Tucker *et al.*, 1992). Experience in two children receiving chloramphenicol succinate i.v. indicated that concomitant administration of rifampicin can reduce peak serum levels of chloramphenicol by 63.8–85.5%, inducing hepatic enzymes which metabolize chloramphenicol (Prober, 1985). Combined treatment by rifampicin and doxycycline results in lowered serum levels of doxycycline, probably by its increased metabolism in liver. This may lead to therapeutic failure when these two drugs are used for treatment of brucellosis (Colmenero *et al.*, 1994). Rifampicin also promotes the glucuronidation of zidovudine in the liver, so if the two drugs are used together for a prolonged period, lower therapeutically active serum levels of zidovudine result. This may have therapeutic consequences (Burger *et al.*, 1993). By the same mechanism rifampicin also markedly reduces serum clarithromycin levels (Wallace *et al.*, 1995).

Other biochemical interactions of doubtful clinical significance have been reported. Early-phase hyperglycemia has been noted in patients with pulmonary tuberculosis taking rifampicin; this may have been due to rifampicin increasing intestinal absorption of glucose; there was no evidence that rifampicin was diabetogenic (Takasu *et al.*, 1982). Rifampicin also increases the cholesterol saturation of bile possibly due to enhanced secretion of cholesterol; theoretically this could predispose patients to cholesterol gall-stones (Von Bergmann *et al.*, 1981). Long-term studies show that combined treatment with rifampicin and isoniazid does not cause changes in vitamin D metabolism (p. 1193).

12 Other side-effects

There have been single case reports of severe exudative conjunctivitis (Cayley and Majumdar, 1976), and Stevens-Johnson syndrome (Nyirenda and Gill, 1977), attributed to rifampicin. A 9-year-old patient developed polyarthritis, rash and hepatitis in association with anti-native DNA antibodies and a positive antinuclear factor after 9 months continuous treatment with rifampicin and ethambutol. It was considered that rifampicin was the most likely cause of this illness (Grennan and Sturrock, 1976).

Clinical circumstances suggested that rifampicin may have caused an organic brain syndrome in a man being treated for pulmonary tuberculosis (Pratt, 1979). There have been four anecdotal case reports suggesting a possible association between rifampicin administration and the rate of growth of lung malignancies (Rodescu *et al.*, 1981; Sebba *et al.*, 1982). This association may be coincidental.

The presence of rifampicin in serum interferes with serum vitamin B_{12} and folate assays. This problem may be overcome either by using a rifampicin-resistant organism in such assays or by collecting specimens for assay from patients just before redosing, when the serum rifampicin level should be low (Cole *et al.*, 1973).

Rifampicin causes a reddish discoloration of the urine and other body fluids such as sputum, sweat and tears, but this is harmless. Plastic contact lenses may also be permanently discolored. Pleural fluid in rifampicin-treated patients may be stained red, and this can be mistaken for blood. Rifampicin overdosage can cause pink-red discoloration of the skin and many tissues, the so-called 'red man syndrome' (Jack *et al.*, 1978). Other symptoms of overdosage described include nausea, vomiting, flushing, abdominal pain, pruritis, angioedema and obtundation. Acute rifampicin overdose is uncommon and three fatalities in the eight reported cases were associated with alcohol intake (Wong *et al.*, 1984).

Clinical Uses of the Drug

1 Tuberculosis

Rifampicin is one of four bactericidal drugs which have important roles in the treatment of tuberculosis. By its unique activity in closed lesions where organisms are multiplying intermittently, rifampicin is particularly useful during the sterilizing phase of treatment (p. 1196). Rifampicin is the most effective companion drug for isoniazid; in developed countries where cost is not a significant factor, these two drugs are always used in combination, unless the *M. tuberculosis* strain is rifampicin-resistant (p. 678). Rifampicin is used in the short-course treatment of tuberculosis and intermittent treatment regimens (Hong *et al.*, 1988). In combination with other drugs, such as ethambutol, streptomycin and/or pyrazinamide, it is also very useful for the treatment of isoniazid-resistant pulmonary tuberculosis (Swai *et al.*, 1988). It may be of value in preventative treatment, although one animal study showed rifabutin (p. 709) to be superior for this purpose (Ji *et al.*, 1993). These, and related problems in the treatment of tuberculosis, are discussed on pp. 1193, 1202. An animal study showed that the antitubercular activity of rifampicin was considerably increased when the drug was encapsulated in egg phosphatidylcholine liposomes (Agarwal *et al.*, 1994).

2 Other mycobacterial infections

Mycobacteria other than tubercle bacilli are markedly heterogenous in their susceptibility to antibiotics (p. 1211), and therefore their drug treatment is often difficult. Rifampicin-containing drug regimens are recommended for the treatment of *M. kansasii* infections (Woods and Washington, 1987; Lillo *et al.*, 1990; Patel *et al.*, 1994) (p. 1216). A regimen of rifampicin, ethambutol and ciprofloxacin had good efficacy for the treatment of *M. avium* complex infections in AIDS patients (Jacobson *et al.*, 1993), but it is now considered that either clarithromycin (p. 648) or azithromycin (p. 657) should be included as the number one drug in the regimen to treat this infection. Ethambutol is the second best drug (p. 1215). Rifampicin may be used as the third drug but rifabutin is preferable as it reduces clarithromycin serum levels to a lesser extent (p. 646). Rifampicin and/or ethambutol are usually included in the treatment regimens for *M. malmoense* infections (Zaugg *et al.*, 1993). Rifampicin in combination with other drugs is usually effective for the treatment of *M. haemophilum* in patients with AIDS (Dever *et al.*, 1992).

Rifampicin has been used with some success to treat infections due to *M. marinum*, although lesions due to this organism often resolve spontaneously (p. 1216). Van Dyke and Lake (1975) treated two patients with an aquarium granuloma with rifampicin and ethambutol (one also with isoniazid) with apparent improvement. This drug combination was of more apparent value for the treatment of a patient reported by Sage and Derrington (1973). This 70-year-old man with lymphosarcoma developed multiple cutaneous lesions due to *M. marinum*; complete resolution of all lesions followed a prolonged course of therapy with rifampicin and ethambutol. Bailey *et al.* (1982) obtained a good clinical response using a rifampicin/ethambutol combination to treat a *M. marinum* infection which involved tendons and joints of the hand; surgical intervention was thereby avoided. Donta *et al.* (1986) described four patients who responded to rifampicin alone or a rifampicin/ethambutol combination, in whom prior treatment with tetracycline, minocycline or doxycycline had been ineffective for their *M. marinum* infection.

3 Leprosy

The treatment of this disease is beset with many of the difficulties which are associated with the treatment of tuberculosis; in both diseases bacterial persistence occurs and drug-resistance develops if monotherapy is used. Moreover, in leprosy, up until 1960 when the technique for cultivating *M. leprae* in the mouse foot-pad was devised, drugs had to be tried empirically in lepromatous patients. The historical aspects of leprosy treatment leading up to the 1981 World Health Organisation (WHO) recommendations (Report, 1982) have been the subject of several reviews (Levy, 1983; Rees, 1983; Waters, 1983).

a Evolution of antileprosy chemotherapy The sulfones, a group of drugs chemically related to the sulfonamides (p. 805), were shown to be effective in leprosy in 1943. After 1947 and until 1971 the simplest sulfone, dapsone (diamino-diphenylsulphone; DDS) was used widely and successfully as monotherapy for leprosy. From the early 1960s relapses amongst patients taking dapsone and failure to respond to dapsone in others, suggested that acquired or secondary resistance to the drug was occurring. This was confirmed by the mouse foot-pad technique in 1964. Clofazimine ('Lamprene') was first used successfully in leprosy in 1962; it kills *M. leprae* at about the same speed as dapsone. No confirmed cases of clofazimine-resistance have been reported (WHO, 1994). Rees *et al.* (1970) first demonstrated that rifampicin was effective against *M. leprae* both in the mouse foot-pad model and in clinical leprosy. It was more rapidly bactericidal than dapsone (p. 679), and it was effective against strains of *M. leprae* resistant to dapsone. Wilkinson *et al.* (1972) used rifampicin to treat 20 patients with lepromatous leprosy; they obtained a good clinical response in 15 patients and considered that a small daily dose of 150 mg of rifampicin was as effective as 450 mg daily. Rees (1975) showed that even lower doses of rifampicin (20 mg daily) were still bactericidal, but as measured by viability of *M. leprae* in the mouse foot-pad test, such doses were not as rapidly killing as one of 600 mg daily. Waters *et al.* (1978) described the daily use of rifampicin in over 100 patients with lepromatous leprosy; they confirmed the rapid bactericidal effect of the drug and noted that sometimes clinical improvement became apparent as early as 14 days after the start of treatment. Strains of *M. leprae* resistant to rifampicin have been confirmed in the mouse foot-pad in a small number of patients who relapsed and had been given the drug as monotherapy or among dapsone-resistant cases treated with rifampicin and dapsone (Report, 1982; WHO, 1994).

By the 1970s dapsone-resistance of *M. leprae* was recognized as a serious and universal problem; additionally, because of the long time (5–20 years or more) taken for the emergence of dapsone-resistance, many more patients were expected to relapse due to dapsone-resistance. Low dosage and irregular treatment with dapsone appeared to be factors in the development of dapsone-resistance. In 1976, the WHO Expert Committee on Leprosy recommended that all active cases of multibacillary leprosy, whether untreated or relapsed, should be treated with at least two effective antileprosy drugs (WHO, 1977). Clofazimine given for the first 4–6 months of treatment, was recommended as the companion drug for dapsone; alternatively dapsone could be combined with rifampicin (300–600 mg daily) for a minimum of 2 weeks to avoid the skin discoloration which occurs in patients with a light-colored skin treated with clofazimine. A combination of rifampicin and clofazimine was recommended for the treatment of patients with disease due to dapsone-resistant *M. leprae*.

Ethionamide and prothionamide, drugs which have been used for the treatment of tuberculosis (p. 1234) have been used for leprosy. In studies in the late 1970s when ethionamide monotherapy was used for lepromatous leprosy, relapses occurred after 6–9 years treatment and ethionamide-resistance was confirmed in the mouse foot-pad. The use of ethionamide and prothionamide for the treatment of leprosy has been studied much less extensively than dapsone, rifampicin and clofazimine (Waters, 1983).

The phenomenon of bacterial persistence had been recognized with *M. leprae*. Although approximately 99.9% of leprosy bacilli are slowly killed by dapsone (dose 50–100 mg daily) and clofazimine in about 3–4 months, and within 3–7 days by rifampicin administered in single doses of 600–1500 mg (p. 679), it had long been known that multibacillary disease could relapse after stopping treatment. It was for this reason, that prolonged and even life-time chemotherapy of lepromatous leprosy was formerly recommended. In 1974 persisting viable leprosy bacilli were detected in patients treated for 10–12 years with dapsone; subsequently drug-susceptible *M. leprae* were isolated from patients treated with rifampicin monotherapy for 5 years (p. 679) and from those treated with clofazimine as monotherapy for 10 years (Report, 1982). Persisters are viable fully drug-susceptible organisms which can survive for many years in a patient despite the presence of bactericidal concentration of an antileprosy drug; presumably persisters are physiologically dormant bacilli.

In 1977 the problem of dapsone-resistance became more serious when primary resistance was first detected i.e. newly diagnosed patients with lepromatous leprosy were confirmed to be infected with dapsone-resistant strains of *M. leprae*. This was subsequently shown to involve many countries in the world, and in some parts up to 40% of strains were resistant (CDC, 1982a).

Because rifampicin is a costly drug and its use is a major economic consideration for developing countries, there was an obvious interest in whether it would be effective against leprosy when given on an intermittent basis. Yawalkar *et al.* (1982) reported the results of a multicenter controlled trial of 93 previously untreated lepromatous leprosy patients; one group of patients was given oral rifampicin 450 mg daily and the other 1200 mg orally monthly in a single dose, and both groups received dapsone 50 mg per day orally. After 6 months treatment, clinical, histopathological and bacteriological regression were satisfactory and practically identical in both groups. The once-monthly schedule was better tolerated than the daily one and complications such as the 'flu' syndrome which have been noted with other intermittent rifampicin regimens (p. 688), did not occur. Also a monthly dose of rifampicin would probably have a negligible effect on dapsone clearance, compared with a daily rifampicin regimen (p. 691). Other studies had also shown that pulse therapy with rifampicin (600 mg on two consecutive days per month) was as effective bacteriologically over 3–5 years as daily dosage in the treatment of sulfone-resistant lepromatous leprosy (Waters, 1983). Warndorff et al. (1982) showed in a small pilot study that 8-weekly doses of 900 mg rifampicin was very effective for paucibacillary leprosy. There had also been a few trials which suggested that combined therapy with dapsone/rifampicin or dapsone/rifampicin/prothionamide may be more effective in removing bacterial persisters, and that such therapy could be given for relatively short periods with a low and acceptable rate of relapse (Waters, 1983).

It was against this background of increasing primary and secondary dapsone-resistance and M. leprae strains exhibiting resistance to dapsone and rifampicin, that a WHO Study Group made recommendations for the treatment of leprosy in 1981 (Report, 1982). The same recommendations were endorsed by WHO in 1993 (WHO, 1994).

b Recommended chemotherapy for leprosy Until recently there were only four suitable drugs. Rifampicin with its high bactericidal activity (p. 679) is expensive but it is effective and non-toxic when given monthly. Clofazimine is also expensive and free of toxicity if a dose of 100 mg daily is not exceeded; it can be administered monthly, thrice-weekly or daily, but has the disadvantage of causing skin discoloration. Ethionamide and prothionamide are expensive and more toxic than dapsone, but their bactericidal activity against M. leprae is better than that of dapsone but not as good as that of rifampicin; their half-lives are short and their bactericidal activity would probably be compromised if they are given intermittently (p. 1237). Dapsone is cheap and weakly bactericidal and serum levels exceed the MIC of M. leprae by a great margin (p. 679) and they remain higher than the MIC for about 10 days (half-life of dapsone about 27 h). The WHO Study Group noted that no drug alone appeared capable of eliminating persisting M. leprae.

For multibacillary (lepromatous) leprosy, a triple-drug regimen is recommended to cope with large potentially dapsone-resistant bacterial populations, which require two additional drugs to prevent emergence of resistance to either one. The regimen consists of rifampicin 600 mg (450 mg if wt <35 kg) once-monthly taken under supervision, plus dapsone 50–100 mg (1–2 mg per kg body weight) daily self administered and clofazimine 300 mg once-monthly supervised and 50 mg daily, self-administered. If clofazimine is unacceptable due to coloration of skin lesions, it can be replaced by 250–375 mg (5–10 mg per kg body wt) self-administered daily doses of ethionamide or prothionamide. However, the acceptability of the latter drug schedule has not been established, and combinations of rifampicin with either ethionamide or prothionamide have been associated with hepatotoxicity in a frequency ranging from 2% to 50% (WHO, 1986). The triple-drug regimen should continue for a minimum of 2 years and whenever possible until skin smears become negative. Nevertheless, there is still some risk of relapse in patients with multibacillary leprosy after this treatment (Lienhardt et al., 1995).

These regimens are inadequate for pulmonary tuberculosis. Moreover, if ethionamide is not included, the regimen is equivalent to rifampicin monotherapy for M. tuberculosis infection, which would lead to rifampicin-resistance (p. 678). Sufficient evidence has now accrued to indicate that the aforementioned multiple-drug regimen is capable of preventing and overcoming dapsone resistance in leprosy (WHO, 1986). The regimen recommended for paucibacillary (tuberculoid) leprosy consists of rifampicin and dapsone, administered in the same dosage schedules as for multibacillary disease, but treatment is only required for 6 months. Although rifampicin alone would probably be effective in this group, dual therapy is recommended for uniformity and to prevent development of rifampicin-resistance in some patients with larger bacterial populations. In general the results of the treatment of leprosy with these regimens have been good; relatively few drug reactions have occurred and patient compliance has been satisfactory (Rangaraj and Rangaraj, 1986; Orege et al., 1987; Hudson, 1989; Pirayavaraporn and Peerapakorn, 1992; Vadher and Lalljee, 1992; Report of a Meeting, 1995).

In developed countries such as USA, clofazimine is not used for lepromatous leprosy, but a regimen of daily rifampicin 600 mg and daily dapsone 100 mg is used for some 3 years or until smear negativity. This then is followed by daily dapsone 100 mg indefinitely. In these countries paucibacillary leprosy is treated by daily dapsone alone for 5 years (Gelber, 1994).

c Future prospects for leprosy treatment Some other drugs may be suitable for the treatment of leprosy. These include minocycline (p. 725), fluoroquinalones such as ofloxacin (p. 1123) and new macrolides such as clarithromycin (p. 648). The use of a combination of rifampicin plus ofloxacin, both given daily, may markedly shorten the therapy of leprosy (WHO, 1994). There is evidence that the combined multidrug treatment plus the use of mycobacterium W vaccine therapy in patients with multibacillary leprosy is more effective than drug treatment alone (Zaheer et al., 1993). Somewhat surprising is a recent report which describes patients with multibacillary leprosy treated either by dapsone alone, dapsone plus rifampicin and a four-drug regimen of dapsone, rifampicin, isoniazid and prothionamide. A 3-year treatment phase was followed by 5-year observation. All three therapies were equally effective (Dietrich et al., 1994).

4 Staphylococcal infections

Rifampicin has been used in staphylococcal infections because of its excellent *in vitro* activity (p. 676), the good response of staphylococcal infections in animals, and its ability to reach intracellular organisms (p. 685). It is always used in combination with another effective anti-staphylococcal drug, otherwise rifampicin-resistant staphylococcal mutants emerge rapidly (p. 676). However, the addition of another anti-staphylococcal agent to rifampicin does not always prevent the emergence of rifampicin-resistant mutants *in vitro*. Resistant mutants have also appeared during treatment of infections in humans with such combinations (p. 676). There have been many anecdotal reports of the value of rifampicin combinations in *Staph. aureus* and *Staph. epidermidis* infections.

Rifampicin was used successfully in combination with fusidic acid or novobiocin to treat infections due to methicillin-resistant *Staph. aureus* (MRSA) strains (Jensen, 1968). A 5-day or 7-day course of novobiocin plus rifampicin eradicated the MRSA carrier state in most patients (Arathoon et al., 1990; Walsh et al., 1993). Oral minocycline/rifampicin plus topical mupirocin has also been successful for this purpose (Darouiche et al., 1991). Studies in animals (Widmer et al., 1990; Chuard et al., 1991) and clinical data (Widmer et al., 1992; Drancourt et al., 1993) indicated that the combination of rifampicin with either a penicillinase-resistant penicillin such as oxacillin or with a quinolone such as ciprofloxacin was effective for the treatment of staphylococcus-infected orthopedic implants. The duration of therapy was 80 days or longer.

In general combinations such as rifampicin/sodium fusidate, rifampicin/novobiocin and rifampicin/ciprofloxacin are best reserved for the treatment of MRSA infections, but in special circumstances they may be justified for the treatment of methicillin-sensitive *Staph. aureus* infections. Dworkin et al. (1989) used ciprofloxacin (initially i.v. then oral) and oral rifampicin for 4 weeks to successfully treat right sided *Staph. aureus* endocarditis in i.v. drug users. Rifampicin was useful in a patient with persistent *Staph. aureus* arthritis after treatment with nafcillin; this was attributed to rifampicin's ability to reach intracellular organisms (Beam, 1979).

The addition of rifampicin to vancomycin therapy in two children with *Staph. aureus* endocarditis also resulted in a clinical response (Faville et al., 1978). Results in a small study of the use of rifampicin with nafcillin for chronic staphylococcal osteomyelitis were encouraging (Norden et al., 1983). Seven of 16 patients with *Staph. aureus* infections treated by combinations of rifampicin with either vancomycin or gentamicin were cured, but rifampicin-resistant strains were isolated from a number of patients in whom this therapy failed (Acar et al., 1983). Cure was obtained in six patients with *Staph. aureus* meningitis treated by a combination of rifampicin and nafcillin or oxacillin (Gordon et al., 1985). Van der Auwera et al. (1983) found that a combination of rifampicin plus oxacillin (or vancomycin) was more effective in 27 patients with *Staph. aureus* infections than treatment with oxacillin (or vancomycin) alone in 29 other patients. Further clinical studies were carried out by this group in Belgium using oral therapy with rifampicin and oxacillin (26 patients) versus oxacillin and a placebo (20 patients). Vancomycin was substituted for oxacillin when the strain of *Staph. aureus* was resistant to oxacillin; statistically there was no difference between the results of treatment in the two groups (Van der Auwera et al., 1984). However, in another trial in which rifampicin in higher dosage (or placebo) was combined with either i.v. oxacillin or i.v. vancomycin, these investigators thought that the addition of rifampicin was only beneficial in severely ill patients with *Staph. aureus* infections (Van der Auwera et al., 1985). Clumeck et al. (1984) used rifampicin with minocycline to treat 25 patients with severe infections due to MRSA strains; daily doses of 600 mg rifampicin and

200–400 mg minocycline given i.v. or orally in two divided doses were used for 5 to 119 days; 19 of 25 infections were cured and in five failure cases, rifampicin-resistant strains emerged. Rifampicin plus either gentamicin or kanamycin was effective for the treatment of endocarditis in two drug addicts, in whom the strains of *Staph. aureus* involved were tolerant to methicillin; these combinations were also effective against the organisms *in vitro* (Suter *et al.*, 1984b).

Ampicillin or amoxycillin, combined with a beta-lactamase inhibitor, has some efficacy in the treatment of MRSA infections in animals (p. 202). In one animal model of MRSA endocarditis ampicillin/sulbactam/rifampicin combination was equally effective to vancomycin for this disease (Chambers *et al.*, 1995).

Rifampicin combinations have been utilized for treatment of *Staph. epidermidis* infections. Although this organism is ordinarily of low virulence, it is a frequent cause of infections associated with indwelling foreign devices (p. 778). Archer *et al.* (1978) used rifampicin with vancomycin and gentamicin to treat successfully a patient with a *Staph. epidermidis* infection of a CSF shunt. Ring *et al.* (1979) used a combination of rifampicin with other antibiotics to cure similar infections in two infants. Oral rifampicin alone was effective in eradicating *Staph. epidermidis* ventriculitis which complicated a CSF shunt in a neonate (Stanley and Balakrishnan, 1982). Studies using *in vitro* models have shown that rifampicin/vancomycin combination was more effective than vancomycin alone in eradication of staphylococcal foreign device-related infections (Blaser *et al.*, 1995). Although various antibiotic combinations, such as gentamicin plus rifampicin plus trimethoprim, may be successful in eradicating shunt infections, in most cases the infected shunt should be removed as part of the treatment (Bayston, 1985). A combination of rifampicin (300 mg 12-hourly) with gentamicin plus vancomycin (or a penicillin or cephalosporin if the strain is sensitive) has been recommended as the treatment for *Staph. epidermidis* endocarditis (Sande and Scheld, 1980). In a retrospective study of 23 patients with prosthetic valve endocarditis caused by MRSA, Karchmer *et al.* (1983) found that more patients were cured by a rifampicin/vancomycin combination than by rifampicin in combination with a beta-lactam antibiotic (p. 258); the addition of rifampicin to vancomycin regimens resulted in an increase in serum bactericidal activity; but rifampicin-resistant strains were selected in two patients who had been treated with combination therapy. Gentamicin has also been added to this regimen (p. 778). Because of the high incidence of prosthetic valve endocarditis due to *Staph. epidermidis*, rifampicin (single dose of 600 mg orally) has been added to nafcillin for prophylaxis in patients undergoing insertion of prosthetic cardiac valves (Sande and Scheld, 1980).

It is apparent from the foregoing that the use of rifampicin combinations for the treatment of staphylococcal infections is still controversial. Whenever rifampicin regimens are used, repeated bacterial culturing of relevant specimens should be undertaken to detect the possible emergence of resistant staphylococcal strains. The selection of rifampicin-resistant *Staph. epidermidis* strains may also be a limiting factor in the use of rifampicin regimens for the treatment of *Staph. aureus* infections, and for the eradication of *Staph. aureus* carriage.

5 Brucellosis

In one animal study rifampicin alone appeared effective for *B. melitensis* infection (Shasha *et al.*, 1994), but in another experiment rifampicin/streptomycin was superior to rifampicin alone (Lang *et al.*, 1993). In adults in an early trial of treatment of patients with *Brucella melitensis* infections, tetracycline or doxycycline given daily for 30 days plus streptomycin daily for 21 days was compared with rifampicin plus doxycycline both given daily for 30 days. The clinical response of both groups of patients was the same but there were less relapses in the first group (2 of 28) compared with the second (7 of 18) (Ariza *et al.*, 1985). In subsequent trials a 6-week course of rifampicin/doxycycline was about as effective as the conventional tetracycline/streptomycin regimen (p. 741). Doxycycline was given in a dosage of 100 mg orally 12-hourly and rifampicin in a dosage of 15 mg per kg orally once-daily (Hall, 1990; Ariza *et al.*, 1992; Morris *et al.*, 1993). However, a more recent trial, involving more patients, showed doxycycline plus rifampicin for 45 days to be inferior to doxycycline (45 days) plus streptomycin (2 weeks). Increased doxycycline inactivation in presence of rifampicin (p. 691) was considered to be a possible factor (Solera *et al.*, 1995). In children a combination of trimethoprim/sulfamethoxazole (10–12 mg per kg of trimethoprim per day and 50–60 mg per kg of sulfamethoxazole per day) plus rifampicin (15–20 mg per kg per day), each administered in two divided doses for 6 weeks, was safe and effective (Khuri-Bulos *et al.*, 1993). Co-trimoxazole alone (p. 871) was less effective (Hall, 1990).

Neurobrucellosis may need a 2- to 4-month course of therapy using i.m. streptomycin, i.v. co-trimoxazole, and nasogastric rifampicin and doxycycline. Streptomycin may be stopped after

2–3 weeks and doxycycline is best omitted in children and pregnant women (McLean *et al.*, 1992). Patients with osteoarticular complications of *B. melitensis* infection usually respond to repeated 4- to 6-week courses of rifampicin plus tetracycline (Mousa *et al.*, 1987). One patient with *B. abortus* endocarditis of the aortic valve recovered after urgent valve replacement and a 3-month course of co-trimoxazole plus rifampicin (Jacobs *et al.*, 1990). When rifampicin is used together with doxycycline for treatment of brucellosis, some patients may have low doxycycline serum levels due to increased drug inactivation (p. 691).

6 Chemoprophylaxis of meningococcal infection

Rifampicin is of no value for treatment of meningococcal meningitis and septicemia, but it has been used successfully in an adult dosage of 300–600 mg daily (according to weight) for 4 days to eradicate meningococci from chronic pharyngeal carriers (Deal and Sanders, 1969; Eickhoff, 1971; Kaiser *et al.*, 1974; Sivonen *et al.*, 1978). This is related to the ability of the drug to produce therapeutically active concentrations in saliva (p. 684). Although penicillin G is excellent for the treatment of meningococcal diseases, it is not satisfactory in eradicating the carrier state. Sulfonamides are not generally suitable for this purpose, as many meningococcal strains are sulfonamide-resistant (p. 808). Minocycline, though effective as a chemoprophylactic agent for meningococcal disease, is associated with a high frequency of vestibular reactions (p. 740). This was confirmed by a trial in an Arctic community; rifampicin was as effective in the eradication of nasopharyngeal carriage of *N. meningitidis* as sequential treatment with minocycline/rifampicin (p. 744), but the latter was associated with more adverse effects (Nicolle *et al.*, 1982b). Although rifampicin has been effective (85–100%) in eradicating meningococci in field trials, rifampicin-resistant strains have been detected in trials in which their presence was sought (Eickhoff, 1975; Chapalain *et al.*, 1994). Meningococcal mutants highly resistant to rifampicin can be easily selected *in vitro* (Ivler *et al.*, 1970), and frequently emerge during treatment *in vivo* (Guttler *et al.*, 1971; Weidmer *et al.*, 1971; Sivonen *et al.*, 1978). Failure to eradicate meningococci has been attributed to one-step development of rifampicin resistance. Rifampicin-resistant meningococci have been found in untreated individuals, but these strains do not persist in a population without continuing rifampicin administration (Eickhoff, 1975; McCormick and Bennett, 1975). Invasive meningococcal disease due to a rifampicin-resistant strain has been described in one child; the onset of disease was 3 days after completing a 2-day course of rifampicin prophylaxis after being a contact of a baby with meningococcal meningitis and septicemia (Cooper *et al.*, 1984). Rifampicin-resistant strains of meningococci may have a decreased virulence (Eickhoff 1971; Levy *et al.*, 1988). Also should widespread rifampicin resistant meningococci occur, the efficacy of penicillin G for the established disease would be unaffected.

For the above reasons, rifampicin has been recommended as the chemoprophylactic agent of choice for meningococcal infections in the USA (McCormick and Bennett, 1975; CDC, 1976). Rifampicin administration to household contacts of meningococcal disease reduces the risk of secondary disease after exposure (Band and Fraser, 1984). Persons at highest risk are household contacts, day-care center contacts, medical personnel who have resuscitated the patient before antibiotics were begun; and persons who had been exposed to the patient's oral secretions through intimate contact or through the sharing of food and beverages (CDC, 1981a). Rifampicin is used for chemoprophylaxis unless the organism is known to be sensitive to sulfadiazine (p. 808). The recommended schedule is rifampicin treatment for 2 days in a dosage of 600 mg twice-daily for adults, 10 mg per kg body weight twice-daily for children, 1 month to 12 years of age, and 5 mg per kg twice-daily for children under 1 month old (Cooke *et al.*, 1989; Jones, 1989; Riedo *et al.*, 1995). Chemoprophylaxis should be given as soon as possible, since one-third of secondary cases occur in the first 4 days after the index case is hospitalized and in the majority within 2 weeks. Despite adequate chemoprophylaxis, secondary cases of meningococcal disease still occur (Cooke *et al.*, 1989; Stuart *et al.*, 1989). It also has been recommended that patients discharged from hospital after treatment for meningococcal disease should receive rifampicin chemoprophylaxis. This decision was based on the assumption that treatment with penicillin G (p. 39) does not eradicate meningococci from the pharynx in every case. However, Weis and Lind (1994) failed to detect meningococci in the throat of 47 patients after they had been treated for meningococcal disease, with penicillin G.

It is possible that with the trend for meningococci showing increasing susceptibility to sulfonamides (88% of strains in the USA were susceptible in 1980), that sulfonamides may again become useful for meningococcal chemoprophylaxis (Nelson, 1982) (p. 822). Chemoprophylaxis of meningococcal disease is also possible by single doses of i.m. ceftriaxone (p. 360) or oral ciprofloxacin (p. 1028) (Cuevas *et al.*, 1995).

7 Prevention of Haemophilus influenzae type b disease

Haemophilus influenzae type b was the most common cause of meningitis in the USA and it was most prevalent in children aged less than 1 year (CDC, 1982b). The situation has now changed because *H. influenzae* type b conjugate vaccines can be used in infants as young as 2 months old (Walter *et al.*, 1994; McIntyre *et al.*, 1995). Invasive *H. influenzae* disease is now rare in children in USA, Australia and other developed countries.

The potentially contagious nature of *H. influenzae* infection was suspected by numerous anecdotal reports of secondary cases occurring amongst household contacts and in closed population groups such as day-care centers. Several studies documented the degree of risk of infection among household contacts of cases during the month following the onset of disease in the index case (Ward *et al.*, 1979; Granoff and Basden, 1980). The risk of secondary disease for contacts of a case of *H. influenzae* meningitis is highest in unvaccinated infants, particularly for those less than 2 years of age; 75% of secondary cases occur within 7 days of the index case (Daum *et al.*, 1986; Fleming *et al.*, 1986). In household contacts the risk is about 600 times greater than the risk in the general population; this is similar to the risk to household contacts of meningococcal infection (p. 697). Contacts of cases with other forms of invasive *H. influenzae* disease, such as epiglottitis, are also considered to have an increased, but less well defined risk of infection. Chemoprophylaxis has been recommended for close contacts of patients with *H. influenzae* disease (CDC, 1982b; Fulginiti, 1982). Clustering of cases of *H. influenzae* infections in day-care centers and nurseries in the USA suggested that children in such facilities may have an increased risk of contracting the infection from other children. This has been borne out by some studies and not by others (CDC, 1986; Makintubee *et al.*, 1987).

Ampicillin (p. 124), cefaclor (p. 278), erythromycin/sulfisoxazole (p. 822) and co-trimoxazole (p. 865) have all been used to attempt to eliminate nasopharyngeal carriage of *H. influenzae*, but none have been uniformly successful (Granoff and Daum, 1980; Horner *et al.*, 1980). Nasopharyngeal carriage of *H. influenzae* can persist following i.v. therapy with chloramphenicol or ampicillin (CDC, 1982b; Li and Wald, 1986), and therefore chemoprophylaxis has also been advocated for the index case to prevent reintroduction of the organism into the household or other closed population group (Nelson, 1982). Rifampicin was considered to be a potentially suitable prophylactic agent because it produces bactericidal concentration against *H. influenzae* in nasopharyngeal secretions (p. 684). However, carriage is unlikely to persist in the index case if the invasive disease is treated by ceftriaxone (p. 360).

When rifampicin was used in a dosage of 10 mg per kg body weight per day, administered once- or twice-daily for 2–3 days, the elimination rate of *H. influenzae* carriage was often ineffective (Granoff and Daum, 1980; Daum *et al.*, 1981; CDC, 1982b; Glode *et al.*, 1983). When a rifampicin regimen of 20 mg per kg body weight (maximum dose 600 mg) was given once-daily for 4 days, carriage of the organism was eradicated in 90–100% of contacts treated. This has been demonstrated in household and day-care center contacts (Granoff and Daum, 1980; Cox *et al.*, 1981; CDC, 1982b, 1986; Murphy *et al.*, 1983; Glode *et al.*, 1985; Gilbert *et al.*, 1991). Moreover, results of trials reported by the Centers for Disease Control (1982b, 1986), indicate that rifampicin also prevents the occurrence of secondary cases of *H. influenzae* infection amongst treated contacts in households and day-care centers. Side-effects of nausea, vomiting, diarrhea, headache and dizziness occurred in 20% of contacts receiving the 20 mg per kg dosage compared with 11% of placebo recipients; orange-coloured urine was noted in 84% of rifampicin recipients (p. 691). Chemoprophylaxis is unlikely to be effective if fewer than 75% of contacts receive rifampicin. The Centers for Disease Control (1986) recommended a prophylactic dosage of 20 mg per kg once-daily (maximum dosage 600 mg per day) for 4 days; the suggested dosage for neonates (aged less than 1 month) was 10 mg per kg once-daily for 4 days. This recommendation still stands, although Green *et al.* (1992) demonstrated that a dosage of 20 mg per kg of body weight per day for only 2 days was also effective. Rifampicin chemoprophylaxis should be given to all members in any household in which a case of invasive *H. influenzae* disease has occurred, and in which another incompletely immunized child younger than 4 years resides; this regimen should be considered strongly for all students and staff in day-care center classrooms in which a case of systemic *H. influenzae* disease has occurred and in which one or more incompletely immunized children younger than 2 years have been exposed. Rifampicin chemoprophylaxis should be instituted as soon as possible; if more than 14 days have elapsed since the last contact with the index case, the benefit of chemoprophylaxis is likely to decrease. The index case (unless treated by ceftriaxone) should also be treated with rifampicin before discharge from hospital. Rifampicin is not recommended for pregnant women because of its teratogenicity in laboratory animals (p. 689). Li and Wald (1986) showed that concurrent treatment of the index patients with rifampicin was as effective as sequential administration in eradicating pharyngeal carriage of *H. influenzae*.

A number of factors may limit the effectiveness of rifampicin chemoprophylaxis (Murphy *et al.*, 1983). There are logistic difficulties in providing prophylaxis when there are many contacts of an index case; failures of prophylaxis are most common in young unvaccinated children, who are at the greatest risk of disease; and rifampicin-resistant strains of *H. influenzae* have emerged after prophylaxis. Other studies of household contacts of patients with invasive *H. influenzae* type b disease suggest that most intrafamilial spread of the organism occurs prior to hospitalization of the index patient and stimulates immunity in contacts older than 2 years. Also, although rifampicin decreases carriage rate, new acquisition of *H. influenzae* continues to occur at a low rate among contacts, even if they have received rifampicin prophylaxis; this may explain reported failures of rifampicin to prevent disease in some household contacts (Glode *et al.*, 1985).

The development of rifampicin-resistant strains has not been a major problem (CDC, 1982b). Murphy *et al.* (1981) recorded the development of resistance in one strain of *H. influenzae* isolated from a child who received prophylaxis because of exposure to a sibling with *H. influenzae* meningitis. Nicolle *et al.* (1982a) had more disturbing findings after community-wide chemoprophylaxis with rifampicin; whereas all strains were rifampicin susceptible before prophylaxis, 10.3% of strains at 1 week and 7.5% of strains at 9 weeks after prophylaxis were rifampicin-resistant. Murphy *et al.* (1983) noted that 22–25% of rifampicin-treated carriers were recolonized with *H. influenzae* 1–4 weeks after rifampicin prophylaxis. Simasathien *et al.* (1980) had a similar experience in a Thailand orphanage where three children had died due to *H. influenzae* meningitis, the causative strain being resistant to ampicillin and chloramphenicol; although rifampicin eradicated carriage of *H. influenzae* from carriers, the overall carriage rate among all children remained unchanged before and after treatment. Boies *et al.* (1982) described the occurrence of *H. influenzae* meningitis 24 days later in a sibling who had received rifampicin prophylaxis in the recommended dosage, beginning 12 h after the onset of meningitis in his sister. Contrary to experience in the USA, serious infection with *H. influenzae* in contacts of an index case were rare in the UK, and doubt was expressed whether rifampicin prophylaxis is required (Davies and Lewis, 1984; Lambert, 1984).

Because the addition of trimethoprim prevents the emergence of rifampicin-resistant *H. influenzae* strains, this combination was tried for *H. influenzae* chemoprophylaxis. Studies in which rifampicin/trimethoprim combinations were used for periods of 2 days showed that they were not dependable for eradication of *H. influenzae* carriage (Daum *et al.*, 1983; Glode *et al.*, 1983).

8 Q fever

One of the tetracyclines is the mainstay of treatment of acute Q fever (p. 748). However, a tetracycline/co-trimoxazole or tetracycline/rifampicin combination, given for prolonged periods, may be of value for the treatment of Q fever endocarditis (Kimbrough *et al.*, 1979; Sawyer *et al.*, 1987).

9 Rhodococcus equi infections in AIDS patients

The combination of erythromycin (p. 620) and rifampicin has been used for these infections (Berkowitz, 1994; Verville *et al.*, 1994). In a model using i.v. infected nude mice, vancomycin monotherapy (p. 782) appeared slightly superior (Nordmann *et al.*, 1992).

10 Cat-scratch disease

This disease, caused by *Bartonella (Rochalimaea) henselae* is usually treated by erythromycin (p. 619), but Golden (1993) reported two cases of severe hepatosplenic cat-scratch disease which responded to rifampicin therapy.

11 Leishmaniasis

Several clinical studies have suggested that rifampicin is effective in the treatment of cutaneous leishmaniasis (Conti and Parenti, 1983). Experience with one patient suggested that isoniazid and rifampicin potentiated each other in this disease (Peters *et al.*, 1981).

12 Fungal infections

Rifampicin and amphotericin B, a combination which may display *in vitro* synergism against some fungi (p. 1252), has been occasionally used to treat some fungal infections.

13 Primary amebic meningoencephalitis

Rifampicin in various combinations with amphotericin B, miconazole and tetracycline may offer the best hope for successful treatment of this disease (p. 1283).

14 Chronic granulomatous disease

Very limited experience suggests that rifampicin, perhaps because of its ability to penetrate into leukocytes (p. 685), may be of value in treating *Staph. aureus* infections in patients with this disease (Lorber, 1980; Hays *et al.*, 1983).

15 Respiratory tract infections

There are a number of reasons why rifampicin should not be used for non-tuberculous respiratory tract infections. Although this drug may be effective for the treatment of diseases such as streptococcal tonsillitis and pneumococcal pneumonia, there are a number of other effective antibiotics, which can be used as alternatives to penicillin G for penicillin-allergic patients (p. 616). The drug may have a possible role in eliminating *Strep. pyogenes* from pharyngeal carriers; in a small study a combination of oral rifampicin with benzathine penicillin seemed more effective treatment than benzathine penicillin alone (Tanz *et al.*, 1983). The large-scale use of this drug for the initial treatment of diseases such as bronchitis and pneumonia is most undesirable because it may mask underlying tuberculosis. Also rifampicin is not effective for the treatment of chronic bronchitis due to *H. influenzae* (Citron and May, 1969). Erythromycin (p. 618) is regarded as the drug of choice for the treatment of Legionnaires' disease, but for severe cases the concomitant administration of rifampicin (1200 mg per day) should be considered. Rifampicin should not be used alone because of the possible emergence of resistant strains (Meyer, 1983).

16 Other infections

Rifampicin in combination with fusidic acid was used to eradicate multiple-antibiotic resistant pneumococci in South Africa (CDC, 1977, 1978) (p. 585). The drug has been used as an adjunct to vancomycin or the cephalosporins such as cefotaxime or ceftriaxone for the treatment of pneumococcal meningitis caused by penicillin G-resistant *Strep. pneumoniae* strains. However, in a rabbit model rifampicin appeared relatively ineffective for this indication (Nau *et al.*, 1994). Rifampicin plus streptomycin have been combined successfully to treat mycetoma (p. 435). Rifampicin has been used successfully to treat meningitis due to *Flavobacterium meningosepticum*, but for this purpose it has usually been combined with other antibiotics, such as erythromycin, vancomycin, gentamicin or co-trimoxazole (Conti and Parenti, 1983).

References.

Abadi FJR, Yakubu DE, Pennington TH (1995). Antimicrobial susceptibility of penicillin-sensitive and penicillin-resistant meningococci. *J Antimicrob Chemother* **35**: 687.

Aber RC, Wennersten C, Moellering RC Jr (1978). Antimicrobial susceptibility of *Flavobacteria*. *Antimicrob Ag Chemother* **14**: 483.

Acar JF, Goldstein FW, Duval J (1983). Use of rifampin for the treatment of serious staphylococcal and Gram-negative bacillary infections. *Rev Infect Dis* **5** (Suppl 3): 502.

Acocella G (1978). Clinical pharmacokinetics of rifampicin. *Clin Pharmacokinet* **3**: 108.

Acocella G (1983). Pharmacokinetics and metabolism of rifampicin in humans. *Rev Infect Dis* **5** (Suppl 3): 428.

Acocella G, Arioli V (1980). Pseudomembranous colitis and rifampicin. *Lancet* **i**: 827.

Acocella G, Conti R (1980). Interaction of rifampicin with other drugs. *Tubercle* **61**: 171.

Acocella G, Scotti R (1976). Kinetic studies on the combination rifampicin-trimethoprim in man. I. Absorption and urinary excretion after administration to healthy volunteers of single doses of the two compounds alone and in combination, and the combination over a period of 1 week. *J Antimicrob Chemother* **2**: 271.

Acocella G, Pagani V, Marchetti M *et al.* (1971). Kinetic studies on rifampicin. *Chemotherapy* **16**: 356.

Acocella G, Hamilton-Miller JMT, Brumfitt W (1977). Can rifampicin use be safely extended? Evidence for non-emergence of resistant strains of *Mycobacterium tuberculosis*. *Lancet* **1**: 740.

Agarwal A, Kendpal H, Gupta HP *et al.* (1994). Tuftsin-bearing liposomes as rifampin vehicles in treatment of tuberculosis in mice. *Antimicrob Ag Chemother* **38**: 588.

Anastasatu C, Bungeteanu Gh, Sibila S (1973). The intermittent chemotherapy of tuberculosis with rifampicin regimens on ambulatory basis. *Scand J Resp Dis* (Suppl 84): 136.

Anderson R (1983). The immunopharmacology of antileprosy agents. *Lepr Rev* **54**: 139.

Aquinas M, Allan WGL, Horsfall PAL *et al.* (1972). Adverse reactions to daily and intermittent rifampicin regimens for pulmonary tuberculosis in Hong Kong. *Brit Med J* **1**: 765.

Arathoon EG, Hamilton JR, Hench CE, Stevens DA (1990). Efficacy of short courses of oral novobiocin-rifampin in eradicating carrier state of methicillin-resistant *Staphylococcus aureus* and *in vitro* killing studies of clinical isolates. *Antimicrob Ag Chemother* **34**: 1655.

Archer GL, Climo MW (1994). Antimicrobial susceptibility of coagulase-negative staphylococci. *Antimicrob Ag Chemother* **38**: 2231.

Archer GL, Tenebaum MJ, Haywood RB III (1978). Rifampicin therapy of *Staphylococcus epidermidis*. Use in infections from indwelling artificial devices. *JAMA* **240**: 751.

Archer GL, Vazquez GL, Johnson JL (1980). Antibiotic prophylaxis of experimental endocarditis due to methicillin-resistant *Staphylococcus epidermidis*. *J Infect Dis* **142**: 725.

Archer GL, Armstrong BC, Kline BJ (1982). Rifampin blood and tissue levels in patients undergoing cardiac valve surgery. *Antimicrob Ag Chemother* **21**: 800.

Ariza J, Gudiol F, Pallarés R *et al.* (1985). Comparative trial of rifampindoxycycline versus tetracycline-streptomycin in the therapy of human brucellosis. *Antimicrob Ag Chemother* **28**: 548.

Ariza J Gudiol F, Pallares R *et al.* (1992). Treatment of human brucellosis with doxycycline plus rifampin or doxycycline plus streptomycin. A randomized, double-blind study. *Ann Intern Med* **117**: 25.

Baciewicz AM, Self TH (1984). Rifampin drug interactions. *Arch Intern Med* **144**: 1667.

Bacon AE, McGrath S, Fekety R, Holloway WJ (1991). *In vitro* synergy studies with *Clostridium difficile*. *Antimicrob Ag Chemother* **35**: 582.

Bailey JP Jr, Stevens SJ, Bell WM *et al.* (1982). *Mycobacterium marinum* infection. A fishy story. *JAMA* **247**: 1314.

Bailey WC, Albert RK, Davidson PT *et al.* (1983). Treatment of tuberculosis and other mycobacterial diseases. *Amer Rev Respir Dis* **127**: 790.

Band JD, Fraser DW (1984). Adverse effects of two rifampicin dosage regimens for the prevention of meningococcal infection. *Lancet* i: 101.

Band JD, Chamberland ME, Platt T *et al.* (1983). Trends in meningococcal disease in the United States, 1975–1980. *J Infect Dis* **148**: 754.

Bannatyne RM, Cheung R (1978). Susceptibility of *Haemophilus influenzae* type b to rifampicin and sulfisoxazole. *Antimicrob Ag Chemother* **13**: 969.

Baron DN, Bell JL (1974). Serum enzyme changes in patients receiving antituberculosis therapy with rifampicin or p-aminosalicyclic acid, plus isoniazid and streptomycin. *Tubercle* **55**: 115.

Baronti A, Lukinovich N (1968). A pilot trial of rifampicin in tuberculosis. *Tubercle* **49**: 180.

Bassi L, Di Berardino L, Perna G, Silvestri LG (1975). Lack of effect of rifampicin on the antibody response to a viral antigen in patients with tuberculosis. *Amer Rev Resp Dis* **112**: 739.

Bassi L, Di Berardino L, Perna G, Silvestri LG (1976). Antibodies against rifampin in patients with tuberculosis after discontinuation of daily treatment. *Amer Rev Resp Dis* **114**: 1189.

Battaner E, Kumar BV (1974). Rifampin: inhibition of ribonucleic acid synthesis after potentiation by amphotericin B in *Saccharomyces cerevisiae*. *Antimicrob Ag Chemother* **5**: 371.

Bayston R (1985). Hydrocephalus shunt infections and their treatment. *J Antimicrob Chemother* **15**: 259.

Beam TR Jr (1979). Sequestration of staphylococci at an inaccessible focus. *Lancet* ii: 227.

Bending MR, Skacel PO (1977). Rifampicin and methadone withdrawal. *Lancet* i: 1211.

Berkowitz FE (1994). The Gram-positive bacilli: a review of the microbiology, clinical aspects, and antimicrobial susceptibilities of a heterogenous group of bacteria. *Pediatr Infect Dis J* **13**: 1126.

Bernard EM, Edwards FF, Kiehn TE *et al.* (1993). Activities of antimicrobial agents against clinical isolates of *Mycobacterium haemophilum*. *Antimicrob Ag Chemother* **37**: 2323.

Bhatnagar N, Getachew E, Straley S *et al.* (1994). Reduced virulence of rifampicin-resistant mutants of *Francisella tularensis*. *J Infect Dis* **170**: 841.

Binda G, Domenichini E, Gottardi A *et al.* (1971). Rifampicin, a general review. *Arzneim Forsch* **21**: 1907.

Blackman HJ, Yoneda C, Dawson CR, Schachter J (1977). Antibiotic susceptibility of *Chlamydia trachomatis*. *Antimicrob Ag Chemother* **12**: 673.

Blajchman MA, Lowry RC, Pettit JE, Stradling P (1970). Rifampicin-induced immune thrombocytopenia. *Brit Med J* **3**: 24.

Blaser J, Vergères P, Widmer AF, Zimmerli W (1995). *In vivo* verification of *in vitro* model of antibiotic treatment of device-related infection. *Antimicrob Ag Chemother* **39**: 1134.

Bloch AB, Cauthen GM, Onorato IM *et al.* (1994). Nationwide suvey of drug-resistant tuberculosis in the United States. *JAMA* **271**: 665.

Bodmer T, Zürcher G, Imboder P, Telenti A (1995). Mutation position and type of substitution in the beta-subunit of the RNA polymerase influence *in vitro* activity of rifamycins in rifampicin-resistant *Mycobacterium tuberculosis*. *J Antimicrob Chemother* **35**: 345.

Boies EG, Granoff DM, Squires JE, Barenkamp SJ (1982). Development of *Haemophilus influenzae* type b meningitis in a household contact treated with rifampicin. *Pediatrics* **70**: 141.

Bolt HM, Kappus H, Bolt M (1974). Rifampicin and oral contraception. *Lancet* i: 1280.

Boman G (1973). Protein binding of rifampicin. A review. *Scand J Resp Dis* (Suppl 84): 40.

Boman G, Hanngren A, Malmborg A *et al.* (1971). Drug interaction: decreased serum concentrations of rifampicin when given with PAS. *Lancet* i: 800.

Borcherding SM, Bastian TL, Self TH *et al.* (1992). Two- and four-day rifampin chemoprophylaxis regimens induce oxidative metabolism. *Antimicrob Ag Chemother* **36**: 1553.

Brook G, Pain A (1987). Major adverse reactions to a short course of daily rifampicin. *Scand J Infect Dis* **19**: 271.

Brouqui P, Raoult D (1990). *In vitro* susceptibility of *Ehrlichia sennetsu* to antibiotics. *Antimicrob Ag Chemother* **34**: 1593.

Buffington GA, Dominguez JH, Piering WF *et al.* (1976). Interaction of rifampicin and glucocorticoids. Adverse effect on renal allograft function. *JAMA* **236**: 1958.

Bullock DW, Webb AJ, Duerden BI, Rotimi V (1981). Bacteraemia due to a rifampicin-resistant strain of *Bacteroides fragilis*. *J Clin Pathol* **34**: 87.

Burger DM, Meenhorst PL, Koks CHW, Beijnen JH (1993). Pharmacokinetic interaction between rifampin and zidovudine. *Antimicrob Ag Chemother* **37**: 1426.

Burman WJ, Cohn DL, Reves RR, Wilson MC (1995). Multifocal cellulitis and monoarticular arthritis as manifestations of *Helicobacter cinaedi* bacteremia. *Clin Infect Dis* **20**: 564.

Bussey HI, Merritt GJ, Hill EG (1984). The influence of rifampin on quinidine and digoxin. *Arch Intern Med* **144**: 1021.

Carper HT, Sullivan GW, Mandell GL (1987). Teicoplanin, vancomycin, rifampicin: *in vivo* and *in vitro* studies with *Staphylococcus aureus*. *J Antimicrob Chemother* **19**: 659.

Carrie F, Roblot P, Bouquet S *et al.* (1994). Rifampin-induced non-responsiveness of giant cell arteritis to prednisolone treatment. *Arch Intern Med* **154**: 1521.

Carter PE, Abadi FJR, Yakubu DE, Pennington TH (1994). Molecular characterization of rifampin-resistant *Neisseria meningitidis*. *Antimicrob Ag Chemother* **38**: 1256.

Cayley FE, Majumdar SK (1976). Ocular toxicity due to rifampicin. *Brit Med J* **1**: 199.

CDC (Center for Disease Control) (1976). Analysis of endemic meningococcal disease by serogroup and evaluation of chemoprophylaxis. *J Infect Dis* **134**: 201.

CDC (Center for Disease Control) (1977). Multiple-antibiotic resistance of pneumococci – South Africa. *MMWR* **26**: 285.

CDC (Center for Disease Control) (1978). Multiple-antibiotic resistance of pneumococci – South Africa. *MMWR* **27**: 1.

CDC (Centers for Disease Control) (1981a). Meningococcal disease – United States, 1981. *MMWR* **30**: 113.

CDC (Centers for Disease Control) (1981b). Drug resistance among Indochinese refugees with tuberculosis. *MMWR* **30**: 273.

CDC (Centers for Disease Control) (1982a). Increase in prevalence of leprosy caused by dapsone-resistant Mycobacterium leprae. *MMWR* **30**: 637.

CDC (Centers for Disease Control) (1982b). Prevention of secondary cases of *Haemophilus influenzae* type b disease. *MMWR* **31**: 672.

CDC (Centers for Disease Control) (1986). ACIP: update: prevention of *Haemophilus influenzae* type b disease. *MMWR* **35**: 170.

Chaisson RE, Schecter GF, Theuer CP *et al.* (1987). Tuberculosis in patients with the acquired immunodeficiency syndrome. Clinical features, response to therapy, and survival. *Am Rev Respir Dis* **136**: 570.

Chambers HF, Kartalija M, Sande M (1995). Ampicillin, sulbactam, and rifampin combination treatment of experimental methicillin-resistant *Staphylococcus aureus* endocarditis in rabbits. *J Infect Dis* **171**: 897.

Chan WC, O'Mahoney MG, Yu DYC, Yu RYH (1975). Renal failure during intermittent rifampicin therapy. *Tubercle* **56**: 191.

Chandler MHH, Toler SM, Rapp RP *et al.* (1990). Multiple-dose pharmacokinetics of concurrent oral ciprofloxacin and rifampin therapy in elderly patients. *Antimicrob Ag Chemother* **34**: 442.

Chapalain J-C, Dusseau J-Y, Perrier-Gros-Claude J-D *et al.* (1994). Effect of rifampicin chemoprophylaxis on the aerobic bacterial flora of the oropharynx. *J Antimicrob Chemother* **33**: 151.

Chuard C, Herrmann M, Vaudaux P *et al.* (1991). Successful therapy of experimental chronic foreign-body infection due to methicillin-resistant *Staphylococcus aureus* by antimicrobial combinations. *Antimicrob Ag Chemother* **35**: 2611.

Citron KM (1972). Tuberculosis-chemotherapy. *Brit Med J* **1**: 426.

Citron KM, May JR (1969). Rifamycin antibiotics in chronic purulent bronchitis. *Lancet* **ii**: 982.

Clark J, Wallace A (1967). The susceptibility of mycobacteria to rifamide and rifampicin. *Tubercle* **48**: 144.

Clumeck N, Marcelis L, Amiri-Lamraski MH, Gordts G (1984). Treatment of severe staphylococcal infections with a rifampicin-minocycline association. *J Antimicrob Chemother* **13** (Suppl C): 17.

Cochran M, Moorhead PJ, Platts M (1975). Permanent renal damage with rifampicin. *Lancet* **i**: 1428.

Cohn JR, Fye DL, Sills JM, Francos GC (1985). Rifampicin-induced renal failure. *Tubercle* **66**: 289.

Cole AJL, Bate J, Gyde OHB (1973). Rifampicin and folate and vitamin B_{12} assays. *Brit Med J* **2**: 53.

Colmenero JD, Fernández-Gallardo LC, Argúndez JAG *et al.* (1994). Possible implications of doxycycline-rifampin interaction for treatment of brucellosis. *Antimicrob Ag Chemother* **38**: 2798.

Commonwealth Department of Health Australia (1982). *Tuberculosis Statistics* Canberra.

Conti R, Parenti F (1983). Rifampin therapy for brucellosis, flavobacterium meningitis, and cutaneous leishmaniasis. *Rev Infect Dis* **5** (Suppl 3): 600.

Cooke RPD, Riordan T, Jones DM, Painter MJ (1989). Secondary cases of meningococcal infection among close family and household contacts in England and Wales, 1984–7. *Brit Med J* **298**: 555.

Cooper ER, Ellison RTIII, Smith GS *et al.* (1984). Rifampin-resistant meningococcal diseases in a prophylaxed contact. In *Abstracts and Program of the 24th Interscience Conference on Antimicrobial Agents and Chemotherapy, Houston, TX* (Abstr. 372). Washington, DC: Society for Microbiology.

Cordonnier D, Muller JM (1972). Acute renal failure after rifampicin. *Lancet* **ii**: 1364.

Council on Drugs (1972). Evaluation of a new antituberculosis agent rifampin (rifadin, rimactane). *JAMA* **220**: 414.

Cox F, Trincher R, Rissing JP *et al.* (1981). Rifampin prophylaxis for contacts of *Haemophilus influenzae* type b disease. *JAMA* **245**: 1043.

Cuevas LE, Kazembe P, Mughogho GK *et al.* (1995). Eradication of nasopharyngeal carriage of *Neisseria meningitidis* in children and adults in rural Africa: a comparison of ciprofloxacin and rifampicin. *J Infect Dis* **171**: 728.

Curci G, Cava FD, Vitalo L (1969). Distribution of rifamycin AMP in blood and cerebro-spinal fluid. *Minerva Medica* **60**: 2399.

Dabbs ER, Yazawa K, Mikami Y *et al.* (1995). Ribosylation by mycobacterial strains as a new mechanism of rifampin inactivation. *Antimicrob Ag Chemother* **39**: 1007.

Daniels NJ, Dover JS, Schachter RK (1984). Interaction between cyclosporin and rifampicin. *Lancet;* **ii**: 639.

Dans PE, McGehee RF Jr, Wilcox C, Finland M (1970). Rifampin: antibacterial activity *in vitro* and absorption and excretion in normal young men. *Amer J Med Sci* **259**: 120.

Darouiche R, Perkins B, Musher D (1990). Levels of rifampin and ciprofloxacin in nasal secretions: correlation with MIC_{90} and eradication of nasopharyngeal carriage of bacteria. *J Infect Dis* **162**: 1124.

Darouiche R, Wright C, Hamill R *et al.* (1991). Eradication of colonization by methicillin-resistant *Staphylococcus aureus* by using oral minocycline-rifampin and topical mupirocin. *Antimicrob Ag Chemother* **35**: 1612.

Darouiche RO, Hamill RJ (1994). Antibiotic penetration of and bactericidal activity within endothelial cells. *Antimicrob Ag Chemother* **38**: 1059.

Daum RS, Glode MP, Goldman DA *et al.* (1981). Rifampin chemoprophylaxis for household contacts of patients with invasive infections due to *Haemophilus influenzae* type b. *J Pediatr* **98**: 485.

Daum RS, Glode MP, Ambrosino D *et al.* (1983). Trimethoprim and rifampin in combination for chemoprophylaxis of household contacts on patients with invasive infections due to *Haemophilus influenzae* type b. *Antimicrob Ag Chemother* **24**: 658.

Daum RS, Granoff DM, Gilsdorf J *et al.* (1986). *Haemophilus influenzae* type b infections in day care attendees: implications for management. *Rev Infect Dis* **8**: 558.

Davies AJ, Lewis DA (1984). Rifampicin in non-tuberculous infections. *Brit Med J* **289**: 3.

Deal WB, Sanders E (1969). Efficacy of rifampin in treatment of meningococcal carriers. *New Engl J Med* **281**: 641.

DeMarais PL, Kocka FE (1995). *Rhodococcus* meningitis in an immunocompetent host. *Clin Infect Dis* **20**: 167.

De Rautlin De La Roy YM, Grignon B, Grollier G *et al.* (1986). Rifampicin resistance in a strain of *Brucella melitensis* after treatment with doxycycline and rifampin. *J Antimicrob Chemother* **18**: 648.

Dever LL, Martin JW, Seaworth B, Jorgensen JH (1992). Varied presentations and responses to treatment of infections caused by *Mycobacterium haemophilum* in patients with AIDS. *Clin Infect Dis* **14**: 1195.

Devine LF, Johnson DP, Hagerman CR *et al.* (1970). Rifampin. Levels in serum and saliva and effect on the meningococcal carrier state. *JAMA* **214**: 1055.

Dickinson JM, Aber VR, Allen BW *et al.* (1974). Assay of rifampicin in serum. *J Clin Path* **27**: 457.

Dietrich M, Gaus W, Kern P, Meyers WM (1994). An international randomized study with long-term follow-up of single versus combination chemotherapy of multibacillary leprosy. *Antimicrob Ag Chemother* **38**: 2249.

Doern GV, Jorgensen JH, Thornsberry C *et al.* (1988). National collaborative study of the prevalence of antimicrobial resistance among clinical isolates of *Haemophilus influenzae*. *Antimicrob Ag Chemother* **32**: 180.

Doble N, Shaw R, Rowland-Hill C *et al.* (1988). Pharmacokinetic study of the interaction between rifampicin and ketoconazole. *J Antimicrob Chemother* **21**: 633.

D'Oliveira JJG (1972). Cerebrospinal fluid concentrations of rifampin in meningeal tuberculosis. *Amer Rev Resp Dis* **106**: 432.

Donald PR, Schoeman JF, O'Kennedy A (1987). Hepatic toxicity during chemotherapy for severe tuberculous meningitis. *Amer J Dis Child* **141**: 741.

Donta ST, Smith PW, Levitz RE, Quintiliani R (1986). Therapy of *Mycobacterium marinum* infections Use of tetracyclines vs rifampin. *Arch Intern Med* **146**: 902.

Drancourt M, Stein A, Argenson JN *et al.* (1993). Oral rifampin plus ofloxacin for treatment of *Staphylococcus*-infected orthopedic implants. *Antimicrob Ag Chemother* **37**: 1214.

Drusano GL, Townsend RJ, Walsh TJ *et al.* (1986). Steady state serum phrmacokinetics of novobiocin and rifampin alone and in combination. *Antimicrob Ag Chemother* **30**: 42.

Drutz DJ, O'Neill SM, Levy L (1974). Viability of blood-borne *Mycobacterium leprae*. *J Infect Dis* **130**: 288.

Dumler JS, Bakken JS (1995). Ehrlichial diseases of humans: emerging tick-borne infections. *Clin Infect Dis* **20**: 1102.

Dunne WM Jr, Mason EO Jr, Kaplan SL (1993). Diffusion of rifampin and vancomycin through a *Staphylococcus epidermidis* biofilm. *Antimicrob Ag Chemother* **37**: 2522.

Dworkin RJ, Lee BL, Sande MA, Chambers HF (1989). Treatment of right-sided *Staphylococcus aureus* endocarditis in intravenous drug users with ciprofloxacin and rifampicin. *Lancet* ii: 1071.

Edelstein PH (1991). Rifampin resistance of *Legionella pneumophila* is not increased during therapy for experimental Legionnaires disease: study of rifampin resistance using a guinea pig model of Legionnaires disease. *Antimicrob Ag Chemother* **35**: 5.

Edelstein PH, Meyer RD (1980). Susceptibility of *Legionella pneumophila* to twenty antimicrobial agents. *Antimicrob Ag Chemother* **18**: 403.

Edwards OM, Courtenay-Evans RJ, Galley JM et al. (1974). Changes in cortisol metabolism following rifampicin therapy. *Lancet* ii: 549.

Eickhoff TC (1971). *In vitro* and *in vivo* studies of resistance to rifampin in meningococci. *J Infect Dis* **123**: 414.

Eickhoff TC (1975). Meningococcal prophylaxis. *JAMA* **234**: 150.

Elansary EH, Earis JE (1983). Rifampicin and adrenal crisis. *Brit Med J* **286**: 1861.

Ellard GA (1980). Combined treatment for lepromatous leprosy. *Lepr Rev* **51**: 199.

Eule H, Werner E, Winsel K, Iwainsky H (1974). Intermittent chemotherapy of pulmonary tuberculosis using rifampicin and isoniazid for primary treatment: the influence of various factors on the frequency of side-effects. *Tubercle* **55**: 81.

Fallon RJ, Lees AW, Allan GW et al. (1975). Probenecid and rifampicin serum levels. *Lancet* ii: 792.

Faville RJ Jr, Zaske DE, Kaplan EL et al. (1978). *Staphylococcus aureus* endocarditis combined therapy with vancomycin and rifampin. *JAMA* **240**: 1963.

Fekety R, O'Connor R, Silva J (1983). Rifampin and pseudomembranous colitis. *Rev Infect Dis* **5** (Suppl 3): 524.

Fleming DW, Cochi SL, Hull HF et al. (1986). Prevention of *Haemophilus influenzae* type b infections in day care: a public health perspective. *Rev Infect Dis* **8**: 568.

Flynn CT, Rainford DJ, Hope E (1974). Acute renal failure and rifampicin: danger of unsuspected intermittent dosage. *Brit Med J* **2**: 482.

Forsgren A, Schmeling D (1977). Effect of antibiotics on chemotaxis of human leukocytes. *Antimicrob Ag Chemother* **11**: 580.

Fournier G, Orgiazzi J, Lenoir B, Dechavanne M (1980). Pseudomembranous colitis probably due to rifampicin. *Lancet* i: 101.

Fox W (1990). Drug combinations and the bioavailability of rifampicin. *Tubercle* **71**: 241.

Franzblau SG (1991). *In vitro* activities of aminoglycosides, lincosamides, and rifamycins against *Mycobacterium leprae*. *Antimicrob Ag Chemother* **35**: 1232.

Fu KP, Lasinski ER, Zoganas HC et al. (1984). Therapeutic efficacy and pharmacokinetic properties of rifampicin in a *Bacteroides fragilis* intra-abdominal abscess. *J Antimicrob Chemother* **14**: 633.

Fulginiti VA (1982). Point: recommendations for rifampin prophylaxis of *Haemophilus* infections by the Committee on Infectious Diseases of the American Academy of Pediatrics. *Pediatr Infect Dis* **1**: 377.

Gabow PA, Lacher JW, Neff TA (1976). Tubulointerstitial and glomerular nephritis associated with rifampicin. *JAMA* **235**: 2517.

Gadaleta MN, Greco M, Saccone C (1970). The effect of rifampicin on mitochondrial RNA polymerase from rat liver. *FEBS Letters* **10**: 54.

Garcia-Arenzana JM, Montes M, Perez-Trallero E (1994). Are rifampin-resistant *Streptococcus pneumoniae* strains a consequence of the increase in cases of tuberculosis? *Clin Infect Dis* **19**: 360.

Gelber RH (1994). Chemotherapy for lepromatous leprosy: recent developments and prospects for the future. *Eur J Clin Microbiol Infect Dis* **13**: 942.

Gibson DH, Fitzgeorge RB, Baskerville A (1983). Antibiotic therapy of experimental airborne Legionnaires' disease. *J Infect* **7**: 210.

Gilbert GL, MacInnes SJ, Guise IA (1991). Rifampicin prophylaxis for throat carriage of *Haemophilus influenzae* type b in patients with invasive disease and their contacts. *Brit Med J* **302**: 1432.

Gill GV (1976). Rifampicin and breakfast. *Lancet* ii: 1135.

Girling DJ (1977). Adverse reactions to rifampicin in antituberculosis regimens. *J Antimicrob Chemother* **3**: 115.

Girling DJ, Fox W (1971). Side effects of intermittent rifampicin. *Brit Med J* **4**: 231.

Girling DJ, Hitze KL (1979). Adverse reactions to rifampicin. *Bull WHO* **57**: 45.

Glode MP, Daum RS, Halsey NA et al. (1983). Rifampin alone and in combination with trimethoprim in chemoprophylaxis for infections due to *Haemophilus influenzae* type b. *Rev Infect Dis* **5** (Suppl 3): 549.

Glode MP, Daum RS, Boies EG et al. (1985). Effect of rifampin chemoprophylaxis on carriage eradication and new acquisition of *Haemophilus influenzae* type b in contacts. *Pediatrics* **76**: 537.

Godfrey-Faussett P, Stoker NG, Scott JAG et al. (1993). DNA fingerprints of *Mycobacterium* tuberculosis do not change during the development of rifampicin resistance. *Tubercle and Lung Disease* **74**: 240.

Golden SE (1993). Hepatosplenic cat-scratch disease associated with elevated anti-*Rochalimaea* antibody titers. *Pediatr Infect Dis J* **12**: 868.

Goldstein RA, Ang UH, Foellmer JW, Janicki BW (1976). Rifampin and cell-mediated immune responses in tuberculosis. *Amer Rev Resp Dis* **113**: 197.

Gordon JJ, Carter DH, Phair JP (1985). Meningitis due to *Staphylococcus aureus*. *Amer J Med* **78**: 965.

Gordon SM, Horsburgh CR Jr, Peloquin CA et al. (1993). Low serum levels of oral antimycobacterial agents in patients with disseminated *Mycobacterium avium* complex disease. *J Infect Dis* **168**: 1559.

Graber CD, Jebaily J, Galphin RL, Doering E (1973). Light chain proteinuria and humoral immunoincompetence in tuberculosis patients treated with rifampin. *Amer Rev Resp Dis* **107**: 713.

Granoff DM, Basden M (1980). *Haemophilus influenzae* infections in Fresno County, California: a prospective study of the effects of age, race, and contact with a case on incidence of disease. *J Infect Dis* **141**: 40.

Granoff DM, Daum RS (1980). Spread of *Haemophilus influenzae* type b: recent epidemiologic and therapeutic considerations. *J Pediatr* **97**: 854.

Grassi GG, Pozzi E (1972). Effect of rifampicin on delayed-hypersensitivity reactions. *J Infect Dis* **126**: 542.

Gray GD, Smith CW, Hollers JC et al. (1983). Rifampin affects polymorpho-nuclear leukocyte interactions with bacterial and synthetic chemotaxins but not interactions with serum-derived chemotaxins. *Antimicrob Ag Chemother* **24**: 777.

Green M, Li KI, Wald ER et al. (1992). Duration of rifampin chemoprophylaxis for contacts of patients infected with *Haemophilus influenzae* type B. *Antimicrob Ag Chemother* **36**: 545.

Grennan DM, Sturrock RD (1976). Polyarthritis, hepatitis and anti-native DNA antibodies after treatment with ethambutol and rifampicin. *Tubercle* **57**: 259.

Grosset J, Leventis S (1983). Adverse effects of rifampin. *Rev Infect Dis* **5** (Suppl 3): 440.

Guebre-Xabier M, Shannon EJ, Kazen R et al. (1995). Early detection of rifampin in human nerve tissue after an oral dose of 600 milligrams. *Antimicrob Ag Chemother* **39**: 1866.

Gupta S, Grieco MH, Siegel I (1975). Suppression of T-lymphocyte rosettes by rifampin. Studies in normals and patients with tuberculosis. *Ann Intern Med* **82**: 484.

Guttler RB, Counts GW, Avent CK, Beaty HN (1971). Effects of rifampin and minocycline on meningococcal carrier rates. *J Infect Dis* **124**: 199.

Hall WH (1990). Modern chemotherapy for brucellosis in humans. *Rev Infect Dis* **12**: 1060.

Hammond GW, Lian CJ, Wilt JC, Ronald AR (1978). Antimicrobial susceptibility of *Haemophilus ducreyi*. *Antimicrob Ag Chemother* **13**: 608.

Hand WL, Boozer RM, King-Thompson NL (1985). Antibiotic uptake by alveolar macrophages of smokers. *Antimicrob Ag Chemother* **27**: 42.

Hartmann G, Honikel KO, Knüsel F, Nüesch J (1967). The specific inhibition of the DNA-directed RNA synthesis by rifamycin. *Biochim Biophys Acta* **145**: 843.

Hays NT, Regelmann WE, Quie PG (1983). The use of rifampin in patients with chronic granulomatous disease of childhood. *Clin Notes* **5** (Suppl 3): 522.

Heifets L (1988). MIC as a quantitative measurement of the susceptibility of

Mycobacterium avium strains to seven antituberculosis drugs. *Antimicrob Ag Chemother* **32**: 1131.

Hendrickse W, McKiernan J, Pickup M, Lowe J (1979). Rifampicin-induced non-responsiveness to corticosteroid treatment in nephrotic syndrome. *Brit Med J* **1**: 306.

Herman RJ, Nakamura K, Wilkinson GR, Wood AJJ (1983). Induction of propranolol metabolism by rifampicin. *Brit J Clin Pharmac* **16**: 565.

Hobby GL, Johnson PM, Boytar-Papirnyik V (1974). Primary drug resistance: a continuing study of drug resistance in tuberculosis in a veteran population within the United States. X. September 1970–September 1973. *Amer Rev Resp Dis* **110**: 95.

Hoeprich PD (1971). Prediction of antimeningococcic chemoprophylactic efficacy. *J Infect Dis* **123**: 125.

Höger PH, Voxbeck K, Seger R, Hitzig WH (1985). Uptake, intracellular activity, and influence of rifampin on normal function of polymorphonuclear leukocytes. *Antimicrob Ag Chemother* **28**: 667.

Holmes IB, Hilson GRF (1972). The effect of rifampicin and dapsone on experimental *Mycobacterium leprae* infections: minimum inhibitory concentrations and bactericidal action. *J Med Microbiol* **5**: 251.

Hong YP, Kim SC, Chang SC *et al.* (1988). Comparison of daily and three intermittent retreatment regimens for pulmonary tuberculosis administered under programme conditions. *Tubercle* **69**: 241.

Hong Kong Tuberculosis Treatment Services/British Medical Research Council (1974). A controlled clinical trial of small daily doses of rifampicin in the prevention of adverse reactions to the drug in a once-weekly regimen of chemotherapy in Hong Kong: Second report. The results at 12 months. *Tubercle* **55**: 193.

Hong Kong Tuberculosis Treatment Services/British Medical Research Council (1975). The influence of age and sex on the incidence of the 'flu' syndrome and rifampicin-dependent antibodies in patients on intermittent rifampicin for tuberculosis. *Tubercle* **56**: 173.

Hong Kong Tuberculosis Treatment Services/Brompton Hospital/British Medical Research Council Investigation (1974). A controlled clinical trial of daily and intermittent regimens of rifampicin plus ethambutol in the treatment of patients with pulmonary tuberculosis in Hong Kong. *Tubercle* **55**: 1.

Hong Kong Tuberculosis Treatment Services/Brompton Hospital/British Medical Research Council (1975). A controlled trial of daily and intermittent rifampicin plus ethambutol in the retreatment of patients with pulmonary tuberculosis: results up to 30 months. *Tubercle* **56**: 179.

Hong Kong Tuberculosis Treatment Services/Singapore Tuberculosis Service/Royal Postgraduate Medical School/Brompton Hospital/British Medical Research Council (1976). Lack of association between rifampicin-dependent antibodies and bacteriological response during intermittent rifampicin treatment. *J Antimicrob Chemother* **2**: 265.

Honore N, Cole ST (1993). Molecular basis of rifampin resistance in *Mycobacterium leprae*. *Antimicrob Ag Chemother* **37**: 414.

Hoogeterp JJ, Mattie H, Krul AM, Van Furth R (1988). The efficacy of rifampicin against *Staphylococcus aureus in vitro* and in an experimental infection in normal and granulocytopenic mice. *Scand J Infect Dis* **20**: 649.

Horner DB, McCracken GH Jr, Ginsburg CM, Zweighaft TC (1980). A comparison of three antibiotic regimens for eradication of *Haemophilus influenzae* type b from the pharynx of infants and children. *Pediatrics* **66**: 136.

Horsburgh CR Jr, Cohn DL, Roberts RB *et al.* (1986). *Mycobacterium avium- M intracellulare* isolates from patients with or without acquired immunodeficiency syndrome. *Antimicrob Ag Chemother* **30**: 955.

Hudson BJ (1989). Tuberculosis and leprosy-provincial implementation of new chemotherapies. *Papua New Guinea Med J* **32**: 1.

Humber DP, Nsanzumuhire H, Aluoch JA *et al.* (1980). Controlled double-blind study of the effect of rifampin on humoral and cellular immune responses in patients with pulmonary tuberculosis and in tuberculosis contacts. *Amer Rev Respir Dis* **122**: 425.

Isley WL (1987). Effect of rifampin therapy on thyroid function tests in a hypothyroid patient on replacement L-thyroxine. *Ann Intern Med* **107**: 517.

Ivler D, Leedom JM, Mathies AW Jr (1970). *In vitro* susceptibility of *Neisseria meningitidis* to rifampicin. *Antimicrob Ag Chemother* **1969**: 473.

Jack DB, Knepil J, McLay WDS, Fergie R (1978). Fatal rifampicin-ethambutol overdosage. *Lancet* **ii**: 1107.

Jacobs F, Abramowicz D, Vercenstracten P *et al.* (1990). *Brucella* endocarditis: the role of combined medical and surgical treatment. *Rev Infect Dis* **12**: 740.

Jacobson RR, Hastings RC (1976). Rifampin-resistant leprosy. *Lancet* **ii**: 1304.

Jacobson MA, Yajko D, Northfelt D *et al.* (1993). Randomized, placebo-controlled trial of rifampin, ethambutol, and ciprofloxacin for AIDS patients with disseminated *Mycobacterium avium* complex infection. *J Infect Dis* **168**: 112.

Jain A, Mehta VL, Kulshresta S (1993). Effect of pyrazinamide on rifampicin kinetics in patients with tuberculosis. *Tubercle and Lung Disease* **74**: 87.

Jensen K (1968). Methicillin-resistant staphylococci. *Lancet* **ii**: 1078.

Jentgens H (1975). Antituberkulotische Therapie mit Ethambutol und Rifampicin in der Schwangerschaft. *Prox Pneumol* **30**: 42.

Jezeguel AM, Orlandi F, Tenconi LT (1971). Changes of the smooth endoplasmic reticulum induced by rifampicin in human and guinea-pig hepatocytes. *Gut* **12**: 984.

Ji B, Truffot-Pernot C, Lacroix C *et al.* (1993). Effectiveness of rifampin, rifabutin, and rifapentine for preventive therapy of tuberculosis in mice. *Am Rev Respir Dis* **148**: 1541.

Jones RB, Ridgway GL, Boulding S, Hunley KL (1983). *In vitro* activity of rifamycins alone and in combination with other antibiotics against *Chlamydia trachomatis*. *Rev Infect Dis* **5** (Suppl 3): 556.

Jones DM (1989). Control of meningococcal disease. Chemoprophylaxis for carriers and some contact groups. *Brit Med J* **298**: 542.

Kaiser AB, Hennekens CH, Saslaw MS *et al.* (1974). Seroepidemiology and chemoprophylaxis of disease due to sulfonamide-resistant *Neisseria meningitidis* in a civilian population. *J Infect Dis* **130**: 217.

Kang SL, Rybak MJ, McGrath BJ *et al.* (1994). Pharmacodynamics of levofloxacin, ofloxacin, and ciprofloxacin, alone and in combination with rifampin, against methicillin-susceptible and -resistant *Staphylococcus aureus* in an *in vitro* infection model. *Antimicrob Ag Chemother* **38**: 2702.

Karchmer AW, Archer GL, Dismukes WE (1983). Rifampin treatment of prosthetic valve endocarditis due to *Staphylococcus epidermidis*. *Rev Infect Dis* **5** (Suppl 3): 543.

Keberle H, Schid K, Meyer-Brunot HG (1968). The metabolic fate of rimactane in the animal and in man In *A Symposium of Rimactane*. Basle: CIBA.

Kemper CA, Havlir D, Hoghighat D *et al.* (1994). The individual microbiologic effect of three antimycobacterial agents, clofazimine, ethambutol, and rifampin, on *Mycobacterium avium* complex bacteremia in patients with AIDS. *J Infect Dis* **170**: 157.

Kenwright S, Levi AJ (1973). Impairment of hepatic uptake of rifamycin antibiotics by probenecid, and its therapeutic implications. *Lancet* **ii**: 1401.

Kerry DW, Hamilton-Miller JMT, Brumfitt W (1975). Trimethoprim and rifampicin: *in vitro* activities separately and in combination. *J Antimicrob Chemother* **1**: 417.

Keshishyan H, Hanna L, Jawetz E (1973). Emergence of rifampiin-resistance in *Chlamydia trachomatis*. *Nature* **244**: 173.

Khuri-Bulos NA, Daoud AH, Azab SM (1993). Treatment of childhood brucellosis: results of a prospective trial on 113 children. *Pediatr Infect Dis J* **12**: 377.

Kimbrough RC, Ormsbee RA, Peacock M *et al.* (1979). Q fever endocarditis in the United States. *Ann Intern Med* **91**: 400.

Kissling M, Bergamini N, Xilinas M (1982). Parenteral rifampicin in tuberculous and severe non-mycobacterial infections. *Chemother* **28**: 229.

Kleinknecht D, Homberg JC, Decroix G (1972). Acute renal failure after rifampicin. *Lancet* **i**: 1238.

Konno K, Oizumi K, Oka S (1973). Mode of action of rifampin on mycobacteria. *Amer Rev Resp Dis* **107**: 1006.

Kreek MJ, Garfield JW, Gutjahr CL, Giusti LM (1976). Rifampin-induced methadone withdrawal. *New Engl J Med* **234**: 1104.

Kristjansson M, Bieluch VM, Byeff PD (1991). *Mycobacterium haemophilum* infection in immunocompromised patients: case report and review of the literature. *Rev Infect Dis* **13**: 906.

Kunin CM, Brandt D, Wood H (1969). Bacteriologic studies of rifampin, a new semisynthetic antibiotic. *J Infect Dis* **119**: 132.

Lakshminarayan S, Sahn SA, Hudson LD (1973). Massive haemolyis caused by rifampicin. *Brit Med J* **2**: 282.

Lambert HP (1984). Prophylaxis in haemophilus meningitis. *Brit Med J* **288**: 739.

Lang R, Shasha B, Rubinstein E (1993). Therapy of experimental murine brucellosis with streptomycin alone and in combination with ciprofloxacin, doxycycline, and rifampin. *Antimicrob Ag Chemother* **37**: 2333.

Langhoff E, Madsen S (1983). Rapid metabolism of cyclosporin and prednisone in kidney transplant patients on tuberculostatic treatment. *Lancet* **ii**: 1303.

Leading Article (1969). New drugs against tuberculosis. *Lancet* **i**: 1081.

Legrand JC, Van der Auwera P, Bailly A *et al.* (1987). Circulating inhibitor of factor VIII during treatment with teicoplanin and rifampicin. *J Antimicrob Chemother* **19**: 850.

Leigh DA (1974). Clinical importance of infections due to *Bacteroides fragilis* and role of antibiotic therapy. *Brit Med J* **3**: 225.

Levy L (1983). Evolution of the modern chemotherapy of leprosy. *Lepr Rev* **54** (Special issue): 69.

Levy L, Shepard CC, Fasal P (1976). The bactericidal effect of rifampicin on *M leprae* in man: (a) single doses of 600, 900 and 1200 mg; and (b) daily doses of 300 mg. *Int J Lepr* **44**: 183.

Levy DI, Del Rio C, Stephens DS (1988). Meningococcemia in identical twins: changes in serum susceptibility after rifampin chemoprophylaxis. *J Infect Dis* **157**: 1064.

Lewis VJ, Thacker WL, Shepard CC, McDade JE (1978). *In vivo* susceptibility of the Legionnaires' disease bacterium to ten antimicrobial agents. *Antimicrob Ag Chemother* **13**: 419.

Li KI, Wald ER (1986). Use of rifampin in *Haemophilus influenzae* type b infections. *Amer J Dis Child* **140**: 381.

Lienhardt C, Jamet P, Sow SO (1995). Risk of relapse in multibacillary leprosy. *Lancet* **345**: 736.

Lillo M, Orengo S, Cernoch P, Harris RL (1990). Pulmonary and disseminated infection due to *Mycobacterium kansasii*: a decade of experience. *Rev Infect Dis* **12**: 760.

Lim I (1995). Susceptibility of *M tuberculosis* isolates in Australia. *Antimicrobials Special Interest Group Newsletter* **2**: 1.

Lobo MC, Mandell GL (1972). Treatment of experimental staphylococcal infection with rifampin. *Antimicrob Ag Chemother* **2**: 195.

Lorber B (1980). Rifampin in chronic granulomatous disease. *New Engl J Med* **303**: 111.

Makintubee S, Istre GR, Ward JI (1987). Transmission of invasive *Haemophilus influenzae* type b disease in day care settings. *J Pediatrics* **111**: 180.

Mandell GL (1983). The antimicrobial activity of rifampin: emphasis on the relation to phagocytes. *Rev Infect Dis* **5** (Suppl 3): 463.

Mandell GL (1994). Delivery of antibiotics by phagocytes. *Clin Infect Dis* **19**: 922.

Mandell GL, Vest TK (1972). Killing of intraleukocytic *Staphylococcus aureus* by rifampin: *in vitro* and *in vivo* studies. *J Infect Dis* **125**: 486.

Martinez E, Muñiz E, Domingo P (1994). Evidence implicating rifampin-independent antiplatelet antibodies in the pathgogenesis of rifampin-induced immune thrombocytopenia. *Clin Infect Dis* **19**: 351.

Maurin M, Gasquet S, Ducco C, Raoult D (1995). MICs of 28 antibiotic compounds for 14 *Bartonella* (formerly *Rochalimaea*). isolates. *Antimicrob Ag Chemother* **39**: 2387.

McAllister WAC, Thompson PJ, Al-Habet SM, Rogers JJ (1983). Rifampicin reduces effectiveness and bioavailability of prednisolone. *Brit Med J* **286**: 923.

McCarty J, Glode MP, Granoff DM, Daum RS (1986). Pathogenicity of a rifampicin-resistant cerebrospinal fluid isolate of *Haemophilus influenzae* type b. *J Pediatrics* **109**: 255.

McClatchy JK, Waggoner RF, Lester W (1969). *In vitro* susceptibility of mycobacteria to rifampin. *Amer Rev Resp Dis* **100**: 234.

McCormick JB, Bennett JV (1975). Public health considerations in the management of meningococcal disease. *Ann Intern Med* **83**: 883.

McCracken GH Jr, Ginsburg CM, Zweighaft TC, Clahsen J (1980). Pharmacokinetics of rifampin in infants and children: relevance to prophylaxis against *Haemophilus influenzae* type b disease. *Pediatrics* **66**: 17.

McLean DR, Russell N, Khan MY (1992). Neurobrucellosis: clinical and therapeutic features. *Clin Infect Dis* **15**: 582.

McIntyre PB, Chey T, Smith WT (1995). The impact of vaccination against invasive *Haemophilus influenzae* type b disease in the Sydney region. *Med J Aust* **162**: 245.

Medoff G (1983). Antifungal action of rifampin. *Rev Infect Dis* **5** (Suppl 3): 614.

Mendelman PM, Roberts MC, Smith AL (1982). Mutation frequency of *Haemophilus influenzae* to rifampin resistance. *Antimicrob Ag Chemother* **22**: 531.

Meyer RD (1983). *Legionella* infections: a review of five years of research. *Rev Infect Dis* **5**: 258.

Miller LP, Crawford JT, Shinnick TM (1994). The *rpo B* gene of *Mycobacterium tuberculosis*. *Antimicrob Ag Chemother* **38**: 805.

Miller WT (1978). Long-term therapy with rifampin and the secondary antibody response to killed influenza vaccine. *Amer Rev Resp Dis* **117**: 605.

Mindermann T, Landolt H, Zimmerli W (1993). Penetration of rifampicin into the brain tissue and cerebral extracellular space of rats. *J Antimicrob Chemother* **31**: 731.

Mitchell I, Wendon J, Fitt S, Williams R (1995). Anti-tuberculous therapy and acute liver failure. *Lancet* **345**: 555.

Morris AB, Brown RB, Sands M (1993). Use of rifampin in non-staphylococcal, nonmycobacterial disease. *Antimicrob Ag Chemother* **37**: 1.

Morris S, Bai GH, Suffys P *et al.* (1995). Molecular mechanisms of multiple drug resistance in clinical isolates of *Mycobacterium tuberculosis*. *J Infect Dis* **171**: 954.

Mousa ARM, Muhtaseb SA, Almudallal DS *et al.* (1987). Osteoarticular complications of brucellosis: a study of 169 cases. *Rev Infect Dis* **9**: 531.

Mouton RP, Mattie H, Swart K *et al.* (1979). Blood levels of rifampicin, desacetyl-rifampicin and isoniazid during combined therapy. *J Antimicrob Chemother* **5**: 447.

Mukerjee P, Schuldt S, Kasik JE (1973). Effect of rifampin on cutaneous hypersensitivity to purified protein derivaties in humans. *Antimicrob Ag Chemother* **4**: 607.

Murdoch JMcC, Speirs CF, Wright N, Wallace ET (1969). Rifampicin. *Lancet* **i**: 1094.

Murphy TV, McCracken GH Jr, Zweighaft TC, Hansen EJ (1981). Emergence of rifampin-resistant *Haemophilus influenzae* after prophylaxis. *J Pediatr* **99**: 406.

Murphy TV, Chrane DF, McCracken GH Jr, Nelson JD (1983). Rifampin prophylaxis v placebo for household contacts of children with *Hemophilus influenzae* type b disease. *Amer J Dis Child* **137**: 627.

Nau R, Prange HW, Menck S *et al.* (1992). Penetration of rifampicin into the cerebrospinal fluid of adults with uninflamed meninges. *J Antimicrob Chemother* **29**: 719.

Nau R, Kaye K, Sachdeva M *et al.* (1994). Rifampin for therapy of experimental pneumococcal meningitis in rabbits. *Antimicrob Ag Chemother* **38**: 1186.

Nelson JD (1982). How preventable is bacterial meningitis. *New Engl J Med* **307**: 1265.

Nessi R, Domenichini E, Fowst G (1973). 'Allergic' reactions during rifampicin treatment: a review of published cases. *Scand J Resp Dis* (Suppl 84): 15.

Nessi R, Bonoldi GL, Redaelli B, Di Filippo G (1976). Acute renal failure after rifampicin: a case report and survey of the literature. *Nephrol* **16**: 148.

Newman R, Doster BE, Muray FJ, Woolpert SF (1974). Rifampin in initial treatment of pulmonary tuberculosis. A US Public Health Service tuberculosis trial. *Amer Rev Resp Dis* **109**: 216.

Nicolle LE, Postl B, Kotelewetz E *et al.* (1982a). Emergence of rifampin-resistant *Haemophilus influenzae*. *Antimicrob Ag Chemother* **21**: 498.

Nicolle LE, Postl B, Kotelewetz E *et al.* (1982b). Chemoprophylaxis for *Neisseria meningitidis* in an isolated arctic community. *J Infect Dis* **145**: 103.

Nilsson BS (1971). Rifampicin: an immunosuppressant? *Lancet* **ii**: 374.

Norden CW, Fierer J, Bryant RE *et al.* (1983). Chronic staphylococcal osteomyelitis; treatment with regimens containing rifampin. *Rev Infect Dis* **5** (Suppl 3): 495.

Nordmann P, Kerestedjian J-J, Ronco E (1992). Therapy of *Rhodococcus equii* disseminated infections in nude mice. *Antimicrob Ag Chemother* **36**: 1244.

Novi C, Bissoli F, Simonati V *et al.* (1980). Rifampin and digoxin: possible drug interaction in a dialysis patient. *JAMA* **244**: 2521.

Nyirenda R, Gill GV (1977). Stevens-Johnson syndrome due to rifampicin. *Brit Med J* **2**: 1189.

O'Brien RJ, Snider DE Jr (1985). Tuberculosis drugs – old and new. *Amer Rev Respir Dis* **131**: 309.

Orege PA, Obura M, Nyawalo JO (1987). Short-course multidrug therapy for leprosy patients in Western Kenya. Preliminary communication. *Lepr Rev* **58**: 263.

O'Reilly RA (1974). Interaction of sodium warfarin and rifampin. Studies in man. *Ann Intern Med* **81**: 337.

O'Reilly RA (1975). Interaction of chronic daily warfarin therapy and rifampin. *Ann Intern Med* **83**: 506.

Outman WR, Levitz RE, Hill DA, Nightingale CH (1992). Intraocular penetration of rifampin in humans. *Antimicrob Ag Chemother* **36**: 1575.

Pasculle AW, Dowling JN, Frola FN *et al.* (1985). Antimicrobial therapy of experimental *Legionella micdadei* pneumonia in guinea pigs. *Antimicrob Ag Chemother* **28**: 730.

Patel KB, Belmonte R, Crowe HM (1995). Drug malabsorption and resistant tuberculosis in HIV-infected patients. *New Engl J Med* **332**: 336.

Patel R, Roberts GD, Keating MR, Paya CV (1994). Infections due to nontuberculous *Mycobacteria* in kidney, heart, and liver transplant recipients. *Clin Infect Dis* **19**: 263.

Pattamasukon P, Pichyangkura C, Fischer GW (1975). Melioidosis in childhood. *J Pediatr* **87**: 133.

Pattyn SR, Dockx P, Rollier MT *et al.* (1976). *Mycobacterium leprae* persisters after treatment with dapsone and rifampicin. *Int J Lepr* **44**: 154.

Pederzoli P, Falconi M, Guaglianone O *et al.* (1985). Rifampicin concentrations in pancreatic juice. *J Antimicrob Chemother* **16**: 129.

Peters W, Lainson R, Shaw JJ *et al.* (1981). Potentiating action of rifampin and isoniazid against *Leishmania mexicana* amazonensis. *Lancet* **i**: 1122.

Philippon AM, Plommet MG, Kazmierczak A *et al.* (1977). Rifampin in the treatment of experimental brucellosis in mice and guinea pigs. *J Infect Dis* **136**: 482.

Piot P, Van Dyck E, Colaert J *et al.* (1979). Antibiotic susceptibility of *Neisseria gonorrhoeae* strains from Europe and Africa. *Antimicrob Ag Chemother* **15**: 535.

Pirayavaraporn C, Peerapakorn S (1992). The measurement of the epidemiological impact of multidrug therapy. *Lepr Rev* **63** (Suppl): 84.

Poole G, Stradling P, Worlledge S (1971). Potentially serious side-effects of high-dose twice-weekly rifampicin. *Brit Med J* **3**: 343.

Poole G, Stradling P, Worlledge S (1973). Side-effects observed during intermittent rifampicin therapy. *Scand J Resp Dis* (Suppl 84): 129.

Poor DM, Self TH, Davis HL (1983). Interaction of rifampin and digitoxin. *Arch Intern Med* **143**: 599.

Powell-Jackson PR, Gray BJ, Heaton RW *et al.* (1983). Adverse effect of rifampicin administration on steroid-dependent asthma. *Amer Rev Respir Dis* **128**: 307.

Powell-Jackson PR, Jamieson AP, Gray BJ *et al.* (1985). Effect of rifampicin administration on theophylline pharmacokinetics in humans. *Amer Rev Respir Dis* **131**: 939.

Pratt TH (1979). Rifampin-induced organic brain syndrome. *JAMA* **241**: 2421.

Prober CG (1985). Effect of rifampin on chloramphenicol levels. *New Engl J Med* **312**: 788.

Proctor RA, Wick P, Hamill RJ *et al.* (1987). *In vitro* studies of antibiotic combinations for multiply-resistant coagulase-negative staphylococci. *J Antimicrob Chemother* **20**: 223.

Pukrittayakamee S, Viravan C, Charoenlarp P *et al.* (1994). Antimalarial effects of rifampin on *Plasmodium vivax* malaria. *Antimicrob Ag Chemother* **38**: 511.

Rangaraj M, Rangaraj J (1986). Experience with multidrug theapy in Sierrra Leone: clinical, operational and managerial analysis. *Lepr Rev* **57** (Suppl 3): 77.

Rees RJW (1975). Rifampicin: investigation of a bactericidal antileprosy drug. *Lepr Rev* **46** (Suppl): 121.

Rees RJW (1983). Chemotherapy of leprosy for control programmes: scientific basis and practical application. *Lepr Rev* **54**: 81.

Rees RJW, Pearson JMH, Waters MFR (1970). Experimental and clinical studies on rifampicin in treatment of leprosy. *Brit Med J* **1**: 89.

Rees RJW, Waters MFR, Pearson JMH *et al.* (1976). Long-term treatment of dapsone-resistant leprosy with rifampicin: clinical and bacteriological studies. *Int J Lepr* **44**: 159.

Report of a Meeting of Physicians and Scientists at the All India Institute of Medical Sciences, New Delhi (1995). Leprosy. *Lancet* **345**: 697.

Report of a WHO Scientific Group (1978). *Neisseria gonorrhoeae* and gonococcal infections. *Wld Hlth Org Techn Rep Ser* 616.

Report of a WHO Study Group (1982). Chemotherapy of leprosy for control programmes. *Wld Hlth Org Tech Rep Ser* 675.

Riedo FX, Plikaytis BD, Broome CV (1995). Epidemiology and prevention of meningococcal disease. *Pediatr Infect Dis J* **14**: 643.

Ring JC, Cates KL, Belani KK *et al.* (1979). Rifampin for CSF shunt infections caused by coagulase-negative staphylococci. *J Pediatr* **95**: 317.

Rodescu D, Abeles H, Zelefsky MN, Williams MH Jr (1981). Accelerated growth of lung cancer in association with rifampicin administration for tuberculosis. *Lancet* **ii**: 983.

Romankiewicz JA, Ehrman M (1975). Rifampicin and warfarin: a drug interaction. *Ann Intern Med* **82**: 224.

Rothwell DL, Richmond DE (1974). Hepatorenal failure with self-initiated intermittent rifampicin therapy. *Brit Med J* **2**: 481.

Ruben FL, Winkelstein A, Fotiadis IG (1974). Immunological responsiveness of tuberculosis patients receiving rifampicin. *Antimicrob Ag Chemother* **5**: 383.

Rupp ME, Archer GL (1994). Coagulase-negative staphylococci: pathogens associated with medical progress. *Clin Infect Dis* **19**: 231.

Sage RE, Derrington AW (1973). Opportunistic cutaneous *Mycobacterium marinum* infection mimicking *Mycobacterium ulcerans* in lymphosarcoma. *Med J Aust* **2**: 434.

Sande MA (1983). The use of rifampin in the treatment of nontuberculous infections: an overview. *Rev Infect Dis* **5** (Suppl 3): 399.

Sande MA, Scheld WM (1980). Combination antibiotic therapy of bacterial endocarditis. *Ann Intern Med* **92**: 390.

Sawyer LA, Fishbein DB, McDade JE (1987). Q fever: current concepts. *Rev Infect Dis* **9**: 935.

Schachter J (1983). Rifampin in chlamydial infections. *Rev Infect Dis* **5** (Suppl 3): 562.

Scharre KA, Eckels DD, Gershwin ME (1981). Depression of colony formation by human thymus-derived lymphocytes with rifampin and other antimicrobial agents. *J Infect Dis* **143**: 832.

Scheld WM (1983). Evaluation of rifampin and other antibiotics against

Listeria monocytogenes in vitro and *in vivo*. *Rev Infect Dis* **5** (Suppl 3): 593.

Sebba L, Beamis JF, Webb-Johnson DC (1982). Lung cancer in patient taking rifampicin. *Lancet* **ii**: 105.

Sensi P (1983). History of the development of rifampin. *Rev Infect Dis* **5** (Suppl 3): 402.

Sensi P, Maggi N, Füresz S, Maffii G (1967). Chemical modifications and biological properties of rifamycins. *Antimicrob Ag Chemother* **1966**: 699.

Seufert CD (1973). Acute renal failure after rifampicin therapy. *Scand J Resp Dis* (Suppl 84): 174.

Shasha B, Lang R, Rubinstein E (1994). Efficacy of combinations of doxycycline and rifampicin in the therapy of experimental mouse brucellosis. *J Antimicrob Chemother* **33**: 545.

Siddiqi SH, Aziz A, Reggiardo Z, Middlebrook G (1981). Resistance to rifampicin and isoniazid in strains of *Mycobacterium tuberculosis*. *J Clin Pathol* **34**: 927.

Siegler DI, Bryant M, Burley DM et al. (1974). Effect of meals on rifampicin absorption. *Lancet* **ii**: 197.

Simasathien S, Duangmani C, Echeverria P (1980). *Haemophilus influenzae* type B resistant to ampicillin and chloramphenicol in an orphanage in Thailand. *Lancet* **ii**: 1214.

Simon GL, Smith RH, Sande MA (1983). Emergence of rifampin-resistant strains of *Staphylococcus aureus* during combination therapy with vancomycin and rifampin: a report of two cases. *Rev Infect Dis* **5** (Suppl 3): 507.

Singapore Tuberculosis Service/British Medical Research Council (1975). Controlled trial of intermittent regimens plus isoniazid for pulmonary tuberculosis in Singapore. *Lancet* **ii**: 1105.

Sippel JE, Mikhail IA, Girgis NI, Youssef HH (1974). Rifampin concentrations in cerebrospinal fluid of patients with tuberculous meningitis. *Amer Rev Resp Dis* **109**: 579.

Sivonen A, Renkonen O-V, Weckström P et al. (1978). The effect of chemoprophylactic use of rifampin and minocycline on rates of carriage of *Neisseria meningitidis* in army recruits in Finland. *J Infect Dis* **137**: 238.

Skolnick JL, Stoler BS, Katz DB, Anderson WH (1976). Rifampin, oral contraceptives, and pregnancy. *JAMA* **236**: 1382.

Small PM, Schecter GF, Goodman PC et al. (1991). Treatment of tuberculosis in patients with advanced human immunodeficiency virus infection. *New Engl J Med* **324**: 289.

Small PM, Shafer RW, Hopewell PC et al. (1993). Exogenous reinfection with multidrug-resistant *Mycobacterium tuberculosis* in patients with advanced HIV infection. *New Engl J Med* **328**: 1137.

Solberg SO, Haltensen A, Digranes A, Hellum KB (1983). Penetration of antibiotics into human leukocytes and dermal suction blisters. *Rev Infect Dis* **5** (Suppl 3): 468.

Solera J, Rodríguez-Zapata M, Geijo P et al. (1995). Doxycycline-rifampin versus doxycycline-streptomycin in treatment of human brucellosis due to *Brucella melitensis*. *Antimicrob Ag Chemother* **39**: 2061.

Staehelin M, Knusel F, Wehrli W (1968). The mechanism of action of rimactane. *A Symposium on Rimactane*. Basle: CIBA.

Stanley TV, Balakrishnan V (1982). Rifampicin in neonatal ventriculitis. *Aust Paediatr J* **18**: 200.

Steiner P, Rao M, Mitchell M, Steiner M (1986). Primary drug-resistant tuberculosis in children Emergence of primary drug-resistant strains of *M tuberculosis* to rifampin. *Am Rev Respir Dis* **134**: 446.

Stern JSM, Stainton-Ellis DM (1977). Rifampicin in pregnancy. *Lancet* **ii**: 604.

Stevens DL, Maier KA, Mitten JE (1987). Effect of antibiotics on toxin production and viability of *Clostridium perfringens*. *Antimicrob Ag Chemother* **31**: 213.

Stone WJ, Waldron JA, Dixon JH Jr et al. (1976). Acute diffuse interstitial nephritis related to chemotherapy of tuberculosis. *Antimicrob Ag Chemother* **10**: 164.

Stottmeier KD (1976). Emergence of rifampin-resistant *Mycobacterium tuberculosis* in Massachusetts. *J Infect Dis* **133**: 88.

Stuart JM, Cartwright KAV, Robinson PM, Noah ND (1989). Does eradication of meningococcal carriage in household contacts prevent secondary cases of meningococcal disease? *Brit Med J* **298**: 569.

Subcommittee of Clinical Trials of the Chemotherapy of Leprosy (THE-LEP). Scientific Working Group of the UNDP/World Bank/WHO Special Programme for Research and Training in Tropical Diseases (1983). THELEP controlled clinical trials in lepromatous leprosy. *Lepr Rev* **54**: 167.

Suter F, Maserati R, Concia E et al. (1984a). Rifampicin in collections of pus: a kinetic study in human abscesses. *J Antimicrob Chemother* **13** (Suppl C): 43.

Suter F, Maserati R, Carnevale G et al. (1984b). Management of staphylococcal endocarditis in drug addicts. Combined therapy with oral rifampicin and amino-glycosides. *J Antimicrob Chemother* **13** (Suppl C): 57.

Swai OB, Aluoch JA, Githui WA et al. (1988). Controlled clinical trial of a regimen of two durations for the treatment of isoniazid-resistant pulmonary tuberculosis. *Tubercle* **69**: 5.

Syvälahti EKG, Pihlajamäki KK, Iisalo EJ (1974). Rifampicin and drug metabolism. *Lancet* **ii**: 232.

Takasu N, Yamada T, Miura H et al. (1982). Rifampin-induced early phase hyper-glycemia in humans. *Amer Rev Respir Dis* **125**: 23.

Tan TQ, Mason EO Jr, Ou C-N, Kaplan SL (1993). Use of intravenous rifampin in neonates with persistent staphylococcal bacteremia. *Antimicrob Ag Chemother* **37**: 2401.

Tanz R, Shulman ST, Willert C et al. (1983). Rifampin treatment for Group A streptococcal carriers. *Clin Res* **31**: 792A.

Tanzil HOK, Chatim A, Utomo RR, Harun H (1972). Sensitivity of various species of nocardia to rifampin *in vitro*. *Amer Rev Resp Dis* **105**: 455.

Tebas P, Ruiz RM, Roman F et al. (1991). Early resistance to rifampicin and ciprofloxacin in the treatment of right sided *Staphylococcus aureus* endocarditis. *J Infect Dis* **163**: 204.

Telenti A, Imboden PM, Marchesi F et al. (1993). Detection of rifampicin-resistance mutations in *Mycobacterium tuberculosis*. *Lancet* **341**: 647.

Thong YH, Rowan-Kelly B, Shepherd C, Ferrante A (1977). Growth inhibition of *Naegleria fowleri* by tetracycline, rifampicin, and micona-zole. *Lancet* **ii**: 876.

Thornsberry C, Baker CN, Kirven LA (1978). *In vitro* activity of antimicrobial agents on Legionnaires' disease bacterium. *Antimicrob Ag Chemother* **13**: 78.

Thornsberry C, Hill BC, Swenson JM, McDougal LK (1983). Rifampin: spectrum of antibacterial activity. *Rev Infect Dis* **5** (Suppl 3): 412.

Torre D, Ferraro G, Fiori GP et al. (1992). Ventriculoatrial shunt infection caused by *Staphylococcus warneri*: case report and review. *Clin Infect Dis* **14**: 49.

Trivedi SS, Desai SG (1988). Primary antituberculosis drug resistance and acquired rifampicin resistance in Gujarat, India. *Tubercle* **69**: 37.

Tsukamura M (1972). The pattern of resistance development to rifampicin in *Mycobacterium tuberculosis*. *Tubercle* **53**: 111.

Tuazon CU, Shamsuddin D, Miller H (1982). Antibiotic susceptibility and synergy of clinical isolates of *Listeria monocytogenes*. *Antimicrob Ag Chemother* **21**: 525.

Tucker RM, Denning DW, Hanson LH et al. (1992). Interaction of azoles with rifampin, phenytoin and carbamazepine: *in vitro* and clinical observatins. *Clin Infect Dis* **14**: 165.

Twum-Barima Y, Carruthers SG (1981). Quinidine-rifampin interaction. *New Engl J Med* **304**: 1466.

Vadher A, Lalljee M (1992). Patient treatment compliance in leprosy. A critical review. *Int J Leprosy* **60**: 587.

Van Assendelft AHW (1985). Leucopenia in rifampicin chemotherapy. *J Antimicrob Chemother* **16**: 407.

Van den Broek PJ (1989). Antimicrobial drugs, microorganisms, and phagocytes. *Rev Infect Dis* **11**: 213.

Van der Auwera P, Meunier-Carpentier F, Klastersky J (1983). Clinical study of combination therapy with oxacillin and rifampin for staphylo-coccal infections. *Rev Infect Dis* **5** (Suppl 3): 515.

Van der Auwera P, Thys JP, Meunier-Carpentier F, Klastersky J (1984). The combination of oxacillin with rifampicin in staphylococcal infections: a review of laboratory and clinical studies of the Institut Jules Bordet. *J Antimicrob Chemother* **13** (Suppl C): 31.

Van der Auwera P, Klastersky J, Thys JP *et al.* (1985). Double-blind, placebo-controlled study of oxacillin combined with rifampin in the treatment of staphylococcal infections. *Antimicrob Ag Chemother* **28**: 467.

Van der Ven AJM, Koopmans PP, Vree TB, Van der Meer JWM (1994). Drug intolerance in HIV disease. *J Antimicrob Chemother* **34**: 1.

Van Dyke JJ, Lake KB (1975). Chemotherapy for aquarium granuloma. *JAMA* **233**: 1380.

Verbist L, Gyselen A (1968). Antituberculous activity of rifampin *in vitro* and *in vivo* and the concentrations attained in human blood. *Amer Rev Resp Dis* **98**: 923.

Verville TD, Huycke MM, Greenfield RA *et al.* (1994). *Rhodococcus equi* infections in humans. 12 cases and review of the literature. *Medicine* **73**: 119.

Von Bergmann K, Fierer J, Mok HYI, Grundy SM (1981). Effect of rifampin on biliary lipids in humans. *Antimicrob Ag Chemother* **19**: 342.

Wake PN, Humphrey C, Walker R (1980). Long-term intravenous rifampicin after massive small bowel resection. *Tubercle* **61**: 109.

Wallace RJ Jr, Dunbar D, Brown BA *et al.* (1994). Rifampin-resistant *Mycobacterium kansasii*. *Clin Infect Dis* **18**: 736.

Wallace RJ Jr, Brown BA, Griffith DE *et al.* (1995). Reduced serum levels of clarithromycin in patients treated with multidrug regimens including rifampin or rifabutin for *Mycobacterium avium* – *M. intracellulare* infection. *J Infect Dis* **171**: 747.

Walsh TJ, Standiford HC, Reboli AC *et al.* (1993). Randomized double-blinded trial of rifampin with either novobiocin or trimethoprim-sulfamethoxazole against methicillin-resistant *Staphylococcus aureus* colonization: prevention of antimicrobial resistance and effect of host factors on outcome. *Antimicrob Ag Chemother* **37**: 1334.

Walter EB, Simmons SS, Clements DA (1994). Anti polyribosylribiol phosphate antibody levels 5 years after a primary series of *Haemophilus influenzae* type b conjugate vaccine. *J Infect Dis* **170**: 1050.

Ward JI, Fraser DW, Baraff LJ, Plikaytis BD (1979). *Haemophilus influenzae* meningitis. A national study of secondary spread in household contacts. *New Engl J Med* **301**: 122.

Warndorff J, Bourland J, Pattyn SR (1982). Follow-up on short-course 2 months' rifampicin treatment of paucibacillary leprosy. *Lep Rev* **53**: 9.

Washington AE, Schultz MG, Cohen ML *et al.* (1982). Treatment of sexually transmitted bacterial and protozoal enteric infections. *Rev Infect Dis* **4**: (Suppl): 864.

Waters MFR (1983). The treatment of leprosy. *Tubercle* **64**: 221.

Waters MFR, Rees RJW, Pearson JMH *et al.* (1978). Rifampicin for lepromatous leprosy: nine years' experience. *Brit Med J* **1**: 133.

Wehrli W (1983). Rifampin: mechanisms of action and resistance. *Rev Infect Dis* **5**: (Suppl 3): 407.

Weidmer CE, Dunkel TB, Pettyjohn FS *et al.* (1971). Effectiveness of rifampicin in eradicating the meningococcal carrier in a relatively closed population: emergence of resistant strains. *J Infect Dis* **124**: 172.

Weis N, Lind I (1994). Pharyngeal carriage of *Neisseria meningitidis* before and after treatment of meningococcal disease. *J Med Microbiol* **41**: 339.

WHO (1977). WHO expert committee on leprosy. *Wld Hlth Org Techn Rep Ser;* 607.

WHO (1986). Implementation of multidrug therapy for leprosy control. *Wkly Epidem Rec* **61**: 189.

WHO (1994). Chemotherapy of Leprosy. Report of a WHO Study Group. *Wld Hlth Org Tech Rep Ser* 847.

Widmer AF, Frei R, Rajacic Z, Zimmerli W (1990). Correlation between *in vivo* and *in vitro* efficacy of antimicrobial agents against foreign body infections. *J Infect Dis* **162**: 96.

Widmer AF, Gaechter A, Ochsner PE, Zimmerli W (1992). Antimicrobial treatment of orthopedic implant-related infections with rifampin combinations. *Clin Infect Dis* **14**: 1251.

Wilkinson FF, Gago J, Santabaya E (1972). Therapy of leprosy with rifampicin. *Int J Lepr* **40**: 53.

Williams DL, Waguespack C, Eisenach K *et al.* (1994). Characterization of rifampin resistance in pathogenic mycobacteria. *Antimicrob Ag Chemother* **38**: 2380.

Wisseman CL Jr, Waddell AD, Walsch WT (1974). *In vitro* studies of the action of antibiotics on *Rickettsia prowazeki* by two basic methods of cell culture. *J Infect Dis* **130**: 564.

Wong P, Bottorff MB, Heritage RW *et al.* (1984). Acute rifampin overdose: a pharmacokinetic study and review of the literature. *J Pediatr* **104**: 781.

Wood MJ (1987). Interactions of antibiotics with other drugs. *J Antimicrob Chemother* **20**: 628.

Woodley CL, Kilburn JO, David HL, Silcox VA (1972). Susceptibility of mycobacteria to rifampin. *Antimicrob Ag Chemother* **2**: 245.

Woods GL, Washington JA II (1987). Mycobacteria other than *Mycobacterium tuberculosis*: review of microbiologic and clinical aspects. *Rev Infect Dis* **9**: 275.

Worlledge S (1973a). The detection of rifampicin-dependent antibodies. *Scand J Resp Dis* (Suppl 84): 60.

Worlledge S (1973b). Correlation between the presence of rifampicin-dependent antibodies and the clinical data. *Scand J Resp Dis* (Suppl 84): 125.

Yagupsky P, Ashkenazi S, Block C (1993). Rifampicin-resistant meningococci causing invasive disease and failure of chemoprophylaxis. *Lancet* **341**: 1152.

Yajko DM, Kirihara J, Sanders C *et al.* (1988). Antimicrobial synergism against *Mycobacterium avium* complex strains isolated from patients with acquired immune deficiency syndrome. *Antimicrob Ag Chemother* **32**: 1392.

Yamada S, Iwai K (1976). Induction of hepatic cortisol-6-hydroxylase by rifampicin. *Lancet* **ii**: 366.

Yamada T, Nagata A, Ono Y *et al.* (1985). Alteration of ribosomes and RNA polymerase in drug-resistant clinical isolates of *Mycobacterium tuberculosis*. *Antimicrob Ag Chemother* **27**: 921.

Yawalkar SJ, McDougall AC, Languillon J *et al.* (1982). Once-monthly rifampicin plus daily dapsone in initial treatment of lepromatous leprosy. *Lancet* **i**: 1199.

Yazawa K, Mikami Y, Maeda A *et al.* (1993). Inactivation of rifampin by *Nocardia brasiliensis*. *Antimicrob Ag Chemother* **37**: 1313.

Yeaman MR, Mitscher LA, Baca OG (1987). *In vitro* susceptibility of *Coxiella burnetii* to antibiotics, including several quinolones. *Antimicrob Ag Chemother* **31**: 1079.

Zackrisson G, Brorson JE, Bjornegard B *et al.* (1985). Susceptibility of *Bordetella pertussis* to doxycycline, cinoxacin, nalidixic acid, norfloxacin, imipenem, mecillinam and rifampicin. *J Antimicrob Chemother* **15**: 629.

Zaheer SA, Mukherjee R, Ramkumar B *et al.* (1993). Combined multidrug and *Mycobacterium W* vaccine therapy in patients with multibacillary leprosy. *J Infect Dis* **167**: 401.

Zaugg M, Salfinger M, Opravil M, Lüthy R (1993). Extrapulmonary and disseminated infections due to *Mycobacterium malmoense*: case report and review. *Clin Infect Dis* **16**: 540.

Zierski M (1973). Clinical aspects of side-effects on intermittent rifampicin regimen. *Scand J Resp Dis* (Suppl 84): 166.

Rifabutin

Description

Similar to rifampicin (p. 676), rifabutin is a derivative of rifamycin S. The most important property of this drug is that it is more active than rifampicin against *Mycobacterium avium* complex *in vitro*, against this organism growing in alveolar macrophages and in experimental animals (O'Brien *et al.*, 1987; Perumal *et al.*, 1987; Saito *et al.*, 1988). Clinical studies have also demonstrated that rifabutin prophylaxis reduced the frequency of disseminated *Mycobacterium avium* complex infection in patients with AIDS and CD4$^+$ counts ≤200/mm^3 (Nightingale *et al.*, 1993).

Sensitive Organisms

1 *Mycobacterium avium* complex

These bacteria, when isolated from both AIDS and non-AIDS patients, are usually rifabutin-sensitive *in vitro*, although there are considerable variations between strains. Rifabutin is usually more active than rifampicin (Horsburgh *et al.*, 1986; O'Brien *et al.*, 1987; Saito *et al.*, 1988). The drug also inhibits the multiplication of this pathogen in activated mouse peritoneal and alveolar macrophages (Perumal *et al.*, 1987; Perronne *et al.*, 1990; Yajko *et al.*, 1991). Rifabutin is also usually active in animals infected by *M. avium* complex and the addition of clofazimine or ethambutol usually results in improved activity (Gangadharam *et al.*, 1987; Saito and Sato, 1989; Furney *et al.*, 1990; Klemens and Cynamon, 1991; Klemens *et al.*, 1994).

In vitro and *in vivo* in animals, rifabutin enhances the activity of clarithromycin against some strains of *M. avium* complex but with other strains the combination is no more active than clarithromycin alone (Fattorini *et al.*, 1995; Furney *et al.*, 1995; Lounis *et al.*, 1995). In AIDS patients with disseminated disease due to *M. avium* complex the gastrointestinal tract appears to be the major route of infection. Rifabutin and sparfloxacin, but not azithromycin, inhibit binding of this organism to intestinal mucosal cells. This inhibition may be one of the mechanisms for the prophylactic effect of rifabutin for *M. avium* complex bacteremia (Bermudez *et al.*, 1994).

2 *Mycobacterium tuberculosis*

This is sensitive to rifabutin. The MICs for rifampicin-sensitive *M. tuberculosis* strains range from 0.03 to 0.06 µg per ml and so rifabutin is some 2- to 20-fold more active than rifampicin against this organism *in vitro*. However, using other methods it has been estimated that rifabutin is usually only some 2.5-fold more active than rifampicin (Chan *et al.*, 1992; Gonzalez-Montaner *et al.*, 1994) although rifabutin is less active than rifampicin against extracellular tuberculous bacilli in pulmonary cavities. This appears to be so because rifabutin produces lower serum and extracellular levels, but it is concentrated into cells (p. 710) (Chan *et al.*, 1992; Sirgel *et al.*, 1993).

There is some cross-resistance between rifabutin and rifampicin, but this is not complete. Usually *M. tuberculosis* strains resistant to 1.0 µg per ml of rifampicin and about 50% of those resistant to 5 µg per ml rifampicin are susceptible to 0.5 µg per ml of rifabutin (Gonzalez-Montaner *et al.*, 1994). Similar to rifampicin, rifabutin-resistance in *M. tuberculosis* is encoded by the rpo *B* gene (p. 678). There, however, is preliminary evidence that *M. tuberculosis* strains, resistant to rifampicin, but sensitive to rifabutin have a different amino acid substitution encoded by the *rpo B* gene, than strains resistant to both drugs. Therefore modern methods such as amplification of the appropriate region of the *rpo B* gene by polymerase chain reaction may identify *M. tuberculosis* strains, which are rifampicin-resistant, but rifabutin-sensitive, within 24 h (Telenti *et al.*, 1993; Miller *et al.*, 1994; Zhang and Young, 1994; Bodmer *et al.*, 1995; Davies 1995). Rifabutin is also active against some strains of *M. tuberculosis* which have developed multiple-drug resistance (Luna-Herrera *et al.*, 1995).

3 Mycobacterium leprae

Rifabutin is more active than rifampicin against this organism when evaluated in mouse-footpad infections or with the BACTEC 460 system (O'Brien *et al.*, 1987; Franzblau, 1991). Rifabutin, when combined with quinolones such as sparfloxacin and clinafloxacin exhibit synergistic activity against *M. leprae* (Dhople and Ibanez, 1993).

4 Other mycobacteria

Rifabutin is effective *in vitro* against *M. kansasii* (O'Brien *et al.*, 1987) and *M. paratuberculosis* (Chiodini, 1990; 1991). The drug is also effective in *M. paratuberculosis* infections in mice (Chiodini *et al.*, 1993).

5 Gram-positive and Gram-negative bacteria

Rifabutin shows a broad spectrum of activity *in vitro* against both Gram-positive and Gram-negative bacteria, similar to rifampicin (p. 676) (O'Brien *et al.*, 1987). Clinical studies with rifabutin for infections caused by these pathogens have not been performed.

6 Chlamydia trachomatis

This is sensitive to rifabutin *in vitro* and resistant strains do not emerge when the organism is grown in presence of subinhibitory concentrations of the drug (Treharne *et al.*, 1989).

7 Toxoplasma gondii

Rifabutin has some activity against this parasite *in vitro* and also in animals *in vivo* (Olliaro *et al.*, 1994). The activity of rifabutin *in vivo* is enhanced by drugs such as pyrimethamine, sulfadiazine or clindamycin (Araujo *et al.*, 1994).

8 Human immunodeficiency virus

Anand *et al.* (1988) reported that rifabutin inhibited the replication of HIV *in vitro*, but others have shown that the drug has no activity against this virus *in vitro* and it did not enhance the antiretroviral drugs such as zidovudine (Birch *et al.*, 1988). It also had no antiviral effect when patients with AIDS-related complex were treated with various doses of rifabutin (Torseth *et al.*, 1989).

Mode of Administration and Dosage

Rifabutin is administered by the oral route. For prophylaxis of *M. avium* complex infections in AIDS patients, an adult dosage of 300 mg rifabutin once-daily is recommended (Nightingale *et al.*, 1993; Gallant *et al.*, 1994; Gordin and Masur, 1994). If rifabutin is included in a three- to four-drug regimen to treat *M. avium* complex bacteremia in AIDS patients a once-daily dosage of 600 mg of rifabutin is now commonly used (Hoy *et al.*, 1990; Benson, 1994; Sullam *et al.*, 1994). However, if rifabutin is combined with clarithromycin, its dose should be usually reduced to 300 mg daily as the concomitant use of clarithromycin markedly elevates rifabutin serum levels (see below) (Griffith *et al.*, 1995). When rifabutin was used in the place of rifampicin in treatment regimens of pulmonary tuberculosis, a daily dose of 150 mg appeared satisfactory (Gonzalez-Montaner *et al.*, 1994).

Serum Levels, Excretion and Body Distribution

Rifabutin is absorbed after oral administration, but compared with rifampicin (p. 682), the serum levels attained are relatively low. The peak serum level, attained in 2–3 h after an oral dose of 300 mg is only approximately 0.4 μg per ml. Doubling the dose to 600 mg, increases the peak serum level to about 0.6 μg per ml. The serum level thereafter falls and 24 h after the dose it is approximately 0.1 μg per ml. The terminal half-life of this drug is as long as 36 h. The drug is incompletely absorbed from the gastrointestinal tract and its bioavailability after oral administration is only 12–20%. After continuous daily administration of rifabutin for 28 days, the area under the curve is lower after 4 weeks, than attained after the first dose, which suggests that rifabutin, similar to rifampicin (p. 688), induces its own drug metabolizing enzymes in the liver (O'Brien *et al.*, 1987; Skinner *et al.*, 1989).The concomitant use of fluconazole results in higher rifabutin serum levels. Clarithromycin also has the same effect but here this is more marked and rifabutin serum levels are nearly doubled. This now appears to be because both flucanazole and clarithromycin inhibit the hepatic metabolism of rifabutin (Fuller *et al.*, 1994; Blaschke and Skinner, 1996; Trapnell *et al.*, 1996). In contrast, combined zidovudine and rifabutin therapy, does not result in altered rifabutin serum levels (Li *et al.*, 1996).

The volume of distribution of rifabutin is very large, suggesting extensive distribution of the drug into tissues (Skinner *et al.*, 1989). Animal studies have shown that the concentrations of rifabutin are much higher in most tissues than in plasma. Tissue levels are particularly high in liver, lung, abdominal adipose tissue and spleen (Battaglia *et al.*, 1991). The concentrations of the drug in cells such as phagocytes are much higher than the serum levels (Van der Auwera *et al.*, 1988).

Some unchanged rifabutin is excreted in the urine and urinary concentrations of the active drug are some 100-fold higher than those in the serum. Two metabolites are also excreted in the urine. The first is 25-deacetyl derivative which is antibacterially as active as rifabutin. The second, 31-hydroxy derivative is 4- to 10-fold less active than the parent compound against mycobacteria. The unchanged drug is also excreted in the bile, where concentrations, similar to those in urine are found (O'Brien *et al.*, 1987; Skinner *et al.*, 1989).

Mode of Action

The mode of action of rifabutin on bacteria is similar to that of rifampicin (p. 685).

Toxicity

The side-effects of rifabutin are similar to those of rifampicin (p. 685). It causes an orange discoloration of urine, tears and skin, which is harmless. In doses of 300 mg daily the drug is well tolerated, but with higher doses nausea, vomiting and sometimes diarrhea may occur (Havlir, 1994). Diarrhea associated with *Clostridium difficile* has occurred in AIDS patients receiving rifabutin (McBride *et al.*, 1994). Hypersensitivity reactions with rash and fever may also result. Hepatotoxicity with elevated liver enzymes has been noted fairly frequently, but this may have often been due to other drugs taken at the time, such as isoniazid (p. 1190) or due to the disease being treated such as *M. avium* complex bacteremia. Neutropenia and thrombocytopenia have also been noted (O'Brien *et al.*, 1987; Havlir, 1994). One patient developed hemolytic anemia during rifabutin therapy which resolved when the drug was withdrawn (Hong Kong/BMRC, 1992). Some patients have developed acute uveitis with severe pain in one or both eyes and transient loss of vision associated with rifabutin therapy (Fuller *et al.*, 1994). This is particularly likely to occur if rifabutin is used together with clarithromycin or fluconazole, drugs which elevate rifabutin serum levels (see above) (Shafran *et al.*, 1994; Dunn *et al.*, 1995; Griffith *et al.*, 1995). The uveitis may be caused by direct rifabutin toxicity or by an immune reaction to protein from dead *M. avium* complex bacteria (Nichols, 1996). In patients treated with both rifabutin and clarithromycin, a diffuse polyarthralgia syndome may also occur (Havlir, 1994; Griffith *et al.*, 1995).

Staphylococcus aureus and *Staph. epidermidis* bacteremias with strains resistant to rifampicin, have occurred in some AIDS patients who had received long-term rifabutin chemoprophylaxis (Wood, 1994).

Like rifampicin (p. 689), rifabutin induces levels of hepatic microsomal enzymes, which causes altered metabolism of oral contraceptives, warfarin, phenytoin, methadone, clarithromycin and zidovudine. However, rifabutin appears to be a weaker inducer of these enzymes than rifampicin (Gallant *et al.*, 1994; Gonzalez-Montaner *et al.*, 1994; Havlir, 1994; Wallace *et al.*, 1995). In particular, rifabutin has only a very minor effect on zidovudine serum levels (Gallicano *et al.*, 1995).

Clinical Uses of the Drug

1 Chemoprophylaxis of M. avium complex bacteremia in AIDS patients

Nightingale *et al.* (1993) conducted two randomized, double-blind, placebo controlled trials with a mean duration of therapy of 223 days in study 1 and 188 days in study 2; there were 590 patients in study 1 and 556 in study 2. In both studies the patients had a previous AIDS-defining illness other than *M. avium* complex bacteremia, a negative tuberculin test and CD4$^+$ lymphocyte count $\leq$200/mm^3. Patients with previous or current mycobacterial infection were excluded.

Patients in both studies were randomly assigned to receive either 300 mg rifabutin daily or placebo. In study 1, *M. avium* complex bacteremia developed in 51 patients (17%) who were receiving placebo and in 24 patients (8%) who received rifabutin. In study 2, bacteremia developed in 51 patients (18%) in the placebo group compared with 24 patients (9%) in the rifabutin group. It was concluded that rifabutin prophylaxis reduced the frequency of disseminated *M. avium* complex infections in these AIDS patients. Fever, fatigue and hospitalizations were reduced by rifabutin. However, overall survival was not affected. Somewhat surprisingly, the breakthrough cases in the rifabutin-treated patients did not have an increased frequency of *M. avium* complex strains resistant to rifabutin.

Because of the results of the above studies, rifabutin in a dosage of 300 mg daily is currently recommended for prophylaxis of *M. avium* complex bacteremia in AIDS patients. This prophylaxis should be only given to AIDS patients if their CD4$^+$ lymphocyte counts are less than 100 per mm^3. Prophylaxis should be life-long unless *M. avium* bacteremia develops. Active mycobacterial disease should be excluded before the initiation of this therapy, but it does not mean that all patients with the above criteria should receive prophylaxis. In some patients it may be preferable to defer prophylaxis and treat *M. avium* bacteremia when it occurs. This may be wiser in patients who are receiving many other drugs and who already have symptoms such as nausea. It may also be best to avoid rifabutin if there is the likelihood of drug interactions. The cost of the drug is another factor. Other drugs are undergoing trials for this purpose and it may soon be recommended that a macrolide such as azithromycin (p. 657) is preferable for prophylaxis of *M. avium* complex bacteremia in AIDS patients (Gallant *et al.*, 1994; Gordin and Masur, 1994; Havlir, 1994; Henderson and Chapman, 1994).

2 Treatment of disseminated disease due to M. avium complex in AIDS patients

Rifabutin may be incorporated in three- or four-drug regimens to treat this disease. In one early study Masur *et al.* (1987) found the combination of rifabutin and clofazimine with or without other antimycobacterial agents not very effective for this purpose. But later Agins *et al.* (1989) and Hoy *et al.* (1990) reported that *M. avium* complex bacteremia cleared in most patients treated by isoniazid, ethambutol, clofazimine and rifabutin. It is now known that isoniazid does not contribute to this treatment regimen, but the triple-drug regimen of rifabutin, clofazimine and ethambutol has been used since then with success (Sullam *et al.*, 1994). Also in regimens where a macrolide such as clarithromycin (p. 648) or azithromycin (p. 657) is used as the number one drug, and ethambutol (p. 648) as the second, rifabutin may be suitable as the third drug, although rifampicin and others such as ciprofloxacin or amikacin are also suitable for this purpose (Benson and Ellner, 1993; Young, 1993 a, b; Benson, 1994). Short-term (14 days) use of rifabutin as a single drug is effective for disseminated *M. avium* complex bacteremia in AIDS patients, and so it should make a significant contribution to combination regimens for the treatment of this disease (Dautzenberg *et al.*, 1996).

3 Pulmonary tuberculosis

In one trial newly diagnosed, drug-sensitive, radiographically active and bacteriologically confirmed pulmonary tuberculosis patients were randomized to receive rifabutin 150 mg daily, rifabutin 300 mg daily or rifampicin, combined with isoniazid for 6 months. All patients also received pyrazinamide and ethambutol for the first 2 months. All three regimens proved effective and well tolerated. It appeared that rifabutin in a daily dosage of 150 mg was as effective as rifampicin in tuberculosis treatment regimens, when this disease was caused by sensitive *M. tuberculosis* strains (Gonzalez-Montaner *et al.*, 1994). Other studies have also confirmed that results of treatment are good if rifabutin 150 mg daily is substituted for rifampicin in standard regimens for the treatment of drug-sensitive pulmonary tuberculosis (Grassi and Peona, 1996).

It is not clear whether rifabutin will have any place in the treatment of tuberculosis caused by rifampicin-resistant *M. tuberculosis* strains. One patient responded to therapy with rifabutin, amikacin, thiacetazone, prothionamide and isoniazid, whose *M. tuberculosis* strain was resistant to streptomycin, isoniazid, ethambutol, rifampicin and pyrazinamide. The strain was rifabutin-sensitive (Gillespie *et al.*, 1990). In another study the *M. tuberculosis* strains were resistant to isoniazid, streptomycin and rifampicin. Initially the response to a rifabutin-containing regimen was good in two patients who had rifabutin-sensitive strains, but later they relapsed and their strains of *M. tuberculosis* became resistant to rifabutin (Hong Kong/BMRC, 1992). In five uncontrolled studies in Algeria, Argentina, France, South Africa and Spain, a total of 270 patients with multidrug-resistant pulmonary tuberculosis (90% of patients had *M. tuberculosis* strains resistant to both isoniazid and rifampicin) were treated by rifabutin-containing regimens. The drug was given in a dosage of 300 or 450 mg daily. Concomitant medications were selected according to the results of *in vitro* susceptibility testing of sputum isolates. Drugs used included kanamycin, ethambutol, pyrazinamide and isoniazid. In the majority of patients, signs and symptoms diminished, but only in one-third of them was there a bacteriologic conversion (Grassi and Peona, 1996).

4 Other mycobacterial infections

Rifabutin may also be used, instead of rifampicin, for the treatment of other mycobacterial infections, mainly in compromised hosts, when the *Mycobacterium* spp., such as *M. kansasii*, is rifabutin-sensitive (Akiyama *et al.*, 1991; Patel *et al.*, 1994). A regimen of clarithromycin, rifabutin and ethambutol is currently being evaluated in the treatment of *M. genavense* infections (Böttger, 1994). Clarithromycin/rifabutin therapy was effective in the treatment of disseminated *M. haemophilum* infection in immunosuppressed animals (Atkinson *et al.*, 1995).

References

Agins BD, Berman DS, Spicehandler D *et al.* (1989). Effect of combined therapy with ansamycin, clofazimine, ethambutol, and isoniazid for. *Mycobacterium avium* infection in patients with AIDS. *J Infect Dis* **159**: 784.

Akiyama H, Maruyama T, Uetake T *et al.* (1991). Systemic infection due to atypical mycobacteria in patients with chronic myelogenous leukemia. *Rev Infect Dis* **13**: 815.

Anand R, Moore JL, Curran JW, Srinivasan A (1988). Interaction between rifabutin and human immunodeficiency virus Type 1: inhibition of replication, cytopathic effect, and reverse transcriptase *in vitro*. *Antimicrob Ag Chemother* **32**: 684.

Araujo FG, Slifer T, Remington JS (1994). Rifabutin is active in murine models of toxoplasmosis. *Antimicrob Ag Chemother* **38**: 570.

Atkinson BA, Bocanegra R, Graybill JR (1995). Treatment of *Mycobacterium haemophilum* infection in a murine model with clarithromycin, rifabutin, and ciprofloxacin. *Antimicrob Ag Chemother* **39**: 2316.

Battaglia R, Salgarollo G, Zini G *et al.* (1991). Absorption, disposition and urinary metabolism of 14 c-rifabutin in rats. *Antimicrob Ag Chemother* **35**: 1391.

Benson CA (1994). Treatment of disseminated disease due to the *Mycobacterium avium* complex in patients with AIDS. *Clin Infect Dis* **18** (Suppl 3): 237.

Benson CA, Ellner JJ (1993). *Mycobacterium avium* complex infection and AIDS: advances in theory and practice. *Clin Infect Dis* **17**: 7.

Bermudez LE, Young LS, Inderlied CB (1994). Rifabutin and sparfloxacin but not azithromycin inhibit binding of *Mycobacterium avium* complex to HT-29 intestinal mucosal cells. *Antimicrob Ag Chemother* **38**: 1200.

Birch C, Tachedjian G, Lucas CR, Gust I (1988). *In vitro* effectiveness of a combination of zidovudine and ansamycin against human immunodeficiency virus. *J Infect Dis* **158**: 895.

Blaschke TF, Skinner MH (1996). The clinical pharmacokinetics of rifabutin (1996).. *Clin Infect Dis* **22** (Suppl 1): 15.

Bodmer T, Zürcher G, Imboden P, Telenti A (1995). Mutation position and type of substitution in the beta-subunit of the RNA polymerase influence *in-vitro* activity of rifamycins in riifampicin-resistant *Mycobacterium tuberculosis*. *J Antimicrob Chemother* **35**: 345.

Böttger EC (1994). *Mycobacterium genavense*: an emerging pathogen. *Eur J Clin Microbiol Infect Dis* **13**: 932.

Chan SL, Yew WW, Ma WK *et al.* (1992). The early bactericidal activity of rifabutin measured by sputum viable counts in Hong Kong patients with pulmonary tuberculosis. *Tubercle and Lung Disease* **73**: 33.

Chiodini RJ (1990). Bacterial activities of various antimicrobial agents against human and animal isolates of *Mycobacterium paratuberculosis*. *Antimicrob Ag Chemother* **34**: 366.

Chiodini RJ (1991). Antimicrobial activity of rifabutin in combination with two and three other antimicrobial agents against strains of *Mycobacterium paratuberculosis*. *J Antimicrob Chemother* **27**: 171.

Chiodini RJ, Kreeger JM, Thayer WR (1993). Use of rifabutin in treatment of systemic *Mycobacterium paratuberculosis* infection in mice. *Antimicrob Ag Chemother* **37**: 1645.

Dautzenberg B, Castellani P, Pellegrin J-L *et al.* (1996). Early bactericidal activity versus that of placebo in treatment of disseminated *Mycobacterium avium* complex bacteremia in AIDS patients. *Antimicrob Ag Chemother* **40**: 1722.

Davies PDO (1995). Tuberculosis. *Curr Opin Infect Dis* **8**: 105.

Dhople AM, Ibanez MA (1993). *In-vitro* activity of three new fluoroquinolones and synergy with ansamycins against *Mycobacterium leprae*. *J Antimicrob Chemother* **32**: 445.

Dunn A-M, Tizer K, Cervia JS (1995). Rifabutin-associated uveitis in a pediatric patient. *Pediatr Infect Dis J* **14**: 246.

Fattorini L, Li B, Piersimoni C *et al.* (1995). *In vitro* and *ex vivo* activities of antimicrobial agents used in combination with clarithromycin, with or without amikacin against *Mycobacterium avium*. *Antimicrob Ag Chemother* **39**: 680.

Franzblau SG (1991). *In vitro* activities of aminoglycosides, lincosamides, and rifamycins against *Mycobacterium leprae*. *Antimicrob Ag Chemother* **35**: 1232.

Fuller JD, Stanfield LED, Craven DE (1994). Rifabutin prophylaxis and uveitis. *New Engl J Med* **330**: 1315.

Furney SK, Roberts AD, Orme IM (1990). Effect of rifabutin on disseminated *Mycobacterium avium* infections in thymectomized, CD4T-cell-deficient mice. *Antimicrob Ag Chemother* **34**: 1629.

Furney SK, Skinner PS, Farrer J, Orme IM (1995). Activities of rifabutin, clarithromycin and ethambutol against two virulent strains of *Mycobacterium avium* in a mouse model. *Antimicrob Ag Chemother* **39**: 786.

Gallant JE, Moore RD, Chaisson RE (1994). Prophylaxis for opportunistic infections in patients with HIV infection. *Ann Intern Med* **120**: 932.

Gallicano K, Sahai J, Swick L *et al.* (1995). Effect of rifabutin on the pharmacokinetics of zidovudine in patients infected with human immunodeficiency virus. *Clin Infect Dis* **21**: 1001.

Gangadharam PRJ, Perumal VK, Jairam BT *et al.* (1987). Activity of rifabutin alone or in combination with clofazimine or ethambutol or both against acute and chronic experimental *Mycobacterium intracellulare* infections. *Am Rev Respir Dis* **136**: 329.

Gillespie SH, Baskerville AJ, Davidson RN *et al.* (1990). The serum rifabutin concentrations in a patient successfully treated for multi-resistant *Mycobacterium tuberculosis* infection. *J Antimicrob Chemother* **25**: 490.

Gonzales-Montaner LJ, Natal S, Yongchaiyud P *et al.* (1994). Rifabutin for the treatment of newly-diagnosed pulmonary tuberculosis: a multi-national, randomized, comparative study versus rifampicin. *Tubercle and Lung Disease* **75**: 341.

Gordin F, Masur H (1994). Prophylaxis of *Mycobacterium avium* complex bacteremia in patients with AIDS. *Clin Infect Dis* **18** (Suppl 3): 223.

Grassi C, Peona V (1996). Use of rifabutin in the treatment of pulmonary tuberculosis. *Clin Infect Dis* **22** (Suppl 1): 50.

Griffith DE, Brown BA, Girard WM, Wallace RJJr (1995). Adverse events associated with high-dose rifabutin in macrolide-containing regimens for the treatment of *Mycobacterium avium* complex lung disease. *Clin Infect Dis* **21**: 594.

Havlir DV (1994). *Mycobacterium avium* complex: advances in therapy. *Eur J Clin Microbiol Infect Dis* **13**: 915.

Henderson HM, Chapman SW (1994). *Mycobacterium avium-intracellulare. Curr Opin Infect Dis* **7**: 225.

Horsburgh CR Jr, Cohn DL, Roberts RB *et al.* (1986). *Mycobacterium avium- M intracellulare* isolates from patients with or without acquired immunodeficiency syndrome. *Antimicrob Ag Chemother* **30**: 955.

Hong Kong Chest Service/British Medical Research Council (1992). A controlled study of rifabutin and an uncontrolled study of ofloxacin in the retreatment of patients with pulmonary tuberculosis resistant to isoniazid, streptomycin and rifampicin. *Tubercle and Lung Disease* **73**: 59.

Hoy J, Mijch A, Sandland M *et al.* (1990). Quadruple-drug therapy for *Mycobacterium avium-intracellulare* bacteremia in AIDS patients. *J Infect Dis* **161**: 801.

Klemens SP, Cynamon MH (1991). *In vivo* activities of newer rifamycin analogs against *Mycobacterium avium* infection. *Antimicrob Ag Chemother* **35**: 2026.

Klemens SP, Grossi MA, Cynamon MH (1994). Comparative *in vivo* activities of rifabutin and rifapentine against *Mycobacterium avium* complex. *Antimicrob Ag Chemother* **38**: 234.

Li RC, Nightingale S, Lewis RC *et al.* (1996). Lack of effect of concomitant zidovudine on rifabutin kinetics in patients with AIDS-related complex. *Antimicrob Ag Chemother* **40**: 1397.

Lounis N, Ji B, Truffot-Pernot C, Grosset J (1995). Selection of clarithromycin-resistant *Mycobacterium avium* complex during combined therapy using the beige mouse model. *Antimicrob Ag Chemother* **39**: 608.

Luna-Herrera J, Reddy MV, Gangadharam PRJ (1995). *In-vitro* and intracellular activity of rifabutin on drug-susceptible and multiple drug-resistant (MDR). tubercle bacilli. *J Antimicrob Chemother* **36**: 355.

Masur H, Tuazon C, Gill V et al (1987). Effect of combined clofazimine and ansamycin therapy on *Mycobacterium avium-Mycobacterium intracellulare* bacteremia in patients with AIDS. *J Infect Dis* **155**: 127.

McBride MO, Coker RJ, Horner PJ *et al.* (1994). Diarrhoea associated with *Clostridium difficile* in AIDS patients receiving rifabutin. *Lancet* **343**: 417.

Miller LP, Crawford JT, Shinnick TM (1994). The *rpo B* gene of *Mycobacterium tuberculosis. Antimicrob Ag Chemother* **38**: 805.

Nichols CW (1996). *Mycobacterium avium* complex infection, rifabutin, and uveitis – is there a connection? *Clin Infect Dis* **22** (Suppl 1): 43.

Nightingale SD, Cameron DW, Gordin FM *et al.* (1993). Two controlled trials of rifabutin prophylaxis against *Mycobacterium avium* complex infection in AIDS. *New Engl J Med* **329**: 828.

O'Brien RJ, Lyle MA, Snider DE Jr (1987). Rifabutin (Ansamycin LM 427): a new rifamycin-S derivative for the treatment of mycobacterial diseases. *Rev Infect Dis* **9**: 519.

Olliaro P, Gorini G, Jabes D *et al.* (1994). *In-vitro* and *in-vivo* activity of rifabutin against *Toxoplasma gondii. J Antimicrob Chemother* **34**: 649.

Patel R, Roberts GD, Keating MR, Paya CV (1994). Infections due to nontuberculous *Mycobacteria* in kidney, heart, and liver transplant recipients. *Clin Infect Dis* **19**: 263.

Perronne C, Gikas A, Truffot-Pernot C *et al.* (1990). Activities of clarithromycin, sulfisoxazole, and rifabutin against *Mycobacterium avium* complex multiplication within human macrophages. *Antimicrob Ag Chemother* **34**: 1508.

Perumal VK, Gangadharam PRJ, Iseman MD (1987). Effect of rifabutin on the phagocytosis and intracellular growth of *Mycobacterium intracellulare* in mouse resident and activated peritoneal and alvealar macrophages. *Am Rev Respir Dis* **136**: 334.

Saito H, Sato K (1989). Activity of rifabutin alone and in combination with clofazimine, kanamycin and ethambutol against *Mycobacterium intracellulare* infections in mice. *Tubercle* **70**: 201.

Saito H, Sato K, Tomioka H (1988). Comparative *in vitro* and *in vivo* activity of rifabutin and rifampicin against *Mycobacterium avium* complex. *Tubercle* **69**: 187.

Shafran SD, Duschênes J, Miller M *et al.* (1994). Uveitis and pseudo-jaundice during a regimen of clarithromycin, rifabutin, and ethambutol. *New Engl J Med* **330**: 438.

Sirgel FA, Botha FJH, Parkin DP *et al.* (1993). The early bactericidal activity of rifabutin in patients with pulmonary tuberculosis measured by sputum viable counts: a new method of drug assessment. *J Antimicrob Chemother* **32**: 867.

Skinner MH, Hsieh M, Torseth J *et al.* (1989). Pharmacokinetics of rifabutin. *Antimicrob Ag Chemother* **33**: 1237.

Sullam PM, Gordin FM, Wynne BA and the Rifabutin Treatment Group (1994). Efficacy of rifabutin in the treatment of disseminated infection due to *Mycobacterium avium* complex. *Clin Infect Dis* **19**: 84.

Telenti A, Imboden P, Marchesi F *et al.* (1993). Direct, automated detection of rifampin-resistant *Mycobacterium tuberculosis* by polymerase chain reaction and single-strand conformation polymorphism analysis. *Antimicrob Ag Chemother* **37**: 2054.

Treharne JD, Yearsley PJ, Ballard RC (1989). *In vitro* studies of *Chlamydia trachomatis* susceptibility and resistance to rifampin and rifabutin. *Antimicrob Ag Chemother* **33**: 1393.

Torseth J, Bhatia G, Harkonen S *et al.* (1989). Evaluation of the antiviral effect of rifabutin in AIDS-related complex. *J Infect Dis* **159**: 1115.

Trapnell CB, Narang PK, Li R, Lavalle JP (1996). Increased plasma rifabutin levels with concomitant fluconazole therapy in HIV-infected patients. *Ann Intern Med* **124**: 573.

Van der Auwera P, Husson M (1989). Influence of rifampicin on motility and adherence of human neutrophils studied *in vitro. J Antimicrob Chemother* **24**: 347.

Van der Auwera P, Matsumoto T, Husson M (1988). Intraphagocytic penetration of antibiotics. *J Antimicrob Chemother* **22**: 185.

Wallace RJ Jr, Brown BA, Griffith DE *et al.* (1995). Reduced serum levels of clarithromycin in patients treated with multidrug regimens including rifampin or rifabutin for *Mycobacterium avium-M. intracellulare* infection. *J Infect Dis* **171**: 747.

Wood CA (1994). Rifampicin-resistant staphylococcal bacteremia in patient with AIDS receiving rifabutin. *Lancet* **343**: 919.

Yajko DM, Nassos PS, Sanders CA, Hadley WK (1991). Effects of antimicrobial agents on survival of *Mycobacterium avium* complex inside alveolar macrophages obtained from patients with human immunodeficiency virus infection. *Antimicrob Ag Chemother* **35**: 1621.

Young LS (1993a). Mycobacterial diseases in the 1990s. *J Antimicrob Chemother* **32**: 179.

Young LS (1993b). Mycobacterial diseases and the compromised host. *Clin Infect Dis* **17** (Suppl 2): 436.

Zhang Y, Young D (1994). Molecular genetics of drug resistance in *Mycobacterium tuberculosis. J Antimicrob Chemother* **34**: 313.

Spectinomycin

Description

Spectinomycin is an aminocyclitol compound which has some structural similarities to the aminocyclitol streptomycin, but it differs by not being an aminoglycoside (p. 428). Spectinomycin was isolated in 1960 from *Streptomyces spectabilis* in the Upjohn Research Laboratories (Mason *et al.*, 1961). It was originally known as actinospectacin and was manufactured as the sulfate salt. Later it was manufactured as the more soluble dihydrochloride salt. Clinical use of this drug has been restricted to the treatment of gonorrhea.

Sensitive Organisms

1 Gram-positive bacteria

Many of these bacteria, such as *Streptococcus pyogenes*, *Strep. pneumoniae* and *Staphylococcus epidermidis*, are usually sensitive. Only a small percentage of *Staph. aureus* and *Strep. viridans* strains are sensitive to concentrations easily obtainable in serum (McCormack and Finland, 1976; Fass and Prior, 1977).

2 Gram-negative bacteria

Spectinomycin has a wide range of activity against these bacteria (Mason *et al.*, 1961; Washington and Yu, 1972; McCormack and Finland, 1976; Fass and Prior, 1977). *Escherichia coli*, *Klebsiella pneumoniae* and the *Enterobacter*, *Salmonella* and *Shigella* spp. are usually sensitive. *Proteus mirabilis* and to a lesser extent other *Proteus* spp. are often sensitive. *Serratia* and *Citrobacter* spp. are sometimes sensitive whilst *Providencia* spp. and *Pseudomonas aeruginosa* are always resistant. A high percentage of the Enterobacteriaceae are inhibited by a concentration of $\leq 128\,\mu$g per ml, a concentration which is easily attainable in the urine with normal spectinomycin doses (Fass and Prior, 1977).

The greatest activity of spectinomycin has been against *Neisseria gonorrhoeae* (Levy *et al.*, 1973; McCormack and Finland, 1976). Nearly all strains of *N. gonorrhoeae* in the USA were inhibited by a concentration of 6.3 μg per ml or less (McCormack and Finland, 1976). Some studies indicated that gonococcal strains relatively resistant to penicillin G showed no increased resistance to spectinomycin (Maness and Sparling, 1973), but others found that there was a weak correlation between their sensitivities (Report, 1978). Gonococcal strains completely resistant to penicillin G without beta-lactamase production were usually sensitive to spectinomycin (p. 14).

Reports on the degree of susceptibility of beta-lactamase-producing gonococcal strains (p. 15) were varied. Such strains of *N. gonorrhoeae* isolated in East Asia were sensitive to 12 μg per ml or less of spectinomycin (Report, 1978). In Japan, beta-lactamase-producing gonococci were equally sensitive to spectinomycin as non-beta-lactamase-producers (Yoshida *et al.*, 1982). Antibiotic susceptibility of beta-lactamase-producing and non-beta-lactamase-producing strains isolated in various South East Asian localities were tested by Ng *et al.* (1983). All isolates were susceptible to spectinomycin (MIC $\leq 32\,\mu$g per ml). In contrast, Herzog *et al.* (1983) found that beta-lactamase-producing gonococcal isolates in London were less sensitive to spectinomycin than those not producing this enzyme. Cohen *et al.* (1983) examined gonococcal isolates collected from patients in the USA. Beta-lactamase-producing and intrinsically penicillin G-resistant strains were slightly more resistant to spectinomycin than penicillin G-susceptible ones.

Gonococci with increased resistance to spectinomycin can be produced *in vitro* by serial passage of the organisms in media containing increasing amounts of the drug (Pedersen *et al.*, 1972). Development of resistance to spectinomycin is of the one-step type, similar to streptomycin (p. 430) and rifampicin (p. 676). Total resistance to spectinomycin results from a chromosomal mutation which affects the ribosomal structure of *N. gonorrhoeae* (Report, 1978), thereby preventing spectinomycin from inhibiting protein synthesis by its action on the ribosome (p. 717). Spectinomycin-resistant strains usually remained sensitive to the aminoglycosides, streptomycin, kanamycin, amikacin, gentamicin, tobramycin and sisomicin (Thornsberry *et al.*, 1977).

During the late 1970s and early 1980s, spectinomycin-resistant *N. gonorrhoeae* strains were reported from several countries, but overall the prevalence of resistant strains was low. They were reported from Holland (Stolz *et al.*, 1975), UK (Easmon *et al.*, 1982, 1984; Ison *et al.*, 1983), USA (Thornsberry *et al.*, 1977; Ashford *et al.*, 1981; Pon *et al.*, 1986) and Australia (Gollow *et al.*, 1986). Later in the 1980s gonococcal strains highly resistant to spectinomycin became more prevalent among USA military personnel stationed in the Republic of Korea (Boslego *et al.*, 1987) and also in USA, where initially most spectinomycin-resistant gonococcal isolates were linked to overseas sources (Zenilman *et al.*, 1987). Spectinomycin therapy failed in patients infected by the resistant strains. Further reports described an increased frequency of spectinomycin-resistant gonococcal strains in Mexico City (Conde-Glez *et al.*, 1988), in the Philippines (Clendennen *et al.*, 1992a) and in Thailand (Clendennen *et al.*, 1992b). These resistant strains were usually also resistant to penicillin G and tetracyclines, but sensitive to cefotaxime and ceftriaxone.

3 Agents causing non-specific urethritis

Etiological agents of this disease include *Chlamydia trachomatis* and *Ureaplasma urealyticum* (pp. 745, 747). Spectinomycin is inactive against *C. trachomatis* but *Ureaplasma urealyticum* is sensitive (Bowie *et al.*, 1976; McCormack and Finland, 1976; Oriel *et al.*, 1977; Report, 1978).

4 Treponema pallidum

Spectinomycin has no curative effect on syphilis (Report, 1978) and used in a single dose it will not abort incubating syphilis but it may prolong the incubation period (McCormack and Finland, 1976).

5 Minimum inhibitory concentrations

The MICs of spectinomycin for a few selected bacterial species are shown in Table I.53. Organisms inhibited by 31.2 μg per ml or less may be considered as sensitive and organisms for which concentrations in excess of 125 μg per ml are required as resistant. Organisms with MICs between these limits belong to an intermediate category (Washington and Yu, 1972).

Serum Levels and Excretion

Spectinomycin is poorly absorbed after oral administration but it is well absorbed from i.m. injection sites. A peak serum level of about 100 μg per ml is attained about 1 h after a 2 g i.m. dose (Wagner *et al.*, 1968). Doubling the dose nearly doubles the serum concentration. A detectable serum level persists for about 8 h after a dose. A mean serum level of 64.3 μg per ml was detected at 1 h in children given an i.m. dose of 40 mg per kg (Rettig *et al.*, 1980). Most of the injected drug (70–80%) is excreted in the urine within 48 h in a microbiologically active form. Urinary concentrations of the active drug may reach 1000 μg per ml. Probenecid does not delay the excretion of spectinomycin. The drug is little bound to serum proteins (Wagner *et al.*, 1968).

Organism	MIC (μg per ml)
Staphylococcus aureus	6.2–25
Streptococcus pneumoniae	12.5–25
Neisseria gonorrhoeae	7.8
Escherichia coli	12.5–50

Table I.53
After Lewis and Clapp (1961)

Mode of Action

Similar to streptomycin (p. 432), spectinomycin acts at the 30S ribosomal subunit (p. 562), thereby inhibiting protein synthesis. Unlike streptomycin, it causes no detectable misreading of the polyribonucleotide code and at high concentration it is not bactericidal to *E. coli* (Davies *et al.*, 1965). In studies using *N. gonorrhoeae*, Ward (1977) showed that spectinomycin was more bactericidal than penicillin G, tetracycline and kanamycin. Spectinomycin also produces alterations in the surface morphology of gonococci, leading to their lysis. This possibly results from the action of spectinomycin on the ribosomes resulting in inhibition of the cytoplasmic membrane proteins and interference with the osmotic integrity of the cell (Ward, 1977).

Toxicity

Spectinomycin given as a single dose once only, appears to be of low toxicity. Willcox (1962) treated 101 patients and observed no side-effects. Its low toxicity has been confirmed by others (Platts, 1970; Duncan *et al.*, 1972). Occasionally patients have noted transient dizziness after the injection (Labowitz *et al.*, 1970). A few patients have developed either transient fever, nausea, headache or moderate discomfort at the injection site. Ototoxicity or nephrotoxicity have not been reported (Savage, 1973). Rarely an erythematous rash has been noted (Pedersen *et al.*, 1972).

When spectinomycin was given in a dose of 2 g four times daily for 21 days to volunteers, no evidence of ototoxicity or nephrotoxicity was detected (Novak *et al.*, 1974).

Spectinomycin is not cross-allergenic with the penicillins.

Clinical Uses of the Drug

1 Gonorrhea

Uncomplicated gonorrhea has been the only clinical indication for the use of spectinomycin. It was given as single-injection therapy in a dose of 2 g (Tiedeman *et al.*, 1965). Results of spectinomycin treatment of uncomplicated gonorrhea caused by non-beta-lactamase-producing strains in both sexes were good and comparable with those obtained by single-injection treatment with penicillin G (Willcox, 1962; Duncan *et al.*, 1972; Pedersen *et al.*, 1972; Judson *et al.*, 1974; Porter and Rutherford, 1977). Anorectal gonorrhea also responded to single-injection treatment with spectinomycin and the drug was used to treat successfully gonococcal proctitis in male homosexual patients (Fiumara, 1978; Fluker *et al.*, 1980; Sands, 1980), but gonococcal infections of the pharynx did not respond to single-dose spectinomycin (McCormack and Finland, 1976; Report, 1978).

Spectinomycin was mainly restricted for the treatment of patients infected with penicillin G-resistant gonococcal strains and for patients allergic to penicillin G. Beta-lactamase-producing *N. gonorrhoeae* strains have become very prevalent in some parts of the world since about 1975 (p. 15) and this has necessitated routine treatment with spectinomycin. The Center for Disease Control (CDC, 1980), therefore, recommended spectinomycin 2 g i.m. for the initial treatment of uncomplicated anogenital gonorrhea in patients who had recently returned from countries such as the Philippines, Singapore and Thailand. Because the prevalence of beta-lactamase-producing gonococci rose above 5%, a level at which it was suggested that spectinomycin should be substituted for penicillin G as first-line treatment, the former drug was used at one sexually transmitted disease clinic in London since the beginning of 1983 (Easmon *et al.*, 1984). In the USA, spectinomycin 2 g i.m. was also recommended for gonorrhea due to chromosomally mediated penicillin-resistant strains (p. 14).

By now spectinomycin-resistant *N. gonorrhoeae* strains have become more prevalent in various parts of the world (p. 716) and spectinomycin is no longer recommended as the preferred single-dose therapy for uncomplicated gonorrhea. Single-dose i.m. ceftriaxone (p. 361), oral cefixime (p. 412), oral ciprofloxacin (p. 1022) or oral ofloxacin (p. 1122) are now preferred. However, in some parts of the world, where spectinomycin-resistant gonococci are uncommon, the drug in a single-dose of 2 g i.m. can still be used for treatment of uncomplicated gonorrhea (Moran and Levine, 1995).

2 Non-specific urethritis

The majority of cases of non-specific (non-gonococcal) urethritis are caused by *Chlamydia trachomatis* and a smaller number are due to *U. urealyticum* (p. 745). A disadvantage of spectinomycin is that it is ineffective against infections due to *C. trachomatis* (p. 716) though infections due to *U. urealyticum* respond (Bowie *et al.*, 1976; McCormack and Finland, 1976).

References

Ashford WA, Potts OW, Adams HJU *et al.* (1981). Spectinomycin-resistant penicillinase-producing *Neisseria gonorrhoeae*. *Lancet* **ii**: 1035.

Boslego JW, Tramont EC, Takafuji ET *et al.* (1987). Effects of spectinomycin use on the prevalence of spectinomycin-resistant and of penicillinase-producing *Neisseria gonorrhoeae*. *New Engl J Med* **317**: 272.

Bowie WR, Alexander ER, Floyd JF *et al.* (1976). Differential response of chlamydial and ureaplasma-associated urethritis to sulphafurazole (sulfisoxazole). and aminocyclitols. *Lancet* **ii**: 1276.

CDC (Center for Disease Control) (1980). Penicillinase-producing *Neisseria gonorrhoeae* – New Mexico, California. *MMWR* **29**: 381.

Clendennen TE III, Hames CS, Kees ES *et al.* (1992a). *In vitro* antibiotic susceptibilities of *Neisseria gonorrhoeae* isolates in the Phillipines. *Antimicrob Ag Chemother* **36**: 277.

Clendennen TE, Echeverria P, Saengeur S *et al.* (1992b). Antibiotic susceptibility survey of *Neisseria gonorrhoeae* in Thailand. *Antimicrob Ag Chemother* **36**: 1682.

Cohen MS, Cooney MH, Blackman E, Sparling PF (1983). *In vitro* antimicrobial susceptibility of penicillinase-producing and intrinsically resistant *Neisseria gonorrhoeae* strains. *Antimicrob Ag Chemother* **24**: 597.

Conde-Glez CJ, Calderón E, Echániz G *et al.* (1988). Serogroup specificity and antimicrobial susceptibilities of *Neisseria gonorrhoeae* isolated in Mexico City. *J Antimicrob Chemother* **21**: 413.

Davies J, Anderson P, Davis BD (1965). Inhibition of protein synthesis by spectinomycin. *Science* **149**: 1096.

Duncan WC, Holder WR, Roberts DP, Knox JM (1972). Treatment of gonorrhoea with spectinomycin hydrochloride: comparison with standard penicillin schedules. *Antimicrob Ag Chemother* **1**: 210.

Easmon CSF, Ison CA, Bellinger CM, Harris JW (1982). Emergence of resistance after spectinomycin treatment for gonorrhoea due to beta-lactamase-producing strain of *Neisseria gonorrhoeae*. *Brit Med J* **284**: 1604.

Easmon CSF, Forster GE, Walker GD *et al.* (1984). Spectinomycin as initial treatment for gonorrhoea. *Brit Med J* **289**: 1032.

Fass RJ, Prior RB (1977). *In vitro* activity of spectinomycin against recent urinary tract isolates. *Antimicrob Ag Chemother* **12**: 551.

Fiumara NJ (1978). The treatment of gonococcal proctitis. An evaluation of 173 patients treated with 4g of spectinomycin. *JAMA* **239**: 735.

Fluker JL, Deherogoda P, Platt DJ, Gerken A (1980). Rectal gonorrhoea in male homosexuals. Presentation and therapy. *Brit J Vener Dis* **56**: 397.

Gollow MM, Blums M, Ismail A (1986). Penicillin-sensitive spectinomycin-resistant *Neisseria gonorrhoeae*. *Med J Aust* **144**: 651.

Herzog C, Ison CA, Easmon CSF (1983). Antimicrobial sensitivity of *Neisseria gonorrhoeae* Comparison of penicillinase producing and non-penicillinase producing strains. *Brit J Vener Dis* **59**: 289.

Ison CA, Littleton K, Shannon KP *et al.* (1983). Spectinomycin resistant gonococci. *Brit Med J* **287**: 1827.

Judson FN, Allaman J, Dans PE (1974). Treatment of gonorrhea. Comparison of penicillin G procaine, doxycycline, spectinomycin and ampicillin. *JAMA* **230**: 705.

Labowitz R, Porter WL, Holloway WJ (1970). The treatment of gonorrhoea with spectinomycin and rifampicin. *Delaware Med J* **42**: 353.

Levy J, Wicher K, Rose NR (1973). *In vitro* susceptibility of *Neisseria gonorrhoeae* to spectinomycin examined by a broth dilution method. *Antimicrob Ag Chemother* **3**: 335.

Lewis C, Clapp HW (1961). Actinospectacin, a new antibiotic. III. *In vitro* and *in vivo* evaluation. *Antibiot Chemother* **11**: 127.

Maness MJ, Sparling PF (1973). Multiple antibiotic resistance due to a single mutation in *Neisseria gonorrhoeae*. *J Infect Dis* **128**: 321.

Mason DJ, Dietz A, Smith RM (1961). Actinospectacin, a new antibiotic. I. Discovery and biological properties. *Antibiot Chemother* **11**: 118.

McCormack WM, Finland M (1976). Drugs five years later. Spectinomycin. *Ann Intern Med* **84**: 712.

Moran JS, Levine WC (1995). Drugs of choice for the treatment of uncomplicated gonococcal infections. *Clin Infect Dis* (Suppl 1): 47.

Ng WS, Chau PY, Ling J *et al.* (1983). Penicillinase-producing *Neisseria gonorrhoeae* isolates from different localities in south east Asia. Susceptibility to 15 antibiotics. *Brit J Vener Dis* **59**: 232.

Novak E, Gray JE, Pfeifer RT (1974). Animal and human tolerance of high-dose intramuscular therapy with spectinomycin. *J Infect Dis* **130**: 50.

Oriel JD, Ridgway GL, Tchamouroff S, Owen J (1977). Spectinomycin hydrochloride in the treatment of gonorrhoea: its effect on associated *Chlamydia trachomatis* infections. *Brit J Vener Dis* **53**: 226.

Pedersen AHB, Wiesner PJ, Holmes KH *et al.* (1972). Spectinomycin and penicillin G in the treatment of gonorrhea. A comparative evaluation. *JAMA* **220**: 205.

Platts WM (1970). 'Trobicin' in the treatment of gonorrhoea. *Med J Aust* **2**: 500.

Pon E, Batchelor RA, Howell HB *et al.* (1986). An unusual case of penicillinase-producing *Neisseria gonorrhoeae* resistant to spectinomycin in California. *Sex Transm Dis* **13**: 47.

Porter IA, Rutherford HW (1977). Treatment of uncomplicated gonorrhoea with spectinomycin hydrochloride (Trobicin). *Brit J Vener Dis* **53**: 115.

Report of a WHO Scientific Group (1978). *Neisseria gonorrhoeae* and gonococcal infections. *Wld Hlth Org Techn Rep Ser* 616.

Rettig PJ, Nelson JD, Kusmiesz H (1980). Spectinomycin therapy for gonorrhea in prepubertal children. *Amer J Dis Child* **134**: 359.

Sands M (1980). Treatment of anorectal gonorrhea infections in men. *JAMA* **243**: 1143.

Savage GM (1973). Spectinomycin related to the chemotherapy of gonorrhea. *Infection* **1**: 227.

Stolz E, Zwart HGF, Michel MF (1975). Activity of eight antimicrobial agents *in vitro* against *N gonorrhoeae*. *Brit J Vener Dis* **51**: 257.

Thornsberry C, Jaffee H, Brown ST *et al.* (1977). Spectinomycin-resistant *Neisseria gonorrhoeae*. *JAMA* **237**: 2405.

Tiedemann JH, Hackney JF, Price EV (1965). Acute gonorrheal urethritis in men. Treatment with spectinomycin sulfate. *JAMA* **191**: 101.

Wagner JG, Novak E, Leslie LG, Metzler CM (1968). Absorption, distribution and elimination of spectinomycin dihydrochloride in man. *Int J Clin Pharmacol* **1**: 261.

Ward ME (1977). The bactericidal action of spectinomycin on *Neisseria gonorrhoeae*. *J Antimicrob Chemother* **3**: 323.

Washington JAII, Yu PKW (1972). *In vitro* antibacterial activity of spectinomycin. *Antimicrob Ag Chemother* **2**: 427.

Willcox RR (1962). Trobicin (actinospectacin). A new injectable antibiotic in the treatment of gonorrhoea. *Brit J Vener Dis* **38**: 150.

Yoshida S-I, Urabe S, Mizuguchi Y (1982). Antibiotic sensitivity patterns of penicillinase-positive and penicillinase-negative strains of *Neisseria gonorrhoeae* isolated in Fukuoka, Japan. *Brit J Vener Dis* **58**: 305.

Zenilman JM, Nims LJ, Menegus MA *et al.* (1987). Spectinomycin-resistant gonococcal infections in the United States, 1985–1986. *J Infect Dis* **156**: 1002.

Tetracyclines

Description

A Classical older tetracyclines

Introduced soon after penicillin G and the sulfonamides, the tetracyclines were once widely used, and still are in some countries. Due to the prevalence of tetracycline-resistant organisms and the availability of effective alternative antibiotics, nowadays tetracyclines are the preferred drugs for a relatively small number of diseases.

Numerous older tetracycline compounds with a similar molecular structure (four benzene rings) and about the same spectrum of activity are available.

1 Chlortetracycline the first tetracycline to be discovered, was isolated from *Streptomyces aureofaciens* in 1944 (Duggar *et al.*, 1948). This is no longer available for oral use.

2 Oxytetracycline derived from *Streptomyces rimosus*, was reported in 1950.

3 Tetracycline first described in 1953, was prepared from chlortetracycline at Lederle laboratories and was also independently derived from oxytetracycline at Pfizer laboratories.

4 Demethylchlortetracycline or demeclocycline was obtained from a mutant of Duggar's original strain of *Streptomyces aureofaciens* and reported in 1957.

5 Methacycline (6-methylene-5-hydroxytetracycline) was prepared in the Pfizer laboratories.

6 Lymecycline (tetracycline-L-methylene-lysine) is a compound of tetracycline and an amino acid (Whitby and Black, 1964). It was developed in Italy and is not available in Australia or the USA.

7 Doxycycline (alpha-6-deoxytetracycline) developed by Pfizer laboratories, is available as both doxycycline monohydrate and doxycycline hyclate. Its main advantage is increased oral absorption and a prolonged serum half-life.

8 Minocycline (7-dimethylamino-6-demethyl-6-deoxytetracycline) (Redin, 1967).

Tetracycline compounds are mainly marketed for oral administration, but preparations of doxycycline and minocycline for i.v. administration are available.

Two more soluble compounds have been introduced specially for parenteral use.

9 Rolitetracycline (pyrrolidino-methyl-tetracycline) (Dimmling, 1960).

10 Rolitetracycline nitrate (pyrrolidino-methyl-tetracycline nitrate) (Kaplan *et al.*, 1960).

B New investigational tetracyclines – glycylcyclines

Two new semisynthetic tetracyclines, named glycylcyclines (CL 329, 998 and CL 331, 002) have been developed. The first is a N, N-dimethylglycylamido derivative of minocycline, also known as DMG-MINO, and the second is 6-demethyl 6-deoxytetracycline (DMG-DMDOT). Information on their *in vitro* activity is available.

These two semisynthetic tetracyclines are more active than tetracycline against Gram-positive cocci such as *Streptococcus pneumoniae*. Activity against *Staphylococcus aureus* is also good, including tetracycline- and methicillin-resistant strains. All enterococci, including multiresistant *Enterococcus faecium* strains, are also susceptible. The glycylcyclines are highly potent against *Neisseria*, *Haemophilus*, *Moraxella* and *Bacteroides* spp. Members of the family Enterobacteriaceae are susceptible and *Pseudomonas aeruginosa* is moderately sensitive. *Chlamydia* spp., *Ureaplasma urealyticum* and the *Mycoplasma* spp. are also susceptible to these new compounds. In general strains of most bacterial species with acquired resistance to tetracyclines are glycylcycline-sensitive (Testa *et al.*, 1993; Eliopoulos *et al.*, 1994; Kenny and Cartwright, 1994; Wise and Andrews, 1994; Tally *et al.*, 1995; Fraise *et al.*, 1995; Whittington *et al.*, 1995). A possible exception is penicillin G-resistant *Strep. pneumoniae*. Whilst some authors have found these to be susceptible to both glycylcyclines, others have reported that strains with intermediate and high-level penicillin G-resistance are only uniformly sensitive to DMG-DMDOT, but that they have increased MICs to DMG-MINO (Weiss *et al.*, 1995).

The information below will largely be confined to tetracycline, doxycycline and minocycline.

Sensitive Organisms

These antibiotics have a wide range of activity.

1 Gram-positive bacteria

Tetracyclines are active against most of these organisms such as *Staph. aureus* (including beta-lactamase-producing strains), *Staph. epidermidis*, *Staph. saprophyticus*, *Strep. pyogenes* (Group A), *Strep. pneumoniae*, *Strep. viridans*, *E. faecalis*, *E. faecium* and also the anaerobic streptococci. Group B streptococci are commonly resistant (see below). Gram-positive bacilli, such as *Bacillus anthracis*, *Clostridium tetani*, *Cl. perfringens* and *Listeria monocytogenes* (Wiggins *et al.*, 1978) are tetracycline-sensitive. *Actinomyces israelii*, the causative organism of human actinomycosis, is sensitive (Holmberg *et al.*, 1977). Minocycline is quite active against the *Nocardia*, most *N. asteroides* strains being inhibited by ≤4 μg per ml, but all other tetracyclines are much less active against this species (Bach *et al.*, 1973; Gutmann *et al.*, 1983; Dewsnup and Wright, 1984). Most strains of *Bacillus cereus* are inhibited by tetracycline (Leading article, 1983).

2 Acquired resistance of Gram-positive bacteria

Most of these bacteria may acquire resistance to tetracyclines and in most cases the resistance determinants are carried on plasmids or within transposons. They code for two principal resistance mechanisms. One of these is energy-dependent removal of the antibiotic from the bacterial cell, mediated by membrane-located efflux proteins. The second mechanism is ribosomal protection and here tetracyclines are unable to prevent attachment of aminoacyl-tRNA to the ribosomal acceptor site (p. 561). A less common third mechanism involves a chemical modification of the tetracycline molecule; the drug here is rendered inactive as an inhibitor of protein synthesis (Chopra, 1986; Poyart-Salmeron *et al.*, 1991; Chopra *et al.*, 1992; Chopra, 1994). Sometimes the tetracycline-resistance determinants can be chromosomally encoded (Nesin *et al.*, 1990).

Staphylococci readily become tetracycline-resistant, so that sensitivity testing is important if these drugs are used for the treatment of staphylococcal infections. With the high usage of tetracyclines in the past, the prevalence of staphylococci resistant to tetracyclines rose in hospitals. In one Boston hospital, of 482 *Staph. aureus* strains isolated, 38.2% were resistant (Sabath, 1969). With the subsequent reduction in consumption of tetracyclines the prevalence of multiresistant *Staph. aureus* strains (resistant to at least three antibiotics including tetracycline) fell in general hospitals, but not in dermatological hospitals or clinics where tetracyclines were commonly used (Rosendal *et al.*, 1977; Ayliffe *et al.*, 1979). During a 3-year period, 14–20% of *Staph. aureus* isolates in Scotland were tetracycline-resistant; resistance was higher in isolates from burns cases, from patients aged over 64 years and from skin isolates (WHO, 1982). Community staphylococci often remained sensitive; in a study of outpatients attending a London hospital the prevalence of tetracycline-resistant *Staph. aureus* strains in 1968 was 6.5% and this had only increased to 8% in 1978 (Hassam *et al.*, 1978). Only 8% of *Staph. aureus* strains isolated from outpatients in Sweden were tetracycline-resistant (Forsgren and Walder, 1982). Tetracycline-resistance was demonstrated in 33.5% of 200 strains of coagulase-negative staphylococci isolated from patients in Ohio, USA (Watanakunakorn, 1984).

Strains of *Strep. pyogenes* (Group A) resistant to tetracycline were first observed in isolates from burns patients in Birmingham, England (Lowbury and Cason, 1954; Lowbury and Hurst, 1956). Kuharic *et al.* (1960) found 20% and Mitchell and Baber (1965) 32% of strains examined to be tetracycline-resistant. Subsequent surveys showed a lower prevalence of resistant strains, possibly resulting from a more selective use of tetracyclines. Kahlmeter and Kamme (1972) found only 6% of *Strep. pyogenes* to be resistant, and Robertson (1973) observed a decrease in the prevalence of resistant strains in south-west Essex from a peak of 35% in 1965 to 9.2% in 1972. The majority of Group A beta-hemolytic streptococci collected in 1972 in Massachusetts were sensitive to tetracyclines (Finland *et al.*, 1976a). A nation-wide survey in Britain during 1975 showed that overall 36% of Group A streptococci were resistant, but the percentage of resistant strains in different localities ranged from 15 to 62 (Report, 1977). Of 100 strains of Group A streptococci isolated from outpatients in Sweden, 17% were resistant to doxycycline (Forsgren and Walder, 1982), but of another 132 strains tested in the USA only 5% were resistant to tetracycline (Bourbeau and Campos, 1982).

Group B hemolytic streptococci are frequently resistant to tetracyclines. In California during 1971–1973, of 607 isolates, 72% were resistant (Anthony and Concepcion, 1975). Similarly, 87.5% of 244 isolates of Group B streptococci during 1970–1975 in Houston, were resistant (Baker *et al.*, 1976). Between 69% and 76% of these bacteria which were tested in Scotland during the years 1978–1980 were tetracycline-resistant; high percentages of streptococci of groups C, G and F were also resistant (Communicable Diseases Scotland, 1981).

Tetracycline-resistant pneumococci were first recognized in Australia in 1962 (Evans and Hansman, 1963). Since that time they have been frequently isolated from patients (Schaedler *et al.*, 1964; Hansman and Andrews, 1967). A survey in the UK during 1975 showed that overall 13% of pneumococci were resistant to tetracyclines, but there was great geographic variation (Report, 1977). In a similar survey during 1977 in the UK, 6.8% of *Strep. pneumoniae* strains studied were resistant to tetracycline (Howard *et al.*, 1978). Pneumococcal strains resistant to tetracyclines appear to be uncommon in the USA (Finland *et al.*, 1976b; Neu, 1978). Tetracycline-resistance was present in only 4% of pneumococci isolated from patients in 1981 at a hospital in Atlanta, USA (Perlino and Lichtenberger, 1984), and in a nationwide survey from 1979 to 1987 it was only 2.9% (Spika *et al.*, 1991). All of 100 pneumococcal isolates from outpatients in Sweden were sensitive to doxycycline (Forsgren and Walder, 1982). These results are in contrast to those obtained in Spain. In a 30-month period prior to December 1981, of 200 clinical isolates of pneumococci, 74% were resistant to tetracycline and 45% were chloramphenicol-resistant (Liñares *et al.*, 1983). Pneumococcal strains have been isolated in South Africa which were resistant to penicillin G and tetracyclines (p.5). Interestingly, other multiply-resistant pneumococci have subsequently been isolated from patients and their contacts in South Africa, which were resistant to tetracyclines, clindamycin, erythromycin and co-trimoxazole, but sensitive to penicillin G (Klugman *et al.*, 1986). Tetracycline- and penicillin G (p.6)- resistant pneumococci are very prevalent in some Eastern European countries such as Hungary (Hryniewicz, 1994). Some penicillin G-resistant pneumococci in the USA are now also tetracycline-resistant (Duchin *et al.*, 1995; Moreno *et al.*, 1995).

Streptococcus viridans, *E. faecalis* and *E. faecium* strains can also acquire tetracycline-resistance (Pepper *et al.*, 1987; Roberts and Hillier, 1990; Bentorcha *et al.*, 1991). The same is true for *L. monocytogenes*, and it appears that this organism can exchange resistance determinants with *E. faecalis* in nature (Poyart-Salmeron *et al.*, 1992; Charpentier *et al.*, 1994, 1995).

Resistance occurs with Gram-positive anaerobic organisms. Strains of *Cl. perfringens* may be resistant to tetracycline (Johnstone and Cockcroft, 1968; Sapico *et al.*, 1972). Chow *et al.* (1975)

found 54% of *Cl. perfringens* strains resistant to tetracycline and comparable percentages were resistant to minocycline and doxycycline. Sutter and Finegold (1976) showed that about 40% of *Cl. perfringens* strains were inhibited by clinically achievable concentrations and a slightly higher percentage of strains were inhibited by minocycline and particularly by doxycycline. In the UK, Brazier *et al.* (1985) reported that 69% of *Cl. perfringens* strains were sensitive to tetracycline; percentages of other *Clostridium* spp. sensitive were *Cl. ramosum* 44%, *Cl. difficile* 84%, *Cl. septicum* 100% and *Cl. tetani* 100%. In resistant strains of *Cl. difficile* the resistance genes are often similar to those found in *E. faecalis* (Hächler *et al.*, 1987). Of the other Gram-positive anaerobes, such as the *Peptococcus, Peptostreptococcus, Eubacterium, Acidamino-coccus, Propionibacterium, Lactobacillus, Bifidobacterium* and *Actinomyces* spp., a variable but significant proportion are resistant to the tetracycline drugs. Overall, doxycycline and minocycline are somewhat more active than tetracycline against these anaerobes, with minocycline being the most active against some *Peptococcus* and *Peptostreptococcus* spp. (Chow *et al.*, 1975; Sutter and Finegold, 1976; Robbins *et al.*, 1987; Roberts, 1991).

3 Gram-negative bacteria

Tetracyclines are active against Enterobacteriaceae such as *Escherichia coli* and the *Enterobacter, Klebsiella, Salmonella, Shigella* and *Yersinia* spp., including *Y. pestis* (CDC, 1994). The latter is more sensitive to doxycycline (MICs 0.25–1.0 µg per ml) than to tetracycline (MICs 0.5–4.0 µg per ml) (Smith *et al.*, 1995). *Serratia marcescens* and the *Proteus* spp. are usually resistant. Although the salmonellae are usually sensitive *in vitro*, tetracycline drugs are not effective for the treatment of infections due to these bacteria. Sometimes minocycline acts synergistically with gentamicin against certain Enterobacteriaceae, in particular against *E. coli* (Fass *et al.*, 1976). *Vibrio cholerae* (both classical and El Tor biotypes) is susceptible. The new *Vibrio cholerae* 0139 Bengal strain which has caused a large epidemic since 1992 in the Indian subcontinent is tetracycline-sensitive, but resistant to co-trimoxazole and furazolidone. It is also resistant to polymyxin B and in this respect it resembles the El Tor biotype (p. 668) (CDC, 1993a; Cholera Working Group, 1993; Waldor and Mekalanos, 1994). The halophilic vibrios, *V. parahaemolyticus, V. aklginolyticus* and *V. hollisae* which cause food-borne gastroenteritis, are nearly always sensitive to tetracycline (Joseph *et al.*, 1978; Morris *et al.*, 1985; French *et al.*, 1989; Abbott and Janda, 1994). *Vibrio vulnificus*, which is associated with septicemia or cellulitis is also sensitive (NIH, 1984, Morris *et al.*, 1985; French *et al.*, 1989; Midani and Rathore, 1994). Non-O Group 1 (non-01) *V. cholerae* strains, which cause gastroenteritis, are sensitive to tetracyclines (Morris *et al.*, 1981).

Most strains of *Campylobacter jejuni* and *C. fetus* are susceptible to the tetracyclines (Chow *et al.*, 1978; Vanhoof *et al.*, 1978) but in Israel about 38% of strains of *C. jejuni* were reported to be resistant (Michel *et al.*, 1983). *Helicobacter pylori* is sensitive to tetracyclines, penicillins, cephalosporins, erythromycin, clarithromycin, clindamycin, rifampicin and usually metronidazole and tinidazole, but resistant to nalidixic acid, trimethoprim and vancomycin (Goodwin *et al.*, 1986; Fennerty, 1994; NIH, 1994). *Helicobacter cinaedi* is doxycycline-sensitive (Burman *et al.*, 1995). *Aeromonas hydrophila* and *Plesiomonas shigelloides* are usually susceptible to the tetracyclines (Holmberg and Farmer, 1984; Janda *et al.*, 1994).

Many other Gram-negative bacteria were also susceptible in the past, but among some of these resistant strains are now common (p. 724). These include *Neisseria meningitidis, Haemophilus influenzae, H. ducreyi, Moraxella catarrhalis, Bordetella pertussis, Francisella tularensis* and *Pasteurella multocida* (Goldstein *et al.*, 1988). *Brucella* spp. are still uniformly tetracycline-sensitive (Robertson *et al.*, 1973; Farrell *et al.*, 1976; Rubinstein *et al.*, 1991). *Neisseria gonorrhoeae* may be sensitive but this varies in different parts of the world (p. 724). Beta-lactamase-producing strains of *N. gonorrhoeae* are often moderately resistant (p. 15). Of 47 strains of *Gardnerella vaginalis*, tested by Balsdon *et al.* (1980) 74% were sensitive to tetracycline. Invariably *P. aeruginosa* is tetracycline-resistant. This is probably mainly due to active efflux of the antibiotic from the bacterial cell, rather than due to decreased permeability (Li *et al.*, 1994). *Burkholderia (Pseudomonas) pseudomallei* is usually susceptible to tetracycline and to minocycline (Eickhoff *et al.*, 1970; Howe *et al.*, 1971; Yamamoto *et al.*, 1990). *Stenotrophomonas maltophilia* is quite sensitive to minocycline and doxycycline (Zuravleff and Yu, 1982). Strains of *Acinetobacter* spp. may be resistant to tetracycline, but most strains are susceptible to minocycline and doxycycline (Maderazo *et al.*, 1975; Kuck, 1976; Montgomerie *et al.*, 1976; Crues *et al.*, 1979). *Legionella pneumophila* is of intermediate sensitivity to tetracycline but it is quite sensitive *in vitro* to doxycycline and minocycline (Thornsberry *et al.*, 1978). Minocycline is effective *in vivo* in guinea pigs infected with this organism (Nash *et al.*, 1978; Yoshida *et al.*, 1985). Doxycycline therapy reduces mortality in guinea pigs infected with *L. micdadei* (Pasculle *et al.*, 1985). The *Bartonella (Rochalimaea)* spp. such as *B. henselae* and *B. quintana* are sensitive to doxycycline (Schwartzman, 1992; Regnery and Tappero, 1995). Their doxycycline MIC is usually $0.12 \mu g$ per ml (Maurin *et al.*, 1995).

Bacteria of the *Bacteroides fragilis* group may be sensitive, but many strains are moderately and others highly resistant to tetracyclines (Martin *et al.*, 1972; Gorbach and Bartlett, 1974). Gentamicin acts synergistically with minocycline against 20% of those *B. fragilis* strains which are sensitive in clinically attainable concentrations (Fass *et al.*, 1976). *Prevotella melaninogenica*, other *Prevotella* spp. and the *Fusobacterium* spp. are more sensitive to tetracycline and even more so to doxycycline and particularly to minocycline (Chow *et al.*, 1975; Sutter and Finegold, 1976). In one *in vivo* study, minocycline was more effective than tetracycline in infections in mice due to some *Fusobacterium* spp. (Hill, 1977).

4 Acquired resistance of Gram-negative bacteria

Tetracycline-resistance is widespread in many aerobic and anaerobic Gram-negative species. The use of tetracyclines in humans and animals has led to the selection of resistant bacteria (Chopra *et al.*, 1981). In most cases this resistance is transferable by plasmids or transposons (p. 459), and it may be multiple against a number of chemotherapeutic agents.

Lewis (1968) found that 24% of *Escherichia coli* strains isolated in UK were resistant to one or more antibiotics, 16% were tetracycline-resistant and in 60% of these, resistance was transferable. In studies on enteropathogenic *E. coli* in the UK, all strains isolated between 1948 and 1951 were susceptible to tetracycline but of those isolated in the years between 1957 and 1960, 1967 and 1968 and 1980 and 1981, 17.5%, 22% and 28.9% were tetracycline-resistant. In over 60% of these tetracycline-resistant strains, resistance was transferable (Slocombe and Sutherland, 1973; Gross *et al.*, 1982). Very similar results were obtained in a study of *E. coli* isolates from hospital patients in Buffalo in the USA. Of 759 strains, 48% were resistant to one or more of ampicillin, chloramphenicol, kanamycin, streptomycin and sulfonamides and multiple resistance occurred in 53% of the resistant strains. Tetracycline-resistant strains accounted for 25% of all strains and 53% of the resistant strains; 79% of tetracycline-resistant strains were resistant to multiple drugs (Camiolo *et al.*, 1975). In other parts of the world enterotoxigenic *E. coli* strains were more resistant; in Thailand 61% were resistant to doxycycline (Echeverria *et al.*, 1984) and about 50% were resistant in Honduras (Sack *et al.*, 1984).

Resistant strains of Enterobacteriaceae have been particularly common in hospitals. In a Boston hospital, 61% of *E. coli* and 62% *Klebsiella*, 58% *Enterobacter*, 91% *Proteus* and 97% *Serratia* spp. strains were tetracycline-resistant (Sabath, 1969). In another survey of *E. coli* strains isolated from patients at a children's hospital in Oklahoma, 25% were highly resistant to tetracycline (MIC $>50 \mu g$ per ml) (Yoshioka *et al.*, 1977). Following administration of the tetracyclines, fecal organisms of the recipients often become resistant to these drugs. Some studies indicated that doxycycline caused a lower percentage of resistant *E. coli* strains in the feces than tetracycline (Bartlett *et al.*, 1975; Alestig and Lidin-Janson, 1975), but others have been unable to show any difference between these drugs with regard either to the emergence of resistant strains or the occurrence of plasmids (Jonsson and Tunevall, 1976). Heimdahl and Nord (1983) found that doxycycline administration decreased the number of aerobic fecal bacteria with little change on the number of anaerobes; but there was a marked increase in doxycycline-resistant aerobes and anaerobes in the oral cavity and colon.

In tetracycline-resistant *E. coli* and other resistant Enterobacteriaceae, the resistance determinants usually reside on plasmids or transposons and they code for similar resistance mechanisms to those found in Gram-positive bacteria (p. 720) (Park and Levy, 1988; Manavathu *et al.*, 1990).

In 1973, 67% of *Shigella* spp. strains tested in Washington were resistant to tetracycline but this fell to 27% in 1976 (Controni *et al.*, 1978). Resistance to tetracycline, often associated with multiple-antibiotic resistance, has been described in *Shigella* isolates in the UK (Frost and Rowe, 1983), Sweden (Hansson *et al.*, 1981) and Lebanon (Uwaydah and Osseiran, 1981). In surveys in the UK, in the period 1974 to 1983 multiple-antibiotic resistant strains of *Sh. dysenteriae*, *Sh. flexneri* and *Sh. boydii* increased progressively from 15% to 69.2% (Gross *et al.*, 1984). Multiply-resistant *Sh. dysenteriae* type 1 strains have now appeared in many developing countries (p. 111). For instance, in Burundi, Africa there has been an epidemic caused by this organism since 1979. The *Sh. dysenteriae* type 1 strains there were resistant to ampicillin, chloramphenicol, nalidixic acid, streptomycin, sulfisoxazole, tetracycline and co-trimoxazole

(Ries *et al.*, 1994). Multiple antibiotic-resistance, including resistance to tetracycline, also occurs with *Salmonella* isolates (Anderson, 1980).

In a study of antibiotic sensitivities of 1156 *V. cholerae* strains from various parts of the world, O'Grady *et al.* (1976) only detected six, all from Indonesia or the Philippines, which had increased resistance to tetracycline (MIC >2 μg per ml). These six strains also showed increased resistance to chloramphenicol, and four had increased resistance to sulfonamides and the other two increased resistance to ampicillin. Subsequently disease outbreaks due to strains of *V. cholerae* 01, biotype El Tor, which were tetracycline-resistant have occurred in Tanzania (Mhalu *et al.*, 1979) and Bangladesh (CDC, 1980). Such strains also developed resistance to multiple antibiotics. An unusual multiresistant *V. cholerae* 01 El Tor appeared in Argentina in 1992. This showed resistance to ampicillin, cephalothin, aztreonam, cefotaxime, sulfisoxazole, gentamicin and kanamycin, but it remained sensitive to tetracyclines (Rossi *et al.*, 1993). However, some strains of this organism from the same South American epidemic, which were isolated in Ecuador in 1992, were also resistant to tetracyclines and chloramphenicol (Threlfall *et al.*, 1993). Some strains of *V. alginolyticus* may also be resistant to tetracycline and these are also resistant to ampicillin and chloramphenicol (Joseph *et al.*, 1978).

A few *N. meningitidis* strains, resistant to tetracycline have been identified. Their tetracycline-resistance determinants were carried on plasmids (Gascoyne-Binzi *et al.*, 1994a). Strains of *N. gonorrhoeae* which are resistant or have a reduced sensitivity to tetracyclines are much more common. The pattern of resistance varies in different parts of the world (Report, 1978). In South-East Asia and the Western Pacific the incidence of *N. gonorrhoeae* strains with reduced sensitivity to tetracyclines has ranged from 30 to 60%. A relatively recent survey in Thailand showed that 70% of gonococcal isolates were tetracycline-resistant (Clendennen *et al.*, 1992). In Mexico City 41.3% of gonococcal strains were resistant to the drug (Conde-Glez *et al.*, 1988). In Belgium, resistance to tetracycline, doxycycline and minocycline was found in 6.3%, 2.5% and 2.5% of strains, respectively; all strains were non-beta-lactamase producers but 17.5% were relatively resistant to penicillin G (Gordts *et al.*, 1982). Beta-lactamase-producing strains often have a reduced susceptibility to tetracyclines (p. 15). Treatment failures with the usual recommended tetracycline regimen for gonorrhea are commonly associated with gonococcal strains with a tetracycline MIC of 1 μg per ml or greater (Karney *et al.*, 1977; Report, 1978). Over 50% of beta-lactamase-producing gonococcal strains isolated in the USA and East Asia had a tetracycline MIC of 1 μg per ml or greater (CDC, 1978; Report 1978). A high percentage of beta-lactamase-producing strains isolated in the USA in 1980 were tetracycline-resistant (Jaffe *et al.*, 1981). A later survey in Baltimore, USA showed that 15% of gonococcal strains had high-level, plasmid-mediated tetracycline-resistance (see above) (Hook *et al.*, 1989). In Liverpool, UK, 20% of gonococcal strains were penicillin- and tetracycline-resistant (Thomas, 1980). Beta-lactamase-producing gonococcal strains isolated in West Africa were usually more sensitive to tetracycline (p. 15). Increased resistance to tetracycline is often associated with increased resistance to other antibiotics such as penicillin G, erythromycin, streptomycin and chloramphenicol, suggesting a common genetic basis (Maness and Sparling, 1973; Maier *et al.*, 1974; Report, 1978). Common chromosomal loci for resistance have been detected for some of these antibiotics (Report, 1978). For instance, genes for high-level resistance to streptomycin and spectinomycin and for low-level resistance to tetracycline and chloramphenicol are linked. In 1985, *N. gonorrhoeae* strains were isolated in the USA with high-level resistance to tetracycline (MIC 24–32 μg per ml) but which remained susceptible to penicillin G, ampicillin, cefotaxime, cefuroxime, cefoxitin, spectinomycin and co-trimoxazole (CDC, 1985). Similar strains were detected in Canada (WHO, 1986).

Neisseria gonorrhoeae with low level of tetracycline-resistance (MICs 0.5–4 μg per ml versus MICs of 0.02–0.2 μg per ml for sensitive strains) arise because of chromosomal mutations. Ribosomal function is affected and this alters the target for the antibiotic (Heritage and Hawkey, 1988). High-level tetracycline-resistance (MICs ≥16.0 μg per ml) is due to the presence of a 25.2 megadalton conjugative plasmid which carries the tetracycline-resistance determinant (Morse *et al.*, 1986; Knapp *et al.*, 1987; Gascoyne *et al.*, 1991; Gascoyne-Binzi *et al.*, 1994b; West *et al.*, 1995).

Non-encapsulated strains of *H. influenzae* may occasionally become resistant to the tetracyclines when these drugs are used for prolonged periods in patients with chronic bronchitis (Gould and Murdoch, 1960). In Australia, four strains of *H. influenzae* type b, which were highly resistant to tetracycline, were isolated from patients (Hansman, 1975). These strains were all resistant to doxycycline but two of them were sensitive to minocycline. In a survey conducted in the UK during 1977, 2.7% of *H. influenzae* strains (two type b and 25 untypable strains) were resistant to tetracycline (Howard *et al.*, 1978). Very similar results were obtained in a 1981 survey in the UK: 3.1% of *H. influenzae* strains (1 type b and 56 non-typable) were tetracycline-resistant (Philpott-Howard and Williams, 1982). Clinical isolates examined at a London hospital in 1981–1982 showed that 5–6% of strains of *H. influenzae* and *H. parainfluenzae* were tetracycline-resistant (Mehtar and Aminiafshar, 1983). In the USA, 6% of *Haemophilus* species (mainly *H. influenzae* and *H. parainfluenzae*) isolated from patients with chronic bronchitis (Kauffman *et al.*, 1979) and in another study only two of 110 clinical isolates from adults (Simon *et al.*, 1980), were tetracycline-resistant. Of 1084 children in Omaha, USA, 34.2% carried non-typable *H. influenzae* strains and 2% *H. influenzae* type b; only one non-typable strain was resistant to tetracycline and to chloramphenicol (Lerman *et al.*, 1979). High rates of tetracycline-resistance have been reported amongst *H. influenzae* isolates in Hong Kong (23%) (Ling *et al.*, 1983), and in Spain (54.4%) where these strains were resistant to multiple antibiotics (p. 114).

Strains of *H. ducreyi* resistant to tetracyclines were isolated in Africa, South-East Asia, Europe, Canada and the USA (Hammond *et al.*, 1980; Kraus *et al.*, 1982; Albritton *et al.*, 1984; Sturm, 1987). These resistant strains possessed a 34-megadalton plasmid (Roberts, 1989). However, many tetracycline-resistant strains of *H. ducreyi* were still sensitive to doxycycline and especially minocycline (Dangor *et al.*, 1990). Tetracycline-resistant *Moraxella catarrhalis* strains have also been described (Brown *et al.*, 1989). The resistance determinants of these appeared to be located on the chromosome and they were not transferable (Roberts *et al.*, 1990, 1991). Some strains of *Aeromonas hydrophila* may also become tetracycline-resistant (Aoki and Takahashi, 1987). *Campylobacter jejuni* and *C. coli* strains can develop resistance to the drug; the resistance-determinants are carried by plasmids (Ng *et al.*, 1987). Strains of *Burkholderia* (*Pseudomonas*) *pseudomallei* resistant to multiple antibiotics, including tetracycline, co-trimoxazole and aminoglycosides have also been reported (Shaefer *et al.*, 1982).

Resistance to tetracycline of Gram-negative anaerobic bacteria, especially *B. fragilis*, has gradually increased. In the UK, only 6% of isolates of *B. fragilis* were tetracycline-resistant in 1973–4, but from 1976 onwards over one-third were resistant (Phillips *et al.*, 1981). Surveys in the USA have detected tetracycline-resistance amongst *B. fragilis* in 63–67% of isolates in the years 1981–1983 (Tally *et al.*, 1985). In France, 63% of *B. fragilis* strains tested were resistant to tetracycline (Acar *et al.*, 1981). In tetracycline-resistant *Bacteroides* spp. strains the resistance-determinants may code for ribosomal protection, or for active reduction of tetracycline accumulation in bacterial cells (Park *et al.*, 1987; Nikolich *et al.*, 1992).

5 Mycobacteria

That tetracyclines have a low degree of activity against *Mycobacterium tuberculosis*, is of no clinical importance. Some biovariants of *M. fortuitum* are quite sensitive (MIC ≤1 μg per ml) to doxycycline, but most strains of *M. chelonae* are resistant to it (Swenson *et al.*, 1985). *Mycobacterium fortuitum* may acquire tetracycline-resistance determinants similar to those found in Gram-positive bacteria (p. 720) and become doxycycline-resistant (Pang *et al.*, 1994). Torres *et al.* (1978) found that a small percentage of strains of *M. marinum* had MICs of 2 μg per ml to either minocycline or doxycycline. Minocycline at a concentration of 6.5 μg per ml may inhibit *M. tuberculosis*, *M. bovis*, *M. kansasii* and *M. intracellulare* (Tsukamura, 1980).

Minocycline in low concentrations is also quite active against *M. leprae*. This has been demonstrated in mice infected by this organism and also in patients with lepromatous leprosy where a daily dose of 100 mg proved to be rapidly bactericidal (Gelber, 1987; Gelber *et al.*, 1991; Ji *et al.*, 1993).

6 Mycoplasma

Mycoplasma pneumoniae is sensitive to all tetracyclines (Rylander and Hallander, 1988; McCormack, 1993). Usually *M. hominis* is also susceptible, but strains with tetracycline-resistance have been more frequently encountered in recent years (Roberts *et al.*, 1985; Cummings and McCormack 1990; McCormack, 1993); *M. genitalium* is tetracycline-sensitive (Renaudin *et al.*, 1992).

7 Ureaplasma urealyticum

This species is usually sensitive (Csonka and Spitzer, 1969), but resistant strains occur naturally (Spaepen *et al.*, 1976; Roberts and Kenny, 1986; Taylor-Robinson and Furr, 1986; Robertson *et al.*, 1988). Evans and Taylor-Robinson (1978) studied 141 *Ureaplasma* strains isolated from men with non-specific urethritis attending London venereal disease clinics between 1973 and 1976, and who had been treated with tetracyclines; 9.9% of these strains were resistant to tetracyclines. They also showed that resistance could be induced *in vitro*. Tetracycline-resistance was reported in 7% of isolates of *U. urealyticum* from males in Washington, USA and these strains were a cause of persistent urethritis (Stimson *et al.*, 1981). In Brazil, 33% of *U. urealyticum* isolates were tetracycline-resistant (Magalhães and Veras, 1984). Evans and Taylor-Robinson (1978) found that all naturally occurring tetracycline-resistant ureaplasmas were sensitive to erythromycin, a different finding to that of Spaepen *et al.* (1976). Comparative studies on the *in vitro* susceptibilities of *U. urealyticum* to various tetracyclines showed that their activity decreased in the order of minocycline, doxycycline and tetracycline (Spaepen *et al.*, 1976; Spaepen and Kundsin, 1977). Nevertheless, when their MICs are related to clinically achievable serum concentrations, all these tetracyclines are comparable in activity and cross-resistance occurs between them.

8 Rickettsiae and Coxiella

Tetracyclines are active against the rickettsiae which cause diseases such as the various typhus fevers. Epidemic typhus is caused by *Rickettsia prowazekii* and scrub typhus by *R. tsutsugamushi*. Murine typhus is caused by *R. typhi* and a newly recognized *R. azadi* (ELB agent) (Radulovic *et al.*, 1995). These organisms also cause the spotted fever group of diseases e.g. *R. rickettsii* causes Rocky Mountain spotted fever, *R. conorii* causes Mediterranean spotted fever and *R. australis* is the causative organism of Queensland tick typhus. Doxycycline with an MIC of 0.1 μg per ml appears more active against these rickettsiae than tetracycline (MIC 0.25 μg per ml) (Raoult *et al.*, 1987b; Raoult and Drancourt, 1991). The action of doxycycline and chloramphenicol on *R. rickettsii* in tissue culture is primarily rickettsiastatic (Wisseman and Ordonez, 1986). Rare strains of *R. tsutsugamushi* may be tetracycline-resistant. These are sensitive to azithromycin *in vitro* (Strickman *et al.*, 1995). *Coxiella burnetii* (the agent causing Q fever) is also sensitive. Isolates from patients with chronic Q fever are less sensitive to doxycycline than isolates from those with acute disease (Yeaman *et al.*, 1989; Raoult *et al.*, 1991).

9 Chlamydiae

Chlamydia trachomatis which causes trachoma and various genital infections (p. 746) is sensitive to tetracycline and even more so to doxycycline and minocycline. The MIC range of doxycycline for this organism is 0.008 to 0.06 μg per ml (Bowie *et al.*, 1978; Beale and Upshon, 1994; Rice *et al.*, 1995). Occasional tetracycline- and doxycycline- resistant strains of *C. trachomatis* have been encountered (Jones *et al.*, 1990). *Chlamydia pneumoniae* is also sensitive to the tetracyclines (Chirgwin *et al.*, 1989; Grayston *et al.*, 1990; Hamerschlag, 1994). *Chlamydia psittaci*, which causes psittacosis, is also susceptible (Khatib *et al.*, 1995).

10 Spirochetes

Tetracycline is active against *Treponema pallidum*, but its MIC against this organism (0.2 μg per ml) is much higher than that of penicillin G (0.0005) (p. 18) (Norris and Edmondson, 1988). The leptospirae are also tetracycline- sensitive (Johnson, 1989), and so is *Borrelia burgdorferi* (Johnson *et al.*, 1987; Nadelman *et al.*, 1993).

11 Miscellaneous

Malarial parasites are susceptible to tetracyclines, and in particular to doxycycline (Pang *et al.*, 1988). Doxycycline and minocycline also show some activity against *Toxoplasma gondii in vitro* and in animals *in vivo* (Chang *et al.*, 1990, 1991). They are also active against *Giardia lamblia in vitro* (Edlind, 1989). Doxycycline and minocycline also show some activity against *Trichomonas vaginalis* and *Entamoeba histolytica*. These drugs are more lipophilic than tetracycline and this may improve their penetration into the cells of these parasites (Katiyar and Edlind, 1991). Minocycline, unlike other tetracyclines also inhibits *Candida albicans* and *C. tropicalis in vitro* (Waterworth, 1974), but *in vivo* there is no difference between the actions of tetracycline and minocycline on vaginal yeast flora (Oriel and Waterworth, 1975). All other fungi are tetracycline-resistant. Doxycycline has a synergistic effect with amphotericin B against *Candida albicans in vitro*, probably because amphotericin B increases cell permeability for doxycycline (Ånséhn *et al.*, 1976). *In vitro*, tetracyclines suppress the growth of *Naegleria fowleri*, the causative agent of primary amebic meningoencephalitis (Thong *et al.*, 1977). The addition of tetracycline to amphotericin B therapy also increases survival of mice with experimental amebic meningoencephalitis (p. 1283).

12 Differences between tetracyclines

There is usually cross-resistance between various tetracyclines and therefore it is only necessary to use one member of the group, such as tetracycline, for sensitivity testing. However, doxycycline and minocycline, differ from the older tetracyclines in a number of respects. Some of these differences have been described in the preceding sections.

Minocycline is more active than other tetracyclines against *Staph. aureus*, being active against a percentage of strains which are resistant to tetracycline (Steigbigel *et al.*, 1968b; Minuth *et al.*, 1974; Chattopadhyay and Harding, 1975). Doxycycline is also active against a proportion of tetracycline-resistant *Staph. aureus* strains (Minuth *et al.*, 1974). Minocycline is more active than tetracycline against penicillin-resistant *Staph. aureus*; of 200 strains, 13.5% were resistant to tetracycline, but susceptible to minocycline (Candanoza and Ellner, 1975). Thirteen methicillin-resistant strains of *Staph. aureus* and *Staph. epidermidis* were found to be resistant to tetracycline and doxycycline but six had a minocycline MIC of ≤2 μg per ml (Minuth *et al.*, 1974). Similarly, Rich and Davidson (1975) found that of 34 cloxacillin-resistant *Staph. aureus* strains isolated from a hospital, one was resistant, one was fully sensitive and the other 32 had MICs in the range of 1.25–2.5 μg per ml for minocycline; all of these strains were resistant to tetracycline. These concentrations of minocycline are just obtainable in the serum after standard doses (p. 731), so that minocycline may have efficacy for infections due to such strains.

Against beta-hemolytic streptococci, minocycline is the most active of the tetracyclines. In one study, 16 of 33 Group A strains were inhibited by tetracycline (MIC ≤2.5 μg per ml) whereas 22 of these were inhibited by minocycline (MIC ≤1.25 μg per ml); the susceptibility of strains from Groups B, C and G were identical (McGill, 1974). Finland *et al.* (1976a) studied 29 Group A, 4 Group B and 2 Group C strains of beta-hemolytic streptococci. The majority were sensitive to all of seven tetracycline drugs tested, but a few strains were sensitive to minocycline (MIC 0.2–1.6 μg per ml), but resistant to other tetracyclines. In another study, minocycline was not found to be as active against *Strep. pyogenes*; with tetracycline-sensitive strains the MICs of minocycline and tetracycline were similar, but with tetracycline-resistant strains although minocycline was more active its MICs were never below 4 μg per ml (Wood *et al.*, 1975). Minocycline is active against tetracycline-sensitive pneumococci (Steigbigel *et al.*, 1968b) and it is usually active against tetracycline-resistant strains in concentrations which are clinically achievable (Wood *et al.*, 1975).

Some Gram-negative organisms resistant to tetracycline are sensitive to minocycline. In a study of 311 clinical isolates of tetracycline-resistant Enterobacteriaceae 48 (24%) were sensitive to minocycline; these included *E. coli*, *Pr. mirabilis*, *Klebsiella*, *Enterobacter* and *Serratia* spp. (Candanoza and Ellner, 1975). The reason for this in the case of *E. coli* appeared to be a difference in bacterial cell penetration; resistance to tetracycline in plasmid bearing cells was due to decreased transport of tetracycline into the cell, but in such cells the transport of minocycline was by a different mechanism (Del Bene and Rogers, 1975). In clinically achievable concentrations minocycline is more active than tetracycline against both tetracycline-sensitive and tetracycline-resistant *Haemophilus* spp. (Wood *et al.*, 1975).

Table I.54
Condensed from Steigbigel *et al.* (1968b)

	MICs (μg per ml)					
	Tetracycline		Doxycycline		Minocycline	
	Range	Median	Range	Median	Range	Median
Gram-positive bacteria						
Staphylococcus aureus	1.6–>100.0	3.1	0.39–>100	1.6	0.39–12.5	0.78
Streptococcus pyogenes	0.19–50.0	0.78	0.09–25.0	0.39	0.09–25.0	0.39
Strepococcus pneumoniae	0.19–3.1	0.39	0.04–0.39	0.19	0.04–0.78	0.09
Enterococcus faecalis	6.3–>100.0	>100.0	1.6–>100.0	50.0	1.6–>100.0	100.0
Gram-negative bacteria						
Escherichia coli	3.1–500.0	12.5	1.6–500.0	12.5	3.1–500.0	6.3
Klebsiella spp.	6.3–500.0	50.0	6.3–300.0	50.0	3.1–500.0	25.0
Neisseria gonorrhoeae	0.39–6.3	0.78	0.09–3.1	0.39	0.19–3.1	0.39
Haemophilus influenzae	3.1–12.5	6.3	1.6–6.3	1.6	1.6–6.3	3.1

13 Minimum inhibitory concentrations

The MICs of the three tetracycline antibiotics against some selected bacterial species are shown in Table I.54. The values are condensed from a study in which the majority of organisms tested were isolated from patients, and therefore also includes strains with acquired tetracycline resistance. For practical purposes organisms inhibited by 1 µg per ml or less can be regarded as highly sensitive, those inhibited by 1–5 µg per ml as intermediate, and those not inhibited by 5 µg per ml as resistant. With doxycycline and minocycline serum levels are lower than with other tetracyclines (p. 729); organisms with an MIC greater than 2–3 µg per ml should be regarded as probably resistant.

Mode of Administration and Dosage

Tetracyclines are usually administered by mouth.

1 Tetracycline

The dosage for children is 25–50 mg per kg body weight per day, given in four divided doses. The adult dosage is 250 mg 6-hourly, or 0.5 g 6-hourly for more serious infections. Dosages larger than 0.5 g 6-hourly are usually of no additional benefit because higher serum levels are not obtained and the excess tetracycline is excreted in the feces.

2 Doxycycline

The usual adult dosage is a single dose of 200 mg (or 100 mg every 12 h) on the first day of treatment, followed by a maintenance dose of 100 mg per day. For severe infections the maintenance dose can be increased to 100 mg 12-hourly. The dosage for children is 4 mg per kg body weight given in two equal doses on the first day, followed by 2.2 mg per kg given as a single daily maintenance dose. The adult dosage of doxycycline for malaria chemoprophylaxis is 100 mg orally daily (Pang et al., 1987; Brown, 1993).

3 Minocycline

The dosage for adults consists of an initial loading dose of 200 mg followed by a maintenance dose of 100 mg every 12 h.

4 Rolitetracycline and rolitetracycline nitrate

The usual daily i.v. dosage of rolitetracycline for adults is 275 mg, and for children 10 mg per kg body weight. The manufacturers recommended that this daily dose should be given as one direct i.v. injection over a period of at least 1 min, but the dose can probably be added to an i.v. flask for a slow infusion, provided that there are no incompatible additives. For the treatment of severe infections the recommended dosage can be doubled for short periods. The usual adult i.m. dosage of rolitetracycline nitrate is a single daily injection of 350 mg, but similarly, this dosage can be doubled for short periods for treatment of severe infections. The i.m. dosage for children is 10 mg per kg per day, but the i.m. use of this preparation is not recommended for children during the first year of life. These parenteral preparations are now rarely used.

5 Parenteral doxycycline and minocycline

Preparations of these drugs suitable for i.v. administration are available. The adult dosage of either drug is 200 mg initially, followed by 100 mg every 12 h. Each dose should be dissolved in 500 or 1000 ml of glucose/saline fluid for slow i.v. infusion over a period of 0.5–1.0 h.

6 Patients with renal failure

Tetracycline therapy should be avoided in such patients, as these drugs may cause further deterioration of renal function (p. 738). In addition, most of the tetracycline compounds accumulate in patients with renal failure if the usual doses are given. Accumulation of tetracycline and rolitetracycline can be avoided in anuric patients by administering individual doses every 3–4 days (Kunin, 1967), but this is not recommended because renal disease may still be aggravated (Ribush and Morgan, 1972).

In contrast, doxycycline which does not accumulate in these patients, appears to be safe in the presence of renal failure (Mérier et al., 1969; Mahon et al., 1970; Whelton et al., 1974). Unlike other tetracyclines, its use, either oral or i.v. is not associated with significant further rises of the blood urea and serum creatinine values in azotemic patients (Little and Bailey, 1970; George and Evans, 1971; Alestig, 1973; Stenbaek et al., 1973; Mahony and Lloyd-Jones, 1975). Doxycycline does not accumulate in the serum of such patients because it is eliminated by an alternate non-renal gastrointestinal pathway (p. 732). Doxycycline has the same effect on mammalian protein synthesis as other tetracyclines (p. 734), but its anti-anabolic effect is rarely manifested in uremic patients, apparently because it does not accumulate to toxic levels (Morgan and Ribush, 1972). Nevertheless, studies by Mahon *et al.* (1976) suggested that doxycycline should be used cautiously in patients with renal failure. They observed that although the serum half-life of doxycycline was only slightly increased and the drug did not accumulate in the plasma compartment of these patients, up to 30% of an administered dose might have accumulated in some other unknown part of the body. Houin *et al.* (1983) confirmed that doxycycline had no deleterious effects on renal function in patients with renal insufficiency. They found that the doxycycline fraction bound to plasma protein and erythrocytes decreased in parallel with renal impairment, presumably due to some endogenous substances displacing doxycycline. It was postulated that the resulting increase in the free fraction of the drug in the blood favored increased hepatic elimination. Houin *et al.* (1983) also found that the amount of doxycycline removed by hemodialysis was negligible.

Evidence concerning the safety of minocycline in patients with impaired renal function is conflicting. Because the drug is excreted in feces and is mainly metabolized in the body and only a small amount is excreted in urine (p. 732), it could be expected that only minor dosage adjustments are required in such patients. Some investigators found that minocycline excretion was not significantly reduced in patients with renal failure (McHenry *et al.*, 1972; Carney *et al.*, 1974). In contrast, Bernard *et al.* (1971) showed that there was a prolongation of the serum half-life of the drug from 18 to 68 h, which was in direct relationship to the severity of the patient's renal failure. In addition, George *et al.* (1973) demonstrated that minocycline administration caused exacerbation of pre-existing renal insufficiency. Welling *et al.* (1975) have further studied the pharmacokinetics of minocycline in patients with renal failure. After a single i.v. infusion of 100 mg minocycline given over 30 min resultant serum levels in patients with normal renal function and those with various grades of renal functional impairment, including two who were essentially anephric, were similar. Although these results suggested that minocycline may be used safely in the presence of mild renal failure, the drug should be used cautiously. In particular, the normal recommended dose of 200 mg per day should not be exceeded because the protein catabolic effect (p. 734) of the drug is dose-dependent, and in such patients a resultant small increase in urea production may be sufficient to aggravate uremia (Carney *et al.*, 1974).

Tetracyclines are slowly removed from the body by hemodialysis, but the rate of removal by peritoneal dialysis is poor (Greenberg and Sanford, 1967). This also applies to doxycycline (Whelton *et al.*, 1974) and minocycline (Carney *et al.*, 1974). The addition of tetracyclines to peritoneal dialysis fluids is not recommended because they are well absorbed from the peritoneal cavity (Kunin, 1967).

7 Patients with liver disease

Tetracyclines should be administered cautiously in such patients, because liver damage may occur as a complication of high-dosage tetracycline therapy (p. 738). Although tetracyclines are excreted in the bile, this is not a major pathway for their excretion (p. 732) and patients with pre-existing liver damage do not appear to be more prone to the toxic effects of tetracyclines (Alestig, 1974).

Serum Levels in Relation to Dosage

1 Tetracycline

Tetracycline, administered orally, produces higher blood levels than oxy- or chlortetracycline (Fig. I.28). Following repeated doses of 250 or 500 mg tetracycline at 6-hourly intervals, the drug accumulates and the serum level gradually increases. With a continuous dosage of 0.5 g tetracycline every 6 h, the serum level stabilizes at about 4–5 μg per ml after about 24 h, which is approximately double the serum level achieved with a dosage of 250 mg orally 6-hourly (Fig. I.27).

Further increase of the dosage to 1 g or more orally every 6 h does not produce significantly higher serum levels. Tetracyclines are better absorbed if the patient is fasting. Compared with the fasting state, serum levels obtained when tetracycline hydrochloride is administered with a meal are reduced by approximately 50% (Welling *et al.*, 1977). The presence of divalent and trivalent

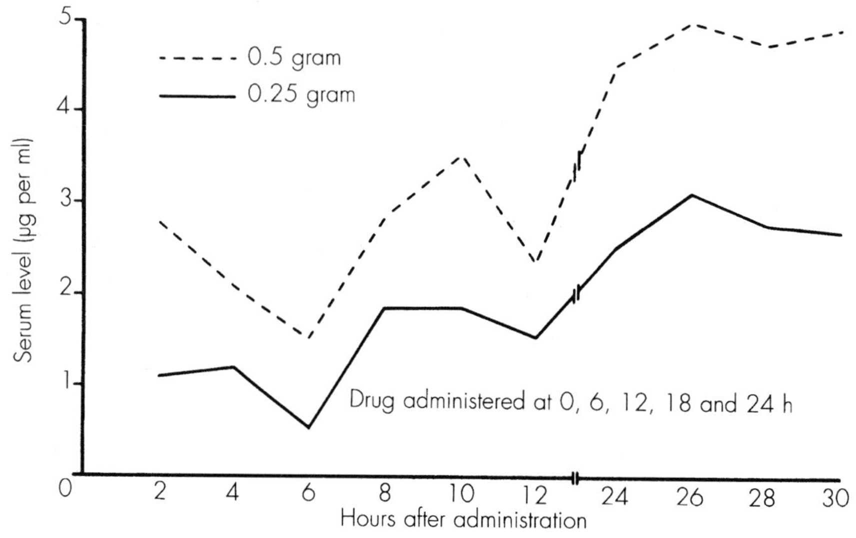

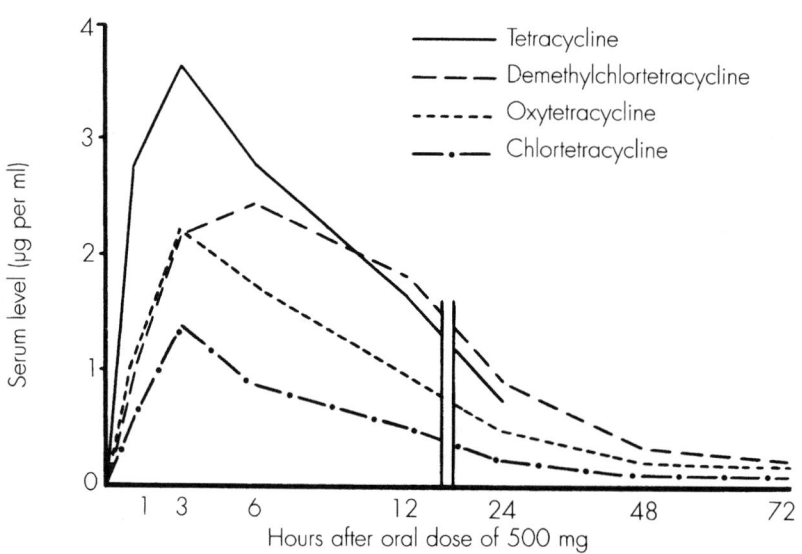

Fig. I.27.

Average serum concentrations following oral administration of 0.25 g and 0.5 g of tetracycline to adults 6-hourly. (Redrawn after Welch, 1954, with permission.)

Fig. I.28.

Mean concentrations of four tetracycline antibiotics in serum of normal subjects after single oral doses of 0.5 g equivalents of their hydrochlorides. (Redrawn after Finland and Garrod, 1960, with permission from the BMJ Publishing Group.)

cations, such as calcium and aluminum, antacids, milk or milk products in the gastrointestinal tract, also reduces absorption of this drug. In addition, simultaneous administration of ferrous sulfate greatly impairs the absorption of tetracycline from the intestinal tract (Neuvonen *et al.* (1970). There is some evidence that cimetidine may reduce the absorption of tetracycline, possibly because tetracycline requires a low gastric pH for dissolution (Cole *et al.*, 1980; Rogers *et al.*, 1980). The serum half-life of tetracycline after oral administration is abut 7 h (Wood *et al.*, 1975).

2 Doxycycline

Doxycycline is almost completely absorbed in the duodenum after oral administration, and it has a more prolonged serum half-life (18–22 h). After oral administration the peak serum level is usually obtained 2–3 h later. Neuvonen *et al.* (1970) obtained a peak serum level of 3.0 μg per ml after an oral dose of 200 mg doxycycline. After an identical dose, Welling *et al.* (1977) detected peak serum levels of 5.0–5.4 μg per ml at 3–4 h in fasted subjects and these levels fell to 2.9–4.0 and 1.3–2.2 μg per ml after 8 and 24 h, respectively. These authors also noted that serum levels of doxycycline were only reduced by 20% if the dose was given with a meal, whereas serum levels of tetracycline were reduced by about 50%. It was estimated that the mean serum doxycycline level obtained on a regimen of 200 mg daily taken on an empty stomach would be 4.4 μg per ml, and this would only drop to 4.0 μg per ml if the drug was taken with meals. All tetracyclines form complexes with metal ions in food but doxycycline complexes are unstable in the acid contents of the stomach, so that this drug enters the duodenum in a free state where it is absorbed. However, metal complexes formed in the alkaline contents of the small bowel, into which doxycycline diffuses as part of its mode of excretion (p. 732), are stable and are not absorbed. This explains why simultaneous ingestion of food does not inhibit the absorption of doxycycline from the upper gastrointestinal tract (Whelton *et al.*, 1974).

The absorption of doxycycline is impaired by the presence of ferrous sulfate (Neuvonen *et al.*, 1970) and by subsalicylate bismuth given simultaneously or 2 h before doxycyline (Ericsson *et al.*, 1982). The bioavailability of doxycycline is not reduced by the concomitant administration of ranitidine, but serum levels of doxycycline are lowered if the drug is taken together with aluminum magnesium hydroxide (Deppermann *et al.*, 1989). Aluminum hydroxide taken orally also lowers the serum levels after i.v. doxycycline administration. This interaction may be due in part to an interference of aluminum ions with the enteric reabsorption of doxycycline (Nguyen *et al.*, 1989). If a patient is treated by both doxycycline and rifampicin (p. 693) the serum doxycycline levels may be lower, presumably due to increased hepatic metabolism of the drug (Colmenero *et al.*, 1994).

When a single oral dose of 0.5 g doxycycline was administered after breakfast, a mean peak serum level of 15.29 µg per ml was obtained at 4 h and this fell to levels of 6.60, 3.42, 1.24 and 1.0 µg per ml after 24, 48, 72 and 96 h, respectively (Adadevoh *et al.*, 1976). The fluorometric method used in this study may have resulted in higher serum levels than those obtained by microbiological assay. Nevertheless, Marlin and Cheng (1979) detected a mean peak serum level of 15.41 µg per ml in volunteers given an oral 600-mg dose of doxycycline as estimated by a microbiological method. After a 200-mg i.v. infusion of doxycycline, a peak serum level of 5–10 µg per ml is usually attained (Alestig, 1973), which falls slowly and levels ranging between 1 and 2 µg per ml persist for 24 h (Klastersky *et al.*, 1972). Gnarpe *et al.* (1976) studied serial serum levels after a 200-mg dose given by infusion over 30–45 min; following this infusion mean serum levels of 8.32, 2.98 and 1.32 µg per ml were obtained at 2, 24 and 48 h, respectively.

3 Minocycline

Similar to doxycycline, minocycline is essentially completely absorbed after oral administration. Its absorption also does not seem to be significantly impaired by administration with food or milk (Smith *et al.*, 1984). After a 150 mg oral dose in adults, an average peak serum level of 2.19 µg per ml is reached in 2 h, which progressively falls to 1.85 µg per ml at 4 h, 1.40 µg per ml at 8 h, and 0.53 µg per ml at 24 h. The drug may be detected in serum for up to 48 h after this single oral dose (Steigbigel *et al.*, 1968a). After an oral loading dose of 200 mg minocycline, peak serum levels occur after 2–4 h and are usually in the range of 2–4 µg per ml (Cartwright *et al.*, 1975; Wood *et al.*, 1975). Following this dose a serum level of about 1 µg per ml is still detectable after 24 h (Cartwright *et al.*, 1975). If after an initial oral dose of 200 mg a dose of 100 mg every 12 h is continued, serum levels are maintained in the range of 2.3–3.5 µg per ml (MacDonald *et al.*, 1973). Very similar results were obtained by Carney *et al.* (1974). When an oral dose of 100 mg minocycline was given twice-daily, peak serum levels were reached after 5 days and these were significantly higher in women (mean 3.4 µg per ml) than in men (mean 2.45 µg per ml) (Fanning *et al.*, 1977). This is probably related to the smaller size of women. A significant inverse correlation has been demonstrated between body surface area and serum concentrations (Bernard *et al.*, 1971; Fanning *et al.*, 1977), but in another study this was not always demonstrable (Gump *et al.*, 1977).

When a 100-mg dose of minocycline dissolved in 200 ml of 5% dextrose in water is infused over 30 min, a mean peak serum level of 8.75 µg per ml is attained immediately after infusion and levels of 3.37, 1.96, 1.32 and 0.81 µg per ml are detected 4, 12, 24 and 36 h later, respectively (Welling *et al.*, 1975). If a dose of 200 mg dissolved in 500 ml is infused daily over a period of 1 h, serum levels of 1–4 µg per ml are maintained (MacDonald *et al.*, 1973). Similar results were obtained when the same dose was infused over 6 h but mean serum level of 6.2 µg per ml was reached immediately on cessation of the infusion (Carney *et al.*, 1974). The serum half-life of minocycline is approximately 13 h (Bernard *et al.*, 1971; Carney *et al.*, 1974; Cartwright *et al.*, 1975).

4 Rolitetracycline and rolitetracycline nitrate

After a single i.v. injection of 275 mg of rolitetracycline, the initial serum level was almost ten times higher than the peak level attained after oral administration of 250 mg of tetracycline. This serum level fell rapidly to about 2–4 µg per ml 2 h after injection. However, therapeutically useful levels were still present in the serum as late as 24 h after the injection (Dimmling, 1960).

After a single i.m. dose of 350 mg of rolitetracycline nitrate, the average serum concentration at 1 h was 3.94 μg per ml, which progressively fell to 2.76 μg per ml at 3 h and 2.4 μg per ml at 6 h. Adequate therapeutic concentrations persisted in serum for at least 24 h (Kaplan *et al.*, 1960).

Excretion

1 Urine

All the tetracyclines are excreted by the kidneys and this occurs solely by glomerular filtration. Urinary excretion accounts for about 20% of an orally administered dose of most of the tetracyclines. More than 50% of a parenterally administered tetracycline is excreted in the urine within 24 h (Kunin *et al.*, 1959; Dimmling, 1960). By comparison only 4–9% of an orally or parenterally administered dose of minocycline (MacDonald *et al.*, 1973; Welling *et al.*, 1975; Wood *et al.*, 1975) and 35–40% of a similarly administered dose of doxycycline (Alestig, 1973; 1974; Mahon *et al.*, 1976) are excreted in the urine. High concentrations of the tetracyclines (about 300 μg per ml) appear in the urine during the first 2 h after an oral dose, and persist for 6–12 h. The rates of excretion of doxycycline and minocycline are slower. Urinary concentrations attained after parenteral administration of the rolitetracyclines are much higher than those attained with any of the oral drugs.

Tetracycline and rolitetracycline accumulate in the body in the presence of renal failure. In contrast doxycycline and probably minocycline do not accumulate in the serum of such patients (p. 728).

2 Bile

Tetracyclines are excreted in bile, where in the absence of biliary obstruction, concentrations reached may be 10–25 times those found in the serum (Barza *et al.*, 1975). High concentrations of doxycycline, up to 14 μg per ml, are attained in bile, but this route of elimination normally only accounts for a small percentage of an administered dose (Mahon *et al.*, 1970; Alestig, 1974). High concentrations (76 μg per ml) of minocycline have been detected in bile (MacDonald *et al.*, 1973).

A large proportion of the tetracyclines excreted in bile is reabsorbed from the intestine.

3 Feces

With the exception of doxycycline and minocycline, the tetracyclines are incompletely absorbed from the gastrointestinal tract and the unabsorbed percentage rises with increased dosage. Fecal concentrations of these tetracyclines may reach 1000 μg per g after oral administration. After parenteral administration, much smaller amounts conveyed by the bile are excreted in the feces.

With doxycycline, that part of an administered dose which is not excreted in the urine is excreted in the feces. Blood-borne doxycycline diffuses across the small bowel wall into the lumen, where cationic chelation occurs preventing absorption (Whelton *et al.*, 1974). The contents of the small bowel, being constantly added to from the stomach and other secretions, easily copes with the binding of successive amounts of doxycycline. Biliary excretion only contributes a small amount to the fecal excretion of doxycycline (see above). In the presence of renal functional impairment increased amounts of doxycycline are excreted in the feces thereby preventing accumulation of the drug in the serum (Alestig, 1974; Whelton *et al.*, 1974; Mahon *et al.*, 1976). For instance, Whelton *et al.* (1974) found that 77% of an orally administered dose given to anephric patients was excreted in the feces.

Despite the fact that minocycline is almost completely absorbed (p. 731), a considerable amount of an orally administered dose is also excreted in the feces (MacDonald *et al.*, 1973). In patients with renal failure the urinary excretion of minocycline is reduced in proportion to renal function (Welling *et al.*, 1975), but it is not clear whether increased fecal excretion or metabolism (see below) prevents accumulation of the drug in the serum of such patients.

4 Inactivation in body

Only relatively small amounts of most tetracyclines are metabolized to bacteriologically inactive derivatives in the liver. Therefore, most of the tetracyclines depend largely on the kidneys and to a lesser extent on the biliary system for their elimination. Although the main non-renal route for excretion of doxycycline is via the gastrointestinal tract (see above), it is possible that a small proportion of the drug is metabolized in the body (Whelton *et al.*, 1974; Mahon *et al.*, 1976). Concomitant administration of barbiturates (Neuvonen and Penttilä, 1974), diphenylhydantoin or carbamazepine (Penttilä *et al.*, 1974) and rifampicin(Colmenero *et al.*, 1994) shortens the serum half-life of doxycycline, suggesting that these drugs, which are inducers of liver enzymes, increase the metabolism of doxycycline. It is also possible that these drugs interfere with the protein binding of doxycycline thereby encouraging its excretion. A small study by Alestig (1974) did not demonstrate an increased metabolism of doxycycline with the concomitant administration of barbiturates. The possibility that doxycycline may be metabolized in man has been rekindled by finding a doxycycline metabolite in animals (Böcker *et al.*, 1982). By comparison, a proportion of an administered dose of minocycline appears to be metabolized in the body (MacDonald *et al.*, 1973) and six metabolites, with some antibacterial activity, have been found in human urine (Nelis and De Leenheer, 1981).

Distribution of the Drugs in Body

All tetracyclines are protein bound to some extent, but quoted figures vary. According to Kunin (1967) tetracycline is about 24% protein bound when estimated by a method of equilibrium dialysis. A higher value of tetracycline binding (65%) has been reported when ultrafiltration was used. Values for doxycycline and minocycline are 82% and 76%, respectively (MacDonald *et al.*, 1973).

Tetracycline penetrates fairly well into body fluids and tissues. Tetracycline can be readily demonstrated in pleural, ascitic, and synovial fluids and cord serum. Tetracycline penetrates well into breast milk, but its bioavailability from this source is low because of chelation with milk (p. 730) (Chow and Jewesson, 1985). It passes into maxillary sinus secretions, where concentrations almost equal to serum levels may be reached if repeated doses are used (Lundberg and Malmborg, 1973, 1974). Most tetracyclines can be detected only in low concentrations in tears and saliva. Following an oral dose of 250 mg tetracycline three times daily, sputum levels in the range of 0.4–2.6 μg per ml have been detected (Ruhen and Tandon, 1976). Tetracyclines penetrate into normal CSF, but to a lesser extent than chloramphenicol (p. 561). The concentration of tetracycline in CSF is about one-tenth of the simultaneous serum concentration. After administration of i.v. rolitetracycline, higher CSF concentrations are obtained in association with high serum levels (p. 731) (Dimmling, 1960).

Doxycycline, and in particular minocycline, are more highly lipid soluble. This lipophilic property is an important factor determining their better tissue penetration. In dogs, lipophilicity of the tetracyclines has been correlated with many of their transport characteristics; it facilitates their transport across lipid-rich cell membranes and, therefore, doxycycline and minocycline penetrate more readily into the brain, eyes and intestinal epithelium. They also penetrate more readily into bacterial cells (Nikaido and Thanassi, 1993).

In humans, concentrations of doxycycline in thoracic duct lymph and peritoneal fluid are maintained at about 75% of simultaneous serum levels (Andersson *et al.*, 1976), and those in colonic tissue and particularly ileal tissue approximate to or exceed the serum level (Höjer and Wetterfors, 1976). The concentration of doxycycline in prostatic tissue may also reach 60% of that in the serum (Eliasson and Malmborg, 1976; Oosterlinck *et al.*, 1976). After i.v. doxycycline 200 mg was given to patients with pleurisy, 2 h later levels as high as 25% of those in the serum were detected in pleural fluid (Lode, 1979). Levels reached in saliva are low. After an oral dose of 600 mg doxycycline, peak salivary concentrations occurred at 8 h and were only 8% of the mean serum level at the time (Marlin and Cheng, 1979). After oral doses of 100 mg daily, mean salivary levels were 0.1–0.5 μg per ml (Heimdahl and Nord, 1983) and such concentrations were unaffected by parotitis (Eneroth *et al.*, 1978). Doxycycline (and minocycline) penetrate fairly well into breast milk (Chow and Jewesson, 1985). Lower concentrations of doxycycline are achieved in bone (Dornbusch, 1976), skin, subcutaneous fat and tendon tissue but levels in muscle are higher (Gnarpe *et al.*, 1976). Therapeutic concentrations of doxycycline may occur in the aqueous humor but CSF concentrations do not exceed 1 μg per ml in subjects with non-inflamed meninges (Andersson and Alestig, 1976). However, Yim *et al.* (1985) detected higher levels in five patients with latent or neurosyphilis; after receiving doxycycline 200 mg twice-daily for 7 days, the mean serum level was 5.8 μg per ml (range 3.6–8.6) and the mean CSF level 1.3 μg per ml (range 0.8–2.0), a mean penetration into the CSF of 26%. In patients with Lyme neuroborreliosis treated with doxycycline 200 mg orally 12-hourly the serum and CSF concentrations 2–3 h after a dose were 7.5 and 1.1 μg per ml, respectively. With a doxycycline dose of 100 mg 12-hourly the CSF concentration at that time was only 0.6 μg per ml (Dotevall and Hagberg, 1989). Penetration of doxycycline (and the older tetracyclines) into sputum is poor (Ruhen and Tandon, 1975, 1976; Hartnett and Marlin, 1976).

MacDonald et al. (1973) showed that minocycline penetrated better into most tissues than all other tetracyclines, and in most instances its tissue levels exceeded simultaneous serum levels. Highest concentrations were found in thyroid, lung, intestinal tract, liver, gallbladder and in bile. Concentrations exceeding those in the serum were obtained in the prostate, uterus, ovaries, fallopian tubes, breast, skin and sinuses, but lower concentrations were found in sweat and sebum. Although minocycline penetrated into the CSF of subjects with non-inflamed meninges better than doxycycline and other tetracyclines, the levels achieved were low (MacDonald et al., 1973; Carney et al., 1974). Minocycline (and to a lesser extent, doxycycline) achieved higher concentrations in tears and saliva than other tetracyclines (Hoeprich and Warshauer, 1974). This probably explains why minocycline is effective for the treatment of meningococcal carriers (p. 744), whilst other tetracyclines are not. Minocycline sputum levels are quite high and may reach 60% of simultaneous serum levels (Ruhen and Tandon, 1975; 1976; Brogan et al., 1977).

Tetracyclines become markedly bound to bones, teeth and neoplasms, causing yellow fluorescence (p. 736).

Mode of Action

Tetracyclines inhibit bacterial protein synthesis. They bind principally to the 30 S subunits of bacteria ribosomes (p. 562) and specifically inhibit the enzyme binding of aminoacyl-t-RNA to the adjacent ribosomal acceptor site (Cundliffe and McQuillen, 1967; Rasmussen et al., 1991). They may also cause alterations in the cytoplasmic membrane (p. 26) thereby allowing leakage of nucleotides and other compounds from the cell. This action would explain the rapid inhibition of DNA replication (which occurs at a site on the membrane) that ensues when cells are exposed to concentrations of tetracycline in excess of that needed for protein inhibition (Pato, 1977). In addition, tetracyclines appear to inhibit adhesion of bacteria to human cells and so render the bacteria less pathogenic. These drugs probably inhibit the synthesis of a specific protein in the bacterial cell surface (Chopra and Hacker, 1986; Schifferli and Beachey, 1988).

In higher concentrations tetracyclines also inhibit mammalian protein synthesis (Beard et al., 1969). This anti-anabolic effect is of clinical significance because it may aggravate pre-existing renal functional impairment (p. 738). In addition, these drugs may interfere with parenteral nutrition in postoperative patients by inhibiting the utilization of amino acids for protein synthesis (Korkeila, 1971).

Toxicity

1 Gastrointestinal side-effects

Nausea, heartburn, epigastric pain, vomiting and diarrhea are more common with tetracyclines than with most other orally administered antibiotics. Diarrhea is probably mainly due to direct chemical irritation of the bowel by unabsorbed tetracyclines (p. 732), but induced changes in bowel flora may also be contributory. Gastrointestinal symptoms usually subside quickly when the tetracycline is stopped. Tetracyclines may also cause antibiotic-associated enterocolitis (see below). Steatorrhea has been reported after tetracycline use and after single 2 g doses of tetracycline 22% of the patients had transient steatorrhea (Mitchell et al., 1982).

It was considered that doxycycline should be less prone to cause these side-effects because of its lower dosage. A few limited studies suggested that gastrointestinal side-effects were indeed less common with doxycycline therapy (Aitchison et al., 1968; Grossan, 1968; Clendinnen, 1974). Minocycline produced more side-effects of all types (including gastrointestinal) in women than in men (Fanning et al., 1977), and this did not appear to be related to the higher serum levels attained in women (p. 731) (Gump et al., 1977). Nausea is the most common gastrointestinal symptom which occurs with minocycline, and this occurred in 40–50% of female volunteers, but vomiting and diarrhea were much less common (Fanning et al., 1977; Gump et al., 1977). One case report suggested that sensitization to a metabolite of tetracycline present in certain foods, as a result of using the drug for growth promotion in stock feeds, led to excessive flatus with alternating diarrhea and constipation (Anthony, 1977).

A number of drugs can lodge in the esophagus and result in local ulceration (Collins et al., 1979). There are numerous reports of tetracycline and doxycycline causing this side-effect (Crowson et al., 1976; Channer and Hollanders, 1981; Geschwind, 1984; Amendola and Spera, 1985; Adverse Drug Reactions, 1994). Many of these patients had taken their capsule or tablet just before retiring to bed; one felt at the time that the capsule 'did not go right down' and several had an associated hiatus hernia. It is postulated that the drug either lodged in the esophagus or had been refluxed from the stomach, and the high acidity of tetracycline in solution caused esophageal ulceration. It is recommended, therefore, that oral tetracyclines should not be given to patients with esophageal obstruction or compression. This side-effect has also been described with clindamycin (p. 594). Studies in volunteers and patients with normal esophageal motility have demonstrated that tablets and capsules can lodge in the esophagus and this is influenced by posture and drink volume. As a result it is advised that capsules and tablets should be taken with at least 100 ml of water during which the patient should be standing if possible (Channer and Virjee, 1982; Hey et al., 1982).

2 Antibiotic-associated colitis

Bacterial overgrowth, by one of several organisms, usually Cl. difficile, may cause this complication (p. 594). Tetracyclines have caused pseudomembranous colitis (Gorbach and Bartlett, 1974). Clostridium difficile-associated diarrhea after doxycycline malaria prophylaxis has been reported (Golledge and Riley, 1995). Colitis due to staphylococcal overgrowth is a rare complication of tetracycline therapy. Tetracycline-resistant staphylococci often appear in the stools of patients treated with a tetracycline, but staphylococcal enterocolitis with severe fulminating diarrhea, dehydration and circulatory collapse is rare (Thaysen and Eriksen, 1956). In this disease superficial necrosis of large areas of intestinal mucosa occurs, and the feces usually contain large numbers of staphylococci. This enterocolitis occurs more commonly as a postoperative complication, and may be associated with either oral or parenteral tetracycline therapy. Lundsgaard-Hansen et al. (1960) reported six cases of staphylococcal enterocolitis with two fatalities, all in surgical patients, who were given i.v. rolitetracycline postoperatively. These authors pointed out that after parenteral tetracycline administration, sufficient tetracycline reaches the intestinal lumen via the bile to inhibit the normal flora, thus predisposing to staphylococcal superinfection. Treatment of staphylococcal enterocolitis consists of stopping tetracycline therapy, administering a reliable anti-staphylococcal agent, such as cloxacillin and fluid replacement. Nowadays tetracyclines are only rarely given to patients postoperatively and this complication has no longer been reported.

3 Candida albicans (Monilia) superinfections

Monilia often increase in the stools of patients treated by tetracycline, but their causal relationship to diarrhea is not well defined. Commercial combinations containing tetracycline and nystatin (p. 1295) or amphotericin B (p. 1245) were manufactured and advertised on the assumption that monilial bowel superinfection was the main cause of tetracycline gastrointestinal side-effects. These antifungal agents effectively prevented monilial overgrowth, but there was little evidence that this had any bearing on gastrointestinal side-effects of tetracycline therapy. The British Tuberculosis Association (Report, 1968) carried out a controlled trial on 111 patients with respiratory infections, using either tetracycline or tetracycline plus nystatin ('Mysteclin'). The frequency of gastrointestinal symptoms was high in both groups before treatment was started. After 10-day treatment 50% of patients in the 'Mysteclin' group and 34% in the tetracycline group had gastrointestinal symptoms, a difference which was not considered significant. The frequency of C. albicans in the stools after 10 days in the 'Mysteclin' group was 9.1%, which was significantly lower than that in the tetracycline group (37.1%), but this was not associated with a reduction in gastrointestinal symptoms. It was concluded that the routine addition of nystatin to tetracycline could not be justified.

Nystatin therapy, however, is indicated when oral or vaginal moniliasis occurs as a complication of the use of the tetracyclines. In debilitated patients treated with tetracyclines or other antibiotics, there is the additional danger that the fungus may spread to involve the bronchi, esophagus and other sites, or even result in a fungemia with widespread dissemination of monilial infection. If the gut is heavily colonized by C. albicans, these organisms may pass through the intestinal wall and cause a temporary fungemia (Krause et al., 1969). For this reason, it was suggested that in severely ill patients, oral nystatin therapy is indicated, whenever it seems that excessive C. albicans proliferation in the gut may lead to disseminated fungemia.

4 Other superinfections

Use of the tetracyclines and other antibiotics may also result in colonization of the respiratory tract and bowel with Gram-negative organisms such as Proteus spp. and Ps. aeruginosa. Usually the presence of these organisms is of no clinical significance, but occasionally they may cause superinfections of the respiratory tract (p. 863).

5 Hypersensitivity reactions

These are uncommon, and usually take the form of urticaria, asthma or facial edema, and contact dermatitis has also been described (Shelley and Heaton, 1973). Rare cases of acute anaphylaxis have occurred (Fellner and Baer, 1965; Furey and Tan, 1969). Copperman (1967) reported two patients who developed hypothermia, apparently due to tetracycline hypersensitivity. The development of lupus erythematous has been observed after the administration of tetracycline (Mull, 1966), but no clear cause and effect relationship has been established. A syndrome of pulmonary infiltrates and eosinophilia has occurred during minocycline therapy (Sitbon et al., 1994).

The Jarisch-Herxheimer reaction (p. 31) may occur when tetracyclines are used to treat spirochetal infections, such as louse-borne relapsing fever and leptospirosis, and other infections such as brucellosis and tularemia. Meptazinol diminishes the Jarish-Herxheimer reaction of relapsing fever (p. 748).

6 Photosensitivity

This side-effect is more common in hot climates. It consists of erythema which if severe may be associated with edema, papules, vesiculation and onycholysis (Bethell, 1977). This is a phototoxic reaction (p. 973), because the rash does not spread to areas of skin not exposed to sun. Demethylchlortetracycline has the greatest propensity to cause this reaction. Photosensitivity has also been reported in patients taking doxycycline (Council on Drugs, 1969; Glette and Sandberg, 1986). According to Ory (1970) any tetracycline may occasionally provoke this reaction. Minocycline may be less likely to cause this side-effect (Allen, 1976). Photo-onycholysis (separation of the nails due to sunlight) due to tetracyclines may rarely occur without an associated skin rash (Lasser and Steiner, 1978).

7 Teeth and other tissue pigmentation and effect on bones

All the tetracyclines are deposited in calcifying areas of bones and teeth and this may cause a yellow discoloration. Teeth discoloration was first noted during an assessment of long-term tetracycline therapy in children with fibrocystic disease (Shwachman et al., 1959). This observation was subsequently confirmed by others (Wallman and Hilton, 1962; Porter et al., 1966). The main disadvantage of tetracycline deposition in teeth is purely a cosmetic one.

Tetracycline may be deposited in the deciduous teeth in children if they receive these drugs early in life, or if their mother is treated by tetracyclines during pregnancy, because these drugs cross the placenta (Kline et al., 1964). The period of mineralization of the anterior deciduous teeth extends from 14 weeks in utero until 2–3 months after birth. However, it appears that deciduous teeth staining is more likely if the mother is treated after the 25th week of gestation (Toaff and Ravid, 1966). Tetracyclines may also produce a life-long discoloration of the permanent teeth if they are administered to children aged less than 6–7 years. Mineralization of these teeth commences about 4–6 months after birth, and it is completed at about the age of 5–6 years. The frequency of tetracycline staining may be particularly high during the first year of life because immature kidneys are unable to excrete these drugs efficiently (Medical News, 1977).

The type of discoloration varies somewhat according to the particular tetracycline used (Weyman, 1965). Chlortetracycline produced grey brown teeth, but tetracycline, oxytetracycline and demethylchlortetracycline caused yellow discoloration. There was some evidence that oxytetracycline caused less discoloration than the other older tetracyclines (Weyman, 1965; Gästrin and Josephson, 1966). Minocycline causes a grey discoloration of teeth (see below). Tooth and bone staining is less common with doxycycline than with most other tetracycline derivatives.

The degree of teeth discoloration depends on the amount of tetracycline administered, and discoloration is usually only obvious in children who have received several courses of these drugs. In one study, only a very mild, cosmetically trivial, darkening of permanent incisor teeth occurred in children who had been given up to five 6-day courses of tetracycline in the first 5 years of life (Grossman et al., 1971). Nevertheless, the degree of discoloration increases with increasing numbers of teeth crown deposits of tetracycline. According to Baker (1975) if there are more than seven tetracycline lines per crown, severe discoloration is unavoidable.

In the past, the frequency of teeth discoloration in children was high. Brearley et al. (1968) examined 1168 Melbourne children aged from 18 months to 7 years, and found teeth discoloration in 20.1% and in 4.0% both discoloration and hypoplasia. Brearley and Storey (1968) examined 1000 deciduous molar teeth extracted from patients attending the pre-school clinic of the Royal Dental Hospital, Melbourne. Fluorescent yellow bands, characteristic of the tetracyclines, were found in 8% of these teeth. They also found that 61% of permanent teeth extracted from patients aged 6–18 years were affected by tetracycline (Baker and Storey, 1970). A similar study from this clinic showed that during 1972, 75% permanent teeth from patients of the same age group had characteristic tetracycline fluorescence (Baker, 1975). In a UK study, Stewart (1973) found that 70% of primary molars, extracted from 505 children aged 3–5 years, were also affected by tetracyclines given during their first 3 years of life. Other authors reported a much lower prevalence of tetracycline discoloration in both deciduous and permanent teeth (Martin and Barnard, 1969). In Belfast, the proportion of children with tetracycline teeth deposits fell from 70% in 1973 to 14.7% in 1982, reflecting decreased tetracycline usage (Kinirons, 1983).

There have been some reports of minocycline causing teeth discoloration in young adults. Poliak et al. (1985) described four such patients who developed areas of grey discoloration of their teeth after receiving the drug for acne for periods of more than 1 year (three patients) but for only 4 weeks in the other patient. The discoloration seemed permanent. Tetracycline seems to cause teeth discoloration by being chelated with free calcium during teeth development up to the age of 7 years. Minocycline caused discoloration in adults by some other mechanism, it complexes poorly with calcium but does chelate with iron to form insoluble complexes (Poliak et al., 1985).

The role of the tetracyclines in the production of defective teeth and enamel hypoplasia has been disputed. Their effect in causing enamel hypoplasia is difficult to assess, because several factors predispose to this condition (McIntosh and Storey, 1970). Enamel hypoplasia associated with tetracycline administration has been most commonly described in premature infants (Wallman and Hilton, 1962), but such hypoplasia is known to occur in association with prematurity, neonatal jaundice and febrile illnesses. Similar hypoplasia has also been described in older children in association with tetracycline therapy, but these children also had suffered from diseases which are known to cause this defect (Witkop and Wolf, 1963). Animal experiments have shown that the tetracyclines per se can cause enamel hypoplasia (McIntosh and Storey, 1970). According to Baker (1975), if there are seven fluorescent tetracycline lines per crown, severe discoloration, enamel hypomineralization and hypoplasia are unavoidable.

The deposition of tetracycline in the bones of infants causes temporary inhibition of bone growth. Administration of tetracycline to premature infants produces a 40% depression of normal skeletal growth, as measured by the inhibition of fibula growth (Cohlan et al., 1963). This effect was rapidly reversible after cessation of tetracycline therapy, and permanent effects on the human skeleton have not been observed. Between 3% and 11% of administered tetracycline becomes incorporated in the inorganic phase of bone. After the use of the drug for years, such as for acne, bones may be visibly colored yellow and be fluorescent. Oklund et al. (1981) found bone levels of 156, 270 and 290 µg per g, respectively, in three such patients and considered that this had no deleterious effect. However, Bhagawan et al. (1982) briefly described a young woman who died due to 'fatty liver of pregnancy' (see below) and who had been using tetracycline previously for acne but not during her pregnancy. She had 60 mg per g of tetracycline in her bone and it was postulated that the release of the drug associated with increased bone metabolism during pregnancy may have precipitated her liver disease.

In view of these side-effects and others which may affect children (see below), there are few reasons for using tetracycline drugs in children aged less than 8 years.

Pigmentation of the skin, nails, sclerae and conjunctivae has been described with minocycline usage (Poliak et al., 1985). A blue-grey discoloration of the skin in sites of cutaneous inflammation, such as acne scars can occur as well as a generalized brown hyperpigmentation, with accentuation in sun-exposed areas. These forms of pigmentation tend to resolve slowly when the drug is stopped. Skin discoloration usually occurs after 3–4 weeks of minocycline treatment (Fenske et al., 1980; Poliak et al., 1985). Single case reports of blue-black pigmentation of the substantia nigra and of other sclerotic plagues have been described after minocycline therapy (Landas et al., 1986). Black pigmentation of the thyroid has been observed at autopsy in five patients who had been taking minocycline for prolonged periods (Attwood and Dennett, 1976; Attwood, 1983; Landas et al., 1986).

8 Teratogenicity

Animal studies have suggested that the tetracyclines may be teratogenic (Leading article, 1965), but there is no evidence that this occurs in humans. The frequency of congenital abnormalities in children whose mothers received tetracycline therapy during pregnancy was no higher than in children whose mothers received penicillin G (Carter and Wilson, 1963).

9 Hepatotoxicity

Rarely a 'hepatitis-like illness' may develop if tetracycline, doxycycline or minocycline is given orally for 10 days in the usual doses. Such complication has also followed i.v. administration of doxycycline. The 'hepatitis' has occasionally been severe, but it usually resolved after the drug was stopped. The excess risk per million for the development of acute symptomatic liver disease resulting in hospitalization after exposure to a 10-day course of tetracycline has been estimated to be only 1.56 cases (Carson et al., 1993).

Of historic interest are fatal cases of liver disease, which occurred, particularly in the early 1960s, when overdosages of the early tetracyclines were given i.v., particularly to pregnant patients. The i.v. dosage for doxycycline and minocycline is the same as the oral dosage (100 mg 12-hourly) because these drugs are completely absorbed from the gastrointestinal tract. However, with tetracycline the oral dosage is 500 mg 6-hourly, yet the i.v. dosage of its equivalent, rolitetracycline is only 275 mg daily (p. 728), as tetracycline is only partially absorbed after oral administration. It appears this was not always understood in the 1960s.

A series of reports indicated that overdosage with i.v. tetracyclines was particularly dangerous during pregnancy (Schultz et al., 1963; Whalley et al., 1964; Dowling and Lepper, 1964; Kunelis et al., 1965). Most of these pregnant patients were treated with i.v. tetracycline for acute pyelonephritis, and in some the daily dose was as high as 3.5–6.0 g. Initial symptoms consisted of nausea, vomiting and fever, which were followed by jaundice. The disease was often severe and was associated with hematemesis and malena, renal failure with acidosis, and in the fatal cases, coma and terminal hypotension. Six fatal cases reported by Schultz et al. (1963) had all received 3.5–6.0 g i.v. tetracycline daily, whereas in the five cases reported by Whalley et al. (1964) which included only one fatality, the daily i.v. tetracycline dosage was only 1–2 g. In fatal cases the liver showed extensive fine vacuolar fatty infiltration, and, in addition, pathological changes were found in the pancreas, kidneys and brain (Whalley et al., 1964; Kunelis et al., 1965).

The findings of Kunelis et al. (1965) were of considerable interest. They described 12 cases of 'fatty liver of pregnancy' associated with the i.v. administration of large doses of tetracycline, but in addition reported four similar cases of 'fatty liver in late pregnancy' in women who had not received tetracycline. 'Tetracycline-induced fatty liver of pregnancy' appears to be a very similar illness to the rare 'acute fatty liver of pregnancy', which may occur during the last trimester, and was first described by Sheehan (1940) as 'idiopathic obstetric acute yellow atrophy'. It is probable that this disease may be associated with several etiological factors, one of which may be the administration of tetracycline in high doses.

A similar syndrome can occur in non-pregnant patients if excessive doses of tetracycline are used (Dowling and Lepper, 1964). There are also isolated reports of fatalities due to 'fatty liver' in non-pregnant adult patients, in whom the tetracycline dose was not excessive (Damjanov et al., 1968; Hanson, 1968). This was described in three children with obstructive uropathy, all of whom received i.v. tetracycline postoperatively and two died (Lloyd-Still et al., 1974). It appears that all patients who developed this complication following normal tetracycline doses had renal functional impairment, which probably resulted in high tetracycline serum levels.

10 Nephrotoxicity

Four types of renal damage due to tetracycline therapy have been described.

a Aggravation of pre-existing renal failure This is an important toxic effect because it is fairly common and often unrecognized (Eastwood et al., 1970; Edwards et al., 1970). In patients with impaired renal function tetracyclines may cause further rises in the blood urea and serum creatinine values (Lew and French, 1966). Associated clinical deterioration may be so severe that peritoneal or hemodialysis may be required, which occasionally has to be continued until renal transplantation is available (Phillips et al., 1974). The known antianabolic effect of the tetracyclines (Shils, 1963) is probably the main cause of this complication (p. 734). These drugs interfere with human protein synthesis, so that the kidneys need to excrete an additional load from amino acid metabolism. Some authors considered that this was the only mechanism by which tetracyclines aggravated azotemia (Van Ypersele de Strihou, 1970), whilst others maintained that they also had a direct toxic effect on the kidneys (Roth et al., 1967; Eastwood et al., 1970). The exact mechanism is difficult to determine in individual patients, and in some, indirect effects of nausea, vomiting, diarrhea and polyuria, caused at times by tetracyclines, may be contributory (Eastwood et al., 1970). Water and salt loss, caused by concomitant diuretic administration, aggravates tetracycline nephrotoxicity (Report, 1972). Doxycycline and possibly minocycline, unlike other tetracyclines, can usually be used safely in patients with renal failure. Nevertheless, even doxycycline should be used cautiously in these patients. Orr et al. (1978)

described a patient whose stable renal failure deteriorated during doxycycline treatment possibly due to impairment of the non-renal excretory pathway for this drug (p. 732).

b   Tetracycline nephrotoxicity associated with 'acute fatty liver'   Features of liver failure usually predominate in this syndrome (p. 738), but renal and electrolyte abnormalities are also often severe (Lew and French, 1966). These authors described a pregnant woman, treated by i.v. tetracycline in a dose of 2–4 g daily, who developed acute hepatic and renal failure without oliguria. They pointed out that this unusual type of renal failure with normal or even increased volumes of urine had been noted in other reported cases (Schultz *et al.*, 1963). In contrast, the acute renal failure which occurs in 'idiopathic fatty liver of pregnancy' without the administration of tetracyclines is usually associated with oliguria. The deterioration of renal function caused by tetracyclines in patients with pre-existing renal damage is not usually associated with oliguria (see above).

c   Demethylchlortetracycline-induced nephrogenic diabetes insipidus and renal failure   First reported by Castell and Sparks (1965), nephrogenic diabetes insipidus is a well recognized side-effect of treatment with demethylchlortetracycline (Roth *et al.*, 1967; Singer and Rotenberg, 1973; Hayek and Ramirez, 1974). In doses of 600–1200 mg per day to adults, demethylchlortetracycline produces a reversible partial nephrogenic diabetes insipidus syndrome in normal subjects. This effect is dose-dependent and a daily dose of 1200 mg consistently induces this syndrome. Polyuria which occurs is vasopressin-resistant. This complication has also been reported in a child who received a high dose of the drug (London *et al.*, 1978). Studies with toad urinary bladders show that demethylchlortetracycline reversibly impairs both antidiuretic hormone (ADH)-induced and cyclic adenosine-$3^1, 5^1$-monophosphate-induced water flow (Singer and Rotenberg, 1973). In human renal medulla, demethylchlortetracycline impairs ADH-stimulated adenylate cyclase (Dousa and Wilson, 1973). The mechanism by which the drug causes natriuresis is unknown but it may act as an aldosterone antagonist and/or have a specific effect on renal tubules (Geheb and Cox, 1980). Because the polyuria induced by demethylchlortetracycline was unresponsive to ADH, Singer and Rotenberg (1973) suggested that the tetracycline may be of value in the treatment of clinical states associated with excessive ADH activity.

There have been numerous reports of effectiveness of demethylchlortetracycline for the treatment of patients with inappropriate secretion of ADH. The drug inhibits the action of ADH in patients with inappropriate hypersecretion of ADH associated with lung carcinoma (De Troyer and Demanet, 1975; Perks *et al.*, 1976; De Troyer, 1977). The response to the drug, similar to that in normal subjects, takes several days so that it is of limited value in acute water intoxication due to excess ADH secretion. Demethylchlortetracycline has also been used with success to treat patients with water retention in congestive cardiac failure who were unresponsive to usual therapy (Cox *et al.*, 1977; Zegers de Beyl *et al.*, 1978). Similarly, it has also been used with effect in a number of patients with alcoholic cirrhosis with sodium and water retention (De Troyer *et al.*, 1976; Carrilho *et al.*, 1977; Kirkpatrick, 1978).

Notwithstanding these successful reports of the efficacy of demethylchlortetracycline in syndromes of excess ADH secretion or for patients with water retention presumed to have inappropriate secretion of ADH, its use for this purpose has been associated with various degrees of renal impairment with elevations of blood urea and serum creatinine values (Roth *et al.*, 1967; De Troyer *et al.*, 1976; Cox *et al.*, 1977; De Troyer, 1977; Zegers de Beyl *et al.*, 1978). Renal impairment was particularly noticeable when demethylchlortetracycline was used to treat patients with cirrhosis and water retention, perhaps because of the tendency for renal failure to occur in such patients (De Troyer *et al.*, 1976; Carrilho *et al.*, 1977; Kirkpatrick, 1978; Miller *et al.*, 1980). In many of these patients azotemia necessitated stopping treatment with demethylchlortetracycline, but the renal failure was usually reversible.

d   Interstitial nephritis   In one report this complication was ascribed to minocycline (Walker *et al.*, 1979). After a course of minocycline in high dosage the patient developed fever, hematuria, proteinuria eosinophilia, polyuria and renal failure. Renal biopsy showed interstitial inflammation. The patient fully recovered. Other antibiotics have been implicated as causes of interstitial nephritis (p. 84).

11 Hematological side-effects   Mild leukopenia can occur with tetracycline therapy, but is rare (Fanning *et al.*, 1977). Tetracycline also very rarely appears to cause vascular purpura, sometimes associated with thrombocytopenia (Kounis, 1975). In these cases a lowered leukocyte ascorbic acid level (see below) may be a contributory factor. Tetracyclines may modify some coagulation factors and cause impaired blood clotting if administered in high doses i.v. (Searcy *et al.*, 1965). There have been several reports of hemolytic anemia attributed to tetracycline. One patient had acute intravascular hemolysis, thrombocytopenia, hypofibrinogenia and transient renal impairment on two occasions after taking oral tetracycline. His serum contained IgG antibody which reacted only with red cells, exposed either *in vivo* or *in vitro* to tetracycline (Simpson *et al.*, 1985).

12 Effects on immune response

There is an increased urinary excretion of vitamin C during tetracycline therapy, leukocytes are thereby depleted of ascorbic acid, and this may interfere with their phagocytic activity (Windsor *et al.*, 1972). In various *in vitro* test systems, some tetracyclines can alter human polymorphonuclear function. Doxycycline can depress leukocyte migration (Forsgren and Schmeling, 1977; Belsheim *et al.*, 1979), but high concentration of the drug is usually necessary to achieve this (Bäck and Norberg, 1984; Glette *et al.*, 1984). With high concentrations of doxycycline or minocycline, chemiluminescence and glucose oxidation of polymorphs are also impaired. It seems that these effects of tetracycline on *in vitro* polymorph functions are due to their divalent cation chelating effect (Glette *et al.*, 1984). The ability of human leukocytes to phagocytose yeasts and bacteria is decreased by tetracycline or doxycycline; this effect may be related to altered surface morphology of granulocytes incubated with tetracyclines (Forsgren and Gnarpe, 1982). Tetracycline, doxycycline and minocycline can suppress phytohemagglutinin-induced lymphocyte transformation *in vitro* (Hauser and Remington, 1982). The clinical significance of these effects is unknown, but they could possibly be important in patients with impaired defence mechanisms.

13 Neurotoxicity

a   Benign intracranial hypertension   This uncommon complication is also known as the 'bulging fontanelle syndrome' in infants. It occurs in infants receiving usual doses of tetracycline, and is characterized by irritability, vomiting and a tense bulging fontanelle. The CSF pressure is raised, but the fluid is otherwise normal (Mull, 1966). All these signs resolve rapidly when the drug is discontinued. There have been several reports of tetracycline or minocycline causing benign intracranial hypertension in both adults and children (Koch-Weser and Gilmore, 1967; Maroon and Mealy, 1971; Pearson *et al.*, 1981; Walters and Gubbay, 1981). This syndrome presents in adults as severe headache and blurring of vision during tetracycline therapy; papilledema is present and often VIth nerve palsies. Most cases have occurred in young adults plus a few in children and the majority had been taking tetracyclines for acne for periods varying from days to months. Meacock and Langton Hewer (1981) described a case in a 63-year-old woman. The mechanism of this side-effect is unknown and the features gradually resolve on withdrawal of the drug.

b   Vestibular disturbance   Minocycline, but not other tetracyclines, can cause reversible dizziness, ataxia, vertigo, tinnitus associated with weakness, nausea and vomiting. Prior to 1974, symptoms of vestibular dysfunction attributed to minocycline were reported at an average rate of 4.5–7.2% (Allen, 1976). Williams *et al.* (1974) reported that 17 (80%) of 19 patients receiving minocycline developed vestibular side-effects. Subsequently a number of small studies in the USA confirmed a high frequency (86–96%) of vestibular symptoms, which in 12–52% were so severe that treatment with the drug had to be stopped, (CDC, 1975; Jacobson and Daniel, 1975). The frequency of vestibular side-effects appeared to be less in the UK (Masterton and Schofield, 1974; CDC, 1976). Side-effects due to minocycline have been studied in controlled trials using volunteers (Fanning *et al.*, 1977; Gump *et al.*, 1977). All toxic effects (including vestibular symptoms) were more common in women, with vestibular side-effects occurring in 70.4% (Fanning *et al.*, 1977). This did not seem to be related to the higher minocycline serum levels which occur in women (p. 731). Most side-effects occurred on the third day of therapy at a time which coincided with peak minocycline serum levels. A second trial showed that there was no significant difference in vestibular symptoms with a daily dose of 150 compared with one of 200 mg minocycline, these occurring at rates of 53.3 and 66.7%, respectively (Gump *et al.*, 1977). Two additional symptoms were observed in this trial, lightheadedness in 53.3% and a feeling of dissociation in about 50% of volunteers. Because of these vestibular side-effects, minocycline is not used widely.

c **Other neurotoxicity** Tetracyclines can produce weak neuromuscular blockade (Snavely and Hodges, 1984). Tetracycline potentiates neuromuscular blockade produced by D-tubarine. This is not consistently reversed by calcium or anticholinesterases. One woman developed four episodes of acute transitory myopia after an injection of tetracycline (Snavely and Hodges, 1984). Sinclair and Phillips (1982) reported a young girl who developed transient myopathy after 2 months treatment with tetracycline for acne.

14 Drug interactions

One patient developed lithium toxicity associated with elevated serum lithium levels when taking tetracycline long-acting capsules (McGennis, 1978). Another patient became pregnant whilst taking an oral contraceptive drug (Bacon and Shenfield, 1980). A causal relationship to tetracycline was presumed in each case. In a minority of patients digoxin is inactivated by gastrointestinal bacteria, and this is reduced by a course of tetracycline or erythromycin. Theoretically, antibiotic administration to such patients may cause a substantial rise in serum digoxin levels (Lindenbaum et al., 1981).

15 Miscellaneous side-effects

There have been a few case reports suggesting that tetracyclines may precipitate lactic acidosis in diabetic patients receiving phenformin (Aro et al., 1978). Tetracyclines also cause reduction in serum B_{12}, B_6 and pantothenic acid levels, and therefore it is possible that long-term therapy with these drugs may cause vitamin deficiencies, particularly in the elderly (Windsor et al., 1972). Tetracycline has been reported to cause pulmonary infiltrates and eosinophilia (Schatz et al., 1981).

Clinical Uses of the Drugs

In the past, tetracyclines were used widely as 'broad spectrum' antibiotics for a wide variety of common infections. Tetracycline-resistance is now common amongst many bacterial species, so that tetracyclines are the drugs of choice for a diminishing list of infections.

1 Respiratory infections

Tetracyclines may still have a place in the management of chronic bronchitis and sinusitis, except in areas where there is a high rate of tetracycline-resistance amongst pneumococci and/or *H. influenzae*. The role of antibiotics for prophylaxis or treatment of chronic bronchitis is not clear-cut (Tager and Speizer, 1975; Hughes 1976; Bates, 1982). Tetracyclines, erythromycin (p. 617), co-trimoxazole (p. 863), ampicillin (p. 123) or amoxycillin (p. 140) have been used in this disease. Newer tetracyclines, doxycycline and minocycline have the advantage of only requiring single- daily- or 12-hourly dosing. Although sputum concentrations of doxycycline are low (p. 734), the drug is usually beneficial in patients with various forms of bronchitis (Swarz, 1977; Chodosh et al., 1988). Higher sputum levels are attained with minocycline (p. 734), but long-term chemoprophylaxis with this drug is contraindicated because of its vestibular side-effects (p. 740). For short-term treatment of acute bronchitis doxycycline is about equally effective to minocycline (Maesen et al., 1989). Nevertheless, tetracyclines (even doxycycline) should be used cautiously in elderly patients who may have occult renal insufficiency (p. 738).

Other drugs are now preferred for the treatment of pneumonia due to staphylococci, streptococci, pneumococci, *H. influenzae* and anaerobes, and for the treatment of streptococcal tonsillitis. Because they cause teeth staining (p. 736), tetracyclines are no longer used in pertussis.

2 Surgical, biliary and urinary tract infections

Because of the high rate of tetracycline-resistance amongst Gram-negative enteric aerobes and anaerobes, tetracyclines alone are not reliable antibiotics for the treatment of peritonitis due to a perforated viscus or to treat or prevent wound infections and other postoperative sepsis. For the same reason, tetracyclines now have a very limited value for the treatment of biliary and urinary tract infections. They should not be used to treat urinary tract infections in patients with impaired renal function, because of their potential nephrotoxicity (p. 738).

3 Brucellosis

A 6-week course of tetracycline 500 mg orally 6-hourly or doxycycline 100 mg orally 12-hourly plus streptomycin 1.0 g i.m. daily for the first 2 weeks is still probably the best treatment for acute brucellosis (Acocella et al., 1989; Cisneros et al., 1990; Lang et al., 1993). A regimen of doxycycline 100 mg 12-hourly plus rifampicin 600–900 mg daily, both for 6 weeks, is also effective (p. 696) (Acocella *et al.*, 1989; Hall, 1990; Montejo *et al.*, 1993). One of the tetracyclines used alone, rifampicin used alone (p. 696) and co-trimoxazole (p. 871) are less effective (Shehabi *et al.*, 1990; Montejo *et al.*, 1993; Robson *et al.*, 1993).

Patients with osteoarticular complications of brucellosis can be treated with the same regimens, but treatment may need to be more prolonged (Mousa *et al.*, 1987). Patients with *Brucella* meningitis or neurobrucellosis have been treated successfully by combining doxycycline with both rifampicin and co-trimoxazole. Some may respond to 6 weeks treatment, but others may need treatment for up to 8 months. For the first 2–3 weeks i.m. streptomycin can also be added to the regimen (Al-Orainey *et al.*, 1987; Bouza *et al.*, 1987; McLean *et al.*, 1992; Al-Eissa, 1995). Tetracycline plus streptomycin and valve replacement has been used successfully to treat *B. abortus* endocarditis (Pazderka and Jones, 1982), but in one case of aortic valve endocarditis, prolonged medical treatment with doxycycline plus rifampicin was successful (Cisneros *et al.*, 1989).

4 Methicillin-resistant Staph. aureus infections

Most *Staph. aureus* strains of this type are sensitive to minocycline, but resistant to all other tetracyclines (p. 727). Limited clinical data indicate that minocycline, administered orally or i.v. may be effective for these infections. Darouiche *et al.* (1991) used a combination of oral minocycline plus rifampicin plus topical mupirocin to successfully eradicate the nasal methicillin-resistant *Staph.* aureus carrier state from patients. Lawlor *et al.* (1990) used oral minocycline 100 mg 12-hourly for 52 days to cure a patient from methicillin-resistant *Staph. aureus* prosthetic valve endocarditis. Of 17 patients with methicillin-resistant *Staph. aureus* or methicillin-resistant *Staph. epidermis* infections such as osteomyelitis or soft tissue infections, 15 were cured with minocycline by Yuk *et al.* (1991). In a study of experimental MRSA endocarditis, minocycline appeared equally effective to vancomycin (Nicolau *et al.*, 1994). As the number of effective drugs for the treatment of systemic methicillin-resistant *Staph. aureus* infections are limited (p. 777), further clinical studies with minocycline are warranted.

5 Bowel infections

a Cholera In this disease correction of dehydration is the most important measure. Controlled studies have demonstrated that oral tetracycline is effective in eradicating vibrios from stools and also in diminishing the volume and duration of diarrhea (Carpenter *et al.*, 1965). Tetracyclines may be useful for prophylactic purposes during a cholera epidemic and for cholera contacts (McCormack *et al.*, 1968). Doxycycline was used prophylactically with apparent success in South Africa (Isaäcson *et al.*, 1974). Two single doses of tetracycline 250 mg (the first given immediately and the other in the evening) reduced the number of severe cases of diarrhea which developed amongst family contacts of cholera cases in Bangladesh (Khan, 1982). A 3-day course of tetracycline has been reported to effectively eliminate the organism from cholera carriers (Joint Study, 1971). A single dose of 1 g tetracycline is effective in the treatment of cholera, but it is associated with asymptomatic bacteriologic relapse (Rabbani *et al.*, 1989). A single oral dose of doxycycline (300 mg for adults) is nearly as effective as 0.5 g tetracycline given every 6 h for 2 days for the treatment of cholera (De *et al.*, 1976). If a daily oral dose of doxycycline is given for 4 days then the results of treatment are as effective as those obtained by tetracycline given 6-hourly for 4 days, the only difference being that feces are cleared of vibrios within 3 days with doxycyline compared with 2 days with tetracycline (Rahaman *et al.*, 1976). Minocycline is also as effective as tetracycline for the treatment of cholera, but similarly it does not clear the feces of vibrios as rapidly as tetracycline (Mazumder *et al.*, 1974). Tetracyclines are of no value in the management of cholera in those parts of the world where tetracycline-resistant strains of *V. cholerae* are encountered (p. 724).

Non-0:1 *V. cholerae* bacteremia may respond to a tetracycline or chloramphenicol (Safrin *et al.*, 1988).

b Shigella dysentery In adults a single oral dose of 2.5 g tetracycline was effective in shigellosis (Pickering *et al.*, 1978). This treatment resulted in a high clinical cure rate and elimination of the organisms (*Sh. flexneri*, *Sh. boydii* and *Sh. sonnei*) from the stools of symptomatic and asymptomatic patients 48 h after therapy. This occurred irrespective of the sensitivity of the organisms, 59% being resistant to tetracycline. Ampicillin (p. 122) or co-trimoxazole (p. 868) are usually the preferred drugs to treat shigellosis. In developing countries many *Shigella* spp. strains are resistant to all these antibiotics and also to nalidixic acid (p. 969).

c **Travelers' diarrhea** In one controlled trial a 100-mg daily dose of doxycycline, given for 3 weeks, was effective in reducing the frequency of travelers' diarrhea amongst Peace Corp volunteers in Kenya (Sack *et al.*, 1978). Tetracyclines were used because the enterotoxigenic strains of *E. coli* in the area were nearly all uniformly sensitive to the drug. Doxycycline was selected because of its once-daily dosage and unique excretion into the bowel (p. 732). In another controlled trial, doxycycline 100 mg twice-weekly to prevent travelers' diarrhea in Peace Corps volunteers in Honduras was not as effective; it was only marginally effective in preventing diarrhea and did not prevent diarrhea secondary to doxycycline-resistant enterotoxigenic *E. coli* strains (Santosham *et al.*, 1981). Other trials in areas where *E. coli* strains resistant to tetracycline were common showed that doxycycline was beneficial because of its action on other organisms (Echeverria *et al.*, 1984; Sack *et al.*, 1984). In these studies travelers' diarrhea caused by doxycycline-resistant strains was not prevented so that protection was not as good as in areas where strains were sensitive. In one study, doxycycline prophylaxis also diminished the severity of the illness (Sack *et al.*, 1984). Doxycycline has been used for short-term prophylaxis (2–5 days) with effect (Freeman *et al.*, 1983). Co-trimoxazole (p. 869), furazolidone (p. 922) and norfloxacin (p. 1067) are also used for prevention and treatment of this disease.

d **Other bowel infections** Tetracycline given orally in a dosage of 250–500 mg every 6 h for 3 days was of only marginal benefit to adults presenting with acute diarrhea due to enterotoxigenic *E. coli* in Bangladesh (Merson *et al.*, 1980).

e **Helicobacter pylori infection** Triple drug therapy of bismuth subcitrate 120 mg four times daily, tetracycline 500 mg four times daily and metronidazole 400 mg three times daily, all given for 2 weeks most consistently heals duodenal ulcers and eradicates *H. pylori* infection. Doxycycline cannot be substituted for tetracycline for this indication. A 1-week treatment with these three drugs has also been successful. Concurrent administration of omeprazole reduces ulcer pain more rapidly but has no effect on ulcer healing (Unge and Gnarpe, 1988; Marshall, 1990; Hosking *et al.*, 1992, 1994; Forbes, 1994). The above regimens eradicate *H. pylori* infection in some 90% of patients (Walsh and Peterson, 1995). If tetracycline is not tolerated and amoxycillin 500 mg four times daily is substituted for it, eradication rate is less. If the above regimen is not tolerated, a 2-week course of omeprazole and amoxycillin can achieve eradication rates of about 80% (p. 142) Forbes, 1994); but sometimes duodenal ulcer may recur in patients in whom *H. pylori* is eradicated due to factors other than reinfection with this organism (Graham, 1995).

A 1-week course of bismuth subcitrate, tetracycline and metronidazole also reliably heals gastric ulcers and eradicates *H. pylori* if the presence of *H. pylori* is demonstrated and if the ulcer has not been caused by the use of non-steroidal anti-inflammatory medications (Sung *et al.*, 1995). There is also a close association between gastric MALT lymphoma and *H. pylori*. Eradication of *H. pylori* by antibiotics may cause regression of the lymphoma (Wotherspoon *et al.*, 1993).

6 Melioidosis

This disease, caused by *Burkholderia* (*Pseudomonas*) *pseudomallei* can either present as subacute pneumonitis or as a fulminating septicemia with a high mortality. Large doses of tetracycline (3 g daily for at least 30 days) were satisfactory for the treatment of subacute pneumonitis (Sponitz *et al.*, 1967). Doxycycline was also effective (Leelarasamee and Bovornkitti, 1989). Everett and Nelson (1975) treated 39 patients with subacute disease including pulmonary melioidosis and found that tetracycline alone or in combination with chloramphenicol (p. 570) were equally effective. For severe forms of this disease either ceftazidime alone or this drug combined with co-trimoxazole are now preferred (p. 378).

7 Nocardiosis

Minocycline has been used with success to treat *N. asteroides* pulmonary infection in five patients who were cardiac allograft recipients (Petersen *et al.*, 1983). A sulfonamide (p. 823) or co-trimoxazole (p. 871) are usually preferred for this disease. Minocycline in combination with co-trimoxazole has been used to treat nocardiosis in AIDS patients. Many such patients are allergic to sulfonamides and drug combinations such as minocycline/imipenem or minocycline/ceftriaxone have been employed for the treatment of these (Kim *et al.*, 1991).

8 Legionellosis

A few anecdotal reports suggest that doxycycline may be effective in Legionnaires' disease (Cunha and Jonas, 1981). Overall, the results of treatment with tetracycline have been variable and erythromycin (p. 618) is best for this infection (Meyer, 1983).

9 Gonorrhea

Tetracyclines were used extensively for the treatment of this disease, but nowadays they are no longer recommended because of the widespread resistance of *N. gonorrhoeae* to these drugs (Karney *et al.*, 1977; Jaffe *et al.*, 1981; CDC, 1993b).

10 Chancroid and granuloma inguinale

Tetracyclines, given for 2 weeks, were effective in these diseases (Willcox, 1977). Minocycline was also effective (Velasco *et al.*, 1972). Due to widespread resistance of *H. ducreyi* to tetracyclines (p. 725), these drugs are no longer recommended for the treatment of chancroid, and erythromycin (p. 620), single-dose ceftriaxone (p. 362), or single-dose azithromycin (p. 658) are preferred. Amoxicillin/clavulanic acid (p. 201) or ciprofloxacin (p. 1022) can also be used (CDC, 1993b).

11 Pelvic inflammatory disease

Many organisms are involved here, such as *N. gonorrhoeae*, *Strep. pyogenes*, Group B streptococci, anaerobic streptococci, *B. fragilis*, Enterobacteriaceae and *Chlamydia trachomatis*. One recommended regimen for this disease is cefoxitin 2 g i.v. 6-hourly (or cefotetan 2 g i.v. 12-hourly) plus doxycycline 100 mg 12-hourly orally or i.v. Patients who quickly improve may be sent home on oral doxycycline only after some 4–7 days to complete a total course of chemotherapy for 10–14 days (p. 45) (Peterson *et al.*, 1990).

12 Bartonella (formerly Rochalimaea) infections

Infections by these bacteria in AIDS patients (bacillary angiomatosis and bacillary peliosis) have most commonly been treated by erythromycin (p. 619). However, milder infections also respond to oral doxycycline (Schwartzman, 1992). One immunocompromised renal transplant patient with opportunistic lung infection due to *Bartonella henselae* responded to prolonged doxycycline therapy (Caniza *et al.*, 1995).

13 Plague (Yersinia pestis infection) and Tularemia (Francisella tularensis infection)

For plague, streptomycin (p. 435) is the preferred drug, but oral tetracycline in a dosage of 0.5–1.0 g 6-hourly for 10 days is also effective. For patients with meningitis or for those with hypotension, who need i.v. antibiotic treatment, chloramphenicol is recommended (Butler, 1994; CDC, 1994). Streptomycin is the drug of choice for tularemia (p. 435) and the alternative drugs, tetracycline and chloramphenicol, are more frequently associated with relapse (CDC, 1983).

14 Chemoprophylaxis of meningococcal infections

Minocycline administered to adults in a dosage of 200 mg initially, then 100 mg 12-hourly for 5 days is moderately effective for the elimination of sulfonamide-resistant meningococci from nasopharyngeal carriers (Devine *et al.*, 1971, 1972; Guttler and Beaty, 1972). A study in Finland indicated that minocycline was nearly as good as rifampicin (p. 697) in eradicating both sulfonamide-sensitive and resistant meningococcal strains (Sivonen *et al.*, 1978). Minocycline-resistant meningococcal strains usually do not emerge after treatment, but the drug only eliminates meningococci from about 60% of carriers. Sequential treatment of carriers with minocycline followed by rifampicin may be more effective (p. 697) (Devine *et al.*, 1973), whilst the simultaneous use of these two drugs may reduce the emergence of rifampicin-resistant meningococci (Munford *et al.*, 1974).

Despite its clinical efficacy, minocycline is not advocated for chemoprophylaxis of meningococcal infections because of its propensity to cause vestibular symptoms (Drew *et al.*, 1976) (p. 740). In the USA rifampicin is preferred (p. 697), but in areas where meningococcal strains are sulfonamide-sensitive, sulfonamides are recommended (p. 822).

15 Actinomycosis and anthrax

Tetracyclines can be used as alternatives to penicillin G for the treatment of these diseases in penicillin-allergic patients.

16 Aeromonas spp. infections

Aeromonas hydrophila, A caviae, A. veronii, A. jandaei and other *Aeromonas* spp. can cause septicemia in patients with severe underlying diseases such as cancer. Most strains are sensitive to tetracycline and this drug or doxycycline, administered orally, can be used to treat milder cases. For severe illness in hospital, a third-generation cephalosporin, such as ceftriaxone, given i.v. is preferred (Janda *et al.*, 1994). *Aeromonas hydrophila* as well as other organisms such as *Vibrio* spp., Enterobacteriaceae and others may be involved in skin and soft tissue infections which may follow water-related injuries e.g. injuries from catfish spine. For serious infections a combination of tetracycline plus a third-generation cephalosporin may be required (Murphey *et al.*, 1992). *Aeromonas* spp. can also cause gastroenteritis, which is usually self-limiting and chemotherapy is not necessary (Jones and Wilcox, 1995).

17 Mycobacterial infections

Both *M. fortuitum* and *M. chelonae* are environmental rapidly growing mycobacteria which only rarely produce lung disease. They often cause cutaneous infections after surgical procedures or accidental penetrating injury, but they can also result in disseminated disease. These mycobacteria may be sensitive to doxycycline, cefoxitin (p. 296), amikacin (p. 506) or sulfonamides (p. 806), but isolates of *M. fortuitum* are much more susceptible to amikacin, doxycycline and sulfonamides than are isolates of *M. chelonae* (Wallace *et al.*, 1983). Recommendation for treatment of infections caused by these bacteria have been made on these *in vitro* findings and limited clinical experience (Wallace *et al.*, 1985). For patients with serious infections, empiric therapy with amikacin (15 mg per kg per day) plus cefoxitin (200 mg per kg per day up to 12 g per day) plus oral probenecid is suggested. This provides two-drug cover except for infrequent isolates which are amikacin- or cefoxitin -resistant. If the isolate is not sensitive to an oral agent this treatment should be continued for at least 12 weeks. If the isolate is cefoxitin-sensitive, this drug may be used alone after 4–8 weeks of combined treatment. If the organism is *M. fortuitum*, the dosage of amikacin can be lowered to reduce toxicity. Should the isolate be susceptible to an oral agent (doxycycline or sulfonamides) one or more of these drugs can be substituted for parenteral therapy after 2–5 weeks. Infections due to *M. marinum* have been reported to respond to tetracyclines but usually rifampicin (p. 692) is the preferred drug if one is required. In two patients reported by Ljungberg *et al.* (1987), doxycycline treatment failed in *M. marinum* infections.

18 Mycoplasma infections

Tetracyclines are effective for the treatment of *Mycoplasma pneumonia* pneumonia (Smith *et al.*, 1967; Foy *et al.*, 1970; McCormack, 1993). In one study, tetracycline was equally effective to erythromycin (p. 619) in reducing the length of illness in pneumonia caused by *M. pneumoniae* (Shames *et al.*, 1970). The organism was cultured from the pharynx of a number of patients following antibiotic treatment, despite a reduction in the duration of their symptoms. *Mycoplasma hominis*, an inhabitant of the genitourinary tract of man, has been implicated as a cause of neonatal central nervous system infections, salpingitis, postpartum fever and septicemia (Bøe *et al.*, 1983; Plummer *et al.*, 1987). Therapy with doxycycline is usually successful. Spencer and Brown (1983) isolated *M. hominis* from the blood of a febrile patient who was a renal transplant recipient. The isolate was resistant to erythromycin but sensitive to tetracycline. Doxycycline therapy was successful.

19 Non-gonococcal urethritis due to Ureaplasma urealyticum

Ureaplasma urealyticum and the *Chlamydia* spp. (see below) are the major causes of this disease. Infection due to both organisms usually respond to the tetracyclines. Dosage regimens of minocycline 100 mg daily or tetracycline 500 mg 6-hourly, each for 7 days are equally effective in eradicating infection due to *Chlamydia* or *Ureaplasma* spp. (Bowie *et al.*, 1980, 1981). But activity of both drugs against *U. urealyticum* was less consistent in another study (Oriel and Ridgway, 1983). Tetracycline-resistant strains of *U. urealyticum* are no longer rare (p. 725). In the USA, treatment with doxycycline 100 mg twice-daily, given orally for 7 days, is recommended concomitant therapy for gonorrhea to treat possible co-existent non-gonococcal urethritis; erythromycin can be substituted if tetracycline is not suitable for the patient (CDC, 1993b). *Ureaplasma*, like *Chlamydia* spp. (see below) have been implicated in an expanding list of infections, including chorioamnionitis, infant pneumonia (Stagno *et al.*, 1981), septicemia and pelvic infection in women (Plummer *et al.*, 1987), septic arthritis in patients with hypogammaglobulinemia (Forgacs *et al.*, 1993) and chronic prostatitis (Brunner *et al.*, 1983). Sometimes the tetracyclines, including minocycline and doxycycline, fail to eradicate *U. urealyticum* from patients because of the presence of resistant strains (Prentice *et al.*, 1976;

Spaepen *et al.*, 1976). Infections due to *U. urealyticum* also respond to the aminocyclitols, streptomycin and spectinomycin (Bowie *et al.*, 1976). *Ureaplasma* are also usually sensitive to erythromycin *in vitro* (p. 610), but not to clindamycin (p. 590) (McCormack, 1993).

20 Chlamydial infections

a Psittacosis Tetracyclines are the most effective drugs against this disease, which is caused by *C. psittaci* (Jawetz, 1969; Yung and Grayson, 1988). A daily dose of 1 g tetracycline for 21 days has been advocated for treatment and prevention of relapse (WHO, 1977). Nowadays doxycycline is most commonly used in a dosage of 100 mg orally 12-hourly or for severe cases the same dosage can be given i.v. (Khatib *et al.*, 1995).

b Lymphogranuloma venereum This is caused by *Chlamydia trachomatis* serovars L1, L2 and L3 and responds to treatment with the tetracyclines (Jawetz, 1969). Treatment is usually required for an average of 2 weeks. Minocycline has been used to treat this disease and it is effective in courses lasting for 15–21 days (Velasco *et al.*, 1972). Recommended treatment in the USA is doxycycline 100 mg twice-daily, given for 3 weeks. Alternative drugs are erythromycin (p. 619) or sulfisoxazole (p. 823) (CDC, 1993b). L1 and L2 serovars can also cause proctitis in homosexual men, which again responds to tetracycline therapy (Bauwens *et al.*, 1995).

c Trachoma Both hyperendemic trachoma and paratrachoma are caused by various serotypes of *C. trachomatis*, previously known as TRIC (trachoma, inclusion body conjunctivitis) agent (Darougar, 1981). Hyperendemic trachoma is transmitted from eye to eye and responds to topical treatment with tetracycline or rifampicin eye ointment given for 5–6 weeks. Oral tetracycline in a dose of 0.75 g twice-daily for 21 days (Dawson *et al.*, 1971) or a daily dose of doxycycline (2.5–4.0 mg per kg body weight) given for 5 days each week for a total of 28 doses in 40 days (Hoshiwara *et al.*, 1973), also result in significant suppression of trachomatous activity. Chloramphenicol eye ointment is not effective. Mass treatment with tetracycline ophthalmic ointment is recommended for children in communities with holoendemic trachoma. The intermittent mass treatment schedule suggested, consisting of twice-daily application of the ointment for 5 consecutive days once a month for 6 months, has a significant but short-lived effect on eye disease (Dawson *et al.*, 1981). When oral doxycycline was added for 5 days treatment each month for 6 months, the healing rates in children were improved. The potential risk of teeth staining in these patients was considered inconsequential and oral doxycycline was recommended for children at risk of developing blindness (Dawson and Schachter, 1985).

Paratrachoma is transmitted sexually and includes TRIC ophthalmia neonatorum in the newborn, inclusion conjunctivitis, TRIC punctuate keratoconjunctivitis and endemic trachoma. These latter eye infections are transmitted to the eyes from infections in the genital tract (cervicitis or urethritis) (see below). Pregnant women who have chlamydial cervicitis or urethritis should be treated with a 1–2 week course of erythromycin (p. 619) and non-pregnant patients with a course of doxycycline. Azithromycin (p. 658) is also effective (Weber and Johnson, 1995). Instillation of tetracycline (1%) or erythromycin (0.5%) ophthalmic ointment within 1 h of birth was recommended to prevent chlamydial and gonococcal ophthalmia neonatorum. Silver nitrate (1% eye drops) have also been used. In a large controlled study Hammerschlag *et al.* (1989) found that all these three agents effectively prevented gonococcal ophthalmia in the newborns, but that such prophylaxis was less effective in preventing chlamydial ophthalmia. Laga *et al.* (1988) performed a controlled study in Nairobi, comparing tetracycline ointment, silver nitrate and placebo for the chemoprophylaxis in newborns from gonococcal and chlamydial ophthalmia neonatorum. Again both agents effectively prevented gonococcal ophthalmia, even if the gonococcal strains were tetracycline-resistant. Chlamydial infection was less well prevented. The authors concluded that ocular prophylaxis at birth should be primarily directed against gonococcal infection. Topical prophylaxis at birth may initially reduce the incidence of neonatal chlamydial conjunctivitis, but it does not reduce ocular transmission or other serious illness in newborns such as neonatal pneumonia. Antenatal case detection appeared to be a more appropriate way to control chlamydia-associated morbidity in both mother and child. As silver nitrate can cause chemical conjunctivitis, tetracycline eye ointment is the preferred treatment.

More recently Isenberg *et al.* (1995) reported results from a large controlled study in Kenya, which compared 2.5% solution of povidone-iodine with silver nitrate and erythromycin ointment for ocular chemoprophylaxis. The povidone-iodine was as effective, less toxic and cheaper in preventing both gonococcal and chlamydial ophthalmia neonatorum. Povidone-iodine has not yet been compared with tetracycline ointment for prophylaxis (Foster and Klaus, 1995).

Erythromycin orally for 2 weeks, should be used to treat established chlamydial conjunctivitis of the newborn, as topical treatment frequently fails to eliminate *C. trachomatis* from the eyes or from the pharynx of such patients (Baum, 1995).

d Non-gonococcal urethritis and other infections *Chlamydia trachomatis* is a major cause of this disease (Schachter, 1978a). Infections by this organism are the most prevalent of all sexually transmitted diseases in the USA (CDC, 1993b). It can cause a wide spectrum of disease including proctitis, conjunctivitis, pharyngitis, cervicitis, salpingitis, epididymitis and pneumonia in infants. Tetracyclines are the most effective drugs for the treatment of non-gonococcal urethritis (Schachter, 1978b). Because a high percentage of patients with gonococcal urethritis also have simultaneous urethral infection with *C. trachomatis* (p. 45), a regimen in which a tetracycline is used to supplement single-dose treatment of gonorrhea is necessary (Ridgway and Oriel, 1984; Stamm *et al.*, 1984). In the USA, doxycycline 100 mg twice-daily, for 7 days is recommended for non-gonococcal urethritis and as concomitant treatment for a single-dose regimen of gonorrhea. For patients in whom tetracyclines are contraindicated or not tolerated for the treatment of chlamydial infections in pregnancy and chlamydial pneumonia in infancy, erythromycin is the recommended alternative drug (CDC, 1993b). Tetracyclines including doxycycline and minocycline administered for 7 days are effective in eradicating *Chlamydia* from the female and male genital tract (Prentice *et al.*, 1976; Kovacs *et al.*, 1989; Toomey and Barnes, 1990; Romanowski *et al.*, 1993).

e Chlamydia pneumoniae respiratory infections This is a new species of *Chlamydia* which causes acute respiratory infections in older children and adults. The disease can be severe in the elderly, but in others it can usually be managed on an outpatient basis. Pneumonia or bronchitis are the most common clinical diseases. Pharyngitis, sinusitis, pericarditis or endocarditis can also occasionally be caused by this organism (Marrie *et al.*, 1990; Grayston, 1992; Ekman *et al.*, 1993; Sundelöf *et al.*, 1993). The most commonly advocated treatment regimen is 2–3 weeks of doxycycline 100 mg 12-hourly for adults, but erythromycin (p. 619) and azithromycin (p. 658) are also effective. For children either erythromycin or clarithromycin (p. 649) can be used (Grayston, 1992; Ekman *et al.*, 1993; Falck *et al.*, 1994; Hammerschlag, 1994). Persistent symptoms of bronchitis may occur in some patients associated with positive cultures for *C. pneumoniae* for several months, despite an adequate course of doxycycline for the acute illness (Hammerschlag *et al.*, 1992).

21 Syphilis

Penicillin G is the best drug for treatment of this disease (p. 46). Accumulating evidence indicates that tetracycline 500 mg four times daily for 14 days is effective treatment for primary and secondary or early latent syphilis (Brown, 1982). Minocycline, in a dose of 100 mg twice-daily for 15 days, also appears to be satisfactory for primary and secondary syphilis (Velasco *et al.*, 1972) as does doxycycline 200 mg daily for 14–28 days (Onoda, 1979; Zenker and Rolfs, 1990). Experience in five patients with latent and neurosyphilis treated with doxycycline 200 mg twice-daily for 21 days, showed that the drug penetrated well into the CSF (p. 733) and suggested that it may be useful for these infections (Yim *et al.*, 1985), but one woman allergic to penicillin with early latent syphilis was treated with two courses of doxycycline. Ten months later she had no serological response and a lumbar puncture demonstrated asymptomatic neurosyphilis (Zenilman *et al.*, 1993). In the USA, tetracycline is recommended for the treatment of primary and secondary syphilis in penicillin-allergic non-pregnant patients. The dosage is 500 mg four times daily for 14 days. Doxycycline 100 mg orally 12-hourly for 2 weeks can also be used. The same regimens can be used for latent syphilis, but if the disease is more than of 12 months duration, the duration of therapy should be 4 weeks. Pregnant patients, children and patients with neurosyphilis, allergic to penicillin, should be treated whenever possible with penicillin G after desensitization (CDC, 1993b; Rolfs, 1995).

22 Yaws

Penicillin G is the preferred drug for this infection, but tetracycline 2 g daily for 5 days seems a satisfactory alternative in penicillin-allergic patients. The efficacy of doxycycline for this infection has not been evaluated (Brown, 1985).

23 Leptospirosis

In studies on soldiers undergoing jungle training in Panama, doxycycline 100 mg twice-daily for 7 days had a therapeutic effect on anicteric leptospirosis and prevented leptospiruria (Takafuji *et al.*, 1984). Penicillin G (p. 48) is also used to treat leptospirosis.

24 Lyme disease

One of the tetracyclines appears to be the most effective treatment for early manifestations, such as erythema migrans, of this disease. One recommendation is doxycycline 100 mg two or three times daily for 20 days (Luft *et al.*, 1989; Luger *et al.*, 1995; Nadelman and Wormser, 1995). Lyme arthritis can also be treated successfully with 1-month courses of oral doxycycline (Steere, 1995). Doxycycline has also been successful for some patients with Lyme meningitis (Dotevall *et al.*, 1988), but i.v. ceftriaxone is now considered superior (Pachner, 1995).

25 Relapsing fever

Louse-borne relapsing fever (an epidemic spirochetal infection due to *Borrelia recurrentis*) responds to single-dose oral treatment with tetracycline 500 mg, doxycycline 100 mg, erythromycin 500 mg, chloramphenicol 500 mg or a single injection of penicillin aluminum monostearate (PAM) (Perine and Teklu, 1983). All of these treatments may invoke the Jarisch-Herxheimer reaction, but in the case of tetracycline this is reduced by meptazinol (p. 736). One of the tetracyclines may be the drug of choice because it more rapidly eliminates *Borrelia spirochetes*, except for pregnant women and children when erythromycin should be used (Warrell *et al.*, 1983). Le (1980) used erythromycin successfully to treat three children with tick-borne relapsing fever (an endemic spirochetal infection due to several *Borrelia spirochetes*).

26 Rickettsial infections

Tetracyclines are the drugs of choice for the treatment of epidemic louse-borne typhus, murine typhus, scrub typhus, tick typhus, Rocky Mountain spotted fever, and Mediterranean spotted fever (Ming-Yuan *et al.*, 1987; Gudiol *et al.*, 1989; Perine *et al.*, 1992). Chloramphenicol is also effective for these diseases, and is sometimes preferred for very severe infections (p. 568). Ciprofloxacin (p. 1031) may also be effective (Gudiol *et al.*, 1989), but rifampicin is not as good as doxycycline (Bella *et al.*, 1991). Louse-borne typhus can be cured by a single dose of doxycycline, 100–200 mg for adults and 50 mg for children (WHO Working Group, 1982), but normally 7–15 days of doxycycline or chloramphenicol is recommended for this disease (Raoult and Drancourt, 1991). Mediterranean spotted fever has also been cured by an abbreviated course of doxycycline. In one trial doxycycline was only continued for 24 h after the patients were afebrile; this form of therapy compared favorably to a standard 7-day doxycycline course (Yagupsky *et al.*, 1987). In another trial 200 mg of doxycycline given 12-hourly on 1 day only was as effective as a classic 10-day course with oral tetracycline for this disease (Bella-Cueto *et al.*, 1987). Some cases of spotted fever, however, can be very severe and result in rapid death, so specific antimicrobial therapy should be administered promptly when the disease is suspected (Yagupsky and Wolach, 1993).

The other rickettsioses require tetracycline treatment for 5–15 days (Raoult and Drancourt, 1991). Trials in Taiwan indicated that doxycycline 200 mg orally once a week was effective for prevention of scrub typhus (Olson *et al.*, 1980). This was confirmed in volunteers exposed to this infection in the laboratory. Scrub typhus needs doxycycline or chloramphenicol therapy for 7–15 days, but for Rocky Mountain spotted fever 5 days of either of these drugs is usually sufficient (Raoult and Drancourt, 1991). Chloramphenicol may be preferred when oral treatment cannot be tolerated or in seriously ill patients. However, failures of chloramphenicol therapy have been noted in recent years. The side-effects of these drugs must be balanced against the severity of the disease (Kelsey, 1979). Because delays in treatment contribute to mortality during endemic periods, early treatment of patients with suspected Rocky Mountain spotted fever is justified (Hattwick *et al.*, 1978; Westerman, 1982; Woodward, 1984; Kirkland *et al.*, 1995).

27 Ehrlichiosis

This is a tick-borne infection caused by small obligate intracellular bacteria of the genus *Ehrlichia*. Two types of this disease occur in the USA: human monocytic ehrlichiosis caused by *Ehrlichia chaffensis*, and human granulocytic ehrlichiosis, caused by an agent closely related to *E. equi*, which is an animal pathogen. Both infections cause undifferentiated fever with leukopenia, thrombocytopenia and elevations in serum aminotransferase levels. Severe infection and mortality are associated with delays in diagnosis and treatment. The treatment of choice is either tetracycline or doxycycline, usually administered for 7 days (CDC, 1995; Dumler and Bakken, 1995; Fishbein and Dennis, 1995; Standaert *et al.*, 1995).

28 Q fever

Acute Q fever is usually a self-limited febrile illness, in which the value of any antibiotic therapy is hard to assess. Many clinicians treat patients with moderately severe disease with tetracyclines (Sawyer *et al.*, 1987; Lieberman *et al.*, 1995).

The most difficult chronic Q fever infection to treat successfully is endocarditis. Prolonged tetracycline therapy has proved to be of some benefit for most patients with this complication, but complete eradication of infection without cardiac surgery was initially unusual (Kristinsson and Bentall, 1967; Laufer *et al.*, 1986). It is now recommended that tetracycline or doxycycline therapy should be continued for some 3 years. Combination chemotherapy has been tried. Doxycycline combined with co-trimoxazole has met with some success (Fernández-Guerrero *et al.*, 1988) and similarly doxycycline plus rifampicin has been tried (Raoult *et al.*, 1987a). However, it now appears that the combination of doxycycline with a fluoroquinolone such as ofloxacin (p. 1126) may be the most effective regimen for the long-term treatment of this disease (Levy *et al.*, 1991; Raoult, 1993). Three years medical treatment with this regimen may cure most patients and valve replacement may only be necessary if there is hemodynamic failure (Raoult, 1993). Currently the combination of hydroxychloroquine 600 mg daily plus doxycycline 200 mg daily is being evaluated for Q fever endocarditis. This combination is bactericidal for *Coxiella burnetii* (Raoult and Marrie, 1995).

Some patients with chronic Q fever have hepatitis, pulmonary disease, arthritis or osteomyelitis, but no cardiac involvement (Brouqui *et al.*, 1993). These usually respond to long-term doxycycline treatment. Some patients may develop Q fever meningititis or meningoence-phalitis as part of acute Q fever. These respond to a 3-week course of doxycycline (Ferrante and Dolan, 1993).

29 Malaria

Because of their activity against malarial parasites, the tetracyclines have been used for treatment of chloroquine-resistant falciparum malaria. This malaria responds rather slowly to tetracycline therapy alone (Clyde *et al.*, 1971), and a regimen of quinine sulfate combined with tetracycline was more successful (Colwell *et al.*, 1972). A regimen of quinine sulfate 600 mg three times daily for 3 days, followed by tetracycline 250 mg four times daily for 10 days, was used (Benson *et al.*, 1972; Colwell *et al.*, 1972). Doxycycline in a dose of 200 mg daily has also been used in these regimens.

Doxycycline in an adult dosage of 100 mg daily is quite effective for both *Plasmodium vivax* and *P. falciparum* chemoprophylaxis. After returning from endemic areas, the drug ideally should be continued for 4 weeks. Doxycycline has little or no activity against the liver stages of *P. vivax*, and therefore it is advisable that a primaquine eradication course be given once the traveller has returned from malarious area (Pang *et al.*, 1987; 1988; Brown, 1993; Shanks *et al.*, 1995).

30 Acne

For mild disease topical keratolytics may suffice, but for more severe acne antibiotics in addition are of value. Tetracycline in an initial daily dosage of 0.5–1.0 g or even 2.0 g is often used and, after improvement occurs, a daily dosage of 0.25–0.5 g may be continued for months or even years. Tetracyclines should be given 1 h before meals to ensure absorption (p. 729). Doxycycline can also be used. Tetracyclines should not be used in children aged less than 8 years or in pregnant women. Treatment with erythromycin (p. 621) or co-trimoxazole is equally effective. Clindamycin, although effective, is not recommended because its long-term use in acne has been associated with the development of pseudomembranous colitis (p. 594). Topical antibiotics have been used with success in acne, particularly in the USA; these include clindamycin, erythromycin and tetracycline (Schachner, 1983). Diarrhea and pseudomembranous colitis have occurred with the use of topical clindamycin.

Topical erythromycin seems safe and some studies have shown it to be as effective as oral tetracycline. Antibiotics act on an anaerobic organism, *Propionibacterium acnes* which colonizes sebaceous follicles. These organisms are active in the conversion of lipids to free fatty acids which may have an inflammatory effect on the follicular wall; they also produce chemotactic substances which draw polymorphic neutrophils into the follicular wall. Long-term use of tetracyclines is usually well tolerated in this disease probably because of the low-dosage used and the age of the patients. Systemic treatment increases the numbers of intestinal bacteria with resistance to tetracycline mediated by plasmids (p. 723), and there is a progressive tendency for this resistance to develop against a number of drugs (Møller *et al.*, 1977). Topical tetracycline, clindamycin and erythromycin treatment can result in the emergence of strains of *Propionibacterium acnes* resistant to the drugs (Brown and Poston, 1983). Because the topical use of antibiotics may predispose to the selection of resistant bacteria, many clinicians believe that this form of treatment should not be used in acne and topical dermatological preparations, other than antibiotics, are preferred (Leading article, 1982).

31 Tropical sprue

Long-term tetracycline administration is beneficial in patients suffering from the disease (Rickles *et al.*, 1972). Most patients show definite improvement after a 4-week course of tetracycline (Tomkins *et al.*, 1974; Simon and Gorbach, 1982). It has been postulated that tropical sprue begins with an acute intestinal infection which leads to small intestinal stasis so that bacterial colonization is encouraged; tetracycline is then thought to eliminate this bacterial overgrowth (Cook, 1984).

32 Whipple's disease

Patients with this disease may respond to treatment with tetracyclines, if penicillin G cannot be used (p. 51).

33 Prevention of microbial colonization of catheters

Slime-producing staphylococci frequently colonize catheters, and when these bacteria are embedded in biofilm, they become resistant to various antibiotics. Using an *in vitro* model Raad *et al.* (1995) showed that when catheters were coated with minocycline plus rifampicin, colonization by *Staph. epidermidis* or *Staph. aureus* was more effectively prevented than when they were coated by other antibiotics such as vancomycin.

34 Rheumatoid arthritis

Minocycline is beneficial for patients with active rheumatoid arthritis. Its mode of action is not understood (Tilley *et al.*, 1995).

References

Abbott SL, Janda JM (1994). Severe gastroenteritis associated with *Vibrio hollisae* infection: report of two cases and review. *Clin Infect Dis* **18**: 310.

Acar JF, Goldstein FW, Kitzis MD, Eyquem MT (1981). Resistance pattern of anaerobic bacteria isolated in a general hospital during a two-year period. *J Antimicrob Chemother* **8** (Suppl D): 9.

Acocella G, Bertrand A, Beytout J (1989). Comparison of three different regimens in the treatment of acute brucellosis: a multicenter multinational study. *J Antimicrob Chemother* **23**: 433.

Adadevoh BK, Ogunnaike IA, Bolodeoku JO (1976). Serum levels of doxycycline in normal subjects after a single oral dose. *Brit Med J* **1**: 880.

Adverse Drug Reactions Advisory Committee (1994). Doxycycline-induced oesophageal ulceration. *Med J Aust* **161**: 490.

Aitchison WRC, Grant IWB, Gould JC (1968). Treatment of acute exacerbations in chronic bronchitis. *Brit J Clin Prac* **22**: 343.

Albritton WL, Maclean IW, Slaney LA *et al.* (1984). Plasmid-mediated tetracycline resistance in *Haemophilus ducreyi*. *Antimicrob Ag Chemother* **25**: 187.

Al-Eissa YA (1995). Clinical and therapeutic features of childhood neurobrucellosis. *Scand J Infect Dis* **27**: 339.

Alestig K (1973). Studies on doxycycline during intravenous and oral treatment with reference to renal function. *Scand J Infect Dis* **5**: 193.

Alestig K (1974). Studies on the intestinal excretion of doxycycline. *Scand J Infect Dis* **6**: 265.

Alestig K, Lidin-Janson G (1975). The effect of doxycycline and tetracycline hydrochloride on the aerobic fecal flora. *Scand J Infect Dis* **7**: 265.

Allen JC (1976). Drugs five years later: minocycline. *Ann Intern Med* **85**: 482.

Al-Orainey IO, Laajam MA, Al-Aska AK, Rajapakse CN (1987). *Brucella* meningitis. *J Infect* **14**: 141.

Amendola MA, Spera TD (1985). Doxycycline-induced esophagitis. *JAMA* **253**: 1009.

Anderson DM (1980). Plasmid studies of *Salmonella typhimurium* phage type 179 resistant to ampicillin, tetracycline, sulphonamides and trimethoprim. *J Hyg Camb* **85**: 293.

Andersson H, Alestig K (1976). The penetration of doxycycline into CSF. *Scand J Infect Dis* (Suppl 9): 17.

Andersson K,-E, Mårdh P-A, Åkerlund M (1976). Passage of doxycycline into extracellular fluid. *Scand J Infect Dis* (Suppl 9): 7.

Ånséhn S, Gramström S, Höjer H *et al.* (1976). *In vitro* effects on *Candida albicans* of amphotericin B combined with other antibiotics. Preliminary observations. *Scand J Infect Dis* (Suppl 9): 62.

Anthony BF, Concepcion NF (1975). Group B streptococcus in a general hospital. *J Infect Dis* **132**: 561.

Anthony HM (1977). Tetracycline sensitivity as a cause of excessive flatus. *Brit Med J* **2**: 1632.

Aoki T, Takahashi A (1987). Class D tetracycline resistance determinants of R plasmids from the fish pathogens *Aeromonas hydrophila*, *Edwardsiella tarda* and *Pasteurella piscicida*. *Antimicrob Ag Chemother* **31**: 1278.

Aro A, Korhonen T, Halinen M (1978). Phenformin-induced lacticacidosis precipitated by tetracycline. *Lancet* **i**: 673.

Attwood HD (1983). A black thyroid and minocycline therapy. *Med J Aust* **1**: 549.

Attwood HD, Dennett X (1976). A black thyroid and minocycline treatment. *Brit Med J* **2**: 1109.

Ayliffe GAJ, Lilly HA, Lowbury EJL (1979). Decline of the hospital staphylococcus? Incidence of multiresistant *Staph aureus* in three Birmingham hospitals. *Lancet* **i**: 538.

Bach MC, Sabath LD, Finland M (1973). Susceptibility of *Nocardia asteroides* to 45 antimicrobial agents *in vitro*. *Antimicrob Ag Chemother* **3**: 1.

Bäck O, Norberg B (1984). The effect of a therapeutic doxycycline concentration on polymorphonuclear leukocyte migration *in vitro*. *Scand J Infect Dis* **16**: 369.

Bacon JF, Shenfield GM (1980). Pregnancy attributable to interaction between tetracycline and oral contraceptives. *Brit Med J* **280**: 293.

Baker CJ, Webb BJ, Barrett FF (1976). Antimicrobial susceptibility of Group B streptococci isolated from a variety of clinical sources. *Antimicrob Ag Chemother* **10**: 128.

Baker KL (1975). Tetracycline-induced tooth changes: part 5. Incidence in extracted first permanent molar teeth: a resurvey after four years. *Med J Aust* **2**: 301.

Baker KL, Storey E (1970). Tetracycline-induced tooth changes: part 3 Incidence in extracted first permanent molar teeth. *Med J Aust* **1**: 109.

Balsdon MJ, Taylor GE, Pead L, Maskell JP (1980). *Corynebacterium vaginale* and vaginitis: a controlled trial of treatment. *Lancet; i*: 501.

Bartlett JG, Bustetter LA, Gorbach SL, Onderdonk AB (1975). Comparative effect of tetracycline and doxycycline on the occurrence of resistant *Escherichia coli* in fecal flora. *Antimicrob Ag Chemother* **7**: 55.

Barza M, Brown RB, Shanks C *et al.* (1975). Relation between lipophilicity and pharmacological behaviour of minocycline, doxycycline, tetracycline and oxytetracycline in dogs. *Antimicrob Ag Chemother* **8**: 713.

Bates J (1982). The role of infection during exacerbation of chronic bronchitis. *Ann Intern Med* **97**: 130.

Baum J (1995). Infections of the eye. *Clin Infect Dis* **21**: 479.

Bauwens JE, Lampe MF, Suchland RJ *et al.* (1995). Infection with *Chlamydia trachomatis* lymphogranuloma venereum serovar L1 in homosexual men with proctitis: molecular analysis of an unusual case cluster. *Clin Infect Dis* **20**: 576.

Beale AS, Upshon PA (1994). Characteristics of murine model of genital infection with *Chlamydia trachomatis* and effects of therapy with tetracyclines, amoxicillin-clavulanic acid, or azithromycin. *Antimicrob Ag Chemother* **38**: 1937.

Beard NS Jr, Armentrout SA, Weisberger AS (1969). Inhibition of mammalian protein synthesis by antibiotics. *Pharmacol Rev* **21**: 213.

Bella F, Espejo E, Uriz S *et al.* (1991). Randomized trial of 5-day rifampin versus 1-day doxycycline therapy for Mediterranean Spotted Fever. *J Infect Dis* **164**: 433.

Bella-Cueto F, Font-Creus B, Seguara-Porta F *et al.* (1987). Comparative, randomized trial of one-day doxycline versus 10-day tetracycline therapy for Mediterranean spotted fever. *J Infect Dis* **155**: 1056.

Belsheim J, Gnarpe H, Persson S (1979). Tetracyclines and host defense mechanisms: interference with leukocyte chemotaxis. *Scand J Infect Dis* **11**: 141.

Benson LE, Siegel AJ, Lynch RE *et al.* (1972). Drug resistance in malaria. *Lancet* **i**: 743.

Bentorcha F, de Cespédés G, Horaud T (1991). Tetracycline resistance heterogeneity in *Enterococcus faecium*. *Antimicrob Ag Chemother* **35**: 808.

Bernard B, Yin EJ, Simon HJ (1971). Clinical pharmacologic studies with minocycline. *J Clin Pharmacol* **11**: 332.

Bethell HJN (1977). Photo-onycholysis caused by demethylchlortetracycline. *Brit Med J* **2**: 96.

Bhagawan BS, Wenk RE, McCartny EF *et al.* (1982). Long-term use of tetracycline. *JAMA* **247**: 2780.

Böcker R, Estler C-J, Weber A (1982). Metabolism of doxycycline. *Lancet* **ii**: 1155.

Bøe Ø, Iversen OE, Mehl A (1983). Septicemia due to *Mycoplasma hominis*. *Scand J Infect Dis* **15**: 87.

Bourbeau P, Campos JM (1982). Current antibiotic susceptibility of Group A beta-hemolytic streptococci. *J Infect Dis* **145**: 916.

Bouza E, de la Torre MG, Parras F *et al.* (1987). Brucellar meningitis. *Rev Infect Dis* **9**: 810.

Bowie WR, Alexander ER, Floyd JF *et al.* (1976). Differential response of chlamydial and ureaplasma-associated urethritis to sulphafurazole (sulfisoxazole). and aminocyclitols. *Lancet* **ii**: 1276.

Bowie WR, Lee CK, Alexander ER (1978). Prediction of efficacy of antimicrobial agents in treatment of infections due to *Chlamydia trachomatis*. *J Infect Dis* **138**: 655.

Bowie WR, Yu JS, Fawcett A, Jones HD (1980). Tetracycline in nongonococcal urethritis. Comparison of 2g and 1g daily for seven days. *Brit J Vener Dis* **56**: 332.

Bowie WR, Alexander ER, Stimson JB *et al.* (1981). Therapy for nongonococcal urethritis. Double-blind randomized comparison of two doses and two durations of minocycline. *Ann Intern Med* **95**: 306.

Brazier JS, Levett PN, Stannard AJ *et al.* (1985). Antibiotic susceptibility of clinical isolates of clostridia. *J Antimicrob Chemother* **15**: 181.

Brearley LJ, Storey E (1968). Tetracycline-induced tooth changes: Part 2. Prevalence, localization and nature of staining in extracted deciduous teeth. *Med J Aust* **2**: 714.

Brearley LJ, Stragis AA, Storey E (1968). Tetracycline-induced tooth changes: Part 1. Prevalence in pre-school children. *Med J Aust* **2**: 653.

Brogan TD, Neale L, Ryley HC *et al.* (1977). The secretion of minocycline in sputum during therapy of bronchopulmonary infection in chronic chest diseases. *J Antimicrob Chemother* **3**: 247.

Brouqui P, Dupont HT, Crancourt M *et al.* (1993). Chronic Q fever. Ninety-two cases from France, including 27 cases without endocarditis. *Arch Intern Med* **153**: 642.

Brown BA, Wallace RJ Jr, Flanagan CW *et al.* (1989). Tetracycline and erythromycin resistance among clinical isolates of *Branhamella catarrhalis*. *Antimicrob Ag Chemother* **33**: 1631.

Brown GV (1993). Chemoprophylaxis of malaria. *Med J Aust* **159**: 187.

Brown JM, Poston SM (1983). Resistance of propionibacteria to antibiotics used in the treatment of acne. *J Med Microbiol* **16**: 271.

Brown ST (1982). Update on recommendations for the treatment of syphilis. *Rev Infect Dis* **4** (Suppl): S873.

Brown ST (1985). Therapy for nonvenerial treponematoses: review of the efficacy of penicillin and consideration of alternatives. *Rev Infect Dis* **7** (Suppl 2): S318.

Brunner H, Weidner W, Schiefer H-G (1983). Studies on the role of *Ureaplasma urealyticum* and *Mycoplasma hominis* in prostatitis. *J Infect Dis* **147**: 807.

Burman WJ, Cohn DL, Reves RR, Wilson ML (1995). Multifocal cellulitis and monoarticular arthritis as manifestations of *Helicobacter cinaedi* bacteremia. *Clin Infect Dis* **20**: 564.

Butler T (1994). *Yersinia* infections: centennial of the discovery of the plague bacillus. *Clin Infect Dis* **19**: 655.

Camiolo SM, Beck ME, Reynard AM (1975). Tetracycline resistance in *Escherichia coli* isolates from hospital patients. *Antimicrob Ag Chemother* **8**: 488.

Candanoza C, Ellner PD (1975). Differences in susceptibility of Enterobacteriaceae and penicillin-resistant *Staphylococcus aureus* to tetracycline and minocycline. *Antimicrob Ag Chemother* **7**: 227.

Caniza MA, Granger DL, WIlson KH *et al.* (1995). *Bartonella hensellae*: etiology of pulmonary nodules in a patient with depressed cell-mediated immunity. *Clin Infect Dis* **20**: 1505.

Carney S, Butcher RA, Dawborn JK, Pattison G (1974). Minocycline excretion and distribution in relation to renal function in man. *Clin Exper Pharmacol Physiol* **1**: 299.

Carpenter CCJ, Wallace CK, Mitra PP *et al.* (1965). Antibiotic therapy in cholera. *Proc Chol Res Symp*, p. 190. US Dept Hlth, Ed, Welfare.

Carrilho F, Bosch J, Arroyo V *et al.* (1977). Renal failure associated with demeclocycline in cirrhosis. *Ann Intern Med* **87**: 195.

Carson JL, Strom BL, Duff A *et al.* (1993). Acute liver disease associated with erythromycins, sulfonamides, and tetracyclines. *Ann Intern Med* **119**: 576.

Carter MP, Wilson F (1963). Antibiotics and congenital malformations. *Lancet* **i**: 1267.

Cartwright AC, Hatfield HL, Yeadon A, London E (1975). A comparison of the bioavailability of minocycline capsules and film-coated tablets. *J Antimicrob Chemother* **1**: 317.

Castell DO, Sparks HA (1965). Nephrogenic diabetes insipidus due to demethylchlortetracycline hydrochloride. *JAMA* **193**: 237.

CDC (Center for Disease Control) (1975). Vestibular reactions to minocycline follow-up. *MMWR* **24**: 55.

CDC (Center for Disease Control) (1976). Vestibular reactions to minocycline – Scotland. *MMWR* **25**: 31.

CDC (Center for Disease Control) (1978). Penicillinase-(beta-lactamase-). producing *Neisseria gonorrhoeae* – worldwide. *MMWR* **27**: 10.

CDC (Center for Disease Control) (1980). *Vibrio cholerae* – Bangladesh. *MMWR* **29**: 119.

CDC (Centers for Disease Control) (1983). Tularemic pneumonia – Tennessee. *MMWR* **32**: 262.

CDC (Centers for Disease Control) (1985). Tetracycline-resistant *Neisseria gonorrhoeae* – Georgia, Pennsylvania, New Hampshire. *MMWR* **34**: 563.

CDC (Centers for Disease Control) (1993a). Imported cholera associated with a newly described toxigenic *Vibrio cholerae* 0139 strain-California, 1993. *JAMA* **270**: 428.

CDC (Centers for Disease Control) (1993b). Sexually transmitted diseases treatment guidelines. *MMWR* **42** (No RR-14): 20; 27; 47; 56.

CDC (Centers for Disease Control) (1994). Human plague-India, 1994. *MMWR* **43**: 689.

CDC (Centers for Disease Control) (1995). Human granulocytic ehrlichiosis – New York, 1995. *MMWR* **44**: 593.

Chang HR, Comte R, Pechére J-C (1990). *In vitro* and *in vivo* effects of doxycycline on *Toxoplasma gondii*. *Antimicrob Ag Chemother* **34**: 775.

Chang HR, Comte R, Piguet P-F, Pechére J-C (1991). Activity of minocycline against *Toxoplasma gondii* infection in mice. *J Antimicrob Chemother* **27**: 639.

Channer KS, Hollanders D (1981). Tetracycline-induced oesophageal ulceration. *Brit Med J* **282**: 1359.

Channer KS, Virjee J (1982). Effect of posture and drink volume on the swallowing of capsules. *Brit Med J* **285**: 1702.

Charpentier E, Gerbaud G, Courvalin P (1994). Presence of the *Listeria* tetracycline resistance gene tet(s). in *Enterococcus faecalis*. *Antimicrob Ag Chemother* **38**: 2330.

Charpentier E, Gerbaud G, Jacquet C *et al.* (1995). Incidence of antibiotic resistance in *Listeria* species. *J Infect Dis* **172**: 277.

Chattopadhyay B, Harding E (1975). *In-vitro* minocycline activity against tetracycline-resistant *Staphylococcus aureus*. *Lancet* i: 405.

Chirgwin K, Roblin PM, Hammerschlag MR (1989). *In vitro* susceptibilities of *Chlamydia pneumoniae* (*Chlamydia* sp. strain TWAR). *Antimicrob Ag Chemother* **33**: 1634.

Chodosh S, Tuck J, Pizzuto D (1988). Comparative trials of doxycycline versus amoxicillin, cephalexin and enoxacin in bacterial infections in chronic bronchitis and asthma. *Scand J Infect Dis* (Suppl 53): 22.

Cholera Working Group, International Centre for Diarrhoeal Diseases Research, Bangladesh (1993). Large epidemic of cholera-like disease in Bangladesh caused by *Vibrio cholerae* 0139 synonym Bengal. *Lancet* **342**: 387.

Chopra I (1986). Genetic and biochemical basis of tetracycline resistance. *J Antimicrob Chemother* **18** (Suppl C): 51.

Chopra I (1994). Tetracycline analogs whose primary target is not the bacterial ribosome. *Antimicrob Ag Chemother* **38**: 637.

Chopra I, Hacker K (1986). Inhibition of K88–mediated adhersion of *Escherichia coli* to mammalian receptors by antibiotics that affect bacterial protein synthesis. *J Antimicrob Chemother* **18**: 441.

Chopra I, Howe TGB, Linton AH *et al.* (1981). The tetracyclines: prospects at the beginning of the 1980s. *J Antimicrob Chemother* **8**: 5.

Chopra I, Hawkey PM, HInton M (1992). Tetracyclines, molecular and clinical aspects. *J Antimicrob Chemother* **29**: 245.

Chow AW, Jewesson PJ (1985). Pharmacokinetics and safety of anti-micirobial agents during pregnancy. *Rev Infect Dis* **7**: 287.

Chow AW, Pattern V, Guze LB (1975). Comparative susceptibility of anaerobic bacteria to minocycline, doxycycline, and tetracycline. *Antimicrob Ag Chemother* **7**: 46.

Chow AW, Pattern V, Bednorz D (1978). Susceptibility of *Campylobacter fetus* to twenty-two antimicrobial agents. *Antimicrob Ag Chemother* **13**: 416.

Cisneros JM, Pachán J, Cuello JA, Martinez A (1989). *Brucella* endocarditis cured by medical treatment. *J Infect Dis* **160**: 907.

Cisneros JM, Viciana P, Colmenero J *et al.* (1990). Multicenter prospective study of treatment of *Brucella melitensis* brucellosis with doxycycline for 6 weeks plus streptomycin for 2 weeks. *Antimicrob Ag Chemother* **34**: 881.

Clendennen TE, Echeverria P, Saengeur S *et al.* (1992). Antibiotic susceptibility survey of *Neisseria gonorrhoeae* in Thailand. *Antimicrob Ag Chemother* **36**: 1682.

Clendinnen IJ (1974). Doxycycline in the treatment of chronic lung infections. *Med J Aust* **1**: 9: .

Clyde DF, Miller RM, DuPont HL, Hornick RB (1971). Antimalarial effects of tetracyclines in man. *J Trop Med* **74**: 238.

Cohlan SQ, Bevelander G, Tiamsic T (1963). Growth inhibition of prematures receiving tetracycline. *Amer J Dis Child* **105**: 453.

Cole JJ, Charles BG, Ravenscroft PJ (1980). Interaction of cimetidine with tetracycline absorption. *Lancet* ii: 536.

Collins FJ, Matthews HR, Baker SE, Strakova J (1979). Drug-induced oesophageal injury. *Brit Med J* **1**: 1673.

Colmenero JD, Fernández-Gallardo LC, Argúndez JAG *et al.* (1994). Possible implications of doxycycline-rifampin interaction for treatment of brucellosis. *Antimicrob Ag Chemother* **38**: 2798.

Colwell EJ, Hickman RL, Kosakal S (1972). Tetracycline treatment of chloroquine-resistant falciparum malaria in Thailand. *JAMA* **220**: 684.

Communicable Diseases Scotland (1981). Tetracycline resistance in beta haemolytic streptococci isolated at Ruchill Hospital, 1978–1980. *CDS Weekly Report* **15** (43): 7.

Conde-Glez CJ, Calderón E, Echániz G *et al.* (1988). Serogroup specificity and antimicrobial susceptibilities of *Neisseria gonorrhoeae* isolated in Mexico City. *J Antimicrob Chemother* **21**: 413.

Controni G, Friedman G, Ficke M (1978). Update of *Shigella* gastro-enteritis: changing patterns of antibiotic resistance, 1964–1976 In *Current Chemotherapy: Proceedings of the 10th International Congress of Chemotherapy, Zurich/Switzerland, 1977* (Siegenthaler W, Lüthy R, eds). p. 169. Washington DC: American Society for Microbiology.

Cook GC (1984). Aetiology and pathogenesis of postinfective tropical malabsorption (Tropical Sprue). *Lancet* i: 721.

Copperman IJ (1967). Hypersensitivity to tetracycline. *Lancet* ii: 610.

Council on Drugs (1969). Evaluation of a new antibacterial agent: doxycycline monohydrate and doxycycline hyclate (vibramycin). *JAMA* **209**: 549.

Cox M, Guzzo J, Morrison G, Singer I (1977). Demeclocycline and therapy of hyponatraemia. *Ann Intern Med* **86**: 113.

Crowson TD, Head LH, Ferrante WA (1976). Esophageal ulcers associated with tetracycline therapy. *JAMA* **235**: 2747.

Crues JVIII, Murray BE, Moellering RC Jr (1979). *In vitro* activity of three tetracycline antibiotics against *Acinetobacter calcoaceticus* subsp ani-tratus. *Antimicrob Ag Chemother* **16**: 690.

Csonka GW, Spitzer RJ (1969). Lincomycin, non-gonococcal urethritis, and mycoplasmata. *Brit J Vener Dis* **45**: 52.

Cummings MC, McCormack WM (1990). Increase in resistance of *Mycoplasma hominis* to tetracyclines. *Antimicrob Ag Chemother* **34**: 2297.

Cundliffe E, McQuillen K (1967). Bacterial protein synthesis: the effects of antibiotics. *J Molec Biol* **30**: 137.

Cunha BA, Jonas M (1981). Legionnaires' disease treated with doxycycline. *Lancet* ii: 1107.

Damjanov I, Arnold R, Faour M (1968). Tetracycline toxicity in a nonpregnant woman. *JAMA* **204**: 934.

Dangor Y, Ballard RC, Miller SD, Koornhof HJ (1990). Antimicrobial susceptibility of *Haemophilus ducreyi*. *Antimicrob Ag Chemother* **34**: 1303.

Darougar S (1981). Chlamydial ocular infection. *J Antimicrob Chemother* **5**: 350.

Darouiche R, Wright C, Hamill R *et al.* (1991). Eradication of colonization by methicillin-resistant *Staphylococcus aureus* by using oral minocy-cline-rifampin and topical mupirocin. *Antimicrob Ag Chemother* **35**: 1612.

Dawson CR, Schachter J (1985). Strategies for treatment and control of blinding trachoma: cost-effectiveness of topical or systemic antibiotics. *Rev Infect Dis* **7**: 768.

Dawson CR, Ostler HB, Hanna L *et al.* (1971). Tetracyclines in the treatment of chronic trachoma in American Indians. *J Infect Dis* **124**: 255.

Dawson CR, Daghfous T, Whitcher J *et al.* (1981). Intermittent trachoma chemotherapy: a controlled trial of topical tetracycline or erythromycin. *Bull Wld Hlth Org* **59**: 91.

De S, Chaudhuri A, Dutta P *et al.* (1976). Doxycycline in the treatment of cholera. *Bull Wld Hlth Org* **54**: 177.

Del Bene VE, Rogers M (1975). Comparison of tetracycline and minocycline transport in *Escherichia coli*. *Antimicrob Ag Chemother* **7**: 801.

Deppermann K-M, Lode H, Höffken G *et al.* (1989). Influence of ranitidine, pirenzepine, and aluminium magnesium hydroxide on the bioavailability of various antibiotics, including amoxicillin, cephalexin, doxycycline, and amoxicillin-clavulanic acid. *Antimicrob Ag Chemother* **33**: 1901.

De Troyer A (1977). Demeclocycline. Treatment for syndrome of inappropriate antidiuretic hormone secretion. *JAMA* **237**: 2723.

De Troyer A, Demanet J-C (1975). Correction of antidiuresis by demeclocycline. *New Engl J Med* **293**: 915.

De Troyer A, Pilloy W, Broeckaert I, Demanet J-C (1976). Demeclocycline treatment of water retention in cirrhosis. *Ann Intern Med* **85**: 336.

Devine LF, Johnson DP, Hagerman CR *et al.* (1971). The effect of minocycline on meningococcal nasopharyngeal carrier state in naval personnel. *Amer J Epidemiol* **93**: 337.

Devine LF, Springer GL, Frazier WE *et al.* (1972). Selective monocycline and rifampin treatment of group C meningococcal carriers in a new naval recruit camp. *Amer J Med Sci* **263**: 79.

Devine LF, Pollard RB, Krumpe PE *et al.* (1973). Field trial of the efficacy of a previously proposed regimen using minocycline and rifampin sequentially for the elimination of meningococci from healthy carriers. *Amer J Epidemiol* **97**: 394.

Dewsnup DH, Wright DN (1984). *In vitro* susceptibility of *Nocardia asteroides* to 25 antimicrobial agents. *Antimicrob Ag Chemother* **25**: 165.

Dimmling T (1960). Experimental and clinical investigations with pyrrolidi-nomethyl tetracycline. *Antibiot Annual 1959–1969*: 350.

Dornbusch K (1976). The detection of doxycycline activity in human bone. *Scand J Infect Dis* (Suppl 9): 47.

Dotevall L, Hagberg L (1989). Penetration of doxycycline into cerebrospinal fluid in patients treated for suspected Lyme neuroborreliosis. *Antimicrob Ag Chemother* **33**: 1078.

Dotevall L, Alestig K, Hanner P *et al.* (1988). The use of doxycycline in nervous system *Borrelia burgdorferi* infection. *Scand J Infect Dis* (Suppl 53): 74.

Dousa TP, Wilson DM (1973). Tetracyclines: interference with ADH-responsive cyclic AMP system in human renal medulla. *Clin Res* **21**: 75.

Dowling HF, Lepper MH (1964). Hepatic reactions to tetracycline. *JAMA* **188**: 307.

Drew TM, Altman R, Black K, Goldfield M (1976). Minocycline for prophylaxis of infection with *Neisseria meningitidis*: high rate of side effects in recipients. *J Infect Dis* **133**: 194.

Duchin JS, Breiman RF, Diamond A *et al.* (1995). High prevalence of multidrug-resistant *Streptococcus pneumoniae* among children in a rural Kentucky community. *Pediatr Infect Dis J* **14**: 745.

Duggar BM *et al.* (1948). Aureomycin: product of continuing search for new antibiotic. *Ann NY Acad Sci* **51**: 177; quoted by Ory (1970).

Dumler JS, Bakken JS (1995). Ehrlichiol diseases of humans: emerging tick-borne infections. *Clin Infect Dis* **20**: 1102.

Eastwood JB, Bailey RR, Curtis JR *et al.* (1970). Tetracycline in renal failure. *Lancet* ii: 39, 262.

Echeverria P, Sack RB, Blacklow NR *et al.* (1984). Prophylactic doxycycline for travelers' diarrhea in Thailand Further supportive evidence of *Aeromonas hydrophila* as an enteric pathogen. *Amer J Epidemiol* **120**: 912.

Edlind TD (1989). Tetracyclines as antiparasitic agents: lipophilic derivatives are highly active against *Giardia lamblia in vitro*. *Antimicrob Ag Chemother* **33**: 2144.

Edwards OM, Huskisson EC, Taylor RT (1970). Azotaemia aggravated by tetracycline. *Brit Med J* **1**: 26.

Eickhoff TC, Bennett JV, Hayes PS, Feeley J (1970). *Pseudomonas pseudomallei*: susceptibility to chemotherapeutic agents. *J Infect Dis* **121**: 95.

Ekman M-R, Grayston JT, Visakorpi R *et al.* (1993). An epidemic of infections due to *Chlamydia pneumoniae* in military conscripts. *Clin Infect Dis* **17**: 420.

Eliasson R, Malmborg A-S (1976). Concentrations of doxycycline in human seminal plasma. *Scand J Infect Dis* (Suppl 9): 32.

Eliopoulos GM, Wennersten CB, Cole G, Moellering RC (1994). *In vitro* activities of two glycylcyclines against Gram-positive bacteria. *Antimicrob Ag Chemother* **38**: 534.

Eneroth C-M, Lundberg C, Malmström L, Ramström G (1978). Antibiotic concentrations in saliva of purulent parotitis. *Scand J Infect Dis* **10**: 219.

Ericsson CD, Feldman S, Pickering LK, Clery TG (1982). Influence of subsalicylate bismuth on absorption of doxycycline. *JAMA* **247**: 2266.

Evans RT, Taylor-Robinson D (1978). The incidence of tetracycline-resistant strains of *Ureaplasma urealyticum*. *J Antimicrob Chemother* **4**: 57.

Evans W, Hansman D (1963). Tetracycline-resistant pneumococcus. *Lancet* i: 451.

Everett ED, Nelson RA (1975). Pulmonary melioidosis Observations in thirty-nine cases. *Amer Rev Resp Dis* **112**: 331.

Falck G, Heyman L, Gnarpe J, Gnarpe H (1994). *Chlamydia pneumoniae* (TWAR): a common agent in acute bronchitis. *Scand J Infect Dis* **26**: 179.

Fanning WL, Gump DW, Sofferman RA (1977). Side-effects of minocycline: a double blind study. *Antimicrob Ag Chemother* **11**: 712.

Farrell ID, Hinchliffe PM, Robertson L (1976). Sensitivity of *Brucella* spp. to tetracycline and its analogues. *J Clin Path* **29**: 1097.

Fass RJ, Ruiz DE, Prior RB, Perkins RL (1976). *In vitro* activity of gentamicin and minocycline alone and in combination against bacteria associated with intra-abdominal sepsis. *Antimicrob Ag Chemother* **10**: 34.

Fellner MJ, Baer RL (1965). Anaphylactic reaction to tetracycline in a penicillin-allergic patient. Immunologic studies. *JAMA* **192**: 997.

Fennerty MB (1994). *Helicobacter pylori*. *Arch Intern Med* **154**: 721.

Fenske NA, Millns JL, Greer KE (1980). Minocycline-induced pigmentation at sites of cutaneous inflammation. *JAMA* **244**: 1103.

Fernández-Guerrero ML, Muelas JM, Arguado JM *et al.* (1988). Q fever endocarditis on porcine bioprosthetic valves. *Ann Intern Med* **108**: 209.

Ferrante MA, Dolan MJ (1993). Q fever meningoencephalitis in a soldier returning from the Persian Gulf war. *Clin Infect Dis* **16**: 489.

Finland M, Garrod LP (1960). Demethylchlortetracycline. *Brit Med J* **2**: 959.

Finland M, Garner C, Wilcox C, Sabath LD (1976a). Susceptibility of beta-hemolytic streptococci to 65 antibacterial agents. *Antimicrob Ag Chemother* **9**: 11.

Finland M, Garner C, Wilcox C, Sabath LD (1976b). Susceptibility of pneumococci and *Haemophilus influenzae* to antibacterial agents. *Antimicrob Ag Chemother* **9**: 274.

Fishbein DB, Dennis DT (1995). Tick-borne diseases- a growing risk. *New Engl J Med* **333**: 452.

Forbes G (1994). *Helicobacter pylori* eradication: who, why and how in 1994? *Med J Aust* **161**: 291.

Forgacs P, Kundsin RB, Margles SW *et al.* (1993). A case of *Ureaplasma urealyticum* septic arthritis in a patient with hypogammaglobulinemia. *Clin Infect Dis* **16**: 293.

Forsgren A, Gnarpe H (1982). The effect of antibacterial agents on the association between bacteria and leukocytes. *Scand J Infect Dis* **33**: 115.

Forsgren A, Schmeling D (1977). Effect of antibiotics on chemotaxis of human leukocytes. *Antimicrob Ag Chemother* **11**: 580.

Forsgren A, Walder M (1982). *Haemophilus influenzae*, Pneumococci, Group A streptococci and *Staphylococcus aureus*: sensitivity of out-patient strains to commonly prescribed antibiotics. *Scand J Infect Dis* **14**: 39.

Foster A, Klaus V (1995). Ophthalmia neonatorum in developing countries. *New Engl J Med* **332**: 600.

Foy HM, Kenny GE, McMahan R *et al.* (1970). *Mycoplasma pneumoniae* pneumonia in an urban area. *JAMA* **214**: 1666.

Fraise AP, Brenwald N, Andrews JM, Wise R (1995). *In-vitro* activity of two glycylcyclines against enterococci resistant to other agents. *J Antimicrob Chemother* **35**: 877.

Freeman LD, Hooper DR, Lathen DF *et al.* (1983). Brief prophylaxis with doxycycline for the prevention of travelers' diarrhea. *Gastroenterology* **84**: 276.

French GL, Woo ML, Hui YW, Chan KY (1989). Antimicrobial susceptibilities of halophilic vibrios. *J Antimicrob Chemother* **24**: 183.

Frost JA, Rowe B (1983). Plasmid-determined antibiotic resistance in *Shigella flexneri* isolated in England and Wales between 1974 and 1978. *J Hyg Camb* **90**: 27.

Furey WW, Tan C (1969). Anaphylactic shock due to oral demethylchlortetracycline. *Ann Intern Med* **70**: 357.

Gascoyne DM, Heritage J, Hawkey PM *et al.* (1991). Molecular evolution of tetracycline-resistance plasmids carrying Tet M found in *Neisseria gonorrhoeae* from different countries. *J Antimicrob Chemother* **28**: 173.

Gascoyne-Binzi DM, Heritage J, Hawkey PM, Sprott MS (1994a). Characterisation of a tet (M)-carrying plasmid from Neisseria meningitidis. *J Antimicrob Chemother* **34**: 1015.

Gascoyne-Binzi DM, Hawkey PM, Heritage J (1994b). The distribution of variants of the Tet M determinant in tetracycline-resistant *Neisseria gonorrhoeae*. *J Antimicrob Chemother* **33**: 1011.

Gästrin U, Josephson S (1966). Tetracyclines and the teeth. *Lancet* **ii**: 492.

Geheb M, Cox M (1980). Renal effects of demeclocycline. *JAMA* **243**: 2519.

Gelber RH (1987). Activity of minocycline in *Mycobacterium leprae*-infected mice. *J Infect Dis* **156**: 236.

Gelber RH, Siu P, Tsang M *et al.* (1991). Effect of low-level and intermittent minocycline therapy on the growth of *Mycobacterium leprae* in mice. *Antimicrob Ag Chemother* **35**: 992.

George CRP, Evans RA (1971). Tetracycline toxicity in renal failure. *Med J Aust* **1**: 1271.

George CRP, Guiness MDG, Lark DJ, Evans RA (1973). Minocycline toxicity in renal failure. *Med J Aust* **1**: 640.

Geschwind A (1984). Oesophagitis and oesophageal ulceration following ingestion of doxycycline tablets. *Med J Aust* **140**: 112.

Gilbert GL (1993). Brucellosis: continuing risk. *Med J Aust* **159**: 147.

Glette J, Sandberg S (1986). Phototoxicity of tetracyclines as related to singlet oxygen production and uptake by polymorphonuclear leukocytes. *Biochem Pharmacol* **35**: 2883.

Glette J Sandberg S, Hopen G, Solberg CO (1984). Influence of tetracyclines on human polymorphonuclear leukocyte function. *Antimicrob Ag Chemother* **25**: 354.

Gnarpe H, Dornbusch K, Hägg O (1976). Doxycycline concentration levels in bone, soft tissue and serum after intravenous infusion of doxycycline. *Scand J Infect Dis* (Suppl 9): 54.

Goldstein EJC, Citron DM, Richwald GA (1988). Lack of *in vitro* efficacy of oral forms of certain cephalosporins, erythromycin and oxacillin against *Pasteurella multocida*. *Antimicrob Ag Chemother* **32**: 213.

Golledge CL, Riley TV (1995). *Clostridium difficile*-associated diarrhoea after doxycycline malaria prophylaxis. *Lancet* **345**: 1377.

Goodwin CW, Blake P, Blincow E (1986). The minimum inhibitory and bactericidal concentrations of antibiotics and anti-ulcer agents against *Campylobacter pyloridis*. *J Antimicrob Chemother* **17**: 309.

Gorbach SL, Bartlett JG (1974). Anaerobic infections (third of three parts). *New Engl J Med* **290**: 1289.

Gordts B, Vanhoof R, Hubrechts JM *et al.* (1982). *In-vitro* activity of 21 antimicrobial agents against *Neisseria gonorrhoeae* in Brussels. *Brit J Vener Dis* **58**: 23.

Gould JC, Murdoch JMcC (1960). The long-term management of chronic bronchitis with antibiotics. *Antibiot Annual 1959–1960*: 190.

Graham JR (1995). *Helicobacter pylori*: human pathogen or simply an opportunist? *Lancet* **345**: 1095.

Grayston JT (1992). Infections caused by *Chlamydia pneumoniae* strain TWAR. *Clin Infect Dis* **15**: 757.

Grayston JT, Campbell LA, Kuo C-C *et al.* (1990). A new respiratory tract pathogen: *Chlamydia pneumoniae* strain TWAR. *J Infect Dis* **161**: 618.

Greenberg PA, Sanford JP (1967). Removal and absorption of antibiotics in patients with renal failure undergoing peritoneal dialysis: tetracycline, chloramphenicol, kanamycin, and colistimethate. *Ann Intern Med* **66**: 465.

Gross RJ, Ward LR, Threlfall EJ *et al.* (1982). Drug resistance among infantile enteropathogenic *Escherichia coli* strains isolated in the United Kingdom. *Brit Med J* **285**: 472.

Gross RJ, Threlfall EJ, Ward LR, Rowe B (1984). Drug resistance in *Shigella dysenteriae*, *S. flexneri* and *S. boydii* in England and Wales: increasing incidence of resistance to trimethoprim. *Brit Med J* **288**: 784.

Grossan M (1968). Management of infections of the ear, nose, and throat with a new tetracycline antibiotic, doxycycline. *Eye, Ear, Nose, Throat Mthly* **47**: 56.

Grossman ER, Walchek A, Freedman H (1971). Tetracyclines and permanent teeth: the relation between dose and tooth colour. *Pediatrics* **47**: 567.

Gudiol F, Pallares R, Carratala J *et al.* (1989). Randomized double-blind evaluation of ciprofloxacin and doxycycline for Mediterranean spotted fever. *Antimicrob Ag Chemother* **33**: 987.

Gump DW, Ashikaga T, Fink TJ, Radin AM (1977). Side effects of minocycline: different dosage regimens. *Antimicrob Ag Chemother* **12**: 642.

Gutmann L, Goldstein FW, Kitzis MD *et al.* (1983). Susceptibility of *Nocardia asteroides* to 46 antibiotics including 22 beta-lactams. *Antimicrob Ag Chemother* **23**: 248.

Guttler RB, Beaty HN (1972). Minocycline in the chemoprophylaxis of meningococcal disease. *Antimicrob Ag Chemother* **1**: 397.

Hächler H, Kayser FH, Berger-Bächi B (1987). Homology of a transferable tetracycline resistance determinant of *Clostridium difficile* with *Streptococcus* (*Enterococcus*) *faecalis* transposon Tn 916. *Antimicrob Ag Chemother* **31**: 1033.

Hall WH (1990). Modern chemotherapy for brucellosis in humans. *Rev Infect Dis* **12**: 1060.

Hammerschlag MR (1994). Antimicrobial susceptibility and therapy of infections caused by *Chlamydia pneumoniae*. *Antimicrob Ag Chemother* **38**: 1873.

Hammerschlag MR, Cummings C, Roblin PM (1989). Efficacy of neonatal ocular prophylaxis for the prevention of chlamydial and gonococcal conjunctivitis. *New Engl J Med* **320**: 769.

Hammerschlag MR, Chirgwin K, Roblin PM *et al.* (1992). Persistent infection with *Chlamydia pneumoniae* following acute respiratory illness *Clin Infect Dis* **14**: 178.

Hammond GW, Slutchuk M, Scatliff J *et al.* (1980). Epidemiologic, clinical laboratory and therapeutic features of an urban outbreak of chancroid in North America. *Rev Infect Dis* **2**: 867.

Hansman D (1975). *Haemophilus influenzae* Type b resistant to tetracycline. *Lancet* **ii**: 893.

Hansman D, Andrews G (1967). Hospital infection with pneumococci resistant to tetracycline. *Med J Aust* **1**: 498.

Hanson GC (1968). A death from tetracycline. *Postgrad Med J* **44**: 870.

Hansson JB, Walder M, Juhlin I (1981). Susceptibility of shigellae to mecillinam, nalidixic acid, trimethoprim, and five other antimicrobial agents. *Antimicrob Ag Chemother* **19**: 271.

Hartnett BJS, Marlin GE (1976). Doxycycline in bronchial secretions. *Med J Aust* **1**: 280.

Hassam ZA, Shaw EJ, Shooter RA (1978). Changes in antibiotic sensitivity in strains of *Staphylococcus aureus*, 1952–78. *Brit Med J* **2**: 536.

Hattwick MAW, Retailliau H, O'Brien RJ *et al.* (1978). Fatal Rocky Mountain spotted fever. *JAMA* **240**: 1499.

Hauser WE Jr, Remington JS (1982). Effect of antibiotics on the immune response. *Amer J Med* **72**: 711.

Hayek A, Ramirez J (1974). Demeclocycline-induced diabetes insipidus. *JAMA* **229**: 676.

Heimdahl A, Nord C-E (1983). Influence of doxycycline on the normal human flora and colonization of the oral cavity and colon. *Scand J Infect Dis* **15**: 293.

Heritage J, Hawkey PM (1988). Tetracycline-resistant *Neisseria gonorrhoeae*. *J Antimicrob Chemother* **22**: 575.

Hey H, Jørgensen F, Sørensen, K *et al.* (1982). Oesophageal transit of six commonly used tablets and capsules. *Brit Med J* **285**: 1717.

Hill GB (1977). Therapeutic evaluation of minocycline and tetracycline for mixed anaerobic infection in mice. *Antimicrob Ag Chemother* **11**: 625.

Hoeprich PD, Warshauer DM (1974). Entry of four tetracyclines into saliva and tears. *Antimicrob Ag Chemother* **5**: 330.

Höjer H, Wetterfors J (1976). Concentration of doxycycline in bowel tissue and postoperative infections. *Scand J Infect Dis* (Suppl 9): 100.

Holmberg K, Nord C-E, Dornbusch K (1977). Antimicrobial *in vitro* susceptibility of *Actinomyces israelii* and *Arachnia propionica*. *Scand J Infect Dis* **9**: 40.

Holmberg SD, Farmer JJIII (1984). *Aeromonas hydrophila* and *Plesiomonas shigelloides* as causes of intestinal infections. *Rev Infect Dis* **6**: 633.

Hook EW III, Brady WE, Reichart CA *et al.* (1989). Determinants of emergence of antibiotic-resistant *Neisseria gonorrhoeae*. *J Infect Dis* **159**: 900.

Hoshiwara I, Ostler HB, Hanna L *et al.* (1973). Doxycycline treatment of chronic trachoma. *JAMA* **224**: 220.

Hosking SW, Ling TKW, Yung MY *et al.* (1992). Randomised controlled trial of short term treatment to eradicate *Helicobacter pylori* in patients with duodenal ulcer. *Brit Med J* **305**: 502.

Hosking SW, Ling TKW, Chung SCS *et al.* (1994). Duodenal ulcer healing by eradication of *Helicobacter pylori* without anti-acid treatment: randomised controlled trial. *Lancet* **343**: 508.

Houin G, Brunner F, Nebout Th *et al.* (1983). The effects of chronic renal insufficiency on the pharmacokinetics of doxycycline in man. *Brit J Clin Pharmac* **16**: 245.

Howard AJ, Hince CJ, Williams JD (1978). Antibiotic resistance in *Streptococcus pneumoniae* and *Haemophilus influenzae*. Report of a study group on bacterial resistance. *Brit Med J* **1**: 1657.

Howe C, Sampath A, Spotnitz M (1971). The *Pseudomallei* group: a review. *J Infect Dis* **124**: 598.

Hryniewicz W (1994). Bacterial resistance in Eastern Europe-selected problems. *Scand J Infect Dis* (Suppl 93): 33.

Hughes D (1976). Chemoprophylaxis in chronic bronchitis. *J Antimicrob Chemother* **2**: 320.

Isaäcson M, Clarke KR, Ellacombe GH *et al.* (1974). The recent cholera outbreak in the South African gold mining industry. A preliminary report. *S Afr Med J* **48**: 2557.

Isenberg SJ, Apt L, Wood M (1995). A controlled trial of povidone-iodine as prophylaxis against ophthalmia neonatorum. *New Engl J Med* **332**: 562.

Jacobson JA, Daniel B (1975). Vestibular reactions associated with minocycline. *Antimicrob Ag Chemother* **8**: 453.

Jaffe HW, Biddle JW, Johnson SR, Wiesner PJ (1981). Infections due to penicillinase-producing *Neisseria gonorrhoeae* in the United States: 1976–1980. *J Infect Dis* **144**: 191.

Janda JM, Guthertz LS, Kokka RP, Shimada T (1994). Aeromonas species in septicemia: laboratory characteristics and clinical observations. *Clin Infect Dis* **19**: 77.

Jawetz E (1969). Chemotherapy of chlamydial infections. *Adv Pharmacol Chemother* **7**: 253.

Ji B, Jamet P, Perani EG *et al.* (1993). Powerful bactericidal activities of clarithromycin and minocycline against *Mycobacterium leprae* in lepromatous leprosy. *J Infect Dis* **168**: 188.

Johnson RC (1989). Isolation techniques for spirochetes and their sensitivity to antibiotics *in vitro* and *in vivo*. *Rev Infect Dis* **11** (Suppl 6): 1505.

Johnson, RC, Kodner C, Russell M (1987). *In vitro* and *in vivo* susceptibility of the Lyme disease spirochete *Borrelia burgdorferi* to four antimicrobial agents. *Antimicrob Ag Chemother* **31**: 164.

Johnstone FRC, Cockcroft WH (1968). *Clostridium welchii* resistance to tetracycline. *Lancet* **i**: 660.

Joint ICMR-GWB-WHO Cholera Study Group, Calcutta, India (1971). Effect of tetracycline on cholera carriers in households of cholera patients. *Bull Wld Hlth Org* **45**: 451.

Jones BL, Wilcox MH (1995). Aeromonas infections and their treatment. *J Antimicrob Chemother* **35**: 453.

Jones RB, Van der Pol B, Martin DH, Shepard MK (1990). Partial characterization of *Chlamydia trachomatis* isolates resistant to multiple antibiotics. *J Infect Dis* **162**: 1309.

Jonsson M, Tunevall G (1976). Selective pressure of tetracyclines on the faecal flora A comparison between tetracycline and doxycycline. *Scand J Infect Dis* (Suppl 9): 89.

Joseph SW, DeBell RM, Brown WP (1978). *In vitro* response to chloramphenicol, tetracycline, ampicillin, gentamicin, and beta-lactamase production by *Halophilic vibrios* from human and environmental sources. *Antimicrob Ag Chemother* **13**: 244.

Kahlmeter G, Kamme C (1972). Tetracycline-resistant Group A streptococci and pneumococci. *Scand J Infect Dis* **4**: 193.

Kaplan MA, Albright H, Buckwalter FH (1960). A new tetracycline antibiotic for parenteral use. *Antibiot Annual 1959–1960*: 365.

Karney WW, Pedersen AHB, Nelson M *et al.* (1977). Spectinomycin versus tetracycline for the treatment of gonorrhea. *New Engl J Med* **296**: 889.

Katiyar SK, Edlind TD (1991). Enhanced antiparasitic activity of lipophilic tetracyclines: role of uptake. *Antimicrob Ag Chemother* **35**: 2198.

Kauffman CA, Bergman AG, Hertz CS (1979). Antimicrobial resistance of haemophilus species in patients with chronic bronchitis. *Amer Rev Respir Dis* **120**: 1382.

Kelsey DS (1979). Rocky Mountain Spotted Fever. *Pediatr Clin North Amer* **26**: 367.

Kenny GE, Cartwright FD (1994). Susceptibilities of *Mycoplasma hominis*, *Mycoplasma pneumoniae*, and *Ureoplasma urealyticum* to new glycylcyclines in comparison with those to older tetracyclines. *Antimicrob Ag Chemother* **38**: 2628.

Khan MU (1982). Efficacy of short course antibiotic prophylaxis in controlling cholera in contacts during epidemic. *J Trop Med Hyg* **85**: 27.

Khatib R, Thirumoorthi MC, Kelly B, Grady KJ (1995). Severe psittacosis during pregnancy and suppression of antibody response with early therapy. *Scand J Infect Dis* **27**: 519.

Kim J, Minamoto GY, Grieco MH (1991). Nocardial infection as a complication of AIDS: report of six cases and review. *Rev Infect Dis* **13**: 624.

Kinirons MJ (1983). Reduction in evidence in children's teeth of use of tetracyclines. *Brit Med J* **287**: 1515.

Kirkland KB, Wilkinson WE, Sexton DJ (1995). Therapeutic delay and mortality in cases of Rocky Mountain spotted fever. *Clin Infect Dis* **20**: 1118.

Kirkpatrick R (1978). Demeclocycline and renal insufficiency. *JAMA* **239**: 616.

Klastersky J, Cappel R, Rens B, Daneau D (1972). Clinical and bacteriological evaluation of intravenous doxycycline in severe hospital infections. *Curr Ther Res* **14**: 49.

Kline AH, Blattner RJ, Lunin M (1964). Transplacental effect of tetracyclines on teeth. *JAMA* **188**: 178.

Klugman KP, Koornhof HK, Kuhnle V *et al.* (1986). Meningitis and pneumonia due to novel multiply resistant pneumococci. *Brit Med J* **292**: 730.

Knapp JS, Zenilman JM, Biddle JW *et al.* (1987). Frequency and distribution in the United States of strains of *Neisseria gonorrhoeae* with plasmid-mediated, high-level resistance to tetracycline. *J Infect Dis* **155**: 819.

Koch-Weser J, Gilmore EB (1967). Benign intracranial hypertension in an adult after tetracycline therapy. *JAMA* **200**: 345.

Korkeila J (1971). Antianabolic effect of tetracyclines. *Lancet* **i**: 974.

Kounis NG (1975). Oxytetracycline-induced thrombocytopenic purpura. *JAMA* **231**: 734.

Kovacs GT, Westcott M, Rusden J *et al.* (1989). A prospective single-blind trial of minocycline and doxycycline in the treatment of genital *Chlamydia trachomatis* infection in women. *Med J Aust* **150**: 483.

Kraus SJ, Kaufman HW, Albritton WL *et al.* (1982). Chancroid therapy: a review of cases confirmed by culture. *Rev Inf Dis* **4** (Suppl): 848.

Krause W, Mathies H, Wulf K (1969). Fungaemia and funguria after oral administration of *Candida albicans*. *Lancet* **i**: 598.

Kristinsson A, Bentall HH (1967). Medical and surgical treatment of Q-fever endocarditis. *Lancet* **ii**: 693.

Kuck NA (1976). *In vitro* and *in vivo* activities of minocycline and other antibiotics against *Acinetobacter* (*Herellea-Mima*). *Antimicrob Ag Chemother* **9**: 493.

Kuharic HA, Roberts CE, Kirby WMM (1960). Tetracycline resistance of Group A beta haemolytic streptococci. *JAMA* **174**: 1779.

Kunelis CT, Peters JL, Edmondson HA (1965). Fatty liver of pregnancy and its relationship to tetracycline therapy. *Amer J Med* **38**: 359.

Kunin CM (1967). A guide to use of antibiotics in patients with renal disease. *Ann Intern Med* **67**: 151.

Kunin CM, Dornbush AC, Finland M (1959). Distribution and excretion of four tetracycline analogues in normal young men. *J Clin Invest* **38**: 1950.

Laga M, Plummer FA, Piot P *et al.* (1988). Prophylaxis of gonococcal and chlamydial ophthalmia neonatorum. A comparison of silver nitrate and tetracycline. *New Engl J Med* **318**: 653.

Landas SK, Schelper RL, Tio FO *et al.* (1986). Black thyroid syndrome: exaggeration of a normal process. *Clin Pathol* **85**: 411.

Lang R, Shasha B, Rubinstein E (1993). Therapy of experimental murine brucellosis with streptomycin alone and in combination with ciprofloxacin, doxycycline, and rifampin. *Antimicrob Ag Chemother* **37**: 2333.

Lasser AE, Steiner MM (1978). Tetracycline photo-onycholysis. *Pediatrics* **61**: 98.

Laufer D, Lew PD, Oberhansli I *et al.* (1986). Chronic Q fever endocarditis with massive splenomegaly in childhood. *J Pediatrics* **108**: 535.

Lawlor MT, Sullivan MC, Levitz RE *et al.* (1990). Treatment of prosthetic valve endocarditis due to methicillin-resistant *Staphylococcus aureus* with minocycline. *J Infect Dis* **161**: 812.

Le CT (1980). Tick-borne relapsing fever in children. *Pediatrics* **66**: 963.

Leading Article (1965). Tetracyclines in pregnancy. *Brit Med J* **1**: 743.

Leading Article (1982). Topical dilemmas in acne treatment. *Lancet* **ii**: 1138.

Leading Article (1983). *Bacillus cereus* as a systemic pathogen. *Lancet* **ii**: 1469.

Leelarasamee A, Bovornkitti S (1989). Melioidosis: review and update. *Rev Infect Dis* **11**: 413.

Lerman SJ, Kucera JC, Brunken JM (1979). Nasopharyngeal carriage of antibiotic-resistant *Haemophilus influenzae* in healthy children. *Pediatrics* **64**: 287.

Levy PY, Drancourt M, Etienne J *et al.* (1991). Comparison of different antibiotic regimens for therapy of 32 cases of Q fever endocarditis. *Antimicrob Ag Chemother* **35**: 533.

Lew HT, French SW (1966). Tetracycline nephrotoxicity and nonoliguric acute renal failure. *Arch Intern Med* **118**: 123.

Lewis MJ (1968). Transferable drug resistance and other transferable agents in strains of *Escherichia coli* from two human populations. *Lancet* **i**: 1389.

Li X-Z, Livermore DM, Nikaido H (1994). Role of efflux pump(s). in intrinsic resistance of *Pseudomonas aeruginosa*: resistance to tetracycline, chloramphenicol, and norfloxacin. *Antimicrob Ag Chemother* **38**: 1732.

Lieberman D, Luberman D, Boldur I *et al.* (1995). Q fever pneumonia in the Negev region of Israel: a review of 20 patients hospitalised over a period of one year. *J Infect* **30**: 135.

Liñares J, Garau J, Dominguez C, Pérez JL (1983). Antibiotic resistance and serotypes of *Streptococcus pneumoniae* from patients with community-acquired pneumococcal disease. *Antimicrob Ag Chemother* **23**: 545.

Lindenbaum J, Rund DG, Butler VP Jr *et al.* (1981). Inactivation of digoxin by the gut flora: reversal by antibiotic therapy. *New Engl J Med* **305**: 789.

Ling J, Chau PY, Leung YK *et al.* (1983). Antibiotic susceptibility of pneumococci and *Haemophilus influenzae* isolated from patients with acute exacerbations of chronic bronchitis: prevalence of tetracycline-resistant strains in Hong Kong. *J Infect* **6**: 33.

Little PJ, Bailey RR (1970). Tetracyclines and renal failure. *NZ Med J* **72**: 183.

Ljungberg B, Christensson B, Grubb R (1987). Failure of doxycycline treatment in aquarium-associated *Mycobacterium marinum* infections. *Scand J Infect Dis* **19**: 539.

Lloyd-Still JD, Grand RJ, Vawter GF (1974). Tetracycline hepatotoxicity in the differential diagnosis of postoperative jaundice. *J Pediatr* **84**: 366.

Lode H (1979). Penetration of antibiotics into the pleural fluid. *J Antimicrob Chemother* **5**: 122.

London AL, Siegel NJ, Zelson JH, Hayslett JP (1978). Nephrogenic diabetes insipidus due to demethylchlortetracycline hydrochloride in a child. *Pediatrics* **61**: 91.

Lowbury EJL, Cason JS (1954). Aureomycin and erythromycin therapy for *Str. pyogenes* in burns. *Brit Med J* **2**: 914.

Lowbury EJL, Hurst L (1956). Atypical anaerobic forms of *Streptococcus pyogenes* associated with tetracycline resistance. *J Clin Path* **9**: 59.

Luft BJ, Gorevic PD, Halperin JJ *et al* (1989). A perspective on the treatment of Lyme borreliosis. *Rev Infect Dis* **11** (Suppl 6): 1518.

Luger SW, Paparone P, Wormser GP *et al.* (1995). Comparison of cefuroxime axetil and doxycycline in treatment of patients with early Lyme disease associated with erythema migrans. *Antimicrob Ag Chemother* **39**: 661.

Lundberg C, Malmborg A-S (1973). Concentration of penicillin V and tetracycline in maxillary sinus secretions after repeated doses. *Scand J Infect Dis* **5**: 123.

Lundberg C, Malmborg A-S (1974). Concentration of penicillin and tetracycline in maxillary sinus secretion after a single dose. *Scand J Infect Dis* **6**: 79.

Lundsgaard-Hansen P, Senn A, Roos B, Waller U (1960). Staphylococcic enterocolitis. Report of six cases with two fatalities after intravenous administration of N-(pyrrolidinomethyl) tetracycline. *JAMA* **173**: 1008.

MacDonald H, Kelly RG, Allen ES *et al.* (1973). Pharmacokinetic studies on minocycline in man. *Clin Pharmacol Ther* **14**: 852.

Maderazo EG, Quintiliani R, Tilton RC *et al.* (1975). Activity of minocycline against *Acinetobacter calcoaceticus* var. *anitratus* (Syn. *Herellea vaginicola*). and *Serratia marcescens*. *Antimicrob Ag Chemother* **8**: 54.

Maesen FPV, Davies BI, Van den Bergh JJAM (1989). Doxycycline and minocycline in the treatment of respiratory infections: a double-blind comparative clinical, microbiological and pharmacokinetic study. *J Antimicrob Chemother* **23**: 123.

Magalhães M, Veras A (1984). Minocycline resistance among clinical isolates of *Ureaplasma urealyticum*. *J Infect Dis* **149**: 117.

Mahon WA, Wittenberg JVP, Tuffnel PG (1970). Studies on the absorption and distribution of doxycycline in normal patients and in patients with severely impaired renal function. *CMAJ* **103**: 1031.

Mahon WA, Johnson GE, Endrenyi L *et al.* (1976). The elimination of tritiated doxycycline in normal subjects and in patients with severely impaired renal function. *Scand J Infect Dis* (Suppl 9): 24.

Mahony JF, Lloyd-Jones D (1975). Serum doxycycline levels after intravenous administration in haemodialysis patients. *Med J Aust* **2**: 673.

Maier TW, Beilstein HR, Zubrzycki L (1974). Multiple antibiotic resistance in *Neisseria gonorrhoeae*. *Antimicrob Ag Chemother* **6**: 22.

Manavathu EK, Fernandez CL, Cooperman BS, Taylor DE (1990). Molecular studies on the mechanism of tetracycline resistance mediated by Tet(0). *Antimicrob Ag Chemother* **34**: 71.

Maness MJ, Sparling PF (1973). Multiple antibiotic resistance due to a single mutation in *Neisseria gonorrhoeae*. *J Infect Dis* **128**: 321.

Marrie TJ, Harczy M, Mann OE *et al.* (1990). Culture negative endocarditis probably due to *Chlamydia pneumoniae*. *J Infect Dis* **161**: 127.

Marlin GE, Cheng S (1979). Pharmacokinetics and tolerability of a single oral 600 mg dose of doxycycline. *Med J Aust* **1**: 575.

Maroon JC, Mealy J Jr (1971). Benign intracranial hypertension. Sequel to tetracycline therapy in a child. *JAMA* **216**: 1479.

Marshall BJ (1990). *Campylobacter pylori*: its link to gastritis and peptic ulcer disease. *Rev Infect Dis* **12** (Suppl 1): 87.

Martin ND, Barnard PD (1969). Prevalence of tetracycline staining in erupted teeth. *Med J Aust* **1**: 1286.

Martin WJ, Gardner M, Washington JAII (1972). *In vitro* antimicrobial susceptibility of anaerobic bacteria isolated from clinical specimens. *Antimicrob Ag Chemother* **1**: 148.

Masterton G, Schofield CBS (1974). Side-effects of minocycline hydrochloride. *Lancet* **ii**: 1139.

Maurin M, Gasquet S, Ducco C, Raoult D (1995). MICs of 28 antibiotic compounds for 14 *Bartonella* (formerly *Rochalimaea*). isolates. *Antimicrob Ag Chemother* **39**: 2387.

Mazumder DNG, Sirkar BK, De SP (1974). Minocycline in the treatment of cholera. A comparison with tetracycline. *Ind J Med Res* **62**: 712.

McCormack WM (1993). Susceptibility of mycoplasmas to antimicrobial agents: clinical implications. *Clin Infect Dis* **17** (Suppl 1): 200.

McCormack WM, Chowdhury AM, Jahangir N *et al.* (1968). Tetracycline prophylaxis in families of cholera patients. *Bull Wld Hlth Org* **38**: 787.

McGennis AJ (1978). Lithium carbonate and tetracycline interaction. *Brit Med J* **1**: 1183.

McGill RET (1974). Minocycline and beta-haemolytic streptococci. *Brit Med J* **3**: 625.

McHenry MC, Gavan TL, Vidt DG *et al.* (1972). Minocycline in renal failure. *Clin Pharmacol Ther* **13**: 146.

McIntosh HA, Storey E (1970). Tetracycline-induced tooth changes, Part 4: discoloration and hypoplasia induced by tetracycline analogues. *Med J Aust* **1**: 114.

McLean DR, Russell N, Khan MY (1992). Neurobrucellosis: clinical and therapeutic features. *Clin Infect Dis* **15**: 582.

Meacock DJ, Langton Hewer R (1981). Tetracycline and benign intracranial hypertension. *Brit Med J* **282**: 1240.

Medical News (1977). Tetracycline stained teeth in children. *JAMA* **237**: 636.

Mehtar S, Aminiafshar S (1983). Antimicrob resistance amongst various types of *Haemophilus* species. *J Antimicrob Chemother* **12**: 565.

Mérier G, Laurencet FL, Rudhardt M *et al.* (1969). Behaviour of doxycycline in renal insufficiency. *Helvetica Medica Acta* **35**: 124.

Merson MH, Sack RB, Islam S *et al.* (1980). Disease due to enterotoxigenic *Escherichia coli* in Bangladeshi adults: clinical aspects and a controlled trial of tetracycline. *J Infect Dis* **141**: 702.

Meyer RD (1983). *Legionella* infections: a review of five years of research. *Rev Infect Dis* **5**: 258.

Mhalu FS, Mmari PW, Ijumba J (1979). Rapid emergence of El Tor *Vibrio cholerae* resistant to antimicrobial agents during first six months of fourth cholera epidemic in Tanzania. *Lancet* **i**: 345.

Michel J, Rogol M, Dickman D (1983). Susceptibility of clinical isolates of *Campylobacter jejuni* to sixteen antimicrobial agents. *Antimicrob Ag Chemother* **23**: 796.

Midani S, Rathore MH (1994). Vibrio species infection of a catfish spine puncture wound. *Pediatr Infect Dis J* **13**: 333.

Miller PD, Linas SL, Schrier RW (1980). Plasma demeclocycline levels and nephrotoxicity. Correlation in hyponatremic cirrhotic patients. *JAMA* **243**: 2513.

Ming-Yuan F, Walker DH, Shu-Rong Y, Qing-Huai L (1987). Epidemiology and ecology of rickettsial diseases in the People's Republic of China. *Rev Infect Dis* **9**: 823.

Minuth JN, Holmes TM, Musher DM (1974). Activity of tetracycline, doxycycline, and minocycline against methicillin-susceptible and resistant staphylococci. *Antimicrob Ag Chemother* **6**: 411.

Mitchell RG, Baber KG (1965). Infections by tetracycline-resistant haemolytic streptococci. *Lancet* **i**: 25.

Mitchell TH, Stamp TCB, Jenkins MV (1982). Steatorrhoea after tetracycline. *Brit Med J* **285**: 780.

Møller JK, Leth Bak A, Stenderup A *et al.* (1977). Changing patterns of plasmid-mediated drug resistance during tetracycline therapy. *Anitmicrob Ag Chemother* **11**: 388.

Montejo JM, Alberola I, Glez-Zarate P *et al.* (1993). Open, randomized therapeutic trial of six antimicrobial regimens in the treatment of human brucellosis. *Clin Infect Dis* **16**: 671.

Montgomerie JZ, Pickett MJ, Yoshimori RN *et al.* (1976). Susceptibility of *Acinobacter calcoaceticus* var. *anitratus* (*Herellea vaginicola*) to minocycline. *Antimicrob Ag Chemother* **10**: 102.

Morgan T, Ribush N (1972). The effect of oxytetracycline and doxycycline on protein metabolism. *Med J Aust* **1**: 55.

Moreno F, Crisp C, Jorgensen JH, Patterson JE (1995). The clinical and molecular epidemiology of bacteremias at a university hospital caused by pneumococci not susceptible to penicillin. *J Infect Dis* **172**: 427.

Morris JG Jr, Willson R, Davis BR *et al.* (1981). Non-O Group 1 *Vibrio cholerae* gastroenteritis in the United States. Clinical, epidemiologic, and laboratory characteristics of sporadic cases. *Ann Intern Med* **94**: 656.

Morris JG Jr, Tenney JH, Drusano GL (1985). *In vitro* susceptibility of pathogenic *Vibrio* species to norfloxacin and six other antimicrobial agents. *Antimicrob Ag Chemother* **28**: 442.

Morse SA, Johnson SR, Biddle JW, Roberts MC (1986). High-level tetracycline resistance in *Neisseria gonorrhoeae* is result of acquisition of streptococcal tet M determinant. *Antimicrob Ag Chemother* **30**: 664.

Mousa ARM, Muhtaseb SA, Almudallal DS *et al.* (1987). Osteoarticular complications of brucellosis: a study of 169 cases. *Rev Infect Dis* **9**: 531.

Mull MM (1966). The tetracyclines, a critical reappraisal. *Amer J Dis Child* **112**: 483.

Munford RS, de Vasconcelos ZJS, Phillips CJ *et al.* (1974). Eradication of carriage of *Neisseria meningitidis* in families: a study in Brazil. *J Infect Dis* **129**: 644.

Murphey DK, Septimus EJ, Waagner DC (1992). Catfish-related injury and infection: report of two cases and review of the literature. *Clin Infect Dis* **14**: 689.

Nadelman RB, Wormser GP (1995). Erythema migrans and early Lyme disease. *Amer J Med* **98** (Suppl 4A): 15.

Nadelman RB, Nowakowski J, Forseter G *et al.* (1993). Failure to isolate *Borrelia burgdorferi* after antimicrobial therapy in culture-documented Lyme borreliosis associated with erythema migrans: report of a prospective study. *Amer J Med* **94**: 583.

Nash P, Sideman L, Pidcoe V, Kleger B (1978). Minocycline in Legionnaires' disease. *Lancet* **i**: 45.

Nelis HJCF, De Leenheer AP (1981). Unique metabolic fate of a tetracycline (minocycline). *Lancet* **ii**: 938.

Nesin M, Svec P, Lupski JR *et al.* (1990). Cloning and nucleotide sequence of a chromosomally encoded tetracycline resistance determinant, tetA(M), from a pathogenic, methicillin-resistant strain of *Staphylococcus aureus*. *Antimicrob Ag Chemother* **34**: 2273.

Neu HC (1978). A symposium on the tetracyclines: a major appraisal. Introduction. *Bull NY Acad Med* **54**: 141.

Neuvonen PJ, Penttilä O (1974). Interaction between doxycycline and barbiturates. *Brit Med J* **1**: 535.

Neuvonen PJ, Gothoni G, Hackman R, Björksten K (1970). Interference of iron with absorption of tetracycline in man. *Brit Med J* **4**: 532.

Ng L-K, Stiles ME, Taylor DE (1987). DNA probes for identification of tetracycline resistance genes in *Campylobacter* species isolated from swine and cattle. *Antimicrob Ag Chemother* **31**: 1669.

Nguyen VX, Nix DE, Gillikin S, Schentag JJ (1989). Effect of oral antacid administration on the pharmacokinetics of intravenous doxycycline. *Antimicrob Ag Chemother* **33**: 434.

Nicolau DP, Freeman CD, Nightingale CH *et al.* (1994). Minocycline versus vancomycin for treatment of experimental endocarditis caused by oxacillin-resistant *Staphylococcus aureus*. *Antimicrob Ag Chemother* **38**: 1515.

Nikaido H, Thanassi DG (1993). Penetration of lipophilic agents with multiple protonation sites into bacterial cells: tetracyclines and fluoroquinolones as examples. *Antimicrob Ag Chemother* **37**: 1393.

Nikolich MP, Shoemaker NB, Salyers AA (1992). A *Bacteroides* tetracycline resistance gene represents a new class of ribosome protection tetracycline resistance. *Antimicrob Ag Chemother* **36**: 1005.

NIH (National Institutes of Health) (1984). Highly invasive new bacterium isolated from US East Coast waters. *JAMA* **251**: 323.

NIH (National Institutes of Health) (1994).Consensus Development Panel on *Helicobacter pylori* in Peptic Ulcer Disease. *Helicobacter pylori* in peptic ulcer disease. *JAMA* **272**: 65.

Norris SJ, Edmondson DG (1988). *In vitro* culture system to determine MICs and MBCs of antimicrobial agents against *Treponema pallidum* subsp. *pallidum* (Nichols strain). *Antimicrob Ag Chemother* **32**: 68.

O'Grady F, Lewis MJ, Pearson NJ (1976). Global surveillance of antibiotic sensitivity of *Vibrio cholerae*. *Bull Wld Hlth Org* **54**: 181.

Oklund SA, Prolo DJ, Gutierrez RV (1981). The significance of yellow bone. Evidence for tetracycline in adult human bone. *JAMA* **246**: 761.

Olson JG, Bourgeois AL, Fang RCY *et al.* (1980). Prevention of scrub typhus. Prophylactic administration of doxycycline in a randomized double blind trial. *Amer J Trop Med Hyg* **29**: 989.

Onada Y (1979). Therapeutic effect of oral doxycycline on syphilis. *Brit J Vener Dis* **55**: 110.

Oosterlinck W, Wallijn, Wijndaele JJ (1976). The concentration of doxycycline in human prostate gland and its role in the treatment of prostatis. *Scand J Infect Dis* (Suppl 9): 85.

Oriel JD, Ridgway GL (1983). Comparison of tetracycline and minocycline in the treatment of non-gonococcal urethritis. *Brit J Vener Dis* **59**: 245.

Oriel JD, Waterworth PM (1975). Effects of minocycline and tetracycline on the vaginal yeast flora. *J Clin Path* **28**: 403.

Orr LJ Jr, Rudisill E Jr, Brodkin R, Hamilton RW (1978). Exacerbation of renal failure associated with doxycycline. *Arch Intern Med* **138**: 793.

Ory EM (1970). The tetracyclines. *Med Clin N Amer* **54**: 1173.

Pachner AR (1995). Early disseminated Lyme disease: Lyme meningitis. *Amer J Med* **98** (Suppl 4A): 30.

Pang LW, Limsomwong N, Boudreau EF, Singharay P (1987). Doxycycline prophylaxis for falciparum malaria. *Lancet* i: 1161.

Pang LW, Limsomwong N, Singharay P (1988). Prophylactic treatment of vivax and falciparum malaria with low-dose doxycycline. *J Infect Dis* **158**: 1124.

Pang Y, Brown BA, Steingrube VA *et al.* (1994). Tetracycline resistance determinants in *Mycobacterium* and *Streptomyces* species. *Antimicrob Ag Chemother* **38**: 1408.

Park BH, Levy SB (1988). The cryptic tetracycline resistance determinant on Tn 4400 mediates tetracycline degradation as well as tetracycline efflux. *Antimicrob Ag Chemother* **32**: 1797.

Park BH, Hendricks M, Malamy MH *et al.* (1987). Cryptic tetracycline resistance determinant (Class F) from *Bacteroides fragilis* mediates resistance in *Escherichia coli* by actively reducing tetracycline accumulation. *Antimicrob Ag Chemother* **31**: 1739.

Pasculle AW, Dowling JN, Frola FN *et al.* (1985). Antimicrobial therapy of experimental *Legionella micdadei* pneumonia in guinea pigs. *Antimicrob Ag Chemother* **28**: 730.

Pato ML (1977). Tetracycline inhibits propogation of deoxyribonucleic acid replication and alters membrane properties. *Antimicrob Ag Chemother* **11**: 318.

Pazderka E, Jones JW (1982). *Brucella abortus* endocartis. Successful treatment of an infected aortic valve. *Arch Intern Med* **142**: 1567.

Pearson MG, Littlewood SM, Bowden AN (1981). Tetracycline and benign intracranial hypertension. *Brit Med J* **282**: 568.

Penttilä O, Neuvonen PJ, Aho K, Lehtovaara R (1974). Interaction between doxycycline and some antiepileptic drugs. *Brit Med J* **2**: 470.

Pepper K, Horaud T, Le Bouguenec C, De Caspédés G (1987). Location of antibiotic resistance markers in clinical isolates of *Enterococcus faecalis* with similar antibiotypes. *Antimicrob Ag Chemother* **31**: 1394.

Perine PL, Teklu B (1983). Antibiotic treatment of louse-borne relapsing fever in Ethopia: a report of 377 cases. *Amer J Trop Med Hyg* **32**: 1096.

Perine PL, Chandler BP, Krause DK (1992). A clinico-epidemiological study of epidemic typhus in Africa. *Clin Infect Dis* **14**: 1149.

Perks WH, Mohr P, Liversedge IA (1976). Demeclocycline in inappropriate ADH syndrome. *Lancet* ii: 1414.

Perlino CA, Lichtenberger CJ (1984). Antibiotic susceptibility and serotype distribution of *Streptococcus pneumoniae*. *Amer Rev Respir Dis* **129**: 1018.

Petersen EA, Nash ML, Mammana RB, Copeland JG (1983). Minocycline treatment of pulmonary nocardiosis. *JAMA* **250**: 930.

Peterson HB, Galaid EI, Zenilman JM (1990). Pelvic inflammatory disease: review of treatment options. *Rev Infect Dis* **12**(Suppl 6): 656.

Phillips I, Warren C, Taylor E *et al.* (1981). The antimicrobial susceptibility of anaerobic bacteria in a London teaching hospital. *J Antimicrob Chemother* **8** (Suppl D): 17.

Phillips ME, Eastwood JB, Curtis JR *et al.* (1974). Tetracycline poisoning in renal failure. *Brit Med J* **2**: 149.

Philpott-Howard J, Williams JD (1982). Increase in antibiotic resistance in *Haemophilus influenzae* in the United Kingdom since 1977: report of study group. *Brit Med J* **284**: 1597.

Pickering LK, DuPont HL, Olarte J (1978). Single-dose tetracycline therapy for shigellosis in adults. *JAMA* **239**: 853.

Plummer DC, Garland SM, Gilbert GL (1987). Bacteraemia and pelvic infection in women due to *Ureaplasma urealyticum* and *Mycoplasma hominis*. *Med J Aust* **146**: 135.

Poliak SC, DiGiovanna JJ, Gross EG *et al.* (1985). Minocycline-associated tooth discoloration in young adults. *JAMA* **254**: 2930.

Porter PJ, Sweeney EA, Golan H, Kass EH (1966). Controlled study of the effect of prenatal tetracycline on primary dentition. *Antimicrob Ag Chemother* **1965**: 668.

Poyart-Salmeron C, Trieu-Cuot P, Carlier C, Courvalin P (1991). Nucleotide sequences specific for Tn 1545–like conjugative transposons in pneumococci and staphylococci resistant to tetracycline. *Antimicrob Ag Chemother* **35**: 1657.

Poyart-Salmeron C, Trieu-Cuot P, Carlier C *et al.* (1992). Genetic basis of tetracycline resistance in clinical isolates of *Listeria monocytogenes*. *Antimicrob Ag Chemother* **36**: 463.

Prentice MJ, Taylor-Robinson D, Csonka GW (1976). Non-specific urethritis. A placebo-controlled trial of minocycline in conjunction with laboratory investigations. *Brit J Vener Dis* **52**: 269.

Raad I, Darouiche R, Hachem R *et al.* (1995). Antibiotics and prevention of microbial colonization of catheters. *Antimicrob Ag Chemother* **39**: 2397.

Rabbani GH, Islam MR, Butler T *et al.* (1989). Single-dose treatment of cholera with furazolidone or tetracycline in a double-blind randomized trial. *Antimicrob Ag Chemother* **33**: 1447.

Radulovic S, Higgins JA, Jaworski DC, Azad AF (1995). *In vitro* and *in vivo* antibiotic susceptibilities of ELB rickettsiae. *Antimicrob Ag Chemother* **39**: 2564.

Rahaman MM, Majid MA, Alam AKMJ, Islam MR (1976). Effects of doxycycline in actively purging cholera patients: a double-blind clinical trial. *Antimicrob Ag Chemother* **10**: 610.

Raoult D (1993). Treatment of Q fever. *Antimicrob Ag Chemother* **37**: 1733.

Raoult D, Drancourt M (1991). Antimicrobial therapy of rickettsial diseases. *Antimicrob Ag Chemother* **35**: 2457.

Raoult D, Marrie T (1995). Q fever. *Clin Infect Dis* **20**: 489.

Raoult D, Etienne J, Massip P *et al.* (1987a). Q fever endocarditis in the South of France. *J Infect Dis* **155**: 570.

Raoult D, Roussellier P, Vestris G, Tamalet J (1987b). *In vitro* antibiotic susceptibility of *Rickettsia rickettsii* and *Rickettsia conorii*: plaque assay and microplaque calorimetric assay. *J Infect Dis* **155**: 1059.

Raoult D, Torres H, Drancourt M (1991). Shell-vial assay: evaluation of a new technique for determining antibiotic susceptibility, tested in 13 isolates of *Coxiella burnetii*. *Antimicrob Ag Chemother* **35**: 2070.

Rasmussen B, Noller HF, Doubresse G *et al.* (1991). Molecular basis of tetracycline action: identification of analogs whose primary target is not the bacterial ribosome. *Antimicrob Ag Chemother* **35**: 2306.

Redin GS (1967). Antibacterial activity in mice of minocycline, a new tetracycline. *Antimicrob Ag Chemother* **1966**: 371; quoted by Steigbigel *et al.* (1968a,b).

Regnery R, Tappero J (1995). Unravelling mysteries associated with cat-scratch disease, bacillary angiomatosis, and related syndromes. *Emerging Infect Dis* **1**: 16.

Renaudin H, Tully JG, Bebear C (1992). *In vitro* susceptibilities of

Mycoplasma genitalium to antibiotics. *Antimicrob Ag Chemother* **36**: 870.

Report of an Ad-Hoc Study Group on Antibiotic Resistance (1977). Tetracycline resistance in pneumococci and Group A streptococci. *Brit Med J* **1**: 131.

Report from the Boston Collaborative Drug Surveillance Program (1972). Tetracycline and drug-attributed rises in blood urea nitrogen. *JAMA* **220**: 377.

Report to the Research Committee of the British Tuberculosis Association by the Clinical Trials Subcommittee (1968). Comparison of side-effects of tetracycline and tetracycline plus nystatin. *Brit Med J* **4**: 411.

Report of a WHO Scientific Group (1978). *Neisseria gonorrhoea* and gonococcal infections. *Wld Hlth Org Tech Rep Ser* 616.

Ribush N, Morgan T (1972). Tetracyclines and renal failure. *Med J Aust* **1**: 53.

Rice RJ, Bhullar V, Mitchell SH *et al.* (1995). Susceptibilities of *Chlamydia trachomatis* isolates causing uncomplicated female genital tract infections and pelvic inflammatory disease. *Antimicrob Ag Chemother* **39**: 760.

Rich G, Davidson J (1975). Minocycline sensitivity related to the phage type of multiply resistant staphylococci. *J Clin Path* **28**: 450.

Rickles FR, Klipstein FA, Tomasini J *et al.* (1972). Long-term follow-up of antiobiotic-treated tropical sprue. *Ann Intern Med* **76**: 203.

Ridgway GL, Oriel JD, (1984). Advantages of adding a course of tetracycline to single dose ampicillin and probenecid in the treatment of gonorrhoea. *Brit J Vener Dis* **60**: 235.

Ries AA, Wells JG, Olivola D *et al.* (1994). Epidemic *Shigella dysenteriae* type 1 in Burundi: panresistance and implications for prevention. *J Infect Dis* **169**: 1035.

Robbins M, Marais R, Felmingham D, Ridgway GL (1987). The *in-vitro* activity of doxycycline and minocycline against anaerobic bacteria. *J Antimicrob Chemother* **20**: 379.

Roberts MC (1989). Plasmid-mediated Tet M in *Haemophilus ducreyi*. *Antimicrob Ag Chemother* **33**: 1611.

Roberts MC (1991). Tetracycline resistance in *Peptostreptococcus* species. *Antimicrob Ag Chemother* **35**: 1682.

Roberts MC, Hillier SL (1990). Genetic basis of tetracycline resistance in urogenital bacteria. *Antimicrob Ag Chemother* **34**: 261.

Roberts MC, Kenny GE (1986). Tet M tetracycline-resistant determinants in *Ureaplasma urealyticum*. *Pediatr Infect Dis* **5** (Suppl): 338.

Roberts MC, Koutsky LA, Holmes KK *et al.* (1985). Tetracycline-resistant *Mycoplasma hominis* strains contain streptococci tet M sequences. *Antimicrob Ag Chemother* **28**: 141.

Roberts MC, Brown BA, Steingrube VA, Wallace RJ Jr (1990). Genetic basis of tetracycline resistance in *Moraxella (Branhamella) catarrhalis*. *Antimicrob Ag Chemother* **34**: 1816.

Roberts MC, Pang Y, Spencer RC *et al.* (1991). Tetracycline resistance in *Moraxella (Branhamella) catarrhalis*: demonstration of two clonal outbreaks by using pulsed-field gel electrophoresis. *Antimicrob Ag Chemother* **35**: 2453.

Robertson JA, Stemke GW, Maclellan SG, Taylor DE (1988). Characterization of tetracycline-resistant strains of *Ureaplasma urealyticum*. *J Antimicrob Chemother* **21**: 319.

Robertson L, Farrell ID, Hinchcliffe PM (1973). the sensitivity of *Brucella abortus* to chemotherapeutic agents. *J Med Microbiol* **6**: 549.

Robertson MH (1973). Tetracycline-resistant beta-haemolytic streptococci in South-West Essex: decline and fall. *Brit Med J* **4**: 84.

Robson JM, Harrison MW, Wood RN *et al.* (1993). Brucellosis: re-emergence and changing epidemiology in Queensland. *Med J Aust* **159**: 153.

Rogers HJ, House FR, Morrison PJ, Bradbrook ID (1980). Interaction of cimetidine with tetracycline absorption. *Lancet* **ii**: 694.

Rolfs RT (1995). Treatment of syphilis, 1993. *Clin Infect Dis* **20** (Suppl 1): 23.

Romanowski B, Talbot H, Stadnyk M *et al.* (1993). Minocycline compared with doxycycline in the tretment of nongonococcal urethritis and mucopurulent cervicitis. *Ann Intern Med* **119**: 16.

Rosendal K, Jessen o, Bentzon MW, Bülow P (1977). Antibiotic policy and spread of *Staphylococcus aureus* strains in Danish hospitals, 1969–1974. *Acta Path Microbiol Scand* **85**: 143.

Rossi A, Galas M, Binztein N *et al.* (1993). Unusual multiresistant *Vibrio cholerae* 01 El Tor in Argentina. *Lancet* **342**: 1172.

Roth H, Beckler KL, Shalhoub RJ, Katz S (1967).Nephrotoxicity of demethylchortetracycline hycrochloride. *Arch Intern Med* **120**: 433.

Rubinstein E, Lang R, Shasha B *et al.* (1991). *In vitro* susceptibility of *Brucella melitensis* to antibiotics. *Antimicrob Ag Chemother* **35**: 1925.

Ruhen RW, Tandon MK (1975). Minocycline, doxycycline and tetracycline levels in serum and bronchial secretions of patients with chronic bronchitis. *Pathology* **7**: 193.

Ruhen RW, Tandon MK (1976). Comparative effectiveness of tetracycline, minocycline and doxycycline in treatment of acute-on-chronic bronchitis. A study based on sputum levels. *Med J Aust* **2**: 151.

Rylander M, Hallander HO (1988). *In vitro* comparison of the activity of doxycycline, tetracycline, erythromycin and a new macrolide, CP 62993, against *Mycoplasma pneumoniae*, *Mycoplasma hominis* and *Ureaplasma urealyticum*. *Scand J Infect Dis* (Suppl 53): 12.

Sabath LD (1969). Current concepts: drug resistance of bacteria. *New Engl J Med* **280**: 91.

Sack DA, Kaminsky DC, Sack RB *et al.* (1978). Prophylactic doxycycline for travelers' diarrhea. Results of a prospective double-blind study of Peace Corps Volunteers in Kenya. *New Engl J Med* **298**: 758.

Sack RB, Santosham M, Froehlich JL (1984). Doxycycline prophylaxis of travelers' diarrhea in Honduras, an area where resistance to doxycycline is common among enterotoxigenic *Escherichia coli*. *Amer J Trop Med Hyg* **33**: 460.

Safrin S, Morrris JG Jr, Adams M *et al.* (1988). Non-0: 1 *Vibrio cholerae* bacteremia: case report and review. *Rev Infect Dis* **10**: 1012.

Santosham M, Sack RB, Froehlich J *et al.* (1981). Biweekly prophylactic doxycycline for travelers' diarrhea. *J Infect Dis* **143**: 598.

Sapico FL, Kwok Y-Y, Sutter VL, Finegold SM (1972). Standardized antimicrobial disc susceptibility testing of anaerobic bacteria: *in vitro* susceptibility of *Clostridium perfringens* to nine antibiotics. *Antimicrob Ag Chemother* **2**: 320.

Sawyer LA, Fishbein DB, McDade JE (1987). Q fever: Current concepts. *Rev Infect Dis* **9**: 935.

Schachner L (1983). The treament of acne: a contemporary review. *Pediatr Clin N Amer* **30**: 501.

Schachter J (1978a). Chlamydial infections (first of three parts). *New Engl J Med* **298**: 428.

Schachter J (1978b). Chlamydial infections (second of three parts). *New Engl J Med* **298**: 490.

Schaedler RW, Choppin PW, Zabriskie JB (1964). Pneumonia caused by tetracycline-resistant pneumococci. *New Engl J Med* **270**: 127.

Schatz M, Wasserman S, Patterson R (1981). Eosinophils and immunologic lung disaease. *Med Clin N Amer* **65**: 1055.

Schifferli DM, Beachey EH (1988). Bacterial adhesion: modulation by antibiotics which perturb protein synthesis. *Antimicrob Ag Chemother* **32**: 1603.

Schultz JC, Adamson JS Jr, Workman WW, Norman TD (1963). Fatal liver disease after intravenous administration of tetracycline in high dosage. *New Engl J Med* **269**: 999.

Schwartzman WA (1992). Infections due to Rochalimaea: the expanding clinical spectrum. *Clin Infect Dis* **15**: 893.

Searcy RL, Simms NM, Foreman JA, Berquist LM (1965). Evaluation of the blood-clotting mechanism in tetracycline-treated patients. *Antimicrob Ag Chemother* **1964**: 179.

Shaefer CF, Trincher RC, Rissing JP (1982). Melioidosis: recrudescence with a strain resistant to multiple antimicrobials. *Amer Rev Respir Dis* **128**: 173.

Shames JM, George RB, Holliday WB *et al.* (1970). Comparison of antibiotics in the treatment of mycoplasmal pneumonia. *Arch Intern Med* **125**: 680.

Shanks GD, Barnett A, Edstein MD, Rickmann KH (1995). Effectiveness of doxycycline combined with primaquine for malaria prophylaxis. *Med J Aust* **162**: 306.

Sheehan HL (1940). the pathology of acute yellow atrophy and delayed chloroform poisoning. *J Obst Gynaec Brit Emp* **47**: 49; quoted by Kunelis *et al.* (1965).

Shehabi A, Shakir K, El-Khateeb M *et al.* (1990). Diagnosis and treatment of 106 cases of human brucellosis. *J Infect***20**: 5.

Shelley WB, Heaton CL (1973). Minocycline sensitivity. *JAMA* **224**: 125.

Shils ME (1963). Renal disease and the metabolic effects of tetracycline. *Ann Intern Med* **58**: 389.

Shwachman H, Fekete E, Kulczycki LL, Foley GE (1959). The effect of long-term antibiotic therapy in patients with cystic fibrosis of the pancreas. *Antiobiot Annual 1958–1959*: 692.

Simon GL, Gorbach SL (1982). Intestinal microflora. *Med Clin N Amer* **66**: 557.

Simon HB, Southwick FS, Moellering RC Jr, Sherman E (1980). *Haemophilus influenzae* in hopitalized adults: current perspectives. *Amer J Med* **69**: 219.

Simpson MB, Pryzbylik J, Innis B, Denham MA (1985). Hemolytic anemia after tetracycline therapy. *New Engl J Med* **312**: 840.

Sinclair D, Phillips C (1982). Transient myopathy apparently due to tetracycline. *New Engl J Med* **307**: 821.

Singer I, Rotenberg D (1973). Demeclocycline-induced nephrogenic diabetes insipidus. *In-vivo* and *in-vitro* studies. *Ann Intern Med* **79**: 679.

Sitbon O, Bidel N, Dussopt C *et al.* (1994). Minocycline pneumonitis and eosinophilia: A report of eight patients. *Arch Intern Med* **154**: 1633.

Sivonen A, Renkonen O-V, Weckström P *et al.* (1978). The effect of chemoprophylactic use of rifampin and minocycline on rates of carriage of *Neisseria meningitidis* in army recruits in Finland. *J Infect Dis* **137**: 238.

Slocombe B, Sutherland R (1973). Transferable antiobiotic resistance in entropathogenic *Escherichia coli* between 1948 and 1968. *Antimicrob Ag Chemother* **4**: 459.

Smith C, Woods CG, Woods MJ (1984). Absorption of minocycline. *J Antimicrob Chemother* **13**: 93.

Smith CB, Friedewald WT, Chanock RM (1967). Shedding of *Mycoplasma pneumoniae* after tetracycline and erythromycin therapy. *New Engl J Med* **276**: 1172.

Smith MD, Vinh DX, Hoa NTT *et al.* (1995). *In vitro* antimicrobial susceptibilities of strains of *Yersinia* pestis. *Antimicrob Ag Chemother* **39**: 2153.

Snavely SR, Hodges GR (1984). The neurotoxicity of antibacterial agents. *Ann Intern Med* **101**: 92.

Spaepen MS, Kundsin RB (1977). Simple, direct broth-disk method for antibiotic susceptibility testing of *Ureaplasma urealyticum. Antimicrob Ag Chemother* **11**: 267.

Spaepen MS, Kundsin RB, Horne HW (1976). Tetracycline-resistant T-*Mycoplasma (Ureaplasma urealyticum)* from patients with a history of reproductive failure. *Antoimicrob Ag Chemother* **9**: 1012.

Spencer RC, Brown CB (1983). Septicaemia in a renal transplant patient due to *Mycoplasma hominis. J Infect* **6**: 267.

Spika JS, Facklam RR, Plikaytis BD *et al.* (1991). Antimicrobial resistance of *Streptococcus pneumoniae* in the United States 1979–1987. *J Infect Dis* **163**: 1273.

Sponitz M, Rudnitsky J, Rambaud JJ (1967). Melioidosis pneumonitis. *JAMA* **202**: 950.

Stagno S, Brasfield DM, Brown MB *et al.* (1981). Infant pneumonitis associated with *Cytomegalovirus, Chlamydia, Pneumocystis,* and *Ureaplasma*: a prospective study. *Pediatrics* **68**: 322.

Stamm WE, Guinan ME, Johnson C *et al.* (1984). Effect of treatment regimens for *Neisseria gonorrhoeae* on simultaneous infection with *Chlamydia trachomatis. New Engl J Med* **310**: 545.

Standaert SM, Dawson JE, Schaffner W *et al.* (1995). Ehrlichiosis in a golf-oriented retirement community. *New Engl J Med* **333**: 420.

Steere AC (1995). Musculoskeletal manifestations of Lyme disease. *Amer J Med* **98** (Suppl 4A): 44.

Steigbigel NH, Reed CW, Finaldn M (1968a). Absorption and excretion of five tetracycline analogues in normal young men. *Amer J Med Sci* **25**: 296.

Steigbigel NH, Reed CW, Finalnd M (1968b). Susceptibility of common pathogenic bacteria to seven tetracycline antibiotics *in vitro. Amer J Med Sci* **225**: 179.

Stenbaek Ø, Myhre E, Berdal BP (1973). The effect of doxycycline on renal function in patients with advanced renal insufficiency. *Scand J Infect Dis* **5**: 199.

Stewart DJ (1973). Prevalence of tetracyclines in children's teeth – Study II: a resurvey after five years. *Brit Med J* **3**: 320.

Stimson JB, Hale J, Bowie WR, Holmes KK (1981). Tetracycline-resistant *Ureaplasma urealyticum*: a cause of persistent nongonopcoccal urethritis. *Ann Intern Med* **94**: 192.

Strickman D, Sheer T, Salata K *et al.* (1995). *In vitro* effectiveness of azithromycin against doxycycline-resistant and -susceptible strains of *Rickettsia tsutsugamushi*, etiological agent of scrub typhus. *Antimicrob Ag Chemother* **39**: 2406.

Sturm AW (1987). Comparison of antimicrobial susceptibility patterns of fifty-seven strains of *Haemophilus ducreyi* isolated in Amsterdam from 1978 to 1985. *J Antimicrob Chemother* **19**: 187.

Su YA, He P, Clewell DB (1992). Characterization of the tet(M). determinant of Tn916: evidence for regulation by transcription attenuation. *Antimicrob Ag Chemother* **36**: 769.

Sundelöf B, Gnarpe J, Gnarpe H *et al.* (1993). *Chlamydia pneumoniae* in Swedish patients. *Scand J Infect Dis* **25**: 429.

Sung JJY, Chung SCS, Ling TKW *et al.* (1995). Antibacterial treatment of gastric ulcers associated with *Helicobacter pylori. New Engl J Med* **332**: 139.

Sutter VL, Finegold SM (1976). Susceptibility of anaerobic bacteria to 23 antimicrobial agents. *Antimicrob Ag Chemother* **10**: 736.

Swarz H (1977). Doxycycline in bronchitis: results of a multicentre study. *Curr Med Res Opin* **5**: 234.

Swenson JM, Wallace RJ Jr, Silcox VA *et al.* (1985). Antimicrobial susceptibility of five subgroups of *Mycobacterium fortuitum* and *Mycobacterium chelonae. Antimicrob Ag Chemother* **28**: 807.

Tager I, Speizer FE (1975). Role of infection in chronic bronchitis. New Engl J Med **292**: 563.

Takafuji ET, Kirkpatrick JW, Miller RN *et al.* (1984). An efficacy trial of doxycycline chemoprophylaxis against leptospirosis. *New Engl J Med* **310**: 497.

Tally FP, Cuchural GJ Jr, Jacobus NV *et al.* (1985). Nationwide study of the susceptibility of the *Baceteroides fragilis* group in the United States. *Antimicrob Ag Chemother* **28**: 675.

Tally FT, Ellestad GA, Testa RT (1995). Glycylcyclines: a new generation of tetracyclines. *J Antimicrob Chemother* **35**: 449.

Taylor-Robinson D, Furr PM (1986). Clinical antibiotic resistance of *Ureaplasma urealyticum. Pediatr Infect Dis* **5**(Suppl): 335.

Testa RT, Petersen PJ, Jacobus NV *et al.* (1993). *In vitro* and *in vivo* antibacterial activities of the glycylcyclines, a new class of semisynthetic tetracyclines. *Antimicrob Ag Chemother* **37**: 2270.

Thaysen EH, Eriksen KR (1956). *Staphylococcal* enteritis following administration of the tetracyclines. *Antibiot Ann 1955–1956:* 867.

Thomas E (1980). Towards better antimicrobial treatment of sexually transmitted diseases. *J Antimicrob Chemother* **6**: 570.

Thong YH, Rowan-Kelly B, Shepherd C, Ferrante A (1977). Growth inhibition of *Naegleria fowleri* by tetracycline, rifamycin, and miconazole. *Lancet* **ii**: 876.

Thormsberry C. Baker CN, Kirven LA (1978). *In vitro* activity of antimicrobial agents on Legionnaires' disease bacterium. *Antimicrob Ag Chemother* **13**: 78.

Threlfall EJ, Said B, Rowe B (1993). Emergence of multiple drug resistance in *Vibrio cholerae* 01 El Tor from Ecuador. *Lancet* **342**: 1173.

Tilley BC, Alarcón GS, Heyse SP *et al.* (1995). Minocycline in rheumatoid arthritis. A 48-week, double-blind, placebo-controlled trial. *Ann Intern Med* **122**: 81.

Toaff R, Ravid R (1966). Tetracyclines and the teeth. *Lancet* **ii**: 281.

Tomkins AM, James WPT, Walters JH, Cole ACE (1974). Malabsorption in overland travellers to India. *Brit Med J* 3: 380.

Toomey KE, Barnes RC (1990). Treatment of *Chlamydia trachomatis* genital infection. *Rev Infect Dis* 12 (Suppl 6): 645.

Torres JR, Sands M, Sanders CV (1978). *In vitro* sensitivity of *Mycobacterium marinum* to minocycline and doxycycline. *Tubercle* 59: 193.

Tsukamura M (1980). *In vitro* antimycobacterial activity of minocycline. *Tibercle* 61: 37.

Unge P, Gnarpe H (1988). Pharmacokinetic, bacteriological and clinical aspects of the use of doxycycline in patients with active duodenal ulcer associated with *Campylobacter pylori*. *Scand J Infect Dis* (Suppl 53): 70.

Uwaydah M, Osseiran M (1981). Susceptibility of recent *Shigella* isolates to mecillinam, ampicillin, tetracycline, chloramphenicol, and cotrimoxazole. *J Antimicrob Chemother* 7: 619.

Vanhoof R, Vanderlinden MP, Dierickx R *et al.* (1978). Susceptibility of *Campylobacter fetus* subsp. *jejuni* to twenty-nine antimicrobial agents. *Antimicrob Ag Chemother* 14: 553.

Van Ypersele de Strihou C (1970). Tetracycline in renal failure. *Lancet* ii: 208.

Velasco JE, Miller AE, Zaias N (1972). Minocycline in the treatment of venereal disease. *JAMA* 220: 1323.

Waldor MK, Mekalanos JJ (1994). Emergence of new cholera pandemic: molecular analysis of virulence determinants in *Vibrio cholerae* 0139 and development of a live vaccine prototype. *J Infect Dis* 170: 278.

Walker RG, Thomson NM, Dowling JP, Chisholm GD (1979). Minocycline-induced acute interstitial nephritis. *Brit Med J* 1: 524.

Wallace RJ Jr, Swenson JM, Silcox VA *et al.* (1983). Spectrum of disease due to rapidly growing mycobacteria. *Rev Infect Dis* 5: 657.

Wallace RJ Jr, Swenson JM, Silcox VA, Bullen MG (1985). Treatment of nonpulmonary infections due to *Mycobacterium fortuitum* and *Mycobacterium chelonei* on the basis of *in vitro* susceptibilities. *J Infect Dis* 152: 500.

Wallman IS, Hilton HB (1962). Teeth pigmented by tetracycline. *Lancet* I: 827.

Walsh JH, Peterson WL (1995). The treatment of *Helicobacter pylori* infection in the management of peptic ulcer disease. *New Engl J Med* 333: 984.

Walters BNJ, Gubbay SS (1981). Tetracycline and benign intracranial hypertension: report of five cases. *Brit Med J* 282: 19.

Warrel DA, Perine PL, Krause DW *et al.* (1983). Pathophysiology and immunology of the Jarisch-Herxheimer-like reaction to louse-borne relapsing fever: comparison of tetracycline and slow-release penicillin. *J Infect Dis* 147: 898.

Watanakunakorn C (1984). Antimicrobial susceptibility of 200 blood isolates of coagulase-negative staphylococci to 20 antimicrobial agents. *Scan J Infect Dis* 16: 345.

Waterworth PM (1974). The effect of minocycline on *Candida albicans*. *J Clin Path* 27: 269.

Weber JT, Johnson RE (1995). New treatments for *Chlamydia trachomatis* genital infection. *Clin Infect Dis* 20 (Suppl 1): 66.

Weiss WJ, Jacobus NV, Petersen PJ, Testa RT (1995). Susceptibility of enterococci, methicillin-resistant *Staphylococcus aureus* and *Streptococcus pneumoniae* to the glycylcyclines. *J Antimicrob Chemother* 36: 225.

Welch H (1954). *Principles and Practice of Antibiotic Therapy* p. 255. New York: Medical Encyclopedia Inc.

Welling PG, Shaw WR, Uman SJ *et al.* (1975). Pharmacokentics of minocycline in renal failure. *Antimicrob Ag Chemother* 8: 532.

Welling PG, Koch PA, Lau CC, Craig WA (1977). Bioavailability of tetracycline and doxycycline in fasted and nonfasted subjects. *Anirmicrob Ag Chemother* 11: 462.

West B, Changalucha J, Grosskurth H *et al.* (1995). Antimicrobial susceptibility, auxotype and plasmid content of *Neisseria gonorrhoeae* in Northern Tanzania: emergence of high level plasmid mediated tetracycline resistance. *Genitourin Med* 71: 9.

Westerman EL (1982). Rocky Mountain spotted fever. A dilemma for the clinician. *Arch Intern Med* 142: 1106.

Weyman J (1965). The clinical appearances of tetracycline staining of the teeth. *Brit Dent J* 118: 289.

Whalley PJ, Adams RH, Combes B (1964). Tetracycline toxicity in pregnancy. *JAMA* 189: 357.

Whelton A, Schach von Wittenau M, Twomey TM *et al.* (1974). Doxycycline pharmacokinetics in the absence of renal function. *Kidney Int* 5: 365.

Whitby JL, Black HJ (1964). Comparison of lymecycline with tetracycline hydrochloride. *Brit Med J* 2: 1491.

Whittington WL, Roberts MC, Hale J, Holmes KK (1995). Susceptibilities of *Neisseria gonorrhoeae* to the glycylcyclines. *Antimicrob Ag Chemother* 39: 1864.

WHO (1977). Chlamydia surveillance. *Wkly Epidem Rec* 52: 230.

WHO (1982). Surveillance of the resistance of *Staphylococcus aureus* to antibiotics. *Wkly Epidem Rec* 57: 265.

WHO (1986). *Neisseria gonorrheae*. Emergence of plasmid-mediated tetracycline-resistant strains. *Wkly epidem Rec* 36: 277.

WHO Working Group on Rickettsial Diseases (1982). Rickettsioses: a continuing disease problem. *Bull WHO* 60: 157.

Wiggins GL, Albritton WL, Feeley JC (1978). Antibiotic susceptibility of clinical isolates of *Listeria monocytogenes*. *Anticrob Ag Chemother* 13: 854,

Wilcox RR (1977). How suitable are available pharmaceuticals for the treatment of sexually transmitted diseases? 2. Conditions presenting as sores or tumours. *Brit J Vener Dis* 53: 340.

Williams DN, Laughlin LW, Yhu-Hsuing Lee (1974). Minocycline: possible vestibular side-effects. *Lancet* ii: 744.

Windsor ACM, Hobbs CB, Treby DA, Cowper RA (1972). Effect of tetracycline on leucocyte ascorbic acid levels. *Brit Med J* 1: 214.

Wise R, Andrews JM (1994). *In vitro* activities of two glycylcyclines. *Antimicrob Ag Chemother* 38: 1096.

Wisseman CL Jr, Ordonex SV (1986). Actions of antibiotics on *Rickettsia rickettsii*. *J Infect Dis* 153: 626.

Witkop CJ, Wolf RO (1963). Hypoplasia and intrinsic staining of enamel following tetracycline therapy. *JAMA* 185: 1008.

Wolfe MS (1982). The treatment of intestinal protozoan infections. *Med Clin N Amer* 66: 707.

Wood MJ, Farrell W, Kattan S, Williams JD (1975). Activity of minocycline and tetracycline against respiratory pathogens related to blood levels. *J Antimicrob Chemother* 1: 323.

Woodward TE (1984). Rocky Mountain spotted fever: epidemiological and early clinical signs are keys to treatment and reduced mortality. *J Infect Dis* 150: 465.

Wotherspoon AC, Doglioni C, Diss TC (1993). Regression of primary low-grade B-cell gastric lymphoma of mucosa-associated lymphoid tissue type after eradication of *Helicobacter pylori*. *Lancet* 342: 575.

Yagupsky P, Wolach B (1993). Fatal Israeli spotted fever in children. *Clin Infect Dis* 17: 850.

Yagupsky P, Gross EM, Alkan M, Bearman JE (1987). Comparison of two dosage schedules of doxycycline in children with rickettsial spotted fever. *J Infect Dis* 155: 1215.

Yamamoto T, Naigowit P, Deysirilert S *et al.* (1990). *In vitro* susceptibility of *Pseudomonas pseudomallei* to 27 antimicrobial agents. *Antimicrob Ag Chemother*, 34: 2027.

Yeaman MR, Roman MJ, Baca OG (1989). Antibiotic susceptibilities of two *Coxiella burnetii* isolates implicated in distinct clinical syndromes. *Antimicrob Ag Chemother* 33: 1052.

Yim CW, Flynn NM, Fitzgerald FT (1985). Penetration of oral doxycycline into the cerebrospinal fluid of patients with latent or neurosyphilis. *Antimicrob Ag Chemother* 28: 347.

Yoshida S, Mizugushi Y, Ohta H, Ogawa M (1985). Effects of tetracyclines on experimental *Legionella pneumophila* infection in guinea-pigs. *J Antimicrob Chemother* 16: 199.

Yoshioka H, Rudoy P, Riley HD Jr, Yoshida K (1977). Antimicrobial susceptibility of *Escherichia coli* isolated at a children's hospital. *Scand J Infect Dis* 9: 207.

Yung AP, Grayson ML (1988). Psittacosis – a review of 135 cases. *Med J Aust* **148**: 228.

Yuk JH, Dignani MC, Harris RL *et al.* (1991). Minocycline as an alterantive antistaphylococcal agent. *Rev Infect Dis* **13**: 1023.

Zegers De Beyl D, Naeije R, De Troyer A (1978). Demeclocycline treatment of water retention in congestive heart failure. *Brit Med J* **1**: 760.

Zenilman JM, Rand S, Barditch P, Rompalo AM (1993). Asymptomatic neurosyphilis after doxycycline therapy for early latent syphilis. *Sex Transm Dis* **20**: 346.

Zenker PN, Rolfs RT (1990). Treatment of syphilis, 1989. *Rev Infect Dis* **12** (Suppl 6): 590.

Zuravleff JJ, Yu VL (1982). Infections caused by *Pseudomonas maltophila* with emphasis on bacteremia: case reports and a review of the literature. *Rev Infect Dis* **4**: 1236.

Vancomycin

Description

Vancomycin was isolated in the Lilly Research Laboratories from *Amycolatopsis orientalis* (previously designated *Streptomyces orientalis*), an organism which was found in soil in Borneo (McCormick *et al.*, 1956). Based on its carbohydrate and peptide content, vancomycin is classified as a glycopeptide antibiotic and it was the first member of this new class (Pfeiffer, 1981). Vancomycin and teicoplanin (p. 791) are the only ones used clinically. Glycopeptide antibiotics have higher molecular weights than penicillins, cephalosporins, tetracyclines, aminoglycosides and macrolides.

When vancomycin was introduced for clinical use in 1958, it was employed for the treatment of staphylococcal infections resistant to available antibiotics. But within 2 years, it was superseded by methicillin (p. 77), and then also by cephalothin (p. 251), drugs which had fewer side-effects. With the spread of methicillin-resistant *Staphylococcus aureus* strains (MRSA) in the late 1970s (p. 77), vancomycin was resurrected for the treatment of infections by these, and other antibiotic-resistant bacteria. Nowadays, the increasing complexity of medical care has led to a growing population of patients at risk of Gram-positive coccal infections. As a result, vancomycin is widely used in intensive care units, for neutropenic patients being treated with myelosuppressive agents, and for infections involving implanted foreign material such as long-term intravenous catheters, prosthetic joints, and prosthetic cardiac valves. Vancomycin also has an important role in the treatment of specific infections such as antibiotic-associated colitis.

Sensitive Organisms

1 Gram-positive bacteria

Vancomycin is highly effective against Gram-positive cocci, such as *Staph. aureus* (including penicillin G- and methicillin-resistant strains), coagulase-negative staphylococci, *Streptococcus pyogenes*, *Strep. pneumoniae*, viridans group streptococci and *Enterococcus faecalis* (Griffith and Peck, 1956).

a   Staphylococcus aureus   In a review of published data since 1956, Watanakunakorn (1984) found that with the exception of a few strains, all isolates of *Staph. aureus*, including those resistant to methicillin, were sensitive to vancomycin. More recent studies have confirmed that vancomycin remains active against all methicillin-sensitive and -resistant strains (Moorhouse et al., 1985; Vedel *et al.*, 1990; Shonekan *et al.*, 1992; Wadsworth *et al.*, 1992; Amsterdam *et al.*, 1994). Results of *in vitro* studies testing vancomycin/rifampicin combinations against *Staph. aureus* have varied (p. 680). By the time-kill curve method, Watanakunakorn and Tisone (1982) showed that vancomycin/gentamicin and vancomycin/tobramycin combinations were synergistic against most methicillin-susceptible and -resistant strains of *Staph. aureus*. *In vitro* synergistic activity has also been demonstrated between vancomycin and imipenem against seven of 30 *Staph. aureus* strains, with additive activity against a further nine strains (Barr *et al.*, 1990).

b   Coagulase-negative staphylococci   Vancomycin is active against coagulase-negative staphylococci. Watanakunakorn (1984) reviewed data published since 1958 and found that vancomycin was active against the majority of strains of *Staph. epidermidis*, *Staph.*

saprophyticus, *Staph. haemolyticus*, *Staph. hominis*, *Staph. warneri* and unspeciated species. Vancomycin has retained its excellent activity against these organisms in more recent studies of isolates from peritoneal dialysis patients (Gruer *et al.*, 1984), neonates (Davies *et al.*, 1986), adult patients (Goldstein *et al.*, 1990; Vedel *et al.*, 1990; Shonekan *et al.*, 1992), and neutropenic patients (Maugein *et al.*, 1990). Sixty strains of *Staph. haemolyticus* studied by Froggatt *et al.* (1989) were all sensitive to vancomycin but the MICs were higher than those of 16 *Staph. epidermidis* strains. Studies investigating *in vitro* synergy between combinations of vancomycin and other antibiotics against coagulase-negative staphylococci have yielded inconsistent results. Against *Staph. epidermidis*, studies have shown combinations of vancomycin/cefazolin and vancomycin/cephalothin (Siebert *et al.*, 1979), vancomycin/cefamandole (Ein *et al.*, 1979), and vancomycin/imipenem (Barr *et al.*, 1990) to be synergistic. In contrast, Lowy *et al.*. (1979) demonstrated antagonism with a vancomycin/cephalothin combination. Similarly, conflicting results have been obtained in *in vitro* testing of combinations of vancomycin with either rifampicin or gentamicin against methicillin-resistant *Staph. epidermidis* (MRSE) strains. Some strains of *Staph. epidermidis* produce an extracellular slime-like substance. Two *in vitro* studies (Evans and Holmes, 1987; Farber *et al.*, 1990) demonstrated increases in the MIC of *Staph. epidermidis* to vancomycin in the presence of this slime.

c Streptococci Group A, C and G streptococci are always sensitive to vancomycin, as are the vast majority of group B streptococci (Watanakunakorn, 1984). Vancomycin has excellent activity against *Strep. pneumoniae*, including penicillin-resistant strains. The MIC of vancomycin was 0.5 μg per ml or less against all penicillin-resistant isolates tested by Goldstein *et al.* (1994). Addition of rifampicin to vancomycin did not result in synergistic activity against these organisms (Barakett *et al.*, 1993). Viridans streptococci are almost always sensitive to vancomycin, including penicillin-resistant strains. For example, 17 of 47 sequential viridans streptococcal blood culture isolates from neutropenic patients were resistant to penicillin but all were sensitive to vancomycin (McWhinney *et al.*, 1993). A combination of vancomycin and rifampicin was synergistic *in vitro* against five of nine nutritionally deficient viridans streptococci tested by Stein and Libertin (1988).

d Enterococci Vancomycin inhibits the growth of *E. faecalis* but is usually not bactericidal in concentrations which can easily be achieved *in vivo* (Harwick *et al.*, 1973). Addition of an aminoglycoside is required for a bactericidal effect, just as an aminoglycoside must be combined with penicillin G to produce bactericidal activity against these organisms. This bactericidal effect is important in the treatment of endocarditis (p. 456). Until the appearance of high-level aminoglycoside-resistance among enterococcal isolates (p. 455), a combination of vancomycin / streptomycin was bactericidal against most strains (Westenfelder *et al.*, 1973), and vancomycin / gentamicin was bactericidal against virtually all strains (Watanakunakorn and Bakie, 1973; Harwick *et al.*, 1974). The majority of enterococcal isolates remain sensitive to vancomycin (Toftee *et al.*, 1984; Perez *et al.*, 1987) but vancomycin-resistant enterococcal isolates have emerged as a significant problem since the late 1980s (see below).

e Gram-positive bacilli Bacillus species, including *B. anthracis*, *B. cereus* and other species are sensitive to this drug (Geraci and Wilson, 1981; Weber *et al.*, 1988). *Listeria monocytogenes* is inhibited by vancomycin (Watanakunakorn, 1984; MacGowan *et al.*, 1990) but *in vitro* studies demonstrate weak bactericidal activity (Appleman *et al.*, 1991). *Corynebacterium* spp., including *C. diphtheriae*, *C. jeikeium* (Gill *et al.*, 1981) and *Corynebacterium* group D2 (Soriano *et al.*, 1987), are vancomycin-senstive. A combination of vancomycin and gentamicin does not exhibit synergistic activity against corynebacteria *in vitro* (Spitzer *et al.*, 1988). The vast majority of clinically important clostridial species, including *Cl. difficile*, *Cl. perfringens*, *Cl. botulinum*, *Cl. septicum* and *Cl. ramosum* strains are vancomycin sensitive (Watanakunakorn, 1984). *Propionibacterium acnes* is sensitive to vancomycin (Pallanza *et al.*, 1983). Of the other Gram-positive anaerobes, the *Actinomyces* spp. may be sensitive as are some, but not all, strains of the *Lactobacillus* spp. (Baker *et al.*, 1983; Watanakunakorn, 1984). *Rhodococcus equi*, a pathogen of immunocompromised patients (p. 782), is usually sensitive to vancomycin (Nordmann and Ronco, 1992).

f Resistant organisms Acquired vancomycin-resistance, a problem that has only appeared in the past 10 years, most commonly involves *Enterococcus* spp., but has also been described in coagulase-negative staphylococci. Some uncommon Gram-positive organisms are intrinsically resistant to vancomycin.

i Enterococci Vancomycin-resistant enterococci had been recognized occasionally in the past (Watanakunakorn, 1984), but larger numbers of isolates were reported in the late 1980s from Europe and the UK (Leclerq *et al.*, 1988; Uttley *et al.*, 1988). Subsequently, resistance appeared in the USA (Frieden *et al.*, 1993; CDC, 1993). Almost all resistant infections have been nosocomially acquired. Affected patients have usually been hospitalized for long periods of time, have received multiple courses of antibiotics (including third-generation cephalosporins or vancomycin) and usually suffer from other serious underlying medical or surgical conditions (Shay *et al.*, 1995). Clusters of infected and colonized patients have been described in specific hospital areas, such as a renal unit (Uttley *et al.*, 1989), an intensive care unit (Karanfil *et al.*, 1992) and oncology wards (Montecalvo *et al.*, 1994; Edmond *et al.*, 1995). Hospital-wide endemic infection and colonization can also occur (Morris *et al.*, 1995). A survey, chiefly of hospitals in the north-east of the USA, noted a 20-fold increase between 1989 and 1993 in the percentage of nosocomial infections caused by vancomycin-resistant enterococci; 13.9% of enterococcal isolates from patients in intensive care units were resistant (CDC, 1993). A more comprehensive USA survey, conducted between October and December 1992, revealed that 4.5% of enterococci were vancomycin-resistant, and 22% of hospitals participating in the survey reported resistant organisms. By March of 1994, this latter figure had increased to 61% (Jones *et al.*, 1995).

At least four patterns of vancomycin-resistance are seen in enterococci. Van A isolates, usually *E. faecium* but occasionally *E. faecalis* or *E. durans*, are resistant to high levels of vancomycin (MIC ≥64 μg per ml) and teicoplanin (MIC ≥64 μg per ml) (Arthur and Courvalin, 1993). Resistance is encoded on plasmids, is inducible in the presence of vancomycin, and is transferable to other enterococci. Enterococci with the Van B phenotype exhibit low to moderate vancomycin resistance (MIC 32–64 μg per ml) but are susceptible to teicoplanin (MIC < 1 μg per ml) (Williamson *et al.*, 1989). These organisms, most commonly strains of *E. faecalis*, are inducibly resistant, and the resistance determinants are usually non-transferable and chromosomally encoded. Van B isolates with plasmid-mediated resistance can also occur (Boyce *et al.*, 1994). Van C-resistance is found in all strains of *E. gallinarum*, an uncommon enterococcal isolate that is intrinsically resistant to low levels of vancomycin (8–32 μg per ml) but sensitive to teicoplanin. Resistance is constituitively expressed, chromosomally mediated and non-transferable (Leclerq *et al.*, 1992). Another uncommon enterococcus, *E. casseliflavus*, bears the Van C-like phenotype and is also intrinsically resistant to vancomycin and sensitive to teicoplanin (Navarro and Courvalin, 1994).

The mechanism of resistance is very complex and has been best characterized in Van A isolates (Arthur and Courvalin, 1993; Walsh, 1993). Plasmids in these isolates contain a cluster of genes that reside on a mobile genetic element – a transposon – within the plasmid. At least seven genes, *vanA*, *vanH*, *vanX*, *vanY*, *vanR*, *vanS* and *vanZ* are involved in mediating resistance. During normal bacterial cell wall synthesis, two D-alanine residues are joined by a bacterial ligase in the cytoplasm to produce the dipeptide D-ala-D-ala. This dipeptide is then added to UDP-muramic acid-tripeptide, a peptidoglycan precursor. *Van A* encodes a novel ligase that attaches a terminal D-lactate molecule to D-alanine, creating a depsipeptide D-ala-D-lac, which is then added to the peptidoglycan precursor in the normal fashion (Arthur *et al.*, 1992a). After the altered peptidoglycan precursor is linked to N-acetyl glucosamine and transported across the bacterial cell membrane, vancomycin cannot bind to this terminal D-lactate residue, but normal cell wall synthesis can still proceed and vancomycin-resistance results. *VanH* encodes a ketoacid reductase which generates the D-lactate subsequently incorporated by the vanA ligase into the peptidoglycan precursor. The product of the *vanX* gene also interferes with normal peptidoglycan synthesis by functioning as a dipeptidase that hydrolyzes the D-ala-D-ala precursor (Reynolds *et al.*, 1994). *VanY* encodes a membrane-associated carboxypeptidase that hydrolyzes the peptidoglycan peptide side-chain to which vancomycin usually binds (Arthur *et al.*, 1994). *VanS* and *vanR* are involved in regulation of the *vanA*, *vanH*, *vanX* and *vanY* gene expression (Arthur *et al.*, 1992b). The function of *vanZ* is unknown.

Similar mechanisms of resistance seem to occur in other resistant enterococci. Genes encoding ligases that are structurally related to the vanA gene product have been detected in Van B and Van C isolates (Evers *et al.*, 1993; Navarro and Courvalin, 1994). The reason why Van A isolates are highly resistant to vancomycin, but Van B and Van C isolates exhibit only moderate or low level resistance, is unknown. Van B and Van C isolates may contain a pool of normal D-ala-D-ala-containing peptidoglycan precursors to which vancomycin can bind and partially inhibit cell wall synthesis (Billot-Klein *et al.*, 1994).

Most vancomycin-resistant enterococci, particularly *E. faecium*, are often resistant to other antibiotics as well. They commonly exhibit intrinsic high-level resistance to penicillin G (p. 10) and ampicillin (p. 108), and plasmid-mediated high-level gentamicin-resistance (p. 455) is also frequent. These organisms may also be resistant to chloramphenicol but a proportion of strains are still sensitive to this drug (p. 555). Many strains are resistant to all commercially available antibiotics (Edmond *et al.*, 1995; Morris *et al.*, 1995: Murray, 1995; Patterson *et al.*, 1995).

A number of *in vitro* studies have investigated the activity of other rarely used or investigational antibiotics against these vancomycin-resistant isolates. Pristinamycin, a streptogramin antibiotic, was active against all 24 vancomycin-resistant *E. faecium* isolates tested by Wade *et al.* (1992); RP 59500, which contains a mixture of pristinamycin IA and pristinamycin IIA, was tested against 72 vancomycin-resistant enterococci (*E. faecalis* – 22, *E. faecium* – 45, *E. casseliflavus* and *E. gallinarum* – 5) by Collins *et al.* (1993a). It was active against all 13 moderately vancomycin-resistant *E. faecium* strains (mean MIC 0.8 µg per ml), but the other 32 highly resistant strains were less sensitive (mean MIC 2.5 µg per ml). Strains of *E. faecalis* were more resistant, with a mean MIC of 22.6 µg per ml; RP 59500 did not exhibit bactericidal activity against either *E. faecium* or *E. faecalis*. Ramoplanin, an investigational lipoglycopeptide antibiotic, inhibited all 43 vancomycin-resistant enterococcal isolates at a concentration of 0.5 µg per ml and time-kill studies demonstrated bactericidal activity (Collins *et al.*, 1993b). Mobarakai *et al.* (1994) also showed ramoplanin to have excellent bactericidal activity against 15 vancomycin-resistant *E. faecium* isolates. Daptomycin, a lipopeptide antibiotic that is not undergoing further development, was also active against these strains. Novobiocin (p. 663), an antibiotic that is rarely used nowadays but has good activity against Gram-positive coccal organisms, inhibited all 60 vancomycin- and ampicillin-resistant *E. faecium* strains at a concentration of ≤2 µg per ml, although MICs were higher when the tests were conducted in 50% serum (French *et al.*, 1993). The drug did not exhibit bactericidal activity by itself, but bactericidal activity could be demonstrated in combination with fluoroquinolone antibiotics (p. 666). Twenty-seven *E. faecalis* isolates tested were resistant to novobiocin. Landman *et al.* (1993) also reported appreciable killing of 12 of 15 resistant *E. faecium* strains with a combination of novobiocin and ciprofloxacin. Bacitracin, a non-absorbable antibiotic (p. 542) was active *in vitro* against some resistant *E. faecium* strains (Eng *et al.*, 1993).

A combination of vancomycin and penicillin G has activity *in vitro* against some vancomycin-resistant enterococci. When either amoxicillin, penicillin G or piperacillin was combined with vancomycin, Leclerq *et al.* (1991) noted synergistic inhibitory activity against 11 vancomycin-resistant *E. faecium* isolates and addition of gentamicin led to bactericidal activity. These isolates were only moderately resistant to penicillin G and none was resistant to high levels of gentamicin. Similar bactericidal activity with a triple combination of penicillin G / vancomycin / gentamicin was reported by Shlaes *et al.* (1991), again with isolates not resistant to high levels of aminoglycoside. The mechanism of synergy is incompletely understood, but probably involves a penicillin binding protein (PBP5) that is usually relatively resistant to inhibition by penicillin G. Expression of vancomycin resistance leads to a reduction in the activity of this PBP, and cell wall synthesis becomes dependent upon other PBPs. In some strains, these PBPs can be inhibited by penicillin G, leading to synergistic activity between vancomycin and penicillin G (Gutmann *et al.*, 1994).

In contrast, Handwerger *et al.* (1992), Fraimow and Venuti (1992) and Cercenado *et al.* (1992) did not demonstrate inhibitory activity with a combination of vancomycin and penicillin G or ampicillin against strains of *E. faecium* that exhibited higher levels of resistance to ampicillin. Addition of gentamicin did not generally lead to bacterial killing, particularly against those strains with high-level resistance to aminoglycosides.

ii Coagulase-negative staphylococci The great majority of coagulase-negative staphylococci remain sensitive to vancomycin. Vancomycin-resistant strains can be selected *in vitro* by passage in gradually increasing concentrations of vancomycin but this resistance is unstable and reversion to sensitivity occurs when vancomycin is removed (Watanakunakorn, 1988). In the early 1980s, isolates of *Staph. epidermidis* with reduced susceptibility to vancomycin were reported (Cherubin *et al.*, 1981; Tuazon and Miller, 1983). Subsequently, there have been a number of reports of clinically significant vancomycin-resistant coagulase-negative staphylococcal infections. Schwalbe *et al.* (1987) described a patient with chronic ambulatory peritoneal dialysis (CAPD)-associated peritonitis from whom *Staph. haemolyticus* was repeatedly isolated despite treatment with vancomycin. The isolate was initially sensitive to vancomycin, but the MIC of subsequent isolates progressively increased and resistant subpopulations of organisms (MIC 128 µg per ml) could be readily selected *in vitro*. *Staphylococcus haemolyticus* infections with low-level resistance to vancomycin have also been reported (Froggatt *et al.*, 1989; Veach *et al.*, 1990; Aubert *et al.*, 1990), mostly in patients treated with prolonged courses of glycopeptides prior to isolation of the resistant organisms. *Staphylococcus epidermidis* with relative resistance to vancomycin has also been reported in two patients with CAPD peritonitis (Sanyal *et al.*, 1993). The mechanism of resistance in coagulase-negative staphylococci is unknown. Resistance is stable in the absence of selective antibiotic pressure but is not plasmid-mediated, and not transferable.

iii   Staphylococcus aureus   Vancomycin-resistance has never been detected in a clinical isolate of *Staph. aureus. In vitro,* isolates of *Staph. aureus* can be selected with 2- to 8-fold increases in MIC by passaging sensitive strains in graded concentrations of vancomycin (Geraci *et al.*, 1957; Grappel *et al.*, 1983; Daum *et al.*, 1992). One of these isolates expressed a novel cytoplasmic protein of unknown function (Daum *et al.*, 1992). Of more concern, Noble *et al.* (1992), were able to transfer vancomycin-resistance genes from a Van A *E. faecalis* isolate to a *Staph. aureus* strain *in vitro* and *in vivo.*

iv   Vancomycin-resistant lactic bacteria   A number of infrequently isolated Gram-positive organisms are intrinsically resistant to vancomycin (Colman and Efstratiou, 1987). These organisms, often confused with viridans streptococci, are collectively known as vancomycin-resistant lactic bacteria (Mackey *et al.*, 1993). *Leuconostoc* spp. (Handwerger *et al.*, 1990), *Pediococcus* spp. (Mastro *et al.*, 1990) and some *Lactobacillus* spp. (Holliman and Bone, 1988) exhibit high-level vancomycin-resistance, although they almost always retain sensitivity to other antibiotics such as penicillins or erythromycin. Alterations in the peptidoglycan precursor leading to reduced binding of vancomycin have been identified in *Lactobacillus casei, Pediococcus pentosaceus* and *Leuconostoc mesenteroides* (Billot-Klein *et al.*, 1994).

v   Other organisms   The Gram-positive bacillus *Erysipelothrix rhusopathiae* is resistant to vancomycin (Gorby and Peacock, 1988). Vancomycin-resistance has been reported among viridans streptococci (Shlaes *et al.*, 1984; Baker and Thornsbury, 1974; Bourgault *et al.*, 1979), but some of these organisms may have been lactobacilli that were incorrectly identified (Thornsbury and Facklam, 1984) (see above).

vi   Tolerance   Tolerance (MBC/MIC ≥32) (p.91) to vancomycin may occur with strains of *Staph. aureus* (Geraci and Wilson, 1981), *Staph. epidermidis* (Geraci and Wilson, 1981), viridans streptococci (Geraci and Wilson, 1981; Meylan *et al.*, 1986), *Strep. bovis* (Geraci and Wilson, 1981) and Group G streptococci (Noble *et al.*, 1980).

2 Gram-negative bacteria

Occasional strains of *Neisseria* spp. may be susceptible to vancomycin (Griffith and Peck, 1956). In some areas up to 14% of gonococcal strains may be sensitive (Miller *et al.*, 1981). The use of vancomycin in modified Thayer-Martin medium, one selective for gonococci, may, therefore, significantly reduce the isolation rate of gonococci (Windall *et al.*, 1980). Results of susceptibility testing of *Flavobacterium* spp. vary with the method used. Vancomycin activity has been demonstrated against these organisms by some investigators (Raimondi *et al.*, 1986), but not by others (Watanakunakorn, 1984; Sader *et al.*, 1995). All other Gram-negative bacteria, including anaerobes (Baker *et al.*, 1983), are resistant.

Table I.55

After Jadeja *et al.* (1983), Watanakunakorn (1984), Moorhouse *et al.* (1985), Wadsworth *et al.* (1992), Amsterdam *et al.* (1994)

Organism	MIC (µg per ml)
Staphylococcus aureus (methicillin-sensitive)	0.25–2.0
Staphylococcus aureus (methicillin-resistant)	0.4–2.0
Coagulase-negative staphylococci	0.39–3.12
Streptococcus pyogenes	0.25–0.5
Streptococcus pneumoniae	0.25–1.0
Viridans group streptococci	0.06–8.0
Enterococcus faecalis	0.2–6.25
Clostridium difficile	1.0–8.0
Listeria monocytogenes	0.625–5.0
Corynebacterium jeikeium	0.20–6.25

3 Other organisms

Mycobacteria and fungi are vancomycin-resistant. *Borrelia burgdorferi*, the cause of Lyme disease, is sensitive *in vitro* (Dever *et al.*, 1993).

4 Minimal inhibitory concentrations

The MICs of vancomycin against some bacterial species are shown in Table I.55. Usually an organism is considered to be vancomycin-resistant if the MIC is 5 μg per ml or higher (Watanakunakorn, 1984).

Mode of Administration and Dosage

1 Parenteral administration

The usual recommended dosage for adults with normal renal function is 2 g i.v. daily, given as 1 g every 12 h or 0.5 g every 6 h. Previous experience has indicated that this dose will effectively treat infections for which vancomycin is being used. Peak serum levels with a dose of 1 g every 12 h are usually between 25 and 40 μg per ml, and trough levels are between 5 and 10 μg per ml. Most of the variability in these levels is related to the patient's weight (Healy *et al.*, 1987), so in order to achieve more uniform blood levels, doses based on body weight can also be used. The normal total daily dose is 30 mg per kg, given as a 6-hourly dose of 7.5 mg per kg or as a 12-hourly dose of 15 mg per kg. In order to overcome the poor CSF penetration of vancomycin (p. 773), higher doses – 15 mg per kg every 6 h – have been used to treat patients with meningitis (Klugman *et al.*, 1995) (p. 779). In obese patients, pharmacokinetic parameters such as volume of distribution and elimination half-life are significantly different from those of patients at or near their normal body weight (Vance-Bryan *et al.*, 1993). A dose of 0.5 g every 6 h or 1 g every 12 h will produce suboptimal peak and trough concentrations, so dosing based on the absolute body weight should be used to calculate initial vancomycin doses in these patients (Moellering *et al.*, 1984).

After the drug is reconstituted in water, the required dose is dissolved in 100–200 ml of 5% dextrose in water or 0.9% saline. This dose is then given by i.v. infusion over a period of at least 60 min (Rotschafer *et al.*, 1982; Moore, 1985). More rapid i.v. infusion can cause side-effects, and it may be prudent to monitor the patient's blood pressure during vancomycin infusion (p. 774). Vancomycin is stable in all commonly used i.v. fluids for at least 24 h, and therefore it can be administered by continuous i.v. infusion, provided that incompatible additives are avoided (Wysocki *et al.*, 1995). However, as for most other antibiotics, intermittent i.v. infusion is the preferred method of administration. Chloramphenicol succinate and methicillin can precipitate in solution with vancomycin (Banner and Ray, 1984). Experience in one patient who had a persistent *Staph. aureus* bacteremia whilst receiving vancomycin, suggested that heparin can inactivate vancomycin if the two agents are administered in a single i.v. line. Tests of the drugs *in vitro* at the concentrations achieved in the i.v. line resulted in precipitate formation and 50–60% reduction of vancomycin activity (Barg *et al.*, 1986). Because serum vancomycin levels may fall precipitously following initiation of cardiopulmonary bypass, a preoperative dose of at least 15 mg per kg must be given to maintain adequate serum levels (Moellering, 1984).

It is worth noting that the value of routine monitoring of serum vancomycin concentrations has recently been questioned (Freeman *et al.*, 1993; Cantu *et al.*, 1994; Moellering, 1994; Saunders, 1995). Such monitoring could be justified if it resulted in maximal therapeutic efficacy with minimal toxicity, but the available evidence does not support this. Higher peak serum levels do not appear to correlate with more successful therapy, nor is there an obvious association between peak levels and either oto- or nephrotoxicity (pp. 775, 776). A minimum trough level of 5 μg per ml is probably necessary for maximal antibacterial effect, but standard doses should readily achieve this. Higher trough levels are seen in association with renal impairment, but are often a consequence of the renal impairment and not necessarily the cause of it. For patients with normal renal function receiving standard vancomycin doses, routine monitoring of serum levels is not essential, although determination of trough levels may be considered (Saunders, 1995). Despite clear evidence of its benefit, serum monitoring should continue in other situations (Moellering, 1994). These include: i) patients also being treated with an aminoglycoside (p. 476) or other nephrotoxic agents, ii) patients with renal failure being treated with infrequent vancomycin doses (p. 769), iii) patients with renal impairment (including those with stable impairment in whom vancomycin doses have been accordingly adjusted, iv) other patients with altered vancomycin pharmacokinetics – preterm infants (see below), burns and pregnant patients (see below) and (possibly) patients with liver disease (p. 771) also pediatric cancer patients (see below), and v) patients receiving higher than normal vancomycin doses, for example in cases of penicillin G-resistant pneumococcal meningitis (p. 779).

Dosage requirements of vancomycin for infants and children vary according to age. In preterm infants, vancomycin clearance is reduced because of immature renal function, but as post-conceptional age increases, renal function improves and higher vancomycin doses are required. The neonate's serum creatinine level should not be used for dosage calculations because it is affected for several weeks after birth by creatinine that has crossed the placenta from the mother. A number of different dosing regimens, based on weight and post-conceptional age, have been suggested (Naqvi et al., 1986; James et al., 1987; Lisby and Nahata, 1987; Hardenbrook et al., 1991). In a prospective validation study of their proposed dosing schedule (James et al., 1987), Koren and James (1987) found that 67% of peak levels and 76% of trough levels in 32 premature infants were within the recommended range. On the basis of a review of published studies, Wandstrat and Phelps (1993) recommended the following doses: post-conceptional age less than 30 weeks – 15 mg per kg once-daily, post-conceptional age 30–34 weeks and weight less than 1.2 kg – 15 mg per kg twice-daily, post-conceptional age 30–42 weeks and weight greater than 1.2 kg – 15 mg per kg three times daily, and post-conceptional age greater than 42 weeks – 10 mg per kg four times daily. Others have proposed dosage regimens based on determination of pharmacokinetic parameters in individual patients because in addition to post-conceptional age and weight, factors such as hypotension, hypoxia, patent ductus arteriosus and use of indomethacin can affect renal function and hence vancomycin clearance. Jarret et al. (1993) found significant differences in dosage requirements (on a mg per kg basis) in preterm infants of a similar post-conceptional age using this individualized approach. Regardless of which approach or dosing regimen is used in preterm infants, vancomycin blood levels should be monitored and doses adjusted accordingly. On the basis of a pharmacokinetic study, Schaad et al. (1980) recommended a dose of 10 mg per kg four times daily in infants and older children.

Malignancy may alter the disposition of vancomycin. In a comparative study of infants and children with and without malignancy, vancomycin clearance rates and dosage requirements were higher in the cancer patients (Chang, 1995). On the basis of this and another study (Chang et al., 1994), a starting dose of 10 mg per kg six times daily was suggested for children with cancer, with further dosing guided by serum vancomycin estimations. Vancomycin clearance was also higher in 35 adult patients with hematologic malignancy, although dosage requirements were not greatly increased (Del Mar Fernandez de Gatta et al., 1993). The mechanism of the increased vancomycin clearance is unknown.

Patients with burns may require higher than normal doses of vancomycin to produce recommended serum concentrations because increases in glomerular filtration, and possibly tubular secretion, lead to increased vancomycin clearance (Brater et al., 1986; Rybak et al., 1990a). Injecting drug users tend to have higher vancomycin clearances (Rybak et al., 1990a) but it is not clear whether higher doses of vancomycin are required in this group. In pregnancy, Salzmann et al. (1987) reported that a dose of 57 mg per kg was required to maintain recommended drug levels in a patient who was 30 weeks pregnant. Increased doses are required because of the increase in volume of distribution and renal clearance and monitoring of serum concentrations is required.

2 Patients with renal failure

Vancomycin accumulates in these patients and a modified dosage schedule with serum level monitoring is necessary. In renal failure the vancomycin half-life is quite variable and may be greatly prolonged up to 17 days (Matzke et al., 1984). Because vancomycin clearance from the serum is linearly related to creatinine clearance, a variety of methods have been developed for determining vancomycin dosage adjustment in patients with impaired renal function. In the nomogram compiled by Moellering et al. (1981a), the total daily dose per kg is adjusted according to the creatinine clearance value. The latter can be estimated, if it cannot be measured directly, by a formula utilizing the patient's age, sex and serum creatinine value (the Cockroft-Gault equation). Matzke et al. (1984) prepared a nomogram for patients with impaired renal function in which, after an initial loading dose of 25 mg per kg, the vancomycin dose remains constant at 19 mg per kg but the dosage interval depends on the creatinine clearance (Fig I.29). This nomogram can be used for initiation of vancomycin therapy for functionally anephric patients on hemodialysis, but not for patients treated with intermittent or continuous peritoneal dialysis (see below). Rodvold et al. (1988), on the basis

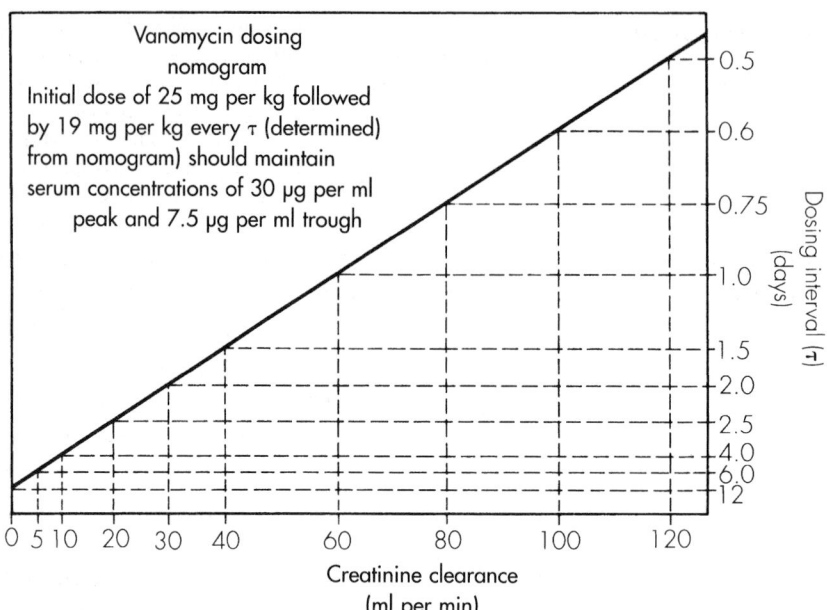

Fig. I.29.

Nomogram for vancomycin dosage in patients with renal failure. (After Matzke *et al.*, 1984, with permission.)

of a detailed pharmacokinetic study in 37 patients with varying degrees of renal impairment, developed the following equation to calculate vancomycin doses: dose (mg per kg per 24 h) = 0.227 × creatinine clearance (ml per min) + 5.67. There is a great variability in vancomycin half-life values in patients with impaired renal function, so that maintenance doses of the drug should be guided by serum levels.

Very little vancomycin is removed from the body by hemodialysis (Lindholm and Murray, 1966; Eykyn *et al.*, 1970). In 29 anephric patients managed by hemodialysis at 3-day intervals, a single 1 g i.v. dose of vancomycin given over a period of 30 min resulted in a mean peak serum level of 48.3 μg per ml which declined to 15 μg per ml within 3–5 h but was still 3.5 μg per ml after 18 days; the mean elimination half-life was 7.5 days (Cunha *et al.*, 1981). A study by Quale *et al.* (1992) suggested that use of newer dialysis membranes with greater permeability to larger molecules (high-flux membranes) altered vancomycin pharmacokinetics. Vancomycin levels post-high-flux membrane dialysis were only 63% of pre-dialysis levels, with low vancomycin levels in the dialysate suggesting binding of vancomycin to the membrane. However, rebound in vancomycin levels occurs after completion of high-flux hemodialysis, so different dosing regimens are probably not required for these patients (Pollard *et al.*, 1994). Patients on hemodialysis should be given an i.v. loading dose of 1 g or 15 mg per kg. A serum level should be measured 5–7 days later, and the vancomycin dose repeated if necessary when the level falls below 5–10 μg per ml.

Peritoneal dialysis also results in minimal clearance of vancomycin (Moellering, 1984). Magera *et al.* (1983) did not find any appreciable change in vancomycin concentrations before, during or after completion of chronic intermittent peritoneal dialysis, and serum levels were maintained above 4 μg per ml for 8 days after a single 1-g i.v. dose. Morse *et al.* (1987) studied four patients undergoing CAPD who received a 15 mg per kg i.v. dose. The mean peak serum vancomycin concentration was 57.1 μg per ml, at 24 h the level was 19.8 μg per ml and 7 days later, the level was still 8.6 μg per ml. The mean terminal elimination half-life was 111 h. The mean dialysate concentration at the end of the initial dwell was 5.8 μg per ml, and subsequent end-dwell dialysate concentrations were greater that 2 μg per ml for most exchanges over a 1 week period. For patients on CAPD, vancomycin doses of 15 mg per kg every 7 days (Krothapalli *et al.*, 1983), or 23 mg per kg initially followed by 17 mg per kg every 7 days (Blevins *et al.*, 1984) have been recommended, but should be guided by serum levels.

In contrast to peritoneal and hemodialysis, some vancomycin is cleared by patients undergoing hemofiltration (Matzke *et al.*, 1986). Continuous hemodiafiltration removes larger amounts of vancomycin (Bellomo *et al.*, 1990), and twice-daily administration of 7.5 mg per kg i.v. was suggested by Santré *et al.* (1993). However, because of patient-to-patient variability resulting from factors such as blood flow rates through the filtration apparatus, monitoring of serum concentrations is necessary to guide dosing.

3 Patients with liver disease

Renal mechanisms account for almost all vancomycin elimination but vancomycin can be detected in feces and bile, indicating that some hepatic clearance also occurs. Brown et al. (1983) found that the vancomycin elimination half-life was prolonged in cancer patients with abnormal liver function, but Rodvold et al. (1988) could not correlate abnormalities in liver function with changes in vancomycin clearance. Dosage adjustment is probably not necessary in patients with liver impairment, but monitoring of serum levels would be prudent.

4 Intraperitoneal administration

Vancomycin can be added to peritoneal dialysis fluid and administered intraperitoneally. The half-life for equilibration of vancomycin into the circulation from the dialysate is 2.8–3 h (Rogge et al., 1985; Baillie et al., 1992) so that approximately 65% and 75% of an intraperitoneal vancomycin dose is absorbed across the peritoneal membrane and into the systemic circulation after 4 and 6-h dwells respectively. In effect, a 2 g dose of vancomycin given intraperitoneally over a 4 h dwell period is equivalent to a 1.3 g dose given i.v.. Absorption is enhanced in the presence of peritonitis (Rubin, 1990). In four CAPD patients given 30 mg per kg of vancomycin intraperitoneally, Morse et al. (1987) found a mean end-dwell dialysate concentration of 610 μg per ml and a mean peak serum concentration of 30.4 μg per ml. Baillie et al. (1992), using a lower intraperitoneal dose of 15 mg per kg, reported a peak serum concentration of 17.8 μg per ml. With lower intraperitoneal doses, such as those used when peritoneal dialysis-associated peritonitis is treated by adding vancomycin to each dialysis bag, much lower levels are obtained – a maintenance dose of 25 mg per liter results in a serum level of 0.27 μg per ml and a dialysate concentration of 10.7 μg per ml at the end of the first dwell, the serum level taking many days to reach 10 μg per ml.

Based on these data, and on the desirability of rapidly achieving adequate serum levels, treatment of CAPD-associated peritonitis should involve the administration of a loading dose of 15–30 mg per kg of vancomycin (given either intravenously or intraperitoneally), after which a maintenance dose (2–30 mg per liter) of vancomycin may be given intraperitoneally with each dialysis exchange (Johnson, 1991).

5 Intrathecal and intraventricular administration

Vancomycin has been administered both intrathecally (Moellering et al.,1981b) and by the intraventricular route (Gump, 1981) because of the variable penetration of vancomycin into the CSF after systemic dosing. Pharmacokinetic parameters are altered by factors such as obstructive hydrocephalus, ventricular CSF shunts, reduced absorption of CSF across the arachnoid villi and concomitant i.v. vancomycin therapy. A wide range of intraventricular doses has been used, from 1–2 to 20 mg per day, but the usual dose is 10–20 mg per day (Luer and Hatton,1993). Reported CSF concentrations have also differed greatly, with significant inter- and intra-patient variability. Ideally, ventricular drug levels should be monitored, aiming for a peak concentration of 30–50 μg per ml (Reesor et al., 1988).

6 Oral administration

Oral vancomycin, in a dosage of 125–500 mg every 6 h for 5–10 days, has been used effectively to treat antibiotic-associated colitis (p. 594). Reconstituted vancomycin is stable for 58 days at room temperature (25°C) and for at least 90 days under refrigeration (4°C) or freezing (0°C) (Mallet et al., 1982). Very little vancomycin is absorbed after oral administration. Fecal levels of 85–540 μg per ml liquid stool were present in two infants given 15–20 mg per kg per day of oral vancomycin, but serum levels were only 0.9–1.05 μg per ml (Schaad et al., 1980). However, some systemic absorption can occur, especially in patients with renal failure in whom vancomycin elimination is decreased. Spitzer and Eliopoulus (1984) noted serum levels between 11.4 and 20.3 μg per ml in a hemodialysis patient with antibiotic-associated colitis given 500 mg four times daily. Bergeron and Boucher (1994) described a leukemic infant with normal renal function who developed antibiotic-associated colitis whilst neutropenic, and was treated with oral vancomycin 1 mg per kg four times daily. A serum level of 28.7 μg per ml was obtained 1 h after dosing in association with a possible hypersensitivity reaction. Absorption probably occurred because of the combined effects of antibiotic-associated colitis, and alterations in mucosal integrity secondary to neutropenia and chemotherapy.

7 Other modes of administration

Vancomycin can be injected intravitreally to treat cases of endophthalmitis. The recommended dose is 1–2 mg, which can repeated after 3–4 days if necessary (Barza, 1989). Vancomycin has also been incorporated into orthopedic bone cement for management of prosthetic joint infections and chronic osteomyelitis (Kuechle *et al.*, 1991), although there is little experience with this technique. Aerosol admininstation of vancomycin has successfully eradicated airway colonization by methicillin-resistant *Staph. aureus* (Weathers *et al.*, 1990).

Serum Levels In Relation To Dosage

In adult volunteers, serum levels 1 h after a 500-mg dose are 13–22 µg per ml, and after a 1-g dose, 25–40 µg per ml (Blouin *et al.*, 1982; Healey *et al.*, 1987; Boeckh *et al.*, 1988). In adults with normal renal function, Healy *et al.* (1987) reported little inter-subject variation in serum levels – a mean level of 33.7 µg per ml 1 h after a 1-g dose with a standard deviation of 3.8 µg per ml and a range between 26.5 and 40.5 µg per ml. Most of the variation could be accounted for by differences in weight of the subjects. There is more variation in the elimination half-life, which ranges from 3 to 13 h, the mean being approximately 6 h (Rotschafer *et al.*, 1982). Healy *et al.* (1987) demonstrated that some vancomycin accumulation occurred in their normal subjects with repeated dosing. Trough levels increased from 5.4 µg per ml to 11.2 µg per ml after five doses of 500 mg given 6-hourly and from 4.9 µg per ml to 7.9 µg per ml after three i.v. 12-hourly doses of 1 g. Continuous infusion of 30 mg per kg over 24 h in 13 patients resulted in a plateau level of 24 ± 6 µg per ml (Wysocki *et al.*, 1995).

Preterm infants do not have fully mature renal systems, and vancomycin clearance is impaired as a result (p. 769)The first dose recommendations for this group were made by Schaad *et al.* (1980) but peak and trough levels were often excessive with the suggested doses (Alpert *et al.*, 1984). Subsequent dosage recommendations have been based on post-conceptional age and weight (p. 769), and generally result in peak levels of 30–40 µg per ml, and trough levels of 5–10 µg per ml (Naqvi *et al.*, 1986; James *et al.*, 1987; Lisby and Nahata, 1987; Hardenbrook *et al.*, 1991)

Schaad *et al.* (1980) also studied vancomycin levels in older infants and children. A 15 mg per kg dose given to seven term infants produced a mean peak level of 29.8 µg per ml, and in infants aged 1–12 months, 10 mg per kg and 15 mg per kg doses resulted in peak levels of 26.1 and 28.0 µg per ml, respectively. Similar levels were noted in children 3–5 years of age given these two doses. Calculated elimination half-lives were 5.9–9.8 h for newborn infants, 4.1 h for older infants and 2.2–3.0 h for children. Serum level monitoring on 11 other patients showed there was no evidence of accumulation with repeated doses.

Because vancomycin administered i.v. is mainly eliminated by the kidneys, higher serum levels are produced in patients with impaired renal function than in those with normal function, if dosage modification is not employed (p. 769). This may also apply to patients with liver disease (p. 771). Pregnant patients or those with burn injuries have higher vancomycin clearances and larger doses are required to produce recommended serum levels (p. 769). After oral administration, only very low serum concentrations are obtained, except in the presence of renal disease plus bowel inflammation (p. 771).

Excretion

1 Urine

Virtually all of an i.v. administered dose of vancomycin is excreted by the kidneys in an unchanged form. This occurs primarily by glomerular filtration but there is evidence that some tubular secretion may occur as well (Moellering, 1984; Rybak *et al.*, 1990a). About 80–90% of an i.v. administered dose can be recovered from the urine during the first 24 h. Urine concentrations of 9–300 µg per ml are maintained for 24 h after a single 0.5-g i.v. dose in healthy adults (Geraci *et al.*, 1957). The prolonged elimination half-life in preterm infants (p. 769) may be related to immaturity of the kidneys, and to a lesser extent possibly to immaturity of the liver.

2 Bile

Geraci *et al.* (1957) found small quantities of vancomycin in the bile and feces after i.v. administration.

3 Feces

After i.v. administration of vancomycin to children, Schaad *et al.* (1980) found fecal concentrations of the drug of 4.1–35.8 µg per g wet stool (mean, 12.5 µg per g).

4 Inactivation in body

Extrarenal (possibly hepatic) excretion of vancomycin may occur to a small extent, because relatively high vancomycin clearances are observed in patients with compromised renal function

(Rotschafer *et al.*, 1982) and there is a prolonged vancomycin half-life in patients with abnormal liver function (p. 769).

Distribution of Drug in the Body

Vancomycin diffuses readily into pleural, pericardial, ascitic and synovial fluids (Geraci *et al.*, 1957). The drug penetrates well into peritoneal dialysate after i.v. administration (Whitby *et al.*, 1987) (p. 771). Vancomycin does not appear to diffuse well into the aqueous humor of the eye (Moellering, 1984). In a study of postmortem tissues from a patient treated with vancomycin until the time of death, good concentrations were found in the kidney, liver, lung, heart and aorta and in an abscess (Torres-R *et al.*,1979). Vancomycin penetrates satisfactorily into mediastinal and cardiac tissues when given as a 15 mg per kg preoperative dose (with or without a supplemental 7.5 mg per kg at the time of cardiopulmonary bypass) (Martin *et al.*, 1994). Vancomycin levels in lung epithelial lining fluid obtained by bronchoalveolar lavage averaged 4.5 µg per ml in 14 critically ill patients being treated with vancomycin (Lamer *et al.*, 1993). Bone penetration has been investigated in 19 patients, five of whom had osteomyelitis, and adequate cancellous and cortical levels were obtained in most specimens (Graziani *et al.*, 1988).

In patients with uninflamed meninges CSF penetration is poor but increases in the presence of meningitis. In 11 adult patients with pneumococcal meningitis treated with vancomycin 7.5 mg per kg every 6 h, median trough levels after 48 h of treatment were 2 and 5.1 µg per ml in CSF and serum respectively. At the end of 10 days of treatment, peak CSF and serum levels were 1.9 and 18.5 µg per ml respectively (Viladrich *et al.*, 1991). When a higher vancomycin dose of 15 mg per kg every 6 h was used in children, the mean CSF level 2–3 h after dosing was 3.3 µg per ml, which was 21% of the mean simultaneously measured serum level (Klugman *et al.*, 1995) (p. 779). Schaad *et al.* (1981) studied three infants treated with i.v. vancomycin who had ventriculoperitoneal shunt infections and a mild CSF pleocytosis; CSF concentrations of vancomycin were 1.2–4.8 µg per ml, which were calculated to be 7–21% (mean 14%) of the concurrent serum levels. In 12 children with ventriculoperitoneal shunt infections treated with i.v. vancomycin (mean dose 55 mg per kg per day), the mean vancomycin level in 27 ventricular fluid specimens was 5.5 µg per ml (McGee *et al.*, 1990). Serum levels were not reported. Ventricular fluid levels correlated with higher CSF protein concentrations and white blood cell counts and lower glucose levels. Levels obtained in CSF may be suboptimal for some infections, so that intrathecal or intraventricular administration may be necessary (p. 771). In contrast to poor penetration into CSF, vancomycin penetrates well into brain tissue itself. Levy *et al.* (1986) found satisfactory brain abscess pus levels in a patient treated with vancomycin for a *Staph. aureus* brain abscess. Vancomycin is about 55% bound to serum proteins (Moellering, 1984), mostly to serum albumin and Ig(CA)A (Sun *et al.*, 1993).

Mode of Action

Vancomycin is bactericidal for most Gram-positive organisms, enterococci being exceptional (p. 764). Resistance of Gram-negative bacilli is due to a permeability barrier provided by porin proteins in the outer membrane (p. 26) (Newsom, 1982). Vancomycin is bound rapidly and irreversibly to the cell walls of sensitive bacteria (Sinha and Neuhaus, 1968), thereby inhibiting cell wall synthesis. Vancomycin is a heptapeptide and its three-dimensional pocket shape is the result of formation of bonds between aromatic amino acid residues. The N-terminal amino acid leucine is critical for the activity of vancomycin. Vancomycin binds by its N-terminal end to the C-terminal D-alanine-D-alanine residues of the peptidoglycan precursor UDP-N-acetylmuramyl pentapeptide at the external surface of the cytoplasmic membrane (p. 26). In the absence of vancomycin, the peptidoglycan precursor is added to the growing peptidoglycan chain by a transglycosylase enzyme, but vancomycin inhibits this reaction, probably due to steric hindrance. Vancomycin also inhibits the transpeptidases and carboxypeptidases that ordinarily cross-link adjacent peptidoglycan chains with pentaglycine side-chains (Nagarajan, 1991). The end result is inhibition of synthesis of the normally rigid cell wall. Lysis of the cell eventually occurs due to the unopposed action of autolysins. Inhibition of cell wall synthesis by vancomycin precedes and is different from the actions of beta-lactam agents on the cell wall (p. 27). Other actions on the cytoplasmic membrane and inhibition of RNA synthesis have been ascribed to vancomycin (Pfeiffer, 1981), but are much less important than actions on the cell wall.

Toxicity

Early preparations, called 'Mississippi mud' because of their appearance, contained many impurities. The frequency of side-effects has been reduced with better purification procedures (Griffith, 1984).

1 Hypersensitivity and related side-effects

A reaction, variably known as the red-man, red man's, red neck or red person's syndrome, is a well-recognized complication of vancomycin infusion (Polk, 1991). It was described soon after vancomycin was first used (Rothenberg, 1959; Spears and Koch, 1960). This reaction comprises any combination of skin itch, skin flushing (most prominent over the upper body), angioedema, hypotension, tachycardia and occasionally muscle aches. The reaction typically begins approximately 30 min after the infusion has started with patients complaining of itch and warmth over the head and chest. Progression of symptoms may occur with development of angioedema, but bronchospasm is not a feature, and hypotension, though not infrequent in closely monitored patients, is rarely clinically significant. The reaction may begin to abate even as the infusion is continued, and almost always resolves completely within 1 h of completion of the infusion.

The red-man syndrome is believed to result from vancomycin-induced histamine release (Polk et al., 1988). This release is non-immunologically mediated. Several studies have demonstrated a correlation between the levels or rate of production of histamine and the occurrence of red-man syndrome in healthy volunteers. Polk et al. (1988) found histamine release to be greater during infusion of a 1000-mg dose than during a 500-mg dose, and the magnitude of the release correlated with the severity of the infusion-related reaction. Similar results were obtained in a study comparing a 1- and 2-h i.v. infusion of vancomycin 1 g (Healy et al., 1990). Pretreatment with antihistamines can reduce the frequency of red-man syndrome; only 8% of healthy volunteers developed the reaction after medication with an H_1 antagonist (hydroxyzine), compared with 92% of placebo recipients. Ranitidine, an H_2 antagonist, did not prevent the development of the syndrome (Sahai et al., 1989). A similar protective effect with antihistamines has also been reported in patients treated with vancomycin (Wallace et al., 1991). However, not all studies have supported a relationship between histamine release and red-man syndrome (Rybak et al., 1992; O'Sullivan et al., 1993), and histamine infusion in normal volunteers does not produce itch or edema so it is possible that other mediators such as bradykinin or serotonin are involved in this reaction.

Red-man syndrome is much more common in healthy volunteers than in patients. Combining the results of six studies, a striking 58 of 66 healthy adult volunteers receiving a 1.0-g i.v. infusion of vancomycin over 60 min have developed red-man syndrome (Polk et al., 1988, 1993; Sahai et al., 1989, 1990; Healy et al., 1990; Rybak et al., 1992). In contrast, the reaction was reported in none of 15 (Rybak et al., 1992), and in only one of 29 (O'Sullivan et al., 1993) patients treated with vancomycin. Reactions may be less common in patients for the following reasons: prior administration of antihistamines for other purposes, depletion of histamine stores in response to acute infection or from prior use of narcotics, or greater difficulty in recognizing the syndrome in ill patients. However, Wallace et al. (1991) reported that eight of 17 patients not pre-treated with antihistamines developed red-man syndrome.

The dose of vancomycin and its rate of infusion also affect the frequency of red-man syndrome. Vancomycin 500 mg i.v. infused over 60 min caused no reactions in 11 healthy adult volunteers compared with reactions in nine of those given 1000 mg (Polk et al., 1988). Similarly, when 1000 mg of vancomycin was infused over 2 h rather than 1 h to ten healthy volunteers, the number developing reactions fell from eight with the shorter infusion to three with the longer infusion (Healy et al., 1990). The incidence of red-man syndrome is highest with the first dose of vancomycin and falls with subsequent doses; Polk et al. (1988) noted that nine of 11 healthy volunteers developed red-man syndrome with the first dose of vancomycin, but only four experienced a reaction after the third dose, and the reaction was less severe. Red-man syndrome is much less common with the other glycopeptide antibiotic teicoplanin (Sahai et al., 1990; Rybak et al., 1992) (p. 795).

If a patient develops red-man syndrome, the infusion time should be extended to 2 h and pre-treatment with an antihistamine may be considered. In the rare patient in whom red-man syndrome still occurs, teicoplanin could be used instead. Vancomycin skin testing (Polk et al., 1993) does not predict the subsequent development of red-man syndrome. Successful vancomycin desensitization has been reported (Lin, 1990; Wong et al., 1994).

The hypotensive effect of i.v. vancomycin seems to be related to the rate of infusion, and has been of most concern in patients given pre- or intraoperative vancomycin. Hypotension is uncommon when vancomycin is infused over 60 min, but was reported in 11 of 25 patients given vancomycin 1 g over 10 min preoperatively (Newfield and Roizen, 1979). Rapid infusions have also been associated with cardiopulmonary arrest (Glicklich and Figura, 1984; Southorn et al., 1986), a grand-mal fit with angioedema of the face and lips (Baillie et al., 1985) and death (McHenry and Gavan, 1983). Romanelli et al. (1993) found that vancomycin infused preoperatively over 30 min did not affect hemodynamic parameters, but doses given intra- and postoperatively resulted in significantly lowered systolic blood pressure and mean arterial pressure. However, the intraoperative dose was infused rapidly in these patients. When vancomycin has been administered more slowly (over 30–60 min) either pre- or postinduction of anesthesia, no significant changes in heart rate or blood pressure have been noted in other studies (Von Kaenel et al., 1993; Rosenberg et al., 1995). Pre- and intraoperative administration of vancomycin appears to be safe, provided the drug is infused over 30–60 min, but potentiation of the hypotensive effect of vancomycin by anesthetic agents being given at the same time can occur. Increased intracranial pressure has also been reported when vancomycin was given as prophylaxis to patients with external ventricular CSF drains (Gaskill and Marlin, 1992).

Some generalized reactions to vancomycin do not have features of the red-man syndrome. Sahai et al. (1988) reported a patient with a severe reaction to vancomycin characterized by fever, hypotension and rash that was not associated with histamine release, and did not abate when the vancomycin infusion rate was slowed. Cole et al. (1985) described a patient with a reaction resembling the red-man syndrome, that developed 30 min after a 1 h infusion with fever, rash, hypertension and pruritis lasting for several hours. True allergic vancomycin reactions, mediated by Ig E, are very uncommon.

2 Local toxicity

Chemical thrombophlebitis is common when vancomycin is administered into a peripheral vein, occurring in up to 13% of patients (Farber and Moellering, 1983). Vancomycin may cause a chemical peritonitis when used in doses of 1 g or greater to treat episodes of CAPD-associated peritonitis (Johnson, 1991). In animal studies, vancomycin is toxic to retinal cells when high doses are injected intravitreally. (Borhani et al., 1993)).

3 Nephrotoxicity

Although long considered to be toxic to kidneys, the true potential of vancomycin to cause kidney damage is not clear. Early reports of nephrotoxicity may have been related to impurities (see above), and more recent information suggests that the nephrotoxicity of vancomycin has been overstated. Other factors that affect renal function, such as other nephrotoxic drugs (particularly aminoglycosides), hypotension and a variety of underlying medical conditions are often present in patients being treated with vancomycin, and these factors confound the interpretation of most studies examining the nephrotoxicity of vancomycin.

In patients receiving vancomycin alone, varying rates of nephrotoxicity have been reported. Nephrotoxicity was not observed in any of 25 patients reported by Sorrell and Collignon (1985), while Farber and Moellering (1983), in a retrospective study, found that only 5% of patients receiving vancomycin alone developed renal impairment, and this was reversible on discontinuation of the drug. A similar figure was obtained by Rybak et al. (1990b) in a prospective study of 168 adult patients with no underlying or predisposing factors that might affect renal function. Higher rates of nephrotoxicity have been noted by other authors: 13% and 19% in two studies of elderly patients (Downs et al., 1989; Goetz and Sayers, 1993) and 15% in cancer patients (Cimino et al., 1987). Dean et al. (1985) detected rises in serum creatinine in two of 19 children treated with vancomycin.

The data on the nephrotoxicity of combined vancomycin and an aminoglycoside are also conflicting. Farber and Moellering (1983) noted renal damage in 35% of patients treated with vancomycin and an aminoglycoside. Pauly et al. (1990) found that 28 of 105 patients (27%) treated with combined vancomycin and an aminoglycoside developed renal impairment, although another nephrotoxic factor was present in 22 of these 28 patients. Rybak et al. (1990b) reported renal impairment in 14 of 63 patients (22%) treated with vancomycin and an aminoglycoside, compared with only eight of 168 patients (5%) receiving vancomycin alone (see above). Other studies do not support a significant nephrotoxic interaction between vancomycin and an aminoglycoside. Neither Mellor et al. (1985) nor Cimino et al. (1987) found evidence of synergistic nephrotoxicity between the two drugs, and Goetz and Sayers (1993) noted only a mild increase in nephrotoxicity with vancomycin and an aminoglycoside (24%) versus vancomycin alone (19%) (see above). In a detailed prospective study of 289 patients, Vance-Bryan et al. (1994) reported an overall rate of vancomycin nephrotoxicity of 13.4%. Nephrotoxicity was significantly more common in patients older than 60 years (18.9%) compared with patients aged less than 60 years (7.8%). Associations were noted with loop diuretic use in the elderly and with amphotericin B use in the younger population. However, aminoglycoside use did not significantly increase the risk of nephrotoxicity in either age group or in the overall population. Goetz and Sayers (1993) performed a meta-analysis of nine other studies published between 1966 and 1991 of adult patients receiving vancomycin plus an aminoglycoside or either agent alone. Of patients receiving vancomycin alone, 8.1% developed renal impairment, compared with 21.4% of those treated with vancomycin and an aminoglycoside. Although this difference was highly significant, 17.1% of patients in five of these studies treated with an aminoglycoside alone developed renal impairment. These authors point out an obvious problem in the interpretation of these non-randomized studies, namely that receipt of combination therapy may be a marker for more serious underlying conditions, and that these conditions, rather than vancomycin, are responsible for nephrotoxicity. The only data on the nephrotoxicity of vancomycin in combination with an aminoglycoside in randomly allocated patients comes from randomized studies of neutropenic patients (EORTC, 1991). Of 370 patients treated with ceftazidime and amikacin, only two developed renal impairment, compared with six of 383 treated with vancomycin plus these two drugs.

Another area of controversy is the role of serum monitoring of vancomycin levels in the prevention of vancomycin-associated nephrotoxicity (p. 775). Some studies have associated high trough levels with the development of nephrotoxicity (Farber and Moellering, 1983; Rybak et al., 1990b; Cimino et al., 1987), but nephrotoxicity has also occurred in patients who have trough serum levels within the normal range. In a critical review of the value of vancomycin levels in general, Cantu et al. (1994) not only question the nephrotoxic potential of vancomycin, but point out that the increased vancomycin levels that may be seen in association with renal impairment have not always preceded an increase in serum creatinine and so may be secondary to the renal impairment and not its primary cause (p. 768).

In summary, although studies on the nephrotoxicity of vancomycin reach different conclusions, the balance of evidence suggests that vancomycin can cause renal impairment. When used alone, and in the absence of other factors that can affect renal function, the rate of nephrotoxicity is of the order of 5% or less. In patients treated with a combination of vancomycin and gentamicin, nephrotoxicity seems to be more common than when either agent is used alone, although whether toxicity is additive or truly synergistic is not established.

4 Ototoxicity

Early reports of tinnitus and deafness complicating vancomycin treatment led to vancomycin developing a reputation as an ototoxic drug. However, many of these early reports described patients being treated with other ototoxic drugs such as streptomycin or erythromycin. It is also possible that earlier preparations of vancomycin were more toxic to the ear, just as these preparations may have been responsible for more hypersensitivity reactions and renal damage.

Although may case reports and small series of cases of deafness related to vancomycin have subsequently appeared in the literature, ototoxicity does not appear to be common. It was not observed in a retrospective study of 98 vancomycin-treated patients (Farber and Moellering, 1983) and of 54 patients monitored prospectively by Sorrell and Collignon (1985), only one of 11 tested patients, who was also being treated with gentamicin, developed unilateral hearing impairment. Mellor et al. (1985) followed 34 patients prospectively and temporary tinnitus and deafness developed in two patients, one of whom also received gentamicin. A recent review of the literature (Brummett and Fox, 1989) concluded that the ototoxicity of vancomycin has been overrated, and that only a very few cases of true vancomycin ototoxicity have occurred. However, an animal study has demonstrated that vancomycin, though not ototoxic itself (Lutz et al., 1991), enhances the ototoxicity of aminoglycosides (Brummett et al., 1990), so vancomycin may be ototoxic when used with aminoglycosides, or possibly with other ototoxic agents.

A relationship between serum levels of vancomycin and ototoxicity has not been established (p. 772). High peak levels of 80 μg per ml were reported to be associated with auditory toxicity in patients with renal failure (Lindholm and Murray, 1966), but high frequency hearing loss and tinnitus have also occurred with peak serum levels as low as 38–40 μg per ml (Sorrell and Collignon, 1985). Given the rarity of vancomycin ototoxicity, it is unlikely that any study will be able to demonstrate an association between higher peak (or trough) levels and increased auditory damage (Cantu et al., 1994).

5 Cutaneous reactions

A variety of cutaneous reactions, not including the red-man syndrome (see above), have been described in patients treated with vancomycin. Early studies reported that 5% of patients developed rashes, most of which were described as erythematous and maculopapular (Farber and Moellering, 1983), but some of these rashes may have been related to impurities in early vancomycin preparations (see above). Other rashes reported to be due to vancomycin include linear IgA bullous dermatosis (Kuechle et al., 1994), exfoliative dermatitis (Forrence and

Goldman, 1990), Stevens–Johnson syndrome (Laurencin *et al.*, 1992), cutaneous vasculitis (Markman *et al.*, 1986) and toxic epidermal necrolysis (Hannah *et al.*, 1990).

6 Hematological toxicity

Vancomycin uncommonly causes neutropenia. Almost all affected patients have been treated with vancomycin for prolonged periods (usually 15–40 days) and neutropenia resolves promptly (within a few days) upon discontinuation of the drug (Koo *et al.*, 1986). In their retrospective study of 94 patients, Farber and Moellering (1983) reported that 2% became neutropenic. An even higher rate of 8% (four of 49 cardiothoracic surgical patients) was reported by Morris and Ward (1991), but general experience would suggest that vancomycin-induced neutropenia is considerably less common than this. There is no clear relationship between serum levels and the development of neutropenia. The neutropenia may be related to the presence of anti-neutrophil antibodies (Domen and Horowitz, 1990). Vancomycin has also been reported as a cause of thrombocytopenia in several patients (Walker and Heaton, 1985; Zenon *et al.*, 1991; Christie *et al.*, 1990).

7 Other side effects

Vancomycin has an unpleasant taste and when administered orally, it may cause nausea (McHenry and Gavan, 1983). Vancomycin overdosage was successfully treated in one patient by hemoperfusion; this man, who was receiving regular hemodialysis, inadvertently received a dose of 500 mg every 6 h (total dose 2.5g). His tinnitus recovered with the associated fall in serum vancomycin levels during hemoperfusion, and high frequency hearing loss recovered after a month (Ahmad *et al.*, 1982).

Clinical Uses of the Drug

1 Methicillin-resistant *Staph. aureus* infections

Prior to the development of the penicillinase-resistant penicillins and other potent anti-staphylococcal agents, vancomycin was used fairly extensively for the treatment of severe *Staph. aureus* infections, such as septicemia and endocarditis. Many clinical studies confirmed that it was effective for these diseases (Geraci *et al.*, 1957, 1958; Kirby *et al.*, 1960). With the spread of MRSA strains, which became progressively resistant to multiple antibiotics in the 1970s (p. 80), vancomycin again became pre-eminent for the treatment of staphylococcal infections. Virtually all strains of MRSA are sensitive to vancomycin (p. 763) though some strains may show tolerance (p. 91). Many publications have attested to the clinical efficacy of vancomycin in serious *Staph. aureus* infections, such as septicemia, endocarditis, pneumonia and cellulitis, due to methicillin- and multiple antibiotic-resistant strains (Cafferkey *et al.*, 1982; Myers and Linnemann, 1982; Sorrell *et al.*, 1982; Craven *et al.*, 1983).

Failure of some MRSA infections to respond to vancomycin has been correlated with the presence of tolerant strains (Sorrell *et al.*, 1982; Faville *et al.*, 1978). Sande and Scheld (1980) recommended that infections caused by vancomycin-tolerant strains should be treated with a combination of vancomycin and rifampicin, although the *in vitro* results of testing combinations of vancomycin with other antibiotics and the therapeutic results of such combinations in patients have been very inconsistent. However, if treatment fails with vancomycin alone, the addition of an aminoglycoside or rifampicin should be considered (Watanakunakorn, 1982).

Response to vancomycin may be delayed in cases of staphylococcal endocarditis. In a study comparing vancomycin with the combination of vancomycin and rifampicin for the treatment of MRSA endocarditis, the median durations of bacteremia and fever were 9 days and 7 days respectively (Levine *et al.*, 1991). No difference was noted between the two treatment groups. In comparison, patients treated with anti-staphylococcal beta-lactam antibiotics for methicillin-sensitive *Staph. aureus* endocarditis have a mean duration of bacteremia of 3 days (Korzeniowski and Sande, 1982). An unexpectedly high failure rate was also observed in 13 intravenous drug users with *Staph. aureus* endocarditis (two methicillin-resistant cases) treated with vancomycin (Small and Chambers, 1990). Five of the 13 patients had complicated courses with persistent or recurrent fevers or positive blood cultures, a much higher failure rate than previously noted in injecting drug users with *Staph. aureus* endocarditis. Time-kill curves for ten clinical isolates demonstrated that vancomycin was less rapidly bactericidal than nafcillin after 24 h incubation. These observations reinforce recommendations that vancomycin should only be used to treat

Staph. aureus endocarditis if the organism is methicillin-resistant, or if there is a strong contraindication to the use of beta-lactam agents in methicillin-sensitive infections (Sande and Scheld, 1980).

There is very little experience in the use of vancomycin for treatment of *Staph. aureus* meningitis. Children with CSF shunt infections (see below) have been successfully treated with i.v. vancomycin (Gump, 1981; Schaad *et al.*, 1981) but because of suboptimal CSF penetration, direct administration into the CSF may be required (p. 771).

2 Coagulase-negative staphylococcal infections

Vancomycin is effective for treatment of infections due to coagulase-negative staphylococci. These organisms, and *Staph. aureus*, are the most common causes of infections of foreign bodies such as prosthetic heart valves, prosthetic joints, vascular graft material, CSF drains and shunts, peritoneal dialysis catheters and long-term indwelling intravenous catheters (Rupp and Archer, 1994). Many of the coagulase-negative staphylococci isolated from foreign body infections produce an extracellular substance called slime, which helps the bacteria adhere to the foreign material and provides protection against host defences such as neutrophils. Slime may also reduce the effectiveness of antibiotics (p. 684). Adjunctive surgery often plays an important role in the management of these infections.

Prosthetic valve endocarditis due to coagulase-negative staphylococci is treated with vancomycin-containing regimens. Surgery is usually required in addition to antibiotic therapy to bring about a cure. A regimen of vancomycin, rifampicin and gentamicin for 2 weeks, followed by another 4 weeks of vancomycin and rifampicin produces the best cure rates (Karchmer *et al.*, 1983). Coagulase-negative staphylococci are also an occasional cause of native valve endocarditis (Badour *et al.*, 1986; Caputo *et al.*, 1987). In comparison with prosthetic valve endocarditis, most isolates from patients with native valve endocarditis are methicillin-sensitive and should be treated with beta-lactam agents, but methicillin-resistant infections do occur. It is unclear whether combination therapy, with addition of either rifampicin or an aminoglocyoside, is superior to vancomycin alone for these latter infections.

Coagulase-negative staphylococci are the commonest cause of peritoneal dialysis-associated peritonitis. Vancomycin is recommended as part of the initial antibiotic regimen for this infection (British Society for Antimicrobial Chemotherapy, 1987; Keane *et al.*, 1993). Although bacteremia is uncommon, a loading dose of vancomycin 15 mg per kg should be given to ensure rapid achievement of satisfactory serum levels. This dose can be given intravenously or added to a dialysis bag and instilled into the peritoneal cavity (p. 771). For subsequent exchanges, vancomycin can be added to dialysis fluid at a concentration of 25 mg per liter, but does not appear to be absolutely necessary. A number of studies have demonstrated the efficacy of this approach (Gruer *et al.*, 1984; Bastani *et al.*, 1987; Boyce *et al.*, 1988). Removal of the peritoneal dialysis catheter is not usually required.

Infections of ventriculoperitoneal and ventriculoatrial shunts usually require removal of the shunt to effect cure, but occasional infections can be treated successfully with antibiotics alone (Younger *et al.*, 1987). For those infections due to coagulase-negative staphylococci, systemic administration of vancomycin may not result in adequate CSF levels, and direct administration of vancomycin into the CSF (either intrathecally, or preferably, into the ventricles) (p. 771) may be necessary (Swayne *et al.*, 1987). Monitoring of CSF levels is recommended in patients treated with intraventricular vancomycin, because the optimal dose and schedule is not known. Addition of rifampicin could be considered if CSF cultures remained positive, but efficacy is unproven.

Coagulase-negative staphylococci are an important cause of infection in newborn infants, particularly in association with infection of implanted devices, and vancomycin has been recommended for these (Munson *et al.*, 1982; Baumgart *et al.*, 1983; Starr, 1985; Noel *et al.*, 1988).

3 Treatment of streptococcal endocarditis and enterococcal infections

The standard treatment of enterococcal endocarditis is a combination of penicillin G or ampicillin with gentamicin (or streptomycin) (p. 42). For patients allergic to penicillins, a vancomycin / aminoglycoside combination is recommended (Bisno *et al.*, 1989). Combination treatment should be continued for 4–6 weeks. Because vancomycin may augment the nephrotoxicity of the aminoglycoside (p. 775), vancomycin levels should be monitored, aiming for peaks of 25–30 and troughs of 5–10 μg per ml, respectively. Vancomycin is also indicated for the treatment of viridans streptococcal endocarditis if the patient is allergic to penicillin G and the cephalosporins (Bisno *et al.*, 1989).

The emergence of resistance in enterococci to penicillins, vancomycin or aminoglycosides poses special problems because of the requirement for combination therapy to achieve bactericidal activity against these organisms (p. 765). If strains demonstrate high-level resistance to both gentamicin and streptomycin, optimal therapy is unknown, but monotherapy with vancomycin could be considered, especially if the isolate is resistant to beta-lactam agents as well (Patterson *et al.*, 1988). Surgery may be required to treat these cases (Eliopoulos, 1993). Endocarditis caused by a vancomycin-resistant enterococcus is a particularly difficult infection to treat. Some *E. faecium* isolates that are vancomycin-resistant and moderately penicillin-resistant can be rendered more susceptible to penicillin with combination vancomycin/penicillin treatment. However, this combination is not bactericical, and addition of an aminoglycoside is required to kill the organisms. For strains that are penicillin-, vancomycin- and high level aminoglycoside-resistant, therapeutic options are few, and the use of novel antibiotics or combinations of antibiotics would have to be considered (p. 766).

4 Diphtheroid infections

Species of *Corynebacterium* (diphtheroids) are usually commensals on the skin and mucous membranes. These organisms can cause infections on foreign bodies or in immunocompromised patients. Examples include bacteremia in neutropenic cancer and leukemia patients (p. 157), prosthetic valve endocarditis, CSF shunt infections, prosthetic joint infections, and occasional infections such as empyema or brain abscesses in normal hosts. Many diphtheroids are resistant to penicillins, and one particular species, *Corynebacterium jeikeium* (previously designated *Corynebacterium* JK), is resistant to almost all antibiotics except vancomycin (Stamm *et al.*, 1979; Gill *et al.*, 1981; Jadeja *et al.*, 1983). Diphtheroid endocarditis, which almost always affects prosthetic valves, should be treated with a combination of vancomycin, gentamicin and rifampicin initially (Geraci and Wilson, 1981). As with infections due to coagulase-negative staphylococci, surgery may be required to adequately deal with foreign body infections caused by diphtheroids.

5 Pneumococcal meningitis

Until recently, almost all pneumococcal isolates were sensitive to penicillin G (p. 5), but penicillin-resistant pneumococci have now become a significant problem in some parts of the world. Some of these isolates are also resistant to third-generation cephalosporins, but all penicillin-resistant pneumococci remain sensitive to vancomycin (p. 764) (Goldstein *et al.*, 1994). Pneumococcal meningitis due to penicillin-resistant organisms is a major therapeutic challenge, and inclusion of vancomycin as part of initial empiric therapy for bacterial meningitis may have to be considered in those areas where penicillin-resistant pneumococci are particularly prevalent (Friedland and McCracken, 1994). Unfortunately, experience with vancomycin in the treatment of pneumococcal meningitis has been disappointing. Viladrich *et al.* (1991) noted treatment failure in four of 11 adult patients treated with vancomycin 7.5 mg per kg every 6 h and dexamethasone. Clearly, if vancomycin is to be used to treat pneumococcal meningitis, patients need to be observed closely, and a repeat lumbar puncture is advisable after 48 h of treatment to determine whether the CSF cultures have become negative. Intrathecal vancomycin has been used in some patients not respondng to i.v. vancomycin (Buzon *et al.*, 1984; Catalan *et al.*, 1994) Combination therapy with vancomycin and ceftriaxone is another option. This combination was more effective than either agent alone against penicillin- and cephalosporin-resistant strains in an animal study (Friedland *et al.*, 1993), while CSF from children treated with a combination of ceftriaxone and vancomycin (at a dose of 15 mg per kg four times a day) achieved greater bactericidal activity against similar strains than ceftriaxone alone (Klugman *et al.*, 1995). Animal studies indicate that administration of dexamethasone reduces the CSF penetration of vancomycin (Paris *et al.*, 1994; Cabellos *et al.*, 1995). However, a mean CSF level of 3.3 μg per ml (21% of simultaneously measured serum levels) could be achieved in children treated with dexamethasone and vancomycin 15 mg per kg four times daily (Klugman *et al.*, 1995) (p. 768).

6 Antibiotic-associated colitis

This complication can occur following the use of most antibiotics; in most patients the mechanism is bowel overgrowth of toxigenic strains of *Cl. difficile*, or less commonly perhaps *Staph. aureus*. Rarely, *Cl. difficile* enterocolitis can occur without prior antibiotic treatment (Hyams *et al.*, 1981). Vancomycin is active against all strains of *Cl. difficile* (p. 764) and numerous studies have attested to the efficacy of vancomycin in treating antibiotic-associated enterocolitis due to *Cl. difficile* (Larson *et al.*, 1978; Keighley *et al.*, 1978; Tedesco *et al.*, 1978; Bartlett *et al.*, 1979; Batts *et al.*, 1980).

In most early studies, oral vancomycin doses of 2 g daily were used for periods of up to 14 days. Fecal concentrations of the drug were often nearly 1000 times the highest MIC of *Cl. difficile* strains isolated (Tedesco *et al.*, 1978). Using an oral dose of 500, 250 or 125 mg 6-hourly, mean daily fecal concentrations were 714, 447, and 351 μg per ml, respectively (Keighley *et al.*, 1978). A dose of 125 mg 6-hourly for 5 days is as effective as higher doses, and is now the recommended dose (Fekety *et al.*, 1984; Fekety *et al.*, 1989). Cholestyramine binds to vancomycin, and should not be used together with vancomycin when the latter drug is given in a total daily dose of only 500 mg (Fekety, 1983). Infants and children have been treated with an oral dose of 500 mg per 1.73m² surface area every 6 h. Despite the proven efficacy of vancomycin, metronidazole is preferred as the drug of first choice for the treatment of this infection (p. 949), chiefly because it is less expensive than vancomycin, but also because of concerns that the use of oral vancomycin may promote the appearance of vancomycin-resistant enterococci in the bowel (Hospital Infection Control Practices Advisory Committee, 1995).

Relapse of antibiotic-associated colitis occurs in up to 20% of patients (George *et al.*, 1979; Bartlett *et al.*, 1980). The mechanism of relapse may involve either re-acquisition of the organism from the environment, or reactivation of spore forms that have persisted in the bowel. Management is problematic (Bartlett, 1994). Another course of the antibiotic that was originally used is tried first. If another relapse occurs, the other of the two first-line antibiotics (either vancomycin or metronidazole) is used. Other strategies tried in this situation have included a prolonged, gradual tapering of the dosage of vancomycin over 1–2 months (Tedesco, 1982), use of intermittent short courses of vancomycin ('pulsing') to kill spores, administration of a fecal enema to reconstitute the bowel flora (Schwan *et al.*, 1984), and concurrent treatment with vancomycin and the non-pathogenic yeast, *Saccharomyces boulardii* (Surawicz *et al.*, 1989). In most cases, administration of the offending antibiotic should be ceased, but is not absolutely essential if the antibiotic must be continued (Fekety, 1983).

Another difficult management problem is the patient with antibiotic-associated colitis who cannot take oral antibiotics. Because i.v. vancomycin only reaches low levels in the feces (p. 772), use of i.v. metronidazole is recommended although treatment failures have been reported (Guzman *et al.*, 1988; Oliva *et al.*, 1989). Another approach is to pass a bowel tube into the cecum by colonoscopy, and to instil vancomycin or metronidazole directly into the large bowel (Pasic *et al.*, 1993).

A variety of other antibiotics are effective therapy for antibiotic-associated colitis. Bacitracin (p. 543) (Dudley *et al.*, 1986) and fusidic acid (p. 585), (Cronberg *et al.*, 1984) have been used. The new glycopeptide teicoplanin (p. 797) was as effective as oral vancomycin in a randomized study of 46 patients (de Lalla *et al.*, 1992).

Extraintestinal *Cl. difficile* infections are very rare – there is one report of a patient with *Cl. difficile* bacteremia who was successfully treated with i.v. vancomycin (Feldman *et al.*, 1995). Vancomycin has also been used effectively in the past to treat staphylococcal enterocolitis (p. 735) but there is some doubt whether *Staph. aureus* has a proven role in antibiotic-associated colitis (George, 1984).

7 Use in neutropenic patients

Gram-positive organisms have re-emerged as a significant cause of infections in neutropenic patients with fever (Wade *et al.*, 1982). The major factor responsible for the shift away from Gram-negative organisms as the predominant neutropenic pathogens has been the widespread use of long-term indwelling central venous catheters, such as the Hickman catheter. In addition, more intensive chemotherapy regimens can produce severe gastrointestinal mucositis, allowing invasion of resident flora, including Gram-positive bacteria, across the disrupted mucosa and into the systemic circulation. Coagulase-negative staphylococci are the commonest cause of Gram-positive sepsis in neutropenic patients. Other Gram-positive pathogens include *Staph. aureus*, viridans streptococci, diphtheroids (notably *C. jeikeium* – p. 779), *Bacillus* species, enterococci, and *Propionibacterium acnes*. With rare exceptions, all these organisms are sensitive to vancomycin.

Organisms normally resident on the skin can colonize long-term central venous catheters, such as the Hickman catheter, and bloodstream infections may result. Gram-positive organisms are the usual cause of these infections. Gram-negative bacteria and fungi are isolated much less frequently. The infection can often be treated successfully with the catheter left in place, although clinically apparent involvement of the subcutaneous tunnel usually requires catheter removal, as does persistence of the bacteremia or fever after 48–72 h of treatment (Press *et al.*, 1984; Smith *et al.*, 1989). Coagulase-negative staphylococci, the commonest cause of these infections, do not usually cause serious morbidity or mortality, but relapses can occur in up to 20% of patients after a course of vancomycin (Raad *et al.*, 1992). Infections due to *Staph. aureus* are more likely to give rise to serious complications, and many would advise catheter removal if this organism is isolated (Dugdale and Ramsey, 1990). Serious infections due to *Bacillus* spp. are a relatively rare but well-recognized cause of bacteremia in neutropenic patients. These infections usually arise from an infected long-term central venous catheter, and may be associated with complications such as pneumonia (Saleh and Schorin, 1987). Bacteremic diphtheroid infections are also usually catheter-related. Vancomycin is the drug of choice for these infections, particularly when *C. jeikeium* is isolated, because this organism is resistant to almost all other agents (Riebel *et al.*, 1986) (p. 764).

Viridans streptococcal infections are an increasingly important cause of sepsis in neutropenic patients (Cohen *et al.*, 1983; Classen *et al.*, 1990)). These organisms arise from the flora of the mouth or gastrointestinal tract. They do not infect intravenous catheters, but are thought to gain access to the bloodstream in association with severe mucositis that complicates some of the more intensive chemotherapeutic regimens, such as those used for induction treatment of acute myelogenous leukemia. Use of prophylactic quinolone agents (p. 1026) may also predispose to these infections, because a substantial reduction in the number of quinolone-sensitive aerobic Gram-negative organisms may allow significant growth of quinolone-resistant viridans streptococci (Elting *et al.*, 1992). Not all viridans streptococci isolated from neutropenic patients are sensitive to penicillin (McWhinney *et al.*, 1993) (p. 764), so vancomycin is the drug of choice for initial treatment of these infections.

Although there is no doubting the benefit of vancomycin for treatment of *proven* Gram-positive infections in neutropenic patients, the role of *empiric* vancomycin therapy in the neutropenic patient with fever is more controversial. A common practice is to add vancomycin if the patient remains febrile 48–72 h after the first-line empiric regimen has been started, even if no Gram-positive infection is proven, or suspected clinically (Rubin *et al.*, 1988). This practice is reasonably well-accepted, and can lead to resolution of the fever in up to 50% of cases (Smith *et al.*, 1990). Whether vancomycin should be included in the initial empiric antibiotic regimen is the subject of ongoing debate. Karp *et al.* (1986) favored initial empiric use of vancomycin, on the basis of fewer secondary Gram-positive infections, more rapid resolution of infectious fever, and fewer total febrile days in patients randomly assigned to vancomycin as part of the initial empiric antibiotic therapy. In contrast, Rubin *et al.* (1988) only used vancomycin when clinically or microbiologically indicated and not as part of the initial empiric regimen. Only 63 of 550 episodes of neutropenic fever required addition of vancomycin and all documented Gram-positive infections were successfully treated. Thus, 'delayed' vancomycin therapy appeared to be safe, presumably because the initial empiric antibiotics provide some Gram-positive cover and because many of the Gram-positive organisms, such as coagulase-negative staphylococci, are less virulent than Gram-negative aerobic organisms. Ramphal *et al.* (1992) supported these observations. A large study of 747 neutropenic, febrile patients also examined this question, by randomizing patients to receive ceftazidime and amikacin, or ceftazidime, amikacin and vancomycin (EORTC, 1991). Not surprisingly, patients with Gram-positive bacteremias receiving initial vancomycin were more likely to respond than those not empirically treated with vancomycin. However, duration of fever did not differ between the two groups, and no patient died of Gram-positive bacteremia during the first 3 days of therapy.

The balance of evidence suggests that vancomycin does not have to be included as part of the initial empiric antibiotic regimen for neutropenic patients with fever, unless the patient is critically ill, there is clinical evidence of a Gram-positive infection such as an inflamed i.v. catheter site, or local rates of Gram-positive infection are especially high. Vancomycin can be added subsequently if there is clinical or microbiological evidence of a Gram-positive infection, or if the fever persists for 48–72 h after institution of broad-spectrum empiric antibiotics.

8 Prophylactic uses

Use of vancomycin to prevent infections is an attractive option for situations where the likelihood of a Gram-positive coccal infection is high, and / or the consequences of such an infection are serious. However, the temptation to use vancomycin in this fashion must be tempered by the realization that the emergence of vancomycin-resistant organisms (p. 764) is likely to be accelerated if vancomycin prophylaxis is administered indiscriminately. The consequences of vancomycin-resistance in *Staph. aureus* are so serious that vancomycin prophylaxis should be limited to certain well-defined situations.

For penicillin-allergic patients, vancomycin is the agent of choice for patients requiring a parenteral agent as prophylaxis against endocarditis (Dajani *et al.*, 1990). It is infused as a 1-g dose given i.v. over 60 min.

For routine perioperative prophylaxis, a first-generation cephalosporin is the preferred prophylactic antibiotic for patients undergoing clean operative procedures (p. 287). Preoperative prophylactic vancomycin is as effective as a first-generation cephalosporin in cardiothoracic surgery (Maki *et al.*, 1992), and has been used to prevent infection in many other surgical settings. Because of concerns about selective antibiotic pressure and emergence of resistance, prophylactic vancomycin should be restricted to operations involving implantation of foreign material such as heart valves or prosthetic joints in institutions with a high rate of infections due to MRSA or coagulase-negative staphylococci (Hospital Infection Control Practices Advisory Committee, 1995). Other patients in whom vancomycin prophylaxis may be considered include those with documented preoperative colonization or infection with MRSA, or those with a long preoperative stay in a ward or unit where rates of MRSA infection or colonization are known to be high.

Numerous other prophylactic uses of vancomycin have been reported. Renal dialysis patients often develop staphylococcal infections of arteriovenous fistulae, and use of weekly vancomycin can reduce the frequency of these infections. Intravenous vancomycin has also been administered prophylactically (not empirically – see above) to neutropenic patients in an attempt to reduce Gram-positive coccal infections, but the benefits of such an approach do not clearly outweigh the risks (Attal *et al.*, 1991; Lamy *et al.*, 1993). Prophylactic vancomycin at the time of insertion did not reduce subsequent colonization or infection rates of subcutaneous tunnelled central venous catheters in cancer patients (Ranson *et al.*, 1990). However, daily installation of a vancomycin-containing solution into similar catheters has been reported to reduce episodes of bacteremia due to vancomycin-susceptible organisms (Schwartz *et al.*, 1990). Finally, oral vancomycin, together with other non-absorbable antimicrobials, has been used to produce total gut decontamination in oncology patients during induction chemotherapy (Levi *et al.*, 1978; Bodey, 1981). The value of adding vancomycin to such a regimen is doubtful (Bender *et al.*, 1979), and for that matter the role of non-absorbable antibiotics in reducing infection in these patients and in intensive care unit patients is not clear-cut (Donnelly, 1993). Nowadays, other approaches, such as administration of quinolone antibiotics (p. 1025) or fluconazole, are used in neutropenic patients.

9 Other infections

Listeria monocytogenes is sensitive *in vitro* to vancomycin, and several patients with *Listeria* infections have been treated successfully with this drug (Zeitlin *et al.*, 1982; Blatt and Zajac, 1991). However, failures of vancomycin have also been reported (Baldassarre *et al.*, 1991; Dryden *et al.*, 1991), and vancomycin cannot be considered as an acceptable anti-*Listeria* agent under any but the most exceptional circumstances.

Rhodococcus equi, a veterinary pathogen, is a rare cause of serious infections in immunocompromised patients, notably those with HIV infection or AIDS (Verville *et al.*, 1994). A combination of erythromycin and rifampicin has been considered the treatment of choice for this infection (p. 620). However, vancomycin has good activity against the organism *in vitro* (Nordman and Ronco, 1992), and in an animal model of *Rhodococcus equi* infection, vancomycin was the single most effective agent (Nordmann *et al.*, 1992). Vancomycin, usually in combination with other antibiotics such as imipenem, has been used successfully to treat several patients with this infection (Rouquet *et al.*, 1991).

Bacillus spp., normally environmental and skin commensals, can cause infections in neutropenic patients (p. 12), and serious soft tissue or eye infections in patients sustaining traumatic injuries involving contact with soil or soil-contaminated objects (Wong and Dolan 1992). Non-anthracis *Bacillus* spp. are not always sensitive to penicillin, and vancomycin is the drug of choice for these infections.

Bacterial endophthalmitis can arise as a postoperative complication, secondary to a penetrating eye injury, or rarely as a metastatic manifestation of a bacteremic infection. Most antibiotics, including vancomycin, penetrate poorly into the vitreous humour, and direct antibiotic administration into the vitreous is required to produce adequate antibiotic levels. Vancomycin, given intravitreally as a 1–2 mg dose, has an important place in the treatment of traumatic and postoperative bacterial endophthalmitis, because coagulase-negative staphylococci, *Bacillus* spp., and *Propionibacterium acnes* are the predominant organisms isolated in these infections (Barza, 1989).

Flavobacterium spp. are environmental Gram-negative organisms that occasionally cause human infections. *Flavobacterium meningosepticum* is a cause of nosocomial outbreaks of neonatal meningitis, and has been isolated (as have other *Flavobacterium* spp.) from hospitalized, often immunosuppressed, patients with bacteraemia, pneumonia and wound infections. Vancomycin is not consistently active against these organisms *in vitro* (p. 767), but has been used successfully in patients with *Flavobacterium meningosepticum* meningitis (Ratner, 1984) and catheter-related bacteraemia (Sader *et al.*, 1995).

Oral vancomycin has been used to treat patients with short-bowel syndrome and other small bowel abnormalities who develop D-lactic acidosis (Stolberg *et al.*, 1982). This complication occurs when carbohydrates that would have been normally digested by bacteria in the small bowel are metabolized by colonic bacteria, leading to excess D-lactic acid production and systemic acidosis.

References

Ahmad R, Raichura N, Kilbane V (1982). Vancomycin: a reappraisal. *Brit Med J* **284**: 1953.

Alpert G, Campos JM, Harris MC et al (1984). Vancomycin dosage in pediatrics reconsidered. *Amer J Dis Child* **138**: 20.

Amsterdam DA, Gorzynski EA, Beam TR, Rotstein C (1994). Susceptibility of bacteraemic isolates of Gram-positive cocci to daptomycin and other antimicrobial agents. *J Antimicrob Chemother* **33**: 1060.

Appleman MD, Cherubin CE, Heseltine PNR, Stratton CW (1991). Susceptibility testing of *Listeria monocytogenes*: a reassessment of bactericidal activity as a predictor for clinical outcome. *Diagn Microbiol Infect Dis* **14**: 311.

Arduino RC, Murray BE (1993). Vancomycin resistance in Gram positive organisms. *Curr Opin Infect Dis* **6**: 715.

Arthur M, Courvalin P (1993). Genetics and mechanisms of glycopeptide resistance in enterococci. *Antimicrob Ag Chemother* **37**: 1563.

Arthur M, Molinas C, Bugg TD et al. (1992a). Evidence for *in vivo* incorporation of D-lactate into peptidoglycan precursors of vancomycin-resistant enterococci. *Antimicrob Ag Chemother* **36**: 867.

Arthur M, Molinas C, Courvalin P (1992b). The vanS-vanR two-component regulatory system controls synthesis of depsipeptide peptidoglycan presursors in *Enterococcus faecium* BM4147. *J Bacteriol* **174**: 2582.

Arthur M, Depardieu F, Snaith HA et al. (1994). Contribution of vanY D.D.-carboxypeptidase to glycopeptide resistance in *Enterococcus faecalis* by hydrolysis of peptidoglylcan precursors. *Antimicrob Ag Chemother* **38**: 1899.

Attal M, Schlaifer D, Rubie H et al. (1991). Prevention of gram-positive infections after bone marrow transplantation by systemic vancomycin: a prospective, randomized trial. *J Clin Oncol* **9**: 865.

Aubert G, Passot S, Lucht F, Dorche G (1990). Selection of vancomycin and teicoplanin-resistant *Staphylococcus haemolyticus* during teicoplanin treatment of *S. epidermidis* infection. *J Antimicrob Chemother* **25**: 491.

Baddour LM, Phillips TN, Bisno AL (1986). Coagulase-negative staphylococcal endocarditis. Occurrence in patients with mitral valve prolapse. *Arch Intern Med* **146**: 119.

Bailie GR, Yu R, Morton R, Waldek S (1985). Vancomycin, red neck syndrome and fits. *Lancet* **ii**: 279.

Baillie GR, Eisele G, Venezia RA et al. (1992). Prediction of serum vancomycin concentrations following intraperitoneal loading doses in continuous ambulatory peritoneal dialysis patients with peritonitis. *Clin Pharmacokinet* **22**: 298.

Baker CN, Thornsberry C (1974). Antimicrobial susceptibility of *Streptococcus mutans* isolated from patients with endocarditis. *Antimicrob Ag Chemother* **5**: 268.

Baker PJ, Slots J, Genco RJ, Evans RT (1983). Minimal inhibitory concentrations of various antimicrobial agents for human oral anaerobic bacteria. *Antimicrob Ag Chemother* **24**: 420.

Baldassarre JS, Ingerman MJ, Nansteel J, Santoro J (1991). Development of *Listeria* meningitis during vancomycin therapy: a case report. *J Infect Dis* **164**: 221.

Banner W Jr, Ray CG (1984). Vancomycin in perspective. *Amer J Dis Child* **138**: 14.

Barakett V, Lesage D, Delisle F *et al.* (1993). Killing kinetics of vancomycin and rifampin tested alone and in combination against penicillin-resistant *Streptococcus pneumoniae*. *Eur J Clin Microbiol Infect Dis* **12**:69.

Barg NL, Supena RB, Fekety R (1986). Persistent staphylococcal bacteremia in an intravenous drug abuser. *Antimicrob Ag Chemother* **29**: 209.

Barr JG, Smyth ETM, Hogg GM (1990). *In vitro* antimicrobial activity of imipenem in combination with vancomycin or teicoplanin against *Staphylococcus aureus* and *Staphylococcus epidermidis*. *Eur J Clin Microbiol Infect Dis* **9**:804.

Bartlett JG (1994). *Clostridium difficile*: history of its role as an enteric pathogen and the current state of knowledge about the organism. *Clin Infect Dis* **18** (Suppl 4): S265.

Bartlett JG, Willey SH, Chang TW, Lowe B (1979). Cephalosporin-associated pseudomembranous colitis due to *Clostridium difficile*. *JAMA* **242**: 2683.

Bartlett JG, Tedesco FJ, Shull S et al. (1980). Symptomatic relapse after oral vancomycin therapy of antibiotic associated pseudomembranous colitis. *Gastroenterology* **78**: 431.

Barza M (1989). Antibacterial agents in the treatment of ocular infections. *Infect Dis Clin N Amer* **3**: 533.

Bastani B, Freer K, Read D et al. (1987). Treatment of gram-positive peritonitis with two intraperitoneal doses of vancomycin in continuous ambulatory peritoneal dialysis patients. *Nephron* **45**: 283.

Batts DH, Martin D, Holmes R et al. (1980). Treatment of antibiotic-associated *Clostridium difficile* diarrhoea with oral vancomycin. *J Pediatr* **97**: 151.

Baumgart S, Hall SE, Campos JM, Polin RA (1983). Sepsis with coagulase-negative staphylococci in critically ill newborns. *Amer J Dis Child* **137**: 461.

Bellomo R, Ernest D, Parkin G, Boyce N (1990). Clearance of vancomycin during continuous arteriovenous hemodiafiltration. *Crit Care Med* **18**: 181.

Bender JF, Schimpff SC, Young VM et al. (1979). Role of vancomycin as a component of oral nonabsorbable antibiotics for microbial suppression in leukemic patients. *Antimicrob Ag Chemother* **15**: 455.

Bergeron L, Boucher FD (1994). Possible red-man syndrome associated with systemic absorption of oral vancomycin in a child with normal renal function. *Ann Pharmacother* **28**: 581.

Billot-Klein D, Gutmann L, Sable S et al. (1994). Modification of peptidoglycan precursors is a common feature of the low-level vancomycin-resistant VANB-type Enterococcus D366 and of the naturally glycopeptide-resistant species *Lactobacillus casei*, *Pediococcus pentosaceus*, *Leuconostoc mesenteroides*, and *Enterococcus gallinarum*. *J Bacteriol* **176**: 2398.

Bisno AL, Dismukes WE, Durack DT et al. (1989). Antimicrobial treatment of infective endocarditis due to viridans streptococci, enterococci and staphylococci. *JAMA* **261**: 1471.

Blatt SP, Zajac RA (1991). Treatment of *Listeria* bacteremia with vancomycin. *Rev Infect Dis* **13**: 181.

Blevins RD, Halstenson CE, Salem NG, Matzke GR (1984). Pharmacokinetics of vancomycin in patients undergoing continuous ambulatory peritoneal dialysis. *Antimicrob Ag Chemother* **25**: 603.

Blouin RA, Bauer LA, Miller DD *et al.* (1982). Vancomycin pharmacokinetics in normal and morbidly obese subjects. *Antimicrob Ag Chemother* **21**: 575.

Bodey GP (1981). Antibiotic prophylaxis in cancer patients: regimens of oral, nonabsorbable antibiotics for prevention of infection during induction of remission. *Rev Infect Dis* **3** (Suppl): 259.

Boeckh M, Lode H, Borner K *et al.* (1988). Pharmacokinetics and serum bactericidal activity of vancomycin alone and in combination with ceftazidime in healthy volunteers. *Antimicrob Ag Chemother* **32**: 92.

Borhani H, Peyman GA, Wafapoor H (1993). Use of vancomycin in vitrectomy infusion and evaluation of retinal toxicity. *Int Ophthalmol* **17**: 85.

Bourgault AM, Wilson WR, Washington JA (1979). Antimicrobial susceptibility of species of viridans streptococci. *J Infect Dis* **140**: 316.

Boyce JM, Opat SM, Chow JW *et al.* (1994). Outbreak of multidrug-resistant *Enterococcus faecium* with transferable vanB class vancomycin resistance. *J Clin Microbiol* **32**: 1148.

Boyce NW, Wood C, Thompson NM *et al.* (1988). Intraperitoneal (IP). vancomycin therapy for CAPD peritonitis: a prospective, randomized comparison of intermittent vs. continuous therapy. *Amer J Kidney Dis* **12**: 304.

Brater DC, Bawdon RE, Anderson SA *et al.* (1986). Vancomycin elimination in patients with burn injury. *Clin Pharmacol Ther* **39**: 631.

British Society for Antimicrobial Chemotherapy (1987). Diagnosis and management of peritonitis in continuous ambulatory peritoneal dialysis. *Lancet* **i**: 845.

Brown N, Ho DHW, Fong K-LL *et al.* (1983). Effects of hepatic function on vancomycin clinical pharmacology. *Antimicrob Ag Chemother* **23**: 603.

Brummett RE, Fox KE (1989). Vancomycin- and erythromycin-induced hearing loss in humans. *Antimicrob Ag Chemother* **33**: 791.

Brummett RE, Fox KE, Jacobs F *et al.* (1990). Augmented gentamicin ototoxicity induced by vancomycin in guinea pigs. *Arch Otolaryngol Head Neck Surg* **116**: 61.

Burdon DW (1984). Treatment of pseudomembranous colitis and antibiotic-associated diarrhoea. *J Antimicrob Chemother* **14** (Suppl D): 103.

Buzon LM, Guerrero A, Romero J *et al.* (1984). Penicillin-resistant *Streptococcus pneumoniae* meningitis successfully treated with vancomycin. *Eur J Clin Microbiol* **3**: 442.

Cabellos C, Martinez-Lacasa J, Martos A *et al.* (1995). Influence of dexamethasone on efficacy of ceftriaxone and vancomycin therapy in experimental pneumococcal meningitis. *Antimicrob Ag Chemother* **39**: 2158.

Cafferkey MT, Hone R, Keane CT (1982). Severe staphylococcal infections treated with vancomycin. *J Antimicrob Chemother* **9**: 69.

Cantu TG, Yamanaka-Yuen NA, Lietman PS (1994). Serum vancomycin concentrations: reappraisal of their clinical value. *Clin Infect Dis* **18**: 533.

Caputo GM, Archer GL, Calderwood SB *et al.* (1987). Native valve endocarditis due to coagulase-negative staphylococci: clinical and microbiologic features. *Amer J Med* **83**: 619.

Catalan MJ, Fernandez JM, Vazquez A *et al.* (1994). Failure of cefotaxime in the treatment of meningitis due to relatively resistant *Streptococcus pneumoniae*. *Clin Infect Dis* **18**: 766.

CDC (Centers for Disease Control) (1993). Nosocomial enterococci resistant to vancomycin – United States, 1989–1993. *MMWR* **42**: 597.

Cercenado E, Eliopoulos GM, Wennersten CB, Moellering RC (1992). Absence of synergistic activity between ampicillin and vancomycin against highly vancomycin-resistant enterococci. *Antimicrob Ag Chemother* **36**: 2201.

Chang D (1995). Influence of malignancy on the pharmacokinetics of vancomycin in infants and children. *Pediatr Infect Dis* **14**: 667.

Chang D, Liem L, Malogolowkin M (1994). A prospective study of vancomycin pharmacokinetics and dosage requirements in pediatric cancer patients. *Pediatr Infect Dis* **13**: 969.

Cherubin CE, Corrado ML, Sierra MF *et al.* (1981). Susceptibility of gram positive cocci to various antibiotics, including cefotaxime, moxalactam and imipenem. *Antimicrob Ag Chemother* **20**: 553.

Christie DJ, van Buren N, Lennon SS, Putnam JL (1990). Vancomycin-dependent antibodies associated with thrombocytopenia and refractoriness to platelet transfusion in patients with leukemia. *Blood* **75**: 518.

Cimino MA, Rotstein C, Slaughter RL, Emrich LJ (1987). Relationship of serum antibiotic concentrations to nephrotoxicity in cancer patients receiving concurrent aminoglycoside and vancomycin therapy. *Amer J Med* **83**: 1091.

Classen DC, Burke JP, Ford CD *et al.* (1990). *Streptococcus mitis* sepsis in bone marrow transplant patients receiving oral antimicrobial prophylaxis. *Amer J Med* **89**: 441.

Cohen J, Donnelly JP, Worsely AM et al (1983). Septicaemia caused by viridans streptococci in neutropenic patients with leukaemia. *Lancet* **ii**: 1452.

Cole DR, Oliver M, Coward RA, Brown CB (1985). Allergy, Red Man syndrome, and vancomycin. *Lancet* **ii**: 280.

Collins LA, Malanoski GJ, Eliopoulos GM *et al.* (1993a). *In vitro* activity of RP59500, an injectable streptogramin antibiotic, against vancomycin-resistant gram-positive organisms. *Antimicrob Ag Chemother* **37**: 598.

Collins LA, Eliopoulos GM, Wennersten CB *et al.* (1993b). *In vitro* activity of ramoplanin against vancomycin-resistant gram-positive organisms. *Antimicrob Ag Chemother* **37**: 1364.

Colman G, Efstratiou A (1987). Vancomycin-resistant leuconostocs, lactobacilli and now pediococci. *J Hosp Infect* **10**: 1.

Craven DE, Kollisch NR, Hsieh CR *et al.* (1983). Vancomycin treatment of bacteremia caused by oxacillin-resistant *Staphylococcus aureus*: comparison with beta-lactam antibiotic treatment of bacteremia caused by oxacillin-sensitive *Staphylococcus aureus*. *J Infect Dis* **147**: 137.

Cronberg S, Castor B, Thoren A (1984). Fusidic acid for the treatment of antibiotic-associated colitis induced by *Clostridium difficile*. *Infection* **12**: 276.

Cunha BA, Quintiliani R, Deglin JM *et al.* (1981). Pharmacokinetics of vancomycin in anuria. *Rev Infect Dis* **3** (Suppl): 269.

Dajani AS, Bisno AL, Chung KJ *et al.* (1990). Prevention of bacterial endocarditis: recommendations by the American Heart Association. *JAMA* **264**: 2919.

Daum RS, Gupta S, Sabbagh R, Milewski WM (1992). Characterization of *Staphylococcus aureus* isolates with decreased susceptibility to vancomycin and teicoplanin: isolation and purification of a constitutively produced protein associated with decreased susceptibility. *J Infect Dis* **166**: 1066.

Davies AJ, Clewett J, Jones A, Marshall R (1986). Sensitivity patterns of coagulase-negative staphylococci from neonates. *J Antimicrob Chemother* **17**: 155.

Dean RP, Wagner DJ, Tolpin MD (1985). Vancomycin/aminoglycoside nephrotoxicity. *J Pediatr* **106**: 861.

de Lalla F, Nicolin R, Rinaldi E *et al.* (1992). Prospective study of oral teicoplanin versus oral vancomycin for therapy of pseudomembranous colitis and *Clostridium difficile*-associated diarrhea. *Antimicrob Ag Chemother* **36**: 2192.

del Mar Fernandez de Gatta M, Fruns I, Hernandez JM *et al.* (1993). Vancomycin pharmacokinetics and dosage requirements in hematologic malignancies. *Clin Pharm* **12**: 515.

Dever LL, Jorgensen JH, Barbour AG (1993). *In vitro* activity of vancomycin against the spirochete *Borrelia burgdorferi*. *Antimicrob Ag Chemother* **37**: 1115.

Domen RE, Horowitz S (1990). Vancomycin-induced neutropenia associated with anti-granulocyte antibodies. *Immunohematol* **6**: 41.

Donnelly JP (1993). Selective decontamination of the digestive tract and its role in antimicrobial prophylaxis. *J Antimicrob Chemother* **31**: 813.

Downs NJ, Neihart RE, Dolezal JM, Hodges GR (1989). Mild nephrotoxicity associated with vancomycin use. *Arch Intern Med* **149**: 1777.

Dryden MS, Jones NF, Phillips I (1991). Vancomycin therapy failure in *Listeria monocytogenes* peritonitis in a patient on continuous ambulatory peritoneal dialysis. *J Infect Dis* **164**: 1239.

Dudley MN, McLaughlin JC, Carrington G *et al.* (1986). Oral bacitracin vs. vancomycin therapy for *Clostridium difficile*-induced diarrhoea A randomized double-blind trial. *Arch Intern Med* **146**: 1101.

Dugdale DC, Ramsey PC (1990). *Staphylococcus aureus* bacteremia in patients with Hickman catheters. *Amer J Med* **89**: 137.

Edmond MB, Ober JF, Weinbaum DL *et al.* (1995). Vancomycin-resistant *Enterococcus faecium* bacteremia: risk factors for infection. *Clin Infect Dis* **20**: 1126.

Ein ME, Smith NJ, Aruffo JF *et al.* (1979). Susceptibility and synergy studies of methicillin-resistant *Staphylococcus epidermidis. Antimicrob Ag Chemother* **16**: 655.

Eliopoulos G M (1993). Aminoglycoside resistant enterococcal endocarditis. *Infect Dis Clin N Amer* **7**: 117.

Elting LS, Bodey GP, Keefe BH (1992). Septicemia and shock syndrome due to viridans streptococci: a case-control study of predisposing factors. *Clin Infect Dis* **14**: 1201.

Eng RHK, Ng K, Smith SM (1993). Susceptibility of resistant *Enterococcus faecium* to unusual antibiotics. *J Antimicrob Chemother* **31**: 609.

EORTC (1991). European Organization for Research and Treatment of Cancer International Antimicrobial Chemotherapy Cooperative group and the National Cancer Institute of Canada-Clinical Trials Group. Vancomycin added to empirical combination antibiotic therapy for fever in granulocytopenic cancer patients. *J Infect Dis* **163**: 951.

Evans RC, Holmes CJ (1987). Effect of vancomycin hydrochloride on *Staphylococcus epidermidis* biofilm associated with silicone elastomer. *Antimicrob Ag Chemother* **31**: 889.

Evers S, Sahm DF, Courvalin P (1993). The vanB gene of vancomycin-resistant *Enterococcus faecalis* V583 is structurally related to genes encoding D-ala:D-ala ligases and glycopeptide-resistance proteins VanA and VanC. *Gene* **124**: 143.

Eykyn S, Phillips I, Evans J (1970). Vancomycin for staphylococcal shunt site infections in patients on regular haemodialysis. *Brit Med J* **3**: 80.

Farber BF, Moellering RC Jr (1983). Retrospective study of the toxicity of preparations of vancomycin from 1974 to 1981. *Antimicrob Ag Chemother* **23**: 138.

Farber BF, Kaplan MH, Clogston AG (1990). *Staphylococcus epidermidis* extracted slime inhibits the antimicrobial action of glycopeptide antibiotics. *J Infect Dis* **161**: 37.

Faville RJ Jr, Zaske DE, Kaplan EL *et al.* (1978). *Staphylococcus aureus* endocarditis. Combined therapy with vancomycin and rifampin. *JAMA* **240**: 1963.

Fekety R (1983). Recent advances in management of bacterial diarrhoea. *Rev Infect Dis* **5**: 246.

Fekety R, Silva J, Buggy B, Deery HG (1984). Treatment of antibiotic-associated colitis with vancomycin. *J Antimicrob Chemother* **14** (Suppl D): 97.

Fekety R, Silva J, Kauffman C *et al.* (1989). Treatment of antibiotic-associated *Clostridium difficile* colitis with oral vancomycin: comparison of two dosage regimens. *Amer J Med* **86**: 15.

Feldman RJ, Kallich M, Weinstein MP (1995). Bacteremia due to *Clostridium difficile*: case report and review of extra-intestinal manifestations. *Clin Infect Dis* **20**: 1560.

Forrence EA, Goldman MP (1990). Vancomycin-associated exfoliative dermatitis. *DICP Ann Pharmacother* **24**: 369.

Fraimow HS, Venuti E (1992). Inconsistent activity of triple combination therapy with vancomycin, ampicillin, and gentamicin against vancomycin-resistant, highly ampicillin-resistant *Enterococcus faecium. Antimicrob Ag Chemother* **36**: 1563.

Freeman CD, Quintiliani R, Nightingale CH (1993). Vancomycin therapeutic drug monitoring; is it necessary? *Ann Pharmacother* **27**: 594.

French P, Venuti E, Fraimow HS (1993). *In vitro* activity of novobiocin against multiresistant strains of *Enterococcus faecium. Antimicrob Ag Chemother* **37**: 2736.

Frieden TR, Munsiff SS, Low DE *et al.* (1993). Emergence of vancomycin resistance in New York City. *Lancet* **342**: 76.

Friedland IR, McCracken GH Jr (1994). Management of infections caused by antibiotic-resistant *Streptococcus pneumoniae. New Engl J Med* **331**: 377.

Friedland IR, Paris M, Ehrett S *et al.* (1993). Evaluation of antimicrobial regimens for treatment of experimental penicillin- and cephalosporin-resistant pneumococcal meningitis. *Antimicrob Ag Chemother* **37**: 1630.

Froggat JW, Johnston JL, Galetto DW, Archer GL (1989). Antimicrobial resistance in nosocomial isolates of *Staphylococcus haemolyticus. Antimicrob Ag Chemother* **33**: 460.

Garrelts JC, Peterie JD (1985). Vancomycin and the 'red man's syndrome'. *New Engl J Med* **312**: 245.

Gaskill SJ, Marlin AE (1992). Vancomycin: its effect on intracranial pressure. *Pediatr Neurosurg* **18**: 139.

George WL (1984). Antimicrobial agent-associated colitis and diarrhoea: historical background and clinical aspects. *Rev Infect Dis* **6**: S208.

George WL, Volpicelli NA, Stiner DB *et al.* (1979). Relapse of pseudomembranous colitis after vancomycin therapy. *New Engl J Med* **301**: 414.

Geraci JE, Wilson WR (1981). Vancomycin therapy for infective endocarditis. *Rev Infect Dis* **3** (Suppl): 250.

Geraci JE, Heilman FR, Nichols DR *et al.* (1957). Some laboratory and clinical experiences with a new antibiotic, vancomycin. *Antibiot Ann 1956–1957*: 90.

Geraci JE, Heilman FR, Nichols DR, Wellman WE (1958). Antibiotic therapy of bacterial endocarditis. VII. Vancomycin for acute Micrococcal endocarditis. *Proc Mayo Clin* **33**: 172.

Gill VJ, Manning C, Lamson M *et al.* (1981). Antibiotic-resistant group JK bacteria in hospitals. *J Clin Microbiol* **13**: 472.

Glicklich D, Figura I (1984). Vancomycin and cardiac arrest. *Ann Intern Med* **101**: 880.

Goetz MB, Sayers J (1993). Nephrotoxicity of vancomycin and aminoglycoside therapy separately and in combination. *J Antimicrob Chemother* **32**: 325.

Goldstein FW, Coutrot A, Sieffer A, Acar JF (1990). Percentages and distributions of teicoplanin- and vancomycin-resistant strains among coagulase-negative staphylococci. *Antimicrob Ag Chemother* **34**: 899.

Goldstein FW, Geslin P, Acar JF, and the French Study Group (1994). Comparative activity of teicoplanin and vancoymcin against 400 penicillin susceptible and resistant *Streptococcus pneumoniae. Eur J Clin Microbiol Infect Dis* **13**: 33.

Gorby GL, Peacock JE (1988). *Erysipelothrix rhusopathiae* endocarditis: microbiologic, epidemiologic, and clinical features of an occupational disease. *Rev Infect Dis* **10**: 317.

Grappel SF, McNichols A, Phillips L, Giovenella A (1983). Characteristics and antibiotic susceptibilities of a vancomycin-resistant mutant of *Staphylococcus aureus*. In *Abstracts and Program of the 23rd Interscience Conference on Antimicrobial Agents and Chemotherapy* (Abstr. 436). Washington, DC: American Society for Microbiology.

Graziani AL, Lawson LA, Gibson GA *et al.* (1988). Vancomycin concentrations in infected and noninfected human bone. *Antimicrob Ag Chemother* **32**: 1320.

Griffith RS (1984). Vancomycin use – an historical review. *J Antimicrob Chemother* **14** (Suppl D): 1.

Griffith RS, Peck FB Jr (1956). Vancomycin, a new antibiotic III Preliminary clinical and laboratory studies. *Antibiot Ann 1955–1956*: 619.

Gruer LD, Bartlett R, Ayliffe GAJ (1984). Species identification and antibiotic sensitivity of coagulase-negative staphylococci from CAPD peritonitis. *J Antimicrob Chemother* **13**: 577.

Gump DW (1981). Vancomycin for treatment of bacterial meningitis. *Rev Infect Dis* **3** (Suppl): 289.

Gutmann L, Al-Obeid S, Billot-Klein D *et al.* (1994). Synergy and resistance to synergy between β-lactam antibiotics and glycopeptide antibiotics against glycopeptide-resistant strains of *Enterococcus faecium. Antimicrob Ag Chemother* **38**: 824.

Guzman R, Kirkpatrick J, Forward K, Lim F (1988). Failure of parenteral metronidazole in the treatment of pseudomembranous colitis. *J Infect Dis* **158**: 1146.

Handwerger S, Horowitz H, Coburn K *et al.* (1990). Infection due to *Leuconostoc* species: six cases and review. *Rev Infect Dis* **12**: 602.

Handwerger S, Perlman DC, Altarac D, McAuliffe V (1992). Concomitant high-level vancomycin and penicillin resistance in clinical isolates of enterococci. *Clin Infect Dis* 14: 655.

Hannah BA, Kimmel PL, Dosa S, Turner ML (1990). Vancomycin-induced toxic epidermal necrolysis. *South Med J* 83: 720.

Hardenbrook GM, Kildoo CW, Gennrich JL *et al.* (1991). Prospective evaluation of a vancomycin dosage guideline for neonates. *Clin Pharm* 10: 129.

Harwick HJ, Kalmanson GM, Guze LB (1973). *In vitro* activity of ampicillin or vancomycin combined with gentamicin or streptomycin against Enterococci. *Antimicrob Ag Chemother* 4: 383.

Harwick HJ, Kalmanson GM, Guze LB (1974). Pyelonephritis. XVII. Comparison of combinations of vancomycin, ampicillin, streptomycin, and gentamicin in the treatment of enterococcal infection in rats. *J Infect Dis* 129: 358.

Healy DP, Polk RE, Garson ML *et al.* (1987). Comparison of steady-state pharmacokinetics of two dosage regimens of vancomycin in normal volunteers. *Antimicrob Ag Chemother* 31: 393.

Healy DP, Sahai JV, Fuller SH, Polk RE (1990). Vancomycin-induced histamine release and 'red man syndrome': comparison of 1- and 2-hour infusions. *Antimicrob Ag Chemother* 34: 550.

Holliman RE, Bone GP (1988). Vancomycin resistance of clinical isolates of lactobacilli. *J Infect* 16: 279.

Hospital Infection Control Practices Advisory Committee (1995). Recommendations for preventing the spread of vancomycin resistance: recommendations of the Hospital Infection Control Practices Advisory Committee (HICPAC). *Amer J Infect Cont* 23: 87.

Hyams JS, Berman MM, Helgason H (1981). Nonantibiotic-associated enterocolitis caused by *Clostridium difficile* in an infant. *J Pediatr* 99: 750.

Jadeja L, Fainstein J, Le Blanc B, Bodey GP (1983). Comparative *in vitro* activities of teichomycin and other antibiotics against JK diphtheroids. *Antimicrob Ag Chemother* 24: 145.

James A, Koren G, Milliken J *et al.* (1987). Vancomycin pharmacokinetics and dose recommendations for preterm infants. *Antimicrob Ag Chemother* 31: 52.

Jarrett RV, Marinkovich GA, Gayle EL *et al.* (1993). Individualized pharmacokinetic profiles to compute vancomycin dosage and dosing interval in preterm infants. *Pediatr Infect Dis J* 12: 156.

Johnson AP, Uttley AHC, Woodford N, George RC (1990). Resistance to vancomycin and teicoplanin: an emerging clinical problem. *Clin Microbiol Rev* 3: 280.

Johnson CA (1991). Intraperitoneal vancomycin administration. *Periton Dial Internat* 11: 9.

Jones RN, Sader HS, Erwin ME *et al.* (1995). Emerging multiply resistant enterococci among clinical isolates. I. Prevalence data from 97 medical center surveillance study in the United States. *Diagn Microbiol Infect Dis* 21: 85.

Karanfil LV, Murphy M, Josephson A *et al.* (1992). A cluster of vancomycin-resistant *Enterococcus faecium* in an intensive care unit. *Infect Control Hosp Epidemiol* 13: 700.

Karchmer AW, Archer GL, Dismukes WE (1983). *Staphylococcus epidermidis* causing prosthetic valve endocarditis: microbiologic and clinical observations as guides to therapy. *Ann Intern Med* 98: 447.

Karp JE, Dick JD, Angelopulos C *et al.* (1986). Empiric use of vancomycin during prolonged treatment-induced granulocytopenia. Randomized, double-blind, placebo-controlled clinical trial in patients with acute leukemia. *Amer J Med* 81: 237.

Keane WF, Everett ED, Golper TA *et al.* (1993). Peritoneal dialysis-related peritonitis treatment recommendations: 1993 update. *Periton Dial Internat* 13: 14.

Keighley MRB, Burdon DW, Arabi Y *et al.* (1978). Randomised controlled trial of vancomycin for pseudomembranous colitis and postoperative diarrhoea. *Brit Med J* 2: 1667.

Kirby WMM, Perry DM, Bauer AW (1960). Treatment of staphylococcal septicemia with vancomycin. Report of thirty-three cases. *New Engl J Med* 262: 49.

Kliegman RM, Fanaroff AA (1984). Necrotizing enterocolitis. *New Engl J Med* 310: 1093.

Klugman KP, Friedland IR, Bradley JS (1995). Bactericidal activity against cephalosporin-resistant *Steptococcus pneumoniae* in cerebrospinal fluid of children with acute bacterial meningitis. *Antimicrob Ag Chemother* 39: 1988.

Koo KB, Bachand RL, Chow AW (1986). Vancomycin-induced neutropenia. *Drug Intell Clin Pharm* 20: 780.

Koren G, James A (1987). Vancomycin dosing in pre-term infants: prospective verification of new recommendations. *J Pediatr* 110: 797.

Korzeniowski O, Sande MA (1982). Combination antimicrobial therapy for *Staphylococcus aureus* endocarditis in patients addicted to parenteral drugs and in non-addicts: a prospective study. *Ann Intern Med* 97: 496.

Krothapalli RK, Senekjian HO, Ayus JC (1983). Efficacy of intravenous vancomycin in the treatment of Gram-positive peritonitis in long-term peritoneal dialysis. *Amer J Med* 75: 345.

Kuechle DK, Landon GC, Musher DM, Noble PC (1991). Elution of vancomycin, daptomycin, and amikacin from acrylic bone cement. *Clin Orthopaed Rel Res* 264: 302.

Kuechle MK, Stegemeir E, Maynard B *et al.* (1994). Drug-induced linear Ig. A bullous dermatosis: report of six cases and review of the literature. *J Amer Acad Dermatol* 30: 187.

Lamer C, DeBeco V, Soler P *et al.* (1993). Analysis of vancomycin entry into pulmonary lining fluid by bronchoalveolar lavage in critically ill patients. *Antimicrob Ag Chemother* 37: 281.

Lamy T, Michelet C, Dauriac C *et al.* (1993). Benefit of prophylaxis by intravenous systemic vancomycin in granulocytopenic patients: a prospective, randomized trial among 59 patients. *Acta Haematol* 90: 109.

Landman D, Mobarakai NK, Quale JM *et al.* (1993). Novel antibiotic regimens against *Enterococcus faecium* resistant to ampicillin, vancomycin, and gentamicin. *Antimicrob Ag Chemother* 37: 1904.

Larson HE, Levi AJ, Borriello SP (1978). Vancomycin for pseudomembranous colitis. *Lancet* ii: 48.

Laurencin CT, Horan RF, Senatus PB *et al.* (1992). Stevens-Johnson-type reaction with vancomycin treatment. *Ann Pharmacother* 26: 1520.

Leclerq R, Derlot E, Duval J, Courvalin P (1988). Plasmid-mediated resistance to vancomycin and teicoplanin in *Enterococcus faecium*. *New Engl J Med* 319: 157.

Leclerq R, Bingen E, Su QH *et al.* (1991). Effects of combinations of β-lactams, daptomycin, gentamicin, and glycopeptides against glycopeptide-resistant enterococci. *Antimicrob Ag Chemother* 35: 92.

Leclerq R, Dutka-Malen S, Duval J, Courvalin P (1992). Vancomycin resistance gene vanC is specific to *Enterococcus gallinarum*. *Antimicrob Ag Chemother* 36: 2005.

Levi JA, Vincent PC, Jennis F *et al.* (1978). Prophylactic oral antibiotics in the management of acute leukaemia. *Med J Aust* 1: 1025.

Levine DP, Fromm BS, Reddy BR (1991). Slow response to vancomycin plus rifampin in methicillin-resistant *Staphylococcus aureus* endocarditis. *Ann Intern Med* 115: 674.

Levy RM, Gutin PH, Baskin DS *et al.* (1986). Vancomycin penetration of brain abscess: case report and review of the literature. *Neurosurgery* 18: 633.

Lin RY (1990). Desensitization in the management of vancomycin hypersensitivity. *Arch Intern Med* 150: 2197.

Liñares J, Perez JL, Garau J *et al.* (1984). Comparative susceptibilities of penicillin-resistant pneumococci to co-trimoxazole, vancomycin, rifampicin and fourteen beta-lactam antibiotics. *J Antimicrob Chemother* 13: 353.

Lindholm DD, Murray JS (1966). Persistence of vancomycin in the blood during renal failure and its treatment by haemodialysis. *New Engl J Med* 274: 1047.

Lisby SM, Nahata MC (1987). Revised dosage guidelines of vancomycin in pediatric patients. *Clin Pharmacol Ther* 43: 197.

Lowy FD, Walsh JA, Mayers MM *et al.* (1979). Antibiotic activity *in vitro* against-methicillin-resistant *Staphylococcus epidermidis* and therapy of an experimental infection. *Antimicrob Ag Chemother* 16: 314.

Luer MS, Hatton J (1993). Vancomycin administration into the cerebrospinal fluid: a review. *Ann Pharmacother* 27: 912.

Lutz H, Lenarz T, Weidauer H et al. (1991). Ototoxicity of vancomycin: an experimental study in guinea pigs. ORL J Otorhinolaryngol 53: 273.

MacGowan AP, Holt HA, Bywater MJ, Reeves DS (1990). In vitro antimicrobial susceptibility of Listeria monocytogenes isolated in the UK and other Listeria species. Eur J Clin Microbiol Infect Dis 9: 767.

Mackey T, Lejeune V, Jannsens M, Wauters G (1993). Identification of vancomycin-resistant lactic bacteria isolated from humans. J Clin Microbiol 31: 2499.

Magera BE, Arroyo JC, Rosansky SJ, Postic B (1983). Vancomycin pharmacokinetics in patients with peritonitis on peritoneal dialysis. Antimicrob Ag Chemother 23: 710.

Maki DG, Bohn MJ, Stolz SM et al. (1992). Comparative study of cefazolin, cefamandole and vancomycin prophylaxis in cardiac and vascular operations. A double-blind, randomized trial. J Thorac Cardiovasc Surg 104: 1423.

Mallet L, Sesin GP, Ericson J, Fraser DG (1982). Storage of vancomycin oral solution. New Engl J Med 307: 445.

Markman M, Lim HW, Bluestein HG (1986). Vancomycin-induced vasculitis. South Med J 79: 382.

Martin C, Alaya M, Mallet M-N et al. (1994). Penetration of vancomycin into mediastinal and cardiac tissues in humans. Antimicrob Ag Chemother 38: 396.

Mastro TD, Spika JS, Lozano P et al. (1990). Vancomycin-resistant Pediococcus acidilactici: nine cases of bacteremia. J Infect Dis 161: 956.

Matzke GR, McGory RW, Halstenson CE, Keane WF (1984). Pharmacokinetics of vancomycin in patients with various degrees of renal function. Antimicrob Ag Chemother 25: 433.

Matzke GR, O'Connell MB, Collins AJ, Keshaviah PER (1986). Disposition of vancomycin during hemofiltration. Clin Pharmacol Ther 40: 425.

Maugein J, Pellegrin JL, Brossard G et al. (1990). In vitro activities of vancomycin and teicoplanin against coagulase-negative staphylococci isolated from neutropenic patients. Antimicrob Ag Chemother 34: 901.

McCormick MH, Stark WM, Pittenger GE et al (1956). Vancomycin, a new antibiotic. I. Chemical and biologic properties. Antibiot Ann 1955–1956: 606.

McElrath MJ, Goldberg D, Neu HC (1986). Allergic cross-reactivity of teicoplanin and vancomycin. Lancet i: 47.

McGee SM, Kaplan SL, Mason EO (1990). Ventricular fluid concentrations of vancomycin in children after intravenous and intraventricular administration. Pediatr Infect Dis J 9: 138.

McHenry MC, Gavan TL (1983). Vancomycin. Pediatr Clin N Amer 30: 31.

McWhinney PHM, Patel S, Whiley RA et al. (1993). Activities of potential therapeutic and prophylactic antibiotics against blood culture isolates of viridans group streptococci from neutropenic patients receiving ciprofloxacin. Antimicrob Ag Chemother 37: 2493.

Mellor JA, Kingdom J, Cafferkey M, Keane CT (1985). Vancomycin toxicity: a prospective study. J Antimicrob Chemother 15: 773.

Meylan PR, Francioli P, Glauser MP (1986). Discrepancies between MBC and actual killing of viridans group streptococci by cell-wall-active antibiotics. Antimicrob Ag Chemother 29: 418.

Miller MA, Parker JW, Rohrer HH (1981). Vancomycin-sensitive Neisseria gonorrhoeae: comment. J Infect Dis 144: 199.

Mobarakai N, Quale JM, Landman D (1994). Bactericidal activities of peptide antibiotics against multidrug-resistant Enterococcus faecium. Antimicrob Ag Chemother 38: 385.

Moellering RC Jr (1984). Pharmacokinetics of vancomycin. J Antimicrob Chemother 14 (Suppl D): 43.

Moellering RC (1994). Monitoring serum vancomycin levels: climbing the mountain because it is there? Clin Infect Dis 18: 544.

Moellering RC Jr, Krogstad DJ, Greenblatt DJ (1981a). Vancomycin therapy in patients with impaired renal function: nomogram for dosage. Ann Intern Med 94: 343.

Moellering RC Jr, Krogstad DJ, Greenblatt DJ (1981b). Pharmacokinetics

of vancomycin in normal subjects and in patients with reduced renal function. Rev Infect Dis 3 (Suppl): 230.

Montecalvo MA, Horowitz H, Gedris C et al. (1994). Outbreak of vancomycin-, ampicillin-, and aminoglycoside-resistant Enterococcus faecium bacteremia in an adult oncology unit. Antimicrob Ag Chemother 38: 1363.

Moore BJ (1985). Vancomycin dosage recommendations. Lancet ii: 39.

Moorhouse EC, Mulvihill TE, Jones L et al. (1985). The in-vitro activity of some antimicrobial agents against methicillin-resistant Staphylococcus aureus. J Antimicrob Chemother 15: 291.

Morris A, Ward C (1991). High incidence of vancomycin-associated leucopenia and neutropenia in a cardiothoracic surgical ward. J Infect 22: 217.

Morris JG, Shay DK, Hebeden JN et al. (1995). Enterococci resistant to multiple antimicrobial agents, including vancomycin. Ann Intern Med 123: 250.

Morse GD, Farolino DF, Apicella MA, Walshe JJ (1987). Comparative study of intraperitoneal and intravenous vancomycin pharmacokinetics during continuous ambulatory peritoneal dialysis. Antimicrob Ag Chemother 31: 173.

Munson DP, Thompson TR, Johnson DE et al. (1982). Coagulase-negative staphylococcal septicemia: experience in a newborn intensive care unit. J Pediatr 101: 602.

Murray BE (1995). What can we do about vancomycin-resistant enterococci? Clin Infect Dis 20: 1134.

Myers JP, Linnemann CC Jr (1982). Bacteremia due to methicillin-resistant Staphylococcus aureus. J Infect Dis 145: 532.

Nagarajan R (1991). Antibacterial activities and modes of action of vancomycin and related glycopeptides. Antimicrob Ag Chemother 35: 605.

Naqvi SH, Keenan WJ, Reichley RM, Fortune KP (1986). Vancomycin pharmacokinetics in small seriously ill infants. Amer J Dis Child 140: 107.

Navarro F, Courvalin P (1994). Analysis of genes encoding D-alanine-D-alanine ligase-related enzymes in Enterococcus casseliflavus and Enterococcus flavescens. Antimicrob Ag Chemother 38: 1788.

Newfield P, Roizen MF (1979). Hazards of rapid administration of vancomycin. Ann Intern Med 91: 581.

Newsom SWB (1982). Leading article. Vancomycin. J Antimicrob Chemother 10: 257.

Nieto M, Perkins HR (1971). The specificity of combination between ristocetins and peptides related to bacterial cell wall mucopeptide precursors. Biochem J 124: 845.

Noble JT, Tyburski MB, Berman M et al. (1980). Antimicrobial tolerance in group G streptococci. Lancet ii: 982.

Noble WC, Virani Z, Cree RGA (1992). Co-transfer of vancomycin and other resistance genes from Enterococcus faecalis NCTC 12201 to Staphylococcus aureus. FEMS Microbiol Lett 93: 195.

Noel GJ, O'Loughlin JE, Edelson PJ (1988). Neonatal Staphylococcus epidermidis right-sided endocarditis: description of five catheterized infants. Pediatr 82: 234.

Nordmann P, Ronco E (1992). In-vitro antimicrobial susceptibility of Rhodococcus equi. J Antimicrob Chemother 29: 383.

Nordmann P, Kerestedjian J-J, Ronco E (1992). Therapy of Rhodococcus equi disseminated infections in nude mice. Antimicrob Ag Chemother 36: 1244.

Oliva SL, Guglielmo J, Jacobs R, Pons VG (1989). Failure of intravenous vancomycin and intravenous metronidazole to prevent or treat antibiotic-associated pseudomembranous colitis. J Infect Dis 159: 1154.

O'Sullivan TL, Ruffing MJ, Lamp KC et al. (1993). Prospective evaluation of red man syndrome in patients receiving vancomycin. J Infect Dis 168: 773.

Pallanza R, Berti M, Goldstein BP et al. (1983). Teichomycin: in-vitro and in-vivo evaluations in comparison with other antibiotics. J Antimicrob Chemother 11: 419.

Paris MM, Hickey SM, Uscher MI et al. (1994). Effect of dexamethasone on therapy of experimental penicillin- and cephalosporin-resistant pneumococcal meningitis. *Antimicrob Ag Chemother* **38**: 1320.

Pasic M, Jost R, Carrel T *et al.* (1993). Intracolonic vancomycin for pseudomembranous colitis. *New Engl J Med* **329**: 583.

Patterson JE, Colodny SM, Zervos MJ (1988). Serious infection due to β-lactamase producing *Streptococcus faecalis* with high-level resistance to gentamicin. *J Infect Dis* **158**: 1144.

Patterson JE, Sweeney AH, Simms M *et al.* (1995). An analysis of 110 serious enterococcal infections. Epidemiology, antibiotic susceptibility, and outcome. *Medicine* **74**: 191.

Pauly DJ, Musa DM, Lestico MR *et al.* (1990). Risk of nephrotoxicity with combination vancomycin-aminoglycoside antibiotic therapy. *Pharmacother* **10**: 378.

Perez JL, Riera L, Valls F *et al.* (1987). A comparison of the *in vitro* activity of seventeen antibiotics against *Streptococcus faecalis*. *J Antimicrob Chemother* **20**: 357.

Pfeiffer RR (1981). Structural features of vancomycin. *Rev Infect Dis* **3** (Suppl): 205.

Polk RE (1991). Anaphylactoid reactions to glycopeptide antiobiotics. *J Antimicrob Chemother* **27** (Suppl B): 17.

Polk RE, Healy DP, Schwartz LB *et al.* (1988). Vancomycin and the red-man syndrome: pharmacodynamics of histamine release. *J Infect Dis* **157**: 502.

Polk RE, Israel D, Wang J *et al.* (1993). Vancomycin skin tests and prediction of 'red man syndrome' in healthy volunteers. *Antimicrob Ag Chemother* **37**: 2139.

Pollard TA, Lampasona V, Akkerman S *et al.* (1994). Vancomycin redistribution: dosing recommendations following high-flux hemodialysis. *Kidney Internat* **45**: 232.

Press OW, Ramsey PG, Larson EB *et al.* (1984). Hickman catheter infections in patients with malignancies. *Medicine* **63**: 189.

Quale JM, O'Halloran JJ, DeVincenzo N, Barth RH (1992). Removal of vancomycin by high-flux hemodialysis membranes. *Antimicrob Ag Chemother* **36**: 1424.

Raad I, Davis S, Khan A *et al.* (1992). Catheter removal affects recurrence of catheter-related coagulase-negative staphylococci bacteremia(CRCNSB). *Infect Cont Hosp Epidemiol* **13**: 215.

Raimondi A, Moosdeen F, Williams JD (1986). Antibiotic resistance pattern of *Flavobacterium meningosepticum*. *Eur J Clin Microbiol Infect Dis* **5**: 461.

Ramphal R, Bolger M, Oblon DJ *et al.* (1992). Vancomycin is not an essential component of the initial empiric treatment regimen for febrile neutropenic patients receiving ceftazidime: a randomized prospective study. *Antimicrob Ag Chemother* **36**: 1062.

Ranson MR, Oppenheim BA, Jackson A *et al.* (1990). Double-blind placebo controlled study of vancomycin prophylaxis for central venous catheter insertion in cancer patients. *J Hosp Infect* **15**: 95.

Ratner H (1984). *Flavobacterium meningosepticum*. *Infect Control* **5**: 237.

Reesor C, Chow AW, Kureishi A, Jewesson P (1988). Kinetics of intraventricular vancomycin in infections of cerebrospinal fluid shunts. *J Infect Dis* **158**: 1142.

Reynolds PE, Depardieu F, Dutka-Malen S *et al.* (1994). Glycopeptide resistance mediated by enterococcal transposon Tn1546 requires production of VanX for hydrolysis of D-alanyl-D-alanine. *Molec Microbiol* **13**: 1065.

Riebel W, Frantz N, Adestein D, Spagnuolo PJ (1986). *Corynebacterium* JK: a cause of nosocomial device-related infection. *Rev Infect Dis* **8**: 42.

Rodvold KA, Blum RA, Fischer JH *et al.* (1988). Vancomycin pharmacokinetics in patients with various degrees of renal function. *Antimicrob Ag Chemother* **32**: 848.

Rogge MC, Johnson CA, Zimmerman SW, Welling PG (1985). Vancomycin disposition during continuous ambulatory peritoneal dialysis: a pharmacokinetic analysis of peritoneal drug transport. *Antimicrob Ag Chemother* **27**: 578.

Romanelli VA, Howie MB, Myerowitz PD *et al.* (1993). Intraoperative and postoperative effects of vancomycin administration in cardiac surgery

patients: a prospective, double-blind, randomized trial. *Crit Care Med* **21**: 1124.

Rosenberg JM, Wahr JA, Smith KA (1995). Effect of vancomycin infusion on cardiac function in patients scheduled for cardiac operation. *J Thorac Cardiovasc Surg* **109**: 561.

Rothenberg HJ (1959). Anaphylactoid reaction to vancomycin. *JAMA* **171**: 1101.

Rotschafer JC, Crossley K, Zaske DE *et al.* (1982). Pharmacokinetics of vancomycin: observations in 28 patients and dosage recommendations. *Antimicrob Ag Chemother* **22**: 391.

Rouquet RM, Clave D, Massip P *et al.* (1991). Imipenem / vancomycin for *Rhodococcus equi* pulmonary infection in HIV-positive patient. *Lancet* **337**: 375.

Rubin J (1990). Vancomycin absorption from the peritoneal cavity during dialysis-related peritonitis. *Periton Dial Internat* **10**: 283.

Rubin M, Hathorn JW, Marshall D *et al.* (1988). Gram-positive infections and the use of vancomycin in 550 episodes of fever and neutropenia. *Ann Intern Med* **108**: 30.

Rupp ME, Archer GL (1994). Coagulase-negative staphylococci: pathogens associated with medical progress. *Clin Infect Dis* **19**: 231.

Rybak MJ, Albrecht LM, Berman JR *et al.* (1990a). Vancomycin pharmacokinetics in burn patients and intravenous drug abusers. *Antimicrob Ag Chemother* **34**: 792.

Rybak MJ, Albrecht LM, Boike SC, Chandrasekar PH (1990b). Nephrotoxicity of vancomycin, alone and with an aminoglycoside. *J Antimicrob Chemother* **25**: 679.

Rybak MJ, Bailey EM, Warbasse LH (1992). Absence of 'red man syndrome' in patients being treated with vancomycin or high-dose teicoplanin. *Antimicrob Ag Chemother* **36**: 1204.

Sader HS, Jones RN, Pfaller MA (1995). Relapse of catheter-related *Flavobacterium meningosepticum* bacteraemia demonstrated by DNA macrorestriction analysis. *Clin Infect Dis* **21**: 997.

Sahai JVS, Polk RE, Schwartz LB *et al.* (1988). Severe reaction to vancomycin not mediated by histamine release and documented by rechallenge. *J Infect Dis* **158**: 1413.

Sahai J, Healy DP, Garris R *et al.* (1989). Influence of antihistamine pretreatment on vancomycin-induced red-man syndrome. *J Infect Dis* **160**: 876.

Sahai J, Healy DP, Shelton MJ *et al.* (1990). Comparison of vancomycin- and teicoplanin-induced histamine release and 'red man syndrome'. *Antimicrob Ag Chemother* **34**: 765.

Saleh RA, Schorin MA (1987). *Bacillus* spp sepsis associated with Hickman catheters in patients with neoplastic disease. *Pediatr Infect Dis J* **6**: 851.

Salzman C, Weingold AB, Simon GL (1987). Increased dose requirements of vancomycin in a pregnant patient with endocarditis. *J Infect Dis* **156**: 409.

Sande MA, Scheld WM (1980). Combination therapy of bacterial endocarditis. *Ann Intern Med* **92**: 390.

Santré C, Leroy O, Simon M *et al.* (1993). Pharmacokinetics of vancomycin during hemodiafiltration. *Intensive Care Med* **19**: 347.

Sanyal D, Williams AJ, Johnson AP, George RC (1993). The emergence of vancomycin resistance in renal dialysis. *J Hosp Infect* **24**: 167.

Saunders NJ (1995). Vancomycin administration and monitoring reappraisal. *J Antimicrob Chemother* **36**: 279.

Schaad UB, McCracken GH Jr, Nelson JD (1980). Clinical pharmacology and efficacy of vancomycin in pediatric patients. *J Pediatr* **96**: 119.

Schaad UB, Nelson JD, McCracken GH Jr (1981). Pharmacology and efficacy of vancomycin for staphylococcal infections in children. *Rev Infect Dis* **3** (Suppl): 282.

Schwalbe RS, Stapleton JT, Gilligan PH (1987). Emergence of vancomycin resistance in coagulase-negative staphylococci. *New Engl J Med* **316**:927.

Schwan A, Sjolin S, Trottestam U, Aronsson B (1984). Relapsing *Clostridium difficile* enterocolitis cured by rectal infusion of normal faeces. *Scand J Infect Dis* **16**: 211.

Schwartz C, Henrickson KJ, Roghmann K, Powell K (1990). Prevention of bacteremia attributed to luminal colonization of tunneled central venous catheters with vancomycin-susceptible organisms. *J Clin Oncol* **8**: 1591.

Shay DK, Maloney SA, Montecalvo M *et al.* (1995). Epidemiology and mortality risk of vancomycin-resistant enterococcal bloodstream infections. *J Infect Dis* **172**: 993.

Shlaes DM, Marino J, Jacobs MR (1984). Infection caused by vancomycin-resistant *Streptococcus sanguis* II. *Antimicrob Ag Chemother* **25**: 527.

Shlaes DM, Etter L, Gutmann L (1991). Synergistic killing of vancomycin-resistant enterococci of classes A, B, and C by combinations of vancomycin, penicillin, and gentamicin. *Antimicrob Ag Chemother* **35**: 776.

Shonekan D, Mildvan D, Handwerger S (1992). Comparative *in vitro* activities of teicoplanin, daptomycin, ramoplanin, vancomycin and PD 127,391 against blood isolates of gram-positive cocci. *Antimicrob Ag Chemother* **36**: 1570.

Siebert WT, Moreland N, Williams TW Jr (1979). Synergy of vancomycin plus cefazolin or cephalothin against methicillin-resistant *Staphylococcus epidermidis*. *J Infect Dis* **139**: 452.

Silva J Jr, Batts DH, Fekety R *et al.* (1981). Treatment of *Clostridium difficile* colitis and diarrhoea with vancomycin. *Amer J Med* **71**: 815.

Silverman DA (1981). Removal of vancomycin by peritoneal dialysis. *New Engl J Med* **304**: 361.

Sinha RK, Neuhaus FC (1968). Reversal of the vancomycin inhibition of peptidoglycan synthesis by cell walls. *J Bacteriol* **96**: 374.

Small PM, Chambers HF (1990). Vancomycin for *Staphylococcus aureus* endocarditis in intravenous drug users. *Antimicrob Ag Chemother* **34**: 1227.

Smith SR, Cheesbrough J, Spearing R, Davies JM (1989). Randomized prospective study comparing vancomycin with teicoplanin in the treatment of infections associated with Hickman catheters. *Antimicrob Ag Chemother* **33**: 1193.

Smith SR, Cheesbrough J, Harding I, Davies JM (1990). Role of glycopeptide antibiotics in the treatment of febrile neutropenic patients. *Brit J Haematol* **76** (Suppl 2): 54.

Soriano F, Ponte C, Santamaria M *et al.* (1987). Susceptibility of urinary isolates of *Corynebacterium* group D2 to fifteen antimicrobials and acetohydroxamic acid. *J Antimicrob Chemother* **20**: 349.

Sorrell TC, Collignon PJ (1985). A prospective study of adverse reactions associated with vancomycin therapy. *J Antimicrob Chemother* **16**: 235.

Sorrell TC, Packham DR, Shanker S *et al.* (1982). Vancomycin therapy for methicillin-resistant *Staphylococcus aureus*. *Ann Intern Med* **97**: 344.

Southorn PA, Plevak DJ, Wright AJ, Wilson WR (1986). Adverse effects of vancomycin administered in the perioperative period. *Mayo Clin Proc* **61**: 721.

Spears RL, Koch R (1960). The use of vancomycin in pediatrics. *Antibiot Ann 1959–1960*: 798.

Spitzer PG, Eliopoulos GM (1984). Systemic absorption of enteral vancomycin in a patient with pseudomembranous colitis. *Ann Intern Med* **100**: 533.

Spitzer PG, Eliopoulos GM, Karchmer AW, Moellering RC (1988). Synergistic activity between vancomycin or teicoplanin and gentamicin or tobramycin against pathogenic diphtheroids. *Antimicrob Ag Chemother* **32**: 434.

Stamm WE, Tompkins LS, Wagner KF *et al.* (1979). Infection due to *Corynebacterium* species in marrow transplant patients. *Ann Intern Med* **91**: 167.

Starr SE (1985). Antimicrobial therapy of bacterial sepsis in the newborn infant. *J Pediatr* **106**: 1043.

Stein DS, Libertin CR (1988). Time kill curve analysis of vancomycin and rifampin alone and in combination against nine strains of nutritionally deficient streptococci. *Diagn Microbiol Infect Dis* **10**: 139.

Stolberg L, Rolfe R, Gitlin N *et al.* (1982). D-lactic acidosis due to abnormal gut flora. *New Engl J Med* **306**: 1344.

Sun H, Maderazo EG, Krussell AR (1993). Serum protein-binding characteristics of vancomycin. *Antimicrob Ag Chemother* **37**: 1132.

Surawicz CM, McFarland LV, Elmer G, Chinn J (1989). Treatment of recurrent *Clostridium difficile* colitis with vancomycin and *Saccharomyces boulardii*. *Amer J Gastroenterol* **84**: 1285.

Swayne R, Rampling A, Newsom SWB (1987). Intraventricular vancomycin for treatment of shunt-associated ventriculitis. *J Antimicrob Chemother* **19**: 249.

Tedesco F, Markham R, Gurwith M *et al.* (1978). Oral vancomycin for antibiotic-associated pseudomembranous colitis. *Lancet* **ii**: 226.

Tedesco FJ (1982). Treatment of recurrent antibiotic-associated pseudomembranous colitis. *Amer J Gastroenterol* **77**: 220.

Thornsberry C, Facklam RR (1984). Vancomycin-resistant streptococci? Probably not. *Antimicrob Newsl* **1**: 63.

Tofte RW, Solliday J, Crossley KB (1984). Susceptibilities of enterococci to twelve antibiotics. *Antimicrob Ag Chemother* **25**: 532.

Torres-R JR, Sanders CV, Lewis AC (1979). Vancomycin concentration in human tissues – preliminary report. *J Antimicrob Chemother* **5**: 475.

Tuazon CU, Miller H (1983). Clinical and microbiologic aspects of serious infections caused by *Staphylococcus epidermidis*. *Scand J Infect Dis* **15**: 347.

Uttley AHC, Collins CH, Naidoo J, George RC (1988). Vancomycin-resistant enterococci. *Lancet* **i**: 57.

Uttley AHC, George RC, Naidoo J *et al.* (1989). High-level vancomycin-resistant enterococci causing hospital infections. *Epidemiol Infect* **103**: 173.

Vance-Bryan K, Guay DRP, Gilliland SS *et al.* (1993). Effect of obesity on vancomycin pharmacokinetic parameters as determined by using a Bayesian forecasting technique. *Antimicrob Ag Chemother* **37**: 436.

Vance-Bryan K, Rotschafer JC, Gilliland SS *et al.* (1994). A comparative assessment of vancomycin-associated nephrotoxicity in the young versus the elderly hospitalized patient. *J Antimicrob Chemother* **33**: 811.

Veach LA, Pfaller MA, Barrett M *et al.* (1990). Vancomycin resistance in *Staphylococcus haemolyticus* causing colonization and bloodstream infection. *J Clin Microbiol* **28**: 2064.

Vedel G, Leruez M, Lemann F *et al.* (1990). Prevalence of *Staphylococcus aureus* and coagulase-negative staphylococci with decreased sensitivity to glycopeptides as assessed by determination of MICs. *Eur J Clin Microbiol Infect Dis* **9**: 820.

Verville TD, Huycke MM, Greenfield RA *et al.* (1994). *Rhodococcus equi* infections of humans: 12 cases and a review of the literature. *Medicine* **73**: 119.

Viladrich PF, Gudiol F, Linares J *et al.* (1991). Evaluation of vancomycin for therapy of adult pneumococcal meningitis. *Antimicrob Ag Chemother* **35**: 2467.

Von Kaenel WE, Bloomfield EL, Amaranath L, Wilde AA (1993). Vancomycin does not enhance hypotension under anesthesia. *Anesth Analg* **76**: 809.

Wade JC, Schimpff SC, Newman KA, Wiernick PH (1982). *Staphylococcus epidermidis*: an increasing cause of infection in patients with granulocytopenia. *Ann Intern Med* **97**: 503.

Wade J, Baillie L, Rolando N, Casewell M (1992). Pristinamycin for *Enterococcus faecium* resistant to vancomycin and gentamicin. *Lancet* **339**: 312.

Wadsworth SJ, Kim K-H, Satishchandran V *et al.* (1992). Development of new antibiotic resistance in methicillin-resistant but not methicillin-susceptible *Staphylococcus aureus*. *J Antimicrob Chemother* **30**: 821.

Walker RW, Heaton A (1985). Thrombocytopenia due to vancomycin. *Lancet* **i**: 932.

Wallace MR, Mascola JR, Oldfield ECIII (1991). Red man syndrome: incidence, etiology, and prophylaxis. *J Infect Dis* **164**: 1180.

Walsh CT (1993). Vancomycin resistance: decoding the molecular logic. *Science* **261**: 308.

Wandstrat TL, Phelps SJ (1993). Vancomycin dosing in neonatal patients: the controversy continues. *Neonat Netw* **13**: 33.

Watanakunakorn C (1982). Treatment of infections due to methicillin-resistant *Staphylococcus aureus*. *Ann Intern Med* **97**: 376.

Watanakunakorn C (1984). Mode of action and *in-vitro* activity of vancomycin. *Antimicrob Ag Chemother* **14** (Suppl D): 7.

Watanakunakorn C (1988). *In vitro* induction of resistance in coagulase negative staphylococci to vancomycin and teicoplanin. *J Antimicrob Chemother* 22:321.

Watanakunakorn C (1990). *In-vitro* selection of resistance of *Staphylococcus aureus* to teicoplanin and vancomycin. *J Antimicrob Chemother* 25: 69.

Watanakunakorn C, Bakie C (1973). Synergism of vancomycin-gentamicin and vancomycin-streptomycin against enterococci. *Antimicrob Ag Chemother* 4: 120.

Watanakunakorn C, Tisone JC (1982). Synergism between vancomycin and gentamicin or tobramycin for methicillin-susceptible and methicillin-resistant *Staphylococcus aureus* strains. *Antimicrob Ag Chemother* 22: 903.

Weathers L, Riggs D, Santeiro M, Weibley RE (1990). Aerosolized vancomycin for treatment of airway colonization by methicillin-resistant *Staphylococcus aureus*. *Pediatr Infect Dis J* 9: 220.

Weber DJ, Saviteer SM, Rutala WA, Thomann CA (1988). *In vitro* susceptibility of *Bacillus* spp. to selected antimicrobial agents. *Antimicrob Ag Chemother* 32: 642.

Westenfelder GO, Paterson PY, Reisberg BE, Carlson GM (1973). Vancomycin-streptomycin synergism in enterococcal endocarditis. *JAMA* 223: 37.

Whitby M, Edwards R, Aston E, Finch RG (1987). Pharmacokinetics of single dose intravenous vancomycin in CAPD peritonitis. *J Antimicrob Chemother* 19: 351.

Williamson RC, Al-Obeid S, Shlaes JC *et al.* (1989). Inducible resistance to vancomycin in *Enterococcus faecium* D366. *J Infect Dis* 159: 1095.

Windall JJ, Hall MM, Washington JA II *et al.* (1980). Inhibitory effects of vancomycin on *Neisseria gonorrhoeae* in Thayer-Martin medium. *J Infect Dis* 142: 775.

Winston DJ, Dudnick DJ, Chapin M *et al.* (1983). Coagulase-negative staphylococcal bacteremia in patients receiving immunosuppressive therapy. *Arch Intern Med* 143: 32.

Wong JT, Ripple RE, Maclean JA *et al.* (1994). Vancomycin hypersensitivity: synergism with narcotics and 'desensitization' by a rapid continuous intravenous protocol. *J Allergy Clin Immunol* 94: 189.

Wong MT, Dalton MJ (1992). Significant infections due to *Bacillus* species following abrasions associated with motor vehicle-related trauma. *Clin Infect Dis* 15: 855.

Wysocki M, Thomas F, Wolff MA *et al.* (1995). Comparison of continuous with discontinuous intravenous infusion of vancomycin in severe MRSA infections. *J Antimicrob Chemother* 35: 352.

Younger JJ, Christensen GD, Bartley DL *et al.* (1987). Coagulase-negative staphylococci isolated from cerebrospinal fluid shunts: importance of slime production, species identification, and shunt removal to clinical outcome. *J Infect Dis* 156: 548.

Zeitlin J, Carvounis CP, Murphy RG, Tortora GT (1982). Graft infection and bacteremia with *Listeria monocytogenes* in a patient receiving hemodialysis. *Arch Intern Med* 142: 2191.

Zenon GJ, Cadle RM, Hamill RJ (1991). Vancomycin-induced thrombocytopenia. *Arch Intern Med* 151: 995.

Teicoplanin

Description

Teicoplanin is a glycopeptide antibiotic (p. 763), chemically related to vancomycin (Bardone *et al.*, 1978), which was obtained by fermenting *Actinoplanes teichomyceticus* (Parenti *et al.*, 1978). Similar to vancomycin (p. 773), teicoplanin binds to, and inhibits, cell wall biosynthesis in susceptible organisms by interfering with the polymerization of peptidoglycan (Somma *et al.*, 1984). Its antibacterial action is restricted to Gram-positive aerobic and anaerobic bacteria (Parenti *et al.*, 1978; Greenwood, 1988).

Sensitive Organisms

1 Staphylococcus aureus

This organism, including penicillin G- and methicillin-resistant strains, is usually about equally sensitive to teicoplanin and vancomycin (p. 763) (Carper *et al.*, 1987; Greenwood, 1988; Gorzynski *et al.*, 1989; Felmingham, 1993). Teicoplanin-resistant strains can be selected *in vitro* by subculturing the organism in media containing a subinhibitory concentration of teicoplanin (Watanakunakorn, 1990). By this method teicoplanin can also select vancomycin-resistant *Staph. aureus* strains and in this respect teicoplanin appears to be a more efficient selective agent than vancomycin itself (Shlaes and Shlaes, 1995).

Strains of *Staph. aureus* resistant to teicoplanin, have also emerged *in vivo* in animals with induced endocarditis, treated by teicoplanin (Kaatz *et al.*, 1990) and in a small number of patients with severe *Staph. aureus* infections treated by the drug (Kaatz *et al.*, 1990; Manquat *et al.*, 1992; Kayser, 1995). A nosocomial spread of methicillin-resistant *Staph. aureus* (MRSA) strains with reduced susceptibility to teicoplanin also occurred in a hospital, involving 12 patients. Four of these had been previously treated by vancomycin, and it appeared that vancomycin might have selected MRSA strains with decreased teicoplanin susceptibility without producing a detectable change in vancomycin sensitivity (Mainardi *et al.*, 1995). This teicoplanin-resistance is constitutive and not plasmid-mediated. It involves a mutation of chromosomal gene. The exact mechanism of *Staph. aureus* resistance to teicoplanin is not known, but resistant strains have a 35 kDa membrane protein and usually also increased levels of penicillin-binding protein, PBP 2. Teicoplanin is less effective than vancomycin at inhibiting peptidoglycan synthesis in resistant strains, suggesting that there are some differences between these two drugs in their mode of action on the cell wall (p. 795) (Kaatz *et al.*, 1990; Daum *et al.*, 1992; Shlaes *et al.*, 1993b; Mainardi *et al.*, 1995).

2 Coagulase-negative staphylococci

These also are usually teicoplanin-sensitive. However, teicoplanin-resistant strains of *Staph. epidermidis* and in particular *Staph. haemolyticus* can be selected *in vitro* by subculturing these organisms in media containing a subinhibitory concentration of teicoplanin. Such resistant strains of *Staph. epidermidis* often have MICs of 64.0 μg per ml and those of *Staph. haemolyticus* ≥128.0 μg per ml (Watanakunakorn, 1988; Biavasco *et al.*, 1991). Strains of *Staph. epidermidis* and *Staph. haemolyticus* with similar degrees of resistance to teicoplanin have also been isolated from clinical specimens (Moore and Speller, 1988; Goldstein *et al.*, 1990; Bannerman *et al.*, 1991). Previous treatment with either vancomycin or teicoplanin often appears to select teicoplanin-resistance in these staphylococci (Maugein *et al.*, 1990). The resistance mechanism in teicoplanin-resistant coagulase-negative staphylococci appears similar to that of resistant *Staph. aureus* (O'Hare and Reynolds, 1992).

3 Streptococci

Groups A, B, C and G streptococci are nearly always sensitive to teicoplanin, the MICs (0.2 μg per ml) often being lower than those for vancomycin (0.8 μg per ml). Viridans streptococci and *Streptococcus bovis* are similarly sensitive (Fainstein *et al.*, 1983; Neu and Labthavikul, 1983; Greenwood, 1988). *Streptococcus pneumoniae*, including penicillin G-resistant strains (p. 5), are always teicoplanin-sensitive. The MICs of teicoplanin for this organism (0.06 μg per ml) are also usually lower than those for vancomycin (0.25 μg per ml) (Rodríguez-Tudela *et al.*, 1992; Goldstein *et al.*, 1994; Klugman, 1994; Lee *et al.*, 1995).

4 Enterococci

Enterococci such as *Enterococcus faecalis*, *E. faecium* and *E. durans* are usually teicoplanin-sensitive, and their MICs are lower for teicoplanin than those of vancomycin (Table I.56) (Fainstein *et al.*, 1983; Pérez *et al.*, 1987; Venditti *et al.*, 1993). *Enterococcus gallinarium* and *E. casseliflavus*, which normally show low-level Van C vancomycin-resistance (p. 765) are usually sensitive to teicoplanin (Leclercq *et al.*, 1992; Dutka-Malen *et al.*, 1994).

Enterococcal isolates, usually *E. faecium*, but occasionally *E. faecalis* or *E. durans*, which have acquired plasmid-mediated inducible and transferable Van A type vancomycin-resistance (p. 765), are also always teicoplanin-resistant. Such *E. faecium* strains, resistant to both drugs, have been detected in hospitals in which teicoplanin has never been used (Noskin *et al.*, 1995). Enterococci with Van B vancomycin-resistance (p. 765) are usually teicoplanin-sensitive (Dutka-Malen *et al.*, 1990; Fantin *et al.*, 1991; Arthur and Courvalin, 1993; Shlaes *et al.*, 1993a). However, in one patient from whom a vancomycin-resistant, but teicoplanin-sensitive (Van B type resistance) strain of *E. faecium* was isolated and who received vancomycin, but not teicoplanin, the *E. faecium* strain became teicoplanin-resistant *in vivo*. It appeared that in this patient the Van B gene mutated to teicoplanin-resistance and that a Van A gene was not acquired (Hayden *et al.*, 1993).

5 Gram-positive bacilli

Listeria monocytogenes and the *Corynebacterium* spp., including *C. jeikeium*, are teicoplanin-sensitive (Neu and Labthavikul, 1983; Greenwood, 1988). So is also *Rhodococcus equi* (Nordman and Ronco, 1992). *Nocardia asteroides* is resistant (Gutmann *et al.*, 1983). Of the anaerobes, the *Clostridia*, including *Cl. perfringens* and *Cl. difficile*, are sensitive as is *Propionibacterium acnes* (Neu and Labthavikul, 1983; Pallanza *et al.*, 1983; Greenwood, 1988). The *Pediococcus*, *Leuconostoc* and *Lactobacillus* spp. and Erysipelothrix rhusopathiae are usually teicoplanin-resistant (Phillips and Golledge, 1992).

6 Gram-negative bacteria

All of these are teicoplanin-resistant (Greenwood, 1988).

7 Minimum inhibitory concentrations

The MICs of some selected bacterial species of teicoplanin, compared with those of vancomycin are shown in Table I.56.

Organism	MICs (μg per ml)	
	Teicoplanin	Vancomycin
Staphylococcus aureus	3.12	3.12
Staphylococcus epidermidis	12.5	3.12
Streptococcus pyogenes	0.2	0.78
Streptococcus pneumoniae	0.2	0.78
Enterococcus faecalis	3.1	3.1
Listeria monocytogenes	0.8	1.6
Corynebacterium jeikeium	1.6	0.8
Clostridium perfringens	0.02–3.2	0.2–6.4

Table I.56
After Fainstein *et al.* (1983), Neu and Labthavikul (1983) and Greenwood (1988)

Mode of Administration and Dosage

1 Adults

Teicoplanin can be given i.m. or i.v. in the same dosage. The usual dosage is 6 mg per kg (usually 400 mg for adults) given once-daily. For i.v. administration this dose is usually dissolved in 100 ml of infusion fluid and administered as a 30-min infusion. For mild infections a dosage of 3 mg per kg (200 mg for adults) daily may be sufficient. For serious infections a dosage of 6 mg per kg is given 12-hourly for the first 2–5 days and thereafter this dosage is administered daily. Sometimes for treatment of serious infections the 6 mg per kg dose 12-hourly can be administered for longer periods. For the treatment of *Staph. aureus* endocarditis a loading regimen of three 12-hourly doses of 12 mg per kg followed by 12 mg per kg every 24 h is recommended (Harding and Garaud, 1988; Nováková *et al.*, 1990; Outman *et al.*, 1990; Phillips and Golledge, 1992; Smithers *et al.*, 1992; Wilson *et al.*, 1993). In patients with severe infections serum level monitoring may help to prescribe an appropriate dosage. Peak serum levels 1 h after an i.v. infusion should be 25–50 μg per ml and the trough levels just prior to next dose should not be less than 20 μg per ml (MacGowan *et al.*, 1992; Phillips and Golledge, 1992; Wilson *et al.*, 1993).

2 Children and neonates

Most commonly a dosage of 10 mg per kg i.v. once-daily is appropriate for children and 6 mg per kg per day for neonates (Lemerle *et al.*, 1988; Tarral *et al.*, 1988). For severe infections such as *Staph. aureus* endocarditis, higher dosages with serum level monitoring may be needed.

3 Patients with renal failure

Teicoplanin dosage should be reduced in these patients. Patients with moderate renal failure (creatinine clearance 10–80 ml per min) should be given approximately half the usual dosage, i.e. 6 mg per kg once every 48 h or 3 mg per kg once every 24 h. Those with severe renal failure (creatinine clearance < 10 ml per min) need approximately one-third of the usual dosage i.e. 6 mg per kg once every 72 h or 2 mg per kg once every 24 h. However, in critically ill patients with renal impairment there is a wide interpatient variations in serum levels of teicoplanin and these are often not predictable from the estimated creatinine clearance. Therefore serum level monitoring is essential (Domart *et al.*, 1987; Falcoz *et al.*, 1987; Bonati *et al.*, 1988).

Hemodialysis does not increase body clearance of teicoplanin, so patients treated this way do not need extra doses (Bonati *et al.*, 1988). Very little teicoplanin is also eliminated by peritoneal dialysis. However, after intraperitoneal administration more than 50% of the drug is absorbed. Peritonitis due to Gram-positive bacteria in patients on peritoneal dialysis may be successfully treated by intraperitoneal teicoplanin. The drug in a dose of 40–50 mg can be added to each 2 liter bag of dialysate for first week of treatment and only to each second bag during the second week. With this regimen serum teicoplanin concentrations reached were less than 10 μg per ml (Bowley *et al.*, 1988; Neville *et al.*, 1988; Guay *et al.*, 1989).

4 Intravenous drug abusers

These often need higher teicoplanin dosage as the renal clearance of the drug is increased, but there is a wide variation between individuals and so the dosage has to be adjusted in each individual and serum levels should be monitored (Rybak *et al.*, 1991).

Serum Levels in Relation to Dosage

Verbist *et al.* (1984) reported the results of single-dose teicoplanin pharmacokinetic studies carried out on six volunteers. Doses of 3 and 6 mg per kg body weight dissolved in saline were given i.v. over a period of 5 min, or a dose of 3 mg per kg was given by i.m. injection. Immediately after i.v. injection, the mean peak values after the 3 and 6 mg per kg doses were 53.48 and 111.81 μg per ml, respectively; these levels fell rapidly in the first 8 h but at 24 h they still exceeded 2 and 4 μg per ml, respectively. After the i.m. injection of 3 mg per kg, a mean peak serum level of 7.12 μg per ml was reached in 2 h and thereafter serum levels followed those attained after an identical i.v. dose, being greater than 2 μg per ml at 24 h. The elimination half-life of the drug was about 47 h. Similar results were obtained by Buniva *et al.* (1988), who gave 400 mg of teicoplanin i.v. over 60 s to volunteers. Plasma concentrations averaged 71.7 μg per ml at 5 min after administration, decreasing to 4.0 μg per ml at 24 h. Other data summarized by

Williams and Grüneberg (1984) showed that after a 200-mg i.m. dose the mean peak serum level in eight volunteers was 7 μg per ml after 4 h; when this dose was repeated every 12 h, this peak rose to 12 μg per ml after the sixth dose. When the drug was continued in a dose of 200 mg daily, trough serum levels were 5.4–7.3 μg per ml from day 2 to day 6.

Del Favero *et al.* (1991) administered single doses of 15, 20 and 25 mg of teicoplanin per kg of body weight to adult volunteers by a 30-min i.v. infusion. Peak levels at the end of the infusion averaged 194, 197 and 253 μg per ml, respectively. Mean concentrations in plasma 24 h after administration were 10.5, 13.6 and 19.8 μg per ml, respectively. Terminal half-lives averaged 88, 83 and 92 h. If multiple doses of teicoplanin are given, both peak and trough serum levels increase, and with a 3 mg per kg daily-dose steady-state serum levels are attained in about 10 days (Carver *et al.*, 1989). In another study a 6 mg per kg dose of teicoplanin was infused i.v. over 30 min to volunteers every 12 h for 5 days and then every 24 h for 9 days. The serum levels after the fourth or fifth dose given 12-hourly at 0.5, 1, and 12 h after the start of the infusion were 72.8, 48.4 and 18.1 μg per ml, respectively. These levels were very similar to those obtained on day 24, i.e. after the last of nine doses given once every 24 h. Therefore it was suggested that for clinical dosing regimens, dosing every 12 h for approximately 48 h should be used, followed by once-daily dosing thereafter (Outman *et al.*, 1990). The steady-state concentrations in the serum increase in proportion to the dose (Smithers *et al.*, 1992). The half-life of teicoplanin in the serum increases after multiple-dose administration (Carver *et al.*, 1989).

Excretion

1 Urine

Most of the parenterally administered dose of teicoplanin is excreted in the urine as the active unchanged drug in 16 days. This accounts for about 83% of the dose given. The renal clearance of the drug is lower than the creatinine clearance, which suggests that there is some tubular reabsorption. After a 400-mg i.v. dose to adults, the urine concentrations of teicoplanin exceed the MICs for susceptible pathogens for at least 24 h (Buniva *et al.*, 1988). In intravenous drug abusers the renal (and non-renal) clearance of teicoplanin is increased (Rybak *et al.*, 1991). In animals both morphine and phenobarbital administration increase renal elimination and hepatic metabolism of the drug (Fan-Havard *et al.*, 1993).

2 Feces

Some 2.7% of i.v. administered dose of active teicoplanin can be recovered from the feces (Buniva *et al.*, 1988). This apparently is excreted into the bowel via the bile.

3 Inactivation in body

Administered teicoplanin, not excreted in urine or feces, appears to be metabolized in the liver. Two metabolites which arise due to hydroxylation of teicoplanin, have been identified. They have some, but reduced activity against Gram-positive bacteria (Bernareggi *et al.*, 1992).

Distribution of the Drug in Body

Teicoplanin is highly (more than 90%) bound to serum proteins. In an *in vitro* study it appeared that this high degree of serum protein binding impaired the bactericidal activity of the drug, compared with that of vancomycin (Bailey *et al.*, 1991), but Dykhuisen *et al.* (1995) reported that *in vivo* in volunteers the serum bactericidal activity of teicoplanin was not impaired by its high degree of protein binding. In another *in vitro* study coagulase-negative staphylococci, multiplying within a clot of human plasma, were shown to be partly protected from inhibition and killing by both vancomycin and teicoplanin. This effect, however, was more pronounced for the highly protein bound teicoplanin (Cunningham and Cheesbrough, 1992).

Teicoplanin penetrates poorly into the CSF, even in patients with bacterial meningitis (Stahl *et al.*, 1987). In patients undergoing cardiac surgery, chemoprophylaxis with teicoplanin 400 mg i.v., at time of induction of anesthesia plus 200 mg 24 h later, was not as effective as flucloxacillin plus tobramycin in preventing sternal wound infections. A teicoplanin regimen 400 mg i.v. at induction of anesthesia, 400 mg at end of cardiopulmonary bypass and 400 mg 24 h after the first dose was no more effective. With both regimens low levels of teicoplanin were found in fat (Wilson *et al.*, 1988a,b). In another study an initial higher i.v. dose of 12 mg per kg body weight was given at the time of induction of anesthesia and a second dose of 400 mg i.v. 24 h later for patients undergoing cardiac surgery. The mean concentrations in serum and tissues were more satisfactory; at the end of cardiopulmonary bypass they were 15 μg per ml in serum, 6 μg per g in fat and 9 μg per g in skin (Wilson *et al.*, 1989). Teicoplanin also readily penetrated into heart tissue (Bergeron *et al.*, 1990).

Teicoplanin is concentrated in phagocytes where it appears to aid the killing of ingested organisms such as *Staph. aureus* (Carlone *et al.*, 1989).

Mode of Action

The mode of action of teicoplanin on bacterial cell walls is similar to that of vancomycin (p. 773), but the additional actions of altering the permeability of the cytoplasmic membrane and impairing RNA synthesis, which occur with vancomycin, have not been described with teicoplanin (Bailey *et al.*, 1991; Dykhuizen *et al.*, 1995).

Toxicity

1 Hypersensitivity and related side-effects

The 'red-man syndrome', which typically occurs with rapid vancomycin i.v. infusions and which results from vancomycin-induced histamine release (p. 774), has occasionally occurred with teicoplanin (Phillips and Golledge, 1992), but most authors have reported that this syndrome does not occur with teicoplanin, even when it was given by rapid i.v. infusions, where the dose was infused over 5 or 30 min. Intramuscular teicoplanin administration also does not cause this syndrome (Verbist *et al.*, 1984; Stille *et al.*, 1988; Smith *et al.*, 1989a; Sahai *et al.*, 1990; Davey and Williams, 1991b). More severe anaphylactoid reactions with rash and hypotension also appear to be much rarer with teicoplanin compared with vancomycin (Smith *et al.*, 1989a; Polk, 1991). Patients who have experienced the 'red-man syndrome' due to vancomycin, usually tolerate teicoplanin with no reactions (Smith *et al.*, 1989b; Polk, 1991).

Milder allergic rashes such as urticaria, may occur with teicoplanin therapy. Bronchospasm has also been occasionally noted (Bibler *et al.*, 1987; Stille *et al.*, 1988; Davey and Williams, 1991b; Rolston *et al.*, 1994). Such reactions are more common with vancomycin (p. 774). Most patients, who had developed allergic rashes due to vancomycin, tolerated teicoplanin subsequently with no reactions (Van Laethem *et al.*, 1984; Schlemmer *et al.*, 1988; Smith *et al.*, 1989b; Wood and Whitby, 1989). However, Grek *et al.* (1991) described a patient who had had a previous allergic rash due to vancomycin, and who developed an immediate rash and severe bronchospasm when teicoplanin was given i.v. at a later date. Conversely de Vries *et al.* (1994) reported a 4-year-old child who had a documented teicoplanin allergy and who subsequently tolerated vancomycin with no reaction.

2 Drug fever

This has occurred during teicoplanin therapy and it has necessitated cessation of treatment in some patients (Greenberg, 1990; Venditti *et al.*, 1992).

3 Local reactions

Phlebitis with i.v. administration and pain at the local site with i.m. therapy do occur with teicoplanin, but these usually are not severe (Davey and Williams, 1991b).

4 Nephrotoxicity

In animals teicoplanin, similar to vancomycin, causes a dose-related nephrotoxicity (Marre *et al.*, 1987). In humans nephrotoxicity appears to be less common with teicoplanin than with vancomycin and this also applies when either of the two drugs are administered together with an aminoglycoside (Smith *et al.*, 1989a; Davey and Williams, 1991b; Van der Auwera *et al.*, 1991). In one clinical trial co-administration of vancomycin plus cyclosporin A was more nephrotoxic than teicoplanin plus cyclosporin A, but among patients receiving vancomycin plus amphotericin B and those treated by teicoplanin plus amphotericin B, deterioration in renal function was equal in both groups (Kureishi *et al.*, 1991).

5 Ototoxicity

Brummett *et al.* (1987) evaluated the potential of teicoplanin for ototoxicity in guinea pigs. No ototoxicity was detected either with teicoplanin alone or when this drug was combined with ethacrynic acid, a diuretic which augments the ototoxicity of many drugs. A few patients receiving high-dose (15 mg per kg per day) teicoplanin therapy developed tinnitus or a mild loss of high-frequency hearing detected by audiograms. The peak teicoplanin serum levels in these patients were 85 μg per ml and trough levels 41 μg per ml (Greenberg, 1990). In general ototoxicity with teicoplanin appears to be rare. Of 3377 patients treated by the drug, 11 developed some degree of ototoxicity but other factors, rather than teicoplanin, might have caused this side-effect in some of these patients (Davey and Williams, 1991b).

6 Hematological side-effects

Leukopenia has occurred during teicoplanin therapy. This appears to be rare and is reversible on cessation of the drug (Del Favero et al., 1989). In one patient who was treated by teicoplanin and rifampicin for severe MRSA infection, a circulating inhibitor of factor VIII appeared, which resulted in bleeding; the role of teicoplanin in production of this complication was uncertain (Legrand et al., 1987). Platelet function and blood coagulation have not been affected by therapeutic serum concentrations of teicoplanin (Agnelli et al., 1987).

7 Other side-effects

Reversible elevations of liver transaminases and bilirubin have occurred in a small number of patients receiving teicoplanin (Smith et al., 1989a; Davey and Williams, 1991b; Kelsey et al., 1992). Mild tremor has also been rarely noted during teicoplanin therapy.

Clinical Uses of the Drug

1 General uses

In general, teicoplanin may be used for indications similar to those for vancomycin (p. 777). Advantages for teicoplanin are the convenient once-daily administration, shorter infusion time i.v., feasibility of i.m. dosing and fewer side-effects. However, it appears that resistant organisms may be more likely to emerge during therapy with this drug, than with vancomycin (p. 791). Teicoplanin currently is also more expensive (Graninger et al., 1995; Kayser, 1995). In most countries, therefore teicoplanin is reserved for infections in patients who do not tolerate vancomycin (Phillips and Golledge, 1992). However, teicoplanin may well be more cost-effective for home antibiotic therapy because of the possibility of rapid i.v. or i.m. administration once-daily (Schaison, 1993; Wilson and Grüneberg, 1994).

2 Methicillin-resistant Staph. aureus infections

Teicoplanin (or vancomycin) are only indicated for MRSA infections or sometimes for methicillin-sensitive Staph. aureus (MSSA) infections, if the patient is allergic to beta-lactam antibiotics. However, in clinical trials the drug has been used for both MRSA and MSSA infections.

In rabbits with induced endocarditis, teicoplanin treatment was comparable with that of nafcillin for infections due to strains of MSSA, and with that of vancomycin for infections due to strains of MRSA (Chambers and Sande, 1984). In another animal study it appeared that high trough teicoplanin concentrations resulted in a better cure of Staph. aureus endocarditis (Chambers and Kennedy, 1990). In a rat model of foreign body MRSA infection, vancomycin was more effective in eradicating the infection than teicoplanin, but a combination of high-dose teicoplanin and rifampicin was also effective (Schaad et al., 1994).

Some studies have suggested that teicoplanin in a dosage of 6 mg per kg 12-hourly for three doses, and then 6 mg per kg body weight once every 24 h may be effective for serious MRSA or MSSA infections (Bibler et al., 1987; de Lalla et al., 1989; Davey and Williams, 1991a; Rolston et al., 1994). However, in one early trial low-dose teicoplanin (400-mg i.v. loading dose followed by 200 mg i.v. daily) was considerably less effective than flucloxacillin for the treatment of MSSA infections (Calain et al., 1987). Also in a trial by Gilbert et al. (1991) when teicoplanin was given in a dosage of 6 mg per kg 12-hourly for three doses, followed by 6 mg per kg every 24 h, to treat Staph. aureus intravascular infections, there was an unexpectedly high number of treatment failures. It is now accepted that for severe Staph. aureus infections, such as septicemia and/or septic arthritis a teicoplanin dosage of 12 mg per kg body weight per day may be needed. For treatment of MRSA endocarditis, the trough teicoplanin serum levels should exceed 20 µg per ml and this is usually achieved by three 12-hourly doses of 12 mg per kg, followed by 12 mg per kg once every 24 h (p. 793) (Martino et al., 1989; Wilson et al., 1993; Graninger et al., 1995). For Staph. aureus endocarditis in i.v. drug abusers higher dosages, determined by serum level monitoring are usually necessary (Ryback et al., 1991; Fortún et al., 1995).

3 Coagulase-negative staphylococcal infections

Similar to vancomycin (p. 778), teicoplanin is effective for these infections. Animal studies showed that it was effective in induced *Staph. epidermidis* endocarditis (Tuazon and Washburn, 1987) and in neutropenic mice infected with *Staph. haemolyticus* (Torney *et al.*, 1991). In humans a relatively small number of patients with *Staph. epidermidis* endocarditis (Presterl *et al.*, 1993), right-sided catheter related *Staph. epidermidis* endocarditis in bone marrow transplant recipients (Martino *et al.*, 1990) and *Staph. epidermidis* bacteremia in patients with cancer (Rolston *et al.*, 1994) have responded to teicoplanin 6–8 mg per kg body weight per day. It is possible that for patients with endocarditis higher doses, similar to those now recommended for this disease caused by *Staph. aureus*, may be needed. Cruciani *et al.* (1992) used a combination of i.v. and intraventricular teicoplanin to treat *Staph. epidermidis* and *Staph. aureus* neurosurgical shunt infections. Two infants received 5 mg of teicoplanin daily, three adults 20 mg daily and another two adults 20 mg every other day intraventricularly. The mean duration of intraventricular therapy was 16 days. All patients were cured and the alternate days schedule of intraventricular administration of teicoplanin was as effective as the once-daily regimen. Peritonitis in peritoneal dialysis patients caused by coagulase-negative staphylococci can also be successfully treated by intraperitoneal teicoplanin (p. 778).

4 Streptococcal and enterococcal infections

Teicoplanin 500 mg every 12 h for the first 2 days and 10 mg per kg body weight every 24 h thereafter for a total of 4 weeks can be considered for the home treatment of *Strep. viridans* or *Strep. bovis* endocarditis. Otherwise penicillin G remains the drug of choice, provided that the strain is sensitive to it (Venditti *et al.*, 1992).

Enterococcal infections, such as those of the urinary tract, septicemia and even endocarditis can be successfully treated with teicoplanin monotherapy (Leport *et al.*, 1989; Martino *et al.*, 1989; Felmingham *et al.*, 1992; Schmit, 1992). An animal study also showed teicoplanin to be more effective than vancomycin for monotherapy in enterococcal endocarditis due to strains with high-level resistance to gentamicin (Eliopoulos *et al.*, 1992), but all this only applies if the enterococcal strain is teicoplanin-sensitive. For patients with endocarditis the addition of an aminoglycoside such as gentamicin or netilmicin may be beneficial, unless the strain shows high-level resistance to all aminoglycosides (Martino *et al.*, 1989). One child who developed *E. faecium* meningitis after neurosurgery, recovered after 14 days of intrathecal teicoplanin (10 mg daily) and i.v. clindamycin, rifampicin and ampicillin. The enterococcal strain was only moderately sensitive to teicoplanin (MIC 4 μg per ml), but resistant to many other antibiotics including ampicillin and vancomycin (Losonsky *et al.*, 1994).

If the *E. faecium* strain is resistant to both vancomycin and teicoplanin, teicoplanin is unlikely to be effective clinically, even when combined with other drugs (Caron *et al.*, 1992). However, *E. faecium* infections caused by teicoplanin-sensitive, but vancomycin-resistant strains are likely to respond to teicoplanin. In one *in vitro* study it was noted that teicoplanin alone (8 μg per ml) was usually bactericidal to such strains at 24 h, but only if these strains lacked high-level gentamicin-resistance. If the latter was present, teicoplanin was inhibitory, but not bactericidal (Hayden *et al.*, 1994).

5 Corynebacterium spp. infections

Similar to vancomycin (p. 779), teicoplanin is likely to be effective in these infections, including those caused by *C. jeikeium* (Martino *et al.*, 1989).

6 Fever in neutropenic patients

If in any unit Gram-positive organism infections are frequent in these patients, then similar to vancomycin (p. 780), teicoplanin can be included in the initial treatment regimen and combinations such as teicoplanin/amikacin/ceftazidime or teicoplanin/ciprofloxacin can be used with success (Del Favero *et al.*, 1987; Kelsey *et al.*, 1992; Kureishi *et al.*, 1991; Menichetti *et al.*, 1994). Once the presence of a Gram-positive infection is confirmed teicoplanin can be continued as monotherapy (Van der Auwera *et al.*, 1991).

7 Antibiotic-associated colitis

Teicoplanin orally in a dosage of 100 mg twice-daily for 10 days appeared to be equally effective to oral vancomycin (p. 779) for the treatment of this disease (de Lalla *et al.*, 1989; de Lalla *et al.*, 1992), but in another trial where a similar dosage (either 50 mg 4 times daily or 100 mg twice-daily) was administered for 7 days only, clinical recurrences were frequent (The Swedish CDAD Study Group, 1994). The formulations of teicoplanin differed in these studies. In the first two trials a parenteral formulation was used, but in the third an oral formulation capsule was employed.

8 Chemoprophylaxis

In the UK and Europe teicoplanin 400 mg i.v. plus gentamicin 120 mg i.v. is now advocated as endocarditis chemoprophylaxis in patients with prosthetic valves undergoing endoscopy, colonoscopy, proctoscopy, sigmoidoscopy or barium enema (p. 44). This dose of teicoplanin alone, instead of erythromycin (p. 617) or clindamycin (p. 44) can also be considered for prophylaxis of endocarditis after dental procedures in penicillin-allergic patients (Shanson et al., 1987; Gould, 1990). Single-dose i.v. teicoplanin, given just before insertion of Hickman catheters also reduced the incidence of Gram-positive organism sepsis in patients with hematological malignancies, especially during the period of neutropenia following cancer chemotherapy (Lim et al., 1991). Teicoplanin in a dose of 800 mg i.v. has also been given 2.5 h before surgery to patients undergoing knee replacement. Regional chemoprophylaxis in such patients has also been tried: 400 mg of teicoplanin in 100 ml of saline was given in a foot vein and an above-knee tourniquet was inflated to 400 mmHg. This regional prophylaxis resulted in higher teicoplanin concentrations in bone, skin, synovia and subcutaneous tissue than was achieved with the 800 mg i.v. dose (de Lalla et al., 1993). The drug may also be suitable for chemoprophylaxis in patients undergoing cardiac surgery (p. 782).

References

Agnelli G, Longetti M, Guerciolini R et al. (1987). Effects of the new glycopeptide antibiotic teicoplanin on platelet function and blood coagulations. Antimicrob Ag Chemother 31: 1609.

Arthur M, Courvalin P (1993). Genetics and mechanisms of glycopeptide resistance in enterococci. Antimicrob Ag Chemother 37: 1563.

Bailey EM, Ryback MJ, Kaatz GW (1991). Comparative effect of protein binding on the killing activities of teicoplanin and vancomycin. Antimicrob Ag Chemother 35: 1089.

Bannerman TL, Wadiak DL, Kloos WE (1991). Susceptibility of Staphylococcus species and subspecies to teicoplanin. Antimicrob Ag Chemother 35: 1919.

Bardone MR, Paternoster M, Coronelli C (1978). Teichomycins, new antibiotics from Actinoplanes teichomyceticus nov. sp. II Extraction and chemical characterization. J Antibiotics 31: 170.

Bergeron MG, Saginur R, Desaulniers D et al. (1990). Concentrations of teicoplanin in serum and atrial appendages of patients undergoing cardiac surgery. Antimicrob Ag Chemother 34: 1699.

Bernareggi A, Borghi A, Borgonovi M et al. (1992). Teicoplanin metabolism in humans. Antimicrob Ag Chemother 36: 1744.

Biavasco F, Giovanetti E, Montanari MP et al. (1991). Development of in-vitro resistance to glycopeptide antibiotics: assessment in staphylococci of different species. J Antimicrob Chemother 27: 71.

Bibler MR, Frame PT, Hagler DN et al. (1987). Clinical evaluation of efficacy, pharmacokinetics and safety of teicoplanin for serious Gram-positive infections. Antimicrob Ag Chemother 31: 207.

Bonati M, Traina GL, Rosina R, Buniva G (1988). Pharmacokinetics of single intravenous dose of teicoplanin in subjects with various degrees of renal impairment. J Antimicrob Chemother 21 (Suppl A): 29.

Bowley JA, Pickering SJ, Scantlebury AJ et al. (1988). Intraperitoneal teicoplanin in the treatment of peritonitis associated with continuous ambulatory peritoneal dialysis. J Antimicrob Chemother 21 (Suppl A): 133.

Brummett RE, Fox KE, Warchol M, Himes D (1987). Absence of ototoxicity of teichomycin A2 in guinea pigs. Antimicrob Ag Chemother 31: 612.

Buniva G, Del Favero A, Bernareggi A et al. (1988). Pharmacokinetics of ^{14}C-teicoplanin in healthy volunteers. J Antimicrob Chemother 21 (Suppl A): 23.

Calain P, Krause K-H, Vaudaux P et al. (1987). Early termination of a prospective, randomized trial comparing teicoplanin and flucloxacillin for treating severe staphylococcal infections. J Infect Dis 155: 187.

Carlone NA, Cuffini AM, Ferrero M et al. (1989). Cellular uptake and intracellular bactericidal activity of teicoplanin in human macrophages. J Antimicrob Chemother 23: 849.

Caron F, Kitzis M-D, Gutmann L et al. (1992). Daptomycin or teicoplanin in combination with gentamicin for treatment of experimental endocarditis due to a highly glycopeptide-resistant isolate of Enterococcus faecium. Antimicrob Ag Chemother 36: 2611.

Carper HT, Sullivan GW, Mandell GL (1987). Teicoplanin, vancomycin, rifampin: in-vivo and in-vitro studies with Staphylococcus aureus. J Antimicrob Chemother 19: 659.

Carver PL, Nightingale CH, Quintiliani R et al. (1989). Pharmacokinetics of single- and multiple-dose teicoplanin in healthy volunteers. Antimicrob Ag Chemother 33: 82.

Chambers HF, Kennedy S (1990). Effects of dosage, peak and trough concentrations in serum, protein binding and bactericidal rate on efficacy of teicoplanin in a rabbit model on endocarditis. Antimicrob Ag Chemother 34: 510.

Chambers HF, Sande MA (1984). Teicoplanin versus nafcillin and vancomycin in the treatment of experimental endocarditis caused by methicillin-susceptible or -resistant Staphylococcus aureus. Antimicrob Ag Chemother 26: 61.

Cruciani M, Navarra A, Di Perri G et al. (1992). Evaluation of intraventricular teicoplanin for the treatment of neurosurgical shunt infections. Clin Infect Dis 15: 285.

Cunningham R, Cheesbrough J (1992). Comparative activity of glycopeptide antibiotics against coagulase-negative staphylococci embedded in fibrin clots. J Antimicrob Chemother 30: 321.

Daum RS, Gupta S, Sabbagh R, Milewski WM (1992). Characterization of Staphylococcus aureus isolates with decreased susceptibility to vancomycin and teicoplanin: isolation and purification of a constitutively produced protein associated with decreased susceptibility. J Infect Dis 166: 1066.

Davey PG, Williams AH (1991a). Teicoplanin monotherapy of serious infections caused by Gram-positive bacteria: a re-evaluation of patients with endocarditis or Staphylococcus aureus bacteraemia from a European open trial. J Antimicrob Chemother 27 (Suppl B): 43.

Davey PG, Williams AH (1991b). A review of safety profile of teicoplanin. J Antimicrob Chemother 27 (Suppl B): 69.

de Lalla F, Privitera G, Rinaldi E et al.(1989). Treatment of Clostridium difficile-associated disease with teicoplanin. Antimicrob Ag Chemother 33: 1125.

de Lalla F, Nicolin R, Rinaldi E et al. (1992). Prospective study of oral teicoplanin versus oral vancomycin for therapy of pseudomembranous colitis and Clostridium difficile-associated diarrhea. Antimicrob Ag Chemother 36: 2192.

de Lalla F, Novelli A, Pellizzer G et al. (1993). Regional and systemic prophylaxis with teicoplanin in monolateral and bilateral total knee replacement procedures: study of pharmacokinetics and tissue penetration. *Antimicrob Ag Chemother* 37: 2693.

Del Favero A, Manichetti F, Guerciolini R et al. (1987). Prospective randomized clinical trial of teicoplanin for empiric combined antibiotic therapy in febrile, granulocytopenic acute leukemia patients. *Antimicrob Ag Chemother* 31: 1126.

Del Favero A, Patoia L, Bucaneva G et al. (1989). Leukopenia with neutropenia associated with teicoplanin therapy. *DICP Ann Pharmacoth* 23: 45.

Del Favero A, Patoia L, Rosina R et al. (1991). Pharmacokinetics and tolerability of teicoplanin in healthy volunteers after single increasing doses. *Antimicrob Ag Chemother* 35: 2551.

de Vries E, van Weel-Sipman MH, Vossen JM (1994). A four-year-old child with teicoplanin allergy but no evidence of cross-reaction with vancomycin. *Pediatr Infect Dis J* 13: 167.

Domart Y, Pierre C, Clair B et al. (1987). Pharmacokinetics of teicoplanin in critically ill patients with various degrees of renal impairment. *Antimicrob Ag Chemother* 31: 1600.

Dutka-Malen S, Leclercq R, Coutant V et al. (1990). Phenotypic and genotypic heterogeneity of glycopeptide resistance determinants in Gram-positive bacteria. *Antimicrob Ag Chemother* 34: 1875.

Dutka-Malen S, Blaimont B, Wauters G, Courvalin P (1994). Emergence of high-level resistance to glycopeptides in *Enterococcus gallinarum* and *Enterococcus casseliflavus*. *Antimicrob Ag Chemother* 38: 1675.

Dykhuizen RS, Harvey G, Stephenson N et al. (1995). Protein binding and serum bactericidal activities of vancomycin and teicoplanin. *Antimicrob Ag Chemother* 39: 1842.

Eliopoulos GM, Thauvin-Eliopoulos C, Moellering RC Jr (1992). Contribution of animal models in the search for efective therapy for endocarditis due to enterococci with high-level resistance to gentamicin. *Clin Infect Dis* 15: 58.

Fainstein V, Le Blanc B, Bodey GP (1983). Comparative *in vitro* study of teichomycin A$_2$. *Antimicrob Ag Chemother* 23: 497.

Falcoz C, Ferry N, Pozet N et al (1987). Pharmacokinetics of teicoplanin in renal failure. *Antimicrob Ag Chemother* 31: 1255.

Fan-Havard P, Koshy Z, Bais RM et al. (1993). Effect of morphine or phenobarbital on teicoplanin elimination pharmacokinetics. *J Antimicrob Chemother* 32: 101.

Fantin B, Leclercq R, Arthur M et al. (1991). Influence of low-level resistance to vancomycin on efficacy of teicoplanin and vancomycin for treatment of experimental endocarditis due to *Enterococcus faecium*. *Antimicrob Ag Chemother* 35: 1570.

Felmingham D (1993). Towards the ideal glycopeptide. *J Antimicrob Chemother* 32: 663.

Felmingham D, Wilson APR, Quintana AI, Grüneberg RN (1992). Enterococcus species in urinary tract infection. *Clin Infect Dis* 15: 295.

Fortún J, Pérez-Molina JA, Añoñ MT et al. (1995). Right-sided endocarditis caused by *Staphylococcus aureus* in drug abusers. *Antimicrob Ag Chemother* 39: 525.

Gilbert DN, Wood CA, Kimbrough RC and The Infectious Diseases Consortium of Oregon. (1991). Failure of treatment with teicoplanin at 6 milligrams/kilogram/day in patients with *Staphylococcus aureus* intravascular infection. *Antimicrob Ag Chemother* 35: 79.

Goldstein FW, Coutrot A, Sieffer A, Acar JF (1990). Percentages and distributions of teicoplanin- and vancomycin- resistant strains among coagulase-negative staphylococci. *Antimicrob Ag Chemother* 34: 899.

Goldstein FW, Geslin P, Acar JF et al. (1994). Comparative activity of teicoplanin and vancomycin against 400 penicillin susceptible and resistant *Streptococcus pneumoniae*. *Eur J Clin Microbiol Infect Dis* 13: 33.

Gorzynski EA, Amsterdam D, Beam TR Jr, Rotstein C (1989). Comparative *in vitro* activities of teicoplanin, vancomycin, oxacillin and other antimicrobial agents against bacteremic isolates of Gram-positive cocci. *Antimicrob Ag Chemother* 33: 2019.

Gould IM (1990). Teicoplanin for prophylaxis of endocarditis after dental bacteraemia. *J Antimicrob Chemother* 25: 501.

Graninger W, Wenisch C, Hasenhündl M (1995). Treatment of staphylococcal infections *Curr Opin Infect Dis* 8 (Suppl 1): 20.

Greenberg RN (1990). Treatment of bone, joint, and vascular-access-associated Gram-positive bacterial infections with teicoplanin. *Antimicrob Ag Chemother* 34: 2392.

Greenwood D (1988). Microbiological properties of teicoplanin. *J Antimicrob Chemother* 21 (Suppl A): 1.

Grek V, Andrien F, Collignon J, Fillet G (1991). Allergic cross-reaction of teicoplanin and vancomycin. *J Antimicrob Chemother* 28: 476.

Guay DRP, Awni WM, Halstenson CE et al. (1989). Teicoplanin pharmacokinetics in patients undergoing continuous ambulatory peritoneal dialysis after intravenous and intraperitoneal dosing. *Antimicrob Ag Chemother* 33: 2012.

Gutmann L, Goldstein FW, Kitzis MD et al. (1983). Susceptibility of *Nocardia asteroides* to 46 antibiotics, including 22 beta-lactams. *Antimicrob Ag Chemother* 23: 248.

Harding I, Garaud J-J (1988). Teicoplanin in the treatment of infections caused by coagulase-negative staphylococci. *J Antimicrob Chemother* 21 (Suppl A): 93.

Hayden MK, Trenholme GM, Schultz JE, Sahm DF (1993). *In vivo* development of teicoplanin resistance in a Van B *Enterococcus faecium* isolate. *J Infect Dis* 167: 1224.

Hayden MK, Koenig GI, Trenholme GM (1994). Bactericidal activities of antibiotics against vancomycin-resistant *Enterococcus faecium* blood isolates and synergistic activities of combinations. *Antimicrob Ag Chemother* 38: 1225.

Kaatz GW, Seo SM, Dorman NJ, Lerner SA (1990). Emergence of teicoplanin resistance during therapy of *Staphylococcus aureus* endocarditis. *J Infect Dis* 162: 103.

Kayser FH (1995). Methicillin and glycopeptide resistance in staphylococci: a new threat? *Curr Opin Infect Dis* 8 (Suppl 1): 7.

Kelsey SM, Weinhardt B, Collins PW, Newland AC (1992). Teicoplanin plus ciprofloxacin versus gentamicin plus piperacillin in the treatment of febrile neutropenic patients. *Eur J Clin Microbiol Infect Dis* 11: 509.

Klugman KP (1994). Activity of teicoplanin and vancomycin against penicillin-resistant pneumococci. *Eur J Clin Microbiol Infect Dis* 13: 1.

Kureishi A, Jewesson PJ, Rubinger M et al. (1991). Double-blind comparison of teicoplanin versus vancomycin in febrile neutropenic patients receiving concomitant tobramycin and piperacillin: effect on cyclosporin A-associated nephrotoxicity. *Antimicrob Ag Chemother* 35: 2246.

Leclercq R, Dutka-Malen S, Duval J, Courvalin P (1992). Vancomycin resistance gene Van C is specific to *Enterococcus gallinarium*. *Antimicrob Ag Chemother* 36: 2005.

Lee H-J, Park J-Y, Jang S-H et al. (1995). High incidence of resistance to multiple antimicrobials in clinical isolates of *Streptococcus pneumoniae* from a University Hospital in Korea. *Clin Infect Dis* 20: 826.

Legrand JC, Van der Auwera P, Bailly A et al. (1987). Circulating inhibitor of factor VIII during teatment with teicoplanin and rifampicin. *J Antimicrob Chemother* 19: 850.

Lemerle S, de La Rocque F, Lamy R et al. (1988). Teicoplanin in combination therapy for febrile episodes in neutropenic and non-neutropenic paediatric patients. *J Antimicrob Chemother* 21 (Suppl A): 113.

Leport C, Perronne C, Massip P et al. (1989). Evaluation of teicoplanin for treatment of endocarditis caused by Gram-positive cocci in 20 patients. *Antimicrob Ag Chemother* 33: 871.

Lim SH, Smith MP, Salooja N et al. (1991). A prospective randomized study of prophylactic teicoplanin to prevent early Hickman catheter-related sepsis in patients receiving intensive chemotherapy for haematological malignancies. *J Antimicrob Chemother* 28: 109.

Losonsky GA, Wolf A, Schwalbe RS et al. (1994). Successful treatment of meningitis due to multiply resistant *Enterococcus faecium* with a combination of intrathecal teicoplanin and intravenous antimicrobial agents. *Clin Infect Dis* 19: 163.

MacGowan AP, McMullin CM, White LO et al. (1992). Serum monitoring of teicoplanin. *J Antimicrob Chemother* 30: 399.

Mainardi J-L, Shlaes DM, Goering RV et al. (1995). Decreased teicoplanin susceptibility of methicillin-resistant strains of Staphylococcus aureus. J Infect Dis 171: 1646.

Manquat G, Croize J, Stahl JP et al. (1992). Failure of teicoplanin treatment associated with an increase in MIC during therapy of Staphylococcus aureus septicaemia. J Antimicrob Chemother 29: 731.

Marre R, Schulz E, Graefe H, Sack K (1987). Teicoplanin: renal tolerance and pharmacokinetics in rats. J Antimicrob Chemother 20: 697.

Martino P, Venditti M, Micozzi A et al. (1989). Teicoplanin in the treatment of Gram-positive-bacterial endocarditis. Antimicrob Ag Chemother 33: 1329.

Martino P, Micozzi A, Venditti M et al. (1990). Catheter-related right-sided endocarditis in bone marrow transplant recipients. Rev Infect Dis 12: 250.

Maugein J, Pellegrin JL, Brossard G et al. (1990). In vitro activities of vancomycin and teicoplanin against coagulase-negative staphylococci isolated from neutropenic patients. Antimicrob Ag Chemother 34: 901.

Menichetti F, Martino P, Bucaneve G et al. (1994). Effects of teicoplanin and those of vancomycin in initial empirical antibiotic regimen for febrile, neutropenic patients with hematologic malignancies. Antimicrob Ag Chemother 38: 2041.

Moore EP, Speller DCE (1988). In-vitro teicoplanin-resistance in coagulase-negative staphyloccci from patients with endocarditis and from a cardiac surgery unit. J Antimicrob Chemother 21: 417.

Neu HC, Labthavikul P (1983). In vitro activity of teichomycin compared with those of other antibiotics. Antimicrob Ag Chemother 24: 425.

Neville LO, Baillod RA, Brumfitt W, Hamilton-Miller JMT (1988). Efficacy and safety of teicoplanin in Gram-positive peritonitis in patients on peritoneal dialysis. J Antimicrob Chemother 21 (Suppl A): 123.

Nordmann P, Ranco E (1992). In-vitro antimicrobial susceptibility of Rhodococcus equi. J Antimicrob Chemother 29: 383.

Noskin GA, Peterson LR, Warren JR (1995). Enterococcus faecium and Enterococcus faecalis bacteremia: acquisition and outcome. Clin Infect Dis 20: 296.

Nováková IRO, Donnelly JP, Verhagen CS, De Pauw BE (1990). Teicoplanin as modification of initial empirical therapy in febrile granulocytopenic patients. J Antimicrob Chemother 25: 985.

O'Hare MD, Reynolds PE (1992). Novel membrane proteins present in teicoplanin-resistant, vancomycin-sensitive, coagulase-negative Staphylococcus spp. J Antimicrob Chemother 30: 753.

Outman WR, Nightingale CH, Sweeney KR, Quintiliani R (1990). Teicoplanin pharmacokinetics in healthy volunteers after administration of intravenous loading and maintenance doses. Antimicrob Ag Chemother 34: 2114.

Pallanza R, Berti M, Goldstein BP et al. (1983). Teichomycin: in-vitro and in-vivo evaluations in comparison with other antibiotics. J Antimicrob Chemother 11: 419.

Parenti F, Beretta G, Berti M, Arioli V (1978). Teichomycins, new antibiotics from Actinoplanes teichomyceticus Nov. Sp. 1. Description of the producer strain, fermentation studies and biological properties. J Antibiotics 31: 276.

Pérez JL, Riera L, Valls F et al. (1987). A comparison of the in-vitro activity of seventeen antibiotics against Streptococcus faecalis. J Antimicrob Chemother 20: 357.

Phillips G, Golledge CL (1992). Vancomycin and teicoplanin: something old, something new. Med J Aust 156: 53.

Polk RE (1991). Anaphylactoid reactions to glycopeptide antibiotics. J Antimicrob Chemother 27 (Suppl B): 17.

Presterl E, Graninger W, Georgopoulos A (1993). The efficacy of teicoplanin in the treatment of endocarditis caused by Gram-positive bacteria. J Antimicrob Chemother 31: 755.

Rodríquez-Tudela JL, López de Felipe F, Martínez-Suárez JV, Fenoll A (1992). Comparative in-vitro activity of four peptide antibiotics against penicillin-resistant Streptococcus pneumoniae isolated from cerebrospinal fluid (CSF). J Antimicrob Chemother 29: 299.

Rolston KVI, Nguyen H, Amos G et al. (1994). A randomized double-blind trial of vancomycin versus teicoplanin for the treatment of Gram-positive bacteremia in patients with cancer. J Infect Dis 169: 350.

Ryback MJ, Lerner SA, Levine DP et al. (1991). Teicoplanin pharmacokinetics in intravenous drug abusers being treated for bacterial endocarditis. Antimicrob Ag Chemother 35: 696.

Sahai J, Healy DP, Shelton MJ et al. (1990). Comparison of vancomycin- and teicoplanin-induced histamine release and 'red man syndrome'. Antimicrob Ag Chemother 34: 765.

Schaad HJ, Chuard C, Vaudaux P et al. (1994). Teicoplanin alone or combined with rifampin compared with vancomycin for prophylaxis and treatment of experimental foreign body infection by methicillin-resistant Staphylococcus aureus. Antimicrob Ag Chemother 38: 1703.

Schaison GS (1993). Cost effectivenessof teicoplanin plus ceftriaxone: a once daily antibiotic regimen. Pediatr Infect Dis J 12: 514.

Schlemmer B, Falkman H, Boudjadja A et al. (1988). Teicoplanin for patients allergic to vancomycin. New Engl J Med 318: 1127.

Schmit JL (1992). Efficacy of teicoplanin for enterococcal infections: 63 cases and review. Clin Infect Dis 15: 302.

Shanson DC, Shehata A, Tadayon M, Harris M (1987). Comparison of intravenous teicoplanin with intramuscular amoxycillin for the prophylaxis of streptococcal bacteraemia in dental patients. J Antimicrob Chemother 20: 85.

Shlaes DM, Shlaes JH (1995). Teicoplanin selects for Staphylococcus aureus that is resistant to vancomycin. Clin Infect Dis 20: 1071.

Shlaes DM, Binczewski B, Rice LB (1993a). Emerging antimicrobial resistance and the immunocompromised host. Clin Infect Dis 17 (Suppl 2): 527.

Shlaes DM, Shlaes JH, Vincent S et al. (1993b). Teicoplanin-resistant Staphylococcus aureus expresses a novel membrane protein and increases expression of penicillin-binding protein 2 complex. Antimicrob Ag Chemother 37: 2432.

Smith SR, Cheesbrough J, Spearing R, Davies JM (1989a). Randomized prospective study comparing vancomycin with teicoplanin in the treatment of infections associated with Hickman catheters. Antimicrob Ag Chemother 33: 1193.

Smith SR, Cheesbrough JS, Makris M, Davies JM (1989b). Teicoplanin administration in patients experiencing reactions to vancomycin. J Antimicrob Chemother 23: 810.

Smithers JA, Kulmala HK, Thompson GA et al. (1992). Pharmacokinetics of teicoplanin upon multiple-dose intravenous administration of 3, 12, and 30 milligrams per kilogram of body weight to healthy male volunteers. Antimicrob Ag Chemother 36: 115.

Somma S, Gastaldo L, Corti A (1984). Teicoplanin, a new antibiotic from Actinoplanes teichomyceticus nov. sp. Antimicrob Ag Chemother 26: 917.

Stahl JP, Croize J, Wolff M et al. (1987). Poor penetration of teicoplanin into cerebrospinal fluid in patients with bacterial meningitis. J Antimicrob Chemother 20: 141.

Stille W, Sietzen W, Dieterich H-A, Fell JJ (1988). Clinical efficacy and safety of teicoplanin. J Antimicrob Chemother 21 (Suppl A): 69.

Tarral E, Jehl F, Tarral A et al. (1988). Pharmacokinetics of teicoplanin in children. J Antimicrob Chemother 21: (Suppl A): 47.

The Swedish CDAD Study Group (1994). Treatment of Clostridium difficile associated diarrhea and colitis with an oral preparation of teicoplanin; a dose finding study. Scand J Infect Dis 26: 309.

Torney HL, Balistreri FJ, Kenny MT, Cheng WD (1991). Comparative therapeutic efficacy of teicoplanin and vancomycin in normal and in neutropenic mice infected with Staphylococcus haemolyticus. J Antimicrob Chemother 28: 261.

Tuazon CU, Washburn D (1987). Teicoplanin and rifampicin singly and in combination in the treatment of experimental Staphylococcus epidermidis endocarditis in the rabbit model. J Antimicrob Chemother 20: 233.

Van der Auwera P, Klastersky J (1987). Bactericidal activity and killing rate of serum in volunteers receiving teicoplanin alone or in combination with oral or intravenous rifampicin. Antimicrob Ag Chemother 31: 1002.

Van der Auwera P, Aoun M, Meunier F (1991). Randomized study of vancomycin versus teicoplanin for the treatment of Gram-positive bacterial infections in immunocompromised hosts. Antimicrob Ag Chemother 35: 451.

Van Laethem Y, Goossens H, Cran S *et al.* (1984). Teicoplanin in severe methicillin-resistant Gram-positive septicemia. In *Abstracts and Program of the 24th Interscience Conference on Antimicrobial Agents and Chemotherapy, Houston, TX* (Abstr. 1219). Washington, DC: American Society for Microbiology.

Venditti M, Gelfusa V, Serra P *et al.* (1992). Four-week treatment of streptococcal native valve endocarditis with high-dose teicoplanin. *Antimicrob Ag Chemother* **36**: 723.

Venditti M, Tarasi A, Gelfusa V *et al.* (1993). Antimicrobial susceptibilities of enterococci isolated from hospitalized patients. *Antimicrob Ag Chemother* **37**: 1190.

Verbist L, Tjandramaga B, Hendrickx B *et al.* (1984). *In vitro* activity and human pharmacokinetics of teicoplanin. *Antimicrob Ag Chemother* **26**: 881.

Watanakunakorn C (1988). *In-vitro* induction of resistance in coagulase-negative staphylococci to vancomycin and teicoplanin. *J Antimicrob Chemother* **22**: 321.

Watanakunakorn C (1990). *In-vitro* selection of resistance of *Staphylococcus aureus* to teicoplanin and vancomycin. *J Antimicrob Chemother* **25**: 69.

Williams AH, Grüneberg RN (1984). Leading article Teicoplanin. *J Antimicrob Chemother* **14**: 441.

Wilson APR, Grüneberg RN (1994). Use of teicoplanin in community medicine. *Eur J Clin Microbiol Infect Dis* **13**: 701.

Wilson APR, Taylor B, Treasure T *et al.* (1988a). Antibiotic prophylaxis in cardiac surgery: serum and tissue levels of teicoplanin, flucloxacillin and tobramycin. *J Antimicrob Chemother* **21**: 201.

Wilson APR, Treasure T, Grüneberg RN *et al.* (1988b). Antibiotic prophylaxis in cardiac surgery: a prospective comparison of two dosage regimens of teicoplanin with a combination of flucloxacillin and tobramycin. *J Antimicrob Chemother* **21**: 213.

Wilson APR, Shankar S, Felmingham D *et al.* (1989). Serum and tissue levels of teicoplanin during cardiac surgery: the effect of a high dose regimen. *J Antimicrob Chemother* **23**: 613.

Wilson APR, Grüneberg RN, Neu H (1993). Dosage recommendations for teicoplanin. *J Antimicrob Chemother* **32**: 792.

Wood G, Whitby M (1989). Teicoplanin in patients who are allergic to vancomycin *Med J Aust* **150**: 668.

Part II

Synthetic Antibacterial and Antiparasitic Drugs

Sulfonamides

Description

The first sulfonamide compound of clinical importance, 'Prontosil rubrum', was synthesized in Germany in 1932, and first used as a chemotherapeutic agent in 1935, initiating a new era in the treatment of infections. It was soon shown that the therapeutic action of this compound depended on its breakdown in the body into an inactive dye and an antibacterial substance called sulfanilamide (p-amino-benzene sulfonamide) which had been synthesized in 1908. Subsequently, by manipulating chemical side-chains, several thousand sulfonamides were synthesized and some of these have clinical uses other than for chemotherapy, such as the oral hypoglycemic agent, tolbutamide. It was observed that sulfanilamide could cause a metabolic acidosis and act as a diuretic, and this was later shown to be due to its sulfamoyl group. Subsequent chemical manipulations of sulfanilamide led to the development of the sulfamoyl diuretics, such as the carbonic anhydrase inhibitors (e.g. acetazolamide), the thiazides and frusemide (Feit, 1975). The history of the sulfonamides has been reviewed by Lerner (1991).

The therapeutic role of sulfonamides alone is steadily diminishing. In combination with other agents such as trimethoprim or pyrimethamine, however, a number of sulfonamides remain clinically relevent. The uses of sulfonamides in such combinations are mostly discussed in the chapter dedicated to the combination agent.

A classification of clinically useful sulfonamides is based on their absorption and excretion patterns and is shown in Table II.1. They may be divided into several groups:

Short-acting sulfonamides. These compounds are readily absorbed from the gastrointestinal tract and are rapidly excreted.

Medium-acting sulfonamides. These are well absorbed from the gastrointestinal tract, but rather more slowly excreted, so that 12-hourly administration is adequate.

Long-acting sulfonamides. Rapidly absorbed from the gastrointestinal tract, but excreted slowly, these can be administered in a once-daily dose.

Ultra-long-acting sulfonamides. Therapeutic serum and urine levels persist for up to 7 days after a single oral dose of 1–2 g of these drugs.

Poorly absorbed sulfonamides. Most of the orally administered dose of these drugs is excreted unchanged in the feces and their action is confined to the gut. These drugs are rarely used nowadays.

Sensitive Organisms

The sulfonamides originally had a wide range of activity, but this range has now been seriously restricted by acquired bacterial resistance. Microorganisms which were originally sensitive to sulfonamides are described first and acquired bacterial resistance is discussed later.

1 Gram-positive bacteria

Cocci, such as *Staphylococcus aureus*, *Staph. saprophyticus*, *Streptococcus pyogenes*, *Strep. pneumoniae* and *Strep. viridans*, are sensitive, but enterococci are resistant. *Stomatococcus mucilaginosus* is variably susceptible (Mitchell *et al.*, 1990). Gram-positive bacilli, such as *Bacillus anthracis*, *Clostridium tetani* and *Cl. perfringens* (*welchii*), are also sensitive. Most strains of *B. cereus* are inhibited by sulfonamides (Leading article, 1983b). The activity of sulfamethoxazole against *Listeria monocytogenes* is variable, some strains being highly susceptible and others being highly resistant (Winslow and Pankey, 1982).

Actinomyces are commonly sulfonamide-sensitive. The *Nocardia*, both *N. asteroides* and *N. brasiliensis*, are usually sensitive, but some strains are resistant to very high sulfonamide concentrations (Bach *et al.*, 1973; Berd, 1973; Dewsnup and Wright, 1984; Wallace *et al.*, 1988; Gombert *et al.*, 1990). If small inocula are used in testing, however, most *Nocardia* isolates are susceptible to sulfonamides (Wallace *et al.*, 1977). Other chemotherapeutic agents, such as ampicillin (Orfanakis *et al.*, 1972), trimethoprim (p. 837) and possibly ciprofloxacin (Gombert *et al.*, 1990), may potentiate the action of sulfonamides against the *Nocardia*.

2 Gram-negative bacteria

Enterobacteriaceae, such as *Escherichia coli*, *Enterobacter*, *Klebsiella*, *Proteus*, *Yersinia*, *Salmonella* and *Shigella* spp., are sulfonamide-susceptible. However, *Providencia* spp. are often resistant (Hawkey, 1984). The pathogenic *Neisseria* (*gonococci* and *meningococci*) are susceptible. *Haemophilus influenzae* type b, including ampicillin-resistant strains (p. 113), are susceptible; this organism can be inhibited by concentrations achievable in saliva (Bannatyne and Cheung, 1978). Often *H. ducreyi* is susceptible to sulfonamides, but the rates of susceptibility vary according to geographical location (Kraus *et al.*, 1982; Dangor *et al.*, 1990). Most strains of *Burkholderia* (formerly *Pseudomonas*) *pseudomallei* are susceptible (Eickhoff *et al.*, 1970). Even some strains of *Ps. aeruginosa* are susceptible. *Legionella pneumophila* is inhibited by sulfadiazine (Lewis *et al.*, 1978). The fastidious, non-oxidative, Gram-negative organisms (termed CDC group NO-1) which are frequently associated with dog and cat bites and appear similar to non-acid producing *Acinetobacter* sp., are susceptible to sulfonamides (Hollis *et al.*, 1993).

Most *Bacteroides fragilis* strains and some other anaerobes may be susceptible to sulfonamides, but the degree of susceptibility depends on the laboratory technique used (Phillips and Warren, 1976) (p. 838). *Gardnerella vaginalis* and *Bacteroides* organisms (other than *B. fragilis*) associated with non-specific vaginitis are resistant to sulfonamides; although they may be inhibited by high concentrations of sulfonamides released by topical vaginal sulfonamide preparations (Jones *et al.*, 1982).

3 Chlamydia

Sulfonamides are active against the serotypes of *Chlamydia trachomatis*, which cause lymphogranuloma venereum, trachoma, inclusion body conjunctivitis and non-specific (chlamydial) urethritis (Toomey and Barnes, 1990). *Chlamydia psittaci* and *C. pneumoniae* (*C. psittaci* strain TWAR) are resistant to sulfonamides (Kuo and Grayston, 1988).

4 Mycobacteria

Long-acting sulfonamides such as sulfamethoxypyridine are bacteriostatic against *M. leprae* (MIC 30 μg per ml) and strains which are resistant to the sulfone, dapsone, are also sulfonamide-resistant (Report, 1982). So-called atypical mycobacteria are very variable in their antibiotic susceptibility patterns. Sulfamethizole, sulfisoxazole, sulfamethoxazole and sulfadimethoxine appear effective against many strains of *Mycobacterium kansasii* and some strains of *M. avium-intracellulare* and *M. fortuitum* (Hejny, 1982). Ahn *et al.* (1987) found that 26 of 28 strains of *M. kansasii* (both wild and treatment-failure isolates) were highly susceptible to sulfamethoxazole (MIC ≤4 μg per ml) *in vitro* and that treatment combinations which included this sulfa had a high cure rate in humans. A number of authors have found the majority of *M. fortuitum* strains to be susceptible to sulfamethoxazole and sulfisoxazole, but *M. chelonae* to be resistant (Wallace *et al.*, 1981; Rodloff, 1982; Swenson *et al.*, 1985).

5 Other microorganisms

Mycoplasma, *Ureaplasma urealyticum* (Toomey and Barnes, 1990), *Treponema*, *Leptospira*, *Rickettsia* and *Coxiella burnetti* are sulfonamide-resistant.

6 Protozoa

Sulfonamides and other related drugs (dapsone, sulfamoxole, sulfamethoxazole, sulfadoxine, sulfadiazine) inhibit *Plasmodium falciparum*, *in vitro*, where infected erythrocytes have been shown to take up more sulfamethoxazole than uninfected erythrocytes, suggesting that the intraparasitic concentrations of these drugs could be much higher than the extracellular concentrations (Zhang and Meshnick, 1991; p. 812). Malarial parasites may become sulfonamide-resistant, however (p. 824). Sulfadiazine, sulfamethoxazole and sulfisoxazole are active against *Toxoplasma gondii* both *in vitro* and *in vivo* (pp. 823, 913), where a synergistic effect has been shown between sulfadiazine combined with pyrimethamine, trimetrexate-glycuronate, and piritrexim; sulfisoxazole combined with pyrimethamine, and trimethoprim combined with sulfamethoxazole (Derouin and Chastang, 1988, 1989; Harris *et al.*, 1988). *In vivo* studies in mice suggest a combination of sulfadiazine and pyrimethamine will result in greater parasite clearance and lower relapse rates than either sulfadiazine, pyrimethamine, or clindamycin given alone (Piketty *et al.*, 1990).

Sulfamoxole, sulfaquinoxaline and dapsone are inhibitory *in vitro* to *Leishmania major* promastigotes (the insect stage) but the mode of activity may not be by the classical route of inhibition of *de novo* folate synthesis and the clinical efficacy of sulfa drugs in leishmaniasis has been questioned (Peixoto and Beverley, 1987). Sulfadiazine may be effective for infections caused by *Acanthomoeba* spp. (Carter *et al.*, 1981). *Pneumocystis carinii* contains dihydropteroate synthetase activity which is inhibited by sulfonamides including sulfamethoxazole, sulfadoxine, dapsone and least by sulfadiazine *in vitro* (Merali *et al.*, 1990). Anti-*Pneumocystis* sulfonamide activity has been confirmed in experimental models of *P. carinii* pneumonia in rats, where sufonamides and sulfones appear to be most active (Walzer *et al.*, 1992a). Improved efficacy was not demonstrated by the addition of a dihydrofolate reductase inhibitor such as trimethoprim or pyrimethamine in this model, however (Walzer *et al.*, 1988, 1992a,b).

7 Fungi

Paracoccidioides brasiliensis (causative agent of South American blastomycosis) is usually sensitive to sulfonamides, but resistant strains occur naturally and strains with acquired resistance may emerge during treatment (Restrepo and Arango, 1980). Sulfadiazine has been used most widely and some authors recommend the combination of trimethoprim and sulfadiazine (cotrimazine) for patients with sulfadiazine-resistant strains (Brummer *et al.*, 1993). Sulfonamides have an effect on infections due to *Histoplasma capsulatum* (Goodwin *et al.*, 1980) and have been used in combination with trimethoprim to treat *H. capsulatum* var. *duboisii* (Loyd *et al.*, 1990).

8 Silver sulfadiazine

At concentrations easily attainable by topical application, it is active against *Ps. aeruginosa* (Rosenkranz and Carr, 1972), although resistance is increasing. It is active against a number of dermatophytes such as the *Microsporum* and *Trichophyton* spp. and *Epidermophyton floccosum* (Speck and Rosenkranz, 1974). At a concentration of 10 μg per ml, it inhibits Herpes simplex virus types 1 and 2 *in vitro* (Chang and Weinstein, 1975b) and prevents acute herpetic keratocojunctivitis in rabbits (Chang and Weinstein, 1975c). Silver sulfadiazine also has activity against *Treponema pallidum* (Chang and Weinstein, 1975a).

9 Acquired resistance

Resistance is now common among many of the bacterial species which are described above as 'classically' sulfonamide-sensitive.

Some strains of all the Gram-positive bacteria are sulfonamide-resistant and resistant strains may also emerge *in vivo* during treatment. Although resistance of Group A beta-hemolytic streptococci to sulfadiazine appeared and spread rapidly among military recruits at the end of World War II, this does not appear to be a continuing problem (Finland *et al.*, 1976; Yourassowsky *et al.*, 1974).

Resistance of Gram-negative organisms to sulfonamides is commonly mediated by plasmids (p. 549). There are only two known genes (*sul I* and *sul II*) encoding plasmid-borne sulfonamide-resistance. Both encode a drug-resistant dihydropteroate synthase enzyme. Among Enterobacteriaceae isolated from several sources around the world, plasmid-mediated resistance to sulfonamides has been shown to be encoded by either *sul I*, *sul II*, or both (Rådström *et al.*, 1991). These genes become stably integrated into transposons and plasmids that are widely disseminated among Gram-negative bacteria. *Sul I* is almost exclusively found on large conjugative plasmids and harbors a site-specific recombination system for the integration of various antibiotic-resistance genes (Sundström *et al.*, 1988). Most known trimethoprim-resistance genes are associated with *sul I*-containing integrons (Sundström and Sköld, 1990; Rådström *et al.*, 1991). *Sul II* is frequently observed on small non-conjugative plasmids where it is genetically linked to a streptomycin-resistance gene (Rådström and Swedberg, 1988). The few strains that carry neither *sul I* or *sul II*, often show low-level resistance to sulfonamides, which is probably chromosomally mediated (Rådström *et al.*, 1991).

Sulfonamide-resistant *E. coli* and all other Enterobacteriaceae are now common, especially in hospitals. In the UK, hospital-acquired infections due to Enterobacteriaceae during the late 1970s to early 1980s had a 50–60% incidence of sulfonamide-resistance (Hamilton-Miller, 1979; Gross *et al.*, 1982). In Oslo, Norway, 35% of all Enterobacteriaceae isolated from hospital-drawn blood cultures in 1989 were resistant to sulfonamides (Scheel and Iverson, 1991). Sulfonamide-resistance is also common in developing countries. In a study which examined fecal *E. coli* isolates from travellers who took no antibiotics prior to, during, or after travel to Mexico, the incidence of sulfonamide-resistant fecal carriage of isolates rose from 55% pre-travel to 100% 6 weeks later (Murray *et al.*, 1990).

The majority of *Shigella* spp. strains are now resistant to sulfonamides. In North America and the UK in the 1960s and 1970s, about 60–80% of clinical isolates were sulfonamide-resistant (Haltalin and Nelson, 1965; Davies *et al.*, 1970; Gordon *et al.*, 1975), while in Sweden during the period 1977–1980, 64% of isolates were resistant (Hansson *et al.*, 1981). These high rates of resistance have persisted throughout the world, with 70–80% resistance (frequently multidrug-resistant) in Bulgaria in 1983–1987 (Bratoeva and John, 1989) and 95% incidence of resistance among Nairobi AIDS patients in 1990–1991 (Kruse *et al.*, 1992).

Resistance to sulfonamides among *Salmonella* spp. is now reasonably common. During the early 1970s in California, 40% of *Salm. typhimurium* and 16.5% of *Salm. typhi* were sulfonamide-resistant (Bissett *et al.*, 1974), but this rate has steadily increased along with multidrug-resistance, including resistance to co-trimoxazole (Ryder *et al.*, 1980; Pilantanapak *et al.*, 1990; p. 841).

O'Grady *et al.* (1976) found sulfonamide-resistance to be relatively uncommon among *Vibrio cholerae* isolates (4 of 1156 strains), but subsequently multiple antibiotic-resistant O-group 1 *V. cholerae* strains have been responsible for outbreaks of disease in Tanzania and Bangladesh. Plasmid-mediated resistance was noted to tetracycline, ampicillin, kanamycin, streptomycin and co-trimoxazole (WHO, 1980). Sulfonamide-resistance among *H. influenzae* has been relatively uncommon with 5.3% resistance in the UK in 1981–1982 and 2.6% resistance in Ireland in 1988 (Mehtar and Aminiafshar, 1983; Howard and Williams, 1989). Wide regional differences exist, however, with up to 64% of isolates in Spain being resistant to co-trimoxazole (Campos *et al.*, 1984; Jorgensen, 1992).

Resistance of *H. ducreyi* to both sulfonamides and tetracyclines is now common throughout the world, but particularly in Africa, Singapore and Thailand (Sng *et al.*, 1982; Dangor *et al.*, 1990). This resistance is mediated by a non-conjugative plasmid closely related to plasmids found in the Enterobacteriaceae (Albritton *et al.*, 1982; Fast *et al.*, 1983).

Sulfonamide-resistant gonococci became common among troops during World War II when these drugs were extensively used for treatment of gonorrhea. Subsequently in many parts of the world, such as South-East Asia, a high percentage of gonococcal strains are resistant to sulfonamides (Report, 1978).

Sulfonamide-resistant meningococci are common in many parts of the world. The definition of resistance has varied in different studies and MIC values of ≥ 10–$100\,\mu g$ per ml have been used. Usually strains with an MIC to sulfadiazine of $< 1\,\mu g$ per ml are regarded as sensitive, those with an MIC of 5–$10\,\mu g$ per ml as partially resistant and strains with an MIC of $\geq 10\,\mu g$ per ml as resistant. Although sulfonamide-resistant meningococci were once thought to release more endotoxin than sensitive strains, this has now been disproven and there is no relationship between sulfonamide-resistance and mortality from meningococcal disease during outbreaks (Anderson *et al.*, 1987). Such resistance is generally plasmid-mediated (Facinelli and Varaldo, 1987), although Kristiansen *et al.* (1990) have described a serogroup B clinical isolate where resistance appeared to be chromosomally mediated. In this latter instance, the responsible gene appeared to be different from the plasmid-borne sulfonamide-resistance genes *sul I* and *sul II* in Enterobacteriaceae and the *Su^r* gene from serogroup C meningococcus (Kristiansen *et al.*, 1990). An increased resistance to sulfonamides was observed during epidemics in World War II and sporadic cases occurred in the 1950s (Peltola, 1983). Resistant meningococci then became prevalent in both military (Millar *et al.*, 1963) and civilian populations in the USA in the early 1960s (Feldman, 1986). In an early US study, 36.9% of strains isolated from civilian patients were sulfadiazine-resistant, but only 3.7% of strains from pharyngeal carriers were resistant, MIC $\geq 100\,\mu g$ per ml (Leedom *et al.*, 1967). After 1969, meningococci of serogroup C replaced those of serogroup B as the most frequent cause of disease in the USA. In the years 1972, 1973 and 1974, 82.3%, 74.4% and 68.9%, respectively, of meningococci were sulfonamide-resistant (Jacobson *et al.*, 1975). In 1975, serogroup B again became the most prevalent serogroup in the USA and, although only 4% of these were sulfonamide-resistant, 27% of all isolates were resistant (CDC, 1976). By 1978, a further shift occurred, so that group B organisms accounted for 49%, group C, 29%, group Y, 8.6%, and the balance belonged to groups W 135 and A (Counts and Petersdorf, 1980). Routine immunization of military recruits against Group C meningococci began in 1971 was very successful. In 1980, group W 135 became the second most prevalent group (21%), causing serious disease in the USA, and surpassing group C (18%). The proportion of meningococcal strains resistant to sulfonamides dropped from 67% in 1970 to 12% in 1980; the proportion of serogroup C strains resistant dropped from 89% to 30% in the same period. Only 8% of group B strains and 4% of group W 135 strains were resistant to sulfonamides in 1980; no resistant Y strains were found (Band et al., 1983). In a Canadian study (Marks et al., 1979), similar to the USA, serogroups B and C were most commonly isolated from ill and asymptomatic subjects; resistance to sulfadiazine (MIC $\geq 10 \mu$g per ml) was present in 6.5% and 39.4% of group B and group C strains, respectively. During 1986–1987, serogroups B and C caused about equal amounts of disease, although there was some geographical variation. Sulfadiazine-resistance (MIC $\geq 32 \mu$g per ml) was noted in 61% of isolates, although among serogroup B isolates 31% were resistant vs 77% of serogroup B isolates (p < 0.001) (Pinner et al., 1991). In Norway, since 1974, approximately 90% of clinical pathogenic strains have been sulfonamide-resistant, while most carrier strains have been susceptible (Kristiansen et al., 1988, 1990).

Meningococci resistant to sulfonamides have been found throughout the world, including Scandinavia (Holmgren and Tunevall, 1973; Salmi et al., 1976; Peltola et al., 1982), Africa (Wright and Plorde, 1970; Peltola, 1983), Brazil (De Morais et al., 1974), UK (WHO, 1971; 1974; Abbott and Graves, 1972; Leading article, 1974a; Fallon, 1983), Spain (WHO, 1979) and Australia (Grigor, 1983). Recent studies have suggested some clonality between geographically distant outbreaks such as those occurring in Scandinavia and Sudan (Salih et al., 1990).

10 Bacterial susceptibility testing

Usually only one sulfonamide is used for these tests and the results obtained are generally applicable to the others. Relative antibacterial activity of various sulfonamides against the 'sensitive bacteria' varies to some extent. Of commonly used short-acting sulfonamides, sulfadiazine appears to have the highest activity against most bacteria. Long-acting sulfonamides are said to have higher in vitro activity against Gram-positive cocci than older compounds. Garrod et al. (1973) tested the in vitro activity of the sulfonamides under standard conditions and concluded that 'there is very little indeed to choose between the antibacterial activities of the more potent sulfonamides'.

11 Synergy with other drugs

Sulfonamides act synergistically with other chemotherapeutic substances against certain pathogens. They may potentiate the action of the polymyxins against Ps. aeruginosa, Proteus spp. and Serratia marcescens and they have a synergistic effect with trimethoprim against many bacteria (p. 842). Similarly, the sulfonamides potentiate the action of pyrimethamine on malarial parasites (McGregor et al., 1963) (pp. 905, 917) and T. gondii (p. 905).

12 Minimum inhibitory concentrations

These vary according to the methods and media used for their estimation, and there are also variations between individual sulfonamides. Table II.3 (p. 844) shows the MICs of sulfamethoxazole and sulfadiazine compared with trimethoprim.

Mode of Administration and Dosage

The sulfonamides are usually administered by mouth.

1 Short-acting sulfonamides

The usual recommended adult dosage for members of this group, such as sulfadiazine, sulfafurazole or sulfadimidine is 2–4 g initially, followed by 4–8 g daily administered in four to six equally divided doses. A dose of 0.5–1.0 g daily may be sufficient for long-term 'suppressive therapy' in chronic urinary tract infection. However, lower doses of sulfadiazine produce effective urinary levels of the drug; this has been utilized in sulfadiazine/trimethoprim combinations for the treatment of urinary tract infections (p. 885). For the treatment of cerebral toxoplasmosis in patients with AIDS, generally 4–6 g daily is required in combination with pyrimethamine (p. 913). Intravenous sulfadiazine dosage is 1–1.5 g every 4 h for adults, or 50 mg per kg every 6 h for children. It should be given by infusion (concentration no greater than 5% sulfadiazine) over at least 10 min. For children aged older than 2 months, an initial dose of 75 mg per kg body weight may be followed by a daily dosage of 150 mg per kg, given in four to six

Table II.1

Classification of sulfonamides

Antibiotic	Advantages/disadvantages and uses
Short-acting sulfonamides	Good gastrointestinal absorption, but rapid excretion
1. Sulfanilamide Sulfacetamide Sulfapyridine Sulfathiazole	Historical interest, rarely used due to low antibacterial activity High solubility; used in eye drops (rarely); low antibacterial activity Used to treat dermatitis herpetiformis Historical interest, rarely used
2. Sulfadiazine/sulfapyrimidine group: Sulfadiazine (sulfapyrimidine) Sulfamerazine (sulfamethylpyrimidine) Sulfadimidine (sulfamezathine, sulfamethazine, sulfadimethylpyrimidine) Silver sulfadiazine	 Potent; excellent CSF penetration; previously 'drug of choice' for meningococcal meningitis; low solubility in urine. No special advantages; rarely used as relatively toxic. Effective and soluble in urine Non-absorbable, topical agent for burns
3. Sulfasomidine (sulfadimethine) Sulfafurazole (sulfisoxazole) Sulfamethizole (sulfamethylthiodiazole)	Soluble in urine; low toxicity; rapidly excreted; useful treatment of UTI Similar to sulfasomidine. Similar to sulfasomidine, but too rapidly excreted for treatment of systemic infections
4. Sulfasalazine ('Salazopyrin')	5-aminosalicylic acid/sulfapyridine conjugate Useful treatment of inflammatory bowel disease
5. Mafenide (marfanil, 'Sulfamylon')	Not inactivated by para-aminobenzoic acid Mafenide acetate cream used in treatment of burns
Medium-acting sulfonamides	
Sulfamethoxazole	Well absorbed; slowly excreted; twice-daily dosing Used in combination with trimethoprim as co-trimoxazole (p. 836)
Long-acting sulfonamides	Rapidly absorbed; slowly excreted; once-daily dosing
1. Sulfamethoxypyridazine	First of the long-acting sulfonamides: serum half-life 40 h.
2. Sulfadimethoxine, sulfaphenazole sulfamethoxydiazine ('Kirocid')	Similar to sulfamethoxypyridazine; sulfamethoxydiazine is less protein bound than other agents in this group (75% versus 90–95%)
3. Sulfasymazine	Serum half-life 26 h; used once or twice-daily for UTI
Ultra-long-acting sulfonamides	Single dose results in therapeutic serum and urine levels for 7 days
1. Sulfadoxine	Used in combination with pyrimethamine ('Fansidar') for treatment of malaria
2. Sulfametopyrazine (sulfalene)	Used as single-dose treatment for UTI
Poorly absorbed sulfonamides	Excreted unchanged in feces; action confined to gut; rarely used.
Sulfaguanadine Succinylsulfathiazole Phthalylsulfathiazole ('Thalazole')	

UTI: Urinary tract infections.

equally divided doses. The total daily dose in children should not exceed 6 g. The adult dosage (including children older than 12 years) of sulfamethizole is 1 g three times daily and, for children aged greater than 2 months, it is 5 mg per kg three times daily. The elimination half-life in infants aged less than 10 days is longer than in adults, but it rapidly decreases during the next 2 weeks to remain at a lower level until the age of 6–8 years. The recommended dosage for children is, therefore, proportionally greater than for adults (Follath, 1979).

The recommended initial dosage of sulfasalazine ('Salazopyrin') is 1–2 g four times daily (the interval between doses should not exceed 8 h), followed by 2 g daily in four divided doses. An enteric coated tablet is available for patients who develop gastrointestinal intolerance. Different doses can be used in certain circumstances (p. 826). The initial dosage of sulfasalazine for children is 40–60 mg per kg body weight daily given in three to six divided doses, followed by a daily maintenance dosage of 40–60 mg per kg, given in four divided doses. Suppositories (500 mg) are generally used in a dose of 1–2 in the morning and evening after defecation, but after 4–5 weeks the dosage may be halved.

2 Medium-acting sulfonamides

The adult oral dosage of sulfamethoxazole is 2 g initially, followed by 1 g two or three times per day (a total daily dose of 3 g should not be exceeded). For children, the initial dose is 50–60 mg per kg body weight and then 25–30 mg per kg twice-daily (a maximum daily pediatric dose of 75 mg per kg should not be exceeded).

3 Long-acting sulfonamides

For adults, an initial dose of 1.0–1.5 g sulfamethoxydiazine is recommended, followed by a single daily dose of 0.5 g given preferably in the morning, after breakfast. Suitable dose reduction is required for children; e.g. for those aged up to 2 years, a quarter of the adult dose, those aged 6–10 years, half the adult dose and those aged 10–14 years, three-quarters of the adult dose. For severe infections in children aged up to 6 years of age (20 kg body weight), 40 mg per kg can be given once and then 20 mg per kg daily.

4 Ultra-long-acting sulfonamides

Sulfadoxine is generally given in combination with pyrimethamine ('Fansidar') where the dose varies depending upon the treatment indication.

5 Poorly absorbed sulfonamides

The adult dosage of phthalylsulfathiazole is 1–12 g daily given in divided doses.

6 Patients with renal failure

It is difficult to formulate dosage schedules for patients with renal failure as individual sulfonamides are excreted by different renal mechanisms and at different rates. Fischer (1972) observed the sulfadimidine clearance in uremic patients to be significantly lower than that in patients with normal renal function. Adam and Dawborn (1970) and Adam *et al.* (1973) in studies on sulfadiazine, sulfamethizole and sulfadimidine found that, with moderate doses, both the free drugs and their conjugated derivatives accumulated in the plasma of uremic patients. In some patients, the high serum levels appeared to cause side-effects. Furthermore, urine concentrations of free sulfonamides were low in uremic patients. These authors concluded that sulfonamides are unlikely to be useful for treatment of urinary tract infections in patients with serum creatinine levels exceeding 5 mg % (0.4 mmol per liter), and that for patients with lesser degrees of renal failure, a reduced sulfonamide dose may be required to avoid toxicity. Sulfonamides, such as sulfafurazole or sulfamethoxazole, which have lower inhibitory concentrations for common urinary pathogens and are less readily conjugated, may be preferable to sulfadimidine for the treatment of urinary tract infections in uremic patients (Adam *et al.*, 1973). Pharmacokinetic studies with sulfadiazine indicate that about 60% of the drug is excreted unchanged via the kidneys and the remainder is eliminated extrarenally. The elimination rate of the drug, which is the sum of the rates of these two processes, is linearly related to the patient's creatinine clearance; the elimination half-life for healthy patients was 10.4 h and that for anuric patients 25.7 h (Reutter *et al.*, 1979). For sulfadiazine the following dosage adjustments are appropriate: GFR > 50–90 ml per min, 0.5–3.0 g twice-daily; GFR 10–50 ml per min, 0.5–3.0 g daily; < 10 ml per min, avoid sulfadiazine use. There are no useful data regarding sulfadiazine use in hemodialysis or peritoneal dialysis. In anuric patients, therefore, the intervals between doses should be extended. In studies of renal transplant recipients, renal elimination of sulfisoxazole was decreased and correlated with creatine clearance (Shermantine *et al.*, 1985).

For treatment of systemic infections, sulfonamides can probably be safely used in most patients with renal disease, but regular estimations of the serum concentrations of both free and acetylated sulfonamide seem advisable. The various sulfonamides are handled by the kidney in different ways (p. 813), and the rate of acetylation of sulfonamides in the body varies in individual patients. For these reasons, in some uremic patients it may be impossible to select a dose which will give adequate serum levels of the free active drug, yet not lead to accumulation of toxic levels of acetylated compounds. The relationship between toxicity and serum levels in the case of the sulfonamides is not well defined, but some patients with a total serum level of greater than 100 µg per ml often show toxic effects (Adam and Dawborn, 1970).

7 Newborn and premature infants

Sulfonamides are contraindicated in these patients (p. 819).

8 Intraperitoneal administration

Sulfadimidine, in a concentration of 100 µg per ml, has been administered intraperitoneally during peritoneal dialysis for 4–5 days without adverse effects (Adam *et al.*, 1973).

Availability

Nearly all the sulfonamides are available as 500-mg *tablets*; some are also available as 250-mg or 1-g *tablets* and as a *pediatric preparation*. Parenteral sulfadiazine and sulfisoxazole diolamine are available in preparations of 250 mg per ml and 400 mg per ml, respectively.

Serum Levels in Relation to Dosage

All sulfonamides, except sulfaguanidine and the other two compounds of that group (p. 810), are well absorbed after oral administration. After absorption, these drugs are partly conjugated with acetate in the liver and the proportion conjugated varies with different sulfonamides. Sulfonamide conjugates are inactive therapeutically and the serum level of the free active (unconjugated) drug is important.

About 60% of sulfadimidine is present in the serum in an active free form after usual therapeutic doses. Following a single oral dose of 4 g of this drug, a peak free drug serum concentration of 80–100 µg per ml is attained after 2–3 h (Fig. II.1). This serum level falls rapidly and the serum half-life is about 2–3 h. Therapeutic levels can be maintained by using an oral dosage of 1 g 6-hourly. Serum levels after parenteral administration are similar, but the peak concentration is achieved more rapidly.

Fig. II.1.
Average free and total sulfadimidine serum concentrations after single oral dose of 4 g in adults. (Redrawn after Bullowa and Ratish, *The Journal of Clinical Investigation*, 1944, **23**:676, by copyright permission of The American Society for Clinical Investigation.)

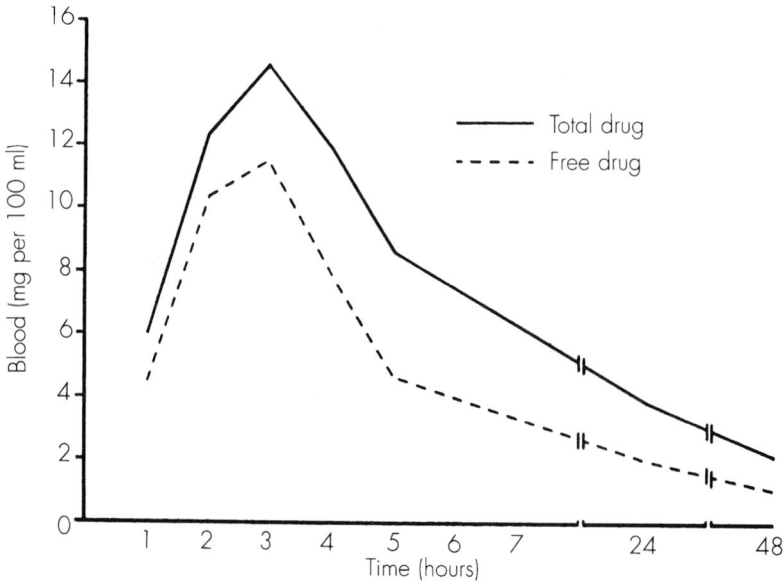

Other short-acting sulfonamides are also well absorbed after oral administration, but differ from sulfadimidine both in the serum levels attained and in the proportion of drug acetylated. Thus, after a 4 g oral dose of sulfadiazine to adults, the peak free drug level is lower (40–60 μg per ml), but about 90–95% is in the active form (Bullowa and Ratish, 1944). When a 400 mg oral dose of sulfadiazine was given to healthy adults, a peak serum level of about 15 μg per ml was reached in 3 h and free drug accounted for 80–90% of the total serum level. The half-life was 12.6 h, but this varied between individuals; after repeated administration some 65% of an oral dose was found in the urine in an unchanged form (Reeves *et al.*, 1979). Sulfisoxazole is highly protein-bound and therefore after a given dose reaches a plasma concentration at least twice that of sulfadiazine. After a 2–4 g oral dose, peak serum concentrations of 110–250 μg per ml are found in 2–4 h. Acetylated sulfisoxazole constitutes about 28–35% of blood and 30% of urine sulfisoxazole levels, with about 95% of a dose being renally excreted in 24 h.

The medium-acting sulfonamide, sulfamethoxazole, is also well absorbed (Fig. II.4, p. 848). Peak serum levels are similar to those obtained with an identical dose of sulfadimidine and 75–85% exists in serum in a free non-acetylated form. In addition, the serum levels of this drug are more prolonged, because it is more slowly excreted by the kidneys.

The long-acting sulfonamides also give high serum levels after oral administration. After a single oral dose of 4 g of sulfamethoxypyridazine to adults, peak total serum levels of 110–118 μg per ml are attained at 5 h and these are maintained for the next 3 h. Very little acetylation occurs during the first 3 h after administration, but subsequently about 5–22% becomes acetylated. Total serum levels of 20–50 μg per ml are still detectable 105 h later (Weinstein *et al.*, 1960). After administration of a 2 g dose of sulfadimethoxine to adults, a total drug level of 50–70 μg per ml is attained in 2 h and this is maintained for 24 h. With an initial dose of 2 g followed by 1.0 g daily in adults, serum levels are maintained in the range 50–100 μg per ml.

The ultra-long-acting sulfonamides, sulfadoxine and sulfametopyrazine, also give high serum levels after oral administration. The serum half-life of the former is 150–200 h and the latter about 65 h. Only a small proportion of these drugs is metabolized; about 5% to the acetyl derivative and 2–3% to the glucuronide (Report, 1984).

Excretion

1 Urine

Free and conjugated sulfonamides are excreted mainly via the kidney. About 73–85% of an orally administered dose of sulfadimidine can be recovered from the urine, but because individuals vary in their ability to acetylate sulfonamides, the proportion which is in a free unconjugated form varies from 15 to 70% (Bullowa and Ratish, 1944).

Sulfonamides and their acetylated conjugates are excreted both by glomerular filtration and tubular secretion. Some of the drug secreted by tubules is reabsorbed. Different sulfonamides and their conjugates are handled by the kidney in different ways. Some compounds, such as sulfafurazole, are rapidly excreted in urine where high concentrations are attained. By contrast, the excretion of the long-acting sulfonamides is slow, so that their serum levels are maintained for long periods and only low concentrations are attained in urine. The long-acting sulfonamides are more extensively bound to serum proteins and the bound fraction is not excreted through the glomeruli. This factor, together with their rate of metabolism, is responsible for the maintenance of prolonged serum levels of the long-acting sulfonamides (Newbould and Kilpatrick, 1960; Reeves *et al.*, 1978). Unmetabolized drugs retain their lipid solubility and may undergo extensive tubular reabsorption, whereas metabolism increases the polarity of the drug molecules making it more hydrophilic and encouraging renal elimination.

The pH of the urine influences the renal clearance of all sulfonamides. Sulfonamide clearance is increased in the presence of alkaline urine (Williams *et al.*, 1968), because sulfonamides are weak acids and their non-ionic tubular reabsorption decreases by alkalinization of the urine (Follath, 1979). This effect is pronounced with the long-acting sulfonamide, sulfasymazine. Furthermore, all the sulfonamides and their acetylated conjugates are more soluble in alkaline urine with the exception of sulfamethizole, which is highly soluble even in acid urine (Peddie and Little, 1979). The solubility in urine of the various sulfonamides and their conjugates varies considerably. Sulfadimidine and its acetylated form are very soluble compared with other sulfonamides, such as sulfadiazine.

2 Bile

Only small amounts of the sulfonamides are excreted via the biliary tract and they are not concentrated in bile.

3 Inactivation in body

A percentage of the absorbed sulfonamide is acetylated in the liver, producing inactive conjugates. Each sulfonamide is acetylated to a different extent. Although the products of acetylation have no antibacterial activity, they retain the toxic potential of the parent sulfonamide. Individuals vary in their capacity to acetylate sulfonamides. Active acetylators of sulfadimidine also rapidly inactivate isoniazid and vice versa, because a similar acetyltransferase enzyme is involved in the processing of both drugs. Patients who, after a test dose of sulfadimidine, have a proportion of acetylated drug less than 25% in the serum, or less than 70% in the urine, may be considered to be slow sulfonamide acetylators and will also usually be slow isoniazid inactivators (Rao *et al.*, 1970) (pp. 1186, 1187).

Some of the sulfonamides are also converted to inactive metabolites in the liver by glucuronidation. This process is particularly marked with sulfadimethoxine, 80% of which is excreted as a very soluble glucuronide in the urine (Busch and Lane, 1967).

Distribution of the Drugs in Body

After absorption the sulfonamides, being lipid-soluble, become widely distributed throughout the body, particularly to extracellular fluids (Wilkinson and Reeves, 1979). The short-acting sulfonamides, especially sulfadiazine, readily penetrate into normal CSF, where this drug may attain a concentration of about half that present in the serum at the time. The drugs also penetrate pleural, peritoneal and synovial fluids (50–80% of serum levels), the aqueous humor of the eye and cross the placenta–fetal serum concentrations reaching 50–90% of those found in maternal blood at the time. High concentrations also occur in saliva and breast milk.

All sulfonamides are bound to serum albumin, but the degree varies. Sulfadiazine is only about 20% protein bound, but most other short-acting sulfonamides, such as sulfadimidine and sulfafurazole, are 40–80% bound. The medium-acting sulfonamide, sulfamethoxazole, is about 65% protein bound. The long-acting sulfonamides are more highly bound, sulfamethoxypyridazine and sulfadimethoxine being about 90% bound, but sulfamethoxydiazine is only about 75% bound. The percentage of each sulfonamide bound to serum proteins is not constant and, similar to the isoxazolyl penicillins (p. 95), decreases as the total serum concentration of the drug increases.

The degree of sulfonamide protein binding influences the rate of renal excretion of these drugs (p. 813). The protein bound drug does not penetrate into some body compartments, such as the subarachnoid space, but this may not apply if the meninges are inflamed. Newbould and Kilpatrick (1960) considered that protein bound sulfonamide has no antibacterial activity and, therefore, higher total serum levels of the newer long-acting, highly protein bound, sulfonamides are required to obtain comparable diffusible concentrations and an equivalent therapeutic effect. Madsen *et al.* (1963) compared the sulfonamide concentration and antibacterial activity in serum of two long-acting sulfonamides, sulfadimethoxine and sulfamethoxypyridazine, with sulfadiazine. These authors found that these three sulfonamides all produced about the same antibacterial activity in the serum. There appeared to be a close correlation between the total sulfonamide concentration and the antibacterial activity regardless of the degree of protein binding. The highly protein bound long-acting sulfonamides also penetrated well into extravascular fluids and exudates, particularly when these were of a high protein content. There are many considerations in assessing the effect of protein binding on antibacterial activity (Rolinson, 1980). A protein bound drug is essentially without antibacterial effect and it is non-diffusible, but this is only a temporary state because when a protein-bound drug dissociates, the drug is available again in active form. The free unbound plasma levels of a drug dictate the free levels in extravascular fluids. The level of free drug after therapeutic doses and how this relates to the MIC of the organism are important factors in determining therapeutic efficacy.

Mode of Action

Folic acid derivatives are essential for purine and ultimately DNA synthesis in both humans and bacteria. Bacterial cells do not generally absorb folic acid and instead synthesize it from para-aminobenzoic acid, whereas humans absorb preformed folic acid from their diet. The sulfonamides, being structurally related to para-aminobenzoic acid, act by inhibiting the bacterial enzyme dihydropteroate synthetase which catalyzes the conversion of para-aminobenzoate to dihydropteroate (Fig. II.2). Not only do the sulfonamides act by competing with para-aminobenzoate, but they take part in the reaction with the formation of pteroate analogs (Hamilton-Miller, 1979). However, these analogs probably contribute very little to the activity of sulfonamide. There is some evidence that this is not the only mode of action for sulfonamides (Gruneberg, 1979; Lacey, 1979, Peixoto and Beverley, 1987). Sulfonamides may possibly also act independently on the enzyme, dihydrofolate reductase, which is affected by trimethoprim

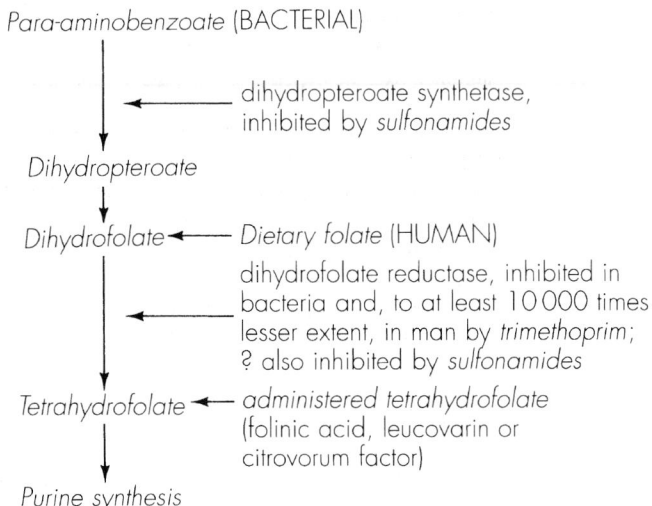

Para-aminobenzoate (BACTERIAL)

dihydropteroate synthetase,
inhibited by *sulfonamides*

Dihydropteroate

Dihydrofolate ◄—— *Dietary folate* (HUMAN)

dihydrofolate reductase, inhibited in
bacteria and, to at least 10 000 times
lesser extent, in man by *trimethoprim*;
? also inhibited by *sulfonamides*

Tetrahydrofolate ◄—— administered tetrahydrofolate
(folinic acid, leucovarin or
citrovorum factor)

Purine synthesis

Fig. II.2
Comparison of human and bacterial
folate metabolism.

(p. 852). Various mechanisms have been implicated for resistance to sulfonamides (Hamilton-Miller, 1979). Chromosomal resistance in Enterobacteriaceae is due to a less susceptible dihydropteroate synthetase, while resistance in staphylococci, pneumococci and gonococci may be due to overproduction of para-aminobenzoate. Plasmid-mediated resistance to sulfonamides, is via the production of drug-resistant dihydropteroate synthetase enzyme (Rådström *et al.*, 1991).

Sulfonamides (and sulfones, such as dapsone, p. 825) also act on malarial parasites by blocking the conversion of para-aminobenzoate. Resistance of malarial parasites to sulfonamides and other antifolate antimalarial drugs may be complex; malarial parasites may be able to synthesize *de novo* active folate cofactors and utilize exogenous intact folate in various forms (Milhous *et al.*, 1985).

Toxicity

1 Gastrointestinal side-effects

Nausea, vomiting and diarrhea were common with earlier compounds such as sulfapyridine, but are uncommon with the newer sulfonamides.

2 Neurological side-effects

Headache and dizziness were commonly reported with the older sulfonamides, but are rare with the newer compounds. In the pre-penicillin era, toxic psychoses due to sulfonamides were well described (Little, 1942). Other disturbances of the nervous system such as drowsiness, fatigue, insomnia, nightmares, confusion, depression, vertigo, ataxia and peripheral neuritis have been reported (Weinstein *et al.*, 1960). Acute encephalopathy and tremulousness, possibly due to sulfadiazine, has been described in a patient with AIDS-related complex who was also being treated with pyrimethamine for refractory *Isospora belli* infection (Young, 1989).

3 Drug fever

This is rare with commonly used short-acting sulfonamides, such as sulfadimidine and sulfafurazole although it was frequent with the earlier sulfonamides. Drug fever has been occasionally observed with the long-acting sulfonamide, sulfamethoxypyridazine (Grieble and Jackson, 1958).

4 Hypersensitivity reactions

The mechanism(s) of idiosyncratic sulfonamide toxicity have not been clearly defined, although a number of authors have demonstrated an association between sulfonamide toxicity and slow acetylator status (with subsequent reduced ability to detoxify oxidative metabolites) (Shear *et al.*, 1986; Rieder *et al.*, 1989). In an *in vitro* assay, lymphocytes from six patients with a history of severe reactions to sulfonamides were compared with those of 20 controls. The lymphocytes of the sulfa-allergic patients demonstrated increased toxicity from sulfonamide metabolites, but not from the drugs themselves (Shear *et al.*, 1986). Rieder *et al.* (1989) found that in the case of sulfamethoxazole hypersensitivity, the hydroxylamine derivative of this agent may be one of the reactive metabolites mediating these reactions. Thus, inherited differences in the rate of toxic metabolite production and detoxification, and the rate of acetylation of the parent drug may contribute to hypersensitivity.

Allergic rashes are fairly frequent complications of sulfonamide therapy. Similar to the penicillins, these usually occur after 1–2 week treatment, but may appear earlier with prior sulfonamide sensitization. The most common types of rashes are maculopapular or urticarial, but erythema nodosum, exfoliative dermatitis or, rarely, Stevens–Johnson syndrome may occur. Photosensitivity can also result. These rashes may be accompanied by features of a serum sickness-like illness such as fever and joint pains (Shear *et al.*, 1986).

Stevens–Johnson syndrome is the most serious form of hypersensitivity reaction to sulfonamides. In its most extensive form, this syndrome consists of erythema multiforme and ulceration of the mucous membranes of the eyes, mouth and urethra, which can be very severe and sometimes fatal. This complication has been described in association with all sulfonamides, but the long-acting ones, sulfamethoxypyridazine and sulfadimethoxine, have been particularly implicated (Salvaggio and Gonzalez, 1959; Rallison *et al.*, 1961; Claxton, 1963). The United States Food and Drug Administration collected reports of 116 cases of Stevens–Johnson syndrome associated with long-acting sulfonamide administration from 1957 to 1965 from all parts of the world (Carroll *et al.*, 1966). This series included 79 children with 20 deaths and 37 adults with 9 deaths. The median time of appearance of this complication was about the tenth day of treatment. Only one patient was known to be rechallenged with the sulfonamide and Stevens–Johnson syndrome promptly recurred. It was estimated that there had been about one or two cases reported for every 10 million doses of these drugs which had been distributed. The report suggested that this syndrome may be more common in children. Nine cases of Stevens–Johnson syndrome in children with three fatalities were reported from one Sydney hospital during the period 1962–1964 (Beveridge *et al.*, 1964).

The risk of Stevens–Johnson syndrome appears to be the main reason why the long-acting sulfonamides did not become more popular for general use (Pryles, 1970). Some authors used these compounds extensively for the treatment of urinary tract infections and did not encounter this complication (Brumfitt, 1970). Drugs other than sulfonamides may also cause this syndrome, and the underlying infection for which the drugs are given may sometimes be responsible for Stevens–Johnson syndrome. A variety of infectious agents, such as *Mycoplasma pneumoniae* and Herpes simplex virus, have an etiological role in this syndrome. The causative role of the sulfonamides is beyond doubt in many cases. Ström (1962) used provocative tests with suspected drugs (sulfonamides and others) in 29 patients who had had Stevens–Johnson syndrome and obtained positive reactions in 19. Lyell (1982) has also drawn attention to other instances where this syndrome appeared to be precipitated by sulfonamides. Cases of agranulocytosis, Stevens–Johnson syndrome, erythema multiforme and toxic epidermal necrolysis with some fatalities have been reported in association with the use of 'Fansidar' (pyrimethamine and sulfadoxine) for malaria (Hornstein and Ruprecht, 1982; Olsen *et al.*, 1982; Whitfield, 1982; CDC, 1985a,b; Selby *et al.*, 1985) and prophylaxis against *P. carinii* pneumonia in patients with AIDS (Navin *et al.*, 1985). Other adverse reactions associated with 'Fansidar' have included serum sickness-type reaction, urticaria, exfoliative dermatitis and hepatitis. As a result indications for the use of this combination were altered and 'Fansidar' is no longer recommended for prophylaxis against malaria or pneumocystis pneumonia (pp. 824, 826). Adverse reactions, including rashes, to co-trimoxazole are more common in patients with AIDS (p. 854). Desensitization to sulfonamides has been reported in both AIDS and non-AIDS patients, with moderate success (Holdsworth, 1981; Taffet and Das, 1982; Finegold, 1985; Hughes *et al.*, 1986; Kreuz *et al*, 1990; Torgovnick and Arsura, 1990; Tenant-Flowers *et al.*, 1991), although Sher *et al.* (1986) described a patient who developed anaphylactic shock during oral desensitization, so caution needs to exercised. Torgovnick and Arsura (1990) described 13 patients with AIDS and sulfonamide-associated cutaneous reactions who underwent oral desensitization – 11 successfully. They used a solution containing either 4 mg per ml of sulfamethoxazole or 5 mg per ml sulfadiazine in which 1 ml was given every 6 h for four doses then, if no reaction was observed, the dose was doubled on the same 6-hourly schedule every 24 h until the desired dose was reached: sulfamethoxazole 1.2 g four times daily, or sulfadiazine 1.5–2 g four times daily.

About 2% of patients receiving sulfasalazine therapy for inflammatory bowel disease (p. 826) develop symptoms that appear to be allergic (Purdy *et al.*, 1984). This is distinct from the non-allergic toxicity of sulfasalazine which is related to the serum sulfapyridine level (p. 827).

Allergic manifestations usually consist of a skin rash (urticaria, macular or diffuse erythema) with or without fever and is not associated with the acetylator phenotype of the patient (p. 1186). Patients with this allergy can be desensitized successfully by starting with a low daily dose of sulfasalazine (1 mg) and gradually increasing it up to 2–3 g per day (Holdsworth, 1981; Taffet and Das, 1982; Purdy et al., 1984). Desensitization should not be attempted in patients with serious reactions to sulfasalazine, such as agranulocytosis, toxic epidermal necrolysis or fibrosing alveolitis. A generalized hypersensitivity reaction associated with fever, arthralgia, lymphadenopathy and hepatitis, can occur with sulfasalazine (p. 818).

Hypersensitivity manifestations following topical sulfonamide therapy are common, and this form of treatment is now only rarely used. Stevens–Johnson syndrome has been described following the use of sulfonamide eye drops (Gottschalk and Stone, 1976).

There is usually cross-allergy between all the sulfonamides and sulfonamide-allergic patients may also be allergic to other drugs of similar structure such as frusemide and hydro-chlorothiazide (and vice versa) (Sullivan, 1991). It is unwise to administer any sulfonamide to a patient with a previous history of allergy to one of these drugs. There is no satisfactory test available for sulfonamide allergy.

5 Hematological side-effects

The most common of these important complications is acute agranulocytosis, although aplastic anemia, megaloblastic anemia and thrombocytopenia have also been described.

Agranulocytosis was reasonably common with the older sulfonamides, such as sulfapyridine, but is rare with currently used drugs. It is reversible and recovery usually occurs within 1 week of stopping the drug. In a survey in Sweden between 1973 and 1978, sulfonamides were one of the most frequent causes of drug-induced leukopenia (Leading article, 1983a). The International Agranulocytosis and Aplastic Anemia Study Group (1989) estimated the relative risk of developing agranulocytosis when co-trimoxazole (sulfamethoxazole/trimethoprim) is used for 3 or more consecutive days to be 12-fold, with the estimated excess risk of of agranulocytosis attributable to the use of co-trimoxazole in a 2-week period to be 1.6 per million (p. 855). The topical use of silver sulfadiazine can cause leukopenia due to the absorption of sulfadiazine, although this effect is usually self-limiting even with continued use of the agent. Leukopenia usually occurs within 2–4 days of commencing sulfadiazine therapy with an estimated frequency of 3–5% (Fraser and Beaulieu, 1979). Usually treatment can be continued if the total leukocyte count is greater than 3000 per cm^2. The sulfapyridine part of sulfasalazine is absorbed (p. 826) and acute agranulocytosis due to this drug has been reported in two patients, both of whom died with septicemia (Thirkettle et al., 1963). Agranulocytosis associated with the use of dapsone in the treatment of dermatitis herpetiformis has been estimated to occur with an increased relative risk of 50-fold, or a total risk of one case per 3000 patient-years of exposure to dapsone (median treatment dose of 100 mg dapsone daily) (Hornsten et al., 1990). Other hematological complications such as hemolytic anemia, alterations in erythrocyte morphology, erythroid hypoplasia and pancytopenia have been described with sulfasalazine. One patient had agranulocytosis, erythroid hypoplasia and bone marrow plasmacytosis due to sulfasalazine (Wheelan et al., 1982).

Fatal aplastic anemia has been attributed to sulfonamides, but less commonly than that due to chloramphenicol. Aplastic anemia and two cases of pure red cell aplasia have been described in association with sulfasalazine therapy (Dunn and Kerr, 1981; Anttila et al., 1985). In the latter case, after recovery from red cell aplasia, the patient was treated with 5-aminosalicylic acid without complications (p. 826).

Acute hemolytic anemia is another rare complication and is sometimes due to prior sensitization to sulfonamides (Weinstein et al., 1960). These drugs can induce hemolysis in patients with glucose-6-phosphate dehydrogenase deficient red cells, producing a 'Heinz body anemia' with intravascular hemolysis and hemoglobinuria. This type of anemia may also occur in the fetus or premature infant whose red cells are normally deficient in glucose-6-phosphate dehydrogenase.

Megaloblastic anemia responding to therapy with folic acid has been described in patients with ulcerative colitis, who were being treated with sulfasalazine (Schneider and Beeley, 1977; Kane and Boots, 1977). Folate deficiency may occur in patients with inflammatory bowel disease and some studies have indicated that sulfasalazine therapy further impairs folate absorption (Halsted et al., 1981). Other investigations suggest that in patients with inactive chronic colitis taking an optimum maintenance dose of 2 g sulfasalazine daily or less, folate deficiency would be rare. However, subclinical tissue depletion could occur with higher doses, particularly if other factors such as deficient dietary intake, severe bowel inflammation, pregnancy, associated hemolysis and small-bowel disease or resection, are present, which increase the likelihood of folate deficiency (Longstreth and Green, 1983).

Thrombocytopenia alone is a rare complication of sulfonamide therapy (Weinstein *et al.*, 1960). In one case induced by sulfisoxazole, an immune mechanism was demonstrated (Hamilton and Sheets, 1978). The patient was a farmer who presumably had become sensitized by drinking cow's milk contaminated by sulfonamides. Thrombocytopenia recurred with a small-challenge dose of sulfisoxazole and a serum factor was detected which caused platelet agglutination in the presence of sulfisoxazole.

Cyanosis due to the formation of either methemoglobin or sulfhemoglobin was fairly common with the earlier sulfonamides, but is now rare with the currently used compounds.

6 Hepatotoxicity

Dujovne *et al.* (1967) reported a patient who developed hepatocellular jaundice after a second course of sulfamethoxazole. The serum transaminase was raised and liver biopsy revealed cell necrosis. Associated eosinophilia suggested hypersensitivity. Liver damage reappeared with a test dose of sulfonamide and the authors noted that the phenomenon had occurred in two other reported cases. They also reviewed 106 cases of sulfonamide hepatotoxicity reported during the preceding 30 years. The majority of these had occurred before 1947, which is probably a reflection of the greater hepatotoxicity of older sulfonamides. There have been a number of case reports of hepatotoxicity associated with sulfasalazine administration (Losek and Werlin, 1981; Smith *et al.*, 1982; Lennard and Farndon, 1983). Losek and Werlin (1981) also reviewed eight previous reports of this complication. Hepatotoxicity appears to be due to sulfapyridine, the major absorbed metabolite of sulfasalazine (p. 826). Associated features commonly include fever, rashes, lymphadenopathy and arthralgia and onset usually after 2–4 weeks latency suggest a hypersensitivity reaction. Liver function tests indicate hepatocellular damage and liver biopsy shows focal inflammation and necrosis. In several patients, features have recurred after challenge with sulfasalazine. Sulfasalazine hypersensitivity may also affect the kidneys and cause pancreatitis and pneumonitis (p. 819). Neurotoxicity, manifested by agitation, confusion, hallucinations and seizures, have also been associated with generalized hypersensitivity reactions in a couple of cases (Smith *et al.*, 1982).

7 Renal damage

Crystalluria causing renal damage is the classic sulfonamide complication which was common with earlier sulfonamides, such as sulfapyridine, because these drugs are excreted in urine in high concentrations, in which the drugs themselves and their acetyl conjugates are relatively insoluble. Crystalluria may cause pain and hematuria, and anuria can occur if the renal pelvis or the ureters become completely occluded. A high fluid intake and alkalinization of urine minimize this side-effect. Currently used short-acting sulfonamides, such as sulfadimidine and sulfafurazole and their acetyl conjugates, are very soluble in urine. Crystalluria and acute renal failure has been particularly described with the use of high-dose sulfadiazine (4–8 g per day) for a number of conditions including the treatment of toxoplasma encephalitis in patients with AIDS (Craft *et al.*, 1977; Arem *et al.*, 1983; Ventura *et al.*, 1989; Simon *et al.*, 1990; Molina *et al.*, 1991). Molina *et al.* (1991) noted an incidence of sulfadiazine-induced crystalluria of 5.4% among their AIDS population treated for cerebral toxoplasmosis during the period 1986–1990. This occurred especially during the first few months of therapy when higher doses of sulfadiazine were often required. Dehydration, with resultant reduced urine output, was an important risk factor. The vast majority of patients respond to urinary alkalinization (since raising the urinary pH from 6.5 to 7.5 allows for a greater than 10-fold increase in sulfadiazine solubility), plus fluid administration, without necessarily discontinuation of sulfadiazine therapy (Fox *et al.*, 1943; Oster *et al.*, 1990). Simon *et al.* (1990), who reported two cases and reviewed the sulfadiazine literature, proposed the following guidelines to avoid sulfadiazine-induced renal toxicity in patients with AIDS:

1. Maintain a fluid intake of >2–3 liters daily;
2. Alkalinize the urine with 6–12 g per day of sodium bicarbonate to maintain urinary pH >7.15
3. Monitor urine for crystalluria and/or hematuria
4. Monitor serum sulfadiazine levels in patients with pre-existing renal insufficiency.

The medium- and long-acting sulfonamides which, being slowly excreted, do not attain high concentrations in the urine, rarely cause crystalluria. Buchanan (1978) reported two patients who developed crystalluria and oliguric renal failure following i.v. co-trimoxazole (sulfamethoxazole/trimethoprim) therapy (p. 857). Both these patients were hypoproteinemic and most of the sulfamethoxazole in their serum was in the free rather than protein bound form. It was postulated that crysalluria ensued secondary to the massive renal load of the free drug. The author recommended that co-trimoxazole should be used with caution in hypoalbuminemic patients. Other forms of renal damage may also occur in association with co-trimoxazole administration (p. 857). Hypersensitivity reactions due to sulfonamide therapy may cause renal damage (p. 815) as may sulfonamide-induced hemolysis and hemoglobinuria (Appel and Neu, 1977). The nephrotic syndrome has been described following topical silver sulfadiazine (SSD) therapy (Owens *et al.*, 1974).

8 Systemic lupus erythematosus and polyarteritis nodosa

Systemic lupus has been observed in patients receiving sulfonamides, particularly the long-acting drugs (Rallison *et al.*, 1961; Alarcon-Segovia, 1969). A lupus-like syndrome has been reported in patients with ulcerative colitis treated with sulfasalazine (Griffiths and Kane, 1977). One such patient developed cardiac tamponade due to lupus-associated effusion (Deboever *et al.*, 1989). The sulfapyridine moiety of sulfasalazine is probably responsible for the lupus syndrome. Polyarteritis nodosa has been reported in patients who had received sulfonamides, but they have a doubtful etiological role in this disease (Rose and Spencer, 1957).

9 Jaundice and kernicterus in the newborn

Sulfonamides compete with a number of substances, including bilirubin, for albumin binding sites. For this reason, infants born to mothers treated with sulfonamides could conceivably develop jaundice with high free serum bilirubin levels or even kernicterus, especially if there is also increased hemolysis. This could also occur in newborn or premature infants treated with sulfonamides. Wadsworth and Suh (1988) investigated 52 antimicrobial agents *in vitro* for their relative bilirubin-displacing activity in pooled cord serum. All seven sulfonamides examined, except sulfamethoxine, revealed high-level bilirubin displacement activity.

10 Cardiomyopathy

This was reported in a 12-year-old African boy, apparently due to sulfonamide hypersensitivity (Macsearraigh and Patel, 1968). A few other cases of apparent sulfonamide-induced 'hypersensitivity myocarditis' have been previously reported (Weinstein *et al.*, 1960).

11 Pulmonary reactions

Pulmonary reactions are associated with the use of a variety of drugs, but such reactions due to sulfonamides are rare (Leading article, 1969; Tydd and Dyer, 1976). Acute syndrome pulmonary eosinophilia usually results, which is characterized by fever, dyspnea, cough, eosinophilia and patchy radiological pulmonary opacities. Symptoms and radiological abnormalities rapidly disappear when the drug is stopped. Sulfasalazine, in addition to this acute syndrome, may produce fibrosing alveolitis or a bronchial asthmatic reaction. Salicylates can also cause pulmonary reactions, and either the salicyclic acid or the sulfonamide component of sulfasalazine may be responsible. The abnormalities again usually disappear when sulfasalazine is stopped (Leading article, 1974b).

12 Teratogenicity

Several sulfonamides can cause fetal abnormalities in experimental animals (Leading article, 1965), but studies of sulfonamide teratogenicity in humans are inconclusive (Sanford, 1993).

13 Infertility

Male infertility is associated with the sulfapyridine component of sulfasalazine, which may result in abnormalities in sperm density and mobility and abnormal sperm morphology (Levi *et al.*, 1979; Toth, 1979). These changes usually revert to normal about 2 months after cessation of sulfasalazine and pregnancy then often ensues in previously infertile couples. Birnie *et al.* (1981) found that 16 of 21 patients taking sulfasalazine for inflammatory bowel disease had abnormalities on examination of their sperm. Cann and Holdsworth (1984) used the other component of sulfasalazine, 5-aminosalicylic acid (p. 826), successfully in one patient with ulcerative colitis without impairment of semen. There may be multiple mechanisms for this complication – toxicity to developing spermatozoa, deficiency in folate, chromium deficiency or an inhibitory effect on prostaglandins E and F (Kirsner and Shorter, 1982).

14 Miscellaneous reactions

Other rare side-effects have been described following sulfonamide administration. Cohen *et al.* (1980) observed a fall in circulating thyroid hormone concentrations in volunteers given co-trimoxazole in standard dosage for 10 days. They suggested that thyroid tests be interpreted cautiously in patients receiving co-trimoxazole and thyroid function should be assessed after long-term treatment. The sulfonamide component of the combination is thought to be responsible for this effect (Cohen *et al.*, 1981). In a study of children receiving continuous low-dose co-trimoxazole for more than a year, however, tests for thyroid hormone levels were normal, (Smellie *et al.*, 1982). Benign intracranial hypertension has also been observed to follow sulfamethoxazole administration in two patients (Ch'ien, 1970). Lisander (1970) reported a patient who on three occasions developed intense myalgia in the arms and legs following the administration of sulfamethoxydiazine. Another patient developed recurrent fever, meningitis, pancreatitis and a leukocytosis in association with administration and re-administration of sulfamethizole (Barrett and Thier, 1963).

Sulfonamides decrease the ability of human neutrophils to kill certain *Candida* spp. and some bacteria, but whether this is of any significance even in patients susceptible to systemic candidiasis is unknown (Lehrer, 1971). In common with other drugs used to treat rheumatoid arthritis, a selective IgA deficiency has been reported with the use of sulfasalazine (Delamere *et al.*, 1983). This has also been noted in children with ulcerative colitis who have received the drug (Savilahti, 1983) – although this does not appear to be clinically relevent since none of these patients had an increased incidence of infections. Sulfasalazine is orange-yellow colored and its use may cause similar coloring of the urine, skin and such items as contact lenses (Riley *et al.*, 1986)

15 Drug interactions

Christensen *et al.* (1963) reported hypoglycemic attacks in several diabetic patients who were treated by both tolbutamide and sulfaphenazole. These patients had greatly increased serum tolbutamide levels and it appeared that sulfaphenazole interfered with oxidation and excretion of tolbutamide. The metabolism by liver microsomal enzymes of other drugs, such as diphenylhydantoin (phenytoin) and warfarin (and tolbutamide), are inhibited by usual therapeutic doses of sulfaphenazole, sulfadiazine and sulfamethizole. Co-trimoxazole also increases the diphenylhydantoin half-life in patients by decreasing its metabolism (Hansen *et al.*, 1975). In contrast, sulfadimethoxine, sulfamethoxypyridazine and sulfamethoxydiazine do not affect phenytoin metabolism.

Reduction in warfarin metabolism associated with concomitant sulfonamide administration may result in potentiation of warfarin-induced anticoagulation (Barnett and Hancock, 1975; Hassall *et al.*, 1975). This often occurs 2–6 days after commencement of sulfa therapy. In some such patients, serum warfarin levels have been found to be low, suggesting that sulfamethoxazole may displace protein bound warfarin, thus increasing both its intrinsic action and its rate of metabolism and excretion. Circumstances in another case also suggested that co-trimoxazole may interact with warfarin by displacing it from its plasma albumin binding sites (Tilstone *et al.*, 1977). These authors considered that co-trimoxazole was not contraindicated in patients receiving warfarin, because this interaction is only likely to occur in patients receiving high warfarin doses and in those who have low plasma albumin concentrations. Subsequently, it was shown that co-trimoxazole causes marked augmentation of warfarin-induced hypoprothrombinemia by a stereoselective interaction of the combination with the levorotatory form of warfarin (O'Reilly and Motley, 1979; O'Reilly, 1980). This causes an increase in the plasma concentration of levorotatory warfarin and a decrease in dextrorotatory warfarin. As levorotatory warfarin is intrinsically more potent than dextrorotatory warfarin, there is a net increase in warfarin activity. Similar interactions occur between warfarin and metronidazole (p. 946). Alcohol can decrease the apparent half-life of sulfadimidine by increasing the amount of its acetylated form in blood and urine. This seems to be due to alcohol increasing the rate of sulfonamide acetylation (p. 814) (Olsen and Mørland, 1978). Experience with five cardiac transplant recipients suggested that i.v. sulfadimidine can cause a marked decrease in serum cyclosporin levels (Wallwork *et al.*, 1983; Jones *et al.*, 1986). Futhermore, concomitant administration of co-trimoxazole and cyclosporin has been associated with an increased incidence of nephrotoxicity, independent of the levels of either drug (Sands and Brown, 1989; p. 859).

Clinical Uses of the Drug

There are now very few specific indications for sulfonamides, because of the wide range of available antibiotics. Emergence of sulfonamide-resistance among many bacterial species has made these drugs unsuitable for the treatment of many diseases, for which they had been used successfully in the past. The combination of sulfonamides with trimethoprim, however, is used for many diseases (p. 860) and the combination of sulfadiazine and pyrimethamine is often used for toxoplasma encephalitis (p. 913). This section describes the clinical use of the sulfonamides alone, or their use in combination with drugs other than trimethoprim (p. 836) or pyrimethamine (p. 905).

1 Urinary tract infections

Sulfonamides alone are often successful for the treatment of acute uncomplicated urinary tract infections due to susceptible pathogens. However, despite their generally low cost, their use for this indication is diminishing due to increasing antibiotic resistance and the availability of effective agents with lower rates of toxicity. Nevertheless, numerous studies have demonstrated the clinical efficacy of sulfonamides in the past (Brumfitt, 1970; Reeves, 1975; Lidin-Janson, 1977; Bergan and Skjerven, 1979). Sulfonamides with medium duration of action (e.g. sulfamethoxazole) are probably preferable to short-acting sulfonamides (e.g. sulfamethizole), although in at least one trial there was no therapeutic difference between these two agents (Bergan and Skjerven, 1979). Similar to other antibiotic agents, single-dose sulfonamide regimens have proved effective for the treatment of acute uncomplicated urinary tract infections (Källenius and Winberg, 1979). Four single-dose regimens: 1 g sulfisoxazole; 2 g sulfisoxazole; trimethoprim 160 mg plus sulfamethoxazole 800 mg or trimethoprim 320 mg plus sulfamethoxazole 1600 mg were given to 117 women with cystitis and resulted in cure rates of 85–95%, with no difference between the regimens (Buckwold et al., 1982). In a review of published studies, Souney and Polk (1982) concluded that sulfisoxazole, trimethoprim/sulfamethoxazole and amoxycillin are all effective as single-dose regimens to treat uncomplicated urinary tract infections in women. Norrby (1990), however, reviewed 28 trials conducted on women with uncomplicated cystitis comparing single-dose or 3-day courses of various antibiotic agents, including regimens which contained sulfamethizole, trimethoprim/sulfamethoxazole and sulfadiazine. With all antibiotic regimens, a single dose was less efficient than a 3-day or ≥5-day treatment in eradicating bacteriuria – although the difference was more pronounced with beta-lactams than trimethoprim-sulfonamide combinations. For these latter combinations no benefits were achieved by increasing the treatment time beyond 5 days. Furthermore, adverse reactions increased markedly for sulfonamide combinations when treatment was given for longer than 3 days (Norrby, 1990). Because the combination of nitrofurantoin (p. 922) and sulfadiazine may be synergistic against some bacteria, it has been used in clinical studies (Reeves et al., 1980). Patients with an acute symptomatic urinary infection received 7 days treatment with either 50 mg nitrofurantoin plus 150 mg sulfadiazine three times daily or 100 mg nitrofurantoin plus 500 mg sulfadiazine three times daily. A cure rate of about 90% was obtained in both groups. Sulfonamides are not usually used for chronic and recurrent infections or in hospital-acquired infections. Furthermore, a randomized trial of meatal care with SSD cream failed to demonstrate any benefit in preventing the development of catheter-associated bacteriuria in short-term catheterized patients (Huth et al., 1992).

2 Respiratory tract infections

These drugs have been used for treatment of Strep. pyogenes throat infections (Alban, 1965), but penicillin G is the drug of choice for these infections and safe, effective alternative antibiotics are available for penicillin-allergic patients. Ampicillin (or amoxycillin) is usually the preferred treatment of otitis media in children, but combinations of a sulfonamide with erythromycin or phenoxymethyl penicillin can be used (Paradise, 1980; Bluestone, 1982). Long-term treatment with sulfisoxazole (75 mg per kg per day for 6 months) was compared with surgical therapy (bilateral insertion of ventilation tubes) for the treatment of chronic otitis media with effusion (otherwise known as serous otitis media or glue ear) in 125 children. Although 67% of the sulfisoxazole-treated group were regarded as treatment failures at 6, 12 and 18 months, the remaining 33% of this group successfully avoided surgery. Since 50% of surgical patients experienced complications after treatment compared with 9% of medical subjects (p < 0.001), the authors recommended a 6-month trial of sulfisoxazole therapy for children with this condition before considering surgical intervention (Bernard et al., 1991). In another trial, sulfisoxazole suspension in a dose of 0.5 g twice-daily proved effective in the prevention of recurrent otitis media in children (Perrin et al., 1974). Liston et al. (1983) also used sulfisoxazole for this purpose; the regimen was 75 mg per kg per day in two divided doses for 3 months. There was a 40% reduction in the rate of otitis media among children receiving sulfisoxazole compared with those receiving placebo. Similar results were obtained by Varsano et al. (1985). Sulfonamides have been used for treatment of pneumococcal pneumonia and other lower respiratory tract bacterial infections, but safer and more effective drugs are available. Sulfonamides are useful for the treatment of some mycobacterial infections (p. 1216).

3 Rheumatic fever chemoprophylaxis

Sulfonamides have been used for this purpose as alternatives to penicillin for penicillin-allergic patients, however, erythromycin (p. 617) is probably a better alternative. Although, the American Heart Association once recommended sulfadiazine 1 g daily as an alternative to penicillin (p. 51) for this purpose (Leading article, 1977), sulfonamides may be unreliable, since sulfonamide-resistant *Strep. pyogenes* strains can emerge.

4 Meningococcal infections

Formerly, sulfonamides were extensively and successfully used for the treatment of meningococcal meningitis and septicemia, for prevention of meningococcal disease in contacts and for eradication of the chronic meningococcal carrier state. Since sulfonamide-resistant meningococci are now common (p. 808) these drugs are usually no longer suitable for these clinical situations (Lennon *et al.*, 1989). Ampicillin, penicillin, chloramphenicol and the third-generation cephalosporins, such as cefotaxime or ceftriaxone, are very effective for these infections. The use of parenteral penicillin G is also probably effective for the prevention of meningococcal disease in contacts, but oral phenoxypenicillin may be ineffective for this purpose (Holten *et al.*, 1970). In general, however, these antibiotics do not achieve sufficiently high concentrations in nasopharygeal secretions to reliably eradicate meningococcal carriage. None of the currently available antibiotics, except perhaps rifampicin (p. 697), minocycline (p. 744), or ciprofloxacin (p. 1028) are as effective in eradicating the nasopharyngeal meningococcal carrier state as the sulfonamides were in the past (Leedom *et al.*, 1965, 1967; Holten *et al.*, 1970). Rifampicin is currently recommended as the chemoprophylactic agent of choice for meningococcal infections in the USA (p. 697), although it will fail to eradicate meningococcus in 10–20% of carriers (Guttler *et al.*, 1971; Kaiser *et al.*, 1974). Minocycline is often avoided because of its associated high incidence of vestibular toxicity and the fact that it is contraindicated in children (p. 736). In some circumstances, such as the localized epidemic of serogroup B sulfonamide-sensitive meningococcal disease which occurred in Alabama during 1975–1976, chemoprophylaxis with sulfonamides can be used with effect (Jacobson *et al.*, 1977). The dose of sulfadiazine for chemoprophylaxis is 1 g twice-daily for adults, 0.5 g twice-daily for children 1–12 years of age, and 0.5 g once-daily for children less than 1 year of age. Treatment is continued for 2 days (CDC, 1981).

5 Bacterial meningitis other than meningococcal

Although the sulfonamides have been combined with chloramphenicol for the treatment of *H. influenzae* meningitis, and occasionally with penicillin G for the treatment of pneumococcal meningitis, there is no evidence that the sulfonamide contributes to the therapeutic success of such treatment. Sulfisoxazole has been used with streptomycin to treat *H. influenzae* meningitis successfully. Although erythromycin/sulfonamide combinations are effective in otitis media (which is often caused by *H. influenzae*) (p. 617), this combination is ineffective in eradicating *H. influenzae* type b from the throat of children who are carriers (Horner *et al.*, 1980). Rifampicin (p. 698) is the preferred chemoprophylaxis for contacts of patients with *H. influenzae* meningitis.

6 Gastrointestinal infections

Both the non-absorbed sulfonamides, such as sulfaguanidine, and the well-absorbed short-acting sulfonamides (e.g. sulfadiazine or sulfadimidine) have been used extensively in the past for treatment of shigella dysentery. These drugs are now rarely useful alone for this disease due to increasing sulfonamide resistance. Resistance to co-trimoxazole, one of the drugs of choice in the treatment of shigellosis, is now common among *Shigella dysentariae* type 1 strains in Africa and Asia, and is increasing in other *Shigella* species, including *S. sonnei*, in the USA and elsewhere (Salam and Bennish, 1991). Sulfonamides have never been useful for treatment of salmonellosis.

The long-acting sulfonamide, sulfadoxine, in a single oral dose of 0.5–2.0 g (according to the patient's age) has been compared with treatment with oral tetracycline 0.25–0.5 g (according to age) 12-hourly for 3 days to reduce transmission of cholera infection among contacts of cholera patients (Deb *et al.*, 1976). Tetracycline was effective in significantly reducing the number of infections from the 2nd to the 6th day, while sulfadoxine was effective from the 3rd to the 6th day after treatment. However, increasing antibiotic resistance among this species is notable. Sulfadimethoxine appears to have some anticryptosporidial activity in one study using a rat model of intestinal cryptosporidiosis, however, the applicability of this data to clinical cryptosporidiosis in humans is uncertain (Rehg *et al.*, 1988).

7 Chlamydial infections

Chlamydia trachomatis and *Ureaplasma urealyticum* are important causes of non-specific (non-gonococcal) urethritis. A number of studies have shown eradication of *C. trachomatis* from both the male urethra and female cervix by a variety of sulfonamides, including sulfisoxazole, sulfamethoxazole and sufafurazole (Bowie *et al*, 1976; Handsfield *et al*., 1976; Johannisson *et al*., 1980; Bowie *et al*., 1982; Stamm *et al*., 1984). Notably, however, Bowie *et al*. (1976) showed that non-gonococcal urethritis caused by *C. trachomatis* responds better to sulfafurazole than that due to *U. urealyticum*, for which sulfonamides are relatively inactive. Conversely, non-gonococcal urethritis due to *U. urealyticum* responds to the aminocyclitols, streptomycin (p. 435) and spectinomycin (p. 717), which are relatively inactive against *C. trachomatis*. A dose of 0.5 g sulfafurazole (sulfisoxazole) four times daily for 10 days was effective for non-specific urethritis in the study by Schachter (1978), but more recent studies of 3–5 day regimens of co-trimoxazole for the treatment of simultaneous infection with *C. trachomatis* and *N. gonorrhoeae* have been notably less successful (Stamm *et al*., 1984; Csangó *et al*., 1984). The treatment of *C. trachomatis* genital infections has been reviewed by Toomey and Barnes (1990). Doxycycline (p. 745), azithromycin (p. 658) or erythromycin are the recommended drugs for uncomplicated urethral, endocervical or rectal *C. trachomatis* infections for adults, with sulfisoxazole 500 mg four times daily for 10 days listed as an inferior alternative by CDC (1993a). Both erythromycin and sulfisoxazole are effective for the treatment of chlamydial pneumonia in infancy (Beem *et al*., 1979), but erythromycin is recommended for this infection (CDC, 1993a). Sulfonamides are effective for the treatment of lymphogranuloma venereum (Willcox, 1977), but doxycycline is preferred (CDC, 1993a). Sulfisoxazole 500 mg four times daily for 21 days is recommended as an alternative treatment to doxycycline (CDC, 1993a). Psittacosis does not respond to sulfonamide therapy. For treatment of trachoma, topical tetracycline or rifampicin eye ointment three times daily for 5 or 6 weeks is usually preferred to topical sulfonamides.

8 Chancroid

Sulfonamide-resistance among strains of *H. ducreyi* is now sufficiently common as to argue against the use of these agents for this disease (Dangor *et al*., 1990; Plourde *et al*., 1992; CDC, 1993a). Rates of resistance to the combination of trimethoprim-sulfamethoxazole (co-trimoxazole, Co-T) vary according to geographical location, but appear to be high in many parts of Africa and the USA (Dangor *et al*., 1990; Plourde *et al*., 1992). Plourde *et al*. (1992) described a 30% rate of culture-proven failure in Co-T-treated versus 3% failure with fleroxacin for the treatment of chancroid in Nairobi. CDC (1993a) no longer recommends Co-T for the treatment of chancroid, but instead suggests azithromycin, ceftriaxone or erythromycin; or as alternative regimens: amoxycillin/clavulanic acid or ciprofloxacin. Sulfonamides are not effective for granuloma inguinale.

9 Nocardiosis

Various drugs have been reported to be effective *in vitro* against the *Nocardia* spp., but these findings correlate variably with clinical results. Sulfonamides remain one of the drugs of choice for nocardiosis, but successful therapy generally requires prolonged treatment with a combination of sulfonamide plus other active agents such as trimethoprim, a second- or third-generation cephalosporin (e.g. cefuroxime or cefotaxime, respectively, imipenem (p. 238), amikacin (p. 515) or minocycline (p. 743) (Orfanakis *et al*., 1972; Berd, 1973; Idriss *et al*., 1975; Krick *et al*., 1975; Kim *et al*., 1991). Many authors now regard trimethoprim–sulfamethoxazole (co-trimoxazole) to be the drug of choice for this infection (Gombert, 1982; p. 871).

10 Toxoplasmosis

In the immunocompetent host, systemic toxoplasmosis does not generally require treatment (McCabe *et al*., 1987). In such patients, infection is usually asymptomatic, often with lymphadenopathy around the head and neck, despite the usual wide dissemination of toxoplasma during acute acquired infection. McCabe *et al*. (1987) reviewed the clinical spectrum of 107 cases of toxoplasma lymphadenopathy and found that the vast majority had no systemic symptoms, no extranodal disease and ran a benign clinical course. Occasionally extranodal involvement occurred, including myocarditis, pneumonitis, encephalitis, chorioretinitis and maternal–fetal transmission, which required treatment in some cases. Central nervous system toxoplasmosis which is commonly due to disease reactivation, rather than acute acquired infection, is often associated with AIDS and other immunocompromising conditions and demands treatment. Sulfonamides, especially the short-acting agent, sulfadiazine, is frequently used in combination with pyrimethamine as the treatment of choice for serious toxoplasma disease (Roth *et al.*, 1971; Mahmoud and Warren, 1977; Luft *et al.*, 1984; p. 913). In this situation sulfadiazine 1–1.5 g four times daily, plus pyrimethamine 100 mg loading dose and then 25 mg daily is generally recommended. A broader discussion of therapy for toxoplasmosis is found in the section covering pyrimethamine (p. 913). A combination of pyrimethamine (25 mg) and sulfadoxine (500 mg) in 'Fansidar' tablets has been used in pregnant women with serological evidence of toxoplasmosis. The usual dose was two tablets weekly for periods of 4–24 weeks. No side-effects were observed and a satisfactory therapeutic effect was considered to be achieved because of a good outcome of pregnancy, and a reduction of toxoplasma antibody titers in the patients (Barbosa and Ferreira, 1978). It has not been established whether co-trimoxazole (p. 874) is effective in toxoplasmosis and most authors do not advocate its use for the treatment of serious disesase (Emerson *et al.*, 1981).

11 Malaria

Historically, Fairley and his co-workers in Cairns, Australia, demonstrated during World War II that sulfonamides have an action upon malarial parasites, and that these drugs are more effective against *P. falciparum* than *P. vivax* infections (Fairley, 1945). It is now known that sulfonamides potentiate the action of pyrimethamine on malarial parasites. McGregor *et al.* (1963) reported that this combination was effective for the treatment of falciparum malaria, which was resistant to pyrimethamine alone. Laing (1964) used the ultra-long-acting sulfonamide, sulfadoxine (then known as sulformethoxine), in field trials in Africa. He found that this drug used by itself in a weekly dose of 0.5 g was just as effective as a schizonticide as when given together with 25 mg pyrimethamine weekly. At that time it was suggested that this sulfonamide may be mainly useful as a suppressive, because its action would be too slow for the treatment of falciparum malaria.

Strains of *P. falciparum* resistant to chloroquine are now widespread in parts of Asia and Oceania over an area extending from central and southern India to Vanuatu, South America and East Africa (Report, 1984; CDC, 1993b). Treatment recommendations for *P. falciparum* acquired from these areas include a combined regimen of quinine plus the long-acting sulfonamide (sulfadoxine)–pyrimethamine combination of 'Fansidar'. 'Fansidar' tablets each contain sulfadoxine 0.5 g and primethamine 25 g. Ampoules (2.5ml) containing 0.5g sulfadoxine and 25 mg pyrimethamine are also available for i.m. administration. One recommended regimen for the treatment of chloroquine-resistant falciparum malaria in adults, particularly presumptive self-treatment, is sulfadoxine (or sulfalene) 15 g plus pyrimethamine 75 mg (3 'Fansidar' tablets) as a single dose (CDC, 1993b), although therapeutic failures of this regimen have been reported (CDC, 1989). However, many physicians give 'Fansidar' after (usually on day 3) administering quinine 600 mg 8-hourly for 3–7 days (10 days if South-East Asia) (Report, 1984; Sanford, 1993; Victorian Drug Usage Advisory Committee, 1994). The corresponding children's doses for presumptive treatment with 'Fansidar' are (pediatric dose weight in kg: number of tablets): 5–10 kg: 0.5 tablet; 11–20 kg: 1 tablet; 21–30 kg: 1.5 tablets; 31–45 kg: 2 tablets; >45 kg: 3 tablets (CDC, 1993b). Treatment with 'Fansidar' alone does not provide a 100% cure rate, even if the parasites are fully sensitive; 10–20% of individuals do not respond, because of vomiting or diarrhea or because of the way they metabolize or eliminate sulfonamides (Report, 1984). Salako *et al.* (1990) have suggested that intramuscular 'Fansidar' results in a similar rate of parasitological cure as the oral preparation when both are given alone for malaria acquired in Nigeria, but that the parenteral preparation was better tolerated. Nevertheless, the oral preparation remains the most popular method of 'Fansidar' administration. 'Fansidar' has not been recommended in pregnancy, because of the possibility of teratogenicity. The regimen of quinine and 'Fansidar' results in a very high cure rate, although some authors have questioned whether, at least in Kenya, this combination is significantly better than quinine alone (Newton *et al.*, 1993). Nevertheless, in Africa, a single i.m. dose of 'Fansidar' may be a suitable alternative to quinine if medical facilities are limited (Simão *et al.*, 1991).

Treatment and prophylaxis with the combination of sulfadoxine–pyrimethamine + mefloquine ('Fansimef') has been successful in many parts of the world, and although resistance has been noted on the Thai-Burmese border and some authors no longer recommend the combination (Nosten *et al.*, 1987), others support its use (Anh *et al.*, 1990; Stürchler *et al.*, 1991; Salako *et al.*, 1992).

Unfortunately 'Fansidar'-resistant *P. falciparum* has now been described in a number of areas, including Thailand and surrounding countries, Vietnam, Burma, Sabah, Papua New Guinea, parts of South America, Africa, including the border region of Kenya–Tanzania (Herzog *et al.*, 1983; Sabchareon *et al.*, 1985; Noel and Morisset, 1986; Ibrahim *et al.*, 1991). In Thailand levels of antifolate-resistance approach 100% (Brown, 1993). Alternative treatment regimens for malaria from these regions include quinine in combination with either doxycycline (100 mg twice-daily for 7 days) or clindamycin (450 mg four times daily for 3 days); mefloquine alone (25 mg per kg) as a single dose or 750 mg immediately followed by 500 mg in 6–8 h; or halofantrine alone (500mg at 0, 6 and 12 h; 25 mg per kg total dose) (Sanford, 1993; CDC, 1990, 1993b) (p. 749).

'Fansidar' is an effective chemosuppressant drug against chloroqine-resistant, 'Fansidar'-sensitive *P. falciparum* strains, being more effective than dapsone–pyrimethamine combinations (Pearlman *et al.*, 1977). *P. vivax* is inherently less sensitive than *P. falciparum* to sulfadoxine, which may explain the disappointing results obtained when 'Fansidar' is used for prophylaxis against pyrimethamine-resistant *P. vivax*. For this reason, when using 'Fansidar' for malaria prophylaxis, appropriate protection against *P. vivax*, *P. ovale* or *P. malariae* requires the combination of 'Fansidar' with a 4-aminoquinolines (chloroquine or amodiaquine) – the usual adult dose being one 'Fansidar' tablet plus chloroquine 300 mg (two tablets) once-weekly (Herwaldt *et al*, 1988). With this regimen, the steady-state serum levels are usually reached by beginning prophylaxis 1–2 weeks before exposure to infection. This also allows time to identify individuals who cannot tolerate sulfonamides. The weekly doses for children are one-eighth of a tablet for those aged 2–11 months, one-quarter of a tablet for those aged 1–3 years, half a tablet for those aged 4–8 years and three-quarters of a tablet for those aged 9–14 years. Prophylaxis with 'Fansidar' for periods up to 2 years has been well tolerated, but it is advisable to perform leukoycte counts every 6 months (Report, 1984; Herwaldt *et al.*, 1988). Studies in the mid-1980s suggested that travellers to Kenya who used a chloroquine-'Fansidar' regimen were six times less likely to acquire *P. falciparum* infections than travellers who used chloroquine alone, and ten times less likely than those who used no prophylaxis (Lobel *et al.*, 1987). However, failures of chloroquine-'Fansidar' chemoprophylaxis have been reported more recently in areas with probable 'Fansidar'-resistant *P. falciparum* such as East Africa and rural Thailand (Herzog *et al.*, 1983; Sabcharoen *et al.*, 1985; Noel and Morisset, 1986; CDC, 1986; Miller *et al.*, 1986a).

In addition to this evidence of 'Fansidar'-failure in some regions, the primary issue which has led to 'Fansidar' no longer being routinely recommended for chemoprophylaxis is its association with fatal cutaneous reactions (erythema multiforme, Stevens–Johnson syndrome or toxic epidermal necrolysis) (Miller *et al.*, 1986b; Pearson and Hewlett, 1987; Herwaldt *et al.*, 1988). Twenty-four patients with cutaneous reactions (incuding seven deaths) have been reported among US travellers and data from CDC suggests that the incidence of fatal cutaneous reactions with prophylactic use of 'Fansidar' is 1 in 11 000 to 1 in 25 000 users (Miller *et al.*, 1986b). Initially this relatively high rate of fatal reactions was considered to be primarily associated with multiple weekly doses and/or the simultaneous administration of chloroquine. However, non-fatal Stevens–Johnson syndrome has been described in at least two patients after single doses of 'Fansidar' and severe cutaneous reactions have occurred in the UK and Scandinavia associated with 'Fansidar' alone without chloroquine (Miller *et al.*, 1986b; Rombo *et al.*, 1985). Severe cutaneous reactions have also been associated with the administration of sulfadoxine alone at doses higher than those found in 'Fansidar' (Taylor, 1968; Hernborg, 1985). In the event of such reactions, the traveler should be advised to discontinue 'Fansidar' immediately.

The combination of dapsone 100 mg + pyrimethamine 12.5 mg ('Maloprim') has been used for malaria prophylaxis, although due to its lack of efficacy against *P. vivax* it has been generally given in combination with chloroquine. However, due to increasing 'Maloprim'-resistance and reports of clinical failures, the lack of a pediatric preparation, and potential toxicities including agranulocytosis and methemoglobinemia (p. 911) it is no longer recommended (Edstein *et al.*, 1988; Shanks *et al.*, 1992; CDC, 1993b; Brown, 1993). 'Maloprim' has no role in the treatment of malaria.

Currently recommended regimens for prophylaxis against chloroquine-resistant *P. falciparum* include: doxycycline 100 mg orally daily (2 mg per kg body weight for children over 8 years of age; not for use in children aged less than 8 years and pregnant women) or mefloquine 250 mg once per week (Brown, 1993; CDC, 1993b, WHO, 1993).

12 Pneumocystis carinii pneumonia

Sulfonamides are active against *P. carinii* in experimental disease in rats (p. 807) and clinically in humans. Co-trimoxazole (trimethoprim–sulfamethoxazole) is the drug of choice for both treatment and prophylaxis against *P. carinii* pneumonia in all immunocompromised patients, including those with AIDS (p. 874). There is an increased incidence of side-effects among patients with HIV infection who are treated with co-trimoxazole (p. 854). Sulfadiazine with pyrimethamine are effective in the treatment and prophylaxis of *P. carinii* pneumonia both in experimental animals and humans. Kirby *et al.* (1971) obtained a satisfactory clinical response when it was used in courses lasting 10–28 days to treat three patients with *P. carinii* pneumonia. A combination of sulfadoxine and pyrimethamine was effective in a small trial to prevent *P. carinii* infection in an orphanage. Treatment at least twice-monthly was recommended for all babies between the ages of 2 and 6 months, who were at risk from this infection (Post *et al.*, 1971). Prophylaxis with 'Fansidar' (p. 879; Table II.4) has been used in AIDS patients (Gottlieb *et al.*, 1984), but generally other regimens are preferred due to concerns regarding the long half-life of sulfadoxine and therefore the potential for severe complications should cutaneous reactions occur (p. 816). Patients who develop side-effects to shorter-acting sulfonamides should therefore avoid sulfadoxine.

13 Ulcerative colitis and Crohn's disease

Sulfasalazine was designed and synthesized in the 1930s as a means of achieving site-specific drug delivery for the treatment of rheumatoid arthritis. The theory was that the 5-aminosalicylic acid component would bind to connective tissue and therefore deliver sulphapyridine to the site of disease and eliminate the bacteria that were considered to be causing the disease (Svartz, 1942, 1948; Editorial, 1987). However, the drug was fortuitously used in a patient with concomitant ulcerative colitis and has subsequently become the mainstay of treating ulcerative colitis (Baron *et al.*, 1962; Leading article, 1986; Editorial, 1987). Since sulfasalazine is poorly absorbed large amounts of active drug (5-aminosalicylic acid) are delivered to the site of inflammation. It is better than placebo in the treatment of mild-moderate active ulcerative colitis and in maintaining remission after an acute attack in adults and children (Gryboski and Hillemeier, 1980; Singleton, 1980; Kirsner and Shorter, 1982; Peppercorn, 1984; Leading article, 1986). In these settings the beneficial effects are dose-related. Sulfasalazine enemas (3 g per day) are effective in the treatment of active distal disease and appear to be as effective as the oral preparation, although the serum concentration of sulfapyridine is not generally greater than 15 μg per ml (Leading article, 1986). Sulfasalazine enemas are particularly useful for patients who suffer nausea, abdominal discomfort or headaches when taking oral sulfasalazine (Serebro *et al.*, 1977; Palmer *et al.*, 1981). Paradoxically, there have been reports of patients in whom oral sulfasalazine has caused an exacerbation of their disease (Schwartz *et al.*, 1982). Sulfasalazine is also better than placebo for the treatment of active colonic Crohn's disease, but its role in active ileal disease is less clear (Leading article, 1986). Furthermore, it does not appear that sulfasalazine maintains remission of inactive Crohn's disease, or after gastrointestinal resection (Summers *et al.*, 1979; Malchow *et al.*, 1984). Sulfasalazine in combination with prednisolone is more effective than sulfasalazine alone in the treatment of active Crohn's disease in terms of faster initial improvement, but there appears to be little difference in disease activity between the two regimens after 16 weeks treatment (Rijk *et al.*, 1991).

The pharmacokinetics of sulfasalazine have been reviewed by Peppercorn (1984). One-quarter to one-third of an oral dose is absorbed in the upper gastrointestinal tract and the drug is detectable in the blood 1–2 h later. Steady-state serum levels are achieved in 24 h. About 10% of the total oral dose is excreted unchanged in the urine. The remainder of absorbed sulfasalazine is excreted unchanged in the bile and, together with the non-absorbed portion of the drug, reaches the distal small intestine and colon. The drug is then split into its two components, 5-aminosalicylate and sulfapyridine, by intestinal bacteria mainly in the colon. Most sulfapyridine is then absorbed and appears in the blood 3–5 h after oral administration where the level varies according to the acetylator status of the patient (p. 814); it is then excreted in the urine either as the free drug or its metabolites. In contrast, 5-aminosalicylate tends to remain in the colon and is excreted unchanged in the feces. However, some is also found in the acetylated form due to gut wall as well as systemic acetylation. Sulfasalazine and its metabolites reach the fetus in concentrations not greatly different from those in the maternal serum, but these concentrations are much less in breast milk (Azad Khan and Truelove, 1979).

The active moiety of sulfasalazine is 5-aminosalicylate and the parent drug only acts as a vehicle for its delivery to distal disease sites in the bowel (Azad Khan *et al.* 1977; Van Hees *et al.*, 1978; Klotz *et al.*, 1980). Additionally, Campieri *et al.* (1981) showed that treatment with 5-aminosalicylic acid 4 g daily given by retention enema was superior to similar treatment with hydrocortisone 100 mg daily. Resin coated tablets containing 5-aminosalicylic acid are now available commercially, which after oral administration remain intact until they reach the colon. The mechanism by which 5-aminosalicylic acid (generic name mesalazine) is beneficial in inflammatory bowel disease remains unclear (Peppercorn, 1984). It has been combined with carrier agents other than sulfapyridine, including the combination of two molecules of mesalazine together (olsalazine). All these preparations (e.g. olsalazine, ipsalazide, balsalazide) deliver 40–60% of available mesalazine to the feces and appear to have a similar therapeutic response, but without the toxicity, including male infertility (Editorial, 1987; Raimundo et al., 1991).

For adults, a dose of 4 g daily is the maximum tolerated by many patients, but a few will tolerate and respond better to doses of 6 g per day. Similarly, some patients tolerate and respond to a higher maintenance dose than 2 g per day (Peppercorn, 1984). The side-effects of sulfasalazine include those of the sulfonamide and those peculiar to sulfasalazine. Apart from the side-effects described in preceding sections, sulfasalazine can also cause an increased heart rate and a bluish skin discoloration; the anionic exchange resin cholestyramine and antibiotics may prevent the breakdown in the gut of sulfasalazine, while sulfasalazine can interfere with the bioavailability of digoxin (Peppercorn, 1984). The common side-effects of sulfasalazine are nausea, vomiting, anorexia and headache; heart-burn, epigastric distress and diarrhea occasionally occur. Common side-effects are directly related to the serum sulfapyridine level and tend to occur in patients receiving 4 g or more per day (Cowan et al., 1977). Most patients, whose ulcerative colitis is maintained in remission, have a serum sulfapyridine concentration greater than 20 μg per ml (Cowan et al., 1977). This level was achieved in rapid acetylators by doses of 3.0–4.0 g sulfasalazine daily, whereas slow acetylators are likely to suffer side-effects at this dosage, because their serum sulfapyridine concentration will rise to over 50 μg per ml. These authors suggested that slow acetylators of sulfapyridine should only be given 2.5–3.0 g of sulfasalazine daily. Studies in 15 children suggest that a dose of 40–70 mg per kg body weight per day can be safely administered; this usually produces serum sulfapyridine levels < 50 μg per ml and a therapeutic response (Goldstein et al., 1979).

Sulfasalazine is an effective drug for treatment of rheumatoid arthritis (Neumann et al., 1983; Pullar et al., 1983; Van der Heijde et al., 1989; Nuver-Zwart et al., 1989) and in this disease sulfapyridine seems to be the active moiety (Pullar et al., 1985). In a double-blind randomized trial comparing the outcome of treatment with sulfasalazine vs hydroxychloroquine in patients with rheumatoid arthritis, sulfasalazine resulted in a clinical response 8 weeks earlier than in the hydroxychloroquine-treated group, although the overall effect at 48 weeks was not significantly different (Nuver-Zwart et al., 1989). Radiographic evidence of erosions was significantly less in the sulfasalazine-treated group after both 24 and 48 weeks of treatment (Van der Heijde et al., 1989). It has been used with success in radiation bowel disease, scleroderma and dermatitis herpetiformis (Peppercorn, 1984).

14 Burns

Certain sulfonamides, applied topically, are of benefit in the management of burns. Mafenide ('Sulfamylon') was used in Germany for the topical therapy of war wounds in the 1940s. Because this topical therapy was effective in suppressing Ps. aeruginosa infection in burned rats, it was used with similar results for the treatment of burns in humans (Lindberg et al., 1965). Many studies have since confirmed that an 11.2% cream of mafenide can significantly reduce sepsis in burned patients (Lowbury et al., 1971; Pegg, 1972). These applications are usually painful and mafenide is absorbed through burned areas. Mafenide and its breakdown products are strong acids and also carbonic anhydrase inhibitors, so that if large quantities of the drug are used, a metabolic acidosis may result, but this is usually compensated for by hyperventilation (Pegg, 1972). Silver nitrate in a 0.5% solution was another popular topical application for burned patients (Lowbury et al., 1971).

The topical use of the compound silver sulfadiazine (SSD; p. 807) has also been very effective for the prevention and treatment of sepsis in burn wounds (Stanford et al., 1969; Lowbury et al., 1971; McDougall, 1972; Sawhney et al., 1989; Monafo and West, 1990; Masterton, 1992). This drug has been used extensively at the Royal Children's Hospital, Melbourne, since 1970, and after 1971 has been combined with 0.2% chlorhexidine. As a result, the incidence of sepsis due to Gram-negative organisms and also that due to Staph. aureus has been considerably reduced (Clarke, 1975). Sawhney et al. (1989) found that while Staph. aureus had been the predominant surface organism isolated from burns patients treated with 1% SSD cream in the early 1980s, Pseudomonas and Klebsiella species became more commonly isolated from such patients in the late 1980s. They found that the incidence of invasive infection and overall mortality was significantly reduced with the use SSD cream. Controlled trials have indicated that 0.5% silver nitrate compresses, 1% SSD cream, and a cream containing 0.5% silver nitrate and 0.2% chlorhexidine digluconate, are all about equally effective in protecting burns from infection. Silver nitrate was, however, less active than the other two preparations against less common Gram-negative bacilli (Lowbury et al., 1976). In one burns unit, sulfonamide-resistant Gram-negative bacilli became predominant during a trial of SSD cream, and the effectiveness of the preparation was reduced such that it became necessary to suspend SSD usage and replace it with silver nitrate and chlorhexidine cream (Lowbury *et al.*, 1976; Bridges and Lowbury, 1977). In another burns unit, *in vitro* tests suggested that extensive use of parenteral gentamicin and replacement of topical mafenide ointments by SSD cream favored the emergence of *Providencia stuartii* over *Ps. aeruginosa* as the predominant colonizing organism (Wenzel *et al.*, 1976). Significant quantities of silver can be absorbed through severe burns treated with SSD cream, but no detrimental effects of high tissue levels have been clearly identified (Wan *et al.*, 1991; Coombs *et al.*, 1992). Current recommendations for the initial care of uninfected burns include either SSD cream (Masterton, 1992), 5% mafenide acetate cream or 0.5% silver nitrate soaks (Sanford, 1993).

15 Umbilical cord care

Silver sulfadiazine cream has been compared with washing with castile soap and triple dye for controlling neonatal bacterial colonization. Triple dye and SSD inhibited bacterial colonization, the former being better for *Staph. aureus*, but SSD was superior in inhibiting Group B streptococci and Gram-negative organisms (Speck *et al.*, 1977).

16 Chronic granulomatous disease

Johnston *et al.* (1975) noted a decrease in the frequency and severity of bacterial infections in four of five children with chronic granulomatous disease, on long-term sulfonamide therapy, which was out of proportion to the anticipated antibacterial effect of the drug. The killing of sulfisoxazole-resistant *E. coli* and *Staph. aureus* by leukocytes of patients with this disease was enhanced in the presence of the sulfonamide. The explanation for this effect of sulfonamides is unknown. Long-term treatment of chronic granulomatous disease with sulfisoxazole or particularly co-trimoxazole has given good results (Van Der Meer and Van den Broek, 1984; Margolis *et al.*, 1990; p. 883).

17 Dermatitis herpetiformis

Prolonged administration of sulfapyridine or the long-acting sulfonamide sulfamethoxypyridazine may be useful for the control of this disease. Sulfapyridine is generally started at 500 mg four times daily and gradually increased to a total of 4–5 g daily. The chemically related drugs, the sulfones (p. 693), such as dapsone (25–50 mg daily initially, increasing to 200 mg daily in some patients), appear to be more effective. For many years sulfapyridine or dapsone were the mainstays of therapy. It is now apparent that the strict adherence to a gluten-free diet will often reduce the need for such treatment and in some cases allow cessation of medication (Katz *et al.*, 1980; Leonard and Fry, 1991). These drugs are also useful for bullous pemphigoid and chronic bullous dermatosis of childhood (Ahmed and Moy, 1982). The mechanism of action of sulfonamides and sulfones in these diseases is unknown.

References

Abbott JD, Graves JFR (1972). Serotype and sulphonamide sensitivity of meningococci isolated from 1966 to 1971. *J Clin Path* **25**: 528.

Adam WR, Dawborn JK (1970). Urinary excretion and plasma levels of sulphonamides in patients with renal impairment. *Aust Ann Med* **19**: 250.

Adam WR, Brown DJ, Hales P, Dawborn JK (1973). The use of sulphadimidine (sulphamethazine) in patients with renal failure. *Med J Aust* **1**: 936.

Ahmed AR, Moy R (1982). Chronic bullous dermatosis of childhood Linear IgA bullous dermatosis. *Amer J Dis Child* **136**: 214.

Ahn CH, Wallace RJ Jr, Steele LC, Murphy DT (1987). Sulfonamide-containing regimens for disease caused by rifampin-resistant *Mycobacterium Kansasii*. *Am Rev Respir Dis* **135**: 10.

Alarcon-Segovia D (1969). Drug-induced lupus syndrome. *Mayo Clin Proc* **44**: 664.

Alban J (1965). Treatment of B-haemolytic streptococcal infection. A study of the pediatric use of sulfamethoxazole. *Amer J Dis Child* **109**: 304.

Albritton WL, Brunton JL, Slaney L, Maclean I (1982). Plasmid-mediated sulfonamide resistance in *Haemophilus ducreyi*. *Antimicrob Ag Chemother* **21**: 159.

Andersen BM, Solberg O, Holten E (1987). Endotoxin release from invasive meningococci related to sulfonamide resistance, serogroup and serotype. *Scand J Infect Dis* **19**: 43.

Anh TK, Kim NV, Arnold K *et al.* (1990). Double-blind studies with mefloquine alone and in combination with sulfadoxine-pyrimethamine in 120 adults and 120 children with falciparum malaria in Vietnam. *Trans Roy Soc Trop Med Hyg* **84**: 50.

Anttila PM, Välimäki M, Pentikäinen PJ (1985). Pure-red-cell aplasia associated with sulphasalazine but not 5-aminosalicylic acid. *Lancet* **ii**: 1006.

Appel GB, Neu HC (1977). The nephrotoxicity of antimicrobial agents (third of three parts). *New Engl J Med* **196**: 784.

Arem R, Garber AJ, Field JB (1983). Sulfonamide-induced hyopglycemia in chronic renal failure. *Arch Intern Med* **143**: 827.

Azad Khan AK, Truelove SC (1979). Placental and mammary transfer of sulphasalazine. *Brit Med J* **2**: 1553.

Azad Khan AK, Piris J, Truelove SC (1977). An experiment to determine the active therapeutic moiety of sulphasalazine. *Lancet* **ii**: 892.

Bach MC, Sabath LD, Finland M (1973). Susceptibility of *Nocardia asteroides* to 45 antimicrobial agents *in vitro*. *Antimicrob Ag Chemother* **3**: 1.

Band JD, Chamberland ME, Platt T *et al.* (1983). Trends in meningococcal disease in the United States, 1975–1980. *J Infect Dis* **148**: 754.

Bannatyne RM, Cheung R (1978). Susceptibility of *Haemophilus influenzae* type b to rifampicin and sulfisoxazole. *Antimicrob Ag Chemother* **13**: 969.

Barbosa JC, Ferreira I (1978). Sulfadoxine-pyrimethamine (Fansidar). in pregnant women with toxoplasma antibody titres In *Current Chemotherapy: Proceedings of the 10th International Congress of Chemotherapy, Zurich/Switzerland, 1977* (Siegenthaler W, Lüthy R, eds) p. 134. Washington DC: American Society for Microbiology.

Barnett DB, Hancock BW (1975). Anticoagulant resistance: an unusual case. *Brit Med J* **1**: 608.

Baron JH, Connell AM, Lennard-Jones JE, Avery Jones F (1962). Sulphasalazine and salicylazosulphadimidine in ulcerative colitis. *Lancet* i: 1094.

Barrett PVD, Thier SO (1963). Meningitis and pancreatitis associated with sulfamethizole. *New Engl J Med* **268**: 36.

Beem MO, Saxon E, Tipple MA (1979). Treatment of chlamydial pneumonia of infancy. *Pediatrics* **62**: 198.

Berd D (1973). *Nocardia brasiliensis* infection in the United States: a report of nine cases and a review of the literature. *Amer J Clin Path* **59**: 254.

Bergan T, Skjerven O (1979). Double blind comparison of short and medium term sulfonamides, sulfamethizole and sulfamethoxazole, in uncomplicated acute urinary infections. *Scand J Infect Dis* **11**: 219.

Bernard, PA, Stenstrom, RJ, Feldman, W *et al.* (1991). Randomized, controlled trial comparing long-term sulfonamide therapy to ventilation tubes for otitis media with effusion. *Pediatrics* **88**: 215.

Beveridge J, Harris M, Wise G, Stevens L (1964). Long-acting sulphonamides associated with Stevens–Johnson syndrome. *Lancet* ii: 593.

Birnie GG, McLeod TIF, Watkinson G (1981). Incidence of sulphasalazine-induced male fertility. *Gut* **22**: 452.

Bissett ML, Abbott SL, Wood RM (1974). Antimicrobial resistance and R factors in *Salmonella* isolated in California (1971–1972). *Antimicrob Ag Chemother* **5**: 161.

Bluestone CD (1982). Otitis media in children: to treat or not to treat? *New Engl J Med* **306**: 1399.

Bowie WR, Alexander ER, Floyd JF *et al.* (1976). Differential response of chlamydial and ureaplasma-associated urethritis to sulphafurazole (sulfisoxazole). and aminocyclitols. *Lancet* ii: 1276.

Bowie WR, Manzon LM, Borrie-Hume CJ *et al.* (1982). Efficacy of treatment regimens for lower urogenital *Chlamydia trachomatis* infection in women. *Amer J Obstet Gynecol* **142**: 125.

Bratoeva MP, John, JJ (1989). Dissemination of trimethoprim-resistant clones of *Shigella sonnei* in Bulgaria. *J Infect Dis* **159**: 648.

Bridges K, Lowbury EJL (1977). Drug resistance in relation to use of silver sulphadiazine cream in a burns unit. *J Clin Path* **30**: 160.

Brown GV (1993). Chemoprophylaxis of malaria. *Med J Aust* **159**: 187.

Brumfitt W (1970). Some basic concepts underlying the chemotherapy of urinary infections. *Aspects of Infection. Proc Symp Auckland, Sydney and Melbourne,* p. 59. Melbourne, Australia: Mercedes Publishing Services.

Brummer E, Castaneda E, Restrepo A (1993). Paracoccidioidomycosis: an update. *Clin Microbiol Rev* **6**: 89.

Buchanan N (1978). Sulphamethoxazole, hypoalbuminaemia, crystalluria, and renal failure. *Brit Med J* **2**: 172.

Buckwold FJ, Ludwig P, Harding GKM *et al.* (1982). Therapy for acute cystitis in adult women. Randomized comparison of single-dose sulfisoxazole vs trimethoprim-sulfamethoxazole. *JAMA* **247**: 1839.

Bullowa JGM, Ratish HD (1944). A therapeutic and pharmacological study of sulfadiazine, monomethylsulfadiazine and dimethylsulfadiazine in lobar pneumonia. *J Clin Invest* **23**: 676.

Busch H, Lane M (1967). *Chemotherapy,* p. 106. Chicago: Year Book Medical Publishers.

Campieri M, Lanfranchi GA, Bazzocchi G *et al.* (1981). Treatment of ulcerative colitis with high-dose 5-aminosalicylic acid enemas. *Lancet* ii: 270.

Campos J, Garcia-Tornel S, Sanfeliu I (1984). Susceptibility studies of

multiply resistant *Haemophilus influenzae* isolated from pediatric patients and contacts. *Antimicrob Ag Chemother* **25**: 706.

Cann PA, Holdsworth CD (1984). Reversal of male infertility on changing treatment from sulphasalazine to 5-aminosalicylic acid. *Lancet* i: 1119.

Carroll OM, Bryan PA, Robinson RJ (1966). Stevens–Johnson syndrome associated with long-acting sulfonamides. *JAMA* **195**: 691.

Carter RF, Cullity GJ, Ojeda VJ *et al.* (1981). A fatal case of meningoencephalitis due to a free-living amoeba of uncertain identity – probably *Acanthamoeba* sp. *Pathology* **13**: 51.

CDC (Center for Disease Control) (1976). Analysis for endemic meningococcal disease by serogroup and evaluation of chemoprophylaxis. *J Infect Dis* **134**: 201.

CDC (Centers for Disease Control) (1981). Meningococcal disease – United States. *MMWR* **30**: 113.

CDC (Centers for Disease Control) (1985a). Adverse reactions to FansidarẀ and updated recommendations for its use in the prevention of malaria. *MMWR* **33**: 713.

CDC (Centers for Disease Control) (1985b). Revised recommendations for preventing malaria in travellers to areas with chloroquine-resistant *Plasmodium falciparum*. *MMWR* **34**: 185.

CDC (Centers for Disease Control) (1986). Need for malaria prophylaxis by travellers to areas with chloroquine-resistant *Plasmodium falciparum*. *MMWR* **35**: 21.

CDC (Centers for Disease Control) (1989). Malaria in travelers returning from Kenya: Failure of self-treatment with pyrimethamine/sulfadoxine. *MMWR* **38**: 363.

CDC (Centers for Disease Control) (1990). Recommendations for the prevention of malaria among travelers. *MMWR* **39**: RR-3.

CDC (Centers for Disease Control) (1993a). Sexually transmitted diseases treatment guidelines. *MMWR* **42**: RR-14.

CDC (Centers for Disease Control) (1993b). *Health Information for International Travel.* Atlanta, Georgia: US Department of Health and Human Services.

Chang TW, Weinstein L (1975a). Inactivation of *Treponema pallidum* by silver sulfadiazine. *Antimicrob Ag Chemother* **7**: 538.

Chang TW, Weinstein L (1975b). *In vitro* activity of silver sulfadiazine against Herpesvirus homins. *J Infect Dis* **132**: 79.

Chang TW, Weinstein L (1975c). Prevention of herpes keratoconjunctivitis in rabbits by silver sulfadiazine. *Antimicrob Ag Chemother* **8**: 677.

Ch'ien LT (1970). Intracranial hypertension and sulfamethoxazole. *New Engl J Med* **283**: 47.

Christensen LK, Hansen JM, Kristensen M (1963). Sulphaphenazole-induced hypoglycaemic attacks in tolbutamide-treated diabetics. *Lancet* ii: 1298.

Clarke AM (1975). Topical use of silver sulphadiazine and chlorhexidine in the prevention of infection in thermal injuries. *Med J Aust* **1**: 413.

Claxton RC (1963). A review of 31 cases of Stevens–Johnson syndrome. *Med J Aust* **1**: 963.

Cohen HN, Beastall GH, Ratcliffe WA *et al.* (1980). Effects on human thyroid function of sulphonamide and trimethoprim combination drugs. *Brit Med J* **281**: 646.

Cohen HN, Pearson DWM, Thomson JA *et al.* (1981). Trimethoprim and thyroid function. *Lancet* i: 676.

Coombs CJ, Wan AT, Masterton JP, *et al.* (1992). Do burn patients have a silver lining? *Burns* **18**: 179.

Counts GW, Petersdorf RG (1980). The wheel within a wheel: meningococcal trends. *JAMA* **244**: 2200.

Cowan GO, Das KM, Eastwood MA (1977). Further studies of sulphasalazine metabolism in the treatment of ulcerative colitis. *Brit Med J* **2**: 1057.

Craft AW, Brocklebank JT, Jackson RH (1977). Acute renal failure and hypoglycaemia due to sulphadiazine poisoning. *Postgrad Med J* **53**: 103.

Csangó PA, Salveson A, Gundersen T *et al.* (1984). Treatment of acute gonococcal urethritis in men with simultaneous infection with *Chlamydia trachomatis*. *Br J Vener Dis* **60**: 95.

Dangor Y, Ballard RC, Miller SD, Koornhof HJ (1990). Antimicrobial susceptibility of *Haemophilus ducreyi. Antimicrob Ag Chemother* **34**: 1303.

Davies JR, Farrant WN, Uttley AHC (1970). Antibiotic resistance of *Shigella sonnei. Lancet* **ii**: 1157.

Deb BC, Sengupta PG, De SP *et al.* (1976). Effect of sulfadoxine on transmission of *Vibrio cholerae* infection among family contacts of cholera patients in Calcutta. *Bull Wld Hlth Org* **54**: 171.

Deboever G, Devogelaere R, Holvoet G (1989). Sulphasalazine-induced lupus-like syndrome with cardiac tamponade in a patient with ulcerative colitis. *Am J Gastroenterol* **84**: 85.

Delamere JP, Farr M, Grindulis KA (1983). Sulphasalazine induced selective IgA deficiency in rheumatoid arthritis. *Brit Med J* **286**: 1547.

De Morais JS, Munford RS, Piri JB *et al.* (1974). Epidemic disease due to sero-group C *Neisseria meningitidis* in São Paulo, Brazil. *J Infect Dis* **129**: 568.

Derouin F, Chastang C (1988). Enzyme immunoassay to assess effect of antimicrobial agents on *Toxoplasma gondii* in tissue culture. *Antimicrob Ag Chemother* **32**: 303.

Derouin F, Chastang C (1989). *In vitro* effects of folate inhibitors on *Toxoplasma gondii. Antimicrob Ag Chemother* **33**: 1753.

Dewsnup DH, Wright DM (1984). *In vitro* susceptibility of *Nocardia asteroides* to 25 antimicrobial agents. *Antimicrob Ag Chemother* **25**: 165.

Dujovne CA, Chan CH, Zimmerman HJ (1967). Sulfonamide hepatic injury. Review of the literature and report of a case due to sulfamethoxazole. *New Engl J Med* **277**: 785.

Dunn AM, Kerr GD (1981). Pure red cell aplasia associated with sulphasalazine. *Lancet* **ii**: 1288.

Editorial (1987). Sulphasalazine: drug or pro-drug? *Lancet* **i**: 1299.

Edstein MD, Veenendaal JR, Rieckmann KH, O'Donoghue M (1988). Failure of dapsone/pyrimethamine plus chloroquine against falciparum malaria in Papua New Guinea. *Lancet* **i**: 237.

Eickhoff TC, Bennett JV, Hayes PS, Feeley J (1970). *Pseudomonas pseudomallei*: susceptibility to chemotherapeutic agents. *J Infect Dis* **121**: 95.

Emerson RG, Jardine DS, Milvenan ES *et al.* (1981). Toxoplasmosis: a treatable neurologic disease in the immunologically compromised patient. *Pediatrics* **67**: 653.

Facinelli B, Varaldo PE (1987). Plasmid-mediated sulfonmide resistance in *Neisseria meningitidis. Antimicrob Ag Chemother* **31**: 1642.

Fairley NH (1945). Chemotherapeutic suppression and prophylaxis in malaria. *Trans Roy Soc Trop Med Hyg* **38**: 311.

Fallon RJ (1983). Meningococcal infections in Scotland, 1982. *Communicable Diseases Scotland Weekly Report* **83/7**: 9.

Fast MV, Nsanze H, Plummer FA *et al.* (1983). Treatment of chancroid A comparison of sulphamethoxazole and trimethoprim-sulphamethoxazole. *Brit J Vener Dis* **59**: 320.

Feit PW (1975). Structure-activity relationships of sulphamoyl diuretics. *Postgrad Med J* (Suppl 6) **51**: 9.

Feldman HA (1986). The meningococcus: a twenty-year perspective. *Rev Infect Dis* **8**: 288.

Finegold I (1985). Oral desensitization to trimethoprim/sulfamethoxazole in a patient with AIDS (Abstr). *J Allergy Clin Immunol* **75**: 137.

Finland M, Garner C, Wilcox C, Sabath LD (1976). Susceptibility of beta-hemolytic streptococci to 65 antibacterial agents. *Antimicrob Ag Chemother* **9**: 11.

Fischer E (1972). Renal excretion of sulphadimidine in normal and uraemic subjects. *Lancet* **ii**: 210.

Follath F (1979). Pharmacokinetics of long half-life antibacterials. *J Antimicrob Chemother* **5** (Suppl B): 97.

Fox, CL, Jensen, OJ, Mudge GH (1943). The prevention of renal obstruction during sulfadiazine therapy. *JAMA* **121**: 1147.

Fraser GL, Beaulieu JT (1979). Leukopenia secondary to sulfadiazine silver. *JAMA* **241**: 1928.

Garrod LP, Lambert HP, O'Grady F (1973). *Antibiotic and Chemotherapy*, 4th edn: p. 14. Edinburgh, London: Churchill Livingstone.

Goldstein PD, Alpers DH, Keating JP (1979). Sulfapyridine metabolites in children with inflammatory bowel disease receiving sulfasalazine. *J Pediatr* **95**: 638.

Gombert ME (1982). Susceptibility of *Nocardia asteroides* to various antibiotics, including new beta-lactams, trimethoprim-sulfamethoxazole, amikacin, and N-formimidoyl thienamycin. *Antimicrob Ag Chemother* **21**: 1011.

Gombert ME, Berkowitz LB, Aulicino TM, du Bouchet L (1990). Therapy of pulmonary nocardiosis in immunocompromised mice. *Antimicrob Ag Chemother* **34**: 1766.

Goodwin RA Jr, Shapiro JL, Thurman GH *et al.* (1980). Disseminated histoplasmosis: clinical and pathologic correlations. *Medicine* **59**: 1.

Gordon RC, Thompson TR, Carlson W *et al.* (1975). Antimicrobial resistance of shigellae isolated in Michigan. *JAMA* **231**: 1159.

Gottlieb MS, Knight S, Mitsuyasu R *et al.* (1984). Prophylaxis of *Pneumocystis carinii* infection in AIDS with pyrimethamine-sulfadoxine. *Lancet* **ii**: 398.

Gottschalk HR, Stone OJ (1976). Stevens–Johnson syndrome from ophthalmic sulfonamide. *Arch Dermatol* **112**: 513.

Grieble HG, Jackson GG (1958). Prolonged treatment of urinary-tract infections with sulfamethoxypyridazine. *New Engl J Med* **258**: 1.

Griffiths ID, Kane SP (1977). Sulphasalazine-induced lupus syndrome in ulcerative colitis. *Brit Med J* **2**: 1188.

Grigor WG (1983). Sulfonamide resistance of meningococci: 1978–1982. *Med J Aust* **1**: 502.

Gross RJ, Ward LR, Threlfall EJ *et al.* (1982). Drug resistance among infantile enteropathogenic *Escherichia coli* strains isolated in the United Kingdom. *Brit Med J* **285**: 472.

Grüneberg RN (1979). The microbiological rationale for the combination of sulphonamides with trimethoprim. *J Antimicrob Chemother* **5** (Suppl B): 27.

Gryboski J, Hillemeier C (1980). Inflammatory bowel disease inchildren. *Med Clin N Amer* **64**: 1185.

Guttler, RB, Counts, GW, Avent, CK, *et al.* (1971). Effects of rifampin and minocycline on meningococcal carriage rates. *J Infect Dis* **124**: 199.

Halsted CH, Gandhi C, Tamura T (1981). Sulfasalazine inhibits the absorption of folates in ulcerative colitis. *New Engl J Med* **305**: 1513.

Haltalin KC, Nelson JD (1965). *In vitro* susceptibility of shigellae to sodium sulfadiazine and to eight antibiotics. *JAMA* **193**: 705.

Hamilton HE, Sheets RF (1978). Sulfisoxazole-induced thrombocytopenic purpura Immunologic mechanism as cause. *JAMA* **239**: 2586.

Hamilton-Miller JMT (1979). Mechanisms and distribution of bacterial resistance to diaminopyrimidines and sulphonamides. *J Antimicrob Chemother* **5** (Suppl B): 61.

Handsfield HH, Alexander ER, Wang SP *et al.* (1976). Differences in the therapeutic response of *Chlamydia*-positive and *Chlamydia*-negative forms of nongonococcal urethritis. *J Amer Vener Dis Assoc* **2**: 5.

Hansen JM, Siersbaek-Nielsen K, Skovsted L *et al.* (1975). Potentiation of warfarin by co-trimoxazole. *Brit Med J* **2**: 684.

Hansson HB, Walder M, Juhlin I (1981). Susceptibility of shigellae to mecillinam, nalidixic acid, trimethoprim, and five other antimicrobial agents. *Antimicrob Ag Chemother* **19**: 271.

Harris C, Salgo MP, Tanowitz HB, Wittner M (1988). *In vitro* assessment of antimicrobial agents against *Toxoplasma gondii. J Infect Dis* **157**: 14.

Hassall C, Feetam CL, Leach RH, Meynell MJ (1975). Potentiation of warfarin by co-trimoxazole. *Lancet* **ii**: 1155.

Hawkey PM (1984). *Providencia stuartii*: a review of a multiply antibiotic-resistant bacterium. *J Antimicrob Chemother* **13**: 209.

Hejný J (1982). A drug sensitivity test strategy for atypical mycobacteria. *Tubercle* **62**: 63.

Hernborg A (1985). Stevens–Johnson syndrome after mass prophylaxis with sulfadoxine for cholera in Mozambique. *Lancet* **ii**: 1072.

Herwaldt BL, Krogstad DJ, Schlessinger PH (1988). Antimalarial agents: specific chemoprophylaxis regimens. *Antimicrob Ag Chemother* **32**: 953.

Herzog C, Kibbler CC, Ellis CJ (1983). Falciparum malaria resistant to chloroquine and Fansidar: implications for prophylaxis. *Brit Med J* **287**: 947.

Holdsworth CD (1981). Sulphasalazine desensitization. *Brit Med J* **282**: 110.

Hollis, D G, Moss, C W, Daneshvar, M I *et al.* (1993). Characterization of Centers for Disease Control group NO-1, a fastidious, nonoxidative, Gram-negative organism associated with dog and cat bites. *J Clin Microbiol* **31**: 746.

Holmgren EB, Tunevall G (1973). Five cases of meningitis due to sulfonamide-resistant meningococci. *Scand J Infect Dis* **5**: 75.

Holten E, Vaage L, Jyssum K (1970). Sulphonamide-resistant meningococci in Norwegian naval recruits. *Scand J Infect Dis* **2**: 111.

Horner DB, McCracken GH Jr, Ginsburg CM, Zweighaft TC (1980). A comparison of three antibiotic regimens for eradication of *Haemophilus influenzae* Type b from the pharynx of infants and children. *Pediatrics* **66**: 136.

Hornstein OP, Ruprecht KW (1982). Fansidar-induced Stevens–Johnson syndrome. *New Engl J Med* **307**: 1529.

Hornsten P, Keisu M, Wiholm BE (1990). The incidence of agranulocytosis during treatment of dermatitis herpetiformis with dapsone as reported in Sweden, 1972 through 1988. *Arch Dermatol* **126**: 919.

Howard AJ, Williams HM (1989). The prevalence of antibiotic resistance in *Haemophilus influenzae* in Ireland. *J Antimicrob Chemother* **24**: 963.

Hughes TE, Almgren TE, McGuffin RE, Omato RJ (1986). Co-trimoxazole desensitization in bone marrow transplantation. *Ann Intern Med* **105**: 148.

Huth TS, Burke JP, Larsen RA *et al.* (1992). Randomized trial of noenatal care with silver sulfadiazine cream for the prevention of catheter-associated bacteriuria. *J Infect Dis* **165**: 14.

Ibrahim ME, Awad-El-Kariem FM, El Hassan IM, El Mubarak ERM (1991). A case of *Plasmodium falciparum* malaria sensitive to chloroquine but resistant to pyrimethamine/sulfadoxine in Sennar, Sudan. *Trans Roy Soc Trop Med Hyg* **85**: 446.

Idriss ZH, Cunningham RJ, Wilfert CM (1975). Nocardiosis in children: report of three cases and review of the literature. *Pediatrics* **55**: 479.

International Agranulocytosis and Aplastic Anemia Study Group (1989). Anti-infective drug use in relation to the risk of agranulocytosis and aplastic anemia. A report from the International Agranulocytosis and Aplastic Anemia Study. *Arch Intern Med* **149**: 1036.

Jacobson JA, Weaver RE, Thornsberry C (1975). Trends in meningococcal disease, 1974. *J Infect Dis* **132**: 480.

Jacobson JA, Chester TJ, Fraser DW (1977). An epidemic of disease due to sero-group B *Neisseria meningitidis* in Alabama: report of an investigation and community-wide prophylaxis with a sulfonamide. *J Infect Dis* **136**: 104.

Johannisson G, Löwhagen G-B, Lycke E (1980). Genital *Chlamydia trachomatis* infection in women. *Obstet Gynecol* **56**: 671.

Johnston RB Jr, Wilfert CM, Buckley RH *et al.* (1975). Enhanced bactericidal activity of phagocytes from patients with chronic granulomatous disease in the presence of sulphisoxazole. *Lancet* **i**: 824.

Jones BM, Kinghorn GH, Geary I (1982). *In vitro* susceptibility of *Gardnerella vaginalis* and *Bacteroides* organisms, associated with nonspecific vaginitis, to sulfonamide preparations. *Antimicrob Ag Chemother* **21**: 870.

Jones DK, Hakim M, Wallwork J *et al.* (1986). Serious interaction between cyclosporin A and sulphadimidine. *Brit Med J* **292**: 728.

Jorgensen JH (1992). Update on mechanisms and prevalence of antimicrobial resistance in *Haemophilus influenzae*. *Clin Infect Dis* **14**: 1119.

Kaiser, AB, Hennekens CH, Saslaw, MS, *et al.* (1974). Seroepidemiology and chemoprophylaxis of disease due to sulfonamide-resistant *Neisseria meningitidis* in a civilian population. *J Infect Dis* **130**: 217.

Källenius G, Winberg J (1979). Urinary tract infections treated with a single dose of short-acting sulfonamide. *Brit Med J* **1**: 1175.

Kane SP, Boots MA (1977). Megaloblastic anaemia associated with sulphasalazine treatment. *Brit Med J* **2**: 1287.

Katz SI, Hall RP III, Lawley TJ, Strober W (1980). Dermatitis herpetiformis: the skin and the gut. *Ann Intern Med* **93**: 857.

Kim, J, Minamoto, G Y Grieco, M H (1991). Nocardial infection as a complication of AIDS: report of six cases and review. *Rev Infect Dis* **13**: 624.

Kirby HB, Kenamore B, Guckian JC (1971). *Pneumocystis carinii* pneumonia treated with pyrimethamine and sulfadiazine. *Ann Intern Med* **75**: 505.

Kirsner JB, Shorter RG (1982). Recent developments in 'nonspecific' inflammatory bowel disease. *New Engl J Med* **306**: 775.

Klotz U, Maier K, Fischer C, Heinkel K (1980). Therapeutic efficacy of sulfasalazine and its metabolites in patients with ulcerative colitis and Crohn's disease. *New Engl J Med* **303**: 1499.

Kraus SJ, Kaufman HW, Albriton WJ *et al.* (1982). Chancroid therapy: a review of cases confirmed by culture. *Rev Infect Dis* **4** (Suppl): 848.

Kreuz W, Gungor T, Lotz C *et al.* (1990). 'Treating through' hypersensitivity to cotrimoxazole in children with HIV infection. *Lancet* **336**: 508.

Krick JA, Stinson EB, Remington JS (1975). *Nocardia* infection in heart transplant patients. *Ann Intern Med* **82**: 18.

Kristiansen, B E, Lind, K W, Mevold, K *et al.* (1988). Meningococcal phenotypic and genotypic characteristics and human antibody levels. *J Clin Microbiol* **26**: 1988.

Kristiansen B E, Rådström P, Jenkins A *et al.* (1990). Cloning and characterization of a DNA fragment that confers sulfonamide resistance in a serogroup B, serotype 15 strain of *Neisseria meningitidis*. *Antimicrob Ag Chemother* **34**: 2277.

Kruse, H, Kariuki, S, Soli, N *et al.* (1992). Multiresistant *Shigella* species from African AIDS patients: antibacterial resistance patterns and application of the E-test for determination of minimum inhibitory concentration. *Scand J Infect Dis* **24**: 733.

Kuo, C C, Grayston, J T (1988). *In vitro* drug susceptibility of *Chlamydia* sp. strain TWAR. *Antimicrob Ag Chemother* **32**: 257.

Lacey RW (1979). Mechanism of action of trimethoprim and sulphonamides: relevance to synergy *in vivo*. *J Antimicrob Chemother* **5** (Suppl B): 75.

Laing ABG (1964). Antimalarial effect of sulphorthodimethoxine (Fanasil). *Brit Med J* **2**: 1439.

Leading Article (1965). Teratogenic effects of sulphonamides. *Brit Med J* **1**: 142.

Leading Article (1969). Lung disease caused by drugs. *Brit Med J* **3**: 729.

Leading Article (1974a). Meningococcal infections. *Brit Med J* **3**: 295.

Leading Article (1974b). Sulphasalazine-induced lung disease. *Lancet* **ii**: 504.

Leading Article (1977). Preventing endocarditis. *Brit Med J* **2**: 1564.

Leading Article (1983a). Drug-induced neutropenia. *Lancet* **ii**: 857.

Leading Article (1983b). *Bacillus cereus* as a systemic pathogen. *Lancet* **ii**: 1469.

Leading article (1986). Suphasalazine in inflammatory bowel disease: recent advances. *N Z Med J* **99**: 757.

Leedom JM, Ivler D, Mathies AW *et al.* (1965). Importance of sulfadiazine resistance in meningococcal disease in civilians. *New Engl J Med* **273**: 1395.

Leedom JM, Ivler D, Mathies AW Jr *et al.* (1967). The problem of sulfadiazine-resistant meningococci. *Antimicrob Ag Chemother* **1966**: 281.

Lehrer RI (1971). Inhibition by sulphonamides of the candidacidal activity of human neutrophils. *J Clin Invest* **50**: 2498.

Lennard TWJ, Farndon JR (1983). Sulphasalazine hepatoxicity after 15 years' successful treatment for ulcerative colitis. *Brit Med J* **287**: 96.

Lennon, D, Voss, L, Sinclair, J *et al.* (1989). An outbreak of meningococcal disease in Auckland, New Zealand. *Pediatr Infect Dis J* **8**: 11.

Leonard JN, Fry L (1991). Treatment and management of dermatitis herpetiformis. *Clin Dermatol* **9**: 403.

Lerner, B H (1991). Scientific evidence versus therapeutic demand: the introduction of the sulfonamides revisited. *Ann Intern Med* **115**: 315.

Levi AJ, Fisher AM, Hughes L, Hendry WF (1979). Male infertility due to sulphasalazine. *Lancet* **ii**: 276.

Lewis VJ, Thacker WL, Shepard CC, McDade JE (1978). *In vivo* susceptibility of the Legionnaires' disease bacterium to ten antimicrobial agents. *Antimicrob Ag Chemother* **13**: 419.

Lidin-Janson G (1977). Sulphonamides in the treatment of acute *Escherichia coli* infection of the urinary tract in women. *Scand J Infect Dis* **9**: 211.

Lindberg RB, Moncrief JA, Switzer WE et al. (1965). The successful control of burn wound sepsis. *J Trauma* **5**: 601.

Lisander B (1970). Myalgia after sulphonamides. *Lancet* **i**: 1062.

Liston TE, Foshee WS, Pierson WD (1983). Sulfisoxazole chemoprophylaxis for frequent otitis media. *Pediatrics* **71**: 524.

Little SC (1942). Nervous and mental effects of the sulfonamides. *JAMA* **119**: 467.

Lobel HO, Roberts JM, Somaini B, Stefffen R (1987). Efficacy of malaria prophylaxis in American and Swiss travelers to Kenya. *J Infect Dis* **155**: 1205.

Longstreth GF, Green R (1983). Folate status in patients receiving maintenance doses of sulfasalazine. *Arch Intern Med* **143**: 902.

Losek JD, Werlin SL (1981). Sulphasalazine hepatotoxicity. *Amer J Dis Child* **135**: 1070.

Lowbury EJL, Jackson DM, Lilly HA et al. (1971). Alternative forms of local treatment for burns. *Lancet* **ii**: 1105.

Lowbury EJL, Babb JR, Bridges K, Jackson DM (1976). Topical chemoprophylaxis with silver sulphadiazine and silver nitrate chlorhexidine creams: emergence of sulphonamide-resistant Gram-negative bacilli. *Brit Med J* **1**: 493.

Loyd JE, Des Prez RM, Goodwin, Jr, RA (1990). *Histoplasma capsulatum*. In *Principles and Practice of Infectious Diseases* 3rd edn (Mandell GL, Douglas RG, Bennet JE, eds). New York: Churchill Livingstone.

Luft BJ, Brooks RG, Conley FK (1984). Toxoplasmic encephalitis in patients with acquired immune deficiency syndrome. *JAMA* **252**: 913.

Lyell A (1982). Sulphonamides and Stevens–Johnson syndrome. *Lancet* **ii**: 1460.

Macsearraigh ETM, Patel KM (1968). Cardiomyopathy as a complication of sulphonamide therapy. *Brit Med J* **3**: 33.

Madsen ST, Øvsthus Ø, Bøe J (1963). Antibacterial activity of long-acting sulfonamides. *Acta Med Scand* **173**: 707.

Mahmoud AAF, Warren KS (1977). Algorithms in the diagnosis and management of exotic diseases. XX. Toxoplasmosis. *J Infect Dis* **135**: 493.

Malchow H, Ewe K, Brandes JW et al. (1984). European Cooperative Crohn's disease study Results of drug treatment. *Gastroenterology*; **86**: 249.

Marks MI, Frasch CE, Shapera RM (1979). Meningococcal colonization and infection in children and their household contacts. *Amer J Epidemiol* **109**: 563.

Margolis DM, Melnick DA, Alling DW et al. (1990). Trimethoprim-sulfamethoxazole prophylaxis in the management of chronic granulomatous disease. *J Infect Dis* **162**: 723.

Masterton JP (1992). Immediate management of the burned patient. *Med J Aust* **156**: 678.

McCabe RE, Brooks RG, Dorfman RF, Remington JS (1987). Clinical spectrum of 107 cases of toxoplasmic lymphadenopathy. *Rev Infect Dis* **9**: 754.

McDougall IA (1972). Use of silver sulphadiazine in treatment of burns at Royal Perth Hospital. *Med J Aust* **1**: 979.

McGregor IA, Williams K, Goodwin LG (1963). Pyrimethamine and sulphadiazine in treatment of malaria. *Brit Med J* **2**: 728.

Mehtar S, Aminiafshar S (1983). Antibiotic resistance amongst various types of Haemophilus species. *J Antimicrob Chemother* **12**: 565.

Merali S, Zhang Y, Sloan D, Meshnick S (1990). Inhibition of *Pneumocystis carinii* dihydropteroate synthetase by sulfa drugs. *Antimicrob Ag Chemother* **34**: 1075.

Milhous WK, Weatherly NF, Bowdre JH et al. (1985). *In vitro* activities of and mechanisms of resistance to antifol antimalarial drugs. *Antimicrob Ag Chemother* **27**: 525.

Millar JW, Siess EE, Feldman HA et al. (1963). *In vivo* and *in vitro* resistance to sulfadiazine in strains of *Neisseria meningitidis*. *JAMA* **186**: 139.

Miller KD, Lobel HO, Pappaioanou M et al. (1986a). Failures of combined chloroquine and Fansidar prophylaxis in American Travellers to East Africa. *J Infect Dis* **154**: 689.

Miller KD, Lobel HO, Satriale et al. (1986b). Severe cutaneous reactions among American travellers using pyrimethamine-sulfadoxine (Fansidar). for malaria prophylaxis. *Amer J Trop Med Hyg* **35**: 451.

Mitchell, P S, Huston, B J, Jones, R N et al. (1990). *Stomatococcus mucilaginosus* bacteremias Typical case presentations, simplified diagnostic criteria, and a literature review. *Diagn Microbiol Infect Dis* **13**: 521.

Molina J-M, Belenfont X, Doco-Lecompte T et al. (1991). Sulfadiazine-induced crystalluria in AIDS patients with toxoplasma encephalitis. *AIDS* **5**: 587.

Monafo WW, West MA (1990). Current treatment recommendations for topical burn therapy. *Drugs* **40**: 364.

Murray, B E, Mathewson, J J, DuPont, H L et al. (1990). Emergence of resistant fecal *Escherichia coli* in travelers not taking prophylactic antimicrobial agents. *Antimicrob Ag Chemother* **34**: 515.

Navin TR, Miller KD, Satriale RF, Lobel HO (1985). Adverse reactions associated with pyrimethamine-sulfadoxine prophylaxis for *Pneumocystis carinii* infections in AIDS. *Lancet* **ii**: 1332.

Neumann VC, Grindulis KA, Hubball S et al. (1983). Comparison between penicillamine and sulphasalazine in rheumatoid arthritis Lees-Birmingham trial. *Brit Med J* **287**: 1099.

Newbould BB, Kilpatrick R (1960). Long-acting sulphonamides and protein-binding. *Lancet* **i**: 887.

Newton CRJC, Winstanley PA, Watkins WM et al. (1993). A single dose of intramuscular sulfadoxine-pyrimethamine as an adjunct to quinine in the treatment of severe malaria: pharmacokinetics and efficacy. *Trans Roy Soc Trop Med Hyg* **87**: 207.

Noel GE, Morisset R (1986). Malaria acquired with double chemical prophylaxis: chloroquine plus Fansidar. *Canada Diseases Weekly Report* **12**: 105.

Norrby, S R (1990). Short-term treatment of uncomplicated lower urinary tract infections in women. *Rev Infect Dis* **12**: 458.

Nosten F, Imvithaya S, Vincenti M et al. (1987). Malaria on the Thai-Burmese border: treatment of 5192 patients with mefloquine-sulfadoxine-pyrimethamine combination. *Bull Wld Health Org* **65**: 891.

Nuver-Zwart H H, Riel van P L, Putte van de L B A, Gribnau F W J (1989). A double-blind comparative study of sulphasalazine and hydroxychloroquine in rheumatoid arthritis: Evidence of an earlier effect of sulphasalazine. *Ann Rheum Dis* **48**: 389.

O'Grady F, Lewis MJ, Pearson NJ (1976). Global surveillance of antibiotic sensitivity of *Vibrio cholerae*. *Bull Wld Hlth Org* **54**: 181.

Olsen H, Mørland J (1978). Ethanol-induced increase in drug acetylation in man and isolated rat liver cells. *Brit Med J* **2**: 1260.

Olsen VV, Loft S, Christensen KD (1982). Serious reactions during malaria prophylaxis with pyrimethamine-sulfadoxine. *Lancet* **ii**: 994.

O'Reilly RA (1980). Stereoselective interaction of trimethoprim-sulfamethoxazole with the separated enantiomorphs of racemic warfarin in man. *New Engl J Med* **302**: 33.

O'Reilly RA, Motley CH (1979). Racemic warfarin and trimethoprim-sulfamethoxazole interaction in humans. *Ann Intern Med* **91**: 34.

Orfanakis MG, Wilcox HG, Smith CB (1972). *In vitro* studies of the combined effects of ampicillin and sulfonamides on *Nocardia asteroides* and results of therapy in four patients. *Antimicrob Ag Chemother* **1**: 215.

Oster, S, Hutchison F, McCabe R (1990). Resolution of acute renal failure in toxoplasmic encephalitis despite continuance of sulfadiazine. *Rev Infect Dis* **12**: 618.

Owens CJ, Yarborough DR III, Brackett NC Jr (1974). Nephrotic syndrome following topically applied sulfadiazine silver therapy. *Arch Intern Med* **134**: 332.

Palmer KR, Goepel JR, Holdsworth CD (1981). Sulphasalazine retention enemas in ulcerative colitis; a double-blind trial. *Brit Med J* **282**: 1571.

Paradise JL (1980). Otitis media in infants and children. *Pediatrics* **65**: 917.

Pearlman EJ, Lampe RM, Thiemanun W, Kennedy RS (1977). Chemosuppressive field trials in Thailand. III. The suppression of *Plasmodium falciparum* and *Plasmodium vivax* parasitemias by a sulfadoxine-pyrimethamine combination. *Amer J Trop Med Hyg* **26**: 1108.

Pearson RD, Hewlett EL (1987). Use of pyrimethamine-sulfadoxine (Fansidar). in prophylaxis against chloroquine-resistant *Plasmodium falciparum* and *Pneumocystis carinii*. *Ann Intern Med* **106**: 714.

Peddie BA, Little PJ (1979). Sulphamethizole in urinary tract infections. *J Antimicrob Chemother* **5**: 195.

Pegg SP (1972). Adult burns: a three-year survey with assessment of sulfamylon. *Med J Aust* **1**: 350.

Peixoto MP, Beverley SM (1987). *In vitro* activity of sulfonamides and sulfones against *Leishmania major* promastigotes. *Antimicrob Ag Chemother* **31**: 1575.

Peltola H (1983). Meningococcal disease: still with us. *Rev Infect Dis* **5**: 71.

Peltola H, Jónsdóttir K, Lystad A *et al.* (1982). Meningococcal disease in Scandinavia. *Brit Med J* **284**: 1618.

Peppercorn MA (1984). Sulfasalazine: pharmacology, clinical use, toxicity, and related new drug development. *Ann Intern Med* **3**: 377.

Perrin JM, Charney E, MacWhinney JB Jr *et al.* (1974). Sulfisoxazole as chemoprophylaxis for recurrent otitis media. A double-blind crossover study in pediatric practice. *New Engl J Med* **291**: 664.

Phillips I, Warren C (1976). Activity of sulfamethoxazole and trimephoprim against *Bacteroides fragilis*. *Antimicrob Ag Chemother* **9**: 736.

Piketty C, Derouin F, Rouveix B, Pocidato J J (1990). *In vivo* assessment of antimicrobial agents against *Toxoplasma gondii* by quantification of parasites in the blood, lungs and brain of infected mice. *Antimicrob Ag Chemother* **34**: 1467.

Pilantanapak, A, Bhumiratana, A, Jayanetra, P *et al.* (1990). Biotinylated probes for epidemiological studies of drug resistance in *Salmonella krefeld*. *J Antimicrob Chemother* **25**: 593.

Pinner RW, Gellin BG, Bibb WF (1991). Meningococcal disease in the United States – 1986. *J Infect Dis* **164**: 368.

Plourde, P J, D'Costa, L J, Agoki, E *et al.* (1992). A randomized, double-blind study of the efficacy of fleroxacin versus trimethoprim-sulfamethoxazole in men with culture-proven chancroid. *J Infect Dis* **165**: 949.

Post C, Fakouhi T, Dutz W *et al.* (1971). Prophylaxis of epidemic infantile pneumocystosis with a sulfadoxine pyrimethamine combination. *Curr Ther Res* **13**: 273.

Pryles CV (1970). The use of sulfonamides in urinary tract infections. *Med Clin N Amer* **54**: 1077.

Pullar T, Hunter JA, Capell HA (1983). Sulphasalazine in rheumatoid arthritis: a double blind comparison of sulphasalazine with placebo and sodium aurothiomalate. *Brit Med J* **287**: 1102.

Pullar T, Hunter JA, Capell HA (1985). Which component of sulphasalazine is active in rheumatoid arthritis?. *Brit Med J* **290**: 1535.

Purdy BH, Philips DM, Summers RW (1984). Desensitization for sulfasalazine skin rash. *Ann Intern Med* **100**: 512.

Rådström P, Swedberg G (1988). RSF1010 and a conjugative plasmid contain sulII, one of two known genes for plasmid-borne sulfonamide resistance dihydropteroate synthase. *Antimicrob Ag Chemother* **32**: 1684.

Rådström P, Swedberg G, Sköld O (1991). Genetic analysis of sulfonamide resistance and its dissemination in Gram-negative bacteria illustrate new aspects of R plasmid evolution. *Antimicrob Ag Chemother* **35**: 1840.

Raimundo AH, Patil DH, Frost PG, Silk DBA (1991). Effects of olsalazine and sulphasalazine on jejunal and ileal water and electrolyte absorption in normal human subjects. *Gut* **32**: 270.

Rallison ML, O'Brien J, Good RA (1961). Severe reactions to long-acting sulfonamides Erythema multiforme exudativum and lupus erythematosus following administration of sulphamethoxypyridazine and sulfadimethoxine. *Pediatrics* **28**: 908.

Rao KVN, Mitchison DA, Nair NGK *et al.* (1970). Sulphadimidine acetylation test for classification of patients as slow or rapid inactivators of isoniazid. *Brit Med J* **3**: 495.

Reeves DS (1975). Laboratory and clinical studies with sulfametopyrazine

as a treatment for bacteriuria in pregnancy. *J Antimicrob Chemother* **1**: 171.

Reeves DS, Bint AJ, Bullock DW (1978). Sulphonamides, co-trimoxazole, and tetracyclines. *Brit Med J* **ii**: 410.

Reeves DS, Broughall JM, Bywater MJ, Holt HA (1979). Pharmacokinetics of tetroxoprim and sulphadiazine in human volunteers. *J Antimicrob Chemother* **5** (Suppl B): 119.

Reeves DS, Morris RW, Watts MR, Reeves RET (1980). Double-blind clinical trials of a nitrofurantoin/sulfadiazine combination at two dosage levels in acute symptomatic urinary infections. *Curr Med Res Opin* **6**: 481.

Rehg JE, Hancock ML, Woodmansee DB (1988). Anticryptosporidial activity of sulfadimethoxine. *Antimicrob Ag Chemother* **32**: 1907.

Report of a WHO Scientific Group (1978). *Neisseria gonorrhoeae* and gonococcal infections. *Wld Hlth Orgn Techn Rep Ser* 616.

Report of a WHO Scientific Group (1984). Advances in malaria chemotherapy. *Wld Hlth Org Tech Rep Ser* **711**: 99.

Report of a WHO Study Group (1982). Chemotherapy of leprosy for control programmes. *Wld Hlth Org Tech Rep Ser* 675.

Restrepo A, Arango MD (1980). *In vitro* susceptibility testing of *Paracoccidioides brasiliensis* to sulfonamides. *Antimicrob Ag Chemother* **18**: 190.

Reutter FW, Vergin H, Sieber R, Ferber H (1979). Pharmacokinetics of tetroxoprim/sulphadiazine in patients with impaired renal function. *J Antimicrob Chemother* **5** (Suppl B): 149.

Rieder MJ, Uetrecht J, Shear NH *et al.* (1989). Diagnosis of sulfonamide hypersensitivity reactions by *in vitro* 'rechallenge' with hydroxylamine metabolites. *Ann Intern Med* **110**: 286.

Rijk MCM, van Hogezand RA, van Lier HJJ, van Tongeren JHM (1991). Sulphasalazine and prednisolone compared with sulphasalazine for treating active Crohn's disease. *Ann Intern Med* **114**: 445.

Riley SA, Flegg PJ, Mandal BK (1986). Contact lens staining due to sulphasalazine. *Lancet* **i**: 972.

Rodloff AC (1982). *In-vitro* susceptibility test of non-tuberculous mycobacteria to sulfamethoxazole, trimethoprim, and combinations of both. *J Antimicrob Chemother* **9**: 195.

Rolinson GN (1980). The significance of protein binding of antibiotics in antibacterial chemotherapy. *J Antimicrob Chemother* **6**: 311.

Rombo L, Stenbeck J, Lobel HO *et al.* (1985). Does chloroquine contribute to the risk of serious adverse reactions to Fansidar? *Lancet* **ii**: 1298.

Rose GA, Spencer H (1957). Polyarteritis nodosa. *Quart J Med* **26**: 43.

Rosenkranz HS, Carr HS (1972). Silver sulfadiazine: effect on the growth and metabolism of bacteria. *Antimicrob Ag Chemother* **2**: 367.

Roth JA, Siegel SE, Levine AS, Berard CW (1971). Fatal recurrent toxoplasmosis in a patient initially infected via a leukocyte transfusion Amer. *J Clin Path* **56**: 601.

Ryder RW, Blake PA, Murlin AC *et al.* (1980). Increase in antibiotic resistance among isolates of salmonella in the United States, 1967–1975. *J Infect Dis* **142**: 485.

Sabcharoen A, Chongsuphajaisiddhi T, Attanath P, *et al.* (1985). *In vitro* susceptibility of *Plasmodium falciparum* collected from pyrimethamine-sulfadoxine sensitive and resistant areas of Thailand. *Bull Wld Hlth Org* **63**: 597.

Salako, LA, Adio, RA, Sowunmi, A, Walker, O (1990). Parenteral sulphadoxine-pyrimethamine (Fansidar®): an effective and safe but under used method of anti-malarial treatment. *Trans Roy Soc Trop Med Hyg* **84**: 641.

Salako LA, Adio RA, Walker O *et al.* (1992). Mefloquine-sulfadoxine-pyrimethamine (Fansimef®, Roche). in the prophylaxis of *Plasmodium falciparum* malaria: a double-blind, comparative, placebo-controlled study. *Ann Trop Med Parasitol* **86**: 575.

Salam MA, Bennish ML (1991). Antimicrobial therapy for shigellosis. *Rev Infect Dis* **13**(Suppl 4): S332.

Salih, M A, Danielsson, D, Backman, A *et al.* (1990). Characterization of epidemic and nonepidemic *Neisseria meningitidis* serogroup A strains from Sudan and Sweden. *J Clin Microbiol* **28**: 1711.

Salmi I, Pettay O, Simula I *et al.* (1976). An epidemic due to sulphonamide-resistant Group A meningococci in the Helsinki area (Finland). Epidemiological and clinical observations. *Scand J Infect Dis* **8**: 249.

Salvaggio J, Gonzalez F (1959). Severe toxic reactions associated with sulfamethoxypyridazine (kynex). *Ann Intern Med* **51**: 60.

Sands M, Brown RB (1989). Interactions of cyclosporine with antimicrobial agents. *Rev Infect Dis* **11**: 691.

Sanford JP (1993). *Guide to Antimicrobial Therapy*. West Bethesda, USA: Antimicrobial Therapy Inc.

Savilahti E (1983). Sulfasalazine induced immunodeficiency. *Brit Med J* **287**: 759.

Sawhney CP, Sharma RK, Rao KR, Kaushish R (1989). Long-term experience with 1% topical silver sulphadiazine cream in the management of burns wounds. *Burns* **15**: 403.

Schachter J (1978). Chlamydial infections (second of three parts). *New Engl J Med* **298**: 490.

Scheel O, Iversen G (1991). Resistant strains isolated from bacteremia patients in northern Norway. *Scand J Infect Dis* **23**: 599.

Schneider RE, Beeley L (1977). Megaloblastic anaemia associated with sulphasalazine treatment. *Brit Med J* **1**: 1638.

Schwartz AG, Targan SR, Saxon A, Weinstein HM (1982). Sulfasalazine-induced exacerbation of ulcerative colitis. *New Engl J Med* **306**: 409.

Selby CD, Ladusans EJ, Smith PG (1985). Fatal multisystemic toxicity associated with prophylaxis with pyrimethamine and sulfadoxine (Fansidar). *Brit Med J* **290**: 113.

Serebro H, Kay S, Javett S, Abrahams C (1977). Sulphasalazine rectal enemas: topical method of inducing remission of active ulcerative colitis affecting rectum and descending colon. *Brit Med J* **2**: 1264.

Shanks GD, Edstein MD, Suriyamongkol V et al. (1992). Malaria chemoprophylaxis using proguanil/dapsone combinations on the Thai-Cambodian border. *Amer J Trop Med Hyg* **46**: 643.

Shear NH, Spielberg SP, Grant DM et al. (1986). Differences in metabolism of sulfonamides predisposing to idiosyncratic toxicity. *Ann Intern Med* **105**: 179.

Sher MA, Suchaz C, Lockey RF (1986). Anaphylactic shock induced by oral desensitization to trimethoprim/sulfamethoxazole (Abstr). *J Allergy Clin Immunol* **77**: 133.

Shermantine M, Gambertoglio J, Amend W et al. (1985). Pharmacokinetics of sulfisoxazole in renal transplant patients. *Antimicrob Ag Chemother* **28**: 535.

Simão F, Macome A, Pateguana F, Schapira A (1991). Comparison of intramuscular quinine for the treatment of falciparum malaria in children. *Trans Roy Soc Trop Med Hyg* **85**: 341.

Simon DI, Brosius F, Rothstein DM (1990). Sulfadiazine crystalluria revisited. The treatment of *Toxoplasma* encephalitis in patients with acquired immunodeficiency syndrome. *Arch Intern Med* **150**: 2379.

Singleton JW (1980). Medical therapy of inflammatory bowel disease. *Med Clin N Amer* **64**: 1117.

Smellie JM, Bantock HM, Thompson BD (1982). Co-trimoxazole and the thyroid. *Lancet* **ii**: 96.

Smith MD, Gibson GE, Rowland R (1982). Combined hepatotoxicity and neurotoxicity following sulphasalazine administration. *Aust NZ J Med* **12**: 76.

Sng EH, Lim AL, Rajan VS et al. (1982). Characteristics of *Haemophilus ducreyi*. A study. *Brit J Vener Dis* **58**: 239.

Souney P, Polk BF (1982). Single-dose antimicrobial therapy for urinary tract infections in women. *Rev Infect Dis* **4**: 29.

Speck WT, Rosenkranz HS (1974). Activity of silver sulphadiazine against dermatophytes. *Lancet* **ii**: 895.

Speck WT, Driscoll JM, Polin RA et al. (1977). Staphylococcal and streptococcal colonization of the newborn infant. Effect of antiseptic cord care. *Amer J Dis Child* **131**: 1005.

Stamm WE, Guinan ME, Johnson C et al. (1984). Effect of treatment regimens for *Neisseria gonorrhoeae* on simultaneous infection with *Chlamydia trachomatis*. *New Engl J Med* **310**: 545.

Stanford W, Rapole BW, Fox CL (1969). Clinical experience with silver sulfadazine, a new topical agent for control of *Pseudomonas* infections in burns. *J Trauma* **9**: 377.

Ström J (1962). The role of drugs in certain febrile mucocutaneous manifestations (syndroma mucocutaneum febrile). as illustrated by provocation of clinical and thrombocyte reactions. *Acta allergologica* **XVII**: 232.

Stürchler D, Handschin J, Mannino S, Mittelholzer M-L (1991). Mefloquine plus sulfadoxine and pyrimethamine. *Lancet* **338**: 51.

Sullivan TJ (1991). Cross-reactions among furosemide, hydrochlorothiazide, and sulfonamides. *JAMA* **265**: 120.

Summers JM, Switz DM, Sessions JT et al. (1979). The National Cooperative Crohn's disease study. Results of drug treatment. *Gastroenterology* **77**: 847.

Sundström, L Skold, O (1990). The dhfrI trimethoprim resistance gene of Tn7 can be found at specific sites in other genetic surroundings. *Antimicrob Ag Chemother* **34**: 642.

Sundström L, Rådström P, Swedberg G, Sköld O (1988). Site-specific recombination promotes linkage between trimethoprim- and sulfonamide-resistance genes. Sequence characterization of *dhfrV* and *sulI* and a recombination active locus of Tn21. *Mol Gen Genet* **213**: 191.

Svartz N (1942). Salazopyrin: a new sulphanilamide preparation. *Acta Med Scand* **110**: 577.

Svartz N (1948). The treatment of 124 cases of ulcerative colitis with salazopyrine and attempts of desensibilization in cases of hypersensitiveness to sulpha. *Acta Med Scand* **130** (Suppl 206): 465.

Swenson JM, Wallace RJ Jr, Silcox VA et al. (1985). Antimicrobial susceptibility of five subgroups of *Mycobacterium fortuitum* and *Mycobacterium chelonae*. *Antimicrob Ag Chemother* **28**: 807.

Taffet SL, Das KM (1982). Desensitization of patients with inflammatory bowel disease due to sulfasalazine. *Amer J Med* **73**: 520.

Taylor GM (1968). Stevens–Johnson syndrome following the use of an ultra-long-acting sulphonamide. *S Afr Med J* **42**: 501.

Tenant-Flowers M, Boyle MJ, Carey D et al. (1991). Sulphadiazine desensitization in patients with AIDS and cerebral toxoplasmosis. *AIDS* **5**: 311.

Thirkettle JL, Gough KR, Read AE (1963). Agranulocytosis associated with sulphasalazine ('Salazopyrin'). therapy. *Lancet* **i**: 1395.

Tilstone WJ, Gray JMB, Nimmo-Smith RH, Lawson DH (1977). Interaction between warfarin and sulphamethoxazole. *Postgrad Med J* **53**: 388.

Toomey KE, Barnes RC (1990). Treatment of *Chlamydia trachomatis* genital infection. *Rev Infect Dis* **12** (Suppl 6): S645.

Torgovnick J, Arsura E (1990). Desensitization to sulfonamides in patients with HIV infection. *Amer J Med* **88**: 548.

Toth A (1979). Male infertility due to sulfasalazine. *Lancet* **ii**: 904.

Tydd TF, Dyer NH (1976). Sulphasalazine lung. *Med J Aust* **1**: 570.

Van der Heijde DM, Van Riel PL, Nuver-Zwart IH et al. (1989). Effects of hydroxychloroquine and sulphasalazine on progression of joint damage in rheumatoid arthritis. *Lancet* **i**: 1036.

Van der Meer JWM, Van den Broek PJ (1984). Present status of the management of patients with defective phagocyte function. *Rev Infect Dis* **6**: 107.

Van Hees PAM, Van Tongeren JHM, Bakker JH, Van Lier HJJ (1978). Active therapeutic moiety of sulphasalazine. *Lancet* **i**: 277.

Varsano I, Volovitz B, Mimouni F (1985). Sulfisoxazole prophylaxis of middle ear effusion and recurrent acute otitis media. *Amer J Dis Child* **139**: 632.

Ventura MG, Wybran J, Farber CM (1989). Sulphadiazine revisited. *J Infect Dis* **160**: 556.

Victorian Drug Usage Advisory Committee (1994). *Antibiotic Guidelines*. Melbourne: Victorian Medical Postgraduate Foundation Inc.

Wadsworth SJ, Suh B (1988). *In vitro* displacement of bilirubin by antibiotics and 2-hydroxybenzoylglycine in newborns. *Antimicrob Ag Chemother* **32**: 1571.

Wallace RJ Jr, Septimus EJ, Musher DM et al. (1977). Disk diffusion susceptibility testing of *Nocardia* species. *J Infect Dis* **135**: 568.

Wallace RJ Jr, Jones DB, Wiss K (1981). Sulfonamide activity against *Mycobacterium fortuitum* and *Mycobacterium chelonei*. *Rev Infect Dis* **3**: 898.

Wallace RJ, Steele LC, Sumter G *et al.* (1988). Antimicrobial susceptibility patterns of *Nocardia asteroides. Antimicrob Ag Chemother* **32**: 1776.

Wallwork J, McGregor CGA, Wells FC *et al.* (1983). Cyclosporin and intravenous sulphadimidine and trimethoprim therapy. *Lancet* **i**: 366.

Walzer, P D, Kim, C K, Foy, J M *et al.* (1988). Inhibitors of folic acid synthesis in the treatment of experimental *Pneumocystis carinii* pneumonia. *Antimicrob Ag Chemother* **32**: 96.

Walzer, P D, Foy, J, Steele, P *et al.* (1992a). Treatment of experimental pneumocystosis: review of 7 years of experience and development of a new system for classifying antimicrobial drugs. *Antimicrob Ag Chemother* **36**: 1943.

Walzer, P D, Foy, J, Steele, P *et al.* (1992b). Activities of antifolate, antiviral, and other drugs in an immunosuppressed rat model of *Pneumocystis carinii* pneumonia. *Antimicrob Ag Chemother* **36**: 1935.

Wan AT, Conyers RA, Coombs CJ, Masterton JP (1991). Dtermination of silver in blood, urine, and tissues of volunteers and burn patients. *Clin Chem* **37**: 1683.

Weinstein L, Madoff MA, Samet CM (1960). The sulphonamides. *New Engl J Med* **263**: 793, 842, 900, 952.

Wenzel RP, Hunting KJ, Osterman CA, Sande MA (1976). *Providencia stuartii*, a hospital pathogen: potential factors for its emergence and transmission. *Amer J Epidemiol* **104**: 170.

Wheelan KR, Cooper B, Stone MJ (1982). Multiple hematologic abnormalities associated with sulfasalazine. *Ann Intern Med* **97**: 726.

Whitfield D (1982). Presumptive fatality due to pyrimethamine-sulfadoxine. *Lancet* **ii**: 1272.

WHO (World Health Organization) (1971). Meningococcal meningitis. *Wkly Epidem Rec* **46**: 381.

WHO (World Health Organization) (1974). Meningococcal meningitis. *Wkly Epidem Rec* **49**: 197.

WHO (World Health Organization) (1979). Meningococcal surveillance. Drug resistance. *Wkly Epidem Rec* **54**: 110.

WHO (World Health Organization) (1980a). Cholera surveillance: multiply antibiotic-resistant O-group 1 *Vibrio cholerae. Wkly Epidem Rec* **22**: 161.

WHO (World Health Organization) (1993). *International Travel and Health* Geneva: WHO.

Wilkinson PJ, Reeves DS (1979). Tissue penetration of trimethoprim and sulphonamides. *J Antimicrob Chemother* **5** (Suppl B): 159.

Willcox RR (1977). How suitable are available pharmaceuticals for the treatment of sexually transmitted diseases? (2) Conditions presenting as sores or tumours. *Brit J Vener Dis* **53**: 340.

Williams DM, Wimpenny J, Asscher AW (1968). Renal clearance of sodium sulphadimidine in normal and uraemic subjects. *Lancet* **ii**: 1058.

Winslow DL, Pankey GA (1982). *In vitro* activities of trimethoprim and sulfamethoxazole against *Listeria monocytogenes. Antimicrob Ag Chemother* **22**: 51.

Wright LJ, Plorde JJ (1970). Group-A sulphadiazine-resistant *Neisseria meningitidis* in Ethiopia. *Lancet* **ii**: 1033.

Young CL (1989). Acute encephalopathy associated with sulfadiazine in a patient with AIDS-related complex. *J Infect Dis* **160**: 163.

Yourassowsky E, Vanderlinden MP, Schoutens E (1974). Sensitivity of *Streptococcus pyogenes* to sulphamethoxazole, trimethoprim, and cotrimoxazole. *J Clin Path* **27**: 897.

Zhang Y, Meshnick SR (1991). Inhibition of *Plasmodium falciparum* dihydropteroate synthetase and growth *in vitro* by sulfa drugs. *Antimicrob Ag Chemother* **35**: 267.

Trimethoprim, Co-trimoxazole (Co-T), and other Trimethoprim Combinations

Description

Trimethoprim or 2,4-diamino-5-(3,4,5-trimethoxybenzyl)-pyrimidine was synthesized in 1956 by Hitchings at the Wellcome Laboratories in the USA (Roth *et al.*, 1962). It has both antibacterial and antimalarial activity, while another diaminopyrimidine, pyrimethamine (p. 905), which was synthesized in 1951 (Russel and Hitchings, 1951), is mainly active against malaria and *Toxoplasma gundii* (pp. 913, 917). Trimethoprim interrupts bacterial purine synthesis and acts in the same metabolic pathway as the sulfonamides (p. 814). The combination of these two drugs, therefore, has a synergistic effect against certain bacteria (Bushby and Hitchings, 1968; Darrell *et al.*,1968). In the period 1968–78, trimethoprim was only available for general clinical use as a mixture with the medium-acting sulfonamide, sulfamethoxazole (p. 810). This was selected for commercial formulations, because its rate of absorption and excretion closely parallels that of trimethoprim. Commercial preparations contain a mixture of sulfamethoxazole and trimethoprim in a fixed ratio of 5:1. The generic name of co-trimoxazole (Co-T) is used to describe this drug combination.

Many of the advantages, originally claimed for Co-T, have been challenged: such as that sequential blockage of bacterial folate synthesis produces synergism; that such synergism occurs *in vivo*; and that its two component drugs protect each other from the development of bacterial resistance (p. 839). Trimethoprim became available for use as a single drug in Finland in 1973 and then in the UK (1979), the USA (1980) and Australia (1982). General review articles regarding Co-T include those by Turnidge (1988, 1989) and Cockerill and Edson (1991).

Sensitive Organisms

Trimethoprim has a wide range of antibacterial activity (Bushby, 1969, 1973; Bach *et al.*, 1973b).

1 Gram-positive aerobic bacteria

Trimethoprim is active against pyogenic cocci such as *Staphylococcus aureus*, including penicillin- and a proportion of methicillin-resistant strains (Seligman, 1973), the majority of *Staph. epidermidis* strains (Jones *et al.*, 1987, and the vast majority of *Streptococcus pyogenes*, *Strep. pneumoniae*, *Strep. viridans* and streptococci in the *milleri* group (Jarvinen *et al.*, 1993; Gomez-Garces *et al.*, 1994; Nissinen *et al.*, 1995b). Trimethoprim is quite active, and Co-T more so, against *Staph. saprophyticus* (Iravani *et al.*, 1985). Co-T has shown good activity against many fluoroquinolone-methicillin-resistant strains of *Staph. aureus* (Aldridge *et al.*, 1992). Studies of world-wide antibiotic-resistance in methicillin-resistant *Staph. aureus* have shown that there are geographical variations in the patterns of resistance. Most strains from the UK and Australia are resistant to trimethoprim, whereas many strains from Europe and the USA are sensitive (Maple *et al.*, 1989). Most *Staph. epidermidis* strains however, can evade the *in vitro* bactericidal activity of Co-T in the presence of low levels of thymidine. Thus, since strains vary in their utilization of thymidine and body tissues vary in thymidine content, there may be a disparity between *in vitro* susceptibility of *Staph. epidermidis* strains and *in vivo* bactericidal activity (Jones *et al.*, 1987).

Enterococci are variable in their *in vitro* susceptibility to trimethoprim (and Co-T) depending upon the concentrations of thymine, thymidine and folates (folate, folinate, dihydrofolate and tetrahydrofolate) in the test media. The presence of small quantities of these compounds which can be taken up by enterococci allow 'bypass' of the dihydrofolate reductase inhibition usually induced by trimethoprim (Hamilton-Miller, 1988). Despite the addition of thymidine phosphorylase to media to convert thymidine to thymine (a less potent inhibitor of trimethoprim activity) for susceptibility testing, results can be variable (Bushby, 1973). Crider and Colby (1985) noted significant variation in susceptibility to Co-T when three different brands of Mueller-Hinton broth were used. Najjar and Murray (1987) also demonstrated inconsistent results when using different batches of the same brand of Mueller-Hinton media (presumably due to minor variations in the amount of exogenous folates). The most accurate susceptibility results appear to be achieved with Oxoid (Isosensitest) agar – probably because this media has tightly controlled levels of 'folates' (Tofte *et al.*, 1984). However, despite the apparent *in vitro* susceptibility of some enterococcal strains to trimethoprim and Co-T, some clinical reports of serious therapeautic failure have raised concerns regarding the *in vivo* efficacy of Co-T. In particular, Goodhart (1984) described two patients with uncomplicated enterococcal urinary infections, who were treated with Co-T but who subsequently developed enterococcal bacteremia despite *in vitro* susceptibility to this antibiotic combination. This apparent disparity between *in vitro* susceptibility and *in vivo* efficacy of Co-T against enterococci has also been demonstrated in two recent *in vivo* animal studies in which Co-T therapy failed against serious enterococcal infections (Grayson *et al.*, 1990; Chenoweth *et al.*, 1990). Thus, Co-T cannot at present be considered acceptable treatment for serious enterococcal infections.

Co-T is active against many Gram-positive bacilli such as *Corynebacterium diphtheriae* and *C. pseudodiphtheriticum* (Manzella *et al.*, 1995). *Rhodococcus equi* is usually susceptible, but Co-T does not appear to be bactericidal against this pathogen (Nordmann and Ronco, 1992). *Arcanobacterium haemolyticum* is usually resistant to Co-T (Carlson *et al.*, 1994). Trimethoprim is bactericidal against most strains of *Listeria monocytogenes* and synergy with sulfamethoxazole has been demonstrated, even when isolates are relatively resistant to sulfamethoxazole alone (Winslow and Pankey, 1982; MacGowan *et al.*, 1990; Appleman *et al.*, 1991). *Bacillus cereus* (Leading article, 1983b) and *Erysipelothrix rhusiopathiae* (Venditti *et al.*, 1990) are resistant.

Some strains of *Nocardia* are susceptible to trimethoprim, but its MIC for this organism varies widely (Bach *et al.*, 1973a; Dewsnup and Wright, 1984). Studies using Co-T usually demonstrate a synergistic effect of this combination against *Nocardia* (Bushby, 1973; Pavillard, 1973; Maderazo and Quintiliani, 1974; Wallace *et al.*, 1982a). The demonstration of this depends on the isolate, duration of incubation and the ratio of the component drugs used (Bennett and Jennings, 1978). Higher doses of trimethoprim than in commercially available Co-T are required to produce synergism and this is usually demonstrable with a trimethoprim/sulfamethoxazole ratio of 1:5 or greater, but not at the usual serum ratio of 1:20 (p. 847). Since trimethoprim reaches higher concentrations in most tissues than in serum, while the concentration of sulfamethoxazole in tissue is 20–50% of the serum level, the ratio of the two drugs in lung or other body tissues may approximate to 1:5 or even less when the usual serum ratios of 1:20 are maintained (Wallace *et al.*, 1982a). Khardori *et al.* (1993) found the MIC_{90} of Co-T against *N. asteroides* to be 4/76 μg per ml (trimethoprim/sulfamethoxazole) and the MIC_{50} against *N. brasiliensis* and *N. caviae* to be 1/19 and 4/76 μg per ml, respectively.

2 Gram-negative aerobic bacteria

Most Enterobacteriaceae are susceptible to trimethoprim. These include *Escherichia coli* and the *Enterobacter*, *Proteus*, *Salmonella*, *Shigella*, *Providencia*, *Citrobacter*, *Hafnia*, *Edwardsiella* and *Arizona* spp. and *Serratia marcescens*. Co-T is active against many enterotoxogenic *E. coli* strains which have been isolated from different geographic locations (DuPont *et al.*, 1978), but the incidence of resistance is increasing (p. 841). *Yersinia enterocolitica* is sensitive to trimethoprim (Gutman *et al.*, 1973; Preston *et al.*, 1994), while *Y. pestis* is sensitive to Co-T (Ai *et al.*, 1973) and probably also to trimethoprim alone, and *Y. pseudotuberculosis* is sensitive to Co-T (Brodie *et al.*, 1973). *Klebsiella* species, including *Kl. rhinoscleromatis* (Perkins *et al.*, 1992), are usually sensitive, but resistant strains were present before trimethoprim became available for clinical use (Hamilton-Miller and Grey, 1975). Co-T is active against many ampicillin-resistant shigellae, which may also be multiply-resistant to tetracyclines, chloramphenicol and sulfonamides (Rodriguez et al., 1978). The Aeromonas species and Plesiomonas shigelloides are usually susceptible to trimethoprim and Co-T (Reinhardt and George, 1985; Kuijper et al., 1989; Burgos et al., 1990; Koehler and Ashdown, 1993). However, susceptibility to trimethoprim and CoT may be overestimated using disk diffusion susceptibility techniques compared with agar dilution, when assessing Aeromonas hydrophila, A. sobria and A. caviae (Koehler and Ashdown, 1993). Campylobacter jejuni, Campylobacter coli and 'Camylobacter upsaliensis' are usually resistant to Co-T (Goossens et al., 1985; Preston et al., 1990). All strains of Helicobacter pylori tested by McNulty et al. (1985) were resistant to sulfamethoxazole and trimethoprim.

Haemophilus influenzae, including ampicillin-resistant strains, is usually (≥94%) sensitive to trimethoprim and when this is combined with sulfamethoxazole, synergism is demonstrable (Kirven and Thornsberry, 1974; Sinai et al., 1978; Kanellakopoulou et al., 1988; Howard and Williams, 1989; Jorgenson et al., 1990; Collignon et al., 1992). Some strains of H. influenzae, while having low inhibitory concentrations to trimethoprim (or Co-T), may require high concentrations of the drug for bactericidal action. Haemophilus ducreyi (including strains resistant to sulfonamides, ampicillin and other antibiotics) has been sensitive to trimethoprim and Co-T (Kraus et al., 1982; McNicol and Ronald, 1984; Dangor et al., 1990a). However, more recently H. ducreyi strains with increased resistance to trimethoprim have been described in some areas of the world including the USA and some parts of Africa (CDC, 1985b; Dangor et al., 1990a; Knapp et al., 1993). Contrary to the findings of early limited studies, most strains of Bordetella pertussis are not susceptible to trimethoprim and Co-T in concentrations which are achievable in vivo (Zackrisson et al., 1983). Pasteurella multocida is quite sensitive. Vibrio cholerae, both classical and El Tor bio-types, are generally susceptible (Northrup et al., 1972; Yamamoto et al., 1995). Brucella spp. (Robertson et al., 1973) and the pathogenic Neisseria (meningococci and gonococci) are moderately resistant to trimethoprim. Moraxella catarrhalis is usually sensitive to Co-T (Slevin et al., 1984; Alvarez et al., 1985; Sweeney et al., 1985; Jorgenson et al., 1990; Wallace et al., 1990), but resistant to trimethoprim (Then, 1982; Fung et al., 1992).

Pseudomonas aeruginosa is resistant to trimethoprim and Co-T due to a permeability barrier but conditions may be such in the urine that trimethoprim may occasionally act synergistically with sulfamethoxazole against this organism (Grey and Hamilton-Miller, 1977). Usually Burkholderia (previously Pseudomonas) cepacia is sensitive to trimethoprim and Co-T (Hamilton et al., 1973; Moody and Young, 1975), although isolates from patients with cystic fibrosis are more frequently Co-T-resistant (Isles et al., 1984; Burns et al., 1989). By comparison, Stenotrophomonas (Xanthomonas) maltophilia is usually resistant to trimethoprim (MIC >32 μg per ml), but the vast majority of strains are sensitive to Co-T (Moody and Young, 1975; Hohl et al., 1991; Garcia-Rodriguez et al., 1991; Vartivarian et al., 1994). Although Burkholderia (previously Pseudomonas) pseudomallei is usually trimethoprim-resistant, some strains are sulfamethoxazole-sensitive and many can be inhibited by therapeutically achievable concentrations of Co-T (Bassett, 1971; Everett and Kishimoto, 1973) – although more recent reports suggest only moderate in vitro susceptibility to Co-T (Dance et al., 1989; Yamamoto et al., 1990); Ps. stutzeri is usually susceptible (Noble and Overman, 1994).

Flavobacterium spp. are resistant to sulfamethoxazole, but sensitive to Co-T (Aber et al., 1978). Co-T is active in vitro against Legionella pneumophila (Thornsberry et al., 1978) and L. micdadei (Myerowitz et al., 1979) and also active in vivo for treatment of guinea-pigs infected with L. pneumophila (Plouffe et al., 1984) or L. micdadei (Pasculle et al., 1985). Bartonella (previously Rochalimaea) spp., including B. henselae and B. quintana, are susceptible in vitro with MIC$_{90}$ of 1 and 5 μg per ml for trimethoprim and sulfamethoxazole, respectively (Maurin et al., 1995). Gardnerella vaginalis is susceptible in vitro to trimethoprim (Kharsany et al., 1993).

3 Anaerobic bacteria

Results of susceptibility testing of these bacteria to trimethoprim and Co-T have been conflicting (Bushby, 1973; Okubadejo et al., 1973; Rosenblatt and Stewart, 1974). Phillips and Warren (1974) showed that Bacteroides fragilis was susceptible to sulfamethoxazole and, when used with trimethoprim, synergism could be demonstrated if greater amounts of trimethoprim than sulfamethoxazole were used, the reverse of the optimum ratio for most bacteria. Phillips and Warren (1976) suggested that previous discrepancies were explicable by differences in techniques. They concluded that true resistance of *B. fragilis* to sulfamethoxazole was rare, and that synergism against *B. fragilis* could be demonstrated if these drugs were combined together in the ratio of their MICs for this organism, as determined by the particular method used. Others have confirmed this (Wust and Wilkins, 1978; Then and Angehrn, 1979; Riley, 1981). *Bacteroides fragilis* is resistant to trimethoprim. All of 28 *B. fragilis* strains investigated by Then and Angehrn (1979), though sensitive to sulfamethoxazole, were resistant to trimethoprim. Other *Bacteroides* spp. are not as frequently sensitive to sulfamethoxazole as *B. fragilis*. *Bacteroides* spp. are commonly resistant to trimethoprim due to decreased susceptibility of their dihydrofolate reductase (p. 852) (Then and Angehrn, 1979). Other anaerobes, such as *Clostridium* spp., are also usually resistant to trimethoprim, though often sensitive to sulfamethoxazole. Wüst and Wilkins (1978) found that despite this, 85% of anaerobes were susceptible to trimethoprim/sulfamethoxazole in a ratio of 1:19 and synergy was most marked when the ratio of these components was near 1:1. Phillips *et al.* (1981) describe similar findings.

4 Other microorganisms

Trimethoprim may have an effect against some true fungi such as *Histoplasma capsulatum* (Macleod, 1970). One *in vitro* study indicated a synergistic effect between trimethoprim and sulfamethoxazole against *Paracoccidioides brasiliensis* despite resistance to trimethoprim and often resistance to sulfamethoxazole (Stevens and Vo, 1982). Trimethoprim has no activity against *Treponema*, *Leptospirae* and *Rickettsia* spp. When tested in cell culture, MICs of trimethoprim and sulfamethoxazole for *Chlamydia trachomatis* are ≥ 64 and $2-128\ \mu g$ per ml, respectively. There was no synergy when trimethoprim was used with sulfamethoxazole, although there was a low degree of potentiation when a ratio of 1:20 was used. The activity of Co-T against *C. trachomatis* appeared to be primarily that of sulfamethoxazole alone (Hammerschlag, 1982). Nevertheless, trimethoprim does cause structural changes in *C. trachomatis* similar to sulfamethoxazole but, in this respect, it is not as potent (Hammerschlag and Vuletin, 1985). Rice *et al.* (1995) noted the MIC range for Co-T against *C. trachomatis* isolates obtained from women with asymptomatic genital infection or pelvic inflammmatory disease to be $0.03-0.25\ \mu g$ per ml, *in vitro*. *Mycobacterium tuberculosis*, *M. haemophilum* and *Mycoplasma* are resistant (Bernard *et al.*, 1993).

5 Malaria parasites

Although these may be sensitive to trimethoprim, albeit to a lesser degree than to pyrimethamine, trimethoprim has no clinical role in the treament of malaria (Winstanley *et al.*, 1995).

6 Comparative antibacterial activity with sulfonamides

Trimethoprim (although having a similar antibacterial spectrum) is more active than the sulfonamides against most bacterial species, with the exception of the *Neisseria*, *Brucella*, *Bacteroides* and *Nocardia* spp. (Table II.3).

7 Acquired resistance

One of the original postulates for Co-T was that the combination would prevent the development of resistance to either of its two component drugs. There are now serious doubts about this concept (Grüneberg, 1979; Lacey, 1982).

If Gram-negative bacteria are passaged in increasing trimethoprim concentrations *in vitro*, drug-resistance develops rapidly (Reisberg *et al.*, 1967). Under certain laboratory conditions, the development of trimethoprim-resistance in Enterobacteriaceae in this way can be prevented by the incorporation of a sulfonamide in the medium (Darrell *et al.*, 1968). It was therefore feared that, if trimethoprim was used as a single drug, trimethoprim-resistance would become prevalent. Trimethoprim has been used alone in Finland since 1973 and in most other countries after 1979. Although the level of trimethoprim-resistance has increased since the early 1970s, evidence to date does not suggest that the use of trimethoprim alone selects resistance. Furthermore, since a high percentage of enterobacteria are sulfonamide-resistant, treatment with Co-T in many instances has been tantamount to treatment with trimethoprim alone.

Soon after the introduction of Co-T more than 20 years ago, trimethoprim-resistance among strains of Gram-negative bacteria was identified, and subsequently resistance has also been noted in Gram-positive bacteria. Worldwide, resistance to Co-T and trimethoprim appears to be increasing, although this rate of increase varies depending on the bacterial species, the types of infection being treated and geography. Some of the most dramatic and disturbing increases in trimethoprim- and Co-T-resistance have been noted in developing countries where Co-T is often freely available with little prescribing control.

The numerous mechanisms of resistance which have been described are generally either plasmid- or chromosome-mediated. Chromosomally mediated mechanisms of resistance include quantitative and qualitative changes in dihydrofolate reductase (DHFR; the target enzyme of trimethoprim), modifications of the pathway for DNA synthesis and alterations in bacterial cell wall permeability to trimethoprim and sulfamethoxazole. Another chromosomal-associated mechanism of low-level resistance is the mutational loss of the ability of some bacteria to methylate deoxyuridylic acid to thymidylic acid, thereby making the bacteria dependent on an external supply of thymine. Thus, the DHFR of the bacteria is not as necessary to regenerate tetrahydrofolate for cell duplication and therefore the cell can afford to have a relatively large fraction of its DHFR inactivated by trimethoprim without interfering in multiplication (Huovinen et al., 1995). Chromosomally mediated resistance mechanisms generally result in low-level resistance to trimethoprim (MIC 4–512 µg per ml). Plasmid- or transposon-mediated resistance is generally manifest by the production of trimethoprim-resistant DHFR which results in high-level resistance to trimethoprim (MIC ≥1000 µg per ml) (Goldstein et al., 1986b; Review, 1990). This latter mechanism of resistance is particularly concerning due to the ready transferability of these resistance determinants. The mechanisms of acquired resistance to trimethoprim are summarized in Table II.2 and have been reviewed by Huovinen et al. (1995).

Low-level resistance (MIC 4–512 µg per ml) usually results from spontaneous mutational events such as decreased permeability and quantitative or qualitative changes in DHFR, where the bacteria then gain a selective growth advantage during therapy. Transferable plasmid-mediated low-level resistance was first described in 1971, but is not common (Lebek and Wiedmer, 1971; Goldstein et al., 1986b; Review, 1990). Trimethoprim-resistance due to decreased cell wall permeability (usually secondary to modification of outer wall proteins) is notable by the presence of cross-resistance to quinolones, chloramphenicol, beta-lactams, sulfonamides and tetracyclines. This type of mutation has been noted in Klebsiella, Enterobacter and Serratia spp. and may be more common than previously assumed (Gutmann et al., 1985).

Mechanism	Resistant organism
Thymine requirement	Enterobacteriaceae Staphylococcus Streptococcus
Impaired antibiotic permeability	Klebsiella Enterobacter Serratia
Altered DHFR[a]	Enterobacteriaceae Staphylococcus
Overproduction of DHFR	Enterobacteriaceae MRSA Haemophilus influenzae
Additional trimethoprim-resistant DHFR[b]	Enterobacteriaceae Vibrio cholerae Acinetobacter Pseudomonas aeruginosa Burkholderia cepacia

Table II.2
Mechanisms of acquired resistance to trimethoprim. (Modified after Goldstein FW, Papadopoulou B, Acar JF, 1986b. The changing pattern of trimethoprim resistance in Paris, with a review of worldwide experience. Rev Infect Dis **8**: 725, with permission from the University of Chicago Press.)

MRSA: methicillin-resistant Staphylococcus aureus.
[a] DHFR: dihydrofolate reductase
[b] Usually plasmid- or transposon-mediated resistance.

High-level resistance (MIC ≥1000 µg per ml) was first identified in 1975 (Breeze *et al.*, 1975) and is generally plasmid- or transposon-mediated. Such transferable resistance has spread to all enterobacterial species and is identified by the production of a variety of new insusceptible DHFR enzymes – at least 15 enzymes (types I-VII) have been described in Gram-negative bacteria (Review, 1990; Towner *et al.*, 1992). A number of transposons have been particularly associated with high-level trimethoprim-resistance. Transposon Tn7, which encodes resistance to spectinomycin, streptomycin and trimethoprim (DHFR Ia) is the most common and best described trimethoprim transposon, being identified in enterobacteria and *V. cholerae*. Transposon Tn4132 encodes trimethoprim-resistance alone (Young and Amyes, 1985). A third group of transposons, Tn402, encode DHFR type II (Shapiro and Sporn, 1977). Several other trimethoprim-resistance transposons have been identified. Fluctuations in the transferability of high-level trimethoprim-resistance are probably due to variations in the transposons jumping from plasmid to plasmid, or in and out of the bacterial chromosome (Review, 1990).

Strains of Enterobacteriaceae resistant to trimethoprim were found before the drug was introduced (Gruneberg and Kolbe, 1969; Reeves *et al.*, 1969, Hamilton-Miller and Gray, 1975). Commonly, resistance to Co-T is assumed to mean resistance to trimethoprim. In the Turku City Hospital, Finland, development of trimethoprim-resistance appeared to be related to total use of trimethoprim, in combination or alone; in 1984, 14 years after the introduction of trimethoprim, trimethoprim-resistance among *E. coli* strains was 34–37%, which was similar to the level of sulfonamide-resistance (40%) (Huovinen *et al.*, 1986). At the Royal Free Hospital in 1985, 24% of all urinary isolates were resistant to trimethoprim which was more than double the rate of resistance in 1981. The incidence of trimethoprim-resistance among strains of *E. coli*, *P. mirabilis*, *Staph. epidermidis* and fecal streptococci was significantly greater than in 1981; although the proportion of Gram-negative strains with high-level trimethoprim-resistance (81%) was similar to the corresponding rate in 1981. Interestingly, resistant isolates were found equally as often in community-acquired urinary infections as those occurring in inpatients (Hamilton-Miller and Purves, 1986). In many hospitals, 15–20% of *E. coli* isolated from urine can be expected to be resistant to trimethoprim (Huovinen *et al.*, 1995). Among nosocomial pathogens such as *E. coli*, *Burkholderia cepacia*, trimethoprim-resistance appears to be due to the production of trimethoprim-resistant DHFR (Burns *et al.*, 1989; Tsakris *et al.*, 1993).

The incidence of trimethoprim-resistant bacteria is especially high in developing countries and has been associated with a significant increase in the relative percentage of high-level resistant bacteria harboring R plasmids and transposons. This increase in resistance is probably related to the increased use of Co-T, trimethoprim and sulfonamides in human and veterinary practice (Goldstein, 1986b; Amyes, 1986). In one study in India, 57% of all bacterial strains were highly resistant to trimethoprim, but a higher proportion of these strains possessed transferable trimethoprim-resistance plasmids than similar isolates from the UK (Young *et al.*, 1986). The resistance rates for *E. coli* are about 44% in Chile and 40% in Thailand, while 76% of *Salmonella* isolates in Brazil are resistant (Murray *et al.*, 1985). In the UK, the proportion of enterobacteria sensitive to trimethoprim has remained high despite increasing use of Co-T, but the trend is of increasing resistance, particularly in hospitals (Leading article, 1980). Co-T-resistance among Enterobacteriaceae is also becoming more common in the USA (Murray *et al.*, 1985; Stamm *et al.*, 1991) and has been associated with the use of Co-T (Pearson *et al.*, 1979; Murray *et al.*, 1982; Stamm *et al.*, 1991). In Finland, meanwhile, the frequency of trimethoprim-resistance among urinary isolates of *E. coli* remained stable at 40% during 1984 to 1988, but the proportion of isolates with high-level resistance (often due to DHFR type I) increased (Heikkila *et al.*, 1990b). Multidrug-resistance, including to Co-T, among *Salmonella* and *Shigella* spp. is now common in many countries such as Spain and countries of the developing world, including Brazil, Peru, Madagascar, Burundi, Indonesia, India and Pakistan (Goldstein *et al.*, 1986a,b; Ling and Chau, 1984; Threlfall *et al.*, 1992; Ries *et al.*, 1994; Ashkenazi *et al.*, 1995; Lima *et al.*, 1995; Mirza *et al.*, 1995). In these regions it appears to be commonly plasmid-mediated high-level resistance (Palenque *et al.*, 1983; CDC, 1987; Delgado and Otero, 1988; Heikkila *et al.*, 1990a; Bennish *et al.*, 1992; Threlfall *et al.*, 1992). An epidemic due to *V. cholerae* El Tor inaba in Thailand was notable for the fact that trimethoprim-resistance was due to a plasmid coding for type II DHFR, rather than the more typical pattern in which type I DHFR (encoded by Tn7) is responsible for such resistance in vibrios (Young and Amyes, 1986; Tabtieng *et al.*, 1989). Yamamoto *et al.* (1995) have reported that *V. cholerae* strains O139, O1 Indian El Tor and Bangladeshi El Tor were highly resistant to multiple agents (streptomycin, sulfamethoxazole and trimethoprim) in 95, 97 and 50%, respectively. Interestingly, Heikkila *et al.* (1990a) noted a dramatic increase in the incidence of trimethoprim-resistance among *Shigella* species isolated from Finnish travellers; in whom resistance increased from 3% of isolates in 1975–1982 to 44%

in 1987–1988. The majority of these later isolates were highly resistant and had detectable type I DHFR. Others have also identified trimethoprim-resistance among 54% *Shigella* isolates causing travelers' diarrhea (Vila *et al.*, 1994). Ashkenazi *et al.* (1995) noted a major increase in Israel in the rate of resistance between 1984 and 1992 among *Shigella* isolates to trimethoprim-sulfamethoxazole, with a shift from 59 to 92% resistance. Notably, *Sh. sonnei*, which accounted for 90% of *Shigella* infections was most likely to be resistant.

The use of trimethoprim or Co-T in cultures can lead to *in vitro* emergence of mutants of some Enterobacteriaceae, which do not utilize the tetrahydrofolate pathway (p. 815) leading to thymidine synthesis (Pinney and Smith, 1973). These strains utilize an exogenous source of thymine or thymidine for DNA synthesis and are unaffected by Co-T which acts on the folate pathway. There is not sufficient thymine or thymidine in normal mammalian tissues, blood or urine for the survival of these mutants. They have been found in patients with urinary, respiratory and wound infections and in salmonellosis (Maskell *et al.*, 1976; Okubadejo and Maskell, 1977; Lacey, 1982). During a 1-month period in 1979, 10% of urine culture isolates of enterococci in Rochester, USA, were found to be thymidine-dependent; the reason for this was not ascertained, but may have been due to overutilization of Co-T (Haltiner *et al.*, 1980). Thymidine-requiring strains have been detected among *Staph. aureus* and *H. influenzae*, as well as the Enterobacteriaceae (Platt *et al.*, 1983). In most instances, the isolation of these mutants from patients has been associated with the administration of Co-T. It is possible that in these situations the breakdown of pus cells and bacteria may act as a source of thymine. Special techniques are required to detect thymine-requiring bacteria and, if they are isolated from a patient, Co-T therapy should be discontinued (Tapsall *et al.*, 1974; Maskell *et al.*, 1976). Infections due to these mutants are rare because their rate of mutation is low and, when thymidine is removed from the environment, the mutants die. They may be less pathogenic than wild strains and they have not caused cross-infection, because thymidine is only found in significant amounts in infected human material (Lacey, 1982).

Trimethoprim-resistant *H. influenzae* are becoming more prevalent, although there are wide regional differences, ranging from less than 1% resistance in the USA, 7% in Europe to 11% in Pakistan (Jorgenson, 1992). Resistance has been higher among non-type b than among type b strains in several studies (Jorgenson, 1992). In Spain, sensitivity tests on *H. influenzae* strains causing invasive infections (meningitis and bacteremia) isolated in the period 1981–1983 revealed that 64% were resistant to Co-T, 50% to ampicillin, 52% to chloramphenicol and 55% to tetracycline, as well as multiple resistance in 45% (Campos *et al.*, 1984). In some strains resistance has been shown to be due to overproduction of chromosomally mediated DHFR (de Groot *et al.*, 1988). *Moraxella catarrhalis*, however, has only rarely been noted to develop resistance to trimethoprim-sulfamethoxazole (Doern, 1995; Nissinen *et al.*, 1995a). *H. ducreyi* resistance to trimethoprim and trimethoprim-sulfamethoxazole has increased dramatically in Central and East Africa, such that Co-T can no longer be recommended for use in the treatment of chancroid in this region (Van Dyck *et al.*, 1994; p. 867).

Among Gram-positive bacteria, the incidence of trimethoprim-resistance is relatively low and has really only become an issue with the appearance of methicillin-resistant *Staph. aureus* (MRSA) which may exhibit low-level trimethoprim-resistance – possibly due to the overproduction of DHFR (Lyon and Skurray, 1987). Such chromosomally mediated resistance has been identified in MRSA strains from Australia, the USA and Europe (Review, 1990; Turnidge *et al.*, 1996). Plasmid-mediated high-level trimethoprim-resistance was identified in 1983 in Australian MRSA isolates (Tennent *et al.*, 1983) and has since been described elsewhere (Coughter *et al.*, 1987). Both low-level chromosomally mediated and high-level plasmid-mediated trimethoprim-resistance has been identified among coagulase-negative staphylococci (Galetto *et al.*, 1987). Trimethoprim-resistance in pneumococci was first reported in 1972 (Howe and Wilson, 1972). Subsequently, Co-T-resistance among pneumococci has been found to vary from region to region, with resistance rates of 0.6%–26% in various areas of the USA, rising to 42% and 44% in Australia and South Africa, respectively (Henderson *et al.*, 1988; Rauch *et al.*,1990; Koornhof *et al.*,1992; Breiman *et al.*, 1994; Hofmann *et al.*, 1995; Collignon and Bell, 1996). Nelson *et al.* (1994) found all highly penicillin-resistant isolates were also resistant to trimethoprim-sulfamethoxazole. Charpentier *et al.* (1995) have, for the first time, described a trimethoprim-resistant isolate of *L. monocytogenes*.

8 Synergy with sulfonamides

Although trimethoprim is a powerful antibacterial drug, when it was first introduced as a component of Co-T, it was mainly considered to be a sulfonamide potentiator. The relevance of synergy between trimethoprim and sulfamethoxazole *in vitro* to the clinical use of Co-T has now been questioned for some infections (Gruneberg, 1979; Lacey, 1982). In urinary tract infections the activity of trimethoprim is dominant over the sulfonamide and potential synergy between them does not occur; the levels of trimethoprim are as effective as Co-T for the treatment of many urinary and respiratory infections (Lacey, 1982). Therefore, there is a good argument for using trimethoprim alone for many infections (p. 839).

Using accepted criteria, trimethoprim and sulfonamides exert a strong synergistic effect against many organisms. When organisms sensitive to both drugs are tested *in vitro*, the addition of a subinhibitory concentration of one often reduces the MIC of the other by about 8-fold or more (Darrell *et al.*, 1968). This potentiation of trimethoprim by sulfonamides and *vice versa* varies with bacterial species and also with individual strains. Darrell *et al.* (1968) found a high degree of potentiation with gonococci and also most strains of *Proteus* spp., but the sulfonamide only potentiated the activity of trimethoprim about 4- to 8-fold against most strains of staphylococci, streptococci, pneumococci, *H. influenzae* and *E. coli*. MacGowan *et al.* (1990) noted *in vitro* synergy between trimethoprim and sufamethoxazole against *L. monocytogenes*. Maximum synergy usually occurs when trimethoprim and sulfamethoxazole are used together in a ratio of their MICs. This ratio is 1:19 for many organisms and is consequently used in Co-T disc testing. Darrell *et al.* (1968) found that some organisms, such as gonococci, were more sensitive to sulfonamides than to trimethoprim so that the optimal ratio was the reverse. Nevertheless, in the USA most *N. gonorrhoeae* strains, when tested against trimethoprim/sulfamethoxazole in a ratio of 1:19, were inhibited by concentrations of 2.5 µg per ml or less of trimethoprim and 47.5 µg per ml or less of sulfamethoxazole (Yoshikawa *et al.*, 1975; Prior *et al.*, 1976). In a study of *Shigella* isolated in Michigan, sulfamethoxazole alone was effective against only 62% of isolates tested, but mixture with trimethoprim in a 20:1 ratio was highly active (Gordon *et al.*, 1975). For *M. fortuitum*, the addition of trimethoprim (to which it is resistant) does not potentiate sulfonamides against sulfonamide-sensitive strains (Wallace *et al.*, 1982b). With some bacterial strains, synergy cannot be demonstrated despite sensitivity to both trimethoprim and sulfonamides (Lewis *et al.*, 1974).

With trimethoprim-sensitive, but sulfonamide-resistant bacteria, sulfonamides do not usually potentiate the action of trimethoprim. With such sulfonamide-resistant bacteria, a synergistic effect can usually be demonstrated *in vitro*, if very high sulfonamide concentrations, which equal or exceed the MICs of the organisms to sulfonamides, are used, however, this finding is of no clinical importance because such high sulfonamide concentrations cannot be used *in vivo*. Synergy with trimethoprim can also be demonstrated against some strains of *Ps. aeruginosa* which are 'moderately resistant to sulfamethoxazole' and, because high concentrations of sulfonamides are attained in urine, this may be of significance in treating urinary tract infections. Similarly, synergy may be attained in the urine of patients with sulfonamide-resistant *E. coli* treated by Co-T (Gruneberg, 1975).

In clinical practice, the sensitivity of organisms to trimethoprim and sulfonamide should be tested separately. If the bacterial species is sensitive to both, a synergistic effect is likely, and treatment may be effective. However, infections due to trimethoprim-sensitive, but sulfonamide-resistant, bacteria also usually respond to the combination and they would probably respond equally well to trimethoprim alone.

9 Synergy with other drugs

Trimethoprim acts synergistically with rifampicin against a wide range of bacteria, particularly Gram-negative bacilli; in addition these two drugs are compatible pharmacologically.

Trimethoprim enhances the activity of the polymyxins against certain bacteria. The combination of a polymyxin, sulfamethoxazole and trimethoprim is more active than combinations of any two of these agents against a variety of Gram-negative bacilli. A combination of trimethoprim and amikacin is synergistic against some Gram-negative bacilli (Parsley *et al.*, 1977). Synergy was demonstrated against most strains of *Kl. pneumoniae*, *S. marcescens* and *E. coli*; trimethoprim had no antibacterial effect on strains of *Ps. aeruginosa* and did not alter the activity of amikacin against them. Gentamicin and Co-T may be synergistic against Co-T-sensitive isolates of *S. marcescens* (Gray *et al.*, 1978). Gentamicin combined with trimethoprim or Co-T is sometimes synergistic against *E. coli* and *Kl. pneumoniae* (Paisley and Washington, 1978). A combination of rifampicin and trimethoprim may have a beneficial effect in experimental *Brucella* infections; this combination may also be synergistic against *H. influenzae in vitro*. The clinical relevence of these *in vitro* synergy findings, however, remains uncertain.

Organism	MIC (µg per ml)	
	Trimethoprim	Sulfamethoxazole
Gram-positive bacteria		
Staphylococcus aureus	0.2	4.0
Streptococcus pyogenes	0.4	100.0
Streptococcus pneumoniae	1.0	32.0
Streptococcus viridans	0.25	8.0
Clostridium perfringens	50.0	16.0
Corynebacterium diphtheriae	0.4	>100.0
Nocardia asteroides	10.0	5.0
Gram-negative bacteria		
Escherichia coli	0.2	8.0
Enterobacter spp.	3.0	>100.0
Klebsiella pneumoniae	0.5	16.0
Citrobacter freundii	0.1	3.0
Proteus spp.	1.0	8.0
Salmonella typhi	0.4	4.0
Salmonella typhimurium	0.3	10.0
Shigella spp.	0.4	4.0
Neisseria gonorrhoeae	12.0	1.6
Neisseria meningitidis	8.0	0.5
Haemophilus influenzae	0.12	>50.0
Bordetella pertussis	1.0–3.0	100.0
Vibrio cholerae	0.8	32.0
Pseudomonas aeruginosa	>100.0	25.0

Table II.3
Compiled from data published by Bushby and Hitchings (1968) and Bushby (1969)

10 Minimum inhibitory concentrations

Table II.3 shows MICs of trimethoprim compared with those of sulfamethoxazole. Trimethoprim is much more active than the sulfonamides against most bacterial species. Acquired bacterial resistance to the sulfonamides is common (p. 807), therefore strains with higher MICs to sulfonamides than those shown in this table will be encountered.

Mode of Administration and Dosage

1 Adults

Until around 1980, trimethoprim was only available for general use as a mixture with sulfamethoxazole. Dosage regimens used for trimethoprim alone are given on pp. 884, 885. The commonly used tablets or capsules of Co-T each contain 80 mg of trimethoprim and 400 mg of sulfamethoxazole, but tablets are also available that contain twice this dosage. The usual adult dosage is two single-strength tablets or one double-strength tablet given 12-hourly after meals. For severe infections, this dosage may be increased to a total of six single-strength tablets per day, given in two or three divided doses. A dosage of one single-strength tablet 12-hourly is sufficient for long-term therapy of chronic bronchial or urinary tract infections. *Pneumocystis carinii* pneumonia generally requires a dose of 15–20 mg per kg per day (trimethoprim component), which equates to approximately two double-strength Co-T tablets every 6 h for a 70 kg adult with normal renal function (pp. 875, 878).

2 Children

A pediatric suspension containing 40 mg trimethoprim and 200 mg sulfamethoxazole per 5 ml is available. The dosages recommended for children are as follows: under 2 years, 20 mg trimethoprim and 100 mg sulfamethoxazole (2.5ml) twice-daily; 2–5 years, 20–40 mg trimethoprim and 100–200 mg sulfamethoxazole (2.5–5.0 ml) twice-daily; and for children aged 6–12 years, 40–80 mg trimethoprim and 200–400 mg sulfamethoxazole (5.0–10.0 ml) twice-daily. Among children with extrahepatic biliary atresia there is appreciable interpatient variability in the disposition of Co-T, such that levels of trimethoprim and sulfamethoxazole may need to be monitored to accurately identify the optimal dose (Lares-Asseff *et al.*, 1994).

3 Newborn and premature infants

The use of Co-T is not recommended for infants during the first 4 weeks of life. Young babies should not be breast-fed by mothers receiving the drug. However, this combination has been occasionally used for treatment of severe infections in 2- to 3-week-old infants without encountering serious toxicity. Roy (1971) suggests that a dose of trimethoprim 8–10 mg per kg per day and sulfamethoxazole 40–50 mg per kg per day may be suitable for infants, but this combination should only be used at this age when absolutely necessary. Sulfonamides may cause kernicterus (p. 819), and, for this reason, it is inadvisable to use trimethoprim/sulfamethoxazole for premature infants or during the first week of life. Despite sulfamethoxazole being a weak displacer of bilirubin, Springer *et al.* (1982) found no bilirubin displacement from albumin with sulfamethoxazole concentrations of up to 300 μg per ml.

4 Patients with renal failure

Both trimethoprim and sulfamethoxazole are excreted via the kidney but, in addition, both drugs are removed by non-renal mechanisms (p. 850). Renal function has little influence on the serum half-life of active sulfamethoxazole until there is severe impairment, but the excretion of sulfonamide metabolites and active trimethoprim is more dependent on renal function (Bergan and Brodwall, 1976). The half-life of total sulfamethoxazole increases rapidly as the creatinine clearance deteriorates below 30–40 ml per min, and it increases rapidly at about 20–25 ml per min for trimethoprim. The half-life of total sulfamethoxazole becomes more prolonged relative to that of trimethoprim (Bergan and Brodwall, 1976), and the half-life of trimethoprim is usually less than that of active sulfamethoxazole (Craig and Kunin, 1973a; Bergan and Brodwall, 1976). There is considerable variation of these half-lives in individual patients with renal failure, being in the range 13.8–46.3 h for trimethoprim and 21.8–50.2 h for active sulfamethoxazole (Craig and Kunin, 1973a).

In patients with mild to moderate degrees of renal impairment, these drugs do not accumulate and usual doses may be given. Patients with a creatinine clearance of 10–30 ml per min may be given an initial full loading dose of both drugs (160 mg trimethoprim and 800 mg sulfamethoxazole) and then half this dose twice-daily (Craig and Kunin, 1973a). In patients with anuria or severe uremia (creatinine clearance less than 10 ml per min), a full loading dose may also be given, followed by half this dose once- or twice-daily. However, in these patients independent adjustment of the dosage of each drug may be advisable, because the serum half-life of total sulfamethoxazole is greatly increased compared with that of trimethoprim. Welling *et al.* (1973) suggest that patients with severe renal failure should receive a normal initial loading dose, and that subsequent 12-hourly doses of sulfamethoxazole and trimethoprim be reduced to one-third and one-half of the usual dose, respectively. Bergan and Brodwall (1976) consider that, because of the possibility of an accumulation of sulfonamide metabolites, Co-T should not be used in patients with a creatinine clearance less than 15 ml per min, unless regular determinations of total sulfonamide serum levels can be made. Both drugs are removed during hemodialysis, and patients undergoing this procedure should receive a full dose before and after dialysis (Craig and Kunin, 1973a).

Even in patients with severe renal failure, urinary levels of both drugs usually exceed those required for the eradication of most urinary pathogens. In patients with severe renal failure, trimethoprim accumulates in the serum to a lesser extent than sulfamethoxazole (because it is more efficiently removed by non-renal mechanisms), but its excretion via the kidney is reduced to a greater extent than that of sulfamethoxazole (Craig and Kunin, 1973a). Thus the sulfamethoxazole/trimethoprim ratio in the urine of uremic patients may approach 19:1, which appears to be optimal for antibacterial synergy against common urinary pathogens (Bushby, 1969; Adam et al., 1973).

Denneberg et al. (1976) used Co-T for long-term treatment of acute and chronic pyelonephritis in 15 patients with impaired renal function in the following dosage schedules: two standard single-strength tablets twice-daily for 6 days, followed by two tablets daily for patients with a creatinine clearance of 30–75 ml per min (serum creatinine 1.3–5.0 mg%); for those with a creatinine clearance of 15–30 ml per min (serum creatinine 5.0–12.0 mg %) two tablets twice-daily for 3 days and then two tablets daily; and for patients with a creatinine clearance of <5.0–15.0 ml per min (serum creatinine >12.0 mg %), some of whom were receiving maintenance hemodialysis, one tablet daily for 3 days and then usually one tablet daily according to serum levels. Patients were treated for periods of up to 2 years; regular serum level monitoring showed that active sulfamethoxazole and trimethoprim levels remained acceptable and their bacteriological and clinical response to treatment was good. Bennett and Craven (1976) treated urinary tract infections in six patients with severe renal failure (creatinine clearance <30 ml per min) by Co-T in a dose of two standard tablets daily for 14 days. Mean serum levels of trimethoprim (3.1 μg per ml) and sulfamethoxazole (65 μg per ml) were higher than normal, but unassociated with adverse effects. Mean urine trimethoprim levels were 28.6 μg per ml and, although in four patients the urine sulfamethoxazole levels were less than 10 μg per ml; bacteriological cure was obtained in all patients.

In studies using i.v. Co-T, Siber et al. (1982) found that the half-life of trimethoprim correlated with the serum creatinine value. Sulfamethoxazole had a similar, but weaker correlation, probably because it is primarily eliminated by hepatic transformation (p. 850). Nevertheless, it appeared that N4-acetyl-sulfamethoxazole, the major metabolite of sulfamethoxazole which is excreted by the kidney, may accumulate in patients with severe renal failure. Siber et al. (1982) proposed that the i.v. doses recommended for maintenance therapy should be given to patients with serum creatinine levels <4 mg % at intervals (hours) equal to the serum creatinine in mg % × 12. For patients with higher levels of serum creatinine, the interval should be 36–48 h.

Because Co-T may cause deterioration in renal function (p. 857), probably due to the high serum concentrations of sulfamethoxazole metabolites, serum concentrations should be determined regularly in patients with a creatinine clearance below 20–30 ml per min (Denneberg et al., 1976). The manufacturers recommend that treatment should be interrupted if the serum level of total sulfamethoxazole exceeds 150 μg per ml and that it should only be recommenced when this level falls below 120 μg per ml.

5 Intravenous administration

A preparation of Co-T suitable for i.v. administration was introduced for general use in the UK in 1974 and subsequently in other countries. It is available in 5-ml ampoules each containing 80 mg trimethoprim and 400 mg sulfamethoxazole for addition to an i.v. infusion; this preparation is not suitable for i.m. or direct i.v. injection. The contents of ampoules should be diluted immediately before use in the following volumes: one ampoule (5 ml) in 125 ml infusion solution, two ampoules (10 ml) in 250 ml and three ampoules (15 ml) in 500 ml infusion solution. Commonly used dextrose and/or sodium chloride i.v. solutions and various dextran solutions are suitable diluents if other additives are not present. The recommended daily dosage is 6 mg trimethoprim and 30 mg sulfamethoxazole per kg body weight, given in two divided doses. The dosage for adults and children aged over 12 years is 10 ml (two ampoules) twice-daily, but this may be increased to 15 ml twice-daily for severe infections. For children, the dosage is 1.25 ml twice-daily for those aged 6 weeks-5 months, 2.5 ml twice-daily for those aged 6 months-5 years and 5.0 ml twice-daily when aged 6–12 years. Where possible, the duration of the infusion should not exceed 1.5 h. This i.v. preparation should only be used when the patient cannot take oral therapy, and it is recommended that it should not be given for more than 3 successive days. Crystalluria and acute renal failure have followed the use of i.v. Co-T in two patients with hypoalbuminemia (p. 818). Nevertheless, this preparation has been used for periods of 10 days to treat patients with septicemias and meningitis and this has been well tolerated (Sabel and Brandberg, 1975; Olcen and Eriksson, 1976).

Serum half-lives for sulfamethoxazole and trimethoprim in neonates are much longer than those of healthy adults (Springer et al., 1982). These authors calculated that the i.v. doses of these drugs for neonates to be optimal therapeutically, and to avoid accumulation, were as follows:

sulfamethoxazole 10 mg and trimethoprim 3 mg per kg body weight as a loading dose and maintenance doses of sulfamethoxazole 3 mg and trimethoprim 1 mg per kg every 12 h. The currently available i.v. Co-T preparation is unsuitable, because the ratio of sulfamethoxazole to trimethoprim is 5:1, so that the individual drugs would need to be used.

6 Intramuscular administration

The intramuscular preparation of Co-T (3 ml contained 160 mg trimethoprim and 800 mg sulfamethoxazole) is now no longer available.

7 Patients with cystic fibrosis

Data obtained from studies of patients with cystic fibrosis receiving Co-T indicate that the elimination half-life of Co-T is shorter and the plasma clearance is greater than in normal subjects (Reed et al., 1984). The authors suggested that increased dosing or decreased dosing intervals are required when giving Co-T to such patients.

8 Contraindications and precautions

Co-T should not be used in patients with severe liver disease, blood dyscrasias, and patients with a history of hypersensitivity to sulfonamides. Siber et al. (1982) used Co-T in 23 patients with hepatocellular damage and/or cholestasis; peak levels and half-lives of trimethoprim, sulfamethoxazole and its acetyl metabolite were not related to liver damage as measured by standard liver function tests. The simultaneous administration of trimethoprim with other 2,4-diaminopyrimidines, such as pyrimethamine or proguanil, should be avoided (Fleming et al., 1974). Because Co-T may interfere with folate metabolism (p. 852), regular full blood examinations should be performed on patients receiving long-term therapy and those who are predisposed to folate deficiency.

Availablility

A Co-trimoxazole

Standard tablets: each containing 80 mg trimethoprim and 400 mg sulfamethoxazole.

Double-strength tablets: each containing 160 mg trimethoprim and 800 mg sulfamethoxazole (e.g. 'Bactrim DS', 'Septrin Forte').

Pediatric suspension: 5 ml containing 40 mg trimethoprim and 200 mg sulfamethoxazole.

Preparation for i.v. use: 5 ml ampoules containing trimethoprim 80 mg and sulfamethoxazole 400 mg in a vehicle containing propylene glycol.

B Trimethoprim

Tablets: each containing 300 mg.

Serum Levels in Relation to Dosage

Trimethoprim is well absorbed after oral administration. After the usual oral dose of 160 mg, a peak serum level of about 2 μg per ml is reached in 1–2 h; this is maintained for about 6 h and then falls progressively. The serum half-life of the drug is about 13 h, and detectable serum levels are still present 24 h after a dose of 160mg (Bushby and Hitchings, 1968). Higher serum levels are attained when this dose is increased (Fig. II.3). When trimethoprim was given in a single daily dose of 300 mg orally at night to eight healthy volunteers for 3 consecutive days, serum concentrations were 3.0, 4.0, 4.7 and 0.96 μg per ml, 12, 36, 60 and 84 h, respectively, after the first dose (Ahlmen and Brorson, 1982).

Sulfamethoxazole is also well absorbed from the gastrointestinal tract. After a 1200-mg oral dose, a peak serum level of about 60 μg per ml of the active drug is attained 2 h after administration, which persists for about 6 h. The serum half-life of this drug is 9–12 h (Fig. II.4).

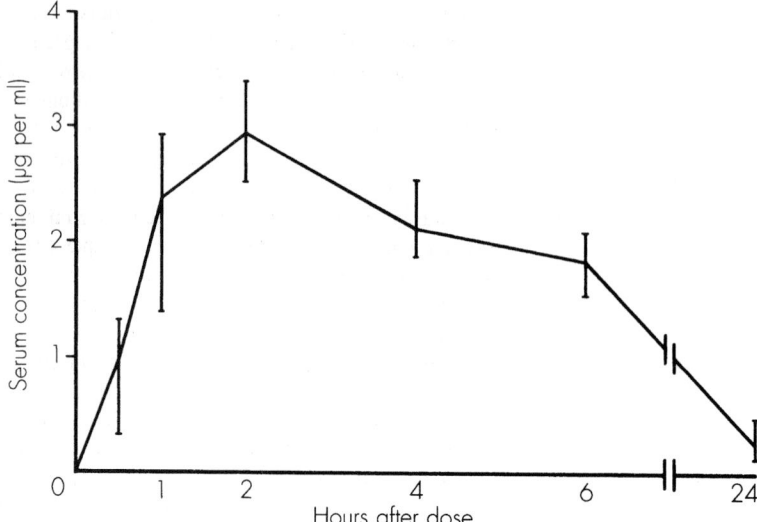

Fig. II.3.

Average trimethoprim serum levels in four volunteers after a 240-mg oral dose. (Redrawn after Brumfitt *et al.*, 1969, with permission.)

Trimethoprim and sulfamethoxazole can be administered simultaneously because their half-lives are almost identical. The administration of these drugs in a 1:5 ratio as Co-T results in their serum levels being in a ratio of about 1:20 to 1:30 when their peak levels are reached at about 2 h. This is the ratio at which maximum synergy occurs against many organisms. After peak levels, this ratio falls gradually to between 1:10 and 1:20 at the end of the dosage interval. In patients with impaired renal function, the ratio at the time of peak serum levels changes from 1:20 to 1:10 after 12 h (Bergan and Brodwall, 1976). Compared with many other antibiotics, serum levels of trimethoprim and sulfamethoxazole are probably not lower in late pregnancy (Chow and Jewesson, 1985).

If the individual dose of Co-T is increased, even up to 12 tablets (960 mg trimethoprim and 4800 mg sulfamethoxazole), peak serum levels of these drugs are increased linearly and their half-lives for elimination from the serum are prolonged (Fass *et al.*, 1977). Yoshikawa and Guze (1976) gave healthy volunteers nine tablets of Co-T (720 mg trimethoprim and 3600 mg sulfamethoxazole) as a single dose; resultant mean serum levels during the first 8 h were 6.12–8.32 μg per ml for trimethoprim and 98–120 μg per ml for sulfamethoxazole, and at 24 h the average levels of trimethoprim and sulfamethoxazole were 2.16 and 31.7 μg per ml, respectively. When a 12-tablet dose of Co-T (960 mg trimethoprim and 4800 mg sulfamethox-

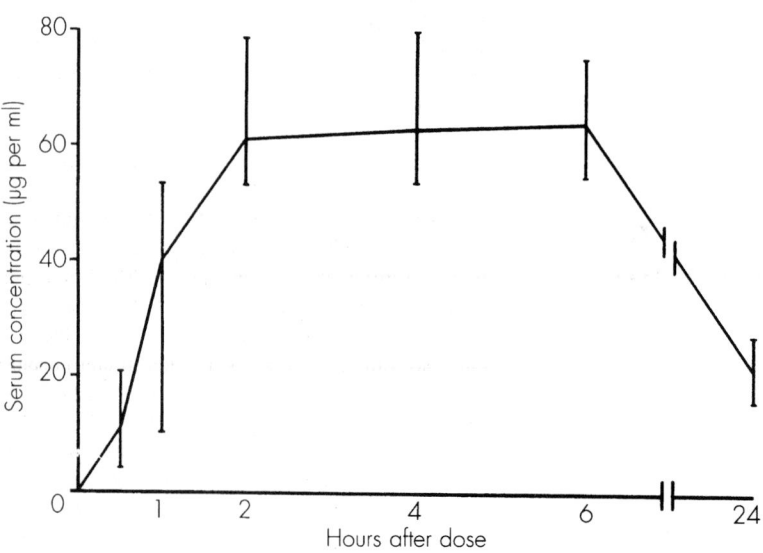

Fig. II.4.

Average serum levels of non-acetylated sulfamethoxazole in four fasting volunteers after a 1200-mg oral dose. (Redrawn after Brumfitt *et al.*, 1969, with permission.)

azole) was given to volunteers, mean peak levels of trimethoprim and sulfamethoxazole at 2–4 h were 6-fold higher than those which occur after a two-tablet dose (Fass *et al.*, 1977). These mean peak serum levels were 9.2, 259.4 and 233.7 μg per ml for trimethoprim, total sulfamethoxazole and free sulfamethoxazole, respectively. Their corresponding elimination half-lives were 16.6, 14.6 and 12.9 h, so that mean serum concentrations at 24 h were approximately 10-fold higher than after a two-tablet dose. In contrast, Stevens *et al.* (1991) who examined the pharmacokinetics of Co-T in 12 healthy adults given the conventional dose for treating *P. carinii* pneumonia (p. 875) of trimethoprim 20 mg per kg of body weight per day and sulfamethoxazole 100 mg per kg per day (divided and administered every 6 h) for 3 days, noted somewhat higher serum levels of trimethoprim and sulfamethoxazole than previously reported. In the seven subjects who completed the study (five withdrew due to toxicity) the mean peak serum concentrations (± SD) of trimethoprim, sulfamethoxazole and N4-acetylsulfamethoxazole after the last dose were 13.6 ± 2.0, 372 ± 64 and 50.1 ± 10.9 μg per ml, respectively. The mean half-lives (± SD) of these agents were 13.6 ± 3.5, 14 ± 2.3 and 18.6 ± 4.3 h respectively. These authors thus claimed that since these levels were at least 2-fold higher than the proposed therapeutic range for the treatment of PCP, and were associated with moderate toxicity (p. 853), consideration of lower dosage regimens of Co-T may be warranted. Subsequently Stevens *et al.* (1993), studied the serum concentrations of trimethoprim and sulfamethoxazole in six healthy volunteers given Co-T at a dose of 12 mg per kg per day (trimethoprim component). Wide intersubject variation in the serum concentrations were noted within the initial 24 h of therapy, such that in some patients this dose would not guarantee therapeutic concentrations against *P. carinii*. Thus, these authors advocate a dose of 15–20 mg per kg per day Co-T (trimethoprim component) for the first 24 h, followed by 12 mg per kg per day for the remainder of therapy. The clinical efficacy of this dosage regimen has not been confirmed, however, suggesting that the routine higher dose of 15–20 mg per kg per day Co-T should probably continue to be used until such clinical studies are available. The pharmacokinetics of trimethoprim-sulfamethoxazole are similar in critically ill and non-critically ill AIDS patients with *P. carinii* infection (Chin *et al.*, 1995). However, among trauma patients with serious Gram-negative infections the half-life of sulfamethoxazole, but not trimethoprim, may be significantly shorter than in non-trauma patients (Hess *et al.*, 1993).

Bushby and Hitchings (1968) studied serum levels in six adult volunteers after an i.v. dose of 100 mg trimethoprim lactate. An average serum level of 1.4 μg per ml was obtained 5 min after injection, 1.0 μg per ml after 3 h and 0.95 μg per ml after 4.5 h. The average serum level was still 0.3 μg per ml at 24 h and the half-life of trimethoprim after i.v. injection was estimated to be 11–12 h. This does not differ significantly from the half-life of this drug after oral administration. Franzén and Brandberg (1976) found that peak serum levels of trimethoprim and sulfamethoxazole immediately after an infusion of Co-T given over a period of 30 min were almost identical to the peak values obtained at 2 h when the same dose was given orally. Grose *et al.* (1979) gave i.v. Co-T to 11 patients with cancer. The administration of 160 mg trimethoprim and 800 mg sulfamethoxazole i.v. over a period of 1 h resulted in mean (± SEM) peak serum levels of trimethoprim of 3.4 (± 0.3) μg per ml and of sulfamethoxazole 46.3 (± 2.7) μg per ml. The serum level was maintained above 2 μg per ml for 4 h in 7 of 11 patients and that of sulfamethoxazole above 20 μg per ml for 8 h in 9 of 11 patients. The serum half-life of trimethoprim was estimated to be 7.7 h. Serum concentrations of both trimethoprim and sulfamethoxazole were higher on day 4 than on day 1 when the above doses were repeated every 8 h. When trimethoprim 240 mg/ sulfamethoxazole 1200 mg was administered i.v. in a volume of 200 ml over a period of 45 min to volunteers every 12 h for 4 days, mean peak serum levels of trimethoprim and sulfamethoxazole were 3.22 and 100 μg per ml, respectively, on day 1 and 5.91 and 178 μg per ml, respectively, on day 4, when a steady state was achieved. Mean serum trough levels at 12 h on days 1 and 4 were 0.8 and 2.6 μg per ml, respectively, for trimethoprim and 37.8 and 78.4 μg per ml, respectively, for sulfamethoxazole. The mean elimination half-lives for trimethoprim and sulfamethoxazole were 16.5 and 14.1 h, respectively (Spicehandler *et al.*, 1982).

Siber *et al.* (1982) studied pharmacokinetics of i.v. Co-T in 37 patients aged 0.2–82 years with various infections. With an 8-hourly dose of 150 mg trimethoprim and 750 mg sulfamethoxazole per m^2 (about 7 mg trimethoprim/35 mg sulfamethoxazole per kg for patients aged 1–10 years and 5 mg trimethoprim/25 mg sulfamethoxazole per kg for patients aged more than 10 years), on day 2 mean peak levels of 7.02 and 148 μg per ml were reached for trimethoprim and sulfamethoxazole, respectively. These peak levels were similar in all age groups, although dosages per weight were higher in children than in adults. This was because the mean half-lives of trimethoprim and sulfamethoxazole increased with age – mean values for trimethoprim and sulfamethoxazole were 9.6 and 10.7 h, respectively. Drug accumulation occurred in all patients but a steady-state was reached in 48–72 h. In 12 patients, peak serum levels after oral administration of Co-T were compared: those after i.v. administration were higher and more reliable. Based on these studies, it was recommended that to achieve peak levels of trimethoprim of 5–10 μg per ml for *P. carinii* pneumonia patients aged 1–10 years a loading dose of 12 mg per kg trimethoprim followed by 7 mg per kg 8-hourly and for those aged older than 10 years, a loading dose of 8 mg per kg followed by a dose of trimethoprim of 5 mg per kg 12-hourly be maintained. Nelson *et al.* (1982) gave i.v. Co-T to 10 children in a dose of 3.3 mg trimethoprim and 16.7 mg sulfamethoxazole per kg by an infusion over 1 h; the serum trimethoprim level increased from a baseline value of 1 μg per ml (they were having an infusion three times daily) to 2.4 μg per ml at the end of the infusion; respective values for sulfamethoxazole were 54 and 106 μg per ml. The ratio of sulfamethoxazole to trimethoprim remained at about 50:1 for 8 h after beginning the infusion. Ardati *et al.* (1979) found a similar serum ratio in children after i.v. Co-T. This differs from the serum ratio of these two drugs of about 12:1 after multiple doses, which Grose *et al.* (1979) found in adults after i.v. Co-T.

Excretion

1 Urine

Unchanged trimethoprim is mainly excreted by non-ionic renal diffusion and this is influenced by pH (Sharpstone, 1969; Craig and Kunin, 1973a). A considerable proportion of orally administered trimethoprim is excreted in the urine unchanged (Bushby and Hitchings, 1968; Bach *et al.*, 1973c). Approximately 10% of the excreted drug is in the form of metabolites with little or no antibacterial activity. Urinary concentrations of about 100 μg per ml after the usual oral dose are approximately 100-fold higher than those attained in serum and remain high for about 24 h. About 40–60% of an orally administered dose of trimethoprim can be recovered from the urine in the active form within 24 h. There is considerable individual variation in the amount of trimethoprim which is excreted as the active drug (Sigel *et al.*, 1973). The amount of active trimethoprim excreted in urine during a 24 h period after i.v. administration varies from 42 to 75% of the administered dose (Bushby and Hitchings, 1968). After an i.v. dose of 240 mg trimethoprim and 1200 mg sulfamethoxazole, 24.7% of the trimethoprim was excreted in the urine in 12 h; urinary concentrations ranged from 19 to 130 μg per ml (Spicehandler *et al.*, 1982).

Sulfamethoxazole is also mainly excreted in the urine, but about 70% of this is in the form of its acetylated and other metabolites. After an i.v. dose of 240 mg trimethoprim and 1200 mg sulfamethoxazole, 9.86% of free sulfamethoxazole was excreted in the urine in 12 h; 46.1% of combined free and N_4-acetylated sulfamethoxazole was excreted in the urine in 12 h; urinary concentrations of free sulfamethoxazole ranged from 40 to 320 μg per ml (Spicehandler *et al.*, 1982). The ratio of sulfamethoxazole to trimethoprim in the urine may vary from 1:1 to 5:1 (Grey and Hamilton-Miller, 1977; Fass *et al.*, 1977). Acidification of the urine results in increased urinary excretion of trimethoprim, but has no significant effect on that of active sulfamethoxazole. By contrast, alkalinization of the urine decreases urinary excretion of trimethoprim and increases the excretion of sulfamethoxazole. In acid urine, the ratio of active sulfamethoxazole to trimethoprim is approximately 1, whereas in alkaline urine the ratio is usually greater than 5 (Craig and Kunin, 1973a).

2 Bile

A small amount of trimethoprim is eliminated via the bile. In patients without biliary obstruction, concentrations of the drug in bile are slightly higher than those in the serum 4 h after a dose, but these fall to levels lower than in the serum 24 h after a dose (Rieder, 1973).

3 Inactivation in body

A significant proportion of administered trimethoprim is converted in the liver to antibacterially inactive metabolites. Five such metabolites have been identified, all of which are excreted in the urine (Sigel *et al.*, 1973).

Distribution of the Drug in Body

After absorption, and due to its lipophilic properties, trimethoprim is rapidly distributed in the body. In animals, tissue levels are usually greater than those in serum, except in brain, skin and fat. Particularly high tissue levels have been found in the kidney and liver (Craig and Kunin, 1973b).

In humans, the drug is equally distributed between plasma and erythrocytes. Concentrations of trimethoprim in most tissues and body fluids, including sputum and pleural fluid, appear to be higher than corresponding serum levels. After a lag time of about 3 h, trimethoprim levels in synovial fluid approach those in the serum and thereafter approximate to them; sulfamethoxazole does not penetrate as readily into synovial fluid (Sattar et al., 1983). Concentrations of trimethoprim in nasal secretion are more than double those of simultaneous serum levels (Ullman et al., 1983). Trimethoprim levels in saliva exceed those in the serum, while sulfamethoxazole, compared with other sulfonamides, such as sulfadiazine, sulfamerazine and sulfamethazine, enters saliva gradually (Kamme et al., 1983). Trimethoprim (and sulfamethoxazole) penetrates well into the middle ear fluid of patients with chronic serous otitis media (Klimek et al., 1980; Krause et al., 1982). Trimethoprim and sulfamethoxazole (to a lesser extent) produce good concentrations in experimental skin blister fluid in human volunteers (Bruun et al., 1981). After Co-T administration, the trimethoprim concentration in sputum is about double that in serum, but the sulfamethoxazole concentration is only about half the serum level (Hughes, 1976). Trimethoprim levels in the kidney can be 20-fold higher than those in the serum, but it is not detectable in the kidney for more than 8 h following cessation of therapy (Bergeron, 1985).

Trimethoprim penetrates well into the CSF of patients with normal meninges after oral and i.v. administration of Co-T (Svedhem and Iwarson, 1979; Bach et al., 1973c; Goodwin et al., 1981; Wang and Prober, 1983) and into the CSF of patients with Gram-negative bacillary meningitis (Levitz et al., 1984). Dudley et al. (1984) studied CSF concentrations obtained after i.v. administration of Co-T to nine patients with normal meninges; a single dose of 5 mg trimethoprim plus 25 mg sulfamethoxazole per kg body weight was infused over approximately 120 min. Peak CSF concentrations of trimethoprim and sulfamethoxazole were 1 and 13.8 µg per ml, respectively; these peaks were reached at 60 and 480 min postinfusion for trimethoprim and sulfamethoxazole, respectively. At 15 h, there was no detectable trimethoprim in the CSF but 4.7 µg per ml of sulfamethoxazole was still present. CSF: serum concentration ratios for trimethoprim were 0.23:0.53 and for sulfamethoxazole 0.2:0.36. Pus obtained from a cerebral abscess of a patient receiving oral Co-T (160 mg trimethoprim, 800 mg sulfamethoxazole) twice-daily had trimethoprim and sulfamethoxazole levels of 1.6 and 15.47 µg per ml, respectively (Greene et al., 1975). Brain tissue from a nocardial brain abscess contained trimethoprim and sulfamethoxazole concentrations of 5.1 and 36 µg per ml, respectively, 6 h after an oral dose of 160 mg trimethoprim and 800 mg sulfamethoxazole (Maderazo and Quintiliani, 1974).

Salmon et al. (1975) studied aqueous humor levels of patients receiving Co-T, who were undergoing cataract surgery. The mean ratios of aqueous humor: sera concentrations for trimethoprim and free sulfamethoxazole were 0.30 and 0.24, respectively. In general, these ratios did not change with the time after the dose or with prolonged dosing with Co-T. Trimethoprim diffuses well into human vaginal fluid, reaching concentrations that sometimes are nearly 3-fold simultaneous serum levels. By contrast, levels of sulfamethoxazole in vaginal fluid are often undetectable or very low after oral treatment with Co-T (Stamey and Condy, 1975). High levels of trimethoprim in vaginal fluid (and prostate) probably result from non-ionic diffusion into these more acid environments. When oral Co-T was given to healthy males, mean levels of 1.0–1.5 µg per ml of trimethoprim were detected in seminal fluid when mean serum levels were 1.8–2.0 µg per ml (Gnarpe and Friberg, 1976). On theoretical grounds, trimethoprim should diffuse well into prostatic tissue (Leading article, 1983a). Only lipid soluble antibiotics are able to cross epithelial membranes and only the unchanged (un-ionized) fraction of the drug is able to pass into prostatic fluid, because the ionized or charged fraction is lipid-insoluble. The degree of ionization of a molecule of a drug is determined by its dissociation constant (pKa) and drugs mainly in the un-ionized state have a high pKa. Trimethoprim is lipid-soluble and has a high pKa of 7.3 indicating that more than half of it is un-ionized and available for diffusion. Therapeutic levels of Co-T have been detected in prostatic tissue obtained at prostatectomy of patients given Co-T (Leading article, 1983a). In some cases the level of trimethoprim in prostatic tissue has been greater than that attained in sera (Meares, 1982). Both trimethoprim and sulfonamides are taken up by human leukocytes in vitro (Climax et al., 1986). This is particularly notable with trimethoprim which is concentrated approximately 3-fold in polymorphonuclear leukocytes (Hand et al., 1987; Hand and King-Thompson, 1990) and monocytes (Hand and King-Thompson, 1989). Trimethoprim penetrates equally into polymorphonuclear leukocytes of normal subjects and those of patients with chronic granulomatous disease; combinations of trimethoprim/sulfamethoxazole and trimethoprim/rifampicin were very effective in killing intracellular *Staph. aureus in vitro* (Jacobs and Wilson, 1983). Trimethoprim appears to be concentrated in the bile of patients with radiologically functioning gallbladders (Morran *et al.*, 1978).

With usual serum concentrations, trimethoprim is 42–46% bound to serum proteins (Schwartz and Ziegler, 1969).

Mode of Action

Trimethoprim interferes with the action of dihydrofolic acid reductase (DHFR), which is an enzyme that converts dihydrofolic to tetrahydrofolic acid – an essential stage in bacterial purine and, ultimately, DNA synthesis. This enzyme acts at a stage which immediately follows the enzyme conversion of para-aminobenzoic acid to dihydrofolic acid, which can be competitively blocked by sulfonamides (p. 814). Originally, it was thought that sulfonamides only had this one site of action and that a sequential action of sulfonamides and trimethoprim explained the synergistic action of this combination against bacteria (Darrell *et al.*, 1968). There are theoretical and experimental objections to a sequential blockage theory (Lacey, 1979, 1982). Harvey (1982) believes that synergy between trimethoprim and sulfamethoxazole occurs because of the cyclic configuration of the folate pathway, i.e. there is not just a simple linear pathway after the formation of dihydrofolate (Fig. II.2, p. 815), but a cyclic pathway. Reaction rates of all enzymes in this cyclic pathway would thus become more sensitive to decreases in substrate concentrations produced by sulfamethoxazole; the cyclic configuration would ensure that the effect of trimethoprim would result in little change in buffering capacity against this decrease, and therefore the two drugs would act synergistically. It is, however, possible that sulfonamides also act independently on the same enzyme, DHFR, which is affected by trimethoprim. This would explain why sometimes synergy can be demonstrated with trimethoprim–sulfamethoxazole, even when the bacteria are sulfonamide-resistant (p. 842) presumably these bacteria are resistant because the sulfonamide was unable to inhibit the conversion of para-aminobenzoic acid, but it was still able to act with trimethoprim on dihydrofolic acid reductase. Various biochemical mechanisms are involved in sulfonamide-resistance (p. 839), so that it cannot be predicted whether a sulfonamide-resistant organism will show synergy. Conversely, if bacteria are fully inhibited by trimethoprim, then the addition of sulfonamides cannot be expected to be of additional benefit. That sulfonamides also bind to dihydrofolate reductase has been disputed (Harvey, 1982).

The sulfonamides do not have an inhibitory effect on human folate metabolism because dihydrofolic acid is obtained directly from dietary folates (Fig. II.2, p. 815). The reduction of dihydrofolic to tetrahydrofolic acid in humans, similar to bacteria, is also catalyzed by DHFR. However, trimethoprim has at least 10 000-fold more inhibitory effect on the bacterial enzyme than on the corresponding mammalian enzyme (Kahn *et al.*, 1968). Nevertheless, it has been postulated that the hematological side-effects of both trimethoprim and sulfamethoxazole may occur because of an effect on human DHFR – both of these drugs inhibit human erythropoiesis *in vitro* and the effect is reversed by the addition of folic acid (Lacey, 1979). However, the situation *in vivo* is less clear. It was predicted from studies of its mode of action that if depression of human folate metabolism due to trimethoprim therapy occurred, it would be reversed by administration of tetrahydrofolate compounds such as folinic acid. In AIDS/ARC patients, however, neutropenia associated with Co-T therapy is not reversed by the co-administration of either folic acid or folinic acid (Jaffe *et al.*, 1983; Bygbjerg *et al.*, 1988; p. 856). On theoretical grounds, the administration of folinic acid should not interfere with the antibacterial action of trimethoprim, because bacteria cannot utilize preformed dihydrofolates or tetrahydrofolates. This has also been confirmed by both bacteriological (Grunberg *et al.*, 1970) and clinical studies (Kahn *et al.*, 1968; Jenkins *et al.*, 1970).

The inhibitory effect of trimethoprim on the DHFR of malarial parasites is about 2000-fold greater than on the human enzyme and trimethoprim can, therefore, be used for treatment of human malaria – although this is rarely used clinically. The chemically related antimalarial drug, pyrimethamine, has a similar mode of action against DHFR of the malarial parasite (p. 911), but this action is about 2000-fold greater than its effect against either the mammalian or bacterial enzymes (Hitchings, 1969). The sulfonamides potentiate the action of both trimethoprim and pyrimethamine against malaria parasites.

A variety of biochemical mechanisms are involved in trimethoprim-resistant bacteria, and may differ in bacterial strains with naturally occurring resistance from those of strains in which resistance is induced *in vitro* (Hamilton-Miller, 1979; Lacey, 1982; Then, 1982). Such mechanisms include poor penetration through the cell envelope, thymine dependence due to altered thymidylate-synthetase, excess production of DHFR and production of trimethoprim-resistant DHFR (p. 840).

While the components of Co-T, trimethoprim and sulfamethoxazole have bacteriostatic activity in clinically achievable concentrations, this combination is bactericidal *in vitro* when synergy is achieved (Bushby, 1969), but when studies are done in media incorporating urine, Co-T is bacteriostatic (Gruneberg, 1979).

Toxicity

In many cases, it is very difficult to separate the side-effects due to the two components of Co-T, trimethoprim and sulfamethoxazole. The reader is, therefore, also referred to the section on side-effects of sulfonamides (p. 815). Overall, the risk of serious side-effects associated with Co-T is small and is similar to that noted with many other antibiotics (Jick and Derby, 1995).

1 Gastrointestinal side-effects

Trimethoprim can cause nausea and diarrhea, and these were common in early clinical studies when doses as high as 1 g daily were given. Nausea has also been commonly reported when the large doses of Co-T required for the treatment of *P. carinii* pneumonia, are used (pp. 875, 878). The usual maximum recommended daily dose of trimethoprim, however, is only 480 mg (six standard tablets of Co-T) with which gastrointestinal side-effects are uncommon. Single oral doses of nine tablets of Co-T (720 mg trimethoprim and 3600 mg sulfamethoxazole) are usually well tolerated (Yoshikawa and Guze, 1976). However, single oral doses of 12 tablets (960 mg trimethoprim and 4800 mg sulfamethoxazole) may cause malaise, nausea, headache and transient oliguria and crystalluria (Fass *et al.*, 1977). Nausea, vomiting, restlessness and headache have also been described in a patient undergoing peritoneal dialysis who was receiving intraperitoneal Co-T 80 mg (trimethoprim component) in each 2 liter exchange, four times daily (Stamatakis *et al.*, 1995).

Following administration of Co-T, the frequency of upper gastrointestinal side-effects has been estimated as about 3% for nausea, vomiting and anorexia, about 0.5% for diarrhea, 0.4% for glossitis and very rarely liver toxicity in patients who are not HIV-infected (Jick, 1982; Lawson and Paice, 1982; Lindgren and Olsson, 1994). Gastrointestinal side-effects are also very infrequent in children (Jick *et al.*, 1984). Pseudomembranous colitis has been described in association with Co-T treatment, similar to most antibacterial drugs; including in two patients receiving Co-T as prophylaxis for *P. carinii* pneumonia (Cameron and Thames, 1977; Pennington, 1980; Rubin and Swartz, 1980; Lawson and Paice, 1982; Gordin *et al.*, 1994).

2 Hypersensitivity reactions

Rashes were observed in 1.6–8% of patients during clinical trials with Co-T (Frisch, 1973; Salter, 1973). Most of these were probably caused by the sulfonamide component, but it is difficult to separate the side-effects of the two individual drugs. Nevertheless, occasionally trimethoprim itself has been implicated as a cause of skin rashes (Gibson, 1982). The frequency of allergic skin rashes in Co-T treated patients is 1.4% (Jick, 1982; Lawson and Paice, 1982). These usually take the form of a toxic erythema, with urticaria and necrotizing vasculitis being infrequent. Skin allergy is generally uncommon in children treated with Co-T (Jick *et al.*, 1984), although Boyce *et al.* (1992) described four children who developed an acute febrile reaction with a generalized erythematous rash after treatment with Co-T. All the other well-known side-effects of sulfonamides (p. 815) can be expected to occur from time to time when the combination is used. Long-acting sulfonamides are more prone to cause Stevens–Johnson syndrome (p. 816), and sulfamethoxazole, the component in co-trimoxazole, is a medium-acting sulfonamide with serum half-life of 9–12 h. Thorpe and Nysenbaum (1978) reported the death of a 48-year-old woman who developed a rash, fever, vomiting and abdominal pain 24 h after taking Co-T; necropsy revealed diffuse gastric and small intestinal hemorrhagic ulceration with diffuse mucosal bullae characteristic of Stevens–Johnson syndrome. Both Salter (1973) and Whittington (1989) have described a number of cases of fatal toxic epidermal necrolysis (Lyell's syndrome) due to Co-T. Other patients have been described with polymorphous rashes and fever in whom microscopic examination of skin lesions showed changes compatible with a necrotizing vasculitis (Wahlin and Rosman, 1976); one such patient also developed reversible renal failure (Ramaiah *et al.*, 1977). One patient was described who developed fever, chills and leukocytosis, simulating sepsis on two occasions after receiving Co-T (Shalit and Levy, 1984). Others have also reported patients where Co-T toxicity manifested as hypotension, mimicking sepsis (Marinac and Stanford, 1993; Nguyen *et al.*, 1993). In a large case-control study to quantify the risk of various drugs being associated with Stevens–Johnson syndrome or toxic epidermal necrolysis, Roujeau *et al.* (1995) found the risk of these skin conditions was increased for Co-T and other sulfonamide-containing antibiotics, with a crude relative risk of 172 (95% confidence interval, 75–396).

Adverse reactions to both Co-T and trimethoprim are more common in patients with acquired immunodeficiency syndrome (AIDS), such that up to 50–60% of AIDS patients will experience adverse reactions of sufficient severity as to require a change in therapy (Lee and Safrin, 1992). These include maculopapular rashes, associated with fever, malaise, often nausea and headache, peripheral cytopenias (neutropenia and thrombocytopenia) and raised hepatic transaminases (Mitsuyasu *et al.*, 1983; Jaffe *et al.*, 1983; Gordin *et al.*, 1984; Lee and Safrin, 1992). In several patients, folinic acid administration was ineffective in preventing cytopenias, or reversing them once established (pp. 852, 876). The reason for this increased rate of hypersensitivity is unclear. No clinical or laboratory parameters are predictive of cutaneous reactions occurring (Roudier *et al.*, 1994). However, various associations including the serum concentrations of trimethoprim and sulfamethoxazole, and metabolites of sulfamethoxazole (Van der Ven *et al.*, 1991) have been proposed, but data are inconclusive. Carr *et al.* (1993) noted AIDS patients with a CD4:CD8 ratio of >0.10 were more likely to develop hypersensitivity, but that once the CD4$^+$ cell count fell below 25×10^6 per liter this risk declined. They proposed that HIV infection of CD4$^+$ lymphocytes or monocytes enhances T lymphocyte sensitivity to Co-T or their metabolites, allowing hypersensitivity to occur; but as CD4$^+$ or CD8$^+$ lymphocyte numbers decline further there are insufficient lymphocytes to produce this response, resulting in a possible reduction in the rate of hypersensitivity in advanced HIV disease. As yet there have been no further studies reported to support this hypothesis. In some cases of Co-T hypersensitivity in AIDS patients, treatment can be carefully continued without apparent ill-effect (Putterman *et al.*, 1990; Kreuz *et al.*, 1990), although in the majority of patients cessation of Co-T is necessary. The concomitant use of corticosteroids with Co-T may reduce the incidence of hypersensitivity reactions (Aguilar *et al.*, 1991). Caumes *et al.* (1994) noted that among patients with severe *P. carinii* pneumonia who are given adjuvant corticosteroids in addition to Co-T (p. 877), the incidence of cutaneous side-effects is significantly less than among those patients who are not treated with corticosteroids (13% vs 47%, respectively; p=0.014); no patients in the steroid-treated group required cessation of Co-T therapy due to side-effects. For reasons that are unclear, the incidence of cutaneous reactions to Co-T among African, Haitian and American black AIDS patients appears to be less than among white AIDS patients (Colebunders *et al.*, 1987). The management of adverse reactions to Co-T among HIV-infected patients has been summarized by Jung and Paauw (1994)

Oral desensitization to trimethoprim-sulfamethoxazole among HIV-infected patients has been investigated by a number of authors with a success rate of 60–96%. The likelihood of success in desensitization does not appear to be related to level of CD4 lymphocyte immunosuppression (Sher *et al.*, 1986; MacLean Smith *et al.*, 1987; Bissuel *et al.*, 1995; Nguyen *et al.*, 1995). Due to the relatively small numbers in most published reports, it is difficult to strongly recommend any one regimen. However, the protocol used by Gluckstein and Ruskin (1995) appears practical, rapid and reasonably effective. In this a freshly prepared 10-fold aqueous dilution of Co-T oral suspension (40 mg trimethoprim and 200 mg sulfamethoxazole in 5 ml) is administered hourly over 4 h, starting with 0.004 mg trimethoprim/ 0.02 mg sulfamethoxazole. Hence at hour 0, 1, 2, 3, and 4 the following doses are administered respectively: 0.004/0.02 mg, 0.04/0.2 mg, 0.4/2 mg, 4/20 mg and 40/200 mg. At hour 5 a single Co-T tablet (160/800 mg) is given. After each dose the patient consumes about 180 ml of water. Histamines or corticosteroids are not routinely necessary. Most desensitizations can be undertaken in the office setting, so long as appropriate resuscitation equipment is available in case of severe anaphylaxis. Anaphylactic shock, however, has been reported during desensitization (Sher *et al.*, 1986). Following successful desensitization Gluckstein and Ruskin (1995) prescribed Co-T 160/800 mg (one double-strength tablet) three times weekly as low-dose chemoproprophylaxis for *P. carinii* pneumonia. With this protocol 86% completed desensitization and 71% were successfully stabilized on long-term Co-T. Other protocols in which desensitization is carried out over a number of days, such as that described by MacLean Smith *et al.* (1987) and Piketty *et al.* (1995), are notable but possibly less convenient. Kreuz *et al.* (1990) has reported successful Co-T desensitization in four children.

3 Hematological side-effects

Because of its mode of action, it was anticipated that trimethoprim might interfere with human folate metabolism and hence hemopoiesis, especially if large doses were given over prolonged periods. The *in vitro* effect of various concentrations of trimethoprim has been studied on human bone marrow cultures. A sensitive indicator which detects the effect of trimethoprim on folate metabolism in such cultures is interference of folate-dependent DNA-thymine synthesis by methylation of deoxyuridylate to thymidylate (Sive et al., 1972; Koutts et al., 1973). Only slight or no effect on folate metabolism was demonstrated by this method in normal bone marrow cells if trimethoprim concentrations used were similar to those attained in serum with usual doses. However, 10-fold greater trimethoprim concentrations produced abnormalities of folate metabolism, which were only partially corrected by folic acid, but were completely corrected by folinic acid in vitro. In vitamin B_{12} or folate-deficient marrow cultures, trimethoprim at therapeutic concentrations caused further disturbance in folate metabolism, which was not corrected by vitamin B_{12} or folic acid, but this was again completely reversed by folinic acid (Koutts et al., 1973). Changes in folate metabolism have also been investigated in patients receiving Co-T by measuring the serum level of tetrahydrofolate, a specific indicator of DHFR activity. These serum levels remain normal in patients with otherwise normal hemopoiesis, if trimethoprim is used in the usual doses (Davis and Jackson, 1973).

Clinical experience with Co-T supports the above experimental observations. If patients without a bone marrow disorder are treated with usual trimethoprim doses, hematological side-effects, although reported, appear to be uncommon (Frisch, 1973; Salter, 1973; Lawson and Henry, 1977; Lawson and Paice, 1982). Reported abnormalities include aplastic anemia (Frisch, 1973), neutropenia (Nielsen et al., 1970; Frisch, 1973; Hawkins et al., 1993), acute agranulocytosis (Evans and Tell, 1969; Palva and Koivisto, 1971), and acute thrombocytopenia (Hammett, 1970; Rickard and Uhr, 1971; Raik and Vincent, 1973; Böse et al., 1974; Hawkins et al., 1993). The International Agranulocytosis and Aplastic Anemia Study Group (1989) estimated the relative risk of developing agranulocytosis when Co-T is used for 3 or more consecutive days to be 12 (95% confidence interval 3.9–40), with the estimated excess risk of agranulocytosis attributable to the use of Co-T in a 2-week period to be 1.6 per million. In this same study the relative risk estimates of aplastic anemia were elevated for Co-T [2.1], sulfonamides without trimethoprim [2.9] and beta-lactams [1.5], but none was statistically significant. Surprisingly, Asmar et al. (1981) reported that in a comparative trial of treatment of children with otitis media with oral Co-T (50 children) and amoxicillin (20 children), the frequencies of neutropenia in the two groups were 34% and 5% respectively; and thrombocytopenia developed in 12% of children treated with Co-T, but in none of those treated by amoxicillin. However, in a subsequent study of 2622 children who received Co-T, there was no report of neutropenia or any other type of blood disorder (Jick et al., 1984). Increased myelosuppression has been observed in granulocytopenic patients treated with Co-T (p. 882).

Thrombocytopenia due to Co-T appears to be more common in patients receiving long-term treatment with diuretics, such as the thiazides or frusemide (Frisch, 1973). Whereas Salter (1973) found thrombocytopenia to be more frequent in patients over 70 years of age, others have observed this complication at all ages (Dickson, 1978). In three patients receiving Co-T, diminished survival of transfused platelets occurred in two and the third developed thrombocytopenia; antibodies against donor platelets coated with Co-T were found in the sera of all cases which were directed against the trimethoprim component only (Claas et al., 1979). Pancytopenia has been described in a 7-month-old baby receiving oral Co-T (Tulloch, 1976). All these toxic effects, which indicate depression of hemopoiesis, appear to be more common following prolonged Co-T therapy (Dawborn et al., 1973). It is possible that some of these reported side-effects have been caused by sulfamethoxazole and not trimethoprim, particularly acute agranulocytosis, a well-known complication of sulfonamides (Palva and Koivisto, 1971). Hemolytic anemia has been rarely observed with Co-T therapy (Frisch, 1973). A patient with typhoid fever and glucose-6-phophate dehydrogenase deficiency developed acute hemolysis when treated with Co-T (Owusu, 1972), but ten infants with the same defect were treated with Co-T for 5 days without hemolysis (Chan and Wong, 1975). Nevertheless, hemolysis is a known complication of sulfonamides in such patients (p. 817).

Jewkes et al. (1970) described a patient who developed megaloblastic erythropoiesis after a 6-month course of Co-T, given in usual doses for chronic bronchitis. Folic acid administration was of no benefit, but the bone marrow reverted to normal within 1 week, despite continued administration of trimethoprim, when folinic acid was given in a daily dose of 60 µg by injection. This appears to be the only case in which megaloblastic changes have followed the administration of standard doses of a Co-T (Frisch, 1973), and even then, in this case, the causative relationship of trimethoprim has been disputed (Girdwood, 1976). In many other patients who have developed megaloblastic anemia while receiving this combination, an alternative explanation has been found for the blood dyscrasia (Girdwood, 1973). Hughes et al. (1975a) administered Co-T for long periods to 11 patients, one for 30 months and the remainder for periods of 3–16 months. At the most, a few of these patients appeared to develop asymptomatic folate depletion as reflected by serial hematological investigations.

If trimethoprim is used in doses higher than normally recommended, bone marrow toxicity may result more commonly. Kahn *et al.* (1968) administered trimethoprim in a daily oral dose of 1.0 g for a period of 4 weeks to 10 adult patients. The same dose of trimethoprim plus 4 g of sulfisoxazole daily was given to 13 other adult patients for periods varying from several months to over 2 years. Hematological abnormalities such as leukopenia, anemia and thrombocytopenia were noted in several patients in both groups, but these abnormalities disappeared about 2 weeks after the drugs were stopped. In one patient thrombocytopenia and leukopenia were reversed by the administration of folinic acid, despite continued administration of trimethoprim. These hematological abnormalities also occur more frequently in patients with severe renal failure, who are treated with usual doses, possibly because they develop high serum levels of both trimethoprim and sulfamethoxazole (p. 845). McPherson and Raik (1970) reported acute thrombocytopenia in two uremic patients, who were treated with usual Co-T doses. Yuill (1973) described megaloblastic anemia in a severely uremic patient receiving this combination, but other factors such as dietary deficiency of folic acid were also contributory. Kobrinsky and Ramsay (1981) described a woman who had undergone bone marrow transplantation for leukemia and who was treated by high doses of i.v. Co-T for *P. carinii* pneumonia; she developed pancytopenia and megaloblastic changes in the bone marrow, which recovered when Co-T was discontinued and treatment with folinic acid was initiated. Co-T is used in high dosage to treat *P. carinii* pneumonia in AIDS patients (p. 874) and this may be a factor in causing an increased frequency of cytopenias in such patients. The value of supplemental folinic acid in preventing or reversing such cytopenias has not been established. Indeed in AIDS patients, folinic acid supplementation appears to be ineffective in reversing Co-T-induced neutropenia and may be associated with a higher rate of therapeutic failure when treating *P. carinii* pneumonia (Jaffe *et al.*, 1983; Bygbjerg *et al.*, 1988; Safrin *et al.*, 1994; p. 852).

Patients with a pre-existing megaloblastic anemia are seriously at risk if treated with Co-T (Annotation, 1973). Trimethoprim aggravates megaloblastic changes and prevents response to either vitamin B_{12} or folic acid (Koutts *et al.*, 1973). In addition, it may cause neutropenia and thrombocytopenia in these patients (Chanarin and England, 1972). The drug is, therefore, contraindicated in all patients with a megaloblastic anemia or in those who may possibly have megaloblastic bone marrow changes such as pregnant women, patients receiving anticonvulsant drugs and those with a raised mean red cell volume. Girdwood (1976) considers that once the folate deficiency is corrected, there is no reason why Co-T should not be used.

In patients with a predisposition to bone marrow depression; for example, those treated with trimethoprim-related drugs such as pyrimethamine (p. 905) and those receiving immunosuppressive drugs, Co-T should be used cautiously. Ansdell *et al.* (1976) described a woman who developed a megaloblastic anemia following a 14-day course of Co-T while taking pyrimethamine for malarial prophylaxis. Hulme and Reeves (1971) reported four renal transplant patients receiving immunosuppressive therapy (prednisolone and azathioprine), who developed a marked leukopenia in association with a course of Co-T, given within the first 60 days after transplantation. Leukopenia was not observed in another ten patients who received identical therapy at a later stage after transplantation. It was concluded that Co-T should be used with caution during the first 60 days after cadaveric renal transplantation. Bradley *et al.* (1980) also described neutropenia or thrombocytopenia in renal allograft recipients when Co-T was given for prolonged periods with azathioprine; this occurred more frequently than in allograft recipients treated with azathioprine alone. In addition, in bone marrow culture, the antifolate action of Co-T enhanced the marrow suppressive effect of 6-mercaptopurine, the active moiety cleaved from azathioprine. A large prospective study confirmed that the frequency of leukopenia in 94 antibiotic-treated patients, who were renal transplant recipients, was greater in the early weeks after transplantation. However, the frequency in a control group treated for urinary infections with antibiotics other than Co-T was not significantly different from those treated with Co-T. In eight patients leukopenia recovered when azathioprine was discontinued, while Co-T was continued. Azathioprine was, therefore, considered to be the cause of leukopenia. This drug is partly excreted by the kidney and the patients who developed leukopenia, although receiving a similar dose of azathioprine as those that did not, had poorer renal function (Hall, 1974). Megaloblastic pancytopenia is more likely in patients treated with methotrexate and Co-T (Govert *et al.*, 1992), probably due to decreased renal clearance of free methotrexate associated with competition for tubular clearance by Co-T (Ferrazzini *et al.*, 1990). Ferrazzini *et al.* (1990) identified a mean 66% increase in systemic exposure to methotrexate when these agents were co-administered. The immunocompromised state plus the high dosage used to treat *P. carinii* pneumonia may be factors causing an increase in the frequency of neutropenia and thrombocytopenia associated with Co-T treatment of patients with AIDS (p. 856). Nevertheless, cytopenias and rashes have not been reported in other types of non-AIDS, immunocompromised patients receiving Co-T for *P. carinii* pneumonia (Jaffe *et al.*,1983).

Despite all these reports, trimethoprim bone marrow toxicity appears to be uncommon. Most of these side-effects can probably be avoided if the known contraindications and precautions are observed. Nevertheless, it would seem advisable to perform regular blood examinations during prolonged or high-dose trimethoprim administration.

As to be expected from its sulfonamide component (p. 818), methemoglobinemia has been described with Co-T treatment (Damergis *et al.*, 1983).

4 Nephrotoxicity

During a 4-year period, Kalowski *et al.* (1973) detected 16 patients who developed deterioration of renal function in association with Co-T treatment; most of these had antecedent renal functional impairment. Co-T-associated renal damage was reversible in most patients when the drug was discontinued, but three developed permanent impairment of renal function. Deterioration in renal function appeared to be due to an acute tubular necrosis, which may have resulted from an accumulation of conjugated sulfamethoxazole metabolites in the presence of renal failure, rather than trimethoprim. The authors recommended that Co-T should not be used in patients with a serum creatinine level greater than 2.0 mg% or 0.17 mmol per liter (creatinine clearance less than 40 ml per min). A subsequent report from the same unit described the simultaneous occurrence of sensitivity rashes in four patients given Co-T, two of whom died; all had underlying renal functional impairment and received an inappropriately high dose of Co-T (Richmond *et al.*, 1979). Bailey and Little (1976) reported four patients whose renal function deteriorated in association with Co-T therapy; one patient had recovering acute oliguric renal failure and the other three had chronic renal failure at the time of Co-T therapy; two of those with chronic disease had further permanent impairment of renal function. Some of the patients reported by these two groups may have received inordinately high doses of Co-T for the state of their renal function. Other studies have not detected deterioration in renal function following the use of Co-T given in suitably reduced dosage to patients with renal disease. Tasker *et al.* (1975) treated urinary or respiratory infections in 20 patients with chronic renal failure with Co-T. Worsening renal function, which occurred in only three of these patients, was not considered to be due to Co-T. The drug has also been given for periods of up to 2 years to patients with chronic renal disease without evidence of deterioration in renal function (Denneberg *et al.*, 1976). Rosenfeld *et al.* (1975) gave prophylactic Co-T to 18 patients with a neurogenic bladder, all of whom had a creatinine clearance value above 50 ml per min; 18 patients were treated for 60–80 days and in seven the period was extended to 330–430 days; there were no significant differences between the creatinine clearance values taken before and after this therapy. Guignard *et al.* (1978) gave Co-T to 16 children for a period of 6 months after urogenital reconstructive surgery. These children had normal renal function preoperatively, and this remained so after treatment. However, findings of Shouval *et al.* (1978) are in direct contrast. They administered Co-T in a dosage of two standard tablets three times daily for periods of 6–8 days; the recipients were two patients who had had decreased creatinine clearance during Co-T therapy 3 months previously, from which they had recovered, and four healthy volunteers. Significant falls in creatinine clearance, rises in serum creatinine values and increases in sodium excretion occurred in all subjects, and all of these changes returned promptly to normal on cessation of the drug. A temporary rise in serum creatinine levels after 5 days treatment with Co-T was noted by Lövestad *et al.* (1976). In 25 patients treated with Co-T by Trollfors *et al.* (1980), two developed decreased glomerular filtration when given doses too high in relation to renal function and, in 21 of 23 others, there was a slight rise in serum creatinine even though they received appropriate doses for their renal function. Smith and Cohen (1994) reported non-oliguric renal failure and hyperkalemia associated with trimethoprim 200 mg twice-daily for urinary tract sepsis in an adult. Interstitial nephritis possibly due to Co-T has also been reported (Saltissi *et al.*, 1979).

Co-T has been associated with the development of a hyperchloremic metabolic acidosis, possibly due to renal tubular acidosis, in children being treated for acute lymphoid leukemia (Murphy, 1992). Similarly, Domingo *et al.* (1995) have described hyperchloremic metabolic acidosis with a normal anion gap due to probable renal tubular acidosis in an an HIV-infected adult receiving Co-T therapy for *P. carinii* pneumonia.

Trimethoprim may also reversibly impair renal excretion of potassium and result in hyperkalemia. Choi *et al.* (1993) reported this phenomenon in an AIDS patient treated with Co-T and demonstrated *in vitro* studies to implicate trimethoprim. Since trimethoprim, amiloride and triamterene are structurally related hetrocyclic bases it is likely that these drugs act in a similar manner in the kidney. Velázquez *et al.* (1993) have demonstrated that in rats trimethoprim acts like amiloride in blocking apical membrane sodium channels in the distal nephron resulting in a reduction in transepithelial voltage and potassium secretion, with resultant hyperkalemia. Greenberg *et al.* (1993) noted that among HIV-infected patients receiving high-dose Co-T for treatment of *P. carinii* pneumonia, the serum potassium increased by 1.1 mmol per liter 9.8 ± 0.5 days after starting Co-T therapy, and in some cases reached life-threatening levels. The hyperkalemia could not be attributed to changes in renal function and steadily returned to normal with cessation of Co-T. Serum potassium should be closely monitored in these patients, particularly 7–10 days after commencing high-dose Co-T therapy. Subsequently, other authors have noted similar problems of hyperkalemia in elderly, non-HIV-infected patients who have been treated with lower routine doses of Co-T (Modest *et al.*, 1994; Pennypacker *et al.*, 1994; Canaday and Johnson, 1994). Alappan *et al.* (1996) prospectively monitored the impact of standard-dose Co-T therapy on serum potassium levels in hospitalized patients in a community-based teaching hospital. A peak serum potassium >5.0 mmol per liter developed in 62.5% patients treated with standard-dose Co-T for various infections; in 21.2% patients severe hyperkalemia (≥ 5.5 mmol per liter) developed. Hyperkalemia was more likely in those patients with pre-existing renal dysfunction.

Deterioration in renal function in association with Co-T therapy has been noted in several renal transplant recipients (Kalowski *et al.*, 1973; Smith *et al.*, 1980). Ringden *et al.* (1984) reported that increases in serum creatinine values during treatment with Co-T of renal transplant recipients occurred in 30 of 41(73%) of those receiving cyclosporin compared with 6 of 46 (13%) receiving azathioprine. They noted less common nephrotoxicity in association with Co-T treatment of bone marrow recipients receiving cyclosporin. Nyberg *et al.* (1984) also described rises in serum creatinine values of renal transplant patients on cyclosporin treatment given trimethoprim alone; they found a similar effect of trimethoprim when these patients were treated with azathioprine. The situation is further confused by the finding that trimethoprim seems to be able to cause a temporary rise in the serum creatinine level without affecting the glomerular filtration rate. This may be caused by competitive inhibition of tubular secretion of creatinine and should not be misinterpreted as deterioration in renal function (Sandberg and Trollfors, 1986).

It seems, therefore, that Co-T can cause renal damage, but this is infrequent and appears to be more common in patients with pre-existing renal disease and in those in whom inappropriately high doses of Co-T are used. Co-T should, therefore, be used cautiously in patients with renal failure.

5 Hepatotoxicity

This is an uncommon complication of Co-T (Lawson and Paice, 1982; Lindgren and Olsson, 1994) and it is probably caused by the sulfonamide component (p. 818). Jaundice is usually mild and cholestatic in type (Stevenson *et al.*, 1978; Nair *et al.*, 1980; Kowdley *et al.*, 1992). In one patient, rechallenge with Co-T caused recurrence of jaundice, which rapidly disappeared when the drug was stopped (Frisch, 1973). Kowdley *et al.* (1992) reported two patients in whom the cholestasis lasted 1–2 years. De Vito (1982) described transient elevation of serum alkaline phosphatase values in two young children, which may have been related to Co-T treatment. Hepatic necrosis in an 80-year-old man (Colucci and Cicero, 1975) and fulminant hepatic failure and hemorrhagic pancreatitis (Alberti-Flor *et al.*, 1989) have also been attributed to Co-T.

6 Aseptic meningitis and encephalitis

Aseptic meningitis associated with Co-T and trimethoprim administration, was first reported by Kremer *et al.* (1983) and has subsequently been described by numerous other authors (Haas, 1984; Biosca *et al.*, 1986; Streiffer and Hudson, 1986; Joffe *et al.*, 1989; Tunkel and Starr, 1990; Harrison *et al.*, 1994; Pashankar *et al.*, 1995). Joffe *et al.* (1989) described three patients with probable Co-T-related meningitis and reviewed the recent literature. Harrison *et al.* (1994) described an HIV-infected adult who developed aseptic meningitis after both Co-T and trimethoprim alone. In this case, and the others reviewed by the authors, all patients had a similar abrupt onset of symptoms, and prompt resolution with cessation of therapy. Encephalitis due to trimethoprim alone has also been reported (Hedlund *et al.*, 1990). The mechanism of the aseptic meningitis is uncertain but most authors favour a hypersensitivity reaction. Other neurological complications such as seizures and coma have been reported occasionally (Theodorou *et al.*, 1995).

7 Pneumonitis

Pneumonitis has been rarely associated with both Co-T (Holdcroft and Ellison, 1991; Kelly *et al.*, 1992) and trimethoprin alone (Higgins and Niklasson, 1990), but probably represents a hypersensitivity reaction. In AIDS patients this may mimic *P. carinii* pneumonia (Holdcroft and Ellison, 1991; Kelly *et al.*, 1992). Kelly *et al.* (1992) described three HIV-infected patients who developed pneumonitis and shock after treatment and rechallange with Co-T, and reviewed the literature regarding this rare side-effect.

8 Miscellaneous side-effects

Various other rare reactions have occurred during Co-T therapy. These include acute rheumatoid arthritis, anaphylaxis, angioneurotic edema, glossitis, severe vasculitis, hypoglycemia, leg paresthesiae, hallucinations, tremor, vertigo, visual disturbances, headache and depression (Hanley, 1969; Frisch, 1973; Borucki *et al.*, 1988; Schattner *et al.*, 1988; McCue and Zandt, 1991; Johnson *et al.*, 1993; Lewis, 1995). Polyneuropathy associated with Co-T therapy has been described in one patient (Grossman *et al.*, 1977), but this may have been a complication of cardiac surgery which was performed on the patient (Vincent, 1977). The significance of these anecdotal reports is not clear.

9 Immunosuppressive effect

Co-T inhibits DNA synthesis in lymphocytes cultured in the presence of phytohemagglutinin. This effect occurs with both trimethoprim and sulfamethoxazole separately, but it is more pronounced with the drug combination (Gaylarde and Sarkany, 1972). Arvilommi *et al.* (1972) demonstrated that Co-T partially suppresses antibody response after tetanus vaccination. Trimethoprim and sulfamethoxazole, individually as well as in combination, inhibit chemiluminescence of human polymorphs in response to phagocytosis (Siegel and Remington, 1982). Somewhat contradictory results were reported by Oleske *et al.* (1983). They found that Co-T and its separate components caused some enhancement in chemotaxis and chemiluminescence of normal polymorphs and this effect was more marked with cells from patients with leukocyte chemotactic and chemiluminescence defects. These observations suggest that Co-T may have some immunosuppressive effects and the recent preliminary literature suggesting a possible role for Co-T in the treatment of Wegener's granulomatosis (p. 883) adds interest to this concept. Neutrophil phagocytosis, random migration and chemotaxis are not affected by trimethoprim and sulfamethoxazole, individually, or in combination (Anderson *et al.*, 1980).

10 Safety in pregnancy

Large doses of trimethoprim are teratogenic in animals. This is to be expected because trimethoprim is a folic acid antagonist (p. 852). The drug has been used in a small number of patients during the first 16 weeks of pregnancy without encountering any fetal malformations. However, folate levels are often marginal in pregnant women. For this reason, the use of Co-T or trimethoprim should be avoided where possible during pregnancy, particularly during the first trimester.

11 Interaction with other drugs

There have been several reports describing the potentiation of warfarin and phenytoin by Co-T (p. 820). The serum half-life of phenytoin may be increased in the presence of Co-T (Wilcox, 1981). One study showed that Co-T given in standard doses could lower thryoid hormone levels, but in another there were no clinically significant changes in these hormone levels in patients taking continuous low-dose Co-T for more than a year. Co-T may cause hyper-phenylalaninemia, but the clinical significance of this is not known (Leeming, 1980). In AIDS patients given either dapsone alone, trimethoprim-dapsone or trimethoprim-sulfamethoxazole for the treatment of *P. carinii* pneumonia, Lee *et al.* (1989) noted a bidirectional drug interaction between trimethoprim and dapsone, resulting in higher concentrations of each agent in the presence of the other. Concomitant administration of trimethoprim-sulfamethoxazole and cyclosporin has been associated with an increased incidence of reversible nephrotoxicity, independent of the levels of cyclosporin or trimethoprim-sulfamethoxazole (Sands and Brown, 1989). Trimethoprim may inhibit the renal clearance of procainamide, resulting in increased procainamide and N-acetyl procainamide plasma concentrations when these agents are administered together (Vlasses *et al.*, 1989).

Clinical Uses of the Drugs

A   Co-trimoxazole (trimethoprim-sulfamethoxazole)

Trimethoprim has been used mainly in combination with sulfamethoxazole as co-trimoxazole (Co-T).

1 Urinary tract infections

Co-T has been used extensively for these diseases. It is effective and superior to either a sulfadimidine or an ampicillin regimen (Reeves et al., 1969), and in other trials, it has produced higher cure rates than cephalexin (Gower and Tasker, 1976) and nitrofurantoin (Lövestad et al., 1976). Co-T is equally effective to nalidixic acid for the treatment of uncomplicated acute urinary tract infections caused by Enterobacteriaceae in young women (Iravini et al., 1981a). Co-T is active against Staph. saprophyticus which, after E. coli, is the second most common cause of urinary tract infection in sexually active young women (Latham et al., 1983). In this respect Co-T has an advantage over nalidixic acid which does not inhibit this organism (p. 967). Co-T, two standard tablets every 12 h for 10 days, was compared with nalidixic acid, 1 g 6-hourly for 7 days, in acute infections in young women; cure rates were the same for both regimens. Neither regimen was associated with the emergence of resistant bacterial mutants in the urine (Iravini et al., 1981a). A 7-day regimen of Co-T is superior to high-dose amoxicillin/clavulanic acid in a single dose for the treatment of uncomplicated urinary tract infection in women (Masterton and Bochsler, 1995). However, a 3-day regimen of Co-T is more effective and less expensive than 3-day regimens of cefadroxil, amoxicillin or nitrofurantoin for the treatment of such infections in women (Hooton et al., 1995). Co-T may, however, be inferior to the fluoroquinolones for the treatment of symptomatic complicated urinary tract infections (Nicolle et al., 1994; p. 1014).

Resistance to Co-T and trimethoprim among common urinary pathogens however, appears to be increasing (Gruneberg, 1990; Stamm et al., 1991). Stamm et al.(1991) noted a 19% incidence of Co-T resistance among isolates collected from women with recurrent urinary tract infections in 1983/4 compared with 5% in 1977/8. Tungsanga et al. (1988) noted a 29% rate of Co-T resistance among E. coli isolates in a double-blind trial comparing Co-T with norfloxacin (p. 841) for the treatment of upper urinary tract infections. This resistance was reflected in a significantly higher bacteriological cure rate and higher (but not statistically significant) clinical cure rate for norfloxacin. Thus Co-T remains an extremely useful agent for the treatment of urinary infections, but increasing Co-T resistance in some regions may erode this position in the future.

Single-dose treatment with Co-T is effective for uncomplicated urinary tract infections in women (Buckwold et al., 1982; Counts et al., 1982; Souney and Polk, 1982; Tolkoff-Rubin et al., 1982a; Fihn et al., 1988). Single doses varying from two to six standard tablets have been used, but usually at least four tablets are recommended. This treatment results in less side-effects than conventional therapy and is more effective than single-dose treatment with ampicillin, amoxycillin or cyclacillin (Souney and Polk, 1982; Gossius and Vorland, 1984; Hooton et al., 1985; Fihn et al., 1988). The efficacy of single-dose (four tablets) and a 10-day course of Co-T was studied in 77 women with cystitis; cure rates were not significantly different, but the 10-day course eliminated enteric bacilli from urethral and vaginal sites more often. In addition, perineal colonization in the 2 weeks after treatment was observed more commonly in women who developed recurrent infections, which were more common during these 2 weeks in women who had received single-dose therapy than 10 days' treatment. There were more side-effects with the longer treatment regimen (Counts et al., 1982). These results were confirmed by Fihn et al. (1988) who found that 10 days treatment resulted in a superior cure rate at 2 weeks compared with that achieved with single-dose therapy; but at the expense of a significantly higher rate of adverse effects (25% vs 12% respectively p=0.009). Factors independently associated with lower cure rates were a history of urinary tract infection within the previous 6 weeks, and the presence of $>10^5$ bacteria per ml in initial midstream urine culture. After controlling for these factors the risk of failure after single-dose treatment was not statistically significantly different from 10 days treatment at 6 weeks (p=0.21). Similarly, Norrby (1990), who reviewed the literature regarding short-term therapy of uncomplicated lower urinary tract infections in women, concluded that although single-dose treatment eradicated bacteriuria less efficiently than treatment for 3 or more days, the difference was less pronounced with Co-T than with beta-lactams. Trienekens et al. (1989) meanwhile, noted no difference in outcome between treatment with 3 and 7 days with Co-T in acute urinary tract infections in non-pregnant females, and Stamm et al. (1987) found a 2-week treatment regimen to be equally as effective as a 6-week regimen in women with pyelonephritis.

Urinary tract infections in women acquired after short-term catheterization often become symptomatic and should be treated. Single-dose therapy appears to be as effective as 10 days therapy in this situation, particularly in women younger than 65 years (Harding et al., 1991). Men with recurrent urinary tract infections are best treated with 6–12 weeks Co-T rather than 1–2 weeks of similar dosage (Smith et al., 1979; Gleckman et al., 1982) and the presence of prostatitis may need specific consideration (p. 862).

Co-T treatment has also been successful in a high proportion of patients with chronic and recurrent urinary tract infections (Nanra et al., 1971; Stratford and Dixson, 1971). Stamm et al. (1991), who studied the natural history of urinary tract infections in 51 infection-prone women in a standardized fashion for a median of 9 years, noted that antibiotic prophylaxis was highly effective in preventing acute cystitis, asymptomatic bacteriuria and acute pyelonephritis, even when used for as long as 5 years. Prophylaxis generally had no long-term impact on the natural history of infection, however, with the rates of infection upon cessation of antibiotics usually returning to the baseline level observed before prophylaxis. Trimethoprim (100 mg daily), Co-T (half a tablet daily) and nitrofurantoin (100 mg daily) were equally effective as prophlylactic agents. Similarly Nicolle et al. (1988) found the continuous use of Co-T for 5 years to be effective in the prevention of recurrent urinary tract infections. Post-coital Co-T prophylaxis (half a tablet) also appears very useful in the infection-prone young women with a history of frequent (two or more annually) urinary tract infections, particularly when they appear to be temporally related to sexual intercourse (Stapleton et al., 1990).

Co-T has been used successfully in a lower dosage (one standard tablet every 1 or 2 nights) for prolonged treatment of patients with chronic bacteriuria (Cattell et al., 1971; O'Grady et al., 1973; Kincaid-Smith et al., 1973; Chinn et al., 1976). A dose of 40 mg trimethoprim plus 200 mg sulfamethoxazole thrice-weekly at bedtime was also effective prophylaxis of recurrent urinary tract infections in women (Harding et al., 1979, 1982; Nicolle et al., 1988). Co-T has compared favorably with other chemotherapeutic agents such as methenamine mandelate (p. 932) and sulfamethoxazole (Harding and Ronald, 1974). Low dose Co-T (one single-strength tablet daily) was more effective than methenamine hippurate (Kalowski et al., 1975) and nitrofurantoin (Stamey et al., 1977; pp. 929, 934), and has similar efficacy to trimethoprim (100 mg) alone (Stamm et al., 1980, 1991). Among patients with recent spinal cord injury undergoing bladder retraining using intermittent catheterization, daily low-dose Co-T (40/200 mg) is superior to placebo in reducing bacteriuria and symptomatic urinary tract infection. However, Co-T-associated adverse effects are relatively common in this population (Gribble and Puterman, 1993). In renal transplant recipients Co-T has been used to prevent urinary tract infections (Tolkoff-Rubin et al., 1982b), but the possibility of renal toxicity due to Co-T (p. 857) and hematological side-effects (p. 854) are important considerations in such patients.

The superiority of Co-T in the prevention of recurrent urinary infections in females without underlying genitourinary diseases has been attributed to its effect of reducing Enterobacteriaceae which colonize the periurethral or vaginal vestibule area and which are responsible for reinfections (Harding and Ronald, 1974; Stamey and Condy, 1975; Stamey et al., 1977). This was thought to be related to the high concentrations of trimethoprim attained in vaginal fluid (p. 851). The importance of periurethral colonization in recurrent urinary tract infection is controversial (Counts et al., 1982; Stapleton et al., 1990). In the study by Stamm et al. (1980) in which nitrofurantoin, trimethoprim and Co-T were compared, both Co-T and trimethoprim eliminated E. coli from rectal, urethral, and vaginal cultures, but nitrofurantoin did not affect rectal carriage and did not reduce the urethral and vaginal carriage of E. coli to the same extent as the other two regimens. Nevertheless, all three drug regimens were equally effective, so that the presence of an active drug in the urine may be as important as prevention of periurethral colonization. These data are further supported by the efficacy of post-coital antibiotic prophylaxis which is known to have only a limited effect on E. coli colonization of these sites and presumably acts by eradicating any transient bacteriuria that may occur after intercourse in some women (Stapleton et al., 1990).

Acute uncomplicated urinary tract infections in children usually respond well to Co-T (Bose et al., 1974). Unlike adults, single-dose antibiotic therapy is not appropriate for children with acute urinary tract infection. In a study of 132 children with acute urinary tract infection who were randomized to receive Co-T in either one dose, two doses daily for 3 days, or two doses daily for 7 days, a significant difference in recurrence rate was noted between the single-dose

(21%), and the 3-day (6%) and 7-day (8%) regimens (Madrigal *et al.*, 1988). For the prevention of reinfections in children, Stansfield (1975) showed that a 6-month course was not superior to a 2-week course of Co-T. In a controlled trial, Ellerstein *et al.* (1977) found that the results of treatment of acute urinary tract infections in children with ampicillin or Co-T were comparable. In a reduced dosage, Co-T is also valuable for long-term suppressive therapy in children with chronic or recurrent urinary tract infections (Hobday, 1971; Lirenman and Arnold, 1973). A dose of 2 mg trimethoprim combined with 10 mg sulfamethoxazole per kg body weight daily has proved effective for this purpose (Smellie *et al.*, 1976, 1978, 1982). These authors noted that during such prophylaxis the number of rectal coliform bacilli was greatly and rapidly reduced, but at least 70% of surviving coliform organisms remained sensitive to the two components of Co-T. When Co-T prophylaxis was stopped, rectal organisms rapidly returned to normal, and they were all again sensitive to trimethoprim and sulfamethoxazole (Gruneberg *et al.*, 1976). The duration of Co-T prophylaxis (for periods of up to 9 years) had no effect on the frequency of trimethoprim-resistant strains of coliform bacteria in the feces of these children. Also such long-term treatment had no effects on renal or hematological function or somatic growth (Smellie *et al.*, 1982). A study involving 30 children with non-obstructive vesicoureteral reflux treated by long-term (mean, 17 months) daily Co-T or nitrofurantoin showed that both drugs were effective in preventing recurrent infection (Holland *et al.*, 1982).

Because trimethoprim diffuses well into prostatic tissue (p. 851), it theoretically should be beneficial in chronic bacterial prostatitis. Disappointingly, treatment of this infection with Co-T has only been successful in 30% of patients, despite adequate dosage for periods as long as 12–16 weeks. Factors, such as alterations in the prostatic secretory function, which could alter the passage of antibiotics into prostatic fluid and the presence of prostatic calculi in chronic prostatitis, may mitigate against success with Co-T treatment (Meares, 1982). The quinolones are now regarded as the treatment of choice for prostatitis (p. 1015). However, Co-T is effective in preventing bacteriuria after prostatectomy (Hills *et al.*, 1976). Bannister *et al.* (1981) showed that a 3-day course of either Co-T or pivmecillinam was also effective for this purpose.

2 Serious infections caused by Gram-negative bacilli

Co-T is a useful combination for the treatment of septicemias due to many Gram-negative bacilli, although it is often used only in certain circumstances. Alone or, less commonly, in combination with polymyxin, it is also often effective for hospital-acquired infections due to bacteria resistant to many other chemotherapeutic agents.

The parenteral preparation of Co-T has been used successfully to treat septicemias due to *E. coli*, *Y. enterocolitica* and *Proteus*, *Klebsiella* and *Enterobacter* species (Noal *et al.*, 1962; Cooper and Wald, 1964; Darrell *et al.*, 1968; Olcen and Eriksson, 1976; Franzén and Brandberg, 1976; Cherchi *et al.*, 1995) and in one young patient with *H. influenzae* septicemia (Franzén and Brandberg, 1976). Therapy has generally consisted of 3–10 days parenteral, followed by oral Co-T. Grose *et al.* (1977) achieved favorable results using oral Co-T to treat oncology patients with infections, many of whom had previously not responded to beta-lactam/aminoglycoside therapy. Schmidt *et al.* (1982) reported the use of i.v. Co-T for the treatment of 22 adults with serious infections due to Gram-negative bacteria; these included pneumonia, meningitis, pyelonephritis, deep-seated abscesses and endocarditis. A dosage of 4–6 mg trimethoprim and 20–30 mg sulfamethoxazole per kg per day was used; in 19 patients, who could be evaluated, 12 were cured. Sattler and Remington (1983) described the successful i.v. use of Co-T in seven other patients with similar infections. Experience with a few infants suggests that Co-T is useful for the treatment and prevention of cholangitis following hepatic portoenterostomy for biliary atresia (Chaudhary and Turner, 1981).

Street and Durack (1988) reviewed the published experience of 62 patients with Co-T in the treatment of infective endocarditis. Most cases were due to either *Coxiella burnetti* (19 cases) or *Pseudomonas* spp. (18 cases; 11 *Burkholderia* (previously *Ps.*) *cepacia*, four *Stenotrophomonas* (previously *Xanthomonas*) *maltophilia*, two *Ps. aeruginosa*, one *Ps. alcaligenes*), with a variety of Gram-negative bacilli and other pathogens being responsible in the remaining cases. Many patients had failed other treatment regimens at the time of commencing Co-T. Sixty of the 62 patients were treated with oral Co-T (often in combination with cardiac surgery) in doses ranging from 240 to 960 mg Co-T (trimethoprim component) daily for a mean duration of 7 weeks. Success rates against *C. burnetti*, *Pseudomonas* spp. and other organisms were 58%, 67% and 60%, respectively. Surgery was performed in a higher proportion of patients with *C. burnetti* and pseudomonal endocarditis (54%) than in patients with endocarditis due to other organisms (28%). Of 21 patients treated with Co-T alone, 11 (52%) were cured, although patients with *B. cepacia* infections were cured more often when Co-T was combined with another drug (six of seven cured) than when it was used alone (one of four cured; p >0.05). Among pathogens in which serum bactericidal titers could be measured (i.e. organisms other than *C. burnetti*), a relationship between higher serum bactericidal titers and successful outcome was noted. The authors concluded that Co-T has a clear role in the treatment of endocarditis secondary to *B. cepacia* and *S. maltophilia*. Conditions other than endocarditis have also been successfully treated with Co-T. Darby (1976) reported a case of an infant girl with an meningomyelocele who developed *B. cepacia* meningitis; this had failed to respond to a variety of antibiotics and eventually responded to oral Co-T. Co-T is frequently used for the treatment of a variety of infections due to *S. maltophilia* (Marshall *et al.*, 1989).

In vitro synergism between Co-T and polymyxin (Rahal *et al.*, 1973; Noriega *et al.*, 1975), and between Co-T and aminoglycoside (Speller, 1973) against *B. cepacia* has been suggested and these combinations have been used clinically by a number of authors with mixed success. *In vitro* synergism between Co-T and polymyxin B against *S. maltophilia* has also been reported (Yu *et al.*, 1978). The *in vitro* synergistic effect of Co-T and polymyxins against Gram-negative bacilli (p. 843) has also been used to treat *Serratia marcescens*, another common nosocomial infection. Thomas *et al.* (1976) used a daily dose of 1600 mg of sulfamethoxazole and 320 mg of trimethoprim orally combined with 100–300 mg of colistin methane sulfonate parenterally to obtain clinical improvement in four of six patients. Possible renal toxicity occurred in two and this combination should be used cautiously because both Co-T (p. 857) and polymyxins (p. 672) can cause nephrotoxicity.

Limited experience has suggested that Co-T may be effective in the treatment of *B. fragilis* infections (Okubadejo, 1974; Hanson and Woods, 1975; Franzén and Brandberg, 1976), but Co-T is not regarded as one of the drugs of first choice for these infections.

Co-T has been used as empiric chemotherapy in granulocytopenic patients (p. 881).

3 Respiratory tract infections

Co-T has been used extensively and successfuly in the treatment of acute bronchitis and bacterial pneumonia. Numerous comparative trials have shown that for the treatment of exacerbations in chronic bronchitis, Co-T has an equal or better effect than tetracycline, doxycycline, ampicillin, amoxycillin, cephalexin and cefaclor (Hughes, 1969; Pines *et al.*, 1969; Renmarker, 1976; Anderson *et al.*, 1981; Hughes, 1983). The common pathogens in bronchitis are pneumococci and *H. influenzae* both of which are generally highly sensitive to Co-T. In 134 Gambian children with severe pneumonia, oral Co-T for 5 days was equally effective as a single i.m. dose of procaine penicillin plus 5 days oral ampicillin, when outcome was assessed after 2 weeks (Campbell *et al.*, 1988). Similarly, Mulholland *et al.* (1995) found comparable efficacy between oral chloramphenicol and Co-T in the treatment of malnourished Gambian children with community-acquired pneumonia. Prolonged treatment with Co-T has also been used in patients with chronic bronchitis, and resistant strains of *H. influenzae* did not emerge (Hughes, 1973; 1983). In acute sinusitis the important pathogens are *Strep. pneumoniae* and *H. influenzae*. Co-T, ampicillin and amoxycillin were shown in one study to be equally effective for the treatment of acute maxillary sinusitis (Hamory *et al.*, 1979). In a randomized controlled trial of decongestant + either 3 days or 10 days of Co-T for acute maxillary sinusitis, no difference in clinical or radiological improvement, or symptomatic relapse or recurrence was noted, suggesting that a 3-day regimen is probably adequate (Williams *et al.*, 1995). However, whether this study had the statistical power to advocate equivalence is open to question (Rosborough *et al.*, 1995; Sawyer *et al.*, 1995; Shahar, 1995). Among HIV-infected children, Co-T prophylaxis for *P. carinii* pneumonia does not reduce the risk of sinusitis, which is most often subacute and recurrent (Mofenson *et al.*, 1995).

Of concern have been the increasing number of reports describing Co-T-resistance among strains of *H. influenzae* and *Strep. pneumoniae*. However, in most areas of the world this has not yet reached a level that would change the usage patterns of Co-T, except in certain specific regions where resistance is very high (p. 842). Co-T-resistance among strains of *H. influenzae* varies with geographical location; ranging from less than 1% in USA (Jorgenson *et al.*, 1990; George *et al.*, 1991) to 5% in Greece (Kanellakopoulou *et al.*, 1988), 7% in Sweden and Europe (Kayser *et al.*, 1990; Olsson *et al.*, 1992) and 11% in Pakistan (Jorgensen, 1992). Co-T-resistance among *Strep. pneumoniae* varies enormously from 0.6% in USA (Spika *et al.*, 1991) and 3% in Sweden (Olsson *et al.*, 1992) to 26% in Spain (Klugman, 1990) and 31% in Pakistan (Mastro *et al.*, 1991; p. 842).

The respiratory tract of patients with chronic bronchitis, who have been treated with antibiotics, is often colonized by Gram-negative bacilli, such as *E. coli* and *Klebsiella* spp. The presence of such organisms in sputum is usually not an indication for specific treatment but, in some debilitated patients, they may cause superinfection evidenced not only by a positive sputum culture, but also by recurrence of fever, worsening of chest signs and increasing amounts of purulent sputum (Weinstein and Musher, 1969). Co-T is effective against most bacteria which cause superinfections in patients with chronic bronchitis including *Klebsiella* spp. Bacteriological studies in patients with lower respiratory tract infections due to *Moraxella catarrhalis* suggest that Co-T, erythromycin or tetracycline may be appropriate antibiotics for treatment (Slevin *et al.*, 1984). Trimethoprim alone may also be effective for the treatment of bronchitis (Brumfitt *et al.*, 1985a; Amyes *et al.*, 1986). In a study of 74 patients with acute bronchitis, 7 days treatment with trimethoprim 200 mg twice-daily was equally effective as Co-T (160 mg trimethoprim component) twice-daily. Neither regimen resulted in the emergence of trimethoprim-resistant bacteria in any significant numbers (Amyes *et al.*, 1986).

Patients infected with HIV are particularly at risk of acquiring bacterial pneumonia, especially when the CD4 lymphocyte count is below 200 per mm^3. Prophylaxis with Co-T is associated with a 67% reduction in confirmed episodes of bacterial pneumonia (p=0.007) (Hirschtick *et al.*, 1995). Overall, the rate of pneumonia due to bacterial pathogens resistant to Co-T in HIV-infected patients appears to be currently <5% (Burack *et al.*, 1994).

4 Otitis media

Comparative trials have indicated that Co-T is equally effective to ampicillin, amoxycillin or cefaclor for the treatrnent of acute otitis media (Marchant and Shurin, 1982; Blumer *et al.*, 1984), including infection due to ampicillin-resistant strains of *H. influenzae* (Schwartz *et al.*, 1982). In the only controlled study of Co-T in the prophylaxis of recurrent acute otitis media, Gaskins *et al.* (1982) demonstrated efficacy. Co-T may be superior to beta-lactams for this indication due to the increasing incidence of beta-lactam resistance among strains of *H. influenzae* and *M. catarrhalis* (Lewin, 1989). In a controlled trial examining Co-T, prednisolone and ibuprofen in the treatment of chronic otitis media (with effusion), Giebink *et al.* (1990) found resolution rates were significantly greater in the Co-T- and prednisolone-treated groups after 2 weeks therapy, but that these differences diminished with longer duration of therapy.

5 Staphylococcal and other Gram-positive coccal infections

Although Co-T is quite effective against staphylococcal infections, other drugs are usually preferred. The combination has been used successfully to treat staphylococcal pneumonia (Darrell *et al.*, 1968), staphylococcal osteomyelitis (Craven *et al.*, 1970) and endocarditis (Bengtsson *et al.*, 1974). However, it appears that Co-T is inferior to vancomycin for the treatment of intravenous drug users with serious *Staph. aureus* infections (Markowitz *et al.*, 1992). In this double-blind, randomized trial of 101 intravenous drug users hospitalized with serious *Staph. aureus* infections (47% methicillin-resistant; 65% bacteremic), cure was achieved in 57 of 58 vancomycin recipients, versus 37 of 43 Co-T recipients (p <0.02). The mean duration of bacteremia was 6.7 days in Co-T recipients and 4.3 days in vancomycin recipients. Importantly, failure occurred only in patients with methicillin-sensitive, Co-T-sensitive *Staph. aureus* strains and mostly in patients with tricuspid valve endocarditis. Thus, these authors concluded that Co-T should be considered an alternative to vancomyin in selected cases of MRSA infection (Markowitz *et al.*, 1992). However, Co-T is markedly inferior to cloxacillin or glycopeptides (vancomycin or teicoplanin) for experimental endocarditis in rabbits due to methicillin-susceptible, or methicillin-resistant *Staph. aureus* (MRSA), respectively. No sterile vegetations were observed in Co-T-treated animals (de Gorgolas *et al.*, 1995).

Intravenous Co-T has been used with success in children with serious infections; these included various soft tissue or skeletal infections caused by one of *Strep. pneumoniae*, *Staph. aureus*, *Strep. pyogenes*, or by one of the Gram-negative bacteria, including *H. influenzae* and *Acinetobacter anitratus*. Also, three children with CSF shunt infection due to coagulase-negative staphylococci were treated successfully (Ardati *et al.*, 1979).

Street and Durack (1988) summarized the published data regarding Co-T treatment of endocarditis due to a variety of Gram-positive pathogens, including *Staph. aureus*, *Staph. epidermidis*, streptococci and micrococcus. Nine of 12 cases were treated successfully, although in five of these cases Co-T was combined with other antibiotics. Olcén and Eriksson (1976) reported two patients with a *Strep. viridans* septicemia who responded to i.v. and then oral Co-T therapy. Seligman *et al.* (1973) treated three patients with *Strep. viridans* endocarditis with oral Co-T; two treated for 4 weeks were cured, but the other patient, who was only treated for 3 weeks, relapsed 3 days after cessation of the drug.

One study showed that although Co-T is effective for *Strep. pyogenes* pharyngitis and tonsillitis, it is inferior to penicillin G (Tricket *et al.*, 1973), which is the preferred drug for this disease.

6 Meningitis

Generally Co-T is not regarded as a first-line agent for the treatment of bacterial meningitis but its good penetration through inflamed meninges (p. 851) makes it a reasonable choice in certain circumstances. There were early reports of the successful use of Co-T to treat a few cases of neonatal meningitis due to *E. coli* (Morzaria *et al.*, 1969; Roy, 1971). Sabel and Brandberg (1975) treated ten infants aged between 8 days and 10 months with meningitis and/or septicemia due to organisms, such as *Morganella morganii*, *E. coli* and *H. influenzae*. Most of these infants had not responded to kanamycin, ampicillin and sulfonamides, but eight responded rapidly to i.v. Co-T. Intravenous Co-T was used to treat four adults and one child with bacterial meningitis due to *N. meningitidis* or *Strep. pneumoniae*. Oral treatment was commenced on the 4th day and was continued for a total of 8 days. In all of these patients clinical recovery was rapid and complete (Farid *et al.*, 1976).

The place of Co-T in the treatment of meningitis has been reviewed (Gates and McCall, 1982; Rahal and Simberkoff, 1982; Levitz and Quintiliani, 1984). Gram-negative bacillary meningitis other than *H. influenzae* is one of the most difficult forms of meningitis to treat successfully and has a mortality of up to 70%. Most cases are related to head trauma, neurosurgery, immunosuppression, or occur in the neonatal period, but they may also be community-acquired, occurring in the elderly and in patients with alcohol-induced hepatic cirrhosis. Third-generation cephalosporins, such as cefotaxime (p. 336) and ceftriaxone (p. 359) are generally the treatments of choice, while chloramphenicol (p. 569) and the aminoglycosides (p. 473) have limitations in the treatment of Gram-negative bacillary meningitis. Co-T yields levels effective against many Gram-negative bacilli, especially *E. coli*, *S. marcescens*, *Klebsiella* spp. and non-aeruginosa pseudomonads, such as *B. cepacia* and *S. maltophilia*. Levitz and Quintiliani (1984) reviewed 33 patients with Gram-negative bacillary meningitis treated with Co-T; bacteriological cure occurred in 26 patients, one patient had *Ps. aeruginosa* infection which was naturally resistant and in another patient an *E. coli* strain resistant to Co-T developed during treatment; the other five patients in whom treatment failed had sensitive organisms. Because of the high activity of cefotaxime and ceftriaxone against *E. coli* and *Klebsiella*, the main indications for Co-T in Gram-negative bacillary meningitis seem to be for infections due to organisms resistant to these cephalosporins, such as *A. calcoaceticus*, *B. cepacia*, *S. maltophilia*, *F. meningosepticum* and some strains of *Serratia* or *Enterobacter* spp. with inducible beta-lactamases (Nguyen and Muder, 1994).

Levitz and Quintiliani (1984) reviewed experience with Co-T in the treatment of other forms of meningitis. Success rate for the treatment of pneumococcal and meningococcal meningitis in developed countries was quite high, but information on the use of Co-T in *H. influenzae* meningitis was scanty. Nevertheless, because of wider experience with penicillin G or chloramphenicol, Co-T was not recommended as initial treatment for these forms of meningitis. However, Co-T has been successfully used to treat *L. monocytogenes* meningitis. Although there have been no comparative trials of Co-T and ampicillin in the treatment of this form of meningitis, success has been reported with sufficient frequency to suggest it to be a reasonable treatment alternative, especially in the beta-lactam-allergic patient (Scheer and Hirschman, 1982; Spitzer *et al.*, 1986; Armstrong and Slater, 1986; Gunther and Philipson, 1988). Also Co-T is an alternative treatment for *Salmonella* meningitis, especially if the species is resistant to ampicillin and chloramphenicol (Levitz and Quintiliani, 1984). Co-T is effective therapy for *Enterobacter* meningitis, when doses of 20mg per kg per day (trimethoprim component) are used. Co-T cured all five patients reported by Wolff *et al.* (1993) and resulted in a superior outcome to third-generation cephalosporins in this setting.

The efficacy of Co-T in the treatment of other bacterial central nervous system infections, such as brain abscesses, remains less clear (Greene *et al.*, 1975). Perioperative Co-T failed to alter the incidence of shunt infection or malfunction in a controlled trial involving patients undergoing ventriculoperitoneal shunt surgery (Wang *et al.*, 1984).

7 Chemoprophylaxis against infections due to N. meningiidis and H influenzae

Co-T is unsatisfactory for the eradication of sulfonamide-resistant meningococci from chronic nasopharyngeal carriers (Feldman, 1973a). It is also not dependable for the eradication of nasopharyngeal carriage of *H. influenzae*. Yogev *et al.* (1978) reported some success using Co-T in the eradication of ampicillin-resistant *H. influenzae* strains from the nasopharynx of children in a chronic care facility, but Granoff *et al.* (1979) found that the combination was ineffective in eliminating carriage in 73% of 26 treated children. Kirven and Thornsberry (1978) performed bacteriological studies on the strains involved in these two trials and provided an explanation for the discrepant results. Although all strains of *H. influenzae* were inhibited by low concentrations of trimethoprim and Co-T, those strains in which prophylaxis failed had higher mean bactericidal concentrations for trimethoprim and Co-T. Rifampicin is recommended for chemoprophylaxis of meningococcal (p. 697) and *H. influenzae* (p. 698) infections.

8 Venereal diseases

a Gonorrhea Although Co-T is effective for the treatment of gonorrhea (Csonka and Knight, 1967; Schofield *et al.*, 1971; Hatos and Tuza, 1972), agents such as penicillin (p. 45), ceftriaxone (p. 361) and ciprofloxacin (p. 1022) are used more frequently. Treatment regimens have varied from single daily doses given for 1–5 days to multiple doses for several days. Cure rates are higher (92–100%) when the daily dose consists of four to six standard-strength tablets rather than one to three tablets (Austin *et al.*, 1973; Lawrence *et al.*, 1973; Svindland, 1973). Effective regimens have been four tablets twice-daily for 2 days (Lawrence *et al.*, 1973; Sattler and Ruskin, 1978), five tablets daily for 4 days (Csonka, 1969) and six tablets daily for 3 days (Austin *et al.*, 1973). Good results have also been obtained by using two five-tablet doses separated by 8 h (Kristensen and From, 1975). This latter regimen also appeared to be satisfactory for rectal gonorrhea in women, and tonsillar gonorrhea which is less responsive to treatment. Other studies indicate that oral Co-T is satisfactory for the treatment of pharyngeal gonorrhea, an infection which does not respond to spectinomycin and cefoxitin (Harrison, 1981; Brunham *et al.*, 1982; CDC, 1982). Single doses of nine tablets of Co-T are feasible for the treatment of gonorrhea, but adverse reactions associated with a 12-tablet dose preclude its use (p. 853). Wulf and Bech-Thomsen (1988) noted no significant difference in efficacy between a 5-day and a 2-day regimen of oral Co-T for the treatment of pharyngeal gonorrhea. The 5-day regimen (ten tablets at once, day 1; five tablets twice-daily, day 2; three tablets twice-daily, days 3–5) resulted in cure in 35 of 36 patients (97%) compared with a cure rate of 44 of 49 patients (90%) for the 2-day regimen (ten tablets at once, day 1; five tablets twice-daily, day 2). A single daily dose of nine standard tablets for 5 days has previously been advocated by the Centers for Disease Control, Atlanta, for the treatment of pharyngeal infections due to penicillinase-producing strains (CDC, 1985a). Current recommendations for uncomplicated gonococcal infections are to use a single dose of either ceftriaxone 250 mg i.m., cefixime 400 mg orally, ciprofloxacin 500 mg orally or ofloxacin 400 mg orally, in addition to a regimen effective against possible co-infection with *C. trachomatis*, such as doxycycline 100 mg twice-daily for 7 days (CDC, 1993).

Lassus and Renkonen (1979) treated patients with uncomplicated gonorrhea by an i.m. dose of 1600 mg sulfamethoxazole plus 320 mg trimethoprim, followed by an oral dose of 2400 mg sulfamethoxazole plus 480 mg trimethoprim 12 h later; 49 of 52 male patients and 37 of 38 female patients were cured. Two other patients with prostatitis due to penicillinase-producing gonococci were cured with cefoxitin plus Co-T in one and Co-T alone in the other (Vandenbroucke-Grauls *et al.*, 1982). A high proportion of penicillin G-resistant *N. gonorrhoeae* strains which do not produce beta-lactamase are resistant to Co-T (p. 838). Co-T is ineffective in syphilis (Csonka, 1969; Lawrence *et al.*, 1973) and its use for gonorrhea will not modify incubating syphilis (Svindland, 1973).

b Chlamydial infections Simultaneous urethral infection with *C. trachomatis* occurs in about 15–20% of heterosexual men with gonococcal urethritis and 25–60% of women with gonorrhea (Stamm *et al.*, 1984). Co-T was initially reported to be ineffective in non-specific urethritis (Csonka, 1969; Carroll and Nicol, 1970), but sulfonamides alone may be effective in this disease when the agent is *C. trachomatis* (p. 823). A number of studies have suggested that various Co-T regimens for gonorrhea may cure simultaneous *C. trachomatis* infection (Brunham *et al.*, 1982; Csango *et al.*, 1984). In another study, chlamydial infection was cured in 30 of 32 patients given Co-T and 27 of 29 given tetracycline but in only 10 of 23 given penicillin. Furthermore, among the *Chlamydia*-positive patients, postgonococcal urethritis in men and cervicitis and salpingitis in women occurred more often after penicillin treatment than the other two regimens (Stamm *et al.*, 1984). *In vitro* data, however, raise some doubts regarding the efficacy of antifolate agents against *Chlamydia* since strains of *C. trachomatis* and *C. psittaci* have been shown to be capable of *de novo* folate synthesis. Certain *C. trachomatis* strains, however, appear to be susceptible to sulfonamides and trimethoprim *in vitro* (Mumtaz *et al.*, 1988; Fan *et al.*, 1992). Doxycycline or azithromycin, however, are the treatment of choice for chlamydial infections (CDC, 1993; pp. 658, 747).

Csonka (1969) reported rapid clinical response to Co-T in three patients with lymphogranuloma venereum. Sulfonamides, with or without trimethoprim, are effective in this disease (Willcox, 1977) and sulfisoxazole 500 mg orally four times daily for 21 days is the recommended alternative treatment to first-line therapy with doxycycline 100 mg twice-daily for 21 days; erythromycin 500 mg four times daily is also a suitable alternative in the USA (CDC, 1993).

c Chancroid Although a variety of antibiotics have previously been used successfully to treat this infection, increasing antibiotic resistance and the association between genital ulcer disease, particularly chancroid, and heterosexual transmission of human immunodeficiency virus (HIV) have resulted in modifications to the recommended treatment regimens. The treatment of chancroid has been well reviewed (Schmid, 1990; Dangor *et al.*, 1990b; Schulte and Schmid, 1995) Although single-dose therapy using either ceftriaxone (p. 362), a quinolone (e.g. ciprofloxacin; p. 1022), or possibly spectinomycin are likely to be curative, single-dose therapy with Co-T is now less effective than 3- or 5-day courses (Schmid, 1990). In fact, due to increasing resistance, Co-T in single or multiple doses, is no longer recommended for the treatment of chancroid (Schulte and Schmid, 1995). Analysis of the outcome of treatment studies in the late 1980s of Co-T or combination trimethoprim-sulfonamide suggested that multi-day treatment courses were more effective than single-dose therapy, with overall cure rates of 98%, 93% and 89% for 5-, 3- and 1-day treatment courses respectively (Schmid, 1990). Importantly, among the single-dose studies the best efficacy was achieved with a trimethoprim dose of >640 mg. However, since 1985, there has been a loss of single-dose efficacy compared with earlier reports from similar regions, e.g. Kenya (Schmid, 1990; Plounde *et al.*, 1992). Co-T resistance among clinical *H. ducreyi* isolates is now reported to be 49% in some African states, with rates of clinical treatment failure with Co-T of 19–47.5% (Bogaerts *et al.*, 1995; Behets *et al.*, 1995; Schulte and Schmid, 1995).

Whether this change is related to an increase in resistance of *H. ducreyi* or to the increasing prevalence of co-existent HIV infection is uncertain (Schmid, 1990). Increasing trimethoprim and Co-T resistance has been demonstrated in a number of countries, although with less certainty in Kenya where this change in single-dose efficacy has been well documented (Taylor *et al.*, 1985; Schmid, 1986; Sturm, 1987; Naamara *et al.*, 1988). Co-existent HIV infection probably has an important impact on chancroid. In the USA where HIV is not as common as in Kenya, 18% of New York City patients with chancroid were also HIV-infected – a rate similar to Kenya (McLaughlin *et al.*, 1989). Infection by *H. ducreyi* may occur in association with up to 15% of primary syphilitic chancres (Leading article, 1982) and in these circumstances Co-T treatment may be advantageous, because it does not mask concomitant syphilis.

The current treatment recommendations for chancroid in the USA are erythromycin 500 mg four times daily for 7 days, ceftriaxome 250 mg i.m. in a single dose, or azithromycin 1 g orally in a single dose (CDC, 1993). Co-T, one double-strength tablet twice-daily for 7 days (CDC, 1989a), is no longer recommended as an alternative.

d   Granuloma venereum (Granuloma inguinale, Donovanosis)   This infection, caused by *Calymmatobacterium granulomatis*, responds to treatment by a number of antibiotics, such as tetracyclines, chloramphenicol, gentamicin and streptomycin. Treatment by Co-T, two standard tablets twice-daily for 10–15 days, also has been reported to be effective in some cases (Garg *et al.*, 1978; Lal and Garg, 1980).

9 *Typhoid fever and other salmonella infections*	It was first reported from Nigeria that Co-T is effective for the treatment of typhoid fever (Akinkugbe *et al.*, 1968). Subsequent reports confirmed this observation (Kamat, 1970; Farid *et al.*, 1970; Wicks and Stamps, 1970; Geddes *et al.*, 1971; Sardesai *et al.*, 1973). Recently observed increases in the incidence of multidrug-resistant *Salmonella* (especially *Salm. typhi*), now pose a threat to the clinical efficacy of Co-T in some regions (p. 841). Nevertheless, results of some early comparative trials in regions where Co-T resistance was uncommon suggested that Co-T is more effective in relieving toxemia in typhoid than chloramphenicol (Kamat, 1970; Sardesai *et al.*, 1973; Hassan *et al.*, 1975), while in others both drugs have been equally effective (Omer, 1975; Uwaydah *et al.*, 1975). Scragg and Rubidge (1971), Snyder *et al.* (1973, 1976) and Ramachandran *et al.* (1978) also examined the efficacy of Co-T and found it to be effective for enteric fevers, but that a proportion of patients (9.5% in the study by Ramachandran *et al.*, 1978) failed to respond to treatment. Butler *et al.* (1982) compared Co-T and chloramphenicol to treat patients with typhoid fever in a trial in Indonesia in 1976–1977; Co-T was more effective in sterilizing the blood, but in other respects the results of treatment were the same for both drugs. These authors reviewed publications on the use of Co-T in typhoid fever; in 31 reports involving 1184 patients there were 38 relapses (3.2%) and 13 deaths (1.1%). The time for defervescence was 3–9 days (median 5.1 days). In 17 of the 31 reports, treatment with Co-T was compared with treatment with chloramphenicol; seven reports found Co-T more favorable, in four they were equally effective, five reports found more prolonged fever with Co-T and one had a higher relapse rate and more prolonged bacteremia with Co-T. Small early studies suggested that chronic carriers of *Salm. typhi* may be less frequent after treatment of typhoid fever with Co-T than chloramphenicol (Geddes *et al.*, 1975; Jonsson, 1976; Ramachandran *et al.*, 1978). On the

basis of all these observations, chloramphenicol (p. 568) and now one of the quinolones (p. 1016) remain the drugs of choice for the treatment of typhoid fever due to sensitive strains, but Co-T is an effective alternative.

Co-T is also a valuable drug for the treatment of typhoid fever due to chloramphenicol-resistant strains. Gilman *et al.* (1975) in Mexico found that orally administered Co-T was equally effective to oral amoxycillin in the treatment of disease due to chloramphenicol-resistant strains, but Co-T produced a more rapid lysis of fever than amoxycillin in infections due to chloramphenicol-sensitive strains. Resistance to chloramphenicol is mediated by an R plasmid (p. 550) and this plasmid also confers resistance to sulfonamides, tetracyclines and streptomycin. It was suggested that probably because of this resistance to sulfonamides, Co-T could not exert synergism against choramphenicol-resistant strains of *Salm. typhi* and therefore trimethoprim alone may be effective for these infections (Gilman *et al.*, 1975). The findings in another, smaller clinical trial in Vietnam are at variance to this (Butler *et al.*, 1977). Co-T was compared with ampicillin for the treatment of patients with infections due to either chloramphenicol-resistant or -sensitive strains of *Salm. typhi*; each drug was given i.v. during the first 3–5 days and then, when improvement occurred, it was given orally. Both drugs were equally effective, but treatment failures were more common in patients with chloramphenicol-sensitive than -resistant strains. Butler *et al.* (1977) demonstrated *in vitro* synergy with Co-T in one-quarter of their chloramphenicol-resistant strains. The differing format of these two trials (Gilman *et al.*, 1975; Butler *et al.*, 1977) probably explains their contrasting results. Co-T is probably also effective for the treatment of typhoid fever caused by chloramphenicol-resistant strains which, in addition, are resistant to ampicillin and amoxicillin.

More recently, Co-T resistance among *Salm. typhi* strains has become so common in some countries such as India and Pakistan that Co-T may, in some regions, be no longer considered appropriate empiric therapy (Rowe *et al.*, 1990; Wallace and Yousif, 1990; Jesudasan and John, 1990; Rao *et al.*, 1993). Rao *et al.* (1993) described a 78% incidence of multidrug-resistance (ampicillin, chloramphenicol, Co-T) among 102 cases with *Salm. typhi* bacteremia in southern India. Seventy-six of these 80 patients did not show a clinical response to conventional antibiotics but were cured with fluroquinolones. Only four of the 80 patients treated with Co-T had an adequate clinical response and continued Co-T therapy. A review of *Salm. typhi* in the UK revealed 38% of patients who were infected in Pakistan had plasmid-mediated multidrug-resistant *Salm. typhi*. (Rowe *et al.*, 1990). These authors suggested that ciprofloxacin may be the best empiric therapy in such patients (p. 1016).

Co-T appears to be a satisfactory drug for the treatment of paratyphoid fever (Franzén *et al.*, 1972) and for septicemias due to other *Salmonella* spp., such as *Salm. typhimurium* (Jafary and Burke, 1970). In India, unlike *Salm. typhi*, most *Salm. paratyphi* strains are Co-T sensitive (Rao *et al.*, 1993). Co-T has been used with effect to treat a small number of patients with *Salmonella* meningitis (Levitz and Quintiliani, 1984). Although it may be useful for cases of meningitis which fail to respond to ampicillin or chloramphenicol (Murphy and Fernald, 1983), the newer cephalosporins, cefotaxime (p. 337) and ceftriaxone (p. 361), may be more appropriate alternative treatments for *Salmonella* meningitis. There is also some evidence that Co-T may eradicate the chronic *Salm. typhi* and *Salm. paratyphi* carrier states (Brodie *et al.*, 1970). Although Chan *et al.* (1973) found that a 2-week course of treatment was unsatisfactory for this purpose, results reported by Pichler *et al.* (1973) using a 3-month course of Co-T appeared promising. The efficacy of any antimicrobial agent in these carrier states is difficult to assess.

Like other antimicrobials, Co-T is probably of little value in *Salmonella* gastroenteritis (Franzén *et al.*, 1972; Kazemi *et al.*, 1973; Ekwall and Jonsson, 1984). Sanchez *et al.* (1993) compared Co-T (160/800 mg) and ciprofloxacin (500 mg) twice-daily for 5 days in a placebo-controlled double-blind trial of empiric therapy of uncomplicated *Salmonella* enteritis. Duration of diarrhea, abdominal pain, or vomiting and time to defervescence were not significantly different between the placebo and treatment groups. Nor was there any difference in the rate of clearance of salmonellae from stools.

10 Shigella infections

The use of Co-T in shigellosis causes a more rapid clinical recovery and shortens the period during which shigellae are excreted (Franzén *et al.*, 1972; Lexomboon *et al.*, 1972). Co-T is equally as effective as ampicillin (p. 122) for the treatment of shigellosis in infants, children, and adults, and it is also effective when the disease is caused by ampicillin-resistant strains (Nelson *et al.*, 1976a,b; Chang *et al.*, 1977; Barada and Guerrant, 1980; Nelson *et al.*, 1982; Yunus *et al.*, 1982). Nelson *et al.* (1982) reviewed the use of Co-T in shigellosis; there were comparative studies of 149 cases and non-comparative studies of 147 cases. Bacteriological and clinical success rates were 90% and Co-T compared favorably with alternate treatments. *Shigella* dysentery, especially that caused by *Sh. sonnei*, is usually a self-limiting disease and chemotherapy is not generally indicated. In contrast to its lack of value for *Salmonella* carriers (p. 868), Co-T is useful for the treatment of carriers of shigellae (Ekwall and Jonsson, 1984).

More recently, however, the widespread emergence of Co-T resistant *Shigella* species has resulted in a substantial diminution in the value of this therapeutic agent (Kagalwalla *et al.*, 1992; Bennish and Salam, 1992). Multiresistant *Shigella* species are most common (>65%) in developing countries such as Thailand (Taylor *et al.*, 1989; Lolekha *et al.*, 1991; Thisyakorn and Rienprayoon, 1992), Bangladesh (Bennish *et al.*, 1992), Bulgaria (Bratoeva and John, 1989), Saudia Arabia (Kagalwalla *et al.*, 1992) and Mexico (Parsonnett *et al.*, 1989). In these countries Co-T can no longer be presumed to be effective and other agents such as pivmecillinam or a fluoroquinolone have been recommended (Salam and Bennish, 1991; Bennish and Salam, 1992). *Shigella* spp. isolated in developed countries remain likely to be susceptible to Co-T and ampicillin. However, special consideration needs to be given to travellers and military personnel who have recently returned from the above listed regions since resistance is common in this patient group (Parsonnett *et al.*, 1989; Tauxe *et al.*, 1990; Heikkila *et al.*, 1990a; Salam and Bennish, 1991; Harnett *et al.*, 1991; Hyams *et al.*, 1991; Bennish and Salam, 1992).

11 Cholera

A 4- or 5-day course of Co-T appears to be as effective as a similar course of tetracycline for the eradication of *V. cholerae*, both classical and El Tor biotypes, from stools of patients with acute cholera (Gharagozloo *et al.*, 1970; Cash *et al.*, 1973). Treatment with Co-T was beneficial for children with severe gastroenteritis due to *V. cholerae* and *V. parahaemolyticus* (Uylangco *et al.*, 1984). Dupont *et al.* (1985) described a patient with a *V. cholerae* infection, who was treated with Co-T, in whom the bacterium persisted in his feces after 8 days treatment; the strain had become resistant due to acquisition of a plasmid which conferred resistance to ampicillin chloramphenicol, sulfonamide and trimethoprim. *V. cholerae* with plasmid-mediated resistance to Co-T has also been reported in an outbreak in Thailand (Tabtieng *et al.*, 1989). Rehydration is the most important measure in the treatment of this disease, but chemotherapy is also of proven value (p. 742).

12 Travelers' diarrhea

Many pathogens can be involved in travelers' diarrhea but enterotoxigenic *E. coli* have been isolated from 40–70% of cases (Gorbach, 1982). Dupont (1982a) demonstrated the efficacy of Co-T (160 mg trimethoprim/800 mg sulfamethoxazole) or trimethoprim (200 mg) given twice-daily for 5 days in a placebo-controlled trial. A reduction in number of unformed stools, and reduced abdominal pain and nausea was noted in *E. coli* diarrhea, shigellosis and diarrhea not associated with an enteropathogen. Subsequently further randomized double-blind trials in Mexico have suggested the most effective treatment regimen is a combination of Co-T and loperamide (4 mg loading dose, 2 mg after each loose stool to a maximum of 16 mg per day) for 3 days; where the Co-T is given as two double-strength tablets loading dose (total 320 mg trimethoprim) followed by one double-strength tablet (160 mg trimethoprim) twice daily for five doses (Ericsson *et al.*, 1990, 1992). Co-T has also been effective in the treatment of acute diarrhea in a Mexican pediatric population where cultures later revealed only 22% of the cases to be due to enterotoxigenic *E. coli* (Oberhelman *et al.*, 1987). However, various rates of expected Co-T efficacy in both treatment and prophylaxis are likely to depend on regional differences in the susceptibility of *E. coli* to this agent. Hyams *et al.* (1991) in their study of US military personnel with diarrhea in the 1991 Persian Gulf War, demonstrated that 39% of *E. coli* infections were Co-T-resistant, but that all isolates were susceptible to fluoroquinolones. In an interesting study, Lester *et al.* (1990) screened the stools of healthy young children (age <3 years) in Boston (USA), Caracas (Venezuala) and Qin Pu (China) and found significantly higher rates of trimethoprim-resistant strains of *E. coli* in Venezuala and China (61–64%) than Boston (3%). The average overall frequency of antibiotic-resistance in Caracas was 3.6-fold greater than in Boston, and that in Qin Pu was 5.3-fold greater. Similarly, Murray *et al.* (1990) has shown that travel, in its own right, to countries such as Mexico is associated with the acquisition of resistant *E. coli* even among healthy travelers who have not used antibiotics.

Both Co-T and to a lesser extent trimethoprim alone, are also highly effective for the prevention of travelers' diarrhea; Co-T in a dosage of 160 mg trimethoprim and 800 mg sulfamethoxazole once- or twice-daily or trimethoprim alone in a dosage of 200 mg daily was effective. Infections by enterotoxigenic *E. coli* and *Shigella* spp. strains were prevented. In Co-T-treated subjects, rashes occurred in 2% and 14% with the once- or twice-daily regimens, respectively, and in 3% of those taking trimethoprim alone (DuPont *et al.*, 1982b, 1983). In the first of these trials, fecal flora of the subjects developed multiple antibiotic-resistance. Co-T in a dosage of 160 mg trimethoprim and 800 mg sulfamethoxazole once-daily has been advocated for the prevention of travelers' diarrhea, but the need for prevention must be balanced against the risks of rashes and severe reactions to Co-T (DuPont *et al.*, 1983). One disadvantage of Co-T for the treatment or prevention of travelers' diarrhea is that it is not active against *Campylobacter* spp. (p. 838). The prevention and treatment of travelers' diarrhea has been reviewed by DuPont and Ericsson (1993).

13 Cyclospora infections

Cyclospora cayetanensis is a coccidian, previously referred to as cyanobacteria or coccidian-like bodies (CLBs), that causes watery diarrhea in both developed and developing countries, but has become particularly notable as a cause of diarrhea in HIV-infected patients. It is presumed to be water-borne and tends to cause diarrhea predominantly in the summer months, which is generally self-limiting in immunocompetent hosts (Wurtz, 1994; Soave and Johnson, 1995). Wurtz *et al.* (1993) and Madico *et al.* (1993) first reported anecdotal success with Co-T therapy. Subsequently Hoge *et al.* (1995) have demonstrated in a plabeo-controlled, double-blind trial in travelers and foreign residents with cyclospora infections in Nepal the efficacy of Co-T. A regimen of 160/800 mg Co-T twice-daily for 7 days resulted in fecal clearance of cyclospora in 29% (Co-T) versus 0% (placebo) after 3 days (p=0.016); while after 7 days therapy 94% Co-T-treated patients had cleared their stools versus 12% of placebo recipients (p<0.0001). Eradication of the pathogen correlated with clinical efficacy and no relapse among Co-T-treated patients was noted in those followed for an additional 7 days. Among HIV-infected patients, however, the rate of relapse appears to be relatively high. Pape *et al.* (1994) noted a high incidence of cyclospora infection among HIV-infected Haitians with diarrhea – clinically their symptoms were indistinguishable from those seen in patients with isosporiasis or cryptosporidiosis. Since both *Cyclospora* and *Cryptosporidia* are acid-fast staining and *Cryptosporidia* do not respond to Co-T (unlike *Isospora*), care must be taken to differentiate these two pathogens (Madico *et al.*, 1993; Soave and Johnson, 1995). Among the 43 patients treated with Co-T 160/800 mg four times daily for 10 days, diarrhea ceased and stool examination was negative within 2.5 days after starting therapy. Recurrent symptomatic cyclosporiasis developed in 12 of 28 patients (43%) followed for ≥1 month, but all responded to a further course of Co-T. Subsequent secondary prophylaxis with Co-T 160/800 mg three times per week was associated with only one recurrence after 7 months. Sifuentes-Osornio *et al.* (1995) have also described the clinical efficacy of Co-T therapy for cyclosporiasis in HIV- and non-HIV-infected patients, but in Mexico City. They noted two HIV-infected patients with acalculous cholecystitis, probably due to *Cyclospora*, which responded to Co-T.

14 Isospora belli infection (coccidiosis)

Infection with the protozoan *Isospora belli* may cause fever, diarrhea and colicky abdominal pain, and is usually self-limited in an immunocompetent host. Enteric infection with *I. belli* is common in patients with AIDS, particularly in some parts of the USA, Latin America, and the Caribbean, and can cause severe diarrhea (De Hovitz *et al.*, 1986; Sorvillo *et al.*, 1990). Treatment with Co-T, one double-strength tablet (160 mg trimethoprim component) four times daily for 10 days, then twice-daily for 3 weeks is effective, but recurrences occur in 50% of cases (Whiteside *et al.*, 1984; De Hovitz *et al.*, 1986). Subsequently Pope *et al.* (1989) have shown that following a 10-day treatment course, prophylaxis with one double-strength tablet three times per week was as effective as prophylaxis with sulfadoxine 500 mg/pyrimethamine 25 mg weekly – both regimens proving superior to placebo.

15 Other bowel infections

In general, it is doubtful whether antibiotics are necessary for the treatment of childhood gastroenteritis in developed countries. In developing countries however, where childhood gastroenteritis is a major cause of mortality, there may be some justification. *Yersinia enterocolitica* is a cause of gastroenteritis, particularly in children, and it is sensitive to trimethoprim (p. 837). In a small placebo-controlled trial, Co-T did not show any benefit in shortening the clinical or bacteriological course of *Y. enterocolitica* gastroenteritis in children (Pai *et al.*, 1984). *Aeromonas* spp. are another cause of gastroenteritis in young children; in most cases the disease is mild and of short duration, but in some cases the clinical course may be severe or protracted. In adults the course tends to be more chronic in nature (Holmberg *et al.*, 1986). These organisms are sensitive to trimethoprim (also to tetracycline, chloramphenicol, third-generation cephalosporins, nitrofurantoin and aminoglycosides) and experience suggests that Co-T is probably of value in severe cases (Gracey *et al.*, 1982; Palfreeman *et al.*, 1983; Kipperman *et al.*, 1984; Holmberg *et al.*, 1986).

16 Brucellosis

Co-T is useful in the treatment of brucellosis (Lal *et al.*, 1970; Farid *et al.*, 1970; Hassan *et al.*, 1971; Daikos *et al.*, 1973), particularly when used in combination with other agents such as tetracycline, rifampicin or streptomycin (McLean *et al.*, 1992; Hall, 1990; Khuri-Bulos *et al.*, 1993; Montejo *et al.*, 1993). Co-T monotherapy has been associated with an unacceptable (30–47%) relapse rate (Ariza *et al.*, 1985; Lubani *et al.*, 1989), although Daikos *et al.* (1973) suggested that the use of high doses (480 mg trimethoprim/2400 mg sulfamethoxazole daily) for a prolonged period (at least 2 months) produced good results. Despite the fact that the optimal treatment regimen for brucellosis is undecided, most authors, including Hall (1990) who recently reviewed the treatment of brucellosis, recommend a combination of Co-T with other agents. Co-T, in doses of 5–10 mg trimethoprim component per kg per day, in combination with rifampicin 15 mg per kg per day for 45 days is recommended for the treatment of acute brucellosis in children younger than 8 years of age (Hall, 1990). Good results were obtained with this combination in two large studies of pediatric brucellosis (Lubani *et al.*, 1989; al-Eissa *et al.*, 1990). Similarly, Khuri-Bulos *et al.* (1993) reported excellent results in childhood brucellosis with the combination of CoT + rifampicin for 6 weeks, but they used a Co-T dose of 10–12 mg per kg per day (trimethoprim component) – relapse after 6 months was noted in only four of 113 children, all of whom responded to repeat therapy with the same agents. Lubani *et al.* (1989) noted comparable results between the combinations of oral rifampicin plus oxytetracycline, rifampicin plus Co-T and oxytetracycline plus Co-T; with relapse rates of 4–8% in patients treated for 3–5 weeks and no relapses after 8 weeks treatment. Combination with streptomycin or gentamicin was associated with few relapses irrespective of duration of treatment. Montejo *et al.* (1993) found little difference in outcome between a variety of treatment regimens studied in a prospective, open, randomized study from 1980 to 1987. However, due to the trial design, conclusions are difficult to draw, especially since one-to-one comparisons between individual treatment groups are complicated by the relatively small number of patients in each group.

Co-T (5 mg trimethoprim component per kg per day) in combination with rifampicin (900 mg per day) for 3 months (± short course corticosteroids) is recommended for the treatment of *Brucella* meningoencephalitis, particularly since good CSF levels can be achieved with oral administration (Hall, 1990). Other authors have reported good results with Co-T plus doxycycline (Roldan *et al.*, 1988; Al-Orainey *et al.*, 1987), but, McLean *et al.* (1992) after reviewing 18 cases of neurobrucellosis, recommended a four-drug regimen of streptomycin, tetracycline, rifampicin and Co-T.

Brucella endocarditis is a rare complication of brucellosis that is associated with a high mortality, possibly because of its apparent predilection for involvement of the aortic valve with common sequelae of myocardial abscess formation (Jacobs *et al.*, 1990). A four-drug combination of Co-T, rifampicin, doxycycline and streptomycin for 8–12 weeks is recommended, but concomitant valve replacement is generally (87%) necessary (Hall, 1990; Jacobs, 1990).

17 Nocardiosis

Nocardia species that are potentially pathogenic for man include *N. asteroides*, *N. farcinica*, *N. brasiliensis*, *N. caviae*, *N. transvalensis* and *N. otitidiscaviarum*; although the first three are the most frequent pathogens (Arduino *et al.*, 1993; Schiff *et al.*, 1993; Farina *et al.*, 1995). Nocardiosis can be an acute, subacute or chronic suppurative infection that ranges from mild cutaneous or pulmonary disease to aggressive and often fatal dissemination, with the clinical presentation and course depending upon the degree of host immune suppression. Pulmonary disease and blood-borne spread to other organs, particularly the central nervous system, are the major clinical manifestations of *N. asteroides* infection. *Nocardia farcinica* is notable for its propensity to cause serious systemic infection in both normal and immunocompromised patients and its greater resistance to many antibacterial agents (Schiff *et al.*, 1993). *Nocardia brasiliensis* more frequently causes infections of the skin and soft tissues such as a mycetoma. Mycetomas are chronic lesions often on the lower extremities with draining sinuses exuding sulfur granules (Smego *et al.*, 1984; Georghiou and Blacklock, 1992). *Nocardia transvalensis*, a rare *Nocardia* species, causes primary pulmonary and disseminated disease mainly in immunosuppressed patients and generally displays greater antimicrobial resistance than other *Nocardia* species, but successful therapy with Co-T has been reported (McNeil *et al.*, 1992; Weinberger *et al.*, 1995).

For many years sulfonamides (sometimes combined with other drugs) were considered the mainstay of treatment for nocardiosis, but the mortality and morbidity of this infection remained unacceptably high (Wallace *et al.*, 1982a). There have now been numerous reports of successful use of Co-T in this disease (Baikie *et al.*, 1970; Pavillard, 1973; Wallace *et al.*, 1982a; Smego *et al.*, 1983, 1984; Berkey and Bodey, 1989; Forbes *et al.*, 1990; McNeil *et al.*, 1992). Maderazo and Quintiliani (1974) described a patient who developed a brain abscess due to *N. asteroides* during therapy with ampicillin and either sulfadiazine or sulfisoxazole for pulmonary nocardiosis. The pulmonary disease responded to this therapy, but the cerebral lesion required surgical excision and a 3-month course of Co-T. Poor penetration of ampicillin and sulfisoxazole into the CSF was demonstrated, but good concentrations of both trimethoprim and sulfamethoxazole were found in brain tissue (p. 851). In addition, these drugs acted synergistically *in vitro* against the organism involved. *In vitro* studies suggest that higher doses of trimethoprim than those available in Co-T are necessary to obtain synergism against this organism, but these higher ratios may be attained in the tissues with the usual treatment (p. 837).

Many authors now consider Co-T to be the drug of choice for nocardiasis (Wallace *et al.*, 1982a; Smego *et al.*, 1983; Smego *et al.*, 1984; Filice and Simpson, 1984; Chapman and Wilson, 1990; Schiff *et al.*, 1993). Experience with 119 cases treated with Co-T was recorded by Smego *et al.* (1983); of 62 cases of systemic nocardiosis, improvement was achieved in 81% and the overall survival rate for patients with disseminated nocardiosis, with or without central nervous system involvement, was 63%. Relapses were common and clinical outcome was related to the duration of therapy. Clinical experience with mycetomas due to *N. brasiliensis* has been excellent, but treatment with Co-T for up to 3 years may be required (Wallace *et al.*, 1982a). It has not been established whether Co-T therapy is superior to treatment with sulfonamides. The general opinion is that sulfonamides may still be useful for cutaneous and pulmonary disease due to *N. brasiliensis*. However, for disseminated and central nervous system infections, Co-T should be used, perhaps combined with other antibiotics to which the organism is susceptible (Wallace *et al.*, 1982a; Smego *et al.*, 1983; 1984). Even though Co-T has now superseded sulfonamides for this disease, resistant strains occasionally occur (Cockerill *et al.*, 1984). Sensitivity tests should always be performed on isolates, plus drug level monitoring in the serum and CSF in serious infections (Smego *et al.*, 1983). Forbes *et al.* (1990), however, noted a good clinical response to Co-T in a patient post-liver transplantion, despite *in vitro* evidence of reduced Co-T susceptibility. Therapy with Co-T produced variable results when used as monotherapy for *N. transvalensis*, but probably remains the first-line agent for this rare infection (McNeil *et al.*, 1992).

A number of Co-T failures have been described, however, particularly in the immunocompromised. Overkamp *et al.* (1992) reported failure of Co-T therapy for the treatment of an *N. asteroides* brain abscess due to a Co-T-sensitive strain in an immunocompromised patient who was treated with Co-T (640 mg trimethoprim component) daily for 2 weeks. King *et al.* (1993) reported a case of cerebral nocardiosis in a renal transplant recipient after the patient had received Co-T (640 mg trimethoprim component) daily for 6 months. The patient responded to re-introduction of the same dose of Co-T. Arduino *et al.* (1993) described nine cases of nocardiosis among renal transplant recipients receiving cyclosporine and prednisolone, four of whom (one cerebral abscess, three pulmonary abscess) were treated with Co-T alone – although the doses were not stated.

Clinical outcome in nocardiosis appears to be related to both Co-T dosage and the duration of therapy. Smego *et al.* (1983) recommends treatment for 3–12 months depending on disease severity and the patient's immune status, with possible indefinite low-dose prophylaxis after completion of successful full-dose therapy, particularly in the immunocompromised. There are no definite guidelines for treatment dosage, however, although 640 mg (trimethoprim component) daily (i.e. four double-strength tablets) has been commonly used for serious infections. Some authors argue for significantly higher Co-T dosages in immunocompromised patients. Wallace *et al.* (1982a) reported the use of 5 mg per kg per day (range 5–10 mg per kg per day; trimethoprim component) for cutaneous nocardiosis and 8 mg per kg per day or higher (range: 4–26 mg per kg per day) for more serious disease such as pulmonary or brain abscesses. Chapman and Wilson (1990) recently summarized the presentation and management of nocardiosis in transplant recipients, however the doses of Co-T used were not described – although reversible nephrotoxicity associated with co-administration of cyclosporine and Co-T was noted. Sanford (1993) recommends 480 mg (trimethoprim component) four times daily for serious *N. asteroides* disease, although this is unreferenced.

18 Plague

Although Co-T is generally not considered a first-line agent for this disease, some studies have suggested that a 5 to 17-day course of Co-T may be effective for the treatment of bubonic plague (Ai et al., 1973; Butler et al., 1974). Subsequently, a small trial was carried out in Vietnam in 1975 in which streptomycin and Co-T treatments for Y. pestis infections were compared. Streptomycin was given i.m. in a dosage of 0.5–1.0 g (depending on the patient's weight) twice-daily for 10 days and Co-T (160 mg trimethoprim, 800 mg sulfamethoxazole, and half this dose for children) was given i.v. for 3–5 days, then orally in the same dose to complete a 10-day course. Patients treated with streptomycin had a shorter median duration of fever and less complications than those treated by Co-T (Butler et al., 1976).

19 Melioidosis

Following early case reports that suggested Co-T was effective against B. pseudomallei (John, 1976; De Buse et al., 1975; Morrison et al., 1979; Fuller et al., 1978), multidrug combinations that include Co-T are now considered to represent conventional therapy by some authors (Shaefer et al., 1983; Leelarasamee and Bovornkitti, 1989; Sookpranee et al., 1992; Chaowagul et al., 1993); although cases of successful monotherapy with Co-T continue to be reported (Worthington and McEniry, 1990). Sookpranee et al. (1992) compared ceftazidime plus Co-T with the 'conventional' therapy of combination chloramphenicol, doxycycline and Co-T, in a prospective, randomized trial of 64 patients in North-Eastern Thailand. Results suggested that the ceftazidime/Co-T combination was more effective in treating severe meliodosis, especially in patients presenting with disseminated septicemic disease; although both regimens were similar in their efficacy in clearing bacteremia within 24 hours (96–97%). All patients in both groups who survived after day 7 were treated with oral doxycycline and/or Co-T for at least 3–6 months; with no relapses during the 9- to 22-month follow-up period.

20 Miscellaneous bacterial infections

Co-T is useful for chemoprophylaxis in infants who have come in contact with whooping cough (Arneil and McAllister, 1977). Co-T and erythromycin were equally effective in eradicating B. pertussis from the nasopharynx of 22 children (Henry et al., 1981). It has also been used with clinical benefit in Whipple's disease (Haeney and Ross, 1978). Because of the in vitro effectiveness of Co-T against susceptible genera of bacteria from burn wounds, it was suggested that it may have potential as a topical agent in burns (Holder, 1981). Oral Co-T, like tetracycline (p. 749), erythromycin (p. 621) and clindamycin (p. 598), has been used successfully in the treatment of acne (Eady et al., 1982). In Australia, Co-T has been used with effect to treat trachoma (Leading article, 1982), but a tetracycline is usually preferred (p. 746).

Co-T has been used with variable efficacy in the treatment of cat-scratch disease (Bogue et al., 1989; Margileth, 1992; Collipp, 1992). Margileth (1992) retrospectively reviewed the management and outcome of 268 patients with cat-scratch disease and found only four drugs to be effective – rifampicin 87%, ciprofloxacin 84%, Co-T (6–8 mg trimethoprim component/kg, two or three times daily for 7 days) 58% and gentamicin 73% effective. In most patients with cat-scratch disease, however, no therapy was required.

21 Mycobacterial diseases

Mycobacterium marinum may be susceptible to Co-T and a number of authors have reported reasonable clinical efficacy (Barrow and Hewitt, 1971; Kelly, 1976; Hugh and Coleman 1981; Iredell et al., 1992). Iredell et al. (1992) reviewed the features of 29 M. marinum infections in Queensland and found that chemotherapy alone was often adequate, especially with deep tissue involvement such as tenosynovitis and arthritis, which was a more common presentation (48%) in this series than previous reports. Monotherapy with Co-T was effective in seven of nine cases, while various combinations of rifampicin, ethambutol and tetracyclines were of similar efficacy.

Serious disease with M. fortuitum has been cured with Co-T. A 16-year-old with M. fortuitum meningitis recovered with a combination of Co-T and isoniazid therapy and surgical removal of an implicated foreign body (Santamaria-Jáuregui et al., 1984). Pacht (1990) successfully treated a 37-year-old male with M. fortuitum lung abscess with a 1-year course of Co-T.

A 64-year-old male with myelodysplastic syndrome and disseminated infection with M. avium complex was improved by therapy with Co-T which was commenced for presumptive (but later disproven) nocardial infection (Chang and Goetz, 1992).

22 Malaria

Trimethoprim has sometimes been used in place of pyrimethamine in combination with quinine and a long-acting sulfonamide to provide triple-drug treatment for chloroquine-resistant falciparum malaria. Trimethoprim in combination with a long-acting sulfonamide alone has also been used successfully for this purpose (Martin and Arnold, 1968). In a comparative trial, Lal (1982) showed that oral Co-T was as effective as oral chloroquine for the treatment of vivax malaria in children, but chloroquine cleared parasitemia faster. The use of Co-T was reported to delay the diagnosis of malaria in two patients (Williams *et al.*, 1982). This can also occur with other antibiotics, such as tetracyclines or clindamycin, which have an effect on malarial parasites. Although a combination of the long-acting sulfonamide, sulfadoxine, and pyrimethamine was once considered optimal for treatment and chemoprophylaxis of chloroquine-resistant falciparum malaria (p. 824), resistance has now increased so markedly in some areas as to warrant the use of other agents such as mefloquine.

23 Toxoplasmosis

Mossner (1969) suggested that Co-T may be effective in the treatment of human toxoplasmosis. There have been a number of anecdotal reports of the efficacy of Co-T in this disease (Norrby *et al.*, 1975; Salter, 1982). Following a retrospective study, Carr *et al.* (1992a) have suggested that low-dose Co-T (one double-strength tablet twice-daily, 2 days per week) given as prophylaxis against *P. carinii* pneumonia in patients with HIV infection is also effective prophylaxis against toxoplasmic encephalitis. Sixty patients given Co-T were compared with 95 patients who received pentamidine (78 aerosolized, 17 intravenous). No patient in the Co-T-treated group and no patient who was seronegative for antibodies to *T. gondii* developed toxoplasmic encephalitis; compared with 12 of 36 seropositive patients in the pentamidine group (p=0.004). Although previously some authors have been cautious in espousing Co-T prophylaxis for toxoplasmic encephalitis, recent recommendations suggest that a regimen of either Co-T or dapsone + pyrimethamine is worthwhile for HIV-infected patients who are seropositive for IgG to *T. gondii* and have a CD4 lymphocyte count <100 per mm^3 (Beaman *et al.* 1992; Richards *et al.*, 1995). Of interest is the report by Zylberberg *et al.* (1995) in which Co-T prophylaxis for *P. carinii* appeared to mask the presence of disseminated toxoplasmosis, which was identified by polymerase chain reaction (PCR) on blood and bronchoalveolar lavage fluid.

Reports on the use of trimethoprim-sulfonamide combinations in animals have been conflicting and these results may not be applicable to humans. In mice, trimethoprim seems to potentiate the action of sulfonamides (Feldman, 1973b; Seah, 1975; Grossman *et al.*, 1978; Nguyen *et al.*, 1978). Grossman and Remington (1979) demonstrated synergy between trimethoprim and sulfamethoxazole against *T. gondii in vitro*, but results of *in vivo* studies in mice were inferior to those obtained by pyrimethamine and sulfadiazine. In squirrel monkeys, sulfonamides alone or in combination with pyrimethamine or trimethoprim were more effective than spiramycin (pp. 633, 823) for toxoplasmosis (Harper *et al.*, 1985). There is currently insufficient evidence to recommend Co-T as an alternative to treatment with a sulfonamide and pyrimethamine (p. 913) for toxoplasmosis.

24 Pneumocystis carinii pneumonia

Pneumocystis carinii was first recognized in 1909 and is thought to initially infect humans in early childhood by the respiratory route (Russell, 1981; Leading article, 1985; Masur, 1992). It was initially presumed to be a protozoan, but more recent studies have shown it to share nucleic acid and structural features with both protozoa and fungi – hence its precise taxonomy remains uncertain (Edman *et al.*, 1988; Stringer *et al*, 1989; Bartlett and Smith, 1991; Masur, 1992). Lung infection with *P. carinii* was originally identified in premature and debilitated infants and now occurs most frequently in the setting of significant immune suppression or deficiency. *Pneumocystis carinii* pneumonia is one of the most common opportunistic infection in patients infected with HIV. Untreated *P. carinii* pneumonia has a 50% mortality in premature or malnourished infants and a 100% mortality in those with impaired immunity (Russell, 1981; Hughes, 1982). *Pneumocystis carinii* pneumonia has been reviewed by Masur (1992).

The investigation of various drugs with activity against *Pneumocystis* was initially limited by the difficulty of cultivating the organism *in vitro* – in fact human *P. carinii* has never been successfully cultured (Bartlett and Smith, 1991; Masur, 1992). Following the reported success of pyrimethamine (p. 916) plus sulfadiazine in a few patients with *P. carinii* pneumonitis, Hughes *et al.* (1974) showed that Co-T was as effective as pentamidine in the treatment of this pneumonitis in the cortisone-treated rat model; also, when given prophylactically, Co-T prevented infection. Hughes *et al.* (1975b) then demonstrated that Co-T was effective treatment for *P. carinii* pneumonitis occurring in children with leukemia. A dose of 20 mg trimethoprim and 100 mg sulfamethoxazole per kg body weight per day was effective and associated with minimal side-effects.

This efficacy was confirmed by Lau and Young (1976) in adults. Subsequently Hughes and colleagues have further documented the therapeutic and prophylactic potential of Co-T in both corticosteroid-treated rats and humans (adults and children) outside the setting of HIV infection (Hughes, 1976, 1977, 1982; Hughes *et al.*, 1978, 1987). Intravenous Co-T is recommended for critically ill patients since the absorption of oral Co-T in these circumstances can be unreliable (Lau and Young, 1976; Miser *et al.*, 1977). The dose and duration of Co-T treatment was initially chosen rather arbitrarily, although Winston *et al.* (1980) aimed to maintain serum trimethoprim and sulfamethoxazole levels above 5 μg per ml and 100 μg per ml, respectively, at 1.5 h post-i.v. dose. Most authors recommend 15–20 μg trimethoprim and 75–100 μg sulfamethoxazole per kg per day, some using the lower dose if administering Co-T i.v. (Winston *et al.*, 1980; Sattler and Remington, 1981; Davey and Masur, 1990; Masur, 1992). Although the monitoring of serum drug levels was once emphasized, the pharmacokinetics of Co-T are now considered so predictable that this is no longer common practice and is only undertaken in special circumstances such as in the setting of significant gastrointestinal or renal dysfunction (Masur, 1992).

Many of the recent studies of Co-T activity have been in AIDS-associated *P. carinii* pneumonia, but in most instances these results appear to also be applicable to non-AIDS-associated *P. carinii* pneumonia; although the duration of therapy and likelihood of relapse is generally greater in AIDS patients. Co-T is the treatment of choice for all patients with *P. carinii* pneumonia who can tolerate it as it appears to be at least as effective as any other agent. It has similar efficacy to parenteral pentamidine isoethionate (p. 876) in the treatment of *P. carinii* pneumonia in patients with non-AIDS malignancies, but Co-T has a lower incidence of serious side-effects, making it the treatment of choice in these patients (Hughes *et al.*, 1978). Knowledge regarding other anti-*P. carinii* pneumonia therapies, however, is based upon trials in AIDS patients.

Similarly, in AIDS-associated *P. carinii* pneumonia, Co-T and pentamidine probably have at least similar efficacies (Klein *et al.*, 1992), although Co-T is preferable to pentamidine. Sattler *et al.* (1988) emphasized this preference, suggesting that there was improved survival, without mechanical support, in AIDS patients treated with Co-T (86%) versus those treated with pentamidine. This finding was not confirmed by Klein *et al.* (1992), who found the two treatments equally effective. The appropriate duration of treatment with Co-T has not been conclusively established, but most clinicians treat non-AIDS *P. carinii* pneumonia for 14 days and AIDS-associated *P. carinii* pneumonia for 21 days – although there are no formal clinical data to support an improvement in efficacy with the longer therapy (Davey and Masur, 1990).

The overal response rate to either Co-T or pentamidine in the treatment of initial episodes of AIDS-associated *P. carinii* pneumonia is generally 60–80% (Masur and Kovacs, 1988; Kovacs and Masur, 1988; Glatt and Chirgwin, 1990). The response rate is somewhat variable, however. First episides of AIDS-associated *P. carinii* pneumonia, especially in patients with mild disease (initial pre-treatment A-a gradient <30 mmHg, or P_aO_2 >70 mmHg, breathing room air) have a response rate of 80–95%, but the response rate is usually 60–80% if the *P. carinii* pneumonia is not HIV-related (Kovacs *et al.*, 1984; Dummer, 1990). Second and subsequent episodes of AIDS-associated *P. carinii* pneumonia have a 60% survival rate (Hughes *et al.*, 1978; Kovacs *et al.*, 1984; Wharton *et al.*, 1986; Leoung *et al.*, 1986; Sattler *et al.*, 1988; Brenner *et al.*, 1987; Garay and Greene, 1989; Dummer, 1990). While most patients improve progressively with Co-T therapy, a transient clinical and radiological worsening is seen in some patients, particularly those with AIDS-associated *P. carinii* pneumonia, during the first 3–5 days of treatment regardless of which agent is used (Montaner *et al.*, 1990; Davey and Masur, 1990). It is hypothesized that this is due to an inflammatory response to the drug-induced death of *Pneumocystis* organisms. In these patients an improvement is generally seen by day 7–10 of therapy. Thus many authors do not consider changing therapeutic agents prior to day 7 of treament (Fischl, 1988; Davey and Masur, 1990). Among patients who fail to respond to initial Co-T or pentamidine therapy, a change to the alternative agent will also be ineffective in 50–90% of cases. If, however, the change in therapy is due to side-effects rather than treatment failure, efficacy remains about 60–80% (Murray *et al.*, 1984; Wolfsy, 1987; Klein *et al.*, 1992). AIDS- and non-AIDS-associated *P. carinii* pneumonia have similar 90-day survival rates, but relapses occur more frequently (20–40%) in AIDS-associated *P. carinii* pneumonia and the second episode carries a higher mortality than the initial bout (Haverkos *et al.*, 1984; Rainer *et al.*, 1987).

Therapy with either Co-T or pentamidine is associated with a significantly higher incidence of side-effects among patients with HIV-associated *P. carinii* pneumonia than in other patients –

greater than 60% in most series (range: 20–85%) (Glatt and Chirgwin, 1990; Davey and Masur, 1990). These generally occur during the 2nd week of treatment, or later. The major side-effects of Co-T (p. 853) are mild-to-severe rash (~50% cases), leukopenia (30–66% cases; which is generally not folinic acid responsive), thrombocytopenia, nausea, vomiting and azotemia. Toxicity may be related to the hydroxylamine metabolite of sulfamethoxazole, but this is controversial (van der Ven et al., 1991; Pozniak et al., 1991). Also controversial is whether the incidence of side-effects is less frequent if serum trimethoprim levels are maintained at <5–$8\,\mu g$ per ml and serum sulfamethoxazole levels at <100–$150\,\mu g$ per ml (Sattler et al., 1988). Generally, adverse reactions are less frequent when lower doses of Co-T are used, such as are given for P. carinii pneumonia prophylaxis (Masur, 1992). Mild toxicity is not necessarily an indication to stop Co-T therapy or avoid Co-T prophylaxis, since some patients can be 'treated through', although this must be done with caution (Gibbons and Lindiver, 1985; Wolfsy, 1987; Sattler et al., 1988; Shafer et al., 1989; Hardy et al., 1992). Furthermore, Hardy et al. (1992) in a prospective trial of Co-T for secondary prophylaxis of P. carinii pneumonia found adverse reactions to Co-T were no more severe or frequent among patients with a history of mild to moderate adverse reactions to Co-T than among patients with no history of such events. Co-T desensitization has been undertaken successfully and is reviewed on p. 854.

Adjunctive folinic acid therapy with Co-T does not alter the frequency of dose-limiting toxicity or time to the occurrence of toxicity (Safrin et al., 1994; Bozzette et al., 1995b). Although the incidence of neutropenia is lower in folinic acid-treated patients (p=0.03), the time to develop this was similar to that noted for placebo-treated group. Notably, however, folinic acid was associated with a higher rate of therapeutic failure (15% vs 0%; p=0.01) and death (11% vs 0%; p=0.06) than placebo. Time to therapeutic failure was shorter (p=0.005) and the probability of death greater (p=0.02) in patients receiving folinic acid, even when adjusted for other relevant variables such as CD4 count and P. carinii pneumonia severity (Safrin et al., 1994).

Parenteral pentamidine isothionate, as noted earlier, is a useful alternative to Co-T for the treatment of P. carinii pneumonia, but is associated with frequent and severe adverse reactions in both patients with, and without, HIV infection (Hughes et al., 1978; Leading article, 1985; Sattler et al., 1988; Conte, 1991). Adverse reactions may be severe and include nephrotoxicity (25–64% cases mild; 3% severe), pancreatitis, hypotension, hypoglycemia (20% cases), hyperglycemia and leukopenia (Drake et al., 1985; Wharton et al., 1986; Sattler et al., 1988). Hypoglycemia is probably due to pancreatic beta-islet cell cytolysis with subsequent hyperinsulinemia (Wharton et al., 1986; Sattler et al., 1988); while hyperglycemia may occur days to weeks after therapy due to permanent islet cell destruction (Drake et al., 1985; Masur, 1992). There appears to be no cross-toxicity for neutropenia between pentamidine and Co-T. Administration of pentamidine i.m. has been abandoned due to localized pain and the development of sterile abscesses. Pentamidine is generally given at a dose of 4 mg per kg by slow i.v. infusion in 100 ml 5% dextrose over 60–90 min.

Alternate therapies for the treatment of P. carinii pneumonia are listed in Table II.3, with the vast majority of studies being conducted in AIDS-associated P. carinii pneumonia. Aerosolized pentamidine may be effective in mild disease but its efficacy, which is less than that of Co-T or parenteral pentamidine, is dependent on the use of a nebulizer ('Respirgard II' or 'Fisoneb') which produces particle sizes of 2–3 μm, such that there is adequate delivery of drug to the lower respiratory tract. Toxicity is less than parenteral pentamidine but relapse rates appear to be high (Montgomery et al., 1987, 1995; Conte et al., 1990; Masur,1992). In a prospective, blinded comparison of 600 mg per day aerosolized pentamidine versus Co-T 15 mg per kg per day (trimethoprim component) for mild to moderate P. carinii pneumonia, a significantly higher (p=0.002) proportion of patients treated with aerosolized pentamidine needed to have their therapy changed due to lack of efficacy compared with Co-T, and the PaO$_2$ improved faster in Co-T-treated patients. However, aerosolized pentamidine was discontinued less often than Co-T because of side-effects (9.4% vs 40%, p <0.001) (Montgomery et al., 1995).

The combination of trimethoprim (15–20 mg per kg per day) and dapsone 100 mg per day is better tolerated and has fewer side-effects than Co-T, and is equally effective for mild-to-moderate first episodes of P. carinii pneumonia (Leoung et al., 1986; Medina et al., 1990). Dapsone (100 mg per day) alone for 21 days, however, appears to be less effective than either standard therapy or trimethoprim-dapsone (Mills et al., 1988). Clindamycin-primaquine combination is effective for mild-to-moderate P. carinii pneumonia, but skin rashes and nausea are reasonably common, and are probably due to the clindamycin (Toma et al., 1989; Ruf and Pohle, 1989; Noskin et al., 1992; Toma et al., 1993). Primaquine can cause methemoglobinuria and hemolysis. Nevertheless, Toma et al. (1993) found no significant difference between clindamycin/primaquine and Co-T in terms of outcome, duration of survival, or incidence or severity of adverse reactions (although there was a trend toward less toxicity with the clindamycin/primaquine combination) in the treament of AIDS-associated *P. carinii* pneumonia. Black *et al.* (1994) treated mild to moderate *P. carinii* pneumonia with clindamycin (900 mg i.v. three times daily, 450 mg orally four times daily or 600 mg three times daily) + primaquine 30 mg daily for a total of 21 days. Response was noted in 55 of 60 (92%) patients, with 46 of 60 (77%) patients completing the full course of therapy. Entirely oral therapy was as effective as initial therapy with i.v. clindamycin. Atovaquone (566C80), a new hydroxynaphthoquinone, is significantly less effective than Co-T for mild to moderate *P. carinii* pneumonia, but has significantly fewer treatment-limiting side-effects (Falloon *et al.*, 1991; Hughes *et al.*, 1993, 1995). The clinical role of atovaquone has been reviewed (Spencer and Goa, 1995). The role of trimethoprim-dapsone, clindamycin-primaquine and atovaquone remains to be clarified, but currently they appear to have a place in the treatment of mild to moderate *P. carinii* pneumonia, especially as alternatives in patients who are intolerant of sulfa drugs.

Other agents which have been used in the treatment of AIDS-associated *P. carinii* pneumonia include trimetrexate (Allegra *et al.*, 1987), difluoromethylornithine [DFMO, eflonithine] (Golden *et al.*, 1984; Paulson *et al.*, 1992) and piritrexim (Masur, 1992). Trimetrexate (p. 878) may have a role in 'salvage therapy' of patients who have failed, or are intolerant, of other agents, but it appears to have a high (60%) relapse rate when used alone (Allegra *et al.*, 1987). In a double-blind study comparing trimetrexate with Co-T for moderate to severe *P. carinii* pneumonia in patients with AIDS, Co-T was more effective: by day 21, failure rates were 20% (Co-T) versus 38% (trimetrexate) (p=0.008); but the cumulative incidence of serious and treatment-terminating side-effects was significantly less with trimetrexate (p<0.001) (Sattler *et al.*, 1994). The therapeutic role of trimetrexate has been reviewed by Fulton *et al.* (1995).

Corticosteroids appear to be useful as early adjunctive therapy in AIDS-associated *P. carinii* pneumonia, to reduce or prevent the early decline in oxygenation commonly seen with the commencement of definitive therapy (Bozzette *et al.*, 1990; Gagnon *et al.*, 1990; Montaner *et al.*, 1990; Special Report, 1990; Nielson *et al.*, 1992). A National Institutes of Health-University of California Expert Panel (Special Report, 1990) reviewed these studies and concluded that corticosteroids were valuable in adults or adolescent (age >13 years) patients with moderate or severe *P. carinii* pneumonia (defined as a pretreatment P_aO_2 <70 mmHg or A-a gradient >35 mmHg while breathing room air) if commenced within 24–72 h of starting specific anti-pneumocystis therapy. Given in this setting, steroids resulted in improved prognosis in terms of both pulmonary function and overall survival. The recommended regimen (Table II.4) is 40 mg oral prednisolone twice-daily, days 1–5; 40 mg daily, days 6–10; 20 mg daily, days 11–21. Intravenous methylprednisolone can be used at 75% of these dosages if parenteral therapy is necessary. This regimen was associated with some oral thrush, perirectal herpes simplex disease and hyperglycemia, but no life-threatening complications. Steroids do not appear to enhance the risk of developing tuberculosis or other AIDS-related diseases in patients with *P. carinii* pneumonia (Martos *et al.*, 1995). Although no studies have examined the role of adjunctive corticosteroid therapy in the treatment of *P. carinii* pneumonia in pregnant women with AIDS or non-AIDS-associated *P. carinii* pneumonia, the Panel believed that such treatment would probably be reasonable assuming the above criteria were met – although no formal recommendation could be made. The role of steroids in mild *P. carinii* pneumonia (P_aO_2 >70 mmHg) and in pediatric patients (age <13 years) remains less uncertain.

Chemoprophylaxis against *P. carinii* pneumonia is worthwhile in all immunosuppressed patients where the risk of developing *P. carinii* pneumonia outweighs the cost and small risk of drug toxicity. Hughes *et al.* (1977) demonstrated the efficacy of Co-T as chemoprophylaxis in a placebo-controlled trial of 160 patients (children and young adults) with either acute lymphoblastic leukemia or other forms of malignancy receiving cytotoxic agents. Co-T was given in a dose of 5 mg trimethoprim/20 mg sulfamethoxazole per kg per day, in two divided doses, for a mean period of about 1 year and significantly reduced the incidence of *P. carinii* pneumonia (17/80 placebo-treated patients developed *P. carinii* pneumonia versus 0/80 Co-T-treated patients). Bacterial sepsis, other forms of pneumonia, upper respiratory tract infection and cellulitis also occurred less frequently in Co-T-treated patients, although the incidence of oral candidiasis was higher in this group. Subsequently, Hughes *et al.* (1987) demonstrated comparable efficacy between Co-T given on 3 consecutive days per week and daily Co-T therapy. Other studies have confirmed the efficacy of Co-T prophylaxis against *P. carinii* pneumonia in the non-AIDS settings (Harris *et al.*, 1980; Wilber *et al.*, 1980) although controlled studies have not been carried out in other at-risk groups. Nevertheless, numerous uncontrolled retrospective series examining other immunocompromised groups suggest that the daily dose recommended by Hughes *et al.* (1977, 1987) for children and that for adults, one double-strength

Table II.4

Drug regimens for the treatment and prophylaxis against *P. carinii* pneumonia. (Adapted from Masur H, 1992. Prevention and treatment of pneumocystis pneumonia. *New Engl J Med* **327**: 1853. With permission of the New England Journal of Medicine, Massachusetts Medical Society.)

Drug	Disease severity	Adult daily dose	Route	Dose interval	Duration of therapy (days
Treatment					
Specific agents[a]					
First line:					
Trimethoprim–sulfamethoxazole[b]	All	15–20 mg per kg 75–100 mg per kg	i.v. or p.o.	6–8 h	14[c]–21[d]
Pentamidine isethionate	All	4 mg per kg	i.v.	24 h	14[c]–21[d]
Second line:					
Trimethoprim + dapsone	Mild/moderate	15–20 mg per kg 100 mg	p.o. p.o.	8 h 24 h	21 21
Clindamycin + primaquine	Mild/moderate	1.8 g 15–30 mg	p.o. p.o.	8 h 24 h	21 21
Trimetrexate	All	45 mg per m²	i.v.	24 h	21
Atovaquone	Mild/moderate	2250 mg	p.o.	8 h	21
Aerosolized pentamidine[e]	Mild	600 mg	Aerosol ('Respirgard')	24 h	21
Adjunctive agents					
Prednisolone	Severe[f]	40 mg[g] 40 mg[g] 20 mg[g]	p.o. p.o. p.o.	12 h 24 h 24 h	5 5 11
Prophylaxis[h]					
Trimethoprim–sulfamethoxazole[b]		160/800 mg	p.o.	24 h	–
Pentamidine isethionate		4 mg 300 mg 60 mg	i.v. Aerosol ('Respirgard II') Aerosol ('Fisoneb')	Monthly Monthly Alternate weekly	– – –
Dapsone		50–100 mg	p.o.	24 h	–
Dapsone + pyrimethamine		200 mg 75 mg	p.o. p.o.	Weekly Weekly	– –
Dapsone + pyrimethamine		50–100 mg 50 mg	p.o. p.o.	24 h Once- or twice-weekly	– –
Pyrimethamine-sulfadoxine		50/100 mg	p.o.	Alternate weekly	–

i.v., intravenous; p.o., oral. [a] Only trimethoprim-sulfamethoxazole and i.v. pentamidine have been extensively studied for non-HIV-associated *P. carinii* pneumonia. [b] Preferred regimen. [c] Treatment duration for non-HIV-associated *P. carinii* pneumonia. [d] Treatment duration for HIV-associated *P. carinii* pneumonia. [e] Some authors believe further confirmatory studies are necessary before this treatment can be formally recommended. [f] Defined as: Initial pre-treatment P_aO_2 <70 mmHg or A-a gradient >30 mmHg (breathing room air). [g] If intravenous therapy is required, use equivalent to 75% of the oral dose. [h] Chemoprophylaxis for HIV-associated *P. carinii* pneumonia is generally life-long.

tablet (160 mg trimethoprim/800 mg sulfamethoxazole) once- or twice-daily is very effective. Whether Co-T should be taken 2, 3 or 7 days per week remains unclear due to insufficient data (Masur, 1992). Dummer (1990) advocates *P. carinii* pneumonia prophylaxis in most transplant patients, but especially heart-lung recipients who are particularly susceptible. In renal transplantation one single-strength Co-T tablet daily has been effective (Higgins *et al.*, 1989). This dosage has also been used in liver transplant recipients, although Dummer (1990) uses a daily dose of two double-strength Co-T tablets daily on an intermittent basis for 7 days of each month in heart, heart-lung and lung transplant recipients – once again, there are no studies to support the use of this regimen. In cardiac transplant recipients Co-T prophylaxis (either as 160/800 mg twice-daily 3 days per week, or daily) is superior to placebo when commenced 14 days after transplantation and continued for 4 months (Olsen *et al.*, 1993). No Co-T recipients developed *P. carinii* pneumonia versus 7 placebo recipients (p <0.005). Both Co-T doses were well tolerated and no patients discontinued therapy due to toxicity. Furthermore, no difference in total leukocyte count, azathioprine dose or number of transplant rejection episodes was noted between Co-T and placebo groups. Insufficient data is available to specify which of the two Co-T regimens is optimal (Olsen *et al.*, 1993). While intermittent inhalation of pentamidine is likely to be effective in transplant patients there have been no formal studies of its use in this setting.

Since approximately 60% of AIDS patients will re-develop *P. carinii* pneumonia within 1 year of their first episode of *P. carinii* pneumonia, regardless of whether they are also receiving antiretroviral agents such as zidovudine (ZDV) (p. 1633), *P. carinii* pneumonia prophylaxis is an important issue (CDC, 1989b, 1992; Simonds *et al.*, 1995). Both primary and secondary prophylaxis with Co-T against AIDS-associated *P. carinii* pneumonia is now the standard against which other regimens are compared (Ioannidis *et al.*, 1996). Nevertheless, the optimal dosage and frequency of administration remains controversial. Fischl *et al.* (1988) in a study of 60 AIDS patients with no past history of *P. carinii* pneumonia (primary prophylaxis), demonstrated the efficacy of one double-strength Co-T tablet twice-daily over placebo in preventing *P. carinii* pneumonia. None of 30 Co-T-treated patients versus 16/30 placebo-treated patients developed *P. carinii* pneumonia over a 2-year follow-up period. Side-effects were common (50%) in the Co-T-treated group, with 17% requiring discontinuation of the drug. These results were supported by two large retrospective studies which administered one double-strength tablet every other day for both primary and secondary prophylaxis (Wormser *et al.*, 1991; Ruskin and LaRiviere, 1991). Co-T twice-daily, three times per week, is better tolerated than similar therapy every day; the addition of folinic acid does not improve Co-T tolerance, regardless of the dosage regimen (Bozzette *et al.*, 1995b). Schneider *et al.* (1995) noted that primary *P. carinii* pneumonia prophylaxis with Co-T 80/400 mg daily had similar efficacy to Co-T 160/800 mg daily, but that the lower dose was less toxic. Whether this study had the statistical power to detect minor differences in efficacy remains uncertain.

Aerosolized pentamidine is effective for both primary and secondary prophylaxis against HIV-associated *P. carinii* pneumonia, although various studies have used a range of dosage regimens and types of nebulizers (Conte *et al.*, 1986; Leoung *et al.*, 1990; Girard *et al.*, 1989; Hirschel *et al.*, 1991; Montaner *et al.*, 1991; Murphy *et al.*, 1991; May *et al.*, 1994; Nielsen *et al.*, 1995). A comparative trial of aerosolized pentamidine (300 mg monthly, 'Respirgard II' nebulizer) and oral Co-T (two regimens: one double-strength tablet daily and one single-strength tablet daily) in HIV-infected patients who had never had *P. carinii* pneumonia, but had significant immunodeficiency (CD4$^+$ cell count <200 cells per μl), demonstrated the superiority of Co-T, with 6 of 71 pentamidine-treated patients developing *P. carinii* pneumonia compared with none in the Co-T-treated group (Schneider *et al.*, 1992). Toxicity requiring cessation of study agent was higher in those patients receiving Co-T, however. Another study which compared Co-T (one double-strength tablet daily) with aerosolized pentamidine ('Respirgard II' nebulizer) for secondary prophylaxis also demonstrated the superiority of Co-T (4% relapses in the Co-T group versus 18% in the pentamidine group) although, again, severe drug-limiting toxicity was more common (27% versus 4%) in the Co-T-treated group (Hardy *et al.*, 1992). These results have been supported by studies by Carr *et al.* (1992b), Martin *et al.* (1992) and Nielsen *et al.* (1995).

Other agents that have been used in various dosages and schedules for *P. carinii* pneumonia prophylaxis include: dapsone alone (Hughes *et al.*, 1990; Kemper *et al.*, 1990; Blum *et al.*, 1992; Bozzette *et al.*, 1995a), dapsone-pyrimethamine combination (Lavelle *et al.*, 1991; Girard *et al.*, 1993; Mallolas *et al.*, 1993; Podzamczer *et al.*, 1995), dapsone with trimethoprim, sulfadoxine with pyrimethamine (Hardy *et al.*, 1987), atovaquone, and oral clindamycin with primaquine (Masur, 1992). In a randomized trial, Bozzette *et al.* (1995a) compared the efficacy of primary *P. carinii* pneumonia prophylaxis with either oral Co-T (160/800 mg daily), oral dapsone (50 mg daily) or aerosolized pentamidine (300 mg monthly via 'Respirgard II' nebulizer) in HIV-infected patients with <200 CD4s who were receiving zidovudine. The 36-month cumulative risks of *P. carinii* pneumonia were 18%, 17% and 21%, respectively (p=0.22). However, among patients entering the study with <100 CD4s, the risk was 33% with aerosolized pentamidine versus 19% and 22% for Co-T and dapsone, respectively (p=0.04). The lowest failure rates were associated with Co-T prophylaxis, while dapsone 50 mg per day did not appear to be as effective as 100 mg per day. Thus, these authors suggest commencing primary *P. carinii* pneumonia prophylaxis with Co-T or high-dose dapsone. Co-T 160/800 mg twice-daily, 3 days per week, is superior to dapsone 100 mg + pyrimethamine 50 mg twice-weekly in preventing *P. carinii* pneumonia: 6 of 96 dapsone/pyrimethamine-treated patients developed *P. carinii* pneumonia (6.9%) versus 0 of 104 Co-T-treated patients (p <0.0001). No differences were noted in the incidence of toxoplasmosis, and similar rates of adverse reactions and mortality were observed between the two treatment groups during follow-up (Podzamczer *et al.*, 1995).

Thus, the Centers for Disease Control, currently recommend Co-T as the agent of choice for both primary and secondary prophylaxis against HIV-associated *P. carinii* pneumonia. Life-long prophylaxis should be considered the standard for HIV-infected patients where the CD4$^+$ T lymphocyte count is <200 cells per μl; for patients with constitutional symptoms such as unexplained persistent fever (>37.8^{0}C) or oropharyngeal candidiasis (unrelated to antibiotic or corticosteroid therapy) for 2 weeks or more, regardless of CD4$^+$; and for patients who have had previous episodes of *P. carinii* pneumonia (CDC, 1992). The current recommendation in adults and adolescents is for one double-strength Co-T tablet daily, 7 days per week (CDC, 1992). Low-dose Co-T prophylaxis regimens have been studied which look promising (Ruskin and LaRiviere, 1991; Stein *et al.*, 1991; Martin *et al.*, 1992; MacGregor *et al.*, 1992; Podzamczer *et al.*, 1995), but CDC currently considers the data to be insufficient to recommend the administration of Co-T fewer than 7 days per week. Co-T may also have the advantage of preventing toxoplasmosis (p. 874; Hardy *et al.*, 1992; CDC, 1992; Schneider *et al.*, 1992; Carr *et al.*, 1992a).

Pneumocystis carinii pneumonia prophylaxis in HIV-infected children has been reviewed, and the current recommended regimen for children ≥4 weeks of age is oral Co-T (150 mg trimethoprim per m^2 per day, plus 750 mg sulfamethoxazole per m^2 per day) in divided doses twice-daily, three times per week on consecutive days (e.g. Monday, Tuesday, Wednesday) (CDC, 1991, 1995). Other acceptable schedules include this same dose administered either every day, or on alternate, rather than consecutive, days; or this same total daily dose as a single dose three times per week on consecutive days. Alternative regimens include oral dapsone 2 mg per kg (not to exceed 100 mg) once-daily, or aerosolized pentamidine (children ≥5 years of age) 300 mg via 'Respirgard II' inhaler monthly (CDC, 1995). Of concern is the fact that there has been no substantial reduction in the incidence of *P. carinii* pneumonia among HIV-infected infants, most likely due to the failure to identify HIV infection before *P. carinii* pneumonia occurs and the limitations in the ability of CD4 measurements to identify children at risk for *P. carinii* pneumonia. Thus, CDC (1995) now recommends the commencement of *P. carinii* pneumonia prophylaxis at 4–6 weeks of age for all children who have been perinatally exposed to HIV; continuation of prophylaxis through 12 months of age for HIV-infected children; and making decisions regarding prophylaxis for HIV-infected children ≥12 months of age based on CD4 measurements and prior history of *P. carinii* pneumonia. A detailed discussion regarding these issues can be found elsewhere (CDC, 1995).

25 Histoplasmosis

Two case reports have suggested that Co-T may have some efficacy in this disease, although it is not the drug of choice (Macleod, 1970; Egere *et al.*, 1978).

26 Q fever

Co-T has been used to treat patients with both acute and chronic Q fever, with mixed success (Freeman and Hodson, 1972; Dathan and Heyworth, 1975; Levy *et al.*, 1991). While there have been reports of successful Co-T therapy in Q fever when combined with tetracyclines, lincomycin or rifampicin (Tobin *et al.*, 1982; pp. 598, 749), there have also been failures with the rifampicin/Co-T combination (p. 699). Street and Durack (1988) reviewed the efficacy of Co-T in the treatment of infective endocarditis, including 19 cases due to *Coxiella burnetti*. Eleven of these 19 patients were cured (eight medically; three medical + surgical therapy) – one with Co-T monotherapy, ten with a combination of Co-T plus other agents such as tetracyclines. In general, tetracyclines (p. 749) have remained the usual preferred drugs for this infection.

27 Chemoprophylaxis in biliary surgery

Morran *et al.* (1978) found a single i.v. dose of Co-T (160 mg trimethoprim and 800 mg sulfamethoxazole) given by infusion over 60 min before operation in patients undergoing biliary surgery was associated with a reduction in the frequency of wound sepsis and pulmonary complications. However, other agents such as second-generation cephalosporins (p. 309) or various other extended-spectrum beta-lactams are now often preferred.

28 Reduction of infection in patients with granulocytopenia

Most infections in granulocytopenic patients with haematologic malignancies are caused by bacteria derived from the patient's respiratory tract or endogenous gastrointestinal flora. The Gram-negative aerobic bacilli *E. coli*, *K. pneumoniae* and *Ps. aeruginosa*, and the Gram-positive cocci such as viridans streptococci, *Staph. aureus* and *Staph. epidermidis* are the frequent bacterial pathogens (Henry, 1984; Bow and Ronald, 1993; Verhoef, 1993). Both absorbable and non-absorbable antibiotics have been used to decrease colonization by new potential pathogens and to suppress endogenous microflora (Young, 1983; Henry, 1984). Antibiotic combinations such as gentamicin and vancomycin often result in 'total decontamination' of the gut, eradicating both aerobic and anaerobic organisms and may be associated with gastrointestinal side-effects (De Vries-Hospers *et al.*, 1981; Hargadon *et al.*, 1981).

The potential value of Co-T prophylaxis was identified by Hughes *et al.* (1977) when he observed that bacterial infections were less frequent in patients with acute leukemia receiving Co-T as prophylaxis after *P. carinii* pneumonitis. Since this time there have been numerous reports of the successful use of Co-T in reducing infection in granulocytopenic patients. The efficacy of antibiotic prophylaxis is based both upon the presence of serum antibiotic levels and upon the concept of 'selective decontamination' of the gut flora – i.e. eradication of pathogenic aerobic flora, particularly Gram-negative bacilli, without disturbing the autochthonous, symbiotic flora which consists largely of anaerobic bacteria (Hargadon *et al.*, 1981; Clasener *et al.*, 1987). The presence of normal anaerobic flora is responsible for what has been termed 'colonization resistance' (De Vries-Hospers *et al.*, 1981; Young, 1983). In concert with host factors, anaerobes limit the growth of aerobes in the gut by some unknown mechanism, perhaps by competing for nutrients. Selective elimination of Enterobacteriaceae and Pseudomonads was demonstrated by De Vries-Hospers *et al.* (1981) in granulocytopenic patients who were given nalidixic acid, Co-T or polymyxin. Yeasts were also eliminated selectively by amphotericin B or nystatin treatment. These antibacterial and antifungal drugs were chosen because they could eliminate Gram-negative aerobic rods and yeasts without affecting anaerobic gut flora. When these authors did bacteriological studies, the selectively decontaminated patients had fewer Gram-negative aerobic rods or yeasts, or both, in the throat and feces. Co-T, compared with non-absorbable drugs, has the advantage of being absorbed and producing serum levels of its components, which are then available to prevent invasion by any surviving Enterobacteriaceae. Despite these findings, the use of these single drugs with activity against *E. coli* and not anaerobes is not adequate alone to avert colonization and infection by pseudomonads (Young, 1983).

Co-T either alone, or in combination with erythromycin, nystatin, or amphotericin has been shown to reduce infection more than non-absorbable antibiotics or untreated controls in neutropenic patients with acute leukemia or malignancy (Enno *et al.*, 1978; Gurwithh *et al.*, 1979; Dekker *et al.*, 1981; Gualitieri *et al.*, 1983; Kauffman *et al.*, 1983; Pizzo *et al.*, 1983; Wade *et al.*, 1983) (EORTC Group, 1984). In granulocytopenic children with leukemia during induction chemotherapy, oral Co-T decreased the frequency of febrile episodes, including bacteremia, but the frequency of oral thrush (without invasive fungal infection) was greater in those receiving Co-T than in the placebo group (Kovatch *et al.*, 1985). Some authors have found Co-T alone to be as effective as Co-T in combination with other agents (Starke *et al.*, 1982), while others disagree. Bow *et al.* (1984) summarized many of the randomized controlled studies using Co-T: Co-T has been used in over 1000 patients with acute leukemia or other bone marrow failure states and has usually been superior to placebo, neomycin plus colistin plus nystatin; it is effective as oral gentamicin with or without oral vancomycin. Co-T alone may be less effective than Co-T plus framycetin plus colistin; Co-T plus vancomycin/ gentamicin appears superior to vancomycin/gentamicin alone; and Co-T plus colistin seems superior over Co-T alone.

Co-T is not only effective in suppressing the aerobic Gram-negative enteric microflora, but has been shown to reduce the morbidity and mortality of infection due to these aerobic Gram-negative bacilli (Riben *et al.*, 1983; Bow *et al.*, 1987). Bow *et al.* (1988) advocate that prophylactic antibiotics should be administered for approximately 1 week before the patient is at risk of neutropenia-related infection; thus permitting sufficient time to eliminate the potentially pathogenic aerobic enteric microflora. Many authors therefore now regard Co-T prophylaxis as the benchmark against which new regimens, such as the fluoroquinolones, should be compared. Nalidixic acid and trimethoprim alone have proved unsatisfactory alternatives to Co-T for infection prophylaxis in neutropenia, possibly because of their more limited antibacterial spectrum (Gurwith et al., 1982; Bow et al., 1984, 1987).

A number of problems with Co-T prophylaxis have now emerged, however. Firstly, variable compliance with regular administration of Co-T has emerged as a significant issue in some studies (Pizzo, 1989). The EORTC Study (1984) only demonstrated a benefit for the Co-T-treated group when non-compliant patients were excluded fom analysis. Toxicity, particularly the suppressive effects on bone marrow and the longer periods of neutropenia observed in patients receiving Co-T prophylaxis, are important (Dekker et al., 1981; Pizzo et al., 1983; Bow et al., 1984; Kovatch et al., 1985). This bone marrow suppressive effect has been attributed to the action of the drug on folic acid metabolism (pp. 855, 856) and the effect on the duration of granulocytopenia may be related to the dosage of Co-T used (Kauffman et al., 1983; EORTC Group, 1984). In this regard ciprofloxacin appears to have less effect on leukocyte recovery than CoT (p. 1026). Among patients recovering from autologous bone marrow transplantation, the time taken to achieve an absolute neutrophil count of $\geq 500 \times 10^9$ per liter was significantly shorter in patients receiving ciprofloxacin than those receiving Co-T (16 days vs 22 days; p=0.006) (Imrie et al., 1995). A number of authors have described an increase in fungal infections, including Aspergillus flavus, with Co-T prophylaxis (Wade et al., 1983; Estey et al., 1984), but this finding has not been confirmed by others (Gurwith et al., 1979; Kauffman et al., 1983). Furthermore, resistant isolates and breakthrough infections have been noted in some Co-T recipients (Dekker et al., 1981; Wilson and Guiney, 1982; Lehtonen and Pelliniemi, 1982; Pizzo et al., 1983; Pizzo, 1983; Gualtieri et al., 1983).

Contrary to all these studies, the double-blind, placebo-controlled trial of Co-T prophylaxis by Ward et al. (1993) in patients with acute leukemia is of interest. In this study, Co-T had no detectable effect on the incidence of fever or documented infection, time to febrile neutropenic episode, the use of antimicrobial therapy or outcome of treatment of the underlying diseases. However, despite the commendable rigor of the trial design which makes the report noteworthy, its relatively small sample size due to early termination resulted in a loss of power to detect statistical differences in bacteremic events between the Co-T and placebo arms (Bow and Ronald, 1993). Thus, further studies are necessary, but given the current interest in fluoroquinolones for prophylaxis (p. 1025), a study of sufficient size using Co-T seems less likely.

In an unblinded, randomized comparison of norfloxacin (400 mg twice-daily) and Co-T (160/800 mg twice-daily), norfloxacin therapy was associated with fewer Gram-negative infections (0/31 versus 4/32), but significantly more Gram-positive bacteremias (17 versus 2, p = 0.003) than patients receiving Co-T therapy (Bow et al., 1988). Presumably this was related to the relative lack of norfloxacin activity against Gram-positive pathogens. Infections observed in Co-T recipients were due to pathogens resistant to this agent. Acquisition of, and infection by, Co-T-resistant Gram-negative bacilli appeared to be a problem for Co-T recipients. Norfloxacin, meanwhile, eliminated aerobic Gram-negative bacilli from the gut in a mean of 5 days, but proved superior for preventing both acquisition of Gram-negative bacilli and infection by these pathogens. Thus, norfloxacin appears to be a safe, well tolerated and effective alternative to Co-T in preventing serious Gram-negative infections, but at a potential cost of more frequent (but generally less serious) Gram-positive infections. Similarly, Dekker et al. (1987) and Verhoef et al. (1989) have found ciprofloxacin to compare very favorably in terms of tolerability and efficacy with Co-T + colistin for prophylaxis. Arning et al. (1990), however, found no significant difference in efficacy between Co-T + colistin, ofloxacin and ciprofloxacin for the prevention of infections in patients with acute leukemia, but noted that both the quinolones were better tolerated. Thus, quinolones now appear to be more popular than Co-T among some authors for prophylaxis in neutropenia.

29 Reduction of infections in patients post-renal transplantation

Long-term prophylaxis with oral Co-T following renal transplantation was investigated in a double-blind, randomized, placebo-controlled trial and found to be effective in reducing infections and minimizing inpatient hospital days with fever (Fox et al., 1990). Prophylaxis was particularly effective in the prevention of urinary tract infections (p < 0.005), bacteremia (p < 0.01) and infections caused by enteric Gram-negative bacilli (p < 0.001), enterococci (p = 0.006) and Staph. aureus (p = 0.01). Prophylaxis did not prevent urinary tract infection associated with urethral catheters in the initial post-transplant period, but reduced the risk of urinary tract infection 3-fold (p < 0.001) after catheter removal. In the early post-transplant period, absorption of Co-T was subnormal and a dosage of two double-strength tablets (320 mg trimethoprim/ 1600 mg sulfamethoxazole) daily was necessary to achieve adequate serum levels, although one double-strength tablet per day appeared to be effective after the initial post-transplant admission. In addition, Co-T provided protection against *P. carinii* pneumonia (p. 874), and infection from *Listeria* and *Nocardia*; was well tolerated, had little discernible effect on the patients' microflora and was cost-effective. Some authors believe that Co-T prophylaxis may be especially important during periods of resistant graft rejection, when the monoclonal antibody Orthoclone OKT3 is used to limit graft rejection. Since renal transplantation programs at the University of Minnesota and Massachusetts General Hospital have used long-term Co-T prophylaxis for many years and have identified few side-effects, Fox *et al.* (1990) suggests prophylaxis for at least 1 year post-transplantation, and probably indefinitely.

30 Reduction of infections in patients with cirrhosis and ascites

In a randomized, placebo-controlled trial of patients with cirrhosis and ascites, one Co-T tablet (double-strength; 160/800 mg) daily, five times per week significantly reduced the risk of developing spontaneous bacterial peritonitis from 27% (placebo) to 3% (Co-T) (p=0.025) in patients followed for a median duration of 90 days. However, there was no difference in the death rate between the two groups (Singh *et al.*, 1995; Nishioka, 1995). The findings of this relatively small study need confirmation before Co-T can be routinely recommended for prophylaxis in this setting.

31 Chronic granulomatous disease

This is characterized by recurrent, often life-threatening, bacterial and mycotic infections. It is caused by the inability of the patient's phagocytes to kill catalase-positive organisms, such as *Staph. aureus*. Long-term prophylaxis with Co-T has resulted in a reduction in infectious episodes, but had no effect on the occurrence of *C. albicans* and *Aspergillus* infections (Weening *et al.*, 1983; Van der Meer and Van den Broek, 1984; Mouy *et al.*, 1989; Margolis *et al.*, 1990). This beneficial effect of Co-T appears to be due to the uptake and concentration of its components in granulocytes (Gmunder and Seger, 1981). Margolis *et al.* (1990) recently reviewed the National Institutes of Health experience with long-term prophylaxis with Co-T in patients with chronic granulomatous disease. Prophylaxis decreased the incidence of non-fungal infections from 7.1 to 2.4 per 100 patient-months in patients with autosomal chronic granulomatous disease and from 15.8 to 6.9 infections per 100 patient-months in X-linked chronic granulomatous disease patients (p = 0.06). However, there was no significant change in the incidence of fungal infections in these patients. Sulfonamides alone may also be effective in this disease (p. 828).

32 Wegener's granulomatosis

A growing number of reports and small series suggest a beneficial effect of Co-T, either alone or as adjunctive therapy to cytotoxics, on both acute and chronic phases of Wegener's granulomatosis (West *et al.*, 1987; Israel, 1988; DeRemee, 1988; Valeriano-Marcet and Spiera, 1991; DeRemee, 1992). Other authors however, have cast doubt on these findings (Hoffman and Fauci, 1992; Hoffman *et al.*, 1992). In some patients Co-T has been supplemented with additional trimethoprim, which Israel (1988) believes to be the more important component of the combination. While the effects of Co-T appear to be suppressive rather than curative, the mechanism of this possible efficacy remains unclear. There is a need for prospective randomized trials to confirm the value of Co-T in this condition.

B Trimethoprim alone

When Co-T was first released, the use of trimethoprim as a single drug was not advocated. It was thought that, without the protective effect of sulfonamides, the use of trimethoprim alone would result in an increase of trimethoprim-resistant strains, and that synergy between the component drugs was essential for therapeutic success. There is little evidence that the use of trimethoprim alone has resulted in an increase in the incidence of trimethoprim-resistant organisms (p. 839). Moreover, although the combination of trimethoprim and sulfamethoxazole suppresses the appearance of resistant mutants *in vitro*, such studies may not be applicable to events *in vivo*. Trimethoprim-resistant mutants selected in this way are often different from those which are isolated from clinical material. Because a high proportion of bacteria are sulfonamide-resistant, treatment with Co-T has, in fact, been equivalent to treatment with trimethoprim alone in many instances. Co-T does not usually produce synergistic inhibition of organisms highly resistant to sulfonamides (p. 842). It is also doubtful whether synergy is a requirement for therapeutic efficacy in many infections, such as those of the urinary tract (p. 843). The concentrations of trimethoprim reached in the body are sufficient to inhibit most pathogens. For these reasons, trimethoprim has been used more widely as a single drug in recent years, with good therapeutic effect and fewer side-effects than Co-T.

1 Urinary tract infections

Early studies using Co-T showed that it was superior to sulfamethoxazole alone for the treatment of these infections (Gruneberg and Kolbe, 1969; Knudsen et al., 1973; Harding and Ronald, 1973). This occurred because many of the bacteria involved were resistant to sulfonamides. Trimethoprim alone has been as effective as Co-T for the treatment of urinary tract infections (Brumfitt and Pursell, 1972; Lacey et al., 1980; Trimethoprim Study Group, 1981; Kasanen and Sundquist, 1982; Keenan et al., 1983; Fihn et al., 1988). Adult dosage regimens of 200–300 mg daily for 5 days have been effective. The Trimethoprim Study Group (1981) demonstrated that cure rates were the same for 7-day regimens of trimethoprim 50, 100 or 200 mg twice-daily or Co-T two standard tablets twice-daily. Asscher and Mackenzie (1982) found that 7-day courses of trimethoprim in doses of 300 mg once-daily or 200 mg twice-daily were equally effective in the treatment of acute urinary infections. Ahlmen and Brorson (1982) gave a single daily dose of 300 mg trimethoprim for 3 consecutive days; urinary concentrations of the drug were in excess of the MICs for most urinary pathogens for up to 5 days after the start of oral treatment.

The efficacy of trimethoprim alone has been compared with other drugs for the treatment of acute urinary tract infections in women. Iravini et al. (1981b) compared trimethoprim 400 mg daily for 14 days and trimethoprim 200 mg daily for 10 days with sulfisoxazole 2 g daily for 10 or 14 days. Results of treatment and rates of recurrence were not significantly different between these drugs, but the higher dose of trimethoprim was associated with a maculopapular rash in 24% of recipients. Trimethoprim (300 mg once-daily for 7 days or 200 mg once-daily for 10 days) was equally as effective as nitrofurantoin (100 mg four times daily for 10 days) (Iravini et al., 1982). In the treatment of acute urinary tract infections, Kasanen and Sundquist (1982) reported that trimethoprim alone is more effective than cephalexin. Guerrant et al. (1981) studied patients who had had recurrent urinary tract infections and who were given either Co-T (trimethoprim 160 mg/ sulfamethoxazole 800 mg) daily or trimethoprim (200 or 100 mg twice-daily) for 4 weeks. All regimens left anaerobes intact and reduced the total aerobic coliform fecal flora. Resistant Enterobacteriaceae did not emerge in the urinary or gastrointestinal tract; there was a slight increase in trimethoprim-resistant organisms of the Pseudomonas and Acinetobacter spp. in patients receiving trimethoprim 200 mg twice-daily compared with those receiving Co-T.

The manufacturers recommend the following regimens for urinary tract infections: for children over 6 years of age half a tablet (150 mg) and for adults one tablet (300 mg) both given once-daily for 7 days. The Australian Guidelines Sub-Committee (1992) recommends for acute urinary tract infections the use of trimethoprim 300 mg daily for 3 days in non-pregnant women; 300 mg daily for 10–14 days in men and 6 mg per kg (maximum 300 mg) daily for 7–10 days in children.

In children with acute urinary tract infection, a 10-day course of trimethoprim alone was equally efficacious as Co-T and achieved a higher cure rate than either sulfamethoxazole or ampicillin alone (Rajkumar et al., 1989). Nolan et al. (1989) found that for uncomplicated urinary tract infections in children, a single dose of trimethoprim resulted in a cure rate at 48 h similar to that achieved with a conventional 7-day course of Co-T. However, similar to other short-course antibiotic regimens in children, there was an unacceptably high recurrence rate at follow-up after 10 days.

Long-term, low-dose trimethoprim prophylaxis has been effective in adult patients with recurrent urinary tract infections (Kasanen et al., 1974; Iwarson and Lidin-Janson, 1979; Svensson et al., 1982; Stamm et al.,1991) (p. 861). A daily dose of 100 mg trimethoprim given at night has been effective and associated with few side-effects. In a comparative trial, trimethoprim was superior to methenamine hippurate and nitrofurantoin in preventing recurrences (Kasanen et al., 1982). Smellie et al. (1982) used long-term trimethoprim effectively for prophylaxis in children with recurrent urinary tract infections. A dose of 2 mg trimethoprim per kg body weight per day was used for a mean period of 7.9 months per child. The effect of trimethoprim prophylaxis on the bowel flora was similar to that of Co-T prophylaxis. Organisms resistant to trimethoprim were found in 16% of rectal swabs from children receiving trimethoprim prophylaxis.

2 Other infections

Trimethoprim has been used successfully to treat patients with enteric fever (*Salm. typhi, Salm. paratyphi* A and B). An adult dosage of 300 mg every 12 h reducing to 200 mg every 12 h after 2–3 days was used, with appropriate dose-reduction for children. Initially 42 of 71 patients were given the drug i.v. as a bolus injection and after 2–3 days this was followed by oral therapy to complete a 14-day course of treatment; 63 of the 71 patients were cured (McKendrick *et al.*, 1981; Gargalianos *et al.*, 1986). Trimethoprim alone has been shown to be equally as effective as Co-T for respiratory tract infections, and to be associated with fewer side-effects in a number of studies (Lacey *et al.*, 1980; Ashford and Downey, 1982). In some studies trimethoprim alone, appears similar in efficacy to Co-T for the treatment of travelers' diarrhea, but is less effective as prophylaxis (p. 869). Trimethoprim has been used alone, 200 mg twice-daily for 5 days, to successfully treat chancroid (Plummer *et al.*, 1983a), however it is significantly less effective if single-dose therapy is used (Dylewski *et al.*, 1985).

C Trimethoprim combined with other sulfonamides

Bernstein (1982) reviewed criteria for selection of sulfonamides for use with trimethoprim and summarized clinical experience with trimethoprim combined with sulfonamides other than sulfamethoxazole. Sulfamoxole is not as active as sulfamethoxazole *in vitro* and there are insufficient data that its combination with trimethoprim is as effective as Co-T clinically (Berstein, 1982; Hughes, 1983; Dylewski *et al.*, 1985). Sulfametrol probably has similar pharmacokinetics to sulfamethoxazole and has been used successfully for the treatment of respiratory, skin and urinary infections and gonorrhea (Berstein, 1982). Various trimethoprim-sulfadiazine combinations have been used to treat respiratory tract infections, non-gonococcal urethritis due to *C. trachomatis* and to cure a 4-month-old child with *Salmonella* meningitis (Briggs and Robinson, 1975). Pharmacokinetic studies after i.v. administration of sulfadiazine indicate certain advantages for sulfadiazine as a partner for trimethoprim compared with sulfamethoxazole; sulfadiazine is less bound to serum proteins, its distribution volume is larger and it gives higher concentrations of active sulfonamide in serum and urine (Mannisto *et al.*, 1982). It seems that trimethoprim/ sulfadiazine combinations may have some theoretical advantage over Co-T, at least for the treatment of urinary tract infections (Bernstein, 1982; Reeves, 1982).

There are very few reports on the clinical use of trimethoprim/sulfadimidine and trimethoprim/ sulfametopyrazine combinations. The former has been used for a variety of infections in eastern Europe (Bernstein, 1982) and the latter for lower respiratory tract infections (Hughes, 1983), all with reported success. Trimethoprim has been combined with a variety of sulfonamides such as sulfamoxole, sufametrole and sulfamethopyrazine to successfully treat chancroid (Dylewski *et al.*, 1986; Schmid, 1990) (p. 823).

D Trimethoprim combined with other drugs

Trimethoprim has previously been used in combination with rifampicin to treat a number of infections; such combinations have been effective for the therapy of urinary tract infections and chancroid, but the combination is not dependable chemoprophylaxis for *H. influenzae* infection (p. 699). A dosage regimen of 900 mg rifampicin plus 240 mg trimethoprim for 4 months followed by 300 mg rifampicin plus 80 mg trimethoprim has been used effectively to treat chronic bacterial prostatitis (Leading article, 1983a).

In comparative trials for the treatment of presumptive bacterial conjunctivitis, there was no difference in clinical efficacy between treatment with trimethoprim/polymyxin B ophthalmic solution and neomycin/polymyxin B/gramicidin ophthalmic solution; but trimethoprim/ polymyxin ophthalmic solution was better than a chloramphenicol one in reducing signs and symptoms (Gibson, 1983). Combinations of trimethoprim and methenamine hippurate have been used in two doses of 100:500 mg and 200:1000 mg, respectively, twice-daily and compared with trimethoprim 200 mg twice-daily and Co-T (two standard tablets twice-daily) to treat urinary tract infections; all regimens were effective, but the ones using trimethoprim and methenamine had fewer side-effects (Seppänen *et al.*, 1983).

E Combinations of other diaminopyrimidines with sulfonamides

Apart from trimethoprim, a number of other diaminopyrimidines have been synthesized, which also affect folic acid synthesis by inhibiting dihydrofolate reductase (p. 852) (Burchall, 1979). Some newer compounds differ from trimethoprim in lipophilicity, *Staph. aureus* antibacterial spectrum and degree of activity and pharmacology (Then *et al.*, 1982). The ability of the diaminopyrimidines to inhibit mammalian or bacterial dihydrofolate reductases differ. For instance, pyrimethamine is a poor antibacterial and its binding to mammalian reductases is considerably greater than trimethoprim; but it binds tightly to protozoal reductases making it an effective antimalarial drug (p.917). Tetroxoprim is another diaminopyrimidine which was marketed for antibacterial indications. Compared with trimethoprim, tetroxoprim is approximately 8- to 16-fold less active against most bacteria and there is also complete cross-resistance between these two compounds and between sulfadiazine and sulfamethoxazole (Bywater *et al.*, 1979). Considering these factors, tetroxoprim has limited clinical relevence and is mostly only of historical interest (Leading article, 1980).

References

Aber RC, Wennersten C, Moellering RC (1978). Antimicrobial susceptibility of Flavobacteria. *Antimicrob Ag Chemother* **14**: 483.

Adam WR, Henning M, Dawborn JK (1973). Excretion of trimethoprim and sulfamethoxazole in patients with renal failure. *Aust NZ J Med* **3**: 383.

Aguilar X, Ruiz J, Clotet B et al. (1991). The use of corticosteroids in the control of the adverse effects of co-trimoxazole in AIDS patients suffering from PCP. *AIDS* **5**: 777.

Ahlmén J, Brorson J-E (1982). Pharmacokinetics of trimethoprim given in single daily doses for three days. *Scand J Infect Dis* **14**: 143.

Ai NV, Hanh ND, Dien PV, Le NV (1973). Co-trimoxazole in bubonic plague. *Brit Med J* **4**: 108.

Akinkugbe OO, Lewis EA, Montefiore D, Okubadejo OA (1968). Trimethoprim and sulphamethoxazle in typhoid. *Brit Med J* **3**: 721.

al-Eissa YA, Kambal AM, al-Nasser MN et al. (1990). Childhood brucellosis: a study of 102 cases. *Pediatr Infect Dis J* **9**: 74.

Al-Orainey IO, Laajam MA, Al-Aska AK, Rajapakse CN (1987). *Brucella* meningitis. *J Infect* **14**: 141.

Alappan R, Perazella MA, Buller GK (1996). Hyperkalemia in hospitalized patients treated with trimethoprim-sulfamethoxazole. *Ann Intern Med* **124**: 316.

Alberti-Flor JJ, Hernandez ME, Ferrer JP et al. (1989). Fulminant liver failure and pancreatitis associated with the use of sulfamethoxazole-trimethoprim. *Gastroenterology* **84**: 1577.

Aldridge KE, Gelfand MS, Schiro DD, Barg NL (1992). The rapid emergence of fluoroquinolone-methicillin-resistant *Staphylococcus aureus* infections in a community hospital. An *in vitro* look at alternative antimicrobial agents. *Diagn Microbiol Infect Dis* **15**: 601.

Allegra CJ, Chabner BA, Tuazon CU et al. (1987). Trimetrexate for the treatment of *Pneumocystis carinii* pneumonia in patients with the acquired immunodeficiency syndrome. *New Engl J Med* **317**: 978.

Alvarez S, Jones M, Holtsclaw-Berk S et al. (1985). *In vitro* susceptibilities and β-lactamase production of 53 clinical isolates of *Branhamella catarrhalis*. *Antimicrob Ag Chemother* **27**: 646.

Amyes SGB (1986). Epidemiology of trimethoprim resistance. *J Antimicrob Chemother* **18** (Suppl C): 215.

Amyes SGB, Doherty CJ, Wonnacott S (1986). Trimethoprim and co-trimoxazole: a comparison of their use in respiratory tract infections. *Scand J Infect Dis* **18**: 561.

Anderson G, Grabow G, Oosthuizen R et al. (1980). Effects of sulfamethoxazole *in vitro*: *in vivo* effects of co-trimoxazole. *Antimicrob Ag Chemother* **17**: 322.

Anderson G, Williams L, Pardoe T, Peel ET (1981). Co-trimoxazole versus cefaclor in acute or chronic bronchitis. *J Antimicrob Chemother* **8**: 487.

Annotation (1973). Co-trimoxazole. *Antimicrob Ag Chemother* **17**: 322.

Ansdell VE, Wright SG, Hutchinson DBA (1976). Megaloblastic anaemia associated with combined pyrimethamine and co-trimoxazole administration. *Lancet* **ii**: 1257.

Appleman MD, Cherubin CE, Heseltine PN, Stratton CW (1991). Susceptibility testing of *Listeria monocytogenes* A reassessment of bactericidal activity as a predictor for clinical outcome. *Diagn Microbiol Infect Dis* **14**: 311.

Ardati KO, Thirumoorthi MC, Dajani AS (1979). Intravenous trimethoprim/

sulfamethoxazole in the treatment of serious infections in children. *J Pediatrics* **95**: 801.

Arduino RC, Johnson PC, Miranda AG (1993). Nocardiosis i renal transplant recipients undergoing immunosuppression with cyclosporine. *Clin Infect Dis* **16**: 505.

Ariza J, Gudiol F, Pallarés R et al. (1985). Comparative trial of co-trimoxazole versus tetracycline-streptomycin in treating human brucellosis. *J Infect Dis* **152**: 1358.

Armstrong RW, Slater B (1986). *Listeria monocytogenes* meningitis treated with trimethoprim-sulfamethoxazole. *Rev Infect Dis* **5**: 712.

Arneil GC, McAllister TA (1977). Whooping-cough in infants: antimicrobial prophylaxis. *Lancet* **ii**: 33.

Arning M, Wolf HH, Aul C et al. (1990). Infection prophylaxis in neutropenic patients with acute leukaemia – a randomized, comparative study with ofloxacin, ciprofloxacin and co-trimoxazole/colistin. *J Antimicrob Chemother* **26** (Suppl D): 137.

Arvilommi H, Vuroi M, Salmi A (1972). Immunosuppression by co-trimoxazole. *Brit Med J* **3**: 761.

Ashford JJ, Downey LJ (1982). A multi-centre study comparing trimethoprim with co-trimoxazole in the treatment of respiratory tract infection in general practice. *Brit J Clin Prac* **36**: 551.

Ashkenazi S, May-Zahav M, Sulkes J et al. (1995). Increasing antimicrobial resistance of *Shigella* isolates in Israel during the period 1984 to 1992. *Antimicrob Ag Chemother* **39**: 819.

Asmar BI, Maqbook S, Dajani AS (1981). Hematologic abnormalities after oral trimethoprim-sulfamethoxazole therapy in children. *Amer J Dis Child* **145**: 1100.

Asscher AW, Mackenzie R (1982). Single vs twice daily dosage in the treatment of urinary tract infections. *J Antimicrob Chemother* **9**: 242.

Austin TW, Brooks GF, Bethel M et al. (1973). Trimethoprim-sulfamethoxazole in the treatment of gonococcal urethritis: clinical and laboratory correlates. *J Infect Dis* **128** (Suppl): 666.

Australian Guidelines Sub-Committee, Victorian Drug Advisory Committee (1992). *Antibiotic Guidelines* 7th edn, pp. 31–33. Moorabbin: Interprint Services Ltd.

Bach MC, Sabath LD, Finland M (1973a). Susceptibility of *Nocardia asteroides* to 45 antimicrobial agents *in vitro*. *Antimicrob Ag Chemother* **3**: 1.

Bach MC, Finland M, Gold O, Wilcox C (1973b). Susceptibility of recently isolated pathogenic bacteria to trimethoprim and sulfamethoxazole separately and combined. *J Infect Dis* **128** (Suppl): 508.

Bach MC, Gold O, Finland M (1973c). Absorbtion and urinary excretion of trimethoprim, sulfamethoxazole, and trimethoprim-sulfamethoxazole: results with single doses in normal young adults and preliminary observations during therapy with trimethoprim-sulfamethoxazole. *J Infect Dis* **128** (Suppl): 584.

Baikie AG, Macdonald CB, Mundy GR (1970). Systemic nocardiosis treated with trimethoprim and sulfamethoxazole. *Lancet* **ii**: 261.

Bailey RR, Little PJ (1976). Deterioration in renal function in association with co-trimoxazole therapy. *Med J Aust* **1**: 914.

Bannister G, Arkell DG, Menday AP (1981). Prostatectomy and prophylaxis. *J Antimicrob Chemother* **7**: 209.

Barada FA Jr, Guerrant RL (1980). Sulfamethoxazole-trimethoprim versus ampicillin in treatment of acute invasive diarrhea in adults. *Antimicrob Ag Chemother* **17**: 961.

Barker J, Healing D, Hutchinson JGP (1972). Characteristics of some co-trimoxazole-resistant Enterobacteriaceae from infected patients. *J Clin Path* **25**: 1086.

Barrow GI, Hewitt M (1971). Skin infection with *Mycobacterium marinum* from a tropical fish tank. *Brit Med J* **2**: 505.

Bartlett MS, Smith JW (1991). *Pneumocystis carinii*, an opportunist in immunocompromised patients. *Clin Microbiol Rev* **4**: 137.

Bassett DCJ (1971). The sensitivity of *Pseudomonas pseudomallei* to trimethoprim and sulfamethoxazole in vitro. *J Clin Path* **24**: 798.

Beaman MH, Luft BJ, Remington JS (1992). Prophylaxis for toxoplasmosis in AIDS. *Ann Intern Med* **117**: 163.

Behets FM, Liomba G, Lule G et al. (1995). Sexually transmitted diseases and human immunodeficiency virus control in Malawi: a field study of genital ulcer disease. *J. Infect Dis* **171**: 451.

Bengtsson E, Svanbom M, Tunevall G (1974). Trimethoprim-sulfamethoxazole treatment in staphylococcal endocarditis and Gram-negative septicaemia. *Scand J Infect Dis* **6**: 177.

Bennett JE, Jennings AE (1978). Factors influencing susceptibility of *Nocardia* species to trimethoprim-sulfamethoxazole. *Antimicrob Ag Chemother* **13**: 624.

Bennett WM, Craven R (1976). Urinary tract infections in patients with severe renal disease. Treatment with ampicillin and trimethoprim-sulfamethoxazole. *JAMA* **236**: 946.

Bennish ML, Salam MA (1992). Rethinking options for the treatment of shigellosis. *J Antimicrob Chemother* **30**: 243.

Bennish, ML, Salam, MA, Hossain MA et al. (1992). Antimicrobial resistance of *Shigella* isolates in Bangladesh, 1983–1990: increasing frequency of strains multiply resistant to ampicillin, trimethoprim-sulfamethoxazole, and nalidixic acid. *Clin Infect Dis* **14**: 1055.

Bergan T, Brodwall EK (1976). The pharmacokinetic profile of co-trimoxazole. *Scand J Infect Dis* (Suppl 8): 42.

Bergeron MG (1985). Therpeutic potential of high renal levels of aminoglycosides in pyelonephritis. *J Antimicrob Chemother* **15**: 4.

Berkey P, Bodey GP (1989). Nocardial infection in patients with neoplastic disease. *Rev Infect Dis* **11**: 407.

Bernard EM, Edwards FF, Kiehn TE et al. (1993). Activities of antimicrobial agents against clinical isolates of *Mycobacterium haemophilum*. *Antimicrob Ag Chemother* **37**: 2323.

Bernstein LS (1982). Combination of trimethoprim with sulfonamides other than sulfamethoxazole. *Rev Infect Dis* **4**: 411.

Biosca M, de la Figuera M, Garcia-Brigado F, Sampol G (1986). Aseptic meningitis due to trimethoprim-sulfamethoxazole. *J Neurol Neurosurg Psychiat* **46**: 332.

Bissuel F, Cotte L, Crapanne JB et al. (1995). Trimethoprim-sulfamethoxazole rechallenge in 20 previously allergic HIV- infected patients after homeopathic. *AIDS* **9**: 407.

Black JR, Feinberg J, Murphy RL et al. (1994). Clindamycin and primaquine therapy for mild-to-moderate episodes of *Pneumocystis carinii* pneumonia in patients with AIDS: AIDS Clinical Trials Group 044. *Clin Infect Dis* **18**: 905.

Blum, R N, Miller, L A, Gaggini, L C et al. (1992). Comparative trial of dapsone versus trimethoprim/sulfamethoxazole for primary prophylaxis of *Pneumocystis carinii* pneumonia. *J AIDS* **5**: 341.

Blumer JL, Bertino JS, Husak MP (1984). Comparison of cefaclor and trimethoprim-sulfamethoxazole in the treatment of acute otitis media. *Pediatr Infect Dis* **3**: 25.

Bogaerts J, Kestens L, Martinez Tello W et al. (1995). Failure of treatment for chancroid in Rwanda is not related to human immunodeficiency virus infection: *in vitro* resistance of *Haemophilus ducreyi* to trimethoprim-sulfamethoxazole. *Clin Infect Dis* **20**: 924.

Bogue CW, Wise JD, Gray GF, Edwards KM (1989). Antibiotic therapy for cat-scratch disease? *JAMA* **262**: 813.

Borucki MJ, Matzke DS, Pollard RB (1988). Tremor induced by trimethoprim-sulfamethoxazole in patients with the acquired immunodeficiency syndrome (AIDS). *Ann Intern Med* **109**: 77.

Böse W, Karama A, Linzenmeier G et al. (1974). Controlled trial of co-trimoxazole in children with urinary-tract infections. Bacteriological efficacy and haematological toxicity. *Lancet* **ii**: 614.

Bow EJ, Ronald AR (1993). Antibacterial chemoprophylaxis in neutropenic patients – where do we go from here? *Clin Infect Dis* **17**: 333.

Bow EJ, Louie TJ, Riben PD et al. (1984). Randomized controlled trial comparing trimemthoprim/sulfamethoxazole and trimethoprim for infection prophylaxis in hospitalized granulocytopenic patients. *Amer J Med* **76**: 223.

Bow EJ, Rayner E, Scott BA, Louie TJ (1987). Selective gut decontamination with nalidixic acid or trimethoprim-sulfamethoxazole for infection prophylaxis in neutropenic cancer patients: relationship of efficacy to antimicrobial spectrum and timing of administration. *Antimicrob Ag Chemother* **31**: 551.

Bow EJ, Rayner E, Louie TJ (1988). Comparison of norfloxacin with co-trimoxazole for infection prophylaxis in acute leukemia The trade-off for reduced Gram-negative sepsis. *Amer J Med* **84**: 847.

Boyce TG, Smidt RG, Edmonson MB (1992). Fever as an adverse reaction to oral trimethoprim-sulfamethoxazole therapy. *Pediatr Infect Dis J* **11**: 772.

Bozzette SA, Sattler FR, Chiu J et al. (1990). A controlled trial of early adjunctive treatment with corticosteroids for *Pneumocystis carinii* pneumonia in the acquired immunodeficiency syndrome California Collaborative Treatment Group. *New Engl J Med* **323**: 1451.

Bozzette SA, Finkelstein DM, Spector SA et al. (1995a). A randomized trial of three antipneumocystis agents in patients with advanced human immunodeficiency virus infection. NIAID AIDS Clinical Trials Group. *New Engl J Med* **332**: 693.

Bozzette SA, Forthal D, Sattler FR et al. (1995b). The tolerance for zidovudine plus thrice weekly or daily trimethoprim- sulfamethoxazole with and without leucovorin for primary prophylaxis in advanced HIV disease. California Collaborative Treatment Group. *Amer J Med* **98**: 177.

Bradley PP, Warden GD, Maxwell JG, Rothstein G (1980). Neutropenia and thrombocytopenia in renal allograft recipients treated with trimethoprim-sulfamethoxazole. *Ann Intern Med* **93**: 560.

Bratoeva MP, John JF Jr (1989). Dissemination of trimethoprim-resistant clones of *Shigella sonnei* in Bulgaria. *J Infect Dis* **159**: 648.

Breeze AS, Sims P, Stacey KA (1975). Trimethoprim-resistant mutants of *E coli* K12: preliminary genetic mapping. *Genet Res* **25**: 207.

Breiman RF, Butler JC, Tenover FC et al. (1994). Emergence of drug-resistant pneumococcal infections in the United States. *JAMA* **271**: 1831.

Brenner M, Ognibene FP, Lack EE et al. (1987). Prognostic factors and life expectancy of patients with acquired immunodeficiency syndrome and *Pneumocystis carinii* pneumonia. *Amer Rev Respir Dis* **136**: 1199.

Briggs AE, Robinson MF (1975). *Salmonella* meningitis treatment with intravenous trimethoprim. *Aust NZ J Med* **5**: 364.

Brodie J, Macqueen IA, Livingstone D (1970). Effects of trimethoprim-sulfamethoxazole on typhoid and *Salmonella* carriers. *Brit Med J* **3**: 318.

Brodie MJ, Boot PA, Girdwood RWA (1973). Severe *Yersinia* pseudotuberculosis infection diagnosed at laparoscopy. *Brit Med J* **4**: 88.

Brumfitt W, Pursell R (1972). Double-blind trial to compare ampicillin, cephalexin, co-trimoxazole and trimethoprim in treatment of urinary infection. *Brit Med J* **2**: 673.

Brumfitt W, Faiers MC, Pursell RE et al. (1969). Bacteriological, pharmacological and clinical studies with trimethoprim-sulfamethoxazole combinations – with particular reference to the treatment of urinary infections. *Postgrad Med J* **45** (Suppl): 56.

Brumfitt W, Hamilton-Miller JMT, Havard CW, Tansley H (1985a). Trimethoprim alone compared to co-trimoxazole in lower respiratory infections: pharmacokinetics and clinical effectiveness. *Scand J Infect Dis* **17**: 99.

Brumfitt W, Smith GW, Hamilton-Miller JMT, Gargan RA (1985b). A clinical comparison between macrodantin and trimethoprim for prophylaxis in women with recurrent urinary infections. *J Antimicrob Chemother* **16**: 111.

Brunham RC, Kuo C-C, Stevens CE, Holmes KK (1982). Treatment of concomitant *Neisseria gonorrhoeae* and *Chlamydia trachomatis* infections in women: comparison of trimethoprim-sulfamethoxazole with ampicillin-probenecid. *Rev Infect Dis* **4**: 491.

Bruun JN, Østby N, Bredesen JE *et al.* (1981). Sulfonamide and trimethoprim concentrations in human serum and skin blister fluid. *Antimicrob Ag Chemother* **19**: 82.

Buckwold FJ, Ludwig P, Harding GKM *et al.* (1982). Therapy for acute cystitis in adult women. Randomized comparison of single-dose sulfisoxazole vs trimethoprim-sulfamethoxazole. *JAMA* **247**: 1839.

Burack JH, Hahn JA, Saint-Maurice D, Jacobson MA (1994). Microbiology of community-acquired bacterial pneumonia in persons with and at risk for human immunodeficiency virus type 1 infection. Implications for rational empiric antibiotic therapy. *Arch Intern Med* **154**: 2589.

Burchall JJ (1979). The development of the diaminopyrimidines. *J Antimicrob Chemother* **5** (Suppl B): 3.

Burgos A, Quindos G, Martinez R *et al.* (1990). *In vitro* susceptibility of *Aeromonas caviae*, *Aeromonas hydrophila* and *Aeromonas sabina* to fifteen antibacterial agents. *Eur J Clin Microbiol Infect Dis* **9**: 413.

Burns JL, Lien DM, Hedin LA (1989). Isolation and characterization of dihydrofolate reductase from trimethoprim-susceptible and trimethoprim-resistant *Pseudomonas cepacia*. *Antimicrob Ag Chemother* **33**: 1247.

Bushby SRM (1969). Combined antibacterial action *in vitro* of trimethoprim and sulphonamides. *Postgrad Med J* **45** (Suppl): 10.

Bushby SRM (1973). Trimethoprim-sulfamethoxazole: *in vitro* microbiological aspects. *J Infect Dis* **128** (Suppl): 442.

Bushby SRM, Hitchings GH (1968). Trimethoprim, a sulphonamide potentiator. *Brit J Pharmacol Chemother* **33**: 72.

Busk HE, Korner B (1980). Trimethoprim resistance in Finland. *Brit Med J* **1**: 1054.

Butler T, Bell WR, Linh NN *et al.* (1974). *Yersinia* pestis infection in Vietnam. I. Clinical and haematological aspects. *J Infect Dis* **129** (Suppl): 78.

Butler T, Levin J, Linh NN *et al.* (1976). *Yersinia pestis* infection in Vietnam. II.-Quantitative blood cultures and detection of endotoxin in the cerebrospinal fluid of patients with meningitis. *J Infect Dis* **133**: 493.

Butler T, Linh NN, Arnold K *et al.* (1977). Therapy of antimicrobial-resistant typhoid fever. *Antimicrob Ag Chemother* **11**: 645.

Butler T, Rumans L, Arnold K (1982). Response of typhoid fever caused by chloramphenicol-susceptible and chloramphenicol-resistant strains of *Salmonella typhi* to treatment with trimethoprim-sulfamethoxazole. *Rev Infect Dis* **4**: 551.

Bygbjerg IC, Lund JT, Hording M (1988). Effect of folic and folinic acid on cytopenia occurring during co-trimoxazole treatment of *Pneumocystis carinii* pneumonia. *Scand J Infect Dis* **20**: 685.

Bywater MJ, Holt HA, Reeves DS (1979). Activity *in vitro* of tetroxoprim-sulphadiazine. *J Antimicrob Chemother* **5** (Suppl B): 51.

Cameron A, Thomas M (1977). Pseudomembranous colitis and co-trimoxazole. *Brit Med J* **1**: 1321.

Campbell H, Byass P, Forgie IM *et al.* (1988). Trial of co-trimoxazole versus procaine penicillin with ampicillin in treatment of community-acquired pneumonia in young Gambian children. *Lancet* **ii**: 1182.

Campos J, Garcia-Tornel S, Sanfeliu I (1984). Susceptibility studies of multiply resistant *Haemophilus influenzae* isolated from pediatric patients and contacts. *Antimicrob Ag Chemother* **25**: 706.

Canaday DH, Johnson JR (1994). Hyperkalemia in elderly patients receiving standard doses of trimethoprim- sulfamethoxazole. *Ann Intern Med* **120**: 437.

Carlson P, Kontiainen S, Renkonen OV (1994). Antimicrobial susceptibility of *Arcanobacterium haemolyticum*. *Antimicrob Ag Chemother* **38**: 142.

Carr A, Tindall B, Brew BJ (1992a). Low dose trimethoprim-sulfamethoxazole prophylaxis for toxoplasmic encephalitis in patients with AIDS. *Ann Intern Med* **117**: 106.

Carr, A, Tindall, B, Penny, R, Cooper DA (1992b). Trimethoprim-sulfamethoxazole appears more effective than aerosolized pentamidine as secondary prophylaxis against *Pneumocystis carinii* pneumonia in patients with AIDS. *AIDS* **6**: 165.

Carr A, Swanson C, Penny R *et al.* (1993). Clinical and laboratory markers of hypersensitivity to trimethoprim-sulfamethoxazole in patients with *Pneumocystis carinii* pneumonia and AIDS. *J Infect Dis* **167**: 180.

Carroll BRT, Nicol CS (1970). Trimethoprim/sulfamethoxazole in the treatment of non-gonococcal urethritis and gonorrhoea. *Brit J Vener Dis* **46**: 31.

Cash RA, Northrup RS, Rahman ASMM (1973). Trimethoprim and sulfamethoxazole in clinical cholera: comparison with tetracycline. *J Infect Dis* **128** (Suppl): 749.

Cattell WR, Chamberlain DA, Fry IK *et al.* (1971). Long-term control of bacteriuria with trimethoprim-sulfamethoxazole. *Brit Med J* **1**: 377.

Caumes E, Roudier C, Rogeaux O, Bricaire F, Gentilini M (1994). Effect of corticosteroids on the incidence of adverse cutaneous reactions to trimethoprim-sulfamethoxazole during treatment of AIDS-associated *Pneumocystis carinii* pneumonia. *Clin Infect Dis* **18**: 319.

CDC (Centers for Disease Control) (1982). Sexually transmitted diseases treatment guidlines. *MMWR* **31**: 39S.

CDC (Centers for Disease Control) (1985a). 1985 STD treatment guidelines. *MMWR* **34** (Suppl): 4S.

CDC (Centers for Disease Control) (1985b). Chancroid – Massachusetts. *MMWR* **34**: 711.

CDC (Centers for Disease Control) (1987). Nationwide dissemination of multiply resistant *Shigella sonnei* following a common-source outbreak. *MMWR* **36**: 633.

CDC (Centers for Disease Control) (1989a). Sexually transmitted diseases treatment guidelines. *MMWR* **38** (Suppl 8): 54.

CDC (Centers for Disease Control) (1989b). Guidelines for prophylaxis against *Pneumocystis carinii* pneumonia for persons infected with human immunodeficiency virus. *MMWR* **38** (Suppl 5): 1.

CDC (Centers for Disease Control) (1991). Guidelines for prophylaxis against *Pneumocystis carinii* pneumonia for children infected with human immunodeficiency virus. *MMWR* **2**: 1.

CDC (Centers for Disease Control) (1992). Recommendations for prophylaxis against *Pneumocystis carinii* pneumonia for adults and adolescents infected with human immunodeficiency virus. *MMWR* **41** (RR 4): 1.

CDC (Centers for Disease Control) (1993). Sexually transmitted diseases treatment guidelines. *MMWR* **42** (Suppl. RR-14): 1.

CDC (Centers for Disease Control) (1995). 1995 revised guidelines for prophylaxis against *Pneumocystis carinii* pneumonia for children infected with or perinatally exposed to human immunodeficiency virus National Pediatric and Family HIV Resource Center and National Center for Infectious Diseases, Centers for Disease Control and Prevention. *MMWR* **44**: 1.

Chan ACH, Forrest CR, Robertson MJ (1973). A fourteen-day treatment of typhoid carriers in Hong Kong with trimethoprim-sulfamethoxazole. *Med J Aust* **1**: 386.

Chan MCK, Wong HB (1975). Glucose-6-phosphate dehydrogenase deficiency and co-trimoxazole. *Lancet* **i**: 410.

Chanarin I, England JM (1972). Toxicity of trimethoprim-sulfamethoxazole in patients with megaloblastic haemopoiesis. *Brit Med J* **1**: 651.

Chang MJ, Dunkle LM, Van Reken D *et al.* (1977). Trimethoprim-sulfamethoxazole compared to ampicillin in the treatment of shigellosis. *Pediatrics* **59**: 726.

Chang, WJ, Goetz, MB (1992). Response to treatment of infection due to *Mycobacterium avium* complex with trimethoprim-sulfamethoxazole. *Clin Infect Dis* **14**: 1267.

Chaowagul W, Suputtamongkol Y, Dance DA *et al.* (1993). Relapse in melioidosis: incidence and risk factors. *J Infect Dis* **168**: 1181.

Chapman SW, Wilson JP (1990). Nocardiosis in transplant recipients. *Semin Resp Infect* **5**: 74.

Charpentier E, Gerbaud G, Jacquet C, Rocourt J, Courvalin P (1995). Incidence of antibiotic resistance in *Listeria* species. *J Infect Dis* **172**: 277.

Chaudray S, Turner RB (1981). Trimethoprim-sulfamethoxazole for cholangitis following hepatic portoenterostomy for biliary atresia. *J Pediatrics* **99**: 656.

Chenoweth CE, Robinson KA, Schaberg DR (1990). Efficacy of ampicillin versus trimethoprim-sulfamethoxazole in a mouse model of lethal enterococcal peritonitis. *Antimicrob Ag Chemother* **34**: 1800.

Cherchi GB, Pacifico L, Cossellu S *et al.* (1995). Prospective study of *Yersinia enterocolitica* infection in thalassemic patients. *Pediatr Infect Dis J* **14**: 579.

Chin TW, Vandenbroucke A, Fong IW (1995). Pharmacokinetics of trimethoprim-sulfamethoxazole in critically ill and non-critically ill AIDS patients. *Antimicrob Ag Chemother* **39**: 28.

Chinn RH, Maskell R, Mead JA, Polak A (1976). Renal stones and urinary infection: a study of antibiotic treatment. *Brit Med J* **2**: 1411.

Choi MJ, Fernandes PC, Patnaik A *et al.* (1993). Trimethoprim-induced hyperkalemia in a patient with AIDS. *New Engl J Med* **328**: 703.

Chow AW, Jewesson PJ (1985). Pharmacokinetics and safety of anti-microbial agents during pregnancy. *Rev Infect Dis* **7**: 287.

Claas FHJ, Van der Meer JWM, Langerak J (1979). Immunological effect of co-trimoxazole on platelets. *Brit Med J* **2**: 898.

Clasener HA, Vollaard EJ, van-Saene HK (1987). Long-term prophylaxis of infection by selective decontamination in leukopenia and in mechanical ventilation. *Rev Infect Dis* **9**: 295.

Climax J, Lenehan TJ, Lambe R *et al.* (1986). Interaction of antimicrobial agents with human peripheral blood leucocytes: uptake and intracellular localization of certain sulphonamides and trimethoprim. *J Antimicrob Chemother* **17**: 489.

Cockerill FR, Edson RS (1991), Trimethoprim – sulfamethoxazole. *Mayo Clin Proc* **66**: 1260.

Cockerill FR, Edson RS, Roberts GD, Waldorf JC (1984). Trimethoprim/sulfamethoxazole-resistant *Nocardia asteroides* causing multiple hepatic abscesses. Successful treatment with ampicillin, amikacin and limited computed tomography-guided needle aspiration. *Amer J Med* **77**: 558.

Colebunders R, Izaley L, Bila K *et al.* (1987). Cutaneous reactions to trimethoprim sulfamethoxazole in African patients with acquired immunodeficiency syndrome. *Ann Intern Med* **107**: 599 .

Collignon PJ, Bell JM (1996). Drug-resistant *Streptococcus pneumoniae*: the beginning of the end for many antibiotics? Australian Group on Antimicrobial Resistance (AGAR). *Med J Aust* **164**: 64.

Collignon, PJ, Bell, JM, MacInnes, SJ *et al.* (1992). A national collaborative study of resistance to antimicrobial agents in *Haemophilus influenzae* in Australian hospitals The Australian Group for Antimicrobial Resistance (AGAR). *J Antimicrob Chemother* **30**: 153.

Collipp PJ (1992). Cat-scratch disease: therapy with trimethoprim-sulfamethoxazole. *Am J Dis Child* **146**: 397.

Colucci CF, Cicero ML (1975). Hepatic necrosis and trimethoprim-sulfamethoxazole. *JAMA* **233**: 952.

Conte JE Jr (1991). Pharmacokinetics of intravenous pentamidine in patients with normal renal function or receiving hemodialysis. *J Infect Dis* **163**: 169.

Conte JE Jr, Upton RA, Phelps RT *et al.* (1986). Use of a specific and sensitive assay to determine pentamidine pharmacokinetics in patients with AIDS. *J Infect Dis* **154**: 923 .

Conte JE Jr, Chernoff D, Feigal DW Jr *et al.* (1990). Intravenous or inhaled pentamidine for treating *Pneumocystis carinii* pneumonia in AIDS: a randomized trial. *Ann Intern Med* **113**: 203.

Cooper RG, Wald M (1964). Successful treatment of *Proteus* septicaemia with a new drug, trimethoprim. *Med J Aust* **2**: 93.

Coughter JP, Johnston JL, Archer GL (1987). Characterization of a staphylococcal trimethoprim resistance gene and its product. *Antimicrob Ag Chemother* **31**: 1027.

Counts GW, Stamm WE, McKevitt M *et al.* (1982). Treatment of cystitis in women with a single dose of trimethoprim-sulfamethoxazole. *Rev Infect Dis* **4**: 484.

Craig WA, Kunin CM (1973a). Trimethoprim-sulfamethoxazole: pharmacodynamic effects of urinary pH and impaired renal function. *Ann Intern Med* **78**: 491.

Craig WA, Kunin CM (1973b). Distribution of trimethoprim-sulfamethoxazole in tissues of rhesus monkeys. *J Infect Dis* **128** (Suppl): 575.

Craven JL, Pugsley DJ, Blowers R (1970). Trimethoprim-sulfamethoxazole in acute osteomyelitis due to penicillin-resistant staphylococci in Uganda. *Brit Med J* **3**: 201.

Crider SR, Colby SD (1985). Suceptibility of enterococci to trimethoprim and trimethoprim-sulfamethoxazole. *Antimicrob Ag Chemother* **27**: 71.

Csángó PA, Salveson A, Gundersen T *et al.* (1984). Treatment of acute gonococcal urethritis in men with simultaneous infection with *Chlamydia trachomatis*. *Brit J Vener Dis* **60**: 95.

Csonka GW, (1969). Therapeutic trial of some genital infections with trimethoprim-sulfamethoxazole. *Postgrad Med J* **45** (Suppl): 77.

Csonka GW, Knight GJ (1967). Therapeutic trial of trimethoprim as a potentiator of sulphonamides in gonorrhoea. *Brit J Vener Dis* **43**: 161.

Daikos GK, Papapolyzos N, Marketos N *et al.* (1973). Trimethoprim-sulfamethoxazole in brucellosis. *J Infect Dis* **128** (Suppl): 731.

Damergis JA, Stoker JM, Abadie JL (1983). Methemglobinemia after sulfamethoxazole and trimethoprim therapy. *JAMA* **249**: 590.

Dance, DA, Wuthiekanun, V, Chaowagul, W *et al.* (1989). The antimicrobial susceptibility of *Pseudomonas pseudomallei*. Emergence of resistance *in vitro* and during treatment. *J Antimicrob Chemother* **24**: 295.

Dangor Y, Ballard RC, Miller SD, Koornhof HJ (1990a). Antimicrobial susceptibility of *Haemophilu ducreyi*. *Antimicrob Ag Chemother* **34**: 1303.

Dangor Y, Ballard RC, Miller SD, Koornhof HJ (1990b). Treatment of chancroid. *Antimicrob Ag Chemother* **34**: 1308.

Darby CP (1976). Treating *Pseudomonas cepacia* meningitis with trimethoprim-sulfamethoxazole. *Amer J Dis Child* **130**: 1365.

Darrell JH,Garrod LP, Waterworth PM (1968). Trimethoprim: laboratory and clinical studies. *J Clin Path* **21**: 202.

Dathan JRE, Heyworth MF (1975). Glomerulonephritis associated with *Coxiella burnetti* endocarditis. *Brit Med J* **1**: 376.

Davey RJ, Masur H (1990). Recent advances in the diagnosis, treatment, and prevention of *Pneumocystis carinii* pneumonia. *Antimicrob Ag Chemother* **34**: 499.

Davis RE, Jackson JM (1973). Trimethoprim/sulfamethoxazole and folate metabolism. *Pathology* **5**: 23.

Dawborn JK, Castaldi PA, Kilgour A *et al.* (1973). The prolonged use of trimethoprim/sulphonamide in urinary infection. *Med J Aust* **1** (Special Suppl): 52.

De Buse PJ, Henderson A, White M (1975). Melioidosis in a child in Papua New Guinea. Successful treatment with kanamycin and trimethoprim-sulfamethoxazole. *Med J Aust* **2**: 476.

De Hovitz JA, Pape JW, Boncy M, Johnson WD, Jr (1986). Clinical manifestations and therapy of *I belli* infection in patients with the acquired immunodeficiency syndrome. *New Engl J Med* **315**: 87.

de Gorgolas M, Aviles P, Verdejo C, Fernandez Guerrero ML (1995). Treatment of experimental endocarditis due to methicillin-susceptible or methicillin-resistant *Staphylococcus aureus* with trimethoprim- sulfamethoxazole and antibiotics that inhibit cell wall synthesis. *Antimicrob Ag Chemother* **39**: 953.

de Groot R, Campos, J, Moseley, SL, Smith AL (1988). Molecular cloning and mechanism of trimethoprim resistance in *Haemophilus influenzae*. *Antimicrob Ag Chemother* **32**: 477.

Dekker AW, Rozenberg-Arska M, Sixma JJ, Verhoef J (1981). Prevention of infection by trimethoprim-sulfamethoxazole plus amphotericin B in patients with acute nonlymphocytic leukaemia. *Ann Intern Med* **95**: 555.

Dekker AW, Rozenberg-Arska M, Verhoef J (1987). Infection prophylaxis in acute leukemia: a comparison of ciprofloxacin with trimethoprim-sulfamethoxazole and colistin. *Ann Intern Med* **106**: 7.

Delgado R, Otero JR (1988). High-level resistance to trimethoprim in *Shigella sonnei* associated with plasmid-encoded dihydrofolate reductase type I. *Antimicrob Ag Chemother* **32**: 1598.

Denneberg T, Ekberg M, Ericson C, Hanson A (1976). Co-trimoxazole in long-term treatment of pyelonephritis with normal and impaired renal function. *Scand. J Infect Dis* (Suppl 8): 61.

DeRemee RA (1988). The treatment of Wegener's granulomatosis with trimethoprim/sulfamethoxazole: illusion or vision? *Arthritis Rheum* **31**: 1068.

DeRemee, RA (1992). Wegeners granulomatosis. *Ann Intern Med* **117**: 619.

De Vito GA Jr (1982). Transient elevation of alkaline phosphatase possibly related to trimethoprim-sulfamethoxazole therapy. *J Pediatrics* **100**: 998.

De Vries-Hospers HG, Sleijfer DT, Mulder NH *et al.* (1981). Bacteriological aspects of selective decontamination of the digestive tract as a method of infection prevention in granulocytopenic patients. *Antimicrob Ag Chemother* **19**: 813.

Dewsnup DH, Wright DN (1984). *In vitro* susceptibility of *Nocardia asteroides* to 25 antimicrobial agents. *Antimicrob Ag Chemother* **25**: 165.

Dickson HG (1978). Trimethoprim-sulfamethoxazole and thrombocytopenia. *Med J Aust* **2**: 5.

Doern GV (1995). Trends in antimicrobial susceptibility of bacterial pathogens of the respiratory tract. *Amer J Med* **99**: 3S.

Domingo P, Ferrer S, Cruz J *et al.* (1995). Trimethoprim-sulfamethoxazole-induced renal tubular acidosis in a patient with AIDS. *Clin Infect Dis* **20**: 1435.

Drake S, Lampasona V, Nicks HL, Schwarzmann SW (1985). Pentamidine isethionate in the treatment of *Pneumocystis carinii* pneumonia. *Clin Pharm* **4**: 507.

Dudley MN, Levitz RE, Quintiliani R *et al.* (1984). Pharmacokinetics of trimethoprim and sulfamethoxazole in serum and cerebrospinal fluid of adult patients with normal meninges. *Antimicrob Ag Chemother* **26**: 811.

Dummer JS (1990). *Pneumocystis carinii* infections in transplant patients. *Semin Resp Infect* **5**: 50.

DuPont HL, Ericsson CD (1993). Prevention and treatment of traveller's diarrhea. *New Engl J Med* **328**: 1821.

DuPont HL, West H, Evans DG *et al.* (1978). Antimicrobial susceptibility of enterotoxigenic *Escherichia coli*. *J Antimicrob Chemother* **4**: 100.

DuPont HL, Evans DG, Rios N *et al.* (1982a). Prevention of travellers' diarrhea with trimethoprim-sulfamethoxazole. *Rev Infect Dis* **4**: 533.

DuPont HL, Rebes RR, Galindo E *et al.* (1982b). Treatment of travellers' diarrhea with trimethoprim/sulfamethoxazole and with trimethoprim alone. *New Engl J Med* **307**: 841.

DuPont HL, Galindo E, Evans DG *et al.* (1983). Prevention of travellers' diarrhoea with trimethoprim-sulfamethoxazole and trimethoprim alone. *Gastroenterology* **84**: 75.

Dupont MJ, Jouvenot M, Couetdic G, Michel-Briand Y (1985). Development of plasmid-mediated resistance in *Vibrio cholerae* during treatment with trimethoprim-sulfamethoxazole. *Antimicrob Ag Chemother* **27**: 280.

Dylewski J, Nsanze H, D'Costa L *et al.* (1985). Trimethoprim sulphamoxazole in the treatment of chancroid Comparison of two single dose treatment regimens with a five day regimen. *J Antimicrob Chemother* **16**: 103.

Dylewski J, D'Costa LJ, Nsanze H, Ronald AR (1986). Single-dose therapy with trimethoprim-sulfametrole for chancroid in females. *Sexually Transmitted Diseases* **13**: 166.

Eady EA, Holland KT, Cunliffe WJ (1982). The use of antibiotics in acne therapy: oral or topical administration? *J Antimicrob Chemother* **10**: 89.

Edman JC, Kovacs JA, Masur H *et al.* (1988). Ribosomal RNA sequence shows *Pneumocystis carinii* to be a member of the Fungi. *Nature* **334**: 519.

Egere JU, Gugnani HC, Okoro AN, Suseelan AV (1978). African histoplasmosis in Eastern Nigeria: report of two culturally proven cases treated with septrin and amphotericin B. *J Trop Med Hyg* **81**: 225.

Ekwall E, Jonsson M (1984). A comparison of the combination pivmecillinam/pivampicillin and co-trimoxazole in the treatment of convalescent carriers of *Salmonella* and *Shigella*. *Scand J Infect Dis* **16**: 99.

Ellerstein NS, Sullivan TD, Baliah T, Neter E (1977). Trimethoprim/sulfamethoxazole and ampicillin in the treatment of acute urinary tract infections in children: a double-blind study. *Pediatrics* **60**: 245.

Enno A, Catovsky D, Darrell J *et al.* (1978). Co-trimoxazole for prevention of infection in acute leukaemia. *Lancet* **ii**: 395.

EORTC International Antimicrobial Therapy Project Group (1984). Trimethoprim/sulfamethoxazole in the prevention of infection in neutropenic patients. *J Infect Dis* **150**: 372.

Ericsson, CD, DuPont, HL, Mathewson, JJ *et al.* (1990). Treatment of traveler's diarrhea with sulfamethoxazole and trimethoprim and loperamide. *JAMA* **263**: 257.

Ericsson, CD, Nicholls, VI, DuPont, HL *et al.* (1992). Optimal dosing of trimethoprim-sulfamethoxazole when used with loperamide to treat traveler's diarrhea. *Antimicrob Ag Chemother* **36**: 2821.

Estey E, Maksymiuk A, Smith T *et al.* (1984). Infection prophylaxis in acute leukemia. Comparative effectiveness of sulfamethoxazole and trimethoprim, ketoconazole, and a combination of the two. *Arch Intern Med* **144**: 1562.

Evans DIK, Tell R (1969). Agranulocytosis after trimethoprim and sulfamethoxazole. *Brit Med J* **1**: 578.

Everett ED, Kishimoto RA (1973). *In vitro* sensitivity of 33 strains of *Pseudomonas pseudomallei* to trimethoprim and sulfamethoxazole. *J Infect Dis* **128** (Suppl): 539.

Falloon J, Kovacs J, Hughes W *et al.* (1991). A preliminary evaluation of 566C80 for the treatment of pneumocystis pneumonia in patients with the acquired immunodeficiency syndrome. *New Engl J Med* **325**: 1534.

Fan H, Brunham RC, McClarty G (1992). Acquisition and synthesis of folates by obligate intracellular bacteria of the genus *Chlamydia*. *J Clin Invest* **90**: 1803.

Farid Z, Hassan A, Wahab MFA, Sanborn WR *et al.* (1970). Trimethoprim-sulfamethoxazole in enteric fevers. *Brit Med J* **3**: 323.

Farid Z, Girgis NI, Yassin W *et al.* (1976). Trimethoprim-sulfamethoxazole and bacterial meningitis. *Ann Intern Med* **84**: 50.

Farina C, Boiron P, Goglio A, Provost F (1995). Human nocardiosis in northern Italy from 1982 to 1992. Northern Italy Collaborative Group on Nocardiosis. *Scand J Infect Dis* **27**: 23.

Fass RJ, Prior RB, Perkins RL (1977). Pharmacokinetics and tolerance of a single twelve-tablet dose of trimethoprim (960 mg) -sulfamethoxazole (4800 mg). *Antimicrob Ag Chemother* **12**: 102.

Feldman HA (1973a). Effects of trimethoprim and sulfisoxazole, alone and in combination, on growth and carriage of *Neisseria meningitidis*. *J Infect Dis* **128**: (Suppl) 723.

Feldman HA (1973b). Effects of trimethoprim and sulfisoxazole alone and in combination on murine toxoplasmosis. *J Infect Dis* **128** (Suppl): 774.

Ferrazzini G, Klein J, Sulh H *et al.* (1990). Interaction between trimethoprim-sulfamethoxazole and methotrexate in children with leukemia. *J Pediatr* **117**: 823.

Fihn SD, Johnson C, Roberts PL *et al.* (1988). Trimethoprim-sulfamethoxazole for acute dysuria in women: a single dose or 10 day course. A double-blind, randomized trial. *Ann Intern Med* **108**: 350.

Filice GA, Simpson GL (1984). Management of *Nocardia* infections. In *Current Clinical Topics in Infectious Disease* (Remington JS, Swartz MN, eds), pp. 49–64. New York: McGraw-Hill.

Fischl MA (1988). Treatment and prophylaxis of *Pneumocystis carinii* pneumonia. *AIDS* **2** (Suppl 1): S143.

Fischl, MA, Dickinson, GM La, VL (1988). Safety and efficacy of sulfamethoxazole and trimethoprim chemoprophylaxis for *Pneumocystis carinii* pneumonia in AIDS. *JAMA* **259**: 1185.

Fleming AF, Warrell DA, Dickmeiss H (1974). Co-trimoxazole and the blood. *Lancet* **ii**: 284.

Forbes GM, Harvey FAH, Philpott-Howard JN *et al.* (1990). Nocardiosis in liver transplantion: variation in presentation, diagnosis and therapy. *J Infect* **20**: 11.

Fox BC, Sollinger HW, Belzer FO, Maki DG (1990). A prospective, randomized, double-blind study of trimethoprim-sulfamethoxazole for prophylaxis of infection in renal transplantation: clinical efficacy, absorption of trimethoprim-sulfamethoxazole, effects on the microflora, and the cost-benefit of prophylaxis. *Am J Med* **89**: 255.

Franzén C, Brandberg A (1976). Co-trimoxazole in cases of Gram-negative septicaemia. *Scand J Infect Dis* (Suppl 8): 96.

Franzén C, Lidin-Janson G, Nygren B (1972 Trimethoprim/sulfamethoxazole in enteric infections. *Scand J Infect Dis* 4: 231.

Freeman R, Hodson ME (1972). Q fever endocarditis treated with trimethoprim and sulfamethoxazole. *Brit Med J* 1: 419.

Frisch JM (1973). Clinical experience with adverse reactions to trimethoprim-sulfamethoxazole. *J Infect Dis* 128 (Suppl): 607.

Fuller PB, Fisk DE, Byrd RB *et al.* (1978). Treatment of pulmonary meliodosis with combination of trimethoprim and sulfamethoxazole. *Chest* 74: 222 .

Fulton B, Wagstaff AJ, McTavish D (1995). Trimetrexate A review of its pharmacodynamic and pharmacokinetic properties and therapeutic potential in the treatment of *Pneumocystis carinii* pneumonia. *Drugs* 49: 563.

Fung, CP, Powell, M, Seymour, A *et al.* (1992). The antimicrobial susceptibility of *Moraxella catarrhalis* isolated in England and Scotland in 1991. *J Antimicrob Chemother* 30: 47.

Gagnon S, Boota AM, Fischl MA (1990). Corticosteroids as adjunctive therapy for severe *Pneumocystis carinii* pneumonia in the acquired immunodeficiency syndrome. A double-blind, placebo-controlled trial. *New Engl J Med* 323: 1444.

Galetto DW, Johnston JL, Archer GL (1987). Molecular epidemiology of trimethoprim resistance among coagulase-negative staphylococci. *Antimicrob Ag Chemother* 31: 1683.

Garay SM, Greene J (1989). Prognostic indicators in the initial presentation of *Pneumocystis carinii* pneumonia. *Chest* 95: 769.

Garcia-Rodriguez JA, Garcia-Sanchez JE, Garcia-Garcia MI *et al.* (1991). Antibiotic susceptibility profile of *Xanthomonas maltophilia*. In vitro activity of beta-lactam/beta-lactamase inhibitor combinations. *Diagn Microbiol Infect Dis* 14: 239.

Garg BR, Lal S, Silvamani S (1978). Efficacy of co-trimoxazole in Donovanosis. A preliminary report. *Brit J Vener Dis* 54: 348.

Gargalianos P, Jackson PT, Herzog C, Geddes AM (1986). Trimethoprim in enteric fever. *J Antimicrob Chemother* 18: 277.

Gaskins JD, Holt RJ, Kyong CU *et al.* (1982). Chemoprophylaxis of recurrent otitis media using trimethoprim/sulfamethoxazole. *Drug Intellig Clin Pharm* 16: 387.

Gates RH, McCall CE (1982). Gram-negative bacillary meningitis. *JAMA* 248: 1217.

Gaylarde PM, Sarkany I (1972). Suppression of thymidine uptake of human lymphocytes by co-trimoxazole. *Brit Med J* 3: 144.

Geddes AM, Fothergill R, Goodall JAD, Dorken PR (1971). Evaluation of trimethoprim-sulfamethoxazole compound in treatment of *Salmonella* infections. *Brit Med J* 3: 451.

Geddes AM, Pugh RNH, Nye FJ (1975). Treatment and follow-up studies with co-trimoxazole in enteric fever and in typhoid carriers. *J Antimicrob Chemother* 1: 51.

George MJ, Kitch B, Henderson FW, Gilligan PH (1991). *In vitro* activity of orally administered antimicrobial agents against *Haemophilus influenzae* recovered from children monitored longitudinally in a group day care center. *Antimicrob Ag Chemother* 35: 1960.

Georghiou PR, Blacklock ZM (1992). Infection with *Nocardia* species in Queensland. A review of 102 clinical isolates. *Med J Aust* 156: 692.

Gharagozloo RA, Naficy K, Mouin M *et al.* (1970). Comparative trial of tetracycline, chloramphenicol and trimethoprim/sulfamethoxazole in eradication of *Vibro cholera* El Tor. *Brit Med J* 4: 281.

Gibbons RB, Lindaver JA (1985). Successful treatment of *Pneumocystis carinii* pneumonia with trimethoprim-sulfamethoxazole in hypersensitive AIDS patients. *JAMA* 253: 1259.

Gibson JR (1982). Recurrent trimethoprim-associated fixed skin eruption. *Brit Med J* 284: 1529.

Gibson JR (1983). Trimethoprim-polymyxin B ophthalmic solution in the treatment of presumptive bacterial conjunctivitis – a multicentre trial of its efficacy versus neomycin-polymyxin B-gramicidin and chloramphenicol ophthalmic solutions. *J Antimicrob Chemother* 11: 217.

Giebink GS, Batalden PB, Le CT *et al.* (1990). A controlled trial comparing three treatments for chronic otitis media with effusion. *Pediatr Infect Dis J* 9: 33.

Gilman RH, Terminel M, Levine MM *et al.* (1975). Comparison of trimethoprim-sulfamethoxazole and amoxycillin in therapy of chloramphenicol-resistant and chloramphenicol-sensitive typhoid fever. *J Infect Dis* 132: 630.

Girard P-M, Landman R, Gaudebout C *et al.* (1989). Prevention of *Pneumocystis carinii* pneumonia relapse by pentamidine aerosol in zidovudine-treated AIDS patients. *Lancet* i: 1348.

Girard PM, Landman R, Gaudebout C *et al.* (1993). Dapsone-pyrimethamine compared with aerosolized pentamidine as primary prophylaxis against *Pneumocystis carinii* pneumonia and toxoplasmosis in children. *New Engl J Med* 328: 1514.

Girdwood RH (1973). Trimethoprim/sulfamethoxazole: long-term therapy and folate levels. *Med J Aust* 1 (Special Suppl): 134.

Girdwood RH (1976). The nature of possible adverse reactions to co-trimoxazole. *Scand J Infect Dis* (Suppl 8): 10.

Glatt AE, Chirgwin K (1990). *Pneumocystis carinii* pneumonia in human immunodeficiency virus-infected patients. *Arch Intern Med* 150: 271.

Gleckman R, Crowley M, Natsios GA (1982). Trimethoprim-sulfamethoxazole treatment of men with recurrent urinary tract infections: a double-blind study utilizing the antibody-coated bacteria technique. *Rev Infect Dis* 4: 449.

Gluckstein D, Ruskin J (1995). Rapid oral desensitization to trimethoprim-sulfamethoxazole (TMP-SMZ): use in prophylaxis for *Pneumocystis carinii* pneumonia in patients with AIDS who were previously intolerant to TMP-SMZ. *Clin Infect Dis* 20: 849.

Gmünder FK, Seger RA (1981). Chronic granulomatous disease: mode of action of sulfamethoxazole/trimethoprim. *Pediatr Res* 15: 1533.

Gnarpe H, Friberg J (1976). The penetration of trimethoprim into seminal fluid and serum. *Scand J Infect Dis* (Suppl 8): 50.

Golden JA, Sjoerdsma A, Santi DV *et al.* (1984). *Pneumocystis carinii* pneumonia treated with a-difluoromethylornithine: a prospective study among patients with the acquired immunodeficiency syndrome. *West J Med* 141: 613.

Goldstein FW, Chumpitaz JC, Guevara JM *et al.* (1986a). Plasmid-mediated resistance to multiple antibiotics in *Salmonella typhi*. *J Infect Dis* 153: 261.

Goldstein FW, Papadopoulou B, Acar JF (1986b). The changing pattern of trimethoprim resistance in Paris, with a review of worldwide experience. *Rev Infect Dis* 8: 725.

Gomez-Garces JL, Alos JI, Cogollos R (1994). Bacteriologic characteristics and antimicrobial susceptibility of 70 clinically significant isolates of *Streptococcus milleri* group. *Diagn Microbiol Infect Dis* 19: 69.

Goodhart GL (1984). *In vivo* v *in vitro* susceptibility of enterococcus to trimethoprim-sulfamethoxazole. *JAMA* 252: 2748.

Goodwin CS, Bucens MC, Davis RE, Norcott TC (1981). High-dose co-trimoxazole and its penetration through uninflamed meninges. *Med J Aust* 2: 24.

Goossens H, De Mol P, Coignau H *et al.* (1985). Comparative *in vitro* activities of aztreonam, ciprofloxacin, norfloxacin, ofloxacin, HR 810 (a new cephalosporin), RU 28965 (a new macrolide), and other agents against enteropathogens. *Antimicrob Ag Chemother* 27: 388.

Gorbach SL (1982). Editorial. Travelers' diarrhoea. *New Engl J Med* 307: 881.

Gordin FM, Simon GL, Wofsy CB, Mills J (1984). Adverse reactions to trimethoprim-sulfamethoxazole in patients with the acquired immunodeficiency syndrome. *Ann Intern Med* 100: 495.

Gordin F, Gibert C, Schmidt ME (1994). *Clostridium difficile* colitis associated with trimethoprim-sulfamethoxazole given as prophylaxis for *Pneumocystis carinii* pneumonia. *Amer J Med* 96: 94.

Gordon RC, Thompson TR, Carlson W *et al.* (1975). Antimicrobial resistance of shigellae isolated in Michigan. *JAMA* 231: 1159.

Gossius G, Vorland L (1984). A randomised comparison of single-dose vs three-day and ten-day therapy with trimethoprim-sulfamethoxazole for acute cystitis in women. *Scand J Infect Dis* 16: 373.

Govert JA, Patton S, Fine RL (1992). Pancytopenia from using trimethoprim and methotrexate. *Ann Intern Med* **117**: 877.

Gower PE, Tasker PRW (1976). Comparative double-blind study of cephalexin and co-trimoxazole in urinary tract infection. *Brit Med J* **1**: 684.

Gracey M, Burke V, Robinson J (1982). Aeromonas-associated gastroenteritis. *Lancet* ii: 1304.

Granoff DM, Gilsdorf J, Gessert C, Basden M (1979). *Haemophilus influenzae* type B disease in a day care center: eradication of carrier state by rifampin. *Pediatrics* **63**: 397.

Gray J, McGhie D, Ball AP (1978). *Serratia marcescens*: a study of the sensitivity of British isolates to antibacterial agents and their combinations. *J Antimicrob Chemother* **4**: 551.

Grayson, ML, Thauvin, EC, Eliopoulos, GM *et al.* (1990). Failure of trimethoprim-sulfamethoxazole therapy in experimental enterococcal endocarditis. *Antimicrob Ag Chemother* **34**: 1792.

Greenberg S, Reiser IW, Chou SY, Porush JG (1993). Trimethoprim-sulfamethoxazole induces reversible hyperkalemia. *Ann Intern Med* **119**: 291.

Greene BM, Thomas FE Jr, Alford RH (1975). Trimethoprim-sulfamethoxazole and brain abscess. *Ann Intern Med* **82**: 812.

Grey D, Hamilton-Miller JMT (1977). Sensitivity of *Pseudomonas aeruginosa* to sulphonamides and trimethoprim and the activity of the combination trimethoprim: sulfamethoxazole. *J Med Microbiol* **10**: 273.

Gribble MJ, Puterman ML (1993). Prophylaxis of urinary tract infection in persons with recent spinal cord injury: a prospective, randomized, double-blind, placebo-controlled study of trimethoprim-sulfamethoxazole. *Amer J Med* **95**: 141.

Grose WE, Bodey GP, Rodriguez V (1977). Sulfamethoxazole-trimethoprim for infections in cancer patients. *JAMA* **237**: 352.

Grose WE, Bodey GP, Loo TL (1979). Clinical pharmacology of intravenously administered trimethoprim-sulfamethoxazole. *Antimicrob Ag Chemother* **15**: 447.

Grossman PL, Remington JS (1979). The effect of trimethoprim and sulfamethoxazole on *Toxoplasma gondii in vitro* and *in vivo*. *Amer J Trop Med Hyg* **28**: 445.

Grossman AB, Braimbridge MV, Ross Russell RW, Smith SE (1977). Acute polyneuropathy possibly associated with co-trimoxazole. *Lancet* ii: 616.

Grossman PL, Krahenbuhl JL, Remington JS (1978). *In vivo* and *in vitro* effects of trimethoprim and sulfamethoxazole on toxoplasma infection. In *Current Chemotherapy. Proceedings of the 10th International Congress of Chemotherapy, Zurich/Switzerland, 1977* (Siegenthaler W, Lüthy R, eds), p. 135. Washington, DC: American Society for Microbiology.

Grunberg E, Prince HN, de Lorenzo WF (1970). The *in vivo* effect of folinic acid (citrovorum factor). on the potentiation of the antibacterial activity of sulfisoxazole by trimethoprim. *J Clin Pharmacol* **10**: 231.

Grüneberg RN (1975). The use of co-trimoxazole in sulphonamide-resistant *Escherichia coli* urinary tract infection. *J Antimicrob Chemother* **1**: 305.

Grüneberg RN (1979). The microbiological rationale for the combination of sulphonamides with trimethoprim. *J Antimicrob Chemother* **5** (Suppl B): 27.

Grüneberg, RN (1990). Changes in the antibiotic sensitivities of urinary pathogens, 1971–1989. *J Antimicrob Chemother*.

Grüneberg RN, Kolbe R (1969). Trimethoprim in the treatment of urinary infections in hospitals. *Brit Med J* **1**: 545.

Grüneberg RN, Smellie JM, Leakey A, Atkin WS (1976). Long-term low-dose co-trimoxazole in prophylaxis of childhood urinary tract infection: bacteriological aspects. *Brit Med J* **2**: 206.

Gualtieri RJ, Donowitz GR, Kaiser DL *et al.* (1983). Double-blind randomized study of prophylactic trimethoprim/sulfamethoxazole in granulocytopenic patients with hematological malignancies. *Amer J Med* **74**: 934.

Guerrant RL, Wood SJ, Krongaard L *et al.* (1981). Resistance among fecal flora of patients taking sulfamethoxazole-trimethoprim or trimethoprim alone. *Antimicrob Ag Chemother* **19**: 33.

Guignard JP, Pippa R, Genton N (1978). Co-trimoxazole and creatinine clearance. *Lancet* i: 712.

Gunther G, Philipson A (1988). Oral trimethoprim as follow-up treatment of meningitis caused by *Listeria monocytogenes*. *Rev Infect Dis* **10**: 53.

Gurwith MC, Brunton JL, Lank BA *et al.* (1979). A prospective controlled investigation of prophylactic trimethoprim/sulfamethoxazole in hospitalized granulocytopenic patients. *Amer J Med* **66**: 248.

Gurwith M, Truog K, Hinthorn D, Liu C (1982). Trimethoprim-sulfamethoxazole and trimethoprim alone for prophylaxis of infection in granulocytopenic patients. *Rev Infect Dis* **4**: 593.

Gutman LT, Wilfert CM, Quan T (1973). Susceptibility of *Yersinia enterocolitica* to trimethoprim-sulfamethoxazole. *J Infect Dis* **128** (Suppl): 538.

Gutmann L, Williamson R, Moreau N *et al.* (1985). Cross-resistance to nalidixic acid, trimethoprim and chloramphenicol associated with alterations in outer membrane proteins of *Klebsiella*, *Enterobacter* and *Serratia*. *J Infect Dis* **151**: 501.

Haas EJ (1984). Trimethoprim-sulfamethoxazole : another cause of recurrent meningitis. *JAMA* **252**: 346.

Haeney MR, Ross IN (1978). Whipple's disease in a female with impaired cell-mediated immunity unresponsive to co-trimoxazole and levamisole therapy. *Postgrad Med J* **54**: 45.

Hall CL (1974). Co-trimoxazole and azathioprine: a safe combination. *Brit Med J* **4**: 15.

Hall, WH (1990). Modern chemotherapy for brucellosis in humans. *Rev Infect Dis* **12**: 1060.

Haltiner RC, Migneault PC, Robertson RG (1980). Incidence of thymidine-dependent enterococci detected on Mueller-Hinton agar with low thymidine content. *Antimicrob Ag Chemother* **18**: 365.

Hamilton J, Burch W, Grimmett G *et al.* (1973). Successful treatment of *Pseudomonas cepacia* endocarditis with trimethoprim-sulfamethoxazole. *Antimicrob Ag Chemother* **4**: 551.

Hamilton-Miller JMT (1979). Mechanisms and distribution of bacterial resistance to diaminopyrimidines and sulphonamides. *J Antimicrob Chemother* **5** (Suppl B): 61.

Hamilton-Miller JMT (1988). Reversal of activity of trimethoprim against gram-positive cocci by thymidine, thymine and 'folates'. *J Antimicrob Chemother* **22**: 35.

Hamilton-Miller JMT, Grey D (1975). Resistance to trimethoprim in *Klebsiella* isolated before its introduction. *J Antimicrob Chemother* **1**: 213.

Hamilton-Miller JMT, Purves D (1986). Trimethoprim resistance and trimethoprim usage in and around the Royal Free Hospital in 1985. *J Antimicrob Chemother* **18**: 643.

Hammerschlag MR (1982). Activity of trimethoprim-sulfamethoxazole against *Chlamydia trachomatis in vitro*. *Rev Infect Dis* **4**: 500.

Hammerschlag MR, Vuletin JC (1985). Ultrastructural analysis of the effect of trimethoprim and sulfamethoxazole on the development of *Chlamydia trachomatis* in cell culture. *J Antimicrob Chemother* **15**: 209.

Hammett JF (1970). Thrombocytopenia following administration of 'bactrim'. *Med J Aust* **2**: 200.

Hamory BH, Sande MA, Sydnor A Jr *et al.* (1979). Etiology and antimicrobial therapy of acute maxillary sinusitis. *J Infect Dis* **139**: 197.

Hand WL, King-Thompson N (1989). The entry of antibiotics into human monocytes. *J Antimicrob Chemother* **23**: 681.

Hand WL, King-Thompson N (1990). Uptake of antibiotics by human polymorphonuclear leukocyte cytoplasts. *Antimicrob Ag Chemother* **34**: 1189.

Hand WL, King-Thompson N, Holman JW (1987).Entry of roxithromycin (RU 965), imipenem, cefotaxime, trimethoprim and metronidazole into human polymorphonuclear leukocytes. *Antimicrob Ag Chemother* **31**: 1553.

Hanley T (1969). Adverse reactions to trimethoprim sulfamethoxazole. *Postgrad Med J* **45** (Suppl): 85.

Hanson GC, Woods RL (1975). Intravenous trimethoprim/sulphadimidine in the treatment of *Bacteroides* septicaemia. *Postgrad Med J* **51**: 105.

Harding GKM, Ronald AR (1973). Efficacy of trimethoprim-sulfamethoxazole in bacteriuria. *J Infect Dis* **128** (Suppl): 641.

Harding GKM, Ronald AR (1974). A controlled study of antimicrobial prophylaxis of recurrent urinary infection in women. *New Engl J Med* **291**: 597.

Harding GKM, Buckwold FJ, Marrie TJ et al. (1979). Prophylaxis of recurrent urinary tract infection in female patients. Efficacy of low-dose, thrice-weekly therapy with trimethoprim-sulfamethoxazole. *JAMA* **242**: 1975.

Harding GKM, Ronald AR, Nicolle LE et al. (1982). Long-term antimicrobial prophylaxis for recurrent urinary tract infection in women. *Rev Infect Dis* **4**: 438.

Harding, GK, Nicolle, LE, Ronald, AR et al. (1991). How long should catheter-acquired urinary tract infection in women be treated? A randomized controlled study. *Ann Intern Med* **114**: 713.

Hardy WD, Wolfe PR, Gottlieb MS et al. (1987). Long-term follow-up of Fansidar prophylaxis for *Pneumocystis carinii* in patients with AIDS [.Abstract TP 232] International Conference on AIDS, Washington, DC, June 1–5.

Hardy WD, Feinberg J, Finkelstein DM et al. (1992). A controlled trial of trimethoprim-sulfamethoxazole or aerosolized pentamidine for secondary prophylaxis of *Pneumocystis carinii* pneumonia in patients with the acquired immunodeficiency syndrome. AIDS Clinical Trials Group Protocol 021. *New Engl J Med* **327**: 1842.

Hargadon MT, Young VM, Schimpff SC et al. (1981). Selective suppression of alimentary tract microbial flora as prophylaxis during granulocytopenia. *Antimicrob Ag Chemother* **20**: 620.

Harnett N, McLeod S, AuYong Y, Krishnan C (1991). Increasing incidence of resistance among shigellae to trimethoprim. *Lancet* **337**: 622.

Harper JS III, London WT, Sever JL (1985). Five drug regimens for treatment of acute toxoplasmosis in squirrel monkeys. *Amer J Trop Med Hyg* **34**: 50.

Harris RE, McCallister JA, Allen SA et al. (1980). Prevention of *Pneumocystis* pneumonia. Use of continuous sulfamethoxazole-trimethoprim therapy. *Amer J Dis Child* **134**: 35.

Harrison MS, Simonte SJ, Kauffman CA (1994). Trimethoprim-induced aseptic meningitis in a patient with AIDS: case report and review. *Clin Infect Dis* **19**: 431.

Harrison WO (1981). Pharyngeal gonorrhea. *JAMA* **246**: 2726.

Harvey RJ (1982). Synergism in the folate pathway. *Rev Infect Dis* **4**: 255.

Hassan A, Erian MM, Farid Z et al. (1971). Trimethoprim-sulfamethoxazole in acute brucellosis. *Brit Med J* **3**: 159.

Hassan A, Hathout S, Safwat Y et al. (1975). A comparative evaluation of the treatment of typhoid fever with co-trimoxazole and chloramphenicol in Egypt. *J Trop Med Hyg* **78**: 50.

Hatos G, Tuza FLC (1972). Treatment of gonorrhoea with trimethoprim-sulfamethoxazole and with rifampicin. *Med J Aust* **1**: 1197.

Haverkos HW, Juranek DD, Pollard RA et al. (1984). Assessment of therapy for *Pneumocystis carinii* pneumonia. PCP therapy project group. *Amer J Med* **76**: 501.

Hawkins T, Carter JM, Romeril KR, Jackson SR, Green GJ (1993). Severe trimethoprim induced neutropenia and thrombocytopenia. *N Z Med J* **106**: 251.

Hedlund J, Aurelius E Andersson J (1990). Recurrent encephalitis due to trimethoprim intake. *Scand J Infect Dis* **22**: 109.

Heikkila E, Siitonen A, Jahkola M et al. (1990a). Increase of trimethoprim resistance among *Shigella* species, 1975–1988: analysis of resistance mechanisms. *J Infect Dis* **161**: 1242.

Heikkila E, Sundstrom L, Huovinen P (1990b). Trimethoprim resistance in *Escherichia coli* isolates from a geriatric unit. *Antimicrob Ag Chemother* **34**: 2013.

Henderson FW, Gilligan PH, Wait K, Goff DA (1988). Nasopharyngeal carriage of antibiotic-resistant pneumococci by children in group day care. *J Infect Dis* **157**: 256.

Henry RL, Dorman DC, Skinner JA, Mellis CM (1981). Antimicrobial therapy in whooping cough. *Med J Aust* **2**: 27.

Henry SA (1984). Chemoprophylaxis of bacterial infections in granulocytopenic patients. *Amer J Med* **76**: 645.

Hess MM, Boucher BA, Laizure SC et al. (1993). Trimethoprim-sulfamethoxazole pharmacokinetics in trauma patients. *Pharmacotherapy* **13**: 602.

Higgins RM, Bloom SL, Hopkin JM et al. (1989). The risks and benefits of low-dose co-trimoxazole prophylaxis for *Pneumocystis pneumonia* in renal transplantation. *Transplantation* **47**: 558 .

Higgins T, Niklasson PM (1990). Hypersensitivity pneumonitis induced by trimethoprim. *Brit Med J* **300**: 1344.

Hills NH, Bultitude MI, Eykyn S (1976). Co-trimoxazole in prevention of bacteriuria after prostatectomy. *Brit Med J* **2**: 498.

Hirschel B, Lazzarin A, Chopard P et al. (1991). A controlled study of inhaled pentamidine for primary prevention of *Pneumocystis carinii* pneumonia. *New Engl J Med* **324**: 1079.

Hirschtick RE, Glassroth J, Jordan MC et al. (1995). Bacterial pneumonia in persons infected with the human immunodeficiency virus. Pulmonary Complications of HIV Infection Study Group. *New Engl J Med* **333**: 845.

Hitchings GH (1969). Species differences among dihydrofolate reductases as a basis for chemotherapy. *Postgrad Med J* **45** (Suppl): 7.

Hobday JD (1971). The prophylactic treatment of recurrent urinary tract infection with sulfamethoxazole-trimethoprim. *Aust Paediat J* **7**: 199.

Hoffman GS, Fauci AS (1992). Wegener's granulomatosis. *Ann Intern Med* **117**: 620.

Hoffman GS, Kerr GS, Leavitt RY et al. (1992). Wegener's granulomatosis: an analysis of 158 patients. *Ann Intern Med* **116**: 488.

Hofmann J, Cetron MS, Farley MM et al. (1995). The prevalence of drug-resistant *Streptococcus pneumoniae* in Atlanta. *New Engl J Med* **333**: 481.

Hoge CW, Shlim DR, Ghimire M et al. (1995). Placebo-controlled trial of co-trimoxazole for cyclospora infections among travellers and foreign residents in Nepal. *Lancet* **345**: 691.

Hohl P, Frei R, Aubry P (1991). *In vitro* susceptibility of 33 clinical case isolates of *Xanthomonas maltophilia*. Inconsistent correlation of agar dilution and of disk diffusion test results. *Diagn Microbiol Infect Dis* **14**: 447.

Holdcroft CJ, Ellison RB (1991). Trimethoprim-sulfamethoxazole reaction simulating *Pneumocystis carinii* pneumonia [letter]. *AIDS* **5**: 1029.

Holder IA (1981). *In vitro* susceptibility of organisms isolated from burns to topical co-trimoxazole. *J Antimicrob Chemother* **7**: 623.

Holland NH, Kazee M, Duff D, McRoberts JW (1982). Antimicrobial prophylaxis in children with urinary tract infection and vesicoureteral reflux. *Rev Infect Dis* **4**: 467.

Holmberg SD, Schell WL, Fanning GR et al. (1986). *Aeromonas* intestinal infections in the United States. *Ann Intern Med* **105**: 683.

Hooton TM, Running K, Stamm WE (1985). Single-dose therapy for cystitis in women. A comparison of trimethoprim-sulfamethoxazole, amoxicillin and cyclacillin. *JAMA* **253**: 387.

Hooton TM, Winter C, Tiu F, Stamm WE (1995). Randomized comparative trial and cost analysis of 3-day antimicrobial regimens for treatment of acute cystitis in women. *JAMA* **273**: 41.

Howard AJ, Williams HM (1989). The prevalence of antibiotic resistance in *Haemophilus influenzae* in Ireland. *J Antimicrob Chemother* **24**: 963. [Published errata appear in *J Antimicrob Chemother* 1990; **25**: 886 and 1991; **28**: 482].

Howe JG, Wilson TS (1972). Co-trimoxazole-resistant pneumococci. *Lancet* **ii**: 184.

Hugh TB, Coleman MJ (1981). 'Fish fanciers' finger': tropical fish-tank granuloma. *Med J Aust* **1**: 614.

Hughes DTD (1969). Single-blind comparative trial of trimethoprim-sulfamethoxazole and ampicillin in the treatment of exacerbations of chronic bronchitis. *Brit Med J* **4**: 470.

Hughes DTD (1973). Use of combinations of trimethoprim and sulfamethoxazole in the treatment of chest infections. *J Infect Dis* **128** (Suppl): 701.

Hughes DTD (1975). The clinical, haematological and bacteriological effects of long-term treatment with co-trimoxazole. *J Antimicrob Chemother* **1**: 55.

Hughes DTD (1983). The use of combinations of trimethoprim and sulphonamides in the treatment of chest infections. *J Antimicrob Chemother* **12**: 423.

Hughes WT (1976). Editorial. Treatment of *Pneumocystis carinii* pneumonitis. *New Engl J Med* **295**: 726.

Hughes WT (1982). Trimethoprim-sulfamethoxazole therapy for *Pneumocystis carinii* pneumonitis in children. *Rev Infect Dis* **4**: 602.

Hughes WT, McNabb PC, Makres TD, Feldman S (1974). Efficacy of trimethoprim and sulfamethoxazole in the prevention and treatment of *Pneumocystis carinii* pneumonitis. *Antimicrob Ag Chemother* **5**: 289.

Hughes WT, Feldman S, Sanyal SK (1975). Treatment of *Pneumocystis carinii* pneumonitis with trimethoprim-sulfamethoxazole. *Can Med Assoc J* **112** (Suppl): 47.

Hughes WT, Kuhn S, Chaudhary S *et al.* (1977). Successful chemoprophylaxis for *Pneumocystis carinii* pneumonitis. *New Engl J Med* **297**: 1419.

Hughes WT, Feldman S, Chaudhary SC *et al.* (1978). Comparison of pentamidine isethionate and trimethoprim-sulfamethoxazole in the treatment of *Pneumocystis carinii* pneumonia. *J Pediatr* **92**: 285.

Hughes WT, Rivera GK, Schell MJ *et al.* (1987). Succesesful intermittent prophylaxis for *Pneumocystis carinii* pneumonitis. *New Engl J Med* **316**: 1627.

Hughes WT, Kennedy W, Dugdale M *et al.* (1990). Prevention of *Pneumocystis carinii* pneumonitis in AIDS patients with weekly dapsone. *Lancet* **336**: 1066.

Hughes W, Leoung G, Kramer F *et al.* (1993). Comparison of atovaquone (566C80). with trimethoprim-sulfametoxazole to treat *Pneumocystis carinii* pneumonia in patients with AIDS. *New Engl J Med* **328**: 1521.

Hughes WT, LaFon SW, Scott JD, Masur H (1995). Adverse events associated with trimethoprim-sulfamethoxazole and atovaquone during the treatment of AIDS-related *Pneumocystis carinii* pneumonia. *J Infect Dis* **171**: 1295.

Hulme B, Reeves DS (1971). Leucopenia associated with trimethoprim-sulfamethoxazole after renal transplantation. *Brit Med J* **3**: 610.

Huovinen P, Pulkkinen L, Helin H-L *et al.* (1986). Emergence of trimethoprim resistance in relation to drug consumption in a Finnish hospital from 1971 through 1984. *Antimicrob Ag Chemother* **29**: 73.

Huovinen P, Sundstrom L, Swedberg G, Skold O (1995). Trimethoprim and sulfonamide resistance. *Antimicrob Ag Chemother* **39**: 279.

Hyams KC, Bourgeois AL, Merrell BR *et al.* (1991). Diarrheal disease during Operation Desert Shield. *New Engl J Med* **325**: 1423.

Imrie KR, Prince HM, Couture F *et al.* (1995). Effect of antimicrobial prophylaxis on hematopoietic recovery following autologous bone marrow transplantation: ciprofloxacin versus co- trimoxazole. *Bone Marrow Transplant* **15**: 267.

International Agranulocytosis and Aplastic Anemia Study Group (1989). Anti-infective drug use in relation to the risk of agranulocytosis and aplastic anemia. A report from the International Agranulocytosis and Aplastic Anemia Study. *Arch Intern Med* **149**: 1036.

Ioannidis JP, Cappelleri JC, Skolnik PR *et al.* (1996). A meta-analysis of the relative efficacy and toxicity of *Pneumocystis carinii* prophylactic regimens. *Arch Intern Med* **156**: 177.

Iredell J, Whitby M, Blacklock Z (1992). *Mycobacterium marinum* infection: epidemiology and presentation in Queensland 1971–1990. *Med J Aust* **157**: 596.

Irivani A, Richard GA, Baer H, Fennell R (1981a). Comparative efficacy and safety of nalidixic acid versus trimethoprim/sulfamethoxazole in treatment of acute urinary tract infections in college-age women. *Antimicrob Ag Chemother* **19**: 598.

Iravani A, Richard GA, Baer H (1981b). Treatment of uncomplicated urinary tract infections with trimethoprim versus sulfisoxazole, with special reference to antibody-coated bacteria and fecal flora. *Antimicrob Ag Chemother* **19**: 842.

Iravani A, Richard GA, Baer H (1982). Trimethoprim once daily vs nitrofurantoin in treatment of acute urinary tract infections in young women, with special reference to periurethral, vaginal and fecal flora. *Rev Infect Dis* **4**: 378.

Iravani A, Welty GS, Newton BR, Richard GA (1985). Effects of changes in pH, medium, and inoculum size on the *in vitro* activity of amifloxacin against urinary isolates of *Staphylococcus saprophyticus* and *Escherichia coli*. *Antimicrob Ag Chemother* **27**: 449.

Isles A, Maclusky I, Corey M *et al.* (1984). *Pseudomonas cepacia* infection in cystic fibrosis: an emerging problem. *J Pediatr* **104**: 206.

Israel HL (1988). Sulfamethoxazole-trimethoprim therapy for Wegener's granulomatosis. *Arch Intern Med* **148**: 2293.

Iwarson S, Lidin-Janson G (1979). Long-term, low-dose trimethoprom prophylaxis in patients with recurrent urinary tract infections. *J Antimicrob Chemother* **5**: 316.

Jacobs F, Abramowicz D, Vereerstraeten P *et al.* (1990). *Brucella* endocarditis: the role of combined medical and surgical treatment. *Rev Infect Dis* **12**: 740.

Jacobs RF, Wilson CB (1983). Intracellular penetration and antimicrobial activity of antibiotics. *J Antimicrob Chemother* **12** (Suppl C): 13.

Jafary MH, Burke GJ (1970). Antibiotics and *Salmonella* excretors. *Brit Med J* **2**: 605.

Jaffe HS, Abrams DI, Ammann AJ *et al.* (1983). Complications of co-trimoxazole in treatment of AIDS-associated *Pneumocystis carinii* pneumonia in homosexual men. *Lancet* **ii**: 1109.

Jarvinen H, Tenovuo J, Huovinen P (1993). *In vitro* susceptibility of *Streptococcus mutans* to chlorhexidine and six other antimicrobial agents. *Antimicrob Ag Chemother* **37**: 1158.

Jenkins GC, Hughes DTD, Hall PC (1970). A haematological study of patients receiving long-term treatment with trimethoprim and sulphonamide. *J Clin Path* **23**: 392.

Jesudasan MV, John TJ (1990). Multi-resistant *Salmonella typhi* in India. *Lancet* **336**: 252.

Jewkes RF, Edwards MS, Grant BJB (1970). Haematological changes in a patient on long-term treatment with a trimethoprim-sulphonamide combination. *Postgrad Med J* **46**: 723.

Jick H (1982). Adverse reactions to trimethoprim-sulfamethoxazole in hospitalized patients. *Rev Infect Dis* **4**: 426.

Jick H, Derby LE (1995). Is co-trimoxazole safe? *Lancet* **345**: 1118.

Jick SS, Jick H, Habakangas JS, Dinan BJ (1984). Co-trimoxazole toxicity in children. *Lancet* **ii**: 631.

Joffe AM, Farley JD, Linden D *et al.* (1989). Trimethoprim-sulfamethoxazole-associated aseptic meningitis: case reports and review of the literature. *Amer J Med* **87**: 332.

John JF Jr (1976). Trimethoprim-sulfamethoxazole therapy of pulmonary melioidosis. *Amer Rev Resp Dis* **114**: 1021.

Johnson JA, Kappel JE, Sharif MN (1993). Hypoglycemia secondary to trimethoprim/sulfamethoxazole administration in a renal transplant patient. *Ann Pharmacother* **27**: 304.

Jones C, Stevens DL, Ojo O (1987). Effects of minimal amounts of thymidine on activity of trimethoprim-sulfamethoxazole against *Staphylococcus epidermidis*. *Antimicrob Ag Chemother* **31**: 144.

Jonsson M (1976). The treatment of typhoid and paratyphoid fevers with co-trimoxazole in a comparative trial with chloramphenicol. *Scand J Infect Dis* (Suppl 8): 81.

Jorgensen JH (1992). Update on mechanisms and prevalence of anti-microbial resistance in *Haemophilus influenzae*. *Clin Infect Dis* **14**: 1119.

Jorgensen JH, Doern GV, Maher LA *et al.* (1990). Antimicrobial resistance among respiratory isolates of *Haemophilus influenzae*, *Moraxella catarrhalis*, and *Streptococcus pneumoniae* in the United States. *Antimicrob Ag Chemother* **34**: 2075.

Jung AC, Paauw DS (1994). Management of adverse reactions to trimethoprim-sulfamethoxazole in human immunodeficiency virus-infected patients. *Arch Intern Med* **154**: 2402.

Kagalwalla AF, Khan SN, Kagalwalla YA *et al.* (1992). Childhood shigellosis in Saudi Arabia. *Pediatr Infect Dis J* **11**: 215.

Kahn SB, Fein SA, Brodsky I (1968). Effects of trimethoprim on folate metabolism in man. *Clin Pharmacol Ther* **9**: 550.

Kalowski S, Nanra RS, Mathew TH, Kincaid-Smith P (1973). Deterioration in renal function in association with co-trimoxazole therapy. *Lancet* i: 394.

Kalowski S, Nanra RS, Friedman A *et al.* (1975). Controlled trial comparing co-trimoxazole and methenamine hippurate in the prevention of recurrent urinary tract infections. *Med J Aust* 1: 585.

Kamat SA (1970). Evaluation of therapeutic efficacy of trimethoprim-sulfamethoxazole and chloramphenicol in enteric fever. *Brit Med J* 3: 320.

Kamme C, Melander A, Nilsson N-I (1983). Serum and saliva concentrations of sulfamethoxazole and trimethoprim in adults and children: relation between saliva concentrations and *in vitro* activity against nasopharyngeal pathogens. *Scand J Infect Dis* 15: 107.

Kanellakopoulou K, Giamarellou H, Avlamis A (1988). Surveillance study of resistance in *Haemophilus* species in Greece. *Eur J Clin Microbiol Infect Dis* 7: 186.

Kasanen A, Sundquist H (1982). Trimethoprim alone in the treatment of urinary tract infections: eight years of experience in Finland. *Rev Infect Dis* 4: 358.

Kasanen A, Toivanen P, Sourander L *et al.* (1974). Trimethoprim in the treatment and long-term control of urinary tract infection. *Scand J Infect Dis* 6: 91.

Kasanen A, Junnila SYT, Kaarsalo E *et al.* (1982). Secondary prevention of recurrent urinary tract infections. Comparison of the effect of placebo, methenamine hipppurate, nitrofurantoin and trimethoprim alone. *Scand J Infect Dis* 14: 293.

Kauffman CA, Liepman MK, Bergman AG, Mioduszewski J (1983). Trimethoprim/sulfamethoxazole prophylaxis in neutropenic patients. Reduction of infections and effect on bacterial and fungal flora. *Amer J Med* 74: 599.

Kayser FH, Morenzoni G, Santanam P (1990). The Second European Collaborative Study on the frequency of antimicrobial resistance in *Haemophilus influenzae*. *Eur J Clin Microbiol Infect Dis* 9: 810.

Kazemi M, Gumpert TG, Marks MI (1973). A controlled trial comparing sulfamethoxazole-trimethoprim, ampicillin, and no therapy in the treatment of salmonella gastorenteritis in children. *J Pediatr* 83: 646.

Keenan TD, Eliot JC, Bishop V *et al.* (1983). Comparison of trimethoprim alone with co-trimoxazole and sulphamethizole for treatment of urinary infections. *New Z Med J* 96: 341.

Kelly JW, Dooley DP, Lattuada CP *et al.* (1992). A severe, unusual reaction to trimethoprim-sulfamethoxazole in patients infected with human immunodeficiency virus. *Clin Infect Dis* 14: 1034.

Kelly R (1976). *Mycobacterium marinum* infection from a tropical fish tank. Treatment with trimethoprim and sulfamethoxazole. *Med J Aust* 2: 681.

Kemper CA, Tucker RM, Lang OS *et al.* (1990). Low-dose dapsone prophylaxis of *Pneumocystis carinii* in AIDS and AIDS-related complex. *AIDS* 4: 1145.

Khardori N, Shawar R, Gupta R *et al.* (1993). *In vitro* antimicrobial susceptibilities of *Nocardia* species. *Antimicrob Ag Chemother* 37: 882.

Kharsany AB, Hoosen AA, Van den Ende J (1993). Antimicrobial susceptibilities of *Gardnerella* vaginalis. *Antimicrob Ag Chemother* 37: 2733.

Khuri-Bulos NA, Daoud AH, Azab SM (1993). Treatment of childhood brucellosis: results of a prospective trial on 113 children. *Pediatr Infect Dis J* 12: 377.

Kincaid-Smith P, Kalowski S, Nanra RS (1973). Co-trimoxazole in urinary tract infection. *Med J Aust* 1 (Special Suppl): 49.

King CT, Chapman SW, Butkus DE (1993). Recurrent Nocardiosis in a renal transplant recipient. *South Med J* 86: 225.

Kipperman H, Ephros M, Lambdin M, White-Rogers K (1984). *Aeromonas* hydrophila: a treatable cause of diarrhea. *Pediatrics* 73: 253.

Kirven LA, Thornsberry C (1974). *In vitro* susceptibility of *Haemophilus influenzae* to trimethoprim-sulfamethoxazole. *Antimicrob Ag Chemother* 6: 869.

Kirven LA, Thornsberry C (1978). Minimum bactericidal concentration of sulfamethoxazole-trimethoprim for *Haemophilus influenzae*: correlation with prophylaxis. *Antimicrob Ag Chemother* 14: 731.

Klein NC, Duncanson FP, Lenox TH *et al.* (1992). Trimethoprim-sulfamethoxazole versus pentamidine for *Pneumocystis carinii* pneumonia in AIDS patients: results of a large prospective randomized treatment trial. *AIDS* 6: 301.

Klimek JJ, Bates TR, Nightingale C *et al.* (1980). Penetration characteristics of trimethoprim-sulfamethoxazole in middle ear fluid of patients with chronic serum otitis media. *J. Pediatrics* 96: 1087.

Klugman KP (1990). Pneumococcal resistance to antibiotics. *Clin Microbiol Rev* 3: 171.

Knapp JS, Back AF, Babst AF *et al.* (1993). *In vitro* susceptibilities of isolates of *Haemophilus ducreyi* from Thailand and the United States to currently recommended and newer agents for treatment of chancroid. *Antimicrob Ag Chemother* 37: 1552.

Knudsen JB, Korner B, Reinicke V *et al.* (1973). Treatment of urinary tract infections with a sulfamethoxazole/trimethoprim compound: a controlled, double blind, clinical trial. *Scand J Infect Dis* 5: 55.

Kobrinsky NL, Ramsay NKC (1981). Acute megaloblastic anemia induced by high-dose trimethoprim-sulfamethoxazole. *Ann Intern Med* 94: 780.

Koehler JM, Ashdown LR (1993). *In vitro* susceptibilities of tropical strains of *Aeromonas* species from Queensland, Australia, to 22 antimicrobial agents. *Antimicrob Ag Chemother* 37: 905.

Koornhof HJ, Wasas A, Klugman K (1992). Antimicrobial resistance in *Streptococcus pneumoniae*: a South African perspective. *Clin Infect Dis* 15: 84.

Koutts J, Van der Weyden MB, Cooper M (1973). Effect of trimethoprim on folate metabolism in human bone marrow. *Aust NZ J Med* 3: 245.

Kovacs JA, Masur H (1988). *Pneumocystis carinii* pneumonia: therapy and prophylaxis. *J Infect Dis* 158: 254.

Kovacs JA, Hiemenz JW, Macher AM *et al.* (1984). *Pneumocystis carinii* pneumonia: a comparison between patients with the acquired immunodeficiency syndrome and patients with other immunodeficiencies. *Ann Intern Med* 100: 663.

Kovatch AL, Wald ER, Albo VC *et al.* (1985). Oral trimethoprim/sulfamethoxazole for prevention of bacterial infection during the induction phase of cancer chemotherapy in children. *Pediatrics* 76: 754.

Kowdley KV, Keeffe EB, Fawaz KA (1992). Prolonged cholestasis due to trimethoprim sulfamethoxazole. *Gastroenterology* 102: 2148.

Kraus SJ, Kaufman HW, Albritton WL *et al.* (1982). Chancroid therapy: a review of cases confirmed by culture. *Rev Infect Dis* 4 (Suppl): 848.

Krause PJ, Owens NJ, Nightingale CH *et al.* (1982). Penetration of amoxicillin, cefaclor, erythromycin-sulfisoxazole and trimethoprim-sulfamethoxazole into the middle ear fluid of patients with chronic serous otitis media. *J Infect Dis* 145: 815.

Kremer I, Ritz R, Brunner F (1983). Aseptic meningitis as an adverse effect of co-trimoxazole. *New Engl J Med* 308: 1481.

Kreuz W, Gungor T, Lotz C *et al.* (1990). 'Treating through' hypersensitivity to co-trimoxazole in children with HIV infection. *Lancet* 336: 508.

Kristensen JK, From E (1975). Trimethoprim-sulfamethoxazole in gonorrhoea. A comparison with pivampicillin combined with probenecid. *Brit J Vener Dis* 51: 31.

Kuijper EJ, Peeters MF, Schoenmakers BS, Zanen HC (1989). Antimicrobial susceptibility of sixty human fecal isolates of *Aeromonas* species. *Eur J Clin Microbiol Infect Dis* 8: 248.

Lacey RW (1979). Mechanism of action in trimethoprim and sulphonamides: relevance to synergy *in vitro*. *J Antimicrob Chemother* 5 (Suppl B): 75.

Lacey RW (1982). Do sulphonamide-trimethoprim combinations select less resistance to trimethoprim than the use of trimethoprim alone? *J Med Microbiol* 15: 403.

Lacey RW, Lord VJ, Gunasekera HKW *et al.* (1980). Comparison of trimethoprim alone with trimethoprim sulfamethoxazole in the treatment of respiratory and urinary infections with particular reference to selection of trimethoprim resistance infections. *Lancet* i: 1270.

Lal H (1982). A comparative trial of oral chloroquine and oral co-trimoxazole in vivax malaria in children. *Amer J Trop Med Hyg* 31: 438.

Lal S, Garg BR (1980). Further evidence of the efficacy of co-trimoxazole in granuloma venerum. *Brit J Vener Dis* **56**: 412.

Lal S, Modawal KK, Fowle ASE et al. (1970). Acute brucellosis treated with trimethoprim and sulfamethoxazole. *Brit Med J* **3**: 256.

Lares-Asseff I, Villegas F, Perez-Guille G et al. (1994). Trimethoprim/sulfamethoxazole kinetics in children with biliary atresia. *Ann Pharmacother* **28**: 404.

Lassus A, Renkonen O-V (1979). Short-term treatment of gonorrhoea with intra-muscular and oral forms of trimethoprim-sulfamethoxazole. *Brit J Vener Dis* **55**: 24.

Latham RH, Running K, Stamm WE (1983). Urinary tract infections in young adult women caused by *Staphylococcus saprophyticus*. *JAMA* **250**: 3063.

Lau WK, Young LS (1976). Trimethoprim-sulfamethoxazole treatment of *Pneumocystis carinii* pneumonia in adults. *New Engl J Med* **295**: 716.

Lavelle J, Falloon J, Morgan A et al. (1991). Weekly dapsone and dapsone/pyrimethamine for pneumocystis pneumonia prophylaxis [Abstract WB2207]. *VII International Conference on AIDS*. Florence, Italy: June 16–21.

Lawrence A, Phillips I, Nicol C (1973). Various regimens of trimethoprim-sulfamethoxazole used in the treatment of gonorrhoea. *J Infect Dis* **128** (Suppl): 673.

Lawson DH, Henry DA (1977). Fatal agranulocytosis attributed to co-trimoxazole therapy. *Brit Med J* **2**: 316.

Lawson DH, Paice BJ (1982). Adverse reactions to trimethoprim-sulfamethoxazole. *Rev Infect Dis* **4**: 429.

Leading Article (1980). Trimethoprim. *Lancet* **i**: 519.

Leading Article (1982). Trachoma control. *Lancet* **i**: 489.

Leading Article (1983a). Chronic bacterial prostatitis. *Lancet* **i**: 393.

Leading Article (1983b). *Bacillus cereus* as a systemic pathogen. *Lancet* **ii**: 1469.

Leading Article (1985). Pneumocystis – an orphan organism? *Lancet* **i**: 676.

Lebek G, Wiedmer E (1971). Empfindlichkeit menschlicher krankeitserreger gegan das kombinations therapeutikum sulfamethoxazol-trimethoprim *in vitro*. *Schweiz Med Wochensch* **101**: 1385.

Lee BL, Safrin S (1992). Interactions and toxicities of drugs used in patients with AIDS. *Clin Infect Dis* **14**: 773.

Lee BL, Medina I, Benowitz NL et al. (1989). Dapsone, trimethoprim, and sulfamethoxazole plasma levels during treatment of *Pneumocystis pneumonia* in patients with the acquired immunodeficiency syndrome (AIDS). Evidence of drug interactions. *Ann Intern Med* **110**: 606.

Leelarasamee A, Bovornkitti S (1989). Melioidosis: review and update. *Rev Infect Dis* **11**: 413.

Leeming RJ (1980). Co-trimoxazole and phenylalanine metabolism. *Lancet* **i**: 255.

Lehtonen O-P, Pelliniemi T-T (1982). Bacterial resistance to trimethoprim-sulfamethoxazole. *New Engl J Med* **307**: 60.

Leoung GS, Mills J, Hopewell PC et al. (1986). Dapsone-trimethoprim for *Pneumocystis carinii* pneumonia in the acquired immunodeficiency syndrome. *Ann Intern Med* **105**: 45.

Leoung GS, Feigal DW Jr, Montgomery AB et al. (1990). Aerosolized pentamidine for prophylaxis against *Pneumocystis carinii* pneumonia – the San Francisco Community Prophylaxis trial. *New Engl J Med* **323**: 769.

Lester SC, del Pilar Pla M, Wang F et al. (1990). The carriage of *Escherichia coli* resistant to antimicrobial agents by healthy children in Boston, in Caracas, Venzuala, and in Qin Pu, China. *New Engl J Med* **323**: 285.

Levitz RE, Quintiliani R (1984). Trimethoprim-sulfamethoxazole for bacterial meningitis. *Ann Intern Med* **100**: 881.

Levitz RE, Dudley MN, Quintiliani R et al. (1984). Cerebrospinal fluid penetration of trimethoprim-sulfamethoxazole in two patients with Gram-negative bacillary meningitis. *J Antimicrob Chemother* **13**: 400.

Levy PY, Drancourt M, Etienne J et al. (1991). Comparison of different antibiotic regimens for therapy of 32 cases of Q fever endocarditis. *Antimicrob Ag Chemother* **35**: 533.

Lewin EB (1989). Role of trimethoprim-sulfamethoxazole in prophylaxis of recurrent otitis media. *Pediatr Infec Dis J* **8**: 730.

Lewis EL, Anderson JD, Lacey RW (1974). A reappraisal of the antibacterial action of co-trimoxazole *in vitro*. *J Clin Path* **27**: 87.

Lewis RJ (1995). Fatal vasculitis following treatment with co-trimoxozole. *Brit J Rheumatol* **34**: 84.

Lexomboon U, Mansuwan P, Duangmani C et al. (1972). Clinical evaluation of co-trimoxazole and furazolidone in treatment of shigellosis in children. *Brit Med J* **3**: 23.

Lima AA, Lima NL, Pinho MC et al. (1995). High frequency of strains multiply resistant to ampicillin, trimethoprim- sulfamethoxazole, streptomycin, chloramphenicol, and tetracycline isolated from patients with shigellosis in northeastern Brazil during the period 1988 to 1993. *Antimicrob Ag Chemother* **39**: 256.

Lindgren A, Olsson R (1994). Liver reactions from trimethoprim. *J Intern Med* **236**: 281.

Ling J, Chau PY (1984). Plasmids mediating resistance to choramphenicol, trimethoprim, and ampicillin in *Salmonella typhi* strains isolated in the Southeast Asian region. *J Infect Dis* **149**: 652.

Lirenman DS, Arnold WJD (1973). Long-term use of trimethoprim-sulfamethoxazole in children with meningomyeloceles and recurrent urinary tract infections. *J Infect Dis* **128** (Suppl): 636.

Lolekha S, Vibulbandhitkit S, Poonyarit P (1991). Response to antimicrobial therapy for shigellosis in Thailand. *Rev Infect Dis* **13** (Suppl 4): S342.

Lövestad A, Sabel G, Stefansson M et al. (1976). Co-trimoxazole and nitrofurantoin in urinary-tract infections: a controlled clinical study. *Scand J Infect Dis* **8** (Suppl): 58.

Lubani MM, Dudin KI, Sharda DC et al. (1989). A multicenter therapeutic study of 1100 children with brucellosis. *Pediatr Infect Dis J* **8**: 75.

Lyon BR, Skurray RA (1987). Antimicrobial resistance of *Staphylococcus aureus*: genetic basis. *Microbiol Rev* **51**: 88.

MacGowan AP, Holt HA, Reeves DS (1990). *In-vitro* synergy testing of nine antimicrobial combinations against *Listeria monocytogenes*. *J Antimicrob Chemother* **25**: 561.

MacGregor R R, Morgan A S, Graziani A L et al. (1992). Efficacy and tolerance of intermittent versus daily co-trimoxazole for PCP prophylaxis in HIV-positive patients. *Amer J Med* **92**: 227.

MacLean Smith R, Iwamoto GK, Richerson HB, Flaherty JP (1987). Trimethoprim-sulfamethoxazole desensitization in the acquired immunodeficiency syndrome. *Ann Intern Med* **106**: 335.

Macleod WM (1970). Treatment of histoplasmosis. *Lancet* **ii**: 363.

Maderazo EG, Quintiliani R (1974). Treatment of nocardial infection with trimethoprim and sulfamethoxazole. *Amer J Med* **57**: 671.

Madico G, Gilman RH, Miranda E, Cabrera L, Sterling CR (1993). Treatment of cyclospora infections with co-trimoxazole. *Lancet* **342**: 122.

Madrigal G, Odio CM, Mohs E et al. (1988). Single dose antibiotic therapy is not as effective as conventional regimens for management of acute urinary tract infections in children. *Pediatr Infect Dis J* **7**: 316.

Mallolas J, Zamora L, Gatell JM et al. (1993). Primary prophylaxis for *Pneumocystis carinii* pneumonia: a randomized trial comparing co-trimoxazole, aerosolized pentamidine and dapsone plus pyrimethamine. *AIDS* **7**: 59.

Männistö PT, Mäntylä R, Mattila J et al. (1982). Comparison of pharmacokinetics of sulphadiazine and sulfamethoxazole after intravenous infusion. *J Antimicrob Chemother* **9**: 461.

Manzella JP, Kellogg JA, Parsey KS (1995). *Corynebacterium pseudodiphtheriticum*: a respiratory tract pathogen in adults. *Clin Infect Dis* **20**: 37.

Maple PA, Hamilton-Miller JM, Brumfitt W (1989). World-wide antibiotic resistance in methicillin-resistant *Staphylococcus aureus*. *Lancet* **i**: 537.

Marchant C, Shurin PA (1982). Antibacterial therapy for acute otitis media: a critical analysis. *Rev Infect Dis* **4**: 506.

Margileth AM (1992). Antibiotic therapy for cat-scratch disease: clinical study of therapeutic outcome in 268 patients and a review of the literature. *Pediatr Infect Dis J* **11**: 474.

Margolis DM, Melnick DA, Alling DW *et al.* (1990). Trimethoprim-sulfamethoxazole prophylaxis in the management of chronic granulomatous disease. *J Infect Dis* **162**: 723.

Marinac JS, Stanford JF (1993). A severe hypersensitive reaction to trimethoprim-sulfamethoxazole in a patient infected with human immunodeficiency virus. *Clin Infect Dis* **16**: 178.

Markowitz N, Quinn EL, Saravolatz LD (1992). Trimethoprim-sulfamethoxazole compared with vancomycin for the treatment of *Staphylococcus aureus* infection. *Ann Intern Med* **117**: 390.

Marshall WF, Keating MR, Anhalt JP *et al.* (1989). *Xanthomonas maltophilia*: an emerging nosocomial pathogen. *Mayo Clin Proc* **64**: 1097.

Martin DC, Arnold JD (1968). Treatment of acute falciparum malaria with sulfalene and trimethoprim. *JAMA* **203**: 476.

Martin M A, Cox P H, Beck K *et al.* (1992). A comparison of the effectiveness of three regimens in the prevention of *Pneumocystis carinii* pneumonia in human immunodeficiency virus-infected patients. *Arch Intern Med* **152**: 523.

Martos A, Podzamczer D, Martinez-Lacasa J, *et al.* (1995). Steroids do not enhance the risk of developing tuberculosis or other AIDS-related diseases in HIV-infected patients treated for *Pneumocystis carinii* pneumonia. *AIDS* **9**: 1037.

Maskell R, Okubadejo OA, Payne RH (1976). Thymine-requiring bacteria associated with co-trimoxazole therapy. *Lancet* **i**: 834.

Masterton RG, Bochsler JA (1995). High-dosage co-amoxiclav in a single dose versus 7 days of co-trimoxazole as treatment of uncomplicated lower urinary tract infection in women. *J Antimicrob Chemother* **35**: 129.

Mastro TD, Ghafoor A, Nomani NK *et al.* (1991). Antimicrobial resistance of pneumococci in children with acute lower respiratory tract infection in Pakistan. *Lancet* **337**: 156.

Masur H (1992). Prevention and treatment of pneumocystis pneumonia. *New Engl J Med* **327**: 1853.

Masur H, Kovacs JA (1988). Treatment and prophylaxis of *Pneumocystis carinii* pneumonia. *Infect Dis Clin N Amer* **2**: 419.

Maurin M, Gasquet S, Ducco C, Raoult D (1995). MICs of 28 antibiotic compounds for 14 *Bartonella* (formerly *Rochalimaea*) isolates. *Antimicrob Ag Chemother* **39**: 2387.

May T, Beuscart C, Reynes J *et al.* (1994). Trimethoprim-sulfamethoxazole versus aerosolized pentamidine for primary prophylaxis of *Pneumocystis carinii* pneumonia: a prospective, randomized, controlled clinical trial. LFPMI Study Group. Ligue Francaise de Prevention des Maladies Infectieuses. *J AIDS* **7**: 457.

McCue JD, Zandt JR (1991). Acute psychoses associated with the use of ciprofloxacin and trimethoprim-sulfamethoxazole. *Amer J Med* **90**: 528.

McKendrick MW, Geddes AM, Farrell ID (1981). Trimethoprim in enteric fever. *Brit Med J* **282**: 364.

McLaughlin M, Wilkes M, Roy MA *et al.* (1989). Risks associated with acquiring chancroid genital ulcerative disease and HIV infection: a case control study. [Abstract No. 615]. In: *Abstracts of the 5th International Conference on AIDS* Ottawa: International Development Research Centre.

McLean DR, Russell N, Khan MY (1992). Neurobrucellosis: clinical and therapeutic features. *Clin Infect Dis* **15**: 582.

McNeil MM, Brown JM, Georghiou PR *et al.* (1992). Infections due to *Nocardia transvalensis*: clinical spectrum and antimicrobial therapy. *Clin Infect Dis* **15**: 453.

McNicol PJ, Ronald AR (1984). The plasmids of *Haemophilus ducreyi*. *J Antimicrob Chemother* **14**: 561.

McNulty CAM, Dent J, Wise R (1985). Susceptibility of clinical isolates of *Campylobacter pyloridis* to 11 antimicrobial agents. *Antimicrob Ag Chemother* **28**: 837.

McPherson VJ, Raik E (1970). Thrombocytopenia following administration of 'Septrin'. *Med J Aust* **2**: 754.

Meares EM Jr (1982). Prostatitis: a review of pharmacokinetics and therapy. *Rev Infect Dis* **4**: 475.

Medina I, Mills J, Leoung G *et al.* (1990). Oral therapy for *Pneumocystis carinii* pneumonia in the acquired immunodeficiency syndrome A controlled trial of trimethoprim-sulfamethoxazole versus trimethoprim-dapsone. *New Engl J Med* **323**: 776.

Mills J, Leoung G, Medina I *et al.* (1988). Dapsone treatment of *Pneumocystis carinii* pneumonia in the acquired immunodeficiency syndrome. *Antimicrob Ag Chemother* **32**: 1057.

Mirza SH, Beeching NJ, Hart CA (1995). The prevalence and clinical features of multi-drug resistant *Salmonella typhi* infections in Baluchistan, Pakistan. *Ann Trop Med Parasitol* **89**: 515.

Miser JS, Savitch J, Bleyer WA (1977). Management of *P. carinii* pneumonia. *New Engl J Med* **296**: 47.

Mitsuyasu R, Groopman J, Volberding P (1983). Cutaneous reaction to trimethoprim-sulfamethoxazole in patients with AIDS and Kaposi's sarcoma. *New Engl J Med* **308**: 1535.

Modest GA, Price B, Mascoli N (1994). Hyperkalemia in elderly patients receiving standard doses of trimethoprim- sulfamethoxazole. *Ann Intern Med* **120**: 437.

Mofenson LM, Korelitz J, Pelton S *et al.* (1995). Sinusitis in children infected with human immunodeficiency virus: clinical characteristics, risk factors, and prophylaxis. National Institute of Child Health and Human Development Intravenous Immunoglobulin Clinical Trial Study Group. *Clin Infect Dis* **21**: 1175.

Montaner JSG, Lawson LM, Levitt N *et al.* (1990). Corticosteroids prevent early deterioration in patients with moderately severe *Pneumocystis carinii* pneumonia and the acquired immunodeficiency syndrome (AIDS). *Ann Intern Med* **113**: 14.

Montaner JSG, Lawson LM, Gervais A *et al.* (1991). Aerosol pentamidine for secondary prophylaxis of AIDS-related *Pneumocystis carinii* pneumonia. *Ann Intern Med* **114**: 948.

Montejo JM, Alberola I, Glez-Zarate P *et al.* (1993). Open, randomized therapeutic trial of six antimicrobial regimens in the treatment of human brucellosis. *Clin Infect Dis* **16**: 671.

Montgomery AB, Debs RJ, Luce JM *et al.* (1987). Aerosolized pentamidine as sole therapy for *Pneumocystis carinii* pneumonia in patients with acquired immunodeficiency syndrome. *Lancet* **ii**: 480.

Montgomery AB, Feigal DW Jr, Sattler F *et al.* (1995). Pentamidine aerosol versus trimethoprim-sulfamethoxazole for *Pneumocystis carinii* in acquired immune deficiency syndrome. *Am J Respir Crit Care Med* **151**: 1068.

Moody MR, Young VM (1975). *In vitro* susceptibility of *Pseudomonas cepacia* and *Pseudomonas maltophilia* to trimethoprim and trimethoprim-sulfamethoxazole. *Antimicrob Ag Chemother* **7**: 836.

Morran C, McNaught W, McArdle CS (1978). Prophylactic co-trimoxazole in biliary surgery. *Brit Med J* **2**: 462.

Morrison RE, Young EJ, Harper WK, Maldonado L (1979). Chronic prostatic melioidosis treated with trimethoprim-sulfamethoxazole. *JAMA* **241**: 500.

Morzaria RN, Walton IG, Pickering D (1969). Neonatal meningitis treated with trimethoprim and sulfamethoxazole. *Brit Med J* **2**: 511.

Mossner G (1969). Clinical results with the combined preparation sulfamethoxazole + trimethoprim. *Proc 6th International Congress Chemother, Tokyo.* A11–2, 250; quoted by *Evaluations on New Drugs* (1971).

Mouy R, Fischer A, Vilmer E *et al.* (1989). Incidence, severity, and prevention of infections in chronic granulomatous disease. *J Pediatr* **114**: 555.

Mulholland EK, Falade AG, Corrah PT *et al.* (1995). A randomized trial of chloramphenicol vs trimethoprim-sulfamethoxazole for the treatment of malnourished children with community-acquired pneumonia. *Pediatr Infect Dis J* **14**: 959.

Mumtaz G, Ridgway GL, Felmingham D (1988). *In vitro* activity of sulfamethoxazole/trimethoprim and sulfadoxine/pyrimethamine against *Chlamydia trachomatis* SA2f in McCoy cell culture. *Eur J Clin Microbiol Infect Dis* **7**: 415.

Murphy JL (1992). Renal tubular acidosis in children treated with trimethoprim-sulfamethoxazole during therapy for acute lymphoid leukemia. *Pediatrics* **89**: 1072.

Murphy R, Lavelle J, Allan J *et al.* (1991). Aerosol pentamidine prophylaxis following *Pneumocystis carinii* pneumonia in AIDS patients. *Amer J Med* **90**: 418.

Murphy TF, Fernald GW (1983). Trimethoprim-sulfamethoxazole therapy for relapses of *Salmonella* meningitis. *Pediatr Infect Dis* **2**: 465.

Murray BE, Rensimer ER, DuPont HL (1982). Emergence of high-level trimethoprim resistance in fecal *Escherichia coli* during oral administration of trimethoprim or trimethoprim-sulfamethoxazole. *New Engl J Med* **306**: 130.

Murray BE, Alvarado T, Kim K-H *et al.* (1985). Increasing resistance to trimethoprim-sulfamethoxazole among isolates of *Escherichia coli* in developing countries. *J Infect Dis* **152**: 1107.

Murray BE, Mathewson JJ, DuPont HL *et al.* (1990). Emergence of resistant fecal *Escherichia coli* in travelers not taking prophylactic antimicrobial agents. *Antimicrob Ag Chemother* **34**: 515.

Murray JF, Felton CP, Garay SM *et al.* (1984). Pulmonary complications of the acquired immunodeficiency syndrome: report of a National, Heart, Lung and Blood Institute Workshop. *New Engl J Med* **310**: 1682.

Myerowitz RL, Pasculle AW, Dowling JN (1979). Opportunistic lung infection due to 'Pittsburgh Pneumonia Agent'. *New Engl J Med* **3**: 953.

Naamara W, Kunimoto DY, D'Costa LJ *et al.* (1988). Treating chancroid with enoxacin. *Genitourin Med* **64**: 189.

Nair SS, Kaplan JM, Levine LH, Geraci K (1980). Trimethoprim-sulfamethoxazole-induced intrahepatic cholestasis. *Ann Intern Med* **92**: 511.

Najjar A, Murray BE (1987). Failure to demonstrate a consistent *in vitro* bactericidal effect of trimethoprim-sulfamethoxazole against enterococci. *Antimicrob Ag Chemother* **31**: 808.

Nanra RS, Anderton JL, Evans M *et al.* (1971). The use of trimethoprim and sulfamethoxazole in the management of chronic and recurrent upper and lower urinary tract infection. *Med J Aust* **1**: 25.

Nelson CT, Mason EO Jr, Kaplan SL (1994). Activity of oral antibiotics in middle ear and sinus infections caused by penicillin-resistant *Streptococcus pneumoniae*: implications for treatment. *Pediatr Infect Dis J* **13**: 585.

Nelson JD, Kusmiesz H, Jackson LH (1976a). Comparison of trimethoprim-sulfamethoxazole and ampicillin therapy for shigellosis in ambulatory patients. *J Pediatr* **89**: 491.

Nelson JD, Kusmiesz H, Jackson LH, Woodman E (1976b). Trimethoprim-sulfamethoxazole therapy for shigellosis. *JAMA* **235**: 1239.

Nelson JD, Kusmiesz H, Shelton S (1982). Oral or intravenous trimethoprim-sulfamethoxazole therapy for shigellosis. *Rev Infect Dis* **4**: 546.

Nguyen BT, Stadtsbaeder S, Horvat F (1978). Comparative effect of trimethoprim and pyrimethamine, alone and in combination with a sulfonamide, on *Toxoplasma gondii*: *in vitro* and *in vivo* studies. In *Current Chemotherapy: Proceedings of the 10th International Congress of Chemotherapy, Zurich/Switzerland, 1977* (Siegenthaler W, Lüthy R, eds), p. 137. Washington DC: American Society for Microbiology.

Nguyen BY, Landucci DL, Cunnion RE *et al.* (1993). A case of hyperdynamic shock caused by trimethoprim-sulfamethoxazole in which no tumor necrosis factor or features of anaphylaxis were detected. *Clin Infect Dis* **17**: 885.

Nguyen MH, Muder RR (1994). Meningitis due to *Xanthomonas maltophilia*: case report and review. *Clin Infect Dis* **19**: 325.

Nguyen MT, Weiss PJ, Wallace MR (1995). Two-day oral desensitization to trimethoprim-sulfamethoxazole in HIV-infected patients. *AIDS* **9**: 573.

Nicolle LE, Harding GK, Thomson M *et al.* (1988). Efficacy of five years of continuous, low-dose trimethoprim-sulfamethoxazole prophylaxis for urinary tract infection. *J Infect Dis* **157**: 1239.

Nicolle LE, Louie TJ, Dubois J *et al.* (1994). Treatment of complicated urinary tract infections with lomefloxacin compared with that with trimethoprim-sulfamethoxazole. *Antimicrob Ag Chemother* **38**: 1368.

Nielsen ML, Laursen H, Strøyer I (1970). Short-term treatment of urinary tract infections with trimethoprim/sulfamethoxazole. *Scand J Infect Dis* **2**: 211.

Nielsen TL, Eeftinck SJ, Jensen BN *et al.* (1992). Adjunctive corticosteroid therapy for *Pneumocystis carinii* pneumonia in AIDS: a randomized European multicenter open label study. *J AIDS* **5**: 726.

Nielsen TL, Jensen BN, Nelsing S *et al.* (1995). Randomized study of sulfamethoxazole-trimethoprim versus aerosolized pentamidine for secondary prophylaxis of *Pneumocystis carinii* pneumonia in patients with AIDS. *Scand J Infect Dis* **27**: 217.

Nishioka SD (1995). Trimethoprim-sulfamethoxazole prophylaxis of spontaneous bacterial peritonitis. *Ann Intern Med* **123**: 810.

Nissinen A, Gronroos P, Huovinen P *et al.* (1995a). Development of beta-lactamase-mediated resistance to penicillin in middle-ear isolates of *Moraxella catarrhalis* in Finnish children, 1978–1993. *Clin Infect Dis* **21**: 1193.

Nissinen A, Leinonen M, Huovinen P *et al.* (1995b). Antimicrobial resistance of *Streptococcus pneumoniae* in Finland, 1987–1990. *Clin Infect Dis* **20**: 1275.

Noall EWP, Sewards HFG, Waterworth PM (1962). Successful treatment of a case of *Proteus septicaemia*. *Brit Med J* **2**: 1101.

Noble RC, Overman SB (1994). *Pseudomonas stutzeri* infection. A review of hospital isolates and a review of the literature. *Diagn Microbiol Infect Dis* **19**: 51.

Nolan T, Lubitz L, Oberklard F (1989). Single dose trimethoprim for urinary tract infection. *Arch Dis Child* **64**: 581.

Nordmann P, Ronco E (1992). *In-vitro* antimicrobial susceptibility of *Rhodococcus equi*. *J Antimicrob Chemother* **29**: 383.

Noriega ER, Rubinstein E, Simberkoff MS, Rahal JJ Jr (1975). Subacute and acute endocarditis due to *Pseudomonas cepacia* in heroin addicts. *Amer J Med* **59**: 29.

Norrby R, Eilard T, Svedhem åA, Lycke E (1975). Treatment of toxoplasmosis with trimethoprim-sulfamethoxazole. *Scand J Infect Dis* **7**: 72.

Norrby SR (1990). Short-term treatment of uncomplicated lower urinary tract infections in women. *Rev Infect Dis* **12**: 458.

Northrup RS, Doyle MA, Feeley JC (1972). *In vitro* susceptibility of E1 Tor and classical *Vibrio cholerae* strains to trimethoprim and sulfamethoxazole. *Antimicrob Ag Chemother* **1**: 310.

Noskin GA, Murphy RL, Black JR, Phair JP (1992). Salvage therapy with clindamycin/primaquine for *Pneumocystis carinii* pneumonia. *Clin Infect Dis* **14**: 183.

Nyberg G, Gäbel H, Althoff P *et al.* (1984). Adverse effect of trimethoprim on kidney function in renal transplant patients. *Lancet* **i**: 394.

Oberhelman RA, Javier de la Cabada F, Garrbay EV *et al.* (1987). Efficacy of trimethoprim-sulfamethoxazole in treatment of acute diarrhoea in a Mexican paediatric population. *J Paediatr* **110**: 960.

O'Grady F, Fry IK, McSherry A, Cattell WR (1973). Long-term treatment of persistent or recurrent urinary tract infection with trimethoprim-sulfamethoxazole. *J Infect Dis* **128** (Suppl): 652.

Okubadejo OA (1974). Susceptibility of *Bacteroides fragilis* to co-trimoxazole. *Lancet* **i**: 1061.

Okubadejo OA, Maskell R (1977). Trimethoprim-resistant coliforms. *Lancet* **ii**: 926.

Okubadejo OA, Green PJ, Payne DJH (1973). *Bacteroides* infection among hospital patients. *Brit Med J* **2**: 212.

Olcen P, Eriksson M (1976). The intravenous infusion of co-trimoxazole in cases of septicaemia: tolerance and results of treatment. *Scand J Infect Dis* (Suppl 8): 91.

Oleske JM, de la Cruz A, Ahdieh H *et al.* (1983). Effects of antibiotics on polymorphonuclear leukocyte chemiluminescence and chemotaxis. *J Antimicrob Chemother* **12** (Suppl C): 35.

Olsen SL, Renlund DG, O'Connell JB *et al.* (1993). Prevention of *Pneumocystis carinii* pneumonia in cardiac transplant recipients by trimethoprim sulfamethoxazole. *Transplantation* **56**: 359.

Olsson LB, Burman LG, Kallings I (1992). Antibiotic susceptibility of upper respiratory tract pathogens in Sweden: a seven year follow-up study including loracarbef Swedish Respiratory Tract Study Group. *Scand J Infect Dis* **24**: 485.

Omer MIA (1975). Trimethoprim-sulfamethoxazole in the treatment of enteric fever. *J Trop Med Hyg* **78**: 162.

Overkamp D, Waldmann B, Lins T et al. (1992). Successful treatment of brain abscess caused by *Nocardia* in an immunocompromised patient after failure of co-trimoxazole. *Infection* **20**: 365.

Owus SK (1972). Acute haemolysis complicating co-trimoxazole therapy for typhoid fever in a patient with G-6-PD deficiency. *Lancet* **ii**: 819.

Pacht E R (1990). *Mycobacterium fortuitum* lung abscess: resolution with prolonged trimethoprim/sulfamethoxazole therapy. *Amer Rev Respir Dis* **141**: 1599.

Pai CH, Gillis F, Toumanen E et al. (1984). Placebo-controlled double-blind evaluation of trimethoprim-sulfamethoxazole treatment of *Yersinia enterocolitica* gastroenteritis. *J Pediatr* **104**: 308.

Paisley JW, Washington JA II (1978). Synergistic activity of gentamicin with trimethoprim or sulfamethoxazole-trimethoprim against *Escherichia coli* and *Klebsiella pneumoniae*. *Antimicrob Ag Chemother* **14**: 656.

Palenque E, Otero JR, Noriega AR (1983). High prevalence on non-epidemic *Shigella sonnei* resistant to co-trimoxazole. *J Antimicrob Chemother* **11**: 196.

Palfreeman SJ, Waters LK, Norris M (1983). *Aeromonas hydrophila* gastroenteritis. *Aust NZ J Med* **13**: 524.

Palva IP, Koivisto O (1971). Agranulocytosis associated with trimethoprim-sulfamethoxazole. *Brit Med J* **4**: 301.

Pape JW, Verdier RI, Boncy M et al. (1994). *Cyclospora* infection in adults infected with HIV. Clinical manifestations, treatment, and prophylaxis. *Ann Intern Med* **121**: 654.

Parsley TL, Provonchee RB, Glicksman C, Zinner SH (1977). Synergistic activity of trimethoprim and amikacin against Gram-negative bacilli. *Antimicrob Ag Chemother* **12**: 349.

Parsonnett J, Greene KD, Gerber AR et al. (1989). *Shigella dysenteriae* type 1 infection in US travellers to Mexico 1988. *Lancet* **ii**: 543.

Pascule AW, Dowling JN, Frola FN et al. (1985). Antimicrobial therapy of experimental *Legionella micdadei* pneumonia in guinea pigs. *Antimicrob Ag Chemother* **28**: 730.

Pashankar D, McArdle M, Robinson A (1995). Co-trimoxazole induced aseptic meningitis. *Arch Dis Child* **73**: 257.

Paulson YJ, Gilman TM, Heseltine PN et al. (1992). Eflornithine treatment of refractory *Pneumocystis carinii* pneumonia in patients with acquired immunodeficiency syndrome. *Chest* **101**: 67.

Pavillard ER (1973). Treatment of nocardial infection with trimethoprim/sulfamethoxazole. *Med J Aust* (Special Suppl) **1**: 65.

Pearson NJ, Towner KJ, McSherry AM et al. (1979). Emergence of trimethoprim-resistant enterobacteria in patients receiving long-term co-trimoxazole for the control of intractable urinary-tract infection. *Lancet* **ii**: 1205.

Pennington CR (1980). Trimethoprim-sulfamethoxazole. Correspondence. *New Engl J Med* **303**: 1533.

Pennypacker LC, Mintzer J, Pitner J (1994). Hyperkalemia in elderly patients receiving standard doses of trimethoprim- sulfamethoxazole. *Ann Intern Med* **120**: 437.

Perkins BA, Hamill RJ, Musher DM et al. (1992). *In vitro* activities of streptomycin and 11 oral antimicrobial agents against clinical isolates of *Klebsiella rhinoscleromatis*. *Antimicrob Ag Chemother* **36**: 1785.

Phillips I, Warren C (1974). Susceptibility of *Bacteroides fragilis* to trimethoprim and sulfamethoxazole. *Lancet* **i**: 827.

Phillips I, Warren C (1976). Activity of sulfamethoxazole and trimethoprim against *Bacteroides fragilis*. *Antimicrob Ag Chemother* **9**: 736.

Phillips I, Warren C, Taylor E et al. (1981). The antimicrobial susceptibility of anaerobic bacteria in a London teaching hospital. *J Antimicrob Chemother* **8** (Suppl D): 17.

Pichler J, Knothe H, Spitzy KH, Vielkind G (1973). Treatment of chronic carriers of *Salmonella typhi* and *Salmonella paratyphi* B with trimethoprim-sulfamethoxazole. *J Infect Dis* **128** (Suppl): 743.

Piketty C, Gilquin J, Kazatchkine MD (1995). Efficacy and safety of desensitization to trimethoprim-sulfamethoxazole in human immunodeficiency virus-infected patients. *J Infect Dis* **172**: 611.

Pines A, Greenfield JSB, Raafat H et al. (1969). Preliminary experience with trimethoprim and sulfamethoxazole in the treatment of purulent chronic bronchitis. *Postgrad Med J* **45** (Suppl): 89.

Pinney RJ, Smith T (1973). Joint trimethoprim and sulfamethoxazole resistance in bacteria infected with R factors. *J Med Microbiol* **6**: 13.

Pizzo PA (1983). Antibiotic prophylaxis in the immunosuppressed patient with cancer. In: *Current Clinical Topics in Infectious Diseases* Vol 4, pp. 153–167 (Remington JS, Swartz MN, eds), New York: McGraw Hill.

Pizzo PA (1989). Considerations for the prevention of infectious complications in patients with cancer. *Rev Infect Dis* **11** (Suppl 7): S1551.

Pizzo PA, Robichaud KJ, Edwards BK et al. (1983). Oral antibiotic prophylaxis in patients with cancer: a double-blind randomized placebo-controlled trial. *J Pediatr* **102**: 125.

Platt DJ, Guthrie AJ, Langan CE (1983). The isolation of thymidine-requiring *Haemophilus influenzae* from the sputum of chronic bronchitic patients receiving trimethoprim. *J Antimicrob Chemother* **11**: 281.

Plouffe JF, Para MF, Bollin GE (1984). Sulfamethoxazole-trimethoprim treatment of guinea pigs infected with *Legionella pneumophila*. *J Infect Dis* **150**: 780.

Plourde PJ, D'Costa LJ, Agoki E et al. (1992). A randomized, double-blind study of the efficacy of fleroxacin versus trimethoprim-sulfamethoxazole in men with culture-proven chancroid. *J Infect Dis* **165**: 949.

Plummer FA, Nsanze H, D'Costa LJ et al. (1983). Short-course and single-dose antimicrobial therapy for chancroid in Kenya: studies with rifampin alone and in combination with trimethoprim. *Rev Infect Dis* **5**: 565.

Podzamczer D, Salazar A, Jimenez J et al. (1995). Intermittent trimethoprim-sulfamethoxazole compared with dapsone-pyrimethamine for the simultaneous primary prophylaxis of *Pneumocystis pneumonia* and toxoplasmosis in patients infected with HIV. *Ann Intern Med* **122**: 755.

Pope JW, Verdier RL, Johnson WD, Jr (1989). Treatment and prophylaxis of *Isopora belli* infection in patients with the acquired immunodeficiency syndrome. *New Engl J Med* **320**: 1044.

Pozniak A, Weinberg J, Macleod G (1991). HIV and co-trimoxazole toxicity. *Lancet* **338**: 760.

Preston MA, Simor AE, Walmsley S et al. (1990). *In vitro* susceptibility of 'Campylobacter upsaliensis' to twenty-four antimicrobial agents. *Eur J Clin Microbiol Infect Dis* **9**: 822.

Preston MA, Brown S, Borczyk AA et al. (1994). Antimicrobial susceptibility of pathogenic *Yersinia enterocolitica* isolated in Canada from 1972 to 1990. *Antimicrob Ag Chemother* **38**: 2121.

Prior RB, Fass RJ, Perkins RL (1976). Regression-line analysis of trimethoprim-sulfamethoxazole activity against *Neisseria gonorrhoeae*. *Amer J Clin Path* **66**: 605.

Putterman C, Rahav G, Shalit M et al. (1990). 'Treating through' hypersensitivity to co-trimoxazole in AIDS patients. *Lancet* **336**: 52.

Rahal JJ, Simberkoff MS (1982). Host defense and antimicrobial therapy in adult Gram-negative bacillary meningitis. *Ann Intern Med* **96**: 468.

Rahal JJ Jr, Simberkoff MS, Hymans PJ (1973). *Pseudomonas cepacia* tricuspid endocarditis: Treatment with trimethoprim, sulfonamide, and polymyxin B. *J Infect Dis* **128** (Suppl): 762.

Raik E, Vincent PC (1973). Thrombocytopenia with combined trimethoprim-sulfamethoxazole and allopurinol therapy. *Med J Aust* **2**: 468.

Rainer CA, Feigal DW, Leoung G et al. (1987). Prognosis and natural history of *Pneumocystis carinii* pneumonia: indicators for early and late survival. International Conference on AIDS, Washington, DC, June 1–5.

Rajkumar S, Saxena Y, Rajagopal V, Sierra MF (1988–89). Trimethoprim in pediatric urinary tract infection. *Child Nephrol Urol* **9**: 77.

Ramachandran S, Godfrey JJ, Lionel NDW (1978). A comparative trial of co-trimoxazole and chloramphenicol in typhoid and paratyphoid fever. *J Trop Med & Hyg* **81**: 36.

Ramaiah RS, Gallagher MA, Biagi RW (1977). Reactions to co-trimoxazole. *Lancet* **i**: 604.

Rao PS, Rajashekar V, Varghese GK et al. (1993). Emergence of multidrug-resistant *Salmonella typhi* in rural southern India. *Amer J Trop Med Hyg* **48**: 108.

Rauch AM, O'Ryan M, Van R et al. (1990). Invasive disease due to multiply resistant *Streptococcus pneumoniae* in a Houston, Texas, day-care center. *Am J Dis Child* **144**: 923.

Reed MD, Stern RC, Bertino JS et al. (1984). Dosing implications of rapid elimination of trimethoprim-sulfamethoxazole in patients with cystic fibrosis. *J Pediatr* **104**: 303.

Reeves D (1982). Sulphonamides and trimethoprim. *Lancet* **ii**: 370.

Reeves DS, Faiers MC, Pursell RE, Brumfitt W (1969). Trimethoprim-sulfamethoxazole: comparative study in urinary infection in hospital. *Brit Med J* **1**: 541.

Reinhardt JF, George WL (1985). Comparative *in vitro* activities of selected antimicrobial agents against *Aeromonas* species and *Plesiomonas shigelloides*. *Antimicrob Ag Chemother* **27**: 643.

Reisberg B, Herzog J, Weinstein L (1967). *In vitro* antibacterial activity of trimethoprim alone and combined with sulphonamides. *Antimicrob Ag Chemother* **1966**: 424.

Renmarker K (1976). A comparative trial of co-trimoxazole and doxycycline in the treatment of acute exacerbations of chronic bronchitis. *Scand J Infect Dis* (Suppl 8): 75.

Review Article (1990). (Amyse SGB, Towner KJ eds). Trimethoprim resistance; epidemiology and molecular aspects. *J Med Microbiol* **31**: 1.

Riben PD, Louie TJ, Lank BA *et al.* (1983). Reduction in mortality from Gram-negative sepsis in neutropenic patients receiving trimethoprim-sulfamethoxazole therapy. *Cancer* **51**: 1587.

Rice RJ, Bhullar V, Mitchell SH *et al.* (1995). Susceptibilities of *Chlamydia trachomatis* isolates causing uncomplicated female genital tract infections and pelvic inflammatory disease. *Antimicrob Ag Chemother* **39**: 760.

Richards FO, Jr, Kovacs JA, Luft BJ (1995). Preventing toxoplasmic encephalitis in persons infected with human immunodeficiency virus. *Clin Infect Dis* **21** (Suppl 1): S49.

Richmond JM, Whitworth JA, Fairley KF, Kincaid-Smith P (1979). Co-trimoxazole nephrotoxicity. *Lancet* **i**: 493.

Rickard KA, Uhr E (1971). Acute thrombocytopenic purpura associated with 'Septrin'. *Med J Aust* **1**: 769.

Rieder J (1973). Excretion of sulfamethoxazole and trimethoprim into human bile. *J Infect Dis* **128** (Suppl): 574.

Ries AA, Wells JG, Olivola D *et al.* (1994). Epidemic *Shigella dysenteriae* type 1 in Burundi: panresistance and implications for prevention. *J Infect Dis* **169**: 1035.

Riley TV (1981). Agar dilution susceptibility of *Bacteroides* spp to sulfamethoxazole and trimethoprim: correlation with a disk diffusion technique. *Antimicrob Ag Chemother* **20**: 731.

Ringdén O, Myrenfors P, Klintmalm G *et al.* (1984). Nephrotoxicity by co-trimoxazole and cyclosporin in transplanted patients. *Lancet* **i**: 1016.

Robertson L, Farrell ID, Hinchliffe PM (1973). The sensitivity of *Brucella abortus* to chemotherapeutic agents. *J Med Microbiol* **6**: 549.

Rodriguez WJ, Kahn WN, Ross S *et al.* (1978). Trimethoprim-sulfamethoxazole in shigellosis. In *Current Chemotherapy: Proceedings of the 10th International Congress of Chemotherapy, Zurich/Switzerland, 1977* (Siegenthaler W, Lüthy R, eds), p. 172. Washington, DC: American Society for Microbiology.

Roldan A, Molina J A, Fernandez A *et al.* (1988). TMP-SMZ in the treatment of brucellar meningitis. *Rev Infect Dis* **10**: 1233.

Rosborough TK, Rierach CA (1995). Three vs 10 days of trimethoprim/sulfamethoxazole for acute maxillary sinusitis. *JAMA* **274**: 1341; discussion 134.

Rosenblatt JE, Stewart PR (1974). Lack of activity of sulfamethoxazole and trimethoprim against anaerobic bacteria. *Antimicrob Ag Chemother* **6**: 93.

Rosenfeld JB, Najenson T, Grosswater Z (1975). Effect of long-term co-trimoxazole therapy on renal function. *Med J Aust* **2**: 546.

Roth B, Falco EA, Hitchings GA, Bushby SRM (1962). 5-benzyl-2,4-diamino-pyrimidines as antibacterial agents I Synthesis and antibacterial activity *in vitro*. *J Med Pharm Chem* **5**: 1103; quoted by Darrell *et al.* (1968).

Roudier C, Caumes E, Rogeaux O *et al.* (1994). Adverse cutaneous reactions to trimethoprim-sulfamethoxazole in patients with the acquired immunodeficiency syndrome and *Pneumocystis carinii* pneumonia. *Arch Dermatol* **130**: 1383.

Roujeau JC, Kelly JP, Naldi L *et al.* (1995). Medication use and the risk of Stevens–Johnson syndrome or toxic epidermal necrolysis. *New Engl J Med* **333**: 1600.

Rowe B, Ward LR, Threlfall EJ (1990). Spread of multi-resistant *Salmonella typhi*. *Lancet* **336**: 1065.

Roy LP (1971). Sulfamethoxazole-trimethoprim in infancy. *Med J Aust* **1**: 148.

Rubin RH, Swartz MN (1980). Trimethoprim-sulfamethoxazole. Correspondence. *New Engl J Med* **303**: 1534.

Ruf B, Pohle HD (1989). Clindamycin/primaquine for *Pneumocystis carinii* pneumonia. *Lancet* **ii**: 626.

Ruskin J, LaRiviere M (1991). Low-dose co-trimoxazole for prevention of *Pneumocystis carinii* pneumonia in human immunodeficiency virus disease. *Lancet* **337**: 468.

Russell NJ (1981). Treatment of *Pneumocystis carinii* pneumonia. *J Antimicrob Chemother* **8**: 87.

Russel PB, Hitchings GH (1951). 2,4-diaminopyrimidines as antimalarials III. 5-aryl-derivatives. *J Amer Chem Soc* **73**: 3763.

Sabel KG, Brandberg åA (1975). Treatment of meningitis and septicaemia in infancy with a sulfamethoxazole/trimethoprim combination. *Acta Paediatr Scand* **64**: 25.

Safrin S, Lee BL, Sande MA (1994). Adjunctive folinic acid with trimethoprim-sulfamethoxazole for *Pneumocystis carinii* pneumonia in AIDS patients is associated with an increased risk of therapeutic failure and death. *J Infect Dis* **170**: 912.

Salam MA, Bennish ML (1991). Antimicrobial therapy for shigellosis. *Rev Infect Dis* **13** (Suppl 4): S332.

Salmon JD, Fowle ASE, Bye A (1975). Concentrations of trimethoprim and sulfamethoxazole in aqueous humour and plasma from regimens of co-trimoxazole in man. *J Antimicrob Chemother* **1**: 205.

Salter AJ (1973). The toxicity profile of trimethoprim/sulfamethoxazole after four years of widespread use. *Med J Aust* (Special Suppl) **1**: 70.

Salter AJ (1982). Trimethoprim-sulfamethoxazole in treatment of severe infections. *Rev Infect Dis* **4**: 338.

Saltissi D, Pusey CD, Rainford DJ (1979). Recurrent acute renal failure due to antibiotic-induced interstitial nephritis. *Brit Med J* **1**: 1182.

Sanchez C, Garcia-Restoy E, Garau J *et al.* (1993). Ciprofloxacin and trimethoprim-sulfamethoxazole versus placebo in acute uncomplicated *Salmonella* enteritis: a double-blind trial. *J Infect Dis* **168**: 1304.

Sandberg T, Trollfors B (1986). Effect of trimethoprim on serum creatinine in patients with acute cystitis. *J Antimicrob Chemother* **17**: 123.

Sands M, Brown RB (1989). Interactions of cyclosporine with antimicrobial agents. *Rev Infect Dis* **11**: 691.

Sanford JP (1993). *Guide to Antimicrobial Therapy*. West Bethesda, USA: Antimicrobial Therapy Inc.

Santamaria-Jaúregui J, Sanz-Hospital J, Berenguer J *et al.* (1984). Meningitis caused by *Mycobacterium fortuitum*. *Amer Rev Respir Dis* **130**: 136.

Sardesai HV, Karandikar RS, Harshe RG (1973). Comparative trial of co-trimoxazole and chloramphenicol in typhoid fever. *Brit Med J* **1**: 82.

Sattar MA, Cawley MID, Holt JE *et al.* (1983). The penetration of trimethoprim and sulfamethoxazole into synovial fluid. *J Antimicrob Chemother* **12**: 229.

Sattler FR, Remington JS (1981). Intravenous trimethoprim-sulfamethoxazole therapy for *Pneumocystis carinii* pneumonia. *Amer J Med* **70**: 1215.

Sattler FR, Remington JS (1983). Intravenous sulfamethoxazole and trimethoprim for serious Gram-negative bacillary infections. *Arch Intern Med* **143**: 1709.

Sattler FR, Ruskin J (1978). Therapy of gonorrhea Comparison of trimethoprim-sulfamethoxazole and ampicillin. *JAMA* **240**: 2267.

Sattler FR, Cowan R, Nielsen DM *et al.* (1988). Trimethoprim-sulfamethoxazole compared with pentamidine for treatment of *Pneumocystis carinii* pneumonia in the acquired immunodeficiency syndrome. A prospective, noncrossover study. *Ann Intern Med* **109**: 280.

Sattler FR, Frame P, Davis R *et al.* (1994). Trimetrexate with leucovorin versus trimethoprim-sulfamethoxazole for moderate to severe episodes of

Pneumocystis carinii pneumonia in patients with AIDS: a prospective, controlled multicenter investigation of the AIDS Clinical Trials Group Protocol 029/031. *J Infect Dis* 170: 165.

Sawyer J, Stryer D, Rydberg M, Polstein B (1995). Three vs 10 days of trimethoprim/sulfamethoxazole for acute maxillary sinusitis. *JAMA* 274: 1341; discussion 134.

Schattner A, Rimon E, Green L *et al.* (1988). Hypoglycemia induced by co-trimoxazole in AIDS. *Brit Med J* 297.

Scheer MS, Hirschman SZ (1982). Oral and ambulatory therapy of *Listeria* bacteremia and meningitis with trimethoprim-sulfamethoxazole. *Mt Sinai J Med* 49: 411.

Schiff TA, McNeil MM, Brown JM (1993). Cutaneous *Nocardia farcinica* infection in a non-immunocompromised patient: case report and review. *Clin Infect Dis* 16: 756.

Schmid GP (1986). The treatment of chancroid. *JAMA* 255: 1757.

Schmid GP (1990). Treatment of chancroid, 1989. *Rev Infect Dis* 12 (Suppl 6): S580.

Schmidt U, Sen P, Kapila R, Louria DB (1982). Clinical evaluation of intravenous trimethoprim-sulfamethoxazole for serious infections. *Rev Infect Dis* 4: 332.

Schneider MM, Hoepelman AI, Eeftinck-Schattenkerk JK *et al.* (1992). A controlled trial of aerosolized pentamidine or trimethoprim-sulfamethoxazole as primary prophylaxis against *Pneumocystis carinii* pneumonia in patients with human immunodeficiency virus infection. *New Engl J Med* 327: 1836.

Schneider MM, Nielsen TL, Nelsing S *et al.* (1995). Efficacy and toxicity of two doses of trimethoprim-sulfamethoxazole as primary prophylaxis against *Pneumocystis carinii* pneumonia in patients with human immunodeficiency virus. Dutch AIDS Treatment Group. *J Infect Dis* 171: 1632.

Schofield CBS, Masterton G, Moffett M, McGill MI (1971). Gonorrhoea in women: treatment with sulfamethoxazole and trimethoprim. *J Infect Dis* 124: 533.

Schulte JM, Schmid GP (1995). Recommendations for treatment of chancroid. *Clin Infect Dis* 20 (Suppl 1): S39.

Schwartz DE, Ziegler WH (1969). Assay and pharmacokinetics of trimethoprim in man and animals. *Postgrad Med J* 45 (Suppl): 32.

Schwartz RH, Rodriguez WJ, Khan WN *et al.* (1982). Trimethoprim-sulfamethoxazole in the treatment of otitis media caused by ampicillin-resistant strains of *Haemophilus influenzae*. *Rev Infect Dis* 4: 514.

Scragg JN, Rubidge CJ (1971). Trimethoprim and sulfamethoxazole in typhoid fever in children. *Brit Med J* 3: 738.

Seah SKK (1975). Chemotherapy in experimental toxoplasmosis: comparison of the efficacy of trimethoprim-sulfur and pyrimethamine-sulfur combinations. *J Trop Med Hyg* 78: 150.

Seligman SJ (1973). *In vitro* susceptibility of methicillin-resistant *Staphylococcus aureus* to sulfamethoxazole and trimethoprim. *J Infect Dis* 128 (Suppl): 543.

Seligman SJ, Madhavan T, Alcid D (1973). Trimethoprim-sulfamethoxazole in the treatment of bacterial endocarditis. *J Infect Dis* 128 (Suppl): 754.

Seppänen J, Sulkava T, Vaalasti T *et al.* (1983). Combination of trimethoprim and methenamine hippurate in the treatment of acute urinary tract infection. *Scand J Infect Dis* 15: 201.

Shaefer CF, Trincher RC, Rissing JP (1983). Melioidosis: recrudescence with a strain resistant to multiple antimicrobials. *Amer Rev Respir Dis* 128: 173.

Shafer RW, Seitzman PA, Tapper ML (1989). Successful prophylaxis of *Pneumocystis carinii* pneumonia with trimethoprim-sulfamethoxazole in AIDS patients with previous allergic reactions. *J AIDS* 2: 389.

Shahar E (1995). Three vs 10 days of trimethoprim/sulfamethoxazole for acute maxillary sinusitis. *JAMA* 274: 1341.

Shalit M, Levy M (1984). Co-trimoxazole reaction simulating sepsis. *J Infect* 9: 291.

Shapiro JA, Sporn P (1977). Tn402: a new transposable element determining trimethoprim resistance that inserts in bacteriophage lambda. *J Bacteriol* 129: 1632.

Sharpstone P (1969). The renal handling of trimethoprim and sulfamethoxazole in man. *Postgrad Med J* 45 (Suppl): 38.

Sher MR, Suchar C, Lockey RF (1986). Anaphylactic shock induced by oral desensitization to trimethoprim-sulfamethoxazole. *J Allergy Clin Immunol* 77: 133 .

Shouval D, Ligumsky M, Ben-Ishay D (1978). Effect of co-trimoxazole on normal creatinine clearance. *Lancet* i: 244.

Siber GR, Gorham CC, Ericson JF, Smith AL (1982). Pharmacokinetics of intravenous trimethoprim-sulfamethoxazole in children and adults with normal and impaired renal function. *Rev Infect Dis* 4: 566.

Siegel JP, Remington JS (1982). Effect of antimicrobial agents on chemiluminescence of human polymorphonuclear leukocytes in response to phagocytosis. *J Antimicrob Chemother* 10: 505.

Sifuentes-Osornio J, Porras-Cortes G, Bendall RP *et al.* (1995). *Cyclospora cayetanensis* infection in patients with and without AIDS: biliary disease as another clinical manifestation. *Clin Infect Dis* 21: 1092.

Sigel CW, Grace ME, Nichol CA (1973). Metabolism of trimethoprim in man and measurement of a new metabolite: a new fluorescence assay. *J Infect Dis* 128 (Suppl): 580.

Simonds RJ, Hughes WT, Feinberg J, Navin TR (1995). Preventing *Pneumocystis carinii* pneumonia in persons infected with human immunodeficiency virus. *Clin Infect Dis* 21 (Suppl 1): S44.

Sinai R, Hammerberg S, Marks MI, Pai CH (1978). *In vitro* susceptibility of *Haemophilus influenzae* to sulfamethoxazole-trimethoprim and cefaclor, cephalexin and cephradine. *Antimicrob Ag Chemother* 13: 861.

Singh N, Gayowski T, Yu VL, Wagener MM (1995). Trimethoprim-sulfamethoxazole for the prevention of spontaneous bacterial peritonitis in cirrhosis: a randomized trial. *Ann Intern Med* 122: 595.

Sive J, Green R, Metz J (1972). Effect of trimethoprim on folate-dependent DNA synthesis in human bone marrow. *J Clin Path* 25: 194.

Slevin NJ, Aitken J, Thornley PE (1984). Clinical and microbiological features of *Branhamella catarrhalis* bronchopulmonary infections. *Lancet* i: 782.

Smego RA Jr, Moeller MB, Gallis HA (1983). Trimethoprim-sulfamethoxazole therapy for *Nocardia* infections. *Arch Intern Med* 143: 711.

Smego RA Jr, Gallis HA (1984). The clinical spectrum of *Nocardia brasiliensis* infection in the United States. *Rev Infect Dis* 6: 164.

Smellie JM, Grüneberg RN, Leakey A, Atkin WS (1976). Long-term low-dose co-trimoxazole in prophylaxis of childhood urinary tract infection: clinical aspects. *Brit Med J* 2: 203.

Smellie JM, Katz G, Grüneberg RN (1978). Controlled trial of prophylactic treatment in childhood urinary-tract infection. *Lancet* ii: 175.

Smellie JM, Grüneberg RN, Normand ICS *et al.* (1982). Trimethoprim-sulfamethoxazole and trimethoprim alone in the prophylaxis of childhood urinary tract infection. *Rev Infect Dis* 4: 461.

Smith EJ, Light JA, Filo RS, Yum MN (1980). Interstitial nephritis caused by trimethoprim-sulfamethoxazole in renal transplant recipients. *JAMA* 244: 360.

Smith GW, Cohen SB (1994). Hyperkalaemia and non-oliguric renal failure associated with trimethoprim. *Brit Med J* 308: 454.

Smith JW, Jones SR, Reed WP *et al.* (1979). Recurrent urinary tract infections in men. Characteristics and response to therapy. *Ann Intern Med* 91: 544.

Snyder MJ, Perroni J, Gonzalez O *et al.* (1973). Trimethoprim-sulfamethoxazole in the treatment of typhoid and paratyphoid fevers. *J Infect Dis* 128 (Suppl): 734.

Snyder MJ, Perroni J, Gonzalez O *et al.* (1976). Comparative efficacy of chloramphenicol, ampicillin, and co-trimoxazole in the treatment of typhoid fever. *Lancet* ii: 1155.

Soave R, Johnson WD Jr (1995). Cyclospora: conquest of an emerging pathogen. *Lancet* 345: 667.

Sookpranee M, Boonma P, Susaengrat W *et al.* (1992). Multicenter prospective randomized trial comparing ceftazidime plus co-trimoxazole with chloramphenicol plus doxycycline and co-trimoxazole for treatment of severe melioidosis. *Antimicrob Ag Chemother* 36: 158.

Sorvillo F, Lieb L, Luiakoshi K, Waterman SH (1990). *I belli* and the acquired immunodeficiency syndrome. *New Engl J Med* 322: 131.

Souney P, Polk BF (1982). Single-dose antimicrobial therapy for urinary tract infections in women. *Rev Infect Dis* **4**: 29.

Special Report The National Institutes of Health-University of California Expert Panel for Corticosteroids as Adjunctive Therapy for Pneumocystis Pneumonia (1990). Consensus statement on the use of corticosteroids as adjunctive therapy for pneumocystis pneumonia in the acquired immunodeficiency syndrome. *New Engl J Med* **323**: 1500.

Speller DCE (1973). *Pseudomonas cepacia* endocarditis treated with cotrimoxazole and kanamycin. *Br Heart J* **35**: 47 .

Spencer CM, Goa KL (1995). Atovaquone A review of its pharmacological properties and therapeutic efficacy in opportunistic infections. *Drugs* **50**: 176.

Spicehandler J, Pollock AA, Simberkoff MS, Rahal JJ Jr (1982). Intravenous pharmacokinetics and *in vitro* bactericidal activity of trimethoprim-sulfamethoxazole. *Rev Infect Dis* **4**: 562.

Spika JS, Facklam RR, Plikaytis BD *et al.* (1991). Antimicrobial resistance of *Streptococcus pneumoniae* in the United States, 1979–1987. The Pneumococcal Surveillance Working Group. *J Infect Dis* **163**: 1273.

Spitzer PG, Hammer SM, Karchmer AW (1986). Treatment of *Listeria monocytogenes* infection with trimethoprim-sulfamethoxazole: Case report and review of literature. *Rev Infect Dis* **8**: 427.

Springer C, Eyal F, Michel J (1982). Pharmacology of trimethoprim-sulfamethoxazole in newborn infants. *J Pediatr* **100**: 647.

Stamatakis MK, Sorkin MI, Moss AH (1995). Toxicity following IP trimethoprim-sulfamethoxazole in a CAPD patient. *Perit Dial Int* **15**: 180.

Stamey TA, Condy M (1975). The diffusion and concentration of trimethoprim in human vaginal fluid. *J Infect Dis* **131**: 261.

Stamey TA, Condy M, Mihara G (1977). Prophylactic efficacy of nitrofurantoin macrocrystals and trimethoprim-sulfamethoxazole in urinary infections. Biologic effects on the vaginal and rectal flora. *New Engl J Med* **296**: 780.

Stamm WE, Counts GW, Wagner KF *et al.* (1980). Antimicrobial prophylaxis of recurrent urinary tract infections. A double-blind, placebo-controlled trial. *Ann Intern Med* **92**: 770.

Stamm WE, Guinan ME, Johnson C *et al.* (1984). Effect of treatment regimens for *Neisseria gonorrhoeae* on simultaneous infection with *Chlamydia trachomatis*. *New Engl J Med* **310**: 545.

Stamm WE, McKevitt M, Counts GW (1987). Acute renal infection in women: treatment with trimethoprim-sulfamethoxazole or ampicillin for two or six weeks. A randomized trial. *Ann Intern Med* **106**: 341.

Stamm WE, McKevitt M, Roberts PL *et al.* (1991). Natural history of recurrent urinary tract infections in women. *Rev Infect Dis* **13**: 77.

Stansfeld JM (1975). Duration of treatment for urinary tract infections in children. *Brit Med J* **3**: 65.

Stapleton A, Latham RH, Johnson C *et al.* (1990). Postcoital antimicrobial prophylaxis for recurrent urinary tract infection. A randomized, double-blind, placebo-controlled trial. *JAMA* **264**: 703.

Starke ID, Donnelly P, Catovsky D *et al.* (1982). Co-trimoxazole alone for prevention of bacterial infection in patients with acute leukaemia. *Lancet* **i**: 5.

Stein D S, Stevens R C, Terry D *et al.* (1991). Use of low-dose trimethoprim-sulfamethoxazole thrice weekly for primary and secondary prophylaxis of *Pneumocystis carinii* pneumonia in human immunodeficiency virus-infected patients. *Antimicrob Ag Chemother* **35**: 1705.

Stevens DA, Vo PT (1982). Synergistic interaction of trimethoprim and sulfamethoxazole on *Paracoccidoides brasiliensis*. *Antimicrob Ag Chemother* **21**: 852.

Stevens RC, Laizure SC, Williams CL *et al.* (1991). Pharmacokinetics and adverse effects of 20 mg per kg per day trimethoprim and 100 mg per kg per day sulfamethoxazole in healthy adult subjects. *Antimicrob Ag Chemother* **35**: 1884.

Stevens RC, Laizure SC, Sanders PL, Stein DS (1993). Multiple-dose pharmacokinetics of 12 milligrams of trimethoprim and 60 milligrams of sulfamethoxazole per kilogram of body weight per day in healthy volunteers. *Antimicrob Ag Chemother* **37**: 448.

Stevenson DK, Christie DL, Haas JE (1978). Hepatic injury in a child caused by trimethoprim-sulfamethoxazole. *Pediatrics* **61**: 864.

Stratford BC, Dixson S (1971). Results of treatment with trimethoprim plus sulfamethoxazole. *Med J Aust* **1**: 526.

Street AC, Durack DT (1988). Experience with trimethoprim-sulfamethoxazole in treatment of infective endocarditis. *Rev Infect Dis* **10**: 915.

Streiffer RH, Hudson JG (1986). Aseptic meningitis and trimethoprim-sulfamethoxazole. *J Fam Pract* **23**: 314.

Stringer SL, Stringer JR, Blase MA *et al.* (1989). *Pneumocystis carinii*: sequence from ribosomal RNA implies a close relationship with fungi. *Exp Parasitol* **68**: 450.

Sturm AW (1987). Comparison of antimicrobial susceptibility patterns of fifty-seven strains of *Haemophilus ducreyi* isolated in Amsterdam from 1978 to 1985. *J Antimicrob Chemother* **19**: 187.

Svedhem A, Iwarson S (1979). Cerebrospinal fluid concentrations of trimethoprim during oral and parenteral treatment. *J Antimicrob Chemother* **5**: 717.

Svensson R, Larsson P, Lincoln K (1982). Low dose trimethoprim prophylaxis in long-term control of chronic recurrent urinary tract infection. *Scand J Infect Dis* **14**: 139.

Svindland HB (1973). Treatment of gonorrhoea with sulfamethoxazole-trimethoprim. Lack of effect on concomitant syphilis. *Brit J Vener Dis* **49**: 50.

Sweeney KG, Verghese A, Needham CA (1985). *In vitro* susceptibilities of isolates from patients from *Branhamella catarrhalis* pneumonia compared with those of colonizing strains. *Antimicrob Ag Chemother* **27**: 499.

Tabtieng R, Wattanasri S, Echeverria P *et al.* (1989). An epidemic of *Vibrio cholerae* el tor Inaba resistant to several antibiotics with a conjugative group C plasmid coding for type II dihydrofolate reductase in Thailand. *Amer J Trop Med Hyg* **41**: 680.

Tapsall JW, Wilson E, Harper J (1974). Thymine dependent strains of *Escherichia coli* selected by trimethoprim-sulfamethoxazole therapy. *Pathology* **6**: 161.

Tasker PRW, MacGregor GA, De Wardener HE *et al.* (1975). Use of co-trimoxazole in chronic renal failure. *Lancet* **i**: 1216.

Tauxe RV, Puhr ND, Wells JG *et al.* (1990). Antimicrobial resistance of *Shigella* isolates in the USA: the importance of international travelers. *J Infect Dis* **162**: 1107.

Taylor DN, Pitarangsi C, Echeverria P *et al.* (1985). Comparative study of ceftriaxone and trimethoprim-sulfamethoxazole for the treatment of chancroid in Thailand. *J Infect Dis* **152**: 1002.

Taylor DN, Bodhidatta L, Brown JE *et al.* (1989). Introduction and spread of multi-resistant *Shigella dysenteriae* I in Thailand. *Amer J Trop Med Hyg* **40**: 77.

Tennent JM, Lyon BR, Gillespie MT *et al.* (1983). Cloning and expression of *Staphylococcus aureus* plasmid-mediating quaternary ammonium resistance in *Escherichia coli*. *Antimicrob Ag Chemother* **27**: 79.

Then RL (1982). Mechanisms of resistance to trimethoprim, the sulfonamides, and trimethoprim-sulfamethoxazole. *Rev Infect Dis* **4**: 261.

Then RL, Angehrn P (1979). Low trimethoprim susceptibility of anaerobic bacteria due to insensitive dihydrofolate reductases. *Antimicrob Ag Chemother* **15**: 1.

Then RL, Böhni E, Angehrn P *et al.* (1982). New analogs of trimethoprim. *Rev Infect Dis* **4**: 372.

Theodorou AA, Barton LL, Rice SA, Rieder MJ (1995). Trimethoprim-sulfamethoxazole-associated central nervous system disease. *Pediatr Infect Dis J* **14**: 76.

Thisyakorn US, Rienprayoon S (1992). Shigellosis in Thai children: epidemiologic, clinical and laboratory features. *Pediatr Infect Dis J* **11**: 213.

Thomas FE Jr, Leonard JM, Alford RH (1976). Sulfamethoxazole-trimethoprim-polymyxin therapy of serious multiple drug-resistant *Serratia* infections. *Antimicrob Ag Chemother* **9**: 201.

Thornsberry C, Baker CN, Kirven LA (1978). *In vitro* activity of antimicrobial agents on Legionnaires' disease bacterium. *Antimicrob Ag Chemother* **13**: 78.

Thorpe JAC, Nysenbaum A (1978). Co-trimoxazole fatality. *Lancet* **i**: 276.

Threlfall EJ, Ward LR, Rowe B *et al.* (1992). Widespread occurrence of multiple drug-resistant *Salmonella typhi* in India. *Eur J Clin Microbiol Infect Dis* **11**: 990.

Tobin MJ, Cahill N, Gearty G *et al.* (1982). Q fever endocarditis. *Amer J Med* **72**: 396.

Tofte RW, Solliday J, Crossley KB (1984). Susceptibilities of enterococci to twelve antibiotics. *Antimicrob Ag Chemother* **25**: 532.

Tolkoff-Rubin NE, Weber D, Fang LST *et al.* (1982a). Single-dose therapy with trimethoprim-sulfamethoxazole for urinary tract infections in women. *Rev Infect Dis* **4**: 444.

Tolkoff-Rubin NE, Cosimi AB, Russell PS, Rubin RH (1982b). A controlled study of trimethoprim-sulfamethoxazole prophylaxis of urinary tract infection in renal transplant recipients. *Rev Infect Dis* **4**: 614.

Toma E, Fournier S, Poisson M *et al.* (1989). Clindamycin with primaquine for *Pneumocystis carinii* pneumonia. *Lancet* **i**: 1046.

Toma E, Fournier S, Dumont M, Bolduc P, Deschamps H (1993). Clindamycin/primaquine versus trimethoprim-sulfamethoxazole as primary therapy for *Pneumocystis carinii* pneumonia in AIDS: a randomized, double-blind pilot trial. *Clin Infect Dis* **17**: 178.

Towner KJ, Amyes SG Young H-K (1992). Classification of plasmid-encoded trimethoprim resistance genes. *J Antimicrob Chemother* **30**: 108.

Trickett PC, Dineen P, Mogabgab W (1973). Trimethoprim-sulfamethoxazole versus penicillin G in the treatment of Group A beta-hemolytic streptococcal pharyngitis and tonsillitis. *J Infect Dis* **128** (Suppl): 693.

Trienekens TA, Stobberingh EE, Winkens RA *et al.* (1989). Different lengths of treatment with co-trimoxazole for acute uncomplicated urinary tract infections in women. *Brit Med J* **299**: 1319.

Trimethoprim Study Group (1981). Comparison of trimethoprim at three dosage levels with co-trimoxazole in the treatment of acute symptomatic urinary tract infection in general practice. *J Antimicrob Chemother* **7**: 179.

Trollfors B, Wahl M, Alestig K (1980). Co-trimoxazole, creatinine and renal function. *J Infect* **2**: 221.

Tsakris A, Johnson AP, Legakis NJ, Tzouvelekis LS (1993). Prevalence of the type I and type II DHFR genes in trimethoprim-resistant urinary isolates of *Escherichia coli* from Greece. *J Antimicrob Chemother* **31**: 665.

Tulloch AL (1976). Pancytopenia in an infant associated with sulfamethoxazole-trimethoprim therapy. *J Pediatr* **88**: 499.

Tungsanga K, Chongthaleong A, Udomsantisuk N *et al.* (1988). Norfloxacin versus co-trimoxazole for the treatment of upper urinary tract infections: a double blind trial. *Scand. J Infect Dis* (Suppl 56): 28.

Tunkel AR, Starr K (1990). Trimethoprim-sulfamethoxazole-associated aseptic meningitis. *Amer J Med* **88**: 696.

Turnidge JD (1988). A reappraisal of co-trimoxazole. *Med J Aust* **148**: 296.

Turnidge JD (1989). Corrigendum: a reappraisal of co-trimoxazole. *Med J Aust* **151**: 355.

Turnidge JD, Nimmo GR, Francis G (1996). Evolution of resistance in *Staphylococcus aureus* in Australian teaching hospitals. Australian Group on Antimicrobial Resistance (AGAR). *Med J Aust* **164**: 68.

Ullmann U, Giebel W, Bamberg P (1983). Concentrations of sulphadiazine and trimethoprim in nasal secretions after co-trimazine administration. *J Antimicrob Chemother* **11**: 89.

Uwaydah M, Matossian R, Balabanian M (1975). Co-trimoxazole compared to chloramphenicol in the treatment of enteric fever. *Scand. J Infect Dis* **7**: 123.

Uylangco C, Santiago L, Pescante M *et al.* (1984). Pivmecillinam, co-trimoxazole and oral mecillinam in gastroenteritis due to *Vibrio* spp. *J Antimicrob Chemother* **13**: 171.

Valeriano-Marset J, Spiera H (1991). Treatment of Wegener's granulomatosis with sulfamethoxazole-trimethoprim. *Arch Intern Med* **151**: 1649.

Vandenbroucke-Grauls CMJE, Rosenberg-Arska M, den Hengst CW, Verhoef J (1982). Prostatitis due to penicillinase-producing *Neisseria gonorrhoeae*. Case reports. *Brit J Vener Dis* **58**: 311.

Van der Meer JWM, Van den Broek PJ (1984). Present stats of the management of patients with defective phagocyte function. *Rev Infect Dis* **6**: 107.

Van der Ven A, Koopmans PP, Vree TB *et al.* (1991). Adverse reactions to co-trimoxazole in HIV infection. *Lancet* **338**: 431.

Van Dyck E, Bogaerts J, Smet H *et al.* (1994). Emergence of *Haemophilus ducreyi* resistance to trimethoprim-sulfamethoxazole in Rwanda. *Antimicrob Ag Chemother* **38**: 1647.

Vartivarian S, Anaissie E, Bodey G, Sprigg H, Rolston K (1994). A changing pattern of susceptibility of *Xanthomonas maltophilia* to antimicrobial agents: implications for therapy. *Antimicrob Ag Chemother* **38**: 624.

Velazquez H, Perazella MA, Wright FS, Ellison DH (1993). Renal mechanism of trimethoprim-induced hyperkalemia. *Ann Intern Med* **119**: 296.

Venditti M, Gelfusa V, Tarasi A *et al.* (1990). Antimicrobial susceptibilities of *Erysipelothrix rhusiopathiae*. *Antimicrob Ag Chemother* **34**: 2038.

Verhoef J (1993). Prevention of infections in the neutropenic patient. *Clin Infect Dis* **17** (Suppl 2): S359.

Verhoef J, Rozenberg-Arska M, Dekker A (1989). Prevention of infection in the neutropenic patient. *Rev Infect Dis* **11** (Suppl 7): S1545.

Vila J, Gascon J, Abdalla S *et al.* (1994). Antimicrobial resistance of *Shigella* isolates causing traveler's diarrhea. *Antimicrob Ag Chemother* **38**: 2668.

Vincent FM (1977). Acute polyneuropathy possibly associated with co-trimoxazole. *Lancet* **ii**: 980.

Vlasses PH, Kosoglou T, Chase SL *et al.* (1989). Trimethoprim inhibition of the renal clearance of procainamide and N-acetylprocainamide. *Arch Intern Med* **149**: 1350.

Wade JC, De Jongh CA, Newman KA *et al.* (1983). Selective antimicrobial modulation as prophylaxis against infection during granulocytopenia: trimethoprim-sulfamethoxazole vs. nalidixic acid. *J Infect Dis* **147**: 624.

Wåhlin A, Rosman N (1976). Skin manifestations with vasculitis due to co-trimoxazole. *Lancet* **ii**: 1415.

Wallace M, Yousif AA (1990). Spread of multi-resistant *Salmonella typhi*. *Lancet* **336**: 1065.

Wallace RJ, Septimus EJ, Williams TW *et al.* (1982a). Use of trimethoprim-sulfamethoxazole for treatment of infections due to *Nocardia*. *Rev Infect Dis* **4**: 315.

Wallace RJ Jr, Wiss K, Bushby MB, Hollowell DC (1982b). *In vitro* activity of trimethoprim and sulfamethoxazole against the nontuberculous mycobacteria. *Rev Infect Dis* **4**: 326.

Wallace RJ, Nash DR, Steingrube VA (1990). Antibiotic susceptibilities and drug resistance in *Moraxella (Branhamella) catarrhalis*. *Amer J Med* **88** (Suppl 5A): 46S.

Wang EEL, Prober CG (1983). Ventricular cerebrospinal fluid concentrations of trimethoprim-sulfamethoxazole. *J Antimicrob Chemother* **11**: 385.

Wang EEL, Prober CG, Hendrick BE *et al.* (1984). Prophylactic sulfamethoxazole and trimethoprim in ventriculoperitoneal shunt surgery. A double-blind, randomized, placebo-controlled trial. *JAMA* **251**: 1174.

Ward TT, Thomas RG, Fye CL *et al.* (1993). Trimethoprim-sulfamethoxazole prophylaxis in granulocytopenic patients with acute leukemia: evaluation of serum antibiotic levels in a randomized, double-blind, placebo-controlled Department of Veterans Affairs Cooperative Study. *Clin Infect Dis* **17**: 323.

Weening RS, Kabel P, Pijman P, Roos D (1983). Continuous therapy with sulfamethoxazole-trimethoprim in patients with chronic granulomatous disease. *J Pediatr* **103**: 127.

Weinberger M, Eid A, Schreiber L *et al.* (1995). Disseminated *Nocardia transvalensis* infection resembling pulmonary infarction in a liver transplant recipient. *Eur J Clin Microbiol Infect Dis* **14**: 337.

Weinstein L, Musher DM (1969). Antibiotic-induced suprainfection. *J Infect Dis* **119**: 662.

Welling PG, Craig WA, Amidon GL, Kunin CM (1973). Pharmacokinetics of trimethoprim and sulfamethoxazole in normal subjects and in patients with renal failure. *J Infect Dis* **128** (Suppl): 556.

West BC, Todd JR, King JW (1987). Wegener's granulomatosis and trimethoprim-sulmethoxazole. *Ann Intern Med* **106**: 840.

Wharton JM, Coleman DL, Wofsy CB *et al.* (1986). Trimethoprim-sulfamethoxazole or pentamidine for *Pneumocystis carinii* pneumonia in the acquired immunodeficiency syndrome. A prospective randomized trial. *Ann Intern Med* **105**: 37.

Whiteside ME, Barkin JS, May RG *et al.* (1984). Enteric coccidiosis among patients with the acquired immunodeficiency syndrome. *Amer J Trop Med* **33**: 1096.

Whittington RM (1989). Toxic epidermal necrolysis and co-trimoxazole. *Lancet* **ii**: 574.

Wicks ACB, Stamps TJ (1970). Trimethoprim-sulfamethoxazole in typhoid. *Brit Med J* **4**: 52.

Wilber RB, Feldman S, Malone WJ *et al.* (1980). Chemoprophylaxis for *Pneumocystis carinii* pneumonitis. Outcome of unstructured delivery. *Amer J Dis Child* **134**: 643.

Wilcox JB (1981). Phenytoin intoxication and co-trimoxazole. *N Z Med J* **94**: 235.

Willcox RR (1977). How suitable are available pharmaceuticals for the treatment of sexually transmitted diseases? (2). Conditions presenting as sores or tumours. *Brit J Vener Dis* **53**: 340.

Williams GR, Law TL, Kennedy DH *et al.* (1982). Delayed diagnosis of malaria. *Brit Med J* **284**: 1616.

Williams JW, Jr, Holleman DR, Jr, Samsa GP, Simel DL (1995). Randomized controlled trial of 3 vs 10 days of trimethoprim/ sulfamethoxazole for acute maxillary sinusitis. *JAMA* **273**: 1015.

Wilson JM, Guiney DG (1982). Failure of oral trimethoprim-sulfamethoxazole prophylaxis in acute leukaemia. Isolation of resistant plasmids from strains of Enterobacteriaceae causing bacteremia. *New Engl J Med* **306**: 16.

Winslow DL, Pankey GA (1982). *In vitro* activities of trimethoprim and sulfamethoxazole against *Listeria monocytogenes*. *Antimicrob Ag Chemother* **22**: 51.

Winstanley PA, Mberu EK, Szwandt IS, Breckenridge AM, Watkins WM (1995). *In vitro* activities of novel antifolate drug combinations against *Plasmodium falciparum* and human granulocyte CFUs. *Antimicrob Ag Chemother* **39**: 948.

Winston DJ, Lau WK, Gale RP, Young LS (1980). Trimethoprim/ sulfamethoxazole for the treatment of *Pneumocystis carinii* pneumonia. *Ann Intern Med* **92**: 762.

Wolff MA, Young CL, Ramphal R (1993). Antibiotic therapy for enterobacter meningitis: a retrospective review of 13 episodes and review of the literature. *Clin Infect Dis* **16**: 772.

Wolfsy CB (1987). Use of trimethoprim-sulfamethoxazole in the treatment of *Pneumocystis carinii* pneumonitis in patients with acquired immunodeficiency syndrome. *Rev Infect Dis* **9** (Suppl 2): S184.

Wormser GP, Horowitz HW, Duncanson FP *et al.* (1991). Low-dose intermittent trimethoprim-sulfamethoxazole for prevention of *Pneumocystis carinii* pneumonia in patients with human immunodeficiency virus infection. *Arch Intern Med* **151**: 688.

Worthington MG, McEniry DW (1990). Chronic meliodosis in a Vietnamese immigrant. *Rev Infect Dis* **12**: 966.

Wulf HC, Bech-Thomsen N (1988). Two-day trimethoprim-sulfamethoxazole treatment of pharyngeal gonorrhea. *Sexually Transmitted Diseases* **15**: 116.

Wurtz R (1994). Cyclospora: a newly identified intestinal pathogen of humans. *Clin Infect Dis* **18**: 620.

Wurtz RM, Kocka FE, Peters CS *et al.* (1993). Clinical characteristics of seven cases of diarrhea associated with a novel acid-fast organism in the stool. *Clin Infect Dis* **16**: 136.

Wüst J, Wilkins TD (1978). Susceptibility of anaerobic bacteria to sulfamethoxazole/trimethoprim and routine susceptibility testing. *Antimicrob Ag Chemother* **14**: 384.

Yamamoto T, Naigowit P, Dejsirilert S *et al.* (1990). *In vitro* susceptibilities of *Pseudomonas pseudomallei* to 27 antimicrobial agents. *Antimicrob Ag Chemother* **34**: 2027.

Yamamoto T, Nair GB, Albert MJ *et al.* (1995). Survey of *in vitro* susceptibilities of *Vibrio cholerae* O1 and O139 to antimicrobial agents. *Antimicrob Ag Chemother* **39**: 241.

Yogev R, Lander HB, David AT (1978). Effect of TMP-SMX on nasopharyngeal carriage of ampicillin-sensitive and ampicillin-resistant *Hemophilus influenzae* type B. *Pediatrics* **93**: 394 .

Yoshikawa TT, Guze LB (1976). Concentrations of trimethoprim-sulfamethoxazole in blood after a single, large oral dose. *Antimicrob Ag Chemother* **10**: 462.

Yoshikawa TT, Miyamoto S, Guze LB (1975). Comparison of *in vitro* susceptibility of *Neisseria gonorrhoeae* to trimethoprim-sulfamethoxazole on three different media. *Antimicrob Ag Chemother* **8**: 515.

Young H-K, Amyes SGB (1985). Characterization of a new transposon-mediated trimethoprim-resistant dihydrofolate reductase. *Biochem Pharmacol* **34**: 4334.

Young H-K, Amyes SGB (1986). Plasmid trimethoprim resistance in *Vibrio cholerae*: migration of type 1 dihydrofolate reductase gene out of the Enterobacteriaceae. *J Antimicrob Chemother* **17**: 697.

Young H-K, Jesudason MV, Koshi G, Amyes SGB (1986). Trimethoprim resistance amongst urinary bacteria in South India. *J Antimicrob Chemother* **17**: 615.

Young LS (1983). Antimicrobial prophylaxis against infection in neutropenic patients. *J Infect Dis* **147**: 611.

Yu VL, Rumans LW, Wing EJ *et al.* (1978). *Pseudomonas maltophilia* causing heroin-associated infective endocarditis. *Arch Intern Med* **138**: 1667.

Yuill GM (1973). Megaloblastic anaemia due to trimethoprim-sulfamethoxazole therapy in uraemia. *Postgrad Med J* **49**: 100.

Yunus M, Rahman ASM, Farooque ASG, Glass RI (1982). Clinical trial of ampicillin v. trimethoprim-sulfamethoxazole in the treatment of shigella dysentery. *J Trop Med & Hyg* **85**: 195.

Zackrisson G, Brorson J-E, Krantz I, Trollfors B (1983). *In-vitro* sensitivity of *Bordetella pertussis*. *J Antimicrob Chemother* **11**: 407.

Zylberberg H, Robert F, Le Gal FA *et al.* (1995). Prolonged isolated fever due to attenuated extracerebral toxoplasmosis in patients infected with human immunodeficiency virus who are receiving trimethoprim-sulfamethoxazole as prophylaxis. *Clin Infect Dis* **21**: 680.

Pyrimethamine

Description

Pyrimethamine was the first of many 2,4-diaminopyrimidines to be synthesized and tested for antimicrobial activity, with trimethoprim being another notable member of this group (p. 836). Unlike trimethoprim, the main value of pyrimethamine is its activity against malaria, toxoplasma and protozoa species (Falco *et al.*, 1951; Symposium, 1952). Until recently, pyrimethamine was mainly considered in combination with sulfadoxine ('Fansidar') as an antimalarial, but the increasing incidence of HIV-associated diseases such as toxoplasmosis, *Pneumocystis carinii* pneumonia and diarrhea due to *Isospora beli* have been associated with a broader use of pyrimethamine, often in combination with non-sulfa compounds such as clindamycin.

Sensitive Organisms

1 Malaria parasites

All malarial (plasmodia) spp. are susceptible to pyrimethamine, although it is mainly effective against *Plasmodium falciparum* and therefore its main therapeutic role is against chloroquine-resistant *Pl. falciparum* strains. *In vitro* susceptibility testing of malaria parasites is difficult, time-consuming and less standardized than similar antibiotic susceptibility testing of bacteria. Furthermore, the correlation between inhibitory concentrations of antimalarials identified *in vitro* and the subsequent *in vivo* antimalarial activity and clinical outcome associated with these agents is less clearly defined than with antibacterial activity. In *Pl. vivax* infections pyrimethamine generally acts only as a suppressant. Among *Pl. falciparum* isolates, pyrimethamine-resistance is defined by some authors as an $IC_{100} \geq 10^{-6}M$, and there appears to be some cross-resistance between pyrimethamine and chlocycloguanil (Peterson *et al.*, 1990b). Lambros *et al.* (1989), who examined *Pl. falciparum* isolates from Malaysian aborigines with relatively little *in vitro* drug-resistance reported that all isolates were susceptible to pyrimethamine with a mean IC_{50} of 21.4 ng per ml (range 9–52 ng per ml), where the IC_{50} represents the inhibitory drug concentration necessary to achieve 50% inhibition of the uptake of radiolabeled hypoxanthine by parasites compared with controls. *In vitro* studies suggest no significant potentiation of antimalarial activity between proguanil (cylcoguanil) and pyrimethamine (Yeo and Rieckmann, 1992). Pyrimethamine is active against asexual erythrocytic forms of *Pl. falciparum*, but has less activity against the tissue forms. It is not gametocidal, but arrests the sporogony of *Pl. falciparum* and *Pl. vivax* in the mosquito. Furthermore, since pyrimethamine acts relatively late in the parasite life-cycle, allowing development to the mature trophozoite stage, pathological effects may ensue despite its activity (White and Krishna, 1989). Since pyrimethamine does not kill the hepatic stages of *Pl. vivax* or *Pl. ovale*, it does not produce radical cure of malaria due to these species.

2 Toxoplasma gondii

The identification of susceptibility of *Toxoplasma gondii* to various antimicrobial agents is limited by difficulties with identifying a suitable *in vitro* assay. Nevertheless, both *in vitro* and *in vivo* studies in mice demonstrate susceptibility of *T. gondii* to pyrimethamine and synergistic antitoxoplasma effect by the combination of pyrimethamine and sulfadiazine (Piketty *et al.*, 1990; Derouin and Chastang, 1989; Derouin *et al.*, 1991, 1992; Israelski *et al.*, 1989; Kovacs *et al.*, 1988; Schoondermark-van de Ven *et al.*, 1995). Israelski *et al.* (1989) identified toxoplasmacidal activity by pyrimethamine at concentrations of ≥ 0.2 µg per ml in an *in vitro* study using trophozoite-infected human foreskin fibroblasts. They also noted marked synergistic activity between pyrimethamine and sulfadiazine, and that the addition of zidovudine interfered with this synergism. Piketty *et al.* (1990) determined the effect of various agents by regularly subculturing blood, lung and brain homogenates from infected mice onto fibroblast tissue cultures to determine the parasitic load. Pyrimethamine (18.5 mg per kg per day) demonstrated antitoxoplasma activity, and synergism was noted with sulfadiazine (p. 809). Pyrimethamine inhibits folic acid metabolism of toxoplasma tachyzoites but has no effect on toxoplasma cysts (Huskinson-Mark *et al.*, 1991; Mariuz *et al.*, 1994). The concentrations of pyrimethamine needed to inhibit or kill *T. gondii* have not been clinically established (Luft and Hafner, 1990). Derouin and Chastang (1989) identified a 50% inhibitory concentration of 0.04 µg per ml pyrimethamine against *T. gondii* grown in fibroblast tissue culture. This compared with 2.3 µg per ml trimethoprim, 0.16 ng per ml trimetrexate-glucuronate and 6.9% piritrexin to produce similar activity. Marked synergism was noted with sulfadiazine and pyrimethamine, trimetrexate-glucuronate, and piritrexin; sulfisoxole and pyrimethamine, and trimethoprim and sulfamethoxazole. Atovaquone and the new macrolides, roxithromycin, azithromycin and clarithromycin, markedly potentiate the anti-toxoplasma activity of both pyrimethamine and sulfadiazine (Derouin *et al.*, 1991; Huskinson-Mark *et al.*, 1991; Araujo *et al.*, 1991, 1992, 1993; Romand *et al.*, 1995).

3 Pneumocystis carinii

This organism is probably susceptible to pyrimethamine, although there have been conflicting data, particularly when the rat model is used (Frenkel *et al.*, 1966; Hughes *et al.*, 1984, 1986; Walzer *et al.*, 1988, 1992). Walzer *et al.* (1992) suggested that the rat model, while being a good system for studying the anti-pneumocystis activity of sulfonamides, has limited value when studying inhibitors of dihydrofolate reductase (DHFR). Nevertheless, *P. carinii* DHFR is inhibited by pyrimethamine and other antifolate agents such as methotrexate and trimetrexate *in vitro* (Broughton and Queener, 1991; Queener, 1991).

4 Isospora belli

This parasite appears to be susceptible to pyrimethamine in humans either when it is used alone or in combination with sulfadoxine, but there are no *in vitro* susceptibility data available (Trier *et al.*, 1974; Weiss *et al.*, 1988b; Pape *et al.*, 1989).

5 Acquired resistance

Resistance to pyrimethamine has been reported in *Pl. vivax*, *Pl. malariae* and *Pl. falciparum*. Strains of *Pl. falciparum* resistant to 'Fansidar' (sulfadoxine/pyrimethamine) have been described in South-East Asia (Thailand, Vietnam, Burma, Sabah), Papua New Guinea, the Amazon, East and West Africa, and Sudan (Herzog *et al.*, 1983; Sabchareon *et al.*, 1985; Noel and Morisset, 1986; Gubler, 1988; Malin and Hall, 1990; Lege-Oguntoye *et al.*, 1990; Ibrahim *et al.*, 1991; Brown, 1993). Antifolate-resistance in *Pl. falciparum* strains found in Thailand approaches 100% (Brown, 1993). Nahlen *et al.* (1989) reported widespread *in vivo* (67%) and *in vitro* (60%) resistance among isolates of *Pl. falciparum* to pyrimethamine among pregnant Nigerian women receiving 25 mg pyrimethamine once-weekly for prophylaxis. Ibrahim *et al.* (1991) described a clinically resistant isolate which was also resistant *in vitro*, with inhibition of schizont maturation detectable only at a sulfadoxine/pyrimethamine concentration of 3000/37.5 pmol. Similarly, in the study reported by Lege-Oguntoye *et al.* (1990), eight isolates underwent schizogony at sulfadoxine/pyrimethamine concentrations of 10 000/125 pmol. Subsequently, Watkins and Mosobo (1993) have suggested that a higher rate of *in vitro* pyrimethamine-resistance is seen in new *Pl. falciparum* infections occuring during the elimination phase of 'Fansidar' after previous treatment. Interestingly, they found no similar evidence for the selection of parasites with reduced sensitivity to sulfadoxine.

The mechanisms of pyrimethamine-resistance among *Pl. falciparum* include changes in the amino acid structure of the DHFR thymidylate synthase enzyme molecule, excess production of DHFR enzyme and chromosomal changes in the DHFR gene. (Zolg *et al.*, 1989, 1990; Snewin *et al.*, 1989; Tanaka *et al.*, 1990; Peterson *et al.*, 1990a, 1991; Thaithong *et al.*, 1992). In particular, the DHFR mutation Asn-108, which acts by interrupting drug binding within the active site of the enzyme, appears to be a common mechanism. Peterson *et al.* (1991) using a mutation-specific polymerase chain reaction assay found 90% of *Pl. falciparum* isolates from a wide section of the Brazilian Amazon where clinical pyrimethamine-resistance is common, contained the Asn-108 codon that confers pyrimethamine-resistance. Some strains of *Pl. falciparum* have further mutations such that they display cross-resistance to both pyrimethamine and cycloguanil (the active metabolite of proguanil) (Peterson *et al.*, 1990a).

While clinical failures have been reported when using pyrimethamine for prophylaxis and treatment of toxoplasmosis and *P. carinii* infections, no *in vitro* or *in vivo* evidence of pyrimethamine-resistance has been reported (Weiss *et al.*, 1988a; Lidman *et al.*, 1989; Girard *et al.*, 1989, 1993; Clotet *et al.*, 1991; Coker *et al.*, 1992; Antinori *et al.*, 1992; Ruf *et al.*, 1993; Podzamczer *et al.*, 1993a, 1993b; Mallolas *et al.*, 1993).

Mode of Administration and Dosage

1 Adults

a Malaria prophylaxis The usual dose of pyrimethamine is 25 mg once-weekly. When pyrimethamine is given in combination with sulfadoxine ('Fansidar') the usual dose of oral preparation is one tablet (500 mg sulfadoxine + 25 mg pyrimethamine) once-weekly commencing 2 weeks prior to exposure, during exposure and for 4–6 weeks after exposure. An alternative regimen is two tablets once every 2 weeks. For both regimens prophylaxis should be given in conjunction with chloroquine. Chemoprophylaxis with pyrimethamine 12.5 mg + dapsone 100 mg ('Maloprim') is given in a dose of one tablet once-weekly for adults and children older than 10 years of age and similar to 'Fansidar' should be given in combination with chloroquine. There is little safety data regarding the use of 'Maloprim' for longer than 12 months.

b Malaria presumptive treatment Adults and children weighing > 45 kg, or those who are older than 14 years, should be treated with three tablets of 'Fansidar' as a single dose (CDC, 1993) for presumptive self-treatment. Alternatively, the parenteral preparation, which can be used i.m. (not i.v.) should be administered to adults (50–70 kg) in a dose of 5–7.5 ml (50–75 mg pyrimethamine). 'Fansidar' is often used in conjunction with quinine sulfate (oral or i.v.). Pyrimethamine alone can be used for the treatment of uncomplicated *Pl. falciparum* infection in a dose of 25 mg once-daily for 2 days, but generally pyrimethamine is given in conjunction with quinine sulfate and sulfadiazine, when it is given in a dose of 25 mg twice-daily for 3 days. If pyrimethamine must be used alone in the treatment of malaria in semi-immune adults, the dose is 50 mg daily for 2 days followed by 25 mg once-weekly for at least 10 weeks. 'Maloprim' should not be used for the definitive treatment of malaria.

c Toxoplasmosis Pyrimethamine is usually combined with either a sulfonamide (e.g. sulfadiazine) or clindamycin for the treatment of toxoplasmosis. In immunocompetent patients the optimum duration of treatment has not been established, but is usually 3–4 weeks. The manufacturer recommends an initial pyrimethamine dose for adults of 50–75 mg daily in conjunction with a sulfonamide for 1–3 weeks, followed by administration of 50% dosage of both agents for a further 4–5 weeks. Other authors suggest for HIV-negative patients a regimen of 100 mg pyrimethamine on day 1, then 25 mg daily in association with 4–6 g daily of sulfadiazine for 4–5 weeks. Frequently HIV-associated cerebral toxoplasmosis relapses if therapy is ceased (p. 915) hence treatment usually consists of an initial period of relatively high dose pyrimethamine therapy followed by life-long suppressive therapy. Some authors suggest 200 mg pyrimethamine on day 1, then 50–75 mg daily in association with sulfadiazine 4–8 gm daily for 3–6 weeks, followed by life-long suppressive therapy of pyrimethamine 50 mg daily and sulfadiazine 2 g daily. Folinic acid 10 mg daily (not folic acid) is often given concurrently (Luft and Hafner, 1990; Luft *et al.*, 1993; Sanford, 1993; Mariuz *et al.*, 1994)).

2 Children

a Malaria prophylaxis Pyrimethamine 0.5 mg/kg once-weekly (up to a maximum of 25 mg) is recommended for children up to 10 years of age, after which an adult dose is appropriate. The usual once-weekly doses are: 4–10 years of age: 12.5 mg; < 4 years of age: 6.25 mg. The chemoprophylaxis regimen for 'Fansidar' is: 9–14 years of age: 0.75 tablet (or 1.5 tablets once every other week); 4–8 years: 0.5 tablet (or 1.0 tablet once every other week); < 4 years: 0.25 tablet (or 0.5 tablets once every other week). Chemoprophylaxis with 'Maloprim' is 0.5 tablet once-weekly for children 5–10 years, usually in combination with chloroquine.

b Malaria presumptive treatment Children's doses for presumptive treatment with 'Fansidar' are (patient weight in kg: number of tablets): 5–10 kg: 0.5 tablet; 11–20 kg: 1 tablet; 21–30 kg: 1.5 tablets; 31–45 kg: 2 tablets; >45 kg: 3 tablets (CDC, 1993). Presumptive treatment with the parenteral preparation of 'Fansidar' (p. 824) should be in the following doses: 4 years: 1–1.5 ml; 5–8 years: 2.5 ml; 9–14 years: 5 ml. As with adults, 'Maloprim' should not be used to treat malaria. Pyrimethamine, when given in conjunction with quinine sulfate and sulfadiazine, is given to children for 3 days in the following doses: 20–40 kg: 25 mg daily; 10–20 kg: 12.5 mg daily; < 10 kg:6.25 mg daily. When pyrimethamine can only be used alone for the treatment of malaria in semi-immune children, the dosage is: 4–10 years: 25 mg once-daily for 2 days followed by 12.5 mg once-weekly for at least 10 weeks.

c Toxoplasmosis The most commonly recommended regimen is pyrimethamine 1–2 mg per kg (up to 100 mg) daily, given in two equally divided doses, for 1–3 days, followed by 0.5–1 mg per kg (up to 25 mg) daily, given in two equally divided doses, together with sulfadiazine 85–200 mg per kg daily, for 4–6 weeks. The duration of therapy may be extended depending on other influencing factors such as the presence of HIV infection (Infectious Diseases Rounds, 1988; p. 915).

3 Newborn and premature infants

Pyrimethamine should be given with caution to newborn infants if folate deficiency is a consideration. 'Fansidar' and 'Maloprim' are contraindicated in children younger than 4 weeks due to their sulfa and sulfone components, respectively. The management of infants with congenital toxoplasmosis is discussed on p. 914.

4 Pregnancy

Pyrimethamine alone and pyrimethamine/sulfadoxine ('Fansidar') are teratogenic in various animal models, probably due to interference in folic acid metabolism. There are no adequate and controlled studies in humans, so that pyrimethamine should only be used during pregnancy where the potential benefits outweigh the risk to the fetus. Nevertheless, pyrimethamine alone or in combination with sulfonamides is used with reasonable success to treat toxoplasmosis during pregnancy (p. 913). 'Fansidar' is contraindicated during pregnancy at term due to the potential for sulfadoxine to cross the placenta and lead to kernicterus in the neonate (p. 819). During pregnancy if 'Fansidar' is given for malaria prophylaxis, or if pyrimethamine is used to treat toxoplasmosis, the concurrent administration of folinic acid (leucovorin) is recommended (especially during the first trimester) to decrease the potential for pyrimethamine-induced hematological toxicity.

5 Patients who are breast-feeding

Pyrimethamine passes transplacentally to the fetus and is excreted in breast milk. Following the maternal ingestion of a single 75-mg dose of pyrimethamine, it is estimated that 3–4 mg may be ingested by a nursing infant during the subsequent 48 h (Clyde et al., 1956). No human problems have been documented, but caution should be exercised, especially if the mother is receiving the higher doses of pyrimethamine often associated with therapy for toxoplasmosis. Contrary to earlier publications (Clyde, 1960), ingestion of pyrimethamine in breast milk by the nursing infant is no longer considered a reliable means of drug administration or effective antimalarial chemoprophylaxis for these infants (Bennett, 1988; Anderson, 1979; p. 910). The American Academy of Pediatrics considers pyrimethamine to be compatible with breast-feeding (Committee on Drugs; 1994).

6 Patients with renal failure

Pyrimethamine is excreted 16–30% unchanged in urine, but metabolites may be excreted for some weeks after administration due to tissue deposition (Bennett et al., 1991; Le Liboux et al., 1991). The serum half-life of pyrimethamine is not altered in end-stage renal failure and no dosage reduction is necessary, even when the glomerular filtration rate (GFR) is <10 ml per min. No dosage supplementation is generally considered necessary after hemodialysis, chronic ambulatory peritoneal dialysis (CAPD) or continuous arteriovenous/venovenous hemofiltration (Bennett et al., 1991; Sanford, 1993). However, Weiss et al. (1988a) have described one patient with AIDS who was treated with 25 mg pyrimethamine daily and intermittent peritoneal dialysis every 4 days for renal failure, in whom pyrimethamine concentrations in the peritoneal dialysate were 75% of the corresponding serum level, and serum concentrations fell from 2313 to 1230 ng per ml (47% decrease) while the patient was undertaking dialysis.

7 Patients with hepatic failure

There are few data regarding the use of pyrimethamine in the setting of hepatic failure. However, pyrimethamine is metabolized by the liver and serum levels may therefore be expected to increase in patients with reduced hepatic clearance (Schmidt et al., 1953; Kumar et al., 1990; McLeod et al., 1992).

8 Patients with folate deficiency

Pyrimethamine, due to its antifolate activity, should be administered with caution to patients with potential folate deficiency. Such patients include those with megaloblastic anemia, malabsorption syndrome, alcoholism, pregnancy and patients receiving other drugs that affect folate levels (e.g. phenytoin, methotrexate). In such patients, folinic acid supplementation may be necessary. Folinic acid rather than folic acid should be used, especially when treating toxoplasmosis, since folic acid can be taken up by *T. gondii* and bypass the pyrimethamine-induced inhibition of DHFR, and therefore lessen pyrimethamine efficacy (Infectious Disease Rounds, 1988).

9 Intramuscular administration

Pyrimethamine is available only in oral form, however, pyrimethamine + sulfadoxine ('Fansidar') is available in a parenteral preparation (2.5 ml contains 25 mg pyrimethamine and 500 mg sulfadoxine) which can be administered by deep i.m. injection. This preparation can not be given intravenously. Parenteral 'Fansidar' is generally used only in severe cases of *Pl. falciparum* malaria when it is usually combined with parenteral quinine. In this situation the usual curative dose for adults weighing 50–70 kg is 5–7.5 ml (2–3 ampoules). The comparable dose for children is: 9–14 years: 5 ml; 5–8 years: 2.5 ml; 4 years: 1–1.5 ml. The combination of pyrimethamine and dapsone ('Maloprim') is available only in oral preparation.

Availability

Pyrimethamine *tablets* contain 25 mg pyrimethamine per tablet.

Combination pyrimethamine + sulfadoxine ('Fansidar') *tablets* each contain 25 mg pyrimethamine + 500 mg sulfadoxine per tablet.

'Fansidar' *ampoules* (2.5 ml) contain 25 mg pyrimethamine + 500 mg sulfadoxine.

Combination pyrimethamine + dapsone ('Maloprim') *tablets* each contain 12.5 mg pyrimethamine + 100 mg dapsone per tablet.

Combination 'Fansidar' + mefloquine ('Fansimef') *tablets* each contain 25 mg pyrimethamine, 500 mg sulfadoxine and 250 mg mefloquine per tablet.

Serum Levels in Relation to Dosage

Pyrimethamine is generally well absorbed after oral administration with peak serum concentrations reached in 2–4 h. The half-life of pyrimethamine in serum varies widely from 20 to 175 h, but most authors report the mean half-life in adults to be approximately 85–90 h (Cavallito et al., 1978; Jones and Ovenell, 1979; Bergqvist et al., 1985; Weiss et al., 1988a; Mansor et al., 1989; Leport et al., 1992). There also appears to be high interpatient variability in the peak serum levels of pyrimethamine after the same dose schedule (Weiss et al., 1988a; Le Liboux et al., 1991; Leport et al., 1992). McLeod et al. (1992) noted peak serum pyrimethamine levels in adults, taken 4 h after an oral dose of 25 mg pyrimethamine, to be 0.9–1.7 µg per ml. Le Liboux et al.(1991), however, who studied 12 healthy volunteers given a single 50 mg oral dose of pyrimethamine, found plasma concentrations peaked at 0.48 ± 0.13 µg per ml after a median duration of 2.5 h post-dose. Plasma pyrimethamine levels subsequently declined slowly, being 0.04 µg per ml, 14 days after administration.

A variablity in serum levels of pyrimethamine has also been noted in patients with AIDS-associated toxoplasma encephalitis. In some such patients, the half-life of pyrimethamine was only 23 h, raising the possibility of variability in the rate of pyrimethamine metabolism or altered hepatic function in these patients. In AIDS patients with acute toxoplasma encephalitis serum concentrations of pyrimethamine 2–5 h after a 25 mg and 50 mg daily dose of pyrimethamine ranged from 0.26 to 1.41 µg per ml and 1.33 to 4.47 µg per ml, respectively. In one patient receiving 25 mg pyrimethamine daily who was studied in detail, the mean peak serum concentration 1 h post-dose was 1.73 µg per ml and mean trough level 23 h post-dose was 0.88 µg per ml (Weiss et al., 1988a).

Combination of pyrimethamine with either sulfadoxine ('Fansidar'), dapsone ('Maloprim') or sulfadoxine + mefloquine ('Fansimef'), does not significantly alter the expected pyrimethamine levels in serum. Peak serum pyrimethamine levels after a single dose of 'Maloprim' (12.5 mg pyrimethamine + 100 mg dapsone) in healthy volunteers were 0.04–0.12 μg per ml (Jones and Ovenell, 1979). Mansor *et al.* (1989) noted that ten healthy male Caucasian volunteers given two 'Fansimef' tablets (total of 50 mg pyrimethamine) achieved peak serum concentrations of pyrimethamine of 0.76 μg per ml, 3.3 ± 2 h after dosing, and that the serum half-life of pyrimethamine was 114 ± 42 h when given in this combination. Studies of pyrimethamine concentrations after 6 months and 2 years of malaria prophylaxis in healthy Caucasian adults taking one 'Fansidar' tablet weekly (500 mg sulfadoxine + 25 mg pyrimethamine) demonstrated mean peak sulfadoxine and pyrimethamine concentrations of 0.85 and 0.95 μg per ml, respectively; mean trough concentrations of 0.28 and 0.36 μg per ml, respectively; and a mean half-life of pyrimethamine of 101 h (4.2 days) (Hellgren *et al.*, 1990, 1991). Such trough concentrations of pyrimethamine are probably inhibitory to *Pl. falciparum* strains susceptible *in vivo* to 'Fansidar' (Hellgren *et al.*, 1990, 1991). In one study, however, there appeared to be significant racial differences in attainable serum concentrations of pyrimethamine during malaria prophylaxis with 'Maloprim', whereby Papua New Guineans had significantly lower serum levels than Caucasians given the same dose (Cook *et al.*, 1986).

Serum concentrations of pyrimethamine in children given the recommended dosage are similar to those found in adults. McLeod *et al.* (1992) examined the levels of pyrimethamine in sera and CSF in 37 infants treated with pyrimethamine for suspected or proven congenital toxoplasmosis. The half-life of pyrimethamine in serum was 64 ± 12 h and did not appear to vary significantly during the first year of life. Serum levels 4 h after administration of a 1 mg per kg daily dose of pyrimethamine to these infants were 1.3 ± 0.5 μg per ml.

Excretion

Pyrimethamine is highly protein bound and is metabolized mostly in the liver and excreted slowly by the kidney. Urinary excretion represents about 20–40% of the dose 7 days after administration (Cavallito *et al.*, 1978; Rudy and Poynor, 1990; Le Liboux *et al.*, 1991). Studies of hepatic elimination of pyrimethamine in isolated rat livers suggest marked impairment of pyrimethamine metabolism during infection with malaria (*Plasmodium berghei*), however there have been no comparable human studies to confirm these findings (Mihaly *et al.*, 1987).

Pyrimethamine is excreted in breast milk (Clyde *et al.*, 1956; Edstein *et al.*, 1986). After a 50–75 mg dose of pyrimethamine, drug concentrations in breast milk are 3.1–3.3 μg per ml, 6 h later and may remain detectable for up to 48 h (Clyde *et al.*, 1956). Edstein *et al.* (1986) estimated that, based on an expected infant ingestion of 1000 ml of breast milk per day, infants probably consume 17–46% of the maternally ingested dose of pyrimethamine over a 9-day period. The American Academy of Pediatrics considers pyrimethamine to be compatible with breast feeding (Committee on Drugs; 1994). Previously, concentrations of pyrimethamine in human breast milk were considered to be sufficient to provide adequate antimalarial prophylaxis for breast-feeding infants in East Africa (Clyde *et al.*, 1956; Clyde, 1960). However, variability of breast milk intake and increasing drug resistance among strains of *Pl. falciparum* and *Pl. vivax* (p. 906) now means that this is an inadequate means of antimalarial prophylaxis for breast-feeding infants (Bennett, 1988).

Distribution of the Drug in Body

Pyrimethamine is 87–94% protein bound, lipophilic and accumulates in kidneys, lung, liver and spleen (Goodman *et al.*, 1990). Pyrimethamine penetration into both CSF and brain tissue is quite reasonable. Weiss *et al.* (1988a) studied four patients with AIDS and acute toxoplasmic encephalitis who were treated with either 25 mg or 50 mg pyrimethamine daily and found the CSF concentrations of pyrimethamine to be 13–27% of the serum concentrations. Similarly in children being treated for congenital toxplasmosis with pyrimethamine, CSF concentrations of pyrimethamine were 10–25% of concomitant serum concentrations (McLeod *et al.*, 1992). In 23 HIV-negative patients given a single 100 mg oral dose of pyrimethamine 12, 24 or 48 h prior to neurosurgery, concentrations of pyrimethamine in brain tissue were noted to be 0.97 μg per g, 1.56 μg per g and 1.02 μg per g, respectively. The ratio of brain:serum pyrimethamine concentrations 12, 24 and 48 h after dosing were 2.5, 5.2 and 4.1, respectively. The estimated half-life of pyrimethamine in brain tissue in this study was 40 h (range: 30–193 h) (Leport *et al.*, 1992). In a further four patients who were given 50 mg oral pyrimethamine, drug concentrations in brain tissue 24 h later were 0.67 ± 0.09 μg per g (Leport *et al.*, 1992).

Studies of the distribution of pyrimethamine into peritoneal fluid are limited, but in one patient with AIDS who was treated with 25 mg pyrimethamine daily and received peritoneal dialysis every 4 days for renal failure, the pyrimethamine concentration in peritoneal dialysate was 75% of the corresponding serum concentration. During dialysis the serum concentration of pyrimethamine fell by 47% from 2.3 μg per ml to 1.2 μg per ml (Weiss *et al.*, 1988a).

Pyrimethamine is excreted in breast milk (p. 910). In patients with a normal hematocrit, the concentration of pyrimethamine in red blood cells is approximately 42% of plasma concentrations with partitioning of pyrimethamine into red blood cells decreasing as plasma albumin concentrations increase (Rudy and Poynor, 1990).

Mode of Action

Pyrimethamine is a folic acid antagonist with a similar mechanism of action as trimethoprim (p. 852). Pyrimethamine binds to DHFR in malaria parasites and mammalian cells, but there is a large differential in the affinity of the drug for malaria DHFR over mammalian DHFR, such that it inhibits DHFR of plasmodia at concentrations significantly below those required to produce inhibition of mammalian enzymes (1400-fold in the rat) (Ferone et al., 1969; Ferone, 1984). Also DHFR is vital for the successful biosynthesis of purines, pyrimidines and certain amino acids (p. 814). Pyrimethamine inhibition of DHFR in malaria parasites is manifested by failure of nuclear division at the time of schizont formation in erythrocytes and liver. Similarly, pyrimethamine inhibits DHFR in T. gondii and P. carinii, although the DHFR enzymes of these two organisms have rather different molecular characteristics (Kovacs et al., 1990).

Toxicity

Toxicity associated with pyrimethamine alone and pyrimethamine in combination with dapsone ('Maloprim') is discussed below, while toxicity associated with the combination of pyrimethamine + sulfadoxine ('Fansidar') is discussed elsewhere (p. 816).

1 Hematologic side-effects

These are uncommon with pyrimethamine doses recommended for malaria prophylaxis, although administration for prolonged periods may result in depression of hematopoiesis due to inhibition of folate metabolism. Use of 'Maloprim' has been associated with significant hematologic toxicity. In a review of adverse reactions to antimalarials, Phillips-Howard and West (1990) identified the rate of serious reactions to 'Maloprim' as 1:9100 prescriptions, and for blood dyscrasias as 1:20 000 prescriptions with a fatality rate of 1:75 000 prescriptions. Such toxicity is possibly dose-related since a higher rate of agranulocytosis has been identified in travellers taking twice the usual recommended dose for antimalarial prophylaxis; i.e. one 'Maloprim' tablet twice-weekly instead of one tablet weekly (Hutchinson et al., 1986; Bruce-Chwatt and Hutchinson, 1984). Hutchinson et al. (1986) speculated that this agranulocytosis may be caused by an idiosyncratic reaction to dapsone exacerbated by the concurrent administration of pyrimethamine. In addition to agranulocytosis, Phillips-Howard and West (1990) also noted that three patients developed cyanosis due to methemoglobinemia secondary to the dapsone component of 'Maloprim'.

The higher doses of pyrimethamine administered in the treatment of toxoplasmosis are not infrequently associated with hematological toxicity, including leucopenia, thrombocytopenia, megaloblstic anemia and pancytopenia. Such toxicity can be reversed by cessation of pyrimethamine therapy or by co-administration of folinic acid (5–20 mg daily). Unlike folinic acid, co-administration of folic acid is likely to reduce the efficacy of pyrimethamine against T. gondii since it may result in 'bypassing' of the inhibition of DHFR induced by pyrimethamine (Infectious Disease Rounds, 1988; Chute et al., 1995).

2 Rashes

Adverse cutaneous reactions associated with pyrimethamine/sulfadiazine and pyrimethamine/clindamycin are common in HIV-infected patients with toxoplasmosis, occurring in 75% and 58% cases, respectively (Caumes et al., 1995). However, the role played by pyrimethamine in these reactions is unclear, given the known association between sulfadiazine and clindamycin and cutaneous reactions (pp. 596, 816).

3 Gastrointestinal effects

High doses of pyrimethamine may be associated with atrophic glossitis, anorexia, vomiting, gastritis, abdominal cramps and diarrhea. Administration of pyrimethamine with meals may reduce the upper gastrointestinal symptoms.

4 Hepatotoxicity

This has been mostly associated with 'Fansidar' at a rate of 1:11,000 'Fansidar' prescriptions. Serious hepatic disorders are less common with 'Maloprim' which occur at a rate of 1:75 000 'Maloprim' prescriptions (Phillips-Howard and West, 1990).

5 Neurotoxicity

High dosages of pyrimethamine have been asociated with a variety of nervous system side-effects including ataxia, tremors, seizures and occasionally with less specific symptoms such as insomnia, depression, fatigue, malaise, headache, lightheadedness and irritability. Marked mental obtundation has been associated with hyperammonemia and carnitine deficiency induced by treatment with pyrimethamine and sulfadiazine (p. 912).

6 Eosinophilia and respiratory toxicity

Marked eosinophilia, including pulmonary eosinophilia, has been associated with administration of 'Maloprim', however, this is generally considered to be due to the dapsone component inducing a 'dapsone syndrome' (Grayson et al, 1988). Nevertheless, reports of pulmonary eosinophilia in patients taking 'Fansidar' or pyrimethamine + chloroquine have raised the possibility that pyrimethamine is responsible for this adverse reaction (Davidson et al, 1988).

7 Nephrotoxicity

Increases in serum creatinine have been noted in some patients treated with pyrimethamine and dapsone. Opravil et al. (1993) studied six healthy volunteers after a single, combined dose of 100 mg pyrimethamine and 200 mg dapsone and noted increases in serum creatinine over a 28 h period post-dose from 81 ± 14 to $102 \pm 16 \mu$mol per liter (p=0.002), with a corresponding reduction in creatinine clearance from 125 ± 27 to 91 ± 26 ml per min (p<0.02), but no change in inulin clearance, blood urea nitrogen or beta 2–microglobulin. All changes were reversible within 21 days and subsequent studies of both pyrimethamine alone and dapsone alone identified pyrimethamine as the agent responsible for the reduction in creatinine clearance. Similar studies in nine HIV-infected males before and after prophylaxis for 1 month with 75 mg pyrimethamine + 200 mg dapsone weekly (i.e. total of four doses) identified an analogous rise in serum creatinine from 69 ± 17 to $87 \pm 32 \mu$mol per liter (p<0.05), but both creatinine and inulin clearances were unchanged. Thus, pyrimethamine appears to reversibly inhibit renal tubular secretion of creatinine without affecting the GFR (Opravil et al., 1993). Hematuria has been reported rarely with pyrimethamine.

8 Immunosuppression

Subtle forms of immunosuppression may be associated with 'Maloprim' administration. Lee and Lau (1988) identified a 64% higher rate of non-specific upper respiratory tract infections in military recruits receiving one 'Maloprim' tablet weekly than those not receiving antimalarial prophylaxis, with the largest monthly differences being recorded during the periods of harder training. They speculated that 'Maloprim' was associated with some degree of immunosuppression, with physical stress possibly having a synergistic effect.

9 Miscellaneous side-effects

Rarely, fever, abnormal skin pigmentation, hyperphenylalaninemia and dryness of the throat have been reported with pyrimethamine therapy (McEnvoy, 1994). Severe confusion, asterixis and mental obtundation has been associated with hyperammonemia and carnitine deficiency in a patient treated with 75 mg pyrimethamine + 6 g sulfadiazine daily for cerebral toxoplasmosis. Correction of the carnitine deficiency with L-carnitine 300 mg daily resulted in prompt normalization of the patient's serum ammonia and mental state. The agent responsible for inducing the carnitine deficiency was not definitely identified, but the authors speculated that the deficiency may have been secondary to either increased urinary carnitine losses induced by pyrimethamine and/or sulfadiazine, or that the metabolites of these agents may bind with carnitine similar to some other drugs (Sekas and Paul, 1993).

10 Drug interactions

Concomitant administration of lorazepam and pyrimethamine has been reported to cause mild hepatic toxicity (Briggs and Briggs, 1974). In vitro studies suggest that pyrimethamine may inhibit tolbutamide metabolism, although the in vivo relevence of these data is less clear (Karbwang et al., 1988). Phenobarbital therapy appears to be associated with a shortening of the pyrimethamine half-life and reduction in serum pyrimethamine concentrations when the two agents are administered concomitantly to children, compared with children treated solely with pyrimethamine (McLeod et al., 1992). Such an effect may be predicted since phenobarbitol induces hepatic enzymes which degrade pyrimethamine. In vitro and animal studies suggest that zidovudine may reduce the efficacy of pyrimethamine in the treatment of toxoplasma encephalitis, but this has yet to be confirmed in clinical studies (Israelski et al., 1989).

Clinical Uses of the Drug

1 Toxoplasmosis

Pyrimethamine is the mainstay and currently the most effective therapy for all forms of toxoplasmosis in adults and children, when it is generally used in combination with other agents such as sulfadiazine or clindamycin (Leport et al., 1988; Cohn et al., 1989; Luft and Hafner, 1990; Dannemann et al., 1992; Luft and Remington, 1992; Luft et al., 1993; Georgiev, 1994; Mariuz et al., 1994). The concentration of pyrimethamine necessary to inhibit or kill toxoplasma tachyzoites has not been clinically established, and importantly, pyrimethamine is inactive against toxoplasma cysts (Luft and Hafner, 1990; Huskinson-Mark et al., 1991; Mariuz et al., 1994). After ingestion of toxoplasma oocytes, the organisms rapidly transform into tachyzoites which multiply in tissue macrophages and disseminate via blood and the lymphatic system to the brain, heart and lungs. In the immunocompetent host the development of immunity is associated with the transformation of tachyzoites into latent cysts (bradyzoites), especially in brain and muscle, which may reactivate at times of reduced host immunity. Thus, most immunocompetent hosts do not develop significant clinical disease and generally do not require treatment. Occasionally primary infection is associated with chorioretinitis, meningoencephalitis, myocarditis or pneumonitis due to unrestrained multiplication of tachyzoites, but such disease usually suggests some degree of host immunosupppression. Congenital infection may result in spontaneous abortion, fetal death or severe disease (hydrocephalus, hepatosplenomegaly with jaundice, chorioretinitis, mental retardation). Treatment is usually with pyrimethamine and sulfadiazine, but the duration of treatment varies depending on the clinical situation.

Outside the setting of AIDS, toxoplasmic encephalitis, carditis and chorioretinitis is generally treated for at least 1 month, often in combination with steroids if chorioretinitis threatens sight (Wilson, 1990a). A typical dosage regimen is pyrimethamine 75 mg per day for 3 days then 25 mg per day thereafter, although higher maintenance doses may be necessary if there is a lack of response. Sulfadiazine is generally given as 2–4 g per day. Some authors advocate using clindamycin (4.8 g per day i.v., or up to 2.4 g per day orally) for chorioretinitis since it is concentrated in the choroid (Lakhanpal et al., 1983). When pyrimethamine is used alone to treat toxoplasma encephalitis, e.g. due to toxicity associated with other agents, high doses should be used (p. 914).

When untreated, the risk of maternal–fetal transmission of T. gondii during primary maternal infection in pregnancy is approximately 50%, but the rate varies with the gestational age at the time of acquisition – 25%, 54%, 65% during first, second and third trimesters, respectively (Stray-Pederson, 1992). Primary toxoplasmosis during the first trimester should not be treated with pyrimethamine (p. 908), instead spiramycin 3 g per day should be used continuously during this period, when it is known to reduce the risk of congenital transmission by more than 50% (Desmonts and Couvreur, 1974; Stray-Pedersen, 1992). Importantly, however, spiramycin does not prevent cerebral toxoplasmosis in immunodeficient mothers since it has relatively poor brain and CSF penetration (Stray-Pedersen, 1992). After the first trimester pyrimethamine 25 mg per day + sulfadiazine 3 g per day may be given for 3–4 weeks, followed by spiramycin 3 g per day for 3 weeks to reduce the risk of congenital transmission. If there is known evidence of placental or fetal infection, this treatment course should be repeated (Stray-Pedersen, 1992).

Hohlfeld et al. (1989) identified the overall risk of fetal infection with toxoplasmosis to be 7% in mothers who acquired the disease during pregnancy and were treated, although the risk varied according to the gestational age at the time of maternal infection, as noted earlier. All women were treated with spiramycin 3 g per day with the mean time of commencement after maternal infection being 29 ± 17 days for continued pregnancies compared with 54 ± 39 days for terminated pregnancies. The majority of pregnancies terminated were on the basis of ultrasonographic evidence of serious neonatal disease. A delay in commencing spiramycin was associated with a higher rate of serious congenital toxoplasmosis. Among the 52 pregnancies that continued, 37 women were treated with a 3-week course of pyrimethamine 50 mg per day plus sulfadiazine 3 g per day, alternating with 3 weeks of spiramycin 3 g per day; six women received pyrimethamine 75 mg per day plus sulfadiazine 1500 mg per day every 10 days until the end of pregnancy and nine women were treated with spiramycin alone. All women treated with pyrimethamine were also given folinic acid. Subsequent follow-up of neonates revealed that such additional treatment with pyrimethamine and sulfadiazine was associated with a significant reduction in severe congenital toxoplasmosis and a relative decrease in the ratio of benign to subclinical toxoplasmosis – although the degree of this benefit has been disputed by Wilson (1990b).

There have been few studies to determine the optimal treatment regimen for newborn infants with congenital toxoplasmosis. In a large national collaborative study to assess the efficacy of pyrimethamine, sulfadiazine plus leukovorin during the first year of life in children with congenital toxoplasmosis, McAuley *et al.*(1994) clearly demonstrated the value of such therapy. Regression of retinal lesions, improved intellectual function, reduction in anticonvulsants and reduction in auditory effects were associated with aggressive drug therapy. Beaman *et al.* (1995) recommend continuous sulfadiazine (50 mg per kg twice-daily), pyrimethamine (2 mg per kg per day for 2 days, then 1 mg per kg per day for 2–6 months, then 1 mg per kg per day three times weekly) plus folinic acid (5 mg three times weekly up to 20 mg per day) for a minimum of 12 months. However, other authors recommend a variety of broadly similar regimens – the common theme being long duration of therapy and the use of pyrimethamine and sulfadiazine. For instances, based on the extensive clinical experience reported by Couvreur *et al.* (1984), Wilson (1990a) recommends pyrimethamine (1 mg per kg per day), sulfadiazine (100 mg per kg per day) plus folinic acid (2 mg per kg per day) for 3 weeks, followed by spiramycin (50–100 mg per kg per day) for 4–5 weeks. Frequently this 2-month treatment course needs to be repeated since Couvreur *et al.* (1984) suggested that the risk of recurrence of chorioretinitis after a single 2-month course was 26% versus 5–8% after 2–5 such courses. Thus, Wilson (1990a) suggests a minimum of 4–6 months therapy, with a longer course for severe disease. Other authors (Hengst, 1992; Stray-Pedersen, 1992) suggest a variety of regimens. For infants with subclinical congenital infection, Stray-Pedersen (1992), recommends repeated cycles of pyrimethamine + sulfadiazine (4 weeks), then spiramycin (6 weeks), for 1 year. Infants with overt congenital infection are treated by Stray-Pedersen (1992) with pyrimethamine plus sulfadiazine for 6 months, then alternating 4 week courses of spiramycin, then pyrimethamine plus sufadiazine, until 1–1.5 years of age.

Although clindamycin is effective in *Toxoplasma* chorioretinitis in older patients, there are no data regarding its use in congenital disease (Lakhanpal *et al.*, 1983). A report by Mitchell *et al.* (1990) of congenital toxoplasmosis occurring in infants perinatally infected with HIV 1 is notable since it raises the possibility of a higher rate of maternal–fetal transmission of *Toxoplasma* in HIV-infected mothers and speculates that the rate of congenital infection may be reduced by chemoprophylaxis with antitoxoplasma therapy of women who are seropositive for antibodies to HIV and *T. gondii*.

In the non-pregnant, immunocompetent host, systemic toxoplasmosis does not generally require treatment (McCabe *et al.*, 1987). In such patients, infection is relatively asymptomatic, often with only lymphadenopathy around the head and neck, despite the usual wide dissemination of toxoplasma during acute acquired infection. McCabe *et al.* (1987) reviewed the clinical spectrum of 107 cases of toxoplasma lymphadenopathy and found that the vast majority had no systemic symptoms, no extranodal disease and the disease had a benign clinical course. Occasionally extranodal involvement occurred, including myocarditis, pneumonitis, encephalitis, chorioretinitis and maternal–fetal transmission, which required treatment in some cases.

There has been a marked increase in the incidence of toxoplasma infections, especially toxoplasma encephalitis, associated with HIV infection. In this setting, toxoplasma encephalitis is almost exclusively due to the reactivation of latent infection. The absence of detectable serum antibody to *T. gondii* in an HIV-infected patient with an intracerebral space-occupying lesion argues very strongly against the diagnosis of toxoplasmic encephalitis (Israelski *et al.*, 1990). Among HIV-infected patients with serious toxoplasmosis the treatment regimen of pyrimethamine 200-mg loading dose then 25–75 mg daily in combination with sulfadiazine 4–8 g per day for 3–6 weeks, followed by maintenance therapy (p. 915) remains the most commonly recommended protocol (Mariuz *et al.*, 1994). This results in a clinical response in 68–95% of patients with toxoplasmic encephalitis (Luft and Remington, 1985; Haverkos, 1987; Leport *et al.*, 1988; Cohn *et al.*, 1989; Cimino *et al.*, 1991; Dannemann *et al.*, 1992), but this high dose regimen is often associated with significant toxicity so that up to 40% of patients require a change in therapy (Haverkos, 1987; Leport *et al.*, 1988; Cohn *et al.*, 1989; Cimino *et al.*, 1991; Dannemann *et al.*, 1992).

Pyrimethamine in combination with clindamycin appears to be a suitable alternative for sulfa-allergic patients. However, although clindamycin is well absorbed orally and has excellent general tissue penetration, brain and CSF concentrations are less predictable (Dannemann *et al.*, 1992). Nevertheless, a number of studies suggest comparable efficacy between pyrimethamine plus clindamycin (oral or i.v.) and pyrimethamine plus sulfadiazine in the treatment of AIDS-associated toxoplasmic encephalitis (Leport *et al.*, 1989; Katlama, 1991; Rolston, 1991; Ruf and Pohle, 1991; Dannemann *et al.*, 1992; Luft *et al.*, 1993). Both Dannemann *et al.* (1992) and Luft *et al.* (1993) used pyrimethamine 75 mg per day orally, but differed in the dose of clindamycin from 1200 mg (initially i.v. then oral) four times daily to 600 mg (oral) four times daily, respectively. Most authors now recommend a dose of 600 mg (oral or i.v.) four times daily for 3–6 weeks, depending on disease severity, before changing to maintenance therapy (Remington and Desmonts, 1990; Remington and Vildé, 1991). Side-effects from clindamycin are reasonably common (p. 594).

Pyrimethamine has been successfully used in combination with the new macrolides, azithromycin and clarithromycin, for acute treatment of toxoplasmic encephalitis. Preliminary data from an AIDS Clinical Trials Group (ACTG)-sponsored study suggested that pyrimethamine 50–75 mg per day in combination with azithromycin 1200–1500 mg per day was effective (Mariuz et al., 1994). Fernandez-Martin et al. (1991) found that pyrimethamine 75 mg per day plus clarithromycin 2 g per day resulted in efficacy comparable with conventional therapy for acute toxoplasmic encephalitis in 13 patients with AIDS, although adverse reactions (mostly mild) occurred in 90% of patients. Notable with this regimen was a 15% incidence of sensorial hearing loss, probably related to clarithromycin.

Atovaquone, a hydroxynapthoquinone, has excellent in vitro and in vivo activity against T. gondii (Araujo et al., 1991), but is associated with a greater than 50% clinical relapse rate when used alone for acute and maintenance therapy (Kovacs, 1992). Combination with pyrimethamine or sulfadiazine has shown significant enhancement of activity in the treatment of murine toxoplasmosis. If these results are confirmed in human studies, this synergism may allow for a useful dose reduction in pyrimethamine or sulfadiazine, with a potential decrease in toxicity (Araujo et al., 1993).

Doxycycline appears to have reasonable in vitro and in vivo activity alone, and in combination with pyrimethamine, against T. gondii (Chang et al., 1990). Hagberg et al. (1993) reported a case of apparent successful therapy with pyrimethamine plus doxycycline for AIDS-associated toxoplasmic encephalitis, however, further clinical studies are necessary before this regimen can be recommended.

The acute management of extraneural AIDS-associated toxoplasmosis is less well studied, but the use of standard pyrimethamine-containing therapeutic regimens for encephalitis appear to be effective. Successful therapy of pulmonary toxoplasmosis has been reported in 50–77% of patients, but long-term maintenance therapy remains important (Mendelson et al., 1987; Oksenhendler et al., 1988; Pomeroy and Felice, 1992).

Since pyrimethamine and other currently available agents are ineffective against toxoplasma tissue cysts, cessation of therapy in the setting of host immunodeficiency, such as with HIV infection, is associated with re-activation of latent disease in up to 80% of patients (Hauser et al., 1982; Navia et al., 1986; Haverkos et al., 1987; Tschirhard and Klaft, 1988; Luft and Remington, 1988; Cohn et al., 1989; Pedrol et al., 1990; Remington and Vildé, 1991; Kovacs, 1995). Thus, life-long maintenance of antitoxoplasma therapy is generally recommended. Until recently, there has been little data to indicate the optimum maintenance protocol, however commonly used regimens are pyrimethamine 25–50 mg per day in combination with either sulfadiazine 2–4 g per day or clindamycin 1200–1800 mg per day in divided doses (Leport et al., 1988; Cohn et al., 1989; Foppa et al., 1991; Remington and Vildé, 1991; Mariuz et al., 1994). Both combinations appear to be equally effective (Cohn et al., 1989). Pedrol et al. (1990) reported success with 'low-dose' intermittent maintenance therapy in which either pyrimethamine (25 mg per day) + sulfadiazine (75 mg per kg per day) or pyrimethamine (25 mg per day) + clindamycin (600 mg four times daily) was given 2 days per week; although the pyrimethamine + clindamycin combination was the less effective of these two regimens. Podzamczer et al. (1995a), however, has demonstrated the superiority of daily over twice-weekly supresive therapy. In a randomized, open, multicenter trial, the daily combination of pyrimethamine 25 mg + sulfadiazine 500 mg four times-daily + folinic acid 15 mg was associated with an estimated cumulative risk of relapse of Toxoplasma encephalitis at 12 months of 6% versus a 30% rate of relapse (p=0.029) for the same dosage regimen administered twice-weekly. Patients receiving the twice-weekly regimen had 1.6 times the adjusted risk for death of patients receiving the daily regimen. No patient developed Pneumocystis carinii pneumonia during the study period.

Experience with pyrimethamine alone for maintenance therapy is either anecdotal or retrospective (Leport et al., 1988; Navia et al., 1986; Cohn et al., 1989; Dannemann et al., 1988; Bhatti and Larson, 1990; De Gans et al., 1992). De Gans et al. (1992) retrospectively analyzed the outcome of 38 AIDS patients given maintenance antitoxoplasma therapy with pyrimethamine alone (25 versus 50 mg per day). Although they did not find a statistically different rate of relapse between the two regimens, they cautiously recommended a dose of 50 mg per day. Nevertheless, given the wide variation in serum pyrimethamine levels both within individuals and between individuals, and documented failures with this regimen, such monotherapy cannot be currently recommended (Weiss *et al.*, 1988a; De Gans *et al.*, 1992). Other potential maintenance therapy options currently under investigation include 'Fansidar' and dapsone (Mariuz *et al.*, 1994).

Primary chemoprophylaxis against toxoplasmic encephalitis is a reasonable consideration for HIV-infected patients who are significantly immunosuppressed (e.g. CD4 lymphocyte count <100–200 per mm^3) and are seropositive for antitoxoplasma antibody. However, there are currently no prospective, randomized trials to determine the optimal regimen. Oral trimethoprim/sulfamethoxazole (160/800 mg daily) is effective in prevention of toxoplasmic encephalitis (Carr *et al.*, 1992; Jacobson *et al.*, 1994; p. 874) and combination pyrimethamine plus dapsone (generally given for prophylaxis against *P. carinii* pneumonia) also provides some protection (Clotet *et al.*, 1991, 1992; Girard *et al.*, 1993; Mariuz *et al.*, 1994). Girard *et al.*(1993) noted that the combination of dapsone (50 mg per day) + pyrimethamine (50 mg per week) given as primary prophylaxis against *P. carinii* pneumonia also significantly prevented first episodes of toxoplasmosis (p=0.018). In this study patients who were seropositive against *T. gondii*, had a CD4 lymphocyte count < 100 per mm^3 and who did not receive dapsone + pyrimethamine, had a 40% greater probability of developing toxoplasmosis after 18 months than those who received pyrimethamine plus dapsone.

Primary prophylaxis with pyrimethamine alone (e.g. 25 mg thrice-weekly) did not appear to be effective in preventing toxoplasmic encephalitis in HIV-infected patients with either CD4 count <200 per mm^3 or AIDS, when studied in a double-blind, placebo-controlled, randomized trial (Jacobson *et al.*, 1994). The results of this trial, however, were probably confounded by a low rate of toxoplasmic encephalitis in the placebo group, possibly due to the concomitant administration of trimethoprim/sulfamethoxazole. These authors suggested that HIV-infected patients receiving trimethoprim/sulfamethoxazole for *P. carinii* pneumonia prophylaxis were unlikely to need additional prophylaxis for toxoplasmic encephalitis. More recently, Leport *et al.* (1996) reported that pyrimethamine 50 mg plus folinic acid 15 mg given three times per week was associated with a similar incidence of toxoplasma encephalitis at 1 year as placebo (12% versus 13%, respectively) and the survival rate was similar. However, in the on-treatment analysis, the incidence of toxoplasmosis was 4% in the pyrimethamine arm versus 12% in the placebo arm (p <0.006). Thus, although pyrimethamine cannot be recommended as first-line prophylaxis for toxoplasma encephalitis in HIV-infected patients, it may be a reasonable alternative among those who are co-trimoxazole-intolerant and at high-risk (CD4 <100 per mm^3).

2 Pneumocystis carinii pneumonia

Various regimens containining pyrimethamine have proven effective for prophylaxis against *P. carinii* pneumonia in HIV-infected patients (p. 879; Table II.4 p. 878). Dapsone (50 mg per day) plus pyrimethamine (50 mg per week) is equal in efficacy to aerosolized pentamidine (300 mg per month) as primary prophylaxis against *P. carinii* pneumonia. Unlike pentamidine, however, this combination also prevents first episodes of toxoplasmosis, albeit at a cost of less tolerability than pentamidine (Girard *et al.*, 1993). Opravil *et al.* (1995a) found similar results using dapsone 200 mg plus pyrimethamine 75 mg once-weekly, but dapsone/pyrimethamine was not tolerated by 30% of patients. However, the efficacy of so-called 'low dose' intermittent therapy with pyrimethamine plus dapsone for *P. carinii* pneumonia prophylaxis, remains controversial. Mallolas *et al.* (1993) found that a low dose regimen of pyrimethamine 25 mg plus dapsone 100 mg weekly was similar in efficacy to trimethoprim/sulfamethoxazole (160 mg/800 mg) given thrice-weekly and once-monthly aerosolized pentamidine for primary *P. carinii* pneumonia prophylaxis. Similarly, dapsone 100 mg plus pyrimethamine 25 mg, both twice-weekly, was effective for primary and secondary *P. carinii* pneumonia prophylaxis in a relatively small uncontrolled study by Clotet *et al.* (1991). In contrast, Antinori *et al.* (1992) (dapsone 100 mg weekly plus pyrimethamine 25 mg twice-weekly), Coker *et al.* (1992) (dapsone 100 mg plus pyrimethamine 25 mg, thrice-weekly) and Podzamczer *et al.* (1993b) (dapsone 100 mg plus pyrimethamine 25 mg, once-weekly) found that low dose dapsone plus pyrimethamine was less effective for primary *P. carinii* pneumonia prophylaxis than co-trimoxazole. Podzamczer *et al.* (1995b) also found dapsone 100 mg plus pyrimethamine 50 mg twice-weekly to be inferior to co-trimoxazole with *P. carinii* pneumonia occurring in 6 of 96 (6.3%) versus 0 of 104 (0%) patients, respectively (p <0.0001). No differences were observed in the incidence of toxoplasmosis. Secondary prophylaxis with pyrimethamine (50–175 mg per week) alone is probably ineffective, since rates of *P. carinii* pneumonia relapse are similar to estimated recurrence rates without prophylaxis (Lidman *et al.*, 1989). Thus, low dose pyrimethamine regimens should only be used with caution based on current data.

Pyrimethamine plus sulfadoxine ('Fansidar') appears to be effective *P. carinii* pneumonia prophylaxis, depending on whether it is given once versus twice per week, although a relatively high rate of serious adverse reactions, probably associated with the sulfadoxine component (pp. 826, 878) has limited its use (Gottlieb *et al.*, 1984; Pearson and Hewlett, 1987; Fischl and Dickinson, 1986; Ruf *et al.*, 1993; Jurado *et al.*, 1994).

Patients receiving maintenance therapy for cerebral toxoplasmosis with combinations containing pyrimethamine (generally 25–50 mg per day) plus sulfadiazine appear to have a lower than expected rate of developing *P. carinii* pneumonia; although prophylaxis failures have been reported, particularly with the maintenance combination of pyrimethamine plus clindamycin (Heald *et al.*, 1991; Cohn *et al.*, 1989; Haverkos, 1987; Girard *et al.*, 1989).

3 Isosporiasis

Isosporiasis, or enteric infection with the protozoan *Isospora belli*, may cause severe diarrhea, especially in patients with AIDS. Although the usual treatment of choice is trimethoprim/sulfamethoxazole, pyrimethamine may be a useful alternative in sulfa-allergic patients. Weiss *et al.* (1988b) reported two patients who responded rapidly to acute therapy with pyrimethamine 50–75 mg per day + folinic acid 10 mg per day for 2–4 weeks, followed by long-term maintenance therapy with pyrimethamine 25 mg per day + folinic acid 5 mg per day. Pape *et al.* (1989) studied 32 Haitian patients with AIDS complicated by *Isospora belli* infection and chronic diarrhea who were treated acutely with trimethoprim/sulfamethoxazole (160/800 mg) four times daily for 10 days, then randomized to receive long-term maintenance therapy with pyrimethamine 25 mg + sulfadoxine 500 mg (one 'Fansidar' tablet) once-weekly, trimethoprim/sulfamethoxazole (160/800 mg) thrice-weekly, or placebo. Pyrimethamine/sulfadoxine and trimethoprim/sulfamethoxazole were equally effective in preventing clinical and parasitological relapse, and were superior to placebo, which was associated with 50% rate of recurrence after less than 2 months.

4 Malaria

Pyrimethamine is effective for the treatment of this disease caused by susceptible strains of *P. falciparum* when used in combination with sulfadoxine ('Fansidar'), and is useful in some regions for chemoprophylaxis when given as 'Fansidar' or 'Maloprim' (pyrimethamine + dapsone). During the 1960s, pyrimethamine given alone was effective as prophylaxis against *P. falciparum* malaria during pregnancy in areas such as Nigeria (Morley *et al.*, 1964). However, a recent study in the same region has demonstrated the clinical ineffectiveness of pyrimethamine (25 mg per week) for supressive and causal prophylaxis (Nahlen *et al.*, 1989). A more detailed discussion regarding the antimalarial uses of pyrimethamine (e.g. 'Fansidar', 'Maloprim') can be found on pp. 824, 825.

5 Mycobacteria

Opravil *et al.* (1995b) noted a lower incidence of mycobacterial diseases among HIV-infected patients receiving dapsone/pyrimethamine prophylaxis for *P. carinii* pneumonia and toxoplasmosis than among those receiving aerosolized pentamidine. Further studies are needed to confirm these observations.

References

Anderson PO (1979). Drugs and breast feeding. *Semin Perinatol* **3**: 271.

Antinori A, Murri R, Tamburrini E *et al.* (1992). Failure of low-dose dapsone-pyrimethamine in primary prophylaxis of *Pneumocystis carinii* pneumonia. *Lancet* **340**: 788.

Araujo FG, Huskinson J, Remington JS (1991). Remarkable *in vitro* and *in vivo* activity of the hydroxynapthoquinone (566C80). against tachyzoites and cysts of *Toxoplasma gondii*. *Antimicrob Ag Chemother* **35**: 293.

Araujo FG, Prokocimer P, Lin T *et al.* (1992). Activity of clarithromycin alone or in combination with other drugs for treatment of murine toxoplasmosis. *Antimicrob Ag Chemother* **36**: 2454.

Araujo FG, Lin T, Remington JS (1993). The activity of atovaquone (566C80). in murine toxoplasmosis is markedly augmented when used in combination with pyrimethamine or sulfadiazine. *J Infect Dis* **167**: 494.

Beaman MH, McCabe RE, Wong S-Y, Remington JS (1995). *Toxoplasma gondii*. In *Principles and Practice of Infectious Diseases* 4th ed (Mandell GL, Bennett JE, Dolin R, eds), p. 2455. New York: Churchill Livingstone.

Bennett PN (ed). (1988). In *Drugs and Human Lactation*. Elsevier: Amsterdam.

Bennett WM, Aronoff GR, Golper TA *et al.* (1991). *Drug Prescribing in Renal Failure. Dosing Guidelines for Adults* 2nd edn. Philadelphia: American College of Physicians.

Bergqvist Y, Eriksson M (1985). Simultaneous determination of pyrimethamine and sulfadoxine in human plasma by high-performance liquid chromatography. *Trans Roy Soc Trop Med Hyg* **79**: 297.

Bhatti N, Larson E (1990). Low-dose alternate-day pyrimethamine for maintenance therapy in cerebral toxoplasmosis complicating AIDS. *J Infect* **21**: 119.

Briggs M, Briggs M (1974). Pyrimethamine toxicity. *Brit Med J* **1**: 40.

Broughton MC, Queener SF (1991). *Pneumocystis carinii* dihydrofolate reductase used to screen potential anti pneumocystis drugs. *Antimicrob Ag Chemother* **35**: 1348.

Brown, GV (1993). Chemoprophylaxis of malaria. *Med J Aust* **159**: 187.

Bruce-Chwatt LJ, Hutchinson DBA (1984). Agranulocytosis associated with Maloprim. *Brit Med J* **288**: 65.

Carr A, Tindall B, Brew BJ *et al.* (1992). Low-dose trimethoprim-sulfamethoxazole prophylaxis for toxoplasmic encephalitis in patients with AIDS. *Ann Intern Med* **117**: 106.

Caumes E, Bocquet H, Guermonprez G *et al.* (1995). Adverse cutaneous reactions to pyrimethamine/sulfadiazine and pyrimethamine/clindamycin in patients with AIDS and toxoplasmic encephalitis. *Clin Infect Dis* **21**: 656.

Cavallito JC, Nichol CA, Brenckman WD *et al.* (1978). Lipid-soluble inhibitors of dihydrofolate reductase I Kinetics, tissue distribution, and extent of metabolism of pyrimethamine, metropine, and etoprine in the rat, dog and man. *Drug Metab Dispos* **6**: 329.

CDC (Centers for Disease Control) (1993). Health information for international travel 1993. Atlanta, Georgia: US Department of Health and Human Services.

Chang HR, Comte R, Pechere JC (1990). *In vitro* and *in vivo* effects of doxycycline on *Toxoplasma gondii*. *Antimicrob Ag Chemother* **34**: 775.

Chute JP, Decker CF, Cotelingam J (1995). Severe megaloblastic anemia complicating pyrimethamine therapy. *Ann Intern Med* **122**: 884.

Cimino C, Lipton RB, Williams A *et al.* (1991). The evaluation of patients with human immunodeficiency virus-related disorders and brain mass lesions. *Arch Intern Med* **151**: 1381.

Clotet B, Sirera G, Romeu J *et al.* (1991). Twice-weekly dapsone-pyrimethamine for preventing PCP and cerebral toxoplasmosis. *AIDS* **5**: 601.

Clotet B, Romeu J, Sirera G (1992). Cerebral toxoplasmosis and prophylaxis for *Pneumocystis carinii* pneumonia. *Ann Intern Med* **117**: 169.

Clyde DF (1960). Prolonged malaria prophylaxis through pyrimethamine in mother's milk. *East Afr Med J* **37**: 659.

Clyde DF, Shute GT, Press J (1956). Transfer of pyrimethamine in human milk. *J Trop Med Hyg* **59**: 277.

Cohn JA, McMeeking A, Cohen W *et al.* (1989). Evaluation of the policy of empiric treatment of suspected *Toxoplasma* encephalitis in patients with the acquired immunodeficiency syndrome. *Amer J Med* **86**: 521.

Coker RJ, Nieman R, McBride M *et al.* (1992). Co-trimoxazole versus dapsone-pyrimethamine for prevention of *Pneumocystis carinii* pneumonia. *Lancet* **340**: 1099.

Committee on Drugs, American Academy of Pediatrics (1994). The transfer of drugs and other chemicals into human milk. *Pediatrics* **93**: 137.

Cook IF, Cochrane JP, Edstein MD (1986). Race-linked differences in serum concentrations of dapsone, monoacetyldapsone and pyrimethamine during malaria prophylaxis. *Trans Roy Soc Trop Med Hyg* **80**: 897.

Couvreur J, Desmonts G, Aron-rosa D (1984). Le pronostic oculaire de la toxoplasmose congenitale: role du traitement. *Ann Pediatr* **31**: 855 .

Dannemann BR, Israelski DM, Remington JS (1988). Treatment of toxoplasmic encephalitis with intravenous clindamycin. *Arch Intern Med* **148**: 2477.

Dannemann B, McCutchan JA, Israelski D *et al.* (1992). Treatment of toxoplasmic encephalitis in patients with AIDS. A randomized trial comparing pyrimethamine plus clindamycin to pyrimethamine plus sulfadiazine. The California Collaborative Treatment Group. *Ann Intern Med* **116**: 33.

Davidson AC *et al.* (1988). Pulmonary toxicity of malaria prophylaxis. *Brit Med J* **297**: 1240.

De Gans J, Portegies P, Reiss P *et al.* (1992). Pyrimethamine alone as maintenance therapy for central nervous system toxoplasmosis in 38 patients with AIDS. *J AIDS* **5**: 137.

Derouin F, Chastang C (1989). *In vitro* effects of folate inhibitors on *Toxoplasma gondii*. *Antimicrob Ag Chemother* **33**: 1753.

Derouin F, Piketty C, Chastang C *et al.* (1991). Anti-toxoplasma effects of dapsone alone and combined with pyrimethamine. *Antimicrob Ag Chemother* **35**: 252.

Derouin F, Almadany R, Chau F *et al.* (1992). Synergistic activity of azithromycin and pyrimethamine or sulfadiazine in acute experimental toxoplasmosis. *Antimicrob Ag Chemother* **36**: 997.

Desmonts G, Couvreur J (1974). Congenital toxoplasmosis: a prospective study of 78 pregnancies. *New Engl J Med* **290**: 1110.

Edstein MD, Veerendaal JR, Newman K, Hyslop R (1986). Excretion of chloroquine, dapsone and pyrimethamine in human milk. *Brit J Clin Pharmacol* **22**: 733.

Falco EA, Goodwin LG, Hithings GH *et al.* (1951). 2: 4-Diaminopyrimidines – a new series of antimalarials. *Brit J Pharmacol Chemother* **6**: 185.

Fernandez MJ, Leport C, Morlat P *et al.* (1991). Pyrimethamine-clarithromycin combination for therapy of acute *Toxoplasma* encephalitis in patients with AIDS. *Antimicrob Ag Chemother* **35**: 2049.

Ferone R (1984). Dihydrofolate reductase. In *Antimicrobial Drugs* Vol II (Peters W, Richards WHG, eds), pp. 207–217. Berlin: Springer Verlag.

Ferone R, Burchall JJ, Hitching GH (1969). *Plasmodium berghei* dihydrofolate reductase: isolation, properties and inhibition by antifolates. *Mol Pharmacol* **5**: 49.

Fischl MA, Dickinson GM (1986). Fansidar prophylaxis of *Pneumocystis carinii* pneumonia in the acquired immunodeficiency syndrome. *Ann Intern Med* **105**: 629.

Foppa CU, Bini T, Gregis G *et al.* (1991). A retrospective study of primary and maintenance therapy of toxoplasmic encephalitis with oral clindamycin and pyrimethamine. *Eur J Clin Microbiol Infect Dis* **10**: 187.

Frenkel JK, Good JT, Schultz JA (1966). Latent *Pneumocystis* infection of rats, relapse and chemotherapy. *Lab Invest* **15**: 1559.

Georgiev VS (1994). Management of toxoplasmosis. *Drugs* **48**: 179.

Girard PM, Lepretre A, Detruchis P *et al.* (1989). Failure of pyrimethamine-clindamycin combination for prophylaxis of *Pneumocystis carinii* pneumonia. *Lancet* **1**: 1459.

Girard PM, Landman R, Gaudebout C *et al.* (1993). Dapsone-pyrimethamine compared with aerosolized pentamidine as primary prophylaxis against *Pneumocystis carinii* pneumonia and toxoplasmosis in HIV infection. The PRIO Study Group. *New Engl J Med* **328**: 1514.

Goodman Gilman A, Rall TW, Nies AS, Taylor P (eds) (1990). Diaminopyrimidines In *The Pharmacological Basis of Therapeutics* 8th edn, p. 985. New York: Pergamon Press.

Gottlieb M, Knight S, Mitsuyasu R *et al.* (1984). Prophylaxis of *Pneumocystis carinii* infection in AIDS with pyrimethamine-sulfadoxine. *Lancet* **ii**: 398.

Grayson ML, Yung AP, Doherty RR (1988). Severe dapsone syndrome due to weekly Maloprim. *Lancet* **i**: 531.

Gubler J (1988). Sulfadoxine-pyrimethamine resistant malaria from west or central Africa. *Brit Med J* **296**: 433.

Hagberg L, Palmertz B, Lindberg J (1993). Doxycycline and pyrimethamine for toxoplasmic encephalitis. *Scand J Infect Dis* **25**: 157.

Hauser WE, Luft BJ, Conley FK, Remington JS (1982). Central nervous system toxoplasmosis in homosexual and heterosexual adults. *New Engl J Med* **307**: 498.

Haverkos HW, Toxoplsma encephalitis study group (1987). Assessment of therapy for toxoplasma encephalitis. *Amer J Med* **82**: 907.

Heald A, Flepp M, Chave JP *et al.* (1991). Treatment for cerebral toxoplasmosis protects against *Pneumocystis carinii* pneumonia in patients with AIDS. The Swiss HIV Cohort Study. *Ann Intern Med* **115**: 760.

Hellgren U, Angel VH, Bergqvist Y *et al.* (1990). Plasma concentrations of sulfadoxine-pyrimethamine and of mefloquine during regular long term malaria prophylaxis. *Trans Roy Soc Trop Med Hyg* **84**: 46.

Hellgren U, Angel VH, Bergqvist Y *et al.* (1991). Plasma concentrations of sulfadoxine-pyrimethamine, mefloquine and its main metabolite after regular malaria prophylaxis for 2 years. *Trans Roy Soc Trop Med Hyg* **85**: 356.

Hengst P (1992). Screening for toxoplasmosis in pregnant women: presentation of a screening programme in the former 'East'-Germany, and the present status in Germany. *Scand J Infect Dis* (Suppl 84): 38.

Herzog C, Kibbler CC, Ellis CJ (1983). *Falciparum malaria* resistant to chloroquine and Fansidar: implications for prophylaxis. *Br Med J* **287**: 947.

Hohlfeld P, Daffos F, Thulliez P *et al.* (1989). Fetal toxoplasmosis: outcome of pregnancy and infant follow-up after *in utero* treatment. *J Pediatr* **115**: 765.

Hughes WT, Smith BL (1984). Efficacy of diaminodiphenyl-sulfone and other drugs in murine *Pneumocystis carinii* pneumonitis. *Antimicrob Ag Chemother* **26**: 436.

Hughes WT, Smith BL, Jacobus DP (1986). Successful treatment and prevention of murine *Pneumocystis carinii* pneumonitis with 4,4'-sulfonybisformanilide. *Antimicrob Ag Chemother* **29**: 509.

Huskinson-MarkJ, Araujo FG, Remington JS (1991). Evaluation of the effect of drugs on the cyst form of *Toxoplasma gondii*. *J Infect Dis* **164**: 170.

Hutchinson DBA, Whiteman PD, Farquhar JA (1986). Agranulocytosis associated with Maloprim: review of cases. *Hum Toxicol* **5**: 221.

Ibrahim ME, Awad-El-Kariem FM, El Hassan IM, El Mubarak ERM (1991). A case of *Plasmodium falciparum* malaria sensitive to chloroquine but resistant to pyrimethamine/sulfadoxine in Sennar, Sudan. *Trans Roy Soc Trop Med Hyg* **85**: 446.

Infectious Disease Rounds (1988). Toxoplasmosis in a premature infant. *Rev Infect Dis* **10**: 624.

Israelski DM, Tom C, Remington JS (1989). Zidovudine antagonizes the action of pyrimethamine in experimental infection with *Toxoplasma gondii*. *Antimicrob Ag Chemother* **33**: 30.

Israelski DM, Dannemann BR, Remington JS (1990). Toxoplasmic encephalitis in patients with AIDS. In *The Medical Management of AIDS* (Sande MA, Volberding PA, eds), p. 241. Philadelphia: WB Saunders.

Jacobson MA, Besch CL, Child C *et al.* (1994). Primary prophylaxis with pyrimethamine for toxoplasmic encephalitis in patients with advanced human immunodeficiency virus disease: results of a randomized trial. *J Infect Dis* **169**: 384.

Jones CR, Ovenell SM (1979). Determination of plasma concentrations of dapsone, monoacetyl dapsone and pyrimethamine in human subjects dosed with maloprim. *J Chromatogr* **163**: 179.

Jurado R, Garcia-Herola A, Garcia-Lazaro M *et al.* (1994). Pyrimethamine/sulfadoxine for prevention of *Pneumocystis carinii* pneumonia in patients infected with the human immunodeficiency virus. *Clin Infect Dis* **19**: 218.

Karbwang J, Back DJ, Bunnag D, Breckenridge AM (1988). Inhibition of tolbutamide metabolism by antimalarial drugs. *Southeast Asian J Trop Med Publ Hlth* **19**: 235.

Katlama C (1991). Evaluation of the efficacy and safety of clindamycin plus pyrimethamine for induction and maintenance of toxoplasmic encephalitis in AIDS. *Eur J Clin Microbiol Infect Dis* **10**: 189.

Kovacs JA (1992). Efficacy of atovaquone in treatment of toxoplasmosis in patients with AIDS. *Lancet* **340**: 637.

Kovacs JA (1995). Toxoplasmosis in AIDS: keeping the lid on. *Ann Intern Med* **123**: 230.

Kovacs JA, Alegra CJ, Swan JC *et al.* (1988). Potent antipneumocystis and antitoxoplasmic activities of piritrexim, a lipid-soluble antifolate. *Antimicrob Ag Chemother* **32**: 430.

Kovacs JA, Allegra CJ, Masur H (1990). Characterization of dihydrofolate reductase of *Pneumocystis carinii* and *Toxoplasma gondii*. *Exp Parasitol* **71**: 60.

Kumar R, Kaushik P, Sharma CB (1990). Studies on the dtermination and degradation of pyrimethamine in mammals. *Biomed Chromatogr* **4**: 165.

Lakhanpal V, Schodket SS, Nirankari VS (1983). Clindamycin in the treatment of toxoplasmic retinochoroiditis. *Amer J Ophthalmol* **95**: 605.

Lambros C, Davis DR, Lewis GJ (1989). Antimalarial drug susceptibility of *Plasmodium falciparum* isolates from forest fringe dwelling aborigines (Orang Asli) of Peninsular Malaysia. *Amer J Trop Med Hyg* **41**: 3.

Le Liboux A, Duquesne H, Montay G *et al.* (1991). Pharmacokinetics of pyrimethamine in healthy young volunteers using a new solid phase extraction/HPLC method. *Eur J Drug Metab Pharmacokinet* **3**: 284.

Lee PS, Lau EYL (1988). Risk of acute non-specific upper respiratory tract infections in healthy men taking dapsone-pyrimethamine for prophylaxis against malaria. *Brit Med J* **296**: 893.

Lege-Oguntoye L, Adagu SI, Werblinska B *et al.* (1990). Resistance of *Plasmodium falciparum* to sulfadoxine-pyrimethamine combination in semi-immune children in Zaria, northern Nigeria. *Trans Roy Soc Trop Med Hyg* **84**: 505.

Leport C, Raffi F, Matheron S *et al.* (1988). Treatment of central nervous system toxoplasmosis with pyrimethamine/sulfadiazine combination in 35 patients with acquired immunodeficiency syndrome. *Amer J Med* **84**: 94.

Leport C, Bastuji GS, Perronne C *et al.* (1989). An open study of the pyrimethamine-clindamycin combination in AIDS patients with brain toxoplasmosis. *J Infect Dis* **160**: 557.

Leport C, Menlemans A, Robine D *et al.* (1992). Levels of pyrimethamine in serum and penetration into brain tissue in humans. *AIDS* **6**: 1040.

Leport C, Chene G, Morlat P *et al.* (1996). Pyrimethamine for primary prophylaxis of toxoplasmic encephalitis in patients with human immunodeficiency virus infection: a double-blind, randomized trial. ANRS 005-ACTG 154 Group Members. Agence Nationale de Recherche sur le SIDA. AIDS Clinical Trial Group. *J Infect Dis* **173**: 91.

Lidman C, Ortqvist A, Lundbergh P *et al.* (1989). *Pneumocystis carinii* pneumonia in Stockholm, Sweden: treatment, outcome, one-year-follow-up and pyrimethamine prophylaxis. *Scand J Infect Dis* **21**: 381.

Luft BJ, Hafner R (1990). Toxoplasmic encephalitis. *AIDS* **4**: 593.

Luft BJ, Remington JS (1985). Toxoplasmosis of the central nervous system. In *Current Clinical Topics in Infectious Diseases* (Remington JS, Swartz WM, eds), p. 315. New York: McGraw-Hill.

Luft BJ, Remington JS (1988). Toxoplasmic encephalitis. *J Infect Dis* **157**: 1.

Luft BJ, Remington JS (1992). Toxoplasmic encephalitis in AIDS. *Clin Infect Dis* **15**: 211.

Luft BJ, Hafner R, Korzun AH *et al.* (1993). Toxoplasmic encephalitis in patients with the acquired immunodeficiency syndrome. *New Engl J Med* **329**: 995.

Malin AS, Hall AP (1990). *Falciparum malaria* resistant to quinine and pyrimethamine-sulfadoxine successfully treated with mefloquine. *Brit Med J* **300**: 1175.

Mallolas J, Zamora L, Gatell JM *et al.* (1993). Primary prophylaxis for *Pneumocystis carinii* pneumonia: a randomized trial comparing cotrimoxazole, aerosolized pentamidine and dapsone plus pyrimethamine. *AIDS* **7**: 59.

Mansor SM, Navaratnam V, Mohamad M *et al.* (1989). Single dose kinetic study of the triple combination mefloquine/sulphadoxine/pyrimethamine (Fansimef). in healthy male volunteers. *Brit J Clin Pharmac* **27**: 381.

Mariuz P, Bosler EM, Luft BJ (1994). Toxoplasmosis in individuals with AIDS. *Infect Dis Clinics N Amer* **8**: 365.

McAuley J, Boyer K, Patel D *et al.* (1994). Early and longitudinal evaluations of treated infants and children and untreated historical patients with congenital toxoplasmosis: The Chicago collaborative treatment trial. *Clin Infect Dis* **18**: 38.

McCabe RE, Brooks RG, Dorfman RF, Remington JS (1987). Clinical spectrum of 107 cases of toxoplasmic lymphadenopathy. *Rev Infect Dis* **9**: 754.

McEnvoy GK (ed). (1994). American Hospital Formulary Service, p. 460. Bethesda, MD: American Society of Hospital Pharmacists.

McLeod R, Mack D, Foss R *et al.* (1992). Levels of pyrimethamine in sera and cerebrospinal and ventricular fluids from infants treated for congenital toxoplasmosis. *Antimicrob Ag Chemother* **36**: 1040.

Mendelson MH, Finkel LJ, Meyers BR *et al.* (1987). Pulmonary toxoplasmosis in AIDS. *Scand J Infect Dis* **19**: 703.

Mihaly GW, Date NM, Veenendaal JR, Newman KT, Smallwood RA (1987). *Biochem Pharmacol* **36**: 2827.

Mitchell CD, Erlich SS, Mastrucci MT *et al.* (1990). Congenital toxoplasmosis occurring in infants perinatally infected with human immunodeficiency virus 1. *Pediatr Infect Dis J* **9**: 512.

Morley D, Woodland M, Cuthbertson WFJ (1964). Controlled trial of pyrimethamine in pregnant women in an African village. *Brit Med J* **i**: 667.

Nahlen BL, Akintunde A, Alakija T *et al.* (1989). Lack of efficacy of pyrimethamine prophylaxis in pregnant Nigerian women. *Lancet* **ii**: 830.

Navia BA, Petito CK, Gold JWM *et al.* (1986). Cerebral toxoplasmosis complicating the acquired immune deficiency syndrome: clinical and neuropathological findings in 27 patients. *Ann Neurol* **19**: 224.

Noel GE, Morisset R (1986). Malaria acquired with double chemical prophylaxis: chloroquine plus Fansidar. *Can Dis Weekly Rep* **12**: 105.

Oksenhendler E, Cadranel J, Sarafati *et al.* (1988). *Toxoplasma gondii* pneumonia in patients with acquired immunodeficiency syndrome. *Amer J Med* **88**: 18.

Opravil M, Keusch G, Luthy R (1993). Pyrimethamine inhibits renal secretion of creatinine. *Antimicrob Ag Chemother* **37**: 1056.

Opravil M, Hirschel B, Lazzarin A *et al.* (1995a). Once-weekly administration of dapsone/pyrimethamine vs aerosolized pentamidine as combined prophylaxis for *Pneumocystis carinii* pneumonia and toxoplasmic encephalitis in human immunodeficiency virus-infected patients. *Clin Infect Dis* **20**: 531.

Opravil M, Pechere M, Lazzarin A *et al.* (1995b). Dapsone/pyrimethamine may prevent mycobacterial disease in immunosuppressed patients infected with the human immunodeficiency virus. *Clin Infect Dis* **20**: 244.

Pape JW, Verdier RI, Johnson WJ (1989). Treatment and prophylaxis of *Isospora belli* infection in patients with the acquired immunodeficiency syndrome. *New Engl J Med* **320**: 1044.

Pearson RD, Hewlett EL (1987). Use of pyrimethamine-sulfadoxine (Fansidar). in prophylaxis against chloroquine-resistant *Plasmodium falciparum* and *Pneumocystis carinii*. *Ann Intern Med* **106**: 714.

Pedrol E, Gonzalez CJ, Gatell JM *et al.* (1990). Central nervous system toxoplasmosis in AIDS patients: efficacy of an intermittent maintenance therapy. *AIDS* **4**: 511.

Peterson DS, Milhous WK, Wellems TE (1990a). Molecular basis of differential resistance to cycloguanil and pyrimethamine in *Plasmodium falciparum* malaria. *Proc Natl Acad Sci USA* **87**: 3018.

Peterson E, Hugh B, Hanson AP, Bjorkman A, Flacks H (1990b). *In vitro* and *in vivo* susceptibility of *Plasmodium falciparum* isolates from Liberia to pyrimethamine, cycloguanil and chlorcycloguanil. *Ann Trop Med Parasitol* **84**: 563.

Peterson DS, Di SS, Povoa M *et al.* (1991). Prevalence of the dihydrofolate reductase Asn-108 mutation as the basis for pyrimethamine-resistant falciparum malaria in the Brazilian Amazon. *Amer J Trop Med Hyg* **45**: 492.

Phillips-Howard PA, West LJ (1990). Serious adverse drug reactions to pyrimethamine-sulfadoxine, pyrimethamine-dapsone and to amodiaquine in Britain. *J R Soc Med*; **83**: 82.

Piketty C, Derouin F, Rouveix B *et al.* (1990). *In vivo* assessment of antimicrobial agents against *Toxoplasma gondii* by quantification of parasites in the blood, lungs, and brain of infected mice. *Antimicrob Ag Chemother* **34**: 1467.

Podzamczer D, Martos A, Ferrer I *et al.* (1993a). Hepatic and pulmonary pneumocystosis during primary prophylaxis for *Pneumocystis carinii* pneumonia with dapsone/pyrimethamine. *Clin Infect Dis* **16**: 000.

Podzamczer D, Santin M, Jimenez J *et al.* (1993b). Thrice-weekly cotrimoxazole is better than weekly dapsone-pyrimethamine for the primary prevention of *Pneumocystis carinii* pneumonia in HIV-infected patients. *AIDS* **7**: 501.

Podzamczer D, Miro JM, Bolao F *et al.* (1995a). Twice-weekly maintenance therapy with sulfadiazine-pyrimethamine to prevent recurrent toxoplasmic encephalitis in patients with AIDS. Spanish Toxoplasmosis Study Group. *Ann Intern Med* **123**: 175.

Podzamczer D, Salazar A, Jimenez J *et al.* (1995b). Intermittent trimethoprim-sulfamethoxazole compared with dapsone-pyrimethamine for the simultaneous primary prophylaxis of *Pneumocystis* pneumonia and toxoplasmosis in patients infected with HIV. *Ann Intern Med* **122**: 755.

Pomeroy C, Felice GA (1992). Pulmonary toxoplasmosis: a review. *Clin Infect Dis* **14**: 863.

Queener SF (1991). Inhibition of *Pneumocystis dihydrofolate* reductase by analogs of pyrimethamine, methotrexate and trimetrexate. *J Protozool* **38**: 154S.

Remington JS, Desmonts G (1990). Toxoplasmosis. In *Infectious Diseases of the Fetus and Newborn Infants*, 3rd edn (Remington JS, Klein JD, eds), p. 89. Philadelphia: WB Saunders.

Remington JS, Vilde JL (1991). Clindamycin for toxoplasma encephalitis in AIDS. *Lancet* **338**: 1142.

Rolston KVI (1991). Treatment of acute toxoplasmosis with oral clindamycin. *Eur J Clin Microbiol Infect Dis* **10**: 181.

Romand S, Bryskier A, Moutot M, Derouin F (1995). *In-vitro* and *in-vivo* activities of roxithromycin in combination with pyrimethamine or sulphadiazine against *Toxoplasma gondii*. *J Antimicrob Chemother* **35**: 821.

Rudy AC, Poynor WJ (1990). Binding of pyrimethamine to human plasma proteins and erythrocytes. *Pharmaceut Res* **7**: 1055.

Ruf B, Pohle HD (1991). Role of clindamycin in the treatment of acute toxoplasmosis of the central nervous system. *Eur J Clin Microbiol Infect Dis* **10**: 183.

Ruf B, Schürmann D, Bergmann F *et al.* (1993). Efficacy of pyrimethamine/sulfadoxine in the prevention of toxoplasmic encephalitis relapses and *Pneumocystis carinii* pneumonia in HIV-infected patients. *Eur J Clin Microbiol Infect Dis* **12**: 325.

Sabcharoen A, Chongsuphajaisiddhi T, Attanath P *et al.* (1985). *In vitro* susceptibility of *Plasmodium falciparum* collected from pyrimethamine-sulfadoxine sensitive and resistant areas of Thailand. *Bull WHO* **63**: 597.

Sanford JP (1993). *Guide to Antimicrobial Therapy*. West Bethesda, USA: Antimicrobial Therapy Inc.

Schmidt LH, Hughes HB, Schmidt IG (1953). The pharmacological properties of 2,4-diamino-5-*p*-chlorophenyl-6-ethylpyrimidine (daraprim). *J Pharmacol Exp Ther* **107**: 92.

Schoondermark-van de Ven E, Vree T, Melchers W *et al.* (1995). *In vitro* effects of sulfadiazine and its metabolites alone and in combination with pyrimethamine on *Toxoplasma gondii*. *Antimicrob Ag Chemother* **39**: 763.

Sekas G, Paul HS (1993). Hyperammonemia and carnitine deficiency in a patient receiving sulfadiazine and pyrimethamine. *Amer J Med* **95**: 112.

Snewin VA, England SM, Sims PF, Hyde JE (1989). Characterisation of the dihydrofolate reductase-thymidylate synthetase gene from human malaria parasites highly resistant to pyrimethamine. *Gene* **76**: 41.

Stray-Pederson B (1992). Treatment of toxoplasmosis in the pregnant mother and newborn child. *Scand J Infect Dis* (Suppl 84): 23.

Symposium (1952). Symposium on Daraprim. *Trans Roy Soc Trop Med Hyg* **46**: 467.

Tanaka M, Gu HM, Bzik DJ, Li WB, Inselburg J (1990). Mutant dihydrofolate reductase-thymidylate synthase genes in pyrimethamine-resistant *Plasmodium falciparum* with polymorphic chromosome duplications. *Mol Biochem Parasitol* **42**: 83.

Thaithong S, Chan SW, Songsomboon S *et al.* (1992). Pyrimethamine resistant mutations in *Plasmodium falciparum*. *Mol Biochem Parasitol* **52**: 149.

Trier JS, Moxey PC, Schimmel EM, Robles E (1974). Chronic intestinal coccidiosis in man: intestinal morphology and response to treatment. *Gastroenterology* **66**: 923.

Tschirlard D, Klaft EC (1988). Disseminated toxoplasmosis in the acquired immunodeficiency syndrome. *Arch Pathol Lab Med* **112**: 1237.

Walzer, P D, Foy, J, Steele, P *et al.* (1992). Activities of antifolate, antiviral, and other drugs in an immunosuppressed rat model of *Pneumocystis carinii* pneumonia. *Antimicrob Ag Chemother* **36**: 1935.

Walzer, P D, Kim, C K, Foy, J M *et al.* (1988). Inhibitors of folic acid synthesis in the treatment of experimental *Pneumocystis carinii* pneumonia. *Antimicrob Ag Chemother* **32**: 96.

Watkins WM, Mosobo M (1993). Treatment of *Plasmodium falciparum* malaria with pyrimethamine-sufadoxine: selective pressure for resistance is a function of long elimination half-life. *Trans Roy Soc Trop Med Hyg* **87**: 75.

Weiss LM, Harris C, Berger M, Tanowitz HB, Wittner M (1988a). Pyrimethamine concentrations in serum and cerebrospinal fluid during treatment of acute *Toxoplasma* encephalitis in patients with AIDS. *J Infect Dis* **157**: 580.

Weiss LM, Perlman DC, Sherman J, Tanowitz H, Wittner M (1988b). *Isospora belli* infection: treatment with pyrimethamine. *Ann Intern Med* **109**: 474.

White NJ, Krishna S (1989). Treatment of malaria: some considerations and limitations of the current methods of assessment *Trans Roy Soc Trop Med Hyg* **83**: 767.

Wilson CB (1990a). Treatment of congenital toxoplasmosis during pregnancy. *J Pediatr* **116**: 1003.

Wilson CB (1990b). Treatment of congenital toxoplasmosis. *Pediatr Infect Dis J* **9**: 682.

Yeo AET, Rieckmann KN (1992). The activity *in vitro* of cycloguanil and pyrimethamine in combination against *Plasmodium falciparum*. *Trans Roy Soc Trop Med Hyg* **86**: 234.

Zolg JW, Plitt JR, Chen GX, Palmer S (1989). Point mutations in the dihydrofolate reductase-thymidylate synthase gene as the molecular basis for pyrimethamine resistance in *Plasmodium falciparum*. *Mol Biochem Parasitol* **36**: 253.

Zolg JW, Chen GX, Plitt JR (1990). Detection of pyrimethamine resistance in *Plasmodium falciparum* by mutation-specific polymerase chain reaction. *Mol Biochem Parasitol* **39**: 257.

Nitrofurans: Nitrofurazone, Furazolidone and Nitrofurantoin

Description

The nitroheterocyclic drugs consist of a primary nitro group joined to a heterocyclic ring. Three groups of these compounds are important in human therapeutics: the nitrothiazoles, nitroimidazoles and nitrofurans. The best known nitrothiazole is niridazole, which is used to treat bilharziasis; it has been used for amebiasis, dracontiasis and strongyloidiasis and is active against a variety of bacteria (Hamilton-Miller and Brumfitt, 1976; Hof et al., 1982). A number of nitroimidazole drugs are of clinical use such as metronidazole (p. 936). Interest was first evoked in the nitrofurans as chemotherapeutic agents in the early 1940s, and since then thousands of nitrofuran compounds have been synthesized (Chamberlain, 1976). The most widely used nitrofurans are nitrofurazone, furazolidone and nitrofurantoin.

1 Nitrofurazone

This is active *in vitro* against *Staphylococcus aureus*, *Streptococcus pyogenes*, *Escherichia coli* and the *Clostridium*, *Salmonella* and *Shigella* spp. It is less active against *Proteus* and *Serratia* spp. and virtually inactive against *Pseudomonas aeruginosa* (Chamberlain, 1976). Nitrofurazone has been mainly used for topical chemotherapy of wounds, burns, skin infections and for skin grafts. A cream and a soluble dressing containing 0.2% nitrofurazone are available commercially. This drug is absorbed from the skin and 1.13% of a daily dose applied to intact skin can be recovered in the urine (Chamberlain, 1976). Nitrofurazone has also been used as a bladder irrigant. Urinary catheters coated with a matrix containing nitrofurazone have been used in an attempt to prevent catheter-associated urinary tract infections (Johnson et al., 1993).

2 Furazolidone

This nitrofuran has *in vitro* activity against *Staph. aureus*, *Strep. pyogenes*, *Enterococcus faecalis*, *E. coli*, *Vibrio cholerae* and the *Clostridium*, *Klebsiella*, *Enterobacter*, *Salmonella*, *Shigella*, *Campylobacter* and *Bacteroides* spp. But the new *Vibrio cholerae* 0139 Bengal strain, which has caused a large epidemic since 1992 in the Indian subcontinent, is furazolidone-resistant (Waldor and Mekalanos, 1994). The drug is also active against trichomonads and *Giardia lamblia* (Chamberlain, 1976). Metronidazole-resistant strains of *Trimchomonas vaginalis* are furazolidone-sensitive (Narcisi and Secor, 1996). Furazolidone can be used for treatment of shigellosis and giardiasis and is available as 100 mg tablets and a suspension containing 25 mg per 5 ml. The dosage for adults is 100 mg four times daily, and appropriately lowered doses are recommended for children. For travelers' diarrhea treatment is given for 5 days, but a course of 7–10 days is required for giardiasis. Dupont et al. (1984) showed that furazolidone was more effective than ampicillin for travelers' diarrhea. They considered that, although co-trimoxazole (p. 860) was superior for treatment of shigellosis and perhaps severe diarrhea due to enterotoxigenic *E. coli* strains, furazolidone may also have a place to treat travelers' diarrhea because of its activity against *Campylobacter* spp. and *Giardia*. Furazolidone was therefore suggested for treatment of diarrhea in settings when laboratory diagnosis of the etiology was not feasible. Furazolidone can also be used for the treatment of cholera, provided that sensitive strains of *V. cholerae* are involved (Rabbani et al., 1991).

It appears that most of orally administered furazolidone is absorbed from the gastrointestinal tract. However, serum and urinary concentrations of the drug are low probably because most furazolidone is rapidly metabolized in tissues (Valadez-Salazar *et al.*, 1989). Side-effects include nausea, vomiting, headache, dizziness, drowsiness, drug fever, rashes and an 'Antabuse' (disulfiram)–like reaction to alcohol.

3 Nitrofurantoin

The sole use of this drug is for treatment of urinary tract infections, because after oral or i.v. administration, therapeutically active concentrations are attained only in urine. It has been available for clinical use in a crystalline form since 1953 and is marketed as 'Furadantin'. A macrocrystalline form has been developed (Hailey and Glascock, 1967), which may produce fewer gastrointestinal side-effects (p. 926), and is marketed with the trade name of 'Macrodantin'. More recently a modified release nitrofurantoin, which consists of 25% macrocrystalline nitrofurantoin and 75% nitrofurantoin monohydrate, has also been developed (nitrofurantoin MR). This is suitable for a twice-daily dosage regimen (Spencer *et al.*, 1994).

The following details only apply to nitrofurantoin.

Sensitive Organisms

1 Gram-negative bacteria

Nitrofurantoin is active against most Gram-negative bacilli, which commonly cause urinary tract infections. Most strains of *E. coli* are sensitive, but *Enterobacter* and *Klebsiella* spp. are less susceptible. Strains of *Proteus* and *Providencia* spp. vary in their sensitivity, but most are moderately resistant. The *Serratia* and *Acinetobacter* spp. and *Ps. aeruginosa* are usually resistant (Alon *et al.*, 1987, London *et al.*, 1993; Beunders, 1994; Thomson *et al.*, 1994).

Other Gram-negative bacteria, which usually do not cause urinary tract infections, such as the *Salmonella*, *Shigella* and *Neisseria* spp. and *Bacteroides fragilis* are also often susceptible to nitrofurantoin (Hamilton-Miller 1975). *Helicobacter pylori* is also sensitive (Simor *et al.*, 1989).

2 Gram-positive bacteria

Nitrofurantoin is active against those Gram-positive cocci which sometimes cause urinary tract infections such as *E. faecalis*, *E. faecium*, *Staph. aureus* and *Staph. epidermidis*. Vancomycin-resistant *E. faecium* strains (p. 765) are usually nitrofurantoin-sensitive (Norris *et al.*, 1995). *Staphylococcus saprophyticus*, an important cause of urinary tract infections in young women, is sensitive to nitrofurantoin (and ampicillin, cephalosporins, tetracyclines, sulfonamides and trimethoprim) but is resistant to nalidixic acid (Hovelius and Mårdh, 1984).

Gram-positive bacteria, such as *Strep. pyogenes*, *Strep. pneumoniae* and *Corynebacterium diphtheriae* are also quite sensitive. These organisms rarely, if ever, cause urinary tract infections and their susceptibility to nitrofurantoin is of little practical importance. Other *Corynebacterium* spp., *Rhodococcus equi* and *Listeria monocytogenes* are usually nitrofurantoin-resistant (Soriano *et al.*, 1995).

3 Acquired resistance

An important property of nitrofurantoin is that usually sensitive microorganisms do not readily become resistant to the drug. Although resistance can be induced *in vitro*, there has been little change in the resistance pattern of bacteria to nitrofurantoin over the years. Cross-resistance can occur between the nitrofurans but there is usually no cross-resistance between them and other chemotherapeutic agents (Alon *et al.*, 1987; London *et al.*, 1993; Beunders, 1994; Thompson *et al.*, 1994).

In 1983, Obaseiki-Ebor reported the isolation of *E. coli* strains in Nigeria which were resistant to aminoglycosides and nitrofurans (nitrofurazone and nitrofurantoin). They showed using laboratory mutants of *E. coli* resistant to aminoglycosides, that the clinical isolates of nitrofuran-resistant *E. coli* were not cross-resistant with aminoglycosides, reflecting differing methods of acquiring resistance in these two groups of antibiotics. Topical use of gentamicin, neomycin and nitrofurazone in Nigeria was probably responsible for the selection of these resistant mutants. Breeze and Obaseiki-Ebor (1983a) studied nitrofurantoin sensitivity of 150 clinical isolates of antibiotic resistant Gram-negative bacteria from patients with urinary tract infections in Edinburgh; 70% showed varying degrees of resistance to nitrofurantoin, 30% of resistant strains being *E. coli* and the remainder being *Klebsiella* or *Proteus* spp. Some of the *E. coli* strains carried plasmids which conferred resistance to nitrofurantoin and nitrofurazone. In some resistant strains, the total resistance was apparently due to a combination of chromosomal and plasmid-borne genes. A reduction in nitrofuran reductase activity was found in nitrofurantoin-resistant strains of *E. coli*, some with chromosomally determined resistance and others carrying plasmids (Breeze and Obaseiki-Ebor, 1983b). However, nitrofurantoin has multiple mechanisms of action on bacteria (p. 925), and this probably explains why emergence of resistance to this agent has been uncommon (McOsker and Fitzpatrick, 1994).

4 Minimum inhibitory concentrations

Bacterial species with an MIC of 32 µg per ml or less can be regarded as highly sensitive to nitrofurantoin. Nitrofurantoin urine concentrations of at least 100 µg per ml can be easily attained with usual therapeutic doses. If the causative enterobacteria are not sensitive to 32 µg per ml or less, the infection often persists or relapses shortly after cessation of treatment (Turck *et al.*, 1967). These authors found that 92% of *E. coli* strains were highly sensitive to the drug, but only 32% of other Gram-negative bacteria were in this category. The usual MIC of nitrofurantoin for *E. coli* is 16 µg per ml, while *Klebsiella aerogenes* is usually only inhibited by 100 µg per ml and *Proteus mirabilis* by 200 µg per ml. The MICs of nitrofurantoin for Gram-positive cocci are lower, being usually 4 µg per ml for *Staph. aureus* and 25 µg per ml for *E. faecalis* (Garrod *et al.*, 1973).

Activity of nitrofurantoin against all bacteria is increased in acid urine. Brumfitt and Percival (1967) demonstrated that the sensitivity of an *E. coli* strain decreased 20-fold when the pH changed from 5.0 to 8.0. Strains of *Pr. mirabilis* are less sensitive to nitrofurantoin than *E. coli* at any pH, and in addition *Proteus* spp. infections make the urine alkaline, further reducing the response of these infections to this drug.

Mode of Administration and Dosage

Nitrofurantoin is usually administered by mouth. Dosage is identical for the crystalline and the macrocrystalline preparations; for adults it is 200–400 mg per day, given in four divided doses, and for children 5–7 mg per kg body weight per day, given in four divided doses. The dosage of nitrofurantoin MR for adults is 100 mg 12-hourly (Spencer *et al.*, 1994).

Acute uncomplicated urinary tract infections due to *E. coli* usually respond well to the lower dose of 200 mg daily. For more severe, chronic or recurrent infections the higher dose of 400 mg daily is advisable, but this high dosage should not be continued for longer than 2 weeks.

For long-term suppressive therapy in adults a single daily dose of 50–100 mg (usually in the evening) is suitable (Brumfitt and Hamilton-Miller, 1995). A long-term prophylactic dosage of 2–4 mg per kg body weight daily has been recommended for children with chronic infections (Marshall and Johnson, 1959). The lower dose of 2 mg per kg body weight per day is advisable if treatment is continued for longer than 3 months.

Nitrofurantoin can be administered i.v. but this is rarely used, and the parenteral preparation is not generally available. A limited study to define clinical indications for i.v. nitrofurantoin was performed by Halliday and Jawetz (1962), who used it in doses of up to 720 mg daily in 10 patients with urinary tract infections. Nowadays, when parenteral treatment is necessary, other drugs are preferred. Intravenous nitrofurantoin is unsuitable for the treatment of systemic infections of any kind.

Availability

Nitrofurantoin ('Furadantin') tablets, each containing 50 or 100 mg.

Nitrofurantoin ('Furadantin') suspension, containing 25 mg per 5 ml.

Nitrofurantoin macrocrystals ('Macrodantin') capsules, each containing 50 or 100 mg.

Serum Levels in Relation to Dosage

Crystalline and macrocrystalline nitrofurantoin preparations are equally well absorbed from the gastrointestinal tract, absorption occurring primarily in the small intestine and is enhanced by food (D'Arcy, 1985). The macrocrystalline form dissolves more slowly and is thus absorbed at a slower rate (Hailey and Glascock, 1967). Despite good absorption, therapeutically active serum levels are not obtained after the usual doses of oral nitrofurantoin (Richards *et al.*, 1955). Its serum half-life in humans with normal renal function is only about 20 min, the drug being both rapidly broken down in the tissues and rapidly excreted in urine (Reckendorf *et al.*, 1962). Nitrofurantoin does not accumulate in the serum of patients with normal renal function if it is continuously administered in the recommended doses. Intravenously administered nitrofurantoin sodium in doses of up to 720 mg per day in adults does not produce therapeutically effective serum levels.

Nitrofurantoin accumulates in the serum of patients with impaired renal function. Loughridge (1962) detected serum levels ranging from 5.1 to 6.5 μg per ml in one patient with uremia (blood urea 300 mg% or 50 mmol per liter), who was receiving 300 mg of oral nitrofurantoin daily. The elevated serum level of nitrofurantoin in this uremic patient was associated with severe toxicity (p. 926). A mean serum level of only 1.8 μg per ml was demonstrated in 12 similarly treated patients with normal renal function. A mean peak serum level of 0.72 μg per ml was reached at 2 h in six healthy volunteers given a single oral dose of 100 mg (Männistö and Lamminsivu, 1982). Newborn and premature infants may also develop toxic serum levels and nitrofurantoin is contraindicated in this age group.

Excretion

1 Urine

Nitrofurantoin is rapidly excreted in urine, where about one-third of an orally or parenterally administered dose appears in a therapeutically active form (Reckendorf et al., 1962). With the usual doses, urine levels are 50–250 μg per ml, provided renal function is normal. There is no difference between excretion patterns of the crystalline and the macrocrystalline forms except that with the macrocrystalline form there is a slower rise of urinary concentrations (Hailey and Glascock, 1967).

Woodruff et al. (1961) studied urinary mechanisms of nitrofurantoin excretion in dogs. The drug is excreted by glomerular filtration, but a small part is also both secreted and reabsorbed by the tubules. Tubular reabsorption is enhanced by acid urine and depressed by alkalinization of urine, the latter yielding higher active nitrofurantoin urine concentrations. Urine acidification therefore increases renal tissue levels of the drug, which may be advantageous when treating pyelonephritis. On the other hand, although alkalinization of the urine increases urine nitrofurantoin concentrations, this is of doubtful value for the treatment of lower urinary tract infections such as cystitis, as the antibacterial effect of the drug is reduced in alkaline urine (Brumfitt and Percival, 1967).

Uremic patients excrete very little nitrofurantoin in the urine, where the levels attained are invariably therapeutically inadequate (Sachs et al., 1968).

2 Bile

Animal studies show that nitrofurantoin is eliminated via the bile, where concentrations about 200-fold higher than those in the serum have been detected. It was noted that nitrofurantoin administration resulted in an increased rate of bile flow (Annotation, 1971).

3 Inactivation in body

In patients with normal renal function a considerable proportion of a dose of nitrofurantoin is inactivated in the body. For this reason, even in patients with renal failure there is only a relatively minor rise in serum levels of the active drug, but these serum levels may cause severe toxicity (Kunin, 1968). Inactivation of nitrofurantoin apparently takes place in all body tissues, but the liver may play a major role. It is not known whether this drug accumulates in patients with liver disease.

Distribution of the Drug in Body

Therapeutically active concentrations of nitrofurantoin are not attained in most body tissues. Tissue levels in the renal medulla are usually about the same as those in the urine (Stamey et al., 1965). About 90% of the drug is bound to serum proteins (Männistö and Lamminsivu, 1982).

Mode of Action

The precise mode of action of nitrofurantoin is not known, but it has several mechanisms of action on bacteria and this may explain why bacterial-resistance to this drug is uncommon (p. 924). The drug inhibits a number of bacterial enzymes. It attacks bacterial ribosomal proteins and this causes complete inhibition of bacterial protein synthesis. Nitrofurantoin may also damage DNA (Chamberlain, 1976; McCalla, 1977; McOsker and Fitzpatrick, 1994).

Toxicity

Adverse reactions to nitrofurantoin have been the subject of a number of reviews. Holmberg *et al.* (1980) analyzed reports of side-effects in Sweden during the period 1966–1976, whilst Penn and Griffin (1982) examined similar reports in the UK and Holland for the periods 1964–1980 and 1975–1980, respectively. D'Arcy (1985) reviewed published reports of reactions and interactions of nitrofurantoin plus information submitted from throughout the world to the major manufacturer of nitrofurantoin, Norwich Eaton Pharmaceuticals in the USA. Using as a denominator for calculation the number of courses of therapy of nitrofurantoin used in the USA since 1953, he estimated the frequency of various nitrofurantoin side-effects (see below).

1 Gastrointestinal side-effects

Anorexia, nausea and vomiting are the most frequent side-effects of nitrofurantoin and are dose-related. They can often be controlled by reducing the dose, but concomitant administration of food or milk is less effective. Nausea and vomiting may sometimes be severe enough to necessitate cessation of treatment, and they occur more commonly in women (Koch-Weser *et al.*, 1971). By comparison, diarrhea is a rare side-effect. Nitrofurantoin induced nausea may result from the action of rapidly absorbed drug on the central nervous system, rather than from gastrointestinal irritation. Intravenously administered nitrofurantoin also causes this effect (Halliday and Jawetz, 1962). Antibiotic-associated diarrhea, caused by toxin producing *Cl. difficile*, has occurred after nitrofurantoin therapy (Hirschhorn *et al.*, 1994).

Some authors have shown that the macrocrystalline form, which is more slowly absorbed, evokes nausea and vomiting less frequently than crystalline nitrofurantoin in patients with a known history of nitrofurantoin intolerance (Hailey and Glascock, 1967). This was also demonstrated by Kalowski *et al.* (1974) in a double-blind study of patients whose past experience with nitrofurantoin was not known. It is possible that these symptoms are related to the rate of absorption of the drug, and thus the more slowly absorbed macrocrystalline form may be less prone to cause nausea and vomiting. Despite its slower rate of absorption macrocrystalline nitrofurantoin appears to be therapeutically equal in efficacy to the older crystalline drug (Hailey and Glascock, 1967; Kalowski *et al.*, 1974). Alternatively, other authors have found that administration of the macrocrystalline form does not prevent nausea, and consider that these symptoms are related more closely to the average serum level rather than to the rate of absorption of the drug (Koch-Weser *et al.*, 1971).

Similar to some other drugs, nitrofurantoin seems to be capable of inducing parotitis. There are several reports of parotitis and enlargement of other salivary glands, often associated with fever, leukocytosis and raised serum amylase values; the onset is often within hours of taking nitrofurantoin and most patients have been elderly (Meyboom *et al.*, 1982; Pellinen and Kalske, 1982; Penn and Griffin, 1982).

Nelis (1983) described an elderly woman who developed pancreatitis and associated jaundice after treatment with nitrofurantoin; her clinical disease recurred following challenge with a single dose of the drug. Another patient who developed acute pancreatitis during nitrofurantoin therapy has been described by Christophe (1994).

2 Hypersensitivity reactions

Compared with gastrointestinal side-effects these are relatively infrequent, and in one large series they were observed in 4.1% of treated patients (Koch-Weser *et al.*, 1971). Common manifestations included skin rashes, eosinophilia and drug fever, which usually subsided rapidly when the drug was stopped. Asthma due to sensitization to the drug has been observed. Anaphylaxis, angioneurotic edema and arthropathy can occur. Stevens–Johnson syndrome and toxic epidermal necrolysis have also been reported (Chan *et al.*, 1990). Allergic reactions comprised about 40% of all adverse reactions due to nitrofurantoin reported in the UK, Sweden and Holland (Penn and Griffin, 1982).

3 Neurotoxicity

A variety of central nervous system reactions have been reported. These include symptoms such as headache, dizziness, depression, confusion, drowsiness, slurred speech and abnormal vision (Penn and Griffin, 1982). Peripheral neuritis is one of the most serious side-effects of nitrofurantoin therapy, and it usually occurs in patients with renal failure who develop toxic serum levels of the drug (Loughridge, 1962). Six cases of nitrofurantoin neuropathy were reported by Ellis (1962). Three patients, in whom the drug was continued, died as a result of progressive polyneuritis, but the other three, in whom therapy was stopped soon after the onset of symptoms, made a slow partial recovery. Symptoms of nitrofurantoin peripheral neuritis usually begin within 45 days of starting treatment, and the clinical course is one of ascending motor and sensory polyneuropathy (Toole and Parrish, 1973). The degree of recovery is usually inversely related to the severity of the neuritis. This complication has also been reported in patients with normal blood urea levels, but who have had marginal renal functional impairment as evidenced by low creatinine clearance values (Craven, 1971). Neuritis may also develop in patients with normal renal function, especially in the elderly, if prolonged courses of nitrofurantoin are used. However, the development of neuritis does not show a consistent relationship to dosage or duration of treatment (Yiannikas et al., 1981). Changes in nerve conduction have been detected without clinical features of neuritis, after a 2-week course of 400 mg nitrofurantoin daily in healthy volunteers (Toole et al., 1968). Peripheral neuritis has comprised 2.2%-14.1% of all adverse reports in the UK, Sweden and Holland (Penn and Griffin, 1982). D'Arcy (1985) calculated the occurrence rate to be 0.0007%. Patients receiving nitrofurantoin should be warned to report early signs of neuritis such as paresthesiae, and in this event the drug should be stopped.

4 Pulmonary reactions

Pulmonary reactions comprised 2–5% of all adverse reactions reported in the UK, Sweden and Holland (Penn and Griffin, 1982) but they were calculated by D'Arcy (1985) to have an occurrence rate of 0.001%. Nitrofurantoin therapy has been associated with three types of pulmonary reaction:

a   Acute pneumonitis   First described in 1962 (Israel and Diamond, 1962), acute pneumonitis is more common in elderly patients, and is characterized by a sudden onset of cough, fever and dyspnea and may simulate acute respiratory infection or pulmonary edema (Hailey et al., 1969; Simonson et al., 1977; Jick et al., 1989; Bryant, 1992). Pulmonary infiltrations may be present on radiological examination of the lungs. Symptoms may become evident within hours or days after starting nitrofurantoin therapy, but in some cases these have only occurred after a prolonged period of treatment. This pneumonitis is probably allergic in nature, and is often accompanied by eosinophilia. Clinical recovery rapidly ensues when the drug is discontinued. However, corticosteroid treatment is beneficial and may be necessary in severe cases (Morgan, 1970). An accelerated and more severe pulmonary reaction typically occurs if the patient is rechallenged with the drug (Murray and Kronenberg, 1965; Murphy, 1966). Acute pneumonitis associated with nitrofurantoin treatment has also been described in a 7-year-old girl (Rantala et al., 1979).

b   Subacute pneumonitis   A subacute reaction was described in a patient who presented with pulmonary symptoms of 1 month duration having taken nitrofurantoin for 1 year (Sollaccio et al., 1966). This patient recovered rapidly when the drug was discontinued and prednisolone was administered. Since that report, many other patients with a subacute reaction have been reported (D'Arcy, 1985).

c   Chronic pulmonary reactions   Five patients described by Rosenow (1968) and another patient reported by Israel et al. (1973), all gradually developed a diffuse interstitial pneumonitis with fibrosis in association with long-term nitrofurantoin therapy. These changes were only partially reversible when the drug was discontinued and corticosteroids were given. In two patients reported by Bäck et al. (1974), long-term nitrofurantoin administration was associated not only with pulmonary fibrosis, but also liver damage and the presence of autoimmune antibodies in the serum. Bone et al. (1976) described another two patients who developed diffuse interstitial lung disease after long-term nitrofurantoin therapy, and who on open-lung biopsy had pathological changes typical of desquamative interstitial pneumonia. Both patients improved considerably with corticosteroid treatment.

There is now ample evidence that nitrofurantoin can cause chronic pulmonary disease characterized by interstitial fibrosis (Robinson, 1983; D'Arcy, 1985; Bryant, 1992). Robinson (1983) described four patients and reviewed the features of 45 other reported patients. All had received the drug for longer than 6 months; common presenting symptoms were dyspnea and a non-productive cough; a few patients had a history suggestive of acute pneumonitis after starting nitrofurantoin; the disease has been described in children but is most common in middle-aged and elderly women. Chest X-rays usually show bilateral patchy basal shadowing or diffuse reticular shadowing and pleural effusions sometimes occur. Various immunological abnormalities are commonly detected, such as circulating antinuclear antibody and elevated gamma globulin levels. Lung histology shows chronic interstitial inflammation and fibrosis. Continuation of nitrofurantoin has led to death, but some patients responded to corticosteroids when still receiving nitrofurantoin. Resolution of the disease usually occurs after ceasing nitrofurantoin therapy and the value of corticosteroids is not established. The mechanisms involved in this reaction seems to be immunological but different from the acute pneumonitis as eosinophilia does not occur. It is possible that nitrofurantoin may directly injure lung tissue through oxidant mechanisms (Boyd et al., 1979; Martin, 1983).

5 Hepatotoxicity

Both acute hepatocellular damage or cholestatic jaundice can on rare occasions be caused by nitrofurantoin administration (Westphal et al., 1994). Ernaelsteen and Williams (1961) reported a patient, who developed prodromal fever, rash and eosinophilia, followed by an intrahepatic obstructive jaundice (confirmed by liver biopsy) similar to chlorpromazine jaundice, in association with nitrofurantoin therapy. Subsequently, Murphy and Innis (1968) reported a 65-year-old patient, who developed a severe toxic hepatitis with jaundice and hemorrhagic manifestations after treatment with nitrofurantoin for 1 month. This patient recovered but required an exchange transfusion to control bleeding. A severe second attack of nitrofurantoin-induced hepatitis can occur as late as 17 years after the first episode (Paiva et al., 1992). Hepatitis caused by this drug occasionally can lead to liver failure necessitating liver transplantation (Mollison et al., 1992; Hebert and Roberts, 1993). Cholestatic hepatitis caused by nitofurantoin can occasionally also be very severe and fatal (Mulberg and Bell, 1993).

Nitrofurantoin, particularly after prolonged administration, may cause chronic active hepatitis (Westphal et al., 1994). In two patients described by Strömberg and Wengle (1976), clinical and biochemical recovery occurred on withdrawal of nitrofurantoin, without treatment with immunosuppressive drugs. Black et al. (1980) reported two other patients with a 'lupoid' form of chronic active hepatitis after prolonged therapy with nitrofurantoin, the features of which also abated after discontinuing the drug. Sharp et al. (1980) reported another five cases of chronic active hepatitis, including two deaths, associated with nitrofurantoin and reviewed 15 other published cases. All patients were women who had taken the drug for periods of 4 weeks to 11 years; most had a low serum albumin, an elevated gamma globulin and antinuclear antibodies. Eighteen patients improved when the drug was withdrawn and cirrhosis occurred in four.

Overall, the incidence of symptomatic nitrofurantoin-induced liver injury has been estimated to be approximately 0.02–0.035%. The liver injury is not due to direct toxicity, but it appears to have an allergic basis (Westphal et al., 1994).

6 Hematological side-effects

Three types of blood disorder have been reported in association with nitrofurantoin therapy. The calculated occurrence rate of these reactions is 0.0004% (D'Arcy, 1985).

a Hemolytic anemia Nitrofurantoin is one of many drugs which can precipitate acute hemolysis in patients with glucose-6-phosphate dehydrogenase deficient red blood cells (D'Arcy, 1985). The drug, therefore, should be used with caution in patients of Mediterranean origin, and it should be avoided in infants under 1 month old, whose red cell enzyme systems are immature. Nitrofurantoin apparently can also precipitate a hemolytic anemia in patients with erythrocytes deficient in other enzymes (D'Arcy, 1985). For instance, Stefanini (1972) described a patient with red blood cells deficient in the enzyme enolase and whose chronic hemolytic anemia was exacerbated by nitrofurantoin.

b Megaloblastic anemia Nitrofurantoin is chemically related to phenytoin, and similarly may cause, albeit rarely, a megaloblastic anemia due to folic acid deficiency, particularly when repeated courses are used (Bass, 1963).

c Bone marrow depression There have been a few reports of leukopenia, thrombocytopenia, agranulocytosis and aplastic anemia associated with nitrofurantoin therapy (D'Arcy, 1985).

7 Miscellaneous side-effects

Nitrofurantoin therapy has rarely been associated with the development of lupus erythematosis (Chapman, 1986). Nitrofurantoin crystalluria was reported in three elderly patients by MacDonald and MacDonald (1976). All of these had urinary catheters and were receiving long-term prophylaxis with nitrofurantoin against urinary infections. Their renal function and urinary output was normal and they were receiving the low recommended dosage. Crystalluria therefore seems to be a rare side-effect of the drug. Benign intracranial hypertension (p. 740) occurred in a 10-month-old child following nitrofurantoin therapy, suggesting a possible causal relationship (Sharma and James, 1974).

Although the nitrofurans, including nitrofurantoin are mutagenic toward mammalian cells by damaging DNA (McCalla, 1977), there is no evidence that they are carcinogenic in humans. Nitrofurantoin crosses the placenta to a very small extent but there is no evidence that it is teratogenic (D'Arcy, 1985).

8 Drug interactions

An 'Antabuse' (disulfiram) reaction to alcohol may be produced by nitrofurans and nitroimidazoles (p. 923) by inhibiting the metabolism of acetaldehyde (Birkett and Pond, 1975), but nitrofurantoin does not cause this reaction (D'Arcy, 1985). One case report suggested that nitrofurantoin caused lowering of the serum phenytoin level (D'Arcy, 1985).

Clinical Uses of the Drug

Nitrofurantoin is only suitable for treatment of urinary tract infections, particularly those caused by *E. coli* (Turck *et al.*, 1967). For uncomplicated acute urinary infections in young girls a 3-day course of nitrofurantoin macrocrystals is just as effective as a 10-day course of treatment (Lohr, 1981). The drug is useful for both acute uncomplicated infections and chronic bacteriuria where it is used as long-term suppressive therapy. For the treatment of acute infections trimethoprim/ sulfamethoxazole is somewhat superior to nitrofurantoin probably because it eliminates *E. coli* from the rectum, urethra and vagina (Hooton *et al.*, 1995). The use of nitrofurantoin for suppressive therapy has the advantage that it does not usually induce resistant strains in the urinary or intestinal tracts. The dose of this drug for suppressive therapy is 50–100 mg once each evening, and this has been highly successful in reducing recurrences of infection (Bailey *et al.*, 1971; Raz and Boger, 1991; Stamm *et al.*, 1991; Bailey, 1993; Brumfitt and Hamilton-Miller, 1995).

The drug can be used for both treatment and prophylaxis of urinary tract infections during pregnancy, because it has been widely used for over 40 years without being implicated as a cause of congenital abnormalities (Sandberg and Brorson, 1991; Pfau and Sacks, 1992; Bint and Hill, 1994; Reeves, 1994). It is also useful for these infections in children (Marshall and Johnson, 1959; Normand and Smellie, 1965). Nitrofurantoin is also suitable as prophylactic treatment of children with recurrent urinary tract infections and urinary tract abnormalities (Brendstrup *et al.*, 1990). This drug is contraindicated for premature babies and infants younger than 1 month (p. 925).

Nitrofurantoin is effective for the treatment of most infections localized to the urinary tract such as urethritis, cystitis and pyelonephritis. Although therapeutically active serum levels are not obtained, it is usually effective for renal infections, because renal medullary and urinary concentrations are almost identical (Stamey *et al.*, 1965). This use of nitrofurantoin in upper urinary tract infections has been questioned (Leading article, 1976, Naumann, 1978). If renal infection is associated with features suggesting a possible Gram-negative septicemia, other drugs such as the third-generation cephalosporins, aminoglycosides, quinolones or trimethoprim, which produce therapeutic serum levels, are indicated. Nitrofurantoin also may not be effective in patients with upper urinary tract infections in whom one kidney has poor function. In such cases, even though overall renal function may be normal, effective concentrations of the drug may not be reached in the urine of kidneys with a unilateral creatinine clearance of less than 20 ml per min. On these grounds nitrofurantoin should be restricted to treatment of lower urinary tract infections in patients with normal renal function (Leading article, 1976). Nitrofurantoin is unsuitable for the treatment of systemic infections such as *E. coli* septicemia.

This drug can be used to treat urinary tract infections caused by Gram-positive cocci such as *E. faecalis*, *Staph. aureus* and *Staph. epidermidis* (McDonald and Lohr, 1994). Other drugs which produce therapeutic serum levels are usually preferred for these infections, particularly for those due to *Staph. aureus*, the presence of which in the urine often reflects disseminated infection.

Nitrofurantoin has been recommended for prophylactic purposes during urinary tract catheterization, other instrumentation and prostatectomy (Johnson *et al.*, 1994). This would be ineffective if *Ps. aeruginosa* or strains of *Proteus* or *Klebsiella* spp. resistant to nitrofurantoin, are introduced. This has been shown to be so with both nitrofurantoin and methenamine hippurate (p. 934).

Nitrofurantoin is contraindicated in all patients with any degree of renal functional impairment (Sachs *et al.*, 1968), because in this situation therapeutic concentrations are not attained in urine, and toxic serum levels may occur (p. 925).

References

Alon U, Davidai G, Berant M, Merzbach D (1987). Five-year survey of changing patterns of susceptibility of bacterial uropathogens to trimethoprim-sulfamethoxazole and other antimicrobial agents. *Antimicrob Ag Chemother* **31**: 126.

Annotation (1971). Nitrofurantoin. *Lancet* **ii**: 1129.

Bäck O, Lundgren R, Wiman L-G (1974). Nitrofurantoin-induced pulmonary fibrosis and lupus syndrome. *Lancet* **i**: 930.

Bailey RR (1993). Management of lower urinary tract infections. *Drugs* **45** (Suppl 3): 139.

Bailey RR, Roberts AP, Gower PE, De Wardener HE (1971). Prevention of urinary tract infection with low-dose nitrofurantoin. *Lancet* **ii**: 1112.

Bass BH (1963). Megaloblastic anaemia due to nitrofurantoin. *Lancet* **i**: 530.

Beunders AJ (1994). Development of antibacterial resistance: the Dutch experience. *J Antimicrob Chemother* **33** (Suppl A): 17.

Bhagwat AG, Warren RE (1969). Hepatic reaction to nitrofurantoin. *Lancet* **ii**: 1369.

Bint AJ, Hill D (1994). Bacteriuria of pregnancy–an update on significance, diagnosis and management. *J Antimicrob Chemother* **33** (Suppl A): 93.

Birkett DJ, Pond SM (1975). Metabolic drug interactions – a critical review. *Med J Aust* **1**: 687.

Black M, Rabin L, Schatz N (1980). Nitrofurantoin-induced chronic active hepatitis. *Ann Intern Med* **92**: 62.

Bone RC, Wolfe J, Sobonya RE *et al.* (1976). Desquamative interstitial pneumonia following long-term nitrofurantoin therapy. *Amer J Med* **60**: 697.

Boyd MR, Catignani GL, Sasame HA *et al.* (1979). Acute pulmonary injury in rats by nitrofurantoin and modification by vitamin E, dietary fat, and oxygen. *Amer Rev Respir Dis* **120**: 93.

Breeze AS, Obaseiki-Ebor EE (1983a). Transferable nitrofuran resistance conferred by R-plasmids in clinical isolates of *Escherichia coli*. *J Antimicrob Chemother* **12**: 459.

Breeze AS, Obaseiki-Ebor EE (1983b). Nitrofuran reductase activity in nitrofurantoin-resistant strains of *Escherichia coli* K12: some with chromosomally determined resistance and others carrying R-plasmids. *J Antimicrob Chemother* **12**: 543.

Brendstrup L, Hjelt K, Petersen KE *et al.* (1990). Nitrofurantoin versus trimethoprim prophylaxis in recurrent urinary tract infection in children. A randomized, double-blind study. *Acta Paediatr Scand* **79**: 1225.

Brumfitt W, Hamilton-Miller JM (1995). A comparative trial of low dose cefaclor and macrocrystalline nitrofurantoin in the prevention of recurrent urinary tract infection. *Infection* **23**: 98.

Brumfitt W, Percival A (1967). Laboratory control of antibiotic therapy in urinary tract infection. *Ann NY Acad Sci* **145**: 329.

Bryant DH (1992). Drug-induced pulmonary disease. *Med J Aust* **156**: 802.

Chamberlain RE (1976). Chemotherapeutic properties of prominent nitrofurans. *J Antimicrob Chemother* **2**: 325.

Chan HL, Stern RS, Arndt KA *et al.* (1990). The incidence of erythema multiforme, Stevens–Johnson syndrome, and toxic epidermal necrolysis. A population-based study with particular reference to reactions caused by drugs among outpatients. *Arch Dermatol* **126**: 43.

Chapman JA (1986). An unusual nitrofurantoin-induced drug reaction. *Ann Allergy* **56**: 16.

Christophe JL (1994). Pancreatitis induced by nitrofurantoin. *Gut* **35**: 712.

Craven RS (1971). Furadantin neuropathy. *Aust NZ J Med* **1**: 246.

D'Arcy PF (1985). Nitrofurantoin. *Drug Intell Clin Pharm* **19**: 540.

DuPont HL, Ericsson CD, Galindo E *et al.* (1984). Furazolidone versus ampicillin in the treatment of traveler's diarrhea. *Antimicrob Ag Chemother* **26**: 160.

Ellis FG (1962). Acute polyneuritis after nitrofurantoin therapy. *Lancet* **ii**: 1136.

Ernaelsteen D, Williams R (1961). Jaundice due to nitrofurantoin. *Gastroenterology* **41**: 590.

Garrod LP, Lambert HP, O'Grady F (1973). *Antibiotic and Chemotherapy* 4th edn, p. 405. Edinburgh and London: Churchill Livingstone.

Hailey FJ, Glascock HW Jr (1967). Gastrointestinal tolerance to a new macrocrystalline form of nitrofurantoin: a collaborative study. *Curr Ther Res* **9**: 600.

Hailey FJ, Glascock HW Jr, Hewitt WF (1969). Pleuropneumonic reactions to nitrofurantoin. *New Engl J Med* **281**: 1087.

Halliday A, Jawetz E (1962). Sodium nitrofurantoin administered intravenously: a limited study to define its clinical indication. *New Engl J Med* **266**: 427.

Hamilton-Miller JMT (1975). Antimicrobial agents acting against anaerobes. *J Antimicrob Chemother* **1**: 273.

Hamilton-Miller JMT, Brumfitt W (1976). Leading article. The versatility of nitro compounds. *J Antimicrob Chemother* **2**: 5.

Hebert MF, Roberts JP (1993). Endstage liver disease associated with nitrofurantoin requiring liver transplantation. *Ann Pharmacother* **27**: 1193.

Hirschhorn LR, Trnka Y, Onderdonk A *et al.* (1994). Epidemiology of community-acquired *Clostridium difficile*-associated diarrhea. *J Infect Dis* **169**: 127.

Hof H, Sticht-Groh V, Müller K-L (1982). Comparative *in vitro* activities of niridazole and metronidazole against anaerobic and microaerophilic bacteria. *Antimicrob Ag Chemother* **22**: 332.

Holmberg L, Boman G, Böttiger LE *et al.* (1980). Adverse reactions to nitrofurantoin. Analysis of 921 Reports. *Amer J Med* **69**: 733.

Hooton TM, Winter C, Tiu F, Stamm WE (1995). Randomized comparative trial and cost analysis of 3-day antimicrobial regimens for treatment of acute cystitis in women. *JAMA* **273**: 41.

Hovelius B, Mårdh P-A (1984). Staphylococcus saprophyticus as a common cause of urinary tract infections. *Rev Infect Dis* **6**: 328.

Israel HL, Diamond P (1962). Recurrent pulmonary infiltration and pleural effusion due to nitrofurantoin sensitivity. *New Engl J Med* **266**: 1024.

Israel KS, Brashear RE, Sharma HM *et al.* (1973). Pulmonary fibrosis and nitrofurantoin. *Amer Rev Resp Dis* **108**: 353.

Jick SS, Jick H, Walker AM, Hunter JR (1989). Hospitalizations for pulmonary reactions following nitrofurantoin use. *Chest* **96**: 512.

Johnson HW, Anderson JD, Chambers GK *et al.* (1994). A short-term study of nitrofurantoin prophylaxis in children managed with clean intermittent catheterization. *Pediatrics* **93**: 752.

Johnson JR, Berggren T, Conway AJ (1993). Activity of nitrofurazone matrix urinary catheter against catheter-associated uropathogens. *Antimicrob Ag Chemother* **37**: 2033.

Kalowski S, Radford N, Kincaid-Smith P (1974). Crystalline and macrocrystalline nitrofurantoin in the treatment of urinary-tract infection. *New Engl J Med* **290**: 385.

Koch-Weser J, Sidel VW, Dexter M *et al.* (1971). Adverse reactions to sulfisoxazole, sulfamethoxazole, and nitrofurantoin. *Arch Intern Med* **128**: 399.

Kunin CM (1968). More on antimicrobials in renal failure. *Ann Intern Med* **69**: 397.

Leading Article (1976). Antibiotic treatment in kidneys of unequal function. *Brit Med J* **1**: 4.

Lohr JA, Hayden GF, Kesler RW *et al.* (1981). Three-day therapy of lower urinary tract infections with nitrofurantoin macrocrystals: a randomized clinical trial. *J Pediatr* **99**: 980.

London N, Nijsten R, v.d. Bogaard A, Stobberingh E (1993). Antibiotic resistance of faecal Enterobacteriaceae isolated from healthy volunteers, a 15-week follow-up study. *J Antimicrob Chemother* **32**: 83.

Loughridge L (1962). Peripheral neuropathy due to nitrofurantoin. *Lancet* **ii**: 1133.

Macdonald JB, Macdonald ET (1976). Nitrofurantoin crystalluria. *Brit Med J* **2**: 1044.

Männistö PT, Lamminsivu U (1982). Nitrofurantoin is highly bound to plasma protein. *J Antimicrob Chemother* **9**: 327.

Marshall M, Johnson SH (1959). Use of nitrofurantoin in chronic and recurrent urinary tract infections in children. *JAMA* **169**: 919.

Martin WJ II (1983). Nitrofurantoin: evidence for the oxidant injury of lung parenchymal cells. *Amer Rev Respir Dis* **127**: 482.

McCalla DR (1977). Biological effects of nitrofurans. *J Antimicrob Chemother* **3**: 517.

McDonald JA, Lohr JA (1994). *Staphylococcus epidermidis* pyelonephritis in a previously healthy child. *Pediatr Infect Dis J* **13**: 1155.

McOsker CC, Fitzpatrick PM (1994). Nitrofurantoin: mechanism of action and implications for resistance development in common uropathogens. *J Antimicrob Chemother* **33** (Suppl A): 23.

Meyboom RHB, Van Gent A, Zinkstok DJ (1982). Nitrofurantoin-induced parotitis. *Brit Med J* **285**: 1049.

Mollison LC, Angus P, Richards M *et al.* (1992). Hepatitis due to nitrofurantoin. *Med J Aust* **156**: 347.

Morgan LK (1970). Nitrofurantoin pulmonary hypersensitivity. *Med J Aust* **2**: 136.

Mulberg AE, Bell LM (1993). Fatal cholestatic hepatitis and multisystem failure associated with nitrofurantoin. *J Pediatr Gastroenterol Nutr* **17**: 307.

Murphy KJ (1966). Pulmonary reaction to nitrofurantoin ('furadantin'). *Med J Aust* **2**: 607.

Murphy KJ, Innis MD (1968). Hepatic disorder and severe bleeding diathesis following nitrofurantoin ingestion. *JAMA* **204**: 396.

Murray MJ, Kronenberg R (1965). Pulmonary reactions simulating cardiac pulmonary edema caused by nitrofurantoin. *New Engl J Med* **273**: 1185.

Narcisi EM, Secor WE (1996). *In vitro* effect of tinidazole and furazolidone on metronidazole-resistant *Trichomonas vaginalis*. *Antimicrob Ag Chemother* **40**: 1121.

Naumann P (1978). The value of antibiotic levels in tissue and in urine in the treatment of urinary tract infections. *J Antimicrob Chemother* **4**: 9.

Nelis GF (1983). Nitrofurantoin-induced pancreatitis: report of a case. *Gastroenterology* **84**: 1032.

Normand ICS, Smellie JM (1965). Prolonged maintenance chemotherapy in the management of urinary infection in childhood. *Brit Med J* **1**: 1023.

Norris AH, Reilly JP, Edelstein PH *et al.* (1995). Chloramphenicol for the treatment of vancomycin-resistant enterococcal infections. *Clin Infect Dis* **20**: 1137.

Obaseiki-Ebor EE (1983). Cross-resistance to nitrofurans of aminoglycoside-aminocyclitol resistant strains of *Escherichia coli*. *J Antimicrob Chemother* **11**: 485.

Paiva LA, Wright PJ, Koff RS (1992). Long-term hepatic memory for hypersensitivity to nitrofurantoin. *Amer J Gastroenterol* **87**: 891.

Pellinen TJ, Kalske J (1982). Nitrofurantoin-induced parotitis. *Brit Med J* **285**: 344.

Penn RG, Griffin JP (1982). Adverse reactions to nitrofurantoin in the United Kingdom, Sweden, and Holland. *Brit Med J* **284**: 1440.

Pfau A, Sacks TG (1992). Effective prophylaxis for recurrent urinary tract infections during pregnancy. *Clin Infect Dis* **14**: 810.

Rabbani GH, Buttler T, Shahrier M *et al.* (1991). Efficacy of a single dose of furazolidone for treatment of cholera in children. *Antimicrob Ag Chemother* **35**: 1864.

Rantala H, Kirvelä O, Anttolainen I (1979). Nitrofurantoin lung in a child. *Lancet* **ii**: 799.

Raz R, Boger S (1991). Long-term prophylaxis with norfloxacin versus nitrofurantoin in women with recurrent urinary tract infection. *Antimicrob Ag Chemother* **35**: 1241.

Reckendorf HK, Castringius RG, Spingler HK (1962). Comparative pharmacodynamcis, urinary excretion and half-life determinations of nitrofurantoin sodium. *Antimicrob Ag Chemother*: 531.

Reeves DS (1994). A perspective on the safety of antibacterials used to treat urinary tract infections. *J Antimicrob Chemother* **33** (Suppl A): 111.

Richards WA, Riss E, Kass EH, Finland M (1955). Nitrofurantoin: clinical and laboratory studies in urinary tract infections. *Arch Intern Med* **96**: 437.

Robinson BWS (1983). Nitrofurantoin-induced interstitial pulmonary fibrosis. Presentation and outcome. *Med J Aust* **1**: 72.

Rosenow EC, De Remee RA, Dines DE (1968). Chronic nitrofurantoin pulmonary reaction. Report of five cases. *New Engl J Med* **279**: 1258.

Sachs J, Geer T, Noell P, Kunin CM (1968). Effect of renal function on urinary recovery of orally administered nitrofurantoin. *New Engl J Med* **278**: 1032.

Sandberg T, Brorson JE (1991). Efficacy of long-term antimicrobial prophylaxis after acute pyelonephritis in pregnancy. *Scand J Infect Dis* **23**: 221.

Sharma DB, James A (1974). Benign intracranial hypertension associated with nitrofurantoin therapy. *Brit Med J* **4**: 771.

Sharp JR, Ishak KG, Zimmerman HJ (1980). Chronic active hepatitis and severe hepatic necrosis associated with nitrofurantoin. *Ann Intern Med* **92**: 14.

Simonson W, Stennett DJ, Hall CA (1977). Nitrofurantoin pneumonitis. *Drug Intel Clin Pharm* **2**: 654.

Simor AE, Ferro S, Low DE (1989). Comparative *in vitro* activities of six new fluoroquinolones and other oral antimicrobial agents against *Campylobacter pylori*. *Antimicrob Ag Chemother* **33**: 108.

Sollaccio PA, Ribaudo CA, Grace WJ (1966). Subacute pulmonary infiltration due to nitrofurantoin. *Ann Intern Med* **65**: 1284.

Soriano F, Zapardiel J, Nieto E (1995). Antimicrobial susceptibilities of *Corynebacterium* species and other non- spore-forming gram-positive bacilli to 18 antimicrobial agents. *Antimicrob Ag Chemother* **39**: 208.

Spencer RC, Moseley DJ, Greensmith MJ (1994). Nitrofurantoin modified release versus trimethoprim or co-trimoxazole in the treatment of uncomplicated urinary tract infection in general practice. *J Antimicrob Chemother* **33** (Suppl A): 121.

Stamey TA, Govan DE, Palmer JM (1965). The localisation and treatment of urinary tract infections: the role of bactericidal urine levels as opposed to serum levels. *Medicine* **44**: 1.

Stamm WE, McKevitt M, Roberts PL, White NJ (1991). Natural history of recurrent urinary tract infections in women. *Rev Infect Dis* **13**: 77.

Stefanini M (1972). Chronic hemolytic anemia association with erythrocyte enolase deficiency exacerbated by ingestion of nitrofurantoin. *Amer J Clin Path* **58**: 408.

Strömberg A, Wengle B (1976). Chronic active hepatitis induced by nitrofurantoin. *Brit Med J* **2**: 174.

Thomson KS, Sanders WE, Sanders CC (1994). USA resistance patterns among UTI pathogens. *J Antimicrob Chemother* **33** (Suppl A): 9.

Toole JF, Parrish ML (1973). Nitrofurantoin polyneuropathy. *Neurology* **23**: 554.

Toole JF, Gergen JA, Hayes DM, Felts JH (1968). Neural effects of nitrofurantoin. *Arch Neurol* **18**: 680.

Turck M, Ronald AR, Petersdorf RG (1967). Susceptibility of Enterobacteriaceae to nitrofurantoin correlated with eradication of bacteriuria. *Antimicrob Ag Chemother* **1996**: 446.

Valadez-Salazar A, Guiscafre-Gallardo H, Sanchez-Garcia S, Múnoz O (1989). Detection of furazolidone in human biological fluids by high performance liquid chromatography. *J Antimicrob Chemother* **23**: 589.

Walder MK, Mekalanos JJ (1994). Emergence of new cholera pandemic: molecular analysis of virulence determinants in *Vibrio cholerae* 0139 and development of live vaccine prototype. *J Infect Dis* **170**: 278.

Westphal JF, Vetter D, Brogard JM (1994). Hepatic side-effects of antibiotics. *J Antimicrob Chemother* **33**: 387.

Woodruff MW, Malvin RL, Thompson IM (1961). The renal transport of nitrofurantoin. Effect of acid-base balance upon its excretion. *JAMA* **175**: 1132.

Yiannikas C, Pollard JD, McLeod JG (1981). Nitrofurantoin neuropathy. *Aust NZ J Med* **11**: 400.

Methenamine Mandelate and Methenamine Hippurate

Description

1 Methenamine (hexamine, hexamethylenetetramine or urotropin)

This drug was introduced into clinical use as a urinary antiseptic as long ago as 1894. The antiseptic action of this cyclic hydrocarbon depends on its hydrolysis to formaldehyde and ammonia. This process takes place in the urine and it only occurs to a significant degree when the urine is acid. *In vitro* studies suggest that an effective bacteriostatic concentration of formaldehyde is likely to be achieved if the urine pH is less than 5.7–5.85 when recommended doses are used (Musher and Griffith, 1974). The drug is thereby entirely dependent for its effect on proper acidification of the urine (Kass, 1955). Formaldehyde is not released while methenamine circulates in the blood.

2 Mandelic acid

Mandelic acid, which was introduced into clinical use by Rosenheim (1935), is another urinary antiseptic which is excreted unchanged in the urine. Although it is promoted as being antibacterial and making urine more acid, it and hippuric acid have only a minimal bacteriostatic effect *in vitro*, and in the doses used there is no evidence that either agent significantly lowers urine pH (Musher and Griffith, 1974; Vainrub and Musher, 1977).

3 Methenamine mandelate and methenamine hippurate

These two drugs are chemical combinations of methenamine with mandelic acid and hippuric acid, respectively. It has been claimed that methenamine hippurate is effective in lower doses than methenamine mandelate and that additional urinary acidification is unnecessary (Gibson, 1970), but the latter has been refuted.

In Australia, methenamine (hexamine) mandelate and methenamine hippurate is available as 'Hexamine', but elsewhere methenamine is available under numerous trade names including 'Mandelamine' (Park-Davis).

Sensitive Organisms

As the antibacterial activity in the urine, produced by these compounds, is due to liberated formaldehyde (to which all microorganisms are susceptible), both methenamine mandelate and hippurate are active against all Gram-positive and Gram-negative bacteria and also against fungi. Urinary tract infections due to urea-splitting organisms, such as *Proteus* spp., will not respond to these agents, because the urine cannot be acidified in the presence of these infections, and therefore formaldehyde is not liberated. The use of acetohydroxamic acid, a urease inhibitor, together with methenamine, has been suggested for the treatment of urinary infections by *Proteus* spp. (Musher *et al.*, 1976). Acquired resistance is not a problem with these compounds because bacteria and fungi do not become resistant to formaldehyde.

Mode of Administration and Dosage

These drugs are administered by the oral route. Enteric-coated tablets are usually used to ensure that formaldehyde is not liberated in the acid-containing stomach.

1 Methenamine mandelate

The dosage for adults is 1.0 g four times daily, and a total daily dose of 6.0 g should not be exceeded. For children aged 6–12 years the dosage is 500 mg four times daily. When methenamine mandelate is used, the urine pH should be ascertained from time to time, and if it is higher than 5.5, additional acidifying agents are recommended. Either ammonium chloride, ascorbic acid or methionine can be used in a dose of 3–6 g daily, but sometimes even higher doses have been used. For instance, Zangwill *et al.* (1962) used doses as high as 8–18g methionine daily for adults, but such doses may cause central nervous system and gastrointestinal disturbances. Some authors, therefore, have preferred ascorbic acid as an acidifying agent (Holland and West, 1963). However, Vainrub and Musher (1977) could not demonstrate any acidification when ascorbic acid was used in a dose of 4.0 g daily. They considered that even if urine acidification were achieved, it would be short-lived, because of renal buffering mechanisms, and a lasting effect on urine pH would only result from doses that produce metabolic acidosis. Excessive fluid intake should be avoided when methenamine mandelate (or hippurate) is used, to prevent dilution of methenamine in the urine and to reduce frequency of micturition, thereby increasing the duration of exposure of bacteria to formaldehyde in the urine.

2 Methenamine hippurate

The usual adult dosage is 1.0 g twice-daily, and for children aged 6–12 years it is 500 mg twice-daily.

3 Patients with renal failure

In these patients, urinary excretion of methenamine salts is impaired, so that these drugs are usually contraindicated. In mild cases of renal functional impairment, it may be possible to use either of the methenamine salts in reduced doses, but with more severe renal failure, toxic serum levels and inadequate urine concentrations result. The additional acid load due to these drugs may be particularly dangerous in uremia (US Public Health, 1968).

Absorption and Excretion

Methenamine mandelate and hippurate are both rapidly absorbed from the gastrointestinal tract (Knight *et al.*, 1952; Gibson, 1970). Antimicrobial activity is not achieved in the blood, as the methenamine moiety does not liberate formaldehyde in serum and mandelic or hippuric acid serum levels are too low to exert any antibacterial effect. Methenamine is rapidly excreted in urine, where some antibacterial activity is demonstrable within 30 min of administration. Pharmacokinetics of methenamine hippurate have been studied in adult volunteers after a single oral dose of 1 g and thereafter twice-daily (Klinge *et al.*, 1982). The mean peak serum level of 35.2 μg per ml was achieved in about 1 h and after 12 h this level had fallen to 4.3 μg per ml; there was no accumulation with repeated doses. The elimination half-life was about 4.3 h. After a single dose, about 82% of the drug is recovered in the urine in 24 h and after continuous twice-daily administration approximately 88% of the dose is excreted within a 12 h dosing interval. Renal clearance is close to creatinine clearance and there is little extrarenal clearance. Urinary concentrations of methenamine hippurate remained above 150 μg per ml, but the pH was not continuously maintained at a level considered low enough to produce sufficient amounts of free formaldehyde.

About 20% of methenamine excreted in the urine is converted to formaldehyde, provided the urine pH is 5.0. At urinary pH levels higher than this, the proportion of formaldehyde liberated is less. Even in an acid medium (pH 5–6), it takes 30–90min to generate inhibitory concentrations of formaldehyde.

The mandelic or hippuric acid moieties are also rapidly excreted in the urine in active unchanged forms by both glomerular filtration and tubular secretion.

Toxicity

Both methenamine salts are generally well tolerated, but some patients develop gastrointestinal side-effects such as nausea, vomiting and diarrhea. High doses or prolonged administration may lead to urinary tract irritation due to liberated formaldehyde. This may result in frequency, dysuria, albuminuria and hematuria. One patient developed generalized edema, urticaria and dyspnea, which appeared to be a reaction to methenamine mandelate (US Public Health, 1968). No evidence of bone marrow depression, liver damage or peripheral neuritis has been observed when these drugs have been used in the recommended doses (Gibson, 1970). The methenamine salts should be avoided in patients with gout, because these drugs may precipitate urate crystals in their urine (US Public Health, 1968). Phototoxicity to methenamine hippurate has been described (Selvaag and Thune, 1994).

Clinical Uses of the Drug

Methenamine mandelate or methenamine hippurate are only suitable for treatment of urinary tract infections. They are rarely used because many other chemotherapeutic agents are available. In addition, the use of drugs such as methenamine, nalidixic acid (p. 975) and nitrofurantoin (p. 929), which produce negligible therapeutic tissue levels, is questionable in anything other than uncomplicated lower urinary tract infections. Because of the time taken to produce antibacterial concentrations of formaldehyde in urine (p. 933), methenamine would not be expected to be effective in upper urinary tract infections.

These drugs may still have a role in chronic bacteriuria, particularly if the infection is caused by highly resistant Gram-negative bacilli or by yeasts, because all such pathogens are susceptible to formaldehyde. Methenamine mandelate has been used successfully for prolonged suppressive therapy (Zangwill et al., 1962; Holland and West, 1963; US Public Health, 1968). The usually recommended doses are used for long-term therapy. Nevertheless, when used as long-term therapy in chronic bacteriuria in men, methenamine mandelate is less successful if underlying genitourinary pathology is present (Freeman et al., 1975). Methenamine hippurate is not as effective as co-trimoxazole (p. 861) or trimethoprim in preventing recurrent urinary tract infections in patients with underlying abnormalities of the urinary tract (Kalowski et al., 1975). Vainrub and Musher (1977) investigated the effect of methenamine mandelate (and ascorbic acid) on bacteriuria in paraplegic and quadraplegic patients. It was of no value in preventing infection in patients with indwelling catheters (to be expected in view of the short duration of the drug in the urine), and in those receiving intermittent catheterization. Similarly, when either methenamine hippurate or nitrofurantoin was given prophylactically to elderly patients at the beginning of long-term catheterization, bacteriuria was only delayed (Kostiala et al., 1982). In patients with bladder neck obstruction and urinary tract infection, treatment prior to and after transuretheral prostatectomy with cefazolin/cephalexin is superior to that by methenamine hippurate (Schönebeck et al., 1980). Even the prophylactic use of methenamine in women with recurrent urinary infeetions without underlying urinary traet abnormalities is in doubt; co-trimoxazole seems to have distinct advantages in this situation (p. 861). It appears that there are very few indications for the use of methenamine and its derivatives.

Reference

Freeman RB, McFate Smith W, Richardson JA et al. (1975). Long-term therapy for chronic bacteriuria in men. US Public Health Service Cooperative Study. Ann Intern Med 83: 133.

Gibson GR (1970). A clinical appraisal of methenamine hippurate in urinary tract infections. Med J Aust 1: 167.

Holland NH, West CD (1963). Prevention of recurrent urinary tract infections in girls. Amer J Dis Child 105: 560.

Kalowski S, Nanra RS, Friedman A et al. (1975). Controlled trial comparing cotrimoxazole and methenamine hippurate in the prevention of recurrent urinary tract infections. Med J Aust 1: 585.

Kass EH (1955). Chemotherapeutic and antibiotic drugs in the management of infections of the urinary tract. Amer J Med 18: 764.

Klinge E, Männistö P, Mäntylä R et al. (1982). Pharmacokinetics of methenamine in healthy volunteers. J Antimicrob Chemother 9: 209.

Knight V, Draper JW, Brady EA, Attmore CA (1952). Methenamine mandelate: antimicrobial activity, absorption and excretion. Antibiot Chemother 2: 615.

Kostiala AAI, Nyrén P, Runeberg L (1982). Effect of nitrofurantoin and methenamine hippurate prophylaxis on bacteria and yeasts in the urine of patients with an indwelling catheter. J Hosp Infect 3: 357.

Musher DM, Griffith DP (1974). Generation of formaldehyde from methenamine: effect of pH and concentration, and antibacterial effect. Antimicrob Ag Chemother 6: 708.

Musher DM, Griffith DP, Templeton GB (1976). Further observations on the potentiation of the antibacterial effect of methenamine by acetohydroxamic acid. J Infect Dis 133: 564.

Rosenheim ML (1935). Mandelic acid in the treatment of urinary infections. Lancet i: 1032; quoted by Zangwill et al. (1962)..

Schönebeck J, Almgård L-E, Boman J (1980). Antibiotics to patients with urinary infections in connection with transurethral prostatectomy. *Scand J Infect Dis* **12**: 129.

Selvaag E, Thune P (1994). Photosensitivity reaction to methenamine hippurate. A case report. *Photodermatol Photoimmunol Photomed* **10**: 259.

US Public Health Service Cooperative Study (1968). Prevention of recurrent bacteriuria with continuous chemotherapy. *Ann Intern Med* **69**: 655.

Vainrub B, Musher DM (1977). Lack of effect of methenamine in suppression of, or prophylaxis against, chronic urinary infection. *Antimicrob Ag Chemother* **12**: 625.

Zangwill DP, Porter PJ, Kaitz AL *et al.* (1962). Antibacterial organic acids in chronic urinary tract infection. *Arch Intern Med* **110**: 801.

Metronidazole

Description

Metronidazole is a nitroimidazole drug (p. 922) similar to tinidazole (p. 959). It has the chemical formula of 1-(beta-hydroxyethyl)-2-methyl-5-nitroimidazole. Following the discovery that azomycin, a nitroimidazole drug isolated from a *Streptomyces* species, was weakly active against *Trichomonas vaginalis*, many similar drugs were synthesized at Rhône-Poulenc Research Laboratories in France. One of these, metronidazole, was very active against experimental *T. vaginalis* infections (Cosar and Julou, 1959), and was soon shown to be useful for the systemic treatment of urogenital trichomoniasis in humans (Durel et al., 1959). Animal studies suggested that it may also be useful in amebiasis (Cosar et al., 1961) and this was subsequently confirmed in humans (Powell *et al.*, 1966). In addition, it was demonstrated to be effective in human *Giardia lamblia* infections (Schneider, 1961).

The observation that metronidazole relieved acute ulcerative gingivitis in a patient being treated for trichomonal vaginitis, led to studies culminating in its use in anaerobic bacterial infections (Shinn, 1962). Subsequently, it was confirmed that the drug was useful for the treatment of Vincent's stomatitis and that it inhibited *Fusobacterium necrophorum* (Davies et al., 1964). Based on experimental infections in mice, Freeman *et al.* (1968) suggested that metronidazole may be useful for the prevention of tetanus and gas gangrene. Finally, Tally *et al.* (1972) showed that metronidazole was useful for the treatment of infections due to *Bacteroides* spp., and since then it has been used for a variety of anaerobic infections.

Sensitive Organisms

1 Protozoa

Metronidazole is active against most anaerobic protozoa. *Trichomonas vaginalis* is usually sensitive (minimum lethal concentrations 0.8–25.0 μg per ml) (Nix *et al.*, 1995). However, resistant strains of this organism are encountered and these may be responsible for treatment failures of *T. vaginalis* infections (Lumsden *et al.*, 1988). Most metronidazole-resistant strains of *T. vaginalis* are also resistant to tinidazole (p. 959), but they are sensitive to furazolidone (p. 922) (Narcisi and Secor, 1996). *Giardia lamblia* is also always metronidazole-sensitive (Boreham *et al.*, 1984; Gordts *et al.*, 1985). *Entamoeba histolytica*, including emetine-resistant strains, is also susceptible and resistant strains have not been encountered (Ravdin and Skilogiannis, 1989; Samuelson *et al.*, 1992; Ravdin, 1995). The less common human pathogen, *Diantamoeba fragilis*, is also sensitive (minimal amebicidal concentration 32 μg per ml) (Chan *et al.*, 1994), as is *Blastocystis hominis* (Telalbasia *et al.*, 1991). The latter probably does not cause human disease (Markell, 1995).

The Microsporidia such as *Enterocytozoon bieneusi*, *Septata intestinalis* and *Encephalitozoon hellem* cause intestinal and other infections in AIDS patients (Ruf and Sandfort, 1994; Weber and Bryan, 1994) and occasionally diarrhea in immunocompetent patients (Sandfort *et al.*, 1994). Some AIDS patients with microsporidiosis have responded temporarily to metronidazole therapy, but in general these parasites appear to be resistant to the drug (Molina *et al.*, 1993; Asmuth *et al.*, 1994; Franssen *et al.*, 1995; He *et al.*, 1996).

2 Gram-negative anaerobic bacteria

The bacteria of the *Bacteroides fragilis* group such as *B. thetaiotaomicron*, *B. ovatus*, *B. uniformis*, *B. eggerthii*, *B. fragilis*, *B. distasonis* and *B. vulgatus* are nearly always metronidazole-sensitive (Sutter and Finegold, 1976; Dubreuil *et al.*, 1984). In most large-scale surveys in the USA and other countries, metronidazole-resistant strains of these bacteria were not detected (Tally *et al.*, 1985; Betriu *et al.*, 1990; Garcia Rodriguez and Garcia Sánchez, 1990; Appleman *et al.*, 1991; Betriu *et al.*, 1992; Phillips *et al.*, 1992; Aldridge *et al.*, 1994; Turgeon *et al.*, 1994), but rarely metronidazole-resistant strains of *B. fragilis* have been detected. Such strains have an MIC for metronidazole higher than 8 μg per ml (Acar *et al.*, 1981). A *B. fragilis* strain resistant to metronidazole, clindamycin and cefoxitin was reported by Brogan *et al.* (1989) and a strain of this organism resistant to metronidazole, co-amoxiclav and imipenem was described by Turner *et al.* (1995).

Metronidazole is also quite active against other Gram-negative anaerobes such as *Prevotella melaninogenica*, *P. disiens*, *P. oralis*, *P. intermedia* and *Fusobacterium* spp. (Appelbaum *et al.*, 1990; Jacobs *et al.*, 1990; Goldstein *et al.*, 1993; Pankuch *et al.*, 1993). Rare relatively resistant strains of *P. melaninogenica* (MIC 32 μg per ml) have been reported (Phillips *et al.*, 1981; Sprott and Kearns, 1988). The *Veillonella* spp. are also susceptible (Goldstein *et al.*, 1993). The facultative anaerobic bacterium, *Actinobacillus actinomyce-temcomitans* is only moderately sensitive to metronidazole and its sensitivity to this drug is increased if it is grown under anaerobic conditions (Pavcic *et al.*, 1992, 1995). *Gardnerella vaginalis*, another facultative anaerobe, is variable in its sensitivity. Its MICs for metronidazole range from 1.0 to >128.0 μg per ml. However, the drugs hydroxy metabolite (p. 942) is more active against this organism, which may explain the its efficacy for the treatment of bacterial vaginosis (p. 947) (Jones *et al.*, 1985; Lossick, 1990; Goldstein *et al.*, 1993; Joesoef and Schmid, 1995). The anaerobic bacteria of the *Mobiluncus* spp. may be metronidazole-sensitive, but the susceptibility may be variable and many strains are resistant (Spiegel, 1987; Goldstein *et al.*, 1993).

The microaerophilic organism, *Helicobacter pylori* is usually sensitive to metronidazole (McNulty *et al.*, 1985; Knapp *et al.*, 1991; Rautelin *et al.*, 1992; Rubinstein *et al.*, 1994). In general, strains with MICs of <4 μg per ml are considered as sensitive, those with MICs of 4–8 μg per ml are intermediate and those with MICs higher than 8 μg per ml as resistant (Knapp *et al.*, 1991; Rautelin *et al.*, 1992; Xia *et al.*, 1994). The MICs of the organism may be estimated by disc diffusion (Xia *et al.*, 1994), agar dilution (Knapp *et al.*, 1991) or by the so-called E test, which is a semi-quantitative variant of the disc diffusion test (Knapp *et al.*, 1991; Goddard and Logan, 1996). The MICs of the organism may differ somewhat with the differing laboratory methods used.

Normally the sensitivity of *H. pylori* to metronidazole is determined under microaerophilic conditions, because *H. pylori* grows best under these circumstances (Van Zwet *et al.*, 1995), but the susceptibility of *H. pylori* strains to metronidazole can be enhanced by anaerobic preincubation (Rubinstein *et al.*, 1994). In addition, metronidazole-resistant strains can become susceptible to the drug after anaerobic incubation in the presence of metronidazole (Van Zwet *et al.*, 1995). It is possible that temporary anaerobic conditions may occur in the antral mucosa which is the ecological niche of *H. pylori*, and this may explain why the classical triple therapy still succeeds in some 68% of patients who have pre-treatment metronidazole-resistant strains of the organism (p. 951).

Metronidazole-resistant *H. pylori* strains can be selected by passaging the organism *in vitro* in presence of subinhibitory concentrations of the drug (Haas *et al.*, 1990; Van Zwet *et al.*, 1994). Pretreatment strains of *H. pylori* in samples obtained by endoscopic biopsy, may frequently be metronidazole-resistant; such resistance probably arose because of the prior use of the drug for other conditions. Such metronidazole resistance varies widely between different populations, but in general it is more common in females than males and it is encountered more frequently in developing compared with developed countries. Such resistance can also appear during chemotherapy of *H. pylori* infection. This is frequent with metronidazole monotherapy and is usually prevented if patient compliance is good and triple therapy with bismuth subcitrate, tetracycline and metronidazole is given for 2 weeks (Anonymous, 1992; Rautelin *et al.*, 1992; Axon, 1993; Noach *et al.*, 1994; Goddard and Logan, 1996).

The mechanism of the metronidazole-resistance of *H. pylori* is not precisely known but resistant strains take up the drug much less effectively than sensitive ones (Lacey *et al.*, 1993). It has also been shown that anaerobiosis abolishes resistance to metronidazole. This resistance may be mediated through the activation of anaerobic metabolic pathways, which may not function at all under microaerophilic conditions and therefore resistance occurs (Smith and Edwards, 1995).

There is evidence that metronidazole or its hydroxymetabolite act synergistically *in vitro* with amoxycillin or tetracycline against most strains of *H. pylori* (Pavcic *et al.*, 1993).

3 Gram-positive anaerobic bacteria

The anaerobic cocci such as the *Peptococcus* and *Peptostreptococcus* spp. are usually metronidazole-sensitive (Dubreuil *et al.*, 1984; Jokipii and Jokipii, 1987). The anaerobic Gram-positive sporing bacilli such as *Clostridium perfringens*, *Cl. tetani*, *Cl. sordelli* and *Cl. septicum* are nearly always susceptible (Brazier *et al.*, 1985; Duerden, 1995). Also *Cl. difficile* is quite sensitive, its MIC being $0.13–0.5\,\mu g$ per ml (Burdon *et al.*, 1979; Chow *et al.*, 1985; Jokipii and Jokipii, 1987).

In contrast, the Gram-positive asporogenous bacilli such as the *Actinomyces*, *Propionibacterium*, *Bifidobacterium* and *Lactobacillus* spp. are usually resistant to this drug, except that *Eubacterium* spp. may be sensitive (Denys *et al.*, 1983; Dubreuil, 1984; Brook and Frazier, 1993; Goldstein *et al.*, 1993).

4 Activity of metronidazole metabolites

Ralph and Kirby (1975b) showed that against *Clostridium* spp., the acid and hydroxy metabolites of metronidazole (p. 942) possess approximately 5% and 30%, respectively, of the activity of the parent compound. When tested against isolates of the *B. fragilis* group, the acid and hydroxy metabolites are bactericidal exhibiting 5% and 65%, respectively, of the inhibitory effect of the parent drug (Haller, 1982; Pendland *et al.*, 1994). Similar findings were reported by O'Keefe *et al.* (1982) who showed that the hydroxy metabolite, though less active than metronidazole, inhibited selected isolates of *B. fragilis*, *Clostridium* spp. and anaerobic cocci at levels within the range of susceptibility. The hydroxy metabolite is very active *in vitro* against *Gardnerella vaginalis*, its MIC being 6.25–25% of that of metronidazole (Balsdon and Jackson, 1981; Easmon *et al.*, 1982). Some strains of *G. vaginalis* which were resistant to metronidazole, were also resistant to its hydroxy metabolite (Jones *et al.*, 1985). These authors also reported that most vaginal isolates of *Prevotella melaninogenica* and *P. oralis* were sensitive to both metronidazole and its hydroxy metabolite. Vaginal isolates of *Mobiluncus* spp. are often resistant to metronidazole, but when sensitive, they are also sensitive to its hydroxy metabolite.

5 Minimum inhibitory concentrations

The majority of *Bacteroides* spp. strains are inhibited *in vitro* by a concentration of $1.0\,\mu g$ per ml of metronidazole (Pendland *et al.*, 1994). The values for *Fusobacterium* and *Clostridium* spp. are both $<4.0\,\mu g$ per ml. These concentrations can easily be attained in serum (p. 940).

Mode of Administration and Dosage

1 Oral administration

Metronidazole is usually administered by this route. The dosage schedule varies according to the infection treated (see clinical uses, p. 946). The drug is available as either 200 mg or 250 mg oral tablets. For adults, the recommended dosage for treatment of urogenital trichomoniasis is a single dose of 2 g or 200–250 mg three-times daily for 7 days, and for giardiasis 2 g daily for 3 days. The adult dosage for treatment of anaerobic infections is 400 or 500 mg three-times daily for 7 days, but Earl *et al.* (1989) reported that an oral dosage of 400 mg 12-hourly was also satisfactory. For severe infections, such as brain abscess, the oral dosage, when tolerated is 500–600 mg 8-hourly (Sjölin *et al.*, 1993). The dosage for acute amebic colitis and amebic liver abscess is 750 mg (or 800 mg) 8-hourly, usually for 10 days (Ravdin, 1995).

The dosage for children is 20–30 mg per kg per day, administered in three divided doses (Sjölin *et al.*, 1993). The biotransformation of metronidazole is markedly impaired in malnourished children and a reduced total daily dosage of only 12 mg per kg has been suggested for these children (Lares-Asseff *et al.*, 1993).

2 Rectal administration

Rectal suppositories for adults may be used whenever oral medication is inappropriate. For treatment of anaerobic infections a 0.5 g or 1 g suppository should be inserted every 8 h for 3 days and thereafter every 12 h.

3 Intravenous administration

This route can be used when the oral or rectal routes are not feasible. Metronidazole solution (500 mg in 100 ml) should be infused i.v. at a rate of 5 ml per min. When used for prophylaxis in adults, a single i.v. dose of 500 mg is given shortly before surgery (p. 949). The equivalent i.v. dose for children is 7.5 mg per kg body weight. For treatment of serious infections the usual adult dosage is 500 mg i.v. 8-hourly, and each dose is infused over 15–30 min. The i.v. dosage for children is 7.5 mg per kg body weight, given every 8 h (Sjölin *et al.*, 1993). For treatment of anaerobic infections in adults an i.v. metronidazole dosage of 500 mg 12-hourly may also be satisfactory (Earl *et al.*, 1989).

4 Patients with renal failure

The main route of clearance of metronidazole and its metabolites is via the kidney (p. 942). Studies on three patients with renal impairment and one anephric patient showed that after a single oral dose of 500 mg metronidazole, the peak serum level and rate of elimination of the drug were not significantly different from normal subjects (McHenry, 1977). In another patient with renal failure, who was treated with an oral dose of 600 mg 8-hourly, there was accumulation of both metronidazole and particularly its metabolites (p. 942). When this patient was undergoing hemodialysis on alternate days, satisfactory serum levels were maintained by an oral dose of 600 mg twice-daily (Ingham *et al.*, 1975b). An i.v. dose of 500 mg every 8 h was given to one patient recovering from acute renal failure and two others receiving hemodialysis; serum concentrations just before the infusion were 7.2, 13.0 and 19.0 μg per ml and peak levels, 30 min after completion of an infusion, were 13.0, 27.0 and 28.0 μg per ml, respectively. These values fell within the ranges found when patients with normal renal function were treated in this way (Eykyn and Phillips, 1976). Other reports, which include estimation of metronidazole metabolites, also indicate that dosage modification is probably unnecessary in patients with renal failure in whom the serum half-life of metronidazole is similar to that of patients with normal renal function (Gabriel *et al.*, 1980; Kreeft *et al.*, 1983; Ljungberg *et al.*, 1984). Nevertheless, metronidazole metabolites accumulate in the blood of patients with impaired renal function, but these have not been definitely associated with adverse effects.

Gabriel *et al.* (1980) showed that hemodialysis removes significant amounts of metronidazole and its hydroxy metabolite (p. 942), and supplemental doses of the drug may be warranted. This was confirmed by Lau *et al.* (1986) who found a mean hemodialysis clearance of metronidazole and its metabolites of 70–110 ml per min, but they thought that dosage supplementation may only be necessary in seriously ill patients. Guay *et al.* (1984) found elimination half-lives of 8.16 and 10.93 h in patients on off-hemodialysis days and those undergoing continuous ambulatory peritoneal dialysis (CAPD), respectively. Both Cassey *et al.* (1983) and Guay *et al.* (1984) concluded that there was no need to adjust metronidazole dosage in patients undergoing CAPD. Peritoneal dialysis accounted only for 8.9% of total body clearance of metronidazole and had a similar insignificant effect on the elimination of its metabolites. After 750 mg of metronidazole was given i.v., peritoneal dialysate concentrations in the first 6-h exchange were in the range of 7.6–11.7 μg per ml (Guay *et al.*, 1984). Bush *et al.* (1983) gave oral metronidazole 400 mg 8-hourly to patients undergoing CAPD; after a 3-day treatment mean concentrations of metronidazole, its hydroxy and its acid metabolite and dialysate were 13.4, 7.9 and 10.2 μg per ml, respectively.

Somogyi *et al.* (1984) investigated metronidazole pharmacokinetics in six patients with acute renal failure; although renal clearance of the drug was virtually absent, non-renal clearance was only marginally depressed; the elimination half-life being 9.9 h. In these patients an i.v. dosage of 500 mg twice-daily produced adequate blood levels of the drug. According to the manufacturers the half-life of metronidazole is unaltered in the presence of anuria and the standard dosage regimen probably needs little modification in renal failure.

5 Patients with liver disease

In patients such as those with obstructive jaundice or alcoholic liver disease, the elimination half-life of the drug and its metabolites are prolonged. A dosage reduction with serum level monitoring is necessary (Farrell *et al.*, 1983; Lau *et al.*, 1987; Plaisance *et al.*, 1988).

6 Use in pregnancy

The manufacturers do not recommend that metronidazole should be given during the first trimester of pregnancy or during lactation; if the drug is used in the second or third trimesters, large single dose treatment should be avoided. There is no evidence that the drug is teratogenic in experimental animals or in humans (Shepard and Fantel, 1977; Piper *et al.*, 1993; Burtin *et al.*, 1995). However, because metronidazole is mutagenic in certain bacterial test systems and it may induce chromosome changes in human lymphocytes (p. 945), its use during pregnancy should be carefully assessed. Visser and Hundt (1984) found that the serum levels and elimination half-lives in pregnant patients after i.v. metronidazole were similar to those reported in non-pregnant patients.

7 Newborn infants

In a study of infants varying in gestational age from 28 to 40 weeks, the elimination half-life was shown to be inversely related to gestational age and ranged from 22.5 to 109 h. A single i.v. dose of 15 mg per kg body weight was proposed; this provides therapeutic serum levels (p. 941) for 48 h in preterm infants and for 24 h in term infants. A lower dosage of 7.5 mg per kg every 12 h was suggested for continuing treatment in the first week of life (Jager-Roman *et al.*, 1982). Higher doses have been used in neonates treated for meningitis (p. 948).

Availability

Tablets: 200 and 400 mg (250 and 500 mg in the USA).

Rectal suppositories containing 500 mg or 1.0 g metronidazole.

Intravenous preparation (0.5%): 500 mg in 100 ml bottles or plastic containers and 100 mg in 20 ml ampoules.

Serum Levels in Relation to Dosage

1 Oral administration

Metronidazole is well absorbed when given by mouth. After a single oral dose of 200 mg, mean serum levels in 12 patients studied by Kane *et al.* (1961a) were 4.8, 4.5, 3.7, 2.9 and 0.8 μg per ml at 1, 2, 4, 8 and 24 h, respectively. Ralph *et al.* (1974) gave metronidazole in single oral doses of 250 and 500 mg to ten adult subjects and mean peak serum levels were 6.2 and 11.5 μg per ml, respectively. However, the rate of absorption in different individuals was quite variable; some developed high serum levels 15 min after administration, whilst in others peak levels occurred at 2–4 h. Other authors used specific high-performance liquid chromatographic methods for the estimation of metronidazole and its metabolites (Houghton *et al.*, 1979; Mattila *et al.*, 1983). After a 400 mg oral dose was given to healthy volunteers, the mean peak serum level was about 10 μg per ml and this gradually fell to about 1.0 μg per ml after 24 h. The hydroxy metabolite appeared in the serum very soon after administration and its peak level at about 6 h was somewhat greater than 1.0 μg per ml; serum levels of metronidazole and its hydroxy metabolite were about the same at 24 h. The acid metabolite was not detected in the serum at any time (Houghton *et al.*, 1979). Volunteers received 500 mg oral metronidazole in the study by Mattila *et al.* (1983). The mean peak serum level at 1.9 h was 9.0 μg per ml and fell to about 4–5 μg per ml at 8 h. There was almost complete absorption after oral administration. A mean peak serum level of 12.3 μg per ml was attained in four adult subjects given a single 750 mg dose of metronidazole (Schwartz and Jeunet, 1976). Following a single oral dose of 2.4 g a mean peak serum level of 44.6 μg per ml (range 19.5–64.5) was obtained at 1 h and after 6 h the mean serum level was still 42 μg per ml (range 19.3–60.5) (McFadzean, 1969).

Wood and Monro (1975) performed serial chemical assays of metronidazole serum levels following a 2.0 g oral dose given to volunteers; the mean peak level at 1 h was 40 μg per ml, and this fell to 32 at 6 h, 5.7 at 24 h and to 0.9 μg per ml at 48 h. When bioassay was used, a mean peak serum level of 81 μg per ml was detected at 2 h, because the latter also estimates active metronidazole metabolites. Urtasun *et al.* (1976) administered large oral doses of 150 mg per kg body weight and serum concentrations of 180–200 μg per ml were obtained at 4 h. Furthermore, Deutsch *et al.* (1975) found a linear relationship between peak serum levels (102–340 μg per ml) when oral doses in the range of 80–190 mg per kg body weight were used. The serum half-life of metronidazole is about 8.5 h (Ralph *et al.*, 1974; Schwartz and Jeunet, 1976; Houghton *et al.*, 1979).

There have been a number of studies using repeated oral doses of metronidazole. Kane *et al.* (1961b) gave two patients a dose of 200 mg 6-hourly for three doses a day, for 7 days; serum levels 2 h after the last dose were in the range of 6.1–9.8 μg per ml and there was no evidence of accumulation of the drug. Higher oral doses were used by Ralph *et al.* (1974) for ten volunteers; dose regimens were 500 mg 4-hourly for four doses per day and 250 mg 6-hourly for three doses a day. Serum levels with both of these dosage schedules increased progressively for the first few doses and then levelled off, with no accumulation evident between 3 and 7 days.

Serum levels 12 h after the last dose each day were 3.9 and 13.1 µg per ml for the 250 mg and 500 mg regimens, respectively. Corresponding levels just prior to the last daily dose were 5.7 and 21.3 µg per ml, respectively. Peak serum levels which occur 1–2 h after administration were not measured, but would have been higher. Measurable serum levels of 0.41 and 0.54 µg per ml were still present in two volunteers 60 and 36 h, respectively, after stopping the drug; the former had received the drug in a dose of 2.0 g daily for 6 days and the latter 750 mg daily for 6 days. A dose of 1 g four times daily was used by Davies (1967) in three patients and this produced serum levels as high as 72.5 µg per ml. Bush *et al.* (1983) gave oral metronidazole 400 mg 8-hourly for 3 days to seven adult patients undergoing CAPD. Two hours after the last dose the mean serum concentrations of metronidazole, its hydroxy and acid metabolites were 16.0, 10.5 and 15.6 µg per ml, respectively. The acid metabolite is usually only found in the blood in the presence of renal failure.

2 Intravenous administration

Ingham *et al.* (1975a) studied serum levels in patients receiving 600 mg metronidazole i.v. over a period of 20 min. Mean levels at 60–90 min were 35.2, at 4 h 33.9 and at 8 h 23.7 µg per ml. Similar levels were observed by Eykyn and Phillips (1976) in 15 adult patients given a 500-mg i.v. dose every 8 h; the drug was infused over a period of 20 min and 30 min after its completion the mean serum level was 27.4 µg per ml; the mean trough concentration, taken just before an infusion, was 15.5 µg per ml. High-performance liquid chromatography methods, which are more specific for metronidazole and its metabolites, have been used in other investigations. Houghton *et al.* (1979) infused 400 mg metronidazole (in 80 ml over a period of 16 min) into ten adult volunteers; peak levels after infusion and declining levels of metronidazole and its hydroxy metabolite were almost identical to those which occurred after a 400-mg oral dose (see above); the elimination half-life was the same (8.3 h). The acid metabolite was not detected in serum. When 500 mg of the drug was infused i.v. over 20 min into six volunteers, very similar results to those following oral administration of the same dose were found (see above) (Mattila *et al.*, 1983). The mean peak serum level after the infusion was 9.4 µg per ml and after 8 h the level was still about 4 µg per ml; the elimination half-life was 7.9 h. After giving four volunteers 500 mg metronidazole i.v. rapidly over 5 min, the peak serum level was about 10 µg per ml immediately afterwards, the hydroxy metabolite appeared very soon in the serum and at about 6 h peaked at around 2 µg per ml, but the acid metabolite only appeared in the serum for a limited time and at very low levels (Nilsson-Ehle *et al.*, 1981).

In newborn infants (1–3 days old), in whom the elimination half-life of metronidazole is prolonged (p. 940), a dose of 15 mg per kg body weight given i.v. by slow injection over 15 min produced peak serum levels of about 20–30 µg per ml. In infants with a gestational age of 28–30 weeks the level was still greater than 20 µg per ml after 48 h and in those with a gestational age of 32–40 weeks the respective level was greater than 6 µg per ml (Jager-Roman *et al.*, 1982).

Kreeft *et al.* (1983) gave 500 mg metronidazole i.v. over a period of 26 min to eight patients with renal insufficiency; serum metronidazole levels were similar to those of five volunteers with normal renal function but metabolite concentrations which peaked at about 12 h were higher; the acid metabolite was 5-fold higher and the hydroxy metabolite 2-fold higher than in normal subjects. In patients undergoing CAPD or those requiring hemodialysis on off-dialysis days, serum levels of metronidazole and its metabolites were measured after they received 750 mg of the drug infused over 20–45 min (Guay *et al.*, 1984). Peak serum levels after infusion were about 10–20 µg per ml and after 24 h were about 1–5 µg per ml. Serum levels of the hydroxy and acid metabolites reached a peak 8–9 h later, being about 3–4 and 1–3 µg per ml, respectively; after 24 h serum levels for both metabolites were about 1–4 µg per ml. Somogyi *et al.* (1984) gave metronidazole i.v. to patients with acute renal failure. In four patients who had received 500 mg (30 min infusion) twice-daily for more than 4 days, the steady-state serum levels of metronidazole, its hydroxy and acid metabolites were 15.3, 17.4 and 1.19 µg per ml, respectively. These studies indicate that there is considerable accumulation in the serum of the hydroxy metabolite and to a lesser extent the acid metabolite of metronidazole, in the presence of renal failure.

3 Rectal administration

After the insertion of a 1 g suppository into volunteers, a mean serum level of 2.3 µg per ml was detected after 1 h and peak levels were usually reached after 4 h with a mean of 10.5 µg per ml (Report, 1975). Greater bioavailability after rectal administration was reported by Ioannides *et al.* (1981); they gave 500-mg suppositories every 8 h to patients who had undergone abdominal or pelvic surgery; when serum concentrations had reached a steady-state a further dose produced a mean peak serum level of 18.5 μg per ml after about 3 h and the level remained above 10 μg per ml for the next 8 h. High serum levels of metronidazole (and lower levels of its hydroxy metabolite) were demonstrated in ten severely ill patients given a 1 g suppository every 8 h (Barker *et al.*, 1983).

4 Vaginal administration

Matilla *et al.* (1983) gave 500 mg metronidazole intravaginally to six volunteers; a peak serum level of only 1.9 μg per ml was reached after 7.7 h.

Excretion

1 Urine

Only a small amount of metronidazole itself is eliminated via the kidneys but the two metabolites are mainly excreted in urine (Lau *et al.*, 1992). Ralph *et al.* (1974) were only able to recover 15–20% of the administered dose in the urine as measured by microbiological assay, suggesting that significant amounts of the drug are excreted as its metabolites. Urinary concentrations of metronidazole during this period were in the range 76.4–115.0 μg per ml after a 500-mg dose. Other studies have used high-performance liquid chromatography methods which are more specific for metronidazole and its metabolites. After giving a 500-mg i.v. dose of metronidazole to volunteers, Nilsson-Ehle *et al.* (1981) found that 43.7% of the dose was eliminated in the urine consisting of the parent drug (7.6%) and its hydroxy (24.1%) and acid (12.0%) metabolites. Bush *et al.* (1983) gave oral metronidazole 400 mg every 8 h for 3 days to patients undergoing CAPD; 2 h after the last dose mean urinary concentrations of metronidazole, its hydroxy and acid metabolites were 31.9, 25.7 and 76.1 μg per ml, respectively; the levels in samples of dialysate taken on the 3rd day were 13.4, 7.9 and 10.2 μg per ml, respectively.

2 Inactivation in body

Metronidazole is metabolized, presumably in the liver, to two oxidation products, the 'alcohol' or 'hydroxy' metabolite and the 'acid' metabolite. The hydroxy metabolite is the major product and is present in considerable amounts in the serum after oral or i.v. administration of the drug (Lau *et al.*, 1992). Serum levels of 2–23 μg per ml of the hydroxy metabolite have been detected (O'Keefe *et al.*, 1982). The acid metabolite is mainly found in the urine but it also has been identified in small amounts in the serum of subjects with normal renal function (Wheeler *et al.*, 1978; Nilsson-Ehle *et al.*, 1981). The hydroxy and acid metabolites accumulate in the sera of patients with renal failure (p. 939). In studies in newborn infants the hydroxy metabolite was not detected in the sera of babies of less than 35 weeks gestation. However, in infants of 28–35 weeks' gestation who had been exposed *in utero* to betamethasone, the hydroxy metabolite was present, suggesting that betamethasone may induce or inactivate metronidazole metabolism in the preterm neonates (Jager-Roman *et al.*, 1982). Experience in single patients suggested that barbiturates (Ioannides *et al.*, 1981) and diphenylhydantoin (Wheeler *et al.*, 1978) might also induce metronidazole metabolism. Other studies show that phenobarbital increased the metabolism of metronidazole and decreased its half-life to 3.5 h (Mead *et al.*, 1982; Gupte, 1983).

3 Feces

Only a small amount of an orally administered dose of metronidazole is excreted in the feces (Schwartz and Jeunet, 1976). Fecal metronidazole and hydroxymetronidazole concentrations are high enough to be bactericidal to *Cl. difficile* when the drug is given orally or i.v. to patients with acute *Cl. difficile* colitis, but these concentrations fall as diarrhea improves and neither substance can be detected in the feces after full recovery (Bolton and Culshaw, 1986).

4 Bile

High levels of the drug have been detected in bile (Knight, 1980; Teasley *et al.*, 1983).

Distribution of the Drug in Body

Concentrations of the drug found in saliva and breast milk are comparable with those found in serum (Gray *et al.*, 1961), whilst lower concentrations are detectable in semen and bone. Therapeutic levels occur in bile and in the CSF (Tally *et al.*, 1972); CSF levels of 13.9 and 11.0 μg per ml with simultaneous serum levels of 15.4 and 8.34 μg per ml, respectively, were detected 2 and 8 h after a 500-mg oral dose in a patient receiving 1.0 g daily for *Fusobacterium* meningitis (O'Grady and Ralph, 1976). In normal volunteers given 2.4 g of metronidazole orally, CSF concentrations 90 min later varied between 6.0 and 22.7 μg per ml, being on the average 43% of the simultaneous serum level (Jokipii et al., 1977). George and Bint (1976) found a concentration of 42 μg per ml in pus aspirated from a brain abscess of a 3-year-old patient, who had received the drug in a dosage of 100 mg four times daily for 1 week. Concentrations of 35.0 and 34.4 μg per ml were detected in abscess cavities of two patients with a brain abscess receiving an oral dose of 400 mg every 8 h, at a time when concurrent serum levels were 11.5 and 35.1 μg per ml, respectively. Abscess cavity concentrations of 20.7 and 45.0 μg per ml were obtained in two other patients receiving 400 and 600 mg, respectively, of the drug by the i.v. route every 8 h (Ingham et al., 1977). In liver abscess pus concentrations of the drug varying from nil to 24.0 μg per ml have been detected after a total oral dose of 5.8 g given over 2 days. A metronidazole level of 24.2 μg per ml was detected in drainage material from a lung empyema of a patient, who had received oral metronidazole in a dose of 400 mg 6-hourly for the previous 3.5 days (Smith and Wellingham, 1976).

Concentrations of metronidazole in middle ear discharge or mucosa of chronic otitis media reach 70% of serum levels (Jokipii and Jokipii, 1981). After the 20-min infusion of 500 mg metronidazole into patients who were undergoing appendicectomy 1 h later, levels of the drug and its hydroxy metabolite in relation to serum levels during the initial 1.25–4.0 h were 60.8% and 103.9% for appendix tissue and 29.0% and 57.0%, for subcutaneous tissue, respectively (Holter et al., 1983). When a single 1.0-g i.v. dose of the drug was given for antibiotic prophylaxis of colorectal surgery, the metronidazole concentration in the colonic wall tissue was 8.9 μg per g 2–3 h after the dose (Martin et al., 1991). After an oral dose of 500 mg metronidazole every 8 h for 5 days to patients undergoing elective gonadal surgery, 8 h after the last dose, tissue levels (μg per g) detected were 14.3 for prostatic tissue, 15.9 for vas deferens, 14.0 for epididymus and 12.5 for testis. Corresponding values after the same dosage with tinidazole were 24.1, 29.1, 22.1 and 18.6 (Viitanen et al., 1985). When metronidazole was given to healthy women in an oral dosage of 400 mg 12-hourly, the peak cervical mucus concentration, attained in 4 h was 5.2 μg per g on the 1st day and 10.3 μg per g on day 5 (Salas-Herrera et al., 1991). After a single i.v. dose of 500 mg of metronidazole, the average concentration of the drug in normal pelvic peritoneal fluid in women was 7.2 μg per ml (Berger et al., 1990).

Studies in three newborn infants given i.v. metronidazole showed that the drug enters the CSF and ascitic fluid in concentrations comparable with those in sera; the hydroxy metabolite was also found in these fluids if it was present in the sera (Jager-Roman et al., 1982). When metronidazole was given to a neonate with meningitis in an oral dosage of 35 mg per kg per day at 6 h intervals, CSF levels estimated 2, 4 and 6 h after a dose were 23.4, 11.4. and 7.4 μg per ml, respectively (Berman et al., 1978). Resultant serum levels and elimination after i.v. metronidazole in pregnant patients is similar to non-pregnant patients and the drug is rapidly transferred across the placenta (Visser and Hundt, 1984).

Ralph et al. (1974) could not detect any binding of metronidazole to serum proteins, whilst Schwartz and Jeunet (1976) using a different technique, found its binding to be less than 15%.

Mode of Action

The mechanism of action of metronidazole has not yet been fully elucidated. Because it inhibits anaerobic protozoa and anaerobic bacteria and because it has limited activity against aerobic organisms (by conventional tests) or vertebrate cells in tissue culture, it was postulated that metronidazole interacts with biochemical pathways found only in obligate anaerobes (Edwards et al., 1973; Ings et al., 1974). However, under strictly anaerobic conditions, metronidazole also has an effect on facultatively anaerobic organisms (see below).

Metronidazole diffuses into aerobic and anaerobic bacteria equally well, but in the former (under aerobic conditions) it remains unchanged whilst in the latter it is reduced. Within the cell the drug is probably reduced to an unstable, and as yet unidentified intermediate by bacterial 'nitroreductases'. In anaerobic bacteria and protozoa this reduction in the nitro group of metronidazole occurs by the pyruvate/ferredoxin oxidoreduatase complex, in which the drug acts as a preferential electron acceptor (Edwards and Mathison, 1970; Edwards et al., 1973; Edwards, 1993a). In this reaction the conversion of pyruvate is catalyzed by the enzyme pyruvate dehydrogenase. This biochemical reaction probably creates a gradient which promotes further uptake of the drug into anaerobic organisms. It was thought that the selective uptake and specificity of metronidazole for anaerobes was related to the low redox potentials achieved in such bacteria, compared with aerobes. Similar low redox potentials can be produced in E. coli and other facultative anaerobes under certain conditions (Sisson and Ingham, 1985). A product of metronidazole reduction, but not the unreduced drug, interacts with DNA and produces cell death (Edwards, 1979, 1993a). Sigeti *et al.* (1983) showed that metronidazole was rapidly bactericidal against *B. fragilis* by an immediate inhibition of DNA synthesis.

Early investigations, using conventional testing methods, indicated that metronidazole was inactive against aerobic and facultatively anaerobic bacteria except in concentrations in excess of those attainable therapeutically. However, by using strict anaerobic conditions, Ingham *et al.* (1980a) demonstrated that not only could various Gram-negative, facultatively anaerobic bacteria (*E. coli*, *Klebsiella* and *Proteus* spp. strains) inactivate metronidazole but they were sensitive to therapeutically attainable concentrations (10 μg per ml). These observations were confirmed by Jackson *et al.* (1984). It is not clear whether this *in vitro* activity of metronidazole against aerobic organisms is relevant in the treatment of infections. Obligate anaerobes in certain infections, such as otogenic cerebral abscess, may lower the oxidation-reduction potential enough for the drug to act against *E. coli*. This could account in part for the rapidity with which both obligate and facultative anaerobes disappear from such abscesses in patients receiving metronidazole (Ingham *et al.*, 1980a). It also may be the reason why metronidazole has sometimes seemed effective in the clinical treatment of some mixed aerobic/anaerobic infections (Eykyn and Phillips, 1976; Willis *et al.*, 1976). Another factor in mixed infections may be that *B. fragilis* and *Prevotella melaninogenica* impede phagocytosis of coliforms by polymorphonuclears (Ingham *et al.*, 1980b); metronidazole by its action of eliminating anaerobes may reduce this effect and allow killing of coliforms. The observation that metronidazole was more rapidly bactericidal for *B. fragilis* in the presence of *E. coli* (Chrystal *et al.*, 1980) was shown to be due to a reduction of the PO$_2$ of the medium by *E. coli* (Ingham *et al.*, 1981), thereby increasing the activity of the drug.

Sindar *et al.* (1982) produced strains of *Cl. perfringens* in the laboratory which were resistant to metronidazole (and tinidazole) and seemed to have absent pyruvate dehydrogenase activity. The resistance in the rare resistant *B. fragilis* strains appears to be due to a different mechanism – a decreased rate of reduction of metronidazole possibly due to lower activity of nitroreductases (Tally and Malamy, 1982). Another study showed that a metronidazole-resistant *B. fragilis* strain had high activity of lactate dehydrogenase which compensated for the decreased activity of pyruvate; ferredoxin oxireductase in the presence of the drug (Narikawa *et al.*, 1991). The metronidazole-resistance genes in *B. fragilis* may be plasmid borne or chromosomally determined (Reysset *et al.*, 1993; Dachs *et al.*, 1995).

The mode of action of metronidazole and the mechanisms of resistance of the microaerophilic organism, *H. pylori*, probably differ from those of anaerobic bacteria. Compared with the anaerobes, *H. pylori* develops resistance to metronidazole, when exposed to it as single drug both *in vitro* and *in vivo*, much more readily (Edwards 1993a,b; Smith and Edwards, 1995) (p. 937).

In studies using strains of *B. fragilis* and *Cl. perfringens*, Ralph and Kirby (1975a) showed that metronidazole is more rapidly bactericidal than penicillin G, carbenicillin or clindamycin.

Toxicity

1 Gastrointestinal side-effects

Occasionally an unpleasant metallic taste in the mouth, a furred tongue, nausea (rarely vomiting) and abdominal pain occur. Doses as high as 180 mg per kg body weight per day, when used in cancer patients as an adjunct to radiotherapy, produced slight but acceptable nausea; higher doses of up to 300 mg per kg body weight per day were progressively less well tolerated and produced severe anorexia, nausea and vomiting, which often persisted for 24–48 h after the last dose (Deutsch *et al.*, 1975). Pseudomembranous colitis was described in two patients in association with metronidazole administration as the sole antimicrobial. In one, *Cl. difficile* was isolated from the feces which was sensitive to metronidazole (Saginur *et al.*, 1980) but in another neither the organism nor its cytotoxin were identified in the patient's feces (Thompson *et al.*, 1981). Antibiotic-associated colitis has been reported with other antibiotics when the *Cl. difficile* isolate was susceptible to the agent implicated. One other case of colitis has been recorded which was due to a metronidazole-resistant strain (Fekety *et al.*, 1984).

2 Leucopenia

A transient and reversible neutropenia has been occasionally observed during metronidazole therapy (Lefebvre and Hesseltine, 1975; Tally *et al.*, 1975; Sanders *et al.*, 1979). Leucopenia has been ascribed to metronidazole in other patients but in two it was used with other drugs that can cause bone marrow depression, azathioprine (McKendrick and Geddes, 1979) and fluorouracil (Windle *et al.*, 1979) and the other patient had disseminated adenocarcinoma (White *et al.*, 1980).

3 Neurotoxicity

Peripheral neuropathy has been described in a number of patients, particularly those who have received prolonged treatment with relatively high doses of metronidazole (Ramsay, 1968; Ursing and Kamme, 1975; Ingham *et al.*, 1975a; Bradley *et al.*, 1977; Bernstein *et al.*, 1980). Peripheral neuropathy is usually relatively mild and full recovery appears to occur when the drug is stopped or the dose decreased. In some patients sensory changes have persisted for months and even years after discontinuation of the drug (Hishon and Pilling, 1977; Karlsson and Hamlyn, 1977; Boyce *et al.*, 1990). Pathological investigations of the patient described by Bradley *et al.* (1977) showed that a major degree of nerve degeneration had occurred.

Clinical circumstances in three patients receiving high doses of metronidazole (in association with radiation for carcinoma) suggested that the drug was responsible for convulsions (Frytak *et al.*, 1978). An adult patient developed confusion, disorientation, cerebellar dysfunction and sensory neuropathy after receiving oral metronidazole 750 mg 6-hourly for 28 days; he fully recovered after withdrawal of the drug but features of the neuropathy persisted for 4 months (Kusumi *et al.*, 1980). A 12-year-old boy developed seizures after receiving the drug i.v. in a dosage of 250 mg 6-hourly; he had prolonged neurological abnormalities after the seizures stopped but he eventually regained his normal status (Bailes *et al.*, 1983). Deafness was reported in association with metronidazole administration in one patient (Hibberd *et al.*, 1984) but the casual relationship has been disputed (Blake and Butt, 1984). One 30-year-old man who had received 21 g of metronidazole over 14 days, developed reversible deafness, tinnitus and ataxia (Lawford and Sorrell, 1994). Metronidazole-associated aseptic meningitis has also been reported. Small doses have caused this complication, for which a hypersensitivity mechanism is likely (Corson and Chretien, 1994).

4 Hypersensitivity

One Asian woman with a history of recurrent vaginitis had previously developed localized erythema while receiving intravaginal metronidazole and nystatin. Later, when treated by oral metronidazole for bacterial vaginosis, she developed chills, fever, generalized erythema, rash and later dyspnea and edema of extremities. She improved after cessation of metronidazole and treatment with methylprednisolone (Knowles *et al.*, 1994).

5 Acute pancreatitis

There are several case reports where an acute pancreatitis occurred during metronidazole therapy. Symptoms usually rapidly subsided on withdrawal of the drug. In some of the patients this complication recurred promptly when metronidazole was readministered (Plotnick *et al.*, 1985; Sanford *et al.*, 1988; Celifarco *et al.*, 1989; Corey *et al.*, 1991). Overall this side-effect of metronidazole appears to be rare (Friedman and Selby, 1990).

6 Mutagenicity and carcinogenicity

Metronidazole can increase the spontaneous mutation rates of certain aerobic bacteria grown *in vitro* (Voogd *et al.*, 1974; Lindmark and Müller, 1976), and urinary metabolites of patients taking metronidazole are also mutagenic when assayed in such bacterial test systems (Speck *et al.*, 1976). Mitelman *et al.* (1976) reported a greater frequency of chromosomal aberrations in the circulating lymphocytes of patients with Crohn's disease receiving long-term metronidazole than in patients with Crohn's disease not treated by the drug or healthy controls. In a later study of such patients they were unable to find evidence of a cytogenetic effect of metronidazole after 4 months treatment; their early findings may have been caused by concomitant administration of sulfasalazine or higher dosage and long treatment with metronidazole (Mitelman *et al.*, 1980). No chromosome-breaking activity could be detected when 12 patients with vaginal trichomoniasis were given metronidazole 200 mg three times daily for 7 days (Hartley-Asp, 1979).

A carcinogenic effect of very high doses of metronidazole in rodents have been reported (Rustia and Shubik, 1972), but this effect has not been confirmed in other experimental animals (Roe, 1977). Moreover, several large retrospective surveys of patients who have been treated with metronidazole in the USA have not shown that they have an increase of cancer (Beard *et al.*, 1979; Friedman, 1980; Danielson *et al.*, 1982; Beard *et al.*, 1988). Roe (1977) has pointed out that the use of metronidazole to eradicate *T. vaginalis* may actually reduce the risk of development of cancer of the uterine cervix. Despite the absence of evidence that metronidazole is carcinogenic or teratogenic in humans, it still seems prudent to avoid its use in the first trimester of pregnancy where possible (p. 939).

7 Interaction with other drugs

Metronidazole can produce the 'Antabuse syndrome' (Taylor, 1964). Similar to disulfiram ('Antabuse'), metronidazole apparently affects the activity of hepatic enzymes involved with the metabolism of ethanol and acetaldehyde. When it is taken with alcohol it produces unpleasant symptoms, probably due to the accumulation of acetaldehyde in the blood (Birkett and Pond, 1975). In addition, a toxic psychosis has been described when metronidazole was given to alcoholic patients receiving disulfiram (Rothstein and Clancy, 1969). There is also the theoretical possibility that the action of metronidazole inhibiting acetaldehyde metabolism may enhance the dangers to the fetus of maternal alcohol ingestion during pregnancy (Dunn *et al.*, 1979). Alcohol ingestion is therefore contraindicated in patients taking metronidazole.

Concomitant administration of metronidazole augments both the hypoprothrombinemic effect and blood levels produced by commercial racemic sodium warfarin (coumadin sodium). O'Reilly (1976) showed that this was a stereoselective interaction in that metronidazole augments the effects of racemic (a mixture of levowarfarin and dextrowarfarin) and S(-)-warfarin (levowarfarin) and not R(+)-warfarin (dextrowarfarin). He suggested that this drug interaction can be lessened and even avoided if racemic warfarin is replaced by R(+)-warfarin (dextrowarfarin). There is some evidence that metronidazole may impair the clearance of phenytoin (Blyden *et al.*, 1988). One 30-year-old woman who had received metronidazole for 6 days, developed an acute dystonic reaction after a single dose of chloroquine (Achumba *et al.*, 1988). In general there are no interactions between metronidazole and the quinolones (Boeckh *et al.*, 1990), but in two patients, who received metronidazole plus pefloxacin (p. 1091), neurotoxicity was observed with confusion, disorientation, slurred speech and extrapyramidal symptoms (Radandt *et al.*, 1992).

8 Other side-effects

Drowsiness, headache, and depression have been reported. The urine of patients taking metronidazole may be colored deep red brown due to the presence of an azometabolite of the drug.

9 Hemolytic-uremic syndrome

Powell *et al.* (1988) reported six children in whom the development of this disease appeared to be related to metronidazole therapy.

Clinical Uses of the Drug

1 Treatment of anaerobic bacterial infections

Most anaerobic infections are acquired from the host's own microflora in the respiratory, gastrointestinal or genital tract, as a result of a breach in the mechanical defence system. They have been particularly implicated in non-traumatic brain abscess, lung and intra-abdominal infections and non-venereal infections of the female genital tract. However, anaerobic bacteria have been recognized with increasing frequency as etiologic agents in a variety of infections (Bartlett, 1983). Many anaerobic infections can be managed by surgery, but others require chemotherapy in combination with surgery. With chemotherapy sometimes anaerobic abscesses (e.g. cerebral or hepatic) may not require surgical drainage. Frequently *B. fragilis*, other anaerobes of the *B. fragilis* group, Prevotella and *Fusobacterium* spp. and other anaerobes are involved in these infections.

Anaerobic infections are often polymicrobial with both anaerobic and aerobic bacteria being involved. Studies in animals and results of some clinical studies in humans suggest that in anaerobic infections there may be a synergistic effect between aerobic and anaerobic bacteria. This may be because anaerobes provide protection for aerobes in a mixed infection by inhibiting their phagocytosis (McGowan and Gorbach, 1981). In many anaerobic infections, therefore, an antibiotic which is active against aerobes is also added to the regimen, despite the fact that metronidazole alone may also be effective in some mixed aerobic/anaerobic infections in humans and animals (p. 944).

a Intra-abdominal infections These usually occur as the result of penetrating trauma or perforation of the gastrointestinal tract due to disease states or surgery. Sepsis results from the release of endogenous gastrointestinal flora the nature of which depends on the site of origin. In the proximal tract there are mainly oral, penicillin-sensitive anaerobes and aerobic coliforms, whilst in the colon there is a high concentration of anaerobic bacteria, particularly *B. fragilis* (Nichols, 1983).

The treatment of intra-abdominal sepsis entails appropriate surgical intervention and the parenteral administration of antibiotics effective against aerobic and anaerobic bacteria. Many other antibiotics, used singly or in combination, are now available for the treatment of these infections and they all appear about equally effective. Other available drugs include chloramphenicol/gentamicin, clindamycin/gentamicin and cefoxitin, cefotetan, imipenem, ticarcillin/clavulanic acid, ampicillin/sulbactam and piperacillin/tazobactam. In some early studies metronidazole, when used alone, appeared satisfactory for these infections (Eykyn and Phillips, 1976; George *et al.*, 1982). However, nowadays an aminoglycoside, such as gentamicin or tobramycin is usually combined with metronidazole for the treatment of intra-abdominal infections (Harding *et al.*, 1984; Fan *et al.*, 1988; Uhari *et al.*, 1992; Gorbach, 1993). Results of treatment are good. Additional cover for Enterococci may be obtained by adding i.v. ampicillin to the metronidazole/aminoglycoside regimen, but this is usually unnecessary. Satisfactory results are also obtained if a third-generation cephalosporin such as cefotaxime, instead of the aminoglycoside, is combined with metronidazole (Aprahamian *et al.*, 1995; Nicolau *et al.*, 1995). Furthermore a quinolone such as ciprofloxacin or pefloxacin may be combined with metronidazole with success for the treatment of these infections (Anonymous, 1990; Yoshioka *et al.*, 1991).

Pyogenic liver abscesses are usually treated by surgical drainage or needle aspiration plus antibiotic regimens similar to those used for intra-abdominal infections. Bäck *et al.* (1978) described a patient with a liver abscess due to *B. fragilis* which appeared to be cured by a 6 week course of oral metronidazole, without surgical drainage.

b Genital infections Bacteria responsible for non-venereal infections of the female genital tract usually originate from the vaginal and endocervical flora and consist of aerobes and anaerobes, with the latter, particularly *Bacteroides* spp. predominating (Sweet, 1981). In various clinical trials, there has been no significant differences in the outcome of treatment of female genital tract infections with combinations of an aminoglycoside with metronidazole, chloramphenicol, clindamycin, cefoxitin or ticarcillin (Bartlett, 1983; Harding *et al.*, 1984). If *Chlamydia trachomatis* infection is suspected, doxycycline should be added to the regimen. In general regimens such as cefoxitin/doxycycline or clindamycin/gentamicin are now favored for the treatment of pelvic inflammatory disease (CDC, 1993).

c Bacterial vaginosis This is a vaginal infection, which produces an increased malodorous vaginal discharge, which is not attributable to uterine infection, *T. vaginalis* or *Candida* spp. infection. This disease is polymicrobial and there is an overgrowth in the vagina of the facultative anaerobe *Gardnerella vaginalis* together with other anaerobic bacteria such as the *Prevotella*, *Bacteroides*, *Mobiluncus*, *Peptococcus* and *Peptostreptococcus* spp. (Lossick, 1990). Bacterial vaginosis may be a sexually transmitted disease. *Gardenella vaginalis* has been isolated from males with urethritis and the organism is often isolated from male sexual partners of females with bacterial vaginosis (Blackwell, 1984). Many studies have shown that oral metronidazole is effective for the treatment of bacterial vaginosis (Balsdon *et al.*, 1980; Spiegel *et al.*, 1980; Blackwell *et al.*, 1983). A regimen of 400–500 mg twice-daily for 7 days has been particularly effective and this is now considered to be the treatment of choice (Joesoef and Schmid, 1995).

Results in some studies indicate that a single oral dose of 2 g metronidazole is also effective (Alawattegama *et al.*, 1984; Jones *et al.*, 1985; Mohanty and Deighton, 1985) whilst in others it has been associated with a higher relapse rate of the infection than a 7-day course (Blackwell *et al.*, 1983; Swedberg *et al.*, 1985). Other less well evaluated treatment options for this disease include clindamycin 300 mg orally 12-hourly for 7 days and topical application of either 0.75% metronidazole gel, 5 g intravaginally 12-hourly or 2% clindamycin cream 5 mg intravaginally at bedtime for 7 days. Pregnant women can be treated by metronidazole in the second and third trimester, but during the first trimester oral or topical clindamycin should be used. Treatment of sexual partners of women with this disease has not been found beneficial in preventing a recurrence of bacterial vaginosis (CDC, 1993; Joesoef and Schmid, 1995). Currently it is recommended that this disease during pregnancy should be treated largely to relieve symptoms

(Joesoef and Schmid, 1995), but there is some evidence that treatment of bacterial vaginosis in pregnancy may also reduce the incidence of preterm delivery (Mcdonald *et al.*, 1994; Hauth *et al.*, 1995).

d   Respiratory infections   Anaerobic bacteria are important etiological agents in necrotizing pneumonia, lung abscess, empyema and aspiration pneumonia (Leading article, 1983). These anaerobes are derived from the oral cavity and whilst some of them are sensitive to penicillin G, some such as *B. fragilis* and many strains of *Prevotella melaninogenica* are not so. Although penicillin G alone may be effective for the treatment of aspiration pneumonia (p. 38), in seriously ill patients antibiotics which are active against these penicillin-resistant organisms should be used (Brook and Finegold, 1980). Clindamycin used as a single drug is satisfactory treatment for these infections (p. 597), but penicillin G/metronidazole combination is also effective.

e   Meningitis and brain abscess   Metronidazole has been used to treat *B. fragilis* meningitis in several newborn infants. After apparent failure of chloramphenicol, Berman *et al.* (1978) gave metronidazole orally in a dose of 30–35 mg per kg per day to a neonate who then recovered but developed hydrocephalus and a neurologic deficit. Law and Marks (1980) reported another neonate who was treated by metronidazole earlier in the course of *B. fragilis* meningitis and who recovered rapidly without sequelae; the drug was given i.v. in a dosage of 30 mg per kg per day in two divided doses for 3 weeks. Also *B. fragilis* meningitis resolved satisfactorily in a 72-year-old woman with metronidazole treatment (Soriano *et al.*, 1986).

Anaerobic bacteria are commonly involved in brain abscesses. Although some cases of cerebritis and multiple brain abscesses have been treated successfully with antibiotics alone, surgical drainage of a brain abscess is usually mandatory (De Louvois, 1983; Mathisen *et al.*, 1984). De Louvois (1978) showed that abscesses of sinusitic origin were mainly due to streptococci, usually *Streptococcus milleri* for which penicillin G alone was adequate. However, such abscesses may contain beta-lactamase-producing strains of *Prevotella* and *Bacteroides* spp. which are resistant to penicillin G (Mathisen *et al.*, 1984). Anaerobic bacteria, particularly *B. fragilis*, are frequently present in temporal lobe abscesses of otitic origin which are penicillin G-resistant (De Louvois, 1978). Oral metronidazole in combination with aspiration and other antibiotics, has been useful in the treatment of a number of adults (Ingham *et al.*, 1977, 1978) and a child (George and Bint, 1976) with a cerebral abscess. A combination of penicillin G and chloramphenicol (p. 40) has often been used to treat cerebral abscesses but for some time now there has been a trend to use penicillin G plus metronidazole (Mathisen *et al.*, 1984). Metronidazole is bactericidal against anaerobes (p. 944) and penetrates well into the brain (p. 943), but it must be combined with a beta-lactam-antibiotic such as penicillin G because facultative bacteria such as streptococci may be metronidazole-resistant. More recently a combination of metronidazole plus a third-generation cephalosporin such as cefotaxime has also been used with success (Donald, 1990; Donald *et al.*, 1990; Sjölin *et al.*, 1993; Gómez *et al.*, 1995).

If cerebral abscesses occur as a result of trauma or are metastatic as part of a septicemia, *Staphylococcus aureus* may be a pathogen, and an effective anti-staphylococcal drug would be required (Donald, 1990). The installation of antibiotics directly into a cerebral abscess is of dubious value (De Louvois, 1983).

f   Osteomyelitis   This disease due to anaerobic bacteria has been classified into three major presentations; an acute hematogenous form usually involving normal bones in young patients; a chronic infection in which anaerobes superinfect a fracture site infected with aerobes; and an indolent infection at the site of indwelling prosthetic device. Metronidazole (plus other antibiotics according to associated pathogens involved) has been recommended for these anaerobic infections if a beta-lactam-resistant organism, such as *B. fragilis*, is involved (Templeton *et al.*, 1983). Oral metronidazole was used to cure osteomyelitis due to *B. fragilis* in a diabetic man in whom treatment with i.v. clindamycin was associated with an incomplete and temporary response (Zimmerman *et al.*, 1980). Metronidazole has been used successfully to treat chronic osteomyelitis due to *Cl. difficile* (Riley and Karthigasu, 1982).

g   Oral and dental infections   Anaerobes are present in the oral and dental indigenous bacterial flora and have a role in infections in these areas. Many anaerobes, such as *Peptostreptococcus*, *Peptococcus*, *Actinomyces*, *Lactobacillus*, *Eubacterum*, *Prevotella* and *Fusobacterium* spp. are involved. For orofacial infections of odontogenic origin penicillin G is the recommended treatment. However, if penicillin G-resistant anaerobic bacteria are involved, a drug such as metronidazole is indicated (Newman, 1984).

h Miscellaneous infections Metronidazole given orally in combination with ampicillin or amoxycillin was successfully used to control *Fusobacterium* endocarditis in a patient who subsequently required valve replacement (Seggie, 1978). The drug was also effective for the treatment in a 23-year-old man with *Cl. bifermentans* endocarditis, who had failed to respond to i.v. penicillin G (Kolander *et al.*, 1989). Monomicrobial *Veillonella* spp. myositis in an immunocompromised patient responded to debridement and metronidazole therapy (Beumont *et al.*, 1995). Oral metronidazole was also effective for the treatment of a *Bacteroides* breast abscess (Hale *et al.*, 1976). Experience in one patient suggested that metronidazole may be useful to treat prostatitis, presumably due to anaerobes (Lockie, 1981). Based on the proposition that anaerobic bacteria are involved in the pathogenesis of glandular fever, metronidazole has been tried as a therapeutic agent. Some studies have shown that this had a beneficial effect (Hedström, 1980; Davidson *et al.*, 1982) but this has not been confirmed by others (Spelman and Newton-John, 1982). There have been several reports of the beneficial effect of metronidazole in reducing the smell of fungating tumors by eliminating anaerobes (Ashford *et al.*, 1980, 1984; Dankert *et al.*, 1981). The drug is also useful in reducing the offensive smell associated with anaerobic infection in axillary abscesses (Leach *et al.*, 1979).

Metronidazole may be useful for the treatment of gas gangrene (Pashby, 1981). In an open trial, patients with tetanus in Indonesia given a 7–10 day course of either i.m. procaine penicillin (76 patients) or metronidazole (97 patients) rectally or orally, the patients receiving metronidazole had a lower mortality and an improved response to treatment (Ahmadsyah and Salim, 1985).

2 Chemoprophylaxis of anaerobic surgical infections

a Obstetric and gynecological surgery An early study involving 202 gynecological patients demonstrated that oral metronidazole was effective in reducing the frequency of postoperative non-clostridial anaerobic pelvic infection (Reports, 1974, 1975). Short-course i.v. metronidazole was also effective in reducing infection following gynecological and obstetric surgery (Khan *et al.*, 1980). Rectally administered metronidazole has been used with equal effectiveness to the i.v. drug in preventing anaerobic infection in gynecological patients (McLean *et al.*, 1983). Nowadays a single i.v. dose of metronidazole is usually given at the time of induction of anesthesia. This may be combined with single dose of ampicillin, cephalothin or cefazolin (Houang *et al.*, 1984; Havekorn, 1987).

b Colorectal surgery and appendicectomy Metronidazole is a useful drug to prevent anaerobic infections after these surgical procedures. It is usually combined with drugs such as gentamicin or cefotaxime which are active against the patient's aerobic Gram-negative microflora. In the past multiple doses of either drug were given and metronidazole was administered iv, orally or rectally (Gillespie and McNaught, 1978; Eykyn *et al.*, 1979; Keighley *et al.*, 1979; Morris *et al.*, 1983). Nowadays usually a single i.v. dose of metronidazole (500 mg or 1.0 g) is given at the time of induction of anesthesia and this is combined with a single dose of gentamicin or cefotaxime (Foster *et al.*, 1986; Haddock *et al.*, 1988; Hall *et al.*, 1989; Rowe-Jones *et al.*, 1990; Martin *et al.*, 1991; Kwok *et al.*, 1993). If at operation an established infection such as peritonitis is already present, then an appropriate course of chemotherapy should be given.

3 Antibiotic-associated colitis

Most antibiotics can produce diarrhea which is usually mild and self-limiting. When diarrhea is severe and persistent it may be associated with colitis and pseudomembrane formation. *Clostridium difficile* is the important cause of pseudomembranous colitis but staphylococci and *Cl. perfringens* type C may be rare causes. *Clostridium difficile* may cause colitis without pseudomembrane; it acts by altering the normal bowel flora resulting in an overgrowth of toxigenic *Cl. difficile* (Fekety, 1983). Pseudomembranous colitis occurred in the pre-antibiotic era and it has been induced by antineoplastic chemotherapy (Fekety *et al.*, 1984). Most commonly used antibiotics given either orally or parenterally have induced *Cl. difficile* colitis, including metronidazole (p. 944). Vancomycin (p. 779), metronidazole and bacitracin (p. 543) have been used successfully to treat antibiotic-associated colitis. Many anecdotal reports indicated that oral metronidazole was useful for this purpose (Dinh *et al.*, 1978; Matuchansky *et al.*, 1978; Pashby *et al.*, 1979; Bolton, 1979; Johnson *et al.*, 1981). Then Cherry *et al.*

(1982) reported the successful use of oral metronidazole in a dosage of 1.5–2 g per day for 7–14 days in 13 consecutive patients with antibiotic-associated pseudomembranous colitis. In 1983, Teasley *et al.* published the results of a prospective randomized trial of metronidazole versus vancomycin for the treatment of *Cl. difficile*-associated diarrhea and colitis. Both drugs were given orally for 10 days, metronidazole 250 mg four times daily and vancomycin 500 mg four times daily. Pseudomembranous colitis was diagnosed after endoscopy in 33 patients; of the remaining patients without these changes, 38 had both *Cl. difficile* culture and cytotoxin and 23 had only culture evidence of *Cl. difficile*. Fifty-two evaluable patients received vancomycin and 42 received metronidazole. There were two treatment failures with metronidazole and nine with vancomycin, and two relapses with metronidazole versus six with vancomycin. It was concluded that both drugs were of equal efficacy in treating this disease. Other authors have confirmed these results (Olson *et al.*, 1994). Wilcox and Howe (1995) in a comparative study found that response and relapse rates were similar in metronidazole and vancomycin-treated patients, but that mean duration of symptoms was shorter in vancomycin-treated patients. Nevertheless, metronidazole should be used for routine treatment of this disease, because it is cheaper and oral vancomycin should be restricted as far as possible because of the recent emergence of vancomycin-resistant *Enterococcus faecium* (p. 765). Vancomycin may be used in severely ill patients (Fekety *et al.*, 1984). For patients who cannot take oral medications, i.v. metronidazole is usually recommended (Bartlett, 1984; Kleinfield *et al.*, 1988), but treatment failures with this have been reported (Guzman *et al.*, 1988; Oliva *et al.*, 1989). Asymptomatic fecal carriage is usually transient and it should not be treated with metronidazole (Johnson *et al.*, 1992).

4 Crohn's disease

Ursing and Kamme (1975) first reported the successful use of metronidazole in five patients with this disease. Subsequently, many patients with Crohn's disease were given the drug, generally with clinical improvement. Bernstein *et al.* (1980) noted improvement in 18 patients with chronic unremitting perineal disease with complete healing occurring in ten. The dosage was 20 mg per kg per day given in three to five divided doses; this had to be decreased in four patients and discontinued in one, all because of peripheral neuritis which was reversible. Subsequently these authors showed that dosage-reduction was associated with exacerbation of disease activity but healing occurred when full dosage was reinstated. The only major side-effect was paresthesiae which occurred in 50% of patients and developed after a mean of 5–6 months of treatment. Treatment continued to be effective for periods as long as 26 months (Brandt *et al.*, 1982). A cooperative study in Sweden established that metronidazole was a useful therapeutic agent in Crohn's disease (Rosén *et al.*, 1982; Ursing *et al.*, 1982). A dose of 800 mg per day of metronidazole was at least as effective as 3 g per day of sulfasalazine (p. 826).

A more recent review also concludes that patients with refractory perineal Crohn's disease and those with Crohn's colitis may benefit from metronidazole (Peppercorn, 1990). It has not been established how metronidazole works in Crohn's disease; it may be related to its antibacterial action or some effect on cell-mediated immunity (Gilat, 1982). Metronidazole does affect the bowel flora in Crohn's disease; Krook *et al.* (1982) showed that after treatment for 1 month or more, there was a selection of less sensitive *Bacteroides* spp. in the feces, but no totally resistant strains were isolated. *Clostridium difficile* has been isolated from the feces of patients with inflammatory bowel disease (Crohn's disease and ulcerative colitis) (Bolton *et al.*, 1980) but a causal relationship has not been established. Bolton and Read (1982) gave metronidazole to two patients with acute toxic dilatation of the colon (one had Crohn's disease and the other ulcerative colitis) with rapid improvement; in both patients *Cl. difficile* and its toxin present in the feces were eradicated after the treatment. Other evidence suggests that *Cl. difficile* causes exacerbation of inflammatory bowel disease only in association with sulfasalazine or other antibiotic therapy (George, 1984).

Many of the perianal lesions of Crohn's disease respond to metronidazole therapy (Van Kruiningen, 1995). A 3-month course of metronidazole also reduces the recurrent rates of this disease in the neoterminal ileum after ileal resection (Rutgeerts *et al.*, 1995).

Metronidazole is not effective in ulcerative colitis (Gilat, 1982; Chapman *et al.*, 1986).

5 Trichomoniasis

Oral administration of metronidazole is highly effective for the treatment of *T. vaginalis* infection of the genitourinary tract in both males and females. To prevent reinfection, the consort should receive treatment concurrently. The usually recommended dose is 200 or 250 mg three times daily for 7 days. Single-dose treatment with 2 g metronidazole orally is also effective (Csonka,

1971; Thin et al., 1979; Hager et al., 1980), but this large single dose causes gastrointestinal side-effects (Nix et al., 1995). A single 1-g dose results in a much lower cure rate (Austin et al., 1982). A single 2-g intravaginal dose of metronidazole is much less effective than a 2-g single dose of the drug given orally (Tidwell et al., 1994). Metronidazole-resistant strains of T. vaginalis are now encountered. Infections due to these may respond to large doses such as 2 g daily for 7 days. There is usually cross-resistance to tinidazole, but not to furazolidone (p. 922). Metronidazole should be avoided during first trimester of pregnancy; patients during this time may respond to intravaginal clotrimazole tablets 100 mg daily for 1–2 weeks.

6 Amebiasis

Metronidazole is a valuable drug for the treatment of all forms of this disease. Recommended adult dosages for treatment of invasive intestinal disease or liver abscess are 750–800 mg orally 8-hourly or 500 mg i.v. 6-hourly for 10 days (Ravdin, 1995). The same treatment is effective for rarer severe E. histolytica infections, such as a brain abscess (Ohnishi et al., 1994) and severe vaginal infection with this parasite (Citronberg and Semel, 1995).

A number of reports have described failed treatment with metronidazole in liver abscess (Pittman, 1973; Fisher et al., 1976; Triger 1978; Harrison et al., 1979; Koutsaimanis et al., 1979). In some patients cure was obtained by adding emetine and sometimes chloroquine as well. It was then recommended that for some forms of amebiasis combination therapy may be needed (Knight, 1980; Wolfe, 1982), but it is now considered that the rather toxic emetine and or chloroquine are rarely if ever necessary in addition to metronidazole. Patients with amebic liver abscess, who respond poorly to metronidazole, need needle aspiration or surgical drainage of the abscess (Thompson et al., 1985; Maltz et al., 1991; Ravdin, 1995). The same applies to amebic liver abscesses in children (Nazir and Moazam, 1993).

If cysts are still present in the feces after apparent cure of amebic dysentery or an amebic liver abscess, then a poorly absorbed, primarily luminal-acting drug, such as diloxanide furoate should also be administered for 10 days (Adams and MacLeod, 1977a,b; Irusen et al., 1992).

7 Giardiasis

The recommended dosage for this infection is 2 g orally once a day, for 3 days. The equivalent dose for children aged 7–10 years is 1 g, for those aged 3–7 years 600 mg, and for those aged 1–3 years, 400 mg. This treatment schedule produces a higher parasitological cure rate than a standard course of quinacrine (mepacrine, 'Atabrine') (Wright et al., 1977). A 5-day course of metronidazole was superior to quinacrine given for 5 days to treat giardiasis in Iran (Kavousi, 1979). Metronidazole also resulted in a higher cure rate than furazolidone (p. 922) in another study (Levi et al., 1977). Single-dose treatment with metronidazole (2.4 g) is not as effective as single-dose treatment with tinidazole (2 g) (p. 962) (Jokipii and Jokipii, 1979) but 2 g metronidazole on 2 consecutive days seems as effective as a single dose of 2 g tinidazole (Kyrönseppä and Pettersson, 1981).

8 Microsporidiosis

Infections by Enterocytozoon spp. in normal hosts cause a self-limiting diarrhea, which requires no treatment (Sandfort et al., 1994). Microsporidia in AIDS patients cause chronic diarrhea and pulmonary, ocular, muscular and renal disease (Weber and Bryan, 1994). Metronidazole therapy has only resulted in transient improvement of diarrhea in some AIDS patients and albendazole appears more effective (Molina et al., 1993; Asmuth et al., 1994). Disseminated infections may also respond to albendazole (De Groote et al., 1995).

9 Helicobacter pylori infection

Triple-drug therapy of bismuth subcitrate 120 mg four times daily, tetracycline 500 mg four times daily and metronidazole 400 mg three times daily, all given for 2 weeks, most consistently heals duodenal ulcers and eradicates H. pylori infection (see tetracyclines, p. 743). Results are still good if the tetracycline dose is reduced to 250 mg four times daily and metronidazole to 400 mg twice-daily (Iser et al., 1994).

The classical higher dose triple therapy eradicates H. pylori from some 90% of patients if the pre-treatment strain is metronidazole-sensitive, but only from some 68% of patients if the strain is metronidazole-resistant. Pretreatment sensitivity testing of the H. pylori strain may therefore be important. However, double therapy with bismuth and tetracycline is successful in less than 68% of patients, which indicates that metronidazole contributes something to therapy even when the pretreatment strain is resistant to this drug (Rautelin et al., 1992; Axon, 1993; Noach et al., 1994; Van Zwet et al., 1995; Goddard and Logan, 1996).

Other regimens which are successful in eradicating *H. pylori* infection include amoxycillin/omeprazole (p. 142) and clarithromycin/omeprazole (p. 649).

10 Rosacea

In a small controlled trial involving 29 patients with rosacea, 6 weeks treatment with metronidazole in an oral dose of 200 mg twice-daily was therapeutically superior to treatment with a placebo (Pye and Burton, 1976). The drug was particularly effective against papules and pustules, but had relatively little effect on the erythema. Later, metronidazole 200 mg or oxytetracycline 250 mg both given twice-daily for 12 weeks were compared; both drugs produced similar improvement (Saihan and Burton, 1980). The mode of action of metronidazole in rosacea is not understood. Topical metronidazole is also beneficial to patients with rosacea (Bleicher *et al.*, 1987; Schmadel and McEvoy, 1990).

References

Acar JF, Goldstein FW, Kitzis MD, Eyquem MT (1981). Resistance pattern of anaerobic bacteria isolated in a general hospital during a two-year period. *J Antimicrob Chemother* **8** (Suppl D): 9.

Achumba JI, Ette EI, Thomas WO, Essien EE (1988). Chloroquine-induced acute dystonic reactions in the presence of metronidazole. *Drug Intell Clin Pharm* **22**: 308.

Adams EB, MacLeod IN (1977a). Invasive amebiasis. I. Amebic dysentery and its complications. *Medicine* **56**: 315.

Adams EB, MacLeod IN (1977b). Invasive amebiasis. II. Amebic liver abscess and its complications. *Medicine* **56**: 325.

Ahmadsyah I, Salim A (1985). Treatment of tetanus: an open study to compare the efficacy of procaine penicillin and metronidazole. *Brit Med J* **291**: 648.

Alawattegama AB, Jones BM, Kinghorn GR *et al.* (1984). Single dose versus seven day metronidazole in *Gardnerella vaginalis* associated non-specific vaginitis. *Lancet* **i**: 1355.

Aldridge KE, Gelfand M, Reller LB *et al.* (1994). A five-year multicenter study of the susceptibility of the *Bacteroides* fragilis group isolates to cephalosporins, cephamins, penicillins, clindamycin, and metronidazole in the United States. *Diagn Microbiol Infect Dis* **18**: 235.

Anonymous (1990). A randomized multicentre trial of pefloxacin plus metronidazole and gentamicin plus metronidazole in the treatment of severe intra-abdominal infections. Report from a Swedish Study Group. *J Antimicrob Chemother* **26** (Suppl B): 173.

Anonymous (1992). Results of a multicentre European survey in 1991 of metronidazole resistance in *Helicobacter pylori*. European Study Group on Antibiotic Susceptibility of *Helicobacter pylori*. *Eur J Clin Microbiol Infect Dis* **11**: 777.

Appelbaum PC, Spangler SK, Jacobs MR (1990). Beta-lactamase production and susceptibilities to amoxicillin, amoxicillin-clavulanate, ticarcillin, ticarcillin-clavulanate, cefoxitin, imipenem, and metronidazole of 320 non-*Bacteroides fragilis Bacteroides* isolates and 129 fusobacteria from 28 US centers. *Antimicrob Ag Chemother* **34**: 1546.

Appleman MD, Heseltine PN, Cherubin CE (1991). Epidemiology, antimicrobial susceptibility, pathogenicity, and significance of *Bacteroides fragilis* group organisms isolated at Los Angeles County – University of Southern California Medical Center. *Rev Infect Dis* **13**: 12.

Aprahamian C, Schein M, Wittmann D (1995). Cefotaxime and metronidazole in severe intra-abdominal infection. *Diagn Microbiol Infect Dis* **22**: 183.

Ashford RFU, Plant GT, Maher J *et al.* (1980). Metronidazole in smelly tumours. *Lancet* **i**: 874.

Ashford R, Plant G, Maher J, Teares L (1984). Double-blind trial of metronidazole in malodorous ulcerating tumours. *Lancet* **i**: 1232.

Asmuth DM, DeGirolami PC, Federman M *et al.* (1994). Clinical features of microsporidiosis in patients with AIDS. *Clin Infect Dis* **18**: 819.

Austin TW, Smith EA, Darwish R *et al.* (1982). Metronidazole in a single dose for the treatment of trichomoniasis. Failure of a 1-g single dose. *Brit J Vener Dis* **58**: 121.

Axon ATR (1993). *Helicobacter pylori* infection. *J Antimicrob Chemother* **32** (Suppl A): 61.

Bäck E, Hermanson J, Wickman M (1978). Metronidazole treatment of liver abscess due to *Bacteroides fragilis*. *Scand J Infect Dis* **10**: 152.

Bailes J, Willis J, Priebe C, Strub R (1983). Encephalopathy with metronidazole in a child. *Amer J Dis Child* **137**: 290.

Balsdon MJ, Jackson D (1981). Metronidazole metabolite and *Gardnerella vaginalis* (*Corynebacterium vaginale*). *Lancet* **i**: 1112.

Balsdon MJ, Taylor GE, Pead L, Maskell R (1980). *Corynebacterium vaginale* and vaginitis: a controlled trial of treatment. *Lancet* **i**: 501.

Barker EM, Aitchison JM, Cridland JS, Baker LW (1983). Rectal administration of metronidazole in severely ill patients. *Brit Med J* **287**: 311.

Bartlett JG (1983). Recent developments in the management of anaerobic infections. *Rev Infect Dis* **5**: 235.

Bartlett JG (1984). Treatment of antibiotic-associated pseudomembranous colitis. *Rev Infect Dis* **6**: 235.

Beard CM, Noller KL, O'Fallon WH *et al.* (1979). Lack of evidence for cancer due to use of metronidazole. *New Engl J Med* **301**: 519.

Beard CM, Noller KL, O'Fallon WM, Kurland LT, Dahlin DC (1988). Cancer after exposure to metronidazole. *Mayo Clin Proc* **63**: 147.

Berger SA, Kupferminc M, Lessing JB *et al.* (1990). Penetration of clindamycin, cefoxitin, and metronidazole into pelvic peritoneal fluid of women undergoing diagnostic laparoscopy. *Antimicrob Ag Chemother* **34**: 376.

Berman BW, King FH, Rubenstein DS, Long SS (1978). *Bacteroides fragilis* meningitis in a neonate successfully treated with metronidazole. *J Pediatr* **93**: 793.

Bernstein LH, Frank MS, Brandt LJ, Boley SJ (1980). Healing of perineal Crohn's disease with metronidazole. *Gastroenterology* **79**: 357.

Betriu C, Campos E, Cabronero C *et al.* (1990). Susceptibilities of species of the *Bacteroides fragilis* group to 10 antimicrobial agents. *Antimicrob Ag Chemother* **34**: 671.

Betriu C, Cabronero C, Gomez M, Picazo JJ (1992). Changes in the susceptibility of *Bacteroides fragilis* group organisms to various antimicrobial agents 1979–1989. *Eur J Clin Microbiol Infect Dis* **11**: 352.

Beumont MG, Duncan J, Mitchell SD, Esterhai JL, Jr, Edelstein PH (1995). *Veillonella myositis* in an immunocompromised patient. *Clin Infect Dis* **21**: 678.

Birkett DJ, Pond SM (1975). Metabolic drug interactions – a critical review. *Med J Aust* **1**: 687.

Blackwell A (1984). Leading article. Anaerobic vaginosis: therapeutic and epidemiological aspects. *J Antimicrob Chemother* **14**: 445.

Blackwell AL, Fox AR, Phillips I, Barlow D (1983). Anaerobic vaginosis (non-specific vaginitis): clinical, microbiological and therapeutic findings. *Lancet* **ii**: 1379.

Blake P, Butt WE (1984). Ototoxicity of metronidazole. *NZ Med J* **97**: 241.

Bleicher PA, Charles JH, Sober AJ (1987). Topical metronidazole therapy for rosacea. *Arch Dermatol* **123**: 609.

Blyden GT, Scavone JM, Greenblatt DJ (1988). Metronidazole impairs clearance of phenytoin but not of alprazolam or lorazepam. *J Clin Pharmacol* **28**: 240.

Boeckh M, Lode H, Deppermann KM *et al.* (1990). Pharmacokinetics and serum bactericidal activities of quinolones in combination with clindamycin, metronidazole, and ornidazole. *Antimicrob Ag Chemother* **34**: 2407.

Bolton RP (1979). *Clostridium difficile*-associated colitis after neomycin treated with metronidazole. *Brit Med J* **2**: 1479.

Bolton RP, Culshaw MA (1986). Faecal metronidazole concentrations during oral and intravenous therapy for antibiotic associated colitis due to *Clostridium difficile*. *Gut* **27**: 1169.

Bolton RP, Read AE (1982). *Clostridium difficile* in toxic megacolon complicating acute inflammatory bowel disease. *Brit Med J* **285**: 475.

Bolton RP, Sherriff RJ, Read AE (1980). *Clostridium difficile* associated diarrhoea: a role in inflammatory bowel disease. *Lancet* **i**: 383.

Boreham PFL, Phillips RE, Shepherd RW (1984). The sensitivity of *Giardia intestinalis* to drugs *in vitro*. *J Antimicrob Chemother* **14**: 449.

Boyce EG, Cookson ET, Bond WS (1990). Persistent metronidazole-induced peripheral neuropathy. *DICP* **24**: 19.

Bradley WG, Karlsson IJ, Rassol CG (1977). Metronidazole neuropathy. *Brit Med J* **2**: 610.

Brandt LJ, Bernstein LH, Boley SJ, Frank MS (1982). Metronidazole therapy for perineal Crohn's disease: a follow-up study. *Gastroenterology* **83**: 383.

Brazier JS, Levett PN, Stannard AJ *et al.* (1985). Antibiotic susceptibility of clinical isolates of clostridia. *J Antimicrob Chemother* **15**: 181.

Brogan O, Garnett PA, Brown R (1989). *Bacteroides fragilis* resistant to metronidazole, clindamycin and cefoxitin. *J Antimicrob Chemother* **23**: 660.

Brook I, Finegold SM (1980). Bacteriology of aspiration pneumonia in children. *Pediatrics* **65**: 1115.

Brook I, Frazier EH (1993). Significant recovery of nonsporulating anaerobic rods from clinical specimens. *Clin Infect Dis* **16**: 476.

Burdon DW, Brown JD, Youngs DJ *et al.* (1979). Antibiotic susceptibility of *Clostridium difficile*. *J Antimicrob Chemother* **5**: 307.

Burtin P, Taddio A, Ariburnu O, Einarson TR, Koren G (1995). Safety of metronidazole in pregnancy: a meta-analysis. *Amer J Obstet Gynecol* **172**: 525.

Bush A, Holt JE, Sankey MG *et al.* (1983). Concentrations of metronidazole and its major metabolites in continuous ambulatory peritoneal dialysate. *J Antimicrob Chemother* **12**: 294.

Cassey JG, Clark DA, Merrick P, Jones B (1983). Pharmacokinetics of metronidazole in patients undergoing peritoneal dialysis. *Antimicrob Ag Chemother* **24**: 950.

Celifarco A, Warschauer C, Burakoff R (1989). Metronidazole-induced pancreatitis. *Am J Gastroenterol* **84**: 958.

CDC (Centers for Disease Control) (1993). Sexually transmitted diseases treatment guidelines. *MMWR* **42** (No RR-14).

Chan FT, Guan MX, Mackenzie AM, Diaz-Mitoma F (1994). Susceptibility testing of *Dientamoeba fragilis* ATCC 30948 with iodoquinol, paromomycin, tetracycline, and metronidazole. *Antimicrob Ag Chemother* **38**: 1157.

Chapman RW, Selby WS, Jewell DP (1986). Controlled trial of intravenous metronidazole as an adjunct to corticosteroids in severe ulcerative colitis. *Gut* **27**: 1210.

Cherry RD, Portnoy D, Jabbari M *et al.* (1982). Metronidazole: an alternate therapy for antibiotic-associated colitis. *Gastroenterology* **82**: 849.

Chow AW, Cheng N, Bartlett KH (1985). *In vitro* susceptibility of *Clostridium difficile* to new β-lactam and quinolone antibiotics. *Antimicrob Ag Chemother* **28**: 842.

Chrystal EJT, Koch RL, McLafferty MA, Goldman P (1980). Relationship between metronidazole metabolism and bactericidal activity. *Antimicrob Ag Chemother* **18**: 566.

Citronberg RJ, Semel JD (1995). Severe vaginal infection with *Entamaoeba histolytica* in a woman who recently returned from Mexico; case report and review. *Clin Infect Dis* **20**: 700.

Corey WA, Doebbeling BN, DeJong KJ, Britigan BE (1991). Metronidazole-induced acute pancreatitis. *Rev Infect Dis* **13**: 1213.

Corson AP, Chretien JH (1994). Metronidazole-associated aseptic meningitis. *Clin Infect Dis* **19**: 974.

Cosar C, Julou L (1959). Activité de l'(hydroxy-2-éthyl).-1-méthyl-2-nitro-5-imidazole (8823 RP). vis-à-vis des infections expérimentales à *Trichomonas vaginalis. Ann Inst Pasteur Paris* **96**: 238.

Cosar C, Ganter P, Julou L (1961). Etude expérimentale du métronidazole (8823 R.P.). Activités trichomonacide et amoebicide. Toxicité et propriétés pharmacologiques générales. *Presse Méd* **69**: 1069.

Csonka GW (1971). Trichomonal vaginitis treated with one dose of metronidazole. *Brit J Vener Dis* **47**: 456.

Dachs GU, Abratt VR, Woods DR (1995). Mode of action of metronidazole and a *Bacteroides fragilis* metA resistance gene in *Escherichia coli*. *J Antimicrob Chemother* **35**: 483.

Danielson DA, Hannan MT, Jick H (1982). Metronidazole and cancer. *JAMA* **247**: 2498.

Dankert J, Holloway Y, Bouma J *et al.* (1981). Metronidazole in smelly gynaecological tumours. *Lancet* **ii** 1295.

Davidson S, Kaplinsky C, Frand M, Rotem J (1982). Treatment of infectious mononucleosis with metronidazole in the pediatric age group. *Scand J Infect Dis* **14**: 103.

Davies AH (1967). Metronidazole in human infections with syphilis. *Brit J Vener Dis* **43**: 197.

Davies AH, McFadzean JA, Squires S (1964). Treatment of Vincent's stomatitis with metronidazole. *Brit Med J* **1**: 1149.

De Groote MA, Visvesvara G, Wilson ML *et al.* (1995). Polymerase chain reaction and culture confirmation of disseminated *Encephalitozoon cuniculi* in a patient with AIDS: successful therapy with albendazole. *J Infect Dis* **171**: 1375.

De Louvois J (1978). The bacteriology and chemotherapy of brain abscess. *J Antimicrob Chemother* **4**: 395.

De Louvois J (1983). Antimicrobial chemotherapy in the treatment of brain abscess. *J Antimicrob Chemother* **12**: 205.

Denys GA, Jerris RC, Swenson JM, Thornsberry C (1983). Susceptibility of *Propionibacterium acnes* clinical isolates to 22 antimicrobial agents. *Antimicrob Ag Chemother* **23**: 335.

Deutsch G, Foster JL, McFadzean JA, Parnell M (1975). Human studies with 'high dose' metronidazole: a non-toxic radiosensitiser of hypoxic cells. *Brit J Cancer* **31**: 75.

Dinh HT, Kernbaum S, Frottier J (1978). Treatment of antibiotic-induced colitis by metronidazole. *Lancet* **i**: 338.

Donald FE (1990). Treatment of brain abscess. *J Antimicrob Chemother* **25**: 310.

Donald FE, Firth JL, Holland IM *et al.* (1990). Brain abscess in the 1980s. *Br J Neurosurg* **4**: 265.

Dubreuil L, Devos J, Neut C, Romond C (1984). Susceptibility of anaerobic bacteria from several French hospitals to three major antibiotics. *Antimicrob Ag Chemother* **25**: 764.

Duerden BI (1995). Role of the reference laboratory in susceptibility testing of anaerobes and a survey of isolates referred from laboratories in England and Wales during 1993–1994. *Clin Infect Dis* **20** (Suppl 2): S180.

Dunn PM, Stewart-Brown S, Peel R (1979). Metronidazole and the fetal alcohol syndrome. *Lancet* **ii**: 144.

Durel P, Roiron V, Siboulet H, Borel LJ (1959). Trial of an anti-trichomonal derivative of imidazole (8823 R.P.). *Comptes Rendus Soc Franç Gyn* **29**: 36.

Earl P, Sisson PR, Ingham HR (1989). Twelve-hourly dosage schedule for oral and intravenous metronidazole. *J Antimicrob Chemother* **23**: 619.

Easmon CSF, Ison CA, Kaye CM *et al.* (1982). Pharmacokinetics of metronidazole and its principal metabolites and their activity against *Gardnerella vaginalis. Brit J Vener Dis* **58**: 246.

Edwards DI (1979). Mechanism of antimicrobial action of metronidazole. *J Antimicrob Chemother* **5**: 499.

Edwards DI (1993a). Nitroimidazole drugs – action and resistance mechanisms. I. Mechanisms of action. *J Antimicrob Chemother* **31**: 9.

Edwards DI (1993b). Nitroimidazole drugs – action and resistance mechanisms. II. Mechanisms of resistance. *J Antimicrob Chemother* **31**: 201.

Edwards DI, Mathison GE (1970). The mode of action of metronidazole against *Trichomonas vaginalis. J Gen Microbiol* **63**: 297.

Edwards DI, Dye M, Carne H (1973). The selective toxicity of antimicrobial nitro-heterocyclic drugs. *J Gen Microbiol* **76**: 135.

Eykyn S, Phillips I (1976). Metronidazole and anaerobic sepsis. *Brit Med J* **2**: 1418.

Eykyn SJ, Jackson BT, Lockhart-Mummery HE, Phillips I (1979). Prophylactic preoperative intravenous metronidazole in elective colorectal surgery. *Lancet* **ii**: 761.

Fan ST, Lau WY, Teoh-Chan CH, Lau KF, Mauracher EH (1988). Once daily administration of netilmicin compared with thrice daily, both in combination with metronidazole, in gangrenous and perforated appendicitis. *J Antimicrob Chemother* **22**: 69.

Farrell G, Zaluzny L, Baird-Lambert J *et al.* (1983). Impaired elimination of metronidazole in decompensated chronic liver disease. *Brit Med J* **287**: 1845.

Fekety R (1983). Recent advances in management of bacterial diarrhoea. *Rev Infect Dis* **5**: 246.

Fekety R, Silva J, Buggy B, Deery HG (1984). Treatment of antibiotic-associated colitis with vancomycin. *J Antimicrob Chemother* **14** (Suppl D): 97.

Fisher LS, Chow AW, Lindquist L, Guze LB (1976). Failure of metronidazole in amebic liver abscess. *Amer J Med Sci* **271**: 65.

Foster MC, Kapila L, Morris DL, Slack RC (1986). A randomized comparative study of sulbactam plus ampicillin vs. metronidazole plus cefotaxime in the management of acute appendicitis in children. *Rev Infect Dis* **8** (Suppl 5): S634.

Franssen FF, Lumeij JT, van Knapen F (1995). Susceptibility of *Encephalitozoon cuniculi* to several drugs in vitro. *Antimicrob Ag Chemother* **39**: 1265.

Freeman WA, McFadzean JA, Whelan JPF (1968). Activity of metronidazole against experimental tetanus and gas gangrene. *J Appl Bact* **31**: 443.

Friedman GD (1980). Cancer after metronidazole. *New Engl J Med* **302**: 519.

Friedman GD, Selby JV (1990). How often does metronidazole induce pancreatitis? *Gastroenterology* **98**: 1702.

Frytak S, Moertel CG, Childs DS, Albers JW (1978). Neurologic toxicity associated with high-dose metronidazole therapy. *Ann Intern Med* **88**: 361.

Gabriel R, Page CM, Collier J *et al.* (1980). Removal of metronidazole by haemodialysis. *Brit J Surg Vol* **67**: 553.

Garcia-Rodriguez JE, Garcia-Sanchez JE (1990). Evolution of antimicrobial susceptibility in isolates of the *Bacteroides fragilis* group in Spain. *Rev Infect Dis* **12** (Suppl 2): S142.

George RH, Bint AJ (1976). Treatment of brain abscess due to *Bacteroides fragilis* with metronidazole. *J Antimicrob Chemother* **2**: 101.

George WL (1984). Antimicrobial agent-associated colitis and diarrhoea: historical background and clinical aspects. *Rev Infect Dis* **6** (Suppl 1): 208.

George WL, Kirby BD, Sutter JL *et al.* (1982). Intravenous metronidazole for treatment of infections involving anaerobic bacteria. *Antimicrob Ag Chemother* **21**: 441.

Gerstner GJ (1982). Chemoprophylaxis for major gynaecological and obstetric surgery. *J Antimicrob Chemother* **10**: 359.

Gilat T (1982). Editorial Metronidazole in Crohn's disease. *Gastroenterology* **83**: 702.

Gillespie G, McNaught W (1978). Prophylactic oral metronidazole in intestinal surgery. *J Antimicrob Chemother* **4** (Suppl C): 29.

Goddard AF, Logan RPH (1996). Antimicrobial resistance and *Helicobacter pyloris. J Antimicrob Chemother* **37**: 639.

Goldstein EJ, Citron DM, Cherubin CE, Hillier SL (1993). Comparative susceptibility of the *Bacteroides fragilis* group species and other anaerobic bacteria to meropenem, imipenem, piperacillin, cefoxitin, ampicillin/sulbactam, clindamycin and metronidazole. *J Antimicrob Chemother* **31**: 363.

Gomez J, Poza M, Martinez M *et al.* (1995). Use of cefotaxime and metronidazole for treating cerebral abscesses. *Clin Infect Dis* **21**: 708.

Gorbach SL (1993). Intraabdominal infections. *Clin Infect Dis* **17**: 961.

Gordts B, Hemelhof W, Asselman C, Butzler J-P (1985). *In vitro* susceptibilities of 25 *Giardia lamblia* isolates of human origin to six commonly used antiprotozoal agents. *Antimicrob Ag Chemother* **28**: 378.

Gray MS, Kane PO, Squires S (1961). Further observations on metronidazole (Flagyl). *Brit J Vener Dis* **37**: 278.

Guay DR, Meatherall RC, Baxter H *et al.* (1984). Pharmacokinetics of metronidazole in patients undergoing continuous ambulatory peritoneal dialysis. *Antimicrob Ag Chemother* **25**: 306.

Gupte S (1983). Phenobarbital and metabolism of metronidazole. *New Engl J Med* **308**: 529.

Guzman R, Kirkpatrick J, Forward K, Lim F (1988). Failure of parenteral metronidazole in the treatment of pseudomembranous colitis. *J Infect Dis* **158**: 1146.

Haas CE, Nix DE, Schentag JJ (1990). *In vitro* selection of resistant *Helicobacter pylori. Antimicrob Ag Chemother* **34**: 1637.

Haddock G, Hansell DT, McArdle CS (1988). Survey of antibiotic prophylaxis in gastrointestinal surgery in Scotland – 5 years on. *J Hosp Infect* **11**: 286.

Hager WD, Brown ST, Kraus SJ *et al.* (1980). Metronidazole for vaginal trichomoniasis. *JAMA* **244**: 1219.

Hale JE, Perinpanayagam RM, Smith G (1976). *Bacteroides*: an unusual cause of breast abscess. *Lancet* **ii**: 70.

Hall C, Curran F, Burdon DW, Keighley MR (1989). A randomized trial to compare amoxycillin/clavulanate with metronidazole plus gentamicin in prophylaxis in elective colorectal surgery. *J Antimicrob Chemother* **24** (Suppl B): 195.

Haller I (1982). *In vitro* activity of the two principal, oxidative metabolites of metronidazole against *Bacteroides fragilis* and related species. *Antimicrob Ag Chemother* **22**: 165.

Harding GKM, Nicolle Le, Haase DA *et al.* (1984). Prospective, randomized, comparative trials in the therapy for intraabdominal and female genital tract infections. *Rev Infect Dis* **6** (Suppl 1): 283.

Harrison HR, Crowe CP, Fulginiti VA (1979). Amebic liver abscess in children: clinical and epidemiologic features. *Pediatrics* **64**: 923.

Hartley-Asp B (1979). Mutagenicity of metronidazole. *Lancet* **i**: 275.

Hauth JC, Goldenberg RL, Andrews WW, DuBard MB, Copper RL (1995). Reduced incidence of preterm delivery with metronidazole and erythromycin in women with bacterial vaginosis. *New Engl J Med* **333**: 1732.

Haverkorn MJ (1987). A comparison of single-dose and multi-dose metronidazole prophylaxis for hysterectomy. *J Hosp Infect* **9**: 249.

He Q, Leitch GL, Visvesvara GS, Wallace S (1996). Effects of nifedipine, metronidazole, and nitric oxide donors on spore germination and cell culture infection of the *Microporidia Encephalitozoon hellem* and *Encephalitozoon intestinalis. Antimicrob Ag Chemother* **40**: 179.

Hedström SA (1980). Treatment of anginose infectious mononucleosis with metronidazole. A controlled clinical and laboratory study. *Scand J Infect Dis* **12**: 265.

Hibberd AD, Nicoll RJ, Macbeth WA (1984). Deafness in an adverse reaction to the prophylactic use of metronidazole. *NZ Med J* **97**: 128.

Hishon S, Pilling J (1977). Metronidazole neuropathy. *Brit Med J* **2**: 832.

Holter O, Bergan T, Flørenes T, Leinebø O (1983). Penetration of metronidazole to tissues. *J Antimicrob Chemother* **11**: 357.

Houang ET, Watson C, Howell R, Chapman M (1984). Ampicillin combined with sulbactam or metronidazole for single-dose chemoprophylaxis in major gynaecological surgery. *J Antimicrob Chemother* **14**: 529.

Houghton GW, Smith J, Thorne PS, Templeton R (1979). The pharmacokinetics of oral and intravenous metronidazole in man. *J Antimicrob Chemother* **5**: 621.

Ingham HR, Selkon JB, Hale JH (1975a). The antibacterial activity of metronidazole. *J Antimicrob Chemother* **1**: 355.

Ingham HR, Rich GE, Selkon JB et al. (1975b). Treatment with metronidazole of three patients with serious infections due to *Bacteroides fragilis*. *J Antimicrob Chemother* **1**: 235.

Ingham HR, Selkon JB, Roxby CM (1977). Bacteriological study of otogenic cerebral abscesses: chemotherapeutic role of metronidazole. *Brit Med J* **2**: 991.

Ingham HR, Selkon JB, Roxby CM (1978). The bacteriology and chemotherapy of otogenic cerebral abscesses. *J Antimicrob Chemother* **4** (Suppl C): 63.

Ingham HR, Hall CJ, Sisson PR et al. (1980a). The activity of metronidazole against facultatively anaerobic bacteria. *J Antimicrob Chemother* **6**: 343.

Ingham HR, Sisson PR, Selkon JB (1980b). Current concepts of the pathogenetic mechanisms of non-sporing anaerobes: chemotherapeutic implications. *J Antimicrob Chemother* **6**: 173.

Ingham HR, Sisson PR, Eisentadt RL et al. (1981). Enhancement of metronidazole by *Escherichia coli* under sub-optimal anaerobic conditions. *J Antimicrob Chemother* **8**: 475.

Ings RMJ, McFadzean JA, Ormerod WE (1974). The mode of action of metronidazole in *Trichomonas vaginalis* and other micro-organisms. *Biochem Pharmacol* **23**: 1421.

Ioannides L, Somogyi A, Spicer J et al. (1981). Rectal administration of metronidazole provides therapeutic plasma levels in postoperative patients. *New Engl J Med* **305**: 1569.

Irusen EM, Jackson TF, Simjee AE (1992). Asymptomatic intestinal colonization by pathogenic *Entamoeba histolytica* in amebic liver abscess: prevalence, response to therapy, and pathogenic potential. *Clin Infect Dis* **14**: 889.

Iser JH, Buttigieg RJ, Iseli A (1994). Low dose, short duration therapy for the eradication of *Helicobacter pylori* in patients with duodenal ulcer. *Med J Aust* **160**: 192.

Jackson D, Salem A, Coombs GH (1984). The *in vitro* activity of metronidazole against strains of *Escherichia coli* with impaired DNA repair systems. *J Antimicrob Chemother* **13**: 227.

Jacobs MR, Spangler SK, Appelbaum PC (1990). Susceptibility of *Bacteroides* non-*fragilis* and *fusobacteria* to amoxicillin, amoxicillin/clavulanate, ticarcillin, ticarcillin/clavulanate, cefoxitin, imipenem and metronidazole. *Eur J Clin Microbiol Infect Dis* **9**: 417.

Jager-Roman E, Doyle PE, Baird-Lambert J et al. (1982). Pharmacokinetics and tissue distribution of metronidazole in the newborn infant. *J Pediatr* **100**: 651.

Joesoef MR, Schmid GP (1995). Bacterial vaginosis: review of treatment options and potential clinical indications for therapy. *Clin Infect Dis* **20** (Suppl 1): S72.

Johnson S, Homann SR, Bettin KM et al. (1992). Treatment of asymptomatic *Clostridium difficile* carriers (fecal excretors) with vancomycin or metronidazole. A randomized, placebo-controlled trial. *Ann Intern Med* **117**: 297.

Johnson TA, Tabbut BR, Page CO (1981). Treatment of antibiotic-associated pseudomembranous colitis with metronidazole. *Amer J Hosp Pharm* **38**: 1034.

Jokipii L, Jokipii AMM (1979). Single-dose metronidazole and tinidazole as therapy for giardiasis: success rates, side effects and drug absorption and elimination. *J Infect Dis* **140**: 984.

Jokipii AMM, Jokipii L (1981). Metronidazole, tinidazole, ornidazole and anaerobic infections of the middle ear, maxillary sinus and central nervous system. *Scand J Infect Dis* (Suppl 26): 123.

Jokipii AM, Jokipii L (1987). Comparative activity of metronidazole and tinidazole against *Clostridium difficile* and *Peptostreptococcus anaerobius*. *Antimicrob Ag Chemother* **31**: 183.

Jokipii AMM, Myllylä VV, Hokkanen E, Jokipii L (1977). Penetration of the blood brain barrier by metronidazole and tinidazole. *J Antimicrob Chemother* **3**: 239.

Jones BM, Geary I, Alawattegama AN et al. (1985). *In-vitro* and *in-vivo* activity of metronidazole against *Gardnerella vaginalis*, *Bacteroides* spp and *Mobiluncus* spp in bacterial vaginosis. *J Antimicrob Chemother* **16**: 189.

Kane PO, McFadzean JA, Squires S et al. (1961a). Absorption and excretion of metronidazole. Part I. Serum concentration and urinary excretion after oral administration. *Brit J Vener Dis* **37**: 273.

Kane PO, McFadzean JA, Squires S (1961b). Absorption and excretion of metronidazole. Part II. Studies on primary failures. *Brit J Vener Dis* **37**: 276.

Karlsson IJ, Hamlyn AN (1977). Metronidazole neuropathy. *Brit Med J* **2**: 832.

Kavousi S (1979). Giardiasis in infancy and childhood: a prospective study of 160 cases with comparison of quinacrine (Atabrine) and metronidazole (Flagyl). *Amer J Trop Med Hyg* **28**: 19.

Keighley MRB, Arabi Y, Alexander-Williams J et al. (1979). Comparison between systemic and oral antimicrobial prophylaxis in colorectal surgery. *Lancet* ii: 894.

Khan MS, Begg HB, Frampton J, Hughes TB (1980). A comparative study of the prophylactic effect of one dose intravenous metronidazole therapy in gynaecological surgery. *Scand J Infect Dis* (Suppl 26): 115.

Kleinfeld DI, Sharpe RJ, Donta ST (1988). Parenteral therapy for antibiotic-associated pseudomembranous colitis. *J Infect Dis* **157**: 389.

Knapp CC, Ludwig MD, Washington JA (1991). *In vitro* activity of metronidazole against *Helicobacter pylori* as determined by agar dilution and agar diffusion. *Antimicrob Ag Chemother* **35**: 1230.

Knight R (1980). The chemotherapy of amoebiasis. *J Antimicrob Chemother* **6**: 577.

Knowles S, Choudhury T, Shear NH (1994). Metronidazole hypersensitivity. *Ann Pharmacother* **28**: 325.

Kolander SA, Cosgrove EM, Molavi A (1989). Clostridial endocarditis. Report of a case caused by *Clostridium bifermentans* and review of the literature. *Arch Intern Med* **149**: 455.

Koutsaimanis KG, Timms PW Ree GH (1979). Failure of metronidazole in a patient with hepatic amebic abscess. *Amer J Trop Med Hyg* **28**: 768.

Kreeft JH, Ogilvie RI, Dufresne LR (1983). Metronidazole kinetics in dialysis patients. *Surgery* **93**: 149.

Krook A, Kjellander J, Danielsson D (1982). Susceptibility of *Bacteroides* species to metronidazole during treatment of patients with Crohn's disease and healthy individuals. *Scand J Infect Dis* **14**: 45.

Kusumi RK, Plouffe JF, Wyatt RH, Fass RJ (1980). Central nervous system toxicity associated with metronidazole therapy. *Ann Intern Med* **93**: 59.

Kwok SP, Lau WY, Leung KL et al. (1993). Amoxycillin and clavulanic acid versus cefotaxime and metronidazole as antibiotic prophylaxis in elective colorectal resectional surgery. *Chemotherapy* **39**: 135.

Kyrönseppä H, Pettersson T (1981). Treatment of giardiasis: relative efficacy of metronidazole as compared with tinidazole. *Scand J Infect Dis* **13**: 311.

Lacey SL, Moss SF, Taylor GW (1993). Metronidazole uptake by sensitive and resistant isolates of *Helicobacter pylori*. *J Antimicrob Chemother* **32**: 393.

Lares-Asseff I, Cravioto J, Santiago P, Perez-Ortiz B (1993). A new dosing regimen for metronidazole in malnourished children. *Scand J Infect Dis* **25**: 115.

Lau AH, Chang CW, Sabatini S (1986). Hemodialysis clearance of metronidazole and its metabolites. *Antimicrob Ag Chemother* **29**: 235.

Lau AH, Evans R, Chang CW, Seligsohn R (1987). Pharmacokinetics of metronidazole in patients with alcoholic liver disease. *Antimicrob Ag Chemother* **31**: 1662.

Lau AH, Lam NP, Piscitelli SC, Wilkes L, Danziger LH (1992). Clinical pharmacokinetics of metronidazole and other nitroimidazole anti-infectives. *Clin Pharmacokinet* **23**: 328.

Law BJ, Marks MI (1980). Excellent outcome of *Bacteroides* meningitis in a newborn treated with metronidazole. *Pediatrics* **66**: 463.

Lawford R, Sorrell TC (1994). Amebic abscess of the spleen complicated by metronidazole-induced neurotoxicity: case report. *Clin Infect Dis* **19**: 346.

Leach JD, Eykyn SJ, Phillips I *et al.* (1979). Anaerobic axillary abscess. *Brit Med J* **2**: 5.

Leading article (1983). Anaerobic infections of the lung. *Lancet* **i**: 800.

Lefebvre Y, Hesseltine HC (1965). The peripheral white blood cells and metronidazole. *JAMA* **194**: 127.

Levi GC, de Avila CA, Neto VA (1977). Efficacy of various drugs for treatment of giardiasis. A comparative study. *Amer J Trop Med Hyg* **26**: 564.

Lindmark DG, Müller M (1976). Antitrichomonad action, mutagenicity and reduction of metronidazole and other nitroimidazoles. *Antimicrob Ag Chemother* **10**: 476.

Ljungberg B, Nilsson-Ehle I, Ursing B (1984). Metronidazole: pharmacokinetic observations in severely ill patients. *J Antimicrob Chemother* **14**: 275.

Lockie ACK (1981). Symptomatic cure of prostatitis with metronidazole. *Lancet* **ii**: 475.

Lossick JG (1990). Treatment of sexually transmitted vaginosis/vaginitis. *Rev Infect Dis* **12** (Suppl 6): S665.

Lumsden WHR, Harrison C, Robertson DHH (1988). Treatment failure in *Trichomonas vaginalis* infections in females. II. *In vitro* estimation of the sensitivity of the organsim to metronidazole. *J Antimicrob Chemother* **21**: 555.

Maltz G, Knauer CM (1991). Amebic liver abscess: a 15-year experience. *Amer J Gastroenterol* **86**: 704.

Markell EK (1995). Is there any reason to continue treating *Blastocystis* infections? *Clin Infect Dis* **21**: 104.

Martin C, Sastre B, Mallet MN *et al.* (1991). Pharmacokinetics and tissue penetration of a single 1000-milligram, intravenous dose of metronidazole for antibiotic prophylaxis of colorectal surgery. *Antimicrob Ag Chemother* **35**: 2602.

Mathisen GE, Meyer RD, George WL *et al.* (1984). Brain abscess and cerebritis. *Rev Infect Dis* **6** (Suppl 1): 101.

Mattila J, Männiströ PT, Mäntylä R *et al.* (1983). Comparative pharmacokinetics of metronidazole and tinidazole as influenced by administration route. *Antimicrob Ag Chemother* **23**: 721.

Matuchansky C, Aries J, Maire P (1978). Metronidazole for antibiotic-associated pseudomembranous colitis. *Lancet* **ii**: 580.

McDonald HM, O'Loughlin JA, Vigneswaran R, Jolley PT, McDonald PJ (1994). Bacterial vaginosis in pregnancy and efficacy of short-course oral metronidazole treatment: a randomized controlled trial. *Obstet Gynecol* **84**: 343.

McFadzean JA (1969). The absorption, distribution and metabolism of metronidazole. *Med Today* **3**: 10.

McGowan K, Gorbach SL (1981). Anaerobes in mixed infections. *J Infect Dis* **144**: 181.

McHenry MC (1977). Use in impaired renal function. Quoted by Roe (1977).

McKendrick MW, Geddes AM (1979). Neutropenia associated with metronidazole. *Brit Med J* **2**: 795.

McLean A, Ioannides-Demos L, Somogyi A *et al.* (1983). Successful substitution of rectal metronidazole administration for intravenous use. *Lancet* **i**: 41.

McNulty CAM, Dent J, Wise R (1985). Susceptibility of clinical isolates of *Campylobacter pyloridis* to 11 antimicrobial agents. *Antimicrob Ag Chemother* **28**: 837.

Mead PB, Gibson M, Schentag JJ, Ziemniak JA (1982). Possible alteration of metronidazole metabolism by phenobarbital. *New Engl J Med* **306**: 1490.

Mitelman F, Hartley-Asp B, Ursing B (1976). Chromosome aberrations and metronidazole. *Lancet* **ii**: 802.

Mitelman F, Strömbeck B, Ursing B *et al.* (1980). No cytogenetic effect of metronidazole. *Lancet* **i**: 1249.

Mohanty KC, Deighton R (1985). Comparison of two different metronidazole regimens in the treatment of *Gardnerella vaginalis* infection with or without trichomoniasis. *J Antimicrob Chemother* **16**: 799.

Molina J-M, Sarfati C, Beauvais B *et al.* (1993). Intestinal microsporidiosis in human immunodeficiency virus-infected patients with chronic unexplained diarrhea: prevalence and clinical and biologic features. *J Infect Dis* **167**: 217.

Morris DL, Hares MM, Voogt RJ *et al.* (1983). Metronidazole need not be combined with an aminoglycoside when used for prophylaxis in elective colorectal surgery. *J Hosp Inf* **4**: 65.

Narcisi EM, Secor WE (1996). *In vitro* effect of tinidzole and furazolidone on metronidazole-resistant *Trichomonas vaginalis*. *Antimicrob Ag Chemother* **40**: 1121.

Narikawa S, Suzuki T, Yamamoto M, Nakamura M (1991). Lactate dehydrogenase activity as a cause of metronidazole resistance in *Bacteroides fragilis* NCTC 11295. *J Antimicrob Chemother* **28**: 47.

Nazir Z, Moazam F (1993). Amebic liver abscess in children. *Pediatr Infect Dis J* **12**: 929.

Newman MG (1984). Anaerobic oral and dental infections. *Rev Infect Dis* **6** (Suppl 1): 107.

Nichols RL (1983). Empiric antibiotic therapy for intraabdominal infections. *Rev Infect Dis* **5** (Suppl): 90.

Nicolau DP, Patel KB, Quintiliani R, Nightingale CH (1995). Cephalosporin-metronidazole combinations in the management of intra-abdominal infections. *Diagn Microbiol Infect Dis* **22**: 189.

Nilsson-Ehle L, Ursing B, Nilsson-Ehle P (1981). Liquid chromatographic assay for metronidazole and tinidazole: pharmacokinetic and metabolic studies in human subjects. *Antimicrob Ag Chemother* **19**: 754.

Nix DE, Tyrrell R, Muller M (1995). Pharmacodynamics of metronidazole determined by a time-kill assay for *Trichomonas vaginalis*. *Antimicrob Ag Chemother* **39**: 1848.

Noach LA, Langenberg WL, Bertola MA (1994). Impact of metronidazole resistance on the eradication of *Helicobacter pylori*. *Scand J Infect Dis* **26**: 321.

O'Grady LR, Ralph ED (1976). Anaerobic meningitis and bacteremia caused by *Fusobacterium* species. *Amer J Dis Child* **130**: 871.

Ohnishi K, Murata M, Kojima H *et al.* (1994). Brain abscess due to infection with *Entamoeba histolytica*. *Amer J Trop Med Hyg* **51**: 180.

O'Keefe JP, Troc KA, Thompson KD (1982). Activity of metronidazole and its hydroxy and acid metabolites against clinical isolates of anaerobic bacteria. *Antimicrob Ag Chemother* **22**: 426.

Oliva SL, Guglielmo BJ, Jacobs R, Pons VG (1989). Failure of intravenous vancomycin and intravenous metronidazole to prevent or treat antibiotic-associated pseudomembranous colitis. *J Infect Dis* **159**: 1154.

O'Reilly RA (1976). The stereoselective interaction of warfarin and metronidazole in man. *New Engl J Med* **295**: 354.

Olson MM, Shanholtzer CJ, Lee JT, Jr, Gerding DN (1994). Ten years of prospective *Clostridium difficile*-associated disease surveillance and treatment at the Minneapolis VA Medical Center, 1982–1991. *Infect Control Hosp Epidemiol* **15**: 371.

Pankuch GA, Jacobs MR, Appelbaum PC (1993). Susceptibilities of 428 gram-positive and -negative anaerobic bacteria to Bay y3118 compared with their susceptibilities to ciprofloxacin, clindamycin, metronidazole, piperacillin, piperacillin-tazobactam, and cefoxitin. *Antimicrob Ag Chemother* **37**: 1649.

Pashby NL (1981). Metronidazole in the treatment of gas gangrene following lower limb amputation. *J Antimicrob Chemother* **8**: 82.

Pashby NL, Bolton RP, Sherriff RJ (1979). Oral metronidazole in *Clostridium difficile* colitis. *Brit Med J* **1**: 1605.

Pavicic MJ, van Winkelhoff AJ, de Graaff J (1992). *In vitro* susceptibilities of *Actinobacillus actinomycetemcomitans* to a number of antimicrobial combinations. *Antimicrob Ag Chemother* **36**: 2634.

Pavicic MJ, Namavar F, Verboom T, van Winkelhoff AJ, de Graaff J (1993). *In vitro* susceptibility of *Helicobacter pylori* to several antimicrobial combinations. *Antimicrob Ag Chemother* **37**: 1184.

Pavicic MJ, van Winkelhoff AJ, Pavivic-Temming YA, de Graaff J (1995). Metronidazole susceptibility factors in *Actinobacillus actinomycetemco-*

mitans. J Antimicrob Chemother **35**: 263.

Pendland SL, Piscitelli SC, Schreckenberger PC, Danziger LH (1994). *In vitro* activities of metronidazole and its hydroxy metabolite against *Bacteroides* spp. *Antimicrob Ag Chemother* **38**: 2106.

Peppercorn MA (1990). Advances in drug therapy for inflammatory bowel disease. *Ann Intern Med* **112**: 50.

Phillips I, Warren C, Taylor E *et al.* (1981). The antimicrobial susceptibility of anaerobic bacteria in a London teaching hospital. *J Antimicrob Chemother* **8** (Suppl D): 17.

Phillips I, King A, Nord CE, Hoffstedt B (1992). Antibiotic sensitivity of the *Bacteroides fragilis* group in Europe European Study Group. *Eur J Clin Microbiol Infect Dis* **11**: 292.

Piper JM, Mitchel EF, Ray WA (1993). Prenatal use of metronidazole and birth defects: no association. *Obstet Gynecol* **82**: 348.

Pittman FE (1973). Treatment of amoebic colitis. *Lancet* ii: 1325.

Plaisance KI, Quintiliani R, Nightingale CH (1988). The pharmacokinetics of metronidazole and its metabolites in critically ill patients. *J Antimicrob Chemother* **21**: 195.

Plotnick BN, Cohen I, Tsang T, Cullinane T (1985). Metronidazole-induced pancreatitis. *Ann Intern Med* **103**: 891.

Powell HR, Davidson PM, McCredie DA, Phair P, Walker RG (1988). Haemolytic-uraemic syndrome after treatment with metronidazole. *Med J Aust* **149**: 222.

Powell SJ, Macleod I, Wilmot AJ, Elsdon-Dew R (1966). Metronidazole in amoebic dysentery and amoebic liver abscess. *Lancet* ii: 1329.

Pye RJ, Burton JL (1976). Treatment of rosacea by metronidazole. *Lancet* i: 1211.

Radandt JM, Marchbanks CR, Dudley MN (1992). Interactions of fluoroquinolones with other drugs: mechanisms, variability, clinical significance, and management. *Clin Infect Dis* **14**: 272.

Ralph ED, Kirby WMM (1975a). Unique bactericidal action of metronidazole against *Bacteroides fragilis* and *Clostridium perfringens. Antimicrob Ag Chemother* **8**: 409.

Ralph ED, Kirby WMM (1975b). Bioassay of metronidazole with either anaerobic or aerobic incubation. *J Infect Dis* **132**: 587.

Ralph ED, Clarke JT, Libke RD *et al.* (1974). Pharmacokinetics of metronidazole as determined by bioassay. *Antimicrob Ag Chemother* **6**: 691.

Ramsay ID (1968). Endocrine ophthalmology. *Brit Med J* **4**: 706.

Rautelin H, Seppala K, Renkonen OV, Vainio U, Kosunen TU (1992). Role of metronidazole resistance in therapy of *Helicobacter pylori* infections. *Antimicrob Ag Chemother* **36**: 163.

Ravdin JI (1995). Amebiasis. *Clin Infect Dis* **20**: 1453.

Ravdin JI, Skilogiannis J (1989). *In vitro* susceptibilities of *Entamoeba histolytica* to azithromycin, CP- 63,956, erythromycin, and metronidazole. *Antimicrob Ag Chemother* **33**: 960.

Report of a Study Group (1974). Metronidazole in the prevention and treatment of *Bacteroides* infections in gynaecological patients. *Lancet* ii: 1540.

Report by a Study Group (1975). An evaluation of metronidazole in the prophylaxis and treatment of anaerobic infections in surgical patients. *J Antimicrob Chemother* **1**: 393.

Reysset G, Haggoud A, Sebald M (1993). Genetic resistance of *Bacteroides* species to 5-nitroimidazole. *Clin Infect Dis* **16** (Suppl 4): 401.

Riley TV, Karthigasu KT (1982). Chronic osteomyelitis due to *Clostridium difficile. Brit Med J* **284**: 1217.

Roe FJC (1977). Metronidazole: review of uses and toxicity. *J Antimicrob Chemother* **3**: 205.

Rosén A, Ursing B, Alm T *et al.* (1982). A comparative study of metronidazole and sulfasalazine for active Crohn's disease: the cooperative Crohn's disease study in Sweden. I. Design and methodologic considerations. *Gastroenterology* **83**: 541.

Rothstein E, Clancy DD (1969). The toxicity of disulfiram combined with metronidazole. *New Engl J Med* **280**: 1006.

Rowe-Jones DC, Peel AL, Kingston RD *et al.* (1990). Single dose cefotaxime plus metronidazole versus three dose cefuroxime plus metronidazole as prophylaxis against wound infection in colorectal surgery: multicentre prospective randomised study. *Brit Med J* **300**: 18.

Rubinstein G, Dunkin K, Howard AJ (1994). The susceptibility of *Helicobacter pylori* to 12 antimicrobial agents, omeprazole and bismuth salts. *J Antimicrob Chemother* **34**: 409.

Ruf B, Sandfort J (1994). Human microsporidiosis. *J Antimicrob Chemother* **34**: 609.

Rustia M, Shubik P (1972). Induction of lung tumours and malignant lymphomas in mice by metronidazole. *J Natl Cancer Inst* **48**: 721.

Rutgeerts P, Hiele M, Geboes K *et al.* (1995). Controlled trial of metronidazole treatment for prevention of Crohn's recurrence after ileal resection. *Gastroenterology* **108**: 1617.

Saginur R, Hawley CR, Bartlett JG (1980). Colitis associated with metronidazole therapy. *J Infect Dis* **141**: 772.

Saihan EM, Burton JL (1980). A double-blind trial of metronidazole versus oxytetracycline therapy for rosacea. *Brit J Dermatol* **102**: 443.

Salas-Herrera IG, Pearson RM, Johnston A, Turner P (1991). Concentration of metronidazole in cervical mucus and serum after single and repeated oral doses. *J Antimicrob Chemother* **28**: 283.

Samuelson JC, Burke A, Courval JM (1992). Susceptibility of an emetine-resistant mutant of *Entamoeba histolytica* to multiple drugs and channel blockers. *Antimicrob Ag Chemother* **36**: 2392.

Sanders CV, Hanna BJ, Lewis AC (1979). Metronidazole in the treatment of anaerobic infections. *Amer Rev Resp Dis* **120**: 337.

Sandfort J, Hannemann A, Gelderblom H *et al.* (1994). *Enterocytozoon bieneusi* infection in an immunocompetent patient who had acute diarrhea and who was not infected with human immunodeficiency virus. *Clin Infect Dis* **19**: 514.

Sanford KA, Mayle JE, Dean HA, Greenbaum DS (1988). Metronidazole-associated pancreatitis. *Ann Intern Med* **109**: 756.

Schmadel LK, McEvoy GK (1990). Topical metronidazole: a new therapy for rosacea. *Clin Pharm* **9**: 94.

Schneider J (1961). Treatment of giardiasis (lambliasis). with metronidazole. *Bull Soc Pathol Exot* **54**: 84.

Schwartz DE, Jeunet F (1976). Comparative pharmacokinetic studies of ornidazole and metronidazole in man. *Chemotherapy* **22**: 19.

Seggie J (1978). *Fusobacterium* endocarditis treated with metronidazole. *Brit Med J* **1**: 960.

Shepard TH, Fantel AG (1977). Is metronidazole teratogenic? *JAMA* **237**: 1617.

Shinn DLS (1962). Metronidazole in acute ulcerative gingivitis. *Lancet* i: 1191.

Sigeti JS, Guiney DG Jr, Davis CE (1983). Mechanism of action of metronidazole on *Bacteroides fragilis. J Infect Dis* **148**: 1083.

Sindar P, Britz ML, Wilkinson RG (1982). Isolation and properties of metronidazole-resistant mutants of *Clostridium perfringens. J Med Microbiol* **15**: 503.

Sisson PR, Ingham HR (1985). Action of metronidazole on facultative anaerobes. *J Infect Dis* **151**: 569.

Sjölin J, Lilja A, Eriksson N, Arneborn P, Cars O (1993). Treatment of brain abscess with cefotaxime and metronidazole: prospective study on 15 consecutive patients. *Clin Infect Dis* **17**: 857.

Smith BJD, Wellingham J (1976). Metronidazole in treatment of empyema. *Brit Med J* **1**: 1074.

Smith MA, Edwards DI (1995). Redox potential and oxygen concentration as factors in the susceptibility of *Helicobacter pylori* to nitroheterocyclic drugs. *J Antimicrob Chemother* **35**: 751.

Somogyi AA, Kong CB, Gurr FW *et al.* (1984). Metronidazole pharmacokinetics in patients with acute renal failure. *J Antimicrob Chemother* **13**: 183.

Soriano F, Aguado JM, Tornero J, Fernandez-Guerrero ML, Gomez-Garces JL (1986). *Bacteroides fragilis* meningitis successfully treated with metronidazole after a previous failure with thiamphenicol. *J Clin Microbiol* **24**: 472.

Speck WTA, Stein AB, Rosenkranz HS (1976). Mutagenicity of metronidazole: presence of several active metabolites in human urine. *J Natl Cancer Inst* **56**: 283.

Spelman DW, Newton-John HF (1982). Metronidazole in the treatment of anginose infectious mononucleosis. *Scand J Infect Dis* **14**: 99.

Spiegel CA (1987). Susceptibility of *Mobiluncus* species to 23 antimicrobial agents and 15 other compounds. *Antimicrob Ag Chemother* **31**: 243.

Spiegel CA, Amsel R, Eschenbach D *et al.* (1980). Anaerobic bacteria in non-specific vaginitis. *New Engl J Med* **303**: 601.

Sprott MS, Kearns AM (1988). Metronidazole-resistant *Bacteroides melaninogenicus*. *J Antimicrob Chemother* **22**: 951.

Sutter VL, Finegold SM (1976). Susceptibility of anaerobic bacteria to 23 antimicrobial agents. *Antimicrob Ag Chemother* **10**: 736.

Swedberg J, Steiner JF, Deiss F *et al.* (1985). Comparison of single-dose vs one-week course of metronidazole for symptomatic bacterial vaginosis. *JAMA* **254**: 1046.

Sweet RL (1981). Treatment of mixed aerobic-anaerobic infections of the female genital tract. *J Antimicrob Chemother* **8** (Suppl D): 105.

Tally FP, Malamy MH (1982). Mechanism of antimicrobial resistance and resitance transfer in anaerobic bacteria. *Scand J Infect Dis* (Suppl 35): 37.

Tally FP, Sutter VL, Finegold SM (1972). Metronidazole versus anaerobes *In vitro* data and initial clinical observations. *Calif Med* **117**: 22.

Tally FP, Sutter VL, Finegold SM (1975). Treatment of anaerobic infections with metronidazole. *Antimicrob Ag Chemother* **7**: 672.

Tally FP, Cuchural GJ Jr, Jacobus NV *et al.* (1985). Nationwide study of the susceptibility of the *Bacteroides fragilis* group in the United States. *Antimicrob Ag Chemother* **28**: 675.

Taylor JAT (1964). Metronidazole: a new agent for combined somatic and psychic therapy of alcoholism. *Bull Los Angeles Neurol Soc* **29**: 158.

Teasley DG, Gerding DN, Olson MM *et al.* (1983). Prospective randomised trial of metronidazole versus vancomycin for *Clostridium difficile*-associated diarrhea and colitis. *Lancet* **ii**: 1043.

Telalbasic S, Pikula ZP, Kapidzic M (1991). *Blastocystis hominis* may be a potential cause of intestinal disease. *Scand J Infect Dis* **23**: 389.

Templeton WC III, Wawrukiewicz A, Melo JC *et al.* (1983). Anaerobic osteomyelitis of long bones. *Rev Infect Dis* **5**: 692.

Thin RN, Symonds MAE, Booker R *et al.* (1979). Double-blind comparison of a single dose and a five-day course of metronidazole in the treatment of trichomoniasis. *Brit J Vener Dis* **55**: 354.

Thompson G, Clark AH, Hare K, Spilg WGS (1981). Pseudomembranous colitis after treatment with metronidazole. *Brit Med J* **282**: 864.

Thompson JE Jr, Forlenza S, Verma R (1985). Amebic liver abscess: a therapeutic approach. *Rev Infect Dis* **7**: 171.

Tidwell BH, Lushbaugh WB, Laughlin MD, Cleary JD, Finley RW (1994). A double-blind placebo-controlled trial of single-dose intravaginal versus single-dose oral metronidazole in the treatment of trichomonal vaginitis. *J Infect Dis* **170**: 242.

Triger DR (1978). Amoebic liver abscess in Wessex – a retrospective survey of 24 cases. *Trop Med Hyg* **81**: 54.

Turgeon P, Turgeon V, Gourdeau M *et al.* (1994). Longitudinal study of susceptibilities of species of the *Bacteroides fragilis* group to five antimicrobial agents in three medical centers. *Antimicrob Ag Chemother* **38**: 2276.

Turner P, Edwards R, Weston V *et al.* (1995). Simultaneous resistance to metronidazole, co-amoxiclav, and imipenem in clinical isolate of *Bacteroides fragilis*. *Lancet* **345**: 1275.

Uhari M, Seppanen J, Heikkinen E (1992). Imipenem-cilastatin vs tobramycin and metronidazole for appendicitis-related infections. *Pediatr Infect Dis J* **11**: 445.

Ursing B, Kamme C (1975). Metronidazole for Crohn's disease. *Lancet* **i**: 775.

Ursing B, Alm T, Bárány F *et al.* (1982). A comparative study of metronidazole and sulfasalazine for active Crohn's disease: the cooperative Crohn's disease study in Sweden. II. Result. *Gastroenterology* **83**: 550.

Urtasun R, Band P, Chapman JD *et al.* (1976). Radiation and high-dose netronidazole in supratnetorial glioblastomas. *New Engl J Med* **234**: 1364.

Van Kruiningen HJ (1995). On the use of antibiotics in Crohn's disease. *J Clin Gastroenterol* **20**: 310.

van Zwet AA, Thijs JC, Schievink-de Vries W, Schiphuis J, Snijder JA (1994). *In vitro* studies on stability and development of metronidazole resistance in *Helicobacter pylori*. *Antimicrob Ag Chemother* **38**: 360.

van Zwet AA, Thijs JC, de Graaf B (1995). Explanations for high rates of eradication with triple therapy using metronidazole in patients harboring metronidazole-resistant *Helicobacter pylori* strains. *Antimicrob Ag Chemother* **39**: 250.

Viitanen J, Haataja H, Männistö PT (1985). Concentrations of metronidazole and tinidazole in male genital tissues. *Antimicrob Ag Chemother* **28**: 812.

Visser AA, Hundt HKL (1984). The pharmacokinetics of a single intravenous dose of metronidazole in pregnant patients. *J Antimicrob Chemother* **13**: 279.

Voogd CE, Van Der Stel JJ, Jacobs JA (1974). The mutagenic action of nitroimidazoles. I. Metronidazole, nimorazole, dimetridazole and ronidazole. *Mutat Res* **26**: 483.

Weber R, Bryan RT (1994). Microsporidial infections in immunodeficient and immunocompetent patients. *Clin Infect Dis* **19**: 517.

Wheeler LA, De Meo M, Halula M *et al.* (1978). Use of high-pressure liquid chromatography to determine plasma levels of metronidazole and metabolites after intravenous administration. *Antimicrob Ag Chemother* **13**: 205.

White CM, Price JJ, Hunt KM (1980). Bone marrow aplasia associated with metronidazole. *Brit Med J* **280**: 647.

Wilcox MH, Howe R (1995). Diarrhea caused by *Clostridium difficile*: response time for treatment with metronidazole and vancomycin. *J Antimicrob Chemother* **36**: 673.

Willis AT, Ferguson IR, Jones PH *et al.* (1976). Metronidazole in prevention and treatment of *Bacteroides* infections after appendicectomy. *Brit Med J* **1**: 318.

Windle R, MacPherson S, Bell PRF (1979). Neutropenia associated with metronidazole. *Brit Med J* **2**: 1219.

Wolfe MS (1982). The treatment of intestinal protozoan infections. *Med Clin N Amer* **66**: 707.

Wood BA, Monro AM (1975). Pharmacokinetics of tinidazole and metronidazole in women after single large oral doses. *Brit J Vener Dis* **51**: 51.

Wright SG, Tomkins AM, Ridley DS (1977). Giardiasis: clinical and therapeutic aspects. *Gut* **18**: 343.

Xia H, Keane CT, Beattie S, O'Morain C (1994). Standardization of disc diffusion test and its clinical significance for susceptibility testing of metronidazole against *Helicobacter pylori*. *Antimicrob Ag Chemother* **38**: 2357.

Yoshioka K, Youngs DJ, Keighley MR (1991). A randomised prospective controlled study of ciprofloxacin with metronidazole versus amoxicillin/clavulanic acid with metronidazole in the treatment of intra-abdominal infection. *Infection* **19**: 25.

Zimmerman J, Silver J, Shapiro M *et al.* (1980). Clindamycin unresponsive anaerobic osteomyelitis treated with oral metronidazole. *Scand J Infect Dis* **12**: 79.

Tinidazole

Description

Tinidazole is a nitroimidazole drug similar to metronidazole (p. 936). It was synthesized in 1969 and *in vitro* it was very effective against *Trichomonas vaginalis* (Howes *et al.*, 1970). Like metronidazole, tinidazole is useful for other parasitic and also anaerobic bacterial infections.

Sensitive Organisms

1 Protozoa

The MIC of tinidazole against *T. vaginalis* is similar to that of metronidazole (p. 936), but its minimum trichomonicidal concentration is lower (Howes *et al.*, 1970; Forsgren and Wallin, 1977). Metronidazole-resistant strains of this parasite are also usually tinidazole-resistant (p. 936) (Sears and O'Hare, 1988), but Hamedi and Studemeister (1992) reported a *T. vaginalis* strain which was resistant to metronidazole but sensitive to tinidazole. The drug is also active against *Entamoeba histolytica* (Simjee *et al.*, 1985) and *Giardia lamblia* (Jokipii and Jokipii, 1980; Boreham *et al.*, 1984).

2 Anaerobic bacteria

Most bacterial species which are sensitive to tinidazole are inhibited by a concentration of 2–4 μg per ml.

a Gram-negative bacteria Most strains of *Bacteroides fragilis*, other members of the *B. fragilis* group, and the *Prevotella*, *Fusobacterium* and *Veillonella* spp. are sensitive (Reynolds *et al.*, 1975; Appelbaum *et al.*, 1978; Bergan, 1985; Jokipii and Jokipii, 1985; Anonymous, 1988). The microaerophilic organism, *Helicobacter pylori*, is usually sensitive, but strains resistant to metronidazole are also tinidazole-resistant. Patients previously exposed to either of these drugs, are more likely to harbor resistant strains (Loo *et al.*, 1992; Banatvala *et al.*, 1994; Rubinstein *et al.*, 1994). Tinidazole and particularly its hydroxy metabolite (p. 960) is quite active against *Gardnerella vaginalis* (Shanker and Munro, 1982; Kharsany *et al.*, 1993). *Mobiluncus curtisii* is usually tinidazole-resistant, but M. mulieris is usually sensitive (Spiegel, 1987).

b Gram-positive bacteria The *Peptococcus*, *Peptostreptococcus*, *Clostridium*, *Lactobacillus* and *Eubacterium* spp. are usually susceptible (Appelbaum and Chatterton, 1978; Olsson-Liljequist and Nord, 1981). *Clostridium difficile* is usually sensitive (Jokipii and Jokipii, 1987). *Actinomyces* and *Propionibacterium* spp. are resistant (Tally *et al.*, 1981; Nord, 1982).

3 Aerobic bacteria

Streptococci, staphylococci and enterobacteria are usually highly resistant. But under anaerobic conditions, the activity of tinidazole against *E. coli*, *Klebsiella* and *Proteus* spp., similar to metronidazole is enhanced (Nord, 1982).

4 Activity of tinidazole metabolites

The hydroxy metabolite (p. 960) is more active than the parent drug against *G. vaginalis* but it is about a quarter as potent against *B. fragilis* and 30-fold less active against *T. vaginalis* (Wood *et al.*, 1982).

Mode of Administration and Dosage

Tinidazole is usually administered by the oral route. The dosage varies according to the infection treated. The dosage for adults with trichomoniasis is a single dose of 2 g. For giardiasis in adults again a single dose of 2 g is recommended. A dose of 50 mg per kg body weight is appropriate as a single dose for children up to a maximum of 2 g. In amebic dysentery the adult dosage is 2 g daily for 2–3 days or 500 mg twice-daily for 5–10 days; for children 50 mg per kg daily (maximum 2 g) for 3 days. Similar doses are recommended for amebic liver abscess. For prevention of postoperative infection in adults a single dose of 2 g is usually given about 12 h before surgery.

Tinidazole is not recommended during the first trimester of pregnancy or for nursing mothers (see metronidazole, p. 939).

Availability

Tablets 500 mg.

Serum Levels in Relation to Dosage

1 Oral administration

Absorption after oral administration, similar to metronidazole, is almost complete. When a single oral dose of 2 g tinidazole was given to female volunteers, a mean serum level of 51 μg per ml was attained at 2 h, and this fell to 19.0 after 24 h, 4.2 after 48 h and 1.3 μg per ml at 72 h (Wood and Monro, 1975). These investigators also estimated metronidazole levels after a 2 g oral dose in a cross-over study; by bioassay metronidazole produced a higher peak level of 81 μg per ml, probably because of the presence of biologically active metabolites (p. 960), but by chemical assay its peak level of 40 μg per ml was lower. Metronidazole serum levels fell much more rapidly 4 h after administration, being one-third of the tinidazole level at 24 h, one-fifth of the tinidazole level at 48 h and undetectable at 72 h. These differences are due to the longer half-life of tinidazole which was estimated to be 12.5 h.

Other pharmacokinetic studies have used high-performance liquid chromatography for tinidazole estimation. Volunteers were given an oral dose of 2 g followed by four doses of 1 g at 24 h intervals. Peak serum levels occurred at about 2 h and mean concentrations on day 1 were 40.0 and 57.6 μg per ml and at the end of the first 24 h, 11.3 and 16.2 μg per ml for males and females, respectively. Following the 1-g tinidazole dose on day 5, about 1 h later mean peak serum levels of 26.3 and 36.2 μg per ml occurred for males and females, respectively. The serum half-life was 12.14 h (Wood et al., 1982).

Excretion

1 Urine

Following a single oral 250-mg dose, approximately 16% of the drug was recovered from the urine in an unchanged form (Taylor et al., 1970). When the drug was given by i.v. infusion, urinary recovery of the unchanged drug was 20–25%. The hydroxymethyl metabolite and its glucuronide conjugate accounted for 2% and another unnamed metabolite accounted for 10% of the dose excreted in the urine. After a 1600-mg i.v. dose urinary concentrations of tinidazole were greater than 10 μg per ml for 3 days (Wood et al., 1982).

2 Inactivation in body

Tinidazole is cleared from the body mainly by metabolism, presumably in the liver, producing a hydroxymethyl derivative, its glucuronide conjugate and two other water-soluble metabolites. Tinidazole is the main drug in the serum where only traces of the hydroxymethyl metabolite are detected (Wood et al., 1982).

3 Bile

Concentrations in bile are similar to those in the serum (Wood et al., 1982).

Distribution of the Drug in Body

Tinidazole (and metronidazole) is secreted in saliva where concentrations approximate to those in the serum at the time (Von Konow and Nord, 1982). Examination of tissues taken at operation demonstrate that the drug penetrates very well into genital tract tissue, abdominal muscle and bowel but not so well into liver and fat. Tinidazole is also secreted in breast milk in high concentrations (Wood *et al.*, 1982). Concentrations of metronidazole and tinidazole in the CSF are 42% and 80%, respectively, of the serum levels; the greater penetrability of tinidazole correlates with its greater lipid solubility (Jokipii and Jokipii, 1981). Concentrations of tinidazole (and metronidazole) in dental alveolar bone are about one-tenth of those obtained in serum (Von Konow and Nord, 1982).

Tinidazole is 21% bound to serum proteins (Taylor *et al.*, 1970).

Toxicity

As with metronidazole (p. 944), side-effects with tinidazole are usually mild and infrequent (Roe, 1985). If the drug is used for more prolonged periods than currently advocated, patients should be carefully observed for side-effects similar to those which have occurred with prolonged metronidazole therapy (p. 945). Nausea, vomiting, anorexia and a metallic or bitter taste in the mouth are the most common side-effects. Malaise, vertigo, pruritus, headache, constipation and skin rashes have been reported. The Australian Adverse Drug Reactions Advisory Committee received ten reports of hypersensitivity reactions, the majority being severe with urticaria, laryngeal edema, hypotension and bronchospasm, occurring in patients given tinidazole. There was the possibility that tartrazine used for coloring the tablets was the cause, and this has now been omitted from tinidazole tablets (McEwen, 1983). Dark urine has been observed in some patients after a single 2-g oral dose (Jones and Enders, 1977; Swami *et al.*, 1977). Tinidazole and metronidazole improve the depressed migration of neutrophil granulocytes which occurs in Crohn's disease but they have no effect on cells from normal people (Gnarpe *et al.*, 1981).

Tinidazole is not recommended for patients with a past history of a blood dyscrasia because, like metronidazole (p. 944), it may cause a leucopenia. Alcohol should be avoided during tinidazole therapy because it may cause the 'Antabuse syndrome' similar to metronidazole (p. 946).

Clinical Uses of the Drug

1 Treatment of anaerobic infections

Similar to metronidazole (p. 946) because of its *in vitro* activity against anaerobes (p. 959), tinidazole has been used for these infections. Packard (1982) summarized the results of uncontrolled trials of the use of the drug alone or with an agent active against aerobes (usually an aminoglycoside) for such infections in 264 patients. Clinical response was good in patients with septicemia, upper respiratory infections and sinusitis, bronchopulmonary infections, osteomyelitis, pelvic infections, septic abortion, intra-abdominal sepsis, cellulitis and post-operative wound infection. Nowadays metronidazole, which can be administered both i.v. or orally, is usually preferred for the treatment of these infections (p. 938).

Tinidazole, in combination with other drugs such as bismuth subcitrate, tetracycline, amoxycillin and omeprazole has been used in various regimens with success for the eradication of *H. pylori* infection (Marshall *et al.*, 1988; Bianchi Poro *et al.*, 1993; Jaup and Norrby, 1995; Saberi-Firoozi *et al.*, 1995). However, most clinicians use metronidazole rather than tinidazole for this indication (p. 951).

Tinidazole has been used in a single oral dose of 2 g to treat bacterial vaginosis (p. 947) with disappointing results (Van Der Meijden, 1983). Results obtained by Mohanty and Deighton (1987), however, were satisfactory when the same single dose of the drug was used.

2 Chemoprophylaxis of anaerobic infections

Tinidazole, similar to metronidazole (p. 949), has been used to prevent anaerobic bacterial infections after surgical and dental procedures. For this purpose, it has usually been given orally 12 h before surgery and sometimes combined with a drug active against aerobic bacteria (Packard, 1982; Dhar *et al.*, 1993a,b). Tinidazole has been useful in preventing infection after colorectal surgery (Packard, 1982; University of Melbourne, 1983; Giercksky and Danialsen, 1990); obstetric and gynecological surgery (Janssens *et al.*, 1982; Packard, 1982; Seligman, 1982; Dhar *et al.*, 1993a,b) and oral surgery (McGregor *et al.*, 1982).

3 Trichomoniasis

Tinidazole is an effective drug when given orally for the treatment of urogenital trichomoniasis in both males and females. Wherever possible the patient's sexual partner should be treated simultaneously to prevent reinfection. A high cure rate was obtained when the drug was given in an oral dose of 150 mg twice-daily for 7 days, or 150 mg three times daily for 5 days. Subsequent to the successful use of single-dose metronidazole treatment for trichomoniasis (p. 950), tinidazole is now also used in this manner. A single oral dose of 2 g tinidazole results in a cure rate usually in excess of 90% (Wallin and Forsgren, 1974; Jones and Enders, 1977; Hillström et al., 1977). Trichomonal infections in men respond to drug treatment better than those in women; Kawamura (1978) found that 1 g tinidazole or 1.5 g metronidazole were equally effective for this purpose. Single-dose therapy has the advantages of being more acceptable to the patient's sexual partner, and of requiring a shorter period for abstinence from sexual intercourse and intake of alcohol. Rarely metronidazole- and tinidazole-resistant strains of T. vaginalis are encountered (pp. 936,959) and infections by these do not respond to treatment by either drug.

4 Giardiasis

Multiple- and single-dose regimens have both been used successfully to treat this disease (p. 951). Andersson et al. (1972) used tinidazole in an oral dose of 150 mg twice-daily for 7 days, and obtained a high cure rate amongst students in Sweden. This 7-day regimen has been found to be slightly more effective than a similar regimen using metronidazole (Levi et al., 1977). Single-dose therapy using 2 g of tinidazole orally has also resulted in cure rates of 90–100% (Farid et al., 1974; Pettersson, 1975; Levi et al., 1977). Single-dose treatment with metronidazole (60 mg per kg body weight to a maximum of 2.4 g) is inferior to treatment with a single dose of tinidazole (50 mg per kg to a maximum dose of 2 g); moreover this single-dose treatment with tinidazole was equally effective to 3 days treatment with metronidazole (50 mg per kg per day, maximum 2 g dose) (Speelman, 1985). Pettersson (1975) used a single oral dose of 1 g to successfully treat children with giardiasis. Gazder and Banerjee (1977) compared single oral doses of 50 mg per kg body weight of tinidazole and metronidazole for the treatment of giardiasis in children; clinical and parasitological cures were much higher in the children treated with tinidazole. Similarly, Welch et al. (1978) found that single doses of 1.0–1.5 g (depending on the patient's weight) of tinidazole was as effective as a 5-day course of metronidazole for eradicating G. lamblia from children aged 6–9 years; the same dose of tinidazole given for 3 consecutive days was somewhat more effective. Patients not cured by a first course of treatment usually respond to a second course of tinidazole.

5 Amebiasis

Similar to metronidazole (p. 951), tinidazole is also effective for the treatment of this disease. For intestinal infection, a dose for adults of 600 mg twice-daily, for a period of 5 or 10 days, has been used (Misra and Laiq, 1974; Joshi and Shah, 1975). Three single daily oral doses of approximately 60 mg per kg body weight have been used for children with intestinal amebiasis; this resulted in a high cure rate and was well tolerated (Scragg and Proctor, 1977). In two studies the efficacy of an oral dose of 2 g tinidazole given for 3 consecutive days has been compared with an identical metronidazole regimen for the treatment of intestinal amebiasis. Both studies showed a cure rate in excess of 90% with tinidazole and one of less than 60% with metronidazole (Swami et al., 1977; Singh and Kumar, 1977). In another trial tinidazole in a dose of 1.0–1.5 g given for 3 consecutive days, or even as a single dose, was somewhat more effective than a 5-day course of metronidazole in clearing E. histolytica from feces of children aged 6–9 years (Welch et al., 1978). Powell and Eldson-Dew (1972) found that more patients continued to pass E. histolytica cysts in stools after tinidazole therapy than after metronidazole therapy.

Hatchuel (1975) used tinidazole in a dose of 800 mg three times daily for 5 days to obtain a high cure rate in patients with an amebic liver abscess. Tinidazole was compared with metronidazole in one small study in which 19 patients with an amebic liver abscess were treated; both drugs were given in a dose of 2 g daily for 2 days. The authors claimed that complete recovery occurred in all ten patients given tinidazole and in only five of nine patients given metronidazole (Khokhani et al., 1977). Others have also recorded the effectiveness of tinidazole given in a dose of 2 g daily for 3–6 days in treating amebic liver abscess (Islam and Hasan, 1978; Quaderi et al., 1978). Despite these reports, there is insufficient data on the use of tinidazole in seriously ill patients with an amebic liver abscess.

One patient with amebic abscess of the spleen responded to two courses of tinidazole, each 2 g daily for 10 days. During the second course a percutaneous aspiration of the abscess was also performed (Lawford and Sorrell, 1994).

References

Andersson T, Forssel J, Sterner G (1972). Outbreak of giardiasis: effect of a new antiflagellate drug, tinidazole. *Brit Med J* **1**: 449.

Anonymous (1988). Belgian Collaborative Study of the *in-vitro* susceptibility of the *Bacteroides fragilis* group. A Belgian Collaborative Study Group. *Eur J Epidemiol* **4**: 360.

Appelbaum PC, Chatterton SA (1978). Susceptibility of anaerobic bacteria to ten antimicrobial agents. *Antimicrob Ag Chemother* **14**: 371.

Banatvala N, Davies GR, Abdi Y *et al.* (1994). High prevalence of *Helicobacter pylori* metronidazole resistance in migrants to east London: relation with previous nitroimidazole exposure and gastroduodenal disease. *Gut* **35**: 1562.

Bergan T (1985). Antibacterial activity and pharmacokinetics of nitroimidazoles. A review. *Scand J Infect Dis* (Suppl 46): 64.

Bianchi Porro G, Parente F, Lazzaroni M (1993). Short and long term outcome of *Helicobacter pylori* positive resistant duodenal ulcers treated with colloidal bismuth subcitrate plus antibiotics or sucralfate alone. *Gut* **34**: 466.

Boreham PFL, Phillips RE, Shepherd RW (1984). The sensitivity of *Giardia intestinalis* to drugs in vitro. *J Antimicrob Chemother* **14**: 449.

Dhar KK, Dhall GI, Ayyagari A (1993a). Tinidazole prophylaxis in elective abdominal hysterectomy. *Int J Gynaecol Obstet* **42**: 121.

Dhar KK, Dhall GI, Ayyagari A (1993b). Single dose tinidazole prophylaxis in vaginal hysterectomy. *Int J Gynaecol Obstet* **42**: 117.

Farid Z, El-Masry NA, Miner WF, Anwar Hassan (1974). Tinidazole in treatment of giardiasis. *Lancet* **ii**: 721.

Forsgren A, Wallin J (1974). Tinidazole – a new preparation for *Trichomonas vaginalis* infections. I. Laboratory evaluation. *Brit J Vener Dis* **50**: 146.

Gazder AJ, Banerjee M (1977). Single-dose treatment of giardiasis in children: a comparison of tinidazole and metronidazole. *Curr Med Res Opin* **5**: 164.

Giercksky KE, Danielsen S (1990). Antimicrobial prophylaxis in upper gastrointestinal, biliary, stomach and oesophageal surgery. *Scand J Infect Dis* (Suppl 70): 45.

Gnarpe H, Belsheim J, Persson S (1981). Influence of nitroimidazole derivatives on leukocyte migration. *Scand J Infect Dis* (Suppl 26): 68.

Hamed KA, Studemeister AE (1992). Successful response of metronidazole-resistant trichomonal vaginitis to tinidazole. A case report. *Sex Transm Dis* **19**: 339.

Hatchuel W (1975). Tinidazole for the treatment of amoebic liver disease. *SA Med J* **49**: 1879.

Hillström L, Pettersson L, Pálsson E (1977). Comparison of ornidazole and tinidazole in single-dose treatment of trichomoniasis in women. *Brit J Vener Dis* **53**: 193.

Howes HL Jr, Lynch JE, Kivlin JL (1970). Tinidazole, a new anti-protozoal agent: effect on *Trichomonas* and other protozoa. *Antimicrob Ag Chemother* **1969**: 261.

Islam N, Hasan M (1978). Tinidazole and metronidazole in hepatic amoebiasis. *J Trop Med Hyg* **81**: 20.

Janssens D, Peeters N, Snauwaert E, Cattersel B (1982). Tinidazole in the prevention of postoperative wound infection after hysterectomy. *J Antimicrob Chemother* **10** (Suppl A): 87.

Jaup BH, Norrby A (1995). Low dose, short-term triple therapy for cure of *Helicobacter pylori* infection and healing of peptic ulcers. *Am J Gastroenterol* **90**: 943.

Jokipii AMM, Jokipii L (1981). Metronidazole, tinidazole, ornidazole and anaerobic infections of the middle ear, maxillary sinus and central nervous system. *Scand J Infect Dis* **26** (Suppl): 123.

Jokipii AM, Jokipii L (1987). Comparative activity of metronidazole and tinidazole against *Clostridium difficile* and *Peptostreptococcus anaerobius*. *Antimicrob Ag Chemother* **31**: 183.

Jokipii L, Jokipii AMM (1980). *In vitro* susceptibility of *Giardia lamblia* trophozoites to metronidazole and tinidazole. *J Infect Dis* **141**: 317.

Jokipii L, Jokipii AMM (1985). Comparative evaluation of the 2-methyl-5-nitroimidazole compounds dimetridazole, metronidazole, secnidazole,

ornidazole, tinidazole, carnidazole, and panidazole against *Bacteroides fragilis* and other bacteria of the *Bacteroides fragilis* group. *Antimicrob Ag Chemother* **28**: 561.

Jones R, Enders P (1977). An evaluation of tinidazole as single-dose therapy for the treatment of *Trichomonas vaginalis*. *Med J Aust* **2**: 679.

Joshii HD, Shah BM (1975). A comparative study of tinidazole and metronidazole in treatment of amoebiasis. *Ind Practit* **28**: 295.

Kawamura N (1978). Metronidazole and tinidazole in a single large dose for treating urogenital infections with *Trichomonas vaginalis* in men. *Brit J Vener Dis* **54**: 81.

Kharsany AB, Hoosen AA, Van den Ende J (1993). Antimicrobial susceptibilities of *Gardnerella vaginalis*. *Antimicrob Ag Chemother* **37**: 2733.

Khokhani RC, Garud AD, Deodhar KP *et al.* (1977). Comparative study of tinidazole and metronidazole in amoebic liver abscess. *Curr Med Res Opin* **5**: 161.

Lawford R, Sorrell TC (1994). Amebic abscess of the spleen complicated by metronidazole-induced neurotoxicity: case report. *Clin Infect Dis* **19**: 346.

Levi GC, De Avila CA, Neto VA (1977). Efficacy of various drugs for treatment of giardiasis. A comparative study. *Amer J Trop Med Hyg* **26**: 564.

Loo VG, Sherman P, Matlow AG (1992). *Helicobacter pylori* infection in a pediatric population: *in vitro* susceptibilities to omeprazole and eight antimicrobial agents. *Antimicrob Ag Chemother* **36**: 1133.

Marshall BJ, Goodwin CS, Warren JR *et al.* (1988). Prospective double-blind trial of duodenal ulcer relapse after eradication of *Campylobacter pylori*. *Lancet* **2**: 1437.

McEwen J (1983). Hypersensitivity reactions to tinidazole (Fasigyn). *Med J Aust* **1**: 498.

McGregor IA, Watson JD, Sweeney G, Sleigh JD (1982). The use of tinidazole in the surgery of oral tumours. *J Antimicrob Chemother* **10** (Suppl A): 173.

Miller MW, Howes HL, English AR (1970). Tinidazole, a potent new antiprotozoal agent. *Antimicrob Ag Chemother* **1969**: 257.

Misra NP, Laiq SM (1974). Comparative trial of tinidazole and metronidazole in intestinal amoebiasis. *Curr Ther Res* **16**: 1255.

Mohanty KC, Deighton R (1987). Comparison of 2 g single dose of metronidazole, nimorazole and tinidazole in the treatment of vaginitis associated with *Gardnerella vaginalis*. *J Antimicrob Chemother* **19**: 393.

Nord CE (1982). Microbiological properties of tinidazole: spectrum, activity and ecological considerations. *J Antimicrob Chemother* **10** (Suppl A): 35.

Olsson-Liljequist B, Nord CE (1981). *In vitro* susceptibility of anaerobic bacteria to nitroimidazoles. *Scand J Infect Dis* (Suppl 26): 42.

Packard RS (1982). Tinidazole: a review of clinical experience in anaerobic infections. *J Antimicrob Chemother* **10** (Suppl A): 65.

Pettersson T (1975). Single-dose tinidazole therapy for giardiasis. *Brit Med J* **1**: 395.

Powell SJ, Elsdon-Dew R (1972). Some new nitro imidazole derivatives: clinical trials in amoebic liver abscess. *Amer J Trop Med Hyg* **21**: 518.

Quaderi MA, Rahman MS, Rahman A, Islam N (1978). Amoebic liver abscess and clinical experiences with tinidazole in Bangladesh. *J Trop Med Hyg* **81**: 16.

Reynolds AV, Hamilton-Miller JMT, Brumfitt W (1975). A comparison of the *in vitro* activity of metronidazole, tinidazole and nimorazole against Gram-negative anaerobic bacilli. *J Clin Path* **28**: 775.

Roe FJ (1985). Safety of nitroimidazoles. *Scand J Infect Dis* (Supp 146): 72.

Rubinstein G, Dunkin K, Howard AJ (1994). The susceptibility of *Helicobacter pylori* to 12 antimicrobial agents, omeprazole and bismuth salts. *J Antimicrob Chemother* **34**: 409.

Saberi-Firoozi M, Massarrat S, Zare S *et al.* (1995). Effect of triple therapy or amoxycillin plus omeprazole or amoxycillin plus tinidazole plus omeprazole on duodenal ulcer healing, eradication of *Helicobacter pylori*, and prevention of ulcer relapse over a 1-year follow-up period: a prospective, randomized, controlled study. *Am J Gastroenterol* **90**: 1419.

Scragg JN, Proctor EM (1977). Tinidazole treatment of acute amoebic dysentery in children. *Amer J Trop Med Hyg* **26**: 824.

Sears SD, O'Hare J (1988). *In vitro* susceptibility of *Trichomonas vaginalis* to 50 antimicrobial agents. *Antimicrob Ag Chemother* **32**: 144.

Seligman SA (1982). Prophylactic oral and intravenous tinidazole in hysterectomy. *J Antimicrob Chemother* **10** (Suppl A): 81.

Shanker S, Munro R (1982). Sensitivity of *Gardnerella vaginalis* to metabolites of metronidazole and tinidazole. *Lancet* i: 167.

Simjee AE, Gathiram V, Jackson TF, Khan BF (1985). A comparative trial of metronidazole v tinidazole in the treatment of amoebic liver abscess. *S Afr Med J* **68**: 923.

Singh G, Kumar S (1977). Short course of single daily dosage treatment with tinidazole and metronidazole in intestinal amoebiasis: a comparative study. *Curr Med Res Opin* **5**: 157.

Speelman P (1985). Single-dose tinidazole for the treatment of giardiasis. *Antimicrob Ag Chemother* **27**: 227.

Spiegel CA (1987). Susceptibility of *Mobiluncus* species to 23 antimicrobial agents and 15 other compounds. *Antimicrob Ag Chemother* **31**: 249.

Swami B, Lavakusulu D, Sitha Devi C (1977). Tinidazole and metronidazole in the treatment of intestinal amoebiasis. *Curr Med Res Opin* **5**: 152.

Tally FP, Goldin B, Sullivan NE (1981). Nitroimidazoles: *in vitro* activity and efficacy in anaerobic infections. *Scand J Infect Dis* (Suppl 26): 46.

Taylor JA Jr, Migliardi JR, Von Wittenau MS (1970). Tinidazole and metronidazole pharmacokinetics in man and mouse. *Antimicrob Ag Chemother* **1969**: 267.

University of Melbourne Colorectal Group (1983). Clinical trial of prophylaxis of wound sepsis in elective colorectal surgery. Cephamandole with tinidazole versus tinidazole alone. *Med J Aust* **2**: 240.

Van der Meijden WI (1983). Treatment of non-specific vaginitis with a single dose of tinidazole. *Scand J Infect Dis* (Suppl 40): 85.

Von Konow L, Nord CE (1982). Concentrations of tinidazole and metronidazole in serum, saliva and alveolar bone. *J Antimicrob Chemother* **10** (Suppl A): 165.

Wallin J, Forsgren A (1974). Tinidazole – a new preparation for *T vaginalis* infections. II. Clinical evaluation of treatment with a single oral dose. *Brit J Vener Dis* **50**: 148.

Welch JS, Rowsell BJ, Freeman C (1978). Treatment of intestinal amoebiasis and giardiasis. Efficacy of metronidazole and tinidazole compared. *Med J Aust* **1**: 469.

Wood BA, Monro AM (1975). Pharmacokinetics of tinidazole and metronidazole in women after single large oral doses. *Brit J Vener Dis* **51**: 51.

Wood BA, Faulkner JK, Monro AM (1982). The pharmacokinetics, metabolism and tissue distribution of tinidazole. *J Antimicrob Chemother* **10** (Suppl A): 43.

Nalidixic Acid and Other Older Quinolones

Description

Nalidixic acid (1-ethyl-l, 4-dihydro-7-methyl-4-oxo-1, 8-naphthyridine-3-carboxylic acid) is one of a series of 1,8-naphthyridine derivatives, which are not chemically related to any other antibacterial agents. These chemotherapeutic drugs were first synthesized by Lesher *et al.* (1962) at the Sterling-Winthrop Research Institute in the USA from a distallate during chloroquine synthesis (Neu, 1987). Nalidixic acid was introduced into clinical use in 1964 and can be regarded as the prototype of the quinolone group of drugs.

Numerous new analogs, which have significantly improved antibacterial spectrum, have been synthesized. Together they are referred to as the quinolones or quinolone carboxylic acids, with the newer agents being fluoroquinolones (Hooper, 1993). Nearly all of the drugs so grouped are either naphthyridine-carboxylic acid or quinoline-carboxylic acid derivatives. These two bicyclic structures have been modified by the addition of different atoms, side-chains or other rings to produce new quinolones. The drugs do not usually show cross-resistance with other antibacterial agents. An expanding list of quinolones have been marketed for clinical use, particularly during the 1980s. Quinolones can be divided into the older derivatives, such as nalidixic acid, oxolinic acid, cinoxacin, flumequine, miloxacin, rosoxacin and pipemidic acid, which have a limited antibacterial spectrum, and the newer fluoroquinolones. These latter agents contain a fluorine atom and a piperazinyl group and include norfloxacin, enoxacin, ciprofloxacin, ofloxacin, pefloxacin, tosufloxacin, temafloxacin and amifloxacin. In addition there are the new generation quinolones such as lomefloxacin or fleroxacin which have sufficiently long half-lives to allow once-daily administration, while others, such as sparfloxacin have enhanced activity against Gram-positive cocci and anaerobes. The newer quinolones are described in subsequent chapters.

Characteristics of the older quinolones: nalidixic acid, oxolinic acid, cinoxacin, flumequine, miloxacin, rosoxacin and pipemidic acid are summarized in Table II.5. Only nalidixic acid ('Negram', Winthrop Laboratories) and cinoxacin ('Cinobac') continue to be marketed, although this latter agent has no useful advantage over other quinolones. The information below applies only to nalidixic acid. Further information regarding the other older quinolones beyond that available in Table II.5 can be found in the 4th edition of this text.

Semsitive Organisms

1 Gram-negative bacteria

Nalidixic acid is active against most of the Enterobacteriaceae, such as *Escherichia coli*, the *Enterobacter*, *Klebsiella*, all *Proteus*, *Citrobacter*, *Morganella*, *Serratia* and *Hafnia* spp. where the MIC_{90} is generally 8–16 μg per ml (Eliopoulos and Eliopoulos, 1989). *Salmonella* and *Shigella* spp. are usually sensitive (Lesher *et al.*, 1962; Newsom *et al.*, 1982; Eliopoulos and Eliopoulos, 1989). *Providencia stuartii* is frequently resistant, with an MIC_{90} of 32 to >128 μg per ml (Hawkey and Hawkey, 1984; Eliopoulos and Eliopoulos, 1989). Enteropathogens such as enteropathogenic, enterotoxigenic and enteroinvasive *E. coli*, *Yersinia enterocolitica* and *Vibrio* spp. are usually susceptible with an MIC_{90} <8 μg per ml (Eliopoulos and Eliopoulos, 1989). *Campylobacter jejuni* is less reliably susceptible to nalidixic acid with an MIC_{90} of 8–256 μg per ml (Walder, 1982; Eliopoulos and Eliopoulos, 1989) but increasing rates of resistance (MIC ≥32 μg per ml) have been noted, including resistance to the fluoroquinolones (p. 970) during the

Table II.5
Older quinolones

Drug	Administration	Absorption, peak serum conc	Antibacterial spectrum	Distribution, excretion	Toxicity	Uses
Nalidixic acid	Oral: 1 g four times daily (adults) 55 mg per kg per day (children)[a]	Good 21–50 µg per ml, 2 h after 1 g dose	Gram-negatives: Enterobacteriaceae *Brucella* *Aeromonas* *Acinetobacter* *Neisseria gonorrhoeae* *Haemophilus influenzae* NOT: *Pseudomonas*, Gram-positives, *Mycoplasma*, *Chlamydia*, anaerobes	93% protein bound; hepatic conjugation; urine conc: 25–250 µg per ml after single 0.5–1 g dose; low tissue conc except in kidney	Gastrointestinal neurotoxicity; skin rash; acidosis; displaces warfarin	UTI *Shigella* dysentary[b]; gut 'decontamination'
Oxolinic acid	Oral: 750 mg twice-daily	Poor 0.8 µg per ml, 2–6 h after 750 mg dose T$_{1/2}$ 6–7 h	Similar to NA, except active against *Staph. aureus*; cross-resistance to NA	80–85% protein bound; urine conc: 9.1 µg per ml after single 750 mg dose; low tissue conc	Similar to NA; CNS stimulation	UTI only; no advantage over NA; no longer available
Cinoxacin	Oral: 250–500 mg twice-daily	Reasonable 15.5 µg per ml, 1 h after 500 mg dose T$_{1/2}$ 1.1–1.6 h	Similar to NA; inducible resistance	16–83% protein bound; 50–60% excreted unchanged in urine; urine conc: 390 µg per ml after single 500 mg dose	Similar to NA; skin rashes 1–3%	UTI only; in USA: 'Cinobac'
Flumequine	Oral: 400 mg four times daily		Similar to oxolinic acid; primary and inducible resistance common		Common (15%)	UTI only; no longer available
Rosoxacin	Oral: 300 mg once (gonorrhea) 150 mg twice-daily × 3 days (chancroid)	Reasonable 6.4 µg per ml, 2 h after 250 mg dose T$_{1/2}$ 5.5 h	Similar to oxolinic acid; active against: *N. gonorrhea*, *H. influenzae*, *H. ducreyi*	70% protein bound; 50% renal excretion over 24 h	Common: 29% with gonorrhea	Gonorrhea and chancroid[c]; no longer available
Pipemidic acid	Oral: 500 mg twice-daily	Good 4.4 µg per ml, 1–2 h after 0.5 g dose T$_{1/2}$ 3.1 h	Similar to NA, except activity against *Staph. aureus* and *Ps. aeruginosa*	30% protein bound; urine conc: 1116 µg per ml after 500 mg dose; 68–88% renal excretion		UTI; otitis media, sinusitis; gut 'decontamination'; no longer available

NA: Nalidixic acid. [a] See text. [b] Other antibiotic agents now generally used in preference. [c] No longer used. Conc: concentration.

past 10 years (Altwegg *et al.*, 1987; Gootz and Martin, 1991; Adler-Mosca *et al.*, 1991; Chatzipanagiotou *et al.*, 1993). *Campylobacter fetus* and *Helicobacter pylori* are resistant to nalidixic acid (Fliegelman *et al.*, 1985). *Aeromonas hydrophila* is usually susceptible (Zemelman *et al.*, 1983). *Brucella* spp. may be susceptible. *Neisseria gonorrhoeae* (including beta-lactamase-producing strains) are generally susceptible (MIC 0.5–2 μg per ml) but resistance has been reported (Report, 1978; Philips, 1987; Stein *et al.*, 1991). Unlike the new fluoroquinolones (p. 982), nalidixic acid has no activity against *Pseudomonas aeruginosa* and other *Pseudomonas* spp. (Eliopoulos and Eliopoulos, 1989). *Haemophilus influenzae* (including beta-lactamase-producing strains) is susceptible, as are most strains of *Acinetobacter* spp. (Newsom *et al.*, 1982), although this has little clinical relevence. *Haemophilus ducreyi* is relatively resistant.

Nalidixic acid-resistant Gram-negative bacilli were previously relatively uncommon in both domiciliary and hospital infections, but this situation may be changing. In the 1960s, there was no apparent increase in resistant strains of *E. coli* (Brumfitt and Pursell, 1971), while in the 1970s and early 1980s nalidixic acid resistance was noted in 9–11.6% of strains of Gram-negative pathogens (Burman, 1977; Newsom *et al.*, 1982)) . Stamey and Bragonje (1976) concluded that among urinary pathogens, with the exception of *Ps. aeruginosa* and Gram-positive cocci, most isolates were susceptible to nalidixic acid, despite the presence of multiple-drug resistance in more than half of the strains. Light *et al.* (1981) found that nalidixic acid-resistant strains of urinary tract isolates of Enterobacteriaceae were most commonly detected in patients who had had prior treatment with the drug, and those with underlying urinary tract abnormalities. In Germany, Austria and Switzerland during 1975–1986, there was no increase in the rate of resistance to nalidixic acid among Enterobacteriaceae (mean rate of resistance 3.7%; MIC_{50} 4 μg per ml, MIC_{90} 8 μg per ml), despite widespread use of 4-quinolones – although there were wide variations in the rates of resistance between different hospitals and between different species (Kresken and Wiedemann, 1988).

One possible explanation for the relatively low frequency of nalidixic acid resistance among Gram-negative bacteria is that such resistance is not mediated by plasmids (p. 969). Therefore, resistance to nalidixic acid is less likely to be transferred in the bowel from one organism to another, and multiply-resistant Enterobacteriaceae remain sensitive to nalidixic acid. In contrast, several unrelated plasmids in *E. coli* have been occasionally noted to confer an increased susceptibility to nalidixic acid by increasing the permeability of the cell wall facilitating an increased uptake of the drug (Crumplin and Smith, 1981). Nalidixic acid also induces less resistance among fecal Gram-negative bacilli than other antimicrobial agents used for urinary tract infections (Stamey and Bragonje, 1976). This may be important if reinfection occurs shortly after therapy, because fecal organisms are usually implicated.

Crumplin and Smith (1975) reported the paradoxical finding that, with susceptible Gram-negative bacteria, when the bactericidal concentration for the strain was exceeded, the bactericidal effect of the drug was reduced and it became relatively bacteriostatic. This phenomenon was explicable by the mode of action of nalidixic acid (p. 971). At the higher concentrations of the drug which were used, RNA and protein synthesis were also inhibited and these are essential for the lethal action of the drug. Contrary to the opinion of Stamey and Bragonje, 1976, Crumplin and Smith (1975) considered that for some bacteria a 1 g oral dose of nalidixic acid may produce a urinary level which is in excess of the bactericidal level and it may be only bacteriostatic; this could favor the emergence of resistant strains. This opinion has not been substantiated by clinical experience.

Nalidixic acid may act synergistically with kanamycin, gentamicin or colistin against most Enterobacteriaceae, whereas with chloramphenicol, tetracycline and nitrofurantoin *in vitro*, antagonism is not infrequent. When it is combined with one of the penicillins or cephalosporins, there is usually neither synergism nor antagonism (Michel *et al.*, 1973). If nalidixic acid is combined with rifampicin, the emergence of resistance of urinary pathogens to either drug is lessened. The clinical relevence of these *in vitro* findings remains uncertain.

Anaerobic Gram-negative bacteria, such as *Bacteroides* and *Fusobacterium* spp., are resistant to nalidixic acid (Goldstein and Citron, 1985; Mitsuhashi, 1988; Eliopoulos and Eliopoulos, 1989).

2 Gram-positive bacteria

Gram-positive bacteria such as *Staphylococcus aureus*, *Streptococcus pneumoniae* and enterococci, are nalidixic acid-resistant (Lesher *et al.*, 1962, Barlow, 1963; Mitsuhashi, 1988; Eliopoulos and Eliopoulos, 1989). Notably, *Staph. saprophyticus*, which is susceptible to most antibiotics used for urinary tract infections, is resistant to nalidixic acid. Anaerobes, such as *Clostridium*, *Eubacterium* and *Lactobacillus* spp., *Actinomyces* spp., *Mobiluncus* spp. and anaerobic cocci, are resistant (generally MIC ≥128 μg per ml) to nalidixic acid (Goldstein and Citron, 1985; Eliopoulos and Eliopoulos, 1989).

3 Chlamydia

Chlamydia trachomatis is resistant to nalidixic acid (Heessen and Muytjens, 1984).

4 Rickettsiaceae and Ehrlichia

Ehrlichia spp. are probably resistant to nalidixic acid. Nalidixic acid was ineffective in eliminating *Ehrlichia risticii* (the cause of Potomac horse fever or equine ehrlichiosis) from macrophages *in vitro* (Rikihisa and Jiang, 1988).

5 Fungi

Nalidixic acid can suppress the growth of *Candida albicans* in concentrations obtained in urine after normal doses of the drug (Sobieski and Brewer, 1976), but has no clinical role in this regard.

6 Plasmodia

Nalidixic acid, unlike the fluoroquinolones, is ineffective *in vitro* in the inhibition of both chloroquine-sensitive and -resistant strains of *Plasmodium falciparum* (Divo *et al.*, 1988).

7 'Acquired' resistance

Similar to other quinolones, resistance to nalidixic acid can occur by a number of mechanisms: most notably due to alterations in DNA gyrase and reduced bacterial permeability. Among Gram-negative pathogens such as *E. coli* and *P. aeruginosa*, alterations in DNA gyrase, with consequent reduction in binding of nalidixic acid are well described. Reduced bacterial permeability, especially in the lipopolysaccharide outer membrane, is most notable for lipophilic quinolones such as nalidixic acid, oxolanic acid and piromidic acid, but has also been noted for fluoroquinolones (Table II.5, p. 966) (Mitsuhashi, 1988; Hooper and Wolfson, 1993a). Unlike beta-lactams and aminoglycosides in which resistance is frequently plasmid-mediated, resistance to quinolones in the clinical setting is generally mediated via chromosomal mutation. Acquisition by susceptible bacteria of new quinolone-resistance genes on plasmids has been demonstrated only in the laboratory (Hooper and Wolfson, 1993a).

The frequency of selection of chromosomally mediated resistant mutants depends on the selecting quinolone, the drug concentration used for selection and the bacterial species and strain (e.g. *P. aeruginosa* and *Staph. aureus* develop resistance mutations more readily than *E. coli*) (Wolfson and Hooper, 1989; Hooper and Wolfson, 1993a). Nalidixic acid selects for resistant *E. coli* reasonably frequently at 8- to 16-fold above the MIC, which is 100- to 1000-fold more frequent than ciprofloxacin, ofloxacin or other quinolones (Chapman *et al.*, 1989; Crumplin and Odell, 1987; Felmington *et al.*, 1988; Hooper *et al.*, 1986, 1987; Smith, 1986; Wolfson *et al.*, 1987). Mutations in DNA gyrase A causing nalidixic acid resistance often result in greater resistance to nalidixic acid (about 128-fold) than to other quinolones such as ciprofloxacin (16- to 32-fold), presumably because these changes are less critical to the activity of these latter agents. Among *E. coli* mutants selected *in vitro* with nalidixic acid, mutations in *gyrA* and *gyrB* appear to be equally common (Nakamura *et al.*, 1989). Clearly, the site of amino acid changes in these gyrases influence the degree of cross-resistance betwen quinolones (Wolfson and Hooper, 1989). Occasionally, isolates have been identified which are resistant to fluoroquinolones, but remain susceptible to nalidixic acid. Alterations in membrane permeability and novel *gyrA* point mutations have been responsible for this unusual pattern of resistance in *E. coli* (Cambau *et al.*, 1993; Moniot-Ville *et al.*, 1991). A broader discussion of resistance mechanisms, particularly as they relate to the therapeautically more important fluoroquinolones, can be found elsewhere (p. 990).

Quinolones vary in their ability to penetrate into bacterial cells (Nagate *et al.*, 1980; Newsom *et al.*, 1982). Differences in the hydrophobicity of quinolones influence their permeability through the outer and inner membranes of Gram-negative bacilli. Hydrophilic quinolones pass through the water-filled porins in the outer membrane of Gram-negative bacilli more readily (Hancock, 1987; Nikaido and Vaara, 1985).

Emergence of nalidixic acid-resistance *in vivo* during the treatment of patients has been observed frequently (Buchbinder *et al.*, 1962; Ronald *et al.*, 1966; Finegold *et al.*, 1967). Underdosing of nalidixic acid and its use to treat complicated urinary tract infections appear to be associated with an increased rate of development of clinical resistance (Cederberg *et al.*, 1974; Preiksaitis *et al.*, 1981; Ronald *et al.*, 1966; Stamey and Bragonje, 1976). Stamey and

Bragonje (1976) found that when adequate dosage was used, resistance to nalidixic acid developed in only 7% of patients, a frequency which is comparable with other effective antimicrobial agents. Among *E. coli* at least, single-step resistance develops rarely ($\leq 10^{-10}$) when the quinolone concentration is at least 8-fold greater than the MIC of the organism – the usual situation in the urine when treating with quinolones (Crumplin and Odell, 1987; Felmingham *et al.*, 1988; Hooper and Wolfson, 1989). Such rates of developing resistance *in vitro* are similar to the frequency at which resistance develops *in vitro* to aminoglycosides. Overall, however, nalidixic acid has *in vitro* resistance frequencies 2- to 3-fold greater than the new quinolones and develops higher levels of resistance (up to 64-fold increases in MIC) than these agents (Milatovic and Braveny, 1987). Spontaneous single-step mutations resulting in resistance are 100- to 1000-fold more likely with nalidixic acid than the fluoroquinolones for many bacterial species, although this difference is less marked with *Ps. aeruginosa* in which the difference is only 10-fold (Cullman *et al.*, 1985; Fernandes *et al.*, 1987; Wolfson *et al.*, 1987). Bacterial strains that develop resistance during serial passage on media with increasing drug concentrations are typically cross-resistant to multiple quinolones and in some cases are also resistant to other classes of drugs such as chloramphenicol, tetracycline, beta-lactams and trimethoprim (Sanders *et al.*, 1984; Gutmann *et al.*, 1985; Traub, 1985; Hooper *et al.*, 1986, 1987; Mouton and Mulders, 1987).

Drug destruction has not been identified as a mechanism of bacterial resistance to quinolones (Wolfson *et al.*, 1989). As noted earlier, plasmid-mediated resistance to quinolones appears to be extremely uncommon (Courvalin, 1990). Although such resistance has been reported among some clinical bacterial isolates, none have been confirmed, nor the mechanism of resistance defined (Panhotra *et al.*, 1985; Munshi *et al.*, 1987; Tanaka *et al.*, 1991; Courvalin, 1990). The fact that quinolones inhibit plasmid conjugation, transfer of conjugating plasmids, and clear some plasmids from their host cells, may provide some explanation for the lack of plasmid-mediated resistance (Hooper *et al.*, 1984; Weisser and Wiedemann, 1985; Courtright *et al.*, 1988; Mehtar *et al.*, 1987). Drugs that inhibit protein synthesis theoretically limit the ability of nalidixic acid to kill bacteria, but not to inhibit DNA synthesis (Deitz *et al.*, 1966). Unlike nalidixic acid, some fluoroquinolones (e.g. ciprofloxacin) are still able to kill *E. coli* in the absence of protein or RNA synthesis (p. 992).

Resistance to nalidixic acid is increasing among many pathogens. In a survey of pathogenic salmonellae isolated across the USA in 1979–1980 and compared with those isolated in 1984–1985, a significant increase in resistance to nalidixic acid ($p < 0.05$) was noted. Interestingly, there was some variation depending on the *Salmonella* species. Overall, resistance to various antibiotics among *Salm. heidelberg* strains decreased during the study period (67% to 35%), while resistance among *Salm. typhimurium* increased significantly from 14% to 26% ($p < 0.01$) (MacDonald *et al.*, 1987). Similarly, anecdotal reports of *Salm. typhimurium* isolated from the Indian subcontinent suggest frequent resistance to nalidixic acid, and although such isolates are generally still susceptible to fluoroquinolones, their MICs to these latter agents are up to 10-fold greater than the MICs for similar nalidixic acid-susceptible strains (Lewin, 1991).

Multiple-antibiotic resistance, including to nalidixic acid, among *Shigella dysenteriae* type I in Bangladesh has increased from 0 to 86% of strains in one study conducted from 1985–1987; but susceptibility to fluoroquinolones was maintained (Munshi *et al.*, 1987; Sen *et al.*, 1988). These authors presented some suggestive, but inconclusive, evidence that this nalidixic acid resistance was plasmid-mediated; although this was doubted by Crumplin (1987). Similarly, Bennish *et al.* (1992) reported an increase in resistance to nalidixic acid from 0.8% in 1986 to 20.2% in 1990 ($p < 0.001$) among *Shigella* spp. isolated in Bangladesh. In particular, 57.9% of *Sh. dysenteriae* type I isolates in 1990 were resistant, generally in association with resistance to ampicillin and trimethoprim-sulfamethoxazole. Clinical treatment options in such situations are consequently somewhat limited. In Thailand in 1988, however, 99–100% of all *Shigella* spp., including *Sh. dysenteriae*, were susceptible to nalidixic acid, despite high rates of resistance to ampicillin, tetracyclines, chloramphenicol and trimethoprim–sulfamethoxazole (Lolekha *et al.*, 1991). These authors reported that in a comparative study, treatment with norfloxacin eradicated *Shigella* spp. from fecal specimens faster than nalidixic acid, however there was no statistically significant difference in clinical response between these two treatment groups ($p > 0.1$). Both nalidixic acid and norfloxacin were more effective than trimethoprim–sulfamethoxazole ($p < 0.01$), probably because only 17% of isolates were susceptible to trimethoprim–sulfamethoxazole. In the Netherlands the incidence of resistance to nalidixic acid among *Shigella* isolates appears to be increasing, but to a lesser extent than in developing countries (Voogd *et al.*, 1992).

Unlike these diarrheal pathogens, *Campylobacter jejuni* strains that have been selected for nalidixic acid resistance *in vitro* often demonstrate significant cross-resistance to newer quinolones (e.g. ciprofloxacin, norfloxacin, temafloxacin). Such resistance was found to be due to reduced DNA gyrase subunit A susceptibility to these agents (Gootz and Martin, 1991). The incidence of resistance to both nalidixic acid and the fluroquinolones appears to be increasing steadily among strains of *C. jejuni* in Europe and Greece (Altwegg *et al.*, 1987; Lariviere *et al.*, 1986; Chatzipanagioutou *et al.*, 1993; Adler-Mosca *et al.*, 1991).

Nalidixic acid resistance in *N. gonorrhoeae* may be due either to mutations in the *gyrA* gene with alterations to DNA gyrase subunit A, or in the case of low-level resistance to nalidixic acid, the change may be in the B subunit of DNA gyrase (Stein *et al.*, 1991).

8 In vitro sensitivities

The MICs of nalidixic acid against some selected bacterial species are presented in the text (pp. 965, 967). For treatment of urinary tract infections, organisms with an MIC of $\leq 16\,\mu$g per ml are regarded as susceptible (Barlow, 1963, Stamey and Bragonje, 1976; Mitsuhashi, 1988; Eliopoulos and Eliopoulos, 1989).

Mode of Administration and Dosage

1 Adults

Nalidixic acid is usually administered by the oral route in a dosage of 4 g daily given in four divided doses. The dose may be reduced to 2 g daily for more prolonged treatment. A single daily dose of 1 g has been used for long-term suppressive therapy of chronic bacteriuria.

2 Children

The drug is not recommended for infants less than 3 months old. For children aged 12 years and under, dosage for initial therapy is 55 mg per kg body weight per day, administered in four divided doses. For prolonged therapy, the total daily dose may be reduced to 33 mg per kg. Caution should be exercised in children less than 6 months of age due to reports of benign intracranial hypertension, especially when nalidixic acid is given in high doses (100–150 mg per kg per day) (p. 972; Mukherjee *et al.*, 1990).

3 Newborn and premature infants

The drug appears to be particularly dangerous in infants under 4 weeks of age. Kemball and Davies (1967) reported a premature infant weighing 1.7 kg, given nalidixic acid in a dose of 60 mg per kg daily, who developed deep sighing respirations, abdominal distension, muscle hypotonia and marked metabolic acidosis 2 days after commencement of treatment. This infant recovered after cessation of nalidixic acid and treatment with sodium bicarbonate. The serum level of the drug 9 h after the last dose was 114 μg per ml, but the urinary level was only 20 μg per ml. Newborn infants apparently conjugate and excrete this drug much more slowly than older children and adults, and the high serum and low urine levels recorded in this case represent a reversal of the characteristic findings in the other age groups.

4 Patients with renal failure

In patients with moderate degrees of renal functional impairment (serum creatinine 4–6 mg% or 0.33–0.5 mmol per liter) treated with usual doses of nalidixic acid, there is no accumulation of the active drug in the body, and adequate urinary concentrations (about 70 μg per ml) of the active drug are usually attained (Stamey *et al.*, 1969). It may, therefore, be feasible to use this drug in ordinary doses for the treatment of urinary tract infections in moderately azotemic patients. However, inactive nalidixic acid metabolites (monoglucuronides) almost certainly accumulate in such patients and may contribute to toxicity. For this reason, treatment with nalidixic acid should be avoided in patients with renal failure whenever possible. Dosage reduction for such patients is not practicable, because this would lead to inadequate urine levels of the active drug. In patients with severe renal failure, therapeutic urinary levels are unlikely to be achieved even with ordinary dosage. Bennett *et al.* (1994) recommend avoiding the use of nalidixic acid when the glomerular filtration rate (GFR) is ≤ 50 ml per min and during all forms of dialysis.

5 Intravenous administration

The sodium salt of nalidixic acid, which is suitable for i.v. administration, is no longer available.

Availability

Nalidixic acid is available as 500 mg *tablets*.

Serum Levels in Relation to Dosage

Early studies showed that serum concentrations could not be predicted after oral administration of nalidixic acid (Buchbinder *et al.*, 1962; Gibbon *et al.*, 1965). Serum levels at 1, 2 and 4h after a single 1.0-g oral dose of nalidixic acid varied widely from patient to patient. Some patients had high serum levels (10–40 μg per ml), but in others, levels of only 1.0–2.0 μg per ml or even lower were recorded (Gibbon *et al.*, 1965). In contrast, studies performed by Stamey *et al.* (1969) showed that adequate serum levels in a range of 21–50 μg per ml were always attained 2 h after a single oral dose of 1 g. Nalidixic acid does not accumulate in the serum of patients with normal renal function if it is administered 6-hourly in the usual recommended doses.

Some nalidixic acid is converted in the body to a hydroxy metabolite, hydroxynalidixic acid, which also has antibacterial activity. Serum levels of the drug, quoted above, include both nalidixic acid and its hydroxy metabolite, the latter accounting for about 30% of biological activity in the serum (Stamey, 1971). Acyl glucuronidation of nalidixic acid occurs in the kidneys (Vree *et al.*, 1992). Overall, metabolism of nalidixic acid is 42% by glucuronidation and 40% hydroxylation (Vree *et al.*, 1988).

Probenecid may prolong the serum half-life of nalidixic acid in healthy adults (Dash and Mills, 1976).

Excretion

Nalidixic acid and its active hydroxy metabolite are both rapidly conjugated in the liver to antibacterially inactive monoglucuronides, which are rapidly excreted via the kidney (Stamey *et al.*, 1969). The drug is actively secreted by the renal tubules. About 85–90% of nalidixic acid excreted by the kidney is in the conjugated inactive form, but the remainder is excreted as unchanged nalidixic acid and its active hydroxy metabolite, producing therapeutically adequate urinary levels. Urine concentrations of these active drugs in adults are in the range of 25–250 μg per ml after a single oral dose of 0.5–1.0 g. These levels remain high (50–500 μg per ml) if a 1-g dose is administered orally every 6h (Buchbinder *et al.*, 1962). The hydroxy metabolite of nalidixic acid accounts for about 85% of the biologically active drug in the urine (Stamey, 1971).

Adequate urine levels of the active drugs are also usually attained in patients with moderate renal failure (Stamey *et al.*, 1969), although nalidixic acid should be avoided when the GFR is ≤50 ml per min (Bennett *et al.*, 1994). Although active nalidixic acid and metabolites do not accumulate in the serum of azotemic patients, their inactive monoglucuronides do and probably contribute to toxicity (Adam and Dawborn, 1971). Nalidixic acid should be administered cautiously to patients with liver disease in whom conjugation of the drug may be impaired. About 4% of orally administered nalidixic acid is not absorbed and is excreted in the feces.

Distribution of the Drug in Body

Even after prolonged administration, animal studies suggest that nalidixic acid does not accumulate in the tissues, where concentrations attained are usually lower than simultaneous serum levels. The kidney is the only organ in which tissue concentrations may exceed serum levels. In patients undergoing elective nephrectomy, renal tissue concentrations exceeded serum levels after treatment for >24 h in seven of 11 patients (Jameson, 1965). There was no difference between renal medullary and cortical tissue levels. Nalidixic acid was also present in the pus of one patient with a perinephric abscess, where the concentration varied from 8 to 24 μg per ml.

The drug is excreted in breast milk (p. 974).

Plasma protein binding of nalidixic acid and its metabolite, 7-hydroxymethyl-nalidixic acid, is 90–95% and 65%, respectively (Stamey, 1971; Vree *et al.*, 1988; Bennett *et al.*, 1994).

Mode of Action

Nalidixic acid inhibits bacterial DNA replication by inhibition of topoisomerase II, or DNA gyrase, causing DNA degradation and inducing filamentation in bacteria (Goss *et al.*, 1964; Winshell and Rosenkranz, 1970; Diver, 1989). These enzymes are required to supercoil strands of bacterial DNA so that they fit in the bacterial cell. In order to introduce negative (underwound) superhelical turns, DNA gyrase must impose a twisting stress and carry out a nicking-closing reaction to relieve the positive winding stress. Quinolones interrupt the function of DNA gyrase in which it breaks and rejoins DNA strands – such that DNA strand-breaking occurs, but the re-joining of broken strands is blocked (Hooper and Wolfson, 1993b). DNA gyrase contains two A and two B subunits. Gyrase A protein mediates the breakage and re-joining of DNA, while gyrase B protein mediates the ATPase activity of the enzyme and therefore functions principally in energy transduction and ATP hydrolysis during gyrase function (Mizuuchi et al., 1978; Hooper and Wolfson, 1993b). Studies by Gellert et al. (1977) and Sugino et al. (1977) suggested that gyrase A subunit was the primary target of nalidixic acid and oxolinic acid, but subsequently, the B subunit has also been shown to be a target (Hooper and Wolfson, 1993b). A bactericidal effect occurs best in the presence of competent ribonucleic acid (RNA) and protein synthesis (Deitz et al., 1966). Inhibition of protein synthesis markedly reduces the ability of nalidixic acid to kill bacteria, even though there is inhibition of DNA synthesis (Deitz et al., 1966). This may occur at high concentrations of nalidixic acid as RNA and protein synthesis may also be inhibited in this setting (Crumplin and Smith, 1975; Stevens, 1980). Similarly, some quinolones that do not inhibit DNA without inhibiting RNA and protein synthesis are only bacteriostatic (Stevens, 1980). To further support these observations, Carret et al. (1991) noted a paradoxical effect for nalidixic acid and pefloxacin whereby bacterial survival was greater in the presence of $5 \times$ MIC than in the presence of $3 \times$ MIC. In contrast, this phenomenon was not noted for the fluoroquinolone, ofloxacin.

Toxicity

1 Gastrointestinal side-effects

Nausea, vomiting or diarrhea are relatively infrequent complications and are usually not severe.

2 Neurotoxicity

This is uncommon and includes visual disturbances, excitement, depression, confusion and hallucinations. In fact, amfenolic acid, a derivative of nalidixic acid was originally developed as a central nervous system stimulant (McMillen and Short, 1978). Headache, giddiness, insomnia, drowsiness, syncope and sensory changes have also been described (Cahal, 1965). Visual disturbances include overbrightness of lights, blurred vision, difficulty in focusing, decreased visual acuity, diplopia and alteration in color perception. Convulsions have occurred in small numbers of patients (Islam and Sreedharan, 1965; Ronald et al., 1966; Fraser and Harrower, 1977; Paul, 1989). Acute reversible psychosis has been observed in a patient treated with large doses of nalidixic acid (Finegold et al., 1967). Similarly, Kremer et al. (1967) described an adult patient with acute glomerulonephritis, who developed a paranoid state after treatment with nalidixic acid for a urinary infection.

Severe neurotoxic reactions due to nalidixic acid have usually occurred when this drug has been used in large doses. It is wise to use it cautiously in patients with pre-existing mental instability, epilepsy and cerebral arteriosclerosis. Among the newer fluoroquinolones, neurological symptoms have been reported in 0.9–7.4% of patients in clinical trials (p. 1008).

3 Intracranial hypertension

This is a rare complication and most reported patients have been infants (Fisher, 1967; Deonna and Guignard, 1974; Mukherjee et al., 1990). Boréus and Sundstrom (1967) described a 6-month-old boy who developed vomiting, a bulging fontanelle, papilledema and widening of the skull sutures a few days after commencement of nalidixic acid in a dosage of 100 mg orally four times a day. This complication was observed on two separate occasions, when this drug was used for the treatment of urinary tract infection, and each time the signs resolved when it was discontinued. The causal relationship between nalidixic acid therapy and increased intracranial pressure was confirmed when the complication was reproduced on a third occasion by the administration of the drug under controlled conditions. Anderson et al. (1971) and Kilpatrick and Ebeling (1982) both described children who developed papilloedema and a VIth nerve palsy which resolved with cessation of nalidixic acid. Mukherjee et al. (1990) reported 12 cases of benign intracranial hypertension after nalidixic acid therapy for acute bacillary dysentary in infants less than 6 months old in Calcutta. These authors attributed the toxicity to the inadvertant use of high doses of nalidixic acid (100–150 mg per kg per day).

4 Myalgia and myopathy

Carmichael and Martin (1988) described a 53-year-old female with moderately severe renal failure who was treated with nalidixic acid 4 g per day for a urinary tract infection and developed severe myalgia and proximal muscle weakness which resolved promptly with cessation of nalidixic acid therapy. Other authors have reported myalgias, weakness and peripheral neuritis (Lane and Mastaglia, 1978; Anonymous, 1972).

5 Metabolic disturbances

Islam and Sreedharan (1965) reported the interesting case of a 14-year-old girl, who took an overdose of nalidixic acid (13 tablets of 500 mg). She developed convulsions, hyperglycemia and glycosuria, which simulated diabetic ketosis, but her plasma ketones were not elevated. Treatment was successful with i.v. fluids without insulin, and the blood glucose returned to normal after 24 h. Convulsions and hyperglycemia may also occur in otherwise healthy people as a result of an idiosyncratic reaction. Fraser and Harrower (1977) reported a 31-year-old woman who developed convulsions and hyperglycemia 2 days after starting nalidixic acid in a dose of 1 g four times daily. This patient had no underlying neurological disease and she recovered after ceasing the drug.

Metabolic acidosis without hyperglycemia has also been ascribed to nalidixic acid overdose. Dash and Mills (1976) described an 18-year-old man who ingested an unknown quantity of nalidixic acid, plus probenecid and a number of other drugs. He became stuporose and had a metabolic acidosis with markedly elevated serum levels of nalidixic acid but a normal plasma glucose. The patient awoke gradually over 21 h, and it was considered that the concomitant administration of probenecid had prolonged the serum half-life of nalidixic acid (p. 996).

Nalidixic acid may cause severe lactic acidosis in some diabetic patients with renal impairment. Phillips *et al.* (1979) described a 62-year-old woman with diabetes and chronic renal impairment. She developed fatal lactic acidosis, hyperglycemia and uremia without ketosis after administration of nalidixic acid. The authors gave nalidixic acid to four healthy volunteers and showed that it increased blood lactate levels after infusion of lactate. They suggested that nalidixic acid may be dangerous in patients with renal impairment and in diabetics who have abnormal lactate metabolism.

6 Skin rashes

Similar to other quinolones (p. 1010), dermatological reactions such as pruritus, rashes (usually urticarial and at times associated with eosinophilia) and severe photosensitivity reactions involving exposed surfaces, have been reported in patients treated with nalidixic acid (Zelickson, 1964; Burry and Crosby, 1966; Mathew, 1966; Baes, 1968; Birkett *et al.*, 1969; Brauner, 1975; Boisvert and Barbeau, 1981). Erythema multiforme and Stevens–Johnson syndrome have also been reported. All skin reactions appear to be reversible with cessation of quinolone therapy. In general, the incidence of such reactions with nalidixic acid is less than with some of the new fluoroquinolones (Hooper and Wolfson, 1993c).

The mechanism(s) of quinolone photosensitivity reactions have not been defined, but nalidixic acid-associated reactions occur after exposure to both ultraviolet (320–400 nm) and visible (>400 nm) light (Brauner, 1975). Animal studies suggest that among various quinolones there appears to be a correlation between ultraviolet A-induced photoinstability and the potential for photosensitivity/phototoxicity (Ferguson and Johnson, 1990; Wagai and Tawara, 1992). Five patients described by Mathew (1966) developed bullous skin eruptions in the summer while receiving nalidixic acid therapy; three had impaired renal function. The bullae slowly resolved 2 weeks to 2 months after cessation of the drug. One of these patients was treated with prednisolone without apparent beneficial effect. Mathew (1966) recommended that nalidixic acid therapy should be avoided during sunny weather, particularly in patients with impaired renal function. All patients receiving nalidixic acid should be warned to avoid sun exposure, and to cease the drug at the first sign of an abnormal skin reaction.

Bilsland and Douglas (1990) described an 43-year-old female who developed a photosensitive bullous rash which mimicked pseudoporphyria after sunbathing under an ultraviolet A sunbed. Interestingly, the patient had used the sunbed only once while taking a 6-day course of nalidixic acid, but used it regularly, 1 week after completing the course, with rash developing after four sunbed sessions. Skin biopsy demonstrated subepidermal bullae with no cellular infiltrate. The blistering healed over 2 weeks with some scarring and persistent skin fragility. Burry and Crosby (1966) considered that the reaction produced by nalidixic acid is a phototoxic reaction (which resembles excessive sunburn and does not spread beyond areas exposed to light), and not a photoallergic reaction (which looks like an allergic skin disease and spreads beyond areas exposed to light). Demethylchlortetracycline causes classical phototoxicity (p. 736), while the sulfonamides (p. 816) cause photoallergy. Brauner (1975) pointed out that nalidixic acid photodermatitis is uncommon; its incubation period is up to several weeks, and reactivity occurs irrespective of dosage and continues even when most of the drug has been cleared from the body. These features suggest photoallergy rather than phototoxicity. However, the fact that for some other quinolones reactions appear to be partly dosage related, suggests that all cutaneous reactions may not be wholly idiosyncratic (Hooper and Wolfson, 1993c). Anaphylactoid reactions with nalidixic acid are extremely uncommon, but have been reported, including cross-reactivity between different quinolones (Valdivieso et al., 1988; Dávila et al., 1993).

7 Arthropathy

Quinolones cause cartilage erosions, non-inflammatory joint effusions and some disorganization of epiphyseal plates in animal studies (p. 1011), however, rheumatologic adverse reactions in humans appear to be very uncommon (Ingham et al., 1977; Adam, 1989; Machida et al., 1990). In a retrospective case-control study by Schaad and Wedgwood-Krucko (1987) of 11 pediatric patients who were followed-up 3–12 years after receiving nalidixic acid for 9–600 days, no difference in skeletal growth or arthralgia was found in the nalidixic acid-treated group compared with controls. Furthermore, in a study of over 200 children treated with nalidixic acid, no clinical or radiographic evidence of arthropathy was detected (Adam, 1989). Thus, nalidixic acid appears to be safe to use in pediatric populations and, indeed, is licenced for such use (p. 970), although some theoretical reservations persist.

8 Hematological side-effects

Hemolytic anemia appears to be a rare, but potentially serious complication of nalidixic acid therapy, particularly in newborn infants and especially those with glucose-6-phosphate dehydrogenase (G6PD) deficiency. Belton and Jones (1965) reported a 2-week-old baby who was not G6PD deficient, who developed a hemolytic anemia, apparently as a result of drinking breast milk while the mother was being treated with nalidixic acid. Mandal and Stevenson (1970) described nalidixic acid-induced hemolytic crises in an older child and an adult both with G6PD deficiency, the latter had an occupational exposure to nalidixic acid dust (Alessio and Morselli, 1972). Coombs'-positive autoimmune hemolytic anemia associated with nalidixic acid therapy has been described in a number of adults, including one case of fatal hemolysis (Gilbertson and Jones, 1972; Tafani et al., 1982). Therefore, it seems that this drug may cause hemolytic anemia by a variety of mechanisms.

Thrombocytopenia has been described in association with nalidixic acid therapy. This complication appears to be rare, but it may be more common in the elderly and in those with impaired renal function (Meyboom, 1984). A number of the fluoroquinolones have been associated with significant hematological toxicity, although the overall incidence is 0.4–5.3% (Hooper and Wolfson, 1993c) (p. 1012).

9 Fetal toxicity

No teratogenic effects have been noted in pregnant animals given nalidixic acid (Ward-McQuaid et al., 1963) and pregnant patients have received this drug without untoward effects (Wren, 1969; Murray, 1981; ADEC, 1992). Some clinicians still have reservations about its use during the first trimester of pregnancy and the manufacturers state that the safety of the drug in the first trimester has not been established. Furthermore, manufacturers caution against the use of nalidixic acid in the days immediately prior to delivery because of the theoretical risk that very high nalidixic acid levels may develop in the neonate immediately after birth due to in utero exposure to maternal nalidixic acid.

10 Drug interactions

Nalidixic acid can displace warfarin and other highly albumin-bound coumarins from their binding sites on serum albumin, so that excess anticoagulation may result if the drug is given to patients stabilized on warfarin (Hoffbrand, 1974; Koch-Weser and Sellers, 1976; Leor et al., 1987).

Nalidixic acid glucuronide conjugates may produce a false positive reaction for glucose in urine with tests utilizing cupric sulfate reagent (Benedict's, Fehling's solution or Clinitest Reagent tablets); colorimetric tests for glucose using glucose oxidase methods (Clinistix or Testape) are unaffected. Diabetic patients should be informed of this if they are treated with nalidixic acid.

Unlike the fluoroquinolones, nalidixic acid does not decrease the clearance of theophylline and is therefore not associated with an increase in serum concentrations of this agent (Prince et *al.*, 1989; p. 1014). Nalidixic acid forms chelation complexes with various metal ions and although no formal study has documented interactions between nalidixic acid and antacids containing metal cations, reports of impaired ciprofloxacin absorption in the presence of antacids (p. 1013) suggest that nalidixic acid absorption may be similarly affected.

Clinical Uses of the Drug

1 Urinary tract infections

Nalidixic acid is useful for treatment of urinary tract infections caused by organisms such as *E. coli* and all species of *Enterobacter*, *Klebsiella* and *Proteus*, although its *in vitro* activity against common pathogens encountered in patients with complicated and/or nosocomial urinary tract infections is significantly less than that of most fluoroquinolones (Naber, 1989). It has been used successfully for the treatment of acute, chronic and recurrent urinary tract infections although the follow-up cure rate in patients with chronic infections, similar to that with other antimicrobial agents, is disappointing (Barlow, 1963; Ward-McQuaid *et al.*, 1963; Gibson and Potts, 1964; Ronald *et al.*, 1966). Increasingly, the use of nalidixic acid has been supplanted by newer, often more active agents, including the fluoroquinolones (pp. 1014, 1066).

Preiksaitis *et al.* (1981) found a similar cure rate with nalidixic acid and cephalexin in the treatment of women with bladder and renal infections, although more relapses occurred in patients with renal infections treated with cephalexin. Similarly, Iravani *et al.* (1981) found that both nalidixic acid and trimethoprim-sulfamethoxazole were equally efficacious for treatment of uncomplicated acute urinary tract infections in young women caused by Gram-negative Enterobacteriaceae. Resistant mutants did not emerge in the urine in either treatment group, however, resistant Enterobacteriaceae were noted to emerge in the feces in 1.1% and 2.3% of nalidixic acid- and trimethoprim-sulfamethoxazole-treated cases, respectively. Nalidixic acid and trimethoprim-sulfamethoxazole eradicated susceptible fecal Enterobacteriaceae in 15% and 22.4%, respectively.

Ferry *et al.* (1987) reported a 90% cure rate in the treatment of females with acute lower urinary tract infections with a 3-day course of low-dose (0.66 g) nalidixic acid in combination with 4 g sodium citrate, although higher rates of nalidixic acid resistance were noted in older patients. Ahlmén *et al.* (1983) found a 3-day course of nalidixic acid to be effective in the treatment of the dysuria-frequency syndrome in women. As noted earlier (p. 967), nalidixic acid is ineffective against infections due to *Staph. saprophyticus*, because these organisms are resistant.

Nalidixic acid in a lower dosage is one of several drugs suitable for long-term suppressive therapy in patients with chronic bacteriuria. Such therapy may prevent recurrent bacteriuria in patients with chronic bacterial prostatitis, but it usually fails to eradicate prostatic infection since it is not excreted into prostatic fluid even when serum levels are high (Stamey, 1971; Leading article, 1983).

Nalidixic acid has been used successfully for the treatment of uncomplicated urinary tract infections in childhood and for the prolonged treatment of children with urinary infections associated with renal tract abnormalities (Kneebone, 1965). However, since resistance to nalidixic acid often emerges during the treatment of complicated urinary sepsis (p. 968), it is best avoided in favor of agents which produce effective blood and tissue levels.

The drug has been used occasionally for the treatment of urinary infections during pregnancy, and no teratogenic effects have been noted (Wren, 1969).

The antibacterial activity of nalidixic acid remains unchanged over the entire pH range of urine, and on this basis alone there is no need to regulate urinary pH when the drug is used to treat urinary infections. However, alkalinization of the urine markedly increases urine levels of the active drug, and, therefore, may enhance its clinical effect (Zinsser, 1970). The absorption of nalidixic acid from the gastrointestinal tract and renal clearance of the active drug both appear to be increased by concomitant administration of sodium bicarbonate (Adam and Dawborn, 1971).

Nalidixic acid should not be used with nitrofurantoin, because these two drugs show antagonism *in vitro*.

2 Systemic infections due to Gram-negative bacilli

Nalidixic acid is not suitable for the reliable treatment of systemic infections, since insufficient tissue levels are generally obtained and resistant strains therefore often develop during therapy. Nevertheless, there are a number of early reports of nalidixic acid use in the treatment of systemic infections. Sharma (1965) reported the successful treatment of four patients with brucellosis with oral nalidixic acid and Hassan *et al.* (1970) described the use of nalidixic acid (60–100mg per kg body weight per day for 10 days) to cure 28 of 32 patients with typhoid or paratyphoid fever; although the average time for patients to become afebrile was 9.5 days.

3 Shigella infections

Early studies indicated that nalidixic acid may be beneficial in the treatment of *Shigella* dysentery (Pesigan and Medado, 1964; Moorhead and Parry, 1965). A higher cure rate was also observed with nalidixic acid, compared with placebo treatment, by Hansson *et al.* (1981). More recent studies also demonstrate the efficacy of nalidixic acid, however, the increasing resistance of *Shigella* strains to nalidixic acid in many developing countries (p. 969) has been associated with a loss of clinical efficacy. A small comparative study of nalidixic acid versus enoxacin for the treatment of bacillary dysentery in Rwanda, in which all isolates were susceptible *in vitro* to both agents, demonstrated similar favorable clinical and bacteriological response (De Mol *et al.*, 1987). Similarly, a comparative study in India of nalidixic acid and norfloxacin demonstrated comparable overall outcome, although the duration of fever, anorexia and abdominal pain were less in the norfloxacin group. As expected, norfloxacin was superior to nalidixic acid in cases where the *Shigella* isolate was resistant *in vitro* to nalidixic acid (Bhattacharya *et al.*, 1991). Rogerie *et al.* (1986) also noted no difference between nalidixic acid and norfloxacin therapy for shigellosis. Lolekha *et al.* (1991) reported a comparative study of nalidixic acid, norfloxacin or trimethoprim-sulfamethoxazole therapy for shigellosis in Thailand in which treatment with norfloxacin eradicated *Shigella* spp. from fecal specimens faster than nalidixic acid, however there was no statistically significant difference in clinical response between these two treatment groups (p > 0.1). Both nalidixic acid and norfloxacin were more effective than trimethoprim–sulfamethoxazole (p < 0.01), probably because only 17% of isolates were susceptible to trimethoprim–sulfamethoxazole.

In a randomized, double-blind trial of 5-day therapy with either nalidixic acid (55 mg per kg per day) or ampicillin (100 mg per kg per day) for childhood shigellosis in Bangladesh, the clinical cure rate was 81% and 77%, respectively, among patients with susceptible strains (Salam and Bennish, 1988). The use of quinolones, either nalidixic acid or particularly the fluoroquinolones, as one- or two-dose therapy for severe shigellosis in young children is now suggested as a treatment option by WHO, since these agents are likely to be effective and the amount of drug given is unlikely to be associated with significant toxicity (Fontaine, 1989).

4 Reduction of bowel flora in patients with granulocytopenia

Nalidixic acid has been used for 'selective decontamination' (selective antimicrobial modulation) of the gut to prevent infection in granulocytopenic patients because, like trimethoprim-sulfamethoxazole (p.881), it suppresses many of the potentially pathogenic aerobes, but preserves the anaerobes (Rozenberg-Arska *et al.*, 1989). In this way, these drugs preserve 'colonization resistance', which by some mechanism prevents microorganisms colonizing body surfaces. In this respect, Wade *et al.* (1983) found nalidixic acid plus nystatin to be not as effective as trimethoprim-sulfamethoxazole plus nystatin in the prevention of infection in granulocytopenic patients. However, a daily regimen using oral neomycin (1 g), amphotericin B (1 g), nalidixic acid (2 g) and polymyxin B (400mg) was effective in reducing infection in such patients, and correlated with the selective elimination of aerobic and facultative anaerobic Gram-negative rods from the gut (Guiot *et al.*, 1983). Veringa and Van der Waaij (1984) showed that antibiotics used for selective decontamination of the gut were rapidly biologically inactivated by intestinal contents in a dose-dependent fashion, but not to the same extent. This may explain why some unabsorbed drugs need to be given in relatively high doses (polymyxin), whereas lower daily doses of some less active drugs (tobramycin) are sufficient. In their experiments, colistin was almost completely inactivated, tobramycin and neomycin were considerably inactivated and temocillin and aztreonam were only partially inactivated; nalidixic acid and trimethoprim were intermediate in their susceptibility to fecal inactivation. Jansen *et al.* (1994) compared the combination of neomycin + polymyxin B sulfate + nalidixic acid with ciprofloxacin 500 mg twice-daily alone for the prevention of bacterial infections in severely myelosuppressed patients (bone marrow transplant recipients or patients post-induction for leukemia). The two regimens proved to be similar in efficacy, but ciprofloxacin therapy was better tolerated. A high incidence of streptococcal infections was noted in both treatment groups.

References

Adam D (1989). Use of quinolones in pediatric patients. *Rev Infect Dis* **11** (Suppl 5): S1113.

Adam WR, Dawborn JK (1971). Plasma levels and urinary excretion of nalidixic acid in patients with renal failure. *Aust NZ J Med* **1**: 126.

ADEC (Australian Drug Evaluation Committee) (1992). *Medicines in Pregnancy* 2nd edn. Canberra: Commonwealth of Australia 1992.

Adler-Mosca H, Lüthy-Hottenstein J, Martinetti Lucchini G *et al.* (1991). Development of resistance to quinolones in five patients with campylobacteriosis treated with norfloxacin or ciptofloxacin. *Eur J Clin Microbiol Infect Dis* **10** 953.

Ahlmén J, Sigurdson J, Wohrm A *et al.* (1983). Effect of a three-day course of nalidixic acid in the frequency-dysuria syndrome with significant bacteriuria in women. *Scand J Infect Dis* **15**: 71.

Alessio L, Morselli G (1972). Occupational exposure to nalidixic acid. *Brit Med J* **4**: 110.

Altwegg M, Burnens A, Zollinger-Iten J, Penner JL (1987). Problems in identification of *Campylobacter jejuni* associated with acquisition of resistance to nalidixic acid. *J Clin Micro* **25**: 1807.

Anderson EE, Anderson B Jr, Nashold BS (1971). Childhood complications of nalidixic acid. *JAMA* **216**: 1023.

Anonymous (1972). Adverse effects of drugs commonly used in the treatment of urinary tract infections: report from the Australian Drug Evaluation Committee. *Med J Aust* **i**: 435.

Baes H (1968). Photosensitivity caused by nalidixic acid. *Dermatologica* **136**: 61.

Barlow AM (1963). Nalidixic acid in infections of urinary tract. *Brit Med J* **2**: 1308.

Belton EM, Jones RV (1965). Haemolytic anaemia due to nalidixic acid. *Lancet* **ii**: 691.

Bennett WM, Aronoff GR, Golper TA (1994). *Drug Prescribing in Renal Failure* 3rd edn. Philadelphia: American College of Physicians.

Bennish ML, Salam MA, Hossain MA *et al.* (1992). Antimicrobial resistance of *Shigella* isolates in Bangladesh, 1983–1990: increasing frequency of strains multiply resistant to ampicillin, trimethoprim–sulfamethoxazole, and nalidixic acid. *Clin Infect Dis* **14**: 1055.

Bhattacharya SK, Bhattacharya MK, Dutta P *et al.* (1991). Randomized clinical trial of norfloxacin for shigellosis. *Amer J Trop Med Hyg* **45**: 683.

Bilsland D, Douglas WS (1990). Sunbed pseudoporphyria induced by nalidixic acid. *Brit J Dermatol* **123**: 547.

Birkett DA, Barretts AM, Stevenson CJ (1969). Phototoxic bullous eruptions due to nalidixic acid. *Brit J Dermatol* **81**: 342.

Boisvert A, Barbeau G (1981). Nalidixic acid-induced photodermatitis after minimal sun exposure. *Drug Intell Clin Pharm* **15**: 126.

Boréus LO, Sundström B (1967). Intracranial hypertension in a child during treatment with nalidixic acid. *Brit Med J* **2**: 744.

Brauner GJ (1975). Bullous photoreaction to nalidixic acid. *Amer J Med* **58**: 576.

Brumfitt W, Pursell R (1971). Observations on bacterial sensitivities to nalidixic acid and critical comments on the 6-centre survey. *Postgrad Med J* **47** (Sept Suppl): 16.

Buchbinder M, Webb JC, Anderson LV, McCabe WR (1962). Laboratory studies and clinical pharmacology of nalidixic acid (WIN 18,320). *Antimicrob Ag Chemother*: 308.

Burman LG (1977). Apparent absence of transferable resistance to nalidixic acid in pathogenic Gram-negative bacteria. *J Antimicrob Chemother* **3**: 509.

Burry JN, Crosby RWL (1966). A case of phototoxicity to nalidixic acid. *Med J Aust* **2**: 698.

Cahal DA (1965). Reactions to nalidixic acid. *Brit Med J* **2**: 590.

Cambau E, Bordon F, Collatz E, Gutmann L (1993). Novel *gyrA* point mutation in astrain of *Escherichia coli* resistant to fluoroquinolones but not to nalidixic acid. *Antimicrob Ag Chemother* **37**: 1247.

Carmichael AJ, Martin AM (1988). Acute painful proximal myopathy associated with nalidixic acid. *Brit Med J* **297**: 742.

Carret G, Flandrois JP, Lobry JR (1991). Biphasic kinetics of bacterial killing by quinolones. *J Antimicrob Chemother* **27**: 319.

Cederberg A, Denneberg AT, Ekberg M, Juhlin I (1974). Nalidixic acid in urinary tract infections with particular reference to the emergence of resistance. *Scand J Infect Dis* **6**: 259.

Chapman JS, Bertasso A, Georgoppapdakou NH (1989). Fleroxacin resistance in *Escherichia coli*. *Antimicrob Ag Chemother* **33**: 239.

Chatzipanagiotou S, Papavasiliou E, Malamou-Lada E (1993). Isolation of *Campylobacter jejuni* strains resistant to nalidixic acid and fluoroquinolones from children with diarrhea in Athens, Greece. *Eur J Clin Microbiol Infect Dis* **12**: 566.

Courtright JB, Turowski DA, Sonstein SA (1988). Alteration of bacterial DNA structure, gene expression, and plsmid encoded antibiotic resistance following exposure to enoxacin. *J Antimicrob Chemother* **21**(Suppl B): 1.

Courvalin P (1990). Plasmid-mediated 4-quinolone resistance: a real or apparent absence? *Antimicrob Ag Chemother* **34**: 681.

Crumplin GC (1987). Plasmid-mediated resistance to nalidixic acid and new 4-quinolones. *Lancet* **ii**: 854.

Crumplin GC, Odell M (1987). Development of resistance to ofloxacin. *Drugs* **34**(Suppl 1): 1.

Crumplin GC, Smith JT (1975). Nalidixic acid: an antibacterial paradox. *Antimicrob Ag Chemother* **8**: 251.

Crumplin GC, Smith JT (1981). The effect of R-factor plasmids on host-cell responses to nalidixic acid I. Increased susceptibility of nalidixic acid-sensitive hosts. *J Antimicrob Chemother* **7**: 379.

Cullman W, Stieglitz M, Baars B, Opferkuch W (1985). Comparative evaluation of recently developed quinolone compounds – with a note on the frequency of resistant mutants. *Chemotherapy* (Basel) **31**: 19.

Dash H, Mills J (1976). Severe metabolic acidosis associated with nalidixic acid overdose. *Ann Intern Med* **84**: 570.

Dávila I, Diez ML, Quirce S *et al.* (1993). Cross-reactivity between quinolones. *Allergy* **48**: 388.

De Mol P, Mets T, Lagasse R *et al.* (1987). Treatment of baciilary dysentery: a comparison between enoxacin and nalidixic acid. *J Antimicrob Chemother* **19**: 695.

Dietz WH, Cook TM, Goss WA (1966). Mechanism of action of nalidixic acid on *Escherichia coli*. *J Bacteriol* **91**: 768.

Deonna T, Guignard JP (1974). Acute intracranial hypertension after nalidixic acid administration. *Arch Dis Child* **49**: 743.

Diver JM (1989). Quinolone uptake by bacteria and bacterial killing. *Rev Infect Dis* **11** (Suppl 5): S941.

Divo AA, Sartorelli AC, Patton CL, Bia FJ (1988). Activity of fluoroquinolone antibiotics against *Plasmodium falciparum in vitro*. *Antimicrob Ag Chemother* **32**: 1182.

Eliopoulos GM, Eliopoulos CT (1989). Quinolone antimicrobial agents: activity *in vitro*. In *Quinolone Antimicrobial Agents* (Wolfson JS, Hooper DC, eds), p. 35. Washington, DC: American Society of Microbiology.

Felmington D, Foxall P, O'Hare MD *et al.* (1988). Resistance studies with ofloxacin. *J Antimicrob Chemother* **22** (Suppl C): 27.

Ferguson J, Johnson BE (1990). Ciprofloxacin-induced photosensitivity: *in vitro* and *in vivo* studies. *Brit J Dermatol* **123**: 9.

Fernandes PB, Hanson CW, Stamm JM *et al.* (1987). The frequency of *in vitro* resistance development to fluoroquinolones and the use of murine pyelonephritis model to demonstrate selection of resistance *in vivo*. *J Antimicrob Chemother* **19**: 449.

Ferry S, Burman LG, Widberg B, Calmenius C (1987). Short-term nalidixic acid plus sodium citrate in acute lower urinary tract infection. *Scand J Infect Dis* **19**: 469.

Finegold SM, Miller LG, Posnick D *et al.* (1967). Nalidixic acid: clinical and laboratory studies. *Antimicrob Ag Chemother* **1966**: 189.

Fisher OD (1967). Nalidixic acid and intracranial hypertension. *Brit Med J* **3**: 370.

Fliegelman RM, Petrak RM, Goodman LJ *et al.* (1985). Comparative *in vitro* activities of twelve antimicrobial agents against *Campylobacter* species. *Antimicrob Ag Chemother* **27**: 429.

Fontaine O (1989). Antibiotics in the management of shigellosis in children: what role for the quinolones. *Rev Infect Dis* **11**: (Suppl 5): S1145.

Fraser AG, Harrower ADB (1977). Convulsions and hyperglycaemia associated with nalidixic acid. *Brit Med J* **2**: 1518.

Gellert M, Mizuuchi K, O'Dea MH *et al.* (1977). Nalidixic acid resistance: a second genetic character involved in DNA gyrase activity. *Proc Natl Acad Sci USA* **74**: 4772.

Gibbon NOK, Benstead JG, Misra GC (1965). A comparative study of the levels of nalidixic acid in plasma and urine and its antibacterial activity in urinary infections in paraplegics. *Postgrad Med J* **41**: 501.

Gibson GR, Potts IF (1964). A clinical trial of nalidixic acid: a new antibacterial substance. *Med J Aust* **2**: 225.

Gilbertson C, Jones DR (1972). Haemolytic anaemia with nalidixic acid. *Brit Med J* **4**: 493.

Goldstein EJC, Citron DM (1985). Comparative activity of the quinolones against anaerobic bacteria isolated at community hospitals. *Antimicrob Ag Chemother* **27**: 657.

Gootz TD, Martin BA (1991). Characterization of high-level quinolone resistance in *Campylobacter jejuni*. *Antimicrob Ag Chemother* **35**: 840.

Goss WA, Dietz WH, Cook TM (1964). Mechanism of action of nalidixic acid on *Escherichia coli*. *J Bacteriol* **88**: 1112.

Guiot HFL, Van den Broek PJ, Van der Meer JWM, Van Furth R (1983). Selective antimicrobial modulation of the intestinal flora of patients with acute nonlymphocytic leukemia: a double-blind, placebo-controlled study. *J Infect Dis* **147**: 615.

Gutmann L, Williamson R, Moreau N *et al.* (1985). Cross-resistance to nalidixic acid, trimethoprim, and chloramphenicol associated with alterations in outer membrane proteins of *Klebsiella, Enterobacter*, and *Serratia*. *J Infect Dis* **151**: 501.

Hancock REW (1987). Role of porins in outer membrane permeability. *J Bacteriol* **169**: 929.

Hansson HB, Barkenius G, Cronberg S, Juhlin I (1981a). Controlled comparison of nalidixic acid or lactulose with placebo in shigellosis. *Scand J Infect Dis* **13**: 191.

Hassan A, Adbel Wahab MF, Farid Z, Rooby ASE (1970). Treatment of typhoid and paratyphoid fever with nalidixic acid. *J Trop Med Hyg* **73**: 145.

Hawkey PM, Hawkey CA (1984). Comparative *in-vitro* activity of quinolone carboxylic acids against Proteeae. *J Antimicrob Chemother* **14**: 485.

Heessen FWA, Muytjens HL (1984). *In vitro* activities of ciprofloxacin, norfloxacin, pipemidic acid, cinoxacin and nalidixic acid against *Chlamydia trachomatis*. *Antimicrob Ag Chemother* **25**: 123.

Hoffbrand BI (1974). Interaction of nalidixic acid and warfarin. *Brit Med J* **2**: 666.

Hooper DC (1993). Introduction. In *Quinolone Antimicrobial Agents* 2nd edn (Hooper DC, Wolfson JS, eds), p. 1. Washington, DC: American Society of Microbiology.

Hooper DC, Wolfson JS (1989). Mode of action of the quinolone antimicrobial agents: review of recent information. *Rev Infect Dis* **11** (Suppl 5): S902.

Hooper DC, Wolfson JS (1993a). Mechanisms of bacterial resistance to quinolones. In *Quinolone Antimicrobial Agents* 2nd edn (Hooper DC, Wolfson JS, eds), p. 97. Washington, DC: American Society of Microbiology.

Hooper DC, Wolfson JS (1993b). Mechanisms of quinolone action and bacterial killing. In *Quinolone Antimicrobial Agents* 2nd edn (Hooper DC, Wolfson JS, eds), p. 53. Washington, DC: American Society of Microbiology.

Hooper DC, Wolfson JS (1993c). Adverse effects. In *Quinolone Antimicrobial Agents* 2nd edn (Hooper DC, Wolfson JS, eds), p. 489. Washington, DC: American Society of Microbiology.

Hooper DC, Wolfson JS, McHugh GL *et al.* (1984). Elimination of plasmid pMG110 from *Escherichia coli* by novobiocin and other inhibitors of DNA gyrase. *Antimicrob Ag Chemother* **25**: 586.

Hooper DC, Wolfson JS, Souza KS *et al.* (1986). Genetic and biochemical characterization of norfloxacin resistance in *Escherichia coli*. *Antimicrob Ag Chemother* **29**: 639.

Hooper DC, Wolfson JS, Ng EY, Swartz MN (1987). Mechanisms of action of and resistance to ciprofloxacin. *Amer J Med* **82**:(Suppl 4A): 12.

Ingham B, Brentnall DW, Dale EA, McFadzean JA (1977). Arthropathy induced by antibacterial fused N-alkyl-4-pyridone-3-carboxylic acids. *Toxicol Lett* **1**: 21.

Iravani A, Richard GA, Baer H, Fennell R (1981). Comparative efficacy and safety of nalidixic acid versus trimethoprim/sulfamethoxazole in treatment of acute urinary tract infections in college-age women. *Antimicrob Ag Chemother* **19**: 598.

Islam MA, Sreedharan T (1965). Convulsions, hyperglycaemia, and glycosuria from overdose of nalidixic acid. *JAMA* **192**: 1100.

Jameson RM (1965). Tissue concentration of nalidixic acid in chronic pyelonephritis. *Brit Med J* **2**: 621.

Jansen J, Cromer M, Akard L *et al.* (1994). Infection prevention in severely myelosuppressed patients: a comparison between ciprofloxacin and a regimen of selective antibiotic modulation of the intestinal flora. *Amer J Med* **96**: 335.

Kemball ML, Davies PA (1967). Nalidixic acid for the newborn. *Brit Med J* **2**: 310.

Kilpatrick C, Ebeling P (1982). Intracranial hypertension in nalidixic acid therapy. *Med J Aust* **1**: 252.

Kneebone GM (1965). A clinical appraisal of nalidixic acid in urinary tract infection in childhood. *Med J Aust* **2**: 947.

Koch-Weser J, Sellers EM (1976). Binding of drugs to serum albumin. (Second of two parts). *New Engl J Med* **294**: 526.

Kremer L, Walton M, Wardle EN (1967). Nalidixic acid and intracranial hypertension. *Brit Med J* **4**: 488.

Kresken M, Wieddemann B (1988). Development of resistance to nalidixic acid and the fluoroquinolones after the introduction of norfloxacin and ofloxacin. *Antimicrob Ag Chemother* **32**: 1285.

Lane RJM, Mastaglia FL (1978). Drug induced myopathies in man. *Lancet* **ii**: 562.

Lariviere LA, Gandreau CL, Turgeon FF (1986). Susceptibility of clinical isolates of *Campylobacter jejuni* to twenty-five antimicrobial agents. *J Antimicrob Chemother* **18**: 681.

Leading Article (1983). Chronic bacterial prostatitis. *Lancet* **i**: 393.

Leor J, Levartowsky D, Sharon C (1987). Interaction between nalidixic acid and warfarin. *Ann Intern Med* **107**: 601.

Lesher GY, Froelich EJ, Gruett MD *et al.* (1962). 1,8-naphthyridine derivatives. A new class of chemotherapeutic agents. *J Med Pharm Chem* **5**: 1063.

Lewin CS (1991). Treatment of multi-resistant *Salmonella* infection. *Lancet* **337**: 47.

Light RB, Ronald AR, Harding G *et al.* (1981). Epidemiologic features of urinary infections due to Enterobacteriaceae resistant to nalidixic acid and trimethoprim. *Scand J Infect Dis* **13**: 195.

Lolekha S, Vibulbandhitkit S, Poonyarit P (1991). Respnse to antimicrobial therapy for shigellosis in Thailand. *Rev Infect Dis* **13**: (Suppl 4): S342.

MacDonald KL, Cohen ML, Hargrett-Bean NT *et al.* (1987). Changes in antimicrobial resistance of *Salmonella* isolated from humans in the United States. *JAMA* **258**: 1496.

Machida M, Kusajima H, Aijima H *et al.* (1990). Toxicokinetic study of norfloxacin-induced arthropathy in juvenile animals. *Toxicol Appl Pharmacol* **105**: 403.

Mandal BK, Stevenson J (1970). Haemolytic crisis produced by nalidixic acid. *Lancet* **i**: 614.

Mathew TH (1966). Nalidixic acid. *Med J Aust* **2**: 243.

McMillen BA, Short PA (1978). Amfonelic acid, a non-amphetamine stimulant, has marked effects on brain dopamine metabolism but not noradrenaline metabolism: associated with differences in neuronal storage systems. *J Pharm Pharmacol* **30**: 464.

Mehtar S, Blakemore PH, Ellis K (1987). Brief report: *in vivo* curing of plasmids from mult-drug-resistant *Serratia marcescens* by ciprofloxacin. *Amer J Med* **82**: (Suppl 4A): 55.

Meyboom RHB (1984). Thrombocytopenia induced by nalidixic acid. *Brit Med J* **289**: 962.

Michel J, Luboshitzky R, Sacks T (1973). Bactericidal effect on combinations of nalidixic acid and various antibiotics on Enterobacteriaceae. *Antimicrob Ag Chemother* **4**: 201.

Milatovic D, Braveny I (1987). Development of resistance during antibiotic therapy. *Eur J Clin Microbiol* **6**: 234.

Mitsuhashi S (1988). Comparative antibacterial activity of new quinolone-carboxylic acid derivatives. *Rev Infect Dis* **10**: (Suppl 1): S27.

Mizuuchi K, O'Dea MH, Gellert M (1978). DNA gyrase: subunit structure and ATPase activity of the purified enzyme. *Proc Natl Acad Sci USA* **75**: 5960.

Moniot-Ville N, Guibert J, Moreau N *et al.* (1991). Mechanisms of quinolone resistance in aclinical isolate of *Escherichia coli* highly resistant to fluoroquinolones but susceptible to nalidixic acid. *Antimicrob Ag Chemother* **35**: 519.

Moorhead PJ, Parry HE (1965). Treatment of Sonne dysentery. *Brit Med J* **2**: 913.

Mouton RP, Mulders SL (1987). Combined resistance to quinolones and beta-lactams after *in vitro* transfer on single drugs. *Chemotherapy* (Basel) **33**: 189.

Mukherjee A, Dutta P, Lahiri M *et al.* (1990). Benign intracranial hypertension after nalidixic acid overdose in infants. *Lancet* **335**: 1602.

Munshi MH, Haider K, Rahaman MM *et al.* (1987). Plasmid-mediated resistance to nalidixic acid in *Shigella dysenteriae* type 1. *Lancet* **ii**: 419.

Murray EDS (1981). Nalidixic acid in pregnancy. *Brit Med J* **282**: 224.

Naber KG (1989). Use of quinolones in urinary tract infections and prostatitis. *Rev Infect Dis* **11** (Suppl 5): S1221.

Nagate T, Komatsu T, Izawa A *et al.* (1980). Mode of action of a new nalidixic acid derivative, AB 206. *Antimicrob Ag Chemother* **17**: 763.

Nakamura S, Nakamura T, Kojima T, Yoshida H (1989). *gyrA* and *gyrB* mutations in quinolone-resistant strains of *Escherichia coli*. *Antimicrob Ag Chemother* **33**: 254.

Neu HC (1987). Ciprofloxacin: an overview and prospective appraisal. *Am J Med* **82** (Suppl 4A): 395.

Newsom SWB, Matthews J, Amphlett M, Warren RE (1982). Norfloxacin and the antibacterial *y* pyridone β carboxylic acids. *J Antimicrob Chemother* **10**: 25.

Nikaido H, Vaara M (1985). Molecular basis of bacterial outer membrane permeability *Microbiol Rev* **49**: 1.

Panhotra BR, Desai B, Sharma PL (1985). Nalidixic acid-resistant *Shigella dysenteriae* I. *Lancet* **i**: 763.

Paul GA (1989). Antibiotic induced convulsions? *N Z Med J* **102**: 538.

Pesigan TP, Medado PM (1964). Clinical evaluation of nalidixic acid in the treatment of shigellosis and salmonellosis. *Int Med* **11**: 123.

Philips I (1987). Quinolones in the treatment of gonnorrhoea. *Quinolones Bull* **2**: 7.

Phillips PJ, Need AG, Thomas DW *et al.* (1979). Nalidixic acid and lactic acidosis. *Aust NZ J Med* **9**: 694.

Preiksaitis JK, Thompson L, Harding GKM *et al.* (1981). A comparison of the efficacy of nalidixic acid and cephalexin in bactiuric women and their effect on fecal and periurethral carriage of Enterobacteriaceae. *J Infect Dis* **143**: 603.

Prince RA, Casabar E, Adair CG *et al.* (1989). Effects of quinolone antimicrobials on theophylline pharmacokinetics. *J Clin Pharmacol* **29**: 650.

Report of a WHO Scientific Group (1978). *Neisseria gonorrhoeae* and gonococcal infections. *Wld Hlth Org Techn Rep Ser* No 616.

Rikihisa Y, Jiang BM (1988). *In vitro* susceptibilities of *Ehrlichia risticii* to eight antibiotics. *Antimicrob Ag Chemother* **32**: 986.

Rogerie F, Ott D, Vandepite J *et al.* (1986). Comparison of norfloxacin and nalidixic acid for treatment of dysentery caused by *Shigella dysenteriae* type 1 in adults. *Antimicrob Ag Chemother* **29**: 883.

Ronald AR, Turck M, Petersdorf RG (1966). A critical evaluation of nalidixic acid in urinary-tract infections. *New Engl J Med* **275**: 1081.

Rosenberg-Arska M, Dekker AW, Verhoef J (1989). Prevention of infections in granulocytopenic patients by fluorinated quinolones. *Rev Infect Dis* **11** (Suppl 5): S1231.

Salam MA, Bennish ML (1988). Therapy for shigellosis I Randomized double-blind trial of nalidixic acid in childhood shigellosis. *J Pediatr* **113**: 901.

Sanders CC, Sanders WE, Goering RV, Werner V (1984). Selection of multiple antibiotic resistance by quinolones, beta-lactams, and aminoglycosides with special reference to cross-resistance between unrelated classes. *Antimicrob Ag Chemother* **26**: 797.

Schaad UB, Wedgwood-Krucko J (1987). Nalidixic acid in children: retrospective matched controlled study for cartilage toxicity. *Infection* **15**: 165.

Sen D, Dutta P, Deb BC, Pal SC (1988). Nalidixic acid resistant *Shigella dysenteriae* type I in Eastern India. *Lancet* **ii**: 911.

Sharma B (1965). Treatment of brucellosis by nalidixic acid. *Lancet* **i**: 1171.

Smith JT (1986). Frequency and expression of mutational resistance to the 4-quinolone antibacterials. *Scand J Infect Dis* **49**: 115.

Sobieski RJ, Brewer AR (1976). Toxicity of nalidixic acid on *Candida albicans*, *Saccharomyces cerevisiae*, and *Kluyveromyces lactis.*. *Antimicrob Ag Chemother* **9**: 485.

Stamey TA (1971). Observations on the clinical use of nalidixic acid. *Postgrad Med J* **47**: (Sept Suppl): 21.

Stamey TA, Bragonje J (1976). Resistance to nalidixic acid. A misconception due to underdosage. *JAMA* **236**: 1857.

Stamey TA, Nemoy NJ, Higgins M (1969). The clinical use of nalidixic acid. A review and some observations. *Investig Urol* **6**: 582.

Stein DC, Danaher RJ, Cook TM (1991). Characterization of a *gyrB* mutation responsible for low-level nalidixic acid resistance in *Neisseria gonorrhoeae*. *Antimicrob Ag Chemother* **35**: 622.

Stevens PJE (1980). Bactericidal effect against *Escherichia coli* of nalidixic acid and four structurally related compounds. *J Antimicrob Chemother* **6**: 535.

Sugino A, Peebles CL, Kreuzer KN *et al.* (1977). Mechanism of action of nalidixic acid: purification of *Escherichia coli* nal A gene product and its relationship to DNA gyrase and novel nicking-closing enzyme. *Proc Natl Acad Sci USA* **74**: 4767.

Tafani O, Mazzoli M, Landini G, Alterini B (1982). Fatal acute immune haemolytic anaemia caused by nalidixic acid. *Brit Med J* **285**: 936.

Tanaka M, Ishii H, Sato K, Osada Y, Nishino T (1991). Characterization of high-level quinolone resistance in methicillin-resistant *Staphylococcus aureus*, In *Program and Abstracts of the 31st Interscience Conference on Antimicrobial Agents and Chemotherapy. Chicago, IL* (Abstr. 308). Washington, DC: American Society for Microbiology.

Traub WH (1985). Incomplete cross-resistance of nalidixic and pipemidic acid-resistant variants of *Serratia marcescens* against ciprofloxacin, enoxacin, and norfloxacin. *Chemotherapy* (Basel) **31**: 34.

Valdivieso R, Pola J, Losada E *et al.* (1988). Severe anaphylactoid reaction to nalidixic acid. *Allergy* **43**: 71.

Veringa EM, Van der Waaij D (1984). Biological inactivation by faeces of antimicrobial drugs applicable in selective decontamination of the digestive tract. *J Antimicrob Chemother* **15**: 605.

Voogd CE, Schot CS, van Leeuwen WJ, van Klingeren B (1992). Monitoring of antibiotic resistance in *Shigella* isolated in the Netherlands 1984–1989. *Eur J Clin Microbiol Infect Dis* **11**: 164.

Vree TB, Wijnands WJ, Baars AM, Hekster YA (1988). Pharmacokinetics of nalidixic acid in man: hydroxyation and glucuronidation. *Pharm Weekl* **10**: 193.

Vree TB, Hekster YA, Anderson PG (1992). Contribution of the human kidney to the metabolic clearance of drugs. *Ann Pharmacother* **26**: 1421.

Wade JC, De Jongh CA, Newman KA *et al.* (1983). Selective antimicrobial modulation as prophylaxis against infection during granulocytopenia: trimethoprim–sulfamethoxazole vs. nalidixic acid. *J Infect Dis* **147**: 624.

Wagai N, Tawara K (1992). Possible direct role of reactive oxygen species in the cause of mouse cutaneous phototoxicity induced by 5 quinolones. *Arch Toxicol* **66**: 392.

Walder M (1982). Epidemiology of *Campylobacter* enteritis. *Scand J Infect Dis* **14**: 27.

Ward-McQuaid JFNC, Jichlinski D, Macis R (1963). Nalidixic acid in urinary infections. *Brit Med J* **2**: 1311.

Weisser J, Wiedemann B (1985). Elimination of plasmids by new 4-quinolones. *Antimicrob Ag Chemother* **28**: 700.

Winshell EB, Rosenkranz HS (1970). Nalidixic acid and the metabolism of *Escherichia coli*. *J Bacteriol* **104**: 1168.

Wolfson JS, Hooper DC (1989). Bacterial resistance to quinolones: mechanisms and clinical importance. *Rev Infect Dis* **11** (Suppl 5): S960.

Wolfson JS, Hooper DC, Ng Ey *et al.* (1987). Antagonism of wild-type and resistant *Escherichia coli* and its DNA gyrase by the tricyclic 4-quinolone analogs ofloxacin and S-25930 stereoisomers. *Antimicrob Ag Chemother* **31**: 1861.

Wolfson JS, Hooper DC, Swartz MN (1989). Mechanisms of action of and resistance to quinolones antimicrobial agents. In *Quinolone Antimicrobial Agents* (Wolfson JS, Hooper DC, eds), p. 5. Washington, DC: American Society of Microbiology.

Wren BG (1969). Subclinical renal infection in pregnancy: pathogenesis and drugs of choice. *Med J Aust* **2**: 895.

Zelickson AS (1964). Phototoxic reaction with nalidixic acid. *JAMA* **190**: 556.

Zemelman R, Dominguez M, Merino C *et al.* (1983). Differential susceptibility of *Aeromonas hydrophila* and Enterobacteriaceae to nalidixic acid. *J Antimicrob Chemother* **12**: 263.

Zinsser HH (1970). Nalidixic acid in acute and chronic urinary tract infections. *Med Clin N Amer* **54**: 1347.

Ciprofloxacin

Description

Ciprofloxacin is a fluoroquinolone (also called 4-quinolone, or quinolone carboxylic acid) which was developed by Bayer Pharmaceuticals for both oral and parenteral use. It is one of the second-generation of quinolones (others include norfloxacin, ofloxacin, pefloxacin and enoxacin) which have substantially enhanced antibacterial activity compared with nalidixic acid. The chemical formula of ciprofloxacin is 1-cyclopropyl-6-fluoro-1,4-dihydro-4-oxo-7-(1-piperazinyl) 3-quinolone carboxylic acid hydrochloride (Wise *et al.*, 1983). Although developed after norfloxacin, the successful widespread clinical experience with ciprofloxacin has resulted in many clinicians regarding it as the classic fluoroquinolone, against which other later generation quinolones are to be compared. Similar to most other second-generation quinolones it has a long half-life allowing twice-daily dosing and good penetration into human cells, thereby providing activity against intracellular pathogens. It has good tissue penetration and high potency against most Gram-negative pathogens with lesser activity against staphylococci and borderline/poor activity against streptococci and anaerobes. In general, ciprofloxacin has 2- to 4-fold greater antimicrobial potency than norfloxacin and considerably greater activity than cephalosporins and aminoglycosides against most Gram-negative bacilli (Sanders *et al.*, 1987; Hooper and Wolfson, 1993b; Moellering, 1993). Neu (1989a) and Mitscher *et al.* (1993) have extensively reviewed the relationship between quinolone structure and *in vitro* activity. Due to the classic status of ciprofloxacin the majority of features which fluoroquinolones have in common will be discussed in this chapter.

Sensitive Organisms

1 Gram-negative bacteria

Ciprofloxacin has excellent activity against the vast majority of enterobacteriaceae (Table II.6, pp. 986, 987), such as *Escherichia coli* and the *Enterobacter, Klebsiella, Proteus, Morganella, Edwardsiella, Providencia, Citrobacter* and *Serratia* species. It is more active than most other antimicrobial agents, including newer agents (Auckenthaler *et al.*, 1986; Samonis *et al.*, 1987; Grüneberg *et al.*, 1988; Mitsuhashi, 1988; Phillips and King, 1988; Bellido and Pechère 1989; Forsgren 1989; Inderlied *et al.*, 1989; Eliopoulos *et al.*, 1990a; Hohl *et al.*, 1990; Mehtar *et al.*, 1990; Barry and Fuchs 1991b; Fuchs *et al.*, 1991; King *et al.*, 1991; Cantón *et al.*, 1992; Bauernfeind, 1993; Eliopoulos and Eliopoulos 1993; Prosser and Beskid, 1995). Among nalidixic acid-resistant strains the activity of ciprofloxacin is generally only slightly diminished (Grüneberg *et al.*, 1988; Barry and Fuchs, 1991b,c). *Serratia marscesens* and *Providentia rettgeri*, however, may be less susceptible and occasionally resistant to ciprofloxacin (Bellido and Pechère, 1989; Eliopoulos *et al.*, 1990b; Mehtar *et al.*, 1990; Fuchs *et al.*, 1991; Visser *et al.*, 1991; Sato *et al.*, 1992; Marshall and Jones, 1993; Wise *et al.*, 1993a,b). *Acinetobacter* species, especially *Acinetobacter calcoaceticus* var *anitratus* and *A. lwoffi* are generally susceptible, although *A. baumanii* has been noted, increasingly, to be relatively resistant (Joly-Guillou and Bergogne-Bérézin, 1992; Seifert *et al.*, 1993; Applebaum *et al.*, 1986; Rolston and Bodey, 1986; Kuah *et al.*, 1994; Wise *et al.*, 1983). Strains of *A. calcoaceticus* var anitratus that are resistant to gentamicin are more likely to have borderline (MIC 2 μg per ml) susceptibility to ciprofloxacin (Shalit *et al.*, 1990; Stiver *et al.*, 1986; Chow *et al.*, 1988b). *Klebsiella rhinoscleromatis* (the probable etiological agent of rhinoscleroma) is extremely susceptible to ciprofloxacin *in vitro* (MIC_{90} 0.008 μg per ml) (Perkins *et al.*, 1992).

The vast majority of enteric pathogens including multiresistant isolates are susceptible to ciprofloxacin including *Salmonella* spp., *Shigella* spp., *Yersinia enterocolitica*, *Aeromonas* spp. (*A. hydrophila*, *A. sobria*, *A. caviae*), *Plesiomonas shigelloides*, *Vibrio cholerae* and *V. parahaemolyticus*, *Edwardsiella* tarda and *Campylobacter* spp. (*C. jejuni*, *C. coli*, *C. fetus*, *C. cincaedi*); although resistance to this latter species appears to be increasing significantly in some regions (p. 993) (Goodman *et al.*, 1984; Fliegelman *et al.*, 1985; Reinhardt and George 1985; Mikhail *et al.*, 1987; Bergan *et al.*, 1988; Ling *et al.*, 1988; Kain and Kelly, 1989; Clark *et al.*, 1990, 1991; Burgos *et al.*, 1990; Pham *et al.*, 1991; Hyams *et al.*, 1991; Sacks *et al.*, 1991; Alós *et al.*, 1992; John *et al.*, 1992; Sjögren *et al.*, 1992; Horiuchi *et al.*, 1993; Newton and Kennedy 1993; Preston *et al.*, 1994; Vila *et al.*, 1994). *Helicobacter pylori* is usually susceptible (McNulty *et al.*, 1985; Simor *et al.*, 1989; Loo *et al.*, 1992) but increasing resistance has been reported in the 1990s. *Gardnerella vaginalis* susceptibility may be borderline with MIC_{90} 2 μg per ml (Kharsany *et al.*, 1993; King *et al.*, 1984).

Flavobacterium spp. including *F. meningosepticum*, are usually susceptible (Husson *et al.*, 1985; Sheridan *et al.*, 1993), while *A. chromobacter xylosoxidans* (also referred to as a *Alcaligenes xylosoxidans*) isolates are often only borderline susceptible or resistant to ciprofloxacin (MIC_{50} 2 μg per ml; MIC_{90} 4 μg per ml) (Legrand and Anaissie, 1992), as are *A. alcaligenes faecalis* (Husson *et al.*, 1985). *Chromobacterium violaceum* is very susceptible to fluoroquinolones, including ciprofloxacin (Aldridge *et al.*, 1988).

Ciprofloxacin is active *in vitro* and *in vivo* against most strains of *Pseudomonas aeruginosa* with a MIC_{90} generally 0.5–1 μg per ml (Applebaum *et al.*, 1986; Auckenthaler *et al.*, 1986; Phillips and King 1988; Bellido and Pechére, 1989; Inderlied *et al.*, 1989; Cooper *et al.*, 1990; Eliopoulos *et al.*, 1990a; Barry and Fuchs, 1991b; Fuchs *et al.*, 1991; Cantón *et al.*, 1992). Eliopoulos and Eliopoulos (1993) noted in their review of the literature (mostly since 1988) that only six of 44 studies reported MIC_{90} >1 μg per ml. Multiply-resistant strains of *Ps. aeruginosa*, including isolates resistant to gentamicin and other aminoglycosides, generally remain susceptible to ciprofloxacin, although the MIC_{90} may rise to 1–2 μg per ml in this latter situation (Ford *et al.*, 1993; Chow *et al.*, 1989; Venezio *et al.*, 1986; Muytjens *et al.*, 1983; Wise *et al.*, 1983; Louie *et al.*, 1991). The clinical circumstances of *Ps. aeruginosa* infection may affect susceptibility. Pascual *et al.* (1993) noted that *Ps. aeruginosa* isolates attached to siliconized latex urinary catheters in biofilms had MBCs of ciprofloxacin 64-fold greater than for the same organism not associated with catheter infection. Isolates of *Ps. aeruginosa* from patients with cystic fibrosis are generally susceptible to ciprofloxacin, although Bosso *et al.* (1989) noted ciprofloxacin susceptibility (defined in this study as < 1 μg per ml) declined from 95% prior to introduction of ciprofloxacin to 86% of isolates more than 1 year after introduction, although the MIC_{90} during this latter period was still 2 μg per ml (Klinger and Aronoff 1985; Bosso *et al.*, 1989; Akaniro *et al.*, 1990). Synergism against some strains of *Ps. aeruginosa* has been reported for combinations of ciprofloxacin + imipenem, ciprofloxacin + aztreonam, and ciprofloxacin + ceftazidime (Bustamante *et al.*, 1987; Giamarellou and Petrikkos 1987; Meyer and Liu, 1988; Bosso *et al.*, 1990; Bustamante *et al.*, 1990; p. 990). Despite these *in vitro* findings of synergy between ciprofloxacin and various antibiotics against *Ps. aeruginosa*, the clinical relevance of these data is yet to be defined, although some authors speculate that in certain difficult clinical situations such as *Ps. aeruginosa* endocarditis, ciprofloxacin + beta-lactam combinations may be worthy of consideration.

Non-*aeruginosa Pseudomonas* species are significantly less susceptible to ciprofloxacin than *Ps. aeruginosa*. *Burkholderia* (previously *Pseudomonas*) *cepacia* isolates are often resistant, with only two of 14 studies reviewed by Eliopoulos and Eliopoulos (1993) reporting an MIC_{90} <4 μg per ml for this species. Subsequently Lewin *et al.* (1993), in a study of 110 routine *B. cepacia* isolates, noted an MIC_{90} 2 μg per ml, but an MIC_{90} 8 μg per ml among 20 isolates from patients with cystic fibrosis. Ford *et al.* (1993) noted similar findings. Kumar *et al.* (1989) identified *in vitro* synergy with combinations of ciprofloxacin + imipenem + rifampicin for 12 of 16 isolates, but the clinical relevance of this finding is uncertain. Generally *Ps. putida* and *Ps. fluorescens* are susceptible to ciprofloxacin with an MIC_{90} 0.25–1 μg per ml (Applebaum *et al.*, 1986; Anaissie *et al.*, 1987; Rolston *et al.*, 1987; Louie *et al.*, 1991; Bauernfeind, 1993), although some resistance has been noted (King *et al.*, 1991). Usually *Ps. acidovorans*, *Ps. stutzeri* and *Ps. putrefaciens* are very susceptible with an MIC_{90} ≤0.5 μg per ml (Applebaum *et al.*, 1986; Cornaglia *et al.*, 1987; King *et al.*, 1991; Louie *et al.*, 1991; Bauernfeind 1993; Ford *et al.*, 1993). *Methylobacterium* species (previously named *Ps. rhodos*, *Ps. rodiora* and *Ps. mesophilica*) generally have an MIC_{90} 1–2 μg per ml (Brown *et al.*, 1992). *Burkholderia* (previously *Pseudomonas*) *pseudomallei* isolates are generally resistant to fluoroquinolones with a ciprofloxacin MIC_{90} 3.1–8 μg per ml (Chau *et al.*, 1986; Ashdown 1988; Winton *et al.*, 1988;

Dance *et al.*, 1989; Yamamoto *et al.*, 1990; Sookpranee *et al.*, 1991). Similarly, *Stenotrophomonas maltophilia* (previously *Xanthomonas maltophilia*) is generally resistant with only four of 24 studies in a recent review reporting MIC_{90} of ciprofloxacin of <4 μg per ml (Eliopoulos and Eliopoulos, 1993). More recent studies have reported similar findings of an MIC_{90} of ciprofloxacin of at least 8 μg per ml (Bauernfeind, 1993; Fass 1993; Ford *et al.*, 1993; Marshall *et al.*, 1993; Marshall and Jones 1993; Pankuch *et al.*, 1994; Vartivarian *et al.*, 1994). The clinical relevance of *in vitro* findings of synergy between ciprofloxacin and extended-spectrum beta-lactamase in some *Stenotrophomonas maltophilia* isolates is uncertain (Chow *et al.*, 1988b).

Brucella species are generally susceptible *in vitro* to the fluoroquinolones with the MIC_{90} of ciprofloxacin against *Brucella melitensis* of 0.5–1.25 μg per ml and for *B. abortus* the MIC_{90} is 1–2 μg per ml (Bosch *et al.*, 1986; Kahn *et al.*, 1989; Qadri *et al.*, 1990; Garciá-Rodriguez *et al.*, 1991; Rubinstein *et al.*, 1991). However, the fluoroquinolones are often not bactericidal, especially against *B. abortus*, and although ciprofloxacin has been clinically efficacious in some situations, this fact may explain the failure of ciprofloxacin in the therapy of experimental murine brucellosis (Garciá-Rodriguez *et al.*, 1991; Shasha *et al.*, 1992). It may also explain a number of therapeutic failures, including those associated with the development of resistance to ciprofloxacin (Acocella *et al.*, 1989; Al-Sibai and Qadri, 1990).

Francisella tularensis is susceptible to fluoroquinolones with a mean MBC of ciprofloxacin of 0.13 μg per ml (range 0.01–0.3 μg per ml) (Syrjälä *et al.*, 1991).

Legionella spp. (including *L. pneumophila*, *L. micdadei*, *L. longbeachae*, *L. bozemanii*, *L. dumoffii*, *L. hackeliae*, *L. wadsworthii*) are very susceptible to ciprofloxacin with an MIC_{90} 0.03–0.5 μg per ml in routine and cell culture assays (Greenwood and Laverick, 1983; Pohlod and Saravolatz, 1986; Moffie and Mouton 1988; Edelstein *et al.*, 1989; Liebers *et al.*, 1989; Edelstein and Edelstein, 1991; Kitsukawa *et al.*, 1991; Gooding *et al.*, 1992; Reda *et al.*, 1994). Ciprofloxacin, unlike pefloxacin, does not exhibit a post-antibacterial effect against *L. pneumophila in vitro* (Rajagopalan-Levasseur *et al.*, 1990), but this appears to have no clinical relevance. Ciprofloxacin is effective in experimental *L. pneumophila* infections in guinea pigs (Fitzgeorge *et al.*, 1985).

Haemophilus influenzae, including multiply-resistant and beta-lactamase-producing strains (including those from patients with cystic fibrosis) is very susceptible to ciprofloxacin with an MIC_{90} ≤0.06–0.25 μg per ml (Barry *et al.*, 1984; King *et al.*, 1984; Collignon *et al.*, 1992; Jorgensen *et al.*, 1988; Swanson *et al.*, 1991; Bongaerts and Hoogkamp-Korstanje, 1993; Hardy, 1991; Cherubin *et al.*, 1992; Cooper *et al.*, 1992; Lehtonen and Huovinen, 1993; Akaniro *et al.*, 1990). Similarly, *Moraxella* (previously *Branhamella*) *catarrhalis*, including beta-lactamase-producing strains, is very susceptible with an MIC_{90} ≤0.03–0.25 μg per ml (Cherubin *et al.*, 1992; Swanson *et al.*, 1991; Bongaerts and Hoogkamp-Korstanje, 1993; Lehtonen and Huovinen, 1993). *Haemophilus ducreyi*, including beta-lactamase-producing and tetracycline-resistant strains, are susceptible to most fluoroquinolones with MIC_{90} of ciprofloxacin being 0.007–0.02 μg per ml (Wall *et al.*, 1985; Sturm, 1987; Motley *et al.*, 1992; Aldridge *et al.*, 1993; Knapp *et al.*, 1993; Van Dyck *et al.*, 1994).

Most *Bordetella* spp. (*Bordetella pertussis* and *B. parapertussis*) are susceptible to fluoroquinolones with ciprofloxacin MIC_{90} ≤0.12 μg per ml, although *B. bronchiseptica* is less susceptible with ciprofloxacin MIC_{90} 1–4 μg per ml (Appleman *et al.*, 1987; Kurzynski *et al.*, 1988; Hoppe and Simon, 1990; Bauwens *et al.*, 1992).

Neisseria meningitidis is extremely susceptible to ciprofloxacin with an MIC < 0.008–0.12 μg per ml (Eliopoulos and Eliopoulos, 1993). *Neisseria gonorrhoea*, including spectinomycin-resistant, beta-lactamase-producing, tetracycline-resistant strains and chromosomally mediated penicillin-resistant strains are very susceptible to ciprofloxacin (MIC_{90} 0.004–0.03 μg per ml), but the incidence of resistance is increasing (p. 993) (Easmon *et al.*, 1987; Segreti *et al.*, 1990; Clendennen *et al.*, 1992; Glatt *et al.*, 1992; Gorwitz *et al.*, 1993; Zenilman *et al.*, 1993; Joesoef *et al.*, 1994; Rice and Knapp, 1994; Blondeau and Yaschuk, 1995). *N. mucosa* is generally susceptible (Anderson and Miller, 1993).

Unusual fastidious Gram-negative pathogens such as *Eikenella corrodens* and *Actinobacillus actinomycetemcomitans* are very susceptible to ciprofloxacin (Goldstein *et al.*, 1986; Goldstein and Citron, 1988; Pavicic *et al.*, 1992). *Pasteurella multocida* is susceptible to all fluoroquinolones including ciprofloxacin (MIC_{90} ≤0.03 μg per ml) (Fass, 1983; Goldstein and Citron, 1988, 1993). Other pathogens frequently isolated in bite wounds such as the anaerobic Gram-negative *Fusobacterium* spp. are generally resistant to ciprofloxacin (MIC_{90} 16–32 μg per ml), while *Prevotella* and *Porphyromonas* spp. have a ciprofloxacin MIC_{90} 2–16 μg per ml (Goldstein and Citron, 1992, 1993). *Veillonella* spp. are susceptible to ciprofloxacin (MIC

≤0.5 μg per ml) (Fernandes *et al.*, 1986; Aldridge, 1994). Overall, however, ciprofloxacin has poor activity against most anaerobes (Fernandes *et al.*, 1986; Watt and Brown, 1986; Goldstein, 1993; Aldridge, 1994). *Bacteroides* spp., including *B. fragilis*, are resistant to ciprofloxacin (MIC$_{90}$ 4 to ≥16 μg per ml) and other similar generation fluoroquinolones, although newer fluoroquinolones appear to have significantly improved activity against anaerobes (pp. 1169, 1172; Fox and Phillips, 1987; Goldstein and Citron, 1992; Phillips *et al.*, 1992; Wexler *et al.*, 1992; Brook, 1993; Goldstein, 1993; Pankuch *et al.*, 1993; Aldridge, 1994; Borobio *et al.*, 1994). *Capnocytophaga* spp. are reasonably susceptible to ciprofloxacin (MIC$_{90}$ 0.25 μg per ml), but less so to other fluoroquinolones, and resistant isolates have been reported (Rummens *et al.*, 1986; Roscoe *et al.*, 1992; Gomez-Garces *et al.*, 1994).

2 Gram-positive bacteria

Staphylococcus aureus and *Staph. epidermidis*, both methicillin-sensitive and -resistant strains, are usually susceptible to ciprofloxacin and ofloxacin – more than to other fluoroquinolones such as norfloxacin or enoxacin. Eliopoulos and Eliopoulos (1993) in their review, noted that most studies reported an MIC$_{90}$ of ciprofloxacin ≤0.5 μg per ml (range 0.25–2 μg per ml) against both *Staph. aureus* and *Staph. epidermidis*. Subsequently other authors have supported these observations (Cohen *et al.*, 1991; Huband *et al.*, 1993). Notable, however, is the recent significant increase in ciprofloxacin-resistance among such staphylococci (p. 994). Other staphylococcal species including *Staph. saprophyticus*, *Staph. hominis*, *Staph. warnerii*, and *Staph. haemolyticus*, regardless of their susceptibility to methicillin, are generally similar or marginally less susceptible to ciprofloxacin (MIC$_{90}$ <0.5–1 μg per ml) (Gorzynski *et al.*, 1989a; Huband *et al.*, 1993; Prosser and Beskid, 1995). Aldridge (1993) and Marshall *et al.* (1993) noted MIC$_{90}$ 0.25–>4 μg per ml against these *Staphylococcus* species. Most fluoroquinolones, except some newer agents (pp. 1169, 1172, 1175), have only borderline activity against *Streptococcus pneumoniae*, most other streptococcal species and enterococci since their MIC$_{90}$ (generally 2–4 μg per ml) is too close to the expected serum concentration (p. 999) to consistently achieve clinical efficacy. These *in vitro* observations are supported by a number of reported clinical failures and 'breakthrough' infections with *Strep. pneumoniae* while receiving ciprofloxacin (Körner *et al.*, 1994; p. 995). Ciprofloxacin is either similar, or more active, than other agents in its class against *Strep. pneumoniae* and other streptococcal species (including *Strep. pyogenes* and *Strep. agalactiae*) with MIC$_{90}$ 1–2 μg per ml (range 0.8–6.2 μg per ml) and 2–4 μg per ml, respectively. No difference in ciprofloxacin susceptibilities have been noted between penicillin-susceptible and -resistant strains of *Strep. pneumoniae* (Fass, 1983; Bassey *et al.*, 1986; Applebaum *et al.*, 1989; Neal *et al.*, 1992; Spangler *et al.*, 1992, 1993; Bongaerts *et al.*, 1993; Yee *et al.*, 1993; Betriu *et al.*, 1994). A number of studies of experimental pneumococcal respiratory infections in mice have highlighted the problems of ciprofloxacin therapy in this situation (Gisby *et al.*, 1991; Azoulay-Dupuis *et al.*, 1991, 1992; Sullivan *et al.*, 1993).

Enterococci are usually resistant to ciprofloxacin with MIC$_{90}$ against *Enterococcus faecalis* generally 2–4 μg per ml, while *E. faecium* is often slightly more resistant with an MIC$_{90}$ 4 μg per ml (Eliopoulos *et al.*, 1984; Pérez *et al.*, 1987; Sahm and Koburov, 1989; Eliopoulos and Eliopoulos 1993). Notably, however, some authors have reported MIC$_{90}$ against both pathogens of 8 to > 32 μg per ml (Gordon *et al.*, 1992; Bongaerts *et al.*, 1993; Venditti *et al.*, 1993). Less common enterococcal spp. (*E. avium*, *E. casseliflavus*, *E. raffinosus*, *E. hirae*) generally require an MIC of 0.5–4 μg per ml, although *E. gallinarum* tends to be more resistant (MIC 2 to >8 μg per ml) (Gordon *et al.*, 1992). Ciprofloxacin activity is similar for both routine and multiply-resistant enterococcal strains, including those resistant to penicillin-aminoglycoside synergy (Sahm and Koburov, 1989). Combinations of ciprofloxacin with novobiocin produces additive activity (French *et al.*, 1993) while combining ciprofloxacin with cell-wall active agents such as ampicillin or vancomycin demonstrates neither synergy or antagonism in most cases (Smith and Eng, 1988). Experimental endocarditis studies in rabbits using a combination of ciprofloxacin and penicillin demonstrated similar efficacy to penicillin alone (Fernandez-Guerrero *et al.*, 1987).

Corynebacteria spp. (including group D2 and *C. jeikeium*) are only moderately susceptible to ciprofloxacin with MIC$_{90}$ 0.5–2 μg per ml, but a wide range of MICs 0.05–128 μg per ml have been reported and resistance has emerged during therapy (Fernández-Roblas *et al.*, 1987; Murphy and Ferguson 1987; Philippon and Bimet, 1990; Martinez-Martinez *et al.*, 1994). Martinez-Martinez *et al.* (1994), however, recently examined 115 coryneform bacteria, and found that *C. jeikeium*, *C. minutissimum*, *C. striatum*, *C. xerosis*, *C. urealyticum* and *Corynebacterium* group 12 had MIC$_{90}$ of ciprofloxacin and ofloxacin of 8 to >16 μg per ml, while *Corynebacterium* group ANF-1 had a MIC_{90} 0.5 µg per ml to both agents. *Corynebacterium pseudodiphtheriticum* (previously *C. hofmannii*) and *Arcanobacterium haemolyticum* (previously *C. haemolyticum*), an infrequent cause of pharyngitis in children and rarely more invasive infections, are generally susceptible to ≤0.5 µg per ml ciprofloxacin (Morris and Guild, 1991; Carlson *et al.*, 1994). *Rhodococcus equi* (previously *Corynebacterium equi*) in relatively small studies appears to be moderately susceptible to ciprofloxacin and sparfloxacin with MIC_{50} 0.25 µg per ml (range 0.12–4 µg per ml) and MBC_{50} 1 µg per ml (range 1–16 µg per ml) for both agents, but it is resistant to other fluoroquinolones (Nordmann and Ronco 1992; Nordmann *et al.*, 1992b). However, studies of disseminated *R. equi* infection in mice demonstrated that ciprofloxacin was ineffective therapy and that combinations including vancomycin produced the best results (Nordmann *et al.*, 1992a).

Listeria monocytogenes is only borderline susceptible to ciprofloxacin (MIC_{90} 2 µg per ml; range 0.5–2 µg per ml) and ofloxacin, and is resistant to other fluoroquinolones, except for some of the newer agents (p. 1173) (Boisivon *et al.*, 1990; MacGowan *et al.*, 1990). However, in experimental *Listeria monocytogenes* infections in mice, therapy with ciprofloxacin proved inferior to ampicillin, suggesting it to be an inappropriate clinical choice for listeriosis (Van Ogtrop *et al.*, 1992).

Nocardia species (*N. asteroides*, *N. brasiliensis*, *N. caviae*) are resistant to most fluoroquinolones, including ciprofloxacin with MIC_{90} of 2–16 µg per ml (Gombert *et al.*, 1987; Southern *et al.*, 1987; Berkey *et al.*, 1988; Wallace *et al.*, 1988b). Furthermore, ciprofloxacin was ineffective therapy for experimental pulmonary *N. asteroides* infection in immunocompromised mice (Gombert *et al.*, 1990). *Erysipelothrix rhusiopathiae* appears to be very susceptible to ciprofloxacin (MIC_{90} 0.06 µg per ml; range ≤0.01–0.06 µg per ml; MBC_{90} 0.12 µg per ml) and less so to pefloxacin (MIC_{90} 0.5 µg per ml), although penicillin and imipenem had the greatest activity in this *in vitro* study (Venditti *et al.*, 1990).

Bacillus species (*B. cereus*, *B. anthracis* and other non-*B. cereus* species) are reasonably susceptible to ciprofloxacin with MIC_{90} 0.06–1 µg per ml (Weber *et al.*, 1988; Doganay and Aydin, 1991).

Ciprofloxacin, similar to ofloxacin, norfloxacin, enoxacin and pefloxacin, has relatively poor activity against Gram-positive anaerobes. The MIC_{90} of ciprofloxacin for *Clostridium* spp. is 1–16 µg per ml, although *Cl. perfringens* and *Cl. tertium* may be more susceptible with MIC_{90} 0.5–8 µg per ml. *Clostridium difficile* is resistant (ciprofloxacin MIC_{90} 8–25 µg per ml) (Chow *et al.*, 1985; Delmee and Avesani, 1986; Clabots *et al.*, 1987; Speirs *et al.*, 1988; Aldridge, 1994). Other Gram-positive anaerobes such as *Peptococcus* and *Peptostreptococcus* spp. (MIC_{90} 2–8 µg per ml), *Propionibacterium* and *Eubacterium* spp. (MIC_{90} 1–16 µg per ml), *Mobiluncus* spp. (MIC_{90} 1–4 µg per ml) and *Actinomyces* spp. (MIC_{90} 8 µg per ml) are resistant (Fernandes *et al.*, 1986; Goldstein and Citron, 1992; Wexler *et al.*, 1992; Eliopoulos and Eliopoulos, 1993; Goldstein, 1993; Pankuch *et al.*, 1993; Aldridge, 1994).

3 Mycobacteria

Ciprofloxacin, similar to various fluoroquinolones, has reasonable activity against *Mycobacteria*. Ciprofloxacin and ofloxacin have similar activity against *Mycobacterium tuberculosis* (MIC_{90} ≤1–2 µg per ml), regardless of the susceptibility of this species to other antituberculous agents (Collins and Uttley, 1985, 1988; Berlin *et al.*, 1987; Davies *et al.*, 1987; Young *et al.*, 1987; Uttley and Collins, 1988; Chen *et al.*, 1989, Leysen *et al.*, 1989; Van Caekenberghe, 1990; Piersimoni *et al.*, 1992; Garcia-Rodriguez and Gomez Garcia, 1993). However, some studies have reported ciprofloxacin MIC_{90} to be 3.2–4.3 µg per ml (Marinis and Legakis, 1985; Gorzynski *et al.*, 1989b). Fluoroquinolones are bactericidal against *M. tuberculosis*, with MBC usually being 2- to 4-fold greater than the MIC (Leysen *et al.*, 1989; Heifets and Lindholm-Levy, 1990). Uttley and Collins (1988) identified *in vitro* antagonism by checkerboard technique between ciprofloxacin and rifampicin but the clinical relevance of this finding is uncertain, especially since this combination was shown to be more effective than rifampicin and isoniazid against *M. tuberculosis* in a mouse model (Chadwick *et al.*, 1989).

The susceptibility of *M. paratuberculosis*, the etiological agent of paratuberculosis in ruminants (Johne's disease) and the organisms isolated from the intestinal tissue of some patients with Crohn's disease, varies from an MIC_{50}/MBC_{50} 0.12/0.5 µg per ml to an MIC ≥5 µg per ml depending on the study examined (Chiodini, 1990; Rastogi *et al.*, 1992). Similarly, the published susceptibility of *M. kansasii* to ciprofloxacin varies widely from MIC_{90} 0.6–100 µg per ml, with a number of large studies suggesting an MIC_{90} 4 µg per ml – i.e. resistant to routinely achievable concentrations of ciprofloxacin (Davies *et al.*, 1987; Collins and Uttley, 1988; Leysen *et al.*, 1989; Hjelm *et al.*, 1992; Garcia-Rodriguez and Gomez Garcia, 1993).

Table II.6a

In vitro susceptibility of various fluoroquinolones

Organism	Typical MIC$_{90}$ µg per ml						
	CPX	NFX	ENX	PFX	FLX	OFX	L-OFX
Gram-negative bacteria							
Escherichia coli	0.015–0.06	0.06–0.12	0.125–0.25	0.125	0.125	0.06–0.125	≤0.06
Enterobacter aerogenes	0.03–0.12	0.25	0.25	0.25	0.12–0.5	0.25	0.125
Enterobacter cloacae	0.03–0.12	0.25	0.5	0.5–2	0.25	0.25–1	0.125
Klebsiella pneumoniae	0.06–0.125	0.25	0.25–1	2	0.5–1	0.25–0.5	0.25
Proteus mirabilis	0.03–0.125	0.06	0.5	0.5–1	0.25–0.5	0.125–0.5	0.25
Proteus vulgaris	≤0.06	0.06	0.5	0.25	0.125–0.25	0.125–0.25	0.25
Morganella morganii	0.015–0.06	0.06–0.125	0.25–0.5	0.5	0.125–0.25	0.25–0.5	0.5
Providentia rettgeri	0.125–1	0.5	1	0.25–0.5	0.5–2	1–2	0.5
Providentia stuartii	0.125–1	0.5–4	0.5–2	4	≤2	0.5–2	0.25
Serratia marcescens	0.25–0.5	0.5–1	0.5–8	1	≤2	1–4	0.5
Citrobacter freundii	0.06–0.12	0.25	0.5–4	0.25–1	0.125–2	0.25–1	0.125
Salmonella spp.	≤0.06	0.06–0.25	0.125–0.25	0.125–0.25	0.125–0.25	0.06–0.125	0.125
Shigella spp.	0.015–0.06	0.015–0.12	0.125–0.25	0.125–0.25	0.125	0.125	0.03–0.125
Yersinia enterocolitica	0.03–0.06	0.06–0.25	0.125–0.5	0.25	0.125	0.125–0.25	0.125
Campylobacter jejuni	0.125–1	0.5–8	0.5–8	0.5–2	0.5	0.25–2	–
Acinetobacter calcoaceticus	1–16	8	4	1	2–16	0.5–16	16
Haemophilus influenzae	0.008–0.06	0.06–0.125	0.125–0.25	0.03–0.125	0.06–0.125	0.03–0.06	0.015
Moraxella catarrhalis	0.03–0.25	0.125–0.25	0.25	0.25	0.125–0.25	0.06–0.125	0.06
Neisseria meningitidis	≤0.008–0.125	0.015–0.03	0.03	0.03	0.03	0.015–0.06	–
Neisseria gonorrhoeae	0.004–0.06	0.03–0.06	0.03–0.125	0.06–0.125	≤0.015–0.125	0.03–0.06	0.015
Pseudomonas aeruginosa	0.25–1	1–2	4–16	4–16	4–8	2–16	8
Burkholderia cepacia	2–>8	16–32	4–8	–	2–>8	4–16	2
Stenotrophomonas maltophilia	4–8	32	16–32	4	4–8	4–≥8	2
Legionella pneumophila	0.015–0.06	0.125–0.25	0.125	0.06	≤0.06	0.03–0.25	0.125
Bacteroides fragilis	4–16	32	32	16	16–32	2–16	2
Gram-positive bacteria							
Staphylococcus aureus (MSSA)	0.25–2	1–4	2–8	0.5–1	1	0.5–2	0.25–0.5
Staphylococcus aureus (MRSA)	0.5–>16	4–>16	2–>8	1	≥16	0.5–≥16	0.5–16
Staphylococcus epidermidis (MSSE)	0.5–1	1–2	1–2	1	1	0.25–1	8
Staphylococcus epidermidis (MRSE)	0.5–≥16	≥4	–	–	≥16	0.5–≥16	8
Streptococcus pneumoniae	1–4	4–16	16	8–32	8–64	2	2
Streptococcus pyogenes	0.5–2	4	4	16	8	2	1
Enterococcus faecalis	1–4	4–8	8	4–8	4–≥8	2–8	2
Enterococcus faecium	4	8–≥16	32	–	≥8	8–16	–
Listeria monocytogenes	1–2	8	8–16	8	≥4	2–8	2
Clostridium perfringens	0.5–2	2	2	1	2	0.5–2	1–64
Clostridium difficile	8–16	128	64	64	16	≥16	–
Peptostreptococcus spp.	4–16	16	16	16	>32	4–16	8
Other bacteria							
Mycoplasma pneumoniae	2	–	–	–	4	1–2	–
Mycoplasma hominis	0.5–2	8	8	4	2–4	1–2	–
Chlamydia pneumoniae	0.5–4	–	–	–	2–4	1	0.5
Chlamydia trachomatis	1–3.1	12.5–16	6.25	–	1.5–4	0.5–1	–
Ureaplasma urealyticum	4	8–>64	16	4	2–4	2	–
Mycobacterium tuberculosis	0.25–2	2–8	8.3	≤1.25	2–6.25	0.5–2.4	0.25–1
Mycobacterium avium complex	>8	≥16	–	–	–	0.5–16	>8

Table II.6b

In vitro susceptibility of various fluoroquinolones

Organism	Typical MIC$_{90}$ µg per ml						
	LOM	TOS	RUF	SPX	TRX	CLX	GPX
Gram-negative bacteria							
Escherichia coli	0.25–0.5	≤0.06	2	0.03–0.06	0.03–0.06	≤0.03	≤0.125
Enterobacter aerogenes	0.5	0.125	64	0.125	0.06–0.125	0.06–0.125	0.5
Enterobacter cloacae	0.5–2	0.125	64	0.25	0.06–0.125	0.03–0.06	0.125–0.25
Klebsiella pneumoniae	2	0.06–0.25	32	0.125–0.25	0.06–0.125	0.06–0.25	0.25
Proteus mirabilis	0.25–1	0.125–0.5	4	0.5	0.25	≤0.015–0.03	0.25–0.5
Proteus vulgaris	0.25	0.25	1	0.5	0.25–0.5	0.015–0.06	0.25–0.5
Morganella morganii	0.25–0.5	0.125	2	0.25–0.5	0.25–2	0.03–0.125	0.125–0.5
Providentia rettgeri	2	0.5	2	0.5	0.5	0.25	0.5–2
Providentia stuartii	2	0.125–1	8	1–2	0.5–2	0.125	0.25–2
Serratia marcescens	1	0.25–2	32	0.5–1	0.5–4	0.125–0.25	1–4
Citrobacter freundii	0.5–1	0.125–0.5	1	0.25–4	0.25–0.5	0.125	0.5–1
Salmonella spp.	0.25	0.03	1	0.06	≤0.03	0.008–0.03	0.125
Shigella spp.	0.125–0.25	0.03	0.5	0.03–0.06	≤0.015–0.06	≤0.008	0.03–0.125
Yersinia enterocolitica	0.125–0.25	0.06	1	0.06	0.03–0.06	≤0.008	0.25
Campylobacter jejuni	0.125–1	0.06	32	0.125–0.25	–	–	–
Acinetobacter calcoaceticus	4–16	16	4	0.03–0.125	8	0.03	16
Haemophilus influenzae	0.06–0.125	≤0.008–0.06	0.5	≤0.015	≤0.03	≤0.06	≤0.06
Moraxella catarrhalis	≤0.03–0.125	≤0.008–0.03	1	≤0.015	0.06	≤0.06	≤0.06
Neisseria meningitidis	≤0.06	≤0.03	0.125	≤0.06	–	≤0.008	0.008
Neisseria gonorrhoeae	≤0.03	≤0.06	0.125	≤0.015	0.003	≤0.008	0.008–≤0.06
Pseudomonas aeruginosa	≥8	0.5–4	8	2–8	1–2	0.25–1	1–8
Burkholderia cepacia	4–>8	0.25–1	–	0.25–2	0.25	0.125	0.5–2
Stenotrophomonas maltophilia	1–16	4	–	0.25–4	0.5–2	0.5–2	1–4
Legionella pneumophila	–	–	–	0.03	0.06	0.015	–
Bacteroides fragilis	32	2	32	2–4	0.5–>8	0.5	2–8
Gram-positive bacteria							
Staphylococcus aureus (MSSA)	1–2	0.125–0.5	2	0.25–0.5	0.03–0.06	0.06	≤0.25
Staphylococcus aureus (MRSA)	1–>16	0.125–8	–	0.25–16	2–4	≤0.015–0.125	0.25–16
Staphylococcus epidermidis (MSSE)	1	0.125	2	0.06–0.5	0.125	0.06	0.25
Staphylococcus epidermidis (MRSE)	>16	8–16	2	0.125–4	2	0.06	8
Streptococcus pneumoniae	8	0.25–0.5	32	0.25–0.5	0.25	0.25	0.25–0.5
Streptococcus pyogenes	8	0.125	–	0.25–0.5	0.25	0.25	0.25–0.5
Enterococcus faecalis	≥8	0.5	16–32	≤0.5–1	1–2	0.125–0.5	0.5–4
Enterococcus faecium	>8	4–8	–	1	2	0.5	8
Listeria monocytogenes	4–8	0.125–0.25	–	1–2	0.25–0.5	0.25–1	–
Clostridium perfringens	2–4	0.25	4	0.125–0.5	0.25	0.125–0.5	1–2
Clostridium difficile	≥32	4	32	4	1	0.25	16–32
Peptostreptococcus spp.	4	0.5	–	1	0.25	0.5	2–4
Other bacteria							
Mycoplasma pneumoniae	4	–	0.5–4	0.125–0.5	–	0.03	–
Mycoplasma hominis	2	–	0.5–4	0.06	–	0.03	–
Chlamydia pneumoniae	4	–	4–8	≤0.25	≤0.06	–	0.5
Chlamydia trachomatis	2–4	0.125–0.25	4–8	0.05	–	0.06	–
Ureaplasma urealyticum	4–8	–	–	0.125–1	–	0.25	–
Mycobacterium tuberculosis	0.5–4	>8	–	0.06–0.5	–	0.25	–
Mycobacterium avium complex	–	>8	–	8	–	>8	–

CPX: ciprofloxacin; NFX: norfloxacin; ENX: enoxacin; PFX: pefloxacin; FLX: fleroxacin; OFX: ofloxacin; L-OFX: levofloxacin; LOM: lomefloxacin; TOS: tosufloxacin; RUF: rufloxacin; SPX: sparfloxacin; TRX: trovafloxacin; CLX: clinafloxacin; GPX: grepafloxacin

MSSA: methicillin-sensitive *Staph. aureus*; MRSA: methicillin-resistant *Staph. aureus*; MSSE: methicillin-sensitive *Staph. epidermidis*; MRSE: methicillin-resistant *Staph. epidermidis*.

– denotes insufficient or inconsistent data.

Compiled from: Auckenthaler *et al.*, 1986; Chin *et al.*, 1986, 1991; Bremner *et al.*, 1988; Ernst and van der Auwera, 1988; Espinoza *et al.*, 1988; Grüneberg *et al.*, 1988; Norrby and Jonsson, 1988; Phillips and King, 1988; Steele-Mortimer and Meier–Ewert, 1988; Wise *et al.*, 1988, 1992, 1993; Barry and Jones, 1989; Gorzynski *et al.*, 1989; Neu *et al.*, 1989, 1992; Segreti *et al.*, 1990; Fuchs *et al.*, 1991; Kenny and Cartwright, 1991a,b; Waites *et al.*, 1991; Canton *et al.*, 1992; Fu, *et al.*; 1992; Goldstein and Citron, 1992; Imada *et al.*, 1992; Nakata *et al.*, 1992; Eliopoulos and Eliopoulos, 1993; Garcia–Rodriguez and Gomez Garcia, 1993; Gooding and Jones, 1993; Murray *et al.*, 1993; Cherubin and Stratton, 1994; Kaku *et al.*, 1994; Neu and Chin,1994; Pankuch *et al.*, 1994, 1995; Roblin *et al.*, 1994; Soriano *et al.*, 1994; Spangler *et al.*, 1994; Wexler *et al.*, 1994; Yew *et al.*, 1994; Baltch *et al.*, 1995; Ji *et al.*, 1995; Prosser and Beskid, 1995; Saito and Gaja, 1995; Zhang *et al.*, 1995.

Rapidly growing mycobacteria such as *M. fortuitum* biovar *fortuitum* are quite susceptible to ciprofloxacin (MIC_{90} 0.125 μg per ml), while biovar *peregrinum* and other biovars are less susceptible (MIC_{90} 1 μg per ml). Similarly, other 'rapid growers' including *M. smegmatis* and *M. chelonae*-like organisms have a ciprofloxacin MIC_{90} 0.5–1 μg per ml, but *M. chelonae* (subspecies *abscessus* and *chelonae*) are generally resistant to ciprofloxacin and other fluoroquinolones with MIC_{90} >8 μg per ml (Wallace *et al.*, 1988a, 1990, 1992; Burns *et al.*, 1990; Garcia Rodriguez and Gomez Garcia, 1993; Khardori *et al.*, 1994). Less common species vary in susceptibility: *M. marinum* and *M. xenopi* are usually susceptible (MIC_{90} ≤2 μg per ml) (Collins and Uttley 1985; Leysen *et al.*, 1989; Forsgren, 1993). *Mycobacterium malmoense* is relatively resistant (MIC_{90} ≥ 2 μg per ml), although combinations of ethambutol with ciprofloxacin, amikacin and rifampicin rendered isolates susceptible (Van Caekenberge, 1990; Hoffner *et al.*, 1993); *M. haemophilum* is resistant (MIC_{90} 8 μg per ml) (Bernard *et al.*, 1993).

Mycobacterium avium–intracellulare complex is relatively resistant to ciprofloxacin and similar fluoroquinolones with MIC_{90} generally ≥4–8 μg per ml, although newer fluoroquinolones appear to be more active (p. 1136) (Fernandes *et al.*, 1989; Leysen *et al.*, 1989; Garcia-Rodriguez and Gomez Garcia, 1993; Klopman *et al.*, 1993). *In vitro* synergism has been noted between ethambutol and ciprofloxacin, and antagonism between rifabutin and ciprofloxacin (Yajko *et al.*, 1988; Hoffner *et al.*, 1989; Kent *et al.*, 1992). Interestingly, Majumdar *et al.* (1992) found liposome-encapsulated ciprofloxacin to be more than 50-fold as effective against intracellular *M. avium–intracellulare* as free drug using a human monocyte/macrophage culture system. In the mouse foot pad model and 'BACTEC' 460 system, ciprofloxacin has no useful activity against *M. leprae*, although some effect has been noted with ofloxacin and sparfloxacin (pp. 1112, 1136) (Banerjee, 1986; Leysen *et al.*, 1989; Garcia-Rodriguez and Gomez Garcia, 1993).

4 Mycoplasmas and Ureaplasmas

Many of the fluoroquinolones, including ciprofloxacin but excluding norfloxacin, are moderately active against *M. hominis* (ciprofloxacin MIC_{90} 0.5–2 μg per ml) while the newer agents sparfloxacin and clinafloxacin (pp. 1136, 1170) have even better activity (Hoban *et al.*, 1989; Kenny *et al.*, 1989; Waites *et al.*, 1991). However, *M. pneumoniae* is only borderline susceptible to ciprofloxacin (MIC_{90} 1–8 μg per ml) (Kenny and Cartwright, 1991b; Waites *et al.*, 1991; Arai *et al.*, 1992). Unlike ofloxacin, however, ciprofloxacin is inactive in the experimental *M. pneumoniae* hamster pneumonia model (Gohara *et al.*, 1993; Arai *et al.*, 1993). *Ureaplasma urealyticum* is less susceptible than *M. hominis* to ciprofloxacin and can, for practical purposes, be regarded as resistant MIC_{90} 1–16 μg per ml (Aznar *et al.*, 1985; Hoban *et al.*, 1989; Kenny *et al.*, 1989; Waites *et al.*, 1991, 1992).

5 Chlamydia

Ciprofloxacin is moderately active against *Chlamydia trachomatis*, including probable tetracycline-resistant strains (MIC_{90} 1–3 μg per ml). *Chlamydia pneumoniae* has a ciprofloxacin MIC in cell assay of 0.5–4 μg per ml (range 0.25–8 μg per ml), and for *C. psittaci* an MIC 0.5–1 μg per ml. The newer fluoroquinolones such as sparfloxacin (p. 1136) are significantly more active against *Chlamydia* spp. with potencies *in vitro* and *in vivo* approaching those of doxycycline and tetracycline (Nagayama *et al.*, 1988; Chirgwin *et al.*, 1989; Hoban *et al.*, 1989; Jones *et al.*, 1990; Segreti et al, 1990; Cooper *et al.*, 1991; Hammerschlag *et al.*, 1992; Nakata *et al.*, 1992; Kimura *et al.*, 1993). Possible treatment failures with ciprofloxacin for *C. trachomatis* genital infections have been reported (Van der Willigen *et al.*, 1992).

6 Rickettsiaceae and Ehrlichiae

Fluoroquinolones, including ciprofloxacin, are active *in vitro* against *Rickettsia* spp. and *Coxiella burnetii*, using various methods including plaque inhibition cell culture assay, the embryonated egg model and animal models. Ciprofloxacin is active *in vitro* against the spotted fever group of *Rickettsia* (*R. rickettsii*, MIC 1 μg per ml; *R. conorii*, MIC 0.25 μg per ml) but activity against the typhus group (*R. typhi* and *R. prowazekii*) and scrub typhus group (*R. tsutsugamushi*) is less known (Raoult *et al.*, 1986a; Raoult and Drancourt, 1991; Jabarit-Aldighieri *et al.*, 1992). McClain *et al.* (1988) found ciprofloxacin to be effective in mice infected with *R. tsutsugamushi*. Eaton *et al.* (1989) and Strand and Stromberg (1990), however, reported successful clinical outcomes treating typhus and scrub typhus with ciprofloxacin (p. 1031). *Coxiella burnetii* is heterogeneously susceptible to fluoroquinolones *in vitro* using the human embryonic lung fibroblast shell vial assay technique, in which Raoult *et al.* (1991) found only five of 13 strains to be susceptible to 1 µg per ml of ciprofloxacin. Other methodologies have suggested the susceptibility of *C. burnetii* to be somewhat strain-dependent (Yeaman *et al.*, 1987; Yeaman and Baca 1990; Raoult *et al.*, 1991). Yeaman *et al.* (1989), however, suggested that combinations of ciprofloxacin + rifampicin have synergistic activity *in vitro* against *C. burnetii*.

Ehrlichia sennetsu, the cause of Sennetsu disease (a mononucleosis-like illness described in South-East Asia) is very susceptible to ciprofloxacin (MIC 0.125 µg per ml) (Brouqui and Raoult, 1990). However, *Ehrlichia chaffensis*, the cause of human ehrlichiosis (previously thought to be caused by *E. canis*) appears to be resistant *in vitro* to ciprofloxacin (MIC 4 µg per ml), although concentrations of ≥2 µg per ml were bacteriostatic. Thus, some discrepancies have been observed in the activity of quinolones against *Ehrlichia* spp. (Brouqui and Raoult, 1992).

7 Giardia lamblia

The fluoroquinolones, including ciprofloxacin, have no useful activity against *G. lamblia*, requiring concentrations of 100 µg per ml to inhibit trophozoite growth *in vitro* (Ikerd and Koletar, 1993).

8 Spirochetes

Ciprofloxacin appears to be active both *in vitro* and in an animal model against at least one strain of *Leptospira interrogans* serogroup *Icterohaemorrhagiae* with an MBC 0.6 µg per ml (Shalit *et al.*, 1989a). These data require further confirmation, however, before ciprofloxacin can be regarded as a suitable therapeutic agent for leptospirosis, especially since quinolones have poor activity against other spirochetal diseases. Ciprofloxacin and ofloxacin have relatively poor activity against *Borrelia burgdorferi in vitro* (MIC_{90} 1 and 2 µg per ml, and MBC_{90} 8 and 8 µg per ml, respectively) (Levin *et al.*, 1993). Fluoroquinolones are ineffective in animal models of *Treponema pallidum* infection and have no role in the treatment of clinical syphilis (CDC, 1993; Peeling and Ronald, 1993).

9 Plasmodia

A number of fluoroquinolones have *in vitro* activity against plasmodia, but ciprofloxacin appears to be the most inhibitory *in vitro* against both chloroquine-susceptible and -resistant strains of *Plasmodium falciparum* at clinically achievable concentrations (Divo *et al.*, 1988; Krishna *et al.*, 1988). Ciprofloxacin is also active against *P. yoelii* in an experimental mouse model (Salmon *et al.*, 1990). Nevertheless, variable and poor clinical responses using norfloxacin and ciprofloxacin, respectively, suggest that fluoroquinolones are unlikely to become major therapeutic agents for malaria (Watt *et al.*, 1991; McLean *et al.*, 1992).

10 Bactericidal activity and post-antibiotic effect

Fluoroquinolones are notable for the fact that MBCs are, with only occasional exceptions, within two dilutions of the MICs for Gram-negative pathogens and 2- to 4-fold the MIC for Gram-positive organisms. This killing occurs very rapidly for Gram-negatives (e.g. ≥3 log_{10} reduction in viable counts within 2 h) and usually somewhat slower for Gram-positive organisms (e.g. 3 log_{10} reduction in 4–8 h) (Chin and Neu, 1984; Espinoza *et al.*, 1988; Fernandes *et al.*, 1988; Fung-Tome *et al.*, 1989; Kaatz and Seo, 1990; Maple *et al.*, 1991; Swanson *et al.*, 1991). Although Eng *et al.* (1991) reported that ciprofloxacin was bactericidal against some slow and non-growing bacteria, this appears to be strain- and species-dependent (Zeiler, 1985; Zeiler and Voigt, 1987; Lewin *et al.*, 1989b; Cooper *et al.*, 1990).

Ciprofloxacin, similar to other fluoroquinolones, exhibits a post-antibiotic effect (PAE) against staphylococci, *Proteus mirabilis*, *Klebsiella pneumoniae*, *S. marcescens*, *Ps. aeruginosa*, *E. coli*, some *B. cepacia* strains, but not *E. faecalis* (Chin and Neu, 1987a; Fuursted, 1987; Davidson *et al.*, 1991; Kumar *et al.*, 1992; Meng *et al.*, 1994). Post-antibiotic effect is defined as the time between the transient exposure of a bacterial culture to an antibiotic and the time at which bacterial growth resumes (Fuursted, 1987; Guan *et al.*, 1992). Variables that affect PAE include the antibiotic type, concentration and duration of antibiotic exposure, the strain and bacterial species under investigation and the culture media used (Eliopoulos and Eliopoulos, 1993). Guan *et al.* (1992) have suggested that quinolone-induced PAE is associated with quinolone inhibition of DNA synthesis rather than via other mechanisms. Ciprofloxacin, ofloxacin and lomefloxacin are similar in producing a PAE of about 2 h in Gram-negative and Gram-positive bacteria exposed for 1 h to antibiotic concentrations 4-fold greater than the MIC (Debbia *et al.*, 1992). Interestingly, ciprofloxacin does not prolong the PAE of other PAE-producing drugs – unlike rifampicin which prolongs PAE in a synergistic fashion combined with other PAE-producing agents (Gudmundsson *et al.*, 1990). The ability of an antibiotic to exhibit a PAE on a particular organism is a theoretically attractive attribute since antibiotic concentrations could fall below the MIC of the organism without regrowth occurring. Given the above caveats regarding *in vitro* variables in testing for PAE, however, the direct applicability of these data to clinical antibiotic choice and usage remains poorly defined.

11 Synergism with other drugs

With a few notable exceptions, most authors have found only occasional synergy between quinolones such as ciprofloxacin, norfloxacin and enoxacin, and either aminoglycosides or beta-lactams. Most commonly these combinations have shown indifferent or additive effects, and only occasionally antagonism. Moody *et al.* (1987) reported that ciprofloxacin combined with azlocillin or ceftizoxime was synergistic *in vitro* against 50% of *Ps. aeruginosa* and *S. marcescens* isolates, and that ciprofloxacin combined with amikacin was synergistic against ≥ 50% of *S. marcescens* and *Staph. aureus* isolates. Subsequent studies in rabbits confirmed the synergistic effect of combining ciprofloxacin and azlocillin against some Enterobacteriaceae and *Ps. aeruginosa*. Similarly, Orlando *et al.* (1990) noted *in vitro* synergy between ciprofloxacin and azlocillin against some strains of *Ps. aeruginosa*, *E. coli* and *Kl. pneumoniae*. However, Haller (1985) found much lower rates of synergy.

Although combinations of ciprofloxacin with aminoglycosides sometimes (≤ 30%) yield synergistic activity against *Ps. aeruginosa*, such synergy is rarely seen against *Stenotrophomonas maltophilia* (Chow *et al.*, 1988a; Eliopoulos & Eliopoulos, 1989; Neu, 1991).

The benefit of combination therapy with ciprofloxacin and rifampicin against *L. pneumophila* infection is unclear. Ciprofloxacin + rifampicin results in suppression of resistance to each agent *in vitro*, but rifampicin has also been shown in broth culture to antagonize the bactericidal activity of ciprofloxacin (Havlicheck *et al.*, 1987; Barker and Farrell, 1990).

In general, combinations of ciprofloxacin with aminoglycosides are additive or indifferent against *Staph. aureus*, and although synergism has been shown with ciprofloxacin + azlocillin against up to 40% of *Staph. aureus* strains, this has little clinical relevence (Chin *et al.*, 1986a,b; Moody *et al.*, 1987). Some studies suggest that rifampicin antagonizes the bactericidal activities of fluoroquinolones against *Staph. aureus in vitro*, however, others report indifference in terms of bactericidal activity. There are no clinical data to suggest that this combination is associated with poorer clinical outcomes (Hackbarth *et al.*, 1986; Fass and Helsel, 1987; Van der Auwera and Joly, 1987; Kaatz *et al.*, 1989; Neu, 1989a; Dworkin *et al.*, 1990). Indifferent activity against enterococci *in vitro* and in animal models has generally been noted with combinations of ciprofloxacin and beta-lactams such as penicillin or ampicillin (Fernandez-Guerrero *et al.*, 1987; Haller, 1987; Ingerman *et al.*, 1987).

Thus although ciprofloxacin + aminoglycoside and ciprofloxacin + beta-lactam synergy is sporadic and relatively infrequent, antagonism between these agents appears to be rare (Eliopoulos and Eliopoulos, 1993). Ciprofloxacin and metronidazole appear to produce additive or indifferent results *in vitro* (Whiting *et al.*, 1987). Overall, combinations of fluoroquinolones with clindamycin, anti-anaerobic penicillins or cephalosporins against anaerobic species such as *Bacteroides fragilis* are only occasionally synergistic and usually indifferent (Esposito *et al.*, 1987a; Whiting *et al.*, 1987, Eliopoulos and Eliopoulos, 1989; Neu, 1989b, 1991; Wolfson and Hooper, 1989c).

Similar to other ciprofloxacin + beta-lactam combinations, there have been mixed results with the combination of ciprofloxacin and imipenem (Bustamante *et al.*, 1987; Chin and Neu, 1987b; Kumar *et al.*, 1989).

In vitro synergy between ciprofloxacin and amikacin, erythromycin, imipenem, rifampicin and or isoniazid against *Mycobacterium tuberculosis* has been reported in 7–41% of isolates, but there are no clinical data to support the proposed benefit of these combinations (Neu, 1991; Casal *et al.*, 1989). Against *Mycobacterium avium*, however, ciprofloxacin and ethambutol demonstrates bactericidal synergy at clinically achievable concentrations, although when ciprofloxacin is combined with rifampicin and ethambutol there is no greater activity than with rifampicin and ethambutol alone (Yajko *et al.*, 1988, 1990).

Despite these numerous *in vitro* studies, there is no reliable evidence of clinical synergy, namely improved clinical outcomes with these various combinations.

12 Acquired resistance

The mechanisms of resistance to ciprofloxacin and other fluoroquinolones are similar to those described for nalidixic acid and other older quinolones (p. 968), however, the incidence of such resistance is significantly lower for fluoroqinolones. Chromosomal mutations affecting DNA gyrase and membrane permeability have been well described (Hooper and Wolfson, 1993b; p. 968). Unlike resistance to beta-lactams and aminoglycosides, plasmid-mediated resistance has been rarely recorded for fluoroquinolones. In the laboratory, as with nalidixic acid, the frequency of selection of chromosomal mutations depends on the selecting quinolone, the quinolone concentration and the media and bacterium used (Wolfson and Hooper, 1989a). By serial passage of organisms on media containing increasing concentrations of the quinolone, one can select for resistance to all fluoroquinolones (Neu, 1988). Resistant mutants of *Ps. aeruginosa*, *Staph. aureus* and some strains of *E. cloacae* and *S. marcescens*, can be more readily selected than mutants of *E. coli* (Duckworth and Williams, 1984; Chantot and Bryskier, 1985; Kumada and Neu, 1985; Scribner *et al.*, 1985; Fernandes *et al.*, 1987; Felmingham *et al.*, 1988; Aldridge *et al.*, 1989; Watanabe *et al.*, 1990). Resistance due to spontaneous single-step chromosomal mutation occurs at a low frequency of $<10^{-9}$ and usually results in a 300-fold lower level of resistance than similar mutations resulting in nalidixic acid resistance (Neu, 1988). This frequency of mutation conferring resistance to ciprofloxacin or norfloxacin is 100- to 1000-fold lower than for nalixidic acid (Hooper *et al.*, 1986). Highly resistant bacteria may contain multiple mutations, presumably contributing in an additive fashion to resistance (Hane and Wood, 1969; Hooper *et al.*, 1986, 1987).

The principal target of quinolone action, DNA gyrase, is composed of two A (GyrA) and two B (GyrB) subunits under the genetic control of *gyrA* and *gyrB* genes, respectively (p. 971). Numerous studies have examined the mechanisms of resistance of various bacterial species. Alterations in subunit A have been reported in *E. coli*, *H. influenzae*, *C. jejuni*, *S. marcescens*, *C. freundii*, *E. aerogenes*, *Kl. pneumoniae*, *Providencia stuartii*, *Acinetobacter calcoaceticus*, *Ps. aeruginosa*, *E. faecalis*, *Staph. aureus*, *Staph. epidermidis* and *B. subtilis* (Rella and Haas, 1982; Setlow *et al.*, 1985; Hirai *et al.*, 1987; Inoue, *et al.*, 1987; Aoyama *et al.*, 1988; Robillard and Scarpa, 1988; Fujimaki *et al.*, 1989; Masecar *et al.*, 1990; Robillard, 1990; Sreedharan *et al.*, 1990, 1991; Gootz and Martin, 1991; Heisig and Wiedemann, 1991; Masecar and Robillard,1991; Nakanishi *et al.*, 1991a,b; Okuda *et al.*, 1991; Segreti *et al.*,1992; Heisig *et al.*, 1994). The majority of information regarding *gyrA* mutants have come from studies of *E. coli* in which single changes in amino acid sequence in the active site of the GyrA subunit have been responsible for the resultant resistance. A commonly observed site of alteration is at position-83 of the A subunit in which the polar amino acid, serine, is changed to leucine or tryptophan (Heisig *et al.*, 1993). Similar changes in serine at position-84 (equivalent to Ser-83 in *E. coli*) GyrA have been noted in quinolone-resistant *Staph. aureus* and *Staph. epidermidis*. Other sites of amino acid changes have also been associated with ciprofloxacin-resistance in *E. coli*. Substituting amino acids that are bulky or non-polar, such as these, presumably interfere with quinolone affinity, binding and action on DNA gyrase; although the exact mechanism by which these amino acid changes confer resistance is not yet known. Notably, however, these studies highlight the fact that quinolones bind specifically with the complex of DNA and DNA gyrases, rather than to DNA gyrase alone (Hooper and Wolfson, 1993b).

Alterations in the GyrB subunit have been associated with quinolone-resistance in isolates of *N. gonorrhoeae* (Stein *et al.*, 1991) and *E. coli* (Yamagishi *et al.*, 1981, 1986), although the site(s) of amino acid changes are less well defined than in *gyrA* mutants. Furthermore, there is currently no proof of an interaction between quinolones and GyrB.

Among *E. coli*, changes in GyrA appear to be associated with higher levels of resistance than with *gyrB* mutations and the relative frequency of *gyrA* and *gyrB* mutants varies depending on the selecting drug, the bacterial strain and the level of resistance selected (Hooper and Wolfson, 1993b).

Hydrophilic quinolones penetrate the outer membrane of Gram-negative bacilli to the periplasmic space through porin protein channels which are filled with water (Hancock, 1987; Nikaido and Vaara, 1985). The characteristics of the porins of a cell are regulated in response to environmental factors such as temperature and growth medium (Lugtenberg *et al.*, 1976; Hall and Silhavey, 1981; Schnaitman and McDonald, 1984).

Studies on *E. coli*, especially involving alterations in the porin OmpF have been associated with both resistance and reduced accumulation of quinolones, and also resistance to structurally unrelated drugs such as tetracycline, chloramphenicol and some beta-lactams (Hooper *et al.*, 1989; Aubert *et al.*, 1992). The genetic control of OmpF and other porins appears to be rather complex. Studies with mutant *E. coli* suggest that at least one operon consisting of at least three genes is involved and the gene expression is altered in response to environmental insults (Rosner *et al.*, 1991). Laboratory and clinical isolates with the highest levels of fluroquinolone-resistance generally have altered DNA gyrase and reduced quinolone permeability (Jacoby and Archer,

1991). The presence of *E. coli* isolates with levels of resistance 2- to 4-fold greater than OmpF mutants, suggest other mechanisms, yet to be clearly defined, are also responsible for resistance to hydrophilic fluoroquinolones, such as norfloxacin and ciprofloxacin (Cohen *et al.*, 1989; Masecar *et al.*, 1990; Young and Hancock, 1992).

Pseudomonas aeruginosa isolates resistant to ciprofloxacin are generally cross-resistant to other quinolones (Rådberg *et al.*, 1990). Dissociated resistance between fluoroquinolones whereby increased ciprofloxacin resistance is not associated with a similar level of resistance to other fluoroquinolones has only occasionally been described (Barry and Fuchs, 1991c; Thomson *et al.*, 1991; Thomson and Sanders, 1994; Chidiac *et al.*, 1995). Chidiac et al (1995), using a rat pneumonia model, demonstrated an *in vivo* correlation between *in vitro* susceptibility and good clinical outcome for fluoroquinolones identified as susceptible compared with fluoroquinolones noted to be resistant *in vitro*.

Kato *et al.* (1988) reported an interesting association between resistance to norfloxacin and resistance to beta-lactam antibiotics in *Bacteroides fragilis,* but the mechanism of this has not been defined. Similarly, Fung-Tomc *et al.* (1993) noted reduced susceptibility to non-quinolone agents imipenem, amikacin and cefepime in *Ps. aeruginosa* isolates which developed ciprofloxacin resistance after exposure *in vitro* to subinhibitory levels of ciprofloxacin. Similar cross-resistance to imipenem has been noted in clinical *Ps. aeruginosa* isolates developing resistance to ciprofloxacin (Aubert *et al.*, 1992). Multiple mechanisms of resistance to ciprofloxacin are often noted in *Ps. aeruginosa* isolates (Diver *et al.*, 1991). In particular, alterations in outer membrane proteins have been noted among strains of *Ps. aeruginosa* with resistance to ciprofloxacin, beta-lactams and aminoglycosides (Legakis *et al.*, 1989).

Drug modification or destruction has not yet been described for quinolones (Jacoby and Archer, 1991). The interaction of quinolones with the inner membrane of Gram-negative bacilli and the role of efflux in quinolone-resistance in these organisms remains complex and incompletely understood (Celesk and Robillard, 1988; Cohen *et al.*, 1988). However, endogenous energy-dependent drug efflux does appear to play some role in ciprofloxacin-resistance in some strains of *Ps. aeruginosa* and other species (McCaffrey *et al.*, 1992; Li *et al.*, 1994). It is uncertain, however, whether quinolone efflux is a mechanism of resistance in Gram-positive bacteria (which lack an outer membrane).

As noted earlier (p. 969) plasmid-mediated quinolone-resistance among clinical isolates has not yet been confirmed, although such resistance has been engineered in laboratory mutants. The ability of quinolones to inhibit plasmid conjugation and eliminate some plasmids from host cells may be responsible for the apparent lack of plasmid-mediated resistance (Courvalin, 1990).

Fungi are intrinsically resistant to quinolones, possibly because they, like other eukaryotes, contain topoisomeriases which are structurally and functionally distinct from the DNA gyrases present in prokaryotic bacteria. Furthermore, little is known regarding quinolone permeability in fungi (Hooper and Wolfson, 1993b).

Clinical resistance to fluoroquinolones has been uncommon, occurring mostly in respiratory pathogens (especially *Ps. aeruginosa* associated with cystic fibrosis) and occasionally in the setting of wound infections due to *S. marcescens, Ps. aeruginosa* and *Staph. aureus* (Neu, 1988).

Eliopoulos and Eliopoulos (1993), in their review of the literature from 1988 to 1993 identified no significant change in overall susceptibilities of Enterobacteriaceae to fluoroquinolones. In Germany, Sweden, Belgium, Holland and the UK during the 1970s, 1980s and early 1990s no change in resistance to ciprofloxacin among Enterobacteriaceae has been reported (Kresken and Wiedemann,1988; Grünberg, 1990; Buirma *et al.*, 1991; Shah *et al.*, 1991; Verbist, 1991; Walder *et al.*, 1994). Nevertheless, some reports have described significant increases in the rates of fluoroquinolone-resistance among Enterobacteriaceae in some regions. In particular, increasing resistance to ciprofloxacin and norfloxacin amongst *E. coli* isolates have been noted in Madrid, Spain, during the period from the late 1980s to early 1990s (Aguiar *et al.*, 1992; Péna *et al.*, 1995).

A significant increase in resistance has been reported among *Ps. aeruginosa* isolates (Kresken and Wiedemann, 1988; MacGowan *et al.*, 1993). MacGowan *et al.* (1993) reviewed the susceptibility of more than 85 000 clinical isolates collected in the UK between 1984 and 1991. Patterns of susceptibility remained largely unchanged among Enterobacteriaceae except for an increase in resistance among *Pseudomonas* spp. (9.6–13% increase) and *Staph. aureus* (6% increase) to ciprofloxacin between 1986 and 1991. Other authors in the UK and Sweden have also noted an increase in ciprofloxacin-resistance among isolates of *Staph. aureus*, coagulase-negative staphylococci, other Gram-positive cocci and *Ps. aeruginosa* (Barry *et al.*, 1990; Fredlund *et al.*, 1990; George *et al.*, 1990).

Not unexpectedly, the development of ciprofloxacin-resistance has often been associated with the increasing use of fluoroquinolones (Chin *et al.*, 1989; Parry *et al.*, 1989; Carratala *et al.*, 1991; Muder *et al.*, 1991; Dostal *et al.*, 1992; Kern *et al.*, 1994; Péna *et al.*, 1995). Kern *et al.* (1994) reported two patients with acute leukemia who developed bacteremia with *E. coli* resistant to fluoroquinolones (including ciprofloxacin) while receiving oral ofloxacin. Péna *et al.* (1995) reported a significant increase in ciprofloxacin-resistant *E. coli* bacteremia in Barcelona, Spain from 0% in 1988 to 7.5% in 1992 (p < 0.01). Prior fluoroquinolone use was the only independent risk factor for ciprofloxacin-resistant *E. coli* bacteremia in this study. Parry *et al.* (1989) noted that a significant increase in resistance to ciprofloxacin among *Pseudomonas* species and staphylococcal species in 1988 was associated with the growing use of fluoroquinolone. In all, 72% of ciprofloxacin-resistant isolates were recovered from patients who had received a fluoroquinolone during the previous month. Significant sources for ciprofloxacin-resistant organisms were soft tissue infection and osteomyelitis (50%) and urinary tract infections associated with instrumentation (26%). Susceptibility to ciprofloxacin among Enterobacteriaceae and other pathogens in this study remained stable from 1984 to 1988. Similarly, Azadian *et al.* (1986), Chin *et al.* (1989) and Cooper *et al.* (1993) all noted the development of resistance to ciprofloxacin in clinical isolates of *Ps. aeruginosa* during treatment with ciprofloxacin.

In a recent study of cirrhotic patients treated with norfloxacin to prevent spontaneous bacterial peritonitis, Dupeyron *et al.* (1994) noted fecal colonization with organisms highly resistant to fluoroquinolones in more than 50% of patients after 14 days therapy. Such data raise concerns regarding the prophylactic use of fluoroquinolones and the potential for selection and dissemination of resistant isolates, especially in the hospital environment.

A significant increase in the rate of resistance to ciprofloxacin has been noted among fecal strains of *Campylobacter jejuni* isolated from pediatric patients in Spain from 1987 (0%) to 1993 (48.8%; MIC ≥4 μg per ml) (Reina *et al.*, 1994). Ciprofloxacin-resistance appears to be increasing in clinical isolates of *C. jejuni* and *C. coli*, with numerous authors reporting both *in vitro* resistance and clinical treatment failure in the USA, UK, Switzerland, Spain, Finland, the Netherlands and Australia (Adler-Mosca *et al.*, 1991; Endtz *et al.*, 1991; Rautelin *et al.*, 1991; Segreti *et al.*, 1992; McIntyre and Lyons, 1993; Sánchez *et al.*, 1994; Tee *et al.*, 1995). Navarro *et al.* (1993) reported a massive increase in ciprofloxacin-resistance among *C. jejuni* and *C. coli* clinical isolates from 7.5% to 57% and 14% to 43%, respectively, between 1989 and 1992 in Barcelona. This change occurred at a time of increased quinolone consumption. Similar rates of resistance have been reported in Madrid (Sánchez *et al.*, 1994). In Finland, ciprofloxacin-resistance among *C. jejuni* and *C. coli* isolates increased from 0% in 1980 to 9% in 1990 (Rautelin *et al.*, 1991). Endtz *et al.* (1991) has associated the increase in quinolone-resistance in human *Campylobacter* isolates in the Netherlands to the widespread use of quinolones in the poultry industry with associated high rates of quinolone-resistance among *Campylobacter* isolated from poultry. Gootz and Martin (1991) and Wang *et al.* (1993) have identified an alteration in the A subunit of DNA gyrase as responsible for ciprofloxacin-resistance in *C. jejuni*.

In comparison, *Shigella* spp. isolated from travelers with diarrhea returning to Spain from a wide range of geographical origins (including Africa, South and Central America and India) demonstrated no resistance to norfloxacin or ciprofloxacin (Vila *et al.*, 1994). Although Ries *et al.* (1994) noted a higher MIC of ciprofloxacin against *Sh. dysenteriae* isolates (MIC 0.25 μg per ml) than either *Sh. flexneri* or *Sh. sonnei* (MIC < 0.06 μg per ml), Vila *et al.* (1994) found all species to be extremely susceptible (MIC < 0.007 μg per ml).

Fluoroquinolone resistance has been rare in salmonellae, although treatment failures associated with development of resistance have been noted (Kresken and Wiedemann, 1988; Howard *et al.*, 1990; Piddock *et al.*, 1990; Hof *et al.*, 1991; Gibb *et al.*, 1991). Heisig (1993) described a multiresistant strain of *Salm. typhimurium* with *gyrA* and *gyrB* mutations, and Rowe *et al.* (1995) have described a number of strains of ciprofloxacin-resistant *Salm. typhi*, mostly cultured from patients who had recently traveled to the Indian subcontinent.

Prior to 1992, almost all strains of *N. gonorrhoeae* were susceptible to fluoroquinolones (ciprofloxacin MIC ≤0.06 μg per ml), however, strains with reduced susceptibility have been increasingly recognized in various states of the USA (CDC, 1993a, 1994; Knapp *et al.*, 1994a, 1994b). In Ohio (1992–1993) 5.6% of isolates had MICs of ciprofloxacin of 0.13–0.25 μg per ml, while in Hawaii (1993–1994) a number of strains with MICs of 2.0 μg per ml of ciprofloxacin were isolated from patients who had potentially acquired infection in South-East Asia. All isolates were susceptible to ceftriaxone and cefixime (CDC, 1994; Knapp *et al.*, 1994a,b). Strains with similar MICs have been reported from Thailand, UK and Australia

(Grandsden *et al.*, 1990; Jephcott and Turner, 1990; Clendennen *et al.*, 1992; Tapsall *et al.*, 1992; Griffith *et al.*, 1996). Decreased susceptibility to ciprofloxacin is associated with cross-resistance to other fluoroquinolones, including ofloxacin, enoxacin, lomefloxacin and norfloxacin (Barry and Jones, 1984). Infections due to isolates with MICs of ciprofloxacin $\geq 2\,\mu$g per ml may not respond to routine doses of ciprofloxacin, although whether lesser degrees of resistance are also associated with a higher incidence of clinical treatment failure is unclear (Knapp *et al.*, 1994a,b). Strains with chromosomally mediated resistance to penicillin and tetracyclines may be expected to be associated with higher levels of resistance to fluoroquinolones; however, this remains to be confirmed (CDC, 1993a; Zenilman *et al.*, 1993).

Widespread resistance to fluoroquinolones has developed among many strains of *Staph. aureus* (particularly methicillin-resistant *Staph. aureus*: MRSA) and coagulase-negative staphylococci throughout the world since the mid-late 1980s with the growing use of these agents (Schaefler, 1989; Shalit *et al.*, 1989b; Ball, 1990; Daum *et al.*, 1990; Dryden *et al.*, 1990; Kotilainen *et al.*, 1990; Raviglione *et al.*, 1990; Smith *et al.*, 1990; Harnett *et al.*, 1991; Wadsworth *et al.*, 1992; Voss *et al.*, 1994; Turnidge *et al.*, 1996). Wadsworth *et al.* (1992) noted a dramatic increase in high-level resistance to ciprofloxacin among MRSA isolates from 2% in 1987 to 52% in 1989. Cross-resistance to enoxacin, fleroxacin, norfloxacin and ofloxacin was also noted. Among methicillin-sensitive *Staph. aureus* (MSSA) isolates during the same period, no increase in resistance was found. Other authors have generally found rates of resistance among MRSA of approximately 80% (range 40–100%) after 1987 (Isaacs *et al.*, 1988; Shalit *et al.*, 1989b; Daum *et al.*, 1990; Peterson *et al.*, 1990; Raviglione *et al.*, 1990; Blumberg *et al.*, 1991; Fung-Tomc *et al.*, 1991; Harnett *et al.*, 1991; Hillery and Reiss-Levy, 1993; Voss *et al.*, 1994; Coronado *et al.*, 1995). Across Europe, more than 80% of MRSA isolates were ciprofloxacin-resistant in 1990–1991 (Voss *et al.*, 1994) and similar rates have been reported in Australia (Hillery and Reiss-Levy, 1993). Raviglione *et al.* (1990) reported an 83% rate of resistance (MIC $> 2\,\mu$g per ml) among MRSA during 1989–1990 and noted that this was associated with prior ciprofloxacin use in approximately 30% of cases. Among MSSA, however, no increase in resistance was noted, with 98.4% susceptible. Shalit *et al.* (1989b) reported similar findings. Blumberg *et al.* (1991) prospectively evaluated the emergence of high-level resistance to ciprofloxacin (MIC_{90} 64 μg per ml) after the introduction of ciprofloxacin use in their hospital in 1988 and noted an increase in resistance from 0% to 79% among MRSA isolates over a 1-year period. High-level ciprofloxacin-resistance also developed in MSSA in this study, increasing to 13.6% during the same period. About half of the patients had a history of previous ciprofloxacin use. Similarly, Weightman and Brass (1993) noted a 7% incidence of ciprofloxacin-resistance among MSSA and Daum *et al.* (1990) noted a 2.5% incidence. A survey conducted by the Centre of Disease Control has demonstrated a 123% increase in the odds of ciprofloxacin-resistance from 1989–90 to 1991–92 among *Staph. aureus*, with isolates of urinary and respiratory tract origin and MRSA most affected. Resistance to ciprofloxacin is now more frequent among nosocomial *Staph. aureus* than among *Ps. aeruginosa* and is increasing rapidly (Coronado *et al.*, 1995).

Nosocomial colonization and disease with ciprofloxacin-resistant coagulase-negative staphylococci (*Staph. epidermidis* and *Staph. haemolyticus*) have been reported in various patient groups, including those with leukemia and those on continuous ambulatory peritoneal dialysis (CAPD) (Dryden *et al.*, 1989; Kotilainen *et al.*, 1990; Kotilainen *et al.*, 1995).

Investigations of newer fluoroquinolones such as sparfloxacin (p. 1135) have shown improved performance against moderately ciprofloxacin-resistant strains of *Staph. aureus* and coagulase-negative staphylococci, but generally complete cross-resistance among highly ciprofloxacin-resistant strains has been noted (Chaudhry *et al.*, 1990; Barry and Fuchs, 1991a,b; Forstall *et al.*, 1991; Maple *et al.*, 1991; Brumfitt and Hamilton-Miller, 1993).

Mutations at the Ser-84 site in DNA gyrase A protein of both *Staph. aureus* and *Staph. epidermidis*, and alterations in fluoroquinolone uptake and efflux in some *Staph. aureus* have been identified in resistant isolates (Sreedharan *et al.*, 1990, 1991; Kaatz *et al.*, 1991; Nakanishi *et al.*, 1991a; Ng *et al.*, 1994). More recently, mutations in *gyrB* gene have also been described in quinolone-resistant *Staph. aureus*, although *gyrA* mutants appear to produce a greater level of resistance and may therefore have a selective advantage in clinical isolates (Ito *et al.*, 1994).

Schaberg *et al.* (1992) noted a significant increase in ciprofloxacin-resistance among clinical enterococcal isolates (especially *E. faecalis* demonstrating high-level gentamicin-resistance) from 0% in 1985–1986 to 24% in 1989–1990 in their institution in Michigan. In comparison, however, Grayson *et al.* (1991) noted little change in the susceptibility of clinical *E. faecium* strains isolated during the 22-year period from 1969 to 1990 at Massachusetts General Hospital,

Boston. Alterations in gyrase A subunit appears to be the major cause of fluoroquinolone-resistance in *E. faecalis* clinical isolates (Nakanishi *et al.*, 1991b).

Among *Strep. pneumoniae* strains, regardless of whether they are susceptible or resistant (MIC $\geq 2 \mu g$ per ml) to penicillin the MIC_{90} of ciprofloxacin was $2 \mu g$ per ml (Mason *et al.*, 1992). Step-wise increases in resistance to ciprofloxacin with cross-resistance to other quinolones can be induced *in vitro*, although with greater difficulty than with group B streptococci (Piddock and Wise, 1988). The borderline activity of ciprofloxacin against most clinical *Strep. pneumoniae* isolates, rather than the development of resistance *per se*, is most likely responsible for the numerous clinical reports of treatment failure and superinfection with this pathogen (Cooper and Lawlor, 1989; Gordon and Kauffman, 1990; Righter, 1990; Lee *et al.*, 1991; Marone and Quadri, 1992).

Mode of Administration and Dosage

1 Oral administration

The usual adult oral dose of ciprofloxacin ranges from 250 mg to 750 mg twice-daily, depending on the type and severity of infection. For infections such as mild to moderate lower respiratory tract, skin and soft tissue, and bone and joint infections, 500 mg twice-daily is generally appropriate. A similar dose is suitable for the treatment of most forms of bacterial infectious diarrhea, except typhoid fever, when higher doses are necessary. A single 500-mg dose is suitable for treatment of uncomplicated genital/rectal *N. gonorrhoeae*, although disseminated or complicated disease requires higher doses for longer durations. The optimum dose for eradication of nasal carriage of *N. meningitidis* is not defined, but regimens include a 500-mg or 750-mg single-dose, 250 mg twice-daily for 2 days, or 500 mg twice-daily for 5 days (AHFS, 1995). Concurrent administration of aluminum and magnesium antacids, or sucralfate may reduce the absorption of ciprofloxacin due to formation of drug-cationic chelate complexes (Preheim *et al.*, 1986; Roberts and Williams 1989; Garrelts *et al.*, 1990; p. 1013). However, calcium carbonate given 2 h prior to oral ciprofloxacin does not alter the bioavailability of ciprofloxacin, in healthy volunteers (Lomaestro and Bailie, 1991). Ciprofloxacin administered via a nasogastric tube as a crushed tablet in suspension, either alone or while receiving enteral feeding, is similar in bioavailability in healthy volunteers to orally administered ciprofloxacin (Yuk *et al.*, 1989a). Administration of ciprofloxacin via jejunostomy tube may result in lower, but generally acceptable, serum concentrations than orally administered drug (Sahai *et al.*, 1991).

2 Intravenous administration

Recommended intravenous doses range from 100 to 400 mg 12-hourly, although 200 mg twice-daily is most commonly used for moderately severe urinary tract infections (Martindale, 1993) and 300–400 mg twice-daily for severe or complicated urinary tract infections, lower respiratory tract infections, skin and soft tissue, and bone and joint infections. For severe systemic infections, especially those due to *Ps. aeruginosa*, *Staph. aureus* or streptococci, a higher daily dose of up to 400 mg 8 hourly i.v. (equivalent to 750 mg twice-daily oral therapy) may be used, although ciprofloxacin is not an optimal agent to treat infections due to these latter two pathogens (Echols 1993; Shah *et al.*, 1994). Among critically ill trauma patients there may be significant variability in ciprofloxacin clearance such that ciprofloxacin doses of 200 mg i.v. 12-hourly may be inadequate, especially if treating *Ps. aeruginosa* or *Staph. aureus* infections (Yuen *et al.*, 1989). Similarly, Dan *et al.* (1994), who examined the pharmacokinetic and serum bactericidal activities of 200 mg, 300 mg and 400 mg i.v. ciprofloxacin suggested that the 200-mg dose was adequate for infections due to Enterobacteriaceae, but that 400 mg twice-daily or even three times daily may be otherwise appropriate. Studies by Catchpole *et al.* (1994) utilizing blister fluid, urine and serum concentrations in healthy volunteers, suggested that ciprofloxacin 400 mg i.v. is more equivalent to 750 mg orally than indicated by plasma pharmacokinetic data.

Forrest *et al.* (1993b) analyzed the outcome of 64 seriously ill patients treated with i.v. ciprofloxacin and found the best predictor of a good clinical and microbiological outcome was the ratio of area-under-the-concentration-time-curve (AUC) for 24 h divided by the MIC of the pathogen being treated (AUC/MIC = AUIC). At an AUIC <125, the probabilities of clinical and microbiological cure were 42 and 26% respectively; while an AUIC >125 was associated with a probability of cure of 80 and 82%, respectively. In a companion article (Forrest *et al.*, 1993a), these authors described a dosing algorithm for i.v. ciprofloxacin based on MIC, patient creatinine clearance and weight, and the AUIC target.

Cardiopulmonary bypass does not significantly alter the disposition of i.v. ciprofloxacin compared with that before and after cardiac surgery (Pryka *et al.*, 1993).

3 Patients with renal failure

The serum half-life of patients with normal renal function is 3–6 h and extends to 6–9 h in patients with end-stage renal function (Boelaert *et al.*, 1985; Bennett *et al.*, 1994; Bindschedler *et al.*, 1988; Drusano *et al.*, 1987). Peak serum levels and times to reach these peaks are not significantly higher even in patients with end-stage renal failure, but the AUC is more than doubled in patients with renal failure, compared with those with good renal function. Drusano *et al.* (1987) recommended a 50% reduction in dose when the glomerular filtration rate (GFR) is less than 20–30 ml per min, but that a 12-hourly dosing schedule should be maintained regardless of renal function due to variations in ciprofloxacin half-life in anephric patients. Similar to other fluoroquinolones, ciprofloxacin is primarily (50–75%) excreted unchanged by the kidneys in healthy individuals (p. 1002). In addition, there is significant proximal tubular secretion, resulting in overall renal excretion of ciprofloxacin exceeding creatinine clearance (Webb *et al.*, 1986; Drusano *et al.*, 1987). Notably, renal excretion is partially blocked by probenecid (Drusano, 1987). In the setting of renal impairment, tubular secretion decreases and there is reasonable correlation between renal and plasma clearance of ciprofloxacin and the creatinine clearance (Richer and LeBel, 1993). Due to the increasing impact of non-renal (e.g. hepatic) clearance of ciprofloxacin in renal failure, however, elimination half-life does not continue to parallel creatinine clearance. Furthermore, due to wide inter-subject variations in the non-renal clearance of ciprofloxacin in patients with similar creatinine clearances, specification of strict dosage regimens in significant renal failure is imprecise. Although the manufacturer suggests that dosage adjustments for oral and i.v. ciprofloxacin in renal failure should be different, there is little clinical data to support this view.

Renal dysfunction does not alter the volume of distribution of ciprofloxacin, nor does it affect the bioavailability of the drug to any extent (Plaisance *et al.*, 1990; Webb *et al.*, 1986). Plaisance *et al.* (1990), studied 21 subjects with a range of renal function, who were given ciprofloxacin 200 mg i.v. and 1 week later 750 mg orally, and found the bioavailability to be 69% for patients with normal renal function and 59.9% in patients with renal insufficiency.

Urine concentrations of ciprofloxacin for up to 24 h after either a 500 mg or 750 mg single oral dose of ciprofloxacin are generally several times the MIC for most urinary pathogens even in patients with significant renal failure, and therefore ciprofloxacin remains a potential therapeutic option for urinary tract infections in patients with impaired renal function (Gasser *et al.*, 1988). Forrest *et al.* (1988) recommend that patients with severe renal failure (creatinine clearance <20 ml per min) should receive two-thirds of the normal oral daily dose and that the dose interval should not be lengthened. Similarly, MacGowan et al (1994) recommend 200 mg i.v. twice-daily in patients with severe sepsis, irrespective of renal function and warn that in some patients lower doses may result in subtherapeutic serum concentrations. In support of these concerns regarding potential underdosing in patients with renal failure, Dibble *et al.* (1987) reported a 29-year-old male with acute renal failure requiring hemodialysis who had *Ps. aeruginosa* septicemia and failed therapy with ciprofloxacin 100 mg twice-daily i.v., which was found to result in low serum levels. The patient eventually responded to ciprofloxacin 300 mg i.v. twice-daily. These authors advocate the use of routine doses of i.v. ciprofloxacin (e.g. 300 mg twice-daily) for serious infections in renal failure. Thus in some cases of serious infection where optimal dosing is vital, therapeutic drug monitoring may be warranted, especially where there is coexistent renal and hepatic failure. In general, most authors recommend that for moderate renal failure (GFR 10–50 ml per min) doses occasionally need to be decreased to 50–75%, while severe renal failure (GFR <10 ml per min) requires a 50% dose reduction (Bennett *et al.*, 1994; Sanford *et al.*, 1995).

Hemodialysis removes only about 2% of the given dose (Boelaert *et al.*, 1985), hence no post-hemodialysis supplementation is necessary. The recommended dosage for patients receiving hemodialysis is 250 mg orally twice-daily; 250 mg thrice-daily in CAPD and 200 mg i.v. twice-daily in continuous arteriovenous or venovenous hemofiltration (Bennett *et al.*, 1994; Sanford *et al.*, 1995).

Chronic ambulatory peritoneal dialysis eliminates only 0.4–1.6% of a dose, and peritoneal dialysate levels are inconsistent (Richer and LeBel, 1993). In patients with end-stage renal failure treated with peritoneal dialysis, only 1% of a single oral ciprofloxacin dose is eliminated in the urine (Shalit *et al.*, 1986). When given in normal daily doses, but as 250 mg four times daily to patients on CAPD, Fleming *et al.* (1987), found the mean plasma concentration to be twice that seen in healthy patients, and dialysate concentrations to be at effective levels in more than half the cases for most pathogens responsible for peritonitis (Fleming *et al.*, 1987). Thus, in patients on CAPD, the dose reduction of oral ciprofloxacin is generally 250 mg 8-hourly, with no additional dose required after or during peritoneal dialysis (Richer and LeBel, 1993; Bennett *et al.*, 1994). When administered intraperitoneally in dialysate, the recommended dose of ciprofloxacin 25 mg per liter will produce dialysate levels after a 4-h cycle of $8.4 \pm 4.6\mu g$ per ml and $3.0\pm3.2\mu g$ per ml after a 12-h cycle; although there is considerable inter-patient variability in transperitoneal absorption. During this period of intraperitoneal administration the mean plasma concentration is approximately $0.5 \pm 0.2 \mu g$ per ml The low serum concentrations reflect efficient non-renal elimination and the large volume of distribution of the drug (Dharmasena *et al.*, 1989). Ciprofloxacin at a dose of 25 mg per liter is stable in dialysate containing both 1.5% and 4.25% dextrose, with 93.4% and 93.7% activity respectively, when stored at 25°C (Kane *et al.*, 1994; p. 1006). Cure of CAPD-associated peritonitis has been achieved with oral ciprofloxacin but relatively high doses (1–2 g per day) were necessary (Fleming *et al.*, 1988). The ingestion of antacids decreases the absorption of oral ciprofloxacin, resulting in serum and dialysate concentrations of 14–50% and 8–33%, respectively, of those observed in subjects not receiving antacids (Golper *et al.*, 1987). Thus, discontinuation of antacids such as aluminum phosphate-binders so commonly prescribed for patients with end-stage renal failure, may be necessary to achieve adequate serum and dialysate concentrations of ciprofloxacin in patients on CAPD (Golper *et al.*, 1987).

4 Patients with hepatic failure

Renal and hepatic mechanisms contribute to the elimination of fluoroquinolones, although the relative predominance of each of these two clearance pathways varies with the fluoro-quinolone. Ciprofloxacin clearance does not appear to be significantly altered in mild to moderate hepatic failure, although currently available data are not extensive. Frost *et al.* (1989b) found the pharmacokinetics of multidose ciprofloxacin to be unaltered in seven patients with cirrhosis, compared with seven matched healthy patients. Fraise and Smith (1990) suggested no change in ciprofloxacin dosage for patients with mild to moderate cirrhosis. Esposito *et al.* (1989) found a moderate increase in serum ciprofloxacin concentrations in patients with severe hepatic cirrhosis, with an increase in elimination half-life of 35% compared with controls. Thus dosage adjustment is probably necessary in severe hepatic failure, but the level of dosage reduction is unclear. The monitoring of serum ciprofloxacin concentrations may be helpful in this situation (Montay and Gaillot, 1990). Nevertheless, caution may need to be exercised, and dosage reduction instituted in patients with combined hepatic and renal failure, since Wenk *et al.* (1988) reported a substantial increase in ciprofloxacin half-life in this setting.

5 Children

Ciprofloxacin is not generally recommended for use in children, but if treatment is necessary, an oral dose of 7.5–15 mg per kg per day or 5–10 mg per kg per day i.v. ciprofloxacin is suggested (Martindale, 1993). Peltola *et al.* (1992), however, found the elimination of ciprofloxacin to be more rapid in 1- to 5-year-old children than in either infants, older children or adults, and that an oral dose of 10–15 mg per kg given thrice-daily (i.e. total daily dose 30–45 mg per kg) may be more appropriate for this 1- to 5-year-old age group. In this study of seven infants aged 5–14 weeks and nine children aged 1–5 years, most of whom were *Salmonella* carriers, who were treated with the above dose of oral ciprofloxacin, the elimination half-life of ciprofloxacin was significantly longer in infants $(2.73 \pm 0.28\,h)$ than it was in children $(1.28 \pm 0.52\,h)$ $(p < 0.001)$. No significant differences in the maximum serum concentrations, or time to maximum concentrations, were noted between the two groups. In one 7-month-old child, who was treated with two doses of ciprofloxacin 15 mg per kg orally, and then after 48 h drug-free period was given a similar dose i.v., the maximum serum concentrations were similar: $11–13\,\mu g$ per ml and $11–15\,\mu g$ per ml, respectively. Thus it appears that ciprofloxacin resembles trimethoprim in that its elimination is more rapid in children than in infants or adults.

6 Ciprofloxacin in pregnancy and lactating women

In pregnant women receiving routine doses of ciprofloxacin (200 mg i.v. every 12 h), serum concentrations of ciprofloxacin are several times lower than those in non-pregnant women. This is probably due to more rapid renal excretion and other elimination mechanisms in pregnant females. To support this view, it is notable that pefloxacin, a fluoroquinolone which is primarily eliminated by hepatic mechanisms, achieves similar serum concentrations in pregnant women as in non-pregnant women (Giamarellou et al., 1989). Thus, in the treatment of serious sepsis in pregnancy in which the use of ciprofloxacin is unavoidable, higher than usual doses may be necessary. Giamarellou et al. (1989) studied pregnant women affected by beta-thalassemia major who underwent termination at 19–25 weeks gestation. Mean ciprofloxacin concentrations 2–4 h after a 200 mg i.v. dose were $0.28 \pm 0.19 \mu g$ per ml in serum and $0.12 \pm 0.06 \mu g$ per ml in amniotic fluid (i.e. 57% of the serum concentration). Breast milk concentrations of ciprofloxacin are 160–214% of serum concentrations between 2–12 h after an oral dose of 750 mg of ciprofloxacin (Giamarellou et al., 1989).

7 Elderly patients

Although one might expect the absorption of fluoroquinolones to be impaired in the elderly due to the presence of ageing-associated diminished gastric acid secretion, gastric emptying time and reduced splanchnic blood flow, no differences have been noted between young and elderly patients in the time after dosing to achieve the maximal serum drug concentrations. However, peak serum concentrations of ciprofloxacin are higher, and the AUCs are larger in the elderly than in healthy young volunteers (Ball et al., 1986; Bayer et al., 1987; Hirata et al., 1989; Naber et al., 1989; Shah et al., 1995). Nevertheless, most authors recommend no dosage adjustment for either i.v. or oral ciprofloxacin in elderly patients with normal renal function, although, due to the expected higher serum concentrations, adverse reactions should be monitored (Guay et al., 1987; LeBel and Bergeron, 1987; Hirata et al., 1989). These authors found that serum concentrations of ciprofloxacin in the elderly were approximately double those in young adult patients after an oral dose of 750 mg twice-daily than after i.v. dosing with 200 mg twice-daily ($C_{max} \mu g$ per ml: 7.6 ± 2.2 versus 3.6 ± 1.0, respectively). No differences in concentrations between genders has been noted (Shah et al., 1995). In the elderly the presence of infection in itself does not alter pharmacokinetics of ciprofloxacin (Hirata et al., 1989; Guay et al., 1987). No dosage adjustment is necessary with concurrent administration of routine doses of ciprofloxacin and rifampicin in elderly patients, since serum concentrations are similar to when each agent is given alone (Chandler et al., 1990).

8 Dosage in cystic fibrosis

Ciprofloxacin, along with most fluoroquinolones, appears to be eliminated faster by patients with cystic fibrosis; probably due to increased total body and non-renal clearance. Therefore, ciprofloxacin has a shorter half-life in patients with cystic fibrosis compared with normal controls (LeBel et al., 1986b; Davis et al., 1987; Pedersen et al., 1987; Strandvik et al., 1989; Christensson et al., 1992; Cogo et al., 1992). The mechanism of this increased clearance is uncertain, but a generalized increase in drug metabolism and/or reduced renal tubular reabsorption has been proposed (Richer and LeBel, 1993). Thus, to achieve the serum concentration of ciprofloxacin expected in normal patients, a higher than usual dosage or a shorter administration interval is often required in patients with cystic fibrosis. Dosages of 750 mg two, three or four times daily are generally required (LeBel et al., 1986b; Reed et al., 1988; Richer and LeBel, 1993). In comparison, however, other authors have found the pharmacokinetics of ciprofloxacin in cystic fibrosis patients to be similar to normal patients and have therefore advocated routine doses of ciprofloxacin of 750 mg orally twice-daily for patients greater than 40kg in body weight (Davis et al., 1987; Stutman et al., 1987; Steen et al., 1989; Christensson et al., 1992). Bioavailability of ciprofloxacin in cystic fibrosis patients appears to be about 70%. Ciprofloxacin pharmacokinetic parameters in sputum appear to be similar to those observed in serum, although the peak concentration occurs 4–5 h after administration and is about one-third of the serum concentration (Smith et al., 1986b; Reed et al., 1988).

Availability

Oral preparation: Ciprofloxacin hydrochloride tablets each contain either 250, 500 or 750 mg of ciprofloxacin.

Parenteral preparation: Ciprofloxacin lactate infusion solution (0.2%) is available in pre-mixed solutions of 100 mg per 50ml and 200 mg per 100ml in 0.9% sodium chloride.

Serum Levels in Relation to Dosage

1 Oral administration

Ciprofloxacin is generally 60–70% absorbed from the gut, mostly from the duodenum and jejunum, but with a variability of 51–88% in some reports. Oral bioavailability is also partially dependent on the dose administered, with wider variations being associated with higher doses (Wingender et al., 1984; Höffken et al., 1985b; Bergan et al., 1986b, 1987; Borner et al., 1986; Drusano et al., 1986b; Plaisance et al., 1987, 1990; Hirata et al., 1989; Sörgel et al., 1991; Lettieri et al., 1992). Plaisance et al. (1987) noted some variation in the availability of 750 mg oral ciprofloxacin given to healthy volunteers, with a range of 375–700 mg of each dose reaching the systemic circulation. The cause of this variability is probably multifactorial, including variable disintegration/dissolution rates and potential variability in the gastrointestinal motility. Administration of ciprofloxacin with food delays the time taken to reach peak serum concentrations but does not alter bioavailability (Ledergerber et al., 1985). Serum half-life increases with increasing dose suggesting the elimination of ciprofloxacin is non-linear. Dose-ranging studies for single oral ciprofloxacin doses of 250, 500, 750 and 1000 mg in healthy male volunteers result in maximum serum concentrations of 0.76, 1.60, 2.54 and 3.38 µg per ml, respectively, 1.0–1.8 h (mean 1.5 h) after dosing. The serum half-life is 4.1 h after 250–500 mg and 6.3–6.9 h after 750–1000 mg (Tartaglione et al., 1986). Serum concentrations 12 and 24 h after each dose are shown in Fig. II.5. Similar findings were noted in the dose-ranging study by Bergan et al. (1987).

Other authors have reported similar results with a maximum serum concentration after 500 mg oral ciprofloxacin of 1.8–2.8 µg per ml, 40 min to 1.3 h after administration, and a half-life of 3.3–5.7 h (Wise et al., 1986, 1988a; Bergan et al., 1987; Eliopoulos, 1988; Wolfson and Hooper, 1989b; Lode et al., 1990a; Lettieri et al., 1992; Paradis et al., 1992; Echols et al., 1994). Similar pharmacokinetics have been noted with lower doses in healthy volunteers (Drusano et al., 1986b). Lettieri et al. (1992) in a single-dose cross-over study, found that 500 mg oral ciprofloxacin produced a similar AUC as 400 mg administered i.v. and that this i.v. dose resulted in a comparable maximum serum concentration as 750 mg given orally. Shah et al. (1994) reported similar findings in their multidose study with 400 mg i.v. ciprofloxacin thrice-daily, producing peak serum concentrations comparable with 750 mg oral ciprofloxacin twice-daily, but finding that the AUC_{24} was similar to 750 mg twice-daily. Echols et al. (1994) found that a 500 mg oral ciprofloxacin dose resulted in nearly equivalent serum bactericidal activity against a spectrum of Gram-negative and Gram-positive pathogens as ciprofloxacin 400 mg i.v. Ciprofloxacin is 16–40% protein bound (Wise et al., 1983; Chin and Neu, 1984; Höffken et al., 1985b; Joos et al., 1985; Bennett et al., 1994).

Pharmacokinetic studies of multidose regimens of ciprofloxacin demonstrate data similar to single-dose trials with either similar or clinically unimportant reduction in terminal half-life and serum clearance (Aronoff et al., 1984; Brumfitt et al., 1984; Gonzalez et al., 1984; LeBel et al.,

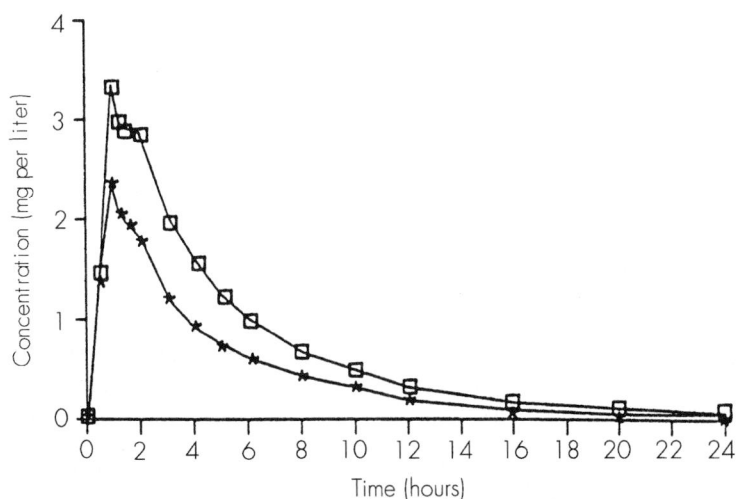

Fig. II.5.
Mean serum ciprofloxin concentrations following single oral doses of 500 mg (*) and 750 mg (□). (From Lettieri et al., 1992, with permission.)

1986a; Israel *et al.*, 1993). Johnson *et al.* (1990) noted a reduction in absorption of oral ciprofloxacin in six patients studied after chemotherapy for hematological malignancies. Mean maximum serum concentration fell from 3.7 μg per ml pre-chemotherapy to 2.0 μg per ml 13 days after chemotherapy in patients treated with 500 mg of oral ciprofloxacin twice-daily. Considerable variability in serum concentrations were noted. Such a reduction in serum concentrations may have clinical implications when treating serious Gram-negative infections in this patient group, and dosage adjustment may need consideration.

Ciprofloxacin is adequately absorbed in patients with diabetic gastroparesis (Marangos *et al.*, 1995). However, the enteric absorption of ciprofloxacin during the immediate postoperative period after major abdominal surgery is erratic, and adequate serum concentrations cannot be assumed (Cohn *et al.*, 1995).

Pregnant women (19–25 weeks gestation) given three doses of 750 mg oral ciprofloxacin have mean serum concentrations of 2.06, 1.06, 0.12 and 0.02 μg per ml, 2, 4, 12, and 24 h after a dose, respectively (Giamarellou *et al.*, 1989). These concentrations are lower than those expected in comparable non-pregnant females – a potentially important consideration when treating nosocomial, or other sepsis in pregnancy.

In children, Peltola *et al.* (1992) found that a single-dose of 15 mg per kg of ciprofloxacin produced mean maximum serum concentrations of 2.1–3.3 μg per ml after a mean of 1–1.2 h in infants 5–14 weeks of age and young children 1–5 years of age. Notably, however, the elimination half-life of ciprofloxacin was significantly (p < 0.001) longer in infants (2.7 ± 0.3 h) than in children (1.3 ± 0.5 hours).

Ball *et al.* (1986) found higher serum levels in elderly subjects associated with an increase in the AUC (p. 998); after an oral 100-mg dose, the peak serum levels in young volunteers and elderly patients at 1–2 h were 0.34 and 0.86 μg per ml, respectively. Other authors also found the peak serum concentration of ciprofloxacin in elderly patients to be up to twice that noted in healthy young volunteers, and the AUC to also be higher in the elderly (Bayer *et al.*, 1987; Hirata *et al.*, 1989; Naber *et al.*, 1989). Among pharmacokinetic studies of elderly patients given 100 mg, 250 mg, 500 mg, 750 mg ciprofloxacin orally, the maximum serum concentrations have been 0.83, 1.47–1.7, 3.24 and 5.87–7.6 μg per ml, respectively, 1.1–1.9 h post-dose. The half-life of oral ciprofloxacin in these patients is 3.5–6.8 h (Ball *et al.*, 1986, LeBel *et al.*, 1986a; Bayer *et al.*, 1987, Guay *et al.*, 1987; Hirata *et al.*, 1989; Nilsson-Ehle and Ljungberg, 1989). Hirata *et al.* (1989) found that factors relating to age and decreasing renal function were more important in determining alterations in the pharmacokinetics of ciprofloxacin in the elderly, than the infectious disease under therapy. Co-administration of either rifampicin or clindamycin with ciprofloxacin does not alter the pharmacokinetic parameters of oral ciprofloxacin in the elderly compared with ciprofloxacin given alone in this group (Chandler *et al.*, 1990; Weinstein *et al.*, 1991).

In patients with cystic fibrosis given oral doses of 500, 750 or 1000 mg of ciprofloxacin, the peak serum concentration and time to peak concentrations are similar to in healthy volunteers (e.g. 2.84 μg per ml [500 mg] and 4.0 μg per ml [750 mg] after 1.55–1.8 h) (LeBel *et al.*, 1986b). However ciprofloxacin elimination may be faster and therefore its half-life shorter, such that an increase in dosage in some patients may be required (p. 998) (Goldfarb *et al.*, 1986; LeBel *et al.*, 1986b; Davis *et al.*, 1987; Pedersen *et al.*, 1987; Stutman *et al.*, 1987; Reed *et al.*, 1988).

Oral administration of a single-dose of 500 mg or 750 mg of ciprofloxacin in patients with renal failure results in peak serum concentrations of 0.81–4.07 (usually 2–2.5) μg per ml following 500 mg and 2.97–4.50 μg per ml post-750 mg, after about 1.5 h – the higher concentrations tend to be associated with lower levels of renal function (Bindschedler *et al.*, 1988; Ebert *et al.*, 1988; Plaisance *et al.*, 1990). Overall bioavailability is essentially unchanged in patients with renal failure compared with those with normal renal function (63.4% versus 69%) (Plaisance *et al.*, 1990). With worsening renal function the AUC approximately doubles, the renal clearance falls to at least one quarter, and elimination half-life is prolonged by about 1.7 times (Gasser *et al.*, 1987a; Ebert *et al.*, 1988). Dosage adjustments for patients with creatinine clearance <20 ml per min have been discussed earlier (p. 996).

Mild and moderate hepatic cirrhosis does not affect ciprofloxacin kinetics (Montay and Gaillot, 1990). However, Esposito *et al.* (1989) found that, compared with mild cirrhosis, severe cirrhosis was associated with a small increase in maximum concentration from 2.03 to 2.74 μg per ml with a prolongation in half-life from 5.18 to 7.0 h and an AUC of 10.9 to 17.7 μg per ml per h after a single 500-mg oral dose. Similarly, Frost *et al.* (1989b) found little difference in ciprofloxacin kinetics between patients with biopsy-proven cirrhosis and normal controls after a single 750-mg oral dose.

2 Intravenous administration

Dose-ranging studies from 25–200 mg reveal a linear increase in the AUC. The terminal elimination half-life is 4–5 h in normal subjects with a total serum clearance of 22.5–25.2 liters per h per 1.73m^2 in studies administering doses of 100–200 mg (Drusano, 1987; Drusano et al., 1986a). Intravenous administration of 200 mg ciprofloxacin by constant-rate infusion over 30 min results in peak serum concentrations of $3.80 \pm 0.62\,\mu\text{g}$ per ml at the end of the infusion, with levels of 0.96, 0.48 and $0.13\,\mu\text{g}$ per ml, 1, 4 and 12 h after infusion, respectively (Drusano et al., 1986a; Drusano, 1987). Under the same circumstances a 100-mg dose resulted in serum concentrations of 2.28, 0.50 and $0.07\,\mu\text{g}$ per ml at the end of the infusion and 1 and 12 h after infusion, respectively (Drusano et al., 1986a). Doses greater than 200 mg may be associated with some non-linearity in serum concentration-time profiles (Drusano et al., 1986a).

With doses of 100–200 mg, the serum levels of drug over 12 h exceed the MIC for 90% of E. coli, Klebsiella, Enterobacter, Serratia and Proteus spp., but fall below the MICs for Ps. aeruginosa and Staph. aureus after 2–4 h (Gonzalez et al.; 1985). Other authors have found similar results in studies of 50, 100, 200 and 250 mg doses of i.v. ciprofloxacin (Wise et al., 1984; Gonzalez et al.; 1985; Höffken et al., 1985b; Dudley et al., 1987; Ljungberg and Nillsson-Ehle, 1988; Lode et al., 1988). The serum concentrations of ciprofloxacin after 300 and 400 mg i.v. are shown in Fig. II.6.

A number of authors have examined the pharmacokinetics of 400 mg ciprofloxacin i.v. and found that 400 mg i.v. thrice-daily produces a similar serum AUC to 750 mg orally twice-daily (Shah et al., 1994). Peak serum concentrations after 400 mg i.v. are similar to those obtained after 750 mg oral ciprofloxacin after both single and multiple dosing. At steady-state, ciprofloxacin 400 mg i.v. thrice-daily may be considered therapeutically equivalent to 750 mg orally twice-daily (see Fig. II.7) (Echols, 1993; Shah et al., 1994). The peak serum concentration of ciprofloxacin immediately after a 1 h infusion of 400 mg is $3.42 \pm 0.80\,\mu\text{g}$ per ml and $4.07 \pm 0.88\,\mu\text{g}$ per ml on day 1 and day 4, respectively; with a total serum clearance of 862 ± 188 and 649 ± 166 ml per min, respectively (Shah et al., 1994). Absolute bioavailability is 80% and is not affected by renal insufficiency (Plaisance et al., 1990; Shah et al., 1994).

Lettieri et al. (1992) described similar results in terms of maximum serum concentrations after 400 mg i.v. over 1 h versus 750 mg orally, but found that 400 mg i.v. was more equivalent to 500 mg orally with respect to AUC. After a 1 h infusion of 300 mg or 400 mg, Lettieri et al. (1992) found the maximum serum concentrations to be 3.2 ± 0.7 and $4.0 \pm 0.6\,\mu\text{g}$ per ml, respectively; with the half-life of ciprofloxacin to be approximately 4.5 h.

Catchpole et al. (1994) found results that differed from those of Shah et al. (1994) in that 400 mg i.v. ciprofloxacin compared with 750 mg oral ciprofloxacin, produced higher serum concentrations (6.7 versus $3.9\,\mu\text{g}$ per ml) but lower AUC (14.2 versus $19.2\,\mu\text{g}$ per ml per h). However, pharmacokinetic data from inflammatory blister fluid suggests equivalence between these two dosing regimens. Regardless of these differences of opinion, the finding by Echols et al. (1994) that both ciprofloxacin 500 mg orally and 400 mg i.v. have nearly equivalent serum bactericidal activity (SBA) against E. coli, Kl. pneumoniae, E. aerogenes, Ps. aeruginosa, Acinetobacter anitratus, H. influenzae, Staph. aureus and Strep. pneumoniae is of interest. However, both regimens have only modest serum bacteriacidal activity against Ps. aeruginosa,

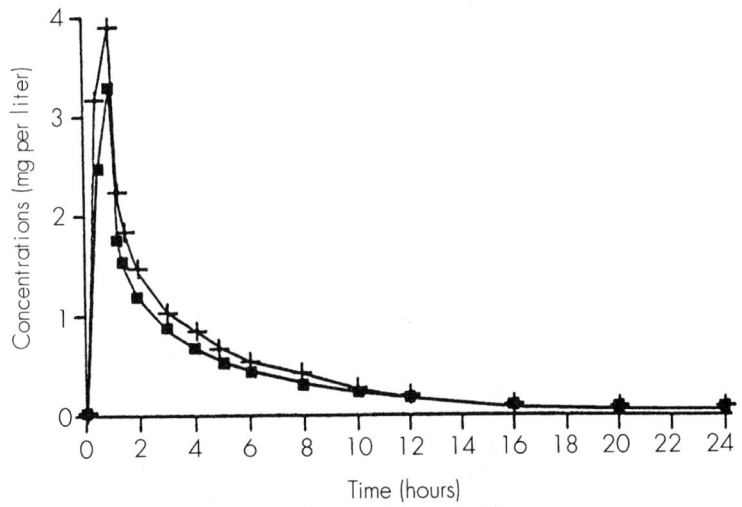

Fig. II.6.

Mean serum ciprofloxacin concentrations following single i.v. doses of 300 mg (■) and 400 mg (+). The duration of infusion was 1 h. (From Lettieri et al., 1992, with permission.)

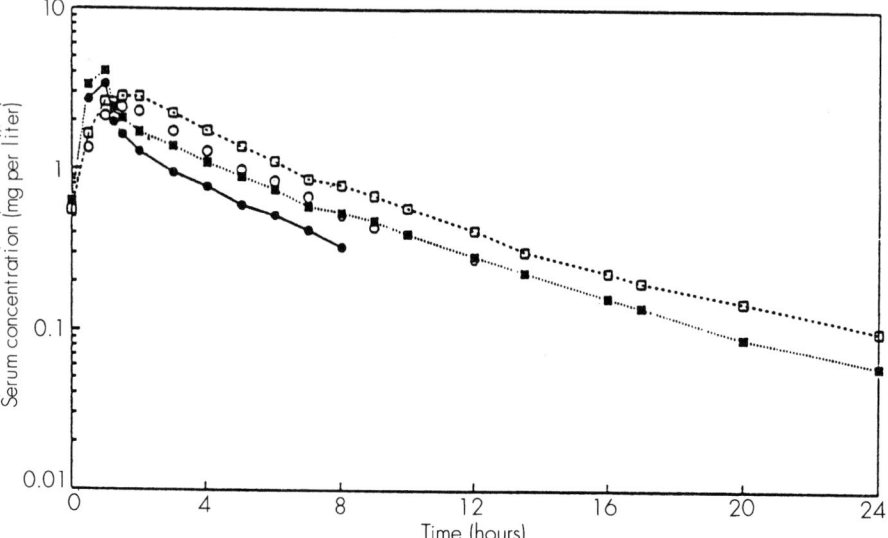

Fig. II.7.

Mean serum concentrations of ciprofloxacin following 400 mg i.v. three times daily (after first dose) (■, after last dose (■) or 750 mg po twice-daily (after first dose (○), after last dose (□), for 4 days. (From Shah *et al.*, 1994, with permission.)

A. anitratus and *Staph. aureus* at peak concentrations, and no activity 8 and 12 h after dosing. Neither regimen exhibits serum bacteriacidal activity against *Strep. pneumoniae*. Other authors have similar concerns regarding the levels achieved with 200 mg i.v. ciprofloxacin for the treatment of anything other than infections caused by Enterobacteriaceae; with much higher doses such as 400 mg i.v. twice- or thrice-daily, being potentially required for the treatment of *Ps. aeruginosa* infections (Dudley *et al.*, 1987; Standiford *et al.*, 1987; Dan *et al.*, 1994). Dan *et al.* (1994) found the serum concentrations achieved even with 400 mg i.v. to result in poor activity against *A. calcoaceticus* var *anitratus* and *Staph. aureus*.

Drusano (1987) studied the pharmacokinetics of ciprofloxacin in patients with various degrees of renal failure given 200 mg i.v. ciprofloxacin. Serum clearances decreased from 26.8 ± 5.7 liters per h per 1.73 m² in normal patients to 15.4 ± 4.3 liters per h per 1.73m² in anephric patients with the mean half-life increasing from 4.3 ± 0.8 h to 8.6 ± 3.3 h, respectively. Regardless of a patient's renal function, serum concentrations at the end of a 200 mg i.v. infusion are similar, varying between 4.1 and 6.3 μg per ml. By 12 h post-infusion, serum concentrations vary from 0.11 μg per ml (normal renal function) to 0.37 μg per ml (severe renal failure). Among the anephric patients there was little variation in serum clearance, but there was very wide variation in terminal elimination half-life: 3.9–13.5 h. It is on the basis of these findings that a 50% reduction in dosage is recommended when renal function declines below 20–30 ml per min (p. 996)

Pharmacokinetics of intravenous ciprofloxacin, metronidazole and clindamycin are not altered when ciprofloxacin is given in combination with each of these agents (Deppermann *et al.*, 1989; Boeckh *et al.*, 1990).

Excretion

Fluoroquinolones vary in their predominant clearance pathways: ofloxacin, temafloxacin and lomefloxacin are predominantly renally cleared; pefloxacin predominantly undergoes hepatic clearance, while drugs which are cleared by a combination of renal and hepatic mechanisms include ciprofloxacin, norfloxacin, enoxacin, fleroxacin and rufloxacin (Karabalut and Drusano, 1993). About one-third to one-half of the serum clearance of ciprofloxacin is by non-renal mechanisms (Lode *et al.*, 1990a; Karabalut and Drusano, 1993).

1 Urine

Ciprofloxacin is primarily (50–75%) excreted unchanged by the kidneys in healthy volunteers. Renal excretion exceeds the creatinine clearance due to significant proximal tubular secretion (Webb *et al.*, 1986; Drusano *et al.*, 1987). Such tubular secretion decreases in the setting of renal failure when renal clearance correlates better with creatinine clearance (Wise *et al.*, 1984; Richer and LeBel, 1993). The percentage urinary recovery of ciprofloxacin in healthy volunteers is slightly higher after i.v. than oral administration (51–57% versus 40–47%, respectively), with more than half of the recovered drug excreted in the first 4 h (Catchpole *et al.*, 1994). By 12–24 h after a single-dose of 400 mg i.v. or 750 mg oral ciprofloxacin, the mean urinary concentration is >26 μg per ml (Catchpole et al., 1994). Parry et al. (1988) identified urinary concentrations of ciprofloxacin of 387 ± 434, 308 ± 197, 52 ± 31 and 20 ± 19 μg per ml, 2, 4, 12 and 24 h, respectively, after a single i.v. dose of 200 mg of ciprofloxacin in six patients. Probenecid blocks proximal tubular excretion and is associated with a reduction in renal clearance of ciprofloxacin by 46% (Wingender et al., 1984).

As might be expected, urinary concentrations of ciprofloxacin taken at later times after administration are somewhat lower. Ciprofloxacin 250 mg orally twice-daily is associated with urine concentrations 6–12 h post-dose of 45 ± 25 to 69 ± 45 μg per ml (Aronoff et al., 1984), while a single-dose of 500 mg of ciprofloxacin results in urine concentrations of 8 μg per ml after 24 h (Davis et al., 1985).

2 Bile

Biliary concentrations of ciprofloxacin are generally 4- to 8-fold greater than simultaneous serum concentrations. Parry et al. (1988) examined the biliary excretion and metabolism of ciprofloxacin in 19 patients undergoing routine cholecystectomy and in six with indwelling biliary drainage catheters. Ciprofloxacin concentrations in common duct bile, gallbladder bile and gallbladder wall were 5.69 ± 4.8 μg per ml, 5.43 ± 3.34 μg per ml and 2.52 ± 1.30 mg per g, respectively, after a single intravenous dose of 200 mg ciprofloxacin given 2.5–3 h prior to cholecystectomy. All these concentrations were at least 4-fold greater than simultaneous serum concentrations. There was an 8-fold increase in gallbladder bile concentrations in patients with normal serum bilirubin who were treated with multiple preoperative doses, although only a modest increase in serum, common bile duct bile and gallbladder wall concentrations were noted. In only two patients were the common bile duct bile and gallbladder bile concentrations less than the peak serum concentrations (0.33–0.68 μg per ml) – both patients had common bile duct obstruction with bilirubin levels of 7 and 12 mg per dl. Nevertheless, these lower concentrations still exceeded the MIC$_{90}$ of most Enterobacteriaceae likely to be pathogens in this situation. Patients with elevated serum bilirubins have lower and delayed peak ciprofloxacin concentrations in common duct bile. The 24 h biliary recovery of ciprofloxacin is only 0.41% of the administered dose. Patients with normal bilirubin values achieve concentrations of 1.95–10.9 and 3.0–16.7 μg per ml in gallbladder bile and common duct bile, respectively. Other authors have found similar results. In patients given oral ciprofloxacin 500 mg 1 h before surgery the serum and common bile duct concentrations are 0.5 and 6.1 μg per ml, respectively, and when this dose is given 2–4 h before operation, the values are 2.5 and 20.2 μg per ml, respectively (Strachan and Thom, 1984). Ciprofloxacin concentrations have been estimated in bile taken by T-tube drainage from patients who have had a cholecystectomy after receiving a single 500-mg dose. Mean peak biliary levels at 4.1 h were 16.0–21.2 μg per ml depending on the assay method used (Brogard et al., 1985). Similarly, Sörgel and Kinzig (1993) have reported biliary concentrations of 16 μg per ml (bile:plasma ratio of 8) after a single oral dose of 500-mg ciprofloxacin.

The concentrations of ciprofloxacin metabolites in common duct bile and gallbladder bile are 4-fold greater than ciprofloxacin concentrations (total metabolites: 21.0 μg per ml and 23.3 μg per ml, respectively). Of these metabolites 83–90% are sulfo ciprofloxacin, the principal fecal metabolite which has less than 5% of the antibacterial activity of ciprofloxacin.

Thus, ciprofloxacin readily achieves therapeutic levels in bile in the presence of a patent or partially obstructed biliary tree – characteristics that no doubt contribute to the efficacy of the drug in clearing *Salmonella* carriage (p. 1018).

3 Inactivation in body

At least four microbiologically active metabolites of ciprofloxacin have been identified and about 15% of an administered dose can be recovered from urine in the form of metabolites and 30–45% as intact ciprofloxacin (Gonzalez et al., 1984). Three of these metabolites have limited microbiological activity of half to one-tenth that of the parent compound (Gonzalez et al., 1985; Karabalut and Drusano, 1993). An increased urinary recovery after repeated doses of ciprofloxacin suggests that there may be some induction of the drug's metabolism with repeated doses (Ledergerber et al., 1985). Ciprofloxacin is metabolized in the liver by alteration to the piperazine side-chain of the ciprofloxacin molecule, with less than 20% of either an i.v. or orally administered dose recoverable as metabolites from urine and feces (Parry et al., 1988; Karabalut and Drusano, 1993). Of metabolites found in bile, Parry et al. (1988) found 83% was sulfo-ciprofloxacin (M2) 13% oxociprofloxacin (M3) and 2% was desethylene-ciprofloxacin (M1).

Phillips *et al.* (1990) demonstrated a 20% reduction in ciprofloxacin microbiologic activity after exposure to ultraviolet A due to photodegradation. Thus, minimal natural sunburn due to this waveband (e.g. naturally or from tanning sunbeds) may be accompanied by a 20% reduction in cutaneous levels of ciprofloxacin. However, given the continuous ciprofloxacin turnover via routine circulation in the skin, the clinical impact of this mechanism of inactivation is likely to be very small, except perhaps were ciprofloxacin is being used to treat skin and soft tissue infections in a sun-exposed area.

4 Feces

A substantial amount of ciprofloxacin (11–30%) is present in the gut after oral administration; on day 7 after a dosage of 500 mg every 12h, a mean value of 891 μg per g is detected in the feces (Brumfitt *et al.*, 1984; Karabalut and Drusano, 1993). Similarly, about 15% of an i.v. dose of ciprofloxacin is recovered in the stool (Lode *et al.*, 1990a). Rohwedder *et al.* (1990) administered 200 mg i.v. ciprofloxacin to five healthy volunteers and five patients with severe renal failure (creatinine clearance 8–16 ml per min) and collected feces for the subsequent 7 days. Among normal volunteers 11.4 ± 2.6% of the dose was recovered, while among the renal failure group, 37.2 ± 12.5% was recovered. Since biliary excretion of ciprofloxacin is less than 1% of administered dose, this mechanism contributes little to the fecal excretion of ciprofloxacin (Parry *et al.*, 1988). The transfer of ciprofloxacin into feces is considered to be by direct transintestinal elimination. This extrarenal elimination is an important factor in ciprofloxacin excretion, especially in severe renal failure. Similarly, Sörgel *et al.* (1989), using a charcoal model for investigation of healthy volunteers, predicted that about 11% of i.v. administered ciprofloxacin was secreted into the gut lumen. Pecquet *et al.* (1990), administered a single oral dose of 750 mg ciprofloxacin to healthy volunteers and found fecal concentrations exceeded 3 mg per g feces and remained generally greater than 0.5 mg per g for at least 4 days. Other authors, however, have noted some variability in fecal concentrations. Brismar *et al.* (1990) gave patients two doses of 750 mg ciprofloxacin orally twice-daily prior to elective colorectal surgery, then a 400-mg i.v. dose at induction of anesthesia and another 400-mg i.v. dose 12h later. Ciprofloxacin concentrations in the colonic mucosa were 2.7–37.8 μg per g of tissue and in the fecal specimens ranged from less than 0.1 to 858 μg per g of feces; although 10 of 21 specimens had concentrations greater than 90 μg per g. This variability is potentially related to the limited fecal sampling method used in this study.

Rubinstein *et al.* (1994, 1995), using a rat model, have shown that approximately 7% of ciprofloxacin is eliminated by a transepithelial process in the small intestine (mostly jejunum) while in the rabbit about 1% is eliminated, mostly in the ileum (Ramon *et al.*, 1994). In rats, ciprofloxacin is neither reabsorbed nor excreted distal to the ileocecal valve, hence the usual concentration process occurs in the large intestine in which reabsorption of water results in very high fecal concentrations of ciprofloxacin (Rubinstein *et al.*, 1994).

Distribution of the Drug in Body

Similar to all fluoroquinolones, ciprofloxacin penetrates well into tissues, with a large volume of distribution which far exceeds the extracellular volume (Wise *et al.*, 1984; Höffken *et al.*, 1985b; Karabalut and Drusano, 1993). Penetration into experimental blister fluid, both inflammatory and non-inflammatory, is similar to, or greater than serum (Crump *et al.*, 1983; Wise *et al.*, 1984; LeBel *et al.*, 1986c). In the non-inflammatory suction blister model, LeBel *et al.* (1986c) compared the penetration of the drug after a single ciprofloxacin dose of 500 mg and after 500 mg thrice-daily for 13 doses. After single and multiple doses ciprofloxacin appeared rapidly in blister fluid (although delayed compared with serum levels) and achieved 88.8 and 84.7% penetration (AUC ratio for blister fluid to serum) and 79.5 and 57.3% penetration based on the maximum concentration of ciprofloxacin, respectively. The mean maximum blister fluid concentrations were 1.75–1.87 μg per ml, 2.3–2.5 h after dosing. Multiple dosing resulted in an increase in steady-state concentration of ciprofloxacin in blister fluid of 0.97 ± 0.57 μg per ml 8 h post-dose. The half-life in blister fluid was similar to that in serum. Lubowski *et al.* (1992) reported similar penetration for both ciprofloxacin and fleroxacin. Wise and Donovan (1987) investigated inflammatory blister fluid under similar dosing conditions and found, due to the longer half-life of ciprofloxacin in inflammatory fluid, ciprofloxacin penetration to be 117%, and after 100 mg i.v. ciprofloxacin penetration was 121%.

Ciprofloxacin exhibits excellent penetration into endothelial and epithelial cell layers with good intracellular antibacterial activity *in vitro* (Chadwick and Mellersh, 1987; Darouiche and Hamill, 1994). Similarly, *in vitro* and *in vivo* studies show marked concentration of ciprofloxacin in human neutrophils with good intracellular antibiotic activity (Easmon and Crane, 1985; Van der Auwera *et al.*, 1988; Garraffo *et al.*, 1991; Yancey *et al.*, 1991; Garcia *et al.*, 1992; Perea *et al.*, 1992). *In vivo* studies by Garraffo *et al.* (1991) demonstrate marked intracellular penetration of ciprofloxacin into human neutrophils with the ratio of intracellular:serum drug concentrations of 3.7, 5.7 and 20, after 1.5 h (time of maximum serum concentration), 12 h and 24 h, respectively, post-dose. Intracellular half-life of ciprofloxacin was prolonged compared with that in serum (6.2 h versus 3.7 h, respectively) (Garraffo *et al.*, 1991).

Penetration into lymphatic fluid, based on comparing the AUC in lymph to that in serum, is about 70% (Bergan *et al.*, 1986a, 1990).

Concentrations reached in saliva range from 30% to 45% of the peak levels in serum (Gonzalez *et al.*, 1984). LeBel *et al.* (1986c) found peak concentrations of ciprofloxacin in saliva of 1.42 ± 0.97 μg per ml after an initial 500 mg oral dose and 1.52 ± 0.86 μg per ml after multiple doses. After 750 mg oral ciprofloxacin twice-daily, steady-state salivary and nasal secretion concentrations are 1.29 ± 1.0 and approximately 1.84 ± 0.91 μg per ml, respectively (Piercy *et al.*, 1989b). Similarly, Darouiche *et al.* (1990), after giving ciprofloxacin 750 mg orally twice-daily for 2 days, found ciprofloxacin concentrations in saliva and nasal secretions to be 1.27 ± 0.31 and 0.27 ± 0.04 μg per ml, respectively, 2 h post-dose and 0.08 and 0.04 μg per ml, respectively, 8 h post-dose. Ciprofloxacin concentrations in nasal secretions far exceed the MIC_{90} for *H. influenzae* and meningococci, but are below the MIC_{90} for methicillin-resistant *Staph. aureus* (p. 984).

Penetration of ciprofloxacin into sputum may be affected by a number of unpredictable factors, hence pulmonary penetration is better measured by analysis of pulmonary components such as bronchial secretions, bronchial mucosa and alveolar macrophages (Bergogne-Bérézin *et al.*, 1986; Winter and Sweeney, 1991). Ciprofloxacin penetrates well into bronchial secretions after i.v. administration with mean peak concentrations of 0.84 ± 0.58 and 1.16 ± 0.86 μg per ml, 1–1.4 h after single and multiple doses of 1.5 mg per kg of ciprofloxacin respectively. The rate of clearance is similar to in serum (Berré *et al.*, 1988). In an assessment of mechanically ventilated patients with nosocomial bronchopneumonia treated with 200 mg i.v. ciprofloxacin 12-hourly for 2 days, Saux *et al.* (1994) found peak and trough concentrations in bronchial secretions to be 0.95 ± 0.51 and 0.21 ± 0.12 μg per ml, respectively. Penetration into bronchial secretions based on a comparison of peak concentrations and AUC was 32% and 55–66%, respectively. This dose resulted in 12 h concentrations in bronchial secretions below the MIC_{90} for the main pathogens responsible for nosocomially-acquired pneumonia. Thus the authors recommended a dose of greater than 200 mg i.v., or more frequent dosing in this clinical setting. Bronchial penetration (AUC bronchial secretions/AUC serum) of oral ciprofloxacin is 46–79% (Davies *et al.*, 1986; Hoogkamp-Korstanje and Klein, 1986; Smith *et al.*, 1986b). Other authors have found ciprofloxacin concentrations in epithelial lining fluid obtained at bronchoscopy of 1.85–2.1 times the serum concentration after 250 mg oral ciprofloxacin twice-daily (Baldwin *et al.*, 1993; Wise *et al.*, 1991). Wise *et al.* (1991) found ciprofloxacin concentrations in alveolar macrophages to be 14- to 18-fold those in serum after 250 mg oral ciprofloxacin given twice-daily.

Ciprofloxacin is concentrated in bronchial mucosa, although the extent of concentration appears to vary according to whether ciprofloxacin levels are measured by high-performance liquid chromotography (HPLC) or microbiological assay – the reason for this difference is not completely understood. Reid *et al.* (1989) found the bronchial mucosa:serum concentration ratios measured by HPLC after single oral doses of ciprofloxacin 250 mg and 750 mg and 200 mg i.v. were 4.97, 2.75 and 6.24, respectively, with mean bronchial tissue concentrations of 2.02, 4.86 and 4.05 μg per g, 3.4, 3.4 and 0.9 h, respectively, after dosing. Similarly, Fabre *et al.* (1991) found concentrations of ciprofloxacin in bronchial mucosa (measured by HPLC) reached 21.6 ± 5.63 μg per g, 2 h after a 30-min infusion of 200 mg ciprofloxacin given twice-daily for 5 days. The mean tissue:plasma concentration ratio was 16.9 ± 5.4. Other authors who have measured ciprofloxacin concentration by microbiologic assay identified similar but less dramatic findings. Winter and Sweeney (1991) for example, found the penetration of ciprofloxacin into bronchial mucosa to be a mean of 162% (range 140–200%). Wise *et al.* (1991) reported similar results. Scaglione *et al.* (1995) noted mean peak concentrations of ciprofloxacin in lung tissue to be 4.2 μg per g, 2 h after the second of two doses of ciprofloxacin 500 mg given 12 h apart.

Ciprofloxacin penetrates well into uninfected pleural fluid. In postoperative patients with continuous pleural drainage who were treated with 1.5 mg per kg i.v. ciprofloxacin thrice-daily, the peak concentrations in pleural fluid 1.5 h after the first and third injections were 0.52 and 0.77 μg per ml and concentrations after 8 h were 0.19 and 0.39 μg per ml, respectively. At steady-state after three doses, the ratio of mean concentration in pleural fluid:serum was 77% after 1 h and 122% after 8 h (Jacobs *et al.*, 1990). Hopf *et al.* (1988) found concentrations of ciprofloxacin in pleural fluid 12 h after 200 mg i.v. ciprofloxacin to be 1.1–1.8 times serum concentrations, depending on the number of doses given. Joseph *et al.* (1994) studied both i.v. and orally administered ciprofloxacin in patients with sterile pleural effusions and empyema. Steady-state ciprofloxacin concentrations in sterile pleural fluid after treatment with 750 mg twice-daily for 3 days of ciprofloxacin were 1.1–1.8 μg per ml with pleural fluid:serum ratio over 4 h of 30–90%. Comparable empyemic pleural fluid concentrations were higher (steady-state concentrations of 1.9–3.4 μg per ml) and pleural fluid:serum ratios of 1.0–2.0 over 5 h.

Fluoroquinolones vary considerably in terms of penetration into CSF, with pefloxacin penetrating best. However, ciprofloxacin achieves approximately 6–37% (generally ~15%) of peak serum concentrations in patients with meningitis and 5–10% of peak serum concentrations in patients without meningitis (Norrby, 1988; Tunkel and Scheld, 1993). Wolff *et al.* (1987) studied 23 patients with bacterial meningitis due to a variety of pathogens who, in addition to treatment with routine regimens, received 200 mg ciprofloxacin i.v. every 12 h for 3 doses between days 2 and 4 of therapy (i.e. early, but not acutely in the disease) and between days 10 and 20 (i.e. at time of cure). Mean CSF concentrations measured 1–6 h after the third dose in each time period were 0.35–0.56 μg per ml (range 0.11–1.20 μg per ml) early in the disease and 0.15–0.27 μg per ml (range 0.11–0.5 μg per ml) at the time of cure (day 10–14). The percentage in the CSF of the peak plasma concentrations were 6.5–16% during the acute stage and 4.5–9.9% during the late stage of the disease. Peak ciprofloxacin concentrations in ventricular fluid measured in four patients occurred between 2 and 4 h after the third dose. Overall CSF concentrations of ciprofloxacin exceeded the MICs for many strains responsible for purulent meningitis, but were insufficient to reliably inhibit *Strep. pneumoniae* or unusual pathogens in this setting such as *Ps. aeruginosa*. Gogos *et al.* (1991) found similar results when treating with two doses of 200 mg i.v. ciprofloxacin, 12-hourly, although their methodology produced less precise data. However these authors also studied patients with non-inflamed meninges where this dosing regimen resulted in CSF concentrations of 0.038–0.178 μg per ml at various times during the 10 h after the second dose. Nau *et al.* (1990) found similar results in patients with non-inflamed meninges. Oral ciprofloxacin (500 mg) achieves reasonably comparable CSF concentrations to 200 mg i.v. ciprofloxacin in both non-inflamed (about 10% penetration) and inflamed meninges (Valainis *et al.*, 1986; Kitzes-Cohen *et al.*, 1988). Overall, therefore, ciprofloxacin penetration in patients with inflamed meninges is lower than that achieved with some sulfonamides and chloramphenicol, but similar or higher than that of penicillin, cephalosporins and aminogylcosides (Sanford *et al.*, 1995).

Ciprofloxacin achieves up to 95% penetration into non-inflammatory peritoneal fluid (Wise and Donovan, 1987). In eight patients with ascites but normal renal function (four malignant; four associated with cardiac failure), Dan *et al.* (1992) found that a single oral dose of 750 mg ciprofloxacin resulted in a mean maximum concentration of 2.6 ± 0.6 μg per ml in ascitic fluid with penetration (based on the ratio of AUC in ascites:AUC serum) of 69 ± 18% – i.e. concentrations well above the MIC of most Enterobacteriaceae.

In the setting of CAPD, oral ciprofloxacin achieves reasonable dialysate penetration with peak concentrations of 1.8–4.5 μg per ml after four doses of 750 mg twice-daily. However, in patients taking oral phosphate-binding aluminum-based antacids, dialysate concentrations were only 8–33% of these values. Importantly, long-dwell exchanges (e.g. 8 h) appear to be necessary to achieve these reasonable dialysate concentrations. The clearance of ciprofloxacin by CAPD is only 2% of the total body clearance (Golper *et al.*, 1987). The antibacterial activity of ciprofloxacin may be reduced in dialysate compared with Isosensitest ('Oxoid') broth, however this is not a cause of treatment failure (Ludlam *et al.*, 1992). In a study of ten CAPD patients with and without active peritonitis, given ciprofloxacin 250 mg four-times daily for 2 days, no difference in ciprofloxacin dialysate kinetics were noted in patients with and without peritonitis. Between patients, dialysate concentrations of ciprofloxacin at the time of bag changes were reasonably large, but intra-patient variability was small. The mean peak dialysate concentration was 2.17 ± 1.63 μg per ml (range 0.66–6.17 μg per ml) using four exchanges per day (Fleming *et al.*, 1987). Although a 50% reduction in dosage is usually recommended in the setting of CAPD (p. 996), a dialysate concentration of ciprofloxacin above 2 μg per ml may be required for some pathogens – in this setting oral doses of greater than 1g per day may be necessary. When mixed in 1.5% and 4.25% dextrose peritoneal dialysate, ciprofloxacin 25 mg per liter is stable for 7 days at 25°C and for 48 h at 37°C (Kane *et al.*, 1994). Intraperitoneal ciprofloxacin (50 mg per liter of dialysate) is effective in the treatment of CAPD peritonitis (Ludlam *et al.*, 1990a,b; p. 1030).

Ciprofloxacin penetrates well into the pancreas, including in the setting of chronic pancreatitis and pancreatic carcinoma (Büchler *et al.*, 1992; Brattström *et al.*, 1988; Isenmann *et al.*, 1994).

The median peak pancreatic tissue concentrations after a single 200-mg i.v. dose of ciprofloxacin is 0.9 mg per kg (range 0.2–0.21 mg per kg) (Büchler *et al.*, 1992). Similar concentrations are likely to be achievable in acute pancreatitis. The mean peak concentration of ciprofloxacin in human allograft pancreatic juice 4 h after a single 500-mg oral dose of ciprofloxacin is 0.5 μg per ml – representing 36% penetration, based on concentration ratios. Ofloxacin achieves higher penetration (92%) and concentrations (2.7 μg per ml) in this setting (Brattström *et al.*, 1988). In patients undergoing gastrointestinal surgery, 200 mg i.v. ciprofloxacin achieves good concentrations in abdominal wall, fat, muscle, peritoneum and gut wall – namely 1.04, 1.94, 1.59 and 3.39 mg per kg, respectively (Silverman *et al.*, 1986). After 400 mg i.v. ciprofloxacin, concentrations in intestinal mucosa are a mean of 11.9 ± 8.9 mg per kg (range: 2.7–37.8 mg per kg) – generally exceeding concentrations in serum (Brismar *et al.*, 1990).

Ciprofloxacin penetrates well into renal cyst fluid in patients with end-stage or advanced polycystic kidney disease with mean ciprofloxacin concentrations of 12.7 μg per ml after 750 mg oral ciprofloxacin twice-daily for 1–14 days (Elzinga *et al.*, 1988).

Penetration of fluoroquinolones into prostate fluid and tissue, and seminal fluid is excellent, making these agents the drugs of choice for treating infections due to susceptible pathogens in these difficult sites (p. 1015). Oral ciprofloxacin 500 mg given 2–3 h before prostatectomy results in a mean prostatic tissue concentration of 3.05 μg per g at a time when the mean serum concentration is about 1.6 μg per ml (Boerema *et al.*, 1984; Hoogkamp-Korstanje *et al.*, 1984). Waldron *et al.* (1986) also found that oral ciprofloxacin produced therapeutic intraprostatic drug levels – often 0.93–2.3 times the corresponding serum concentrations. After 750 mg ciprofloxacin therapeutic prostate tissue concentrations are attainable for up to 9 h after the dose (Dan *et al.*, 1986). After 200 mg i.v. ciprofloxacin the median concentrations in prostatic tissue 1–2.5 h after the dose are 1.7–1.87 mg per kg (1.9–2.6 times the plasma concentration) (Naber, 1993). Seminal fluid concentrations 4 and 12 h after 200 mg of i.v. ciprofloxacin are 2.53 and 0.61–0.70 μg per ml, respectively (i.e. 5.8–9.4 times the corresponding serum concentration) (Naber, 1993).

Irrespective of the route of administration, ciprofloxacin concentrations in gynecologic tissues are 2- to 5-fold greater than the corresponding serum concentrations (Cho *et al.*, 1984; Dalhoff and Weuta, 1987). By 12 h after a 500 mg oral dose of ciprofloxacin, mean concentrations in ovary, uterus, endometrium, myometrium and fallopian tube are 0.28, 0.49, 0.23, 0.34 and 0.36 mg per kg, respectively (Dalhoff and Weuta, 1987).

Ciprofloxacin has excellent penetration into human heart tissue, including heart valves, myocardium and mediastinal fat. Mertes *et al.* (1990) examined tissue concentrations in patients treated with a single 400-mg i.v. dose of ciprofloxacin and in patients who received 750 mg orally twice-daily for 2 days, followed by a single 400-mg i.v. dose prior to cardiac surgery. Both regimens produced similar tissue concentrations, except that in the latter treatment group higher heart valve levels were achieved. After a single 400-mg i.v. dose of ciprofloxacin, peak myocardial concentrations of 31.6 ± 25.0 μg per g were achieved after 1 h, while peak concentrations in heart valves of 5.8 ± 3.2 μg per g occurred slightly later (1–3 h post-dose). In mediastinal fat the peak concentrations were lower (3.1 ± 3.8 μg per g) and occurred later (3–5 h). In all cases ciprofloxacin levels remained higher than the MICs for the commonly susceptible pathogens for at least 8 h. Pryka *et al.* (1993) noted little difference in the pharmacokinetics and distribution of i.v. ciprofloxacin during cardiopulmonary bypass surgery compared with these parameters before and after surgery.

Excellent bone concentrations of ciprofloxacin are achieved after both oral and i.v. administration. After an oral dose of 750 mg, peak concentrations of 1.4 ± 1 μg per g in bone are achieved in patients with osteomyelitis. After 1g dosing in patients without osteomyelitis, ciprofloxacin concentrations in bone are 1.6 ± 0.6 μg per g; while muscle concentrations are even higher (Fong *et al.*, 1986).

Licitra *et al.* (1987) noted excellent ciprofloxacin penetration into soft tissue in 22 patients (mean concentration 1.75-fold greater than that in serum) with soft tissue infections treated with 750 mg oral ciprofloxacin twice-daily. Mean concentrations in soft tissue from the margins of the infected areas 1 and 11 h after dosing were 3.3–4.0 and 1.26–1.89 μg per g, respectively. Aigner and Dalhoff (1986) also noted excellent penetration (1.8–3.3 times serum) into skin and muscle. Similarly, ciprofloxacin penetrates synovial fluid and tissue well with Bosseray *et al.* (1992) noting ciprofloxacin concentrations in these sites of 0.6–1.2 and 0.6–2.3 times, respectively, the plasma concentration.

High doses of ciprofloxacin are required to achieve adequate concentrations in aqueous humor. Sweeney *et al.* (1990) noted ciprofloxacin concentrations in aqueous humor of 2.8–12.1% of the corresponding serum concentrations in patients treated with a single-dose of either 1g or 1.5g of ciprofloxacin, 1–4 h before elective cataract removal. Aqueous humor concentrations exceeded 0.5 μg per ml, 2.5 h post-dose in both these treatment groups, but a further group treated with a single oral dose of 500 mg ciprofloxacin had levels insufficient to reliably inhibit *Ps. aeruginosa*. Higher aqueous humor concentrations are noted with repeated dosing (Sweeney *et al.*, 1990). In summarizing the literature, Barza (1993) found ciprofloxacin achieved peak concentrations in aqueous humor compared with serum concentrations of 6–33% (generally 10–20%) and 10–20% for vitreous humor. Topically applied 0.3% solutions of ciprofloxacin and norfloxacin (given as two drops 90 min and 30 min preoperatively) achieve mean concentrations in the aqueous humor of 0.057–0.072 μg per ml, although a number of patients have had undetectable concentrations. Similarly applied ofloxacin achieves concentrations of 0.34 μg per ml suggesting it to be superior for this form of administration (Donnenfeld *et al.*, 1994). Topical ciprofloxacin achieves reasonable penetration into corneal tissue (Price *et al.*, 1995).

Ciprofloxacin penetrates well into head and neck tissues with peak concentrations of 150–190%, 100–150% and 45% those of serum in tonsil tissue, sinus mucosa and saliva, respectively (Barza, 1988). Penetration into nasal secretions of 73–90%, based on AUC tissue:AUC serum, can be expected (Ullmann *et al.*, 1986; Barza, 1991) (p. 1005).

Mode of Action

Fluoroquinolones such as ciprofloxacin are similar to nalidixic acid in their mode of action (p. 971). Both GyrA and GyrB are targets for fluoroquinolones in which they bind with the DNA gyrase-DNA complex, rather than to DNA gyrase alone. Disrupting DNA gyrase function results in decreased introduction of negative supercoils in DNA and therefore an increase in subsequent DNA damage (Hooper and Wolfson, 1993b). Variations in the antibacterial potency of different fluoroquinolones have often, but not always, correlated with differences in inhibition of the appropriate DNA gyrase. Other factors such as cell permeability to fluoroquinolones affect drug potency (Domagala *et al.*, 1986; Wolfson *et al.*, 1987; p. 991). As noted earlier, fluoroquinolones inhibit plasma conjugation and encourage plasmid elimination from bacteria (p. 992).

Quinolones initially kill bacteria rapidly but for some bacteria their activity lessens *in vitro* when the viable cell count is about 10^4 below the initial inoculum, or in some circumstances when bacteria are in a stationary phase of growth. Thus, quinolone bactericidal activity, depending on the bacterial species, is cell cycle-specific, although this appears to be less so for ciprofloxacin and ofloxacin, at least against Gram-negative organisms (Eng *et al.*, 1991; Hooper and Wolfson, 1993b). Bacterial killing tends to increase in rate and magnitude with increasing quinolone concentrations, however, above a maximum of 30- to 60-fold above the MIC, the so called 'Eagle' effect may occur for some fluoroquinolones, with a reduction in killing similar to the effect seen in some bacterial strains with excess penicillin concentration (p. 9). Drugs such as chloramphenicol and rifampicin inhibit protein synthesis and are known to reduce bacterial killing by some quinolones, suggesting that some protein synthesis in addition to quinolone interference with DNA gyrase activity is necessary for cell death (Crumplin *et al.*, 1984; Deitz *et al.*, 1966). Interestingly, protein synthesis inhibitors such as rifampicin and chloramphenicol, while abolishing the bactericidal activity of nalidixic acid and norfloxacin have only partial effect on fluoroquinolones such as ciprofloxacin, pefloxacin, ofloxacin and lomefloxacin (Lewin and Amyes, 1990; Lewin *et al.*, 1989a; Smith, 1984). Thus these latter fluoroquinolones presumably possess other mechanisms of killing. In addition, anaerobic conditions inhibit fluoroquinolone killing, while oxygen reverses this effect (Lewin *et al.*, 1991).

Toxicity

Fluoroquinolones appear to be associated with relatively few side-effects, although a wide range of incidents have been reported (Radandt *et al.*, 1992; Matsuno *et al.*, 1995). Manufacturers' data suggest that the rate of all adverse events is up to 19% for oral and 29% for i.v. ciprofloxacin; with 7.1%, 8.6% and 3.4% regarded as probable, possible and remotely related reactions, respectively. Only 1.5–3.5% of patients have reactions sufficiently severe to require cessation of therapy (AHFS, 1995; Schacht *et al.*, 1989; Ball 1986; Smith 1987; Arcieri *et al.*, 1989; Rahm and Schacht 1989; Halkin 1988). Other authors have reported little difference in systemic toxicity between multiple dosing of either i.v. or oral administration of ciprofloxacin (Thorsteinsson *et al.*, 1989, 1990). In their review, Hooper and Wolfson (1993a) noted that among most trials comparing fluoroquinolones with non-quinolone agents, there were generally no differences in the rate of toxicity between fluoroquinolones and the other agents. While six trials reported a lower incidence of toxicity in the fluoroquinolone-treated group, seven studies reported a higher incidence of side-effects in this group. Thus, depending on variables such as treatment population, the fluoroquinolone under study, the dose used, the condition being treated, other co-morbidities and the comparison non-quinolone, some differences in toxicity rates may be encountered. Some fluoroquinolones, such as fleroxacin and temafloxacin, are associated with higher rates of toxicity (pp. 1104, 1144).

There is generally cross-allergy between various quinolones, hence newer fluoroquinolones are contraindicated in patients with a history of allergy to any fluoroquinolone, including old analogs such as nalidixic acid and cinoxacin. The frequency of adverse reactions for both i.v. and oral fluoroquinolones appears to increase with dose and duration of treatment, with generally no differences detected between single-dose regimens (Arcieri et al., 1989; Hooper and Wolfson 1989; Stahlmann 1990; Norrby and Pernet 1991; Bennish et al., 1992; Saginur et al., 1992). In particular, photosensitivity reactions appear to be associated with increasing dose (Stahlmann 1990). The most common adverse reactions reported to the manufacturer are gastrointestinal symptoms, central nervous system disturbance, injection site reactions, eosinophilia and abnormal liver function tests, with variable strength of the association between these symptoms and ciprofloxacin therapy.

1 Gastrointestinal side-effects

Nausea, vomiting, diarrhea, fever and abdominal discomfort have been reported in 2–15% of patients treated with ciprofloxacin (Ramirez et al., 1985; Scully et al., Rahm and Schacht 1989; Stahlmann, 1990; AHFS, 1995). These are generally transient and mild, but are more common with higher dose. In some cases, nausea and vomiting is due to theophylline toxicity associated with concomitant fluoroquinolone-theophylline administration (p. 1014). Other symptoms such as dry mouth, bad taste, dysphagia, painful oral mucosa, oral candidiasis, gastric irritation, ileus, flatulence, gastrointestinal bleeding, pancreatitis and intestinal perforation have all been reported by the manufacturer but are generally rare, occurring in less than 1% of patients (AHFS, 1995). Pseudomembranous colitis due to *Cl. difficile* has been associated with ciprofloxacin and other fluoroquinolones, although this is quite uncommon (Dan and Samra 1989; Bates *et al.*, 1990; Cain and O'Connor 1990; Hillman *et al.*, 1990; O'Keeffe and Tillotson 1990; Golledge *et al.*, 1992; Manzione 1992; McFarland *et al.*, 1995). Loo et al., (1985) noted an 11% incidence of minor abnormalities in liver function tests associated with oral ciprofloxacin, however manufacturers' data suggest an incidence of increased AST and ALT of only 2%, and elevated bilirubin and gamma GT in less than 1% or patients (AHFS, 1995). Severe hepatic failure has been associated with ciprofloxacin, norfloxacin and ofloxacin, but appears to be rare (<1 in 2.5 million). The mechanisms of such hepatitis is unclear, including whether it is due to an allergic hepatitis (Grassmick *et al.*, 1992; Fuchs *et al.*, 1994; Pfeiffer and Reiter 1994; Villeneuve *et al.*, 1995).

2 Neurotoxicity

Central nervous system toxicity associated with fluoroquinolones, including ciprofloxacin, has been reported in 0.9–7.4% of patients (Rahm and Schacht 1989; Christ, 1990). Most common symptoms include mild headache and dizziness, but insomnia, nightmares, somnolence, mood alteration (agitation, anxiety, depression), hallucinations, delirium, acute psychosis, unsteady gait/ataxia, paresthesia, impaired driving and depersonalization have all been reported by the manufacturer and others (Altés *et al.*, 1989; McCue and Zandt 1991; Gray *et al.*, 1994; AHFS, 1995; Mulhall and Bergmann, 1995). Similar to nalidixic acid, but probably less frequent in incidence, benign intracranial hypertension has been reported with ciprofloxacin (Winrow and Supramaniam, 1990) (p. 972). Worsening myesthenia gravis has been noted in a number of patients with infections being treated with ciprofloxacin, although whether this was truly an adverse reaction to ciprofloxacin is not definite (Moore *et al.*, 1988; Mumford and Ginsberg 1990). Aoun et al. (1992) reported the development of peripheral neuropathy in a patient with a past history of vincristine therapy who was treated with a prolonged course of pefloxacin. Symptoms improved with cessation of pefloxacin, but recurred with recommencement of ofloxacin. Transient acute hemiparesis has been reported in one patient with lymphoblastic leukemia following ciprofloxacin therapy. This recurred following rechallenge, but resolved with cessation of ciprofloxacin (Rosolen *et al.*, 1994). Zehnder et al. (1995) have described two patients who developed painful dysesthesia possibly associated with ciprofloxacin.

Seizures have been reported both in patients with a history of epilepsy and/or structural lesions in the central nervous system, and those without such predisposing factors. Nalidixic acid, norfloxacin, ciprofloxacin, ofloxacin, enoxacin and temafloxacin have all been implicated (Islam and Sreedharan, 1965; Davies *et al.*, 1984; Simpson and Brodie, 1985; Arcieri *et al.*, 1986; Wang *et al.*, 1988; Fass *et al.*, 1987; Raoof *et al.*, 1987a; Anastasio *et al.*, 1988; Janknegt 1990; Schacht *et al.*, 1989; Slavich *et al.*, 1989; Tack and Smith, 1989; Norrby and Pernet, 1991; O'Mahony and FitzGerald 1991). Concurrent administration of ciprofloxacin (and other fluoroquinolones, especially enoxacin) with theophylline results in theophylline accumulation (p. 1014) and can predispose to the development of seizures (Davies *et al.*, 1984; Arcieri *et al.*, 1986; Ball 1986; Raoof *et al.*, 1987a). Similarly, the concurrent administration of non-steroidal anti-inflammatory agents such as fenbufen with fluoroquinolones may be associated with an increased incidence of central nervous system adverse reaction such as convulsions, but data are limited (Christ 1990; Janknegt 1990). Non-steroidal anti-inflammatory agents may augment the ability of fluoroquinolones to antagonize the binding of the inhibitory neurotransmitter gamma-aminobutyric acid (GABA) to central nervous system receptors, but the details of how these changes result in altered seizure threshold and the impact of differences between various fluoroquinolones and non-steroidal anti-inflammatory agents in their seizure-inducing potential need further definition (Christ 1990; Halliwell *et al.*, 1991; De Salla *et al.*, 1993; Davey *et al.*, 1994). Akahane *et al.* (1989) have proposed that the epileptogenic activity of quinolones relates to the GABA-like structures of substituents at their seven positions which act as GABA receptor antagonists. In mice, quinolones with an unsubstituted piperazine moiety at the seven positions, such as enoxacin, norfloxacin, ciprofloxacin and pipemidic acid were most likely to promote seizures in a dose-dependant manner. Akahane *et al.* (1994) have also suggested that 4-biphenyl-acetic acid (BPAA), a metabolite of fenbufen, enhances the interaction of quinolones with the GABA receptor. Unlike nalidixic acid, ciprofloxacin does not impair brain glucose uptake, while neither agent alters brain blood flow or oxygen metabolism in studies of healthy volunteers studied by positive emission tomography (Bednarczyk *et al.*, 1994).

Eosinophilic meningitis, presumably as a manifestation of allergy, has also been associated with ciprofloxacin therapy (Asperilla and Smego, 1989).

3 Hypersensitivity reactions and rashes

Mild transient rash occurs in 0.4–4% of patients and other cutaneous reactions including pruritus, urticaria, erythema nodosum, hyperpigmentation occur in less than 1% (Halkin 1988; Schacht *et al.*, 1988; Rahm and Schacht 1989; Stahlmann 1990; AHFS, 1995). Severe (including fatal) anaphylaxis, anaphylactoid reactions and glottic angioedema have been reported in both HIV-infected and uninfected patients (Davis *et al.*, 1989; Peters and Pinching 1989; Wurtz *et al.*, 1989; Miller *et al.*, 1991; Assouad *et al.*, 1995; Vidal *et al.*, 1995). Davis *et al.* (1989) calculated that the rate of such reactions was probably about 1.2 per 100 000 prescriptions. Slama (1990) described a serum sickness-like illness associated with ciprofloxacin in which a 56-year-old man developed polyarthralgias, myalgia, fever, generalized urticarial eruption, joint effusions and abnormal liver function tests after commencing oral ciprofloxacin 500 mg twice-daily. Symptoms resolved with cessation of ciprofloxacin and commencement of steroid therapy, but the patient was not rechallenged. Guharoy (1994) described a similar, but less convincing, case of possible ciprofloxacin-associated serum sickness.

Erythema multiforme/Stevens–Johnson Syndrome, toxic epidermal necrolysis, Henoch-Schonlein purpura and lobular panniculitis have been reported rarely by the manufacturer and others (Rodriguez *et al.*, 1990; Tham *et al.*, 1991; AHFS, 1995; Gamboa *et al.*, 1995). Cutaneous vasculitis associated with ciprofloxacin administration has been reported and appears to resolve with cessation of therapy (Stubbings *et al.*, 1992; Choe *et al.*, 1989).

Photosensitivity reactions have been reported with most fluoroquinolones, although the incidence appears to be higher with pefloxacin, lomefloxacin and fleroxacin (Ball 1986; Desplaces *et al.*, 1986; Jensen *et al.*, 1987b; Ferguson *et al.*, 1988; Halkin, 1988; Jungst and Mohr, 1988; Bowie *et al.*, 1989; Gonzales *et al.*, 1989; Granowitz, 1989; Schacht *et al.*, 1989; Stahlmann, 1990; Norrby, 1991; Rizk, 1992; Iravani 1993). Burdge *et al.* (1995) surveyed adult patients with cystic fibrosis who were treated with oral ciprofloxacin and noted a 52% incidence of photosensitivity symptoms associated with usage of this agent. The vast majority of these patients who used a an ultraviolet A-blocking sunscreen noted valuable prevention of these symptoms. Although this high incidence may be related to the presence of cystic fibrosis, it is noteworthy. The mechanism of ciprofloxacin-associated photosensitivity is uncertain, but possibly relates to differences in ultraviolet A-induced photoinstability. Although such reactions appear to be idiosyncratic in most cases, data suggesting some association with higher fluoroquinolone doses and longer duration courses raises doubts about this concept (Petri and Tronnier, 1986; Bowie *et al.*, 1989; Ferguson and Johnson, 1990; Stahlmann 1990; Matsumoto *et al.*, 1992). Intravenous ciprofloxacin is associated with phlebitis in about 2% of patients (Hooper and Wolfson, 1993a).

4 Arthropathy

As noted in the chapter on nalidixic acid (p. 974), studies in rats and beagles showing cartilage erosions, non-inflammatory joint effusions and inhibition of cartilaginous embryonic limb bud growth associated with quinolone administration have raised concerns regarding the use of these agents in pregnancy and in prepubertal children (Ingham *et al.*, 1977; Tatsumi *et al.*, 1978; Corrado *et al.*, 1987; Monk and Campoli-Richards, 1987; Schlüter, 1987; Christ *et al.*, 1988). Such studies suggest that the arthropathy in weight-bearing joints is dose-related and varies with the quinolone under investigation and the animal species studied (Schaad and Wedgwood, 1992). Nevertheless, a number of clinical studies have cast doubt on the likelihood of these effects in children, at least with nalidixic acid (p. 974). Ciprofloxacin appears to be relatively safe in most studies, although Raeburn *et al.* (1987) reported that one of 30 children with cystic fibrosis who were treated with ciprofloxacin 1500 mg per day, developed arthropathy which resolved with cessation of ciprofloxacin therapy. Other studies of ciprofloxacin use in this situation have not noted significant problems, although pefloxacin was reportedly associated with a 14% incidence of arthralgia and joint swelling, and 45% incidence of arthropathy in 15- to 20-year old patients with cystic fibrosis (Black *et al.*, 1990; Hooper and Wolfson, 1993a). Thus, some variability depending on the fluoroquinolone, may exist. Schaad *et al.* (1991) and Danisovicová *et al.* (1994) used magnetic resonance imaging to examine for arthropathy in children with cystic fibrosis who had been treated with either ciprofloxacin or ofloxacin, but found no evidence for arthropathogenicity. Similarly, Pradhan *et al.* (1995) found no magnetic resonance imaging evidence of arthropathy in 58 children treated with ciprofloxacin 15–25 mg per kg for 9–16 days. Schaad *et al.* (1992) found no autopsy evidence of arthropathology in two cystic fibrosis patients who had received prolonged treatment with high dose courses of ciprofloxacin premortem. Similarly, Berkovitch *et al.* (1994) found no increase in risk of malformations or musculoskeletal problems among children born to women who had been treated with either ciprofloxacin or norfloxacin during the first trimester of pregnancy. Ciprofloxacin therefore appears to be safe in children but, as always, the potential benefits of such treatment need to be weighed against the possible risks.

In general, other musculoskeletal symptoms such as arthralgia, back pain, tenosynovitis and joint stiffness have been reported by the manufacturer in less than 1% of patients treated with ciprofloxacin (McEwan and Davey 1988; AHFS, 1995). Achilles tendinitis, including rupture, has been reported in patients treated with pefloxacin, ofloxacin and ciprofloxacin (Rose *et al.*, 1990; Lee and Collins 1992; Ribard *et al.*, 1992).

The administration of ciprofloxacin to neonates may be associated with the development of a greenish discoloration of teeth. Lumbiganon *et al.* (1991) noted this possible side-effect in two of five neonates treated with ciprofloxacin 10–40 mg per kg per day for *Klebsiella* sepsis, who were followed-up at 12–23 months of age. In other respects the teeth appeared to be normal.

5 Renal side-effects

Impaired renal function with elevated serum creatinine, interstitial nephritis, dysuria, polyuria and albuminuria has been reported by the manufacturer and others in $\leq$ 1% of patients receiving ciprofloxacin (Gonski, 1991). Acute renal failure has been noted after an overdose of ciprofloxacin in which a 29-year-old female ingested 21g of ciprofloxacin tablets (George *et al.*, 1991). Acute interstitial nephritis has been reported with ciprofloxacin and norfloxacin therapy, and is the commonest serious renal adverse reaction of fluoroquinolones (Boelaert *et al.*, 1986; Rippelmeyer and Synhavsky 1988; Hootkins *et al.*, 1989; Allon *et al.*, 1990; Helmink and Benediktsson, 1990; Rastogi *et al.*, 1990; Simpson *et al.*, 1991; Bailey *et al.*, 1992; Ortiz *et al.*, 1992; Connor *et al.*, 1994; Rosado *et al.*, 1994). It may occur alone, or as a component of a generalized allergic reaction with lymphocyte and/or eosinophilic infiltration of the renal interstitium (Rippelmeyer and Synhavsky 1988; Helmink and Benediktsson, 1990; Ortiz *et al.*, 1992). Lo *et al.* (1993) described five patients with cancer who developed acute renal failure following treatment with ciprofloxacin, and reviewed an additional 15 cases from the literature. No characteristic clinical or laboratory findings were identifiable, with the diagnosis being made only on renal biopsy. In all but one case, the dose of ciprofloxacin ranged from 200 mg i.v. twice-daily to 750 mg orally thrice-daily. The duration of antibiotic therapy before the onset of acute renal failure was 3–16 days, except in one case of attempted suicide in which anuria and acute renal failure occured within 24 h. Of the 20 patients reviewed, the type of acute renal failure was noted in 18: 13 were non-oliguric, five were oliguric/anuric. Urinalysis was little help except when there was significant eosinophiluria, however its absence does not exclude the possibility of interstitial nephritis (Lo *et al.*, 1993). Potential predisposing factors appear to include: age older than 60 years, recent or concomitant administration of other potentially nephrotoxic agents, and reduced patient hydration (Lucena *et al.*, 1995). Acute tubular necrosis and recurrent hematuria have each been reported in one patient (Gerritsen *et al.*, 1987; Jungst and Mohr, 1988; Ball 1986), and Shih *et al.* (1995) have described two patients who developed necrotizing renal vasculitis following ciprofloxacin therapy.

Crystalluria, generally associated with high doses and alkaline urine (and hence reduced quinolone solubility), has been occasionally reported with ciprofloxacin and norfloxacin, but not with other fluoroquinolones (Swanson *et al.*, 1983; Thorsteinsson *et al.*, 1986; Wang *et al.*, 1988; Schaeffer, 1987; Campoll-Richards *et al.*, 1988; Schacht *et al.*, 1989; Tack and Smith, 1989; Norrby and Pernet, 1991; Rizk, 1992). Interestingly, Thorsteinsson *et al.* (1986) noted crystalluria in five of six healthy volunteers treated with 1000 mg of ciprofloxacin in combination with sodium bicarbonate which alkalinized the urine, but no crystalluria when the same dose of ciprofloxacin was given with the urine acidifier ammonium chloride. In the setting of renal transplantation, the pharmacokinetic parameters of cyclosporin and the risk of cyclosporin nephrotoxicity do not appear to be altered by concomitant ciprofloxacin therapy despite occasional case reports suggesting the contrary (Avent *et al.*, 1988; Lang *et al.*, 1989; p. 1013).

6 Hematologic side-effects

Hematologic toxicity occurs in 0.4–5.3% of patients treated with fluoroquinolones; with norfloxacin more commonly implicated. Leukopenia (0.06–3.3%), eosinophilia, anemia (0.4–0.6%), thrombocytosis and thrombocytopenia have all been reported by the manufacturer and others, but are reversible (Patoia *et al.*, 1987; Halkin 1988; Hooper and Wolfson, 1993a; Teh and McKendrick 1993). Castaman and Rodeghiero (1994) described two cases of severe but temporary acquired von Willebrand syndrome associated with ciprofloxacin therapy. Ciprofloxacin and norfloxacin have rarely been reported to interact with warfarin to increase prothrombin time, although the mechanism is unclear (Linville and Matanin 1989; Mott *et al.*, 1989; Jolson *et al.*, 1991).

7 Endocrine side-effects

Although ciprofloxacin is an inhibitor of the metabolism of a number of drugs (p. 1013), no alterations in testosterone or cortisol concentrations were noted in healthy male volunteers treated with ciprofloxacin 500 mg twice-daily for 4 days (Waite *et al.*, 1989). Ciprofloxacin can cause a false positive reaction for glucose (pseudoglycosuria) when urine is tested with the 'BM-Test-7' (Boehringer-Mannheim) urine test which is based on a specific glucose oxidase/peroxidase reaction. This false reaction is thought to be due to a ciprofloxacin metabolite since solutions of ciprofloxacin do not produce an abnormal result (Drysdale *et al.*, 1988).

8 Hepatotoxicity

Increased serum concentrations of AST and ALT have been noted in about 2% of patients, while less than 1% have developed increases in alkaline phosphatase and other enzymes in patients treated with ciprofloxacin. The manufacturer reports that rarely, fulminant and occasionally fatal hepatic failure has occurred in patients being treated with ciprofloxacin. Lopez-Navidad *et al.* (1990) described a patient with presumed norfloxacin-associated hepatitis, in whom a liver biopsy demonstrated moderate steatosis with small foci of centrilobular necrosis with scattered eosinophilic bodies and ceroid-laden macrophages. Aggarwal and Gurka (1995) described a patient who developed possible ciprofloxacin-associated cholestasis.

9 Ototoxicity

Despite some initial concerns regarding potential ciprofloxacin-associated ototoxicity in animals, a number of detailed studies have shown no evidence that ciprofloxacin is associated with any ototoxicity (Bagger-Sjöbäck and Spångberg 1989; Claes *et al.*, 1991). Ciprofloxacin may rarely be associated with tinnitus (Paul and Brown, 1995).

10 Immune modulation

Therapeutic doses of fluoroquinolones do not appear to be associated with measurable changes in immune function, although some animal studies have suggested a suppressive effect when very high doses were given. *In vitro* studies suggest no direct effect of phagocytic cell function, immunoglobulin production, lymphocyte proliferation, bone-marrow proliferation or secretion of interferon gamma, but the *in vivo* situation is less clear, with some authors reporting a depression of bone marrow graft uptake in mice treated with high doses of ciprofloxacin (Somekh *et al.*, 1989; Shalit, 1991; Rubinstein and Shalit, 1993; Jimenez-Valera *et al.*, 1995). Riesbeck *et al.* (1994) found that cyclosporin-dependent inhibition of both interleukin-2 and interferon-gamma expression *in vitro* is counteracted by high concentrations of ciprofloxacin.

11 Drug interactions

Numerous authors have reviewed the observed drug interactions between fluoroquinolones and various agents, which can be broadly classified as either pharmacokinetic or pharmacodynamic (Davey 1988; Davies and Maesen 1989; Polk 1989; Janknegt 1990; Stein 1991; Radandt et al., 1993). Pharmacokinetic interactions are observed when one drug interferes with absorption, distribution or elimination of another drug. However, when one drug increases or decreases the potency of another drug, this is referred to as a pharmacodynamic interaction (Davey 1988). Both forms of interactions are noted with fluoroquinolones, as with many antibiotics. Clinically it is generally more helpful to discuss these interactions in terms of the uses of these other agents. Some fluoroquinolones such as ciprofloxacin, norfloxacin, and ofloxacin can inhibit cytochrome P-450 and therefore result in increased serum concentration of some drugs (e.g. caffeine and theophylline; p. 1014) (Rodvold and Piscitelli, 1993; Radandt et al., 1992).

Sucralfate and antacids containing aluminum, calcium, or magnesium cause a clinically-significant reduction in absorption of ciprofloxacin, as does ferrous sulfate and zinc-containing multivitamins (Höffken et al., 1985a, 1988; Fleming et al., 1986; Preheim et al., 1986; Nix et al., 1989, 1990; Polk et al., 1989; Yuk et al., 1989b; Flor et al., 1990; Garrelts et al., 1990; Le Pennec et al., 1990; Radandt et al., 1992). Frost et al. (1992) found that when ciprofloxacin was given with calcium carbonate, bioavailability was reduced to about 60% of control values, while with aluminum hydroxide the relative bioavailability was 15%. Preheim et al. (1986) found antacids reduced peak and trough serum concentrations of ciprofloxacin to approximately one-third of levels noted without antacids in 20 elderly patients, and affected clinical efficacy. Similarly, bismuth subsalicylate appears to affect ciprofloxacin bioavailability (Rambout et al., 1994). Calcium carbonate administered 2 h before ciprofloxacin, however, does not alter relative bioavailability of ciprofloxacin and the H2 antagonists, cimetidine and ranitidine, do not affect ciprofloxacin bioavailability (Lomaestro and Baillie 1991, 1993; Radandt et al., 1992).

Although food does not generally reduce the oral bioavailability of fluoroquinolones, dairy products (milk and yoghurt) with a high calcium content may interfere with fluoroquinolone bioavailability, reducing ciprofloxacin absorption by 30–36% (Neuvonen et al., 1991; Kivistö et al., 1992; Neuvonen and Kivistö 1992; Nix, 1993; Hoogkamer and Kleinbloesem, 1995). However, ciprofloxacin bioavailability is not altered significantly by a 'standard' or high-fat/high-calcium breakfast (Frost et al., 1989a). The co-administration of ciprofloxacin and ofloxacin with the enteral feeding solution 'Ensure' is associated with a reduction in the bioavailability of these agents (ciprofloxacin – 72% bioavailability; ofloxacin – 90% bioavailability) compared with co-administration of these antibiotics with water. This effect may be due to the concentration of calcium and magnesium in 'Ensure' and has important implications in the clinical setting (Mueller et al., 1994). Notably, however, pancreatic enzyme supplements when co-administered with ciprofloxacin to patients with cystic fibrosis, do not influence the pharmacokinetics of oral ciprofloxacin (Mack et al., 1991). The absorption of ciprofloxacin may, however, be reduced after cytotoxic chemotherapy (Johnson et al., 1990).

Concurrent administration of ciprofloxacin and cyclosporin (cyclosporin A) does not appear to alter the pharmacokinetics of cyclosporin and no dosage adjustment is generally needed (Lang et al., 1989; Krüger et al., 1990; Hoey and Lake 1994). Although a number of anecdotal reports have suggested a potential interaction between ciprofloxacin and cyclosporin A, Hoey and Lake (1994) in their review of the literature, concluded that there was no pharmacokinetic or pharmacodynamic interaction on the basis of controlled studies.

Concurrent i.v. administration of azlocillin and ciprofloxacin results in higher and more prolonged concentrations of ciprofloxacin in serum, but no change in azlocillin concentrations. Thus clinicians need to be aware of a possible increased risk of ciprofloxacin toxicity in this situation (Barriere et al., 1990). Probenecid inhibits the renal tubular secretion of ciprofloxacin and some other fluoroquinolones, thereby reducing renal elimination and increasing serum concentrations of fluoroquinolones (Shimada et al., 1983; Weidekamm et al., 1987; Wijnands et al., 1988; Davies and Maesen 1989; Jaehde et al., 1995). For agents such as ciprofloxacin, pefloxacin and enoxacin, with significant non-renal elimination, the effect of probenecid on serum concentrations is less significant (Radant et al., 1992).

Fluoroquinolones, including ciprofloxacin, may occasionally interact with warfarin to result in prolongation of the prothrombin time (Jolson et al., 1991; Linville et al., 1991). Jolson et al. (1991) reviewed 18 reports of this possible interaction to the US Food and Drug Administration (FDA) and proposed three possible mechanisms. The first and most likely explanation is the inhibition of warfarin elimination. Other potential mechanisms include the displacement of warfarin from protein-binding sites and the inhibition by fluoroquinolones of vitamin K-producing bowel flora; although these latter two explanations appear less likely. Overall, however, this interaction appears to be rare (Nix, 1993).

Co-administration of ciprofloxacin and quinidine does not alter the pharmacokinetics or ECG parameters associated with quinidine, and no dosage adjustment is necessary (Bleske *et al.*, 1990). Some premedicant agents such as paravertum, used prior to abdominal surgery, reduce peak serum ciprofloxacin concentrations after oral administration to less than half of the concentrations found in the control groups and prolong the ciprofloxacin half-life. Temazepam, however, does not affect the pharmacokinetics of oral ciprofloxacin (Morran *et al.*, 1989).

Fluoroquinolones such as ciprofloxacin, norfloxacin and enoxacin significantly reduce theophylline clearance (30% reduction in clearance – ciprofloxacin; norfloxacin – 10% reduction), resulting in increased serum concentrations such that careful monitoring of theophylline levels during co-administration is warranted (Raoof *et al.*, 1987b; Wijnands *et al.*, 1987; Schwartz *et al.*, 1988; Wijnands and Vree, 1988; Polk, 1989; Prince *et al.*, 1989; Robson 1992). The mechanism of this interaction is due to the competition of quinolones for cytochrome P-450–related isoenzymes, resulting in decreased demethylation of theophylline. In contrast, ofloxacin and lomefloxacin, do not affect theophylline concentrations (pp. 1121, 1150) (Wijnands and Vree 1988; Sarkar *et al.*, 1990; Robson 1992). Grasela and Dreis (1992) reviewed the 48 reports of adverse events reported to the US FDA in patients receiving concomitant therapy with ciprofloxacin or norfloxacin, and theophylline. The mean age of these patients was 68 years while the mean percent change in theophylline concentrations after commencement of a quinolone was 114% (range 32–308%). Approximately one-third of these patients suffered seizures, most likely due to the elevated theophylline levels observed.

Ciprofloxacin, similar to other fluoroquinolones that reduce theophylline metabolism, also significantly increase the half-life of caffeine by delaying the conversion of caffeine to paraxanthine and therefore reducing the total body clearance of caffeine. Thus, symptoms of caffeine toxicity may be noted when these two drugs are co-administered (Stille *et al.*, 1987; Harder *et al.*, 1989; Healy *et al.*, 1989). In addition, caffeine may alter the kinetics of ciprofloxacin.

Concomitant administration of ciprofloxacin with either metronidazole or clindamycin in humans does not alter the concentrations of these agents (Boeckh *et al.*, 1990; Ludwig *et al.*, 1990). Although some case reports have suggested an increased incidence of neurotoxicity when either ciprofloxacin or pefloxacin are given concomitantly with metronidazole, these observations need further confirmation (Lucet *et al.*, 1988; Semel and Allen, 1989).

Clinical Uses of the Drug

1 Urinary tract infection

The antibacterial spectrum and pharmacokinetics of fluoroquinolones, including ciprofloxacin, make these ideal agents for the treatment of urinary tract sepsis, since almost all achieve urinary concentrations of greater than $8\ \mu g$ per ml for at least 24 h – thus inhibiting the vast majority of urinary pathogens including *Ps. aeruginosa* (Norrby 1993). Drug concentrations in renal tissue and prostate are high, especially compared with concurrent levels in serum (p. 1007). However, not all fluoroquinolones reliably achieve adequate serum concentrations to treat complicated urinary tract sepsis in which septicemia is more likely. In his review of the literature Norrby (1993) found that no major differences in efficacy between various fluoroquinolones when given for 3 days or more for uncomplicated cystitis, with failure rates of only 2.5–8.2%. Some differences in outcome may be found between various fluoroquinolones when they are used as single-dose therapy. In this setting failure rates range from 2.9 to 40%, depending on the agent and dose (Ode *et al.*, 1987; Preheim *et al.*, 1987; Ryan *et al.*, 1987; Backhouse and Mathews, 1989; Petersen *et al.*, 1990; von Balen *et al.*, 1990). Optimal results are generally obtained with treatment for 3–7 days. Iravani *et al.* (1995), in a comparison of multiple oral dosage regimens, found ciprofloxacin 100 mg twice-daily for 3 days was the minimum effective dose for the treatment of uncomplicated urinary tract infection in women, resulting in 93% bacteriologic eradication and 93% clinical success at the end of therapy. Single-dose oral therapy with either 100 mg or 250 mg ciprofloxacin results in cure in 84–89% of women with uncomplicated urinary tract infections (Garlando *et al.*, 1987). However, Iravani (1993) found single-dose therapy with fleroxacin 400 mg to be inferior to a 7-day course of either oral fleroxacin 200 mg once-daily or ciprofloxacin 250 mg twice-daily, with bacteriologic cure rates at 5–9 days post-therapy of 88%, 96% and 96% respectively (p < 0.05). By 4–6 weeks after therapy, however, the rates of bacteriologic cure (89–93%) were comparable in all three treatment groups. For most uncomplicated urinary tract infections, however, other agents such as trimethoprim alone, trimethoprim–sulfamethoxazole or beta-lactams are preferred, and fluoroquinolones are reserved for the treatment of infections due to resistant pathogens, recurrent urinary tract infections recalcitrant to treatment with other agents, and complicated urinary tract infection. For complicated urinary tract sepsis, including pyelonephritis, therapy for 7–14 days with either ciprofloxacin, enoxacin, fleroxacin, lomefloxacin, norfloxacin or ofloxacin, results in failure rates (persistent infection or reinfection 5–12 days after completion of therapy) of 1.5–22% (generally ≤10%). Such outcomes are generally better than the failure rates achieved by other agents such as trimethoprim–sulfamethoxazole or beta-lactams, including ceftazidime (Sabbaj *et al.*, 1985; Gasser *et al.*, 1987b; Preheim *et al.*, 1987; Allais *et al.*, 1988; Cox 1989a, 1992; Childs 1990; Sandberg *et al.*, 1990; Norrby 1993). Also, Pfau and Sacks (1994) found post-coital prophylaxis with a single-dose of either ofloxacin 100 mg, ciprofloxacin 125 mg or norfloxacin 200 mg to be effective in preventing recurrent UTIs in females. Van der Wall *et al.* (1992) found prophylaxis with either ciprofloxacin 250 mg daily or ciprofloxacin 500 mg twice-daily to be effective in preventing catheter-associated urinary tract infections in a double-blind, placebo-controlled trial in surgical patients requiring 3–14 days temporary postoperative bladder drainage. At catheter removal 75% of placebo recipients were bacteriuric compared with 11% of ciprofloxacin-treated patients. Nevertheless, the relative infrequency of symptomatic urinary tract infections in this setting, its usual ease of effective therapy, and concerns regarding the potential development of ciprofloxacin resistance argue against such prophylaxis. In chronically catheterized patients such as paraplegic and quadriplegic patients, short-course (e.g. 5 days) ciprofloxacin is effective in treating urinary tract infections, but does not prevent the prompt re-development of bacteriuria in about two-thirds of patients 14 days post-therapy (Stannard *et al.*, 1990). Ciprofloxacin 500 mg twice-daily for 7–10 days produced a comparable clinical response to parenteral aminoglycoside (usually gentamicin) used for a similar period in chronically catheterized patients. Although ciprofloxacin resulted in a superior bacteriological response at day 5–9 post-therapy, the response 1 month later was almost identical between the two treatments. The emergence of ciprofloxacin resistance was noted in 62% of patients who did not show any bacteriological response (Fang *et al.*, 1991). Chronic suppressive therapy with ciprofloxacin 100 mg orally nightly is effective in preventing symptomatic urinary tract infections in patients with spinal cord lesions and neurogenic bladder, without the development of super-colonization with ciprofloxacin-resistant pathogens (Bierring-Sørensen *et al.*, 1994). Fluoroquinolones including ciprofloxacin, appear to be useful either i.v. or orally, for prophylaxis in urological surgery such as transurethral prostatectomy (Murdoch *et al.*, 1987; Kanaiyalal *et al.*, 1988; Charton *et al.*, 1989; Christensen *et al.*, 1989; Cox 1989b; Gombert *et al.*, 1989; Hellsten *et al.*, 1989; Mandell, 1991). George *et al.* (1995) described a patient with bilateral emphysematous pyelonephritis who was cured with a combination of antibiotics, including ciprofloxacin; however, surgical management is generally necessary for this serious condition.

2 Prostatitis and epididymoorchitis

Fluoroquinolones such as ciprofloxacin have revolutionized the treatment of prostatitis, which previously had been difficult to cure with agents such as trimethoprim–sulfamethoxazole or beta-lactams. Nevertheless, despite well over 30 clinical studies of fluoroquinolone efficacy in this condition, a comparison of clinical results remains difficult due to differences in study methodology and clinical definitions, including variable use of diagnostic techniques such as the standard four-specimen technique for localizing infection to the prostate (Meares and Stamey 1968). Furthermore, many studies combine the treatment results for acute and chronic prostatitis rather than reporting them separately. Naber (1993) analyzed only those studies that met appropriate criteria and suggested that norfloxacin 400 mg twice-daily (generally 2–4 weeks), ciprofloxacin 500 mg twice-daily (generally 3–4 weeks), ofloxacin 200–300 mg twice-daily (generally 3–6 weeks) and other fluoroquinolones such as enoxacin, temafloxacin and rufloxacin are effective therapy, with rates of bacteriological cure generally greater than 75% for both acute and chronic infection (Weidner *et al.*, 1987a; Andriole 1991; Naber 1993).

Low-dose, short-term (e.g. ≤2 weeks) therapy appears to be associated with a higher rate of relapse. Thus, chronic bacterial prostatitis, especially when due to *E. coli* and other Enterobacteriaceae, is best treated for 4–6 weeks with a fluoroquinolone such as ciprofloxacin 500 mg twice-daily or norfloxacin 400 mg twice-daily. Other fluoroquinolones (e.g. ofloxacin, fleroxacin) possibly have similar efficacy but good comparable clinical studies are needed. The dosage and duration of therapy for prostatitis due to *Ps. aeruginosa* or enterococci is less clear, but considering known *in vitro* susceptibility data regarding these pathogens, more prolonged fluoroquinolone therapy in high dose would be justifiable. Whether the shorter duration of treatment (e.g. 2 weeks) is acceptable for acute prostatitis is uncertain, but many clinicians take a conservative approach due to the possibility of acute-on-chronic disease and therefore treat for 4–6 weeks. Follow-up assessment 6 months after completion of treatment is always wise.

Few studies have formally examined the efficacy of fluoroquinolones in the treatment of epididymitis and epididymo-orchitis, but the known antibacterial spectrum and pharmacokinetics of fluoroquinolones suggest them to be a potentially appropriate therapeutic choice. Ciprofloxacin, pefloxacin and ofloxacin have proven efficacy (Weidner et al., 1987b; Costa et al., 1991). Humphreys and Speller (1989) reported three patients with acute epididymo-orchitis caused by Ps. aeruginosa who were cured with ciprofloxacin (500–750 mg twice-daily after initial i.v. therapy in two cases) for 8–14 days. Costa et al. (1991) successfully treated 18 of 20 men with acute epididymitis with pefloxacin 800 mg daily for 21–42 days. The current CDC (1993b) recommendation for treatment of epididymitis is ceftriaxone 250 mg i.m. single-dose + doxycycline 100 mg twice-daily for 10 days, but ofloxacin 300 mg orally twice-daily for 10 days is a suitable alternative to this combination.

3 Bacterial diarrhea and enteric fever

Fluoroquinolones have generally excellent in vitro activity against the majority of gastro-intestinal bacterial pathogens such as Salmonella spp., Shigella spp., C. jejuni, Aeromonas hydrophila, Vibrio spp., Yersinia enterocolitica and E. coli, and are therefore logical candidates for use in the setting of bacterial diarrhea (p. 982). Fluoroquinolones such as ciprofloxacin and norfloxacin achieve concentrations in feces of 185–2220 μg per g and 207–2716 μg per g of stool, respectively, in healthy volunteers after routine oral doses (Brumfitt et al., 1984; Cofsky et al., 1984). A number of double-blind, randomized trials have shown the superiority of ciprofloxacin 500 mg twice-daily for 5 days over either trimethoprim–sulfamethoxazole or placebo as empiric treatment for acute diarrhea due to Campylobacter, Shigella, Salmonella or unidentified pathogens (Pichler et al., 1987; Goodman et al., 1990).

a Shigellosis Fluoroquinolones such as norfloxacin and ciprofloxacin are superior to nalidixic acid and other antibiotics in the treatment of shigellosis. Ericsson et al. (1987) found the average duration of diarrhea after commencing ciprofloxacin therapy to be 28 h compared with 84 h in patients receiving placebo for shigellosis. In a double-blind, randomized trial comparing a 5-day course of ciprofloxacin 500 mg twice-daily with ampicillin 500 mg four-times daily in 121 adults hospitalized for shigellosis in Bangladesh, Bennish et al. (1990) found there was resolution or marked improvement in symptoms in 95% of ciprofloxacin-treated patients versus 88% ampicillin-treated patients with ampicillin-sensitive stains and 43% of ampicillin-resistant strains. Overall, bacteriologic cure was more common in the ciprofloxacin-treated group (p < 0.025) and these patients had a mean of 63% the number of stools experienced by the ampicillin-treated group (p = 0.004). Subsequently Bennish et al. (1992) have shown that a single 1g dose of ciprofloxacin is effective therapy for patients with Shigella species other than Sh. dysenteriae type 1, but this is inferior to a 5-day course of 500 mg twice-daily (40% failure rate versus 0%, respectively) for treating patients infected with ciprofloxacin-sensitive Sh. dysenteriae type 1. Similarly, Gottuzo et al. (1989) found single-dose norfloxacin therapy was equivalent to a 5-day course of trimethoprim–sulfamethoxazole in mild disease, but none of these patients had Sh. dysenteriae type 1. Other authors have also advocated the use of 1g single-dose ciprofloxacin for shigellosis (Williams and Richards 1990; Bhattacharya et al., 1992). One- or two-dose regimens have particular appeal in the treatment of shigellosis in children, when the potential risks associated with fluoroquinolone use in this age group are considered by some authors to be outweighed by the potential benefits of effective therapy (Fontaine, 1989). In adults, Murphy et al. (1993) have shown that the administration of loperamide (4 mg immediately then 2 mg after each loose bowel action to a maximum of 16 mg per day) + ciprofloxacin 500 mg twice-daily for 3 days, significantly shortens the duration of diarrhea compared with patients treated with ciprofloxacin alone.

b Salmonellosis and enteric fever Counter to previous conventional teaching in which antibiotic therapy was not considered clinically useful in treating intestinal salmonellosis, ciprofloxacin and other fluoroquinolones have been shown by some authors to be beneficial (DuPont et al., 1987a,b; Pichler et al., 1987; López-Brea et al.,1989). Both the duration of diarrheal illness and fecal shedding of Salmonella may be reduced with ciprofloxacin therapy (Hudson et al., 1985; Dirdl et al., 1986; Pichler et al., 1987). In particular, Pichler et al. (1987) noted a reduction in diarrhea duration from 3.4 days (placebo) to 1.9 days (ciprofloxacin therapy). In comparison, however, Sánchez et al. (1993) found little difference in clinical efficacy between a 5-day treatment course of ciprofloxacin (500 mg twice-daily), trimethoprim–sulfamethoxazole (160/800 mg twice-daily) or placebo in a comparative double-blind trial of empiric treatment of uncomplicated non-typhi Salmonella enteritis, suggesting some doubt regarding the benefit of fluoroquinolones. However, the definition of cure in this study was more restrictive than that used by Pichler *et al.* (1987). Furthermore, this study explicitly excluded patients with severe disease or who were at risk of bacteremia, and deliberately chose patients with a short clinical history prior to study entry. Other studies, although not placebo-controlled, have suggested good clinical efficacy with ciprofloxacin 500 mg twice-daily for 7 days for the treatment of outbreaks of multiresistant non-enteric *Salm. heidelberg* and 5–7 days therapy for *Salm. enteritidis* (Barnass *et al.*, 1990; Willocks *et al.*, 1990; Leigh 1992). The management of institutional outbreaks of *Salmonella* gastroenteritis, including the use of ciprofloxacin, has been reviewed by Lightfoot *et al.* (1990). Jacobson *et al.* (1989) reported success with 750 mg twice-daily for 1–8 months in the treatment of non-typhoidal bacteremia in four patients with AIDS.

Ciprofloxacin has also proven effective against empyema and neonatal brain abscesses due to *Salm. enteritidis*; lung abscesses, recurrent bacteremia and neonatal meningitis due to *Salm. typhimurium*, and meningitis in a neonate due to *Salm. paratyphi* A (Zumla *et al.*, 1988; Ragunathan *et al.*, 1990; Murdoch *et al.*, 1991; Albrecht *et al.*, 1992; Bhutta *et al.*, 1992; Wessalowski *et al.*, 1993). Cheesebrough *et al.* (1991) reported excellent results in the use of ciprofloxacin in 33 children with non-*typhi Salmonella* bacteremia in Zaire, with no significant short-term adverse effects.

Ciprofloxacin is effective therapy for *Salm. typhi* bacteremia when given as 500 mg twice-daily for 14 days (Ramirez *et al.*, 1985) – resulting in defervescence after 4–5 days. Comparative studies between ciprofloxacin and trimethoprim–sulfamethoxazole, and ciprofloxacin and ceftriaxone in the treatment of enteric fever due to *Salm. typhi* or *Salm. paratyphi* have demonstrated the superiority of ciprofloxacin (Limson and Littaua 1989; Wallace *et al.*, 1993). In a randomized, non-blinded study of uncomplicated enteric fever (28 *Salm. typhi*, nine *Salm. paratyphi* A, three *Salm. paratyphi* B) in which all isolates were susceptible to ciprofloxacin and trimethoprim–sulfamethoxazole, Limson and Littaua (1989) found all 20 patients treated with ciprofloxacin 500 mg twice-daily for 10 days were clinically and bacteriologically cured, compared with 18 of 20 patients treated with trimethoprim–sulfamethoxazole (160/800 mg) twice-daily for 14 days. The two trimethoprim–sulfamethoxazole failures subsequently responded to ciprofloxacin. Wallace *et al.* (1993) compared ciprofloxacin 500 mg twice-daily for 7 days with ceftriaxone 3 g i.m./i.v. daily for 7 days in the treatment of *Salm. typhi* bacteremia in an open randomized trial in Bahrain. Clinical failure was noted in none of 20 ciprofloxacin-treated patients versus six of 22 (27%) ceftriaxone-treated patients (five of these six patients had persistent fevers for ≥7 days; p = 0.01). The mean duration of fever was 4 days for ciprofloxacin-treated patients versus approximately 5 days for ceftriaxone-treated patients (p = 0.04). All ceftriaxone failures responded clinically to ciprofloxacin within 48 h. All isolates were susceptible to both agents, but seven of 12 strains examined in detail were resistant to ampicillin, chloramphenicol and trimethoprim.

Other authors have described excellent rates of cure in open, non-comparative studies of either oral, or combination i.v./oral, ciprofloxacin treatment for 10–14 days in enteric fever (Eykyn and Williams 1989; Stanley *et al.*, 1989). Courses of ciprofloxacin shorter than 10–14 days may also be effective. In a randomized, prospective study of *Salm. typhi* bacteremia, Uwaydah *et al.* (1992) compared 500 mg or 750 mg oral ciprofloxacin twice-daily for 7 days, or for 2 days following defervescence, whichever was greater. Among the 34 patients treated with 500 mg twice-daily, fever subsided in 4.9 ± 1.7 days versus 5.2 ± 2.2 days in the 28 patients treated with 750 mg twice-daily (p = 0.54). Treatment for 7–10 days was adequate for 57 of the 62 patients (93%), but five patients required treatment for more than 10 days – all patients were cured. All patients requiring treatment for ≥10 days had prolonged fever (≥10 days) before presentation and commencement of therapy. This study suggests that ciprofloxacin 500 mg twice-daily is adequate treatment for typhoid fever but the duration of treatment may need to be individualized depending on the duration of pre-treatment symptoms and time to defervescence. Other authors have reported promising results with 5–7 days ciprofloxacin therapy in small studies. Given current information, however, optimal results in all patients are achieved with 10–14 days treatment (Carbon *et al.*, 1987; Chew *et al.*, 1992; Alam *et al.*, 1995).

Similar to non-typhoidal salmonellosis, ciprofloxacin has proven effective in the treatment of severe typhoid in children (Dawood *et al.*, 1991; Dutta *et al.*, 1993). Dutta *et al.* (1993) treated 18 children (mean 6.4 years; range 1.5–9.5 years) with life-threatening *Salm. typhi* bacteremia with i.v. ciprofloxacin (10 mg per kg per day), followed by oral ciprofloxacin for 14 days, or 7 days after the patient became afebrile. Children regained consciousness within a mean of 2 days, were afebrile within a mean of 3.3 days and cure was achieved in 17 patients (94%). One child who was severely malnourished died 24 h after ciprofloxacin therapy was commenced. These results appear promising in comparison with standard chloramphenicol therapy in this setting –

especially considering the increasing emergence of chloramphenicol resistance among *Salm. typhi* strains which necessitate the use of alternative regimens (p. 550; Panigrahi *et al.*, 1991; Rowe *et al.*, 1992).

Ciprofloxacin appears to be safe when given during pregnancy for multiply-resistant *Salm. typhi* infection. Koul *et al.* (1995) described seven patients, all in the second or third trimester of pregnancy, with multiresistant *Salm. typhi* infection who were successfully treated with ciprofloxacin. Fever resolved in 4–7 days. All pregnancies carried to term and healthy babies with no congenital abnormalities were delivered. Manufacturer reports of 130 women, mostly with first trimester of pregnancies who accidentally received ciprofloxacin note that none of these babies had any congenital abnormalities (Koul *et al.*, 1995).

Other fluoroquinolones such as pefloxacin and ofloxacin also appear to be effective in typhoid fever (Hajji *et al.*, 1988; Wang *et al.*, 1989). Thus, fluoroquinolones should now be considered the drugs of choice where resistant *Salm. typhi* is common.

Among patients infected with *Salm. typhi*, approximately 1–5% become chronic carriers, compared with less than 1% of patients infected with other *Salmonella* spp. (Buchwald and Blaser 1984; Pithie and Woods 1990). Ciprofloxacin and norfloxacin are effective in eradicating non-typhoidal salmonellae and *Salm. typhi* in chronic carriers (Hudson *et al.*, 1985; Sammalkorpi *et al.*, 1987; Ferreccio *et al.*, 1988; Gotuzzo *et al.*, 1988; Damjanovic *et al.*, 1990; Eng *et al.*, 1990). In a placebo-controlled trial, norfloxacin 400 mg twice-daily for 4 weeks cleared *Salm. typhi* from 78% of carriers, regardless of the presence or absence of cholelithiasis (Gotuzzo *et al.*, 1988). Other authors have found similar results with ciprofloxacin (Hudson *et al.*, 1985; Ferreccio *et al.*, 1988). Ferreccio *et al.* (1988) cleared carriage of *Salm. typhi* in 10 of 12 patients treated with 750 mg ciprofloxacin twice-daily for 28 days and followed for 1 year. In comparison to these positive findings, Neill *et al.* (1991) found less promising results in clearance of *Salm. java* carriage. In a randomized, placebo-controlled double-blind trial of ciprofloxacin 750 mg twice-daily for 14 days versus placebo, commenced on day 9 of infection, in 15 health-care workers with *Salm. java* diarrhea, these authors found all eight ciprofloxacin recipients showed eradication of *Salm. java* within 7 days of commencing ciprofloxacin versus one of seven placebo recipients. However, four of eight ciprofloxacin-recipients relapsed with positive stool cultures 14–21 days after therapy. The explanation for these findings is unclear, including whether the delay in commencing treatment (day 9) or lower total duration of treatment (i.e. 14 days versus 28 days) were relevant factors. Nevertheless, this study suggests that the efficacy of ciprofloxacin for treatment of patients with enteric fever and *Salm. typhi* carrier state cannot necessarily be directly extrapolated to carriage with non-typhoidal salmonellae. The optimal dosage and duration of ciprofloxacin therapy for chronic *Salmonella* carriage has not been defined, with doses ranging from 750 to 1500 mg per day for 2–4 weeks. Overall clearance rates vary between 90 and 100%. Most authors, however, favor 750 mg twice-daily for 2–4 weeks (Hudson *et al.*, 1985; Diridal *et al.*, 1986; Sammalkorpi *et al.*, 1987; Lähdevirta, 1989).

c Travelers' diarrhea Fluoroquinolones such as ciprofloxacin, norfloxacin and ofloxacin are effective against so-called "travelers' diarrhea", including the commonest pathogen, enterotoxigenic *E. coli* (ETEC), and other pathogens such as *Shigella*, *Salmonellae* and *Plesiomonas* spp. A 5-day treatment course of ciprofloxacin 500 mg twice-daily is at least as effective as trimethoprim–sulfamethoxazole (160/800 mg twice-daily) in this setting, reducing the average duration of diarrhea from 81 h (placebo) to 30 h (trimethoprim–sulfamethoxazole) and 27 h (ciprofloxacin) for all pathogens (DuPont *et al.*, 1987b; Ericsson *et al.*, 1987). The duration of diarrhea secondary to enterotoxigenic *E. coli* was reduced from 84 h (placebo) to 23 h (ciprofloxacin). Lower doses (250 mg twice-daily for 3 days) have also proven effective (Wiström *et al.*, 1992). More recently, Salam *et al.* (1994), reported the success of 500 mg single-dose ciprofloxacin therapy compared with placebo in reducing the duration and severity of diarrhea in travelers. In this study the mean duration of diarrhea was reduced from 50–53 h (placebo) to 21–25 h (ciprofloxacin) (p < 0.0001).

In a randomized, double-blind, placebo-controlled trial in US military personnel in Egypt of ciprofloxacin alone (500 mg twice-daily for 3 days; 50 patients) versus ciprofloxacin + loperamide (4 mg immediately then 2 mg after each loose bowel motion to a maximum of 16 mg per day; 54 patients) for treatment of travelers' diarrhea, where enterotoxigenic *E. coli* was the most common pathogen identified (57%), Taylor *et al.* (1991) found ciprofloxacin + loperamide was clinically no better than ciprofloxacin alone. In a similar study conducted in Thailand comparing a single 750-mg dose of ciprofloxacin + placebo versus a single 750-mg dose of ciprofloxacin + loperamide versus 500 mg ciprofloxacin twice-daily for 3 days + loperamide, in a population where 41% of travelers' diarrhea was due to *Campylobacter* spp, 18% *Salmonellae* and only 6% were secondary to enterotoxigenic *E. coli*, total duration of diarrhea did not vary significantly between the three treatment groups. However, a lower cumulative number of loose bowel actions were noted at 48 and 72 h among the patients treated with ciprofloxacin + loperamide compared with patients in the ciprofloxacin alone group (p = 0.01). Thus the addition of loperamide in this situation may provide a small symptomatic benefit (Petruccelli *et al.*, 1992).

Therapy with norfloxacin or ofloxacin for 3 days is also effective (Wiström *et al.*, 1989; DuPont *et al.*, 1992). Thus, fluoroquinolones should be considered the drugs of choice for the empiric treatment of severe diarrhea in adults from regions such as South-East Asia, South America and Africa, where trimethoprim–sulfamethoxazole-resistant strains of enterotoxigenic *E. coli* and *Shigella* are known to be common (Murray 1986).

Prophylaxis with ciprofloxacin (250–500 mg per day) or norfloxacin (400 mg per day) is effective in reducing the incidence of travelers' diarrhea by up to 88–94% in studies undertaken in Mexico, Morocco and Nepal (Johnson *et al.*, 1986; Rademaker *et al.*, 1989; Scott *et al.*, 1990; Wiström and Norrby 1990; Parry *et al.*, 1994).

d   Cholera   In a randomized, double-blind treatment trial of moderate-severe cholera in Peruvian adults, ciprofloxacin 250 mg once-daily for 3 days was comparable in clinical and bacteriologic efficacy, and safety, with standard therapy with teracycline 500 mg four-times daily for 3 days. A good/excellent outcome was achieved in 84% and 89%, respectively. Ciprofloxacin may therefore represent an alternative to tetracyclines in areas where multiresistant strains of *V. cholerae* O1 are common (Gotuzzo *et al.*, 1995). Interestingly, a single 250 mg dose of ciprofloxacin did not prevent *V. cholerae* O1 infection or diarrhea among household contacts of patients with proven cholera in Peru. However, this study was statistically underpowered to show anything more than a major therapeutic effect, since it was conducted during a period of low transmissibility. Nevertheless, any perceived benefits of such antibiotic use would need to be weighed against the potential risks of encouraging the development of ciprofloxacin-resistant strains (Echevarria *et al.*, 1995).

e   Acute diarrhea of unknown etiology   Empiric treatment of adults with acute diarrhea of unknown etiology with norfloxacin 400 mg twice-daily or three times daily for 5 days results in clinical cure in 89–91%, compared with 78% cure with trimethoprim–sulfamethoxazole (DuPont *et al.*, 1987a). Similar results have been noted with ciprofloxacin (Goodman *et al.*, 1990). The presence of fecal leukocytes is associated with a higher cure rate, presumably because they are indicative of the presence of an invasive bacterial pathogen (Harris *et al.*, 1972). Anecdotal reports suggest that ciprofloxacin is effective therapy for *Aeromonas hydrophila* gastroenteritis (Nathwani *et al.*, 1991), while norfloxacin (3-day course) is effective in clearing intestinal carriage of *Aeromonas* spp., *Plesiomonas shigelloides* and *Vibrio* spp; although the effect on clinical outcome is less clear (Lolekha *et al.*, 1988). Ciprofloxacin has proven effective in limited studies of *Yersinia enterocolitica* infection (Hoogkamp-Korstanje 1987; Read and Barry 1990).

Ciprofloxacin is effective in reducing the severity and duration of diarrhea due to *Campylobacter jejuni*. Pichler *et al.* (1987) noted a reduction in duration of diarrhea from 2.2 days for 11 placebo-treated patients to 1.1 days for 19 ciprofloxacin-treated patients (p < 0.01). However, increasing reports of *in vitro* resistance to ciprofloxacin, including its development during therapy, and associated clinical treatment failures raises doubts about the long term usefulness of fluoroquinolones for intestinal campylobacteriosis (p. 993; Rao 1991).

4 Osteomyelitis

The excellent bone penetration of fluoroquinolones such as ciprofloxacin, ofloxacin and pefloxacin, in association with their antibacterial spectrum of activity make them ideal agents for use against osteomyelitis due to Enterobacteriaceae, and most *Ps. aeruginosa* strains. Some caution is generally required however, when considering their use for osteomyelitis secondary to *Staph. aureus* (Norrby 1989; Lew and Waldvogel 1993). Ciprofloxacin, generally in a dose of 750 mg twice-daily for greater than 2 months, results in clinical and bacteriological success after 6 months follow-up in about 61–80% of patients with osteomyelitis due to *Ps. aeruginosa* or *Staph. aureus*; although when used alone, the emergence of resistant *Staph. aureus* strains has been noted (p. 994) (Greenberg *et al.*, 1987a; Desplaces and Acar 1988; Swedish Study Group, 1988; Hoogkamp-Korstanje *et al.*, 1989; Norrby, 1989; Wispelwey and Scheld 1990).

A number of studies of ciprofloxacin use against osteomyelitis have combined outcome results from patients with both Gram-positive and Gram-negative pathogens, and patients with and without diabetes. Nix *et al.* (1987) noted resolution or improvement in 84% of patients with osteomyelitis in non-diabetics, 79% in patients with infections in diabetics and a good microbiological outcome in 75%. Greenberg *et al.* (1987b) found 24 of 26 patients with osteomyelitis without a prosthesis, responded initially to ciprofloxacin therapy, but after 1 year of follow-up only 14 of 22 were cured (64%), while the others either failed treatment or relapsed. Infection with MRSA was commonly associated with treatment failure or relapse. However, variables such as whether the osteomyelitis is acute or chronic, the adequacy of bone debridement and vascular supply, the presence of foreign bodies such as joint prothesis or fixation devices, presence of sensory neuropathy and the susceptibility profile of the infecting pathogen(s) all impact on the success of fluoroquinolone therapy in this setting. For instance, in the study by Peterson *et al.* (1989) of 29 patients with lower limb osteomyelitis in association with peripheral vascular disease and/or diabetes, long-term (about 90 days) oral ciprofloxacin 750–1000 mg twice-daily resulted in 1 year clinical success of 65%, with bacteriological eradication of *Staph. aureus* of only 57%, but 83% for *Ps. aeruginosa*. However, caution is required in interpreting these results, since cure of osteomyelitis with antibiotics alone and no debridement of infected bone is often extremely difficult in patients with diabetes (Grayson *et al.*, 1994; Grayson, 1995).

Gentry and Rodriguez (1990) compared oral ciprofloxacin monotherapy with directed parenteral treatment in a randomized trial of 59 patients in which all infections were surgically debrided, foreign bodies removed and bone biopsy cultures were taken to optimize choice of antibiotics. Although the 2-year success rate was 77% for oral ciprofloxacin versus 79% for conventional parenteral treatment, persistent infection with *Staph. aureus* was a problem for some ciprofloxacin-treated patients. Other authors have shown similar efficacy with oral ciprofloxacin, ofloxacin and pefloxacin against Gram-negative pathogens but with some limitations for treatment of staphylococcal infections (Greenberg *et al.*, 1987b; Desplaces and Acar 1988; Ketterl *et al.*, 1988; Dellamonica *et al.*, 1989; Lew and Waldvogel 1990; Gentry and Rodriguez-Gomez 1991). New agents, such as sparfloxacin, with greater activity against *Staph. aureus* than ciprofloxacin, may provide more reliable activity in osteomyelitis due to staphylococci, especially if given in combination with rifampicin (Lew and Waldvogel 1993).

Among studies that have examined the efficacy of ciprofloxacin for osteomyelitis due to Gram-negative pathogens such as *Ps. aeruginosa*, 750 mg twice-daily for 6–24 weeks is generally recommended and results in long-term cure rates of 61–65%. These studies include a combination of both acute and chronic osteomyelitis in a variety of anatomic sites (Gilbert *et al.*, 1987; Lesse *et al.*, 1987; Swedish Study Group 1988).

Few authors have studied the efficacy of ciprofloxacin purely in acute osteomyelitis. In 20 selected patients with acute and subacute *Ps. aeruginosa* osteomyelitis treated with 750 mg twice-daily for 4–17 weeks (mean 12 weeks) and followed for a mean of 27 months, cure was achieved in 19 of 20 patients (95%) (Dan *et al.*, 1990). In a small study of selected patients, Brouqui *et al.* (1995) cured nine of nine patients with *Ps. aeruginosa*-infected osteosynthetic material with a combination of ceftazidime and ciprofloxacin but without removal of the prosthetic material. A variety of therpeutic protocols were used, but generally treatment consisted of ceftazidime 3 g per day i.v. and ciprofloxacin 750 mg orally twice-daily for 6 weeks, then the same ciprofloxacin dose for a further 6 months. Widmer *et al.* (1992) has also reported success with combination of fluoroquinolones + rifampicin therapy in a small study of orthopaedic device-related infections due to staphylococci or streptococci in which the implant was not removed. However, cure is generally only achievable with removal of the foreign body. Otherwise, long-term suppressive is currently advocated.

No large studies have investigated the efficacy of ciprofloxacin in the treatment of septic arthritis, however, numerous clinical reports of successful therapy, especially with Gram-negative pathogens such as salmonellae have encouraged their use in this setting (Greenberg *et al.*, 1987a; Diaz Tejeiro *et al.*, 1989; Praet *et al.*, 1989; Widmer *et al.*, 1990). Ciprofloxacin was ineffective in a patient with systemic lupus erythematosus and septic arthritis due to *Mycoplasma hominis*. However, cure was achieved with a combination of temafloxacin plus doxycycline, arthroscopic drainage, discontinuation of corticosteroid therapy and i.v. infusions of immunoglobulin (Clough *et al.*, 1992).

5 Soft tissue and skin infections

Fluoroquinolones such as ciprofloxacin and ofloxacin are suitable for the treatment of skin and soft tissue infections due to Gram-negative pathogens, including *Ps. aeruginosa*, but are generally not the optimal choice for Gram-positive pathogens such as *Staphylococcus* or *Streptococcus* spp. (Wood and Logan 1986; Gentry 1993). Numerous non-comparative open studies of oral ciprofloxacin 500–750 mg twice-daily for 5–10 days for the treatment of wound infections, abscesses, cellulitis and infected ulcers due to a variety of Gram-positive and/or Gram-negative pathogens suggest an overall efficacy of 77–81% and a superinfection rate of about 8% (Fass, 1986; Scully and Neu, 1986; Wood and Logan 1986; Licitra et al., 1987; Valainis et al., 1987; Greenberg et al., 1987a; Pien and Yamane, 1987; Self et al., 1987; Gorkiewicz-Petkow et al., 1988; Peterson et al., 1989; Valtonen et al., 1989; Gentry 1993). However, the non-comparative study design, lack of observer blinding and small patient numbers in many of these studies make the formulation of specific recommendations difficult.

Randomized, prospective and generally double-blind trials of hospitalized patients with difficult-to-treat soft tissue/skin infections comparing sequential i.v. then oral (500–750 mg twice-daily) ciprofloxacin with cephalosporins such as cefotaxime or ceftazidime suggest reasonably comparable efficacy of approximately 75–85% (Parish and Asper 1987; Perez-Ruvalcaba et al., 1987; Ramirez-Ronda et al., 1987; Dominguez et al., 1989; Fass et al., 1989; Gentry et al., 1989; Gentry and Koshdel 1989; Tice et al., 1990). In a number of these studies vancomycin and anti-anaerobic antibiotics were given in combination with these agents if Gram-positive or anaerobic pathogens were identified; alternatively, patients with these infections were excluded (Gentry and Koshdel 1989; Gentry et al., 1989; Tice et al., 1990). Treatment failures were generally associated with the presence of chronic infection in both treatment groups. Ciprofloxacin has proven effective for infections occurring in the setting of peripheral vascular disease, diabetes, oncology and geriatric populations which are traditionally more difficult to treat (Parish and Asper 1987; Haron et al., 1989; Peterson et al., 1989; Yangco et al., 1989). Ofloxacin (200–400 mg twice-daily) has shown similar efficacy to ciprofloxacin in comparable clinical trials. However, the predominance of open, non-randomized, non-comparative studies limit the formulation of specific recommendations (Fritzen et al., 1986; Gentry et al., 1989; Lentino et al., 1991). Oral ciprofloxacin (generally 750 mg twice-daily for 7–14 days) is effective in the treatment of nail puncture wounds of the foot in which infection with Ps. aeruginosa is common (Raz and Miron, 1995).

Pathogens commonly identified as failing treatment with either ciprofloxacin or ofloxacin are Staph. aureus (especially MRSA), coagulase-negative staphylococci, enterococci, and some resistant strains of Ps. aeruginosa (Scully and Neu, 1986; Oppenheim et al., 1989; Peterson et al., 1989; Kotilainen et al., 1990; Gentry 1993). Nevertheless, the convenience of oral fluoroquinolones in the treatment of soft tissue and skin infections (especially due to Gram-negative pathogens) are important clinical and economic features favoring the increasing use of these agents in this setting.

6 Sexually transmitted diseases

For bacterial sexually transmitted diseases other than uncomplicated gonorrhea, fluoroquinolones are not the drugs of first choice, however, they are recommended as alternative regimens for chancroid, chlamydia and some cases of pelvic inflammatory disease (CDC, 1993b).

a Chlamydia infection The treatment of urethritis and sexually transmitted diseases due to C. trachomatis is complicated by a number of factors. Firstly, the biphasic life cycle of the pathogen in which the elementary body (the infectious intracellular form) is metabolically inert and therefore not susceptible to antibiotics which require protein or DNA synthesis for activity is an important feature. Secondly, in the host cell the reticulate body of the organism multiples inside a membrane-bound inclusion, which must be penetrated by the antibiotic if it is to be effective. In addition, Chlamydia's long life cycle of 48–72 h means that adequate drug concentrations must be maintained for a number of days. Thus, prolonged treatment courses are generally needed to achieve suitable efficacy (Pocidalo, 1990; Peeling and Ronald, 1993). An exception to this is the new macrolide azithromycin, where a single 1-g dose achieves excellent efficacy and is now the drug of choice for this condition in many countries (Stamm, 1991; CDC 1993b). In vitro susceptibility testing techniques for Chlamydia are not standardized, however, the newer fluoroquinolones such as sparfloxacin and tosufloxacin appear to be more active than agents such as ciprofloxacin or norfloxacin (Ehret and Judson, 1988; Peeling and Ronald, 1993). Ciprofloxacin is associated with cure rates of 45–81% for genital chlamydial infections, with some authors claiming that higher doses (e.g. 750–1000 mg twice-daily) for longer periods (e.g. 7–14 days) are associated with better outcomes (Fong et al., 1987; Ahmed-Jushuf et al., 1988; Bishoff and Bishoff, 1989; Hooton et al., 1990). Ciprofloxacin is similar to doxycycline (100 mg twice-daily for 7 days) in efficacy when there is mixed infection with C. trachomatis and Ureaplasma urealyticum, but doxycycline is superior in patients with chlamydial infections alone (Fong *et al.*, 1987). In fact, Hooton *et al.* (1990) found the recurrence rate of *C. trachomatis* was so common (38–52%) with ciprofloxacin therapy that they concluded that doses as high as 2 g daily were inadequate for the treatment of chlamydial urethritis in men. Better rates of cure (90–100%) have been achieved with ofloxacin (generally 200–300 mg twice-daily for 7 days), while the efficacy of fleroxacin appears to be between that of ciprofloxacin and ofloxacin. Single-dose therapy with ciprofloxacin or fleroxacin is not effective against *C. trachomatis* genital infections (Avonts *et al.*, 1988; Lassus *et al.*, 1988; Peeling and Ronald, 1993).

b　Gonorrhea　Not surprisingly, given the excellent *in vitro* activity of fluoroquinolones against *N. gonorrhoeae* (p. 983), agents such as ciprofloxacin, norfloxacin, fleroxacin and ofloxacin are very effective as single-dose therapy for gonococcal infections, with cure rates approaching 100% (Lassus *et al.*, 1989; Hook *et al.*, 1993; Peeling and Ronald, 1993). Ciprofloxacin is generally associated with ratios of serum concentration to MIC_{90} of ≥100-fold. The clinical experience with fluoroquinolones and gonorrhea has been well summarized by Peeling and Ronald (1993). The usual recommended regimens include single-dose treatment with either oral ciprofloxacin 500 mg, ofloxacin 400 mg, cefixime 400 mg or intramuscular ceftriaxone 125 mg, which are effective against both penicillinase-producing and tetracycline-resistant *N. gonorrhoeae* (CDC, 1993b). Hook *et al.* (1993) found that oral ciprofloxacin 250 mg cured 100% of women with cervical gonorrhea versus 99% treated with ceftriaxone, and that both regimens were 100% effective for difficult-to-treat sites such as pharyngeal and rectal infection. Coker *et al.* (1989) and Bryan *et al.* (1990) found similar results, including among HIV-infected patients. Fluoroquinolones for longer treatment periods are also effective against disseminated gonococcal infection and gonococcal arthritis (Ramirez *et al.*, 1985). Echols *et al.* (1994) note in their review that 250 mg single-dose ciprofloxacin results in similar excellent efficacy as 500 mg for uncomplicated gonorrhoea, including extragenital sites of infection. Nevertheless, resistance to fluoroquinolones among *N. gonorrhoeae* strains and associated clinical treatment failure is being reported increasingly in some regions (Tapsall *et al.*, 1992; CDC, 1994; p. 993). Since at least one-third of patients with genital gonococcal infections will have concomitant chlamydial infection, a 7-day course of doxycycline 100 mg twice-daily is also recommended (CDC, 1993b; Peeling and Ronald, 1993).

c　Chancroid　Due to the increasing resistance of *H. ducreyi* to various antibiotics (p. 867), CDC (1993b) recommends treatment with either a single-dose of oral azithromycin 1g or i.m. ceftriaxone 250 mg, or a 7-day course of erythromycin 500 mg four-times daily. Alternative regimens include ciprofloxacin 500 mg twice-daily for 3 days or amoxicillin 500 mg plus clavulanic acid 125 mg thrice-daily for 7 days (CDC, 1993b). The combination of increasing antibiotic resistance and the fact that cure rates are lower in HIV-infected patients make such routine regimens less reliable, especially in regions where HIV infection is common (MacDonald *et al.*, 1989; Dangor *et al.*, 1990; Schmid, 1990; Peeling and Ronald, 1993; Tyndall *et al.*, 1993; Bogaerts *et al.*, 1995). *In vitro*, *H. ducreyi* is very susceptible to fluoroquinolones (p. 983) and no fluoroquinolone-resistance has yet been reported. One or two oral doses of ciprofloxacin (500 mg or 1-g single-dose) is effective, but more reliable results (100%) are achieved with 500 mg twice-daily for 3 days (Naamara *et al.*, 1987; Bodhidatta *et al.*, 1988; Ballard *et al.*, 1989). In a double-blind randomized trial comparing single-dose ciprofloxacin (500 mg) and a 3-day regimen (500 mg twice-daily) with a 3-day regimen of trimethoprim–sulfamethoxazole (160/800 mg twice-daily) for the treatment of chancroid in Nairobi males attending a sexually transmitted disease clinic, Naamara *et al.* (1987) found the 3-day ciprofloxacin regimen eradicated *H. ducreyi* and resulted in rapid clinical improvement in all 40 patients, with no treatment failures. Bacteriologic and clinical failure was noted in two of 41 patients treated with single-dose ciprofloxacin and three of 41 patients treated with trimethoprim–sulfamethoxazole. All patients with buboes noted resolution. Similarly, Bogaerts *et al.* (1995) have noted excellent rates of cure in Rwanda with a single dose of ciprofloxcain 500 mg in a setting where HIV infection is common. In Thailand, Bodhidatta *et al.* (1988) found single-dose therapy with 500 mg ciprofloxacin produced similar excellent efficacy (98–100%) to two doses of 500 mg, 12 h apart in culture-positive Thai men. Notably, however, this study was undertaken at a time when HIV infection was less of a problem than it is currently in South-East Asia.

Fleroxacin (200 mg or 400 mg) single-dose therapy is 83–100% effective overall, with lower rates in HIV-positive patients (MacDonald *et al.*, 1989; Miller *et al.*, 1989; Plourde *et al.*, 1991). The lack of emergence of resistance to fluoroquinolones and the efficacy of single-dose or short-course treatment make these agents a useful treatment option against chancroid.

d Syphilis The fluoroquinolones are ineffective against *Trepenoma pallidum* in animals (p. 989) and have no role in the clinical treatment of syphilis in humans. Targeted therapy against this pathogen therefore needs to be considered in mixed sexually transmitted infections where fluoroquinolones are likely to be selected for use against other diseases such as gonorrhoea or chancroid.

e Pelvic inflammatory disease Most treatment of pelvic inflammatory disease is empiric since accurate identification of the pathogen(s) involved is often inadequate. The majority of infections (60–80%) include *N. gonorrhoeae* and/or *C. trachomatis*, while Enterobacteriaceae and anaerobes are also common (Mardh and Lowing, 1990; CDC, 1993b; Peeling and Ronald, 1993). The continued recommendation by the CDC is combination treatment with either cefoxitin (or cefotetan) + 14 days treatment with doxycycline, or clindamycin + gentamicin. Ofloxacin 400 mg orally twice-daily for 14 days + clindamycin 450 mg orally four-times daily, or metronidazole 500 mg twice-daily for 14 days is recommended as an alternative regimen in the outpatient setting. Ciprofloxacin monotherapy has been prospectively studied in at least five randomized clinical trials of pelvic inflammatory disease, when cure rates of 82–100% were noted. However, variability in diagnostic criteria and identification of responsible pathogens in these studies, the lack of ciprofloxacin activity against anaerobes and the variable efficacy of ciprofloxacin against *C. trachomatis* augur some caution when considering the use of ciprofloxacin monotherapy for this disease (Apuzzio *et al.*, 1989; Crombleholme *et al.*, 1989; Heinonen *et al.*, 1989; Hoyme *et al.*, 1989; Fishbach *et al.*, 1991). Crombleholme *et al.* (1989) reported clinical resolution in 31 of 33 (94%) patients treated with ciprofloxacin monotherapy compared with 34 of 35 (97%) treated with a combination of clindamycin + gentamicin. In all cases *N. gonorrhoeae* was eradicated, but ciprofloxacin failed to clear one of seven cases with *C. trachomatis* and was less effective in eradicating bacterial vaginosis-associated organisms. Clinical response was comparable in the two treatment groups.

Ofloxacin appears to be more effective than ciprofloxacin, achieving cure rates of 97–100%, especially when combined with amoxicillin-clavulanic acid to provide adequate anaerobic cover (Verhoest *et al.*, 1989; Judlin *et al.*, 1991; Wendel *et al.*, 1991). However, outside the outpatient setting when the excellent oral absorption of fluoroquinolones such as ofloxacin is an important consideration, there appears to be little reason to change from the tried-and-trusted combinations recommended by CDC (1993b).

7 Respiratory tract infections

The excellent activity of ciprofloxacin and other fluoroquinolones against potential respiratory pathogens such as *H. influenzae*, *Moraxella catarrhalis*, *Legionella* spp., *Kl. pneumoniae*, *Enterobacter* species, *E. coli* and most strains of *Ps. aeruginosa*, makes these agents an appropriate choice for the treatment of Gram-negative respiratory infections, including nosocomial pneumonia (p. 981). However, efficacy against *Burkholderia cepacia* and *Acinetobacter* spp. is limited (p. 982). Ofloxacin, and especially sparfloxacin, are more active against *Mycoplasma pneumoniae*, *Chlamydia pneumoniae* and *Mycobacterium tuberculosis* than ciprofloxacin (pp. 1112, 1136). The generally high penetration of fluoroquinolones into sputum and excellent penetration into respiratory secretions and pulmonary tissue are an important characteristic. As noted earlier (p. 1005), however, the activity of ciprofloxacin and ofloxacin against Gram-positive respiratory pathogens such as *Strep. pneumoniae*, *Strep. pyogenes*, and *Staph. aureus* are borderline, while sparfloxacin is more reliable against streptococcal spp. (p. 1135). Indeed, pneumococcal bacteremia and meningitis have occurred during ciprofloxacin treatment (Cooper and Lawlor, 1989; Lee *et al.*, 1991; Körner *et al.*, 1994). Numerous comparative and open clinical studies of oral ciprofloxacin 500–750 mg twice-daily, or 100–200 mg i.v. twice-daily followed by oral therapy, have demonstrated clinical efficacy of generally 80–98% in acute and chronic bronchitis and/or pneumonia (Ernst *et al.*, 1986; Gleadhill *et al.*, 1986; Hoogkampe-Korstanje and Klein, 1986; Crysanthopoulos *et al.*, 1987; Bantz *et al.*, 1987; Fass, 1987; Kobayashi, 1987; Lode *et al.*, 1987; Wollschlager *et al.*, 1987; Salvati *et al.*, 1988; Haddow *et al.*, 1989; Levine *et al.*, 1989; Schmidt *et al.*, 1989; Trenholme *et al.*, 1989; Davey, 1991; Thys *et al.*, 1991; Scully, 1993). In this disease, oral ciprofloxacin 500–750 mg twice-daily appears to have clinical efficacy comparable with trimethoprim–sulfamethoxazole, doxycycline, ampicillin, cephalexin, cefamandole, cefaclor, amoxicillin or amoxicillin–clavulanate, with superior efficacy (90–100%) against most Gram-negative infections (Gleadhill *et al.*, 1986; Bantz *et al.*, 1987; Wollschlager *et al.*, 1987; Peterson *et al.*, 1988; Chodosh *et al.*, 1989; Pederson, 1989; Schmidt *et al.*, 1989; Quenzer *et al.*, 1990; Chodosh, 1991). Persistence and relapse with *Ps. aeruginosa*, including the development of ciprofloxacin-resistance has been well described (Fass, 1987; Jensen *et al.*, 1987a; Chodosh *et al.*, 1989; Peloquin *et al.*, 1989; Chodosh, 1991). Nevertheless, ciprofloxacin has proven effective in most patient groups, including smokers, the elderly and patients with chronic hepatitis. Esposito *et al.* (1987b) reported success in 19 of 20 patients with bronchitis treated with oral ciprofloxacin 250 mg twice-daily who had severe impairment of liver function secondary to chronic hepatitis, cirrhosis or neoplasm. Prolonged ciprofloxacin therapy appears to be successful for the treatment of *Ps. aeruginosa* lung abscess (Lubitz, 1990).

In comparison with imipenem or ceftazidime, ciprofloxacin 100–200 mg i.v. twice-daily changing to oral therapy when improved, has comparable or better clinical efficacy (71–100%; generally 91–100%) in seriously ill patients with nosocomial or community-acquired pneumonia or bronchitis (Lode *et al.*, 1987, 1990b; Haddow *et al.*, 1989; Khann and Basir, 1989; Levine *et al.*, 1989; Menon *et al.*, 1989; Trenholme *et al.*, 1989). Higher doses, such as 400 mg i.v. twice-daily, would often now be considered more appropriate but there are no specific data to support this. However, persistence of *Ps. aeruginosa* strains, including the development of resistance, remains a potential problem with intravenous ciprofloxacin – a problem that higher doses and combinations of ciprofloxacin with other agents may help to avoid.

Fink *et al.* (1994) compared monotherapy with ciprofloxacin (400 mg i.v. 8-hourly) versus imipenem (1000 mg i.v. 8-hourly) in a prospective, randomized, double-blind, multicentre trial of 312 patients with severe pneumonia. The majority of these patients had Gram-negative pathogens, required mechanical ventilation (79%) and had nosocomial pneumonia (78%). Ciprofloxacin-treated patients had a significantly higher clinical response rate than did imipenem-treated patients (69% versus 56%; p = 0.02), and bacteriological eradication was also marginally higher (69% versus 59%; p = 0.07). Eradication of Enterobacteriaceae was most notable for ciprofloxacin compared with imipenem (93% versus 65%; p = 0.0009). Failure to eradicate *Ps. aeruginosa* and the development of resistance in this species during treatment was comparable in the two treatment groups. Similarly, comparable rates of eradication were noted for other pathogens such as *Strep. pneumoniae* and *Staph. aureus* (almost all were methicillin susceptible). Seizures were more common in the imipenem-treated group. Although the authors concluded that monotherapy with either ciprofloxacin or imipenem is a safe and effective initial strategy in patients with severe pneumonia (except when *Ps. aeruginosa* is isolated), it should be noted that the trial required that all pretreatment isolates were susceptible to both study agents. Thus, depending on the local incidence of various nosocomial pathogens and their patterns of resistance, combination therapy, at least including vancomycin, should generally be considered (Wood, 1994).

In the limited clinical studies available, i.v. ciprofloxacin appears to be effective for *Legionella pneumonia*, but whether the addition of ciprofloxacin to erythromycin improves the outcome in severe legionellosis as advocated by Winter *et al.* (1988) remains uncertain (Hooper *et al.*, 1988; Winter *et al.*, 1988; Unertl *et al.*, 1989). Unertl *et al.* (1989) reported ten patients with severe *Legionella pneumonia* (four *L. pneumophila*; six other *Legionella* species) who were generally treated with 200 mg i.v. twice-daily for 7–31 days (median 12 days). Treatment was successful in eight of ten cases, usually with improvement within a few days. Of the two non-responders, one had already failed prior erythromycin and rifampicin, and eventually died. The other patient had an orthotopic liver transplant, failed 9 days ciprofloxacin therapy, but responded to erythromycin. Of concern is the case reported by Kurz *et al.* (1988) in which a patient with severe *Legionella* pneumonia deteriorated despite 6 days therapy with 200 mg ciprofloxacin i.v. twice-daily (albeit ciprofloxacin was started late in the clinical illness).

Intravenous ciprofloxacin may be effective against *Bordetella bronchiseptica* pneumonia in patients with AIDS, although failures have also been reported (Chauncey and Schaberg, 1990; Amador *et al.*, 1991; Ng *et al.*, 1992; de la Fuente *et al.*, 1994). Ciprofloxacin was also effective in one case of pneumonia due to *Flavobacterium meningosepticum* in a neonate with renal failure (Humphreys *et al.*, 1989).

Thus, due to the availability of other effective agents, ciprofloxacin is not generally recommended for empiric treatment of community-acquired bronchitis/pneumonia, but it may be an appropriate choice for the treatment of nosocomial Gram-negative or multiresistant pneumonia.

Ofloxacin has similar efficacy and limitations as ciprofloxacin in the treatment of lower respiratory tract infections (Kromann-Andersen *et al.*, 1988; Scully, 1993). In addition, satisfactory responses in patients with community-acquired non-lobar pneumonia due to *M. pneumoniae* have been reported (Forsberg *et al.*, 1989; Scully, 1993). Due to the weak activity of pefloxacin against *Strep. pneumoniae*, this agent is best considered only for pneumonia due to Gram-negative or possibly *Legionella* pneumonia (p. 983). Lomefloxacin, tosufloxacin, temafloxacin, rufloxacin and fleroxacin are reasonably comparable with ciprofloxacin in efficacy but data is far more limited (Kosmidis, 1991; Lindsay *et al.*, 1992). Sparfloxacin, due to its improved activity against *Strep. pneumoniae* and long half-life allowing once-daily treatment, appears to have activity comparable with ofloxacin in limited studies of bronchitis and pneumonia (Scully, 1993; pp. 1123, 1140).

8 Respiratory infections in cystic fibrosis

The elimination of fluoroquinolones such as ciprofloxacin and ofloxacin in patients with cystic fibrosis is increased, such that higher doses (e.g. ciprofloxacin 500–750 mg thrice-daily; ofloxacin 400–600 mg twice-daily) are generally recommended (p. 998). As in other clinical conditions, oral ciprofloxacin provides comparable, or better, efficacy than the intravenous preparation, assuming adequate absorption. However, malabsorption is an important consideration in patients with cystic fibrosis. For susceptible pathogens, oral ciprofloxacin (generally 500 mg thrice-daily or 750 mg twice-daily or thrice-daily for 2–3 weeks) provides clinical efficacy (62–100%) comparable with combination intravenous regimens such as azlocillin + tobramycin, but most studies have been relatively small and/or open trials (Bosso *et al.*, 1987, 1989; Shalit *et al.*, 1987; Goldfarb *et al.*, 1987; Rubio, 1987; Scully *et al.*, 1987; Grenier, 1989; Strandvik *et al.*, 1989; LeBel, 1991). However, as expected in cystic fibrosis, infections due to *Ps. aeruginosa* and other pseudomonal species such as *Burkholderia cepacia* are often difficult to treat successfully and the development of resistance has been a problem – especially with prolonged treatment courses (e.g. >3 weeks) (Hodson *et al.*, 1987; Shalit *et al.*, 1987; Schaad *et al.*, 1989; Strandvik *et al.*, 1989). Shalit *et al.* (1987) noted 45% of *Ps. aeruginosa* isolates had developed resistance after 2 weeks treatment. However, this issue is complicated since persistence of respiratory colonization with *Ps. aeruginosa* is not infrequent despite clinical improvement with treatment. Comparable outcomes are achieved with both 750 mg twice-daily and 1000 mg twice-daily regimens. Scully (1993) recommends that courses of ciprofloxacin should be limited to 10–20 days and that ciprofloxacin should not be used to treat consecutive exacerbations.

Valerius *et al.* (1991) have found that chronic respiratory colonization with *Ps. aeruginosa* can be prevented by the early institution of oral ciprofloxacin and aerosol inhalations of colistin twice-daily for 3 weeks, once *Ps. aeruginosa* colonization of sputum is first detected. In this study, 26 patients who had never received anti-pseudomonal antibiotic therapy were randomized to receive either no chemotherapy, or oral ciprofloxacin (250–750 mg twice-daily) and inhalation of colistin 10^6 IU twice-daily for 3 weeks whenever *Ps. aeruginosa* was isolated from routine sputum cultures. Chronic *Ps. aeruginosa* colonization occurred in significantly fewer treated versus untreated patients, however the authors did not comment on whether this reduction in colonization translated into fewer, less severe pneumonic exacerbations sufficient to warrant the widespread use of this regimen.

Ofloxacin appears to be comparable with ciprofloxacin in the treatment of this patient group, despite its inferior *in vitro* anti-pseudomonal activity (Jensen *et al.*, 1987b; Scully *et al.*, 1991).

As in other clinical situations, the use of ciprofloxacin has been largely avoided in children younger than 12 years due to concerns regarding potential drug toxicity (p. 1011). However, Rubio (1990) treated a small number of children with cystic fibrosis with ciprofloxacin 20 mg per kg twice-daily for 21–76 days and noted no short-term evidence of arthropathy attributable to ciprofloxacin therapy.

9 Prevention of infection in neutropenic patients

While selective decontamination of the gastrointestinal tract with trimethoprim–sulfamethoxazole or nalidixic acid have produced mixed results in terms of potential benefit, fluoroquinolones have a number of favorable features that may overcome some of the limitations of these agents. Their excellent activity against greater than 90% of Enterobacteriaceae and *Ps. aeruginosa*, lack of anti-anaerobic activity, high fecal concentrations after oral administration, and lack of myelosuppression allow true selective decontamination and potential maintenance of 'colonization resistance', with suppression of aerobic Gram-negative bowel flora and preservation of anaerobes (Bergan *et al.*, 1986c; Reeves, 1986; Nord, 1988; van Saene *et al.*, 1988; Edlund and Nord, 1989; Meijer-Severs *et al.*, 1990; Imrie *et al.*, 1995). In the comprehensive summary of the literature to 1993 by Winston (1993b), fluoroquinolones (norfloxacin, ciprofloxacin, ofloxacin) were superior to placebo, trimethoprim–sulfamethoxazole and vancomycin + polymyxin in preventing the acquisition of Enterobacteriaceae and *Ps. aeruginosa*. Exceptions were non-*aeruginosa Pseudomonas* spp. and *Acinetobacter* spp. which colonized in fluoroquinolone-treated patients, but few infections were noted. Ciprofloxacin, norfloxacin, ofloxacin, pefloxacin and enoxacin have all been studied in patients receiving either conventional chemotherapy for hematologic malignancy or undergoing bone marrow transplantation. In the vast majority of these studies the patients receiving fluoroquinolone prophylaxis had fewer microbiologically proven infections than did control patients, with an overall incidence of 40% versus 59%, respectively. Fluoroquinolones were most effective in preventing Gram-negative bacteremia but had no significant impact on the number of Gram-positive bacteremias (19% fluoroquinolone-treated versus 35% controls). When Gram-negative bacteremia did occur, it was generally with fluoroquinolone-resistant *Ps. aeruginosa* or other *Pseudomonas* spp. (Cruciani *et al.*, 1989; Liang *et al.*, 1990; Archimbaud *et al.*, 1991; Kern and Kurrle, 1991). Most Gram-positive bacteremias in this setting are due to viridans group streptococci, coagulase negative staphylococci or MRSA – thus correlating with the poor activity of fluoroquinolones against these pathogens. Interestingly, no increase in the incidence of fungal infections has been noted and fluoroquinolones are generally well tolerated (Karp *et al.*, 1986; Dekker *et al.*, 1987; Bow *et al.*, 1988; Winston *et al.*, 1990; Archimbaud *et al.*, 1991; Kern and Kurrle, 1991; Talbot *et al.*, 1993). Jansen *et al.* (1994) recently found prophylaxis with ciprofloxacin 500 mg twice-daily to be superior to combination neomycin 250 mg four times daily + polymyxin B 100 mg four times daily + nalidixic acid 1000 mg twice-daily in severely neutropenic patients in terms of the overall incidence of bacteremia; although streptococcal bacteremias were frequent in both treatment arms. Side-effects were also similar in both treatment groups, but compliance with ciprofloxacin was better. Lew *et al.* (1995) found ciprofloxacin and trimethoprim–sulfamethoxazole to be equally safe and effective in the prevention of bacterial infections in bone marrow transplant patients when the overall infection rate was used as the primary endpoint, but trimethoprim–sulfamethoxazole prophylaxis was associated with a higher incidence of *Cl. difficile* colitis and infections caused by Gram-negative bacilli. Also, Imrie *et al.* (1995) found that antibiotic prophylaxis with ciprofloxacin resulted in more rapid neutrophil recovery than prophylaxis with trimethoprim–sulfamethoxazole following autologous bone marrow transplantation.

Studies comparing fluoroquinolones have produced conflicting results with some suggesting ciprofloxacin or ofloxacin to be superior to norfloxacin, some favoring norfloxacin, and others finding no difference between ciprofloxacin, ofloxacin and trimethoprim–sulfamethoxazole + colistin for preventing infection (Karp *et al.*, 1988; Maschmeyer *et al.*, 1988; Arning *et al.*, 1990; D'Antonio *et al.*, 1991; The GIMEMA infection program, 1991; Winston, 1993a). Most recently, D'Antonio *et al.* (1994) found ciprofloxacin 500 mg twice-daily to be superior to ofloxacin 300 mg twice-daily and pefloxacin 400 mg twice-daily in the prevention of bacterial infections in a randomized trial of neutropenic patients with hematological malignancies. In this trial all patients also received fluconazole 150 mg daily to prevent fungal infection.

Overall, the most common dose of ciprofloxacin used for prophylaxis in neutropenic patients has been 500 mg twice-daily.

Although combinations of a fluoroquinolone with agents with Gram-positive activity (e.g. erythromycin, roxythromycin, penicillin) reduce the incidence of streptococcal bacteremia, staphylococcal bacteremia remains a problem unless vancomycin is used. However, most clinicians have concerns regarding the routine use of i.v. vancomycin as prophylaxis, due to the growing emergence of vancomycin-resistant nosocomial pathogens such as vancomycin-resistant enterococci (pp. 764–5).

10 Treatment of febrile neutropenic patients

Monotherapy with i.v. ciprofloxacin in febrile neutropenic patients is effective, but has been associated with a higher incidence of Gram-positive superinfections than that noted with routine combinations such as an anti-pseudomonal penicillin + an aminoglycoside, or ceftazidime monotherapy (Bayston *et al.*, 1989; Lim *et al.*, 1990; Meunier *et al.*, 1991; Johnson *et al.*, 1992). However, when fluoroquinolones are used in combination with agents with Gram-positive cover, the outcomes have been good. Ciprofloxacin + azlocillin, piperacillin or penicillin have produced similar outcomes (33–59% response rate to documented infections) to a combination of an aminoglycoside + anti-pseudomonal beta-lactam (piperacillin, azlocillin, ceftazidime) in a number of studies (42–52% response) (Flaherty *et al.*, 1989; Kelsey *et al.*, 1990; Philpott-Howard *et al.*, 1990; Hyatt *et al.*, 1991; Samuelsson *et al.*, 1992). In one trial, ciprofloxacin + netilmicin was as effective as piperacillin + netilmicin, but this fluoroquinolone-aminoglycoside combination would not usually be expected to avoid the potential problem of propensity for Gram-positive infections (Chan *et al.*, 1989). Teicoplanin + ciprofloxacin was significantly more effective than gentamicin + piperacillin in one study in which infection with *Staph. epidermidis* was common (Kelsey *et al.*, 1992). The better toxicity profile of ciprofloxacin over aminoglycosides has led some clinicians to view ciprofloxacin as an aminoglycoside substitute, but more clinical data is required before this can be assumed. Furthermore, the high cost of i.v. ciprofloxacin compared with most aminoglycosides needs to be balanced against the potential theoretic benefits of reduced toxicity and the large clinical experience of reliable and generally predictable activity of aminoglycosides in serious situations such as Gram-negative bacteremia.

A number of studies have examined the role of oral fluoroquinolones (ciprofloxacin or pefloxacin) as empiric outpatient therapy for febrile neutropenic patients, with promising results. However, more experience is necessary before this treatment modality can be recommended in place of routine inpatient treatment with parenteral antibiotics (Haron *et al.*, 1989; Rubenstein *et al.*, 1990; Gardembas-Pain *et al.*, 1991).

11 Endocarditis

Despite promising data from animal studies regarding the efficacy of ciprofloxacin and other fluoroquinolones against endocarditis secondary to *Ps. aeruginosa*, *Enterobacter aerogenes*, *E. coli*, *Staph. epidermidis* and *Staph. aureus*, there are relatively little human data available (Fernandez-Guerrero *et al.*, 1988; Kaatz *et al.*, 1989; Rouse *et al.*, 1990; Yeaman and Bayer, 1993). Most notable, has been the open, non-randomized study by Dworkin *et al.* (1989) in which 10 intravenous drug addicts with *Staph. aureus* tricuspid valve endocarditis were treated predominantly with an oral combination of ciprofloxacin 750 mg twice-daily + rifampicin 600 mg daily for 3–4 weeks, after a brief course of intravenous antibiotics. All 10 patients were cured at 4 week follow-up post-therapy. Regardless of these excellent results, the fact that right-sided endocarditis is generally more easily cured than at other sites, the small number of patients in the trial and the fact that therapy with ciprofloxacin alone has been associated with the rapid development of resistance in *Staph. aureus* in such high inoculum infections, all raise concerns regarding the application of these results to other clinical situations (Gomez-Jimenez *et al.*, 1989; Trucksis *et al.*, 1991). In particular, ciprofloxacin-resistance has been frequently noted in MRSA strains (p. 994). Thus, such oral regimens have not gained widespread acceptance in the treatment of endocarditis.

Ciprofloxacin is only partially effective in endocarditis secondary to *Ps. aeruginosa*, but long-term oral suppressive therapy has been used successfully (Breuer *et al.*, 1988; Daikos *et al.*, 1988; Uzun *et al.*, 1992).

Ciprofloxacin appears to be useful in the treatment of acute and chronic Q fever when given in combination with doxycycline + rifampicin. Effective long-term suppressive therapy with ciprofloxacin alone has also been reported (Yebra *et al.*, 1990). Levy *et al.* (1991). compared various antibiotic combinations in the treatment of chronic Q fever endocarditis and found doxycycline (100 mg twice-daily) in combination with either ofloxacin (200 mg twice-daily) or pefloxacin (400 mg daily) resulted in reduction in mortality. However, these combinations did not decrease the need for cardiac valve replacement and did not achieve eradication of *C. burnetii* from cardiac tissue despite up to 12 months therapy. Thus, the recommended duration of such antibiotic therapy is 24–36 months, in addition to the frequent need for valve replacement (Levy *et al.*, 1991; Yeaman and Bayer, 1993).

Cases of successful therapy with ciprofloxacin for endocarditis due to *Erysipelothrix rhusiopathiae*, *Serratia* spp., vancomycin-resistant *Corynebacterium* spp. and *Haemophilus aphrophilus* have been reported (Barnass *et al.*, 1991; Ena *et al.*, 1991; MacGowan *et al.*, 1991; Dawson and White, 1992).

12 Meningitis

Fluoroquinolones penetrate well into CSF (p. 1006) but very few human studies have examined their role in the treatment of meningitis. The limited/poor activity of these agents against pneumococci, staphylococci and *L. monocytogenes* mean currently available fluoroquinolones are inappropriate first-line empiric therapy in patients with meningitis of unknown etiology, and are unlikely to supplant conventional regimens of beta-lactams or chloramphenicol. Indeed, pneumonococcal meningitis has been noted in a patient while receiving i.v. ciprofloxacin (Righter, 1990). Nevertheless, fluoroquinolones have a potentially important role in the treatment of meningitis due to multiresistant Gram-negative pathogens such as *Ps. aeruginosa*, or difficult-to-treat Gram-negative pathogens such as salmonellae. No comparative studies of fluor-oquinolone activity in meningitis have been undertaken, however, case reports of ciprofloxacin and pefloxacin usage suggest good efficacy (73–90%) in most Gram-negative meningitis patients (Norrby, 1988; Schönwald *et al.*, 1989; Segev *et al.*, 1990; Modai, 1991; Tunkel and Scheld, 1993). Schönwald *et al.* (1989) treated 20 patients with trauma, surgery-related, or pneumonia-associated bacterial meningitis with ciprofloxacin 200 mg i.v. twice-daily for 10 days. Pathogens included *E. coli*, *P. mirabilis*, *Kl. pneumoniae*, *Ps. aeruginosa*, *E. cloacae* and

A. calcoaceticus. Two patients received concomitant penicillin and cefotaxime. Eighteen patients (90%) were cured.

Case reports of successful ciprofloxacin therapy in ventriculitis and meningitis due to *Ps. aeruginosa, Salm. typhimurium, E. cloacae, E. coli* and *Flavobacterium meningosepticum* are notable (Isaacs *et al.*, 1986; Millar *et al.*, 1986; Norrby, 1988; Bannon *et al.*, 1989; Ragunathan *et al.*, 1990; Goepp *et al.*, 1992; Green *et al.*, 1993). A 4-week course of oral ciprofloxacin has also been used to successfully treat a brain abscess due to *H. parainfluenzae* following a two week course of i.v. ceftriaxone (Visvanathan and Jones, 1991).

Newer fluoroquinolones such as levofloxacin and temafloxacin which have improved activity against pneumococci compared with ciprofloxacin, all show promise in rabbit meningitis models, but clinical human experience is currently lacking (Nau *et al.*, 1995).

Ciprofloxacin is 92–96% effective in clearing nasopharyngeal carriage of *N. meningitidis* with doses ranging from single-doses of 500–750 mg to 250 mg twice-daily (Renkonen *et al.*, 1987; Dworzack *et al.*, 1988; Gaunt and Lambert, 1988; Pugsley *et al.*, 1988). In a placebo-controlled trial of army recruits in Finland in which 56 with positive nasopharyngeal cultures were treated with ciprofloxacin and 53 were treated with placebo, nasopharyngeal carriage was reduced by 96% at day 8 versus 13% for placebo. Similarly, the results of single-dose regimens (500–750 mg) are impressive and given their simplicity, are clinically more attractive. In a placebo-controlled, randomized, double-blinded study of single-dose ciprofloxacin 750 mg, Dworzack *et al.* (1988) found 96% of ciprofloxacin-treated patients remained culture-negative 21 days post-dose compared with 9% among placebo recipients. Gaunt and Lambert (1988) found similar results with a single 500 mg dose during an outbreak of group C meningococcal meningitis at a military training camp. Cuevas *et al.* (1995), in a large comparative study in Malawi, found eradication rates to be similar for rifampicin, ciprofloxacin and ceftriaxone. Given these data, single-dose therapy with either 500 mg or 750 mg oral ciprofloxacin is a reasonable alternative to rifampicin for the clearance of meningococcal carriage. Oral ciprofloxacin should theoretically be effective in the elimination of nasopharyngeal carriage of *H. influenzae* (p. 983) but there are no clinical trials to confirm this hypothesis.

13 Staphylococcal infections

Ciprofloxacin has been used in the treatment of *Staph. aureus* infections, especially MRSA, but as noted elsewhere (p. 994), this should be discouraged due to the ready development of fluoroquinolone-resistance in this species. A number of authors who treated patients with MRSA infection and/or colonization with ciprofloxacin 750 mg twice-daily for 5–21 days obtained bacteriologic eradication in 40–79% of cases and clinical cure or improvement in up to 91% of patients (Mulligan *et al.*, 1987; Piercy *et al.*, 1989a; Smith *et al.*, 1989). Ciprofloxacin-resistant strains developed in about 16–33% of cases and were associated with treatment failure (Mulligan *et al.*, 1987; Piercy *et al.*, 1989a). Eradication of *Staph. aureus* occurs in 82–100% when rifampicin 600 mg per day is combined with ciprofloxacin 500–750 mg twice-daily and clinical resolution/improvement may be up to 90% (Smith *et al.*, 1989; Cheong *et al.*, 1992).

Righter (1987) found treatment with combination (i.v./oral) ciprofloxacin of patients requiring hospitalization with moderate-severe *Staph. aureus* infections was associated with a 29% clinical and 71% bacteriological failure rate, although all isolates remained susceptible to ciprofloxacin.

Ciprofloxacin is initially effective in suppressing MRSA carriage in hemodialysis patients, but after 2 or 3 months, the rate of post-treatment nasal carriage is comparable with control patients (33% versus 30%, respectively) (Chow and Yu, 1992).

14 Empiric treatment of bacteremia

Ciprofloxacin (i.v. then oral) has been used as empiric therapy for unspecified bacteremia, with up to 94% clinical efficacy. However, the incidence of Gram-negative infection in these studies is an important feature in determining the likely outcome with this agent. In an open study of ciprofloxacin-susceptible Gram-negative bacteremias, i.v. ciprofloxacin 200 mg twice-daily was equivalent to a combination of i.v. and oral ciprofloxacin therapy in terms of bacteriological eradication (94% versus 96%) and clinical cure (92% versus 93%, respectively) (Ganji *et al.*, 1989). Further information regarding the use of ciprofloxacin in bacteremia associated with specific infections can be found in the appropriate section in this chapter. Due to the possibility of Gram-positive bacteremia, ciprofloxacin monotherapy is generally inappropriate empiric therapy for clinical septicemia.

15 Otitis and sinusitis

Ciprofloxacin and other similar fluoroquinolones have proven to be a major advance in the treatment of malignant otitis externa. *Pseudomonas aeruginosa* is the responsible pathogen in more than 98% of malignant otitis externa, which involves infection of the external ear canal, mastoid and base of skull, generally in elderly patients with diabetes mellitus or immunosuppression (Grandis and Yu, 1993). Prolonged therapy with aminoglycosides and anti-pseudomonal penicillins is associated with a 15–30% mortality and high rates of toxicity, but oral ciprofloxacin therapy is associated with a greater than 90% rate of success with little toxicity or development of antibiotic-resistance (Joachims *et al.*, 1988, Leggett *et al.*, 1988; Rubin and Yu, 1988; Fairley and Glover, 1989; Hickey *et al.*, 1989; Osborne *et al.*, 1989; Sade *et al.*, 1989; Lang *et al.*, 1990a; Levy *et al.*, 1990; Levenson *et al.*, 1991). Although there have been no prospective comparative studies with ciprofloxacin and older regimens such as i.v. beta-lactams + aminoglycoside, oral monotherapy with ciprofloxacin 750 mg twice-daily for 6–12 weeks is generally recommended (Barza, 1991; Grandis and Yu, 1993). Rubin *et al.* (1989) advocate the addition of rifampicin 600 mg twice-daily to this regimen, however this has not been confirmed by other authors. Clinical efficacy has also been reported with oral ciprofloxacin in the treatment of auricular perichondritis due to *Ps. aeruginosa* (Noel *et al.*, 1989).

Oral ciprofloxacin is reported to have clinical efficacy in open non-comparative treatment studies of chronic middle ear infections, but the heterogeneous nature of this condition and variations in trial methodology and definitions make an accurate assessment of the value of ciprofloxacin in these circumstances difficult (Piccirillo and Parnes, 1989; Van de Heyning, 1988). Nevertheless, Lang *et al.* (1992) reported an 86% rate of initial clinical cure, among 21 children with chronic suppurative otitis media without cholesteatoma who were treated with oral ciprofloxacin 30 mg per kg per day for a mean of about 17 days – although one-third had a recurrence. Similarly, Legent *et al.* (1994) found ciprofloxacin to be superior to amoxicillin–clavulanate in an open randomized trial of chronic suppurative otitis media in adults.

Notable is the study by Esposito *et al.* (1990b) which demonstrated that topical ciprofloxacin (two drops [250 mg per ml] twice-daily) was at least equally, if not more, effective than oral ciprofloxacin (250 mg twice-daily for 5–10 days) or a combination of oral + topical ciprofloxacin in 60 patients with chronic otitis media. These data support the widely held doubts about the role of systemic therapy in uncomplicated otorrhea. Despite the frequent isolation of *Ps. aeruginosa* from chronically draining ears, its pathogenicity and the therapeutic role of fluoroquinolones in this setting remains unestablished.

Despite the excellent penetration of fluoroquinolones into the nasal and sinus mucosa (p. 1008), their weak activity against the Gram-positive pathogens commonly causing acute sinusitis, and the ready availability of other highly-active agents, argues against their use as first-line therapy. Similarly, there is little rationale for using fluoroquinolones in the treatment of acute pharyngotonsillitis, despite a number of studies demonstrating reasonable efficacy of both ciprofloxacin and ofloxacin (Esposito *et al.*, 1990a; Grandis and Yu, 1993).

16 Ocular infections

Studies in rabbits suggest that systemically administered ciprofloxacin penetrates the aqueous and vitreous humor to a similar extent, regardless of the presence or absence of infection, and also reach good concentrations in ocular tissues such as the cornea, iris, choroid, retina and sclera (Barza, 1993) (p. 1007). Vitreal penetration of fluoroquinolones is better than beta-lactam agents, aminoglycosides and clindamycin given as a single-dose, and there appears to be no difference in penetration between diabetic and non-diabetic patients (Barza, 1989; El Baba *et al.*, 1992). Penetration of other fluoroquinolones such as pefloxacin, ofloxacin and norfloxacin are roughly similar and the degree of penetration for all fluoroquinolones increases with repeated dosing (Barza, 1993).

Few studies have examined the clinical use of fluoroquinolones for the treatment of ocular infections in humans. Topical ciprofloxacin (3 mg per ml) for 3 days was superior to placebo, and equivalent to tobramycin (3 mg per ml), when both were given for 7 days for the treatment of bacteriologically proven conjunctivitis (Leibowitz, 1991a). Similar results have been noted with ofloxacin and norfloxacin (Gwon, 1992; Miller *et al.*, 1992). Topical ciprofloxacin (3 mg per ml; 0.3%) appears to be as effective in the treatment of bacterial keratitis as a fortified mixture of cefazolin and an aminoglycoside in a non-randomized comparative study (Leibowitz 1991b). Notably, 17% of ciprofloxacin-treated patients developed a white precipitate on the cornea which sometimes disappeared during continued therapy but lead to discontinuation in one patient.

Gonococcal keratoconjunctivitis has been successfully treated with oral norfloxacin 1200 mg for 1 to 3 days (Kostelyn *et al.*, 1989).

Despite this evidence in favor of fluoroquinolone use, there seems to be little reason to use fluoroquinolones in preference to an aminoglycoside unless the ocular pathogen is aminoglycoside-resistant. The empiric treatment of bacterial endophthalmitis should continue to be by direct intravitreal injection of agents such as vancomycin and an aminoglycoside to achieve immediate high antibiotic concentrations, with fluoroquinolones being potentially used as adjunctive treatment (Barza, 1993).

17 Peritonitis associated with CAPD

Oral ciprofloxacin compares favorably to intraperitoneal vancomycin and netilmicin in the treatment of CAPD-associated peritonitis, except when the pathogens are coagulase-negative staphylococci. Tapson *et al.* (1990) compared oral ciprofloxacin 500 mg at each dialysate exchange (i.e. four doses daily; total 2 g per day) with intraperitoneal vancomycin (15 mg per liter dialysate) + netilmicin (15 mg per liter in alternate bags) in a prospective, randomized comparison of the treatment of 50 consecutive episodes of CAPD peritonitis in 35 patients. Cure was achieved in 76% and 72%, respectively, with all six failures in the ciprofloxacin-treated group being due to Gram-positive cocci (five coagulase-negative staphylococci; one diphtheroid). Ciprofloxacin levels in dialysate were maintained at $>2\mu g$ per liter in the vast majority of cases. Bennett-Jones *et al.* (1990) and Fleming *et al.* (1990) also found comparable, although less impressive, results. Notably, the majority of failures and relapses were due to staphylococcal species.

Intraperitoneal ciprofloxacin (50 mg per liter dialysate for 7 days) is effective in 83% of cases with mean serum and dialysate concentrations of $1.1\mu g$ per liter and $10\mu g$ per liter, respectively (Ludlam *et al.*, 1990a). Friedland *et al.* (1990) found similar results when comparing empiric treatment with intraperitoneal ciprofloxacin 20 mg per liter dialysate to intraperitoneal vancomycin 12.5 mg per liter dialysate + gentamicin 4 mg per liter dialysate. Dryden *et al.* (1991) achieved 79% success when treating with 25 mg per liter dialysate for 5 days. These and other authors argue that the high drug levels achievable with intraperitoneal ciprofloxacin improve efficacy against Gram-positive cocci and therefore warrant the use of the intraperitoneal route rather than oral administration (Friedland *et al.*, 1990; Ludlam *et al.*, 1990a,b; Dryden *et al.*, 1991). Nevertheless, since coagulase-negative staphylococci are often the predominant cause of CAPD-associated peritonitis, and are not infrequently resistant to ciprofloxacin (p. 994), some caution is necessary when using either intraperitoneal or oral ciprofloxacin in this setting (Ludlam *et al.*, 1990a,b; Wilcox and Finch 1990).

18 Intra-abdominal and biliary tract infections

Ciprofloxacin and other fluoroquinolones, due to their spectrum of antibiotic activity and excellent biliary, hepatic and peritoneal penetration (pp. 1006–7), have proven effective in the treatment of spontaneous bacterial peritonitis, biliary sepsis and other intra-abdominal sepsis (Houwen *et al.*, 1987; Lonka and Pedersen, 1987; Smith, 1991; Sung *et al.*, 1995; Solomkin *et al.*, 1996). However, they should be used in combination with agents with anti-anaerobic activity, and depending on the clinical situation, anti-enterococcal activity. Fluoroquinolones also appear to be effective in preventing infections in selected patients with cirrhotic liver disease, where either norfloxacin 400 mg daily or ciprofloxacin 750 mg once-weekly has been shown to provide effective prophylaxis against spontaneous bacterial peritonitis compared with untreated patients (Soriano *et al.*, 1991; Rolachon *et al.*, 1995). Of concern, however, is a study by Dupeyron *et al.* (1994) which demonstrated the emergence of fluoroquinolone resistance among fecal organisms isolated from 16 of 31 patients given norfloxacin prophylaxis for spontaneous bacterial peritonitis. These authors advocate that such prophylaxis should therefore not be routinely given to cirrhotic patients with ascites. However, using the lower dose of ciprofloxacin (750 mg once-weekly) for 6 months, Rolachon *et al.* (1995) noted no development of resistant isolates.

Intravenous ciprofloxacin appears to be as effective as third-generation cephalosporins in preoperative antibiotic prophylaxis for biliary tract sepsis and colorectal surgery. However, except for drug allergy, there are no compelling reasons to use fluoroquinolones in preference to current routine regimens (Kujath, 1989; Görtz *et al.*, 1990; McArdle, 1994).

Ciprofloxacin and other fluoroquinolones alone and in combination with other agents such as H2 blockers, have proven generally disappointing in the treatment of gastric dyspepsia and peptic ulceration associated with *H. pylori* infection, with frequent emergence of fluoroquinolone-resistance (Glupczynski *et al.*, 1987; Stone *et al.*, 1988; Mertens *et al.*, 1989; Forsmark *et al.*, 1990).

19 Brucellosis

Ciprofloxacin monotherapy for *Brucella melitensis* infection results in good initial clinical improvement, but appears to be associated with a relatively high rate of relapse compared with routine therapy with rifampicin + doxycycline. Nevertheless, larger clinical studies are necessary to confirm this observation. In a small prospective, randomized study of ten patients with *B. melitensis* infection (mostly diagnosed by positive serology) in which six patients received 750–1000 mg oral ciprofloxacin twice-daily versus four patients treated with rifampicin 600 mg per day + doxycycline 100 mg twice-daily (all treated for 6 weeks), Lang *et al.* (1990b) found five of the six ciprofloxacin-treated patients relapsed after initial improvement compared with no relapses among the patients treated with rifampicin + doxycycline. Patients relapsed 1–3 weeks after cessation of ciprofloxacin therapy, but all responded to rifampicin + doxycycline therapy.

Al-Sibai *et al.* (1992) also examined the efficacy of ciprofloxacin monotherapy in a prospective, non-randomized study of brucellosis caused by *B. melitensis*. Serious cases with central nervous system involvement, endocarditis, severe renal dysfunction, disease in pregnant females or children <16 years age were excluded. Sixteen patients (seven acute systemic disease; nine arthritis-discitis) were treated with ciprofloxacin, with doses ranging between 500 mg twice-daily for 12 weeks (one patient) to 750 mg thrice-daily for 6 weeks (12 patients). In 50% of patients there was at least one positive culture for *B. melitensis*. A clinical response was seen in all patients within 5 days of treatment. One patient remained bacteremic after 3 weeks therapy, but responded to rifampicin + tetracycline. However, four patients (25%) developed recurrence or relapse within 8–32 weeks after treatment cessation. Doganay and Aygen (1992) found similar results in an open study of 14 patients treated with ciprofloxacin 500 mg thrice-daily for 3–6 weeks in which three patients relapsed. Although these rates of relapse are comparable with the outcome reported in other trials of treatment for brucellosis (10–41%), the regimen of tetracycline or doxycycline + streptomycin generally yields relapse rates of ≤ 10% (Acocella *et al.*, 1989; Hall, 1990). Thus, further studies of ciprofloxacin therapy are necessary, but the present literature suggests that ciprofloxacin may be a promising alternative for inclusion in treatment combinations.

20 Cat-scratch disease

Ciprofloxacin appears to be effective in the treatment of cat-scratch disease, which is caused by *Bartonella* (previously *Rochalimaea*) *henselae*. Holley (1990) described five adults with probable cat-scratch disease who improved within a few days of commencing ciprofloxacin 500 mg twice-daily; none relapsed. Margileth (1992) also found ciprofloxacin to be effective in a retrospective review of patients treated for cat-scratch disease. Lucey *et al.* (1992) described two immunocompetent patients with *B. henselae* bacteremia in which the isolates were studied *in vitro* and found to be inhibited by 2μg per ml ciprofloxacin and 4μg per ml norfloxacin, but to be resistant to nalidixic acid.

21 Rickettsial diseases

Ciprofloxacin is similar in efficacy to doxycycline in the treatment of Mediterranean Spotted Fever which is caused by *Rickettsia conorii*. Raoult *et al.* (1986b) initially described the cure of five patients with *R. conorii* infection treated with ciprofloxacin. Subsequently Gudiol *et al.* (1989) compared 2-day courses of ciprofloxacin 500 mg twice-daily (19 patients) with doxycycline 100 mg twice-daily (24 patients) in a prospective, randomized, double-blind study of non-severe disease. The doxycycline-treated group defervesced significantly faster than the ciprofloxacin-treated group (2.5 versus 3.8 days; p = 0.037), but all patients were cured. The role of ciprofloxacin in severe disease or in patients with severe prognostic features is less clear. Case reports also suggest that ciprofloxacin 500 mg twice-daily is effective in the treatment of murine typhus (caused by *R. typhi*) and scrub typhus (caused by *R. tsutsugamushi*) (Eaton *et al.*, 1989; Strand and Strömberg, 1990).

22 Mycobacterial infections

a   Tuberculosis   Ciprofloxacin and ofloxacin have reasonable *in vitro* activity against many strains of *Mycobacterium tuberculosis* (pp. 985, 1112). However, because of its longer half-life, ofloxacin has been most studied clinically. The efficacy of ciprofloxacin or ofloxacin in combination antituberculous regimens is difficult to assess but overall rates of sputum clearance of acid-fast bacilli of 15–90% after 4 months therapy have been described (Tsukamura *et al.*, 1985; Besozzi *et al.*, 1991; Scully, 1993). Kennedy *et al.* (1993) demonstrated that ciprofloxacin alone (750 mg daily) has better early bactericidal activity in sputum over 7 days than isoniazid (300 mg per day). In an interesting study these authors also compared the efficacy of a standard antituberculous regimen (rifampicin + isoniazid + pyrazinamide + ethambutol) with a regimen of ciprofloxacin 750 mg per day + rifampicin 600 mg per day + isoniazid 300 mg per day in 20 adults in Tanzania with pulmonary tuberculosis, where all isolates were fully susceptible to all study agents. Overall, the ciprofloxacin-containing regimen (nine patients) was inferior to the routine regimen in its sterilizing ability, with a culture conversion rate of 67% at 2 months compared with 100% for the routine regimen. Analysis of these data based on the presence of HIV infection however, revealed that both regimens were comparable in activity in HIV-negative patients, but that in HIV-positive patients, the rate of culture conversion at 4 months was significantly worse for the ciprofloxacin-containing regimen (0/4) compared with the routine regimen (4/4) (p = 0.03). The difference in overall response to the two regimens was therefore mainly due to poor response to the ciprofloxacin-containing regimen in HIV-infected patients.

Ciprofloxacin (16 mg per kg per day for 9 months) in combination with cycloserine and kanamycin was effective in curing a 5-year-old boy with multiresistant extrapulmonary tuberculosis in one case report (Hussey et al., 1992).

Thus, fluoroquinolones have a role as potential second-line agents in the treatment of tuberculosis, especially when isolates are resistant to first-line drugs (p. 1200).

b Mycobacterium avium complex Among the currently available fluoroquinolones, ciprofloxacin and sparfloxacin have the greatest activity against *Mycobacterium avium–intracellulare*, with 25–50% of isolates inhibited (Young et al., 1987; Yajko et al., 1988; Leysen et al., 1989). Ciprofloxacin-containing regimens are effective against *M. avium–intracellulare* infections in patients with AIDS, with defervescence and reduction in other infection-related symptoms, but toxicity is significant. The combination ciprofloxacin + ethambutol + rifampicin + amikacin + clofazime led to a reduction in bacteremia and symptoms after 2 weeks therapy, but relapse of infection after discontinuation of therapy was common (Chiu et al., 1990; Benson et al., 1991; de Lalla et al., 1992; Kemper et al., 1992; Winston, 1993b).

In a randomized, placebo-controlled, cross-over study of patients with AIDS and *M. avium–intracellulare* infection, treatment with ciprofloxacin 750 mg per day + ethambutol + rifampicin was compared with placebo for 8 weeks. Patients were then crossed over to the opposite treatment regimen for another 8 weeks. A significant decrease in the intensity of bacteremia and a reduction in clinical symptoms were noted during treatment but dose-limiting toxicity was significantly worse in the treated group and there was no difference in survival overall (Jacobson et al., 1993). Gordon et al. (1993) noted a clearance of mycobacteremia in 35% of HIV-infected patients with disseminated *M. avium–intracellulare* infection treated with rifampicin (600 mg per day + clofazamine (100 mg per day) + ciprofloxacin (750 mg twice-daily) + ethambutol (800 mg per day) but observed that although serum drug levels were often below those expected, this did not correlate with therapeutic failure.

c Other mycobacteria Cavitating lung disease due to *M. fortuitum* has been successfully treated with ofloxacin alone (300–600 mg daily) and a prolonged course of combination therapy with ciprofloxacin (750 mg twice-daily) + minocycline (100 mg per day) proved effective in a case of disseminated *M. fortuitum* (Ichiyama and Tsukamura, 1987; Burns et al., 1990; Yew et al., 1990). Similarly, ciprofloxacin is effective in some cases of *M. chelonae* infection, but its use should be based on known susceptibility data since Wallace et al. (1992) found that less than 20% of isolates had an MIC $\leq 2\,\mu g$ per ml (McWhinney et al., 1992; Singh and Yu, 1992; Zahid et al., 1994).

23 Miscellaneous conditions

Ciprofloxacin 750 mg twice-daily is ineffective in the treatment of chloroquine-resistant falciparum malaria, despite achieving adequate plasma and intraerythrocyte concentrations (Watt et al., 1991). Ciprofloxacin (250–500 mg twice-daily for 4 weeks) appears to be effective therapy for rhinoscleroma in which *Kl. rhinoscleromatis* or ozena is cultured, with better outcome than treatment with rifampicin + trimethoprim–sulfamethoxazole (Borgstein et al., 1993; Avery et al., 1995). Van Furth et al. (1992) reported the cure of two patients with malakoplakia (a chronic granulomatis condition involving the genitourinary tract and other organs) with ciprofloxacin 500 mg twice-daily. Ciprofloxacin 250 mg twice-daily for 5 weeks resulted in the cure of a 14-year-old Thai girl with cervical lymphadenitis due to *Burkholderia pseudomallei* which was susceptible *in vitro* to ciprofloxacin (Lumbiganon and Sookpranee, 1992). On the basis of a small number of case reports, ciprofloxacin appears to be effective against tularemia (Enderlin et al., 1994; Risi et al., 1995) (p. 1069).

References

Acocella G, Berstrand A, Beytout J *et al.* (1989). Comparison of three different regimens in the treatment of acute brucellosis: a multicenter multinational study. *J Antimicrob Chemother* **23**: 433.

Adler-Mosca H, Luthy-Hottenstein J, Martinetti Lucchini G *et al.* (1991). Development of resistance to quinolones in five patients with campylobacteriosis treated with norfloxacin or ciprofloxacin. *Eur J Clin Microbiol Infect Dis* **10**: 953.

Aggarwal A, Gurka J (1995). Probable ciprofloxacin induced cholestasis. *Aust N Z J Med* **25**: 541.

Aguiar JM, Chacon J, Canton R, Baquero F (1992). The emergence of highly fluoroquinolone-resistant *Escherichia coli* in community-acquired urinary tract infections. *J Antimicrob Chemother* **29**: 349.

AHFS (1995). *American Hospital Formulary Service – Drug Information* (McEnvoy GK, ed). Bethesda, USA: American Society of Health-System Pharmacists.

Ahmed-Jushuf IH, Arya OP, Hobson D *et al.* (1988). Ciprofloxacin treatment of chlamydial infections of urogenital tracts of women. *Genitourin Med* **64**: 14.

Aigner KR, Dalhoff A (1986). Penetration activities of ciprofloxacin into muscle, skin and fat following oral administration. *J Antimicrob Chemother* **18**: 644.

Akahane K, Sekiguchi M, Une T *et al.* (1989). Structure-epileptogenicity relationship of quinolones with special reference to their interaction with gamma-aminobutyric acid receptor sites. *Antimicrob Ag Chemother* **33**: 1704.

Akahane K, Kimura Y, Tsutomi Y, Hayakawa I (1994). Possible intermolecular interaction between quinolones and biphenylacetic acid inhibits gamma-aminobutyric acid receptor sites. *Antimicrob Ag Chemother* **38**: 2323.

Akaniro JC, Vidaurre CE, Stutman HR *et al.* (1990). Comparative *in vitro* activity of a new quinolone, fleroxacin, against respiratory pathogens from patients with cystic fibrosis. *Antimicrob Ag Chemother* **34**: 1880.

Al-Sibai MB, Hussain Qadri SM (1990). Development of ciprofloxacin resistance in *Brucella melitensis*. *J Antimicrob Chemother* **25**: 302.

Al-Sibai MB, Halim MA, El-Shaker MM *et al.* (1992). Efficacy of ciprofloxacin for treatment of *Brucella melitensis* infections. *Antimicrob Ag Chemother* **36**: 150.

Alam MN, Haq SA, Das KK *et al.* (1995). Efficacy of ciprofloxacin in enteric fever: comparison of treatment duration in sensitive and multidrug-resistant *Salmonella*. *Amer J Trop Med Hyg* **53**: 306.

Albrecht H, Stellbrink HJ, Fenske S *et al.* (1992). *Salmonella typhimurium* lung abscesses in an HIV-infected patient: successful treatment with oral ciprofloxacin. *AIDS* **6**: 1400.

Aldridge KE (1992). *In vitro* antistaphylococcal activities of two investigative fluoroquinolones, CI-960 and WIN 57273, compared with those of ciprofloxacin, mupirocin (pseudomonic acid), and peptide-class antimicrobial agents. *Antimicrob Ag Chemother* **36**: 851.

Aldridge KE (1994). Increased activity of a new chlorofluoroquinolone, BAYy 3118, compared with activities of ciprofloxacin, sparfloxacin, and other antimicrobial agents against anaerobic bacteria. *Antimicrob Ag Chemother* **38**: 1671.

Aldridge KE, Valainis GT, Sanders CV (1988). Comparison of the *in vitro* activity of ciprofloxacin and 24 other antimicrobial agents against clinical strains of *Chromobacterium violaceum*. *Diagn Microbiol Infect Dis* **10**: 31.

Aldridge KE, Henderberg A, Sanders CV (1989). Mutational frequency of gram-positive and gram-negative bacteria to resistance to lomefloxacin and other quinolones. *Rev Infect Dis* **11** (Suppl 5): S974.

Aldridge KE, Cammarata C, Martin DH (1993). Comparison of the *in vitro* activities of various parenteral and oral antimicrobial agents against endemic *Haemophilus ducreyi*. *Antimicrob Ag Chemother* **37**: 1986.

Allais JM, Preheim LC, Cuevas TA *et al.* (1988). Randomized, double-blind comparison of ciprofloxacin and trimethoprim–sulfamethoxazole for complicated urinary tract infections. *Antimicrob Ag Chemother* **32**: 1327.

Allon M, Lopez EJ, Min KW (1990). Acute renal failure due to ciprofloxacin. *Arch Intern Med* **150**: 2187.

Alos JI, Gomez GJ, Cogollos R *et al.* (1992). Susceptibilities of ampicillin-resistant strains of *Salmonella* other than *S. typhi* to 10 antimicrobial agents. *Antimicrob Ag Chemother* **36**: 1794.

Altés J, Gasco J, de Antonio J *et al.* (1989). Ciprofloxacin and delirium. *Ann Intern Med* **110**: 170.

Amador C, Chiner E, Calpe JL *et al.* (1991). Pneumonia due to *Bordetella bronchiseptica* in a patient with AIDS. *Rev Infect Dis* **13**: 771.

Anaissie E, Fainstein V, Miller P *et al.* (1987). *Pseudomonas putida*. Newly recognized pathogen in patients with cancer. *Amer J Med* **82**: 1191.

Anastasio GE, Menscer D, Little JM (1988). Norfloxacin and seizures. *Ann Intern Med* **109**: 169.

Anderson MD, Miller LK (1993). Endocarditis due to *Neisseria mucosa*. *Clin Infect Dis* **16**: 184.

Andriole VT (1991). Use of quinolones in treatment of prostatitis and lower urinary tract infections. *Eur J Clin Microbiol Infect Dis* **10**: 342.

Aoun M, Jacquy C, Debusscher L *et al.* (1992). Peripheral neuropathy associated with fluoroquinolones. *Lancet* **340**: 127.

Aoyama H, Sato K, Fujii T *et al.* (1988). Purification of *Citrobacter freundii* DNA gyrase and inhibition by quinolones. *Antimicrob Ag Chemother* **32**: 104.

Appelbaum PC, Spangler SK, Sollenberger L (1986). Susceptibility of non-fermentative gram-negative bacteria to ciprofloxacin, norfloxacin, amifloxacin, pefloxacin and cefpirome. *J Antimicrob Chemother* **18**: 675.

Appelbaum PC, Spangler SK, Crotty E *et al.* (1989). Susceptibility of penicillin-sensitive and -resistant strains of *Streptococcus pneumoniae* to new antimicrobial agents, including daptomycin, teicoplanin, cefpodoxime and quinolones. *J Antimicrob Chemother* **23**: 509.

Appleman ME, Hadfield TL, Gaines JK, Winn RE (1987). Susceptibility of *Bordetella pertussis* to five quinolone antimicrobic drugs. *Diagn Microbiol Infect Dis* **8**: 131.

Apuzzio JJ, Stankiewicz R, Ganesh V *et al.* (1989). Comparison of parenteral ciprofloxacin with clindamycin-gentamicin in the treatment of pelvic infection. *Amer J Med* **87** (Suppl 5A): 148S.

Arai S, Gohara Y, Kuwano K *et al.* (1992). Antimycoplasmal activities of new quinolones, tetracyclines, and macrolides against *Mycoplasma pneumoniae*. *Antimicrob Ag Chemother* **36**: 1322.

Arai S, Gohara Y, Akashi A *et al.* (1993). Effects of new quinolones on *Mycoplasma pneumoniae*-infected hamsters. *Antimicrob Ag Chemother* **37**: 287.

Archimbaud E, Guyotat D, Maupas J *et al.* (1991). Pefloxacin and vancomycin versus gentamicin, colistin sulphate and vancomycin for prevention of infection in granulocytopenic patients; a randomized double-blind study. *Eur J Cancer* **27**: 174.

Arcieri GM, Becker N, Esposito B *et al.* (1989). Safety of intravenous ciprofloxacin. A review. *Amer J Med* **87** (Suppl 5A): 92S.

Arcieri GR, August N, Becker C *et al.* (1986). Clinical experience with ciprofloxacin in the USA. *Eur J Clin Microbiol* **5**: 220.

Arning M, Wolf HH, Aul C *et al.* (1990). Infection prophylaxis in neutropenic patients with acute leukaemia – a randomized, comparative study with ofloxacin, ciprofloxacin and co-trimoxazole/colistin. *J Antimicrob Chemother* **26** (Suppl D): 137.

Aronoff GE, Kenner CH, Sloan RS, Pottratz ST (1984). Multiple-dose ciprofloxacin kinetics in normal subjects. *Clin Pharmacol Ther* **36**: 384.

Arya O, Hobson D, Hart CA *et al.* (1986). Evaluation of ciprofloxacin 500 mg twice daily for one week in treating uncomplicated gonococcal, chlamydial, and non-specific urethritis in men. *Genitourin Med* **62**: 170.

Ashdown LR (1988). *In vitro* activities of the newer beta-lactam and quinolone antimicrobial agents against *Pseudomonas pseudomallei*. *Antimicrob Ag Chemother* **32**: 1435.

Asperilla MO, Smego RJ (1989). Eosinophilic meningitis associated with ciprofloxacin. *Amer J Med* **87**: 589.

Assouad M, Willcourt RJ, Goodman PH (1995). Anaphylactoid reactions to ciprofloxacin. *Ann Intern Med* **122**: 396.

Aubert G, Pozzetto B, Dorche G (1992). Emergence of quinolone-imipenem cross-resistance in *Pseudomonas aeruginosa* after fluoroquinolone therapy. *J Antimicrob Chemother* **29**: 307.

Auckenthaler R, Michea HM, Pechère JC (1986). *In-vitro* activity of newer quinolones against aerobic bacteria. *J Antimicrob Chemother* **17** (Suppl B): 29.

Avent CK, Krinsky D, Kirklin JK *et al.* (1988). Synergistic nephrotoxicity due to ciprofloxacin and cyclosporine. *Amer J Med* **85**: 452.

Avery RK, Salman SD, Baker AS (1995). Rhinoscleroma treated with ciprofloxacin: a case report. *Laryngoscope* **105**: 854.

Avonts D, Fransen L, Vielfont J *et al.* (1988). Treating uncomplicated gonococcal infection with 250mg or 100mg ciprofloxacin in a single oral dose. *Genitourin Med* **64**: 134.

Azadian BS, Bendig JW, Samson DM (1986). Emergence of ciprofloxacin-resistant *Pseudomonas aeruginosa* after combined therapy with ciprofloxacin and amikacin. *J Antimicrob Chemother* **18**: 771.

Aznar J, Caballero MC, Lozano MC *et al.* (1985). Activities of new quinoline derivatives against genital pathogens. *Antimicrob Ag Chemother* **27**: 76.

Azoulay-Dupuis E, Bedos JP, Vallee E *et al.* (1991). Antipneumococcal activity of ciprofloxacin, ofloxacin, and temafloxacin in an experimental mouse pneumonia model at various stages of the disease. *J Infect Dis* **163**: 319.

Azoulay-Dupuis E, Vallee E, Veber B *et al.* (1992). *In vivo* efficacy of a new fluoroquinolone, sparfloxacin, against penicillin-susceptible and -resistant and multiresistant strains of *Streptococcus pneumoniae* in a mouse model of pneumonia. *Antimicrob Ag Chemother* **36**: 2698.

Backhouse CI, Matthews JA (1989). Single-dose enoxacin compared with 3-day treatment for urinary tract infections. *Antimicrob Ag Chemother* **33**: 877.

Bagger-Sjöbäck D, Spangberg ML (1989). Does ciprofloxacin affect the inner ear? A preliminary report. *Scand J Infect Dis* (Suppl 60): 28.

Bailey JR, Trott SA, Philbrick JT (1992). Ciprofloxacin-induced acute interstitial nephritis. *Am J Nephrol* **12**: 271.

Baldwin DR, Wise R, Andrews JM *et al.* (1993). Comparative bronchoalveolar concentrations of ciprofloxacin and lomefloxacin following oral administration. *Respir Med* **87**: 595.

Ball AP, Fox C, Ball ME *et al.* (1986). Pharmacokinetics of oral ciprofloxacin, 100 mg single dose, in volunteers and elderly patients. *J Antimicrob Chemother* **17**: 629.

Ball P (1986). Ciprofloxacin: an overview of adverse experiences. *J Antimicrob Chemother* **18** (Suppl D): 187.

Ball P (1990). Emergent resistance to ciprofloxacin amongst *Pseudomonas aeruginosa* and *Staphylococcus aureus*: clinical significance and therapeutic approaches. *J Antimicrob Chemother* **26** (Suppl F): 165.

Ballard RC, Duncan MO, Fehler HG *et al.* (1989). Treating chancroid; summary of studies in southern Africa. *Genitourin Med* **65**: 54.

Baltch AL, Smith RP, Ritz W (1995). Inhibitory and bactericidal activities of levofloxacin, ofloxacin, erythromycin, and rifampin used singly and in combination against *Legionella pneumophila*. *Antimicrob Ag Chemother* **39**: 1661.

Banerjee DK (1986). Ciprofloxacin (4-quinolone). and *Mycobacterium leprae*. *Lepr Rev* **57**: 159.

Bannon MJ, Strutchfield PR, Weinling AM, Damjanovic V (1989). Ciprofloxacin in neonatal *Enterobacter cloacae* septicaemia. *Arch Dis Child* **64**: 1388.

Bantz PM, Goote J, Peters-Hartel W *et al.* (1987). Low-dose ciprofloxacin in respiratory tract infections. A randomized comparison with doxycycline in general practice. *Amer J Med* **82** (Suppl 4A): 208.

Barker JE, Farrell ID (1990). The effects of single and combined antibiotics on the growth of *Legionella pneumophila* using time-kill studies. *J Antimicrob Chemother* **26**: 45.

Barnass S, Franklin J, Tabaqchali S (1990). The successful treatment of multiresistant nonenteric salmonellosis with seven day oral ciprofloxacin. *J Antimicrob Chemother* **25**: 299.

Barnass S, Holland K, Tabaqchali S (1991). Vancomycin-resistant *Corynebacterium* species causing prosthetic valve endocarditis successfully treated with imipenem and ciprofloxacin. *J Infect* **22**: 161.

Barriere SL, Catlin DH, Orlando PL *et al.* (1990). Alteration in the pharmacokinetic disposition of ciprofloxacin by simultaneous administration of azlocillin. *Antimicrob Ag Chemother* **34**: 823.

Barry AL, Fuchs PC (1991a). Anti-staphylococcal activity of temafloxacin, ciprofloxacin, ofloxacin and enoxacin. *J Antimicrob Chemother* **28**: 695.

Barry AL, Fuchs PC (1991b). *In vitro* activities of sparfloxacin, tosufloxacin, ciprofloxacin, and fleroxacin. *Antimicrob Ag Chemother* **35**: 955.

Barry AL, Fuchs PC (1991c). Cross-resistance and cross-susceptibility between fluoroquinolone agents. *Eur J Clin Microbiol Infect Dis* **10**: 1013.

Barry AL, Jones RN (1984). Cross-resistance among cinoxacin, ciprofloxacin, DJ-6783, enoxacin, nalidixic acid, norfloxacin, and oxolinic acid after *in vitro* selection of resistant populations. *Antimicrob Ag Chemother* **25**: 775.

Barry AL, Jones RN (1989). *In-vitro* activities of temafloxacin, tosufloxacin (A-61827). and five other fluoroquinolone agents. *J Antimicrob Chemother* **23**: 527.

Barry AL, Jones RN, Thornsberry C *et al.* (1984). Antibacterial activities of ciprofloxacin, norfloxacin, oxolinic acid, cinoxacin and nalidixic acid. *Antimicrob Ag Chemother* **25**: 633.

Barry AL, Fuchs PC, Pfaller MA *et al.* (1990). Prevalence of fluoroquinolone-resistant bacterial isolates in four medical centers during the first quarter of 1990. *Eur J Clin Microbiol Infect Dis* **9**: 906.

Barza M (1988). Pharmacokinetics and efficacy of the new quinolones in infections of the eye, ear, nose, and throat. *Rev Infect Dis* **10** (Suppl 1): S241.

Barza M (1989). Antibacterial agents in the treatment of ocular infections. *Infect Dis Clin North Am* **3**: 533.

Barza M (1991). Use of quinolones for treatment of ear and eye infections. *Eur J Clin Microbiol Infect Dis* **10**: 296.

Barza M (1993). Treatment of eye infections. In: *Quinolone Antimicrobial Agents*. 2nd edn. (Hooper DC, Wolfson JS, eds), p. 423. Washington, DC: American Society of Microbiology.

Bassey CM, Baltch AL, Smith RP (1986). Comparative antimicrobial activity of enoxacin, ciprofloxacin, amifloxacin, norfloxacin and ofloxacin against 177 bacterial isolates. *J Antimicrob Chemother* **17**: 623.

Bates CJ, Wilcox MH, Spencer RC *et al.* (1990). Ciprofloxacin and *Clostridium difficile* infection. *Lancet* **336**: 1193.

Bauernfeind A (1993). Comparative *in-vitro* activities of the new quinolone, Bay y 3118, and ciprofloxacin, sparfloxacin, tosufloxacin, CI-960 and CI-990. *J Antimicrob Chemother* **31**: 505.

Bauwens JE, Spach DH, Schacker TW *et al.* (1992). *Bordetella bronchiseptica* pneumonia and bacteremia following bone marrow transplantation. *J Clin Microbiol* **30**: 2474.

Bayer A, Gajewska A, Stephens M *et al.* (1987). Pharmacokinetics of ciprofloxacin in the elderly. *Respiration* **51**: 292.

Bayston KF, Want S, Cohen J (1989). A prospective, randomized comparison of ceftazidime and ciprofloxacin as initial empiric therapy in neutropenic patients with fever. *Amer J Med* **87** (Suppl 5A): 269S.

Bednarczyk EM, Adler LP, Remler B *et al.* (1994). Assessment of the effects of ciprofloxacin and nalidixic acid on cerebral blood flow and metabolism in healthy subjects by positron emission tomography. *Pharmacotherapy* **14**: 153.

Beermann DH, Scholl W, Wingender D *et al.* (1986). Metabolism of ciprofloxacin in man. In: *1st International Ciprofloxacin Workshop, Leverkusen 1985* (Neu HC, Weuta H, eds), pp. 141–146. Amsterdam: Excerpta Medica.

Bellido F, Pechère JC (1989). Laboratory survey of fluoroquinolone activity. *Rev Infect Dis* **11** (Suppl 5): S919.

Bennett WM, Aronoff GR, Golper TA (1994). *Drug Prescribing in Renal Failure* 3rd edn. Philadelphia: American College of Physicians.

Bennett-Jones DN, Russell GI, Barrett A (1990). A comparison between oral ciprofloxacin and intra-peritoneal vancomycin and gentamicin in the treatment of CAPD peritonitis. *J Antimicrob Chemother* **26** (Suppl F): 73.

Bennish ML, Salam MA, Haider R *et al.* (1990). Therapy for shigellosis. II. Randomized, double-blind comparison of ciprofloxacin and ampicillin. *J Infect Dis* **162**: 711.

Bennish ML, Salam MA, Khan WA *et al.* (1992). Treatment of shigellosis: III. Comparison of one- or two-dose ciprofloxacin with standard 5-day therapy. A randomized, blinded trial. *Ann Intern Med* **117**: 727.

Benson CA, Kessler HA, Pottage JJ *et al.* (1991). Successful treatment of acquired immunodeficiency syndrome-related *Mycobacterium avium* complex disease with a multiple drug regimen including amikacin. *Arch Intern Med* **151**: 582.

Bergan T (1990). Extravascular penetration of ciprofloxacin A review. *Diagn Microbiol Infect Dis* **13**: 103.

Bergan T, Engeset A, Olszewski W *et al.* (1986a). Pharmacokinetics of ciprofloxacin in peripheral lymph and skin blisters. *Eur J Clin Microbiol* **4**: 458.

Bergan T, Thorsteinsson SB, Kolstad IM, Johnsen S (1986b). Pharmacokinetics of ciprofloxacin after intravenous and increasing oral doses. *Eur J Clin Microbiol* **5**: 187.

Bergan T, Delin C, Johansen S *et al.* (1986c). Pharmacokinetics of ciprofloxacin and effect of repeated dosage on salivary and fecal microflora. *Antimicrob Ag Chemother* **29**: 298.

Bergan T, Thorsteinsson SB, Solberg R *et al.* (1987). Pharmacokinetics of ciprofloxacin: intravenous and increasing oral doses. *Amer J Med* **82** (Suppl 4A): 97.

Bergan T, Lolekha S, Cheong MK *et al.* (1988). Effect of recent antibacterial agents against bacteria causing diarrhoea. *Scand J Infect Dis* (Suppl 56): 7.

Bergogne-Bérézin E, Berthelot G, Even P *et al.* (1986). Penetration of ciprofloxacin into bronchial secretions. *Eur J Clin Microbiol* **5**: 197.

Berkey P, Moore D, Rolston K (1988). *In vitro* susceptibilities of *Nocardia* species to newer antimicrobial agents. *Antimicrob Ag Chemother* **32**: 1078.

Berkovitch M, Pastuszak A, Gazarian M *et al.* (1994). Safety of the new quinolones in pregnancy. *Obstet Gynecol* **84**: 535.

Berlin OGW, Young LS, Bruckner DA (1987). *In-vitro* activity of six fluorinated quinolones against *Mycobacterium tuberculosis*. *J Antimicrob Chemother* **19**: 611.

Bernard EM, Edwards FF, Kiehn TE *et al.* (1993). Activities of antimicrobial agents against clinical isolates of *Mycobacterium haemophilum*. *Antimicrob Ag Chemother* **37**: 2323.

Berré J, Thys JP, Husson M *et al.* (1988). Penetration of ciprofloxacin in bronchial secretions after intravenous administration. *J Antimicrob Chemother* **22**: 499.

Besozzi G, Colombo F, Montellini PV *et al.* (1991). Use of ofloxacin in mycobacterial lung infections. *Amer Rev Respir Dis* **143**: 119.

Betriu C, Gomez M, Sanchez A *et al.* (1994). Antibiotic resistance and penicillin tolerance in clinical isolates of Group B streptococci. *Antimicrob Ag Chemother* **38**: 2183.

Bhattacharya SK, Bhattacharya MK, Dutta D *et al.* (1992). Single-dose ciprofloxacin for shigellosis in adults. *J Infect* **25**: 117.

Bhutta ZA, Farooqui BJ, Sturm AW (1992). Eradication of a multiple drug resistant *Salmonella paratyphi* A causing meningitis with ciprofloxacin. *J Infect* **25**: 215.

Biering-Sørensen F, Hoiby N, Nordenbo A *et al.* (1994). Ciprofloxacin as prophylaxis for urinary tract infection: prospective, randomized, crossover, placebo controlled study in patients with spinal cord lesion. *J Urol* **151**: 105.

Bindschedler M, Koelz A, Stalder H, Follath F (1988). Pharmacokinetics of ciprofloxacin in patients with normal and impaired renal function. *Rev Infect Dis* **10** (Suppl 1): S110.

Bishoff W, Bishoff H (1989). *Chlamydia trachomatis* urethritis; clinical efficacy of ciprofloxacin. *Rev Infect Dis* **11** (Suppl 5): S1283.

Black A, Redmond AO, Steen HJ *et al.* (1990). Tolerance and safety of ciprofloxacin in paediatric patients. *J Antimicrob Chemother* **26** (Suppl F): 25.

Blackhouse CL, Matthews JA (1989). Single-dose enoxacin compared with 3-day treatment for urinary tract infections. *Antimicrob Ag Chemother* **33**: 877.

Bleske BE, Carver PL, Annesley TM *et al.* (1990). The effect of ciprofloxacin on the pharmacokinetic and ECG parameters of quinidine. *J Clin Pharmacol* **30**: 911.

Blondeau JM, Yaschuk Y (1995). *In vitro* activities of ciprofloxacin, cefotaxime, ceftriaxone, chloramphenicol, and rifampin against fully susceptible and moderately penicillin-resistant *Neisseria meningitidis*. *Antimicrob Ag Chemother* **39**: 2577.

Blumberg HM, Rimland D, Carroll DJ *et al.* (1991). Rapid development of ciprofloxacin resistance in methicillin-susceptible and -resistant *Staphylococcus aureus*. *J Infect Dis* **163**: 1279.

Bodhidatta L, Taylor DN, Chitwarakorn A *et al.* (1988). Evaluation of 500- and 1000-mg doses of ciprofloxacin for the treatment of chancroid. *Antimicrob Ag Chemother* **32**: 723.

Boeckh M, Lode H, Deppermann KM *et al.* (1990). Pharmacokinetics and serum bactericidal activities of quinolones in combination with clindamycin, metronidazole, and ornidazole. *Antimicrob Ag Chemother* **34**: 2407.

Boelaert J, Yalcke Y, Schurgers M *et al.* (1985). The pharmacokinetics of ciprofloxacin in patients with impaired renal function. *J Antimicrob Chemother* **16**: 87.

Boelaert J, de Jaegere PP, Daneels R *et al.* (1986). Case report of renal failure during norfloxacin therapy. *Clin Nephrol* **25**: 272.

Boerema JBJ, Kraay WVD, Dalhoff A (1984). The concentration of ciprofloxacin in human prostatic tissue and prostatic fluid. *4th Medit Congr Chemother* Abstr. No. 625.

Bogaerts J, Kestens L, Martinez Tello W *et al.* (1995). Failure of treatment for chancroid in Rwanda is not related to human immunodeficiency virus infection: *in vitro* resistance of *Haemophilus ducreyi* to trimethoprim–sulfamethoxazole. *Clin Infect Dis* **20**: 924.

Boisivon A, Guiomar C, Carbon C (1990). *In vitro* bactericidal activity of amoxicillin, gentamicin, rifampicin, ciprofloxacin and trimethoprim–sulfamethoxazole alone or in combination against *Listeria monocytogenes*. *Eur J Clin Microbiol Infect Dis* **9**: 206.

Bongaerts GP, Hoogkamp-Korstanje J (1993). *In vitro* activities of BAY Y3118, ciprofloxacin, ofloxacin, and fleroxacin against gram-positive and gram-negative pathogens from respiratory tract and soft tissue infections. *Antimicrob Ag Chemother* **37**: 2017.

Borgstein J, Sada E, Cortes R (1993). Ciprofloxacin for rhinoscleroma and ozena. *Lancet* **342**: 122.

Borner K, Höffken G, Lode H *et al.* (1986). Pharmacokinetics of ciprofloxacin in healthy volunteers after oral and intravenous administration. *Eur J Clin Microbiol* **5**: 179.

Borobio MV, Conejo M, Ramirez E *et al.* (1994). Comparative activities of eight quinolones against members of the *Bacteroides fragilis* group. *Antimicrob Ag Chemother* **38**: 1442.

Bosch J, Liñares J, López de Goicoechea MJ *et al.* (1986). *In-vitro* activity of ciprofloxacin, ceftriaxone and five other antimicrobial agents against 95 strains of *Brucella melitensis*. *J Antimicrob Chemother* **17**: 459.

Bosseray A, Leclercq P, Manquat G *et al.* (1992). Penetration of ciprofloxacin into synovial fluid after oral dosing. *J Antimicrob Chemother* **30**: 874.

Bosso JA (1989). Use of ciprofloxacin in cystic fibrosis patients. *Amer J Med* **87** (Suppl 5A): 123S.

Bosso JA, Black PG, Matsen JM (1987). Ciprofloxacin versus tobramycin plus azlocillin in pulmonary exacerbations in adult patients with cystic fibrosis. *Amer J Med* **82**: 180.

Bosso JA, Allen JE, Matsen JM (1989). Changing susceptiblity of *Pseudomonas aeruginosa* isolates from cystic fibrosis patients with the clinical use of newer antibiotics. *Antimicrob Ag Chemother* **33**: 526.

Bosso JA, Saxon BA, Matsen JM (1990). *In vitro* activities of combinations of aztreonam, ciprofloxacin, and ceftazidime against clinical isolates of *Pseudomonas aeruginosa* and *Pseudomonas cepacia* from patients with cystic fibrosis. *Antimicrob Ag Chemother* **34**: 487.

Bouza E, Diaz LM, Bernaldo DQJ *et al.* (1989). Ciprofloxacin in patients with bacteremic infections. The Spanish Group for the Study of Ciprofloxacin. *Amer J Med* **87** (Suppl 5A): 228S.

Bow EJ, Rayner E, Louie TJ (1988). Comparison of norfloxacin with co-trimoxazole for infection prophylaxis in acute leukemia. The trade-off for reduced gram-negative sepsis. *Amer J Med* **84**: 847.

Bowie WR, Willetts V, Jewesson PJ (1989). Adverse reactions in a dose-ranging study with a new long acting fluoroquinolone, fleroxacin. *Antimicrob Ag Chemother* **33**: 1778.

Brattström C, Malmborg AS, Tyden G (1988). Penetration of ciprofloxacin and ofloxacin into human allograft pancreatic juice. *J Antimicrob Chemother* **22**: 213.

Bremner DA, Dickie AS, Singh KP (1988). *In-vitro* activity of fleroxacin compared with three other quinolones. *J Antimicrob Chemother* **22** (Suppl D): 19.

Breuer J, Bragman SG, Sahatlevan MD *et al.* (1988). The possible role of ciprofloxacin in the treatment of endocarditis caused by *Pseudomonas aeruginosa*. *J Infect* **16**: 106.

Brismar B, Edlund C, Malmborg AS *et al.* (1990). Ciprofloxacin concentrations and impact of the colon microflora in patients undergoing colorectal surgery. *Antimicrob Ag Chemother* **34**: 481.

Brogard J-M, Jehl F, Monteil H *et al.* (1985). Comparison of high-pressure fluid chromatography and microbiological assay for the determination of biliary elimination of ciprofloxacin in humans. *Antimicrob Ag Chemother* **28**: 311.

Brook I (1993). *In vivo* efficacies of quinolones and clindamycin for treatment of infections with *Bacteroides fragilis* and/or *Escherichia coli* in mice: correlation with *in vitro* susceptibilities. *Antimicrob Ag Chemother* **37**: 997.

Brouqui P, Raoult D (1990). *In vitro* susceptibility of *Ehrlichia* sennetsu to antibiotics. *Antimicrob Ag Chemother* **34**: 1593.

Brouqui P, Raoult D (1992). *In vitro* antibiotic susceptibility of the newly recognized agent of ehrlichiosis in humans, *Ehrlichia chaffeensis*. *Antimicrob Ag Chemother* **36**: 2799.

Brouqui P, Rousseau MC, Stein A *et al.* (1995). Treatment of *Pseudomonas aeruginosa*-infected orthopedic prostheses with ceftazidime-ciprofloxacin antibiotic combination. *Antimicrob Ag Chemother* **39**: 2423.

Brown WJ, Sautter RL, Crist AJ (1992). Susceptibility testing of clinical isolates of *Methylobacterium* species. *Antimicrob Ag Chemother* **36**: 1635.

Brumfitt W, Hamilton-Miller JMT (1993). Incomplete cross-resistance between ciprofloxacin and sparfloxacin in staphylococci, with a note on selection pressure due to clinical use of ciprofloxacin. *J Antimicrob Chemother* **31**: 610.

Brumfitt W, Franklin I, Grady D *et al.* (1984). Changes in the pharmacokinetics of ciprofloxacin and fecal flora during administration of a 7-day course to human volunteers. *Antimicrob Ag Chemother* **26**: 757.

Bryan JP, Hira SK, Brady W *et al.* (1990). Oral ciprofloxacin versus ceftriaxone for the treatment of urethritis from resistant *Neisseria gonorrhoeae* in Zambia. *Antimicrob Ag Chemother* **34**: 819.

Büchler M, Malfertheiner P, Friess H *et al.* (1992). Human pancreatic tissue concentration of bactericidal antibiotics. *Gastroenterology* **103**: 1902.

Buchwald DS, Blaser MJ (1984). A review of human salmonellosis II: duration of excretion following infection with nontyphi salmonella. *Rev Infect Dis* **6**: 345.

Buirma RJ, Horrevorts AM, Wagenvoort JH (1991). Incidence of multiresistant gram-negative isolates in eight Dutch hospitals The 1990 Dutch Surveillance Study. *Scand J Infect Dis* (Suppl 78): 35.

Burdge DR, Nakeilna EM, Rabin HR (1995). Photosensitivity associated with ciprofloxacin use in adult patients with cystic fibrosis. *Antimicrob Ag Chemother* **39**: 793.

Burgos A, Quindos G, Martinez R, Rojo P, Cisterna R (1990). *In vitro* susceptibility of *Aeromonas caviae*, *Aeromonas hydrophila* and *Aeromonas* sobria to fifteen antibacterial agents. *Eur J Clin Microbiol Infect Dis* **9**: 413.

Burns DN, Rohatgi PK, Rosenthal R *et al.* (1990). Disseminated *Mycobacterium fortuitum* successfully treated with combination therapy including ciprofloxacin. *Amer Rev Respir Dis* **142**: 468.

Bustamante CI, Drusano GL, Wharton RC *et al.* (1987). Synergism of the combinations of imipenem plus ciprofloxacin and imipenem plus amikacin against *Pseudomonas aeruginosa* and other bacterial pathogens. *Antimicrob Ag Chemother* **31**: 632.

Bustamante CI, Wharton RC, Wade JC (1990). *In vitro* activity of ciprofloxacin in combination with ceftazidime, aztreonam, and azlocillin against multiresistant isolates of *Pseudomonas aeruginosa*. *Antimicrob Ag Chemother* **34**: 1814.

Cain DB, O'Connor ME (1990). Pseudomembranous colitis associated with ciprofloxacin. *Lancet* **336**: 946.

Campoli-Richards DM, Monk JP, Price A *et al.* (1988). Ciprofloxacin A review of its antibacterial activity, pharmacokinetic properties and therapeutic use. *Drugs* **35**: 373.

Cantón E, Peman J, Jimenez MT *et al.* (1992). *In vitro* activity of sparfloxacin compared with those of five other quinolones. *Antimicrob Ag Chemother* **36**: 558.

Carbon C, Weber P, Levy M *et al.* (1987). Short-term ciprofloxacin therapy for typhoid fever. *J Infect Dis* **155**: 833.

Carlson P, Kontiainen S, Renkonen OV (1994). Antimicrobial susceptibility of *Arcanobacterium haemolyticum*. *Antimicrob Ag Chemother* **38**: 142.

Carratala J, Corbella X, Dominguez A *et al.* (1991). Development of resistance to ciprofloxacin during therapy for a *Pseudomonas aeruginosa* lung abscess. *Rev Infect Dis* **13**: 764.

Casal M, Rodriguez F, Gutierrez J, Ruiz P (1989). Effect *in vitro* of the new quinolones in combination with antimycobacterial agents. *Rev Infect Dis* **11** (Suppl 5): 1042.

Castaman G, Rodeghiero F (1994). Acquired transitory von Willebrand syndrome with ciprofloxacin. *Lancet* **343**: 492.

Catchpole C, Andrews JM, Woodcock J *et al.* (1994). The comparative pharmacokinetics and tissue penetration of single-dose ciprofloxacin 400 mg iv and 750 mg po. *J Antimicrob Chemother* **33**: 103.

CDC (Centers for Disease Control) (1993a). Sentinel surveillance for antimicrobial resistance in *Neisseria gonorrhoeae* – United States, 1988–1991. *MMWR* **42** (SS3): 29.

CDC (Centers for Disease Control) (1993b). Sexually transmitted diseases treatment guidelines. *MMWR* **42** (Suppl RR-14): 1.

CDC (Centers for Disease Control) (1994). Decreased susceptibility of *Neisseria gonorrhoeae* to fluoroquinolones – Ohio and Hawaii, 1992–1994. *MMWR* **43**: 325.

Celesk RA, Robillard NJ (1989). Factors influencing the accumulation of ciprofloxacin in *Pseudomonas aeruginosa*. *Antimicrob Ag Chemother* **33**: 1921.

Chadwick M, Nicholson G, Gaya H (1989). Combination chemotherapy with ciprofloxacin for infection with *Mycobacterium tuberculosis* in mouse models. *Amer J Med* **87** (Suppl 5A): 35S.

Chadwick PR, Mellersh AR (1987). The use of a tissue culture model to assess the penetration of antibiotics into epithelial cells. *J Antimicrob Chemother* **19**: 211.

Chan CC, Oppenheim BA, Anderson H *et al.* (1989). Randomized trial comparing ciprofloxacin plus netilmicin versus piperacillin plus netilmicin for empiric treatment of fever in neutropenic patients. *Antimicrob Ag Chemother* **33**: 87.

Chandler MH, Toler SM, Rapp RP *et al.* (1990). Multiple-dose pharmacokinetics of concurrent oral ciprofloxacin and rifampin therapy in elderly patients. *Antimicrob Ag Chemother* **34**: 442.

Chantot JE, Bryskier A (1985). Antibacterial activity of ofloxacin and other 4-quinolone derivatives: *in-vitro* and *in-vivo* comparison. *J Antimicrob Chemother* **16**: 475.

Charton M, Mombet A, Praponich D (1989). Ideal duration of pefloxacin prophylaxis or urinary tract infection following transurethral resection of the prostate. *Rev Infect Dis* **11** (Suppl 5): 1345.

Chau PY, Ng WS, Leung YK *et al.* (1986). *In vitro* susceptibility of strains of *Pseudomonas pseudomallei* isolated in Thailand and Hong Kong to some newer beta-lactam antibiotics and quinolone derivatives. *J Infect Dis* **153**: 167.

Chaudhry AZ, Knapp CC, Sierra MJ *et al.* (1990). Antistaphylococcal activities of sparfloxacin (CI-978; AT-4140), ofloxacin, and ciprofloxacin. *Antimicrob Ag Chemother* **34**: 1843.

Chauncey JB, Schaberg DR (1990). Interstitial pneumonia caused by *Bordetella bronchiseptica* in a heart transplant patient. *Transplantation* **49**: 917.

Cheesbrough JS, Mwema FI, Green SD et al. (1991). Quinolones in children with invasive salmonellosis. *Lancet* **338**: 127.

Chen CH, Shih JF, Lindholm LP et al. (1989). Minimal inhibitory concentrations of rifabutin, ciprofloxacin, and ofloxacin against *Mycobacterium tuberculosis* isolated before treatment of patients in Taiwan. *Amer Rev Respir Dis* **140**: 987.

Cheong I, Zin Z, Tan SC et al. (1992). Combined ciprofloxacin/rifampicin therapy in methicillin-resistant *Staphylococcus aureus* (MRSA). infection. *Med J Aust* **157**: 71.

Cherubin CE, Stratton CW (1994). Assessment of the bactericidal activity of sparfloxacin, ofloxacin, levofloxacin, and other fluoroquinolones compared with selected agents of proven efficacy against *Listeria monocytogenes*. *Diagn Microbiol Infect Dis* **20**: 21.

Cherubin CE, Eng RH, Smith SM, Tan EN (1992). A comparison of antimicrobial activity of ofloxacin, L-ofloxacin, and other oral agents for respiratory pathogens. *Diagn Microbiol Infect Dis* **15**: 141.

Chew SK, Monteiro EH, Lim YS et al. (1992). A 7-day course of ciprofloxacin for enteric fever. *J Infect* **25**: 267.

Chidiac C, Roussel-Delvallez M, Guery B, Beaucaire G (1995). Should *Pseudomonas aeruginosa* isolates resistant to the fluorinated quinolones be tested for the others. Studies with an experimental model of pneumonia. *Antimicrob Ag Chemother* **39**: 677.

Childs SJ (1990). Intravenous and oral ciprofloxacin versus intravenous ceftazidime for the treatment of severe urinary tract infections. *Diagn Microbiol Infect Dis* **13**: 161.

Chin N-X, Neu HC (1984). Ciprofloxacin, a quinolone carboxylic acid compound active against aerobic and anaerobic bacteria. *Antimicrob Ag Chemother* **25**: 319.

Chin N-X, Neu HC (1987a). Post-antibiotic suppressive effect of ciprofloxacin against gram-positive and gram-negative bacteria. *Amer J Med* **82** (Suppl 4A): 58.

Chin N-X, Neu HC (1987b). Synergy of imipenem – a novel carbapenem, and rifampin and ciprofloxacin against *Pseudomonas aeruginosa*, *Serratia marcescens* and *Enterobacter* species. *Chemotherapy* **33**: 183 .

Chin N-X, Jules K, Neu HC (1986a). Synergy of ciprofloxacin and azlocillin *in vitro* and in a neutropenic mouse model of infection. *Eur J Clin Microbiol* **5**: 23.

Chin NX, Brittain DC, Neu HC (1986b). *In vitro* activity of Ro 23–6240, a new fluorinated 4-quinolone. *Antimicrob Ag Chemother* **29**: 675.

Chin NX, Clynes N, Neu HC (1989). Resistance to ciprofloxacin appearing during therapy. *Amer J Med* **87** (Suppl 5A): 28S.

Chin N-X, Gu J-W, Yu K-W et al. (1991). *In vitro* activity of sparfloxacin. *Antimicrob Ag Chemother* **35**: 567.

Chiodini RJ (1990). Bactericidal activities of various antimicrobial agents against human and animal isolates of *Mycobacterium paratuberculosis*. *Antimicrob Ag Chemother* **34**: 366.

Chirgwin K, Roblin PM, Hammerschlag MR (1989). *In vitro* susceptibilities of *Chlamydia pneumoniae* (*Chlamydia* sp. strain TWAR). *Antimicrob Ag Chemother* **33**: 1634.

Chiu J, Nussbaum J, Bozzette S et al. (1990). Treatment of disseminated *Mycobacterium avium* complex infection in *AIDS* with amikacin, ethambutol, rifampin, and ciprofloxacin. California Collaborative Treatment Group. *Ann Intern Med* **113**: 358.

Cho N, Fukunaga K, Kunii K (1984). Laboratory and clinical studies on Bay 0 9867; antibacterial activity, pharmacokinetics, and clinical evaluations in obstetrics and gynecology. *4th Medit Congr Chemother* Abstr. No. 636.

Chodosh S (1991). Use of quinolones for the treatment of acute exacerbations of chronic bronchitis. *Amer J Med* **91** (Suppl 6A): 93S.

Chodosh S, Tuck J, Stottmeier KD et al. (1989). Comparison of ciprofloxacin with ampicillin in acute infectious exacerbations of chronic bronchitis. A double-blind crossover study. *Amer J Med* **87** (Suppl 5A): 107S.

Choe U, Rothschild BM, Laitman L (1989). Ciprofloxacin-induced vasculitis. *New Engl J Med* **320**: 257.

Chow AW, Cheng N, Bartlett KH (1985). *In vitro* susceptibility of *Clostridium difficile* to new β-lactam and quinolone antibiotics. *Antimicrob Ag Chemother* **28**: 842.

Chow AW, Wong J, Bartlett KH et al. (1989). Cross-resistance of *Pseudomonas aeruginosa* to ciprofloxacin, extended-spectrum beta-lactams, and aminoglycosides and susceptibility to antibiotic combinations. *Antimicrob Ag Chemother* **33**: 1368.

Chow AW, Wong J, Bartlett KH (1988a). Synergistic interactions of ciprofloxacin and extended-spectrum beta-lactams or aminoglycosides against multiply drug-resistant *Pseudomonas maltophilia*. *Antimicrob Ag Chemother* **32**: 782.

Chow AW, Wong J, Bartlett KH (1988b). Synergistic interactions of ciprofloxacin and extended spectrum beta-lactams or aminoglycosides against *Acinetobacter calcoaceticus* ss. *anitratus*. *Diagn Microbiol Infect Dis* **9**: 213.

Chow JW, Yu VL (1992). Failure of oral ciprofloxacin in suppressing *Staphylococcus aureus* carriage in haemodialysis patients. *J Antimicrob Chemother* **29**: 88.

Christ W (1990). Central nervous system toxicity of quinolones: human and animal findings. *J Antimicrob Chemother* **26** (Suppl B): 219.

Christ W, Lehnert T, Ulbrich B (1988). Specific toxicologic aspects of the quinolones. *Rev Infect Dis* **10** (Suppl 1): S141.

Christensen MM, Nielson KT, Knes J, Madsen PO (1989). Single-dose preoperative prophylaxis in transurethral prostatic surgery. *Amer J Med* **87** (Suppl 5A): 258.

Christensson BA, Nilsson EI, Ljungberg B et al. (1992). Increased oral bioavailability of ciprofloxacin in cystic fibrosis patients. *Antimicrob Ag Chemother* **36**: 2512.

Clabots CR, Shanholtzer CJ, Peterson LR, Gerding DN (1987). *In vitro* activity of efrotomycin, ciprofloxacin, and six other antimicrobials against *Clostridium difficile*. *Diagn Microbiol Infect Dis* **6**: 49.

Claes J, Govaerts PJ, Van dHP et al. (1991). Lack of ciprofloxacin ototoxicity after repeated ototopical application. *Antimicrob Ag Chemother* **35**: 1014.

Clark RB, Lister PD, Arneson RL et al. (1990). *In vitro* susceptibilities of *Plesiomonas shigelloides* to 24 antibiotics and antibiotic-beta-lactamase-inhibitor combinations. *Antimicrob Ag Chemother* **34**: 159.

Clark RB, Lister PD, Janda JM (1991). *In vitro* susceptibilities of *Edwardsiella tarda* to 22 antibiotics and antibiotic-beta-lactamase-inhibitor agents. *Diagn Microbiol Infect Dis* **14** : 173.

Clendennen TE, Echeverria P, Saengeur S et al. (1992). Antibiotic susceptibility survey of *Neisseria gonorrhoeae* in Thailand. *Antimicrob Ag Chemother* **36**: 1682.

Clough W, Cassell GH, Duffy LB et al. (1992). Septic arthritis and bacteremia due to *Mycoplasma* resistant to antimicrobial therapy in a patient with systemic lupus erythematosus. *Clin Infect Dis* **15**: 402.

Cofsky RD, DuBouchet L, Landesman SH (1984). Recovery of norfloxacin in feces after administration of a single oral dose to human volunteers. *Antimicrob Ag Chemother* **26**: 110.

Cogo R, Rimoldi R, Mattina R, Imbimbo BP (1992). Steady-state pharmacokinetics of rufloxacin in elderly patients with lower respiratory tract infections. *Ther Drug Monit* **14**: 36.

Cohen MA, Huband MD, Mailloux GB et al. (1991). *In vitro* activity of sparfloxacin (CI-978, AT-4140, and PD 131501). A quinolone with high activity against gram-positive bacteria. *Diagn Microbiol Infect Dis* **14**: 403.

Cohen SP, Hooper DC, Wolfson JS et al. (1988). Endogenous active efflux of norfloxacin in susceptible *Escherichia coli*. *Antimicrob Ag Chemother* **32**: 1187.

Cohen SP, McMurry LM, Hooper DC et al. (1989). Cross-resistance to fluoroquinolones in multiple antibiotic resistant (Mar). *Escherichia coli* selected by tetracycline and chloramphenicol: decreased drug accumulation associated with membrane changes in addition to OmpF reduction. *Antimicrob Agents Chemother* **33**: 1318.

Cohn SM, Cohn KA, Rafferty MJ et al. (1995). Enteric absorption of ciprofloxacin during the immediate postoperative period. *J Antimicrob Chemother* **36**: 717.

Coker DM, Ahmed JI, Arya OP *et al.* (1989). Evaluation of single dose ciprofloxacin in the treatment of rectal and pharyngeal gonorrhoea. *J Antimicrob Chemother* **24**: 271.

Collignon PJ, Bell JM, MacInnes SJ *et al.* (1992). A national collaborative study of resistance to antimicrobial agents in *Haemophilus influenzae* in Australian hospitals. The Australian Group for Antimicrobial Resistance (AGAR). *J Antimicrob Chemother* **30**: 153.

Collins CH, Uttley AHC (1985). In-vitro susceptibility of mycobacteria to ciprofloxacin. *J Antimicrob Chemother* **16**: 575.

Collins CH, Uttley AH (1988). In-vitro activity of seventeen antimicrobial compounds against seven species of mycobacteria. *J Antimicrob Chemother* **22**: 857.

Connor JP, Curry JM, Selby TL, Perlmutter AD (1994). Acute renal failure secondary to ciprofloxacin use. *J Urol* **151**: 975.

Cooper B, Lawlor M (1989). Pneumococcal bacteremia during ciprofloxacin therapy for pneumococcal pneumonia. *Amer J Med* **87**: 475.

Cooper MA, Andrews JM, Ashby JP *et al.* (1990). In-vitro activity of sparfloxacin, a new quinolone antimicrobial agent. *J Antimicrob Chemother* **26**: 667.

Cooper MA, Baldwin D, Matthews RS *et al.* (1991). In-vitro susceptibility of *Chlamydia pneumoniae* (TWAR) to seven antibiotics. *J Antimicrob Chemother* **28**: 407.

Cooper MA, Andrews JM, Wise R (1992). In-vitro activity of PD 131628, a new quinolone antimicrobial agent. *J Antimicrob Chemother* **29**: 519.

Cooper MA, Andrews JM, Wise R (1993). Ciprofloxacin resistance developing during treatment of malignant otitis externa. *J Antimicrob Chemother* **32**: 163.

Cornaglia G, Pompei R, Dainelli B *et al.* (1987). In vitro activity of ciprofloxacin against aerobic bacteria isolated in a southern European hospital. *Antimicrob Ag Chemother* **31**: 1651.

Coronado VG, Edwards JR, Culver DH, Gaynes RP (1995). Ciprofloxacin resistance among nosocomial *Pseudomonas aeruginosa* and *Staphylococcus aureus* in the United States. National Nosocomial Infections Surveillance (NNIS) System. *Infect Control Hosp Epidemiol* **16**: 71.

Corrado ML, Struble WE, Peter C *et al.* (1987). Norfloxacin; review of safety studies. *Amer J Med* **82** (Suppl 6B): 22–26.

Costa P, Louis JF, Mottet N *et al.* (1991). Acute epididymitis and pefloxacin in monoantibiotic therapy. *Eur J Clin Microbiol Infect Dis* Special issue: 626.

Courvalin P (1990). Plasmid-mediated 4-quinolone resistance: a real or apparent absence? *Antimicrob Ag Chemother* **34**: 681.

Cox CE (1989a). Sequential intravenous and oral ciprofloxacin versus intravenous ceftazidime in the treatment of complicated urinary tract infections. *Amer J Med* **87** (Suppl 5A): 157S.

Cox CE (1989b). Comparison of intravenous ciprofloxacin and intravenous cefotaxime for antimicrobial prophylaxis in transurethral surgery. *Amer J Med* **87** (Suppl 5A): 252S.

Cox CE (1992). A comparison of the safety and efficacy of lomefloxacin and ciprofloxacin in the treatment of complicated or recurrent urinary tract infections. *Amer J Med* **92** (Suppl 14A): 82S.

Crombleholme WR, Schachter J, Ohm SM *et al.* (1989). Efficacy of single-agent therapy for the treatment of acute pelvic inflammatory disease with ciprofloxacin. *Amer J Med* **87** (Suppl 5A): 142S.

Cruciani M, Concia E, Navarra A *et al.* (1989). Prophylactic co-trimoxazole versus norfloxacin in neutropenic children-perspective randomized study. *Infection* **17**: 65.

Crump B, Wise R, Dent J (1983). Pharmacokinetics and tissue penetration of ciprofloxacin. *Antimicrob Ag Chemother* **24**: 784.

Crumplin GC, Kenwright M, Hirst T (1984). Investigations into the mechanisms of action of the antibacterial agent norfloxacin. *J Antimicrob Chemother* **13** (Suppl B): 9.

Crysanthopoulos CJ, Skoutelis AT, Starakis JC *et al.* (1987). Use of intravenous ciprofloxacin in respiratory tract infections and biliary sepsis. *Amer J Med* **82** (Suppl 4A): 357.

Cuevas LE, Kazembe P, Mughogho GK, Tillotson GS, Hart CA (1995). Eradication of nasopharyngeal carriage of *Neisseria meningitidis* in children and adults in rural Africa: a comparison of ciprofloxacin and rifampicin. *J Infect Dis* **171**: 728.

D'Antonio D, Iacone A, Fioritoni G *et al.* (1991). Antibacterial prophylaxis in granulocytopenic patients: a randomized study of ofloxacin versus norfloxacin. *Curr Ther Res* **50**: 304.

D'Antonio D, Piccolomini R, Iacone A *et al.* (1994). Comparison of ciprofloxacin, ofloxacin and pefloxacin for the prevention of the bacterial infection in neutropenic patients with haematological malignancies. *J Antimicrob Chemother* **33**: 837.

Daikos GL, Kathpalia SB, Lolans VT *et al.* (1988). Long-term oral ciprofloxacin: experience in the treatment of incurable infective endocarditis. *Amer J Med* **84**: 786.

Dalhoff A, Weuta H (1987). Penetration of ciprofloxacin into gynecologic tissues. *Amer J Med* **82**: 133.

Damagala JM, Hanna LD, Heifetz CL *et al.* (1986). New structure-activity relationships of the quinolone antibacterials using the target enzyme. The development and application of a DNA gyrase assay. *J Med Chem* **29**: 394.

Damjanovic V, Williets TH, Glynne TD *et al.* (1990). Eradication of *Salmonella* by oral ciprofloxacin in food handlers. *Lancet* **335**: 974.

Dan M, Samra Z (1989). *Clostridium difficile* colitis associated with ofloxacin therapy. *Amer J Med* **87**: 479.

Dan M, Golomb J, Gorea A *et al.* (1986). Concentration of ciprofloxacin in human prostatic tissue after oral administration. *Antimicrob Ag Chemother* **30**: 88.

Dan M, Siegman IY, Pitlik S *et al.* (1990). Oral ciprofloxacin treatment of *Pseudomonas aeruginosa* osteomyelitis. *Antimicrob Ag Chemother* **34**: 849.

Dan M, Zuabi T, Quassem C, Rotmensch HH (1992). Distribution of ciprofloxacin in ascitic fluid following administration of a single oral dose of 750 milligrams. *Antimicrob Ag Chemother* **36**: 677.

Dan M, Poch F, Quassem C, Kitzes R (1994). Comparative serum bactericidal activities of three doses of ciprofloxacin administered intravenously. *Antimicrob Ag Chemother* **38**: 837.

Dance DA, Wuthiekanun V, Chaowagul W *et al.* (1989). The antimicrobial susceptibility of *Pseudomonas pseudomallei*. Emergence of resistance *in vitro* and during treatment. *J Antimicrob Chemother* **24**: 295.

Dangor Y, Ballard RC, Miller SD, Koornhof HJ (1990). Treatment of chancroid. *Antimicrob Ag Chemother* **34**: 1308.

Danisovicova A, Brezina M, Belan S *et al.* (1994). Magnetic resonance imaging in children receiving quinolones: no evidence of quinolone-induced arthropathy. A multicenter survey. *Chemotherapy* **40**: 209.

Darouiche R, Perkins B, Musher D *et al.* (1990). Levels of rifampin and ciprofloxacin in nasal secretions: correlation with MIC_{90} and eradication of nasopharyngeal carriage of bacteria. *J Infect Dis* **162**: 1124.

Darouiche RO, Hamill RJ (1994). Antibiotic penetration of and bactericidal activity within endothelial cells. *Antimicrob Ag Chemother* **38**: 1059.

Daum TE, Schaberg DR, Terpenning MS *et al.* (1990). Increasing resistance of *Staphylococcus aureus* to ciprofloxacin. *Antimicrob Ag Chemother* **34**: 1862.

Davey PG (1988). Overview of drug interactions with the quinolones. *J Antimicrob Chemother* **22** (Suppl C): 97.

Davey PG (1991). Efficacy of temafloxacin versus ciprofloxacin or amoxicillin for lower respiratory tract infections in smokers and the elderly. *Amer J Med* **91** (Suppl 6A): 101S.

Davey PG, Charter M, Kelly S *et al.* (1994). Ciprofloxacin and sparfloxacin penetration into human brain tissue and their activity as antagonists of $GABA_A$ receptor of rat vagus nerve. *Antimicrob Ag Chemother* **38**: 1356.

Davidson RJ, Zhanel GG, Phillips R *et al.* (1991). Human serum enhances the postantibiotic effect of fluoroquinolones against *Staphylococcus aureus*. *Antimicrob Ag Chemother* **35**: 1261.

Davies BI, Maesen FP (1989). Drug interactions with quinolones. *Rev Infect Dis* **11** (Suppl 5): S1083.

Davies BI, Maesen FPV, Teengs JP (1984). Serum and sputum concentrations of enoxacin after single oral dosing in a clinical and bacteriological study. *J Antimicrob Chemother* **14** (Suppl C): 83–89.

Davies BI, Maesen FPV, Baur C (1986). Ciprofloxacin in the treatment of acute exacerbation of chronic bronchitis. *Eur J Clin Microbiol* **5**: 226.

Davies S, Sparham PD, Spencer RC (1987). Comparative *in-vitro* activity of five fluoroquinolones against mycobacteria. *J Antimicrob Chemother* **19**: 605.

Davis H, McGoodwin E, Reed TG (1989). Anaphylactoid reactions reported after treatment with ciprofloxacin. *Ann Intern Med* **111**: 1041.

Davis RL, Koup JR, Williams-Warren J *et al.* (1985). Pharmacokinetics of three oral formulations of ciprofloxacin. *Antimicrob Ag Chemother* **28**: 74.

Davis RL, Koup JR, Williams WJ *et al.* (1987). Pharmacokinetics of ciprofloxacin in cystic fibrosis. *Antimicrob Ag Chemother* **31**: 915.

Dawood ST, Uwaydah AK, Hroob A (1991). Treatment of multiresistant *Salmonella typhi* with intravenous ciprofloxacin. *Pediatr Infect Dis J* **10**: 343.

Dawson SJ, White LA (1992). Treatment of *Haemophilus aphrophilus* endocarditis with ciprofloxacin. *J Infect* **24**: 317.

De Salla A, Zappala M, Chimirri A *et al.* (1993). Quinolones potentiate cefazolin-induced seizures in DBA/2 mice. *Antimicrob Ag Chemother* **37**: 1497.

De la Fuente J, Albo C, Rodriguez A *et al.* (1994). *Bordetella bronchiseptica* pneumonia in a patient with AIDS. *Thorax* **49**: 719.

de Lalla F, Maserati R, Scarpellini P *et al.* (1992). Clarithromycin-ciprofloxacin-amikacin for therapy of *Mycobacterium avium–Mycobacterium intracellulare* bacteremia in patients with AIDS. *Antimicrob Ag Chemother* **36**: 1567.

Debbia EA, Pesce A, Schito GC (1992). *In vitro* assessment of the postantibiotic effect of lomefloxacin against gram-positive and gram-negative pathogens. *Amer J Med* **92** (Suppl 4A): 45S.

Deitz WH, Cook TM, Goss WA (1966). Mechanism of action of nalidixic acid on *Escherichia coli*. III. Conditions required for lethality. *J Bacteriol* **91**: 768.

Dekker AW, Rozenberg-Arska M, Verhoef J (1987). Infection prophylaxis in acute leukemia; a comparison of ciprofloxacin with trimethoprim–sulfamethoxazole and colistin. *Ann Intern Med* **106**: 7.

Dellamonica P, Bernard E, Etesse H *et al.* (1989). Evaluation of pefloxacin, ofloxacin and ciprofloxacin in the treatment of thirty-nine cases of chronic osteomyelitis. *Eur J Clin Microbiol Infect Dis* **8**: 1024.

Delmee M, Avesani V (1986). Comparative *in vitro* activity of 7 quinolones against 100 clinical isolates of *Clostridium difficile*. *Antimicrob Ag Chemother* **29**: 374.

Deppermann KM, Boeckh M, Grineisen S *et al.* (1989). Combination effects of ciprofloxacin, clindamycin, and metronidazole intravenously in volunteers. *Amer J Med* **87** (Suppl 5A): 46S.

Desplaces N, Acar JF (1988). New quinolones in the treatment of joint and bone infections. *Rev Infect Dis* **10** (Suppl 1): S179.

Desplaces N, Gutmann L, Carlet J *et al.* (1986). The new quinolones and their combinations with other agents for therapy of severe infections. *J Antimicrob Chemother* **17** (Suppl A): 25–39.

Dharmasena D, Roberts DE, Coles GA, Williams JD (1989). Pharmacokinetics of intraperitoneal ciprofloxacin in patients on CAPD. *J Antimicrob Chemother* **23**: 253.

Diaz Tejeiro R, Diez J, Maduell F *et al.* (1989). Successful treatment with ciprofloxacin of multiresistant salmonella arthritis in a renal transplant recipient. *Nephrol Dial Transplant* **4**: 390.

Dibble JB, Acomb C, Campbell L *et al.* (1987). Dosage of intravenous ciprofloxacin. *J Antimicrob Chemother* **20**: 454.

Diridal G, Pichler H, Wolf D (1986). Treatment of chronic salmonella carriers with ciprofloxacin. *Eur J Clin Microbiol* **5**: 260.

Diver JM, Schollaardt T, Rabin HR *et al.* (1991). Persistence mechanisms in *Pseudomonas aeruginosa* from cystic fibrosis patients undergoing ciprofloxacin therapy. *Antimicrob Ag Chemother* **35**: 1538.

Divo AA, Sartorelli AC, Patton CL *et al.* (1988). Activity of fluoroquinolone antibiotics against *Plasmodium falciparum in vitro*. *Antimicrob Ag Chemother* **32**: 1182.

Doganay M, Aydin N (1991). Antimicrobial susceptibility of *Bacillus anthracis*. *Scand J Infect Dis* **23**: 333.

Doganay M, Aygen B (1992). Use of ciprofloxacin in the treatment of brucellosis. *Eur J Clin Microbiol Infect Dis* **11**: 74.

Domagala JM, Hanna LD, Heifetz CL *et al.* (1986). New structure-activity relationships of the quinolone antibacterials using the target enzyme. The development and application of a DNA gyrase assay. *J Med Chem* **29**: 394.

Dominguez J, Palma F, Vega ME *et al.* (1989). Brief report: Prospective, controlled, randomized non-blind comparison of intravenous/oral ciprofloxacin with intravenous ceftazidime in the treatment of skin or soft-tissue infections. *Amer J Med* **87**: 136.

Donnenfeld ED, Schrier A, Perry HD *et al.* (1994). Penetration of topically applied ciprofloxacin, norfloxacin, and ofloxacin into the aqueous humor. *Ophthalmology* **101**: 902.

Dostal RE, Seale JP, Yan BJ (1992). Resistance to ciprofloxacin of respiratory pathogens in patients with cystic fibrosis. *Med J Aust* **156**: 20.

Drusano GL (1987). An overview of the pharmacology of intravenously administered ciprofloxacin. *Amer J Med* **82** (Suppl 4A): 339.

Drusano GL, Plaisance KI, Forrest A *et al.* (1986a). Dose ranging study and constant infusion evaluation of ciprofloxacin. *Antimicrob Ag Chemother* **30**: 440.

Drusano GL, Standiford HC, Plaisance K *et al.* (1986b). Absolute oral bioavailability of ciprofloxacin. *Antimicrob Ag Chemother* **30**: 444.

Drusano GL, Weir M, Forrest A *et al.* (1987). Pharmacokinetics of intravenously administered ciprofloxacin in patients with various degrees of renal function. *Antimicrob Ag Chemother* **31**: 860.

Dryden MS, Ludlam HA, Phillips I (1990). 4-Quinolone resistant staphylococci. *J Antimicrob Chemother* **26**: 448.

Dryden MS, Wing AJ, Phillips I (1991). Low dose intraperitoneal ciprofloxacin for the treatment of peritonitis in patients receiving continuous ambulatory peritoneal dialysis (CAPD). *J Antimicrob Chemother* **28**: 131.

Drysdale L, Gilbert L, Thomson A *et al.* (1988). Pseudoglycosuria and ciprofloxacin. *Lancet* **2**: 961.

Duckworth GJ, Williams JD (1984). Frequency of appearance of resistant variants to norfloxacin and nalidixic acid. *J Antimicrob Chemother* **13** (Suppl B): 33.

Dudley MN, Mandler HD, Gilbert D *et al.* (1987). Pharmacokinetics and pharmacodynamics of intravenous ciprofloxacin. Studies *in vivo* and in an *in vitro* dynamic model. *Amer J Med* **82**: 363.

Dupeyron C Mangeney N, Sedrati L *et al.* (1994). Rapid emergence of quinolone resistance in cirrhotic patients treated with norfloxacin to prevent spontaneous bacterial peritonitis. *Antimicrob Agents Chemother* **38**: 340.

DuPont HL (1993). Use of the quinolones for treatment and prophylaxis of bacterial and gastrointestinal infections. In *Quinolone Antimicrobial Agents* 2nd edn (Hooper DC, Wolfson JS, eds), p. 329. Washington, DC: American Society of Microbiology.

DuPont HL, Corrado ML, Sabbaj J (1987a). Use of norfloxacin in the treatment of acute diarrheal disease. *Amer J Med* **82** (Suppl 6B): 79.

DuPont HL, Ericsson CD, Robinson A, Johnson PC (1987b). Current problems in antimicrobial therapy for bacterial enteric infection. *Amer J Med* **82** (Suppl 4A): 324.

DuPont HL, Ericsson CD, Mathewson JJ, DuPont MW (1992). Five versus three day of ofloxacin therapy for travellers' diarrhea: a placebo-controlled study. *Antimicrob Ag Chemother* **36**: 87.

Dutta P, Rasaily R, Saha MR *et al.* (1993). Ciprofloxacin for treatment of severe typhoid fever in children. *Antimicrob Ag Chemother* **37**: 1197.

Dworkin R, Modin G, Kunz S *et al.* (1990). Comparative efficacies of ciprofloxacin, pefloxacin, and vancomycin in combination with rifampin in a rat model of methicillin-resistant *Staphylococcus aureus* chronic osteomyelitis. *Antimicrob Ag Chemother* **34**: 1014.

Dworkin RJ, Lee BL, Sande MA *et al.* (1989). Treatment of right-sided *Staphylococcus aureus* endocarditis in intravenous drug users with ciprofloxacin and rifampicin. *Lancet* **ii**: 1071.

Dworzack DL, Sanders CC, Horowitz EA *et al.* (1988). Evaluation of single-dose ciprofloxacin in the eradication of *Neisseria meningitidis* from nasopharyngeal carriers. *Antimicrob Ag Chemother* **32**: 1740.

Easmon CS, Crane JP (1985). Uptake of ciprofloxacin by human neutrophils. *J Antimicrob Chemother* **16**: 67.

Easmon CS, Woodford N, Ison CA (1987). The activity of the 4 quinolone Ro 23 6240 and the cephalosporins Ro 15 8074 and Ro 19 5247 against penicillin sensitive and resistant gonococci. *J Antimicrob Chemother* **19**: 761.

Eaton M, Cohen MT, Shlim DR *et al.* (1989). Ciprofloxacin treatment of typhus. *JAMA* **262**: 772.

Ebert SC, Graversen PH, Madsen PO (1988). Pharmacokinetics of ciprofloxacin in patients with impaired renal function. *Rev Infect Dis* **10** (Suppl 1): S110.

Echevarria J, Seas C, Carrillo C *et al.* (1995). Efficacy and tolerability of ciprofloxacin prophylaxis in adult household contacts of patients with cholera. *Clin Infect Dis* **20**: 1480.

Echols R, Weinstein MP, O'Keeffe B *et al.* (1994). Comparative crossover assessment of serum bactericidal activity and pharmacokinetics of ciprofloxacin and ofloxacin. *J Antimicrob Chemother* **33**: 111.

Echols RM (1993). The selection of appropriate dosages for intravenous ciprofloxacin. *J Antimicrob Chemother* **31**: 783.

Echols RM, Heyd A, O'Keeffe BJ, Schacht P (1994). Single-dose ciprofloxacin for the treatment of uncomplicated gonorrhea: a worldwide summary. *Sex Transm Dis* **21**: 345.

Edelstein PH, Edelstein MA (1991). *In vitro* activity of azithromycin against clinical isolates of *Legionella* species. *Antimicrob Ag Chemother* **35**: 180.

Edelstein PH, Gaudet EA, Edelstein MA (1989). *In vitro* activity of lomefloxacin (NY-198 or SC 47111), ciprofloxacin, and erythromycin against 100 clinical *Legionella* strains. *Diagn Microbiol Infect Dis* **12** (Suppl 3): 93S.

Edlund C, Nord CE (1989). Suppression of the oropharyngeal and gastrointestinal microflora by ciprofloxacin: microbiological and clinical consequences. *Scand J Infect Dis* (Suppl 60): 98.

Ehret JM, Judson FN (1988). Susceptibility testing of *Chlamydia trachomatis*: from eggs to monoclonal antibodies. *Antimicrob Ag Chemother* **32**: 1295.

El Baba FZ, Trousdale MD, Gauderman WJ *et al.* (1992). Intravitreal penetration of oral ciprofloxacin in humans. *Ophthalmology* **99**: 483.

Eliopoulos GM (1988). New quinolones: pharmacology, pharmacokinetics, and dosing in patients with renal insufficiency. *Rev Infect Dis* **10** (Suppl 1): S102.

Eliopoulos GM, Eliopoulos CT (1989). Ciprofloxacin in combination with other antimicrobials. *Amer J Med* **87** (Suppl 5A): 17S.

Eliopoulos GM, Eliopoulos CT (1993). Activity *in vitro* of the quinolones. In *Quinolone Antimicrobial Agents* 2nd edn (Hooper DC, Wolfson JS, eds), p. 161. Washington, DC: American Society of Microbiology.

Eliopoulos GM, Gardella A, Moellering RC Jr (1984). *In vitro* activity of ciprofloxacin, a new carboxyquinoline antimicrobial agent. *Antimicrob Ag Chemother* **25**: 331.

Eliopoulos GM, Klimm K, Grayson ML (1990a). *In vitro* activity of sparfloxacin (AT-4140; CI-978; PD 131501), a new antimicrobial agent. *Diagn Microbiol Infect Dis* **13**: 345.

Eliopoulos GM, Klimm K, Rice LB *et al.* (1990b). Comparative *in vitro* activity of WIN 57273, a new fluoroquinolone antimicrobial agent. *Antimicrob Ag Chemother* **34**: 1154.

Elzinga LW, Golper TA, Rashad AL *et al.* (1988). Ciprofloxacin activity in cyst fluid from polycystic kidneys. *Antimicrob Ag Chemother* **32**: 844.

Ena J, Amador C, Parras F *et al.* (1991). Ciprofloxacin as an effective antibacterial agent in serratia endocarditis. *J Infect* **22**: 103.

Enderlin G, Morales L, Jacobs RF, Cross JT (1994). Streptomycin and alternative agents for the treatment of tularemia: review of the literature. *Clin Infect Dis* **19**: 42.

Endtz HP, Ruijs GJ *et al.* (1991). Quinolone resistance in campylobacter isolated from man and poultry following the introduction of fluoroquinolones in veterinary medicine. *J Antimicrob Chemother* **27**: 199.

Eng RH, Smith SM, Lo W *et al.* (1990). Eradication of non-typhi *Salmonella* colonization by ciprofloxacin: implications for health care workers and institutionalized patients. *Amer J Med* **89**: 386.

Eng RH, Padberg FT, Smith SM *et al.* (1991). Bactericidal effects of antibiotics on slowly growing and nongrowing bacteria. *Antimicrob Ag Chemother* **35**: 1824.

Ericsson CD, Johnson PC, Dupont HL *et al.* (1987). Ciprofloxacin or trimethoprim–sulfamethoxazole as initial therapy for travelers' diarrhea A placebo-controlled, randomized trial. *Ann Intern Med* **106**: 216.

Ernst F, van der Auwera P (1988). *In vitro* activity of fleroxacin (Ro 23–6240), a new fluor-quinolone, and other agents, against *Mycobacterium* spp. *J Antimicrob Chemother* **21**: 501.

Ernst JA, Sy ER, Colon-Lucca H *et al.* (1986). Ciprofloxacin in the treatment of pneumonia. *Antimicrob Ag Chemother* **29**: 1088.

Espinoza AM, Chin NX, Novelli A *et al.* (1988). Comparative *in vitro* activity of a new fluorinated 4-quinolone, T-3262 (A-60969). *Antimicrob Agents Chemother* **32**: 663–670.

Esposito S, Gupta A, Thadepalli H (1987a). *In vitro* synergy of ciprofloxacin and three other antibiotics against *Bacteriodes fragilis*. *Drugs Exp Clin Res* **13**: 489.

Esposito S, Galante D, Bianchi W *et al.* (1987b). Efficacy and safety of oral ciprofloxacin in the treatment of respiratory tract infections associated with chronic hepatitis. *Amer J Med* **82**: 211.

Esposito S, Miniero M, Barba D, Sagnelli E (1989). Pharmacokinetics of ciprofloxacin in impaired liver function. *International J Clin Pharmacol Res* **9**: 37.

Esposito S, D'Errico G, Montanaro C (1990a). Oral ciprofloxacin for treatment of acute bacterial pharyngotonsillitis. *J Chemother* **2**: 108.

Esposito S, D'Errico G, Montanaro C (1990b). Topical and oral treatment of chronic otitis media with ciprofloxacin. A preliminary study. *Otolaryngol Head Neck Surg* **116**: 557.

Eykyn SJ, Williams H (1987). Treatment of multiresistant *Salmonella typhi* with oral ciprofloxacin. *Lancet* **ii**: 1407.

Fabre D, Bressolle F, Gomeni R *et al.* (1991). Steady-state pharmacokinetics of ciprofloxacin in plasma from patients with nosocomial pneumonia: penetration of the bronchial mucosa. *Antimicrob Ag Chemother* **35**: 2521.

Fairley J, Glover GW (1989). Treating malignant otitis with oral ciprofloxacin. *Brit Med J* **299**: 794.

Fang GD, Brennen C, Wagener M *et al.* (1991). Use of ciprofloxacin versus use of aminoglycosides for therapy of complicated urinary tract infection: prospective, randomized clinical and pharmacokinetic study. *Antimicrob Ag Chemother* **35**: 1849.

Fass RJ (1983). *In vitro* activity of ciprofloxacin (Bay 0 9867). *Antimicrob Ag Chemother* **24**: 568.

Fass RJ (1986). Treatment of skin and soft tissue infections with oral ciprofloxacin. *J Antimicrob Chemother* **18** (Suppl D): 153.

Fass RJ, (1987). Efficacy and safety of oral ciprofloxacin in the treatment of serious respiratory infections. *Amer J Med* **82** (Suppl 4A): 202.

Fass RJ (1993). *In vitro* activity of Bay y 3118, a new quinolone. *Antimicrob Ag Chemother* **37**: 2348.

Fass RJ, Helsel VL (1987). *In vitro* antistaphylococcal activity of pefloxacin alone and in combination with other antistaphylococcal drugs. *Antimicrob Ag Chemother* **31**: 1457.

Fass R J, Plouffe JF, Russell JA (1989). Intravenous/oral ciprofloxacin versus ceftazidime in the treatment of serious infections. *Amer J Med* **87** (Suppl 5A): 164–168.

Felmingham D, Robbins MJ, Foxall P *et al.* (1988). *In vitro* activity, postantibiotic effect, and resistance studies with amifloxacin. *Rev Infect Dis* **11** (Suppl 5): S952.

Ferguson J, Johnson BE (1990). Ciprofloxacin-induced photosensitivity, *in vitro* and *in vivo* studies. *Brit J Dermatol* **123**: 9.

Ferguson J, McIntosh J, Walker EM (1988). Ciprofloxacin-induced photosensitivity *in vitro* and *in vivo* studies. *J Invest Dermatol* **91**: 385.

Fernandes PB, Shipkowitz N, Bower R *et al.* (1986). *In-vitro* and *in-vivo* potency of five new fluoroquinolones against anaerobic bacteria. *J Antimicrob Chemother* **18**: 693.

Fernandes PB, Hanson CW, Stamm JM *et al.* (1987). The frequency of *in-vitro* resistance development to fluoroquinolones and the use of murine pyelonephritis model to demonstrate selection of resistance *in vivo*. *J Antimicrob Chemother* **19**: 449.

Fernandes PB, Chu DTW, Swanson RN *et al.* (1988). A-61827 (A-60969), a new fluoronaphthyridine with activity against both aerobic and anaerobic bacteria. *Antimicrob Ag Chemother* **32**: 27–32.

Fernandes PB, Hardy DJ, McDaniel D *et al.* (1989). *In vitro* and *in vivo* activities of clarithromycin against *Mycobacterium avium*. *Antimicrob Ag Chemother* **33**: 1531.

Fernandez-Guerrero M, Rouse MS, Henry NK *et al.* (1987). *In vitro* and *in vivo* activity of ciprofloxacin against enterococci isolated from patients with infective endocarditis. *Antimicrob Ag Chemother* **31**: 430.

Fernandez-Guerrero M, Rouse M, Henry N *et al.* (1988). Ciprofloxacin therapy of experimental endocarditis caused by methicillin-susceptible or methicillin-resistant *Staphylococcus aureus*. *Antimicrob Ag Chemother* **32**: 747.

Fernandez-Roblas R, Prieto S, Santamaria M *et al.* (1987). Activity of nine antimicrobial agents against *Corynebacterium* group D2 strains isolated from clinical specimens and skin. *Antimicrob Ag Chemother* **31**: 821.

Ferreccio C, Morris JG, Valdivieso C *et al.* (1988). Efficacy of ciprofloxacin in the treatment of chronic typhoid carriers. *J Infect Dis* **157**: 1235.

Fink MP, Snydman DR, Niederman MS *et al.* (1994). Treatment of severe pneumonia in hospitalized patients: results of a multicenter, randomized, double-blind trial comparing intravenous ciprofloxacin with imipenem-cilastatin. The Severe Pneumonia Study Group. *Antimicrob Ag Chemother* **38**: 547.

Fishbach F, Deckardt R, Graeff H *et al.* (1991). Comparison of ciprofloxacin/metronidazole versus cefoxitin/doxycycline in the treatment of pelvic inflammatory disease. *Eur J Clin Microbiol Infect Dis* Special Issue: 402.

Fitzgeorge RB, Gibson DH, Jepras R, Baskerville A (1985). Studies on ciprofloxacin therapy of experimental Legionnaires'disease. *J Infect* **10**: 194.

Flaherty JP, Waitley D, Edlin B *et al.* (1989). Multicenter, randomized trial of ciprofloxacin plus azlocillin versus ceftazidime plus amikacin for empiric treatment of febrile neutropenic patients. *Amer J Med* **87** (Suppl 5A): 278S.

Fleming LW, Moreland TA, Stewart WK *et al.* (1986). Ciprofloxacin and antacids. *Lancet* **ii**: 294.

Fleming LW, Moreland TA, Scott AC *et al.* (1987). Ciprofloxacin in plasma and peritoneal dialysate after oral therapy in patients on continuous ambulatory peritoneal dialysis. *J Antimicrob Chemother* **19**: 493.

Fleming LW, Phillips G, Moreland TA *et al.* (1988). Treatment of CAPD peritonitis with oral ciprofloxacin. In *Abstracts of the 2nd International Symposium on New Quinolones, Geneva* p. 261.

Fleming LW, Phillips G, Stewart WK *et al.* (1990). Oral ciprofloxacin in the treatment of peritonitis in patients on continuous ambulatory peritoneal dialysis. *J Antimicrob Chemother* **25**: 441.

Fliegelman RM, Petrak RM, Goodman LJ *et al.* (1985). Comparative *in vitro* activities of twelve antimicrobial agents against *Campylobacter* species. *Antimicrob Ag Chemother* **27**: 429.

Flor S, Guay DRP, Opsahl JA, Tack K, Matzke GR (1990). Effects of magnesium-aluminium hydroxide and calcium cardonate antacids on bioavailability of ofloxacin. *Antimicrob Ag Chemother* **34**: 2436.

Fong IW, Ledbetter WH, Vandenbroucke AC *et al.* (1986). Ciprofloxacin concentrations in bone and muscle after oral dosing. *Antimicrob Ag Chemother* **29**: 405.

Fong IW, Linton W, Simbul M *et al.* (1987). Treatment of nongonococcal urethritis with ciprofloxacin. *Amer J Med* **82**: 311.

Fontaine O (1989). Antibiotics in the management of shigellosis in chidren: what role for the quinolones. *Rev Infect Dis* **11** (Suppl 5): S1145.

Ford AS, Baltch AL, Smith RP *et al.* (1993). *In-vitro* susceptibilities of *Pseudomonas aeruginosa* and *Pseudomonas* spp to the new fluoroquinolones clinafloxacin and PD 131628 and nine other antimicrobial agents. *J Antimicrob Chemother* **31**: 523.

Forrest A, Weir M, Plaisance KI *et al.* (1988). Relationships between renal function and disposition of oral ciprofloxacin. *Antimicrob Ag Chemother* **32**: 1537.

Forrest A, Ballow CH, Nix DE *et al.* (1993a). Development of a population pharmacokinetic model and optimal sampling strategies for intravenous ciprofloxacin. *Antimicrob Ag Chemother* **37**: 1065.

Forrest A, Nix DE, Ballow CH *et al.* (1993b). Pharmacodynamics of intravenous ciprofloxacin in seriously ill patients. *Antimicrob Ag Chemother* **37**: 1073.

Forsberg P, Maller R, Nilsson L (1989). Comparative study of oral ofloxacin and erythromycin in the treatment of pneumonia. *Rev Infect Dis* **11** (Suppl 5): S1229.

Forsgren A (1989). Overview of Scandinavian *in vitro* studies with ciprofloxacin. *Scand J Infect Dis* (Suppl 60): 16.

Forsgren A (1993). Antibiotic susceptibility of *Mycobacterium marinum*. *Scand J Infect Dis* **25**: 779.

Forsmark CE, Wilcox CM, Cello JP *et al.* (1990). Ciprofloxacin in the treatment of *Helicobacter pylori* in patients with gastritis and peptic ulcer. *J Infect Dis* **162**: 998.

Forstall GJ, Knapp CC, Washington JA (1991). Activity of new quinolones against ciprofloxacin-resistant staphylococci. *Antimicrob Ag Chemother* **35**: 1679.

Fox AR, Phillips I (1987). The antibiotic sensitivity of the *Bacteroides fragilis* group in the United Kingdom. *J Antimicrob Chemother* **20**: 477.

Fraise AP, Smith SP (1990). Ciprofloxacin in combined renal and hepatic impairment. *J Antimicrob Chemother* **25**: 297.

Fredlund H, Bjoreman M, Kjellander J *et al.* (1990). A 10-year survey of clinically significant blood culture isolates and antibiotic susceptibilities from adult patients with hematological diseases at a major Swedish hospital. *Scand J Infect Dis* **22**: 381.

French P, Venuti E, Fraimow HS (1993). *In vitro* activity of novobiocin against multiresistant strains of *Enterococcus faecium*. *Antimicrob Ag Chemother* **37**: 2736.

Friedland JS, Iveson TJ, Fraise AP *et al.* (1990). A comparison between intraperitoneal ciprofloxacin and intraperitoneal vancomycin and gentamicin in the treatment of peritonitis associated with continuous ambulatory peritoneal dialysis (CAPD). *J Antimicrob Chemother* **26** (Suppl F): 77.

Fritzen T, Marx E, Uy J (1986). Treatment of surgical infections with a modern quinolone; therapy of soft tissue infections and pneumonia with ofloxacin. *Infection* **14** (Suppl 4): 293.

Frost RW, Carlson JD, Dietz AJ *et al.* (1989a). Ciprofloxacin pharmacokinetics after a standard or high-fat/high-calcium breakfast. *J Clin Pharmacol* **29**: 953.

Frost RW, Lettieri JT, Kiol G, Shamblen EC, Lasseter KC (1989b). The effect of cirrhosis on the steady-state pharmacokinetics of oral ciprofloxacin. *Clin Pharmacol Ther* **45**: 608.

Frost RW, Lasseter KC, Noe AJ *et al.* (1992). Effects of aluminum hydroxide and calcium carbonate antacids on the bioavailability of ciprofloxacin. *Antimicrob Ag Chemother* **36**: 830.

Fu KP, Lafredo SC, Foleno B *et al.* (1992). *In vitro* and *in vivo* antibacterial activities of levofloxacin (l-ofloxacin), an optically active ofloxacin. *Antimicrob Ag Chemother* **36**: 860.

Fuchs PC, Barry AL, Pfaller MA *et al.* (1991). Multicenter evaluation of the *in vitro* activities of three new quinolones, sparfloxacin, CI-960, and PD 131,628, compared with the activity of ciprofloxacin against 5252 clinical bacterial isolates. *Antimicrob Ag Chemother* **35**: 764.

Fuchs S, Simon Z, Brezis M (1994). Fatal hepatic failure associated with ciprofloxacin. *Lancet* **343**: 738.

Fujimaki K, Fujii T, Aoyama H *et al.* (1989). Quinolone resistance in clinical isolates of *Serratia marcescens*. *Antimicrob Ag Chemother* **33**: 785.

Fung-Tomc J, Huczko E, Gradelski E *et al.* (1991). Emergence of homogeneously methicillin-resistant *Staphylococcus aureus*. *J Clin Microbiol* **29**: 2880.

Fung-Tomc J, Kolek B, Bonner DP (1993). Ciprofloxacin-induced, low-level resistance to structurally unrelated antibiotics in *Pseudomonas aeruginosa* and methicillin-resistant *Staphylococcus aureus*. *Antimicrob Ag Chemother* **37**: 1289.

Fung-Tome JJ, Desiderio JV, Tsai YH *et al.* (1989). *In vitro* and *in vivo* antibacterial activities of BMY 40062, a new fluoronaphthyridone. *Antimicrob Ag Chemother* **33**: 906–914.

Fuursted K (1987). Post-antibiotic effect of ciprofloxacin on *Pseudomonas aeruginosa*. *Eur J Clin Microbiol* **6**: 271.

Gamboa F, Rivera JM, Gomez Mateos JM, Gomez-Gras E (1995). Ciprofloxacin-induced Henoch-Schonlein purpura. *Ann Pharmacother* **29**: 84.

Gangji D, Jacobs F, de JJ *et al.* (1989). Randomized study of intravenous versus sequential intravenous/oral regimen of ciprofloxacin in the treatment of gram-negative septicemia. *Amer J Med* **87** (Suppl 5A): 206S.

Garcia I, Pascual A, Perea EJ (1992). Effect of several antimicrobial agents on ciprofloxacin uptake by human neutrophils. *Eur J Clin Microbiol Infect Dis* **11**: 260.

Garcia-Rodriguez JA, Gomez Garcia AC (1993). *In-vitro* activities of quinolones against mycobacteria. *J Antimicrob Chemother* **32**: 797.

García-Rodriguez JA, García Sánchez JE, Trujillano I (1991). Lack of effective bactericidal activity of new quinolones against *Brucella* spp. *Antimicrob Ag Chemother* **35**: 765.

Gardembas-Pain M, Desablens B, Sensebe L *et al.* (1991). Home treatment of febrile neutropenia; an empirical oral antibiotic regimen. *Ann Oncol* **2**: 485.

Garlando F, Rietiker S, Tauber MG *et al.* (1987). Single-dose ciprofloxacin at 100 versus 250 mg for treatment of uncomplicated urinary tract infections in women. *Antimicrob Ag Chemother* **31**: 354.

Garraffo R, Jambou D, Chichmanian RM *et al.* (1991). *In vitro* and *in vivo* ciprofloxacin pharmacokinetics in human neutrophils. *Antimicrob Ag Chemother* **35**: 2215.

Garrelts JC, Godley PJ, Peterie JD *et al.* (1990). Sucralfate significantly reduces ciprofloxacin concentrations in serum. *Antimicrob Ag Chemother* **34**: 931.

Gasser TC, Ebert SC, Graversen PH *et al.* (1987a). Ciprofloxacin pharmacokinetics in patients with normal and impaired renal function. *Antimicrob Ag Chemother* **31**: 709.

Gasser TC, Graversen PH, Madsen PO (1987b). Treatment of complicated urinary tract infections with ciprofloxacin. *Amer J Med* **82** (Suppl 4A): 278.

Gasser TC, Ebert SC, Graverson PH *et al.* (1988). Pharmacokinetics of ciprofloxacin in patients with impaired renal function. *Rev Infect Dis* **10** (Supp 1): S110.

Gaunt PN, Lambert BE (1988). Single dose ciprofloxacin for the eradication of pharyngeal carriage of *Neisseria meningitidis*. *J Antimicrob Chemother* **21**: 489.

Gentry LO (1993). Treatment of skin and soft tissue infections with quinolone antimicrobial agents. In *Quinolone Antimicrobial Agents* 2nd edn (Hooper DC, Wolfson JS, eds), p. 413. Washington, DC: American Society of Microbiology.

Gentry LO, Koshdell A (1989). Intravenous/oral ciprofloxacin versus intravenous ceftazidine in the treatment of serious Gram-negative infections of the skin and skin structure. *Amer J Med* **87** (Suppl 5A): 132S.

Gentry LO, Rodriguez GG (1990). Oral ciprofloxacin compared with parenteral antibiotics in the treatment of osteomyelitis. *Antimicrob Ag Chemother* **34**: 40.

Gentry LO, Rodriguez-Gomez G (1991). Ofloxacin versus parenteral therapy for chronic osteomyelitis. *Antimicrob Ag Chemother* **35**: 538.

Gentry LO, Rodriguez-Gomez G, Zeluff BJ *et al.* (1989). A comparative evaluation of oral ofloxacin versus intravenous cefotaxime therapy for serious skin and skin structure infection. *Amer J Med* **87** (Suppl 6C): 57.

George J, Chakravarthy S, John GT, Jacob CK (1995). Bilateral emphysematous pyelonephritis responding to nonsurgical management. *Am J Nephrol* **15**: 172.

George MJ, Dew R3, Daly JS (1991). Acute renal failure after an overdose of ciprofloxacin. *Arch Intern Med* **151**: 620.

George RC, Ball LC, Norbury PB (1990). Susceptibility to ciprofloxacin of nosocomial gram-negative bacteria and staphylococci isolated in the UK. *J Antimicrob Chemother* **26** (Suppl F): 145.

Gerritsen WR, Peters A, Henry FC *et al.* (1987). Ciprofloxacin induced nephrotoxicity. *Nephrol Dial Transplant* **2**: 382.

Giamarellou H, Petrikkos G (1987). Ciprofloxacin interactions with imipenem and amikacin against multiresistant *Pseudomonas aeruginosa*. *Antimicrob Ag Chemother* **31**: 959.

Giamarellou H, Kolokythas E, Petrikkos G *et al.* (1989). Pharmacokinetics of three newer quinolones in pregnant and lactating women. *Amer J Med* **87** (Suppl 5A): 49S.

Gibb AP, Lewin CS, Garden OJ (1991). Development of quinolone resistance and multiple antibiotic resistance in *Salmonella bovismorbificans* in a pancreatic abscess. *J Antimicrob Chemother* **28**: 318.

Gilbert DN, Tice AD, Marsh PK *et al.* (1987). Oral ciprofloxacin therapy for chronic contiguous osteomyelitis caused by aerobic gram-negative bacilli. *Amer J Med* **82**: 254.

Gisby J, Wightman BJ, Beale AS (1991). Comparative efficacies of ciprofloxacin, amoxicillin, amoxicillin-clavulanic acid, and cefaclor against experimental *Streptococcus pneumoniae* respiratory infections in mice. *Antimicrob Ag Chemother* **35**: 831.

Glatt AE, Cummings M, McCormack W (1992). *In vitro* activity of temafloxacin compared with those of other agents against 100 clinical isolates of *Neisseria gonorrhoeae*. *Antimicrob Ag Chemother* **36**: 1131.

Gleadhill IC, Ferguson W, Lowry RC (1986). Efficacy and safety of ciprofloxacin in patients with respiratory infections in comparison with amoxicillin. *J Antimicrob Chemother* **18** (Suppl D): 133.

Glupczynski Y, Labbe M, Burette A *et al.* (1987). Treatment failure of ofloxacin in *Campylobacter pylori* infection. *Lancet* **i**: 1096.

Goepp JG, Lee CK, Anderson T *et al.* (1992). Use of ciprofloxacin in an infant with ventriculitis. *J Pediatr* **121**: 303.

Gogos CA, Maraziotis TG, Papadakis N *et al.* (1991). Penetration of ciprofloxacin into human cerebrospinal fluid in patients with inflamed and non-inflamed meninges. *Eur J Clin Microbiol Infect Dis* **10**: 511.

Gohara Y, Arai S, Akashi A *et al.* (1993). *In vitro* and *in vivo* activities of Q-35, a new fluoroquinolone, against *Mycoplasma pneumoniae*. *Antimicrob Ag Chemother* **37**: 1826.

Goldfarb J, Wormser GP, Inchiosa MJ *et al.* (1986). Single-dose pharmacokinetics of oral ciprofloxacin in patients with cystic fibrosis. *J Clin Pharmacol* **26**: 222.

Goldfarb J, Stern RC, Reed MD *et al.* (1987). Ciprofloxacin monotherapy for acute pulmonary exacerbations of cystic fibrosis. *Amer J Med* **82**: 174.

Goldstein EJ (1993). Patterns of susceptibility to fluoroquinolones among anaerobic bacterial isolates in the United States. *Clin Infect Dis* **16** (Suppl 4): S377.

Goldstein EJ, Citron DM (1988). Comparative activities of cefuroxime, amoxicillin-clavulanic acid, ciprofloxacin, enoxacin, and ofloxacin against aerobic and anaerobic bacteria isolated from bite wounds. *Antimicrob Ag Chemother* **32**: 1143.

Goldstein EJ, Citron DM (1992). Comparative activity of ciprofloxacin, ofloxacin, sparfloxacin, temafloxacin, CI-960, CI-990, and WIN 57273 against anaerobic bacteria. *Antimicrob Ag Chemother* **36**: 1158.

Goldstein EJ, Citron DM (1993). Comparative susceptibilities of 173 aerobic and anaerobic bite wound isolates to sparfloxacin, temafloxacin, clarithromycin, and older agents. *Antimicrob Ag Chemother* **37**: 1150.

Goldstein EJ, Citron DM, Vagvolgyi AE, Gombert ME (1986). Susceptibility of *Eikenella corrodens* to newer and older quinolones. *Antimicrob Ag Chemother* **30**: 172.

Golledge CL, Carson CF, O'Neill GL *et al.* (1992). Ciprofloxacin and *Clostridium difficile*-associated diarrhoea. *J Antimicrob Chemother* **30**: 141.

Golper TA, Hartstein AI, Morthland VH *et al.* (1987). Effects of antacids and dialysate dwell times on multiple-dose pharmacokinetics of oral ciprofloxacin in patients on continuous ambulatory peritoneal dialysis. *Antimicrob Ag Chemother* **31**: 1787.

Gombert ME, Aulicino TM, duBouchet L *et al.* (1987). Susceptibility of *Nocardia asteroides* to new quinolones and beta-lactams. *Antimicrob Ag Chemother* **31**: 2013.

Gombert ME, duBouchet L, Aulicino TM *et al.* (1989). Intravenous ciprofloxacin versus cefotaxime prophylaxis during transurethral surgery. *Amer J Med* **87** (Suppl 5A): 250S.

Gombert ME, Berkowitz LB, Aulicino TM *et al.* (1990). Therapy of pulmonary nocardiosis in immunocompromised mice. *Antimicrob Ag Chemother* **34**: 1766.

Gomez-Garces JL, Alos JI, Sanchez J, Cogollos R (1994). Bacteremia by multidrug-resistant *Capnocytophaga sputigena. J Clin Microbiol* **32**: 1067.

Gomez-Jimenez J, Ribera E, Almirante B *et al.* (1989). Ciprofloxacin resistance and staphylcoccal endocarditis. *Lancet* **ii**: 1525.

Gonski PN (1991). Ciprofloxacin-induced renal failure in an elderly patient. *Med J Aust* **154**: 638.

Gonzales JP, Henwood JM (1989). Pefloxacin A review of its antibacterial activity, pharmacokinetic properties and therapeutic use. *Drugs* **37**: 628.

Gonzales MA, Uribe F, Moisen SD *et al.* (1984). Multiple-dose pharmacokinetics and safety of ciprofloxacin in normal volunteers. *Antimicrob Ag Chemother* **26**: 741.

Gonzalez MA, Moranchel AH, Duran S *et al.* (1985). Multiple-dose pharmacokinetics of ciprofloxacin administered intravenously to normal volunteers. *Antimicrob Ag Chemother* **28**: 235.

Gooding BB, Jones RN (1993). *In vitro* antimicrobial activity of CP-99,219, a novel azabicyclo-naphthyridone. *Antimicrob Ag Chemother* **37**: 349.

Gooding BB, Erwin ME, Barrett MS *et al.* (1992). Antimicrobial activities of two investigational fluoroquinolones (CI-960 and E4695). against over 100 *Legionella* sp. isolates. *Antimicrob Ag Chemother* **36**: 2049.

Goodman LJ, Fliegelman RM, Trenholme GM, Kaplan RL (1984). Comparative *in vitro* activity of ciprofloxacin against *Campylobacter* spp and other bacterial enteric pathogens. *Antimicrob Ag Chemother* **25**: 504.

Goodman LJ, Trenholme GM, Kaplan RL *et al.* (1990). Empiric antimicrobial therapy of domestically acquired acute diarrhea in urban adults. *Arch Intern Med* **150**: 541.

Gootz TD, Martin BA (1991). Characterization of high-level quinolone resistance in *Campylobacter jejuni. Antimicrob Ag Chemother* **35**: 840.

Gordon JJ, Kauffman CA (1990). Superinfection with *Streptococcus pneumoniae* during therapy with ciprofloxacin. *Amer J Med* **89**: 383.

Gordon S, Swenson JM, Hill BC *et al.* (1992). Antimicrobial susceptibility patterns of common and unusual species of enterococci causing infections in the United States. Enterococcal Study Group. *J Clin Microbiol* **30**: 2373.

Gordon SM, Horsburgh CJ, Peloquin CA *et al.* (1993). Low serum levels of oral antimycobacterial agents in patients with disseminated *Mycobacterium avium* complex disease. *J Infect Dis* **168**: 1559.

Gorkiewicz-Petkow A, Weuta H, Jablonska S *et al.* (1988). Bacterial infections of the skin treated with ciprofloxacin. *Infection* **16** (Suppl 1): 55.

Görtz G, Boese-Landgraf J, Hopfenmuller W *et al.* (1990). Ciprofloxacin as single-dose antibiotic prophylaxis in colorectal surgery. Results of a randomized, double-blind trial. *Diagn Microbiol Infect Dis* **13**: 181.

Gorwitz RJ, Nakashima AK, Moran JS *et al.* (1993). Sentinel surveillance for antimicrobial resistance in *Neisseria gonorrhoeae* – United States, 1988–1991. The Gonococcal Isolate Surveillance Project Study Group. *MMWR* **42**: 29.

Gorzynski EA, Amsterdam D, Beam TJ *et al.* (1989a). Comparative *in vitro* activities of teicoplanin, vancomycin, oxacillin, and other antimicrobial agents against bacteremic isolates of gram-positive cocci. *Antimicrob Ag Chemother* **33**: 2019.

Gorzynski EA, Gutman SI, Allen W (1989b). Comparative antimycobacterial activities of difloxacin, temafloxacin, enoxacin, pefloxacin, reference fluoroquinolones, and a new macrolide, clarithromycin. *Antimicrob Ag Chemother* **33**: 591.

Gotuzzo E, Oberhelman RA, Maguina C *et al.* (1989). Comparison of single-dose treatment with norfloxacin and standard 5-day treatment with trimethoprim–sulfamethoxazole for acute shigellosis in adults. *Antimicrob Ag Chemother* **33**: 1101.

Gotuzzo E, Seas C, Echevarria J *et al.* (1995). Ciprofloxacin for the treatment of cholera: a randomized, double-blind, controlled clinical trial of a single daily dose in Peruvian adults. *Clin Infect Dis* **20**: 1485.

Gotuzzo EJ, Guerra G, Benavente L *et al.* (1988). Use of norfloxacin to treat chronic typhoid carriers. *J Infect Dis* **137**: 1221.

Grandis JR, Yu VL (1993). Treatment of infections of the ears, nose and throat and nasal carriage. In *Quinolone Antimicrobial Agents* 2nd edn (Hooper DC, Wolfson JS, eds), p. 363. Washington, DC: American Society of Microbiology.

Granowitz EV (1989). Photosensitivity rash in a patient being treated with ciprofloxacin. *J Infect Dis* **160**: 910.

Gransden WR, Warren CA, Phillips I *et al.* (1990). Decreased susceptibility of *Neisseria gonorrhoeae* to ciprofloxacin. *Lancet* **335**: 51.

Grasela TJ, Dreis MW (1992). An evaluation of the quinolone-theophylline interaction using the Food and Drug Administration spontaneous reporting system. *Arch Intern Med* **152**: 617.

Grassmick BK *et al.* (1992). Fulminant hepatic failure possibly related to ciprofloxacin. *Ann Pharmacother* **26**: 636.

Gray KJ, Allen KD, Ridgway EJ (1994). Impairment of driving by ciprofloxacin. *Brit Med J* **309**: 542.

Grayson ML (1995). Diabetic foot infections: Antimicrobial therapy. *Infect Dis Clin N America* **9**: 143.

Grayson ML, Eliopoulos GM, Wennersten CB *et al.* (1991). Increasing resistance to beta-lactam antibiotics among clinical isolates of *Enterococcus faecium*: a 22-year review at one institution. *Antimicrob Ag Chemother* **35**: 2180.

Grayson ML, Gibbons GW, Habershaw GM *et al.* (1994). Ampicillin/ sulbactam versus imipenem/cilastatin in the treatment of limb-threatening foot infections in diabetic patients. *Clin Infect Dis* **18**: 683.

Green SD, Ilunga F, Cheesbrough JS *et al.* (1993). The treatment of neonatal meningitis due to gram-negative bacilli with ciprofloxacin: evidence of satisfactory penetration into the cerebrospinal fluid. *J Infect* **26**: 253.

Greenberg RN, Kennedy DJ, Reilly PM *et al.* (1987a). Treatment of bone, joint, and soft-tissue infections with oral ciprofloxacin. *Antimicrob Ag Chemother* **31**: 151.

Greenberg RN, Tice AD, Marsh PK *et al.* (1987b). Randomized trial of ciprofloxacin compared with other antimicrobial therapy in the treatment of osteomyelitis. *Amer J Med* **82**: 266.

Greenwood D, Laverick A (1983). Activities of newer quinolones against legionella group organisms. *Lancet* **ii**: 279.

Grenier B (1989). Use of the new quinolones in cystic fibrosis. *Rev Infect Dis* **11** (Suppl 5): S1245.

Griffith JM, Barclay LM, de Petra V *et al.* (1996). High-level ciprofloxacin-resistant *Neisseria gonorrhoeae* and heterosexually acquired infections in Victoria. *Med J Aust* **164**: 125.

Grüneberg RN (1990). Changes in the antibiotic sensitivities of urinary pathogens, 1971–1989. *J Antimicrob Chemother* **26** (Suppl F): 3.

Grüneberg RN, Felmingham D, O'Hare MD *et al.* (1988). The comparative *in-vitro* activity of ofloxacin. *J Antimicrob Chemother* **22** (Suppl C): 9.

Guan L, Blumenthal RM, Burnham JC (1992). Analysis of macromolecular biosynthesis to define the quinolone-induced postantibiotic effect in *Escherichia coli. Antimicrob Ag Chemother* **36**: 2118.

Guay DR, Awni WM, Peterson PK *et al.* (1987). Pharmacokinetics of ciprofloxacin in acutely ill and convalescent elderly patients. *Amer J Med* **82** (Suppl 4A): 124.

Gudiol F, Pallares R, Carratala J *et al.* (1989). Randomized double-blind evaluation of ciprofloxacin and doxycycline for Mediterranean spotted fever. *Antimicrob Ag Chemother* **33**: 987.

Gudmundsson S, Erlendsdottir H, Gottfredsson M *et al.* (1990). The postantibiotic effect induced by antimicrobial combinations. *Scand J Infect Dis* (Suppl 74): 80.

Guharoy SR (1994). Serum sickness secondary to ciprofloxacin use. *Vet Hum Toxicol* **36**: 540.

Gwon A (1992). Ofloxacin vs tobramycin for the treatment of external ocular infection. Ofloxacin Study Group II. *Arch Ophthalmol* **110**: 1234.

Hackbarth CJ, Chambers HF, Sande MA (1986). Serum bactericidal activity of rifampin in combination with other antimicrobial agents against *Staphylococcus aureus. Antimicrob Ag Chemother* **29**: 611.

Haddow A, Greene S, Heinz G *et al.* (1989). Ciprofloxacin (intravenous/

oral). versus ceftazidime in lower respiratory tract infections. *Amer J Med* **87** (Suppl 5A): 113S.

Hajji M, Mdaghri NE, Benbachir M *et al.* (1988). Prospective randomized comparative trial of pefloxacin versus cotrimoxazole in the treatment of typhoid fever in adults. *Eur J Clin Microbiol Infect Dis* **7**: 361.

Halkin H (1988). Adverse effects of the fluoroquinolones. *Rev Infect Dis* **10** (Suppl 1): S258.

Hall MN, Silhavey TJ (1981). The *ompB* locus and the regulation of the major outer membrane porin proteins of *Escherichia coli* K12. *J Mol Biol* **146**: 23.

Hall WH (1990). Modern chemotherapy for brucellosis in humans. *Rev Infect Dis* **12**: 1060.

Haller I (1985). Comprehensive evaluation of ciprofloxacin-aminoglycoside combinations against Enterobacteriaceae and *Pseudomonas aeruginosa* strain. *Antimicrob Ag Chemother* **28**: 663.

Haller I (1987). Evaluation of ciprofloxacin alone and in combination with other antibiotics in a murine model of thigh muscle infection. *Amer J Med* **82**: 76.

Halliwell RF, Davey PG, Lambert JJ (1991). The effects of quinolones and NS*AIDS* upon GABA-evoked currents recorded from rat dorsal root ganglion neurones. *J Antimicrob Chemother* **27**: 209.

Hammerschlag MR, Hyman CL, Roblin PM (1992). *In vitro* activities of five quinolones against *Chlamydia pneumoniae*. *Antimicrob Ag Chemother* **36**: 682.

Hancock REW (1987). Role of porins in outer membrane permeability. *J Bacteriol* **169**: 929.

Hane MW, Wood TH (1969). Escherichia coli K-12 mutants resistant to nalidixic acid: genetic mapping and dominance studies. *J Bacteriol* **99**: 238.

Harder S, Fuhr U, Staib AH *et al.* (1989). Ciprofloxacin-caffeine: a drug interaction established using *in vivo* and *in vitro* investigations. *Amer J Med* **87** (Suppl 5A): 89S.

Hardy DJ (1991). Activity of temafloxacin and other fluoroquinolones against typical and atypical community-acquired respiratory tract pathogens. *Amer J Med* **91** (Suppl 6A): 12S.

Harnett N, Brown S, Krishnan C (1991). Emergence of quinolone resistance among clinical isolates of methicillin-resistant *Staphylococcus aureus* in Ontario, Canada. *Antimicrob Ag Chemother* **35**: 1911.

Haron E, Rolston KVI, Cunningham C *et al.* (1989). Oral ciprofloxacin therapy for infections in cancer patients. *J Antimicrob Chemother* **24**: 955.

Harris JC, DuPont HL, Hornick RB (1972). Fecal leukocytes in diarrheal illness. *Ann Intern Med* **76**: 697.

Havlicheck D, Saravolatz L, Pohlod D (1987). Effect of quinolones and other antimicrobial agents on cell-associated *Legionella pneumophila*. *Antimicrob Ag Chemother* **31**: 1529.

Healy DP, Polk RE, Kanawati L *et al.* (1989). Interaction between oral ciprofloxacin and caffeine in normal volunteers. *Antimicrob Ag Chemother* **33**: 474.

Heifets LB, Lindholm-Levy P (1990). MICs and MBCs of Win 57273 against *Mycobacterium avium* and *M. tuberculosis*. *Antimicrob Ag Chemother* **34**: 770.

Heinonen PK, Teisala K, Aine R *et al.* (1989). Intravenous and oral ciprofloxacin in the treatment of proven pelvic inflammatory disease. A comparison with doxycycline and metronidazole. *Amer J Med* **87** (Suppl 5A): 152S.

Heisig P (1993). High-level fluoroquinolone resistance in a *Salmonella typhimurium* isolate due to alterations in both gyrA and gyrB genes. *J Antimicrob Chemother* **32**: 367.

Heisig P, Wiedemann B (1991). Use of a broad-host-range *gyrA* plasmid for genetic characterization of fluoroquinolone-resistant gram-negative bacteria. *Antimicrob Ag Chemother* **35**: 2031.

Heisig P, Schedletzky H, Falkenstein-Paul H (1993). Mutations in the gyrA gene of a highly fluoroquinolone-resistant clinical isolate of *Escherichia coli*. *Antimicrob Ag Chemother* **37**: 696.

Heisig P, Tzouvelekis L, Vatopoulos A, Legakis N (1994). Ciprofloxacin resistance in enterobacterial clinical isolates. *J Antimicrob Chemother* **33**: 887.

Hellsten S, Forsgren A, Bjork T *et al.* (1989). Use of ciprofloxacin in patients undergoing transurethral prostatic surgery. *Scand J Infect Dis* (Suppl 60): 104.

Helmink R, Benediktsson H (1990). Ciprofloxacin induced allergic interstitial nephritis. *Nephron* **55**: 432.

Hickey SA, Ford GR, O'Connor AF *et al.* (1989). Treating malignant otitis with oral ciprofloxacin. *Brit Med J* **299**: 550.

Hillery SJ, Reiss-Levy EA (1993). Increasing ciprofloxacin resistance in MRSA. *Med J Aust* **158**: 861.

Hillman RJ, Rao GG, Harris JR *et al.* (1990). Ciprofloxacin as a cause of *Clostridium difficile*-associated diarrhoea in an HIV antibody-positive patient. *J Infect* **21**: 205.

Hirai K, Suzue S, Irikura T, Iyobe S, Mitsuhashi S (1987). Mutations producing resistance to norfloxacin in *Pseudomonas aeruginosa*. *Antimicrob Ag Chemother* **31**: 582.

Hirata CA, Guay DR, Awni WM *et al.* (1989). Steady-state pharmacokinetics of intravenous and oral ciprofloxacin in elderly patients. *Antimicrob Ag Chemother* **33**: 1927.

Hjelm U, Kaustova J, Kubin M, Hoffner SE (1992). Susceptibility of *Mycobacterium kansasii* to ethambutol and its combination with rifamycins, ciprofloxacin and isoniazid. *Eur J Clin Microbiol Infect Dis* **11**: 51.

Hoban D, DeGagne P, Witwicki E (1989). *In vitro* activity of lomefloxacin against *Chlamydia trachomatis*, *Neisseria gonorrhoeae*, *Haemophilus ducreyi*, *Mycoplasma hominis*, and *Ureaplasma urealyticum*. *Diagn Microbiol Infect Dis* **12** (Suppl 3): 83S.

Hodson ME, Roberts CM, Butland RJ *et al.* (1987). Oral ciprofloxacin compared with conventional intravenous treatment for *Pseudomonas aeruginosa* infection in adults with cystic fibrosis. *Lancet* **i**: 235.

Hoey LL, Lake KD (1994). Does ciprofloxacin interact with cyclosporine? *Ann Pharmacother* **28**: 93.

Hof H, Ehrhard I, Tschape H (1991). Presence of quinolone resistance in a strain of *Salmonella typhimurium*. *Eur J Clin Microbiol Infect Dis* **10**: 747.

Höffken G, Borner K, Glatzel PD *et al.* (1985a). Reduced enteral absorption of ciprofloxacin in the presence of antacids. *Eur J Clin Microbiol* **4**: 345.

Höffken G, Lode H, Prinzing C *et al.* (1985b). Pharmacokinetics of ciprofloxacin after oral and parenteral administration. *Antimicrob Ag Chemother* **27**: 375.

Höffken G, Lode H, Wiley R *et al.* (1988). Pharmacokinetic and bioavailability of ciprofloxacin and ofloxacin: effect of food and antacid intake. *Rev Infect Dis* **10** (Suppl 1): S138.

Hoffner SE, Kratz M, Olsson LB *et al.* (1989). *In-vitro* synergistic activity between ethambutol and fluorinated quinolones against *Mycobacterium avium* complex. *J Antimicrob Chemother* **24**: 317.

Hoffner SE, Hjelm U, Kallenius G (1993). Susceptibility of *Mycobacterium malmoense* to antibacterial drugs and drug combinations. *Antimicrob Ag Chemother* **37**: 1285.

Hohl P, Luthy HJ, Zollinger IJ *et al.* (1990). *In vitro* activities of fleroxacin, cefetamet, ciprofloxacin, ceftriaxone, trimethoprim–sulfamethoxazole, and amoxicillin-clavulanic acid against rare members of the family Enterobacteriaceae primarily of human (clinical) origin. *Antimicrob Ag Chemother* **34**: 1605.

Holley HP, Jr (1991). Successful treatment of cat-scratch disease with ciprofloxacin. *JAMA* **265**: 1563.

Hoogkamer JF, Kleinbloesem CH (1995). The effect of milk consumption on the pharmacokinetics of fleroxacin and ciprofloxacin in healthy volunteers. *Drugs* **49** (Suppl 2): 346.

Hoogkamp-Korstanje JAA (1987). Antibiotics in *Yersinia enterocolitica* infections. *J Antimicrob Chemother* **20**: 123.

Hoogkamp-Korstanje JAA, Klein SJ (1986). Ciprofloxacin in acute exacerbations of chronic bronchitis. *J Antimicrob Chemother* **18**: 407.

Hoogkamp-Korstanje JAA, Van Oort HJ, Schipper JJ, Van der Wal T (1984). Intraprostatic concentration of ciprofloxacin and its activity against urinary pathogens. *J Antimicrob Chemother* **14**: 641.

Hoogkamp-Korstanje JAA, van Bottenburg HA, van Bruggan J *et al.* (1989). Treatment of chronic osteomyelitis with ciprofloxacin. *J Antimicrob Chemother* **23**: 427.

Hook E, Jones RB, Martin DH et al. (1993). Comparison of ciprofloxacin and ceftriaxone as single-dose therapy for uncomplicated gonorrhea in women. Antimicrob Ag Chemother 37: 1670.

Hooper DC, Wolfson JS (1989). Treament of genitourinary infections with fluoroquinolones: clinical efficacy in genital infections and adverse effects. Antimicrob Ag Chemother 33: 1662.

Hooper DC, Wolfson JS (1993a). Adverse effects. In Quinolone Antimicrobial Agents 2nd edn (Hooper DC, Wolfson JS, eds), p. 489. Washington, DC: American Society of Microbiology.

Hooper DC, Wolfson JS (1993b). Mechanisms of bacterial resistance to quinolones. In Quinolone Antimicrobial Agents 2nd edn (Hooper DC, Wolfson JS, eds), p. 97. Washington, DC: American Society of Microbiology.

Hooper DC, Wolfson JS, Souza KS et al. (1986). Genetic and biochemical characterization of norfloxacin resistance in Escherichia coli. Antimicrob Ag Chemother 29: 639.

Hooper DC, Wolfson JS, Ng EY, Swartz MN (1987). Mechanisms of action of and resistance to ciprofloxacin. Amer J Med 82 (Suppl 4A): 12.

Hooper DC, Wolfson JS, Souza KS et al. (1989). Mechanisms of quinolone resistance in Escherichia coli: characterization of nfxB and cfxB, two mutant resistance loci decreasing norfloxacin accumulation. Antimicrob Ag Chemother 33: 283.

Hooper TL, Gould FK, Swinburn CR et al. (1988). Ciprofloxacin; a preferred treatment for Legionella infections in patients receiving cyclosporin A. J Antimicrob Chemother 22: 952.

Hootkins RA, Fenves AZ, Stephens MK (1989). Acute renal failure secondary to oral ciprofloxacin therapy a presentation of three cases and a review of the literature. Clin Nephrol 32: 75.

Hooton TM, Rogers ME, Medina TG et al. (1990). Ciprofloxacin compared with doxycycline for nongonococcal urethritis. Ineffectiveness against Chlamydia trachomatis due to relapsing infection. JAMA 264: 1418.

Hopf G, Böcker R, Esther CJ, Radtke HJ, Floh W (1988). Concentration of ciprofloxacin in human serum, lung and pleural tissues and fluids during and after lung surgery. Infection 16: 29.

Hoppe JE, Simon CG (1990). In vitro susceptibilities of Bordetella pertussis and Bordetella parapertussis to seven fluoroquinolones. Antimicrob Ag Chemother 34: 2287.

Horiuchi S, Inagaki Y, Yamamoto N et al. (1993). Reduced susceptibilities of Shigella sonnei strains isolated from patients with dysentery to fluoroquinolones. Antimicrob Ag Chemother 37: 2486.

Houwen RH, Bijleveld CM, de VHH (1987). Ciprofloxacin for cholangitis after hepatic portoenterostomy. Lancet i: 1367.

Howard AJ, Joseph TD, Bloodworth LL et al. (1990). The emergence of ciprofloxacin resistance in Salmonella typhimurium. J Antimicrob Chemother 26: 296.

Hoyme UB, Buhler K, Krasemann C et al. (1989). Ciprofloxacin in therapy for uncomplicated salpingitis. Rev Infect Dis 11 (Suppl 5): S1279.

Huband MD, Cohen MA, Meservey MA et al. (1993). In vitro antibacterial activities of PD 138312 and PD 140248, new fluoronaphthyridines with outstanding gram-positive potency. Antimicrob Ag Chemother 37: 2563.

Hudson SJ, Ingham HR, Snow MH (1985). Treatment of Salmonella typhi carrier state with ciprofloxacin. Lancet i: 1047.

Humphreys H, Speller DC (1989). Acute epididymo-orchitis caused by Pseudomonas aeruginosa and treated with ciprofloxacin. J Infect 19: 257.

Humphreys H, Lovering A, White LO et al. (1989). Flavobacterium meningosepticum infection, in a 32-day-old child on acute peritoneal dialysis, treated with ciprofloxacin. J Antimicrob Chemother 23: 292.

Hussey G, Kibel M, Parker N (1992). Ciprofloxacin treatment of multiply drug-resistant extrapulmonary tuberculosis in a child. Pediatr Infect Dis J 11: 408.

Husson MO, Izard D, Bouillet L, Leclerc H (1985). Comparative in vitro activity of ciprofloxacin against non-fermenters. J Antimicrob Chemother 15: 457.

Hyams KC, Bourgeois AL, Merrell BR et al. (1991). Diarrheal disease during Operation Desert Shield. New Engl J Med 325: 1423.

Hyatt DS, Rogers TR, McCarthy DM et al. (1991). A randomized trial of ciprofloxacin plus azlocillin versus netilmicin plus azlocillin for the empirical treatment of fever in neutropenic patients. J Antimicrob Chemother 28: 324.

Ichlyama S, Tsukamura M (1987). Ofloxacin and the therapy of pulmonary disease due to Mycobacterium fortuitum. Chest 92: 1110.

Ikerd TR, Koletar SL (1993). In-vitro activity of ciprofloxacin, temafloxacin, azithromycin, clarithromycin and metronidazole against Giardia lamblia. J Antimicrob Chemother 31: 615.

Imada T, Miyazaki S, Nishida M et al. (1992). In vitro and in vivo antibacterial activities of a new quinolone, OPC-17116. Antimicrob Ag Chemother 36: 573.

Imrie KR, Prince HM, Couture F et al. (1995). Effect of antimicrobial prophylaxis on hematopoietic recovery following autologous bone marrow transplantation: ciprofloxacin versus co-trimoxazole. Bone Marrow Transplant 15: 267.

Inderlied CB, Lancero MG, Bermudez LM, Young LS (1989). In vitro activity of lomefloxacin as compared with ciprofloxacin. Diagn Microbiol Infect Dis 12 (Suppl 3): 17S.

Ingerman M, Pitsakis PG, Rosenberg A et al. (1987). Beta-lactamase production in experimental endocarditis due to aminoglycoside-resistant Streptococcus faecalis. J Infect Dis 155: 1226.

Ingham B, Brentnall DW, Dale EA et al. (1977). Arthropathy induced by antibacterial fused N-alkyl-4-pyridine-3-carboxylic acids. Toxicol Lett 1: 21.

Inoue Y, Sata K, Fujii T et al. (1987). Some properties of subunits of DNA gyrase from Pseudomonas aeruginosa PAO1 and its nalidixic acid-resistant mutant. J Bacteriol 169: 2322.

Iravani A (1993). Multicenter study of single-dose and multiple-dose fleroxacin versus ciprofloxacin in the treatment of uncomplicated urinary tract infections. Amer J Med 94 (Suppl 3A): 89S.

Iravani A, Tice AD, McCarty J et al. (1995). Short-course ciproflox treatment of acute uncomplicated urinary tract infection in women. The minimum effective dose. The Urinary Tract Infection Study Group. Arch Intern Med 155: 485.

Isaacs D, Slack MPE, Wilkinson AR, Westwood AW (1986). Successful treatment of Pseudomonas ventriculitis with ciprofloxacin. J Antimicrob Chemother 17: 535.

Isaacs RD, Kunke PJ, Cohen RL, Smith JW (1988). Ciprofloxacin resistance in epidemic methicillin-resistant Staphylococcus aureus. Lancet ii: 843.

Isenmann R, Friess H, Schlegel P et al. (1994). Penetration of ciprofloxacin into the human pancreas. Infection 22: 343.

Islam MA, Sreedharan T (1965). Convulsions, hyperglycaemia and glycosuria from overdose of nalidixic acid. JAMA 192: 1000–1001.

Israel D, Gillum JG, Turik M et al. (1993). Pharmacokinetics and serum bactericidal titers of ciprofloxacin and ofloxacin following multiple oral doses in healthy volunteers. Antimicrob Ag Chemother 37: 2193.

Ito H, Yoshida H, Bogaki-Shonai M et al. (1994). Quinolone resistance mutations in the DNA gyrase gyrA and gyrB genes of Staphylococcus aureus. Antimicrob Ag Chemother 38: 2014.

Jabarit-Aldighieri N, Torres H, Raoult D (1992). Susceptibility of Rickettsia conorii, R. rickettsii, and Coxiella burnetii to PD 127,391, PD 131,628, pefloxacin, ofloxacin, and ciprofloxacin. Antimicrob Ag Chemother 36: 2529.

Jacobs F, Marchal M et al. (1990). Penetration of ciprofloxacin into human pleural fluid. Antimicrob Ag Chemother 34: 934.

Jacobson MA, Hahn SM, Gerberding JL et al. (1989). Ciprofloxacin for Salmonella bacteremia in the acquired immunodeficiency syndrome (AIDS). Ann Intern Med 110: 1027.

Jacobson MA, Yajko D, Northfelt D et al. (1993). Randomized, placebo-controlled trial of rifampin, ethambutol, and ciprofloxacin for AIDS patients with disseminated Mycobacterium avium complex infection. J Infect Dis 168: 112.

Jacoby GA, Archer GL (1991). Mechanisms of bacterial resistance to antimicrobial agents. New Engl J Med 324: 601.

Jaehde U, Sorgel F, Reiter A et al. (1995). Effect of probenecid on the distribution and elimination of ciprofloxacin in humans. Clin Pharmacol Ther 58: 532.

Janknegt R (1990). Drug interactions with quinolones. *J Antimicrob Chemother* **26** (Suppl D): 7.

Jansen J, Cromer M, Akard L *et al.* (1994). Infection prevention in severely myelosuppressed patients: a comparison between ciprofloxacin and a regimen of selective antibiotic modulation of the intestinal flora. *Amer J Med* **96**: 335.

Jensen T, Pedersen SS, Hoiby N *et al.* (1987a). Efficacy of oral fluoroquinolones versus conventional intravenous antipseudomonal chemotherapy in treatment of cystic fibrosis. *Eur J Clin Microbol* **6**: 618.

Jensen T, Pedersen SS, Nielsen CH *et al.* (1987b). The efficacy and safety of ciprofloxacin and ofloxacin in chronic *Pseudomonas aeruginosa* infection in cystic fibrosis. *J Antimicrob Chemother* **20**: 585.

Jephcott AE, Turner A (1990). Ciprofloxacin resistance in gonococci. *Lancet* **335**: 165.

Ji B, Lounis N, Truffot-Pernot C, Grosset J (1995). *In vitro* and *in vivo* activities of levofloxacin against *Mycobacterium tuberculosis*. *Antimicrob Ag Chemother* **39**: 1341.

Jimenez-Valera M, Sampedro A, Moreno E, Ruiz-Bravo A (1995). Modification of immune response in mice by ciprofloxacin. *Antimicrob Ag Chemother* **39**: 150.

Joachims HZ, Danimo J, Raz R (1988). Malignant external otitis, treatment with fluoroquinolones. *Am J Otolaryngol* **9**: 102.

Joesoef MR, Knapp JS, Idajadi A *et al.* (1994). Antimicrobial susceptibilities of *Neisseria gonorrhoeae* strains isolated in Surabaya, Indonesia. *Antimicrob Ag Chemother* **38**: 2530.

John JJ, Atkins LT, Maple PA *et al.* (1992). Activities of newer fluoroquinolones against *Shigella sonnei*. *Antimicrob Ag Chemother* **36**: 2346.

Johnson EJ, MacGowan AP, Potter MN *et al.* (1990). Reduced absorption of oral ciprofloxacin after chemotherapy for haematological malignancy. *J Antimicrob Chemother* **25**: 837.

Johnson PC, Ericsson CD, Morgan DR *et al.* (1986). Lack of emergence of resistant fecal flora during successful prophylaxis of travellers' diarrhea with norfloxacin. *Antimicrob Ag Chemother* **30**: 671.

Johnson PR, Liu YJ, Tooth JA (1992). A randomized trial of high-dose ciprofloxacin versus azlocillin and netilmicin in the empirical therapy of febrile neutropenic patients. *J Antimicrob Chemother* **30**: 203.

Jolson HM, Tanner LA, Green L *et al.* (1991). Adverse reaction reporting of interaction between warfarin and fluoroquinolones. *Arch Intern Med* **151**: 1003.

Joly-Guillou ML, Bergogne-Bérézin E (1992). *In-vitro* activity of sparfloxacin, pefloxacin, ciprofloxacin and temafloxacin against clinical isolates of *Acinetobacter* spp. *J Antimicrob Chemother* **29**: 466.

Jones RB, Van dPB, Martin DH *et al.* (1990). Partial characterization of *Chlamydia trachomatis* isolates resistant to multiple antibiotics. *J Infect Dis* **162**: 1309.

Joos B, Ledergerber B, Flepp M *et al.* (1985). Comparison of high pressure liquid chromatography and bioassay for determination of ciprofloxacin in serum and urine. *Antimicrob Ag Chemother* **27**: 353.

Jorgensen JH, Doern GV, Thornsberry C *et al.* (1988). Susceptibility of multiply resistant *Haemophilus influenzae* to newer antimicrobial agents. *Diagn Microbiol Infect Dis* **9**: 27.

Joseph J, Vaughan LM, Basran GS (1994). Penetration of intravenous and oral ciprofloxacin into sterile and empyemic human pleural fluid. *Ann Pharmacother* **28**: 313.

Judlin P, Scheffler C, Dailloux M *et al.* (1991). Shorter duration of treatment in chlamydial pelvic infections with ofloxacin–amoxicillin–clavulanate, compared with doxycycline-amoxicillin–clavulanate. *Eur J Clin Microbiol Infect Dis* Special Issue: 314.

Jungst G, Mohr R (1988). Overview of postmarketing experience with ofloxacin in Germany. *J Antimicrob Chemother* **22** (Suppl C): 167.

Kaatz GW, Seo SM (1990). WIN 57273, a new fluoroquinolone with enhanced *in vitro* activity *versus* Gram-positive pathogens. *Antimicrob Ag Chemother* **34**: 1376.

Kaatz GW, Seo SM, Barriere SL *et al.* (1989). Ciprofloxacin and rifampin, alone and in combination, for therapy of experimental *Staphylococcus aureus* endocarditis. *Antimicrob Ag Chemother* **33**: 1184.

Kaatz GW, Seo SM, Ruble CA (1991). Mechanisms of fluoroquinolone resistance in *Staphylococcus aureus*. *J Infect Dis* **163**: 1080.

Kain KC, Kelly MT (1989). Antimicrobial susceptibility of *Plesiomonas shigelloides* from patients with diarrhea. *Antimicrob Ag Chemother* **33**: 1609.

Kaku M, Ishida K, Irifune K *et al.* (1994). *In vitro* and *in vivo* activities of sparfloxacin against *Mycoplasma pneumoniae*. *Antimicrob Ag Chemother* **38**: 738.

Kanaiyalal DM, Abrams PH, White LO (1988). A double-blind comparative trial of short-term orally administered enosacin in the prevention of urinary infection after elective transurethral prostatectomy; a clinical and pharmacokinetic study. *J Urol* **139**: 1232.

Kane MP, Bailie GR, Moon DG, Siu I (1994). Stability of ciprofloxacin injection in peritoneal dialysis solutions. *Amer J Hosp Pharm* **51**: 373.

Karabalut N, Drusano GL (1993). Pharmacokinetics of the quinolone antimicrobial agents. In *Quinolone Antimicrobial Agents* 2nd edn (Hooper DC, Wolfson JS, eds), p. 195. Washington, DC: American Society of Microbiology.

Karp JE, Menz WG, Hendricksen C *et al.* (1986). Oral norfloxacin for prevention of gram-negative bacterial infections in patients with acute leukemia and granulocytopenia. A randomized double-blind placebo-controlled trial. *Ann Intern Med* **106**: 1.

Karp JE, Dick JD, Merz WG (1988). Systemic infection and colonization with and without prophylactic norfloxacin use over time in the granulocytopenic, acute leukemia patient. *Eur J Clin Oncol* **24** (Suppl 1): S5.

Kato N, Miyauchi M, Muto Y *et al.* (1988). Emergence of fluoroquinolone resistance in *Bacteroides fragilis* accompanied by resistance to beta-lactam antibiotics. *Antimicrob Agents Chemother* **32**: 1437.

Kelsey SM, Wood ME, Shaw E *et al.* (1990). A comparative study of intravenous ciprofloxacin and benzylpenicillin versus netilmicin and piperacillin for the empirical treatment of fever in neutropenic patients. *J Antimicrob Chemother* **25**: 149.

Kelsey SM, Weinhardt B, Collins PW, Newland AC (1992). Teicoplanin plus ciprofloxacin versus gentamicin plus piperacillin in the treatment of febrile neutropenic patients. *Eur J Clin Microbiol Infect Dis* **11**: 509.

Kemper CA, Meng TC, Nussbaum J *et al.* (1992). Treatment of *Mycobacterium avium* complex bacteremia in *AIDS* with a four-drug oral regimen. Rifampin, ethambutol, clofazimine, and ciprofloxacin. The California Collaborative Treatment Group. *Ann Intern Med* **116**: 466.

Kennedy N, Fox R, Kisyombe GM *et al.* (1993). Early bactericidal and sterilizing activities of ciprofloxacin in pulmonary tuberculosis. *Amer Rev Respir Dis* **148**: 1547.

Kenny GE, Cartwright FD (1991a). Susceptibilities of *Mycoplasma hominis* and *Ureaplasma urealyticum* to two new quinolones, sparfloxacin and WIN 57273. *Antimicrob Ag Chemother* **35**: 1515.

Kenny GE, Cartwright FD (1991b). Susceptibility of *Mycoplasma pneumoniae* to several new quinolones, tetracycline, and erythromycin. *Antimicrob Ag Chemother* **35**: 587.

Kenny GE, Hooton TM, Roberts MC *et al.* (1989). Susceptibilities of genital mycoplasmas to the newer quinolones as determined by the agar dilution method. *Antimicrob Ag Chemother* **33**: 103.

Kent RJ, Bakhtiar M, Shanson DC (1992). The *in-vitro* bactericidal activities of combinations of antimicrobial agents against clinical isolates of *Mycobacterium avium*-intracellulare. *J Antimicrob Chemother* **30**: 643.

Kern W, Kurrle E (1991). Ofloxacin versus trimethoprim–sulfamethoxazole for prevention of infection in patients with acute leukemia and granulocytopenia. *Infection* **19**: 73.

Kern WV, Markus A, Andriof E (1994). Bacteremia due to fluoroquinolone-resistant *Escherichia coli* in two immunocompromised patients. *Eur J Clin Microbiol Infect Dis* **13**: 161.

Ketterl R, Beckurts T, Stubinger B, Claudi B (1988). Use of ofloxacin in open fractures and in the treatment of post-traumatic osteomyelitis. *J Antimicrob Chemother* **22** (Suppl C): 159.

Khan EA, Basir R (1989). Sequential intravenous-oral administration of ciprofloxacin vs ceftazidime in serious bacterial respiratory tract infections. *Chest* **96**: 528.

Khan MY, Dizon M, Kiel FW (1989). Comparative *in vitro* activities of ofloxacin, difloxacin, ciprofloxacin, and other selected antimicrobial agents against *Brucella melitensis. Antimicrob Ag Chemother* 33: 1409.

Khardori N, Nguyen H, Rosenbaum B *et al.* (1994). *In vitro* susceptibilities of rapidly growing mycobacteria to newer antimicrobial agents. *Antimicrob Ag Chemother* 38: 134.

Kharsany AB, Hoosen AA, Van dEJ (1993). Antimicrobial susceptibilities of *Gardnerella vaginalis. Antimicrob Ag Chemother* 37: 2733.

Kimura M, Kishimoto T, Niki Y *et al.* (1993). *In vitro* and *in vivo* antichlamydial activities of newly developed quinolone antimicrobial agents. *Antimicrob Ag Chemother* 37: 801.

King A, Shannon K, Phillips I (1984). The *in-vitro* activity of ciprofloxacin compared with that of norfloxacin and nalidixic acid. *J Antimicrob Chemother* 13: 325.

King A, Bethune L, Phillips I (1991). The *in-vitro* activity of tosufloxacin, a new fluorinated quinolone, compared with that of ciprofloxacin and temafloxacin. *J Antimicrob Chemother* 28: 719.

Kitsukawa K, Hara J, Saito A (1991). Inhibition of *Legionella pneumophila* in guinea pig peritoneal macrophages by new quinolone, macrolide and other antimicrobial agents. *J Antimicrob Chemother* 27: 343.

Kitzes-Cohen R, Miler A, Gilboa A, Harel D (1988). Penetration of ciprofloxacin into cerebrospinal fluid. *Rev Infect Dis* 10 (Suppl): S256.

Kivistö KT *et al.* (1992). Inhibition of norfloxacin absorption by dairy products. *Antimicrob Ag Chemother* 36: 489.

Klinger JD, Aronoff SC (1985). Antimicrobial effects of cefotaxime as studied by the potentiometric measurement of lipoic acid reduction in *Escherichia coli* cultures. *J Antimicrob Chemother* 15: 679.

Kljucar S, Heimesaat M, von PE *et al.* (1989). Efficacy and safety of higher-dose intravenous ciprofloxacin in severe hospital-acquired infections. *Amer J Med* 87 (Suppl 5A): 52S.

Klopman G, Wang S, Jacobs MR *et al.* (1993). Anti-*Mycobacterium avium* activity of quinolones: *in vitro* activities. *Antimicrob Ag Chemother* 37: 1799.

Knapp JS, Back AF, Babst AF *et al.* (1993). *In vitro* susceptibilities of isolates of *Haemophilus ducreyi* from Thailand and the United States to currently recommended and newer agents for treatment of chancroid. *Antimicrob Ag Chemother* 37: 1552.

Knapp JS, Ohye R, Neal SW *et al.* (1994a). Emerging *in vitro* resistance to quinolones in penicillinase-producing *Neisseria gonorrhoeae* strains in Hawaii. *Antimicrob Ag Chemother* 38: 2200.

Knapp JS, Washington JA, Doyle LJ *et al.* (1994b). Persistence of *Neisseria gonorrhoeae* strains with decreased susceptibilities to ciprofloxacin and ofloxacin in Cleveland, Ohio, from 1992 through 1993. *Antimicrob Ag Chemother* 38: 2194.

Kobayashi H (1987). Clinical efficacy of ciprofloxacin in the treatment of patients with respiratory infection in Japan. *Amer J Med* 82 (Suppl 4A): 169.

Kosmidis J (1991). A double-blind study of once-daily temafloxacin in the treatment of bacterial lower respiratory tract infections. *J Antimicrob Chemother* 28 (Suppl C): 73.

Kostelyn P, Bogaerts J, Stevens AM *et al.* (1989). Treatment of adult gonococcal keratoconjunctivitis with oral norfloxacin. *Amer J Ophthalmol*; 108: 515.

Kotilainen P, Nikoskelainen J, Huovinen P (1990). Emergence of ciprofloxacin-resistant coagulase-negative staphylococcal skin flora in immunocompromised patients receiving ciprofloxacin. *J Infect Dis* 161: 41.

Kotilainen P, Huovinen S, Jarvinen H *et al.* (1995). Epidemiology of the colonization of inpatients and outpatients with ciprofloxacin-resistant coagulase-negative staphylococci. *Clin Infect Dis* 21: 685.

Koul PA, Wani JI, Wahid A (1995). Ciprofloxacin for multiresistant enteric fever in pregnancy. *Lancet* 346: 307.

Körner RJ, Reeves DS, MacGowan AP (1994). Dangers of oral fluoroquinolone treatment in community acquired upper respiratory tract infections. *Brit Med J* 308: 191.

Kresken M, Wiedemann B (1988). Development of resistance to nalidixic acid and the fluoroquinolones after the introduction of norfloxacin and ofloxacin. *Antimicrob Ag Chemother* 32: 1285.

Krishna S, Davis TM, Chan PC *et al.* (1988). Ciprofloxacin and malaria. *Lancet* i: 1231.

Kromann-Andersen B, Sommer P, Pers C *et al.* (1988). Ofloxacin compared with ciprofloxacin in the treatment of complicated lower urinary tract infections. *J Antimicrob Chemother* 22 (Suppl C): 143.

Krüger HU, Schuler U, Proksch B *et al.* (1990). Investigation of potential interaction of ciprofloxacin with cyclosporine in bone marrow transplant recipients. *Antimicrob Ag Chemother* 34: 1048.

Kuah BG, Kumarasinghe G, Doran J, Chang HR (1994). Antimicrobial susceptibilities of clinical isloates of *Acinetobacter baumannii* from Singapore. *Antimicrob Ag Chemother* 38: 2502.

Kujath P (1989). Antibiotic prophylaxis in biliary tract surgery Ciprofloxacin versus ceftriaxone. *Amer J Med* 87 (Suppl 5A): 255S.

Kumada T, Neu HC (1985). *In-vitro* activity of ofloxacin, a quinolone carboxylic acid compared to other quinolones and other antimicrobial agents. *J Antimicrob Chemother* 16: 563.

Kumar A, Wofford MR, Gordon RC (1989). Ciprofloxacin, imipenem and rifampicin: *in-vitro* synergy of two and three drug combinations against *Pseudomonas cepacia. J Antimicrob Chemother* 23: 831.

Kumar A, Hay MB, Maier GA *et al.* (1992). Post-antibiotic effect of ceftazidime, ciprofloxacin, imipenem, piperacillin and tobramycin for *Pseudomonas cepacia. J Antimicrob Chemother* 30: 597.

Kurz RW, Graninger W, Egger TP *et al.* (1988). Failure of treatment of legionella pneumonia with ciprofloxacin. *J Antimicrob Chemother* 22: 389.

Kurzynski TA, Boehm DM, Rott PJ *et al.* (1988). Antimicrobial susceptibilities of *Bordetella* species isolated in a Multicenter Pertussis Surveillance Project. *Antimicrob Ag Chemother* 32: 137.

Lähdevirta J (1989). Ciprofloxacin in the elimination of enteric *Salmonella* carriage stage. *Scand J Infect Dis* (Suppl 60): 112.

Lang J, Finaz dVJ, Garraffo R *et al.* (1989). Cyclosporine (cyclosporin A). pharmacokinetics in renal transplant patients receiving ciprofloxacin. *Amer J Med* 87 (Suppl 5A): 82S.

Lang R, Goshen S, Kitzes CR *et al.* (1990a). Successful treatment of malignant external otitis with oral ciprofloxacin: report of experience with 23 patients. *J Infect Dis* 161: 537.

Lang R, Raz R, Sacks T *et al.* (1990b). Failure of prolonged treatment with ciprofloxacin in acute infections due to *Brucella melitensis. J Antimicrob Chemother* 26: 841.

Lang R, Goshen S, Raas RA *et al.* (1992). Oral ciprofloxacin in the management of chronic suppurative otitis media without cholesteatoma in children: preliminary experience in 21 children. *Pediatr Infect Dis J* 11: 925.

Lassus A, Renkonen OV, Ellmen J (1988). Fleroxacin vs standard therapy in gonococcal urethritis. *J Antimicrob Chemother* 22 (Suppl D): 223.

Lassus A, Karppinen L, Ingervo L *et al.* (1989). Ciprofloxacin versus amoxycillin and probenecid in the treatment of uncomplicated gonorrhoea. *Scand J Infect Dis* (Suppl 60): 58.

LeBel M (1991). Fluoroquinolones in the treatment of cystic fibrosis: a critical appraisal. *Eur J Clin Microbiol Infect Dis* 10: 316.

LeBel M, Bergeron MG (1987). Pharmacokinetics in the elderly Studies on ciprofloxacin. *Amer J Med* 82 (Suppl 4A): 108.

LeBel M, Barbeau G, Bergeron MG, Roy D, Vallée F (1986a). Pharmacokinetics of ciprofloxacin in elderly subjects. *Pharmacother* 6: 87.

LeBel M, Bergeron MG, Vallee F *et al.* (1986b). Pharmacokinetics and pharmacodynamics of ciprofloxacin in cystic fibrosis patients. *Antimicrob Ag Chemother* 30: 260.

LeBel M, Vallee F, Bergeron MG (1986c). Tissue penetration of ciprofloxacin after single and multiple doses. *Antimicrob Ag Chemother* 29: 501.

Ledergerber B, Bettex J-D, Joos B *et al.* (1985). Effect of standard breakfast on drug absorption and multiple-dose pharmacokinetics on ciprofloxacin. *Antimicrob Ag Chemother* 27: 350.

Lee BL, Padula AM, Kimbrough RC *et al.* (1991). Infectious complications with respiratory pathogens despite ciprofloxacin therapy. *New Engl J Med* 325: 520.

Lee WT, Collins JF (1992). Ciprofloxacin associated bilateral achilles tendon rupture. *Aust N Z J Med* 22: 500.

Legakis NJ, Tzouvelekis LS, Makris A *et al.* (1989). Outer membrane alterations in multiresistant mutants of *Pseudomonas aeruginosa* selected by ciprofloxacin. *Antimicrob Ag Chemother* **33**: 124.

Legent F, Bordure P, Beauvillain C, Berche P (1994). Controlled prospective study of oral ciprofloxacin versus amoxycillin/clavulanic acid in chronic suppurative otitis media in adults. *Chemotherapy* **40** (Suppl 1): 16.

Leggett JM, Prendergast K (1988). Malignant external otitis; the use of oral ciprofloxacin. *J Laryngol Otal* **102**: 53.

Legrand C, Anaissie E (1992). Bacteremia due to *Achromobacter xylosoxidans* in patients with cancer. *Clin Infect Dis* **14**: 479.

Lehtonen L, Huovinen P (1993). Susceptibility of respiratory tract pathogens in Finland to cefixime and nine other antimicrobial agents. *Scand J Infect Dis* **25**: 373.

Leibowitz HM (1991a). Antibacterial effectiveness of ciprofloxacin 03% ophthalmic solution in the treatment of bacterial conjunctivitis. *Amer J Ophthalmol* **112**: 29S.

Leibowitz HM (1991b). Clinical evaluation of ciprofloxacin 03% ophthalmic solution for treatment of bacterial keratitis. *Amer J Ophthalmol* **112**: 34S.

Leigh DA (1992). The treatment of a large outbreak of acute bacterial gastroenteritis with ciprofloxacin. *J Antimicrob Chemother* **30**: 733.

Lentino JR, Augustinsky JB, Weber TM *et al.* (1991). Therapy of serious skin and soft tissue infections with ofloxacin administered by intravenous and oral route. *Chemotherapy* **37**: 70.

LePennec MP, Kitzis MD, Terdjman M *et al.* (1990). Possible interaction of ciprofloxacin with ferrous sulphate. *J Antimicrob Chemother* **25**: 184.

Lesse AJ, Freer C, Salata RA *et al.* (1987). Oral ciprofloxacin therapy for gram-negative bacillary osteomyelitis. *Amer J Med* **82**: 247.

Lettieri JT, Rogge MC, Kaiser L *et al.* (1992). Pharmacokinetic profiles of ciprofloxacin after single intravenous and oral doses. *Antimicrob Ag Chemother* **36**: 993.

Levenson MJ, Parister SC, Dolitsky J, Bindra G (1991). Ciprofloxacin; drug of choice in the treatment of malignant external otitis (MEO). *Laryngoscope* **101**: 821.

Levin JM, Nelson JA, Segreti J *et al.* (1993). *In vitro* susceptibility of *Borrelia burgdorferi* to 11 antimicrobial agents. *Antimicrob Ag Chemother* **37**: 1444.

Levine DP, McNeil P, Lerner SA (1989). Randomized, double-blind comparative study of intravenous ciprofloxacin versus ceftazidime in the treatment of serious infections. *Amer J Med* **87** (Suppl 5A): 160.

Levy PY, Drancourt M, Etienne J *et al.* (1991). Comparison of different antibiotic regimens for therapy of 32 cases of Q fever endocarditis. *Antimicrob Ag Chemother* **35**: 533.

Levy R, Shpitzer T, Shvero J, Pitlik SD (1990). Oral ofloxacin as treatment of malignant external otitis; a study of 17 cases. *Laryngoscope* **100**: 548.

Lew D, Waldvogel F (1993). Use of quinolones for treatment of osteomyelitis and septic arthritis. In *Quinolone Antimicrobial Agents* 2nd edn (Hooper DC, Wolfson JS, eds), p. 371. Washington, DC: American Society of Microbiology.

Lew MA, Kehoe K, Ritz J *et al.* (1995). Ciprofloxacin versus trimethoprim/sulfamethoxazole for prophylaxis of bacterial infections in bone marrow transplant recipients: a randomized, controlled trial. *J Clin Oncol* **13**: 239.

Lewin C, Doherty C, Govan J (1993). *In vitro* activities of meropenem, PD 127391, PD 131628, ceftazidime, chloramphenicol, co-trimoxazole, and ciprofloxacin against *Pseudomonas cepacia*. *Antimicrob Ag Chemother* **37**: 123.

Lewin CS, Amyes SGB (1990). Conditions required for the bactericidal activity of pefloxacin and fleuoxacin against *Escherichia coli* KL16. *J Med Microbiol* **32**: 83.

Lewin CS, Amyes SGB, Smith JT (1989a). Bactericidal activity of enoxacin and lomefloxacin against *Escherichia coli* KL16. *Eur J Clin Microbiol Infect Dis* **8**: 731–733.

Lewin CS, Morrissey I, Smith JT (1989b). Role of oxygen in the bactericidal action of the 4-quinolones. *Rev Infect Dis* **11** (Suppl 5): S913.

Lewin CS, Morrissey I, Smith JT (1991). The mode of action of quinolones; the paradox in activity in th anaerobic environment. *Eur J Clin Microbiol Infect Dis* **10**: 240.

Leysen DC, Haemers A, Pattyo SR (1989). *Mycobacteria* and the new quinolones. *Antimicrob Ag Chemother* **33**: 1.

Li X-Z, Livermore DM, Nikaido H (1994). Role of efflux pump (s). in intrinsic resistance of *Pseudomonas aeruginosa*: resistance to teracycline, chloramphenicol and norfloxacin. *Antimicrob Ag Chemother* **38**: 1732.

Liang RHS, Yung RWH, Chau TK (1990). Ofloxacin versus co-trimoxazole for prevention of infection in neutropenic patients following cytotoxic chemotherapy. *Antimicrob Ag Chemother* **34**: 215.

Licitra CM, Brooks RG, Sieger BE (1987). Clinical efficacy and levels of ciprofloxacin in tissue in patients with soft tissue infection. *Antimicrob Ag Chemother* **31**: 805.

Liebers DM, Baltch AL, Smith RP *et al.* (1989). Susceptibility of *Legionella pneumophila* to eight antimicrobial agents including four macrolides under different assay conditions. *J Antimicrob Chemother* **23**: 37.

Lightfoot NF, Ahmad F, Cowden J (1990). Management of institutional outbreaks of *Salmonella* gastroenteritis. *J Antimicrob Chemother* **26** (Suppl F): 37.

Lim SH, Smith MP, Goldstone AH, Machin SJ (1990). A randomized prospective study of ceftazidime and ciprofloxacin with or without teicoplanin as an empiric antibiotic regimen for febrile neutropenic patients. *Br J Haematol* **76** (Suppl 2): 41.

Limson BM, Littaua RT (1989). Comparative study of ciprofloxacin versus cotrimoxazole in the treatment of salmonella enteric fever. *Infection* **17**: 105.

Lindsay G, Scorer HJ, Carnegie CM (1992). Safety and efficacy of temafloxacin versus ciprofloxacin in lower respiratory tract infections: a randomized, double-blind trial. *J Antimicrob Chemother* **30**: 89.

Ling J, Kam KM, Lam AW, French GL (1988). Susceptibilities of Hong Kong isolates of multiply resistant *Shigella* spp to 25 antimicrobial agents, including ampicillin plus sulbactam and new 4-quinolones. *Antimicrob Ag Chemother* **32**: 20.

Linville D, Emory C, Graves L (1991). Ciprofloxacin and warfarin interaction. *Amer J Med* **90**: 765.

Linville T, Matanin D (1989). Norfloxacin and warfarin. *Ann Intern Med* **110**: 751.

Ljungberg B, Nilsson-Ehle I (1988). Pharmacokinetics of intravenous ciprofloxacin at three different doses. *J Antimicrob Chemother* **22**: 715.

Lo WK, Rolston KV, Rubenstein EB *et al.* (1993). Ciprofloxacin-induced nephrotoxicity in patients with cancer. *Arch Intern Med* **153**: 1258.

Lode H, Wiley R, Hoffken G *et al.* (1987). Prospective randomized controlled study of ciprofloxacin versus imipenem-cilastatin in severe clinical infections. *Antimicrob Ag Chemother* **31**: 1491.

Lode H, Höffken G, Olschewski P *et al.* (1988). Comparative pharmacokinetics of intravenous ofloxacin and ciprofloxacin. *J Antimicrob Chemother* **22** (Suppl C): 73.

Lode H, Hoffken G, Boeckk M *et al.* (1990a). Quinolone pharmacokinetics and metabolism. *J Antimicrob Chemother* **26** (Suppl B): 41.

Lode H, Wiley E, Olschewski P *et al.* (1990b). Prospective randomized clinical trials of new quinolones versus beta-lactam antibiotics in lower respiratory tract infections. *Scand J Infect Dis* (Suppl 68): 50.

Lolekha S, Patanacharoen S, Thanangkul B, Vibulbandhitkit S (1988). Norfloxacin versus co-trimoxazole in the treatment of acutre bacterial diarrhea: a placebo controlled study. *Scand J Infect Dis* (Suppl 56): 35.

Lomaestro BM, Bailie GR (1991). Effect of staggered dose of calcium on the bioavailability of ciprofloxacin. *Antimicrob Ag Chemother* **35**: 1004.

Lomaestro BM, Bailie GR (1993). Effect of multiple staggered doses of calcium on the bioavailability of ciprofloxacin. *Ann Pharmacother* **27**: 1325.

Lonka L, Pedersen RS (1987). Ciprofloxacin for cholangitis. *Lancet* **ii**: 212.

Loo PS, Ridgway GL, Oriel JD (1985). Single dose ciprofloxacin for treating gonococcal infections in men. *Genitourin Med* **61**: 302.

Loo VG, Sherman P, Matlow AG (1992). *Helicobacter pylori* infection in a pediatric population: *in vitro* susceptibilities to omeprazole and eight antimicrobial agents. *Antimicrob Ag Chemother* **36**: 1133.

López-Brea M; Jimenez ML, Lopez Lavid MC *et al.* (1989). Norfloxacin vs trimethoprim–sulfamethoxazole in the treatment of salmonella gastro-enteritis. *Rev Infect Dis* **11** (Suppl 5): S1153.

López-Navidad A, Domingo P, Cadafalch J, Farrerons J (1990). Nor-floxacin-induced hepatotoxicity. *J Hepatol* **11**: 277.

Louie A, Baltch AL, Ritz WJ *et al.* (1991). Comparative *in-vitro* susceptibilities of *Pseudomonas aeruginosa, Xanthomonas maltophilia,* and *Pseudomonas* spp to sparfloxacin (CI-978, AT-4140, PD131501). and reference antimicrobial agents. *J Antimicrob Chemother* **27**: 793.

Lubitz RM (1990). Resolution of lung abscess due to *Pseudomonas aeruginosa* with oral ciprofloxacin: case report. *Rev Infect Dis* **12**: 757.

Lubowski TJ, Nightingale C, Sweeney K *et al.* (1992). Penetration of fleroxacin and ciprofloxacin into skin blister fluid: a comparative study. *Antimicrob Ag Chemother* **36**: 651.

Lucena MI, Marquez M, Velasco JL, Andrade RJ (1995). Acute renal failure attributable to ciprofloxacin in a patient with the acquired immunodefi-ciency syndrome. *Arch Intern Med* **155**: 114.

Lucet JC, Tilly H, Lerebours G *et al.* (1988). Neurological toxicity related to pefloxacin. *J Antimicrob Chemother* **21**: 811.

Lucey D, Dolan MJ, Moss CW *et al.* (1992). Relapsing illness due to *Rochalimaea henselae* in immunocompetent hosts: implication for therapy and new epidemiological associations. *Clin Infect Dis* **14**: 683.

Ludlam HA, Barton I, White L *et al.* (1990a). Intraperitoneal ciprofloxacin for the treatment of peritonitis in patients receiving continuous ambula-tory peritoneal dialysis (CAPD). *J Antimicrob Chemother* **25**: 843.

Ludlam H, Dryden M, Barton I *et al.* (1990b). Short course ciprofloxacin therapy for CAPD peritonitis. *J Antimicrob Chemother* **26**: 162.

Ludlam H, Johnston L, Hopkins P (1992). Susceptibility testing of bacteria recovered from patients with peritonitis complicating continuous ambula-tory peritoneal dialysis. *Antimicrob Ag Chemother* **36**: 1097.

Ludwig E, Graber H, Szekely E, Csiba A (1990). Metabolic interactions of ciprofloxacin. *Diagn Microbiol Infect Dis* **13**: 135.

Lugtenberg B, Peters R, Bernheimer H, Berendsen W (1976). Influence of cultural conditions and mutations on the composition of the outer membrane proteins of *Escherichia coli*. *Mol Gen Genet* **147**: 251.

Lumbiganon P, Sookpranee T (1992). Ciprofloxacin therapy for localized melioidosis. *Pediatr Infect Dis J* **11**: 418.

Lumbiganon P, Pengsaa K, Sookpranee T (1991). Ciprofloxacin in neonates and its possible adverse effect on the teeth. *Pediatr Infect Dis J* **10**: 619.

MacDonald KS, Cameron DW, D'Costa L *et al.* (1989). Evaluation of fleroxacin (RO-23–6240). as single-oral dose therapy of culture-proven chancroid in Nairobi, Kenya. *Antimicrob Ag Chemother* **33**: 612.

MacGowan AP, Holt HA, Bywater MJ, Reeves DS (1990). *In vitro* antimicrobial susceptibility of *Listeria monocytogenes* isolated in the UK and other *Listeria* species. *Eur J Clin Microbiol Infect Dis* **9**: 767.

MacGowan AP, Reeves DS, Wright C *et al.* (1991). Tricuspid valve infective endocarditis and pulmonary sepsis due to *Erysipelothrix rhusiopathiae* successfully treated with high doses of ciprofloxacin but complicated by gynaecomastia. *J Infect* **22**: 100.

MacGowan AP, Brown NM, Holt HA *et al.* (1993). An eight-year survey of the antimicrobial susceptibility patterns of 85,971 bacteria isolated from patients in a district general hospital and the local community. *J Antimicrob Chemother* **31**: 543.

MacGowan AP, White LO, Brown NM *et al.* (1994). Serum ciprofloxacin concentrations in patients with severe sepsis being treated with ciprofloxacin 200 mg iv bd irrespective of renal function. *J Antimicrob Chemother* **33**: 1051.

Mack G, Cooper PJ, Buchanan N (1991). Effects of enzyme supplementa-tion on oral absorption of ciprofloxacin in patients with cystic fibrosis. *Antimicrob Ag Chemother* **35**: 1484.

Majumdar S, Flasher D, Friend DS *et al.* (1992). Efficacies of liposome-encapsulated streptomycin and ciprofloxacin against *Mycobacterium avium–M. intracellulare* complex infections in human peripheral blood monocyte/macrophages. *Antimicrob Ag Chemother* **36**: 2808.

Mandell LA (1991). Role of quinolones in surgical prophylaxis. *Eur J Microbiol Infect Dis* **10**: 368.

Manzione NC (1992). A note of caution on empiric use of ciprofloxacin for diarrhea. *Arch Intern Med* **152**: 213.

Maple PAC, Hamilton-Miller MT, Brumfitt W (1991). Differing activities of quinolones against ciprofloxacin-susceptible and ciprofloxacin-resist-ant, methicillin-resistant *Staphylococcus aureus*. *Antimicrob Ag Chem-other* **35**: 345.

Marangos MN, Skoutelis AT, Nightingale CH *et al.* (1995). Absorption of ciprofloxacin in patients with diabetic gastroparesis. *Antimicrob Ag Chemother* **39**: 2161.

Mardh PA, Lowing C (1990). Treatment of chlamydial infections. *Scand J Infect Dis* (Suppl 68): 23.

Margileth AM (1992). Antibiotic therapy for cat-scratch disease: clinical study of therapeutic outcome in 268 patients and a review of the literature. *Pediatr Infect Dis J* **11**: 474.

Marinis E, Legakis NJ (1985). *In-vitro* activity of ciprofloxacin against clinical isolates of mycobacteria resistant to antimycobacterial drugs. *J Antimicrob Chemother* **16**: 527.

Marone C, Quadri F (1992). Beware of ciprofloxacin in acute otitis media. *Brit Med J* **305**: 870.

Marshall SA, Jones RN (1993). *In vitro* activity of DU-6859a, a new fluorocyclopropyl quinolone. *Antimicrob Ag Chemother* **37**: 2747.

Marshall SA, Jones RN, Murray PR *et al.* (1993). *In-vitro* comparison of DU-6859a, a novel fluoroquinolone, with other quinolones and oral cephalosporins tested against 5086 recent clinical isolates. *J Antimicrob Chemother* **32**: 877.

Martindale The Extra Pharmacopoeia 30th edn (1993). (Reynolds JEF, ed) London, UK: The Pharmaceutical Press.

Martinez-Martinez L, Suarez AI, Ortega MC, Perea EJ (1994). Comparative *in vitro* activities of new quinolones against coryneform bacteria. *Antimicrob Ag Chemother* **38**: 1439.

Maschmeyer G, Haralambie E, Guas W *et al.* (1988). Ciprofloxacin and norfloxacin for selective decontamination in patients with severe granulocytopenia. *Infection* **16**: 98.

Masecar BL, Robillard NJ (1991). Spontaneous quinolone resistance in *Serratia marcescens* due to a mutation in *gyrA*. *Antimicrob Ag Chemother* **35**: 898.

Masecar BL, Celesk RA, Robillard NJ (1990). Analysis of acquired ciprofloxacin resistance in a clinical strain of *Pseudomonas aeruginosa*. *Antimicrob Ag Chemother* **34**: 281.

Mason EJ, Kaplan SL, Lamberth LB *et al.* (1992). Increased rate of isolation of penicillin-resistant *Streptococcus pneumoniae* in a children's hospital and *in vitro* susceptibilities to antibiotics of potential therapeutic use. *Antimicrob Ag Chemother* **36**: 1703.

Matsumoto M, Kojima K, Nagano H *et al.* (1992). Photostability and biological activity of fluoroquinolones substituted at the 8 position after UV irradiation. *Antimicrob Ag Chemother* **36**: 1715.

Matsuno K, Kunihiro E, Yamatoya O *et al.* (1995). Surveillance of adverse reactions due to ciprofloxacin in Japan. *Drugs* **49** (Suppl 2): 495.

McArdle CS (1994). Oral prophylaxis in biliary tract surgery. *J Antimicrob Chemother* **33**: 200.

McCaffrey C, Bertasso A, Pace J *et al.* (1992). Quinolone accumulation in *Escherichia coli, Pseudomonas aeruginosa,* and *Staphylococcus aureus*. *Antimicrob Ag Chemother* **36**: 1601.

McClain JB, Joshi B, Rice R (1988). Chloramphenicol, gentamicin, and ciprofloxacin against murine scrub typhus. *Antimicrob Ag Chemother* **32**: 285.

McCue JD, Zandt JR (1991). Acute psychoses associated with the use of ciprofloxacin and trimethoprim–sulfamethoxazole. *Amer J Med* **90**: 528.

McEwan SR, Davey PG (1988). Ciprofloxacin and tenosynovitis. *Lancet* **ii**: 900.

McFarland LV, Bauwens JE, Melcher SA *et al.* (1995). Ciprofloxacin-associated *Clostridium difficile* disease. *Lancet* **346**: 977.

McIntyre M, Lyons M (1993). Resistance to ciprofloxacin in *Campylo-bacter* spp. *Lancet* **341**: 188.

McLean KL, Hitchman D, Shafran SD (1992). Norfloxacin is inferior to chloroquine for falciparum malaria in northwestern Zambia; a comparative clinical trial. *J Infect Dis* **165**: 904.

McNulty CAM, Dent J, Wise R (1985). Susceptibility of clinical isolates of *Campylobacter pyloridis* to 11 antimicrobial agents. *Antimicrob Ag Chemother* **28**: 837.

McWhinney PH, Yates M, Prentice HG et al. (1992). Infection caused by *Mycobacterium chelonae*: a diagnostic and therapeutic problem in the neutropenic patient. *Clin Infect Dis* **14**: 1208.

Meares EM, Stamey TA (1968). Bacteriologic localization patterns in bacterial prostatitis and urethritis. *Invest Urol* **5**: 492.

Mehtar S, Drabu YJ, Blakemore PH (1990). The *in-vitro* activity of piperacillin/tazobactam, ciprofloxacin, ceftazidime and imipenem against multiple resistant gram-negative bacteria. *J Antimicrob Chemother* **25**: 915.

Meijer-Severs GJ, van Santen E, de Vries-Hospers HG (1990). Low-dose ciprofloxacin for selective decontamination of the digestive tract in human volunteers. *Eur J Clin Microbiol Infect Dis* **9**: 285.

Meng X, Nightingale CH, Sweeney KR, Quintiliani R (1994). Loss of bactericidal activities of quinolones during the post-antibiotic effect induced by rifampicin. *J Antimicrob Chemother* **33**: 721.

Menon L, Ernst JA, Sy ER et al. (1989). Sequential intravenous/oral ciprofloxacin compared with intravenous ceftazidime in the treatment of serious lower respiratory tract infections. *Amer J Med* **87** (Suppl 5A): 119S.

Mertens JCC, Dekker W, Ligtvoet EEJ, Blok P (1989). Treatment failure of norfloxacin against *Campylobacter pylori* and chronic gastritis in patients with nonulcerative dyspepsia. *Antimicrob Ag Chemother* **33**: 256.

Mertes PM, Voiriot P, Dopff C et al. (1990). Penetration of ciprofloxacin into heart valves, myocardium, mediastinal fat, and sternal bone marrow in humans. *Antimicrob Ag Chemother* **34**: 398.

Meunier F, Zinner SH, Gaya H et al. (1991). Prospective randomized evaluation of ciprofloxacin versus piperacillin plus amikacin for empiric antibiotic therapy of febrile granulocytopenic cancer patients with lymphomas and solid tumors. The European Organization for Research on Treatment of Cancer International Antimicrobial Therapy Cooperative Group. *Antimicrob Ag Chemother* **35**: 873.

Meyer RD, Liu S (1988). *In vitro* synergy studies with ciprofloxacin and selected beta-lactam agents and aminoglycosides against multidrug-resistant *Pseudomonas aeruginosa*. *Diagn Microbiol Infect Dis* **11**: 151.

Mikhail IA, Bourgeois AL, Hyams KC et al. (1987). *In vitro* activity of ciprofloxacin compared to trimethoprim–sulfamethoxazole against *Campylobacter* spp., *Shigella* spp. and Enterotoxigenic *Escherichia coli* causing travellers' diarrhea in Egypt. *Scand J Infect Dis* **19**: 479.

Millar MR, Bransby ZM, Tompkins DS et al. (1986). Ciprofloxacin for *Pseudomonas aeruginosa* meningitis. *Lancet* **i**: 1325.

Miller I, Vogel R, Cook TJ et al. (1992). Topically administered norfloxacin compared with topically administered gentamicin for the treatment of external ocular bacterial infections. *Amer J Ophthalmol* **113**: 638.

Miller MS, Gaido F, Rourk MJ et al. (1991). Anaphylactoid reactions to ciprofloxacin in cystic fibrosis patients. *Pediatr Infect Dis J* **10**: 164.

Miller SD, da L Exposto F, Dangor Y et al. (1989). A dose finding study of fleroxacin in the treatment of chancroid. *Rev Infect Dis* **11** (Suppl 5): S1310.

Mitscher LA, Devasthale P, Zavod R (1993). Structure-activity relationships. In *Quinolone Antimicrobial Agents* 2nd edn. (Hooper DC, Wolfson JS, eds), p. 3. Washington, DC: American Society of Microbiology.

Mitsuhashi S (1988). Comparative antibacterial activity of new quinolone-carboxylic acid derivatives. *Rev Infect Dis* **10** (Suppl 1): S27.

Modai J (1991). Potential role of fluoroquinolones in the treatment of bacterial meningitis. *Eur J Clin Microbiol Infect Dis* **10**: 291.

Moellering RC, Jr (1993). Quinolone antimicrobial agents: overview and conclusions. In *Quinolone Antimicrobial Agents* 2nd edn (Hooper DC, Wolfson JS, eds), p. 527. Washington, DC: American Society of Microbiology.

Moffie BG, Mouton RP (1988). Sensitivity and resistance of *Legionella pneumophila* to some antibiotics and combinations of antibiotics. *J Antimicrob Chemother* **22**: 457.

Monk J P, Campoli-Richards DM (1987). Ofloxacin A review of its

antibacterial activity, pharmacokinetic properties and therapeutic use. *Drugs* **33**: 346.

Montay G, Gaillot J (1990). Pharmacokinetics of fluoroquinolones in hepatic failure. *J Antimicrob Chemother* **26** (Suppl B): 61.

Moody JA, Gerding DN, Peterson LR (1987). Evaluation of ciprofloxacin's synergism with other agents by multiple *in vitro* methods. *Amer J Med* **82** (Suppl 4A): 44.

Moore B, Safani M, Keesey J (1988). Possible exacerbation of myasthenia gravis by ciprofloxacin. *Lancet* **i**: 882.

Morran C, McArdle C, Pettitt L et al. (1989). Pharmacokinetics of orally administered ciprofloxacin in abdominal surgery. *Amer J Med* **87** (Suppl 5A): 86S.

Morris A, Guild I (1991). Endocarditis due to *Corynebacterium pseudodiphtheriticum*: five case reports, review, and antibiotic susceptibilities of nine strains. *Rev Infect Dis* **13**: 887.

Motley M, Sarafian SK, Knapp JS et al. (1992). Correlation between *in vitro* antimicrobial susceptibilities and beta-lactamase plasmid contents of isolates of *Haemophilus ducreyi* from the United States. *Antimicrob Ag Chemother* **36**: 1639.

Mott FE, Murphy S, Hunt V (1989). Ciprofloxacin and warfarin. *Ann Intern Med* **111**: 542.

Muder RR, Brennen C, Goetz AM et al. (1991). Association with prior fluoroquinolone therapy of widespread ciprofloxacin resistance among gram-negative isolates in a Veterans Affairs medical center. *Antimicrob Ag Chemother* **35**: 256.

Mueller BA, Brierton DG, Abel SR, Bowman L (1994). Effect of enteral feeding with 'Ensure' on oral bioavailabilities of ofloxacin and ciprofloxacin. *Antimicrob Ag Chemother* **38**: 2101.

Mulhall JP, Bergmann LS (1995). Ciprofloxacin-induced acute psychosis. *Urology* **46**: 102.

Mulligan ME, Ruane PJ, Johnston L et al. (1987). Ciprofloxacin for eradication of methicillin-resistant *Staphylococcus aureus* colonization. *Amer J Med* **82**: 215.

Mumford CJ, Ginsberg L (1990). Ciprofloxacin and myasthenia gravis. *Brit Med J* **301**: 818.

Murdoch DA, Badenoch DE, Gatchalian ER (1987). Oral ciprofloxacin as prophylaxis in transurethral surgery. *Brit J Urol* **60**: 153.

Murdoch MB, Peterson LR (1991). Nontyphoidal *Salmonella* pleuro-pulmonary infections. *Arch Intern Med* **151**: 196.

Murphy GS, Bodhidatta L, Echeverria P et al. (1993). Ciprofloxacin and loperamide in the treatment of bacillary dysentery. *Ann Intern Med* **118**: 582.

Murphy PG, Ferguson WP (1987). *Corynebacterium* jeikeium (group JK). resistance to ciprofloxacin emerging during therapy. *J Antimicrob Chemother* **20**: 922.

Murray BE (1986). Resistance of *Shigella, Salmonella*, and other selected enteric pathogens to antimicrobial agents. *Rev Infect Dis* **8**: S172.

Murray PR, Bratcher JL, Niles AC, Hampton CM (1993). *In vitro* activity of nine fluoroquinolone antibiotics against 200 strains of enterococci. *Diagn Microbiol Infect Dis* **16**: 83.

Muytjens H, Van der Ros-Van de Repe J, Van Veldhuizen G (1983). Comparative activities of ciprofloxacin (Bay 0 9867), norfloxacin, pipemidic acid, and nalidixic acid. *Antimicrob Ag Chemother* **24**: 302.

Naamara W, Plummer FA, Greenblatt RM et al. (1987). Treatment of chancroid with ciprofloxacin A prospective, randomized clinical trial. *Amer J Med* **82**: 317.

Naber KG (1993). Role of quinolones in treatment of chronic bacterial prostatitis. In *Quinolone Antimicrobial Agents* 2nd edn (Hooper DC, Wolfson JS, eds), p. 285. Washington, DC: American Society of Microbiology.

Naber KG, Sorgel F, Kees F, et al. (1989). Pharmacokinetics of ciprofloxacin in young (healthy volunteers) and elderly patients, and concentrations in prostatic fluid, seminal fluid, and prostatic adenoma tissue following intravenous administration. *Amer J Med* **87** (Suppl 5A): 57S.

Nagayama A, Nakao T, Taen H (1988). *In vitro* activities of ofloxacin and four other new quinoline-carboxylic acids against *Chlamydia trachomatis*. *Antimicrob Ag Chemother* **32**: 1735.

Nakanishi N, Yoshida S, Wakebe H *et al.* (1991a). Mechanisms of clinical resistance to fluoroquinolones in *Staphylococcus aureus*. *Antimicrob Ag Chemother* **35**: 2562.

Nakanishi N, Yoshida S, Wakebe H *et al.* (1991b). Mechanisms of clinical resistance to fluoroquinolones in *Enterococcus faecalis*. *Antimicrob Ag Chemother* **35**: 1053.

Nakata K, Maeda H, Fujii A *et al.* (1992). *In vitro* and *in vivo* activities of sparfloxacin, other quinolones, and tetracyclines against *Chlamydia trachomatis*. *Antimicrob Ag Chemother* **36**: 188.

Nathwani D, Laing RB, Harvey G *et al.* (1991). Treatment of symptomatic enteric aeromonas hydrophila infection with ciprofloxacin. *Scand J Infect Dis* **23**: 653.

Nau R, Prange HW, Martell J *et al.* (1990). Penetration of ciprofloxacin into the cerebrospinal fluid of patients with uninflamed meninges. *J Antimicrob Chemother* **25**: 965.

Nau R, Schmidt T, Kaye K *et al.* (1995). Quinolone antibiotics in therapy of experimental pneumococcal meningitis in rabbits. *Antimicrob Ag Chemother* **39**: 593.

Navarro F, Miro E, Mirelis B *et al.* (1993). *Campylobacter* spp antibiotic susceptibility. *J Antimicrob Chemother* **32**: 906.

Neal TJ, O'Donoghue MA, Ridgway EJ *et al.* (1992). *In-vitro* activity of ten antimicrobial agents against penicillin-resistant *Streptococcus pneumoniae*. *J Antimicrob Chemother* **30**: 39.

Neill MA, Opal SM, Heelan J *et al.* (1991). Failure of ciprofloxacin to eradicate convalescent fecal excretion after acute salmonellosis: experience during an outbreak in health care workers. *Ann Intern Med* **114**: 195.

Neu HC (1988). Bacterial resistance to fluoroquinolones. *Rev Infect Dis* **10** (Suppl 1): S57.

Neu HC (1989a). Chemical evolution of the fluoroquinolone antimicrobial agents. *Amer J Med* **87** (Suppl 6C): 2S.

Neu HC (1989b). Synergy of fluoroquinolones with other antimicrobial agents. *Rev Infect Dis* **11** (Suppl 5): S1025.

Neu HC (1991). Synergy and antagonism of combinations with quinolones. *Eur J Clin Microbiol Infect Dis* **10**: 255.

Neu HC, Chin NX (1994). *In vitro* activity of the new fluoroquinolone CP-99,219. *Antimicrob Ag Chemother* **38**: 2615.

Neu HC, Novelli A, Chin NX (1989). Comparative *in vitro* activity of a new quinolone, AM-1091. *Antimicrob Ag Chemother* **33**: 1036.

Neu HC, Fang W, Gu F-W, Chin N-X (1992). *In vitro* activity of OPC-17116. *Antimicrob Ag Chemother* **36**: 1310.

Neuvonen PJ, Kivistö KT (1992). Milk and yoghurt do not impair the absorption of ofloxacin. *Br J Clin Pharmacol* **33**: 346.

Neuvonen PJ *et al.* (1991). Interference of dairy products with the absorption of ciprofloxacin. *Clin Pharmacol Ther* **50**: 498.

Newton JJ, Kennedy CA (1993). Wound infection due to *Aeromonas* sobria. *Clin Infect Dis* **17**: 1082.

Ng EYW, Trucksis M, Hooper DC (1994). Quinolone resistance mediated by *norA*: physiologic characterization and relationship to *flqB*, a quinolone resistance locus on the *Staphylococcus aureus* chromosome. *Antimicrob Ag Chemother* **38**: 1345.

Ng VL, Boggs JM, York MK *et al.* (1992). Recovery of *Bordetella bronchiseptica* from patients with AIDS. *Clin Infect Dis* **15**: 376.

Nikaido H, Vaara M (1985). Molecular basis of bacterial outer membrane permeability. *Microbiol Rev* **49**: 1.

Nilsson-Ehle I, Ljungberg B (1989). Influence of age on the pharmacokinetics of ciprofloxacin. *Scand J Infect Dis* (Suppl 60): 23.

Nix DE (1993). Drug-drug interactions with fluoroquinolone antimicrobial agents. In *Quinolone Antimicrobial Agents* 2nd edn (Hooper DC, Wolfson JS, eds), p. 245. Washington, DC: American Society of Microbiology.

Nix DE, Cumbo TJ, Kuritzky P *et al.* (1987). Oral ciprofloxacin in the treatment of serious soft tissue and bone infections Efficacy, safety, and pharmacokinetics. *Amer J Med* **82**: 146.

Nix DE, Watson WA, Leuer ME *et al.* (1989). Effects of magnesium antacids and ranitidine on the absorption of ciprofloxacin. *Clin Pharmacol Ther* **46**: 700.

Nix DE, Wilton JH, Ronald B *et al.* (1990). Inhibition of norfloxacin absorption by antacids. *Antimicrob Ag Chemother* **34**: 432.

Noel SB, Scallan P, Meadors MC, Meek TJ (1989). Treatment of *Pseudomonas aeruginosa* auricular perichondritis with oral ciprofloxacin. *Dermatol Surg Oncol* **6**: 633.

Nord CE (1988). Effect of new quinolones on the human gastrointestinal microflora. *Rev Infect Dis* **10** (Suppl 1): S193.

Nordmann P, Ronco E (1992). *In-vitro* antimicrobial susceptibility of *Rhodococcus equi*. *J Antimicrob Chemother* **29**: 383.

Nordmann P, Kerestedjian JJ, Ronco E (1992a). Therapy of *Rhodococcus equi* disseminated infections in nude mice. *Antimicrob Ag Chemother* **36**: 1244.

Nordmann P, Rouveix E, Guenounou M, Nicolas MH (1992b). Pulmonary abscess due to a rifampin and fluoroquinolone resistant *Rhodococcus equi* strain in a HIV infected patient. *Eur J Clin Microbiol Infect Dis* **11**: 557.

Norrby SR (1988). 4-Quinolones in the treatment of infections of the central nervous system. *Rev Infect Dis* **10** (Suppl 1): S253.

Norrby SR (1989). Ciprofloxacin in the treatment of acute and chronic osteomyelitis: a review. *Scand J Infect Dis* (Suppl 60): 74.

Norrby SR (1991). Side-effects of quinolones; comparisons between quinolones and other antibiotics. *Eur J Clin Microbiol Infect Dis* **10**: 378.

Norrby SR (1993). Treatment of urinary tract infections with quinolone antimicrobial agents. In *Quinolone Antimicrobial Agents* 2nd edn (Hooper DC, Wolfson JS, eds), p. 273. Washington, DC: American Society of Microbiology.

Norrby SR, Jonsson M (1988). Comparative *in vitro* activity of PD 127,391, a new fluorinated 4-quinolone derivative. *Antimicrob Ag Chemother* **32**: 1278.

Norrby SR, Pernet AG (1991). Assessment of adverse events during drug development: experience with temafloxacin. *J Antimicrob Chemother* **20** (Suppl C): 111.

O'Keeffe BJ, Tillotson GS (1990). Ciprofloxacin and pseudomembranous colitis. *Lancet* **336**: 1509.

O'Mahony MS, FitzGerald MX (1991). Cystic fibrosis and seizures. *Lancet* **338**: 259.

Ode B, Walder M, Forsgren A (1987). Failure of single dose of 100 mg ofloxacin in lower urinary tract infections in females. *Scand J Infect Dis* **19**: 877.

Okuda J, Okamoto S, Takahata M, Nishino T (1991). Inhibitory effects of ciprofloxacin and sparfloxacin on DNA gyrase purified from fluoroquinolone-resistant strains of methicillin-resistant *Staphylococcus aureus*. *Antimicrob Ag Chemother* **35**: 2288.

Oppenheim BA, Hartley JW, Lee W *et al.* (1989). Outbreak of coagulase negative staphylococcus highly resistant to ciprofloxacin in a leukaemia unit. *Brit Med J* **299**: 294.

Orlando PL, Barriere SL, Hindler JA, Frost RW (1990). Serum bactericidal activity from intravenous ciprofloxacin and azlocillin given alone and in combination to healthy subjects. *Diagn Microbiol Infect Dis* **13**: 93.

Ortiz A, Plaza JJ and Egido J (1992). Ciprofloxacin-associated tubulointerstitial nephritis with linear tubular basement membrane deposits. *Nephron* **60**: 248.

Osborne JE, Blair RL, Davey P (1989). Successful treatment of malignant otitis externa with oral ciprofloxacin. *J Infect* **18**: 298.

Panigrahi D, Roy P, Sehgal R (1991). Ciprofloxacin for typhoid fever. *Lancet* **338**: 1601.

Pankuch GA, Jacobs MR, Appelbaum PC (1993). Susceptibilities of 428 gram-positive and -negative anaerobic bacteria to Bay y3118 compared with their susceptibilities to ciprofloxacin, clindamycin, metronidazole, piperacillin, piperacillin-tazobactam, and cefoxitin. *Antimicrob Ag Chemother* **37**: 1649.

Pankuch GA, Jacobs MR, Appelbaum PC (1994). Susceptibilities of 123 *Xanthomonas maltophilia* strains to clinafloxacin, PD 131628, PD 138312, PD 140248, ciprofloxacin, and ofloxacin. *Antimicrob Ag Chemother* **38**: 369.

Pankuch GA, Jacobs MR, Appelbaum PC (1995). Activity of CP99,219 compared with DU-6859a, ciprofloxacin, ofloxacin, levofloxacin, lomefloxacin, tosufloxacin, sparfloxacin and grepafloxacin against penicillin-susceptible and -resistant pneumococci. *J Antimicrob Chemother* **35**: 230.

Paradis D, Vallee F, Allard S *et al.* (1992). Comparative study of pharmacokinetics and serum bactericidal activities of cefpirome, ceftazidime, ceftriaxone, imipenem, and ciprofloxacin. *Antimicrob Ag Chemother* **36**: 2085.

Parish LC, Asper R (1987). Systemic treatment of cutaneous infections. A comparative study of ciprofloxacin and cefotaxime. *Amer J Med* **82**: (4A): 227.

Parry H, Howard AJ, Galpin OP, Hassan SP (1994). The prophylaxis of travellers' diarrhoea, a double blind placebo controlled trial of ciprofloxacin during a Himalayan expedition. *J Infect* **28**: 337.

Parry MF, Smego DA, Digiovanni MA (1988). Hepatobiliary kinetics and excretion of ciprofloxacin. *Antimicrob Ag Chemother* **32**: 982.

Parry MF, Panzer KB, Yukna ME (1989). Quinolone resistance Susceptibility data from a 300-bed community hospital. *Amer J Med* **87** (Suppl 5A): 12S.

Pascual A, Martinez-Martinez L, Ramirez de Arellano E, Perea EJ (1993). Susceptibility to antimicrobial agents of *Pseudomonas aeruginosa* attached to siliconized latex urinary catheters. *Eur J Clin Microbiol Infect Dis* **12**: 761.

Patoia L, Guerciolini R, Menichetti F *et al.* (1987). Norfloxacin and neutropenia. *Ann Intern Med* **107**: 788.

Paul J, Brown NM (1995). Tinnitus and ciprofloxacin. *Brit Med J* **311**: 232.

Pavicic MJ *et al.* (1992). *In vitro* susceptibilities of *Actinobacillus actinomycetemcomitans* to a number of antimicrobial combinations. *Antimicrob Ag Chemother* **36**: 2634.

Pecquet S, Ravoire S, Andremont A (1990). Faecal excretion of ciprofloxacin after a single oral dose and its effect on faecal bacteria in healthy volunteers. *J Antimicrob Chemother* **26**: 125.

Pedersen SS (1989). Clinical efficacy of ciprofloxacin in lower respiratory tract infections. *Scand J Infect Dis* (Suppl 60): 89.

Pedersen SS, Jensen T, Hvidberg EF (1987). Comparative pharmacokinetics of ciprofloxacin and ofloxacin in cystic fibrosis patients. *J Antimicrob Chemother* **20**: 575.

Peeling RW, Ronald AR (1993). Use of quinolones in sexually transmitted diseases. In *Quinolone Antimicrobial Agents* 2nd edn (Hooper DC, Wolfson JS, eds), p. 299. Washington, DC: American Society of Microbiology.

Peloquin CA, Cumbo TJ, Nix DE *et al.* (1989). Evaluation of intravenous ciprofloxacin in patients with nosocomial lower respiratory tract infections. Impact of plasma concentrations, organism, minimum inhibitory concentration, and clinical condition on bacterial eradication. *Arch Intern Med* **149**: 2269.

Peltola H, Vaarala M, Renkonen OV *et al.* (1992). Pharmacokinetics of single-dose oral ciprofloxacin in infants and small children. *Antimicrob Ag Chemother* **36**: 1086.

Péna C, Albareda JM, Pallares R *et al.* (1995). Relationship between quinolone use and emergence of ciprofloxacin-resistant *Escherichia coli* in bloodstream infections. *Antimicrob Ag Chemother* **39**: 520.

Perea EJ, Garcia I, Pascual A (1992). Comparative penetration of lomefloxacin and other quinolones into human phagocytes. *Amer J Med* **92** (Suppl 4A): 48S.

Pérez JL, Riera L, Valls F *et al.* (1987). A comparison of the *in-vitro* activity of seventeen antibiotics against Streptococcus faecalis. *J Antimicrob Chemother* **20**: 357.

Pérez-Ruvalcaba JA, Quintero-Perez NP, Morales-Reyes JJ *et al.* (1987). Double-blind comparison of ciprofloxacin with cefotaxime in the treatment of skin and skin structure infections. *Amer J Med* **82** (4A): 242.

Perkins BA, Hamill RJ, Musher DM *et al.* (1992). *In vitro* activities of streptomycin and 11 oral antimicrobial agents against clinical isolates of *Klebsiella rhinoscleromatis*. *Antimicrob Ag Chemother* **36**: 1785.

Peters B, Pinching AJ (1989). Fatal anaphylaxis associated with ciprofloxacin in a patient with AIDS related complex. *Brit Med J* **298**: 605.

Peterson LR, Lissack LM, Canter K *et al.* (1989). Therapy of lower extremity infections with ciprofloxacin in patients with diabetes mellitus, peripheral vascular disease, or both. *Amer J Med* **86**: 801.

Peterson LR, Quick JN, Jensen B *et al.* (1990). Emergence of ciprofloxacin resistance in nosocomial methicillin-resistant *Staphylococcus aureus* isolates Resistance during ciprofloxacin plus rifampin therapy for methicillin-resistant *S. aureus* colonization. *Arch Intern Med* **150**: 2151.

Peterson PK, Stein D, Guay DR *et al.* (1988). Prospective study of lower respiratory tract infections in an extended-care nursing home program: potential role of oral ciprofloxacin. *Amer J Med* **85**: 164.

Petri H, Tronnier H (1986). Efficacy of enoxacin in the treatment of bacterial infections of the skin with regards to photosensitization. *Infection* **14** (Suppl 3): S213.

Petruccelli BP, Murphy GS, Sanchez JL *et al.* (1992). Treatment of traveler's diarrhea with ciprofloxacin and loperamide. *J Infect Dis* **165**: 557.

Pfau A, Sacks TG (1994). Effective postcoital quinolone prophylaxis of recurrent urinary tract infections in women. *J Urol* **152**: 136.

Pfeiffer M, Reiter C (1994). Who is withholding information? *Lancet* **343**: 1163.

Pham JN, Bell SM, Lanzarone JY (1991). Biotype and antibiotic sensitivity of 100 clinical isolates of *Yersinia enterocolitica*. *J Antimicrob Chemother* **28**: 13.

Philippon A, Bimet F (1990). *In vitro* susceptibility of *Corynebacterium* group D2 and *Corynebacterium* jeikeium to twelve antibiotics. *Eur J Clin Microbiol Infect Dis* **9**: 892.

Phillips G, Johnson BE, Ferguson J (1990). The loss of antibiotic activity of ciprofloxacin by photodegradation. *J Antimicrob Chemother* **26**: 783.

Phillips I, King A (1988). Comparative activity of the 4-quinolones. *Rev Infect Dis* **10** (Suppl 1): S70.

Phillips I, King A, Nord CE, Hoffstedt B (1992). Antibiotic sensitivity of the *Bacteroides fragilis* group in Europe European Study Group. *Eur J Clin Microbiol Infect Dis* **11**: 292.

Philpott-Howard JV, Barker KF, Wade JJ *et al.* (1990). Randomized multicentre study of ciprofloxacin and azlocillin versus gentamicin and azlocillin in the treatment of febrile neutropenic patients. *J Antimicrob Chemother* **26** (Suppl F): 89.

Piccirillo JE, Parnes SM (1989). Ciprofloxacin for the treatment of chronic ear disease. *Laryngoscope* **99**: 510.

Pichler HET, Diridl G, Sticler K, Wolf D (1987). Clinical efficacy of ciprofloxacin compared with placebo in bacterial diarrhea. *Amer J Med* **82** (Suppl 4A): 329.

Piddock LJ, Wise R (1988). The selection and frequency of streptococci with decreased susceptibility to ofloxacin compared with other quinolones. *J Antimicrob Chemother* **22** (Suppl C): 45.

Piddock LJV, Whale K, Wise R (1990). Quinolone resistance in salmonella: clinical experience. *Lancet* **335**: 1459.

Pien FD, Yamane KK (1987). Ciprofloxacin treatment of soft tissue and respiratory infections in a community outpatient practice. *Amer J Med* **82** (Suppl 4A): 236.

Piercy EA, Barbaro D, Luby JP *et al.* (1989a). Ciprofloxacin for methicillin-resistant *Staphylococcus aureus* infections. *Antimicrob Ag Chemother* **33**: 128.

Piercy EA, Bawdon RE, Mackowiak PA (1989b). Penetration of ciprofloxacin into saliva and nasal secretions and effect of the drug on the oropharyngeal flora of ill subjects. *Antimicrob Ag Chemother* **33**: 1645.

Piersimoni C, Morbiducci V, Bornigia S *et al.* (1992). *In vitro* activity of the new quinolone lomefloxacin against *Mycobacterium tuberculosis*. *Amer Rev Respir Dis* **146**: 1445.

Pithie AD, Wood MJ (1990). Treatment of typhoid fever and infectious diarrhoea with ciprofloxacin. *J Antimicrob Chemother* **26** (Suppl F): 47.

Plaisance KI, Drusano GL, Forrest A *et al.* (1987). Effect of dose size on bioavailability of ciprofloxacin. *Antimicrob Ag Chemother* **31**: 956.

Plaisance KI, Drusano GL, Forrest A *et al.* (1990). Effect of renal function on the bioavailability of ciprofloxacin. *Antimicrob Ag Chemother* **34**: 1031.

Plourde PJ, D'Costa LJ, Agoki E *et al.* (1991). A randomized double blind study of the efficacy of fleroxacin vs trimethoprim–sulfamethoxazole in male prostitutes with culture-proven chancroid. *J Infect Dis* **165**: 949.

Pocidalo JJ (1990). Use of fluoroquinolones for intracellular pathogens. *Rev Infect Dis* **11**: S979.

Pohlod DH, Saravolatz LD (1986). Activity of quinolones against *Legionellaceae. J Antimicrob Chemother* **17**: 540.

Polk RE (1989). Drug-drug interactions with ciprofloxacin and other fluoroquinolones. *Amer J Med* **87** (Suppl 5A): 76S.

Polk RE, Healy DP, Sahai J *et al.* (1989). Effect of ferrous sulfate and multivitamins with zinc on absorption of ciprofloxacin in normal volunteers. *Antimicrob Ag Chemother* **33**: 1841.

Pradhan KM, Arora NK, Jena A, Susheela AK, Bhan MK (1995). Safety of ciprofloxacin therapy in children: magnetic resonance images, body fluid levels of fluoride and linear growth. *Acta Paediatr* **84**: 555.

Praet JP, Peretz A, Goossens H *et al.* (1989). Salmonella septic arthritis: additional 2 cases with quinolone treatment. *J Rheumatol* **16**: 1610.

Preheim LC, Cuevas TA, Roccaforte JS *et al.* (1986). Ciprofloxacin and antacids. *Lancet* **ii**: 48.

Preheim LC, Cuevas TA, Roccaforte JS *et al.* (1987). Oral ciprofloxacin in the treatment of elderly patients with complicated urinary tract infections due to trimethoprim/sulfamethoxazole-resistant bacteria. *Amer J Med* **82**: 295.

Preston MA, Brown S, Borczyk AA *et al.* (1994). Antimicrobial susceptibility of pathogenic *Yersinia enterocolitica* isolated in Canada from 1972 to 1990. *Antimicrob Ag Chemother* **38**: 2121.

Price FW, Jr, Whitson WE, Collins KS, Gonzales JS (1995). Corneal tissue levels of topically applied ciprofloxacin. *Cornea* **14**: 152.

Prince RA, Casabar E, Adair CG *et al.* (1989). Effect of quinolone antimicrobials on theophylline pharmacokinetics. *J Clin Pharmacol* **29**: 650.

Prosser BL, Beskid G (1995). Multicenter *in vitro* comparative study of fluoroquinolones against 25 129 gram-positive and gram-negative clinical isolates. *Diagn Microbiol Infect Dis* **21**: 33.

Pryka RD, Rodvold KA, Ting W *et al.* (1993). Effects of cardiopulmonary bypass surgery on intravenous ciprofloxacin disposition. *Antimicrob Ag Chemother* **37**: 2106.

Pugsley MP, Dworzack DL, Roccaforte JS *et al.* (1988). An open study of the efficacy of a single dose of ciprofloxacin in eliminating the chronic nasopharyngeal carriage of *Neisseria meningitidis. J Infect Dis* **157**: 852.

Qadri SM, Al-Sediary S, Ueno Y (1990). Antibacterial activity of lomefloxacin against *Brucella melitensis. Diagn Microbiol Infect Dis* **13**: 277.

Quenzer RW, Davis RL, Neidhart MM (1990). Prospective randomized study comparing the efficacy and safety of ciprofloxacin with cefaclor in the treatment of patients with purulent bronchitis. *Diagn Microbiol Infect Dis* **13**: 143.

Radandt JM, Marchbanks CR, Dudley MN (1992). Interactions of fluoroquinolones with other drugs: mechanisms, variability, clinical significance, and management. *Clin Infect Dis* **14**: 272.

Rådberg G, Nilsson LE, Svensson S (1990). Development of quinolone-imipenem cross resistance in *Pseudomonas aeruginosa* during exposure to ciprofloxacin. *Antimicrob Ag Chemother* **34**: 2142.

Rademaker CM, Hoepelman IM, Wolfhagen MJ *et al.* (1989). Results of a double-blind placebo-controlled study using ciprofloxacin for prevention of travellers' diarrhea. *Eur J Clin Microbiol Infect Dis* **8**: 690.

Raeburn JA, Govan JRW, McCrae WM (1987). Ciprofloxacin therapy in cystic fibrosis. *J Antimicrob Chemother* **20**: 295.

Ragunathan PL, Potkins DV, Watson JG *et al.* (1990). Neonatal meningitis due to *Salmonella typhimurium* treated with ciprofloxacin. *J Antimicrob Chemother* **26**: 727.

Rahm V, Schacht P (1989). Safety of ciprofloxacin A review. *Scand J Infect Dis* (Suppl 60): 120.

Rajagopalan-Levasseur P, Dournon E, Dameron G *et al.* (1990). Comparative postantibacterial activities of pefloxacin, ciprofloxacin, and ofloxacin against intracellular multiplication of *Legionella pneumophila* serogroup 1. *Antimicrob Ag Chemother* **34**: 1733.

Rambout L, Sahai J, Gallicano K *et al.* (1994). Effect of bismuth subsalicylate on ciprofloxacin bioavailability. *Antimicrob Ag Chemother* **38**: 2187.

Ramirez CA, Bran JL, Mejia CR *et al.* (1985). Open, prospective study of the clinical efficacy of ciprofloxacin. *Antimicrob Ag Chemother* **28**: 128.

Ramirez-Ronda CH, Saavedra S, Rivera-Vazquez CR (1987). Comparative, double-blind study of oral ciprofloxacin and intravenous cefotaxime in skin and skin structure infections. *Amer J Med* **82** (4A): 220.

Ramon J, Dantery S, Farinoti R, Carbon C, Rubinstein E (1994). Intestinal elimination of ciprofloxacin in rabbits. *Antimicrob Ag Chemother* **38**: 757.

Rao RG (1991). Development of spontaneous resistance to ciprofloxacin in a strain of *Campylobacter jejuni. J Antimicrob Chemother* **28**: 317.

Raoof S, Wollschlager C, Khan E (1987a). Treatment of respiratory tract infections with ciprofloxacin. *J Antimicrob Chemother* **18** (Suppl D): 139.

Raoof S, Wollschlager C, Khan FA (1987b). Ciprofloxacin increases serum levels of theophylline. *Amer J Med* **82** (Suppl 4A): 115.

Raoult D, Drancourt M (1991). Antimicrobial therapy of rickettsial diseases. *Antimicrob Ag Chemother* **35**: 2457.

Raoult D, Gallais H, De MP *et al.* (1986a). Ciprofloxacin therapy for Mediterranean spotted fever. *Antimicrob Ag Chemother* **30**: 606.

Raoult D, Roussellier P, Galicher V *et al.* (1986b). *In vitro* susceptibility of *Rickettsia conorii* to ciprofloxacin as determined by suppressing lethality in chicken embryos and by plaque assay. *Antimicrob Ag Chemother* **29**: 424.

Raoult D, Torres H, Drancourt M (1991). Shell-vial assay: evaluation of a new technique for determining antibiotic susceptibility, tested in 13 isolates of *Coxiella burnetii. Antimicrob Ag Chemother* **35**: 2070.

Rastogi N, Goh KS, Labrousse V (1992). Activity of clarithromycin compared with those of other drugs against *Mycobacterium paratuberculosis* and further enhancement of its extracellular and intracellular activities by ethambutol. *Antimicrob Ag Chemother* **36**: 2843.

Rastogl S, Atkinson LD, McCarthy JT (1990). Allergic nephropathy associated with ciprofloxacin. *Mayo Clin Proc* **65**: 987.

Ratcliffe NT, Smith JT (1985). Norfloxacin has a novel bactericidal mechanism unrelated to that of other 4-quinolones. *J Pharm Pharmacol* **37**: 92P.

Rautelin H, Renkonen OV, Kosunen TU (1991). Emergence of fluoroquinolone resistance in *Campylobacter jejuni* and *Campylobacter coli* in subjects from Finland. *Antimicrob Ag Chemother* **35**: 2065.

Raviglione MC, Boyle JF, Mariuz P *et al.* (1990). Ciprofloxacin-resistant methicillin-resistant *Staphylococcus aureus* in an acute-care hospital. *Antimicrob Ag Chemother* **34**: 2050.

Raz R, Miron D (1995). Oral ciprofloxacin for treatment of infection following nail puncture wounds of the foot. *Clin Infect Dis* **21**: 194.

Read RC, Barry RE (1990). Relapsing yersinia infection. *Brit Med J* **300**: 1694.

Reda C, Quaresima T, Pastoris MC (1994). *In-vitro* activity of six intracellular antibiotics against *Legionella pneumophila* strains of human and environmental origin. *J Antimicrob Chemother* **33**: 757.

Reed MD, Stern RC, Myers CM *et al.* (1988). Lack of unique ciprofloxacin pharmacokinetic characteristics in patients with cystic fibrosis. *J Clin Pharmacol* **28**: 691.

Reeves DS (1986). The effect of quinolone antibacterials on the gastrointestinal flora compared with that of other antibacterials. *J Antimicrob Chemother* **18** (Suppl D): 89.

Reid TM, Gould IM, Golder D *et al.* (1989). Respiratory tract penetration of ciprofloxacin. *Amer J Med* **87** (Suppl 5A): 60S.

Reina J, Ros MJ, Serra A (1994). Susceptibilities to 10 antimicrobial agents of 1220 *Campylobacter* strains isolated from 1987 to 1993 from feces of pediatric patients. *Antimicrob Ag Chemother* **38**: 2917.

Reinhardt JF, George WL (1985). Comparative *in vitro* activities of selected antimicrobial agents against *Aeromonas* species and *Plesiomonas shigelloides. Antimicrob Ag Chemother* **27**: 643.

Rella M, Haas D (1982). Resistance of *Pseudomonas aeruginosa* PAO to nalidixic acid and low levels of beta-lactam antibiotics: mapping of chromosomal genes. *Antimicrob Ag Chemother* **22**: 242.

Renkonen OV, Sivonen A, Visakorpi R (1987). Effect of ciprofloxacin on carrier rate of *Neisseria meningitidis* in army recruits in Finland. *Antimicrob Ag Chemother* **31**: 962.

Ribard P, Audisio F, Kahn M-F *et al.* (1992). Seven Achilles tendinitis including three complicated by rupture during fluoroquinolone therapy. *J Rheumatol* **19**: 1479.

Rice RJ, Knapp JS (1994). Antimicrobial susceptibilities of *Neisseria gonorrhoeae* strains representing five distinct resistance phenotypes. *Antimicrob Ag Chemother* **38**: 155.

Richer M, LeBel M (1993). Pharmacokinetics of fluoroquinolones in selected populations. In *Quinolone Antimicrobial Agents* 2nd edn (Hooper DC, Wolfson JS, eds), p. 225. Washington, DC: American Society of Microbiology.

Ries AA, Wells JG, Olivola MD *et al.* (1994). Epidemic *Shigella dysenteriae* type 1 in burundi: panresistance and implications for prevention. *J Infect Dis* **169**: 1035.

Riesbeck K, Gullberg M, Forsgren A (1994). Evidence that the antibiotic ciprofloxacin counteracts cyclosporine-dependent suppression of cytokine production. *Transplantation* **57**: 267.

Righter J (1987). Ciprofloxacin treatment of *Staphylococcus aureus* infections. *J Antimicrob Chemother* **20**: 595.

Righter J (1990). Pneumococcal meningitis during intravenous ciprofloxacin therapy. *Amer J Med* **88**: 548.

Rippelmeyer DJ, Synhavsky A (1988). Ciprofloxacin and allergic interstitial nephritis. *Ann Intern Med* **109**: 170.

Risi GF, Pombo DJ (1995). Relapse of tularemia after aminoglycoside therapy: case report and discussion of therapeutic options. *Clin Infect Dis* **20**: 174.

Rizk E (1992). The US clinical experience with lomefloxacin, a new once daily fluoroquinolone. *Amer J Med* **92** (Suppl 4A): 1305.

Roberts DE, Williams JD (1989). Ciprofloxacin in renal failure. *J Antimicrob Chemother* **23**: 820.

Robillard NJ (1990). Broad-host-range gyrase A gene probe. *Antimicrob Ag Chemother* **34**: 1889.

Robillard NJ, Scarpa AL (1988). Genetic and physiological characterization of ciprofloxacin resistance in *Pseudomonas aeruginosa* PAO. *Antimicrob Ag Chemother* **32**: 535.

Roblin PM, Montalban G, Hammerschlag MR (1994). *In vitro* activities of OPC-17116, a new quinolone; ofloxacin; and sparfloxacin against *Chlamydia pneumoniae*. *Antimicrob Ag Chemother* **38**: 1402.

Robson RA (1992). The effects of quinolones on xanthine pharmacokinetics. *Amer J Med* **92** (Suppl 4A): 22S.

Røder BL, Gutschik E (1989). *In-vitro* activity of ciprofloxacin combined with either fusidic acid or rifampicin against *Staphylococcus aureus*. *J Antimicrob Chemother* **23**: 347.

Rodriguez E, Martinez JA, Torres M *et al.* (1990). Lobular panniculitis associated with ciprofloxacin. *Brit Med J* **300**: 1468.

Rodvold KA, Piscitelli SC (1993). New oral macrolide and fluoroquinolone antibiotics: an overview of pharmacokinetics, interactions, and safety. *Clin Infect Dis* **17** (Suppl 1): S192.

Rohwedder RW, Bergan T, Thorsteinsson SB, Scholl H (1990). Transintestinal elimination of ciprofloxacin. *Diagn Microbiol Infect Dis* **13**: 127.

Rolachon A, Cordier L, Bacq Y *et al.* (1995). Ciprofloxacin and long-term prevention of spontaneous bacterial peritonitis: results of a prospective controlled trial. *Hepatology* **22**: 1171.

Rolston KVI, Bodey GP (1986). *In vitro* susceptibility of *Acinetobacter* species to various antimicrobial agents. *Antimicrob Ag Chemother* **30**: 769.

Rolston KV, Anaissie EA, Bodey GP (1987). *In-vitro* susceptibility of *Pseudomonas* species to fifteen antimicrobial agents. *J Antimicrob Chemother* **19**: 193.

Rosado LJ, Siskind MS, Copeland JG (1994). Acute interstitial nephritis in a cardiac transplant recipient receiving ciprofloxacin. *J Thorac Cardiovasc Surg* **107**: 1364.

Roscoe DL, Zemcov SJ, Thornber D *et al.* (1992). Antimicrobial susceptibilities and beta-lactamase characterization of *Capnocytophaga* species. *Antimicrob Ag Chemother* **36**: 2197.

Rose TF, Ellis-Pegler R, Collins J, Small M (1990). Oral pefloxacin mesylate in the treatment of continuous ambulatory peritoneal dialysis associated peritonitis: an open non-comparative study. *J Antimicrob Chemother* **25**: 853.

Rosner JL, Chai T-J, Foulds J (1991). Regulation of OmpF porin expression by salicylate in *Escherichia coli*. *J Bacteriol* **173**: 5631.

Rosolen A, Drigo P, Zanesco L (1994). Acute hemiparesis associated with ciprofloxacin. *Brit Med J* **309**: 1411.

Rouse MS, Wilcox RM, Henry NK *et al.* (1990). Ciprofloxacin therapy of experimental endocarditis caused by methicillin-resistant *Staphylococcus epidermidis*. *Antimicrob Ag Chemother* **34**: 273.

Rowe B, Ward LR, Threlfall EJ (1992). Ciprofloxacin and typhoid fever. *Lancet* **339**: 740.

Rowe B, Ward LR, Threlfall EJ (1995). Ciprofloxacin-resistant *Salmonella typhi* in the UK. *Lancet* **346**: 1302.

Rubenstein E, Rolston K, Escalante C *et al.* (1990). Ambulatory treatment of fever in neutropenic patients. *J Cancer Res Clin Oncol* **116** (Suppl): 1150.

Rubin J, Yu VL (1988). Malignant external otitis: insights into pathogenesis, clinical manifestations, diagnosis, and therapy. *Amer J Med* **85**: 391.

Rubin J, Stoehr G, Yu VL *et al.* (1989). Efficacy of oral ciprofloxacin plus rifampin for treatment of malignant external otitis. *Arch Otolaryngol Head Neck Surg* **115**: 1063.

Rubinstein E, Shalit I (1993). Effects of the quinolones on the immune system. In *Quinolone Antimicrobial Agents* 2nd edn (Hooper DC, Wolfson JS, eds), p. 519. Washington, DC: American Society of Microbiology.

Rubinstein E, Lang R, Shasha B *et al.* (1991). *In vitro* susceptibility of *Brucella melitensis* to antibiotics. *Antimicrob Ag Chemother* **35**: 1925.

Rubinstein E, St JL, Ramon J *et al.* (1994). The intestinal elimination of ciprofloxacin in the rat. *J Infect Dis* **169**: 218.

Rubinstein E, Dautrey S, Farinoti R *et al.* (1995). Intestinal elimination of sparfloxacin, fleroxacin and ciprofloxacin in rats. *Antimicrob Ag Chemother* **39**: 99.

Rubio TT (1987). Ciprofloxacin: comparative data in cystic fibrosis. *Amer J Med* **82**: 185.

Rubio TT (1990). Ciprofloxacin in the treatment of *Pseudomonas* infection in children with cystic fibrosis. *Diagn Microbiol Infect Dis* **13**: 153.

Rummens JL, Gordts B, Van LH (1986). *In vitro* susceptibility of *Capnocytophaga* species to 29 antimicrobial agents. *Antimicrob Ag Chemother* **30**: 739.

Ryan JL, Berenson CS, Greco TP *et al.* (1987). Oral ciprofloxacin in resistant urinary tract infections. *Amer J Med* **82**: 303.

Sabbaj J, Hoagland VL, Shih WJ (1985). Multiclinic comparative study of norfloxacin and trimethoprim–sulfamethoxazole for treatment of urinary tract infections. *Antimicrob Ag Chemother* **27**: 297.

Sacks LV, Labriola AM, Gill VJ *et al.* (1991). Use of ciprofloxacin for successful eradication of bacteremia due to *Campylobacter* cinaedi in a human immunodeficiency virus-infected person. *Rev Infect Dis* **13**: 1066.

Sade J, Lang R, Goshen S *et al.* (1989). Ciprofloxacin treatment of malignant external otitis. *Amer J Med* **87** (Suppl 5A): 138S.

Saginur R, Nicolle LE, Canadian Infectious Disease Society Clinical Trials Study Group (1992). Single dose compared with 3-day norfloxacin treatment of uncomplicated urinary tract infection in women. *Arch Intern Med* **152**: 1233.

Sahai J, Memish Z, Conway B (1991). Ciprofloxacin pharmacokinetics after administration via a jejunostomy tube. *J Antimicrob Chemother* **28**: 936.

Sahm DF, Koburov GT (1989). *In vitro* activities of quinolones against enterococci resistant to penicillin-aminoglycoside synergy. *Antimicrob Ag Chemother* **33**: 71.

Saito A, Gaja M (1995). *In vitro* and *in vivo* activities of sparfloxacin in *Legionella* infections. *Drugs* **49** (Suppl 2): 250.

Salam I, Katelaris P, Leigh-Smith S, Farthing MJ (1994). Randomised trial of single-dose ciprofloxacin for travellers' diarrhoea. *Lancet* **344**: 1537–9.

Salmon D, Deloron P, Gaudin C *et al.* (1990). Activities of pefloxacin and ciprofloxacin against experimental malaria in mice. *Antimicrob Ag Chemother* **34**: 2327.

Salvati F, Zubiani M, Antilli A *et al.* (1988). Ciprofloxacin in the oral treatment of severe respiratory tract infections. *Rev Infect Dis* **10** (Suppl 1): 220.

Sammalkorpi K, Lahdevirta J, Makela T *et al.* (1987). Treatment of chronic *Salmonella* carriers with ciprofloxacin. *Lancet* **ii**: 164.

Samonis G, Ho DH, Gooch GF *et al.* (1987). *In vitro* susceptibility of *Citrobacter* species to various antimicrobial agents. *Antimicrob Ag Chemother* **31**: 829.

Samuelsson J, Nilsson PG, Wahlin A *et al.* (1992). A pilot study of piperacillin and ciprofloxacin as initial therapy for fever in severely neutropenic leukemia patients. *Scand J Infect Dis* **24**: 467.

Sánchez C, Garcia RE, Garau J *et al.* (1993). Ciprofloxacin and trimethoprim–sulfamethoxazole versus placebo in acute uncomplicated *Salmonella enteritis*: a double-blind trial. *J Infect Dis* **168**: 1304.

Sánchez R, Fernández-Baca V, Díaz MD *et al.* (1994). Evolution of susceptibilities of *Campylobacter* spp to quinolones and macrolides. *Antimicrob Ag Chemother* **38**: 1879.

Sandberg T, Englund G, Lincoln K, Nilsson LG (1990). Randomized double-bling study of norfloxacin and cefadroxil in the treatment of acute pyelonephritis. *Eur J Clin Microbiol Infect Dis* **9**317.

Sanders CC, Sanders WE, Goering RV (1987). Overview of preclinical studies with ciprofloxacin. *Amer J Med* **82** (Suppl 4A): 2.

Sanford JP, Gilbert DN, Sande MA (1995). Guide to antimicrobial therapy 25th edn. Dallas, USA: Antimicrobial Therapy, Inc.

Sarkar M, Polk RE, Guzelian PS *et al.* (1990). *In vitro* effect of fluoroquinolones on theophylline metabolism in human liver microsomes. *Antimicrob Ag Chemother* **34**: 594.

Sato K, Hoshino K, Tanaka M *et al.* (1992). Antimicrobial activity of DU-6859, a new potent fluoroquinolone, against clinical isolates. *Antimicrob Ag Chemother* **36**: 1491.

Saux P, Martin C, Mallet MN *et al.* (1994). Penetration of ciprofloxacin into bronchial secretions from mechanically ventilated patients with nosocomial bronchopneumonia. *Antimicrob Ag Chemother* **38**: 901.

Scaglione F, Mezzetti M, Arcidiacono MM *et al.* (1995). Penetration of pefloxacin and ciprofloxacin into lung tissue. *J Antimicrob Chemother* **35**: 557.

Schaad UB, Wedgwood J (1992). Lack of quinolone-induced arthropathy in children. *J Antimicrob Chemother* **30**: 414.

Schaad UB, Wedgwood-Krucko K, Guenin U *et al.* (1989). Anti-pseudomonal therapy in cystic fibrosis; aztreonam and amikacin vs ceftazidime and amikacin administered intravenously, followed by oral ciprofloxacin. *Eur J Clin Microbiol* **8**: 858.

Schaad UB, Stoupis C, Wedgwood J *et al.* (1991). Clinical, radiologic and magnetic resonance monitoring for skeletal toxicity in pediatric patients with cystic fibrosis receiving a three-month course of ciprofloxacin. *Pediatr Infect Dis J* **10**: 723.

Schaad UB, Sander E, Wedgwood J *et al.* (1992). Morphologic studies for skeletal toxicity after prolonged ciprofloxacin therapy in two juvenile cystic fibrosis patients. *Pediatr Infect Dis J* **11**: 1047.

Schaberg DR, Dillon WI, Terpenning MS *et al.* (1992). Increasing resistance of enterococci to ciprofloxacin. *Antimicrob Ag Chemother* **36**: 2533.

Schacht P, Arcieri G, Brandte J *et al.* (1988). World-wide clinical data on efficacy and safety of ciprofloxacin. *Infection* **16** (Suppl 1): S29.

Schacht P, Arcieri G, Hullmann R (1989). Safety of oral ciprofloxacin An update based on clinical trial results. *Amer J Med* **87** (Suppl 5A): 98S.

Schaeffer AJ (1987). Multiclinic study of norfloxacin for treatment of complicated or uncomplicated urinary tract infections. *Amer J Med* **82** (Suppl 6B): 53.

Schaefler S (1989). Methicillin-resistant strains of *Staphylococcus aureus* resistant to quinolones. *J Clin Microbiol* **27**: 335.

Schlüter G (1987). Ciprofloxacin: review of potential toxicologic effects. *Amer J Med* **82** (Suppl 4A): 91.

Schmid GP (1990). Treatment of chancroid, 1989. *Rev Infect Dis* **12** (Suppl 6): S580.

Schmidt EW, Zimmermann I, Ritzerfeld W *et al.* (1989). Controlled prospective study of oral amoxicillin/clavulanate vs ciprofloxacin in acute exacerbations of chronic bronchitis. *J Antimicrob Chemother* **24** (Suppl B): 185.

Schnaitman CA, McDonald GA (1984). Regulation of outer membrane protein synthesis in *Escherichia coli* K-12: deletion of *ompC* affects expression of the OmpF protein. *J Bacteriol* **159**: 555.

Schönwald S, Beus I, Lisic M *et al.* (1989). Ciprofloxacin in the treatment of gram-negative bacillary meningitis. *Amer J Med* **87** (Suppl 5A): 248S.

Schwartz J, Jauregui L, Lettieri J *et al.* (1988). Impact of ciprofloxacin on theophylline clearance and steady-state concentrations in serum. *Antimicrob Ag Chemother* **32**: 75.

Scott DA, Haberberger RL, Thornton SA, Hyams KG (1990). Norfloxacin for the prophylaxis of travellers' diarrhea in US military personnel. *Am J Trop Med Hyg* **42**: 160.

Scribner RK, Welch DF, Marks MI (1985). Low frequency of bacterial resistance to enoxacin *in vitro* and in experimental pneumonia. *J Antimicrob Chemother* **16**: 597.

Scully BE (1993). Therapy of respiratory tract infections with quinolone antimicrobial agentts. In *Quinolone Antimicrobial Agents* 2nd edn (Hooper DC, Wolfson JS, eds), p. 339. Washington, DC: American Society of Microbiology.

Scully BE, Neu HC (1986). Oral ciprofloxacin therapy of infection caused by multiply resistant bacteria other than *Pseudomonas aeruginosa*. *J Antimicrob Chemother* **18** (Suppl D): 179.

Scully BE, Neu HC, Parry MF, Mandell W (1986). Oral ciprofloxacin therapy of infections due to *Pseudomonas aeruginosa*. *Lancet* **i**: 819.

Scully BE, Nakatomi M, Ores C *et al.* (1987). Ciprofloxacin therapy in cystic fibrosis. *Amer J Med* **82**: 196.

Scully BE, Clynes N, Neu HC (1991). Oral ofloxacin therapy of infections due to multiply-resistant bacteria. *Diag Microbiol Infect Dis* **14**: 435.

Segev, S, Rosen N, Joseph G *et al.* (1990). Pefloxacin efficacy in gram negative bacillary meningitis. *J Antimicrob Chemother* **26** (Suppl B): 187.

Segreti J, Hirsch DJ, Harris AA *et al.* (1990). *In vitro* activity of tosufloxacin (A-61827; T-3262) against selected genital pathogens. *Antimicrob Ag Chemother* **34**: 971.

Segreti J, Gootz TD, Goodman LJ *et al.* (1992). High-level quinolone resistance in clinical isolates of *Campylobacter jejuni*. *J Infect Dis* **165**: 667.

Seifert H, Baginski R, Schulze A *et al.* (1993). Antimicrobial susceptibility of *Acinetobacter* species. *Antimicrob Ag Chemother* **37**: 750.

Self PL, Zeluff BA, Sollo D, Gentry LO (1987). Use of ciprofloxacin in the treatment of serious skin and skin structure infections. *Amer J Med* **82** (Suppl 4A): 239.

Semel JD, Allen N (1989). Combination effects of ciprofloxacin, clindamycin, and metronidazole intravenously in volunteers. *South Med J* **84**: 465.

Setlow JK, Cabrera-Juárez E, Albritton WL *et al.* (1985). Mutations affecting gyrase in *Haemophilus influenzae*. *J Bacteriol* **164**: 525.

Shah A, Lettieri J, Kaiser L, Echols R, Heller AH (1994). Comparative pharmacokinetics and safety of ciprofloxacin 400 mg iv thrice daily versus 750 mg po twice daily. *J Antimicrob Chemother* **33**: 795.

Shah A, Lettieri J, Nix D, Wilton J, Heller AH (1995). Pharmacokinetics of high-dose intravenous ciprofloxacin in young and elderly and in male and female subjects. *Antimicrob Ag Chemother* **39**: 1003.

Shah PM, Asanger R, Kahan FM (1991). Incidence of multi-resistance in gram-negative aerobes from intensive care units of 10 German hospitals. *Scand J Infect Dis* (Suppl 78): 22.

Shalit I (1991). Immunological aspects of new quinolones. *Eur J Clin Microbiol Infect Dis* **10**: 262.

Shalit I, Greenwood RB, Marks MI *et al.* (1986). Pharmacokinetics of single-dose oral ciprofloxacin in patients undergoing chronic ambulatory peritoneal dialysis. *Antimicrob Ag Chemother* **30**: 152.

Shalit I, Stutman HR, Marks MI *et al.* (1987). Randomized study of two dosage regimens of ciprofloxacin for treating chronic bronchopulmonary infection in patients with cystic fibrosis. *Amer J Med* **82**: 189.

Shalit I, Barnea A, Shahar A (1989a). Efficacy of ciprofloxacin against *Leptospira interrogans* serogroup icterohaemorrhagiae. *Antimicrob Ag Chemother* **33**: 788.

Shalit I, Berger SA, Gorea A *et al.* (1989b). Widespread quinolone resistance among methicillin-resistant *Staphylococcus aureus* isolates in a general hospital. *Antimicrob Ag Chemother* **33**: 593.

Shalit I, Dan M, Gutman R *et al.* (1990). Cross resistance to ciprofloxacin and other antimicrobial agents among clinical isolates of *Acinetobacter calcoaceticus* biovar anitratus. *Antimicrob Ag Chemother* **34**: 494.

Shasha B, Lang R, Rubinstein E (1992). Therapy of experimental murine brucellosis with streptomycin, co-trimoxazole, ciprofloxacin, ofloxacin, pefloxacin, doxycycline, and rifampin. *Antimicrob Ag Chemother* **36**: 973.

Sheridan RL, Ryan CM, Pasternack MS *et al.* (1993). Flavobacterial sepsis in massively burned pediatric patients. *Clin Infect Dis* **17**: 185.

Shih DJ, Korbet SM, Rydel JJ, Schwartz MM (1995). Renal vasculitis associated with ciprofloxacin. *Am J Kidney Dis* **26**: 516.

Shimada J, Yamaji T, Ueda Y *et al.* (1983). Mechanism of renal excretion of AM-715, a new quinolone carboxylic acid derivative, in rabbits, dogs, and humans. *Antimicrob Ag Chemother* **23**: 1.

Silverman SH, Johnson M, Burdon DW *et al.* (1986). Pharmacokinetics of single dose intravenous ciprofloxacin in patients undergoing gastrointestinal surgery. *J Antimicrob Chemother* **18**: 107.

Simor AE, Ferro S, Low DE (1989). Comparative *in vitro* activities of six new fluoroquinolones and other oral antimicrobial agents against *Campylobacter pylori*. *Antimicrob Ag Chemother* **33**: 108.

Simpson J, Watson AR, Mellersch A *et al.* (1991). Typhoid fever ciprofloxacin and renal failure. *Arch Dis Child* **66**: 1083.

Simpson KJ and Brodie MJ (1985). Convulsions related to enoxacin. *Lancet* **ii**: 161.

Singh N, Yu VL (1992). Successful treatment of pulmonary infection due to *Mycobacterium chelonae*: case report and review. *Clin Infect Dis* **14**: 156.

Sjögren E, Kaijser B, Werner M (1992). Antimicrobial susceptibilities of *Campylobacter jejuni* and *Campylobacter coli* isolated in Sweden: a 10-year follow-up report. *Antimicrob Ag Chemother* **36**: 2847.

Slama TG (1990). Serum sickness-like illness associated with ciprofloxacin. *Antimicrob Ag Chemother* **34**: 904.

Slavich IL, Gleffe RF, Haas EJ (1989). Grand mal epileptic seizures during ciprofloxacin therapy. *JAMA* **261**: 558.

Smith CR (1987). The adverse effects of fluoroquinolones. *J Antimicrob Chemother* **19**: 709.

Smith JA (1991). Treatment of intra-abdominal infections with quinolones. *Eur J Clin Microbiol Infect Dis* **10**: 330.

Smith JT (1984). Awakening the slumbering potential of the 4-quinolone antibacterials. *Pharm J* **233**: 299.

Smith MJ, Hodson ME, Batten JC (1986a). Ciprofloxacin in cystic fibrosis. *Lancet* **i**: 1103.

Smith MJ, White LO, Bowyer H *et al.* (1986b). Pharmacokinetics and sputum penetration of ciprofloxacin in patients with cystic fibrosis. *Antimicrob Ag Chemother* **30**: 614.

Smith SM, Eng RH (1988). Interaction of ciprofloxacin with ampicillin and vancomycin for Streptococcus faecalis. *Diagn Microbiol Infect Dis* **9**: 239.

Smith SM, Eng RH, Tecson TF (1989). Ciprofloxacin therapy for methicillin-resistant *Staphylococcus aureus* infections or colonizations. *Antimicrob Ag Chemother* **33**: 181.

Smith SM, Eng RH, Bais P *et al.* (1990). Epidemiology of ciprofloxacin resistance among patients with methicillin-resistant *Staphylococcus aureus*. *J Antimicrob Chemother* **26**: 567.

Solomkin JS, Reinhart HH, Dellinger EP *et al.* (1996). Results of a randomized trial comparing sequential intravenous/oral treatment with ciprofloxacin plus metronidazole to imipenem/cilastatin for intra-abdominal infections. The Intra-Abdominal Infection Study Group. *Ann Surg* **223**: 303.

Somekh E, Lev B, Schwartz E *et al.* (1989). The effect of ciprofloxacin and pefloxacin on bone marrow engraftment in the spleen of mice. *J Antimicrob Chemother* **23**: 247.

Sookpranee T, Sookpranee M, Mellencamp MA *et al.* (1991). *Pseudomonas pseudomallei*, a common pathogen in Thailand that is resistant to the bactericidal effects of many antibiotics. *Antimicrob Ag Chemother* **35**: 484.

Soriano F, Fernandez-Roblas R, Lopez JC *et al.* (1994). Comparative *in-vitro* activity of rufloxacin with five other antimicrobial agents against bacterial enteric pathogens. *J Antimicrob Chemother* **34**: 157.

Soriano G, Guarner C, Teixidó M *et al.* (1991). Selective intestinal decontamination prevents spontaneous bacterial peritonitis. *Gastroenterology* **100**: 477.

Southern PM Jr, Kutscher AE, Ragsdale R, Luttrell B (1987). Susceptibility *in vitro* of *Nocardia* species to antimicrobial agents. *Diagn Microbiol Infect Dis* **8**: 119.

Sörgel F, Kinzig M (1993). Pharmacokinetics of gyrase inhibitors, Part 2: Renal and hepatic elimination pathways and drug interactions. *Amer J Med* **94** (Suppl 3A): 56S.

Sörgel F, Naber KG, Jaehde U *et al.* (1989). Gastrointestinal secretion of ciprofloxacin. Evaluation of the charcoal model for investigations in healthy volunteers. *Amer J Med* **87** (Suppl 5A): 62S.

Sörgel F, Naber KG, Kinzig M *et al.* (1991). Comparative pharmacokinetics of ciprofloxacin and temafloxacin in humans: a review. *Amer J Med* **91** (Suppl 6A): 51S.

Spangler SK, Jacobs MR, Appelbaum PC (1992). Susceptibilities of penicillin-susceptible and -resistant strains of *Streptococcus pneumoniae* to RP 59500, vancomycin, erythromycin, PD 131628, sparfloxacin, temafloxacin, win 57273, ofloxacin, and ciprofloxacin. *Antimicrob Ag Chemother* **36**: 856.

Spangler SK, Jacobs MR, Pankuch GA *et al.* (1993). Susceptibility of 170 penicillin-susceptible and penicillin-resistant pneumococci to six oral cephalosporins, four quinolones, desacetylcefotaxime, Ro 23–9424 and RP 67829. *J Antimicrob Chemother* **31**: 273.

Spangler SK, Jacobs MR, Appelbaum PC (1994). Activity of CP 99,219 compared with those of ciprofloxacin, grepafloxacin, metronidazole, cefoxitin, piperacillin, and piperacillin-tazobactam against 489 anaerobes. *Antimicrob Ag Chemother* **38**: 2471.

Speirs G, Warren RE, Rampling A (1988). *Clostridium tertium* septicemia in patients with neutropenia. *J Infect Dis* **158**: 1336.

Sreedharan S, Oram M, Jensen B *et al.* (1990). DNA gyrase *gyrA* mutations in ciprofloxacin-resistant strains of *Staphylococcus aureus*: close similarity with quinolone resistance mutations in *Escherichia coli*. *J Bacteriol* **172**: 7260.

Sreedharan S, Pterson LR, Fisher LM (1991). Ciprofloxacin resistance in coagulase-positive and -negative staphylococci: role of mutations at serine 84 in the DNA gyrase A protein of *Staphylococcus aureus* and *Staphylococcus epidermidis*. *Antimicrob Ag Chemother* **35**: 2151.

Stahlmann R (1990). Safety profile of the quinolones. *J Antimicrob Chemother* **26** (Suppl D): 31.

Stamm WE (1991). Azithromycin in the treatment of uncomplicated genital chlamydial infections. *Amer J Med* **91** (Suppl 3A): 19S.

Standiford HC, Drusano GL, Forrest A *et al.* (1987). Bactericidal activity of ciprofloxacin compared with that of cefotaxime in normal volunteers. *Antimicrob Ag Chemother* **31**: 1177.

Stanley PJ, Flegg PJ, Mandal BK *et al.* (1989). Open study of ciprofloxacin in enteric fever. *J Antimicrob Chemother* **23**: 789.

Stannard AJ, Sharples SJ, Norman PM *et al.* (1990). Ciprofloxacin therapy of urinary tract infections in paraplegic and tetraplegic patients: a bacteriological assessment. *J Antimicrob Chemother* **26** (Suppl F): 13.

Steele-Mortimer O, Meier-Ewert H (1988). *In-vitro* activity of fleroxacin against *Chlamydia trachomatis*. *J Antimicrob Chemother* **22** (Suppl D): 65.

Steen HJ, Scott EM, Stevenson MI *et al.* (1989). Clinical and pharmacokinetic aspects of ciprofloxacin in the treatment of acute exacerbations of pseudomonas infection in cystic fibrosis patients. *J Antimicrob Chemother* **24**: 787.

Stein DC, Danaher RJ, Cook TM (1991). Characterization of a *gyrB* mutation responsible for low-level nalidixic acid resistance in *Neisseria gonorrhoeae*. *Antimicrob Ag Chemother* **35**: 622.

Stein GE (1991). Drug interactions with fluoroquinolones. *Amer J Med* **91** (Suppl 6A): 81S.

Stille W, Harder S, Mieke S *et al.* (1987). Decrease of caffeine elimination in man during co-administration of 4-quinolones. *J Antimicrob Chemother* **20**: 729.

Stiver HG, Bartlett KH, Chow AW (1986). Comparison of susceptibility of gentamicin-resistant and -susceptible *Acinetobacter anitratus* to 15 alternative antibiotics. *Antimicrob Ag Chemother* **30**: 624.

Stone JW, Wise R, Donovan IA, Gearty J (1988). Failure of ciprofloxacin to eradicate *Campylobacter pylori* from the stomach. *J Antimicrob Chemother* **22**: 92.

Strachan CJL, Thom BT (1984). Excretion of intravenous and orally administered ciprofloxacin in biliary disease. *4th Medit Congr Chemother* Abstr. No. 622.

Strand O, Stromberg A (1990). Ciprofloxacin treatment of murine typhus. *Scand J Infect Dis* **22**: 503.

Strandvik B, Hjelte L, Lindblad A *et al.* (1989). Comparison of efficacy and tolerance of intravenously and orally administered ciprofloxacin in cystic fibrosis patients with acute exacerbations of lung infection. *Scand J Infect Dis* (Suppl 60): 84.

Stubbings J, Sheehan DR, Walton S (1992). Cutaneous vasculitis due to ciprofloxacin. *Brit Med J* **305**: 29.

Sturm AW (1987). Comparison of antimicrobial susceptibility patterns of fifty-seven strains of *Haemophilus ducreyi* isolated in Amsterdam from 1978 to 1985. *J Antimicrob Chemother* **19**: 187.

Stutman HR, Shalit I, Marks MI *et al.* (1987). Pharmacokinetics of two dosage regimens of ciprofloxacin during a two-week therapeutic trial in patients with cystic fibrosis. *Amer J Med* **82** (Suppl 4A): 142.

Sullivan MC, Cooper BW, Nightingale CH *et al.* (1993). Evaluation of the efficacy of ciprofloxacin against *Streptococcus pneumoniae* by using a mouse protection model. *Antimicrob Ag Chemother* **37**: 234.

Sung JJ, Lyon DJ, Suen R *et al.* (1995). Intravenous ciprofloxacin as treatment for patients with acute suppurative cholangitis: a randomized, controlled clinical trial. *J Antimicrob Chemother* **35**: 855.

Swanson BN, Boppana VK, Vlasses PH *et al.* (1983). Norfloxacin disposition after sequentially increasing oral doses. *Antimicrob Ag Chemother* **23**: 284.

Swanson RN, Hardy DJ, Chu DTW *et al.* (1991). Activity of temafloxacin against respiratory pathogens. *Antimicrob Ag Chemother* **35**: 423.

Swedish Study Group (1988). Therapy of acute and chronic gram-negative osteomyelitis with ciprofloxacin. Report from a Swedish Study Group. *J Antimicrob Chemother* **22**: 221.

Sweeney G, Fern AI, Lindsay G *et al.* (1990). Penetration of ciprofloxacin into the aqueous humour of the uninflamed human eye after oral administration. *J Antimicrob Chemother* **26**: 99.

Syrjälä H, Schildt R, Räisäinen S (1991). *In vitro* susceptibility of *Francisella tularensis* to fluoroquinolones and treatment of tularemia with norfloxacin and ciprofloxacin. *Eur J Clin Microbiol Infect Dis* **10**: 68.

Tack KJ, Smith JA (1989). The safety profile of ofloxacin. *Amer J Med* **87** (Suppl 6C): 78S.

Talbot GH, Cassileth PA, Paradiso L *et al.* (1993). Oral enoxacin for infection prevention in adult acute non-lymphocyte leukemia. *Antimicrob Ag Chemother* **37**: 474.

Tapsall JW, Shultz TR, Lovett R *et al.* (1992). Failure of 500 mg ciprofloxacin therapy in male urethral gonorrhoea. *Med J Aust* **156**: 143.

Tapson JS, Orr KE, George JC *et al.* (1990). A comparison between oral ciprofloxacin and intraperitoneal vancomycin and netilmicin in CAPD peritonitis. *J Antimicrob Chemother* **26** (Suppl F): 63.

Tartaglione TA, Raffalovich AC, Poyner WS *et al.* (1986). Pharmacokinetics and tolerance of ciprofloxacin after sequential increasing oral doses. *Antimicrob Ag Chemother* **29**: 62.

Tatsumi H, Senda H, Yatera S *et al.* (1978). Toxicological studies on pipemidic acid V effect on diarthrodial joints of experimental animals. *J Toxicol Sci* **3**: 357.

Taylor DN, Sanchez JL, Candler W *et al.* (1991). Treatment of travelers' diarrhea: ciprofloxacin plus loperamide compared with ciprofloxacin alone. A placebo-controlled, randomized trial. *Ann Intern Med* **114**: 731.

Tee W, Mijch A, Wright E, Yung A (1995). Emergence of multidrug resistance in *Campylobacter jejuni* isolates from three patients infected with human immunodeficiency virus. *Clin Infect Dis* **21**: 634.

Teh C, McKendrick M (1993). Ciprofloxacin-induced thrombocytopenia. *J Infect* **27**: 213.

Tham TC, Allen G, Hayes D *et al.* (1991). Possible association between toxic epidermal necrolysis and ciprofloxacin. *Lancet* **338**: 522.

The GIMENA Infection Program (1991). Prevention of bacterial infection in neutropenic patients with hematologic malignancies. A randomized, multicenter trial comparing norfloxacin with ciprofloxacin. The GIMEMA Infection Program Gruppo Italiano Malattie Ematologiche Maligne dell'Adulto. *Ann Intern Med* **115**: 7.

Thomson KS, Sanders CC (1994). Dissociated resistance among fluoroquinolones. *Antimicrob Ag Chemother* **38**: 2095.

Thomson KS, Sanders CC, Hayden ME (1991). *In vitro* studies with five quinolones: evidence for changes in relative potency as quinolone resistance rises. *Antimicrob Ag Chemother* **35**: 2329.

Thorsteinsson SB, Bergan T, Oddsdottir S *et al.* (1986). Crystalluria and ciprofloxacin, influence of urinary pH and hydration. *Chemotherapy* **33**: 448.

Thorsteinsson SB, Rahm V, Bergan T (1989). Tolerance of intravenous ciprofloxacin. *Scand J Infect Dis* (Suppl 60): 116.

Thorsteinsson SB, Bergan T, Rahm V, Rohwedder RW (1990). Safety of intravenous ciprofloxacin in healthy volunteers after multiple dosing. A review. *Diagn Microbiol Infect Dis* **13**: 191.

Thys JP, Jacobs F, Byl B (1991). Role of quinolones in the treatment of bronchopulmonary infections, particularly pneumococcal and community-acquired pneumonia. *Eur J Clin Microbiol Infect Dis* **10**: 304.

Tice AD, Marsh PK, Craven PC (1990). Comparison of intravenous ciprofloxacin with ceftazidime in the treatment of serious soft tissue infections. *Diagn Microbiol Infect Dis* **13**: 165.

Trenholme GM, Schmitt BA, Spear J *et al.* (1989). Randomized study of intravenous/oral ciprofloxacin versus ceftazidime in the treatment of hospital and nursing home patients with lower respiratory tract infections. *Amer J Med* **87** (Suppl 5A): 116S.

Trucksis M, Hooper DC, Wolfson JS (1991). Emerging resistance to fluoroquinolones in staphylococci: an alert. *Ann Intern Med* **114**: 424.

Tsukamura M, Nakamura E, Yoshii S *et al.* (1985). Therapeutic effect of a new antibacterial substance ofloxacin (DL 8280) on pulmonary tuberculosis. *Amer Rev Respir Dis* **131**: 352.

Tunkel AR, Scheld WM (1993). Treatment of bacterial meningitis. In *Quinolone Antimicrobial Agents* 2nd edn (Hooper DC, Wolfson JS, eds), p. 381. Washington, DC: American Society of Microbiology.

Turnidge JD, Nimmo GR, Francis G (1996). Evolution of resistance in *Staphylococcus aureus* in Australian teaching hospitals. Australian Group on Antimicrobial Resistance (AGAR). *Med J Aust* **164**: 68.

Tyndall M, Malisa M, Plummer FA *et al.* (1993). Ceftriaxone no longer predictably cures chancroid in Kenya. *J Infect Dis* **167**: 469.

Ullmann U, Giebel W, Dalhoff A, Koeppe P (1986). Single and multiple dose pharmacokinetics of ciprofloxacin. *Eur J Clin Microbiol* **5**: 193.

Unertl KE, Lenhart FP, Forst H *et al.* (1989). Ciprofloxacin in the treatment of legionellosis in critically ill patients including those cases unresponsive to erythromycin. *Amer J Med* **87** (Suppl 5A): 128S.

Uttley AHC, Collins CH (1988). *In vitro* activity of ciprofloxacin in combination with standard antituberculous drugs against *Mycobacterium tuberculosis*. *Tubercle* **69**: 193.

Uwaydah AK, al SH, Matar I (1992). Randomized prospective study comparing two dosage regimens of ciprofloxacin for the treatment of typhoid fever. *J Antimicrob Chemother* **30**: 707.

Uzun O, Akalin HE, Unal S *et al.* (1992). Long-term oral ciprofloxacin in the treatment of prosthetic valve endocarditis due to *Pseudomonas aeruginosa*. *Scand J Infect Dis* **24**: 797.

Valainis G, Thomas D, Pankey G (1986). Penetration of ciprofloxacin into cerebrospinal fluid. *Eur J Clin Microbiol* **5**: 206.

Valainis GT, Pankey GA, Katner HP *et al.* (1987). Ciprofloxacin in the treatment of bacterial skin infections. *Amer J Med* **82** (Suppl 4A): 230.

Valerius NH, Koch C, Hoiby N (1991). Prevention of chronic *Pseudomonas aeruginosa* colonisation in cystic fibrosis by early treatment. *Lancet* **338**: 725.

Valtonen V, Karppinen L, Kariniemi A-L (1989). A comparative study of ciprofloxacin and conventional therapy in the treatment of patients with chronic lower leg ulcers infected with *Pseudomonas aeruginosa* or other gram-negative rods. *Scand J Infect Dis* (Suppl 60): 79.

Van Caekenberghe D (1990). Comparative *in-vitro* activities of ten fluoroquinolones and fusidic acid against *Mycobacterium* spp. *J Antimicrob Chemother* **26**: 381.

Van de Heyning PH, Pattyn SR, Valcke HD et al. (1988). Use of ciprofloxacin in chronic suppurative otitis. *Rev Infect Dis* **10** (Suppl 1): S250.

Van der Auwera P, Joly P (1987). Comparative *in-vitro* activities of teicoplanin, vancomycin, coumermycin and ciprofloxacin, alone and in combination with rifampicin or LM 427, against *Staphylococcus aureus*. *J Antimicrob Chemother* **19**: 313.

Van der Auwera P, Matsumoto T, Husson M (1988). Intraphagocytic penetration of antibiotics. *J Antimicrob Chemother* **22**: 185.

Van der Willigen AH, van Rijsoord-Vos T, Wagenvoort JH et al. (1992). Antimicrobial susceptibility and serotyping of *Chlamydia trachomatis* strains isolated before and after treatment with ciprofloxacin and doxycycline. *Eur J Clin Microbiol Infect Dis* **11**: 561.

Van Dyck E, Bogaerts J, Smet H et al. (1994). Emergence of *Hemophilus ducreyi* resistance to trimethoprim–sulfamethoxazole in Rwanda. *Antimicrob Ag Chemother* **38**: 1647.

van der Wall E, Verkooyen RP, Mintjes-deGroot J et al. (1992). Prophylactic ciprofloxacin for catheter-associated urinary-tract infection. *Lancet* **339**: 946.

van Furth R, van't Wout JW, Wertheimer PA, Zwartendijk J (1992). Ciprofloxacin for treatment of malakoplakia. *Lancet* **339**: 148.

van Ogtrop ML, Mattie H, Sekh BR et al. (1992). Comparison of the antibacterial efficacies of ampicillin and ciprofloxacin against experimental infections with *Listeria monocytogenes* in hydrocortisone-treated mice. *Antimicrob Ag Chemother* **36**: 2375.

van Saene HKF, Lemmens SE, van Saene JJM (1988). Gut decontamination by oral ofloxacin and ciprofloxacin in healthy volunteers. *J Antimicrob Chemother* **22** (Suppl C): 127.

Vartivarian S, Anaissie E, Bodey G et al. (1994). A changing pattern of susceptibility of *Xanthomonas maltophilia* to antimicrobial agents: implications for therapy. *Antimicrob Ag Chemother* **38**: 624.

Venditti M, Gelfusa V, Tarasi A et al. (1990). Antimicrobial susceptibilities of *Erysipelothrix rhusiopathiae*. *Antimicrob Ag Chemother* **34**: 2038.

Venditti M, Tarasi A, Gelfusa V et al. (1993). Antimicrobial susceptibilities of enterococci isolated from hospitalized patients. *Antimicrob Ag Chemother* **37**: 1190.

Venezio FR, Tatarowicz W, DiVincenzo CA et al. (1986). Activity of ciprofloxacin against multiply resistant strains of *Pseudomonas aeruginosa*, *Staphylococcus epidermidis*, and group JK corynebacteria. *Antimicrob Ag Chemother* **30**: 940.

Verbist L (1991). Incidence of multi-resistance in gram-negative bacterial isolates from intensive care units in Belgium: a surveillance study. *Scand J Infect Dis* (Suppl 78): 45.

Verhoest P, Fernandez H, Boulanger JC et al. (1989). Use of ofloxacin plus amoxicillin-clavulanic acid for the treatment of acute genital tract infections. *Rev Infect Dis* **11** (Suppl 5): S1307.

Vidal C, Suarez J, Martinez M, Gonzalez-Quintela A (1995). Ciprofloxacin-induced glottic angioedema. *Postgrad Med J* **71**: 318.

Vila J, Gascon J, Abdalla S et al. (1994). Antimicrobial resistance of *Shigella* isolates causing traveller's diarrhea. *Antimicrob Ag Chemother* **38**: 2668.

Villeneuve JP, Davies C, Cote J (1995). Suspected ciprofloxacin-induced hepatotoxicity. *Ann Pharmacother* **29**: 257.

Visser MR, Rozenberg AM, Beumer H et al. (1991). Comparative *in vitro* antibacterial activity of sparfloxacin (AT-4140; RP 64206), a new quinolone. *Antimicrob Ag Chemother* **35**: 858.

Visvanathan K, Jones PD (1991). Ciprofloxacin treatment of *Haemophilus paraphrophilus* brain abscess. *J Infect* **22**: 306.

von Balen EAM, Touw-Otten FWMM, de Meiker RA (1990). Single dose pefloxacin versus five-days treatment with norfloxacin in uncomplicated cystitis in women. *J Antimicrob Chemother* **26** (Suppl B).153.

Voss A, Milatovic D, Wallrauch-Schwarz C et al. (1994). Methicillin-resistant *Staphylococcus aureus* in Europe. *Eur J Clin Microbiol Infect Dis* **13**: 50.

Wadsworth SJ, Kim KH, Satishchandran V et al. (1992). Development of new antibiotic resistance in methicillin-resistant but not methicillin-susceptible *Staphylococcus aureus*. *J Antimicrob Chemother* **30**: 821.

Waite NM, Edwards DJ, Arnott WS et al. (1989). Effects of ciprofloxacin on testosterone and cortisol concentrations in healthy males. *Antimicrob Ag Chemother* **33**: 1875.

Waites KB, Duffy LB, Schmid T et al. (1991). In vitro susceptibilities of *Mycoplasma pneumoniae*, *Mycoplasma hominis*, and *Ureaplasma urealyticum* to sparfloxacin and PD 127391. *Antimicrob Ag Chemother* **35**: 1181.

Waites KB, Crouse DT, Cassell GH (1992). Antibiotic susceptibilities and therapeutic options for *Ureaplasma urealyticum* infections in neonates. *Pediatr Infect Dis J* **11**: 23.

Walder M, Karlsson E, Nilsson B (1994). Sensitivity of 880 blood culture isolates to 24 antibiotics. *Scand J Infect Dis* **26**: 67.

Waldron R, Arkell DG, Wise R, Andrews JM (1986). The intraprostatic penetration of ciprofloxacin. *J Antimicrob Chemother* **17**: 544.

Wall RA, Mabey DCW, Bello CSS, Felmingham D (1985). The comparative *in-vitro* activity of twelve-4-quinolone antimicrobials against *Haemophilus ducreyi*. *J Antimicrob Chemother* **16**: 165.

Wallace MR, Yousif AA, Mahroos GA et al. (1993). Ciprofloxacin versus ceftriaxone in the treatment of multiresistant typhoid fever. *Eur J Clin Microbiol Infect Dis* **12**: 907.

Wallace RJ, Nash DR, Tsukamura M et al. (1988a). Human disease due to *Mycobacterium smegmatis*. *J Infect Dis* **158**: 52.

Wallace RJ, Steele LC, Sumter G et al. (1988b). Antimicrobial susceptibility patterns of *Nocardia asteroides*. *Antimicrob Ag Chemother* **32**: 1776.

Wallace RJ, Bedsole G, Sumter G et al. (1990). Activities of ciprofloxacin and ofloxacin against rapidly growing mycobacteria with demonstration of acquired resistance following single-drug therapy. *Antimicrob Ag Chemother* **34**: 65.

Wallace RJ, Brown BA, Onyi GO (1992). Skin, soft tissue, and bone infections due to *Mycobacterium chelonae chelonae*: importance of prior corticosteroid therapy, frequency of disseminated infections, and resistance to oral antimicrobials other than clarithromycin. *J Infect Dis* **166**: 405.

Wang C, Sabbaj J, Corrado M et al. (1988). World-wide clinical experience with norfloxacin; efficacy and safety. *Scand J Infect Dis* (Suppl 48): 81.

Wang F, Gu X-J, Zang M-F, Tay T-Y (1989). Treatment of typhoid fever with norfloxacin. *J Antimicrob Chemother* **23**: 785.

Wang Y, Huang WM, Taylor DE (1993). Cloning and nucleotide sequence of the *Campylobacter jejuni* gyrA gene and characterization of quinolone resistance mutations. *Antimicrob Ag Chemother* **37**: 457.

Watanabe M, Kotera Y, Yosue K et al. (1990). *In vitro* emergence of quinolone-resistant mutants of *Escherichia coli*, *Enterobacter cloacae*, and *Serratia marcescens*. *Antimicrob Ag Chemother* **34**: 173.

Watt B, Brown FV (1986). Is ciprofloxacin active against clinically important anaerobes? *J Antimicrob Chemother* **17**: 605.

Watt G, Shanks GD, Edstein MD et al. (1991). Ciprofloxacin treatment of drug-resistant falciparum malaria. *J Infect Dis* **164**: 602.

Webb DB, Roberts DE, Williams JD, Asscher AW (1986). Pharmacokinetics of ciprofloxacin in healthy volunteers and patients with impaired kidney function. *J Antimicrob Chemother* **18** (Suppl D): 83.

Weber DJ, Saviteer SM, Rutala WA et al. (1988). *In vitro* susceptibility of *Bacillus* spp to selected antimicrobial agents. *Antimicrob Ag Chemother* **32**: 642.

Weidekamm E, Portmann R, Suter K et al. (1987). *Antimicrob Ag Chemother* **31**: 1909.

Weidner W, Schiefer HG, Dalhoff A (1987a). Treatment of chronic bacterial prostatitis with ciprofloxacin Results of a one-year follow-up study. *Amer J Med* **82**: 280.

Weidner W, Schiefer HG, Garbe C (1987b). Acute non-gonococcal epididymitis. Etiological and therapeutic aspects. *Drugs* **34** (Suppl): 145.

Weightman NC, Brass AS (1993). Ciprofloxacin-resistant methicillin-sensitive *Staphylococcus aureus*. *J Antimicrob Chemother* **31**: 179.

Weinstein MP, Deeter RG, Swanson KA *et al.* (1991). Crossover assessment of serum bactericidal activity and pharmacokinetics of ciprofloxacin alone and in combination in healthy elderly volunteers. *Antimicrob Ag Chemother* **35**: 2352.

Wendel GD, Cox SM, Bawdon R *et al.* (1991). A randomized trial of ofloxacin versus cefoxitin and doxycycline in the outpatient treatment of acute salpingitis. *Am J Obstet Gynecol* **164**: 1390.

Wenk M, Birdschedler M, Koelz A *et al.* (1988). Pharmacokinetics of ciprofloxacin in patients with normal and impaired renal function. *Rev Infect Dis* **10** (Supp 1): S110.

Wessalowski R, Thomas L, Kivit J *et al.* (1993). Multiple brain abscesses caused by *Salmonella enteritidis* in a neonate: successful treatment with ciprofloxacin. *Pediatr Infect Dis J* **12**: 683.

Wexler HM, Molitoris E, Finegold SM (1992). *In vitro* activities of three of the newer quinolones against anaerobic bacteria. *Antimicrob Ag Chemother* **36**: 239.

Wexler HM, Molitoris E, Finegold SM (1994). *In vitro* activity of grepafloxacin (OPC-17116). against anaerobic bacteria. *Diagn Microbiol Infect Dis* **19**: 129.

Whiting JL, Cheng N, Chow AW (1987). Interactions of ciprofloxacin with clindamycin, metronidazole, cefoxitin, cefotaxime, and mezlocillin against gram-positive and gram-negative anaerobic bacteria. *Antimicrob Ag Chemother* **31**: 1379.

Widmer AF, Colombo VE, Gachter A *et al.* (1990). *Salmonella* infection in total hip replacement: tests to predict the outcome of antimicrobial therapy. *Scand J Infect Dis* **22**: 611.

Widmer AF, Gaechter A, Ochsner PE *et al.* (1992). Antimicrobial treatment of orthopedic implant-related infections with rifampin combinations. *Clin Infect Dis* **14**: 1251.

Wijnands WJ, Vree TB (1988). Interaction between the fluoroquinolones and the bronchodilator theophylline. *J Antimicrob Chemother* **22** (Suppl C): 109.

Wijnands WJA, Vree TB, van Herwaarden CLA (1986). The influence of quinolone derivatives on theophylline clearance. *Brit J Clin Pharmacol* **22**: 677.

Wilcox MH, Finch RG (1990). Ciprofloxacin and CAPD peritonitis. *J Antimicrob Chemother* **26**: 447.

Williams HM, Richards J (1990). Single-dose ciprofloxacin for shigellosis. *Lancet* **335**: 1343.

Willocks LJ, Thompson C, Emmanuel FX *et al.* (1990). Hospital outbreak of *Salmonella enteritidis* infection treated with ciprofloxacin. *Lancet* **335**: 1404.

Wingender W, Graefe K-H, Gau W, Förster D *et al.* (1984). Pharmacokinetics of ciprofloxacin after oral and intravenous administration in healthy volunteers. *Eur J Clin Microbiol* **3**: 355.

Winrow AP, Supramaniam G (1990). Benign intracranial hypertension after ciprofloxacin administration. *Arch Dis Child* **65**: 1165.

Winston DJ (1993a). Prophylaxis and treatment of infection in the bone marrow transplant recipient. In *Current Clinical Topics in Infectious Diseases* Vol 13 (Remington JS, Swartz MN, eds), pp. 293–321. Boston, USA: Blackwell Scientific Publications Inc.

Winston DJ (1993b). Use of quinolone antimicrobial agents in immunocompromised patients. In *Quinolone Antimicrobial Agents* 2nd edn (Hooper DC, Wolfson JS, eds), p. 435. Washington, DC: American Society of Microbiology.

Winston DJ, Ho WG, Bruckner DA *et al.* (1990). Ofloxacin versus vancomycin/polymyxin for prevention of infections in granulocytopenic patients. *Amer J Med* **88**: 36.

Winter J, Sweeney G (1991). Reproducibility of the measurement of ciprofloxacin concentration in bronchial mucosa. *J Antimicrob Chemother* **27**: 329.

Winter JH, McCartney C, Bingham J *et al.* (1988). Ciprofloxacin in the

treatment of severe Legionnaire's disease. *Rev Infect Dis* **10** (Suppl 1): S218.

Winton MD, Everett ED, Dolan SA (1988). Activities of five new fluoroquinolones against *Pseudomonas pseudomallei*. *Antimicrob Ag Chemother* **32**: 928.

Wise R, Donovan IA (1987). Tissue penetration and metabolism of ciprofloxacin. *Amer J Med* **82** (Suppl 4A): 103.

Wise R, Andrews JM, Edwards LJ (1983). *In vitro* activity of Bay 0 9867, a new quinoline derivative compared with those of other antimicrobial agents. *Antimicrob Ag Chemother* **23**: 559.

Wise R, Lockley RM, Webberly M, Dent J (1984). Pharmacokinetics of intravenously administered ciprofloxacin. *Antimicrob Ag Chemother* **26**: 208.

Wise R, Lister D, McNulty CA *et al.* (1986). The comparative pharmacokinetics of five quinolones. *J Antimicrob Chemother* **18** (Suppl D): 71.

Wise R, Ashby JP, Andrews JM (1988a). *In vitro* activity of PD 127,391, an enhanced-spectrum quinolone. *Antimicrob Ag Chemother* **32**: 1251.

Wise R, Griggs D, Andrews JM (1988b). Pharmacokinetics of the quinolones in volunteers: a proposed dosing schedule. *Rev Infect Dis* **10** (Suppl 1): S83.

Wise R, Baldwin DR, Andrews JM *et al.* (1991). Comparative pharmacokinetic disposition of fluoroquinolones in the lung. *J Antimicrob Chemother* **28** (Suppl C): 65.

Wise R, Andrews JM, Matthews R, Wolstenholme M (1992). The *in-vitro* activity of two new quinolones: rufloxacin and MF 961. *J Antimicrob Chemother* **29**: 649.

Wise R, Andrews JM, Brenwald N (1993a). The *in-vitro* activity of Bay y 3118, a new chlorofluoroquinolone. *J Antimicrob Chemother* **31**: 73.

Wise R, Andrews JM, Brenwald N (1993b). The *in-vitro* activity of OPC-17116, a new 5-methyl substituted quinolone. *J Antimicrob Chemother* **31**: 497.

Wispelwey B, Scheld WM (1990). Ciprofloxacin in the treatment of *Staphylococcus aureus* osteomyelitis. A review. *Diagn Microbiol Infect Dis* **13**: 169.

Wiström J, Norrby R (1990). Antibiotic prophylaxis of travellers' diarrhoea. *Scand J Infect Dis* (Suppl 70): 111.

Wiström J, Jertborn M, Hedström SA *et al.* (1989). Short-term self-treatment of travellers' diarrhea with norfloxacin: a placebo-controlled study. *J Antimicrob Chemother* **23**: 905.

Wiström J, Gentry LO, Palmgren AC *et al.* (1992). Ecological effects of short-term ciprofloxacin treatment of travellers' diarrhoea. *J Antimicrob Chemother* **30**: 693.

Wolff M, Boutron L, Singlas E *et al.* (1987). Penetration of ciprofloxacin into cerebrospinal fluid of patients with bacterial meningitis. *Antimicrob Ag Chemother* **31**: 899.

Wolfson JS, Hooper DC (1989a). Bacterial resistance to quinolones: mechanisms and clinical importance. *Rev Infect Dis* **11** (Suppl 5): S960.

Wolfson JS, Hooper DC (1989b). Comparative pharmacokinetics of ofloxacin and ciprofloxacin. *Amer J Med* **87** (Suppl 6C): 31S.

Wolfson JS, Hooper DC (1989c). Fluoroquinolone antimicrobial agents. *Clin Micro Rev* **2**: 378.

Wolfson JS, Hooper DC, Ng EY *et al.* (1987). Antagonism of wild-type and resistant *Escherichia coli* and its DNA gyrase by the tricyclic 4-quinolone analogs ofloxacin and S-25930 stereoisomers. *Antimicrob Ag Chemother* **31**: 1861.

Wolfson JS, Hooper DC, Shih DJ *et al.* (1989). Isolation and characterization of an *Escherichia coli* strain exhibiting partial tolerance to quinolones. *Antimicrob Ag Chemother* **33**: 705.

Wollschlager CM, Raoof S, Khan FA *et al.* (1987). Controlled, comparative study of ciprofloxacin versus ampicillin in treatment of bacterial respiratory tract infections. *Amer J Med* **82**: 164.

Wood CA (1994). Treatment of severe pneumonia with ciprofloxacin or imipenem. *Antimicrob Ag Chemother* **38**: 1871.

Wood MJ, Logan MN (1986). Oprofloxacin for soft tissue infections. *J Antimicrob Chemother* **18** (Suppl D): 159.

Wurtz RM, Abrams D, Becker S *et al.* (1989). Anaphylactoid drug reactions to ciprofloxacin and rifampicin in HIV-infected patients. *Lancet* i: 955.

Yajko DM, Kirihara J, Sanders C *et al.* (1988). Antimicrobial synergism against *Mycobacterium avium* complex strains isolated from patients with acquired immune deficiency syndrome. *Antimicrob Ag Chemother* **32**: 1392.

Yajko DM, Sanders CA, Nassos PS *et al.* (1990). *In vitro* susceptibility of *Mycobacterium avium* complex to the new fluoroquinolone sparfloxacin (CI-978; AT-4140). and comparison with ciprofloxacin. *Antimicrob Ag Chemother* **34**: 2442.

Yamagishi J, Furutami Y, Inoue S *et al.* (1981). New nalidixic acid resistance mutations related to deoxyribonucleic acid gyrase activity. *J Bacteriol* **148**: 450.

Yamagishi J, Yoshida H, Yamayoshi M, Nakamura S (1986). Nalidixic acid-resistant mutations of the *gyrB* gene of *Escherichia coli*. *Mol Gen Genet* **204**: 367.

Yamamoto T, Naigowit P, Dejsirilert S *et al.* (1990). *In vitro* susceptibilities of *Pseudomonas pseudomallei* to 27 antimicrobial agents. *Antimicrob Ag Chemother* **34**: 2027.

Yancey RJ, Sanchez MS, Ford CW (1991). Activity of antibiotics against *Staphylococcus aureus* within polymorphonuclear neutrophils. *Eur J Clin Microbiol Infect Dis* **10**: 107.

Yangco BG, Kenyon VS, Halkias KD *et al.* (1989). Oral ciprofloxacin treatment of infections in geriatric patients. *Clin Ther* **1**: 503.

Yeaman MR, Baca OG (1990). Unexpected antibiotic susceptibility of a chronic isolate of *Coxiella burnetii*. *Ann N Y Acad Sci* **590**: 297.

Yeaman MR, Bayer AS (1993). Treatment of experimental and human bacterial endocarditis with quinolone antimicrobial agents. In *Quinolone Antimicrobial Agents* 2nd edn (Hooper DC, Wolfson JS, eds), p. 397. Washington, DC: American Society of Microbiology.

Yeaman MR, Mitscher LA, Baca OG (1987). *In vitro* susceptibility of *Coxiella burnetii* to antibiotics, including several quinolones. *Antimicrob Ag Chemother* **31**: 1079.

Yeaman MR, Roman MJ, Baca OG (1989). Antibiotic susceptibilities of two *Coxiella burnetii* isolates implicated in distinct clinical syndromes. *Antimicrob Ag Chemother* **33**: 1052.

Yebra M, Ortigosa J, Albarran F *et al.* (1990). Ciprofloxacin in a case of Q fever endocarditis. *New Engl J Med* **323**: 614.

Yee YC, Thornsberry C, Brown SD *et al.* (1993). A comparative study of the *in-vitro* activity of cefepime and other antimicrobial agents against penicillin-susceptible and penicillin-resistant *Streptococcus pneumoniae*. *J Antimicrob Chemother* **31** (Suppl B): 13.

Yew WW, Kwan SYL, Wong PC *et al.* (1990). Ofloxacin and imipenem in the treatment of *Mycobacterium fortuitum* and *Mycobacterium chelonae* lung infections. *Tubercle* **71**: 131.

Yew WW, Piddock LJ, Li MS *et al.* (1994). *In-vitro* activity of quinolones and macrolides against mycobacteria. *J Antimicrob Chemother* **34**: 343.

Young LS, Berlin OGW, Inderlied CB (1987). Activity of ciprofloxacin and other fluorinated quinolones against *Mycobacteria*. *Amer J Med* **82** (Suppl 4A): 23.

Young M, Hancock RE (1992). Fluoroquinolone supersusceptibility mediated by outer membrane protein OprH overexpression in *Pseudomonas aeruginosa*: evidence for involvement of a nonporin pathway. *Antimicrob Ag Chemother* **36**: 2365.

Yuen GJ, Drusano GL, Plaisance K *et al.* (1989). Ciprofloxacin pharmacokinetics in critically ill trauma patients. *Amer J Med* **87** (Suppl 5A): 70S.

Yuk JH, Nightingale CH, Sweeney KR *et al.* (1989a). Relative bioavailability in healthy volunteers of ciprofloxacin administered through a nasogastric tube with and without enteral feeding. *Antimicrob Ag Chemother* **33**: 1118.

Yuk JH, Nightingale CN, Quintiliani R (1989b). Ciprofloxacin levels when receiving sucralfate. *JAMA* **262**: 901.

Zahid MA, Klotz SA, Goldstein E, Bartholomew W (1994). *Mycobacterium chelonae* (*M. chelonae* subspecies *chelonae*): report of a patient with a sporotrichoid presentation who was successfully treated with clarithromycin and ciprofloxacin. *Clin Infect Dis* **18**: 999.

Zehnder D, Hoigne R, Neftel KA, Sieber R (1995). Painful dysaesthesia with ciprofloxacin. *Brit Med J* **311**: 1204.

Zeiler HJ (1985). Evaluation of the *in vitro* bactericidal action of ciprofloxacin on cells of *Escherichia coli* in the logarithmic and stationary phases of growth. *Antimicrob Ag Chemother* **28**: 524.

Zeiler HJ, Voigt WH (1987). Efficacy of ciprofloxacin in stationary-phase bacteria *in vivo*. *Amer J Med* **82**: 87.

Zenilman JM, Neumann T, Patton M *et al.* (1993). Antibacterial activities of OPC-17116, ofloxacin, and ciprofloxacin against 200 isolates of *Neisseria gonorrhoeae*. *Antimicrob Ag Chemother* **37**: 2244.

Zhang YY, Wang F, Zhang JD *et al.* (1995). *In vitro* antibacterial activity of levofloxacin. *Drugs* **49** (Suppl 2): 274.

Zumla A, Lewis D, Brown J (1988). Ciprofloxacin treatment of recurrent *Salmonella typhimurium* septicaemia in a splenectomized and immunosuppressed patient. *J Antimicrob Chemother* **21**: 809.

Zweerink MM, Edison A (1986). Inhibition of *Micrococcus luteus*. DNA gyrase by norfloxacin and 10 other quinolone carboxylic acids. *Antimicrob Ag Chemother* **29**: 598–601.

Norfloxacin

Description

Norfloxacin was synthesized at the Kyorin Central Research Laboratory in Japan (Ito *et al.*, 1980). It is a fluorinated quinolone carboxylic acid derivative which has the chemical formula of 1-ethyl-6-fluoro-1, 4-dihydro-4-oxo-7-(1-piperazinyl)-3-quinoline carboxylic acid. The antibacterial spectrum of norfloxacin is very similar to that of enoxacin but generally the drug is less active than ciprofloxacin (p. 986; Table II.6). Since the distribution of norfloxacin is more limited than that of ciprofloxacin it is used primarily to treat infections associated with the gastrointestinal or genitourinary systems. This chapter focuses on the differences between norfloxacin and other quinolones such as ciprofloxacin.

Sensitive Organisms

1 Gram-negative bacteria

The activity of norfloxacin against Gram-negative bacili is similar to, or less than, that of ciprofloxacin (p. 981). Most Enterobacteriaceae are sensitive, including *Escherichia coli*, the *Enterobacter*, *Klebsiella*, *Salmonella*, *Shigella*, *Arizona* and *Citrobacter* spp. Of the *Proteeae*, *Proteus mirabilis*, *Pr. vulgaris*, *Morganella morganii* and *Providencia rettgeri* are quite susceptible (MIC_{90} 0.06–0.25 μg per ml); as are *Serratia* spp. (MIC_{90} 0.5 μg per ml), while *Providencia stuartii* is less frequently so (MIC_{90} 4 μg per ml) (Downs *et al.*, 1982; Neu and Labthavikul,1982; King *et al.*, 1982; Norrby and Jonsson, 1983; Newsom, 1984; King and Phillips, 1986; Bassey *et al.*, 1986; Auckenthaler *et al.*, 1986; Goldstein, 1987; Wolfson and Hooper, 1988; Rao *et al.*, 1993). The activity of norfloxacin against Enterobacteriaceae is comparable with that of cefotaxime (p. 320; King *et al.*, 1982). *Campylobacter jejuni* and *C. coli* are susceptible to norfloxacin and other fluoroquinolones, although resistance is increasing (Lariviere *et al.*, 1986; Sanchez *et al.*, 1994; Sjogren *et al.*, 1992; Wretlind *et al.*, 1992; p. 982). *Helicobacter pylori*, however, is only moderately susceptible (MIC_{90} 1μg per ml) (Shungu *et al.*, 1987; Hupertz *et al.*, 1988; Glupczynski *et al.*, 1988; Mertens *et al.*, 1989). *Aeromonas* spp. (MIC_{90} 0.016 μg per ml) and *Plesiomonas shigelloides* ($MIC \leq 0.1$ μg per ml) are quite sensitive (Reinhardt and George, 1985; Kain and Kelly, 1989; Olsson-Liljequist and Mollby, 1990). *Yersinia enterocolitica* and *Pasteurella multocida* are susceptible. *Vibrio* spp. are very sensitive: *V. cholerae* MIC_{90} 0.016 μg per ml, *V. parahaemolyticus* MIC_{90} 0.25 μg per ml and *V. vulnificus* MIC_{90} 0.063 μg per ml; including strains with plasmids coding for various patterns of multiresistance to tetracycline, ampicillin, chloramphenicol and co-trimoxazole (Morris *et al.*, 1985; Olsson-Liljequist and Mollby, 1990). *Flavobacterium* spp. are usually resistant, as are *Acinetobacter* spp. – especially strains which are also resistant to gentamicin (Stiver *et al.*, 1986). *Gardnerella vaginalis* is usually resistant (MIC_{90} 16 μg per ml) (King and Phillips, 1986).

Most strains of *Pseudomonas aeruginosa*, including strains resistant to gentamicin, are susceptible to norfloxacin (Downs *et al.*, 1982; King and Phillips, 1986; Bassey *et al.*, 1986; Auckenthaler *et al.*, 1986; Goldstein, 1987). Its activity against *Ps. aeruginosa* is often superior to that of gentamicin, amikacin, ticarcillin, azlocillin, mezlocillin, cefoperazone, ceftazidime, cefotaxime, ceftizoxime, ceftriaxone and moxalactam, and similar to that of tobramycin (Forward *et al.*, 1983; Leigh and Emmanuel, 1984). *Burkholderia* (previously *Pseudomonas*) *cepacia* may be sensitive, but *Stenotrophomonas maltophilia* is resistant (Neu and Labthavikul,1982; Bassey *et al.*, 1986; Auckenthaler *et al.*, 1986). *Burkholderia* (previously *Pseudomonas*) *pseudomallei* is also resistant to most fluoroquinolones (Winton *et al.*, 1988).

Haemophilus influenzae (including beta-lactamase-producing strains), *Neisseria meningitidis* and *N. gonorrhoeae* (including beta-lactamase-producing strains) are all very susceptible, although resistance in this latter species is increasing (pp. 993, 1063) (King *et al.*, 1982; Khan *et al.*, 1981; King and Phillips, 1986; Auckenthaler *et al.*, 1986; Bogaerts *et al.*, 1986; Ponticas *et al.*, 1989; Slaney *et al.*, 1990; Clendennen *et al.*, 1992a,b). Norfloxacin, like ciprofloxacin, is active against *H. ducreyi*. *Bordetella pertussis* is susceptible (MIC$_{90}$ 0.25 µg per ml) (Zackrisson *et al.*, 1985; Appleman *et al.*, 1987; Kurzynski *et al.*, 1988). *Legionella* spp. are susceptible to norfloxacin (*L. pneumophila*: MIC$_{90}$ 0.125µg per ml) (Greenwood and Laverick, 1983; Moffie and Mouton, 1988).

Francisella tularensis is susceptible to clinically achievable concentrations of many fluoroqunolones, including norfloxacin (mean MIC 0.24 µg per ml) and ciprofloxacin (mean MIC 0.13 µg per ml), with associated reports of clinical efficacy (Syrjala *et al.*, 1991; p. 1032).

Eikenella corrodens is generally susceptible to <2 µg per ml norfloxacin, ciprofloxacin , ofloxacin and enoxacin (Goldstein *et al.*, 1986). However, norfloxacin has poor activity against most anaerobes, including *Bacteroides* and *Fusobacterium* spp., and is generally inferior to ciprofloxacin (Goldstein and Citron, 1985; Edlund and Nord, 1986; Goldstein, 1993).

2 Gram-positive bacteria

Norfloxacin is less active against *Staphylococcus aureus*, *Staph. epidermidis* and *Staph. saprophyticus* (MIC$_{90}$ 2 µg per ml) than ciprofloxacin (p. 984), and *Streptococcus faecalis* and *Strep. pneumoniae* are often resistant (MIC$_{90}$ 4–8 µg per ml) (Neu and Labthavikul, 1982; Auckenthaler *et al.*, 1986; Murray *et al.*, 1993). Methicillin-resistant strains of *Staph. aureus* are usually sensitive to norfloxacin, but less so than methicillin-sensitive strains, and resistance is emerging in many regions (p. 994; Corrado *et al.*, 1983; Harnett *et al.*, 1991; Chang *et al.*, 1994). Viridans group streptococci are resistant (Chin and Neu, 1983; Goldstein, 1987). Similar to the situation with ciprofloxacin, norfloxacin activity *in vitro* against *Strep. pyogenes* and other beta-hemolytic streptococci (Groups B, C, and G) is borderline or resistant with MIC$_{90}$ 2–16 µg per ml (King *et al.*, 1982; Chin and Neu, 1983; Corrado *et al.*, 1983; Goldstein, 1987). Norfloxacin is generally less active than ciprofloxacin against both penicillin-sensitive and penicillin-resistant strains of *Strep. pneumoniae* (MIC$_{90}$ 2–16 µg per ml) (Gombert and Aulicino, 1984; Auckenthaler *et al.*, 1986; Goldstein, 1987). *Listeria monocytogenes* is generally resistant (MIC$_{90}$ 8 µg per ml), as are *Nocardia* spp. (MIC$_{90}$ 64 µg per ml) (Auckenthaler *et al.*, 1986; Macgowan *et al.*, 1990). Ciprofloxacin is more active *in vitro* than norfloxacin against *Corynebacterium* group D2 (Fernández-Roblas *et al.*, 1987). *Clostridium* spp., including *Cl. difficile* and anaerobic cocci, are resistant (King *et al.*, 1982; Goldstein and Citron, 1985; Delmee and Avesani, 1986; Edlund and Nord, 1986).

3 Other organisms

Ureaplasma urealyticum and *Chlamydia trachomatis* are resistant to norfloxacin (MIC 8 to >64 µg per ml and 12.5–16 µg per ml, respectively) (Heessen and Muytjens, 1984; Aznar *et al.*, 1985; Nakata *et al.*, 1992). Norfloxacin has some activity against *Coxiella burnetii in vitro*, but ciprofloxacin is significantly more active *in vitro* and *in vivo* (Yeaman *et al.*, 1989; p. 988).

Norfloxacin has moderate *in vitro* activity against *Mycobacterium tuberculosis* (MIC 2–8 µg per ml) but the better *in vitro* activity and wider *in vivo* distribution of ciprofloxacin and ofloxacin make these the preferred clinical agents (pp. 985, 1112) (Fenlon and Cynamon, 1986; Berlin *et al.*, 1987; Young *et al.*, 1987; Davies *et al.*, 1987; Garcia-Rodriguez and Gomez Garcia, 1993). *Mycobacterium fortuitum* has MIC$_{90}$ of 2 µg per ml, but *M. kansasii*, *M. xenopi* and *M. chelonae* are relatively resistant (MIC$_{90}$ 4–8 µg per ml), and *M. avium* complex strains are resistant (MIC$_{90}$ ≥16 µg per ml) (Gay *et al.*, 1984; Davies *et al.*, 1987; Young *et al.*, 1987; Goldstein, 1987). Norfloxacin has poor activity against *M. leprae* (Franzblau and White, 1990).

Similar to ciprofloxacin (p. 989), norfloxacin has some *in vitro* activity against *Plasmodium falciparum* but the clinical relevence of this is not clear (Divo *et al.*, 1988; Sarma, 1989; Wyler, 1989; p. 1069).

4 Acquired resistance

Issues and mechanisms associated with acquired resistance to norfloxacin are similar to those described for ciprofloxacin (p. 990). Similar to ciprofloxacin, a number of studies have correlated the increased use of fluroquinolones with increasing emergence of norfloxacin-resistance and cross-resistance with other fluoroquinolones among many species (Perez-Trallero *et al.*, 1993; Dupeyron *et al.*, 1994; Neu, 1988; Desgrandchamps and Munzinger, 1989; Kresken and Wiedemann, 1988). Alterations in the A subunit of DNA gyrase, altered outer membrane permeability and active efflux mechanisms have been described as mechanisms of norfloxacin-resistance in various species (Hooper *et al.*, 1989; Gootz and Martin, 1991; Moniot-Ville *et al.*, 1991; Nakanishi *et al.*, 1991a,b; Alarcon *et al.*, 1993; Li *et al.*, 1994; Tanaka *et al.*, 1994a; Yoshida *et al.*, 1994).

Increasing rates of norfloxacin-resistance have been described among strains of *Campylobacter* spp. (especially *C. jejuni*), methicillin-resistant *Staph. aureus*, *Ps. aeruginosa* and *N. gonorrheae* (Smith, 1986; Yeung and Dillon, 1990; Adler-Mosca *et al.*, 1991; Harnett *et al.*, 1991; Rautelin *et al.*, 1991; Wretlind *et al.*, 1992; Baird, 1993; Chang et al, 1994; Sanchez *et al.*, 1994; Tanaka *et al.*, 1994b).

5 *In vitro sensitivities*

The MICs of norfloxacin against selected bacterial species are shown in Table II.6, pp. 986–7).

Mode of Administration and Dosage

1 *Oral administration*

Norfloxacin is available only in oral preparation. The recommended adult dosage is 400 mg twice-daily.

2 *Patients with renal failure*

In patients with impaired renal function, the elimination rate of norfloxacin is reduced and the serum half-life increases as creatinine clearance or the glomerular filtration rate (GFR) decreases (Fillastre *et al.*, 1984; Hughes *et al.*, 1984). The normal serum half-life of 3.75 h is prolonged to 8–9 h in end-stage renal disease. However, even in severe renal impairment, urinary concentrations of norfloxacin exceed 4 μg per ml which is the MIC_{90} for the least susceptible urinary pathogens (Hughes *et al.*, 1984). Opinions vary with regard to the severity of renal impairment below which reduction of norfloxacin dosage is necessary; however, once the creatinine clearance falls below 20–30 ml per min the dose should be halved to 400 mg daily (Fillastre *et al.*, 1984; Hughes *et al.*, 1984; Stein, 1987; Eliopoulos, 1988; Bennett et al, 1994). Since the half-life of norfloxacin is not influenced by hemodialysis, no post-dialysis supplementation is necessary (Fillastre *et al.*, 1984, 1990; Lau *et al.*, 1994). Unlike Fillastre *et al.* (1984), however, Bennett *et al.* (1994) recommend avoidance of norfloxacin in patients with GFR <10 ml per min and therefore patients on any form of dialysis.

Availability

Norfloxacin is available as 400-mg *tablets*. No i.v. preparation is available.

3 *Patients with hepatic failure*

In a small study of three patients with hepatic dysfunction due to acute hepatitis B, the pharmacokinetics of norfloxacin were not significantly different to those in healthy volunteers, suggesting that no dosage allteration is necessary in this setting (Eandi *et al.*, 1983).

4 *Elderly patients*

No dosage adjustment is necessary in elderly patients other than that required for renal impairment of GFR <30 ml per min (Kelly *et al.*, 1988; MacGowan *et al.*, 1988; Norrby and Ljungberg, 1989; Lepage *et al.*, 1991).

Serum Levels in Relation to Dosage

After oral administration, 30–40% of the norfloxacin dose is rapidly absorbed and peak serum levels occur in 1-2h (Wise, 1984; Stein, 1987). The serum half-life of norfloxacin is 3.75 h (Wise *et al.*, 1986). Overall, norfloxacin is absorbed slightly slower than ciprofloxacin and ofloxacin (Wise *et al.*, 1986). Absorption is only slightly delayed if the drug is given with food rather than in the fasting state. After single doses of 200, 400, 800, 1200 and 1600 mg, mean peak serum levels occurring 1–2h later are 0.75, 1.58, 2.41, 3.15 and 3.87 μg per ml, respectively (Shimada *et al.*, 1983; Adhami *et al.*, 1984; Wise *et al.*, 1986). The reason why there is not a proportionate increase in serum levels with doses higher than 800 mg is unclear, but less of the drug may be absorbed with higher doses. Absorption of norfloxacin may continue for up to 4 h at least.

Norfloxacin is only about 14% protein bound and is highly lipid soluble (Stein, 1987). There is no significant accumulation of norfloxacin with repeated oral doses of 200 mg thrice-daily (Wise,1984). Similar to ciprofloxacin, the absorption of norfloxacin is significantly reduced when it is given with milk or yoghurt, with mean peak serum concentrations of 50–60% of those achieved when norfloxacin is given with water (Kivisto et al., 1992; Minami et al., 1993).

The presence of acute diarrhea does not significantly alter the pharmacokinetics of norfloxacin, except that the time to peak serum concentrations is delayed. Other parameters such as the peak serum concentration, total area-under-the-serum-concentration-curve (AUC), serum half-life and rate of elimination are similar to that found when intestinal function is normal (Bergan et al., 1988).

Excretion

1 Urine

The main method of excretion for norfloxacin is via the kidneys, and about 24–30% of a dose is excreted unchanged in the urine (Swanson et al.,1983; Zeiler et al., 1988). Administration of probenicid greatly reduces the urinary clearance of norfloxacin but has little effect on serum concentrations of norfloxacin (Shimada et al., 1983). Urine exretion is therefore due to a combination of glomerular filtration and active renal tubular secretion (Stein, 1987). Peak urine concentrations occur 1–2 h after oral administration. After doses of 200, 400, 800, 1200 and 1600 mg, peak urinary concentrations of 200, 478, 697, 992 and 1045 µg per ml, respectively, are reached. Usually urine concentrations of norfloxacin are 100–300 times the simultaneous serum concentration and exceed the MIC of most urinary pathogens for 12–24 h (Swanson et al.,1983). Wise et al. (1986) found the mean urine concentration 12–24 h after a 400-mg dose was 8.5 µg per ml. Crystals of the drug have been detected microscopically in the urine of volunteers who received the two high doses but only when the urine pH values exceeded 7 0 (Wise, 1984). The effect of renal dysfunction on serum norfloxacin concentrations and dosing has been discussed (p. 1063).

2 Bile

The liver is a major site of norfloxacin metabolism with some metabolites being microbiologically active. Biliary excretion, however, is not a major site of norfloxacin elimination (Wise, 1984; Stein, 1987). The concentration of norfloxacin in gallbladder bile after a single oral dose of 400 mg given prior to elective cholecystectomy for non-obstructive disorders is 0.6–15.6 µg per ml in healthy patients, with a mean bile/serum ratio of 7.0 (Dan et al., 1987b).

3 Feces

In healthy volunteers, after a single 400-mg oral dose, 8.3–53.3% of the dose is recovered from the feces in the subsequent 48-h period. Peak concentrations in fecal specimens are in the range of 207–2715 µg per g, 23–36 h after dosing (Cofsky et al.,1984; Edlund et al., 1987).

4 Inactivation in body

The drug is metabolized in the liver and six metabolites have been described, some of which are microbiologically active. The major urinary metabolite M-1 (3-oxo-1-piperazinyl) constitutes less than 20% of the parent compound. Similar to cinoxacin, but unlike nalidixic acid and oxolinic acid, norfloxacin is not conjugated (Ozaki et al., 1981; Wise, 1984).

Distribution of the Drug in Body

Norfloxacin is widely distributed in the many tissues, achieving concentrations slightly less than, or similar to, those obtained with ciprofloxacin (p.1004). Penetration into the exudate of experimental blisters is such that peak concentrations of 1 µg per ml are achieved after a 400-mg dose, which is about 67% of the peak serum level. These data suggest that a dose of 800 mg or more would be necessary to treat systemic infections caused by susceptible pathogens, and infections due to less susceptible strains (e.g. MIC 2 µg per ml) may require even higher doses. Thus, in such circumstances, alternative fluoroquinolones such as ciprofloxacin are generally recommended (Adhami et al., 1984; Wise et al., 1986). Similar to ciprofloxacin, norfloxacin achieves excellent penetration into the renal tract, prostate and seminal fluid (Bologna et al., 1983; Dan et al., 1987a; Netto et al., 1988). The ratio of tissue:serum concentrations reached in the kidney and prostate after oral norfloxacin are about 6.6 and 1.7, respectively (Bergeron et al., 1985). Concentrations of 0.3–1.73 µg per g of prostatic tissue have been reported after a single 400-mg dose, with mean peak concentrations of 1.63 µg per g (range 0.75–3.30 µg per g) after two doses (Dan *et al.*, 1987a; Netto *et al.*, 1988). In epididymal tissue, mean concentrations of 3.4 ± 2.0 μg per g (range 1.4–9.6 μg per g) have been noted after multiple dosing (Blondin *et al.*, 1991). These concentrations exceed the MICs of most urinary tract pathogens.

A single 400-mg dose of norfloxacin prior to elective laparotomy results in mean drug concentrations in abdominal wall muscle tissue of 0.87 μg per g (range <0.1–2.3 μg per g), which represents a mean ratio of the muscle:serum concentrations of 0.8 (Dan *et al.*, 1989). As noted earlier (p. 1064), norfloxacin concentrations in gallbladder bile and gallbladder tissue after a single oral dose of 400 mg given prior to elective cholecystectomy for non-obstructive disorders are 0.6–15.6 μg per ml and 1.8 μg per g, respectively, in healthy patients (Dan *et al.*, 1987a). Norfloxacin concentrations are somewhat less in tonsillar and sinus tissues, where mean levels of 0.5 μg per ml have been reported (Stein, 1987). Norfloxacin has been detected in umbilical cord blood and amniotic fluid, but not in maternal milk (Wise, 1984). Norfloxacin is 14% protein bound (Swanson *et al.*, 1983; Stein, 1987).

Topically applied norfloxacin eye drops (0.3%) achieve a mean concentration in aqueous humor of 0.06–0.14 μg per ml, which is comparable with those observed with ciprofloxacin, but significantly less than that achieved with ofloxacin (Donnenfeld *et al.*, 1994; Leeming *et al.*, 1994). Bron *et al.* (1992) noted the concentration of norfloxacin in the cornea to be 15.5 ± 2.1 μg per g after five drops of 0.3% topical solution.

Mode of Action

The mode of action of norfloxacin is similar to that of ciprofloxacin (p. 1008).

Toxicity

The side-effects reported with norfloxacin are similar to those described for ciprofloxacin (p. 1008). Overall, norfloxacin is relatively safe with the rate of adverse experiences being only about 3%. Nausea, headache, dizziness, rash, elevation of liver enzymes and eosiniphilia are the most commonly reported adverse effects (Wang, 1986; Corrado *et al.*, 1987b). Among neutropenic patients given norfloxacin prophylaxis, the rate of adverse effects was 5.5%, which is less than with other agents used for this purpose (Rubinstein *et al.*, 1994).

Fluoroquinolones, although not recommended in pregnancy, were not associated with any increased risk of malformations or musculoskeletal abnormalities in a small study of 38 women accidentally treated with either norfloxacin or ciprofloxacin in the first trimester, mostly for urinary tract infections (Berkovitch *et al.*, 1994). However, more pregnancies in the quinolone-treated group resulted in cesarean delivery due to reported fetal distress without a clear reason, compared with the control group.

Norfloxacin is less likely to be associated with phototoxicity than some other fluoroquinolones, but is occasionally associated with photosensitivity (Ferguson and Johnson, 1993; pp. 973, 1010). A possible case of acantholytic bullous eruption has been reported after norfloxacin (Ramsay *et al.*, 1993). Similar to ciprofloxacin, norfloxacin has occasionally been associated with the development of hepatitis; in one of these reports the patient was a known carrier of hepatitis C (Lopez-Navidad *et al.*, 1990; Davoren and Mainstone, 1993). Occasionally *Cl. difficile*-associated diarrhea has been reported after norfloxacin (Ehrenpreis *et al.*, 1990). Neurological complications include seizures and exacerbation of myesthenia gravis (Anastasio *et al.*, 1988; Rauser *et al.*, 1990). Jeandel *et al.* (1989) described a patient with acute, self-limited arthritis following norfloxacin. Other side-effects such as neutropenia, transient renal failure, nephrotic syndrome, interstitial nephritis, hematuria and albuminuria have all been reported (Patoia *et al.*, 1987; Boelaert *et al.*, 1986; Wolfson and Hooper, 1991; Hestin *et al.*, 1995).

The absorption of norfloxacin is significantly reduced when it is given with milk or yoghurt, compared with when it is given with water (p. 1064) (Kivisto *et al.*, 1992; Minami *et al.*, 1993). Similarly, the concomitant administration of norfloxacin with calcium-, magnesium- and aluminum-containing antacids, ferrous sulfate or zinc sulfate significantly reduces norfloxacin absorption, such that these agents should be avoided if clinically reliable norfloxacin concentrations are to be achieved (Noyes and Polk, 1988; Nix *et al.*, 1990; Campbell *et al.*, 1992; Lehto *et al.*, 1994). Sucralfate also reduces norfloxacin absorption but, as one would expect, this effect is less the longer the period between norfloxacin and sucralfate dosing (Parpia *et al.*, 1989; Lehto and Kivisto, 1994).

Norfloxacin interferes with theophylline metabolism to a much lesser extent than other fluoroquinolones such as ciprofloxacin, enoxacin and pefloxacin (p. 1014), so that clinically significant theophylline toxicity (which presents with seizures in one-third of cases), is less common than with these other agents (Bowles *et al.*, 1988; Sano *et al.*, 1988; Davis *et al.*, 1989; Green and Clark, 1989; Prince *et al.*, 1989; Radandt *et al.*, 1992; Grasela and Dreis, 1992).

Nevertheless, caution should be exercised when co-administering norfloxacin and theophylline. Norfloxacin has little effect on caffeine metabolism (Harder *et al.*, 1988).

Despite the case report by Thomson *et al.* (1988) of an increase in cyclosporin levels when norfloxacin and cyclosporin were given together, other authors who have studied this combination in a larger number of patients have found no alteration in cyclosporin levels or evidence of nephrotoxicity (Jadoul *et al.*, 1989; Robinson *et al.*, 1990). Norfloxacin has been reported by the US Food and Drug Administration as occasionally enhancing the anticoagulant effect of warfarin (similar to ciprofloxacin) (Linville and Matanin, 1989; Jolson *et al.*, 1991; p. 1013), although Rocci *et al.* (1990) found no such effect in their study of ten healthy volunteers.

Clinical Uses of the Drug

1 Urinary tract infections

As with other fluoroquinolones, norfloxacin has excellent activity against virtually all bacterial urinary pathogens (Greenwood *et al.*, 1984; p. 1061). After a single oral dose of 400 mg norfloxacin, high urinary concentrations are maintained for at least 24h (Wise, 1984). For uncomplicated urinary infections in women, norfloxacin 400 mg twice-daily for 3–7 days is associated with greater efficacy and a lower rate of relapse than single-dose therapy; with 3-day treatment courses being generally preferred (Andriole, 1991; Saginur and Nicolle, 1992; Iravani *et al.*, 1995). Rates of bacteriological and clinical cure of 93–98%, 5–9 days post-treatment, and 83–90% 4–6 weeks post-treatment can be expected (Malinverni and Glauser, 1988; Neringer *et al.*, 1992; Nicolle *et al.*, 1993; Pummer, 1993; Arav-Boger *et al.*, 1994; Iravani *et al.*, 1995). Three-day and single-dose therapy are probably equivalent in efficacy against *E. coli*, but single-dose therapy is less effective against other pathogens, especially *Staph. saprophyticus* (Saginur and Nicolle, 1992). Three- to 7-day therapy with norfloxacin has similar efficacy to other fluoroquinolones such as ciprofloxacin, ofloxacin, lomefloxacin and fleroxacin (Goldstein *et al.*, 1987; Stein *et al.*, 1987; Neringer *et al.*, 1992; Nicolle *et al.*, 1993; Pfau and Sacks, 1993; Pummer, 1993; Iravani *et al.*, 1995; pp. 1014, 1105, 1121), and has similar or superior efficacy to trimethoprim–sulfamethoxazole, trimethoprim alone or amoxycillin (Panichi *et al.*, 1983; Haase *et al.*, 1984; Leigh *et al.*, 1984; Vogel *et al.*, 1984; Goldstein *et al.*, 1985; Sabbaj *et al.*, 1985; Ewer *et al.*, 1988; Wong *et al.*, 1988; Chan *et al.*, 1989; Seidmon *et al.*, 1990). Since urinary infections in males are frequently associated with underlying abnormalities such as prostatitis, norfloxacin and other fluoroquinolones are useful therapeutic agents in this setting (Sabbaj *et al.*, 1986; Corrado et al., 1987a; p. 1067). For complicated urinary infections 7–14 day therapy with norfloxacin 400 mg twice-daily is superior to 200 mg twice-daily, trimethoprim–sulfamethoxazole 160 mg/800 mg twice-daily, cefadroxil 1 g twice-daily and some parenteral antibiotics, with short-term rates of bacteriological cure of 90–99 %. Norfloxacin has similar efficacy to ciprofloxacin, fleroxacin and lomefloxacin, although fleroxacin is generally associated with higher rates of adverse reactions (Cherubin and Stilwell, 1986; Anonymous, 1987; Tungsanga *et al.*, 1988; Sandberg *et al.*, 1990; Schaeffer and Anderson, 1992; Childs, 1993; Hoepelman *et al.*, 1993; Pittman *et al.*, 1993). As might be expected, cure rates with norfloxacin are lower among patients with complicated infections associated with long-standing structural urinary tract abnormalities such as neurogenic bladder (Sheehan *et al.*, 1988; Waites *et al.*, 1991).

Postcoital prophylaxis with single doses of either 200 mg norfloxacin, 100 mg ofloxacin, or 125 mg ciprofloxacin is highly effective in women suffering from recurrent urinary infections and is a cost-effective option to long-term prophyaxis in some patients (Pfau and Sacks, 1994). For long-term prophylaxis of women with recurrent urinary infections, norfloxacin 200 mg daily is superior to placebo and either nitrofurantoin 50 mg or 100 mg daily (Nicolle *et al.*, 1989; Brumfitt *et al.*, 1991; Raz and Boger, 1991). In a study comparing norfloxacin 200 mg daily with nitrofuratoin 50 mg daily, the 6-month symptom-free rates were 81% versus 65%, respectively, and bacteriological cure rates were 92% versus 71%, respectively (Raz and Boger, 1991). Nevertheless, the additional cost of norfloxacin over nitrofuratoin needs to be balanced against any potential clinical benefit. Postoperative prophylaxis with norfloxacin 200 mg daily is effective in reducing the rate of catheter-associated bacteriuria following reconstructive gynecologic surgery (Verbrugh *et al.*, 1988) and may reduce the incidence of bladder neck strictures following transurethral resection of the prostate (Hammarsten and Lindqvist, 1993).

2 Prostatitis

Similar to ciprofloxacin (p. 1015), norfloxacin 400 mg twice-daily for 4–6 weeks is effective therapy for bacterial prostatitis, including cases which have failed to respond to other agents such as trimethoprim–sulfamethoxazole and carbenicillin (Sabbaj *et al.*, 1986; Schaeffer and Darras, 1990; Naber, 1991).

3 Gonorrhea and other sexually transmitted diseases

Norfloxacin, like ciprofloxacin and some other fluoroquinolones, is effective in a variety of dosages against penicillinase-producing and non-penicillinase-producing *N. gonorrhoeae* infections (Crider *et al.*, 1984; Lee and Wong, 1988). A single oral dose of 800 mg cures 99–100% of patients with gonococcal urethritis, cervicitis and anorectal infection, and is as effective as 2 g i.m. spectinomycin and superior to 2.5 g oral thiamphenicol for penicillinase-producing *N. gonorrhoeae* cervicitis or urethritis. Similarly, this norfloxacin regimen is as effective as 3.5 g ampicillin + 1 g probenicid for non-penicillinase-producing *N. gonorrhaoae* infections (Romanowski, 1986; Romanowski *et al.*, 1986; Bogaerts et al, 1987; Kaplowitz *et al.*, 1987; Lee and Wong, 1988). However, as noted earlier (p. 1022), the current Centers for Disease Control (CDC) recommended regimens include single-dose treatment with either oral ciprofloxacin 500 mg, ofloxacin 400 mg, cefixime 400 mg or i.m. ceftriaxone 125 mg for both penicillinase-producing *N. gonorrhoeae* and tetracycline-resistant *N. gonorrhoeae* infections (CDC, 1993). A single oral dose of norfloxacin 1200 mg is as effective for adult gonococcal keratoconjunctivitis as 1200 mg daily for 3 days (Kestelyn *et al.*, 1989). Increasing reports of fluoroquinolone-resistance among clinical gonococcal isolates are a concern (p. 993).

A single dose of 800 mg norfloxacin appears to be effective in the treatment of chancroid, but given the findings of studies with ciprofloxacin (p. 1022), longer courses of 3 days duration may be warranted (Ariyarit *et al.*, 1988). Norfloxacin, unlike ciprofloxacin, is not currently recommended by CDC for the treatment of chancroid (CDC, 1993).

Norfloxacin 400 mg twice-daily for 10 days is ineffective in eradicating *Chlamydia trachomatis* among men with non-gonococcal urethritis but is more effective (56%) in those in whom *Ureaplasma urealyticum* is the responsible pathogen (Bowie *et al.*, 1986).

4 Bacterial diarrhea and enteric fever

Similar to ciprofloxacin and other fluoroquinolones, norfloxacin is effective in the prevention and treatment of a wide variety of enteric infections (p. 1016).

In doses of 400 mg twice-daily norfloxacin is comparable with, or generally better than, trimethoprim–sulfamethoxazole for the empiric treatment of bacterial diarrhea, particularly in regions where multidrug-resistance is common (Dupont *et al.*, 1987; Lolekha *et al.*, 1988; Wistrom *et al.*, 1989; Hyams *et al.*, 1991; Wistrom *et al.*, 1992). In a double-blind, placebo-controlled study of travelers' diarrhea in which a 3-day course of norfloxacin 400 mg twice-daily was commenced once specific diagnostic criteria had been met, Mattila *et al.* (1993) found the overall duration of diarrhea was reduced from 3.3 days in the placebo group to 1.2 days in the norfloxacin-treated group. Similar dramatic reductions in diarrheal duration were noted when the causative pathogens were identified to be *Salmonella*, *Campylobacter jejuni* or enterotoxigenic *E. coli*. Furthermore, the rate of full clinical recovery was greater among norfloxacin recipients (87% versus 47%, p < 0.001), with no significant adverse effects noted. Wistrom *et al.* (1989) found similar impressive results demonstrating the efficacy of norfloxacin in the treatment of travelers' diarrhea. Norfloxacin 400 mg daily is also effective in preventing diarrhea among travelers visiting a variety of developing countries (Dupont *et al.*, 1986; Johnson *et al.*, 1986; Wistrom *et al.*, 1987; Scott *et al.*, 1990). In a randomized, placebo-controlled, double-blind study of prophylaxis with norfloxacin 200 mg twice-daily, the incidence of diarrhea was much less among norfloxacin recipients (6/56 norfloxacin versus 20/59 placebo recipients, p = 0.0006) and the duration of diarrhea was 1 day versus 3.6 days for placebo recipients. Similar findings were noted by Scott *et al.* (1990) among US military personnel serving in Egypt. To avoid overuse of antibiotics, prophylaxis against travelers' diarrhea should probably be restricted to patients with immunodeficiencies, inflammatory bowel disease, reduced gastric acidity or serious illnesses which would be significantly worsened by concomitant diarrhea.

Norfloxacin (800 mg single dose or 400 mg twice-daily for 3 days) is similar to, or better than, trimethoprim–sulfamethoxazole (5-day course) or nalidixic acid for the treatment of diarrhea due to *Shigella* spp., particularly in areas where resistance to these latter antibiotics is prevalent (p. 842). Norfloxacin shortens the course of diarrhea and reduces shedding of the pathogen, thereby preventing spread of infection (Rogerie *et al.*, 1986; Gotuzzo *et al.*, 1989; Lolekha *et al.*, 1991; Bhattacharya *et al.*, 1991, 1992; Bassily *et al.*, 1994).

Norfloxacin appears to be similar to ciprofloxacin in its efficacy against diarrhea due to various *Salmonella* spp., including *Salm. typhi* and *Salm. paratyphi*; but there are far fewer studies of norfloxacin than ciprofloxacin in the treatment of acute salmonellosis (Sarma and Durairaj, 1991). For clearance of fecal carriage of *Salmonella*, norfloxacin appears to be very comparable with other fluoroquinolones, such as ciprofloxacin, although there have been few direct comparative studies. In a double-blind, placebo-controlled trial of norfloxacin 400 mg twice-daily for 28 days versus placebo in the clearance of *Salm. typhi* carriage, 11 of 12 norfloxacin recipients had negative stool and bile cultures for *Salm. typhi* compared with none of 12 placebo recipients. Subsequently 11 placebo recipients were treated with norfloxacin, of whom seven cleared their fecal carriage of *Salm. typhi*. Thus, overall, 78% of patients treated with norfloxacin cleared their fecal *Salmonella* carriage (Gotuzzo *et al.*, 1988). Clearance rates of non-typhi *Salmonella* spp. such as *Salm. typhimurium* and *Salm. enteritidis* have in some studies, however, been less impressive (Carlstedt *et al.*, 1990; Nagler *et al.*, 1994). Nevertheless, other anecdotal reports suggest good efficacy in clearing non-typhoidal carriage (Cherubin and Kowalski, 1990). A 30-day course of norfloxacin 400 mg twice-daily was effective in clearing fecal *Salmonella* carriage among nine AIDS patients with recurrent clinical salmonellosis (Heseltine *et al.*, 1988).

Norfloxacin is superior to trimethoprim–sulfamethoxazole and placebo in the treatment of patients with proven cholera – reducing stool output, duration of diarrhea, fluid requirements and excretion of *V. cholerae* (Lolekha *et al.*, 1988; Bhattacharya *et al.*, 1990).

5 Prevention of infection in neutropenic patients

The effective role of norfloxacin, ciprofloxacin and other fluoroquinolones in the prevention of Gram-negative infections in neutropenic patients following cytotoxic therapy has been discussed in detail in the chapter on ciprofloxacin (p. 1025). A dose of 400 mg twice-daily is most commonly used. In comparative studies, norfloxacin is more effective than placebo and better tolerated than a vancomycin/polymyxin combination or other non-absorbable regimens for this purpose (Winston *et al.*, 1986, 1987; Karp *et al.*, 1987; Schmeiser *et al.*, 1988; Nemet *et al.*, 1989). Norfloxacin prophylaxis is also effective in patients undergoing bone marrow transplantation; but similar to oncology patients, Gram-positive infections remain a problem (Bow *et al.*, 1988; Cruciani *et al.*, 1989; Giuliano *et al.*, 1989; Menichetti *et al.*, 1989; Classen *et al.*, 1990; Broun *et al.*, 1994). In one comparison of prophylaxis with norfloxacin 400 mg twice-daily with ciprofloxacin 500 mg once-daily in neutropenic patients with hematologic malignancies, ciprofloxacin therapy was associated with a significantly lower incidence of fever (p=0.01) and a lower rate of microbiologically documented infection, although this did not reach statistical significance (p=0.058). Nevertheless documented Gram-negative infections were significantly less in the ciprofloxacin-treated group (p=0.03), but there were no differences in the rates of fever of unknown origin or mortality (GIMEMA Infection Program, 1991).

6 Prophylaxis in non-neutopenic patients

a Intensive care patients The value of gastrointestinal decontamination among non-neutropenic patients in intensive care units with regimens containing norfloxacin remains unclear. Cerra *et al.* (1992), in a prospective, randomized, double-blind, placebo-controlled trial of intensive care unit patients with hypermetabolism, compared norfloxacin 400 mg suspension thrice-daily + nystatin 1 million units every 6 h with matching placebo solutions administered via nasogastric tube within 48 h of admission to the intensive care unit and continued for at least 5 days. Patients who underwent selective gut decontamination experienced significant reduction in the incidence of nosocomial infections and a reduced length of stay, but there was no associated decrease in progressive organ failure, adult respiratory distress syndrome, or mortality. Aerdts *et al.* (1991), in a prospective, randomized trial with blinded comparison of patients requiring prolonged mechanical ventilation, studied the effect of norfloxacin + polymyxin E + amphotericin applied topically in the oropharynx and stomach plus i.v. cefotaxime during the initial 5 days of intensive care unit admission to two other regimens that did not include topical prophylaxis. Although a reduced incidence of acquired colonization of oropharynx and stomach and lower respiratory tract infection was noted with this prophylaxis regimen, there was no difference in mortality. Other studies which claim a reduction in morbidity and mortality among surgical intensive care unit patients receiving norfloxacin-containing decontamination regimens have been either not blinded or not randomized (Ulrich *et al.*, 1989; Tetteroo *et al.*, 1993). These possible benefits must be balanced against the potential to encourage the emergence of fluoroquinolone-resistant pathogens in the intensive care unit setting.

b Cirrhosis and ascites Prophylaxis with norfloxacin 400 mg once- or twice-daily is effective in preventing spontaneous bacterial peritonitis among patients with cirrhosis and low protein ascites (Gines et al., 1990; Hoefs, 1990; Soriano et al., 1991, 1992; Salmeron et al., 1992). This effect is predominantly due to a reduction in the rate of infection due to aerobic Gram-negative bacilli. Gines et al. (1990) found the overall probability of bacterial peritonitis after prophylaxis with 400 mg daily for 1 year was 20% in the norfloxacin-treated group compared with 68% in the placebo group (p = 0.006), but that the probability of peritonitis due to Gram-negative bacilli was 3% compared with 60%, respectively (p=0.001). Despite these findings there was no significant reduction in the number of hospitalizations, episodes of hepatic encephalopathy or mortality among the norfloxacin-treated group. Other authors using similar norfloxacin-containing regimens have found similar or more impressive results (Salmeron et al., 1992; Soriano et al., 1991). Soriano et al. (1991) also found a general decrease in the incidence of extraperitoneal infections and the rate of overall mortality among norfloxacin-treated patients; however these differences did not reach statistical significance compared with placebo. In another study of cirrhotic patients with ascites who were treated with 400 mg twice-daily or placebo for 7 days beginning immediately after emergency gastroscopy, there was a significantly lower incidence of infections (10% versus 37%, p=0.001), bacteremia and/or bacterial peritonitis (3.3% versus 16.9%, p<0.05) and urinary infections (0% versus 18.6%, p=0.001) in the norfloxacin-treated group. Once again, however, there was no statistically significant decrease in mortality, but the cost of antibiotic treatment was 62% less than that incurred in the control group, suggesting such norfloxacin prophylaxis may be cost-effective in some cases (Soriano et al., 1991). Given the experience in neutropenic patients where long-term prophylaxis has led to a shift in the spectrum of infecting pathogens to a higher incidence of Gram-positive infections, there are concerns that a similar shift may occur with norfloxacin in spontaneous bacterial peritonitis, with more infections due to *Strep. pneumoniae*, other streptococcal species and enterococci (Schubert et al., 1991). Whether norfloxacin prophylaxis should become routine in all cirrhotic patients with ascites currently therefore remains uncertain (Hoefs, 1990; Schubert et al., 1991).

c Prevention of biliary stent obstruction Preliminary reports suggest that a combination of norfloxacin and ursodeoxycholic acid may prevent the occlusion of biliary stents inserted to relieve obstructive jaundice, but larger confirmatory studies are needed (Barrioz et al., 1994; Wilcox, 1994).

7 Ocular infections

Topical 0.3% norfloxacin drops are clinically and microbiologically similar in activity to topical chloramphenicol, gentamicin or tobramycin, and superior to placebo, for acute bacterial conjunctivitis and/or blepharitis (Jacobson et al., 1988; Huber-Spitzy et al., 1991; Miller et al., 1992a,b,c). In particular, topical 0.3% norfloxacin drops have proven effective in *Pseudomonas* ulcerative keratitis (Vajpayee et al., 1991). Preoperative norfloxacin eyedrops are no better than placebo in preventing bacterial contamination of anterior chamber aspirates after extracapsular cataract surgery, suggesting that the value of such preoperative treatment may be debatable (Chitkara et al., 1994).

8 Malaria

Norfloxacin 400–800 mg twice-daily for 3 days has some limited *in vivo* activity against *P. falciparum*. However, in a prospective, randomized, comparative trial of norfloxacin 400 mg twice-daily for 3 days versus standard course chloroquine in semi-immune adults with symptomatic falciparum malaria in northwestern Zambia (where chloroquine-resistance is common), norfloxacin was markedly inferior to chloroquine such that the trial was terminated early (cure rates: 100% chloroquine; 40% norfloxacin, p<0.001) (McClean et al., 1992; Triapathi et al., 1993). Similarly, in Kenyan children norfloxacin is not an effective treatment for P. falciparum malaria (Havemann et al., 1992). These findings are consistent with those of similar studies using other fluoroquinolones (Deloran et al., 1991; Watt et al., 1991; p. 1032).

9 Other infections

Although ciprofloxacin and norfloxacin are not the drugs of first choice for the treatment of tularemia, they have proven effective in at least six cases (Enderlin et al., 1994).

References

Adhami ZN, Wise R, Weston D, Crump B (1984). The pharmacokinetics and tissue penetration of norfloxacin. *J Antimicrob Chemother* **13**: 87.

Adler-Mosca H, Luthy-Hottenstein J, Martinet-Lucchini G et al. (1991). Development of resistance to quinolones in five patients with campylobacteriosis treated with norfloxacin or ciprofloxacin. *Eur J Clin Microbiol Infect Dis* **10**: 953.

Aerdts SJ, van Dalen R, Clasener HA et al. (1991). Antibiotic prophylaxis of respiratory tract infection in mechanically ventilated patients. A prospective, blinded, randomized trial of the effect of a novel regimen. *Chest* **100**: 783.

Alarcon T, Pita J, Lopez-Brea M, Piddock LJ (1993). High level quinolone resistance amongst clinical isolates of *Escherichia coli* and *Klebsiella pneumoniae* from Spain. *J Antimicrob Chemother* **32**: 605.

Anastasio GD, Menscer D, Little JM, Jr (1988). Norfloxacin and seizures. *Ann Intern Med* **109**: 169.

Andriole VT (1991). Use of quinolones in treatment of prostatitis and lower urinary tract infections. *Eur J Clin Microbiol Infect Dis* **10**: 342.

Anonymous (1987). Coordinated multicenter study of norfloxacin versus trimethoprim–sulfamethoxazole treatment of symptomatic urinary tract infections. The Urinary Tract Infection Study Group. *J Infect Dis* **155**: 170.

Appelbaum PC, Spangler SK, Sollenberger L (1986). Susceptibility of non fermentative gram negative bacteria to ciprofloxacin, norfloxacin, amifloxacin, pefloxacin and cefpirome. *J Antimicrob Chemother* **18**: 675.

Appleman ME, Hadfield TL, Gaines JK, Winn RE (1987). Susceptibility of *Bordetella pertussis* to five quinolone antimicrobic drugs. *Diagn Microbiol Infect Dis* **8**: 131.

Arav-Boger R, Leibovici L, Danon YL (1994). Urinary tract infections with low and high colony counts in young women. Spontaneous remission and single-dose vs multiple-day treatment. *Arch Intern Med* **154**: 300.

Ariyarit C, Mokamukkul B, Chitwarakorn A et al. (1988). Clinical and microbiological efficacy of a single dose of norfloxacin in the treatment of chancroid. *Scand J Infect Dis* (Suppl 56): 55.

Auckenthaler R, Michea-Hamzehpour M, Pechere JC (1986). *In vitro* activity of newer quinolones against aerobic bacteria. *J Antimicrob Chemother* **17** (Suppl B): 29.

Aznar J, Caballero MC, Lozano MC et al. (1985). Activities of new quinoline derivatives against genital pathogens. *Antimicrob Ag Chemother* **27**: 76.

Baird RW (1993). Development of clinically significant resistance to norfloxacin given for *Campylobacter* diarrhoea. *Med J Aust* **158**: 503.

Barrioz T, Ingrand P, Besson I et al. (1994). Randomised trial of prevention of biliary stent occlusion by ursodeoxycholic acid plus norfloxacin. *Lancet* **344**: 581.

Bassey CM, Baltch AL, Smith RP (1986). Comparative antimicrobial activity of enoxacin, ciprofloxacin, amifloxacin, norfloxacin and ofloxacin against 177 bacterial isolates. *J Antimicrob Chemother* **17**: 623.

Bassily S, Hyams KC, el-Masry NA et al. (1994). Short-course norfloxacin and trimethoprim–sulfamethoxazole treatment of shigellosis and salmonellosis in Egypt. *Amer J Trop Med Hyg* **51**: 219.

Bennett WM, Aronoff GR, Golper TA (1994). *Drug Prescribing in Renal Failure* 3rd edn. Philadelphia: American College of Physicians.

Bergan T, Lolekha S, Cheong MK et al. (1988). Consequences of diarrhoeal disease on the pharmacokinetics of norfloxacin. *Scand J Infect Dis* (Suppl 56): 11.

Bergeron MG, Thabet M, Roy R et al. (1985). Norfloxacin penetration into human renal and prostatic tissues. *Antimicrob Ag Chemother* **28**: 349.

Berkovitch M, Pastuszak A, Gazarian M et al. (1994). Safety of the new quinolones in pregnancy. *Obstet Gynecol* **84**: 535.

Berlin OG, Young LS, Bruckner DA (1987). *In vitro* activity of six fluorinated quinolones against *Mycobacterium tuberculosis*. *J Antimicrob Chemother* **19**: 611.

Bhattacharya MK, Nair GB, Sen D et al. (1992). Efficacy of norfloxacin for shigellosis: a double-blind randomised clinical trial. *J Diarrhoeal Dis Res* **10**: 146.

Bhattacharya MK, Bhattacharya SK, Paul M et al. (1994). Shigellosis in Calcutta during 1990–1992: antibiotic susceptibility pattern and clinical features. *J Diarrhoeal Dis Res* **12**: 121.

Bhattacharya SK, Bhattacharya MK, Dutta P et al. (1990). Double-blind, randomized, controlled clinical trial of norfloxacin for cholera. *Antimicrob Ag Chemother* **34**: 939.

Bhattacharya SK, Bhattacharya MK, Dutta P et al. (1991). Randomized clinical trial of norfloxacin for shigellosis. *Amer J Trop Med Hyg* **45**: 683.

Blondin C, Costa P, Bressolle F et al. (1991). Norfloxacin concentrations in plasma and human epididymal tissue after repeated oral administration. *J Antimicrob Chemother* **27**: 392.

Boelaert J, de Jaegere PP, Daneels R et al. (1986). Case report of renal failure during norfloxacin therapy. *Clin Nephrol* **25**: 272.

Bogaerts J, Vandepitte J, Van Dyck E et al. (1986). *In vitro* antimicrobial sensitivity of *Neisseria gonorrhoeae* from Rwanda. *Genitourin Med* **62**: 217.

Bogaerts J, Martinez-Tello W, Verbist L et al. (1987). Norfloxacin versus thiamphenicol for treatment of uncomplicated gonorrhea in Rwanda. *Antimicrob Ag Chemother* **31**: 434.

Bologna M, Vaggi L, Forchetti CM, Martini E (1983). Bactericidal intraprostatic concentrations of norfloxacin. *Lancet* **ii**: 280.

Bow EJ, Rayner E, Louie TJ (1988). Comparison of norfloxacin with cotrimoxazole for infection prophylaxis in acute leukemia. The trade-off for reduced gram-negative sepsis. *Amer J Med* **84**: 847.

Bowie WR, Willetts V, Sibau L (1986). Failure of norfloxacin to eradicate *Chlamydia trachomatis* in nongonococcal urethritis. *Antimicrob Ag Chemother* **30**: 594.

Bowles SK, Popovski Z, Rybak MJ et al. (1988). Effect of norfloxacin on theophylline pharmacokinetics at steady state. *Antimicrob Ag Chemother* **32**: 510.

Bron AM, Pechinot A, Garcher C et al. (1992). Ocular penetration of topically applied norfloxacin 03% in the rabbits and in humans. *J Ocul Pharmacol* **8**: 241.

Broun ER, Wheat JL, Kneebone PH et al. (1994). Randomized trial of the addition of gram-positive prophylaxis to standard antimicrobial prophylaxis for patients undergoing autologous bone marrow transplantation. *Antimicrob Ag Chemother* **38**: 576.

Brumfitt W, Hamilton-Miller JM, Smith GW, al-Wali W (1991). Comparative trial of norfloxacin and macrocrystalline nitrofurantoin (Macrodantin). in the prophylaxis of recurrent urinary tract infection in women. *Quart J Med* **81**: 811.

Campbell NR, Kara M, Hasinoff BB et al. (1992). Norfloxacin interaction with antacids and minerals. *Brit J Clin Pharmacol* **33**: 115.

Carlstedt G, Dahl P, Niklasson PM et al. (1990). Norfloxacin treatment of salmonellosis does not shorten the carrier stage. *Scand J Infect Dis* **22**: 553.

Cerra FB, Maddaus MA, Dunn DL et al. (1992). Selective gut decontamination reduces nosocomial infections and length of stay but not mortality or organ failure in surgical intensive care unit patients. *Arch Surg* **127**: 163.

CDC (Centers for Disease Control) (1993). Sexually transmitted diseases treatment guidelines. *MMWR* **42** (Suppl RR-14): 1.

Chan MK, Wong WT, Cheng IK (1989). A double-blind controlled trial of norfloxacin versus cotrimoxazole in the treatment of urinary tract infections. *Br J Clin Practice* **43**: 61.

Chang SC, Hsieh WC, Luh KT (1994). Fluoroquinolone resistance among methicillin-resistant staphylococci after usage of fluoroquinolones other than ciprofloxacin in Taiwan. *Diagn Microbiol Infect Dis* **19**: 143.

Cherubin C, Stilwell S (1986). Norfloxacin versus parenteral therapy in the treatment of complicated urinary tract infections and resistant organisms. *Scand J Infect Dis* (Suppl 48): 32.

Cherubin CE, Kowalski J (1990). Nontyphoid *Salmonella* carrier state treated with norfloxacin. *Am J Gastroenterol* **85**: 100.

Childs SJ (1993). Fleroxacin versus norfloxacin for oral treatment of serious urinary tract infections. *Amer J Med* **94** (3A): 105S.

Chin N-X, Neu HC (1983). *In vitro* activity of enoxacin, a quinolone carboxylic acid, compared with those of norfloxacin, new β-lactams, aminoglycosides, and trimethoprim. *Antimicrob Ag Chemother* **24**: 754.

Chitkara DK, Manners T, Chapman F et al. (1994). Lack of effect of preoperative norfloxacin on bacterial contamination of anterior chamber aspirates after cataract surgery. Brit J Ophthalmol 78: 772.

Classen DC, Burke JP, Ford CD et al. (1990). Streptococcus mitis sepsis in bone marrow transplant patients receiving oral antimicrobial prophylaxis. Amer J Med 89: 441.

Clendennen T,E, Hames CS, Kees ES et al. (1992a). In vitro antibiotic susceptibilities of Neisseria gonorrhoeae isolates in the Philippines. Antimicrob Ag Chemother 36: 277.

Clendennen TE, Echeverria P, Saengeur S et al. (1992b). Antibiotic susceptibility survey of Neisseria gonorrhoeae in Thailand. Antimicrob Ag Chemother 36: 1682.

Cofsky RD, DuBouchet L, Landesman SH (1984). Recovery of norfloxacin in feces after administration of a single oral dose to human volunteers. Antimicrob Ag Chemother 26: 110.

Corrado ML, Cherubin CE, Shulman M (1983). The comparative activity of norfloxacin with other antimicrobial agents against Gram-positive and Gram-negative bacteria. J Antimicrob Chemother 11: 369.

Corrado ML, Grad C, Sabbaj J (1987a). Norfloxacin in the treatment of urinary tract infections in men with and without identifiable urologic complications. Amer J Med 82 (Suppl. 6B): 70.

Corrado ML, Struble WE, Peter C et al. (1987b). Norfloxacin: review of safety studies. Amer J Med 82 (Suppl. 6B): 22.

Crider SR, Colby SD, Miller LK et al. (1984). Treatment of penicillin-resistant Neisseria gonorrhoeae with oral norfloxacin. New Engl J Med 311: 137.

Cruciani M, Concia E, Navarra A et al. (1989). Prophylactic co-trimoxazole versus norfloxacin in neutropenic children–perspective randomized study. Infection 17: 65.

Dan M, Golomb J, Gorea A et al. (1987a). Penetration of norfloxacin into human prostatic tissue following single-dose oral administration. Chemotherapy 33: 240.

Dan M, Serour F, Gorea A et al. (1987b). Concentration of norfloxacin in human gallbladder tissue and bile after single-dose oral administration. Antimicrob Ag Chemother 31: 352.

Dan M, Serour F, Gorea A, Krispin M, Berger SA (1989). Penetration of norfloxacin into abdominal wall muscle tissue. Infection 17: 249.

Davies S, Sparham PD, Spencer RC (1987). Comparative in vitro activity of five fluoroquinolones against mycobacteria. J Antimicrob Chemother 19: 605.

Davis RL, Kelly HW, Quenzer RW et al. (1989). Effect of norfloxacin on theophylline metabolism. Antimicrob Ag Chemother 33: 212.

Davoren P, Mainstone K (1993). Norfloxacin-induced hepatitis. Med J Aust 159: 423.

Delmee M, Avesani V (1986). Comparative in vitro activity of seven quinolones against 100 clinical isolates of Clostridium difficile. Antimicrob Ag Chemother 29: 374.

Deloran P, Lepers JP, Raharimalala L et al. (1991). Pefloxacin for falciparum malaria: only modest success. Ann Intern Med 114: 874.

Desgrandchamps D, Munzinger J (1989). Increasing rates of in vitro resistance to ciprofloxacin and norfloxacin in isolates from urine specimens. Antimicrob Ag Chemother 33: 595.

Divo AA, Sartorelli AC, Patton CL, Bia FJ (1988). Activity of fluoroquinolone antibiotics against Plasmodium falciparum in vitro. Antimicrob Ag Chemother 32: 1182.

Donnenfeld ED, Schrier A, Perry HD et al. (1994). Penetration of topically applied ciprofloxacin, norfloxacin, and ofloxacin into the aqueous humor. Ophthalmology 101: 902.

Downs J, Andriole VT, Ryan JL (1982). In vitro activity of MK-0366 against clinical urinary pathogens including gentamicin-resistant Pseudomonas aeruginosa. Antimicrob Ag Chemother 21: 670.

Dupeyron C, Mangeney N, Sedra L et al. (1994). Rapid emergence of quinolone resistance in cirrhotic patients treated with norfloxacin to prevent spontaneous bacterial peritonitis. Antimicrob Ag Chemother 38: 340.

DuPont HL, Ericsson CD, Johnson PC, Cabada FJ (1986). Antimicrobial agents in the prevention of travelers' diarrhea. Rev Infect Dis 8 (Suppl 2): S167.

DuPont HL, Corrado ML, Sabbaj J (1987). Use of norfloxacin in the treatment of acute diarrheal disease. Amer J Med 82 (6B): 79.

Eandi M, Viano I, DiNola F et al. (1983). Pharmacokinetics of norfloxacin in healthy volunteers and patients with renal and hepatic damage. Eur J Clin Microbiol 2: 253.

Edlund C, Nord CE (1986). Comparative in vitro activities of ciprofloxacin, enoxacin, norfloxacin, ofloxacin and pefloxacin against Bacteroides fragilis and Clostridium difficile. Scand J Infect Dis 18: 149.

Edlund C, Lidbeck A, Kager L, Nord CE (1987). Comparative effects of enoxacin and norfloxacin on human colonic microflora. Antimicrob Ag Chemother 31: 1846.

Ehrenpreis ED, Lievens MW, Craig RM (1990). Clostridium difficile-associated diarrhea after norfloxacin. J Clin Gastroenterol 12: 188.

Eliopoulos GM (1988). New quinolones: pharmacology, pharmacokinetics, and dosing in patients with renal insufficiency. Rev Infect Dis 10 (Suppl 1): S102.

Enderlin G, Morales L, Jacobs RF, Cross JT (1994). Streptomycin and alternative agents for the treatment of tularemia: review of the literature. Clin Infect Dis 19: 42.

Ewer TC, Bailey RR, Gilchrist NL et al. (1988). Comparative study of norfloxacin and trimethoprim for the treatment of elderly patients with urinary tract infection. N Z Med J 101: 537.

Fenlon CH, Cynamon MH (1986). Comparative in vitro activities of ciprofloxacin and other 4 quinolones against Mycobacterium tuberculosis and Mycobacterium intracellulare. Antimicrob Ag Chemother 29: 386.

Ferguson J, Johnson BE (1993). Clinical and laboratory studies of the photosensitizing potential of norfloxacin, a 4-quinolone broad-spectrum antibiotic. Br J Dermatol 128: 285.

Fernandez-Roblas R, Prieto S, Santamaria M, Ponte C, Soriano F (1987). Activity of nine antimicrobial agents against Corynebacterium group D2 strains isolated from clinical specimens and skin. Antimicrob Ag Chemother 31: 821.

Fillastre JP, Hannedouche Th, Leroy A, Humbert G (1984). Pharmacokinetics of norfloxacin in renal failure. J Antimicrob Chemother 14: 439.

Fillastre JP, Leroy A, Moulin B et al. (1990). Pharmacokinetics of quinolones in renal insufficiency. J Antimicrob Chemother 26 (Suppl B): 51.

Forward KR, Harding GKM, Gray GJ et al. (1983). Comparative activities of norfloxacin and fifteen other antipseudomonal agents against gentamicin-susceptible and -resistant Pseudomonas aeruginosa strains. Antimicrob Ag Chemother 24: 602.

Franzblau SG, White KE (1990). Comparative in vitro activities of 20 fluoroquinolones against Mycobacterium leprae. Antimicrob Ag Chemother 34: 229.

Garcia-Rodriguez JA, Gomez-Garcia AC (1993). In vitro activities of quinolones against mycobacteria. J Antimicrob Chemother 32: 797.

Gay JD, De Young DR, Roberts GD (1984). In vitro activities of norfloxacin and ciprofloxacin against Mycobacterium tuberculosis. M. avium complex, M. chelonei, M. fortuitum, and M. kansasii. Antimicrob Ag Chemother 26: 94.

Gines P, Rimola A, Planas R et al. (1990). Norfloxacin prevents spontaneous bacterial peritonitis recurrence in cirrhosis: results of a double-blind, placebo-controlled trial. Hepatology 12: 716.

Giuliano M, Pantos A, Gentile G et al. (1989). Effects on oral and intestinal microfloras of norfloxacin and pefloxacin for selective decontamination in bone marrow transplant patients. Antimicrob Ag Chemother 33: 1709.

Glupczynski Y, Delmee M, Bruck C et al. (1988). Susceptibility of clinical isolates of Campylobacter pylori to 24 antimicrobial and anulcer agents. Eur J Epidemiol 4: 154.

Goldstein EJ (1987). Norfloxacin, a fluoroquinolone antibacterial agent Classification, mechanism of action, and in vitro activity. Amer J Med 82: 3.

Goldstein EJ (1993). Patterns of susceptibility to fluoroquinolones among anaerobic bacterial isolates in the United States. Clin Infect Dis 16 (Suppl 4): S377.

Goldstein EJ, Citron DM, Vagvolgyi AE, Gombert ME (1986). Susceptibility of Eikenella corrodens to newer and older quinolones. Antimicrob Ag Chemother 30: 172.

Goldstein EJ, Alpert ML, Najem A *et al.* (1987). Norfloxacin in the treatment of complicated and uncomplicated urinary tract infections. A comparative multicenter trial. *Amer J Med* **82** (6B): 65.

Goldstein EJC, Citron DM (1985). Comparative activity of the quinolones against anaerobic bacteria isolated at community hospitals. *Antimicrob Ag Chemother* **27**: 657.

Goldstein EJC, Alpert ML, Ginsberg BP (1985). Norfloxacin versus trimethoprim–sulfamethoxazole in the therapy of uncomplicated, community-acquired urinary tract infections. *Antimicrob Ag Chemother* **27**: 422.

Gombert ME, Aulicino TM (1984). Susceptibility of multiply antibiotic resistant pneumococci to the new quinolone antibiotics nalidixic acid, coumermycin, and novobiocin. *Antimicrob Ag Chemother* **26**: 933.

Gootz TD, Martin BA (1991). Characterization of high level quinolone resistance in *Campylobacter jejuni*. *Antimicrob Ag Chemother* **35**: 840.

Gotuzzo E, Guerra JG, Benavente L *et al.* (1988). Use of norfloxacin to treat chronic typhoid carriers. *J Infect Dis* **157**: 1221.

Gotuzzo E, Oberhelman RA, Maguina C *et al.* (1989). Comparison of single-dose treatment with norfloxacin and standard 5-day treatment with trimethoprim–sulfamethoxazole for acute shigellosis in adults. *Antimicrob Ag Chemother* **33**: 1101.

Grasela TH, Jr, Dreis MW (1992). An evaluation of the quinolone-theophylline interaction using the Food and Drug Administration spontaneous reporting system. *Arch Intern Med* **152**: 617.

Green L, Clark J (1989). Fluoroquinolones and theophylline toxicity: norfloxacin. *JAMA* **262**: 2383.

Greenwood D, Laverick A (1983). Activities of newer quinolones against *Legionella* group organisms. *Lancet* **ii**: 279.

Greenwood D, Osman M, Goodwin J *et al.* (1984). Norfloxacin: activity against urinary tract pathogens and factors influencing the emergence of resistance. *J Antimicrob Chemother* **13**: 315.

Haase DA, Harding GKM, Thomson MJ *et al.* (1984). Comparative trial of norfloxacin and trimethoprim–sulfamethoxazole in the treatment of women with localized, acute, symptomatic urinary tract infections and antimicrobial effect on periurethral and fecal microflora. *Antimicrob Ag Chemother* **26**: 481.

Hammarsten J, Lindqvist K (1993). Norfloxacin as prophylaxis against urethral strictures following transurethral resection of the prostate: an open, prospective, randomized study. *J Urol* **150**: 1722.

Harder S, Staib AH, Beer C *et al.* (1988). 4-quinolones inhibit biotransformation of caffeine. *Eur J Clin Pharmacol* **35**: 651.

Harnett N, Brown S, Krishnan C (1991). Emergence of quinolone resistance among clinical isolates of methicillin resistant *Staphylococcus aureus* in Ontario, Canada. *Antimicrob Ag Chemother* **35**: 1911.

Havemann K, Bhibi P, Hellgren U, Rombo L (1992). Norfloxacin is not effective for treatment of *Plasmodium falciparum* infection in Kenya. *Trans R Soc Trop Med Hyg* **86**: 586.

Heessen FWA, Muytjens HL (1984). *In vitro* activities of ciprofloxacin, norfloxacin, pipemidic acid, cinoxacin and nalidixic acid against *Chlamydia trachomatis*. *Antimicrob Ag Chemother* **25**: 123.

Heseltine PN, Causey DM, Appleman MD, Corrado ML, Leedom JM (1988). Norfloxacin in the eradication of enteric infections in AIDS patients. *Eur J Cancer Clin Oncol* **24** (Suppl 1): S25.

Hestin D, Hanesse B, Frimat L *et al.* (1995). Norfloxacin-induced nephrotic syndrome. *Lancet* **345**: 732.

Hoefs JC (1990). Spontaneous bacterial peritonitis: prevention and therapy. *Hepatology* **12**: 776.

Hoepelman IM, Havinga WH, Benne RA *et al.* (1993). Safety and efficacy of lomefloxacin versus norfloxacin in the treatment of complicated urinary tract infections. *Eur J Clin Microbiol Infect Dis* **12**: 343.

Hooper DC, Wolfson JS, Souza KS, *et al.* (1989). Mechanisms of quinolone resistance in *Escherichia coli*: characterization of nfxB and cfxB, two mutant resistance loci decreasing norfloxacin accumulation. *Antimicrob Ag Chemother* **33**: 283.

Huber-Spitzy V, Arocker Mettinger E, Baumgartner I (1991). Efficacy of norfloxacin in bacterial conjunctivitis. *Eur J Ophthalmol* **1**: 69.

Hughes PJ, Webb DB, Asscher AW (1984). Pharmacokinetics of norfloxacin (MK 366). in patients with impaired kidney function – some preliminary results. *J Antimicrob Chemother* **13** (Suppl B): 55.

Hupertz V, Carr H, Czinn SJ (1988). Susceptibility of *Campylobacter pylori* isolated from pediatric and adult patients to seven new quinolone antibiotics and nalidixic acid. *Chemotherapy* **34**: 341.

Hyams KC, Bourgeois AL, Merrell BR *et al.* (1991). Diarrheal disease during Operation Desert Shield. *New Engl J Med* **325**: 1423.

Iravani A, Tice AD, McCarty J *et al.* (1995). Short-course ciproflox treatment of acute uncomplicated urinary tract infection in women. The minimum effective dose. The Urinary Tract Infection Study Group. *Arch Intern Med* **155**: 485.

Ito A, Hirai K, Inoue M *et al.* (1980). *In vitro* antibacterial activity of AM-715, a new nalidixic acid analog. *Antimicrob Ag Chemother* **17**: 103.

Jacobson JA, Call NB, Kasworm EM *et al.* (1988). Safety and efficacy of topical norfloxacin versus tobramycin in the treatment of external ocular infections. *Antimicrob Ag Chemother* **32**: 1820.

Jadoul M, Pirson Y, van Ypersele de Strihou C (1989). Norfloxacin and cyclosporine – a safe combination. *Transplantation* **47**: 747.

Jeandel C, Manciaux MA, Bannwarth B *et al.* (1989). Arthritis induced by norfloxacin. *J Rheumatol* **16**: 560–.

Johnson PC, Ericsson CD, Morgan DR *et al.* (1986). Lack of emergence of resistant fecal flora during successful prophylaxis of traveler's diarrhea with norfloxacin. *Antimicrob Ag Chemother* **30**: 671.

Jolson HM, Tanner LA, Green L, Grasela TH, Jr (1991). Adverse reaction reporting of interaction between warfarin and fluoroquinolones. *Arch Intern Med* **151**: 1003.

Kain KC, Kelly MT (1989). Antimicrobial susceptibility of *Plesiomonas shigelloides* from patients with diarrhea. *Antimicrob Ag Chemother* **33**: 1609.

Kaplowitz LG, Vishniavsky N, Evans T *et al.* (1987). Norfloxacin in the treatment of uncomplicated gonococcal infections. *Amer J Med* **82** (6B): 35.

Karp JE, Merz WG, Hendricksen C *et al.* (1987). Oral norfloxacin for prevention of gram-negative bacterial infections in patients with acute leukemia and granulocytopenia. A randomized, double-blind, placebo-controlled trial. *Ann Intern Med* **106**: 1.

Kelly JG, Deaney NB, Lavan J, Noel J (1988). Chronic dose urinary and serum pharmacokinetics of norfloxacin in the elderly. *Brit J Clin Pharmacol* **26**: 787.

Kestelyn P, Bogaerts J, Stevens AM *et al.* (1989). Treatment of adult gonococcal keratoconjunctivitis with oral norfloxacin. *Am J Ophthalmol* **108**: 516.

Khan MY, Siddiqui Y, Gruninger RP (1981). Comparative *in vitro* activity of Mk-0366 and other selected oral antimicrobial agents against *Neisseria gonorrhoeae*. *Antimicrob Ag Chemother* **20**: 265.

King A, Phillips I (1986). The comparative *in vitro* activity of eight newer quinolones and nalidixic acid. *J Antimicrob Chemother* **18** (Suppl D): 1.

King A, Warren C, Shannon K, Phillips I (1982). *In vitro* antibacterial activity of norfloxacin (MK-0366). *Antimicrob Ag Chemother* **21**: 604.

Kivistö KT *et al.* (1992). Inhibition of norfloxacin absorption by dairy products. *Antimicrob Ag Chemother* **36**: 489.

Kresken M, Wiedemann B (1988). Development of resistance to nalidixic acid and the fluoroquinolones after the introduction of norfloxacin and ofloxacin. *Antimicrob Ag Chemother* **32**: 1285.

Kurzynski TA, Boehm DM, Rott-Petri JA *et al.* (1988). Antimicrobial susceptibilities of *Bordetella* species isolated in a Multicenter Pertussis Surveillance Project. *Antimicrob Ag Chemother* **32**: 137.

Lariviere LA, Gaudre CL, Turgeon FF (1986). Susceptibility of clinical isolates of *Campylobacter jejuni* to twenty-five antimicrobial agents. *J Antimicrob Chemother* **18**: 681.

Lau AH, Tang I, Fitzloff J, Jain R (1994). Hemodialysis removal of norfloxacin. *Chemotherapy* **40**: 369.

Lee CT, Wong EC (1988). Norfloxacin in the treatment of gonorrhea due to penicillinase and non-penicillinase producing *Neisseria gonorrheae*: a review. *Scand J Infect Dis* (Suppl 56): 49.

Leeming JP, Diamond JP, Trigg R et al. (1994). Ocular penetration of topical ciprofloxacin and norfloxacin drops and their effect upon eyelid flora. Brit J Ophthalmol 78: 546.

Lehto P, Kivisto KT (1994). Effect of sucralfate on absorption of norfloxacin and ofloxacin. Antimicrob Ag Chemother 38: 248.

Lehto P, Kivisto KT, Neuvonen PJ (1994). The effect of ferrous sulphate on the absorption of norfloxacin, ciprofloxacin and ofloxacin. Brit J Clin Pharmacol 37: 82.

Leigh DA, Emmanuel FXS (1984). The treatment of Pseudomonas aeruginosa urinary tract infections with norfloxacin. J Antimicrob Chemother 13 (Suppl B): 85.

Leigh DA, Smith EC, Marriner J (1984). Comparative study using norfloxacin and amoxycillin in the treatment of complicated urinary tract infections in geriatric patients. J Antimicrob Chemother 13 (Suppl B): 79.

Lepage JY, Caillon J, Malinowsky JM et al. (1991). Pharmacokinetics of norfloxacin in the elderly. Fundam Clin Pharmacol 5: 203.

Li XZ, Livermore DM, Nikaido H (1994). Role of efflux pump(s). in intrinsic resistance of Pseudomonas aeruginosa: resistance to tetracycline, chloramphenicol, and norfloxacin. Antimicrob Ag Chemother 38: 1732.

Linville T, Matanin D (1989). Norfloxacin and warfarin. Ann Intern Med 110: 751.

Lolekha S, Patanacharoen S, Thanangkul B, Vibulbandhitkit S (1988). Norfloxacin versus co-trimoxazole in the treatment of acute bacterial diarrhoea: a placebo controlled study. Scand J Infect Dis (Suppl 56): 35.

Lolekha S, Vibulbandhitkit S, Poonyarit P (1991). Response to antimicrobial therapy for shigellosis in Thailand. Rev Infect Dis 13 (Suppl 4): S342.

Lopez-Navidad A, Domingo P, Cadafalch J, Farrerons J (1990). Norfloxacin-induced hepatotoxicity. J Hepatol 11: 277.

MacGowan AP, Greig MA, Clarke EA et al. (1988). The pharmacokinetics of norfloxacin in the aged. J Antimicrob Chemother 22: 721.

MacGowan AP, Holt HA, Bywater MJ, Reeves DS (1990). In vitro antimicrobial susceptibility of Listeria monocytogenes isolated in the UK and other Listeria species. Eur J Clin Microbiol Infect Dis 9: 767.

Malinverni R, Glauser MP (1988). Comparative studies of fluoroquinolones in the treatment of urinary tract infections. Rev Infect Dis 10 (Suppl 1): S153.

Mattila L, Peltola H, Siitonen A et al. (1993). Short-term treatment of traveler's diarrhea with norfloxacin: a double-blind, placebo-controlled study during two seasons. Clin Infect Dis 17: 779.

McClean KL, Hitchman D, Shafran SD (1992). Norfloxacin is inferior to chloroquine for falciparum malaria in northwestern Zambia: a comparative clinical trial. J Infect Dis 165: 904.

Menichett F, Felicini R, Bucaneve G et al. (1989). Norfloxacin prophylaxis for neutropenic patients undergoing bone marrow transplantation. Bone Marrow Transplantation 4: 489.

Mertens JC, Dekker W, Ligtvoet EE, Blok P (1989). Treatment failure of norfloxacin against Campylobacter pylori and chronic gastritis in patients with nonulcerative dyspepsia. Antimicrob Ag Chemother 33: 256.

Miller IM, Wittreich JM, Cook T, Vogel R (1992a). The safety and efficacy of topical norfloxacin compared with chloramphenicol for the treatment of external ocular bacterial infections. The Norfloxacin-Chloramphenicol Ophthalmic Study Group. Eye 6: 111.

Miller IM, Wittreich J, Vogel R, Cook TJ (1992b). The safety and efficacy of topical norfloxacin compared with placebo in the treatment of acute, bacterial conjunctivitis. The Norfloxacin-Placebo Ocular Study Group. Eur J Ophthalmol 2: 58.

Miller IM, Vogel R, Cook TJ, Wittreich J (1992c). Topically administered norfloxacin compared with topically administered gentamicin for the treatment of external ocular bacterial infections. The Worldwide Norfloxacin Ophthalmic Study Group. Am J Ophthalmol 113: 638.

Minami R, Inotsume N, Nakano M et al. (1993). Effect of milk on absorption of norfloxacin in healthy volunteers. J Clin Pharmacol 33: 1238.

Moffie BG, Mouton RP (1988). Sensitivity and resistance of Legionella pneumophila to some antibiotics and combinations of antibiotics. J Antimicrob Chemother 22: 457.

Moniot-Ville N, Guibert J, More N et al. (1991). Mechanisms of quinolone resistance in a clinical isolate of Escherichia coli highly resistant to fluoroquinolones but susceptible to nalidixic acid. Antimicrob Ag Chemother 35: 519.

Morris JG Jr, Tenney JH, Drusano GL (1985). In vitro susceptibility of pathogenic Vibrio species to norfloxacin and six other antimicrobial agents. Antimicrob Ag Chemother 28: 442.

Murray PR, Bratcher JL, Niles AC, Hampton CM (1993). In vitro activity of nine fluoroquinolone antibiotics against 200 strains of enterococci. Diagn Microbiol Infect Dis 16: 83.

Naber KG (1991). The role of quinolones in the treatment of chronic bacterial prostatitis. Infection 19 (Suppl 3): S170.

Nagler JM, Van-de-Vijvere M, Levy J, Mertens AH (1994). Salmonella gastroenteritis: longterm follow-up of an outbreak after treatment with norfloxacin or co-trimoxazole. J Antimicrob Chemother 34: 291.

Nakanishi N, Yoshida S, Wakebe H, Inoue M, Mitsuhashi S (1991a). Mechanisms of clinical resistance to fluoroquinolones in Enterococcus faecalis. Antimicrob Ag Chemother 35: 1053.

Nakanishi N, Yoshida S, Wakebe H et al. (1991b). Mechanisms of clinical resistance to fluoroquinolones in Staphylococcus aureus. Antimicrob Ag Chemother 35: 2562.

Nakata K, Maeda H, Fujii A et al. (1992). In vitro and in vivo activities of sparfloxacin, other quinolones, and tetracyclines against Chlamydia trachomatis. Antimicrob Ag Chemother 36: 188.

Nemet D, Kalenic S, Badanjak A et al. (1989). Prevention of gram-negative bacterial infection in granulocytopenic patients: a randomized study comparing oral norfloxacin with gentamycin. Bone Marrow Transplantation 4 (Suppl 3): 105.

Neringer R, Forsgren A, Hansson C, Ode B (1992). Lomefloxacin versus norfloxacin in the treatment of uncomplicated urinary tract infections: three-day versus seven-day treatment. The South Swedish Lolex Study Group. Scand J Infect Dis 24: 773.

Netto NR, Jr, Palma PC, Srulzon GB, Cortado PL, Fonseca RC (1988). Concentrations of norfloxacin in prostatic tissues following oral administration in patients with benign prostatic hyperplasia. Int Urol Nephrol 20: 47.

Neu HC (1988). Bacterial resistance to fluoroquinolones. Rev Infect Dis 10 (Suppl 1): S57.

Neu HC, Labthavikul P (1982). In vitro activity of norfloxacin, a quinolinecarboxylic acid compared with that of beta-lactams, aminoglycosides, and trimethoprim. Antimicrob Ag Chemother 22: 23.

Newsom SWB (1984). The antimicrobial spectrum of norfloxacin. J Antimicrob Chemother 13 (Suppl B): 25.

Nicolle LE, Harding GK, Thompson M et al. (1989). Prospective, randomized, placebo-controlled trial of norfloxacin for the prophylaxis of recurrent urinary tract infection in women. Antimicrob Ag Chemother 33: 1032.

Nicolle LE, DuBois J, Martel AY et al. (1993). Treatment of acute uncomplicated urinary tract infections with 3 days of lomefloxacin compared with treatment with 3 days of norfloxacin. Antimicrob Ag Chemother 37: 574.

Nix DE, Wilton JH, Ronald B et al. (1990). Inhibition of norfloxacin absorption by antacids. Antimicrob Ag Chemother 34: 432.

Norrby SR, Jonsson M (1983). Antibacterial activity of norfloxacin. Antimicrob Ag Chemother 23: 15.

Norrby SR, Ljungberg B (1989). Pharmacokinetics of fluorinated 4-quinolones in the aged. Rev Infect Dis 11 (Suppl 5): S1102.

Noyes M, Polk RE (1988). Norfloxacin and absorption of magnesium-aluminum. Ann Intern Med 109: 168.

Olsson-Liljequist B, Mollby R (1990). In vitro activity of norfloxacin and other antibacterial agents against gastro intestinal pathogens isolated in Sweden. APMIS 98: 150.

Ozaki T, Uchida H, Irikura T (1981). Studies on metabolism of AM-715 in humans by high performance liquid chromatography. Chemotherapy (Japan); 29 (Suppl 4): 128.

Panichi G, Pantosti A, Testore GP (1983). Norfloxacin (MK-0366). treatment of urinary tract infections in hospitalized patients. *J Antimicrob Chemother* **11**: 589.

Parpia SH, Nix DE, Hejmanowski LG et al. (1989). Sucralfate reduces the gastrointestinal absorption of norfloxacin. *Antimicrob Ag Chemother* **33**: 99.

Patoia L, Guerciolini R, Menichet F, Bucaneve G, Del Favero A (1987). Norfloxacin and neutropenia. *Ann Intern Med* **107**: 788.

Perez-Trallero E, Urbieta M, Jimenez D, Garcia-Arenzana JM, Cilla G (1993). Ten year survey of quinolone resistance in *Escherichia coli* causing urinary tract infections. *Eur J Clin Microbiol Infect Dis* **12**: 349.

Pfau A, Sacks TG (1993). Single dose quinolone treatment in acute uncomplicated urinary tract infection in women. *J Urol* **149**: 532.

Pfau A, Sacks TG (1994). Effective postcoital quinolone prophylaxis of recurrent urinary tract infections in women. *J Urol* **152**: 136.

Pittman W, Moon JO, Hamrick LC, Jr et al. (1993). Randomized double-blind trial of high- and low-dose fleroxacin versus norfloxacin for complicated urinary tract infection. *Amer J Med* **94** (3A): 101S.

Ponticas S, Shungu DL, Gill CJ (1989). Comparative *in vitro* activity of norfloxacin against resistant *Neisseria gonorrhoeae*. *Eur J Clin Microbiol Infect Dis* **8**: 626.

Prince RA, Casabar E, Adair CG et al. (1989). Effect of quinolone antimicrobials on theophylline pharmacokinetics. *J Clin Pharmacol* **29**: 650.

Pummer K (1993). Fleroxacin versus norfloxacin in the treatment of urinary tract infections: a multicenter, double-blind, prospective, randomized, comparative study. *Amer J Med* **94** (3A): 108S.

Radandt JM, Marchbanks CR, Dudley MN (1992). Interactions of fluoroquinolones with other drugs: mechanisms, variability, clinical significance, and management. *Clin Infect Dis* **14**: 272.

Ramsay B, Woodrow D, Cream JJ (1993). An acantholytic bullous eruption after norfloxacin. *Brit J Dermatol* **129**: 500.

Rao PS, Rajashekar V, Varghese GK, Shivananda PG (1993). Emergence of multidrug resistant *Salmonella typhi* in rural southern India. *Amer J Trop Med Hyg* **48**: 108.

Rauser EH, Ariano RE, Anderson BA (1990). Exacerbation of myasthenia gravis by norfloxacin. *DICP* **24**: 207.

Rautelin H, Renkonen OV, Kosunen TU (1991). Emergence of fluoroquinolone resistance in *Campylobacter jejuni* and *Campylobacter coli* in subjects from Finland. *Antimicrob Ag Chemother* **35**: 2065.

Raz R, Boger S (1991). Long-term prophylaxis with norfloxacin versus nitrofurantoin in women with recurrent urinary tract infection. *Antimicrob Ag Chemother* **35**: 1241.

Reinhardt JF, George WL (1985). Comparative *in vitro* activities of selected antimicrobial agents against *Aeromonas* species and *Plesiomonas shigelloides*. *Antimicrob Ag Chemother* **27**: 643.

Robinson JA, Venezio FR, Costanzo-Nordin MR et al. (1990). Patients receiving quinolones and cyclosporine after heart transplant. *J Heart Transplant* **9**: 30.

Rocci ML, Jr, Vlasses PH, Distlerath LM et al. (1990). Norfloxacin does not alter warfarin's disposition or anticoagulant effect. *J Clin Pharmacol* **30**: 728.

Rogerie F, Ott D, Vandepitte J et al. (1986). Comparison of norfloxacin and nalidixic acid for treatment of dysentery caused by *Shigella dysenteriae* type 1 in adults. *Antimicrob Ag Chemother* **29**: 883.

Romanowski B (1986). Norfloxacin in the therapy of gonococcal infections. *Scand J Infect Dis* (Suppl 48): 40.

Romanowski B, Wood H, Draker J, Tsianco MC (1986). Norfloxacin in the therapy of uncomplicated gonorrhea. *Antimicrob Ag Chemother* **30**: 514.

Rubinstein E, Potgieter P, Davey P, Norrby SR (1994). The use of fluoroquinolones in neutropenic patients – analysis of adverse effects. *J Antimicrob Chemother* **34**: 7.

Sabbaj J, Hoagland VL, Shih WJ (1985). Multiclinic comparative study of norfloxacin and trimethoprim–sulfamethoxazole for treatment of urinary tract infections. *Antimicrob Ag Chemother* **27**: 297.

Sabbaj J, Hoagland VL, Cook T (1986). Norfloxacin versus co-trimoxazole in the treatment of recurring urinary tract infections in men. *Scand J Infect Dis* (Suppl 48): 48.

Saginur R, Nicolle LE (1992). Single-dose compared with 3-day norfloxacin treatment of uncomplicated urinary tract infection in women. Canadian Infectious Diseases Society Clinical Trials Study Group. *Arch Intern Med* **152**: 1233.

Salmeron JM, Tito L, Rimola A et al. (1992). Selective intestinal decontamination in the prevention of bacterial infection in patients with acute liver failure. *J Hepatol* **14**: 280.

Sanchez R, Fernandez-Baca V, Diaz MD et al. (1994). Evolution of susceptibilities of *Campylobacter* spp to quinolones and macrolides. *Antimicrob Ag Chemother* **38**: 1879.

Sandberg T, Englund G, Lincoln K, Nilsson LG (1990). Randomised double-blind study of norfloxacin and cefadroxil in the treatment of acute pyelonephritis. *Eur J Clin Microbiol Infect Dis* **9**: 317.

Sano M, Kawakatsu K, Ohkita C et al. (1988). Effects of enoxacin, ofloxacin and norfloxacin on theophylline disposition in humans. *Eur J Clin Pharmacol* **35**: 161.

Sarma PS (1989). Norfloxacin: a new drug in the treatment of falciparum malaria. *Ann Intern Med* **111**: 336.

Sarma PS, Durairaj P (1991). Randomized treatment of patients with typhoid and paratyphoid fevers using norfloxacin or chloramphenicol. *Trans R Soc Trop Med Hyg* **85**: 670.

Schaeffer AJ, Anderson RU (1992). Efficacy and tolerability of norfloxacin vs ciprofloxacin in complicated urinary tract infection. *Urology* **40**: 446.

Schaeffer AJ, Darras FS (1990). The efficacy of norfloxacin in the treatment of chronic bacterial prostatitis refractory to trimethoprim–sulfamethoxazole and/or carbenicillin. *J Urol* **144**: 690.

Schmeiser T, Kurrle E, Arnold R et al. (1988). Norfloxacin for prevention of bacterial infections during severe granulocytopenia after bone marrow transplantation. *Scand J Infect Dis* **20**: 625.

Schubert ML, Sanyal AJ, Wong ES (1991). Spontaneous bacterial peritonitis: prevention and therapy Antibiotic prophylaxis for prevention of spontaneous bacterial peritonitis? *Gastroenterology* **101**: 550.

Scott DA, Haberberger RL, Thornton SA, Hyams KC (1990). Norfloxacin for the prophylaxis of travelers' diarrhea in US military personnel. *Amer J Trop Med Hyg* **42**: 160.

Seidmon EJ, Krisch EB, Truant AL et al. (1990). Treatment of recurrent urinary tract infection with norfloxacin versus trimethoprim–sulfamethoxazole. *Urology* **35**: 187.

Sheehan GJ, Harding GK, Haase DA et al. (1988). Double-blind, randomized comparison of 24 weeks of norfloxacin and 12 weeks of norfloxacin followed by 12 weeks of placebo in the therapy of complicated urinary tract infection. *Antimicrob Ag Chemother* **32**: 1292.

Shimada J, Yamaji T Ueda Y et al. (1983). Mechanism of renal excretion of AM-715, a new quinolonecarboxylic acid derivative, in rabbits, dogs, and humans. *Antimicrob Ag Chemother* **23**: 1.

Shungu DL, Nalin DR, Gilman RH et al. (1987). Comparative susceptibilities of *Campylobacter pylori* to norfloxacin and other agents. *Antimicrob Ag Chemother* **31**: 949.

Sjogren E, Kaijser B, Werner M (1992). Antimicrobial susceptibilities of *Campylobacter jejuni* and *Campylobacter coli* isolated in Sweden: a 10 year follow up report. *Antimicrob Ag Chemother* **36**: 2847.

Slaney L, Chubb H, Ronald A, Brunham R (1990). *In vitro* activity of azithromycin, erythromycin, ciprofloxacin and norfloxacin against *Neisseria gonorrhoeae*, *Haemophilus ducreyi*, and *Chlamydia trachomatis*. *J Antimicrob Chemother* **25** (Suppl A): 1.

Smith SM (1986). *In vitro* comparison of A 56619, A 56620, amifloxacin, ciprofloxacin, enoxacin, norfloxacin, and ofloxacin against methicillin-resistant *Staphylococcus aureus*. *Antimicrob Ag Chemother* **29**: 325.

Soriano G, Guarner C, Teixido M et al. (1991). Selective intestinal decontamination prevents spontaneous bacterial peritonitis. *Gastroenterology* **100**: 477.

Soriano G, Guarner C, Tomas A et al. (1992). Norfloxacin prevents bacterial infection in cirrhotics with gastrointestinal hemorrhage. *Gastroenterology* **103**: 1267.

Stein GE (1987). Review of the bioavailability and pharmacokinetics of oral norfloxacin. *Amer J Med* **82** (6B): 18.

Stein GE, Mummaw N, Goldstein EJ *et al.* (1987). A multicenter comparative trial of three-day norfloxacin vs ten-day sulfamethoxazole and trimethoprim for the treatment of uncomplicated urinary tract infections. *Arch Intern Med* **147**: 1760.

Stiver HG, Bartlett KH, Chow AW (1986). Comparison of susceptibility of gentamicin resistant and susceptible '*Acinetobacter anitratus*' to 15 alternative antibiotics. *Antimicrob Ag Chemother* **30**: 624.

Swanson BN, Boppana VK, Vlasses PH *et al.* (1983). Norfloxacin disposition after sequentially increasing oral doses. *Antimicrob Ag Chemother* **23**: 284.

Syrjala H, Schildt R, Raisainen S (1991). *In vitro* susceptibility of *Francisella tularensis* to fluoroquinolones and treatment of tularemia with norfloxacin and ciprofloxacin. *Eur J Clin Microbiol Infect Dis* **10**: 68.

Tanaka M, Fukuda H, Hirai K *et al.* (1994a). Reduced uptake and accumulation of norfloxacin in resistant strains of *Neisseria gonorrhoeae* isolated in Japan. *Genitourin Med* **70**: 253.

Tanaka M, Kumazawa J, Matsumoto T, Kobayashi I (1994b). High prevalence of *Neisseria gonorrhoeae* strains with reduced susceptibility to fluoroquinolones in Japan. *Genitourin Med* **70**: 90.

Tetteroo GW, Wagenvoort JH, Mulder PG *et al.* (1993). Decreased mortality rate and length of hospital stay in surgical intensive care unit patients with successful selective decontamination of the gut. *Crit Care Med* **21**: 1692.

The GIMEMA Infection Program (1991). Prevention of bacterial infection in neutropenic patients with hematologic malignancies. A randomized, multicenter trial comparing norfloxacin with ciprofloxacin. The GIMEMA Infection Program. Gruppo Italiano Malattie Ematologiche Maligne dell'Adulto. *Ann Intern Med* **115**: 7.

Thomson DJ, Menkis AH, McKenzie FN (1988). Norfloxacin-cyclosporine interaction. *Transplantation* **46**: 312.

Tripathi KD, Sharma AK, Valecha N, Kulpati DD (1993). Curative efficacy of norfloxacin in falciparum malaria. *Indian J Med Res* **97**: 176.

Tungsanga K, Chongthaleong A, Udomsantisuk N *et al.* (1988). Norfloxacin versus co-trimoxazole for the treatment of upper urinary tract infections: a double blind trial. *Scand J Infect Dis* (Suppl 56): 28.

Ulrich C, Harinck de Weerd JE, Bakker NC *et al.* (1989). Selective decontamination of the digestive tract with norfloxacin in the prevention of ICU-acquired infections: a prospective randomized study. *Intensive Care Med* **15**: 424.

Vajpayee RB, Gupta SK, Angra SK, Munjal A (1991). Topical norfloxacin therapy in *Pseudomonas* corneal ulceration. *Cornea* **10**: 268.

Verbrugh HA, Mintjes de Groot AJ, Andriesse R *et al.* (1988). Postoperative prophylaxis with norfloxacin in patients requiring bladder catheters. *Eur J Clin Microbiol Infect Dis* **7**: 490.

Vogel R, Deaney NB, Round EM *et al.* (1984). Norfloxacin, amoxycillin, cotrimoxazole and nalidixic acid. A summary of 3-day and 7-day therapy studies in the treatment of urinary tract infections. *J Antimicrob Chemother* **13** (Suppl B): 113.

Waites KB, Canupp KC, DeVivo MJ (1991). Efficacy and tolerance of norfloxacin in treatment of complicated urinary tract infection in outpatients with neurogenic bladder secondary to spinal cord injury. *Urology* **38**: 589.

Wang C, Sabbaj J, Corrado M, Hoagland V (1986). World-wide clinical experience with norfloxacin: efficacy and safety. *Scand J Infect Dis* (Suppl 48): 81.

Watt G, Shanks GD, Edstein MD *et al.* (1991). Ciprofloxacin treatment of drug-resistant falciparum malaria. *J Infect Dis* **164**: 602.

Wilcox MH (1994). Preventing biliary stent occlusion. *Lancet* **344**: 1087.

Winston DJ, Ho WG, Nakao SL *et al.* (1986). Norfloxacin versus vancomycin/polymyxin for prevention of infections in granulocytopenic patients. *Amer J Med* **80**: 884.

Winston DJ, Ho WG, Champlin RE *et al.* (1987). Norfloxacin for prevention of bacterial infections in granulocytopenic patients. *Amer J Med* **82** (Suppl 6B): 40.

Winton MD, Everett ED, Dolan SA (1988). Activities of five new fluoroquinolones against *Pseudomonas pseudomallei*. *Antimicrob Ag Chemother* **32**: 928.

Wise R (1984). Norfloxacin – a review of pharmacology and tissue penetration. *J Antimicrob Chemother* **13** (Suppl B): 59.

Wise R, Lister D, McNulty CA *et al.* (1986). The comparative pharmacokinetics of five quinolones. *J Antimicrob Chemother* **18** (Suppl D): 71.

Wistrom J, Norrby SR, Burman LG *et al.* (1987). Norfloxacin versus placebo for prophylaxis against travellers' diarrhoea. *J Antimicrob Chemother* **20**: 563.

Wistrom J, Jertborn M, Hedstrom SA *et al.* (1989). Short-term self-treatment of travellers' diarrhoea with norfloxacin: a placebo-controlled study. *J Antimicrob Chemother* **23**: 905.

Wistrom J, Jertborn M, Ekwall E *et al.* (1992). Empiric treatment of acute diarrheal disease with norfloxacin A randomized, placebo-controlled study. Swedish Study Group. *Ann Intern Med* **117**: 202.

Wolfson JS, Hooper DC (1988). Norfloxacin: a new targeted fluoroquinolone antimicrobial agent. *Ann Intern Med* **108**: 238.

Wolfson JS, Hooper DC (1991). Overview of fluoroquinolone safety. *Amer J Med* **91** (Suppl 6A): 153.

Wong WT, Chan MK, Li MK *et al.* (1988). Treatment of urinary tract infections in Hong Kong: a comparative study of norfloxacin and co-trimoxazole. *Scand J Infect Dis* (Suppl 56): 22.

Wretlind B, Stromberg A, Ostlund L *et al.* (1992). Rapid emergence of quinolone resistance in *Campylobacter jejuni* in patients treated with norfloxacin. *Scand J Infect Dis* **24**: 685.

Wyler DJ (1989). Fluoroquinolones for malaria: the newest kid on the block? *Ann Intern Med* **111**: 269.

Yeaman MR, Roman MJ, Baca OG (1989). Antibiotic susceptibilities of two *Coxiella burnetii* isolates implicated in distinct clinical syndromes. *Antimicrob Ag Chemother* **33**: 1052.

Yeung KH, Dillon JR (1990). Norfloxacin resistant *Neisseria gonorrhaeae* in North America. *Lancet* **336**: 759.

Yoshida T, Muratani T, Iyobe S, Mitsuhashi S (1994). Mechanisms of high level resistance to quinolones in urinary tract isolates of *Pseudomonas aeruginosa*. *Antimicrob Ag Chemother* **38**: 1466.

Young LS, Berlin OG, Inderlied CB (1987). Activity of ciprofloxacin and other fluorinated quinolones against mycobacteria. *Amer J Med* **82** (Suppl 4A): 23.

Zackrisson G, Brorson J-E, Björnegård B *et al.* (1985). Susceptibility of *Bordetella pertussis* to doxycycline, cinoxacin, nalidixic acid, norfloxacin, imipenem, mecillinam and rifampicin. *J Antimicrob Chemother* **15**: 629.

Zeiler HJ, Beermann D, Wingender W *et al.* (1988). Bactericidal activity of ciprofloxacin, norfloxacin and ofloxacin in serum and urine after oral administration to healthy volunteers. *Infection* **16** (Suppl 1): S19.

Enoxacin

Description

Enoxacin was discovered by screening pipemidic acid analogs (p. 965) (Matsumoto *et al.*, 1980). Its chemical formula is l-ethyl-6- fluoro-I, 4-dihydro-4-oxo-7 piperazinyl)-I, 8-naphthyridine-3-carboxylic acid.

Sensitive Organisms

Overall, the *in vitro* activity of enoxacin is comparable with norfloxacin or lomefloxacin (p. 1147) but inferior to other fluoroquinolones such as ciprofloxacin (p. 981) and ofloxacin (p. 1111) (Chin and Neu, 1983; Bauernfeind and Ullmann, 1984; Reeves *et al.*, 1984; Siporin and Towse, 1984, Guimaraes and Noone, 1986; Henwood and Monk, 1988; Weinstein, 1988; Ismaeel and Tayeb, 1993).

1 Gram-negative bacteria

Against Gram-negative organisms enoxacin has greater activity than the older quinolones, such as nalidixic, oxolinic and pipemidic acids, and its activity is also superior to cephalexin, ampicillin and carbenicillin, but is comparable with gentamicin, amikacin, tobramycin and cefotaxime (Shimizu *et al.*, 1980; Vanhoof *et al.*, 1986).

Enoxacin is active against most Enterobacteriaceae, but *Citrobacter freundii* and *Serratia marcescens* (MIC$_{90}$ 4 µg per ml) are less susceptible (Kouno *et al.*, 1983; Bauernfeind and Ullmann, 1984; Reeves *et al.*, 1984; Siporin and Towse, 1984; Fernandes *et al.*, 1986; Henwood and Monk, 1988). *Shigella* isolates resistant to ampicillin or chloramphenicol are sensitive to enoxacin, although enoxacin is less active against *Sh. sonnei* than either ciprofloxacin, sparfloxacin or temafloxacin (Chartrand *et al.*, 1983; John *et al.*, 1992). *Proteus vulgaris* and *Morganella morganii* are more susceptible than *Pr. mirabilis*, *Providencia rettgeri* or *Providencia stuartii* (Hawkey and Hawkey, 1984). Many members of the Enterobacteriaceae which are multiply-resistant to other antibiotics, such as the aminoglycosides, extended-spectrum penicillins (e.g. ticarcillin, piperacillin), third-generation cephalosporins (cefotaxime, ceftazidime) and chloramphenicol, are susceptible to enoxacin and other fluoroquinolnes (Chartrand *et al.*, 1983; Chin and Neu, 1983; Rudrick *et al.*, 1984).

Yersinia enterocolitica, *Pasteurella multocida*, *Vibrio parahaemolyticus* and *Acinetobacter calcoaceticus* (var. *anitratus* and *lwoffi*) are usually susceptible to enoxacin; as are *Aeromonas hydrophila* and *Plesiomonas shigelloides* (Shimizu *et al.*, 1980; Chin and Neu, 1983; Bauernfiend and Ullmann, 1984; Reinhardt and George, 1985). Enoxacin has variable activity against *Campylobacter* spp., although *C. jejuni* is generally susceptible (Chartrand *et al.*, 1983; Nakamura *et al.*, 1983; Chin and Neu, 1984; Taylor *et al.*, 1985). *Gardnerella vaginalis* is usually enoxacin-resistant (Wise *et al.*, 1984a). Enoxacin is quite active against *Legionella* spp. (Fallon and Brown, 1985).

Although the majority of *Pseudomonas aeruginosa* strains are susceptible to enoxacin, the superior activity of ciprofloxacin against this species argues for its preferential use against infections due to this pathogen (p. 982). The susceptibility of *Ps. putida*, *Burkholderia* (previously *Pseudomonas*) *cepacia* and *Stenotrophomonas maltophilia* to enoxacin is variable and often poor, while *Flavobacterium* spp. are only borderline susceptible (Shimizu *et al.*, 1980; Chartrand *et al.*, 1983; Kouno *et al.*, 1983).

Haemophilus influenzae (including beta-lactamase-producing strains and chloramphenicol-resistant strains), *H. parainfluenzae* and *B. pertussis* are usually susceptible to enoxacin (Chartrand *et al.*, 1983; Chin and Neu, 1983; Appleman *et al.*, 1987; Machka *et al.*, 1988).

Usually *H.ducreyi* is susceptible (Hoban *et al.*, 1984) (p. 1080). The drug also has excellent activity against *Neisseria gonorrhoeae* (including beta-lactamase-producing strains) (MIC_{90} 0.08–0.16 μg per ml), *N. meningitidis* and *Moraxella catarrhalis* (Chin and Neu, 1983; Wise *et al.*, 1984a; Aznar *et al.*, 1985; Shapiro *et al.*, 1987; Jephcott and Gough, 1988).

Similar to norfloxacin, enoxacin has poor *in vitro* activity against anaerobes such *Bacteroides* and *Fusobacterium* spp. (Goldstein and Citron, 1985; Goldstein, 1993). *Eikenella corrodens* is susceptible to enoxacin (MIC < 2μg per ml) (Goldstein *et al.*, 1986).

2 Gram-positive bacteria

Enoxacin has reasonable activity against *Staphylococcus aureus* (including methicillin-resistant strains) and *Staph. epidermidis*, but is inferior to ciprofloxacin and ofloxacin (Barry and Jones, 1989; Barry and Fuchs, 1991a). Streptococci (Groups A, B, C and G), *Streptococcus pneumoniae* and viridans group streptococci are usually moderately resistant (Chartrand *et al.*, 1983; Chin and Neu, 1983; Bauernfeind and Ullmann, 1984; Reeves *et al.*, 1984; Wise *et al.*, 1984a; Henry *et al.*, 1985). Among staphylococcal strains resistant to enoxacin, cross-resistance against most other fluoroquinolones is usual (Chang *et al.*, 1994). Enoxacin is the least active of the fluoroquinolones against enterococci (Muranaka and Greenwood, 1988; Murray *et al.*, 1993). *Lysteria monocytogenes* and other *Listeria* spp. are also usually enoxacin-resistant (MIC_{90} 8–16 μg per ml) (Chin and Neu, 1983; MacGowan *et al.*, 1990).

Enoxacin has poor *in vitro* activity against Gram-positive anaerobes such as *Clostridium* spp., including *Cl. difficile* (MIC_{90} 64μg per ml) (Reeves *et al.*, 1984; Goldstein and Citron, 1985; Edlund and Nord, 1986; Goldstein, 1993).

3 Other organisms

Mycoplasma pneumoniae (Fallon and Brown, 1985), *Chlamydia trachomatis* and *Ureaplasma urealyticum* are resistant (Aznar *et al.*, 1985). Enoxacin and norfloxacin have only limited activity against *Mycoplasma hominis* (MIC_{90} 8 μg per ml), compared with ciprofloxacin; while MIC_{90} against *U. urealyticum* is generally 2-fold greater (Kenny *et al.*, 1989).

Enoxacin and norfloxacin are similar in their weak activity, compared with ciprofloxacin, against most mycobacteria, including *Mycobacterium tuberculosis* and *M. avium* complex (p. 1062) (Davies *et al.*, 1987; Young *et al.*, 1987). Enoxacin and norfloxacin are inactive against *M. leprae* (Franzblau and White, 1990).

Similar to ciprofloxacin and norfloxacin, enoxacin has some *in vitro* activity against *Plasmodium falciparum*; however, this has no clinical relevence (Divo *et al.*, 1988).

4 Acquired resistance

Many strains which are highly resistant to nalidixic acid are often susceptible to enoxacin and other fluoroquinolones, but cross-resistance between fluoroquinolones is usually complete (Shimizu *et al.*, 1980; Nakamura *et al.*, 1983; Duncan *et al.*, 1984; Piddock *et al.*, 1986; Barry and Fuchs, 1991b). Other issues regarding resistance are similar to those encountered with norfloxacin (p. 1062) and ciprofloxacin (p. 990).

5 In vitro sensitivities

The MICs of enoxacin against selected bacterial species are shown in Table II.6, pp. 986–987. There are no major differences between the MICs and MBCs of enoxacin (Chin and Neu, 1983).

Mode of Administration and Dosage

1 Oral administration

The usual oral regimen of enoxacin is either a single daily dose of 400 mg, or 200 mg twice-daily. For uncomplicated cystitis a single dose of 400 mg or 200 mg twice-daily for 3 days is generally recommended. Complicated urinary infections and respiratory infections generally require 400 mg twice-daily for 7–14 days.

2 Patients with renal failure

The elimination half-life of enoxacin increases with worsening renal function. The average steady-state plasma concentration in uremic patients treated with oral enoxacin 200 mg twice-daily for 7 days is 4.07 μg per ml (Bury *et al.*, 1987). With severe renal impairment the half-life of enoxacin doubles compared with normal volunteers (Nix *et al.*, 1988). Thus, when the creatinine clearance falls below 20–30 ml per min the dosage interval for enoxacin should be doubled, or the dose halved (Nix *et al.*, 1988), in a manner similar to that recommended for ciprofloxacin and norfloxacin (Fillastre *et al.*, 1990). Hemodialysis does not remove significant amounts of enoxacin or its major metabolite oxo-enoxacin (Nix *et al.*, 1988).

3 Elderly patients

Oral bioavailability of enoxacin in the elderly is similar to that in younger adults (Marchbanks *et al.*, 1990). The plasma half-life of enoxacin and its oxo-metabolite are also similar to that in younger patients, being 6.1 and 6.7h, respectively. However, older age is associated with a smaller volume of distribution and higher peak serum concentrations (Marchbanks *et al.*, 1990). No alteration in enoxacin dosing is necessary for the elderly compared with younger patients, except when there is renal impairment (Wise *et al.*, 1987, Dobbs et al, 1987).

Availability

Enoxacin is available as 200 mg and 400 mg *tablets* ('Penetrex': Rhone-Poulenc Roer). Presently no i.v. preparation is commercially available.

Serum Levels in Relation to Dosage

Enoxacin is rapidly absorbed after oral administration, but there is individual variation. In adult volunteers, peak serum levels are reached in 0.5–3.0 h and are about 1.2, 2.1, 4.0, 4.6, 3.8 and 8.2 μg per ml after single doses of 200, 400, 800, 1000, 1200 and 1600 mg, respectively. Some enoxacin is still present in serum 12h following a dose, so that with repeated drug administration, serum concentrations increase; a steady-state is achieved by the 3rd day. The serum elimination half-life is 3.4–6.8 h (Wolf *et al.*, 1984; Wise *et al.*, 1986; Chang *et al.*, 1988; Somogyi and Bochner, 1988). Absolute oral bioavailability is about 89% and is independent of the dose administered (Chang *et al.*, 1988; Marchbanks *et al.*, 1990). Due to a dose-dependent decrease in enoxacin renal clearance, total body clearance decreases and elimination half-life increases with increasing dose (Chang *et al.*, 1988). When 400 mg twice-daily was given to volunteers, a steady-state was reached within 4 days, with an average minimum serum concentration (at 12h) of 1.25 ± 0.59 μg per ml and the average peak concentration (1.5h after the dose) was 3.53 ± 0.92 μg per ml (Tsuei *et al.*, 1984). Thus, enoxacin pharmacokinetics are characterized by first-order elimination, large volume of distribution and dose-dependent increase of half-life (Chang *et al.*, 1988). Davies *et al.* (1984) gave 600 mg enoxacin orally to patients with chronic bronchitis; a peak serum level occurred at about 2.3 h after dosing and averaged 3.7 μg per ml. Similar results were obtained by Wise *et al.* (1984b) using this dosage in volunteers.

Gastric acidity is important for maximal enoxacin absorption. Abolition of gastric acidity by agents such as ranitidine, reduce the oral bioavailability of enoxacin by about 26% (Lebsack *et al.*, 1992). Furthermore, antacids such as magnesium-aluminum hydroxide reduce bioavailability by 50 to 73% when given 2h and 30 min before enoxacin, respectively (Toothaker, 1989; p. 1079). The extent of enoxacin absorption and rate of elimination is not altered by co-administration with food; however, a carbohydrate meal delays the time to peak serum concentration by about 0.9 h (Somogyi *et al.*, 1987).

Excretion

1 Urine

The kidneys are the main route of excretion for enoxacin and 30–80% of an administered dose is excreted over a 72 h period; urinary concentrations are 10- to 100-fold higher than serum levels and remain high for 24 h (Wolf *et al.*, 1984; Naber 1985). Enoxacin is eliminated predominantly as unchanged drug by the kidney, with peak urine concentrations of 460–690 μg per ml and 1200–1300 μg per ml after 200 mg and 800 mg doses (either oral or i.v.), respectively. Urine concentrations remain above 20μg per ml for 24h after a 200 mg dose (Chang *et al.*, 1988). Renal clearance of enoxacin is by glomerular filtration ($17 \pm 8\%$) and tubular secretion ($83 \pm 8\%$) (Somogyi and Bochner, 1988).

2 Inactivation in body

Enoxacin is metabolized at the piperazinyl ring to form oxo-, amino-, formyl- and acetyl-compounds. The major metabolite is the oxo-form which is found in the serum in concentrations about one-tenth that of the parent compound. In the urine it accounts for about 15% of the amount of parent enoxacin recovered. The oxo-form has microbiological activity of about one-tenth that of the parent compound. The other metabolites are not found in serum and only as traces in urine (Wise *et al.*, 1984b).

Distribution of the Drug in Body

Serum protein binding of enoxacin is 35–40% (Nakamura *et al.*, 1983). Enoxacin penetrates well into experimental blister fluid in humans (Wise *et al.*, 1984b, 1986). After oral administration, good levels are found in saliva, tonsillar tissue, sinus mucosa, nasal secretion and middle ear effusions (Baba, 1984; Sundberg and Eden, 1990). Sputum penetration is good with concentrations ranging from mean trough levels of 1.75 µg per ml to mean peak concentrations of 7.12 µg per ml after 200 mg orally twice-daily for 7 days (Dobbs *et al.*, 1988; Wijnands *et al.*, 1988). Other authors have found lower mean peak concentrations of 2.2 to 4.0 µg per ml after 400–600 mg dose schedules (Fong *et al.*, 1987). Lung penetration is also good with concentrations of 3.2–13.1 µg per ml after two oral doses of 400 mg enoxacin, representing a mean lung:serum ratio of 4.2 (Newsom *et al.*, 1989).

Enoxacin achieves mean concentrations of 4.1 ± 1.2 µg per g in the prostate after oral doses of 200 mg twice-daily for 3 days prior to prostatectomy – these are more than twice the comparable serum concentrations (Rannikko and Malmborg, 1986). Similarly, Bergeron *et al.* (1988) found the mean ratios of enoxacin concentration in prostatic tissue over concentration in serum to be 1.4 ± 0.2. In kidney after oral doses of 400 mg twice-daily, the mean concentrations 3 and 12 h after dosing are 13.9 µg per g and 9.7–14.4 µg per g, respectively (Charton and Timbal, 1990). Similarly, Malmborg and Rannikko (1988) found renal enoxacin concentrations to be about 3.2–3.8 times the serum concentration.

Enoxacin penetrates well into pelvic tissues, achieving mean concentrations of 1.8–3.0 µg per g in myometrium, fallopian tubes and cervix after 600 mg given either as a single oral dose or as three 200-mg oral doses 12 h apart (Bates and Elder, 1988).

Enoxacin, like other fluoroquinolones, penetrates well into both normal and infected bone, achieving mean concentrations of 1.0–1.3 µg per g (Fong *et al.*, 1988). Penetration into cancellous bone is significantly better than into cortical bone, with penetration rates of 82% versus 40%, respectively (Fong *et al.*, 1988).

Mode of Action

The mode of activity for enoxacin is similar to that of other fluoroquinolones such as ciprofloxacin (p. 1008).

Toxicity

Enoxacin-associated side-effects are similar to those encountered with other fluoroquinolones (Stahlmann, 1990; p. 1008) and include: photosensitivity rash, headache, dizziness, nausea, convulsions, hallucinations, depression, nausea and anorexia (Davies *et al.*, 1984; Tsuei *et al.*, 1984; Wolf *et al.*, 1984; Thomas and Ellis-Pegler, 1985; Petri and Tronnier, 1986; Kawabe *et al.*, 1989; Kang *et al.*, 1993; Izu *et al.*, 1992). Possible acute cholestatic hepatic injury associated with enoxacin has also been reported (Amitrano *et al.*, 1993).

Among the commonly used fluoroquinolones, enoxacin is the strongest inhibitor of theophylline and caffeine metabolism (probably due to inhibition of cytochrome P-450) followed by tosufloxacin, ciprofloxacin, and pefloxacin; while fleroxacin, ofloxacin, rufloxacin and sparfloxacin have little effect (Wijnands *et al.*, 1984, 1985; Beckmann *et al.*, 1987; Staib *et al.*, 1987; Stille *et al.*, 1987; Parent and LeBel, 1991; Robson, 1992; Sorgel and Kinzig, 1993). A 50% reduction in theophylline dose during co-administration with enoxacin results in the maintenance of stable serum theophylline concentrations (Koup *et al.*, 1990). Theophylline does not, however, alter fluoroquinolone pharmacokinetics (Wijnands *et al.*, 1987).

As noted earlier (p. 1078) ranitidine and antacids reduce the oral bioavailability of enoxacin by their effect in reducing gastric acidity (Toothaker, 1989; Grasela *et al.*, 1989; Lebsack *et al.*, 1992). However, intravenous enoxacin may be co-administered with intensive aluminum-magnesium hydroxide antacid regimens without significant effect on enoxacin levels (Nix *et al.*, 1993). Food and dairy products do not alter the oral absorption of enoxacin (Lehto and Kivisto, 1995). Enoxacin does not appear to affect the hypoprothrombinemic response produced by warfarin (Toon *et al.*, 1987).

Clinical Uses of the Drug

Since enoxacin has similar, or less, activity than other fluoroquinolones such as ciprofloxacin or norfloxacin and when used in high doses it is associated with a reasonably high rate of side-effects, there is little to recommend its use in preference to these other agents. Nevertheless, given its reasonable clinical activity in some infections and practical issues such as its cost, enoxacin may be a suitable treatment choice in certain circumstances

1 Urinary tract infection

Enoxacin is effective therapy for uncomplicated urinary infections – in comparative trials enoxacin achieves clinical improvement or cure in 67–96% cases (Thomas and Ellis-Pegler, 1985; Kamidono et al., 1984; Bailey and Peddie, 1985; Backhouse and Matthews, 1989; Childs, 1989; Donabedian et al., 1995). Single-dose 400 mg enoxacin is equivalent to single-dose 600 mg trimethoprim in women with bacterial cystitis, but enoxacin has disappointing efficacy against infections due to Staph. saprophyticus (Bailey et al., 1987). Similarly, enoxacin 200 mg twice-daily for 3 days results in similar clinical and bacteriological rates of cure as cefuroxime axetil 125 mg twice-daily for 7 days (Brumfitt et al., 1993). Enoxacin 400 mg twice-daily for 14 days is comparable in clinical efficacy, but superior in bacteriological efficacy, to co-trimoxazole (160/800 mg twice-daily for 14 days) for the treatment of complicated urinary tract infections (Cox et al., 1989). Other open, non-comparative studies have demonstrated good enoxacin efficacy in complicated urinary infections, in both young and elderly patients (Foot et al., 1988; Huttunen et al., 1988)

Enoxacin is probably effective therapy for bacterial prostatitis, but limitations in the design of reported trials make conclusions difficult (Andriole, 1991; Naber, 1991).

2 Sexually transmitted diseases

Enoxacin, in a variety of dosage regimens, including a single oral dose of 200, 400 or 600 mg; two doses of 400 mg 4 h apart, and 200 mg or 400 mg twice-daily for 2 days, is effective against gonorrhea. This latter regimen of 200 mg or 400 mg twice-daily for 2 days is effective against anal and pharyngeal gonorrhea – two sites which have been generally more difficult to cure (Notowicz et al., 1984; Tegelberg-Stassen et al., 1986; van der Willigen et al., 1987; Bakhtiar and Samarasinghe, 1988; Siboulet et al., 1988; Romanowski et al., 1989; Covino et al., 1993). A single oral dose of 400 mg enoxacin is equal in efficacy to a single i.m. dose of 250 mg ceftriaxone for uncomplicated anogenital gonorrhea, with cure rates of 95–100% (Albrecht et al., 1989; Pabst et al., 1989; Covino et al., 1993).

Enoxacin 400 mg twice-daily for three doses is as effective as a single dose of 640/3200 mg trimethoprim/sulfamethoxazole in the treatment of chancroid in Kenya. Both regimens resulted in improvement or cure in 91–94% (Naamara et al., 1988). However, as noted on p. 1022 longer treatment courses (e.g. 3 days) with fluoroquinolones are recommended, especially in regions where rates of co-infection with HIV are high.

3 Bacterial diarrhea

Similar to other fluoroquinolones, enoxacin 400 mg twice-daily for 10–14 days is very effective treatment for typhoid fever (Ahmed et al., 1992; Ruanguan et al., 1994). As might be expected, enoxacin is similar in efficacy to nalidixic acid for the treatment of bacillary dysentary due to multiresistant (but quinolone-sensitive) Shigella spp. (De Mol et al., 1987).

4 Respiratory tract infection

Enoxacin, like other fluoroquinolones, is effective against Gram-negative respiratory infections, but has unreliable activity against Gram-positive pathogens and is therefore an inappropriate choice for the treatment of routine community-acquired pneumonia where these latter pathogens generally predominate (Thys et al., 1991). In limited studies in which Strep. pneumoniae infection was not common, the success rate of enoxacin (usually 400 mg twice-daily for 7–14 days) for the treatment of lower respiratory tract infections is about 85% (Thys et al., 1989; Philip-Joet et al., 1988). Enoxacin is similar in efficacy to amoxycillin for the treatment of acute exacerbations of chronic bronchitis due to susceptible Gram-negative pathogens (Prigogine et al., 1988); however its clinical efficacy against infections due to Ps. aeruginosa is often suboptimal despite doses of 600 mg twice-daily (Wijnands et al., 1986). Enoxacin has been used successfully in combination with co-trimoxazole to cure a case of pneumonia due to Mycobacterium fortuitum (Sears et al., 1991).

5 Other infections

Similar to other fluoroquinolones (p. 1025), enoxacin markedly reduces colonic colonization with Enterobacteriaceae, and is effective prophylaxis against infections in immunocompromised patients (Edlund *et al.*, 1987; Maschmeyer, 1993; Talbot *et al.*, 1993). In a double-blind, placebo-controlled trial of oral enoxacin in adult patients with acute non-lymphocytic leukemia, significantly fewer patients receiving enoxacin developed Gram-negative bacteremia or infection at any site, than those receiving placebo (Talbot *et al.*, 1993). Enoxacin has been used to treat otitis media, tonsillitis and sinusitis (Baba, 1984), but is not recommended for these infections.

References

Ahmed A, Salahuddin N, Ahsan T *et al.* (1992). Enoxacin in the treatment of typhoid fever. *Clin Ther* **14**: 825.

Albrecht LM, Rybak MJ, Schubiner HH, Weiner LM (1989). Single dose enoxacin for the treatment of uncomplicated urogenital gonorrhea. *Sex Transm Dis* **16**: 114.

Amitrano L, Gigliotti T, Guardascione MA, Ascione A (1993). Acute cholestatic liver injury induced by enoxacin. *J Hepatol* **18**: 139.

Andriole VT (1991). Use of quinolones in treatment of prostatitis and lower urinary tract infections. *Eur J Clin Microbiol Infect Dis* **10**: 342.

Appleman ME, Hadfield TL, Gaines JK, Winn RE (1987). Susceptibility of *Bordetella pertussis* to five quinolone antimicrobic drugs. *Diagn Microbiol Infect Dis* **8**: 131.

Aznar J, Caballero MC, Lozano MC *et al.* (1985). Activities of new quinoline derivatives against genital pathogens. *Antimicrob Ag Chemother* **27**: 76.

Baba S (1984). Clinical evaluation of enoxacin in the treatment of infections in the field of otorhinolaryngology. *4th Medit Congr Chemother* Abstr. No. 763.

Backhouse CI, Matthews JA (1989). Single-dose enoxacin compared with 3-day treatment for urinary tract infection. *Antimicrob Ag Chemother* **33**: 877.

Bailey RR, Peddie BA (1985). Enoxacin for the treatment of urinary tract infections. *NZ Med J* **98**: 286.

Bailey RR, Gorrie SI, Peddie BA, Davies PR (1987). Double blind, randomised trial comparing single dose enoxacin and trimethoprim for treatment of bacterial cystitis. *N Z Med J* **100**: 618.

Bakhtiar M, Samarasinghe PL (1988). Enoxacin as one day oral treatment of men with anal or pharyngeal gonorrhoea. *Genitourin Med* **64**: 364.

Barry AL, Fuchs PC (1991a). Anti-staphylococcal activity of temafloxacin, ciprofloxacin, ofloxacin and enoxacin. *J Antimicrob Chemother* **28**: 695.

Barry AL, Fuchs PC (1991b). Cross-resistance and cross-susceptibility between fluoroquinolone agents. *Eur J Clin Microbiol Infect Dis* **10**: 1013.

Barry AL, Jones RN (1989). *In-vitro* activities of temafloxacin, tosufloxacin (A-61827). and five other fluoroquinolone agents. *J Antimicrob Chemother* **23**: 527.

Bates SA, Elder MG (1988). An evaluation of pelvic tissue concentrations after oral administration of enoxacin. *J Antimicrob Chemother* **21** (Suppl B): 79.

Bauernfeind A, Ullman U (1984). *In-vitro* activity of enoxacin, ofloxacin, norfloxacin and nalidixic acid. *Antimicrob Ag Chemother* **14**: 33.

Beckmann J, Elsasser W, Gundert-Remy U, Hertrampf R (1987). Enoxacin–a potent inhibitor of theophylline metabolism. *Eur J Clin Pharmacol* **33**: 227.

Bergeron MG, Roy R, Lessard C, Foucault P (1988). Enoxacin penetration into human prostatic tissue. *Antimicrob Ag Chemother* **32**: 1433.

Brumfitt W, Hamilton-Miller JM, Walker S (1993). Enoxacin relieves symptoms of recurrent urinary infections more rapidly than cefuroxime axetil. *Antimicrob Ag Chemother* **37**: 1558.

Bury RW, Becker GJ, Kincaid-Smith PS *et al.* (1987). Elimination of enoxacin in renal disease. *Clin Pharmacol Ther* **41**: 434.

Chang SC, Hsieh WC, Luh KT (1994). Fluoroquinolone resistance among methicillin-resistant staphylococci after usage of fluoroquinolones other than ciprofloxacin in Taiwan. *Diagn Microbiol Infect Dis* **19**: 143.

Chang T, Black A, Dunky A *et al.* (1988). Pharmacokinetics of intravenous and oral enoxacin in healthy volunteers. *J Antimicrob Chemother* **21** (Suppl B): 49.

Charton M, Timbal Y (1990). *In vivo* diffusion of enoxacin in healthy renal and adenomatous prostate tissue in man. *Eur Urol* **17**: 252.

Chartrand SA, Scribner RK, Weber AH *et al.* (1983). *In vitro* activity of Cl–919 (AT-2266), an oral antipseudomonal compound. *Antimicrob Ag Chemother* **23**: 658.

Childs SJ (1989). Tissue penetration and clinical efficacy of enoxacin in urinary tract infections. *Clin Pharmacokinet* **16** (Suppl 1): 32.

Chin N-X, Neu HC (1983). *In vitro* activity of enoxacin, a quinolone carboxylic acid, compared with those of norfloxacin, new beta-lactams, aminoglycosides, and trimethoprim. *Antimicrob Ag Chemother* **24**: 754.

Covino JM, Smith BL, Cummings MC *et al.* (1993). Comparison of enoxacin and ceftriaxone in the treatment of uncomplicated gonorrhea. *Sex Transm Dis* **20**: 227.

Cox CE, Drylie DM, Klimberg I *et al.* (1989). A multicenter, double-blind, trimethoprim-sulfamethoxazole controlled study of enoxacin in the treatment of patients with complicated urinary tract infections. *J Urol* **141**: 575.

Davies BI, Maesen FPV, Teengs JP (1984). Serum and sputum concentrations of enoxacin after single oral dosing in a clinical and bacteriological study. *Antimicrob Ag Chemother* **14** (Suppl C): 83.

Davies S, Sparham PD, Spencer RC (1987). Comparative *in-vitro* activity of five fluoroquinolones against mycobacteria. *J Antimicrob Chemother* **19**: 605.

De Mol P, Mets T, Lagasse R *et al.* (1987). Treatment of bacillary dysentery: a comparison between enoxacin and nalidixic acid. *J Antimicrob Chemother* **19**: 695.

Divo AA, Sartorelli AC, Patton CL, Bia FJ (1988). Activity of fluoroquinolone antibiotics against *Plasmodium falciparum in vitro*. *Antimicrob Ag Chemother* **32**: 1182.

Dobbs BR, Gazeley LR, Campbell AJ, Edwards IR (1987). The effect of age on the pharmacokinetics of enoxacin. *Eur J Clin Pharmacol* **33**: 101.

Dobbs BR, Gazeley LR, Stewart IA, Edwards IR (1988). Pharmacokinetics and sputum penetration of enoxacin after twice daily oral dosing for seven days. *J Antimicrob Chemother* **21** (Suppl B): 61.

Donabedian H, O'Donnell E, Drill C *et al.* (1995). Prevention of subsequent urinary tract infections in women by the use of anti-adherence antimicrobial agents: a double-blind comparison of enoxacin with co-trimoxazole. *J Antimicrob Chemother* **35**: 409.

Duncan IBR, Skulnick M, Marshall PW (1984). *In vitro* activity of enoxacin against aminoglycoside-resistant Gram-negative bacilli and other clinical isolates. *J Antimicrob Chemother* **14** (Suppl C): 1.

Edlund C, Nord CE (1986). Comparative *in vitro* activities of ciprofloxacin, enoxacin, norfloxacin, ofloxacin and pefloxacin against *Bacteroides fragilis* and *Clostridium difficile*. *Scand J Infect Dis* **18**: 149.

Edlund C, Lidbeck A, Kager L, Nord CE (1987). Comparative effects of enoxacin and norfloxacin on human colonic microflora. *Antimicrob Ag Chemother* **31**: 1846.

Fallon RJ, Brown WM (1985). *In-vitro* sensitivity of legionellas, meningococci and mycoplasmas to ciprofloxacin and enoxacin. *J Antimicrob Chemother* **15**: 787.

Fernandes CJ, Munro R, Toohey M et al. (1986). In vitro antibacterial activity of enoxacin (CI-919). *Pathology* **18**: 240.

Fillastre JP, Leroy A, Moulin B et al. (1990). Pharmacokinetics of quinolones in renal insufficiency. *J Antimicrob Chemother* **26** (Suppl B): 51.

Fong IW, Vandenbroucke A, Simbul M (1987). Penetration of enoxacin into bronchial secretions. *Antimicrob Ag Chemother* **31**: 748.

Fong IW, Rittenhouse BR, Simbul M, Vandenbroucke AC (1988). Bone penetration of enoxacin in patients with and without osteomyelitis. *Antimicrob Ag Chemother* **32**: 834.

Foot M, Williams G, Want S et al. (1988). An open study of the safety and efficacy of enoxacin in complicated urinary tract infections. *J Antimicrob Chemother* **21** (Suppl B): 97.

Franzblau SG, White KE (1990). Comparative *in vitro* activities of 20 fluoroquinolones against *Mycobacterium leprae*. *Antimicrob Ag Chemother* **34**: 229.

Goldstein EJ (1993). Patterns of susceptibility to fluoroquinolones among anaerobic bacterial isolates in the United States. *Clin Infect Dis* **16** (Suppl 4): S377.

Goldstein EJ, Citron DM, Vagvolgyi AE, Gombert ME (1986). Susceptibility of *Eikenella corrodens* to newer and older quinolones. *Antimicrob Ag Chemother* **30**: 172.

Goldstein EJC, Citron DM (1985). Comparative activity of the quinolones against anaerobic bacteria isolated at community hospitals. *Antimicrob Ag Chemother* **27**: 657.

Grasela TH, Jr, Schentag JJ, Sedman AJ et al. (1989). Inhibition of enoxacin absorption by antacids or ranitidine. *Antimicrob Ag Chemother* **33**: 615.

Guimaraes MA, Noone P (1986). The comparative *in-vitro* activity of norfloxacin, ciprofloxacin, enoxacin and nalidixic acid against 423 strains of Gram-negative rods and staphylococci isolated from infected hospitalised patients. *J Antimicrob Chemother* **17**: 63.

Hawkey PM, Hawkey CA (1984). Comparative *in-vitro* activity of quinolone carboxylic acids against Proteeae. *J Antimicrob Chemother* **14**: 485.

Henry D, Skidmore AG, Ngui-Yen J et al. (1985). *In vitro* activities of enoxacin, ticarcillin plus clavulanic acid, aztreonam, piperacillin, and imipenem and comparison with commonly used antimicrobial agents. *Antimicrob Ag Chemother* **28**: 259.

Henwood JM, Monk JP (1988). Enoxacin A review of its antibacterial activity, pharmacokinetic properties and therapeutic use. *Drugs* **36**: 32.

Hoban D, Grabowski M, Urias B et al. (1984). Antibacterial activity of enoxacin (C1-919). *4th Medit Congr Chemother* Abstr. No. 700.

Huttunen M, Kunnas K, Saloranta P (1988). Enoxacin treatment of urinary tract infections in elderly patients. *J Antimicrob Chemother* **21** (Suppl B): 105.

Ismaeel NA, Tayeb OS (1993). Comparative antimicrobial activity of lomefloxacin, norfloxacin, ofloxacin, ciprofloxacin and enoxacin against >500 bacterial isolates. *Microbios* **74**: 147.

Izu R, Gardeazabal J, Gonzalez M et al. (1992). Enoxacin-induced photosensitivity: study of two cases. *Photodermatol Photoimmunol Photomed* **9**: 86.

Jephcott AE, Gough K (1988). *In-vitro* activity of enoxacin against gonococcal isolates in comparison with that of five other antibiotics. *J Antimicrob Chemother* **21** (Suppl B): 43.

John JF Jr, Atkins LT, Maple PA, Bratoeva M (1992). Activities of newer fluoroquinolones against *Shigella sonnei*. *Antimicrob Ag Chemother* **36**: 2346.

Jones RM (1989). *In-vitro* antimicrobial activity of enoxacin and its metabolites. *J Antimicrob Chemother* **23**: 658.

Kamidono S, Nishiura T, Ishigami J (1984). Randomized multicentre double blind studies of enoxacin and pipemidic acid in acute uncomplicated cystitis and complicated urinary tract infection. *4th Medit Congr Chemother* Abstr. No. 759.

Kang JS, Kim TH, Park KB et al. (1993). Enoxacin photosensitivity. *Photodermatol Photoimmunol Photomed* **9**: 159.

Kawabe Y, Mizuno N, Sakakibara S (1989). Photoallergic reaction caused by enoxacin. *Photodermatol* **6**: 57.

Kenny GE, Hooton TM, Roberts MC et al. (1989). Susceptibilities of genital mycoplasmas to the newer quinolones as determined by the agar dilution method. *Antimicrob Ag Chemother* **33**: 103.

Kouno K, Inoue M, Mitsuhashi S (1983). *In vitro* and *in vivo* antibacterial activity at AT-2266. *Antimicrob Ag Chemother* **24**: 78.

Koup JR, Toothaker RD, Posvar E, Sedman AJ, Colburn WA (1990). Theophylline dosage adjustment during enoxacin coadministration. *Antimicrob Ag Chemother* **34**: 803.

Lebsack ME, Nix D, Ryerson B et al. (1992). Effect of gastric acidity on enoxacin absorption. *Clin Pharmacol Ther* **52**: 252.

Lehto P, Kivisto KT (1995). Effects of milk and food on the absorption of enoxacin. *Br J Clin Pharmacol* **39**: 194.

MacGowan AP, Holt HA, Bywater MJ, Reeves DS (1990). *In vitro* antimicrobial susceptibility of *Listeria monocytogenes* isolated in the UK and other *Listeria* species. *Eur J Clin Microbiol Infect Dis* **9**: 767.

Machka K, Balg H, Braveny I (1988). *In vitro* activity of new antibiotics against *Haemophilus influenzae*. *Eur J Clin Microbiol Infect Dis* **7**: 812.

Malmborg AS, Rannikko S (1988). Enoxacin distribution in human tissues after multiple oral administration. *J Antimicrob Chemother* **21** (Suppl B): 57.

Marchbanks CR, Mikolich DJ, Mayer KH et al. (1990). Pharmacokinetics and bioavailability of intravenous-to-oral enoxacin in elderly patients with complicated urinary tract infections. *Antimicrob Ag Chemother* **34**: 1966.

Maschmeyer G (1993). Use of the quinolones for the prophylaxis and therapy of infections in immunocompromised hosts. *Drugs* **45** (Suppl 3): 73.

Matsumoto J-I, Miyamoto T, Minamida A et al. (1980). Structure-activity relationships of 4-oxo-1, 8-naphthyridine-3-carboxylic acids including AT-2266, a new oral antipseudomonal agent. In *Current Chemotherapy and Infectious Disease* Vol 1 (Nelson JD, Grassi C, eds), p. 454. Washington, DC: American Society for Microbiology.

Muranaka K, Greenwood D (1988). The response of *Streptococcus faecalis* to ciprofloxacin, norfloxacin and enoxacin. *J Antimicrob Chemother* **21**: 545.

Murray PR, Bratcher JL, Niles AC, Hampton CM (1993). *In vitro* activity of nine fluoroquinolone antibiotics against 200 strains of enterococci. *Diagn Microbiol Infect Dis* **16**: 83.

Naamara W, Kunimoto DY, D'Costa LJ, et al. (1988). Treating chancroid with enoxacin. *Genitourin Med* **64**: 189.

Naber KG (1991). The role of quinolones in the treatment of chronic bacterial prostatitis. *Infection* **19** (Suppl 3): S170.

Naber KG, Sorgel F, Gutzler F, Bartosik-Wich B (1985). *In vitro* activity, pharmacokinetics, clinical safety and therapeutic efficacy of enoxacin in the treatment of patients with complicated urinary tract infections. *Infection* **13**: 219.

Nakamura S, Minimi A, Katae H et al. (1983). *In vitro* antibacterial properties of AT-2266, a new pyridonecarboxylic acid. *Antimicrob Ag Chemother* **23**: 641.

Newsom SW, Eden CG, Wells FC, Meredith P (1989). Penetration of enoxacin into lung tissue. *J Antimicrob Chemother* **23**: 113.

Nilsson-Ehle I, Ljungberg B (1991). Quinolone disposition in the elderly Practical implications. *Drugs Aging* **1**: 279.

Nix DE, Schultz RW, Frost RW *et al.* (1988). The effect of renal impairment and haemodialysis on single dose pharmacokinetics of oral enoxacin. *J Antimicrob Chemother* **21** (Suppl B): 87.

Nix DE, Lebsack ME, Chapelsky M *et al.* (1993). Effect of oral antacids on disposition of intravenous enoxacin. *Antimicrob Ag Chemother* **37**: 775.

Notowicz A, Stolz E, Van Kingeren B (1984). A double blind study comparing two dosages of enoxacin for the treatment of uncomplicated urogenital gonorrhoea. *J Antimicrob Chemother* **14** (Suppl C): 91.

Pabst KM, Siegel NA, Smith S *et al.* (1989). Multicenter, comparative study of enoxacin and ceftriaxone for treatment of uncomplicated gonorrhea. *Sex Transm Dis* **16**: 148.

Parent M, LeBel M (1991). Meta-analysis of quinolone-theophylline interactions. *DICP* **25**: 191.

Petri H, Tronnier H (1986). Efficacy of enoxacin in the treatment of bacterial infections of the skin with regards to photosensitization. *Infection* **14** (Suppl 3): S213.

Philip-Joet F, Nourrit J, Frances Y, Arnaud A (1988). Enoxacin in the treatment of lower respiratory tract infections. *J Antimicrob Chemother* **21** (Suppl B): 125.

Piddock LJ, Diver JM, Wise R (1986). Cross-resistance of nalidixic acid resistant Enterobacteriaceae to new quinolones and other antimicrobials. *Eur J Clin Microbiol* **5**: 411.

Prigogine T, Glupczynski Y, Carpiaux JP *et al.* (1988). Enoxacin in acute exacerbations of chronic bronchitis: a comparison with amoxycillin. *J Antimicrob Chemother* **21** (Suppl B): 131.

Rannikko S, Malmborg A-S (1986). Enoxacin concentration in human prostatic tissue after oral administration. *J Antimicrob Chemother* **17**: 123.

Reeves DS, Bywater MJ, Holt HA (1984). The activity of enoxacin against clinical bacterial isolates in comparison with that of five other agents, and factors affecting that activity. *J Antimicrob Chemother* **14** (Suppl C): 7.

Reinhardt JF, George WL (1985). Comparative *in vitro* activities of selected antimicrobial agents against *Aeromonas* species and *Plesiomonas shigelloides*. *Antimicrob Ag Chemother* **27**: 643.

Robson RA (1992). The effects of quinolones on xanthine pharmacokinetics. *Amer J Med* **92**: 22S.

Romanowski B, Hardy JS, Rafter MS, Draker J (1989). Enoxacin in the therapy of anal and pharyngeal gonococcal infections. *Sex Transm Dis* **16**: 190.

Ruanguan W, Kunming Y, Qiong S (1994). Antibiotic therapy for typhoid fever. *Chemotherapy* **40**: 61.

Rudrick JT, Cavalieri SJ, Britt EM (1984). *In vitro* activities of enoxacin and 17 other antimicrobial agents against multiply resistant Gram-negative bacteria. *Antimicrob Ag Chemother* **6**: 97.

Scheife RT, Cramer WR, Decker EL (1993). Photosensitizing potential of ofloxacin. *Int J Dermatol* **32**: 413.

Sears MR, van der Linden A, Pollock M (1991). *Mycobacterium fortuitum* pneumonia–treatment with enoxacin and cotrimoxazole. *N Z Med J* **104**: 407.

Shapiro MA, Heifetz CL, Sesnie JC (1987). Comparative *in-vitro* activity of enoxacin against penicillinase- and non-penicillinase-producing *Neisseria gonorrhoeae*. *Sex Transm Dis* **14**: 111.

Shimizu M, Takase S, Nakamura H *et al.* (1980). AT-2266, a new oral antipseudomonal agent. In *Current Chemotherapy and Infectious Disease* Vol 1 (Nelson JD, Grassi C, eds), p. 451. Washington DC: American Society for Microbiology.

Siboulet A, Bohbot JM, Catalan F (1988). Enoxacin in the treatment of sexually transmitted diseases. *J Antimicrob Chemother* **21** (Suppl B): 119.

Siporin C, Towse G (1984). Enoxacin: worldwide *in-vitro* activity against 22451 clinical isolates. *J Antimicrob Chemother* **14** (Suppl C): 47.

Somogyi AA, Bochner F (1988). The absorption and disposition of enoxacin in healthy subjects. *J Clin Pharmacol* **28**: 707.

Somogyi AA, Bochner F, Keal JA *et al.* (1987). Effect of food on enoxacin absorption. *Antimicrob Ag Chemother* **31**: 638.

Sorgel F, Kinzig M (1993). Pharmacokinetics of gyrase inhibitors, Part 2: Renal and hepatic elimination pathways and drug interactions. *Amer J Med* **94**: 56S.

Stahlmann R (1990). Safety profile of the quinolones. *J Antimicrob Chemother* **26** (Suppl D): 31.

Staib AH, Stille W, Dietlein G *et al.* (1987). Interaction between quinolones and caffeine. *Drugs* **34** (Suppl 1): 170.

Stille W, Harder S, Mieke S *et al.* (1987). Decrease of caffeine elimination in man during co-administration of 4- quinolones. *J Antimicrob Chemother* **20**: 729.

Sundberg L, Eden T (1990). Penetration of enoxacin into middle ear effusion. *Acta Otolaryngol (Stockh)* **109**: 438.

Talbot GH, Cassileth PA, Paradiso L *et al.* (1993). Oral enoxacin for infection prevention in adults with acute nonlymphocytic leukemia. The Enoxacin Prophylaxis Study Group. *Antimicrob Ag Chemother* **37**: 474.

Taylor DE, Ng LK, Lior H (1985). Susceptibility of *Campylobacter* species to nalidixic acid, enoxacin, and other DNA gyrase inhibitors. *Antimicrob Ag Chemother* **28**: 708.

Tegelberg-Stassen MJ, van der Willigen AH, van der Hoek JC *et al.* (1986). Treatment of uncomplicated urogenital gonorrhoea in women with a single dose of enoxacin. *Eur J Clin Microbiol* **5**: 395.

Thomas MG, Ellis-Pegler RB (1985). Enoxacin treatment of urinary tract infections. *J Antimicrob Chemother* **15**: 759.

Thys JP, Jacobs F, Motte S (1989). Quinolones in the treatment of lower respiratory tract infections. *Rev Infect Dis* **11** (Suppl 5): S1212.

Thys JP, Jacobs F, Byl B (1991). Role of quinolones in the treatment of bronchopulmonary infections, particularly pneumococcal and community-acquired pneumonia. *Eur J Clin Microbiol Infect Dis* **10**: 304.

Toon S, Hopkins KJ, Garstang FM *et al.* (1987). Enoxacin-warfarin interaction: pharmacokinetic and stereochemical aspects. *Clin Pharmacol Ther* **42**: 33.

Toothaker RD (1989). Enoxacin absorption and elimination characteristics. *Clin Pharmacokinet* **16** (Suppl 1): 52.

Tsuei SE, Darragh AS, Brick I (1984). Pharmacokinetics and tolerance of enoxacin in healthy volunteers administered at a dosage of 400 mg twice daily for 14 days. *Antimicrob Ag Chemother* **14**: 71.

van der Willigen AH, van der Hoek JC, Wagenvoort JH *et al.* (1987). Comparative double-blind study of 200- and 400-mg enoxacin given orally in the treatment of acute uncomplicated urethral gonorrhea in males. *Antimicrob Ag Chemother* **31**: 535.

Vanhoof R, Hubrechts JM, Roebben E *et al.* (1986). Antibacterial activity of enoxacin: comparison with aminoglycosides, beta- lactams and other antimicrobial agents. *J Antimicrob Chemother* **17**: 297.

Weinstein MP (1988). Comparative *in vitro* activity of lomefloxacin and other antimicrobials against 597 microorganisms causing bacteremia. *Diagn Microbiol Infect Dis* **11**: 195.

Wijnands WJA, Van Herwaarden CLA, Vree TB (1984). Enoxacin raises plasma theophylline concentrations. *Lancet* **ii**: 108.

Wijnands WJ, Vree TB, van Herwaarden CL (1985). Enoxacin decreases the clearance of theophylline in man. *Br J Clin Pharmacol* **20**: 583.

Wijnands WJ, van Griethuysen AJ, Vree TB *et al.* (1986). Enoxacin in lower respiratory tract infections. *J Antimicrob Chemother* **18**: 719.

Wijnands WJ, Vree TB, Baars AM, van Herwaarden CL (1987). Steady-state kinetics of the quinolone derivatives ofloxacin, enoxacin, ciprofloxacin and pefloxacin during maintenance treatment with theophylline. *Drugs* **34** (Suppl 1): 159.

Wijnands WJ, Vree TB, Baars AM, van Herwaarden CL (1988). Pharmacokinetics of enoxacin and its penetration into bronchial secretions and lung tissue. *J Antimicrob Chemother* **21** (Suppl B): 67.

Wise R, Andrews JM, Danks G (1984a). *In-vitro* activity of enoxacin (C1–919), a new quinoline derivative, compared with that of other antimicrobial agents. *J Antimicrob Chemother* **13**: 237.

Wise R, Lockley R, Webberly M, Adhami ZN (1984b). The pharmacokinetics and tissue penetration of enoxacin and norfloxacin. *J Antimicrob Chemother* **14** (Suppl C): 75.

Wise R, Lister D, McNulty CA, Griggs D, Andrews JM (1986). The comparative pharmacokinetics of five quinolones. *J Antimicrob Chemother* **18** (Suppl D): 71.

Wise R, Baker SL, Misra M, Griggs D (1987). The pharmacokinetics of enoxacin in elderly patients. *J Antimicrob Chemother* **19**: 343.

Wolf R, Eberl R, Dunky A *et al.* (1984). The clinical pharmacokinetics and tolerance of enoxacin in healthy volunteers. *J Antimicrob Chemother* **14** (Suppl C): 63.

Young LS, Berlin OG, Inderlied CB (1987). Activity of ciprofloxacin and other fluorinated quinolones against mycobacteria. *Amer J Med* **82** (Suppl 4A): 23.

Pefloxacin

Description

Pefloxacin (perfloxacine) was developed by Rhône-Poulenc and has the chemical formula of l-ethyl-6-fluoro-1,4-dihydro-4-oxo-7(4-methyl-1-piperazinyl)-quinoline-3-carboxylic acid. Overall, the antibacterial spectrum of pefloxacin is similar to that of norfloxacin (p. 1061) and enoxacin (p. 1076), but it is less than ciprofloxacin (p. 981) (Van Caekenberghe and Pattyn, 1984; Clarke et al., 1985; Ligtvoet and Wickerhoff-Minoggio, 1985; Auckenthaler et al., 1986; King and Phillips, 1986a,b). Although pefloxacin has little clinical advantage over these other fluoroquinolones, its good penetration of the central nervous system is notable, but there are only limited clinical data available to support its use for treatment of infections of the central nervous system (p. 1092).

Sensitive Organisms

1 Gram-negative bacteria

The *in vitro* activity of pefloxacin against most Enterobacteriaceae is greater than that of nalidixic acid, ampicillin, amikacin, gentamicin and ceftazidime; approximately equivalent to enoxacin, ofloxacin, norfloxacin and cefotaxime, but is less than the activity of ciprofloxacin (Ligtvoet and Wickerhoff-Minogio, 1985; Jones et al., 1986; King and Phillips, 1986a; Yourassowsky et al. 1986; Geogopoulos et al., 1988; Gruneberg et al., 1988; Phillips and King, 1988; Gonzalez and Henwood, 1989; Van der Auwera et al., 1989). It is also quite active against *Aeromonas* and *Plesiomonas* spp. (Gruneberg et al., 1988; Kuijper et al., 1989). *Yersinia enterocolitica* are generally susceptible, but ciprofloxacin has greater activity (Hoogkamp-Korstanje, 1987). *Campylobacter jejuni* is usually sensitive, but *Helicobacter pylori* is only moderately susceptible, similar to norfloxacin and enoxacin (Glupczynski et al., 1988; Van der Auwera et al., 1989). *Acinetobacter* spp. are generally less susceptible to pefloxacin than to ciprofloxacin, ofloxacin and sparfloxacin (Joly-Guillou and Bergogne-Bérézin, 1986, 1992). *Gardnerella vaginalis* is often resistant (King and Phillips, 1986a).

Similar to other fluoroquinolones (p. 983) pefloxacin has excellent activity against *N. gonorrhoeae*, including penicillinase-producing strains and those with chromosomally mediated penicillin-resistance (Jones et al., 1986; King and Phillips, 1986a,b; Phillips and King, 1988; van der Willigen et al., 1990). It is also very active against *Haemophilus ducreyi* (Rutanarugsa et al., 1990; Sturm, 1987). *Haemophilus influenzae* and *H. parainfluenzae* are very susceptible to pefloxacin; however, the MIC_{90} for ofloxacin, and especially ciprofloxacin, are generally one or two dilutions lower (e.g. 0.03–0.06 μg per ml) (Quentin et al., 1988). *Moraxella catarrhalis* is very susceptible (Phillips and King, 1988).

Pefloxacin has reasonable *in vitro* activity against *Francisella tularensis*, but is less active than either ciprofloxacin or norfloxacin (Syrjala et al., 1991). Pefloxacin and enoxacin have relatively poor *in vitro* activity against *Bordetella pertussis* and *B. parapertussis*, especially compared with ciprofloxacin (Hoppe and Simon, 1990). *Brucella melitensis* is generally susceptible to pefloxacin and other fluoroquinolones (Qadri et al., 1989).

Pefloxacin is active *in vitro* and *in vivo* in guinea pigs against *Legionella pneumophila*, but unlike ofloxacin and ciprofloxacin, it appears to exhibit a prolonged post-antibacterial effect *in vitro* (Dournon et al., 1986; Rajagopalan-Levasseur et al., 1990).

Pseudomonas aeruginosa and some other *Pseudomonas* spp. are reasonably susceptible to pefloxacin (MIC_{50}/MIC_{90} 1/8 μg per ml), but notably less than to ciprofloxacin (Clarke et al.,

1985; Phillips and King, 1988; Gonzalez and Henwood, 1989). Pefloxacin has poor activity against *Burkholderia* (*Pseudomonas*) *pseudomallei* (Cheong *et al.*, 1987).

Of the anaerobes, *Bacteroides fragilis*, *Prevotella melaninogenica* and the *Fusobacterium* and *Mobiluncus* spp. are generally resistant (Delmee and Avesani, 1986; Edlund and Nord, 1986; Jones *et al.*, 1986; King and Phillips, 1986a, 1986b).

2 Gram-positive bacteria

Staphylococcus aureus (including beta-lactamase-producing and methicillin-resistant strains), *Staph. epidermidis* and *Staph. saprophyticus* are usually susceptible. In general, pefloxacin has activity comparable with ciprofloxacin and ofloxacin against *Staph. aureus*. *Streptococcus pneumoniae*, *Strep. pyogenes*, *Strep. viridans*, enterococci and Groups B, C, D and G streptococci are relatively resistant (MIC$_{90}$ 8–32 µg per ml) compared with ciprofloxacin (Ligtvoet and Wickerhoff-Minogio, 1985; Yourassowsky *et al.*, 1986; King and Phillips, 1986a,b; Phillips and King, 1988; Gruneberg *et al.*, 1988; Van der Auwera *et al.*, 1989). Some *in vitro* studies suggest more rapid killing of staphylococci when pefloxacin is combined with oxacillin or vancomycin compared with each agent alone; however, there are no data to indicate that this observation has any clinical relevance (Fass and Helsel, 1987). Although pefloxacin has some *in vitro* activity against the Gram-positive bacillus *Erysipelothrix rhusiopathiae* (MBC$_{90}$ 4 µg per ml) it is inferior to ciprofloxacin (MBC$_{90}$ 0.12 µg per ml) and penicillin (MBC$_{90}$ 0.06 µg per ml) (Venditti *et al.*, 1990). *Nocardia* spp. are resistant, as is *Listeria monocytogenes* (MIC$_{90}$ 8 µg per ml) (Eliopoulos and Eliopoulos, 1993; Farina *et al.*, 1995).

Gram-postive anaerobes such as are *Eubacterium*, *Peptococcus*, *Peptostreptococcus* and *Clostridium* (including *Cl. difficile*) species are pefloxacin-resistant (King and Phillips, 1986b; Gruneberg *et al.*, 1988; Van der Auwera *et al.*, 1989; Eliopoulos and Eliopoulos, 1993).

3 Mycobacteria

The *in vitro* activity of pefloxacin against *Mycobacterium tuberculosis*, *M. bovis*, *M. xenopi*, *M. kansasii* is inferior to that of ciprofloxacin and ofloxacin (which are generally associated with a MIC of ≤1.25 µg per ml), but is similar to the activity of enoxacin and norfloxacin (Davies *et al.*, 1987; Texier-Maugein *et al.*, 1987; Gorzynski *et al.*, 1989; pp. 1062, 1077). Pefloxacin has bactericidal activity against *M. leprae* in experimentally infected mice, but is inferior to ofloxacin, temafloxacin and especially sparfloxacin (Pattyn, 1987; Gelber *et al.*, 1992).

4 Rickettsia and Coxiella burnetii

Similar to ciprofloxacin and ofloxacin, pefloxacin has *in vitro* activity against the spotted fever rickettsioses, *Rickettsia conorii* and *R. rickettsii*, which cause Mediterranean spotted fever and Rocky Mountain spotted fever, respectively (Raoult *et al.*, 1987; Jabarit-Aldighieri *et al.*, 1992). Similarly, these fluoroquinolones also have *in vitro* activity against some strains of *Coxiella burnetii*, but their clinical therapeutic role is less clear (p. 1094) (Raoult *et al.*, 1989; Yeaman *et al.*, 1989; Keren *et al.*, 1994).

5 Plasmodia

Pefloxacin, more than ciprofloxacin, has *in vivo* activity against experimental *Plasmodium yoelii* in mice and both agents have activity against *Plasmodium falciparum in vitro* (Divo *et al.*, 1988; Salmon *et al.*, 1990). Clinically, however, pefloxacin has only modest activity against *Plasmodium falciparum*, and at a dose of 400 mg twice-daily for 3 days is insufficient to reliably cure *P. falciparum* malaria (p. 1094) (Deleron *et al.*, 1991).

6 Acquired resistance

Similar to other fluoroquinolones (p. 990), resistance to pefloxacin due to altered DNA gyrase and outer membrane permeability among some Gram-negative species such as *Enterobacter cloacae* and *Ps. aeruginosa* has been described and appears to be increasing in incidence in some institutions (Lucain *et al.*, 1989; Michea-Hamzehpour *et al.*, 1991; Shalit *et al.*, 1992).

7 Minimum inhibitory concentrations

The MICs of pefloxacin against selected bacterial species are shown in Table II.6, pp. 986–987.

Mode of Administration and Dosage

1 Oral administration

The usual recommended oral dose of pefloxacin is 400 mg twice-daily, taken with meals to avoid gastrointestinal disturbance. Occasionally an initial loading dose of 800 mg may be appropriate to promptly attain steady-state serum concentrations. Doses of up to 1200 mg daily have been used.

2 Intravenous administration

Intravenous and oral dosing of pefloxacin is generally the same. Parenteral pefloxacin should be administered as a 1-h i.v. infusion mixed in 5% dextrose solution, rather than in normal saline which results in drug precipitation.

3 Patients with renal failure

Since pefloxacin is extensively metabolized and cleared by non-renal mechanisms (less than 20% of the drug is recoverable in the urine as unmodified pefloxacin) pharmacokinetic parameters are unaltered, or only minimally altered, in patients with renal impairment (Eliopoulos, 1988; Fillastre *et al.*, 1990; Bressolle *et al.*, 1994). Although pefloxacin levels remain relatively unchanged, reduced renal function is associated with an accumulation of the N-oxide metabolite which lacks antibacterial activity (Jungers *et al.*, 1987). The metabolite N-demethylpefloxacin (norfloxacin) also accumulates, but serum levels of this appear to be too low to be clinically important. Thus, no dosage adjustment is necessary for pefloxacin in patients with renal failure (Fillastre *et al.*, 1990). Haemodialysis does not remove pefloxacin – hence, no supplementary dose is necessary post-dialysis (Montay *et al.*, 1985).

Pefloxacin is associated with good bidirectional diffusion across the peritoneal membrane and so therapeutic concentrations are achieved in dialysate after i.v. and oral administration to patients undergoing continuous ambulatory peritoneal dialysis (CAPD). Futhermore 400 mg pefloxacin added to each 6-hourly bag of dialysate results in both therapeutic dialysate and serum concentrations, suggesting that systemic pefloxacin therapy could be administered by the intraperitoneal route in these patients (Schmit *et al.*, 1991). Interestingly, the half-life of pefloxacin in these patients is 18.8–19.9 h, which is longer than that noted for uremic patients on hemodialysis – suggesting that once-daily dosing of 400 mg (i.v., oral, or intraperitoneal) may be adequate in this setting (Schmit *et al.*, 1991; Nikolaidis *et al.*, 1991). Rose *et al.* (1990a) treated CAPD patients who had peritonitis with 400 mg oral pefloxacin twice-daily for 10 or 21 days with good clinical success, although two patients developed *Achilles tendonitis* (p. 1091) while receiving this higher dose.

4 Patients with hepatic failure

The presence of hepatic cirrhosis is associated with a significant prolongation of the half-life of pefloxacin to 35.1 ± 19 h and an 18% reduction in the volume of the drug distribution, due to reduced drug metabolism. Furthermore, the half-life is longer in patients with ascites or jaundice than in similar patients without these complications (Danan *et al.*, 1985; Westphal and Brogard, 1993). Galtier *et al.* (1993) noted wide variability between patients, but reported an even longer half-life of 46.3 ± 42.5 h. In patients with liver disease of grade B or C severity according to the Child-Pugh classification, total body pefloxacin clearance may be 30% of normal values (Galtier *et al.*, 1993). The penetration of pefloxacin into ascites after a single oral 400-mg dose is estimated to be 68 ± 26%. Following three 400-mg oral doses every 12 h, the mean trough ascitic fluid concentration is 6.1 ± 3.1 μg per ml (range 2.0–10.2) (Montay and Gaillot, 1990). These authors recommend a once-daily oral or i.v. dose of 400 mg (8 mg per kg) pefloxacin in patients with hepatic failure. If serum drug concentrations cannot be readily monitored during treatment, an alternative fluoroquinolone which is not so dependent on hepatic metabolism for clearance, and therefore does not require dosage adjustment in these circumstances (e.g. ciprofloxacin; p. 997), may be used.

Availability

Pefloxacin is available in some European countries ('Peflacin', 'Perflacine'), but is currently investigational in the USA and is not available in Australia.

Serum Levels in Relation to Dosage

1 Oral administration

Pefloxacin is rapidly absorbed from the gastrointestinal tract, with near 100% bioavailability, and plasma pefloxacin concentrations increase in a dose-dependent manner when single oral or i.v. doses of 200 to 800 mg are given to healthy volunteers. Single oral doses of 200 or 400 mg achieve mean maximum concentrations after 1–1.5 h of 2.5 and 4.3 μg per ml, respectively (Gonzalez and Henwood, 1989). Similarly, Montay et al. (1984) noted peak serum levels of 3.77–3.84 μg per ml about 1 h after an oral dose of 400 mg to healthy volunteers; while Webberley et al. (1987) noted even higher peak serum concentrations of 6.6 μg per ml after the same dose. Repeated oral doses of 400 mg twice-daily are associated with an increase in peak and trough serum concentrations to 7.9–10 μg per ml and 3.8 μg per ml, respectively, after approximately 48 h. Under these circumstances the elimination half-life increases from 7.2–12.3 h (generally 10.5 h after a single dose) to 14.8–15.4 h, suggesting saturation of the clearance pathway of pefloxacin (p. 1089) (Montay et al., 1984; Frydman et al., 1986; Wise et al., 1986; Gonzalez and Henwood, 1989; Lode et al., 1990). A number of metabolites of pefloxacin have been described and two of them, pefloxacin N-oxide and N-desmethyl pefloxacin (norfloxacin) have been found in human serum; the former has very little antibacterial activity, but norfloxacin is very active. Most of the activity (84%) in serum is due to unchanged pefloxacin, which is 20–30% protein-bound (Montay et al., 1984).

2 Intravenous administration

The pharmacokinetics of i.v. and orally administered pefloxacin are similar (Maesen et al., 1985; Lode et al., 1990). When repeated doses of 400 mg pefloxacin i.v. twice-daily are given to healthy volunteers, the peak serum levels immediately after the first infusion for pefloxacin and its metabolites norfloxacin and pefloxacin-N-oxide are 5.8, 0.10 and 0.09 μg per ml, respectively; with mean trough serum levels at 12 h of 1.49, 0.07 and 0.14, respectively. After the tenth dose, the mean peak levels are 9.55, 0.28 and 0.42, respectively, and mean trough serum levels 4.22, 0.22 and 0.39 μg per ml, respectively. The mean serum elimination half-life is 11 h, but this increases to nearly 15 h after repeated doses. Similar to after oral administration, there is a gradual accumulation of the drug (Frydman et al.,1985; Wise et al., 1986, 1988). Petitjean et al. (1993) found similar results when comparing i.v. 400 mg twice-daily to a single 800-mg dose in healthy volunteers. Mean peak concentrations were 7.42 and 12.11 μg per ml, respectively, while mean trough concentrations at 24 h were 1.93 and 2.77 μg per ml, respectively.

3 Pregnant and lactating women

Pefloxacin 400 mg i.v. every 12 h for two doses results in maternal serum concentrations of 2.65–4.31 μg per ml and amniotic fluid concentrations of 1.97–2.74 μg per ml. Among lactating women given three doses of 400 mg oral pefloxacin twice-daily, breast milk concentrations 2, 4, 6, 9, 12 and 24 h after dosage administration are 3.54, 3.43, 2.93, 2.24, 1.79, and 0.88 μg per ml, respectively. Thus, pefloxacin achieves reasonable concentrations in amniotic fluid and quite high levels in breast milk (Giamarellou et al., 1989a).

Excretion

1 Urine

The minor difference in structure between pefloxacin and norfloxacin alters the half-life and renal handling of pefloxacin such that, unlike norfloxacin which is secreted by the renal tubule, there is a net renal tubular reabsorption of pefloxacin (Karabalut and Drusano, 1993). Renal clearance of pefloxacin is low, varying from 7.5 to 21.9 ml per min with various doses. Urinary excretion of pefloxacin and its metabolites accounts for 31–59% of the pefloxacin dose (Montay et al., 1984; Frydman et al., 1986; Lode et al., 1990).

2 Bile

Biliary excretion of pefloxacin and its metabolites accounts for 20–30% of an oral dose (Bressolle et al., 1994). Biliary concentrations after a 800 mg i.v. dose are 2- to 3-fold greater than the serum concentrations, with the peak biliary concentrations reached about 4 h post-dose (Wittke and Adam, 1989; Bressolle *et al.*, 1994). After a 400-mg oral dose gallbladder bile concentrations of 83 μg per ml can be expected 12 h post-dose if there is no biliary obstruction (Bressolle *et al.*, 1994; p. 1090).

3 Inactivation in body

Non-renal clearance is the main elimination pathway for pefloxacin, with the liver being the predominant organ of metabolism (Lode *et al.*, 1990; Bressolle *et al.*, 1994). Five metabolites have been identified, of which four are measurable in human urine – N-desmethyl-pefloxacin [norfloxacin], pefloxacin-N-oxide, oxo-norfloxacin and oxo-pefloxacin (Montay *et al.*, 1984; Outman and Nightingale, 1989). As noted earlier, the two primary metabolites are pefloxacin-N-oxide, which is inactive, and norfloxacin (Jones, 1989).

4 Feces

Fecal concentrations of pefloxacin after repeated oral dosing of 400 mg twice-daily are high – approximately 645μg per g (Janin *et al.*, 1987).

Distribution of the Drug in Body

Intravenous and oral pefloxacin achieve about 70% penetration into experimentally induced blister fluid (Wise et al, 1986; Webberley *et al.*, 1987). Salivary concentrations of pefloxacin are generally 0.61–0.70 of serum levels after a single dose, but following repeated oral doses of 400 mg twice-daily the saliva levels closely relate to the serum concentrations; being 3.46 μg per ml on day 1 and 7.54 μg per ml on day 7. Under this latter dosing regimen, fecal concentrations of pefloxacin on day 8 are about 645 μg per g (Janin *et al.*, 1987). However, van de Leur *et al.* (1995) found median fecal concentrations of only 187 μg per g after administering the same dose of 400 mg twice-daily to neutropenic patients.

Pefloxacin penetrates well into the maxillary sinus cavity and nasal secretions in the setting of chronic maxillary sinusitis, and in fact accumulates in inflamed sinus fluid. Mean sinus aspirate concentrations taken 3, 6, 9, 12 h after two 400 mg doses 12 h apart are 6.92, 3.74, 3.47, 2.82 μg per ml, respectively. At the same time intervals, concentrations in nasal secretions are 9.05, 3.71, 3.20, 2.85 μg per ml (Petrikkos *et al.*, 1992).

Pefloxacin penetrates both inflamed and un-inflamed meninges well, achieving concentrations in CSF and brain tissue superior to those of ciprofloxacin (Norrby, 1988). Relative rank order among the commonly used fluoroquinolones in terms of CSF penetration is: pefloxacin (~50%), which is greater than that of ofloxacin and ciprofloxacin (~20–30%) (Scheld, 1989). Wolff *et al.* (1984) studied the diffusion of pefloxacin into CSF of 15 patients with bacterial meningitis or ventriculitis, who were being treated with other antibiotics. Three doses of pefloxacin were administered at 12 h intervals as a 1 h i.v. infusion in 11 patients and orally in the other four; individual doses of 7.5 mg per kg were used in seven patients and 15 mg per kg in the other eight. Mean peak serum levels were obtained immediately after i.v. infusion or 2 h after oral intake; concentrations of pefloxacin in CSF were measured 2h after the third i.v. dose and 4h after the third oral dose. The mean peak and trough serum levels after an i.v. dose of 7.5 mg per kg were 10.28 and 3.54 μg per ml, respectively; and the mean CSF concentration was 4.8 μg per ml. The comparable serum values after the i.v. 15 mg per kg regimen were 20.15 and 8.21 μg per ml; and the mean CSF concentration was 8.3 μg per ml. After oral administration of the low dose, peak and trough serum levels were 8.2–10 μg per ml and 3.5–6.8 μg per ml, respectively, while CSF concentrations were 3.0–3.8 μg per ml. With the higher oral dose, the peak serum levels were 21.24 μg per ml and CSF concentrations were 10.17 μg per ml. In seven patients tested after cure of their meningitis, pefloxacin CSF levels were 2.7–6.4 and 6.0–7.5 μg per ml after the low and high doses, respectively (Wolff *et al.*, 1984).

Dow *et al.* (1986) gave 400 mg pefloxacin by a 1-h infusion to nine subjects (aged 17–66 years) with hydrocephalus and measured CSF levels via a ventricular drain. Mean peak serum levels for pefloxacin and norfloxacin were 8.54 and 0.17 μg per ml and the peak concentrations in the CSF 5–6 h after the start of the infusion were 2.97 and 0.1–0.2 μg per ml, respectively. After this peak in the CSF, the CSF/serum ratio was 0.6 and the CSF elimination half-life for pefloxacin was 13.4h, suggesting that accumulation in the CSF was unlikely.

Segev *et al.* (1990a) studied 16 patients with acute Gram-negative meningitis (in 14 cases this was a complication of neurosurgical operations; three were children) to whom pefloxacin 800 mg twice-daily i.v. was administered for a mean of 11 days to adult patients. Mean CSF pefloxacin concentrations were 8.8 ± 5.0 μg per ml, which were approximately 5-fold greater than the mean

MBC of the responsible pathogens. Clinical outcome was good (p. 1092). From rather limited data, pefloxacin appears to penetrate well into brain tissue. In a study of 30 patients with brain tumors who were treated with various pefloxacin dosage regimens prior to surgery, brain tissue concentrations ranged from 3.28 to 4.50 μg per g. Tumor concentrations, however, were known to be 2- to 3-fold higher than surrounding unaffected brain (Korinek et al., 1988).

Pefloxacin penetration into uninfected heart valves and myocardium is good. Mean aortic valve concentrations 4, 8, 12 and 24 h after a single 800-mg i.v. dose are 6.08, 7.29, 4.64, 2.23 mg per g, respectively, while mitral valve concentrations are similar. Mean myocardial concentrations at the same time intervals are 20.1, 17.8, 10.7 and 9.2 mg per g, respectively. Thus the valve:plasma pefloxacin concentration ratio varies between 0.65 and 1.33; while the myocardium:plasma ratio varies between 1.70 and 4.00 during the 24 h post-dose period (Brion et al., 1986).

Like other fluoroquinolones, pefloxacin penetrates well into bone. When the drug is given in a dosage of 400 mg 12-hourly i.v. for 48 h, followed by oral treatment, bone biopsies taken after at least 7 days treatment and 2 h after the last dose contain pefloxacin levels of 2–10 μg per g of bone (Dellamonica et al., 1986; Bressolle et al., 1994).

When 400 mg of the drug is either infused i.v. over 60 min or taken orally, peak sputum levels in patients with chronic bronchitis are reached in 2.3 and 3.26 h, respectively, with mean values of 3.83 and 4.56 μg per ml, respectively (Maesen et al., 1985). Bonmarchand et al. (1989) reported mean pefloxacin concentrations in bronchial secretions taken from intubated patients with chronic obstructive pulmonary disease treated with six doses of 400 mg i.v. twice-daily, to vary between 6.5 and 11.1 μg per ml. Mean pefloxacin concentrations in alveolar macrophages and epithelial lining fluid obtained by bronchoalveolar lavage from ten healthy volunteers were 106 and 88 μg per ml, respectively. This 13- to 16-fold accumulation of pefloxacin over that found in serum may support the use of the drug against intracellular bacterial pulmonary pathogens (Panteix et al., 1994).

Biliary concentrations of pefloxacin may be 2- to 3-fold more than the serum concentrations, with the peak biliary concentrations reached about 4 h post-dose (Wittke and Adam, 1989; Bressolle et al., 1994). Following a single 400-mg oral dose in patients without biliary obstruction, gallbladder bile concentrations of 83 μg per ml can be expected 12 h post-dose (Bressolle et al., 1994). However, lower concentrations may be expected if there is biliary obstruction. Pefloxacin, like ciprofloxacin, achieves concentrations in pancreatic juice of 100% those in serum following a single oral dose of 400 mg – mean peak pancreatic juice concentrations of 4.6 μg per ml can be expected (Malmborg et al., 1990). Studies on patients undergoing elective gastrointestinal surgery or biliary surgery who were given pefloxacin 400 mg i.v. prior to surgery, suggest wide variability in peritoneal fluid concentrations, but levels of 2 μg per ml can be expected for at least 4 h after the dose (Webberley et al., 1989). Ascitic fluid penetration of pefloxacin is about 68% after a single 400-mg oral dose in patients with cirrhosis, and significant drug accumulation occurs in ascites following repeated dosing (Cardey et al., 1987; p. 1087).

Similar to other fluoroquinolones, pefloxacin concentrations in prostate and ejaculate fluids are probably high, but there are only limited data available (Bressolle et al., 1994). Mean pefloxacin concentrations of 101.5 μg per g are achieved in renal parenchyma following a single i.v. 800 mg dose – this being approximately 10-fold more than the plasma concentration (Varini et al., 1992). Pefloxacin penetration into dialysate in CAPD patients receiving oral pefloxacin is complete, with excellent bidirectional diffusion.

Similar to ciprofloxacin (p. 1007), pefloxacin penetrates well into gynecological tissues, including myometrium, ovary and fallopian tubes, exceeding the MIC_{90} for many common bacterial pathogens implicated in gynecologic infections (Bouvet et al., 1992).

Pefloxacin diffuses well into uninfected aqueous humor, achieving concentrations of 0.75, 1.45, 1.04 and 0.86 μg per ml, 2, 6, 12, 24 h, respectively, after a 1 h infusion of 400 mg (Salvanet et al., 1986). Giamarellou et al. (1993) found pefloxacin penetration into aqueous humor to be superior to that of ciprofloxacin and ofloxacin, with concentrations of 1.04–7.80 μg per ml achievable after two i.v. doses of 400 mg or 800 mg – representing 21–48% of serum levels. Pefloxacin penetration into the vitreous humor is also good, with mean concentrations of 1.37 μg per ml measurable 6 h after an oral 400-mg dose (Oncel and Peyman, 1993).

Mode of Action

The mode of action is similar to that of other fluoroquinolones (p. 1008).

Toxicity

Toxicities associated with pefloxacin are similar to those reported for other fluoroquinolones (Halkin, 1988; Christ, 1990; p. 1008). In a review of spontaneous notifications to the manufacturer of potential pefloxacin toxicity from 1985 to 1990, skin and musculoskeletal toxicities were most commonly reported (Simon and Guyot, 1990). Photosensitivity has been noted in 0.6% patients during clinical trials, and is related to the dose and duration of pefloxacin therapy, and the amount of sun exposure. Pefloxacin, fleroxacin and lomefloxacin appear to be more likely to cause phototoxicity than other fluoroquinolones (Scheife et al., 1993). Case reports of photoonycholysis associated with pefloxacin and ofloxacin therapy have been described (Baran and Brun, 1986); while blue-black pigmentation of the legs has been noted with pefloxacin therapy (Le Cleach et al., 1995). Similar to ciprofloxacin (p. 1010), however, pefloxacin has been associated with occasional reports of angioedema, sometimes with other symptoms of anaphylactoid reaction such as dyspnea. Arthralgia was the most frequently reported musculoskeletal side-effect in the review and was noted in 0.6% of patients during clinical trials. Other authors have described case reports of severe polyarthropathy in adolescents in which pefloxacin may have been implicated (Le Loet et al., 1991; Chevalier et al., 1992). Achilles tendinitis, including rupture, have been reported in patients treated with pefloxacin, ofloxacin and ciprofloxacin (Rose et al., 1990a; Ribard et al., 1992; p. 1011).

Psychiatric and CNS reactions have been noted in 1.2% of patients treated with pefloxacin in clinical trials. Convulsions have been reported after both i.v. and oral pefloxacin, while a pre-existing history of epilepsy or intracerebral lesions was noted in only some of these patients (Lucet et al., 1988). Chapuis et al. (1993) reported a number of cases in which grand mal seizures developed in patients with hepatic cirrhosis who were treated with the usual pefloxacin dose of 400 mg twice-daily and had no other apparent predisposing factors. Elevated pefloxacin levels were demonstrated in a number of these patients. No recurrence of seizures were observed after pefloxacin withdrawal. These cases reaffirm the need to reduce the dose of pefloxacin (or carefully monitor levels) in cirrhotic patients due to their reduced ability to metabolize pefloxacin (pp. 1087, 1089).

Less severe symptoms such as insomnia and vertigo have also been described (Simon and Guyot, 1990). Aoun et al. (1992) reported a patient who developed a severe peripheral neuropathy, possibly associated with pefloxacin therapy. The paresthesia resolved dramatically with cessation of pefloxacin, but recurred with the commencement of ofloxacin, and later with the recommencement of pefloxacin. The authors speculated that the patient's prior treatment with vinca alkaloids for Hodgkin's disease may have potentiated the development of fluoroquinolone-induced peripheral neuropathy.

Gastrointestinal symptoms such as nausea and indigestion have been reported in about 7% patients in clinical trials. Clostridium difficile diarrhea has occurred, as with most antibiotics. Reversible thrombocytopenia (rarely <20 000) and, less frequently, neutropenia have been reported (Simon and Guyot, 1990). In vitro studies by Pallavicini et al. (1989) suggest no inhibition of myelopoiesis by either pefloxacin or ofloxacin, but other studies are less conclusive (Somekh et al., 1989).

Pefloxacin has been reported to cause cataracts, azoospermia and testicular damage in dogs, although the human implications of these findings are unclear (Mayer, 1987; Christ et al., 1988).

Similar to other fluoroquinolones (p. 1014), pefloxacin decreases the metabolic clearance of theophylline, resulting in elevated theophylline levels when these drugs are co-administered (Wijnands et al., 1986, 1987; Robson, 1992). In a comparative study, Wijnands et al. (1986) noted that total body clearance of theophylline was significantly decreased by enoxacin (63.6%), ciprofloxacin (30.4%) and pefloxacin (29.4%). Unlike the NSAID, fenbufen, which appears to increase the terminal half-life of ciprofloxacin, ketoprofen does not alter the pharmacokinetics of either pefloxacin or ofloxacin in humans (Fillastre et al., 1993).

Absorption of all fluoroquinolones are reduced by antacids and sucralfate, while cimetidine (but not newer H_2-inhibitors) reduces the clearance of pefloxacin due to its effect on liver metabolism (Davies and Maesen, 1989; Jaehde et al., 1994). To ensure adequate absorption, pefloxacin should be given at least 2 h before antacids containing magnesium and aluminum hydroxide (Jaehde et al., 1994).

Rifampicin significantly increases the plasma clearance of pefloxacin when these drugs are co-administered in humans, but this inductive effect is not sufficient to always require an adjustment in pefloxacin dose. However, measurement of pefloxacin levels may be advisable in some clinical situations (Humbert et al., 1991).

Clinical Uses of the Drug

1 Meningitis and other central nervous system infections

Pefloxacin penetrates well into CSF of patients with meningitis, and probably achieves reasonable levels in brain tissue (Scheld, 1989; Modai, 1991; p. 1089). Pefloxacin cured 13 of 16 patients with Gram-negative bacillary meningitis when administered in doses of 800 mg i.v. twice-daily for 11 ± 4 days. In 14 of these 16 patients infection was a complication of neurosurgical operations and all but two of these 16 patients had received prior unsuccessful therapy. Nine of these infections were due to *Ps. aeruginosa* or *Acinetobacter calcoaceticus* (Segev *et al.*, 1990a). It is unclear how many of these patients had also been described in an earlier report by Segev *et al.* (1989) of successful pefloxacin therapy. Modai (1991) treated 11 adults with bacterial meningitis with doses of either 400 mg twice- or thrice-daily, or 800 mg twice-daily. Of seven patients treated with pefloxacin alone, six were cured, but one continued to grow *E. coli* despite 9 days pefloxacin therapy. Four patients were treated with combinations of pefloxacin and various other agents. Overall, eight of the 11 (73%) patients were cured, while lack of success was due to superinfection, reinfection, or treatment failure in each of the other three patients, respectively. Case reports have described therapeutic success with pefloxacin in the treatment of *Morganella morganii* meningitis in an adult, and ventriculitis due to *Klebsiella pneumoniae* in a neonate (Isaacs and Ellis-Pegler, 1987; Linder *et al.*, 1994).

2 Osteomyelitis

Similar to ciprofloxacin (p. 1019), pefloxacin is effective treatment for acute and chronic osteomyelitis, but the rate of success is dependent on the infecting pathogen, since resistance develops readily in pathogens such as staphylococci and *Ps. aeruginosa* (Desplaces and Acar, 1988). Desplaces *et al.* (1986) used pefloxacin for a mean period of 6 months to successfully treat 17 of 20 patients with chronic staphylococcal osteomyelitis; in the three failures, resistant strains emerged (two *Staph. aureus* and one coagulase-negative staphylococcus). Subsequently, they also reported cures among 14 other patients with chronic staphylococcal osteomyelitis (mean follow-up 1.9 years) by using a combination of pefloxacin and rifampicin for 6 months (Desplaces and Acar, 1988). For Gram-negative or polymicrobial bone and joint infections, the same authors reported that pefloxacin in combination with either aminoglycosides (15 patients) or beta-lactam antibiotics (three patients) was curative in 16 of 18 patients.

Pefloxacin has also been used by Dellamonica *et al.* (1986, 1989) to treat chronic osteomyelitis. Fifteen patients in whom the pathogens were *Staph. aureus* (5), *Ps. aeruginosa* (5), *Serratia* spp. (3), *Pr. mirabilis* (1) and mixed infection with *Enterococcus faecalis* and *Escherichia coli* (1) were given 400 mg 12-hourly i.v. for 48 h, then oral treatment in the same dosage. In 11 patients treated for 6 months and followed for up to 14 months, therapy was successful. In two patients fistulae closed, but there was only limited follow-up and additionally there were two failures. Subsequently Dellamonica *et al.* (1990) also described some success with pefloxacin (generally 400 mg twice-daily) for 2.5–6 months in the treatment of 13 patients with foreign body-associated chronic osteomyelitis. However, seven of the 13 required either removal of the foreign body (prosthesis, orthopaedic wire or nail) or some drainage surgery to achieve a satisfactory outcome. The authors noted that the risk of failure with the development of resistance among the infecting pathogen(s) was greater if the foreign body was not removed.

3 Respiratory tract infections

Pefloxacin has only moderate efficacy in the treatment of routine pneumonia or bronchitis, mainly due to its limited activity against *Strep. pneumoniae* and *Staph. aureus* (Maesen *et al.*, 1987). Maesen *et al.* (1985) gave 400 mg of the drug orally twice-daily to 43 patients with exacerbations of chronic bronchitis; 34 (79%) showed clinical improvement by day 11 and this fell to 65% 7 days later. All strains of *H. influenzae* and *Moraxella catarrhalis* were eradicated by the treatment, but eight infections caused by *Strep. pneumoniae* and three caused by *Ps. aeruginosa* were unaffected. These results correlated with the resistance of these organisms, which increased during therapy; mode MICs for the pre- and post-treatment strains of *Strep. pneumoniae* were 4 and 16 μg per ml and the corresponding values for *Ps. aeruginosa* were 2 and 16 μg per ml, respectively.

In patients with pneumonia due to predominantly Gram-negative pathogens (e.g. nosocomial pneumonia in intensive care units), the rate of cure/improvement with pefloxacin 400 mg twice-daily is 66–90%, and is roughly comparable with ceftazidime or imipenem (Lauwers *et al.*,

1986; Martin *et al.*, 1988; Thys *et al.*, 1989; Giamarellou *et al.*, 1990; Grassi *et al.*, 1990; Potgieter, 1990; Vanderdonckt, 1990). In patients with cystic fibrosis, however, resistance develops reasonably readily in *Ps. aeruginosa* isolates (Grenier, 1989). In one retrospective study, pefloxacin, either alone or in combination with rifampicin and/or erythromycin, demonstrated reasonable clinical efficacy in the treatment of severe Legionnaires' disease (Dournon *et al.*, 1990).

4 Urinary tract infections and sexually transmitted disease

Similar to other fluoroquinolones, pefloxacin is effective in the treatment of cystitis and complicated urinary tract infections, but appears to offer no particular advantage over more commonly used agents such as norfloxacin (p. 1066), ciprofloxacin (p. 1014) or ofloxacin (p. 1121), and may have a higher rate of side-effects (Boerema *et al.*, 1986; Chan *et al.*, 1990; Petersen *et al.*, 1990; van Balen *et al.*, 1990; Andriole, 1991; Timmerman *et al.*, 1992; Jardin and Cesana, 1995). Similarly, pefloxacin is effective therapy for bacterial prostatitis (approximately 74% cure rate) but in one study 22.5% patients suffered side-effects (Guibert *et al.*, 1990).

Clinical data regarding the efficacy of pefloxacin in gonococcal infections is limited compared with other fluoroquinolones, and although comparable cure rates have been reported, pefloxacin is not generally recommended for treatment of this disease (Ball *et al.*, 1990; Tio *et al.*, 1990; Cheong *et al.*, 1992; Moran and Levine, 1995).

5 Peritonitis associated with continuous ambulatory peritoneal dialysis (CAPD)

Similar to ciprofloxacin (p. 1030), pefloxacin is effective in the treatment of peritonitis due to Gram-negative pathogens, but clinical experience is less extensive with pefloxacin than with ciprofloxacin (Ragnaud *et al.*, 1987; Benzakour *et al.*, 1988; Nikolaidis, 1990; Rose *et al.*, 1990a,b; Lye *et al.*, 1993). As might be expected, clinical outcomes are relatively poor when treating CAPD peritonitis due to Gram-positive pathogens such as staphylococci (Rose *et al.*, 1990b). However, oral pefloxacin plus intraperitoneal vancomycin had similar efficacy to intraperitoneal vancomycin plus gentamicin in one prospective, randomized study of patients with CAPD-associated peritonitis – although the pefloxacin-treated group had a higher incidence of nausea and vomiting (Lye *et al.*, 1993).

6 Bacteraemia and other serious infections

Pefloxacin, either alone or in combination with a variety of other agents, has proven to be effective therapy (approximately 70–80%) for Gram-negative bacteraemia, including nosocomially acquired infections. As expected, therapeutic failures are generally due to methicillin-resistant staphylococci or *Ps. aeruginosa* (Lauwers *et al.*, 1986; Bernard *et al.*, 1990; Limson *et al.*, 1990; Potgieter, 1990). In two limited studies pefloxacin was found to be comparable with ceftazidime in the treatment of a variety of infections, including soft tissue sepsis, bronchopneumonia and urinary tract infections, but its rate of adverse reactions may be higher (Giamarellou *et al.*, 1989b; Segev *et al.*, 1990b). Nevertheless, there are no data to recommend pefloxacin ahead of ciprofloxacin in these settings.

Pefloxacin plus metronidazole was similar in efficacy to gentamicin plus metronidazole in an open, randomized, multicenter trial of 184 evaluable patients with proven intra-abdominal sepsis (cured/improved rate: 90% versus 80%, respectively) (Swedish Study Group, 1990). Pefloxacin achieves high biliary concentrations (pp. 1088, 1090) and compared favorably with ampicillin+ gentamicin in one study of bacteriologically proven cholecystitis or cholangitis (98% versus 96% cured, respectively) (Chacon *et al.*, 1990).

7 Gastrointestinal infections

Similar to ciprofloxacin (p. 1016) and norfloxacin (p. 1068), pefloxacin is highly effective in the treatment of acute typhoid fever and clearance of typhoid carriage in both adults and children, but there have been no direct comparisons between these fluoroquinolones to recommend pefloxacin ahead of the other agents (Hajji *et al.*, 1988; Cristiano *et al.*, 1989, 1995; Ait-Khaled *et al.*, 1990; DuPont, 1993; Gendrel *et al.*, 1993; Raymond *et al.*, 1994). In a prospective, randomized trial of 42 adults with bacteriologically confirmed typhoid who were treated with 14 days therapy of either pefloxacin 400 mg twice-daily or co-trimoxazole 160/800 mg twice-daily, faster resolution of fever and gastrointestinal and neurological symptoms was noted in the pefloxacin-teated group, but the overall cure rate and incidence of carriage was similar in the two groups (Hajji *et al.*, 1988). Ait-Khaled *et al.* (1990), however, found a 7-day course of pefloxacin 400 mg twice-daily in adults to result in a 95% rate of clinical cure.

In children, 12 mg per kg per day for 7 days has been effective for severe salmonellosis for those who failed with initial conventional antibiotic therapy (Gendrel *et al.*, 1993). Two doses of pefloxacin 12 mg per kg (day 1 and 4) was effective in clearing non-typhoidal *Salmonella* carriage in 13 of 15 children, compared with clearance from only 1 of 6 controls, in a small non-randomized study by Raymond *et al.* (1994).

In a non-randomized study of Madagascan children with multiresistant *Shigella* dysentery (*Sh. dysenteriae*, *Sh. flexneri*, *Sh. sonnei*), single-dose therapy with pefloxacin 20 mg per kg was similar in efficacy to three once-daily doses of pefloxacin 12 mg per kg – no adverse articular effects were noted during 3–9 months follow-up (Guyon *et al.*, 1994).

8 Prevention and treatment of infection in neutropenic patients

Pefloxacin (400 mg twice-daily) appears to be inferior to ciprofloxacin (pp. 1025, 1026) and possibly ofloxacin, in its efficacy in preventing infections in neutropenic patients, but may be superior to norfloxacin (Meunier, 1990; D'Antonio *et al.*, 1992, 1994). The emergence of Gram-positive infections remains a potential problem, although this is significantly reduced by the co-administration of penicillin V 500 mg twice-daily, especially in terms of streptococcal species (International Antimicrobial Therapy Cooperative Group of the European Organization for Research and Treatment of Cancer, 1994). In another study, oral pefloxacin + vancomycin was significantly better than gentamicin + colistin sulphate + vancomycin in preventing bacteraemia in granulocytopenic patients (Archimbaud *et al.*, 1991). Similar to norfloxacin, pefloxacin (either i.v. or oral) is effective in selectively decontaminating the alimentary tract of Gram-negative bacilli in healthy volunteers and bone marrow transplant recipients (Nord, 1988; Giuliano *et al.*, 1989; Vollaard *et al.*, 1990). Pefloxacin is generally effective therapy for neutropenic sepsis, especially in combination with agents with better Gram-positive activity, such as piperacillin or amoxycillin/clavulanic acid (Cajozzo *et al.*, 1990; Gardembas-Pain *et al.*, 1991; Kattan *et al.*, 1992). This latter combination may be suitable for home-based oral therapy in selected patients (Gardembas-Pain *et al.*, 1991).

9 Other infections and conditions

Pruna *et al.* (1992) described three patients with nephrotic syndrome due to idiopathic minimal change nephropathy or focal and segmental glomerulosclerosis where their proteinuria markedly diminished after treament with pefloxacin 400 mg twice-daily for 15–30 days. Subsequently, however, other authors have found no benefit in a total of 13 patients, but reported a high rate (50%) of side-effects, often sufficient to require cessation of pefloxacin therapy (Geffriaud-Ricouard *et al.*, 1993; Aigrain *et al.*, 1993). Thus, there are currently no confirmed data to recommend the use of pefloxacin in this condition.

Pefloxacin has been used in combination with other agents in the treatment of tuberculosis, but its clinical efficacy is difficult to determine (Rao, 1995). Pefloxacin appears to have some clinical efficacy in small uncontrolled studies of patients with lepromatous leprosy (N'Deli *et al.*, 1990; Ji and Grosset, 1991). Pefloxacin 800 mg per day in combination with rifampicin 300 mg per day and valve replacement cured one patient with prosthetic valve endocarditis due to *Coxiella burnetii* (Cacoub *et al.*, 1991).

Pefloxacin, similar to other fluoroquinolones, has proven ineffective in the treatment of experimental murine brucellosis (*Brucella melitensis*) (Shasha *et al.*, 1992), Micozzi *et al.* (1990) reported one patient in whom *Brucella melitensis* endocarditis was cured with pefloxacin. However, the larger clinical experience with ciprofloxacin (p. 1031) in treating brucellosis suggests that its use may currently be preferred when considering a fluoroquinolone in this clinical setting.

In a double-blind comparison, pefloxacin was similar in efficacy to cefazolin as prophylaxis in elective cardiovascular surgery (Auger *et al.*, 1990). However, the use of fluoroquinolones for surgical prophylaxis should generally be avoided, to minimize the emergence of resistance to these valuable agents.

Despite encouraging *in vitro* data, pefloxacin has shown only modest efficacy against *Plasmodium falciparum* malaria, and at a dose of 400 mg twice-daily for 3 days is insufficient to reliably cure this disease. In a study of 22 Madagascan patients (mainly adults) treated with this dose, 16 were initially cleared of parasitemia, but seven relapsed by day 14 – thus only nine patients (41%) were cured (Deloron *et al.*, 1991).

References

Aigrain EJ, Brun P, Bennasr S, Loirat C (1993). Side-effects of pefloxacin in idiopathic nephrotic syndrome. *Lancet* **342**: 438.

Ait-Khaled A, Zidane L, Amrane A, Aklil R (1990). The efficacy and safety of pefloxacin in the treatment of typhoid fever in Algeria. *J Antimicrob Chemother* **26** (Suppl B): 181.

Andriole VT (1991). Use of quinolones in treatment of prostatitis and lower urinary tract infections. *Eur J Clin Microbiol Infect Dis* **10**: 342.

Aoun M, Jacquy C, Debusscher L *et al.* (1992). Peripheral neuropathy associated with fluoroquinolones. *Lancet* **340**: 127.

Archimbaud E, Guyotat D, Maupas J *et al.* (1991). Pefloxacin and vancomycin vs gentamicin, colistin sulphate and vancomycin for prevention of infections in granulocytopenic patients: a randomised double-blind study. *Eur J Cancer* **27**: 174.

Auckenthaler R, Michéa-Hamzehpur M, Pechère JC (1986). *In-vitro* activity of newer quinolones against aerobic bacteria. *J Antimicrob Chemother* **17** (Suppl B): 29.

Auger P, Leclerc Y, Pelletier LC, Blain R, Phillips R (1990). Double-blind comparison of pefloxacin and cefazolin as prophylaxis in elective cardiovascular surgery. *J Antimicrob Chemother* **26** (Suppl B): 75.

Ball M, Kanga JM, Meilo H, Debeugny B (1990). Treatment of acute gonococcal urethritis in men with a single dose of 800 mg pefloxacin. *Brit J Clin Pract* **44**: 140.

Baran R, Brun P (1986). Photoonycholysis induced by the fluoroquinolones pefloxacine and ofloxacine. Report on two cases. *Dermatologica* **173**: 185.

Benzakour M, Lagarde C, Benevent D *et al.* (1988). Peritonitis during continuous ambulatory peritoneal dialysis. Treatment with pefloxacin: first results and pharmacokinetics. *Nephron* **50**: 175.

Bernard E, Durant J, Elbaze P, Dellamonica P (1990). Pefloxacin in the treatment of septicaemia: three years' experience. *J Antimicrob Chemother* **26** (Suppl B): 97.

Berthoux F, Alamartine E, Lambert C (1994). More about pefloxacin and nephrotic syndrome. *Nephrol Dial Transplant* **9**: 1838.

Boerema JBJ, Pauwels R, Scheepers J, Crombach W (1986). Efficacy and safety of pefloxacin in the treatment of patients with complicated urinary tract infections. *J Antimicrob Chemother* **17**: 103.

Bonmarchand G, Gres JJ, Lerebours G *et al.* (1989). Penetration of pefloxacin into bronchial secretions. *Antimicrob Ag Chemother* **33**: 391.

Bouvet O, Bressolle F, Courtieu C, Galtier M (1992). Penetration of pefloxacin into gynaecological tissues. *J Antimicrob Chemother* **29**: 579.

Bressolle F, Goncalves F, Gouby A, Galtier M (1994). Pefloxacin clinical pharmacokinetics. *Clin Pharmacokinet* **27**: 418.

Brion N, Lessana A, Mosset F *et al.* (1986). Penetration of pefloxacin in human heart valves. *J Antimicrob Chemother* **17** (Suppl B): 89.

Cacoub P, Wechsler B, Chapelon C *et al.* (1991). Q-fever endocarditis and treatment with the fluoroquinolones. *Arch Intern Med* **151**: 816, 818.

Cajozzo A, Carbone R, Carotenuto M *et al.* (1990). Pefloxacin in the antibacterial treatment of immunodepressed patients. *J Chemother* **2**: 185.

Cardey J, Silvain C, Bouquet S *et al.* (1987). Oral pharmacokinetics and ascitic fluid penetration of pefloxacin in cirrhosis. *Eur J Clin Pharmacol* **33**: 469.

Chacon JP, Criscuolo PD, Kobata CM *et al.* (1990). Prospective randomized comparison of pefloxacin and ampicillin plus gentamicin in the treatment of bacteriologically proven biliary tract infections. *J Antimicrob Chemother* **26** (Suppl B): 167.

Chan PC, Cheng IK, Chan MK, Wong WT (1990). Clinical experience with pefloxacin in patients with urinary tract infections. *Brit J Clin Pract* **44**: 564.

Chapuis L, Cadranel JF, Nordmann P *et al.* (1993). Grand mal seizures as a complication of treatment with pefloxacin in patients with cirrhosis. A report of three cases. *J Hepatol* **19**: 383.

Cheong LL, Chan RK, Nadarajah M (1992). Pefloxacin and ciprofloxacin in the treatment of uncomplicated gonococcal urethritis in males. *Genitourin Med* **68**: 260.

Cheong YM, Joseph PG, Koay AS (1987). *In-vitro* susceptibility of *Pseudomonas pseudomallei* isolated in Malaysia to some new cephalosporins and a quinolone. *Southeast Asian J Trop Med Public Hlth* **18**: 94.

Chevalier X, Albengres E, Voisin MC *et al.* (1992). A case of destructive polyarthropathy in a 17-year-old youth following pefloxacin treatment. *Drug Saf* **7**: 310.

Christ W (1990). Central nervous system toxicity of quinolones: human and animal findings. *J Antimicrob Chemother* **26** (Suppl B): 219.

Christ W, Lehnert T, Ulbrich B (1988). Specific toxicologic aspects of the quinolones. *Rev Infect Dis* **10** (Suppl 1): S141.

Clarke AM, Zemcov SJV, Campbell ME (1985). *In-vitro* activity of pefloxacin compared to enoxacin, norfloxacin, gentamicin and new beta-lactams. *J Antimicrob Chemother* **15**: 39.

Cristiano P, Morelli G, Briante V *et al.* (1989). Clinical experience with pefloxacin in the therapy of typhoid fever. *Infection* **17**: 86.

Cristiano P, Imparato L, Carpinelli C *et al.* (1995). Pefloxacin versus chloramphenicol in the therapy of typhoid fever. *Infection* **23**: 103.

D'Antonio D, Iacone A, Fioritoni G *et al.* (1992). Comparison of norfloxacin and pefloxacin in the prophylaxis of bacterial infection in neutropenic cancer patients. *Drugs Exp Clin Res* **18**: 141.

D'Antonio D, Piccolomini R, Iacone A *et al.* (1994). Comparison of ciprofloxacin, ofloxacin and pefloxacin for the prevention of the bacterial infection in neutropenic patients with haematological malignancies. *J Antimicrob Chemother* **33**: 837.

Danan G, Montay G, Cunci R, Erlinger S (1985). Pefloxacin kinetics in cirrhosis. *Clin Pharmacol Ther* **38**: 439.

Davies BI, Maesen FP (1989). Drug interactions with quinolones. *Rev Infect Dis* **11** (Suppl 5): S1083.

Davies S, Sparham PD, Spencer RC (1987). Comparative *in-vitro* activity of five fluoroquinolones against mycobacteria. *J Antimicrob Chemother* **19**: 605.

Dellamonica P, Bernard E, Etesse H, Garraffo R (1986). The diffusion of pefloxacin into bone and the treatment of osteomyelitis. *J Antimicrob Chemother* **17**: 93.

Dellamonica P, Bernard E, Etesse H *et al.* (1989). Evaluation of pefloxacin, ofloxacin and ciprofloxacin in the treatment of thirty-nine cases of chronic osteomyelitis. *Eur J Clin Microbiol Infect Dis* **8**: 1024.

Dellamonica P, Etesse-Carsenti H, Bernard E *et al.* (1990). Pefloxacin in the treatment of bone infections associated with foreign material. *J Antimicrob Chemother* **26** (Suppl B): 199.

Delmee M, Avesani V (1986). Comparative *in vitro* activity of seven quinolones against 100 clinical isolates of *Clostridium difficile*. *Antimicrob Ag Chemother* **29**: 374.

Deloron P, Lepers JP, Raharimalala L *et al.* (1991). Pefloxacin for falciparum malaria: only modest success. *Ann Intern Med* **114**: 874.

Desplaces N, Acar JF (1988). New quinolones in the treatment of joint and bone infections. *Rev Infect Dis* **10** (Suppl 1): S179.

Desplaces N, Gutmann L, Carlet J *et al.* (1986). The new quinolones and their combinations with other agents for therapy of severe infections. *J Antimicrob Chemother* **17** (Suppl A): 25.

Divo AA, Sartorelli AC, Patton CL, Bia FJ (1988). Activity of fluoroquinolone antibiotics against *Plasmodium falciparum in vitro*. *Antimicrob Ag Chemother* **32**: 1182.

Dournon E, Rajagopalan P, Vilde JL, Pocidalo JJ (1986). Efficacy of pefloxacin in comparison with erythromycin in the treatment of experimental guinea pig legionellosis. *J Antimicrob Chemother* **17**: 41.

Dournon E, Mayaud C, Wolff M *et al.* (1990). Comparison of the activity of three antibiotic regimens in severe Legionnaires' disease. *J Antimicrob Chemother* **26** (Suppl B): 129.

Dow J, Chazal J, Frydman AM *et al.* (1986). Transfer kinetics of pefloxacin into cerebro-spinal fluid after one hour iv infusion of 400 mg in man. *J Antimicrob Chemother* **17**: 81.

DuPont HL (1993). Quinolones in *Salmonella typhi* infection. *Drugs* **45** (Suppl 3): 119.

Edlund C, Nord CE (1986). Comparative *in vitro* activities of ciprofloxacin, enoxacin, norfloxacin, ofloxacin and pefloxacin against *Bacteroides fragilis* and *Clostridium difficile*. *Scand J Infect Dis* **18**: 149.

Eliopoulos GM (1988). New quinolones: pharmacology, pharmacokinetics, and dosing in patients with renal insufficiency. *Rev Infect Dis* **10** (Suppl 1): S102.

Eliopoulos GM, Eliopoulos CT (1993). Activity *in vitro* of the quinolones. In *Quinolone Antimicrobial Agents* 2nd edn (Hooper DC, Wolfson JS, eds), p. 161, Washington, DC: American Society of Microbiology.

Farina C, Boiron P, Goglio A, Provost F (1995). Human nocardiosis in northern Italy from 1982 to 1992. Northern Italy Collaborative Group on Nocardiosis. *Scand J Infect Dis* **27**: 23.

Fass RJ, Helsel VL (1987). *In vitro* antistaphylococcal activity of pefloxacin alone and in combination with other antistaphylococcal drugs. *Antimicrob Ag Chemother* **31**: 1457.

Fillastre JP, Leroy A, Moulin B *et al.* (1990). Pharmacokinetics of quinolones in renal insufficiency. *J Antimicrob Chemother* **26** (Suppl B): 51.

Fillastre JP, Leroy A, Borsa-Lebas F *et al.* (1993). Lack of effect of ketoprofen on the pharmacokinetics of pefloxacin and ofloxacin. *J Antimicrob Chemother* **31**: 805.

Frydman AM, Le Roux Y, Lefebvre MA *et al.* (1985). Pharmacokinetics of pefloxacin after repeated intravenous and oral administration (400 mg bid). in young healthy volunteers. *J Antimicrob Chemother* **17**: 65.

Frydman AM, Le Roux Y, Lefebvre MA *et al.* (1986). Pharmacokinetics of pefloxacin after repeated intravenous and oral administration (400 mg bid). in young healthy volunteers. *J Antimicrob Chemother* **17** (Suppl B): 65.

Galtier M, Bressolle F, de la Coussaye JE *et al.* (1993). Multiple-dose pharmacokinetics of pefloxacin in patients with hepatocellular deficiency. *Clin Pharmacokinet* **25**: 415.

Gardembas-Pain M, Desablens B, Sensebe L *et al.* (1991). Home treatment of febrile neutropenia: an empirical oral antibiotic regimen. *Ann Oncol* **2**: 485.

Geffriaud-Ricouard C, Jungers P, Chauveau D, Grunfeld JP (1993). Inefficacy and toxicity of pefloxacin in focal and segmental glomerulosclerosis with steroid-resistant nephrotic syndrome. *Lancet* **341**: 1475.

Gelber RH, Iranmanesh A, Murray L *et al.* (1992). Activities of various quinolone antibiotics against *Mycobacterium leprae* in infected mice. *Antimicrob Ag Chemother* **36**: 2544.

Gendrel D, Raymond J, Legall MA *et al.* (1993). Use of pefloxacin after failure of initial antibiotic treatment in children with severe salmonellosis. *Eur J Clin Microbiol Infect Dis* **12**: 209.

Georgopoulos A, Breyer S, Georgopoulos M *et al.* (1988). In-vitro activity of fleroxacin. *J Antimicrob Chemother* **22** (Suppl D): 25.

Giamarellou H, Kolokythas E, Petrikkos G *et al.* (1989a). Pharmacokinetics of three newer quinolones in pregnant and lactating women. *Amer J Med* **87**: 49S.

Giamarellou H, Perdikaris G, Galanakis N *et al.* (1989b). Pefloxacin versus ceftazidime in the treatment of a variety of gram- negative-bacterial infections. *Antimicrob Ag Chemother* **33**: 1362.

Giamarellou H, Mandragos K, Bechrakis P *et al.* (1990). Pefloxacin versus imipenem in the therapy of nosocomial lung infections of intensive care unit patients. *J Antimicrob Chemother* **26** (Suppl B): 117.

Giamarellou H, Kanellas D, Kavouklis E *et al.* (1993). Comparative pharmacokinetics of ciprofloxacin, ofloxacin and pefloxacin in human aqueous humour. *Eur J Clin Microbiol Infect Dis* **12**: 293.

Ginsburg C, Toledano D, Deray G *et al.* (1994). Pefloxacin as first-line treatment in nephrotic syndrome. *Nephrol Dial Transplant* **9**: 335.

Giuliano M, Pantosti A, Gentile G *et al.* (1989). Effects on oral and intestinal microfloras of norfloxacin and pefloxacin for selective decontamination in bone marrow transplant patients. *Antimicrob Ag Chemother* **33**: 1709.

Glupczynski Y, Delmee M, Bruck C *et al.* (1988). Susceptibility of clinical isolates of *Campylobacter pylori* to 24 antimicrobial and anti-ulcer agents. *Eur J Epidemiol* **4**: 154.

Gonzalez JP, Henwood JM (1989). Pefloxacin A review of its antibacterial activity, pharmacokinetic properties and therapeutic use. *Drugs* **37**: 628.

Gorzynski EA, Gutman SI, Allen W (1989). Comparative antimycobacterial activities of difloxacin, temafloxacin, enoxacin, pefloxacin, reference fluoroquinolones, and a new macrolide, clarithromycin. *Antimicrob Ag Chemother* **33**: 591.

Grassi C, Catena E, de Iola G *et al.* (1990). Pefloxacin in lower respiratory tract infections. *J Antimicrob Chemother* **26** (Suppl B): 103.

Grenier B (1989). Use of the new quinolones in cystic fibrosis. *Rev Infect Dis* **11** (Suppl 5): S1245.

Gruneberg RN, Felmingham D, O'Hare MD *et al.* (1988). The comparative in-vitro activity of ofloxacin. *J Antimicrob Chemother* **22** (Suppl C): 9.

Guibert J, Boutelier R, Guyot A (1990). A clinical trial of pefloxacin in prostatitis. *J Antimicrob Chemother* **26** (Suppl B): 161.

Guyon P, Cassel-Beraud AM, Rakotonirina G, Gendrel D (1994). Short-term pefloxacin therapy in Madagascan children with shigellosis due to multiresistant organisms. *Clin Infect Dis* **19**: 1172.

Hajji M, el Mdaghri N, Benbachir M *et al.* (1988). Prospective randomized comparative trial of pefloxacin versus cotrimoxazole in the treatment of typhoid fever in adults. *Eur J Clin Microbiol Infect Dis* **7**: 361.

Halkin H (1988). Adverse effects of the fluoroquinolones. *Rev Infect Dis* **10** (Suppl 1): S258.

Hoban DJ (1989). Comparative *in vitro* activity of quinolones. *Clin Invest Med* **12**: 10.

Hoogkamp-Korstanje JA (1987). Antibiotics in *Yersinia enterocolitica* infections. *J Antimicrob Chemother* **20**: 123.

Hoppe JE, Simon CG (1990). *In vitro* susceptibilities of *Bordetella pertussis* and *Bordetella parapertussis* to seven fluoroquinolones. *Antimicrob Ag Chemother* **34**: 2287.

Humbert G, Brumpt I, Montay G *et al.* (1991). Influence of rifampin on the pharmacokinetics of pefloxacin. *Clin Pharmacol Ther* **50**: 682.

International Antimicrobial Therapy Cooperative Group of the European Organization for Research and Treatment of Cancer (1994). *JAMA* **272**: 1183.

Isaacs RD, Ellis-Pegler RB (1987). Successful treatment of *Morganella morganii* meningitis with pefloxacin mesylate. *J Antimicrob Chemother* **20**: 769.

Jabarit-Aldighieri N, Torres H, Raoult D (1992). Susceptibility of *Rickettsia conorii*, *R. rickettsii*, and *Coxiella burnetii* to PD 127,391, PD 131,628, pefloxacin, ofloxacin, and ciprofloxacin. *Antimicrob Ag Chemother* **36**: 2529.

Jaehde U, Sorgel F, Stephan U, Schunack W (1994). Effect of an antacid containing magnesium and aluminum on absorption, metabolism, and mechanism of renal elimination of pefloxacin in humans. *Antimicrob Ag Chemother* **38**: 1129.

Janin N, Meugnier H, Desnottes JF *et al.* (1987). Recovery of pefloxacin in saliva and feces and its action on oral and fecal floras of healthy volunteers. *Antimicrob Ag Chemother* **31**: 1665.

Jardin A, Cesana M (1995). Randomized, double-blind comparison of single-dose regimens of rufloxacin and pefloxacin for acute uncomplicated cystitis in women. French Multicenter Urinary Tract Infection-Rufloxacin Group. *Antimicrob Ag Chemother* **39**: 215.

Ji B, Grosset J (1991). Ofloxacin for the treatment of leprosy. *Acta Leprol* **7**: 321.

Joly-Guillou ML, Bergogne-Berezin E (1986). *In vitro* activity of antimicrobial agents against *Acinetobacter calcoaceticus*. *Drugs Exp Clin Res* **12**: 949.

Joly-Guillou ML, Bergogne-Berezin E (1992). *In-vitro* activity of sparfloxacin, pefloxacin, ciprofloxacin and temafloxacin against clinical isolates of *Acinetobacter* spp. *J Antimicrob Chemother* **29**: 466.

Jones BM, Geary I, Lee ME, Duerden BI (1986). Activity of pefloxacin and thirteen other antimicrobial agents *in vitro* against isolates from hospital and genitourinary infections. *J Antimicrob Chemother* **17**: 739.

Jones RN (1989). Antimicrobial activity and interaction of pefloxacin and its principal metabolites Collaborative Antimicrobial Susceptibility Testing Group. *Eur J Clin Microbiol Infect Dis* **8**: 551.

Jungers P, Ganeval D, Hannedouche T *et al.* (1987). Steady-state levels of pefloxacin and its metabolites in patients with severe renal impairment. *Eur J Clin Pharmacol* **33**: 463.

Karabalut N, Drusano GL (1993). Pharmacokinetics of the quinolone antimicrobial agents. In *Quinolone Antimicrobial Agents* 2nd edn (Hooper

DC, Wolfson JS, eds), p. 195. Washington, DC: American Society of Microbiology.

Kattan J, Droz JP, Ribrag V *et al.* (1992). Non-nephrotoxic empiric antimicrobial therapy in febrile neutropenic cancer patients. *Eur J Cancer* **28A**: 867.

Keren G, Keysary A, Goldwasser R, Rubinstein E (1994). The inhibitory effect of fluoroquinolones on *Coxiella burnetii* growth in *in-vitro* systems. *J Antimicrob Chemother* **33**: 1253.

King A, Phillips I (1986a). The comparative *in-vitro* activity of eight newer quinolones and nalidixic acid. *J Antimicrob Chemother* **18** (Suppl D): 1.

King A, Phillips I (1986b). The comparative *in-vitro* activity of pefloxacin. *J Antimicrob Chemother* **17** (Suppl B): 1.

Korinek AM, Montay G, Bianchi A *et al.* (1988). Penetration of pefloxacin into brain tissue. *Rev Infect Dis* **10** (Suppl 1): S257.

Kuijper EJ, Peeters MF, Schoenmakers BS, Zanen HC (1989). Antimicrobial susceptibility of sixty human fecal isolates of *Aeromonas* species. *Eur J Clin Microbiol Infect Dis* **8**: 248.

Lauwers S, Vincken W, Naessens A, Pierard D (1986). Efficacy and safety of pefloxacin in the treatment of severe infections in patients hospitalized in intensive care units. *J Antimicrob Chemother* **17** (Suppl B): 111.

Le Loet X, Fessard C, Noblet C *et al.* (1991). Severe polyarthropathy in an adolescent treated with pefloxacin. *J Rheumatol* **18**: 1941.

Ligtvoet EEJ, Wickerhoff-Minoggio T (1985). *In-vitro* activity of pefloxacin compared with six other quinolones. *J Antimicrob Chemother* **16**: 485.

Limson BM, Pena AC, Garvez MD (1990). Monotherapy with pefloxacin in multidrug-resistant nosocomial gram-negative bacteraemia. *J Antimicrob Chemother* **26** (Suppl B): 91.

Linder N, Dagan R, Kuint J *et al.* (1994). Ventriculitis caused by *Klebsiella pneumoniae* successfully treated with pefloxacin in a neonate. *Infection* **22**: 210.

Lode H, Hoffken G, Boeckk M *et al.* (1990). Quinolone pharmacokinetics and metabolism. *J Antimicrob Chemother* **26** (Suppl B): 41.

Lucain C, Regamey P, Bellido F, Pechere JC (1989). Resistance emerging after pefloxacin therapy of experimental *Enterobacter cloacae* peritonitis. *Antimicrob Ag Chemother* **33**: 937.

Lucet JC, Tilly H, Lerebours G *et al.* (1988). Neurological toxicity related to pefloxacin. *J Antimicrob Chemother* **21**: 811.

Lye WC, Lee EJ, van der Straaten J (1993). Intraperitoneal vancomycin/oral pefloxacin versus intraperitoneal vancomycin/gentamicin in the treatment of continuous ambulatory peritoneal dialysis peritonitis. *Perit Dial Int* **13** (Suppl 2): S348.

Maesen FP, Davies BI, Teengs JP (1985). Pefloxacin in acute exacerbations of chronic bronchitis. *J Antimicrob Chemother* **16**: 379.

Maesen FP, Davies BI, Geraedts WH, Baur C (1987). The use of quinolones in respiratory tract infections. *Drugs* **34** (Suppl 1): 74.

Malmborg AS, Brattstrom C, Tyden G (1990). Penetration of pefloxacin into human allograft pancreatic juice. *J Antimicrob Chemother* **25**: 393.

Martin C, Gouin F, Fourrier F *et al.* (1988). Pefloxacin in the treatment of nosocomial lower respiratory tract infections in intensive care patients. *J Antimicrob Chemother* **21**: 795.

Mayer DG (1987). Overview of toxicological studies. *Drugs* **34** (Suppl 1): 150.

Meunier F (1990). Prevention of infections in neutropenic patients with pefloxacin. *J Antimicrob Chemother* **26** (Suppl B): 69.

Michea-Hamzehpour M, Lucain C, Pechère JC (1991). Resistance to pefloxacin in *Pseudomonas aeruginosa*. *Antimicrob Ag Chemother* **35**: 512.

Micozzi A, Venditti M, Gentile G *et al.* (1990). Successful treatment of *Brucella melitensis* endocarditis with pefloxacin. *Eur J Clin Microbiol Infect Dis* **9**: 440.

Modai J (1991). Potential role of fluoroquinolones in the treatment of bacterial meningitis. *Eur J Clin Microbiol Infect Dis* **10**: 291.

Montay G, Gaillot J (1990). Pharmacokinetics of fluoroquinolones in hepatic failure. *J Antimicrob Chemother* **26** (Suppl B): 61.

Montay G, Goueffon Y, Roquet F (1984). Absorption, distribution, metabolic fate, and elimination of pefloxacin mesylate in mice, rats, dogs, monkeys, and humans. *Antimicrob Ag Chemother* **25**: 463.

Montay G, Jacquot C, Bariety J *et al.* (1985). Pharmacokinetics of pefloxacin in renal insufficiency. *Eur J Clin Pharmacol* **29**: 345.

Moran JS, Levine WC (1995). Drugs of choice for the treatment of uncomplicated gonococcal infections. *Clin Infect Dis* **20** (Suppl 1): S47.

N'Deli L, Guelpa-Lauras CC, Perani EG, Grosset JH (1990). Effectiveness of pefloxacin in the treatment of lepromatous leprosy. *Int J Lepr Other Mycobact Dis* **58**: 12.

Nikolaidis P (1990). Newer quinolones in the treatment of continuous ambulatory peritoneal dialysis (CAPD). related infections. *Perit Dial Int* **10**: 127.

Nikolaidis P, Walker SE, Dombros N *et al.* (1991). Single-dose pefloxacin pharmacokinetics and metabolism in patients undergoing continuous ambulatory peritoneal dialysis (CAPD). *Perit Dial Int* **11**: 59.

Nord CE (1988). Effect of new quinolones on the human gastrointestinal microflora. *Rev Infect Dis* **10** (Suppl 1): S193.

Norrby SR (1988). 4-Quinolones in the treatment of infections of the central nervous system. *Rev Infect Dis* **10** (Suppl 1): S253.

Oncel M, Peyman GA (1993). Intravitreal penetration of oral pefloxacin in humans. *Int Ophthalmol* **17**: 217.

Outman WR, Nightingale CH (1989). Metabolism and the fluoroquinolones. *Amer J Med* **87**: 37S.

Pallavicini F, Antinori A, Federico G *et al.* (1989). Influence of two quinolones, ofloxacin and pefloxacin, on human myelopoiesis *in vitro*. *Antimicrob Ag Chemother* **33**: 122.

Panteix G, Harf R, Desnottes JF *et al.* (1994). Accumulation of pefloxacin in the lower respiratory tract demonstrated by bronchoalveolar lavage. *J Antimicrob Chemother* **33**: 979.

Pattyn SF (1987). Activity of ofloxacin and pefloxacin against *Mycobacterium leprae* in mice. *Antimicrob Ag Chemother* **31**: 671.

Petersen EE, Wingen F, Fairchild KL *et al.* (1990). Single dose pefloxacin compared with multiple dose co-trimoxazole in cystitis. *J Antimicrob Chemother* **26** (Suppl B): 147.

Petitjean O, Pangon B, Brion N *et al.* (1993). Pharmacokinetics and bactericidal activities of one 800-milligram dose versus two 400-milligram doses of intravenously administered pefloxacin in healthy volunteers. *Antimicrob Ag Chemother* **37**: 737.

Petrikkos G, Goumas P, Moschovakis E, Giamarellou H (1992). Penetration of pefloxacin into maxillary sinus cavity and nasal secretions. *Eur J Clin Microbiol Infect Dis* **11**: 828.

Phillips I, King A (1988). Comparative activity of the 4-quinolones. *Rev Infect Dis* **10** (Suppl 1): S70.

Potgieter PD (1990). Pefloxacin therapy for nosocomial infections in the intensive care unit. *J Antimicrob Chemother* **26** (Suppl B): 83.

Pruna A, Metivier F, Akposso K *et al.* (1992). Pefloxacin as first-line treatment in nephrotic syndrome. *Lancet* **340**: 728.

Qadri SM, Akhtar M, Ueno Y, al-Sibai MB (1989). Susceptibility of *Brucella melitensis* to fluoroquinolones. *Drugs Exp Clin Res* **15**: 483.

Quentin R, Koubaa N, Cattier B *et al.* (1988). *In vitro* activities of five new quinolones against 88 genital and neonatal *Haemophilus* isolates. *Antimicrob Ag Chemother* **32**: 147.

Ragnaud JM, Roche-Bezian MC, Dupon M, Wone C (1987). Management of peritonitis related to chronic ambulatory peritoneal dialysis (CAPD) using two daily intraperitoneal injections of 400 mg pefloxacin. *Chemioterapia* **6**: 481.

Rajagopalan-Levasseur P, Dournon E, Dameron G *et al.* (1990). Comparative postantibacterial activities of pefloxacin, ciprofloxacin, and ofloxacin against intracellular multiplication of *Legionella pneumophila* serogroup 1. *Antimicrob Ag Chemother* **34**: 1733.

Rao S (1995). An uncontrolled trial of pefloxacin in the retreatment of patients with pulmonary tuberculosis. *Tuber Lung Dis* **76**: 219.

Raoult D, Roussellier P, Vestris G *et al.* (1987). Susceptibility of *Rickettsia conorii* and *R rickettsii* to pefloxacin, *in vitro* and *in ovo*. *J Antimicrob Chemother* **19**: 303.

Raoult D, Yeaman MR, Baca OG (1989). Susceptibility of *Coxiella burnetii* to pefloxacin and ofloxacin *in ovo* and in persistently infected L929 cells. *Antimicrob Ag Chemother* **33**: 621.

Raymond J, Moulin F, Badoual J, Gendrel D (1994). Eradication of convalescent-phase *Salmonella* carriage in children with two oral doses of pefloxacin. *Eur J Clin Microbiol Infect Dis* **13**: 307.

Ribard P, Audisio F, Kahn MF *et al.* (1992). Seven Achilles tendinitis including three complicated by rupture during fluoroquinolone therapy. *J Rheumatol* **19**: 1479.

Robson RA (1992). The effects of quinolones on xanthine pharmacokinetics. *Amer J Med* **92**: 22S.

Rose TF, Bremner DA, Collins J *et al.* (1990a). Plasma and dialysate levels of pefloxacin and its metabolites in CAPD patients with peritonitis. *J Antimicrob Chemother* **25**: 657.

Rose TF, Ellis-Pegler R, Collins J, Small M (1990b). Oral pefloxacin mesylate in the treatment of continuous ambulatory peritoneal dialysis associated peritonitis: an open non-comparative study. *J Antimicrob Chemother* **25**: 853.

Rutanarugsa A, Vorachit M, Polnikorn N, Jayanetra P (1990). Drug resistance of *Haemophilus ducreyi*. *Southeast Asian J Trop Med Public Hlth* **21**: 185.

Salmon D, Deloron P, Gaudin C *et al.* (1990). Activities of pefloxacin and ciprofloxacin against experimental malaria in mice. *Antimicrob Ag Chemother* **34**: 2327.

Salvanet A, Fisch A, Lafaix C *et al.* (1986). Pefloxacin concentrations in human aqueous humour and lens. *J Antimicrob Chemother* **18**: 199.

Scheife RT, Cramer WR, Decker EL (1993). Photosensitizing potential of ofloxacin. *Int J Dermatol* **32**: 413.

Scheld WM (1989). Quinolone therapy for infections of the central nervous system. *Rev Infect Dis* **11** (Suppl 5): S1194.

Schmit JL, Hary L, Bou P *et al.* (1991). Pharmacokinetics of single-dose intravenous, oral, and intraperitoneal pefloxacin in patients on chronic ambulatory peritoneal dialysis. *Antimicrob Ag Chemother* **35**: 1492.

Segev S, Barzilai A, Rosen N *et al.* (1989). Pefloxacin treatment of meningitis caused by gram-negative bacteria. *Arch Intern Med* **149**: 1314.

Segev S, Rosen N, Joseph G *et al.* (1990a). Pefloxacin efficacy in gram-negative bacillary meningitis. *J Antimicrob Chemother* **26** (Suppl B): 187.

Segev S, Rosen N, Pitlik SD *et al.* (1990b). Pefloxacin versus ceftazidime in therapy of soft tissue infections in compromised patients. *J Antimicrob Chemother* **26** (Suppl B): 193.

Shalit I, Haas H, Berger SA (1992). Susceptibility of *Pseudomonas aeruginosa* to fluoroquinolones following four years of use in a tertiary care hospital. *J Antimicrob Chemother* **30**: 149.

Shasha B, Lang R, Rubinstein E (1992). Therapy of experimental murine brucellosis with streptomycin, co-trimoxazole, ciprofloxacin, ofloxacin, pefloxacin, doxycycline, and rifampin. *Antimicrob Ag Chemother* **36**: 973.

Simon J, Guyot A (1990). Pefloxacin: safety in man. *J Antimicrob Chemother* **26** (Suppl B): 215.

Somekh E, Douer D, Shaked N, Rubinstein E (1989). *In vitro* effects of ciprofloxacin and pefloxacin on growth of normal human hematopoietic progenitor cells and on leukemic cell lines. *J Pharmacol Exp Ther* **248**: 415.

Sturm AW (1987). Comparison of antimicrobial susceptibility patterns of fifty-seven strains of *Haemophilus ducreyi* isolated in Amsterdam from 1978 to 1985. *J Antimicrob Chemother* **19**: 187.

Swedish Study Group (1990). A randomized multicentre trial of pefloxacin plus metronidazole and gentamicin plus metronidazole in the treatment of severe intra-abdominal infections. Report from a Swedish Study Group. *J Antimicrob Chemother* **26** (Suppl B): 173.

Syrjala H, Schildt R, Raisainen S (1991). *In vitro* susceptibility of *Francisella tularensis* to fluoroquinolones and treatment of tularemia with norfloxacin and ciprofloxacin. *Eur J Clin Microbiol Infect Dis* **10**: 68.

Texier-Maugein J, Mormede M, Fourche J, Bebear C (1987). *In vitro* activity of four fluoroquinolones against eighty-six isolates of myco-bacteria. *Eur J Clin Microbiol* **6**: 584.

Thys JP, Jacobs F, Motte S (1989). Quinolones in the treatment of lower respiratory tract infections. *Rev Infect Dis* **11** (Suppl 5): S1212.

Timmerman C, Hoepelman I, de Hond J *et al.* (1992). Open, randomized comparison of pefloxacin and cefotaxime in the treatment of complicated urinary tract infections. *Infection* **20**: 34.

Tio TT, Sindhunata IR, Wagenvoort JH *et al.* (1990). Pefloxacin compared with cefotaxime for treating men with uncomplicated gonococcal urethritis. *J Antimicrob Chemother* **26** (Suppl B): 141.

Van der Auwera P, Grenier P, Glupczynski Y, Pierard D (1989). *In-vitro* activity of lomefloxacin in comparison with pefloxacin and ofloxacin. *J Antimicrob Chemother* **23**: 209.

van Balen FA, Touw-Otten FW, de Melker RA (1990). Single-dose pefloxacin versus five-days treatment with norfloxacin in uncomplicated cystitis in women. *J Antimicrob Chemother* **26** (Suppl B): 153.

Van Caekenberghe DL, Pattyn SR (1984). *In vitro* activity of ciprofloxacin compared with those of other new fluorinated piperazinyl-substituted quinoline derivatives. *Antimicrob Ag Chemother* **25**: 518.

van de Leur JJ, Vollaard EJ, Janssen AJ, Dofferhoff AS (1995). Concentration of pefloxacin in feces during infection prophylaxis in neutropenic patients. *Antimicrob Ag Chemother* **39**: 1182.

van der Willigen AH, Degener JE, Vogel M *et al.* (1990). *In vitro* activities of seven quinolone derivatives against *Neisseria gonorrhoeae*. *Arznei-mittelforschung* **40**: 684.

Vanderdonckt J (1990). Comparison of pefloxacin with ceftazidime in severe bronchopulmonary infections. *J Antimicrob Chemother* **26** (Suppl B): 111.

Varini C, Dami A, Valenza T *et al.* (1992). Pefloxacin penetration of renal parenchyma. *J Antimicrob Chemother* **29**: 86.

Venditti M, Gelfusa V, Tarasi A *et al.* (1990). Antimicrobial susceptibilities of *Erysipelothrix rhusiopathiae*. *Antimicrob Ag Chemother* **34**: 2038.

Vollaard EJ, Clasener HA, Janssen AJ (1990). Decontamination of the bowel by intravenous administration of pefloxacin. *J Antimicrob Chemother* **26**: 847.

Webberley JM, Andrews JM, Ashby JP *et al.* (1987). Pharmacokinetics and tissue penetration of orally administered pefloxacin. *Eur J Clin Microbiol* **6**: 521.

Webberley JM, Donovan IA, Ashby JP *et al.* (1989). Intraperitoneal penetration of pefloxacin. *Rev Infect Dis* **11** (Suppl 5): S1294.

Westphal JF, Brogard JM (1993). Clinical pharmacokinetics of newer antibacterial agents in liver disease. *Clin Pharmacokinet* **24**: 46.

Wijnands WJ, Vree TB, van Herwaarden CL (1986). The influence of quinolone derivatives on theophylline clearance. *Brit J Clin Pharmacol* **22**: 677.

Wijnands WJ, Vree TB, Baars AM, van Herwaarden CL (1987). Steady-state kinetics of the quinolone derivatives ofloxacin, enoxacin, cipro-floxacin and pefloxacin during maintenance treatment with theophylline. *Drugs* **34** (Suppl 1): 159.

Wise R, Lister D, McNulty CA *et al.* (1986). The comparative pharmacoki-netics of five quinolones. *J Antimicrob Chemother* **18** (Suppl D): 71.

Wise R, Griggs D, Andrews JM (1988). Pharmacokinetics of the quinolones in volunteers: a proposed dosing schedule. *Rev Infect Dis* **10** (Suppl 1): S83.

Wittke RR, Adam D (1989). Diffusion of pefloxacin in the biliary tract. *Rev Infect Dis* **11** (Suppl 5): S1297.

Wolff M, Regnier B, Daldoss C *et al.* (1984). Penetration of pefloxacin into cerebrospinal fluid of patients with meningitis. *Antimicrob Ag Chemother* **26**: 289.

Yeaman MR, Roman MJ, Baca OG (1989). Antibiotic susceptibilities of two *Coxiella burnetii* isolates implicated in distinct clinical syndromes. *Antimicrob Ag Chemother* **33**: 1052.

Yourassowsky E, Van der Linden MP, Crokaert F, Glupczynski Y (1986). *In-vitro* activity of pefloxacin compared to other antibiotics. *J Antimicrob Chemother* **17** (Suppl B): 19.

Fleroxacin

Description

Fleroxacin (Ro 23–6240, AM 833) is different from other fluoroquinolones such as ciprofloxacin or ofloxacin, since it is a trifluorinated quinolone having three fluorine atoms rather than one, attached to the quinolone ring system. It is a 6,8-difluoro-1-(2-fluorethyl)-1,4-dihydro-7-(4-methyl-1-piperazinyl)-4-oxo-3-quinolonine carboxylic acid which was developed by Hoffmann-LaRoche Ltd (Stuck *et al.*, 1992). Clinical experience with fleroxacin for gonorrhea and urinary tract infections suggests activity comparable with other fluoroquinolones, while its use in other conditions looks promising, but further data are required. A major advantage of fleroxacin is its long half-life allowing once-daily dosing. However, it appears to have a higher rate of adverse side-effects than other fluoroquinolones – the clinical importance of which need to be weighed against the potential benefits of once-daily therapy. Many of the side-effects appear to be dose-related.

Sensitive Organisms

Similar to other fluoroquinolones, fleroxacin has a broad spectrum of *in vitro* activity; however, this is generally less than that of ciprofloxacin, sparfloxacin and tosufloxacin; roughly comparable with ofloxacin and norfloxacin; and possibly superior to enoxacin, lomefloxacin, and pefloxacin – although data vary considerably regarding these latter agents (Chin *et al.*, 1986; Hirai *et al.*, 1986; Fass and Helsel, 1987; Aoyama *et al.*, 1988; Bremner *et al.*, 1988; Georgopoulos *et al.*, 1988; Machka and Braveny, 1988; Paganoni *et al.*, 1988; Verschraegen *et al.*, 1988; Barry and Fuchs, 1991; Beskid and Prosser, 1993; Prosser and Beskid, 1995).

1 Gram-negative bacteria

*Enterobacter*iaciae are very susceptible, with a mean MIC_{90} of less than 0.5 μg per ml for the majority of species. *Providencia stuartii*, *Pr. rettgeri*, and *Salmonella* spp. are less susceptible, but still exhibit MIC_{90} of generally less than 2 μg per ml. *Serratia marcescens* may be relatively resistant with a mean MIC_{90} of 3.4 μg per ml noted (Chin *et al.*, 1986; Hirai *et al.*, 1986; Manek *et al.*, 1986; Bremner *et al.*, 1988; Georgopoulos *et al.*, 1988; Paganoni *et al.*, 1988; Barry and Fuchs, 1991; Arman *et al.*, 1994; Prosser and Beskid, 1995). Other Gram-negative bacteria such as *Haemophilus*, *Moraxella*, *Neisseria*, *Aeromonas*, *Bordetella*, *Acinetobacter*, *Vibrio* and *Legionella* spp. and *Brucella melitensis* and *Pleisiomonas shigelloides* are susceptible. *Campylobacter* spp. are less susceptible (MIC_{90} 1–2 μg per ml), while *Alcaligenes* spp. are resistant (MIC_{90} 4–8 μg per ml). *Helicobacter pylori* is resistant (MIC_{90} 4 μg per ml) (Hupertz *et al.*, 1988; Simor *et al.*, 1989). Compared with ciprofloxacin, fleroxacin has relatively poor activity against *Pseudomonas aeruginosa*, with many reports of MIC_{90} >8 μg per ml. Similarly, most other *Pseudomonas* spp. and *Stenotrophomonas* (*Xanthomonas*) *maltophilia* are often resistant (Hohl *et al.*, 1987; Le Saux *et al.*, 1987; Abeck *et al.*, 1988; Aoyama *et al.*, 1988; Paganoni *et al.*, 1988; Hoppe and Simon, 1990; Barry and Fuchs, 1991; Bongaerts and Hoogkamp-Korstanje, 1993; Rice and Knapp, 1994; Prosser and Breskid, 1995).

Similar to many other fluoroquinolones, fleroxacin has poor activity against Gram-negative anaerobes such as *Bacteroides fragilis*, other members of the *B. fragilis* group and *Fusobacterium* spp. (Chin *et al.*, 1986; Georgopoulos *et al.*, 1988; Griggs *et al.*, 1989; Balfour *et al.*, 1995).

In vitro studies of combining fleroxacin with either aminoglycosides, beta-lactams, rifampicin, metronidazole or clindamycin demonstrate indifference against *Enterobacteriaceae* or *Ps. aeruginosa* (Zhang and Neu, 1991; Neu and Chin, 1993).

2 Gram-positive bacteria

In general, fleroxacin has anti-staphylococcal activity roughly comparable with, or slightly less than, ciprofloxacin. Methicillin-susceptible *Staphylococcus aureus* and coagulase-negative staphylococci are generally susceptible, while methicillin-resistant staphylococci are more likely to be resistant. Generally *Staph. saprophyticus* are resistant (mean MIC_{90} 3.7 μg per ml) compared with ciprofloxacin (mean MIC_{90} 0.7 μg per ml) (Pohlod *et al.*, 1988; Paganoni *et al.*, 1988; Bannerman *et al.*, 1991; Prosser and Breskid, 1995). Fleroxacin has poor activity against streptococcal species, including *Streptococcus pneumoniae* and *Strep. pyogenes*, compared with ciprofloxacin. Enterococci are generally resistant, as is *Listeria monocytogenes* (MIC_{90} 4 to >16 μg per ml). *Corynebacterium diphtheriae* and *C. jeikeium* are often susceptible (MIC_{90} 1–2 μg per ml). *Nocardia asteroides* is resistant (MIC_{90} 64 μg per ml) (Chin *et al.*, 1986; Manek *et al.*, 1986; Aoyama *et al.*, 1988; Digranes *et al.*, 1988; Georgopoulos *et al.*, 1988; Paganoni *et al.*, 1988; Barry and Jones, 1989; Barry and Fuchs, 1991; Bongaerts and Hoogkamp-Korstanje, 1993).

Anaerobic Gram-positive bacteria such as *Clostridium* spp., *Propionibacterium acnes*, *Peptostreptococcus* spp. and *Peptococcus* spp. are generally resistant to fleroxacin (Chin *et al.*, 1986; Aoyama *et al.*, 1988; Paganoni *et al.*, 1988; Balfour *et al.*, 1995).

3 Mycobacteria

Fleroxacin activity against Mycobacteria spp. is roughly comparable with that of norfloxacin or enoxacin, but is less than that of ciprofloxacin or ofloxacin (Young *et al.*, 1987; Khardori *et al.*, 1989). Fleroxacin MIC_{90} against *Mycobacterium tuberculosis* and *M. bovis* are 2–6.25 μg per ml; *M. kansasii*, 3–4 μg per ml and *M. fortuitum*, 2–6.25 μg per ml. Other mycobacterial species such as *M.avium* complex, *M. chelonae*, *M. marinum*, *M. scrofulaceum* and *M. xenopi* are generally resistant *in vitro*, although these latter three species were susceptible in one study (Ernst and van der Auwera, 1988; Salfinger *et al.*, 1988; Tomioka *et al.*, 1991).

4 Chlamydia, Mycoplasma, Ureaplasma and Coxiella burnetii

Fleroxacin has only borderline activity against *Mycoplasma hominis*, *Ureaplasma urealyticum* and *Chlamydia pneumoniae* (mean MIC 2–4 μg per ml); being less active than ciprofloxacin and especially tetracyclines (Krausse and Ullmann, 1988; Steele-Mortimer and Meier-Ewert, 1988). *Mycoplasma pneumoniae* is relatively resistant with MIC_{90} 4 μg per ml *in vitro* (Kenny and Cartwright, 1991) Fleroxacin concentrations of 1 μg per ml are 100% inhibitory to *Coxiella burnetii in vitro* (Keren *et al.*, 1994).

5 Acquired resistance

Similar to other fluoroquinolones (p. 990), resistance to fleroxacin is increasing among some species, especially *Ps. aeruginosa* and methicillin-resistant *Staph. aureus* (Waites *et al.*, 1994; Balfour *et al.*, 1995). As expected (p. 994), cross-resistance between fleroxacin and other fluoroquinolones is generally complete. Resistance to fleroxacin *in vitro* emerges at a rate of 10^{-7} to 10^{-11}, depending on the organism, the fleroxacin concentrations and the *in vitro* conditions (Chin *et al.*, 1986; Stobberingh *et al.*, 1987; Aoyama *et al.*, 1988; Chapman *et al.*, 1989). In one study of experimental methicillin-susceptible *Staph. aureus* endocarditis in rabbits, resistance to fleroxacin at concentrations 5- and 10-fold the MIC developed in the test strain of *Staph. aureus* in 73% and 27% of cases, respectively, with resistant isolates found mainly in the vegetations (Kaatz *et al.*, 1991). These data reinforce the contention that fleroxacin and some other fluoroquinolones should not be used as first-line therapeutic agents for serious *Staph. aureus* infections.

6 Minimum inhibitory concentrations

The MICs of fleroxacin against selected bacterial species are shown in Table II.6, pp. 986–987.

Mode of Administration and Dosage

1 Oral administration

The usual recommended dose of oral fleroxacin for mild-to-moderate infections such as uncomplicated urinary tract infections is 200 mg once-daily. For more severe infections such as typhoid, gonorrhea, complicated urinary tract infections or lower respiratory tract infections a dose of 400 mg once-daily is recommended. Fleroxacin can be taken with or without food.

2 Intravenous administration

Intravenous fleroxacin is administered in similar doses to oral fleroxacin, with 200 mg given over 0.5 h and 400 mg administered over 1 h in 5% dextrose.

3 Patients with renal failure

Reduction in fleroxacin dosage from the usual dose of 400 mg once-daily to 400 mg every 36 h is recommended for patients with moderate renal impairment (glomerular filtration rate [GFR] 10–30 ml per min). In patients with severe renal failure (GFR <10 ml per min) a dose of fleroxacin 400 mg every 48 h is considered appropriate (Singlas et al., 1990). Alternatively, however, Weidekamm (1993) recommends that patients with a GFR of <40 ml per min should be given a normal loading dose (i.e. 400 mg), but should then receive maintenance doses that are 50% reduced (i.e. 200 mg per day). Stuck et al. (1989) argues for a similar dosage adjustment to Weidekamm (1993), but only after the GFR has declined to 20–30 ml per min. For patients undergoing hemodialysis a 400 mg dose should be given at the end of dialysis if the patient is being dialyzed every 2 days (Singlas et al., 1990). Continuous ambulatory peritoneal dialysis (CAPD) is responsible for only about 8% of total fleroxacin clearance (p. 1102). Thus, the dosage adjustment for patients receiving CAPD should be the same as for an undialyzed patient with a GFR <10 ml per min – namely a loading dose of 400 mg + maintenance 200 mg per day (Stuck et al., 1989).

4 Patients with hepatic failure

Although no change in fleroxacin loading dose is necessary in patients with impaired liver function, a 50% reduction in fleroxacin maintenance dose (i.e. 200 mg daily instead of 400 mg per day) is recommended for those patients with hepatic failure and associated ascites (Blouin et al., 1992).

Availability

Fleroxacin ('Megalone', 'Quinidis') is available in Europe, but is currently investigational in the USA, and is not available in Australia. It is available in 200-mg and 400-mg *tablets*, and in an *i.v. preparation* of 400 mg in 100 ml solution.

Serum Levels in Relation to Dosage

1 Oral administration

Fleroxacin is characterized by a long elimination half-life, allowing once-daily administration. The serum protein binding of fleroxacin is 32% (Nakashima et al., 1988). Oral absorption is virtually complete in healthy volunteers, with maximum serum concentrations and area-under-the-plasma-fleroxacin-concentration-curve (AUC) increasing in a linear manner with increasing dose (at least with doses of up to 800 mg per day). Due to this excellent bioavailability, serum fleroxacin concentrations are nearly identical for oral and i.v. doses. After single oral doses of 100, 200, 400 or 800 mg fleroxacin, maximum serum concentrations of 1.6, 2.3–2.9, 4.4–6.8, and 7.0 μg per ml, respectively, are generally attained within 0.7–2.2 h (Weidekamm et al., 1987; Wise et al., 1987; De Lepeleire et al., 1988; Nakashima et al., 1988; Sörgel et al., 1988a; Heim-Duthoy et al., 1990; Balfour et al., 1995). Due to the presence of microbiologically active metabolites, bioassay will generally overestimate the fleroxacin concentrations in serum compared with those measured by high-performance liquid chromotography (HPLC) or other methods (Griggs et al., 1988). Consistent with a mean plasma elimination half-life of 9–15 h (generally 9–10 h), steady-state plasma fleroxacin concentrations are reached by the 3rd day of repeated once-daily dosing, with peak and trough concentrations of 6.7–7.0 and 1.4–1.6 μg per ml, respectively, expected after once-daily doses of 400 mg (Panneton et al., 1988; Balfour et al., 1995). Following multiple dosing of 800 or 1200 mg fleroxacin on 10 consecutive days, the mean steady-state trough levels are 2.4 and 4.2 μg per ml, respectively, while peak concentrations increase from 9.35 μg per ml on day 1 to 11.2 μg per ml on day 10 after 800 mg per day, and increase from 11.9 to 13.5 μg per ml, respectively, after 1200 mg per day. Thus a 1.3 rate of accumulation occurs at these high doses (800–1200 mg per day), presumably due to saturation of elimination pathways. Unlike ciprofloxacin, probenicid does not affect the renal elimination of fleroxacin and therefore does not increase its serum concentrations (Weidekamm et al., 1987, 1988; Panneton et al., 1988; p. 1003). Single-dose fleroxacin pharmacokinetics are similar in bacteremic patients to those in healthy controls (Schrenzel et al., 1994). Similarly, steady-state fleroxacin pharmacokinetics in patients with skin and soft tissue infections are also similar to those in healthy volunteers (Heim-Duthoy et al., 1990).

The oral bioavailability of fleroxacin is not substantially affected by the intake of a light meal, or a fat- and calcium-rich breakfast (Nakashima *et al.*, 1988; Bertino *et al.*, 1994). Although co-administration of calcium-containing antacids do not alter fleroxacin bioavailability, aluminum and magnesium-containing antacids and sucralfate result in approximately a 25% reduction in maximum serum fleroxacin concentrations and AUC – less than for other fluoroquinolones (Lubowski *et al.*, 1992b; Balfour *et al.*, 1995; pp. 1013, 1065).

2 Intravenous administration

Peak serum fleroxacin concentrations of $2.9 \pm 1.2\,\mu g$ per ml are achieved immediately after a single 100 mg i.v. infusion (Weidekamm *et al.*, 1987). In comparison, single i.v. and oral doses of 400 mg fleroxacin produce peak serum concentrations of 5.75 and $4.31\,\mu g$ per ml, respectively (Nightingale, 1993). Similarly, i.v. and oral doses of 400 mg fleroxacin daily for 5 days produce comparable steady-state serum concentrations: peak levels are 8.1 versus $7.0\,\mu g$ per ml, respectively; while trough levels are 1.2 versus $1.2\,\mu g$ per ml (Nightingale, 1993; Balfour *et al.*, 1995).

3 Elderly patients

Taburet *et al.* (1990) found that age alone does not significantly alter the pharmacokinetics of fleroxacin, and they therefore recommended that no dosage adjustment is necessary in elderly patients. However, if there is associated renal impairment, dose reduction is necessary when the patient's creatinine clearance is <30 ml per min (Taburet *et al.*, 1990; p. 1101). Other authors have questioned these recommendations, noting that the half-life was 20–60% longer and the AUC higher in the elderly patients studied by Taburet *et al.* (1990), and that dose reduction may be necessary in some cases, especially if the patient has low body weight or possibly chronic heart failure (Stuck *et al.*, 1992; Balfour *et al.*, 1995).

4 Patients with renal failure

Renal impairment has no impact on the complete gastrointestinal absorption of fleroxacin. However, total clearance of fleroxacin and its metabolites falls in parallel with decreasing GFR since fleroxacin is primarily eliminated by the kidney (p. 1103; Singlas *et al.*, 1990; Stuck *et al.*, 1989; Weidekamm, 1993). Regardless of the degree of renal impairment, the bioavailability and therefore the peak serum concentration of fleroxacin, and the time after the dose at which this is attained (generally 1.5–2 h) do not change significantly. Extrarenal clearance of fleroxacin remains reasonably constant regardless of the severity of renal dysfunction. In uremic patients there is accumulation of fleroxacin metabolites, *N*-demethyl-fleroxacin and *N*-oxide-fleroxacin, due to reduced urinary elimination and the AUC for fleroxacin increases (Fillastre *et al.*, 1990; Singlas *et al.*, 1990).

In patients with end-stage renal failure, the peak serum fleroxacin concentration after a 400-mg dose is about $6.8\,\mu g$ per ml, but this is attained 3.3 h post-dose and the half-life of the drug lengthens to $25 \pm 3\,h$. Hemodialysis clears fleroxacin and its metabolites readily; in fact fleroxacin clearance by hemodialysis is similar to the usual plasma clearance found in healthy controls, with a serum half-life of 10.4 h. Thus, patients undergoing hemodialysis should be given a dose at the end of dialysis (p. 1101) (Singlas *et al.*, 1990).

It is known that CAPD is responsible for only about 8% of total fleroxacin clearance since penetration of unchanged fleroxacin into peritoneal dialysate is low. Thus, the dosage adjustment for fleroxacin should be the same as for an undialyzed patient with a GFR <10 ml per min (p. 1101). Importantly, the duration of dialysis dwell time influences fleroxacin penetration, with the dialysate:serum ratio increasing from 0.52 to 0.71 with increasing dwell time. Therapeutic concentrations of fleroxacin are therefore achievable in peritoneal dialysate (Stuck *et al.*, 1989).

5 Patients with hepatic failure

In a study comparing the pharmacokinetics of i.v. and oral fleroxacin 400 mg in healthy volunteers with those in cirrhotic patients with and without ascites, Blouin *et al.* (1992) found fleroxacin was completely absorbed and achieved similar peak serum concentrations in all three study groups. Liver impairment alone did not significantly affect fleroxacin pharmacokinetics, but patients with concomitant ascites demonstrated reduced systemic and renal clearance of fleroxacin (and its metabolites; p. 1103), such that the half-life of fleroxacin was approximately doubled. Thus, a normal commencement dose of fleroxacin is given to patients with compromised liver function, but a 50% reduction in fleroxacin maintenance dose is recommended for those patients with associated ascites (p. 1101). These findings are consistent with the predominant renal excretion of fleroxacin (p. 1103).

6 Pregnant and lactating women

Compared with healthy male volunteers, the time to reach maximum serum fleroxacin concentrations in breast-feeding women given a single oral 400-mg dose is doubled (mean 2.4 ± 1.9 h), and the total clearance is reduced by about 25%. The mean maximum serum concentration is 5.6 μg per ml. In breast milk the mean maximum concentration is 3.5 μg per ml; being achieved 2.6 h after dose administration. Fleroxacin penetration into breast milk is about 62% (p. 1104) (Dan et al., 1993).

7 Cystic fibrosis

In patients with cystic fibrosis, fleroxacin is absorbed more slowly and renal clearance is higher than in normal subjects. Although the plasma half-life is reduced, this reduction is insufficient to warrant dosage adjustment in these patients (Mimeault et al., 1989, 1990).

Excretion

Elimination of fleroxacin is by both renal (60–87%) and non-renal (13–40%) mechanisms (Nakashima et al., 1988; Stuck et al., 1992). Fleroxacin is 32% protein bound (Nakashima et al., 1988).

1 Urine

Excretion of unchanged fleroxacin accounts for the majority of renal elimination. After a single oral 400-mg dose of fleroxacin, 50–77% is excreted unchanged in the urine over a 3-day period, while approximately 5–7% is in the form of N-demethyl-fleroxacin and 4–6% is N-oxide-fleroxacin (Griggs et al., 1988; Nakashima et al., 1988; Panneton et al., 1988; Sörgel et al., 1988b; Stuck et al., 1989). Renal clearance of fleroxacin includes glomerular filtration and both some tubular secretion and reabsorption, while the clearance of fleroxacin metabolites is by glomerular filtration and secretion (Weidekamm et al., 1987; Stuck et al., 1992). Urine concentrations of unchanged fleroxacin are roughly 100-fold greater than the concomitant serum concentrations. After doses of 100 mg, 200 mg, and 400 mg, the mean urine concentrations sustained over 24 h are approximately 50, 100 and 150 μg per ml, respectively. Steady-state (day 3 and later) urine concentrations after repeated dosing of 200 mg or 400 mg twice-daily, are about 200 and 300 μg per ml, respectively (Nakashima et al., 1988). Compared with pefloxacin, urinary concentrations of fleroxacin are approximately 2- to 3-fold higher for at least 48 h post-dose (De Lepeleire et al., 1988). Probenecid decreases the renal clearance and urinary recovery of fleroxacin and results in an increase in elimination half-life and AUC (Shiba et al., 1990).

2 Bile

The extent of bilary excretion of fleroxacin has not been extensively investigated. However, in one study of bile obtained by T-tube following cholecystectomy in patients receiving 800 mg once-daily fleroxacin for 5 days, the percentage of unchanged drug was <1% in six of nine patients; while in three patients up to 16.5% was recovered in bile (Hayton et al., 1990). How these data relate to biliary concentrations in healthy subjects is uncertain.

3 Inactivation in body

Fleroxacin is metabolized in the liver by N-demethylation to N-demethyl-fleroxacin, which is microbiologically active, and by N-oxidation to N-oxide-fleroxacin, which is inactive (Griggs et al., 1988; Sörgel et al., 1988b). The extent of metabolism of fleroxacin appears to be similar to that of ciprofloxacin (p. 1003), but is greater than it is for ofloxacin (p. 1117) and less than for pefloxacin (p. 1089) and enoxacin (p. 1078) (Sörgel et al., 1988b).

4 Feces

Following a single 200-mg dose of fleroxacin after a meal, 3% is recovered in the feces over 3 days. The peak fecal concentration after a single 200-mg dose is on day 2 when it is about 27 μg per g. The total of all fecal and urinary recovery is about 96% of the dose. Repeated doses of 400 mg twice-daily fleroxacin result in fecal drug concentrations of 100–160 μg per g (Nakashima et al., 1988).

Distribution of the Drug in Body

Fleroxacin penetrates readily into suction-induced blister fluid, with concentrations increasing significantly with repeated doses. Mean peak blister fluid concentrations after a single dose of 400 mg or 800 mg are 3.7 and 7.7 μg per ml, respectively; while concentrations after similar once-daily therapy for 5 days are 5.7 and 12.3 μg per ml, respectively. Panneton et al. (1988) found fleroxacin penetration to be greater than 100%, based on comparison of the AUC in blister fluid to that in plasma. Lubowski *et al.* (1992a), however, calculated the penetration into interstitial fluid to be 74–92%, based on the ratio of peak drug concentrations or AUC in blister fluid to those in serum.

Fleroxacin concentrations in saliva are about 40% of total serum concentrations (60% of free serum fleroxacin), suggesting rapid secretion into saliva (Nakashima *et al.*, 1988). Fleroxacin penetrates well into nasal secretions, tears (69%) and sweat (43%) (Sörgel *et al.*, 1988a). Following a single 400-mg dose of fleroxacin, the mean maximum concentration in breast milk is 3.5 μg per ml, which occurs about 2.6 h after administration. Based on a comparison of AUC_{milk} versus AUC_{plasma} fleroxacin penetration into breast milk is 62%. Among breast-fed children who drink breast milk at an average of 150 ml per kg of body weight per day, the maximum daily ingested dose of fleroxacin is ≤10 mg (Dan *et al.*, 1993).

Fleroxacin penetrates well into bronchial mucosa, with the mean percentage penetration being 158% in one study of 20 patients undergoing bronchoscopy after receiving 400 mg fleroxacin daily for 4 days (Wise *et al.*, 1988). Lung concentrations 8 h after a 400-mg dose are 8.9 ± 7.7 μg per g (Portmann and Weidekamm, 1992). Following a 200-mg dose of fleroxacin 1–2 h prior to surgery, mean drug concentrations in maxillary sinus mucosa and tonsillar tissue are 2.6 μg per g and 3.3 μg per g, respectively; being similar to simultaneous serum levels (Baba *et al.*, 1988).

Fleroxacin concentrations in T-tube bile collected from cholecystectomized patients treated with 800 mg once-daily for 5 days were high, with a median peak concentration of 22.1 μg per ml in one study. These concentrations were 2- to 3-fold greater than those in plasma and the ratio of $AUC_{bile/plasma}$ was 1.3–9.9 (Hayton *et al.*, 1990).

Fleroxacin concentrations in seminal and prostatic fluid are reasonably high, with prostatic fluid concentrations of about 30% of plasma levels 2–4 h post-dose. Fleroxacin is concentrated by a median ratio of 1.7 times the plasma levels in seminal fluid, but levels in prostatic adenoma tissue are similar to concomitant plasma concentrations (Kees *et al.*, 1988; Naber *et al.*, 1988). In fallopian tube and ovary 6 h after a 600-mg dose, the concentrations are 6.3 and 9.6 μg per ml, while levels in myometrium are similar (Portmann *et al.*, 1989; Portmann and Weidekamm, 1992).

Fleroxacin penetrates well into muscle, but not fat (Cakmakci *et al.*, 1992; Portmann and Weidekamm, 1992). Following a 400-mg dose of fleroxacin, bone concentrations are somewhat variable but achieve mean values of 3.68, 4.22, 2.36, 2.47, and 1.91 μg per g after 2, 4, 8, 12 and 24 h, respectively, following this dose. These are generally comparable with, or slightly higher, than those concomitantly measured in serum (Weidekamm and Portmann, 1993). Synovial fluid concentrations are 2.97, 4.50, 2.24 μg per ml, 2, 4 and 12 h, respectively, after a single 400-mg oral dose of fleroxacin (Weidekamm and Portmann, 1993).

Penetration into aqueous humor and ocular lens is relatively poor with ratios of 0.1–0.4 compared with plasma (Weidekamm and Portmann, 1993).

Mode of Action

The mode of action of fleroxacin is similar to that of other fluoroquinolones (p. 1008).

Toxicity

In a large review of the safety of fleroxacin in clinical trials, the overall rate of adverse effects among patients treated with 200 mg or 400 mg daily oral fleroxacin was 20% and 21%, respectively; and the incidence with i.v. fleroxacin was also about 20%. However, among patients treated with a single 200-mg dose, adverse reactions occured in 7.5%, compared with 26% among patients treated with multiple doses. The most frequent side-effects were gastrointestinal (11%), especially nausea, and neurological (9%), mainly insomnia, headache and dizziness. In this review, there were no side-effects not previously reported with other fluoroquinolones. However, the rates of adverse reactions increased markedly among patients receiving fleroxacin doses greater than 400 mg daily: 44% with 600 mg daily, and 67% with 800 mg daily. The nature of adverse events was similar to those with lower doses, except that photosensitization became more common with higher doses: 5% and 16% with 600 mg and 800 mg daily, respectively. In doses of 400 mg daily the rate of side-effects with fleroxacin appeared in this review to be generally comparable with those of ciprofloxacin, norfloxacin or ofloxacin, although two studies found norfloxacin to have fewer side-effects. Importantly, all so-called serious adverse reactions were reversible, and mostly consisted of insomnia, headache, dizziness and nausea (Geddes, 1993). Other authors, however, have noted a lower rate of reactions with ciprofloxacin than fleroxacin in comparative studies (Balfour *et al.*, 1995). Since short-term fleroxacin does not appear to alter cerebral blood flow, glucose or oxygen metabolism, these factors are unlikely to be the explanation for fleroxacin-associated neurological adverse effects (Gardner et al., 1991). Hallucinations, seizures, psychosis and increased intracranial pressure occur rarely (Balfour et al., 1995).

In a double-blind, dose-ranging study of oral fleroxacin using 400, 600, or 800 mg once-daily for 7 days in an ambulatory setting, Bowie et al. (1989a) noted an overall rate of adverse reactions of 84% and severe reactions in 48%, with the incidence being dose-related. Insomnia, nightmares and photosensitivity reactions resulting in desquamation were notable, although photosensitivity was correlated with doses of 600 or 800 mg daily and with outdoor occupation. All photosensitized patients had some desquamation and some required treatment with silver sulfadiazine. Photosensitivity is typically characterized by transient acute sunburn and is dependent on the extent and intensity of ultraviolet-light exposure, dosage regimen and skin type (Balfour et al., 1995). In a study of 27 healthy volunteers, Scheife et al. (1993) found the hierarchy of phototoxic risk among fluoroquinolones to be: fleroxacin >> lomefloxacin, pefloxacin >> ciprofloxacin > enoxacin, norfloxacin, ofloxacin.

Manufacturer's data suggest a rate of adverse reactions of 33% with multiple oral doses of 200-mg per day, 26.8% with 400 mg per day, and 22.7% with i.v. 400 mg per day. Achilles tendinitis has been reported in 0.08% fleroxacin-treated patients (Balfour et al., 1995). Among healthy volunteers, fleroxacin 800 mg daily for 3 consecutive days is not associated with any nephrotoxic side-effects (Mondorf et al., 1988).

Thus, some clinicians remain wary of using fleroxacin in clinical circumstances where very high doses of drug may be necessary, such as osteomyelitis, endocarditis or meningitis. However, there are few clinical data regarding the use of fleroxacin in these settings anyway. Furthermore, possibly in part because of the dose-related nature of fleroxacin toxicity, the usual recommended doses of fleroxacin are limited to 200 mg or 400 mg daily (p. 1100).

Unlike some other fluoroquinolones, fleroxacin has little effect on the pharmacokinetics of theophylline or caffeine (Seelmann et al., 1989; Soejima et al., 1989; Parent et al., 1990; Parent and LeBel, 1991; Sörgel and Kinzig, 1993b). Nor does fleroxacin significantly alter the anticoagulant effect of warfarin (Sörgel and Kinzig, 1993a). Concomitant administration of cimetidine with fleroxacin reduces total systemic clearance of fleroxacin by about 25% due to interaction with cytochrome P-450 metabolism (Portmann, 1993), but ranitidine has no significant effect on the absorption or clearance of fleroxacin (Sörgel and Kinzig, 1993a). Since the renal elimination of fleroxacin is mostly by filtration rather than active secretion, the co-administration of probenicid (an agent that competes with antibiotics for active secretion) has no significant clinical effect on the fleroxacin pharmacokinetics (Nightingale, 1993; p. 1101). Rifampicin increases the metabolic clearance of fleroxacin by about 28% when given in doses of 600 mg rifampicin and 400 mg fleroxacin, but this effect on the half-life and AUC of fleroxacin is generally not clinically significant (Schrenzel et al., 1993).

Compared with other fluoroquinolones, aluminum- or magnesium-containing antacids and sucralfate have a less marked effect on the absorption of fleroxacin, with a reduction of approximately 25%. Calcium-containing antacids do not significantly affect the absorption of fleroxacin (Shiba et al., 1989; Lubowski et al., 1992; Nightingale, 1993; Balfour et al., 1995).

Clinical Uses of the Drug

1 Urinary tract infections

Fleroxacin in doses of either 200 mg or 400 mg once-daily is effective therapy for uncomplicated urinary tract infections, with bacteriological and clinical cure rates of 86–100% (generally about 90%) and 75–100% (generally about 85%), respectively. As with other antibiotic regimens for these infections, 3- or 7-day treatment regimens result in higher bacteriological cure rates with lower rates of relapse than single-dose regimens (p. 1014). Single-dose fleroxacin 400 mg is significantly more effective than a single dose of amoxycillin 3g, with bacteriological and clinical cure rates of 97% versus 56% and 94% versus 49%, respectively. However, fleroxacin 400 mg per day for 7 days is similar in efficacy to ciprofloxacin 250 mg twice-daily for the same treatment duration, and a 10-day fleroxacin course produces similar results to norfloxacin 400 mg twice-daily for 10 days. However, in this latter comparative study the rate of fleroxacin-associated adverse reactions was significantly higher than that encountered with norfloxacin (Moller et al., 1988; Iravani, 1993; Pummer, 1993; Whitby et al., 1993; Balfour et al., 1995)

For complicated urinary tract infections, including pyelonephritis, a 7- to 14-day course of 200 mg or 400 mg fleroxacin is bacteriologically effective in about 90% of patients; although at least one study suggested that the 400-mg regimen may result in a lower rate of relapse. Seven to 10 days of therapy with fleroxacin 200 mg per day or 400 mg per day is similar in efficacy to norfloxacin 400 mg twice-daily or ofloxacin 200 mg twice-daily (Bernstein-Hahn *et al.*, 1989; Wolfhagen *et al.*, 1990; Childs, 1993; Gelfand *et al.*, 1993; Naber and Sigl, 1993; Pittman *et al.*, 1993; Pummer, 1993; Balfour *et al.*, 1995). Similarly, i.v. fleroxacin 400 mg once-daily and ceftazidime (0.5–2g thrice-daily or 1–2g twice-daily) appear to have comparable efficacy against complicated urinary infections with susceptible pathogens (Cox, 1993).

2 Gastrointestinal infections

In a double-blind, randomized, placebo-controlled trial of fleroxacin 400 mg once-daily for either 1 or 2 days in patients with travelers' diarrhea, fleroxacin was superior to placebo, but there was no difference in outcome between treatment for 1 or 2 days. Adverse reactions (mostly headache and insomnia) were more common in the fleroxacin-treated patients (Steffen *et al.*, 1993). Butler *et al.* (1993) found similar results in a large placebo-controlled trial in Thailand comparing a 400-mg single-dose regimen to 400 mg daily for 3 days. Patients with shigellosis, cholera or *Vibrio parahemolyticus* infection showed clinical and bacteriological response, but patients with salmonellosis showed only a bacteriological response. Thus, a single dose of 400 mg fleroxacin appears to be effective empiric self-treatment for travelers' diarrhea.

In the treatment of typhoid fever, a 7-day course of fleroxacin 400 mg daily was similar to a 14-day treatment regimen in bacteriological (96–97%) and clinical (83–100%) efficacy, and both were comparable with a 14-day course of chloramphenicol 50 mg per kg per day (85% bacteriological, 82% clinical efficacy). However, the time to defervescence was shorter for fleroxacin-treated patients. Relapse occurred in 17% of patients treated with fleroxacin for 7 days, 6% who received chloramphenicol, and in none who received 10–14 days fleroxacin therapy – suggesting that fleroxacin should be given for at least 10 days to prevent relapse (Arnold *et al.*, 1993).

3 Sexually transmitted disease

Single-dose therapy with 400 mg fleroxacin is 99–100% effective for uncomplicated gonococcal urethritis and anorectal and pharyngeal gonorrhea, being comparable in efficacy with ceftriaxone. However, fleroxacin is associated with a significantly higher rate of side-effects than ceftriaxone (Lassus *et al.*, 1988, 1992; Smith *et al.*, 1993; Moran and Levine, 1995). The increasing reports of fluoroquinolone-resistance among some strains of *Neisseria gonorrhoeae* in certain regions raise concerns regarding the future efficacy of fleroxacin and other fluoroquinolones (p. 993).

Some studies and manufacturer's data suggest that fleroxacin, especially in doses of ≥400 mg per day, may be effective against *Chlamydia trachomatis* infections, although the study by Bowie *et al.* (1989) was less convincing and highlighted the problem of fleroxacin-associated side-effects at these high doses (Pust *et al.*, 1988; Bowie *et al.*, 1989b; Balfour *et al.*, 1995). Thus, fleroxacin cannot be relied upon to treat chlamydial sexually transmitted diseases.

In East Africa single-dose therapy with 400 mg fleroxacin was superior to a 3-day course of trimethoprim–sulfamethoxazole 160/800 mg twice-daily for culture-proven chancroid (*Haemophilus ducreyi*) in HIV negative patients, with cure rates of 97% versus 70%, respectively (MacDonald *et al.*, 1989; Plourde *et al.* 1992). Notably in this region, however, resistance to trimethoprim–sulfamethoxazole is known to be high (p. 867). Due to the added difficulty of curing chancroid in HIV-infected patients, Tyndall *et al.* (1993) conducted an open study which compared a single 400-mg fleroxacin dose for HIV negative patients, with a regimen of 400 mg per day for 5 days for HIV-infected patients with chancroid. Among the HIV negative men 55 of 58 were clinically and microbiologically cured, while the 5-day treatment regimen resulted in 20 of 22 evaluable patients being cured; both regimens were well tolerated. Despite these findings, fleroxacin is not currently recommended as first-line therapy for chancroid (Schulte and Schmid, 1995).

4 Bone and joint infections

Small, open-label, non-comparative studies of fleroxacin 400 mg daily for 2–12 weeks, suggest clinical efficacy of 54–77% for osteomyelitis and generally lower rates for septic arthritis. Notably, only 26% of patients enrolled in these studies were subsequently evaluable. Adverse reactions occurred in 28% of patients with 8% requiring cessation of therapy in one study (Liu *et al.*, 1992; Green, 1993; Putz, 1993). Thus, the clinical experience with fleroxacin for the treatment of such infections is limited.

5 Respiratory tract infections

Multiple once-daily doses of either oral or i.v. fleroxacin 400 mg are bacteriologically effective in 84–96% of selected patients with acute-on-chronic bronchitis and 84–100% with non-pneumococcal pneumonia or tracheobronchitis (Chodosh, 1993; Farkas, 1993; Ulmer, 1993; Balfour et al., 1995). However, these promising results are somewhat misleading as they do not necessarily reflect the likely outcome if fleroxacin is used as empiric therapy in these situations, since most studies excluded cases with fleroxacin-resistant pathogens (e.g. Strep. pneumoniae) or where no pathogen was isolated. In fact, only 27–46% of enrolled patients were subsequently analyzed for efficacy in these studies. Nevertheless, fleroxacin compared favorably to amoxycillin for exacerbations of chronic bronchitis with clinical cure rates of 90–95% versus 76–82%, respectively (Chodosh, 1993; Ulmer, 1993). For non-pneumococcal lower respiratory tract infections, i.v. fleroxacin 400 mg daily resulted in clinical cure in 88% versus 82% for ceftazidime, although there was insufficient statistical power to state that the two treatment regimens were equivalent (Farkas, 1993). Thus, in certain clinical situations, especially where the pathogen is known to be sensitive to fluoroquinolones, fleroxacin may be a convenient and effective antibiotic choice.

6 Skin and soft tissue infections

Oral fleroxacin 400 mg daily appears to be similar in clinical and bacteriological efficacy (72–90%) to amoxicillin/clavulanate potassium 500 mg/125 mg thrice-daily for skin and soft tissue infections in a number of relatively small, randomized, generally open-label, multicenter trials. However, the statistical power in these studies was insufficient to confirm equivalence (Smith and Nichols, 1993; Powers, 1993; Tassler, 1993). Fleroxacin 400 mg i.v. daily appeared comparable with i.v. ceftazidime (variable doses), with clinical cure rates of 82% and 73%, respectively; however, less than half of the patients enrolled in this unblinded study were included in the analysis of efficacy – thus weakening the conclusions that can be drawn. Notably, fleroxacin-treated patients experienced approximately twice the rate of adverse reactions reported by the ceftazidime-treated group (Parish and Jungkind, 1993). Although fleroxacin activity against infections due to Staph. aureus and Ps. aeruginosa appeared to be satisfactory in these studies, an assumption of reliable clinical efficacy cannot be made based on the currently available data, especially knowing the limited in vitro activity of fleroxacin against these pathogens.

References

Abeck D, Johnson AP, Dangor Y, Ballard RC (1988). Antibiotic susceptibilities and plasmid profiles of Haemophilus ducreyi isolates from southern Africa. J Antimicrob Chemother 22: 437.

Aoyama H, Inoue M, Mitsuhashi S (1988). In-vitro and in-vivo antibacterial activity of fleroxacin, a new fluorinated quinolone. J Antimicrob Chemother 22 (Suppl D): 99.

Arman D, Willke A, Tural D (1994). In vitro activity of eight antibiotics against Salmonella and Shigella species. Eur J Epidemiol 10: 345.

Arnold K, Hong CS, Nelwan R et al. (1993). Randomized comparative study of fleroxacin and chloramphenicol in typhoid fever. Amer J Med 94: 195S.

Baba S, Mori Y, Maruo T (1988). Penetration of fleroxacin into maxillary sinus mucosa and palatine tonsil. J Antimicrob Chemother 22 (Suppl D): 195.

Balfour JA, Todd PA, Peters DH (1995). Fleroxacin. A review of its pharmacology and therapeutic efficacy in various infections. Drugs 49: 794.

Bannerman TL, Wadiak DL, Kloos WE (1991). Susceptibility of Staphylococcus species and subspecies to fleroxacin. Antimicrob Ag Chemother 35: 2135.

Barry AL, Fuchs PC (1991). In vitro activities of sparfloxacin, tosufloxacin, ciprofloxacin, and fleroxacin. Antimicrob Ag Chemother 35: 955.

Barry AL, Jones RN (1989). In-vitro activities of temafloxacin, tosufloxacin (A-61827). and five other fluoroquinolone agents. J Antimicrob Chemother 23: 527.

Bernstein-Hahn L, Barclay CA, Iribarren MA et al. (1989). Treatment of complicated urinary tract infections with fleroxacin: a dose-finding study. Rev Infect Dis 11 (Suppl 5): S1359.

Bertino JS, Jr, Nafziger AN, Wong M et al. (1994). Effect of a fat- and calcium-rich breakfast on pharmacokinetics of fleroxacin administered in single and multiple doses. Antimicrob Ag Chemother 38: 499.

Beskid G, Prosser BL (1993). A multicenter study on the comparative in vitro activity of fleroxacin and three other quinolones: an interim report from 27 centers. Amer J Med 94: 2S.

Blouin RA, Hamelin BA, Smith DA et al. (1992). Fleroxacin pharmacokinetics in patients with liver cirrhosis. Antimicrob Ag Chemother 36: 632.

Bongaerts GP, Hoogkamp-Korstanje JA (1993). In vitro activities of BAY Y3118, ciprofloxacin, ofloxacin, and fleroxacin against gram-positive and gram-negative pathogens from respiratory tract and soft tissue infections. Antimicrob Ag Chemother 37: 2017.

Bowie WR, Willetts V, Jewesson PJ (1989a). Adverse reactions in a dose-ranging study with a new long-acting fluoroquinolone, fleroxacin. Antimicrob Ag Chemother 33: 1778.

Bowie WR, Willetts V, Megran DW (1989b). Dose-ranging study of fleroxacin for treatment of uncomplicated Chlamydia trachomatis genital infections. Antimicrob Ag Chemother 33: 1774.

Bremner DA, Dickie AS, Singh KP (1988). In-vitro activity of fleroxacin compared with three other quinolones. J Antimicrob Chemother 22 (Suppl D): 19.

Butler T, Lolekha S, Rasidi C et al. (1993). Treatment of acute bacterial diarrhea: a multicenter international trial comparing placebo with fleroxacin given as a single dose or once daily for 3 days. Amer J Med 94: 187S.

Cakmakci M, Gossweiler L, Schilling J et al. (1992). Penetration of fleroxacin into human lung, muscle, and fat tissue. Drugs Exp Clin Res 18: 299.

Chapman JS, Bertasso A, Georgopapadakou NH (1989). Fleroxacin resistance in Escherichia coli. Antimicrob Ag Chemother 33: 239.

Childs SJ (1993). Fleroxacin versus norfloxacin for oral treatment of serious urinary tract infections. Amer J Med 94: 105S.

Chin NX, Brittain DC, Neu HC (1986). In vitro activity of Ro 23–6240, a new fluorinated 4-quinolone. Antimicrob Ag Chemother 29: 675.

Chodosh S (1993). Efficacy of fleroxacin versus amoxicillin in acute exacerbations of chronic bronchitis. Amer J Med 94: 131S.

Cox CE (1993). Comparison of intravenous fleroxacin with ceftazidime for treatment of complicated urinary tract infections. Amer J Med 94: 118S.

Dan M, Weidekamm E, Sagiv R et al. (1993). Penetration of fleroxacin into breast milk and pharmacokinetics in lactating women. Antimicrob Ag Chemother 37: 293.

De Lepeleire I, Van Hecken A, Verbesselt R et al. (1988). Comparative oral pharmacokinetics of fleroxacin and pefloxacin. J Antimicrob Chemother 22: 197.

Digranes A, Benonisen E, Salveson A, Zahm F (1988). In vitro studies of fleroxacin (Ro 23–6240), a new trifluorinated quinolone derivative. Chemotherapy 34: 401.

Ernst F, van der Auwera P (1988). In vitro activity of fleroxacin (Ro 23–6240), a new fluor-quinolone, and other agents, against Mycobacterium spp. J Antimicrob Chemother 21: 501.

Farkas SA (1993). Intravenous fleroxacin versus ceftazidime in the treatment of acute nonpneumococcal lower respiratory tract infections. Amer J Med 94: 142S.

Fass RJ, Helsel VL (1987). In vitro activity of RO 23–6240 (AM-833): a new fluoroquinolone. Diagn Microbiol Infect Dis 6: 293.

Fillastre JP, Leroy A, Moulin B et al. (1990). Pharmacokinetics of quinolones in renal insufficiency. J Antimicrob Chemother 26 (Suppl B): 51.

Gardner SF, Green JA, Bednarczyk EM et al. (1991). An assessment of cerebral blood flow and metabolism after fleroxacin therapy. J Clin Pharmacol 31: 151.

Geddes AM (1993). Safety of fleroxacin in clinical trials. Amer J Med 94: 201S.

Georgopoulos A, Breyer S, Georgopoulos M et al. (1988). In-vitro activity of fleroxacin. J Antimicrob Chemother 22 (Suppl D): 25.

Gelfand MS, Simmons BP, Craft RB et al. (1993). A sequential study of intravenous and oral fleroxacin in the treatment of complicated urinary tract infection. Amer J Med 94 (Suppl 3A): 126S.

Green SL (1993). Efficacy of oral fleroxacin in bone and joint infections. Amer J Med 94: 174S.

Griggs DJ, Wise R, Kirkpatrick B, Ashby JP (1988). The metabolism and pharmacokinetics of fleroxacin in healthy subjects. J Antimicrob Chemother 22 (Suppl D): 191.

Griggs DJ, Piddock LJ, Wise R (1989). The killing action of fleroxacin upon Bacteroides fragilis. J Antimicrob Chemother 23: 53.

Hayton WL, Vlahov V, Bacracheva N et al. (1990). Pharmacokinetics and biliary concentrations of fleroxacin in cholecystectomized patients. Antimicrob Ag Chemother 34: 2375.

Heim-Duthoy K, Peltier G, Awni W (1990). Steady-state pharmacokinetics of fleroxacin in patients with skin and skin structure infections. Antimicrob Ag Chemother 34: 922.

Hirai K, Aoyama H, Hosaka M et al. (1986). In vitro and in vivo antibacterial activity of AM-833, a new quinolone derivative. Antimicrob Ag Chemother 29: 1059.

Hohl P, von Graevenitz A, Zollinger-Iten J (1987). Fleroxacin (Ro 23–6240): activity in vitro against 355 enteropathogenic and non-fermentative gram-negative bacilli and Legionella pneumophila. J Antimicrob Chemother 20: 373.

Hoppe JE, Simon CG (1990). In vitro susceptibilities of Bordetella pertussis and Bordetella parapertussis to seven fluoroquinolones. Antimicrob Ag Chemother 34: 2287.

Hupertz V, Carr H, Czinn SJ (1988). Susceptibility of Campylobacter pylori isolated from pediatric and adult patients to seven new quinolone antibiotics and nalidixic acid. Chemotherapy 34: 341.

Iravani A (1993). Multicenter study of single-dose and multiple-dose fleroxacin versus ciprofloxacin in the treatment of uncomplicated urinary tract infections. Amer J Med 94: 89S.

Kaatz GW, Seo SM, Barriere SL et al. (1991). Development of resistance to fleroxacin during therapy of experimental methicillin-susceptible Staphylococcus aureus endocarditis. Antimicrob Ag Chemother 35: 1547.

Kees F, Naber KG, Schumacher H, Grobecker H (1988). Penetration of fleroxacin into prostatic secretion and prostatic adenoma tissue. Chemotherapy 34: 437.

Kenny GE, Cartwright FD (1991). Susceptibility of Mycoplasma pneumoniae to several new quinolones, tetracycline, and erythromycin. Antimicrob Ag Chemother 35: 587.

Keren G, Keysary A, Goldwasser R, Rubinstein E (1994). The inhibitory effect of fluoroquinolones on Coxiella burnetii growth in in-vitro systems. J Antimicrob Chemother 33: 1253.

Khardori N, Rolston K, Rosenbaum B et al. (1989). Comparative in vitro activity of twenty antimicrobial agents against clinical isolates of Mycobacterium avium complex. J Antimicrob Chemother 24: 667.

Krausse R, Ullmann U (1988). Comparative in vitro activity of fleroxacin (RO 23–6240). against Ureaplasma urealyticum and Mycoplasma hominis. Eur J Clin Microbiol Infect Dis 7: 67.

Lassus A, Renkonen OV, Ellmen J (1988). Fleroxacin versus standard therapy in gonococcal urethritis. J Antimicrob Chemother 22 (Suppl D): 223.

Lassus A, Abath Filho L, Santos Junior MF, Belli L (1992). Comparison of fleroxacin and penicillin G plus probenecid in the treatment of acute uncomplicated gonococcal infections. Genitourin Med 68: 317.

Le Saux NM, Slaney LA, Plummer FA et al. (1987). In vitro activity of ceftriaxone, cefetamet (Ro 15–8074), ceftetrame (Ro 19- 5247; T-2588), and fleroxacin (Ro 23–6240; AM-833) versus Neisseria gonorrhoeae and Haemophilus ducreyi. Antimicrob Ag Chemother 31: 1153.

Liu YC, Cheng DL, Liu CY et al. (1992). Clinical evaluation of fleroxacin in the treatment of bone and joint infections. Southeast Asian J Trop Med Publ Hlth 23: 514.

Lubowski TJ, Nightingale C, Sweeney K et al. (1992a). Penetration of fleroxacin and ciprofloxacin into skin blister fluid: a comparative study. Antimicrob Ag Chemother 36: 651.

Lubowski TJ, Nightingale CH, Sweeney K, Quintiliani R (1992b). Effect of sucralfate on pharmacokinetics of fleroxacin in healthy volunteers. Antimicrob Ag Chemother 36: 2758.

MacDonald KS, Cameron DW, D'Costa L et al. (1989). Evaluation of fleroxacin (RO 23–6240). as single-oral-dose therapy of culture-proven chancroid in Nairobi, Kenya. Antimicrob Ag Chemother 33: 612.

Machka K, Braveny I (1987). Comparative in vitro activity of RO 23–6240 (fleroxacin), a new 4-quinolone derivative. Eur J Clin Microbiol 6: 482.

Manek N, Andrews JM, Wise R (1986). In vitro activity of Ro 23–6240, a new difluoroquinolone derivative, compared with that of other antimicrobial agents. Antimicrob Ag Chemother 30: 330.

Mimeault J, Ruel M, Bergeron MG et al. (1989). Pharmacokinetics of fleroxacin in patients with cystic fibrosis. Rev Infect Dis 11 (Suppl 5): S1253.

Mimeault J, Vallee F, Seelmann R et al. (1990). Altered disposition of fleroxacin in patients with cystic fibrosis. Clin Pharmacol Ther 47: 618.

Moller BR, Kaspersen P, Mamsen A et al. (1988). Fleroxacin in the treatment of uncomplicated acute cystitis in women. J Antimicrob Chemother 22 (Suppl D): 215.

Mondorf AW, Buch A, Steinbacher G et al. (1988). Renal tolerance of fleroxacin in healthy volunteers. J Antimicrob Chemother 22 (Suppl D): 179.

Moran JS, Levine WC (1995). Drugs of choice for the treatment of uncomplicated gonococcal infections. *Clin Infect Dis* 20 (Suppl 1): S47.

Naber KG, Sigl G (1993). Fleroxacin versus ofloxacin in patients with complicated urinary tract infection: a controlled clinical study. *Amer J Med* 94: 114S.

Naber KG, Sorgel F, Kees F et al. (1988). *In-vitro* activity of fleroxacin against isolates causing complicated urinary tract infections and concentrations in seminal and prostatic fluid and in prostatic adenoma tissue. *J Antimicrob Chemother* 22 (Suppl D): 199.

Nakashima M, Kanamaru M, Uematsu T et al. (1988). Clinical pharmacokinetics and tolerance of fleroxacin in healthy male volunteers. *J Antimicrob Chemother* 22 (Suppl D): 133.

Neu HC, Chin NX (1993). *In vitro* activity of fleroxacin in combination with other antimicrobial agents. *Amer J Med* 94: 9S.

Nightingale CH (1993). Overview of the pharmacokinetics of fleroxacin. *Amer J Med* 94: 38S.

Paganoni R, Herzog C, Braunsteiner A, Hohl P (1988). Fleroxacin: *in-vitro* activity worldwide against 20,807 clinical isolates and comparison to ciprofloxacin and norfloxacin. *J Antimicrob Chemother* 22 (Suppl D): 3.

Panneton AC, Bergeron MG, LeBel M (1988). Pharmacokinetics and tissue penetration of fleroxacin after single and multiple 400- and 800-mg-dosage regimens. *Antimicrob Ag Chemother* 32: 1515.

Parent M, LeBel M (1991). Meta-analysis of quinolone-theophylline interactions. *DICP* 25: 191.

Parent M, St-Laurent M, LeBel M (1990). Safety of fleroxacin coadministered with theophylline to young and elderly volunteers. *Antimicrob Ag Chemother* 34: 1249.

Parish LC, Jungkind DL (1993). Systemic antimicrobial therapy for skin and skin structure infections: comparison of fleroxacin and ceftazidime. *Amer J Med* 94: 166S.

Pittman W, Moon JO, Hamrick LC, Jr et al. (1993). Randomized double-blind trial of high- and low-dose fleroxacin versus norfloxacin for complicated urinary tract infection. *Amer J Med* 94: 101S.

Plourde PJ, D'Costa LJ, Agoki E et al. (1992). A randomized, double-blind study of the efficacy of fleroxacin versus trimethoprim-sulfamethoxazole in men with culture-proven chancroid. *J Infect Dis* 165: 949.

Pohlod DJ, Saravolatz LD, Somerville MM (1988). *In-vitro* susceptibility of staphylococci to fleroxacin in comparison with six other quinolones. *J Antimicrob Chemother* 22 (Suppl D): 35.

Portmann R (1993). Influence of cimetidine on fleroxacin pharmacokinetics. *Drugs* 45 (Suppl 3): 471.

Portmann R, Weidekamm E (1992). Penetration of fleroxacin into human and animal tissues. *Chemotherapy* 38: 145.

Portmann R, Hansz C, Stiglmayer R, Weidekamm E (1989). Fleroxacin concentrations in myometrium, ovary and fallopian tube. *J Antimicrob Chemother* 23: 662.

Powers RD (1993). Open trial of oral fleroxacin versus amoxicillin/clavulanate in the treatment of infections of skin and soft tissue. *Amer J Med* 94: 155S.

Prosser BL, Beskid G (1995). Multicenter *in vitro* comparative study of fluoroquinolones against 25 129 gram-positive and gram-negative clinical isolates. *Diagn Microbiol Infect Dis* 21: 33.

Pummer K (1993). Fleroxacin versus norfloxacin in the treatment of urinary tract infections: a multicenter, double-blind, prospective, randomized, comparative study. *Amer J Med* 94: 108S.

Putz PA (1993). A pilot study of oral fleroxacin given once daily in patients with bone and joint infections. *Amer J Med* 94: 177S.

Pust RA, Ackenheil-Koppe HR, Weidner W, Meier-Ewert H (1988). Clinical efficacy and tolerance of fleroxacin in patients with urethritis caused by *Chlamydia trachomatis*. *J Antimicrob Chemother* 22 (Suppl D): 227.

Rice RJ, Knapp JS (1994). Antimicrobial susceptibilities of *Neisseria gonorrhoeae* strains representing five distinct resistance phenotypes. *Antimicrob Ag Chemother* 38: 155.

Salfinger M, Hohl P, Kafader FM (1988). Comparative *in-vitro* activity of fleroxacin and other 6-fluoroquinolones against mycobacteria. *J Antimicrob Chemother* 22 (Suppl D): 55.

Scheife RT, Cramer WR, Decker EL (1993). Photosensitizing potential of ofloxacin. *Int J Dermatol* 32: 413.

Schrenzel J, Dayer P, Leemann T et al. (1993). Influence of rifampin on fleroxacin pharmacokinetics. *Antimicrob Ag Chemother* 37: 2132.

Schrenzel J, Cerruti F, Herrmann M et al. (1994). Single-dose pharmacokinetics of oral fleroxacin in bacteremic patients. *Antimicrob Ag Chemother* 38: 1219.

Schulte JM, Schmid GP (1995). Recommendations for treatment of chancroid, 1993. *Clin Infect Dis* 20 (Suppl 1): S39.

Seelmann R, Mahr G, Gottschalk B et al. (1989). Influence of fleroxacin on the pharmacokinetics of theophylline. *Rev Infect Dis* 11 (Suppl 5): S1100.

Shiba K, Saito A, Shimada J et al. (1989). Interactions of fleroxacin with dried aluminium hydroxide gel and probenecid. *Rev Infect Dis* 11 (Suppl 5): S1097.

Shiba K, Saito A, Shimada J et al. (1990). Renal handling of fleroxacin in rabbits, dogs, and humans. *Antimicrob Ag Chemother* 34: 58.

Simor AE, Ferro S, Low DE (1989). Comparative *in vitro* activities of six new fluoroquinolones and other oral antimicrobial agents against *Campylobacter pylori*. *Antimicrob Ag Chemother* 33: 108.

Singlas E, Leroy A, Sultan E et al. (1990). Disposition of fleroxacin, a new trifluoroquinolone, and its metabolites. Pharmacokinetics in renal failure and influence of haemodialysis. *Clin Pharmacokinet* 19: 67.

Smith JW, Nichols RL (1993). Comparison of oral fleroxacin with oral amoxicillin/clavulanate for treatment of skin and soft tissue infections. *Amer J Med* 94: 150S.

Soejima R, Niki Y, Sumi M (1989). Effect of fleroxacin on serum concentrations of theophylline. *Rev Infect Dis* 11 (Suppl 5): S1099.

Sörgel F, Kinzig M (1993a). Pharmacokinetics of gyrase inhibitors, Part 1: basic chemistry and gastrointestinal disposition. *Amer J Med* 94 (Suppl 3A): 44S.

Sörgel F, Kinzig M (1993b). Pharmacokinetics of gyrase inhibitors, Part 2: Renal and hepatic elimination pathways and drug interactions. *Amer J Med* 94 (Suppl 3A): 56S.

Sörgel F, Metz R, Naber K et al. (1988a). Pharmacokinetics and body fluid penetration of fleroxacin in healthy volunteers. *J Antimicrob Chemother* 22 (Suppl D): 155.

Sörgel F, Seelmann R, Naber K et al. (1988b). Metabolism of fleroxacin in man. *J Antimicrob Chemother* 22 (Suppl D): 169.

Steele-Mortimer O, Meier-Ewert H (1988). *In-vitro* activity of fleroxacin against *Chlamydia trachomatis*. *J Antimicrob Chemother* 22 (Suppl D): 65.

Steffen R, Jori J, DuPont HL et al. (1993a). Treatment of travellers' diarrhoea with fleroxacin: a case study. *J Antimicrob Chemother* 31: 767.

Steffen R, Jori R, DuPont HL et al. (1993b). Efficacy and toxicity of fleroxacin in the treatment of travelers' diarrhea. *Amer J Med* 94: 182S.

Stobberingh EE, Houben AW, van Boven CP (1987). *In vitro* evaluation of Ro 23–6240, a new fluorinated 4-quinolone. *Chemotherapy* 33: 197.

Stuck AE, Frey FJ, Heizmann P et al. (1989). Pharmacokinetics and metabolism of intravenous and oral fleroxacin in subjects with normal and impaired renal function and in patients on continuous ambulatory peritoneal dialysis. *Antimicrob Ag Chemother* 33: 373.

Stuck AE, Kim DK, Frey FJ (1992). Fleroxacin clinical pharmacokinetics. *Clin Pharmacokinet* 22: 116.

Taburet AM, Devillers A, Thomare P et al. (1990). Disposition of fleroxacin, a new trifluoroquinolone, and its metabolites. Pharmacokinetics in elderly patients. *Clin Pharmacokinet* 19: 80.

Tassler H (1993). Comparative efficacy and safety of oral fleroxacin and amoxicillin/clavulanate potassium in skin and soft tissue infections. *Amer J Med* 94: 159S.

Tomioka H, Sato K, Saito H (1991). Comparative *in vitro* and *in vivo* activity of fleroxacin and ofloxacin against various mycobacteria. *Tubercle* 72: 176.

Tyndall MW, Plourde PJ, Agoki E *et al.* (1993). Fleroxacin in the treatment of chancroid: an open study in men seropositive or seronegative for the human immunodeficiency virus type 1. *Amer J Med* **94**: 85S.

Ulmer W (1993). Fleroxacin versus amoxicillin in the treatment of acute exacerbation of chronic bronchitis. *Amer J Med* **94**: 136S.

Verschraegen G, Claeys G, Van den Abeele AM (1988). Comparative *in vitro* activity of the new quinolone fleroxacin (RO 23–6240). *Eur J Clin Microbiol Infect Dis* **7**: 63.

Waites K, Rand K, Jenkins S *et al.* (1994). Multicenter *in vitro* comparative study of fluoroquinolones after four years of widespread clinical use. *Diagn Microbiol Infect Dis* **18**: 181.

Weidekamm E (1993). Pharmacokinetics of fleroxacin in renal impairment. *Amer J Med* **94**: 70S.

Weidekamm E, Portmann R (1993). Penetration of fleroxacin into body tissues and fluids. *Amer J Med* **94**: 75S.

Weidekamm E, Portmann R, Suter K *et al.* (1987). Single- and multiple-dose pharmacokinetics of fleroxacin, a trifluorinated quinolone, in humans. *Antimicrob Ag Chemother* **31**: 1909.

Weidekamm E, Portmann R, Partos C, Dell D (1988). Single and multiple dose pharmacokinetics of fleroxacin. *J Antimicrob Chemother* **22** (Suppl D): 145.

Whitby M, Brown P, Silagy C, Rana C (1993). Comparison of fleroxacin and amoxicillin in the treatment of uncomplicated urinary tract infections in women. *Amer J Med* **94**: 97S.

Wise R, Kirkpatrick B, Ashby J, Griggs DJ (1987). Pharmacokinetics and tissue penetration of Ro 23–6240, a new trifluoroquinolone. *Antimicrob Ag Chemother* **31**: 161.

Wise R, Honeybourne D, Andrews JM, Ashby JP (1988). The penetration of fleroxacin into bronchial mucosa. *J Antimicrob Chemother* **22**: 203.

Wolfhagen MJHM, Hoepelman AIM, Verhoef J (1990). Double-blind, dose-range-finding study of fleroxacin (RO23-6240; AM-833) for treatment of complicated urinary tract infections. *Antimicrob Ag Chemother* **34**: 409.

Young LW, Berlin OGW, Inderlied CB (1987). Activity of ciprofloxacin and other fluorinated quinolones against mycobacteria. *Amer J Med* **82** (Suppl 4A): 23.

Zhang YX, Neu HC (1991). Fleroxacin combined with rifampin. *Diagn Microbiol Infect Dis* **14**: 23.

Ofloxacin

Description

Ofloxacin was synthesized at Daiichi Seiyaku Company, Japan, and has the chemical formula: 9-fluoro-3-methyl-10-(4-methyl-1-piperazinyl)-7-oxo-2,3-dihydro-7H-pyrido-(1,2,3-de)1,4-benzoxazine-6-carboxylic acid (Sato *et al.*, 1982). The antibacterial spectrum of ofloxacin is similar to norfloxacin and enoxacin, but there are some differences, including activity against *Mycobacterium tuberculosis* (Sato *et al.*, 1982; Van Caekenberghe and Pattyn, 1984; Chantot and Bryskier, 1985; Forsgren, 1985; Goossens *et al.*, 1985; Kumada and Neu, 1985).

Sensitive Organisms

The *in vitro* activity of ofloxacin is generally comparable with, or less than, that of ciprofloxacin (p. 981); although a number of studies have suggested that in terms of overall breadth of activity against a wide variety of pathogens, ofloxacin may be superior. Against some Gram-negative species such as *Pseudomonas aeruginosa*, however, ofloxacin is frequently inferior to ciprofloxacin. Against common Gram-positive and -negative pathogens, ofloxacin is similar to, or more active than, other fluoroquinolones such as norfloxacin, fleroxacin or enoxacin (Aukenthaler *et al.*, 1986; Bassey *et al.*, 1986; Grüneberg *et al.*, 1988; Cantón *et al.*, 1992; Sanders, 1992a; Jones *et al.*, 1994; Prosser and Beskid, 1995).

1 Gram-negative bacteria

Ofloxacin is very active against the Enterobacteriaceae, such as *Escherichia coli*, the *Enterobacter*, *Klebsiella*, *Proteus*, *Salmonella*, *Shigella*, *Serratia* and *Citrobacter* spp. and *Morganella morganii*. Compared with the other Enterobacteriaceae, *Citrobacter*, *Providencia* (especially *P. stuartii*) and *Serratia* spp. are not quite as susceptible. As with other fluoroquinolones, ofloxacin is active against Enterobacteriaceae which are resistant to nalidixic acid, ampicillin and cephalexin. However, ciprofloxacin (p. 981) is generally more active than ofloxacin against Enterobacteriaceae. *Acinetobacter calcoaceticus*, *Alcaligenes faecalis* and *Flavobacterium* meningosepticum are susceptible, but less so than the Enterobacteriaceae. *Aeromonas*, *Plesiomonas* and *Campylobacter* spp., *Vibrio cholerae* and *Yersinia enterocolitica* are quite sensitive. Ciprofloxacin is more active against enteric pathogens than ofloxacin (p. 982), but ofloxacin appears to be very active against the vast majority of pathogens that are associated with spontaneous bacterial peritonitis (Sader *et al.*, 1995). *Helicobacter pylori* and *Gardnerella vaginalis* are often susceptible (King *et al.*, 1985; Bassey *et al.*, 1986; King and Phillips, 1986a,b; Kumada and Neu, 1986; Monk and Campoli-Richards, 1987; Glupczynski *et al.*, 1988; McNulty and Dent, 1988; Phillips and King, 1988; Burgos *et al.*, 1990; Todd and Faulds, 1991; Sanders, 1992a).

Pseudomonas aeruginosa is often sensitive, but not to the same degree as it is to ciprofloxacin (p. 982), which is often more potent by up to three dilutions. Ofloxacin is generally as potent as gentamicin against *Ps. aeruginosa*, and 2- to 3-fold more potent than aztreonam or cefotaxime. Ofloxacin has less activity against other species such as *Burkholderia cepacia*, *B. pseudomallei* or *Stenotrophomonas* (previously *Xanthomonas*) *maltophilia*, which are generally resistant (Winton *et al.*, 1988; Yamagishi *et al.*, 1993; Pankuch *et al.*, 1994; Ristow *et al.*, 1995). *Haemophilus influenzae*, *Neisseria gonorrhoeae* (including ampicillin-resistant strains) and *N. meningitidis* are very susceptible to ofloxacin, but ciprofloxacin is generally more active (Clendennen *et al.*, 1992a,b; Zenilman *et al.*, 1993; Joesoef *et al.*, 1994; Rice and Knapp, 1994). Ofloxacin is similar in activity to norfloxacin and enoxacin against *Bordetella pertussis* (MIC_{90} 0.25–0.5 μg per ml) but, once again, ciprofloxacin is more active (MIC_{90} 0.06 μg per ml);

B. parapertussis tends to be 2- to 4-fold less susceptible to the fluoroquinolones (Appleman *et al.*, 1987; Kurzynski *et al.*, 1988; Hoppe and Simon, 1990). Ofloxacin is active against *Brucella melitensis* (MIC$_{90}$ 0.02 µg per ml), *Eikenella corrodens* (MIC$_{90}$ 0.03 µg per ml), *H. ducreyi* and *Moraxella catarrhalis* (Wall *et al.*, 1985; Aukenthaler *et al.*, 1986; Goldstein *et al.*, 1986; Phillips and King, 1988; Khan *et al.*, 1989; Cantón *et al.*, 1992; Prosser and Beskid, 1995).

Legionella pneumophila is susceptible (MIC$_{90}$ 0.03–0.25 µg per ml) and the drug is effective in experimental *L. pneumophila* pneumonia in guinea-pigs (Saito *et al.*, 1985; Rajagopalan-Levasseur *et al.*, 1990; Baltch *et al.*, 1995). Ofloxacin is significantly less active than either ciprofloxacin, norfloxacin or pefloxacin against *Francisella tularensis* (Syrjala *et al.*, 1991), but *Yersinia pestis* is susceptible (MIC$_{90}$ 0.25 µg per ml) (Smith *et al.*, 1995).

Anaerobic Gram-negative bacteria such as *Bacteroides fragilis*, *Fusobacterium* and *Prevotella* spp. may be borderline susceptible to ofloxacin (MIC$_{90}$ 4–8 µg per ml), but other *Bacteroides* spp. are usually resistant (Fernandes *et al.*, 1986; Grüneberg *et al.*, 1988; Goldstein and Citron, 1992; Goldstein, 1993; Borobio *et al.*, 1994; Appelbaum, 1995).

2 Gram-positive bacteria

Ofloxacin has broadly similar, but slightly inferior, activity to ciprofloxacin against most Gram-positive pathogens. *Staphylococcus aureus*, *Staph. epidermidis* and *Streptococcus pneumoniae* (including penicillin-resistant strains) are usually susceptible, or borderline susceptible, but ofloxacin has unreliable activity against hemolytic streptococci (Groups A, B, C and G) and viridans streptococci (King *et al.*, 1985; Mazzulli *et al.*, 1990; Spangler *et al.*, 1992; McWhinney *et al.*, 1993; Pankuch *et al.*, 1995). Ofloxacin is generally active (MIC$_{90}$ 0.5 µg per ml) against methicillin-resistant *Staph. aureus*, although its activity is less than that of sparfloxacin (p. 984). However, among strains that are clearly resistant to ciprofloxacin or ofloxacin, cross-resistance among the fluoroquinolones is generally complete (Chantot and Bryskier, 1985; Mraovic and Canic-Radojlovic, 1986; Smith *et al.*, 1986; Chaudry *et al.*, 1990; Van der Auwera *et al.*, 1990; Barry and Fuchs, 1991; Maple *et al.*, 1991; Eliopoulos, 1995). Enterococci should generally be considered resistant (MIC$_{90}$ 4–8 µg per ml), as should *Listeria monocytogenes* (MIC$_{90}$ 8 µg per ml) (MacGowan *et al.*, 1990; Murray *et al.*, 1993; Cherubin and Stratton, 1994). *Corynebacterium* group D2 and *Bacillus anthracis* are generally susceptible (Soriano *et al.*, 1987; Doganay and Aydin, 1991).

Gram-positive anaerobes, such as *Peptococcus* spp., may be borderline susceptible (MIC$_{90}$ ≤ 8 µg per ml), but *Actinomyces* spp. are resistant. *Clostridium perfringens* are often susceptible to ofloxacin and ciprofloxacin (MIC$_{90}$ 0.5 µg per ml), but other *Clostridia* spp. are generally resistant (Goldstein and Citron, 1992; Goldstein, 1993; Appelbaum, 1995). In particular, *Cl. difficile* is usually resistant to ofloxacin (MIC$_{90}$ 16–32 µg per ml) (Delmee and Avesani, 1986;).

3 Mycobacteria

Ofloxacin has similar, or occasionally slightly greater, *in vitro* activity against *M. tuberculosis* (MIC$_{90}$ 0.63–2.4 µg per ml; generally <1 µg per ml) than ciprofloxacin, and may have good clinical efficacy (p. 1123; Tsukamura, 1985; Berlin *et al.*, 1987; Davies *et al.*, 1987b; Gorzynski *et al.*, 1989; Yew *et al.*, 1990a, 1994a; Garcia-Rodriguez and Gomez-Garcia, 1993; Jacobs, 1995). Other authors, using the BACTEC radiometric culture method, have found among the available fluoroquinolones, sparfloxacin to have the greatest activity, followed by ciprofloxacin then ofloxacin (Rastogi and Goh, 1991).

Among the atypical mycobacteria, some strains of *M. avium* complex may be susceptible, but considerable variability has been reported with MIC$_{90}$ 0.5–16 µg per ml (Fenlon and Cynamon, 1986; Johnson and Roberts, 1987; Hoffner *et al.*, 1989; Jacobs, 1995). Ofloxacin is active against *M. fortuitum* and may exhibit some post-antibiotic effect *in vitro* (Casal *et al.*, 1987; Tsui *et al.*, 1993; Garcia-Rodriguez and Gomez-Garcia, 1993). *Mycobacterium kansasii* is susceptible to ofloxacin (MIC$_{90}$ 0.5 µg per ml), but *M. haemophilum* is relatively resistant to fluoroquinolones with MIC$_{90}$ of 8, 8 and 4 µg per ml, for ofloxacin, ciprofloxacin and sparfloxacin, respectively (Bernard *et al.*, 1993; Garcia-Rodriguez and Gomez-Garcia, 1993; Witzig and Franzblau, 1993). *Mycobacterium chelonae* and *M. scrofulaceum* are resistant (Texier-Maugein *et al.*, 1987). Ofloxacin is active against *M. leprae in vitro*, in experimental animal models and in some clinical trials of patients with lepromatous leprosy (Franzblau, 1989; Gelber *et al.*, 1992)

4 Mycoplasma and Chlamydia

Mycoplasma pneumoniae and *M. hominis* are susceptible to ofloxacin (MIC$_{90}$ 1–2 µg per ml), but sparfloxacin has greater activity (p. 1136; Kenny and Cartwright, 1991a,b; Kaku *et al.*, 1994; Ishida *et al.*, 1994). *Ureaplasma urealyticum* may be borderline susceptible (MIC$_{90}$ 2 µg per ml), but other authors have reported resistance (MIC$_{90}$ 8–25 μg per ml) (Schachter and Moncada, 1989; Kenny and Cartwright, 1991b). *Chlamydia trachomatis* is often susceptible (MIC 0.5–1 μg per ml), as is *C. pneumoniae* (mean MIC 0.7 μg per ml), but sparfloxacin is significantly more active (p. 1137; Schachter and Moncada, 1989; Hammerschlag *et al.*, 1992; Nakata *et al.*, 1992; Lefevre *et al.*, 1993; Rice *et al.*, 1995).

5 Rickettsia and Coxiella burnetii

Ofloxacin appears to be active against *Coxiella burnetii in vitro* at clinically achievable concentrations, although there may be some heterogeneity in this susceptibility (Raoult *et al.*, 1989, 1991; Yeaman *et al.*, 1989). *Rickettsia rickettsii* and *R. conorii* are susceptible to ofloxacin (MIC 1 μg per ml) but ciprofloxacin, pefloxacin and especially sparfloxacin appear to be more active (Jabarit-Aldighieri *et al.*, 1992).

6 Borrelia burgdorferi

Ofloxacin has limited activity against *Borrelia burgdorferi* (MIC$_{90}$ 2–4 μg per ml; MBC$_{90}$ 8 μg per ml) *in vitro* (Mursic *et al.*, 1987; Levin *et al.*, 1993).

7 Acquired resistance

Since the introduction of fluoroquinolones, the development of resistance to ofloxacin has been generally uncommon, except in certain species such as *Pseudomonas*, *Acinetobacter*, *Citrobacter*, *Stenotrophomonas*, *Providencia* and some staphylococcal species (Cheng *et al.*, 1987; Hoban *et al.*, 1993; Jones *et al.*, 1994; Waites *et al.*, 1994). Strains of *Shigella sonnei* with MICs to sparfloxacin, ciprofloxacin and ofloxacin, 16- to 32-fold higher than those noted among typical strains have been reported from patients with enteritis in Japan in recent years. Nevertheless, all these isolates had MICs of <2 μg per ml ofloxacin (i.e. clinically achievable concentrations). This resistance appears to be due to alterations in DNA gyrase subunit A gene (Horiuchi *et al.*, 1993).

As noted previously (p. 993), prophylaxis of cirrhotic patients with norfloxacin to prevent spontaneous bacterial peritonitis has been associated with a change in the fecal ecology to include a substantial increase in fluoroquinolone-resistant Gram-negative and Gram-positive organisms (Dupeyron *et al.*, 1994). Among patients with leukemia given oral ofloxacin for prophylaxis against Gram-negative sepsis, a notable increase in the incidence of bacteremia due to fluoroquinolone-resistant *E. coli* was noted from <0.5% in 1988–89 and 0.8% in 1990–91 to 4.5% in 1992–93 (p < 0.01) at one institution (Kern *et al.*, 1994a). Similarly, reasonably high rates of ofloxacin-resistance have been noted among strains of *Helicobacter pylori* following treatment with oral ofloxacin (Glupczynski *et al.*, 1987).

One strain of *Proteus vulgaris* has been described which had multiple mechanisms of ofloxacin-resistance, including alterations of DNA gyrase and outer membrane proteins as well as possibly active drug efflux (Ishii *et al.*, 1991). As noted for ciprofloxacin (p. 993), isolates of *N. gonorrhoeae* with increased resistance to ofloxacin have been noted in various countries in South-East and East Asia, Hawaii and some mainland states of the USA, with associated treatment failure (Kam *et al.*, 1993; CDC, 1994, 1995; Knapp *et al.*, 1994). Tanaka-Bandoh *et al.* (1995) have reported an increase in the rate of resistance to ofloxacin in *B. fragilis* from 42% of strains in 1989 to 81% in 1992.

Similar to the situation with ciprofloxacin (p. 994), resistance to ofloxacin has been noted mostly in methicillin-resistant *Staph. aureus* (MRSA), rather than methicillin-susceptible *Staph. aureus* (Shalit *et al.*, 1989). Among these strains of ofloxacin- or ciprofloxacin-resistant *Staph. aureus*, cross-resistance with other fluoroquinolones is usually complete (Aldridge *et al.*, 1992b). Such resistance is generally due to mutations in the *gyrA* gene with alterations in DNA gyrase (Hori *et al.*, 1993). In one study, the introduction of ciprofloxacin on an unrestricted basis into a large community hospital, was followed by the rapid emergence during the subsequent 18-month period of high-level fluoroquinolone-resistance among MRSA (Aldridge *et al.*, 1992a). Increasing resistance to ofloxacin has been noted among strains of group A streptococci in some institutions (Betriu *et al.*, 1993). Among *Enterococcus faecalis* strains resistant to fluoroquinolones such as ofloxacin, alterations in the gyrase A subunit have been noted to be the major contibutor to fluoroquinolone-resistance (Nakanishi *et al.*, 1991; p. 991).

The development of resistance to fluoroquinolones such as ofloxacin, ciprofloxacin and sparfloxacin has been noted in clinical strains of *M. tuberculosis* which have developed stepwise multidrug-resistance (Rastogi *et al.*, 1992).

8 Minimum inhibitory concentrations	The MICs of ofloxacin against selected bacterial species are shown in Table II.6, pp. 986–987.

Mode of Administration and Dosage

1 Oral administration	The usual recommended dose is 400 mg once- or twice-daily, with the higher dose used for urinary tract or lower respiratory infections. A daily dose of 400 mg is recommended for nongonococcal urethritis and cervicitis, while a single 400-mg dose may be sufficient for uncomplicated gonorrhea. The empiric treatment of sexually acquired epididymitis generally requires 300 mg twice-daily for 10 days. Acute pelvic inflammatory disease often requires 400 mg twice-daily for 14 days; usually in combination with an agent with activity against anaerobes such as clindamycin or metronidazole. Treatment of travelers' diarrhea generally consists of 300 mg twice-daily for 3 days (Martindale, 1993; AHFS, 1996).
2 Intravenous administration	Infusions of ofloxacin i.v. should be administered slowly over a 60-min period to avoid the risk of hypotension with more rapid or bolus delivery. Doses are generally similar to those recommended with the oral preparation as the formulations show bioequivalence. Thus doses are: i.v. ofloxacin 200–400 mg 12-hourly, with the higher dose necessary for complicated urinary tract infections, and a regimen of 300 mg twice-daily being usual for prostatitis (Todd and Faulds, 1991; AHFS, 1996).
3 Ophthalmic administration	The dosage of ofloxacin ophthalmic solution recommended by the manufacturer for conjunctivitis is one or two drops in the affected eye every 2–4 h while awake for 2 days, then one or two drops, four-times daily for up to an additional 5 days (AHFS, 1996).
4 Patients with renal failure	In patients with end-stage renal failure, the half-life of ofloxacin increases from 5–8 h to 28–37 h (p. 116). For patients with a glomerular filtration rate (GFR) of 10–50 ml per min the usual daily dose of ofloxacin (400 mg per day) should be reduced by 50%, while patients with a GFR of <10ml per min should receive 25–50% the usual dose at an unchanged dosing interval of twice-daily (i.e. 100–200 mg per day) (Bennett et al., 1994; AHFS, 1996). Other authors do not advocate dosage reduction until the GFR is <30 per ml per min (Eliopoulos, 1988). Patients undergoing hemodialysis should receive 100 mg twice-daily; but some authors suggest a loading dose of 200 mg followed by 100 mg daily. No additional supplemental doses are required after dialysis (Dörfler et al., 1987; Lameire et al., 1991; Bennett et al., 1994). Patients receiving continuous ambulatory peritoneal dialysis (CAPD) should receive doses similar to patients with GFR <10ml per min. Continuous arteriovenous or venovenous hemofiltration removes some ofloxacin, hence the recommended dose is 300 mg daily (Bennett et al., 1994; AHFS, 1996).
5 Patients with hepatic failure	Among patients with alcoholic cirrhosis and ascites, renal clearance is reduced and the elimination half-life of ofloxacin is increased (p. 117). Thus, an oral dose of ofloxacin 200 mg twice-daily has been recommended for such patients with bacterial peritonitis (Silvain et al., 1989).
6 Pregnant and lactating women and children	Similar to other fluoroquinolones (pp. 997, 1011), ofloxacin is not generally administered to children, adolescents, or pregnant women (Todd and Faulds, 1991; Giamarellou et al., 1989).
7 Elderly patients	Pharmacokinetic parameters for elderly patients are generally considered to be similar to those found in younger controls, so that no dosage adjustment is necessary for older age unless there is concomitant renal dysfunction – in which case the degree of dose reduction is dictated by the severity of the renal failure (Norrby and Ljungberg, 1989; Flor, 1989; Lamp et al., 1992).

Molinarno *et al.* (1992), however, recommends a possible 50% reduction in ofloxacin dose for patients older than 75 years due to altered ofloxacin pharmacokinetics in this age group (p. 1117).

Availability

Ofloxacin is available in the USA as 'Floxin' (Ortho Pharmaceuticals Corp.), 'Flobacin' (Sigma-Tau), 'Tarwid' (Hoechst) in 200-, 300- and 400-mg *tablets*.

Ofloxacin is also available in some countries as an *i.v. preparation* in concentrations of 4 mg per ml, 20 mg per ml, 40 mg per ml (200 mg in 50ml; 40 mg in 100ml).

An *ophthalmic solution* of 3 mg per ml (0.3%) is available (Allergan Pharmaceuticals).

Serum Levels in Relation to Dosage

1 Oral administration

Ofloxacin has excellent oral bioavailability with 95–100% absorption, and is notable for its low protein binding (25%), extensive body distribution, negligible metabolism, and near exclusive renal elimination. The serum elimination half-life is 5–8 (generally 7) h (Lockley *et al.*, 1984; Leroy *et al.*, 1987; Lode *et al.*, 1987, 1990; Bennett *et al.*, 1994; Todd and Faulds, 1995).

Mean maximum serum concentrations are reached at 0.7–2 h (generally about 1.2 h) after oral administration (Lockley *et al.*, 1984; Leroy *et al.*, 1987; Flor, 1989; Marchbanks *et al.*, 1992). Co-administration of ofloxacin with food delays the time to maximum serum concentration, but does not alter the extent of absorption (Leroy *et al.*, 1987; Höffken *et al.*, 1988). Mean peak serum concentrations after a single doses of 100, 200, 300, 400 or 600 mg are 1.0–1.3, 1.6–2.2, 2.8–4.6, 3.2–4.3 and 6.7–10.7 µg per ml, respectively (see Fig. II.8) (Lockley *et al.*, 1984; Verho *et al.*, 1985; Wise *et al.*, 1986; Leroy *et al.*, 1987; Lode *et al.*, 1987; Wise and Lockley, 1988; Bitar *et al.*, 1989; Flor, 1989; Yuk *et al.*, 1991; Marchbanks *et al.*, 1992). Maximum serum concentrations and area-under-the-plasma-concentration-curve (AUC) are linearly related to dose (oral or i.v.) when doses are 100–600 mg, with steady-state achieved after two to four doses at 12-hourly intervals (Verho *et al.*, 1985; Lode *et al.*, 1987, 1988; De Bernadis *et al.*, 1988; Farinotti *et al.*, 1988; Flor, 1989). Multiple doses of ofloxacin 300 mg twice-daily for 3–14 days result in peak and trough levels of 3.3–5.9 µg per ml and 1.0–1.4 µg per ml, respectively, in healthy volunteers; while doses of 200 or 400 mg twice-daily result in steady-state maximum serum levels of 3 and 5.0 ± 1.0 µg per ml, respectively (Dagrosa *et al.*, 1986; Monk and Campoli-Richards, 1987; Flor, 1989; Warlich *et al.*, 1990).

In a number of small comparative studies between ofloxacin and ciprofloxacin, ofloxacin appears to achieve a slightly higher peak serum concentration than ciprofloxacin. After a single oral 200-mg dose of either ofloxacin, ciprofloxacin or norfloxacin, peak concentrations are 2.3, 1.1

Fig. II.8.
Mean plasma concentrations of ofloxacin during the 24 h following oral administration of 100, 300 and 600 mg to normal subjects. (From Flor S, 1989. Pharmacokinetics of ofloxacin. An overview. *Amer J Med* **87**:24S. Copyright 1989 by Excerpta Medica Inc.)

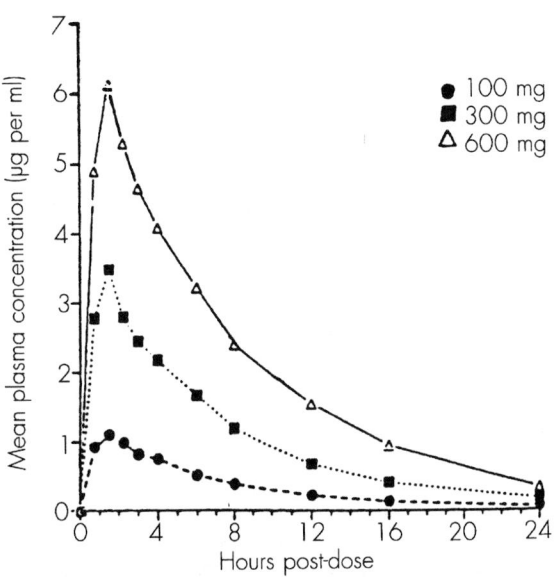

and 0.8 μg per ml, respectively, and AUC are 15.86, 3.57 and 3.28 μg per ml per h, respectively (Beermann *et al.*, 1984). Similarly Echols *et al.* (1994) compared the levels achieved with oral ofloxacin 400 mg versus ciprofloxacin 400 mg, and the same dose administered i.v. Mean peak serum concentrations achieved after i.v. ofloxacin or ciprofloxacin were 5.44 versus 4.48 μg per ml, respectively; while after oral administration the levels were 4.44 versus 2.45 μg per ml, respectively. The authors commented, however, that the generally greater *in vitro* activity of ciprofloxacin meant that in terms of antibacterial activity against most pathogens, this difference in achievable serum concentrations was unlikely to be associated with any difference in clinical effect. Other studies in which the doses used were not so exactly comparable, have found broadly similar results, with higher ofloxacin levels on a milligram for milligram basis (Lockley *et al.*, 1984; Wise *et al.*, 1986; Monk and Campoli-Richards, 1987; Lode *et al.*, 1990).

Oral ofloxacin absorption is slightly reduced during the 2–3 days immediately following cytotoxic chemotherapy for hematological malignancy, resulting in reduction in the expected peak serum concentrations; nevertheless, these are generally still therapeutic against most common pathogens. Rates of absorption have generally returned to pre-chemotherapy values by day 5–7 post-chemotherapy (Brown *et al.*, 1993).

2 Intravenous administration

Following i.v. ofloxacin administration, maximum serum concentrations are reached at the end of a 30-min or 60-min infusion. Compared with oral administration, the maximum serum concentrations achieved after i.v. administration may be up to 50% higher, but distribution and elimination pharmacokinetics are similar regardless of the means of administration, hence overall plasma concentrations after this initial peak are comparable with those reported after oral ofloxacin (Lode *et al.*, 1987; Farinotti *et al.*, 1988; Flor, 1989; Lode *et al.*, 1988; Yuk *et al.*, 1991; Guay *et al.*, 1992). For example, peak serum concentrations after a 400-mg once-daily i.v. dose of ofloxacin are 8.1 ± 2.1 μg per ml (Walstad *et al.*, 1995). Steady-state is generally reached within 24–36 h (Farinotti *et al.*, 1988). This bioequivalence between oral and i.v. ofloxacin supports the interchangeability of both routes of administration (Flor, 1989; Yuk *et al.*, 1991). Compared with ciprofloxacin administered i.v. in doses of either 100 or 200 mg, ofloxacin achieves higher and more long-lasting concentrations in serum (see Fig. II.8) due to the higher elimination rate (both renal and extrarenal) of ciprofloxacin. However, the clinical relevance of this finding is unclear (Lode *et al.*, 1988).

Total body clearance of ofloxacin appears to be lower (>50%) in patients requiring mechanical ventilation, such as in the intensive care setting, than in healthy volunteers. The elimination half-life, peak and trough serum concentrations and AUC were all noted to increase in this setting in one small study; but the explanation for these changes remains unclear and is possibly multifactorial (Martin *et al.*, 1991).

3 Patients with renal failure

Since ofloxacin is primarily eliminated by the kidney (p. 1117), reduction in renal function is linearly related to increases in the elimination half-life of ofloxacin and therefore significant increases in ofloxacin levels. In severely uremic patients the terminal half-life increases from the normal 5–8 h to 37 h (approximately 6- to 9-fold increase). However, renal impairment does not alter the availability of the drug, the volume of distribution or the non-renal clearance; although in some cases (especially when GFR <30ml per min) the time to reach peak serum concentrations may be increased (Fillastre *et al.*, 1987; Höffler and Koeppe, 1987; Bandai *et al.*, 1989; Lameire *et al.*, 1991).

Neither hemodialysis nor CAPD remove clinically significant amounts of ofloxacin. After an initial 200-mg oral dose followed by 100 mg per day for 10 days, Kampf *et al.* (1992) found serum peak and trough concentrations to be 3.1 μg per ml and 1.6 μg per ml, respectively – levels roughly comparable with those achieved with oral doses of 300–400 mg in healthy volunteers. Kampf *et al.* (1990, 1992) found that hemodialysis achieved a fractional removal of ofloxacin of 21.5%, but that this was significantly below the 30–50% which is considered the lower limit for the definition of drug dialisability. Wide variations in half-life, maximum serum concentrations and time to achieve these peaks are noted in patients undergoung hemodialysis (White *et al.*, 1988). In addition, hemodialysis removes only slight amounts of the metabolite desmethyl ofloxacin (White *et al.*, 1988).

Ofloxacin given intraperitoneally in patients undergoing CAPD is almost completely absorbed after an 8-h dwell regardless of the presence or absence of peritonitis. Peritoneal clearance accounts for only about one-tenth of total serum clearance under these circumstances. A single dose of 200 mg in the first bag of three 2-liter × 8-h exchanges provides adequate serum and peritoneal concentrations for more than 24 h in patients undergoing CAPD (Cheng *et al.*, 1993). After an oral dose of 300 mg ofloxacin, peak serum concentrations of 2.44 μg per ml are achieved 3.7 h later, but peritoneal fluid concentrations undergo cyclical changes with each change of solutions, reaching > 0.5 μg per ml after 2 h of equilibration. CAPD per exchange removes < 2% of the total ofloxacin dose (Chan *et al.*, 1987). Kampf *et al.* (1991) found that the elimination of ofloxacin from dialysate was significantly faster in patients with peritonitis compared with those without peritonitis. Intraperitoneal ofloxacin 20 mg per 2 liters every 6 h resulted in mean peritoneal fluid concentrations at the end of each exchange of >3 μg per ml.

The optimal dosing of oral ofloxacin to achieve good peritoneal concentrations in CAPD is not precisely defined. However, Chan *et al.* (1988b) described two small open studies: one in which a single oral dose of 400 mg was followed by 200 mg daily for 7 days; and the second in which 400 mg oral ofloxacin was followed by 300 mg daily for 10 days. The cure rate was 50% versus 83%, respectively, and with the second dosing regimen mean serum trough levels plateaued at 6 μg per ml on day 10 and the mean peritoneal effluent ofloxacin levels all exceeded 3 μg per ml.

4 Patients with hepatic failure

Among patients with alcoholic cirrhosis, ascitic fluid penetration is about 80% after the first oral dose of ofloxacin and concentrations equal corresponding plasma concentrations after 10 h, without significant ascitic accumulation of ofloxacin (Silvain *et al.*, 1989). Renal clearance is significantly reduced in patients with ascites, probably due to alteration in tubular secretion of ofloxacin. This occurs regardless of the presence of normal serum creatinine concentrations, and is responsible for an increased elimination half-life. These pharmacokinetic changes do not always correlate with changes in hepatic function tests. A secondary peak in serum ofloxacin concentrations may be seen 4–6 h after dosing, possibly due to either enterohepatic circulation or biphasic gastric emptying of ofloxacin (Silvain *et al.*, 1989; Montay and Gaillot, 1990; Orlando *et al.*, 1992).

5 Elderly patients

Molinarno *et al.* (1992) found mild prolongation of the elimination half-life in geriatric patients (8.5 h versus 6.2 h in younger controls), with AUC and peak plasma concentrations in elderly patients exceeding those in young healthy volunteers (peak concentrations: 4.7 versus 2.7 μg per ml, respectively). Other authors have noted that alteration in ofloxacin pharmacokinetics is mainly associated with changes in renal function rather than simply aging (Flor, 1989; Lamp *et al.*, 1992).

6 Pregnant women

Two doses of ofloxacin 400 mg i.v. every 12 h results in maternal serum concentrations of between 0.07 and 0.68 μg per ml, with amniotic fluid concentrations of 0.13 to 0.25 μg per ml (Giamarellou *et al.*, 1989). However, ofloxacin, like other fluoroquinolones should be avoided in pregnancy (p. 997).

Excretion

1 Urine

Ofloxacin is mainly eliminated unchanged in the urine, with 70–90% of a dose recoverable after 24–48 h and only minimal amounts (<4%) as metabolites. The renal clearance of ofloxacin is linearly related to the creatinine clearance, being 10.2–12.0 liters per h after oral dosing in healthy humans (Lode *et al.*, 1987, 1988, 1990; Marchbanks *et al.*, 1992). Very high urinary levels are therefore achieved with usual therapeutic doses (p. 1119).

2 Inactivation in body

Serum protein binding of ofloxacin is about 30% (Chantot and Bryskier, 1985). Ofloxacin is not metabolized to any large extent, but is excreted unchanged in the urine. In fact, ofloxacin undergoes less biotransformation than other commonly available fluoroquinolones. Desmethylo-floxacin and ofloxacin *N*-oxide are the two major metabolites, but these account for only about 6% of the total dose (Borner and Lode, 1986; Eliopoulos, 1988; Lode *et al.*, 1987, 1990). Desmethyl ofloxacin has significant antimicrobial activity, although less than ofloxacin (White *et al.*, 1987).

3 Feces

Fecal elimination accounts for only about 4% of an ofloxacin dose after 48 h, and about 8% after 7 days (Ichihara *et al.*, 1984; Lode *et al.*, 1990; Wong and Flor, 1990).

Distribution of the Drug in Body

Similar to ciprofloxacin and other fluoroquinolones, ofloxacin penetrates well into blister fluid. After a 600-mg oral dose, penetration is up to 125%, with a mean peak level of 5.2 μg per ml reached in experimental human blister fluid at 5.3 h (Lockley *et al.*, 1984; Kalager *et al.*, 1986; Wise *et al.*, 1986; Wise and Lockley, 1988). After more commonly used doses of 200 mg twice-daily for 3.5 days, Warlich *et al.* (1990) noted blister fluid concentrations to be 0.94 -1.1 μg per ml 12 h after dosing, suggesting good skin penetration.

Ofloxacin levels in saliva are comparable with those in serum after a 300-mg oral dose. Although the time to achieve peak concentrations in saliva is slightly delayed compared with serum, the overall pharmacokinetic correlations are sufficiently similar that some authors advocate the use of salivary ofloxacin concentrations as a less invasive alternative to measuring serum ofloxacin levels when monitoring ofloxacin absorption (Koizumi *et al.*, 1994; Fujita *et al.*, 1995). Ofloxacin also penetrates well into nasal secretions and tissues, including cartilage and mucosa, and the tonsils (Barza, 1988; Van Landuyt *et al.*, 1988; Wise and Lockley, 1988; Tolsdorff, 1993a). Similarly, middle ear concentrations after a single 400-mg dose 3–7 h prior to tympanoplasty are good, being 2.2 μg per g in mucous membrane and bone (Thorn, 1987; Barza, 1988; Tolsdorff, 1993b).

Peak ofloxacin concentrations in tears after oral dosing are about 60% those in serum (Barza, 1988). After a single oral dose of 400 mg ofloxacin, the mean ratios of aqueous humor to plasma concentrations are 0.18, 0.35, 0.45. 0.69 and 1.43, after a duration post-dose of 2, 6, 12, 24 and 48 h, respectively (Fisch *et al.*, 1987). Ocular lens concentrations, however, are generally low (Fisch *et al.*, 1987). Giamarellou *et al.* (1993) and von Gunten *et al.* (1994) have found similar results with aqueous humor concentrations 2 h after an oral dose of 200 mg of 0.38 μg per ml and after 400 mg of 0.44–2.27 μg per ml. Comparable penetration is noted with i.v. ofloxacin. Ofloxacin penetration is superior to that of ciprofloxacin, but less than that of pefloxacin (Giamarellou *et al.*, 1993). Topical 0.3% ofloxacin eyedrops generally achieve higher aqueous humor concentrations than other commonly available fluoroquinolone drops: when instilled six times at 3-hourly intervals, mean aqueous humor concentrations of 0.53 μg per ml can be expected, or lower concentrations with less frequent administration (Donnenfeld *et al.*, 1994; Tang-Liu *et al.*, 1994; von Gunten *et al.*, 1994). Minimal systemic absorption or toxicity occurs with topical administration (Borrmann *et al.*, 1992).

Ofloxacin administered either i.v. or orally, pentrates well into bronchial secretions, lung tissue and pleural fluid. Among patients with purulent exacerbations of chronic respiratory disease, Davies *et al.* (1987a) noted sputum ofloxacin concentrations of 2.7, 6.1 and 6.3 μg per ml after single doses of either 400 mg, 600 mg, or 800 mg, respectively. Similar concentrations have been reported in bronchial secretions obtained at bronchoscopy (Symonds *et al.*, 1988; Perea, 1990). Among patients with tuberculous pleural effusions treated with oral ofloxacin 300 mg once-daily, pleural fluid concentrations of 3.82–4.21 μg per ml can be expected 2–4 h post-dose (Yew *et al.*, 1991). Mean lung tissue levels after 200 mg oral ofloxacin are 2.17 μg per g, representing a mean lung tissue/serum concentration ratio of 2.6–3.9, depending on the number of doses given and whether the lung is diseased (Perea, 1990; Serour *et al.*, 1991). Davey *et al.* (1991) noted wide variations in bronchial mucosa levels after single and multiple dosing with 200 mg ofloxacin, with concentrations of 1.3–15.5 μg per g and 1.7–21.0 μg per g, respectively. Similarly, 2 h after a single oral dose of 600 mg, Wijnands *et al.* (1988) noted mean lung tissue concentrations of 17.7 ± 9.2 μg per g. Couraud *et al.* (1987) reported similar results. Good intracellular penetration can be expected with high ofloxacin concentrations in alveolar macrophages, epithelial cells and fibroblasts (Perea, 1990; Walstad *et al.*, 1995).

Ofloxacin penetrates well into myocardium, heart valves and sternal bone, but relatively poorly into mediastinal fat. One hour after a single dose of i.v. 400 mg ofloxacin, peak concentrations in myocardium and heart valves are 8.9 and 5.0 μg per g, respectively. After multiple 200-mg oral doses of ofloxacin twice-daily, concentrations 9–10 h post-dose in myocardium, heart valve, sternal bone marrow and mediastinal fat are 5.92, 1.57, 2.56 and 0.67 μg per g, respectively (Mertes *et al.*, 1992).

Similar to other fluoroquinolones, ofloxacin penetrates well into bone. During total hip replacement surgery for osteoarthritis, tissue concentrations measured approximately 1.5, 4 and 12 h after a single 200-mg i.v. dose were 0.64, 0.86 and 0.59 μg per g, respectively, in cortical bone; 1.70, 1.47 and 0.99 μg per g, respectively, in cancellous bone; and 1.38, 2.19 and 2.18 μg per g, respectively, in cartilage (Meissner *et al.*, 1990).

Regardless of the presence or absence of meningitis, ofloxacin (both oral and i.v.) penetrates sufficiently well into CSF to be clinically effective against typical Gram-negative pathogens such as *N. meningitidis*, *H. influenzae* and *E. coli*. In general, however, inadequate bactericidal titers are obtained against *Strep. pneumoniae*, *Staph. aureus* and *Listeria monocytogenes* (Stubner *et al.*, 1986; Bitar *et al.*, 1989). Concentrations in CSF may be up to 50–60% of those in serum after 200 mg oral ofloxacin twice-daily among patients with meningitis (Stahl *et al.*, 1986). Among 22 patients with purulent meningitis treated concurrently with conventional antibiotics and ofloxacin, concentrations of ofloxacin in CSF were 0.96–1.80 μg per ml, depending on sample time after three successive i.v. doses of 200 mg ofloxacin (Pioget *et al.*, 1989). As might be expected, studies of patients without purulent meningitis have shown lower CSF concentrations of ofloxacin. Among patients with acute lymphoblastic leukemia receiving ofloxacin for bowel decontamination, Anders *et al.* (1987) reported mean CSF ofloxacin concentrations of 0.33 ± 0.12 μg per ml, although the timing of these samples in relation to dosing was unclear. Due to concerns about the possibility of obtaining sub-therapeutic CSF concentrations with doses of 200 mg ofloxacin, Nau *et al.* (1994) measured CSF concentrations in six patients with occlusive hydrocephalus caused by various cerebrovascular diseases, treated with a single 400-mg i.v. dose of ofloxacin, in which the CSF was obtained from an external ventriculostomy. A mean peak CSF concentration of 2.04 μg per ml was obtained 0.5–4h post-dose. The overall penetration of ofloxacin into CSF, as expressed by the ratios of the AUCs, was 0.59–0.81 (mean 0.65).

High urine concentrations of ofloxacin are readily achieved. Following oral administration of a single dose of 200 mg, average urine concentrations are 220 μg per ml and 34 μg per ml after 0–6h and 12–24h, respectively (AHFS, 1996). After a 600-mg dose, mean urine ofloxacin concentrations 0–4h, 4–8h, 8–12h, 12–24h and 24–48h later are 141.3, 46.4, 11.2, 6.7 and 2.2 μg per ml, respectively (Wise *et al.*, 1986; Wise and Lockley, 1988). Excellent renal tissue levels are also easily obtained. After a single 300-mg ofloxacin dose, renal parenchyma concentrations are 19.2–22.1 μg per g (di Silverio *et al.*, 1987). After administration of a single oral dose of 200 mg ofloxacin only 9.7% is recoverable in peritoneal dialysate and 10.1% in hemodialysis dialysate (Flor, 1989). Similar to ciprofloxacin (p. 1007), ofloxacin penetrates well into prostatic tissue/fluid and ejaculate. After a single 400-mg oral dose of ofloxacin prior to transurethral prostatectomy, prostatic tissue concentrations are similar to, or higher than, those in serum (Fujita and Munakata, 1988). Di Silverio *et al.* (1987) noted prostate concentrations of 10.6 μg per g after a single 300 mg dose of ofloxacin. Ofloxacin concentrations in ejaculate collected from healthy volunteers treated with 400 mg per day for 3.5 days are about 2.5 μg per ml – notably sperm motility is not affected by ofloxacin concentrations up to 4.5 μg per ml (Schramm, 1986). Naber *et al.* (1993) noted median concentrations of ofloxacin in prostatic fluid among healthy volunteers treated with 400 mg to be about one-third that in plasma; while in ejaculate and seminal fluid the concentrations were about twice those of plasma.

Weissenbacher *et al.* (1984) found concentrations of 0.36–2.6 μg per g in uterine muscle after oral ofloxacin, while concentrations of 1.6–21.6 μg per ml have been noted in vaginal fluid after oral ofloxacin 200 mg twice-daily (Tartaglione *et al.*, 1988).

Biliary penetration of ofloxacin is good (Kazmierczak *et al.*, 1987; Pederzoli *et al.*, 1987; Chin *et al.*, 1990). After seven oral doses of 200 mg twice-daily, peak common duct bile concentrations 7.5h after the first dose and 14h after the seventh dose were 6.6 μg per ml and 12.0 μg per ml, respectively; while mean concentrations in gallbladder wall were 5.3 μg per ml, 6h after the seventh dose (Kazmierczak *et al.*, 1987). Chin *et al.* (1990) found similar results after ofloxacin 400 mg i.v. 12-hourly, with bile and gallbladder concentrations of 6.0 ± 7.9 μg per ml and 3.1 ± 2.9 μg per g, respectively. Penetration of ofloxacin into human allograft pancreatic juice is about 92% that of serum with concentrations of 2.7 μg per ml after 3.6h post-dose (Brattstrom *et al.*, 1988). Similar penetration was noted by Pederzoli *et al.* (1987) among non-transplant patients who had pancreatic fistulae. Fecal concentrations of ofloxacin are 30–65 μg per g (average generally 38–44 μg per g) after 200 mg oral ofloxacin given 12 hourly (Midtvedt, 1987; AHFS, 1996). Other authors have reported fecal concentrations as high as 300 μg per g (AHFS, 1996).

Mode of Action

Ofloxacin acts in a similar manner to other fluoroquinolones such as ciprofloxacin (p. 1008).

Toxicity

The overall rate of adverse reactions reported for ofloxacin in clinical trials is 2.4–12.3%, which compares favorably to other fluoroquinolones such as ciprofloxacin (Koverech *et al.*, 1986; Halkin, 1988; Jüngst and Mohr, 1987, 1988; Tack and Smith, 1989; Berning *et al.*, 1995;

Rubinstein *et al.*, 1994; p. 1008). Side-effects are similar to those reported with other fluoroquinolones including gastrointestinal symptoms (mostly nausea 3.5%), rashes, dizziness (1.2%), headache (1.4%), insomnia (1.8%) and general pruritis (0.9%), which are usually mild to moderate, and are generally rapidly reversible (Tack and Smith, 1989). In only about 0.5–1.7% of patients is cessation of therapy necessary due to adverse reactions (Koverech *et al.*, 1986; Fostini *et al.*, 1988; Halkin, 1988). The incidence of adverse reactions does not appear to increase with patient age (Tack and Smith, 1989). Laboratory abnormalities are uncommon, but include reduced neutrophil count (not true neutropenia; 0.98%), hypoglycemia (0.91%), eosinophilia (0.88%), relative lymphocytosis (0.74%) and elevated liver transaminases (0.69%) (Tack and Smith, 1989). Post-marketing studies in Germany have noted rare reports of hallucinations, psychotic reaction and shock, which were not noted in earlier clinical trials (Jüngst and Mohr, 1988). When ofloxacin (800 mg per day) is given in combination with pyrazinamide (1500 mg per day) as prophylaxis against tuberculosis, the reported rate of adverse effects in one unblinded study was high, with 14 of 16 health care workers discontinuing prophylaxis after less than 6 months (Horn *et al.*, 1994).

Toxicologic evaluation of ofloxacin demonstrates that it has only low toxicologic potential (Davis and McKenzie, 1989). Ofloxacin overdose appears, from limited data, to be relatively benign. A patient who accidentally received 3 g ofloxacin i.v. (peak serum ofloxacin level: 39.3 μg per ml) experienced only moderate/severe central nervous system symptoms, which resolved within 9 h (Kohler *et al.*, 1991).

In addition to the above general side-effects, the following have also been described:

1 Gastrointestinal side-effects

Ofloxacin-associated *Clostridium difficile* diarrhea has been reported rarely (Jüngst and Mohr, 1988; Dan and Samra, 1989).

2 Neurotoxicity

Idiopathic intracranial hypertension has been associated with ofloxacin therapy in one case report; the adverse effect resolved spontaneously with cessation of ofloxacin (Getenet *et al.*, 1993). There have also been case reports of ofloxacin being associated with exacerbations of myasthenia gravis and Guillain-Barré syndrome (Azevedo *et al.*, 1993; Schmidt *et al.*, 1993). Insomnia is a common side-effect, and has been especially noted in children and in patients treated with a combination of ofloxacin and cycloserine for multidrug-resistant TB (Yew *et al.*, 1993; Upton, 1994). Ofloxacin-associated psychosis and delirium have also been described (Zaudig and von Bose, 1987; Zaudig *et al.*, 1989; Fennig and Mauas, 1992).

3 Hypersensitivity reactions and rashes

Similar to ciprofloxacin, hypersensitivity vasculitis, including one fatal case, has been reported in association with ofloxacin therapy by the manufacturer and a number of authors (Huminer *et al.*, 1989; Pace and Gatt, 1989). Ofloxacin has only a low potential to cause phototoxic reactions in humans, being comparable in risk to norfloxacin, and slightly better than ciprofloxacin (Scheife *et al.*, 1993). Ofloxacin has been associated with a fixed drug eruption in one case report (Kawada *et al.*, 1994).

4 Arthropathy

Ofloxacin therapy has been associated with Achilles tendonitis in both rats and humans (Kato *et al.*, 1995). In one study of seven cases with Achilles tendonitis during therapy with either ofloxacin or pefloxacin, three patients ruptured the tendon (Ribard *et al.*, 1992).

5 Renal side-effects

Renal failure has been only rarely reported in association with ofloxacin therapy (Espiriu and Walton, 1995).

6 Immune modulation

Ofloxacin therapy (600 mg per day for 10 days) does not affect T or B lymphocyte numbers, or the concentration of plasma interferon gamma or serum immunoglobulins in elderly patients (Munno *et al.*, 1990).

7 Drug interactions

Ofloxacin does not impair hepatic metabolism of drugs to any major extent (Davey, 1988). Gregoire *et al.* (1987) noted that co-administration of ofloxacin with theophylline for 1 day did not change theophylline clearance, but that co-administration for 4 days resulted in a statistically significant decrease (12.1%) in clearance; but that despite this, there were no increase in clinical adverse reactions. Thus, although there is statistically an interaction between ofloxacin and methylxanthines such as theophylline or caffeine, this is not clinically significant and no dosage alteration of these latter compounds is necessary during co-administration (Fourtillan *et al.*, 1986; Wijnands and Vree, 1988; Harder *et al.*, 1989; Tack and Smith, 1989; Wijnands *et al.*, 1989; Marchbanks 1993). In this regard, ofloxacin appears to be roughly comparable with lomefloxacin and fleroxacin (Parent and LeBel, 1991).

Co-administration of food reduces peak serum ofloxacin concentrations by 20% compared with fasting conditions and the time to reach maximum concentration is prolonged by about 1 h, however there is no alteration to the overall extent of absorption or elimination rate of ofloxacin (Dudley *et al.*, 1991). Milk and yoghurt, however, do not impair the rate or extent of ofloxacin absorption (Dudley *et al.*, 1991; Neuvonen and Kivisto, 1992). Ofloxacin absorption is significantly less affected by the co-administration of the enteral feeding product ('Ensure') than ciprofloxacin (p. 1013), although relative bioavailability is 90 ± 8.3% compared with co-administration with water (Mueller *et al.*, 1994).

Overall ofloxacin absorption is not significantly impaired by the co-administration of calcium carbonate or aluminum phosphate, although it may be delayed and possibly slightly reduced by co-administration of magnesium-aluminum hydroxide – nevertheless this effect is somewhat less than that observed with other fluoroquinolones (Maesen *et al.*, 1987; Flor *et al.*, 1990; Akerele and Okhamafe, 1991; Sánchez Navarro *et al.*, 1994). Regardless of these findings, separating the administration of ofloxacin and these antacids by 2 h would seem prudent. Similarly, concurrent administration of sucralfate and ofloxacin reduces ofloxacin bioavailability by about 61%, but no such reduction occurs if the ofloxacin is given 2 h prior to sucralfate (Kawakami *et al.*, 1994; Lehto and Kivistö, 1994).

The absorption of ciprofloxacin, norfloxacin and ofloxacin is significantly reduced by the co-administration of ferrous sulfate, although ofloxacin is less affected than the other agents, with a reduction of AUC and peak plasma concentrations of 25% and 36%, respectively. Thus, ferrous sulfate and these fluoroquinolones should not be administered together (Lehto *et al.*, 1994).

Ofloxacin may occasionally interact with warfarin to significantly prolong prothrombin time, so careful monitoring of prothrombin time is necessary if these drugs are administered concurrently (Leor and Matetzki, 1988; Baciewicz *et al.*, 1993).

Co-administration of either amoxycillin or the non-steroidal anti-inflammatory agent, ketprofen, does not alter the pharmacokinetics of ofloxacin (Fillastre *et al.*, 1993; Paintaud *et al.*, 1993). Although not really a drug interaction, clinicians should be aware that ofloxacin may result in a false positive screen for urinary porphyrins. This interference in the screening test is thought to be due to an overlap in the emission fluorescence spectra of ofloxacin and urinary porphyrins at the wavelength 600 nm. The use of high-performance liquid chromatography (HPLC) to separate ofloxacin from urinary porphyrins should help avoid the possibility of making a false-positive diagnosis (Schoenfeld and Mamet, 1994).

Clinical Uses of the Drug

Overall, ofloxacin has clinical activity roughly comparable with ciprofloxacin, for which there is more clinical experience, but ofloxacin offers the potential advantage of being less likely to interact with other concomitantly administered agents such as theophylline, caffeine and fenbufen (p. 1014). Since there have been few head-to-head comparisons, the clinician is left to choose between ofloxacin and ciprofloxacin based on their clinical experience. Against pathogens susceptible to both agents such as *H. influenzae*, Gram-negative cocci and Enterobacteriaceae both agents appear comparable, although ofloxacin may be inferior to ciprofloxacin against infections due to *Ps. aeruginosa*. Unlike ciprofloxacin, ofloxacin is effective in genitourinary infections due to *Chlamydia trachomatis*. The clinical use of oral and i.v. ofloxacin has been previously reviewed by a number of authors and hence the following discussion will summarize clinically useful data and draw comparisons with ciprofloxacin for which the clinical uses have already been discussed in depth (p. 1014) (Monk and Campoli-Richards, 1987; Graninger *et al.*, 1990; Kanellakopoulou and Giamarellou, 1990; Mouton *et al.*, 1990; Regamey and Steinbach-Lebbin, 1990; Todd and Faulds, 1991; Eron and Gentry, 1992; Sanders, 1992b; Bassaris *et al.*, 1995; Giamarellou, 1995).

1 Urinary tract infection and prostatitis

Ofloxacin is very effective in the treatment of both complicated and uncomplicated urinary tract infection, especially those due to Gram-negative pathogens. Cure rates of ≥89% can generally be expected for uncomplicated urinary tract infection (Cox, 1989, 1991; Cox *et al.*, 1992; Sanders,

1992b; Spencer and Cole, 1992; Raz *et al.*, 1994). A 3-day course of ofloxacin 200 mg daily is similar in efficacy to a 7-day course of co-trimoxazole 160/800 mg twice-daily among women with uncomplicated urinary tract infection, with an 89% cure rate 5 weeks post-treatment. Similar to other agents, however, single dose therapy with ofloxacin is generally inferior in efficacy to longer duration regimens, although some authors have reported success (Ode *et al.*, 1987; Raz *et al.*, 1988; Hooton *et al.*, 1989, 1991). Postcoital prophylaxis with either 100 mg ofloxacin, 200 mg norfloxacin or 125 mg ciprofloxacin is highly effective for pre- and postmenopausal women with recurrent urinary tract infections (Pfau and Sacks, 1994). In a small head-to-head comparison, a 7-day course of ofloxacin 100 mg twice-daily demonstrated similar efficacy to a 7-day course of ciprofloxacin 250 mg twice-daily (63% cure in both groups) among patients with infection associated with structural or functional abnormalities of the urinary tract (Kromann-Andersen *et al.*, 1988). Other authors have reported approximately 75% clinical efficacy with ofloxacin 200 mg daily for 7–10 days in complicated urinary sepsis (Rugendorff, 1987; Schalkhauser, 1990). Similarly, other small studies have found encouraging results in which ofloxacin is comparable with various regimens of fleroxacin or rufloxacin for complicated urinary tract infections (Mattina *et al.*, 1993; Naber and Sigl, 1993; McCue *et al.*, 1995; Zorbas *et al.*, 1995). A single dose of oral ofloxacin 600 mg 4–12 h prior to transurethral surgery in males appeared to provide effective prophylaxis against urinary sepsis in one small study in which it was compared with a single dose of i.m. cefotaxime (Madsen *et al.*, 1995).

Similar to other fluoroquinolones, ofloxacin has shown excellent activity in the treatment of prostatitis, although there are fewer data available than for ciprofloxacin (Sanders, 1992b; p. 1015).

2 Bacterial diarrhea and enteric fever

Similar to ciprofloxacin (p. 1016), ofloxacin 200–400 mg (generally 300 mg) twice-daily for 7–14 days is highly effective against multiresistant typhoid fever and in clearing fecal carriage (Loffler and Grafvon Westphalen, 1986; Wang *et al.*, 1989; Sabbour and Osman, 1990; DuPont, 1993; Khan *et al.*, 1994). In an open, randomized comparison of short-course treatment of uncomplicated enteric fever (mostly *Salm. typhi*) in Vietnam: oral ofloxacin 200 mg twice-daily for 5 days versus i.v. ceftriaxone 3 g once-daily for 3 days, ofloxacin was significantly superior to ceftriaxone (100% versus 72% cure, respectively) (Smith *et al.*, 1994). Similarly, Tran *et al.* (1995) also reported excellent results with short-course ofloxacin therapy for multiresistant typhoid in a paired, open, randomized study comparing ofloxacin 15 mg per kg per day for 3 days with 10 mg per kg per day for 5 days, in which 65% of subjects were ≤ 14 years age. Both treatments were completely effective except for one treatment failure in a patient who took one dose only.

A 3-day regimen of ofloxacin 300 mg twice-daily is as effective as a 5-day regimen, and superior to placebo, in the treatment of patients with both culture-positive and culture-negative travelers' diarrhea (DuPont *et al.*, 1992). Rates of clinical cure and microbiologic eradication are generally 89–95% and 96%, respectively. In a Norwegian study of acute bacterial enteritis, a 3-day regimen of ofloxacin 400 mg once-daily was effective therapy for acute bacterial enteritis, however the cure rates were lower than those reported for travelers' diarrhea (Halstensen *et al.*, 1995b).

3 Sexually transmitted diseases

a Gonorrhea Ofloxacin 400 mg orally in a single dose is recommended by CDC as an alternative to ceftriaxone (p. 361), cefixime (p. 412) or ciprofloxacin (p. 1022) for the treatment of uncomplicated gonococcal infection (CDC, 1993). Numerous studies with such a regimen have reported a clinical cure rate of >95% – comparable with that expected with ceftriaxone (Richmond *et al.*, 1988; Black *et al.*, 1989; Lutz, 1989; Covino *et al.*, 1990; Smith *et al.*, 1991; Ridgway, 1995; Sivayathorn, 1995). Various studies have identified a ≥ 88% cure rate with this dose for pharyngeal or rectal gonococcal infection (Black *et al.*, 1989; CDC, 1993; Moran and Levine, 1995). Of major concern is the growing number of reports of fluoroquinolone-resistant gonococcal infections from South-East Asia, Australia, Hong Kong, Britain and the USA (CDC, 1995; p. 993).

b Chlamydia and Ureaplasma infection In situations where doxycycline or azithromycin is inappropriate for the treatment of chlamydial sexually transmitted disease in men and women, ofloxacin 300 mg orally twice-daily for 7 days is recommended as a suitable alternative regimen (Oriel, 1989; CDC, 1993; Weber and Johnson, 1995). Single-dose therapy with ofloxacin, however, is not reliable against chlamydial sexually transmitted diseases and longer courses such as that recommended above, have been slightly less effective than doxycycline in some reports, but not in others (Boslego *et al.*, 1988; Batteiger *et al.*, 1989; Kitchen *et al.*, 1990; Mogabgab *et al.*, 1990; Faro *et al.*, 1991; Hooton *et al.*, 1992; Sivayathorn, 1995). Ofloxacin 200–300 mg twice-daily for 7 days also appears to be effective treatment for urethritis due to *Ureaplasma* infection (Mogabgab *et al.*, 1990; Moller *et al.*, 1990).

c   Chancroid   Fluoroquinolones are highly effective against chancroid, with single doses of ofloxacin 400 mg, ciprofloxacin 500 mg or norfloxacin 800 mg all being curative but longer courses may be better (Sivayathorn, 1995; p. 1022).

d   Syphilis   Similar to other fluoroquinolones, ofloxacin has no role in the treatment of syphilis.

4 Respiratory tract infections

Overall, clinical trials of ofloxacin suggest a response rate of about 77–89% in pneumonia and 87–95% in open and comparative studies of acute exacerbations of chronic bronchitis. Bacterial eradication of susceptible pathogens such as *Moraxella catarrhalis* or *H. influenzae* is often 85–94%, but is only about 70% for pneumococci. Various studies, many of insufficient size to statistically confirm equivalence of efficacy, have suggested that ofloxacin in doses of 200–400 mg twice-daily for 7–10 days has clinical efficacy reasonably comparable with ciprofloxacin, amoxicillin, amoxicillin/clavulanate, erythromycin and doxycycline for lower respiratory tract infections, including acute exacerbations of chronic bronchitis and bronchiectasis; but superior efficacy than co-trimoxazole (Lam *et al.*, 1986, 1989; Maesen *et al.*, 1986; Stocks *et al.*, 1989; Ball, 1990; Khajotia *et al.*, 1990; Punakivi *et al.*, 1990; Rademaker *et al.*, 1990; Boye and Gaustad, 1991; Petermann, 1991; Polubiec *et al.*, 1994; Kawahara *et al.*, 1995). In a small dose-comparison study, ofloxacin 200 mg twice-daily appeared to be similar in efficacy to 200 mg thrice-daily for the treatment of respiratory tract infections, but larger studies will be necessary to accurately define the optimal dosing regimen in this setting (Sawae *et al.*, 1995). Due to concerns about the efficacy of ofloxacin against pneumococci, Gaillat *et al.* (1994) compared penicillin G plus ofloxacin to erythromycin plus amoxicillin/clavulanate in the treatment of community-acquired pneumonia in which *Strep. pneumoniae* constituted about half of the identifiable pathogens. As might be expected, no difference in efficacy was noted. For infections due to *Ps. aeruginosa*, ofloxacin doses of 800 mg twice-daily have been used by some authors (Meek *et al.*, 1989). Among older children with cystic fibrosis, ofloxacin has been used to treat infective exacerbations of respiratory disease, but more data is available regarding ciprofloxacin in this setting (Grenier, 1989; LeBel, 1991; p. 1025).

Ofloxacin 400 mg twice-daily has been effective in the treatment of lower respiratory tract infections due to *Chlamydia pneumoniae* in four patients, and may be a suitable alternative to erythromycin in some patients (Lipsky *et al.*, 1990). Despite *in vitro* susceptibility, ofloxacin therapy has been ineffective in some cases of pneumonia due to *Legionella pneumophila* (Salord *et al.*, 1993).

5 Mycobacterial infections

a   Tuberculosis   In an early clinical study, ofloxacin was given to 19 patients with chronic cavitary lung tuberculosis in single doses of 300 mg daily for 8 months. All of these patients had disease due to isoniazid-resistant strains and all but one strain were also resistant to rifampicin. In 17 of the 19 patients other anti-tuberculosis drugs were also given, but because the strains were resistant to most of them, treatment with ofloxacin was virtually monotherapy. A decrease in the amount of tubercle bacilli in the sputum occurred in almost all patients, with complete clearance in five. As might be expected, ofloxacin-resistant strains of *M. tuberculosis* appeared in patients who did not show negative conversion (Tsukamura *et al.*, 1985). Subsequently, a number of studies have demonstrated the clinical efficacy of fluoroquinolones, especially ofloxacin and ciprofloxacin, in the management of tuberculosis (Kohno *et al.*, 1992; Yew *et al.*, 1994b; p. 1031). Discussion regarding the role of ofloxacin in anti-tuberculous regimens can be found on p. 1200.

b   Leprosy   Ofloxacin has demonstrated impressive activity against *M. leprae* in laboratory studies and in clinical trials (Ji and Grosset, 1991; Gelber, 1994; Ji *et al.*, 1994). Among 24 patients with newly diagnosed lepromatous leprosy three treatment regimens were studied: monotherapy with either ofloxacin 400 mg daily or ofloxacin 800 mg daily, and combination therapy with ofloxacin 400 mg daily + dapsone 100 mg daily + clofazimine 50 mg daily + clofazimine 300 mg once every 28 days. The patients in all three groups demonstrated dramatic clinical improvement and marked reduction in viable *M. leprae* organisms as measured by inoculation into mouse footpads. Mild to moderate hepatotoxicity (elevated glutamic pyruvic transaminase) was noted in four patients after 28 days therapy, but all returned to normal after trial completion. Clinical improvement, bactericidal activity and hepatotoxicity did not differ significantly among the treatment groups (Ji *et al.*, 1994). Although further studies will be necessary to confirm these clinical findings, ofloxacin appears to be a potentially exciting new treatment option for leprosy.

c Other mycobacterial infections   Ofloxacin, either as monotherapy or in combination with amikacin, is effective treatment for sternotomy wound infections due to *M. fortuitum* (Yew *et al.*, 1989a,b, 1990b). Although various dosage regimens have been used, Yew *et al.* (1990b) found 600 mg once-daily for about 3–6 months to be effective as monotherapy. Combination oral ofloxacin plus systemic and intraventricular amikacin has also been used to cure a ventriculoatrial shunt infection due to *M. fortuitum* (Chan *et al.*, 1991).

6 Osteomyelitis

Similar to other fluoroquinolones, ofloxacin is effective in the treatment of acute and chronic osteomyelitis, especially when it is due to Gram-negative pathogens. However, efficacy against Gram-positive infections such as those due to staphylococcal species is somewhat less reliable (overall cure rate about 67–85%) (Ketterl *et al.*, 1988; Dellamonica *et al.*, 1989; Gentry and Rodriguez-Gomez, 1991). In a relatively small randomized study comparing ofloxacin 400 mg twice-daily for 8 weeks with prolonged parenteral antibiotic therapy (either cefazolin or ceftazidime for an average of 4 weeks) for the treatment of biopsy-confirmed non-prosthesis osteomyelitis, the long-term response to therapy was 14 of 19 (74%) for ofloxacin versus 12 of 14 (86%) for parenteral therapy. Infecting pathogens included *Staph. aureus* (40%), *Enterococcus* spp. (3%), *Ps. aeruginosa* (15%) and other Gram-negative pathogens (42%), but of the four relapses among the ofloxacin-treated group, three were due to *Staph. aureus*. Although the authors suggest that these two modes of therapy are equivalent in efficacy, there was insufficient statistical power in this study to make this claim. Nevertheless, these findings are notable, given the difficulty in undertaking such clinical studies on osteomyelitis. In an interesting study, Drancourt *et al.* (1993) found that long-term therapy with a combination of rifampicin 900 mg daily plus ofloxacin 200 mg thrice-daily (600 mg per day) and timely removal of the prosthesis, may be effective in a reasonable proportion of patients with susceptible *Staphylococcus*-infected orthopedic implants. Patients with hip prosthesis infections were treated for 6 months with removal of any unstable prostheses after 5 months of treatment; patients with knee prosthesis infections were treated for 9 months with removal of the prosthesis after 6 months of treatment, and patients with infected bone plates were treated for 6 months with removal of the plate after 3 months in some cases. The choice of these various treatment algorithms appeared to be somewhat arbitrary and possibly open to some clinician bias. Among the evaluable 51 patients, four had side-effects such that they were not evaluable for treatment efficacy, while 35 of the remaining 47 patients (74%) were cured 6 months after therapy – implying an overall success rate based on intention-to-treat of 69%. These results are encouraging compared with previously published data on treatment of these difficult infections.

7 Soft tissue and skin infections

Similar to ciprofloxacin (p. 1020), ofloxacin appears to have reasonable activity against skin and soft tissue infections due to Gram-negative pathogens, but its activity against Gram-positive infections such as those due to staphylococci and streptococci is less certain. Data regarding the use of ofloxacin in this setting are less comprehensive than those available for ciprofloxacin (Gentry *et al.* 1989; Gentry, 1991; Cruciani and Bassetti, 1994; Liu *et al.*, 1995).

8 Nasal carriage of Neisseria meningitidis

Similar to ciprofloxacin (p. 1028), a single dose of ofloxacin 400 mg appears to be highly effective (97.2%) in eradicating nasal carriage of *N. meningitidis* (Gilja *et al.*, 1993; Halstensen *et al.*, 1995a).

9 Prevention of infection in neutropenic patients

Among neutropenic oncology patients, prophylaxis with ofloxacin 300 mg twice-daily is superior to trimethoprim/sulfamethoxazole 160/800 mg twice-daily in preventing febrile episodes, incidence of Gram-negative bacteremia and rate of drug-associated skin rashes (Liang *et al.*, 1990). In this study no patient in either group had documented Gram-positive bacteremia. Other authors have found either similar results, or no difference between these regimens (Arning *et al.*, 1990; Kern *et al.*, 1991; Sawada *et al.*, 1991). Oral ofloxacin prophylaxis also appears to be superior to prophylaxis with oral vancomycin plus polymyxin in this setting, and to be effective single-drug prophylaxis in bone marrow recipients (Winston *et al.*, 1990; Schmeiser *et al.*, 1993). Due to concerns regarding potential 'break through' bacteremia with Gram-positive pathogens among patients receiving ofloxacin prophylaxis (p. 1026), Kern *et al.* (1994b) examined the additional benefit of oral roxithromycin (150 mg twice-daily) prophylaxis in adults with acute leukemia and bone marrow transplant recipients receiving concomitant ofloxacin prophylaxis. Among patients receiving both agents, significantly fewer patients developed bacteremia with viridans group streptococci, but the incidence of bacteremia due to other pathogens and the overall incidence of febrile episodes were otherwise comparable between the two treatment groups. However, adverse reactions were more common among the patients receiving both agents (p=0.05); hence these authors do not recommend the routine addition of roxythromycin prophylaxis to that of ofloxacin, unless there is thought to be a high risk of streptococcal infection. In comparisons of ciprofloxacin, ofloxacin and pefloxacin in this setting; however, ciprofloxacin appears to be associated with lower rates of colonization with resistant Gram-negative bacilli than ofloxacin, or especially pefloxacin (D'Antonio *et al.*, 1994)

10 Treatment of febrile neutropenic patients

Oral ofloxacin 400 mg twice-daily may be similar in efficacy to routine, broad-spectrum combination parenteral antibiotic therapy (e.g. amikacin plus either carbenicillin, cloxacillin or piperacillin) for the treatment of neutropenic febrile patients, with success rates of about 77% versus 73%, respectively (Malik *et al.*, 1992). Subsequently, the same authors in a multicenter, prospective, randomized trial, demonstrated an 83% response among cancer patients with fever and neutropenia who self-administered oral ofloxacin. Two patients died before they could be hospitalized, but among the 15% who were admitted, the vast majority responded to parenteral therapy (Malik *et al.*, 1994). In a later study, about 21% of patients randomized to outpatient therapy with oral ofloxacin 400 mg twice-daily required hospitalization, but mortality rates were comparable between inpatients and outpatients (2% versus 4%, respectively) (Malik *et al.*, 1995). Thus, among low-risk neutropenic febrile patients (e.g. those who are expected to have neutropenia of short duration), outpatient management with oral ofloxacin may be a reasonable treatment option, although some authors believe further studies are needed to confirm these findings (Kromery, 1995).

11 Otitis and sinusitis

Ofloxacin 200 mg twice-daily for 12–39 days has proven effective in the treatment of malignant otitis externa due to *Ps. aeruginosa* (Levy *et al.*, 1990) and in the treatment of chronic sinusitis and chronic otitis media (Gehanno and Cohen, 1993).

12 Ocular infections

Topical 0.3% ofloxacin results in greater intracorneal penetration than do similar doses of either ciprofloxacin or norfloxacin, but there are more clinical data regarding the efficacy of ciprofloxacin in the treatment of ulcerative keratitis than there are for ofloxacin currently (Barza, 1991; Diamond *et al.*, 1995). Topical ofloxacin 0.3% is comparable in efficacy with a fortified solution of 1.5% tobramycin plus 10% cefazolin for the treatment of bacterial keratitis (O'Brien *et al.*, 1995). Topical ofloxacin 0.3% appears to have similar efficacy to either topical gentamicin 0.3% or tobramycin 0.3% in the treatment of external ocular infection due to a variety of Gram-positive and Gram-negative pathogens (Gwon, 1992a,b). Furthermore, topical ofloxacin results in superior penetration into aqueous humor than does tobramycin and is effective in sterilizing the external ocular adnexa (Barza *et al.*, 1991; Kirsch *et al.*, 1995).

13 Peritonitis associated with CAPD

Compared with ciprofloxacin (p. 1030), there are fewer data regarding the efficacy of ofloxacin in the treatment of CAPD-associated peritonitis. A regimen of oral ofloxacin 400 mg initially, followed by 300 mg daily for 10 days resulted in a 1- and 2-month cure rate of 83%, in which staphylococcal species constituted the vast majority of identified pathogens. Ofloxacin diffused well into dialysate and no patients had to discontinue therapy due to side-effects (Chan *et al.*, 1988a). Chan *et al.* (1990) found similar results in a study in which they compared this ofloxacin regimen with intraperitoneal cephalothin plus tobramycin, or oral ofloxacin plus rifampicin. Notably, however, other authors have found monotherapy with ofloxacin, albeit in doses of only

200 mg daily for 10 days, to be inadequate for the empiric treatment of peritonitis, with cure rates of only 67% (Gucek *et al.*, 1994).

14 Intra-abdominal and biliary tract infections

Among patients with cirrhosis and gastrointestinal hemorrhage from ruptured esophageal varices, a 10-day prophylactic course of ofloxacin 400 mg per day was associated with a significant reduction in infections compared with patients receiving no prophylaxis; however, there was no difference in 2-week survival (Blaise *et al.*, 1994). Of concern, however, is the report by Dupeyron *et al.* (1994) (p. 1113) which demonstrated the rapid emergence of quinolone-resistance among fecal organisms in cirrhotic patients treated with norfloxacin prophylaxis to prevent spontaneous bacterial peritonitis. Clearly, long-term prophylaxis with ofloxacin in this setting is likely to carry similar implications.

A 3-week course of oral ofloxacin 400 mg per day was effective in curing an HIV-infected patient with spontaneous peritonitis due to *Yersinia enterocolitica* (Flament-Saillour *et al.*, 1994).

15 Brucellosis

Ofloxacin 400 mg in combination with rifampicin 600 mg each once-daily for 6 weeks is similar in efficacy to a 6-week course of doxycycline 200 mg plus rifampicin 600 mg once-daily in the treatment of *Brucella melitensis* infection, regardless of the presence of complications of the disease. Therapeutic failures were reported in only about 3% patients treated with either regimen, but 43% in the doxycycline/rifampicin group complained of gastric discomfort compared with 6.5% in the ofloxacin/rifampicin group (Akova *et al.*, 1993).

16 Miscellaneous conditions

Clinical efficacy has been reported with oral ofloxacin in the treatment of a case of Q-fever endocarditis (Raffi, 1989). Two patients with postoperative sternotomy infections due to *Nocardia asteroides* have been successfully treated with oral ofloxacin 400–600 mg daily (Yew *et al.*, 1991).

References

AHFS (1996). *American Hospital Formulary Service – Drug Information* (McEnvoy GK, ed), Bethesda, USA: American Society of Health-System Pharmacists.

Akerele JO, Okhamafe AO (1991). Influence of oral co-administered metallic drugs on ofloxacin pharmacokinetics. *J Antimicrob Chemother* **28**: 87.

Akova M, Uzun O, Akalin HE *et al.* (1993). Quinolones in treatment of human brucellosis: comparative trial of ofloxacin-rifampin versus doxycycline-rifampin. *Antimicrob Ag Chemother* **37**: 1831.

Aldridge KE, Gelfand MS, Schiro DD, Barg NL (1992a). The rapid emergence of fluoroquinolone-methicillin-resistant *Staphylococcus aureus* infections in a community hospital. An *in vitro* look at alternative antimicrobial agents. *Diagn Microbiol Infect Dis* **15**: 601.

Aldridge KE, Jones RN, Barry AL, Gelfand MS (1992b). *In vitro* activity of various antimicrobial agents against *Staphylococcus aureus* isolates including fluoroquinolone- and oxacillin-resistant strains. *Diagn Microbiol Infect Dis* **15**: 517.

Anders CU, Hofeler H, Schmidt CG (1987). Concentration of the quinolone ofloxacin in the cerebrospinal fluid. *Amer J Med* **83**: 1006.

Appelbaum PC (1995). Quinolone activity against anaerobes: microbiological aspects. *Drugs* **49** (Suppl 2): 76.

Appleman ME, Hadfield TL, Gaines JK, Winn RE (1987). Susceptibility of *Bordetella pertussis* to five quinolone antimicrobic drugs. *Diagn Microbiol Infect Dis* **8**: 131.

Arning M, Wolf HH, Aul C *et al.* (1990). Infection prophylaxis in neutropenic patients with acute leukaemia – a randomized, comparative study with ofloxacin, ciprofloxacin and co- trimoxazole/colistin. *J Antimicrob Chemother* **26** (Suppl D): 137.

Auckenthaler R, Michéa-Hamzehpur M, Pechère JC (1986). *In-vitro* activity of newer quinolones against aerobic bacteria. *J Antimicrob Chemother* **17** (Suppl B): 29.

Azevedo E, Ribeiro JA, Polonia J, Pontes C (1993). Probable exacerbation of myasthenia gravis by ofloxacin. *J Neurol* **240**: 508.

Baciewicz AM, Ashar BH, Locke TW (1993). Interaction of ofloxacin and warfarin. *Ann Intern Med* **119**: 1223.

Ball P (1990). Overview of experience with ofloxacin in respiratory tract infection. *Scand J Infect Dis* (Suppl 68): 56.

Baltch AL, Smith RP, Ritz W (1995). Inhibitory and bactericidal activities of levofloxacin, ofloxacin, erythromycin, and rifampin used singly and in combination against *Legionella pneumophila*. *Antimicrob Ag Chemother* **39**: 1661.

Bandai H, Tsubakihara Y, Yamato E *et al.* (1989). Pharmacokinetics of ofloxacin in severe chronic renal failure. *Clin Ther* **11**: 210.

Barry AL, Fuchs PC (1991). Anti-staphylococcal activity of temafloxacin, ciprofloxacin, ofloxacin and enoxacin. *J Antimicrob Chemother* **28**: 695.

Barza M (1988). Pharmacokinetics and efficacy of the new quinolones in infections of the eye, ear, nose, and throat. *Rev Infect Dis* **10** (Suppl 1): S241.

Barza M (1991). Use of quinolones for treatment of ear and eye infections. *Eur J Clin Microbiol Infect Dis* **10**: 296.

Bassaris H, Akalin E, Calangu S *et al.* (1995). A randomised, multinational study with sequential therapy comparing ciprofloxacin twice daily and ofloxacin once daily. *Infection* **23**: 227.

Bassey CM, Baltch AL, Smith RP (1986). Comparative antimicrobial activity of enoxacin, ciprofloxacin, amifloxacin, norfloxacin and ofloxacin against 177 bacterial isolates. *J Antimicrob Chemother* **17**: 623.

Batteiger BE, Jones RB, White A (1989). Efficacy and safety of ofloxacin in the treatment of nongonococcal sexually transmitted disease. *Amer J Med* **87**: 75S.

Beermann D, Wingender W, Zeiler HJ *et al.* (1984). Comparative pharmacokinetics of three new quinolone carboxylic acid antibiotics after oral administration in healthy volunteers. *J Clin Pharmacol* **24**: 403.

Bennett WM, Aronoff GR, Golper TA (1994). *Drug Prescribing in Renal Failure* 3rd edn. Philadelphia: American College of Physicians.

Berlin OG, Young LS, Bruckner DA (1987). *In-vitro* activity of six fluorinated quinolones against *Mycobacterium tuberculosis*. *J Antimicrob Chemother* **19**: 611.

Bernard EM, Edwards FF, Kiehn TE *et al.* (1993). Activities of antimicrobial agents against clinical isolates of *Mycobacterium haemophilum*. *Antimicrob Ag Chemother* **37**: 2323.

Berning SE, Madsen L, Iseman MD, Peloquin CA (1995). Long-term safety of ofloxacin and ciprofloxacin in the treatment of mycobacterial infections. *Amer J Respir Crit Care Med* **151**: 2006.

Betriu C, Sanchez A, Gomez M *et al.* (1993). Antibiotic susceptibility of group A streptococci: a 6-year follow-up study. *Antimicrob Ag Chemother* **37**; 1717.

Bitar N, Claes R, Van der Auwera P (1989). Concentrations of ofloxacin in serum and cerebrospinal fluid of patients without meningitis receiving the drug intravenously and orally. *Antimicrob Ag Chemother* **33**: 1686.

Black JR, Long JM, Zwickl BE *et al.* (1989). Multicenter randomized study of single-dose ofloxacin versus amoxicillin- probenecid for treatment of uncomplicated gonococcal infection. *Antimicrob Ag Chemother* **33**: 167.

Blaise M, Pateron D, Trinchet JC *et al.* (1994). Systemic antibiotic therapy prevents bacterial infection in cirrhotic patients with gastrointestinal hemorrhage. *Hepatology* **20**: 34.

Borner K, Lode H (1986). Biotransformation von ausgewählten Gyrasehemmern. *Infection* **14** (Suppl 1): 54.

Borobio MV, Conejo M, Ramirez E *et al.* (1994). Comparative activities of eight quinolones against members of the *Bacteroides fragilis* group. *Antimicrob Ag Chemother* **38**: 1442.

Borrmann L, Tang-Liu DD, Kann J *et al.* (1992). Ofloxacin in human serum, urine, and tear film after topical application. *Cornea* **11**: 226.

Boslego JW, Hicks CB, Greenup R *et al.* (1988). A prospective randomized trial of ofloxacin vs doxycycline in the treatment of uncomplicated male urethritis. *Sex Transm Dis* **15**: 186.

Boye NP, Gaustad P (1991). Double-blind comparative study of ofloxacin (Hoe 280). and trimethoprim-sulfamethoxazole in the treatment of patients with acute exacerbations of chronic bronchitis and chronic obstructive lung disease. *Infection* **19** (Suppl 7): S388.

Brattstrom C, Malborg AS, Tyden G (1987). Penetration of ciprofloxacin and ofloxacin into pancreatic juice. *Chemioterapia* **6**: 295.

Brown NM, White LO, Blundell EL *et al.* (1993). Absorption of oral ofloxacin after cytotoxic chemotherapy for haematological malignancy. *J Antimicrob Chemother* **32**: 117.

Burgos A, Quindos G, Martinez R *et al.* (1990). *In vitro* susceptibility of *Aeromonas caviae*, *Aeromonas hydrophila* and *Aeromonas sobria* to fifteen antibacterial agents. *Eur J Clin Microbiol Infect Dis* **9**: 413.

Cantón E, Peman J, Jimenez MT *et al.* (1992). *In vitro* activity of sparfloxacin compared with those of five other quinolones. *Antimicrob Ag Chemother* **36**: 558.

Casal M, Rodriguez F, Villalba R *et al.* (1987). *In vitro* susceptibility of *Mycobacterium fortuitum*, *Mycobacterium chelonae* and *Mycobacterium avium* against some quinolones. *Chemioterapia* **6**: 431.

CDC (Centers for Disease Control) (1993). Sexually transmitted diseases treatment guidelines. *MMWR* **42** (Suppl RR-14): 1.

CDC (Centers for Disease Control) (1994). Decreased susceptibility of *Neisseria gonorrhoeae* to fluoroquinolones – Ohio and Hawaii, 1992–1994. *MMWR* **43**: 325.

CDC (Centers for Disease Control) (1995). Fluoroquinolone resistance in *Neisseria gonorrhoeae* – Colorado and Washington, 1995. *MMWR* **44**: 761.

Chan KH, Mann KS, Seto WH (1991). Infection of a shunt by *Mycobacterium fortuitum*: case report. *Neurosurgery* **29**: 472.

Chan MK, Chau PY, Chan WW (1987). Ofloxacin pharmacokinetics in patients on continuous ambulatory peritoneal dialysis. *Clin Nephrol* **28**: 277.

Chan MK, Chau PY, Chan WW (1988a). Oral treatment of peritonitis in CAPD patients with ofloxacin. *Nephrol Dial Transplant* **3**: 194.

Chan MK, Chau PY, Chan WW (1988b). Oral treatment of peritonitis in CAPD patients with two dosage regimens of ofloxacin. *J Antimicrob Chemother* **22**: 371.

Chan MK, Cheng IK, Ng WS (1990). A randomized prospective trial of three different regimens of treatment of peritonitis in patients on continuous ambulatory peritoneal dialysis. *Amer J Kidney Dis* **15**: 155.

Chantot JF, Bryskier A (1985). Antibacterial activity of ofloxacin and other 4-quinolone derivatives: *in-vitro* and *in-vivo* comparison. *J Antimicrob Chemother* **16**: 475.

Chaudhry AZ, Knapp CC, Sierra-Madero J, Washington JA (1990). Antistaphylococcal activities of sparfloxacin (CI-978; AT-4140), ofloxacin, and ciprofloxacin. *Antimicrob Ag Chemother* **34**: 1843.

Cheng AF, Li MK, Ling TK, French GL (1987). Emergence of ofloxacin-resistant *Citrobacter freundii* and *Pseudomonas maltophilia* after ofloxacin therapy. *J Antimicrob Chemother* **20**: 283.

Cheng IK, Chau PY, Kumana CR *et al.* (1993). Single-dose pharmacokinetics of intraperitoneal ofloxacin in patients on continuous ambulatory peritoneal dialysis. *Perit Dial Int* **13** (Suppl 2): S383.

Cherubin CE, Stratton CW (1994). Assessment of the bactericidal activity of sparfloxacin, ofloxacin, levofloxacin, and other fluoroquinolones compared with selected agents of proven efficacy against *Listeria monocytogenes*. *Diagn Microbiol Infect Dis* **20**: 21.

Chin A, Okamoto MP, Gill MA *et al.* (1990). Intraoperative concentrations of ofloxacin in serum, bile fluid, and gallbladder wall tissue. *Antimicrob Ag Chemother* **34**: 2354.

Clarke AM, Zemcov SJV, Campbell ME (1985). *In vitro* activity of pefloxacin compared to enoxacin, norfloxacin, gentamicin and new beta-lactams. *J Antimicrob Chemother* **15**: 39.

Clendennen TE III, Hames CS, Kees ES *et al.* (1992a). *In vitro* antibiotic susceptibilities of *Neisseria gonorrhoeae* isolates in the Philippines. *Antimicrob Ag Chemother* **36**: 277.

Clendennen TE, Echeverria P, Saengeur S *et al.* (1992b). Antibiotic susceptibility survey of *Neisseria gonorrhoeae* in Thailand. *Antimicrob Ag Chemother* **36**: 1682.

Cornett JB, Wagner RB, Dobson RA *et al.* (1985). *In vitro* and *in vivo* antibacterial activities of the fluoroquinolone WIN 49375 (Amifloxacin). *Antimicrob Ag Chemother* **27**: 4.

Couraud L, Fourtillan JB, Saux MC *et al.* (1987). Diffusion of ofloxacin into human lung tissue. *Drugs* **34** (Suppl 1): 37.

Covino JM, Cummings M, Smith B *et al.* (1990). Comparison of ofloxacin and ceftriaxone in the treatment of uncomplicated gonorrhea caused by penicillinase-producing and non-penicillinase-producing strains. *Antimicrob Ag Chemother* **34**: 148.

Cox CE (1989). Ofloxacin in the management of complicated urinary tract infections, including prostatitis. *Amer J Med* **87**: 61S.

Cox CE (1991). Parenteral ofloxacin in treatment of pyelonephritis. *Urology* **37**: 16.

Cox CE, Gentry LO, Rodriguez-Gomez G (1992). Multicenter open-label study of parenteral ofloxacin in treatment of pyelonephritis in adults. *Urology* **39**: 453.

Cruciani M, Bassetti D (1994). The fluoroquinolones as treatment for infections caused by gram-positive bacteria. *J Antimicrob Chemother* **33**: 403.

D'Antonio D, Piccolomini R, Iacone A *et al.* (1994). Comparison of ciprofloxacin, ofloxacin and pefloxacin for the prevention of the bacterial infection in neutropenic patients with haematological malignancies. *J Antimicrob Chemother* **33**: 837.

Dagrosa EE, Verho M, Malerczyk V *et al.* (1986). Multiple-dose pharmacokinetics of ofloxacin, a new broad-spectrum antimicrobial agent. *Clin Ther* **8**: 632.

Dan M, Samra Z (1989). Clostridium difficile colitis associated with ofloxacin therapy. *Amer J Med* **87**: 479.

Davey PG (1988). Overview of drug interactions with the quinolones. *J Antimicrob Chemother* **22** (Suppl C): 97.

Davey PG, Precious E, Winter J (1991). Bronchial penetration of ofloxacin after single and multiple oral dosage. *J Antimicrob Chemother* **27**: 335.

Davies BI, Maesen FP, Geraedts WH, Baur C (1987a). Penetration of ofloxacin from blood to sputum. *Drugs* **34** (Suppl 1): 26.

Davies S, Sparham PD, Spencer RC (1987b). Comparative *in-vitro* activity of five fluoroquinolones against mycobacteria. *J Antimicrob Chemother* **19**: 605.

Davis GJ, McKenzie BE (1989). Toxicologic evaluation of ofloxacin. *Amer J Med* **87**: 43S.

De Bernardis E, Bonaccorsi S, Carlino S et al. (1988). Pharmacokinetics and tissue distribution of ofloxacin in human subjects during a multiple dose regimen. *Int J Clin Pharmacol Res* **8**: 239.

Dellamonica P, Bernard E, Etesse H et al. (1989). Evaluation of pefloxacin, ofloxacin and ciprofloxacin in the treatment of thirty-nine cases of chronic osteomyelitis. *Eur J Clin Microbiol Infect Dis* **8**: 1024.

Delmee M, Avesani V (1986). Comparative *in vitro* activity of seven quinolones against 100 clinical isolates of *Clostridium difficile*. *Antimicrob Ag Chemother* **29**: 374.

di Silverio F, Cruciani E, Ferrone G et al. (1987). Tissue levels of ofloxacin in the urogenital system. *Chemioterapia* **6**: 120.

Diamond JP, White L, Leeming JP et al. (1995). Topical 03% ciprofloxacin, norfloxacin, and ofloxacin in treatment of bacterial keratitis: a new method for comparative evaluation of ocular drug penetration. *Brit J Ophthalmol* **79**: 606.

Doganay M, Aydin N (1991). Antimicrobial susceptibility of *Bacillus anthracis*. *Scand J Infect Dis* **23**: 333.

Donnenfeld ED, Schrier A, Perry HD et al. (1994). Penetration of topically applied ciprofloxacin, norfloxacin, and ofloxacin into the aqueous humor. *Ophthalmology* **101**: 902.

Dörfler A, Schulz W, Burkhardt F, Zichner M (1987). Pharmacokinetics of ofloxacin in patients on haemodialysis treatment. *Drugs* **34** (Suppl 1): 62.

Drancourt M, Stein A, Argenson JN et al. (1993). Oral rifampin plus ofloxacin for treatment of Staphylococcus-infected orthopedic implants. *Antimicrob Ag Chemother* **37**: 1214.

Dudley MN, Marchbanks CR, Flor SC, Beals B (1991). The effect of food or milk on the absorption kinetics of ofloxacin. *Eur J Clin Pharmacol* **41**: 569.

Dupeyron C, Mangeney N, Sedrati L et al. (1994). Rapid emergence of quinolone resistance in cirrhotic patients treated with norfloxacin to prevent spontaneous bacterial peritonitis. *Antimicrob Ag Chemother* **38**: 340.

DuPont HL (1993). Quinolones in *Salmonella typhi* infection. *Drugs* **45** (Suppl 3): 119.

DuPont HL, Ericsson CD, Mathewson JJ et al. (1992). Five versus three days of ofloxacin therapy for travelers' diarrhea: a placebo-controlled study. *Antimicrob Ag Chemother* **36**: 87.

Echols R, Weinstein MP, O'Keeffe B et al. (1994). Comparative crossover assessment of serum bactericidal activity and pharmacokinetics of ciprofloxacin and ofloxacin. *J Antimicrob Chemother* **33**: 111.

Eliopoulos GM (1988). New quinolones: pharmacology, pharmacokinetics, and dosing in patients with renal insufficiency. *Rev Infect Dis* **10** (Suppl 1): S102.

Eliopoulos GM (1995). *In vitro* activity of fluoroquinolones against gram-positive bacteria. *Drugs* **49** (Suppl 2): 48.

Eron LJ, Gentry LO (1992). Oral ofloxacin for infections caused by bacteria resistant to oral antimicrobial agents. *Diagn Microbiol Infect Dis* **15**: 435.

Espiritu J, Walton T (1995). Acute renal failure due to ofloxacin. *W V Med J* **91**: 16.

Farinotti R, Trouvin JH, Bocquet V et al. (1988). Pharmacokinetics of ofloxacin after single and multiple intravenous infusions in healthy subjects. *Antimicrob Ag Chemother* **32**: 1590.

Faro S, Martens MG, Maccato M et al. (1991). Effectiveness of ofloxacin in the treatment of *Chlamydia trachomatis* and *Neisseria gonorrhoeae* cervical infection. *Amer J Obstet Gynecol* **164**: 1380.

Fenlon CH, Cynamon MH (1986). Comparative *in vitro* activities of ciprofloxacin and other 4-quinolones against *Mycobacterium tuberculosis* and *Mycobacterium intracellulare*. *Antimicrob Ag Chemother* **29**: 386.

Fennig S, Mauas L (1992). Ofloxacin-induced delirium. *J Clin Psychiat* **53**: 137.

Fernandes PB, Shipkowitz N, Bower RR et al. (1986). *In-vitro* and *in-vivo* potency of five new fluoroquinolones against anaerobic bacteria. *J Antimicrob Chemother* **18**: 693.

Fernandez-Roblas R, Prieto S, Santamaria M et al. (1987). Activity of nine antimicrobial agents against *Corynebacterium* group D2 strains isolated from clinical specimens and skin. *Antimicrob Ag Chemother* **31**: 821.

Fillastre JP, Leroy A, Humbert G (1987). Ofloxacin pharmacokinetics in renal failure. *Antimicrob Ag Chemother* **31**: 156.

Fillastre JP, Leroy A, Borsa-Lebas F et al. (1993). Lack of effect of ketoprofen on the pharmacokinetics of pefloxacin and ofloxacin. *J Antimicrob Chemother* **31**: 805.

Fisch A, Lafaix C, Salvanet A et al. (1987). Ofloxacin in human aqueous humour and lens. *J Antimicrob Chemother* **20**: 453.

Flament-Saillour M, de Truchis P, Risbourg M, Nordmann P (1994). *Yersinia enterocolitica* peritonitis in a patient infected with the human immunodeficiency virus. *Clin Infect Dis* **18**: 655.

Flor S (1989). Pharmacokinetics of ofloxacin. An overview. *Amer J Med* **87**: 24S.

Flor S, Guay DR, Opsahl JA et al. (1990). Effects of magnesium-aluminum hydroxide and calcium carbonate antacids on bioavailability of ofloxacin. *Antimicrob Ag Chemother* **34**: 2436.

Forsgren A (1985). Comparative *in vitro* activity of three new quinolone antibiotics against recent clinical isolates. *Scand J Infect Dis* **17**: 91.

Fostini R, Girelli M, Dalle Vedove P et al. (1988). Safety profile of ofloxacin in elderly patients. *Drugs Exp Clin Res* **14**: 393.

Fourtillan JB, Granier J, Saint-Salvi B et al. (1986). Pharmacokinetics of ofloxacin and theophylline alone and in combination. *Infection* **14** (Suppl 1): S67.

Franzblau SG (1989). Drug susceptibility testing of *Mycobacterium leprae* in the BACTEC 460 system. *Antimicrob Ag Chemother* **33**: 2115.

Fujita K, Munakata A (1988). Serum and prostatic tissue concentrations of ofloxacin. *Clin Ther* **10**: 32.

Fujita K, Matsuoka N, Takenaka I et al. (1995). Pharmacokinetics of ofloxacin – measurement of drug concentration in saliva of patients with impaired renal function. *Drugs* **49** (Suppl 2): 312.

Gaillat J, Bru JP, Sedallian A (1994). Penicillin G/ofloxacin versus erythromycin/amoxicillin-clavulanate in the treatment of severe community-acquired pneumonia. *Eur J Clin Microbiol Infect Dis* **13**: 639.

Garcia I, Bodey GP, Fainstein V et al. (1984). *In vitro* activity of Win 49375 compared with those of other antibiotics in isolates from cancer patients. *Antimicrob Ag Chemother* **26**: 421.

Garcia-Rodriguez JA, Gomez Garcia AC (1993). *In-vitro* activities of quinolones against mycobacteria. *J Antimicrob Chemother* **32**: 797.

Gehanno P, Cohen B (1993). Effectiveness and safety of ofloxacin in chronic otitis media and chronic sinusitis in adult outpatients. *Eur Arch Otorhinolaryngol* **250** (Suppl 1): S13.

Gelber RH (1994). Chemotherapy of lepromatous leprosy: recent developments and prospects for the future. *Eur J Clin Microbiol Infect Dis* **13**: 942.

Gelber RH, Iranmanesh A, Murray L et al. (1992). Activities of various quinolone antibiotics against *Mycobacterium leprae* in infected mice. *Antimicrob Ag Chemother* **36**: 2544.

Gentry LO (1991). Review of quinolones in the treatment of infections of the skin and skin structure. *J Antimicrob Chemother* **28** (Suppl C): 97.

Gentry LO, Rodriguez-Gomez G (1991). Ofloxacin versus parenteral therapy for chronic osteomyelitis. *Antimicrob Ag Chemother* **35**: 538.

Gentry LO, Rodriguez-Gomez G, Zeluff BJ et al. (1989). A comparative evaluation of oral ofloxacin versus intravenous cefotaxime therapy for serious skin and skin structure infections. *Amer J Med* **87**: 57S.

Getenet JC, Croisile B, Vighetto A *et al.* (1993). Idiopathic intracranial hypertension after ofloxacin treatment. *Acta Neurol Scand* **87**: 503.

Giamarellou H (1995). Activity of quinolones against gram-positive cocci: clinical features. *Drugs* **49** (Suppl 2): 58.

Giamarellou H, Kolokythas E, Petrikkos G *et al.* (1989). Pharmacokinetics of three newer quinolones in pregnant and lactating women. *Amer J Med* **87**: 49S.

Giamarellou H, Kanellas D, Kavouklis E *et al.* (1993). Comparative pharmacokinetics of ciprofloxacin, ofloxacin and pefloxacin in human aqueous humour. *Eur J Clin Microbiol Infect Dis* **12**: 293.

Gilja OH, Halstensen A, Digranes A *et al.* (1993). Use of single-dose ofloxacin to eradicate tonsillopharyngeal carriage of *Neisseria meningitidis*. *Antimicrob Ag Chemother* **37**: 2024.

Glupczynski Y, Labbe M, Burette A *et al.* (1987). Treatment failure of ofloxacin in *Campylobacter pylori* infection. *Lancet* **i**: 1096.

Glupczynski Y, Delmee M, Bruck C *et al.* (1988). Susceptibility of clinical isolates of *Campylobacter pylori* to 24 antimicrobial and anti-ulcer agents. *Eur J Epidemiol* **4**: 154.

Goldstein EJ (1993). Patterns of susceptibility to fluoroquinolones among anaerobic bacterial isolates in the United States. *Clin Infect Dis* **16** (Suppl 4): S377.

Goldstein EJ, Citron DM (1992). Comparative activity of ciprofloxacin, ofloxacin, sparfloxacin, temafloxacin, CI-960, CI-990, and WIN 57273 against anaerobic bacteria. *Antimicrob Ag Chemother* **36**: 1158.

Goldstein EJ, Citron DM, Vagvolgyi AE, Gombert ME (1986). Susceptibility of *Eikenella corrodens* to newer and older quinolones. *Antimicrob Ag Chemother* **30**: 172.

Goossens H, De Mol P, Coignau H *et al.* (1985). Comparative *in vitro* activities of aztreonam, ciprofloxacin, norfloxacin, ofloxacin, HR 810 (a new cephalosporin), RU 28965 (a new macrolide), and other agents against enteropathogens. *Antimicrob Ag Chemother* **27**: 388.

Gorzynski EA, Gutman SI, Allen W (1989). Comparative antimycobacterial activities of difloxacin, temafloxacin, enoxacin, pefloxacin, reference fluoroquinolones, and a new macrolide, clarithromycin. *Antimicrob Ag Chemother* **33**: 591.

Graninger W, Presterl E, Walzl B *et al.* (1990). Intravenous ofloxacin in severe infections. *J Antimicrob Chemother* **26** (Suppl D): 123.

Gregoire SL, Grasela TH, Jr, Freer JP, Tack KJ, Schentag JJ (1987). Inhibition of theophylline clearance by coadministered ofloxacin without alteration of theophylline effects. *Antimicrob Ag Chemother* **31**: 375.

Grenier B (1989). Use of the new quinolones in cystic fibrosis. *Rev Infect Dis* **11** (Suppl 5): S1245.

Grüneberg RN, Felmingham D, O'Hare MD *et al.* (1988). The comparative *in-vitro* activity of ofloxacin. *J Antimicrob Chemother* **22** (Suppl C): 9.

Guay DR, Opsahl JA, McMahon FG *et al.* (1992). Safety and pharmacokinetics of multiple doses of intravenous ofloxacin in healthy volunteers. *Antimicrob Ag Chemother* **36**: 308.

Gucek A, Bren AF, Lindic J *et al.* (1994). Is monotherapy with cefazolin or ofloxacin an adequate treatment for peritonitis in CAPD patients? *Adv Perit Dial* **10**: 144.

Gwon A (1992a). Ofloxacin vs tobramycin for the treatment of external ocular infection. Ofloxacin Study Group II. *Arch Ophthalmol* **110**: 1234.

Gwon A (1992b). Topical ofloxacin compared with gentamicin in the treatment of external ocular infection. Ofloxacin Study Group. *Brit J Ophthalmol* **76**: 714.

Halkin H (1988). Adverse effects of the fluoroquinolones. *Rev Infect Dis* **10** (Suppl 1): S258.

Halstensen A, Gilja OH, Digranes A *et al.* (1995a). Single dose ofloxacin in the eradication of pharyngeal carriage of *Neisseria meningitidis*. *Drugs* **49** (Suppl 2): 399.

Halstensen A, Voltersvik P, Gossius G *et al.* (1995b). Double-blind comparison of ofloxacin for 3 days and placebo in acute bacterial enteritis. *Drugs* **49** (Suppl 2): 454.

Hammerschlag MR, Hyman CL, Roblin PM (1992). *In vitro* activities of five quinolones against *Chlamydia pneumoniae*. *Antimicrob Ag Chemother* **36**: 682.

Harder S, Fuhr U, Staib AH, Wolff T (1989). Ciprofloxacin-caffeine: a drug interaction established using *in vivo* and *in vitro* investigations. *Amer J Med* **87**: 89S.

Hoban DJ, Jones RN, Harrell LJ *et al.* (1993). The North American component (the United States and Canada) of an International Comparative MIC trial monitoring ofloxacin resistance. *Diagn Microbiol Infect Dis* **17**: 157.

Höffler D, Koeppe P (1987). Pharmacokinetics of ofloxacin in healthy subjects and patients with impaired renal function. *Drugs* **34** (Suppl 1): 51.

Hoffner SE, Kratz M, Olsson-Liljequist B *et al.* (1989). *In-vitro* synergistic activity between ethambutol and fluorinated quinolones against *Mycobacterium avium* complex. *J Antimicrob Chemother* **24**: 317.

Hooton TM, Latham RH, Wong ES *et al.* (1989). Ofloxacin versus trimethoprim-sulfamethoxazole for treatment of acute cystitis. *Antimicrob Ag Chemother* **33**: 1308.

Hooton TM, Johnson C, Winter C *et al.* (1991). Single-dose and three-day regimens of ofloxacin versus trimethoprim–sulfamethoxazole for acute cystitis in women. *Antimicrob Ag Chemother* **35**: 1479.

Hooton TM, Batteiger BE, Judson FN *et al.* (1992). Ofloxacin versus doxycycline for treatment of cervical infection with *Chlamydia trachomatis*. *Antimicrob Ag Chemother* **36**: 1144.

Hoppe JE, Simon CG (1990). *In vitro* susceptibilities of *Bordetella pertussis* and *Bordetella parapertussis* to seven fluoroquinolones. *Antimicrob Ag Chemother* **34**: 2287.

Hori S, Ohshita Y, Utsui Y, Hiramatsu K (1993). Sequential acquisition of norfloxacin and ofloxacin resistance by methicillin-resistant and -susceptible *Staphylococcus aureus*. *Antimicrob Ag Chemother* **37**: 2278.

Horiuchi S, Inagaki Y, Yamamoto N *et al.* (1993). Reduced susceptibilities of *Shigella sonnei* strains isolated from patients with dysentery to fluoroquinolones. *Antimicrob Ag Chemother* **37**: 2486.

Horn DL, Hewlett D, Jr, Alfalla C *et al.* (1994). Limited tolerance of ofloxacin and pyrazinamide prophylaxis against tuberculosis. *New Engl J Med* **330**: 1241.

Höffken G, Lode H, Wiley R *et al.* (1988). Pharmacokinetic snad bioavailability of ciprofloxacin and ofloxacin: effect of food and antacid intake. *Rev Infect Dis* **10** (Suppl 1): S138.

Huminer D, Cohen JD, Majadla R, Dux S (1989). Hypersensitivity vasculitis due to ofloxacin. *Brit Med J* **299**: 303.

Ichihara N, Tachizawa H, Tsumura M *et al.* (1984). Phase I study on DL-8280. *Chemotherapy (Tokyo)*; **32** (Suppl 1): 118.

Ishida K, Kaku M, Irifune K *et al.* (1994). *In-vitro* and *in-vivo* activity of a new quinolone AM-1155 against *Mycoplasma pneumoniae*. *J Antimicrob Chemother* **34**: 875.

Ishii H, Sato K, Hoshino K *et al.* (1991). Active efflux of ofloxacin by a highly quinolone-resistant strain of *Proteus vulgaris*. *J Antimicrob Chemother* **28**: 827.

Jabarit-Aldighieri N, Torres H, Raoult D (1992). Susceptibility of *Rickettsia conorii*, *R rickettsii*, and *Coxiella burnetii* to PD 127,391, PD 131,628, pefloxacin, ofloxacin, and ciprofloxacin. *Antimicrob Ag Chemother* **36**: 2529.

Jacobs MR (1995). Activity of quinolones against mycobacteria. *Drugs* **49** (Suppl 2): 67.

Jacobus NV, Tally FP, Barza M (1984). Antimicrobial spectrum of Win 49375. *Antimicrob Ag Chemother* **26**: 104.

Ji B, Grosset J (1991). Ofloxacin for the treatment of leprosy. *Acta Leprol* **7**: 321.

Ji B, Perani EG, Petinom C *et al.* (1994). Clinical trial of ofloxacin alone and in combination with dapsone plus clofazimine for treatment of lepromatous leprosy. *Antimicrob Ag Chemother* **38**: 662.

Joesoef MR, Knapp JS, Idajadi A *et al.* (1994). Antimicrobial susceptibilities of *Neisseria gonorrhoeae* strains isolated in Surabaya, Indonesia. *Antimicrob Ag Chemother* **38**: 2530.

Johnson SM, Roberts GD (1987). *In vitro* activity of ciprofloxacin and ofloxacin against the *Mycobacterium avium-intracellulare* complex. *Diagn Microbiol Infect Dis* **7**: 89.

Jones RN, Hoban DJ (1994). North American (United States and Canada).

comparative susceptibility of two fluoroquinolones: ofloxacin and ciprofloxacin. A 53-medical-center sample of spectra of activity. North American Ofloxacin Study Group. *Diagn Microbiol Infect Dis* **18**: 49.

Jones RN, Kehrberg EN, Erwin ME, Anderson SC (1994). Prevalence of important pathogens and antimicrobial activity of parenteral drugs at numerous medical centers in the United States, I. Study on the threat of emerging resistances: real or perceived? Fluoroquinolone Resistance Surveillance Group. *Diagn Microbiol Infect Dis* **19**: 203.

Jüngst G, Mohr R (1987). Side effects of ofloxacin in clinical trials and in postmarketing surveillance. *Drugs* **34** (Suppl 1): 144.

Jüngst G, Mohr R (1988). Overview of postmarketing experience with ofloxacin in Germany. *J Antimicrob Chemother* **22** (Suppl C): 167.

Kaku M, Ishida K, Irifune K *et al.* (1994). *In vitro* and *in vivo* activities of sparfloxacin against *Mycoplasma pneumoniae*. *Antimicrob Ag Chemother* **38**: 738.

Kalager T, Digranes A, Bergan T, Rolstad T (1986). Ofloxacin: serum and skin blister fluid pharmacokinetics in the fasting and non-fasting state. *J Antimicrob Chemother* **17**: 795.

Kam KM, Lo KK, Lai CF *et al.* (1993). Ofloxacin susceptibilities of 5667 *Neisseria gonorrhoeae* strains isolated in Hong Kong. *Antimicrob Ag Chemother* **37**: 2007.

Kam KM, Lo KK, Ho NK, Cheung MM (1995). Rapid decline in penicillinase-producing *Neisseria gonorrhoeae* in Hong Kong associated with emerging 4-fluoroquinolone resistance. *Genitourin Med* **71**: 141.

Kampf D, Borner K, Pustelnik A (1990). Pharmacokinetics of ofloxacin and adequacy of maintenance dose for patients on haemodialysis. *J Antimicrob Chemother* **26** (Suppl D): 61.

Kampf D, Borner K, Hain H, Conrad W (1991). Multiple-dose-kinetics of ofloxacin after intraperitoneal application in CAPD patients. *Perit Dial Int* **11**: 317.

Kampf D, Borner K, Pustelnik A (1992). Multiple dose kinetics of ofloxacin and ofloxacin metabolites in haemodialysis patients. *Eur J Clin Pharmacol* **42**: 95.

Kanellakopoulou K, Giamarellou H (1990). Clinical experience with parenteral and oral ofloxacin in severe infections. *Scand J Infect Dis* (Suppl 68): 64.

Kato M, Takada S, Kashida Y, Nomura M (1995). Histological examination on Achilles tendon lesions induced by quinolone antibacterial agents in juvenile rats. *Toxicol Pathol* **23**: 385.

Kawada A, Hiruma M, Morimoto K *et al.* (1994). Fixed drug eruption induced by ciprofloxacin followed by ofloxacin. *Contact Dermatitis* **31**: 182.

Kawahara S, Watanabe Y, Matsuka Y *et al.* (1995). Inhibitory effect of ofloxacin on acute exacerbations of chronic respiratory tract infections in comparison with erythromycin. *Drugs* **49** (Suppl 2): 414.

Kawakami J, Matsuse T, Kotaki H *et al.* (1994). The effect of food on the interaction of ofloxacin with sucralfate in healthy volunteers. *Eur J Clin Pharmacol* **47**: 67.

Kazmierczak A, Pechinot A, Duez JM *et al.* (1987). Biliary tract excretion of ofloxacin in man. *Drugs* **34** (Suppl 1): 39.

Kenny GE, Cartwright FD (1991a). Susceptibilities of *Mycoplasma hominis* and *Ureaplasma urealyticum* to two new quinolones, sparfloxacin and WIN 57273. *Antimicrob Ag Chemother* **35**: 1515.

Kenny GE, Cartwright FD (1991b). Susceptibility of *Mycoplasma pneumoniae* to several new quinolones, tetracycline, and erythromycin. *Antimicrob Ag Chemother* **35**: 587.

Kern W, Kurrle E (1991). Ofloxacin versus trimethoprim-sulfamethoxazole for prevention of infection in patients with acute leukemia and granulocytopenia. *Infection* **19**: 73.

Kern WV, Andriof E, Oethinger M *et al.* (1994a). Emergence of fluoroquinolone-resistant *Escherichia coli* at a cancer center. *Antimicrob Ag Chemother* **38**: 681.

Kern WV, Hay B, Kern P *et al.* (1994b). A randomized trial of roxithromycin in patients with acute leukemia and bone marrow transplant recipients receiving fluoroquinolone prophylaxis. *Antimicrob Ag Chemother* **38**: 465.

Ketterl R, Beckurts T, Stubinger B, Claudi B (1988). Use of ofloxacin in open fractures and in the treatment of post-traumatic osteomyelitis. *J Antimicrob Chemother* **22** (Suppl C): 159.

Khajotia R, Drlicek M, Vetter N (1990). A comparative study of ofloxacin and amoxycillin/clavulanate in hospitalized patients with lower respiratory tract infections. *J Antimicrob Chemother* **26** (Suppl D): 83.

Khan MA, Hayat Z, Sadick A (1994). Ofloxacin in the treatment of typhoid fever resistant to chloramphenicol and amoxicillin. *Clin Ther* **16**: 815.

Khan MY, Dizon M, Kiel FW (1989). Comparative *in vitro* activities of ofloxacin, difloxacin, ciprofloxacin, and other selected antimicrobial agents against *Brucella melitensis*. *Antimicrob Ag Chemother* **33**: 1409.

King A, Phillips I (1986a). The comparative *in-vitro* activity of pefloxacin. *J Antimicrob Chemother* **17** (Suppl B): 1.

King A, Phillips I (1986b). The comparative *in-vitro* activity of eight newer quinolones and nalidixic acid. *J Antimicrob Chemother* **18** (Suppl D): 1.

King A, Shannon K, Phillips I (1985). The *in-vitro* activities of enoxacin and ofloxacin compared with that of ciprofloxacin. *J Antimicrob Chemother* **15**: 551.

Kirsch LS, Jackson WB, Goldstein DA, Discepola MJ (1995). Perioperative ofloxacin vs. tobramycin: efficacy in external ocular adnexal sterilization and anterior chamber penetration. *Can J Ophthalmol* **30**: 11.

Kitchen VS, Donegan C, Ward H *et al.* (1990). Comparison of ofloxacin with doxycycline in the treatment of non-gonococcal urethritis and cervical chlamydial infection. *J Antimicrob Chemother* **26** (Suppl D): 99.

Knapp JS, Ohye R, Neal SW *et al.* (1994). Emerging *in vitro* resistance to quinolones in penicillinase-producing *Neisseria gonorrhoeae* strains in Hawaii. *Antimicrob Ag Chemother* **38**: 2200.

Kohler RB, Arkins N, Tack KJ (1991). Accidental overdose of intravenous ofloxacin with benign outcome. *Antimicrob Ag Chemother* **35**: 1239.

Kohno S, Koga H, Kaku M *et al.* (1992). Prospective comparative study of ofloxacin or ethambutol for the treatment of pulmonary tuberculosis. *Chest* **102**: 1815.

Koizumi F, Ohnishi A, Takemura H *et al.* (1994). Effective monitoring of concentrations of ofloxacin in saliva of patients with chronic respiratory tract infections. *Antimicrob Ag Chemother* **38**: 1140.

Koverech A, Picari M, Granata F *et al.* (1986). Safety profile of ofloxacin: the Italian data base. *Infection* **14** (Suppl 4): S335.

Krcmery V Jr (1995). The use of quinolones as therapy in granulocytopenic cancer patients. Comparison with other antimicrobials. *Drugs* **49** (Suppl 2): 139.

Kromann-Andersen B, Sommer P, Pers C *et al.* (1988). Ofloxacin compared with ciprofloxacin in the treatment of complicated lower urinary tract infections. *J Antimicrob Chemother* **22** (Suppl C): 143.

Kumada T, Neu HC (1985). *In-vitro* activity of ofloxacin, a quinolone carboxylic acid compared to other quinolones and other antimicrobial agents. *J Antimicrob Chemother* **16**: 563.

Kurzynski TA, Boehm DM, Rott-Petri JA *et al.* (1988). Antimicrobial susceptibilities of *Bordetella* species isolated in a Multicenter Pertussis Surveillance Project. *Antimicrob Ag Chemother* **32**: 137.

Lam WK, Chau PY, So SY *et al.* (1986). A double-blind randomized study comparing ofloxacin and amoxicillin in treating infective episodes in bronchiectasis. *Infection* **14** (Suppl 4): S290.

Lam WK, Chau PY, So SY *et al.* (1989). Ofloxacin compared with amoxycillin in treating infective exacerbations in bronchiectasis. *Respir Med* **83**: 299.

Lameire N, Rosenkranz B, Malerczyk V *et al.* (1991). Ofloxacin pharmacokinetics in chronic renal failure and dialysis. *Clin Pharmacokinet* **21**: 357.

Lamp KC, Bailey EM, Rybak MJ (1992). Ofloxacin clinical pharmacokinetics. *Clin Pharmacokinet* **22**: 32.

LeBel M (1991). Fluoroquinolones in the treatment of cystic fibrosis: a critical appraisal. *Eur J Clin Microbiol Infect Dis* **10**: 316.

Lefevre JC, Escaffre MC, Courdil M, Lareng MB (1993). *In vitro* evaluation of activities of azithromycin, clarithromycin and sparfloxacin against *Chlamydia trachomatis*. *Pathol Biol (Paris)*; **41**: 313.

Lehto P, Kivisto KT (1994). Effect of sucralfate on absorption of norfloxacin and ofloxacin. *Antimicrob Ag Chemother* **38**: 248.

Lehto P, Kivisto KT, Neuvonen PJ (1994). The effect of ferrous sulphate on the absorption of norfloxacin, ciprofloxacin and ofloxacin. *Brit J Clin Pharmacol* **37**: 82.

Leor J, Matetzki S (1988). Ofloxacin and warfarin. *Ann Intern Med* **109**: 761.

Leroy A, Borsa F, Humbert G *et al.* (1987). The pharmacokinetics of ofloxacin in healthy adult male volunteers. *Eur J Clin Pharmacol* **31**: 629.

Levin JM, Nelson JA, Segreti J *et al.* (1993). *In vitro* susceptibility of *Borrelia burgdorferi* to 11 antimicrobial agents. *Antimicrob Ag Chemother* **37**: 1444.

Levy R, Shpitzer T, Shvero J, Pitlik SD (1990). Oral ofloxacin as treatment of malignant external otitis: a study of 17 cases. *Laryngoscope* **100**: 548.

Liang RH, Yung RW, Chan TK *et al.* (1990). Ofloxacin versus co-trimoxazole for prevention of infection in neutropenic patients following cytotoxic chemotherapy. *Antimicrob Ag Chemother* **34**: 215.

Ligtvoet EEJ, Wickerhoff-Minoggio T (1985). *In-vitro* activity of pefloxacin compared with six other quinolones. *J Antimicrob Chemother* **16**: 485.

Lipsky BA, Tack KJ, Kuo CC *et al.* (1990). Ofloxacin treatment of *Chlamydia pneumoniae* (strain TWAR) lower respiratory tract infections. *Amer J Med* **89**: 722.

Liu HH, Bolash NK, McAnany ME, Lynch RA (1995). Susceptibility of bacterial isolates from complicated skin and skin structure infections to cefazolin, imipenem-cilastatin, ciprofloxacin and ofloxacin. *Drugs* **49** (Suppl 2): 215.

Lockley MR, Wise R, Dent J (1984). The pharmacokinetics and tissue penetration of ofloxacin. *J Antimicrob Chemother* **14**: 647.

Lode H, Hoffken G, Olschewski P *et al.* (1987). Pharmacokinetics of ofloxacin after parenteral and oral administration. *Antimicrob Ag Chemother* **31**: 1338.

Lode H, Hoffken G, Olschewski P *et al.* (1988). Comparative pharmacokinetics of intravenous ofloxacin and ciprofloxacin. *J Antimicrob Chemother* **22** (Suppl C): 73.

Lode H, Hoffken G, Boeckk M *et al.* (1990). Quinolone pharmacokinetics and metabolism. *J Antimicrob Chemother* **26** (Suppl B): 41.

Loffler A, Grafvon Westphalen H (1986). Successful treatment of chronic Salmonella excretor with ofloxacin. *Lancet* **i**: 1206.

Lutz FB, Jr (1989). Single-dose efficacy of ofloxacin in uncomplicated gonorrhea. *Amer J Med* **87**: 69S.

MacGowan AP, Holt HA, Bywater MJ, Reeves DS (1990). *In vitro* antimicrobial susceptibility of *Listeria monocytogenes* isolated in the UK and other *Listeria* species. *Eur J Clin Microbiol Infect Dis* **9**: 767.

Madsen PO, Malek GH, Kahn JB (1995). Single dose UTI prophylaxis in transurethral surgery. Oral ofloxacin vs parenteral cefotaxime. *Drugs* **49** (Suppl 2): 480.

Maesen FP, Davies BI, Baur C, Sumajow CA (1986). Clinical, microbiological and pharmacokinetic studies on ofloxacin in acute purulent exacerbations of chronic respiratory disease. *J Antimicrob Chemother* **18**: 629.

Maesen FP, Davies BI, Geraedts WH, Sumajow CA (1987). Ofloxacin and antacids. *J Antimicrob Chemother* **19**: 848.

Malik IA, Abbas Z, Karim M (1992). Randomised comparison of oral ofloxacin alone with combination of parenteral antibiotics in neutropenic febrile patients. *Lancet* **339**: 1092.

Malik IA, Khan WA, Aziz Z, Karim M (1994). Self-administered antibiotic therapy for chemotherapy-induced, low-risk febrile neutropenia in patients with nonhematologic neoplasms. *Clin Infect Dis* **19**: 522.

Malik IA, Khan WA, Karim M, Aziz Z, Khan MA (1995). Feasibility of outpatient management of fever in cancer patients with low-risk neutropenia: results of a prospective randomized trial. *Amer J Med* **98**: 224.

Maple PA, Hamilton-Miller JM, Brumfitt W (1991). Differing activities of quinolones against ciprofloxacin-susceptible and ciprofloxacin-resistant, methicillin-resistant *Staphylococcus aureus*. *Antimicrob Ag Chemother* **35**: 345.

Marchbanks CR (1993). Drug-drug interactions with fluoroquinolones. *Pharmacotherapy* **13**: 23S.

Marchbanks CR, Dudley MN, Flor S, Beals B (1992). Pharmacokinetics and safety of single rising doses of ofloxacin in healthy volunteers. *Pharmacotherapy* **12**: 45.

Martin C, Lambert D, Bruguerolle B *et al.* (1991). Ofloxacin pharmacokinetics in mechanically ventilated patients. *Antimicrob Ag Chemother* **35**: 1582.

Martindale The Extra Pharmacopoeia 30th edn (1993). (Reynolds JEF, ed), London: The Pharmaceutical Press.

Mattina R, Cocuzza CE, Cesana M (1993). Rufloxacin once daily versus ofloxacin twice daily for treatment of complicated cystitis and upper urinary tract infections. Italian Multicentre UTI Rufloxacin Group. *Infection* **21**: 106.

Mazzulli T, Simor AE, Jaeger R *et al.* (1990). Comparative *in vitro* activities of several new fluoroquinolones and beta-lactam antimicrobial agents against community isolates of *Streptococcus pneumoniae*. *Antimicrob Ag Chemother* **34**: 467.

McCue JD, Gaziano P, Orders D (1995). A randomised controlled trial of ofloxacin 200 mg 4 times daily or twice daily vs ciprofloxacin 500 mg twice daily in elderly nursing home patients with complicated UTI. *Drugs* **49** (Suppl 2): 368.

McNulty CA, Dent JC (1988). Susceptibility of clinical isolates of *Campylobacter pylori* to twenty-one antimicrobial agents. *Eur J Clin Microbiol Infect Dis* **7**: 566.

McWhinney PH, Patel S, Whiley RA *et al.* (1993). Activities of potential therapeutic and prophylactic antibiotics against blood culture isolates of viridans group streptococci from neutropenic patients receiving ciprofloxacin. *Antimicrob Ag Chemother* **37**: 2493.

Meek JC, Maesen FP, Davies BI (1989). A prospective study of ofloxacin in acute exacerbations of chronic respiratory disease associated with *Pseudomonas aeruginosa*. *J Antimicrob Chemother* **24**: 447.

Meissner A, Borner K, Koeppe P (1990). Concentrations of ofloxacin in human bone and in cartilage. *J Antimicrob Chemother* **26** (Suppl D): 69.

Mertes PM, Jehl F, Burtin P *et al.* (1992). Penetration of ofloxacin into heart valves, myocardium, mediastinal fat, and sternal bone marrow in humans. *Antimicrob Ag Chemother* **36**: 2493.

Midtvedt T (1987). Influence of ofloxacin on the faecal flora. *Drugs* **34** (Suppl 1): 154.

Mogabgab WJ, Holmes B, Murray M *et al.* (1990). Randomized comparison of ofloxacin and doxycycline for *Chlamydia* and *Ureaplasma* urethritis and cervicitis. *Chemotherapy* **36**: 70.

Molinaro M, Villani P, Regazzi MB *et al.* (1992). Pharmacokinetics of ofloxacin in elderly patients and in healthy young subjects. *Eur J Clin Pharmacol* **43**: 105.

Moller BR, Herrmann B, Ibsen HH *et al.* (1990). Occurrence of *Ureaplasma urealyticus* and *Mycoplasma hominis* in non-gonococcal urethritis before and after treatment in a double-blind trial of ofloxacin versus erythromycin. *Scand J Infect Dis* (Suppl 68): 31.

Monk JP, Campoli-Richards DM (1987). Ofloxacin A review of its antibacterial activity, pharmacokinetic properties and therapeutic use. *Drugs* **33**: 346.

Montay G, Gaillot J (1990). Pharmacokinetics of fluoroquinolones in hepatic failure. *J Antimicrob Chemother* **26** (Suppl B): 61.

Moran JS, Levine WC (1995). Drugs of choice for the treatment of uncomplicated gonococcal infections. *Clin Infect Dis* **20** (Suppl 1): S47.

Mouton Y, Leroy O, Beuscart C *et al.* (1990). Efficacy of intravenous ofloxacin: a French multicentre trial in 185 patients. *J Antimicrob Chemother* **26** (Suppl D): 115.

Mraovic M, Canic-Radojlovic M (1986). The activity of ofloxacin against methicillin-resistant *Staphylococcus aureus*. *Infection* **14** (Suppl 4): S231.

Mueller BA, Brierton DG, Abel SR, Bowman L (1994). Effect of enteral feeding with ensure on oral bioavailabilities of ofloxacin and ciprofloxacin. *Antimicrob Ag Chemother* **38**: 2101.

Munno I, Arpinelli F, Benedetti M *et al.* (1990). The effect of ofloxacin on the immune system of elderly patients. *J Antimicrob Chemother* **25**: 455.

Murray PR, Bratcher JL, Niles AC, Hampton CM (1993). *In vitro* activity of nine fluoroquinolone antibiotics against 200 strains of enterococci. *Diagn Microbiol Infect Dis* **16**: 83.

Mursic VP, Wilske B, Schierz G *et al.* (1987). *In vitro* and *in vivo* susceptibility of *Borrelia burgdorferi*. *Eur J Clin Microbiol* **6**: 424.

Naber KG, Sigl G (1993). Fleroxacin versus ofloxacin in patients with complicated urinary tract infection: a controlled clinical study. *Amer J Med* **94**: 114S.

Naber KG, Kinzig M, Sorgel F, Weigel D (1993). Penetration of ofloxacin into prostatic fluid, ejaculate and seminal fluid. *Infection* **21**: 98.

Nakanishi N, Yoshida S, Wakebe H *et al.* (1991). Mechanisms of clinical resistance to fluoroquinolones in *Enterococcus faecalis*. *Antimicrob Ag Chemother* **35**: 1053.

Nakata K, Maeda H, Fujii A *et al.* (1992). *In vitro* and *in vivo* activities of sparfloxacin, other quinolones, and tetracyclines against *Chlamydia trachomatis*. *Antimicrob Ag Chemother* **36**: 188.

Nau R, Kinzig M, Dreyhaupt T *et al.* (1994). Kinetics of ofloxacin and its metabolites in cerebrospinal fluid after a single intravenous infusion of 400 milligrams of ofloxacin. *Antimicrob Ag Chemother* **38**: 1849.

Neuvonen PJ, Kivisto KT (1992). Milk and yoghurt do not impair the absorption of ofloxacin. *Brit J Clin Pharmacol* **33**: 346.

Norrby SR, Ljungberg B (1989). Pharmacokinetics of fluorinated 4-quinolones in the aged. *Rev Infect Dis* **11** (Suppl 5): S1102.

O'Brien TP, Maguire MG, Fink NE *et al.* (1995). Efficacy of ofloxacin vs cefazolin and tobramycin in the therapy for bacterial keratitis Report from the Bacterial Keratitis Study Research Group. *Arch Ophthalmol* **113**: 1257.

Ode B, Walder M, Forsgren A (1987). Failure of a single dose of 100 mg ofloxacin in lower urinary tract infections in females. *Scand J Infect Dis* **19**: 677.

Oriel JD (1989). Use of quinolones in chlamydial infection. *Rev Infect Dis* **11** (Suppl 5): S1273.

Orlando R, Sawadogo A, Miglioli PA *et al.* (1992). Oral disposition kinetics of ofloxacin in patients with compensated liver cirrhosis. *Chemotherapy* **38**: 1.

Pace JL, Gatt P (1989). Fatal vasculitis associated with ofloxacin. *Brit Med J* **299**: 658.

Paintaud G, Alvan G, Hellgren U, Nilsson-Ehle I (1993). Lack of effect of amoxycillin on the absorption of ofloxacin. *Eur J Clin Pharmacol* **44**: 207.

Pankuch GA, Jacobs MR, Appelbaum PC (1994). Susceptibilities of 123 *Xanthomonas maltophilia* strains to clinafloxacin, PD 131628, PD 138312, PD 140248, ciprofloxacin, and ofloxacin. *Antimicrob Ag Chemother* **38**: 369.

Pankuch GA, Jacobs MR, Appelbaum PC (1995). Activity of DU-6859a, ciprofloxacin, ofloxacin, levofloxacin, sparfloxacin and OPC-17116 against 112 penicillin-susceptible and -resistant pneumococci. *Drugs* **49** (Suppl 2): 235.

Parent M, LeBel M (1991). Meta-analysis of quinolone-theophylline interactions. *DICP* **25**: 191.

Pederzoli P, Falconi M, Bassi C *et al.* (1989). Ofloxacin penetration into bile and pancreatic juice. *J Antimicrob Chemother* **23**: 805.

Perea EJ (1990). Ofloxacin concentrations in tissues involved in respiratory tract infections. *J Antimicrob Chemother* **26** (Suppl D): 55.

Petermann W (1991). Ofloxacin in lower respiratory tract infections. *Infection* **19** (Suppl 7): S372.

Pfau A, Sacks TG (1994). Effective postcoital quinolone prophylaxis of recurrent urinary tract infections in women. *J Urol* **152**: 136.

Phillips I, King A (1988). Comparative activity of the 4-quinolones. *Rev Infect Dis* **10** (Suppl 1): S70.

Pioget JC, Wolff M, Singlas E *et al.* (1989). Diffusion of ofloxacin into cerebrospinal fluid of patients with purulent meningitis or ventriculitis. *Antimicrob Ag Chemother* **33**: 933.

Pohlod DJ, Saravolatz LD (1984). *In vitro* susceptibilities of 393 recent clinical isolates to WIN 49375 cefotaxime, tobramycin and piperacillin. *Antimicrob Ag Chemother* **25**: 377.

Polubiec A, Jorasz I, Pietrzak J *et al.* (1994). A randomized study comparing low dose ciprofloxacin and ofloxacin in the treatment of lower respiratory tract infections. *Infection* **22**: 62.

Prosser B La T, Beskid G (1995). Multicenter *in vitro* comparative study of fluoroquinolones against 25,129 Gram-positive and Gram-negative clinical isolates. *Diagn Microbiol Infect Dis* **21**: 33.

Punakivi L, Keistinen T, Backman R *et al.* (1990). Oral ofloxacin once daily and doxycycline in the treatment of acute exacerbations of chronic bronchitis. *Scand J Infect Dis* (Suppl 68): 41.

Rademaker CM, Sips AP, Beumer HM *et al.* (1990). A double-blind comparison of low-dose ofloxacin and amoxycillin/clavulanic acid in acute exacerbations of chronic bronchitis. *J Antimicrob Chemother* **26** (Suppl D): 75.

Raffi F (1989). Q-fever endocarditis. *Lancet* **ii**: 1336.

Rajagopalan-Levasseur P, Dournon E, Dameron G *et al.* (1990). Comparative postantibacterial activities of pefloxacin, ciprofloxacin, and ofloxacin against intracellular multiplication of *Legionella pneumophila* serogroup 1. *Antimicrob Ag Chemother* **34**: 1733.

Raoult D, Yeaman MR, Baca OG (1989). Susceptibility of *Coxiella burnetii* to pefloxacin and ofloxacin in ovo and in persistently infected L929 cells. *Antimicrob Ag Chemother* **33**: 621.

Raoult D, Torres H, Drancourt M (1991). Shell-vial assay: evaluation of a new technique for determining antibiotic susceptibility, tested in 13 isolates of *Coxiella burnetii*. *Antimicrob Ag Chemother* **35**: 2070.

Rastogi N, Goh KS (1991). *In vitro* activity of the new difluorinated quinolone sparfloxacin (AT-4140). against *Mycobacterium tuberculosis* compared with activities of ofloxacin and ciprofloxacin. *Antimicrob Ag Chemother* **35**: 1933.

Rastogi N, Ross BC, Dwyer B *et al.* (1992). Emergence during unsuccessful chemotherapy of multiple drug resistance in a strain of *Mycobacterium tuberculosis*. *Eur J Clin Microbiol Infect Dis* **11**: 901.

Raz R, Genesin J, Gonen E *et al.* (1988). Single low-dose ofloxacin for the treatment of uncomplicated urinary tract infection in young women. *J Antimicrob Chemother* **22**: 945.

Raz R, Rottensterich E, Leshem Y, Tabenkin H (1994). Double-blind study comparing 3-day regimens of cefixime and ofloxacin in treatment of uncomplicated urinary tract infections in women. *Antimicrob Ag Chemother* **38**: 1176.

Regamey C, Steinbach-Lebbin C (1990). Severe infections treated with intravenous ofloxacin: a prospective clinical multicentre Swiss study. *J Antimicrob Chemother* **26** (Suppl D): 107.

Ribard P, Audisio F, Kahn MF *et al.* (1992). Seven Achilles tendinitis including three complicated by rupture during fluoroquinolone therapy. *J Rheumatol* **19**: 1479.

Rice RJ, Knapp JS (1994). Susceptibility of *Neisseria gonorrhoeae* associated with pelvic inflammatory disease to cefoxitin, ceftriaxone, clindamycin, gentamicin, doxycycline, azithromycin, and other antimicrobial agents. *Antimicrob Ag Chemother* **38**: 1688.

Rice RJ, Bhullar V, Mitchell SH, Bullard J, Knapp JS (1995). Susceptibilities of *Chlamydia trachomatis* isolates causing uncomplicated female genital tract infections and pelvic inflammatory disease. *Antimicrob Ag Chemother* **39**: 760.

Richmond SJ, Bhattacharyya MN, Maiti H *et al.* (1988). The efficacy of ofloxacin against infection caused by *Neisseria gonorrhoeae* and *Chlamydia trachomatis*. *J Antimicrob Chemother* **22** (Suppl C): 149.

Ridgway GL (1995). Quinolones in sexually transmitted diseases Global experience. *Drugs* **49** (Suppl 2): 115.

Ristow TA, Peterson LR, Kahn JB (1995). *In vitro* activity of ofloxacin, ciprofloxacin, and cefoperazone alone and in combination against *Xanthomonas maltophilia*. *Drugs* **49** (Suppl 2): 246.

Rubinstein E, Potgieter P, Davey P, Norrby SR (1994). The use of fluoroquinolones in neutropenic patients – analysis of adverse effects. *J Antimicrob Chemother* **34**: 7.

Rugendorff EW (1987). Open randomised comparison of ofloxacin and norfloxacin in the treatment of complicated urinary tract infections. *Drugs* **34** (Suppl 1): 91.

Sabbour MS, Osman LM (1990). Experience with ofloxacin in enteric fever. *J Chemother* **2**: 113.

Sader HS, Runyon BA, Erwin ME, Jones RN (1995). Antimicrobial activity of 11 newer and investigational drugs tested against aerobic isolates from spontaneous bacterial peritonitis. *Diagn Microbiol Infect Dis* **21**: 105.

Saito A, Sawatari K, Fukuda Y *et al.* (1985). Susceptibility of *Legionella pneumophila* to ofloxacin *in vitro* and in experimental legionella pneumonia in guinea pigs. *Antimicrob Ag Chemother* **28**: 15.

Salord JM, Matsiota-Bernard P, Staikowsky F *et al.* (1993). Unsuccessful treatment of *Legionella pneumophila* infection with a fluoroquinolone. *Clin Infect Dis* **17**: 518.

Sanchez Navarro A, Martinez Cabarga M, Dominguez-Gil Hurle A (1994). Oral absorption of ofloxacin administered together with aluminum. *Antimicrob Ag Chemother* **38**: 2510.

Sanders CC (1992a). Review of preclinical studies with ofloxacin. *Clin Infect Dis* **14**: 526.

Sanders WE, Jr (1992b). Oral ofloxacin: a critical review of the new drug application. *Clin Infect Dis* **14**: 539.

Sato K, Matsuura Y, Inoue M *et al.* (1982). *In vitro* and *in vivo* activity of DL-8280, a new oxazine derivative. *Antimicrob Ag Chemother* **22**: 548.

Sawada H, Tashima M, Okuma M (1991). Use of ofloxacin in prevention and treatment of secondary infections in hematological malignancies. *Chemotherapy* **37** (Suppl 1): 25.

Sawae Y, Ninomiya K, Takaki K *et al.* (1995). A comparative study of ofloxacin twice and three times daily in the treatment of respiratory tract infections. *Drugs* **49** (Suppl 2): 430.

Schachter J, Moncada JV (1989). *In vitro* activity of ofloxacin against *Chlamydia trachomatis*. *Amer J Med* **87**: 14S.

Schalkhauser K (1990). Comparison of iv ofloxacin and piperacillin in the treatment of complicated urinary tract infections. *J Antimicrob Chemother* **26** (Suppl D): 93.

Scheife RT, Cramer WR, Decker EL (1993). Photosensitizing potential of ofloxacin. *Int J Dermatol* **32**: 413.

Schmeiser T, Kern WV, Hay B *et al.* (1993). Single-drug oral antibacterial prophylaxis with ofloxacin in BMT recipients. *Bone Marrow Transplant* **12**: 57.

Schmidt S, Cordt-Schlegel A, Heitmann R (1993). Guillain-Barre syndrome during treatment with ofloxacin. *J Neurol* **240**: 506.

Schoenfeld N, Mamet R (1994). Interference of ofloxacin with determination of urinary porphyrins. *Clin Chem* **40**: 417.

Schramm P (1986). Ofloxacin: concentration in human ejaculate and influence on sperm motility. *Infection* **14** (Suppl 4): S274.

Serour F, Dan M, Gorea A *et al.* (1991). Penetration of ofloxacin into human lung tissue following a single oral dose of 200 milligrams. *Antimicrob Ag Chemother* **35**: 380.

Shalit I, Berger SA, Gorea A, Frimerman H (1989). Widespread quinolone resistance among methicillin-resistant *Staphylococcus aureus* isolates in a general hospital. *Antimicrob Ag Chemother* **33**: 593.

Silvain C, Bouquet S, Breux JP *et al.* (1989). Oral pharmacokinetics and ascitic fluid penetration of ofloxacin in cirrhosis. *Eur J Clin Pharmacol* **37**: 261.

Sivayathorn A (1995). The use of fluoroquinolones in sexually transmitted diseases in Southeast Asia. *Drugs* **49** (Suppl 2): 123.

Smith BL, Cummings MC, Covino JM *et al.* (1991). Evaluation of ofloxacin in the treatment of uncomplicated gonorrhea. *Sex Transm Dis* **18**: 18.

Smith MD, Duong NM, Hoa NT *et al.* (1994). Comparison of ofloxacin and ceftriaxone for short-course treatment of enteric fever. *Antimicrob Ag Chemother* **38**: 1716.

Smith MD, Vinh DX, Nguyen TT *et al.* (1995). *In vitro* antimicrobial susceptibilities of strains of *Yersinia pestis*. *Antimicrob Ag Chemother* **39**: 2153.

Smith SM (1986). *In vitro* comparison of A-56619, A-56620, amifloxacin, ciprofloxacin, enoxacin, norfloxacin, and ofloxacin against methicillin-resistant *Staphylococcus aureus*. *Antimicrob Ag Chemother* **29**: 325.

Soriano F, Ponte C, Santamaria M *et al.* (1987). Susceptibility of urinary isolates of *Corynebacterium* group D2 to fifteen antimicrobials and acetohydroxamic acid. *J Antimicrob Chemother* **20**: 349.

Spangler SK, Jacobs MR, Appelbaum PC (1992). Susceptibilities of penicillin-susceptible and -resistant strains of *Streptococcus pneumoniae* to RP 59500, vancomycin, erythromycin, PD 131628, sparfloxacin, temafloxacin, win 57273, ofloxacin, and ciprofloxacin. *Antimicrob Ag Chemother* **36**: 856.

Spencer RC, Cole TP (1992). Ofloxacin versus trimethoprim and co-trimoxazole in the treatment of uncomplicated urinary tract infection in general practice. *Brit J Clin Pract* **46**: 30.

Stahl JP, Croize J, Lefebvre MA *et al.* (1986). Diffusion of ofloxacin into the cerebrospinal fluid in patients with bacterial meningitis. *Infection* **14** (Suppl 4): S254.

Stocks JM, Wallace RJ, Jr, Griffith DE *et al.* (1989). Ofloxacin in community-acquired lower respiratory infections A comparison with amoxicillin or erythromycin. *Amer J Med* **87**: 52S.

Stubner G, Weinrich W, Brands U (1986). Study of the cerebrospinal fluid penetrability of ofloxacin. *Infection* **14** (Suppl 4): S250.

Symonds J, Javaid A, Bone M, Turner A (1988). The penetration of ofloxacin into bronchial secretions. *J Antimicrob Chemother* **22** (Suppl C): 91.

Syrjala H, Schildt R, Raisainen S (1991). *In vitro* susceptibility of *Francisella tularensis* to fluoroquinolones and treatment of tularemia with norfloxacin and ciprofloxacin. *Eur J Clin Microbiol Infect Dis* **10**: 68.

Tack KJ, Smith JA (1989). The safety profile of ofloxacin. *Amer J Med* **87**: 78S.

Tanaka-Bandoh K, Kato N, Watanabe K, Ueno K (1995). Antibiotic susceptibility profiles of *Bacteroides fragilis* and *Bacteroides thetaiotaomicron* in Japan from 1990 to 1992. *Clin Infect Dis* **20** (Suppl 2): S352.

Tang-Liu DD, Schwob DL, Usansky JI, Gordon YJ (1994). Comparative tear concentrations over time of ofloxacin and tobramycin in human eyes. *Clin Pharmacol Ther* **55**: 284.

Tartaglione TA, Johnson CR, Brust P *et al.* (1988). Pharmacodynamic evaluation of ofloxacin and trimethoprim-sulfamethoxazole in vaginal fluid of women treated for acute cystitis. *Antimicrob Ag Chemother* **32**: 1640.

Texier-Maugein J, Mormede M, Fourche J, Bebear C (1987). *In vitro* activity of four fluoroquinolones against eighty-six isolates of mycobacteria. *Eur J Clin Microbiol* **6**: 584.

Thorn V (1987). Tissue concentrations of ofloxacin in the middle ear. *Clin Ther* **9**: 523.

Todd PA, Faulds D (1991). Ofloxacin A reappraisal of its antimicrobial activity, pharmacology and therapeutic use. *Drugs* **42**: 825.

Tolsdorff P (1993a). Penetration of ofloxacin into nasal tissues. *Infection* **21**: 66.

Tolsdorff P (1993b). Tissue and serum concentrations of ofloxacin in the ear region following a single daily oral dose of 400 mg. *Infection* **21**: 63.

Tran TH, Bethell DB, Nguyen TT *et al.* (1995). Short course of ofloxacin for treatment of multidrug-resistant typhoid. *Clin Infect Dis* **20**: 917.

Tsui SY, Yew WW, Li MS *et al.* (1993). Postantibiotic effects of amikacin and ofloxacin on *Mycobacterium fortuitum*. *Antimicrob Ag Chemother* **37**: 1001.

Tsukamura M (1985). *In vitro* antituberculosis activity of a new antibacterial substance ofloxacin (DL 8280). *Amer Rev Respir Dis* **13**: 348.

Tsukamura M, Nakamura E, Yoshii S, Amano H (1985). Therapeutic effect of a new antibacterial substance ofloxacin (DL 8280). on pulmonary tuberculosis. *Amer Rev Respir Dis* **131**: 352.

Upton C (1994). Sleep disturbance in children treated with ofloxacin. *Brit Med J* **309**: 1411.

Van Caekenberghe DL, Pattyn SR (1984). *In vitro* activity of ciprofloxacin compared with those of other new fluorinated piperazynyl-substituted quinoline derivatives. *Antimicrob Ag Chemother* **25**: 518.

Van der Auwera P, Godard C, Denis C *et al.* (1990). *In vitro* activities of new antimicrobial agents against multiresistant *Staphylococcus aureus* isolated from septicemic patients during a Belgian national survey from 1983 to 1985. *Antimicrob Ag Chemother* **34**: 2260.

Van Landuyt HW, Gordts B, D'Hondt G (1988). Pharmacokinetic evaluation of ofloxacin in serum and tonsils. *J Antimicrob Chemother* **22** (Suppl C): 81.

Verho M, Malerczyk V, Dagrosa E, Korn A (1985). Dose linearity and other pharmacokinetics of ofloxacin: a new, broad-spectrum antimicrobial agent. *Pharmatherapeutica* **4**: 376.

von Gunten S, Lew D, Paccolat F *et al.* (1994). Aqueous humor penetration of ofloxacin given by various routes. *Am J Ophthalmol* **117**: 87.

Waites K, Rand K, Jenkins S *et al.* (1994). Multicenter *in vitro* comparative study of fluoroquinolones after four years of widespread clinical use. *Diagn Microbiol Infect Dis* **18**: 181.

Wall RA, Mabey DC, Bello CS, Felmingham D (1985). The comparative *in-vitro* activity of twelve 4-quinolone antimicrobials against *Haemophilus ducreyi. J Antimicrob Chemother* **16**: 165.

Walstad RA, Vilsvik JS, Thurmann-Nielsen E, Rolstad T (1995). The pharmacokinetics and distribution of ofloxacin into the lower respiratory tract. *Drugs* **49** (Suppl 2): 344.

Wang F, Gu XJ, Zhang MF, Tai TY (1989). Treatment of typhoid fever with ofloxacin. *J Antimicrob Chemother* **23**: 785.

Warlich R, Korting HC, Schafer-Korting M, Mutschler E (1990). Multiple-dose pharmacokinetics of ofloxacin in serum, saliva, and skin blister fluid of healthy volunteers. *Antimicrob Ag Chemother* **34**: 78.

Weber JT, Johnson RE (1995). New treatments for *Chlamydia trachomatis* genital infection. *Clin Infect Dis* **20** (Suppl 1): S66.

Weissenbacher ER, Gutschow K, Adam D, Mavinova N (1984). Serum and tissue concentrations of ofloxacin in obstetrical and gynecological infections. *4th Medit Congr Chemother* Abstr. No. 756.

White LO, MacGowan AP, Lovering AM *et al.* (1987). A preliminary report on the pharmacokinetics of ofloxacin, desmethyl ofloxacin and ofloxacin N-oxide in patients with chronic renal failure. *Drugs* **34** (Suppl 1): 56.

White LO, MacGowan AP, Mackay IG, Reeves DS (1988). The pharmacokinetics of ofloxacin, desmethyl ofloxacin and ofloxacin N-oxide in haemodialysis patients with end-stage renal failure. *J Antimicrob Chemother* **22** (Suppl C): 65.

Wijnands GJ, Vree TB, Janssen TJ, Guelen PJ (1989). Drug-drug interactions affecting fluoroquinolones. *Amer J Med* **87**: 47S.

Wijnands WJ, Vree TB (1988). Interaction between the fluoroquinolones and the bronchodilator theophylline. *J Antimicrob Chemother* **22** (Suppl C): 109.

Wijnands WJ, Vree TB, Baars AM *et al.* (1988). The penetration of ofloxacin into lung tissue. *J Antimicrob Chemother* **22** (Suppl C): 85.

Winston DJ, Ho WG, Bruckner DA *et al.* (1990). Ofloxacin versus vancomycin/polymyxin for prevention of infections in granulocytopenic patients. *Amer J Med* **88**: 36.

Winton MD, Everett ED, Dolan SA (1988). Activities of five new fluoroquinolones against *Pseudomonas pseudomallei. Antimicrob Ag Chemother* **32**: 928.

Wise R, Lockley MR (1988). The pharmacokinetics of ofloxacin and a review of its tissue penetration. *J Antimicrob Chemother* **22** (Suppl C): 59.

Wise R, Lister D, McNulty CA *et al.* (1986). The comparative pharmacokinetics of five quinolones. *J Antimicrob Chemother* **18** (Suppl D): 71.

Witzig RS, Franzblau SG (1993). Susceptibility of *Mycobacterium kansasii* to ofloxacin, sparfloxacin, clarithromycin, azithromycin, and fusidic acid. *Antimicrob Ag Chemother* **37**: 1997.

Wong FA and Flor SC (1990). The metabolism of ofloxacin in humans. *Drug Metabolism Disposition* **B18**: 1103.

Yamagishi Y, Fujita J, Takigawa K *et al.* (1993). Clinical features of *Pseudomonas cepacia* pneumonia in an epidemic among immunocompromised patients. *Chest* **103**: 1706.

Yeaman MR, Roman MJ, Baca OG (1989). Antibiotic susceptibilities of two *Coxiella burnetii* isolates implicated in distinct clinical syndromes. *Antimicrob Ag Chemother* **33**: 1052.

Yew WW, Kwan SY, Ma WK *et al.* (1989a). Combination of ofloxacin and amikacin in the treatment of sternotomy wound infection. *Chest* **95**: 1051.

Yew WW, Kwan SY, Ma WK *et al.* (1989b). Single daily-dose ofloxacin monotherapy for *Mycobacterium fortuitum* sternotomy infection. *Chest* **96**: 1150.

Yew WW, Kwan SY, Ma WK *et al.* (1990a). *In-vitro* activity of ofloxacin against *Mycobacterium tuberculosis* and its clinical efficacy in multiply resistant pulmonary tuberculosis. *J Antimicrob Chemother* **26**: 227.

Yew WW, Kwan SY, Ma WK *et al.* (1990b). Ofloxacin therapy of *Mycobacterium fortuitum* infection: further experience. *J Antimicrob Chemother* **25**: 880.

Yew WW, Wong PC, Kwan SY *et al.* (1991). Two cases of *Nocardia asteroides* sternotomy infection treated with ofloxacin and a review of other active antimicrobial agents. *J Infect* **23**: 297.

Yew WW, Piddock LJ, Li MS *et al.* (1994a). *In-vitro* activity of quinolones and macrolides against mycobacteria. *J Antimicrob Chemother* **34**: 343.

Yew WW, Wong PC, Lee J, Chau CH (1994b). Ofloxacin and pulmonary tuberculosis. *Chest* **105**: 1624.

Yew WW, Wong CF, Wong PC *et al.* (1993). Adverse neurological reactions in patients with multidrug-resistant pulmonary tuberculosis after coadministration of cycloserine and ofloxacin. *Clin Infect Dis* **17**: 288.

Yuk JH, Nightingale CH, Quintiliani R, Sweeney KR (1991). Bioavailability and pharmacokinetics of ofloxacin in healthy volunteers. *Antimicrob Ag Chemother* **35**: 384.

Zaudig M, von Bose M (1987). Ofloxacin-induced psychosis. *Brit J Psychiatry* **151**: 563.

Zaudig M, von Bose M, Weber MM *et al.* (1989). Psychotoxic effects of ofloxacin. *Pharmacopsychiatry* **22**: 11.

Zenilman JM, Neumann T, Patton M, Reichart C (1993). Antibacterial activities of OPC-17116, ofloxacin, and ciprofloxacin against 200 isolates of *Neisseria gonorrhoeae. Antimicrob Ag Chemother* **37**: 2244.

Zorbas P, Giamarellou H, Staszewska-Pistoni M *et al.* (1995). Comparison of two oral ofloxacin regimens for the treatment of bacteriuria in elderly subjects. *Drugs* **49** (Suppl 2): 384.

Sparfloxacin

Description

Sparfloxacin (AT-4140, CI-978, PD 131501) is a fluoroquinolone with broad spectrum antibacterial activity. It has the chemical formula 5-amino-1-cyclopropyl-7-(cis-3,5-dimethylpiperazin-1-yl)-6,8-difluoro-1,4-dihydro-4-oxoquinolone-3-carboxylic acid. The main potential advantages of sparfloxacin over older fluoroquinolones is its improved activity against Gram-positive pathogens (such as *Streptococcus pneumoniae* and *Staphylococcus aureus*), *Mycobacteria* and *Chlamydia* spp., and its long half-life that allows once-daily dosing (Richard and Gutmann, 1992).

Sensitive Organisms

1 Gram-negative bacteria

Overall, sparfloxacin is less active than ciprofloxacin, but more active than ofloxacin against Enterobacteriaceae, with $MIC_{90} \leq 1$ μg per ml (generally ≤ 0.5 μg per ml). Against *Pseudomonas aeruginosa* it is 2- to 4-fold less active than ciprofloxacin, but is either similar in activity, or up to 2-fold more active, than afloxacin with a MIC_{90} 2–8 μg per ml. Sparfloxacin is very active against *Haemophilus influenzae* (regardless of beta-lactamase production), *Moraxella catarrhalis* and *Neisseria gonorrheae* with $MIC_{90} \leq 0.015$ μg per ml, *Yersinia enterocolitica* (MIC_{90} 0.06 μg per ml) and *Haemophilus ducreyi*. Such activity against *H. influenzae* is comparable with that of trovafloxacin and clinafloxacin. Sparfloxacin has greater activity than ciprofloxacin against *Acinetobacter calcoaceticus* (MIC_{90} 0.03–0.06 μg per ml), *Flavobacterium* spp. (MIC_{90} 0.25 μg per ml), and *Stenotrophomonas* (previously *Xanthomonas*) *maltophilia* (MIC_{90} 0.25–4 μg per ml). The activity of sparfloxacin against *Klebsiella pneumoniae* is similar to that of trovafloxacin (Doebbeling *et al.*, 1990; Eliopoulos *et al.*, 1990; Rolston *et al.*, 1990; Chin *et al.*, 1991; Louie *et al.*, 1991a; Akaniro *et al.*, 1992; Canton *et al.*, 1992; Lefevre *et al.*, 1992; Joly-Guillou and Bergogne-Berezin,1992; Qadri *et al.*, 1992; Aldridge *et al.*, 1993; Bauernfeind, 1993; Vartivarian *et al.*, 1994; Baquero and Canton, 1996). Sparfloxacin has similar, or superior, activity to ciprofloxacin and ofloxacin against *Legionella pneumophila* (Nakamura *et al.*, 1989; Saito and Gaja, 1995).

Generally, sparfloxacin and ciprofloxacin are very active against *Shigella sonnei* (MIC_{90} 0.016 and 0.008 μg per ml, respectively), but Horiuchi *et al.* (1993) have identified strains of *Sh. sonnei* from patients with dysentery which are relatively resistant to sparfloxacin, ciprofloxacin and ofloxacin, with MICs 16- to 32-fold higher than those typically obtained (John *et al.*, 1992).

Sparfloxacin is more active than ciprofloxacin and tosufloxacin, but inferior to clinafloxacin, against *Gardnerella vaginalis* (MIC_{90} 0.25 μg per ml) (Bauernfeind, 1993). Sparfloxacin is active ($MIC_{90} \leq 1$ μg per ml) against the majority of aerobic and anaerobic pathogens encountered in bite wounds, except for fusobacteria (MIC_{90} 16 μg per ml) and some *Prevotella* spp. (Goldstein and Citron, 1993; Goldstein *et al.*, 1995). Sparfloxacin has reasonable activity against *Bacteroides fragilis* with $MIC_{90} \leq 2$–4 μg per ml and similar, or slightly inferior, activity against other *Bacteroides* spp. (Chin *et al.*, 1991; Goldstein and Citron, 1992; Goldstein, 1993; Borobio *et al.*, 1994).

2 Gram-positive bacteria

Sparfloxacin is 4- to 10-fold more active than ofloxacin or ciprofloxacin against methicillin-sensitive *Staph. aureus*, *Staph. epidermidis*, most *Strep. pneumoniae* and *Strep. pyogenes* (MIC_{90}

0.25–0.5 μg per ml). Furthermore, the MBCs for sparfloxacin against these pathogens are 2- to 8-fold lower than those of ciprofloxacin. Clinafloxacin and trovafloxacin generally have better activity than sparfloxacin against methicillin-susceptible strains of *Staph. aureus*. Sparfloxacin is superior to levofloxacin, inferior to clinafloxacin, but is broadly comparable with trovafloxacin, tosufloxacin and grepafloxacin against penicillin-susceptible and -resistant pneumococci. Such anti-pneumococcal activity is generally independent of the presence of penicillin-resistance among this species, although penicillin-resistant isolates are more likely to also exhibit higher fluoroquinolone MICs. Sparfloxacin is also active against macrolide-resistant strains of *Strep. pneumoniae* (Pankuch *et al.*, 1995; Baquero and Canton, 1996). Sparfloxacin is more active than most other fluoroquinolones against ciprofloxacin- and methicillin-resistant *Staph. aureus* with MIC_{90} 8 μg per ml, but this is above the usually achievable serum concentrations of sparfloxacin, and therefore cross-resistance among all fluoroquinolones in this situation can be assumed for practical purposes (Forstall *et al.*, 1991; Bauernfeind, 1993; Brumfitt and Hamilton-Miller, 1993). Sparfloxacin is 2- to 4-fold more active than ciprofloxacin against *Enterococcus faecalis* ($MIC_{90} \leq 0.5$ μg per ml) and has borderline activity against *Listeria monocytogenes* (MIC_{90} 1–2 μg per ml). Sparfloxacin has reasonable activity against *Strep. milleri* (MIC_{90} 0.5 μg per ml), but poor activity ($MIC_{90} > 64$ μg per ml) against vancomycin-resistant strains of *E. faecalis* and *E. faecium*. The susceptibility of *Corynebacterium jeikeium* and other *Corynebacterium* spp. to sparfloxacin appears to be somewhat variable, with some authors noting resistance ($MIC_{90} > 16$ μg per ml) and others reporting susceptibility (MIC 0.06–0.25 μg per ml). *Rhodococcus equi* is generally susceptible to sparfloxacin (Eliopoulos *et al.*, 1990; Rolston *et al.*, 1990; Chin *et al.*, 1991; Louie *et al.*, 1991b; Richard and Gutmann, 1991; Akaniro *et al.*, 1992; Canton *et al.*, 1992; Nordmann and Ronco, 1992; Bauernfeind, 1993; Murray *et al.*, 1993; Rotstein *et al.*, 1993; Cherubin and Stratton, 1994; Martinez-Martinez *et al.*, 1994; Michelet *et al.*, 1994; Freeman *et al.*, 1995; Baquero and Canton, 1996).

Sparfloxacin has somewhat varied activity against Gram-positive anaerobes such as *Clostridium perfringens* (MIC_{90} 0.5 μg per ml), *Clostridium* spp. (MIC_{90} 4–8 μg per ml), *Cl. difficile* (MIC_{90} 4 μg per ml) and *Peptococcus* spp. (MIC_{90} 2 μg per ml) – being generally inferior to clinafloxacin (Goldstein and Citron, 1992; Bauernfeind, 1993).

3 Mycobacteria

While ofloxacin, ciprofloxacin, clinafloxacin, levofloxacin and tosufloxacin have MIC_{90} values of 0.5, 0.25, 0.25, 0.25 and > 8 μg per ml, respectively, against strains of *Mycobacterium tuberculosis* that are fully sensitive to conventional agents, the MIC_{90} for sparfloxacin is generally 0.06 μg per ml, (although occasionally MIC_{90} of 0.5 μg per ml has been reported). Nevertheless, sparfloxacin is the most bactericidal of these agents. However, similar to other fluoroquinolones, sparfloxacin activity is less impressive against multiresistant ($\geq$ five drugs) strains of *M. tuberculosis* where the MIC_{90} is 1 μg per ml (Rastogi and Goh, 1991; Garcia-Rodriguez and Gomez Garcia, 1993; Yew *et al.*, 1994; Jacobs, 1995). Studies in mice suggest that on a weight to weight basis, sparfloxacin is 6- to 8-fold more active against *M. tuberculosis* than ofloxacin (Ji *et al.*, 1991; Lalande *et al.*, 1993).

Sparfloxacin has excellent *in vivo* activity against *M. leprae* and may have a higher therapeutic index than ofloxacin. Given the pharmacokinetics of sparfloxacin, a dose of 200 mg daily should be suitable for clinical studies (Franzblau *et al.*, 1993).

Against *M. kansasii* and *M. scrofulaceum*, sparfloxacin is notably more active than other fluoroquinolones, with MIC_{90} 0.06–2.0 and 1 μg per ml, respectively. Sparfloxacin has activity comparable with clinafloxacin against *M. fortuitum* with MIC_{90} 2 μg per ml. However, similar to all currently available fluoroquinolones, sparfloxacin activity against *M. avium* complex and *M. chelonae* is limited, with $MIC_{90} \geq 8$ μg per ml. Similarly, ciprofloxacin, ofloxacin and sparfloxacin are only moderately active against *M. haemophilum*, with an MIC_{90} 4–8 μg per ml (Bernard *et al.*, 1993; Klopman *et al.*, 1993; Witzig and Franzblau, 1993; Yew *et al.*, 1994).

4 Chlamydia and Mycoplasma

Sparfloxacin is significantly more active than ciprofloxacin, ofloxacin or lomefloxacin against both tetracycline-susceptible and -resistant strains of *Mycoplasma hominis* (MIC_{90} 0.03–0.06 μg per ml), and *Ureaplasma urealyticum* (MIC 0.125–1 μg per ml) (Kenny and Cartwright, 1991b; Lefevre *et al.*, 1992; Perea *et al.*, 1996). Sparfloxacin has approximately 8- to 10-fold greater activity against *M. pneumoniae* (MIC_{90} 0.125–0.5 μg per ml) than ofloxacin or ciprofloxacin; but erythromycin is better ($MIC_{90} < 0.008$ μg per ml) (Nakamura *et al.*, 1989; Kenny and Cartwright, 1991a; Waites *et al.*, 1991). In the experimental pulmonary *M. pneumoniae* infection model in Syrian golden hamsters, sparfloxacin is as effective as erythromycin when given orally at 15 mg per kg twice-daily for 5 days – a dose that results in serum levels similar to those achieved in humans (Kaku *et al.*, 1994).

Sparfloxacin (MIC_{90} 0.25 μg per ml) is more active than ciprofloxacin and ofloxacin (MIC_{90} 1 μg per ml) against *Chlamydia pneumoniae*; being 5- to 6-fold more active *in vitro* than erythromycin (Hammerschlag *et al.*, 1992; Kimura *et al.*, 1993; Roblin *et al.*, 1994; Baquero and Canton, 1996). Sparfloxacin has good activity (MIC_{50} 0.03 μg per ml) against *C. psittaci* (Nakamura *et al.*, 1989). Sparfloxacin is more active than either tosufloxacin, lomefloxacin, ciprofloxacin, ofloxacin, fleroxacin, enoxacin or norfloxacin against *C. trachomatis*, with MIC_{90} 0.05 μg per ml and similar MBC (Nakata *et al.*, 1992; Perea *et al.*, 1996).

Mode of Administration and Dosage

The *in-vitro* MICs of sparfloxacin against some selected bacterial species are shown in Table II.6 (pp. 986–987).

1 Oral administration

The usual recommended dose of sparfloxacin for serious infections is 400 mg on day 1, followed by 200 mg once-daily. For less serious infections such as uncomplicated urinary tract sepsis, a loading dose of 200 mg, followed by 100 mg daily is generally recommended. Duration of therapy varies with the indication, with single-dose therapy suitable for gonococcal urethritis and uncomplicated cystitis, and 7- to 14-day treatment for complicated urinary sepsis and respiratory tract infections.

2 Patients with renal failure

Dosage reduction of sparfloxacin is generally only necessary when the glomerular filtration rate (GFR) falls below 10 ml per min, at which time a 400-mg loading dose followed by 200 mg daily every second day is recommended (Fillastre *et al.*, 1994; Montay, 1996).

3 Patients with liver failure

Since the pharmacokinetics of sparfloxacin are not significantly altered in patients with cirrhosis or hepatic failure without cholestasis, no dosage adjustment is necessary in this patient population and routine doses should be given (Montay, 1996; p. 1138).

4 Elderly patients

No dosage adjustment of sparfloxacin is necessary in the elderly unless there is concomitant renal failure (Bergan, 1995, Montay, 1996).

Serum Levels in Relation to Dosage

1 Oral administration

Sparfloxacin is readily absorbed after oral administration, with mean serum concentrations of 0.9–1.0 μg per ml, 1 h after a routine loading dose of 400 mg and a mean peak serum concentration of 1.2 μg per ml is achieved 3–5 h post-dose; although significant interpatient variability has been noted (Montay, 1996). Montay (1996) has speculated that this variability may be due to a combination of factors such as active intestinal absorption and secretion of sparfloxacin and the fact that sparfloxacin is potentially absorbed from the full length of the intestinal tract from duodenum to the colon. The half-life of sparfloxacin is 16–20 h (Montay *et al.*, 1994; Montay, 1996). Food does not affect the absorption and pharmacokinetics of sparfloxacin (Shimada *et al.*, 1993). After single oral doses of 200, 400, 600 or 800 mg the peak serum concentration is 0.71 ± 0.16, 1.18 ± 0.28, 1.65 ± 0.58 and 1.97 ± 0.62 μg per ml, respectively. Thus, there is a slight, but clinically insignificant, decrease in sparfloxacin bioavailability with increasing dose, probably due to a reduction in drug absorption. After repeated dose administration, steady-state concentrations are achieved after the second dose and pharmacokinetic data are consistent with single dose data. Subsequent to a loading dose of 200, 400, 600 or 800 mg sparfloxacin on day 1, followed by once-daily doses of 100, 200, 300 or 400 mg, respectively, the minimum serum levels are 0.25 μg per ml (200/100), 0.30 μg per ml (400/200), 0.59 μg per ml (600/300) and 0.65 μg per ml (800/400, respectively (Johnson *et al.*,

1992; Montay *et al.*, 1994; Montay, 1996). The long half-life of sparfloxacin makes it suitable for once-daily dosing.

The pharmacokinetics of sparfloxacin in the elderly is similar to that noted in younger patients with comparable renal function (Montay, 1996).

2 Serum concentrations in renal failure

Lower renal and non-renal sparfloxacin clearances are observed in patients with renal failure and the metabolite sparfloxacin glucuronide accumulates. Levels of conjugated sparfloxacin in plasma are approximately 4- to 10-fold higher in patients with chronic renal failure than in healthy volunteers. After a single 400-mg dose of sparfloxacin in patients with a GFR of either 10–30 ml per min or < 10 ml per min, peak serum concentrations are comparable: 1.43 and 1.31 µg per ml, respectively; being achieved 4 h post-dose. Under these circumstances, the half-life of the drug increases to 34.9 and 38.5 h, respectively. Thus, following the usual 400-mg loading dose, a doubling of the dosage interval to 200 mg every second day is necessary (Fillastre *et al.*, 1994; Montay, 1996).

3 Serum concentrations in hepatic failure

The mean peak serum sparfloxacin level after a single 400-mg dose in patients with cirrhosis (but no cholestasis or ascites) is 1.68 µg per ml, 5 h post-dose; the half-life is 22.3 h. There appears to be no relationship between the severity of hepatic insufficiency and sparfloxacin clearance. Thus, since these pharmacokinetic parameters are similar to those noted in healthy volunteers, no dosage reduction is necessary (Montay, 1996).

Excretion

1 Urine

Renal excretion of unchanged sparfloxacin plays a minor role in the drug's pharmacokinetics. Following a single 400-mg oral dose of sparfloxacin, 8.8% of the dose is recovered in urine during the 52 h post-dose (Johnson *et al.*, 1992). Similarly, during the 72 h post-dose, urinary excretion of unchanged sparfloxacin accounts for 9–14% of the given dose and urinary excretion of glucuronide accounts for 28–36%. Urinary concentrations of sparfloxacin are 10–50 µg per ml when the drug is administered 300 mg daily (Shimada *et al.*, 1993; Montay, 1996).

2 Bile

Biliary excretion of sparfloxacin and of its glucuronide is relatively minor, being about 13%. Following a single 400-mg dose of sparfloxacin, biliary excretion of free drug and its glucuronide account for about 1.5 and 11.5% of the administered dose, respectively (Wittke *et al.*, 1992; Montay, 1996). The enterohepatic circulation does not appear to play a significant role in reabsorption.

3 Inactivation in body

Sparfloxacin is eliminated primarily by non-renal mechanisms, including hepatic biotransformation, biliary excretion and possibly transluminal secretion across the enteric mucosa. Sparfloxacin undergoes metabolism to a glucuronide form which is detectable in plasma at about 30–40% of the unchanged sparfloxacin concentration, and in urine and bile at 2- to 3-fold and 4- to 20-fold the unchanged sparfloxacin concentration, respectively (Shimada *et al.*, 1993; Montay, 1996).

4 Feces

Within 72 h of a single oral 200-mg dose, excretion of unchanged sparfloxacin in feces accounts for about 50–56% of a dose (Nakashima *et al.*, 1991; Shimada *et al.*, 1993). Fecal concentrations of sparfoxacin following an initial 400-mg loading dose and subsequent 200 mg daily, are 759.6 ± 484 and 476.4 ± 239.7 µg per g on day 2 and 8, respectively (Ritz *et al.*, 1994).

Distribution of the Drug in Body

Sparfloxacin achieves a high degree of penetration into most tissues, except for the central nervous system. Sparfloxacin is about 37–45% protein bound (Shimada *et al.*, 1993; Montay, 1996). Following a single 400-mg oral dose of sparfloxacin, the mean peak concentration in cantharides-induced inflammatory fluid is 1.3 μg per ml after a mean duration of 5 h post-dose. Thus, overall sparfloxacin penetration into inflammatory fluid is 117% and the mean elimination half-life from this fluid is 19.7 h (Johnson *et al.*, 1992). Skin penetration of sparfloxacin is good with skin:plasma ratios of 1.00 at 4 h (time of peak plasma concentration) and 1.39 at 5 h. Following single oral doses of 100 or 200 mg, concentrations in skin of 0.56 and 0.82–1.31 μg per g, respectively, can be expected (Nogita and Ishibashi, 1991). Sparfloxacin achieves excellent penetration into human polymorphonuclear leukocytes *in vitro* (Garcia *et al.*, 1992).

Sparfloxacin achieves high concentrations in respiratory and sinus tissues. Following an oral loading dose of 400 mg followed by 200 mg daily, mean concentrations of sparfloxacin (2.5 to 5 h after dosing) in bronchial mucosa, epithelial lining fluid and alveolar macrophages are 4.4 μg per g, 15.0 μg per ml and 53.7 μg per g, respectively. The mean sparfloxacin concentration in maxillary sinus mucosa, 2–5 h after a single 400-mg dose, is 5.8 μg per g (Wise and Honeybourne, 1996)

Shimada *et al.* (1993) has summarized many of the studies published in Japanese regarding the tissue distribution of sparfloxacin. High concentrations are achieved in sputum, pleural fluid, skin, lung, prostate, gynecological tissues, breast milk and otolaryngological tissues. Salivary concentrations are 66–70% of plasma levels, while CSF penetration appears to be somewhat limited with CSF:plasma concentration ratios of only 0.25–0.35. Sparfloxacin achieves concentrations in bile and gallbladder of 7.1- to 83-fold the concurrent serum levels.

In rabbits, sparfloxacin achieves very good penetration into the ocular vitreous (54%), cornea (76%) and lens (36%) (Cochereau-Massin *et al.*, 1993).

Mode of Action

Sparfloxacin has a similar mechansim of action to other fluoroquinolones (Piddock and Zhu, 1991; p. 1008).

Toxicity

Sparfloxacin has a similar rate of adverse reactions as ciprofloxacin and other commonly used fluoroquinolones. In a review of 2081 adult patients participating in a Phase III clinical trial of sparfloxacin in community-acquired, lower respiratory tract infections, sparfloxacin (200- or 400-mg loading dose then 100 or 200 mg daily; i.e. 200/100 mg and 400/200 mg) had a similar incidence of adverse events as the comparator agents (Rubinstein, 1996). The overall rates of drug-related adverse reactions for sparfloxacin 400/200 mg versus comparators and 200/100 mg versus the comparator (amoxycillin/clavulanic acid) were 13.7 versus 17.7%, and 9.5 versus 13.2%, respectively. However, many of these reported reactions were very minor; discontinuation of the antibacterial agent because of drug-related adverse reactions occured in 1.6 versus 1.6%, and 1.1 versus 1.1%, respectively. Adverse reactions affecting the nervous system were reported in 5.7% of the sparfloxacin group, with insomnia and other sleep disorders the most common events. Phototoxicity was noted in 2.0% of sparfloxacin recipients, with the average delay in onset being 6.3 ± 4.5 days (range 1–14 days) after commencing sparfloxacin. Mostly this consisted of erythema on the face and hands which lasted an average of 6.4 ± 4.2 days. The incidence of phototoxicity associated with sparfloxacin appears to be higher than that observed with ciprofloxacin and ofloxacin but less than that reported for fleroxacin, pefloxacin, enoxacin and nalidixic acid. Most importantly, features of the hemolytic–uremic syndrome such as that associated with temafloxacin (p. 1144) have not been reported (Ramsay and Obershkova, 1974; Bowie *et al.*, 1989; Davey, 1989; Wolfson and Hooper, 1991; Rubinstein, 1996).

Sparfloxacin does not produce neuromuscular blockade or potentiate the effect of neuromuscular relaxants such as pancuronium bromide or alcuronium as do some other agents, such as tetracyclines and the aminoglycosides (Paradelis *et al.*, 1995). Although sparfloxacin was noted in preclinical studies to prolong the electrocardiographic QT interval in dogs, this effect has not been noted to be of clinical significance in subsequent human studies, where a mean prolongation of only 3% has been reported (Jaillon *et al.*, 1996).

Sparfloxacin does not alter the pharmacokinetics of theophylline or interfere with the cytochrome P-450 system (Takagi *et al.*, 1991; Shimada *et al.*, 1993, Mizuki *et al.*, 1996). The concomitant administration of aluminum hydroxide and sparfloxacin results in reduced peak concentrations of the latter by 22%, although this effect is less than noted with many other fluoroquinolones. Co-administration of sucralfate and sparfloxacin reduces sparfloxacin bioavailability by 44% (Zix *et al.*, 1996). Similarly, ferrous sulfate reduces the absorption of sparfloxacin (Kanemitsu *et al.*, 1995). Sparfloxacin clearance is not altered by the concurrent administration of probenicid, suggesting a lack of tubular secretion of sparfloxacin (Shimada *et al.*, 1993).

Clinical Uses of the Drug

1 Respiratory tract infections

A 400-mg loading dose of sparfloxacin followed by 200 mg once-daily (400/200 mg) for 7–14 days is effective in the treatment of community-acquired pneumonia, with rates of clinical efficacy of about 88% (Richard and Gutmann, 1992; Gialdroni Grassi and Brumpt, 1995; Aubier *et al.*, 1996; Portier *et al.*, 1996). In trials comparing this dose of sparfloxacin with either amoxycillin/clavulanic acid, erythromycin or amoxycillin administered at recommended doses, efficacy with sparfloxacin was 88.3% compared with 84.1% in patients receiving the comparator agent. Notably, sparfloxacin was effective in 88.9% of patients with pneumococcal pneumonia (Aubier *et al.*, 1996). Portier *et al.* (1996) compared sparfloxacin 400/200 mg with amoxycillin 1 g thrice-daily plus ofloxacin 200 mg twice-daily for 10 days in a randomized, double-blind study of community-acquired pneumonia. Overall efficacy was comparable at 91.9% versus 81.5%, respectively, in evaluable patients at the end of treatment.

Sparfloxacin is also effective when treating acute exacerbations of chronic obstructive lung disease. In randomized, double-blind comparative trials in patients with acute exacerbations of chronic obstructive lung disease, Allegra *et al.* (1996) found 7–14 days therapy with sparfloxacin 200/100 mg to be comparable with amoxycillin/clavulanic acid (500 mg/125 mg) thrice-daily. Clinical efficacy at the end of treatment and at follow-up was 87.3 and 78.9% for sparfloxacin, and 88.8 and 79.8% for amoxycillin/clavulanic acid, respectively. Less than one-third of patients in this study had a pathogen cultured from sputum – of these, 24–28% grew *Strep. pneumoniae*. At follow-up, *Ps. aeruginosa* and *Strep. pneumoniae* accounted for seven of the eight sparfloxacin bacteriological failures, although these strains were susceptible to sparfloxacin. However, a comparable rate of bacteriological failure due to *Strep. pneumoniae* was also noted in the amoxycillin/clavulanic acid group.

2 Urinary tract infections

In a double-blind, randomized, multicenter study of complicated urinary tract infections, a sparfloxacin 200-mg loading dose followed by 100 mg daily was comparable in clinical efficacy with ciprofloxacin 500 mg twice-daily, when both agents were given for 10–14 days. Rates of clinical and bacteriological cure at the end of treatment were 88.6 versus 85.4% and 72.6 versus 81.4%, respectively. Differences in the rate of bacteriological cure were related to persisting pathogens that included Enterobacteriaceae, *Ps. aeruginosa* and enterococci which exhibited only moderate susceptibility to sparfloxacin. However, this difference was less marked at follow-up when rates of bacteriological cure were 62.9% for sparfloxacin and 67.4% for ciprofloxacin (Naber *et al.*, 1996). Other authors have found higher rates of clinical success with sparfloxacin when higher daily doses (e.g. 200 or 300 mg daily) are used (Kawada *et al.*, 1991)

3 Sinusitis

A 400-mg loading dose of sparfloxacin followed by 200 mg daily for 5 days is comparable with oral cefuroxime axetil 250 mg twice-daily for 8 days in the treatment of purulent sinusitis in which *H. influenzae* and *Strep. pneumoniae* were the most commonly cultured pathogens. At the end of treatment, clinical success was noted in 82.6 versus 83.2%, respectively (Gehanno *et al.*, 1996).

4 Sexually transmitted diseases

A single dose of sparfloxacin 200 mg is comparable in clinical efficacy with a single dose of ciprofloxacin 250 mg for men with acute gonococcal urethritis, where both agents result in 98–99% cure at follow-up. Notably, however, the rate of post-gonococcal urethritis was 26% in both groups, although *C. trachomatis* was isolated in only 4% of patients at enrolment (Moi *et al.*, 1996).

In a double-blind, randomized study of males with non-gonococcal urethritis, Phillips *et al.* (1996) compared the efficacy of a sparfloxacin 200-mg loading dose followed by 100 mg daily for either 2 or 6 additional days with doxycycline 200 mg once-daily for 7 days. The overall rates of success at the end of treatment and at follow-up were comparable in each of the three treatment groups. However, among patients with *Ureaplasma urethritis* and urethritis of unknown etiology, the rate of relapse/possible reinfection at the follow-up visit was markedly lower in the 7-day sparfloxacin group compared with either of the other two groups. In comparison, however, the rates of relapse/possible reinfection for chlamydial urethritis were similar in each group, with >95% rates of eradication. A 7-day course of sparfloxacin 400/200 mg appears to be a suitable regimen for the treatment of non-gonococcal urethritis (Phillips *et al.*, 1996).

5 Leprosy

Recent studies suggest that sparfloxacin, similar to ofloxacin, may have a useful future role in the treatment of leprosy (Waters, 1993; Chan *et al.*, 1994). Chan *et al.* (1994) treated nine previously untreated patients with lepromatous leprosy with sparfloxacin 200 mg once-daily for 12 weeks, with efficacy monitored both clinically, by morphological index, mouse footpad infectivity and the radiorespirometric activity of *M. leprae* organisms obtained from serial biopsy specimens. Most patients showed clinical improvement within 2 weeks of treatment, and after 4 weeks of treatment all patients had a morphological index of zero, specimens from most patients were non-infectious for mice and the median decrease in radiorespirometric activity was >99%. Clinical improvement occurred earlier than is usually observed with World Health Organisation-recommended multidrug regimens of rifampicin, dapsone and clofazimine. Thus, sparfloxacin 200 mg daily appears to be rapidly bactericidal *against M. leprae* in humans, with activity similar to that noted previously with ofloxacin (p. 1123).

6 Other infections

Sparfloxacin and clinafloxacin are both effective in the treatment of experimentally induced endocarditis in rabbits due to ampicillin-resistant *E. faecalis*, but no human data are available (Vazquez *et al.*, 1993). Similarly, in a rat model of endocarditis due to penicillin-resistant streptococci, sparfloxacin was very effective, while ceftriaxone failed *in vivo* (Entenza *et al.*, 1994). Sparfloxacin has also shown promise in the prophylaxis and treatment of experimental foreign-body infections in a guinea pig model caused by quinolone-susceptible strains of methicillin-resistant *Staph. aureus* (Cagni *et al.*, 1995). The clinical relevence of these animal studies is yet to be defined.

References

Akaniro JC, Stutman HR, Arguedas AG, Vargas OM (1992). *In vitro* activity of sparfloxacin (AT-4140), a new quinolone agent, against invasive isolates from pediatric patients. *Antimicrob Ag Chemother* **36**: 255.

Aldridge KE, Cammarata C, Martin DH (1993). Comparison of the in vitro activities of various parenteral and oral antimicrobial agents against endemic *Haemophilus ducreyi*. *Antimicrob Ag Chemother* **37**: 1986.

Allegra L, Konietzko N, Leophonte P *et al.* (1996). Comparative safety and efficacy of sparfloxacin in the treatment of acute exacerbations of chronic obstructive pulmonary disease: a double-blind, randomised, parallel, multicentre study. *J Antimicrob Chemother* **37** (Suppl A): 93.

Aubier M, Lode H, Gialdroni-Grassi G *et al.* (1996). Sparfloxacin for the treatment of community-acquired pneumonia: a pooled data analysis of two studies. *J Antimicrob Chemother* **37** (Suppl A): 73.

Baquero F, Canton R (1996). *In-vitro* activity of sparfloxacin in comparison with currently available antimicrobials against respiratory tract pathogens. *J Antimicrob Chemother* **37** (Suppl A): 1.

Bauernfeind A (1993). Comparative *in-vitro* activities of the new quinolone, Bay y 3118, and ciprofloxacin, sparfloxacin, tosufloxacin, CI-960 and CI-990. *J Antimicrob Chemother* **31**: 505.

Bergan T (1995). Quinolones in the elderly. *Drugs* **49** (Suppl 2): 112.

Bernard EM, Edwards FF, Kiehn TE *et al.* (1993). Activities of antimicrobial agents against clinical isolates of *Mycobacterium haemophilum*. *Antimicrob Ag Chemother* **37**: 2323.

Borobio MV, Conejo M, Ramirez E, Suarez AI, Perea EJ (1994).

Comparative activities of eight quinolones against members of the *Bacteroides* fragilis group. *Antimicrob Ag Chemother* **38**: 1442.

Bowie WR, Willetts V, Jewwsson PJ (1989). Adverse reactions in a dose ranging study with a new long acting fluoroquinolone, fleroxacin. *Antimicrob Ag Chemother* **33**: 1778.

Brumfitt W, Hamilton-Miller JM (1993). Incomplete cross-resistance between ciprofloxacin and sparfloxacin in staphylococci, with a note on selection pressure due to clinical use of ciprofloxacin. *J Antimicrob Chemother* **31**: 610.

Cagni A, Chuard C, Vaudaux PE *et al.* (1995). Comparison of sparfloxacin, temafloxacin, and ciprofloxacin for prophylaxis and treatment of experimental foreign-body infection by methicillin- resistant *Staphylococcus aureus*. *Antimicrob Ag Chemother* **39**: 1655.

Canton E, Peman J, Jimenez MT *et al.* (1992). *In vitro* activity of sparfloxacin compared with those of five other quinolones. *Antimicrob Ag Chemother* **36**: 558.

Chan GP, Garcia-Ignacio BY, Chavez VE *et al.* (1994). Clinical trial of sparfloxacin for lepromatous leprosy. *Antimicrob Ag Chemother* **38**: 61.

Cherubin CE, Stratton CW (1994). Assessment of the bactericidal activity of sparfloxacin, ofloxacin, levofloxacin, and other fluoroquinolones compared with selected agents of proven efficacy against *Listeria monocytogenes*. *Diagn Microbiol Infect Dis* **20**: 21.

Chin N-X, Gu J-W, Yu K-W *et al.* (1991). *In vitro* activity of sparfloxacin. *Antimicrob Ag Chemother* **35**: 567.

Cochereau-Massin I, Bauchet J, Marrakchi-Benjaafar S *et al.* (1993). Efficacy and ocular penetration of sparfloxacin in experimental streptococcal endophthalmitis. *Antimicrob Ag Chemother* 37: 633.

Davey PG (1989). Post marketing surveillance of the quinolones. *Rev Infect Dis* 11 (Suppl 5): S1402.

Doebbeling BN, Pfaller MA, Bale MJ, Wenzel RP (1990). Comparative *in vitro* activity of the new quinolone sparfloxacin (CI-978, AT-4140) against nosocomial Gram-negative bloodstream isolates. *Eur J Clin Microbiol Infect Dis* 9;298.

Eliopoulos G M, Klimm K, Grayson M L (1990). *In vitro* activity of sparfloxacin (AT-4140, CI-978, PD 131501): a new quinolone antimicrobial. *Diagn Microbiol Infect Dis* 13: 345.

Entenza JM, Blatter M, Glauser MP, Moreillon P (1994). Parenteral sparfloxacin compared with ceftriaxone in treatment of experimental endocarditis due to penicillin-susceptible and -resistant streptococci. *Antimicrob Ag Chemother* 38: 2683.

Fillastre JP, Montay G, Bruno R *et al.* (1994). Pharmacokinetics of sparfloxacin in patients with renal impairment. *Antimicrob Ag Chemother* 38: 733.

Forstall GJ, Knapp CC, Washington JA (1991). Activity of new quinolones against ciprofloxacin-resistant staphylococci. *Antimicrob Ag Chemother* 35: 1679.

Franzblau SG, Parrilla ML, Chan GP (1993). Sparfloxacin is more bactericidal than ofloxacin against *Mycobacterium leprae* in mice. *Int J Lepr Other Mycobact Dis* 61: 66.

Freeman C, Robinson A, Cooper B *et al.* (1995). *In vitro* antimicrobial susceptibility of glycopeptide-resistant enterococci. *Diagn Microbiol Infect Dis* 21: 47.

Garcia I, Pascual A, Guzman MC, Perea EJ (1992). Uptake and intracellular activity of sparfloxacin in human polymorphonuclear leukocytes and tissue culture cells. *Antimicrob Ag Chemother* 36: 1053.

Garcia-Rodriguez JA, Gomez Garcia AC (1993). *In-vitro* activities of quinolones against mycobacteria. *J Antimicrob Chemother* 32: 797.

Gehanno P, Berche P and the Sinusitis Study Group (1996). Sparfloxacin versus cefuroxime axetil in the treatment of acute purulent sinusitis. *J Antimicrob Chemother* 37 (Suppl A): 105.

Gialdroni Grassi G, Brumpt I (1995). Sparfloxacin empirical therapy in community-acquired pneumonia Results of a meta-analysis of 2 comparative studies. *Drugs* 49 (Suppl 2): 406.

Goldstein EJ (1993). Patterns of susceptibility to fluoroquinolones among anaerobic bacterial isolates in the United States. *Clin Infect Dis* 16 (Suppl 4): S377.

Goldstein EJ, Citron DM (1992). Comparative activity of ciprofloxacin, ofloxacin, sparfloxacin, temafloxacin, CI-960, CI-990, and WIN 57273 against anaerobic bacteria. *Antimicrob Ag Chemother* 36: 1158.

Goldstein EJ, Citron DM (1993). Comparative susceptibilities of 173 aerobic and anaerobic bite wound isolates to sparfloxacin, temafloxacin, clarithromycin, and older agents. *Antimicrob Ag Chemother* 37: 1150.

Goldstein EJC, Nesbit CA, Citron DM (1995). Comparative *in vitro* activities of azithromycin, Bay y 3118, levofloxacin, sparfloxacin, and 11 other antimicrobial agents against 194 aerobic and anaerobic bite wound isolates. *Antimicrob Ag Chemother* 39: 1097.

Hammerschlag MR, Hyman CL, Roblin PM (1992). *In vitro* activities of five quinolones against *Chlamydia pneumoniae*. *Antimicrob Ag Chemother* 36: 682.

Horiuchi S, Inagaki Y, Yamamoto N *et al.* (1993). Reduced susceptibilities of *Shigella sonnei* strains isolated from patients with dysentery to fluoroquinolones. *Antimicrob Ag Chemother* 37: 2486.

Jacobs MR (1995). Activity of quinolones against mycobacteria. *Drugs* 49 (Suppl 2): 67.

Jaillon P, Morganroth J, Brumpt I *et al.* (1996). Overview of electrocardiographic and cardiovascular safety data for sparfloxacin. *J Antimicrob Chemother* 37 (Suppl A): 161.

Ji B, Truffot-Pernot C, Grosset J (1991). *In vitro* and *in vivo* activities of sparfloxacin (AT-4140) against *Mycobacterium tuberculosis*. *Tubercle* 72: 181.

John JF, Jr, Atkins LT, Maple PA, Bratoeva M (1992). Activities of newer fluoroquinolones against *Shigella sonnei*. *Antimicrob Ag Chemother* 36: 2346.

Johnson JH, Cooper MA, Andrews JM, Wise R (1992). Pharmacokinetics and inflammatory fluid penetration of sparfloxacin. *Antimicrob Ag Chemother* 36: 2444.

Joly-Guillou ML, Bergogne-Berezin E (1992). *In-vitro* activity of sparfloxacin, pefloxacin, ciprofloxacin and temafloxacin against clinical isolates of *Acinetobacter* spp. *J Antimicrob Chemother* 29: 466.

Kaku M, Ishida K, Irifune K *et al.* (1994). *In vitro* and *in vivo* activities of sparfloxacin against *Mycoplasma pneumoniae*. *Antimicrob Ag Chemother* 38: 738.

Kanemitsu K, Hori S, Yanagawa A, Shimada J (1995). Effect of ferrous sulfate on the absorption of sparfloxacin in healthy volunteers and rats. *Drugs* 49 (Suppl 2): 352.

Kawada Y, Kumamoto Y, Aso Y *et al.* (1991). Comparative study of sparfloxacin and enoxacin in complicated urinary tract infections. *Chemotherapy* 39 (Suppl 4): 571.

Kenny G E, Cartwright F D (1991a). Susceptibility of *Mycoplasma pneumoniae* to several new quinolones, tetracycline, and erythromycin. *Antimicrob Ag Chemother* 35: 587.

Kenny GE, Cartwright FD (1991b). Susceptibilities of *Mycoplasma hominis* and *Ureaplasma urealyticum* to two new quinolones, sparfloxacin and WIN 57273. *Antimicrob Ag Chemother* 35: 1515.

Kimura M, Kishimoto T, Niki Y, Soejima R (1993). *In vitro* and *in vivo* antichlamydial activities of newly developed quinolone antimicrobial agents. *Antimicrob Ag Chemother* 37: 801.

Klopman G, Wang S, Jacobs MR *et al.* (1993). Anti-*Mycobacterium avium* activity of quinolones: *in vitro* activities. *Antimicrob Ag Chemother* 37: 1799.

Lalande V, Truffot-Pernot C, Paccaly-Moulin A *et al.* (1993). Powerful bactericidal activity of sparfloxacin (AT-4140). against *Mycobacterium tuberculosis* in mice. *Antimicrob Ag Chemother* 37: 407.

Lefevre JC, Bauriaud R, Gaubert E *et al.* (1992). *In vitro* activity of sparfloxacin and other antimicrobial agents against genital pathogens. *Chemotherapy* 38: 303.

Louie A, Baltch AL, Ritz WJ, Smith RP (1991a). Comparative *in-vitro* susceptibilities of *Pseudomonas aeruginosa*, *Xanthomonas maltophilia*, and *Pseudomonas* spp to sparfloxacin (CI-978, AT- 4140, PD131501) and reference antimicrobial agents. *J Antimicrob Chemother* 27: 793.

Louie A, Baltch AL, Ritz WJ, Smith RP (1991b). *In vitro* activity of sparfloxacin and six reference antibiotics against gram-positive bacteria. *Chemotherapy* 37: 275.

Martinez-Martinez L, Suarez AI, Ortega MC, Perea EJ (1994). Comparative *in vitro* activities of new quinolones against coryneform bacteria. *Antimicrob Ag Chemother* 38: 1439.

Michelet C, Avril JL, Cartier F, Berche P (1994). Inhibition of intracellular growth of *Listeria monocytogenes* by antibiotics. *Antimicrob Ag Chemother* 38: 438.

Mizuki Y, Fujiwara I, Yamaguchi T (1996). Pharmacokinetic interactions related to the chemical structures of fluoroquinolones. *J Antimicrob Chemother* 37 (Suppl A): 41.

Moi H, Morel P, Gianotti B *et al.* (1996). Comparative efficacy and safety of single oral doses of sparfloxacin versus ciprofloxacin in the treatment of acute gonococcal urethritis in men. *J Antimicrob Chemother* 37 (Suppl A): 115.

Montay G (1996). Pharmacokinetics of sparfloxacin in healthy volunteers and patients: a review. *J Antimicrob Chemother* 37 (Suppl A): 27.

Montay G, Bruno R, Vergniol JC *et al.* (1994). Pharmacokinetics of sparfloxacin in humans after single oral administration at doses of 200, 400, 600, and 800 mg. *J Clin Pharmacol* 34: 1071.

Murray PR, Bratcher JL, Niles AC, Hampton CM (1993). *In vitro* activity of nine fluoroquinolone antibiotics against 200 strains of enterococci. *Diagn Microbiol Infect Dis* 16: 83.

Naber KG, Di Silverio F, Geddes A, Guibert J (1996). Comparative efficacy of sparfloxacin versus ciprofloxacin in the treatment of complicated urinary tract infection. *J Antimicrob Chemother* 37 (Suppl A): 135.

Nakamura S, Minami A, Najata K *et al.* (1989). *In vitro* and *in vivo* antibacterial activities of AT-4140, a new broad-spectrum quinolone. *Antimicrob Ag chemother* **33**: 1167.

Nakashima M, Kanamaru M, Uematsu T and Takiguchi Y (1991). Phase I study of pyridone carboxylic acid antibacterial agent, sparfloxacin. *Rinshou Iyaku* **7**: 1639.

Nakata K, Maeda H, Fujii A *et al.* (1992). *In vitro* and *in vivo* activities of sparfloxacin, other quinolones, and tetracyclines against *Chlamydia trachomatis*. *Antimicrob Ag Chemother* **36**: 188.

Nogita T, Ishibashi Y (1991). The penetration of sparfloxacin into human plasma and skin tissues. *J Antimicrob Chemother* **28**: 313.

Nordmann P, Ronco E (1992). *In-vitro* antimicrobial susceptibility of *Rhodococcus equi*. *J Antimicrob Chemother* **29**: 383.

Pankuch GA, Jacobs MR, Appelbaum PC (1995). Activity of CP99,219 compared with DU-6859a, ciprofloxacin, ofloxacin, levofloxacin, lomefloxacin, tosufloxacin, sparfloxacin and grepafloxacin against penicillin-susceptible and -resistant pneumococci. *J Antimicrob Chemother* **35**: 230.

Paradelis AG, Kouvelas D, Pangalis A *et al.* (1995). Absence of neuromuscular blocking activity of sparfloxacin. *Drugs* **49** (Suppl 2): 291.

Perea EJ, Aznar J, Garcia-Iglesias MC, Pascual A (1996). Comparative *in-vitro* activity of sparfloxacin against genital pathogens. *J Antimicrob Chemother* **37** (Suppl A): 19.

Phillips I, Dimian C, Barlow D *et al.* (1996). A comparative study of two different regimens of sparfloxacin versus doxycycline in the treatment of non-gonococcal urethritis in men. *J Antimicrob Chemother* **37** (Suppl A): 123.

Piddock LJ, Zhu M (1991). Mechanism of action of sparfloxacin against and mechanism of resistance in gram-negative and gram-positive bacteria. *Antimicrob Ag Chemother* **35**: 2423.

Portier H, May Th, Proust A, the French Study Group (1996). Comparative efficacy of sparfloxacin in comparison with amoxycillin plus ofloxacin in the treatment of community-acquired pneumonia. *J Antimicrob Chemother* **37** (Suppl A): 83.

Qadri SM, Ueno Y, Burns JJ *et al.* (1992). *In vitro* activity of sparfloxacin (CI-978), a new broad-spectrum fluoroquinolone. *Chemotherapy* **38**: 99.

Ramsay CA, Obershkova E (1974). Photosensitivity from nalidixic acid. *Brit J Dermatol* **91**: 523.

Rastogi N, Goh KS (1991). *In vitro* activity of the new difluorinated quinolone sparfloxacin (AT-4140) against *Mycobacterium tuberculosis* compared with activities of ofloxacin and ciprofloxacin. *Antimicrob Ag Chemother* **35**: 1933.

Richard P, Gutmann L (1992). Sparfloxacin and other new fluoroquinolones. *J Antimicrob Chemother* **30**: 739.

Ritz M, Lode H, Fassbender M *et al.* (1994). Multiple-dose pharmacokinetics of sparfloxacin and its influence on fecal flora. *Antimicrob Ag Chemother* **38**: 455.

Roblin PM, Montalban G, Hammerschlag MR (1994). *In vitro* activities of OPC-17116, a new quinolone; ofloxacin; and sparfloxacin against *Chlamydia pneumoniae*. *Antimicrob Ag Chemother* **38**: 1402.

Rolston KV, Nguyen H, Messer M *et al.* (1990). *In vitro* activity of sparfloxacin (CI-978; AT-4140) against clinical isolates from cancer patients. *Antimicrob Ag Chemother* **34**: 2263.

Rotstein C, Amsterdam D, Beam TR *et al.* (1993). *In vitro* activity of sparfloxacin, ciprofloxacin, ofloxacin, and other antibiotics against bloodstream isolates of gram-positive cocci. *Diagn Microbiol Infect Dis* **17**: 85.

Rubinstein E (1996). Safety profile of sparfloxacin in the treatment of respiratory tract infections. *J Antimicrob Chemother* **37** (Suppl A): 145.

Saito A, Gaja M (1995). *In vitro* and *in vivo* activities of sparfloxacin in *Legionella* infections. *Drugs* **49** (Suppl 2): 250.

Shimada J, Nogita T, Ishibashi Y (1993). Clinical pharmacokinetics of sparfloxacin. *Clin Pharmacokinet* **25**: 358.

Takagi K, Yamaki K, Nadai M *et al.* (1991). Effect of a new quinolone, sparfloxacin, on the pharmacokinetics of theophylline in asthmatic patients. *Antimicrob Ag Chemother* **35**: 1137.

Vartivarian S, Anaissie E, Bodey G, Sprigg H, Rolston K (1994). A changing pattern of susceptibility of *Xanthomonas maltophilia* to antimicrobial agents: implications for therapy. *Antimicrob Ag Chemother* **38**: 624.

Vazquez J, Perri MB, Thal LA *et al.* (1993). Sparfloxacin and clinafloxacin alone or in combination with gentamicin for therapy of experimental ampicillin-resistant enterococcal endocarditis in rabbits. *J Antimicrob Chemother* **32**: 715.

Waites KB, Duffy LB, Schmid T *et al.* (1991). *In vitro* susceptibilities of *Mycoplasma pneumoniae*, *Mycoplasma hominis*, and *Ureaplasma urealyticum* to sparfloxacin and PD 127391. *Antimicrob Ag Chemother* **35**: 1181.

Waters MF (1993). Chemotherapy of leprosy–current status and future prospects. *Trans Roy Soc Trop Med Hyg* **87**: 500.

Wise R, Honeybourne D (1996). A review of the penetration of sparfloxacin into the lower respiratory tract and sinuses. *J Antimicrob Chemother* **37** (Suppl A): 57.

Wittke RR, Fabian W, Leperlier C *et al.* (1992). Biliary concentrations of sparfloxacin and its glucuronide in man. In *Proceedings of the Fourth International Symposium on New Quinolones, München, Germany.* (Abstr. 96).

Witzig RS, Franzblau SG (1993). Susceptibility of *Mycobacterium kansasii* to ofloxacin, sparfloxacin, clarithromycin, azithromycin, and fusidic acid. *Antimicrob Ag Chemother* **37**: 1997.

Wolfson JS, Hooper DC (1991). Overview of fluoroquinolone safety. *Amer J Med* **91** (Suppl 6A): 153.

Yew WW, Piddock LJ, Li MS *et al.* (1994). *In-vitro* activity of quinolones and macrolides against mycobacteria. *J Antimicrob Chemother* **34**: 343.

Zix JA, Geerdes-Fenge HF, Rau M *et al.* (1996). Sparfloxacin: interaction with sucralfate and cisapride. In *Program and Abstracts of the 36th Interscience Conference on Antimicrobial Agents and Chemotherapy, New Orleans* (Abstr. A10). Washington, DC: American Society for Microbiology.

Temafloxacin

Description

Temafloxacin (6-fluoro-7-piperazino-4-quinolone) was developed by Abbott Laboratories and gained marketing approval by the FDA in early 1992 for use in the treatment of acute bacterial exacerbations of chronic bronchitis and pneumonia, skin and soft tissue infections, uncomplicated and complicated urinary tract infections and prostatitis. In June 1992, however, after about 5 months clinical use, the drug was voluntarily withdrawn due to a high rate of reported adverse reactions. These reactions, termed by Blum et al. (1994) as the 'temafloxacin syndrome' are worthy of some discussion since there are some features that may be potentially associated, albeit at a markedly lower rate, with some other fluoroquinolones. In addition, the toxicity associated with temafloxacin highlight some of the difficulties in drug marketing since uncommon, even serious, side-effects may escape detection despite the usual rigorous pre-market testing.

Temafloxacin is a new fluoroquinolone with a broad range of activity against Gram-positive as well as Gram-negative pathogens and some anaerobes. In particular, its activity against *Streptococcus pneumoniae*, *Staphylococcus aureus*, *Legionella* and *Mycoplasma* spp. meant it was likely to be more reliable for respiratory tract and skin/soft tissue infections than other fluoroquinolones (Hardy et al., 1987; Gorzynski et al., 1989; Bryan et al., 1990; Bille and Glauser, 1991; Finegold et al., 1991; Jacobs, 1991; King et al., 1991; Pankey, 1991; Segreti et al., 1989; Segreti, 1991; Swanson et al., 1991; Glatt et al., 1992).

Temafloxacin has excellent bioavailability, with about 80–93% absorption, high water solubility, low protein binding (about 26%) and peak serum concentrations obtained 2–3 h after an oral dose. The half-life is 7–8 h and more than 60% of an administered dose is excreted unchanged in the urine within 48 h, with fecal elimination and biliary excretion accounting for 24% and 3%, respectively (Dudley, 1991; Pankey, 1991; Sorgel et al., 1991; Granneman et al., 1991a,b, 1992a,b; Granneman, 1992; Granneman and Mukherjee, 1992; Sorgel et al., 1992a). With the exception of the central nervous system, temafloxacin has excellent tissue and body fluid penetration (Pankey, 1991; Sörgel, 1992). Initially reported toxicities and drug interactions were similar to those generally associated with other fluoroquinolones such as ciprofloxacin (Norrby and Pernet, 1991; Pankey, 1991; Ruff et al., 1991; Granneman et al., 1992c; Mahr et al., 1992; Millar et al., 1992; Sorgel et al., 1992b). Recommended oral doses were 400 or 600 mg twice-daily, or occasionally once-daily for less severe infections (Pankey, 1991). Clinical studies demonstrated rates of efficacy in the treatment of lower respiratory tract infections of 90–100%, skin and soft tissue infections of >90%, urinary tract infections of >95%, prostatitis of ≥ 84% and excellent activity against gonococcal and non-gonococcal (other than syphilis) sexually transmitted diseases (Davies et al., 1990; Cox and Childs, 1991; Cox, 1991; Davey, 1991; Iravani, 1991a,b; Kosmidis, 1991; Mogadgab, 1991; Naber et al., 1991; Pankey, 1991; Parish and Jungkind, 1991; Carbon et al., 1992; Lindsay et al., 1992).

Temafloxacin was withdrawn after new and serious adverse reactions were reported at a frequency of about one per 3500 patients treated. By the time of withdrawal an estimated 189 000 prescriptions had been issued. In general, clinical trial programs can only be expected to detect adverse reactions at a frequency of about one per 1000 patients or higher, although studies using high doses may be useful in identifying dose-dependent adverse reactions. Due to the fact that only small doses of temafloxacin are necessary to induce serious reactions, early identification of the potential drug toxicity was unlikely (Norrby and Lietman, 1993).

Blum et al. (1994) reviewed all adverse-event reports for temafloxacin submitted to the FDA and summarized the findings of a detailed analysis of 95 patients with hemolysis and other organ system dysfunction, which they subsequently termed as constituting probable 'temafloxacin syndrome'. These patients typically presented with fever, chills, hemolysis and jaundice about 6.4 days after starting temafloxacin. New-onset renal dysfunction was noted in 57% cases, with about two-thirds of these patients requiring dialysis. Other findings included coagulopathy (35% cases), hepatic dysfunction (51% cases), central nervous system complications in two patients, and death in two patients. A history of previous quinolone use was associated with the rapid development of hemolysis after only one dose of temafloxacin, suggesting that immune hemolytic anemia, most likely due to immune complex formation, was a possible explanation for the adverse reaction. In comparison, 70% of patients with no history of quinolone use did not develop hemolysis until after 5 days temafloxacin therapy (mean 7.3 days) – this being consistent with the time required to develop a primary immune response. Interestingly, the core structure of fluoroquinolones has some similarities with those of quinine and quinidine – both of which are known to cause hemolytic anemia and thrombocytopenia by immune complex mechanisms. Indeed, temafloxacin-dependent red cell antibodies have been detected in some patients who developed hemolysis and renal dysfunction following temafloxacin ingestion (Deamer et al., 1993; Blum et al., 1994; Maguire et al., 1994)

Importantly, the one per 3500 incidence of serious adverse reactions with temafloxacin is much higher than that found with other fluoroquinolones, such as ciprofloxacin (one per 17 000 patients treated), norfloxacin (one per 25 000 patients treated) or ofloxacin (one per 33 000 patients treated) (Norrby and Lietman, 1993).

References

Bille J, Glauser MP (1991). *In-vitro* activity of temafloxacin for gram-positive pathogens. *J Antimicrob Chemother* **28** (Suppl C): 9.

Blum MD, Graham DJ, McCloskey CA (1994). Temafloxacin syndrome: review of 95 cases. *Clin Infect Dis* **18**: 946.

Bryan JP, Waters C, Sheffield J *et al.* (1990). *In vitro* activities of tosufloxacin, temafloxacin, and A-56620 against pathogens of diarrhea. *Antimicrob Ag Chemother* **34**: 368.

Carbon C, Leophonte P, Petitpretz P *et al.* (1992). Efficacy and safety of temafloxacin versus those of amoxicillin in hospitalized adults with community-acquired pneumonia. *Antimicrob Ag Chemother* **36**: 833.

Cox CE (1991). Oral temafloxacin compared to norfloxacin for the treatment of complicated urinary tract infections. *Amer J Med* **91**: 129S.

Cox CE, Childs SJ (1991). Treatment of chronic bacterial prostatitis with temafloxacin. *Amer J Med* **91**: 134S.

Davey PG (1991). Efficacy of temafloxacin versus ciprofloxacin or amoxicillin for lower respiratory tract infections in smokers and the elderly. *Amer J Med* **91**: 101S.

Davies BI, Maesen FP, Gubbelmans HL, Cremers HM (1990). Temafloxacin in acute purulent exacerbations of chronic bronchitis. *J Antimicrob Chemother* **26**: 237.

Deamer RL, Prichard JG, Koenker N *et al.* (1993). Temafloxacin-induced hemolytic anemia and renal failure. *Clin Pharm* **12**: 380.

Dudley MN (1991). A review of the pharmacokinetic profile of temafloxacin. *J Antimicrob Chemother* **28** (Suppl C): 55.

Finegold SM, Molitoris E, Reeves D, Wexler HM (1991). *In-vitro* activity of temafloxacin against anaerobic bacteria: a comparative study. *J Antimicrob Chemother* **28** (Suppl C): 25.

Glatt AE, Cummings M, McCormack W (1992). *In vitro* activity of temafloxacin compared with those of other agents against 100 clinical isolates of *Neisseria gonorrhoeae*. *Antimicrob Ag Chemother* **36**: 1131.

Gorzynski EA, Gutman SI, Allen W (1989). Comparative antimycobacterial activities of difloxacin, temafloxacin, enoxacin, pefloxacin, reference fluoroquinolones, and a new macrolide, clarithromycin. *Antimicrob Ag Chemother* **33**: 591.

Granneman GR (1992). Pharmacokinetics of temafloxacin after multiple oral administration. *Clin Pharmacokinet* **22** (Suppl 1): 14.

Granneman GR, Mukherjee D (1992). The effect of food on the bioavailability of temafloxacin. A review of 3 studies. *Clin Pharmacokinet* **22** (Suppl 1): 48.

Granneman GR, Braeckman R, Kraut J *et al.* (1991a). Temafloxacin pharmacokinetics in subjects with normal and impaired renal function. *Antimicrob Ag Chemother* **35**: 2345.

Granneman GR, Carpentier P, Morrison PJ, Pernet AG (1991b). Pharmacokinetics of temafloxacin in humans after single oral doses. *Antimicrob Ag Chemother* **35**: 436.

Granneman GR, Carpentier P, Morrison PJ, Pernet AG (1992a). Pharmacokinetics of temafloxacin in humans after multiple oral doses. *Antimicrob Ag Chemother* **36**: 378.

Granneman GR, Mahr G, Locke C *et al.* (1992b). Pharmacokinetics of temafloxacin in patients with liver impairment. *Clin Pharmacokinet* **22** (Suppl 1): 24.

Granneman GR, Stephan U, Birner B *et al.* (1992c). Effect of antacid medication on the pharmacokinetics of temafloxacin. *Clin Pharmacokinet* **22** (Suppl 1): 83.

Hardy DJ, Swanson RN, Hensey DM *et al.* (1987). Comparative antibacterial activities of temafloxacin hydrochloride (A- 62254). and two reference fluoroquinolones. *Antimicrob Ag Chemother* **31**: 1768.

Iravani A (1991a). Comparative, double-blind, prospective, multicenter trial of temafloxacin versus trimethoprim-sulfamethoxazole in uncomplicated urinary tract infections in women. *Antimicrob Ag Chemother* **35**: 1777.

Iravani A (1991b). Treatment of uncomplicated urinary tract infections with temafloxacin. *Amer J Med* **91**: 124S.

Jacobs MR (1991). Evaluation of the bactericidal activity of temafloxacin. *Amer J Med* **91**: 31S.

King A, Bethune L, Phillips I (1991). The *in-vitro* activity of temafloxacin compared with other antimicrobial agents. *J Antimicrob Chemother* **27**: 769.

Kosmidis J (1991). A double-blind study of once-daily temafloxacin in the treatment of bacterial lower respiratory tract infections. *J Antimicrob Chemother* **28** (Suppl C): 73.

Lindsay G, Scorer HJ, Carnegie CM (1992). Safety and efficacy of temafloxacin versus ciprofloxacin in lower respiratory tract infections: a randomized, double-blind trial. *J Antimicrob Chemother* **30**: 89.

Maguire RB, Stroncek DF, Gale E, Yearlsey M (1994). Hemolytic anemia and acute renal failure associated with temafloxacin-dependent antibodies. *Amer J Hematol* **46**: 363.

Mahr G, Sorgel F, Granneman GR *et al.* (1992). Effects of temafloxacin and ciprofloxacin on the pharmacokinetics of caffeine. *Clin Pharmacokinet* **22** (Suppl 1): 90.

Millar E, Coles S, Wyld P, Nimmo W (1992). Temafloxacin does not potentiate the anticoagulant effect of warfarin in healthy subjects. *Clin Pharmacokinet* **22** (Suppl 1): 102.

Mogabgab WJ (1991). Single-dose oral temafloxacin versus parenteral ceftriaxone in the treatment of gonococcal urethritis/cervicitis. *Amer J Med* **91**: 145S.

Naber KG, Boerema JB, Bischoff W *et al.* (1991). An assessment of temafloxacin in the treatment of chronic bacterial prostatitis. *J Antimicrob Chemother* **28** (Suppl C): 87.

Norrby SR, Lietman PS (1993). Safety and tolerability of fluoroquinolones. *Drugs* **45** (Suppl 3): 59.

Norrby SR, Pernet AG (1991). Assessment of adverse events during drug development: experience with temafloxacin. *J Antimicrob Chemother* **28** (Suppl C): 111.

Pankey GA (1991). Temafloxacin: an overview. *Amer J Med* **91**: 166S.

Parish LC, Jungkind DL (1991). Systemic antimicrobial therapy in skin and skin structure infections: comparison of temafloxacin and ciprofloxacin. *Amer J Med* **91**: 115S.

Ruff F, Santais MC, Callens E *et al.* (1991). Effect of temafloxacin on the pharmacokinetics of theophylline. *Amer J Med* **91**: 76S.

Segreti J (1991). *In vitro* activity of temafloxacin against pathogens causing sexually transmitted diseases. *Amer J Med* **91**: 24S.

Segreti J, Kessler HA, Kapell KS, Trenholme GM (1989). *In vitro* activities of temafloxacin (A-62254). and four other antibiotics against *Chlamydia trachomatis*. *Antimicrob Ag Chemother* **33**: 118.

Sorgel F (1992). Penetration of temafloxacin into body tissues and fluids. *Clin Pharmacokinet* **22** (Suppl 1): 57.

Sörgel F, Naber KG, Kinzig M *et al.* (1991). Comparative pharmacokinetics of ciprofloxacin and temafloxacin in humans: a review. *Amer J Med* **91**: 51S.

Sorgel F, Granneman GR, Mahr G *et al.* (1992a). Hepatobiliary elimination of temafloxacin. *Clin Pharmacokinet* **22** (Suppl 1): 33.

Sorgel F, Mahr G, Granneman GR *et al.* (1992b). Effects of two quinolone antibacterials, temafloxacin and enoxacin, on theophylline pharmacokinetics. *Clin Pharmacokinet* **22** (Suppl 1): 65.

Swanson RN, Hardy DJ, Chu DT *et al.* (1991). Activity of temafloxacin against respiratory pathogens. *Antimicrob Ag Chemother* **35**: 423.

Lomefloxacin

Description

Lomefloxacin (SC-47111, NY-198) is a difluoroquinolone that was synthesized by Hokuriku and Seiyaku and Co. Ltd in Japan and is licensed to GD Searle and Co. for development. Its chemical formula is 1-ethyl-6,8-difluoro-1,4-dihydro-7-(3-methyl-1-piperazinyl)-4-oxoquinoline-3-carboxylic acid. The antibacterial spectrum of lomefloxacin is roughly comparable with norfloxacin but it has better tissue penetration and its longer half-life allows it to be given once-daily. Lomefloxacin appears to be effective in the treatment of urinary tract and respiratory tract infections (although it has limited activity against *Streptococcus pneumoniae*) and it does not interact with theophylline (p. 1014). Whether these advantages are sufficient to result in widespread use, given the more recent development of other fluoroquinolones with broader spectrum of activity and similar once-daily dosing, remains to be determined (pp. 1172, 1175).

Sensitive Organisms

Lomefloxacin has antibacterial activity broadly similar to norfloxacin, enoxacin and fleroxacin; is similar or inferior to ofloxacin, but is 2- to 8-fold less active than ciprofloxacin (Jones *et al.*, 1988; Weinstein, 1988; Wise *et al.*, 1988; Aldridge *et al.*, 1989; Clarke and Zemcov, 1989; Inderlied *et al.*, 1989; Robbins *et al.*, 1989; Shah *et al.*, 1989; Stratton and Weeks, 1989; Sun *et al.*, 1989; Mayer and Ellal, 1992). In terms of antibacterial spectrum, lomefloxacin has no advantage over these latter two agents and is inferior in spectrum to many of the newer fluoroquinolones. The *in vitro* MICs of lomefloxacin against some selected bacterial species are shown in Table II.6 (pp. 986–987).

1 Gram-negative bacteria

Lomefloxacin has excellent activity against Enterobacteriaceae ($MIC_{90} \leq 0.50 \mu g$ per ml), *Haemophilus influenzae* ($MIC_{90} \leq 0.125 \mu g$ per ml), *Moraxella catarrhalis* and *Neisseria gonorrhoae* (both $MIC_{90} \leq 0.03 \mu g$ per ml). Lomefloxacin is active against most diarrheal pathogens. However, it has only moderate to poor activity against *Acinetobacter* spp. (MIC_{90} $4 \mu g$ per ml), *Pseudomonas aeruginosa* (MIC_{90} $8 \mu g$ per ml), *Citrobacter freundii* and *Providentia rettgeri*. It has poor activity against *Stenotrophomonas* (previously *Xanthomonas*) *maltophilia* (MIC_{90} $16 \mu g$ per ml) and *Burkholderia cepacia* (MIC_{90} $16 \mu g$ per ml). Lomefloxacin has good *in vitro* activity against *Vibrio* spp. ($MIC_{90} \leq 0.06 \mu g$ per ml) and *Legionella* spp. ($MIC_{90} \leq 0.06–1 \mu g$ per ml), but variable activity against *Campylobacter jejuni* ($MIC_{90} \leq 0.1–4 \mu g$ per ml) (Chin *et al.*, 1988; Aldridge *et al.*, 1989; Clarke and Zemcov, 1989; Dubois and Joly, 1989; Edelstein *et al.*, 1989; Forward *et al.*, 1989; Hoban *et al.*, 1989b; Robbins *et al.*, 1989; Segreti *et al.*, 1989; Simor *et al.*, 1989; Felmingham and Robbins, 1992; Jones *et al.*, 1994; Prosser and Beskid, 1995). Lomefloxacin is active against *Bordetella pertussis* and *B. parapertussis* (MIC_{90} $0.125 \mu g$ per ml), and against *Brucella melitensis* with 99% of strains inhibited by $\leq 0.5 \mu g$ per ml (Hoppe and Simon, 1990; Qadri *et al.*, 1990).

Lomefloxacin has poor activity against Gram-negative anaerobes such as *Bacteroides* spp. (MIC_{90} $16 \mu g$ per ml) (Robbins *et al.*, 1989).

Some authors have been able to readily isolate drug-resistant mutants to lomefloxacin, especially among strains of *Ps. aeruginosa*, while others have claimed low rates of single-step resistance (Chambers *et al.*, 1991; Mayer and Ellal, 1992). Similar to other agents in this class, lomefloxacin is subject to cross-resistance with other fluoroquinolones (Barry and Fuchs, 1991).

2 Gram-positive bacteria

Similar to norfloxacin, but sometimes inferior to ofloxacin and ciprofloxacin, lomefloxacin has reasonable activity against methicillin-susceptible strains of *Staph. aureus* and *Staph. epidermidis* (MIC_{90} 1–2 μg per ml), but activity is variable against methicillin-resistant strains. Notably, lomefloxacin has limited activity against *Strep. pneumoniae* (MIC_{90} 8 μg per ml), *Strep. pyogenes* (MIC_{90} 8 μg per ml), other streptococci (MIC_{90} >8 μg per ml), enterococci (MIC_{90} 8 μg per ml) and *Listeria monocytogenes* (MIC_{90} 8 μg per ml). Lomefloxacin is generally at least two dilutions less active than sparfloxacin against Gram-positive species (Wise *et al.*, 1988; Aldridge *et al.*, 1989; Hoban *et al.*, 1989b; Canton *et al.*, 1992; Murray *et al.*, 1993; Spangler *et al.*, 1993; Cerubin and Stratton, 1994; Pankuch *et al.*, 1995; Prosser and Beskid, 1995).

Lomefloxacin has generally limited activity against Gram-positive anaerobes such as *Clostridium perfringens* (MIC_{90} 2 μg per ml), *Clostridium difficile* (MIC_{90} 32 μg per ml) and *Reptostreptoccus* spp. (MIC_{90} 4 μg per ml) (Robbins *et al.*, 1989).

3 Mycobacteria

Lomefloxacin has broadly similar *in vitro* activity against *Mycobacterium tuberculosis* as ciprofloxacin and ofloxacin, with MIC range of 0.5–4 μg per ml, but it is inferior to these agents against other *Mycobacteria* spp. (Banerjee *et al.*, 1992; Piersimoni *et al.*, 1992). Lomefloxacin has some activity in *M. leprae*-infected mice, but this is inferior to that of ofloxacin and sparfloxacin (Gelber *et al.*, 1992).

4 Chlamydia and Mycoplasma

Lomefloxacin has only moderate activity against *Mycoplasma pneumoniae* (MIC_{90} 4 μg per ml), *Chlamydia trachomatis* (MIC_{90} 2–4 μg per ml), *M. hominis* (MIC_{90} 2–8 μg per ml) and *Ureaplasma urealyticum* (MIC_{90} 8 μg per ml) (Hoban *et al.*, 1989a; Kenny *et al.*, 1989; Robbins *et al.*, 1989; Talbot and Romanowski, 1989; Kenny and Cartwright, 1991; Ishida *et al.*, 1994). Sparfloxacin and some of the other newer fluoroquinolones are significantly more active against these pathogens than lomefloxacin (Nakata *et al.*, 1992).

Mode of Administration and Dosage

1 Oral administration

The usual dose of lomefloxacin is 400 mg once-daily (or occasionally twice-daily), except in Japan where 200 mg thrice-daily is often used. Generally, single dose 200–400 mg is adequate for gonococcal urethritis or cervicitis, while 3–7 days therapy is sufficient for uncomplicated urinary tract infections; 7–14 days therapy for complicated urinary sepsis and respiratory tract infections, and longer courses are necessary for prostatitis (Wadworth and Goa, 1991).

2 Patients with renal failure

Since lomefloxacin is primarily eliminated in the urine, dosage reduction is necessary in patients with renal dysfunction. In patients with a glomerular filtration rate (GFR) > 30 ml per min, the usual dose of lomefloxacin 400 mg once-daily is appropriate, but when the GFR is < 30 ml per min the dose should be reduced to 200 mg per day. Hemodialysis has little effect on serum lomefloxacin concentrations and no additional dosage adjustment is necessary in these patients (Blum *et al.*, 1990; Leroy *et al.*, 1990; Nilsen *et al.*, 1992).

3 Patients with liver failure

Liver failure *per se* does not affect lomefloxacin pharmacokinetics and hence no dosage adjustment is necessary in patients with cirrhosis and/or hepatic failure. However, a reduction in renal function is not uncommon in patients with hepatic failure, and under these circumstances, dosage reduction may be needed (Lebrec *et al.*, 1992).

4 Elderly patients

Although there are some changes in the pharmacokinetics of lomefloxacin associated with aging, these are insufficient to require any dosage adjustment in this population, unless renal dysfunction is present (Blum *et al.*, 1990; Cowling *et al.*, 1991; Schentag and Goss, 1992)

Serum Levels in Relation to Dosage

1 Oral administration

The absolute bioavailability of lomefloxacin is greater than 95%, with the drug rapidly absorbed after oral administration. Plasma half-life of lomefloxacin is 7–8 h (Hunt and Adams, 1989; Mant, 1992). Increases in the peak serum concentrations and area-under-the-concentration-time-curve (AUC) are proportional to increases in dose, being a linear relationship over a dose range of 100–800 mg. Following single doses of 100, 400 or 800 mg lomefloxacin, peak serum concentrations of 0.9–1.1, 3.0–5.2 and 7.0–7.7 μg per ml, respectively, are achieved 1–1.5 h post-dose (Morrison et al., 1988; Stone et al., 1988; Freeman et al., 1993). Trough and peak serum levels after 5- to 7-day multidose regimens of either 400, 600 or 800 mg once-daily are 0.27–0.31 and 2.8–4.7 μg per ml, 0.40–0.49 and 5.02–5.31 μg per ml, and 0.53–0.56 and 5.42–5.99 μg per ml, respectively. After similar duration regimens of 200 or 400 mg twice-daily, trough and peak levels are 0.49–0.72 and 2.12–2.73 μg per ml, and 0.64–1.56 and 3.77–5.36 μg per ml, respectively (Gros and Carbon, 1990; Hunt and Adams, 1989; Mant, 1992). The presence of respiratory infection does not alter these pharmacokinetics (Freeman et al., 1993). The absorption of lomefloxacin is delayed when the drug is taken at the same time as food, with a delay in the time to peak serum concentrations. However, peak serum concentrations and the amount of lomefloxacin absorbed following either a carbohydrate or high-fat meal is similar to that expected when the drug is taken after an overnight fast (Hooper et al., 1990).

2 Patients with renal failure

There is a roughly linear correlation between lomefloxacin serum and renal clearances and creatinine clearance. Compared with patients with renal function of > 40 ml per min GFR, the mean half-life of lomefloxacin in patients with GFR 10–40 ml per min and ≤ 10 ml per min increases from 7–8 to 20.9 and 38–44.25 h, respectively. However, no significant differences in peak serum concentration or time to peak concentration are noted, regardless of the level of renal dysfunction. In patients with GFR < 30 ml per min given 200 mg once-daily, serum peak and trough levels of 4–6 and 1–3 μg per ml, respectively, can be expected. Interestingly, non-renal lomefloxacin clearance also decreases with declining renal function. Hemodialysis has no effect on serum lomefloxacin levels, with < 3% of a dose recovered in dialysis fluid, and as noted earlier, no dosage adjustment is necessary in these patients (Blum et al., 1990; Leroy et al., 1990; Blum, 1992; Nilsen et al., 1992).

3 Patients with hepatic failure

Lebrec et al. (1992) studied the pharmacokinetics of a single oral dose of 400 mg lomefloxacin in 12 patients with hepatic cirrhosis of varying degrees of severity. The mean peak serum concentration in these patients was 3.9 ± 1.2 μg per ml; the mean time to this peak was 2.1 ± 2.6 h and the mean elimination half-life was 9.2 h. In patients with cirrhosis there was a decrease in total drug clearance, which was only 60% that found in healthy volunteers. Mean non-renal lomefloxacin clearance was 41% of the total, with no correlation noted betwen the level of non-renal clearance and either hepatic insufficiency or plasma bilirubin. These authors suggest that the main changes in lomefloxacin clearance are due to changes in renal function associated with cirrhosis, rather than cirrhosis per se. Thus, as noted earlier (p. 1148), no dosage adjustment is necessary in patients with liver dysfunction unless there is associated renal impairment.

Excretion

1 Urine

Both renal and non-renal mechanisms are associated with the elimination of lomefloxacin, but the vast majority of the drug (60–85%) is excreted unchanged in urine (Blum et al., 1990; Morrison et al., 1988; Leroy et al., 1990). Metabolites of lomefloxacin have been recovered in urine, but these constitute < 5% of an oral dose and do not appear to have any significant antibacterial activity (Stone et al., 1988; Freeman et al., 1993).

2 Bile

Some biliary elimination takes place but there have been only limited studies to quantify the amount of lomefloxacin in bile (p. 1150).

3 Inactivation in body

Lomefloxacin is thought to undergo limited metabolism in the liver, although this probably accounts for less than 20% of a lomefloxacin dose (Leroy *et al.*, 1990; Freeman *et al.*, 1993)

4 Feces

Following 400 mg once-daily lomefloxacin for 4 days, drug is detectable in feces for up to 6 days after the last dose, with concentrations of up to 42 μg per g present on day 1 and levels of 1.7–8.3 μg per g on days 5–6 (Leigh *et al.*, 1991). Other authors have found fecal concentrations of 203 μg per g, when receiving 400 mg lomefloxacin once-daily (Edlund *et al.*, 1990). Overall, only about 9% of an ingested dose is eliminated unchanged in feces (Nakashima *et al.*, 1988)

Distribution of the Drug in Body

Lomefloxacin is approximately 15% protein-bound and therefore achieves reasonable tissue penetration (Wise *et al.*, 1988; Freeman *et al.*, 1993). Lomefloxacin achieves about 100% penetration (based on AUC ratio) into inflammatory blister fluid after both single- and multiple-dose regimens. Mean peak blister fluid levels following both single and multiple doses of 400 mg are 3.2–3.5 μg per ml after 2.7 h post-dose. The elimination half-life is similar in blister fluid to that in serum (Stone *et al.*, 1988; Kavi *et al.*, 1989).

Saliva concentrations of lomefloxacin are up to 37% those in serum, or about 0.6 μg per ml (Edlund *et al.*, 1990; Leigh *et al.*, 1991). In one study the concentration of lomefloxacin in bile, 2–4 h after a single 200-mg dose was 1.75 μg per ml (Shimizu, 1988).

Lomefloxacin penetrates well into respiratory tissues and secretions. Following a single 400-mg dose of lomefloxacin, the mean concentration in bronchial secretions (obtained at bronchoscopy) is 2.78 μg per ml, 1 h post-dose. The ratio between bronchial and simultaneous serum concentrations is 89%, 1 and 2 h post-dose. Results are similar after multiple doses (Bergogne-Berezin and Muller-Serieys, 1992). Among elderly patients with chronic obstructive airways disease treated with lomefloxacin 400 mg once-daily, the peak concentration in purulent, expectorated sputum is 4.3 μg per ml, 3.1 h post-dose. At the end of the 24-h dosing interval, the concentration of lomefloxacin in sputum can still be expected to be 1.7 μg per ml. Thus, penetration into sputum, based on a comparison of sputum and serum AUC, is about 120% (Kovarik *et al.*, 1992). The median bronchial mucosa concentration following a regimen of 400 mg once-daily for 4 days is 5.0 μg per g (177% penetration), while the concentration in alveolar macrophages is about 20 times that in serum (Baldwin *et al.* 1990, 1993).

Urine concentrations of lomefloxacin are at least 27.2–34.3 μg per ml about 1.7 h after multiple once-daily doses of 400 mg (Leigh *et al.*, 1991). Other authors (Morrison *et al.*, 1988) have reported higher urinary concentrations with mean values during the 4 h after a 100- or 800-mg dose to be 104 and 713 μg per ml, respectively. In addition, these latter authors also noted urinary levels of 120 μg per ml lomefloxacin, 12–24 h after a 400-mg dose. Prostatic concentrations of lomefloxacin are 6.5 ± 2.7 μg per g (representing a ratio of tissue:serum concentration of 1.53), following a single preoperative oral dose of 400 mg (Leroy *et al.*, 1992). Other authors have found broadly similar results (Kovarik *et al.*, 1990; Klimberg *et al.*, 1992).

The concentration of lomefloxacin in bone following a single dose of 400 mg is 70% of that in serum (On *et al.*, 1992).

Mode of Action

Lomefloxacin has a similar mode of action to other fluoroquinolones.

Toxicity

The rate of adverse reactions associated with lomefloxacin is similar to that associated with other fluoroquinolones. Most commonly reported side-effects include nausea (3.7%), diarrhea (1.4%), photosensitivity (2.4%), headache (3.2%), and dizziness (2.3%). Scheife *et al.* (1993) have suggested that the hierarchy of phototoxic risk among the fluoroquinolones is fleroxacin >> lomefloxacin, pefloxacin >> ciprofloxacin > enoxacin, norfloxacin, ofloxacin. The rate of these reactions in elderly patients appears to be no higher than that observed in younger patients. Laboratory abnormalities are uncommon, with alterations in hepatic function tests (0.1–0.4%), monocytosis (0.4%), thrombocytopenia (0.1%), decreased hemoglobin (0.1%) and elevated urea (0.2%) most reported (Rizk, 1992; Correia and Delgado, 1994; Poh-Fitzpatrick, 1994).

Unlike some fluoroquinolones, lomefloxacin does not alter the pharmacokinetics of theophylline or caffeine (Nix *et al.*, 1989; LeBel *et al.*, 1990; Wijnands *et al.*, 1990; Healy *et al.*, 1991; Upton, 1991). The lack of interaction with theophylline may be a useful feature when considering the use of lomefloxacin in the treatment of respiratory tract infections in patients with chronic lung diseases who require concomitant theophylline therapy.

Furosemide reduces the renal clearance of lomefloxacin and co-administration of these two agents may result in elevation of serum lomefloxacin levels (Sudoh *et al.*, 1994).

Similar to other fluoroquinolones, the absorption of lomefloxacin (as measured by reduction in AUC) is impaired by the co-administration of aluminum- and magnesium-containing antacids (40% reduction), ferrous sulfate (26% reduction) and sucralfate (51% reduction). The co-administration of ranitidine, omeprazole, calcium carbonate or milk with lomefloxacin does not affect the bioavailability of the latter (Shimada *et al.*, 1992; Freeman *et al.*, 1993; Lehto and Kivisto, 1994; Stuht *et al.*, 1995).

Clinical Uses of the Drug

1 Urinary tract infections and prostatitis

Some authors have found lomefloxacin 400 mg once-daily to be more effective than norfloxacin 400 mg twice-daily for the treatment of uncomplicated urinary tract infections, with clinical success reported in 99.1 % versus 93.5%, respectively (p=0.002). Bacteriologic response, however, was similar: 98.2 versus 96.3% (Iravani, 1992; Rizk, 1992). Other studies have demonstrated a 3-day course of lomefloxacin or norfloxacin to have similar efficacy in uncomplicated urinary tract infection with rates of cure after 5–9 days and 4–6 weeks of 91–95% and 87–89%, respectively (Nicolle *et al.*, 1993). Neringer *et al.* (1992) compared a 3-day or a 7-day course of lomefloxacin with a 7-day course of norfloxacin – all three regimens had comparable results, but phototoxicity was more common in the two lomefloxacin-treated groups. In another study, a 7- to 10-day course of lomefoxacin 400 mg once-daily was similar in efficacy to trimethoprim/sulfamethoxazole 160/800 mg twice-daily for the treatment of uncomplicated urinary tract infection (Andrade-Villanueva *et al.*, 1992).

A 10- to 14-day course of lomefloxacin 400 mg once-daily has been compared with norfloxacin 400 mg twice-daily and ciprofloxacin 500 mg twice-daily in a number of randomized, controlled trials of patients with complicated or recurrent urinary tract infections. Lomefloxacin was superior to norfloxacin in rates of bacteriological eradication (91.3 versus 78.4%, respectively, p=0.015), but the clinical outcomes were similar. Similar duration courses of once-daily lomefloxacin has similar efficacy to twice-daily ciprofloxacin (Cox, 1992). The overall rate of clinical cure/improvement with lomefloxacin in this setting is generally 88–99%, although lower rates have been reported (Rizk, 1992; Hoepelman *et al.*, 1993). Lomefloxacin 400 mg once-daily appears to be superior, at least in terms of bacterial eradication, to trimethoprim/sulfamethoxazole 160/800 mg twice-daily when both are given for 14 days to patients with pyelonephritis and other forms of complicated urinary tract sepsis (Mouton *et al.*, 1992; Nicolle *et al.*, 1994).

When given 2–6 h prior to transurethral surgery, lomefloxacin 400 mg proved to be effective (98.6%) prophylaxis against postoperative infections, and was comparable with preoperative i.m. cefotaxime (Klimberg *et al.*, 1992). Costa (1994) and Charton *et al.* (1992) have also found lomefloxacin to be effective prophylaxis against bacteriuria in patients undergoing laser ablation of the prostate.

2 Respiratory tract infections

Lomefloxacin 400 mg once-daily is superior to cefaclor 250 mg thrice-daily when both are given for 7–10 days in the treatment of acute exacerbations of chronic bronchitis. Rates of bacterial eradication 1–4 days after completion of treatment were 82 versus 63%, respectively (p< 0.001), while clinical success was noted in 80% of patients receiving lomefloxacin versus 65% in the cefaclor-treated group (p=0.002) (Gotfried and Ellison, 1992). Similarly, lomefloxacin is superior to oral amoxycillin in this setting (Grassi *et al.*, 1992). Once-daily 400 mg lomefloxacin appears to have efficacy comparable with 400 mg twice-daily in patients with chronic bronchitis due to Gram-negative pathogens – hence the once-daily dose is preferred (Kemper and Kohler, 1992). Given the poor *in vitro* activity of lomefloxacin against *Strep. pneumoniae*, respiratory tract infections in which this pathogen is proven or likely, should probably be treated with agents which have more reliable anti-pneumococcal activity, such as penicillin or a cephalosporin.

3 Other infections

In a double-blind, placebo-controlled trial of lomefloxacin 400 mg once-daily for 5 days in the treatment of community-acquired bacterial diarrhea (85% due to *Campylobacter* spp.), lomefloxacin eradicated *Campylobacter* spp. in 75% cases but did not alter clinical outcome. In addition, 25% of *Campylobacter* isolates developed resistance and 33% of patients developed side-effects (Ellis-Pegler *et al.*, 1995).

A number of limited studies have suggested that lomefloxacin has efficacy in the treatment of gonococcal and non-gonococcal urethritis and cervicitis; ear/nose/throat infections and biliary tract infections; but further data are necessary before lomefloxacin can be recommended for the treatment of these conditions (Wadsworth and Goa, 1991).

References

Aldridge KE, Henderberg A, Gebbia K *et al.* (1989). Lomefloxacin, a new fluoroquinolone. Studies on *in vitro* antimicrobial spectrum, potency, and development of resistance. *Diagn Microbiol Infect Dis* **12**: 221.

Andrade-Villanueva J, Flores-Gaxiola A, Lopez-Guillen P *et al.* (1992). Comparison of the safety and efficacy of lomefloxacin and trimethoprim/sulfamethoxazole in the treatment of uncomplicated urinary tract infections: results from a multicenter study. *Amer J Med* **92**: 71S.

Baldwin DR, Honeybourne D, Andrews JM *et al.* (1990). Concentrations of oral lomefloxacin in serum and bronchial mucosa. *Antimicrob Ag Chemother* **34**: 1017.

Baldwin DR, Wise R, Andrews JM *et al.* (1993). Comparative bronchoalveolar concentrations of ciprofloxacin and lomefloxacin following oral administration. *Respir Med* **87**: 595.

Banerjee DK, Ford J, Markanday S (1992). *In-vitro* activity of lomefloxacin against pathogenic and environmental mycobacteria. *J Antimicrob Chemother* **30**: 236.

Barry AL, Fuchs PC (1991). Cross-resistance and cross-susceptibility between fluoroquinolone agents. *Eur J Clin Microbiol Infect Dis* **10**: 1013.

Bergogne-Berezin E, Muller-Serieys C, Kafe H (1992). Penetration of lomefloxacin into bronchial secretions following single and multiple oral administration. *Amer J Med* **92**: 8S.

Blum RA (1992). Influence of renal function on the pharmacokinetics of lomefloxacin compared with other fluoroquinolones. *Amer J Med* **92**: 18S.

Blum RA, Schultz RW, Schentag JJ (1990). Pharmacokinetics of lomefloxacin in renally compromised patients. *Antimicrob Ag Chemother* **34**: 2364.

Canton E, Peman J, Jimenez MT *et al.* (1992). *In vitro* activity of sparfloxacin compared with those of five other quinolones. *Antimicrob Ag Chemother* **36**: 558.

Chambers ST, Peddie BA, Robson RA *et al.* (1991). Antimicrobial effects of lomefloxacin *in vitro*. *J Antimicrob Chemother* **27**: 481.

Charton M, Mombet A, Gattegno B (1992). Urinary tract infection prophylaxis in transurethral surgery: oral lomefloxacin versus parenteral cefuroxime. *Amer J Med* **92**: 118S.

Cherubin CE, Stratton CW (1994). Assessment of the bactericidal activity of sparfloxacin, ofloxacin, levofloxacin, and other fluoroquinolones compared with selected agents of proven efficacy against *Listeria monocytogenes*. *Diagn Microbiol Infect Dis* **20**: 21.

Chin NX, Novelli A, Neu HC (1988). *In vitro* activity of lomefloxacin (SC-47111; NY-198), a difluoroquinolone 3- carboxylic acid, compared with those of other quinolones. *Antimicrob Ag Chemother* **32**: 656.

Clarke AM, Zemcov SJ (1989). Comparative *in vitro* activity of lomefloxacin, a new difluoroquinolone. *Eur J Clin Microbiol Infect Dis* **8**: 164.

Correia O, Delgado L, Barros MA (1994). Bullous photodermatosis after lomefloxacin. *Arch Dermatol* **130**: 808.

Costa FJ (1994). Lomefloxacin prophylaxis in visual laser ablation of the prostate. *Urology* **44**: 933.

Cowling P, Rogers S, McMullin CM *et al.* (1991). The pharmacokinetics of lomefloxacin in elderly patients with urinary tract infection following daily dosing with 400 mg. *J Antimicrob Chemother* **28**: 101.

Cox CE (1992). A comparison of the safety and efficacy of lomefloxacin and ciprofloxacin in the treatment of complicated or recurrent urinary tract infections. *Amer J Med* **92**: 82S.

Dubois J, Joly JR (1989). *In vitro* activity of lomefloxacin (SC 47111 or NY-198). against isolates of *Legionella* spp. *Diagn Microbiol Infect Dis* **12**: 89S.

Edelstein PH, Gaudet EA, Edelstein MA (1989). *In vitro* activity of lomefloxacin (NY-198 or SC 47111), ciprofloxacin, and erythromycin against 100 clinical *Legionella* strains. *Diagn Microbiol Infect Dis* **12**: 93S.

Edlund C, Brismar B, Nord CE (1990). Effect of lomefloxacin on the normal oral and intestinal microflora. *Eur J Clin Microbiol Infect Dis* **9**: 35.

Ellis-Pegler RB, Hyman LK, Ingram RJ, McCarthy M (1995). A placebo controlled evaluation of lomefloxacin in the treatment of bacterial diarrhoea in the community. *J Antimicrob Chemother* **36**: 259.

Felmingham D, Robbins MJ (1992). *In vitro* activity of lomefloxacin and other antimicrobials against bacterial enteritis pathogens. *Diagn Microbiol Infect Dis* **15**: 339.

Forward KR, Degagne PA, Bartlett KR (1989). The comparative activity of lomefloxacin (SC-47111, NY-198). and other orally absorbable agents against *Haemophilus influenzae* and *Branhamella catarrhalis*. *Diagn Microbiol Infect Dis* **12**: 437.

Freeman CD, Nicolau DP, Belliveau PP, Nightingale CH (1993). Lomefloxacin clinical pharmacokinetics. *Clin Pharmacokinet* **25**: 6.

Gelber RH, Iranmanesh A, Murray L *et al.* (1992). Activities of various quinolone antibiotics against *Mycobacterium leprae* in infected mice. *Antimicrob Ag Chemother* **36**: 2544.

Gotfried MH, Ellison WT (1992). Safety and efficacy of lomefloxacin versus cefaclor in the treatment of acute exacerbations of chronic bronchitis. *Amer J Med* **92**: 108S.

Grassi C, Albera C, Pozzi E (1992). Lomefloxacin versus amoxicillin in the treatment of acute exacerbations of chronic bronchitis: an Italian multicenter study. *Amer J Med* **92**: 103S.

Gros I, Carbon C (1990). Pharmacokinetics of lomefloxacin in healthy volunteers: comparison of 400 milligrams once daily and 200 milligrams twice daily given orally for 5 days. *Antimicrob Ag Chemother* **34**: 150.

Healy DP, Schoenle JR, Stotka J, Polk RE (1991). Lack of interaction between lomefloxacin and caffeine in normal volunteers. *Antimicrob Ag Chemother* **35**: 660.

Hoban D, DeGagne P, Witwicki E (1989a). *In vitro* activity of lomefloxacin against *Chlamydia trachomatis, Neisseria gonorrhoeae, Haemophilus ducreyi, Mycoplasma hominis*, and *Ureaplasma urealyticum. Diagn Microbiol Infect Dis* **12**: 83S.

Hoban D, Grabowski M, Koss J, Weselowski V (1989b). Lomefloxacin, a new difluoroquinolone: *in vitro* activity against Gram- positive and Gram-negative bacteria. *Diagn Microbiol Infect Dis* **12**: 77S.

Hoepelman IM, Havinga WH, Benne RA *et al.* (1993). Safety and efficacy of lomefloxacin versus norfloxacin in the treatment of complicated urinary tract infections. *Eur J Clin Microbiol Infect Dis* **12**: 343.

Hooper WD, Dickinson RG, Eadie MJ (1990). Effect of food on absorption of lomefloxacin. *Antimicrob Ag Chemother* **34**: 1797.

Hoppe JE, Simon CG (1990). *In vitro* susceptibilities of *Bordetella pertussis* and *Bordetella parapertussis* to seven fluoroquinolones. *Antimicrob Ag Chemother* **34**: 2287.

Hunt TL, Adams MA (1989). Pharmacokinetics and safety of lomefloxacin following multiple doses. *Diagn Microbiol Infect Dis* **12**: 181.

Inderlied CB, Lancero MG, Bermudez LM, Young LS (1989). *In vitro* activity of lomefloxacin as compared with ciprofloxacin. *Diagn Microbiol Infect Dis* **12**: 17S.

Iravani A (1992). Efficacy of lomefloxacin as compared to norfloxacin in the treatment of uncomplicated urinary tract infections in adults. *Amer J Med* **92**: 75S.

Ishida K, Kaku M, Irifune K *et al.* (1994). *In-vitro* and *in-vivo* activity of a new quinolone AM-1155 against *Mycoplasma pneumoniae. J Antimicrob Chemother* **34**: 875.

Jones RN, Aldridge KE, Barry AL *et al.* (1988). Multicenter *in vitro* evaluation of lomefloxacin (NY-198, SC-47111), including tests against nearly 7000 bacterial isolates and preliminary recommendations for susceptibility testing. *Diagn Microbiol Infect Dis* **10**: 221.

Jones RN, Sader HS, Erwin ME (1994). Update of lomefloxacin *in vitro* activity and spectrum. A multicenter trial testing contemporary pathogens following Food and Drug Administration validation guidelines. Lomefloxacin Activity Study Group. *Diagn Microbiol Infect Dis* **20**: 93.

Kavi J, Stone J, Andrews JM *et al.* (1989). Tissue penetration and pharmacokinetics of lomefloxacin following multiple doses. *Eur J Clin Microbiol Infect Dis* **8**: 168.

Kemper P, Kohler D (1992). A double-blind study of two dosage regimens of lomefloxacin in bacteriologically proven exacerbations of chronic bronchitis of Gram-negative etiology. *Amer J Med* **92**: 98S.

Kenny GE, Cartwright FD (1991). Susceptibility of *Mycoplasma pneumoniae* to several new quinolones, tetracycline, and erythromycin. *Antimicrob Ag Chemother* **35**: 587.

Kenny GE, Hooton TM, Roberts MC *et al.* (1989). Susceptibilities of genital mycoplasmas to the newer quinolones as determined by the agar dilution method. *Antimicrob Ag Chemother* **33**: 103.

Klimberg IW, Childs SJ, Madore RJ, Klimberg SR (1992). A multicenter comparison of oral lomefloxacin versus parenteral cefotaxime as prophylactic agents in transurethral surgery. *Amer J Med* **92**: 121S.

Kovarik JM, de Hond JA, Hoepelman IM *et al.* (1990). Intraprostatic distribution of lomefloxacin following multiple-dose administration. *Antimicrob Ag Chemother* **34**: 2398.

Kovarik JM, Hoepelman AI, Smit JM *et al.* (1992). Steady-state pharmacokinetics and sputum penetration of lomefloxacin in patients with chronic obstructive pulmonary disease and acute respiratory tract infections. *Antimicrob Ag Chemother* **36**: 2458.

LeBel M, Vallee F, St-Laurent M (1990). Influence of lomefloxacin on the pharmacokinetics of theophylline. *Antimicrob Ag Chemother* **34**: 1254.

Lebrec D, Gaudin C, Benhamou JP (1992). Pharmacokinetics of lomefloxacin in patients with cirrhosis. *Amer J Med* **92**: 41S.

Lehto P, Kivisto KT (1994). Different effects of products containing metal ions on the absorption of lomefloxacin. *Clin Pharmacol Ther* **56**: 477.

Leigh DA, Harris C, Tait S *et al.* (1991). Pharmacokinetic study of lomefloxacin and its effect on the faecal flora of volunteers. *J Antimicrob Chemother* **27**: 655.

Leroy A, Fillastre JP, Humbert G (1990). Lomefloxacin pharmacokinetics in subjects with normal and impaired renal function. *Antimicrob Ag Chemother* **34**: 17.

Leroy A, Humbert G, Fillastre JP, Grise P (1992). Penetration of lomefloxacin into human prostatic tissue. *Amer J Med* **92**: 12S.

Mant TG (1992). Multiple-dose pharmacokinetics of lomefloxacin: rationale for once-a-day dosing. *Amer J Med* **92**: 26S.

Mayer KH, Ellal JA (1992). Lomefloxacin: microbiologic assessment and unique properties. *Amer J Med* **92**: 58S.

Morrison PJ, Mant TG, Norman GT *et al.* (1988). Pharmacokinetics and tolerance of lomefloxacin after sequentially increasing oral doses. *Antimicrob Ag Chemother* **32**: 1503.

Mouton Y, Ajana F, Chidiac C *et al.* (1992). A multicenter study of lomefloxacin and trimethoprim/sulfamethoxazole in the treatment of uncomplicated acute pyelonephritis. *Amer J Med* **92**: 87S.

Murray PR, Bratcher JL, Niles AC, Hampton CM (1993). *In vitro* activity of nine fluoroquinolone antibiotics against 200 strains of enterococci. *Diagn Microbiol Infect Dis* **16**: 83.

Nakashima M, Uematsu T, Takiguchi Y *et al.* (1988). Phase I study on NY-198. *Chemotherapy* **36** (Suppl 2): 201.

Nakata K, Maeda H, Fujii A *et al.* (1992). *In vitro* and *in vivo* activities of sparfloxacin, other quinolones, and tetracyclines against *Chlamydia trachomatis. Antimicrob Ag Chemother* **36**: 188.

Neringer R, Forsgren A, Hansson C, Ode B (1992). Lomefloxacin versus norfloxacin in the treatment of uncomplicated urinary tract infections: three-day versus seven-day treatment. The South Swedish Lolex Study Group. *Scand J Infect Dis* **24**: 773.

Nicolle LE, Dubois J, Martel AY *et al.* (1993). Treatment of acute uncomplicated urinary tract infections with 3 days of lomefloxacin compared with treatment with 3 days of norfloxacin. *Antimicrob Ag Chemother* **37**: 574.

Nicolle LE, Louie TJ, Dubois J *et al.* (1994). Treatment of complicated urinary tract infections with lomefloxacin compared with that with trimethoprim-sulfamethoxazole. *Antimicrob Ag Chemother* **38**: 1368.

Nilsen OG, Saltvedt E, Walstad RA, Marstein S (1992). Single-dose pharmacokinetics of lomefloxacin in patients with normal and impaired renal function. *Amer J Med* **92**: 38S.

Nix DE, Norman A, Schentag JJ (1989). Effect of lomefloxacin on theophylline pharmacokinetics. *Antimicrob Ag Chemother* **33**: 1006.

On A, Nightingale C H, Quintiliani R *et al.* (1992). Lomefloxacin concentrations in bone after a single oral dose. *Amer J Med* **92** (Suppl 41): 155.

Pankuch GA, Jacobs MR, Appelbaum PC (1995). Activity of CP99,219 compared with DU-6859a, ciprofloxacin, ofloxacin, levofloxacin, lomefloxacin, tosufloxacin, sparfloxacin and grepafloxacin against penicillin-susceptible and -resistant pneumococci. *J Antimicrob Chemother* **35**: 230.

Piersimoni C, Morbiducci V, Bornigia S *et al.* (1992). *In vitro* activity of the new quinolone lomefloxacin against *Mycobacterium tuberculosis. Amer Rev Respir Dis* **146**: 1445.

Poh-Fitzpatrick MB (1994). Lomefloxacin photosensitivity. *Arch Dermatol* **130**: 261.

Prosser BL, Beskid G (1995). Multicenter *in vitro* comparative study of fluoroquinolones against 25 129 gram-positive and gram-negative clinical isolates. *Diagn Microbiol Infect Dis* **21**: 33.

Qadri SM, al-Sedairy S, Ueno Y (1990). Antibacterial activity of lomefloxacin against *Brucella melitensis. Diagn Microbiol Infect Dis* **13**: 277.

Rizk E (1992). The US clinical experience with lomefloxacin, a new once-daily fluoroquinolone. *Amer J Med* **92**: 130S.

Robbins MJ, Baskerville AJ, Sanghrajka M *et al.* (1989). Comparative *in vitro* activity of lomefloxacin, a difluoro-quinolone. *Diagn Microbiol Infect Dis* **12**: 65S.

Scheife RT, Cramer WR, Decker EL (1993). Photosensitizing potential of ofloxacin. *Int J Dermatol* **32**: 413.

Schentag JJ, Goss TF (1992). Quinolone pharmakokinetics in the elderly. *Amer J Med* **92** (Suppl 4A): 335.

Segreti J, Nelson JA, Goodman LJ *et al.* (1989). *In vitro* activities of lomefloxacin and temafloxacin against pathogens causing diarrhea. *Antimicrob Ag Chemother* **33**: 1385.

Shah PM, Muller S, Kipp J, Stille W (1989). *In vitro* activity of lomefloxacin (NY-198 or SC 47111).. *Diagn Microbiol Infect Dis* **12**: 97S.

Shimada J, Shiba K, Oguma T *et al.* (1992). Effect of antacid on absorption of the quinolone lomefloxacin. *Antimicrob Ag Chemother* **36**: 1219.

Shimizu T (1988). Biliary excretion of NY-198 (a new oral antimicrobial agent). and its clinical application. *Chemotherapy* **36**(Suppl 2): 1188.

Simor AE, Ferro S, Low DE (1989). Comparative *in vitro* activities of six new fluoroquinolones and other oral antimicrobial agents against *Campylobacter pylori*. *Antimicrob Ag Chemother* **33**: 108.

Spangler SK, Jacobs MR, Appelbaum PC (1993). Comparative activity of the new fluoroquinolone Bay y3118 against 177 penicillin susceptible and resistant pneumococci. *Eur J Clin Microbiol Infect Dis* **12**: 965.

Stone JW, Andrews JM, Ashby JP *et al.* (1988). Pharmacokinetics and tissue penetration of orally administered lomefloxacin. *Antimicrob Ag Chemother* **32**: 1508.

Stratton CW, Weeks LS (1989). Bactericidal activity of lomefloxacin SC 47111 (NY-198). and ciprofloxacin against selected pathogens. *Diagn Microbiol Infect Dis* **12**: 29S.

Stuht H, Lode H, Koeppe P *et al.* (1995). Interaction study of lomefloxacin and ciprofloxacin with omeprazole and comparative pharmacokinetics. *Antimicrob Ag Chemother* **39**: 1045.

Sudoh T, Fujimura A, Shiga T *et al.* (1994). Renal clearance of lomefloxacin is decreased by furosemide. *Eur J Clin Pharmacol* **46**: 267.

Sun ZM, Maskell JP, Sehgal SC, Williams JD (1989). In-vitro activity of lomefloxacin (SC-47111). and other quinolones. *Infection* **17**: 165.

Talbot H, Romanowski B (1989). *In vitro* activities of lomefloxacin, tetracycline, penicillin, spectinomycin, and ceftriaxone against *Neisseria gonorrhoeae* and *Chlamydia trachomatis*. *Antimicrob Ag Chemother* **33**: 2049.

Upton RA (1991). Pharmacokinetic interactions between theophylline and other medication (Part I). *Clin Pharmacokinet* **20**: 66.

Wadworth AN, Goa KL (1991). Lomefloxacin A review of its antibacterial activity, pharmacokinetic properties and therapeutic. *Drugs* **42**: 1018.

Weinstein MP (1988). Comparative *in vitro* activity of lomefloxacin and other antimicrobials against 597 microorganisms causing bacteremia. *Diagn Microbiol Infect Dis* **11**: 195.

Wijnands GJ, Cornel JH, Martea M, Vree TB (1990). The effect of multiple-dose oral lomefloxacin on theophylline metabolism in man. *Chest* **98**: 1440.

Wise R, Andrews JM, Ashby JP, Matthews RS (1988). *In vitro* activity of lomefloxacin, a new quinolone antimicrobial agent, in comparison with those of other agents. *Antimicrob Ag Chemother* **32**: 617.

Tosufloxacin

Description

Tosufloxacin (A-61827, T-3262) is the the tosylate salt of A-60969 which was developed by Toyama Chemical Co. Ltd. and is marketed by Abbott Laboratories. It is another of the newer fluoroquinolones developed with a broad spectrum of activity against Gram-negative, Gram-positive and anaerobic organisms and *Chlamydia* spp. Due to concerns regarding potential toxicity, tosufloxacin is not available in the USA, but it is available in Japan, the Philippines and some South-East Asian countries. Although tosufloxacin displays good *in vitro* activity compared with many other fluoroquinolones, its generally lower serum levels may potentially impact on its clinical efficacy (Fujimaki *et al.*, 1988; Barry and Fuchs, 1991; Appelbaum, 1995).

Tosufloxacin inhibits 90% of Enterobacteriaceae at a concentration of ≤ 0.25 μg per ml; being comparable with sparfloxacin and trovafloxacin, 2- to 4-fold more active than ofloxacin, but generally less active (2- to 8-fold) than ciprofloxacin. Tosufloxacin is more active than ciprofloxacin against *Acinetobacter* spp. and *Stenotrophomonas* (previously *Xanthomonas*) *maltophilia*, but most importantly, is inferior to ciprofloxacin in its activity against *Pseudomonas aeruginosa*. Tosufloxacin activity against *Burkholderia pseudomallei* is similar to ciprofloxacin in being borderline, with MIC_{90} 3.1 μg per ml. Most *Haemophilus influenzae*, *Moraxella catarrhalis* and *Neisseria gonorrhoeae* strains are inhibited by ≤ 0.008 μg per ml. Tosufloxacin is similar to, or more active than, ciprofloxacin or norfloxacin against pathogens that cause diarrhea such as *Salmonella* spp., *Shigella* spp., *Campylobacter* spp., *Aeromonas hydrophila* and *Vibrio* spp. (Espinoza *et al.*, 1988; Fujimaki *et al.*, 1988; Barry and Jones, 1989; Arguedas *et al.*, 1990; Bryan *et al.*, 1990; Glick *et al.*, 1990; Segreti *et al.*, 1990; Yamamoto *et al.*, 1990; Barry and Fuchs, 1991; King *et al.*, 1991; Cooper *et al.*, 1992; Neu and Chin, 1994; Srimuang *et al.*, 1995).

Tosufloxacin is superior to ciprofloxacin and either comparable with, or slightly better than, grepafloxacin against Gram-positive pathogens. The MIC_{90} values against *Streptococcus pneumoniae*, *Strep. pyogenes*, viridans streptococci and methicillin-susceptible *Staphylococcus aureus* are 0.25–0.5, 0.12, 0.5 and 0.12 μg per ml, respectively. However, its activity against methicillin-resistant *Staph. aureus* and *Staph. epidermidis* strains is less impressive, with MIC_{90} values of 8 and 16 μg per ml, respectively (Espinoza *et al.*, 1988; Neu *et al.*, 1992). Among ciprofloxacin-resistant, methicillin-resistant *Staph. aureus* strains, cross-resistance among fluoroquinolones is generally complete (Maple *et al.*, 1991). Tosufloxacin (MIC_{90} 0.25 μg per ml) is comparable with trovafloxacin in its activity against *Strep. pneumoniae*, including penicillin-resistant strains (Pankuch *et al.*, 1995). Although not good, tosufloxacin has some activity against enterococci, while the MIC_{90} for tosufloxacin against *Listeria monocytogenes* is 0.12 μg per ml (Fujimaki *et al.*, 1988; Barry and Fuchs, 1991; King *et al.*, 1991). Tosufloxacin is more active than ciprofloxacin or other commonly available fluoroquinolones against *Nocardia* spp., but against most species other than *N. farcinica*, where the MIC_{90} is 0.57 μg per ml, the MIC_{90} is above the readily achievable serum concentrations of tosufloxacin. Given this fact and the known difficulties with susceptibility testing of *Nocardia*, further studies will be necessary before tosufloxacin can be considered a treatment option for disease caused by these pathogens (Yazawa *et al.*, 1989).

Similar to sparfloxacin, grepafloxacin and temafloxacin, tosufloxacin has 'intermediate' activity against most anaerobes, being inferior to highly active agents such as clinafloxacin and trovafloxacin, but superior to other fluoroquinolones such as ciprofloxacin, ofloxacin, pefloxacin, lomefloxacin and levofloxacin. In one study that assessed a wide variety of anaerobes including, *Bacteroides fragilis* group, beta-lactamase-producing non-*B. fragilis* group *Bacter-*

oides spp., beta-lactamase-producing fusobacteria and beta-lactamase-negative anaerobe spp., tosufloxacin was active against 94%, 85%, 89% and 100%, respectively (Appelbaum *et al.*, 1991; Jacobs *et al.*, 1992; Nord *et al.*, 1992; Appelbaum, 1995)

Tosufloxacin has activity broadly comparable with sparfloxacin and grepafloxacin against *Chlamydia psittaci, C. trachomatis* and *C. pneumoniae* with MICs that range from 0.03 to 0.125 µg per ml, although some authors have found sparfloxacin to be slightly more active than tosufloxacin. This anti-chlamydial activity is superior to that of ciprofloxacin, ofloxacin, fleroxacin and erythromycin, but is inferior to that of minocycline and doxycycline which have MIC values of 0.015–0.03 µg per ml (Maeda *et al.*, 1988; Segreti *et al.*, 1990; Nakata *et al.*, 1992; Kimura *et al.*, 1993).

Interestingly, tosufloxacin may have some *in vitro* activity against *Leptospira interrogans*, although the MBC appears to be approximately 10- to 100-fold greater than the MIC (Takashima *et al.*, 1993).

Tosufloxacin has relatively poor activity against most non-tuberculous *Mycobacteria* spp., being generally comparable or inferior to ciprofloxacin, sparfloxacin and clinafloxacin (Bauernfeind, 1993).

The *in vitro* MICs of tosufloxacin against some selected bacterial species are shown in Table II.6 (pp. 986–987).

Preliminary pharmacokinetics studies demonstrate mean peak serum concentrations after 300, 600 and 900 mg of 1.2, 1.9 and 2.8 µg per ml, respectively. Serum half-life is 5.6–6.9 h (Kinzig *et al.*, 1991). Following a 450-mg oral dose of tosufloxacin on the day prior to prostatectomy for benign prostatic hypertrophy, and 150 mg immediately before surgery, mean prostatic tissue concentrations 2, 4 and 6 h post-dose were 0.35, 0.58 and 0.22 µg per g. Serum concentrations taken at the same times post-dose are 0.38, 0.43 and 0.24 µg per ml, respectively (Uchibayashi *et al.*, 1992). In a small, open, comparative study of patients with non-gonococcal urethritis, tosufloxacin 150 mg thrice-daily resulted in clinical efficacy comparable with doxycycline 100 mg twice-daily 21 days after commencing therapy (Tanaka *et al.*, 1994). Further toxicity and clinical efficacy data regarding tosufloxacin is needed.

References

Appelbaum PC (1995). Quinolone activity against anaerobes: microbiological aspects. *Drugs* **49** (Suppl 2):76.

Appelbaum PC, Spangler SK, Jacobs MR (1991). Susceptibilities of 394 *Bacteroides fragilis*, non-*B fragilis* group *Bacteroides* species, and *Fusobacterium* species to newer antimicrobial agents. *Antimicrob Ag Chemother* **35**:1214.

Arguedas AG, Akaniro JC, Stutman HR, Marks MI (1990). *In vitro* activity of tosufloxacin, a new quinolone, against respiratory pathogens derived from cystic fibrosis sputum. *Antimicrob Ag Chemother* **34**:2223.

Barry AL, Fuchs PC (1991). *In vitro* activities of sparfloxacin, tosufloxacin, ciprofloxacin, and fleroxacin. *Antimicrob Ag Chemother* **35**:955.

Barry AL, Jones RN (1989). *In-vitro* activities of temafloxacin, tosufloxacin (A-61827). and five other fluoroquinolone agents. *J Antimicrob Chemother* **23**:527.

Bauernfeind A (1993). Comparative *in-vitro* activities of the new quinolone, Bay y 3118, and ciprofloxacin, sparfloxacin, tosufloxacin, CI-960 and CI-990. *J Antimicrob Chemother* **31**:505.

Bryan JP, Waters C, Sheffield J *et al.* (1990). *In vitro* activities of tosufloxacin, temafloxacin, and A-56620 against pathogens of diarrhea. *Antimicrob Ag Chemother* **34**:368.

Cooper MA, Andrews JM, Wise R (1992). *In-vitro* activity of tosufloxacin, a new quinolone antibacterial agent. *J Antimicrob Chemother* **29**:639.

Espinoza AM, Chin NX, Novelli A, Neu HC (1988). Comparative *in vitro* activity of a new fluorinated 4-quinolone, T-3262 (A- 60969). *Antimicrob Ag Chemother* **32**:663.

Fujimaki K, Noumi T, Saikawa I *et al.* (1988). *In vitro* and *in vivo* antibacterial activities of T-3262, a new fluoroquinolone. *Antimicrob Ag Chemother* **32**:827.

Glick EJ, Segreti J, Goodman LJ, Trenholme GM (1990). *In vitro* activity of tosufloxacin against bacterial enteric pathogens. *Diagn Microbiol Infect Dis* **13**:333.

Jacobs MR, Spangler SK, Appelbaum PC (1992). beta-Lactamase production and susceptibility of US and European anaerobic gram-negative bacilli to beta-lactams and other agents. *Eur J Clin Microbiol Infect Dis* **11**:1081.

Kimura M, Kishimoto T, Niki Y, Soejima R (1993). *In vitro* and *in vivo* antichlamydial activities of newly developed quinolone antimicrobial agents. *Antimicrob Ag Chemother* **37**:801.

King A, Bethune L, Phillips I (1991). The *in-vitro* activity of tosufloxacin, a new fluorinated quinolone, compared with that of ciprofloxacin and temafloxacin. *J Antimicrob Chemother* **28**:719.

Kinzig M, Kuye O, Sorgel F *et al.* (1991). Pharmacokinetics of rising doses of tosufloxacin. In: *Proceedings of the 17th International Congress of Chemotherapy, Berlin, 1991* (Abstr. 380.)

Maeda H, Fujii A, Nakata K *et al.* (1988). *In vitro* activities of T-3262, NY-198, fleroxacin (AM-833; RO 23–6240), and other new quinolone agents against clinically isolated *Chlamydia trachomatis* strains. *Antimicrob Ag Chemother* **32**:1080.

Maple PA, Hamilton-Miller JM, Brumfitt W (1991). Differing activities of quinolones against ciprofloxacin-susceptible and ciprofloxacin-resistant, methicillin-resistant *Staphylococcus aureus*. *Antimicrob Ag Chemother* **35**:345.

Nakata K, Maeda H, Fujii A *et al.* (1992). *In vitro* and *in vivo* activities of sparfloxacin, other quinolones, and tetracyclines against *Chlamydia trachomatis*. *Antimicrob Ag Chemother* **36**:188.

Neu HC, Chin NX (1994). *In vitro* activity of the new fluoroquinolone CP-99,219. *Antimicrob Ag Chemother* **38**:2615.

Neu HC, Fang W, Gu JW, Chin NX (1992). *In vitro* activity of OPC-17116. *Antimicrob Ag Chemother* **36**:1310.

Nord CE, Lindmark A, Persson I, Runow C (1992). Susceptibility of anaerobic bacteria to tosufloxacin. *Eur J Clin Microbiol Infect Dis* **11**:263.

Pankuch GA, Jacobs MR, Appelbaum PC (1995). Activity of CP99,219 compared with DU-6859a, ciprofloxacin, ofloxacin, levofloxacin, lomefloxacin, tosufloxacin, sparfloxacin and grepafloxacin against penicillin-susceptible and -resistant pneumococci. *J Antimicrob Chemother* **35**:230.

Segreti J, Hirsch DJ, Harris AA *et al.* (1990). *In vitro* activity of tosufloxacin (A-61827; T-3262) against selected genital pathogens. *Antimicrob Ag Chemother* **34**:971.

Srimuang S, Fugpholngam V, Asvanich K *et al.* (1995). *In vitro* activity of tosufloxacin against *Pseudomonas pseudomallei*, *Salmonella* spp and other Enterobacteriaceae. *Drugs* **49** (Suppl 2):260.

Takashima I, Ngoma M, Hashimoto N (1993). Antimicrobial effects of a new carboxyquinolone drug, Q-35, on five serogroups of *Leptospira interrogans*. *Antimicrob Ag Chemother* **37**:901.

Tanaka M, Matsumoto T, Kumazawa J *et al.* (1994). Tosufloxacin in the treatment of non-gonococcal urethritis, including *Chlamydia trachomatis*. *Clin Ther* **16**:819.

Uchibayashi T, Hisazumi H, Kanayama J, Kumano K (1992). Diffusion of tosufloxacin into prostatic tissue. *Chemotherapy* **38**:150.

Yamamoto T, Naigowit P, Dejsirilert S *et al.* (1990). *In vitro* susceptibilities of *Pseudomonas pseudomallei* to 27 antimicrobial agents. *Antimicrob Ag Chemother* **34**:2027.

Yazawa K, Mikami Y, Uno J (1989). *In vitro* susceptibility of *Nocardia* spp to a new fluoroquinolone, tosufloxacin (T-3262). *Antimicrob Ag Chemother* **33**:2140.

Levofloxacin

Description

Levofloxacin (DR-3355, CAS 100986–85–4) is the optical S-(-) isomer of ofloxacin which has been developed by the Daiichi Seiyaku Pharmaceutical Co. Ltd, in Japan. Its chemical formula is (-)-(S)-9-fluoro-2,3-dihydro-3-methyl-10-(4-methyl-1-piperazinyl)-7-oxo-7H-pyrido[1,2,3-de] [1,4]benzoxazine-6-carboxylic acid hemihydrate. Ofloxacin is a racemic mixture, but the S-isomer has antibacterial activity 32- to 128-fold more potent than the R-isomer – hence most of the antibacterial activity of ofloxacin is due to the S-isomer. Levofloxacin has been developed to take advantage of this antibacterial potency while requiring only about half the usual dose of ofloxacin to achieve similar efficacy, but potentially with an improved toxicity profile (Une *et al.*, 1988; Tanaka *et al.*, 1992; Inage *et al.*, 1992; Davis and Bryson, 1994; Nakamori *et al.*, 1995).

Levofloxacin looks to be a potentially promising agent; however the vast majority of initial pharmacokinetic and clinical efficacy studies have been undertaken in Japanese subjects and further data from other population groups is needed to better identify the optimal dosage regimens – many of these studies are currently in progress.

Sensitive Organisms

Overall, MIC_{90} values for levofloxacin are about 50% lower than those observed for ofloxacin against Gram-negative and Gram-positive bacteria, and about 3- to 4-fold lower than ciprofloxacin against methicillin-susceptible and methicillin-resistant *Staphylococcus aureus*. However, ciprofloxacin is approximately twice as active as levofloxacin, based on MIC_{90} values, against Gram-negative bacteria, especially *Pseudomonas aeruginosa*. Similar to ofloxacin, levofloxacin demonstrates some *in vitro* post-antibiotic effect against various strains of *Escherichia coli* and *Staph. aureus* (Houston and Jones, 1994). The *in vitro* MICs of levofloxacin against selected bacterial species are shown in Table II.6 (pp. 986–987).

1 Gram-negative bacteria

Levofloxacin is about 2-fold more active than ofloxacin and generally 2- to 4-fold less active than ciprofloxacin against most Enterobacteriaceae and *Ps. aeruginosa*. The MIC_{90} of levofloxacin against *Ps. aeruginosa* is generally 4–8 µg per ml. Similarly, levofloxacin is comparable with, or one- or two dilutions inferior to ciprofloxacin in its activity against *Haemophilus influenzae*, *Neisseria gonorrhoeae* and *Moraxella catarrhalis*, with MIC_{90} values of 0.015 – 0.06 µg per ml (Fu *et al.*, 1992; Dholakia *et al.*, 1994; Yamane *et al.*, 1994; Zhang *et al.*, 1995). Similar levofloxacin activity has been noted against Gram-negative pathogens isolated from cancer patients – a clinical setting in which levofloxacin may have a future role (Dholakia *et al.*, 1994). Levofloxacin has good activity against both *Pasteurella* spp. and *Eikenella corrodens* with MIC_{90} values of 0.015 µg per ml (Goldstein *et al.*, 1995). The MIC_{90} of levofloxacin against *Legionella pneumophila* is 0.125 µg per ml, compared with 0.25 µg per ml for ofloxacin (Baltch *et al.*, 1995).

Levofloxacin is slightly more active against *Bacteroides fragilis* than ciprofloxacin with an MIC_{90} 2 µg per ml; but in general, levofloxacin can only be considered to have low activity against anaerobes *Fusobacterium* spp. are resistant (MIC_{90} 64 µg per ml) (Fu *et al.*, 1992; Appelbaum, 1995).

2 Gram-positive bacteria

Levofloxacin is about 2-fold more active than ciprofloxacin against penicillin-susceptible and -resistant *Streptococcus pneumoniae* (MIC_{90} 2 µg per ml) and 2- to 4-fold more active against methicillin-susceptible *Staph. aureus* (MIC$_{90}$ 0.5 μg per ml). Activity against methicillin-resistant *Staph. aureus* is less impressive with MIC$_{90}$ 16 μg per ml. Concentrations of 1–2 μg per ml inhibit 90% of streptococci, while the MIC$_{90}$ against *Enterotoccus faecalis* is generally no better than 2 μg per ml. Indeed, Hayden *et al.* (1995) found only 39% of vancomycin-susceptible and 11% vancomycin-resistant strains of enterococci were susceptible to <2 mg per ml levofloxacin. Levofloxacin has variable activity against *Listeria monocytogenes* (MIC$_{90}$ 2–8 μg per ml) and is poorly active against *Corynebacterium jeikeium* (MIC$_{90}$ >64 μg per ml) (Fu *et al.*, 1992; Cherubin and Stratton, 1994; Dholakia *et al.*, 1994; Yamane *et al.*, 1994; Pankuch *et al.*, 1995a,b; Zhang *et al.*, 1995).

Studies in mice suggest that levofloxacin may be more active *in vivo* than ciprofloxacin against *Strep. pneumoniae* (Fu *et al.*, 1992). Similarly, in a rabbit model of pneumococcal meningitis levofloxacin was superior to ciprofloxacin (Nau *et al.*, 1995).

Levofloxacin has variable activity against Gram-positive anaerobes, with MIC$_{90}$ 8 μg per ml against *Peptostreptococcus* spp. and broadly similar activity against *Clostridium* spp. (Fu *et al.*, 1992; Appelbaum, 1995; Goldstein *et al.*, 1995).

3 Mycobacteria

In vivo studies of *M. tuberculosis* suggest that levofloxacin activity is comparable with that produced by a 2-fold greater dosage of ofloxacin, although the MIC$_{90}$ values for both drugs are similar at 1 μg per ml. Sparfloxacin has better activity with MIC$_{90}$ 0.5 μg per ml (Ji *et al.*, 1995). Other authors have found similar findings *in vitro* (Mor *et al.*, 1994; Yew *et al.*, 1994). Rifampicin and isoniazid were more active than levofloxacin in a murine model of tuberculosis, but there was little difference in activity between levofloxacin and ethambutol or pyrazinamide (Klemens *et al.*, 1994). Levofloxacin (MIC 0.75 μg per ml) has 2-fold greater bactericidal activity against *Mycobacterium leprae* than ofloxacin (Dhople and Ibanez, 1995).

4 Mycoplasma

Levofloxacin is active aginst *Mycoplasma fermentans*, the *Mycoplasma* spp. isolated in patients with HIV infection, with MIC$_{90}$ 0.078 μg per ml (Hayes *et al.*, 1993).

Mode of Administration and Dosage

1 Oral administration

The optimal dosage of levofloxacin for various patient populations has yet to be determined, but most Japanese studies have used 100 mg thrice-daily (occasionally 200 mg thrice-daily) for the treatment of a variety of infections, including respiratory, skin, enteral, biliary, genitourinary, obstetric/gynecology and eye infections. The usual duration of treatment is single-dose therapy for women with uncomplicated cystitis, 3–5 days for other urinary tract sepsis or gonococcal urethritis and 7–14 days therapy for most other indications except for prostatitis, when longer courses may be needed (Davis and Bryson, 1994).

2 Patients with renal failure

Since levofloxacin is mainly excreted unchanged in the urine (p. 1160) serum levels are sensitive to changes in renal function. Thus, dosage reduction is required in patients with renal impairment. In Japanese patients, doses are reduced as follows: glomerular filtration rate (GFR) 40–70 ml per min, 100 mg twice-daily; GFR 20–40 ml per min, 100 mg daily; GFR <20 ml per min, 100 mg every 48 h (Saito *et al.*, 1992a; Davis and Bryson, 1994).

No information is available regarding the need for any dosage adjustment in the elderly or in patients with hepatic failure.

Serum Levels in Relation to Dosage

1 Oral administration

Oral bioavaolability of levofloxacin is nearly 100% and following single doses of either 50, 100 or 200 mg, peak serum concentrations of 0.57, 0.86–1.36 and 2.04–3.42 μg per ml, respectively, are achieved after 0.8–2.4 h. Co-administration of food has little effect on the absorption of levofloxacin. Following multiple doses of 200 mg thrice-daily for 7 days, mean steady-state trough and peak levels are 1.05–1.39 µg per ml and 3.15–3.35 µg per ml, respectively. The plasma elimination half-life of levofloxacin is approximately 4–7 h (Nakashima *et al.*, 1992; Davis and Bryson, 1994; Nakamori *et al.*, 1995).

Chien *et al.* (1996) reported that after a single oral dose of either 750 mg or 1000 mg levofloxacin to healthy volunteers, the mean peak serum concentrations are 7.1 and 8.9 µg per ml, respectively. When the same dose is given daily for 7 days, mean peak serum levels are 8.6 µg per ml (750 mg) and 11.8 µg per ml (1000 mg). In this study the serum half-life of levofloxacin was 7.7–8.8 h.

In a phase I, double-blind, randomized, placebo-controlled trial to evaluate the pharmacokinetics and safety of levofloxacin in asymptomatic HIV-infected males, pharmacokinetic parameters were found to be similar to those obtained in healthy subjects. Single- and multidose studies of 350 mg thrice-daily demonstrated that single-dose and multidose parameters are similar, except for the peak levels achieved in plasma, where concentrations of 4.79 and 6.92 µg per ml, respectively, were noted. The half-life of levofloxacin in this study was 6.5 ± 1.6 h (Goodwin *et al.*, 1994).

2 Patients with renal failure

Gisdon *et al.* (1996) studied the pharmacokinetics of a single 500-mg oral dose of levofloxacin in five groups of patients with various degrees of renal impairment: GFR 50–80 ml per min, 20–49 ml per min, 10–19 ml per min, hemodialysis and continuous ambulatory peritoneal dialysis (CAPD). The mean peak serum concentrations of levofloxacin for each of these five groups were 7.5, 7.1, 8.2, 5.7 and 6.9 µg per ml, respectively; while the half-life of levofloxacin was 9, 27, 35, 76 and 51 h in each group, respectively. Only about 12% of a levofloxacin dose is removed by either hemodialysis or CAPD.

Excretion

1 Urine

Levofloxacin is mainly excreted unchanged in the urine, with 80–86% recovered within 24 h post-dose. Thus, high urinary levels of levofloxacin, several times the MIC_{90} for most urinary pathogens, can be expected (Nakashima *et al.*, 1992).

2 Bile

Biliary concentrations of levofloxacin 2–4, 4–6 and 6–12 h after a single oral dose of 100 mg levofloxacin are 1.2–2.4, 1.3–3.5 and 1.3–2.4 µg per ml, respectively (Hukagawa and Noga, 1992)..

3 Inactivation in body

Levofloxacin undergoes only very limited metabolism and is largely excreted unchanged in the urine (Davis and Bryson, 1994).

4 Feces

Approximately 2% of a levofloxacin dose is eliminated in the feces (Nakashima *et al.*, 1992). In healthy volunteers treated with levofloxacin 200 mg thrice-daily, fecal drug concentrations 3 days post-dose are 50–100 µg per ml (Inagaki *et al.*, 1992; Davis and Bryson, 1994).

Distribution of the Drug in Body

Most studies regarding the distribution of levofloxacin have been done in Japanese subjects. Protein binding of levofloxacin is estimated to be 47–52% (Okazaki *et al.*, 1991). Lung penetration of levofloxacin is good. In a small study of patients with respiratory tract infections who were treated with 200 mg levofloxacin once-daily for 7 days, the mean peak concentration in sputum was 4.36 µg per ml, 4 h post-dose, while 8, 12 and 24 h post-dose the levels were 1.68, 0.91 and 0.25 µg per ml, respectively (Nakamori *et al.*, 1995).

Levofloxacin readily penetrates gallbladder tissue and bile; 2–3 h after a single 100-mg oral dose of levofloxacin, concentrations in gallbladder and adipose tissue are 0.34–1.59 and 0.07–0.26 µg per g, respectively, at a time when serum concentrations are 0.20–1.05 µg per ml. Biliary concentrations may be somewhat variable in this situation with levels ranging from 1.8 to 12.2 µg per ml in gallbladder bile and 1.4 to 5.8 µg per ml in common duct bile (Hukagawa and Noga, 1992). Other authors have noted similar biliary concentrations (Tanimura *et al.*, 1992).

Penetration of levofloxacin into uterine and adnexal tissues appears to be good, with concentrations of 1.2–2.2 µg per g achieved after a single 100-mg dose (Cho *et al.*, 1992). Levofloxacin also penetrates well into the testis, epididymis and semen. Following a single oral 200-mg dose 2 h prior to surgery in patients with prostate cancer, tissue concentrations in testis and epididymis were 4.73 and 3.6 µg per g, respectively. In healthy male volunteers given 100 mg thrice-daily for 13 days, levofloxacin levels in semen were 1.19–1.32 µg per ml, representing a semen/serum ratio of 1.12–1.26 (Saito *et al.*, 1992b).

Mode of Action

Levofloxacin has a similar mode of action to other fluoroquinolones (p. 1008).

Toxicity

Doses of 200–600 mg levofloxacin per day appear to be well tolerated with side-effects largely consisting of those noted with all fluoroquinolones, such as abdominal discomfort, anorexia, occasionally diarrhea and central nervous system effects, including headache. The phototoxic potential of levofloxacin is similar to that of ofloxacin and ciprofloxacin in studies in mice (Wagai *et al.*, 1992). Transient elevation of liver function tests, eosinophilia and leukopenia have been described occasionally. Overall, levofloxacin appears to have fewer side-effects than ofloxacin (Davis and Bryson, 1994; Kawai, 1995).

The concurrent administration of levofloxacin with magnesium- and aluminum-containing antacids reduces the bioavailability of levofloxacin by 15–52% (Tanaka *et al.*, 1993; Tanigawara *et al.*, 1995). However, co-administration of a single dose of levofloxacin and one of the Chinese medicines Hotyuekki-to, Rikkunshi-to or Juzen-taiho-to does not appear to alter the pharmacokinetics of levofloxacin (Hasegawa *et al.*, 1995). Levofloxacin does not appear to significantly alter the clearance of theophylline, although patients receiving this combination should be monitored carefully for signs of theophylline toxicity (Marchbanks, 1993).

Clinical Uses of the Drug

Clinical experience with levofloxacin looks promising based on published Japanese studies, but similar studies in other populations, who may have different dose requirements, are needed.

1 Urinary tract infections and prostatitis

Various Japanese studies of levofloxacin 100–200 mg thrice-daily for 3–14 days suggest rates of clinical efficacy of 85–100% in the treatment of uncomplicated and complicated urinary tract infections. Richard *et al.* (1996) found levofloxacin 250 mg daily for 10 days to have similar efficacy to either ciprofloxacin 500 mg twice-daily for 10 days, or lomefloxacin 400 mg daily for 14 days, in the treatment of acute pyelonephritis.

Results also look promising for levofloxacin in the treatment of acute and chronic prostatitis, epididymitis and gonococcal and chlamydial urethritis (Davis and Bryson, 1994). In a small open study of 23 patients with acute epididymitis treated with levofloxacin 100 mg two- or three-times daily for 14 days, overall clinical efficacy was 100% (Saito *et al.*, 1992b). A 5-day course of 300 mg per day levofloxacin was effective in a small study of gonococcal urethritis (Osato *et al.*, 1991).

2 Respiratory tract infections

In a number of small, open, non-comparative studies, levofloxacin appears to be effective in the treatment of respiratory tract infections when used in doses ranging from 200 mg once-daily to 200 mg thrice-daily (Davis and Bryson, 1994). In one study, treatment of 12 patients with various lower respiratory tract infections with levofloxacin 200 mg once-daily for 7–14 days, resulted in 100% efficacy (Nakamori *et al.*, 1995). Other authors using various regimens, including 100–200 mg thrice-daily, have found less satisfactory results with approximately only 50% patients classified as having a 'good' or 'excellent' clinical outcome. As might be expected, knowing the *in vitro* activity of levofloxacin, the rate of *Ps. aeruginosa* eradication was low in the 300 mg per day group, but approached 75% in patients receiving 200 mg thrice-daily (Kawai, 1995; Odagiri, 1995; Shishido *et al.*, 1995). In one of the largest studies reported, Sato *et al.* (1995) examined the efficacy of either 300 or 600 mg per day in 87 patients who were managed either as outpatients (300 mg per day for 3 days) or as inpatients (200 mg thrice-daily for 7 days). Eradication of responsible pathogens was noted in 80% cases by day 7, and among patients with pneumonia, clinical efficacy was noted in about 89% cases.

A 7- to 14-day course of levofloxacin 500 mg once-daily appears to be as effective as ceftriaxone (1–2 g per day)/cefuroxime (500 mg twice-daily) for community-acquired pneumonia, and cefaclor 250 mg twice-daily for acute exacerbatiuons of chronic bronchitis (File *et al.*, 1996; Habib *et al.*, 1996).

3 Biliary tract infections

Among 11 patients with biliary tract infections (six cholecystitis; three cholangitis; cholecystocholangitis and liver abscess) treated with levofloxacin 100–200 mg thrice-daily for 3–14 days, clinical outcome was good in eight patients (73%) and fair in the remainder (Tanimura *et al.*, 1992).

4 Other infections

Non-comparative studies of levofloxacin 100 mg thrice-daily for soft tissue and skin infections, obstetric and gynecological infections and ear, nose and throat infections (occasionally requiring 200 mg thrice-daily) have demonstrated overall clinical efficacy in about 80–92% cases (Davis and Bryson, 1994). Levofloxacin 500 mg once-daily for 7 days appears to have efficacy comparable with ciprofloxacin 500 mg twice-daily for 7 days in the treatment of skin and skin structure infections, with reported rates of cure/improvement in 96.1% versus 93.5% cases, respectively (Nicodemo *et al.*, 1996).

In one Japanese study of 22 patients with obstetric and gynecological infections, the clinical efficacy of levofloxacin 200–600 mg daily for 3–14 days was 95% (Cho *et al.*, 1992). In a study of 114 patients with bacterial enteritis, levofloxacin 200–300 mg per day for 3–5 days was associated with a clinical cure rate of 97% (Davis and Bryson, 1994).

References

Appelbaum PC (1995). Quinolone activity against anaerobes: microbiological aspects. *Drugs* **49** (Suppl 2): 76.

Baltch AL, Smith RP, Ritz W (1995). Inhibitory and bactericidal activities of levofloxacin, ofloxacin, erythromycin, and rifampin used singly and in combination against *Legionella pneumophila. Antimicrob Ag Chemother* **39**: 1661.

Cherubin CE, Stratton CW (1994). Assessment of the bactericidal activity of sparfloxacin, ofloxacin, levofloxacin, and other fluoroquinolones compared with selected agents of proven efficacy against *Listeria monocytogenes. Diagn Microbiol Infect Dis* **20**: 21.

Chien SC, Chow AT, Fowler C *et al.* (1996). Double-blind evaluation of the safety and pharmacokinetics (PK). of multiple oral once-daily 750 mg and 1 g doses of levofloxacin (LVFX). in healthy volunteers. In *Program and Abstracts of the 36th Interscience Conference on Antimicrobial Agents and Chemotherapy, New Orleans* (Abstr. A14). Washington, DC: American Society for Microbiology.

Cho N, Araki H, Kimura T *et al.* (1992). Pharmacokinetic and clinical evaluation of levofloxacin in obstetrics and gynecology. *Jpn J Antibiot* **45**: 270.

Davis R, Bryson HM (1994). Levofloxacin A review of its antibacterial activity, pharmacokinetics and therapeutic efficacy. *Drugs* **47**: 677.

Dholakia N, Rolston KV, Ho DH *et al.* (1994). Susceptibilities of bacterial isolates from patients with cancer to levofloxacin and other quinolones. *Antimicrob Ag Chemother* **38**: 848.

Dhople AM, Ibanez MA (1995). *In vitro* activity of levofloxacin, singly and in combination with rifamycin analogs, against *Mycobacterium leprae. Antimicrob Ag Chemother* **39**: 2116.

File TM, Segreti J, Dunbar L *et al.* (1996). A multcenter, randomized study comparing the efficacy and safety of IV/PO levofloxacin (LVFX) vs ceftriaxone/cefuroxime axetil (CC) in the treatment of adults, with community-acquired pneumonia (CAP). In *Program and Abstracts of the 36th Interscience Conference on Antimicrobial Agents and Chemotherapy, New Orleans* (Abstr. LM1). Washington, DC: American Society for Microbiology.

Fu KP, Lafredo SC, Foleno B *et al.* (1992). *In vitro* and *in vivo* antibacterial activities of levofloxacin (l-ofloxacin), an optically active ofloxacin. *Antimicrob Ag Chemother* **36**: 860.

Gisdon LG, Curtin CR, Chien SC *et al.* (1996). The pharmacokinetics (PK). of levofloxacin (LVFX) in subjects with renal impairment, and in subjects receiving hemodialysis or continuous ambulatory peritoneal dialysis. In *Program and Abstracts of the 36th Interscience Conference on Antimicrobial Agents and Chemotherapy, New Orleans* (Abstr. A13). Washington, DC: American Society for Microbiology.

Goldstein EJ, Nesbit CA, Citron DM (1995). Comparative *in vitro* activities of azithromycin, Bay y 3118, levofloxacin, sparfloxacin, and 11 other oral antimicrobial agents against 194 aerobic and anaerobic bite wound isolates. *Antimicrob Ag Chemother* **39**: 1097.

Goodwin SD, Gallis HA, Chow AT *et al.* (1994). Pharmacokinetics and safety of levofloxacin in patients with human immunodeficiency virus infection. *Antimicrob Ag Chemother* **38**: 799.

Habib MP, Gentry LO, Rodriguez-Gomez G *et al.* (1996). A multicenter randomized study comparing the efficacy and safety of oral levofloxacin (LVFX) vs cefoclor (C) in the treatment of acute bacterial exacerbations of chronic bronchitis (ACECB). In *Program and Abstracts of the 36th Interscience Conference on Antimicrobial Agents and Chemotherapy, New Orleans* (Abstr. LM2). Washington, DC: American Society for Microbiology.

Hasegawa T, Yamaki K, Muraoka I *et al.* (1995). Effects of traditional Chinese medicines on pharmacokinetics of levofloxacin. *Antimicrob Ag Chemother* **39**: 2135.

Hayden MK, Matushek MG, Trenholme GM (1995). Comparison of the *in vitro* activity of levofloxacin and other antimicrobial agents against vancomycin-susceptible and vancomycin-resistant *Enterococcus* species. *Diagn Microbiol Infect Dis* **22**: 349.

Hayes MM, Foo HH, Kotani H *et al.* (1993). *In vitro* antibiotic susceptibility testing of different strains of *Mycoplasma fermentans* isolated from a variety of sources. *Antimicrob Ag Chemother* **37**: 2500.

Houston AK, Jones RN (1994). Postantibiotic effect of DU-6859a and levofloxacin as compared with ofloxacin. *Diagn Microbiol Infect Dis* **18**: 57.

Hukagawa H, Noga K (1992). A study on the concentrations of levofloxacin in the gallbladder tissue and bile of patients. *Jpn J Antibiot* **45**: 253.

Inagaki Y, Nakaya R, Chida T, Hashimoto S (1992). The effect of levofloxacin, an optically-active isomer of ofloxacin, on fecal microflora in human volunteers. *Jpn J Antibiot* **45**: 241.

Inage F, Kato M, Yoshida M *et al.* (1992). Lack of nephrotoxic effects of the new quinolone antibacterial agent levofloxacin in rabbits. *Arzneimittelforschung* **43**: 395.

Ji B, Lounis N, Truffot-Pernot C, Grosset J (1995). *In vitro* and *in vivo* activities of levofloxacin against *Mycobacterium tuberculosis*. *Antimicrob Ag Chemother* **39**: 1341.

Kawai T (1995). Clinical evaluation of levofloxacin 200 mg 3 times daily in the treatment of bacterial lower respiratory tract infections. *Drugs* **49** (Suppl 2): 416.

Klemens SP, Sharpe CA, Rogge MC, Cynamon MH (1994). Activity of levofloxacin in a murine model of tuberculosis. *Antimicrob Ag Chemother* **38**: 1476.

Marchbanks CR (1993). Drug-drug interactions with fluoroquinolones. *Pharmacotherapy* **13**: 23S.

Mor N, Vanderkolk J, Heifets L (1994). Inhibitory and bactericidal activities of levofloxacin against *Mycobacterium tuberculosis in vitro* and in human macrophages. *Antimicrob Ag Chemother* **38**: 1161.

Nakamori Y, Miyashita Y, Nakatani I, Nakata K (1995). Levofloxacin: penetration into sputum and once-daily treatment of respiratory tract infections. *Drugs* **49** (Suppl 2): 418.

Nakashima M, Uematsu T, Kanamaru M *et al.* (1992). Phase I study of levofloxacin, (S).-(-).-ofloxacin. *Jpn J Clin Pharmacol Ther* **23**: 515.

Nau R, Schmidt T, Kaye K, Froula JL, Tauber MG (1995). Quinolone antibiotics in therapy of experimental pneumococcal meningitis in rabbits. *Antimicrob Ag Chemother* **39**: 593.

Nicodemo AC, Robledo JA, Jasovich A, Neto W (1996). A multicenter, randomized study comparing the efficacy and safety of oral levofloxacin (LVFX) vs. ciprofloxacin (CIP) in the treatment of skin and skin structure infections. In *Program and Abstracts of the 36th Interscience Conference on Antimicrobial Agents and Chemotherapy, New Orleans* (Abstr. LM4). Washington, DC: American Society for Microbiology.

Odagiri S (1995). Levofloxacin in patients with severe respiratory tract infection. *Drugs* **49** (Suppl 2): 426.

Okazaki O, Kojima C, Hakusui H *et al.* (1991). Enantioselective disposition of ofloxacin in humans. *Antimicrob Ag Chemother* **35**: 2106.

Osato K, Katsukawa C, Makino M (1991). Treatment of gonococcal urethritis. *Jpn J Antibiot* **44**: 1206.

Pankuch GA, Jacobs MR, Appelbaum PC (1995a). Activity of CP99,219 compared with DU-6859a, ciprofloxacin, ofloxacin, levofloxacin, lomefloxacin, tosufloxacin, sparfloxacin and grepafloxacin against penicillin-susceptible and -resistant pneumococci. *J Antimicrob Chemother* **35**: 230.

Pankuch GA, Jacobs MR, Appelbaum PC (1995b). Activity of DU-6859a, ciprofloxacin, ofloxacin, levofloxacin, sparfloxacin and OPC-17116 against 112 penicillin-susceptible and -resistant pneumococci. *Drugs* **49** (Suppl 2): 235.

Richard GA, Klimberg IN, Fowler C *et al.* (1996). A combined analysis of two studies comparing levofloxacin (LVFX). with two other fluoroquinolones for the treatment of acute pyelonephritis (pyelo). In *Program and Abstracts of the 36th Interscience Conference on Antimicrobial Agents and Chemotherapy, New Orleans* (Abstr. LM3). Washington, DC: American Society for Microbiology.

Saito A, Oguchi K, Harada Y *et al.* (1992a). Pharmacokinetics of levofloxacin in patients with impaired renal function. *Chemotherapy* **40** (Suppl 3): 188.

Saito I, Suzuki A, Saiko Y *et al.* (1992b). Acute nongonococcal epididymitis–pharmacological and therapeutic aspects of levofloxacin. *Hinyokika Kiyo* **38**: 623.

Sato A, Ogawa H, Iwata M *et al.* (1995). Clinical efficacy of levofloxacin in elderly patients with respiratory tract infections. *Drugs* **49** (Suppl 2): 428.

Shishido H, Furukawa K, Nagai H *et al.* (1995). Oral levofloxacin 600 mg and 300 mg daily doses in difficult-to-treat respiratory infections. *Drugs* **49** (Suppl 2): 433.

Tanaka K, Iwamoto M, Maesaki S *et al.* (1992). Laboratory and clinical studies of levofloxacin. *Jpn J Antibiot* **45**: 548.

Tanaka M, Kurata T, Fujisawa C *et al.* (1993). Mechanistic study of inhibition of levofloxacin absorption by aluminum hydroxide. *Antimicrob Ag Chemother* **37**: 2173.

Tanigawara Y, Nomura H, Kagimoto N *et al.* (1995). Premarketing population pharmacokinetic study of levofloxacin in normal subjects and patients with infectious diseases. *Biol Pharm Bull* **18**: 315.

Tanimura H, Ohnishi H, Okamura T *et al.* (1992). Chemotherapy of biliary tract infections (XXXVII). Excretion into bile and gallbladder tissue levels of levofloxacin and its clinical effect in biliary tract infections. *Jpn J Antibiot* **45**: 557.

Une T, Fujimoto T, Sato K *et al.* (1988). *In vitro* activity of DR-3355, an optically active ofloxacin. *Antimicrob Ag Chemother* **32**: 1336.

Wagai N, Yoshida M, Takayama S (1992). Phototoxic potential of the new quinolone antibacterial agent levofloxacin in mice. *Arzneimittelforschung* **42**: 404.

Yamane N, Jones RN, Frei R *et al.* (1994). Levofloxacin *in vitro* activity: results from an international comparative study with ofloxacin and ciprofloxacin. *J Chemother* **6**: 83.

Yew WW, Piddock LJ, Li MS *et al.* (1994). *In-vitro* activity of quinolones and macrolides against mycobacteria. *J Antimicrob Chemother* **34**: 343.

Zhang YY, Wang F, Zhang JD *et al.* (1995). *In vitro* antibacterial activity of levofloxacin. *Drugs* **49** (Suppl 2): 274.

Rufloxacin

Description

Rufloxacin (MF 934), or 9-fluoro-10-(-methyl) piperazinyl-7-oxo-2,3-dihydro-7H-pyrido-(1,2,3, de) (1,4) benzothiazine-6-carboxylic acid, and its N-desmethylated derivative (MF 922), have antibacterial activity against a broad spectrum of pathogens, although generally less than that of ciprofloxacin and norfloxacin . Due its spectrum of activity and very long half-life, it has been considered as a once-daily agent for urinary tract and respiratory infections (Wise et al., 1992).

Sensitive Organisms

1 Gram-negative bacteria

The *in vitro* MICs of rufloxacin against some selected bacterial species are shown in Table II.6 (pp. 986–987).

Rufloxacin is active against most Enterobacteriaceae and some strains of *Pseudomonas aeruginosa* (MIC_{90} 1–8 μg per ml), but *Klebsiella* spp., *Serratia* spp and *Enterobacter* spp. are relatively resistant (MIC_{90} 32, 32 and 64 μg per ml, respectively). Gram-negative respiratory pathogens such as *Haemophilus influenzae* and *Moraxella catarrhalis* are susceptible (MIC_{90} 0.5–1 μg per ml), unlike *Streptococcus pneumoniae*. *Neisseria gonorrhoeae* strains are susceptible (MIC_{90} 0.12 μg per ml). Rufloxacin is more active than nalidixic acid, but generally has less *in vitro* activity than ciprofloxacin, norfloxacin, ofloxacin or pefloxacin. Against bacterial enteric pathogens such as *Shigella*, *Salmonella* spp., *Yersinia* spp. and *Aeromonas*, norfloxacin has ≥8-fold more activity than rufloxacin. Nevertheless, the high fecal concentrations of rufloxacin after a single dose mean that bowel concentrations remain above the MIC of the most common enteropathogens for up to 1 week (p. 1166). *Brucella melitensis* is resistant (MIC_{90} 4–8 μg per ml). Any bacterial strains that demonstrate resistance to other fluoroquinolones exhibit cross-resistance with rufloxacin. *Bacteroides fragilis* spp. are resistant (Ravizzola *et al.*, 1989; Wise *et al.*, 1992; Qadri *et al.*, 1993a,b; Soriano *et al.*, 1994).

2 Gram-positive bacteria

Rufloxacin has reasonable to fair activity against methicillin-susceptible *Staphylococcus aureus* and *Staph. epidermidis* (MIC_{90} 2 μg per ml), but *Strep. pneumoniae*, *Enterococcus* spp. and Group A and B streptococci are resistant (MIC_{90} 16–32 μg per ml). *Clostridium perfringens*, *Cl. difficile* and other *Clostridium* spp. are resistant with MIC_{50} of 4, 32 and 8 μg per ml, respectively (Wise *et al.*, 1992; Qadri *et al.*, 1993b).

3 Chlamydia and Mycoplasma

Rufloxacin has only moderate activity against *Chlamydia trachomatis* and *C. pneumoniae* (MIC_{90} 4–8 μg per ml), being inferior to ciprofloxacin in this regard (Wise *et al.*, 1992). Rufloxacin and ciprofloxacin have similar activity against mycoplasmas, including *Mycoplasma pneumoniae* and *M. hominis*, with MIC_{90} 0.5–4 μg per ml (Furneri *et al.*, 1994;)

Mode of Administration and Dosage

1 Oral administration

In patients with normal renal function, the usual recommended regimen of rufloxacin is a single oral loading dose of 400 mg, followed by 200 mg once-daily for various durations depending on the indication (Perry *et al.* 1993).

2 Patients with renal failure

Although no dosage adjustment is necessary with moderate renal impairment (glomerular filtration rate [GFR] > 30 ml per min), patients with a GFR of < 30 ml per min should have the dose interval prolonged to 48 h to avoid excessive drug accumulation. In patients undergoing dialysis (hemodialysis and continuous amulatory peritoneal dialysis (CAPD)) the elimination half-life of rufloxacin is not significantly different to that of controls, probably due to clearance by dialysis (Perry *et al.*, 1993).

3 Patients with hepatic failure

Liver impairment itself does not appear to alter the pharmacokinetics of rufloxacin and therefore no alteration in dosage is necessary with liver dysfunction, unless there is concomitant renal impairment, when dosage reduction may be necessary (Triger *et al.*, 1993).

4 Elderly patients

The elimination half-life of rufloxacin appears to be similar in the elderly to that noted in young healthy volunteers, however, plasma levels may be 80% higher. Thus, although no dosage adjustment is necessary due to old age alone, carefully monitoring of drug levels should be considered in this patient group (Cogo *et al.*, 1992).

Serum Levels in Relation to Dosage

The measurement of serum concentrations of rufloxacin may be partly dependent on the method used since high-performance liquid chromatography (HPLC) measures rufloxacin alone, while microbiologic assays will tend to measure the combined activity of both rufloxacin and its *N*-desmethylated derivative. Thus, serum concentrations measured by bioassay may be recorded as slightly higher than those measured by HPLC (Imbimbo *et al.*, 1991; Wise *et al.*, 1991).

The oral bioavailability of rufloxacin in humans is uncertain (Kisicki *et al.*, 1992). However, following a single 400-mg oral dose of rufloxacin in healthy volunteers, mean peak plasma concentrations of 4.4 μg per ml measured by bioassay can generally be expected about 1.9 h post-dose; although wide intersubject variations may be noted. In comparison, Imbimbo *et al.* (1991) found peak serum concentrations of rufloxacin following a 400-mg dose to be 2.56–2.74 μg per ml, 3.8–4.0 h post-dose, using an HPLC assay. These single-dose studies suggest the mean elimination half-life of rufloxacin to be 28.2–38.9 h (Imbimbo *et al.*, 1991; Wise *et al.*, 1991). Higher serum concentrations have been found following multiple doses. A regimen of 400-mg oral loading dose, followed by 200 mg daily for 9 days, results in a mean peak serum concentration after the initial dose of 3.35 μg per ml, 2–3 h post-dose (i.e. reasonably comparable with that found by Wise *et al.*, 1991), and a maximum serum concentration at the end of treatment of 4.51 μg per ml. Serum concentrations following a regimen of a 600-mg loading dose plus a 300-mg daily dose subsequently, are 4.54 μg per ml, 2–3 h post-loading dose, and 7.20 μg per ml at the end of treatment. In this study, the elimination half-life was found to be 40.0–44.0 h (Kisicki *et al.*, 1992). Others studying slightly different dosing regimens have found broadly similar results (Mattina *et al.*, 1991; Rimoldi *et al.*, 1992; Segre *et al.*, 1992). Segre *et al.* (1992) found the pharmacokinetics of rufloxacin to be linear in the dose range of 100–400 mg, but to be less linear above oral doses of 800 mg.

Excretion

1 Urine

Overall, about 20–25% of a single 400-mg dose of rufloxacin is excreted in the urine in the 48 h post-dose, with approximately 7% being excreted in the 24–48 h post-dose period. After 72 h, 27 ± 12% of the dose will be excreted in the urine. Mean concentrations of rufloxacin in urine 0–6, 6–12, 12–24 and 48 h following such a dose are 22.0–28.0 μg per ml, 19.8–23.4 μg per ml, 26.7–27.7 μg per ml and 47.1–53.6 μg per ml, respectively (Imbimbo *et al.*, 1991; Privitera *et al.*, 1993). After multidosing regimens of a 400- or 600-mg loading dose followed by a 200- or 300-mg daily dose for 9 days, 49.6 to 51.1% of the total administered dose is excreted in the urine. Urine concentrations 0–2 h, 12–24 h and 3 days after the last dose of the 400/200 mg and 600/300 mg regimens were 43.07 and 85.69 μg per ml, 60.24 and 70.25 μg per ml, and 29.75 and 36.19 μg per ml, respectively. Rufloxacin probably undergoes some renal tubular reabsorption (Kisicki *et al.*, 1992).

2 Bile

Biliary excretion is about 0.9% during the 72 h after a single 400 mg oral dose of rufloxacin (Imbimbo *et al.*, 1991; Privitera *et al.*, 1993). Privitera *et al.* (1993) found no traces of the *N*-desmethyl metabolite of rufloxacin in bile after a 400-mg oral dose.

3 Inactivation in body

Rufloxacin undergoes a modest amount of metabolism, probably in the liver, and small amounts of the *N*-desmethyl metabolite (about 1.1–1.8% of the given dose) is recoverable in the urine (Imbimbo *et al.*, 1991; Kisicki *et al.*, 1992; Privitera *et al.*, 1993).

Distribution of the Drug in Body

Rufloxacin is approximately 64% protein-bound (Wise *et al.*, 1991). Following a single oral dose of 400 mg, the mean peak concentration in inflammatory fluid is 3.2 μg per ml (measured by bioassay), 3.5 h post-dose; representing about 90% penetration (Wise *et al.*, 1991). The same single oral dose of rufloxacin results in a peak serum level of 3.56 μg per ml and is concentrated in bronchial mucosa, alveolar macrophages and respiratory epithelial lining cells 1.8-, 21.6- and 7.7-fold (as measured by AUC ratios). These concentrations exceed the MIC_{90} for most respiratory pathogens except *Strep. pneumoniae*, where only alveolar macrophages achieve reliably adequate concentrations against this pathogen (Wise *et al.*, 1993). Prostatic penetration of rufloxacin is excellent with prostate:plasma and prostatic fluid:plasma concentration ratios of 1.9 and 1.5, respectively, following two preoperative doses: 400 mg 16 h prior and 200 mg 5 h prior to surgery (Boerema *et al.*, 1991a).

Rufloxacin achieves excellent biliary concentrations: after a single 400-mg oral dose of rufloxacin to 12 patients with extrahepatic cholestasis, a mean biliary concentration of 8.24 ± 7.16 μg per ml was noted 4.2 ± 3.5 h post-dose. Thus, the MICs of most common biliary tract pathogens will be exceeded (Privitera *et al.*, 1993). Mean fecal concentrations of rufloxacin 2 and 7 days after a single 400 mg oral dose are 94 ± 73 and 19 ± 17 μg per g (Marco *et al.*, 1995).

In rabbits, rufloxacin has been shown to reach therapeutically useful concentrations in the aqueous and vitreous humor (Nucci *et al.*, 1992).

Mode of Action

Rufloxacin has a similar mode of action to other fluoroquinolones (p. 1008).

Toxicity

Headache, nervousness, dizziness, insomnia, abdominal discomfort, flatulence, nausea and postprandial vomiting have been reported in some studies (Boerema *et al.*, 1991b; Mattina *et al.*, 1991; Kisicki *et al.*, 1992; Klietmann *et al.*, 1993; Perry *et al.*, 1993).

In one study of patients with chronic bronchitis who were treated with rufloxacin, the number of adverse events in patients receiving both rufloxacin and theophylline was no higher than that noted in patients receiving rufloxacin alone – suggesting no major clinically significant interaction beween these two agents (Klietmann *et al.*, 1993).

Similar to the situation with other fluoroquinolones, antacid suspensions containing magnesium hydroxide and aluminum hydroxide reduce the bioavailability of rufloxacin to 64% of control values when given within 5 min of rufloxacin. Administration of antacid 4 h after rufloxacin slightly reduces absorption, resulting in about 87% bioavailability compared with controls (Lazzaroni *et al.*, 1993).

Clinical Uses of the Drug

1 Urinary tract infections and prostatitis

In a randomized, double-blind comparison of single-dose regimens of rufloxacin 400 mg (n=226) and pefloxacin 800 mg (n=237) for uncomplicated cystitis in women, rates of bacteriological cure and clinical resolution were 88 versus 84% and 85 versus 84%, respectively. Among clinically assessable patients at 4 weeks follow-up, 89 and 88%, respectively, remained cured. Potentially drug-related adverse events occurred in 19% of the rufloxacin-treated patients and in 18% of the perfloxacin-treated patients. Thus, unlike other agents in which single-dose therapy is generally less effective than longer duration regimens, the long half-life of rufloxacin may be an advantage (Jardin and Cesana, 1995). Other rather small studies also suggest that rufloxacin is effective in the treatment of urinary tract infections. Rufloxacin (400-mg loading dose, plus

200 mg daily) was comparable with ofloxacin 300 mg twice-daily when given for a median of 8 days for complicated cystitis and upper urinary tract infections, with rates of bacterial elimination of 90% and 81%, respectively. At 2 weeks follow-up there were no recurrences in the rufloxacin group compared with 17% of the ofloxacin patients (Mattina *et al.*, 1993). Similarly, a 10-day course of once-daily rufloxacin 200 mg (after a 400-mg loading dose) appeared to be comparable with twice-daily ciprofloxacin 500 mg in the treatment of acute uncomplicated pyelonephritis. Bacteriological and clinical success rates were 55.6% versus 58.8%, and 74% versus 71%, respectively – although these outcomes are lower than what would be expected from other studies of fluoroquinolones (p. 1014) (Bach *et al.*, 1995).

In an open study of 27 patients with chronic bacterial prostatitis, a 4-week course of rufloxacin (400-mg loading dose followed by 200 mg daily) was associated with a 92% rate of clinical success (cure or improvement) and 79% rate of bacterial eradication 1 month after treatment. Among patients with persistent infections, *Enterococcus faecalis* and *Staph. epidermidis* were the responsible pathogens; which is notable since rufloxacin generally has limited activity against these species (Boerema *et al.*, 1991b).

2 Respiratory tract infections

Rufloxacin appears to be effective in the treatment of exacerbations of chronic bronchitis. In a double-blind, randomized study comparing a 10-day outpatient course of two dosage regimens of oral rufloxacin once-daily (a 400-mg load followed by 200 mg daily, or a 300-mg load followed by 150 mg daily) versus amoxicillin 500 mg orally thrice-daily, clinical success rates were comparable in the three groups: 94, 95 and 98%, respectively. Pretreatment cultures were positive in 139 of the 192 enrolled patients, with the most frequently isolated pathogens being *Strep. pneumoniae*, *Moraxella catarrhalis* and *H. influenzae*. Rates of bacteriological success at the end of treatment were similar: 93, 95 and 91%, respectively. Notably, the rate of bacteriological failure at follow-up from pneumococcal infection was 18% in both rufloxacin groups versus 5% in the amoxicillin group. Given the higher serum concentrations achieved with the 400/200 mg rufloxacin schedule, the authors recommended this dosing regimen over the lower dose combination for the treatment of exacerbations of chronic bronchitis (Klietmann *et al.*, 1993). Dirksen *et al.* (1991) also found the 400/200 mg rufloxacin 10-day regimen to be effective in a small open study of patients with acute exacerbations of chronic bronchitis.

3 Prevention of infection in neutropenic patients

Similar to norfloxacin, a single 400-mg dose of rufloxacin is very effective in the selective decontamination of feces of Gram-negative organisms. Given the long duration of reasonable rufloxacin levels in feces, a once-weekly daily dose may be sufficient to achieve useful selective decontamination in neutropenic patients (Marco *et al.*, 1995). Further clinical studies are necessary to demonstrate the efficacy of rufloxacin in this setting.

References

Bach D, van den Berg-Segers A, Hubner A *et al.* (1995). Rufloxacin once daily versus ciprofloxacin twice daily in the treatment of patients with acute uncomplicated pyelonephritis. *J Urol* **154**: 19.

Boerema JB, Bach D, Jol C, Pahlmann W (1991a). Penetration of rufloxacin into human prostatic tissue and fluid. *J Antimicrob Chemother* **28**: 547.

Boerema JB, Bischoff W, Focht J, Naber KG (1991b). An open multicentre study on the efficacy and safety of rufloxacin in patients with chronic bacterial prostatitis. *J Antimicrob Chemother* **28**: 587.

Cogo R, Rimoldi R, Mattina R, Imbimbo BP (1992). Steady-state pharmacokinetics of rufloxacin in elderly patients with lower respiratory tract infections. *Ther Drug Monit* **14**: 36.

Dirksen M, Focht J, Boerema J (1991). Rufloxacin once daily in acute exacerbations of chronic bronchitis. *Infection* **19**: 297.

Furneri PM, Bisignano G, Cerniglia G *et al.* (1994). *In vitro* antimycoplasmal activities of rufloxacin and its metabolite MF 922. *Antimicrob Ag Chemother* **38**: 2651.

Imbimbo BP, Broccali G, Cesana M *et al.* (1991). Inter- and intrasubject

variabilities in the pharmacokinetics of rufloxacin after single oral administration to healthy volunteers. *Antimicrob Ag Chemother* **35**: 390.

Jardin A, Cesana M (1995). Randomized, double-blind comparison of single-dose regimens of rufloxacin and pefloxacin for acute uncomplicated cystitis in women. French Multicenter Urinary Tract Infection-Rufloxacin Group. *Antimicrob Ag Chemother* **39**: 215.

Kisicki JC, Griess RS, Ott CL *et al.* (1992). Multiple-dose pharmacokinetics and safety of rufloxacin in normal volunteers. *Antimicrob Ag Chemother* **36**: 1296.

Klietmann W, Cesana M, Rondel RK, Focht J (1993). Double-blind, comparative study of rufloxacin once daily versus amoxicillin three times a day in treatment of outpatients with exacerbations of chronic bronchitis. *Antimicrob Ag Chemother* **37**: 2298.

Lazzaroni M, Imbimbo BP, Bargiggia S *et al.* (1993). Effects of magnesium-aluminum hydroxide antacid on absorption of rufloxacin. *Antimicrob Ag Chemother* **37**: 2212.

Marco F, Gimenez MJ, Jimenez de Anta MT et al. (1995). Comparison of rufloxacin and norfloxacin effects on faecal flora. *J Antimicrob Chemother* **35**: 895.

Mattina R, Bonfiglio G, Cocuzza CE et al. (1991). Pharmacokinetics of rufloxacin in healthy volunteers after repeated oral doses. *Chemotherapy* **37**: 389.

Mattina R, Cocuzza CE, Cesana M (1993). Rufloxacin once-daily versus ofloxacin twice-daily for treatment of complicated cystitis and upper urinary tract infections. Italian Multicentre UTI Rufloxacin Group. *Infection* **21**: 106.

0,444,444,Nucci P, Lombardo N, Cremonesi F et al. (1992). Ocular pharmacokinetics of rufloxacin a new fluoroquinolone antibiotic. *Clin Ter* **140**: 563.

Perry G, Mant TG, Morrison PJ et al. (1993). Pharmacokinetics of rufloxacin in patients with impaired renal function. *Antimicrob Ag Chemother* **37**: 637.

Privitera G, Nicastro G, Imbimbo BP et al. (1993). Biliary excretion of rufloxacin in humans. *Antimicrob Ag Chemother* **37**: 2545.

Qadri SM, Ayub A, Ueno Y, Saldin H (1993a). Susceptibility of *Salmonella typhi* and *Brucella melitensis* to the new fluoroquinolone rufloxacin (MF 934). *Chemotherapy* **39**: 311.

Qadri SM, Ueno Y, Postle G et al. (1993b). Comparative activity of the new fluoroquinolone rufloxacin (MF 934) against clinical isolates of gram-negative and gram-positive bacteria. *Eur J Clin Microbiol Infect Dis* **12**: 372.

Ravizzola G, Pinsi G, Pirali F et al. (1989). Rufloxacin (MF-934): *in vitro* and *in vivo* antibacterial activity. *Drugs Exp Clin Res* **15**: 11.

Rimoldi R, Fioretti M, Albrici A, Imbimbo BP (1992). Pharmacokinetics of rufloxacin once daily in patients with lower respiratory tract infections. *Infection* **20**: 89.

Segre G, Cerretani D, Moltoni L, Urso R (1992). Pharmacokinetics of rufloxacin in healthy volunteers. *Eur J Clin Pharmacol* **42**: 101.

Soriano F, Fernandez-Roblas R, Lopez JC et al. (1994). Comparative *in-vitro* activity of rufloxacin with five other antimicrobial agents against bacterial enteric pathogens. *J Antimicrob Chemother* **34**: 157.

Triger DR, Granai F, Woodcock J et al. (1993). Multiple-dose pharmacokinetics of rufloxacin in patients with cirrhosis. *Hepatology* **18**: 847.

Wise R, Johnson J, O'Sullivan N et al. (1991). Pharmacokinetics and tissue penetration of rufloxacin, a long acting quinolone antimicrobial agent. *J Antimicrob Chemother* **28**: 905.

Wise R, Andrews JM, Matthews R, Wolstenholme M (1992). The *in-vitro* activity of two new quinolones: rufloxacin and MF 961. *J Antimicrob Chemother* **29**: 649.

Wise R, Andrews J, Imbimbo BP et al. (1993). The penetration of rufloxacin into sites of potential infection in the respiratory tract. *J Antimicrob Chemother* **32**: 861.

Clinafloxacin

Description

Clinafloxacin (AM-1091, CI-960, PD127391), or 7-(3-amino-1-pyrrolidinyl)-8-chloro-1-cyclo-propyl-6-fluoro-1,4-dihydro-4-oxo-3-quinolone carboxylic acid hydrochloride, is a new fluoroquinolone with impressive broad spectrum *in vitro* activity against Gram-positive, Gram-negative and anaerobic bacteria. Notably, this increased activity against Gram-positive species and anaerobes has not been associated with a loss of activity against Enterobacteriaceae and *Pseudomonas aeruginosa* (Neu *et al.*, 1989; Fuchs *et al.*, 1991).

Clinafloxacin is 2-fold more active than ciprofloxacin and 2- to 32-fold more active than ofloxacin against Enterobacteriaceae; roughly comparable with ciprofloxacin against *Enterobacter* spp., *Citrobacter* spp., and *Klebsiella* spp., and similar to, or occasionally marginally less active than, ciprofloxacin against *Ps. aeruginosa* (MIC_{90} 0.5–1 μg per ml), including aminoglycoside-resistant isolates. Notably, clinafloxacin is often active against imipenem- and gentamicin-resistant Gram-negative pathogens such as *Burkholderia cepacia* and *Stenotrophomonas* (previously *Xanthomonas*) *maltophilia* (MIC_{90} 0.12 and ≤0.5–2 μg per ml, respectively), including some strains that are ciprofloxacin-resistant. Clinfloxacin is highly active (MIC_{90} ≤0.06 μg per ml) against *Haemophilus influenzae*, *Neisseria gonorrhoeae*, *N. meningitidis*, *Moraxella cartarrhalis* and *Brucella melitensis*. Clinafloxacin is active against strains of *N. gonorrhoeae* (MIC_{90} 0.016 μg per ml) with reduced susceptibility (MIC_{90} 0.25 μg per ml) to ciprofloxacin, but its MIC is about 8-fold higher than for ciprofloxacin-susceptible strains. The highest clinafloxacin MICs, however, are generally noted for *Achromobacter xylosoxidans*, *Flavobacterium* spp. and some strains of *Burkholderia cepacia*. Overall, against non-enteric Gram-negative bacilli, clinafloxacin is more active than either ciprofloxacin, or especially sparfloxacin (King *et al.*, 1988; Norrby and Jonsson, 1988; Wise *et al.*, 1988; Neu *et al.*, 1989; Rolston *et al.*, 1990; Barrett *et al.*, 1991; Cohen *et al.*, 1991; Fuchs *et al.*, 1991; Qadri *et al.*, 1992; Ford *et al.*, 1993; Qadri and Ueno, 1993; Pankuch *et al.*, 1994; Carlyn *et al.*, 1995; Cormican *et al.*, 1995; Garcia-Rodriguez and Garcia Sanchez, 1995).

Clinafloxacin is very active against *Legionella pneumophila* and other *Legionella* spp. with an MIC_{90} 0.015 μg per ml – this activity is 2- to 4-fold greater than that of ciprofloxacin, substantially greater than that of erythromycin (MIC_{90} 0.5 μg per ml), and approaches that of rifampicin (MIC_{90} 0.008 μg per ml) (Gooding *et al.*, 1992).

Clinafloxacin is very active against *Staphylococcus aureus*, *Staph. epidermidis*, *Streptococcus pneumoniae* and hemolyic streptococci with MIC_{90}s of 0.06, 0.06, 0.25 and 0.25 μg per ml, respectively. Studies of experimental penicillin- and cephalosporin-resistant pneumococcal meningitis in a rabbit meningitis model suggest reasonable *in vivo* clinafloxacin activity (Friedland *et al.*, 1993). Clinafloxacin activity against *Enterococcus faecalis* and *E. faecium* is slightly less than for other Gram-positive cocci with MIC_{90} 0.5 μg per ml (occasionally 2 μg per ml). In one study, the *in vitro* activity of clinafloxacin against strains of multiresistant *E. faecium* appeared to be substantially improved when clinafloxacin was combined with ampicillin, but these findings are yet to be confirmed (Burney *et al.*, 1994). *In vivo* studies of clinafloxacin in an experimental ampicillin-resistant enterococcal endocarditis rabbit model suggested that clinafloxacin has potentially useful activity against serious enterococcal infections (Vazquez *et al.*, 1993). Methicillin-resistant *Staph. aureus* (MRSA) are generally very susceptible (MIC_{90} ≤0.015 μg per ml), while the MIC_{90} for *Listeria moncytogenes* is 1 μg per ml. Against ciprofloxacin-resistant (MIC_{90} ≥32 μg per ml) staphylococci, clinafloxacin inhibits 95% of isolates at 2 μg per ml. However, studies of spontaneous mutations among these isolates suggest that the future potential for developing cross-resistance against clinafloxacin remains a concern.

In vivo animal studies and studies monitoring the resistance patterns of clinical MRSA isolates support this concern (Forstall *et al.*, 1991; Kaatz *et al.*, 1992; Harrington *et al.*, 1995). Unlike ciprofloxacin, ofloxacin and sparfloxacin, clinafloxacin is active against the majority of *Corynebacterium* spp. (MIC$_{90}$ 1 μg per ml) (Martinez-Martinez *et al.*, 1994). Overall, clinafloxacin is 4- to 8-fold more active against Gram-positive cocci, and 2- to 8-fold more active against *Listeria monocytogenes* than ciprofloxacin (Norrby and Jonsson, 1988; Wise *et al.*, 1988; Neu *et al.* 1989; Barry and Fuchs, 1991; Cohen *et al.*, 1991, 1995; Fuchs *et al.*,1991; Miranda *et al.*, 1992; Shonekan *et al.*, 1992; Perri *et al.*, 1993; Forstall *et al.*, 1994)

Clinafloxacin displays excellent activity against anaerobes, with MIC$_{90}$ 0.5, 0.5–2, ≤0.5 and ≤0.5 μg per ml against *Bacteroides fragilis* group, *Bacteroides* spp., *Clostridia* spp.and peptococci/peptostreptococci, respectively. *Clostridium difficile* is susceptible to 0.25 μg per ml clinafloxacin *in vitro*. Among the anaerobes, no relationship between resistance to clindamycin, cefoxitin or piperacillin and resistance to fluoroquinolones has been noted (Neu *et al.*, 1989; Barrett *et al.*, 1991; Goldstein and Citron, 1992; Barry *et al.*, 1993; Borobio *et al.*, 1994; Wexler *et al.*, 1994; Appelbaum, 1995).

Clinafloxacin is very active against *Mycoplasma pneumoniae*, *M. hominis*, *U. urealyticum* and *Chlamydia trachomatis* with MIC$_{90}$ of 0.03, 0.03, 0.25 and 0.06 μg per ml, respectively (Wise *et al.*, 1988; Waites *et al.*, 1991). Similarly clinafloxacin has good *in vitro* activity against *Rickettsia rickettsii* and *R. conorii* (MIC ≤0.25 μg per ml) and lesser activity against *Coxiella burnetii* (MIC ≤1 μg per ml) (Jabarit-Aldighieri *et al.*, 1992).

Clinafloxacin is similar to ciprofloxacin, and to a lesser extent ofloxacin, in its activity against *Mycobacterium tuberculosis* (MIC$_{90}$ 0.125–2 μg per ml); however, cross-resistance to fluoroquinolones has been noted in some isolates collected from patients receiving long-term unsuccessful therapy with ofloxacin. *Mycobacterium fortuitum* may be susceptible to clinafloxacin (MIC$_{90}$ 2 μg per ml), but other non-tuberculous *Mycobacteria* spp. are generally resistant (MIC$_{90}$ >8 μg per ml), although some authors have reported reasonable *in vitro* activity aginst *M. avium* complex (Wise *et al.*, 1988; Barrett *et al.*, 1992; Yew *et al.*, 1994).

The *in vitro* MICs of clinafloxacin against selected bacterial species are shown in Table II.6 (p. 987).

Small human pharmacokinetic studies suggest that following oral doses of clinafloxacin 100 mg or 200 mg, peak serum concentrations of 0.89 and 2.5 μg per ml, respectively, can be expected with an elimination half-life of 6 h (Dorr *et al.*, 1991). Tack *et al.* (1995) found serum peak and trough concentrations of 1.68–1.93 and 0.12–0.65 μg per ml, respectively, after 200 mg i.v., and levels of 1.72–1.85 and 0.87–0.92 μg per ml after 200 mg orally. In one patient receiving clinifloxacin 200 mg i.v. every 12 h, the peak serum concentration was 1.93 μg per ml at 1 h post-infusion, with a CSF concentration of 0.43 μg per ml at 2 h post-infusion. Trough serum and CSF concentrations were 0.12 and 0.16 μg per ml, respectively.

Clinafloxacin has been used in doses of 100 mg or 200 mg orally twice-daily, or 200–400 mg i.v. twice-daily (Tack *et al.*, 1995). Initial limited clinical experience using clinafloxacin in an emergency-use program for serious infections due to difficult-to-treat infections such as pneumonia due to *Pseudomonas* spp., *Stenotrophomonas maltophilia* and *Burkholderia cepacia S. maltophilia* meningitis, endocarditis and a variety of other conditions resulted in cure in seven of 11 patients. Reported side-effects in this study included diplopia, tremulousness, apprehension, confusion and photosensitive skin rash (Tack *et al.*, 1995). Possible interaction between clinafloxacin and theophylline has been reported (Matuschka and Vissing, 1995).

Despite the very promising *in vitro* susceptibility profile of clinafloxacin, the future clinical role of this drug remains unclear until further pharmacokinetic and toxicity studies are completed.

References

Appelbaum PC (1995). Quinolone activity against anaerobes: microbiological aspects. *Drugs* **49** (Suppl 2): 76.

Barrett MS, Jones RN, Erwin ME *et al.* (1991). Antimicrobial activity evaluations of two new quinolones, PD127391 (CI-960 and AM-1091) and PD131628. *Diagn Microbiol Infect Dis* **14**: 389.

Barrett MS, Jones RN, Erwin ME, Koontz FP (1992). CI-960 (PD127391 or AM-1091), sparfloxacin, WIN 57273, and isepamicin activity against clinical isolates of *Mycobacterium avium–intracellularae* complex, *M. chelonae*, and *M. fortuitum*. *Diagn Microbiol Infect Dis* **15**: 169.

Barry AL, Fuchs PC (1991). Antistaphylococcal activity of the fluoroquinolones CI-960, PD 131628, sparfloxacin, ofloxacin and ciprofloxacin. *Eur J Clin Microbiol Infect Dis* **10**: 168.

Barry AL, Fuchs PC, Citron DM *et al.* (1993). Methods for testing the susceptibility of anaerobic bacteria to two fluoroquinolone compounds, PD 131628 and clinafloxacin. *J Antimicrob Chemother* **31**: 893.

Borobio MV, Conejo M, Ramirez E *et al.* (1994). Comparative activities of eight quinolones against members of the *Bacteroides fragilis* group. *Antimicrob Ag Chemother* **38**: 1442.

Burney S, Landman D, Quale JM (1994). Activity of clinafloxacin against multidrug-resistant *Enterococcus faecium. Antimicrob Ag Chemother* **38**: 1668.

Carlyn CJ, Doyle LJ, Knapp CC *et al.* (1995). Activities of three investigational fluoroquinolones (BAY y 3118, DU-6859a, and clinafloxacin) against *Neisseria gonorrhoeae* isolates with diminished susceptibilities to ciprofloxacin and ofloxacin. *Antimicrob Ag Chemother* **39**: 1606.

Cohen MA, Huband MD, Mailloux GB *et al.* (1991). *In vitro* antibacterial activities of the fluoroquinolones PD 117596, PD 124816, and PD 127391. *Diagn Microbiol Infect Dis* **14**: 245.

Cohen MA, Yoder SL, Huband MD *et al.* (1995). *In vitro* and *in vivo* activities of clinafloxacin, CI-990 (PD 131112), and PD 138312 versus enterococci. *Antimicrob Ag Chemother* **39**: 2123.

Cormican MG, Marshall SA, Jones RN (1995). Cross-resistance analysis for DU-6859a, a new fluoroquinolone, compared to six structurally similar compounds (ciprofloxacin, clinafloxacin, fleroxacin, levofloxacin, ofloxacin, and sparfloxacin). *Diagn Microbiol Infect Dis* **21**: 51.

Dorr MB, Webb CL, Bron N, Vassoss AB (1991). Single-dose tolerance and pharmacokinetics of CI-960 (PD 127391). in healthy volunteers. In *Program and Abstracts of the 31st Interscience Conference on Antimicrobial Agents and Chemotherapy, Chicago, IL.* (Abstr. 1151). p. 291. Washington, DC: American Society for Microbiology.

Ford AS, Baltch AL, Smith RP, Ritz W (1993). *In-vitro* susceptibilities of *Pseudomonas aeruginosa* and *Pseudomonas* spp to the new fluoroquinolones clinafloxacin and PD 131628 and nine other antimicrobial agents. *J Antimicrob Chemother* **31**: 523.

Forstall GJ, Knapp CC, Washington JA (1991). Activity of new quinolones against ciprofloxacin-resistant staphylococci. *Antimicrob Ag Chemother* **35**: 1679.

Forstall GJ, Knapp CC, Washington JA (1994). Bactericidal activities of DU-6859a and clinafloxacin (CI-960) against staphylococci. *Antimicrob Ag Chemother* **38**: 1868.

Friedland IR, Paris M, Ehrett S *et al.* (1993). Evaluation of antimicrobial regimens for treatment of experimental penicillin- and cephalosporin-resistant pneumococcal meningitis. *Antimicrob Ag Chemother* **37**: 1630.

Fuchs PC, Barry AL, Pfaller MA *et al.* (1991). Multicenter evaluation of the *in vitro* activities of three new quinolones, sparfloxacin, CI-960, and PD 131,628, compared with the activity of ciprofloxacin against 5252 clinical bacterial isolates. *Antimicrob Ag Chemother* **35**: 764.

Garcia-Rodriguez JA, Garcia Sanchez JE, Trujillano I *et al.* (1995). Susceptibilities of *Brucella melitensis* isolates to clinafloxacin and four other new fluoroquinolones. *Antimicrob Ag Chemother* **39**: 1194.

Goldstein EJ, Citron DM (1992). Comparative activity of ciprofloxacin, ofloxacin, sparfloxacin, temafloxacin, CI-960, CI-990, and WIN 57273 against anaerobic bacteria. *Antimicrob Ag Chemother* **36**: 1158.

Gooding BB, Erwin ME, Barrett MS *et al.* (1992). Antimicrobial activities of two investigational fluoroquinolones (CI-960 and E4695). against over 100 *Legionella* sp isolates. *Antimicrob Ag Chemother* **36**: 2049.

Harrington GD, Zarins LT, Ramsey MA *et al.* (1995). Susceptibility of ciprofloxacin-resistant staphylococci and enterococci to clinafloxacin. *Diagn Microbiol Infect Dis* **21**: 27.

Jabarit-Aldighieri N, Torres H, Raoult D (1992). Susceptibility of *Rickettsia*

conorii, R. rickettsii, and *Coxiella burnetii* to PD 127,391, PD 131,628, pefloxacin, ofloxacin, and ciprofloxacin. *Antimicrob Ag Chemother* **36**: 2529.

Kaatz GW, Seo SM, Lamp KC *et al.* (1992). CI-960, a new fluoroquinolone, for therapy of experimental ciprofloxacin- susceptible and -resistant *Staphylococcus aureus* endocarditis. *Antimicrob Ag Chemother* **36**: 1192.

King A, Boothman C, Phillips I (1988). The *in-vitro* activity of PD127,391, a new quinolone. *J Antimicrob Chemother* **22**: 135.

Martinez-Martinez L, Suarez AI, Ortega MC, Perea EJ (1994). Comparative *in vitro* activities of new quinolones against coryneform bacteria. *Antimicrob Ag Chemother* **38**: 1439.

Matuschka PR, Vissing RS (1995). Clinafloxacin-theophylline drug interaction. *Ann Pharmacother* **29**: 378.

Miranda AG, Wanger AR, Singh KV, Murray BE (1992). Comparative *in vitro* activity of PD 127391, a new fluoroquinolone agent, against susceptible and resistant clinical isolates of gram-positive cocci. *Antimicrob Ag Chemother* **36**: 1325.

Neu HC, Novelli A, Chin NX (1989). Comparative *in vitro* activity of a new quinolone, AM-1091. *Antimicrob Ag Chemother* **33**: 1036.

Norrby SR, Jonsson M (1988). Comparative *in vitro* activity of PD 127,391, a new fluorinated 4-quinolone derivative. *Antimicrob Ag Chemother* **32**: 1278.

Pankuch GA, Jacobs MR, Appelbaum PC (1994). Susceptibilities of 123 *Xanthomonas maltophilia* strains to clinafloxacin, PD 131628, PD 138312, PD 140248, ciprofloxacin, and ofloxacin. *Antimicrob Ag Chemother* **38**: 369.

Perri MB, Chow JW, Zervos MJ (1993). *In vitro* activity of sparfloxacin and clinafloxacin against multidrug- resistant enterococci. *Diagn Microbiol Infect Dis* **17**: 151.

Qadri SM, Ueno Y (1993). Susceptibility of *Brucella melitensis* to the new fluoroquinolone PD 131628: comparison with other drugs. *Chemotherapy* **39**: 128.

Qadri SM, Abo-Askar H, Ueno Y (1992). Antibacterial activity of the new quinolone CI-960 (PD 127391) against clinical isolates at a major tertiary care center in Saudi Arabia. *Chemotherapy* **38**: 92.

Rolston KV, Ho DH, LeBlanc B, Bodey GP (1990). *In vitro* activity of PD127,391, a new quinolone against bacterial isolates from cancer patients. *Chemotherapy* **36**: 365.

Shonekan D, Mildvan D, Handwerger S (1992). Comparative *in vitro* activities of teicoplanin, daptomycin, ramoplanin, vancomycin, and PD127,391 against blood isolates of gram-positive cocci. *Antimicrob Ag Chemother* **36**: 1570.

Tack KJ, McGuire NM, Eiseman IA (1995). Initial clinical experience with clinafloxacin in the treatment of serious infections. *Drugs* **49** (Suppl 2): 488.

Vazquez J, Perri MB, Thal LA *et al.* (1993). Sparfloxacin and clinafloxacin alone or in combination with gentamicin for therapy of experimental ampicillin-resistant enterococcal endocarditis in rabbits. *J Antimicrob Chemother* **32**: 715.

Waites KB, Duffy LB, Schmid T *et al.* (1991). *In vitro* susceptibilities of *Mycoplasma pneumoniae, Mycoplasma hominis,* and *Ureaplasma urealyticum* to sparfloxacin and PD 127391. *Antimicrob Ag Chemother* **35**: 1181.

Wexler HM, Molitoris E, Reeves D, Finegold SM (1994). *In-vitro* activity of clinafloxacin (CI-960) and PD 131628-2 against anaerobic bacteria. *J Antimicrob Chemother* **34**: 579.

Wise R, Ashby JP, Andrews JM (1988). *In vitro* activity of PD 127,391, an enhanced-spectrum quinolone. *Antimicrob Ag Chemother* **32**: 1251.

Yew WW, Piddock LJ, Li MS *et al.* (1994). *In-vitro* activity of quinolones and macrolides against mycobacteria. *J Antimicrob Chemother* **34**: 343.

Trovafloxacin

Description

Trovafloxacin (CP-99,219), 7-(3-azabicyclo[3,1,0]hexyl)-naphthyridone is a new fluoroquinolone with a broad spectrum of activity against Gram-positive and Gram-negative bacteria and can be differentiated from other commonly available agents such as ciprofloxacin, norfloxacin and ofloxacin, by its greater activity against many clinically important Gram-positive pathogens such as steptococci, including *Streptococcus pneumoniae*. The 1-*N* substitution of trovafloxacin is identical to that of tosufloxacin, namely a difluorinated structure that enhances activity against some ciprofloxacin-resistant strains. Trovafloxacin is signficantly more active against methicillin-resistant, ciprofloxacin-susceptible staphylococci (MIC_{90} $\leq 0.25\,\mu g$ per ml) than either ciprofloxacin or sparfloxacin, but has less activity against methicillin-resistant, ciprofloxacin-resistant strains. Against these latter strains, trovafloxacin is the most active fluoroquinolone of those currently studied, but relatively high concentrations are required for inhibition (MIC_{90} $8-16\,\mu g$ per ml). Compared with ciprofloxacin and sparfloxacin it is 32-fold and 4-fold, respectively, more active against *Strep. pneumoniae*, including strains resistant to penicillin and erythromycin (MIC_{90} $\leq 0.25\,\mu g$ per ml). Preliminary *in vivo* studies using a rabbit meningitis model, suggested promising activity for trovafloxacin against penicillin-resistant pneumococcal meningitis (Paris *et al.*, 1995; Kim *et al.*, 1996). Trovafloxacin is also very active against *Strep. pyogenes* and *Enterococcus faecalis* (MIC_{90} $\leq 0.5\,\mu g$ per ml) and against *Listeria monocytogenes* (MIC_{90} $0.25-0.5\,\mu g$ per ml). However, *in vitro* studies suggest that trovafloxacin is only bacteriostatic against intracellular vancomycin-resistant *E. faecium* (Herrera-Insua *et al.*, 1996). Against the less common pathogens such as *Leuconostoc* spp. and *Pediococcus* spp. trovafloxacin is also active (Eliopoulos *et al.*, 1993; Gooding and Jones, 1993; Gootz *et al.*, 1994; Neu and Chin, 1994; Pankuch *et al.*, 1995; Endtz *et al.*, 1996; Cohen *et al.*, 1996).

Trovafloxacin is comparable with sparfloxacin and tosufloxacin, but generally less active than ciprofloxacin, against common Gram-negative pathogens such as *Escherichia coli*, *Enterobacter* spp., *Klebsiella* spp. and *Citrobacter* spp. with MIC_{90} $\leq 0.5\,\mu g$ per ml. Although activity against *Salmonella* spp. and *Shigella* spp. is comparable with ciprofloxacin (MIC_{90} $\leq 0.03\,\mu g$ per ml), *Morganella morgagnii*, *Serratia marcescens* and *Pseudomonas aeruginosa* are less susceptible to trovafloxacin, with MIC_{90} of 2, 4 and $1-2\,\mu g$ per ml, respectively. Activity against *Neisseria gonorrhoeae*, *Moraxella catarrhalis* and *Haemophilus influenzae* is excellent with MIC_{90} of 0.003, 0.06 and $0.03\,\mu g$ per ml, respectively. Notably, trovafloxacin maintains activity (MIC_{90} $0.25\,\mu g$ per ml) against ciprofloxacin-resistant (MIC_{90} $2\,\mu g$ per ml) strains of *N. gonorrhoeae*. Trovafloxacin has good activity against *Chlamydia pneumoniae* (MIC_{50} $\leq 0.06\,\mu g$ per ml) and *Legionella pneumophila*. (MIC_{90} $0.06\,\mu g$ per ml) (Gooding and Jones, 1993; Gootz *et al.*, 1994; Neu and Chin, 1994; Child *et al.*, 1995; Jones, 1995; Knapp *et al.*, 1995; van Rijsoort-Vos *et al.*, 1995; Dubois and St Pierre, 1996). Other authors have found even better *in vitro* activity against *Legionella* spp., and in the experimental guinea pig pneumonia model, 100% of animals survived after treatment with trovafloxacin (Millas *et al.*, 1996).

Trovafloxacin has generally excellent activity against most clinically significant anaerobe groups, with an overall MIC_{50} and MIC_{90} of 0.25 and $1\,\mu g$ per ml, respectively. Using a breakpoint of $2.0\,\mu g$ per ml, 99.6% of strains are susceptible. Against all anaerobes trovafloxacin is significantly superior to ciprofloxacin, and against important pathogens such as *Bacteroides fragilis* MIC_{90} of $0.39-0.5\,\mu g$ per ml can be expected (Gootz *et al.*, 1994; Spangler *et al.*, 1994; Appelbaum, 1995).

The *in vitro* MICs of trovafloxacin against selected bacterial species are shown in Table II.6 (p. 987).

Trovafloxacin has very promising *in vitro* and *in vivo* activity against *Toxoplasma gondii*. Trovafloxacin protected 100% of *T. gondii*-infected mice against death at concentrations of 100 and 200 mg per kg per day and 90% of mice at 50 mg per kg per day. Homogenates of brain, liver and spleen from previously infected mice failed to kill healthy mice following subinoculation with this tissue – suggesting elimination of viable parasites (Khan *et al.*, 1996).

Pharmacokinetic studies using single doses of 30, 100, 300, 600 and 1000 mg trovafloxacin in healthy volunteers, demonstrate that the drug is rapidly absorbed, with mean peak concentrations of 0.3, 1.5, 4.4, 6.6 and 10.1 µg per ml attained approximately 1 h after dosing. The terminal half-life is approximately 9.9 ± 2.5 h and appears to be independent of the dose. Although some variability has been noted, peak serum concentrations and AUC increase linearly with dose. Compared with oral ciprofloxacin 500 mg, the half-life and AUC for trovafloxacin 300 mg are about 2-fold longer and 4-fold greater, respectively, than those of ciprofloxacin. Trovafloxacin is about 70% protein-bound and only 8% of the administered dose is recoverable unchanged in urine. Renal clearance of trovafloxacin is generally constant regardless of dose. Although maximum attainable urine concentrations of trovafloxacin are lower than those obtained with other fluoroquinolones, the urine concentrations achieved after 100-mg and 300-mg doses are sufficient to inhibit most Gram-negative urinary pathogens (Teng *et al.*, 1995).

No clinically significant changes in biochemical or hematological parameters have been noted across the 30- to 1000-mg dose range, but some adverse events have been reported in subjects receiving 300–1000 mg per day. The most frequent of these have been lightheadedness, nausea and vomiting (Teng *et al.*, 1995). Trovafloxacin does not significantly interact with warfarin (Teng *et al.*, 1996), and although concomitant administration of trovafloxacin and caffeine is associated with a 15% increase in peak serum caffeine levels, these changes do not appear to be clinically significant (LeBel *et al.*, 1996).

Trovafloxacin penetrates well into alveolar macrophages, respiratory epithelial lining fluid and bronchial mucosa (Andrews *et al.*, 1996).

Given these data, trovafloxacin 100 mg or 300 mg once-daily may to be a suitable agent for many lower respiratory tract, skin/soft tissue and urinary tract infections.

References

Andrews JM, Brenwald NP, Wise R, Honeybourne D (1996). Concentrations of trovafloxacin in lung tissue. In *Program and Abstracts of the 36th Interscience Conference on Antimicrobial Agents and Chemotherapy, New Orleans* (Abstr. A4). Washington, DC: American Society for Microbiology.

Appelbaum PC (1995). Quinolone activity against anaerobes: microbiological aspects. *Drugs* **49** (Suppl 2): 76.

Child J, Andrews J, Boswell F *et al.* (1995). The *in-vitro* activity of CP 99,219, a new naphthyridone antimicrobial agent: a comparison with fluoroquinolone agents. *J Antimicrob Chemother* **35**: 869.

Cohen MA, Huband MD, Gage JW, Yoder SL (1996). *In vitro* activity of clinafloxacin, trovafloxacin, and ciprofloxacin. In *Program and Abstracts of the 36th Interscience Conference on Antimicrobial Agents and Chemotherapy, New Orleans* (Abstr. E85). Washington, DC: American Society for Microbiology.

Dubois J, St Pierre C (1996). An *in vitro* susceptibility study of trovafloxacin against *Legionella* spp. In *Program and Abstracts of the 36th Interscience Conference on Antimicrobial Agents and Chemotherapy, New Orleans* (Abstr. E75). Washington, DC: American Society for Microbiology.

Eliopoulos GM, Klimm K, Eliopoulos CT *et al.* (1993). *In vitro* activity of CP-99,219, a new fluoroquinolone, against clinical isolates of gram-positive bacteria. *Antimicrob Ag Chemother* **37**: 366.

Endtz HP, Mouton JW, Den JG *et al.* (1996). Comparative *in-vitro* activity of trovafloxacin (CP-99,219), a new fluoroquinolone, and other antibiotics against 458 Gram-positive strains isolated from patients with endocarditis and other bloodstream infections. In *Program and Abstracts*

of the 36th Interscience Conference on Antimicrobial Agents and Chemotherapy, New Orleans* (Abstr. E83). Washington, DC: American Society for Microbiology.

Gooding BB, Jones RN (1993). *In vitro* antimicrobial activity of CP-99,219, a novel azabicyclo-naphthyridone. *Antimicrob Ag Chemother* **37**: 349.

Gootz TD, Brighty KE, Anderson MR *et al.* (1994). *In vitro* activity of CP-99,219, a novel 7-(3-azabicyclo[310]hexyl) naphthyridone antimicrobial. *Diagn Microbiol Infect Dis* **19**: 235.

Herrera-Insua I, Jacques-Palaz K, Murray BE, Rakita RM (1996). Intracellular activity of trovafloxacin (CP-99,219) against vancomycin-susceptible (VSEF) and vancomycin-resistant (VREF) *Enterococcus faecium*. In *Program and Abstracts of the 36th Interscience Conference on Antimicrobial Agents and Chemotherapy, New Orleans* (Abstr. E78). Washington, DC: American Society for Microbiology.

Jones RN (1995). *In vitro* antimicrobial activity of CP-99,219, a new 7-azabicyclonaphthyridone. *Drugs* **49** (Suppl 2): 205.

Khan AA, Slifer T, Araujo FG, Remington JS (1996). Trovafloxacin is active against *Toxoplasma gondii*. In *Program and Abstracts of the 36th Interscience Conference on Antimicrobial Agents and Chemotherapy, New Orleans* (Abstr. E74). Washington, DC: American Society for Microbiology.

Kim YS, Liu QX, Chow LL, Täuber MG (1996). Tovafloxacin (TV) is effective in penicillin (PCN) resistant *S. pneumoniae* (SP) meningitis in rabbits. In *Program and Abstracts of the 36th Interscience Conference on Antimicrobial Agents and Chemotherapy, New Orleans* (Abstr. B37). Washington, DC: American Society for Microbiology.

Knapp JS, Neal SW, Parekh MC, Rice RJ (1995). *In vitro* activity of a new fluoroquinolone, CP-99,219, against strains of *Neisseria gonorrhoeae*. *Antimicrob Ag Chemother* **39**: 987.

LeBel M, Teng R, Dogolo LC *et al.* (1996). The effect of steady-state trovafloxacin on the steady-state pharmacokinetics of caffeine in healthy subjects. In *Program and Abstracts of the 36th Interscience Conference on Antimicrobial Agents and Chemotherapy, New Orleans* (Abstr. A1). Washington, DC: American Society for Microbiology.

Millas E, Lazaro MA, Bermejo M *et al.* (1996). *In vivo* activity of trovafloxacin (CP-116,517) against *Legionella pneumophila* in an experimental guinea pig pneumonia model. In *Program and Abstracts of the 36th Interscience Conference on Antimicrobial Agents and Chemotherapy, New Orleans* (Abstr. E76). Washington, DC: American Society for Microbiology.

Neu HC, Chin NX (1994). *In vitro* activity of the new fluoroquinolone CP-99,219. *Antimicrob Ag Chemother* **38**: 2615.

Pankuch GA, Jacobs MR, Appelbaum PC (1995). Activity of CP99,219 compared with DU-6859a, ciprofloxacin, ofloxacin, levofloxacin, lomefloxacin, tosufloxacin, sparfloxacin and grepafloxacin against penicillin-susceptible and -resistant pneumococci. *J Antimicrob Chemother* **35**: 230.

MM, Hickey SM, Trujillo M *et al.* (1995). Evaluation of CP-99,219, a new fluoroquinolone, for treatment of experimental penicillin- and cephalosporin-resistant pneumococcal meningitis. *Antimicrob Ag Chemother* **39**: 1243.

Spangler SK, Jacobs MR, Appelbaum PC (1994). Activity of CP 99,219 compared with those of ciprofloxacin, grepafloxacin, metronidazole, cefoxitin, piperacillin, and piperacillin-tazobactam against 489 anaerobes. *Antimicrob Ag Chemother* **38**: 2471.

Teng R, Harris SC, Nix DE *et al.* (1995). Pharmacokinetics and safety of trovafloxacin (CP-99,219), a new quinolone antibiotic, following administration of single oral doses to healthy male volunteers. *J Antimicrob Chemother* **36**: 385.

Teng R, Apseloffl G, Vincent J *et al.* (1996). Effect of trovafloxacin (CP-99,219). on the pharmacokinetics and pharmacodynamics of warfarin in healthy male subjects. In *Program and Abstracts of the 36th Interscience Conference on Antimicrobial Agents and Chemotherapy, New Orleans* (Abstr. 2). Washington, DC: American Society for Microbiology.

van Rijsoort-Vos JH, Stolz E, Verbrugh HA, Kluytmans JA (1995). *In-vitro* activity of a new quinolone (CP-99,219) compared with ciprofloxacin, pefloxacin, azithromycin and penicillin against *Neisseria gonorrhoeae*. *J Antimicrob Chemother* **36**: 215.

Grepafloxacin

Description

Grepafloxacin (OPC-17116) is a new fluoroquinolone with the chemical structure (+)-1-cyclo-propyl-6-fluoro-1,4-dihydro-5-methyl-7-(3-methyl-1-piperazinyl)-4-oxo-3-quinolone carboxylic acid hydrochloride. In comparison with earlier fluoroquinolones, grepafloxacin has enhanced activity against Gram-positive cocci such as *Streptococcus pneumoniae*, *Enterococcus* species and some strains of methicillin-resistant *Staphylococcus aureus*, but generally less activity than ciprofloxacin against many Gram-negative pathogens. Notably, grepafloxacin does not generally inhibit methicillin-resistant, ciprofloxacin-resistant strains of *Staph. aureus* or *Staph. epidermidis*. The MIC_{90} of grepafloxacin against Enterobacteriaceae, *Staph. aureus* and *Strep. pneumoniae* are ≤ 0.25, ≤ 0.25 and $0.5 \mu g$ per ml, respectively. *Haemophilus influenzae* and *Moraxella catarrhalis* are more susceptible with MIC_{90} of $\leq 0.03 \mu g$ per ml. Grepafloxacin is less active against *Pseudomonas aeruginosa* than ciprofloxacin (MIC_{90} $1 \mu g$ per ml versus $0.25 \mu g$ per ml, respectively), but more active against *Chlamydia* spp. (MIC_{90} ≤ 0.12 versus $\leq 2 \mu g$ per ml, respectively) (Imada *et al.*, 1992; Neu *et al.*, 1992; Sader *et al.*, 1992; Wise *et al.*, 1993; Pankuch *et al.*, 1995).

Grepafloxacin has intermediate activity against anaerobes, being similar to sparfloxacin, but generally having MICs one or two doubling dilutions lower than those obtained with ciprofloxacin. Against a broad range of anaerobes the MIC_{50} and MIC_{90} of grepafloxacin is 2 and $16 \mu g$ per ml, respectively Using a breakpoint of $2 \mu g$ per ml, grepafloxacin inhibits 83% of *Bacteroides fragilis* spp., compared with 6% and 0% for ciprofloxacin and fleroxacin, respectively. However, against other *B. fragilis* group anaerobes, grepafloxacin inhibits only 39% of strains (Spangler *et al.*, 1994; Wexler *et al.*, 1994); Appelbaum, 1995). Grepafloxacin is 2- to 20-fold more active *in vitro* than norfloxacin, ofloxacin, tosufloxacin and ciprofloxacin against a wide variety of common and rare *Nocardia* species, with MIC_{90} of 0.6 to $20 \mu g$ per ml (Yazawa and Mikami, 1995). The clinical efficacy of grepafloxacin in the treatment of *Nocardia* infections is yet to be determined.

The *in vitro* MICs of grepafloxacin against selected bacterial species are shown in Table II.6 (p. 987).

Grepafloxacin appears to be rapidly absorbed from the gastrointestinal tract. After a single 400-mg oral dose of grepafloxacin given to six healthy male volunteers, the mean peak plasma concentration was $1.5 \mu g$ per ml after a mean of 2.0 h post-dose. In experimentally induced blister fluid, penetration is 133–181%, with peak concentrations of $1.1 \mu g$ per ml attained after a mean of 4.8 h, but wide inter- and intrasubject variation may be noted. The mean elimination half-life in plasma is 5.2 h. Plasma and exudate concentrations generally exceed $0.5 \mu g$ per ml for more than 10–12 h after a single oral dose. Compared with ciprofloxacin and ofloxacin, excretion of grepafloxacin in urine is low, with 8.3% of the total dose recoverable from urine (Child *et al.*, 1995). Animal studies suggest that the main route of excretion is probably in the feces, possibly via the bile or by transmucosal excretion (Akiyama *et al.*, 1991). Based on the study by Child *et al.* (1995), once- or twice-daily dosage of grepafloxacin should be adequate to treat systemic infections caused by susceptible bacterial pathogens.

In preliminary reports, a 14-day course of grepafloxacin 300 mg daily is comparable with ofloxacin 200 mg thrice-daily in the treatment of pneumonia and chronic respiratory tract infections. Among patients with chronic respiratory tract infections, rates of clinical and bacteriological efficacy were 90.3% versus 90.7%, and 72.9% versus 84.2%, respectively. Adverse reactions were more common in the grepafloxacin-treated group (8.3% versus 4.1%) (Kobayashi, 1996a). Higher rates of clinical and bacteriological cure were noted in both treatment groups in patients with pneumonia (Kobayashi, 1996b). Grepafloxacin 300 mg daily may also be comparable with ofloxacin 200 mg thrice-daily in the treatment of obstetric and gynecological infections and skin and skin structure infections (Arata, 1996; Matsuda, 1996). A single 400-mg dose of grepafloxacin is as effective as a single dose of cefixime 400 mg in the treatment of uncomplicated gonococcal urethritis in males, with similar rates of clinical (99% versus 97%) and bacteriological cure (Hook *et al.*, 1996).

References

Akiyama H, Koike M, Nii S *et al.* (1991). OPC-17116, an excellently tissue penetrative new quinolone: pharmacokinetic profiles in animals and antibacterial activities of metabolites. In *Abstracts and Program of the 31st Interscience Conference on Antimicrobial Agents and Chemotherapy, Chicago, IL,* (Abstr. 1477). Washington, DC: American Society for Microbiology.

Appelbaum PC (1995). Quinolone activity against anaerobes: microbiological aspects. *Drugs* **49** (Suppl 2): 76.

Arata J (1996). A multicenter, double-blind comparative study of grepafloxacin (GPFX) versus ofloxacin in the treatment of skin and skin structure. In *Abstracts and Program of the 36th Interscience Conference on Antimicrobial Agents and Chemotherapy, New Orleans* (Abstr. LM17). Washington, DC: American Society for Microbiology.

Child J, Andrews JM, Wise R (1995). Pharmacokinetics and tissue penetration of the new fluoroquinolone grepafloxacin. *Antimicrob Ag. Chemother* **39**: 513.

Hook EW, Martin DH, Jones RB *et al.* (1996). The efficacy and safety of grepafloxacin (GREP) 400 mg single dose compared to cefixime (CFX). 400 mg single dose in the treatment of uncomplicated gonococcal urethritis in males. In *Abstracts and Program of the 36th Interscience Conference on Antimicrobial Agents and Chemotherapy, New Orleans* (Abstr. LM19). Washington, DC: American Society for Microbiology..

Imada T, Miyazaki S, Nishida M, Yamaguchi K, Goto S (1992). *In vitro* and *in vivo* antibacterial activities of a new quinolone, OPC-17116. *Antimicrob Ag Chemother* **36**: 573.

Kobayashi H (1996a). A multicenter, double-blind comparative study of grepafloxacin (GPFX) versus ofloxacin in the treatment of chronic tract respiratory infection. In *Abstracts and Program of the 36th Interscience Conference on Antimicrobial Agents and Chemotherapy, New Orleans* (Abstr. LM15). Washington, DC: American Society for Microbiology.

Kobayashi H (1996b). A multicenter, double-blind comparative study of grepafloxacin (GPFX) versus ofloxacin in the treatment of pneumonia. In *Abstracts and Program of the 36th Interscience Conference on Antimicrobial Agents and Chemotherapy, New Orleans* (Abstr. LM18). Washington, DC: American Society for Microbiology.

Matsuda S (1996). A multicenter, double-blind comparative study of grepafloxacin (GPFX) versus ofloxacin in the treatment of obstetric and gynecological infection. In *Abstracts and Program of the 36th Interscience Conference on Antimicrobial Agents and Chemotherapy, New Orleans* (Abstr. LM16). Washington, DC: American Society for Microbiology.

Neu HC, Fang W, Gu F-W, Chin N-X (1992). *In vitro* activity of OPC-17116. *Antimicrob Ag Chemother* **36**: 1310.

Pankuch GA, Jacobs MR, Appelbaum PC (1995). Activity of CP99,219 compared with DU-6859a, ciprofloxacin, ofloxacin, levofloxacin, lomefloxacin, tosufloxacin, sparfloxacin and grepafloxacin against penicillin-susceptible and -resistant pneumococci. *J Antimicrob Chemother* **35**: 230.

Sader HS, Erwin ME, Jones RN (1992). *In vitro* activity of OPC-17116 compared to other broad spectrum fluoroquinolones. *Eur J Clin Microbiol Infect Dis* **11**: 372.

Spangler SK, Jacobs MR, Appelbaum PC (1994). Activity of CP 99,219 compared with those of ciprofloxacin, grepafloxacin, metronidazole, cefoxitin, piperacillin, and piperacillin-tazobactam against 489 anaerobes. *Antimicrob Ag Chemother* **38**: 2471.

Wexler HM, Molitoris E, Finegold SM (1994). *In vitro* activity of grepafloxacin (OPC-17116) against anaerobic bacteria. *Diagn Microbiol Infect Dis* **19**: 129.

Wise R, Andrews JM, Brenwald N (1993). The *in-vitro* activity of OPC-17116, a new 5-methyl substituted quinolone. *J Antimicrob Chemother* **31**: 497.

Yazawa K, Mikami Y (1995). *In-vitro* antimicrobial activity of the new fluoroquinolone, grepafloxacin, against pathogenic *Nocardia* spp. *J Antimicrob Chemother* **35**: 541.

Part III

Drugs mainly for
Tuberculosis

Isoniazid

Description

Isoniazid, isonicotinic acid hydrazide or INAH was discovered independently in 1952 at both Squibb and Roche Laboratories (Bernstein *et al.*, 1952; Fox, 1953). Animal studies showed that isoniazid was a very potent antituberculosis drug, and subsequent clinical trials confirmed its high efficacy for the treatment of human tuberculosis (An Interim Report, 1952). Isoniazid is relatively non-toxic and cheap, and despite the development of other drugs, it remains a most valuable drug for the treatment of tuberculosis.

Sensitive Organisms

1 Mycobacterium tuberculosis

Isoniazid is highly active against *Mycobacterium tuberculosis*, most strains being inhibited by 0.05–0.20 μg per ml (Ad Hoc Committee, 1995). Strains are considered to be isoniazid-sensitive if the MIC is 0.20 μg per ml or less.

Isoniazid-resistant strains of *M. tuberculosis* can be readily produced *in vitro*, and these also occur *in vivo* if this drug is used singly for treatment of tuberculosis. In an early clinical trial in which 173 patients were treated by isoniazid alone, resistant tubercle bacilli were found in 11% of patients at the end of the first month, in 52% at the end of the second, and in 71% at the end of the third month (An Interim Report, 1952). The reason for this is that small numbers of naturally occurring drug-resistant mutants appear regularly during replication in *M. tuberculosis* populations; the larger the bacterial population and the more active its replication, the more drug-resistant mutants it will produce (Dutt and Stead, 1982). If only one antituberculosis drug is used to treat the disease, selection and multiplication of these drug-resistant mutants occurs. Fortunately naturally occurring resistance of one antituberculosis drug is independent of resistance to any other drug. This means that the likelihood of mutants resistant to two antituberculosis drugs occurring, is rare. The selection of resistant bacilli is easily avoided if two bactericidal antituberculosis drugs are used from the commencement of treatment. Antituberculosis drugs have been graded according to their ability to prevent emergence of isoniazid-resistant organisms; rifampicin has high activity, ethambutol and streptomycin moderate activity whilst pyrazinamide and thiacetazone have low activity. This ability to prevent emergence of drug-resistance has no bearing on early bactericidal or sterilizing activities of these drugs (see below) (Mitchison, 1985).

The differing actions of antituberculosis drugs, which are dependent on the metabolic activity of organisms and their environmental pH, provides a theoretical basis for modern tuberculosis chemotherapy (Fox, 1978; Dutt and Stead, 1982). Tubercle bacilli are only susceptible to drugs when they are replicating. They multiply actively in areas where the oxygen tension is high, such as extracellularly in pulmonary cavitary lesions. The large numbers of bacilli which are present in the neutral or slightly alkaline environment of such cavities are rapidly eliminated by isoniazid, rifampicin and streptomycin. Streptomycin is only active against this extracellular population; although it penetrates into macrophages it may be less effective because of intracellular acidity (Crowle *et al.*, 1984). In these lesions ethambutol and para-aminosalicylic acid (PAS) were considered only to have a bacteriostatic action. However, it seems that, similar to other antibiotics, the designation of whether a drug is bacteriostatic or bactericidal may vary with the criteria used. Jindani *et al.* (1980) investigated the bactericidal activity of drugs in patients with pulmonary tuberculosis by counting viable bacilli during the first 14 days of treatment. The most rapid fall occurred in the first 2 days probably due to killing of actively growing bacilli; during this period isoniazid had the greatest bactericidal activity followed by ethambutol and rifampicin with lesser activity; streptomycin, thiacetazone and pyrazinamide were only just bactericidal. After this early bactericidal activity, the bactericidal effect of these drugs was the same as determined by the rate of fall of counts of viable bacilli during the remainder of the 14-day period. That ethambutol was bactericidal in this study was contrary to early *in vitro* studies which indicated that it was a bacteriostatic drug. Subsequently, Crowle *et al.* (1985) demonstrated that ethambutol is mycobactericidal in human macrophages at clinically attainable concentrations.

Bacilli which multiply in macrophages or closed caseous lesions where the oxygen tension is low, are selectively killed by rifampicin and more slowly by isoniazid. Pyrazinamide usually has no activity in cavities or in the neutral environment of closed caseous lesions, but it is specifically active in the acidic interior of macrophages (p. 1219). The population of organisms which are in an acid environment may increase due to inflammatory response and thereby be available to the bactericidal action of pyrazinamide (Mitchison, 1985). A reduction in inflammatory response and a rise in pH may be reasons why pyrazinamide has little sterilizing activity after the first 2 months of short-course regimens. Rifampicin has a unique activity in closed lesions against organisms that are multiplying intermittently. Isoniazid appears to be less active than rifampicin or pyrazinamide against slowly or intermittently multiplying bacilli inside macrophages or closed caseous lesions. Ethambutol penetrates both the extracellular and intracellular environments of tuberculous lesions and can deter selection of resistant mutants.

Strains of *M. tuberculosis* resistant to isoniazid may be isolated from patients who have not received pervious treatment with this drug. Such primary drug-resistance was relatively rare in developed countries such as Britain, North America and Australia, and in these areas it did not appear to be increasing in incidence until about the mid-1980s (Miller *et al.*, 1966; Hobby *et al.*, 1974; Commonwealth, 1982; CDC, 1983a).

Primary drug-resistance to isoniazid and other antituberculosis drugs was higher in developing countries of South-East Asia, Africa, the Philippines and Latin America (Dutt and Stead, 1982). A substantial proportion of Indo-Chinese refugees in the USA with pulmonary tuberculosis had primary resistance to isoniazid and streptomycin (CDC, 1981). A high proportion of strains with primary resistance to isoniazid were detected in isolates from patients entering the USA from Haiti (Pitchenik *et al.*, 1982). Studies on *M. tuberculosis* isolates acquired in Korea showed an increased incidence of primary resistance to isoniazid, streptomycin, rifampicin and ethambutol (Carpenter *et al.*, 1982). Primary drug-resistance was more frequent amongst Asian than European patients in the UK (Yates *et al.*, 1982). One heterogenous group of strains of the tubercle bacillus has been called *Mycobacterium africanum* because of its laboratory characteristics which vary between *M. tuberculosis* and *M. bovis* (Collins *et al.*, 1984; Baril *et al.*, 1995). *Mycobacterium africanum* is widespread in Africa and comprises 15–90% of *M. tuberculosis* strains depending on the area studied. A feature of *M. africanum* has been frequent primary resistance to thiacetazone (p. 1238), but primary resistance to isoniazid, streptomycin, ethionamide, ethambutol and rifampicin has occurred in varying frequency in African countries (Toure, 1982). *Mycobacterium bovis* is usually sensitive to isoniazid, streptomycin, ethambutol and rifampicin, but resistant to pyrazinamide (Dankner *et al.*, 1993).

Secondary (acquired) drug-resistance to isoniazid develops in patients who have been treated with the drug, either singly or in combination with other drugs, and the treatment has been inappropriate or inadequate. It is usually manifested clinically as failed chemotherapy or a relapse. Some patients, particularly immigrants regarded as having primary drug-resistance, may have had acquired resistance; the prior use of antituberculosis drugs may not have been ascertained or it may not have been known to the patient. Conversely, resistance to antituberculosis drugs can develop not only in the strain that caused the initial disease, but also as a result of reinfection with a new strain of *M. tuberculosis* that is drug-resistant (Small *et al.*, 1993).

During the last decade there has been a marked increase in many parts of the world in the number of patients with tuberculosis. This has been particularly noticeable in sub-Saharan Africa, South-East Asia, Latin America and Western Pacific regions (Raviglione *et al.*, 1995). Tuberculosis and deaths from the disease are still prevalent in most countries of Eastern Europe and the former USSR (Raviglione *et al.*, 1994). In Australia (Dawson *et al.*, 1995) and the UK (Davies, 1995) there was only a minor increase in this disease during this time. In Western Europe there was some increase of the disease in some countries and decrease in others (CDC, 1993; Raviglione *et al.*, 1995), but in the USA from 1985 through 1992, the number of cases of tuberculosis increased by some 20% (Ellner *et al.*, 1993; Cantwell *et al.*, 1994).

Co-infection with HIV is a risk factor for progression of dormant tuberculosis infection to clinical disease. Also once infected with a new strain of *M. tuberculosis*, the HIV-infected person is much more likely to develop clinical disease. These factors appear to be largely responsible for the increase of tuberculosis in developing countries such as sub-Saharan Africa, South-East Asia, Latin America and Western Pacific regions (Harries, 1990; Narain *et al.*, 1992; Snider and Montagne, 1994). Co-infection with HIV has also been an important factor for the increase of tuberculosis in the USA (Chaisson *et al.*, 1987; Burwen *et al.*, 1995; Castro, 1995; Raviglione *et al.*, 1995). Studies in both New York City and San Francisco, USA, using conventional epidemiological and also molecular methods, indicated that approximately two-thirds of the patients infected with HIV acquired tuberculosis due to recent transmission rather than due to reactivation of remote infection. This to a somewhat lesser degree also applied to patients with tuberculosis who did not have HIV infection (Alland *et al.*, 1994; Hamburg and Frieden, 1994; Small *et al.*, 1994). Other factors causing an increase in tuberculosis, identified in the USA, include immigration from high-prevalence countries, increase in alcohol and drug abuse and outbreaks in congregative facilities (Ellner *et al.*, 1993; Cantwell *et al.*, 1994; McKenna *et al.*, 1995; Zaza *et al.*, 1995). The homeless population in the USA also appears to be a risk group for both HIV infection and tuberculosis (Zalopa *et al.*, 1994). In Eastern Europe poor living conditions, malnutrition and lack of crucial antituberculosis drugs appear to have caused the increased mortality and prevalence of the disease (Raviglione *et al.*, 1994).

Overall, the World Health Organisation predicted that the number of new cases of tuberculosis in the world will increase from 7.5 million in 1990 to 8.8 million in 1995 and to 10.2 million in the year 2000. Deaths attributed to tuberculosis were predicted to rise from 2.5 million in 1990 to 3.5 million by 2000. In industrialized countries most of the affected individuals are over 50 years of age but in the developing world, over 75% of tuberculosis infections occur in individuals below the age of 50 years (Dolin *et al.*, 1994; Editorial, 1994).

As the prevalence of tuberculosis increased during recent years, the isolation of isoniazid-resistant strains of *M. tuberculosis* also increased. Moreover, many strains of this organism were detected, which were resistant to isoniazid and also other antituberculosis drugs. Strains resistant to both of the best antituberculosis drugs, isoniazid and rifampicin, are referred to as multidrug-resistant, but many such strains have been resistant to other drugs as well, such as ethambutol, streptomycin, pyrazinamide and others (Riley, 1993; Bloch *et al.*, 1994; Jacobs, 1994; Sepkowitz *et al.*, 1994; Shafer *et al.*, 1995). The extent of isoniazid- and multidrug-resistant tuberculosis has been extensively studied in the USA.

Bloch *et al.* (1994) reported the sensitivities of *M. tuberculosis* strains collected from patients nationwide in the USA during the first quarter of 1991. Of the 3307 isolates tested for susceptibility to isoniazid and/or rifampicin, 315 (9.5%) were resistant to one or both drugs (with or without resistance to other drugs). A total of 187 strains (5.7%) were resistant to isoniazid, 114 (3.4%) to both isoniazid and rifampicin and 14 (0.4%) resistant to rifampicin only. The 114 multidrug-resistant isolates were reported from 13 states, but New York City accounted for 61.4% of the nation's multidrug-resistant isolates. In a study in New York City, *M. tuberculosis* strains were collected during April 1991 and 466 of these were tested; 26% of isolates were resistant to isoniazid and another 19% were resistant to both isoniazid and rifampicin (Frieden *et al.*, 1993). Other authors have also reported an increased prevalence of multidrug-resistant *M. tuberculosis* isolates in New York City in 1991, compared with 1987 (Sepkowitz *et al.*, 1994; Shafer *et al.*, 1995). Outbreaks of multidrug-resistant tuberculosis during 1990–1991 also occurred in New York State prisons (Valway *et al.*, 1994). Nosocomial transmission of multidrug-resistant tuberculosis also occurred to hospital staff and other patients, particularly those infected with HIV (Pearson *et al.*, 1992; Coronado *et al.*, 1993; Haas and Des Prez, 1994; Sepkowitz *et al.*, 1995).

The usual reasons for increased resistance to isoniazid- and multidrug-resistant *M. tuberculosis* isolates in New York City and elsewhere appeared to be an increased use of non-observed outpatient therapy of the disease with resultant poor compliance with treatment, homelessness, crowding in shelters and jails and impact of co-infection with HIV. Intravenous narcotic drug abuse appears to be a risk factor for tuberculosis in itself, but it often co-exists with other social factors and HIV-infection. The most common errors of management of these patients was the addition of one drug only to a clinically failing regimen, before results of sensitivity tests were available. This often amounted to further monotherapy and so further drug-resistance developed (Frieden *et al.*, 1993; Mahmoudi and Iseman, 1993; Bellin, 1994; Perlman *et al.*, 1995). Malabsorption of isoniazid and/or rifampicin can occur in AIDS patients, and this can also lead to drug-resistance (Patel *et al.*, 1995).

Initially it appeared that most of the patients with drug-resistant tuberculosis had acquired (secondary) drug-resistance due to inadequate therapy. However, the distinction between primary and secondary drug resistance is no longer clear-cut as exogenous reinfection with a resistant strain of *M. tuberculosis* can occur during or after treatment of the disease caused originally by a sensitive strain, particularly in AIDS patients (Small *et al.*, 1993; Horn *et al.*, 1994; Shafer *et al.*, 1995). Alland *et al.* (1994) used DNA fingerprinting and conventional epidemiological methods in New York City to distinguish recently transmitted tuberculosis from reactivation of latent disease. Recently transmitted disease accounted for approximately 40% of all patients and for almost two-thirds of drug-resistant cases. Similarly, in another study in New York City it was demonstrated that the majority of multidrug-resistant cases represented primary progressive disease due to recently transmitted isolates (Saloman *et al.*, 1995).

From 1992 through 1994, however, there was 21% decrease in the reported cases of tuberculosis in New York City. There was an even greater decreases in the number (44%) and proportion (30%) of patients who had multidrug-resistant tuberculosis. This decrease largely happened in the groups who very likely acquired the infection recently. These included the poor, some racial and ethnic minorities, patients with multidrug-resistant tuberculosis and those co-infected with AIDS. The reasons for this decrease in tuberculosis as such as well as resistant tuberculosis, appeared to be more frequent use of directly observed therapy (p. 1200), efforts to reduce the spread of the disease in institutions such as hospitals, shelters and jails and the initial use of at least four drugs for the treatment regimen (p. 1200) (Frieden *et al.*, 1995). Similarly, Weis *et al.* (1994) in North Texas, USA, demonstrated that the administration of tuberculosis chemotherapy under direct observation led to significant reductions in the frequency of drug resistance and relapse of the disease. Nationwide, in the USA from 1992 through 1994, the number of tuberculosis cases reported annually decreased by 8.7% because of similar measures as those implemented in New York City (see above) (CDC, 1995b). Based on test results for 28 states in the USA, 8% of *M. tuberculosis* strains were resistant to isoniazid and 2% were resistant to both isoniazid and rifampicin in 1994 (CDC, 1995a).

In the UK *M. tuberculosis* strains resistant to isoniazid and streptomycin have been detected, particularly in the elderly, but resistance to rifampicin as well has been uncommon. Co-infection with HIV has not yet been a major factor in the development of drug-resistant tuberculosis in the UK (Uttley and Pozniak, 1993; Davies 1994; 1995). Resistance in *M. tuberculosis* to isoniazid and streptomycin, and in some cases to rifampicin as well has been reported from France, and in some patients co-infection with HIV was a factor (Heym *et al.*, 1994). In Italy a higher proportion of AIDS patients, than in other industrialized countries, developed tuberculosis (Girardi *et al.*, 1994) and the *M. tuberculosis* strains were not uncommonly resistant to isoniazid and less commonly to rifampicin as well (Monno *et al.*, 1993). A high initial and acquired drug-resistance (to isoniazid, rifampicin and other antituberculosis drugs) has been reported in patients with pulmonary tuberculosis in Turkey (Tahaoglu *et al.*, 1994). The extent of antituberculosis drug-resistance in Eastern Europe and the former USSR is not well known, but a high resistance rate has been reported from West Kazakhstan – 20% of *M. tuberculosis* strains were resistant to isoniazid, 19% to rifampicin, 45% to ethambutol and 66% to streptomycin (Burns *et al.*, 1994). In Australia antituberculosis drug-resistance is still relatively uncommon, compared with that in some other countries. During 1989–1992 streptomycin-resistance was detected in 7.6% of isolates, isoniazid resistance in 8.4%, rifampicin-resistance was rare and fewer than 1.0% of isolates were resistant to isoniazid and rifampicin in combination (Dawson *et al.*, 1995; Lim, 1995). However, in 1993, 1.5% of isolates were resistant to both isoniazid and rifampicin (Gilbert, 1996).

In a study in Ryadh, Saudi Arabia, drug-resistance to isoniazid was most common (19.4%) followed to that by rifampicin and streptomycin. The prevalence of primary and acquired rifampicin-resistance was 3 and 33.7%, respectively (Al-Orainey *et al.*, 1989). In Korea the resistance of *M. tuberculosis* isolates to one or more antituberculosis drugs was as high as 48% in 1980, but this decreased to 25.3% and this decrease coincided with increase in treatment efficacy (Kim and Hong, 1992).

It may be expected that isoniazid and other antituberculosis drug-resistance may be high in developing countries, especially in Africa, where there is frequent co-infection of tuberculosis and HIV (Narain *et al.*, 1992). Rodier *et al.* (1993) found a high rate of resistance to most antituberculosis drugs (71.4% to isoniazid, 68.8% to ethambutol, 67.5% to streptomycin and 51.9% to rifampicin) from patients in Djibouti in the Horn of Africa, but in a study from Zambia only 5% of isolates were resistant to isoniazid and rifampicin resistance was not detected. All these patients had both tuberculosis and HIV infection (Elliott *et al.*, 1993). In another study in the same country drug-resistance was also uncommon: only 2% of isolates were resistant to isoniazid alone and 2.4% to streptomycin alone. Only one isolate (0.1%) was resistant to rifampicin (Drobniewski *et al.*, 1994). Resistance to isoniazid and other antituberculosis drugs was also rare in Zaire (Perriëns *et al.*, 1995). Similarly, isolates of *M. tuberculosis*, resistant to isoniazid and other drugs were uncommon in Kenya (Hawken *et al.*, 1993). In contrast, there was high drug-resistance of *M. tuberculosis* isolates in Ghana: 27% to isoniazid, 23% to streptomycin and 29% to thiacetazone. Primary drug-resistance to rifampicin, pyrazinamide or ethambutol was not observed (Van der Werf *et al.*, 1989).

Isoniazid- and/or streptomycin-resistant strains of *M. tuberculous* occur in India, but rifampicin-resistance is probably less frequent (Tub Res Centre, Madras/Nat Tub Inst, Bangalore, 1986; Santha *et al.*, 1989; Gangadharam, 1994). Haitian immigrants entering the USA, with pulmonary tuberculosis, underwent drug susceptibility studies between 1991–1993 (Malone *et al.*, 1994) and again a new cohort of immigrants were similarly screened in 1994 (Rusnak *et al.*, 1995). In both studies the *M. tuberculosis* isolates showed approximately 20% resistance to isoniazid and infrequent resistance to streptomycin and ethambutol. Only one patient in the second study had combined isoniazid/rifampicin-resistance. In general, however, our current knowledge about the nature and extent of drug-resistance of *M. tuberculosis* in the developing world is incomplete. Obviously in these countries it is not possible to carry out routine sensitivity tests for all new patients with tuberculosis ((Shimao, 1987; Nunn and Felten, 1994).

There is still incomplete understanding of the mode of action of isoniazid on *M. tuberculosis* (p. 1187) and so the mechanisms involved in isoniazid-resistance are also not completely known (Jacobs, 1994). Rapid reliable methods for detection of isoniazid-resistance such as polymerase chain reaction (PCR) and single-strand conformation polymorphism (SSCP) analysis are not yet very accurate for detection of isoniazid-resistance. These methods only detect isoniazid resistance with about 78% efficacy, whilst they have 97% success in detecting rifampicin-resistance (p. 678) (Altamirano *et al.*, 1994; Heym *et al.*, 1994; Rouse *et al.*, 1995). There are some known genetic markers in strains of isoniazid-resistant *M. tuberculosis*. For instance, the catalase-peroxidase enzyme of *M. tuberculosis*, encoded by the *kat G* gene, mediates susceptibility to isoniazid and this gene is deleted or mutated in some, but not all, highly isoniazid-resistant isolates (MIC $\geq 1.0\,\mu g$ per ml). However, isolates with low-level isoniazid resistance rarely have a deletion of the *kat G* gene (Stoeckle *et al.*, 1993; Cockerill *et al.*, 1995; Ferrazoli *et al.*, 1995; Pretorius *et al.*, 1995). In addition, a mutation in the *inh A* gene, which encodes an enoyl acid reductase involved in mycolyc acid biosynthesis, can be detected in some isoniazid-resistant *M. tuberculosis* strains. This finding is in keeping with the hypothesis that isoniazid inhibits an enzyme involved in biosynthesis of mycolic acid for the mycobacterial cell wall (Quémard *et al.*, 1991; Morris *et al.*, 1995; Rouse *et al.*, 1995). However, these two mechanisms do not account for all isoniazid-resistant isolates, and so other unknown resistance mechanisms are also involved (Jacobs, 1994; Zhang and Young, 1994; Rouse *et al.*, 1995).

Bacille Calmette-Guérin (BCG) organisms are usually susceptible to the major antituberculosis drugs including isoniazid. A persisting finger infection due to accidental inoculation with BCG has been described which was caused by a strain resistant to isoniazid (Lorber *et al.*, 1977).

2 Atypical mycobacteria

Organisms of this group (p. 1211) are usually isoniazid-resistant. In comparison with *M. tuberculosis*, the frequency of naturally occurring resistance to antituberculosis drugs is much higher in wild strains of *M. kansasii*, *M. avium* complex and *M. fortuitum* (Hejný, 1982) (p. 1211). Isoniazid plus streptomycin show synergistic activity *in vitro* and *in vivo* in animals against *M. avium* complex, but the clinical significance of this is not clear (Reddy *et al.*, 1994). Of these mycobacteria, *M. kansasii* and *M. xenopi* are the most sensitive to antimicrobial agents and both may be sensitive to isoniazid (David, 1981; Weber *et al.*, 1989). In *in vitro* testing against *M. kansasii*, a combination of streptomycin and isoniazid was better than streptomycin, isoniazid or ethambutol, used alone or in any other combination (Tsang *et al.*, 1978). Other studies indicate that triple-drug combinations including rifampicin are more effective against this organism (p. 1211). Isoniazid is inactive against *M. ulcerans*.

Mode of Administration and Dosage

1 Daily administration

Isoniazid is nearly always administered by the oral route; it is very soluble in water and practically insoluble in lipid solvents. Factors which influence the absorption of isoniazid from the upper gastrointestinal tract have been discussed by Männistö *et al.* (1982). Both food and antacids reduce its bioavailability. All types of food, especially those containing carbohydrates, impair absorption of isoniazid both in slow and rapid acetylators (p. 1186). This may be partly due to delay in gastric emptying but it is more likely to be due to the formation of unabsorbable condensation products between isoniazid and various sugars. It is therefore advisable to administer isoniazid in the fasting state. Isoniazid should also be given at least 1 h before, or 2 h after, the administration of antacids, such as aluminum hydroxide (Hurwitz and Schlozman, 1974). This effect is not due to decreased acidity in the stomach as H_2 blockers such as cimetidine and ranitidine do not impair isoniazid absorption. Isoniazid bioavailability is also unaffected by the antacids in didanosine tablets when the two medications are administrated simultaneously to HIV-infected patients (Gallicano *et al.*, 1994). However, malabsorption of isoniazid can occur in AIDS patients, especially if they have enteropathy and this can lead to inadequate treatment of tuberculosis and emergence of drug-resistance (Patel *et al.*, 1995).

The usual adult dosage of isoniazid is 5 mg per per kg body weight per day (maximum 300 mg daily) which is commonly given as a single dose. For severely ill patients with miliary disease or tuberculosis meningitis, this dose may be doubled for the first few weeks of treatment. In children a dosage of 10–20 mg per per kg per day is recommended (Ad Hoc Committee, 1995). For most children the daily dosage of 10 mg per per kg (300 mg maximum) is sufficient (CDC, 1980b), and the higher dosage of 20 mg per per kg per day is appropriate for the treatment of severe disease such as tuberculous meningitis (Donald *et al.*, 1987).

When the drug is administered daily, it is not necessary to determine whether patients are slow or rapid inactivators of isoniazid (p. 1186), because with usual daily doses results of treatment have been satisfactory in both groups (Ellard, 1984).

2 Intermittent administration

Regimens of thrice-weekly, twice-weekly or once-weekly administration of antituberculosis drugs, given under close supervision, have been introduced in an attempt to obviate the unreliable self-administration of these drugs over prolonged periods, particularly in developing countries (Fox and Mitchison, 1975). Intermittent chemotherapy is equally as effective as daily drug administration (p. 1183); it is usually cheaper and sometimes may be less toxic. The dose of isoniazid for twice- and thrice-weekly regimens in adults is 15 mg per per kg body weight (maximum 900 mg). For children this is 20–40 mg per per kg body weight (maximum 900 mg) (Castelo *et al.*, 1989; Cohn *et al.*, 1990; Ad Hoc Committee, 1995). The clinical efficacy of twice-weekly regimens containing isoniazid is usually not affected by the patient's acetylator phenotype (Ellard, 1984).

Although the antituberculosis drug ethambutol (p. 1213) can be administered safely and effectively in increased doses once a week, there have been difficulties in adapting isoniazid to such a regimen (Ellard, 1984). For instance, isoniazid used in a dose of 13–17 mg per per kg once-weekly was unsatisfactory, because resistant organisms emerged in some patients, especially in those who were rapid isoniazid inactivators (p. 1186) (Tub Chemother Centre, 1973b; WHO Prague, 1977). Similarly, once-weekly regimens of ethambutol plus isoniazid (15 mg per per kg) (Tuberculosis Research/Madras, 1981) and rifampicin plus isoniazid (Singapore/BMRC, 1977) were unsatisfactory due to the poor efficacy of isoniazid in rapid inactivators. Alternatively, increasing the once-weekly isoniazid dose to 30 mg per per kg body weight may cause acute toxicity, especially in patients who inactivate the drug slowly. Where it is practicable to investigate the patient's inactivator status, streptomycin plus isoniazid could be administered once-weekly to slow inactivators and twice-weekly to rapid inactivators (Fox, 1968; WHO Prague, 1977). Slow-release isoniazid formulations (either enteric-coated tablets or isoniazid-matrix preparations) were developed in an attempt to overcome these difficulties. Pharmacological studies in humans (Ellard *et al.*, 1972, 1973; Sarma *et al.*, 1975) and a trial on Indian patients with tuberculosis (Santha *et al.*, 1976), indicated that the administration of a slow-release preparation of isoniazid (matrix isoniazid) once-weekly was feasible. Matrix isoniazid in a dose of 35 mg per per kg body weight in slow inactivators and 50 mg per per kg in rapid inactivators, produces peak serum levels similar to those obtained with a non-toxic dose of ordinary isoniazid (15 mg per per kg) in slow inactivators; matrix isoniazid in a lower dose of 30 mg per per kg in rapid inactivators, however, produced substantially lower serum levels (Sarma *et al.*, 1975). A 6-month trial of matrix isoniazid in Indian patients with tuberculosis in a dose of 50 mg per per kg for rapid inactivators (27 patients) and 35 mg per per kg for slow inactivators (37 patients), each given weekly with streptomycin 1 g, demonstrated that these regimens were tolerated by most patients (Santha *et al.*, 1976). Other studies using a slow-release form of matrix isoniazid in Czechoslovakian patients resulted in an unacceptable level of adverse reactions in both rapid and slow inactivators (WHO Prague, 1977). There is also considerable individual variation among rapid inactivators, and therefore one standard isoniazid slow-release formula and dosage may not be suitable for all patients who inactivate the drug rapidly.

3 Patients with renal failure

Some active isoniazid is excreted via the kidney, so that the drug accumulates and some dosage reduction may be necessary in patients with moderate or severe renal failure (Kovnat et al., 1973). Significant amounts of isoniazid are removed by peritoneal dialysis and hemodialysis (Bennett et al., 1977). Cheigh (1977) recommended that the usual dose of 300 mg per day may be given to patients with mild renal failure and to patients undergoing dialysis; those with severe disease not receiving dialysis or those who are slow acetylators should be given 200–300 mg per day. However, Usuda and Sekine (1978) found that most patients on dialysis treated with customary doses of isoniazid developed peripheral neuritis (p. 1189); they considered that a safe effective dose of isoniazid was 5 mg per per kg per day, three times per week for patients on dialysis. It has also been recommended that where possible the dose of isoniazid should be adjusted according to monitored serum levels in patients with renal disease. Mitchison and Ellard (1980) disagreed with these views; they believed that there was no justification for giving renal failure patients less than the standard dosage of 300 mg daily, particularly since 200 mg per day was less efficacious and peripheral neuropathy could be prevented by giving vitamin B_6 (p. 1189). They also considered that serum monitoring of isoniazid levels which require special expertise, was not essential. The half-life of isoniazid in slow acetylators is only increased by about 30% in the event of almost complete renal failure; this is unlikely to cause significantly elevated toxicity, so that isoniazid dosage reduction or determination of acetylator phenotype are unnecessary in patients with impaired renal function (Ellard, 1984). However, Cheung et al. (1993) described encephalopathy in three dialysis patients treated by usual isoniazid doses. This resolved in all patients when the drug was ceased and in two patients confusion recurred on rechallenge with isoniazid. Serum isoniazid levels were not measured.

4 Pregnant patients

Isoniazid can be safely used in pregnant patients (Ludford et al., 1973; Schaefer et al., 1975). Supplemental pyridoxine therapy is recommended for them (p. 1189).

5 Parenteral administration

A solution containing 100 mg per ml suitable for i.m. or i.v. administration is available; this is effective and it is only rarely used, when oral administration is not feasible.

Serum Levels in Relation to Dosage

Isoniazid is very well absorbed from the gastrointestinal tract, and the peak serum level is reached 1–2 h after administration. After a single large dose of 12.5 mg per per kg body weight (800–1000 mg in an adult), the peak level is 10–15 μg per ml. A similar peak serum level is attained by all patients at this time, but 4–6 h after administration serum levels differ according to whether the subject is a rapid or slow isoniazid inactivator. In the former, serum levels at 6 h approach zero, whilst in the latter a level of 5 μg per ml is still present (Fig. III.1). The serum half-life of isoniazid in slow inactivators is 2–4 h and that in rapid inactivators 0.5–1.5 h (Bennett et al., 1977).

Evans et al. (1960) studied isoniazid serum levels in 484 subjects 6 h after the administration of a single dose of 9.8–10 mg per per kg body weight. The frequency distribution curve for these values showed two peaks, separated by a trough (an antimode) at 2.5 μg per ml. Persons with serum isoniazid concentrations less than this value (most commonly about 1.0 μg per ml) were classified as rapid inactivators, whereas those with serum levels higher than 2.5 (most commonly 4.5 μg per ml) as slow inactivators.

Serum levels are lower with the smaller doses which are commonly used for daily chemotherapy, and halving the dose approximately halves the serum levels. For instance, after the usual adult dose of 5 mg per per kg body weight (usually 300 mg), the peak serum level is approximately 5 μg per ml, 1–2 h after administration (Ad Hoc Committee, 1995).

After a 300-mg dose to adults in the fasting state, a peak serum level of about 7 μg per ml occurs; after 8 h the level is usually above 1 μg per ml in slow acetylators, but it is negligible in rapid acetylators. Following this dose, the peak serum level of acetyl isoniazid (p. 1186) reaches about 4 μg per ml and is about 2 μg per ml after 8 h in rapid acetylators; these levels are halved in slow acetylators (Männistö et al., 1982). Serum levels after i.m. administration are similar to those after oral administration in children (Olson et al., 1981).

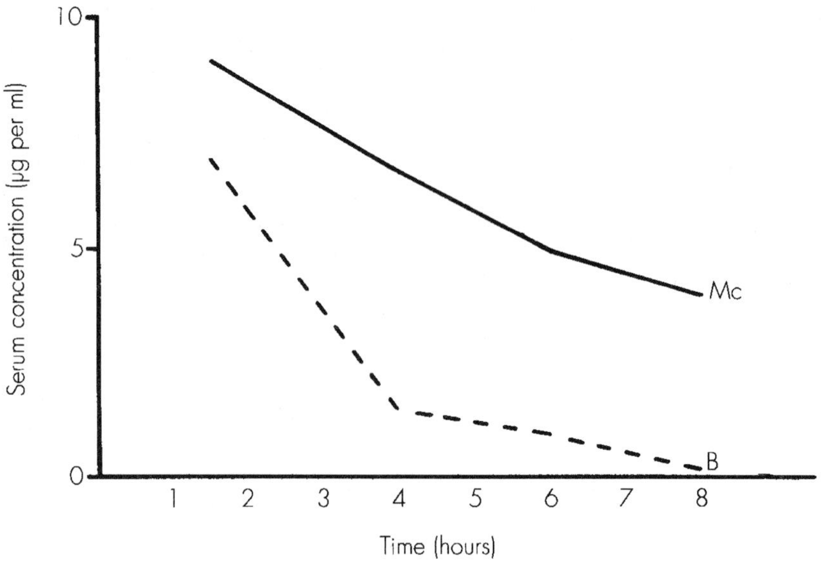

Fig. III.1.
Serum concentrations in patients after a single 800-mg isoniazid dose (Mc-slow inactivator; B-rapid inactivator). (Redrawn after Short, 1962, with permission.)

The serum half-life in slow acetylators is about 3.8 h and this is prolonged to 4.9 h in patients with renal failure (Mitchison and Ellard, 1980). The serum half-life is shorter in rapid acetylators due to the more rapid inactivation of the drug (see above).

Excretion

1 Urine

Some unchanged active isoniazid is excreted via the kidney, and the amount excreted in the first 1–2 h after administration is about the same in all subjects. Slow inactivators excrete about 10-fold more active isoniazid in the urine compared with rapid inactivators from about the 6th hour after administration (Short, 1962). Approximately 70% of administered isoniazid is excreted via the kidney, but most of this is in an inactive form. The main inactive substances excreted are acetyl isoniazid and isonicotinic acid, but there are others such as hydrazones of isoniazid (Robson and Sullivan, 1963) (see below). Fast inactivators excrete approximately 94% of isoniazid as acetyl isoniazid and its metabolites and only 2.8% and 3.6% as free isoniazid and isoniazid hydrazone conjugates, respectively. In contrast, slow inactivators excrete almost 37% of the drug as either free isoniazid or its hydrazone conjugates and only 63% as acetyl isoniazid and its metabolites of isonicotinic acid and monoacetylhydrazine (Mitchell *et al.*, 1976).

2 Inactivation in body

The metabolism of isoniazid has been extensively studied in man and animals (Hughes, 1953; Ellard, 1984). The main method by which it is inactivated in man is acetylation in the liver by an enzyme N-acetyl transferase which converts it to acetyl isoniazid, which in turn is split to form monoacetylhydrazine and isonicotinic acid; monoacetylhydrazine is then acetylated to diacetylhydrazine and isonicotinic acid is conjugated to form isonicotinylglycine. Isoniazid is also partly conjugated directly to form acid-labile hydrazones. Non-acetylated isoniazid is excreted in the urine, either unchanged or as its hydrazone conjugates. The rate at which humans acetylate isoniazid is genetically controlled, and accordingly they can be broadly classified as slow or rapid isoniazid inactivators or acetylators (Peters *et al.*, 1965). Slow inactivators are autosomal homozygous recessives, and rapid inactivators either heterozygous or homozygous dominants (Evans *et al.*, 1960; Harris, 1963). The acetylation rate is about 5-fold greater in heterozygous rapid inactivators and about 10-fold greater in homozygous rapid inactivators than in slow inactivators (Ellard, 1984). The amount of isoniazid acetylation metabolites in the urine reflects the acetylator status of the person (see below). Isoniazid and sulfonamides are acetylated in the liver by similar enzymatic processes, and so an individual is either a slow or rapid inactivator of both of these drugs (Rao *et al.*, 1970) (p. 814). Over 90% of Orientals are genetically rapid inactivators compared with only 45% black and white Americans (Mitchell *et al.*, 1976). There were an equal number of slow and fast inactivators in Australia (Birkett and Pond, 1975). There have been many studies to determine the proportion of the two acetylator phenotypes in different parts of the world (Ellard, 1984). Some 50–60% of subjects of South Indian, European or Negro origin are slow acetylators; among the Chinese, Eskimos and Japanese the proportion of slow acetylators varies from 5% to 22%.

In clinical practice when the drug is administered daily, there is little need to determine the patient's inactivator status (p. 1183). On theoretical grounds it may be expected that rapid inactivators would require higher doses of isoniazid. When isoniazid was combined with PAS in standard doses, clinical results were not influenced by the patient's isoniazid inactivation phenotype (Harris, 1963). Also in children with primary tuberculosis, in whom isoniazid was used as a single drug for preventive treatment (p. 1201), results were about the same in both phenotype groups (Mount *et al.*, 1961). Nevertheless, peripheral neuritis due to isoniazid (p. 1189) appears to be related to high serum levels of the active drug, and is more common in slow isoniazid inactivators (Evans *et al.*, 1960; Harris, 1963).

If isoniazid is included in once-weekly intermittent regimens, to ensure its effectiveness, it is important to determine the patient's inactivator status (p. 1186). Several simple laboratory methods have been described for this purpose (Ellard, 1984).

Higher active isoniazid serum levels were demonstrated when PAS and isoniazid are administered together, suggesting that PAS may inhibit isoniazid acetylation (Lauener and Favez, 1959). This was not confirmed by others (Robson and Sullivan, 1963).

When a 20 mg dose of prednisolone was administered with isoniazid (10 mg per per kg), serum isoniazid levels were reduced by 25% in slow inactivators and by 40% in rapid inactivators (Sarma *et al.*, 1980). This appeared to be due to enhancement of both the rate of acetylation and the renal clearance of isoniazid in slow inactivators and only due to increased renal clearance in rapid inactivators. Rifampicin (p. 691), a known inducer of hepatic microsomal enzymes, did not affect isoniazid serum levels when used concomitantly in a dose of 12 mg per per kg. However, when rifampicin, isoniazid and prednisolone were used together, rifampicin counteracted the prednisolone effect of lowering isoniazid serum levels in rapid inactivators, presumably by inducing enzymes which catabolize prednisolone. This effect of rifampicin did not occur in slow inactivators. These drug interactions may be very complex, because isoniazid may have a marginal effect of lowering rifampicin serum levels (p. 691). In the study by Sarma *et al.* (1980) prednisolone had no effect on the therapeutic response of patients, but this could be a factor if isoniazid was used in lower doses.

Distribution of the Drug in Body

After absorption isoniazid is widely distributed in body fluids and tissues (Harris, 1963; Robson and Sullivan, 1963). Concentrations of the drug in the CSF of normal patients and those with tuberculous meningitis are approximately the same as those in the serum (Forgan-Smith *et al.*, 1973). Adequate concentrations of isoniazid occur in pleural effusions, saliva and in all body tissues and are similar to serum levels (Gurumurthy *et al.*, 1990; Ad Hoc Committee, 1995). The drug readily penetrates into caseous tissue, and by its entry into macrophages it has some activity against intracellular tubercle bacilli (Hand *et al.*, 1983; Dhillon and Mitchison, 1989). It easily crosses the placenta and is excreted in human milk. Serum protein binding is less than 10% (Bennett *et al.*, 1977).

Mode of Action

Isoniazid has a bactericidal action on *M. tuberculosis*, but how this occurs, is still not fully understood (Jacobs, 1994). The drug has been reported to affect virtually every aspect of mycobacterial metabolism. Isoniazid inhibits the synthesis of mycolic acids in *M. tuberculosis* by affecting an enzyme mycolase synthetase, which is unique for mycobacteria; but this cannot be assumed to be the main mechanism of its action (Takayama *et al.*, 1972; Wang and Takayama, 1972; Quémard *et al.*, 1991). Some genetic markers have been detected in a proportion of isoniazid-resistant *M. tuberculosis* strains (p. 1183), but these findings do not completely explain the resistance mechanisms nor the mode of action of the drug.

Toxicity

Isoniazid has relatively low toxicity and can be used safely in pregnancy (p. 1185).

1 Gastrointestinal side-effects

These are very uncommon, but nausea, vomiting and diarrhea may occur if very large doses, such as 20 mg per per kg body weight per day are given (Robson and Sullivan, 1963). Matrix isoniazid preparations may also cause gastrointestinal symptoms (Parthasarathy *et al.*, 1976).

2 Hypersensitivity reactions

These are uncommon with isoniazid and are more frequent with streptomycin (p. 423), PAS (p. 1225) and thiacetazone (p. 1239). Manifestations are diverse, but they usually take the form of fever and a maculopapular rash. Such reactions due to isoniazid and also due to rifampicin may be more frequent in HIV-infected patients (Chaisson et al., 1987; Small et al., 1991). These may be minor and self-limiting so that therapy need not be interrupted. With more severe reactions the drug must be stopped. Often reactions occur when two or more antituberculosis drugs are being used at the same time. In this situation all drug therapy should cease and the drug causing the reaction should be established by sequential challenge (Girling, 1982). Drug challenge should be carried out in the order of drugs with an increasing likelihood of causing a reaction, isoniazid having the least propensity. Suggested challenge doses and the order of challenge are shown in Table III.1.

Smaller challenge doses (1/10 of those for day 1) are recommended if the reaction was severe. If there is no reaction to challenge doses, the drug can be continued in full dosage. If isoniazid is incriminated, and the reaction is not serious, then in contrast to PAS (p. 1226), desensitization is advisable because the drug is valuable. Desensitization is accomplished by giving a course of gradually increasing doses of the drug over several weeks until the full dose is reached. The course can be started by using the largest challenge dose which does not cause a reaction; doses are then given twice-daily and increments can be a doubling of the previous dose, but if reactions occur, slower increases should be employed. During desensitization, two other effective antituberculosis drugs to which the patient is not hypersensitive, should also be administered to prevent the emergence of acquired drug-resistance (p. 1179). Desensitization may be done under corticosteroid cover if the reaction is severe or if the patient is hypersensitive to more than one drug. Corticosteroids may be used also to allow rapid desensitization if the severity of the patient's disease requires that the drug be resumed rapidly. Isoniazid and other antituberculosis drugs may be continued in the usual doses and reactions may be suppressed by corticosteroids. The dose of corticosteroids is gradually reduced over about 2 months. This form of desensitization may be employed in patients severely ill with tuberculous meningitis, in whom isoniazid is essential. Desensitization should not be attempted (even under corticosteroid cover) in patients with severe exfoliative dermatitis (Girling, 1982).

One patient who developed acute meningoencephalitis on readministration of isoniazid and in whom hypersensitivity meningitis was postulated as the cause, has been described (Garagusi et al., 1976). Stevens–Johnson syndrome associated with isoniazid administration and which recurred when a test dose of the drug was given after the patient had fully recovered, has also been described (Bomb et al., 1976). Febrile reactions without other manifestations of hypersensitivity occurring 1–3 weeks after commencement of treatment have been described when isoniazid was used alone for preventive treatment (Davis and Stoler, 1977). Coombs' positive hemolytic anemia, vasculitis, and neutropenia have been ascribed to isoniazid (Jenkins et al., 1980; Young et al., 1982).

3 Neurotoxicity

This is due to the effects of isoniazid on the vitamin B_6 group (pyridoxine) metabolism. The B_6 group is rapidly converted in the body to the coenzymes pyridoxal phosphate and pyridoxamine phosphate, which are essential for protein metabolism. Vitamin B_6 is also a cofactor in the production of amines which act as synaptic transmitters in various brain areas, and it is also

Table III.1.

Challenge doses and order of drug challenge for detecting hypersensitivity to antituberculosis drugs. (After Girling, 1982.)

| Drug | Challenge doses | |
	Day 1	Day 2
Isoniazid	50 mg	300mg
Rifampicin	75 mg	300 mg
Pyrazinamide	250 mg	1.0 g
Ethionamide, prothionamide	125 mg	375 mg
Cycloserine	125 mg	250 mg
Ethambutol	100 mg	500 mg
PAS	1.0 g	5.0 g
Thiacetazone	25 mg	50 mg
Streptomycin and other aminoglycosides	125 mg	500 mg

necessary for the formation of the inhibitory transmitter gamma-aminobutyric acid (Snider, 1980). Isoniazid can cause vitamin B_6 deficiency by the formation of hydrazones which inhibit the conversion of pyridoxine to pyridoxal phosphate and which also inactivate the latter. Isoniazid has a further action of lowering effective tissue and serum levels of pyridoxine through the formation of these isoniazid-pyridoxine hydrazones, which are rapidly excreted by the kidney (Miller et al., 1980; Atkins, 1982).

Peripheral neuropathy may occur during isoniazid therapy. In the early stages this is characterized by parasthesiae in the 'stocking-glove' distribution but it may progress to sensory loss and muscle paralysis. Neuropathy is more likely if high doses of isoniazid are used (Snider, 1980). It is uncommon in patients treated by the recommended doses of isoniazid (300 mg daily or 15 mg per per kg two or three times per week). Patients who may be mildly pyridoxine-deficient are also at a greater risk of developing peripheral neuropathy; these include pregnant women, cancer patients, uremic patients, malnourished patients, chronic alcoholics, patients with chronic liver disease and the aged (Snider, 1980; Girling, 1982). Numerous studies have demonstrated that peripheral neuropathy is more common in slow acetylators of isoniazid (p. 1186) (Snider, 1980). Isoniazid-induced neuropathy can be prevented (even with high-dosage isoniazid therapy) by small doses of pyridoxine such as 10–25 mg per day. High doses of pyridoxine should be avoided because of the possibility that they may reduce the antibacterial activity of isoniazid. If neuropathy develops it can be treated successfully by pyridoxine doses of 100–200 mg daily, without interrupting isoniazid administration (Girling, 1982). Pyridoxine is not routinely given to patients taking the recommended isoniazid dosage because peripheral neuropathy is uncommon and if it occurs, it is easily recognized and treated. Supplemental pyridoxine (10 mg per day) is usually given to malnourished patients, pregnant patients, alcoholics and aged patients; patients with uremia and diabetes, diseases which may also predispose to neuropathy, are often given pyridoxine to avoid diagnostic confusion (Bailey et al., 1983). Snider (1980) also suggests that pyridoxine should be routinely administered to patients with a seizure disorder, because pyridoxine deficiency can cause convulsions, some seizure disorders are pyridoxine-responsive and anti-epileptic drugs may lead to pyridoxine deficiency. In the USA a tablet containing isoniazid and 10 mg of vitamin B_6 has been available for this purpose. Atkins (1982) showed that pregnant patients taking isoniazid who were also given supplemental doses of vitamin B_6 of 52–60 mg per day, had adequate serum pyridoxal phosphate levels. They did not ascertain the minimum dosage of vitamin B_6 to maintain these levels.

Psychosis, confusion, coma, convulsions and death may occur if toxic serum levels of isoniazid are attained, such as in accidental poisoning, attempted suicide, or rarely with ordinary doses in uremic patients (p. 1185). A dose of 2–3 g is potentially toxic and 10–15 g produces a high fatality rate (Sievers et al., 1982). These symptoms do not usually occur if the drug is used in its recommended dosage. Acute toxicity is extremely rare if dosage does not exceed about 17 mg per per kg per day, and since peak concentrations of isoniazid attained in slow acetylators only exceed those in rapid acetylators by about 25%, the risk of such toxicity is probably similar in the two phenotypes (Ellard, 1984). Other features of isoniazid poisoning are nausea, vomiting, hypotension, leukocytosis, hyperpyrexia and respiratory distress. Metabolic changes consisting of acidosis, ketonuria, hyperglycemia and mild hyperkalemia also occur because of complex alterations in pyridoxine metabolism. Interference with the formation of the inhibitory neurotransmitter gamma-aminobutyric acid, may partly explain the intractable seizures caused by isoniazid intoxication (Miller et al., 1980). Isoniazid overdosage has been reported to respond promptly to therapy with pyridoxine (Wason et al., 1981; Sievers et al., 1982). Pyridoxine is given by slow i.v. injection or i.v. infusion in a dose equal to the estimated overdose of isoniazid. A dose of 5 g pyridoxine i.v. has been recommended for isoniazid overdosage even if seizures have not occurred or the amount of isoniazid ingested is unknown (Sievers et al., 1982).

In Indian patients, doses of 30 mg per kg of matrix isoniazid are well tolerated. Higher doses of this preparation caused dizziness, which was dose-related, late in onset and usually present even 24 h later (Parthasarathy et al., 1976). When the matrix preparation was given to Indian patients in doses of 50 and 36 mg per kg to rapid and slow inactivators, respectively, the dose had to be modified in a small number because of giddiness (Santha et al., 1976).

Minor neurotoxic symptoms, such as muscle twitchings, restlessness and insomnia, may occur with ordinary isoniazid doses. The drug may also precipitate convulsions in stabilized epileptics (see above) and urinary retention in the elderly. Convulsions respond to anticonvulsants and i.v. pyridoxine in a dose of 100 mg (Girling, 1982). Loss of memory, sometimes quite disabling, has also been noted (Leading article, 1969).

Pellagra (niacin deficiency) may occur as a side-effect of isoniazid unless supplementary vitamin B_6 is given. This may be due to the inhibition of an enzyme (kynureninase) which is involved in the synthesis of nicotinamide nucleotide from tryptophan. Isoniazid interferes with pyridoxal phosphate (see above) which is a cofactor for kynureninase. Bender and Russell-Jones (1979) described a patient, a vegan treated by isoniazid who developed pellagra despite adequate vitamin B_6 supplements, and who recovered after treatment with 150 mg nicotinamide daily. They attributed the onset of pellagra to a marginal intake of tryptophan and niacin in a strict vegetarian even though vitamin B_6 was given with isoniazid.

4 Hepatoxicity

Originally it was considered that liver damage due to isoniazid was rare, mild and transient. It is now apparent that isoniazid frequently causes asymptomatic hepatoxicity and that it is an occasional cause of severe clinical hepatitis. Prior to the widespread use of isoniazid for preventive therapy, hepatotoxicity was probably attributed to other antituberculosis drugs, all of which, with the possible exception of streptomycin, can cause hepatitis.

The risk of developing clinical hepatitis, particularly fatal hepatitis, during what was once regarded as standard chemotherapy of tuberculosis based on isoniazid, was very small. In the period 1953–1973, a large number of clinical trials using various regimens containing isoniazid, were carried out in Europe, Asia Minor, India, Africa, the Pacific and the Far East. The companion drugs used were streptomycin, PAS and thiacetazone. Hepatitis was uncommon and in general the incidence was less than 2%, but routine liver function tests were only performed in a small number of trials. Many cases of hepatitis were probably not due to drug therapy. In drug-induced cases of hepatitis, PAS or thiacetazone seemed more likely causes than isoniazid; the incidence of hepatitis was higher when PAS and thiacetazone were used than when isoniazid was given alone or with streptomycin (Girling, 1978).

When rifampicin (p. 686) became available as a first-line antituberculosis drug, there was concern that a rifampicin/isoniazid combination might be more hepatotoxic. Some early relatively small studies seemed to confirm this (Lees et al., 1971; Lal et al., 1972; Ravikrishnan et al., 1977). Severe hepatotoxicity was also described in children treated by an isoniazid/rifampicin combination (Casteels-van Daele et al., 1975; Bistritzer et al., 1980). In the USA, the reported rate of hepatotoxicity for adults receiving isoniazid/rifampicin was 3.9% or less and that for children 3.2% (Cross et al., 1980; CDC, 1980c; O'Brien et al., 1983). Most of the children who showed hepatotoxicity had received doses in excess of those recommended for isoniazid (10 mg per per kg) and rifampicin (15 mg per per kg) (Donald et al., 1987). The risk of hepatotoxicity from combined isoniazid/rifampicin therapy is higher in elderly than in young patients, and routine liver function test monitoring may be prudent in older patients and also in younger patients if they develop symptoms (Van den Brande et al., 1995). Cross et al. (1980) also concluded that in the absence of clinically significant and persistent pretreatment abnormalities of liver function tests, rifampicin and isoniazid are not contraindicated in alcoholic patients.

It is now generally accepted that the combination of isoniazid/rifampicin causes hepatitis more commonly than either drug given alone, and if the drugs are given singly, isoniazid is more frequently hepatotoxic than rifampicin (Westphal et al., 1994; Lee, 1995). Rare cases of acute liver failure necessitating liver transplantation have occurred from combined isoniazid/rifampicin therapy (Mitchell et al., 1995).

Isoniazid-associated hepatitis occurs in patients receiving this drug alone for preventive treatment (p. 1201). Garibaldi et al. (1972) reported 19 cases of hepatitis amongst 2321 positive tuberculin reactors receiving isoniazid prophylactically. Thirteen of these were jaundiced and two died. Clinical features and pathological findings were indistinguishable from those found in viral hepatitis. In a matched control group of 2154 subjects who were not taking isoniazid, only one case of hepatitis occurred during the same 9-month period. Moss et al. (1972) reported five and Maddrey and Boitnott (1973) reported another 14 patients with hepatitis associated with isoniazid preventive therapy. In the latter study three patients died from liver failure; on rechallenge of three other patients with isoniazid, two developed an accelerated recurrence of severe liver disease and the other only an elevated serum transaminase. Liver histology showed hepatocellular injury similar to viral hepatitis and there was no evidence of cholestasis.

Isoniazid-associated hepatitis, although described, is a rare occurrence in children (Stein and Liang, 1979; Starke and Correa, 1995). However, fatal hepatic necrosis presumably due to isoniazid preventive therapy was reported in a 15-year-old girl (Vanderhoof and Ament, 1976) and another 16-year-old female developed the same complication but she was treated successfully by liver transplantation (Palusci et al., 1995).

Chronic liver disease resulting from isoniazid therapy, although reported, appears to be rare (Graham and Dundas, 1979). In an international controlled trial using isoniazid for preventive treatment, 20 838 subjects were given a dose of 300 mg daily and 6991 a placebo; the risk of hepatitis caused or exacerbated by isoniazid was estimated to be 5.2 per 1000 subjects; the risk increased from 2.8 in subjects aged less than 35 years to 7.7 per 1000 in those aged 55 years or more. Three patients with hepatitis died (0.4 per 1000) all of whom continued isoniazid after liver function abnormality had been recognized (Riska, 1976). In the USA the overall frequency of overt hepatitis with isoniazid is approximately 1%, but the risk increases in older age groups particularly in those aged greater than 35 years (Black, 1974; Kopanoff et al., 1978; Bailey et al., 1983). The probability of developing hepatitis during a 1-year treatment with isoniazid in the USA, estimated per 1000 subjects, was 0 for those aged less than 20 years, 2.4 for those aged 20–34 years and 19.2 for those aged 50–64 years (Comstock and Edwards, 1975). Hepatitis can occur at any time during isoniazid therapy, but it is more common in the first 2 months of treatment (Black, 1974; Mitchell et al., 1976), and drinking alcohol seems to increase the risk (Riska, 1976; Kopanoff et al., 1978). The case fatality rate of isoniazid hepatitis is not known but it has been estimated to be 0.7% for all age groups (Comstock, 1981).

Isoniazid frequently causes hepatotoxicity as evidenced by abnormalities of serum enzymes, particularly the SGOT. About 12% of adult tuberculin-positive hospital employees receiving isoniazid developed moderately raised SGOT levels, compared with a control group in New Orleans (Bailey et al., 1974). Of 1000 patients receiving isoniazid preventive treatment for 1 year who had their liver function evaluated clinically and biochemically at monthly intervals, 222 (22.2%) had at least one elevated SGOT level during the course of treatment and in 47 asymptomatic persons isoniazid therapy was discontinued because of consistent elevations 5-fold greater than normal. Another 17 had symptoms in association with elevated SGOT levels and therapy was stopped in these patients as well. No patients were seriously ill and there were no deaths. Of the 47 asymptomatic patients with high SCOT levels 42 had these within the first 6 months of therapy. In patients over 40 years of age SGOT elevation (with or without symptoms) leading to cessation of therapy, was more frequent (Byrd et al., 1979). Abnormalities in SGPT values were also detected in 10% of adolescents receiving isoniazid; these occurred without jaundice usually within the first 10 weeks of isoniazid administration; treatment was continued in all patients(except one who had a very high SGPT level) and transaminase levels fell spontaneously (Litt et al., 1976).

Similarly, 25 of 369 children (6.8%) receiving isoniazid preventive treatment developed a raised SGOT level 2 months after medication was begun. They had no other evidence of hepatotoxicity and in 21 of these children isoniazid administration was continued and the SGOT levels soon decreased (Beaudry et al., 1974). SGOT determinations were performed at 6–20 weeks and after a therapeutic course on 116 children (including 50 under 10 years old) receiving isoniazid therapy for tuberculous infections; increases were only found in five children at 6–20 weeks but not after completion of therapy (Rapp et al., 1979). Other studies have also indicated that an asymptomatic rise in the SGOT may occur in 10–20% of patients given isoniazid preventive therapy (American Thoracic Society, 1974; Bailey et al., 1983). Such rises in liver enzymes are less common in children, compared with adults (Starke, 1988; Starke and Correa, 1995).

Because of the definite risk of hepatitis, the number of indications for isoniazid preventive treatment have been reduced (p. 1201). If symptoms or signs of hepatitis occur during isoniazid preventive treatment, the drug should be discontinued (Romero, 1994). If such symptoms or signs develop during treatment of tuberculosis and biochemical tests confirm that there is liver injury, hepatotoxic drugs such as isoniazid, rifampicin and pyrazinamide should be stopped. If treatment cannot be interrupted, drugs which cause no liver damage such as ethambutol, streptomycin and ofloxacin can be substituted. Once the liver function tests normalize, the potentially hepatotoxic drugs can be reintroduced one at a time to identify the offending agent and to determine the optimal regimen to complete therapy (O'Brien, 1989; Barnes and Barrows, 1993).

The value of routine monitoring of liver function tests in detecting hepatitis has been controversial. However, most clinicians now advocate monthly monitoring of serum transaminase values for persons at a high risk of developing hepatitis – those aged over 35 years, those who drink alcohol daily, patients taking other potentially hepatotoxic drugs and patients with a history of liver disease. Isoniazid should be ceased in these patients if the transaminase value exceeds three times the upper limit of normal. The drug can be tried again if the tests return to normal (O'Brien, 1989; Barnes and Barrows, 1993), but all patients receiving isoniazid as preventive therapy or as part of regimen for treatment should be questioned at monthly intervals about symptoms or signs of hepatitis or other toxic effects. Liver function tests should be performed if there are any symptoms. If the enzyme level exceeds 3- to 5-fold the normal value, the decision to continue isoniazid should be reconsidered (Bailey et al., 1983). Also selective biochemical monitoring of children receiving isoniazid and rifampicin is warranted. This includes children with severe tuberculosis and those receiving higher than recommended doses of the drugs. Bi-weekly monitoring of liver function tests during the first 2 months of treatment and less frequent monitoring thereafter has been suggested (O'Brien *et al.*, 1983; Donald *et al.*, 1987). Other factors associated with increased risk of isoniazid-induced hepatitis include chronic liver disease, injection drug abuse and the risk may also be higher in post-pubertal black and Hispanic women (Jordan *et al.*, 1991; Ad Hoc Committee, 1995). Isoniazid and/or rifampicin hepatotoxicity also appears to be more common in HIV-infected patients, but this does not mean that these drugs should not be used in this patient population when they are indicated (Chaisson *et al.*, 1987; Small *et al.*, 1991).

The exact mechanism of isoniazid hepatotoxicity is not yet defined. Earlier suggestions that a hypersensitivity reaction was involved (Maddrey and Boitnott, 1973) have been disputed. Mitchell *et al.* (1976) noted that there was no correlation between SGOT levels and isoniazid induced antinuclear antibodies (see below), antibodies to isoniazid were not detected and associated features of hypersensitivity, such as a rash or eosinophilia, were uncommon. In addition, the variable and often prolonged period of treatment with isoniazid before evidence of hepatotoxicity is not usual with hypersensitivity. Mitchell *et al.* (1976) suggested that acetylhydrazine (a metabolite of isoniazid, p. 1186) may act as a hepatotoxin because this substance is split to form monoacetylhydrazine which in turn could be converted to a potent acylating agent which produces liver necrosis. They also provided evidence that rapid inactivators (p. 1186) were more prone to liver disease, probably because they metabolized more isoniazid to acetylhydrazine than slow inactivators. However, rapid acetylators also acetylate monoacetylhydrazine to a non-toxic substance which is excreted in similar proportions in both slow and rapid acetylators (Girling, 1978; Ellard *et al.*, 1981). Moreover, a number of studies have shown that the inactivator status is not a risk factor in isoniazid hepatotoxicity (Riska, 1976; Dickinson *et al.*, 1977; Girling, 1978; Bailey *et al.*, 1979; Pilheu *et al.*, 1979; Ellard, 1984; Jenner and Ellard, 1989).

However, if isoniazid is used together with rifampicin, the risk of hepatotoxicity is increased (p. 1190). There is some evidence that rifampicin induces the metabolism of isoniazid and as a result of this another isoniazid metabolite, hydrazide, is produced, which is hepatotoxic. Higher free hydrazine plasma levels appear to occur in slow rather than in rapid acetylators of isoniazid (Gangadharam, 1986).

5 Acute pancreatitis

This complication occurred in two patients with tuberculosis who were treated for tuberculosis with isoniazid, rifampicin and pyrazinamide. Pancreatitis in both patients resolves when antituberculosis drugs were stopped, but pancreatitis rapidly recurred when isoniazid alone was recommenced (Chan *et al.*, 1994a; Rabassa *et al.*, 1994).

6 Miscellaneous side-effects

Good *et al.* (1965) described seven patients who developed pain and contractures in the shoulders and arms, which appeared to be associated with isoniazid therapy. Acute arthritis, associated with fever and periorbital edema has been described in a woman after a 9-day treatment with isoniazid; subsequently this arthritis rapidly recurred after one dose of isoniazid (Periman and Venkataramani, 1975). Antinuclear antibodies occur in a large proportion of tuberculous patients treated with isoniazid for prolonged periods. This is usually asymptomatic but an occasional patient may develop overt systemic lupus erythematosus (Alarcón-Segovia *et al.*, 1969, 1971). Patients who develop this type of systemic lupus erythematosus are predominantly of the slow acetylator phenotype; the drug itself and not its metabolites appears to cause deposition of immune complexes by inhibiting the C4 component of the complement system (Sim *et al.*, 1984). Experience in a few patients suggests that isoniazid may be a rare cause of pure red cell aplasia (Claiborne and Dutt, 1985).

Theoretically, there has been some concern that isoniazid may be carcinogenic because it can induce neoplasms in albino mice (Leading article, 1966). However, there have been no indications of an increased risk of cancer in follow-up studies of patients who were treated with isoniazid 10–20 years previously (Stott *et al.*, 1976; Costello and Snider, 1980).

A diffuse interstitial nephritis, with similar features to that described with penicillin G (p. 32) and methicillin (p. 84), has been observed in two patients, which may have been due to isoniazid and/or ethambutol therapy (Stone *et al.*, 1976). Isoniazid has been implicated as a cause of pubertal gynecomastia (Leading article, 1976).

Tager *et al.* (1985) confirmed previous observations that tuberculin skin tests may revert to negative in patients given preventive treatment with isoniazid; this was especially so if the initial positive reaction was relatively small and reversions were not stable in all cases.

7 Drug interactions

Inhibition of diphenylhydantoin (phenytoin) metabolism and associated diphenylhydantoin toxicity may occur due to isoniazid, particularly in slow inactivators in whom blood levels of isoniazid are relatively high (p. 1185) (Kutt *et al.*, 1970). When the two drugs are used together, serum phenytoin levels should be measured (Ad Hoc Committee, 1995). Probably by a similar mechanism of inhibiting hepatic microsomal enzymes, isoniazid can interfere with the metabolism of the anticonvulsant drug carbamazepine, resulting in carbamazepine toxicity (Block, 1982; Valsalan and Cooper, 1982). Experience with one patient suggested that in addition to isoniazid decreasing the clearance of carbamazepine, carbamazepine being a microsomal enzyme inducing agent, can increase the formation of toxic isoniazid metabolites and thereby increase the risk of isoniazid hepatotoxicity (Wright *et al.*, 1982). Isoniazid has also been reported to interfere with the metabolism of primidone ('Mysoline') and certain barbiturates (Bourgeois *et al.*, 1982). Isoniazid administration may be associated with reduced ketaconazole serum levels (p. 1370).

Symptoms similar to those of histamine poisoning have been observed in patients in Sri Lanka taking isoniazid after eating various types of fish (Uragoda and Kottegoda, 1977; Uragoda, 1978, 1980). During spoilage of scromboid fish (skipjack and tuna) bacteria convert histidine to histamine; isoniazid probably precipitates a histamine reaction by inhibiting the enzyme diamine oxidase (histaminase) which is involved in histamine metabolism. Symptoms including palpitations, erythema, red eyes, headache, vomiting, wheezing, sweating, loose motions, urticaria and itching appear within minutes of eating the fish and pass away within a few hours. Ordinary cooking fails to destroy histamine in food. In one patient histamine-induced hypotension may have contributed to hemiplegia (Senanayake *et al.*, 1978). Similar clinical features have been described immediately after eating cheese in patients taking isoniazid. This has also been ascribed to rapid gastrointestinal absorption of histamine from cheese, the inactivation of which is prevented by isoniazid's inhibition of histaminase (Uragoda and Lodha, 1979). In other reports of these cheese/isoniazid reactions, in which one was associated with a hypertensive episode, they were considered to be due to inhibition of the enzyme monoamine oxidase (Kent Smith and Durack, 1978; Lejonc *et al.*, 1979; Toutoungi *et al.*, 1985). Isoniazid is closely related to some of the monoamine oxidase inhibitors, such as iproniazid, which have been used in certain mental illnesses. These drugs can cause hypertensive crises in patients who partake of substances rich in monoamines especially tyramine, such as cheese and red wine. Whatever the biochemical mechanism is, patients who experience flushing with isoniazid should be advised to avoid taking cheese and probably other food and beverages rich in monoamines.

One case report has suggested that isoniazid administration may enhance the anticoagulant activity of warfarin (Rosenthal *et al.*, 1977). Reports that isoniazid and rifampicin may affect vitamin D metabolism have not been borne out by long-term studies (Williams *et al.*, 1985).

8 Paradoxical enlargement or development of intracranial tuberculoma

This has occasionally happened despite administration of appropriate therapy including isoniazid. This does not represent failure of antituberculosis therapy; the likely explanation is an interaction between the host's immune response and the direct effects of mycobacterial products. Some patients may die, some may need surgical intervention and some may have residual neurological abnormalities (Afghani and Lieberman, 1994).

Clinical Uses of the Drug

1 Treatment of active pulmonary tuberculosis

The treatment of pulmonary tuberculosis changed considerably some 20 years ago in respect to both the duration and the drugs used. Moreover, since it was considered that there was little risk of contacts becoming infected once effective chemotherapy had begun, most patients with tuberculosis were managed as outpatients (Glassroth *et al.*, 1980). The purpose of tuberculosis chemotherapy is to sterilize lesions quickly and completely. This entails the administration of bactericidal antituberculosis drugs in combinations which eliminate large rapidly multiplying populations of tubercle bacilli, thereby preventing emergence of resistant organisms (p. 1179); this is followed by the sterilization of lesions by appropriate drugs which act on less active and intermittently dividing bacillary populations (Dutt and Stead, 1982). However, during the last decade the number of patients with tuberculosis in many countries has increased and new problems, such as multidrug-resistant disease have developed (p. 1181).

a Evolution of antituberculosis chemotherapy The modern short-course chemotherapy of tuberculosis evolved as a result of many carefully controlled clinical trials throughout the world. D'Esopo (1982) reviewed some of the critical ones. Soon after the development of streptomycin (p. 428) in 1944, clinical trials showed that it was highly effective for tuberculosis but bacterial resistance became a major problem. The same applied to PAS (p. 1224) after its introduction in 1946. Trials began in 1948 and subsequently, demonstrated that the non-bactericidal drug PAS, used singly, or with streptomycin, did not improve efficacy of therapy but largely prevented the development of streptomycin-resistance. The availability of isoniazid in 1952 was a major advance in antituberculosis therapy. Used singly, bacterial-resistance occurred rapidly (p. 1179), but availability of isoniazid did enable combinations of three drugs to be used. In general, combinations of the three drugs were not superior to any combination of two drugs. The three-drug regimen was more effective for very advanced cavitary pulmonary disease. It then became apparent that not only could antituberculosis drugs suppress the disease but they could sterilize open cavities. For this to be realized, it was necessary to give chemotherapy for 2 years. Standard therapy became streptomycin, isoniazid and PAS for 2–4 months, or longer if bacteriological conversion (see below) had not occurred; this was followed by maintenance therapy with an isoniazid/PAS combination to complete a 2-year course. Problems were that streptomycin regimens required injections and this drug had appreciable toxicity; PAS was often nauseating in the doses required and was not taken by many patients – leading to the development of isoniazid-resistance.

When ethambutol (p. 1211) became available in the late 1960s some of these problems were solved; it deterred development of resistance to the other drugs and was better tolerated by patients. Ethambutol was often used with isoniazid in triple-drug regimens during the first 3 months, either replacing streptomycin to avoid injections, or more commonly as a substitute for poorly tolerated PAS. Nevertheless, treatment with an isoniazid/ethambutol combination for 18–24 months was still necessary for cure and often resulted in poor patient compliance. Trials in developing countries showed that 12-month drug regimens were also useful. For instance, in the early 1960s in Madras intermittent administration (see below) of streptomycin and isoniazid given twice-weekly for 12 months, achieved good results (D'Esopo, 1982).

Pyrazinamide (p. 1219) was introduced as an antituberculosis drug in 1952. Although it was recognized to be a bactericidal drug, for a period it was relegated to the status of a second-line drug mainly because of its apparent toxicity. The special sterilizing action of pyrazinamide (p. 1220) and the unique properties of rifampicin (p. 692), were utilized later to make possible chemotherapeutic regimens of 6 months or less (see below). Rifampicin (p. 676) became available for the treatment of tuberculosis in the late 1960s. This was another bactericidal drug, but similar to all other antituberculosis drugs, its use singly resulted in the emergence of resistant strains (p. 678). For a period of time rifampicin was only regarded as another first-line antituberculosis drug. When it was used in standard treatment regimens as a replacement for PAS, results were at least equal but maintenance therapy with isoniazid and rifampicin produced fewer side-effects and less interruptions to treatment than maintenance with isoniazid and PAS. In many countries standard chemotherapy then became isoniazid and rifampicin for 18 months plus streptomycin or ethambutol for the first 2–4 months. In the USA initial triple therapy was not always employed; the most frequently used regimen was isoniazid and ethambutol for 18 months. Streptomycin was added if there was extensive cavitary disease or if drug-resistant disease was a consideration. This regimen was still recommended in the USA when rifampicin could not be used (Bailey et al., 1983). However, it was soon recognized that rifampicin and isoniazid were as effective as any three-drug regimen for the treatment of extensive cavitary disease (Bailey et al., 1977). Other trials in the USA showed that a regimen of daily rifampicin and isoniazid for 20 weeks followed after sputum cultures became negative by daily isoniazid plus ethambutol for 1 year, was very effective (Long et al., 1979). Such regimens lasting no longer than 12–18 months then became acceptable in the USA (CDC, 1980a). Similarly, after initial therapy with isoniazid, rifampicin and ethambutol, continuation therapy for 1 year with daily isoniazid and ethambutol was just as effective as daily isoniazid and rifampicin for the same period (Lees et al., 1977).

b Intermittent chemotherapy This was introduced to improve patient compliance and to reduce the cost of treatment. It is suitable for outpatients in urban areas who require fully supervised treatment. Drugs are administered two or three times per week. Such regimens have been used effectively in developing countries since the early 1960s. Intermittent regimens were usually preceded by 2–3 months of daily triple therapy. Two commonly used intermittent therapies were streptomycin (1 g i.m.) plus isoniazid (15 mg per per kg) twice-weekly (Fox, 1971; BMRC, 1973; WHO, 1975) or PAS (12 g) and isoniazid (15 mg per per kg) twice-weekly (Tub Chemother Centre, 1973a). It was confirmed in Czechoslovakia that after an initial course of triple chemotherapy for 6–13 weeks, continuation therapy with twice-weekly streptomycin and isoniazid for a total duration of 12 months was just as effective as a similar regimen lasting for a total of 18 months (WHO Prague, 1976, 1977). Isoniazid plus rifampicin (Singapore/ BMRC, 1975, 1977) and isoniazid and ethambutol (Albert et al., 1976) have been used successfully in twice-weekly regimens after initial daily triple-drug therapy. When twice-weekly isoniazid (15 mg per per kg) and ethambutol (45 mg per per kg) were used after an initial 2-week course of daily streptomycin, ethambutol and isoniazid, for a course of total duration of 12 months, results were less satisfactory than those obtained with the highly effective daily isoniazid/ethambutol regimen (Tuberculosis Research/Madras, 1981).

Intermittent chemotherapy can be combined with short-course chemotherapy for tuberculosis, provided the patient can tolerate the first-line antituberculosis drugs and there is no drug resistance to them (p. 1180). The regimen most widely accepted is daily isoniazid, rifampicin, pyrazinamide for 2 months followed by twice-weekly treatment with isoniazid (900 mg) and rifampicin (600 mg) for a further 4 months. Streptomycin i.m. and/or oral ethambutol may be added to the regimen during the first 1–2 months if there is any likelihood of isoniazid resistance. Some authors have started intermittent chemotherapy as early as the third week of treatment, but pyrazinamide cannot be omitted at that stage; this drug should be continued either daily or intermittently in a dose of 4 g twice-weekly until the end of 2 months chemotherapy and then intermittent isoniazid/rifampicin continued for a further 4 months (Hong Kong/BMRC, 1981; Zierski et al., 1981; Singapore/BMRC, 1985; Castelo et al., 1989; Cohn et al., 1990; Chaulk et al., 1995). A combination formulation of isoniazid, rifampicin and pyrazinamide has been available which is equally efficacious and safe compared with giving the three drugs in separate tablets (Geiter et al., 1987; Hong Kong/BMRC, 1989; Singapore/BMRC, 1991).

If intermittent therapy for pulmonary tuberculosis is started with isoniazid, rifampicin and pyrazinamide from the beginning, without daily therapy at all, results appear marginally less satisfactory. The results of treatment are improved if for the first 2 months intermittent streptomycin 1.0 g i.m. or oral ethambutol 2 g twice-weekly is used in addition (Davidson, 1990; Hong Kong/BMRC, 1991). However, a regimen of four drugs (isoniazid 600 mg, rifampicin 600 mg, pyrazinamide 2.75 g plus ethambutol 2g), given intermittently three times per week throughout the course of 6 months of treatment is quite satisfactory for adults (Barnes and Barrows, 1993; Ad Hoc Committee, 1995).

In developed countries such as the USA, Australia etc. the short course regimens (see below) are now preferred. If there is a need to directly observe therapy, intermittent therapy is advantageous and can start with four drugs right from start, or an initial daily therapy can be given for 2–8 weeks. For this the drugs used should be those described above (Grosset, 1989; Davidson, 1990; Snider and La Montagne, 1994; Ad Hoc Committee, 1995). If there are no drug reactions, drug-resistance and the drugs are actually taken under observation, results of treatment in normal hosts are excellent, but if an intermittent regimen is inadequately supervised, results of treatment may be poor (Gangadharam, 1994).

For pulmonary tuberculosis in children, isoniazid, rifampicin and pyrazinamide daily for 2 months followed by isoniazid and rifampicin twice-weekly for another 4 months again is satisfactory. Intermittent administration can commence as soon as the 3rd week, but pyrazinamide should be included in the regimen for the first 2 months (Abernathy, 1989; Starke and Correa, 1995). However, one pediatric suspension combining isoniazid, rifampicin and pyrazinamide was rather unstable and unsatisfactory (Seifart et al., 1991). If possible, ethambutol should be avoided in children as it is hard to monitor visual acuity in this age group (p. 1214). Pediatric tuberculosis can be treated by isoniazid plus rifampicin only, provided the M. tuberculosis strain is sensitive to these drugs. However, if pyrazinamide is not used initially, treatment for total of 9–12 months is necessary (Pineda et al., 1993).

c Short-course chemotherapy Since the early 1970s a series of carefully planned, controlled studies were carried out in several areas of the world to demonstrate methodically that certain drug regimens are effective for short-course chemotherapy. Most of these were under the auspices of the British Medical Research Council (Fox and Mitchison, 1975; Fox, 1978). In particular, these studies revealed that the combination of isoniazid and rifampicin is effective both for an immediate bactericidal effect and for a sterilizing action. That therapy containing these two drugs for a period of only 9 months could be effective, was only slowly accepted. Short-course chemotherapy did not receive general approval in the USA until 1980 (CDC, 1980a). Advantages of short-course chemotherapy are numerous; it is cheaper, there is less chronic drug toxicity, patient co-operation is greater, there is less hazard to them if they default early from treatment, and the period of follow-up after treatment can be reduced.

The experimental studies which provide a theoretical basis for short-course chemotherapy have been summarized by Grosset (1978). There are two important drug actions in short-course chemotherapy; the bactericidal action which results in the death of actively dividing bacilli, and the sterilizing action whereby bacilli which are metabolizing only very slowly or irregularly, are eliminated. The most effective drug combinations for sterilization are isoniazid plus rifampicin and isoniazid plus pyrazinamide. These drugs have individual bactericidal actions which vary according to the pathological situation and enable the rapid sterilization of lesions (p. 1179). Failure to eliminate bacilli in closed caseous lesions or within macrophages where they divide intermittently or only occasionally, is the reason for late relapses after therapy; these drug-sensitive bacilli remain dormant during therapy (persisters) and multiply after the treatment course is finished. The best index of the bactericidal activity of a drug regimen is the rate of elimination of bacilli from the sputum; this is usually assessed by obtaining negative cultures (conversion) within 2 months of starting therapy (Fox, 1978). The bacteriological relapse rate after the end of chemotherapy is the best index of sterilizing activity and for a regimen to be acceptable this should not be greater than 5% (95% success rate) (CDC, 1980a).

Short-course chemotherapy is now an established method for the treatment of pulmonary tuberculosis, and courses lasting 9 months were just as effective even for advanced disease, as the former standard regimens of 18–24 months. Initially in the UK, France and the USA standard therapy with 9-month regimens were adopted (Fox, 1978; A Controlled trial, 1980; CDC, 1980a,b). The regimens consisted of daily rifampicin and isoniazid to which either ethambutol or streptomycin was added for the first 2 months. Neither streptomycin nor ethambutol contributed significantly to the efficacy of this regimen, except in cases harboring isoniazid-resistant bacilli (Stead and Dutt, 1982).

Results comparable with those obtained with 9-month regimens can also be achieved with 6-month regimens. The use of rifampicin and pyrazinamide in both daily and intermittent regimens have made this possible. This initially was particularly applicable to developing countries, which had already been using 12-month regimens (see above), where there was a need for shorter less expensive courses of treatment. Studies in East Africa and Zambia (East African/ BMRC, 1972, 1973, 1974) showed that 6-month regimens using streptomycin, isoniazid together with pyrazinamide or rifampicin had success rates of 90% and 95% respectively. A trial in the USA demonstrated the inadequacy of a 6-month regimen of rifampicin and isoniazid, which had a 9% relapse rate (Snider et al., 1984). Successful regimens have entailed the use of an initial intensive therapy phase with four bactericidal drugs. In Singapore, streptomycin 0.75 g i.m. and oral therapy with isoniazid 300 mg, rifampicin 450 or 600 mg and pyrazinamide 1.5 or 2.0 g daily were used; the higher doses of rifampicin and pyrazinamide were given to patients weighing 50 kg or more. When these four drugs were given for 2 months and then followed by continuation therapy with daily isoniazid and rifampicin, with or without pyrazinamide for another 4 months, the regimen was highly effective (Singapore/BMRC, 1981).

British Thoracic Association (1982) also demonstrated that 6-month regimens of isoniazid and rifampicin, supplemented for the first 2 months by streptomycin + pyrazinamide or by ethambutol + pyrazinamide, were as effective as a 9-month daily regimen of isoniazid + rifampicin. However, further trials have shown that the inclusion of streptomycin or ethambutol during the first 2 months of treatment is only important to cover the possibility of isoniazid resistance. Excellent results are obtained in pulmonary tuberculosis by 6-month daily administration of isoniazid plus rifampicin, but during the first 2 months of treatment daily pyrazinamide should be added. This regimen can also be adapted for intermittent therapy, and such daily or intermittent therapy is now used in most developed countries such as the USA, UK and Australia (Grosset, 1989; O'Brien, 1989; Combs et al., 1990; Algerian Working Group/ BMRC, 1991; Blom-Bülow, 1991; Barnes and Barrows, 1993; Davies, 1994).

To be effective these 6-month treatments require full supervision. The effectiveness of short-course chemotherapy depends very much on the patients adherence to treatment (Chan et al., 1994b). These regimens would also be ideal for developing countries, but they may be too expensive. Further studies in Africa showed that for a 6-months regimen, 2 months of isoniazid, rifampicin + pyrazinamide was necessary followed by 4 months of isoniazid + rifampicin (East and Central African/BMRC, 1983, 1986). Cheaper regimens need at least 8 months treatment. For instance daily isoniazid + thiacetazone (p. 1239) or isoniazid + ethambutol can be used after an initial 2 months intensive phase with the four bactericidal drugs. However, in these regimens the continuation phase must be prolonged to 6 months to achieve comparable results (Fox, 1978; Third East African/BMRC, 1980).

The situation with short-course chemotherapy has been summarized by the WHO (Report, 1982). There are now a number of regimens of 6–9 months duration that are highly effective, of low toxicity, and well tolerated. Some are daily regimens, others intermittent after an initial intensive daily phase, and some intermittent throughout. In addition, they are nearly as effective in patients with strains initially resistant to isoniazid or streptomycin, or even to both drugs, as in patients with sensitive strains. A high proportion of patients are cured even within the first 3 months, which is an advantage for those who default from treatment. The regimen chosen for short-term chemotherapy will vary from country to country. If cost is not a factor then 6-month regimens including rifampicin throughout will usually be selected. In developing countries cheaper regimens are recommended by the WHO. One such regimen is daily thiacetazone and isoniazid for 12 months, often supplemented by streptomycin in the initial intensive phase (Report, 1982). This may no longer be appropriate for patients in Africa, where tuberculosis and HIV infection often coexist, because thiacetazone frequently causes serious cutaneous reactions in HIV-infected patients (p. 1239) (Nunn et al., 1991; Van der Ven et al., 1994).

Attempts to shorten antituberculosis chemotherapy to less than 6 months have, in general, been disappointing. Regimens consisting of daily streptomycin, isoniazid, rifampicin and pyrazinamide for 2 months followed by a continuation phase for 2 months of daily isoniazid and rifampicin with or without pyrazinamide, have had a high relapse rate (East Africa/BMRC, 1978, 1981; Singapore/BMRC, 1981). In Agra, India, regimens of 3 months daily streptomycin, rifampicin, isoniazid and pyrazinamide were compared with 4.5-month regimens during the additional 1.5 months of which either streptomycin, isoniazid and pyrazinamide were given twice-weekly or rifampicin and isoniazid were given 6 days per week. The relapse rates after 12 months for these three regimens were 6%, 7% and 2%, respectively (Mehrotra et al., 1981, 1984). Subsequently, in Madras, 5 and 7-month regimens were tried with and without rifampicin. Rifampicin, streptomycin, isoniazid and pyrazinamide were given daily for 2 months, followed by streptomycin, isoniazid and pyrazinamide twice-weekly for either 3 months or 5 months; a third regimen was the same as the 7-month one but rifampicin was not included. None of the patients who had received a 7-month regimen had a bacteriological relapse whereas the relapse rate was 5% in those who had a 5-month treatment. This trial showed that rifampicin was not essential in short-course chemotherapy if the organisms were sensitive, but it was important if there was initial resistance to isoniazid, especially if there was also resistance to streptomycin. This Madras trial also showed that corticosteroids did not influence the response to chemotherapy (Tuberculosis Research/Madras, 1983). Further studies of short-course therapy in Madras in which streptomycin, rifampicin, isoniazid and pyrazinamide were used daily for 3 months, resulted in a high relapse rate (Tripathy, 1983; Tub Res Centre, Madras, 1986; Balasubramanian et al., 1990).

d   Special clinical problems   There are clinical situations in which antituberculosis chemotherapy should be designed for the particular problems of the individual. These include patients with coexisting medical conditions such as silicosis, diabetes, cancer, organ transplantation, chronic alcoholism and complicated pulmonary tuberculosis such as empyema. In general, the same antituberculosis therapy as for normal hosts is suitable, but the regimen often has to be prolonged for a total of 9–12 months (CDC, 1980b; Stead and Dutt, 1982). Co-infection of tuberculosis and HIV is considered separately (p. 1198). In patients with organ transplantation rifampicin, due to liver enzyme induction, lowers the serum levels of corticosteroids and cyclosporine (p. 690). The problem can often be overcome by increasing the dosage of these drugs, but in some patients adequate cyclosporine levels may be very hard to attain. In such cases a four-drug regimen of streptomycin, isoniazid, pyrazinamide and ethambutol is used for the first 2 months, followed by isoniazid + ethambutol for another 16 months. If rifampicin is omitted, shorter regimens are not effective (Muñoz et al., 1995).

Therapy of tuberculosis should be modified in pregnancy and in patients with hepatitis or impending liver failure. Isoniazid and ethambutol, both being well tolerated by the mother and fetus, have been recommended for use in pregnancy (Glassroth et al., 1980). Rifampicin can aso be used safely (Bailey et al., 1983), but pyrazinamide is not recommended in the USA because the data about this drug are considered to be insufficient. However, in other countries pyrazinamide has been used during pregnancy with no ill effects. Therefore a 6-month regimen is possible for pregnant patients, but if pyrazinamide is not used, 9- to 12-month regimens are necessary. A combination of isoniazid and ethambutol (plus streptomycin for multibacillary cavitary cases) has been recommended for patients with severe liver disease (Stead and Dutt, 1982). The American Thoracic Society recommended the use of streptomycin and ethambutol for patients with hepatic failure, with the cautious administration of isoniazid or rifampicin if a third drug is required (Bailey et al., 1983). These drugs constitute what was once standard therapy (p. 1194) and treatment for 18–24 months is required to obtain satisfactory results. However, therapy is usually modified as clinical circumstances change.

e Sputum smear-negative cases Patients considered to have active pulmonary tuberculosis on radiographic grounds, but without acid fast bacilli on microscopic examination of sputum, are a group for which treatment may be modified. This is an important group because in most countries, both developing and technically advanced, in at least half the patients the diagnosis of pulmonary tuberculosis is never confirmed bacteriologically (Fox, 1978). Because the chance of detecting bacilli by smear depends on their concentration in sputum, which in turn is closely dependent on the character and extent of the underlying lesion, and untreated smear-negative patients seem to have a better prognosis, it has been assumed that such patients would require less treatment than smear-positive ones (Leading article, 1980). This has been investigated by clinical trials. In Hong Kong, three different regimens were used to treat smear-positive and smear-negative patients (five smears): streptomycin, isoniazid, rifampicin and pyrazinamide for 2 months; the same regimen for 3 months; or a standard regimen of streptomycin, isoniazid and PAS daily for 3 months followed by a further 9 month treatment usually with streptomycin and isoniazid twice-weekly. Relapse rates in patients who had initial positive sputum smears were unacceptable for the regimens lasting 2 or 3 months only. These relapse rates for the smear-negative group were 11% and 7% for the short-courses, respectively and 2% for the 12-month regimen during 60 months (Hong Kong/Madras/BMRC, 1981, 1984). Patients with smear-negative pulmonary disease have also been treated successfully with 6 months therapy consisting of daily isoniazid and rifampicin for 1 month followed by the same drugs twice-weekly for 5 months (Dutt et al., 1983; 1990).

f Tuberculosis and HIV infection Ultimately HIV infection has a profound effect on cell-mediated immunity, so this infection predisposes patients to tuberculosis. Reactivation of latent tuberculosis is likely, but in areas where tuberculosis is common, such as New York City in the USA and in Africa, HIV infected patients can also acquire tuberculosis infection. In the USA, in patients with AIDS, tuberculosis is more common among intravenous drug abusers (Chaisson and Slutkin, 1989; Rosenheim, 1990; Horner and Moss, 1991).

Tuberculosis can present at any time during HIV infection, but many cases present early. The early cases are ones with pulmonary tuberculosis with fairly typical features of the disease. Cases presenting later usually still have largely pulmonary disease, but chest radiographs are usually atypical; the middle and lower lobes are often affected whilst the upper lobes are spared, hilar and mediastinal lymphadenopathy is common and cavitation is uncommon.

Extrapulmonary foci in this group are also common (Chaisson et al., 1987; Chaisson and Slutkin, 1989; Horner and Moss, 1991; Girardi et al., 1994). In atypical cases the diagnosis will usually be suspected in areas where tuberculosis is common, but it may be overlooked where the disease is rare. Sputum smears and smears from other involved sites, such as the CSF, are often positive, but there is the problem of differentiating M. tuberculosis from other mycobacteria such as M. avium complex which cause disease in HIV-positive patients. However, in one study from a hospital, where M. avium complex infections were common in HIV-infected patients, the predictive value of the acid-fast bacilli smear for M. tuberculosis was 92% for expectorated sputum specimens, 71% for induced sputum specimens and 71% for bronchoalveolar lavage specimens (Yajko et al., 1994). Therefore empiric therapy should often be commenced pending the results from culture and sensitivities. It is sometimes possible to isolate tubercle bacilli from blood cultures and a direct smear of the blood buffy coat may also be positive (Rosenheim, 1990). Polymerase chain reaction may also detect M. tuberculosis in the blood of patients with pulmonary tuberculosis (Schluger et al., 1994).

The treatment of tuberculosis in HIV-infected patients may be complicated by multidrug-resistant M. tuberculosis infection (p. 1181), but if the M. tuberculosis strain is sensitive to first-line drugs, the treatment used does not differ greatly from that employed for other patients, except that most commonly a 9-month, rather than 6-month regimen has been used. This consists of isoniazid 300 mg daily, rifampicin (600 mg daily or 450 mg daily for persons weighing <50 kg), pyrazinamide 20–30 mg per per kg per day and usually also ethambutol 15 mg per per kg per day, each administered daily for first 2 months. Thereafter isoniazid and rifampicin should be administered either daily or intermittently for at least another 7 months. More prolonged treatment may be indicated if bacteriologic conversion is delayed or if treatment is interrupted because of non-compliance or adverse reactions. At present it is unresolved whether after successful completion of tuberculosis treatment in AIDS patients, there should be life-long isoniazid chemoprophylaxis (Chaisson and Slutkin, 1989; Horner and Moss, 1991; Small *et al.*, 1991; Hopewell, 1992).

In Africa in both HIV-positive children and adults, the standard isoniazid/thiacetazone regimen is ineffective and it also causes severe cutaneous hypersensitivity reactions. Treatment with isoniazid, rifampicin, pyrazinamide ,and ethambutol daily for 2 months, followed by rifampicin plus isoniazid twice-weekly for 4 months is satisfactory, but the relapse rate is further reduced if the last two drugs are continued for further 6 months (Hawken *et al.*, 1993; Luo *et al.*, 1994; Perriëns *et al.*, 1995). In an area such as sub-Saharan Africa, where both HIV and tuberculosis are common, it is likely that reinfection may occur after successful therapy of tuberculosis. Again it is unresolved whether lifelong maintenance therapy should be used in HIV-infected patients after the successful treatment for tuberculosis. This may not be practicable in most African countries (Daley, 1993).

Surveys in New York City have shown that both HIV-exposed or HIV-infected children develop tuberculosis much more commonly than comparable aged children in the general population. Some are infected by multiresistant strains (Drucker *et al.*, 1994; Gutman *et al.*, 1994). If their *M. tuberculosis* strain is sensitive to first-line drugs, a treatment regimen, similar to that used for adults in USA, should be effective. The duration of treatment should be 9–12 months (Starke and Correa, 1995).

Extrapulmonary tuberculosis infections are common in AIDS patients and often large tuberculous abscesses develop in them. They may be located in liver, spleen, abdominal wall, psoas muscle, mediastinum and peripancreatic area. Diagnosis is usually made by examining material obtained by CT guided aspiration. This procedure also often helps therapeutically, but in some patients surgical drainage may be needed. For splenic abscesses, splenectomy may be the best treatment. Some patients, but not all recover after these procedures plus appropriate antituberculosis drug therapy (Johnson *et al.*, 1990; Pedro-Botet *et al.*, 1991; Wolff *et al.*, 1991; Lupatkin *et al.*, 1992).

Tuberculous meningitis has not been very common in AIDS patients; it is likely to respond to similar regimens which are employed to treat this disease in other patients (p. 1201) (Parsons, 1989).

g Drug-resistant tuberculosis Modified chemotherapy is necessary for the treatment of pulmonary tuberculosis due to possible drug-resistant strains. The frequency of such strains varies not only from country to country but sometimes within geographic areas of one nation (p. 1181). The possibility of isoniazid-resistance should be considered in patients in whom therapy has failed or who have relapsed after a course of treatment, those who have received isoniazid preventive therapy, and those who may have acquired infection in an area with a high prevalence of isoniazid-resistance or due to contact with a patient with a resistant strain (Dutt and Stead, 1982). In these situations if a two-bactericidal drug regimen is used, such as isoniazid plus rifampicin, and the bacterial strain involved is resistant to isoniazid, such therapy is likely to lead to rifampicin-resistance as well (p. 678). It is essential to use at least two bactericidal drugs to both of which the bacilli are sensitive.

In areas of the USA where the prevalence of primary drug-resistance to isoniazid and/or streptomycin is high, treatment with other drugs to which the organisms are rarely resistant, such as rifampicin and ethambutol, is recommended. This combination was also used for treatment of a community outbreak of tuberculosis in the USA due to *M. tuberculosis* strains resistant to isoniazid, streptomycin and PAS (Reves *et al.*, 1981). Similarly, because a high proportion of isolates from Indochinese refugees are resistant to isoniazid and streptomycin, it has been recommended that initial therapy should consist of isoniazid, rifampicin and ethambutol until results of drug-susceptibility tests are known (CDC, 1981). Ethambutol is not recommended in this regimen for children whose visual acuity cannot be monitored; in these circumstances either PAS (200–300 mg per per kg up to 12 g daily) or streptomycin (20 mg per per kg up to 1 g daily) should be used in its place (CDC, 1980b).

In the clinical situations described above, where primary drug-resistance to isoniazid (and possibly other drugs) is a possibility, the development of further resistance can be reliably prevented by commencing treatment with four bactericidal drugs, streptomycin, rifampicin, isoniazid and pyrazinamide (Stead and Dutt, 1982). Trials in which these four drugs have been given for an initial intensive phase followed by a continuation phase with a two-drug regimen containing rifampicin and pyrazinamide or streptomycin have been unsuccessful for the treatment of patients with pretreatment drug-resistance to isoniazid or to isoniazid and streptomycin (see above) (Singapore/BMRC, 1981; Hong Kong/BMRC, 1981). Dutt and Stead (1982) used the four-drug regimen in cases of suspected isoniazid-resistance for 6–8 weeks until the results of susceptibility tests were available. Isoniazid and rifampicin were then continued in patients with bacilli sensitive to isoniazid. If isoniazid-resistance was confirmed then streptomycin, rifampicin and pyrazinamide are continued for a total of 9 months or at least 6 months beyond the time of bacteriological conversion. In this continuation phase these drugs can be administered twice-weekly viz; streptomycin 1 g, isoniazid 900 mg, rifampicin 600 mg and pyrazinamide 45–50 mg per per kg body weight.

It has been much more difficult to treat pulmonary tuberculosis due to multiresistant strains of *M. tuberculosis* which have emerged in various parts of the world more recently (p. 1181). Here the strains are resistant to both isoniazid and rifampicin and often also to other first-line drugs. The results of treatment in the USA initially were poor, especially if the patients also had HIV infection. Many patients died, many remained chronically ill with sputum positive for *M. tuberculosis*. Others required lung resection in addition to chemotherapy and there were also additional problems such as nosocomial spread of the disease to other patients and staff (Fischl *et al.*, 1992; Frieden *et al.*, 1993; Goble *et al.*, 1993; Chapman and Henderson, 1994; Young and Wormser, 1994; Menzies *et al.*, 1995). However, more recent reports indicate improvement. Rapid recognition of such cases and isolation procedures have stopped the nosocomial spread of multidrug-resistant tuberculosis (McGowan, 1995). Also the use of directly observed therapy significantly reduced the frequency of primary drug-resistance, acquired drug-resistance and it improved the results of treatment (Weis *et al.*, 1994; Frieden *et al.*, 1995). Also Telzak *et al.* (1995) described quite satisfactory results of treatment of multidrug-resistant tuberculosis in patients without HIV infection in New York City, although some of the patients still required lung resections.

There were two major problems with treatment of multidrug-resistant tuberculosis, as reported in the early studies. First of all culture of *M. tuberculosis* often required 4–6 weeks and it took an additional 2–4 weeks to obtain data on drug susceptibility. The automated BACTEC system can identify mycobacteria in about 2 weeks and drug sensitivity tests take an additional 4–7 days (Iseman, 1993; Jacobs, 1994). Rapid techniques, which can immediately identify drug-resistance are not yet available in routine microbiology laboratories (Snider and La Montagne, 1994), but the more rapid identification and sensitivity testing by the BACTEC system is certainly valuable and it allows clinicians to prescribe the best chemotherapy much earlier.

Finally many patients received appropriate chemotherapy too late. Quite often during the period when sensitivities were not yet known, only first-line drugs were prescribed and the *M. tuberculosis* strains were not infrequently resistant to all of them. When a regimen was clinically failing, sometimes only one second-line drug was added and then the strain rapidly became resistant to that drug as well (Riley, 1993). In areas where multidrug-resistant tuberculosis is common, often isoniazid, rifampicin, pyrazinamide and ethambutol should be used initially plus three second-line drugs, so that initially the patient receives at least two drugs to which the *M. tuberculosis* strain is still sensitive (Iseman, 1993). The available second-line drugs include a quinolone (ciprofloxacin or ofloxacin) (pp. 1031, 1123), PAS (p. 1226), ethionamide (p. 1236), cycloserine (p. 1230), capreomycin (p. 1233), and one of the aminoglycosides such as streptomycin (p. 434), kanamycin (p. 446) or amikacin (p. 515). Multidrug-resistant strains can be resistant to streptomycin, but they are usually sensitive to kanamycin and amikacin. In two more recent reports, the survival of patients with multidrug-resistant tuberculosis, mainly in HIV-infected patients, was much improved and this was largely due to inclusion of second-line drugs in the regimen for initial treatment. Most patients received initially at least two drugs to which their *M. tuberculosis* strain was still sensitive. In addition susceptibility results were available within 4 weeks (Salomon *et al.*, 1995; Turett *et al.*, 1995). Prolonged treatment, up to 24 months or longer is often necessary in these patients if their isolates are resistant to isoniazid and rifampicin and other first-line drugs. Injectable drugs are stopped after 4–6 months and then three oral medications are used for 24 more months after their sputum culture becomes negative (Iseman, 1993).

2 Treatment of extrapulmonary tuberculosis

These forms of tuberculosis should be treated in the same way as pulmonary tuberculosis. The bactericidal drugs can be delivered to the kidneys, spine, peritoneum, pericardium and meninges as easily as to the lung. In miliary and meningeal disease, although lesions are numerous, they are tiny and easily penetrated by the drugs (Dutt and Stead, 1982). Tuberculous meningitis is treated by isoniazid, rifampicin, pyrazinamide and usually streptomycin as well for 3 months and then by isoniazid and rifampicin for further 9 months or longer. A total duration of treatment for 12 months is probably sufficient. Intrathecal streptomycin is not necessary. Some clinicians use corticosteroids in addition to chemotherapy and they may improve the outcome (Dutt and Stead, 1989; Parsons, 1989; Kent et al., 1993; Kumarvelu et al., 1994). Miliary tuberculosis in adults is often treated by isoniazid, rifampicin and ethambutol for 9 months, but for the first 2 months pyrazinamide is added (Kim et al., 1990). Therapy for children is similar but duration of treatment for 6 months is usually sufficient (Hussey et al., 1991).

Since 1978, a 9-month regimen of isoniazid and rifampicin (largely twice-weekly therapy) has been used to treat extrapulmonary tuberculosis in Arkansas in the USA (Dutt and Stead, 1982). This treatment has been used successfully for more than 200 patients. If for the first 2 months streptomycin is added, the total duration of treatment can be only 6 months (Dutt and Stead, 1989). In renal tuberculosis apart from the drainage of large collections of pus and renal reconstruction, surgery has been largely eliminated. Short-course chemotherapy for genitourinary tuberculosis has been described in the UK (Gow, 1979, 1981). This has consisted of daily isoniazid, rifampicin and pyrazinamide for 2 months, followed by daily isoniazid, and rifampicin for another 2–4 months, depending on the severity of the disease. Apart from reconstructive procedures, the need for surgery was virtually eliminated. Garcia-Rodriguez et al. (1994) described good results in genitourinary tuberculosis by combining isoniazid, rifampicin and ethambutol for 12 months.

When the data were reviewed 36 months after commencing treatment, a study in the UK indicated that 9 months' treatment for tuberculosis of lymph nodes with isoniazid and rifampicin, supplemented initially by ethambutol for 8 weeks, was as effective as a regimen in which rifampicin and isoniazid were used for 18 months (British Thoracic Society, 1985). Tuberculous pericarditis responds to the classical 6-month chemotherapy (p. 1195) and the concomitant use of corticosteroids produces rapid initial improvement (Strang, 1994). Tuberculosis of bones and joints including vertebral disease, was often treated for some 12 months (Pouchot et al., 1988), but more recently the classical 6-months chemotherapy has been shown to be effective (Dutt and Stead, 1989; Muradali et al., 1993). If tuberculosis involves a prosthetic joint, chemotherapy may need to be more prolonged and the prosthesis often has to be removed (Tokumoto et al., 1995). In tuberculous peritonitis and other forms of abdominal tuberculosis 12 months isoniazid plus rifampicin is often sufficient, supplemented in first 2–3 months by pyrazinamide and ethambutol (Jakubowski et al., 1988). Congenital tuberculosis responds well to isoniazid, rifampicin and streptomycin, or other drugs if required, but diagnosis is often overlooked and this contributes to a high mortality (Abughali et al., 1994).

In developing countries where the cost of drugs may be an important consideration, as with pulmonary tuberculosis (p. 1197), longer regimens with less expensive drugs may be used for treatment of extrapulmonary diseases.

3 Preventive treatment of tuberculosis

This was formerly regarded as chemoprophylaxis. Isoniazid should only be used as a single drug for this purpose. Treatment with isoniazid is valuable in preventing subsequent tuberculous morbidity in primary tuberculosis, in contacts, tuberculin reactors and in those with presumed inactive disease (Leading article, 1974a). This reduction in tuberculosis risk is life-long when the risk of exogenous reinfection is virtually negligible (Comstock et al., 1979; Hsu, 1984). This use of isoniazid alone has only rarely led to the emergence of resistant M. tuberculosis strains. Presumably isoniazid acts in preventive treatment by diminishing the relatively small bacterial population which is present in new infections and healed lesions. Isoniazid is given as a single daily dose, usually for a period of 12 months. Preventive therapy for more than 1 year is not advantageous. Indeed, a large study in Eastern Europe showed that shorter duration of treatment is also effective; in a 5-year follow-up, two-thirds of the preventive value of isoniazid therapy resulting from 1 year of treatment was achieved with a 24-week regimen (International Union, 1982).

Previously preventive treatment with isoniazid was offered to any person who was judged to be at risk of developing active tuberculosis. The risk of liver damage due to isoniazid, particularly in persons over 35 years of age (p. 1190) has resulted in controversy and conflicting views in the USA on the benefits and risk of isoniazid preventive therapy for certain groups of tuberculin reactors (Comstock, 1981; Stead, 1981; Taylor et al., 1981). Nevertheless, in the USA isoniazid treatment has been recommended for various categories of persons in whom the risk of developing side-effects is thought to be smaller than the risk of developing tuberculosis

(American Thoracic Society, 1974, 1976; Farer, 1982). The following recommendations in order of priority, were made by the American Thoracic Society and the Centers for Disease Control and other authors (Bailey *et al.*, 1983; McGlynn *et al.*, 1986; Starke, 1989; Pape *et al.*, 1993; Ad Hoc Committee, 1995; McAnulty *et al.*, 1995; Menzies *et al.*, 1995; Mohle-Boetani *et al.*, 1995). Isoniazid preventative therapy should be given to persons with HIV infection who have a significant reaction to a tuberculin skin test. In addition, preventive therapy should be considered for HIV-infected persons who are tuberculin-negative, but who live in areas where tuberculosis is common. In HIV-infected patients isoniazid preventive therapy should last at least 12 months.

Other groups to whom isoniazid preventive therapy should be given include: household members and other close associates of potentially infectious tuberculosis cases (the risk of developing tuberculosis being greater in young children and adolescents); newly infected persons (those who have had a tuberculin skin test conversion within the past 2 years); persons with significant reactions to tuberculin skin test and abnormal chest X-rays, not previously treated by adequate chemotherapy; persons with significant reactions to tuberculin skin test and who are in special clinical situations (silicosis, diabetes mellitus, prolonged therapy with adrenocorticosteroids, immunosuppressive therapy, some hematologic and reticuloendothelial diseases, such as leukemia or Hodgkin's disease, chronic hemodialysis, associated substantial rapid weight loss or chronic under nutrition); and tuberculin skin test reactors under 35 years of age with none of the above risk factors. Tuberculin testing and isoniazid preventive treatment may also have to be considered for health-care workers who commonly treat tuberculosis patients, but isolation procedures may be more important.

Preventive treatment is contraindicated in patients with a history of previous isoniazid hepatitis or other severe adverse reactions or those with acute liver disease of any etiology, but isoniazid can be given to hepatitis B carriers. Special precautions are advised for patients aged greater than 35 years (p. 1190), those receiving concurrent long-term medication to avoid drug interactions (p. 1193), those taking alcohol daily or with chronic liver disease, those with peripheral neuropathy or conditions predisposing to it (p. 1189) and during pregnancy and breast feeding. Although isoniazid can be given safely during pregnancy (p. 1185), preventive therapy is usually delayed until delivery unless the patient is likely to have been recently infected. There is no evidence of adverse effects of isoniazid on nursing infants.

In Australia preventive therapy is much less commonly given to HIV-infected patients. Most of them live in areas where tuberculosis is uncommon and previous vaccination with bacille Calmette-Guérin (BCG) makes interpretation of tuberculin tests difficult. However, preventive therapy is usually given to those HIV-infected patients who have immigrated from countries where tuberculosis is common. Also in the UK and many other countries, preventive treatment with isoniazid is used less commonly, except in children aged under 6 years, an age group with a very low risk of isoniazid hepatitis. Tuberculin skin tests may revert to normal in patients given isoniazid (p. 1193). Currently isoniazid preventative therapy is only rarely used in developing countries (FitzGerald, 1995).

Preventive treatment with isoniazid has been used to eradicate tuberculosis in isolated rural communities. In one such trial, all active cases were identified and treated conventionally, whilst healthy tuberculin reactors were given isoniazid. Such use of isoniazid was considered to be beneficial (Furcolow and Deuschle, 1973). An intermittent regimen has also been used for preventive treatment. Isoniazid in a dose of 10 mg per per kg body weight (maximum 600 mg) and ethambutol 30 mg per per kg (maximum 2000 mg) given three times per week to Eskimo patients over the age of 10 years for a period of 18 months, was very successful (Grzybowski *et al.*, 1976; Dorken *et al.*, 1984).

Difficulties arise in the management of patients who cannot tolerate isoniazid or who may be infected with isoniazid-resistant organisms. The use of isoniazid preventive treatment in patients infected with isoniazid-resistant organisms has resulted in failures (CDC, 1978). Results of a study in which expert opinion was canvassed in the USA and decision analysis was used, concluded that where the infecting bacilli are known to be or have a high probability of being isoniazid-resistant, preventive therapy with rifampicin alone or in combination with isoniazid or ethambutol may be effective (Koplan and Farer, 1980). However, the efficacy of rifampicin for preventive treatment has not been demonstrated. In an outbreak of isoniazid-resistant tuberculosis involving children, rifampicin has been used empirically for preventive treatment (CDC, 1983b). One contact (the wife) of an index patient with isoniazid-resistant tuberculosis, has been described in whom rifampicin prophylaxis failed and her infection was caused by a rifampicin-resistant strain (Livengood *et al.*, 1985). Answers concerning dosage and duration of rifampicin preventive therapy, its possible side-effects and the risk of development of rifampicin-resistant organisms, are awaited. It is possible that a very short course of treatment as used for smear-negative tuberculosis (p. 1198) could be adapted for preventive treatment in outbreaks due to isoniazid-resistant organisms (Farer, 1982).

4 Other mycobacterial infections

Many mycobacteria other than tubercle bacilli are capable of causing human disease (p. 1211). For the treatment of *M. kansasii* infections, drug regimens containing rifampicin have been the most successful (Pezzia *et al.*, 1981), and therapy consisting of rifampicin, isoniazid and ethambutol for about 2 years have been suggested (Bass and Hawkins, 1983). The American Thoracic Society recommended rifampicin plus isoniazid plus ethambutol or streptomycin for a period of 18–24 months (Bailey *et al.*, 1983). A study by Ahn *et al.* (1983) suggested that chemotherapy for 12 months may be sufficient for initial treatment of pulmonary disease due to *M. kansasii*; 40 patients were given rifampicin, isoniazid and ethambutol daily for 12 months, supplemented by streptomycin twice-weekly for the first 3 months; only one patient relapsed 6 months after completing chemotherapy. Isoniazid, even combined with other drugs, is ineffective for treatment of infections caused by *M. avium* complex (p. 712), but the drug in combination with rifampicin and ethambutol is effective in *M. xenopi* infections (Weber *et al.*, 1989). Isoniazid is also usually effective for the treatment of persistent local or the more rare disseminated infection due to BCG vaccination. Even when these complications occur in patients receiving BCG immunotherapy for malignancy, they respond rapidly to isoniazid (Aungst *et al.*, 1975; Sparks, 1976). One physician, who developed a persisting ulcer on her finger after accidental inoculation with BCG despite isoniazid treatment, had an infection with a strain resistant to isoniazid; the infection rapidly healed when treatment was changed to ethambutol and rifampicin (Lorber *et al.*, 1977).

References

Abernathy RS (1989). Tuberculosis in children and its management. *Semin Respir Infect* **4**: 232.

Abughali N, Van der Kuyp F, Annable W, Kumar ML (1994). Congenital tuberculosis. *Pediatr Infect Dis J* **13**: 738.

A Controlled Trial by the British Thoracic Association (3rd report). (1980). Short-course chemotherapy in pulmonary tuberculosis. *Lancet* i: 1182.

Ad Hoc Committee of the Scientific Assembly on Microbiology, Tuberculosis, and Pulmonary Infections (1995). Treatment of tuberculosis and tuberculosis infection in adults and children. *Clin Infect Dis* **21**: 9.

Afghani B, Lieberman JM (1994). Paradoxical enlargement or development of intracranial tuberculomas during therapy: case report and review. *Clin Infect Dis* **19**: 1092.

Ahn CH, Lowell JR, Ahn SS *et al.* (1983). Short-course chemotherapy for pulmonary disease caused by *Mycobacterium kansasii*. *Amer Rev Respir Dis* **128**: 1048.

Alarcón-Segovia D, Fishbein E, Betancourt VM (1969). Antibodies to nucleo-protein and to hydrazide-altered soluble nucleoprotein in tuberculous patients receiving isoniazid. *Clin Exp Immunol* **5**: 429.

Alarcón-Segovia D, Fishbein E, Alcalá H (1971). Isoniazid acetylation rate and development of antinuclear antibodies upon isoniazid treatment. *Arthritis Rheum* **14**: 748.

Albert RK, Sbarbaro JA, Hudson LD, Iseman M (1976). High-dose ethambutol; its role in intermittent chemotherapy. *Amer Rev Respir Dis* **114**: 699.

Algerian Working Group/British Medical Research Council Cooperative Study (1991). Short-course chemotheapy for pulmonary tuberculosis under routine programme conditions: a comparison of regimens of 28 and 36 weeks duration in Algeria. *Tubercle* **72**: 88.

Alland D, Kalkut GE, Moss AR *et al.* (1994). Transmission of tuberculosis in New York city. *New Engl J Med* **330**: 1710.

Al-Orainey IO, Saeed ES, El-Kassimi FA, Al-Shareef N (1989). Resistance to antituberculous drugs in Riyadh, Saudi Arabia. *Tubercle* **70**: 207.

Altamirano M, Marostenmaki J, Wong A *et al.* (1994). Mutation of the catalase-peroxidase gene from isoniazid-resistant *Mycobacterium tuberculosis* isolates. *J Infect Dis* **169**: 1162.

American Thoracic Society (1974). Preventive therapy of tuberculous infection. *Amer Rev Respir Dis* **110**: 371.

American Thoracic Society (1976). Guidelines for the investigation and management of tuberculosis contacts. *Amer Rev Respir Dis* **114**: 459.

An Interim Report of the Medical Research Council by their Tuberculosis Chemotherapy Trials Committee (1952). The treatment of pulmonary tuberculosis with isoniazid. *Brit Med J* **2**: 735.

Atkins JN (1982). Maternal plasma concentration of pyridoxal phosphate during pregnancy: adequacy of vitamin B_6 supplementation during isoniazid therapy. *Amer Rev Respir Dis* **126**: 714.

Aungst CW, Sokal JE, Jager BV (1975). Complications of BCG vaccination in neoplastic disease. *Ann Intern Med* **82**: 666.

Bailey WC, Weill H, deRouen TA *et al.* (1974). The effect of isoniazid on transaminase levels. *Ann Intern Med* **81**: 200.

Bailey WC, Raleigh JW, Turner JAP (1977). Treatment of mycobacterial disease. *Amer Rev Respir Dis* **115**: 185.

Bailey WC, Dickinson S, Hirschowitz BI, Hodgkin MM (1979). Isoniazid acetylation and hepatitis. *Bull Int Un Tuberc* **54**: 47.

Bailey WC, Albert RK, Davidson PT *et al.* (1983). Treatment of tuberculosis and other mycobacterial diseases. *Amer Rev Respir Dis* **127**: 790.

Balasubramanian R, Sivasubramanian S, Vijayan VK *et al.* (1990). Five year results of a 3-month and two 5-month regimens for the treatment of sputum-positive pulmonary tuberculosis in South India. *Tubercle* **71**: 253.

Baril L, Caumes E, Truffot-Pernot C *et al.* (1995). Tuberculosis caused by *Mycobacterium africanum* associated with involvement of the upper and lower respiratory tract, skin, and mucosa. *Clin Infect Dis* **21**: 653.

Barnes PF, Barrows SA (1993). Tuberculosis in the 1990s. *Ann Intern Med* **119**: 400.

Bass JB Jr, Hawkins EL (1983). Treatment of disease caused by nontuberculous mycobacteria. *Arch Intern Med* **143**: 1439.

Beaudry PH, Brickman HF, Wise MB, MacDougall D (1974). Liver enzyme disturbances during isoniazid chemoprophylaxis in children. *Amer Rev Respir Dis* **110**: 581.

Bellin E (1994). Failure of tuberculosis control A prescription for change. *JAMA* **271**: 708.

Bender DA, Russell-Jones R (1979). Isoniazid-induced pellagra despite vitamin-B$_6$ supplementation. *Lancet* **ii**: 1125.

Bennett WM, Singer I, Golper T *et al.* (1977). Guidelines for drug therapy in renal failure. *Ann Intern Med* **86**: 754.

Bernstein J, Lott WA, Steinberg BA, Yale HL (1952). Chemotherapy of experimental tuberculosis-isonicotinic acid by hydrazide (nydrazid). and related compounds. *Amer Rev Tuberc* **65**: 357; quoted by Robson and Sullivan (1963).

Birkett DJ, Pond SM (1975). Metabolic drug interactions – a critical review. *Med J Aust* **1**: 687.

Bistritzer T, Barzilay Z, Jonas A (1980). Isoniazid-rifampicin-induced fulminant liver disease in an infant. *J Pediatr* **97**: 480.

Black M (1974). Editorial. Isoniazid and the liver. *Amer Rev Respir Dis* **110**: 1.

Bloch AB, Cauthen GM, Onorato IM *et al.* (1994). Nationwide survey of drug-resistant tuberculosis in the United States. *JAMA* **271**: 665.

Block SH (1982). Carbamezepine – isoniazid interaction. *Pediatrics* **69**: 494.

Blom-Bülow B (1991). Dosing regimens in the treatment of tuberculosis. *Scand J Infect Dis* (Suppl 74): 258.

Bomb BS, Purohit SD, Bedi HK (1976). Stevens-Johnson syndrome caused by isoniazid. *Tubercle* **57**: 229.

Bourgeois BFD, Dodson WE, Ferrendelli JA, Mallinckrodt E (1982). Isoniazid and other drugs. *Pediatrics* **70**: 824.

British Medical Research Council Co-operative Study (1973). Co-operative controlled trial of a standard regimen of streptomycin, PAS and isoniazid and three alternative regimens of chemotherapy in Britain. *Tubercle* **54**: 99.

British Thoracic Association (1982). A controlled trial of six months' chemotherapy in pulmonary tuberculosis. Second report: results during the 24 months after the end of chemotherapy. *Amer Rev Respir Dis* **126**: 460.

British Thoracic Society Research Committee (1985). Short course chemotherapy for tuberculosis of lymph nodes: a controlled trial. *Brit Med J* **290**: 1106.

Burns DN, Gellert GA, Crone RK (1994). Tuberculosis in eastern Europe and the former Soviet Union: how concerned should we be? *Lancet* **343**: 1445.

Burwen DR, Bloch AB, Griffin LD *et al.* (1995). National trends in the concurrence of tuberculosis and acquired immunodeficiency syndrome. *Arch Intern Med* **155**: 1281.

Byrd RB, Horn BR, Solomon DA, Griggs GA (1979). Toxic effects of isoniazid in tuberculosis chemoprophylaxis. *JAMA* **241**: 1239.

Cantwell MF, Snider DE Jr, Cauthen GM, Onorato IM (1994). Epidemiology of tuberculosis in the United States, 1985 through 1992. *JAMA* **272**: 535.

Carpenter JL, Covelli HD, Avant ME *et al.* (1982). Drug-resistant *Mycobacterium tuberculosis* in Korean isolates. *Amer Rev Respir Dis* **126**: 1092.

Casteels-Van Daele M, Igodt-Ameye L, Corbeel L, Eeckels R (1975). Hepatotoxicity of rifampicin and isoniazid in children. *J Pediatr* **86**: 739.

Castelo A, Jardim JRB, Goihman S *et al.* (1989). Comparison of daily and twice-weekly regimens to treat pulmonary tuberculosis. *Lancet* **ii**: 1173.

Castro KG (1995). Tuberculosis as an opportunistic disease in persons infected with human immunodeficiency virus. *Clin Infect Dis* **21** (Suppl 1): 66.

CDC (Center for Disease Control) (1978). Follow-up on drug-resistant tuberculosis – Mississippi. *MMWR* **27**: 355.

CDC (Center for Disease Control) (1980a). Guidelines for short-course tuberculosis chemotherapy. *MMWR* **29**: 97.

CDC (Center for Disease Control) (1980b). Follow-up on guidelines for short-course tuberculosis chemotherapy. *MMWR* **29**: 183.

CDC (Center for Disease Control) (1980c). Adverse drug reactions among children treated for tuberculosis. *MMWR* **29**: 589.

CDC (Centers for Disease Control) (1981). Drug resistance among Indochinese refugees with tuberculosis. *MMWR* **30**: 273.

CDC (Centers for Disease Control) (1983a). Primary resistance to antituberculosis drugs – United States. *MMWR* **32**: 521.

CDC (Centers for Disease Control) (1983b). Interstate outbreak of drug-resistant tuberculosis involving children – California, Montana, Nevada, Utah. *MMWR* **32**: 516.

CDC (Centers for Disease Control) (1993). Tuberculosis – Western Europe, 1974–1991. *MMWR* **42**: 628.

CDC (Centers for Disease Control and Prevention) (1995a). Laboratory practices for diagnosis of tuberculosis – United States, 1994. *JAMA* **274**: 787.

CDC (Centers for Disease Control and Prevention) (1995b). Tuberculosis morbidity – United States, 1994. *JAMA* **274**: 788.

Chaisson RE, Slutkin G (1989). Tuberculosis and human immunodeficiency virus infection. *J Infect Dis* **159**: 96.

Chaisson RE, Schecter GF, Theuer CP *et al.* (1987). Tuberculosis in patients with the acquired immunodeficiency syndrome. Clinical features, response to therapy, and survival. *Amer Rev Respir Dis* **136**: 570.

Chan KL, Chan HS, Lui SF, Lai KN (1994a). Recurrent acute pancreatitis induced by isoniazid. *Tubercle Lung Dis* **75**: 383.

Chan SL, Wong PC, Tam CM (1994b). 4-, 5- and 6- month regimens containing isoniazid, rifampicin, pyrazinamide and steptomycin for treatment of pulmonary tuberculosis under program conditions in Hong Kong. *Tubercle Lung Dis* **75**: 245.

Chapman SW, Henderson HM (1994). New and emerging pathogens – multiply resistant *Mycobacterium tuberculosis*. *Curr Opin Infect Dis* **7**: 231.

Chaulet P (1987). Compliance with anti-tuberculosis chemotherapy in developing countries. *Tubercle* **68** (Suppl): 19.

Chaulk CP, Moore-Rice K, Rizzo R, Chaisson RE (1995). Eleven years of community-based directly observed therapy for tuberculosis. *JAMA* **274**: 945.

Cheigh JS (1977). Drug administration in renal failure. *Amer J Med* **62**: 555.

Cheung WC, Lo CY, Lo WK *et al.* (1993). Isoniazid induced encephalopathy in dialysis patients. *Tubercle Lung Dis* **74**: 136.

Claiborne RA, Dutt AK (1985). Isoniazid-induced pure red cell aplasia. *Amer Rev Respir Dis* **131**: 947.

Cockerill FR III, Uhl JR, Temesgen Z *et al.* (1995). Rapid identification of a point mutation of the *Mycobacterium tuberculosis* catalase-peroxidase (*kat G*). gene associated with isoniazid resistance. *J Infect Dis* **171**: 240.

Cohn DL, Catlin BJ, Peterson KL *et al.* (1990). A 62-dose, 6-month therapy for pulmonary and extrapulmonary tuberculosis A twice-weekly, directly observed and cost-effective regimen. *Ann Intern Med* **112**: 407.

Collins CH, Yates MD, Grange JM (1984). Names for mycobacteria. *Brit Med J* **288**: 463.

Combs DL, O'Brien RJ, Geiter LJ (1990). USPHS tuberculosis short-course chemotherapy trial 21: effectiveness, toxicity, and acceptability. The report of final results. *Ann Intern Med* **112**: 397.

Commonwealth Department of Health Australia (1982). *Tuberculosis Statistics*. Canberra: Australian Government Publishing Service.

Comstock GW (1981). Evaluating isoniazid preventive therapy: the need for more data. *Ann Intern Med* **94**: 817.

Comstock GW, Edwards PQ (1975). Editorial The competing risks of tuberculosis and hepatitis for adult tuberculin reactors. *Amer Rev Respir Dis* **111**: 573.

Comstock GW, Baum C, Snider DE Jr (1979). Isoniazid prophylaxis among Alaskan Eskimos: a final report of the Bethel isoniazid studies. *Amer Rev Respir Dis* **119**: 827.

Coronado VG, Beck-Sague CM, Hutton MD *et al.* (1993). Transmission of multidrug-resistant *Mycobacterium tuberculosis* among persons with human immunodeficiency virus infection in an urban hospital: epidemiologic and restriction fragment length polymorphism analysis. *J Infect Dis* **168**: 1052.

Costello HD, Snider DE Jr (1980). The incidence of cancer among participants in a controlled, randomized isoniazid preventive therapy trial. *Amer J Epidemiol* **111**: 67.

Cross FS, Long MW, Banner AS, Snider DE Jr (1980). Rifampicin-isoniazid therapy of alcoholic and nonalcoholic tuberculous patients in a US public health service cooperative therapy trial. *Amer Rev Respir Dis* **122**: 349.

Crowle AJ, Sbarbaro JA, Judson FN *et al.* (1984). Inhibition by streptomycin of tubercle bacilli within cultured human macrophages. *Amer Rev Respir Dis* **130**: 839.

Crowle AJ, Sbarbaro JA, Judson FN, May MH (1985). The effect of ethambutol on tubercle bacilli within cultured human macrophages. *Amer Rev Respir Dis* **132**: 742.

Daley CL (1993). Tuberculosis recurrence in Africa: true relapse or reinfection? *Lancet* **342**: 756.

Dankner WM, Waecker NJ, Essey MA *et al.* (1993). *Mycobacterium bovis* infections in San Diego: a clinicoepidemiologic study of 73 patients and a historical review of a forgotten pathogen. *Medicine* **72**: 11.

David HL (1981). Basis for lack of drug susceptibility of atypical mycobacteria. *Rev Infect Dis* **3**: 878.

Davidson PT (1990). Treating tuberculosis: what drugs, for how long? *Ann Intern Med* **112**: 393.

Davies PDO (1994). Tuberculosis in the elderly. *J Antimicrob Chemother* **34** (Suppl A): 93.

Davies PDO (1995). Tuberculosis. *Curr Opin Infect Dis* **8**: 105.

Davis RS, Stoler BS (1977). Febrile reactions to INH. *New Engl J Med* **297**: 337.

Dawson DJ, Cheah DF, Chew WK *et al.* (1995). Tuberculosis in Australia, 1989–1992. Bacteriologically confirmed cases and drug resistance. *Med J Aust* **162**: 287.

D'Esopo ND (1982). Clinical trials in pulmonary tuberculosis. *Amer Rev Respir Dis* **125**: 85.

Dhillon J, Mitchison DA (1989). Activity and penetration of antituberculosis drugs in mouse peritoneal macrophages infected with *Mycobacterium microti* OV254. *Antimicrob Ag Chemother* **33**: 1255.

Dickinson DS, Bailey WC, Hirschowitz BI (1977). The effect of acetylation status on isoniazid (INH) hepatitis. *Amer Rev Respir Dis* **115** (Suppl): 395.

Dolin PJ, Raviglione MC, Kochi A (1994). Global tuberculosis incidence and mortality during 1990–2000. *Bull Wld Hlth Org* **72**: 213.

Donald PR, Schoeman JF, O'Kennedy A (1987). Hepatic toxicity during chemotherapy for severe tuberculous meningitis. *Amer J Dis Child* **141**: 741.

Dorken E, Grzybowski S, Enarson DA (1984). Ten year evaluation of a trial of chemoprophylaxis against tuberculosis in Frobisher Bay, Canada. *Tubercle* **65**: 93.

Drobniewski F, Kahenya G, Msiska R *et al.* (1994). Drug resistance is not the principal barrier to effective control of tuberculosis in Zambia. *J Infect Dis* **169**: 1180.

Drucker E, Alcabes P, Bosworth W, Sckell B (1994). Childhood tuberculosis in the Bronx, New York. *Lancet* **343**: 1482.

Dutt AK, Stead WW (1982). Medical perspective: present chemotherapy for tuberculosis. *J Infect Dis* **146**: 698.

Dutt AK, Stead WW (1989). Treatment of extrapulmonary tuberculosis. *Semin Respir Infect* **4**: 225.

Dutt AK, Moers D, Thomas C, Stead WW (1983). Short-course chemotherapy for six months in smear-negative pulmonary and pleural tuberculosis. *Amer Rev Respir Dis* (Suppl): **127**: 192.

Dutt AK, Moers D, Stead WW (1990). Smear-negative, culture-positive pulmonary tuberculosis. Six-month chemotherapy with isoniazid and rifampin. *Amer Rev Respir Dis* **141**: 1232.

East African/British Medical Research Councils (1972). Controlled clinical trial of short-course (6-month) regimens of chemotherapy for treatment of pulmonary tuberculosis. *Lancet* **i**: 1079.

East African/British Medical Research Councils (1973). Controlled clinical trial of four short-course (6-month) regimens of chemotherapy for treatment of pulmonary tuberculosis. Second report. *Lancet* **i**: 1331.

East African/British Medical Research Councils (1974). Controlled clinical trial of four short-course (6-month) regimens of chemotherapy for treatment of pulmonary tuberculosis. Third report. *Lancet* **ii**: 237.

East African/British Medical Research Councils (1978). Controlled clinical trial of five short-course (4-month) chemotherapy regimens in pulmonary tuberculosis. *Lancet* **ii**: 334.

East African/British Medical Research Councils Study (1981). Controlled clinical trial of five short-course (4-month) chemotherapy regimens in pulmonary tuberculosis. Second report of the 4th study. *Amer Rev Respir Dis* **123**: 165.

East and Central African/British Medical Research Council Fifth Collaborative Study (1983). Controlled clinical trial of 4 short-course regimens of chemotherapy (three 6-month and one 8-month) for pulmonary tuberculosis. *Tubercle* **64**: 153.

East and Central African/British Medical Research Council Fifth Collaborative Study (1986). Controlled clinical trial of 4 short-course regimens of chemotherapy (three 6-month and one 8-month) for pulmonary tuberculosis: final report. *Tubercle* **67**: 5.

Editorial (1994). The global challenge of tuberculosis. *Lancet* **344**: 277.

Ellard GA (1984). The potential clinical significance of the isoniazid acetylator phenotype in the treatment of pulmonary tuberculosis. *Tubercle* **65**: 211.

Ellard GA, Aber VR, Gammon PT *et al.* (1972). Pharmacology of some slow-release preparations of isoniazid of potential use in intermittent treatment of tuberculosis. *Lancet* **i**: 340.

Ellard GA, Gammon PT, Polansky F *et al.* (1973). Further studies on the pharmacology of a slow-release matrix preparation of isoniazid (Smith & Nephew HS 82) of potential use in the intermittent treatment of tuberculosis. *Tubercle* **54**: 57.

Ellard GA, Girling DJ, Nunn AJ (1981). The hepatotoxicity of isoniazid among the three acetylator phenotypes. *Amer Rev Respir Dis* **123**: 568.

Ellner JJ, Hinman AR, Dooley SW *et al.* (1993). Tuberculosis symposium: emerging problems and promise. *J Infect Dis* **168**: 537.

Elliott AM, Halwiindi B, Hayes RJ *et al.* (1993). The impact of human immunodeficiency virus on presentation and diagnosis in tuberculosis in a cohort study in Zambia. *J Trop Med Hyg* **96**: 1.

Evans DAP, Manley KA, McKusick VA (1960). Genetic control of isoniazid metabolism in man. *Brit Med J* **2**: 485.

Farer LS (1982). Chemoprophylaxis. *Amer Rev Respir Dis* **125**: 102.

Ferrazoli L, Palaci M, da Silva Telles MA *et al.* (1995). Catalase expression, kat G, and MIC of isonizid for *Mycobacterium tuberculosis* isolates from São Paulo, Brazil. *J Infect Dis* **171**: 237.

Fischl MA, Daikos GL, Uttamchandani RB *et al.* (1992). Clinical presentation and outcome of patients with HIV infection and tuberculosis caused by multi-drug resistant bacilli. *Ann Intern Med* **117**: 184.

FitzGerald JM (1995). The downside of isoniazid chemoprophylaxis. *Lancet* **345**: 404.

Forgan-Smith R, Ellard GA, Newton D, Mitchison DA (1973). Pyrazinamide and other drugs in tuberculous meningitis. *Lancet* **ii**: 374.

Fox HH (1952–53). The chemical attack on tuberculosis. *Trans NY Acad Sci* **15**: 234.

Fox W (1968). Changing concepts in the chemotherapy of pulmonary tuberculosis. *Amer Rev Respir Dis* **97**: 767.

Fox W (1971). General considerations in intermittent drug therapy of pulmonary tuberculosis. *Postgrad Med J* **47**: 729.

Fox W (1978). The current status of short-course chemotherapy. *Bull Int Un Tuberc* **53**: 268.

Fox W, Mitchison DA (1975). Short-course chemotherapy for pulmonary tuberculosis. *Amer Rev Respir Dis* **111**: 325.

Frieden TR, Sterling T, Pablos-Mendez A *et al.* (1993). The emergence of drug-resistant tuberculosis in New York City. *New Engl J Med* **328**: 521.

Frieden TR, Fujiwara PI, Washko RM, Hamburg MA (1995). Tuberculosis in New York City – turning the tide. *New Engl J Med* **333**: 229.

Furcolow ML, Deuschle KW (1973). Modern tuberculosis control. A six-year follow-up in an Appalachian community. *Amer Rev Respir Dis* **107**: 253.

Gallicano K, Sahai J, Zaror-Behrens G, Pakuts A (1994). Effect of antacids in didanoside tablet on bioavailability of isoniazid. *Antimicrob Ag Chemother* **38**: 894.

Gangadharam PRJ (1986). Isoniazid, rifampin, and hepatotoxicity. *Amer Rev Respir Dis* **133**: 963.

Gangadharam PRJ (1994). Chemotherapy of tuberculosis under program conditions. *Tubercle Lung Dis* **75**: 241.

Garagusi VF, Neefe LI, Mann O (1976). Acute meningoencephalitis association with isoniazid administration. *JAMA* **235**: 1141.

Garcia-Rodriguez JA, Garcia Sánchez JE, Bellido JLM *et al.* (1994). Genitourinary tuberculosis in Spain: review of 81 cases. *Clin Infect Dis* **18**: 557.

Garibaldi RA, Drusin RE, Ferebee SH, Gregg MB (1972). Isoniazid-associated hepatitis. Report of an outbreak. *Amer Rev Respir Dis* **106**: 357.

Geiter LJ, O'Brien RJ, Combs DL, Snider DE Jr (1987). United States public health tuberculosis therapy trial 21: preliminary results of an evaluation of a combination tablet of isoniazid, rifampin and pyrazinamide. *Tubercle* **68** (Suppl): 41.

Gilbert GL (1996). Multidrug-resistant tuberculosis: prevention is better than cure. *Med J Aust* **164**: 121.

Girardi E, Antonucci G, Armignocco O *et al.* (1994). Tuberculosis and AIDS: a retrospective, longitudinal, multicentre study of Italian AIDS patients. *J Infect* **28**: 261.

Girling DJ (1978). The hepatic toxicity of antituberculosis regimens containing isoniazid, rifampicin and pyrazinamide. *Tubercle* **59**: 13.

Girling DJ (1982). Adverse effects of antituberculosis drugs. *Curr Therap* **23**: 101.

Glassroth J, Robins A, Snider DE Jr (1980). Medical progress: tuberculosis in the 1980s. *New Engl J Med* **302**: 1441.

Goble M, Iseman MD, Madsen LA *et al.* (1993). Treatment of 171 patients with pulmonary tuberculosis resistant to isoniazid and rifampin. *New Engl J Med* **328**: 527.

Good AE, Green RA, Zarafonetis CJD (1965). Rheumatic symptoms during tuberculosis therapy. A manifestation of isoniazid toxicity? *Ann Intern Med* **63**: 800.

Gow JG (1979). The management of patients suffering from genito-urinary tuberculosis by short-course chemotherapy and early surgery. A several year review. *Bull Int Un Tuberc* **54**: 298.

Gow JG (1981). The management of genitourinary tuberculosis. *J Antimicrob Chemother* **7**: 590.

Graham WGB, Dundas R (1979). Isoniazid-related liver disease Occurrence with portal hypertension, hypoalbuminaemia, and hypersplenism. *JAMA* **242**: 353.

Grosset J (1978). The sterilizing value of rifampicin and pyrazinamide in experimental short-course chemotherapy. *Tubercle* **59**: 287.

Grosset JH (1989). Present status of chemotherapy for tuberculosis. *Rev Infect Dis* **11** (Suppl 2): 347.

Grzybowski S, Galbraith JD, Dorken E (1976). Chemoprophylaxis trial in Canadian Eskimos. *Tubercle* **57**: 263.

Gurumurthy P, Rahman F, Narayana ASL, Sarma GR (1990). Salivary levels of isoniazid and rifampicin in tuberculous patients. *Tubercle* **71**: 29.

Gutman LT, Moyle J, Zimmer B, Tian C (1994). Tuberculosis in human immunodeficiency virus-exposed or -infected United States children. *Pediatr Infect Dis J* **13**: 963.

Haas DW, Des Prez RM (1994). Tuberculosis and acquired immunodeficiency syndrome: a historical perspective on recent developments. *Amer J Med* **96**: 439.

Hamburg MA, Frieden TR (1994). Tuberculosis transmission in the 1990s. *New Engl J Med* **330**: 1750.

Hand WL, King-Thompson NL, Steinberg TH (1983). Interaction of antibiotics and phagocytes. *J Antimicrob Chemother* **12** (Suppl C): 1.

Harries AD (1990). Tuberculosis and human immunodeficiency virus infection in developing countries. *Lancet* **335**: 387.

Harris HW (1963). Current concepts of the metabolism of antituberculous agents. *Ann NY Acad Sci* **106**: 43.

Hawken M, Nunn P, Gathua S *et al.* (1993). Increased recurrence of tuberculosis in HIV-1-infected patients in Kenya. *Lancet* **342**: 332.

Hejný J (1982). A drug sensitivity strategy for atypical mycobacteria. *Tubercle* **62**: 63.

Heym B, Honoré N, Truffot-Pernot C *et al.* (1994). Implications of multidrug resistance for the future of short-course chemotherapy of tuberculosis: a molecular study. *Lancet* **344**: 243.

Hobby GL, Johnson PM, Boytar-Papirnyik V (1974). Primary drug resistance: a continuing study of drug resistance in tuberculosis in a veteran population within the United States. X. September 1970–September 1973. *Amer Rev Respir Dis* **110**: 95.

Hong Kong Chest Service/British Medical Research Council (1981). Controlled trial of four thrice-weekly regimens and a daily regimen all given for 6 months for pulmonary tuberculosis. *Lancet* i: 171.

Hong Kong Chest Service/British Medical Research Council (1989). Acceptability, compliance, and adverse reactions when isoniazid, rifampin, and pyrazinamide are given as a combined formulation or separately during three-times-weekly antituberculosis chemotherapy. *Amer Rev Respir Dis* **140**: 1618.

Hong Kong Chest Service/British Medical Research Council (1991). Controlled trial of 2, 4, and 6 months of pyrazinamide in 6-month, three-times-weekly regimens for smear-positive pulmonary tuberculosis, including an assessment of a combined preparation of isonizid, rifampin, and pyrazinamide. *Amer Rev Respir Dis* **143**: 700.

Hong Kong Chest Service/Tuberculosis Research Centre, Madras/British Medical Research Council (1981). A controlled trial of 2-month, 3-month, and 12-month regimens of chemotherapy for sputum-smear-negative pulmonary tuberculosis: the results at 30 months. *Amer Rev Respir Dis* **124**: 138.

Hong Kong Chest Service/Tuberculosis Research Centre, Madras/British Medical Research Council (1984). A controlled trial of 2-month, 3-month, and 12-month regimens of chemotherapy for sputum-smear-negative pulmonary tuberculosis. Results at 60 months. *Amer Rev Respir Dis* **130**: 23.

Hopewell PC (1992). Impact of human immunodeficiency virus infection on the epidemiology, clinical features, management, and control of tuberculosis. *Clin Infect Dis* **15**: 540.

Horn DL, Hewlett D Jr, Haas WH *et al.* (1994). Superinfection with rifampin-isoniazid-streptomycin-ethambutol (RISE)- resistant tuberculosis in three patients with AIDS: confirmation by polymerase chain reaction fingerprinting. *Ann Intern Med* **121**: 115.

Horner PJ, Moss FM (1991). Tuberculosis in HIV infection. *Int J STD AIDS* **2**: 162.

Hsu KHK (1984). Thirty years after isoniazid Its impact on tuberculosis in children and adolescents. *JAMA* **251**: 1283.

Hughes HB (1953). On the metabolic fate of isoniazid. *J Pharmacol Exp Ther* **109**: 444.

Hurwitz A, Schlozman DL (1974). Effects of antacids on gastrointestinal absorption of isoniazid in rat and man. *Amer Rev Respir Dis* **109**: 41.

Hussey G, Chisholm T, Kibel M (1991). Miliary tuberculosis in children: a review of 94 cases. *Pediatr Infect Dis J* **10**: 832.

International Union Against Tuberculosis Committee on Prophylaxis (1982). Efficacy of various durations of isoniazid preventative therapy for tuberculosis: five years of follow-up in the IUAT trial. *Bull Wld Hlth Org* **60**: 555.

Iseman MD (1993). Treatment of multidrug-resistant tuberculosis. *New Engl J Med* **329**: 784.

Jacobs RF (1994). Multiple-drug-resistant tuberculosis. *Clin Infect Dis* **19**: 1.

Jakubowski A, Elwood RK, Enarson DA (1988). Clinical features of abdominal tuberculosis. *J Infect Dis* **158**: 687.

Jenkins PF, Williams TDM, Campbell IA (1980). Neutropenia with each standard antituberculosis drug in the same patient. *Brit Med J* **280**: 1069.

Jenner PJ, Ellard GA (1989). Isoniazid-related hepatotoxicity: a study of the effect of rifampicin administration on the metabolism of acetylisoniazid in man. *Tubercle* **70**: 93.

Jindani A, Aber VF, Edwards EA, Mitchison DA (1980). The early bactericidal activity of drugs in patients with pulmonary tuberculosis. *Amer Rev Respir Dis* **121**: 939.

Johnson SC, Stamm CP, Hicks CB (1990). Tuberculous psoas muscle abscess following chemoprophylaxis with isoniazid in a patient with human immunodeficiency virus infection. *Rev Infect Dis* **12**: 754.

Jordan TJ, Lewit EM, Montgomery RL, Reichman LB (1991). Isoniazid as preventative therapy in HIV-infected intravenous drug abusers. A decision analysis. *JAMA* **265**: 2987.

Kent SJ, Crowe SM, Yung A *et al.* (1993). Tuberculous meningitis: a 30-year review. *Clin Infect Dis* **17**: 987.

Kent Smith C, Durack DT (1978). Isoniazid and reaction to cheese. *Ann Intern Med* **88**: 520.

Kim JH, Langsten AA, Gallis HA (1990). Miliary tuberculosis: epidemiology, clinical manifestations, diagnosis, and outcome. *Rev Infect Dis* **12**: 583.

Kim SJ, Hong YP (1992). Drug resistance of *Mycobacterium tuberculosis* in Korea. *Tubercle Lung Dis* **73**: 219.

Kopanoff DE, Snider DE Jr, Caras GJ (1978). Isoniazid-related hepatitis. A US Public Health Service cooperative suveillance study. *Amer Rev Respir Dis* **117**: 991.

Koplan JP, Farer LS (1980). Choice of preventive treatment of isoniazid-resistant tuberculosis infection. Use of decision analysis and the delphi technique. *JAMA* **244**: 2736.

Kovnat P, Labovitz E, Levison SP (1973). Antibiotics and the kidney. *Med Clin N Amer* **57**: 1045.

Kumarvelu S, Prasad K, Khosla A *et al.* (1994). Randomized controlled trial of dexamethasone in tuberculous meningitis. *Tubercle Lung Dis* **75**: 203.

Kutt H, Brennan R, Dehejia H, Verebely K (1970). Diphenylhydantoin intoxication. A complication of isoniazid therapy. *Amer Rev Respir Dis* **101**: 377.

Lal S, Singhal SN, Burley DM, Crossley G (1972). Effect of rifampicin and isoniazid on liver function. *Brit Med J* **1**: 148.

Lauener H, Favez G (1959). The inhibition of isoniazid inactivation by means of PAS and benzoyl-PAS in man. *Amer Rev Respir Dis* **80**: 26.

Leading Article (1966). Isoniazid: How much a carcinogen? *Lancet* **ii**: 1452.

Leading Article (1969). Isoniazid and loss of memory. *Brit Med J* **1**: 461.

Leading Article (1974). Chemoprophylaxis against tuberculosis. *Brit Med J* **4**: 63.

Leading Article (1976). Pubertal gynaecomastia. *Brit Med J* **1**: 1238.

Leading Article (1980). Smear-negative pulmonary tuberculosis. *Tubercle* **61**: 113.

Lee WM (1995). Drug-induced hepatotoxicity. *New Engl J Med* **333**: 1118.

Lees AW, Allan GW, Smith J *et al.* (1971). Toxicity from rifampicin plus isoniazid and rifampicin plus ethambutol therapy. *Tubercle* **52**: 182.

Lees AW, Allan GW, Smith J, Tyrrell WF (1977). Ethambutol plus isoniazid compared with rifampicin plus isoniazid in antituberculosis continuation treatment. *Lancet* **i**: 1232.

Lejonc JL, Gusmini D, Brochard P (1979). Isoniazid and reaction to cheese. *Ann Intern Med* **91**: 793.

Lim I (1995). Susceptibility of *M tuberculosis* isolates in Australia. *ASIG Newsletter* **2**: 1.

Litt IF, Cohen MI, McNamara H (1976). Isoniazid hepatitis in adolescents. *J Pediatr* **89**: 133.

Livengood JR, Sigler TG, Foster LR *et al.* (1985). Isoniazid-resistant tuberculosis. A community outbreak and report of a rifampicin prophylaxis failure. *JAMA* **235**: 2847.

Long MW, Snider DE Jr, Farer LS (1979). US public health service cooperative trial of three rifampicin-isoniazid regimens in treatment of pumonary tuberculosis. *Amer Rev Respir Dis* **119**: 879.

Lorber B, Vonderheid EC, Swenson RM, Cundy KR (1977). Failure of isoniazid to cure localised BCG infection. *JAMA* **238**: 55.

Ludford J, Doster B, Woolpert SF (1973). Effect of isoniazid on reproduction. *Amer Rev Respir Dis* **108**: 1170.

Luo C, Chintu C, Bhat G *et al.* (1994). Human immunodeficiency virus type-1 infection in Zambian children with tuberculosis: changing seroprevalence and evaluation of a thiacetazone-free regimen. *Tubercle Lung Dis* **75**: 110.

Lupatkin H, Bräu N, Flomenberg P, Simberkoff MS (1992). Tuberculous abscesses in patients with AIDS. *Clin Infect Dis* **14**: 1040.

Maddrey WC, Boitnott JK (1973). Isoniazid hepatitis. *Ann Intern Med* **79**: 1.

Mahmoudi A, Iseman MD (1993). Pitfalls in the care of patients with tuberculosis. *JAMA* **270**: 65.

Malone JL, Paparello SF, Malone JD *et al.* (1994). Drug susceptibility of *Mycobacteirum tuberculosis* isolates from recent Haitian migrants: correlation with clinical response. *Clin Infect Dis* **19**: 938.

Männistö P, Mäntylä R, Klinge E *et al.* (1982). Influence of various diets on the bioavailability of isoniazid. *J Antimicrob Chemother* **10**: 427.

McAnulty JM, Fleming DW, Hawley MA, Baron RC (1995). Missed opportunities for tuberculosis prevention. *Arch Intern Med* **155**: 713.

McGlynn KA, Lustbader ED, Sharrar RG *et al.* (1986). Isoniazid prophylaxis in hepatitis B carriers. *Amer Rev Respir Dis* **134**: 666.

McGowan JEJr (1995). Nosocomial tuberculosis: new progress in control and prevention. *Clin Infect Dis* **21**: 489.

McKenna MT, McCray E, Onorato I (1995). The epidemiology of tuberculosis among foreign-born persons in the United States, 1986–1993. *New Engl J Med* **332**: 1071.

Mehrotra ML, Gautam KD, Chaube CK (1981). Shortest possible acceptable effective ambulatory chemotherapy in pulmonary tuberculosis: preliminary report 1. *Amer Rev Respir Dis* **124**: 239.

Mehrotra ML, Gautam KD, Chaube CK (1984). Shortest possible acceptable effective chemotherapy in ambulatory patients with pulmonary tuberculosis, Part II. Results during the 24 months after the end of chemotherapy. *Amer Rev Respir Dis* **129**: 1016.

Menzies D, Fanning A, Yuan L, Fitzgerald M (1995). Tuberculosis among health care workers. *New Engl J Med* **332**: 92.

Miller AB, Tall R, Fox W *et al.* (1966). Primary drug resistance in pulmonary tuberculosis in Great Britain: Second national survey, 1963. *Tubercle* **47**: 92.

Miller AB, Robinson A, Percy AK (1980). Acute isoniazid poisoning in childhood. *Amer J Dis Child* **134**: 290.

Mitchell I, Wendon J, Fitt S, Williams R (1995). Anti-tuberculous therapy and acute liver failure. *Lancet* **345**: 555.

Mitchell JR, Zimmerman HJ, Ishak KG *et al.* (1976). Isoniazid liver injury: clinical spectrum, pathology, and probable pathogenesis. *Ann Intern Med* **84**: 181.

Mitchison DA (1985). Mechanisms of drug action in short-course chemotherapy. *Bull Int Un Ag Tuberc* **60**: 34.

Mitchison DA, Ellard GA (1980). Tuberculosis in patients having dialysis. *Brit Med J* **280**: 1533.

Mohle-Boetani JC, Miller B, Halpern M *et al.* (1995). School-based screening for tuberculous infection. A cost-benefit analysis. *JAMA* **274**: 613.

Monno L, Angarano G, Carbonara S *et al.* (1993). Current problems in treating tuberculosis in Italian HIV-infected patients. *Tubercle Lung Dis* **74**: 280.

Morris S, Bai GH, Suffys P *et al.* (1995). Molecular mechanisms for multiple drug resistance in clinical isolates of *Mycobacterium tuberculosis*. *J Infect Dis* **171**: 954.

Moss JD, Lewis JE, Knauer CM (1972). Isoniazid-associated hepatitis. A study of five cases. *Amer Rev Respir Dis* **106**: 849.

Mount FW, Anastasiades AA, Schnack GA (1961). Control study of biologically active isoniazid in serum of children with primary tuberculosis. *Amer Rev Respir Dis* **83**: 173.

Muñoz P, Palomo J, Muéoz R *et al.* (1995). Tuberculosis in heart transplant recipients. *Clin Infect Dis* **21**: 398.

Muradali D, Gold WL, Wellend H, Becker E (1993). Multifocal osteoarticular tuberculosis: report of four cases and review of management. *Clin Infect Dis* **17**: 205.

Narain JP, Raviglione MC, Kochi A (1992). HIV-associated tuberculosis in developing countries: epidemiology and strategies for prevention. *Tubercle Lung Dis* **73**: 311.

Nunn P, Felten M (1994). Surveilance of resistance to antituberculosis drugs in developing countries. *Tubercle Lung Dis* **75**: 163.

Nunn P, Kubuga D, Gathua S *et al.* (1991). Cutaneous hypersensitivity reactions due to thiacetazone in HIV-1 seropositive patients treated for tuberculosis. *Lancet* **337**: 627.

O'Brien RJ (1989). Present chemotherapy of tuberculosis. *Semin Respir Infect* **4**: 216.

O'Brien RJ, Long MW, Cross FS *et al.* (1983). Hepatotoxicity from isoniazid and rifampicin among children treated for tuberculosis. *Pediatrics* **72**: 491.

Olson WA, Pruitt AW, Dayton PG (1981). Plasma concentration of isoniazid in children with tuberculous infection. *Pediatrics* **67**: 876.

Palusci VJ, O'Hare D, Lawrence RM (1995). Hepatotoxicity and transaminase measurement during isoniazid chemoprophylaxis in children. *Pediatr Infect Dis J* **14**: 144.

Pape JW, Jean SS, Ho JL *et al.* (1993). Effect of isoniazid prophylaxis on incidence of active tuberculosis and progression of HIV infection. *Lancet* **342**: 268.

Parsons M (1989). Leading article The treatment of tuberculous meningitis. *Tubercle* **70**: 79.

Parthasarathy R, Devadatta S, Fox W *et al.* (1976). Studies of immediate adverse reactions to different doses of a slow-release preparation of isoniazid. *Tubercle* **57**: 115.

Patel KB, Belmonte R, Crowe HM (1995). Drug malabsorption and resistant tuberculosis in HIV-infected patients. *New Engl J Med* **332**: 336.

Pearson ML, Jereb JA, Frieden TR *et al.* (1992). Nosocomial transmission of multidrug-resistant *Mycobacterium tuberculosis*: a risk to patients and health care workers. *Ann Intern Med* **117**: 191.

Pedro-Botet J, Maristany MT, Miralles R *et al.* (1991). Splenic tuberculosis in patients with AIDS. *Rev Infect Dis* **13**: 1069.

Periman P, Venkataramani TK (1975). Acute arthritis induced by isoniazid. *Ann Intern Med* **83**: 667.

Perlman DC, Salomon N, Perkins MP *et al.* (1995). Tuberculosis in drug users. *Clin Infect Dis* **21**: 1253.

Perriëns JH, St Louis ME, Mukadi YB *et al.* (1995). Pulmonary tuberculosis in HIV-infected patients in Zaire. A controlled trial of treatment for either 6 or 12 months. *New Engl J Med* **332**: 779.

Peters JH, Miller KS, Brown P (1965). Studies on the metabolic basis for the genetically determined capacities for isoniazid inactivation in man. *J Pharmacol Exp Ther* **150**: 298.

Pezzia W, Raleigh JW, Bailey MC *et al.* (1981). Treatment of pulmonary disease due to *Mycobacterium kansasii*: recent experience with rifampicin. *Rev Infect Dis* **3**: 1035.

Pilheu JA, de Salvo NC, Manchinu I *et al.* (1979). Incidence of hepatic disturbance connected with the use of isoniazid, and its speed of inactivation. *Bull Int Un Tuberc* **54**: 48.

Pineda PR, Leung A, Muller NL *et al.* (1993). Intrathoracic paediatric tuberculosis: a report of 202 cases. *Tubercle Lung Dis* **74**: 261.

Pitchenik AE, Russell BW, Cleary T *et al.* (1982). The prevalence of tuberculosis and drug resistance among Haitians. *New Engl J Med* **307**: 162.

Posniak AL, MacLeod GA, Ndlovu D *et al.* (1995). Clinical and chest radiographic features of tuberculosis associated with human immunodeficiency virus in Zimbabwe. *Amer J Respir Crit Care Med* **152**: 1556.

Pouchot J, Vinceneux P, Barge J *et al.* (1988). Tuberculosis of the sacroiliac joint: clinical features, outcome, and evaluation of closed needle biopsy in 11 consecutive cases. *Amer J Med* **84**: 622.

Pretorius GS, Van Helden PD, Sirgel F *et al.* (1995). Mutations in *kat G* gene sequences in isoniazid-resistant clinical isolates of *Mycobacterium tuberculosis* are rare. *Antimicrob Ag Chemother* **39**: 2276.

Quémard A, Lacave C, Lanéelle G (1991). Isoniazid inhibition of mycolic acid synthesis by cell extracts of sensitive and resistant strains of *Mycobacterium aurum*. *Antimicrob Ag Chemother* **35**: 1035.

Rabassa AA, Trey G, Shukla U *et al.* (1994). Isoniazid-induced acute pancreatitis. *Ann Intern Med* **121**: 433.

Rao KVN, Mitchison DA, Nair MGK *et al.* (1970). Sulphadimidine acetylation test for classification of patients as slow or rapid inactivators of isoniazid. *Brit Med J* **3**: 495.

Rapp RS, Campbell RW, Howell JC, Kendig EL Jr (1979). Isoniazid hepatotoxicity in children. *Amer Rev Respir Dis* **118**: 794.

Raviglione MC, Rieder HL, Styblo K *et al.* (1994). Tuberculosis trends in Eastern Europe and the former USSR. *Tubercle Lung Dis* **75**: 400.

Raviglione MC, Snider DEJr, Kochi A (1995). Global epidemiology of tuberculosis. *JAMA* **273**: 220.

Ravikrishnan KP, Muller BF, Neuhaus A (1977). Toxicity to isoniazid and rifampin in active tuberculosis patients. *Amer Rev Respir Dis* **115** (Suppl): 405.

Reddy MV, Srinivasan S, Gangadharam PRJ (1994). *In vitro* and *in vivo* synergistic effect of isoniazid with streptomycin and clofazimine against *Mycobacteriuma avium* complex (MAC). *Tubercle Lung Dis* **75**: 208.

Report of a Joint IUAT/WHO Study Group (1982). Tuberculosis control. *Tubercle* **63**: 157.

Reves R, Blakey D, Snider DE Jr, Farer LS (1981). Transmission of multiple drug-resistant tuberculosis: report of a school and community outbreak. *Amer J Epidemiol* **113**: 423.

Riley LW (1993). Drug-resistant tuberculosis. *Clin Infect Dis* **17** (Suppl 2): 442.

Riska N (1976). Hepatitis cases in isoniazid treated groups and in a control group. *Bull Int Un Tuberc* **51**: 203.

Robson JM, Sullivan FM (1963). Antituberculosis drugs. *Pharmacol Rev* **15**: 169.

Rodier G, Gravier P, Sévre J-P *et al.* (1993). Multidrug-resistant tuberculosis in the Horn of Africa. *J Infect Dis* **168**: 523.

Romero JR (1994). Pediatric tuberculosis. *Curr Opin Infect Dis* **7**: 374.

Rosenheim M (1990). Problems of diagnosis and therapy. *Bull Int Un Tub Lung Dis* **65**: 35.

Rosenthal AR, Self TH, Baker ED, Linden RA (1977). Interaction of isoniazid and warfarin. *JAMA* **238**: 2177.

Rouse DA, Li Z, Bai G-H, Morris SL (1995). Characterization of the *kat G* and *inh A* genes of isoniazid-resistant clinical isolates of *Mycobacterium tuberculosis*. *Antimicrob Ag Chemother* **39**: 2472.

Rusnak J, Sartin JS, Pace E *et al.* (1995). Drug susceptibility of *Mycobacterium tuberculosis* isolates from a cohort of Haitian migrants evaluated in 1994. *Clin Infect Dis* **21**: 1066.

Salomon N, Perlman DC, Friedman P *et al.* (1995). Predictors and outcome of multidrug-resistant tuberculosis. *Clin Infect Dis* **21**: 1245.

Santha T, Fox W, Nazareth O *et al.* (1976). Study of adverse reactions to a once-weekly regimen of streptomycin plus a slow-release preparation of isoniazid in high dosage for six months. *Tubercle* **57**: 123.

Santha T, Nazareth O, Krishnamurthy MS *et al.* (1989). Treatment of pulmonary tuberculosis with short course chemotherapy in South India-5-year follow up. *Tubercle* **70**: 229.

Sarma GR, Kailasam S, Mitchison DA *et al.* (1975). Studies of serial plasma isoniazid concentrations with different doses of a slow-release preparation of isoniazid. *Tubercle* **56**: 314.

Sarma GR, Kailasam S, Nair NGK *et al.* (1980). Effect of prednisolone and rifampin on isoniazid metabolism in slow and rapid inactivators of isoniazid. *Antimicrob Ag Chemother* **18**: 661.

Schaefer G, Zervoudakis IA, Fuchs FF, David S (1975). Pregnancy and pulmonary tuberculosis. *Obstet Gynecol* **46**: 706.

Schluger NW, Condos R, Lewis S, Rom WN (1994). Amplification of DNA of *Mycobacterium tuberculosis* from peripheral blood of patients with pulmonary tuberculosis. *Lancet* **344**: 232.

Seifart HI, Parkin DP, Donald PR (1991). Stability of isoniazid, rifampin and pyrazinamide in suspensions used for the treatment of tuberculosis in children. *Pediatr Infect Dis J* **10**: 827.

Senanayake N, Vyravanathan S, Kanagasuriyam S (1978). Cerebrovascular accident after a 'skipjack' reaction in a patient taking isoniazid. *Brit Med J* **2**: 1127.

Sepkowitz KA, Telzak EE, Recalde S *et al.* (1994). Trends in the susceptibility of tuberculosis in New York City, 1987–1991. *Clin Infect Dis* **18**: 755.

Sepkowitz KA, Friedman CR, Hafner A *et al.* (1995). Tuberculosis among urban health care workers: a study using restriction fragment length polymorphism typing. *Clin Infect Dis* **21**: 1098.

Shafer RW, Small PM, Larkin C *et al.* (1995). Temporal trends and transmission patterns during the emergence of multidrug-resistant tuberculosis in New York City: a molecular epidemiologic assessment. *J Infect Dis* **171**: 170.

Shimao T (1987). Drug resistance in tuberculosis control. *Tubercle* **68** (Suppl): 5.

Short EI (1962). Studies on the inactivation of isonicotinyl acid hydrazide in normal subjects and tuberculous patients. *Tubercle* **43**: 33.

Sievers ML, Herrier RN, Chin L, Picchioni AL (1982). Treatment of isoniazid overdose. *JAMA* **247**: 583.

Sim E, Gill EW, Sim RB (1984). Drugs that induce systemic lupus erythematosus inhibit complement component C4. *Lancet* **ii**: 422.

Singapore Tuberculosis Service/British Medical Research Council (1975). Controlled trial of intermittent regimens of rifampicin plus isoniazid for pulmonary tuberculosis in Singapore. *Lancet* **ii**: 1105.

Singapore Tuberculosis Service/British Medical Research Council (1977). Controlled trial of intermittent regimens of rifampin plus isoniazid for pulmonary tuberculosis in Singapore. The results up to 30 months. *Amer Rev Respir Dis* **116**: 807.

Singapore Tuberculosis Service/British Medical Research Council (1981). Clinical trial of six-month and four-month regimens of chemotherapy in the treatment of pulmonary tuberculosis: the results up to 30 months. *Tubercle* **62**: 95.

Singapore Tuberculosis Service/British Research Council (1985). Clinical trial of three 6-month regimens of chemotherapy given intermittently in the continuation phase in the treatment of pulmonary tuberculosis. *Amer Rev Respir Dis* **132**: 374.

Singapore Tuberculosis Service/British Medical Research Council (1991). Assessment of a daily combined preparation of isoniazid, rifampin, and pyrazinamide in a controlled trial of three 6-month regimens for smear-positive pulmonary tuberculosis. *Amer Rev Respir Dis* **143**: 707.

Small PM, Schecter GF, Goodman PC *et al.* (1991). Treatment of tuberculosis in patients with advanced human immunodeficiency virus infection. *New Engl J Med* **324**: 289.

Small PM, Shafer RW, Hopewell PC *et al.* (1993). Exogenous reinfection with multidrug-resistant *Mycobacterium tuberculosis* in patients with advanced HIV infection. *New Engl J Med* **328**: 1137.

Small PM, Hopewell PC, Singh SP *et al.* (1994). The epidemiology of tuberculosis in San Francisco A population-based study using conventional and molecular methods. *New Engl J Med* **330**: 1703.

Snider DE Jr (1980). Pyridoxine supplementation during isoniazid therapy. *Tubercle* **61**: 191.

Snider DE Jr, La Montagne JR (1994). The neglected global tuberculosis problem: a report of the 1992 world congress on tuberculosis. *J Infect Dis* **169**: 1189.

Snider DE Jr, Long MW, Cross FS, Farer LS (1984). Six-months isoniazid-rifampicin therapy for pulmonary tuberculosis Report of a United States public health service cooperative trial. *Amer Rev Respir Dis* **129**: 573.

Sparks FC (1976). Hazards and complications of BCG immunotherapy. *Med Clin N Amer* **60**: 499.

Starke JR (1988). Modern approach to the diagnosis and treatment of tuberculosis in children. *Pediatr Clin N Amer* **35**: 441.

Starke JR (1989). Prevention of tuberculosis. *Semin Respir Infect* **4**: 318.

Starke JR, Correa AG (1995). Management of mycobacterial infection and disease in children. *Pediatr Infect Dis J* **14**: 455.

Stead WW (1981). Isoniazid prophylaxis. *Ann Intern Med* **95**: 393.

Stead WW, Dutt AK (1982). Chemotherapy for tuberculosis today. *Amer Rev Respir Dis* **125**: 94.

Stein MT, Liang D (1979). Clinical hepatotoxicity of isoniazid in children. *Pediatrics* **64**: 499.

Stoeckle MY, Guan L, Riegler N *et al.* (1993). Catalase-peroxidase gene sequences in isoniazid-sensitive and -resistant strains of *Mycobacterium*

tuberculosis from New York City. *J Infect Dis* **168**: 1063.

Stone WJ, Waldron JA, Dixon JH Jr *et al.* (1976). Acute diffuse interstitial nephritis related to chemotherapy of tuberculosis. *Antimicrob Ag Chemother* **10**: 164.

Stott H, Peto J, Stephens R *et al.* (1976). An assessment of the carcinogenicity of isoniazid in patients with pulmonary tuberculosis. *Tubercle* **57**: 1.

Strang JIG (1994). Rapid resolution of tuberculous pericardial effusions with high dose prednisolone and anti-tuberculosis drugs. *J Infect* **28**: 251.

Tager IB, Kalaidjian R, Baldini L, Rocklin RE (1985). Variability in the intra-dermal and *in vitro* lymphocyte responses to PPD in patients receiving isoniazid chemoprophylaxis. *Amer Rev Respir Dis* **131**: 214.

Tahaoglu K, Kizkin O, Karagöz T *et al.* (1994). High initial and acquired drug resistance in pulmonary tuberculosis in Turkey. *Tubercle Lung Dis* **75**: 324.

Takayama K, Wang L, David HL (1972). Effect of isoniazid on the *in vivo* mycolic acid synthesis, cell growth, and viability of *Mycobacterium tuberculosis*. *Antimicrob Ag Chemother* **2**: 29.

Taylor WC, Aronson MD, Delbanco TL (1981). Should young adults with a positive tuberculin test take isoniazid? *Ann Intern Med* **94**: 808.

Telzak EE, Sepkowitz K, Alpert P *et al.* (1995). Multidrug-resistant tuberculosis in patients without HIV infection. *New Engl J Med* **333**: 907.

Third East African/British Medical Research Council Study (1980). Controlled clinical trial of four short-course regimens of chemotherapy for the duration in the treatment of pulmonary tuberculosis. Second report. *Tubercle* **61**: 59.

Tokumoto JAN, Follanslee SE, Jacobs RA (1995). Prosthetic joint infection due to *Mycobacterium tuberculosis*: report of three cases. *Clin Infect Dis* **21**: 134.

Toure IM (1982). The situation with regard to *Mycobacterium africanum* in West Africa. *Bull Int Un Tuberc* **57**: 234.

Toutoungi M, Carroll RLA, Enrico J-F, Perey L (1985). Cheese, wine and isoniazid. *Lancet* **ii**: 671.

Tripathy SP (1983). Controlled clinical trial of a 3-month and two 5-month regimens in pulmonary tuberculosis, second Madras short-course study. *Bull Int Un Tuberc* **58**: 97.

Trivedi SS, Desai SG (1988). Primary antituberculosis drug resistance and acquired rifampicin resistance in Gujarat, India. *Tubercle* **69**: 37.

Tsang AY, Bentz Rr, Schork MA, Sodeman TM (1978). Combined vs. single-drug studies of susceptibilities of *Mycobacterium kansasii* to isoniazid, streptomycin, and ethambutol. *Amer J Clin Path* **70**: 816.

Tuberculosis Chemotherapy Centre, Madras (1973a). Controlled comparison of oral twice-weekly and oral daily isoniazid plus PAS in newly diagnosed pulmonary tuberculosis. *Brit Med J* **2**: 7.

Tuberculosis Chemotherapy Centre, Madras (1973b). A controlled comparison of two fully supervised once-weekly regimens in the treatment of newly diagnosed pulmonary tuberculosis. *Tubercle* **54**: 23.

Tuberculosis Research Centre, Madras-600031, India (1981). Ethambutol plus isoniazid for the treatment of pulmonary tuberculosis – a controlled trial of four regimens. *Tubercle* **61**: 13.

Tuberculosis Research Centre (1983). Study of chemotherapy regimens of 5 and 7 months duration and the role of corticosteroids in the treatment of sputum-positive patients with pulmonary tuberculosis in South India. *Tubercle* **64**: 73.

Tuberculosis Research Centre, Madras, and National Tuberculosis Institute, Bangalore (1986). A controlled clinical trial of 3- and 5- month regimens in the treatment of sputum-positive pulmonary tuberculosis in South India. *Am Rev Respir Dis* **134**: 27.

Turett GS, Telzak EE, Torian LV *et al.* (1995). Improved outcomes for patients with multi-drug resistant tuberculosis. *Clin Infect Dis* **21**: 1238.

Uragoda CG (1978). Histamine poisoning in tuberculosis patients on ingestion of tropical fish. *Amer J Trop Med Hyg* **81**: 243.

Uragoda CG (1980). Histamine poisoning in tuberculous patients after ingestion of tuna fish. *Amer Rev Respir Dis* **121**: 157.

Uragoda CG, Kottegoda SR (1977). Adverse reactions to isoniazid in ingestion of fish with a high histamine content. *Tubercle* **58**: 83.

Uragoda CG, Lodha SC (1979). Histamine intoxication in a tuberculous patient after ingestion of cheese. *Tubercle* **60**: 59.

Usuda Y, Sekine O (1978). Chemotherapy of tuberculosis in patients on dialysis. In *Current Chemotherapy: Proceedings of the 10th International Congress of Chemotherapy, Zurich/Switzerland, 1977* (Siegenthaler W, Lüthy R, eds), p. 241. Washington, DC: American Society for Microbiology.

Uttley AHC, Pozniak A (1993). Resurgence of tuberculosis. *J Hosp Infect* **23**: 249.

Valsalan VC, Cooper GL (1982). Carbamazepine intoxication caused by interaction with isoniazid. *Brit Med J* **285**: 261.

Valway SE, Greifinger RB, Papania M *et al.* (1994). Multidrug-resistant tuberculosis in the New York State prison system, 1990–1991. *J Infect Dis* **170**: 151.

Van den Brande P, Van Steenbergen W, Vervoort G, Demedts M (1995). Aging and hepatotoxicity of isoniazid and rifampin in pulmonary tuberculosis. *Amer J Respir Crit Care Med* **152**: 1705.

Vanderhoof JA, Ament ME (1976). Fatal hepatic necrosis due to isoniazid chemoprophylaxis in a 15-year-old girl. *J Pediatr* **88**: 867.

Van der Ven AJM, Koopmans PP, Vree TB, Van der Meer JWM (1994). Drug intolerance in HIV disease. *J Antimicrob Chemother* **34**: 1.

Van der Werf TS, Groothuis DG, van Klingeren B (1989). High initial drug resistance in pulmonary tuberculosis in Ghana. *Tubercle* **70**: 249.

Wang L, Takayama K (1972). Relationship between the uptake of isoniazid and its action on the *in vivo* mycolic acid synthesis in *Mycobacterium tuberculosis*. *Antimicrob Ag Chemother* **2**: 438.

Wason S, Lacouture PG, Lovejoy FH Jr (1981). Single high-dose pyridoxine treatment for isoniazid overdose. *JAMA* **246**: 1102.

Weber J, Mettang T, Staerz E *et al.* (1989). Pulmonary disease due to *Mycobacterium xenopi* in a renal allograft recipient: report of a case and review. *Rev Infect Dis* **11**: 964.

Weis SE, Slocum PC, Blais FX *et al.* (1994). The effect of directly observed therapy on the rates of drug resistance and relapse in tuberculosis. *New Engl J Med* **330**: 1179.

Westphal JF, Vetter D, Brogard JM (1994). Hepatic side-effects of antibiotics. *J Antimicrob Chemother* **33**: 387.

WHO (1975). Tuberculosis control: progress of the new strategy. *WHO Chron* **29**: 123.

WHO Collaborating Centre for Tuberculosis Chemotherapy, Prague (1976). A study of two twice-weekly and a once-weekly continuation regimen of tuberculosis chemotherapy, including a comparison of two durations of treatment. 1. First report: the results at 18 months. *Tubercle* **57**: 235.

WHO Collaborating Centre for Tuberculosis Chemotherapy, Prague (1977). A study of two twice-weekly and a once-weekly continuation regimen of tuberculosis chemotherapy, including a comparison of two durations of treatment. 2. Second report: the results at 36 months. *Tubercle* **58**: 129.

Williams SE, Wardman AG, Taylor GA *et al.* (1985). Long term study of the effect of rifampicin and isoniazid on vitamin D metabolism. *Tubercle* **66**: 49.

Wolff MJ, Bitran J, Northland RG, Levy IL (1991). Splenic abscesses due to *Mycobacterium tuberculosis* in patients with AIDS. *Rev Infect Dis* **13**: 373.

Wright JM, Stokes EF, Sweeney VP (1982). Isoniazid-induced carbamazepine toxicity and vice versa. *New Engl J Med* **307**: 1325.

Yajko DM, Nassos PS, Sanders CA *et al.* (1994). High predictive value of the acid-fast smear for *Mycobacterium tuberculosis* despite the high prevalence of *Mycobacterium avium* complex in respiratory specimens. *Clin Infect Dis* **19**: 334.

Yates MD, Collins CH, Grange JM (1982). 'Classical' and 'Asian' variants of *Mycobacterium tuberculosis* isolated in South East England 1977–1980. *Tubercle* **62**: 55.

Young EJ, Fainstein J, Musher DM (1982). Drug-induced fever: cases seen in the evaluation of unexplained fever in a general hospital population. *Rev Infect Dis* **4**: 69.

Young LS, Wormser GP (1994). The resurgence of tuberculosis. *Scand J Infect Dis* (Suppl 93): 9.

Zaza S, Blumberg HM, Beck-Sagué C *et al.* (1995). Nosocomial transmission of *Mycobacterium tuberculosis*: role of health care workers in outbreak propagation. *J Infect Dis* **172**: 1542.

Zhang Y, Young D (1994). Molecular genetics of drug resistance in *Mycobacterium tuberculosis*. *J Antimicrob Chemother* **34**: 313.

Zierski M, Bek E, Long MW, Snider DE Jr (1981). Short-course (6-month) cooperative tuberculosis study in Poland: results 30 months after completion of treatment. *Amer Rev Respir Dis* **124**: 249.

Zolopa AR, Hahn JA, Gorter R *et al.* (1994). HIV and tuberculosis infection in San Francisco's homeless adults. *JAMA* **272**: 455.

Ethambutol

Description

This drug was discovered at Lederle Laboratories in 1961, when randomly selected synthetic compounds were being tested for antituberculosis activity. Chemically, it is dextro-2, 2'-(ethylenediimino)-di-1–butanol dihydrochloride, and it has a high degree of antituberculosis activity (Thomas *et al.*, 1961). Ethambutol is a useful drug for the treatment of both human tuberculosis and for infections caused by other mycobacteria.

Activity Against Mycobacteria

Ethambutol is only active against mycobacteria, all other bacteria being completely resistant (Wilson, 1967).

1 Mycobacterium tuberculosis

This is highly sensitive and the MIC is usually 1–2 μg per ml and seldom higher than 5 μg per ml (Karlson, 1961). Strains with an MIC of 8 μg per ml are considered as sensitive, but those with higher MICs are resistant. Ethambutol is often active against *M. tuberculosis* strains resistant to isoniazid and other antituberculosis drugs (Robson and Sullivan, 1963). Ethambutol-resistant *M. tuberculosis* strains can be readily produced *in vitro* (Hobby and Lenert, 1972), and if it is used in the treatment of human tuberculosis without an adequate companion drug or drugs, resistant strains emerge *in vivo* (Crofton, 1971). Primary ethambutol-resistance is still relatively uncommon in developed countries, but during the last decade it has been encountered with increasing frequency. In the USA, some 50% of multidrug-resistant *M. tuberculosis* strains (strains resistant to both isoniazid and rifampicin, p. 1181) have been also ethambutol-resistant (Bloch *et al.*, 1994). In Australia during the years 1988–1991, only some 1% of *M. tuberculosis* isolates were resistant to this drug (Lim, 1995). Ethambutol-resistant strains of *M. tuberculosis* appear to have changes in their cell walls which lead to altered permeability or transport of the drug into the bacterial cell (Sareen and Khuller, 1990).

    Mycobacterium bovis is usually ethambutol-sensitive (Dankner *et al.*, 1993).

2 Mycobacterium avium complex

Only about 40% of strains of these bacteria are moderately ethambutol-sensitive (MICs 2.0–4.0 μg per ml). Others are resistant with MICs of 8.0 μg per ml or higher (Dutt and Stead, 1979; Hawkins *et al.*, 1986; Heifets *et al.*, 1986; Horsburgh *et al.*, 1986; Inderlied *et al.*, 1987; Hoffner *et al.*, 1989; Kemper *et al.*, 1994). If used as a single drug in AIDS patients with *M. avium* bacteremia, ethambutol achieves some reduction in the level of bacteremia in 4 weeks and in this respect it is superior to rifampicin and clofazamine (Kemper *et al.*, 1994), but ethambutol is not as active as the macrolides, clarithromycin (p. 644) and azithromycin (p. 654). When combined with either of these macrolides or with rifampicin, rifabutin, ciprofloxacin, amikacin or streptomycin in a two- , or more effectively, a three-drug regimen ethambutol exhibits synergistic activity against *M. avium* complex both *in vitro* and *in vivo* (Etzkorn *et al.*, 1986; Yajko *et al.*, 1988, 1991; Hoffner *et al.*, 1989; 1990).

3 Other mycobacteria

Mycobacterium kansasii can cause pulmonary or disseminated disease in AIDS patients or more usually pulmonary disease in other patients. This organism is often susceptible to rifampicin and ethambutol; some strains may be sensitive to isoniazid as well (Kuze *et al.*, 1981; Yates and

Collins, 1981; Carpenter and Parks, 1991; Bamberger *et al.*, 1994; Moreno *et al.*, 1994). Hejný (1982) found *M. kansasii* also to be sensitive to other antituberculosis drugs such as ethionamide and cycloserine and also to some other drugs such as erythromycin and sulfonamides.

A species closely related to the *M. avium* complex, *M. malmoense*, may also cause pulmonary disease; strains tested by Banks *et al.* (1983) were sensitive to streptomycin, ethambutol, ethionamide and thiacetazone but resistant to isoniazid, rifampicin, para-aminosalicylic acid (PAS), pyrazinamide and cycloserine. However, Hoffner *et al.* (1993) found most strains of this organism to be resistant or moderately resistant to any single drug, but combinations of ethambutol with ciprofloxacin, amikacin and rifampicin, rendered most isolates susceptible to the combined drugs.

Mycobacterium scrofulaceum, a common cause of lymphadenitis in children, is often sensitive to rifampicin and ethambutol and to a lesser extent to streptomycin and kanamycin (Kuze *et al.*, 1981). *Mycobacterium xenopi* is often susceptible to commonly used antituberculous drugs such as isoniazid, streptomycin and rifampicin (David, 1981). In a study of seven clinical isolates, varying numbers were susceptible to all antituberculous drugs, but streptomycin, kanamycin, ethionamide, and cycloserine inhibited the majority of isolates (Simor *et al.*, 1984). The rapidly growing mycobacteria, *M. fortuitum* and *M. chelonae*, which cause cutaneous, pulmonary and disseminated disease, are resistant to all antituberculous drugs (Kuze *et al.*, 1981; Hejný, 1982); but they may be sensitive to sulfonamides (p. 806), doxycycline (p. 725), amikacin (p. 506), erythromycin (p. 610) or cefoxitin (p. 296). *Mycobacterium simiae*, which can produce pulmonary and less commonly disseminated disease, is resistant to all of the standard antimycobacterial drugs except cycloserine and ethionamide (Weiszfeiler *et al.*, 1981; Rose *et al.*, 1982; Huminer *et al.*, 1993). *Mycobacterium asiaticum* has been reported to be a possible cause of pulmonary disease; this mycobacterium was sensitive to cycloserine and ethionamide but resistant to PAS, isoniazid, rifampicin and thiacetazone (Blacklock *et al.*, 1983). Sensitivity to ethambutol was variable (Woods and Washington, 1987). Surgery may be required for the pulmonary disease or lymphadenitis resulting from these mycobacterial infections.

Mycobacterium marinum is not an uncommon cause of superficial infections (swimming pool or fish tank granuloma). This organism is usually resistant to most antituberculosis drugs but it may be sensitive to ethambutol (Barrow and Hewitt, 1971; Sage and Derrington, 1973), rifampicin (p. 67) and co-trimoxazole. One strain isolated in Denmark was sensitive to rifampicin, ethambutol, cycloserine, ethionamide, prothionamide, viomycin, kanamycin, capreomycin and co-trimoxazole, but resistant to streptomycin and PAS (Engbaek *et al.*, 1980). All four strains of *M. marinum* tested by Yates and Collins (1981) were sensitive to rifampicin and ethambutol. Some strains of *M. szulgai* are ethambutol-sensitive, but others are resistant (Maloney *et al.*, 1987). Most *M. gordonae* isolates are sensitive to isoniazid, PAS, ethambutol, rifampicin, cycloserine, kanamycin, streptomycin and kanamycin (Weinberger *et al.*, 1992). Usually *M. haemophilum* is sensitive to rifampicin, but resistant to ethambutol, isoniazid and streptomycin (Woods and Washington, 1987).

Mycobacterium ulcerans is an important cause of disabling cutaneous ulceration in tropical and semi-tropical areas. Although some strains may be sensitive to ethambutol, streptomycin (p. 428) is the only antibiotic to which this organism is consistently sensitive. In the absence of secondary bacterial infection it is doubtful whether any chemotherapeutic agents are of value for infections due to *M. ulcerans*, and surgical excision and skin grafting are the best forms of treatment (Report, 1970; Radford, 1975). Sometimes streptomycin and dapsone with or without ethambutol has been combined with surgery (Woods and Washington, 1987).

Mode of Administration and Dosage

1 Daily chemotherapy

Ethambutol is administered by the oral route. The dosage is 15–25 mg per kg body weight per day, administered in one dose. The higher daily dose of 25 mg per kg is usually not used for longer than 2 months, when it is lowered to 15 mg per kg to reduce the frequency of ocular complications (Hong Kong/BMRC, 1981). The dose recommended in the USA is 15 mg per kg per day and ethambutol is not usually advised for children whose visual acuity cannot be monitored (CDC, 1980a,b). If absolutely necessary, the lower dosage of 15 mg per kg per day can be used in children with caution (Ad Hoc Committee, 1995).

2 intermittent chemotherapy

Ethambutol is suitable for use in regimens whereby chemotherapy is given intermittently for the treatment of tuberculosis (p. 1195). Dosages utilized in such regimens have been 70 mg per kg body weight (Hong Kong/BMRC, 1984) or 90 mg per kg once-weekly (Tuberculosis Research/ Madras, 1981), 45 mg per kg twice-weekly (Tuberculosis Research/Madras, 1981; Hong Kong/ BMRC, 1978; 1979), 50 mg per kg once- or twice-weekly (Zierski and Bek, 1980) and 15 mg per kg thrice-weekly (Hong Kong/BMRC, 1981).

3 Patients with renal failure

As ethambutol is largely excreted via the kidneys (see below), these patients need dosage reduction (Kovnat et al., 1973). The normal serum half-life of ethambutol of 4 h is doubled in end-stage renal disease (Bennett et al., 1977). Recommended dosage schedules for patients with renal failure are daily oral doses of 25–15, 15–7.5 and 5 mg per kg for those with creatinine clearance values of 50–25, 25–10 and less than 10 ml per min, respectively. A dose of 5 mg per kg per day is recommended for patients undergoing hemodialysis or peritoneal dialysis, although significant amounts of the drug are removed by both forms of dialysis (Cheigh, 1977). The need for a special dosage schedule for dialysis patients was disputed by Mitchison and Ellard (1980); although the average serum levels attained after several days of this dosage would probably be similar to those following a dosage of 25 mg per kg per day in patients with normal renal function, concentrations in the first 1 or 2 days would be much lower and patients who are dialyzed three times a week may not be getting effective therapy. They suggested that larger doses of ethambutol should only given 4–6 h before each dialysis. The pre-dialysis ethambutol dose should be 25 mg per kg for patients being dialyzed three times or more per week, the dose being increased to 45 mg per kg for twice-weekly dialysis and 90 mg per kg for once-weekly dialysis. However, all these dosage recommendations can only be approximate guides, and serum level monitoring is necessary to adjust the dosage of ethambutol in all patients with renal failure (Varughese et al., 1986).

Serum Levels in Relation to Dosage

Ethambutol is well absorbed after oral administration, and following a dose of 25 mg per kg body weight, a peak serum level of about 5 μg per ml is reached in approximately 4 h (Peets et al., 1965). Doubling the dose doubles the peak serum level (Place and Thomas, 1963). Thereafter, the serum level slowly falls and 24 h after the dose it is usually less than 1.0 μg per ml. Administration with food does not impair absorption. In the absence of renal disease ethambutol does not accumulate if daily doses of 25 mg per kg are used (Place and Thomas, 1963). Some AIDS patients, treated for *M. avium* complex disease, may absorb ethambutol and other antimycobacterial agents such as rifampicin (p. 683) poorly from the gastrointestinal tract and low serum levels may result (Gordon et al., 1993).

Excretion

1 Urine

Most of absorbed ethambutol (about 80%) is excreted via the kidneys as the active unchanged drug. This excretion occurs within 24 h of administration (Place and Thomas, 1963), and high concentrations of the active drug are attained in urine.

2 Inactivation in body

Some 8–15% of absorbed ethambutol is converted to various inactive metabolites, and these are also excreted in the urine (Peets et al., 1965). The rate of ethambutol metabolism is similar in all individuals and it is not altered after prolonged administration.

3 Feces

Unabsorbed ethambutol, about 20% of an oral dose, is excreted unchanged in the feces.

Distribution of the Drug in Body

Detailed data about the distribution of ethambutol in various body fluids and tissues are unavailable, but as the drug is therapeutically effective, it presumably reaches infected tissues in sufficient concentrations. Ethambutol enters the red blood cells, where it accumulates against a concentration gradient (Peets et al., 1965). Erythrocytes may therefore serve as a depot for the drug. In animals ethambutol is widely distributed to most body tissues except brain (Kelly et al., 1981; Liss et al., 1981).

Ethambutol does not enter the CSF of patients with normal meninges (Place *et al.*, 1969), though very low levels have been detected by some investigators (Pilheu *et al.*, 1971). In patients with tuberculous meningitis, some ethambutol enters the CSF and with a daily dose of 25 mg per kg, CSF concentrations of 1–2 μg per ml have been reported (Place *et al.*, 1969; Bobrowitz, 1972). Studies in one pregnant patient showed that the ethambutol concentrations reached in placental and cord blood and amniotic fluid were similar to the concentrations in maternal blood (Shneerson and Francis, 1979). The serum protein binding of ethambutol is less than 10% (Bennett *et al.*, 1977).

Mode of Action

Studies with *M. smegmatis* indicate that ethambutol inhibits the biosynthesis of a structurally and biologically important cell wall polysaccharide named arabinogalactan, although it probably also has other actions on the biosynthesis of the cell walls of mycobacteria (Takayama and Kilburn, 1989; Silve *et al.*, 1993; Mikušová *et al.*, 1995). The synergy between ethambutol and other drugs is well documented (p. 1211), and is presumed to occur because ethambutol enables the other drugs to enter via the damaged cell wall into the cells of mycobacteria (Deng *et al.*, 1995).

Early studies indicated that ethambutol had a bacteriostatic action against tubercle bacilli, but in later *in vitro* studies and some clinical studies it has been shown to be bactericidal (p. 1180). It penetrates both extracellular and intracellular environments of tuberculosis lesions and can deter the selection of resistant mutants by other antituberculosis drugs (p. 1180).

Toxicity

In general, ethambutol is a well tolerated drug.

1 Ocular complications

Retrobulbar neuritis is the main complication of ethambutol therapy. Symptoms include blurred vision, central scotomata and color blindness, but sometimes the only change is constriction of visual fields. These changes are usually completely reversible if treatment is stopped (Clarke *et al.*, 1972), though defective color vision may persist for a prolonged period (Lees *et al.*, 1971). If the drug is continued after the onset of symptoms, optic atrophy with permanent impairment of vision may result. Rarely a hemorrhagic retinopathy has been observed.

Ocular complications due to ethambutol appear to be dose-related (Leibold, 1966). Previously when a dosage as high as 50 mg per kg per day was used, this complication occurred in 15% of patients, but with a dosage of 25 mg per kg per day continued longer than 2 months, it occurred in about 5% of patients. Aquinas and Citron (1972) treated 40 patients with daily rifampicin, ethambutol and capreomycin. Ethambutol was used in a dosage of 25 mg per kg per day for 6 months and severe retrobulbar neuritis was observed in two patients, one of whom developed hemorrhagic retinopathy. These patients still had evidence of persistent eye damage 18 months after the drug was stopped. If ethambutol is used in a dosage of 25 mg per kg for 60 days only, and then 15 mg per kg per day (as currently recommended), ocular complications are infrequent and commonly mild, but occasionally these can be severe. The only changes usually noted with such dosage regimens are diminution of visual acuity and red-green color blindness, in most cases both completely reversible (Wilson, 1967). An ethambutol dosage of 15 mg per kg daily has little or no visual toxicity (Snider *et al.*, 1984). The intermittent ethambutol regimens of either 45 mg per kg twice-weekly or 90 mg per kg once-weekly also appear quite safe (Hong Kong, 1974), but even with these regimens a very small percentage of patients can develop dimness of vision which is usually reversible (Tuberculosis Research/Madras, 1981).

Ocular complications sometimes can arise many months after the drug is started, but the total dose of ethambutol administered appears to have no relation to the frequency of these side-effects (Adel, 1969).

Patients treated by ethambutol should be instructed to report all ocular symptoms, which usually precede abnormalities in tests of visual function. Girling (1982) did not consider that such tests are necessary during ethambutol administration. Others have suggested that base-line ophthalmological tests should be performed before treatment is started (Leading article, 1973) and testing of visual fields, visual acuity and color discrimination, every 6 weeks has been recommended by some.

2 Peripheral neuritis

This is a rare side-effect. Tugwell and James (1972) described three patients who developed this complication during ethambutol therapy. One patient was treated by large doses (50 mg per kg per day) and also developed optic neuritis, but the other two patients received ethambutol in doses of less than 20 mg per kg per day. Two of these patients were also receiving isoniazid, but it appeared that isoniazid was not responsible for this complication, because the neuritis only improved in all three patients when ethambutol was discontinued. Although this complication is rare, it is important to recognize that ethambutol as well as isoniazid (p. 1189) can cause peripheral neuropathy.

3 Nephrotoxicity

Circumstances relating to the occurrence and recovery of renal failure in two patients suggested that ethambutol may rarely cause direct toxic damage to the kidneys (Collier et al., 1976). A diffuse interstitial nephritis with similar features to that described with penicillin G (p. 32) and methicillin (p. 84) has been observed in two patients, which may have been due to isoniazid and/or ethambutol therapy (Stone et al., 1976).

4 Other side-effects

Allergic reactions with ethambutol appear to be very rare. Hypersensitivity, manifested by fever, rash, hypotension and liver damage, attributable to ethambutol, has only been reported in a couple of patients (Kerremans et al., 1981). Elevated serum uric acid levels occur in about two-thirds of patients treated with ethambutol; generalized arthralgia and acute gout has been observed in association with hyperuricemia (Postlethwaite et al., 1972; Khanna et al., 1984).

Polyarthritis, rash and hepatitis, associated with anti-native DNA antibodies and positive antinuclear factor, have been described in a 9-year-old boy after 7 months of continuous treatment with rifampicin and ethambutol (Grennan and Sturrock, 1976). It was considered that rifampicin was more likely to be the cause of these side-effects (p. 691). Jaundice and abnormal liver function tests in one elderly patient which occurred three times in association with ethambutol administration, suggests that this drug may be a rare cause of hepatotoxicity (Gulliford et al., 1986). Thrombocytopenia appeared to be induced by ethambutol in one patient (Prasad and Mukerji, 1989).

False-positive phentolamine tests for phaechromocytoma have been observed in patients receiving ethambutol, presumably because of some interaction between these substances (Gabriel, 1972).

Ethambutol is not teratogenic in animals and clinical experience has confirmed that it can be administered safely to pregnant patients (Brock and Roach, 1981).

Clinical Uses of the Drug

1 Treatment of tuberculosis

The past and present roles of ethambutol in the treatment of tuberculosis are described on pp. 1194, 1195. Originally it was a first-line drug used in regimens combined with streptomycin and isoniazid which lasted 18–24 months. Later it was successfully used in shorter regimens lasting 12–18 months. Nowadays it is included in the 6-months regimen of treatment with isoniazid and rifampicin to which pyrazinamide is added for the first 2 months. Ethambutol probably contributes very little to such short-course chemotherapy, unless the patient is harboring isoniazid-resistant bacilli. The drug is also very suitable for use in certain regimens in which chemotherapy is given intermittently.

The main use for ethambutol is as a reserve drug for the treatment of patients with particular problems. These include patients with diabetes, pregnancy or severe liver disease and those with disease due to suspected or proven resistance to antituberculosis drugs. But some multidrug-resistant M. tuberculosis strains are also ethambutol-resistant (p. 1181).

2 Preventive treatment of tuberculosis

An intermittent regimen using isoniazid plus ethambutol has been used successfully for this purpose (p. 1202). A combination of isoniazid, rifampicin and ethambutol has also been suggested for such treatment if it is suspected that the M. tuberculosis strain is isoniazid-resistant (Steinberg et al., 1988).

3 Mycobacterium avium complex infections

Bacteremia due to this organism in AIDS patients is now usually treated by one of the macrolides such as clarithromycin (p. 648) or azithromycin (p. 657) as the first drug in the regimen, ethambutol as the second drug and the third can be rifabutin (p. 712), ciprofloxacin or one of the other drugs. If the macrolides are considered to be too expensive, regimens of ethambutol, rifabutin plus ciprofloxacin can also be successful. *Mycobacterium avium* complex infections in lungs, terminal ileum and other sites in AIDS patients can also be treated with the same drugs, as can pulmonary disease in non-AIDS patients (Bass, 1986; Etzkorn *et al.*, 1986; Schneebaum *et al.*, 1987; Agins *et al.*, 1989; Meduri and Stein, 1992; Heurlin and Petrini, 1993).

4 Other mycobacterial infections

In non-AIDS patients *M. kansasii* pulmonary infections usually respond to rifampicin plus ethambutol (p. 692); sometimes isoniazid is also added to this regimen (Wolinsky, 1992). Disseminated disease and/or pulmonary disease in HIV-infected patients is treated in the same way, perhaps adding another drug such as streptomycin or pyrazinamide to the regimen. Such infections also occur in organ transplant recipients, who are treated similarly, but the treatment in these latter two groups of patients is often unsuccessful (Carpenter and Parks, 1991; Bamberger *et al.*, 1994; Moreno *et al.*, 1994; Patel *et al.*, 1994; Parenti *et al.*, 1995; Witzig *et al.*, 1995).

Although antituberculous drugs have been tried in *M. scrofulaceum* infections, surgical excision of cervical lymphadenitis is usually successful (Schaad *et al.*, 1979; Woods and Washington, 1987). An occasional cause of pulmonary disease in humans, *M. xenopi* is often susceptible to antituberculosis drugs (p. 1212) and may respond to therapy with isoniazid, rifampicin and streptomycin (Bass and Hawkins, 1983; Wolinsky, 1992). Doxycycline (p. 745), amikacin (p. 516), cefoxitin (p. 309), sulfonamides (p. 809) and erythromycin (p. 621) may be useful for the treatment of infections due to *M. fortuitum* and *M. chelonae*. Wallace *et al.* (1983) suggested that because of the frequent susceptibility of *M. fortuitum* to doxycycline and sulfonamides, empiric oral therapy could be instituted for patients with this infection prior to obtaining susceptibility results, but because *M. chelonae* is usually resistant to these oral drugs, parenteral therapy with amikacin and cefoxitin should be used. The place of chemotherapy in the treatment of *M. simiae* infections has not yet been established (Rose *et al.*, 1982; Bell *et al.*, 1983; Woods and Washington, 1987; Huminer *et al.*, 1993). Pulmonary disease due to *M. asiaticum* in two patients appeared to respond to treatment with rifampicin and ethambutol, even though the strains were resistant *in vitro* to rifampicin and probably ethambutol (Blacklock *et al.*, 1983). Granulomata caused by *M. marinum* do not usually require chemotherapy because they resolve spontaneously, but in some circumstances, such as delayed resolution, treatment with rifampicin and ethambutol has been successful (Engbaek *et al.*, 1980) (p. 692).

The best regimen for treatment of disseminated *M. gordonae* infections has not been determined, but ethambutol and rifampicin are usually used together with other drugs (Weinberger *et al.*, 1992). Infections of *M. szulgae* are usually treated by rifampicin, isoniazid and ethambutol, with streptomycin or capreomycin serving as a fourth or substitute drug (Maloney *et al.*, 1987; Woods and Washington, 1987). The best regimen for the treatment of *M. malmoense* infections has not been established (Woods and Washington, 1987; Henriques *et al.*, 1994).

5 Nocardia brasiliensis infections

Ethambutol has been reported to be effective in the treatment of mycetomas (actinomycetomas) caused by this organism (Borelli and Leal, 1969; Berd, 1973).

References

Adel A (1969). Ophthalmological side-effects of ethambutol. *Scand J Respir Dis* (Suppl 69): 55.

Ad Hoc Committee on the Scientific Assembly on Microbiology, Tuberculosis and Pulmonary Infections (1995). Treatment of tuberculosis and tuberculosis infection in adults and children. *Clin Infect Dis* 21: 9.

Agins BD, Berman DS, Spicehandler D *et al.* (1989). Effect of combined therapy with ansamycin, clofazamine, ethambutol, and isoniazid for *Mycobacterium avium* infection in patients with AIDS. *J Infect Dis* **159**: 784.

Aquinas M, Citron KM (1972). Rifampicin, ethambutol and capreomycin in pulmonary tuberculosis, previously treated with both first and second line

drugs: the results of 2 years chemotherapy. *Tubercle* **53**: 153.

Bamberger DM, Driks MR, Gupta MR *et al.* (1994). *Mycobacterium kansasii* among patients infected with human immunodeficiency virus in Kansas City. *Clin Infect Dis* **18**: 395.

Banks J, Smith AP, Jenkins PA (1983). *Mycobacterium malmoense* – problems with treatment and diagnosis – case report. *Tubercle* **64**: 217.

Barksdale L, Kim K (1977). Mycobacteria. *Bacteriol Rev* **41**: 217.

Barrow GI, Hewitt M (1971). Skin infection with *Mycobacterium marinum* from a tropical fish tank. *Brit Med J* **1**: 505.

Bass JB Jr (1986). *Mycobacterium avium–intracellulare*-rational therapy of chronic pulmonary infection? *Amer Rev Respir Dis* **134**: 431.

Bass JB R, Hawkins EL (1983). Treatment of disease caused by nontuberculous mycobacteria. *Arch Intern Med* **143**: 1439.

Bell RC, Higuchi JH, Donovan WN *et al.* (1983). Mycobacterium simiae Clinical features and follow up of twenty-four patients. *Amer Rev Respir Dis* **127**: 35.

Bennett WM, Singer I, Golper T *et al.* (1977). Guidelines for drug therapy in renal failure. *Ann Intern Med* **86**: 754.

Berd D (1973). *Nocardia brasiliensis* infection in the United States: a report of nine cases and a review of the literature. *Amer J Clin Pathol* **59**: 254.

Blacklock ZM, Dawson DJ, Kane DW, McEvoy D (1983). *Mycobacterium asiaticum* as a potential pulmonary pathogen for humans. *Amer Rev Respir Dis* **127**: 241.

Bloch AB, Cauthen GM, Onorato IM *et al.* (1994). Nationwide survey of drug-resistant tuberculosis in the United States. *JAMA* **271**: 665.

Bobrowitz ID (1972). Ethambutol in tuberculous meningitis. *Chest* **61**: 629.

Borelli D, Leal J (1969). Mycetoma by *Nocardia brasiliensis* successfully treated with ethambutol. *Trans Roy Soc Med Hyg* **63**: 881; quoted by Berd (1973).

Brock PG, Roach M (1981). Antituberculous drugs in pregnancy. *Lancet* **i**: 43.

Carpenter JL, Parks JM (1991). *Mycobacterium kansasii* infections in patients positive for human immunodeficiency virus. *Rev Infect Dis* **13**: 789.

CDC (Center for Disease Control) (1980a). Guidelines for short-course tuberculosis chemotherapy. *MMW Rep* **29**: 97.

CDC (Center for Disease Control) (1980b). Follow-up on guidelines for short-course tuberculosis chemotherapy. *MMW Rep* **29**: 183.

Cheigh JS (1977). Drug administration in renal failure. *Amer J Med* **62**: 555.

Clarke GBM, Cuthbert J, Cuthbert RJ, Lees AW (1972). Isoniazid plus ethambutol in the initial treatment of pulmonary tuberculosis. *Brit J Dis Chest* **66**: 272.

Collier J, Joekes AM, Philalithis PE, Thompson FD (1976). Two cases of ethambutol nephrotoxicity. *Brit Med J* **2**: 1105.

Crofton J (1971). Problems of drug resistance in tuberculosis – the newer antituberculosis drugs. *Postgrad Med J* **47**: 748.

Dankner WM, Waeckner NJ, Essey MA *et al.* (1993). *Mycobacterium bovis* infections in San Diego: a clinicoepidemiologic study of 73 patients and a historical review of a forgotten pathogen. *Medicine* **72**: 11.

David HL (1981). Basis for lack of drug susceptibility of atypical mycobacteria. *Rev Infect Dis* **3**: 878.

Deng L, Mikusová K, Robuck KG *et al.* (1995). Recognition of multiple effects of ethambutol on metabolism of mycobacterial cell envelope. *Antimicrob Ag Chemother* **39**: 694.

Dutt AK, Stead WW (1979). Long-term results of medical treatment in *Mycobacterium intracellulare* infection. *Amer J Med* **67**: 449.

Engbaek HC, Thormann J, Vergmann B (1980). Aquarium-borne *Mycobacterium marinum* granulomas. *Scand J Infect Dis* **12**: 74.

Etzkorn ET, Aldarondo S, McAllister CK *et al.* (1986). Medical therapy of *Mycobacterium avium–intracellulare* pulmonary disease. *Amer Rev Respir Dis* **134**: 442.

Gabriel R (1972). Ethambutol and a false-positive screening test for phaeochromocytoma. *Brit Med J* **3**: 332.

Girling DJ (1982). Adverse effect of antituberculosis drugs. *Curr Therap* **23**: 101.

Gordon SM, Horsburgh CRJr, Peloquin CA *et al.* (1993). Low serum levels of oral antimycobacterial agents in patients with disseminated *Mycobacterium avium* complex disease. *J Infect Dis* **168**: 1559.

Grennan DM, Sturrock RD (1976). Polyarthritis, hepatitis and anti-native DNA antibodies after treatment with ethambutol and rifampicin. *Tubercle* **57**: 259.

Gulliford M, Mackay AD, Prowse K (1986). Cholestatic jaundice caused by ethambutol. *Brit Med J* **292**: 866.

Hawkins CC, Gold JWM, Whimbey E *et al.* (1986). *Mycobacterium avium* complex infections in patients with the acquired immunodeficiency syndrome. *Ann Intern Med* **105**: 184.

Heifets LB, Iseman MD, Lindholm-Levy PJ (1986). Ethambutol MICs and MBCs for *Mycobacterium avium* complex and *Mycobacterium tuberculosis*. *Antimicrob Ag Chemother* **30**: 927.

Hejný J (1982). A drug sensitivity strategy for atypical mycobacteria. *Tubercle* **62**: 63.

Henriques B, Hoffner SE, Petrini B *et al.* (1994). Infection with *Mycobacteirum malmoense* in Sweden: report of 221 cases. *Clin Infect Dis* **18**: 596.

Heurlin N, Petrini B (1993). Treatment of non-tuberculous mycobacterial infections in patients without AIDS. *Scand J Infect Dis* **25**: 619.

Hobby GL, Lenert TF (1972). Observations on the action of rifampin and ethambutol alone and in combination with other antituberculous drugs. *Amer Rev Respir Dis* **105**: 292.

Hoffner SE, Kratz M, Olsson-Lijequist B *et al.* (1989). *In vitro* synergistic activity between ethambutol and fluorinated quinolones against *Mycobacterium avium* complex. *J Antimicrob Chemother* **24**: 317.

Hoffner SE, Svenson SB, Beezer AE (1990). Microcalorimetric studies of the initial interaction between antimycobacterial drugs and *Mycobacterium avium*. *J Antimicrob Chemother* **25**: 353.

Hoffner SE, Hjelm U, Källenius G (1993). Susceptibility of *Mycobacterium malmoense* to antibacterial drugs and drug combinations. *Antimicrob Ag Chemother* **37**: 1285.

Hong Kong Chest Service/British Medical Research Council (1978). Controlled trial of 6-month and 8-month regimens in the treatment of pulmonary tuberculosis. *Amer Rev Respir Dis* **118**: 219.

Hong Kong Chest Service/British Medical Research Council (1979). Controlled trial of 6-month and 8-month regimens in the treatment of pulmonary tuberculosis: the results up to 24 months. *Tubercle* **60**: 201.

Hong Kong Chest Service/British Medical Research Council (1981). Controlled trial of four thrice-weekly regimens and a daily regimen all given for 6 months for pulmonary tuberculosis. *Lancet* **i**: 171.

Hong Kong Chest Service/British Medical Research Council (1984). Study of a fully supervised programme of chemotherapy for pulmonary tuberculosis given once weekly in the continuation phase in the rural areas of Hong Kong. *Tubercle* **65**: 5.

Hong Kong Tuberculosis Treatment Services/Brompton Hospital/British Medical Research Council Investigation (1974). A controlled clinical trial of daily and intermittent regimens of rifampicin plus ethambutol in the retreatment of patients with pulmonary tuberculosis in Hong Kong. *Tubercle* **55**: 1.

Horsburgh CR Jr, Cohn DL, Roberts RB *et al.* (1986). *Mycobacterium avium-M intracellulare* isolates from patients with or without acquired immunodeficiency syndrome. *Antimicrob Ag Chemother* **30**: 955.

Huminer D, Dux S, Samra Z *et al.* (1993). *Mycobacterium simiae* infection in Israeli patients with AIDS. *Clin Infect Dis* **17**: 508.

Inderlied CB, Young LS, Yamada JK (1987). Determination of *in vitro* susceptibility of *Mycobacterium avium* complex isolates to antimycobacterial agents by various methods. *Antimicrob Ag Chemother* **31**: 1697.

Karlson AG (1961). The *in vitro* activity of ethambutol (dextro-2,2'-[ethylenedi-iminol]-DI-1-butanol). against tubercle bacilli and other microorganisms. *Amer Rev Respir Dis* **84**: 905.

Kelly RG, Kaleita E, Eisner HJ (1981). Tissue distribution of (14C). ethambutol in mice. *Amer Rev Respir Dis* **123**: 689.

Kemper CA, Havlir D, Haghighat D *et al.* (1994). The individual microbiologic effect of three antimycobacterial agents, clofazimine, ethambutol, and rifampin, on *Mycobacterium avium* complex bacteremia in patients with AIDS. *J Infect Dis* **170**: 157.

Kerremans A, Majoor CLH, Gribnau FWJ (1981). Hypersensitivity to ethambutol. *Tubercle* **62**: 215.

Khanna BK, Gupta VP, Singh MP (1984). Ethambutol-induced hyperuricaemia. *Tubercle* **65**: 195.

Kovnat P, Labovitz E, Levison SP (1973). Antibiotics and the kidney. *Med Clin N Amer* **57**: 1045.

Kuze F, Kurasawa T, Bando K *et al.* (1981). *In vitro* and *in vivo* susceptibility of atypical mycobacteria to various drugs. *Rev Infect Dis* **3**: 885.

Leading Article (1973). Rifampicin or ethambutol in the routine treatment of tuberculosis. *Brit Med J* **4**: 568.

Lees AW, Allan GW, Smith J *et al.* (1971). Toxicity from rifampicin plus isoniazid and rifampicin plus ethambutol therapy. *Tubercle* **52**: 182.

Leibold JE (1966). The ocular toxicity of ethambutol and its relation to dose. *Ann NY Acad Sci* **135**: 904.

Lichtenstein IH, MacGregor RR (1983). Mycobacterial infections in renal transplant recipients: report of five cases and review of the literature. *Rev Infect Dis* **5**: 216.

Lim I (1995). Susceptibility of *M tuberculosis* isolates in Australia. *ASIG Newsletter* **2**: 1.

Liss RH, Letourneau RJ, Schepis JP (1981). Distribution of ethambutol in primate tissues and cells. *Amer Rev Respir Dis* **123**: 529.

Maloney JM, Gregg CR, Stephens DS *et al.* (1987). Infections caused by *Mycobacterium szulgai* in humans. *Rev Infect Dis* **9**: 1120.

Meduri GU, Stein DS (1992). Pulmonary manifestations of acquired immunodeficiency syndrome. *Clin Infect Dis* **14**: 98.

Mikušová K, Slayden RA, Besra GS, Brennan PJ (1995). Biogenesis of the mycobacterial cell wall and the site of action of ethambutol. *Antimicrob Ag Chemother* **39**: 2484.

Mitchison DA, Ellard GA (1980). Tuberculosis in patients having dialysis. *Brit Med J* **1**: 1186.

Moreno F, Sharkey-Mathis PK, Mokulis E, Smith JA (1994). *Mycobacterium kansasii* pericarditis in patients with AIDS. *Clin Infect Dis* **19**: 967.

Parenti DM, Symington JS, Keiser J, Simon GL (1995). *Mycobacterium kansasii* bacteremia in patients infected with human immunodeficiency virus. *Clin Infect Dis* **21**: 1001.

Patel R, Roberts GD, Keating MR, Paya CV (1994). Infections due to nontuberculous mycobacteria in kidney, heart, and liver transplant recipients. *Clin Infect Dis* **19**: 263.

Peets EA, Sweeney WM, Place VA, Buyske DA (1965). The absorption, excretion and metabolic fate of ethambutol in man. *Amer Rev Respir Dis* **91**: 51.

Pilheu JA, Maglio F, Cetrangolo R, Pleus AD (1971). Concentrations of ethambutol in the cerebrospinal fluid after oral administration. *Tubercle* **52**: 117.

Place VA, Thomas JP (1963). Clinical pharmacology of ethambutol. *Amer Rev Respir Dis* **87**: 901.

Place VA, Pyle MM, De la Huerga J (1969). Ethambutol in tuberculous meningitis. *Amer Rev Respir Dis* **99**: 783.

Postlethwaite AE, Bartel AG, Kelley WN (1972). Hyperuricemia due to ethambutol. *New Engl J Med* **286**: 761.

Prasad R, Mukerji PK (1989). Ethambutol-induced thrombocytopenia. *Tubercle* **70**: 211.

Radford AJ (1975). *Mycobacterium ulcerans* in Australia. *Aust NZ J Med* **5**: 162.

Report II of the Uganda Buruli Group (1970). Clinical features and treatment of pre-ulcerative buruli lesions. *Brit Med J* **1**: 390.

Robson JM, Sullivan FM (1963). Antituberculosis drugs. *Pharmacol Rev* **15**: 169.

Rose HD, Dorff GJ, Lauwasser M, Sheth NK (1982). Pulmonary and disseminated *Mycobacterium simiae* infection in humans. *Amer Rev Respir Dis* **126**: 1110.

Sage RE, Derrington AW (1973). Opportunistic cutaneous *Mycobacterium marinum* infection mimicking *Mycobacterium ulcerans* in lympho-sarcoma. *Med J Aust* **2**: 434.

Sareen M, Khuller GK (1990). Cell wall and membrane changes associated with ethambutol resistance in *Mycobacterium tuberculosis* H$_{37}$ Ra. *Antimicrob Ag Chemother* **34**: 1773.

Schaad UB, Votteler TP, McCracken GH Jr, Nelson JD (1979). Management of atypical mycobacterial lymphadenitis in childhood: a review based on 380 cases. *J Pediatr* **95**: 356.

Schneebaum CW, Novick DM, Chabon AB *et al.* (1987). Terminal ileitis associated with *Mycobacterium avium–intracellulare* infection in a homosexual man with acquired immune deficiency syndrome. *Gastroenterology* **92**: 1127.

Shneerson JM, Francis RS (1979). Ethambutol in pregnancy – foetal exposure. *Tubercle* **60**: 167.

Silve G, Valero-Guillen P, Quemard A *et al.* (1993). Ethambutol inhibition of glucose metabolism in mycobacteria: a possible target of the drug. *Antimicrob Ag Chemother* **37**: 1536.

Simor AE, Salit IE, Vellend H (1984). The role of *Mycobacterium xenopi* in human disease. *Amer Rev Respir Dis* **129**: 435.

Snider DE Jr, Long MW, Cross FS, Farer LS (1984). Six-months isoniazid-rifampicin therapy for pulmonary tuberculosis. Report of a United States public health service cooperative trial. *Amer Rev Respir Dis* **129**: 573.

Steinberg JL, Nardell EA, Kass EH (1988). Antibiotic prophylaxis after exposure to antibiotic-resistant *Mycobacterium tuberculosis*. *Rev Infect Dis* **10**: 1208.

Stone WJ, Waldron JA, Dixon JH Jr *et al.* (1976). Acute diffuse interstitial nephritis related to chemotherapy of tuberculosis. *Antimicrob Ag Chemother* **10**: 164.

Takayama K, Kilburn JO (1989). Inhibition of synthesis of arabinogalactan by ethambutol in Mycobacterium smegmatis. *Antimicrob Ag Chemother* **33**: 1493.

Thomas JP, Baughn CO, Wilkinson RG, Shepherd RG (1961). A new synthetic compound with antituberculous activity in mice: ethambutol (dextro-2,2'-[ethylenediiminol]-DI-1–butanol).. *Amer Rev Respir Dis* **83**: 891.

Tuberculosis Research Centre, Madras-600031, India (1981). Ethambutol plus isoniazid for the treatment of pulmonary tuberculosis – a controlled trial of four regimens. *Tubercle* **61**: 13.

Tugwell P, James SL (1972). Peripheral neuropathy with ethambutol. *Postgrad Med J* **48**: 667.

Varughese A, Brater DC, Benet LZ, Lee CSC (1986). Ethambutol kinetics in patients with impaired renal function. *Amer Rev Respir Dis* **134**: 34.

Wallace RJ Jr, Swenson JM, Silcox VA *et al.* (1983). Spectrum of disease due to rapidly growing mycobacteria. *Rev Infect Dis* **5**: 657.

Weinberger M, Berg SL, Feuerstein IM *et al.* (1992). Disseminated infection with *Mycobacterium gardonae*: report of a case and critical review of the literature. *Clin Infect Dis* **14**: 1229.

Weiszfeiler JG, Karasseva J, Karczag E (1981). *Mycobacterium simiae* and related mycobacteria. *Rev Infect Dis* **3**: 1040.

Wilson TM (1967). Current therapeutics CCXL – Capreomycin and ethambutol. *Practitioner* **199**: 817.

Witzig RS, Fazal BA, Mera RM *et al.* (1995). Clinical manifestations and implications of coinfection with *Mycobacterium kansasii* and human immunodeficiency virus type 1. *Clin Infect Dis* **21**: 77.

Wolinsky E (1992). Mycobacterial diseases other than tuberculosis. *Clin Infect Dis* **15**: 1.

Woods GL, Washington JA II (1987). Mycobacteria other than *Mycobacterium tuberculosis*: review of microbiologic and clinical aspects. *Rev Infect Dis* **9**: 275.

Yajko DM, Kirihara J, Sanders C *et al.* (1988). Antimicrobial synergism against *Mycobacterium avium* complex strains isolated from patients with acquired immune deficiency syndrome. *Antimicrob Ag Chemother* **32**: 1392.

Yajko DM, Nassos PS, Sanders CA, Hadley WK (1991). Effects of antimicrobial agents on survival of *Mycobacterium avium* complex inside alveolar macrophages obtained from patients with human immunodeficiency virus infection. *Antimicrob Ag Chemother* **35**: 1621.

Yates MD, Collins CH (1981). Sensitivity of opportunist mycobacteria to rifampicin and ethambutol. *Tubercle* **62**: 117.

Zierski M, Bek E (1980). Side-effects of drug regimens used in short-course chemotherapy for pulmonary tuberculosis. A controlled clinical study. *Tubercle* **61**: 41.

Pyrazinamide

Description

Pyrazinamide, a derivative of nicotinamide, was synethetized in 1952 and shown to possess a high degree of antituberculosis activity in man (Yeager *et al.*, 1952). Previously regarded as a reserve drug, pyrazinamide now has an important role, particularly in the short-course treatment of tuberculosis (p. 1195).

Activity Against Mycobacteria

Pyrazinamide has a relatively low activity against *Mycobacterium tuberculosis*. The usual MIC is 20 μg per ml if this is tested at an acid pH of 5.5 (Stottmeier *et al.*, 1968), but pyrazinamide is almost completely inactive against *M. tuberculosis* at a neutral pH (Robson and Sullivan, 1963; Salfinger and Heifets, 1988). *In vivo* studies show that pyrazinamide is an effective bactericidal antituberculosis drug, and it has a specific sterilizing action against *M. tuberculosis* in the intracellular environment of macrophages (p. 1180). The acid environment presumably in some way makes *M. tuberculosis* more susceptible to pyrazinamide. Paradoxically, other *in vitro* studies and studies of the activity of the drug against intracellularly growing *M. tuberculosis* have shown that pyrazinamide is only very weakly bactericidal (Rastogi *et al.*, 1988; Heifets and Lindholm-Levy, 1990), but *in vivo* in a murine model pyrazinamide had some activity against *M. tuberculosis* infection if the MIC of the strain was 256 μg per ml or lower (Klemens *et al.*, 1996). *Mycobacterium bovis* is resistant (Dankner *et al.*, 1993). As with other antituberculosis drugs, resistance to pyrazinamide develops rapidly if it is used alone to treat human tuberculosis. Pyrazinamide-resistant *M. tuberculosis* strains are still uncommon, but some multidrug-resistant strains are now also resistant to this drug (p. 1181).

Other mycobacteria are usually pyrazinamide-resistant.

Mode of Administration and Dosage

1 Daily administration

Pyrazinamide is administered by the oral route in a single daily dose of 25–30 mg per kg body weight. Common adult daily doses which are used are 1.5 g (weight less than 50 kg), 2.0 g (weight 50–74 kg) and 2.5 g (weight 75 kg or more) (British Thoracic Association, 1982; Corbella *et al.*, 1995).

2 Intermittent administration

Pyrazinamide is suitable for intermittent therapy of tuberculosis (p. 1184). The recommended dosages are 45 mg per kg three times per week or 70 mg per kg twice-weekly (Girling, 1982). Common adult regimens given as a single dose in clinical trials are 2.0 or 2.5 g three times per week and 3.0 or 3.5 g twice-weekly, with the higher dose being used for patients weighing more than 50 kg (Hong Kong/BMRC, 1979).

3 Patients with liver disease and renal failure

As pyrazinamide is hepatotoxic (p. 1221) it would be best avoided in patients with liver diseases, but if it is essential to use it in such patients, its serum levels should be monitored and dosage adjusted, as the drug is metabolized in the liver (p. 1220). As very little pyrazinamide is excreted as such via the kidney (see below), the drug can probably be given in the normal dosage to patients with renal failure, but again it may be best to avoid its use in these patients, as its metabolites may accumulate in the serum and these may be toxic.

Serum Levels in Relation to Dosage

The absorption of pyrazinamide from the gastrointestinal tract is rapid and virtually complete. Peak serum levels occur within 2 h; these and the urinary excretion of pyrazinamide and its metabolite pyrazinoic acid are proportional to the dose used, over a range of 0.5–3.0 g pyrazinamide (Ellard, 1969). Peak serum levels in one subject reached 33 μg per ml after 1.5 g and 59 μg per ml after 3.0 g of pyrazinamide; these then fell exponentially during the period 3–48 h after administration, with a serum half-life of 9–10 h. If pyrazinamide is given in a dosage of 0.5 g three times daily, a serum concentration of 5 μg per ml is maintained for about 90% of the time, but a level of 20 μg per ml is only briefly reached. When a dose of 3.0 g is given every second day, serum levels of 30 μg per ml or higher are maintained for 7 h, but a level of 5 μg per ml is only present for about 23 h.

The co-administration of pyrazinamide and rifampicin results in slightly lower serum levels of rifampicin, but this is not important clinically (Jain et al., 1993).

Excretion

1 Urine

About 3–4% of administered pyrazinamide is excreted as such in the urine and 30–41% as pyrazinoic acid (Ellard, 1969; Ellard and Haslam, 1976). Urinary concentrations of pyrazinamide, similar to serum levels, reach a peak in about 2 h then fall exponentially from 3- to 48-h after a dose. The half-life of the drug in the urine is about 9 h. The ratio of urinary to serum concentrations of pyrazinamide after a single dose is fairly constant; after a dose of 1.5 g urinary concentrations are about 44% higher and after 3.0 g about 85% higher.

Approximately 98% of pyrazinamide filtered by the kidneys is reabsorbed but very little pyrazinoic acid appears to be reabsorbed. Urinary levels of pyrazinoic acid after a single dose of pyrazinamide reach a maximum after about 12 h and fall exponentially from 16–50 h.

2 Bile

Animal experiments suggest that pyrazinamide may also be excreted and concentrated in the bile (Stottmeier et al., 1968).

3 Inactivation in body

Pyrazinamide (pyrazinoic acid amide) is metabolized to pyrazinoic acid by the hepatic microsomal enzyme pyrazinamide deamidase, and pyrazinoic acid is further metabolized to 5–hydroxypyrazinoic acid by xanthine oxidase. The failure to recover the whole of an administered dose of pyrazinamide from the urine suggests that there may be other metabolites (Ellard and Haslam, 1976). Pyrazinamide accumulates in jaundiced patients receiving the usual doses (Stottmeier et al., 1968).

Distribution of the Drug in Body

Animal studies have shown that tissue concentrations of 15–20 μg per g may be attained in the liver, lungs and kidneys, but concentrations reached in other tissues, such as the spleen, bone marrow and skeletal muscle, are much less. Pyrazinamide apparently penetrates the cell wall of macrophages, indicating that it may have a high activity against phagocytosed tubercle bacilli (Stottmeier et al., 1968). A pyrazinamide concentration of 15 μg per g of lung tissue was demonstrated in one patient treated for pulmonary tuberculosis (Stottmeier et al., 1968).

Pyrazinamide appears to penetrate into the CSF, at least in patients with tuberculous meningitis. In such patients the peak CSF concentrations 1.5–2.5 h after each dose averaged 50 μg per ml which was identical or even higher to the serum concentration at the time (Forgan-Smith et al., 1973; Ellard et al., 1987; Donald and Seifart, 1988).

Mode of Action

The precise mechanism of action of pyrazinamide on tubercle bacilli is not known. Its metabolite which is less active in vitro may possibly be involved in the in vivo activity of the drug. Pyrazinamide-susceptible strains of M. tuberculosis are known to produce an enzyme pyrazinamidase, which converts pyrazinamide into pyrazinoic acid. This enzyme generated product may have high antibacterial activity in an acid environment and pyrazinamide itself may not have any activity at all. Pyrazinoic acid also appears to accumulate within macrophages and it appears to lower the pH within these cells and this probably increases its antimycobacterial activity. It is also possible that pyrazinoic acid is transported more efficiently than pyrazinamide itself into the mycobacterial cell (Heifets *et al.*, 1989; Salfinger *et al.*, 1990; Speirs *et al.*, 1995).

Toxicity

1 Hepatotoxicity

This is the most important toxic effect of this drug. Hepatotoxicity first became evident in the USA when pyrazinamide was used as a first-line drug for tuberculosis in the 1950s (McDermott *et al.*, 1954). In these early studies a high dosage of 40–50 mg per kg body weight per day was used. Results of A United States Public Health Service Trial (1959) indicated that hepatotoxicity was related to the use of such high dosage. As a result of these and similar studies, the use of pyrazinamide as a first-line drug for tuberculosis was abandoned (Girling, 1978). Later it became apparent that the reputation of pyrazinamide as a toxic drug had been exaggerated because of the circumstances in which it had been used (Fox and Mitchison, 1975). Apart from being used in high dosage for prolonged periods, it was often used with other toxic drugs such as ethionamide (p. 1236) and/or cycloserine (p. 1228) in retreatment regimens, and it was frequently given to middle-aged or elderly patients who are more vulnerable to toxic effects. When pyrazinamide was used in later studies in other countries, hepatic toxicity was not a major problem (Girling, 1978). If used in a moderate daily dosage of 20–30 mg per kg body weight, combined with streptomycin or streptomycin plus para-aminosalicylic acid (PAS), toxicity was not marked. Moreover, even when pyrazinamide was used in high dosage in intermittent regimens (maximum of 90 mg per kg weekly) combined with streptomycin or streptomycin plus isoniazid, hepatotoxicity was uncommon.

Pyrazinamide has now been used extensively in short-course chemotherapy in many countries and there have been no reports of a high incidence of serious toxicity (Fox, 1978). These have included many studies (p. 1196) in which pyrazinamide has been given together with isoniazid and rifampicin; these regimens have been well tolerated and the addition of pyrazinamide to the other two drugs has not increased the incidence of hepatitis. It is now generally accepted that pyrazinamide, if used in the proper doses, has a small risk of hepatotoxicity (Dutt and Stead, 1982; Girling, 1982). It is probably not necessary to perform routine liver function tests during antituberculosis therapy unless the patient has liver disease or may be more prone to liver damage (p. 1191). Girling (1982) pointed out that transient and symptomless increases in serum hepatic enzyme levels are usual during the early weeks of treatment, whatever the drug regimen, and alone is not an indication to interrupt therapy. If symptoms of hepatitis or grossly elevated transaminase levels are detected then all drugs should be stopped and if the liver damage is drug-induced it usually resolves quickly. Treatment with the same drugs can often be resumed uneventfully but monitoring of liver function is then essential.

Pyrazinamide hepatotoxicity is normally considered to be a direct, dose-related toxic effect (Girling, 1978), but Corbella *et al.* (1995) reported a patient with pyrazinamide-induced hepatitis for which the rechallenge data suggested a hypersensitivity mechanism.

2 Arthralgia

The other main side-effect of pyrazinamide is arthralgia associated with raised serum uric acid levels. In the earliest report on the use of pyrazinamide in pulmonary tuberculosis, Yeager *et al.* (1952) noted the occurrence of pain and restricted joint movement without evidence of arthritis in a quarter of patients treated. Cullen *et al.* (1956) observed that the serum uric acid was elevated in patients receiving pyrazinamide and some of these developed clinical gout. The hyperuricemic effect of pyrazinamide has been confirmed by numerous studies. Arthralgia has occurred with varying frequency amongst patients receiving pyrazinamide in antituberculous regimens (p. 1194). Some studies have shown that arthralgia is more common when the drug is given daily than when given intermittently (Hong Kong/BMRC, 1976, 1978). In the more recent short-course regimens using pyrazinamide, only a small percentage of patients developed arthralgia, though the percentage may be higher amongst patients treated in India (Tuberculous Research Centre, 1983). One study suggested that the patients who develop arthralgia had higher serum uric acid concentrations than those who do not (Hong Kong/BMRC, 1976); this was not confirmed by others (Jenner *et al.*, 1981). Acute gouty arthritis has only rarely been observed in association with pyrazinamide therapy and the arthralgia which occurs differs from gout in a number of respects. The joints most frequently affected by pyrazinamide arthralgia are the shoulders, knees and fingers; symptoms and signs are mild and arthralgia is usually self-limiting; aspirin has a small beneficial effect but not allopurinol (Horsfall *et al.*, 1979).

In clinical trials in India using short-course regimens for pulmonary tuberculosis containing pyrazinamide and rifampicin, the incidence of arthralgia was appreciably less in patients who received rifampicin than those who did not; this was also demonstrated in a small study carried out to investigate this association (Sarma *et al.*, 1983). This was in contrast to previous experience in Hong Kong and Singapore, where the incidence of arthralgia and hyperuricemia with regimens containing pyrazinamide was uninfluenced by rifampicin administration (Jenner *et al.*, 1981).

Pyrazinamide suppresses the urinary excretion of uric acid by attenuating its tubular secretion, and this is mediated by its metabolite, pyrazinoic acid (Guttman *et al.*, 1969). After a 3-g dose of pyrazinamide the urinary excretion of uric acid is maximally suppressed for 24 h and partially reduced for a further 24 h (Ellard and Haslam, 1976). Sarma *et al.* (1983) showed that after a dose of pyrazinamide the renal excretion of uric acid at 5 h was less than 40% of the pre-drug administration value, and it returned nearly to pretreatment levels at 24 h. They also observed that rifampicin enhanced the renal excretion of uric acid, both in the presence and in the absence of pyrazinamide, and also that of pyrazinoic acid. It was postulated that this effect of rifampicin leads to a decrease of the deposition of uric acid in joints and thereby a lower incidence of arthralgia. Rifampicin did not affect serum uric acid levels, presumably because these were already saturated by the effect of pyrazinamide and would continue to be maintained by mobilization of uric acid from the tissues despite the uricosuric effect of rifampicin. This effect of rifampicin may be due to inhibition of tubular reabsorption of uric acid and pyrazinoic acid.

A number of complex interactions occur when pyrazinamide and probenecid are given to patients with gout (Yü *et al.*, 1977). Pretreatment with pyrazinamide results in prolongation of the half-life of probenecid. As the rate of probenecid metabolism is decreased, its uricosuric action tends to be prolonged and the effect of pyrazinamide is lessened. After probenecid-induced uricosuria, pyrazinamide has a greater effect in suppressing urate excretion; this may be because it lessens the capacity of probenecid to inhibit tubular urate reabsorption while it continues to exert an inhibition on tubular urate secretion. When pyrazinamide and probenecid are co-administered, urinary excretion of urate depends on the relative doses and the times at which the drugs are administered.

3 Gastrointestinal side-effects

Anorexia and nausea and less commonly vomiting may occur in the absence of hepatotoxicity, but liver function tests should be performed in these circumstances.

4 Hypersensitivity reactions

Cutaneous hypersensitivity reactions and photosensitivity are rare, but pyrazinamide commonly causes flushing (Girling, 1982).

5 Other side-effects

Rarely pyrazinamide has caused thrombocytopenia (Jain *et al.*, 1988) and one 2-year-old boy developed convulsions which appeared to be caused by the drug (Herlevsen *et al.*, 1987).

Clinical Uses of the Drug

Previously, because of an exaggerated fear of its hepatotoxicity, pyrazinamide was not regarded as a first-line drug (McDermott *et al.*, 1954; Zorini *et al.*, 1958), and it was relegated to the position of a reserve drug for the retreatment of tuberculosis due to resistant strains (Horsfall, 1972). As a result of many more recent clinical trials, pyrazinamide is now accepted as a very valuable drug for the treatment of tuberculosis. It is a bactericidal drug which has a unique sterilizing action (p. 1191), and when used in the recommended dosage it is of low toxicity. Pyrazinamide has been particularly effective in short-course regimens for the treatment of tuberculosis, in which it can be given either daily or intermittently. It is usually given for the first 2 months together with at least isoniazid and rifampicin, and the last two drugs are then continued alone for further 4 months (p. 1196). Pyrazinamide is also used in regimens to treat patients with drug-resistant *M. tuberculosis* strains (p. 1199).

References

A United States Public Health Service Tuberculosis Therapy Trial (1959). Hepatic toxicity of pyrazinamide used with isoniazid in tuberculosis patients. *Amer Rev Respir Dis* **80**: 371.

British Thoracic Association (1982). A controlled trial of six months chemotherapy in pulmonary tuberculosis. Second report: results during the 24 months after the end of chemotherapy. *Amer Rev Respir Dis* **126**: 460.

Corbella X, Vadillo M, Cabellos C *et al.* (1995). Hypersensitivity hepatitis due to pyrazinamide. *Scand J Infect Dis* **27**: 93.

Cullen JH, Early LJA, Fiore JM (1956). The occurrence of hyperuricemia during pyrazinamide-isoniazid therapy. *Amer Rev Tuberc* **74**: 289.

Dankner WM, Waecker NJ, Essey MA *et al.* (1993). *Mycobacterium bovis* infections in San Diego: a clinicoepidemiologic study of 73 patients and a historical review of a forgotten pathogen. *Medicine* **72**: 11.

Donald PR, Seifart H (1988). Cerebrospinal fluid pyrazinamide concentrations in children with tuberculous meningitis. *Pediatr Infect Dis J* **7**: 469.

Dutt AK, Stead WW (1982). Medical perspective: present chemotherapy for tuberculosis. *J Infect Dis* **146**: 698.

Ellard GA (1969). Absorption, metabolism and excretion of pyrazinamide in man. *Tubercle* **50**: 144.

Ellard GA, Haslam RM (1976). Observations on the reduction of the renal elimination of urate in man caused by the administration of pyrazinamide. *Tubercle* **57**: 97.

Ellard GA, Humphries MJ, Gabriel M, Teoh R (1987). Penetration of pyrazinamide into the cerebrospinal fluid in tuberculous meningitis. *Brit Med J* **294**: 284.

Forgan-Smith R, Ellard GA, Newton D, Mitchison DA (1973). Pyrazinamide and other drugs in tuberculous meningitis. *Lancet* **ii**: 374.

Fox W (1978). The current status of short-course chemotherapy. *Bull Int Un Tuberc* **53**: 268.

Fox W, Mitchison DA (1975). Short-course chemotherapy for pulmonary tuberculosis. *Amer Rev Respir Dis* **111**: 325.

Girling DJ (1978). The hepatic toxicity of antituberculosis regimens containing isoniazid, rifampicin and pyrazinamide. *Tubercle* **59**: 13.

Girling DJ (1982). Adverse effect of antituberculosis drugs. *Curr Therap* **23**: 101.

Guttman AB, Yü TF, Berger L (1969). Renal function in gout III. Estimation of tubular secretion and reabsorption of uric acid by use of pyrazinamide (pyrazinoic acid). *Amer J Med* **47**: 575.

Heifets LB, Lindholm-Levy PJ (1990). Is pyrazinamide bactericidal against *Mycobacterium tuberculosis*? *Am Rev Respir Dis* **141**: 250.

Heifets LB, Flory MA, Lindholm-Levy PJ (1989). Does pyrazinoic acid as an active moiety of pyrazinamide have specific activity against *Mycobacterium tuberculosis*? *Antimicrob Ag Chemother* **33**: 1252.

Herlevsen P, Nielsen C, Pedersen JT (1987). Convulsions after treatment with pyrazinamide. *Tubercle* **68**: 145.

Hong Kong Chest Service/British Medical Research Council (1978). Controlled trial of 6-month and 8-month regimens in the treatment of pulmonary tuberculosis. *Amer Rev Respir Dis* **118**: 219.

Hong Kong Chest Service/British Medical Research Council (1979). Controlled trial of 6-month and 8-month regimens in the treatment of pulmonary tuberculosis: the results up to 24 months. *Tubercle* **60**: 201.

Hong Kong Tuberculosis Treatment Services/British Medical Research Council (1976). Adverse reactions to short-course regimens containing streptomycin, isoniazid, pyrazinamide and rifampicin in Hong Kong. *Tubercle* **57**: 81.

Horsfall PAL (1972). Treatment of resistant pulmonary tuberculosis in Hong Kong with regimens of second-line drugs. *Tubercle* **53**: 166.

Horsfall PAL, Plummer J, Allan WGL *et al.* (1979). Double blind controlled comparison of aspirin, allopurinol and placebo in the management of arthralgia during pyrazinamide administration. *Tubercle* **60**: 13.

Jain A, Mehta VL, Kulshresta S (1993). Effect of pyrazinamide on rifampicin kinetics in patients with tuberculosis. *Tubercle Lung Dis* **74**: 87.

Jain VK, Vardhan H, Prakash OM (1988). Pyrazinamide induced thrombocytopenia. *Tubercle* **69**: 217.

Jenner PJ, Ellard GA, Allan WGL *et al.* (1981). Serum uric acid concentrations and arthralgia among patients treated with pyrazinamide-containing regimens in Hong Kong and Singapore. *Tubercle* **62**: 175.

Klemens SP, Sharpe CA, Cynamon MH (1996). Activity of pyrazinamide in a murine model against *Mycobacterium tuberculosis* isolates with various levels of *in vitro* susceptibility. *Antimicrob Ag Chemother* **40**: 14.

McDermott W, Ormond L, Muschenheim C *et al.* (1954). Pyrazinamide-isoniazid in tuberculosis. *Amer Rev Tuberc* **69**: 319.

Rastogi N, Potar M-C, David HL (1988). Pyrazinamide is not efective against intracellularly growing *Mycobacterium tuberculosis*. *Antimicrob Ag Chemother* **32**: 287.

Robson JM, Sullivan FM (1963). Antituberculosis drugs. *Pharmacol Rev* **15**: 169.

Salfinger M, Heifets LB (1988). Determination of pyrazinamide MICs for *Mycobacterium tuberculosis* at different pHs by the radiometric method. *Antimicrob Ag Chemother* **32**: 1002.

Salfinger M, Crowle AJ, Reller LB (1990). Pyrazinamide and pyrazinoic acid activity against tubercle bacilli in cultured human macrophages and in the BACTEC system. *J Infect Dis* **162**: 201.

Sarma GR, Acharyulu GS, Kannapiran M *et al.* (1983). Role of rifampicin in arthralgia induced by pyrazinamide. *Tubercle* **64**: 93.

Speirs RJ, Welch JT, Cynamon MH (1995). Activity of n-propyl pyrazinoate against pyrazinamide-resistant *Mycobacterium tuberculosis*: investigations into mechanism of action of and mechanism of resistance to pyrazinamide. *Antimicrob Ag Chemother* **39**: 1269.

Stottmeier KD, Beam RE, Kubica GP (1968). The absorption and excretion of pyrazinamide. *Amer Rev Respir Dis* **98**: 70.

Tuberculosis Research Centre (1983). Study of chemotherapy regimens of 5 and 7 months duration and the role of corticosteroids in the treatment of sputum-positive patients with pulmonary tuberculosis in South India. *Tubercle* **64**: 73.

Yeager RL, Munroe WGC, Dessau FI (1952). Pyrazinamide (aldinamide). in the treatment of pulmonary tuberculosis. *Amer Rev Tuberc* **65**: 523; quoted by McDermott *et al.* (1954)..

Yü TF, Perel J, Berger L *et al.* (1977). The effect of the interaction of pyrazinamide and probenecid on urinary uric acid excretion in man. *Amer J Med* **63**: 723.

Zorini AO, Spina G, De Simoni GE (1958). Clinical and biological investigations on the new antituberculosis drugs (pyrazinamide and cycloserine). *Dis Chest* **34**: 27.

Para-aminosalicylic Acid

Description

Para-aminosalicylic acid (PAS) was discovered as a result of a deliberate search for antituberculosis drugs. In 1941 Bernheim showed that salicylic and benzoic acids increase the oxygen consumption of the tubercle bacillus, and it was concluded that these acids were oxidized by the bacilli as metabolites. Subsequently Lehmann (1946) investigated many derivatives of these acids and discovered PAS, and showed that it was beneficial for the treatment of human tuberculosis. This antituberculous action was confirmed by many trials (D'Esopo, 1982) and for a period PAS was a standard first-line drug for the treatment of tuberculosis (p. 1194). In technically advanced countries PAS is now rarely used, except as one drug in a regimen for treatment of multidrug-resistant tuberculosis (p. 1200). In some developing countries, where the cost of drugs is an important factor, it may still have a place for treatment of the disease caused by sensitive strains of *Mycobacterium tuberculosis*.

Activity Against Mycobacteria

Sensitive strains of *M. tuberculosis* are inhibited by concentrations of PAS ranging from 0.5 to 2.0 μg per ml. Strains with an MIC higher than 2.0 μg per ml for practical purposes are considered resistant.

Primary drug-resistance to PAS did occur, but when the drug was still commonly used in developed countries, resistance to it in those areas was uncommon and usually less than 2% (Miller *et al.*, 1966; Hobby *et al.*, 1974; Stottmeier and Baker, 1977; Pien *et al.*, 1982). In certain developing countries, such as in South-East Asia, newly isolated strains of *M. tuberculosis* are more frequently resistant to PAS and other drugs.

Other mycobacteria (p. 1211) are usually resistant to PAS (Kuze *et al.*, 1981).

Mode of Administration and Dosage

1 Oral administration

Usually PAS is administered by this route, and is available either as the sodium or calcium salt. The former is commonly used, but the latter may be more suitable for patients needing sodium restriction.

The total daily adult dose ranges from 10 to 15 g and this is administered as a single dose or in two divided doses. The most common adult dosage used is 12 g daily. The exact dose prescribed depends on the weight of the patient and the patient's tolerance of the drug. If PAS is selected as a companion drug to isoniazid for intermittent therapy (p. 1195), it is usually administered in a dosage of 10–12 g twice-weekly (Tub Chem Centre, 1973).

The dosage for children is 150 mg per kg body weight, up to 12 g daily.

2 Intravenous administration

The i.v. route of administration is now rarely used. The usual daily dose was 15 g dissolved in 500 ml, which was infused over 2–4 h. Thrombophlebitis and hypersensitivity reactions (p. 1225) were common problems with this mode of administration (Sattler, 1962).

3 Patients with renal failure

If the drug is used in patients with renal failure, dosage reduction is necessary (Kovnat et al., 1973). However, it should be avoided in these patients because it might aggravate uremic gastrointestinal symptoms and acidosis (Cheigh, 1977). In end-stage renal disease the serum half-life of PAS is extended to 23 h. Significant amounts of PAS are removed by hemodialysis (Bennett et al., 1977).

Serum Levels in Relation to Dosage

It is known that PAS is well absorbed from the gastrointestinal tract. In adults after an oral dose of 4 g, a peak serum level of 7–8 μg per ml is reached in 1–2 h (Way et al., 1948). Thereafter, the serum level falls and after 6 h it is less than 1 μg per ml; the serum half-life being 0.75 h.

Excretion

1 Urine

In the urine PAS is rapidly excreted by both glomerular filtration and tubular secretion. Approximately 85% of the dose can be recovered from the urine within 7 h of oral administration (Way et al., 1948). Only 14–33% of the total dose is excreted in the urine as the active unchanged drug (Robson and Sullivan, 1963). The remainder is excreted as metabolites such as acetyl-PAS, para-aminosalicyluric acid and other conjugated amines.

Probenecid can partially block the renal tubular secretion of PAS and therefore enhance the serum levels of the drug (Boger and Pitts, 1950).

2 Inactivation in body

Like the sulfonamides (p. 814), PAS appears to be metabolized in the liver mainly by acetylation and inactive acetylated compounds are excreted in the urine (Harris, 1963). In contrast to isoniazid (p. 1186), phenotypic variation in PAS metabolism has not been demonstrated.

Distribution of the Drug in Body

After absorption PAS is well distributed to various body fluids and tissues, but it does not penetrate into the CSF of patients with uninflamed meninges. Studies in animals have shown that it penetrates readily into caseous tissue (Robson and Sullivan, 1963). The serum protein binding of PAS is 60–70% (Bennett et al., 1977).

Mode of Action

The mechanism of action of PAS on *M. tuberculosis* is probably similar to the mode of action of sulfonamides on bacteria (p. 814); PAS is a bacteriostatic drug.

Toxicity

1 Gastrointestinal irritation

Preparations of PAS are bulky and unpleasant to take, and gastrointestinal symptoms are experienced by almost every patient to some degree. Symptoms include nausea, vomiting, anorexia, abdominal cramps and diarrhea. Diarrhea may be severe enough to cause steatorrhea, malabsorption, secondary folic acid deficiency and megaloblastic anemia (Girling, 1982). Various PAS preparations have been made available to attempt to reduce gastrointestinal side-effects. Nevertheless, in some patients the drug has to be withdrawn because of intractable symptoms. In aqueous solution PAS is unstable and may polymerize to form toxic compounds; such solutions should not be used if they are darker in color than a freshly prepared solution.

2 Hypersensitivity reactions

These occur in about 5–10% of patients and usually become evident during the first 5 weeks of treatment. When streptomycin, isoniazid and PAS were used together, it was sometimes difficult to know which drug was causing the reaction (p. 1188). Cross-sensitivity may also occur between these three drugs, and apparently PAS can trigger reactions to streptomycin and isoniazid (Thompson, 1969). In a study of 7492 patients receiving antituberculosis therapy in Cape Town, drug reactions occurred in 9%, PAS was the most common cause of these (including hepatitis) compared with streptomycin, isoniazid, ethionamide and ethambutol (Rossouw and Saunders, 1975).

The most common manifestations of PAS hypersensitivity are fever, conjunctivitis, rash and pruritus. The rash is usually morbilliform, sometimes urticarial and rarely takes the form of exfoliative dermatitis (Simpson and Walker, 1960; Thompson, 1969; Rossouw and Saunders, 1975). The blood film may show an eosinophilia or atypical monocytes. Less common manifestations include lymphadenopathy, hepatosplenomegaly and joint pains. Pulmonary infiltrates associated with eosinophilia, similar to those produced by sulfonamides (p. 819), have also been observed. Other rare, probably allergic manifestations include encephalopathy and myocarditis (Thompson, 1969), and a syndrome resembling lupus erythematosus has been described (Masel, 1967). Anaphylaxis is rare.

Hepatitis which can be fatal has also been ascribed to PAS and appears to be due to hypersensitivity (Simpson and Walker, 1960; Rossouw and Saunders, 1975). This hepatitis usually becomes apparent within the first 3 months of PAS treatment and is commonly preceded by features of hypersensitivity to the drug, described above. This is in contrast to the hepatitis which occurs with other antituberculosis drugs such as rifampicin (p. 686), isoniazid (p. 1190), pyrazinamide (p. 1221) and ethionamide (p. 1236), which are much less commonly associated with allergic manifestations. It is quite possible that a percentage of cases in which hepatotoxicity was ascribed to PAS were due to isoniazid used concomitantly (p. 1190).

If severe hypersensitivity reactions to PAS, such as 'hepatitis' or exfoliative dermatitis, occur, the drug should be stopped, and large doses of corticosteroids administered in conjunction with other antituberculosis drugs. In patients with milder reactions all tuberculosis chemotherapy is usually stopped, and when the reaction subsides the offending drug is identified by administering small test doses of each drug separately (p. 1188).

Nowadays desensitization (p. 1188) is no longer recommended for PAS hypersensitivity. In this situation it is simpler and safer to discontinue PAS and substitute another antituberculosis drug.

3 Hematological side-effects

Rarely, PAS may cause neutropenia or acute agranulocytosis. It may also precipitate acute hemolytic anemia in patients with glucose-6–phosphate dehydrogenase deficiency. In addition, MacGibbon et al. (1960) reported a patient who developed an acute autoimmune hemolytic anemia associated with renal failure due to PAS sensitivity. Mild hypoprothrombinemia (due to salicylate) and thrombocytopenia are rare side-effects (Girling, 1982).

4 Renal failure

Renal failure is a rare complication of PAS therapy, and in most cases it has probably occurred in association with hemolysis (MacGibbon et al., 1960) or hypersensitivity reactions (Sattler, 1962).

5 Hypokalemia

The uncommon occurrence of hypokalemia in patients receiving PAS therapy is largely due to gastrointestinal disturbances caused by this drug (McIntyre, 1953).

6 Sodium overload

Fluid retention due to excess sodium may occur in patients suffering from heart disease if the sodium salt of PAS is used. This problem may be obviated by administering the calcium salt.

7 Goiter

Thyroid enlargement or even myxedema have been observed on rare occasions after a prolonged course of PAS.

Clinical Uses of the Drug

For many years PAS was one of the first-line drugs for the treatment of tuberculosis (p. 1194). In developed countries the main drugs for the treatment of this disease are now isoniazid, rifampicin, pyrazinamide and ethambutol, and PAS is only indicated for treatment of multidrug-resistant tuberculosis (p. 1200). It may have a continuing place in some developing countries because of its cheapness.

Also PAS has been used as one of the drugs in the intermittent chemotherapy regimens for tuberculosis (p. 1195). In India it was shown that PAS (0.2 g per kg body weight) and isoniazid (15 mg per kg body weight) administered twice-weekly were about as effective as a standard PAS/isoniazid combination administered daily to patients with pulmonary tuberculosis (Tub Chem Centre, 1973). So-called bacteriostatic drugs, such as PAS and ethambutol, do not contribute to short-course chemotherapy (p. 1195) in patients with drug-sensitive bacilli (Fox, 1978).

References

Bennett WM, Singer I, Golper T *et al.* (1977). Guidelines for drug therapy in renal failure. *Ann Intern Med* **86**: 754.

Boger WP, Pitts FW (1950). Influence of p-(di-n-propylsulfamyl)-benzoic acid, 'benemid', on para-aminosalicylic acid (PAS). plasma concentrations. *Ann Rev Tuberc Pulm Dis* **61**: 862.

Cheigh JS (1977). Drug administration in renal failure. *Amer J Med* **62**: 555.

D'Esopo ND (1982). Clinical trials in pulmonary tuberculosis. *Amer Rev Respir Dis* **125**: 85.

Fox W (1978). The current status of short-course chemotherapy. *Bull Int Un Tuberc* **53**: 268.

Girling DJ (1982). Adverse effect of antituberculosis drugs. *Curr Therapy* **23**: 101.

Harris HW (1963). Current concepts of the metabolism of anti-tuberculous agents. *Ann NY Acad Sci* **106**: 43.

Hobby GL, Johnson PM, Boytar-Papirnyik V (1974). Primary drug resistance: a continuing study of drug resistance in tuberculosis in a veteran population within the United States. X. September 1970–September 1973. *Amer Rev Respir Dis* **110**: 95.

Kovnat P, Labovitz E, Levison SP (1973). Antibiotics and the kidney. *Med Clin N Amer* **57**: 1045.

Kuze F, Kurasawa T, Bando K *et al.* (1981). *In vitro* and *in vivo* susceptibility of atypical mycobacteria to various drugs. *Rev Infect Dis* **3**: 885.

Lehmann J (1946). Para-aminosalicylic acid in the treatment of tuberculosis. *Lancet* **i**: 15.

MacGibbon B, Loughridge L, Hourihane DO'B, Boyd DW (1960). Autoimmune haemolytic anaemia with acute renal failure due to phenacetin and p-aminosalicylic acid. *Lancet* **i**: 7.

Masel MA (1967). A lupus-like reaction to antituberculosis drugs. *Med J Aust* **2**: 738.

McIntyre PA (1953). Hyopkalaemia occurring during para-aminosalicylic acid therapy. *Bull Johns Hopkins Hosp* **92**: 210.

Miller AB, Tall R, Fox W *et al.* (1966). Primary drug resistance in pulmonary tuberculosis in Great Britain: Second national survey, 1963. *Tubercle* **47**: 92.

Pien FD, Ang KS, Cohen HI (1982). Primary antituberculosis drug resistance in Hawaii 1977–1981. *Amer Rev Respir Dis* **126**: 928.

Robson JM, Sullivan FM (1963). Antituberculosis drugs. *Pharmacol Rev* **15**: 169.

Rossouw JE, Saunders SJ (1975). Hepatic complications of antituberculous therapy. *Quart J Med* **44**: 1.

Sattler A (1962). The present status of PAS in tuberculosis therapy. *Amer Rev Respir Dis* **85**: 927.

Simpson DG, Walker JH (1960). Hypersensitivity to para-aminosalicylic acid. *Amer J Med* **29**: 297.

Stottmeier KD, Baker S (1977). Primary drug-resistant tuberculosis in Massachusetts, 1975/76. *New Engl J Med* **296**: 823.

Thompson JE (1969). The management of hypersensitivity reactions to antituberculosis drugs. *Med J Aust* **2**: 1058.

Tuberculosis Chemotherapy Centre, Madras (1973). Controlled comparison of oral twice-weekly and oral daily isoniazid plus PAS in newly diagnosed pulmonary tuberculosis. *Brit Med J* **2**: 7.

Way EL, Smith PK, Howie DL *et al.* (1948). The absorption, distribution, excretion and fate of para-aminosalicylic acid. *J Pharmacol Exp Ther* **93**: 368.

Cycloserine

Description

Cycloserine was isolated by independent investigators from cultures of *Streptomyces orchidaceus* (Harned *et al.*, 1955), and *Streptomyces garyphalus* (Harris *et al.*, 1955). The drug is a crystalline substance of low molecular weight with a chemical structure of D-4–amino-S-isoxazolidone.

Sensitive Organisms

1 Mycobacterium tuberculosis

This is sensitive to cycloserine, and strains which have become resistant to streptomycin, isoniazid and rifampicin (p. 1181) usually remain cycloserine-sensitive (Robson and Sullivan, 1963). Most *M. tuberculosis* strains are inhibited by cycloserine in a concentration of 10–20 μg per ml. Strains with MICs higher than 40 μg per ml are considered to be resistant. Strains of *M. tuberculosis* resistant to cycloserine emerge if this drug is used singly for the treatment of tuberculosis (Storey and McLean, 1957).

2 Other mycobacteria

Mycobacterium kansasii and *M. avium* complex may be sensitive to cycloserine (p. 1211).

3 Other bacteria

Staphylococcus aureus and Gram-negative enteric bacilli are cycloserine-sensitive to a variable degree (Hoeprich, 1964). *Escherichia coli* is the most susceptible; *Proteus* and *Klebsiella* spp. are more resistant and *Pseudomonas aeruginosa* is highly resistant (Murdoch *et al.*, 1966). This now has no clinical significance.

Mode of Administration and Dosage

Cycloserine can only be administered by the oral route. For the treatment of tuberculosis, it is always given with one or two other antituberculosis drugs. The dosage is 10–20 mg per kg per day. The maximum daily dosage of cycloserine for adults is 1.0 g administered in two divided doses. Many patients may not tolerate this dosage for prolonged periods and it may be necessary to reduce the daily dosage to 0.75 g or even 0.5 g.

Appropriate doses for children are a quarter of the adult dose for those aged less than 2 years and a half of the adult dose for those aged 2–10 years.

Cycloserine should be avoided in patients with impaired renal function, but if it is used, the dosage should be reduced and serum levels monitored.

Serum Levels in Relation to Dosage

Cycloserine is well absorbed after oral administration. Following a 250-mg oral dose, the peak serum level of about 10 μg per ml is attained in 3–4 h (Storey and McLean, 1957; Truant, 1958). Doubling the dose doubles the peak serum level. Thereafter, the serum concentration falls rapidly, but some drug is still detectable after 12 h. With repeated doses of cycloserine, there is slight accumulation of the drug during the first 3 days of treatment (Storey and McLean, 1957).

Excretion

1 Urine

About 60–70% of orally administered cycloserine is excreted by glomerular filtration in the urine in an unchanged active form. This excretion is not affected by probenecid. Most of the administered dose is excreted in urine during the first 24 h (Robson and Sullivan, 1963). High concentrations of active cycloserine are attained in urine. The drug given in usual doses will accumulate in patients with impaired renal function, because it is only slowly excreted in such patients.

2 Inactivation in body

It appears that about 35% of administered cycloserine is metabolized in the body. The metabolites have not been identified (Storey and McLean, 1957).

3 Feces

Cycloserine is almost completely absorbed after oral administration, and only negligible amounts are excreted in the feces.

Distribution of the Drug in Body

After absorption from the gastrointestinal tract, cycloserine becomes widely distributed throughout the body. It penetrates well into the normal CSF where concentrations may approximate to those attained in serum (Storey and McLean, 1957). In animals the drug reaches significant concentrations in lymph, amniotic fluid and the fetal circulation (Anderson et al., 1956).

Mode of Action

Cycloserine interferes with bacterial cell wall synthesis, but its mechanism of action differs from that of the penicillins (p. 25). During the early stages of cell wall synthesis D-alanine molecules are linked together. Cycloserine, being a structural analog of D-alanine, acts as a competitive antagonist of the enzymes which link D-alanine molecules in the bacterial cell wall (Strominger et al., 1959; Strominger and Tipper, 1965). In some cycloserine-resistant bacteria, similar to the tetracyclines (p. 720), the resistance is due to a reduced uptake of the drug into the cell (Clark and Young, 1977).

Toxicity

1 Neurotoxicity

This is the most important toxic effect of cycloserine. Psychotic disturbances such as excitement, aggression, confusion and depression are not infrequent. In addition, headache, drowsiness, tremor and convulsions may occur. For these reasons the drug should be avoided in patients with mental instability or epilepsy. With a dosage of 0.5 g twice-daily, about 8% of patients have been reported to develop convulsions (Storey and McLean, 1957). These complications of cycloserine appear to be dose-related and their frequency is much higher if a peak serum level of 30 μg per ml is exceeded. Convulsions and other neurotoxic manifestations are less common if a smaller daily dose of 0.5 g is used (Storey and McLean, 1957). These toxic effects disappear when the drug is stopped. Rarely, peripheral neuritis may result from cycloserine therapy.

Markedly reduced levels of CSF calcium and magnesium have been found in patients taking large doses of cycloserine and these changes may contribute to the toxicity of the drug (Murdoch, 1967). Neurotoxicity almost certainly results from a direct effect of the drug on the nervous system and the administration of various vitamins is unlikely to be beneficial. However, both pyridoxine and nicotinamide have been used to prevent these complications with apparent success (Swash et al., 1972).

2 Other side-effects

Rarely, drug fever, rashes (Kirshner, 1958) and cardiac arrhythmias have been reported. Murdoch et al. (1966) treated 27 pregnant women with cycloserine without evidence of teratogenicity.

Clinical Uses of the Drug

Cycloserine now only has a role for the treatment of patients with tuberculosis, whose *M. tuberculosis* strains are resistant to several first-line drugs (multiresistant-tuberculosis) (p. 1200). Under such circumstances cycloserine should always be combined with at least one and preferably two drugs to which the *M. tuberculosis* strain is still sensitive.

References

Anderson RC, Worth HM, Welles JS *et al.* (1956). Pharmacology and toxicology of cycloserine. *Antibiot Chemother* **6**: 360.

Clark VL, Young FE (1977). Inducible resistance to D-cycloserine in *Bacillus subtilis* 168. *Antimicrob Ag Chemother* **11**: 871.

Harned RL, Hidy PH, Labaw EK (1955). Cycloserine I. A preliminary report. *Antib Chemo* **5**: 204; quoted by Storey and McLean (1957).

Harris DA, Ruger M, Reagan MA *et al.* (1955). Discovery, development, and antimicrobial properties of D-4-amino-3-isoxazolidone (oxamycin), a new antibiotic produced by *Streptomyces garyphalus* n. Sp. *Antib Chemo* **5**: 183; quoted by Storey and McLean (1957).

Hoeprich PD (1964). Alanine: cycloserine antagonism. I. Significance of phenomenon in testing susceptibility to cycloserine. *Amer J Clin Pathol* **41**: 140.

Kirshner JJ (1958). Cycloserine with isoniazid in chronic pulmonary tuberculosis. *Antibiotic Annual* 1957–58: 627.

Murdoch JMcC, Geddes AM, Tulloch WS *et al.* (1966). The problem of pyelonephritis. A four-year study of a pyelonephritis unit. *Practitioner* **196**: 800.

Murdoch JMcC (1967). Panel discussion: clinical aspects of the therapy of systemic and urinary Gram-negative infections. *Ann NY Acad Sci* **145**: 354.

Robson JM, Sullivan FM (1963). Antituberculosis drugs. *Pharmacol Rev* **15**: 169.

Storey PB, McLean RL (1957). A current appraisal of cycloserine. *Antibiot Med Clin Ther* **4**: 223.

Strominger JL, Tipper DJ (1965). Bacterial cell wall synthesis and structure in relation to the mechanism of action of penicillins and other antibacterial agents. *Amer J Med* **39**: 708.

Strominger JL, Threnn RH, Scott SS (1959). Oxamycin, a competitive antagonist of the incorporation of D-alanine into a uridine nucleotide in *Staphylococcus aureus*. *J Amer Chem Soc* **81**: 3803.

Swash M, Roberts AJ, Murnaghan DJ (1972). Reversible pellagra-like encephalopathy with ethionamide and cycloserine. *Tubercle* **53**: 132.

Truant JP (1958). Studies on the *in vitro* and *in vivo* effect of cycloserine and isoniazid on tubercle bacilli. *Antibiotic Annual* 1957–58: 630.

Capreomycin

Description

Capreomycin, a polypeptide antibiotic (p. 667), was isolated from *Streptomyces capreolus* in 1960. It consists of four microbiologically active compounds which are named capreomycin IA, IB, IIA and IIB (Herr and Redstone, 1966). For clinical purposes capreomycin is used as the sulfate.

Activity Against Mycobacteria

Capreomycin is only active against mycobacteria. *Mycobacterium tuberculosis* is moderately sensitive and its MIC is usually $10\,\mu$g per ml. Strains of *M. tuberculosis* with an MIC of up to $40\,\mu$g per ml can still be regarded as sensitive. Tubercle bacilli which have become resistant to isoniazid, streptomycin, rifampicin, para-aminosalicylic acid (PAS), ethambutol, cycloserine and ethionamide, usually remain capreomycin-sensitive. Cross-resistance may occur between capreomycin and viomycin and between capreomycin and kanamycin (Sutton *et al.*, 1966; Drug Commentary, 1973). Capreomycin-resistant variants of *M. tuberculosis* can be readily selected *in vitro* (Sutton *et al.*, 1966), and they also develop readily *in vivo* if the drug is used as a single agent for the treatment of tuberculosis (Wilson, 1967). Primary drug-resistance to capreomycin has been uncommon in the USA (CDC, 1983). The drug has a bacteriostatic action against *M. tuberculosis*.

Capreomycin may show *in vitro* activity against some other mycobacteria such as *M. kansasii* (Sutton *et al.*, 1966). The *M. avium* complex is relatively resistant; MICs ranging from 20 to $80\,\mu$g per ml and MBCs are much higher (Heifets and Lindholm-Levy, 1989; Le Conte *et al.*, 1994).

Mode of Administration and Dosage

1 Adults

Capreomycin is administered by the i.m. route. The usual dosage is 15–20 mg per kg per day given as a single daily injection. A common adult daily dose is 1.0 g, which is usually given for 2–4 months, thereafter it is reduced to 1.0 g two or three times per week for the remainder of the course of treatment.

In some treatment regimens the daily dose for adults has been adjusted according to age. The dose is 1.0 g for patients under 50 years, 0.75 g for those aged 50–59 years and 0.5 g for those aged 60 years or more (Andrews *et al.*, 1974).

2 Children

A dosage of 15–30 mg per kg per day may be suitable for children but there is insufficient data on the use of capreomycin in this age group.

3 Patients with renal failure

Capreomycin accumulates in these patients, so that a reduced dosage and serum level monitoring is necessary. A similar dose reduction to that advocated for streptomycin (p. 431) may be used because the two drugs are excreted by the kidney in a similar manner (Black *et al.*, 1966).

Serum Levels in Relation to Dosage

Capreomycin is not absorbed after oral administration, but it is well absorbed from i.m. injection sites. A peak serum level of 30–35 µg per ml is attained 1–2 h after an i.m. injection of 1.0 g in adults. Thereafter, the serum concentration gradually falls, being 10 µg per ml at 6 h, and usually less than 1.0 µg per ml at 24 h (Black et al., 1966; Morse et al., 1966). These serum concentrations are similar to those attained after an i.m. injection of 1.0 g of streptomycin (p. 431). Capreomycin does not accumulate in the serum of patients with normal renal function, when repeated daily doses of 1.0 g are given for prolonged periods.

Excretion

1 Urine

About 50–60% of an administered dose of capreomycin is excreted by glomerular filtration, producing high concentrations of the active unchanged drug in the urine (Black et al., 1966). Most of this is excreted during the first 12 h after the dose.

2 Bile

Animal studies suggest that small amounts may be eliminated via the bile (Black et al., 1966).

3 Inactivation in body

Capreomycin not excreted in the urine is probably inactivated in the body.

Distribution of the Drug in Body

The distribution of capreomycin in various body fluids and tissues has not been studied. The drug probably does not penetrate into the CSF of patients with normal meninges.

Mode of Action

The mode of action of capreomycin is apparently unknown. It has a bactericidal action against tubercle bacilli similar to streptomycin (p. 432) i.e. it is active in a medium which is neutral or has a slightly alkaline pH such as is found extracellularly in cavities (Stead and Dutt, 1982).

Toxicity

1 Nephrotoxicity

This appears to be the most serious toxic effect of capreomycin therapy (Garfield et al., 1966; Miller et al., 1966; Hesling, 1969). Many patients develop proteinuria and casts; red and white cells may be detected in their urine. If only these changes occur, capreomycin may be continued cautiously in a reduced dosage. If there is a rise in blood urea and serum creatinine, the drug should be stopped. Capreomycin can also cause renal tubular dysfunction with alkalosis and potassium, calcium and magnesium depletion. Patients with this complication may develop lethargy, muscular weakness and tetany (Hesling, 1969), in which case the drug should be discontinued and correction of electrolyte disturbances may be needed.

When the drug has only been used for periods of 4–6 months in the retreatment of tuberculosis, hypokalemia has been uncommon. Aquinas and Citron (1972) monitored serum potassium regularly; during 6 months therapy two of 36 patients with capreomycin-induced hypokalemia were detected and both responded rapidly to oral potassium. Andrews et al. (1974) did not observe any electrolyte changes when capreomycin was used for 4 months in a dosage adjusted for age.

2 Ototoxicity

Capreomycin-treated patients may develop vertigo, tinnitus or deafness. These are uncommon, provided that the drug is not given to patients with pre-existing hearing loss or to patients with renal functional impairment. Elderly patients are more prone to ototoxicity and should not receive prolonged therapy. Three of 36 patients in Hong Kong who were treated with capreomycin for 6 months developed deafness or tinnitus (Aquinas and Citron, 1972), but these symptoms were not observed in 33 British patients treated for 4 months (Andrews et al., 1974).

3 Hepatotoxicity

Transient abnormalities in liver function tests have been noted during capreomycin therapy, but in most cases these were probably caused by companion drugs such as isoniazid or PAS (Browning and Donnerberg, 1966; Miller *et al.*, 1966). Serious hepatotoxicity has not been reported.

4 Other side-effects

Leucopenia has been observed, but appears to be rare. Eosinophilia is more common and sometimes is associated with hypersensitivity rashes or drug fever (Miller *et al.*, 1966). Capreomycin does not appear to be cross-allergenic with streptomycin (Wilson, 1969).

Clinical Uses of the Drug

Capreomycin is an effective antituberculosis drug, but because of its toxicity, it is only used for the treatment of patients with suspected or proven drug-resistance (p. 1199). When used for this purpose it must always be combined with at least one other drug to which the organism is sensitive. Aquinas and Citron (1972) used capreomycin to treat 35 patients in Hong Kong; daily rifampicin and ethambutol were given for 2 years, supplemented by daily capreomycin in a dose of 15 mg per kg of body weight for the first 6 months; sputum cultures of 33 of the 36 patients rapidly became negative and remained so during the 2 years of chemotherapy. Andrews *et al.* (1974) also used these three drugs to treat 33 patients with isoniazid-resistant pulmonary tuberculosis in Britain; daily rifampicin and ethambutol were given for 2 years and daily capreomycin in a dosage adjusted for age (p. 1231) for the first 4 months; all patients receiving this therapy had negative sputum cultures after treatment for 6 months, 1 year and 2 years.

References

Andrews RH, Jenkins PA, Marks J *et al.* (1974). Treatment of isoniazid-resistant pulmonary tuberculosis with ethambutol, rifampicin and capreomycin: a co-operative study in England and Wales. *Tubercle* **55**: 105.

Aquinas M, Citron KM (1972). Rifampicin, ethambutol, and capreomycin in pulmonary tuberculosis, previously treated with both first and second line drugs: the results of 2 years' chemotherapy. *Tubercle* **53**: 153.

Black HR, Griffith RS, Peabody AM (1966). Absorption, excretion and metabolism of capreomycin in normal and diseased states. *Ann NY Acad Sci* **135**: 974.

Browning RH, Donnerberg RL (1966). Capreomycin-experiences in patient acceptance and toxicity. *Ann NY Acad Sci* **135**: 1057.

CDC (Centers for Disease Control) (1983). Primary resistance to antituberculosis drugs – United States. *MMWR* **32**: 521.

Drug Commentary (1973). Evaluation of a new antituberculous agent. Capreomycin sulfate (capastat sulfate). *JAMA* **223**: 179.

Garfield JW, Jones JM, Cohen NL *et al.* (1966). The auditory, vestibular and renal effects of capreomycin in humans. *Ann NY Acad Sci* **135**: 1039.

Heifets L, Lindholm-Levy P (1989). Comparison of bactericidal activities of streptomycin, amikacin, kanamycin, and capreomycin against *Mycobacterium avium* and *M tuberculosis*. *Antimicrob Ag Chemother* **33**: 1298.

Herr EB Jr, Redstone MO (1966). Chemical and physical characterization of capreomycin. *Ann NY Acad Sci* **135**: 940.

Hesling CM (1969). Treatment with capreomycin, with special reference to toxic effects. *Tubercle* (March Suppl): 39.

Le Conte P, Le Gallou F, Potel G *et al.* (1994). Pharmacokinetics, toxicity, and efficacy of liposomal capreomycin in disseminated *Mycobacterium avium* beige mouse model. *Antimicrob Ag Chemother* **38**: 2695.

Miller JD, Popplewell AG, Landwehr A, Greene ME (1966). Toxicology studies in patients on prolonged therapy with capreomycin. *Ann NY Acad Sci* **135**: 1047.

Morse WC, Sproat EF, Arrington CW, Hawkins JA (1966). *M tuberculosis in vitro* susceptibility and serum level experiences with capreomycin. *Ann NY Acad Sci* **135**: 983.

Stead WW, Dutt AK (1982). Chemotherapy for tuberculosis today. *Amer Rev Respir Dis* **125**: 94.

Sutton WB, Gordee RS, Wick WE, Stanfield LV (1966). *In vitro* and *in vivo* laboratory studies on the antituberculous activity of capreomycin. *Ann NY Acad Sci* **135**: 947.

Wilson TM (1967). Current therapeutics. CCXL. – Capreomycin and ethambutol. *Practitioner* **199**: 817.

Wilson TM (1969). Capreomycin, ethambutol and rifampicin. Clinical experience in Manchester. *Scand J Respir Dis* (Suppl 69): 33.

Ethionamide and Prothionamide

Description

Ethionamide (2–ethyl thioisonicotinamide) is a derivative of isonicotinic acid, which was synthetized in France in 1956, and soon after shown to be an effective antituberculosis agent. Subsequently the n-propyl derivative of ethionamide, prothionamide, which has similar *in vitro* activity, was used for the treatment of tuberculosis because it was thought to be less toxic. In the few comparative studies of these two drugs, prothionamide appears to be better tolerated than ethionamide. For the treatment of tuberculosis and leprosy, ethionamide and prothionamide have usually been regarded as interchangeable. Jenner *et al.* (1984) found that ethionamide has a pharmacological advantage over prothionamide, but this may not have any clinical significance. Most of the following information relating to ethionamide also applies to prothionamide.

Activity Against Mycobacteria

Ethionamide is active against *Mycobacterium tuberculosis*. The MIC is usually 10 μg per ml and most strains are inhibited by 10–20 μg per ml. Ethionamide-resistant strains of *M. tuberculosis* can rapidly be induced *in vitro* and they also emerge *in vivo* if the drug is used as a single agent for the treatment of human tuberculosis (Robson and Sullivan, 1963). Strains of *M. tuberculosis* which have become resistant to drugs, such as isoniazid, streptomycin and para-aminosalicylic acid (PAS), remain ethionamide-sensitive, but ethionamide may show cross-resistance with thiacetazone (Today's Drugs, 1968).

Primary drug-resistance was monitored in the USA during the period March 1975 through September 1982. Drug-resistance to antituberculosis drugs (including ethionamide) was higher in some ethnic groups, such as Asians and Hispanics and in some geographic areas, such as the USA – Mexico border area; for ethionamide the overall drug-resistance rate was 1.1%. An ethionamide-resistance rate of 7.2% was found in patients presenting to the Cook County Hospital in Chicago in 1980/81 (Greene and Muthuswamy, 1982). *Mycobacterium africanum* may be resistant (p. 1180). Ethionamide has a bacteriostatic action against *M. tuberculosis*.

In kinetic studies using animals, depending on the dosage used, ethionamide has bacteriostatic and bactericidal activity against *M. leprae* (Shepard *et al.*, 1976). Ethionamide shows significant bactericidal activity against *M. leprae* in mice when it is administered continuously but if administered intermittently it only has a prolonged bacteriostatic effect (Colston *et al.*, 1980). As a bactericidal drug ethionamide is almost as powerful as rifampicin against *M. leprae*; the MIC for ethionamide against the organism is about 0.05 μg per ml, and its peak serum level exceeds this MIC by about 45-fold (Ellard, 1980). Resistance to ethionamide (confirmed in the mouse footpad) has been detected in strains isolated from patients in whom the drug was used as monotherapy (Report, WHO, 1982). Some strains of *M. ulcerans* are sensitive to ethionamide (Radford, 1975). The *M. avium* complex strains, especially if they are isolated from AIDS patients, may also be ethionamide-sensitive (Horsburgh *et al.*, 1986).

Mode of Administration and Dosage

Ethionamide is administered by the oral route in a dosage of 15–30 mg per kg body weight per day. The maximum daily adult dose is 1.0 g, but many patients cannot tolerate this, and more commonly a smaller daily dose of 500–750 mg is prescribed. A dosage of 250–375 mg daily (5–10 mg per kg) is recommended for the treatment of leprosy (p. 1237). Ethionamide is often given as a single daily dose, prior to retiring at night or with the main meal, to minimize gastrointestinal side-effects. Alternatively, it can be given in two divided doses.

Serum Levels in Relation to Dosage

Wide discrepancies have been reported in the serum concentrations after the oral administration of ethionamide (Weinstein et al., 1962). The use of poorly absorbed enteric-coated ethionamide tablets in the past may have been the explanation for these differences.

Robson and Sullivan (1963) found that after an oral dose of 1.0 g, a peak serum concentration of about 20 μg per ml was attained in 3 h. Thereafter, the serum level slowly fell and the drug was undetectable 20–24 h after the dose. Jenner et al. (1984) used a more sensitive high pressure liquid chromatographic method to perform pharmacological studies on nine volunteers. After oral doses of 250 mg ethionamide and 250 mg prothionamide, peak serum levels (1–2 μg per ml) were attained at about 2 h; from the rapid decline in levels from 4 to 8 h, half-lives of 2.1 and 1.8 h were calculated for ethionamide and prothionamide, respectively. Ethionamide was eliminated from the body slightly more slowly than prothionamide and during the 8 h period following dosing, serum concentrations of ethionamide were approximately 1.8-fold higher than those of prothionamide. Serum concentrations of their sulfoxide metabolites (see below) were lower than those of the parent drugs, and levels of ethionamide sulfoxide were substantially higher than those of prothionamide. In a later study Jenner and Smith (1987) found that the serum levels of ethionamide and prothionamide after oral administration were very similar and concluded that the minor differences reported were of no clinical significance.

Excretion

1 Urine

The excretion of ethionamide and prothionamide closely correlates with concomitant serum levels; but only small amounts are excreted in the urine. After an oral dose, approximately 0.16% of ethionamide and 0.08% of prothionamide are recovered in the urine; corresponding proportions of their sulfoxides excreted are about 1.2% and 0.4%, respectively (Jenner et al., 1984).

3 Feces

After oral dosing, less than 0.1% of ethionamide or prothionamide are excreted in the feces, suggesting good absorption or conversion in the gut wall to metabolites (Jenner et al., 1984).

4 Inactivation in body

Both ethionamide and prothionamide are metabolized in the body to sulfoxides, but interconversion takes place between each drug and its metabolite. The sulfoxides are active against *M. tuberculosis* similar to their parent drugs and activity in leprosy may result from a summation of the activities of the unchanged drugs and their sulfoxide metabolites. Sulfoxides are then converted to inactive metabolites (Jenner et al., 1984).

Distribution of the Drug in Body

After absorption ethionamide appears to be widely distributed in the body. It penetrates well into the CSF both in patients with tuberculous meningitis and in those with normal meninges, and CSF concentrations approximate to serum levels at the time (Hughes et al., 1962). Animal studies indicate that ethionamide is quickly distributed to various organs in the body, such as the liver, kidneys and spleen (Hamilton et al., 1962).

Mode of Action

Ethionamide inhibits mycolic acid synthesis as does isoniazid (p. 1187). However, their modes of action are not identical and therefore there is no cross-resistance between the two drugs (Quémard et al., 1992).

Toxicity

1 Gastrointestinal side-effects

Symptoms such as a metallic taste, nausea, vomiting, anorexia, abdominal pain and sometimes diarrhea are very common, and occur to some degree in the majority of patients treated by ethionamide (Weinstein et al., 1962; Schwartz, 1966). Such symptoms are often severe enough to necessitate cessation of treatment. These disturbances may be partly due to an effect of the drug on the central nervous system because parenterally administered ethionamide also causes gastrointestinal symptoms (Today's Drugs, 1968). Prothionamide is probably a little less prone to cause these disturbances.

Fox *et al.* (1969) performed a study amongst African patients to compare side-effects of ethionamide and prothionamide after a single dose of each drug as large as 1.75 g. The principal side-effects of both drugs were gastrointestinal, giddiness and headache; males had more side-effects due to ethionamide than prothionamide, but there were no differences in females; there were more side-effects in females than in males with both drugs.

2 Hepatoxicity

Liver damage due to ethionamide is relatively uncommon. Jaundice usually of the hepatocellular type with a raised SGOT may occur (Phillips and Tashman, 1963). It is not known whether hepatotoxicity is due to a hypersensitivity reaction or to a direct toxic effect of the drug on the liver. Following cessation of ethionamide, the jaundice usually resolves, but it reappears if the drug is resumed (Pernod, 1965). Rifampicin may potentiate hepatotoxicity caused by ethionamide or prothionamide; a 13% incidence of hepatitis occurred in 54 patients with multibacillary leprosy treated by a combination of dapsone + rifampicin + ethionamide or prothionamide (10 mg per kg per day); recovery resulted when treatment with dapsone alone was continued and hepatitis did not recur when rifampicin alone was added to the therapy (Cartel *et al.*, 1983). In a subsequent study by these authors (Cartel *et al.*, 1985), another 110 similar patients were given the same drugs, but ethionamide/prothionamide was given in a lower dosage of 5 mg per kg per day; hepatotoxicity occurred in patients but jaundice was only observed in 11% of them compared with 71% in the previous study. Investigations by Baohong *et al.* (1984) also suggested that the simultaneous administration of rifampicin may have contributed to hepatotoxicity which was observed in leprosy patients treated with prothionamide.

3 Neurotoxicity

Various types of mental disturbances may be caused by ethionamide, such as depression (Weinstein *et al.*, 1962), intense anxiety (Lees, 1967) and acute psychosis (Lees, 1965; Narang, 1972). In addition, dizziness, visual disturbances and peripheral neuritis have been reported (Lees, 1965). A pellagra-like encephalopathy has also been described in three patients receiving ethionamide therapy and two of these patients also developed a myelopathy. All three patients improved when ethionamide was stopped, but they were also treated by nicotinamide and other group B vitamins (Swash *et al.*, 1972). These authors considered that vitamin therapy had aided recovery, and suggested that nicotinamide should be administered to patients receiving ethionamide if any alteration of intellectual function occurs during therapy.

4 Other side-effects

Excessive salivation, gynecomastia, skin rashes, photodermatitis, acne and alopecia have been described in association with ethionamide therapy (Today's Drugs, 1968). There are a few reports indicating that ethionamide can cause goiter and less commonly hypothyroidism (Drucker *et al.*, 1984).

5 Teratogenicity

The drug is teratogenic in experimental animals and its use during human pregnancy is not advised.

Clinical Uses of the Drug

1 Tuberculosis

Although it is effective for tuberculosis, because of its toxicity, ethionamide was only used as a reserve drug for retreatment of patients in whom former standard chemotherapy (p. 1200) had failed (Schwartz, 1966). For this purpose it was used successfully in combination with cycloserine (Riddell *et al.*, 1960) and/or pyrazinamide (Horsfall, 1972). Because of the development of safer effective drugs, ethionamide has only a very limited role in the chemotherapy of tuberculosis, especially in developed countries. Ethionamide was added as a fifth drug to the four bactericidal drugs, streptomycin, isoniazid, rifampicin and pyrazinamide in trials of 3- and 4.5-month short-course regimens; its addition was of no benefit and ethionamide-containing regimens were associated with a greater percentage of adverse reactions (p. 1235). Bacteriostatic drugs such as ethionamide, ethambutol and cycloserine may be required in treatment regimens only if there is multiple drug-resistance affecting two bactericidal drugs or the use of some of these bactericidal drugs is precluded by side-effects (Stead and Dutt, 1982) (p. 1200).

2 Leprosy

Ethionamide/prothionamide is one of the four bactericidal drugs which are available for the treatment of this disease. It was recommended by the WHO Study Group in 1981, to be used in the multidrug regimen for the treatment of multibacillary leprosy. Ethionamide/prothionamide 250–375 mg daily, self-administered, is the alternative to clofazimine if the patient finds clofazimine unacceptable due to skin pigmentation (p. 693). Because of their side-effects (p. 1235), ethionamide or prothionamide, however, should be substituted for clofazimine only if this is absolutely necessary (WHO, 1994).

References

Baohong JI, Jiakun C, Chenmin W, Guang X (1984). Hepatotoxicity of combined therapy with rifampicin and daily prothionamide for leprosy. *Lepr Rev* **55**: 283.

Cartel J-L, Millan J, Guelpa-Lauras CC, Grosset JH (1983). Hepatitis in leprosy patients treated by a daily combination of dapsone, rifampin, and a thiomide. *Int J Lepr* **51**: 461.

Cartel J-L, Naudillon Y, Artus JC *et al.* (1985). Hepatotoxicity of the daily combination of 5mg per kg prothionamide + 10mg per kg rifampin. *Int J Lepr* **53**: 15.

Colston MJ, Hilson GRF, Lancaster RD (1980). Intermittent chemotherapy of experimental leprosy in mice. *Amer J Trop Med Hyg* **29**: 103.

Drucker D, Eggo MC, Salit IE, Burrow GN (1984). Ethionamide-induced goitrous hypothyroidism. *Ann Intern Med* **100**: 837.

Ellard GA (1980). Combined treatment for lepromatous leprosy. *Lepr Rev* **51**: 199.

Fox W, Robinson KK, Tall R *et al.* (1969). A study of acute intolerance to ethionamide, including a comparison with prothionamide, and of the influence of a vitamin B-complex additive in prophylaxis. *Tubercle* **50**: 125.

Greene AB, Muthuswamy P (1982). Primary drug resistance in tuberculosis in a black urban population. *Amer Rev Respir Dis* **125**: 172.

Hamilton EJ, Eidus L, Little E (1962). A comparative study *in vivo* of isoniazid and alpha-ethylthioisonicotinamide. *Amer Rev Respir Dis* **85**: 407.

Horsburgh CR Jr, Cohn DL, Roberts RB *et al.* (1986). *Mycobacterium avium–M intracellulare* isolates from patients with or without acquired immunodeficiency syndrome. *Antimicrob Ag Chemother* **30**: 955.

Horsfall PAL (1972). Treatment of resistant pulmonary tuberculosis in Hong Kong with regimens of second line drugs. *Tubercle* **53**: 166.

Hughes IE, Smith H, Kane PO (1962). Ethionamide: its passage into the cerebrospinal fluid in man. *Lancet* **i**: 616.

Jenner PJ, Smith SE (1987). Plasma levels of ethionamide and prothionamide in a volunteer following intravenous and oral dosages. *Lepr Rev* **58**: 31.

Jenner PJ, Ellard GA, Gruer PJK, Aber VR (1984). A comparison of the blood levels and urinary excretion of ethionamide and prothionamide in man. *Antimicrob Ag Chemother* **13**: 267.

Lees AW (1965). Ethionamide, 750 mg daily, plus isoniazid, 450 mg daily, in previously untreated cases of pulmonary tuberculosis. *Amer Rev Respir Dis* **92**: 966.

Lees AW (1967). Ethionamide, 500 mg daily, plus isoniazid, 500 mg or 300 mg daily in previously untreated patients with pulmonary tuberculosis. *Amer Rev Respir Dis* **95**: 109.

Narang RK (1972). Acute psychotic reaction probably caused by ethionamide. *Tubercle* **53**: 137.

Pernod J (1965). Hepatic tolerance of ethionamide. *Amer Rev Respir Dis* **92**: 39.

Phillips S, Tashman H (1963). Ethionamide jaundice. *Amer Rev Respir Dis* **87**: 896.

Quémard A, Lanéelle G, Lacave C (1992). Mycolic acid synthesis: a target for ethionamide in mycobacteria? *Antimicrob Ag Chemother* **36**: 1316.

Radford AJ (1975). Mycobacterium ulcerans in Australia. *Aust NZ J Med* **5**: 162.

Report of a WHO Study Group (1982). Chemotherapy of leprosy for control programmes. *Wld Hlth Org Techn Rep Serv* No. 675.

Riddell RW, Stewart SM, Somner AR (1960). Ethionamide. *Brit Med J* **2**: 1207.

Robson JM, Sullivan FM (1963). Antituberculosis drugs. *Pharmacol Rev* **15**: 169.

Schwartz WS (1966). Comparison of ethionamide with isoniazid in original treatment cases of pulmonary tuberculosis. *Amer Rev Respir Dis* **93**: 685.

Shepard CC, Ellard GA, Levy L *et al.* (1976). Experimental chemotherapy in leprosy. *Bull Wld Hlth Org* **53**: 425.

Stead WW, Dutt AK (1982). Chemotherapy for tuberculosis today. *Amer Rev Respir Dis* **125**: 94.

Swash M, Roberts AH, Murnaghan DJ (1972). Reversible pellagra-like encephalopathy with ethionamide and cycloserine. *Tubercle* **53**: 132.

Today's Drugs (1968). Drugs for tuberculosis. *Brit Med J* **3**: 664.

Weinstein HJ, Hallett WY, Sarauw AS (1962). The absorption and toxicity of ethionamide. *Amer Rev Respir Dis* **86**: 576.

WHO (1994). Chemotherapy of Leprosy. Report of a WHO Study Group. *WHO Tech Rep Ser* 847.

Thiacetazone

Description

Thiacetazone is one of many thiosemicarbazones discovered by Domagk and his co-workers in Germany in 1946. Of several compounds from this group exhibiting antituberculosis activity, thiacetazone was the most promising for human therapeutics. Initially it was considered to be too toxic for widespread clinical use (Hinshaw and McDermott, 1950). However, because there was a need for another cheap and effective antituberculosis drug in developing countries, it was tried with success initially in East Africa. Thiacetazone still has a place in the treatment of tuberculosis in developing countries where cost is a factor; it is rarely used in technically advanced countries.

Activity Against Mycobacteria

Thiacetazone is quite active against *M. tuberculosis*, most strains being inhibited by a concentration of 1.0 µg per ml. Pretreatment strains in various parts of the world may vary in their degree of sensitivity to thiacetazone. For instance, strains isolated in East Africa are usually more sensitive (MIC 0.4 µg per ml), than those found in Southern India, Hong Kong and Singapore (Citron, 1972; Ellard *et al.*, 1974). One type of tubercle bacillus with certain laboratory characteristics is called *M. tuberculosis africanum* (p. 1180). This bacillus is found in some areas of Africa and it is frequently resistant to thiacetazone, so that regimens containing this drug are unsuitable for treatment (WHO, 1975). *Mycobacterium africanum* also shows secondary resistance to other drugs used for tuberculosis (p. 1180). As with other antituberculosis drugs, thiacetazone-resistance may emerge in patients during treatment unless at least one other effective drug is used concurrently (East African/BMRC, 1970). Thiacetazone has a bacteriostatic action on *M. tuberculosis*.

Although the MIC of thiacetazone against *M. leprae* is 0.2 µg per ml, the drug only has a bacteriostatic action against this organism (Ellard, 1980).

Mode of Administration and Dosage

Thiacetazone is administered by the oral route, as a single daily dose of 150 mg to adults. The size of the individual dose appears to be critical; larger doses cause toxicity whilst lower doses are often ineffective (Citron, 1972). In children or underweight adults, daily doses of 25, 50 and 100 mg have been given to those weighing less than 10 kg, 10–20 kg and 20–40 kg, respectively; this approximates to a dose of 3–5 mg per kg per day (Pearson, 1978). Thiacetazone in a dose of 450 mg is suitable for intermittent chemotherapy and this is well tolerated (Fox *et al.*, 1974).

Absorption and Excretion

Thiacetazone is well absorbed following oral administration. After a 150-mg dose to adults, a peak serum level of 1–2 µg per ml is attained 4–5 h later. Doubling the dose approximately doubles the serum concentrations, but when a dose as high as 600 mg is given the peak level is attained at 5 h or later. The serum half-life of the drug is approximately 12 h (Ellard *et al.*, 1974). Jenner *et al.* (1984), using a high-performance liquid chromatography method to investigate pharmacokinetics, had similar findings. After daily oral doses of 150 mg, peak serum levels at 4 h averaged 1.76 µg per ml and trough levels at 24 h averaged 0.6 µg per ml.

About 20% of an orally administered thiacetazone dose is excreted in the urine in an unchanged form. Some metabolites of the drug are also eliminated via the kidney (Ellard *et al.*, 1974). Thiacetazone would presumably accumulate in patients with renal failure.

Toxicity

1 Gastrointestinal side-effects

Thiacetazone can cause symptoms such as nausea, vomiting or diarrhea, their frequency and severity being similar to those caused by para-aminosalicylic acid (PAS) (p. 1225) (Miller *et al.*, 1966).

2 Hepatotoxicity

Severe liver damage with jaundice, resulting in occasional fatalities, apparently due to thiacetazone has been reported (Miller *et al.*, 1966). However, most of these patients had also received isoniazid simultaneously (p. 1190).

3 Hematological side-effects

Bone marrow depression, thrombocytopenia and agranulocytosis have been caused by thiacetazone therapy (Miller *et al.*, 1966). Hemolytic anemia has also been reported and according to Masel and Johnston (1968) minor degrees of hemolysis can be commonly detected in patients receiving the drug.

4 Ototoxicity

Symptoms such as dizziness, vertigo, ataxia, tinnitus and even deafness can result from thiacetazone therapy. This drug also potentiates streptomycin ototoxicity (Miller *et al.*, 1966; Pearson, 1978).

5 Hypersensitivity

Rashes, often trivial, frequently occur during thiacetazone therapy and fatal exfoliative dermatitis has been described occasionally (Ferguson *et al.*, 1971). When a thiacetazone rash is observed, it is advisable to stop the drug. Severe hypersensitivity rashes due to thiacetazone are frequent in HIV-infected patients (Nunn *et al.*, 1991; Van der Ven *et al.*, 1994).

6 Side-effects in different ethnic groups

The frequency of rashes varies widely in different geographical areas. In one large international study rashes were found to be common in patients from Singapore and Malaysia, less common in those from Czechoslovakia and non-existent in patients from Ethiopia (Ferguson *et al.*, 1971). Gastrointestinal irritation and ototoxicity are more common in patients from Hong Kong than in those from Africa (Miller *et al.*, 1966). In a study of toxic effects of a daily isoniazid/thiacetazone regimen (supplemented by streptomycin in the first 2 months) used for 10 years in Nigeria, 14% of patients developed reactions which in 11% were sufficient to require a change of treatment; giddiness and rashes were the most common effects (Pearson, 1978). These differences probably result from environmental factors and from variations in recording and interpretation of side-effects. The patient's ethnic origin *per se* does not appear to be an important factor, because if patients from different racial groups are treated together in one hospital, the frequency of side-effects in all groups is about the same (Miller *et al.*, 1972).

Nevertheless, it has been suggested that sample population groups should be investigated for thiacetazone toxicity prior to its widespread use in a new community.

Clinical Uses of the Drug

1 Pulmonary tuberculosis

Because of its cheapness, thiacetazone has been extensively used as a first-line drug, usually in combination with isoniazid, for the treatment of pulmonary tuberculosis in many countries, particularly in Asia and Africa. In some areas of Africa, where HIV infection is now common, it is hard to use it because these patients often develop serious reactions (see above). It is only rarely used in developed countries where other less toxic drugs are readily available. Isoniazid 300 mg and thiacetazone 150 mg given in one daily dose in a single tablet has been recommended as effective and of low toxicity for patients weighing 35 kg or more (WHO, 1975). Results with this therapy are improved if i.m. streptomycin in a dose of 1 g daily is added during the first 8 weeks of treatment (East African/BMRC, 1970, 1973). A comparative trial of thiacetazone 150 mg and isoniazid 300 mg in one daily dose and a combination of PAS 12 g with isoniazid

300 mg daily in divided doses was carried out on 72 selected patients with pulmonary tuberculosis in Nigeria.

Thiacetazone was equally effective to PAS as a companion drug for isoniazid and was preferable because of its relative cheapness and once-daily administration (Onadeko and Sofowora, 1975). Thiacetazone regimens have not been satisfactory in some countries. In Singapore, a combination of thiacetazone 150 mg + isoniazid 300 mg daily was found to be rather ineffective and too toxic, and a second regimen, which contained streptomycin 1 g daily in addition for the first 6 months, although effective, was also too toxic (Singapore/Brompton Hospital/BMRC, 1971, 1974). Nevertheless, the WHO in 1982 (p. 1197) recommended a cheaper regimen for use in developing countries, consisting of daily thiacetazone and isoniazid for 12 months, often supplemented by streptomycin in the initial intensive phase.

This drug has also been used in regimens for intermittent chemotherapy (p. 1195) of pulmonary tuberculosis in East Africa. Thiacetazone 450 mg plus isoniazid 15 mg per kg body weight given twice-weekly has been used to complete a 2-year course after an initial phase of streptomycin 1 g with thiacetazone 150 mg plus isoniazid 300 mg daily for 4 or 8 weeks (East African/BMRC, 1974b). These regimens were fairly effective but somewhat inferior to continuation therapy with a daily regimen of these drugs.

Short-course regimens (p. 1197) for the treatment of pulmonary tuberculosis which contain thiacetazone, have not been satisfactory (East African/BMRC, 1972; 1974a). It may have a place in some short-course regimens in the continuation phase of treatment with isoniazid after an intensive initial phase of treatment with four bactericidal drugs.

2 Leprosy

Thiacetazone has been used with dapsone and rifampicin to treat leprosy (Rees et al., 1979) but it is only bacteriostatic and less effective than other drugs. It is currently not recommended for the treatment of leprosy (WHO, 1994).

References

Citron KM (1972). Tuberculosis-chemotherapy. *Brit Med J* **1**: 426.

East African/British Medical Research Council Fifth Thiacetazone Investigation (1970). Isoniazid with thiacetazone (thioacetazone) in the treatment of pulmonary tuberculosis in East Africa – fifth investigation. *Tubercle* **51**: 123.

East African/British Medical Research Councils (1972). Controlled clinical trial of short-course (6-month). regimens of chemotherapy for treatment of pulmonary tuberculosis. *Lancet* **i**: 1079.

East African/British Medical Research Council Fifth Thiacetazone Investigation – Third Report (1973). Isoniazid with thiacetazone (thioacetazone). in the treatment of pulmonary tuberculosis in East Africa. Third report of fifth investigation. *Tubercle* **54**: 169.

East African/British Medical Research Councils (1974a). Controlled clinical trial of four short-course (6-month) regimens of chemotherapy for treatment of plumonary tuberculosis. Third report. *Lancet* **ii**: 237.

East African/British Medical Research Council Intermittent Thiacetazone Investigation (1974b). A pilot study of two regimens of intermittent thiacetazone plus isoniazid in the treatment of pulmonary tuberculosis in East Africa. *Tubercle* **55**: 211.

Ellard GA (1980). Combined treatment for lepromatous leprosy. *Lepr Rev* **51**: 199.

Ellard GA, Dickinson JM, Gammon PT, Mitchison DA (1974). Serum concentrations and antituberculosis activity of thiacetazone. *Tubercle* **55**: 41.

Ferguson GC, Nunn AJ, Fox W et al. (1971). A second international co-operative investigation into thiacetazone side-effects: rashes on two thiacetazone-containing regimens. *Tubercle* **52**: 166.

Fox W et al. (1974). A study of adverse reactions to high dosage intermittent thiacetazone. *Tubercle* **55**: 29.

Hinshaw HC, McDermott W (1950). Thiosemicarbazone therapy of tuberculosis in humans. *Amer Rev Tuberc* **61**: 145.

Jenner PJ, Ellard GA, Swai OB (1984). A study of thiacetazone blood levels and urinary excretion in man, using high performance liquid chromatography. *Lepr Rev* **55**: 121.

Masel MA, Johnston NG (1968). Haemolytic anaemia in a patient taking thiacetazone. *Med J Aust* **2**: 840.

Miller AB, Fox W, Tall R (1966). An international co-operative investigation into thiacetazone (thioacetazone) side-effects. *Tubercle* **47**: 33.

Miller AB, Nunn AJ, Robinson DK et al. (1972). A second international co-operative investigation into thiacetazone side-effects. *Bull Wld Hlth Org* **47**: 211.

Nunn P, Kibuga D, Gathua S et al. (1991). Cutaneous hypersensitivity reactions due to thiacetazone in HIV-1 seropositive patients treated for tuberculosis. *Lancet* **337**: 627.

Onadeko BO, Sofowora EO (1975). Comparative trial of thiacetazone with isoniazid and paraaminosalicylic acid (PAS) with isoniazid in the treatment of pulmonary tuberculosis in Nigerians. *J Trop Med Hyg* **78**: 201.

Pearson CA (1978). Thiacetazone toxicity in the treatment of tuberculosis patients in Nigeria. *Amer J Trop Med Hyg* **81**: 238.

Rees RJ W, Pearson JMH, Waters MFR (1979). Studies on the bacteriology, epidemiology and prevention of dapsone resistance in leprosy. *Bull Int Un Tuberc* **54**: 365.

Singapore Tuberculosis Services/Brompton Hospital/British Medical Research Council Investigation (1971). A controlled clinical trial of the role of thiacetazone-containing regimens in the treatment of pulmonary tuberculosis in Singapore. *Tubercle* **52**: 88.

Singapore Tuberculosis Services/Brompton Hospital/British Medical

Research Council Investigation (1974). A controlled trial of the role of thiacetazone-containing regimens in the treatment of pulmonary tuberculosis in Singapore: Second report. *Tubercle* **55**: 251.

Van der Ven AJM, Koopmans PP, Vree TB, Van der Meer JWM (1994). Drug intolerance in HIV disease. *J Antimicrob Chemother* **34**: 1.

WHO (1975). Tuberculosis control: progress of the new strategy. *WHO Chron* **29**: 123.

WHO (1994). Report of a WHO Study Group. Chemotherapy of Leprosy. *WHO Technical Report Series* 847.

Viomycin

Description

This is a polypeptide antibiotic (p. 667), which has been used as a reserve drug for the treatment of drug-resistant tuberculosis since 1950. Viomycin is now only very rarely prescribed, because there are safer and more effective drugs available. For this reason only a brief outline of this drug is included.

The activity of viomycin against *Mycobacterium tuberculosis* is only about one-quarter that of streptomycin (Robson and Sullivan, 1963). It is usually active against organisms resistant to streptomycin and other antituberculosis drugs with the exception that it shows complete cross-resistance with capreomycin (McClatchy *et al.*, 1977).

Viomycin is administered by the i.m. route. After a 1 g dose in adults the serum levels attained and the excretion patterns of this drug are similar to those of streptomycin (p. 431).

The toxic effects of viomycin are like those of capreomycin (p. 1232); nephrotoxicity with associated electrolyte imbalance and ototoxicity being the main ones. Viomycin appears to be more toxic than capreomycin.

To avoid toxicity, viomycin is usually only administered in an adult dose of 1.0–2.0 g daily for short periods of 2 or 3 weeks. Thereafter, the dose is reduced to 2.0 g twice-weekly (Pyle, 1970).

For treatment of tuberculosis, the drug is always administered in conjunction with two or even more other antituberculosis drugs. However, the combination of viomycin with other nephrotoxic and ototoxic drugs such as streptomycin, kanamycin and capreomycin should be avoided.

References

McClatchy JK, Kanes W, Davidson PT, Moulding TS (1977). Cross-resistance in *M tuberculosis* to kanamycin, capreomycin and viomycin. *Tubercle* **58**: 29.

Pyle MM (1970). Ethambutol and viomycin. *Med Clin N Amer* **54**: 1317.

Robson JM, Sullivan FM (1963). Antituberculosis drugs. *Pharmacol Rev* **15**: 169.

Part IV

Antifungal Drugs

Amphotericin B (AMB)

Description

Despite its inherent toxicity and the continued development of potent imidazole drugs, amphotericin B (AMB) remains the drug of choice for systemic treatment of invasive fungal infections. It was developed and introduced into clinical mangement prior to the use of rigorous clinical trials to examine efficacy and safety of new therapeutic agents.

One of the polyene group of antibiotics produced by several different species of *Streptomyces*, AMB is characterized by a macrocylic lactone ring with a series of conjugated double bonds (Hamilton-Miller, 1973, Kotler-Brajtburg *et al.*, 1979). It is produced by *Streptomyces nodosus* which was first isolated in the Orinoco river valley in Venezuela and reports of its antifungal activity were first published in 1956 (Dutcher, 1968). It was initially developed as an oral agent by Squibb, but despite administration of large oral doses efficacy was extremely poor. This observation led to the development of particulate suspensions for i.v. administration and associated improved efficacy.

Virtually insoluble in aqueous solutions at physiologic pH, AMB is unstable at the extremes of pH and forms soluble salts in both acidic and basic environments. It is supplied for parenteral administration as a colloidal suspension using sodium desoxycholate (41mg) as a dispersing agent and sodium phosphate (25.2mg) as a buffer for each 50-mg AMB dose.

A more water-soluble methyl ester derivative of AMB was developed (Mechlinski and Schaffner, 1972). It produced comparatively higher serum levels in animals and initially appeared to be less nephrotoxic than the AMB-desoxycholate suspension (Keim *et al.*, 1976). *In vitro*, this AMB methyl ester had slightly lower activity than AMB against pathogenic fungi (Howarth *et al.*, 1975). In certain experimental murine infections, it was also less effective than the parent compound (Bonner *et al.*, 1975; Lawrence and Hoeprich, 1976; Gadesbusch *et al.*, 1976), but the dose regimens employed may not have been adequate (Lawrence *et al.*, 1980). The ester had an antiviral effect against some viruses (Jordan and Seet, 1978), and it had been used successfully to treat a couple of patients with severe fungal infections (Hoeprich, 1978). However, a leukoencephalopathy consisting of progressive neurologic dysfunction and diffuse white matter degeneration was described in patients treated with AMB-methyl ester (Ellis *et al.*, 1982). Although a causal relationship between AMB, its ester or other contaminating polyenes and this leukoencephalopathy has not been established (Hoeprich, 1982), further clinical studies with the methyl ester form of AMB have been terminated.

Because dose-limiting toxicity often results in suboptimal clinical efficacy, particularly in immunocompromised hosts, two approaches have been utilized to improve the therapeutic index of AMB – the development of less toxic preparations of AMB, and improved methods of delivery of AMB directly to target organs (intranasal, intracavitary, intraperitoneal etc). See section on administration of AMB (p. 1255).

Entrapment of AMB in liposomes reduces both the acute infusional toxicity and the nephrotoxicity observed with AMB-desoxycholate solutions. It is thought the reduction in toxicity is the result of different affinities of AMB to the ergosterol in fungal membranes (high affinity), the lipids in the carrier, and cholesterol in human cell membranes (low affinity) (Lopez-Berenstein,1989). When AMB is delivered in a lipid carrier formulation, AMB-lipid complexes are formed and are present in equilibrium with free AMB. The extent of complex formation is dependant on the concentration of both AMB and the lipid carrier, as well as the affinity of AMB to the lipid in the carrier. The concentration of free AMB in the aqueous phase will depend primarily on the affinity of the lipid carrier, the higher the affinity, the lower the concentration of aqueous phase AMB. There is a selective transfer of AMB from the high affinity lipid carrier to the 'target' cell membranes by a diffusion process through an aqueous phase of free AMB.

Toxicity to cells is therefore dependant on availability of a critical concentration of AMB in the aqueous phase and is differential for human and fungal cells (Brajtburg *et al.*, 1990b, Jullien *et al.*, 1989).

There is no single lipid vehicle and the characteristics of the liposomal carrier/vehicle (chemical composition, charge, size, structure, and mode of preparation) can modify the physiochemical, biological and pharmacological properties of both the liposomes and the carried drug (Brajtburg *et al.*, 1990b). Whether the use of liposomes improves the therapeutic index of AMB is not yet known. It was initially thought that delivery of AMB in a liposomal preparation altered the disposition of the drug, resulting in significantly higher AMB concentrations in liver and spleen (Lopez-Berenstein 1984), but no significant difference in organ distribution of AMB was found 24 h after i.v. administration of the liposomal preparation of AMB and the commercial AMB-desoxycholate in mice in other studies. (Szoka *et al.*,1987).

There are a number of liposomal preparations of AMB that have been tested in humans. These include amphotericin B-lipid complex (ABLC, 'Abelcet'), amphotericin B-liposome ('AmBisome') and amphotericin B-colloidal dispersion (ABCD, 'Amphocil') also known as amphotericin B cholesteryl sulfate complex ('Amphotec'). It is clear that these preparations have different pharmacokinetic properties and studies are required to determine whether differences in serum concentrations of AMB have any clinical significance. It is still unknown whether tissue concentrations of AMB are more important than serum concentrations. There is insufficient clinical data to recommend definite doses of lipid formulations of AMB and duration of treatment for the management of serious invasive fungal infections, as no large comparative clinical trials have been performed. Some animal studies suggest that the lipid formulations have reduced efficacy compared with AMB-desoxycholate when administered in equivalent doses (3- to 4-fold higher doses of the lipid formulations are required for equivalent activity). In one study, liposomal AMB had 4- to 8-fold less activity than AMB-desoxycholate in the setting of murine candidiasis (both systemic candidiasis and localized candidiasis) (Pahls and Schaffner, 1994). Because of the differences in pharmacokinetic properties of each of the lipid vehicles for administration of AMB, individual controlled studies will be required to examine efficacy and safety, so optimal recommendations of dose and duration of therapy can be developed. See pharmacokinetic section for further discussion of comparative pharmacokinetics of liposomal preparations of AMB (p. 1259).

Sensitive Organisms

In vitro susceptibility testing of fungal isolates from studies performed over the last 40 years are difficult to compare because of changing methodology and lack of standardization of the tests used. The proposed standard for antifungal susceptibility testing of yeasts has recently been developed by the National Committee for Clinical Laboratory Standards (NCCLS) and released in 1992 (Reference method for broth dilution antifungal susceptibility testing for yeasts) and provides a uniform method for *in vitro* testing of yeasts that is reproducible and allows comparison across studies. It is likely that a correlation between *in vitro* susceptibility testing and *in vivo* efficacy will exist, once the best techniques are selected. Antifungal susceptibility testing using a microbroth dilution method has shown a good correlation with *in vivo* outcome of antifungal treatment of murine experimental hematogenous candidiasis, regardless of the immune status of the mice. *In vitro* resistance to AMB was predictive of lack of *in vivo* activity (Anaisse *et al.*, 1994). A significant correlation between *in vitro* antifungal testing based on the NCCLS method and *in vivo* response to fluconazole treatment in murine cryptococcosis has also been shown (Velez *et al.*, 1993) However, no correlation between *in vitro* antifungal susceptibility testing and clinical outcome in humans was found in a large study comparing AMB and fluconazole for the treatment of candidemia (Rex *et al.*, 1995). Currently, it is probably not appropriate to predict clinical outcome on the basis of MIC data and knowledge of achievable serum levels of the antifungal agent. A standardized reference method for antifungal susceptibility testing of filamentous fungi is still to be developed. An excellent review of the issues pertaining to antifungal susceptibility testing has been published (Rex *et al.*, 1993).

Assessment of the effect of lipid complexing of AMB on antifungal potency has been documented by comparing AMB-desoxycholate with ABCD *in vitro* against a number of clinical isolates (Table IV.2) Hanson *et al.* (1992) showed variable effects on *in vitro* activity of AMB by lipid complexing in the ABCD preparation. In about one-third of comparisons between formulations of AMB, there was a large decrease in activity (4-fold or more) and for some isolates there was enhanced activity for the lipid preparation. 'AmBisome' has been shown to be 4- to 8-fold less active than AMB-desoxycholate both *in vitro* (99% reduction in log cfu/ml) and *in vivo* animal model of murine candidiasis when compared at equal doses. (Pahls and Schaffner, 1994)

Another study revealed similar minimum inhibitory concentrations (MICs) and minimum fungicidal concentrations (MFCs) for AMB-desoxycholate and 'AmBisome', but a significantly reduced fungicidal activity for 'AmBisome' based on time-kill studies (Van Etten *et al.*, 1993).

The classification of many fungi has also changed in recent years. The obsolete name has been placed in brackets after the currently used term, as many *in vitro* susceptibility tests and clinical efficacy reports are published using the older terminology.

1 Pathogenic yeasts

Cryptococcus neoformans is usually sensitive (Espinel-Ingroff *et al.*, 1991; Barchiesi *et al.*, 1994). Isolates from patients experiencing recurrent cryptococcal meningitis after treatement with AMB do not show any reduction in susceptibility (Casadevall *et al.*, 1993). Isolates of *Hansenula anomala* are susceptible to AMB (Klein *et al.*, 1988).

It has been generally accepted that *Candida albicans* is quite sensitive. Other *Candida* spp. such as *C. tropicalis* are sensitive to a lesser degree (Stieritz *et al.*, 1973). *Candida (Torulopsis) glabrata* is also susceptible. Acquired resistance of isolates of *C. albicans* (MIC >2 µg per ml) has been reported (Dick 1980), but is relatively rare. *Candida tropicalis*, *C. parapsilosis*, *C. kefyr* and *C. guillermondii* have developed AMB-resistance during prolonged treatment in the immunocompromised host (Dick *et al.* 1985, Drutz *et al.* 1978, Merz *et al.* 1979, Pappagiannis *et al.* 1979) *Candida lusitaniae* is often resistant to AMB (Hadfield *et al.*, 1987). Comparison of the activity of free and liposomal AMB in the murine candidiasis model, reveals that liposomal AMB is 4- to 8-fold less potent than conventional AMB (Pahls and Schaffner, 1994).

Fungi of the genus *Trichosporon*, *T. beigelii*, have MICs of AMB of 0.14–0.58 µg per ml, but the minimum fungicidal concentration for AMB range from 4.62 to >18.5 µg per ml (Walsh *et al.*, 1992). In addition, both AMB and liposossmal AMB were found to be ineffective in the persistently neutropenic rabbit model of disseminated trichosporonosis, with no *in vivo* antifungal activity demonstrated (Walsh *et al.*, 1992).

2 Dimorphic fungi

Blastomyces dermatitidis, *Paracoccidioides brasiliensis*, *Histoplasma capsulatum* and *Coccidioides immitis* are all sensitive to AMB. In one *in vitro* study of clinical isolates at least one-fifth of *C. immitis* strains were considered to be resistant (Hoeprich and Huston, 1975), but in experimental murine infections AMB in clinically attainable concentrations was uniformly effective against *C. immitis* strains, including some of those studied by Hoeprich and Huston (Collins and Pappagianis, 1977). In the murine model of coccidioidomycosis AMB was compared with ABCD and found to be 3- to 4-fold more efficacious, but 5- to 8-fold more toxic (Clemons and Stevens, 1991). In the murine model of blastomycosis, AMB was superior to 'AmBisome' at equivalent 1 mg per kg dosages, however curative doses (7.5 mg per kg) of 'AmBisome' could be administered without toxicity, revealing a significantly improved therapeutic index of AMB when administered as a liposomal preparation (Clemons and Stevens, 1993). Finally, in the murine model of histoplasmosis, liposomal AMB was as efficacious as conventional AMB at equivalent doses in immunodeficient mice (Graybill and Bocanegra, 1995). Up to 60% of clinical isolates of *Penicillium marneffei* are sensitive to AMB; the rest were moderately sensitive or considered resistant (Supparatpinyo *et al.*, 1993).

3 Molds or filamentous fungi

Aspergillus spp. are usually sensitive (Denning *et al.*, 1992). The causative organisms of chromoblastomycosis (*Phialophora* spp. and *Cladosporium carrionii*) are usually resistant, but *Sporothrix schenckii* is usually sensitive. Species of the genera which cause zygomycosis such as *Mucor*, *Rhizopus*, *Absidia*, *Basidiobolus* and *Conidiobolus*, are often sensitive. For instance, Eng *et al.* (1981) showed that all of 25 clinical isolates from zygomycosis (*Mucor*, *Rhizopus*, *Absidia* and *Cunninghamella*) were susceptible to AMB when tested in the presence of serum. However, *in vitro* testing of the Mucoraceae (*Mucor*, *Rhizopus* and *Absidia*) have produced contradictory results, possibly due to strain variation or differences in methodology; although results of studies in animals and humans support an *in vivo* effect of AMB (Lehrer *et al.*, 1980). The *in vitro* susceptibility of 13 *Basidiobolus* and three *Conidiobolus* isolates to AMB was tested by Yangco *et al.* (1984), and only 50% of *Basidiobolus* spp. were susceptible to AMB, while two of three *Conidiobolus* isolates were susceptible.

Fungal mycetoma (eumycetoma) caused by organisms, such as *Madurella* spp., *Pseudallescheria (Petriellidium) boydii (Monosporium apiospermum)* and *Cephalosporium recifei*, are usually resistant. The dermatophytes or ringworm fungi, such as *Microsporum*, *Trichophyton* and *Epidermophyton* spp. are usually resistant. *Scedosporium inflatum* and *Scedosporium apiospermum* are resistant to AMB (Salkin *et al.*, 1988).

4 Actinomycetes and actinomyces

Aerobic bacteria of the *Nocardia* and *Actinomadura* spp., which also cause mycetoma (actinomycetoma) are AMB-resistant. Various other anaerobic or microaerophilic bacteria of the *Actinomyces* spp., which cause actinomycosis and which can be confused with mycetoma, are also resistant.

5 Prototheca spp

These organisms which appear to be achloric algae and resemble fungi can be rare causes of human infection (protothecosis), characterized by chronic, persistent granulomata which may be localized to the skin or disseminated (Nosanchuk and Greenberg, 1973). *Prototheca* spp. are usually sensitive to AMB (Segal *et al.*, 1976).

6 Naegleria

These ameboflagellates, in particular *Naegleria fowleri*, which is one of the main causes of primary amebic meningoencephalitis in humans, are usually sensitive to AMB with MICs in the range of <0.018–0.078 μg per ml (Lee *et al.*, 1979, Smego and Durack, 1984).

7 Acanthamoebae

Fresh water amebae, such as *Acanthamoeba polyphaga* and *A. castellanii*, can cause suppurative corneal and intraocular infections resembling those due to fungi. These protozoa are susceptible *in vitro* to AMB (Nagington and Richards, 1976).

8 Leishmania

Using an *in vitro* test system, Berman and Wyler (1980) showed that AMB eliminated 90–100% of the mammalian form (amastigotes) of *Leishmania tropica* and *L. donovani,* and it was also toxic to the extracellular forms of these parasites (promastigotes). It is active *in vitro* against *L. mexicana* (Coombs *et al.*, 1983). Intravenously administered AMB, particularly if entrapped in liposomes, is parasiticidal in rodent visceral leishmaniasis (New *et al.*, 1981). The activity of ABCD was greater than conventional AMB in the hamster model of visceral leishmaniasis, probably due to improved delivery of AMB to the site of infection, the macrophages (Berman *et al.*, 1992).

9 Malaria parasites

Amphotericin B is active *in vitro* against chloroquine-sensitive and chloroquine-resistant *Plasmodium falciparum* parasites (Pfaller and Krogstad, 1981).

10 Hepatitis B virus

In concentrations as low as 5 μg per ml AMB causes ultrastructural and biochemical changes in hepatitis B virus particles, possibly through an interaction with cholesterol in the hepatitis B surface antigen molecule (Kessler *et al.*, 1981). In concentrations of 10 μg per ml AMB produced a 60% reduction in HBsAg production in a human hepatoma cell line. The inhibition of HBsAg production was non-specific (Pottage and Kessler, 1985). The clinical relevance of these observations is unknown.

11 Synergism and antagonism with other drugs

The action of AMB on the cytoplasmic membrane may render yeast cells more susceptible to 5-flucytosine (Medoff *et al.*, 1971). Alternatively, synergy may result from a sequential action of AMB and 5-flucytosine on yeast cells (Beggs, 1986). Together these two drugs frequently exert an *in vitro* synergistic effect against *Candida* spp. (Shadomy *et al.*, 1975). Synergy has been demonstrated when the strain is resistant to 5-flucytosine (Montgomerie *et al.*, 1975). These two drugs usually have an enhanced effect when used to treat experimental infections due to *Candida albicans* in mice (Ravinovich *et al.*, 1974), and in neutropenic rabbits (Thaler *et al.*, 1988b). Other investigators, using different methodology, have not been able to demonstrate synergy between AMB and 5-flucytosine (Dupont and Drouhet, 1979). The combination of AMB and 5-flucytosine also shows *in vitro* synergism against a proportion of isolates of *Cryptococcus neoformans* (Shadomy *et al.*, 1975) and enhanced efficacy in cryptococcal murine infections (Block and Bennett, 1973). Synergism is not demonstrable with all isolates of yeast-like organisms, and *in vitro* antagonism has sometimes been demonstrated when the two drugs have been used against *C. albicans* (Hoeprich and Finn, 1972) and *C. neoformans* (Hamilton and Elliot, 1975). *In vitro* synergism of AMB with 5-flucytosine has been demonstrated with some clinical isolates of *Aspergillus* (Kitahara *et al.*, 1976a), but others have not been able to confirm such synergy (Lauer *et al.*, 1978; Hughes *et al.*, 1984a). In a murine model of systemic aspergillosis, these two drugs produce better results than the use of either drug alone (Arroyo *et al.*, 1977), and in a rabbit model of *Aspergillus fumigatus* endocarditis the combination of AMB and 5-flucytosine effected eradication of Aspergillus from cardiac vegetations in 30% of animals (Longman and Martin, 1987).

Theoretically, AMB and the azoles were thought to be antagonistic, due to the action of AMB and the other polyene antifungal drugs which bind to the ergosterol in the fungal cytoplasmic membrane and the action of the azoles which inhibit the synthesis of ergosterol resulting in the disappearance of ergosterol from the cell membrane. Results have been conflicting when AMB has been combined with imidazole drugs in *in vitro* susceptibility studies and animal models of mycoses.

In general, results of antifungal susceptibility testing have revealed antagonism between the azoles and AMB against most fungi tested. *In vitro* antagonism using AMB with either clotrimazole or miconazole against *Candida* spp. (including *C. albicans*, *C. kefyr (pseudotropicalis)* and *C. glabrata (Torulopsis glabrata)* was demonstrated by Cosgrove *et al.* (1978). This *in vitro* antagonism of the polyene effect by azoles (miconazole, ketoconazole, itraconazole and fluconazole) on *C. albicans* was confirmed in other studies (Brajtburg *et al.*, 1982; Polak, 1987; Martin *et al.*, 1994; Petrou *et al.*, 1991). Antagonism between AMB with miconazole or econazole has also been shown with *Candida albicans* and *Cryptococcus neoformans* (Dupont and Drouhet. 1979). In contrast, *in vitro* testing by Odds (1982) against *Candida* spp. and *C. neoformans* using combinations of AMB, 5-flucytosine, ketoconazole and miconazole, indicated that combinations which included AMB and ketoconazole were usually synergistic. However AMB-susceptible *C. albicans* becomes resistant to the drug after growth in the presence of ketoconazole; and this is associated with a parallel decrease in cellular ergosterol (Sud and Feingold, 1983). However, *in vitro* tests using ketoconazole with AMB against *H. capsulatum* and *C. neoformans* failed to show antagonism (Graybill *et al.*, 1980). Ketoconazole antagonized the fungicidal effect of AMB *in vitro* on *Aspergillus fumigatus* (Schaffner and Frick, 1985), but in another study ketoconazole did not alter the *in vitro* activity of AMB against *Aspergillus* spp. (Hughes *et al.*, 1984a).

It appears that discrepancies in the demonstration of antagonism and synergy *in vitro* when using AMB and the imidazole drugs in combination may be explained by variations in the assay conditions employed. Brajtburg *et al.* (1982) showed that combinations of AMB with miconazole or ketoconazole could be more, equally or less potent against *C. albicans* than the use of the agents alone, and the variability in potency depended on the experimental conditions used. Smith *et al.* (1983b) confirmed that depending on the period of incubation of the culture, either *in vitro* synergy or antagonism between ketoconazole and AMB against *C. neoformans* could be demonstrated. The lipophilic azole drugs (itraconazole, ketoconazole and miconazole) are able to reduce the fungicidal activity of subsequently added AMB, but preincubation of *C. albicans* with fluconazole did not produce any significant effect on the fungicidal activity of AMB (Scheven *et al.*, 1995). Ketoconazole, itraconazole and miconazole have a long postantifungal effect compared with fluconazole which has a short-lasting antifungal effect of 0.5–2 h (Mikami *et al.*, 1992). This suggests that the length of the postantifungal effect may be related to antagonism demonstrated between the azoles and subsequently applied AMB (Sheven *et al.*, 1995).

Animal models of mycoses have also been used to examine the effects of combination therapy with AMB and the azole drugs. Immunosuppressed mice infected with *Aspergillus fumigatus* and treated with a combination of AMB and ketoconazole or pretreated with ketoconazole and subsequently treated with AMB (Schaffner and Frick, 1985) had the beneficial effects of AMB abolished. A similar observation of antagonism was noted between AMB and itraconazole, whether it was used concurrently or sequentially, for the treatment of aspergillosis in immunosuppressed mice (Schaffner *et al.*,1993). Although, no antagonism could be demonstrated for the combination of fluconazole and AMB in the immunosuppressed rabbit model of invasive aspergillosis, fluconazole did not augment the antifungal activity of AMB (George *et al.* 1993). In the murine model of invasive candidiasis in both immunocompromised and immunocompetent mice, combinations of AMB and fluconazole were not antagonistic, and in some doses were considered additive (Sugar *et al.*, 1995). In addition the combination of AMB and saperconazole and DO870 was not antagonistic in this candidiasis model (Sugar *et al.*, 1994, Atkinson *et al.*, 1994). The addition of ketoconazole to subtherapeutic doses of AMB in a rabbit model increased the killing of cryptococci in the CSF (Perfect and Durack, 1982). In murine pulmonary cryptococcosis, an AMB and ketoconazole combination was as effective as ketoconazole alone but, after more prolonged treatment, the results suggested that this combination may be antagonistic (Iwen *et al.*, 1984). Combinations

Table IV.1

Compiled from data published by Bergan and Vangdal, (1983), Yangco et al. (1984), Vartian et al. (1985), Adam et al. (1986), Hussain Qadri, et al. (1986), Ando and Takatori, (1987), Dixon and Polak, (1987), Marcon et al. (1987), Haron et al. (1988), Iwatsu, (1988), Schmitt et al. (1988a), Mahul et al. (1989), Reuben et al. (1989), Wong et al. (1989), Gallis et al. (1990), McGinnis and Rinaldi (1991), Morace et al. (1991), Sands et al. (1991), Hernandez Molina et al. (1992), Martin et al. (1992), Penn et al. (1992), Sekhon et al. (1992a,b, 1993, 1994), Brummer et al. (1993), Casadevall et al. (1993), Anaisse et al. (1994), Kontoyianis et al. (1994), Espinel-Ingroff et al. (1995, 1996), Lau et al. (1995), and van Eldere et al. (1996)

Organism	MIC (μg per ml) range	
	Broth	Agar
Yeast		
Candida species		
C. albicans	0.25–1	0.06–>4
C. guilliermondii	0.156	0.12–1
C. krusei	0.078–0.312	0.06–2
C. parapsilosis	0.078–0.625	0.25–2
C. tropicalis	0.078–0.312	0.12–2
C. kefyr (pseudotropicalis)		0.25–0.5
C. lusitaniae	0.3125–2.5	0.12–1
C. rugosa	0.29–1.16	0.008–0.5
C. glabrata (Torulopsis glabrata)	0.039–0.156	0.06–1
Blastoschizomyces capitatus	0.1–0.5	
Cryptococcus neoformans	<0.14–0.29	
Hansenula anomala	0.78–1.56	
Malassezia furfur	0.6–2.5	
Rhodotorula rubra	0.1–1	0.5
Trichosporon beigelii	0.14–0.58	
Dimorphic fungi		
Histoplasma capsulatum	<4.0	
Blastomyces dermatitidis	0.05–0.78	
Coccidioides immitis	0.5–1.0	
Paracoccidioides brasiliensis	0.2–0.5	
Penicillium marneffei	3.125–25 (yeast form)	0.25–4.0
	0.78–1.56 (myceliel form)	
Sporothrix schenckii	0.5–16	
Mold		
Aspergillus		
A. fumigatus	0.25–1	
A. flavus	0.5–16	
A. niger	0.4–0.8	
Hyphomycetes		
Acremonium spp.	1	
Fusarium spp.	1.56–100	
Pseudallescheria boydii	0.5–16	
Pythium insidiosum		50–100
Paecilomyces spp.		50
Scedosporium prolificans (inflatum)		>18
Scytalidium spp.	<0.1	
Dermatophytes		
Trichophyton spp.	5.6–>100	
Microsporum spp.	1.8	
Epidermophyton spp.	1.47–>100	

Cont.

Table IV.1
Continued

Organism	MIC (µg per ml) range	
	Broth	Agar
Zygomycetes		
Absidia corymbifera		0.39–100
Rhizomucor pusillus		0.1–2.5
Rhizopus arrhizus (oryzae)		0.5–>100
Cunninghamella bertholletiae		12.5–50
Conidiobolus spp.	0.098–0.39	
Basidiobolus spp.	0.098–12.5	
Dematiaceous fungi		
Alternaria alternata	3.2	3.9
Bipolaris spp.	<0.14–2.31	
Cladosporium carrionii		2.5–>32
Curvularia lunata	1.56	
Dactylaria spp.		0.35
Exophiala jeanselmei		6–>32
Exserohilum spp.		<0.14–1.16
Fonsecaea pedrosoi		8–>32
Phialophora spp.		1.56–>100
Wangiella dermatitidis		1–>32
Algae		
Prototheca wickerhamii	0.4	

Table IV.2
Comparative MIC and MFC ranges observed with different formulations of AMB. Compiled and adapted from Hanson (1992).

	AMB-desoxycholate		ABCD	
	MIC µg per ml	MFC µg per ml	MIC µg per ml	MFC µg per ml
Candida albicans	0.5–2.0	1.0–>16	1.0–2.0	1.0–>16
Candida tropicalis	1.0–2.0	8.0	1.0	1.0–8.0
Candida parapsilosis	0.5–2.0	1.0–8.0	1.0	4.0–>16
Candida glabrata	1.0–2.0	1.0–4.0	4.0–8.0	4.0–>16
Cryptococcus neoformans	0.5–4.0	1.0–>16	0.5–1.0	0.5–1.0
Aspergillus fumigatus	2.0	2.0–4.0	4.0–8.0	4.0–8.0
Aspergillus flavus	4.0	4.0–>16	4.0–>16	4.0–>16
Aspergillus niger	1.0	1.0–4.0	1.0–4.0	2.0–4.0
Aspergillus terreus	1.0	16	16	>16
Sporothrix schenckii	2.0	4.0	>16	>16
Rhizopus spp.	2.0	2.0	>16	>16
Blastomyces dermatitidis	0.5	1.0	<0.125–0.5	0.5
Coccidioides immitis	0.5–1.0	2.0–16	0.125–0.25	>16
Histoplasma capsulatum	0.25	0.25–0.5	<0.125	<0.125–0.25
Paracoccidioides brasiliensis	1.0–2.0	1.0–2.0	0.5–1.0	0.5–1.0

of AMB with itraconazole or SCH 39304 were also found to be additive or synergistic in animal models of cryptococcosis (Albert *et al.*, 1991; Van Cutsem *et al.*, 1992). Comparison of animal model data for the combination of azoles and AMB is difficult, because of the different infection models used.

Studies with *N. fowleri* have shown variable results when AMB was combined with miconazole. No synergism was shown in mice infected with amebae isolated from one patient (Stevens *et al.*, 1981) but *in vitro* studies on another strain isolated from a patient did show synergism (Seidel *et al.*, 1982).

Rifampicin (rifampin) is normally inactive against fungi, but acts synergistically with AMB, because the latter increases the fungal cytoplasmic membrane permeability and penetration of rifampicin into the cell (Battaner and Kumar, 1974). Once inside the cell, rifampicin inhibits fungal RNA synthesis most likely by inhibiting ribosomal RNA, rather than inhibition of the DNA-dependent RNA polymerase which occurs in bacteria (Medoff, 1983). A combination of AMB and rifampicin is synergistic *in vitro* against *Aspergillus* spp. (Kitahara *et al.*, 1976a; Hughes *et al.*, 1984a), *Candida* spp. (Edwards *et al.*, 1980), *C. immitis* (Huppert *et al.*, 1976), *C. neoformans* (Fujita and Edwards, 1981), *H. capsulatum* and *B. dermatitidis* (Kobayashi *et al.*, 1974), and *Rhizopus* spp (Christenson *et al.*, 1987). This combination is also more effective than AMB alone for murine infections due to *A. fumigatus* (Arroya *et al.*, 1977), *H. capsulatum* and *B. dermatitidis* (Kitahara *et al.*, 1976b), but not for those due to *C. immitis* (Huppert *et al.*, 1976).

However, in one report, the addition of rifampicin to AMB did not enhance survival of athymic mice infected with *H. capsulatum* and may have even been deleterious, possibly due to an immunosuppressive effect of rifampicin (Williams *et al.*, 1979). Other workers have been unable to confirm the *in vitro* synergism of AMB and rifampicin against *C. albicans* in experimental infections of mice, guinea pigs or neutropenic rabbits (Ernst *et al.*, 1983; Graybill and Ahrens, 1983; Thaler *et al.*, 1988b). In mice infected with *N. fowleri*, AMB and rifamycin act synergistically (Thong *et al.*, 1979). Synergy of AMB and rifampin was demonstrated *in vitro* for the majority of clinical isolates of *Rhizopus* species tested and possible *in vivo* synergy was seen in a diabetic girl with *Rhizopus* pneumonia not responding to AMB alone (Christenson *et al.*, 1987).

Tetracyclines act synergistically with AMB *in vitro* against *H. capsulatum* (Kwan *et al.*, 1972) and this combination is also more effective in murine coccidioidomycosis (Huppert *et al.*, 1974). Both tetracycline and its analog minocycline, also act synergistically with AMB against *N. fowleri in vitro* (Lee *et al.*, 1979); additionally, tetracycline in conjunction with AMB increases the survival rate of mice infected with *N. fowleri* (Thong *et al.*, 1978). Minocycline enhances the activity of AMB against *Candida* spp., *C. glabrata* and *C. neoformans* (Lew *et al.*, 1978) and *Aspergillus* spp. (Hughes *et al.*, 1984b).

Notwithstanding these *in vitro* observations of synergistic effects of AMB and other drugs, drug combinations should be carefully assessed before use in any fungal infection (Medoff and Kobayashi, 1975).

12 Acquired resistance

Apart from odd reports of *Candida* spp. developing resistance to AMB during treatment (Pappagianis *et al.*, 1979), acquired resistance to AMB of usually sensitive fungi has been regarded as an infrequent problem in clinical practice. When chronic *C. albicans* oral infections failed to respond to topical AMB, strains involved were shown to retain sensitivity to the drug and failure was ascribed to various host factors influencing the course of the infection (Holbrook and Kippax, 1979). The failure to detect AMB-resistant strains may be attributable to a lack of routine sensitivity testing, on the premise that yeasts are universally susceptible to AMB (Dick *et al.*, 1980). They examined 1372 yeast strains which were isolated from patients in Baltimore, USA and resistance to AMB (and nystatin) was only detected in three species, *C. albicans, C. tropicalis* and *C. glabrata*. Resistance to these polyenes (7.4% of all 747 fungal strains) was only found in strains isolated from oncology patients. It is possible that long-term therapy with antibiotics and polyenes, the use of cytoxic agents (known mutagens) and the rapid growth of fungi in association with granulocytopenia, may all have contributed to the emergence of resistance.

It is now apparent that acquired resistance to AMB is not as rare as previously thought. Further surveys on usually sensitive fungi are indicated and sensitivity testing is advisable whenever serious fungal infections are not responding as expected to AMB. A strong association between the decreased *in vitro* susceptibility to AMB of *Candida* spp. and subsequent poor clinical outcome has been demonstrated in immunocompromised patients with fungemia. (Powderly *et al.* 1988) A fatal outcome was observed in all patients infected with a yeast isolate with an MIC for AMB >8 μg per ml. In addition, it has been suggested that the NCCLS reference method may not be sensitive enough to detect AMB-resistance in yeasts (Rex *et al.* 1993).

The development of resistance to AMB has been documented in *Cryptococcus neoformans* from an AIDS patient. In the post-treatment isolate in which relative resistance to AMB was seen, a defect in sterol delta 8→7 isomerase was found (Kelly *et al.*, 1994).

13 Tolerance

A phenomenon similar to that which may occur when the penicillins are tested *in vitro* against some bacteria has also been observed with AMB. Seidenfeld *et al.* (1983) showed that although growth of *Candida parapsilosis* was inhibited by concentrations of AMB of < 0.4 μg per ml minimal fungicidal concentrations of AMB were over 32-fold higher. Tolerance was not demonstrated with other *Candida* spp., *C. glabrata* or *C. neoformans* strains which were tested, and the significance of this observation is unknown.

14 Minimum inhibitory concentrations

Table IV.1.shows the MICs of AMB against some selected fungal species. Fungi with MICs of less than 1.0 μg per ml are considered highly sensitive to this drug. Comparative MIC and MFC ranges observed with different formulations of AMB for some selected fungi are shown in Table IV.2.

Mode of Administration and Dosage

1 Intravenous administration

Because AMB is poorly absorbed after oral administration (Louria, 1958) and from i.m. sites, it is given i.v. for the treatment of systemic fungal infections. To avoid side-effects, it is given by slow infusion. Vials of lyophilized powder containing 50 mg AMB are reconstituted by the addition of 10 ml water for injection to produce a concentration of 5 mg per ml. This is then further diluted 1 in 50 with 5% dextrose, to produce a 0.1 mg per ml concentration. Reconstitution with saline or the addition of other antibiotics must be avoided, because precipitation of AMB may result. The addition of heparin, hydrocortisone and sodium bicarbonate does not appear to cause precipitation (Trissel, 1994). For adults, the daily dose is usually dissolved in 1000 ml of 5% dextrose and delivered over 4–6 h. When tolerated, rapid infusion of AMB over 1 h has been used successfully (Tarala and Smith, 1980), but this can rarely cause cardiac arrest. Commercial preparations of 5% dextrose usually have a pH of about 4.2. If the pH is less than 4.2, the dextrose should be suitably buffered before it is used to dilute the concentrated solution of AMB. Infusion of AMB by a central venous catheter enables smaller volumes to be administered and avoids peripheral thrombophlebitis. Since AMB is in the form of a colloid suspension, membrane filters should not be used in the infusion line because they may remove significant amounts of the drug.

There is no general agreement on optimal dosage schedules for i.v. AMB. Doses recommended by the manufacturers are often those which were determined by early investigators and are usually the largest daily doses which patients can tolerate without undue toxicity. Several other regimens have been suggested using lower doses mainly as a result of anecdotal clinical experience. Similarly, there is very little objective data on the optimal duration of therapy for fungal infections. There are many factors which can influence the outcome of therapy with AMB. These include the pathological changes in the host, immune competence of the patient and the effect of AMB on this, vagaries of susceptibility testing of fungi and the sensitivity of the fungus to AMB. These problems and the rationale of various regimens for i.v. AMB have been reviewed (Polak, 1979; Medoff and Kobayashi, 1980).

At the commencement of therapy, it is recommended that a test dose of 0.25–1 mg dissolved in 25–50 ml of 5% dextrose be given over 30–60 min. Earlier recommendations suggested the daily infusion dose should be increased by 5–10mg per day, until the 'optimal' dose is reached. The dose recommended by the manufacturers is 1.0–1.5 mg per kg body weight per day, or 50–100 mg for adults; but a daily dose of 1.5 mg per kg should never be exceeded. Many patients cannot tolerate this dose because of side-effects, and in particular, nephrotoxicity. Some patients may not even tolerate a 1-mg test dose, developing chills, fever and hypotension. An initial dose as low as 0.1 mg may be necessary, which can be gradually increased as tolerance develops (Medoff and Kobayashi, 1980). Slow step-wise increases in dose may delay achievement of therapeutic concentrations, because of the time taken for the drug to equilibrate in the peripheral body compartment. After 4 days of gradually increasing doses, serum levels of AMB would not exceed 0.2 μg per ml for over 14 h of the 24 h day (Atkinson and Bennett, 1978). The recommendation for patients with systemic fungal disease is to administer 0.5–0.6 mg per kg AMB from the onset of therapy, after the initial 1-mg test dose. Others have suggested that AMB should first be given in a test dose of 1–5 mg over 2–6 h and then on each subsequent day the dose can be doubled, until the desired dosage is reached. For seriously ill patients, the following accelerated schedule is recommended: the 1-mg test dose can be followed immediately by 0.25 mg per kg body weight and 0.5 mg per kg can be given on subsequent days (Medoff and Kobayashi, 1980).

The tendency nowadays is to use reduced dose schedules of AMB to avoid toxicity. Current experience indicates that these are just as efficacious as those using maximally tolerated doses. Drutz et al. (1968) advocated that the dosage of AMB should be adjusted in individual patients according to the in vitro sensitivity of the fungus involved. They manipulated the daily i.v. dose to produce, 1 h after infusion, a peak serum level of about twice the MIC for the fungus. Such treatment was given for 10 weeks to each of 15 patients who had cryptococcosis, histoplasmosis or blastomycosis, with satisfactory results and little toxicity. These authors suggested that a daily AMB dose of 1.0 mg per kg may be too large and the total duration of therapy may be the important factor. Medoff and Kobayashi (1980) believe that it is seldom necessary to use more than 0.5 mg per kg per day of AMB. They also point out that very low dose regimens, such as a total dose of 100–200 mg of AMB given over 7–10 days, have been used for some Candida infections (perhaps the drug's non-lethal fungistatic effect at low dosage and its potentiation of the host immune systems may be the basis of its effectiveness in low dosage). Bindschadler and Bennett (1969) considered that alternate day therapy with AMB was better tolerated, and they showed that minimum serum levels of the drug obtained with daily infusion were not significantly different from those when double the recommended dose was given on alternate days. The manufacturers caution that the maximum daily dose of 1.5 mg per kg should not be exceeded in alternate day therapy. A comparatively low dose of 0.5 mg per kg body weight has been used on alternate days (Polak, 1979). Combined therapy with AMB and flucytosine may also allow the use of lower doses of AMB. The duration of therapy for serious fungal infections will vary with the clinical situation. Most patients are given a total dose of 1.5–2.0 g of AMB administered over 6–12 weeks (Medoff and Kobayashi, 1980), but the total dose of the drug used is often determined by nephrotoxicity. Baley et al. (1984) treated ten premature infants with systemic fungal infections by recommended doses of AMB (maximum dose 1.0 mg per kg per day) plus 5-flucytosine (100–150 mg per kg per day). Of these, seven infants developed nephrotoxicity temporally related to the administration of AMB; and six died. These authors recommended limiting the maximum maintenance dose of AMB to 0.5 mg per kg per day in very low birthweight infants.

Solutions of AMB are sensitive to light, but there is no appreciable loss of activity of the drug in a 5% dextrose solution at room temperature and in the presence of conventional fluorescent lighting for periods of 8–24 h (Hoeprich and Huston, 1978).

'AmBisome' is indicated for patients with severe systemic mycoses (including Candida, Aspergillus and Cryptococcus infections). It is administered over 30–60 min, and treatment is instituted at 1 mg per kg per day with stepwise increases to 5 mg per kg per day as required. For disseminated cryptococcal infection in HIV-infected patients, the recommended dose is 3 mg per kg per day for up to 6 weeks. For visceral leishmaniasis in immunocompetent or immunocompromised patients, the recommended dose is 1.0–1.5 mg per kg per day for 21 days. Finally, 'AmBisome' has been licensed for the indication of antifungal prophylaxis in liver transplant recipients, at a dose of 1 mg per kg per day.

'Abelcet' is indicated for the managment of severe systemic fungal infections in patients who have not responded to AMB-desoxycholate, or who have developed intolerance to AMB infusions, or AMB-induced nephrotoxicity. Following an initial test dose of 1.0 mg over 15 min, the recommended dose is 5 mg per kg per day infused over 2 h.

'Amphocil' or 'Amphotec' is indicated for the treatment of severe systemic or deep mycoses particularly aspergillosis in cases where toxicity or renal failure precludes the use of appropriate doses of AMB, and in cases where prior systemic antifungal therapy has failed. Therapy is initiated at 1.0 mg per kg daily, and increased to the recommended dose of 3.0–4.0 mg per kg per day infused over 60–90 min.

2 Patients with renal failure

Renal failure may be caused by AMB in which case the drug may have to be discontinued. In patients with pre-existing renal failure it should be avoided, if possible, because it may aggravate their disease. If AMB therapy is imperative in such patients, it can be administered in the usual dosage. The excretion and serum concentrations of this drug are unaffected by renal failure (Bindschadler and Bennett, 1969). Even in anephric patients, the decline in serum levels of AMB is similar to that in patients with normal renal function. Hemodialysis does not remove AMB (Feldman *et al.*, 1973; Block *et al.*, 1974). Nevertheless, there is a risk of ventricular fibrillation in anuric patients given AMB by rapid infusion.

3 Intrathecal and intraventricular administration

These modes of administration may be used in combination with i.v. therapy for the treatment of coccidioidal meningitis and some cases of candida and cryptococcal meningitis (Medoff and Kobayashi, 1980).

The drug may be injected into the lumbar theca or the cisterna magna. Lumbar theca administration is not appropriate for treatment of ventriculitis as there is poor distribution to the ventricles. For intrathecal administration, AMB is reconstituted with sterile water to produce a concentration of 0.25 mg (250 μg) per ml. An initial dose of 25–50 (μg is given after dilution with 10–20ml of CSF. Usual doses are 0.05–0.25 mg daily or the dose can gradually be increased to 0.5–1.0 mg given two to three times per week. This will be determined by the patient's tolerance, as radicular pain, headache and vomiting commonly occur after administration. A dose of 0.5–1.0 mg up to three times per week is recommended for coccidioidal and cryptococcal meningitis, 0.1–0.5 mg daily for 10 days with systemic therapy for *Candida* intraventricular shunt infections, and 0.05–0.4 mg three times per week with systemic therapy for a *Rhizopus* brain abscess has been used successfully. (Wen *et al.*, 1992). The use of hydrocortisone in doses of 20–50 mg intrathecally have been advocated to reduce the adverse effects during intrathecal administration of AMB (Labadie and Hamilton *et al.*, 1986).

Severe arachnoiditis can follow this procedure. Animal studies suggest that this complication could be minimized if AMB was administered in 10% dextrose in water and the patient was placed in the Trendelenburg position after intrathecal injection (Alazraki *et al.*, 1974). However this method does not avoid arachnoiditis and may cause more neurological complications (Drutz and Catanzaro, 1978). Intrathecally administered AMB is diluted by newly formed CSF and is probably taken up by the arachnoid villi. A 0.3-mg dose produces peak levels of 0.6–0.8 μg per ml which fall to 0.2–0.3 μg per ml after 24 h and the drug is basically undetectable after 48 h.

It is preferable to administer AMB in similar doses intraventricularly, because the drug will distribute well into the lumbar CSF unless there is an obstruction to CSF flow. This is usually done using a subcutaneous Ommaya reservoir when prolonged therapy is required (Diamond and Bennett, 1973; Posner, 1973). If an Ommaya reservoir is *in situ*, specimens of CSF for laboratory tests should be taken by lumbar puncture, because fluid from the reservoir often shows low cell counts and normal protein and glucose values, which do not reflect the findings in the lumbar CSF (Goldstein *et al.*, 1972; Holt *et al.*, 1972).

Complications are associated with the administration of AMB into the lateral ventricle by means of these prostheses, such as ventricular hemorrhage, obstruction or bacterial infection (Diamond and Bennett, 1973). In one report of persistent cryptococcal meningitis despite 4 months treatment, the infection resolved after a Rickham reservoir was removed, suggesting that it was the cause of persistent cryptococcal infection (Schonheyder *et al.*, 1980). In two patients receiving 0.5 mg AMB intraventricularly by means of an Ommaya reservoir, mean ventricular concentrations of the drug taken via the reservoir after flushing were 1.7, 0.24 and 0–16 μg per ml at 4, 24 and 48 h, respectively. Simultaneous lumbar concentrations were lower, but still detectable after 48 h (Craven *et al.*, 1983).

4 Intraperitoneal administration

For the purpose of either treatment or prevention of *Candida* infection during peritoneal dialysis, AMB can be added to peritoneal dialysis fluid. The recommended dose is 1.0 mg added to 1000 ml of dialysis fluid (a concentration of 1.0 μg per ml), although concentrations of 2–4 μg per ml have been used safely (Bayer *et al.*, 1976b). After a test dose of 10 mg, a dose of 25 mg AMB in 250 ml 5% dextrose containing 25 mg hydrocortisone, delivered intraperitoneally every 48 h, has been used to treat fungal peritonitis. With this dosage, AMB seemed to accumulate in peritoneal fluid with pre-dose trough levels rising from 1.6 to 2.2 μg per ml to peak levels 4 h after infusion of 2.5–3.6 μg per ml. Simultaneous serum levels of AMB were 15–33% of the peritoneal levels, but the pharmacokinetics in the patient studied may have been influenced by the presence of ascites (Rahko *et al.*, 1983). Chemical peritonitis following intraperitoneal administration of AMB at a concentration of 2.5 mg per liter has been reported (Coronel *et al.*, 1993)

5 Bladder instillation or irrigation

Wise *et al.* (1973,1982) treated patients with *Candida* bladder infections by daily instillations of sterile water containing AMB in a concentration of 50 μg per ml, via continuous flow (42 ml per h) through a triple lumen indwelling urethral catheter, for a mean of 5 days. No evidence of drug toxicity was observed, and treatment was stopped when the urine was clear of microscopic *Candida* organisms. Eradication of candiduria occurs in 80–93% of patients (Wise *et al.*, 1982; Jacobs *et al.*, 1994), and was similar for those with and without indwelling catheters. In contrast, other investigators have suggested that concentrations as low as 10 μg per ml should suffice for infection confined to the bladder (Fisher *et al.*, 1982). Fong *et al.*, (1991) evaluated the fungicidal activity of AMB in urine and found a correlation between the rapidity and completeness of killing and increasing concentration of AMB. At 5 μg per ml, complete killing was seen after 4 h. Complete killing was achieved after 2 h with AMB concentrations greater than 100 μg per ml. The current recommendation is to instil 200–300 ml of 5–10 mg per liter AMB solution by a triple lumen urethral catheter with cross-clamping for 60–90 min at regular intervals. This irrigation technique should be used for no longer than 2 days (Sanford,1993).

6 Intra-articular administration

This may sometimes be indicated for the treatment of coccidioidal arthritis, articular sporotrichosis or mycetoma. Doses of 5–15 mg have been injected into joint spaces.

7 Aerosol administration

This mode of administration has been proposed for chemoprophylaxis of pulmonary aspergillosis in neutropenic patients. An efficient nebulizer and good technique would mean nebulized AMB could reach the distal airways and sinuses in sufficient concentrations to inhibit growth of the *Aspergillus* spores. Studies in the rat model reveal mean concentrations in lung tissue of 2.79 μg per g after a single aerosol dose of 1.6 mg per kg of AMB and 9.88 μg per g after 4 doses. The aerosol route was more efficient than intraperitoneal administration of drug for delivery of AMB to the lungs in the rat. The drug was undetectable in serum, liver, kidney and brain. The elimination half-life of AMB from the lungs was 4.8 days (Niki *et al.*,1990). For inhalation, 10 mg of AMB preparation for intravenous use is diluted in sterile water to a total volume of 5 ml and nebulized with the 'Respirgard' II nebulizer for 15–20 min twice-daily (Beyer *et al.*, 1993). This regimen was used in bone marrow transplant patients during the neutropenic phase to prevent invasive aspergillosis in an uncontrolled study, so efficacy could not be assessed (Beyer *et al.*, 1993). Side-effects of the AMB inhalations included unpleasant taste, nausea and vomiting, and were more severe in patients with severe mucositis. In addition, clinically significant bronchospasm, increase in cough and dyspnea was described in several patients in one series (Dubois *et al.*, 1995).

8 Intracavitary administration

Pulmonary aspergilloma, which often form in pre-existing fibrotic lung cavities, are often difficult to control with systemic treatment and surgery is associated with significant morbidity and mortality. A catheter can be placed in the cavity and 50 mg AMB instilled into the cavity each day, followed 12 h later with instillation of N-acetylcysteine and overnight continuous low pressure suction. A total of 500–800 mg AMB has been used primarily to control hemoptysis in these patients (Cochrane *et al.*, 1991). An alternative method of intracavitary administration of AMB was described by Munk *et al.* (1993) as a substitute for repeated injections. They prepared an AMB gelatin mixture by dissolving 6 g of oxoid laboratory standard gelatin in 8.5 ml of sterile water using a hot water bath at 40°C. Immediately before injection, 15 mg AMB was then dissolved in this mixture and drawn up in a syringe that had been warmed in the hot water bath. A needle was placed in the mycetoma cavity under computed tomographic or fluoroscopic guidance and the viscous mixture injected rapidly as it solidifies quickly. This single administration resulted in complete resolution of three out of four pulmonary aspergillomas within 3 months, with no evidence of recurrence at 6–18 months (Munk *et al.*, 1993).

9 Topical therapy

Amphotericin B is available as a lotion, cream and ointment for the treatment of cutaneous candidal infections and as lozenges for the treatment of oral candidiasis. Tablets and a suspension are also available for oral administration to treat gastrointestinal candidiasis.

For otic administration AMB is prepared by adding water for injection to AMB parenteral preparation to make a concentration of 0.25%, and administered at a dose of one to two drops three times daily. This was prescribed for *Aspergillus fumigatus* otitis externa in an HIV-infected patient, with resolution in 2–3 weeks (Kintzel *et al.*, 1994).

10 Intralesional infiltration

Iwatsu (1988) reported that intralesional AMB administration was effective for the treatment of cutaneous alternariosis. Amphotericin B 50 mg was dissolved in 10 ml distilled water, and then diluted with 4 volumes of 0.5% procaine hydrochloride (final AMB concentration 1 mg per ml). One ml of procaine-AMB solution was then injected into the lesion twice-weekly for 10 injections. After each injection a painful local reaction with erythema and edema was noted.

Availability

1   Amphotericin B ('Fungizone', Bristol-Myers Squibb Pharmaceuticals Pty Ltd; Apothecon).
Vials containing lyophilized powder, providing 50 mg amphotericin B and 41 mg sodium desoxycholate and 20.2 mg sodium phosphate as a buffer, which is ready for reconstitution in 10 ml sterile water for injection.

2. Amphotericin B ('Fungilin', Bristol-Myers Squibb Pharmaceuticals Pty Ltd).

a   *Lozenges*: 10 mg.
b   *Oral suspension*: 100 mg per ml.
c   *Lotion, cream and ointment*: 3%.

3   Liposomal amphotericin B ('AmBisome', Nexstar).
Vials containing amphotericin B 50 mg encapsulated in the biolayer of liposomes consisting of approximately 213 mg hydrogenated soy phosphatidylcholine, 52 mg cholesterol, 84 mg distearoylphosphatidylglycerol, 0.64 mg alpha tocopherol plus 900 mg sucrose and 27 mg sodium succinate hexahydrate.

4   Amphotericin B lipid complex (ABLC; 'Abelcet', Liposome Company).
Vials (20 ml), each ml containing amphotericin B 5.0 mg.
L-alpha-dimyristoylphosphatidylcholine(DMPC) 3.4 mg.
L-alpha-dimysistoylphosphatidylglycerol (DMPG) 1.5 mg, and sodium chloride 9.0 mg.

5   Amphotericin B colloidal dispersion (ABCD; 'Amphocil', Sequus Pharmaceuticals) also known as Amphotericin B cholesteryl sulfate complex ('Amphotec', Sequus Pharmaceuticals).
Vials of lyophilized product providing 5 mg per ml of AMB.
A 10 ml vial contains AMB 50 mg, sodium cholesteryl sulfate 26.4 mg, tromethemine 5.64 mg, disodium edetate dihydrate 0.372 mg, and lactose monohydrate 950 mg.

Serum Levels in Relation to Dosage

If an AMB dose of 0.65 mg per kg is given by i.v. infusion over a period of 4–6 h, a peak serum level (C_{max}) of 1.8–3.5 μg per ml is reached during the first hour after infusion (Louria, 1958). This level is maintained for 6–8 h, and then gradually falls to about half the peak level 20 h after the infusion. Trough levels are generally 0.2–0.5 μg per ml (Christianson *et al.*,1985). The drug does not accumulate in the serum if this dose is used daily (Bindschadler and Bennett, 1969). Alternate day doses of 25–105 mg result in serum concentrations of 1.0–2.4 μg per ml AMB, and the serum concentrations are not influenced by alternate day dosing (Bindschadler and Bennett, 1969). Dose proportionality exists up to doses of 50 mg, after which serum concentrations are lower than predicted on the basis of linearity (Daneshmend *et al.*, 1983).

After an AMB infusion, there is a rapid initial elimination of the drug (half-life 24–48 h) and a slow elimination half life of 15 days. A three-compartment pharmacokinetic model has been suggested by Atkinson and Bennett (1978) – a central compartment and rapidly and slowly equilibrating peripheral compartments of the body. They postulated that the central compartment is likely to be the total blood volume, and the rapidly equilibrating peripheral compartment is probably the extravascular compartment consisting of interstitial fluid of tissues with discontinuous capillaries such as liver, spleen and intestine. The slowly equilibrating peripheral extravascular compartment probably consists of the interstitial fluid of tissues with continuous capillaries, such as skeletal muscle and skin. After a course of AMB, the drug disappears from the serum and urine very slowly (3–7 weeks). The AMB blood levels are not influenced by renal or hepatic failure (Daneshmend and Warnock,1983), and hemodialysis does not reduce blood levels. Clearance of AMB was measured at 3–5% of the creatinine clearance in four patients receiving AMB and requiring hemodialysis (Block *et al.*, 1974). The mean serum concentration of AMB may be higher 1 h after the rapid infusion of AMB (45 min) but are no different at 18 and 42 h post-infusion when compared with the 4–6 h infusion times (Fields *et al.*,1971).

Pregnancy does not appear to affect the pharmacokinetics of AMB. The mean peak and trough concentrations of AMB (2.60 µg per ml and 0.32 µg per ml, respectively) were similar in a group of pregnant women compared with a group of non-pregnant women. The increased glomerular filtration rate (GFR) seen in pregnancy does not appear to increase elimination of AMB (McCoy *et al.*, 1980).

In children aged between 4 months and 14 years, a marked variation in peak serum AMB concentrations of 0.78–10.02 µg per ml was measured after doses ranging from 0.25–1.0 mg per kg. The peak serum AMB concentration was 2.9 ± 2.8 µg per ml, and the mean total clearance, volume of distribution, and elimination half-life were 0.46 ± 0.20 ml per min per kg, 0.76 ± 0.52 liters per kg, and 18.1 ± 6.6 h. There was no correlation between AMB dose on a mg per kg basis, infusion rate, patient age and peak serum concentration. Total clearance of AMB was inversely proportional to age, with decreasing AMB clearance with increasing age. No increased toxicity was observed in the older age group (Benson and Nahata,1989). Serum concentrations in a premature infant given AMB in doses of 0.5 mg per kg per day and 1.0 mg per kg on alternate days were similar to those obtained in older patients given the same dosage (Ward *et al.*, 1983).

Absorption of AMB from the gastrointestinal tract is poor. If large oral doses of 1.6–5.0 g per day are administered to adults, serum levels ranging from 0.04 to 0.05 µg per ml have been measured (Louria, 1958). However, up to 9% of AMB in a dose of 10 mg four times per day was absorbed in cancer patients (Ching *et al.*,1983). When AMB is used orally in doses of 2–5 g daily for decontamination of the gastrointestinal tract, the serum concentrations remain below 0.5 µg per ml (Janknegt *et al.*, 1992).

Excretion

1 Urine

Only 2–5% of a total daily dose of AMB is excreted in the urine as the active drug within 24 h of administration (Atkinson and Bennett, 1978). It is thought that excretion of AMB in the urine occurs by glomerular filtration. Excretion is restricted by the high level of protein binding (>90%). Pre-existing renal dysfunction has no effect on AMB excretion (Bindschadler and Bennett, 1969) with the total clearance of AMB in individuals with impaired renal function measured at 17–40 ml per min (Janknegt *et al.*, 1992). Dose reduction is not required for patients with renal dysfunction, as far as serum levels of AMB is concerned, however, due consideration to AMB-induced nephrotoxicity is warranted. No data are available on the pharmacokinetics and tissue accumulation following long-term administration of AMB in patients with renal impairment.

2 Bile

In monkeys (Lawrence *et al.*, 1980) and in dogs (Craven *et al.*, 1979), AMB is excreted in the bile. In the dog it accounts for <20% of the total excretion of the drug. The median concentration of AMB in bile of autopsied cancer patients who had received AMB-desoxycholate up to 72 h prior to death was 7.3 µg per ml and was estimated to be from 0.8–14.6% of the daily dose of AMB. This confirms that biliary excretion contributes to AMB elimination up to 15% of the daily dose (Collette *et al.*,1989).

3 Inactivation in the body

The metabolic fate of the major portion of an administered dose of AMB is unknown. No metabolites have been identified in human or animal studies. Some of the drug is stored in the body, because after treatment is stopped, serum concentrations continue to fall slowly over several weeks. In one study AMB was still detectable in liver, spleen and kidney as long as 1 year after completion of therapy (Benson and Nahata, 1988).

Distribution of the Drug in Body

The estimated volume of distribution of AMB is 4 liters per kg. It is highly protein bound in serum particularly to beta-lipoproteins (Brajtburg *et al.*, 1984). The mean protein binding is 91–95% (Daneshmend and Warnock,1983).

Tissue concentrations of AMB have been measured by high-performance liquid chromotography (HPLC) in two autopsy studies of cancer patients who had received known total doses of

AMB-desoxycholate for invasive fungal infections. Higher concentrations were recovered from liver and spleen compared with lungs and kidneys. The range of recovery as a percentage of the total dose of AMB received was 27.5%(17.5–40%) for the liver, 5.2%(1–14%) for spleen, 3.2%(0.4–13%) for lungs, 1.5%(0.6–4%) for kidneys and <1% for pancreas, heart, muscle, brain, fat, esophagus and thyroid (Collette *et al.*, 1989). The range of recovery of AMB from tissues was remarkably consistent across studies, measured at 15.8–50.8% of the total dose administered in one study (Christiansen *et al.* 1985) and 23–51.3% in another (Collette *et al.*, 1989). It is apparent that the liver is the major site of storage of AMB, with suggested reversible binding to cholesterol in the cell membranes. Only a small proportion of AMB is bioavailable in tissues despite high tissue concentrations. The measured amount of bioactive AMB was only 20–40% of the extractable drug as measured by HPLC. This bioactivity increased to 60–80% when the bioassay was performed on methanolic extracts, suggesting that the AMB is strongly bound to cholesterol in the cell membranes (Collette *et al.* 1989). Neither study was able to demonstrate any metabolism of AMB. A third autopsy study compared the tissue distribution of AMB following administration entrapped in small liposomes (ampholiposomes, not commercially available) or AMB complexed with desoxycholate, and found no detectable alteration in the tissue distribution despite considerable differences in pharmacokinetics (Collette *et al.*, 1991).

After i.v. infusion, concentrations of AMB in body fluids are low compared with serum levels. In patients with uninflamed meninges CSF levels are 30- to 50-fold lower than simultaneous serum levels (Louria, 1958). In seven patients with cryptococcal meningitis studied by Utz *et al.* (1975), the drug was not detected in the CSF of four patients and was less than 10% of the serum values in the other three patients. In neonates, the CSF concentrations of AMB were 40–90% of the corresponding serum concentration, compared with the 2–4% of serum levels observed in adults (Benson and Nahata, 1988). Meningeal AMB levels may be higher than corresponding CSF levels according to animal data (Perfect and Durack,1985). In peritoneal, pleural and joint fluids less than 50% of serum levels are achieved (Polak, 1979). Bindschadler and Bennett (1969) using a microbiological assay demonstrated a pleural fluid concentration of $1.0 \,\mu g$ per ml in one patient, whose simultaneous serum level was $1.8 \,\mu g$ per ml. Using HPLC, others have also shown good penetration of pleural fluid with levels of $0.7–1.04 \,\mu g$ per ml achieved continuously over 24 h following daily i.v. dosing of 70 mg AMB (Kutty and Neicheril, 1987). It is known that AMB crosses the placenta producing levels in cord blood and amniotic fluid which are lower than maternal serum levels (Ismail and Lerner, 1982). Dean *et al.* (1994) measured AMB levels in cord serum, infant serum and placental tissue at delivery, 30 days after the last dose of AMB was administered and found similar levels of $0.20–0.24 \,\mu g$ per ml in all three sites. This means significant AMB tissue concentrations persist for over 30 days following completion of therapy. A level of less than $0.5 \,\mu g$ per ml was detected in human aqueous humor when the serum level was $0.6 \,\mu g$ per ml after i.v. administration of 0.8 mg per kg body weight (Richards *et al.*, 1969). Lower levels of AMB were found in the aqueous and vitreous humors of two patients with orbital zygomycosis after i.v. administration. The amount of penetration of the drug may be related to the degree of eye inflammation (Fisher *et al.*, 1983). In dogs, the drug penetrates into bronchial secretions poorly (Pennington *et al.*, 1974).

The pharmacokinetics of the lipid complexes of AMB are complicated by the fact that most assays do not distinguish between the free AMB concentrations and the lipid-complexed or protein-bound AMB, making interpretation of serum and tissue levels of the drug problematic. There is only limited information on the serum and tissue concentrations following administration of the different formulations of AMB, and there are no data concerning the concentration of AMB complexed to lipid or liposome-encapsulated, AMB bound to protein and free AMB, to enable an understanding of the therapeutic and toxic effects of these agents in comparison with AMB-desoxycholate.

Amphotericin B lipid complex (ABLC) is derived from the first liposomal preparation of AMB developed by Lopez-Berestein and contains a 7:3 molar ratio of dimyristoyl phosphatidylcholine and dimyristoyl phosphatidylglycerol, but the ratio of AMB:lipid is much higher in ABLC. The concentration of AMB is 33 mol% (Janknegt *et al.*, 1992). Because of its large size, ABLC is rapidly removed by the reticuloendotheliel system, resulting in significantly lower blood levels than AMB-desoxycholate, and a corresponding large volume of distribution and small area-under-the-concentration-time-curve (AUC). A single-dose pharmacokinetic study in healthy male volunteers compared low doses of AMB-desoxycholate and ABLC. At 0.25 mg per kg, the C_{max} of AMB following ABLC administration was $0.2 \,\mu g$ per ml – only 20% of the corresponding C_{max} for AMB-desoxycholate of $0.98 \,\mu g$ per ml. The elimination half-life was 26.9 h for ABLC and 50 h for AMB-desoxycholate, and the volume of distribution and clearance were greater for ABLC than AMB-desoxycholate (Kan *et al.*, 1991).

Liposomal AMB is a liposomal formulation of AMB with a concentration of 50 mg AMB/350 mg lipid. This corresponds to a concentration of 10 mol% (Janknegt *et al.*, 1992). Pharmacokinetic data for liposomal AMB is limited. Peak serum AMB concentrations of 6.0 μg per ml and 12.6 μg per ml were measured after administration of 50-mg and 80-mg doses of liposomal AMB respectively in heart transplant patients (Katz *et al.*, 1990). Trough serum concentrations at 24 h were 1.7 μg per ml and 2.3 μg per ml. The higher serum levels of total AMB than those predicted for an equivalent dose of AMB-desoxycholate were confirmed by Tollemar *et al.* (1990) who measured C_{max} of 2.2–20.3 μg per ml and trough concentrations of 0.36–1.07 μg per ml following doses of liposomal AMB ranging from 0.9 to 2.5 mg per kg. Autopsy examination of tissue concentrations of AMB following a total dose of 900–3428 mg liposomal AMB revealed 14–23% of the administered dose was recovered from the liver, 1–6% from the spleen and less than 1% recovered from lung and kidney (Tollemar *et al.*, 1990). In mice, an equivalent dose comparison study of the pharmacokinetics of liposomal AMB and AMB-desoxycholate revealed a C_{max} of 8 μg per ml and 1.5 μg per ml respectively following a 1 mg per kg dose. The higher serum concentrations of AMB also disappeared more slowly, with the first- and second-phase half-lifes of 1.6 and 17 h for liposomal AMB and 0.5 and 11 h for AMB-desoxycholate. Tissue concentrations

Table IV.3

Characteristics of each of the commercially available lipid formulations of AMB, and their relevant pharmacokinetics. Adapted from De Marie *et al.* (1994), and compiled from data from Amphotericin B lipid complex ('Abelcet') Product Information, Kan *et al.* (1991), Janknegt *et al.* (1992), Hay (1994), De Marie *et al.* (1994), Amantea *et al.* (1995).

	AMB_{DOC} Amphotericin B-desoxycholate 'Fungizone'	ABLC Amphotericin B-lipid complex 'Abelcet'	Liposomal AMB Amphotericin B-liposome 'AmBisome'	ABCD Amphotericin B-colloidal dispersion 'Amphocil' 'Amphotec'
Manufacturer	Bristol-Myers Squibb	The Liposome Company	Nexstar	Sequus Pharmaceuticals
Lipids	Desoxycholate	DMPC/DMPG	HPC/Chol/DSPG	Cholesteryl sulphate
Mol % AMB	34	35	10	50
Size (μm)	<0.4	1.6–11	0.08	0.12
Target dose (mg per kg)	0.5–1.5	1–4	1–4	1–5
C_{max} compared with 'Fungizone'	equivalent	lower 20%	higher	lower
Dose (mg per kg)	0.25	5	5	4
C_{max} (μg per ml)	0.98	1.7	35.9	2.8
AUC (μg . min per ml)	8.67	9.5	523	10.5
Clearance (ml. kg per h)	10	211	960 ml per min	112
Half-life (h) second phase	50.0	173.4	32	29.8
Distribution	Liver, spleen lung, kidney	RES spleen, liver, lung	RES liver, spleen lung kidney	Liver

DMPC: Dimyristoylphosphatidyl choline; DMPG: dimyristoylphosphatidyl glycerol; HPC: hydrogenated phosphatidyl choline; Chol: cholesterol; DSPG: distearoylphosphatidyl glycerol; C_{max}: peak serum concentration; total AMB levels measured, therefore cannot distinguish between circulating lipid-complexed AMB and free AMB; RES: reticuloendotheliel system.

of AMB revealed higher liver and spleen levels, but comparable lung and kidney concentrations for the liposomal AMB'-treated animals (Gondal *et al.*, 1989).

Amphotericin B-colloidal dispersion is a complex of AMB and cholesteryl sulfate in a 1:1 molar ratio. When AMB is administered as ABCD in a single dose to the rat, nearly 100% of AMB was recovered from the rat liver 30 min after dosing. In addition, pharmacokinetic studies in dogs and rats showed reduced peak plasma levels of AMB and reduced delivery to the major target organ for toxicity, the kidney, was observed. The rapid and extensive hepatic uptake of AMB when administered as ABCD suggests that the liver may act as a reservoir for AMB. There was no evidence of increased toxicity in the reticuloendothelial system (Fielding *et al.*, 1991, 1992). Single dose pharmacokinetics in healthy male volunteers in doses of 0.25–1.5 mg per kg revealed dose linearity for the C_{max} and AUC. The total clearance remained constant and the third-phase half-life, but not the first- and second-phase half-lives, increased with higher doses (Sanders *et al.*, 1991). Multiple-dose pharmacokinetic analysis of escalating doses of ABCD was performed in patients undergoing bone marrow transplantion. The pharmacokinetics were best described by a two-compartment model, with an initial rapid decline with distribution to rapidly equilibrating tissues, followed by a prolonged terminal phase. Both the plasma clearance and the volume of distribution increased with increasing doses of ABCD, suggesting a saturable binding site in the central volume compartment.

Finally, some investigators have suggested that delivery of AMB-desoxycholate in fat emulsion prepared commercially for parenteral nutrition ('Intralipid' 20%) reduces the toxicity without impairing efficacy associated with AMB-desoxycholate dissolved in 5% dextrose, and reduces

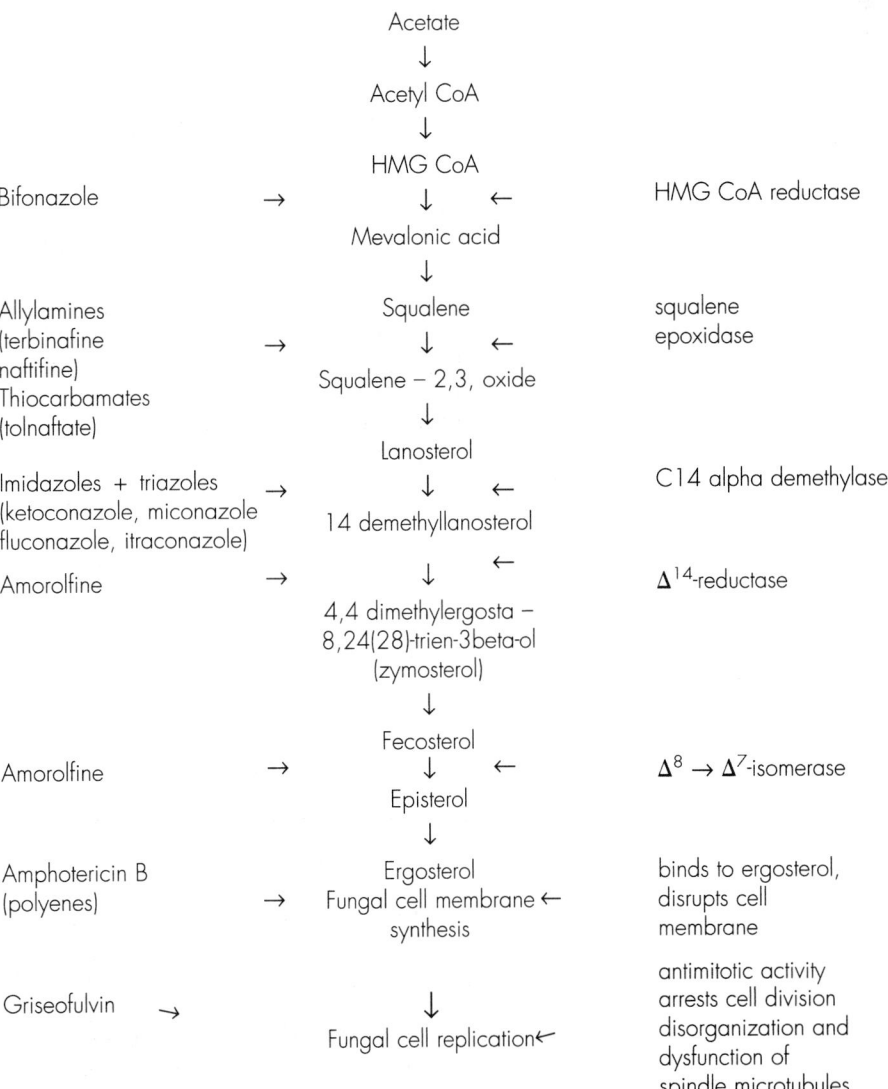

Fig. IV.1.
Mechanism of action of antifungal drugs. This figure is referred to throughout Section IV. (Modified from Gupta *et al.*, 1994, with permission.)

cost compared with liposomal preparations. Kirsch *et al.* (1988) initally demonstrated equipotency of the fat emulsion and dextrose delivery systems for the treatment of murine systemic candidiasis. The AMB-fat emulsion treatment was associated with reduced nephrotoxicity and red cell toxicity. Caillot *et al.* (1994) performed a controlled trial comparing AMB-desoxycholate infused in 'Intralipid' or dextrose in patients with hematological malignancies and neutropenic fever or documented fungal infection. They demonstrated a modification in pharmacokinetics of AMB by infusion in fat emulsion. Peak serum concentrations of AMB were lower and the trough concentrations were significantly lower in the group receiving AMB in 'Intralipid'. Significant reductions in peak (50%) and trough AMB concentrations and AUC, as well as increased volume of distribution and total clearance of AMB when infused in 20% 'Intralipid' were confirmed in a study of HIV-infected patients and neutropenic patients (Chavenet *et al.*, 1992; Heinemann *et al.*, 1995; Ayestaran *et al.*, 1996). These studies showed a significant reduction in toxicity for AMB delivered in a fat emulsion. Washington *et al.* (1993) have stressed the importance of AMB associated with the oil droplets in the emulsion for efficacy and have suggested that >95% AMB precipitates, but is still taken up by the reticuloendotheliel system.

Mode of Action

There appears to be at least two effects of AMB on fungal cytopalsmic membranes. The first is the insertion of AMB into the fungal cytoplasmic membrane and the formation of aggregates bound closely to sterols such as ergosterol. This causes depolarization of the membrane and an increase in the cytoplasmic membrane permeability to protons and monovalent cations (Fig. IV.1). At low AMB concentrations the potassium channel activity is increased, resulting in reversible fungistatic activity (Hsu,1993). At higher AMB concentrations 40–105 nm pores are formed in the cytoplasmic membrane disrupting the osmotic integrity with leakage of intracellular potassium and other molecules. This impairs fungal viability. Brajtburg *et al.* (1990a) have proposed that the effects of AMB can be divided into three separate dose-dependent stages: stimulation, permeabilization and lethality. Stimulatory effects on cells of the immune system were seen at concentrations of AMB below those required for changes in permeability, and lethality occurred at AMB concentrations higher than those required to induce changes in cell permeability. Lethality of fungal cells is not due to changes in cell permeability alone.

The second effect of AMB is fungal cell damage caused by AMB auto-oxidation whch is probably the major cause of cell death. Auto-oxidation of AMB bound to membrane components results in formation of free radicals. Cell injury induced by AMB can be modified by extracellular catalase, hypoxia or pro-oxidants such as ascorbic acid (Brajtburg *et al.*,1989, Brajtburg *et al.*, 1990a). In addition, AMB may potentiate the antifungal effect of 5–fluorocytosine and other drugs, by facilitating their penetration through the fungal cytoplasmic membrane (Kwan *et al.*, 1972).

The plasma membrane of the mammalian cell also contains sterols, mainly cholesterol, while the fungal plasma membrane contains mainly ergosterol (Gale, 1973). Mammalian cells are less susceptible than yeast cells to AMB because the drug has a higher affinity for ergosterol than cholesterol (Kotler-Brajtburg *et al.*, 1974). Most of the toxic effects of AMB in humans are probably caused by similar actions on human cell cytoplasmic membranes (HsuChen and Feingold, 1973). For instance, human red blood cells can be destroyed by AMB *in vitro*, because the drug binds to sterol groups on the surface of erythrocytes (Carter and McCarthy, 1966) and AMB-induced hemolysis involves oxidative cell damage (Brajtburg *et al.* 1985). AMB can injure human neutrophils *in vitro*, by a similar mechanism (Supapidhayakul *et al.*, 1981). The lethal AMB-induced cell injury appeared to be associated with both ion movement and oxidative effects in experiments in isolated perfused rat kidneys (Brezis *et al.*, 1984). The toxic and therapeutic effects of AMB are contingent on competitive interactions between sterol-containing cell membranes of the host and the parasite and components of blood, such as lipoproteins and proteins (Brajtburg *et al.*, 1984).

To gain access to the ergosterol in the fungal cytoplasmic cell membrane, AMB must traverse the rigid cell wall which is composed of beta-1,3-glucans and chitin. The contribution, if any, of the beta-1,3-glucans in inhibiting access to ergosterol as a cause of AMB resistance is not known (Gale, 1986). Most AMB-resistant fungi have either quantitative or qualitative alterations in the sterol composition of the cytoplasmic membrane, some with reduced and some with increased ergosterol content (Woods *et al.*, 1974; Athar and Winner 1971; Hamilton-Miller 1972; Kim *et al.*, 1975). The type and quantity of sterols in the fungal cell membrane will determine the level of interaction of AMB with the cytoplasmic membrane. HsuChen and Feingold (1974) reported two forms of resistance in *C. albicans*. One resisted both the AMB-induced increased permeability and leakage of intracellular contents and killing (type 1) and the other resisted only the AMB-induced killing (type 2). They proposed that type 1 resistance was associated with a decreased interaction between AMB and the cytoplasmic membrane; and that in type 2 resistance the AMB interacted with the cell membrane but the critical step resulting in lethality failed to occur (HsuChen and Feingold,1974). The development of resistance to oxidative-dependant cell damage is probably the second mehanism of resistance to AMB. The susceptibility of *C. albicans* to AMB-induced killing is also linked to cellular catalase levels (Sokol-Anderson *et al.* 1988).

Toxicity

1 Infusion-related adverse events

These include headache, fever, chills, malaise, muscle and joint pain, nausea, vomiting and hypotension, and occur in 50–90% of patients receiving infusions over 4–6 h. Hyperthermia (temperature >40°C) may be marked (Bennett, 1974). It has been shown by *in vitro* studies of AMB suspensions at a concentration of 1.0 μg per ml, that the mechanism responsible for the chills and fever is the induction of prostaglandin E_2 synthesis by mononuclear cells. A placebo-controlled trial of ibuprofen, a potent inhibitor of prostaglandin synthesis, demonstrated a reduction in the incidence and severity of chill reactions associated with AMB infusions, from 69% to 15% (Gigliotti *et al.*, 1987). Antipyretic, antiemetic and antihistamine drugs can be used to provide some symptomatic relief, as can the addition of hydrocortisone to the infusion solution for reduction in febrile reactions (Maddux and Barriere, 1980). Tynes *et al.* (1963) were able to demonstrate a statistically significant reduction in chills, fever and vomiting in individuals given 25 mg hydrocortisone as a premedication. There was no increased benefit observed when 50 mg hydrocortisone was used. In a prospective multicenter surveillance study of adverse effects experienced in the first 7 days of AMB therapy, infusion-related adverse effects were experienced by 71% (282 of 397) of patients. This study also compared the incidence of infusion-related adverse effects associated with different pretreatment regimens aimed at preventing these side-effects. These regimens most commonly included acetaminophen, diphenhydramine, corticosteroid and heparin, and were similar to no pretreatment for the prevention of infusion-related adverse effects (Goodwin *et al.*, 1995).

Several investigators have examined the effect of infusion rates of AMB on the incidence and severity of AMB toxicity in small studies (Cruz *et al.*, 1992; Ellis *et al.*, 1992; Oldfield *et al.*, 1990). Rapid infusions (45 min to 1 h) were evaluated for safety in individuals with no evidence of renal impairment. Oldfield and colleagues (1990) found no difference in the overall incidence in side-effects between the !-h and 4-h infusions of AMB when maintenance doses of 0.3–0.5 mg per kg per day had already been reached. In another study of the entire incremental dosing period and maintenance dosing, rapid infusions were not associated with any increased toxicity than the conventional 4-h infusions (Cruz *et al.*, 1992). Ellis *et al.* (1992) found a greater incidence and severity of infusional reactions in the 45-min infusion group compared with a group who received a 4-h infusion, but they found that tolerance to toxicity developed in the first 5–7 days of treatment, so that the incidence and severity of side-effects were similar by day 7. Finally, Nicholl *et al.* (1995) demonstrated that patients with leukemia or undergoing bone marrow transplant without evidence of renal and cardiac dysfunction, tolerated a 2-h infusion equally as well as a 4-h infusion, with no statistical significance between the rate of infusion-related adverse events. Generally these studies have enrolled small numbers of patients and excluded those patients at increased risk of adverse reactions. It would be advisable to avoid rapid infusions in those with cardiovascular or renal disease, especially in the first week after initiation of therapy.

Thrombophlebitis is a common problem, and occurred in 5% patients observed for the first 7 days only, in a multicenter surveillance study (Goodwin *et al.*, 1995). Recommendations made to minimize the thrombophlebitic reaction include the rotation of infusion sites, avoidance of tissue infiltration of the AMB solution, use of a central venous catheter and avoidance of infusion times of less than 4 h. A tendency for peripheral vein thrombosis has been observed if concentrations of AMB greater than 0.1 mg per ml are infused (Tarala and Smith, 1980). The addition of heparin at a dose of 500–1000 units/liter is also recommended to reduce thrombophlebitis. However, there are no controlled data to support this strategy. In the surveillance study performed by Goodwin *et al.* (1995) there was no reduction in the incidence of thrombophlebitis in those patients who had heparin added to AMB infusion.

The liposomal preparations of AMB are also associated with acute infusional toxicity, albeit to a lesser degree. In a phase I study using doses up to 1.5 mg per kg of ABCD, acute adverse reactions were reasonably frequent – nausea (53%), headache (46%), thrombophlebitis (35%), vomiting (20%) and chills (20%) (Sanders *et al.*, 1991). Mild somnolence was reported in 75%

of healthy volunteers who received 0.5 mg per kg ABLC in a phase I study (Kan *et al.*, 1991). Acute infusional toxicity was experienced by 68% of bone marrow transplant patients with invasive fungal infections, who were enrolled in a phase I study of escalating doses of ABCD from 0.5–8 mg per kg per day. The maximum tolerated dose was 7.5 mg per kg (Bowden *et al.*, 1996). When AMB is diluted in 'Intralipid' 20% to a concentration of 1 g per liter and administered over 8 h, the infusion is well tolerated. However, when the concentration was increased to 2 g per liter and infused over 2 h, acute infusional toxicity was observed in neutropenic patients with proven candidemia (Caillot *et al.*, 1993).

2 Nephrotoxicity

This is the most important side-effect of parenteral AMB. Some impairment of renal function occurs in almost all patients treated. The GFR falls by about 40% soon after commencing therapy in nearly all patients. After repeated doses, it frequently stabilizes at 20–60% of normal, where it stays throughout the course of therapy (Medoff and Kobayashi, 1980). Nephrotoxicity results in rises in levels of the blood urea and serum creatinine, and the appearance of red and white cells, albumin and casts in the urine. If the patient's GFR deteriorates below the above levels, and the blood urea rises above 16.7 mmol per liter or the serum creatinine above 0.17 mmol per liter, the drug should be stopped for 2–5 days. Although nephrotoxicity frequently dictates duration of treatment, AMB can usually be continued until the above limits of renal function are reached (Forgan-Smith and Darrell, 1974). Biochemical evidence of nephrotoxicity occured in 27% of 194 patients with cryptococcal meningitis treated with either 4 or 6 weeks of AMB 0.3 mg per kg per day plus flucytosine (Stamm *et al.*, 1987). Renal function appears to return to normal some months after cessation of AMB (Medoff and Kobayashi, 1980; Maddux and Barriere, 1980). Permanent renal impairment is uncommon unless the total dose of AMB exceeds 4–5 g. Irreversible renal failure may also occur if large doses of the drug are used (Takacs *et al.*, 1963).

The mechanism of AMB nephrotoxicity has been extensively studied. It has a direct vasoconstrictive effect on afferent renal arterioles, which reduces renal blood flow and consequently glomerular blood flow. This causes a dose-dependant reduction in GFR. In addition, there is impaired proximal and distal tubular reabsorption of electrolytes with associated potassium and bicarbonate wasting. There is an increased clearance of uric acid by the proximal tubule. AMB-induced renal tubular acidosis occurs more frequently in patients who have received a total dose of 0.5–1.0 g or more. It is usually reversible after therapy has been discontinued. Irreversible tubular lesions have been reported (McCurdy *et al.*, 1968; Burgess and Birchall, 1972). Potassium supplements are required for about one-quarter of patients receiving AMB, because of the excessive renal losses (Medoff and Kobayashi, 1980). Hypokalemia was observed in 30% of HIV-infected patients receiving liposomal AMB 3 mg per kg per day (Coker *et al.*, 1993). Mild to moderate hypomagnesemia may also result from AMB therapy, due to a tubular defect in magnesium reabsorption. Barton *et al.* (1984) observed hypomagnesemia and increased fractional excretion of magnesium in ten patients by the second week of AMB therapy. The lowest levels and largest fractional excretions of magnesium occurred in the 4th week and thereafter did not alter with continuing AMB therapy. Data relating to three patients about 1 year after AMB was discontinued suggested that this complication was reversible. The authors recommended that serum levels of magnesium should be monitored routinely during AMB therapy.

Studies in rats to elucidate the mechanisms responsible for reductions in renal blood flow and GFR in response to AMB infusions revealed a rapid 50% reduction in renal blood flow during the AMB infusion, which returned to baseline at the end of the infusion. However, the accompanying reduction in creatinine clearance during the AMB infusion continued to decrease to less than 50% of baseline, after the infusion ceased. Salt loading was found to have a protective effect against AMB nephrotoxicity, and theophylline administration also inhibited the acute renal responses by maintaining renal blood flow. It was proposed from this study that calcium influx into cells was responsible for the acute changes in renal blood flow and GFR in response to AMB (Sabra and Branch, 1991). Others have proposed that an activation of the intrarenal regulatory mechanism called tubuloglomerular feedback, which regulates proximal and distal tubule delivery of ions, contributes to AMB-induced renal toxicity (Branch, 1988). Salt loading appears to minimize the decreases in GFR in chronic AMB-induced nephrotoxicity in rats, and salt depletion appears to potentiate the nephrotoxic effects (Feely *et al.*, 1981; Ohnishi *et al.*, 1989; Tollins and Raij, 1988). Clinical evidence to support the use of sodium supplementation for the prevention of AMB-induced nephrotoxicity is anecdotal and comes from retrospective studies and prospective observational studies (Heidemann *et al.*, 1983; Branch, 1988). Although no prospective randomized trials of salt loading have been performed, there is probably sufficient evidence to advocate a pretreatment infusion of 0.5–1 liter of 0.9% saline over 30 min prior to administration of AMB. If vomiting is a problem, the sodium supplementation should be increased. Patients with mild renal impairment are not adversely affected by sodium supplementation. Heidemann *et al.* (1992) found that i.v. administered flucytosine in 0.9% saline had a significant but small effect in reduction of AMB-induced nephrotoxicity in rats that was independent of saline administration. Animal experiments (Bennett, 1974) and some uncontrolled studies in humans (Rosch *et al.*, 1976) indicated that concomitant administration of i.v. mannitol could reduce AMB nephrotoxicity. This was not confirmed in a double-blind study conducted by Bullock *et al.* (1976).

The possibility of severe AMB nephrotoxicity should not preclude its use in patients with potentially fatal systemic fungal infections if this is the only suitable drug available. Temporary severe renal failure may be treated by dialysis and even irreversible renal failure may be successfully managed (Symmers, 1973). Several strategies to reduce the AMB-induced nephrotoxicity have been suggested and include slow infusion of AMB, administration of AMB at double the daily dose on alternate days (little evidence for reduced nephrotoxicity), pre-treatment sodium loading and administration of AMB in liposomal formulations. Renal function sparing effects of ABCD have been documented in a multiple dose escalating study (Amantea *et al.*, 1995). There was no net change in renal function over the duration of ABCD treatment (up to 8 mg per kg per day) for the study population as 20% of patients had a greater than 30% increase in creatinine clearance and 20% had greater than 30% decline in creatinine clearance. There was no association with ABCD exposure or combination with potentially nephrotoxic drugs and the changes in creatinine clearance. In patients with invasive fungal infections who received ABLC over 21–121 weeks, in a cumulative dose of 22.3–73.6 g, the mean serum creatinine increased by 0.5 mg per dl, from 1.0 mg per dl to 1.5 mg per dl, and about half the patients required potassium replacement (Kline *et al.*, 1995). In rats, the concentration of AMB in kidneys was 7-fold lower in ABCD-treated animals than in AMB-desoxycholate treated rats. It has been postulated that AMB bound to low density lipoproteins is resposible for the nephrotoxicity (Barwicz *et al.* 1991) and the greater affinity of lipid-carrier formulations of AMB for high density lipoproteins may explain the lower amount of AMB found in the kidney, and consequently the less nephrotoxicity observed (Amantea *et al.*, 1995). Infusing AMB-desoxycholate in 20% 'Intralipid' was associated with a significant reduction in nephrotoxicity in a controlled trial. Greater than 50% decrease in creatinine clearance was seen in 66% of patients receiving AMB-desoxycholate in 5% dextrose and 33% of those receiving AMB-desoxycholate in 20% 'Intralipid' (Caillot *et al.*, 1994). Safety data from a phase II/III trial examining 133 episodes of therapy with liposomal AMB in doses up to 5 mg per kg per day, showed a 15% incidence of development of renal impairment, and 18% incidence of hypokalemia, but also revealed that one-third of patients with an initially abnormal serum creatinine recovered normal serum creatinine during treatment with liposomal AMB (Meunier *et al.*, 1991).

3 Hematological side-effects

A normochromic, normocytic anemia occurs in about 75% of patients receiving prolonged AMB therapy. The hematocrit frequently falls to a stable value of 22–35% (Medoff and Kobayashi, 1980). Anemia results primarily from a direct suppressive effect on the bone marrow (Hoeprich, 1992). Reduced erythropoiesis, may secondarily result from inhibition of renal erythropoietin production (MacGregor *et al.*, 1978). In a controlled study, Lin *et al.* (1990) determined that AMB suppresses the erythropoietin response to anemia, noting that erythropoietin levels remained constant or declined during therapy with AMB, and increased in response to anemia within 2 weeks of cessation of AMB. Red cell production usually returns to normal several months after cessation of treatment and only occasionally anemia is severe enough to require blood transfusion. Drutz *et al.* (1968) reported two patients in whom a pure red blood cell aplasia developed during AMB therapy. There have been reports of reversible thrombocytopenia thought to be due to a suppressive effect of AMB on platelet production (Chan *et al.*, 1982). A reduced platelet recovery has been reported in some patients who receive simultaneous platelet transfusions and AMB, and may be due to an effect of AMB on platelet membrane glycoproteins (Sloand *et al.*, 1994). In a trial of treatment for cryptococcal meningitis, 11% of 194 patients treated with AMB 0.3 mg per kg per day plus flucytosine 150 mg per kg per day for 4–6 weeks developed thrombocytopenia and 15% developed leukopenia (Stamm *et al.*, 1987). Leukopenia secondary to treatment with AMB alone appears to be rare. AMB interferes with the chemotactic and random migration of human neutrophils (Marmer *et al.*, 1981; Rank *et al.*, 1981). Miconazole, AMB and ketoconazole all can cause suppression of granulocyte progenitor cells in tissue culture (Meeker *et al.*, 1983). The clinical significance of these observations is not known.

4 Neurotoxicity

This is infrequent with i.v. AMB therapy. A case of severe demyelinating peripheral neuropathy has been reported (Haber and Joseph, 1962). Cases of fatal leukoencephalopathy have also been reported in association with i.v. AMB (Devinsky *et al.*, 1987; Walker and Rosenblum, 1992). A well documented case of AMB-induced leukoencephalopathy evolved 2 months after the development of acute hepatorenal failure in a patient receiving AMB for cryptococcal meningitis. A CT brain scan revealed multifocal white matter lesions, and brain biopsy showed changes of demyelination. Minor improvement occurred with low dose corticosteroid treatment (Liu *et al.*, 1995). Three children undergoing bone marrow transplantation, receiving high-dose amphotericin B developed encephalopathy, leukoencephalopathy and parkinsonism. Of these, one recovered without deficit, one improved with residual intellectual impairment and one died from other causes and had leukoencephalopathy on postmortem examination (Mott *et al.*, 1995). These cases were similar to the syndrome of progressive dementia, akinesia, mutism and sphincter dysfunction which complicated treatment with i.v. AMB-methyl ester described by Ellis *et al.* (1982). Postmortem examinations revealed a diffuse non-inflammatory leukoencephalopathy. The exact role of AMB-methyl ester in the development of leukoencephalopathy was not clearly established. *In vitro* and *in vivo* studies suggest that AMB is significantly more neurotoxic than AMB-methyl ester (Racis *et al.*, 1990; Reuhl *et al.*, 1993).

Intrathecal administration can cause local and radicular pain, paresthesiae, nerve palsies, transient paraplegia, convulsions, bladder dysfunction, impotence, visual disturbances and a chemical meningitis (headache and meningismus). Intraventricular administration is less likely to cause chemical meningitis. In addition, myelopathy, delirium, parkinsonism, ventriculitis and tinnitus have been reported (Wen *et al.*, 1992). Fisher and Dewald (1983) described a patient who developed persistent parkinsonism following the successful treatment of cryptococcal meningitis with i.v. and intrathecal AMB, and parkinsonism has also been described after amphotericin B and cytosine arabinoside (Kulkantrakorn *et al.*, 1996). It has been suggested that intrathecal administration of AMB may cause direct vascular injury to the spinal cord (Carnevale *et al.*, 1980). Doses as low as 0.5 mg may cause spinal cord injury. If transient symptoms of spinal cord dysfunction occur, the indications, dose, dosing interval and route of administration should be reviewed.

5 Cardiovascular side-effects

Cardiac arrest has been reported with a rapid AMB infusion in which 28 mg of the drug was infused over 40 min (Hildick-Smith *et al.*, 1964). Reports of cardiac failure during AMB therapy may be explained by associated circulatory overload and reports of arrhythmias by associated hypokalemia which commonly occurs due to renal tubular loss (Maddux and Barriere, 1980). In contrast, there is a potential danger of hyperkalemia with rapid infusion of AMB in anuric patients. Craven and Gremillion (1985) described an anuric patient who developed hyperkalemia (up to 8 mEq (mmol) per liter) and ventricular fibrillation during rapid infusion of high-dose AMB (1.4 mg per kg over 45 min) on two occasions. The peak serum AMB concentration at the end of the infusion was 6.7 µg per ml. This complication was avoided by either prolonging the AMB infusion (3 h) or concurrent hemodialysis. Only a slight rise in serum potassium and lower AMB serum levels (mean 1.7 µg per ml) were observed in eight patients with normal renal function who were given 0.7 mg per kg AMB over 45 min. Reports of ventricular fibrillation during AMB infusion have occurred mainly in patients with severe renal impairment and hyperkalemia who received large AMB doses over short infusion times. In contrast, there is a report of ventricular tachycardia following test doses of 1 mg and 0.1 mg AMB in a patient with chronic renal failure receiving dialysis (Cimolai *et al.*, 1987). Bowler *et al.* (1992) did not observe significant asymptomatic ventricular dysrhythmias in patients with preserved renal function (creatinine clearances greater than 25 ml per min) who received doses of AMB up to 0.9 mg per kg in rapid infusions of 1 h. Ventricular fibrillation resulting in death has been described in a patient with no renal impairment on day 7 of treatment with liposomal AMB 3 mg per kg. At autopsy there was no evidence of ischemic heart disease (Aguado *et al.*, 1993). Cardiopulmonary toxicity has also been reported with the use of liposomal AMB (formulated by Lopez-Berenstein and colleagues) in a 22-year-old with hepatosplenic candidiasis. Reproducible hypoxia, decreased cardiac output and increased pulmonary artery pressure occurred with each infusion of 5 mg per kg over 50 min. No cardiac effects were noted with a reduced dose and slower rate of infusion (Levine *et al.*, 1991). There is another case report of an individual receiving liposomal AMB 3 mg per kg in a 3-h infusion who developed ventricular fibrillation and died on day 7 of treatment. Autopsy revealed no evidence of myocardial infarction or renal failure (Aguado *et al.*, 1993).

Malignant hypertension during infusion of AMB at a dose of 0.3 mg per kg has been documented in two patients on two to three separate occasions. The hypertension required control with a nitroprusside infusion (Dukes and Perfect, 1990; Omizo *et al.*, 1993). Bradycardia and significant heart rate decreases occurred in 7% of children on AMB, temporally related to AMB administration. The mean drop in heart rate was from 104 to 62 beats per min and were first noted on day 3–7 of treatment (Levy *et al.*, 1995).

6 Pulmonary reactions

Transient dyspnea may be one of the general reactions which occur during early therapy with i.v. AMB. Severe, and occasionally lethal, acute pulmonary reactions characterized by acute dyspnea, hypoxemia and radiological changes of interstitial infiltrates have been described in patients receiving concomitant AMB and leukocyte transfusions (Wright *et al.*, 1981). It was postulated that they may be due to an interaction of AMB and transfused leukocytes in lung tissue. Since reactions occurred commonly during or shortly after an infusion of AMB that followed a leukocyte transfusion, Wright *et al.* (1981) advised that i.v. AMB infusions should be given more slowly and temporally separated as far as practical from a leukocyte transfusion. Other investigators have refuted this causal relationship of AMB and leukocytes in causing these pulmonary changes (Dana *et al.*, 1981; De Gregorio *et al.*, 1981; Forman *et al.*, 1981; Bow *et al.*, 1984). Nevertheless, studies *in vitro* and an *in vivo* model show that AMB can induce aggregation of polymorphonuclear leukocytes and increase pulmonary leukostasis (Berliner *et al.*, 1985). The acute pulmonary toxicity (sudden onset of dyspnea and tightness of the chest) has also been observed during infusion of 3 mg per kg liposomal AMB in at least two patients and resolved within minutes of stopping the infusion (Arning *et al.*, 1995).

7 Hepatotoxicity

Liver function abnormalities are rarely detected during AMB therapy. Acute liver failure has been reported (Carnecchia and Kurtzke, 1960). This complication is so rare that doubt has been cast on its relation to AMB therapy (Bennett, 1974).

Transient elevations in transaminases were seen in 40% of healthy volunteers in a phase I study of ABLC (0.5 mg per kg) (Kan *et al.*, 1991), 38% of immunocompromised patients after liposomal AMB treatment (Meunier *et al.*, 1991) and in 44% of HIV-infected patients with cryptococcosis receiving 3 mg per kg per day of 'AmBisome' (Coker *et al.*, 1993).

8 Allergic reactions

Anaphylaxis has been noted but is rare, and has been reported for both AMB-desoxycholate and liposomal AMB (Bates *et al.*, 1995). Hypersensitivity rashes are uncommon (Lorber *et al.*, 1976). Anaphylactic reactions (hypotension, erythema, fever, bronchospasm and facial edema) have been reported within 30 min of infusing liposomal AMB in two patients receiving their first dose. Both patients tolerated AMB-desoxycholate without allergic reaction (Laing *et al.*, 1994). An additional three patients who received liposomal AMB as antifungal prophylaxis during the neutropenic period following bone marrow transplantation, experienced allergic reactions (flushing, erythema, dyspnea, and headache) related to the infusion of the drug (Tollemar *et al.*, 1993) Descriptions of acute allergic reactions including bronchospasm, dyspnea and tachypnea have been reported more commonly in individuals with a history of acute asthma or chronic obstructive lung disease (Murray, 1974).

9 Effect on fetus

There have been no studies performed to evaluate teratogenicity, carcinogenicity or the effect on fertility. Pregnant patients given AMB for serious fungal infections, have given birth to normal infants (Ismail and Lerner, 1982; Cohen, 1987), and both mother and infant have tolerated AMB therapy well (Dean *et al.*, 1994). The drug crosses the placenta and its safety during the first trimester of pregnancy has not been determined conclusively, but there are no reports of teratogenicity. Abnormal neonatal renal function has been described and is generally transient (Dean *et al.*, 1994). It is unknown whether AMB is excreted in breast milk.

10 Effects on the immune system

Both immunostimulatory and immunosuppressive effects have been described. *In vitro*, AMB can suppress human lymphocyte transformation (Roselle and Kauffman, 1978). The lymphocyte suppression was shown to be the result of induction of suppressor cells in normal volunteers exposed to levels of AMB achievable in human serum. This was associated with an increased production of prostaglandin E_2 synthesis (Stewart *et al.*, 1981). In animals, the drug can enhance the number of antibody-producing cells and augment delayed type hypersensitivity reactions and cell-mediated immunity (Medoff and Kobayashi, 1980). *In vitro* studies have shown that AMB decreases natural killer cell and antibody-dependent cellular cytotoxic activity (Hauser and Remington, 1983). Effects on neutrophil function include reduced chemotaxis, inhibition of phagocytosis and decreased random migration (Chan and Ballish,1978; Rank *et al.*,1981; Yasui *et al.*, 1988). It is only speculative whether these effects have any clinical significance.

Clinical Uses of the Drug

1 Cryptococcosis

Infection with *Cryptococcus neoformans* predominantly occurs in AIDS patients with declining CD4 cell counts, in those with organ transplantation, Hodgkin's lymphoma, sarcoidosis, patients given corticosteroid therapy and some otherwise healthy individuals. The onset of clinical manifestations due to cryptococcosis may be insidious or acute, and infection may affect almost any part of the body, but the meninges and the lungs are most frequently involved. The course of the infection may be indolent or rapidly progressive and correlates with the degree of immunosuppression in the host. Pulmonary lesions may be asymptomatic, and in the absence of concomitant immunodeficiency will generally resolve spontaneously without antifungal therapy (Kerkering *et al.*, 1981). Often, sputum cultures are negative and a biopsy is required for diagnostic purposes. A total excision biopsy will be curative if there is no extrapulmonary infection. If a cryptococcal lung abscess is the only manifestation, it can usually be satisfactorily treated by surgery alone (Hammerman *et al.*, 1973a). The situation is different in compromised hosts in whom antifungal treatment is always indicated for pulmonary disease because of the increased risk of dissemination (Kerkering *et al.*, 1981).

Management of cryptococcal meningitis in the non-AIDS patient, includes the use of AMB and 5-flucytosine (Bennett *et al.*, 1979). A prospective study by Utz *et al.* (1975) on 20 patients with disseminated cryptococcosis (15 with confirmed meningitis) indicated that a regimen using these two drugs was effective and was associated with reduced AMB nephrotoxicity. AMB was given in a dose of 20 mg daily with 5-flucytosine orally in a dose of 150 mg per kg per day for 6 weeks. Others have obtained encouraging results using low doses of AMB and 5-flucytosine to treat cryptococcal meningitis (Schroter *et al.*, 1976; Tobias *et al.*, 1976). Subsequently, Bennett *et al.* (1979) performed a prospective multicenter randomized controlled trial in 50 patients with cryptococcal meningitis. AMB alone (0.4 mg per kg per day for 42 days, followed by 0.8 mg per kg on alternate days for 28 days) was compared with AMB (0.3 mg per kg per day) combined with 5-flucytosine (150 mg per kg per day in four divided doses) for 6 weeks. The combination cured or improved 67% of patients compared with a 41% cure or improved rate for AMB alone. The combination also produced fewer relapses and more rapid sterilization of the CSF. Less nephrotoxicity was observed in the combination group than in the AMB alone group, probably due to the lower dose of AMB utilized. One of the criticisms of this study was the lack of comparison with a dose of AMB commonly used in routine practice (0.5–0.6 mg per kg per day). Adverse reactions to 5-flucytosine occurred in one-third of patients and resulted in premature discontinuation of the drug in 20%. As a result of this study, combination therapy has been recommended for the treatment of cryptococcal meningitis (Bennett *et al.* 1979; Medoff and Kobayashi, 1980). The risk of flucytosine accumulation as renal impairment due to AMB develops can be reduced, by initiating therapy at 75–100 mg per kg per day and continuing doses that maintain flucytosine levels between 25 to 60 μg per ml (Francis and Walsh, 1992). The duration of therapy should be dictated by the individual patient response, and continued until cultures are negative for 4 weeks and CSF glucose is normal. A minimum treatment course is 6 weeks, although some non-immunocompromised patients have been cured after 4 weeks of therapy with combination AMB and 5-flucytosine (Dismukes *et al.*, 1987). Relapses are reasonably common in immunocompromised patients and usually occur in the first year after therapy (Dismukes *et al.*, 1980). Failure of therapy occurs in 25% of those with no obvious predisposing factors and up to 55% of immunocompromised patients. Poor prognostic features for failure of therapy include a high CSF opening pressure, a low CSF glucose level, less than 20 leukocytes per ml of CSF, a positive India ink smear, the isolation of cryptococci from other sites, particularly blood, and high cryptococcal antigen titers in the serum and CSF (Diamond and Bennett, 1974).

Intraventricular or intrathecal administration of AMB is rarely required in cryptococcal meningitis. Diamond and Bennett (1973) recommended that it should be reserved for patients who fail to respond to i.v. therapy or show severe reactions to this form of treatment. Indications for direct administration of AMB into the CSF have not been determined by controlled trials.

Treatment of cryptococcal meningitis in AIDS patients is associated with 20–30% failure rates, high rates of treatment-associated toxicity, and relapse occurs in up to 60% without chronic suppressive therapy (Powderly, 1992). Because of the treatment-related toxicity due to 5-flucytosine (bone marrow suppression) and AMB nephrotoxicity, alternative approaches to treatment have been evaluated. Larsen *et al.* (1990) compared oral fluconazole 400 mg per day with the combination of AMB 0.7 mg per kg per day and 5-flucytosine 150 mg per kg per day orally in a small randomized trial. Combination therapy resulted in clinical and mycological cure in 100% (six out of six patients) compared with a 43% response rate for fluconazole (six out of 14 patients). More rapid sterilization of CSF was achieved with combination therapy.

A larger multicenter, randomized study compared AMB 0.3–0.7 mg per kg per day with or without 5-flucytosine with fluconazole 200 mg per day in 194 AIDS patients with cryptococcal meningitis (Saag *et al.*, 1992). Clinical and mycological response rates were low (40% for AMB, and 34% for fluconazole) but clinical improvement, without mycological response was noted in 67% for AMB and 60% of fluconazole recipients. Sterilization of the CSF appeared to be more rapid in the AMB group. This may have been due to the low treatment doses of both AMB and fluconazole chosen for this study. There was no statistical difference between responses rates of the two regimens, which has resulted in the use of the better tolerated fluconazole for primary treatment of cryptococcal meningitis particularly in mild cases, in many centers.

However, concern about the time to sterilization of CSF, has led many investigators to recommend initial treatment of cryptococcal meningitis to include AMB 0.7–1.0 mg per kg per day with or without 5-flucytosine 75–100 mg per kg per day, for 6–10 weeks (White and Armstrong, 1994). This regimen (AMB 1 mg per kg plus 5-flucytosine 100–150 mg per kg) was reported to produce mycological cure rates of 93% in one study of 31 patients. Renal toxicity occurred in 25% of the patients (de Lalla *et al.*, 1995). The combination of AMB 0.3 mg per kg per day plus 5-flucytosine 150 mg per kg per day for 6 weeks was compared with oral itraconazole 200 mg twice-daily, and the combination was found to be significantly superior (deGans *et al.*, 1992). Liposomal AMB ('AmBisome') has also been reported to be effective for treatment of unresponsive cryptococcal meningitis in AIDS (Coker *et al.*, 1991). In a follow-up open study of liposomal AMB 3 mg per kg daily for the primary treatment of cryptococcosis in patients with AIDS, the cure rate was 61%, with an additional 17% of patients with improvement of clinical symptoms (Coker *et al.*, 1993). A randomized open-label comparison of AMB 0.7 mg per kg daily for 2 weeks followed by 1.2 mg per kg three-times weekly, and ABLC in ascending dose cohorts of 1.2 mg per kg, 2.5 mg per kg and 5.0 mg per kg once-daily for 2 weeks followed by 5 mg per kg thrice-weekly was performed in 55 AIDS patients with first-episode cryptococcal meningitis. There was no significant difference in clinical or mycological response rates, but ABLC was significantly better tolerated than AMB with reduced bone marrow and renal toxicity. However, at the end of treatment, 42% ABLC recipients remained CSF-culture positive, compared with 12% AMB recipients. The sample size was inadequate to address significant differences in efficacy, but the trend is worrisome and the lack of demonstrable dose-response for ABLC should be evaluated in larger studies (Sharkey *et al.*, 1996).

Suppressive therapy starting after successful completion of primary treatment and continuing for life is important to prevent relapse of infection. Weekly infusions of 1 mg per kg AMB was the most commonly used regimen (Zuger *et al.*, 1988) prior to the results of a large multicenter AIDS Clinical Trials Group study comparing the weekly infusions of AMB 1 mg per kg and oral fluconazole 200 mg per day. Fluconazole maintenance therapy was significantly superior to AMB in prevention of relapse (37% relapse in the AMB group and 2% in the fluconazole group). Fluconazole was also better tolerated than AMB (Powderly *et al.* 1992).

2 Candidiasis

Systemic candidiasis   The incidence of infection due to *Candida* spp. has increased over the last 20–30 years, due to more widespread use of antibiotics, the increased use of indwelling intravenous catheters, and new therapeutics which allow individuals to experience more severe immunosuppression for longer durations (e.g., transplantation, cancer chemotherapy) as well as HIV infection. *Candida lusitaniae* is commonly resistant to AMB, and other species, namely *C. albicans*, *C. guilliermondii*, *C. tropicalis* and *C. glabrata* may be relatively resistant. It is important to know which of the *Candida* spp. is causing the infection under treatment.

a Fungemia There has been a dramatic increase in the incidence of candidemia since the 1980s, with 10–15% of hospital-acquired blood-stream infections due to *Candida* (Pfaller and Wenzel, 1992). The management of candidemia has been controversial until recently.

Immunocompetent patients with candidemia associated with an indwelling catheter have been noted to have spontaneous resolution of the fungemia following removal of the catheter (Ellis and Spivack, 1967). However, it is imperative to exclude disseminated disease (cutaneous lesions, arthritis, osteomyelitis, endophthalmitis and endocarditis), which often proves difficult, as complications may not manifest until late. There is now a consensus that all patients with candidemia, whether immunocompetent or immunocompromised, with catheter-associated fungemia or not, with persistent candidemia or a single isolation from blood cultures, should be treated with antifungal therapy. Rex *et al.* (1994) performed a randomized controlled trial comparing the efficacy and safety of i.v. AMB 0.5–0.6 mg per kg per day and oral fluconazole 400 mg per day for a minimum of 14 days after the last positive blood culture, in patients without neutropenia (50% had recent surgery, 30% had cancer) There was no statistically significant difference in effectiveness between the two groups. The treatment was judged successful in 79% of AMB recipients and 70% of fluconazole recipients. There was significantly more renal toxicity and hypokalemia in the AMB group, and a comparable rate of hepatotoxicity between the two groups. The majority of isolates in this study were *Candida albicans*.

Amphotericin B is indicated for infections due to all *Candida* spp. known to have reduced susceptibility to the azole antifungal agents. In this large study, 30% of patients were found to have endophthalmitis before the end of therapy, and patients with candidemia had a 36% mortality rate (Rex *et al.*, 1994). Neither the optimal duration of therapy nor the appropriate total dose of AMB is known. At least a 14-day treatment duration or a total dose of 500–1000 mg of AMB is empirically recommended for candidemia without complications. No prospective studies have been performed to determine the total dose required (Bennett *et al.*, 1978; Gauto *et al.*, 1977). Removal of the indwelling i.v. catheter is recommended and the new catheter should not be inserted over a guidewire in the site of the original potentially infected catheter. Prolonged duration of candidemia and increased morbidity and mortality are associated with failure to remove the indwelling catheter (Eppes *et al.*, 1989; Lecciones *et al.*, 1992).

In neutropenic patients, and those with acute sepsis and worsening conditions AMB should be used as initial therapy. In neutropenic patients, the isolation of *Candida* spp. from blood cultures should be considered indicative of disseminated disease (Swerdloff *et al.*, 1993). In this setting, there is a high mortality rate of 50%. Intravenous AMB at a dose of 0.6–0.8 mg per kg per day should be instituted promptly, as prognosis is related to the interval between onset of clinical symptoms, diagnosis of fungemia and commencement of therapy (Lecciones *et al.*, 1992) and AMB should be continued until the patient has received a total dose of 1–2 g (Crislip and Edwards, 1989). Fungemia in severely immunocompromised patients is frequently caused by *Candida* isolates that are relatively resistant to AMB, (MIC > 0.8 μg per ml) and clinical response to AMB 1 mg per kg per day was observed more often in patients whose isolates had an MIC of less than 0.8 μg per ml (Powderly *et al.*, 1988). In neutropenic patients with proven candidemia and no evidence of tissue invasion, treatment with AMB diluted in 'Intralipid' 20% administered at a mean dose of 1 mg per kg per day plus flucytosine was successful in 13 of 14 (93%) episodes (Caillot *et al.*, 1993). The same general principles of treatment of disseminated candidiasis apply to organ transplant recipients, burns patients and the postoperative patient with multiple risk factors for disseminated candidiasis.

Combined AMB and 5-flucytosine has been used to treat a case of *Candida* fungemia associated with an aortocoronary graft (Eilard *et al.*, 1976). Fungemia due to *C. lusitaniae* requires attention to the *in vitro* susceptibility test results, as many isolates are resistant to AMB. Yinnon *et al.* (1992) report a case of *C. lusitaniae* fungemia associated with central venous catheter infection in a neonate. The infant developed urinary tract involvement and did not respond to 2 weeks of i.v. AMB. In a retrospective review of candidemia in low birthweight neonates, Butler *et al.* (1990) using prompt treatment with AMB rapidly escalating to a daily dose of 1 mg per kg, reported an overall mortality rate of 22%. They found that neonates with uncomplicated central intravascular catheter-associated candidemia were effectively treated with catheter removal and a total dose of AMB between 10 and 15 mg per kg. Neonates with disseminated disease had a higher mortality and required a total dose of AMB between 25 and 30 mg per kg.

Hepatosplenic candidiasis occurs in patients who experienced an episode of prolonged neutropenia secondary to chemotherapy, usually for acute leukemia. Cure rates with AMB have been low. Residual candidiasis has been noted at autopsy in individuals who received 2 g of AMB, and some patients have required up to 9 g AMB for cure (Thaler *et al.*, 1988a; Helton *et al.*, 1986). Liposomal AMB has been used successfully for this syndrome (Lopez-Berestein *et al.*, 1987). Clinical and mycological response rates of 76% were attained with liposomal AMB 0.7–5 mg per kg per day treatment for invasive candidiasis in immunocompromised patients who had persistent fungal infection or toxicity after conventional AMB (Ringden *et al.*, 1991), and 58% of patients with systemic candidiasis who received ABCD at doses of 3 mg per kg per day in an open non-comparative trial (Oppenheim *et al.*, 1995).

b   Endocarditis   *Candida* spp. are the most common cause of fungal endocarditis which usually occurs after cardiac surgery (Seelig *et al.*, 1979). Infections associated with i.v. heroin use or damaged valves are commonly due to *C. parapsilosis*, whereas the majority of patients with infection associated with a prosthetic valve have *C. albicans* infection (Bennett, 1978). *Candida* endocarditis is treated with a combination of AMB, 0.6–0.8 mg per kg per day and immediate surgery to remove the infected valve (native or prosthetic). After removal of the infected valve AMB should be continued for 6–10 weeks to reduce the likelihod of relapse (Crislip and Edwards,1989). Seelig *et al.* (1979) summarized 29 cases of candidal endocarditis which had been cured by therapy with AMB alone or with other antifungal agents. Most of the patients underwent surgery with debridement of cardiac vegetations, replacement of homograft or prosthetic valves or insertion of a prosthesis in addition to chemotherapy. *Candida* prosthetic valve endocarditis is associated with a high mortality rate. Immediate removal of the infected prosthesis, irrigation of the infected site with AMB (1.0 g per liter of Ringer's solution), followed by a 6- to 8-week course of i.v. AMB has been recommended (Crislip and Edwards, 1989). Dual therapy with AMB and 5-flucytosine is now commonly used to treat endocarditis.

Experience by Wain *et al.* (1979) indicates that in the management of candidal endocarditis following homograft valve replacement, initial intensive chemotherapy using AMB and 5-flucytosine, with late reoperation when indicated, appears to give better results than immediate excision of the infected valve. Fass and Perkins (1971) described successful treatment of a patient with *Candida* endocarditis associated with an aortic valve prosthesis, by the use of AMB with 5-flucytosine and surgical removal of the prosthesis. Such combined therapy in association with removal of vegetations and insertion of a valve prosthesis was used to cure a case of *C. parapsilosis* endocarditis (Martin *et al.* 1979). Others have described persistence of viable fungal organisms in vegetations following prolonged courses of AMB (Utley *et al.*, 1975; Rubinstein *et al.*, 1974) suggesting poor penetration of vegetations by AMB. The *in vitro* antifungal activity of AMB on *C. albicans* in human fibrin clots was assessed and concentrations up to 18.5 μg per ml (not achievable in clinical practice) were unable to sterilize the clots (Smith *et al.*, 1983a). These observations and reports of relapse of *Candida* endocarditis years after apparent medical cure, lend support to the combined medical and surgical approach to this infection. Patients should be monitored closely for 2 years post-treatment for evidence of relapse.

c   Urinary tract infection   Candiduria may represent colonization or infection. The prevalence of candiduria in hospitalized patients was found to be 20% in one study (Goldberg *et al.*, 1979). Approximately 10% of patients with candidemia will have the urinary tract identified as the source, but development of candidemia is a rare complication of candiduria and occurs in patients with significant urinary tract pathology, obstruction, and patients with nephrostomy tubes, or after major urinary tract surgery (Ang *et al.*, 1993).

Candida spp. may cause cystitis, pyelonephritis, papillary necrosis, perinephric abscess, and fungus ball formation (Crislip and Edwards,1989). Risk factors for the development of *Candida* urinary tract infections include use of indwelling Foley catheters, diabetes mellitus and broad-spectrum antibiotics. For the majority of individuals, candiduria is urinary catheter-related, is asymptomatic and responds to removal of the catheter. If the catheter cannot be removed, or invasive cystitis is demonstrated, AMB bladder washes are usually effective. There are no prospective, controlled trials to determine the most effective treatment for uncomplicated funguria. When administered systemically AMB is minimally excreted in the urine, so AMB urinary lavage is the most commonly employed therapy for uncomplicated funguria. It is instilled either intermittently or by continuous infusion. Details of the case reports of either intermittent or continous irrigation of AMB in the management of candidal urinary tract infections can be found in a review by Gubbins *et al.* (1993). Instillation of 200–300 ml of AMB solution at a concentration of 5–10 μg per ml, by a triple lumen urethral catheter for no longer than 2 days is the currently recommended treatment (Sanford,1993). Continuous bladder irrigation with 50 μg per ml AMB over 24 h for 2 days was more effective in eradicating candiduria than intermittent bladder irrigation with 10 mg

AMB in 100 ml (Trinh *et al.*, 1995). Others have suggested that bladder washouts of AMB (50 μg per ml) for 3–5 days allows the localization of the infection. Persistent candiduria after twice-daily bladder washouts by continous infusion suggests renal candidiasis (Hsu and Ukleja, 1990; Hsu and Chang, 1995). Symptomatic cystitis has been successfully treated with single-dose AMB 0.3 mg per kg i.v., or oral fluconazole, and itraconazole (Zervos *et al.*, 1994).

If upper urinary tract *Candida* infection is suspected, or if the patient is neutropenic or a renal transplant recipient, i.v. AMB at doses used for disseminated candidiasis should be instituted. Flucytosine is excreted in high doses in the urine but there is concern about development of resistance when it is used as sole therapy. Fluconazole also achieves high urinary concentrations and may be a useful alternative. Fungus balls require surgical removal. Keller *et al.* (1977) used AMB and 5-flucytosine in association with surgery successfully to treat an infant who had *C. albicans* renal fungus balls and *C. albicans* arthritis.

d Meningitis *Candida* meningitis is uncommon and is usually a complication of disseminated candidiasis. It is more common in the newborn than adults (Bayer *et al.*,1976a). Parenchymal brain involvement in the form of microabscesses distributed most commonly along the middle cerebral artery is also associated with disseminated candidiasis. Diagnosis is most often made at autopsy. Treatment with i.v. AMB 0.6–1 mg per kg per day and oral 5-flucytosine is indicated for these conditions. *Candida* meningitis can also result from infection of a ventricular shunt. Successful eradication of fungal infection often includes removal of the shunt in addition to systemic antifungal therapy. Roe and Haynes (1972) reported a child who recovered from *C. albicans* meningitis after 43 days therapy with AMB alone; however, the addition of 5-flucytosine may be beneficial in *Candida* meningitis (Chesney *et al.*, 1979; Smego *et al.*, 1984b). Chesney *et al.* (1976) successfully treated two children with *C. albicans* meningitis using i.v. AMB for 9–13 days with 6–9 weeks of oral 5-flucytosine, while Smego *et al.* (1984a) effectively managed two infants with severe combined immunodeficiency and *C. albicans* meningitis with AMB and 5-flucytosine in one child and AMB and ketoconazole in the other child.

Smego *et al.* (1984b) reviewed the clinical outcome of 17 patients with *Candida* meningitis reported in the medical literature. Eleven patients were aged 12 months or less, seven were neonates. Following dual therapy with AMB and 5-flucytosine, 15 patients improved and 14 were cured. A cure rate of 75–100% was achieved for the combination of AMB and 5-flucytosine, compared with 87% for AMB alone. Smego *et al.* (1984b) recommend combination AMB and 5-flucytosine for the treatment of *Candida* meningitis. The rarity of this infection precludes a prospective controlled trial to prove a clinical advantage of combination therapy over AMB alone. The role of intrathecal administration of AMB is not clearly defined so it should be reserved for severe cases, not reponding to systemic therapy. The exception to this is the management of *Candida* meningitis associated with an infected shunt, because AMB does not reach adequate CSF concentrations when given by the i.v. route. Nguyen and Yu (1995) reviewed their experience of neurosurgery-related *Candida* meningitis, and found treatment with AMB (0.5 mg per kg) and 5-flucytosine (minimum 75 mg per kg) daily was effective therapy. Although numbers were small and the review was retrospective, they noted a fluconazole treatment failure, and i.v. AMB + intrathecal AMB was inferior to combination AMB + 5-flucytosine.

e Bone and joint infections Osteomyelitis due to *Candida* species localizes predominantly in the axial skeleton (vertebrae and intervertebral discs) in adults, and occurs primarily as a result of hematogenous dissemination. In children the long bones are more frequently affected. *Candida* arthritis occurs most frequently as a consequence of disseminated candidiasis, but can also occur from joint surgery and the use of prostheses, from sternotomy wound infections, from intra-articular injection of steroids or in i.v. heroin users (Bennett, 1978). The most common pathogens are *C. albicans* followed by *C. tropicalis* and other *Candida* spp. The management of *Candida* osteomyelitis includes i.v. AMB and assessment for the need for surgical debridement. Vertebral osteomyelitis rarely requires debridement; however, sternal osteomyelitis should be surgically debrided. AMB is the drug of choice, due to the lack of controlled, comparative studies. The dose and duration of AMB treatment is not known; however, Gathe *et al.* (1987) recommended a total dose of 1–1.5 g, after a review of all reported cases of *Candida* osteomyelitis. There have been rare reports of *Candida* osteomyelitis which have resolved without treatment (Edwards *et al.*, 1975).

Arthritis due to *Candida* species is uncommon. The monoarthritis produced by direct inoculation of *Candida* colonizing skin either by trauma or surgery is more common in older adults, than hematogenously disseminated candidiasis seen in the immunocompromised host and manifests as mono- or polyarthritis. Intravenous AMB, combined with joint aspiration and washouts is the mainstay of treatment for *Candida* arthritis in adults and children (Fainstein *et al.*, 1982). This therapeutic approach may be supplemented by intra-articular injections of AMB. Systemic and intra-articular AMB has also been of clinical value for neonates with *C. albicans* arthritis (Pittard *et al.*, 1976; Ward *et al.*, 1983).

f Pulmonary infection Bronchopulmonary candidiasis is uncommon, and usually occurs in one of two forms. A focal or diffuse bronchopneumonia can develop secondary to spread of organisms from the endobronchial tree, or hematogenous seeding of the lungs can result in a diffuse infiltrative or nodular appearance in the lungs. *Candida* pulmonary infections usually occur in severely immunocompromised patients who tend to be colonized by *Candida* spp. prior to invasive disease. For this reason it is important to make a diagnosis on biopsy specimens, rather than compatible radiographic appearances and isolation of *Candida* spp. from sputum or bronchoscopy specimens. The appropriate treatment in the immunocompromised patient with invasive candidiasis, in whom the pulmonary manifestations probably represent more widespread invasive disease, is intravenous AMB 0.5–1.0 mg per kg per day. The duration of treatment will be dictated by clinical response and the resolution of the immunosuppression, generally a total dose of 1–1.5 g. Schiffman *et al.* (1982) described the successful treatment of a diabetic patient with a *C. albicans* lung abscess with an AMB-5-flucytosine combination.

g Peritonitis *Candida* peritonitis occurs as a complication of abdominal surgery, ruptured abdominal viscus or continuous ambulatory peritoneal dialysis (CAPD). Intravenous AMB is indicated for treatment of *Candida* peritonitis associated with a ruptured abdominal viscus, particularly in infants in whom hematogenous dissemination is common. For the patient who has *Candida* spp. isolated from a drain tube following abdominal surgery, colonization should be considered, and evidence for active infection sought. *Candida* peritonitis associated with CAPD has been successfully managed with the instillation of AMB at a concentration of 2–4 μg per ml in the dialysate fluid (Bayer *et al.*, 1976b). Removal of the indwelling Tenckhoff catheter in addition to systemic AMB is often required to cure the fungal infection (Bastani and Westervelt, 1986). Peritoneal lavage with AMB (1 μg per ml) was used successfully to treat peritonitis due to *C. tropicalis* in a 14-year-old girl, who was a renal transplant recipient (Bortolussi *et al.*, 1975). Intraperitoneal AMB and/or short duration low-dose systemic AMB treatment was useful for adult patients with unremitting *Candida* peritonitis (Bayer *et al.*, 1976b).

h Ocular candidiasis Infection of the eye occurs either by hematogenous dissemination or direct inoculation. There have been increasing reports of endophthalmitis associated with candidemia, with 12–28% of patients developing this complication (Ellard, 1987; Brooks, 1989). Fungal infection originates in the chorioretinal area, and progresses to involve the vitreous. The majority of cases are due to *Candida albicans*, but recently cases due to other *Candida* spp. have been reported (e.g. *Candida tropicalis*) in association with catheter-related candidemia (Cohen and Montgomerie, 1993). The treatment of choice for *Candida* endophthalmitis is i.v. AMB. The role of vitrectomy in the management of fungal endophthalmitis is controversial, with proponents reporting improved visual acuity in those that undergo therapeutic vitrectomy combined with systemic AMB (Pflugfelder and Flynn,1992). Isolated *Candida* chorioretinitis, not involving the vitreous has been reported to heal spontaneously, and endogenous *Candida* endophthalmitis without evidence of systemic disease may be successfully treated with vitrectomy and intravitreal AMB (Brod *et al.*,1990). Two patients with *Candida* endophthalmitis have been successfully treated with a single intravitreal injection of 5 μg AMB, without adverse effects (Stern *et al.*, 1977; Perraut *et al.*, 1981), but in a series of cases of postsurgical *C. parapsilosis* endophthalmitis reported by Stern *et al.* (1985), repeated intravitreal injections of AMB and vitrectomy were required to resolve the infection.

Keratitis caused by *Candida* spp. manifests as a corneal ulcer and usually occurs following the use of topical steroids, or damage to the surface of the cornea. Topical ocular use of AMB 0.05–0.15% solution (prepared from the i.v. formulation) is effective and well tolerated in patients with superficial to medium depth keratitis. The AMB drops are administered hourly around the clock for the first 7 days, then hourly while the patient is awake, for up to 12 weeks depending on the severity of the infection (Foster, 1992).

Superficial candidiasis

a Mucous membrane infections

i *Oral candidiasis* In immunocompetent patients, an episode of oral thrush precipitated by a course of antibiotics, or inhaled oral steroids is self-limiting and responds rapidly to topical nystatin or clotrimazole. In the immunocompromised patient, cancer patients receiving chemotherapy and AIDS patients, widespread use of the azole drugs has resulted in fluconazole-resistant candidiasis. Some AIDS patients may have persistent fluconazole-sensitive candidiasis which does not respond to increasing doses of fluconazole. These patients require intermittent courses of i.v. AMB. For intermittent treatment of oral thrush AMB lozenges (one lozenge sucked four times a day have been used effectively.

ii *Candida esophagitis* In the immunocompromised patient, resolution of symptomatic disease is achieved with ketoconazole or fluconazole orally. In the AIDS patient, recurrent disease and the need for chronic courses of the oral azole drugs often culminates in fluconazole resistence and the need to treat symptomatic disease with a short course of i.v. AMB, 0.3 mg per kg daily or 0.6 mg per kg on alternate days (Medoff, 1987). In all patients with severe disease or those unable to take oral medications AMB is indicated.

iii *Vaginal candidiasis* A common infection in women, vulvovaginitis primarily due to *Candida albicans*, responds readily to topical treatment with nystatin, clotrimazole, miconazole or the newer azole drugs and the oral azole drugs ketoconazole, itraconazole or fluconazole, in the majority of cases. A small number of women experience chronic *Candida* vaginitis that responds partially to the topical antifungals and relapse once therapy stops. These women require 6-month courses of oral azole drugs. AMB is rarely required for control.

b Cutaneous candidiasis Superficial infections of both skin and nails giving rise to *Candida* folliculitis, *Candida* balanitis, intertrigo, paronychia, and onychomycosis, are generally mild to moderate infections which respond to topical agents such as nystatin, clotrimazole, miconazole and the newer azole drugs. Affected areas are treated twice-daily for 7 days. Severe infections or those reponding poorly to topical agents may require systemic treatment with one of the azole drugs. Also AMB lotion or cream can be used for intertrigo, nappy or diaper rash in addition to attempts to keep the area free of chronic moisture. The application of AMB lotion to the nail beds may be used for mild cases of *Candida* paronychia. Prolonged or repeated courses of topical or systemic antifungals is often required.

c Chronic mucocutaneous candidiasis This syndrome is characterized by chronic *Candida* infections of the skin, nails and mucous membranes that persist despite adequate antifungal therapy and occur in individuals with a variety of T cell function abnormalities. Severity of the syndrome varies and isolated skin and nail infections may be controlled by topical antifungal agents. As the *Candida* infection progresses, short courses of AMB i.v. or the azole antifungal agents are indicated. Infection regularly recurs and treatment is often required for months or years (Rosenblatt and Steihm, 1983). Esophageal or laryngeal candidiasis may occur in chronic mucocutaneous candidiasis. Aerosolized AMB (5 mg three times daily for 21 days) has been used successfully to treat *Candida* laryngitis. For most patients treatment of *Candida* laryngitis and esophagitis requires 2–4 weeks AMB i.v. at a dose of 0.7 mg per kg per day (Kobayashi *et al.*, 1980).

d Prevention of invasive candidiasis and other opportunistic fungal disease in patients with neoplastic diseases or transplant recipients Invasive fungal infections are an important cause of morbidity and mortality in patients with neoplastic disorders and patients undergoing transplantation. These patients have prolonged periods of neutropenia, receive broad spectrum antiobiotics or high-dose steroids, or other immunocompromising regimens which predispose the individual to colonization and subsequent dissemination of opportunistic fungi such as *Candida* spp. The use of antibiotics encourages the overgrowth of *Candida* spp. in the gastrointestinal tract and cytotoxic drugs cause mucosal damage providing access to the systemic circulation for dissemination of *Candida* organisms.

Preventative strategies trialled to date include prophylaxis, empiric therapy and secondary prophylaxis. Nystatin, ketoconazole, AMB, itraconazole and fluconazole have all been studied and fluconazole appears to be most effective and least toxic. In neutropenic and febrile neutropenic patients, AMB significantly reduces the rate of invasive fungal infections and has the advantage of activity against fluconazole-resistant *C. krusei, C. glabrata* and the filamentous fungi.

Conflicting and very limited information on the efficacy of prophylactic strategies for the prevention of candidal infections is available. A controlled study by Ezdinli *et al.* (1979) in which patients with hematological malignancies received oral AMB, 50 mg four times per day, or placebo revealed a reduction in invasive candidiasis found at autopsy from 24% in the placebo group, to 5% in the AMB group. In contrast, no difference in the rate of upper gastrointestinal tract colonization by *Candida* was found in a controlled study of oral AMB 800 mg per day, as prophylaxis with co-trimoxazole for leukemic patients undergoing remission induction chemotherapy (Dekker *et al.*, 1981). However, there was no disseminated *Candida* infections in either group, probably due to the administration of nystatin to both groups. Pizzo *et al.* (1982) evaluated the strategy of empiric AMB in addition to antibiotic therapy for patients undergoing cytotoxic chemotherapy with prolonged fever and neutropenia. In a daily dose of 0.5 mg per kg i.v., AMB appeared to prevent fungal superinfections. A comparison of fluconazole and AMB 500 mg orally, four times per day, in neutropenic patients, revealed equivalent efficacy in preventing invasive candidiasis. However, fluconazole was better tolerated (Menichetti *et al.*, 1994).

There have been two controlled trials of low dose i.v. AMB (0.1 mg per kg per day) for the prevention of invasive fungal disease. The first found no significant reduction in the rate of invasive disease, despite a significant reduction in the rate of oropharyngeal colonization of yeast (Perfect *et al.*, 1992), but the second did show a reduction in the frequency of invasive mycoses and the requirement for empiric AMB for febrile neutropenia (Riley *et al.*, 1992). Liposomal AMB at a dosage of 1 mg per kg per day, administered as prophylaxis when the neutrophil count decreased to $<500 \times 10^9$ per liter in bone marrow transplant recipients, was not associated with a significant reduction in proven fungal infections in a placebo-controlled trial. However, the number of patients enrolled was small, and there was a trend to reduced fungal infections (Tollemar *et al.*, 1993). In another placebo-controlled trial in liver transplant recipients, liposomal AMB at a dosage of 1 mg per kg daily for 5 days following transplantation, significantly reduced the incidence of invasive fungal infections, but did not prolong survival (Tollemar *et al.*, 1995).

Empiric administration of AMB to persistently febrile neutropenic patients is a strategy that allows early treatment for clinically occult fungal infection and also provides prophylaxis for those individuals at high risk for invasive mycoses. This approach is supported by both non-randomized studies (Stein *et al.*, 1982; Holleran *et al.*, 1985) and randomized trials (Pizzo *et al.*, 1982; EORTC, 1989) which consistently showed a significant reduction in fungal infections, in particular candidiasis. The subset of patients who derived most benefit from AMB in the EORTC study were those with less than 100 neutrophils per μl, and those who did not receive antifungal prophylaxis. Empiric AMB is usually instituted at a dose of 0.5–0.6 mg per kg per day. This dose appears to be inadequate for the pre-emptive treatment or prevention of invasive aspergillosis, trichosporonosis, or infection due to *Fusarium* spp. (Walsh *et al.*, 1991).

There are problems in assessing the results of trials of antifungal therapy in the prevention of invasive candidiasis and other mycoses, due to different dose regimens used, the paucity of placebo-controlled studies, and the different criteria selected by investigators for evaluation of the intervention. The most widely used drugs for prophylaxis are AMB, ketoconazole, fluconazole and itraconazole. The Working Party of the British Society for Antimicrobial Chemotherapy (1993) has published their recommendations for chemoprophylaxis for candidosis and aspergillosis. They recommend the use of fluconazole 50 mg per day orally in combination with selective digestive tract decontamination as primary prophylaxis for neutropenia, initiated when the neutrophil count falls below 1000 per μl and stopped when the neutrophil count is greater than 500 per μl or if empiric systemic AMB is given.

3 Aspergillosis

Inhalation of spores of *Aspergillus fumigatus* and other less common aspergilli such as *A. flavus*, *A. nidulans*, *A. niger*, *A. terreus*, *A. oryzae*, and *A. sydowi* can result in various pulmonary disorders, from colonization, allergy and tissue invasion. *Aspergillus* is a ubiquitous mold. Allergic aspergillosis comprises the syndromes of extrinsic allergic alveolitis, (malt worker's lung, farmer's lung), extrinsic asthma (baker's asthma) and allergic bronchopulmonary asthma due to *Apergillus fumigatus*. Treatment of these syndromes is symptomatic with bronchodilators, and with oral corticosteroids (Evans, 1979; Patterson *et al.*, 1982). The use of aerosolized antifungal agents for control of this disease has not been successful (Glimp and Bayer, 1981). For the other two forms of pulmonary aspergillosis, invasive aspergillosis and aspergilloma, AMB has been used with variable results.

Invasive aspergillosis is life-threatening and occurs primarily in the immunocompromised host (leukemia/lymphoma, bone marrow transplant, liver transplant, chronic granulomatous disease and AIDS). Acute rapidly progressive pneumonitis due to *Aspergillus* spp occurs in patients with prolonged and severe neutropenia (less than 100 cells per μl). These patients are also at risk for mucosal invasion of the nose or paranasal sinuses by *Aspergillus* which can spread to contiguous structures and invade blood vessels causing thrombosis and tissue necrosis. Cerebral vascular involvement will result in cerebral infarction with progression to cerebral abscess. Response to treatment varies with the type of host and antifungal regimen used. Extremely poor response rates of 5–10% have been seen in bone marrow transplant patients, aplastic anemia and liver transplant recipients treated with AMB for at least 14 days. Amphotericin B is effective in 60–70% of leukemia patients who recover from neutropenia, and heart and renal transplant recipients (Denning and Stevens, 1990; Burton *et al.*,1972; Pennington, 1976). Aisner *et al.*, (1977) argued for aggressive attempts to establish an early diagnosis of aspergillosis, thereby allowing early treatment with AMB, and improved outcome.

Denning and Stevens (1990) have reviewed the management of the varied clinical manifestations of aspergillosis in detail. Most cases of aspergillosis are treated initially as a presumptive diagnosis, particularly in patients with prolonged severe neutropenia. The 'gold standard' of primary treatment for invasive aspergillosis is AMB at a dose of 1–1.25 mg per kg per day. This dose is often poorly tolerated because of AMB-induced nephrotoxicity compounded by the use of other nephrotoxic agents, but the target dose should be 0.8–1.0 mg per kg per day. The overall response rate for AMB has been reported from 30 to 35% in an intention to treat analsysis (Denning, 1994) to 55% in Denning and Stevens' review of published cases.

The lipid-associated AMB preparations have been studied in patients with aspergillosis, in an attempt to reduce nephrotoxicity but still deliver adequate AMB to the sites of infection. liposomal B (5 mg per kg per day) therapy was associated with a 67% (four of six cases) response rate in documented cases of invasive aspergillosis in neutropenic patients, 32% response rate for proven invasive pulmonary aspergillosis in immunocompromised patients (Ringden *et al.*, 1991) and a 44% (11 of 25 cases) response rate in unconfirmed cases empirically treated (Chopra *et al.*,1992). The clinical efficacy of ABCD for the treatment of invasive aspergillosis was reported as 16% cure rate and 19% improvement in a trial utilizing 4 mg per kg per day, and the response rate appeared to correlate with the degree and duration of neutropenia (Oppenheim *et al.*, 1995). There are no data published on the efficacy of ABLC for the treatment of invasive aspergillosis, and there are also no controlled trial data available comparing the efficacy of AMB and the liposomal preparations of AMB.

In patients with prolonged and profound neutropenia AMB has been used empirically to treat presumptive occult fungal infection. In this situation the dose used is 0.5–0.6 mg per kg and continued until neutropenia resolves. Unfortunately, many patients develop invasive pulmonary aspergillosis while receiving AMB 0.5–0.6 mg per kg per day. Patients with symptoms or signs consistent with invasive aspergillosis should undergo extensive diagnostic procedures to document infection, even in the setting of neutrophil recovery. If invasive aspergillosis is confirmed, some authorities recommend that a total dose of 1.5–2 g AMB be administered, while others recommend that treatment should continue until a clinical and radiological response is achieved (Denning, 1994). Patients who recover from an episode of aspergillosis have a greater than 50% chance of relapse during another period of cytotoxic chemotherapy-induced neutropenia, and should receive empiric systemic AMB as secondary prophylaxis. This should be instituted either at the onset of a neutropenic fever (Robertson and Larson, 1988) or at the start of cytotoxic chemotherapy. Karp *et al.* (1988) successively used prophylactic AMB at a dose of 1 mg per kg in combination with 5-flucytosine, initiated 48 h after cytotoxic chemotherapy and continued until neutrophil recovery to prevent relapse of invasive aspergillosis.

Because of the poor overall efficacy achieved using AMB alone, and the potential synergy with 5-flucytosine against *Aspergillus* spp. observed *in vitro* and in animal models, combination therapy with these two drugs has been examined. Codish *et al.* (1979) combined AMB and 5-flucytosine successfully to treat a case of *Aspergillus* pneumonia, and good response rates were also obtained in leukemia patients (58%) and renal transplant patients (82%) (Denning and Stevens, 1990). Theoretical concerns about prolonging recovery time of cytotoxic chemotherapy-induced neutropenia have not been justified by clinical observation, if serum levels of 5-flucytosine are maintained in the therapeutic range. It has been suggested that the combination of AMB and 5-flucytosine would have a role in the management of cerebral or meningeal aspergillosis where the penetration of AMB into the brain is poor, and endocarditis because the penetration of AMB into vegetations is also poor, but the tissue penetration of 5-flucytosine is good (Denning, 1994). The combination of rifampin and AMB has been shown to be synergistic both *in vitro* and in animal models, but this combination has practical problems in the clinical setting, due to rifampin induction of the P-450 enzyme system, and the subsequent metabolism of cyclosporin and other drugs. Itraconazole has been shown to be effective for the treatment of invasive aspergillosis (Denning *et al.*, 1989), but there has not been a controlled trial comparing its efficacy with AMB. Itraconazole is useful oral therapy to complete a course of treatment for aspergillosis initiated with AMB.

The risk of development of invasive pulmonary aspergillosis is proportional to the duration of neutropenia and peaks at 70% risk after 34 days of neutropenia (Gerson *et al.*, 1984) and response to therapy also appears to be related to the duration of neutropenia, with greater efficacy of AMB achieved in those with shorter episodes of profound neutropenia (Denning and Stevens, 1990). Recent randomized placebo-controlled studies have confirmed the lack of efficacy of fluconazole for the prophylaxis of aspergillosis in bone marrow transplant and leukemia patients (Winston *et al.*, 1993; Goodman *et al.*, 1992). The increasing use of fluconazole for antifungal prophylaxis during neutropenia is likely to result in an increased incidence of aspergillosis and the importance of other forms of prophylaxis such as intranasal and aerosolized AMB for the prevention of invasive pulmonary aspergillosis. In non-randomized studies of the intranasal administration of AMB using historical controls, this delivery of AMB was thought to reduce the frequency of invasive aspergillosis (Meunier-Carpenter *et al.*, 1984; Jeffrey *et al.*, 1991). Meunier (1989) documented a statistically significant reduction in cases of invasive aspergillosis in a prospective randomized trial of AMB nasal spray, 10 mg three times daily; but a randomized study revealed that intranasal administration of AMB aerosol reduced the nasal colonization with aspergillus, but did not reduce the incidence of invasive aspergillosis (Cushing *et al.*, 1991).

Aerosol application of AMB has been shown to prevent invasive pulmonary aspergillosis in animal models, (Schmitt *et al.*, 1988b) and in non-randomized trials in humans (Conneally *et al.*, 1990; Beyer *et al.*, 1993). A prospective randomized trial of prophylactic AMB 10 mg aerosol inhaled twice-daily versus no inhalation, in patients with prolonged neutropenia, failed to detect any reduction in the incidence of possible, probable or proven invasive pulmonary aspergillosis at the interim analysis. Larger numbers of patients will be required to be randomized to definitively rule out any prophylactic efficacy for this strategy (Behre *et al.*, 1995). Theoretically, delivery of the AMB to the alveoli where the aspergillus conidia are located would seem to be most appropriate, and this is more effectively achieved by aerosolization than by systemic administration (Niki *et al.*, 1990). Another uncontrolled study of oral intraconazole 200 mg per day and nasal AMB 10 mg per day showed a reduction in aspergillosis infections using historical controls from the one institution (Todeschini *et al.*, 1993). McWhinney *et al.* (1993) evaluated their experience of aspergillosis in bone marrow transplantation over 13 years and found graft rejection was a significant predisposing risk factor for the development of invasive aspergillosis, and recommended i.v. AMB (1 mg per kg every 3rd day) prophylaxis in patients with graft rejection.

Aspergillomas occur as a late complication of invasive pulmonary aspergillosis (primary) or follow colonization of pre-existing pulmonary cavities (secondary). Up to 10% of aspergillomas resolve without treatment (Hammerman *et al.*, 1973b). One prospective study determined that systemic AMB was no more effective than regular pulmonary toilet alone (Hammerman *et al.*, 1974). However, systemic AMB is indicated for those with locally invasive disease (chronic necrotizing aspergillosis) and systemic symptoms (Binder *et al.*, 1982). Surgical resection is often recommended for pulmonary aspergillomas, particularly when associated with a chronic cough and hemoptysis (Evans, 1979), but surgery may not be possible because of underlying chronic pulmonary disease. Hargis *et al.* (1980) obtained improvement in four of six patients with symptomatic pulmonary aspergillomas by the use of percutaneous instillation of intracavitary AMB. The initial dose was 5 mg diluted in 10–20ml of 5% dextrose and subsequent daily doses were increased by 10 mg per day until 50 mg was reached. Thereafter 50 mg was instilled two to three times per week to a total dose of 500 mg. Alternative approaches to repeated injections which increase the risk of complications are the instillation of an intracavitary catheter for instillation of daily AMB 50 mg (Cochrane *et al.*, 1991) and the instillation into the cavity of a gel containing AMB (Munk *et al.*, 1993). (See intracavitary instillation, p. 1256)

There is an increasing incidence of invasive aspergillosis in AIDS patients, 50% of whom will not have the characteristic risk factors of neutropenia and administration of high-dose corticosteroids. The majority of patients will be severely immunocompromised with CD4 cell counts below 50 per μl. (Lorthelary *et al.*, 1993). As in other immunocompromised hosts, the diagnosis is often difficult to confirm antemortem and histological diagnosis is often replaced with presumptive diagnosis on culture of bronchoalveolar lavage. Treatment with AMB or intraconazole is generally not associated with good response rates. In AIDS patients with advanced disease, AMB is poorly tolerated and oral itraconazole has erratic absorption in this population, requiring the availability of measurement of serum levels. Lortholary *et al.* (1993) were unable to correlate clinical outcome with serum levels of itraconazole, but the numbers were small. Patients with AIDS should receive chronic suppressive therapy following recovery from invasive aspergillosis with intraconazole or AMB for life.

Aspergillus endocarditis, which usually occurs after open-heart surgery, has a high mortality due to delayed diagnosis as blood cultures are rarely positive. Treatment with medical therapy alone is almost always unsuccessful. As AMB poorly penetrates vegetations, the combined use of AMB and 5-flucytosine may be of benefit. There are no data available on the penetration of 5-flucytosine or intraconazole into cardiac vegetations. Denning and Stevens (1990) review of published cases of *Aspergillus* endocarditis found that 43% of patients survived following a combined medical and surgical approach to therapy with valve replacement. One patient with *Aspergillus* endocarditis was cured with a combination of surgery, AMB, and long-term therapy with 5-flucytosine (Carrizosa *et al.*, 1974).

Aspergillus osteomyelitis is a rare infection acquired either hematogenously following surgery or trauma, or by direct extension from sinus or cerebral disease. Immunocompetent patients have better response rates to therapy with AMB, and a combined medical and surgical approach is associated with improved outcome. Because AMB poorly penetrates bone, surgical intervention is recommended (Denning and Stevens, 1990). The addition of 5-flucytosine to AMB treatment appears effective (Tack *et al.*, 1982), possibly due to the good bone penetration of 5-flucytosine.

4 Histoplasmosis

Although AMB remains an effective treatment for histoplasmosis, it may be replaced by itraconazole for the management of mild cases (p. 1435). Acute pulmonary histoplasmosis does not usually require specific treatment, but if symptomatic and the patient is intolerant of azoles, then low total doses of AMB (150–500 mg) have been used successfully (Sarosi *et al.*, 1979). If the acute pulmonary infection is associated with acute respiratory distress syndrome, or if symptomatic acute disease persists for more than 2–3 weeks in adults, AMB 0.7–1.0 mg per kg daily for 2–3 weeks is recommended (Goodwin and Des Prez, 1978). In infants and children, acute histoplasmosis may be severe and has a greater tendency to dissemination. Fosson and Wheeler (1975) used AMB in six children with acute disease and obtained a favorable response. A maximum daily dose (1 mg per kg per day) was reached rapidly by the 3rd day and was continued for short periods of 7–19 days. Therapy with AMB is always required for disseminated histoplasmosis, especially in the immune compromised host, as mortality rates observed in untreated patients are greater than 80%. The recommended adult total dose of 35–40 mg per kg body weight achieved clinical cure in 90% of patients (Sarosi *et al.*, 1971), while for infants 1 mg per kg per day for 6 weeks is recommended (Goodwin and Des Prez, 1978). A lower dose of 25–35 mg per day for adults, a dose tailored to provide a serum concentration of twice the MIC of the organism has been used (Drutz *et al.*, 1968).

Wheat *et al.* (1990) have reviewed disseminated histoplasmosis in AIDS, and report AMB as highly effective with responses in 80% patients. Clinical responses were observed in half the patients within 5 days of starting induction treatment with AMB. Total doses of 1–2 g or 15 mg per kg body weight have been used in induction regimens (McKinsey *et al.*, 1989; Wheat *et al.*, 1990). Without chronic suppressive treatment after successful induction therapy, 60–80% of patients will relapse (Wheat *et al.*, 1990). AMB administered as 50–80 mg weekly or bi-weekly, has been associated with low relapse rates of 3–19% in small open series, and appears to be more effective than ketoconazole with reported relapse rates of 50% (Wheat *et al.*, 1990; McKinsey *et al.*, 1989, 1992). McKinsey *et al.*, (1992) recommend bi-weekly AMB maintenance treatment, via a peripheral catheter because of its efficacy and tolerability at this dosing interval. There is an extremely high rate of central venous catheter-related bacteremias and thrombophlebitis associated with long-term catheter placement in the AIDS patients. Wheat *et al.* (1990) recommend a maintenance regimen of AMB 50 mg weekly after completion of an induction regimen of 15 mg per kg body weight. Itraconazole may replace AMB for maintenance treatment, and in some cases primary treatment of AIDS, in particular in those with central nervous system involvement (Wheat, 1994).

African histoplasmosis responds to AMB given i.v. (Egere *et al.*, 1978). This disease, due to *Histoplasma duboisii*, is usually localized causing subacute granuloma of the skin or bone, but dissemination can occur.

5 Blastomycosis

The description of a self-limited pulmonary blastomycosis has resulted in a difference of opinion concerning treatment of acute pulmonary infection, with some authors recommending withholding treatment and observation for 2 weeks (Sarosi *et al.*, 1986; Bradsher, 1992) and others recommending treatment for all patients because of the risk of acute pulmonary exacerbations and chronic extrapulmonary disease (Chapman, 1995). The drug of choice is AMB for immunocompromised patients, those with severe life-threatening disease or central nervous system infection. The rates of cure without relapse associated with at least 1 g AMB, range from 78 to 91%, from five large series (Bradsher,1988). A total dose of 1.5–2.0 g is recommended to prevent relapse. In one series, two of 30 patients treated with 1.5 g AMB relapsed compared with five of 19 patients who received smaller doses (Parker *et al.*, 1969). Immunocompromised patients should receive at least 1 g AMB, followed by at least 6 months of oral azole therapy (Pappas *et al.*, 1993). Powell and Schuit (1979) advocate that all children with blastomycosis should be treated with AMB, and not observed for self-limiting infection. Ketoconazole has been shown to be effective for treatment of blastomycosis in immunocompetent hosts (responses of 80–90%) (p. 1375), and itraconazole has shown excellent results also. No comparative trials with AMB have been performed. Itraconazole will replace AMB for the primary treatment of uncomplicated non life-threatening blastomycosis in the immunocompetent host (p. 1436).

6 Coccidioidomycosis

Therapy is usually not required for most patients with primary pulmonary infection, unless the patient has a severe symptomatic infection, persistent symptoms for greater than 6 weeks, or underlying disease or immunodeficiency which is associated with an increased risk of chronic or disseminated disease. Treatment of persistent coccidioidal pneumonia or chronic progressive cavitary pulmonary disease has traditionally been with i.v. AMB 1–1.5 mg per kg per day initially, then 1–1.5 mg per kg three times weekly to a total dose of 1–2.5 g (Drutz, 1983) in combination with assessment for the need of surgical removal of cavitary disease. In pulmonary coccidioidomycosis the recommended total dose is arbitrary, ranging from 0.5 to 2.5 g, depending on disease severity. There are currently no controlled trials comparing AMB with the azole drugs which are more tolerable for the long courses of therapy required (6–12 months), and show promise in open non-comparative studies. Extrapulmonary disease always requires treatment. Disseminated disease is subject to spontaneous exacerbations and remissions, so that the effect of chemotherapy may be difficult to assess. Immunocompromised HIV-infected patients with reticulonodular pulmonary infiltrates are usually acutely unwell and should be treated with i.v. AMB. Even with this treatment, 70% patients in one series died with a median survival of 1 month (Galgiani and Ampel, 1990).

One form of dissemination, meningitis, is uniformly fatal within 2 years without treatment (Drutz and Catanzaro, 1978). Management of coccidioidal meningitis presents special problems. AMB penetrates poorly into CSF, and obstruction of the flow of CSF causing non-communicating hydrocephalus may occur. Because of the difficulty in eradication of this infection, therapy may be required for years or for life. Direct administration of AMB into the CSF is recommended in addition to i.v. AMB (0.5–1.0 g). Administration by the lumbar route involves suspension of 0.5 mg AMB in 5 ml of hypertonic saline and the patient tilted on a table to ensure delivery of the drug to the basilar area. Hydrocortisone 25 mg is commonly co-administered to reduce the local reactions and complications which limit this form of treatment. Injections of AMB into the cisterna magna deliver AMB closest to the main site of infection, the basilar meninges, but are hazardous because of the development of drug-related arachnoiditis or neurotoxicity. Therefore AMB is usually administered intraventricularly by means of an Ommaya reservoir. This reservoir is particularly useful when there is evidence of spread to the ventricular system and obstruction of CSF flow. Dosage and duration of intraventricular therapy depend on the response of the infection, but in some cases suppressive therapy given directly into the CSF may be needed for years or for life (Drutz and Catanzaro, 1978; Bouza *et al.*, 1981). Treatment regimens begin with doses of 0.01 mg and gradual dose escalation to 1.5 mg as tolerated. The AMB is administered three times weekly for either 3 months or until the CSF leukocyte count is less than 10 cells per mm^3, then reduced to once-weekly for several months, and gradually tapered to once every 1–6 weeks. The CSF is regularly reviewed for evidence of relapse, at which time the frequency of intrathecal administrations would be increased again. Therapy is continued for at least 1 year after normalization of CSF parameters (Holeman and Johnson, 1976).

Chronic articular coccidiodal arthritis is managed with systemic chemotherapy with either i.v. AMB or one of the azole drugs, combined with synovectomy, immobilization and intra-articular AMB (Greenman *et al.*, 1975). For large joints, doses of 15–50 mg have been instilled intra-articularly three times a week for 2 weeks, then weekly for 6 weeks, followed by intra-articular injections every 2 weeks for 4 months (Aidem, 1968). Doses of 5–15 mg injected into joint spaces is generally recommended.

7 Paracoccidioidomycosis

This mycosis, restricted to Latin America and South America, is difficult to treat and AMB alone is not curative. Treatment with AMB is reserved for those with severe disease or those not responding to oral therapy, and total doses of 1.2–3.0 g have been employed. This is followed by maintenance sulphonamide or azole therapy (principally ketoconazole or itraconazole). Response rates to AMB with sulphonamide or ketoconazole therapy are 65–70%, with a high mortality rate of up to 25–30% (Dillon *et al.*, 1986; Goldani and Sugar, 1996). The response rate to AMB 0.5–0.75 mg per kg daily for 3–4 months is 47% and without sulfonamide maintenance treatment the relapse rate is 38% (Brummer *et al.*, 1993). Itraconazole is the drug of choice for patients with both mild and severe disease, although some authors advocate early aggressive treatment with AMB (Goldani and Sugar, 1996) (p. 1437).

8 Penicillium marneffei infections

This fungus, endemic to South-East Asia and Southern China, causes infections in both immunocompetent and immunocompromised hosts. It is a common opportunistic infection in HIV-infected individuals in these areas. Treatment with AMB to a total cumulative dose of 40 mg per kg was associated with a 75% response rate in AIDS patients (Supparatpinyo *et al.*, 1992).

Lau *et al.* (1992) described a case of recurrent disseminated *Penicillium marneffei* infection in a 17-year-old boy with a natural killer cell defect, who despite repeated prolonged courses of AMB (total dose >5 g), had progressive disease. All bone, lymph node and soft tissue masses resolved on oral fluconazole therapy.

9 Mucormycosis (zygomycosis, phycomycosis)

The name zygomycosis designates all fungal infections by two orders of the class Zygomycetes (Phycomycetes), namely the Mucorales and the Entomophthorales. Mucormycosis is a severe disease, occurs in compromised hosts, and principally affects rhinocerebral, pulmonary or gastrointestinal blood vessels. Disseminated disease usually results from progression of infection from the lungs to multiple organs, and occurs in the severely immunocompromised patient such as acute leukemia, bone marrow transplantation or diabetes, and is associated with a high mortality rate. A cutaneous form is usually associated with minor trauma and diabetes, although a well documented outbreak due to contaminated elastic bandages has been reported (Gartenberg *et al.*, 1978; Lehrer *et al.*, 1980).

Mucormycosis may be caused by seven pathogenic families of the order Mucorales; the Mucoraceae, Cunninghamellaceae, Saksenaeaceae, Mortierellaceae, Syncephalastracae, Apophysomyceae and Thamnidiceae. The Mucoraceae includes the genera *Absidia*, *Mucor*, *Rhizomucor* and *Rhizopus*, which are the most commonly isolated causes of mucormycosis. Invasive mucormycosis is relatively refractory to medical treatment alone, and successful treatment requires reversal of the underlying predisposing condition (acidosis in the diabetic, neutropenia or immunosuppression in the transplant or leukemic patient), aggressive surgical debridement of necrotic tissue and systemic antifungal therapy (Parfrey, 1986; Rinaldi, 1989; Weinberg *et al.*, 1993; Kontoyianis *et al.*, 1994). Invasive mucormycosis manifests as rhinocerebral disease (includes oculomycosis), pulmonary disease, or rarely, central nervous system disease. To date AMB remains the most reliable agent for the mucormycoses.

Following a 1-mg test dose, the dose of AMB should be escalated rapidly until 0.70–1.0 mg per kg is reached. Most patients will require doses of 0.7–1.0 mg per kg continued until stabilization of the disease process, when alternate day AMB administration at the same dose is started. The duration of treatment required is not known and should be individualized to the patient's clinical response. Hamill *et al.* (1983) recommend that after an accumulated dose of 1500 mg AMB, biopsy specimens should be taken after each 500–750 mg increment. If there is histological evidence of continued infection, surgical debridement and AMB therapy should be continued. Although there is *in vitro* data suggesting synergistic activity against *Rhizopus* species for AMB and rifampin (Christenson *et al.*, 1987) there is no evidence that the addition of rifampin or flucytosine is useful for the clinical management of mucormycosis. Liposomal AMB has been used sucessfully to treat rhinocerebral mucormycosis, in one case with 3 mg per kg alternate days for 8 months (Ericsson *et al.*, 1993), and 3 mg per kg per day for 4 weeks in another case (Munckhof *et al.*, 1993) combined with extensive surgical debridement. In general, the outcome of infection with a member of the Mucorales (e.g. *Cunninghamella* spp.) is discouraging, even with treatment with high dose AMB and extensive surgical debridement, and reversal of the underlying cause of immunosuppression (Cohen-Abbo *et al.*, 1993).

Short courses using lower doses of i.v. AMB have been used with good results to treat children with cutaneous and gastrointestinal mucormycosis (Dennis *et al.*, 1980), and patients with primary cutaneous involvement secondary to trauma, may require only local debridement and topical AMB. Systemic AMB should be administered if there is any progression of infection beyond the skin.

Entomophthoromycosis is a fungal infection caused by Zygomycetes of the order Entomophthorales due to the genera *Basidiobolus* and *Conidiobolus*. This infection most commonly occurs in tropical Africa and Asia, usually in otherwise healthy persons. Disease due to *Basidiobolus* causes non-necrotic painless subcutaneous lesions which may regress spontaneously, but are usually slowly progressive. Disease due to *Conidiobolus* is manifest as nodular swelling which originates from around the nose and spreads to contiguous areas, resulting in generalized facial swelling without constitutional symptoms (Martinson, 1972). Although AMB has been used for the treatment of entomophthoromycosis, its activity *in vivo* has not been compared with other active agents including the azoles. Yangco *et al.* (1984) found AMB effective by *in vitro* testing for *Conidiobolus* infections but not as effective for entomophthoromycosis due to *Basidiobolus*, but *in vitro* susceptibility testing may not be reliable.

10 Fusarium infections

Fusarium species cause life-threatening disseminated infections in severely immunocompromised patients, and are associated with poor outcome in the persistently neutropenic patient. They are also the most common cause of fungal keratitis. In the murine model of fusarial infection, AMB administered intraperitoneally in doses up to 2 mg per kg daily, was not effective in treating disseminated fusarium infection, despite *in vitro* susceptibility to AMB of 1.56 μg per ml (Anaisse *et al.*, 1992). Successful outcome in human infections is primarily related to recovery from neutropenia. In high dosage (1 mg per kg per day), AMB is the treatment of choice, but is usually not effective in persistently neutropenic patients. Amphotericin B lipid complex administered at a dose of 5 mg per kg to a severely neutropenic patient with disseminated *Fusarium* infection, successfully controlled the infection with resolution of clinical symptoms and signs, while the patient remained neutropenic (<100 neutrophils per ml). There was no recurrence of infection during the consolidation course of chemotherapy 1 month later during which neutropenia occurred again (Wolff and Ramphal, 1995). Ellis *et al.* (1994) report the development of localized cutaneous *Fusarium* infection without evidence of wider dissemination, in a bone marrow transplant patient during the period of profound neutropenia. A successful outcome was achieved with initial AMB 1 mg per kg per day for 1 week, followed by liposomal AMB 3 mg per kg per day for 4 weeks, granulocyte-macrophage colony stimulating factor (GM-CSF) to aid neutrophil recovery, and surgical excision of the fungal lesion.

11 Trichosporon infections

Infection with *Trichosporon beigelii* has been reported with increasing frequency over the last 10 years, in severely immunocompromised patients with hematologic malignancies, especially those with prolonged profound neutropenia (Hoy *et al.*, 1986). Infection due to *Blastoschizomyces capitatus* (*Trichosporon capitatum*) is much less common. Although *in vitro* testing of *T. beigelii* isolates suggest susceptibility to AMB, *in vivo* responses to AMB treatment have been uniformly disappointing in the retrospective studies reported (Hoy *et al.*, 1986; Walsh *et al.*, 1986). However, Walsh *et al.*, (1990) reported some *T. beigelii* isolates which were inhibited, but not killed by clinically achievable concentrations of AMB, and animal studies (persistently neutropenic rabbit model of trichosporonosis) have shown that maximally tolerated doses of AMB (1.2 mg per kg), AMB plus 5-flucytosine, and liposomal AMB (5 mg per kg) had no *in vivo* antifungal effect (Walsh *et al.*, 1992). Successful treatment of invasive disseminated disease with *T. beigelii* with AMB appears to be primarily related to recovery of neutropenia (Hoy *et al.*, 1986).

Trichosporon beigelii endocarditis has been reported in non-immunocompromised patients, although it is a rare cause of fungal endocarditis. The combination of AMB and 5-flucytosine was used to treat a patient with a *T. beigelii* prosthetic valve endocarditis, in whom the diagnosis was delayed and the patient died. Combinations of AMB with 5-flucytosine and rifampicin were synergistic against the isolate cultured (Marier *et al.*, 1978). Brahn and Leonard (1982) described another patient with aortic valve infection due to *T. beigelii,* who recovered after prosthetic valve replacement and treatment with AMB and 5-flucytosine. Martinez Lacasa *et al.* (1991) described a case of *T. beigelii* endocarditis who survived for 4 years with prolonged multiple courses of AMB, combined with two prosthetic valve replacements, but died of multiple septic complications of the infection. Postoperative infection with *T. beigelii* causing endophthalmitis, was unsuccessfully treated with AMB and the patient lost the sight in the involved eye (Sheikh *et al.*, 1974).

Disseminated infection with *Blastoschizomyces capitatus* (*Trichosporon capitatum*) developed in a neutropenic patient with acute leukemia, and an allogeneic bone marrow transplant complicated by graft-versus-host disease, who was treated with fluconazole 150 mg daily for oropharyngeal candidiasis. Treatment with AMB, initially at 0.5 mg per kg, then increased to 1 mg per kg daily failed to control the infection in this persistently neutropenic patient (Liu *et al.*, 1990). Treatment of disseminated infection with *Blastoschizomyces capitatus* also appears to depend on neutrophil recovery.

12 Infections due to Pseudallescheria boydii (Petriellidium boydii, and asexual spore form Scedosporium apiospermum)

Infection generally follows penetrating trauma and results in localized infection of bone, subcutaneous tissue, joint or the eye with extension to the central nervous system. In the profoundly neutropenic patient, disseminated pseudallescheriasis resembles aspergillosis. This fungus is resistant to clinically achievable concentrations of both AMB and 5-flucytosine (Lutwick *et al.*, 1976) and surgical drainage and debridement of necrotic tissue is the mainstay of treatment in localized disease in the non-immunocompromised patient. Miconazole is considered the drug of choice for treatment of *Pseudallescheria boydii* (p. 1454). Hayden *et al.* (1977) described a boy with a monoarticular arthritis of the knee due to *Pseudallescheria boydii*, which responded to treatment with intra-articular injections of AMB. A series of cases of endophthalmitis due to *Pseudallescheria boydii* reported by McGuire *et al.* (1991) revealed that the majority were exogenous infections. Twelve of the 17 patients received AMB, and five of the 12 were changed to miconazole after poor response or microbiological identification of the fungus. Of those that received AMB as the sole systemic antifungal agent, six patients survived with either enucleation of the eye or significant visual defect.

13 Chromoblastomycosis (Chromomycosis)

This fungal disease which occurs most commonly in tropical and subtropical regions, is caused by dematiaceous fungi such as *Fonsecaea pedrosoi*, *Cladosporium carrionii*, and *Phialophora verrucosa*. It is difficult to treat and the causative fungi are often resistant to AMB. There have been reports of successful treatment using i.v. AMB (Gugnani *et al.*, 1978), and it has been administered both i.v., topically and intralesionly (Restrepo, 1994). 5-Flucytosine (p. 1312) may be effective in this disease, and is synergistic in combination with AMB. Recommended treatment in adults is AMB 50 mg i.v. on alternate days, with 5-flucytosine 70–100 mg per kg in four divided doses daily, for a total duration of 6–12 months (Restrepo, 1994).

14 Phaeohyphomycosis

There are four forms of phaehyphomycosis – superficial infection, cutaneous or corneal disease, subcutaneous infection and systemic disease (Fader and McGinnis (1988). It can be caused by many of the dematiaceous fungi. Infections caused by *Bipolaris* and *Exserhilum* have been reviewed by Adam *et al.* (1986) and include disseminated disease in the immunocompromised host characterized by vascular invasion and tissue necrosis, osteomyelitis, meningoencephalitis, sinusitis, peritonitis in association with continuous ambulatory peritoneal dialysis, keratitis and allergic bronchopulmonary disease. For these infections, AMB is the treatment of choice and treatment should include surgical debridement of locally invasive disease. *Wangiella dermatitidis* (*Exophiala dermatitidis*, *Phialophora dermatitidis*) usually causes skin and subcutaneous infections, and rarely causes bacteremia, pulmonary disease and endocarditis. Vartian *et al.* (1985) reported a case of native valve endocarditis, treated with AMB, ketoconazole and rifampin for 8 weeks. However, relapse occurred 5 months later, valve replacement and AMB for 2 months controlled the infection, until *W. dermatitidis* was isolated from a lumbar disc space. Although AMB, rifampin and ketoconazole were resumed they were unable to eradicate the infection. Cases of *Phialophora parasitica* have been reviewed by Wong *et al.* (1989) and treatment with AMB elicited poor or no response. Cutaneous and subcutaneous disease due to *Exophiala* species should be managed with surgical excision, while the most effective treatment for deep-seated infection is uncertain. Case reports of successful treatment with AMB, 5-flucytosine and ketoconazole have been reviewed by Sudduth *et al.* (1992). Cutaneous alternariosis was eradicated with intralesional AMB 1 mg per ml twice-weekly over 5 weeks, in an elderly woman who presented with symptoms of 5 years duration (Iwatsu, 1988).

15 Sporotrichosis

Combined with surgical resection, AMB is recommended for systemic, articular, or pulmonary forms of sporotrichosis. Potassium iodide was found to be ineffective for pulmonary and systemic disease, and AMB alone cured only 35% of cases reported in the literature. Total surgical resection is the most effective therapy for pulmonary sporotrichosis (Pluss and Opal, 1986). Total doses of AMB between 2 and 3 g are recommended as primary therapy or in treatment failures. However, medical therapy alone has been disappointing in the majority of cases (Pluss and Opal, 1986). Unfortunately, AMB is not effective for the milder cutaneous or lymphocutaneous infections, which usually respond to orally administered potassium iodide. Itraconazole is recommended for those that are intolerant or resistant to potassium iodide (Sarosi *et al.*, 1979, Restrepo 1994) (p. 1438).

16 Hansenula anomala infection

The organism is a yeast belonging to the class Ascomycetes, and is a rare cause of infection. Reports in the literature suggest it causes a fungemia, often catheter-related, in immunocompromised patients. An outbreak in a neonatal intensive care unit involved eight neonates (Murphy *et al.*, 1986). Most patients respond to either AMB alone, or AMB plus 5-flucytosine. The total dose of AMB required for response varied from 132 mg in catheter-related fungemia, to 2 g in a patient with endocarditis. Removal of an infected venous catheter may also be important in determining outcome (Haron *et al.*, 1988; Klein *et al.*, 1988; Sekhon *et al.*, 1992b).

17 Paecilomyces sp. infections

Infections caused by this species are rare and usually associated with immunosuppression or the presence of a foreign body. Treatment has been disappointing, especially for endocarditis which is almost always fatal. Williamson *et al.* (1992) reported a case of *Paecilomyces varioti* soft tissue infection in a child with chronic granulomatous disease, who was cured following AMB treatment for 7 weeks (total dose 40 mg per kg) then oral itraconazole for 1 year.

18 Protothecosis

This rare human infection caused by the unicellular algae, *Prototheca wickerhamii* or *Prototheca zopfi*, is usually manifest as cutaneous infection or olecranon bursitis, and is associated with trauma, or exposure to contaminated water (Cochran *et al.*, 1986). Olecranon bursitis was successfully treated with intrabursal instillation of AMB at a dose of 2 mg once-weekly for 6 weeks (Cochran *et al.*, 1986). Some cases of cutaneous protothecosis have responded to i.v. AMB alone, but surgical excision is also recommended (Vanezio *et al.*, 1982). *Prototheca wickerhamii* peritonitis in a patient undergoing chronic ambulatory peritoneal dialysis was successfully treated with Tenckhoff catheter removal, i.v. AMB and oral doxycycline (Sands *et al.*, 1991).

19 Primary amebic meningoencephalitis

This infection, due to *Naegleria fowleri*, is usually rapidly fatal, and of the hundred cases described there have only been five survivors (Seidel *et al.*, 1982; Poungvarin and Jariya, 1991). Of these patients, four were treated with i.v. AMB and one of these received AMB intrathecally. More recent reports confirm that even with early initiation of treatment with i.v. and intraventricular AMB the disease is usually fatal (Stevens *et al.*, 1981). The fourth patient to survive received high doses of AMB both i.v. and intrathecally plus miconazole i.v. and intrathecally, plus oral rifampicin, and the fifth patient received the combination of i.v. AMB 0.5 mg per kg per day for 14 days, and 1 month of oral rifampicin and ketoconazole. Chemotherapy using AMB, rifampicin, miconazole, and tetracycline in various combinations, and given intraventricularly when feasible has been recommended for this disease (Thong, 1982).

20 Leishmaniasis

Visceral leishmaniasis (Kala-azar) is an important opportunistic infection in the immunocompromised host, including HIV-infected individuals, in whom the response rate to antimony is less than 75% and the relapse rate is as high as 40% (Montalban *et al.*, 1990). Patients who have failed to respond to pentavalent antimonial compounds, or in whom drug-resistance has developed, can be successfully treated with AMB 0.5 mg per kg daily or 1 mg per kg alternate days for up to 8 weeks (Moskovskij and Southgate, 1971). In a randomized trial comparing the efficacy of AMB and pentamidine for leishmaniasis unresponsive to antimony, AMB treatment was associated with a 98% cure rate at 6 months following completion of therapy (Mishra *et al.*, 1992). Also AMB is an effective alternative for those individuals who have failed or relapsed following antimony treatment for mucocutaneous leishmaniasis (American cutaneous leishmaniasis) due to *L. mexicana* or *L. braziliansis*. A dose of 0.5 mg per kg daily or 1 mg per kg alternate days to a total dose of 1.5–2 g is indicated (Crofts, 1976). Liposomal AMB and ABCD have been shown to have superior efficacy and reduced toxicity in recent studies (Croft *et al.*, 1991; Davidson *et al.*, 1991), and the recommended regimen for 'Amphocil' (ABCD) is 2 mg per kg per day for 7 days. No relapses occurred in 12 months follow-up (Dietze *et al.*, 1995). Seaman *et al.* (1995) have suggested that the optimal regimen of liposomal AMB for visceral leishmaniasis complicated by relapse after antimony treatment or resistance to antimony is administration of 4 mg per kg on days 0,3,6,8,10 and 13. Amphotericin B lipid complex has also been used successfully (apparent 100% cure rate) at a dose of 3 mg per kg per day for 5 days in patients who did not respond or relapsed after 4–8 weeks of pentavalent antimony therapy (Sunder and Murray, 1996).

References

Adam RD, Paquin ML, Petersen EA *et al.* (1986). Phaeohyphomycosis caused by the fungal genera *Bipolaris* and *Exserohilum*. A report of 9 cases and review of the literature. *Medicine* **65**: 203.

Aguado JM, Hidalgo M, Moya I *et al.* (1993). Ventricular arrhythmias with conventional and liposomal amphotericin. *Lancet* **342**: 1239.

Aidem HP (1968). Intra-articular amphotericin B in the treatment of coccidioidal arthritis of the knee. *J Bone Joint Surg* **50A**: 1663.

Aisner J, Schimpff SC, Wiernik PH (1977). Treatment of invasive aspergillosis: relation of early diagnosis and treatment to response. *Ann Intern Med* **86**: 539.

Alazraki NP, Fierer J, Halpern SE, Becker RW (1974). Use of a hyperbaric solution for administration of intrathecal amphotericin B. *New Engl J Med* **290**: 641.

Albert MM, Graybill JR, Rinaldi MG (1991). Treatment of murine cryptococcal meningitis with an SCH 39304-amphotericin B combination. *Antimicrob Ag Chemother* **35**: 1721.

Amantea MA, Bowden RA, Forrest A *et al.* (1995). Population pharmacokinetics and renal function sparing effects of amphotericin B colloidal dispersion in patients receiving bone marrow transplants. *Antimicrob Ag Chemother* **39**: 2042.

Anaisse EJ, Hachem R, Legrand C *et al.* (1992). Lack of activity of amphotericin B in systemic murine fusarial infection. *J Infect Dis* **165**: 1155.

Anaisse EJ, Karyotakis NC, Hachem R *et al.* (1994). Correlation between *in vitro* and *in vivo* activity of antifungal agents against *Candida* species. *J Infect Dis* **170**: 384.

Ando N, Takatori K (1987). Keratomycosis due to *Alternaria alternata* corneal transplant infection. *Mycopathologia* **100**: 17.

Ang BSP, Telenti A, King B *et al.* (1993). Candidemia from a urinary tract source. Microbiological aspects and clinical significance. *Clin Infect Dis* **17**: 662.

Arning M, Heer-Sonderhoff AH, Wehmeier A, Schneider W (1995). Pulmonary toxicity during infusion of liposomal amphotericin B in two patients with acute leukemia. *Eur J Clin Microbiol Infect Dis* **14**: 41.

Arroyo J, Medoff G, Kobayashi GS (1977). Therapy of murine aspergillosis with amphotericin B in combination with rifampin or 5-fluorocytosine. *Antimicrob Ag Chemother* **11**: 21.

Athar MA, Winner HI (1971). The development of resistance by *Candida* species to polyene antibiotics *in vitro*. *J Med Microbiol* **4**: 505.

Atkinson AJ Jr, Bennett JE (1978). Amphotericin B pharmacokinetics in humans. *Antimicrob Ag Chemother* **13**: 271.

Atkinson AJ Jr, Bindschadler DD (1969). Pharmacokinetics of intrathecally administered amphotericin B. *Amer Rev Respir Dis* **99**: 917.

Atkinson BA, Bocanegra R, Colombo AL, Graybill JR (1994). Treatment of disseminated *Torulopsis glabrata* infection with DO870 and amphotericin B. *Antimicrob Ag Chemother* **38**: 1604.

Ayestaran A, Lopez RM, Montoro JB *et al.* (1996). Pharmacokinetics of conventional formulation versus fat emulsion of amphotericin B in a group of patients with neutropenia. *Antimicrob Ag Chemother* **40**: 609.

Baley JE, Kliegman RM FanaroffAA (1984). Disseminated fungal infections in very low-birthweight infants: therapeutic toxicity. *Pediatrics* **73**: 153.

Barchiesi F, Colombo AL, McGough DA, Rinaldi MG (1994). Comparative study of broth macrodilution and microdilution techniques for *in vitro* antifungal susceptibility for yeasts by using the National Committee for Clinical Laboratory Standards proposd guidelines. *J Clin Microbiol* **32**: 2494.

Barst RJ, Prince AS, Neu HC (1981). *Aspergillus* endocarditis in children: case report and review of the literature. *Pediatrics* **68**: 73.

Barton CH, Pahl M, Vaziri ND, Cessario T (1984). Renal magnesium wasting associated with amphotericin B therapy. *Amer J Med* **77**: 471.

Barwicz J, Gareau R, Audet A *et al.* (1991). Inhibition of the interaction between lipoproteins and amphotericin B by some delivery systems. *Biochem Biophys Res Commun* **181**: 722.

Bastani B, Westervelt FB (1986). Persistence of *Candida* despite seemingly adequate systemic and intraperitoneal amphotericin B treatment in a patient on CAPD. *Amer J Kid Dis* **8**: 265.

Bates CM, Carey PB, Hind CR (1995). Anaphylaxis due to liposomal amphotericin (AmBisome). *Genitourin Med* **71**: 414.

Battaner E, Kumar BV (1974). Rifampin: inhibition of ribonucleic acid synthesis after potentiation by amphotericin B in *Saccharomyces cerevisiae*. *Antimicrob Ag Chemother* **5**: 371.

Bayer AS, Edwards JE, Seidel JS *et al.* (1976a). *Candida* meningitis: Report of seven cases and review of the English literature. *Medicine* **55**: 477.

Bayer AS, Blumenkrantz MJ, Montgomerie JZ *et al.* (1976b). *Candida* peritonitis Report of 22 cases and review of the English literature. *Amer J Med* **61**: 832.

Beggs WH (1986). Mechanisms of synergistic interactions between amphotericin B and flucytosine. *J Antimicrob Chemother* **17**: 402.

Behre GF, Schwartz S, Lenz K *et al.* (1995). Aerosol amphotericin B inhalations for prevention of invasive pulmonary aspergillosis in neutropenic cancer patients. *Ann Hematol* **71**: 287.

Bennett JE (1974). Chemotherapy of systemic mycoses (first of two parts). *New Engl J Med* **290**: 30.

Bennett JE (1978). Diagnosis and management of candidiasis in the immunosuppressed host. *Scand J Infect Dis* (Suppl 16): 83.

Bennett JE, Dismukes WE, Duma RJ *et al.* (1979). A comparison of amphotericin B alone and combined with flucytosine, in the treatment of cryptococcal meningitis. *New Engl J Med* **301**: 126.

Benson JM, Nahata MC (1988). Clinical use of systemic antifungal agents. *Clin Pharm* **7**: 424.

Benson JM, Nahata MC (1989). Pharmacokinetics of amphotericin B in children. *Antimicrob Ag Chemother* **33**: 1989.

Bergan T, Vangdal M (1983). *In vitro* activity of antifungal agents against yeast species. *Chemotherapy* **29**: 104.

Berliner S, Weinberger M, Ben-Bassat M *et al.* (1985). Amphotericin B causes aggregation of neutrophils and enhances pulmonary leukostasis. *Amer Rev Respir Dis* **132**: 602.

Berman JD, Wyler DJ (1980). An *in vitro* model for investigation of chemotherapeutic agents in leishmaniasis. *J Infect Dis* **142**: 83.

Berman JD, Ksionski G, Chapman WL *et al.* (1992). Activity of amphotericin B cholesterol dispersion (Amphocil) in experimental visceral leishmaniasis. *Antimicrob Ag Chemother* **36**: 1978.

Beyer J, Barzen G, Risse G *et al.* (1993). Aerosol amphotericin B for prevention of invasive pulmonary aspergillosis. *Antimicrob Ag Chemother* **37**: 1367.

Binder RE, Faling LJ, Pugatch RD *et al.* (1982). Chronic necrotizing aspergillosis: A discrete clinical entity. *Medicine* **61**: 109.

Bindschadler DD, Bennett JE (1969). A pharmacologic guide to the clinical use of amphotericin B. *J Infect Dis* **120**: 427.

Block ER, Bennett JE (1973). The combined effect of 5-fluorocytosine and amphotericin B in the therapy of murine cryptococcosis. *Proc Soc Exp Biol Med* **142**: 476.

Block ER, Bennett JE, Livoti LG *et al.* (1974). Flucytosine and amphotericin B: Hemodialysis effects on the plasma concentration and clearance. *Ann Intern Med* **80**: 613.

Bonner DP, Tewari RP, Solotorovsky M *et al.* (1975). Comparative chemotherapeutic activity of amphotericin B and amphotericin B methyl ester. *Antimicrob Ag Chemother* **7**: 724.

Bortolussi RA, MacDonald MRA, Bannatyne RM, Arbus GS (1975). Treatment of *Candida* peritonitis by peritoneal lavage with amphotericin. *Brit J Pediatr* **87**: 987.

Bouza E, Dreyer JS, Hewitt WL, Meyer RD (1981). Coccidioidal meningitis. An analysis of thirty-one cases and review of the literature. *Medicine* **60**: 139.

Bow EJ, Schroeder M-L, Louie TJ (1984). Pulmonary complications in patients receiving granulocyte transfusions and amphotericin B. *Can Med Assoc J* **130**: 593.

Bowden RA, Cays M, Gooley T *et al.* (1996). Phase I study of Amphotericin B Colloidal Dispersion for the treatment of invasive fungal infections after marrow transplant. *J Infect Dis* **173**: 1208.

Bowler WA, Weiss PJ, Hill HA *et al.* (1992). Risk of ventricular dysrhythmias during 1-hour infusions of amphotericin B in patients with preserved renal function. *Antimicrob Ag Chemother* **36**: 2542.

Bradsher RW (1988). Blastomycosis. *Inf Dis Clin N Amer* **2**: 877.

Bradsher RW (1992). Blastomycosis. *Clin Infect Dis* **14** (Suppl 1): S82.

Brahn E, Leonard PA (1982). *Trichosporon cutaneum* endocarditis. *Amer J Clin Pathol* **78**: 792.

Brajtburg J, Kobayashi D, Medoff G, Kobayashi GS (1982). Antifungal action of amphotericin B in combination with other polyene or imidazole antibiotics. *J Infect Dis* **146**: 138.

Brajtburg J, Elberg S, Bolard J *et al.* (1984). Interaction of plasma proteins and lipoproteins with amphotericin B. *J Infect Dis* **149**: 986.

Brajtburg J, Elberg S, Schwartz DR *et al.* (1985). Oxidative damage in erythrocyte lysis induced by amphotericin B. *Antimicrob Ag Chemother* **27**: 172.

Brajtburg J, Elberg S, Kobayashi GS, Medoff G (1989). Effects of ascorbic acid on the antifungal action of amphotericin B. *J Antimicrob Chemother* **24**: 333.

Brajtburg J, Powderly W, Kobayashi GS, Medoff G (1990a). Amphotericin B: Current understanding of mechanisms of action. *Antimicrob Ag Chemother* **34**: 183.

Brajtburg J, Powderly W, Kobayashi GS, Medoff G (1990b). Amphotericin B: Delivery systems. *Antimicrob Ag Chemother* **34**: 381.

Branch RA (1988). Prevention of amphotericin B-induced renal impairment. *Arch Intern Med* **148**: 2389.

Brandsberg JW, French ME (1972). *In vitro* susceptibility of isolates of *Aspergillus fumigatus* and *Sporothrix schenckii* to amphotericin B. *Antimicrob Ag Chemother* **2**: 402.

Brezis M, Rosen S, Silva P *et al.* (1984). Polyene toxicity in renal medulla: injury mediated by transport activity. *Science* **224**: 66.

Brod RD, Flynn HW, Clarkson JG *et al.* (1990). Endogenous *Candida* endophthalmitis: Management without amphotericin B. *Ophthalmology* **97**: 666.

Brooks RG (1989). Prospective study of *Candida* endophthalmitis in hospitalized patients with candidemia. *Arch Intern Med* **149**: 2226.

Brummer E, Castaneda E, Restrepo A (1993). Paracoccidioidomycosis: an update. *Clin Microbiol Rev* **6**: 89.

Bullock WE, Luke RG, Nuttall CE, Bhathena D (1976). Can mannitol reduce amphotericin B nephrotoxicity? Double-blind study and description of a new vascular lesion in kidneys. *Antimicrob Ag Chemother* **10**: 555.

Burgess JL, Birchall R (1972). Nephrotoxicity of amphotericin B, with emphasis on changes in tubular function. *Amer J Med* **53**: 77.

Burton JR, Zachery JB, Bessin R *et al.* (1972). Aspergillosis in four renal transplant recipients. *Ann Intern Med* **77**: 383.

Butler KM, Rench MA, Baker CJ (1990). Amphotericin B as a single agent in the treatment of systemic candidiasis in neonates. *Pediatr Infect Dis J* **9**: 51.

Caillot D, Casasnovas O, Solary E *et al.* (1993). Efficacy and tolerance of an amphotericin B lipid (Intralipid) emulsion in the treatment of candidemia in neutropenic patients. *J Antimicrob Chemother* **31**: 161.

Caillot D, Reny G, Solary E *et al.* (1994). A controlled trial of the tolerance of amphotericin B infused in dextrose or in Intralipid in patients with haematological malignancies. *J Antimicrob Chemother* **33**: 603.

Cantrill HL, Rodman WP, Ramsay RC, Knobloch WH (1980). Postpartum candida endophthalmitis. *JAMA* **243**: 1163.

Carnecchia BM, Kurtzke JF (1960). Fatal toxic reaction to amphotericin B in cryptococcal meningo-encephalitis. *Ann Intern Med* **53**: 1027.

Carnevale NT, Galgiani JN, Stevens DA *et al.* (1980). Amphotericin-induced myelopathy. *Arch Intern Med* **140**: 1189.

Carrizosa J, Levison ME, Lawrence T, Kaye D (1974). Cure of *Aspergillus ustus* endocarditis on a prosthetic valve. *Arch Intern Med* **133**: 486.

Carter W, McCarthy KS (1966). Molecular mechanisms of antibiotic action. *Ann Intern Med* **64**: 1087.

Casadevall A, Spitzer ED, Webb D, Rinaldi MG (1993). Susceptibilities of serial *Cryptococcus neoformans* isolates from patients with recurrent cryptococcal meningitis to amphotericin B and fluconazole. *Antimicrob Ag Chemother* **37**: 1383.

Chan CK, Ballish E (1978). Inhibition of granulocyte phagocytosis of *Candida albicans* by amphotericin B. *Can J Microbiol* **24**: 363.

Chan CP, Tuazon CU, Lessin LS (1982). Amphotericin B-induced thrombocytopenia. *Ann Intern Med* **96**: 332.

Chapman SW (1995). *Blastomyces dermatitidis*. In: *Principles and Practice of Infectious Diseases* 4th edn (Mandell GL, Bennett JE, Dolin R, eds), p. 2353. New York: Churchill Livingstone.

Chavanet PY, Garry I, Charlier N *et al.* (1992). Trial of glucose versus fat emulsion in preparation of amphotericin for use in HIV infected patients with candidiasis. *Brit Med J* **305**: 921.

Chesney PJ, Teets KC, Mulvihill JJ *et al.* (1976). Successful treatment of *Candida* meningitis with amphotericin B and 5-fluorocytosine in combination. *J Pediatr* **89**: 1017.

Chesney PJ, Justman RA, Bogdanowicz WM (1979). *Candida* meningitis in newborn infants: A review and report of combined amphotericin B-flucytosine therapy. *Johns Hopkins Med J* **72**: 1468.

Ching MS, Raymond K, Bury RW *et al.* (1983). Absorption of orally administered amphotericin B lozenges. *Brit J Clin Pharmacol* **16**: 106.

Chopra R, Fielding A, Goldstone AH (1992). Successful treatment of fungal infections in neutropenic patients with liposomal amphotericin (AmBisome) – a report on 40 cases from a single centre. *Leukemia Lymphoma* **7**: 73.

Christenson JC, Shalit I, Welch DF *et al.* (1987). Synergistic action of amphotericin B and rifampin against *Rhizopus* species. *Antimicrob Ag Chemother* **31**: 1775.

Christiansen KJ, Bernard EM, Gold JWM, Armstrong D (1985). Distribution and activity of Amphotericin B in humans. *J Infect Dis* **152**: 1037.

Cimolai N, Gill MJ, Church D (1987). *Saccharomyces cerevisiae* fungemia: case report and review of the literature. *Diagn Microbiol Infect Dis* **8**: 113.

Clemons KV, Stevens DA (1991). Comparative efficacy of amphotericin B colloidal dispersion and amphotericin deoxycholate suspension in treatment of murine coccidioidomycosis. *Antimicrob Ag Chemother* **35**: 1829.

Clemons KV, Stevens DA (1993). Therapeutic efficacy of a liposomal formulation of amphotericin B (AmBisome) against murine blastomycosis. *J Antimicrob Chemother* **32**: 465.

Cochran RK, Pierson CL, Sell TL, Palella T (1986). Prototrophic olecranon bursitis: Treatment with intrabursal Amphotericin B. *Rev Infect Dis* **8** 952.

Cochrane LJ, Morano JU, Norman JR, Mansel JJ (1991). Use of intracavitary amphotericin B in a patient with aspergilloma and recurrent hemoptysis. *Amer J Med* **90**: 654.

Codish SD, Tobias JS, Hannigan M (1979). Combined amphotericin B-flucytosine therapy in *Aspergillus* pneumonia. *JAMA* **241**: 2418.

Cohen I (1987). Absence of congenital infection and teratogenesis in three children born to mothers with blastomycosis and treated with amphotericin B during pregnancy. *Pediatr Infect Dis J* **6**: 76.

Cohen M, Montgomerie JZ (1993). Hematogenous endophthalmitis due to *Candida tropicalis*: Report of two cases and review. *Clin Infect Dis* **17**: 270.

Cohen-Abbo A, Bozeman PM, Patrick CC (1993). *Cunninghamella* infections: review and report of two cases of *Cunninghamella* pneumonia in immunocompromised children. *Clin Infect Dis* **17**: 173.

Coker R, Tomlinson D, Harris J (1991). Successful treatment of cryptococcal meningitis with liposomal amphotericin B after failure of treatment with fluconazole and conventional amphotericin B. *AIDS* **5**: 231.

Coker RJ, Viviani M, Gazzard BG *et al.* (1993). Treatment of cryptococcosis with liposomal amphotericin B (AmBisome) in 23 patients with AIDS. *AIDS* **7**: 829.

Collette N, Van der Auwera P, Pascual Lopez A *et al.* (1989). Tissue concentrations and bioactivity of amphotericin B in cancer patients treated with amphotericin B-deoxycholate. *Antimicrob Ag Chemother* **33**: 362.

Collette N, Van der Auwera P, Meunier F *et al.* (1991). Tissue distribution and bioactivity of amphotericin B administered in liposomes to cancer patients. *J Antimicrob Chemother* **27**: 535.

Collins MS, Pappagianis D (1977). Uniform susceptibility of various strains of *Coccidioides immitis* to amphotericin B. *Antimicrob Ag Chemother* **11**: 1049.

Conneally E, Cafferky MT, Daly PA *et al.* (1990). Nebulized amphotericin B as prophylaxis against invasive aspergillosis in granulocytopenic patients. *Bone Marrow Transplant* **5**: 403.

Coombs GH, Hart DT, Capaldo J (1983). *Leishmania mexicana*: drug sensitivities of promastigotes and transforming amastigotes. *J Antimicrob Chemother* **11**: 151.

Coronel F, Martin-Rabaden P, Romero J (1993). Chemical peritonitis after intraperitoneal administration of amphotericin B in a fungal infection of the catheter subcutaneous tunnel. *Peritoneal Dial Int* **13**: 161.

Cosgrove RF, Beezer AE, Miles RJ (1978). *In vitro* studies of amphotericin B in combination with the imidazole antifungal compounds clotrimazole and miconazole. *J Infect Dis* **138**: 681.

Craven PC, Gremillion DH (1985). Risk factors of ventricular fibrillation during rapid amphotericin B infusion. *Antimicrob Ag Chemother* **27**: 868.

Craven PC, Ludden TM, Drutz DJ *et al.* (1979). Excretion pathways of amphotericin B. *J Infect Dis* **140**: 329.

Craven PC, Graybill JR, Jorgensen JH *et al.* (1983). High-dose ketoconazole for treatment of fungal infections of the central nervous system. *Ann Intern Med* **98**: 160.

Crislip MA, Edwards JE (1989). Candidiasis. *Infect Dis Clin N Amer* **3**: 103.

Croft SL, Davidson RN, Thornton EA *et al.* (1991). Liposomal amphotericin B in the treatment of visceral leishmaniasis. *J Antimicrob Chemother* **28** (Suppl B): 111.

Crofts M AJ (1976). Use of amphotericin B in mucocutaneous leishmaniasis. *J Trop Med Hyg* **79**: 111.

Cruz JM, Peacock JE, Loomer L *et al.* (1992). Rapid intravenous infusion of amphotericin B: A pilot study. *Amer J Med* **93**: 123.

Cushing D, Bustamante C, Devlin A *et al.* (1991). *Aspergillus* infection prophylaxis: amphotericin nasal spray, a double-blind trial. In *Program*

and Abstracts of the 31st Interscience Conference on Antimicrobial Agents and Chemotherapy, Chicago, p. 222. Washington, DC: American Society for Microbiology.

Dana BW, Durie BGM, White RF, Huestis DW (1981). Concomitant administration of granulocyte transfusions and amphotericin B in neutropenic patients: absence of significant pulmonary toxicity. *Blood* **57**: 90.

Daneshmend TK, Warnock DW (1983). Clinical pharmacokinetics of systemic antifungal drugs. *Clin Pharmacokinet* **8**: 17.

Davidson RN, Croft SL, Scott A *et al.* (1991). Liposomal amphotericin B in drug-resistant visceral leishmaniasis. *Lancet* **337**: 1061.

Dean JL, Wolf JE, Ranzini AC, Laughlin MA (1994). Use of amphotericin B in pregnancy: Case report and review. *Clin Infect Dis* **18**: 364.

de Gans J, Portegies P, Tiessens G *et al.* (1992). Itraconazole compared with amphotericin B plus flucytosine in AIDS patients with cryptococcal meningitis. *AIDS* **6**: 185.

De Gregorio MW, Lee WMF, Ries CA (1981). Pulmonary reactions associated with amphotericin B and leukocyte transfusions. *New Engl J Med* **305**: 585.

Dekker AW, Rozenberg-Arska M, Sixma JJ, Verhoef J (1981). Prevention of infection by trimethoprim-sulfamethoxazole plus amphotericin B in patients with acute nonlymphocytic leukaemia. *Ann Intern Med* **95**: 555.

de Lalla F, Pellizzer G, Vaglia A *et al.* (1995). Amphotericin B as primary therapy for cryptococcosis in patients with AIDS: reliability of relatively high doses administered over a relatively short period. *Clin Infect Dis* **20**: 263.

De Marie S, Janknegt R, Bakker-Woudenberg AJM (1994). Clinical use of liposomal and lipid-complexed amphotericin B. *J Antimicrob Chemother* **33**: 907.

Denning DW (1994). Treatment of invasive aspergillosis. *J Infect* **28** (Suppl1): 25.

Denning DW, Stevens DA (1990). Antifungal and surgical treatment of invasive aspergillosis: review of 2121 published cases. *Rev Infect Dis* **12**: 1147.

Denning DW, Tucker RM, Hanson LH, Stevens DA (1989). Treatment of invasive aspergillosis with itraconazole. *Amer J Med* **86**: 791.

Denning DW, Hanson LH, Perlman AM, Stevens DA (1992). *In vitro* susceptibility and synergy studies of *Aspergillus* species to conventional and new agents. *Diagn Microbiol Infect Dis* **15**: 21.

Dennis JE, Rhodes KH, Cooney DR, Roberts GD (1980). Nosocomial rhizopus infection (zygomycosis) in children. *J Pediatr* **96**: 824.

Devinsky O, Lemann W, Evans AC *et al.* (1987). Akinetic mutism in a bone marrow transplant recipient following total-body irradiation and amphotericin B chemoprophylaxis. A positron emission tomographic and neuropathologic study. *Arch Neurol* **44**: 414.

Diamond RD, Bennett JE (1973). A subcutaneous reservoir for intrathecal therapy of fungal meningitis. *New Engl J Med* **288**: 186.

Diamond RD, Bennett JE (1974). Prognostic factors in cryptococcal meningitis. A study in 111 cases. *Ann Intern Med* **80**: 176.

Dick JD, Merz WG, Saral R (1980). Incidence of polyene-resistant yeasts recovered from clinical specimens. *Antimicrob Ag Chemother* **18**: 158.

Dick JD, Rosengard BR, Merz WG *et al.* (1985). Fatal disseminated candidiasis due to amphotericin B resistant *Candida guilliermondii*. *Ann Intern Med* **102**: 68–69.

Dietze R, Fagundes SM, Brito EF *et al.* (1995). Treatment of kala-azar in Brazil with Amphocil (amphotericin B cholesterol dispersion). for 5 days. *Trans Roy Soc Trop Med Hyg* **89**: 309.

Dillon NL, Sampaio SAP, Habermann MC *et al.* (1986). Delayed results of treatment of paracoccidioidomycosis with amphotericin B plus sulfonamides versus amphotericin B alone. *Rev Inst Med Trop Sao Paulo* **28**: 265.

Dismukes WE, Bennett JE, Drutz DJ *et al.* (1980). Criteria for evaluation of therapeutic response to antifungal drugs. *Rev Infect Dis* **2**: 535.

Dismukes WE, Cloud G, Gallis HA *et al.* (1987). Treatment of cryptococcal meningitis with combination amphotericin B and flucytosine for four as compared with six weeks. *New Engl J Med* **317**: 334.

Dixon DM, Polak A (1987). *In vitro* and *in vivo* drug studies with three agents of central nervous system phaeohyphomycosis. *Chemotherapy* 33: 129.

Drutz D (1983). Amphotericin B in the treatment of coccidioidomycosis. *Drugs* 26: 337.

Drutz DJ, Catanzaro A (1978). State of the art Coccidioidomycosis. *Amer Rev Respir Dis* 117: 727.

Drutz DJ, Lehrer RI (1978). Development of amphotericin B resistant *Candida tropicalis* in a patient with defective leukocyte function. *Amer J Med Sci* 276: 77.

Drutz DJ, Spickard A, Rogers DE, Koenig MG (1968). Treatment of disseminated mycotic infections A new approach to amphotericin B therapy. *Amer J Med* 45: 405.

Dubois J, Bartter T, Gryn J, Pratter MR (1995). The physiologic effects of inhaled amphotericin B. *Chest* 108: 599.

Dukes CS, Perfect JR (1990). Amphotericin B-induced malignant hypertensive episodes. *J Infect Dis* 161: 588.

Dupont B, Drouhet E (1979). *In vitro* synergy and antagonism of antifungal agents against yeast-like fungi. *Postgrad Med J* 55: 683.

Dutcher JD (1968). The discovery and development of amphotericin B. *Dis Chest* 54: 40.

Editorial (1976). Direct fungal infection of the eye and its prevention. *Brit J Ophthal* 60: 605.

Edwards JE Jr, Turkel SB, Elder HA *et al.* (1975). Hematogenous *Candida* osteomyelitis. Report of three cases and review of the literature. *Amer J Med* 59: 89.

Edwards JE Jr, Morrison J, Henderson DK, Montgomerie JZ (1980). Combined effect of amphotericin B and rifampin on *Candida* species. *Antimicrob Ag Chemother* 17: 484.

Egere JU, Gugnani HC, Okoro AN, Suseelan AV (1978). African histoplasmosis in Eastern Nigeria: report of two culturally proven cases treated with septrin and amphotericin B. *J Trop Med Hyg* 81: 225.

Eilard T, Beskow D, Norrby R *et al.* (1976). Combined treatment with amphotericin B and flucytosine in severe fungal infections. *J Antimicrob Chemother* 2: 239.

Ellard AJ (1987). Isolation of fungi in blood cultures: A review of fungal infections in the western part of Sweden, 1970–1982. *Scand J Infect Dis* 19: 145.

Ellis CA, Spivack ML (1967). The significance of candidemia. *Ann Intern Med* 67: 511.

Ellis ME, Al-Hokail AA, Clink HM *et al.* (1992). Double-blind randomized study of the effect of infusion rates on toxicity of amphotericin B. *Antimicrob Ag Chemother* 36: 172.

Ellis ME, Clink H, Younge D, Hainau B (1994). Successful combined surgical and medical treatment of *Fusarium* infection after bone marrow transplantation. *Scand J Infect Dis* 26: 225.

Ellis WG, Sobel RA, Nielsen SL (1982). Leukoencephalopathy in patients treated with amphotericin B methyl ester. *J Infect Dis* 146: 125.

Eng RHK, Person A, Mangura C *et al.* (1981). Susceptibility of *Zygomycetes* to amphotericin B, miconazole and ketoconazole. *Antimicrob Ag Chemother* 20: 688.

EORTC International Antimicrobial Therapy Cooperative Group (1989). Empiric antifungal therapy in febrile granulocytopenic patients. *Amer J Med* 86: 668.

Eppes SC, Troutman JL, Gutman LT (1989). Outcome of treatment of candidemia in children whose central venous catheters were removed or retained. *Pediatr Infect Dis J* 8: 99.

Ericsson M, Anniko M, Gustafsson H *et al.* (1993). A case of chronic progressive rhinocerebral mucormycosis treated with liposomal amphotericin B and surgery. *Clin Infect Dis* 16: 585.

Ernst JD, Rusnak M, Sande MA (1983). Combination antifungal chemotherapy for experimental disseminated candidiasis: lack of correlation between *in vitro* and *in vivo* observations with amphotericin B and rifampin. *Rev Infect Dis* (Suppl 3): 626.

Espinel-Ingroff A, Kerkering TM, Goldson PR, Shadomy S (1991). Comparison study of broth macrodilution and microdilution antifungal susceptibility tests. *J Clin Microbiol* 29: 1089.

Espinel-Ingroff A, Dawson K, Pfaller M *et al.* (1995). Comparative and collaborative evaluation of standardization of antifungal susceptibility testing for filamentous fungi. *Antimicrob Ag Chemother* 39: 314.

Espinel-Ingroff A, Pfaller M, Erwin ME, Jones RN (1996). Interlaboratory evaluation of Etest method for testing antifungal susceptibilities of pathogenic yeasts to five antifungal agents by using casitone agar and solidified RPMI 1640 medium with 2% glucose. *J Clin Microbiol* 34: 848.

Evans CC (1979). Management of pulmonary disorders caused by the inhalation of aspergillus spores. *J Antimicrob Chemother* 5: 335.

Ezdinli EZ, O'Sullivan DD, Wasser LP *et al.* (1979). Oral amphotericin for candidiasis in patients with hematologic neoplasms. *JAMA* 242: 258.

Fader RC, McGinnis MR (1988). Infections caused by dematiaceous fungi: chromoblastomycosis and phaeohyphomycosis. *Infect Dis Clin N Amer* 2: 925.

Fainstein V, Gilmore C, Hopfer RL *et al.* (1982). Septic arthritis due to *Candida* species in patients with cancer: report of five cases and review of the literature. *Rev Infect Dis* 4: 78.

Fass RJ, Perkins RL (1971). 5-Fluorocytosine in the treatment of cryptococcal and *Candida* mycoses. *Ann Intern Med* 74: 535.

Feely J, Heidemann H, Gerkens J *et al.* (1981). Sodium depletion enhances nephrotoxicity of amphotericin B. *Lancet* i: 1422.

Feldman HA, Hamilton JD, Gutman RA (1973). Amphotericin B therapy in an anephric patient. *Antimicrob Ag Chemother* 4: 302.

Fielding RM, Smith PC, Wang LH *et al.* (1991). Comparative pharmacokinetics of amphotericin B after administration of a novel colloidal delivery system, ABCD, and a conventional formulation to rats. *Antimicrob Ag Chemother* 35: 1208.

Fielding RM, Singer AW, Wang LH *et al.* (1992). Relationship of pharmacokinetics and drug distribution in tissues to increased safety of amphotericin B colloidal dispersion in dogs. *Antimicrob Ag Chemother* 36: 299.

Fields BT, Bates JH, Abernathy RS (1971). Effect of rapid intravenous infusion on serum concentrations of amphotericin B. *Appl Microbiol* 22: 615.

Fisher JF, Dewald J (1983). Parkinsonism associated with intraventricular amphotericin B. *J Antimicrob Chemother* 12: 97.

Fisher JF, Chew WH, Shadomy S *et al.* (1982). Urinary tract infections due to *Candida albicans*. *Rev Infect Dis* 4: 1107.

Fisher JF, Taylor AT, Clark J *et al.* (1983). Penetration of amphotericin B into the human eye. *J Infect Dis* 147: 164.

Fong IW, Cheng PC, Hinton NA (1991). Fungicidal effect of amphotericin B in urine: *in vitro* study to assess feasibility of bladder washout for localization of site of candiduria. *Antimicrob Ag Chemother* 35: 1856.

Forgan-Smith R, Darrell JH (1974). Amphotericin pharmacophobia and renal toxicity. *Brit Med J* 1: 244.

Forman SJ, Robinson GV, Wolf JI *et al.* (1981). Pulmonary reactions associated with amphotericin B and leukocyte transfusions. *New Engl J Med* 305: 584.

Fosson AR, Wheeler WE (1975). Short-term amphotericin B treatment of severe childhood histoplasmosis. *J Pediatr* 86: 32.

Foster CS (1992). Fungal keratitis. *Infect Dis Clin N Amer* 6: 851.

Francis P, Walsh TJ (1992). Evolving role of of flucytosine in immunocompromised patients: New insights into safety, pharmacokinetics, and antifungal therapy. *Clin Infect Dis* 15: 1003.

Fujita NK, Edwards JE Jr (1981). Combined *in vitro* effect of amphotericin B and rifampin on *Cryptococcus neoformans*. *Antimicrob Ag Chemother* 19: 196.

Gadebusch HH, Pansy F, Klepner C, Schwind R (1976). Amphotericin B and amphotericin B methyl ester ascorbate 1 Chemotherapeutic activity against *Candida albicans*, *Cryptococcus neoformans*, and *Blastomyces dermatitidis* in mice. *J Infect Dis* 134: 423.

Gale EF (1973). Perspectives in chemotherapy. *Brit Med J* 4: 33.

Gale EF (1986). Nature and development of phenotypic resistance to amphotericin B in *Candida albicans*. *Adv Microb Physiol* 27: 278.

Galgiani JN, Ampel NM (1990). Coccidioidomycosis in human immunodeficiency virus-infected patients. *J Infect Dis* 162: 1165.

Gallis HA, Drew RH, Pickard WW(1990). Amphotericin B: 30 years of clinical experience. *Rev Infect Dis* **12**: 308.

Gartenberg G, Bottone EJ, Keusch GT *et al.* (1978). Hospital-acquired mucormycosis (*Rhizopus rhizopodiformis*). of skin and subcutaneous tissue Epidemiology, mycology and treatment. *New Engl J Med* **299**: 1115.

Gathe JC, Harris RL, Garland B *et al.* (1987). *Candida* osteomyelitis. Report of five cases and review of the literature. *Amer J Med* **82**: 927.

Gauto A, Law EJ, Holder IA, MacMillan BG (1977). Experience with amphotericin B in the treatment of systemic candidiasis in burn patients. *Amer J Surg* **133**: 174.

George D, Kordick D, Miniter P *et al.* (1993). Combination therapy in experimental invasive aspergillosis. *J Infect Dis* **168**: 692.

Gerson, SL, Talbot GH, Hurwitz S *et al.* (1984). Prolonged granulocytopenia: the major risk factor for invasive aspergillosis in patients with acute leukemia. *Ann Intern Med* **100**: 345.

Gigliotti F, Shenep JL, Lott L, Thornton D (1987). Induction of prostaglandin synthesis as the mechanism responsible for the chills and fever produced by infusing amphotericin B. *J Infect Dis* **156**: 784.

Glimp RA, Bayer AS (1981). Fungal pneumonias: Part 3 Allergic bronchopulmonary aspergillosis. *Chest* **80**: 85.

Goldani LZ, Sugar AM (1995). Paracoccidioidomycosis and AIDS: an overview. *Clin Infect Dis* **21**: 1275.

Goldberg PK, Kozinn PJ, Wise GJ *et al.* (1979). Incidence and significance of candiduria. *JAMA* **241**: 582.

Goldstein E, Winship MJ, Pappagianis D (1972). Ventricular fluid and the management of coccidioidal meningitis. *Ann Intern Med* **77**: 243.

Gondal JA, Swartz RP, Ralunan A (1989). Therapeutic evaluation of free and liposome-encapsulated amphotericin B in the treatment of systemic candidiasis in mice. *Antimicrob Ag Chemother* **33**: 1544.

Goodman JL, Winston DJ, Greenfield RA *et al.* (1992). A controlled trial of fluconazole to prevent fungal infections in patients undergoing bone marrow transplantation. *New Engl J Med* **326**: 845.

Goodwin RA Jr, Des Prez RM (1978). State of the art histoplasmosis. *Amer Rev Respir Dis* **117**: 929.

Goodwin SD, Cleary JD, Walawander CA *et al.* (1995). Pretreatment regimens for adverse events related to infusion of amphotericin B. *Clin Infect Dis* **20**: 755.

Graybill JR, Ahrens J (1983). Interaction of rifampin with other antifungal agents in experimental murine candidiasis. *Rev Infect Dis* **5** (Suppl 3): 620.

Graybill JR Bocanegra R (1995). Liposomal amphotericin B therapy of murine histoplasmosis. *Antimicrob Ag Chemother* **39**: 1885.

Graybill JR, Williams DM, Van Cutsem E, Drutz DJ (1980). Combination therapy of experimental histoplasmosis and cryptococcosis with amphotericin B and ketoconazole. *Rev Infect Dis* **2**: 551.

Greenman R, Becker J, Campbell G *et al.* (1975). Coccidioidal synovitis of the knee. *Arch Intern Med* **135**: 526.

Gubbins PO, Piscitelli SC, Danziger LH (1993). Candidal urinary tract infections: A comprehensive review of their diagnosis and management. *Pharmacotherapy* **13**: 110.

Gugnani HC, Egere JU, Suseelan AV *et al.* (1978). Chromomycosis caused by *Phialophora pedrosoi* in Eastern Nigeria. *J Trop Med* **81**: 210.

Gupta AK, Sander DM, Shear NH (1994). Antifungal agents: An overview Part II. *J Amer Acad Dermatol* **30**: 11.

Haber RW, Joseph M (1962). Neurological manifestations after amphotericin B therapy. *Brit Med J* **1**: 230.

Hadfield TL, Smith MB, Winn RE *et al.* (1987). Mycoses caused by *Candida lusitaniae*. *Rev Infect Dis* **9**: 1006.

Halloran WM, Wilbur JR, DeGregario MW (1985). Empiric amphotericin B therapy with acute leukemia. *Rev Infect Dis* **7**: 619.

Hamill R, Oney LA, Crane LR (1983). Successful therapy for rhinocerebral mucormycosis with associated bilateral brain abscesses. *Arch Intern Med* **143**: 581.

Hamilton JD, Elliott DM (1975). Combined activity of amphotericin B and 5-fluorocytosine against *Cryptococcus neoformans in vitro* and *in vivo* in mice. *J Infect Dis* **131**: 129.

Hamilton-Miller JMT (1972). Sterols from polyene-resistant mutants of *Candida albicans*. *J Gen Microbiol* **73**: 201.

Hamilton-Miller JMT (1973). Chemistry and biology of the polyene macrolide antibiotics. *Bacteriol Rev* **37**: 166.

Hammerman KJ, Powell KE, Christianson CS *et al.* (1973a). Pulmonary cryptococcosis: clinical forms and treatment. *Amer Rev Respir Dis* **108**: 1116.

Hammerman KJ, Christianson CS, Huntington I *et al.* (1973b). Spontaneous lysis of aspergillomata. *Chest* **64**: 697.

Hammerman KJ, Sarosi GA, Tosh FE (1974). Amphotericin B in the treatment of saprophytic forms of pulmonary aspergillosis. *Amer Rev Respir Dis* **109**: 57.

Hanson LH, Stevens DA (1992). Comparison of antifungal activity of amphotericin B deoxycholate suspension with that of amphotericin B cholesteryl sulfate colloidal dispersion. *Antimicrob Ag Chemother* **36**: 486.

Hargis JI, Bone RC, Stewart J *et al.* (1980). Intracavitary amphotericin B in the treatment of symptomatic pulmonary aspergillomas. *Amer J Med* **68**: 389.

Haron E, Anaissie E, Dumphy F *et al.* (1988). *Hansenula anomala* fungemia. *Rev Infect Dis* **10**: 1182.

Hauser WE Jr, Remington JS (1983). Effect of amphotericin B on natural killer cell activity *in vitro*. *J Antimicrob Chemother* **11**: 257.

Hay RJ (1994). Liposomal amphotericin B, AmBisome. *J Infect* **28** (Suppl): 35.

Hayden G, Lapp C, Loda F (1977). Arthritis caused by *Monosporium apiospermum* treated with intra-articular amphotericin B. *Amer J Dis Child* **131**: 927.

Heidemann HT, Gerkens JF, Spickard WA *et al.* (1983). Amphotericin B nephrotoxicity in humans decreased by salt repletion. *Amer J Med* **75**: 476.

Heidemann HT, Brune KH, Sabra R, Branch RA (1992). Acute and chronic effects of flucytosine on amphotericin B nephrotoxicity in rats. *Antimicrob Ag Chemother* **36**: 2670–2675.

Heinemann V, Kahny B, Debus A *et al.* (1994). Pharmacokinetics of liposomal amphotericin B (AmBisome) versus other lipid-based formulations. *Bone Marrow Transplant* **14**(Suppl 5): S8.

Helton WS, Carriw J, Zaveruha PA *et al.* (1986). Diagnosis and treatment of splenic fungal abscesses in immunosuppressed patients. *Arch Surg* **121**: 580.

Hernandez Molina JM, Llosa J, Martinez Brocal A, Ventosa A (1992). *In vitro* activity of cloconazole, sulconazole, butoconazole, isoconazole, fenticonazole, and five other antifungal agents against clinical isolates of *Candida albicans* and *Candida* spp. *Mycopathologia* **118**: 15.

Hildick-Smith G, Blank H, Sarkany I (1964). *Fungus Diseases and Their Treatment*, p. 403. London: J & A Churchill.

Hoeprich PD (1978). New antifungal drugs in the therapy of systemic mycoses. *Scand J Infect Dis* (Suppl 16): 74.

Hoeprich PD (1982). Amphotericin B methyl ester and leukoencephalopathy: the other side of the coin. *J Infect Dis* **146**: 173.

Hoeprich PD (1992). Clinical use of Amphotericin B and derivatives: Lore, mystique, and fact. *Clin Infect Dis* **14** (Suppl): S114.

Hoeprich PD, Finn PD (1972). Activity of combinations of antifungal agents against *Candida albicans* and *Cryptococcus neoformans* (abstract). In *Proceedings of the 72nd Meeting of the American Society for Microbiology*, p. 135. Washington, DC: American Society for Microbiology.

Hoeprich PD, Huston AC (1975). Susceptibility of *Coccidioides immitis*, *Candida albicans* and *Cryptococcus neoformans* to amphotericin B, flucytosine and clotrimazole. *J Infect Dis* **132**: 133.

Hoeprich PD, Huston AC (1978). Stability of four antifungal antimicrobials *in vitro*. *J Infect Dis* **137**: 87.

Holbrook WP, Kippax R (1979). Sensitivity of *Candida albicans* from patients with chronic oral candidiasis. *Postgrad Med J* **55**: 692.

Holeman CW, Johnson P (1976). Long-term follow-up of amphotericin treated coccidioidal meningitis patients. In *Proceedings of the 21st Annual Meeting of the Coccidioidomycosis Study Group*. Abstract 1 (Stevens DA ed).

Holleran WM, Wilbur JR, De Gregorio MW (1985). Empiric amphotericin B therapy in patients with acute leukemia. *Rev Infect Dis* **7**: 619.

Holt JE, Gray JE, Lerner WL (1972). Coccidioidal meningitis. *Ann Intern Med* **77**: 814.

Howarth WR, Tewari RP, Solotorovsky M (1975). Comparative *in vitro* antifungal activity of amphotericin B and amphotericin B methyl ester. *Antimicrob Ag Chemother* **7**: 58.

Hoy J, Hsu K-C, Rolston K *et al.* (1986). *Trichosporon beigelii* infection: A review. *Rev Infect Dis* **8**: 959.

Hsu CCS, Chang R-H (1995). Two-day continuous bladder irrigation with amphotericin B. *Clin Infect Dis* **20**: 1570.

Hsu CCS, Ukleja B (1990). Clearance of *Candida* colonizing the urinary bladder by a two-day amphotericin B irrigation. *Infection* **18**: 280.

HsuChen CC, Feingold DS (1973). Selective membrane toxicity of the polyene antibiotics: studies on natural membranes. *Antimicrob Ag Chemother* **4**: 316.

HsuChen CC, Feingold DS (1974). Two types of resistance to polyene antibiotics in *Candida albicans*. *Nature* **251**: 656.

Hsu S, Burnette RR (1993). The effect of amphotericin B on the K channel activity of MDCK cells. *Biochem Biophys Acta* **1152** 189.

Hughes CE, Harris C, Moody JA *et al.* (1984a). *In vitro* activities of amphotericin B in combination with four antifungal agents and rifampin against *Aspergillus* spp. *Antimicrob Ag Chemother* **25**: 560.

Hughes CE, Harris C, Peterson LR, Gerding DN (1984b). Enhancement of the *in vitro* activity of amphotericin B against *Aspergillus* spp by tetracycline analogs. *Antimicrob Ag Chemother* **26**: 840.

Huppert M, Sun SH, Vukovich KR (1974). Combined amphotericin B-tetracycline therapy for experimental coccidioidomycosis. *Antimicrob Ag Chemother* **5**: 473.

Huppert M, Pappagianis D, Sun SH *et al.* (1976). Effect of amphotericin B and rifampin against *Coccidioides immitis in vitro* and *in vivo*. *Antimicrob Ag Chemother* **9**: 406.

Hussain Qadri SMH, Flournoy DJ, Qadri SGM, Ramirez EG (1986). Susceptibility of clinical isolates of yeasts to anti-fungal agents. *Mycopathologia* **95**: 183.

Huston AC, Hoeprich PD (1978). Comparative susceptibilities of four kinds of pathogenic fungi to amphotericin B and amphotericin B methyl ester. *Antimicrob Ag Chemother* **13**: 905.

Ismail MA, Lerner SA (1982). Disseminated blastomycosis in a pregnant woman. *Amer Rev Respir Dis* **126**: 350.

Iwatsu T (1988). Cutaneous alternariosis. *Arch Dermatol* **124**: 1822.

Iwen PC, Miller NG, McFadden HW Jr (1984). Treatment of murine pulmonary cryptococcosis with ketoconazole and amphotericin B. *J Infect Dis* **149**: 650.

Jacobs LG, Skidmore EA, Cardoso LA, Ziv F (1994). Bladder irrigation with amphotericin B for treatment of fungal urinary tract infections. *Clin Infect Dis* **18**: 313.

Jagdis FA, Hoeprich PD, Lawrence RM, Schaffner CP (1977). Comparative pharmacology of amphotericin B and amphotericin B methyl ester in the nonhuman primate, *Macaca mulatta*. *Antimicrob Ag Chemother* **12**: 582.

Janknegt R, de Marie S, Bakker-Woudenberg IAJM, Crommelin DJA (1992). Liposomal and lipid formulations of amphotericin B. *Clin Pharmacokinet* **23** (4): 279.

Jeffrey GM, Beard MEJ, Ikram RB *et al.* (1991). Intranasal amphotericin B reduces the frquency of invasive aspergillosis in neutropenic patients. *Amer J Med* **90**: 685.

Jones BR (1975). Principles in the management of oculomycosis. *Trans Am Acad Ophthalmol Otolaryngol* **70**: OP-15.

Jones BR, Clayton YM, Oji EO (1979). Recognition and chemotherapy of oculomycosis. *Postgrad Med J* **55**: 525.

Jordan GW, Seet EC (1978). Antiviral effects of amphotericin B methyl ester. *Antimicrob Ag Chemother* **13**: 199.

Jullien S, Contrpois A, Sligh JE (1989). Study of the effects of liposomal amphotericin B on *Candida albicans*, *Cryptococcus neoformans* and erythrocytes by using small unilamellar vesicles prepared from saturated phosspsolipids. *Antimicrob Ag Chemother* **33**: 345.

Kan VL, Bennett JE, Amantea MA *et al.* (1991). Comparative safety, tolerance, and pharmacokinetics of amphotericin B lipid complex and amphotericin B deoxycholate in healthy male volunteers. *J Infect Dis* **164**: 418.

Karp JE, Burch PA, Merz WG (1988). An approach to intensive antileukemia therapy in patients with previous invasive aspergillosis. *Amer J Med* **85**: 203.

Katz NM, Pierce PF, Anzock RA *et al.* (1990). Liposomal amphotericin B for treatment of pulmonary aspergillosis in a heart transplant patient. *J Heart Transplant* **9**: 14.

Keim GR Jr, Sibley PL, Yoon YH *et al.* (1976). Comparative toxicological studies of amphotericin B methyl ester and amphotericin B in mice, rats, and dogs. *Antimicrob Ag Chemother* **10**: 687.

Keller MA, Sellers BB Jr, Melish ME *et al.* (1977). Systemic candidiasis in infants. A case presentation and literature review. *Amer J Dis Child* **131**: 1260.

Kelly SL, Lamb DC, Taylor M *et al.* (1994). Resistance to amphotericin B associated with defective sterol delta 8→7 isomerase in a *Cryptococcus neoformans* strain from an AIDS patient. *FEMS Microbiol Lett* **122**: 39.

Kerkering TM, Duma RJ, Shadomy S(1981).The evolution of pulmonary cryptococcosis: Clinical implications from a study of 41 patients with and without compromising host factors. *Ann Intern Med* **94**: 611.

Kessler HA, Dixon J, Howard CR *et al.* (1981). Effect of amphotericin B on hepatitis B virus. *Antimicrob Ag Chemother* **20**: 826.

Kim SJ, Kwon-Chung KW, Milne GWA *et al.* (1975). Relationship between polyene resistance and sterol compositions in *Cryptococcus neoformans*. *Antimicrob Ag Chemother* **7**: 99.

Kintzel PE, Trausch DE, Copfer AL (1994). Otic administration of amphotericin B 0.25% in sterile water. *Ann Pharmacother* **28**: 333.

Kirsch R, Goldstein R, Tarloff J *et al.* (1988). An emulsion formulation of amphotericin B improves the therapeutic index when treating systemic murine candidiasis. *J Infect Dis* **158**: 1065.

Kitahara M, Seth VK, Medoff G, Kobayashi GS (1976a). Activity of amphotericin B, 5-fluorocytosine, and rifampin against six clinical isolates of aspergillus. *Antimicrob Ag Chemother* **9**: 915.

Kitahara M, Kobayashi GS, Medoff G (1976b). Enhanced efficacy of amphotericin B and rifampicin combined in treatment of murine histoplasmosis and blastomycosis. *J Infect Dis* **133**: 663.

Klein AS, Tortora GT, Malowits R, Greene WH (1988). *Hansenula anomala*: a new fungal pathogen Two case reports and a review of the literature. *Arch Intern Med* **148**: 1210.

Kline S, Larsen TA, Fieber L *et al.* (1995). Limited toxicity of prolonged therapy with high doses of amphotericin B lipid complex. *Clin Infect Dis* **21**: 1154.

Kobayashi GS, Cheung SC, Schlessinger D, Medoff G (1974). Effects of rifampicin derivatives, alone and in combination with amphotericin B, against *Histoplasma capsulatum*. *Antimicrob Ag Chemother* **5**: 16.

Kobayashi RH, Rosenblatt HM, Carney JM *et al.* (1980). *Candida* esophagitis and laryngitis in chronic mucocutaneous candidiasis. *Pediatrics* **66**: 380.

Kontoyianis DP, Vartivarian S, Anaissie EJ *et al.* (1994). Infections due to *Cunninghamella bertholletiae* in patients with cancer: report of three cases and review. *Clin Infect Dis* **18**: 925.

Kotler-Brajtburg J, Medoff G, Kobayashi GS *et al.* (1979). Classification of polyene antibiotics according to chemical structure and biological effects. *Antimicrob Ag Chemother* **15**: 716.

Kovacs JA, Kovacs AA, Polis M *et al.* (1985). Cryptococcosis in the acquired immunodeficiency syndrome. *Ann Intern Med* **103**: 533.

Kulkantrakorn K, Selhorst JB, Petruska PJ (1996). Cytosine arabinoside and amphotericin B-induced parkinsonism. *Ann Neurol* **39**: 413.

Kutty K, Neicheril JC (1987). Treatment of pleural blastomycosis: penetration of amphotericin B into the pleural fluid. *J Infect Dis* **156**: 689.

Kwan CN, Medoff G, Kobayashi S *et al.* (1972). Potentiation of the antifungal effects of antibiotics by amphotericin B. *Antimicrob Ag Chemother* **2**: 61.

Labadie EL, Hamilton RH (1986). Survival improvement in coccidioidal meningitis by high-dose intrathecal amphotericin B. *Arch Intern Med* **146**: 2013.

Laing RBS, Milne LJR, Leen CLS *et al.* (1994). Anaphylactic reactions to liposomal amphotericin. *Lancet* **344**: 682.

Larsen RA, Leal M, Chan L (1990). Fluconazole compared with amphotericin B plus flucytosine for cryptococcal meningitis in AIDS. *Ann Intern Med* **113**: 183–187.

Lau GKK, Kumana CR, Wong KL *et al.* (1992). Disseminated *Penicillium marneffei* infection responding to treatment with oral fluconazole. *J Hong Kong Med Assoc* **44**: 176.

Lau YL, Yuen KY, Lee CW, Chan CF (1995). Invasive *Acremonium falciforme* infection in a patient with severe combined immunodeficiency. *Clin Infect Dis* **20**: 197.

Lauer BA, Reller L~B, Schroter GPJ (1978). Susceptibility of *Aspergillus* to 5-fluorocytosine and amphotericin B alone and in combination. *J Antimicrob Chemother* **4**: 375.

Lawrence RM, Hoeprich PD (1976). Comparison of amphotericin B and amphotericin B methyl ester: efficacy in murine coccidioidomycosis and toxicity. *J Infect Dis* **133**: 168.

Lawrence RM, Hoeprich PD, Jagdis FA *et al.* (1980). Distribution of doubly radiolabelled amphotericin B methyl ester and amphotericin B in the non-human primate, *Macaca mulatta. J Antimicrob Chemother* **6**: 241.

Lecciones JA, Lee JW, Navarro EE *et al.* (1992). Vascular catheter associated fungemia in patients with cancer: analysis of 155 episodes. *Clin Infect Dis* **14**: 875.

Lee KK, Karr SL Jr, Wong MM, Hoeprich PD (1979). *In vitro* susceptibilities of *Naegleria fowleri* strain HB-I to selected antimicrobial agents, singly and in combination. *Antimicrob Ag Chemother* **16**: 217.

Lehrer RI, Howard DH, Sypherd PS *et al.* (1980). Mucor mycosis. *Ann Intern Med* **93**: 93.

Levine SJ, Walsh TJ, Martinez A *et al.* (1991). Cardiopulmonary toxicity after liposomal amphotericin B infusion. *Ann Intern Med* **114**: 664.

Levy M, Domoratzki J, Koren G (1995). Amphotericin-induced heart-rate decrease in children. *Clin Pediatrics* **34**: 358.

Lew MA, Beckett KM, Levin MJ (1978). Combined activity of minocycline and amphotericin B *in vitro* against medically important yeasts. *Antimicrob Ag Chemother* **14**: 465.

Lin AC, Goldwasser E, Bernard EM, Chapman SW (1990). Amphotericin B blunts erythropoietin response to anemia. *J Infect Dis* **161**: 348.

Liu KL, Herbrecht R, Bergerat JP, Koenig H, Waller J, Oberling F (1990). Disseminated *Trichosporon capitatum* infection in a patient with acute leukemia undergoing bone marrow transplantation. *Bone Marrow Transplantation* **6**: 219.

Liu JS, Chang YY, Chen WH, Chen SS (1995). Amphotericin B-induced leukoencephalopathy in a patient with cryptococcal meningitis. *J Formosan Med Assoc* **94**: 432.

Longman LP, Martin MV (1987). A comparison of the efficacy of itraconazole, amphotericin B and 5-fluorocytosine in the treatment of *Aspergillus fumigatus* endocarditis in the rabbit. *J Antimicrob Chemother* **20**: 719.

Lopez-Berestein G (1989). Liposomes in infectious diseases: present and future. *Curr Clin Topic Infect Dis* **10**: 241.

Lopez-Berestein G, Rosenblum MG, Mehta R (1984). Altered tissue distribution of amphotericin B by liposomal encapsulation: comparison of normal mice to mice infected with *Candida albicans. Cancer Drug Delivery* **1**: 199.

Lopez-Berestein G, Fainstein V, Hopfer R *et al.* (1985). Liposomal amphotericin B for the treatment of system fungal infections in patients with cancer: a preliminary study. *J Infect Dis* **151**: 704.

Lopez-Berestein G, Bodey GP, Frankel LS *et al.* (1987). Treatment of hepatosplenic candidiasis with liposomal amphotericin B. *J Clin Oncol* **5**: 310–317.

Lorber B, Cutler C, Barry WE (1976). Allergic rash due to amphotericin B. *Ann Intern Med* **84**: 54.

Lortholary O, Meyohas M-C, Dupont B *et al.* (1993). Invasive aspergillosis in patients with acquired immunodeficiency syndrome: report of 33 cases. *Amer J Med* **95**: 177.

Lou P, Kazdan J, Bannatyne RM, Cheung R (1977). Successful treatment of *Candida* endophthalmitis with a synergistic combination of amphotericin B and rifampin. *Amer J Ophthalmol* **83**: 12.

Louria DB (1958). Some aspects of the absorption, distribution, and excretion of amphotericin B in man. *Antibiot Med Clin Ther* **5**: 295.

Lutwick LI, Galgiani IN, Johnson RH, Stevens DA (1976). Visceral fungal infections due to *Petriellidium boydii (Allescheria boydii). In vitro* drug sensitivity studies. *Amer J Med* **61**: 632.

MacGregor RR, Bennett JE, Erslev AJ (1978). Erythropoietin concentration in amphotericin B-induced anemia. *Antimicrob Ag Chemother* **14**: 270.

Maddux MS, Barriere SL (1980). A review of complications of amphotericin-B therapy: recommendations for prevention and management. *Drug Intell Clin Pharm* **14**: 177.

Mahul P, Piens M-A, Guyotat D *et al.*, (1988). Disseminated *Geotrichum capitatum* infection in a patient with acute myeloid leukemia. *Mycoses* **32**: 573.

Marcon MJ, Durrell DE, Powell DA, Buesching WJ (1987). *In vitro* activity of systemic antifungal agents against *Malassezia furfur. Antimicrob Ag Chemother* **31**: 951.

Marier R, Zakhireh B, Downs J *et al.* (1978). *Trichosporon cutaneum* endocarditis. *Scand J Infect Dis* **10**: 255.

Marmer DJ, Fields BT Jr, France GL, Steele RW (1981). Ketoconazole, amphotericin B, and amphotericin B methyl ester: comparative *in vitro* and *in vivo* toxicological effects on neutrophil function. *Antimicrob Ag Chemother* **20**: 660.

Martin E, Pancoast SJ, Neu HC (1979). *Candida parapsilosis* endocarditis: medical and surgical care. *Ann Intern Med* **91**: 870.

Martin E, Parras P, Lozano MC (1992). *In vitro* susceptibility of 245 yeast isolates to amphotericin B, 5-fluorocytosine, ketoconazole, fluconazole and itraconazole. *Chemother* **38**: 335.

Martin E, Maier F, Bhakdi S (1994). Antagonistic effects of fluconazole and 5-fluorocytosine on candidacidal action of amphotericin B in human serum. *Antimicrob Ag Chemother* **38**: 1331.

Martinez-Lacasa J, Mana J, Niubo R *et al.* (1991). Long-term survival of a patient with prosthetic valve endocarditis due to *Trichosporon beigelii. Eur J Clin Microbiol Infect Dis* **10**: 756.

Martinson FD (1972). Clinical epidemiological and therapeutic aspects of entomophthoromycosis. *Ann Soc Belg Med Trop* **52**: 329–342.

McCoy MJ, Ellenburg JF, Killam AP (1980). Coccidioidomycosis complicating pregnancy. *Amer J Obstet Gynecol* **137**: 739.

McCurdy DK, Frederic M, Elkinton JR (1968). Renal tubular acidosis due to amphotericin B. *New Engl J Med* **278**: 124.

McGinnis MR, Rinaldi MG (1991). Antifungal drugs: Mechanisms of action, drug resistance, susceptibility testing, and assays of activity in biological fluids. In *Antibiotics in Laboratory Medicine* 3rd edn (Lorian V, ed), p. 198. Baltimore: Williams and Wilkins.

McGuire TW, Bullock JD, Bullock D *et al.* (1991). Fungal endophthalmitis: An experimental study with review of 17 human ocular cases. *Arch Ophthalmol* **109**: 1289.

McKinsey DS, Gupta MR, Riddler SA *et al.* (1989). Long-term amphotericin B therapy for disseminated histoplasmosis in patients with the acquired immunodeficiency syndrome (AIDS). *Ann Intern Med* **111**: 655.

McKinsey DS, Gupta MR, Driks MR *et al.* (1992). Histoplasmosis in patients with AIDS: Efficacy of maintenance amphotericin B. *Amer J Med* **92**: 225.

McWhinney PHM, Kibbler CC, Hamon MD *et al.* (1993). Progress in the diagnosis and management of aspergillosis in bone marrow transplantation: 13 years experience. *Clin Infect Dis* **17**: 397.

Mechlinski W, Schaffner CP (1972). Polyene macrolide derivatives 1 N-acylation and esterification reactions with amphotericin B. *J Antibiot* (Tokyo) **25**: 256.

Medoff G (1983). Antifungal action of rifampin. *Rev Infect Dis* **5** (Suppl3): S614.

Medoff G (1987). Controversial areas in antifungal chemotherapy: Short-course and combination therapy with amphotericin B. *Rev Infect Dis* **9**: 403.

Medoff G, Kobayashi GS (1975). Amphotericin B Old drug, new therapy. *JAMA* **232**: 619.

Medoff G, Kobayashi GS (1980). Strategies in the treatment of systemic fungal infections. *New Engl J Med* **302**: 145.

Medoff G, Comfort M, Kobayashi GS (1971). Synergistic action of amphotericin B and 5-fluorocytosine against yeast-like organisms. *Proc Soc Exp Biol Med* **138**: 571.

Meeker TC, Siegel MS, Shiota FM *et al.* (1983). Toxicity of amphotericin B, miconazole and ketoconazole to human granulocyte progenitor cells *in vitro*. *Antimicrob Ag Chemother* **23**: 169.

Menichetti F, Del Favero A, Martino P *et al.* (1994). Preventing fungal infection in neutropenic patients with acute leukemia: fluconazole compared with oral amphotericin B. The GIMEMA Infection Program. *Ann Intern Med* **120**: 913.

Merz WG, Sandford GR (1979). Isolation and characterization of a polyene resistant variant of *Candida tropicalis*. *J Clin Microbiol* **9**: 677.

Meunier F (1989). New methods for delivery of antifungal agents. *Rev Infect Dis* **11** (Suppl 7): S1605.

Meunier F, Prentice HG, Ringden O (1991). Liposomal amphotericin B (AmBisome): safety data from a phase II/III clinical trial. *J Antimicrob Chemother* **28** (SupplB): 83.

Meunier-Carpentier F Snoeck R, Gerain J *et al.* (1984). Amphotericin B nasal spray as prophylaxis against aspergillosis in patients with neutropenia. *New Engl J Med* **311**: 1056.

Mikami Y, Scalarone GM, Kurita N *et al.* (1995). Synergistic postantifungal effect of flucytosine and fluconazole on *Candida albicans*. *J Med Vet Mycol* **30**: 197.

Mishra M, Biswas UK, Jha DN, Khan AB (1992). Amphotericin B versus pentamidine in antimony-unresponsive kala-azar. *Lancet* **340**: 1256.

Montalban C, Calleja JL, Erice A *et al.* (1990). Visceral leishmaniasis in patients infected with human immunodeficiency virus. Co-operative Group for the study of leishmaniasis in AIDS. *J Infect* **21**: 261.

Montgomerie JZ, Edwards JE Jr, Guze LB (1975). Synergism of amphotericin B and 5-fluorocytosine for *Candida* species. *J Infect Dis* **132**: 82.

Morace G, Manzara S, Dettori G (1991). *In vitro* susceptibility of 119 yeast isolates to fluconazole, 5-fluorocytosine, amphotericin B and ketoconazole. *Chemotherapy* **37**: 23.

Moskovskij SD, Southgate BA (1971). Clinical aspects of leishmaniasis with special reference to the USSR. *Bull World Health Org* **44**: 491.

Mott SH, Packer RJ, Vezina LG *et al.* (1995). Encephalopathy woth parkinsonian features in children following bone marrow transplantation and high-dose amphotericin B. *Ann Neurol* **37**: 810.

Munk PL, Vellet AD, Rankin RN *et al.* (1993). Intracavitary aspergilloma: Transthoracic percutaneous injection of amphotericin gelatin solution. *Radiology* **188**: 821.

Munckhof W, Jones R, Tosolini FA *et al.* (1993). Cure of *Rhizopus* sinusitis in a liver transplant recipient with liposomal amphotericin B. *Clin Infect Dis* **16**: 183.

Murphy N, Buchanan CR, Damjanovic V *et al.* (1986). Infection and colonization of neonates by *Hansenula anomala*. *Lancet* **i**: 291.

Murray HW (1974). Allergic reactions to amphotericin B. *New Engl J Med* **290**: 693.

Nagington J, Richards JE (1976). Chemotherapeutic compounds and acanthamoebae from eye infections. *J Clin Path* **29**: 648.

National Committee for Clinical Laboratory Standards (1992). Reference method for broth dilution antifungal susceptibility testing for yeasts: proposed standard M27-P. Villanova, PA: NCCLS, 1992.

New RRC, Chance ML, Heath S (1981). Antileishmanial activity of amphotericin and other antifungal agents entrapped in liposomes. *J Antimicrob Chemother* **8**: 371.

Nguyen MH, Yu VL(1995). Meningitis caused by *Candida* species: an emerging problem in neurosurgical patients. *Clin Infect Dis* **21**: 323.

Nicholl TA, Nimmo CR, Shepherd JD *et al* (1995). Amphotericin B infusion-related toxicity: comparison of two- and four-hour infusions. *Ann Pharmacother* **29**: 1081.

Niki Y, Bernard EM, Schmitt HJ *et al.* (1990). Pharmacokinetics of aerosol amphotericin B in rats. *Antimicrob Ag Chemother* **34**: 29.

Nosanchuk JS, Greenberg RD (1973). Protothecosis of the olecranon bursa caused by achloric algae. *Amer J Clin Pathol* **59**: 567.

Odds FC (1982). Interactions among amphotericin B, 5-fluorocytosine, ketoconazole, and miconazole against pathogenic fungi *in vitro*. *Antimicrob Ag Chemother* **22**: 763.

Ohnishi A, Ohnishi T, Stevenhead W *et al.* (1989). Sodium status influences chronic amphotericin B nephrotoxicity in rats. *Antimicrob Ag Chemother* **33**: 1222.

Oldfield EC, Garst PD, Hostettler C *et al.* (1990). Randomized, double-blinded trial of 1- versus 4-hour amphotericin B infusion durations. *Antimicrob Ag Chemother* **34**: 1402.

Omizo MKN, Bryant RE, Loveless MO (1993). Amphotericin B-induced malignant hypertension. *Clin Infect Dis* **17**: 817.

Oppenheim BA, Herbrecht R, Kusne S (1995). The safety and efficacy of Amphotericin B Colloidal Dispersion in the treatment of invasive mycoses. *Clin Infect Dis* **21**: 1145.

Pahls S, Schaffner A (1994). Comparison of the activity of free and liposomal amphotericin B *in vitro* and in a model of systemic and localized murine candidiasis. *J Infect Dis* **169**: 1057.

Pappagianis D, Collins MS, Hector R, Remington J (1979). Development of resistance to amphotericin B in *Candida lusitaniae* infecting a human. *Antimicrob Ag Chemother* **16**: 123.

Pappas PG, Threlkeld MG, Bedsole GD *et al.* (1993). Blastomycosis in immunocompromised patients. *Medicine* **72**: 311.

Parfrey NA (1986). Improved diagnosis and prognosis of mucormycosis. A clinicopathologic study of 33 cases. *Medicine* **65**: 113.

Parker JD, Doto IL, Tosh FE (1969). A decade of experience with blastomycosis and its treatement with amphotericin B. *Amer Rev Respir Dis* **99**: 895.

Patterson R, Greenberger PA, Radin RC, Roberts M (1982). Allergic bronchopulmonary aspergillosis: staging as an aid to management. *Ann Intern Med* **96**: 286.

Penn CC, Goldstein E, Bartholomew WR (1992). *Sporothrix schenckii* meningitis in a patient with AIDS. *Clin Infect Dis* **15**: 741.

Pennington JE (1976). Successful treatment of *Aspergillus* pneumonia in hematologic neoplasia. *New Engl J Med* **29S**: 42.

Pennington JE, Block ER, Reynolds HY (1974). 5-Fluorocytosine and amphotericin B in bronchial secretions. *Antimicrob Ag Chemother* **6**: 324.

Perfect JR, Durack DT (1982). Treatment of experimental cryptococcal meningitis with amphotericin B, 5-fluorocytosine, and ketoconazole. *J Infect Dis* **146**: 429.

Perfect JR, Durack DT (1985). Comparison of amphotericin B and *N-d*-ornithyl amphotericin B methyl ester in experimental cryptococcal meningitis and *Candida albicans* endocarditis with pyelonephritis. *Antimicrob Ag Chemother* **28**: 751.

Perfect JR, Klotman ME, Gilbert CC *et al.* (1992). Prophylactic intravenous amphotericin B in neutropenic autologous bone marrow transplant recipients. *J Infect Dis* **165**: 891.

Perraut LE Jr, Perraut LE, Bleiman B, Lyons J (1981). Successful treatment of *Candida albicans* endophthalmitis with intravitreal amphotericin B. *Arch Ophthalmol* **99**: 1565.

Petrou MA, Rogers TR (1991). Interactions *in vitro* between polyenes and imidazoles against yeast. *J Antimicrob Chemother* **27**: 491.

Pfaller MA, Krogstad DJ (1981). Imidazole and polyene activity against chloroquine-resistant *Plasmodium falciparum*. *J Infect Dis* **144**: 372.

Pfaller MA, Wenzel R (1992). Impact of the changing epidemiology of fungal infections in the 1990s. *Eur J Clin Microbiol Infect Dis* **11**: 287.

Pflugfelder SC, Flynn HW (1992). Infectious endophthalmitis. *Inf Dis Clin N Amer* **6**: 859.

Pittard WB III, Thullen JD, Fanaroff AA (1976). Neonatal septic arthritis. *J Pediatr* **88**: 621.

Pizzo PA, Robichaud KJ, Gill FA, Witebsky FG (1982). Empiric antibiotic and antifungal therapy for cancer patients with prolonged fever and granulocytopenia. *Amer J Med* **72**: 101.

Pluss JL, Opal SM (1986). Pulmonary sporotrichosis: Review of treatment and outcome. *Medicine* **65**: 143.

Polak A (1979). Pharmacokinetics of amphotericin B and flucytosine. *Postgrad Med J* **55**: 667.

Polak A (1987). Combination therapy of experimental candidiasis, cryptococcosis, aspergillosis and wangiellosis in mice. *Chemotherapy* **33**: 381.

Posner JB (1973). Editorial. Reservoirs for intraventricular chemotherapy. *New Engl J Med* **288**: 212.

Pottage JC, Kessler HA, (1985). Inhibition of *in vitro* HBsAg production by amphotericin B and ketoconazole. *J Med Virol* **16**: 275.

Poungvarin N, Jariya P (1991). The fifth nonlethal case of primary amoebic meningoencephalitis. *J Med Assoc Thai* **74**: 112.

Powderly WG (1992). Therapy for cryptococcal meningitis in patients with AIDS. *Clin Infect Dis* **14** (Suppl 1): S54.

Powderly WG, Kobayashi GS, Herzig GP, Medoff G (1988). Amphotericin B-resistant yeast infection in severely immunocompromised patients. *Amer J Med* **84**: 826.

Powderly WG, Saag MS, Cloud GA *et al.* (1992). A controlled trial of fluconazole or amphotericin B to prevent relapse of cryptococcal meningitis in patients with the acquired immunodeficiency syndrome. *New Engl J Med* **326**: 793.

Powell DA, Schuit KE (1979). Acute pulmonary blastomycosis in children: clinical course and follow-up. *Pediatrics* **63**: 736.

Racis SP, Plescia OJ, Geller HM, Schaffner CP (1990). Comparative toxicities of amphotericin B and its monomethyl ester derivative on glial cells in culture. *Antimicrob Ag Chemother* **34**: 1360.

Rahko PS, Davey WP, Wheat J, Bartlett M (1983). Treatment of *Torulopsis glabrata* peritonitis with intraperitoneal amphotericin B. *JAMA* **249**: 1187.

Rank EL, Hopfer RL, Williams RP (1981). Amphotericin B causes a decrease in human leucocyte migration. *J Antimicrob Chemother* **8**: 497.

Ravinovich S, Shaw BD, Bryant T, Donta ST (1974). Effect of 5-fluorocytosine and amphotericin B on *Candida albicans* infection in mice. *J Infect Dis* **130**: 28.

Restrepo A (1994). Treatment of tropical mycoses. *J Amer Acad Dermatol* **31**: S91.

Reuben A, Anaissie E, Nelson PE *et al.* (1989). Antifungal susceptibility of 44 clinical isolates of *Fusarium* species determined by using a broth microdilution method. *Antimicrob Ag Chemother* **33**: 1647.

Reuhl KR, Vapiwala M, Ryzlak MT, Schaffner CP (1993). Comparative neurotoxicities of amphotericin B and its mono-methyl ester derivative in rats. *Antimicrob Ag Chemother* **37**: 419.

Rex JH, Pfaller MA, Rinaldi MG *et al.* (1993). Antifungal susceptibility testing. *Clin Microbiol Rev* **6**: 367.

Rex JH, Bennett JE, Sugar AM *et al.* (1994). A randomized trial comparing fluconazole with amphotericin B for the treatment of candidemia in patients without neutropenia. *New Engl J Med* **331**: 1325.

Rex JH, Pfaller MA, Barry AL *et al.* Mycoses Study Group, and Candidemia Study Group (1995). Antifungal susceptibility testing of isolates from a randomized, multicenter trial of fluconazole versus amphotericin B as treatment of nonneutropenic patients with candidemia. *Antimicrob Ag Chemother* **39**: 40.

Richards AB, Jones BR, Whitwell J, Clayton YM (1969). Corneal and intraocular infection by *Candida albicans* treated with 5-fluorocytosine. *Trans Ophthal Soc UK* **29**: 867.

Riley D, Beatty P, Pavia A, Evans TG (1992). Prophylactic use of low-dose amphotericin (AMB) in bone marrow transplant (BMT) patients (Abstract no 620). In *Program and Abstracts of the 32nd Interscience Conference on Antimicrobial Agents and Chemotherapy*, p. 214. Washington, DC: American Society for Microbiology.

Rinaldi MG (1989). Zygomycosis. *Infect Dis Clin N Amer* **3**: 19.

Ringden O, Meunier F, Tollemar J *et al.* (1991). Efficacy of amphotericin B encapsulated in liposomes (AmBisome). in the treatment of invasive fungal infections in immunocompromised patients. *J Antimicrob Chemother* **28** (Suppl B): 73.

Robertson MJ, Larson RA (1988). Recurrent fungal pneumonias in patients with acute nonlymphocytic leukemia undergoing multiple courses of intensive chemotherapy. *Amer J Med* **84**: 233.

Roe DC, Haynes RE (1972). *Candida albicans* meningitis successfully treated with amphotericin B. *Amer J Dis Child* **124**: 926.

Rosch JM, Pazin GJ, Fireman P (1976). Reduction of amphotericin B nephrotoxicity with mannitol. *JAMA* **235**: 1995.

Roselle GA, Kauffman CA (1978). Amphotericin B and 5-fluorocytosine: *in vitro* effects on lymphocyte function. *Antimicrob Ag Chemother* **14**: 398.

Rosenblatt HM, Steihm ER (1983). Therapy for chronic mucocutaneous candidiasis. *Amer J Med* **74**: 20.

Rubinstein E, Noriega ER, Simberkoff MS *et al.* (1974). Tissue penetration of amphotericin B in candida endocarditis. *Chest* **66**: 376.

Saag MS, Powderly WG, Cloud GA *et al.* (1992). Comparison of amphotericin B with fluconazole in the treatment of acute AIDS-associated cryptococcal meningitis. *New Engl J Med* **326**: 83.

Sabra R, Branch RA (1991). Mechanisms of amphotericin B-induced decrease in glomerular filtration rate in rats. *Antimicrob Ag Chemother* **35**: 2509.

Salkin IF, McGinnis MR, Dykstra MJ, Rinaldi MG (1988). *Scedosporium inflatum*, an emerging pathogen. *J Clin Microbiol* **26**: 498.

Sanders SW, Buchi KN, Goddard MS *et al.* (1991). Single dose pharmacokinetics and tolerance of a cholesteryl-sulfate complex of amphotericin B administered to healthy volunteers. *Antimicrob Ag Chemother* **35**: 1029.

Sands M, Poppel D, Brown R (1991). Peritonitis due to *Prototheca wickerhamii* in a patient undergoing chronic ambulatory peritoneal dialysis. *Rev Infect Dis* **13**: 376.

Sanford JP (1993). The enigma of candiduria: Evolution of bladder irrigation with Amphotericin B for management-from anecdote to dogma and a lesson from Machiavelli. *Clin Infect Dis* **16**: 145.

Sarosi GA, Voth DW, Dahl BA *et al.* (1971). Disseminated histoplasmosis: results of long-term follow-up. *Ann Intern Med* **75**: 511.

Sarosi GA, Armstrong D, Barbee RA *et al.* (1979). Treatment of fungal diseases *Amer Rev Respir Dis* **120**: 1393.

Sarosi GA Davies SF, Phillips JR (1986). Self-limited blastomycosis: A report of 39 cases. *Semin Respir Infect* **1**: 40.

Schaffner A, Bohler A (1993). Amphotericin-B refractory aspergillosis after itraconazole- evidence for significant antagonism. *Mycoses* **36**: 421.

Schaffner A, Frick PG (1985). The effect of ketoconazole on amphotericin B in a model of disseminated aspergillosis. *J Infect Dis* **151**: 902.

Scheven M, Schwegler F (1995). Antagonistic interactions between azoles and amphotericin B with yeasts depend on azole lipophilia for special test conditions *in vitro*. *Antimicrob Ag Chemother* **39**: 1779.

Schiffman RL, Scott Johnson T, Weinberger SE *et al.* (1982). *Candida* lung abscess: successful treatment with amphotericin B and 5-flucytosine. *Amer Rev Respir Dis* **125**: 766.

Schmitt HJ, Bernard EM, Andrade J *et al.* (1988a). MIC and fungicidal activity of terbinafine against clinical isolates of *Aspergillus* spp. *Antimicrob Ag Chemother* **32**: 780.

Schmitt HJ, Bernard EM, Hauser M, Armstrong D (1988b). Aerosol amphotericin B is effective for prophylaxis and therapy in a rat model of pulmonary aspergillosis. *Antimicrob Ag Chemother* **32**: 1676.

Schonheyder H, Thestrup-Pedersen K, Esmann V, Stenderup A (1980). Cryptococcal meningitis: complications due to intrathecal treatment. *Scand J Infect Dis* **12**: 155.

Schroter GPJ, Temple DR, Husberg BS *et al.* (1976). Cryptococcosis after renal transplantation: report of ten cases. *Surgery* **79**: 268.

Seabury JH, Dascomb HE (1960). Experience with amphotericin B. *Ann NY Acad Sci* **89**: 202.

Seaman J, Boer C, Wilkinson R *et al.* (1995). Liposomal amphotericin B (AmBisome) in the treatment of complicated Kala-azar under field conditions. *Clin Infect Dis* **21**: 188.

Seelig MS, Kozinn PJ, Goldberg P, Berger AR (1979). Fungal endocarditis: patients at risk and their treatment. *Postgrad Med J* **55**: 632.

Segal E, Padhye AA, Ajello L (1976). Susceptibility of *Prototheca* species to antifungal agents. *Antimicrob Ag Chemother* **10**: 75.

Seidel JS, Harmatz P, Visvesvara G S *et al.* (1982). Successful treatment of primary amebic meningoencephalitis. *New Engl J Med* **306**: 346.

Seidenfeld SM, Cooper BH, Smith JW *et al.* (1983). Amphotericin B tolerance: a characteristic of *Candida parapsilosis* not shared by other *Candida* species. *J Infect Dis* **147**: 116.

Sekhon AS, Padhye AA, Garg AK (1992a). *In vitro* sensitivity of *Penicillium marneffei* and *Pythium insidiosum* to various antifungal agents. *Eur J Epidemiol* **8**: 427.

Sekhon AS, Kowalewska-Grochowska J, Garg AK, Vaudry W (1992b). *Hansenula anomala* fungemia in an infant with gastric and cardiac complications with a review of the literature. *Eur J Epidemiol* **8**: 305.

Sekhon AS, Garg AK Padhye AA, Hamir Z (1993). *In vitro* susceptibility of myceliel and yeast forms of *Penicillium marneffei* to amphotericin B, fluconazole, 5-fluorocytosine and itraconazole. *Eur J Epidemiol* **9**: 553.

Sekhon AS, Padhye AA, Garg AK *et al.* (1994). *In vitro* sensitivity of medically significant *Fusarium* species to various antimycotics. *Chemotherapy* **40**: 239.

Shadomy S, Wagner G, Espinel-Ingroff A, Davis BA (1975). *In vitro* studies with combinations of 5-fluorocytosine and amphotericin B. *Antimicrob Ag Chemother* **8**: 117.

Sharkey PK, Graybill JR, Johnson ES *et al.* (1996). Amphotericin B lipid complex compared with amphotericin B in the treatment of cryptococcal meningitis in patients with AIDS. *Clin Infect Dis* **22**: 315.

Sheikh HA, Mahgoub S, Badi K (1974). Postoperative endophthalmitis due to *Trichosporon cutaneum. Brit J Ophthalmol* **58**: 591.

Sloand EM, Kumar P, Yu M, Klein HG (1994). Effect of amphotericin B and fluconazole on platelet membrane glycoproteins. *Transfusion* **34**: 415.

Smego RA, Durack DT (1984). *In vitro* susceptibility testing of *Naegleria fowleri* to ketoconazole, Bay n 7133, and allopurinol riboside. *J Parasit* **70**: 317.

Smego RA Jr, Devoe PW, Sampson HA *et al.* (1984a). *Candida* meningitis in two children with severe combined immunodeficiency. *J Pediatr* **104**: 902.

Smego RA Jr, Perfect JR, Durack DT (1984b). Combined therapy with amphotericin B and 5- fluorocytosine for *Candida* meningitis. *Rev Infect Dis* **6**: 791.

Smith BM, Hoeprich PD, Huston AC *et al.* (1983a). Activity of two polyene and two imidazole antimycotics on *Candida albicans* in human fibrin clots. *J Lab Clin Med* **102**: 126.

Smith D, McFadden HW Jr, Miller NG (1983b). Effect of ketoconazole and amphotericin B on encapsulated and non-encapsulated strains of *Cryptococcus neoformans. Antimicrob Ag Chemother* **24**: 851.

Sokol-Anderson M, Sligh JE, Elberg S *et al.* (1988). Role of cell defense against oxidative damage in the resistance of *Candida albicans* to the killing effect of amphotericin B. *Antimicrob Ag Chemother* **32**: 702.

Stamm AM, Diasio RB, Dismukes WE *et al.* (1987). Toxicity of amphotericin B plus flucytosine in 194 patients with cryptococcal meningitis. *Amer J Med* **83**: 236.

Stein RS, Kayser J, Flexner JM (1982). Clinical value of empirical amphotericin B in patients with acute myelogenous leukemia. *Cancer* **50**: 2247.

Stern GA, Fetkenhour CL, O'Grady RB (1977). Intravitreal amphotericin B treatment for *Candida* endophthalmitis. *Arch Ophthalmol* **95**: 89.

Stern WH, Tamura E, Jacobs RA *et al.* (1985). Epidemic postsurgical *Candida parapsilosis* endophthalmitis. *Ophthalmology* **92**: 1701.

Stevens AR, Shulman ST, Lansen TA *et al.* (1981). Primary amoebic meningoencephalitis: a report of two cases and antibiotic and immunologic studies. *J Infect Dis* **143**: 193.

Stewart SJ, Spangaolo PH, Ellner JJ (1981). Generation of suppressor T lymphocytes and monocytes by amphotericin B. *Immunol* **127**: 135–139.

Stieritz DD, Law EJ, Holder 1A (1973). Speciation and amphotericin B sensitivity studies on blood isolates of *Candida* from burned patients. *J Clin Path* **26**: 405.

Sud IJ, Finegold DS (1983). Effects of ketoconazole on the fungicidal action of amphotericin B on *Candida albicans. Antimicrob Ag Chemother* **23**: 185.

Sudduth EJ, Crumbley AJ, Farrar WE (1992). Phaeohyphomycosis due to *Exophiala* species: Clinical spectrum of disease in humans. *Clin Infect Dis* **15**: 639.

Sugar AM, Salibian M, Goldani LZ (1994). Saperconazole therapy of murine disseminated candidiasis: efficacy and interactions with amphotericin B. *Antimicrob Ag Chemother* **38**: 371.

Sugar AM, Hitchcock CA, Troke PF, Picard M (1995). Combination therapy of murine invasive candidiasis with fluconazole and amphotericin B. *Antimicrob Ag Chemother* **39**: 598.

Sunder S, Murray HW (1996). Cure of antimony-unresponsive Indian visceral leishmaniasis with amphotericin B lipid complex. *J Infect Dis* **173**: 762.

Supapidhayakul S-R, Kizlaitis LR, Andersen BR (1981). Stimulation of human and canine neutrophil metabolism by amphotericin B. *Antimicrob Ag Chemother* **19**: 284.

Supparatpinyo K, Chiewchanvit S, Hirunsri P *et al.* (1992). *Penicillium marneffei* infection in patients infected with human immunodeficiency virus. *Clin Infect Dis* **14**: 871.

Supparatpinyo K, Nelson KE, Merz WG *et al.* (1993). Response to antifungal therapy by human immunodeficiency virus-infected patients with disseminated *Penicillium marneffei* infections and *in vitro* susceptibilities of isolates from clinical specimens. *Antimicrob Ag Chemother* **37**: 2407.

Swerdloff JN, Filler SG, Edwards JE (1993). Severe candidal infections in neutropenic patients. *Clin Infect Dis* **17** (Suppl 2): S457.

Symmers WStC Sen (1973). Amphotericin pharmacophobia. *Brit Med J* **4**: 460.

Szoka FC, Milholland D, Barza M (1987). Effect of lipid composition and liposome size on toxicity and *in vitro* fungicidal activity of liposome-intercalated amphotericin B. *Antimicrob Ag Chemother* **31**: 421.

Tack KJ, Rhame FS, Brown B, Thompson RC Jr (1982). Aspergillus osteomyelitis. Report of four cases and review of the literature. *Amer J Med* **73**: 295.

Takacs FJ, Tomkiewicz ZM, Merrill JP (1963). Amphotericin B nephrotoxicity with irreversible renal failure. *Ann Intern Med* **59**: 716.

Tarala RA, Smith JD (1980). Cryptococcosis treated by rapid infusion of amphotericin B. *Brit Med J* **281**: 28.

Thaler M, Behram P, Shawker TH *et al.* (1988a). Hepatic candidiasis in cancer patients: The evolving picture of the syndrome. *Ann Intern Med* **108**: 100.

Thaler M, Bacher J, O'Leary T, Pizzo PA (1988b). Evaluation of single-drug and combination antifungal therapy in an experimental model of candidiasis in rabbits with prolonged neutropenia. *J Infect Dis* **158**: 80.

Thong YH (1982). Chemotherapy for primary amebic meningoencephalitis. *New Engl J Med* **306**: 1295.

Thong YH, Rowan-Kelly B, Ferrante A, Shepherd C (1978). Synergism between tetracycline and amphotericin B in experimental amoebic meningoencephalitis. *Med J Aust* **1**: 663.

Thong YH, Rowan-Kelly B, Ferrante A (1979). Treatment of experimental *Naegleria* meningoencephalitis with a combination of amphotericin B and rifamycin. *Scand J Infect Dis* **11**: 151.

Tobias JS, Wrigley PFM, Shaw E (1976). Combination antifungal therapy for cryptococcal meningitis. *Postgrad Med J* **52**: 305.

Todenschini G, Murari C, Bonesi R *et al.* (1993). Oral intraconazole plus nasal amphotericin B for prophylaxis of invasive aspergillosis in patients with haematological malignancies. *Eur J Clin Microbiol Infect Dis* **12**: 614.

Tollemar J, Ringden O, Tyden G (1990). Liposomal amphotericin B (AmBisome) treatment in solid organ transplant recipients: efficacy and safety evaluation. *Clin Transplant* **4**: 167.

Tollemar J, Ringden O, Andersson S *et al.* (1993). Randomized, double-blind study of liposomal amphotericin B (AmBisome). prophylaxis of invasive fungal infections in bone marrow transplant recipients. *Bone Marrow Transplant* **12**: 577.

Tollemar J, Hockerstedt K, Ericzon B *et al.* (1995). Liposomal amphotericin B prevents invasive fungal infections in liver transplant recipients. A randomized placebo-controlled trial. *Transplant* **59**: 45.

Tollins JP and Raij L (1988). Chronic amphotericin B nephrotoxicity in the rat, protective effect of prophylactic salt loading. *Amer J Kidney Dis* **11**: 313.

Tremblay C, Barza M, Fiore C, Szoka F (1984). Efficacy of liposome-intercalated amphotericin B in the treatment of systemic candidiasis in mice. *Antimicrob Ag Chemother* **26**: 170.

Trinh T, Simonian J, Vigil S, Chin D, Bidair M (1995). Continuous versus intermittent bladder irrigation of amphotericin B for the treatment of candiduria. *J Urol* **154**: 1032.

Trissel LA (1994). In *Handbook on Injectable Drugs* 8th edn, p. 67. Bethesda MD, USA: American Society of Hospital Pharmacists.

Tynes BS, Utz JP, Bennett JE, Alling DW (1963). Reducing amphotericin B reactions. A double blind study. *Amer Rev Respir Dis* **87**: 264.

Utley JR, Mills J, Roe BB (1975). The role of valve replacement in the treatment of fungal endocarditis. *J Thorac Cardiovasc Surg* **69**: 255.

Utz JP, Garriques IL, Sande MA *et al.* (1975). Therapy of cryptococcosis with a combination of flucytosine and amphotericin B. *J Infect Dis* **132**: 368.

Valero G, Graybill JR (1995). Successful treatment of cryptococcal meningitis with amphotericin B colloidal dispersion: report of four cases. *Antimicrob Ag Chemother* **39**: 2588.

Van Cutsem J, Van Gerven F, de Backer P, Zaman R (1992). Therapy of meningeal and disseminated cryptococcosis. *Chemotherapy* **38** (Suppl 1): 57.

van Eldere J, Jooston L, Verhaeghe A, Surmont I (1996). Fluconazole and amphotericin B antifungal susceptibility testing by National Committee for Clinical Laboratory Standards Broth Macrodilution method compared with E-test and semi-automated broth microdilution test. *J Clin Microbiol* **34**: 842.

Van Etten EWM, Van den Heuvel-de Groot C, Bakker-Woudenberg IAJM (1993). Efficacies of amphotericin B-desoxycholate (Fungizone), liposomal amphotericin B (AmBisome) and fluconazole in the treatment of systemic candidosis in immunocompetent and leucopenic mice. *J Antimicrob Chemother* **32**: 723.

Vanezio FR, Lavoo E, Williams JE *et al.* (1982). Progressive cutaneous protothecosis. *Amer J Clin Pathol* **77**: 485.

Vartian CV, Shlaes DM, Padhye AA, Ajello L (1985). *Wangiella dermatitidis* endocarditis in an intravenous drug user. *Amer J Med* **78**: 703.

Velez JD, Allendoerfer R, Luther M *et al.* (1993). Correlation of *in vitro* azole susceptibility with *in vivo* response in a murine model of cryptococcal meningitis. *J Infect Dis* **168**: 508.

Wain W, Ahmed M, Thompson RL, Yacoub M (1979). The role of chemotherapy in the management of fungal endocarditis following homograft valve replacement. *Postgrad Med J* **55**: 629.

Walker RW, Rosenblum MK (1992). Amphotericin B-associated leukoencephalopathy. *Neurol* **42**: 2005.

Walsh TJ, Newman KR, Moody M *et al.* (1986). Trichosporonosis in patients with neoplastic disease. *Medicine* **65**: 268.

Walsh TJ, Melcher GP, Rinaldi MG *et al.* (1990). *Trichosporon beigelii*, an emerging pathogen resistant to amphotericin B. *Brit J Clin Microbiol* **28**: 1616.

Walsh TJ, Lee J, Lecciones J *et al.* (1991). Empiric therapy with amphotericin B in febrile granulocytopenic patients. *Rev Infect Dis* **13**: 496.

Walsh TJ, Lee JW, Melcher GP *et al.* (1992). Experimental *Trichosporon* infection in persistently granulocytopenic rabbits: Implications for pathogenesis, diagnosis, and treatment of an emerging opportunistic mycosis. *J Infect Dis* **166**: 121.

Ward RM, Sattler FR, Dalton AS Jr (1983). Assessment of antifungal therapy in an 800–gram infant with candidal arthritis and osteomyelitis. *Pediatrics* **72**: 234.

Washington C, Lance M, Davis SS (1993). Toxicity of amphotericin B emulsion formulations. *J Antimicrob Chemother* **31**: 806.

Weinberg WG, Wade BH, Cierny G *et al.* (1993). Invasive infection due to *Apophysomyces elegans* in immunocompetent hosts. *Clin Infect Dis* **17**: 881.

Wen DY, Bottini AG, Hall WA, Haines SJ (1992). The intraventricular use of antibiotics. *Neurosurg Clin N Amer* **3**: 343.

Wheat LJ, Slama TG, Zeckel ML (1985). Histoplasmosis in the acquired immune deficiency syndrome. *Amer J Med* **78**: 203.

Wheat LJ, Connolly-Stringfield PA, Baker RL *et al.* (1990). Disseminated histoplasmosis in the acquired immunodeficiency syndrome: Clinical findings, diagnosis and treatment, and review of the literature. *Medicine* **69**: 361.

Wheat J (1994). Histoplasmosis and coccidiomycosis in individuals with AIDS. A clinical review. *Infect Dis Clinics N Amer* **8**: 467.

White MH, Armstrong D (1994). Cryptococcosis. *Infect Dis Clin N Amer* **8**: 383.

Williams DM, Graybill JR, Drutz DJ (1979). Experimental chemotherapy of histoplasmosis in nude mice. *Amer Rev Respir Dis* **120**: 837.

Williamson PR, Kwon-Chung KJ, Gallin JI (1992). Successful treatment of *paecilomyces varioti* infection in a patient with chronic granulomatous disease and a review of *Paecilomyces* species infections. *Clin Infect Dis* **14**: 1023.

Winston DJ, Chandresakar PH, Lazarus HM *et al.* (1993). Fluconazole prophylaxis of fungal infections in patients with acute leukemia. *Ann Intern Med* **118**: 495.

Wise GJ, Wainstein S, Goldberg P, Kozinn PJ (1973). *Candidal* cystitis. Management by continuous bladder irrigation with amphotericin B. *JAMA* **224**: 1636.

Wise GJ, Kozinn PJ, Goldberg P (1982). Amphotericin B as a urologic irrigant in the management of noninvasive candiduria. *J Urol* **128**: 82.

Wolff MA, Ramphal R (1995). Use of amphotericin B lipid complex for treatment of disseminated cutaneous *Fusarium* infection in a neutropenic patient. *Clin Infect Dis* **20**: 1568.

Wong PW, Ching WTW, Kwon-Chung KJ, Meyer RD (1989). Disseminated *Phialophora parasitica* infection in humans: Case report and review. *Rev Infect Dis* **11**: 770.

Woods RA, Bard M, Jackson IE, Drutz DJ (1974). Resistance to polyene antibiotics and correlated sterol changes in two isolates of *Candida tropicalis* from a patient with an amphotericin B-resistant funguria. *J Infect Dis* **129**: 53.

Working Party of the British Society for Antimicrobial Chemotherapy (1993). Chemoprophylaxis for candidosis and aspergillosis in neutropenia and transplantation: a review and recommendations. *J Antimicrob Chemother* **32**: 5.

Wright DG, Robichaud KJ, Pizzo PA, Deisseroth AB (1981). Lethal pulmonary reactions associated with the combined use of amphotericin B and leukocyte transfusions. *New Engl J Med* **304**: 1185.

Yangco BG, Okafor JI, TeStrake D (1984). *In vitro* susceptibilities of human and wild-type isolates of *Basidiobolus* and *Conidiobolus* species. *Antimicrob Ag Chemother* **25**: 413.

Yasui K, Masuda M, Matsuoka T *et al.* (1988). Miconazole and amphotericin B alter polymorphonuclear leukocyte functions and membrane fluidity in similar fashions. *Antimicrob Ag Chemother* **32**: 1864.

Yinnon AM, Woodin KA, Powell KP (1992). *Candida lusitaniae* infection in the newborn: case report and review of the literature. *Pediatr Infect Dis J* **11**: 878.

Zervos MJ, Silverman J, Meunier F (1994). Fluconazole and fungal infections: a review. *Infect Dis Clin Pract* **3**: 94.

Zuger A, Schuster M, Simberkoff MS *et al.* (1988). Maintenance amphotericin B for cryptococcal meningitis in the acquired immunodeficiency syndrome (AIDS). *Ann Intern Med* **109**: 592.

Nystatin

Description

Nystatin, like amphotericin B and natamycin, is a polyene antifungal antibiotic. It was isolated from *Streptomyces noursei* in 1950 and originally named fungicidin (Hazen and Brown, 1951). Nystatin is not a single chemical compound, but a mixture of closely related substances (Chowdhry, 1976). It is a yellow powder which is insoluble in water and only sparingly soluble in methanol and ethanol. The drug was further developed by Squibb Research Laboratories (Dutcher *et al.*, 1954), and it was first approved by the US Food and Drug Administration in 1955 for treatment of vaginal candidiasis. Nystatin is a toxic and insoluble polyene, which is unsuitable for parenteral administration. It is used topically for the treatment of superficial infections.

Sensitive Organisms

Nystatin has no activity against bacteria, but it has a wide spectrum of antifungal activity. Yeasts such as *Candida albicans* and the other *Candida* spp., and *Cryptococcus neoformans* are susceptible. Using an agar dilution methodology, the MICs of nystatin for *C. albicans* are 0.5–2 μg per ml, for *C. glabrata* 1.0–2.0 μg per ml, other *Candida* spp. 2.0 μg per ml, and for *Cryptococcus neoformans* 2.0 μg per ml (Bergan and Vangdal, 1983). Molds or filamentous fungi, such as *Aspergillus, Trichophyton, Epidermophyton* and *Microsporum* spp., are usually sensitive. The same applies to most of the dimorphic fungi, such as *Histoplasma capsulatum, Blastomyces dermatitidis, Coccidioides immitis* and others. Fungi of the genus *Trichosporon* are sensitive, as are *Rhodotorula* spp., and *Blastoschizomyces capitatus* (*Geotrichum capitatum*). The MICs of nystatin against these sensitive fungi are usually in the range 1.56–6.25 μg per ml (Hazen and Brown, 1951; Hussain Qadri *et al.*, 1986).

Nystatin inhibits HIV-1 replication in H9 cells, and decreases reverse transcriptase activity by 85% at 10 μg per ml. The activity was comparable with zidovudine and amphotericin B (Selvam *et al.*, 1993). Nystatin has also shown activity against other lipid-enveloped RNA and DNA viruses.

Nystatin-resistant *Candida* strains can be produced in the laboratory (Woods, 1971; Nobre *et al.*, 1980). In one study of over 2000 clinical isolates of *Candida* spp., no nystatin-resistant variants were found (Athar and Winner, 1971). However, these authors showed that after gradual exposure to increased nystatin concentrations *in vitro*, nystatin-resistance could be induced in isolates of seven *Candida* species. These nystatin-resistant strains were cross-resistant to other polyene antibiotics such as amphotericin B and natamycin. Such resistant variants were less pathogenic. More recently, nystatin-resistance has been identified from clinical specimens (Dick *et al.*, 1980). Of 747 fungal strains isolated from oncology patients in Baltimore, 7.4% were found to be resistant to nystatin; resistance only occurred in strains of *C. albicans, C. tropicalis* and *C. glabrata*. Dube *et al.* (1994) described the increased isolation of nystatin-resistant *Candida* rugosa in the burns intensive care unit following the introduction of the routine use of nystatin prophylaxis.

Absorption of the Drug

Nystatin is poorly absorbed from the gastrointestinal tract. After a very large oral dose (10 million units), some nystatin can be detected in the serum, but with the usual recommended oral doses, there is insufficient absorption to produce a systemic chemotherapeutic effect. Some absorption must occur to explain the infrequent cases of allergic dermatitis, Stevens–Johnson syndrome and fixed drug eruption that have been reported.

Liposomal nystatin (multilamellar vesicles containing 500 μg nystatin per 10 mg phospholipids) is as effective as free nystatin against yeasts and molds *in vitro*. The MICs obtained for liposomal nystatin were either identical or lower than the corresponding MIC for nystatin against a wide range of fungi (Mehta *et al.*, 1987a). This observation is in contrast to the comparison between MICs for amphotericin B and liposomal amphotericin B (Hopfer *et al.*, 1984). *In vitro*, the liposomal preparation appears to protect human erythrocytes from the toxicity of the free nystatin (Mehta *et al.*, 1987a). Liposome encapsulation provides a parenteral preparation of nystatin that had markedly reduced toxicity and improved therapeutic efficacy in the murine model of systemic candidiasis (Mehta *et al.*, 1987b).

The pharmacokinetics of single doses of liposomal nystatin (0.25, 0.5, 0.75 and 1.0 mg per kg i.v.) were evaluated in HIV-infected patients. The drug was administered at 2 mg per min and the initial plasma concentration of nystatin ranged from 3.7 to 9 μg per ml over the four dose cohorts. The area-under-the-concentration-time-curve (AUC) increased from 452 μg.min per ml for the 0.25 mg per kg cohort to 1263 μg.min per ml for the 1.0 mg per kg cohort. The clearance rate of nystatin from blood of 0.6–1.0 ml.kg per min did not appear to vary significantly with increasing dose (Rios *et al.*, 1993).

Mode of Action

Nystatin, like amphotericin B (pp. 1261–2), acts by by binding to a specific sterol in the cytoplasmic membrane of sensitive fungi, induces excessive permeability of the plasma membrane allowing leakage of essential molecules including potassium. Nystatin, presumably by its action of making the cytoplasmic membrane more permeable, potentiates the entry of 5-flucytosine and tetracycline into *C. albicans* cells (Aszalos, 1975).

Toxicity

Mild nausea, vomiting, and diarrhea may occur following the administration of oral doses of nystatin exceeding 5 million units (Cohen, 1982).

Allergic contact dermatitis, Stevens–Johnson syndrome and fixed drug eruptions have been reported due to oral and topical nystatin (Wasilewski, 1970; Cosky, 1971; Pareek, 1980; De Groot and Conemans, 1990; Garty, 1991). A generalized, slightly pruritic, maculopapular rash associated with a swollen tongue, developed 3 days after commencing nystatin tablets 500 000 units four times daily in a non-atopic woman with aphthous ulcers. She required oral and topical corticosteroid medication for resolution. Skin biopsy suggested a drug reaction, and rechallenge, as well as patch testing confirmed that the reaction was due to nystatin (Quirce *et al.*, 1991). Both the cream and ointment formulations are well tolerated and adverse reactions are extremely rare even during prolonged use. When nystatin is combined in formulations with ethlyenediamine, a contact allergic dermatitis can develop at the site of application. Patch testing has shown the reaction is to the ethylenediamine component (Freeman, 1986).

No animal reproduction studies have been performed to establish the safety of nystatin in pregnancy. Nystatin should therefore be used in pregnancy only when absolutely needed.

Clinical Uses, Administration and Dosage

1 Preparations available

There are many preparations of this drug, such as oral tablets (500 000 units), an oral suspension (100 000 units per ml) and a powder for oral suspension, and pastilles (lozenges) containing 200 000 units nystatin. For the treatment of intestinal candidiasis (including oropharyngeal candidiasis) doses of 400 000 to 1 million units four times daily are administered, until resolution of the infection and for 48 h thereafter. In neonates, the dose is 100 000 units four times daily. For vulvovaginal candidiasis, vaginal tablets or foam pessaries (100 000 units), vaginal cream 100 000 units per 4–5 g are inserted high in the vagina daily for 14 days. Other topical preparations available include cream, ointment and powder in a concentration of 100 000 units per g and are applied to affected ares of skin three to four times per day. The eye should be avoided. In addition, creams and ointments are marketed in which nystatin is combined with antibiotics such as bacitracin, neomycin and polymyxin B, as well as steroids such as triamcinolone acetonide. One milligram of nystatin is equivalent to 3500 units.

2 Skin infections

Topical nystatin is suitable for the treatment of superficial *Candida* spp. infections, including diaper dermatitis and angular cheilitis. Topical nystatin applied three to four times daily for 7–10 days is usually effective, and symptomatic improvement usually occurs within 1–3 days (Rezabeck and Friedman, 1992). Topical nystatin cream (100 000 units per g) alone was as effective as combined oral nystatin suspension (100 000 units four times daily) and topical nystatin therapy for 10 days as treatment of diaper dermatitis due to *Candidia albicans*. Mycologic eradication of the skin rash occurred in 78%, but there was no difference in the eradication of *C. albicans* from skin or gastrointestinal tract between infants treated with the combined oral and topical therapy and those treated with topical nystatin alone (Munz *et al.*, 1982). Dermatophyte infections respond poorly.

3 Oral candidiasis ('thrush')

There are multiple regimens used for the treatment of oropharyngeal candidiasis, and include up to 10–15 ml of the suspension swished around the mouth in an attempt to cover all mucosal surfaces and then swallowed for esophageal exposure. Local treatment of oral candidiasis in patients receiving radiotherapy and/or chemotherapy for cancer of the head and neck is often less effective than in other immunocompromised patients. Nystatin 100 000 units four times daily for 3 weeks effected a clinical cure in 63% patients, of whom two-thirds relapsed (Holst, 1984). In infants and newborns with oral candidosis, oral ketoconazole suspension (20 mg per ml) had significantly greater efficacy, and more rapid therapeutic effect than nystatin (100 000 unit per ml) (Boon *et al.*, 1989). In Zairian AIDS patients with oropharyngeal or esophageal candidiasis, nystatin suspension 200 000 units 'swish and swallow' four times daily was significantly less effective than ketoconazole and gentian violet was more effective than nystatin for oral thrush (Nyst *et al.*, 1992). Nystatin is often used intermittently for oropharyngeal candidiasis, because of the concern over development of azole-resistance associated with chronic azole use. Treatment and suppressive doses of 500 000 units five times daily are generally required for adults with HIV infection. Some investigators recommend oral nystatin suspension for primary prophylaxis of mucocutaneous candidiasis in HIV-infected infants.

4 Vaginal candidiasis

This usually responds well to a 14-day course of nystatin pessaries, inserted high in the vagina, daily. The Nystatin Multicenter Study Group (1986) determined that a combined approach of nystatin administered both as an intravaginal pessary 100 000 units and oral tablets (3 000 000 units daily in three divided doses) for 1 week was significantly superior to intravaginal treatment with nystatin alone. These results are in contrast to other studies which failed to demonstrate that suppressing the intestinal reservoir of *Candida* spp. results in improved response rates for candidal vaginitis treatment (Milne and Warnock, 1979). Comparison of oral ketoconazole (400 mg per day for 5 days) and nystatin pessaries (100 000 units twice-daily for 7 days) for the treatment of vaginal candidosis, revealed no difference in response rate (80–87%), but a higher relapse rate in the nystatin-treated group (Salem *et al.*, 1989). The azole antifungal agents have replaced topical nystatin as the agent of first choice for vulvovaginal candidiasis, because of improved antifungal efficacy, shorter treatment regimens and better patient compliance.

5 Prophylaxis

The prophylactic use of nystatin in immunocompromised patients has often been disappointing. Several studies have been published that reveal the efficacy of nystatin suspension for antifungal prophylaxis in both adults and children is questionable (Williams *et al.*, 1977; Carpentieri *et al.*, 1978; De Gregario *et al.*, 1982; Barrett, 1984; Buchanan *et al.*, 1985). Oral forms of the drug are often unpalatable and patient compliance poor (Young, 1982; Gombert *et al.*, 1987; Reents *et al.*, 1993). The dose of nystatin and method of administration is not consistent across studies, making comparisons of efficacy inappropriate. Oral nystatin has been used as a prophylactic strategy to try to prevent systemic candidiasis in patients with hematologic malignancy and in cancer patients undergoing induction chemotherapy. DeGregorio *et al.* (1982) evaluated the use of nystatin prophylaxis during induction chemotherapy for acute leukemia, and found that nystatin did not reduce the risk of oropharyngeal or systemic candidiasis.

Ketoconazole has been compared with nystatin suspension for antifungal prophylaxis in cancer patients. In bone marrow transplant patients, ketoconazole was significantly more effective in preventing fungal infections in one study, but was no more effective than nystatin in another study (Hann *et al.*,1982; Shepp *et al.*, 1985), and in patients with hematological malignancy ketoconazole prevented more mucocutaneous candidal infections, but not systemic fungal infections (Jones *et al.*, 1984; Turhan *et al.*,1987). A comparison of oral fluconazole 3 mg per kg per day, nystatin 50 000 units per kg four times daily and oral amphotericin B 25 mg per kg four times daily for the prevention of fungal infection in pediatric patients with hematological or other malignancy, revealed the systemically absorbed fluconazole was significantly superior to the non-absorbed polyenes with reduction in fungal infections overall from 8.4% to 2.1%. However, there was no difference in clinical outcome or the rate of fungal colonization between the two groups (Ninane, 1994). A similar prospective randomized study was performed in adults at high risk of neutropenia, and fluconazole was more effective than the non-absorbed polyenes for the prevention of orophayngeal candidiasis, but equally effective for the prevention of other systemic fungal infections (Philpott Howard *et al.*, 1993). Comparable good efficacy for prevention of oropharyngeal candidiasis between clotrimazole troches and nystatin suspension has been established in renal transplant patients given 15 ml nystatin (100 000 units per ml) six times daily by the swish and swallow maneuver, and orthoptic liver transplant patients given 500 000 units four times daily (Gombert *et al.*, 1987; Ruskin *et al.*, 1992).

Up to 30% of burn patients become colonized with *Candida* spp. and are put at significant risk of *Candida* sepsis. Desai *et al.* (1992) reviewed their experience before and after the institution of nystatin prophylaxis (5–10 ml by 'swish and swallow' technique four times daily, and topical application of nystatin ointment to burn wounds with other topical antibiotics) in all burns patients. They noted a significant reduction in colonization, wound infection and sepsis from *Candida* spp. following the introduction of this strategy. This was confirmed in another retrospective study, in which the topical use of nystatin was associated with a significant decrease in fungal colonization and infection of burn wounds and 50% reduction in fungemia. However, an increase in colonization and sepsis from nystatin-resistant *C. rugosa* was observed with 75% cases of *Candida* spp. sepsis due to *C. rugosa* after the introduction of nystatin prophylaxis, compared with none prior to its institution (Dube *et al.*, 1994).

Among very low birthweight infants, mucocutaneous candidiasis is a significant risk factor for the development of invasive candidiasis. In a randomized, controlled study in very low birthweight infants, nystatin suspension 100 000 units in each side of the mouth every 8 h, significantly reduced the incidence of colonization and sepsis with *Candida* spp. (Sims *et al.*, 1988). However, another prospective study by Faix *et al.* (1989) revealed that nystatin therapy of established mucocutaneous candidiasis did not prevent the development of invasive candidiasis. Nevertheless, in an outbreak of *C. parapsilosis* infection in a neonatal intensive care unit, selective decontamination of the digestive tract with nystatin 100 000 units administered four times daily to all neonates in the unit until all surveillance site cultures were negative for 2 weeks, was an effective strategy in controlling the outbreak (Damjanovic *et al.*, 1993).

In critically ill surgical and trauma patients, the prophylactic use of nystatin 2 million units every 6 h administered via a nasogastric tube, significantly reduced the incidence of yeast colonization but not the incidence of yeast sepsis compared with no antifungal prophylaxis. The effect of nystatin was not different to that of clotrimazole or ketoconazole in this prospective randomized study which lacked statistical power to determine a difference between the individual agents (Savino *et al.*, 1994). Cerra *et al.* (1992), evaluated gut decontamination with an antibiotic and nystatin versus placebo for the prevention of nosocomial infections in a similar group of patients. Although they found that gut decontamination significantly reduced the number of fungal infections, it did not reduce the number of patients developing infection or overall mortality. Although the optimal dose of nystatin for selective gut decontamination has not been established, it is known that initially 12 million units per day is required to achieve nystatin concentrations of greater than 20 μg per ml in feces (for antifungal activity against yeast), with a subsequent decrease to 4 million units daily (Hofstra *et al.*, 1979). Placing patients on selective bowel decontamination with an oral quinolone and nystatin prior to the time of liver transplantation and continued for 4 weeks post-transplantation effectively reduced the incidence of fungal infections compared with historical controls (Gorensek *et al.*, 1993).

Zaruba *et al.* (1991) reported a reduction in the incidence of fungal peritonitis in continuous ambulatory peritoneal dialysis patients by the administration of nystatin during the period patients received antibiotics.

References

Aszalos A (1975). Differential potentiation by nystatin of the effect of antibiotics on yeast and mammalian cells. *Antimicrob Ag Chemother* **7**: 754.

Athar MA, Winner HI (1971). The development of resistance by *Candida* species to polyene antibiotics *in vitro*. *J Med Microbiol* **4**: 505.

Barrett AP (1984). Evaluation of nystatin in prevention and elimination of oropharyngeal *Candida* in immunosuppressed patients. *Oral Surg* **58**: 148.

Bergan T, Vangdal M (1989). *In vitro* activity of antifungal agents against yeast species. *Chemother* **29**: 104.

Boon JM, Lafeber HN, 't Mannetje AH *et al.* (1989). Comparison of ketoconazole suspension and nystatin in the treatment of newborns and infants with oral candidosis. *Mycoses* **32**: 312.

Buchanan AG, Riben PD, Rayner EN *et al.* (1985). Nystatin prophylaxis of fungal colonization and infection in granulocytopenic patients: correlation of colonization and clinical outcome. *Clin Invest Med* **8**: 139.

Carpentieri U, Haggard ME, Lockhart LH *et al.* (1978). Clinical experience in prevention of candidiasis by nystatin in children with acute lymphocytic leukemia. *J Pediatr* **92**: 593.

Cerra FB, Maddeus MA, Dunn DL *et al.* (1992). Selective gut decontamination reduces nosocomial infections and length of stay but not mortality or organ failure in surgical intensive care patients. *Arch Surg* **127**: 163.

Chowdhry BZ (1976). Antifungal agents. *J Antimicrob Chemother* **2**: 102.

Cohen J (1982). Antifungal chemotherapy. *Lancet* **ii**: 532.

Cosky RJ (1971). Contact dermatitis due to nystatin. *Arch Dermatol* **103**: 228.

Damjanovic V, Connolly CM, van Saene HKF *et al.* (1993). Selective decontamination with nystatin for control of a *Candida* outbreak in a neonatal intensive care unit. *J Hosp Infect* **24**: 245.

DeGregorio MW, Lee WM, Ries CA (1982). *Candida* infections in patients with acute leukemia: ineffectiveness of nystatin prophylaxis and relationship between oropharyngeal and systemic candidiasis. *Cancer* **50**: 2780.

De Groot AC, Conemans JM (1990). Nystatin allergy. *Dermatol Clin* **8**: 153.

Desai MH, Rutan RL, Heggars JP, Herndon DN (1992). *Candida* infection with and without nystatin prophylaxis. An 11-year experience with patients with burn injury. *Arch Surg* **127**: 159.

Dick JD, Merz WG, Saral R (1980). Incidence of polyene-resistant yeasts recovered from clinical specimens. *Antimicrob Ag Chemother* **18**: 158.

Dube MP, Heseltine PNR, Rinaldi MG *et al.* (1994). Fungemia and colonization with nystatin-resistant *Candida rugosa* in a burn unit. *Clin Infect Dis* **18**: 77.

Dutcher JD, Boyack G, Fox S (1954). The preparation and properties of crystalline fungicidin (nystatin). *Antibiot Annual* **1953–54**, p 191.

Faix RG, Kovarik SM, Shaw TR, Johnson RV (1989). Mucocutaneous candidiasis among very low birth weight (less than 1500 grams) infants in intensive care nurseries: a prospective study. *Pediatr* **83**: 101.

Freeman S (1986). Allergy to Kenacomb cream. *Med J Aust* **145**: 361.

Garty B-Z (1991). Stevens–Johnson syndrome associated with nystatin treatment. *Arch Dermatol* **127**: 741.

Gombert ME, duBouchet L, AulicinoTM, Butt KMH (1987). A comparative trial of clotrimazole troches and oral nystatin suspension in recipients of renal transplants. Use in prophylaxis of oropharyngeal candidiasis. *JAMA* **258**: 2553.

Gorensek MJ, Carey WD, Washington JA *et al.* (1993). Selective bowel decontamination with quinolones and nystatin reduces gram negative and fungal infections in orthoptic liver transplant recipients. *Cleve Clin J Med* **60**: 139.

Hann IM, Corringham R, Keaney M *et al.* (1982). Ketoconazole versus nystatin plus amphotercicin B for fungal prophylaxis in severely immunocompromised patients. *Lancet* **i**: 826.

Hazen EL, Brown R (1951). Fungicidin, an antibiotic produced by a soil actinomycete. *Proc Soc Exp Biol* **76**: 93.

Hofstra W, De Vries-Hospers HG, van der Waaij D (1979). Concentration of nystatin in feces after oral administration of various doses of nystatin. *Infection* **7**: 166.

Holst E (1984). Natamycin and nystatin for treatment of oral candidiasis during and after radiotherapy. *J Prosthet Dent* **51**: 226.

Hopfer RL, Mills K, Mehta R *et al.* (1984). *In vitro* antifungal activities of amphotericin B and liposome-encapsulated amphotericin B. *Antimicrob Ag Chemother* **25**: 387.

Hussain Qadri SMH, Flournoy DJ, Qadri SGM, Ramirez EG (1986). Susceptibility of clinical isolates of yeasts to anti-fungal agents. *Mycopathologia* **95**: 183.

Jones PG, Kauffman CA, McAuliffe LS *et al.* (1984). Efficacy of ketoconazole vs nystatin in prevention of fungal infections in neutropenic patients. *Arch Intern Med* **144**: 549.

Mehta RT, Hopfer RL, Gunner LA, Juliano RL, Lopez-Berestein G (1987a). Formulation, toxicity, and antifungal activity of liposome-encapsulated nystatin as therapeutic agent for systemic candidiasis. *Antimicrob Ag Chemother* **31**: 1897.

Mehta RT, Hopfer RL, McQueen T *et al.* (1987b). Toxicity and therapeutic effects in mice of liposome-encapsulated nystatin for systemic fungal infections. *Antimicrob Ag Chemother* **31**: 1901.

Milne JD, Warnock DW (1979). Effect of simultaneous oral and vaginal treatment on the rate of cure and relapse in vaginal candidosis. *Brit J Vener Dis* **55**: 362.

Munz D, Powell KR, Pai CH (1982). Treatment of candidal diaper dermatitis: a double-blind placebo-controlled comparison of topical nystatin with topical plus oral nystatin. *J Pediatr* **101**: 1022.

Ninane J (1994). A multicentre study of fluconazole versus oral polyenes in the prevention of fungal infection in children with hematological and oncological malignancies. Multicentre Study Group. *Eur J Clin Microbiol Infect Dis* **13**: 330.

Nobre GN, Pereira A, Coias R, Cordeiro J (1980). *In vitro* development of resistance to nystatin by *Candida albicans* and *Torulopsis glabrata*. *J Gen Microbiol* **118**: 263.

Nyst MJ, Perriens JH, Kimputu L *et al.* (1992). Gentian violet, ketoconazole and nystatin in oropharyngeal and esophageal candidiasis in Zairian AIDS patients. *Ann Soc Belg Med Trop* **72**: 45.

Nystatin Multicenter Study Group (1986). Therapy of candidal vaginitis: The effect of eliminating intestinal *Candida*. *Amer J Obstet Gynecol* **155**: 651.

Pareek SS (1980). Nystatin-induced fixed eruption. *Brit J Dermatol* **103**: 679.

Philpott Howard JN, Wade JJ, Mufti GJ *et al.* (1993). Randomized comparison of oral fluconazole versus oral polyenes for the prevention of fungal infection in patients at risk of neutropenia. Multicentre Study Group. *J Antimicrob Chemother* **31**: 973.

Quirce S, Parra F, Lazaro M *et al.* (1991). Generalized dermatitis due to oral nystatin. *Contact Dermatitis* **25**: 197.

Reents S, Goodwin D, Singh V (1993). Antifungal prophylaxis in immunocompromised hosts. *Ann Pharmacother* **27**: 53.

Rezabek GH, Friedman AD (1992). Superficial fungal infections of the skin Diagnosis and current treatment recommendations. *Drugs* **43**: 674.

Rios A, Rosenblum M, Crofoot G *et al.* (1993). Pharmacokinetics of liposomal nystatin in patients with Human Immunodeficiency Virus infection. *J Infect Dis* **168**: 253.

Ruskin JD, Wood RP, Bailey MR *et al.* (1992). Comparative trial of oral clotrimazole and nystatin for oropharyngeal candidiasis prophylaxis in orthoptic liver transplant patients. *Oral Surg Oral Med Oral Pathol* **74**: 567.

Salem HT, Salah M, Farid A *et al.* (1989). Oral versus local treatment of vaginal candidosis. *Int J Obstet Gynecol* **30**: 57.

Savino JA, Agarwal N, Wry P *et al.* (1994). Routine prophylactic antifungal agents (clotrimazole, ketoconazole, and nystatin) in nontransplant/nonburned critically ill surgical and trauma patients. *J Trauma* **36**: 20.

Selvam MP, Blay RA, Geyer S *et al.* (1993). Inhibition of HIV-1 replication in H9 cells by nystatin-A compared with other antiviral agents. *AIDS Res Hum Retroviruses* **9**: 475.

Shepp DH, Klosterman A, Siegal MS, Meyers JD (1985). Comparative trial of ketoconazole and nystatin for prevention of fungal infection in neutropenic patients in a protective environment. *J Infect Dis* **152**: 1257.

ME, Yoo Y, You H, Salminen C, Walther FJ (1988). Prophylactic oral nystatin and fungal infections in very-low-birthweight infants. *Amer J Perinatol* **5**: 33.

Turhan A, Connors JM, Klimo EF (1987). Ketoconazole versus nystatin as prophylaxis against fungal infection for lymphoma patients receiving chemotherapy. *Amer J Clin Oncol* **10**: 355.

Wasilewski C (1970). Allergic contact dermatitis from nystatin. *Arch Dermatol* **102**: 216.

Williams C, Whitehouse JA, Lister TA, Wrigley PFM (1977). Oral anticandidal prophylaxis in patients undergoing chemotherapy for acute leukemia. *Med Pediatr Oncol* **3**: 275.

Woods RA (1971). Nystatin-resistant mutants of yeast: alterations of sterol content. *J Bacteriol* **108**: 69.

Young LS (1982). The outlook for antifungal prophylaxis in the compromised host. *J Antimicrob Chemother* **9**: 338.

Zaruba K, Peters J, Jungbluth H (1991). Successful prophylaxis for fungal peritonitis in patients on continuous ambulatory peritoneal dialysis: six years experience. *Amer J Kidney Dis* **17**: 43.

Natamycin (Pimaricin)

Description

Natamycin is a tetrene polyene antifungal agent, isolated from *Streptomyces natalensis* (Struyk *et al.*, 1958). It is a highly toxic polyene, and is unsuitable for systemic treatment. It has limited treatment applications and is used mainly for mycotic keratitis caused by *Fusarium* spp. or *Acremonium* spp. and other molds. It has not been extensively evaluated either *in vitro* or *in vivo*.

Sensitive Organisms

Natamycin has a wide spectrum of antifungal activity. Yeasts such as *Cryptococcus neoformans, Candida albicans* and other *Candida* spp., are sensitive. Filamentous fungi, such as *Aspergillus* spp., *Acremonium* spp., and *Cunninghamella* spp. are sensitive, with MICs less than 4 μg per ml. *Fusarium* spp. and *Pseudallescheria boydii* are also susceptible to natamycin (Reuben *et al.*, 1989; Rotowa *et al.*, 1990). Natamycin topical drops at a concentration of 50 mg per ml were effective in the rabbit model of experimental keratitis due to *Aspergillus fumigatus* (Garcia de Lomas *et al.*, 1985).

The dermatophytes *Epidermophyton, Microsporum* and *Trichophyton* spp. are moderately resistant, and in comparison with other antifungal agents used for dermatomycoses, natamycin was the least effective *in vitro* (Macura, 1993). *Alternaria alternata* is suceptible with an MIC of 2 μg per ml (Ando and Takatori, 1987), but an isolate of *Paecilomyces lilanicus* causing keratomycosis was resistant (Gordon and Norton, 1985). Most of the dimorphic fungi such as *Histoplasma capsulatum, Blastomyces dermatitidis, Coccidioides immitis* and *Sporothrix schenckii* are also sensitive. The majority of sensitive fungi are inhibited by natamycin concentrations of 1–10 μg per ml (Struyk *et al.*, 1958). Acquired fungal resistance to this drug has not been seen.

Unlike other polyene antifungal agents, natamycin is active against *Trichomonas vaginalis* (Struyk *et al.*, 1958). Natamycin has no antibacterial activity.

Natamycin possesses some *in vitro* cysticidal activity against amebic cysts of *Acanthamoeba* (Osato *et al.*, 1991).

Absorption of the Drug

No pharmacokinetic data for humans are available. Animal pharmacokinetics have shown a peak plasma level of 40 μg per ml following administration of 7.5 mg per kg i.v. (Korteweg *et al.*, 1961).

After topical administration natamycin penetrates into corneal tissue, as demonstrated in rabbits. Corneal levels of natamycin were higher than amphotericin B, and were also greater when the cornea was debrided compared with intact epithelium (O'Day *et al.*, 1986). However, as the drug is water insoluble, it penetrates into ocular tissues poorly.

Mode of Action

The mode of action of natamycin is similar to that of the other polyenes (p. 1261).

Toxicity

There is minimal toxicity from the topical use of natamycin. It may cause minor irritation. Vomiting and diarrhea may occur if an oral dosage higher than 600 mg daily is given (Newcomer *et al.*, 1960). No oral formulation is currently available.

Clinical Uses, Administration and Dosage

Topical preparations only are available. Natamycin is marketed as a 5% ophthalmic suspension and a 2% cream is also available. Vaginal pessaries containing 25 mg natamycin are used for the treatment of trichomonal and candidal vaginitis. The suspension for inhalation is prepared to provide a 2.5% concentration. Other skin and otic ointments are marketed in which natamycin is combined with neomycin and hydrocortisone.

1 Keratomycosis

Combination antifungal therapy including topical natamycin has been used successfully for the treatment of keratitis due to *Alternaria alternata* (Ando and Takatori, 1987), *Exophiala jeanselmei* (al Hedaith and al Kaff, 1993), *Pseudallescheria boydii* (Mills and Garrett, 1992), *Acanthameba polyphaga* (Jackson et al., 1986), and *Aspergillus oryzae* (Stenson et al., 1982). The recommended dose of the 5% natamycin ophthalmic suspension is one drop instilled in the conjunctiva every 1–2 h for the first 3–4 days, followed by one drop 6–8 times daily. Therapy is continued in responding patients for 14–21 days.

2 Oral candidiasis

Natamycin is effective for oral candidiasis. In children with hematological malignancy, 2.5% natamycin drops administered in a dose of 6–20 drops four times daily for up to 8 weeks, produced complete resolution in 80%, without side-effects (Moszczenska, 1989).

3 Vaginal candidiasis

Although it has been established that topical natamycin vaginal cream in doses of 25 mg, 50 mg and 100 mg or vaginal tablet 100 mg, administered once-daily for 6 days has good efficacy for vulvovaginal candidiasis (cure rates of 86–97%), this treatment is associated with a high recurrence rate of 30% (Buch and Skytte-Christensen, 1982; Christensen and Buch, 1982). The recommended dose is one 25-mg pessary inserted nightly for 20 days or twice-daily for 10 days. Natamycin is not considered a first-line therapy for vaginal candidiasis.

4 Aerosol therapy for bronchopulmonary aspergillosis

Administation of natamycin by aerosol has been used for pulmonary aspergillosis. Edward and La Touche (1964) treated ten patients, using natamycin as a 2.5% suspension diluted in an alkaline agent, and administered 2.5 mg doses by aerosol two or three times a day. These authors observed clinical improvement in seven of the ten patients after 6 weeks of therapy. Nebulized natamycin 5 mg twice-daily for 1 year was evaluated in a placebo-controlled trial to determine if it had a steroid sparing effect in patients with allergic bronchopulmonary aspergillosis. After 1 year, there was no evidence of any benefit conferred by nebulized natamycin (Currie et al., 1990).

5 Other fungal infections

A case of cutaneous alternariosis of the epidermal type has been reported to be successfully treated with topical natamycin (Higashi and Asada, 1973).

References

al Hedaith SS, al Kaff AS (1993). *Exophiala jeanselmei* keratitis. *Mycoses* **36**: 97.

Ando N, Takatori K (1987). Keratomycosis due to *Alternaria alternata* corneal transplant infection. *Mycopathologica* **100**: 17.

Buch A, Skytte-Christensen E (1982). Treatment of vaginal candidosis with natamycin and effect of treating the partner at the same time. *Acta Obstet Gynecol Scand* **61**: 393.

Christensen ES, Buch A (1982). Vaginal *Candida albicans* treated with three different concentrations of natamycin (Pimafucin) for 6 days. *Acta Obstet Gynecol Scand* **61**: 325.

Currie DC, Lueck C, Milburn HJ et al. (1990). Controlled trial of natamyin in the treatment of allergic bronchopulmonary aspergillosis. *Thorax* **45**: 447.

Edwards G, La Touche CJP (1964). The treatment of bronchopulmonary mycoses with a new antibiotic – pimaricin. *Lancet* **I**: 1349.

Garcia de Lomas J, Fons MA, Nogueira JM et al. (1985). Chemotherapy of *Aspergillus fumigatus* keratitis: an experimental study. *Mycopathologia* **89**: 135.

Gordon MA, Norton SW (1985). Corneal transplant infection by *Paecilomyces lilanicus*. *Sabouraudia* **23**: 295.

Higashi N, Asada Y (1973). Cutaneous alternariosis with mixed infection of *Candida albicans*. Report of a patient responding to natamycin. *Arch Dermatol* **108**: 558.

Jackson TN, Heinze JB, Tuxen J, Weiner JM (1986). Successful medical treatment of a corneal ulcer due to *Acanthamoeba polyphaga*. *Aust NZ J Ophthalmol* **14**: 139.

Korteweg GC, Szabo KLH, Rutten AMG, Hoogerheide JC (1961). Some pharmacological properties of pimaricin and possible clinical application of this antifungal antibiotic. *Antibiot Chemother* **2**: 261.

Macura AB (1993). *In vitro* susceptibility of dermatophytes to antifungal drugs: a comparison of two methods. *Int J Dermatol* **32**: 533.

Mills R, Garrett G (1992). *Pseudallescheria boydii* keratitis. *Aust NZ J Med* **20**: 253.

Moszczenska A (1989). The use of 2.5% natamycin, as orally administered drops, in the treatment of fungal infections of the oral cavity in children with chronic blood diseases. *J Int Med Res* **17**: 82.

Newcomer VD, Sternberg TH, Wright ET *et al.* (1960). The treatment of systemic mycoses with orally administered pimaricin: preliminary report. *Ann NY Acad Sci* **89**: 240.

O'Day DM, Head WS, Robinson RD, Clanton JA (1986). Corneal penetration of topical amphotericin B and natamycin. *Curr Eye Res* **5**: 877.

Osato MS, Robinson NM, Wilhelmus WR, Jones DB (1991). *In vitro* evaluation of antimicrobial compounds for cysticidal activity against *Acanthamoeba*. *Rev Infect Dis* **13** (Suppl 5): 431.

Reuben A, Anaissie E, Nelson PE *et al.* (1989). Antifungal susceptibility of 44 clinical isolates of *Fusarium* species determined by using a broth microdilution method. *Antimicrob Ag Chemother* **33**: 1647.

Rotowa NA, Shadomy HJ, Shadomy S (1990). *In vitro* activities of polyene and imidazole antifungal agents against unusual opportunistic fungal pathogens. *Mycoses* **33**: 203.

Stenson S, Brookner A, Rosenthal S (1982). Bilateral endogenous scleritis due to *Aspergillus oryzae*. *Ann Ophthalmol* **14**: 67.

Struyk AP, Hoette 1, Drost G *et al.* (1958). Pimaricin, a new antifungal antibiotic. *Antibiot Annual 1957–1958*: 878.

Flucytosine (5-Fluorocytosine; 5-FC)

Description

Flucytosine is used primarily in combination with amphotericin B or fluconazole for the treatment of serious disseminated infections due to yeasts and yeast-like fungi. Concern over the emergence of drug-resistance has limited the use of flucytosine as montherapy. The drug is a water soluble, fluorinated pyrimidine, which was synthesized in 1957 at Roche Laboratories as a cytosine antimetabolite for the treatment of leukemia. The drug proved ineffective for this purpose, as it was not cytotoxic, but it was discovered to have antifungal activity (Grunberg *et al.*, 1964).

Sensitive Organisms

Compared with amphotericin B, flucytosine has a relatively narrow spectrum of antifungal activity. (Kitahara *et al.*, 1976; Bennett, 1977).

1 Pathogenic yeasts

In vitro, flucytosine is usually active against *Cryptococcus neoformans*, *Candida albicans*, other *Candida* spp., such as *C. krusei*, *C. tropicalis*, *C. lusitaniae*, *C. parapsilosis*, and *C. (Torulopsis) glabrata* (Shadomy *et al.*, 1973; Galgiani *et al.*, 1987; Hadfield *et al.*, 1987; Fromtling *et al.*, 1993; Anaissie *et al.*, 1994). *Candida rugosa* isolates were found to have MICs <10 μg per ml, but flucytosine was not fungicidal against any isolate (Dube *et al.*, 1994). Flucytosine is effective in experimental murine infections due to *Cryptococcus neoformans* and *Candida albicans* (Medoff and Kobayashi, 1980) It also prevents experimental *C. albicans* endocarditis in rabbits (Demierre and Freedman, 1979). *Trichosporon beigelii* may be flucytosine-sensitive (Hajjeh and Blumberg,1995).

Published results on the prevalence of resistance of naturally occurring yeasts to flucytosine vary. With *Cryptococcus neoformans*, it was of the order of 1–2% (Bennett, 1977; Medoff and Kobayashi, 1980), but more recent surveys show the prevalence at 22% (Chin *et al.*, 1989). Natural resistance in strains of *C. albicans* was higher and there was also geographical variation in the prevalence of natural resistance (Francis and Walsh, 1992). In some surveys, 7–8% of pre-treatment isolates of *C. albicans*, *C. glabrata* and unspeciated *Candida* were resistant to flucytosine. Higher proportions of resistance (22%) were seen in species other than *C. albicans*, as *C. tropicalis* and *C. krusei* were generally less sensitive. Resistance to flucytosine was reported in 23% *C. parapsilosis* isolates from ocular infections (Segal *et al.*, 1975). In addition, about one-third of resistant isolates of *C. albicans* were completely resistant with an MIC ≥1000 μg per ml (Medoff and Kobayashi, 1980). The remainder of the *C. albicans* strains could be inhibited by low flucytosine concentrations, but were capable of multiplying after prolonged incubation (Normark and Schonebeck, 1972). Other studies showed that 37% of *C. albicans* isolates were partially resistant to flucytosine, and that such strains had a mutation which conferred partial resistance when in a heterozygous state. Partially resistant strains could give rise to strains which were homozygous and had a high level of resistance to flucytosine (Whelan *et al.*, 1981; DeFever *et al.*, 1982). The percentage of naturally resistant strains of *C. albicans* varies widely in the world. In Europe, 4.5–11 7%, Africa, 21.6%, and in North America, 12–50% of strains have been reported as resistant by different investigators (Auger *et al.*, 1979; Stiller *et al.*, 1982).

There is also variation in the susceptibility of *C. albicans* to flucytosine when its two serotypes are examined separately. Serotype B strains are more frequently isolated from black persons in Africa, and are commonly resistant to flucytosine (85%) than serotype A strains (1%) which are more common in Europe and appear to have a different cell wall ultrastructure (Montplaisir *et al.*, 1976). In further studies on *C. albicans* isolates from white European patients, 90–96% were serotype A (resistance in 0.6–2.5%) and 4–10% serotype B (resistance in 78.5–81%). In the USA and Canada, 50–67.7% and 74.3%, respectively, were serotype A and the remainder were serotype B. Additionally, sensitivity studies to flucytosine on isolates in the USA and Canada showed 6.9% and 11.3%, respectively, of serotype A strains and 28% and 49.7%, respectively, of serotype B strains to be resistant. In the USA and Canada, *C. albicans* isolates from black people were 40% and 46% serotype A, respectively, and the remainder serotype B, whereas 77% of isolates from black African women were serotype A. In black Canadian patients of West Indian origin, all *C. albicans* isolates of serotype A were sensitive to flucytosine while 40% of the serotype B strains were resistant (Auger *et al.*, 1979; Stiller *et al.*, 1982).

2 Molds or filamentous fungi

Aspergillus spp. are occasionally sensitive to flucytosine, but in general they are moderately or highly resistant (Holt and Newman, 1973). Of seven *Aspergillus* strains tested by Steer *et al.* (1972), three had an MIC of 3.9 µg per ml or less and the remainder had an MIC greater than 100 µg per ml. Denning *et al.* (1992) found that 35% of 60 *Aspergillus* isolates had an MIC less than 12.5 µg per ml, but no fungicidal activity has been documented for flucytosine. Only marginally beneficial effects occur with the use of flucytosine in experimental *Aspergillus* infections in mice (Medoff and Kobayashi, 1980). One *in vitro* study showed that amphotericin B and flucytosine were synergistic against 23% of *Aspergillus* spp. strains, and a similar percentage of strains exhibited *in vitro* antagonism (Denning *et al.*, 1992).

The *Fusarium* spp. are also flucytosine-resistant (Merz *et al.*, 1988; Sekhon *et al.*, 1994). The causative agents of chromoblastomycosis (also called chromomycosis) and phaeohyphomycosis, such as the *Phialophora, Cladosporium*, and *Exophila* spp., are usually flucytosine-sensitive (Vandevelde *et al.*, 1972; Block *et al.*, 1973; Francis and Walsh, 1992; Sudduth *et al.*, 1992; Gold *et al.*, 1994). Flucytosine has no consistent *in vitro* or *in vivo* activity against the Mucoraceae, the important group causing mucormycosi (Lehrer *et al.*, 1980; Medoff and Kobayashi, 1980). Entomophthorales are resistant to flucytosine (Yangco *et al.*, 1984). The *Madurella* spp. and all the dermatophytes such as the *Microsporum, Trichophyton* and *Epidermophyton* spp. are resistant.

3 Dimorphic fungi

Blastomyces dermatitidis, Paracoccidioides brasiliensis, Histoplasma capsulatum and *Coccidioides immitis* are resistant to flucytosine (Shadomy, 1969). The drug has no efficacy in experimental murine infections due to *H. capsulatum* and *B. dermatitidis* (Medoff and Kobayashi, 1980). *Penicillium marneffei*, which causes disseminated disease in HIV-infected individuals, is susceptible to flucytosine (Sekhon *et al.*, 1993; Supparatpinyo *et al.*, 1993). *Sporothrix (Sporotrichum) schenckii* is usually completely resistant, but occasional moderately susceptible strains have been isolated (Vandevelde *et al.*, 1972).

4 Actinomycetes and Actinomyces

Flucytosine has no effect on these bacteria or on any other bacteria.

5 Synergism with other drugs

Flucytosine may act synergistically with amphotericin B against strains of *Candida* and *Aspergillus* spp., and *Cryptococcus neoformans*. Amphotericin B and flucytosine may act synergistically against *C. albicans* strains which are resistant to both drugs when tested singly against such strains (Conly *et al.*, 1992), but Martin *et al.* (1994) showed that under certain *in vitro* testing conditions, flucytosine can antagonize the fungicidal activity of amphotericin B against *C. albicans* strains sensitive to both drugs. However, in the experimental model of candidiasis in rabbits with prolonged neutropenia, the combination of amphotericin B and flucytosine was the only regimen able to eradicate renal candidiasis (Thaler *et al.*, 1988). Amphotericin B and flucytosine were found to be synergistic or indifferent in animal models of aspergillosis (Arroyo *et al.*, 1977; Polak *et al.*, 1982, Longman and Martin, 1987).

Synergy is often demonstrated when flucytosine is combined with imidazole drugs against yeasts. Weak inhibitory concentrations of clotrimazole may enhance the action of flucytosine against some *Candida* strains. In one study, flucytosine and ketoconazole were usually additive or synergistic when tested against strains of *C. albicans, C. parapsilosis, C. tropicalis* and *C. glabrata* (Beggs and Sarosi, 1982). In the treatment of cryptococcal meningitis in mice, a flucytosine and ketoconazole combination produced results superior to those achieved by either agent used alone (Craven and Graybill, 1984). Fluconazole and flucytosine was found to be synergistic in the murine model of cryptococcosis (Allendoerfer *et al.*, 1991) and the combination of itraconazole and flucytosine was synergistic in murine candidiasis and was either synergistic or additive in about half the mice with disseminated aspergillosis in another study (Polak, 1987).

6 Acquired resistance

Strains of *Candida* spp. and *Cryptococcus neoformans* resistant to flucytosine can be readily induced *in vitro* by successive culture in the presence of increasing concentrations of the drug (Holt and Newman, 1973). Fungi resistant to flucytosine frequently arise *in vivo* during treatment with the drug. Almost two-thirds of isolates from patients receiving flucytosine alone become resistant (Medoff and Kobayashi, 1980). Such secondary resistance has occurred during treatment for cryptococcosis (Sugarman and Pesanti, 1980), and for *Candida* infections (Cartwright *et al.*, 1972; Sugarman and Pesanti,1980). For this reason, flucytosine is almost never used as a single agent in clinical situations. It is most commonly combined with amphotericin B (Francis and Walsh, 1992) or fluconazole (Graybill, 1992).

Table IV.4

Compiled from data published by Yangco *et al.* (1984), Ando and Takatori (1987), Dixon and Polak (1987), Haron *et al.* (1988), Wong *et al.* (1989), Patterson *et al.* (1990), Morace *et al.* (1991), Braun and Kauffman (1992), Denning *et al.* (1992), Martin *et al.* (1992), Sekhon *et al.* (1992, 1993), Weber and Polak (1992), Dube *et al.* (1994), Lau *et al.* (1995)

Organism	MIC (µg per ml) range	
	Broth	Agar
Yeast		
Candida species		
C. albicans	0.04–1.56	0.12–8
C. guilliermondii	0.19	0.24
C. krusei	1.56–25	0.12–4
C. parapsilosis	0.19–1.56	0.25–5
C. tropicalis	0.04->100	0.12–4
C. lusitaniae	0.04	0.12–1
C. rugosa	<10	
C. glabrata (Torulopsis glabrata)	0.04–0.39	0.12–4
Blastoschizomycs capitatum	0.04	
Cryptococcus neoformans	0.04–3.12	
Hansenula anomala	0.1	
Malassezia furfur	>100	
Rhodotorula rubra	0.2	
Penicillium marneffei	<0.195–0.78	
Trichosporon beigelii	1.56->100	
Mold		
Aspergillus spp.	<12.5->25	
Acremonium spp.		>32
Alternaria alternata	100	
Cladosporium spp.		3–10
Dactylaria spp.		>100
Phialophora parasitica	12.5	
Pseudallecheria boydii		>50
Pythium insidiosum	25->100	
Wangiella dermatitidis		10–100
Conidiobolus spp.	200	
Basidiobolus spp.	>200	

7 Minimum inhibitory concentrations

Table IV.4 shows the MICs of flucytosine against selected fungal species. Fungi with MICs of 6.25 μg per ml or less are regarded as highly sensitive to this drug and those with an MIC greater than 25 μg per ml are usually regarded as resistant (Medoff and Kobayashi, 1980). Because testing methods are not standardized (p. 1246), others regard an MIC > 12.5 μg per ml after 48 h incubation as resistant (Shadomy, 1969; Stiller et al., 1982). When the therapeutic effect of flucytosine is tested in experimental murine candidiasis, there is a correlation between in vitro susceptibility and in vivo response, but this is not absolute and only has a limited predictive value (Stiller et al., 1983). Highly resistant variants (MICs greater than 1000 μg per ml) of all these fungi can occur with previous exposure to the drug.

Mode of Administration and Dosage

1 Oral administration in adults and older children

Flucytosine is usually administered by the oral route in a dose of 150 mg per kg per day, given in four divided doses at intervals of 6 h. In some patients, particularly those with concomitant HIV infection. the dose may have to be lowered to 100 mg per kg per day to avoid bone marrow toxicity (Francis and Walsh, 1992; Powderly, 1993; Larsen et al., 1994).

2 Infants and young children

Usually infants and young children are treated with a flucytosine dose of 50–100 mg per kg per day, administered orally in four divided doses. Duration of treatment has ranged from 21 to 44 days (Ward et al.,1983; Leibovitz et al., 1992). Some authors have administered the total daily dose once-daily to patients in this age group. Monitoring of serum flucytosine levels may be necessary in infants and young children (Baly et al., 1990; Zenker et al., 1991).

3 Patients with renal failure

Patients with renal failure need a reduced dose schedule, because the drug is excreted almost entirely by glomerular filtration. Various methods have been devised to calculate the correct dose for these patients, aiming to maintain serum concentrations within the optimum therapeutic range of 25–100 μg per ml (MacLeod et al., 1979; Shaunak and Cohen, 1991; Francis and Walsh, 1992). The 6-h interval between doses can be maintained and the individual doses can be reduced according to declining creatinine clearance: 27.5 mg per kg every 6 h for a creatinine clearance of 40–49 ml per min; 18.5 and 9.5 mg per kg every 6 h for creatinine clearances of 20–29 ml per min and less than 10 ml per min, respectively. Alternatively, the interval between doses may be doubled when the creatinine clearance is 20–40 ml per min, and quadrupled when it is less than 20 ml per min. Another method uses the usual individual doses, but the normal 6-hourly interval between doses is increased by multiplying it by the value of the serum creatinine in mg%. For example, an adult with moderate renal failure (serum creatinine 4 mg%) would be given flucytosine once every 24 (6 × 4) h (Dawborn et al., 1973). Nevertheless, serum level monitoring is advisable in patients with renal failure, and the peak serum flucytosine level should be maintained below 100 μg per ml. The drug is removed from the body by hemodialysis and its clearance rate is the same as that of creatinine. In patients treated by maintenance hemodialysis every 48–72 h, therapeutic non-toxic serum levels of flucytosine can usually be maintained by administering single doses of 25–30 mg per kg body weight after each dialysis (Block et al., 1974).

4 Patients with liver disease

Flucytosine is administered in the usual recommended doses, as hepatic function does not influence serum levels of flucytosine (Block, 1973).

5 Intravenous administration

An i.v. preparation (1%) of flucytosine has been available for use when oral administration is not feasible. The dose for i.v. administration is the same as that used for the oral route. A quarter of the total daily dose should be given by short infusion (20–40 min), every 6 h. The manufacturers recommend that this infusion solution should be stored at a temperature between 15°C and 20°C. When tested by bioassay, flucytosine remains stable in distilled water, human serum and 5% dextrose for up to 7 days (Hoeprich and Huston, 1978).

6 Intrathecal administration

Flucytosine has been used intrathecally on rare occasions to treat patients with cryptococcal meningitis, but there are virtually no indications for this form of therapy. A 10 ml dose of the 1% solution was administered to adults twice-weekly without producing chemical meningitis or other side-effects (Roche, 1972).

7 Topical administration to the eyes

The drug can be used in eye-drops (1.5%) which are non-irritating. This may be effective for corneal lesions, but intraocular penetration is poor. Intravitreal injection of 100 μg flucytosine produced no detectable ocular adverse reactions in the rabbit (Yoshizumi and Silverman, 1985).

Availability

Tablets: 500 mg and 250 mg flucytosine

Intravenous formulation: 250 ml normal saline containing 2.5 g of flucytosine

Serum Levels in Relation to Dosage

More than 90% of an oral dose of flucytosine is absorbed. After an oral dose of 2 g in an adult, a peak serum level of about 45 μg per ml is reached within 2–6 h (Fig. IV.2) (Daneshmend and Warnock, 1983). This level gradually declines over the next 6 h, but some drug is still detectable 24 h after the dose. In patients with normal renal function, there is a slight accumulation of the drug during the first 4 days of treatment, but thereafter mean or peak serum levels remain much the same, even if therapy is continued for months. Peak serum levels are reached in a shorter period of 1–2 h in patients who have already received the drug for several days (Block and Bennett, 1972). With normal renal function, the optimal serum level range of 25–100 μg per ml can be achieved with a dose of 37.5 mg per kg given every 6 h. Absorption of flucytosine can be delayed by food and antacids, but peak serum levels are not significantly reduced (Francis and Walsh, 1992).

After an i.v. infusion of 2 g of flucytosine over 15 min, levels similar to those achieved after oral administration are obtained, but the peak level (about 50 μg per ml) is reached immediately after the infusion (Wade and Sudlow, 1972).

A dose of 20 mg per kg given i.v. every 6 h or a dose of 25 mg per kg was given orally every 6 h to a premature infant, serum concentrations obtained were similar to those seen in adults who received a 2 g dose orally every 6 h (Ward *et al.*, 1983).

Irrespective of the route of administration, the half-life of the drug is 3–5 h. It is prolonged in patients with impaired renal function, and is about 85 h in anephric patients (Norrby and Eilard, 1978; Polak, 1979). Flucytosine is removed by hemodialysis and its clearance increases proportionally to the blood flow through the dialyzer. Peritoneal dialysis is less effective in removing flucytosine (Polak, 1979).

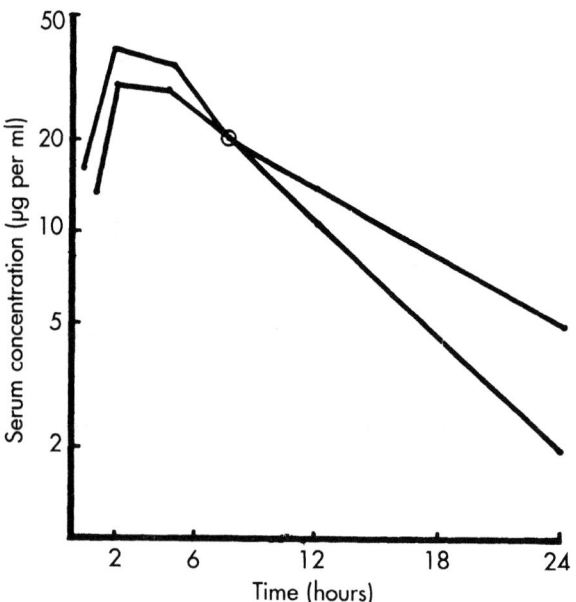

Fig. IV.2.
Blood levels of flucytosine in two patients after single oral doses of 2 g. (Redrawn after Koechlin *et al.*, 1966, with permission.)

Excretion

1 Urine

The majority of an oral dose of flucytosine (85–95%) is excreted unchanged via the kidneys by glomerular filtration (Wade and Sudlow, 1972). Very high urine levels of the active drug (>1000 μg per ml) are attained in patients with normal renal function. Patients with impaired renal function have lower urine concentrations (Davies and Reeves, 1971).

2 Inactivation in body

A small amount of the drug is converted to 5-fluorouracil in the body and raised serum levels of this metabolite may account for the hematological toxicity associated with flucytosine (Diasio *et al.*, 1978). Metabolic degradation may be more significant in patients with renal disease.

3 Feces

Unabsorbed flucytosine, usually less than 10%, is excreted unchanged in the feces (Koechlin *et al.* 1966).

Distribution of the Drug in Body

Flucytosine is well distributed in body fluids and tissues. Tissue levels in liver, kidney, spleen, heart and lung are equal or greater than serum levels at the time (Utz, 1972; Hoeprich *et al.*, 1987). The drug penetrates well into the CSF, where levels of 71–85% of the concomitant serum concentration have been attained (Polak, 1979). Flucytosine penetrates well into infected exudates of peritoneum and joints (Bennett, 1977). Synovial fluid levels measured concurrently with serum levels in a premature infant receiving flucytosine 25 mg per kg per day were 39.6 μg per ml and 47.5 μg per ml respectively (Weisse *et al.*, 1993). In dogs, it also penetrates well into bronchial secretions (Pennington *et al.*, 1974). Effective concentrations of flucytosine have been measured in saliva and bone, although lower than the concomitant serum level (Polak, 1979). In one human study, a level of 10 μg per ml of flucytosine was found in the aqueous humor when the serum level was 50 μg per ml (Richards *et al.*, 1969). Levels of 10–40 μg per ml have been detected in the aqueous humor of patients receiving flucytosine in an oral dose of 200 mg per kg per day (Jones, 1975). The flucytosine concentration in amniotic fluid was 168 μg per ml and corresponding cord blood concentration was 64.7 μg per ml, in a woman with cryptococcal meningitis of 21 weeks gestation (Stafford *et al.*, 1983). Binding of flucytosine to serum proteins is negligible (Block *et al.*, 1974).

Mode of Action

There are at least two mechanisms of action of flucytosine (Wain and Polak, 1979; Waldorf and Polak, 1983; Chouini-Lalanne *et al.*, 1989). The drug enters the fungal cell via a permease system that recognizes several purines in addition to the natural analog, cytosine. Inside the cell, flucytosine is rapidly deaminated by an enzyme called cytosine deaminase to the antimetabolite 5-fluorouracil. 5-Fluorouracil competes with uracil, interferes with pyrimidine metabolism and incorporation into the fungal RNA, resulting in inhibition of protein synthesis. Cytosine deaminase is either absent or has minimal activity in mammalian cells. The second mechanism is the conversion of flucytosine into 5-fluorodeoxyuridine monophosphate by the enzyme uridine monophosphate pyrophosphorylase, and the subsequent inhibition of thymidylate synthetase and interference with DNA synthesis.

Acquired resistance of a strain of *C. parapsilosis* appeared to be due to a genetic block of cytosine deaminase (Hoeprich *et al.*, 1974), but several mechanisms may be involved in such resistance (Polak and Wain, 1979). In *C. albicans* a decrease in the amount of the enzyme UMP pyrophosphorylase (which converts 5-fluorouracil to 5-fluorouridine monophosphate) may be the mechanism of resistance to flucytosine (Whelan and Kerridge, 1984). Cytosine arabinoside is a competitive inhibitor of flucytosine (Bennett, 1974).

Flucytosine can be both fungistatic and fungicidal, the effect being dependent on the concentration of the drug and the time of incubation used in the test system (Medoff and Kobayashi, 1980). The synergistic effect of amphotericin B and flucytosine against some fungi results from an action of amphotericin B on the plasma membrane (p. 1262), which allows greater penetration of flucytosine.

Toxicity

It was thought that the absence of cytosine permease in mammalian cells would mean the host cells would not be exposed to the effects of 5-fluorouracil, and therefore the administration of flucytosine would not be associated with significant toxicity. However, using gas chromatography-mass-spectrophotometry, it was demonstrated that serum levels of flucytosine of 100 ng per ml were present for up to 6 h following a 2 g single oral dose of flucytosine. It was postulated that Gram-negative bacteria in the gastrointestinal tract deaminate flucytosine to fluorouracil (Diasio *et al.*, 1978). Harris *et al.* (1986) provided experimental evidence that the enzyme or enzymes responsible for the deamination of flucytosine to 5-fluorouracil by the intestinal microflora, can be induced by chronic exposure to flucytosine, and Malet-Martino *et al.* (1991) correlated the number of gastrointestinal Gram-negative bacteria with the amount of urinary fluorouracil metabolites, using ^{19}F magnetic resonance spectroscopy. It is apparent that flucytosine toxicity (in particular myelosuppression and hepatotoxicity) is associated with elevated serum flucytosine levels greater than 100 µg per ml in most patients (Stamm *et al.*, 1987). Amphotericin B is generally used in combination with flucytosine, and commonly causes nephrotoxicity which in turn significantly prolongs the half-life of flucytosine with resulting elevated serum levels. Francis and Walsh (1992) found the combination of flucytosine 150 mg per kg per day and amphotericin B 0.5–1.0 mg per kg per day often resulted in serum flucytosine levels greater than 100 µg per ml in patients with initially normal renal function. It is therefore important to monitor serum levels of flucytosine during therapy, and maintain them between 25 and 100 µg per ml. Serum levels of flucytosine should be measured twice-weekly. The trough level is measured immediately prior to dosing and the peak level is measured 2 h after an oral dose and 30 min after i.v. administration (British Society for Antimicrobial Chemotherapy Working Party, 1991).

1 Gastrointestinal side-effects

Nausea and diarrhea may be caused by oral flucytosine, but are uncommon (6%) and dose-related. More severe symptoms may occur such as vomiting, abdominal pain and copious diarrhea. In these cases proctosigmoidoscopic findings are usually normal (Bennett, 1977). Ulcerating enterocolitis has been described with total resolution on cessation of the drug (White and Traube, 1982) One fatal case resembled acute ulcerative colitis with multiple intestinal perforations and peritonitis (Robertson *et al.*, 1974).

2 Hypersensitivity reactions

Skin rashes have occasionally been observed, and a photosensitive skin rash has been described (Shelley and Sica, 1983). Anaphylaxis to flucytosine has also been reported in a patient with AIDS (Kotani *et al.*, 1988).

3 Hematological side-effects

Many patients with serious fungal infections also have underlying hematologic disorders. In addition, flucytosine is often administered in conjunction with other drugs such as amphotericin B, immunosuppressive agents and corticosteroids. For these reasons, it has been difficult to assess possible effects of flucytosine on the bone marrow. However, there are reports indicating that flucytosine can cause marrow toxicity, and leukopenia and thrombocytopenia have been reported in 6% of patients taking flucytosine (Bennett, 1977), and recent studies have correlated myelosuppression with serum levels of flucytosine greater than 125 µg per ml (Stamm *et al.*, 1987; Francis and Walsh, 1992).

Meyer and Axelrod (1974) reported a fatal case of aplastic anemia resulting from flucytosine therapy. Record *et al.* (1971) treated three patients with *Candida* endocarditis, two of whom died from bone marrow depression. Recent amphotericin B administration was probably contributory in one case, but in the other patient, amphotericin B was discontinued 3 months prior to the onset of marrow depression, and therefore this complication was attributed to flucytosine. Bryan and McFarland (1978) described a patient who developed fatal bone marrow aplasia after a short course of flucytosine, combined with amphotericin B for cryptococcal meningitis, but this patient also had multiple myeloma. Anemia (Utz *et al.*, 1969), neutropenia (Davies and Reeves, 1971), thrombocytopenia (Weese and Schope, 1972) and eosinophilia (Stanton and Sanderson, 1974) have been associated with flucytosine therapy, and bone marrow suppression occurred in 22% patients in a study of treatment for cryptococcal meningitis with amphotericin B and flucytosine (Stamm *et al.*, 1987).

Kauffman and Frame (1977) reported bone marrow toxicity in four of 15 patients with serious fungal infections treated with flucytosine, but three had renal insufficiency and two had received concomitant amphotericin B. Maximum serum levels of flucytosine preceding leukopenia in three patients were in the range 125–200 µg per ml. Leukopenia was readily reversed when the flucytosine dosage, and subsequently serum levels, were lowered. One patient with acute renal failure and prolonged high levels of flucytosine (maximum 500 µg per ml) developed marrow aplasia and died of bacterial sepsis. Studies with larger patient numbers have indicated that isolated flucytosine levels higher than 100 μg per ml, which are quickly corrected by dose reduction, are usually not associated with bone marrow toxicity. However, this toxicity was encountered more frequently if peak flucytosine levels exceeded 100 μg per ml for 2 weeks or longer (Dismukes *et al.*, 1987; Stamm *et al.*, 1987). High serum levels of the drug are likely to occur if the patient has renal failure, or if amphotericin B is used concomitantly and causes impairment of renal function. In the presence of renal failure serum levels of flucytosine should be monitored more frequently. In rapidly progressive renal failure, very high levels of flucytosine can occur and persist, despite cessation of the drug. In this situation dialysis is recommended to remove accumulated flucytosine (Kauffman and Frame, 1977). Regular full blood examinations should be performed on all patients receiving flucytosine. In patients with HIV infection, the concomitant use of zidovudine and other myelosuppressive drugs may potentiate flucytosine-induced bone marrow toxicity (Powderly, 1993).

Studies on human and murine bone marrow cultures show that flucytosine inhibits granulocyte-monocyte and erythroid precursor cells and suggested that hemopoietic toxicity is mediated through cellular metabolism of the drug. Uracil reversed these inhibitory effects on the bone marrow (Koeffler and Golde, 1979). The metabolite of flucytosine, 5-fluorouracil may be responsible for some of its toxicity.

Although myelosuppression appears to be related to high flucytosine levels in most patients, there are reports of idiosyncratic reactions to flucytosine that are clearly not related to elevated serum levels. These include eosinophilia, leukopenia and thrombocytopenia (Utz *et al.*, 1975; Eilard *et al.*,1974; Stamm *et al.*, 1987; Francis and Walsh, 1992).

4 Hepatotoxicity

Transient liver enlargement with associated elevation of hepatic transaminase levels has been noted in a few patients (Steer *et al.*, 1972). Abnormal liver function is readily reversible. Extensive liver cell necrosis together with fatal bone marrow depression have been reported in two patients (Record *et al.*, 1971), but this appears to be very rare. It is advisable to monitor liver function tests regularly in patients receiving this drug. Flucytosine is not contraindicated in patients with pre-existing liver disease. Both hepatotoxicity and hemopoietic toxicity are probably dose-related and more likely to occur when high serum levels (> 100 μg per ml) are attained for a period of 2 or more weeks (Stamm *et al.*, 1987).

5 Nephrotoxicity

This has not been ascribed to flucytosine therapy, and the drug apparently can be used safely in patients with pre-existing uremia, provided appropriate dosage adjustments are made (p. 1307). In the rat, flucytosine was shown to significantly increase renal blood flow and increase creatinine clearance. It is unknown whether this improvement in renal function is observed in humans (Heidemann and Brune, 1991). Spurious elevations in serum creatinine without a concomitant rise in blood urea nitrogen have been described in patients taking flucytosine, when their blood was examined by a Kodak 'Ektachem' analyzer (Kennedy *et al.*, 1989; Mitchell, 1984; Herrington *et al.*, 1984; Mitchell *et al.*, 1985).

6 Effect on fetus

Philpot and Lo (1972) treated a woman in early pregnancy with flucytosine without apparent ill-effect to the fetus. Similar experience has been recorded by Schonebeck and Segerbrand (1973), who used the drug successfully for the treatment of *Candida* fungemia in a woman during the 4th month of pregnancy. However, the safety of flucytosine during pregnancy, especially the first trimester, has not been established. The drug is teratogenic in rats at doses of 40 mg per kg per day, but not rabbits and monkeys.

7 Drug interactions

The antifungal effect of flucytosine may be inhibited by the concomitant administration of cytosine arabinoside (Product Information Flucytosine), but studies by Wingfield (1987) did not find significant antagonism of flucytosine activity by cytosine arabinoside.

Clinical Uses of the Drug

1 Cryptococcosis

In the past some patients with disseminated cryptococcal infection were cured by flucytosine alone, especially if they could not tolerate amphotericin B (Vandevelde *et al.*, 1972; Tolentino and Barrone, 1976; Fusner and McClain, 1979). Nowadays, flucytosine is mainly used as an adjunct to either amphotericin B (p. 1268) or fluconazole (p. 1399) for the treatment of cryptococcal meningitis and other systemic cryptococcal infections. Frequent adjustments to the dosage of flucytosine are necessary if renal function is impaired due to amphotericin B. Unless limited by toxicity, amphotericin B/flucytosine combination treatment should be continued for 4 weeks in otherwise healthy patients, but for 6 weeks in those with immunosuppression or malignancies (Dismukes *et al.*, 1987; White *et al.*, 1992). In HIV-infected patients, the amphotericin B/flucytosine combination has also been used wth success, especially for treatment of cryptococcal meningitis (Shaunak and Cohen, 1991; Graybill, 1992; Dismukes, 1993; Powderly, 1993). The addition of flucytosine to amphotericin B is not always necessary. For instance, in one retrospective study in AIDS patients, the addition of flucytosine appeared to offer no additional therapeutic benefit and the use of this drug was associated with a greater number of side-effects, especially cytopenias (Chuck and Sande, 1989). Fluconazole alone (p. 1398) or fluconazole plus flucytosine have also been used with success for the treatment of cryptococcal meningitis in AIDS patients. The combination appears superior (Larsen *et al.*, 1994).

2 Candidiasis

This infection, if disseminated or involving deep tissues, particularly in neutropenic patients, may be treated by a combination of amphotericin B and flucytosine (p. 1270). Chronic infections such as candidal endophthalmitis and endocarditis may need surgery in addition to medical therapy. Hepatosplenic candidiasis, candidal meningitis and peritonitis can also be treated with combination amphotercicn B and flucytosine, but some will respond to amphotericin B (p. 1270) or fluconazole (p. 1400) used alone. Combination amphotericin B and flucytosine is preferable if these infections are caused by *C. tropicalis, C. parapsilosis, C. krusei* or *C. glabrata,* which are less susceptible to amphotericin B than *C. albicans* (Tsui and Liang, 1991; Zenker *et al.*, 1991; Francis and Walsh, 1992; Graybill, 1992; Cohen and Montgomerie, 1993; Flynn *et al.*, 1995). Systemic candidal infections associated with use of peripheral venous catheters in neonates are also usually treated with a combination of i.v. amphotericin B plus oral flucytosine (Leibovitz *et al.*, 1992). Flucytosine and fluconazole was used successfully to treat osteomyelitis due to *C. lusitaniae* in a premature infant (Oleinik *et al.*, 1993).

For candidal urinary tract infections, flucytosine was used as a single drug with success for *Candida* pyelonephritis (Steer *et al.*, 1972) and for urinary candidiasis in children secondary to neurological bladder disease (Lines,1976). Nowadays, because of its toxicity and the possible emergence of flucytosine-resistant *Candida* spp. strains, one of the oral azoles, such as fluconazole, are preferred for this indication (p. 1402) (Fisher *et al.*, 1995).

As a single agent, flucytosine has been reported to cure *Candida* fungemia (Eilard *et al.*, 1974), including fungemia in an infant aged 9 weeks (Burnell, 1971), *Candida* pulmonary mycetoma (Firkin, 1974) and *Candida* thyroiditis (Robinson *et al.*, 1975). In addition, flucytosine has been reported to be effective in *C. albicans* arthritis (Lindstrom and Lindholm, 1973), *C. parapsilosis* arthritis (Imbeau *et al.*, 1977) and *Candida* osteomyelitis (Edwards *et al.*, 1975). *Candida* peritonitis in a patient receiving hemodialysis resolved after treatment with oral flucytosine (Phillips *et al.*, 1973). Another patient with end-stage renal failure managed by peritoneal dialysis and who also developed *Candida* peritonitis was effectively managed by a continuous 5-day peritoneal lavage containing 50 μg per ml of flucytosine (Holdsworth *et al.*, 1975). It is difficult to determine the place, if any, of flucytosine as a single drug for the treatment of *Candida* infections from such anecdotal case reports.

3 Chromoblastomycosis

This disease has been successfully treated by flucytosine. Vandevelde *et al.* (1972) found a 90-day course of flucytosine to be effective in two patients with long-standing disease in whom amphotericin B therapy had failed. Gugnani *et al.* (1978) used a combination of amphotericin B and flucytosine to treat one patient and used flucytosine orally and topically as a 10% cream twice-daily to cure another. Combined therapy may prove more effective (p. 1282). Lopes *et al.* (1978) also showed that chromoblastomycosis due to *Fonsecaea pedrosoi* responded rapidly to flucytosine, but the fungus can develop resistance. They recommend a combination of flucytosine with i.v. amphotericin B. Another case that did not respond to ketoconazole alone, was successfully managed with the combination of ketoconazole and flucytosine (Silber *et al.*, 1983).

4 Phaeohyphomycosis

This disease is caused by black-pigmented molds and the infection involves the skin and subcutaneous tissues, sinuses, lungs and bones. The treatment of choice appears to be itraconazole (p. 1437) (Graybill, 1992) but this disease, when caused by *Exophiala* spp., has also responded to combined i.v. amphotericin B and oral flucytosine therapy (Kenney *et al.*, 1992; Sudduth *et al.*, 1992; Gold *et al.*, 1994). Cutaneous phaehyphomycosis due to *Exophiala jeanselmei* was successfully treated with flucytosine in a renal transplant patient (Hachisuka *et al.*, 1990).

5 Aspergillosis and fusariosis

Invasive aspergillosis in compromised hosts such as those with neutropenia, organ transplantation and AIDS, often responds poorly to antifungal therapy. However, the disease may respond in neutropenic patients if their cytopenia improves. Aspergillosis is usually treated by either amphotericin B (p. 1275) or itraconazole (p. 1433), but when the response is poor, flucytosine may be added to either of the above agents. It is uncertain how much benefit there is from such combination therapy with flucytosine (Francis and Walsh, 1992; Hummel *et al.*, 1992; George *et al.*, 1992; Denning, 1994; Khoo and Denning, 1994). In a review of over 2000 cases of invasive aspergillosis reported in the literature, Denning and Stevens (1990) reported that of the 64 patients treated with the combination of amphotericin B and flucytosine, 60% of leukemic patients, and over 80% of renal transplant and non-immunocompromised patients responded. Although *Fusarium* spp. are usually flucytosine-resistant, some compromised hosts with disseminated fusariosis have responded to combined amphotericin B and flucytosine therapy (Merz *et al.*, 1988). Peritonitis due to *Fusarium* spp. in patients undergoing chronic ambulatory peritoneal dialysis was unsucessfully treated with flucytosine alone, but resolved rapidly on removal of the Tenckhoff catheter (Chiaridia *et al.*, 1990).

6 Other fungal infections

Disseminated *Penicillium marneffei* infections in HIV-infected patients have been usually treated by either amphotericin B (p. 1280) or itraconazole (p. 1437). This fungal pathogen is sensitive to flucytosine, but combination therapy with flucytosine has not been employed (Supparatpinyo *et al.*, 1993). Infections caused by *Trichosporon beigelii*, such as endocarditis in patients with prosthetic heart valves, or bloodstream infection in patients with burns have usually been treated by amphotericin B, but flucytosine has also been added to the treatment regimen in some cases (Keay *et al.*, 1991; Hajjeh and Blumberg, 1995).

References

Allendoerfer R, Marquis AJ, Rinaldi MG, Graybill JR (1991). Combined therapy with fluconazole and flucytosine in murine cryptococcal meningitis. *Antimicrob Ag Chemother* **35**: 726–729.

Anaisse EJ, Karyotakis NC, Hachem R *et al.* (1994). Correlation between *in vitro* and *in vivo* activity of antifungal agents against *Candida* species. *J Infect Dis* **170**: 384–389.

Ando N, Takatori K (1987). Keratomycosis due to *Alternaria alternata* corneal transplant infection. *Mycopathologia* **100**: 17–22.

Arroyo J, Medoff G, Kobayashi GS (1977). Therapy of murine aspergillosis with amphotericin B in combination with rifampin or 5-fluorocytosine. *Antimicrob Ag Chemother* **11**: 21–25.

Auger P, Dumas C, Joly J (1979). A study of 666 strains of *Candida albicans*: correlation between serotype and susceptibility of 5-fluorocytosine. *J Infect Dis* **139**: 590.

Baley JE, Meyers C, Klugman RM *et al.* (1990). Pharmacokinetics, outcome of treatment, and toxic effects of amphotericin B and 5-fluorocytosine in neonates. *J Pediatrics* **116**: 791.

Beggs WH, Sarosi GA (1982). Combined activity of ketoconazole and 5-fluorocytosine on potentially pathogenic yeasts. *Antimicrob Ag Chemother* **21**: 355.

Bennett JE (1974). Chemotherapy of systemic mycoses (second of two parts). *New Engl J Med* **290**: 320.

Bennett JE (1977). Flucytosine. *Ann Intern Med* **86**: 319.

Block ER (1973). Effect of hepatic insufficiency on 5-fluorocytosine concentrations in serum. *Antimicrob Ag Chemother* **3**: 141.

Block ER, Bennett JE (1972). Pharmacological studies with 5-fluorocytosine. *Antimicrob Ag Chemother* **1**: 476.

Block ER, Jennings AE, Bennett JE (1973). Experimental therapy of cladosporiosis and sporotrichosis with 5-fluorocytosine. *Antimicrob Ag Chemother* **3**: 95.

Block ER, Bennett JE, Livoti LG *et al.* (1974). Flucytosine and amphotericin B: hemodialysis effects on the plasma concentration and clearance. Studies in man. *Ann Intern Med* **80**: 613.

Braun DK, Kauffman CA (1992). *Rhodotorula* fungaemia: a life-threatening complication of indwelling central venous catheters. *Mycoses* **35**: 305.

British Society for Antimicrobial Chemotherapy Working Party (1991). Laboratory monitoring of antifungal chemotherapy. *Lancet* **337**: 1577–1580.

Bryan CS, McFarland JA (1978). Cryptococcal meningitis Fatal marrow aplasia from combined therapy. *JAMA* **239**: 1068.

Burnell RH (1971). Systemic candidiasis in an infant treated with 5-fluorocytosine. *Med J Aust* **2**: 859.

Cartwright RY, Shaldon C, Hall GH (1972). Urinary candidiasis after renal transplantation. *Brit Med J* **2**: 351.

Chiaradia V, Schinella D, Pascoli L *et al.* (1990). Fusarium peritonitis in peritoneal dialysis: report of 2 cases. *Microbiologica* **13**: 77–78.

Chin CS, Cheong YM, Wong YH (1989). 5-fluorocytosine resistance in clinical isolates of *Cryptococcus neoformans*. *Med J Malaysia* **44**: 194–198.

Chouini-Lalenne N, Malet-Martino MC, Martino R, Michel G (1989). Study of the metabolism of flucytosine in *Aspergillus* species by ^{19}F nuclear magnetic resonance spectroscopy. *Antimicrob Ag Chemother* **33**: 1939.

Chuck SL, Sande MA (1989). Infections with *Cryptococcus neoformans* in the acquired immunodeficiency syndrome. *New Engl J Med* **321**: 794.

Cohen M, Montgomerie JZ (1993). Hematogenous endophthalmitis due to *Candida tropicalis*: report of two cases and review. *Clin Infect Dis* **17**: 270.

Conly J, Rennie R, Johnson J *et al.* (1992). Disseminated candidiasis due to amphotericin B-resistant *Candida albicans*. *J Infect Dis* **165**: 761.

Craven PC, Graybill JR (1984). Combination of oral flucytosine and ketoconazole as therapy for experimental cryptococcal meningitis. *J Infect Dis* **149**: 584.

Daneshmend TK, Warnock DW (1983). Clinical pharmacokinetics of systemic antifungal drugs. *Clin Pharmacokinet* **8**: 17.

Davies RR, Reeves DS (1971). 5-Fluorocytosine and urinary candidiasis. *Brit Med J* **1**: 577.

Dawborn JK, Page MD, Schiavone DJ (1973). Use of 5-fluorocytosine in patients with impaired renal function. *Brit Med J* **4**: 382.

DeFever KS, Whelan WL, Rogers AL *et al.* (1982). *Candida albicans* resistance to 5-fluorocytosine: frequency of partially resistant strains among clinical isolates. *Antimicrob Ag Chemother* **22**: 810.

Demierre G, Freedman LR (1979). Experimental endocarditis prophylaxis of *Candida albicans* infections by 5-fluorocytosine in rabbits. *Antimicrob Ag Chemother* **16**: 252.

Denning DW (1994). Treatment of invasive aspergillosis. *J Infect* **28** (Suppl 1): 25.

Denning DW, Stevens DA (1990). Antifungal and surgical treatment of invasive aspergillosis: Review of 2121 published cases. *Rev Infect Dis* **12**: 1147–1201.

Denning DW, Hanson LH, Perlman AH, Stevens DA (1992). *In vitro* susceptibility and synergy studies of *Aspergillus* species to conventional and new agents. *Diagn Microbiol Infect Dis* **15**: 21.

Diasio RB, Lakings DE, Bennett JE (1978). Evidence for conversion of 5-fluorocytosine to 5-fluorouracil in humans: possible factor in 5-fluorocytosine clinical toxicity. *Antimicrob Ag Chemother* **14**: 903–908.

Dismukes WE (1993). Management of cryptococcosis. *Clin Infect Dis* **17** (Suppl 2): 507.

Dismukes WE, Cloud G, Gallis HA *et al.* (1987). Treatment of cryptococcal meningitis with combination amphotericin B and flucytosine for four as compared with six weeks. *New Engl J Med* **317**: 334.

Dixon DM, Polak A (1987). *In vitro* and *in vivo* drug studies with three agents of central nervous system phaeohyphomycosis. *Chemotherapy* **33**: 129–140.

Dube MP, Heseltine PN, Rinaldi MG, Evans S, Zawacki B (1994). Fungemia and colonization with nystatin-resistant *Candida rugosa* in a burn unit. *Clin Infect Dis* **18**: 77–82.

Edwards JE Jr, Turkel SB, Elder HA *et al.* (1975). Hematogenous *Candida* osteomyelitis Report of three cases and review of the literature. *Amer J Med* **59**: 89.

Eilard T, Alestig K, Wahlen P (1974). Treatment of disseminated candidiasis with 5-fluorocytosine. *J Infect Dis* **130**: 155.

Firkin FC (1974). Therapy of deep-seated fungal infections with 5-fluorcytosine. *Aust NZ J Med* **4**: 462.

Fisher JF, Newman CL, Sobel JD (1995). Yeast in the urine: solutions for a budding problem. *Clin Infect Dis* **20**: 183.

Flynn PM, Shenep JL, Crawford R, Hughes WT (1995). Use of abdominal computed tomography for identifying disseminated fungal infection in pediatric cancer patients. *Clin Infect Dis* **20**: 964.

Francis P, Walsh TJ (1992). Evolving role of flucytosine in immunocompromised patients: new insights into safety, pharmacokinetics, and antifungal therapy. *Clin Infect Dis* **15**: 1003.

Fromtling RA, Galgioni JN, Pfaller MA *et al.* (1993). Multicenter evaluation of broth macrodilution antifungal susceptibility test for yeasts. *Antimicrob Ag Chemother* **37**: 39.

Fusner JE, McClain KL (1979). Disseminated lymphonodular cryptococcosis treated with 5- fluorocytosine. *J Pediatr* **94**: 599.

Galgiani JN, Reiser J, Brass C *et al.* (1987). Comparison of relative susceptibilities of *Candida* species to three antifungal agents as determined by unstandardized methods. *Antimicrob Ag Chemother* **31**: 1343.

George D, Kordick D, Miniter P *et al.* (1993). Combination therapy in experimental invasive aspergillosis. *J Infect Dis* **168**: 692.

Gold WL, Vellend H, Salit I E *et al.* (1994). Successful treatment of systemic and local infections due to *Exophila* species. *Clin Infect Dis* **19**: 339.

Graybill JR (1992). Future directions of antifungal chemotherapy. *Clin Infect Dis* **14** (Suppl 1): 170.

Grunberg E, Titsworth E, Bennett M (1964). Chemotherapeutic activity of 5-fluorocytosine. *Antimicrob Ag Chemother* **1963**: 556; quoted by Holt and Newman (1973).

Gugnani HC, Egere JU, Suseelan AV *et al.* (1978). Chromomycosis caused by *Phialophoria pedrosoi* in Eastern Nigeria. *J Trop Med Hyg* **81**: 208.

Hadfield TL, Smith MB, Winn RE *et al.* (1987). Mycoses caused by *Candida lusitaniae*. *Rev Infect Dis* **9**: 1006.

Hajjeh RA, Blumberg HM (1995). Bloodstream infection due to *Trichosporon beigelii* in a burn patient: case report and review of therapy. *Clin Infect Dis* **20**: 913.

Haron E, Anaissie E, Dumphy F, McCredie K, Fainstein V (1988). *Hansenula anomala* fungemia. *Rev Infect Dis* **10**: 1182.

Harris BE, Manning BW, Federle, TW, Diasio RB (1986). Conversion of 5-fluorocytosine to 5-fluorouracil by human intestinal microflora. *Antimicrob Ag Chemother* **29**: 44.

Hachisuka H, Matsumoto T, Kusuhara M *et al.* (1990). Cutaneous phaeohyphomycosis caused by *Exophiala jeanselmei* after renal transplantation. *Int J Dermatol* **29**: 198–200.

Heidemann HT, Brune KH (1991). Effect of flucytosine on renal function in the rat. *Mycoses* **34**: 401–404.

Herrington D, Drusaoo GL, Smalls U, Staniford HC (1984). False elevation in serum creatinine levels. *JAMA* **252**: 2962.

Hoeprich PD, Huston AC (1978). Stability of four antifungal antimicrobics *in vitro*. *J Infect Dis* **137**: 87.

Hoeprich PD, Ingraham J, Kleker E, Winship MJ (1974). Development of resistance to 5-fluorocytosine in *Candida parapsilosis* during therapy. *J Infect Dis* **130**: 112.

Hoeprich PD, Merry JM, Gunther R, Franti CE (1987). Entry of five antifungal agents into the ovine lung. *Antimicrob Ag Chemother* **31**: 1234.

Holdsworth SR, Atkins RC, Scott DF, Jackson R (1975). Management of *Candida* peritonitis by prolonged peritoneal lavage containing 5-fluorocytosine. *Clin Nephrol* **4**: 157.

Holt RJ, Newman RL (1973). The antimycotic activity of 5-fluorocytosine. *J Clin Path* **26**: 167.

Hummel M, Thalmann U, Jautzke G *et al.* (1992). Fungal infections following heart transplantations. *Mycoses* **35**: 23.

Imbeau SA, Hanson J, Langejans G, D'Alessio D (1977). Flucytosine treatment of *Candida* arthritis. *JAMA* **238**: 1395.

Jones B R (1975). Principles in the management of oculomycosis. *Trans Amer Acad Ophthalmol Otolaryngol* **70**: OP-15.

Kauffman CA, Frame PT (1977). Bone marrow toxicity associated with 5-fluorocytosine therapy. *Antimicrob Ag Chemother* **11**: 244.

Keay S, Denning DW, Stevens DA (1991). Endocarditis due to *Trichosporon beigelii*: *in vitro* susceptibility of isolates and review. *Rev Infect Dis* **13**: 383.

Kennedy CA, Goetz MB, Mathisen G (1989). Artifactual elevation of the serum creatinine in patients receiving flucytosine for cryptococcal meningitis. *J Infect Dis* **160**: 1090–1091.

Kenney RT, Kuon-Chung KJ, Waytes AT *et al.* (1992). Successful treatment of systemic *Exophiala dermatitidis* infection in a patient with chronic granulomatous disease. *Clin Infect Dis* **14**: 235.

Khoo SH, Denning DW(1994). Invasive aspergillosis in patients with AIDS. *Clin Infect Dis* **19** (Suppl 1): 41.

Kitahara M, Seth VK, Medoff G, Kobayashi GS (1976). Antimicrobial susceptibility testing of six clinical isolates of *Aspergillus*. *Antimicrob Ag Chemother* **9**: 908.

Koechlin BA, Rubio F, Palmer S *et al.* (1966). The metabolism of 5-fluorocytosine-2^{14}C and of cytosine-^{14}C in the rat and the disposition of 5-fluorocytosine-2^{14}C in man. *Biochem Pharmacol* **15**: 435.

Koeffler HP, Golde DW (1979). 5-Fluorocytosine: inhibition of hemato-poieses *in vitro* and reversal of inhibition by uracil. *J Infect Dis* **139**: 438.

Kotani S, Hirose S, Niiya K, Kubonishi I, Miyoshi I (1988). Anaphylaxis to flucytosine in a patient with AIDS. *JAMA* **260**: 3275–3276.

Larsen RA, Bozzette SA, Jones BE *et al.* (1994). Fluconazole combined with flucytosine for treatment of cryptococcal meningitis in patients with AIDS. *Clin Infect Dis* **19**: 741.

Lau YL, Yuen KY, Lee CW, Chan CF (1995). Invasive *Acremonium falciforme* infection in a patient with severe combined immunodeficiency. *Clin Infect Dis* **20**: 197–198.

Lehrer Rl, Howard DH, Sypherd PS *et al.* (1980). Mucormycosis. *Ann Intern Med* **93**: 93.

Leibovitz E, Iuster-Reicher A, Amitai M, Mogilner B (1992). Systemic candidal infections associated with use of peripheral venous catheters in neonates: a 9-year experience. *Clin Infect Dis* **14**: 485.

Lindstrom FD, Lindholm T (1973). *Candida albicans* arthritis treated with flucytosine. *Ann Intern Med* **79**: 131.

Lines D (1976). Childhood urinary candidiasis successfully treated with 5-fluorocytosine. *Aust Pediatr J* **12**: 49.

Longman LP, Martin MV (1987). A comparison of the efficacy of itraconazole, amphotericin B and 5-fluorocytosine in the treatment of *Aspergillus fumigatus* endocarditis in the rabbit. *J Antimicrob Chemother* **20**: 719–724.

Lopes CF, Alvarenga RJ CiSalpeno EO *et al.* (1978). Six years experience in treatment of chromomycosis with 5-fluorocytosine. *Int J Dermatol* **17**: 414–418.

MacLeod SM, Ti TY, Williams RB, Sellers EM (1979). Parenteral 5-fluorocytosine for candidiasis. *Drug Intell Clin Pharm* **13**: 72.

Marcon MJ, Durrell DE, Powell DA, Buesching WJ (1987). *In vitro* activity of systemic antifungal agents against *Malassezia furfur*. *Antimicrob Ag Chemother* **31**: 951–953.

Martin E, Parras P, Lozano MC (1992). *In vitro* susceptibility of 245 yeast isolates to amphotericin B, 5-fluorocytosine, ketoconazole, fluonazole and itraconazole. *Chemotherapy* **38**: 335–339.

Martin E, Maier F, Bhakdi S (1994). Antagonistic effects of fluconazole and 5-fluorocytosine on candidacidal action of amphotericin B in human serum. *Antimicrob Ag Chemother* **38**: 1331.

Malet-Martino MC, Martino R, de Forni M *et al.* (1991). Flucytosine conversion to fluorouracil in humans: does a correlation with gut flora exist? A report of 2 cases using fluorine-19 magnetic resonance spectroscopy. *Infection* **19**: 178–180.

Medoff G, Kobayashi GS (1980). Strategies in the treatment of systemic fungal infections. *New Engl J Med* **302**: 145.

Merz WG, Karp JE, Hoagland M *et al.* (1988). Diagnosis and successful treatment of fusariosis in the compromised host. *J Infect Dis* **158**: 1046.

Meyer R, Axelrod JL (1974). Fatal aplastic anaemia resulting from flucytosine. *JAMA* **228**: 1573.

Mitchell EK (1984). Flucytosine and false elevation of serum creatinine level. *Ann Intern Med* **101**: 278.

Mitchell RT, Marshall LH, Lefkowitz LB, Stratton CW (1985). Falsely elevated serum creatinine levels secondary to the presence of 5-fluor-ocytosine. *Amer J Clin Pathol* **84**: 251–253.

Montplaisir S, Nabarra B, Drouhet E (1976). Susceptibility and resistance of *Candida* to 5-fluorocytosine in relation to the cell wall ultrastructure. *Antimicrob Ag Chemother* **9**: 1028.

Morace G, Manzara S, Dettori G (1991). *In vitro* susceptibility of 119 yeast isolates to fluconazole, 5-fluorocytosine, amphotericin B and ketocona-zole. *Chemotherapy* **37**: 23.

Normark S, Schonebeck J (1972). *In vitro* studies of 5-fluorocytosine resistance in *Candida albicans* and *Torulopsis glabrata*. *Antimicrob Ag Chemother* **2**: 144.

Norrby R, Eilard T (1978). Treatment of opportunistic systemic mycoses. *Scand J Infect Dis* (Suppl 16): 59.

Oleinik EM, Della-Latta P, Rinaldi MG, Saiman L (1993). *Candida lusitaniae* osteomyelitis in a premature infant. *Amer J Perinatol* **10**: 313.

Patterson TF, Andriole VT, Zervos MJ *et al.* (1990). The epidemiology of pseudallescheriasis complicating transplantation: Nosocomial and com-munity-acquired infection. *Mycoses* **33**: 297.

Pennington JE, Block ER, Reynolds HY (1974). 5-Fluorocytosine and amphotericin B in bronchial secretions. *Antimicrob Ag Chemother* **6**: 324.

Phillips I, Eykyn S, MacGregor GA, Jones NF (1973). *Candida* peritonitis treated with 5-fluorocytosine in a patient receiving hemodialysis. *Clin Nephrol* **1**: 271.

Philpot CR, Lo D (1972). Cryptococcal meningitis in pregnancy. *Med J Aust* **2**: 1005.

Polak A (1979). Pharmacokinetics of amphotericin B and flucytosine. *Postgrad Med J* **55**: 667.

Polak A (1987). Combination therapy of experimental candidiasis, crypto-coccosis, aspergillosis and wangiellosis in mice. *Chemotherapy* **33**: 381–395.

Polak A, Wain WH (1979). The effect of 5-fluorocytosine on the blastospores and hyphae of *Candida albicans*. *J Med Microbiol* **12**: 83.

Polak A, Scholer HJ, Wall M (1982). Combination therapy of experimental candidiasis, cryptococcosis and aspergillosis in mice. *Chemotherapy* **28**: 461–479.

Powderly WG (1993). Cryptococcal meningitis and AIDS. *Clin Infect Dis* **17**: 837.

Record CO, Skinner JM, Sleight P, Speller DCE (1971). *Candida* endocarditis treated with 5-fluorocytosine. *Brit Med J* **1**: 262.

Richards AB, Jones BR, Whitwell J, Clayton YM (1969). Corneal and intraocular infection by *Candida albicans* treated with 5-fluorocytosine. *Trans Ophthal Soc UK* **29**: 867.

Robertson DM, Riley FC, Hermans PE (1974). Endogenous *Candida* oculomycosis Report of two patients treated with flucytosine. *Arch Ophthalmol* **91**: 33.

Robinson MF, Forgan-Smith WR, Craswell PW (1975). *Candida* thyroiditis treated with 5-fluorocytosine. *Aust NZ J Med* **5**: 472.

Roche Products Ltd (1972). Data sheet on 5-fluorocytosine Roche Research Department, Roche Products Ltd, Welwyn Garden City, Herts, UK.

Schonebeck J, Segerbrand E (1973). *Candida albicans* septicaemia during first half of pregnancy successfully treated with 5-fluorocytosine. *Brit Med J* **4**: 337.

Sekhon AS, Padhye AA, Garg AK (1992). *In vitro* sensitivity of *Penicillium marneffei* and *Pythium insidiosum* to various antifungal agents. *Eur J Epidemiol* **8**: 427.

Sekhon AS, Garg AK, Padhye AA, Hamir Z (1993). *In vitro* susceptibility of myceliel and yeast forms of *Penicillium marneffei* to amphotericin B, fluconazole, 5-fluorocytosine and itraconazole. *Eur J Epidemiol* **9**: 553–558.

Sekhon AS, Padhye AA, Garg AK *et al.* (1994). *In vitro* sensitivity of medically significant *Fusarium* species to various antimycotics. *Chem-otherapy* **40**: 239.

Segal E, Romano A, Eylan E, Stein R (1975). Experimental and clinical studies of 5-fluorocytosine activity in *Candida* ocular infections. I. *In vitro* activity of 5-fluorocytosine on *Candida* species isolated from ocular infections. *Chemotherapy* **21**: 358–366.

Shadomy S (1969). *In vitro* studies with 5-fluorocytosine. *Appl Microbiol* **17**: 871.

Shadomy S, Kirchoff CB, Ingroff AE (1973). *In vitro* activity of 5-fluorocytosine against *Candida* and *Torulopsis* species. *Antimicrob Ag Chemother* **3**: 9.

Shaunak S, Cohen J (1991). Clinical management of fungal infection in patients with AIDS. *J Antimicrob Chemother* **28** (Suppl A): 67.

Shelley WB, Sica PA (1983). Disseminated sporotrichosis of skin and bone cured with 5-fluorocytosine: Photosensitivity as a complication. *J Amer Acad Dermatol* **8**: 229–235.

Silber JG, Gombert ME, Green K *et al.* (1983). Treatment of chromomycosis with ketoconazole and 5-fluorocytosine. *J Amer Acad Dermatol* **8**: 236–238.

Stafford CR, Fisher JF, Fadel HE *et al.* (1983). Cryptococcal meningitis in pregnancy. *Obstet Gynecol* **62** (Suppl): 35–37.

Stamm AM, Diasio RB, Dismukes WE *et al.* (1987). Toxicity of amphotericin B plus flucytosine in 194 patients with cryptococcal meningitis. *Amer J Med* **83**: 236.

Stanton KG, Sanderson CR (1974). The treatment of systemic cryptococcosis with 5-fluorocytosine. *Aust NZ J Med* **4**: 262.

Steer PL, Marks Ml, Klite PD, Eickhoff TC (1972). 5-Fluorocytosine: an oral antifungal compound. A report on clinical and laboratory experience. *Ann Intern Med* **76**: 15.

Stiller RL, Bennett JE, Scholer HJ *et al.* (1982). Susceptibility to 5-fluorocytosine and prevalence of serotype in 402 *Candida albicans* isolates from the United States. *Antimicrob Ag Chemother* **22**: 482.

Stiller RL, Bennett JE, Scholer HJ *et al.* (1983). Correlation of *in vitro* susceptibility test results with *in vivo* response: flucytosine therapy in a systemic candidiasis model. *J Infect Dis* **147**: 1070.

Sudduth EJ, Crumbley AJ III, Farrar WE (1992). Phaeohyphomycosis due to *Exophiala* species: clinical spectrum of disease in humans. *Clin Infect Dis* **15**: 639.

Sugarman B, Pesanti E (1980). Treatment failures secondary to *in vivo* development of drug resistance by microorganism. *Rev Infect Dis* **2**: 153.

Supparatpinyo K, Nelson KE, Merz WG *et al.* (1993). Response to antifungal therapy by human immunodeficiency virus-infected patients with disseminated *Penicillium marneffei* infections and *in vitro* susceptibilities of isolates from clinical specimens. *Antimicrob Ag Chemother* **37**: 2407.

Thaler M, Bacher J, O'Leary T, Pizzo PA (1988). Evaluation of single-drug and combination antifungal therapy in an experimental model of candidiasis in rabbits with prolonged neutropenia. *J Infect Dis* **158**: 80–88.

Tolentino P, Borrone C (1976). Multiple lymphonodular cryptococcosis cured by 5-fluorocytosine. *Scand J Infect Dis* **8**: 61.

Tsui E, Liang R (1991). Successful treatment of focal hepatic candidiasis in a patient with acute myeloid leukemia. *Scand J Infect Dis* **23**: 267.

Utz JP (1972). Editorial Flucytosine. *New Engl J Med* **286**: 777.

Utz JP, Tynes BS, Shadomy HJ *et al.* (1969). 5-Fluorocytosine in human cryptococcosis. *Antimicrob Ag Chemother* **1968**: 344.

Utz JP, Garriques IL, Sande MA *et al.* (1975). Therapy of cryptococcosis with a combination of flucytosine and amphotericin B. *J Infect Dis* **132**: 368–373.

Vandevelde AG, Mauceri AA, Johnson JE III (1972). 5-Fluorocytosine in the treatment of mycotic infections. *Ann Intern Med* **77**: 43.

Wade DN, Sudlow G (1972). The kinetics of 5-fluorocytosine elimination in man. *Aust NZ J Med* **2**: 153.

Wain WH, Polak A (1979). The effect of flucytosine on the germination of *Candida albicans*. *Postgrad Med J* **55**: 671.

Waldorf AR, Polak A (1983). Mechanisms of action of 5-fluorocytosine. *Antimicrob Ag Chemother* **23**: 79.

Ward RM, Sattler FR, Dalton AS Jr (1983). Assessment of antifungal therapy in an 800–gram infant with candidal arthritis and osteomyelitis. *Pediatrics* **72**: 234.

Weber S, Polak A (1992). Susceptibility of yeast isolates from defined German patient groups to 5-fluorocytosine. *Mycoses* **35**: 163.

Weese WC, Schope RW (1972). 5-Fluorocytosine therapy. *Ann Intern Med* **77**: 1003.

Weisse ME, Person DA, Berkenbaugh JT (1993). Treatment of *Candida* arthritis with flucytosine and amphotericin. *B J Perinatol* **13**: 402–404.

Whelan WL, Kerridge D (1984). Decreased activity of UMP pyrophosphorylase associated with resistance to 5-fluorocytosine in *Candida albicans*. *Antimicrob Ag Chemother* **26**: 570.

Whelan WL, Beneke ES, Rogers AL, Soll DR (1981). Segregation of 5-fluorocytosine-resistant variants by *Candida albicans*. *Antimicrob Ag Chemother* **19**: 1078.

White CA, Traube J (1982). Ulcerating enteritis associated with flucytosine therapy. *Gastroenterology* **83**: 1127–1129.

White M, Cirrincione C, Blevins A, Armstrong D (1992). Cryptococcal meningitis: outcome in patients with AIDS and patients with neoplastic disease. *J Infect Dis* **165**: 960.

Wingfield HJ (1987). Absence of fungistatic antagonism between flucytosine and cytarabine *in vitro* and *in vivo*. *J Antimicrob Chemother* **20**: 523–527.

Wong PW, Ching WTW, Kwon-Chung KJ, Meyer RD (1989). Disseminated *Phialophora parasitica* infection in humans: Case report and review. *Rev Infect Dis* **11**: 770–775.

Yangco BG, Okafor JI, TeStrake D (1984). *In vitro* susceptibilities of human and wild-type isolates of *Basidiobolus* and *Conidiobolus* species. *Antimicrob Ag Chemother* **25**: 413–416.

Yoshizumi MO, Silverman C (1985). Experimental intravitreal 5-fluorocytosine. *Ann Ophthalmol* **17**: 58–61.

Zenker PN, Rosenberg EM, Van Dyke RB *et al.* (1991). Successful medical treatment of presumed *Candida* endocarditis in critically infants. *J Pediatrics* **119**: 472.

Griseofulvin

Description

Griseofulvin is a metabolic product of *Penicillium griseofulvum* discovered in 1939 (Oxford *et al.*, 1939), but it was not investigated further at that time because it lacked antibacterial activity. Although it was shown in 1947 that griseofulvin protected plants from fungal infections, its potential for the treatment of human infections was not realized until Gentles (1958) demonstrated that oral griseofulvin was effective in experimental *Microsporum canis* infection of guinea pigs. It was soon shown that the drug was also effective in human ringworm infections (Williams *et al.*, 1958; Blank *et al.*, 1959). Griseofulvin is effective treatment of dermatophyte infections, particularly those involving the skin, hair or nails. However, newer drugs with improved therapeutic efficacy, lower rates of relapse and less toxicity are relegating griseofulvin to second-line treatment.

Sensitive Organisms

1 Dermatophytes

These fungi include the *Microsporum, Trichophyton* and *Epidermophyton* spp., and are highly sensitive to griseofulvin. Strains of dermatophytes resistant to the drug have been produced *in vitro* (Roth, 1960–61).

2 Other fungi

Griseofulvin has no activity against other filamentous fungi such as *Aspergillus* and *Phialophora* spp. The drug has no effect against yeasts such as *Cryptococcus neoformans*, and *Candida* spp., or against dimorphic fungi such as *Blastomyces dermatitidis, Paracoccidioides brasiliensis, Histoplasma capsulatum, Sporothrix schenckii* and *Coccidioides immitis* (Roth, 1960–61).

3 Bacteria

Griseofulvin has no activity against *Actinomyces* and *Nocardia* spp., and is also inactive against all other bacteria.

4 Minimum inhibitory concentrations

Determination of the MICs of griseofulvin using a broth dilution test in microtiter plates for recent clinical isolates of dermatophytes from patients with tinea unguium yielded a range of MICs of 0.5–3 μg per ml for *Tricophyton rubrum*, and 2–10 μg per ml for *T. mentagrophytes*. (Korting *et al.*, 1995). There is only one report of *in vitro* resistance to *T. rubrum* and corresponding clinical failure of griseofulvin therapy. An MIC of 3 μg per ml was considered a resistant isolate (Artis *et al.*, 1981). Using a cut-off of 3 μg per ml to identify relative resistance, at least one-third of *T. rubrum* isolates from the German multicenter study would be considered resistant (Korting *et al.*, 1995).

Mode of Administration and Dosage

Two preparations of griseofulvin are available for administration by the oral route – microsize crystals and ultramicrosize crystals.

1 Adults

The dose of the microsize preparation is 0.5–1 g daily administered in one or two divided doses. For difficult chronic infections, such as fungal paronychia, a dose as high as 0.5 g three times per day, has been used (Davies *et al.*, 1967). The absorption of microsize griseofulvin is enhanced by administration with a high-fat meal, but this is often not practical in the clinical situation. Recommended adult doses of the ultramicrosize preparation are 330–660 mg daily. The duration of therapy depends on the site of infection.

2 Children

The daily dose of microsize griseofulvin is 10 mg per kg body weight, administered in one or two divided doses. A commonly used dose for children is 125 mg twice-daily. Ginsburg *et al.* (1983) recommend a 15 mg per kg dose of the microsize preparation for children with superficial fungal infections, and this should be administered with whole milk or other food containing fat, to ensure optimum bioavailability. Grin and Nadazdin (1965) demonstrated that the optimal dose for children suffering from favus, a *T. schoenleinii* infection, was 25 mg per kg per day.

The recommended dose for the ultramicrosize preparation is 5.5 mg per kg body weight per day.

3 Patients with renal failure

Griseofulvin can be given in the usual doses to such patients, because it does not accumulate in the presence of renal impairment.

4 Pregnancy

As griseofulvin is teratogenic and embryotoxic in rats, dogs, cats and mice, its use is not recommended in pregnancy. Sperm abnormalities have been induced in griseofulvin-treated mice and it is recommended that males do not father children during treatment with griseofulvin, or within 6 months of completion of therapy (De Carli and Larizza, 1988). Rosa *et al.* (1987) suggested the possibility of griseofulvin teratology with conjoined twins because the only conjoined twins (two pairs) on the US Food and Drug Administration teratology information system had been born to women exposed to griseofulvin in first-trimester pregnancy. The overall incidence of birth defects in women with first-trimester exposure to griseofulvin was 1 in 16, implying most pregnancy outcomes following first-trimester exposure to griseofulvin will be normal, but there was an estimated relative risk of 2.5 (95% CI 1.01–6.1) for spontaneous abortion. Knudsen (1987) and Metneki and Czeizel (1987) were unable to support the proposal for conjoined twinning related to griseofulvin teratology.

It is unknown whether griseofulvin is excreted in breast milk and the safety of griseofulvin in neonates has not been established.

Availability

Microsize particle preparation: 250 mg and 500 mg tablets.

Ultramicrosize particle preparation: 125 mg, 165 mg, 250 mg, and 330 mg tablets.

Suspension: 125 mg per 5 ml

Serum Levels in Relation to Dosage

After oral administration of 1.0 g of the microsize preparation to adults, a peak serum level of 1–2 μg per ml is reached in about 4 h in most patients. The level is slightly lower 8 h after administration, and at 12 h it is about half the peak serum level. There is considerable individual variation in the serum levels obtained after griseofulvin administration. Crounse (1961) studied 27 adult patients, each of whom received 1.0 g of the drug orally. Serum levels at 4 h ranged from 0 to 3.75 μg per ml, and at 8 h from 0.25 to 3.75 μg per ml. The mean values were 1.31 and 1.10 μg per ml at 4 h and 8 h, respectively. Crounse (1961) repeated these experiments over several months, and showed that patients who had high serum levels would consistently show high levels when retested, and those with low levels would consistently show low levels. After repeated administration of 500 mg of microsize griseofulvin daily, mean serum levels plateau after the third dose at 1.5 μg per ml. The elimination half-life is 9.5–42 h (Lin and Symchowicz, 1975). Ultramicrosize griseofulvin is almost completely absorbed and, according to the manufacturers, the bioavailability after a 330-mg tablet is the same as that of an equivalent dose (500 mg) of the microsize preparation.

If griseofulvin is taken with a fatty meal instead of in the fasting state, serum levels are approximately double. It appears that the presence of fat in the gut in some way enhances griseofulvin absorption (Crounse, 1961). The bioavailability of microsized or ultramicrosized griseofulvin was compared in healthy volunteers who were given a fatty meal after administration of the griseofulvin. A minor increase only in the mean peak plasma level and the AUC were observed for the ultramicrosize formulation, suggesting co-administration of griseofulvin with food will reduce the difference in bioavailability between the two types of formulation (Bijanzadeh *et al.*, 1990).

Ginsburg *et al.* (1983) studied bioavailability of griseofulvin in 23 children (aged 19 months–11 years) with tinea capitis or tinea corporis when given the microsize preparation as an oral suspension (125 mg per ml). Considerable variation in serum concentrations was observed in fasting patients. Other patients were given the drug with 120 ml of homogenized milk. After a 10 mg per kg dose, mean peak serum concentrations of 1.29 and 0.34 μg per ml were attained at 4 h in non-fasting and fasting children, respectively. Serum levels were also higher 6 h after the dose in children who received drug and milk concomitantly. Of the fasting patients, 31 % had no drug detected in serum at any time after ingestion, whereas griseofulvin was present in serum for at least 4 h in all children who received the drug with milk. After 15 mg per kg body weight doses administered with milk, the mean peak serum level at 4 h was 1.03 μg per ml and mean levels at 0.5, 2, 6 and 24 h were 0.28, 0.96, 0.92 and 0.43 μg per ml, respectively. Levels at 0.5 and 24 h were higher than attained with 10 mg per kg doses, whereas those at 1 through 6 h were similar with the two dosages. In seven of ten of the fed children given 15 mg per kg, griseofulvin serum levels greater than 1 μg per ml were achieved (a level quoted to be necessary to achieve cure in tinea capitis). The authors recommended a 15 mg per kg daily dose for children to be administered with milk or other fat-containing food.

Excretion

1 Urine

Renal excretion does not play a significant role in the elimination of the active drug; less than 1 % of an administered dose of griseofulvin appears in the urine in an unchanged form (Roth,1960–61).

2 Inactivation in body

Most absorbed griseofulvin is inactivated in the liver by dealkylation; the inactive metabolite, 6-desmethylgriseofulvin, is then excreted in the urine, some of it as a glucuronide conjugate. Griseofulvin inactivation in rats is enhanced by barbiturates, which induce the hepatic enzymes involved (Busfield *et al.*, 1964). Concomitant administration of griseofulvin and a barbiturate may reduce the efficacy of griseofulvin therapy, and lowering of griseofulvin serum levels has been demonstrated in volunteers when this drug combination was used (Busfield *et al.*, 1963). This effect may not be due to stimulated griseofulvin metabolism in man, but because phenobarbital reduces the absorption of the drug (Lin and Symchowicz, 1975).

3 Feces

A considerable proportion of the administered dose of the microsize preparation appears unchanged in feces. This could be due to incomplete absorption, or to complete absorption of the drug followed by biliary excretion, or both (Lin and Symchowicz, 1975).

Distribution of the Drug in Body

In animals griseofulvin is distributed widely in body fluids and tissues and it is concentrated in liver, fat, and skeletal muscle (Roth, 1960–61).

Gentles *et al.* (1959) postulated that griseofulvin is deposited in the keratinous layer of the epidermis and also in newly formed keratin of hair shafts. They confirmed this in guinea pigs by demonstrating the presence of the drug in hair after oral therapy. Griseofulvin is concentrated in keratin precursor cells where it exerts its antifungal effect; this includes the stratum corneum of the skin, the nails and hair. Levels of the drug in the skin exceed those reached in the serum. Griseofulvin is also secreted in sweat and this is probably the major route of griseofulvin delivery to the stratum corneum (Shah *et al.*, 1972). New keratin formed during treatment with griseofulvin is resistant to invasion by fungus, but the drug does not destroy fungus which has infected the outer keratin layers. The rate of penetration of griseofulvin through the layers of skin varied from detection of griseofulvin at the base of the stratum corneum at 48–72 h, at the lower quarter of the horny layer at 6–12 days and the middle layer of the horny layer at 12–19 days from initial ingestion. The level of griseofulvin in keratin was 3 ng per mg in 8 h following ingestion and reach 12–22 ng per mg in 2–4 days (Shah *et al.*, 1974).

Schafer-Korting (1987) examined the penetration of griseofulvin into skin blister fluid in the rat model, as a more reliable indicator of griseofulvin activity at the site of action. Maximum concentrations in skin blister fluid were attained 60 min after i.v. administration of griseofulvin and the level of unbound (active) drug in skin blister fluid was several fold lower than the concentration of total drug in excised skin. The latter concentration had been used as a guide for *in vitro* susceptibility of dermatophytes.

Mode of Action

Griseofulvin impairs fungal growth, resulting in distortion of hyphae. It is a fungistatic drug which is active only against growing cells. Susceptibility of fungi appears to be related to binding of griseofulvin to RNA. The drug interferes with microtubules of the mitotic spindle and cytoplasmic microtubules. Since microtubules are involved in the transport of secretory material through the cytoplasm to the periphery of the cell, destruction of microtubules may lead to impaired processing of newly synthesized cell wall constituents at the growing tips of hyphae (Borgers, 1980).

Toxicity

1 Gastrointestinal side-effects

These are the most common side-effects and include nausea, vomiting, diarrhea, heartburn, flatulence, angular stomatitis, glossodynia, thirst and a black-furred tongue.

2 Neurotoxicity

Headache is a frequent side-effect (up to 15% of treated patients), but it often disappears as therapy is continued. Other rare side-effects are irritability, fatigue, confusion, impaired co-ordination, peripheral neuritis, paresthesias of hands and feet after prolonged therapy, vertigo and blurred vision. Lecky (1990), described a case of peripheral neuropathy manifest as paresthesias of all fingers followed by numbness of the feet, and absent ankle jerks, which developed after 6 months on griseofulvin. Nerve conduction studies revealed a severe motor and sensory neuropathy which resolved over 4 months after cessation of the drug.

3 Hypersensitivity

Cutaneous adverse effects are varied and uncommon. Maculopapular, urticarial or photo-sensitivity rashes occur in a small percentage of patients, and these disappear when the drug is stopped (Kojima *et al.*, 1988; Kawabe *et al.*, 1988). Serum sickness and angioneurotic edema are rare. A Kawasaki-like syndrome, toxic epidermal necrolysis (fatal in one case), erythema multiforme and a fixed drug reaction precipitated by griseofulvin have all been reported (Amita *et al.*, 1993; Mion *et al.*, 1990; Rustin *et al.*, 1989; Boudghene-Stambouli and Merad-Boudia, 1989; Taylor and Duffill, 1988). Subacute cutaneous lupus erythematosus lesions occurred in several patients with circulating antibodies to SSA/Ro and SSB/La antigens. It is thought griseofulvin may be synergistic with the anti-SSA/Ro antibodies in the production of this syndrome (Miyagawa and Sakamoto, 1989; Miyagawa *et al.*, 1990). Systemic lupus erythematosus is a contraindication for griseofulvin therapy. Griseofulvin induced a severe generalized vesiculobullous eruption in a man with chronic benign familial pemphigus (Meffert *et al.*, 1995).

4 Renal side-effects

Albuminuria and cylindruria without evidence of renal insufficiency have been described. There is a report of membranous glomerulopathy and nephrotic syndrome in a 16-year-old male who also appeared to develop evidence of systemic lupus erythematosus after treatment with griseofulvin (Bonilla-Felix *et al.*, 1995). Interstitial nephritis manifest as hematuria, pyuria and eosinophiluria with renal impairment associated with chronic griseofulvin therapy for onychomycosis has also been reported (Haskell *et al.*, 1990).

5 Hematological side-effects

Leukopenia and neutropenia have been reported rarely. Isolated erythroid hypoplasia causing severe anemia induced by long-term griseofulvin has been reported (Haskell *et al.*, 1990).

6 Other

Myositis and a proximal myopathy secondary to griseofulvin treatment have been reported (Deo *et al.*, 1994; Davidson, 1995). Hepatotoxicity is infrequent, generally mild and usually reversible on cessation of the drug. Pre-existing liver disease may be exacerbated by griseofulvin, and severe liver disease or hepatocellular failure are contraindications to treatment with this drug.

7 Interference with porphyrin metabolism

Griseofulvin has an effect on the porphyrin metabolism of normal subjects. This does not have any clinical significance, because it does not produce symptoms or abnormalities in liver function tests (Rimington *et al.*, 1963). Griseofulvin may aggravate acute intermittent porphyria (Redeker *et al.*, 1964). Berman and Franklin (1965) described a woman aged 43 years with this form of porphyria, whose disease was acutely exacerbated following a 10-day course of griseofulvin. Established porphyria is a contraindication to treatment with griseofulvin.

8 Drug interactions

Griseofulvin may reduce the anticoagulant effect of warfarin, presumably by acting as an inducer of its hepatic metabolism (Cullen and Catalano, 1967). A weak, but on occasions severe, 'disufiram-like' reaction which manifests as vomiting, diarrhea, flushing, tachycardia, and hypotension, can can occur due to an interaction of griseofulvin and alcohol (Fett and Vukov, 1994). Patients should be warned of the potential of griseofulvin to enhance the effects of alcohol. Concomitant administration of barbiturates diminishes the absorption of griseofulvin (Cartwright, 1978). Reports to adverse drug reaction committees in the UK and Netherlands have suggested that there may be an interaction between oral contraceptives and griseofulvin (Van Dijke and Weber, 1984), and Shenfield (1993) reported that the plasma concentration of oral contraceptives may be reduced by the induction of hepatic metabolism by griseofulvin, and this could result in impaired effectiveness of the oral contraceptive and potential breakthrough bleeding or pregnancy. Griseofulvin also significantly reduces serum salicylate concentrations (Phillips *et al.*, 1993).

9 Carcinogenicity

Chronic griseofulvin administration to mice induces development of multiple hepatomas; however, this does not appear to have significance for human exposures (De Carli and Larizza, 1988).

Clinical Uses of the Drug

Griseofulvin is only useful for the treatment of dermatophyte infections of the skin, hair and nails, i.e. tinea corporis, tinea pedis, tinea cruris, tinea barbae, tinea capitis and tinea unguium (onychomycosis). It is not effective against *Candida* spp. infections.

Mild forms of tinea can be treated by topical antifungal agents, but for severe forms of tinea and infections involving the face, hands, hair and nails, oral griseofulvin became the preferred treatment. Its role is now diminishing with the advent of more potent agents such as terbinafine and itraconazole. The response to griseofulvin in a particular infection depends upon the rate of keratinization and time necessary for desquamation of infected keratinized structures. A minimum of 4 weeks treatment is recommended. Infections of the palms and soles require 4–8 weeks, fingernails 4–6 months and toenails 6–12 months treatment.

Tinea capitis responds poorly to topical treatment, but 90% cases will respond to griseofulvin 500 mg daily in adults and 250 mg daily in children (Laude *et al.*, 1982). Comparable efficacy (cure rates of 88%) between griseofulvin 500 mg daily and itraconazole 100 mg daily for 6 weeks was demonstrated in a controlled trial of treatment of tinea capitis in children; however, itraconazole appeared to be better tolerated by the children (Lopez-Gomez *et al.*, 1994). Tinea corporis is often successfully managed with topical therapy, and systemic treatment with griseofulvin is indicated for widespread disease or when granulomatous lesions occur. Cure rates of 60% have been reported with griseofulvin (Artis *et al.*, 1981), compared with 80% for itraconazole and 75–90% for terbinafine (De Doncker and Cauwenbergh, 1992; Villars and Jones, 1989; Lachapelle *et al.*, 1992). Tinea cruris and tinea pedis are also generally managed with topical antifungal agents, with griseofulvin reserved for resistant cases. Symptomatic improvement may take up to 6 weeks and clinical cure may not occur before 6 months. Terbinafine 125 mg twice-daily was found to be significantly superior to griseofulvin 250 mg twice-daily for chronic moccasin type tinea pedis with mycological cure rates of 88% and 45% respectively (Savin, 1989; Hay *et al.*, 1991), and a 4-week course of itraconazole 100 mg daily was superior to griseofulvin 500 mg daily for tinea pedis (Wishart, 1994).

Griseofulvin 1 g per day for 3–15 months for tinea unguium of the toenails resulted in a clinical cure of 16% of patients, probably due to poor penetration of the nail (Weitzman and Summerbell, 1995). Griseofulvin (1000 mg per day of microsized formulation) for 48 weeks was compared with terbinafine (250 mg per day) for 24 weeks for the treatment of severe dermatophyte infection of the toenails. At 48 weeks, cure rates were not significantly different (67% terbinafine and 56% griseofulvin); however, terbinafine-treated patients maintained the cure rate at 60% 6 months later, while those treated with griseofulvin had a cure rate of 39%

(Hofmann *et al.*, 1995). Another study with similar results compared a shorter 16-week course of terbinafine 250 mg per day, with a 52-week course of griseofulvin 500 mg per day. Terbinafine was significantly more effective than griseofulvin with mycological cure rates of 84% and 45% respectively (Faergemann *et al.*, 1995). A comparison of ultramicrosized griseofulvin 660–990 mg daily (resulting in higher plasma and skin tissue levels of griseofulvin) and itraconazole 100 mg daily for tinea unguium, did not reveal a significant difference in clinical response; however, it did reveal a significant difference in cessation of treatment for adverse reactions favoring itraconazole (Korting *et al.*, 1993). Comparable efficacy for microsize griseofulvin and itraconazole for onychomycosis was also demonstrated by Piepponen *et al.* (1992). For fingernail dermatophytosis, terbinafine 250 mg daily (cure rate of 76%) was shown to be significantly superior to microsized griseofulvin 500 mg daily (cure rate of 39%) after 12-weeks treatment (Haneke *et al.*, 1995). Terbinafine, therefore, has superior long-term efficacy as a theraputic agent for toenail onychomycosis and requires a shorter duration of treatment, which will increase patient compliance.

Scholz and Meinhof (1991) performed susceptibility testing on a large number of isolates of *T. rubrum* and concluded that *in vitro* resistance or susceptibility did not reliably explain the therapeutic effect of griseofulvin. Hay (1979) studied 50 patients with chronic dermatophyte infections (48 due to *T. rubrum*) which had not responded to griseofulvin and topical antifungal therapy. *In vitro* resistance to griseofulvin was not detected and immunological studies suggested that therapeutic failure may have been due to deficiencies in the hosts' defence mechanisms. About 80–90% of chronic or recurrent dermatophyte infections are due to *T. rubrum*, and it has been shown that infection with these organisms is associated with decreased delayed-type hypersensitivity reactions to trichophyton antigen, but normal responses to other antigens, and suppressed immune responses (Weitzman and Summerbell, 1995). There are anecdotal case reports of griseofulvin-resistant tinea capitis infection due to *Microsporum canis* that responded to itraconazole (Lukacs *et al.*, 1994). Therapy with fungicidal drugs such as terbinafine or itraconazole with their shorter duration of necessary treatment, improved therapeutic efficacy, reduced relapse rate and reduced toxicity may be preferable to griseofulvin for nail dermatophyte infection (Roberts, 1994).

Griseofulvin 500 mg three times daily for 12 months has been used successfully in several patients with eumycetoma due to *Madurella mycetomatis* who have not responded to ketoconazole (Restrepo, 1994). A renal transplant patient developed a hyalohyphomycosis caused by *Paecilomyces lilacinus* which localized to the forearm, and was successfully treated with griseofulvin 500 mg daily for 6 weeks (Castro *et al.*, 1990). Cutaneous disease due to *Hendersonula toruloidea* responds poorly to griseofulvin, and MICs are greater than 100 μg per ml (Greer and Gutierrez, 1987; Kotrajaras *et al.*, 1988).

References

Amita DB, Danon YL, Garty BZ (1993). Kawasaki-like syndrome associated with griseofulvin treatment. *Clin Exp Dermatol* **18**: 389.

Artis WM, Odle BM, Jones HE (1981). Griseofulvin-resistant dermatophytosis correlates with *in vitro* resistance. *Arch Dermatol* **117**: 16.

Berman A, Franklin RL (1965). Precipitation of acute intermittent porphyria by griseofulvin therapy. *JAMA* **192**: 1005.

Bijanzadeh M, Mahmoudian M, Salehian P *et al.* (1990). The bioavailability of griseofulvin from microsized and ultramicrosized tablets in nonfasting volunteers. *Ind J Physiol Pharmacol* **34**: 157.

Blank H, Smith JG Jr, Roth FJ Jr, Zaias N (1959). Griseofulvin for the systemic treatment of dermatomycoses. *JAMA* **171**: 2168.

Bonilla-Felix M, Verani R, Vanasse LG, Hebert A (1995). Nephrotic syndrome related to systemic lupus erythematosus after griseofulvin therapy. *Pediatr Nephrol* **9**: 478.

Borgers M (1980). Mechanism of action of antifungal drugs, with special reference to the imidazole derivatives. *Rev Infect Dis* **2**: 520.

Boudghene-Stambouli O, Merad-Boudia A (1989). Fixed drug eruption induced by griseofulvin. *Dermatologica* **179**: 92.

Busfield D, Child KJ, Atkinson RM, Tomich EG (1963). An effect of phenobarbitone on blood-levels of griseofulvin in man. *Lancet* **ii**: 1042.

Busfield D, Child KJ, Tomich EG (1964). An effect of phenobarbitone on griseofulvin metabolism in the rat. *Brit J Pharmacol* **22**: 137.

Cartwright RY (1978). Use of antibiotics. *Brit Med J* **2**: 108.

Castro LG, Salebian A, Sotto MN (1990). Hyalohyphomycosis by *Paecilomyces lilacinus* in a renal transplant patient and a review of human *Paecilomyces* species infections. *J Med Vet Mycol* **28**: 15.

Crounse RG (1961). Human pharmacology of griseofulvin: the effect of fat intake on gastrointestinal absorption. *J Invest Dermatol* **37**: 529.

Cullen SI, Catalano PM (1967). Griseofulvin-warfarin antagonism. *JAMA* **199**: 582.

Davidson BK (1995). Myositis associated with griseofulvin therapy. *Am Family Physician* **52**: 1277.

Davies RR, Everall JD, Hamilton E (1967). Mycological and clinical evaluation of griseofulvin for chronic onychomycosis. *Brit Med J* **3**: 464.

De Carli L, Larizza L (1988). Griseofulvin. *Mutation Res* **195**: 91.

De Doncker P, Cauwenbergh G (1992). Management of fungal skin infections with 15 days of itraconazole treatment: a worldwide review. *Brit J Clin Pract* **71** (Suppl): 118.

Deo A, Mehta HG, Biniyala R et al. (1994). Proximal myopathy associated with griseofulvin therapy. *J Assoc Phys India* **42**: 85.

Faergemann J, Anderson C, Hersle K et al. (1995). Double-blind, parallel-group comparison of terbinafine and griseofulvin in the treatment of toenail onychomycosis. *J Amer Acad Dermatol* **32**: 750.

Fett DL, Vukov LF (1994). An unusual case of severe griseofulvin-alcohol interaction. *Ann Emerg Med* **24**: 95.

Gentles JC (1958). Experimental ringworm in guinea pigs: oral treatment with griseofulvin. *Nature* **182**: 476.

Gentles JC, Barnes MT, Fantes KH (1959). Presence of griseofulvin in hair of guinea-pigs after oral administration. *Nature* **183**: 256.

Ginsburg CM, McCracken GH Jr, Petruska M, Olsen K (1983). Effect of feeding on bioavailability of griseofulvin in children. *J Pediatr* **102**: 309.

Greer DL, Gutierrez MM (1987). Tinea pedis caused by *Hendersonula toruloidea* A new problem in dermatology. *J Amer Acad Dermatol* **16**: 1111.

Grin EI, Nadazdin M (1965). Experimental investigation into the therapeutic effect of griseofulvin in favus caused by *Trichophyton schoenleinii. Bull Wld Hlth Org* **33**: 183.

Haneke E, Tausch I, Brautigam M et al. (1995). Short-duration treatment of fingernail dermatophytosis: a randomized, double-blind study with terbinafine and griseofulvin. LAGOS III Study Group. *J Amer Acad Dermatol* **32**: 72.

Haskell LP, Mennemyer RP, Greenman R, Pelczar C (1990). Isolated erythroid hypoplasia and renal insufficiency induced by long-term griseofulvin therapy. *South Med J* **83**: 1327.

Hay RJ (1979). Failure of treatment in chronic dermatophyte infections. *Postgrad Med J* **55**: 608

Hay RJ, Logan RA, Moore MK et al. (1991). A comparative study of terbinafine versus griseofulvin in 'dry-type' dermatophyte infections. *J Amer Acad Dermatol* **24**: 243.

Hofmann H, Brautigam M, Weidinger G, Zaun H (1995). Treatment of toenail onychomycosis. A randomized, double-blind study with terbinafine and griseofulvin. LAGOS II Study Group. *Arch Dermatol* **131**: 919.

Kawabe Y, Mizuno N, Miwa N, Sakakibara S (1988). Photosensitivity induced by griseofulvin. *Photo-Dermatol* **5**: 272.

Knudsen LB (1987). No association between griseofulvin and conjoined twinning. *Lancet* **ii**: 1097.

Kojima T, Hasegawa T, Ishida H et al. (1988). Griseofulvin-induced photodermatitis- report of six cases. *J Dermatol* **15**: 76.

Korting HC, Schafer-Korting M, Zienicke H et al. (1993). Treatment of tinea unguium with medium and high doses of ultramicrosize griseofulvin compared with that with itraconazole. *Antimicrob Ag Chemother* **37**: 2064.

Korting HC, Ollert M, Abeck D, German Collaborative Dermatophyte Drug Susceptibility Study Group (1995). Results of German multicenter study of antimicrobial susceptibilities of *Trichophyton rubrum* and *Trichophyton mentagrophytes* strains causing tinea unguium. *Antimicrob Ag Chemother* **39**: 1206.

Kotrajaras R, Chongsathien S, Rojanavanich V et al. (1988). *Hendersonula toruloidea* infection in Thailand. *Int J Dermatol* **27**: 391.

Lachapelle JM, De Doncker P, Tennstedt D et al. (1992). Itraconazole compared with griseofulvin in the treatment of tinea corporis/cruris and tinea pedis/manus: an interpretation of the clinical results of all completed studies with respect to the pharmacokinetic profile. *Dermatol* **184**: 45.

Laude TA, Shah BR, Lynfield Y (1982). Tinea capitis in Brooklyn. *Amer J Dis Child* **136**: 1047.

Lecky BR (1990). Griseofulvin-induced neuropathy. *Lancet* **i**: 230.

Lin C, Symchowicz S (1975). Absorption, distribution, metabolism, and excretion of griseofulvin in man and animals. *Drug Metab Rev* **4**: 75.

Lopez-Gomez S, Del Palacio A, Van Cutsem J et al. (1994). Itraconazole versus griseofulvin in the treatment of tinea capitis: a double-blind randomized study in children. *Int J Dermatol* **33**: 743.

Lukacs A, Korting HC, Lindner A (1994). Successful treatment of griseofulvin-resistant tinea capitis in infants. *Mycoses* **37**: 451.

Meffert JJ, Davis BM, Campbell JC (1995). Bullous drug eruption to griseofulvin in a man with Hailey-Hailey disease. *Cutis* **56**: 279.

Metneki J, Czeizel A (1987). Griseofulvin teratology. *Lancet* **i**: 1042.

Mion G, Verdon R, Le Gulluche Y et al. (1990). Fatal toxic epidermal necrolysis after griseofulvin. *Lancet* **ii**: 1331.

Miyagawa S, Sakamuto K (1989). Adverse reactions to griseofulvin in patients with circulating anti-SSA/Ro and SSB/La autoantibodies. *Amer J Med* **87**: 100.

Miyagawa S, Okuchi T, Shiomi Y, Sakamoto K (1990). Subacute cutaneous lupus erythematosus lesions precipitated by griseofulvin. *J Amer Acad Dermatol* **21**: 343.

Oxford AE, Raistrick H, Simonart P (1939). Studies in the biochemistry of microorganisms. LX. Griseofulvin, C17 H17 O6 Cl, a metabolic product of Penicillium griseofulvum Diercks. *Biochem J* **33**: 240; quoted by Roth (1960).

Phillips KR, Wideman SD, Cochran EB, Becker JA (1993). Griseofulvin significantly decreases serum salicylate concentrations. *Pediatr Infect Dis J* **12**: 350.

Piepponen T, Blomqvist K, Brandt H et al. (1992). Efficacy and safety of itraconazole in the long-term treatment of onychomycosis. *J Antimicrob Chemother* **29**: 195.

Redeker AG, Sterling RE, Bronow RS (1964). Effect of griseofulvin in acute intermittent porphyria. *JAMA* **188**: 466.

Restrepo A (1994). Treatment of tropical mycoses. *J Amer Acad Dermatol* **31**: S91.

Rimington C, Morgan PN, Nicholls K et al. (1963). Griseofulvin administration and porphyrin metabolism. *Lancet* **ii**: 318.

Roberts DT (1994). Oral therapeutic agents in fungal nail disease. *J Amer Acad Dermatol* **31**: S78.

Rosa FW, Hernandez C, Carlo WA (1987). Griseofulvin teratology, including two thoracopagus conjoined twins. *Lancet* **i**: 171.

Roth FJ Jr (1960–61). Griseofulvin. *Ann NY Acad Sci* **89**: 247.

Rustin MH, Bunker CB, Dowd PM, Robinson TW (1989). Erythema multiforme due to griseofulvin. *Brit J Dermatol* **120**: 455.

Savin R (1989). Successful treatment of chronic tinea pedis (mocassin type). with terbinafine (Lamisil). *Clin Exp Dermatol* **14**: 116.

Schafer-Korting M (1987). Pharmacokinetics of griseofulvin in blood and skin suction blister fluid of rats. *Drug Metab Disposit* **15**: 374.

Scholz R, Meinhof W (1991). Susceptibility of *Trichophyton rubrum* to griseofulvin. *Mycoses* **34**: 411.

Shah VP, Riegelman S, Epstein WL (1972). Determination of griseofulvin in skin, plasma and sweat. *J Pharm Sci* **61**: 634.

Shah VP, Riegelman S, Epstein WL (1974). Griseofulvin absorption, metabolism and excretion In *The Diagnosis and Treatment of Fungal Infections* (Robinson HM, ed), p. 315. Springfield, Illinois: CC Thomas.

Shenfield GM (1993). Oral contraceptives. Are drug interactions of clinical significance? *Drug Safety* **9**: 21.

Taylor B, Duffill M (1988). Toxic epidermal necrolysis from griseofulvin. *J Amer Acad Dermatol* **19**: 565.

Van Dijke CPH, Weber JCP (1984). Interaction between oral contraceptives and griseofulvin. *Brit Med J* **288**: 1125.

Villars V, Jones TC (1989). Clinical efficacy and tolerability of terbinafine (Lamisil)- a new topical and systemic fungicidal drug for treatment of dermatomycoses. *Clin Exp Dermatol* **14**: 124.

Weitzman I, Summerbell RC (1995). The dermatophytes. *Clin Microbiol Rev* **8**: 240.

Williams DI, Marten RH, Sarkany I (1958). Oral treatment of ringworm with griseofulvin. *Lancet* **ii**: 1212.

Wishart JM (1994). A double blind study of itraconazole vs griseofulvin in patients with tinea pedis and tinea manus. *NZ Med J* **107**: 126.

Naftifine

Description

Naftifine is a first-generation allylamine derivative with the chemical structure of *(E)-N-Cinnamyl-N-methyl(1-naphthylmethyl)amine* hydrochloride. It was first described in 1974 and became commercially available in 1985 (Stutz, 1988).

Its primary mode of action is specific and selective inhibition of squalene epoxidase resulting in depletion of ergosterol in fungal cell membranes and intracellular accumulation of squalene. In comparison with terbinafine, naftifine has inferior *in vitro* potency as a sterol synthesis inhibitor.

Sensitive Organisms

The *in vitro* inhibitory effects of naftifine are pH-dependent with maximal activity observed at neutral pH (Ryder *et al.*, 1984).

1 Pathogenic yeast

The susceptibility of *Candida* spp. to naftifine varies widely with an MIC of 1.56 to >100 μg per ml. The activity of naftifine against *Candida albicans, C. parapsilosis, C. krusei* and *C. tropicalis* appeared to be poor for the majority of isolates tested (Georgopoulos *et al.*, 1981).

2 Molds or filamentous fungi

Naftifine is fungicidal against dermatophytes, with MICs in the range of 0.1–0.2 μg per ml (Georgopoulos *et al.*, 1981). Naftifine inhibited 99% of dermatophytes including *Trichophyton rubrum, T. mentagrophytes, Microsporum canis, Epidermophyton floccosum* at concentrations less than 1.0 μg per ml, and was the most potent agent compared with griseofulvin, natamycin and several azole drugs (Macura, 1993). In the guinea pig model of trichophytosis, naftifine 1% cream produced a 100% response rate. It did not result in complete clinical cure although it did produce a dose-dependent improvement in clinical signs (Petranyi *et al.*, 1981). Naftifine also showed good activity against *Aspergillus* spp. with MICs in the range of 0.8–12.5 μg per ml, and *Sporothrix schenckii* with MICs of 0.8 and 1.5 μg per ml (Georgopoulos *et al.*, 1981).

Mode of administration and dose

Indications and recommended doses

Tinea corporis and tinea cruris: 1% cream applied to affected areas once daily OR
1% gel applied to affected areas twice daily for 2–4 weeks

Tinea pedis: 1% cream applied once daily OR
1% gel applied twice daily for 4–6 weeks

Availability

Topical preparations: 1% cream (naftifine hydrochloride with benzyl alcohol)
1% gel (naftifine hydrochloride with alcohol)

Absorption of the Drug

There is no oral formulation. Systemic absorption following topical administration of naftifine 1% cream or gel to normal intact skin of healthy volunteers is negligible, amounting to about 3–6% of the dose. Approximately 40–60% of an absorbed dose is excreted in urine as unchanged drug and its metabolites, and the remaining 40–60% is eliminated as metabolites by biliary excretion in the feces. Metabolism occurs by at least two mechanisms, oxidation of the phenyl and naphthyl rings and *N*-dealkylation.

Naftifine readily penetrates the epidermis after topical application and inhibitory concentrations of naftifine for *T. rubrum* and *T. mentagrophytes* persist in the stratum corneum for at least 24 h following a single application of the drug, and possibly up to 5 days (Meinicke *et al.*, 1984, Stoughton *et al.*, 1989). The concentration of naftifine in the stratum corneum reaches 300 times the MIC for most dermatophytes (Stoughton *et al.*, 1989).

Mode of Action

Naftifine is a reversible squalene epoxidase inhibitor, an enzyme that is responsible for conversion of squalene to lanosterol (see Figs IV.1, IV.3). Inhibition of squalene epoxidase results in depletion of membrane ergosterol and intracellular accumulation of squalene. Although accumulation of squalene causes alterations in membrane properties of susceptible fungi, this does not appear to be responsible for the fungicidal action of naftifine. Inhibition of phospholipid and glycoprotein synthesis occur consequent to the accumulation of squalene (Petranyi *et al.*, 1984; Ryder, 1988). *In vitro* morphological studies of *Candida* organisms after exposure to naftifine reveal changes of cytoplasmic accumulation of lipid particles, alteration of the plasma membrane and thickening of the cell wall (Georgopapadakou and Bertasso, 1992). There appears to be a differential effect of naftifine on dermatophytes and *Candida* species, with a total block of ergosterol synthesis resulting in fungicidal activity in dermatophytes compared with reduced ergosterol synthesis in *Candida* spp. and residual sterol synthesis by another pathway. The greater *in vitro* activity in dermatophytes is not due to differential penetration of the cell envelope, but due to higher affinity for the squalene epoxidase enzyme, and greater susceptibility of filamentous growth secondary to squalene accumulation (Favre and Ryder, 1996). This differential specificity for squalene epoxidase correlates with *in vitro* activity. Naftifine is highly selective for fungal sterol biosynthesis compared with mammalian sterol biosynthesis (Ryder, 1985).

Toxicity

The topical administration of both the 1% cream and 1% gel is well tolerated. Transient burning and stinging at the site of application occurs in about 5% of treated patients. Other mild to moderate local adverse effects include erythema, local irritation with dryness and itching, which occur infrequently. Allergic contact dermatitis has also been described (Senff *et al.*, 1989; Willa-Craps *et al.*, 1995).

Clinical Uses of the Drug

Topical application of naftifine is effective and well tolerated as treatment for superficial fungal infections

1 Dermatophyte infections

Comparisons with econazole and clotrimazole reveal a more rapid mycological eradication and earlier symptomatic response in patients with tinea corporis, tinea cruris and tinea pedis treated with 1% naftifine (Haas *et al.*, 1985; Kagawa, 1985; Millikan *et al.*, 1988; Smith *et al.*, 1990). Naftifine 1% cream applied twice-daily for 4 weeks as treatment for tinea corporis and tinea cruris resulted in resolution in 19% of patients at 1 week compared with 4% of econazole treated patients at the same time point. At the end of 4 weeks treatment naftifine was as effective as econazole with 80% of patients with both mycological and clinical responses, although there was

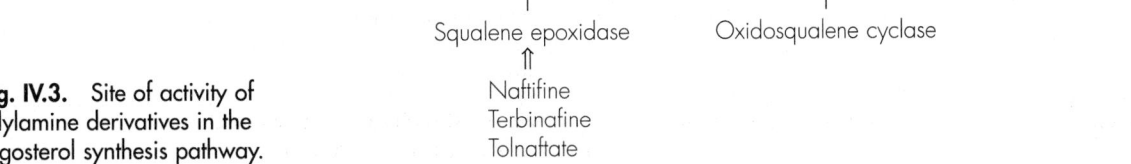

Fig. IV.3. Site of activity of allylamine derivatives in the ergosterol synthesis pathway.

a trend to greater efficacy in the naftifine group (Millikan *et al.*, 1988). A similar trend to greater rates of mycologically cure and earlier resolution of clinical symptoms and signs noted as early as 2 weeks of treatment was achieved in patients with tinea pedis randomized to naftifine 1% cream applied twice-daily for 4 weeks compared with clotrimazole 1% cream, although the differences were not statistically different (Naftifine Pediatric Study Group, 1990). Significant differences in treatment success were noted for the post-treatment review of patients with tinea pedis favoring naftifine 1% cream applied twice-daily compared with clotrimazole cream (Smith *et al.*, 1990). Significantly higher cure rates were produced by 1% naftifine compared with 1% clotrimazole/betamethasone dipropionate cream in patients with tinea pedis treated for 4 weeks. The superior efficacy was evident from week 1 (33% versus 24% cure), to week 4 (68% versus 50% cure), and persisted throughout 4 weeks of post-treatment follow-up (73% versus 45% remained cured). Relapse rates significantly favored naftifine (7%) compared with 36% for clotrimazole/betamethasone 2 weeks post-treatment. There was no difference in the time to resolution of clinical signs and symptoms (Smith *et al.*, 1992). It has been suggested that naftifine may possess anti-inflammatory properties (Tronnier, 1987; Jung, 1987), and a study in patients with clinically diagnosed fungal infection of the skin, naftifine was equivalent to clotrimazole / 1% hydrocortisone with respect to clinical resolution of symptoms, and to mycological efficacy in those patients subsequently confirmed to have a dermatomycosis (Evans *et al.*, 1993) Similar rates of mycological and clinical efficacy have been achieved with once-daily versus twice-daily application of the gel or cream formulation (Meinicke *et al.*, 1984; Polemann, 1985; Smith *et al.*, 1990).

Naftifine cream has also proved efficacious in the management of chronic dermatomycoses, often due to *Trichophyton rubrum* that were resistant to therapy with griseofulvin, topical azoles or ciclopirox olamine (Rosen *et al.*, 1991).

References

Evans EG, James IG, Seaman RA, Richardson MD (1993). Does naftifine have anti-inflammatory properties? A double-blind comparative study with 1% clotrimazole/1% hydrocortisone in clinically diagnosed fungal infection of the skin. *Brit J Dermatol* **129**: 437.

Favre B, Ryder NS (1996). Characterization of squalene epoxidase activity from the dermatophyte *Trichophyton rubrum* and its inhibition by terbinafine and other antimycotic agents. *Antimicrob Ag Chemother* **40**: 443.

Georgopapadakou NH, Bertasso A (1992). Effects of squalene epoxidase inhibitors in *Candida albicans*. *Antimicrob Ag Chemother* **36**: 1779.

Georgopoulos A, Petranyi G, Mieth H, Drews J (1981). *In vitro* activity of naftifine, a new antifungal agent. *Antimicrob Ag Chemother* **19**: 386.

Haas PJ, Tronnier H, Weidenger G (1985). Naftifine in tinea pedis. Double-blind comparison with clotrimazole. *Mykosen* **28**: 33.

Jung EG (1987). The anti-inflammatory efficacy of naftifine as evaluated from the erythema response to ultraviolet light. *Mykosen* **30** (Suppl 1): 88.

Kagawa S (1985). Comparative clinical trial of naftifine and clotrimazole in tinea pedum, tinea cruris and tinea corporis. *Mykosen* **28** (Suppl 1): 82.

Macura AB (1993). *In vitro* susceptibility of dermatophytes to antifungal drugs: a comparison of two methods. *Int J Dermatol* **32**: 533.

Meinicke K, Striegel C, Weidenger G (1984). Treatment of dermatomycoses with naftifine. Therapeutic efficacy after once-a-day and twice-a-day application. *Mykosen* **27**: 608.

Millikan LE, Galen WK, Gewirtzman GB *et al.* (1988). Naftifine cream 1 percent versus econazole cream 1 percent in the treatment of tinea cruris and tinea corporis. *J Amer Acad Dermatol* **18**: 52.

Naftifine Podiatric Study Group (1990). Naftifine cream 1% versus clotrimazole cream 1% in the treatment of tinea pedis. *J Amer Podiatr Med Assoc* **80**: 314.

Petranyi G, Georgopoulos A, Mieth H (1981). *In vivo* antimycotic activity of naftifine. *Antimicrob Ag Chemother* **19**: 390.

Petranyi G, Ryder NS, Stutz A (1984). Allylamine derivatives: a new class of synthetic antifungal agents inhibiting squalene epoxidase. *Science* **224**: 1239.

Polemann G (1985). Antimycotic efficacy of naftifine after once-daily application. *Mykosen* **28** (Suppl 1): 113.

Rosen T, Fischer M, Orengo I *et al.* (1991). Naftifine treatment of resistant dermatophytosis. *Int J Dermatol* **30**: 590.

Ryder NS (1985). Specific inhibition of fungal sterol biosynthesis by SF 86–327, a new allylamine antimycotic agent. *Antimicrob Ag Chemother* **27**: 252.

Ryder NS (1988). Mechanism of action and biochemical selectivity of allylamine antimycotic agents. *Ann NY Acad Sci* **544**: 208.

Ryder NS, Seidl G, Troke PF (1984). Effect of the antimycotic drug naftifine on growth and sterol biosynthesis in *Candida albicans*. *Antimicrob Ag Chemother* **25**: 483.

Senff H, Tholen S, Stieler W, Reinel D, Hausen BM (1989). Allergic contact dermatitis to naftifine. Report of two cases. *Dermatologica* **178**: 107.

Smith EB, Wiss K, Hanifin JM *et al.* (1990). Comparison of once-daily and twice-daily naftifine cream regimens with twice-daily clotrimazole in the treatment of tinea pedis. *J Amer Acad Dermatol* **22**: 1116.

Smith EB, Breneman DL, Griffith RF *et al.* (1992). Double-blind comparison of naftifine cream and clotrimazole/betamethasone dipropionate cream in the treatment of tinea pedis. *J Amer Acad Dermatol* **26**: 125.

Stoughton RB, Sefton J, Zeleznick L (1989). *In vitro* and *in vivo* cutaneous penetration and antifungal activity of naftifine. *Cutis* **44**: 333.

Stutz A (1988). Synthesis and structure-activity correlations within allylamine antimycotics. *Ann NY Acad Sci* **544**: 46.

Tronnier H (1987). Inflammatory dermatomycoses – comparative study of naftifine and a combination of a corticosteroid and an imidazole derivative. *Mykosen* **30** (Suppl 1): 7.

Willa-Craps C, Wyss M, Elsner P (1995). Allergic contact dermatitis from naftifine. *Contact Derm* **32**: 369.

Terbinafine

Description

Terbinafine is a synthetic naphthalenemethanamine with the chemical structure (E)-*N*-(6,6-Dimethyl-2-hepten-4-ynyl)-*N*-methyl-1-naphthalenemethanamine hydrochloride. It is an allylamine derivative structurally related to naftifine, with fungicidal actvity against dermatophytes and is 10- to 100-fold more potent than the first-generation allylamine naftifine. It is highly lipophilic, and concentrates in the stratum corneum, sebum and hair follicles. Terbinafine is available in both an oral formulation and a topical preparation, and has excellent therapeutic efficacy in the management of cutaneous dermatophytosis and onychomycosis.

Sensitive Organisms

1 Pathogenic yeast

Cryptococcus neoformans appears to be susceptible to terbinafine, with MICs in the range of 1.0–4.0 μg per ml (Balfour and Faulds, 1992). The activity of terbinafine against yeast is variable, with *Candida albicans* (yeast form), *C. tropicalis* and *C. glabrata* relatively resistant, and the myceliel form of *C. albicans* more susceptible (Balfour and Faulds, 1992). The inhibitory activity of terbinafine against *C. albicans* was inferior to that of clotrimazole and econazole, with MICs of 6.25–100 μg per ml. It is considered to be fungistatic (Petranyi *et al.*, 1987a). Topically administered terbinafine has some activity in the guinea pig model of cutaneous candidiasis; however, the efficacy of terbinafine is inferior to that of clotrimazole. In the rat model of vaginal candidiasis, terbinafine was less effective than miconazole in eradication of *C. albicans*. (Petranyi *et al.*, 1987b). *Pityrosporum ovale* and *P. orbiculare,* as well as the hyphal form *Malassezia furfur,* are all susceptible to terbinafine (Balfour and Faulds, 1992).

2 Dimorphic fungi

Terbinafine is fungicidal for *Histoplasma capsulatum, Blastomyces dermatitidis* (Shadomy *et al.,* 1985). Good *in vitro* activity has been shown for terbinafine against *Sporothrix schenckii* with MICs in the range of 0.1–0.4 μg per ml (Petranyi *et al.*, 1987a). However, in the murine model of sporotrichosis, terbinafine was no more effective than no treatment (Kan and Bennett, 1988).

3 Molds or filamentous fungi

Terbinafine is highly active *in vitro* against *Aspergillus* spp., with superior activity to amphotericin B against *A. niger* and *A. flavus,* but inferior activity against *A. fumigatus.* Terbinafine is fungicidal at concentrations close to the MIC against *Aspergillus* spp. (Petranyi *et al.*, 1987a; Schmitt *et al.*, 1988). Despite this fungicidal activity, terbinafine displayed no activity in the rat model of pulmonary aspergillosis (Schmitt *et al.*, 1990). Although *in vitro* susceptibility testing revealed excellent activity against the demitaceous fungi, *Cladiosporium bantianum, Wangiella dermatitidis,* and *Dactylaria constricta,* terbinafine showed no *in vivo* activity in a murine model (Dixon and Polak, 1987).

Terbinafine has shown excellent *in vitro* fungicidal activity against the dermatophyte genera, with MIC ranges of 0.0015–0.006 μg per ml for *Trichophyton* spp., 0.006–0.01 μg per ml for *Microsporum* spp., and 0.0015–0.006 μg per ml for *Epidermophyton* spp. (Petranyi *et al.*, 1987a; Korting *et al.*, 1995). The *in vitro* activity was confirmed in the guinea pig model of dermatophytosis, in which topical administration of terbinafine cleared infection with *T. mentagrophytes* and *M. canis* at concentrations of 0.03–1%. The efficacy of orally administered terbinafine was comparable with griseofulvin for *M. canis* infections (Petranyi *et al.*, 1987b).

4 Pneumocystis carinii

Terbinafine exhibited high activity against *Pneumocytis carinii* both *in vitro* and *in vivo*. The concentration required to eliminate over 80% of trophozoites compared with control within 72 h was 0.4 μg per ml, and for elimination of over 80% of cysts was 0.8 μg per ml (Cirioni *et al.*, 1995). Terbinafine also showed excellent activity against cyst forms *in vitro*, when compared with co-trimoxazole and pentamidine, and was effective *in vivo* in the treatment of *P. carinii* in immunosuppressed rats clearing the infection in 97% of rats (Contini *et al.*, 1994).

5 Protozoa

Terbinafine inhibits the *in vitro* proliferation and sterol synthesis by promastigotes of *Leishmania mexicana* (Goad *et al.*, 1985), and amastigotes (Berman and Gallalee, 1987). Terbinafine also exhibits potent antiproliferative activity against both the epimastigotes and amastigotes of *Trypanosoma cruzi,* and the intracellular destruction of the intracellular amastigotes is rapid with terbinafine (Urbina *et al.*, 1988).

6 Bacteria

Terbinafine has some *in vitro* activity against common skin bacteria such as *Staphylococcus aureus, Streptococcus faecalis, Propionibacterium acnes,* and some Gram-negative bacteria *Escherichia coli* and *Pseudomonas aeruginosa* (Nolting and Brautigam, 1992).

7 Synergism with other drugs

Synergistic effects of terbinafine and ketoconazole was demonstrated against both forms of the parasite *T. cruzi* (Urbina *et al.*, 1988), and this observation was confirmed in the murine model of Chagas' disease (Maldonado *et al.*, 1993). Mevinolin (lovastatin) combined with terbinafine had only additive effects on intracellular amastigotes *in vitro* (Urbina *et al.*, 1993).

8 Acquired resistance

Development of resistance to terbinafine in organisms originally susceptible has not been reported to date.

9 Minimum inhibitory concentrations

The MICs for a variety of fungi can be found in Table IV.5.

Mode of administration and dose

Indications and recommended doses

Superficial dermatomycosis
Tinea pedis, tinea manuum: oral terbinafine 250 mg daily for 2–4 weeks
1% cream applied to affected areas once- or twice-daily for 1–2 weeks (moccasin-type tinea pedis 2–4 weeks)

Tinea corporis, tinea cruris: oral terbinafine 250 mg daily for 2–4 weeks
1% cream applied once- or twice-daily for 1–2 weeks

Onychomycosis: oral terbinafine 250 mg daily for 12 weeks

Cutaneous candidiasis: 1% cream applied once- or twice-daily for 1–2 weeks

Children:	Weight	Oral terbinafine dose
	<20 kg	62.5 mg daily
	20–40 kg	125 mg daily
	>40 kg	250 mg daily

Table IV.5.

Compiled from data published by Shadomy *et al.* (1985), Dixon and Polak (1987), Petranyi *et al.* (1987a), Scmitt *et al.* (1988), Wong *et al.* (1989), Balfour and Faulds, (1992)

Organism	MIC (µg per ml) range	
	Broth	Agar
Yeast		
Candida spp.		
C. albicans (yeast form)		6.25–100
C. albicans (myceliel form)	0.098–0.78	
C. guilliermondii		6.25–100
C. krusei		50–100
C. parapsilosis	0.1–3.13	
C. tropicalis		10–128
C. kefyr (pseudotropicalis)		0.5–50
C. glabrata		>100
Cryptococcus neoformans	0.25–2	
Histoplasma capsulatum	<0.05–2.0	
Blastomyces dermatitidis	<0.05–0.39	
Malassezia furfur		0.2–0.8
Sporothrix schenkii	0.1–0.4	
Mold		
Aspergillus spp.	0.8–1.6	
A. fumigatus	0.8–1.6	
A. flavus	0.025–0.4	
A. niger	0.025–0.04	
Dematiaceous fungi		
Cladosporium spp.		0.012–1
Curvularia spp.	0.25–5	
Dactylaria soo.		0.01–0.03
Fonsecaea pedrosoi		<0.06–2.0
Phialophora verrucosa		<0.06–2.0
Phialophora parasitica	0.10	
Wangiella dermatitidis		0.001–0.025
Zygomycetes		
Mucor spp.		64–>128
Rhizopus spp		64–>128
Hyphomycetes		
Acremonium spp.		1.0–4.0
Fusarium spp.		32–>64
Hendersonula toruloidea	1.0–4	
Paecilomyces spp.		8.0–64
Pseudallescheria boydii		32–>64
Scopulariopsis brevicaulis	0.8	
Dermatophytes		
Trichophyton spp.	0.0015–0.006	
Microsporum spp.	0.006–0.01	
Epidermophyton spp.	0.0015–0.006	

1 Patients with renal failure

Renal insufficiency causes a prolonged elimination half-life and elevated peak plasma concentrations and area-under-the-concentration-time-curve (AUC) of terbinafine. It is recommended that patients with impaired renal function (creatinine clearance less than 50 ml per min or a serum creatinine greater than 0.3 mmol per liter) should receive half the normal dose of terbinafine. It is unknown whether terbinafine is hemodialyzed or eliminated by peritoneal dialysis, and there is no experience with the drug in individuals with a creatinine clearance of less than 20 ml per min reported.

2 Patients with hepatic insufficiency

In patients with pre-existing chronic stable hepatic impairment, the dose of terbinafine should be half the usual dose, as the plasma clearance of the drug is reduced by 30%. In addition, terbinafine may cause hepatic dysfunction, so regular monitoring of hepatic function is recommended. Terbinafine should be discontinued in individuals with evidence of increasing hepatic dysfunction.

3 Topical

Affected areas are applied with 1% terbinafine once- or twice-daily. The duration of treatment depends on the type and site of infection. Recommended treatment courses are included above.

Availability

Oral formulation: 250 mg tablets

Topical preparation: 1% cream (10 mg per g)

Serum Levels in Relation to Dose

The pharmacokinetics of terbinafine were studied in ten healthy male volunteers. After a single oral dose of 250 mg in the fasting state, the drug was rapidly absorbed with a mean peak plasma terbinafine concentration of 1.34 μg per ml which occurred 1.5 h post-dosing. There was a biphasic decline in plasma levels (Kovarik *et al.*, 1995). Multiple-dose pharmacokinetics revealed a 20% increase in the peak plasma terbinafine concentration over 2 weeks of daily dosing with 250 mg with a mean peak plasma concentration of 1.62 μg per ml on day 16. There was only a further 3% increase from 2 to 4 weeks. Trough concentrations rose slowly over the duration of dosing, with wide intersubject variability, and terbinafine accumulated about 2-fold over 4 weeks. The absorption of terbinafine does not appear to be affected by food (Stephen *et al.*, 1987). Steady-state is reached after 10–14 days (Villars and Jones, 1990). The mean half-life is about 17 days. There appear to be three disposition phases, the initial biphasic disposition with mean half-lifes of 1.7 h and 28.7 h after 28 days dosing, and the terminal disposition with a half-life of 16.5 days which probably represents the slow return of terbinafine to the central compartment from the peripheral tissues (Kovarik *et al.*, 1995, Zehander *et al.*, 1994).

Humbert *et al.* (1995), determined the plasma pharmacokinetics of terbinafine and its major metabolites after a single dose of 125 mg in healthy volunteers. The carboxybutyl metabolites achieved the highest plasma concentrations (2.4 times terbinafine). All the metabolites appeared to have similar half-lives (about 25 h). Three major metabolites identified in plasma following multiple dosing in another study also had plasma concentration time profiles similar to that of terbinafine. The ratio of metabolite to terbinafine AUC after 4 weeks dosing was 1.08, 1.25 and 1.38, and in this study, the half-life of each metabolite was about twice that of terbinafine (Kovarik *et al.*, 1995).

The pharmacokinetics of terbinafine in the elderly are not significantly different to those observed in younger normal volunteers (Jensen, 1989). In patients with hepatic insufficiency, the plasma clearance was reduced by about 30% resulting in moderate increases in the AUC, but no effect on the peak plasma concentration (Jensen, 1990). Renal dysfunction caused a prolongation of the terbinafine plasma elimination half-life and a marked increase in the AUC and peak plasma concentrations (Jensen, 1990).

Penetration of terbinafine into the systemic circulation following topical administration of 1% cream is minimal, and represents less than 5% of a dose. Detectable concentrations of terbinafine in plasma (<0.011 μg per ml) occurred in normal volunteers who had terbinafine applied topically for 8 days under occlusion. In patients with pityriasis versicolor treated twice-daily with 1% cream for 4 weeks, the maximum plasma terbinafine concentration achieved was 0.025 μg per ml (Dykes *et al.*, 1990). In healthy volunteers who received topical applications of 1% terbinafine cream for 1, 3, 5, or 7 days, skin biopsy evaluation of terbinafine levels revealed the peak concentration in the stratum corneum did not increase with multiple applications, but terbinafine concentrations above the MIC for dermatophytes persisted in the stratum corneum after cessation of application for longer durations with increased number of applications (Hill *et al.*, 1992).

Excretion

1 Urine

Clearance of terbinafine is essentially non-renal with no intact terbinafine eliminated via renal excretion. The major metabolites identified in pharmacokinetic studies are further bio-transformed prior to elimination (Kovarik *et al.*, 1995). Following a single administration of radiolabeled drug, 80% of the total radioactivity in plasma comprises terbinafine and its metabolites, and only 14% of the administered dose is excreted in the urine over 48 h as terbinafine or one of its five major metabolites. Total radioactivity excreted in the urine over 48 h is 57% of the administered dose, implying many more metabolites are present in urine (Humbert *et al.*, 1995).

2 Inactivation in the body

Terbinafine is extensively biotransformed, and 15 metabolites have been identified to date (Kovarik *et al.*, 1995). N-Demethylation, N-oxidation, oxidation and hydrolysis and conjugation are the metabolic processes involved, and utilize less than 5% of the hepatic cytochrome P-450 capacity (Jensen, 1989; Schuster 1985).

3 Feces

Approximately 20% of an administered oral dose of radiolabeled terbinafine is excreted in feces (Jensen, 1989).

Distribution of the Drug in Body

Terbinafine is strongly bound to plasma proteins (99%) (Jensen, 1990). The distribution of terbinafine in high concentration to skin, hair and nails has been established in several studies (Faergemann *et al.*, 1991; Lever *et al.*, 1990; Kovarik *et al.*, 1995). The concentrations are highest in sebum and hair and are several fold higher than those in plasma, with concentrations of 1 μg per g achieved in stratum corneum from the sole of the foot, and nail (Kovarik *et al.*, 1995). Stratum corneum concentrations of 10 μg per ml were achieved in another pharmacokinetic study utilizing a similar study design, but the stratum corneum was sampled from the back in that study (Faergemann *et al.*, 1993). Penetration of terbinafine into stratum corneum, nails and hair appears to occur by both diffusion from plasma through dermis/epidermis and via sebum to hair and skin (Lever, 1990). Concentrations of terbinafine achieved after administration of 250 mg daily to normal volunteers were 0.1–10 μg per ml in plasma, 45 μg per ml in sebum, and 2.6 μg per g in hair. There is no detectable terbinafine in sweat (Faergemann *et al.*, 1991). Concentrations of terbinafine increase in the stratum corneum, dermis/epidermis and hair over 12-day dosing, whereas sebum concentrations peak on day 2 of dosing (Balfour and Faulds, 1992). Fungicidal concentrations of terbinafine persist in stratum corneum and sebum for 2–3 weeks after stopping the drug (Faergemann *et al.*, 1991). A recent study revealed terbinafine concentrations greater than the MIC for most dermatophytes persisted in the stratum corneum for 7 weeks after completing a 7-day course of terbinafine 250 mg daily (Faergemann *et al.*, 1994).

In patients with onychomycosis receiving either 250 mg terbinafine once-daily or 125 mg twice-daily, terbinafine was first detected in distal toe nail clippings, a mean of 7.8 weeks (3–18 weeks) after starting treatment, which was much faster than would be anticipated if terbinafine was solely taken up by newly formed nail. Thus terbinafine appears to diffuse into formed nail plate. The mean concentration of terbinafine in nail clippings was 0.25–0.55 ng per mg and did not increase during treatment. In addition, the pharmacokinetics of terbinafine were similar in normal fingernails compared with infected nails. The kinetics of the major metabolite, demethylterbinafine are similar to that of the parent compound (Finlay, 1992). Faergemann *et al.* (1994) and Schatz *et al.* (1995) found levels of terbinafine of 0.5 μg per g in nails after 7 days treatment with 250 mg daily, and these levels were still above the MIC at 0.2 μg per g 3 months later, indicating that shorter courses of treatment may have similar efficacy as those currently recommended.

Following intraperitoneal administration of 20 mg per kg to rats, serum terbinafine concentrations at 30 min were 1.0–1.25 µg per ml. At 2 h, terbinafine concentrations in the lung were 5.9–6.1 µg per g and similar concentrations were found in the liver, spleen and kidneys (Schmitt et al., 1990).

Mode of Action

Terbinafine reversibly inhibits squalene epoxidase, a key enzyme in ergosterol biosynthesis, resulting in accumulation of intracellular squalene, and a blockade of *de novo* sterol synthesis with diminished membrane ergosterol content. The allylamines do not significantly affect other enzyme steps in sterol biosynthesis and are specific for squalene epoxidase (see Figs IV.1, p. 1261 and IV.3, p. 1325). The inhibitory effect is pH-dependent and is maximal at neutral pH (Ryder, 1985). It is highly selective with much greater inhibitory activity against fungal than mammalian squalene oxidase (Ryder and Dupont, 1985). Terbinafine is the most potent squalene epoxidase inhibitor of the allylamines and thiocarbamate antifungal agents, and it has a similar affinity for the squalene epoxidase of *Trichophyton rubrum* and *C. albicans,* which correlates with its wide range of *in vitro* activity (Favre and Ryder, 1996). The action of terbinafine is fungicidal against dermatophytes, molds and some yeast, and cell death is associated with intracellular accumulation of squalene, and the susceptibility of filamentous growth to the disturbances in membrane composition (Ryder, 1989; Favre and Ryder, 1996). In contrast, the fungistatic activity in *C. albicans* appears to be due to diminished ergosterol content (Ryder, 1989). The mechanism of action in protozoa also appears to be inhibition of sterol biosynthesis (Goad et al., 1985).

Toxicity

1 Gastrointestinal side-effects

The most commonly reported adverse events associated with terbinafine therapy in clinical trials are gastrointestinal and include nausea, vomiting, abdominal cramps and discomfort, flatulence, diarrhea and mouth ulcers. Terbinafine appears to delay gastric emptying and the gastrointestinal effects of this occur in about 5% of those receiving the drug (Villars and Jones, 1989). Overall, terbinafine is well tolerated, however. Taste disturbance (perversion or loss) is an uncommon side-effect which is estimated to occur in 0.13% of patients (Beutler et al., 1993). In a well documented case, a total loss of taste occurred during 6 weeks treatment with 250 mg daily. Taste for salt and bitter substances disappeared first, followed by loss of sweet and sour taste 1 week later. Taste sensations returned in the same order as they had disappeared, from 2 to 5 weeks after cessation of terbinafine (Juhlin, 1992). There are similar reports of loss of taste and taste distortion, also associated with discoloration of the tongue (Ottervanger and Stricker, 1992; Beutler et al., 1993).

2 Rash and hypersensitivity reactions

Urticaria, pruritus, erythema multiforme, photosensitive skin rash and hypersensitivity have all been reported. Stevens–Johnson syndrome, and a fixed drug eruption have also been associated with terbinafine therapy (Carstens et al., 1994; Rzany et al., 1994; McGregor and Rustin, 1994; Munn and Russell Jones, 1995; Todd et al., 1995; Wach et al., 1995). Redness and stinging or pruritus may occur at the site of topical application of the cream formulation, but rarely require treatment discontinuation.

3 Hepatic effects

Transient increases in liver function tests (hepatic transaminases), hepatitis, cholestatic hepatitis with jaundice, and mixed cholestatic-hepatocellular hepatitis have all been reported in association with terbinafine treatment, but appear to be quite uncommon (Lowe et al., 1993; van 't Wout et al., 1994).

4 Hematologic effects

Neutropenia and agranulocytosis have been reported rarely. Generally no significant hematological adverse events occur (Villars and Jones; 1989, Kovacs et al., 1994).

5 Central nervous system effects

Headache, dizziness, lethargy and sedation have all been reported rarely.

6 Endocrine effects

Because terbinafine binds weakly to cytochrome P-450 enzymes (type 1 binding), and does not inhibit their activity, it should not interfere with steroid hormone production to a clinically significant effect (Schuster, 1985). Terbinafine 500 mg daily for 8 days had no effect on plasma testosterone levels in healthy male volunteers (Effendy and Krause, 1989).

7 Other adverse effects

Erectile dysfunction developed in one patient taking terbinafine 250 mg daily, and this resolved when the drug was ceased (Hull and Vismer, 1992).

8 Effect on the fetus

Teratogenicity and fertility studies in animals suggest no adverse effects; however, there is no clinical outcome experience in pregnant women reported as yet. Terbinafine has been detected in breast milk in two women given single oral doses of 500 mg (Stephen et al., 1987). It is recommended that oral terbinafine not be used by pregnant or breastfeeding women until more information is available.

9 Drug interactions

The effect of terbinafine (125 mg twice-daily for 1 week) on the clearance of antipyrine in normal volunteers was negligible, suggesting a lack of effect on hepatic drug metabolism (Seyffer et al., 1989). In contrast to ketoconazole, administration of terbinafine reduced caffeine clearance by 20%, which is thought to be due to competitive type 1 binding to hepatic microsomes (Wahllander and Paumgartner, 1989; Balfour and Faulds, 1992). At a 50 μmolar concentration terbinafine inhibited the metabolism by human liver microsomes of tolbutamide and ethoxycoumarin by less than 5%, and ethinylestradiol by 35% (Back et al., 1989). Terbinafine does not inhibit the hepatic metabolism of cyclosporin in vitro, and a randomized study in normal male volunteers determined that terbinafine does not significantly alter the absorption, metabolism or the elimination of cyclosporin (Back et al., 1989; Back and Tjia, 1991; Shah et al., 1993; Long et al., 1994). Drug interactions reported for terbinafine are decreased elimination of terbinafine when co-administered with cimetidine 400 mg twice-daily, and an increase in elimination occurs when pretreatment with rifampicin is administered (Jensen et al., 1990).

Clinical Uses of the Drug

Limited randomized controlled study data are available to establish a comparative role for terbinafine in the management of cutaneous infections caused by dermatophytes, Candida species and other less common skin pathogens.

1 Dermatophyte infections

In placebo-controlled trials of terbinafine 250 mg daily for 6 weeks as treatment of tinea pedis, or 2 weeks as treatment for tinea pedis or tinea manuum, terbinafine was clinically and mycologically effective in 65 and 71% of patients respectively (Savin and Zaias, 1990; White et al., 1990). Oral terbinafine in doses of 250–500 mg daily, for 3–6 weeks produced mycological eradication in 90% and was a clinically effective treatment in 78–85% of patients pooled from 24 studies (Villars and Jones, 1990). When the data are examined according to etiological organism, mycological cure and clinical efficacy rates were 90–95% for oral and 80–90% for topical treatment of infections due to T. rubrum, T. mentagrophytes, and E. floccosum, but were lower for oral treatment (86%) and topical treatment (50%) of M. canis infections (Balfour and Faulds, 1992). Farag et al. (1994) demonstrated that 1 week of treatment with 250 mg daily was just as effective for the treatment of tinea cruris and tinea corporis, compared with results from other studies.

Comparative studies with griseofulvin 500–1000 mg, revealed terbinafine 250–500 mg daily for 6 weeks was significantly more effective for the treatment of tinea pedis and tinea manuum with efficacy rates of 71–88% compared with 35–45% for griseofulvin treated patients (Savin, 1989, 1990; Hay et al., 1991). For the treatment of tinea corporis and tinea cruris, terbinafine 250–500 mg for 6 weeks was as effective as griseofulvin 500–1000 mg daily with clinical and mycological efficacy rates of 77–87% for terbinafine and 73–82% for griseofulvin (Cole and Stricklin, 1989; del Palacio Hernanz et al., 1990). Terbinafine 250 mg was also more effective than ketoconazole 200 mg daily for up to 6 weeks for the treatment of tinea corporis, and itraconazole 100 mg daily for treatment of tinea imbricata in randomized controlled trials (de Wit, 1990; Budimulja et al., 1994). Terbinafine 250 mg per day for 2 weeks was significantly more effective both clinically and mycologically than itraconazole 100 mg per day as treatment for tinea pedis (De Keyser et al., 1994), but was as effective as 100 mg itraconazole daily for 4 weeks as treatment of plantar-type tinea pedis, with cure rates of 69% for terbinafine and 67% for itraconazole at week 8 review (Hay *et al.*, 1995).

Terbinafine effectively cured 93% of children with tinea capitis using 4 weeks treatment with oral dosing (Jones, 1995). Terbinafine 125 mg daily for 6 weeks effectively cured all children with tinea capitis in a small pilot study. The time to mycological eradication appeared to be related to baseline severity of infection, with 58% of children culture negative after 3 weeks treatment (Nejjam *et al.*, 1995).

Terbinafine 1% cream is also an effective treatment for dermatophytosis (tinea corporis, tinea cruris, tinea pedis), with mycological eradication rates of 86–89% achieved in placebo-controlled studies using applications of the cream either once- or twice-daily for periods of 1–2 weeks. The effectiveness of treatment from a clinical perspective was rated as successful (complete resolution of clinical signs and symptoms) in 78–85% of cases (Millikan, 1990; Greer and Jolly, 1990; Smith *et al.*, 1990; Evans *et al.*, 1991, 1992; Berman *et al.*, 1992). Evans *et al.* (1994) determined that a single topical application of terbinafine 1% cream was as effective as topical treatment administered for 3, 5 or 7 days.

Terbinafine 1% cream applied twice-daily for 1 week is significantly more effective than 1% clotrimazole applied twice-daily for 4 weeks in the treatment of tinea pedis. Mycological cure rates for terbinafine were 94% at 4 weeks and 97% at 6 weeks compared with 73% at 4 weeks and 84% at 6 weeks for clotrimazole-treated patients. Terbinafine treatment also produced a significantly better clinical efficacy, judged in association with mycological eradication with 90% of patients effectively treated compared with 59% for clotrimazole at week 4 (Evans *et al.*, 1993).

Relapse rates of dermatophyte infections following completion of a course of terbinafine treatment are extremely low and range from 0% during short-term (4 weeks) follow-up to 6% in long-term follow-up of 6–15 months (Villars and Jones, 1989, Savin, 1989).

2 Superficial candidiasis

Orally administered terbinafine 250–500 mg daily for 2–4 weeks resulted in mycological eradication with resolution of clinical symptoms and signs in 60% of patients (Villars and Jones, 1990), in contrast to the 80% clinical efficacy and 93% mycological eradication for topical terbinafine treatment for *Candida* skin infections (Villars and Jones, 1990; Kagawa, 1989). Terbinafine 250 mg twice-daily was as effective as ketoconazole 200 mg daily for 4 weeks in the treatment of cutaneous candidiasis with mycological cure rates of 82% in the terbinafine group and 73% in the ketoconazole group (Jung *et al.*, 1994).

3 Onychomycosis

Terbinafine is an effective treatment for dermatophyte onychomycosis, achieving clinical and mycological cure rates of 90–100% for fingernail infections and 70–100% for toenail infections (Allen *et al.*, 1989; Goodfield *et al.*, 1989; Zaias and Serrano, 1989; Rakosi, 1990; Baudraz-Rousselet *et al.*, 1992). In a placebo-controlled trial of oral terbinafine 250 mg daily for 12 weeks, 29% of toenail infections were mycologically cured at the end of treatment and this proportion increased to 82% 36 weeks after completion of treatment. For fingernail infections, 71% were mycologically cured at the end of treatment and this proportion did not change at the week 48 follow-up visit. Clinical cure (unaffected full normal nail growth) occurred in 69% of toenail infections and 71% of fingernail infections (Goodfield *et al.*, 1992). Van der Schroeff *et al.* (1992) established that the duration of therapy with terbinafine 250 mg for toenail onychomycosis could be reduced to 3 months without compromising efficacy rates of 71–79%; however, a 6-week course gave inferior results, achieving only 40% efficacy. Relapse rates of 0% in the short term and 10% after long-term follow-up are comparable with those observed after treatment for skin dermatophytosis (Villars and Jones, 1989).

Terbinafine 250 mg daily for 24 weeks exhibited superior therapeutic efficacy to microsized griseofulvin 1000 mg daily for 48 weeks in the treatment of toenail onychomycosis. At 48 weeks, cure rates of 67% for terbinafine and 56% for griseofulvin were not statistically different. However, at 72 weeks, the clinical cure rate for terbinafine was 60% compared with 39% for griseofulvin, and the mycological eradication was 81% for terbinafine and 62% for griseofulvin (Hofmann *et al.*, 1995). A shorter course of terbinafine 250 mg daily for 16 weeks was also established as a significantly superior regimen to griseofulvin 500 mg daily for up to 52 weeks for the treatment of toenail onychomycosis with clinical and mycological cure rates of 42% for terbinafine and 2% for griseofulvin (Faergemann *et al.*, 1995).

Terbinafine 250 mg daily for 12 weeks was significantly more effective in the treatment of toenail onychomycosis than itraconazole 200 mg daily, with mycological eradiaction achieved in

92% compared with 67% of itraconazole-treated patients (Brautigam *et al.*, 1995). Intermittent terbinafine treatment (500 mg daily for 1 week every month) was equivalent to intermittent itraconazole treatment (400 mg daily for 1 week every month) but both intermittent treatments were inferior to continuous therapy with terbinafine 250 mg daily with mycological cures at 6 months after the end of treatment of 80% versus 75% versus 94% respectively. The differences were not statistically significant. Toenail infections were treated for 4 months and fingernail infections were treated for 2 months (Tosti *et al.*, 1996).

The efficacy of terbinafine for the treatment of onychomycosis due to non-dermatophytes was not as impressive. The mycological and clinical cure rates for patients treated with terbinafine 250 mg daily for up to 48 weeks were 70% and 54% for *C. albicans,* 85% and 63% for *C. parapsilosis,* and 43% of *Scopulariopsis brevicaulis* infections. Relapse rates were also higher than those seen for dermatophyte onychomycosis and were 45% for *C. albicans* and 13% for *C. parapsilosis* infections (Nolting *et al.*, 1994).

4 Pityriasis versicolor

This superficial infection caused by *Pityrosporum orbiculare* or *P. ovale (Malassezia furfur),* does not respond to oral terbinafine. However, topical terbinafine 1% cream produces a mycological eradication in 85% patients and clinical efficacy in 80% (Jones, 1990). Terbinafine 1% cream was found to be as effective as bifonazole 1% cream in a randomized study of treatment for 4 weeks for pityriasis versicolor with efficacy rates of 100% and 95% respectively (Aste *et al.*, 1991).

5 Other cutaneous infections

Terbinafine 250 mg daily for 6 weeks was effective treatment for a case of black piedra of the scalp, caused by *Piedraia hortae* which was susceptible to terbinafine (Gip, 1994).

In patients with superficial staphylococcal pyoderma, the administration of 1% terbinafine cream produced mycological eradication of the bacteria in 97% of patients (compared with 100% treated with 0.1% gentamicin sulphate cream) and there was no significant difference in clinical outcome between the two treatment groups. The apparent antibacterial activity of terbinafine makes it a suitable agent for mixed bacterial and fungal infections such as otomycosis and athlete's foot (Nolting and Brautigam, 1992).

Cutaneous sporotrichosis resolved in five of five patients treated with oral terbinafine 250 mg daily, and a rapid clinical response was noted with three patients culture negative at 8 weeks of treatment and the remaining two patients becoming culture negative at 12 and 32 weeks (Hull and Vismer, 1992).

References

Allen BR, Cowley N, Dawber R *et al.* (1989). Oral terbinafine: effective in the treatment of chronic nail dermatophytosis. *Brit J Dermatol* **121** (Suppl 34): 16.

Aste N, Pau M, Pinna AL *et al.* (1991). Clinical efficacy and tolerability of terbinafine in patients with pityriasis versicolor. *Mycoses* **34**: 353.

Back DJ, Tjia JF (1991). Comparative effects of the antimycotic drugs ketoconazole, fluconazole, itraconazole and terbinafine on the metabolism of cyclosporin by human liver microsomes. *Brit J Clin Pharmacol* **32**: 624.

Back DJ, Stevenson P, Tjia JF (1989). Comparative effects of two antimycotic agents, ketoconazole and terbinafine on the metabolism of tolbutamide, ethinyloestradiol, cyclosporin and ethoxycoumarin by human liver microsomes *in vitro*. *Brit J Clin Pharmacol* **28**: 166.

Balfour JA, Faulds D (1992). Terbinafine A review of tis pharmacodynamic and pharmacokinetic properties, and therapeutic potential in superficial mycoses. *Drugs* **43**: 259.

Baudraz-Rosselet F, Rakosi T, Wili PB, Kenzelmann R (1992). Treatment of onychomycosis with terbinafine. *Brit J Dermatol* **126** (Suppl 39): 40.

Berman JD, Gallalee JV (1987). *In vitro* antileishmanial activity of

inhibitors of steroid biosynthesis and combinations of antileishmanial agents. *J Parasitol* **73**: 671.

Berman B, Ellis C, Leyden J *et al.* (1992). Efficacy of a 1-week, twice-daily regimen of terbinafine 1% cream in the treatment of interdigital tinea pedis. *J Amer Acad Dermatol* **26**: 956.

Beutler M, Hartmann K, Kuhn M, Gartmann J (1993). Taste disorders and terbinafine. *Brit Med J* **307**: 26.

Brautigam M, Nolting S, Schopf RE, Weidinger G (1995). Randomised double blind comparison of terbinafine and itraconazole for treatment of toenail infection. Seventh Lamisil German Onychomycosis Study Group. *Brit Med J* **311**: 919.

Budimulja U, Kuswadji K, Bramono S *et al.* (1994). A double-blind, randomized, stratified controlled study of the treatment of tinea imbricata with oral terbinafine or itraconazole. *Brit J Dermatol* **130** (Suppl 43): 29.

Carstens J, Wendelboe P, Sogaard H, Thestrup-Pederson K (1994). Toxic epidermal necrolysis and erythema multiforme following therapy with terbinafine. *Acta Derm-Venereol* **74**: 391.

Cirioni O, Giacometti A, Balducci M *et al.* (1995). *In-vitro* activity of terbinafine, atovaquone and co-trimoxazole against *Pneumocystis carinii*. *J Antimicrob Chemother* **36**: 740.

Cole GW, Stricklin GA (1989). A comparison of new oral antifungal terbinafine, with griseofulvin as therapy for tinea corporis. *Arch Dermatol* **125**: 1537.

Contini C, Manganaro M, Romani R *et al.* (1994). Activity of terbinafine against *Pneumocystis carinii in vitro* and its efficacy in the treatment of experimental pneumonia. *J Antimicrob Chemother* **34**: 727.

del Palacio Hernanz A, Lopez Gomez S, Gonzalez Lastra F, Moreno Palancar P, Iglesias Diez L (1990). A comparative double-blind study of terbinafine (Lamisil) and griseofulvin in tinea corporis and tinea cruris. *Clin Exp Dermatol* **15**: 210.

De Keyser P, De Backer M, Massart DL, Westelinck KJ (1994). Two-week oral treatment of tinea pedis, comparing terbinafine (250 mg/day) with itraconazole (100 mg/day): a double-blind, multicentre study. *Brit J Dermatol* **130** (Suppl 43): 22.

de Wit RFE (1990). A randomized double-blind multicentre comparative study of Lamisil® (terbinafine). versus ketoconazole in tinea corporis. *J Dermatol Treat* **1** (Suppl 2): 41.

Dixon DM, Polak A (1987). *In vitro* and *in vivo* drug studies with three agents of central nervous system phaeohyphomycosis. *Chemotherapy* **33**: 129–140.

Dykes PJ, Thomas R, Lever L, Marks R (1990). Pharmacokinetics of topically applied terbinafine: results from studies in healthy volunteer subjects and patients with pityriasis versicolor. *J Dermatol Treat* **1** (Suppl 2): 19.

Effendy I, Krause W (1989). *In vivo* effects of terbinafine and ketoconazole on testosterone plasma levels in healthy males. *Dermatologica* **178**: 103.

Evans EGV, James IGV, Joshipura RC (1991). Two week treatment of tinea pedis with terbinafine (Lamisil) 1% cream: a placebo-controlled study. *J Dermatol Treatment* **2**: 95.

Evans EGV, James IGV, Joshipura RC (1992). One week treatment of tinea corporis and tinea cruris with terbinafine (Lamisil) 1% cream: a placebo-controlled study. *J Dermatol Treat* **3**: 181.

Evans EGV, Dodman B, Williamson DM *et al.* (1993). Comparison of terbinafine and clotrimazole in treating tinea pedis. *Brit Med J* **307**: 645.

Evans EG, Seaman RA, James IG (1994). Short-duration therapy with terbinafine 1% cream in dermatophyte skin infections. *Brit J Dermatol* **130**: 83.

Faergemann J, Zehander H, Jones T, Maibach I (1991). Terbinafine levels in serum, stratum corneum, dermis-epidermis (without stratum corneum), hair, sebum and eccrine sweat. *Acta Derm Venereol Stockh* **71**: 322.

Faergemann J, Zehender H, Denouel J, Millerioux L (1993). Levels of terbinafine in plasma, stratum corneus, dermis-epidermis (without stratum corneum), sebum, hair and nails during and after 250 mg terbinafine orally once per day for four weeks. *Acta Derm Venereol Stockh* **73**: 305.

Faergemann J, Zehender H, Millerioux L (1994). Levels of terbinafine in plasma, stratum corneum, dermis-epidermis (without stratum corneum), sebum, hair and nails during and after 250 mg terbinafine orally once daily for 7 and 14 days. *Clin Exp Dermatol* **19**: 121.

Faergemann J, Anderson C, Hersle K *et al.* (1995). Double-blind, parallel-group comparison of terbinafine and griseofulvin in the treatment of toenail onychomycosis. *J Amer Acad Dermatol* **32**: 750.

Farag A, Taha M, Halim S (1994). One-week therapy with oral terbinafine in cases of tinea cruris/corporis. *Brit J Dermatol* **131**: 684.

Favre B, Ryder NS (1996). Characterization of squalene epoxidase activity from the dermatophyte *Trichophyton rubrum* and its inhibition by terbinafine and other antimycotic agents. *Antimicrob Ag Chemother* **40**: 443.

Finlay AY (1992). Pharmacokinetics of terbinafine in the nail. *Brit J Dermatol* **126** (Suppl 39): 28.

Gip L (1994). Black piedra: the first case treated with terbinafine (Lamisil). *Brit J Dermatol* **130** (Suppl 43): 26.

Goad LJ, Holtz GG, Beach DH (1985). Effect of the allylamine antifungal drug SF-86327 on the growth and sterol synthesis of *Leishmania mexicana mexicana* promastigotes. *Biochem Pharmacol* **34**: 3785.

Goodfield MJD, Rowell NR, Forster RA *et al.* (1989). Treatment of dermatophyte infection of the finger- and toe-nails with terbinafine (SF 86–327, Lamisil), an orally active fungicidal agent. *Brit J Dermatol* **121**: 753.

Goodfield MJD, Andrew L, Evans EGV (1992). Short term treatment of dermatophyte onychomycosis with terbinafine. *Brit Med J* **304**: 1151.

Greer DL, Jolly HW Jr (1990). Treatment of tinea cruris with topical terbinafine. *J Amer Acad Dermatol* **23**: 800.

Hay RJ, Logan RA, Moore MK *et al.* (1991). A comparative study of terbinafine versus griseofulvin in 'dry-type' dermatophyte infections. *J Amer Acad Dermatol* **24**: 243.

Hay RJ, McGregor JM, Wuite J *et al.* (1995). A comparison of 2 weeks of terbinafine 250 mg/day with 4 weeks of itraconazole 100 mg/day in plantar-type tinea pedis. *Brit J Dermatol* **132**: 604.

Hill S, Thomas R, Smith SG, Finlay AY (1992). An investigation of the pharmacokinetics of topical terbinafine (Lamisil) 1% cream. *Brit J Dermatol* **127**: 396.

Hofmann H, Brautigam M, Weidinger G, Zaun H (1995). Treatment of toenail onychomycosis. A randomised, double-blind study with terbinafine and griseofulvin. LAGOS II Study Group. *Arch Dermatol* **131**: 919.

Hull PR, Vismer HF (1992). Treatment of cutaneous sporotrichosis with terbinafine. *Brit J Dermatol* **126** (Suppl 39): 51.

Humbert H, Cabiac MD, Denouel J, Kirkesseli S (1995). Pharmacokinetics of terbinafine and of its five main metabolites in plasma and urine, following a single oral dose in healthy subjects. *Biopharmaceutics Drug Disposition* **16**: 685.

Jensen JC (1989). Clinical pharmacokinetics of terbinafine (Lamisil). *Clin Exp Dermatol* **14**: 110.

Jensen JC (1990). Pharmacokinetics of Lamisil® in humans. *J Dermatol Treat* **1** (Suppl 2): 15.

Jones TC (1990). Treatment of dermatomycoses with topically applied allylamines: naftifine and terbinafine. *J Dermatol Treat* **1** (Suppl 2): 29.

Jones TC (1995). Overview of the use of terbinafine (Lamisil) in children. *Brit J Dermatol* **132**: 683.

Juhlin L (1992). Loss of taste and terbinafine. *Lancet* **339**: 1483.

Jung EG, Haas PJ, Brautigam M, Weidinger G (1994). Systemic treatment of skin candidosis: a randomized comparison of terbinafine and ketoconazole. *Mycoses* **37**: 361.

Kagawa S (1989). Clinical efficacy of terbinafine in 629 Japanese patients with dermatomycosis. *Clin Exp Dermatol* **14**: 114.

Kan VL, Bennett JE (1988). Efficacies of four antifungal agents in experimental murine sporotrichosis. *Antimicrob Ag Chemother* **32**: 1619.

Korting HC, Ollert M, Abeck D, German Collaborative Dermatophyte Drug Susceptibility Study Group (1995). Results of German Multicenter study of antimicrobial susceptibilities of *Trichophyton rubrum* and *Trichophyton mentagrophytes* strains causing tinea unguium. *Antimicrob Ag Chemother* **39**: 1206.

Kovacs MJ, Alshammari S, Guenther L, Bourcier M (1994). Neutropenia and pancytopenia associated with oral terbinafine. *J Amer Acad Dermatol* **31**: 806.

Kovarik JM, Mueller EA, Zehender H *et al.* (1995). Multiple-dose pharmacokinetics and distribution in tissue of terbinafine and metabolites. *Antimicrob Ag Chemother* **39**: 2738.

Lever LR, Dykes PJ, Thomas R, Finlay AY (1990). How orally administered terbinafine reaches the stratum corneum. *J Dermatol Treat* **1** (Suppl 2): 23.

Long CC, Hill SA, Thomas RC *et al.* (1994). Effect of terbinafine on the pharmacokinetics of cyclosporin in humans. *J Invest Dermatol* **102**: 740.

Lowe G, Green C, Jennings P (1993). Hepatitis associated with terbinafine treatment. *Brit Med J* **306**: 248 .

Maldonado RA, Molina J, Payares G, Urbina JA (1993). Experimental chemotherapy with combinations of ergosterol biosynthesis inhibitors in murine models of Chagas' disease. *Antimicrob Ag Chemother* **37**: 1353.

McGregor JM, Rustin MH (1994). Terbinafine and erythema multiforme. *Brit J Dermatol* **131**: 587.

Millikan LE (1990). Efficacy and tolerability of topical terbinafine on the treatment of tinea cruris. *J Amer Acad Dermatol* **23**: 795.

Munn SE, Russell Jones R (1995). Terbinafine and fixed drug eruption. *Brit J Dermatol* **133**: 815.

Nejjam F, Zagula M, Cabiac MD *et al.* (1995). Pilot study of terbinafine in children suffering from tinea capitis: evaluation of efficacy, safety and pharmacokinetics. *Brit J Dermatol* **132**: 98.

Nolting S, Brautigam M (1992). Clinical relevance of the antibacterial activity of terbinafine: a contralateral comparison between 1% terbinafine cream and 0.1% gentamicin sulphate cream in pyoderma. *Brit J Dermatol* **126** (Suppl 39): 56.

Nolting S, Brautigam M, Weidinger G (1994). Terbinafine in onychomycosis with involvement by non-dermatophytic fungi. *Brit J Dermatol* **130** (Suppl 43): 16.

Ottervanger JP, Stricker BHCh (1992). Loss of taste and terbinafine. *Lancet* **340**: 728.

Petranyi G, Meingassner JG, Mieth H (1987a). Antifungal activity of the allylamine derivative terbinafine *in vitro*. *Antimicrob Ag Chemother* **31**: 1365.

Petranyi G, Meingassner JG, Mieth H (1987b). Activity of terbinafine in experimental fungal infections of laboratory animals. *Antimicrob Ag Chemother* **31**: 1558.

Rakosi T (1990). Terbinafine and onychomycosis. *Dermatologica* **181**: 174.

Ryder NS (1985). Specific inhibition of fungal sterol biosynthesis by SF 86–327, a new allylamine antimycotic agent. *Antimicrob Ag Chemother* **27**: 252.

Ryder NS (1989). The mechanism of action of terbinafine. *Clin Exp Dermatol* **14**: 98.

Ryder NS, Dupont MC (1985). Inhibition of squalene epoxidase by allylamine antimycotic compounds. A comparative study of the fungal and mammalian enzymes. *Biochem J* **230**: 765.

Rzany B, Mockenhaupt M, Gehring W, Schopf E (1994). Stevens-Johnson syndrome after terbinafine therapy. *J Amer Acad Dermatol* **30**: 509.

Savin R (1989). Successful treatment of tinea pedis (moccasin type) with terbinafine (Lamisil). *Clin Exp Dermatol* **14**: 116.

Savin RC (1990). Oral terbinafine versus griseofulvin in the treatment of moccasin-type tinea pedis. *J Amer Acad Dermatol* **23**: 807.

Savin RC, Zaias N (1990). Treatment of chronic mocassin-type tinea pedis with terbinafine: a double-blind, placebo-controlled trial. *J Amer Acad Dermatol* **23**: 804.

Schatz F, Brautigam M, Dobrowolski E *et al.* (1995). Nail incorporation kinetics of terbinafine in onychomycosis patients. *Clin Exp Dermatol* **20**: 377.

Schmitt HJ, Bernard EM, Andrade J *et al.* (1988). MIC and fungicidal activity of terbinafine against clinical isolates of *Aspergillus* spp. *Antimicrob Ag Chemother* **32**: 780.

Schmitt HJ, Andrade J, Edwards F *et al.* (1990). Inactivity of terbinafine in a rat model of pulmonary aspergillosis. *Eur J Clin Microbiol Infect Dis* **9**: 832.

Schuster I (1985). The interaction of representative members from two classes of antimycotics – the azoles and the allylamines – with cytochromes P-450 in steroidogenic tissues and liver. *Xenobiotica* **15**: 529.

Seyffer R, Eichelbaum M, Jensen JC, Klotz U (1989). Antipyrine metabolism is not affected by terbinafine, a new antifungal agent. *Eur J Clin Pharmacol* **37**: 231.

Shadomy S, Espinel-Ingroff A, Gebhart RJ (1985). *In vitro* studies with SF 86–327, a new orally active allylamine derivative. *J Med Vet Mycol* **23**: 125.

Shah IA, Whiting PH, Omar G *et al.* (1993). The effects of retinoids and terbinafine on the human hepatic microsomal metabolism of cyclosporin. *Brit J Dermatol* **129**: 395.

Smith EB, Noppakun N, Newton RC (1990). A clinical trial of topical terbinafine (a new allylamine antifungal) in the treatment of tinea pedis. *J Amer Acad Dermatol* **23**: 790.

Stephen A, Czok R, Male O (1987). Terbinafine: initial clinical results In *Recent Trends in the Discovery, Development and Evaluation of Antifungal Agents* (Fromtling RA, ed), p. 511. Barcelona: JR Prous Science Publishers.

Todd P, Halpern S, Munro DD (1995). Oral terbinafine and erythema multiforme. *Clin Exp Dermatol* **20**: 247.

Tosti A, Piraccini BM, Stinchi C *et al.* (1996). Treatment of dermatophyte nail infections: an open randomized study comparing intermittent terbinafine therapy with continuous terbinafine treatment with intermittent itraconazole therapy. *J Amer Acad Dermatol* **34**: 595.

Urbina JA, Lazardi K, Aguirre T *et al.* (1988). Antiproliferative synergism of the allylamine SF 86–327 and ketoconazole on epimastigotes and amastigotes of *Trypanosoma (Schizotrypanum) cruzi*. *Antimicrob Ag Chemother* **32**: 1237.

Urbina JA, Lazardi K, Marchan E *et al.* (1993). Mevinolin (Lovastatin). potentiates the antiproliferative effects of ketoconazole and terbinafine against *Trypanosoma (Schizotrypanum) cruzi: In vitro* and *in vivo* studies. *Antimicrog Ag Chemother* **37**: 580.

van der Schroeff JG, Cirkel PKS, Crijns MB *et al.* (1992). A randomized treatment duration-finding study of terbinafine in onychomycosis. *Brit J Dermatol* **126** (Suppl 39): 36.

van 't Wout JW, Hermann WA, de Vries RA, Stricker BH (1994). Terbinafine-associated hepatic injury. *J Hepatol* **21**: 115.

Villars V, Jones TC (1989). Clinical efficacy and tolerability of terbinafine (Lamisil) – a new topical and systemic fungicidal drug for treatment of dermatomycoses. *Clin Exp Dermatol* **14**: 124.

Villars V, Jones TC (1990). Present status of the efficacy and tolerability of terbinafine (Lamisil©) used systemically in the treatment of dermatomycoses of skin and nails. *J Dermatol Treat* **1** (Suppl 2): 33.

Wach F, Stolz W, Hein R, Landthaler M (1995). Severe erythema anulare centrifugum-like psoriatic drug eruption induced by terbinafine. *Arch Dermatol* **131**: 960.

Wahllander A, Paumgartner G (1989). Effect of ketoconazole and terbinafine on the pharmacokinetics of caffeine in healthy volunteers. *Eur J Clin Pharmacol* **37**: 279.

White JE, Perkins P, Evans EGV (1990). Successful treatment of chronic tinea pedis and tinea manuum with Lamisil© (terbinafine). *Brit J Dermatol* **123** (Suppl 37): 30.

Wong PW, Ching WTW, Kwon-Chung KJ, Meyer RD (1989). Disseminated *Phialophora parasitica* infection in humans: Case report and review. *Rev Infect Dis* **11**: 770–775.

Zaias N, Serrano L (1989). The successful treatment of finger *Trichophyton rubrum* onychomycosis with oral terbinafine. *Clin Exp Dermatol* **14**: 120.

Zehender H, Cabiac MD, Denouel J *et al.* (1994). Elimination kinetics of terbinafine from human plasma and tissues following multiple-dose administration, and comparison with 3 main metabolites. *Drug Invest* **8**: 203.

Tolnaftate

Description

Tolnaftate is a thiocarbamate derivative, which has the chemical name *O*-2 naphthyl *m, N*-dimethylthiocarbanilate. It has excellent activity against dermatophytes and is available for topical use in numerous preparations, most of which are available over the counter.

Sensitive Organisms

The *in vitro* activity of tolnaftate against dermatophytes is excellent with MICs in the range of 0.1–0.4 μg per ml for *Trichophyton* spp., 0.1 μg per ml for *Epidermophyton floccosum*, and 0.1 μg per ml for *Microsporum canis* (Georgopoulos *et al.*, 1981). This *in vitro* activity was confirmed in a guinea pig model of trichophytosis (Weber and Balish, 1985), with 84% mycological eradication and 79% clinical cure achieved with once-daily application of tolnaftate for 7 days (Petranyi *et al.*, 1981). The activity of tolnaftate against *Aspergillus* spp. is variable and ranges from 0.1 to >100 μg per ml (Georgopoulos *et al.*, 1981). Maher *et al.* (1982) determined the tolnaftate MIC for over 100 mold isolates from cases of otitis externa (including *Aspergillus* spp., *Penicillium* spp., *Alternaria* spp. and *Cladosporium* spp.) was less than 0.1 μg per ml, and tolnaftate was equipotent with clotrimazole, but was more potent than natamycin, polymyxin B sulfate or iodochlorhydroxyquin.

Tolnaftate has no activity against *Candida* species (Weinstein *et al.*, 1965; D'Arcy and Scott, 1978; Iwata *et al.*, 1989), and no antibacterial activity (Iwata *et al.*, 1989).

Mode of Administration and Dose

Tolnaftate is indicated for tinea pedis and tinea cruris:
1% cream, solution and powder is applied twice-daily for 2–6 weeks.

It is recommended that tolnaftate application should be extended at least 2 cm beyond the visible edge of the tinea lesion, and the cream or lotion should be rubbed gently into the area (Pierard *et al.*, 1996).

Availability

Topical formulation: 1% lotion, cream, aerosol spray and powder

Mode of Action

Tolnaftate selectively and specifically inhibits fungal squalene epoxidase, in a manner similar to the allylamine antifungal agents, terbinafine and naftifine (Barrett-Bee *et al.*, 1986) (see Figs IV.1, p. 1261, and IV.3, p. 1325). In *Trichophyton mentagrophytes* cells, tolnaftate caused a dose-dependent inhibition of ergosterol biosynthesis and accumulation of squalene. Complete inhibition was achieved at concentrations of 0.1 μg per ml. In contrast, the activity in *Candida albicans* and *Candida parapsilosis* was notably lower and incomplete inhibition only was achieved at concentrations of 100 μg per ml. The activity of tolnaftate on sterol biosynthesis was enhanced in a cell-free system of *C. albicans*, suggesting tolnaftate may not penetrate the cell envelope of *Candida* spp. well (Barrett-Bee *et al.*, 1986; Ryder *et al.*, 1986). The comparative potency of the thiocarbamates and allylamines for the microsomal squalene epoxidase of *T. rubrum* and *C. albicans* can be explained by the affinity of the antifungal agent for the squalene epoxidase. Tolnaftate has a much higher specificity for the *T. rubrum* squalene epoxidase than the enzyme of *C. albicans* (Favre and Ryder, 1996).

Toxicity

Local reactions are rare, but include skin irritation and contact dermatitis (Gellin *et al.*, 1972; Emmett and Marrs, 1973; Lang and Goos, 1985; Gonzalez Perez *et al.*, 1995).

Clinical Uses of the Drug

1 Surperficial dermatomycosis

Tolnaftate 1% cream applied twice-daily for 3 or 4 weeks is equally effective as clotrimazole 1% cream for the treatment of tinea pedis, tinea corporis and tinea cruris due to *T. rubrum*, *T. mentagrophytes* and *E. floccosum*. Mycological eradication was demonstrated in 93% of tolnaftate-treated patients and clinical cure was achieved in 53–70% of patients in small studies. No relapse was documented in the 4 weeks after treatment (Hall-Smith, 1974; Male, 1974; Keczkes *et al.*, 1975). Equivalent mycological and clinical efficacy (65–70%) was documented for tolnaftate 1% cream, 3% undecylenic acid and 20% zinc undecylenate as a cream (Battistini *et al.*, 1983). Tolnaftate 2% cream and ointment was compared with oxiconazole nitrate 1% cream applied twice-daily for 4 weeks as treatment for tinea infections and was found to be significantly inferior, both clinically and mycologically, to oxiconazole in one study, and to have equivalent clinical and mycological efficacy in another randomized study (Jegasothy and Pakes, 1991). A randomized, controlled study of 10% tea-tree oil cream, 1% tolnaftate cream and placebo determined that although tea-tree oil and tolnaftate had similar efficacy in resolving clinical symptoms of tinea pedis, 1% tolnaftate cream was significantly more effective in achieving a mycological cure (85% versus 30%) (Tong *et al.*, 1992).

Topical treatment with ointment containing 2% tolnaftate and 20% urea for the treatment of onychomycosis produced a clinical response in 70% of patients. Short-course treatment was ineffective (Ishii *et al.*, 1983).

References

Barrett-Bee KJ, Lane AC, Turner RW (1986). The mode of antifungal action of tolnaftate. *J Med Vet Mycol* **24**: 155.

Battistini F, Cordero C, Urcuyo FG *et al.* (1983). The treatment of dermatophytoses of the glabrous skin: a comparison of undecylenic acid and its salt versus tolnaftate. *Int J Dermatol* **22**: 388.

D'Arcy PF, Scott EM (1978). Antifungal agents. *Prog Drug Res* **22**: 93.

Emmett EA, Marrs JM (1973). Allergic contact dermatitis from tolnaftate. *Arch Dermatol* **108**: 98.

Favre B, Ryder NS (1996). Characterization of squalene epoxidase activity from the dermatophyte *Trichophyton rubrum* and its inhibition by terbinafine and other antimycotic agents. *Antimicrob Ag Chemother* **40**: 443.

Gellin GA, Maibach HI, Wachs GN (1972). Contact allergy to tolnaftate. *Arch Dermatol* **106**: 715.

Georgopoulos A, Petranyi G, Mieth H, Drews J (1981). *In vitro* activity of naftifine, a new antifungal agent. *Antimicrob Ag Chemother* **19**: 386.

Gonzalez Perez R, Aguirre A, Oleaga JM *et al.* (1995). Allergic contact dermatitis from tolnaftate. *Contact Dermatitis* **32**: 173.

Hall-Smith P (1974). Dermatomycoses: a brief history of therapy and initial results with clotrimazole. *Postgrad Med J* **50** (Suppl 1): 70.

Ishii M, Hamada T, Asai Y (1983). Treatment of onychomycosis by ODT therapy with 20% urea ointment and 2% tolnaftate ointment. *Dermatologica* **167**: 273.

Iwata K, Yamashita T, Uehara H (1989). *In vitro* and *in vivo* activities of piretrate (M-732) a new antidermatophytic thiocarbamate. *Antimicrob Ag Chemother* **33**: 2118.

Jegasothy BV, Pakes GE (1991). Oxiconazole nitrate: Pharmacology, efficacy, and safety of a new imidazole antifungal agent. *Clin Ther* **13**: 126.

Keczkes K, Leighton I, Good CS (1975). Topical treatments of dermatophytoses and candidoses. *Practitioner* **214**: 412.

Lang E, Goos M (1985). Combined allergy to tolnaftate and nystatin. *Contact Derm* **12**: 182.

Maher A, Bassiouny A, Moawad MK, Hendawy DS (1982). Otomycosis: An experimental evaluation of six antimycotic agents. *J Laryngol Otol* **96**: 205.

Male O (1974). A double-blind comparison of clotrimazole and tolnaftate therapy of superficial dermatophytoses. *Postgrad Med J* **50** (Suppl 1): 75.

Petranyi G, Georgopoulos A, Mieth H (1981). *In vivo* antimycotic activity of naftifine. *Antimicrob Ag Chemother* **19**: 390.

Pierard GE, Arrese JE, Pierard-Franchimond C (1996). Treatment and prophylaxis of tinea infections. *Drugs* **52**: 209.

Ryder NS, Frank I, Dupont M-C (1986). Ergosterol biosynthesis inhibition by the thiocarbamate antifungal agents tolnaftate and tolciclate. *Antimicrob Ag Chemother* **29**: 858.

Tong MM, Altman PM, Barnetson RS (1992). Tea-tree oil in the treatment of tinea pedis. *Australas J Dermatol* **33**: 145.

Weber J, Balish E (1985). Antifungal therapy of dermatophytosis in guinea pigs and congenitally athymic mice. *Mycopathologia* **90**: 47.

Weinstein MJ, Oden EM, Moss E (1965). Antifungal properties of tolnaftate *in vitro* and *in vivo*. *Antimicrob Ag Chemother* **1964**: 595.

Amorolfine

Description

Amorolfine is a synthetic morpholine which inhibits ergosterol biosynthesis. Its chemical name is *cis*-4-[(RS)-3-[4-(1,1-dimethylpropyl)phenyl]-2-methylpropyl]-2,6-dimethyl morpholine hydrochloride. It has fungicidal and fungistatic activity *in vitro* against dermatophytes, some dematiaceous and filamentous fungi and some yeasts. It is available as a 5% nail lacquer and it is indicated for onychomycosis.

Sensitive Organisms

1 Pathogenic yeast

Amorolfine has activity against *Cryptococcus neoformans* with MICs in the range of 0.001–8 μg per ml (Haria and Bryson, 1995). The antifungal activity against yeast is variable, and dependant on strain, incubation temperature and method of assessment of *in vitro* activity. The reported MIC range for *Candida* species is from 0.001 to >100 μg per ml (Odds *et al.*, 1984; Haria and Bryson, 1995). The susceptibility of *Candida albicans* and *C. tropicalis* is lower when tested at 37°C compared with 25°C (Odds, 1993). Using relative inhibition factors or relative growth assays, *C. albicans* appears to be the least susceptible of *Candida* spp. to amorolfine (Odds *et al.*, 1984; Odds, 1992). Studies in the rat model of vaginal candidiasis reveal 1% amorolfine applied intravaginally twice-daily for 3 days completely eradicated *C. albicans*. A dose-dependant effect was noted for increasing concentrations from 0.01% (Polak, 1992).

2 Dimorphic fungi

Amorolfine has good *in vitro* activity against *Histoplasma capsulatum* and *Blastomyces dermatitidis* (Haria and Bryson, 1995).

3 Moulds and filamentous fungi

Amorolfine has potent activity against dermatophytes, and exhibits primary fungicidal activity against most strains (Clayton, 1994). Potent activity against other filamentous fungi which cause onychomycosis, *Scopulariopsis* spp. and *Scytalidium* spp. has also been demonstrated (Clayton, 1994). The efficacy of the topical application of amorolfine for cutaneous infection due to *Trichophyton mentagrophytes* was tested in the guinea pig model. Amorolfine at a concentration of 0.01% completely cleared fungal lesions, and the activity was superior to the azoles, but inferior to terbinafine on a comparative concentration basis (Haria and Bryson, 1995). No *in vivo* activity of amorolfine was demonstrated in a murine model of infection with *Cladosporium* spp., *Wangiella dermatitidis,* or *Dactylaria constricta* despite good *in vitro* activity (Dixon and Polak, 1987).

4 Protozoa

Amorolfine was demonstrated to have potent *in vitro* activity against *Leishmania donovani* that was superior to the standard antileishmanial drugs (Gebre-Hiwot and Frommel, 1993).

5 Synergism with other drugs

The combination of griseofulvin, ketoconazole, itraconazole and terbinafine with amorolfine produced a slight increase in fungistatic activity compared with amorolfine alone, and was consistent for *T. mentagrophytes*. Synergy was demonstrated in the murine model of dermatophytosis for combinations of amorolfine with griseofulvin, itraconazole, fluconazole and terbinafine (Polak, 1993a).

6 Acquired resistance

There are no reports of the development of resistance to amorolfine, and post-treatment MIC values in a trial of increasing concentrations of amorolfine cream for dermatomycoses did not reveal any development of resistance (del Palacio *et al.*, 1992a).

7 Minimum inhibitory concentrations

The MICs for a wide variety of fungi are shown in Table IV.6. They were generally performed using agar dilution methods, and reveal the potent *in vitro* activity against most fungi. However, *in vivo* testing of amorolfine in animal models document the lack of activity when amorolfine is given systemically. This inactivity has been postulated to be due to extensive protein binding or to rapid metabolism (Haria and Bryson, 1995).

Table IV.6

Compiled from data published by Polak (1983), Espinel-Ingroff *et al.* (1984), Shadomy *et al.* (1984), Dixon and Polak (1987), Martin *et al.* (1992), Clayton (1994)

Organism	MIC (μg per ml) range
Yeast	
Candida species	
C. albicans	0.001–>100
C. guilliermondii	0.1–2
C. krusei	0.05–10
C. parapsilosis	0.02–100
C. tropicalis	0.001–>100
C. glabrata	0.06–>100
Cryptococcus neoformans	<0.001–8
Histoplasma capsulatum	0.063
Blastomyces dermatitidis	0.13–0.5
Malassezia furfur	0.005–0.5
Sporothrix schenckii	0.63–0.5
Mold	
Aspergillus spp.	
A. fumigatus	16–>128
A. flavus	30–>128
A. niger	3–>100
Dematiaceous fungi	
Cladosporium spp.	0.006–1
Dactylaria spp.	0.01–0.03
Wangiella dermatitidis	0.001–0.025
Agents of onychomycosis	
Scopulariopsis brevicaulis	0.03–5
Acremonium spp.	0.25–2
Fusarium spp.	0.3–100
Dermatophytes	
Trichophyton spp.	0.001–0.13
Microsporum spp.	0.001–0.13
Epidermophyton spp.	0.003–6.2
Scytalidium spp.	0.1–1

Mode of Administration and Dose

Indications and recommended doses

Superficial dermatomycosis: 0.25% cream applied to affected areas once-daily for 2–6 weeks.

Onychomycosis: 5% nail lacquer applied to affected nails once-weekly. Continue weekly applications until nail is regenerated and affected areas cured. Fingernails generally require 6 months and toenails require 12 months.

Availability

Topical formulation: 0.25% amorolfine cream
5% nail lacquer

Serum Levels in Relation to Dose

Less than 0.5 ng equivalents per ml (detection limit) of intact drug was detected in plasma samples from normal volunteers following a single dose of 0.5 g of 0.25% radiolabeled amorolfine cream to intact or stripped skin (Roncari *et al.*, 1992). No amorolfine was detected in the plasma of 19 patients randomized to receive amorolfine 5% nail lacquer either once- or twice-weekly (Reinel, 1992).

Excretion

Elimination of amorolfine is very slow. Following application of a single 0.5 g dose of radiolabeled amorolfine, approximately 7% of the dose was excreted in urine and feces over 3 weeks (Roncari *et al.*, 1992).

Distribution of the Drug in Body

A single dose of 0.5 g of radiolabeled amorolfine 0.25% cream was applied to both intact and stripped skin of healthy volunteers for 24 h, after which the remaining drug was removed and the skin stripped with adhesive tape to assess the percutaneous absorption of amorolfine. The mean percutaneous absorption of amorolfine was estimated to be 8–10% of the dose applied topically (Roncari *et al.*, 1992).

The amorolfine lacquer builds a non-water soluble film which contains a high concentration of amorolfine on the nail plate after topical application, that remains in place for 1 week. The drug then penetrates into the nail plate rapidly. An *in vitro* study using a porcine hoof horn revealed concentrations of amorolfine far above the MIC for dermatophytes within 6 h of application, and this concentration continued to increase during the 1 week of the study. After 7 days, almost 2% of an applied dose of 500 μg had penetrated under the nail (Pittrof *et al.*, 1992). Permeation rates of 5% amorolfine through the nail ranged from 20–100 mg per cm^2 per h in an *in vitro* assay (Franz, 1992). Polak (1993b) reported amorolfine was detected in the nail earlier and in higher concentrations than either terbinafine or itraconazole.

Mode of Action

Amorolfine inhibits two reactions in the ergosterol pathway, sterol-$\triangle^{14}$-reductase (which converts 14-demethyl lanosterol to zymosterol) and sterol-$\triangle^7$-$\triangle^8$-isomerase (which converts fecosterol to episterol), thereby depleting fungal membrane ergosterol content, and producing an accumulation of 24-methylene ignosterol in the plasma membrane (see Fig. IV.1, p. 1261). It is thought that the antifungal activity is due to inhibition of $\triangle^{14}$ reductase (Georgopapadakou and Walsh, 1996). Amorolfine has also been reported to cause intracellular accumulation of squalene in *Trichophyton* cells, but not in *Candida albicans* (Polak, 1988). This is in keeping with a differential inhibitory effect on the squalene epoxidase from *T. rubrum* and *C. albicans* (Favre and Ryder,1996). Severe ultrastructural changes in both *C. albicans* and *T. mentagrophytes* following exposure to varying concentrations of amorolfine have been demonstrated, and include thickening of cell walls and accumulation of electron dense structures in the cell wall and cytoplasm (Muller *et al.*, 1992; Nishiyama *et al.*, 1992).

Toxicity

1 Local adverse reactions

Local adverse reactions to the topical application of amorolfine cream occurred in 5–7% of patients in clinical trials, and 2.5–3% discontinued trial medication. The most commonly reported local reactions include burning, itching, erythema, local pain, weeping, and scaling (del Palacio *et al.*, 1992b). Infrequent reports of edema, blistering, eczematous reaction and dermatitis have been observed. No systemic adverse events have been reported.

The nail lacquer is well tolerated. Approximately 1% of patients treated either once- or twice-weekly reported mild local irritation (Reinel, 1992).

2 Effect on the fetus

Animal studies reveal exposure to high doses of amorolfine resulted in embryotoxicity. It is unknown whether amorolfine is excreted in breast milk in humans.

Clinical Uses of the Drug

1 Superficial dermatomycoses

Amorolfine 0.25% cream is effective for the treatment of tinea pedis, tinea corporis and tinea cruris. In a dose-finding study of amorolfine cream for the treatment of dermatomycoses, del Palacio et al. (1992b) evaluated concentrations of 0.125%, 0.25% and 0.5% applied once-daily for about 4 weeks. There was no significant difference in mycological eradication rates at 1 week after completion of treatment (81%, 81% and 85%). These results were confirmed in a second study that included bifonazole 1% cream as a comparator. Mycological cure was achieved in 88%, 92%, 91% and 92% of the patients randomized to amorolfine cream 0.125%, 0.25% and 0.5% and bifonazole 1% respectively. The cream was applied once-daily for 4 weeks (Nolting et al., 1992). From these studies amorolfine 0.25% cream was chosen for commercial development. Subgroup analysis from these studies determined there was no statistical difference in response according to pathogen (T. rubrum, T. mentagrophytes, E. floccosum, and M. canis), body area or concentration of amorolfine. In addition, amolforine spray in two concentrations (0.5% and 2%) was compared with 0.5% cream for tinea pedis. Mycological cure was documented in 95% of patients randomized to spray, regardless of concentration, and 87% of those randomized to 0.5% cream (Nolting et al., 1993).

2 Onychomycosis

A comparison of amorolfine nail lacquer at concentrations of 2% and 5% applied once-weekly for 6 months as treatment of mild onychomycosis (less than 80% of the nail surface area affected), revealed a superior cure rate (based on clinical and mycological efficacy) for the 5% lacquer, although the failure rate in both groups was equivalent. By 3 months after the end of treatment, there was no significant difference in the rate of negative mycology cultures between the two groups (Lauharanta, 1992). Another study compared efficacy of the 5% nail lacquer applied once-weekly with a twice-weekly application for 6 months. There was a non-statistically significant trend to superior cure rates for the twice-weekly application (52% versus 46%), which was more evident for fongernail infections than toenail infections. The failure rate was about 30% (Reinel and Clarke, 1992). The response to topical amorolfine nail lacquer is higher when the onychomycosis has been present for shorter durations prior to treatment, with a 19% response rate for onychomycosis of greater than 5 years duration, compared with a 50% response for infection of less than 5 years (Zaug and Bergstraesser, 1992). In non-comparative studies of the 5% lacquer applied once-weekly, eradication rates for infection due to T. rubrum were generally lower than T. mentagrophytes and C. albicans, and fingernails responded better than toenails (Zaug, 1993; Haria and Bryson, 1995).

One study evaluated combination therapy for onychomycosis, and compared griseofulvin 1000 mg daily with amorolfine 5% nail lacquer applied twice-weekly for 2 months with griseofulvin alone. Mycological cure rates at 2 months were 42% and 13% respectively, suggesting significantly improved efficacy for the combination. The patients were then randomized to monotherapy for another 4 months and amorolfine produced higher cure rates (67% versus 45%). The study design does not allow conclusions to be drawn in respect of the comparative efficacy of the combination and amorolfine alone (Lauharanta et al., 1993).

3 Vulvoaginal candidosis

There has been one randomized study of single-dose treatment for vaginal candidosis comparing two doses of amorolfine (50 mg and 100 mg vaginal tablets) with clotrimazole (500 mg). Partners of trial participants were also treated with the corresponding cream. Mycological eradication assessed 1 week later was achieved in 90% of the 50 mg amorolfine group, 95% of the 100 mg amorolfine group and 93% of the clotrimazole group. Long-term follow-up (4 weeks) revealed greater efficacy for amorolfine (80–84% cured) compared with clotrimazole (67% cured). There was a 10% relapse rate for amorolfine treated patients compared with 25% for clotrimazole (del Palacio et al., 1991). There is no commercially available vaginal tablet formulation.

References

Clayton YM (1994). Relevance of broad-spectrum and fungicidal activity of antifungals in the treatment of dermatomycoses. *Brit J Dermatol* **130** (Suppl 43): 7.

del Palacio A, Sanz F, Garcia-Bravo M *et al.* (1991). Single dose treatment of vaginal candidosis: randomised comparison of amorolfine (50 mg and 100 mg) and clotrimazole (500 mg) in patients with vulvovaginal candidosis. *Mycoses* **34**: 85.

del Palacio A, Lopez-Gomez S, Garcia-Bravo M *et al.* (1992a). Experience with amorolfine in the treatment of dermatomycoses. *Dermatol* **184** (Suppl 1): 25.

del Palacio A, Gip L, Bergstraesser M, Zaug M (1992b). Dose-finding study of amorolfine cream (0.125%, 0.25%, and 0.5%) in the treatment of dermatomycoses. *Clin Exp Dermatol* **17** (Suppl 1): 50.

Dixon DM, Polak A (1987). *In vitro* and *in vivo* drug studies with three agents of central nervous system phaeohyphomycosis. *Chemotherapy* **33**: 129.

Espinel-Ingroff A, Shadomy S, Gebhart RJ (1984). *In vitro* studies with R51, 211 (itraconazole). *Antimicrob Ag Chemother* **26**: 5.

Favre B, Ryder NS (1996). Characterization of squalene epoxidase activity from the dermatophyte *Trichophyton rubrum* and its inhibition by terbinafine and other antimycotic agents. *Antimicrob Ag Chemother* **40**: 443.

Franz TJ (1992). Absorption of amorolfine through human nail. *Dermatol* **184** (Suppl 1): 18.

Gebre-Hiwot A, Frommel D (1993). The *in-vitro* anti-leishmanial activity of inhibitors of ergosterol biosynthesis. *J Antimicrob Chemother* **32**: 837.

Georgopapadakou NH, Walsh TJ (1996). Antifungal agents: Chemotherapeutic targets and immunologic strategies. *Antimicrob Ag Chemother* **40**: 279.

Haria M, Bryson HM (1995). Amorolfine A review of its pharmacological properties and therapeutic potential in the treatment of onychomycosis and other superficial fungal infections. *Drugs* **49**: 103.

Lauharanta J (1992). Comparative efficacy and safety of amorolfine nail lacquer 2% versus 5% once weekly. *Clin Exp Dermatol* **17** (Suppl 1): 41.

Lauharanta J, Zaug M, Polak A *et al.* (1993). Combination of amorolfine with griseofulvin: *in vitro* activity and clinical results in onychomycosis. *JAMA SE Asia* **9** (Suppl 4): 23.

Muller J, Polak-Wyss A, Melchinger W (1992). Influence of amorolfine on the morphology of *Candida albicans* and *Trichophyton mentagrophytes*. *Clin Exp Dermatol* **17** (Suppl 1): 18.

Nishiyama Y, Asagi Y, Hiratani T *et al.* (1992). Morphological changes associated with growth inhibition of *Trichophyton mentagrophytes* by amorolfine. *Clin Exp Dermatol* **17** (Suppl 1): 13.

Nolting S, Sernig G, Friedrich HK *et al.* (1992). Double-blind comparison of amorolfine and bifonazole in the treatment of dermatomycoses. *Clin Exp Dermatol* **17** (Suppl 1): 56.

Nolting S, Reinel D, Semig G *et al.* (1993). Amorolfine spray in the treatment of foot mycoses (a dose-finding study). *Brit J Dermatol* **129**: 170.

Odds FC (1992). Antifungal susceptibility testing of *Candida* spp by relative growth measurement at single concentrations of antifungal agents. *Antimicrob Ag Chemother* **36**: 1727.

Odds FC (1993). Effects of temperature on anti-*Candida* activities of antifungal antibiotics. *Antimicrob Ag Chemother* **37**: 685.

Odds FC, Webster CE, Abbott AB (1984). Antifungal relative inhibition factors: BAY 1–9139, bifonazole, butoconazole, isoconazole, itraconazole (R 51,211), oxiconazole, Ro 14–4767/002, sulconazole, terconazole, and vibunazole (BAY n-7133) compared *in vitro* with nine established antifungal agents. *J Antimicrob Chemother* **14**: 105.

Pittrof F, Gerhards J, Emi W, Klecak G (1992). Loceryl nail lacquer – realization of a new galenical approach to onychomycosis therapy. *Clin Exp Dermatol* **17** (Suppl 1): 26.

Polak A (1983). Antifungal activity *in vitro* of Ro 14–4767/002. *Sabouraudia* **21**: 205.

Polak A (1988). Mode of action of dimethylmorpholine derivatives. *Ann NY Acad Sci* **544**: 221.

Polak A (1992). Preclinical data and mode of action of amorolfine. *Clin Exp Dermatol* **17** (Suppl 1): 8.

Polak, A (1993a). Combination of amorolfine with various antifungal drugs in dermatophytosis. *Mycoses* **36**: 43.

Polak A (1993b). Kinetics of amorolfine in human nails. *Mycoses* **36**: 101.

Reinel D (1992). Topical treatment of onychomycosis with amorolfine 5% nail lacquer: comparative efficacy and tolerability of once and twice weekly use. *Dermatol* **184** (Suppl 1): 21.

Reinel D, Clarke C (1992). Comparative efficacy and safety of amorolfine nail lacquer 5% in onychomycosis, once-weekly versus twice-weekly. *Clin Exp Dermatol* **17** (Suppl 1): 44.

Roncari G, Ponelle C, Zumbrennen R *et al.* (1992). Percutaneous absorption of amorolfine following a single topical application of an amorolfine cream formulation. *Clin Exp Dermatol* **17** (Suppl 1): 33.

Shadomy S, Espinel-Ingroff A, Kerkering TM (1984). *In-vitro* studies with four new antifungal agents: BAY n 7133, bifonazole (BAY n 4502), ICI 153,066 and Ro 14–4767/002. *Sabourauradia* **22**: 7.

Zaug M (1993). Amorolfine nail lacquer: once-weekly application in onychomycosis. *JAMA SE Asia* **9** (Suppl 4): 19.

Zaug M, Bergstraesser M (1992). Amorolfine in the treatment of onychomycoses and dermatomycoses (an overview). *Clin Exp Dermatol* **17** (Suppl 1): 1.

Ciclopirox Olamine

Description

Ciclopirox is a substituted hydroxypyridone and ciclopirox olamine is the ethanolamine salt of ciclopirox. It has a broad spectrum of antifungal activity including dermatophytes, yeasts and molds. It has the chemical name 2-aminoethanol salt of 6-cyclohexyl-1-hydroxy-4-methyl-2-pyridone. It is available as a topical formulation for the treatment of dermatophytosis, cutaneous candidiasis and tinea versicolor.

Sensitive Organisms

1 Pathogenic yeast

Ciclopirox olamine has activity against *Cryptococcus neoformans* with an MIC range of 0.9–3.9 μg per ml (Jue *et al.*, 1985). *Candida albicans* and other *Candida* spp. are susceptible to ciclopirox olamine with an MIC range of 0.9–3.9 μg per ml. The *in vitro* antifungal activity differs according to inoculum size, growth medium used and the addition of human or bovine serum albumin to the media (Jue *et al.*, 1985). Moderate activity against *Pitryosporum ovale* and *P. orbiculare (Malassezia furfur)* has been documented (Jue *et al.*, 1985).

2 Dimorphic fungi

Both *Blastomyces dermatitidis* and *Histoplasma capsulatum* are susceptible to ciclopirox olamine (Jue *et al.*, 1985).

3 Molds or filamentous fungi

The dermatophytes are all susceptible to ciclopirox olamine with MICs in the range of 0.9–3.9 μg per ml for *T. mentagrophytes*, 0.5–3.9 μg per ml for *T. rubrum*, 0.9–1.9 μg per ml for *E. floccosum*, and 0.5–3.9 μg.ml for *Microsporum canis* (Jue *et al.*, 1985; Hanel *et al.*, 1988; Korting *et al.*, 1995). The activity was moderate against *Aspergillus* spp. (MIC 1.9–15.6 μg per ml), *Pseudallescheria boydii* (MIC 7.8 μg per ml), and was poor against *Fusarium* spp. (MIC 31 μg per ml. Good activity was noted for *Madurella* spp. (MIC 1.9–3.9 μg per ml), *Penicillium* spp. (MIC 1.9 μg per ml), *Fonsecaea pedrosoi*, *Exophiala jeanselmei* and *Cladosporium carrionii* (MIC 1.9–7.8 μg per ml).

4 Bacteria

Ciclopirox olamine has activity against both Gram-positive and Gram-negative bacteria. *Staphylococcus aureus*, *Streptococcus* spp., *Klebsiella pneumoniae*, *Listeria monocytogenes*, *Bacillus* spp., and *Shigella flexneri* are inhibited by concentrations of 15.6 μg per ml or below. *Salmonella* spp., *Escherichia coli*, *Enterobacter cloacae*, and *Corynebacterium diphtheriae* require concentrations up to 32 μg per ml for inhibition (Jue *et al.*, 1985). *Trichomonas vaginalis* and *Mycoplasma* spp. were inhibited by ciclopirox olamine concentrations of 7.8–100 μg per ml (Jue *et al.*, 1985). In He La cell cultures, *Chlamydia trachomatis* and *C. psittaci* are inhibited by 10 μg per ml ciclopirox olamine (Jue *et al.*, 1985).

Mode of Administration and Dose

Indications and recommended doses
Tinea pedis, tinea corporis, tinea cruris: 1% cream or lotion applied twice-daily for 4 weeks.
Tinea (pityriasis) versicolor: 1% cream or lotion applied twice-daily for 2 weeks.
Cutaneous candidiasis: 1% cream or lotion applied twice-daily for 4 weeks.

Availability

Topical formulation: 1% cream, 1% lotion

Absorption of the Drug

Approximately 1.3% of a dose of 1% ciclopirox olamine cream applied topically to the skin is absorbed into the systemic circulation, with peak serum concentrations of 0.01 µg per ml achieved 6 h after application. Vaginal application of 5 g ciclopirox olamine cream for 1 week in women with vaginitis was associated with 15–20% absorption into the systemic circulation. In contrast, Coppi *et al.* (1993) found a low intravaginal absorption of ciclopirox olamine in women, and an intravaginal bioavailability of 2% in rabbits. The drug is highly protein bound. Metabolism of absorbed drug is rapid and is primarily by glucuronidation. The half-life is 1.7 h. Renal excretion of ciclopirox olamine as metabolites is the primary route of elimination. Fecal excretion is negligible (Jue *et al.*, 1985).

Penetration of ciclopirox olamine into skin structures has been evaluated using skin from human cadavers, and levels of 70–600 µg per ml have been documented in the upper dermis within 1–2 h after topical application, and 20–30 µg per ml were noted in the dermis. Studies using radiolabeled 1% ciclopirox olamine cream reveal penetration into stratum corneum of 0.8–1.6% of the dose 1.5–6 h after application. It also penetrates into hair, hair follicles, and sebaceous glands. Penetration through the fingernail has also been documented by the demonstration of antifungal activity against *T. mentagrophytes* on the underside of the nail after topical application to the upper side (Jue *et al.*, 1985).

Mode of Action

Ciclopirox olamine accumulates in *Candida albicans* to concentrations up to 200-fold that of the surrounding culture medium, and the primary site of action appears to be the cell membrane (Sakurai *et al.*, 1978). Ciclopirox olamine interferes with the uptake and accumulation of essential substrates and/or ions required for cell membrane synthesis. *In vitro* tests have shown ciclopirox olamine blocks transmembrane transport of leucine, and at a concentration of 20 µg per ml, ciclopirox olamine causes over 90% inhibition of the intracellular accumulation of leucine. At higher concentrations, further perturbation of membrane function occurs, with leakage of potassium ions (Jue *et al.*, 1985). It has also been suggested that ciclopirox olamine inhibits the arichidonic acid cascade with some resultant anti-inflammatory activity (Jue *et al.*, 1985). Ciclopirox olamine has also been shown to significantly reduce the adherence of *C. albicans* to both buccal and vaginal epitheliel cells at subinhibitory concentrations (Braga *et al.*, 1992).

Toxicity

Local reactions were reported in 1–4% of patients enrolled in the open and controlled studies, and included irritation, burning, itching, redness, and pain. These were mild and transient (Jue *et al.*, 1985; Bogaert *et al.*, 1986). Contact dermatitis has also been described (Goitre *et al.*, 1986).

Clinical Uses of the Drug

1 Superficial dermatomycosis

Ciclopirox olamine 1% cream was significantly superior to placebo for the treatment of dermatophytoses, with clinical and mycological cure rates of 50–60% (Sehgal, 1976; Kligman *et al.*, 1985; Bogaert *et al.*, 1986). Bioequivalence between the 1% cream and the 1% lotion formulations of ciclopirox olamine has been demonstrated in tinea pedis (Aly *et al.*, 1989).

Randomized studies with clotrimazole 1% cream revealed comparable activity using 4-week twice-daily administration treatment regimens. Mycological eradication was generally achieved in 85–100% of those treated with ciclopirox olamine, and clinical cure was observed in 80% (Jue *et al.*, 1985; Bogaert *et al.*, 1986). Improvement in clinical symptoms generally occurs during the first week of treatment and the majority of patients usually respond by the third week of treatment. Clinical resolution was achieved in 70% with tinea pedis, 65–95% with tinea cruris, and 65–75% with tinea corporis (Jue *et al.*, 1985). There was no difference in clinical or mycological efficacy of ciclopirox olamine 1% cream and ciclopirox 1%-hydrocortisone 1% cream in a randomized, double-blind study (Lassus *et al.*, 1988). Equivalent efficacy was demonstrated for ciclopirox olamine 1% spray and fentaconazole 2% spray applied once-daily for 2–4 weeks, although there was a high rate (30%) of clinical deterioration following cessation of ciclopirox olamine treatment (Altmeyer *et al.*, 1990).

2 Cutaneous candidiasis

Ciclopirox olamine 1% cream is an effecive agent for cutaneous candidiasis. Mycological eradication occurred in 85% of patients and the clinical response occurred in 68–100% of patients treated in open or controlled studies. In two small uncontrolled studies of cutaneous candidiasis, the clinical cure rate was low at 20–30%, although the majority of patients experienced some improvement in clinical signs and symptoms (Jue *et al.*, 1985).

3 Onychomycosis

The application of ciclopirox olamine 1% lotion plus cream to nails infected with *T. rubrum* several times daily for an average of 13 weeks resulted in 57% clinical resolution 6 weeks after the end of treatment (Jue *et al.*, 1985). Onychomycosis due to *Hendersonula toruloidea* was successfully treated with avulsion of the infected nail and topical treatment with 1% ciclopirox olamine (Rollman and Johansson, 1987).

4 Tinea (pityriasis) versicolor

Clinical and mycological cure was achieved in 49% of patients treated in a placebo-controlled trial of ciclopirox olamine 1% cream applied twice-daily for 14 days (Cullen *et al.*, 1985). Comparable and superior activity has been noted for ciclopirox olamine 1% cream applied twice-daily for 14 days when used in controlled studies with clotrimazole 1% cream of treatment of tinea versicolor, and there is a suggestion of a more rapid onset of clinical improvement for those treated with ciclopirox olamine. Clinical and mycological resolution occurred in 77–88% of patients with tinea versicolor treated with ciclopirox olamine 1% cream, compared with 45% treated with clotrimazole 1% cream (Cullen *et al.*, 1985; Jue *et al.*, 1985).

5 Vaginal candidiasis

Open studies using 50 g of vaginal 1% ciclopirox olamine cream inserted once-daily for 1–2 weeks demonstrated mycological cure rates of 72–91%. Comparative studies with 1% miconazole cream revealed comparable activity both mycologically and clinically (Jue *et al.*, 1985).

References

Altmeyer P, Nolting S, Kuhlwein A *et al.* (1990). Effect of fenticonazole spray in cutaneous mycosis: a double-blind clinical trial versus cyclopyroxolamine spray. *J Int Med Res* **18**: 61.

Aly R, Maibach HI, Bagatell FK *et al.* (1989). Ciclopirox olamine lotion 1% bioequivalence to ciclopirox olamine cream 1% and clinical efficacy in tinea pedis. *Clin Ther* **11**: 290.

Bogaert H, Cordero C, Ollague W *et al.* (1986). Multicentre double-blind clinical trials of ciclopirox olamine cream 1% in the treatment of tinea corporis and tinea cruris. *J Int Med Res* **14**: 210.

Braga PC, Piatti G, Conti E, Vignali F (1992). Effects of subinhibitory concentrations of ciclopirox on the adherence of *Candida albicans* to human buccal and vaginal epitheliel cells. *Arzneim Forsch* **42**: 1368.

Coppi G, Silingardi S, Girardello R *et al.* (1993). Pharmacokinetics of ciclopirox olamine after vaginal application to rabbits and patients. *J Chemother* **5**: 302.

Cullen SI, Frost P, Jacobson C *et al.* (1985). Treatment of tinea versicolor with a new antifungal agent, ciclopirox olamine cream 1%. *Clin Ther* **7**: 574.

Goitre M, Bedello PG, Cane D *et al.* (1986). Contact dermatitis due to cyclopyroxolamine. *Contact Derm* **15**: 94.

Hanel H, Raether W, Dittmar W (1988). Evaluation of fungicidal action *in vitro* and in a skin model considering the influence of penetration kinetics of various standard antimycotics. *Ann NY Acad Sci* **544**: 329.

Jue SG, Dawson GW, Brogden RN (1985). Ciclopirox olamine 1% cream A preliminary review of its antimicrobial activity and therapeutic use. *Drugs* **29**: 330.

Kligman AM, Bogaert H, Cordero C *et al.* (1985). Evaluation of ciclopirox olamine cream for the treatment of tinea pedis: multicenter, double-blind comparative studies. *Clin Ther* **7**: 409.

Korting HC, Ollert M, Abeck D *et al.* (1995). Results of German Multicenter Study of antimicrobial susceptibilities of *Trichophyton rubrum* and *Trichophyton mentagrophytes* strains causing tinea unguium. *Antimicrob Ag Chemother* **39**: 1206.

Lassus A, Nolting KS, Savopoulos C (1988). Comparison of ciclopirox olamine 1% cream with ciclopirox 1%-hydrocortisone acetate 1% cream in the treatment of inflamed superficial mycoses. *Clin Ther* **10**: 594.

Rollman O, Johansson S (1987). *Hendersonula toruloidea* infection: successful response of onychomycosis to nail avulsion and topical ciclopiroxolamine. *Acta Dermato-Venereologica* **67**: 243.

Sakurai K, Sakaguchi T, Yamaguchi H, Iwata K (1978). Mode of action of 6-cyclohexyl-1-hydroxy-4-methyl-2-(1H).-pyridone ethanolamine salt (Hoe 296). *Chemotherapy* **24**: 68.

Sehgal VN (1976). Ciclopirox: a new topical pyrodonium antimycotic agent A double-blind study in superficial dermatomycoses. *Brit J Dermatol* **95**: 83.

Clotrimazole

Description

Clotrimazole is an imidazole derivative (bis-phenyl-2-chlorophenyl-1-imidazolyl-methane) which was synthesized in the Bayer Research Laboratories in Germany in 1967 (Plempel *et al.*, 1969). It was the first imidazole derivative developed as an antimycotic agent. Although clotrimazole has a broad spectrum of antifungal and antibacterial activity, its pharmacokinetic profile and toxicity observed following oral dosing mean that clinical use of this drug is currently limited to the topical treatment of superficial fungal infections.

Sensitive Organisms

Clotrimazole has a wide range of antimycotic activity, most fungi pathogenic to man being susceptible (Plempel *et al.*, 1969; Burgess and Bodey, 1972). Its activity against some of these (*Coccidioides immitis, Candida albicans, Cryptococcus neoformans*) is much greater than that of amphotericin B or of flucytosine (Hoeprich and Huston, 1975).

1 Pathogenic yeasts

Cryptococcus neoformans is usually sensitive (Holt and Newman, 1972b). *Candida albicans*, other *Candida* spp., such as *C. tropicalis* and *C. (Torulopsis) glabrata*, are all susceptible (Burgess and Bodey, 1972).

2 Dimorphic fungi

Blastomyces dermatitidis, Paracoccidioides brasiliensis, Histoplasma capsulatum and *Coccidioides immitis* are all susceptible to clotrimazole with MICs between 0.2 and 3.13 μg per ml (Shadomy *et al.*, 1971). *Sporothrix schenckii* is susceptible to clotrimazole.

3 Molds or filamentous fungi

Dermatophytes such as the *Microsporum, Trichophyton* and *Epidermophyton* spp. which cause superficial infections, are highly susceptible to clotrimazole. Molds, such as *Aspergillus* spp., have a wide range of susceptibilities from 0.1 to 10 μg per ml (Bassiouny *et al.*, 1986). The drug has no consistent *in vitro* or *in vivo* activity against the *Mucoraceae* (Lehrer *et al.*, 1980). Filamentous fungi of the *Cladosporium* spp. (Bassiouny *et al.*, 1986) and *Phialophora* spp. are susceptible, but the *Madurella* spp. may be clotrimazole-resistant.

4 Nocardia spp

Compared with the true fungi, this genus is considerably less sensitive to clotrimazole. The drug has also only limited activity against other bacteria (Holt and Newman, 1972b).

5 Naegleria

The ameboflagellate *Naegleria fowleri* which causes primary amebic meningoencephalitis is sensitive to clotrimazole *in vitro* (Jamieson and Anderson, 1974), but it is ineffective in protecting mice against the infection (Jamieson, 1975).

6 Acanthamoeba

Clotrimazole was shown to be the most effective drug against the trophozoite form of *Acanthamoeba* with MIC ranging from 0.19 to 1.55 μg per ml (Driebe *et al.*, 1988).

Table IV.7
Compiled from data published by
Plempel (1969), Holt (1974), Kusunoki
and Harada (1984), Bassiouny et al.
(1986)

Organism	MIC (μg per ml) range	
	Broth	Agar
Candida **species**	0.1–1.56	
C. albicans	0.1–>10	
C. glabrata (Torulopsis glabrata)	0.2–>12.5	0.1–0.5
Dermatophytes		
Trichophyton spp.	0.03–1	0.1–10
Microsporum spp.	0.06–4	0.1–2
Epidermophyton spp.	0.03–0.06	0.1–2

7 Bacteria and protozoa

Strains of *Staphylococcus aureus*, *Streptococcus pyogenes*, and coryneform bacteria associated with skin infections are all susceptible to clotrimazole, while Gram-negative bacilli such as *Escherichia coli*, *Klebsiella pneumoniae*, *Proteus mirabilis* and *Pseudomonas aeruginosa* are all resistant (MIC >50 μg per ml) (Waitz *et al.*, 1971; Jones *et al.*, 1989). In addition, the *Bacteroides* spp. associated with bacterial vaginosis (*Bacteroides melaninogenicus-B oralis* group) are highly susceptible to clotrimazole (Jones *et al.*, 1989). Clotrimazole is also active against some isolates of *Trichomonas vaginalis*.

8 Synergy with other drugs

Weak or partially inhibitory concentrations of clotrimazole may enhance the antifungal activity of both amphotericin B and flucytosine against some strains of *C. albicans* and *C. tropicalis* (Beggs *et al.*, 1976). Others have demonstrated antagonism using clotrimazole with amphotericin B (p. 1249) (Cosgrove *et al.*, 1978).

9 Acquired resistance

It has been difficult to induce clotrimazole-resistant strains of *Candida* and *Aspergillus* spp. *in vitro*. Waitz *et al.* (1971) produced clotrimazole-resistant *Candida* strains using prolonged incubation times, but normal sensitivity reappeared on subculture in drug-free media. It is not known whether resistant strains of other fungi may emerge more readily. Emergence of resistant strains of sensitive fungi during treatment has not been observed (Holt and Newman, 1972a,b; Fong *et al.*, 1993).

10 Minimum inhibitory concentrations

The MICs of clotrimazole against various pathogenic fungal species are shown in Table IV.7.

Mode of Administration and Dosage

Clotrimazole is suitable for topical chemotherapy of dermatophyte or superficial fungal infections. It is used as a 1% cream for the treatment of superficial and vaginal fungal infections, and as vaginal tablets (100 mg, 500 mg) for the treatment of vaginal candidiasis.

For dermatophyte infections, the 1% cream, lotion, or solution is applied topically to the affected area twice-daily. Duration of therapy for tinea pedis or tinea corporis is 4–8 weeks, and for tinea cruris is 2–4 weeks.

For the treatment of vulvovaginal candidiasis, several regimens are effective. These include the insertion of two 100-mg vaginal tablets once-daily for 3 consecutive days; one 100-mg vaginal tablet inserted once-daily for 7 consecutive days; single-dose therapy with one 500-mg vaginal tablet containing lactic acid; the insertion of 5 g of 1% clotrimazole cream intravaginally once-daily for 7–14 days.

For the prevention or treatment of oropharyngeal candidiasis, buccal troches (10 mg) are retained in the mouth and dissolved over 15–30 min, then swallowed. The troches are administered five times daily for 14 days.

There is no parenteral preparation because the drug is poorly soluble in water. Because of problems with toxicity, and the poor pharmacologic profile, the oral preparation of clotrimazole was withdrawn from development. In clinical trials clotrimazole was used in doses ranging from 60 mg per kg body weight per day (Oberste-Lehn *et al.*, 1969; Weuta, 1974) to 200 mg per kg per day (Marget and Adam, 1971). Doses higher than 100 mg per kg per day were poorly tolerated in adults. Dosage regimens used in children varied from 60 to 120 mg per kg body weight per day.

Availability

Oral lozenges: 10 mg

Vaginal tablets: 100 mg and 500 mg.

Cream for vaginal use: 1% (10 mg per g) and 2% (20 mg per g).

Cream, lotion or topical solution: 1%.

Combination creams: Betamethasone dipropionate 0.05%/clotrimazole 1%

Serum Levels in Relation to Dosage

Clotrimazole is nearly completely absorbed after oral administration. After a dose of 20 mg per kg body weight, peak serum levels of 0.5–1.5 μg per ml may be obtained, but there is wide individual variation. The serum half-life is 4.5–6.0 h (Plempel, 1979). After a 500-mg single oral dose of radioactively labeled clotrimazole, peak concentrations of radioactivity reached 5 μg per ml; however, only 1% of the radioactivity was unchanged clotrimazole and the rest was metabolites which have no antifungal activity (Ritter, 1985). Single-dose radiolabeled clotrimazole administered to eight volunteers (mean 27 mg per kg dose) resulted in peak radioactivity of 15 μg per ml 3 h post-ingestion, and most of the radioactivity was attributed to metabolites (Duhm *et al.*, 1974). Low serum concentrations are due to pronounced first-pass hepatic metabolism, which also occurs with drug absorbed after topical or vaginal administration (Ritter *et al.*, 1982). Continued administration of the drug over several days usually resulted in a progressive decline in serum concentrations (Burgess and Bodey, 1972). Clotrimazole is a potent inducer of hepatic microsomal enzymes, resulting in accelerated metabolism of the drug with increased duration of therapy (Bennett, 1974; Ritter *et al.*, 1982). There is individual variation with the extent of this enzyme induction. As with isoniazid, there are slow inactivators of clotrimazole, in whom, after 3 weeks treatment, there is only a slight or no reduction in serum levels. In those who are rapid inactivators, only traces of microbiologically active drug are detectable in the serum after about 1 week treatment (Plempel, 1979; Ritter *et al.*, 1982).

Absorption of clotrimazole into the systemic circulation after vaginal application of either a 100-mg tablet or 1% cream is between 3 and 10%, with the maximum radioactivity concentration related to clotrimazole of 0.03 μg per ml reached at 1–3 days after administration (Ritter *et al.*, 1982). However, subsequent studies determined that the majority of the radiactivity was due to metabolites. Negligible amounts of clotrimazole are present in the circulation following vaginal application of 100–200 mg clotrimazole tablets or 1–2% cream. Nevertheless, vaginal fluid concentrations ranged from 14 to 3300 μg per ml at 24 h after administration and remained at 1–25 μg per ml at 72 h. Following a single administration of a 500-mg tablet formulated with lactic acid, mean vaginal fluid levels of 68 000 μg per ml were measured at 24 h and 2 000 μg per ml at 72 h (range <15–13 230) At the same time, serum levels of clotrimazole were less than 0.01 μg per ml (Ritter *et al.*, 1982).

Following application of 1% cream or solution of ^{14}C clotrimazole to healthy skin, no radioactivity could be detected in serum, and less than 0.05% of applied activity was excreted in the urine. Although there is minimal absorption of clotrimazole or its metabolites through the skin following topical application, concentrations of clotrimazole in the epidermis exceed the MICs of most dermatophytes and *Candida* spp. (Duhm *et al.*, 1974). In the rabbit model of *Candida albicans* keratitis, clotrimazole was found to penetrate into the cornea after topical application, and after debridement of the corneal epithelium, it penetrated into the aqueous humor (Behrens-Baumann *et al.*, 1990).

Excretion

1 Urine

Very little of the active drug is excreted by the kidney. Less than 1% of an administered dose can be recovered from the urine (Burgess and Bodey, 1972). Urinary concentrations of the active drug are as low as 0.01–0.3 μg per ml (Holt and Newman, 1972b).

2 Bile and other routes

It is uncertain whether clotrimazole is excreted in the active form in humans by any other route such as the bile (Marget and Adam, 1971). In animals a considerable quantity is excreted in the feces, sweat and other body secretions (Marget and Adam, 1969). In rats administered 30 mg per kg of a radiolabeled dose either orally or i.v., 90% of the radioactivity was eliminated in feces and only 2–4% in urine, and intraduodenal administration revealed 80% excretion in bile (Ritter *et al.*, 1982).

3 Inactivation in body

The drug is rapidly and extensively metabolized to microbiologically inactive compounds.

Distribution of the Drug in Body

Autoradiographs of rats given radiolabeled clotrimazole i.v. revealed highest radioactivity concentrations in liver, adipose tissue, adrenals and skin 6 h after administration (Ritter *et al.*, 1982). Clotrimazole does not penetrate well into the CSF even when meninges are inflamed. Concentrations of 0.5–1.0 µg per g of the active drug have been detected in muscle and fatty tissue. The drug is about 50% bound to serum proteins (Plempel *et al.*, 1979).

Mode of Action

At least two distinct mechanisms are involved with the imidazole antifungal agents (Plempel, 1979; Sud and Feingold, 1981). At low concentrations, clotrimazole exerts a fungistatic effect on susceptible fungi. This is due to partial inhibition of de novo synthesis of sterols for cell membrane production which only occurs in actively growing organisms. This action differs from that of amphotericin B which affects preformed membrane components. Clotrimazole (as with the other azole drugs) specifically inhibits demethylation of lanosterol, one of the biochemical steps to production of the major fungal sterol ergosterol. Accumulation of lanosterol may act as an additional negative feedback control of ergosterol synthesis. Depletion of ergosterol from the cytoplasmic membrane results in structural alterations which allow efflux of ions and cytoplasmic material essential for maintenance of fungus integrity (Haller, 1985) (see Fiv. IV.1, p. 1261). If imidazole drugs are used at high concentrations, they are fungicidal to susceptible fungi. There is a concentration-dependent scale of inhibition of sterol synthesis, with reduction of fungal growth observed at low concentrations and complete inhibition at the MIC and fungicidal effects observed at 5- to 10-fold the MIC (Haller, 1985). Using time-killing tests, Lefler and Stevens (1984) demonstrated that ketoconazole may also kill *C. albicans* at lower concentrations than miconazole or clotrimazole. Hyphae and pseudomycelia of *C. albicans* are 100-fold more susceptible to the inhibitory action of clotrimazole than yeast cells (Haller *et al.*, 1985).

Recent work has shown that clotrimazole is a potent and specific inhibitor of the movement of calcium and potassium ions across the plasma membrane. It is an inhibitor of the calcium-activated potassium channel and has been shown to prevent potassium loss and cell dehydration of sickled erythrocytes, making it a potentially useful agent for sickle cell disease (Stuart *et al.*, 1994; Rifai *et al.*, 1995). Benzaquen *et al.* (1995) demonstrated the action of clotrimazole was inhibition of ion transport, causing depletion of intracellular calcium stores and alteration of the early mitogenic signals, resulting in inhibition of cell proliferation. The rate of cell proliferation is reversibly inhibited by clotrimazole in a dose-dependent manner. Clotrimazole administered daily to severe combined immunodeficiency mice previously inoculated with melanoma cells, was shown to significantly reduce the number of lung metastases. Panayi (1995) discussed the results of a small controlled trial of clotrimazole 80 mg per kg orally daily versus ketoprofen for the treatment of rheumatoid arthritis. They determined that clotrimazole effectively reduced clinical and laboratory markers of disease activity, which was also associated with cortisol secretion stimulation, but at a cost of a high rate of intolerable gastrointestinal side-effects. The authors were left uncertain as to whether the antiproliferative effect of clotrimazole or the stimulation of cortisol had led to the reduction in disease activity. The antiproliferative effects of clotrimazole may result in a renaissance for this drug, if the dose can be reduced sufficiently to remove the intolerable side-effects.

Toxicity

1 Gastrointestinal side-effects

Anorexia, nausea, vomiting, abdominal pain and diarrhea may occur in patients taking oral clotrimazole, and may be quite pronounced (Goldstein and Hoeprich, 1972; Weuta, 1974). In one study 60% of patients receiving 1.5 g every 6 h were unable to tolerate the drug because of gastrointestinal side-effects (Burgess and Bodey, 1972).

2 Hepatotoxicity

Many patients treated with oral clotrimazole show abnormalities in liver function tests such as serum bilirubin, serum aspartate transaminase (AST) and serum alkaline phosphatase elevations (Weuta, 1974). These usually resolve when the drug is stopped. Up to 15% of patients receiving clotrimazole lozenges have elevated AST levels.

3 Other side-effects

Excessive drowsiness and disorientation have been described (Cartwright et al., 1972) and depression and other mental disturbances have been reported. Normal volunteers receiving 1.5 g or 40 mg per kg experienced a weak sedative effect, and a slowing of reflex time in visual and acoustic tests was recorded (Weuta, 1974).

4 Side-effects due to topical therapy

Clotrimazole cream is usually well tolerated, but local effects such as burning, irritation, erythema, urticaria or pruritus have been recorded in 2.7% patients (Spiekermann and Young, 1976). Up to 15% of patients experienced burning after administration of clotrimazole cream in one study (Clayton and Connor, 1974). Contact allergic dermatitis occurs rarely, and manifests as erythema, edema and vesicles in the areas where the drug has been applied topically (Roller, 1978; Kalb and Grossman, 1985; Baes, 1995). When patch testing has been performed, cross-reactivity with other imidazoles used as topical agents is rarely observed (Kalb and Grossman, 1985; Raulin and Frosch, 1988). Connubial contact sensitization to clotrimazole occurred in a man, whose wife received repeated courses of clotrimazole pessaries for vulvovaginitis, when he was prescribed 1% clotrimazole cream. Acute dermatitis with erythema, edema, vesicles and pruritus over the genital area, upper thighs and abdomen occurred 3 days later, and resolved on cessation of the topical medication (Valsecchi et al., 1994). If irritation or sensitization occurs, the drug should be stopped.

The 1% clotrimazole cream applied topically to the eye produces a mild conjunctival reaction and is poorly tolerated by patients with normal corneal sensation. (Driebe et al., 1988).

5 Pregnancy

Small amounts of clotrimazole are absorbed from the vagina, and although there have been no reports of resultant harm to the developing fetus, its use is not recommended in first trimester of pregnancy. A prescription survey revealed a relative risk of 1.4 (95% confidence limits 1.1–1.6) for spontaneous abortion following exposure to clotrimazole in the first trimester of pregnancy; however, further studies should elucidate whether this is a true association or not (Rosa et al., 1987). No adverse effects of intravaginal clotrimazole have been reported with use in the second and third trimester. It is unknown whether clotrimazole is excreted in breast milk.

6 Drug interactions

FK506 is an immunosuppressant used following organ transplantation. Co-administration of clotrimazole and FK506 resulted in a significant increase in the AUC of FK506, with no effect on the FK506 half-life, and elevated serum creatinine levels in a liver transplant patient. It was suggested that clotrimazole competes with FK506 for binding sites of the enterocyte P-450 enzyme system, decreasing the metabolism of FK506, and allowing greater absorption of the drug. The dose of the immunosuppressant drug may need to be reduced to avoid toxicity (Mieles et al., 1991).

Clinical Uses of the Drug

Because of its side-effects and unreliability in maintaining effective serum levels, clotrimazole is no longer recommended for the treatment of systemic fungal infections. It is useful for the management of the following superficial fungal infections.

1 Candida infections

Clotrimazole applied as a 1% cream is very effective (comparable with nystatin) for the treatment of cutaneous candidiasis which commonly occurs on intertrigenous areas of the skin (Zaias, 1975) and also for candidal balanitis (Waugh et al., 1978). Topically applied clotrimazole cream may also be of benefit in chronic mucocutaneous candidiasis (Pazin et al., 1979).

Vaginal candidiasis may be treated by application of the 1% vaginal cream for 6 successive days, or the application of the 2% vaginal cream for 3 successive days. Clotrimazole vaginal tablets are effective alternatives for the treatment of vaginal candidiasis. The recommended schedules are either to use one vaginal tablet (100 mg) daily for 6 days or two tablets daily for 3 days. The shorter course is equally effective (Masterton et al., 1977). A single 500-mg clotrimazole pessary appears to produce equivalent results as regimens of longer duration (Milsom and Forssman, 1982; Cohen, 1984; Floyd and Hodgson, 1986). A comparison of the 3-day regimen of two 100-mg vaginal tablets daily compared with a single administration of 500 mg revealed a clinical and mycological cure rate of 89% and 77% respectively at 5–10 days following treatment, and 74% and 65% respectively at 4 weeks (Lebherz et al., 1985). Oral itraconazole 200 mg daily for 3 days was determined to be as effective as intravaginal clotrimazole 200 mg for 3 days as treatment of acute vaginal candidiasis, and considered more tolerable (Tobin et al., 1992; Stein and Mummaw, 1993). Single-dose fluconazole 150 mg was also found to be as effective and better tolerated than intravaginal clotrimazole (Boag et al., 1991; Patel et al., 1992; Sobel et al., 1995).

Unfortunately, 10–20% of treated women experience recurrent vaginal candidiasis, and this is not due to the development of resistance to clotrimazole in C. albicans (Fong et al., 1993). In women with no reversible predisposing conditions, prophylactic regimens are recommended. Clotrimazole 500 mg vaginal tablet can be administered on day 7 and day 21 of the menstrual cycle, then monthly on day 21 of the cycle (or postmenstrually) for periods of 3–6 months (Roth et al., 1990; Kinghorn, 1991). Intermittent intravaginal clotrimazole was more effective than itraconazole as suppressive therapy for recurrent candidal vaginitis (Fong, 1992). In contrast, a study evaluating cost-effectiveness and women's preference determined that empiric treatment with a 500-mg single dose was superior to the cyclical monthly prophylactic administration of 500-mg vaginal tablets (Fong, 1994). The single dose application is not recommended for severe vulvovaginal candidiasis.

Buccal troches (10 mg) have been used three to five times per day to control chronic oral candidiasis in immunosuppressed patients (Kirkpatrick and Alling, 1978), to treat oral candidiasis successfully in patients with neoplastic disease (Schechtman et al., 1984) and to prevent oral candidiasis in patients with hematological malignancies, and renal transplant recipients (Owens et al., 1984; Cuttner et al., 1986; Gombert et al., 1987). Recently, oral fluconazole was found to be superior to clotrimazole troches for the prevention of fungal infections in neutropenic patients (Ellis et al., 1994). Clotrimazole has been given to infants with oral candidiasis, either brushed onto the oral mucosa or sucked into the mouth via a pacifier (Montello et al., 1979; Mansour and Gelfand, 1981).

Clotrimazole troches were found to be as effective as oral fluconazole for the treatment of oral candidiasis in HIV-infected individuals, but fluconazole effected a mycological cure more often (Pons et al., 1993; Sangeorzan et al., 1994). One small study showed fluconazole to be superior to clotrimazole troches (Koletar et al., 1990).

Oral clotrimazole was of value for chronic mucocutaneous candidiasis. Leikin et al. (1976) controlled skin and mucosal lesions in an 11-year-old girl by continuous treatment with an oral dose of 120 mg per kg body weight per day (1 g twice-daily). An intolerable frequency of side-effects was associated with orally administered clotrimazole for some patients with chronic mucocutaneous candidiasis (Higgs, 1974). Effectiveness combined with minimal side-effects was accomplished in some patients by using oral clotrimazole intermittently (Ipp et al., 1977; Meade, 1977). Clotrimazole has been replaced by oral ketoconazole and fluconazole for this indication.

2 Trichomonas vaginitis

This infection can be effectively treated by clotrimazole vaginal tablets (100 mg per day) for 6 days (Lohmeyer, 1974). The cure rate is low compared with treatment with oral metronidazole (p. 950). However, it is the treatment of choice for symptomatic infection in the first trimester of pregnancy. Krieger et al. (1985) revealed that concentrations of clotrimazole >100 μg per ml were required to kill some Trichomonas vaginalis isolates, and that resistance to clotrimazole correlated with increasing resistance to metronidazole. Local clotrimazole therapy also has the disadvantage that it cannot prevent renewed infection arising from the urethra and Bartholin's glands. Jones et al. (1989) showed that strains of bacterial species associated with bacterial vaginosis (Gardnerella vaginalis, Bacteroides spp., Mobiluncus spp.) were susceptible to clotrimazole. Because of its antibacterial spectrum, clotrimazole may be suitable for the treatment of mixed bacterial and fungal infections, or the empiric treatment of vaginal discharge.

3 Superficial dermatophyte infections

Various forms of tinea caused by dermatophytes, such as Microsporum canis, Trichophyton mentagrophytes, T. rubrum, T. verrucosum and Epidermophyton floccosum, respond equally well to 1% clotrimazole cream as to Whitfield's ointment and tolnaftate cream (Clayton and Connor, 1974; Gip, 1974; Comaish, 1974; Male, 1974). However, griseofulvin, itraconazole or oral terbinafine is preferred for those dermatophyte infections for which topical therapy is not suitable. Clotrimazole 1% cream applied for 4 weeks was found to be inferior to 1 week of 1% terbinafine cream for tinea pedis (73.1% versus 93.5% mycological cure rates respectively) (Evans, 1994). A study of experimental dermatophytosis due to *T. mentagrophytes* in guinea pigs comparing clotrimazole cream with the combination of hydrocortisone and clotrimazole revealed more rapid resolution in the combination cream group (Shankland and Richardson, 1990). The combination has been used topically for the treatment of tinea pedis, tinea cruris and tinea corporis and favorable results were achieved when compared with 1% clotrimazole cream alone (Katz *et al.*, 1984). Tinea versicolor (caused by *Pityrosporum orbicularis*, also called *Malassezia furfur*) and erythrasma (caused by *Cornyebacterium minutissimum*) also respond to treatment with 1% clotrimazole lotion or solution (Alchorne *et al.*, 1987; Tham, 1987).

4 Keratomycosis

Because of its *in vitro* activity against *Candida*, *Aspergillus*, and *Fusarium* spp., 1% clotrimazole in sterile peanut oil has been recommended for this eye infection. It is applied to the eye every 2–4 h for up to 6 weeks. Topical clotrimazole 1% has been used successfully for the treatment of *Acanthamoeba* keratitis, which is often associated with contact lens use. It is recommended that neomycin-polymixin B-gramicidin be used in addition to clotrimazole (Driebe *et al.*, 1988). However, not all cases respond to topical clotrimazole and surgical therapy with corneal grafts (Dougherty *et al.*, 1994).

References

Alchorne MMA, Paschoalick RC, Forjaz MH (1987). Comparative study of tioconazole and clotrimazole in the treatment of Tinea versicolor. *Clin Ther* 9: 360.

Baes H (1995). Contact dermatitis from clotrimazole. *Contact Derm* 32: 187.

Bassiouny A, Kamel T, Moawad MK, Hindawy DS (1986). Broad spectrum antifungal agents in otomycosis. *J Laryngol Otol* 100: 867.

Beggs WH, Sarosi GA, Steele NM (1976). Inhibition of potentially pathogenic yeastlike fungi by clotrimazole in combination with 5-fluorocytosine or amphotericin B. *Antimicrob Ag Chemother* 9: 863.

Behrens-Baumann W, Klinge B, Uter W (1990). Clotrimazole and bifonazole in the topical treatment of *Candida* keratitis in rabbits. *Mycoses* 33: 567.

Bennett JE (1974). Chemotherapy of systemic mycoses (second of two parts). *New Engl J Med* 290: 320.

Benzaquen LR, Brugnara C, Byers HR *et al.* (1995). Clotrimazole inhibits cell proliferation *in vitro* and *in vivo*. *Nat Med* 1: 534.

Boag FC, Houang ET, Westrom R *et al.* (1991). Comparison of vaginal flora after treatment with a clotrimazole 500 mg vaginal pessary or a fluconazole 150 mg capsule for vaginal candidosis. *Genitourin Med* 67: 232.

Burgess MA, Bodey GP (1972). Clotrimazole (Bay b 5097): *In vitro* and clinical pharmacological studies. *Antimicrob Ag Chemother* 2: 423.

Cartwright RY, Shaldon C, Hall GH (1972). Urinary candidiasis after renal transplantation. *Brit Med J* 2: 351.

Clayton YM, Connor BL (1973). Comparison of clotrimazole, Whitfield's ointment and Nystatin ointment for the topical treatment of ringworm infections, pityriasis versicolor, erythrasma and candidiasis. *Brit J Dermatol* 89: 297.

Clayton YM, Connor BL (1974). Clinical trial of clotrimazole in the treatment of superficial fungal infections. *Postgrad Med J* 50 (July Suppl): 66.

Cohen L (1984). Single dose treatment of vaginal candidosis: comparison of clotrimazole and isoconazole. *Brit J Vener Dis* 60: 42.

Comaish JS (1974). Double-blind comparisons of clotrimazole with Whitfield's and nystatin ointments. *Postgrad Med J* 50 (Suppl): 73.

Cosgrove RF, Beezer AE, Miles RJ (1978). *In vitro* studies of amphotericin B in combination with the imidazole antifungal compounds of clotrimazole and miconazole. *J Infect Dis* 138: 681.

Cuttner J, Troy KM, Funaro L *et al.* (1986). Clotrimazole treatment for prevention of oral candidiasis in patients with acute leukemia undergoing chemotherapy. *Amer J Med* 81: 771.

Dougherty PJ, Binder PS, Mondino BJ, Glasgow BJ (1994). *Acanthamoeba* sclerokeratitis. *Am J Ophthalmol* 117: 475.

Driebe WT, Stern GA, Epstein RJ *et al.* (1988). *Acanthamoeba* keratitis Potential role for topical clotrimazole in combination therapy. *Arch Ophthalmol* 106: 1196.

Duhm B, Maul W, Medenwald H *et al.* (1974). The pharmacokinetics of clotrimazole-^{14}C. *Postgrad Med J* 50 (July Suppl): 13.

Ellis ME, Clink H, Ernst P *et al.* (1994). Controlled study of fluconazole in the prevention of fungal infections in neutropenic patients with haematological malignancies and bone marrow transplant recipients. *Eur J Clin Microbiol Infect Dis* 13: 3.

Evans EG (1994). A comparison of terbinafine (Lamisil) 1% cream given for one week with clotrimazole (Canesten) 1% cream given for four weeks, in the treatment of tinea pedis. *Brit J Dermatol* 130 (Suppl43): 12.

Floyd R, Hodgson C (1986). One-day treatment of vulvovaginal candidiasis with a 500 mg clotrimazole vaginal tablet compared with a three-day regimen of two 100 mg vaginal tablets daily. *Clin Ther* 8: 181.

Fong IW (1992). The value of chronic suppressive therapy with itraconazole versus clotrimazole in women with recurrent vaginal candidiasis. *Genitourin Med* 68: 374.

Fong IW (1994). The value of prophylactic (monthly) clotrimazole versus empiric self-treatment in recurrent vaginal candidiasis. *Genitourin Med* 70: 124.

Fong IW, Bannatyne RM, Wong P (1993). Lack of *in vitro* resistance of *Candida albicans* to ketoconazole, itraconazole and clotrimazole in women treated for recurrent vaginal candidiasis. *Genitourin Med* 69: 44.

Gip L (1974). The topical therapy of pityriasis versicolor with clotrimazole. *Postgrad Med J* 50 (Suppl): 59.

Goldstein E, Hoeprich PD (1972). Problems in the diagnosis and treatment of systemic candidiasis. *J Infect Dis* 125: 190.

Gombert ME, du Bouchet L, Aulicino TM, Butt KMH (1987). A comparative trial of clotrimazole troches and oral nystatin suspension in recipients of renal transplants. Use in prophylaxis of oropharyngeal candidiasis. *JAMA* 258: 2553.

Gugnani HC, Nzelibe FK, Osunkwo IC (1986). Onychomycosis due to *Hendersonula toruloidea* in Nigeria. *J Med Vet Mycol* **24**: 239.

Haller I (1985). Mode of action of clotrimazole: Implications for therapy. *Amer J Obstet Gynecol* **152**: 939.

Higgs JM (1974). The use of clotrimazole in the treatment of chronic mucocutaneous candidiasis. *Postgrad Med J* **50** (Suppl): 57.

Hoeprich PD, Huston AC (1975). Susceptibility of *Coccidioides immitis*, *Candida albicans* and *Cryptococcus neoformans* to amphotericin B, flucytosine and clotrimazole. *J Infect Dis* **132**: 133.

Holt RJ (1974). Laboratory and clinical studies with clotrimazole. *Postgrad Med J* **50** (July Suppl): 24.

Holt RJ, Newman RL (1972a). Urinary candidiasis after renal transplantation. *Brit Med J* **2**: 714.

Holt RJ, Newman R L (1972b). Laboratory assessment of the antimycotic drug clotrimazole. *J Clin Path* **25**: 1089.

Ipp MM, Boxall L, Gelfand EW (1977). Clotrimazole intermittent therapy in chronic mucocutaneous candidiasis. *Amer J Dis Child* **131**: 305.

Jamieson A (1975). Effect of clotrimazole on *Naegleria fowleri*. *J Clin Path* **28**: 446.

Jamieson A, Anderson K (1974). Primary amoebic meningoencephalitis. *Lancet* **i**: 261.

Jones BR, Clayton YM, Oji EO (1979). Recognition and chemotherapy of oculomycosis. *Postgrad Med J* **55**: 625.

Jones BM, Geary I, Lee ME, Duerden BI (1989). Comparison of the *in vitro* activities of fenticonazole, other imidazoles, metronidazole, and tetracycline against organisms associated with bacterial vaginosis and skin infections. *Antimicrob Ag Chemother* **33**: 970.

Kalb RE, Grossman ME (1985). Contact dermatitis to clotrimazole. *Cutis* **36**: 240.

Katz HI, Bard J, Cole GW *et al.* (1984). SCH 370 (clotrimazole-betamethasone dipropionate) cream in patients with tinea cruris or tinea corporis. *Cutis* **34**: 183.

Kinghorn GR (1991). Vulvovaginal candidiasis. *J Antimicrob Chemother* **28** (Suppl A): 59.

Kirkpatrick CH, Alling DW (1978). Treatment of chronic oral candidiasis with clotrimazole troches A controlled clinical trial. *New Engl J Med* **299**: 1201.

Koletar SL, Russell JA, Fass RJ, Plouffe JF (1990). Comparison of oral fluconazole and clotrimazole troches as treatment for oral candidiasis in patients infected with human immunodeficiency virus. *Antimicrob Ag Chemother* **34**: 2267.

Krieger JN, Dickins CS, Rein MF (1985). Use of time-kill technique for susceptibility testing of *Trichomonas vaginalis*. *Antimicrob Ag Chemother* **27**: 332.

Kusunoki T, Harada S (1984). Comparison of the *in vitro* antifungal activities of clotrimazole, miconazole, econazole and exalamide against clinical isolates of dermatophytes. *J Dermatol* **11**: 277.

Lebherz T, Guess E, Wolfson N (1985). Efficacy of single- versus multiple-dose clotrimazole therapy in the management of vulvovaginal candidiasis. *Amer J Obstet Gynecol* **152**: 965.

Lefler E, Stevens DA (1984). Inhibition and killing of *Candida albicans in vitro* by five imidazoles in clinical use. *Antimicrob Ag Chemother* **25**: 450.

Lehrer Rl, Howard DH, Sypherd PS *et al.* (1980). Mucormycosis. *Ann Intern Med* **93**: 93.

Leikin S, Parrott R, Randolph J (1976). Clotrimazole treatment of chronic mucocutaneous candidiasis. *J Pediatr* **88**: 864.

Lohmeyer H (1974). Treatment of candidiasis and trichomoniasis of the female genital tract. *Postgrad Med J* **50** (Suppl): 78.

Male O (1974). A double-blind comparison of clotrimazole and tolnaftate therapy of superficial dermatophytoses. *Postgrad Med J* **50** (Suppl): 75.

Mansour A, Gelfand EW (1981). A new approach to the use of antifungal agents in infants with persistent oral candidiasis. *J Pediatr* **98**: 161.

Marget W, Adam D (1969). First experience with the broad-spectrum antimycotic BAY b 5097. *Med Klin* **64**: 1235.

Marget W, Adam D (1971). BAY B 5097, a new orally applicable antifungal substance with broadspectrum activity Preliminary clinical and laboratory experiences in children. *Acta Paediatr Scand* **60**: 341.

Masterton G, Napier lR, Henderson JN, Roberts JE (1977). Three-day clotrimazole treatment in candidal vulvovaginitis. *Brit J Vener Dis* **53**: 126.

Meade RH III (1977). Treatment of chronic mucocutaneous candidiasis. *Ann Intern Med* **86**: 314.

Mieles L, Venkataramanan R, Yokoyama I, Warty VJ, Starzel TE (1991). Interaction between FK506 and clotrimazole in a liver transplant recipient. *Transplantation* **52**: 1086–1087.

Milsom I, Forssman L (1982). Treatment of vaginal candidosis with a single 500 mg clotrimazole pessary. *Brit J Vener Dis* **58**: 124.

Montello JM, Darby MH, Faubel K, August CS (1979). Clotrimazole by thumb. *New Engl J Med* **301**: 1005.

Oberste-Lehn H, Baggesen 1, Plempel M (1969). First clinical experience in systemic mycoses with a new oral antimycotic. *Dtsch Med Wochenschr* **94**: 1365.

Owens NJ, Nightingale CH, Schweizer RT *et al.* (1984). Prophylaxis of oral candidiasis with clotrimazole troches. *Arch Intern Med* **144**: 290.

Panayi GS (1995). Treating rheumatoid arthritis with clotrimazole. *Nat Med* **1**: 977.

Patel HS, Peters MD, Smith CL (1992). Is there a role for fluconazole in the treatment of vulvovaginal candidiasis? *Ann Pharmacother* **26**: 350.

Pazin GJ, Nagel JE, Friday GA, Fireman P (1979). Topical clotrimazole treatment of chronic mucocutaneous candidiasis. *J Pediatr* **94**: 322.

Plempel M (1979). Pharmacokinetics of imidazole antimycotics. *Postgrad Med J* **55**: 662.

Pons V, Greenspan D, Debruin M (1993). Therapy for oropharyngeal candidiasis in HIV-infected patients: a randomized, prospective multi-center study of oral fluconazole versus clotrimazole troches. *J AIDS* **6**: 1311.

Raulin C, Frosch PJ (1988). Contact allergy to imidazole antimycotics. *Contact Dermatitis* **18**: 76.

Rifai N, Sakamotot M, Law T *et al.* (1995). HPLC measurement, blood distribution, and pharmacokinetics of oral clotrimazole, potentially useful antisickling agent. *Clin Chem* **41**: 387.

Ritter W (1985). Pharmacokinetic fundamentals of vaginal treatment with clotrimazole. *Amer J Obstet Gynecol* **7**: 945.

Ritter W, Patzschke K, Krause U, Stettendorf S (1982). Pharmacokinetic fundamentals of vaginal treatment with clotrimazole. *Chemotherapy* **28** (Suppl 1): 37.

Roller JA (1978). Contact allergy to clotrimazole. *Brit Med J* **2**: 737.

Rosa FW, Baum C, Shaw M (1987). Pregnancy outcomes after first-trimester vaginitis drug therapy. *Obstet Gynecol* **69**: 751.

Roth AC, Milsom I, Forssman L, Wahlen P (1990). Intermittent prophylactic treatment of recurrent vaginal candidiasis by postmenstrual application of a 500 mg clotrimazole vaginal tablet. *Genitourin Med* **66**: 357.

Sangeorzan JA, Bradley SF, He X *et al.* (1994). Epidemiology of oral candidiasis in HIV-infected patients: colonization, infection, treatment, and emergence of fluconazole resistance. *Amer J Med* **97**: 339.

Schechtman LB, Funaro L, Robin T *et al.* (1984). Clotrimazole treatment of oral candidiasis in patients with neoplastic disease. *Amer J Med* **76**: 91.

Shadomy S (1971). *In vitro* and fungal activity of clotrimazole. *Infect Immun* **4**: 143.

Shankland GS Richardson MD (1990). Comparative *in-vivo* activity of clotrimazole and a clotrimazole/hydrocortisone combination in the treatment of experimental dermatophytosis in guinea pigs. *J Antimicrob Chemother* **25**: 825.

Sobel JD, Brooker D, Stein GE *et al.* (1995). Single dose fluconazole compared with conventional clotrimazole topical therapy of *Candida* vaginitis. Fluconazole Vaginitis Study Group. *Amer J Obstet Gynecol* **172**: 1263.

Spiekermann PH, Young MD (1976). Clinical evaluation of clotrimazole. *Arch Dermatol* **112**: 350.

Stein GE, Mummaw N (1993). Placebo-controlled trial of itraconazole for treatment of acute vaginal candidiasis. *Antimicrog Ag Chemother* **37**: 89.

Stuart J, Mojiminiyi FB, Stone PC, Culliford SJ, Ellory JC (1994). Additive *in vitro* effects of anti-sickling drugs. *Brit J Hematol* **86**: 820.

Sud IJ, Feingold DS (1981). Heterogeneity of action mechanisms among antimycotic imidazoles. *Antimicrob Ag Chemother* **20**: 71.

Sud IJ, Feingold DS (1982). Action of antifungal imidazoles on *Staphylococcus aureus*. *Antimicrob Ag Chemother* **22**: 470.

Tham SN (1987). Treatment of Pityriasis versicolor: Comparison of sulconazole nitrate 1% solution and clotrimazole 1% solution. *Australas J Dermatol* **28**: 123.

Tobin JM, Loo P, Granger SE (1992). Treatment of vaginal candidosis: a comparative study of the efficacy and acceptability of itraconazole and clotrimazole. *Genitourin Med* **68**: 36.

Valsecchi R, Pansera B, Di Landro A, Cainelli T (1994). Connubial contact sensitization to clotrimazole. *Contact Dermatitis* **30**: 248.

Waitz JA, Moss EL, Weinstein MJ (1971). Chemotherapeutic evaluation of clotrimazole [Bay b5097,1(0-chloro-α-α-diphenylbenzyl). imidazole]. *Appl Microbiol* **22**: 891.

Waugh MA, Evans EGV, Nayyar KC, Fong R (1978). Clotrimazole (canesten) in the treatment of candidal balanitis in men. *Brit J Vener Dis* **54**: 184.

Weuta H (1974). Clinical studies with oral clotrimazole. *Postgrad Med J* **50** (July Suppl): 45.

Zaias N (1975). Clotrimazole and miconazole. *Proceedings of the Third International Conference on the Mycoses, Sao Paulo, 27–29 August 1974*. PAHO, WHO Scientific Publication No304, p 241.

Ketoconazole

Description

Clinical research with ketoconazole began in 1977. It was marketed in the USA in 1981, and subsequently in other countries (Janssen and Symoens, 1983; Lewis *et al.*, 1984). It is structurally related to clotrimazole and miconazole, and similarly has a wide spectrum of antifungal activity. It has the advantage of being effective when administered by the oral route. Treatment-associated toxicity has led to the development of newer orally bioavailable azole compounds.

Ketoconazole was developed at Janssen Pharmaceutica Research Laboratories in Belgium (Heeres *et al.*, 1979). It has the chemical formula *cis*-1-acetyl-4-[4-{(2-(2,4-dichlorophenyl)-2-(1*H*-imidazol-1-ylmethyl)-1,3-dioxolan-4-yl) methoxy} phenyl] piperazine.

Sensitive Organisms

Table IV.8 shows that ketoconazole has activity against a large variety of fungi. For many of these species, published MICs have a wide range. Broth dilution susceptibility testing for ketoconazole and the other imidazole antifungal agents is difficult to interpret and compare across studies because of different methodology and the influence of inoculum effect (Galgani and Stevens, 1978; Cook *et al.*, 1990), the composition of the medium (Doern *et al.*, 1986; Morace *et al.*, 1991), the pH of the medium (Minagawa *et al.*, 1983) and the duration and temperature of incubation (Stevens, 1984). There is also the problem of reading the MIC due to a lack of clear visual endpoint (Odds, 1979). Also in the case of *Candida albicans*, there are differences in susceptibility to ketoconazole depending on whether the yeast or mycelial form of the fungus is tested. Pseudomycelial forms are more susceptible (Borgers *et al.*, 1983). Germ tube formation and elongation is a prerequisite for mycelial formation. Ketoconazole (and miconazole) inhibit germ tube elongation in *C. albicans* and this action correlates more closely with the *in vivo* efficacy of ketoconazole than MIC determinations by conventional methods (Johnson *et al.*, 1984). In addition, *in vivo* activity may not be predicted by *in vitro* testing (Heel, 1982; Shadomy *et al.*, 1985).

1 Pathogenic yeasts

Cryptococcus neoformans, and *Candida* spp. are usually sensitive to ketoconazole (Hernandez Molina *et al.*, 1992; Martin *et al.*, 1992). Some investigators have described a bimodal pattern of response to ketoconazole for *C. albicans* in susceptibility testing (Espinel-Ingroff *et al.*, 1984; Hussain Qadri *et al.*, 1986; Hernandez Molina *et al.*, 1992). No cross-resistance to other imidazole agents has been found (Hernandez Molina *et al.*, 1992). The drug had a beneficial effect on experimental *Candida* and *C. neoformans* infections in animals (Heel, 1982; Van Cutsem, 1983). Low-dose oral ketoconazole protects against experimental candidal vaginitis in rats (Sobel and Muller, 1984). *Pityrosporum orbicularis* (*Malassezia furfur*) is also sensitive and ketoconazole is protective against experimental rabbit tinea versicolor (Faergemann, 1984).

2 Dimorphic fungi

Blastomyces dermatitidis, *Coccidioides immitis*, *Histoplasma capsulatum*, *Histoplasma duboisii* and *Paracoccidioides brasiliensis* are all usually susceptible. Shadomy *et al.* (1985) found that *B. dermatitidis*, *C. immitis*, and *H. capsulatum* were uniformly susceptible to ketoconazole, the majority of strains being inhibited by a concentration <0.39 µg per ml. In addition, *P. brasiliensis* is highly susceptible to ketoconazole (San-Blas *et al.*, 1993). Ketoconazole has been shown to be efficacious in murine models of blastomycosis (Lefler *et al.*, 1985), fungistatic in murine coccidioidomycosis (Hoeprich and Merry, 1985) and histoplasmosis (Polak and Dixon, 1987). *Sporothrix schenckii* may be sensitive, but results may vary with the *in vitro* test employed (Shadomy *et al.*, 1985).

3 Molds or filamentous fungi

Some strains of *Aspergillus* spp. may be sensitive, as may be the agents which cause chromoblastomycosis (*Cladosporium, Fonsecaea* and *Phialophora* spp.). Its action against the Zygomycetes of the order Mucorales, such as the genera *Cunninghamella Rhizopus, Absidia* and *Mucor*, is poor (Eng *et al.*, 1981). Zygomycetes of the order Entomophthorales of the genera *Basidiobolus* and *Conidiobolus* are sometimes sensitive (Drouhet and Dupont, 1983; Van Cutsem, 1983; Yangco *et al.*, 1984). *Fusarium* spp. are generally resistant to ketoconazole (Reuben *et al.*, 1989). *Madurella* spp. and *Pseudallescheria* (*Petriellidium*) *boydii*, which are causes of eumycetoma, may be sensitive to ketoconazole. It is active against many strains of the dermatophytes (*Microsporum, Trichophyton* and *Epidermophyton* spp.).

4 Actinomycetes

Bacteria of this group, *Actinomadura, Nocardia* and *Streptomyces* spp., are usually resistant (Heel, 1982; Martin, 1982).

5 Other bacteria and protozoa

Like the other imidazole drugs. ketoconazole has some *in vitro* activity against certain Gram-positive bacteria. such as *Staphylococcus aureus* and *Staph. epidermidis*, however the activity is not sufficient to be of clinical relevance. (Heeres *et al.*, 1979). Ketoconazole has also been found to be inhibitory to *Helicobacter pylori* (causative agent of chronic atrophic gastritis) with an MIC range of 8–128 µg per ml (von Recklinghausen *et al.*, 1992). No *in vivo* effect has been documented to date. Conflicting results have been reported for the activity of ketoconazole against isolates of *Trichomonas vaginalis*. Minimal *in vitro* activity was demonstrated by Sears and O'Hare (1988) compared with comparable activity with metronidazole demonstrated in another study which used smaller inoculum of trichomonads (Sugarman and Mummaw,1988)

6 Malaria

Ketoconazole is active *in vitro* against chloroquine-susceptible and chloroquine-resistant *Plasmodium falciparum* strains (Pfaller and Krogstad, 1981).

7 Leishmania

The drug has antileishmanial activity *in vitro* against *Leishmania tropica* in human macrophages (Berman, 1981), but was ineffective against *L. major* and *L. mexicana* in the murine model of cutaneous leishmaniasis (Weinrauch and El-On, 1984).

8 Trypanosomes

Ketoconazole protects mice against death caused by infection with *Trypanosoma cruzi* (the cause of Chagas' disease) and it also inhibits the intracellular multiplication of amastigotes *in vitro* (McCabe *et al.*, 1983, 1984).

9 Ameba

Ketoconazole has an amebicidal effect on *Naegleria fowleri* with an MIC of 0.3 µg per ml (Smego and Durack, 1984).

10 Viruses

Antiviral activity against herpes simplex virus 1 (HSV-1) and HSV-2 was demonstrated for ketoconazole in a yield reduction assay. Synergistic activity with acyclovir was also demonstrated (Pottage *et al.*, 1986). Clinical efficacy of ketoconazole as a prophylactic agent against HSV-2 infections was suggested in a report of cessation of 2-weekly recurrences of genital HSV for the 5 months duration of ketoconazole treatment for vulvovaginal candidiasis (Tkach and Rinaldi, 1983). No other clinical studies have been performed to evaluate a role, if any, for ketoconazole in recurrent HSV infections. Hepatitis B surface antigen production in a chronically infected hepatoma cell line has also been shown to be inhibited by ketoconazole (Pottage and Kessler, 1985). The mechanism of action of this antifungal agent on viral replication is unknown.

11 Synergy with other drugs

The combination of ketoconazole and amphotericin B may be synergistic, additive, or antagonistic *in vitro* (p. 1249), and in animal models against a variety of fungi. In experimental murine cryptococcosis and histoplasmosis, the combination of amphotericin B and ketoconazole produced a modest additive effect (Graybill *et al.*, 1980a). Significant antagonism has been demonstrated for the combination of ketoconazole and amphotericin B, or pretreatment with ketoconazole and subsequent treatment with amphotericin B in the murine model of aspergillosis (Suger, 1995). Ketoconazole plus flucytosine has synergistic *in vitro* fungistatic activity against *Candida* spp., but no fungicidal activity (Beggs and Sarosi, 1982; Hughes *et al.*, 1986). The combination is also additive or moderately synergistic in the murine model of candidiasis (Polak *et al.*, 1982), and additive in murine cryptococcosis. Unlike miconazole, ketoconazole does not show synergy with rifampicin against *Candida* spp. (Moody *et al.*, 1980). Also the addition of rifampicin to ketoconazole was of little benefit in the treatment of murine candidiasis (Graybill and Ahrens, 1983).

Lovastatin is synergistic with ketoconazole against *Trypanosoma cruzi*, both *in vitro* and in the murine model of Chagas' disease (Urbina *et al.*, 1993). Ketoconazole has also been shown to be synergistic with terbinafine in the murine model of *T. cruzi* infection, with the combination able to eradicate the parasitemia (Maldonado *et al.*, 1993).

12 Acquired resistance

Reports of apparent ketoconazole resistance (Horsburgh *et al.*, 1982; Church *et al.*, 1982) have been attributed to varying results obtained by differing laboratory methodology on pretreatment and post-treatment isolates (Levine, 1982) and to the lack of a standard to define resistance (Blatchford *et al.*, 1982; Odds, 1982). Nevertheless, Warnock *et al.* (1983), using germ tube growth, showed that mycelial formation of a particular *C. albicans* strain was not inhibited to the same degree as other clinical isolates. The strain was isolated from a child with chronic mucocutaneous candidiasis which had not responded to ketoconazole. Two other patients with chronic mucocutaneous candidiasis, who had both received prolonged courses of oral ketoconazole, appeared to develop highly resistant *C. albicans* strains associated with clinical relapse (Horsburgh and Kirkpatrick,1983). Furthermore, when the three strains described by Horsburgh and Kirkpatrick (1983) and by Warnock *et al.* (1983) were tested by three different laboratory methods, they were shown to be less sensitive to ketoconazole than other strains tested; however, pretreatment strains were not available for comparison. *Candida* strains resistant to ketoconazole were isolated from two patients with AIDS treated with the drug for prolonged periods (Tavitian *et al.*, 1986). O'Connor and Sobel (1986) evaluated vaginal isolates of *C. albicans* prior to treatment, and following long-term therapy with ketoconazole in 115 women with recurrent vulvovaginal candidiasis and were unable to demonstrate acquisition of resistance in those who received either low-dose long-term treatment or cyclical therapy. There was no evidence for selection of ketoconazole-resistant *Candida* spp. other than *C. albicans* either. When ketoconazole was given as prophylaxis to immunocompromised patients the emergence of *C. glabrata* strains was reported in three studies; however, this observation was not seen in other ketoconazole prophylaxis studies (Odds, 1993). Acquired resistance to ketoconazole appears to be infrequent.

13 Minimum inhibitory concentrations

There is a lack of correlation between the MIC of ketoconazole for pretreatment isolates and clinical response following treatment (Shadomy *et al.*, 1985) and results of ketoconazole therapy in a systemic candidiasis animal model (Polak *et al.*, 1985). In addition, interpretation of the MICs of ketoconazole is clouded by methodology (see p. 1358). An example is the difference in susceptibility of *C. glabrata* when tested with the agar dilution method (highly sensitive) and broth dilution method (resistant). *In vivo*, ketoconazole does not appear to be effective for *C. glabrata* infection in immunocompetent or immunocompromised mice, which correlates with the broth microdilution tests and not the agar dilution method (Nobre *et al.*, 1989). Caution is recommended when interpreting ketoconazole MICs and predicting clinical response. The MICs of ketaconazole are shown in Table IV.8 below.

Table IV.8

Compiled from data published by Heel (1982), Faergemann (1984), Gebhart *et al.* (1984), Hoeprich and Merry (1984), Yangco *et al.* (1984), Sugar and Stevens (1985); Adam *et al.* (1986), Dixon and Polak (1987), Marcon *et al.* (1987), Polak and Dixon (1987), Okeke and Gugnani (1987), Haron *et al.* (1988), Iwatsu (1988), Wong *et al.* (1989), Patterson *et al.* (1990), Morace *et al.* (1991), Hernandez Molina *et al.* (1992), Martin *et al.* (1992), Sekhon *et al.* (1992), Naqvi *et al.* (1993), Venugopal *et al.* (1993)

Organism	MIC (µg per ml) range	
	Broth	Agar
Yeast		
Candida spp.		0.02–80
C. albicans	0.04–100	0.0037–2
C. guilliermondii	0.39	0.0075–0.06
C. krusei	0.19–3.12	0.0037–0.25
C. parapsilosis	0.04–0.39	0.0037–0.12
C. tropicalis	0.04–12.5	0.0037–8
C. kefyr (pseudotropicalis)		0.5–1
C. lusitaniae	0.04	0.0037–8
C. rugosa		12.5
C. glabrata (Torulopsis glabrata)	0.19–12.5	0.0037–0.12
Blastoschizomyces capitatum	0.78	
Cryptococcus neoformans	0.2–50	0.1–32
Hansenula anomala	0.39	
Malassezia furfur	0.02–0.5	0.05–4
Trichosporon beigelii	0.09–0.78	
Dimorphic fungi		
Histoplasma capsulatum	0.05–0.2	0.1–5
Blastomyces dermatitidis	0.05–3.13	0.1–2
Coccidioides immitis	0.05–0.39	0.1–8
Paracoccidioides brasiliensis		0.002–0.1
Penicillium marneffei	<0.195–0.39	
Sporothrix schenckii	0.2	0.5–1.0
Mold		
Aspergillus spp.		
A. fumigatus	<10	1–100
A. flavus	<2.5	1
A. niger	<1.25	
Dematiaceous fungi		
Alternaria alternata		7.8
Bipolaris spp.	0.1–3.2	
Cladosporium spp.		0.02–0.08
Cladosporium carrionii		0.05–2.0
Dactylaria spp.		2.5–5
Exophiala jeanselmei	1–5	0.1
Exserohilum spp.	0.2–3.2	
Fonsecaea pedrosoi		0.05–1.56
Phialophora parasitica	0.1	
Phialophora verrucosa		0.1
Wangiella dermatitidis		0.075–0.15
Zygomycetes		
Mucor spp.	<0.07	
Rhizopus spp.	<10	
Conidiobolus spp.	0.195–1.56	
Basidiobolus spp.	<0.098–1.56	
Dermatophytes	0.06–4	
Trichophyton spp.		0.00001–128
Microsporum spp.		0.1–63
Epidermophyton spp.		0.1–8
Hyphomycetes		
Pseudallescheria boydii		1.56–3.12
Madurella spp.	0.01–5	
Pythium insidiosum	<0.195–50	

Mode of Administration and Dosage

1 Oral administration

Ketoconazole is administered by the oral route. The recommended dose for adults is 200 mg (one tablet) daily, which may be increased to 400 mg daily if a clinical response is not achieved. Daily doses of 800 mg have been used when usual doses have failed to produce adequate serum levels or a therapeutic effect (Drouhet and Dupont, 1983). The safety of the drug has not been adequately studied in children, but reduced doses adjusted according to weight have been used in some studies. Recommended doses for children weighing 20 kg or less, 20–40 kg, and greater than 40 kg are 50, 100 and 200 mg daily, respectively (Heel, 1982). There is no pediatric preparation available. It is necessary to crush or break 200 mg tablets. A dose of 3 mg per kg per day has been used for neonatal patients (Tudehope and Rigby, 1983).

Absorption of ketoconazole is poor in patients with renal failure as indicated by levels measured in six patients on continuous ambulatory peritoneal dialysis (CAPD) (Chapman and Warnock, 1983). Reduced absorption has also been noted in bone marrow transplant recipients, neutropenic patients with hematological malignancies (Hann et al., 1982a; Stockley et al., 1986), as well as AIDS patients who have a high prevalence of gastric achlorhydria (Lake-Bakaar et al., 1988).

2 Patients with renal failure

Dosage adjustment is not necessary in patients with renal failure as the drug is excreted in the urine in only small amounts (Graybill and Drutz, 1980; Brass et al., 1982; Heel, 1982). The half-life of ketoconazole in patients undergoing hemodialysis was comparable with that of healthy volunteers (Brass et al., 1982). Clearance of ketoconazole by hemodialysis is small compared with hepatic clearance by metabolism (Brass et al., 1982). In patients with renal failure on CAPD, the serum half-life was 2.4 h and peritoneal clearance was less than 1 ml per min. The peritoneal penetration of ketoconazole was 3.4% of serum concentration at 5 h (Johnson et al., 1985).

3 Patients with liver disease

Preliminary studies on a few patients with mild liver dysfunction showed no significant change in serum levels compared with normal subjects (Heel, 1982), but one patient with hepatic insufficiency had persistently high ketoconazole serum levels (Brass et al., 1982). Because of the drug's potential to cause hepatotoxicity, it should be avoided in patients with liver disease.

4 Use in pregnancy

Ketoconazole crosses the placenta, is embryotoxic and teratogenic in rats. It should not be used in pregnant women unless expected benefits outweigh potential risks. Ketoconazole is excreted in human breast milk, and it has been estimated that infant exposure to ketoconazole from breast milk amounts to about 0.4% of that expected from therapeutic doses administered directly to the infant (Moretti et al., 1995).

Availability

Tablets: 200 mg.

Liquid shampoo: 20 mg per g ketoconazole and sodium chloride; 6 ml sachets, or 60 ml, 100 ml, bottles.

Cream: 2% ketoconazole in aqueous cream containing propylene glycol, stearyl and cetyl alcohols, sorbitan, monostearate, polysorbate 60, isopropyl myristate, sodium bisulfite, polysorbate 80 and water, 30 g.

Serum Levels in Relation to Dosage

There is wide intra- and inter-individual variation in serum levels following oral administration of the same dose of ketoconazole (Drouhet and Dupont, 1983). Some of the inter-individual variation may be due to factors which affect gastric acidity, as the dissolution of ketoconazole tablets and subsequent absorption is dependent on pH. Carlson et al. (1983) showed that ketoconazole tablets dissolve more rapidly and completely at pH of 2–3 (85% dissolution at 30 min), than pH of 6 (10% dissolution at 1 h). The bioavailability of oral ketoconazole is thus dependent on the pH of the gastric contents. Bioavailability of oral ketoconazole is 76% in healthy volunteers (Van Tyle, 1984)

When a 200-mg dose of ketoconazole is given to healthy subjects before breakfast, peak serum concentrations of 3.0–4.5 μg per ml are reached at 2 h. After a dose of 400 mg the peak serum level was about 7 μg per ml. (Heel, 1982). Similar mean peak levels of 3.6 μg per ml at 2 h after a 200-mg dose, and mean peak levels at 3 h of 6.5 μg per ml after a 400-mg dose, were obtained by Daneshmend *et al.* (1981, 1983).

Somewhat lower levels have been reported in other studies. Mean peak serum concentrations at 1–2 h for doses of 50, 100 and 200 mg were 1.0, 1.60 and 2.75 μg per ml, respectively, in a trial conducted by Brass *et al.* (1982). After a 200-mg dose, Graybill and Drutz (1980) described a 2 μg per ml peak at 2–4 h, which fell to 1 and <0.4 μg per ml, at 8 and 24 h, respectively. In patients with advanced malignancy, a 200-mg dose of ketoconazole resulted in levels of 1.7 at 2 h, 0.9 at 6 h and 0.7 μg per ml at 8 h. When this dose was continued every 6 h, serum concentrations rose after 3–4 days and remained consistently above 1 μg per ml (Maksymiuk *et al.*, 1982). Higher and more prolonged serum levels associated with an increased half-life value have also been observed on the fifth day compared with the first day when ketoconazole was given to volunteers in a dosage of 200 mg 12-hourly (Daneshmend *et al.*, 1983).

Higher serum levels result from higher oral doses, as can be seen in Table IV.9. Sugar *et al.* (1987) showed there was minimal benefit in administering ketoconazole in doses greater than 1200 mg daily, as there was no significant increase in serum concentrations beyond this dose. The pharmacokinetics of the drug are dose-dependent, i.e. the half-life and area-under-the-serum concentration-time-curve increase disproportionately with increasing dose both in single-dose studies (Daneshmend *et al.*, 1984; Huang *et al.*, 1986) and multiple-dose studies (Daneshmend *et al.*, 1983). The observation of dose-dependency has been attributed to the first-pass metabolism in the liver or the gastrointestinal tract which becomes saturable at the higher doses.

Table IV.9

Serum levels after single- and multiple-ketoconazole doses of 200–1200 mg. Compiled from Graybill and Drutz (1980), Brass *et al.* (1982), Craven *et al.* (1983), Huang *et al.* (1986), Stockley *et al.* (1986), Sugar *et al.* (1987).

Dose	Time to serum level measurement (h)	Serum concentration mean (range) μg per ml
200 mg single dose in normal volunteers	2	3.26
	8	0.34
	24	0.01
200 mg single dose in hematological malignancy	2	3.2 (0.4–5.5)
	12	<0.5
	24	undetectable
400 mg single dose in normal volunteers	2	9.6
	8	2.0
	24	0.03
400 mg single dose in hematological malignancy	2	4.6 (1.4–10.4)
	18	<0.5
	24	undetectable
400 mg chronic dosing	2	5.18
	8	4.45
	24	1.07
600 mg single dose	2	7.95 (3.4–14.0)
	24	0.14 (0.1–0.2)
800 mg single dose	2	20.9
	8	8.71
	24	0.21
800 mg chronic dosing	2	9.19
	8	7.10
	24	1.72
1200 mg single dose	4	15.6
	24	2.4
1200 mg chronic dosing	2	8.69
	8	11.58
	24	4.24

Serum levels of ketoconazole after initial stabilization, remain unchanged following daily administration for months (Drouhet and Dupont, 1983). Unlike clotrimazole, ketoconazole does not appear to induce hepatic microsomal enzymes to accelerate its own metabolism (Brass *et al.*, 1982).

The drug has been administered to children (2–12 years), either as a commercially prepared suspension (no longer available) or as crushed tablets in apple sauce. After a 5 mg per kg dose, mean peak serum levels were observed 1 and 2 h after administration by suspension and crushed tablets, respectively. Mean levels for the crushed tablets at 1, 2, 4 and 6 h were 2.3, 2.6, 0.99, and 0.46 µg per ml, respectively. Higher mean levels were obtained with the suspension with corresponding values of 4.4, 4.1, 1.7 and 0.8 µg per ml at the same time points (Ginsburg *et al.*, 1983). It has been suggested that mixing crushed ketoconazole with apple sauce may reduce its absorption (Daneshmend and Warnock, 1988). The administration of ketoconazole suspension 3 mg per kg three times daily did not produce therapeutic serum ketoconazole levels compared with 8–10 mg per kg administered once-daily in children (Bardare *et al.*, 1984). These authors suggested ketoconazole tablets given twice-daily produced lower peak serum concentrations but shorter periods of time during which the serum concentration of ketoconazole was less than 0.5 µg per ml, compared with once-daily dosing.

Stockley *et al.* (1986) showed a striking variation in ketoconazole pharmacokinetics in immunocompromised patients administered either 200 mg or 400 mg daily, and unlike previous pharmacokinetic studies revealed that the AUC and half-life increased proportionately with dose in this patient group. Importantly, they determined there was inadequate ketoconazole levels from 12 h after a 200-mg dose and 18 h after a 400-mg dose, suggesting that higher doses were needed in these patients with invasive fungal infections.

Serum concentrations of ketoconazole decline in a biexponential fashion after oral dosing. There is an initial rapid elimination phase with half-life values of 1.7 and 2.2 h following doses of 200 and 400 mg, respectively. This is followed by a slower phase which occurs at serum concentrations below 0.1 µg per ml which has half-life values of 8.1 and 9.6 h, following oral doses of 200 and 400 mg respectively (Daneshmend and Roberts, 1982; Heel, 1982).

Ketoconazole is rapidly absorbed from the gastrointestinal tract, and the bioavailability is influenced by gastric pH. Conflicting results concerning the influence of food on bioavailability have been reported, but the recommendation by the manufacturer is to administer the once-daily dose with food. In a study by Mannisto *et al.* (1982) absorption of ketoconazole was found to be decreased when it was ingested immediately after breakfast (low in fat content), and a non-significant effect of meals on the absorption of ketoconazole was demonstrated by Brass *et al.* (1982). Further studies of ketoconazole absorption were carried out by Daneshmend *et al.* (1984) over a wider single-dose range (200–800 mg) in the fasting state and at the end of a standard breakfast. They determined that food did not reduce absorption or alter peak serum concentrations, but did increase the time to achieve maximum serum concentrations. With 400- and 600-mg doses, food appeared to enhance absorption but this did not occur with 800-mg doses. Finally, Lelawongs *et al.* (1988) found that food (both high-fat and high-carbohydrate) significantly decreased the rate of absorption, and the type of food will affect the extent of absorption of 200 mg ketoconazole (reduced maximum concentration after a high-carbohydrate meal).

Sufficient gastric acidity is required for dissolution of the ketoconazole and the transformation of ketoconazole into a hydrochloride salt, and subsequent absorption (Van Tyle, 1984). A significant reduction in bioavailability of ketoconazole is associated with an increase in gastric pH. Concurrent cimetidine or ranitidine (H_2-receptor antagonists) administration resulted in a 95% reduction in AUC and a significant reduction in peak serum concentration of ketoconazole to 0.5–0.6 µg per ml in normal volunteers (Blum *et al.*, 1991; Piscitelli *et al.*, 1991). Concomitant administration of agents which reduce gastric secretion should be avoided. Antacids, anticholinergic drugs and histamine H_2-receptor blockers should not be given until at least 2 h after ketoconazole administration (Van der Meer *et al.*, 1980). Didanosine, which contains an alkaline buffer, also should be separated from ketoconazole dosing by 2 h (see p. 1720). To improve absorption in achlorhydric individuals, the 200-mg ketoconazole tablet can be dissolved in 4 ml of 0.2*N* hydrochloric acid solution and administered via a plastic straw to avoid contact with the teeth and damage to tooth enamel. A glass of water should be ingested directly after the ketoconazole solution. This approach did not improve absorption in healthy subjects and is generally unpalatable (Daneshmend and Warnock, 1988). Variable responses in enhancing ketoconazole absorption have been observed by the use of dilute hydrochloric acid (Lake-Bakaar *et al.*, 1988) and glutamic acid capsules, which are no longer commercially available (Lelawongs *et al.*, 1988). 'Coca-Cola Classic' with a pH of 2.5 was found to effectively increase the absorption of ketoconazole by 50%

in normal volunteers rendered achlorhydric by omeprazole, suggesting ketoconazole absorption may be enhanced in achlorhydric individuals by taking the medication with an acidic beverage. This strategy was not successful in 20% of volunteers (Chin *et al.*, 1995). Sugar *et al.* (1992) examined the ability of various beverages to disintegrate and dissolve ketoconazole tablets and determined the carbonated beverages were the most effective and orange juice the least effective. However, absorption of ketoconazole was not evaluated.

Co-administration of ketoconazole and sucralfate, which does not alter gastric acidity, was also associated with a 20% decrease in ketoconazole bioavailability, and it is recommended that ketoconazole is administered at least 2 h prior to sucralfate dosing (Piscitelli *et al.*, 1991, Carver *et al.*, 1994).

Systemic absorption of ketoconazole was evaluated following insertion of ketoconazole as a vaginal pessary. Negligible absorption was measured after intravaginal insertion of 400 mg, 800 mg, and 1200 mg ketoconazole, with area-under-the-plasma-concentration-time-curves of 0.27–0.52 mg per ml.h in healthy volunteers without vaginal infection (Ene *et al.*, 1984).

Excretion

1 Urine

About 13% of an administered dose is excreted in the urine, of which only 2–4% is in an unchanged form (Heel, 1982). In a chronic dosing study of 200 mg daily for 1–6 months. Badcock *et al.* (1987) measured the excretion of unchanged drug for 24 h after the last dose at a mean of 0.22% (range 0.02–0.49%). With high daily doses of 1200 mg, urine concentrations of 6 μg per ml may occur (Graybill and Craven, 1983).

2 Bile

Very little active ketoconazole is excreted by this route (Graybill and Drutz, 1980), however bile is the major route of excretion of the inactive metabolites of ketoconazole (Van Tyle, 1984)

3 Feces

This is the major route of excretion (about 57% of a dose), consisting of 20–65% of the unchanged drug and the rest as metabolites.

4 Inactivation in body

It has been suggested that ketoconazole undergoes first-pass metabolism, and that transient saturation of hepatic metabolizing capacity occurs. This would explain the disproportionate increase in serum levels seen with increasing doses (Van Tyle, 1984). In the liver, ketoconazole is extensively metabolized and the resultant metabolites have no antifungal activity. The major metabolic pathways are oxidation and degradation of the imidazole and piperazine rings, oxidative O-dealkylation and and aromatic hydroxylation of the phenyl ring (Heel,1982).

Distribution of the Drug in Body

Ketoconazole is 99% protein bound in whole blood, only 1% as free drug in plasma, 84% bound to plasma proteins and 15% bound to cell membranes and cell constituents of red blood cells (Heel, 1982).

After an oral dose of 200 mg, ketoconazole is detectable in saliva, sebum and cerumen (Heel, 1982). In human volunteers given 400 mg ketoconazole daily, palmar stratum corneum obtained after 7–14 days treatment contained up to 14 μg per g of ketoconazole. The drug appears in sweat within 1 h of administration and remains at similar concentrations of 0.014–0.323 μg per ml for 14 days. Eccrine sweat rapidly transports ketoconazole across the blood–skin barrier, where it binds to keratinocytes and surface lipids (Harris *et al.*, 1983). Ketoconazole persists in skin at therapeutic concentrations for up to 10 days after 200 mg daily for 10 days (Daneshmend and Warnock, 1988). Salivary concentrations of 2.43 and 0.3 μg per ml occur 1 and 2 h after a 200-mg dose, but thereafter it is undetectable, and peak salivary concentrations after a 400-mg dose were 0.12 μg per ml which became undetectable at 24 h (Brass *et al.*, 1982; Force and Nahata, 1995).

Tissue from an amputated finger of a child with coccidioidomycosis was assayed 2 h after administration of ketoconazole. Uninfected bone, soft tissue and infected bone had no detectable ketoconazole, but tendon had a concentration of 2.0 μg per g and infected skin 10.7 μg per g (Brass *et al.*, 1982). In contrast, ketoconazole concentration of 2.5 μg per g in a biopsy of bone has been reported (Drouhet and Dupont, 1983). There is limited penetration into joint fluid. Brass *et al.* (1982) detected concentrations of 0.06 and 1.04 μg per ml in joint fluid samples at 2 and 8 h, respectively, after a 200 mg dose. Peak and trough levels of 0.8 and < 0.4 μg per ml, respectively, were detected in synovial fluid of a patient receiving 400 mg ketoconazole daily (Fainstein *et al.*, 1982). Ketoconazole diffuses into aqueous and vitreous humors, with concentrations of 0.7 and 0.35 μg per ml following dosing with ketoconazole at 600 mg daily (O'Day *et al.*, 1985). Vitreous ketoconazole concentration 8 h after a 600-mg dose was 0.92 μg per ml, at 14 days treatment with 600 mg ketoconazole daily (Goodman and Stern, 1987). Peritoneal penetration is poor so that drug concentrations reached in dialysis fluid of patients undergoing CAPD are negligible (Chapman and Warnock, 1983).

Penetration of ketoconazole into the CSF after oral doses of 200 and 400 mg is poor. In three patients without meningeal inflammation, ketoconazole was undetectable in the CSF after 200 or 400 mg doses. In patients with inflamed meninges, CSF concentrations ranged from undetectable to 0.24 μg per ml after a 200-mg dose, and from undetectable to 0.85 μg per ml after 400 mg of ketoconazole. There appears to be no correlation between concomitant serum and CSF levels (Brass *et al.*, 1982) nor administered dose and CSF levels (Sugar *et al.*, 1987). Low CSF concentrations after a 400-mg dose were also reported by Jorgensen *et al.* (1981). Higher levels (2 μg per ml or more) were found in the CSF of a patient with *C. albicans* meningitis 4–8 h after receiving 400 mg twice-daily for 30 days (Fibbe *et al.*, 1980). In contrast to these disappointing results, better penetration into the lumbar and ventricular CSF, lasting for 8 h after administration, occurs in patients with coccidioidal meningitis given larger doses of ketoconazole. Mean ventricular fluid (from CSF reservoirs) and lumbar concentrations ranged from 0.05 to 1.65 μg per ml after a 800-mg and 1200-mg doses, with no drug detectable at 24 h. Lumbar CSF concentrations were higher than simultaneous ventricular levels. Calculations utilizing simultaneous serum level values indicated that the penetration of ketoconazole from serum into lumbar CSF (5.4%) was higher than penetration into ventricular CSF (1.9%). These CSF concentrations were dependent on serum concentrations and on CSF protein levels. In addition, lumbar: ventricular ratios of ketoconazole were not higher in patients with obstructive hydrocephalus (Craven *et al.*, 1983). In another study of high dose ketoconazole for coccidioidal meningitis, 113 of 168 CSF samples removed from 35 patients had no detectable ketoconazole. No patient receiving less than 1200 mg daily had ketoconazole detected in CSF within 12 h of administration of dose, 5.2% of those receiving 1200–1600 mg and 4.8% of those receiving >1600 mg daily had CSF levels >1 μg per ml (Sugar *et al.*, 1987).

Concentrations of ketoconazole in the urine are low and vary with the dose administered. They range from 0.25–1.15 μg per ml after 400 mg, 1.0–1.6 μg per ml after 600 mg, and 3.8–4.2 μg per ml after 800–1200 mg (Graybill *et al.*, 1983). Ketoconazole penetrates into vaginal tissue with concentrations proportional to concomitant serum levels (Heykants *et al.*, 1982), and penetrates poorly into seminal fluid (Daneshmend and Warnock, 1988).

Administration of a single dose of 2% ketoconazole cream produced 7- to 14-fold greater drug concentrations in the human stratum corneum than application of the same dose of 2% miconazole. The ketoconazole concentrations then decreased linearly over 8 h, and had consistently superior bioactivity per microgram of drug compared with topical miconazole (Pershing *et al.*, 1994). Ketoconazole is not absorbed appreciably systemically following topical application to skin.

Mode of Action

At low concentrations ketoconazole, similar to the other azole antifungal agents, has a fungistatic effect on susceptible fungi by inhibiting sterol synthesis in the cell membrane. It inhibits the 14 alpha-demethylation of lanosterol resulting in reduction in ergosterol synthesis (see Fig. IV.1, p. 1261). It differs from its antifungal analogs in that at higher concentrations it is not usually fungicidal to susceptible fungi. Ketoconazole can exert a fungicidal effect at very high concentrations, but such high levels are usually unattainable in tissues after oral dosing (Borgers *et al.*, 1983).

Ketoconazole at low concentrations has a potent effect in inhibiting pseudomycelium formation of *C. albicans*, and is 100-fold more potent than miconazole (Borgers *et al.*, 1979). This may be of clinical significance because pseudomycelial, rather than yeast forms of *C. albicans*, predominate in candidiasis. *In vitro* experiments suggest that ketoconazole may be synergistic with host defence cells against fungi (Borgers *et al.*, 1983), although Johnson *et al.* (1986) determined that ketoconazole had no effect on neutrophil phagocytosis or killing of *C. albicans*.

Ketoconazole has also been shown to competitively inhibit calmodulin activity at concentrations in the micromolar range and this may contribute to the efficacy of ketoconazole in the treatment of inflammatory skin diseases (Hegeman *et al.*, 1993).

Ketoconazole may inhibit thromboxane synthetase resulting in decreased thromboxane B2 levels. This has been observed in two studies in which ketoconazole appeared to effectively prevent acute respiratory distress syndrome in surgical patients at risk of this complication (Frazee and Neidig, 1995).

Toxicity

Ketoconazole is a drug of comparatively low toxicity. Gastrointestinal and endocrinological toxicity appears to be dose-related and reversible. The maximum tolerable dose of ketoconazole is 800 mg per day (Sugar *et al.*, 1987).

1 Gastrointestinal side-effects

The most frequent adverse effects are nausea and vomiting. Reported prevalence of gastrointestinal side-effects vary from 3% (Heel, 1982) to 20–43% (De Felice *et al.*, 1982; Dismukes *et al.*, 1983; Graybill and Craven, 1983; Sugar *et al.*, 1987). In some instances, nausea has been reduced by giving the drug with meals (Symoens *et al.*, 1980). Nausea occurred in six of 23 patients given a higher dose of 200 mg 6-hourly (Maksymiuk *et al.*, 1982). Often nausea and vomiting resolve spontaneously without discontinuing therapy. Abdominal pain, anorexia, diarrhea, flatulence and discoloration of the tongue have been reported. Ketoconazole appears to be well tolerated in children (Heel, 1982).

2 Hepatotoxicity

Abnormalities of liver function tests have been reported commonly during ketoconazole therapy (Petersen *et al.*, 1980; Firebrace, 1981; Heiberg and Svejgaard, 1981; Macnair *et al.*, 1981; Catanzaro *et al.*, 1982; De Felice *et al.*, 1982; Drouhet and Dupont, 1983; Horsburgh and Kirkpatrick, 1983). These abnormalities do not appear to correlate with daily dose, cumulative dose of ketoconazole or duration of treatment (Dismukes *et al.*, 1983; Graybill and Craven, 1983; Stricker *et al.*, 1986). The hepatic reaction appears to be idiosyncratic, usually without any evidence of hypersensitivity.

Hepatic reactions reported during ketoconazole therapy have been reviewed by Janssen and Symoens (1983), Lewis *et al.* (1984) and Lake-Bakaar *et al.* (1987). These reviews established that transient, asymptomatic and reversible elevations of serum transaminases or alkaline phosphatase may occur at any time during ketoconazole treatment, and occur in 5–10% of patients. The incidence of symptomatic, potentially serious hepatitis is about 1 in 12 000–15 000 in individuals receiving ketoconazole. Ketoconazole-induced hepatitis appears to be more common in women over 40 years of age, and occurrs mainly during the first few months of treatment, but is rare during the first 7–10 days of treatment. Hepatic reactions have also been reported in children. Acute hepatocellular injury occured in just over half of those with hepatic reactions, primarily cholestatic abnormalities were noted in 15% and the remainder had a mixed pattern. Recovery from symptomatic ketoconazole-induced hepatitis can take from 1 week to 6 months after cessation of the drug, and liver function test abnormalities may become more pronounced in the first 2 weeks after stopping ketoconazole in some cases. There are several reports of both fatal and non-fatal fulminant hepatitis in patients with symptomatic hepatic reactions who continued taking ketoconazole (Lewis *et al.*,1984; Duarte *et al.*, 1984; Svedhem, 1984; Bercoff *et al.*, 1985). In addition, liver transplantation was required in a case of ketoconazole-induced fulminant hepatitis (Knight *et al.*, 1991). Another case of prolonged jaundice following ketoconazole-induced injury required prednisolone for resolution of jaundice (Benson *et al.*, 1988). The role of corticosteroid treatment in drug-induced hepatic injury is not well established. Recurrent liver damage can occur with rechallenge with ketoconazole (Van Parys *et al.*, 1987).

Liver function tests should be performed before starting treatment with ketoconazsole to exclude asymptomatic hepatitis. Liver function tests should be repeated after 10 days of treatment, then every 2 weeks of ongoing therapy with ketoconazole. Therapy should be discontinued if hepatic abnormalities are detected and the patient develops any symptoms of hepatitis, or the serum transaminases increase significantly (>3-fold) above normal (Lake-Bakaar, 1987). Whether therapy should be continued in the presence of asymptomatic, mildly abnormal liver function tests depends on assessment of the severity of the hepatic reaction and assessment of requirement for ketoconazole treatment for the fungal infection. Any liver function test abnormality should alert the physician that frequent monitoring of the patient for continued rise in the hepatic enzymes is required.

3 Endocrine effects

Ketoconazole interferes with the cytochrome P-450 enzyme system in the testis, ovary, and adrenal gland and has a greater effect on testosterone secretion than cortisol secretion. The hormonal changes appear to be dose-dependent (Sonino, 1987). It blocks testosterone synthesis with significant decreases in total and free testosterone levels after a single dose of 200 mg (Graybill and Craven, 1983; Grosso et al., 1983; Pont et al., 1983, 1984). There is only a transient block of testosterone synthesis (<24 h) when daily doses of 200–400 mg are used. Reduced serum and salivary testosterone levels on a long-term basis result in end-organ effects with daily doses of 400 mg or more (Schurmeyer and Nieschlag, 1982; Graybill and Craven, 1983). Males often develop tender gynecomastia at these doses (De Felice et al., 1981; Catanzaro et al., 1982; Dismukes et al., 1983; Stevens et al., 1983) as well as decreased libido, oligospermia, and loss of hair. High daily doses of ketoconazole (800–1200 mg) cause more prolonged blockage of testosterone synthesis, and with prolonged therapy, gynecomastia is more common than with lower doses, (21% in those receiving >400 mg daily) and azospermia and impotence can occur (Pont et al., 1984; Sugar et al., 1987). In one study, gynecomastia appeared within 6 months of the onset of treatment in the majority of patients, but can develop up to 32 months after the onset of treatment. It can persist for up to 12 months (Sugar et al., 1987). These effects seem reversible on cessation of treatment. The effect on testosterone synthesis appears to correlate with the ketoconazole serum level (Pont et al., 1984). Elevated pretreatment serum testosterone levels in three women with acne fell to the normal range after 3 months of treatment with ketoconazole 300 mg twice-daily (Ghetti et al., 1986). A raised estradiol:testosterone serum ratio was demonstrated in volunteers receiving ketoconazole and in patients receiving long-term therapy (Pont et al., 1985). The ability of ketoconazole to interfere with both gonadal and adrenal synthesis of androgens has been utilized in the treatment of progressive prostate cancer (Allen et al., 1983; Trachtenberg and Pont, 1984), precocious puberty in boys (Holland et al., 1985) and hirsutism (Carvalho et al., 1985). Ketoconazole is generally not used as the sole treatment in prostate cancer, because decreases in serum testosterone are not sustained, and the gastrointestinal side-effects, gynecomastia and impotence are poorly tolerated (Sonino, 1987).

In five of 20 female patients with blastomycosis, who were treated with an oral ketoconazole dose of 400 mg daily, menses which were otherwise normal occurred more frequently. This resolved spontaneously in three women and resolution occurred in the other two when the dosage was reduced to 200 mg daily. Serum estrogen and progesterone levels measured in four of the women were normal and the mechanism of this apparent side-effect is not clear (Bradsher et al., 1985).

Ketoconazole transiently blocks cortisol secretion and the adrenal response to corticotrophin is blunted in patients receiving 800–1200 mg daily (Pont et al., 1984). Despite the observation that some patients have greatly reduced serum cortisol values throughout the day, basal cortisol levels are generally not affected and clinical features of hypoadrenalism are rarely seen in patients receiving high daily doses of ketoconazole for the treatment of fungal infection (Graybill and Craven, 1983; Pont et al., 1984). However, White and Kendall-Taylor (1985), using ketoconazole in a daily dose of 1200 mg to treat patients with prostate cancer, described persistent anorexia and malaise in five patients associated with a blunted cortisol response, within 2 days of starting treatment, and hyperpigmentation in one patient after 3 months treatment. Pillans et al. (1985) also described a patient with prostate cancer who developed hyponatremia and confusion when treated by ketoconazole in a dose of 600 mg daily for 2.5 months. Adrenal insufficiency developed in the third week of treatment with ketoconazole 800 mg daily for pulmonary blastomycosis, and these symptoms completely resolved within days of cessation of the drug (Tucker et al., 1985). The frequency with which relative corticosteroid deficiency occurs in high-dose ketoconazole therapy is yet to be determined.

Ketoconazole has been used successfully for control of hypercortisolism in patients with Cushing's syndrome, adrenal adenomas and adrenal carcinomas (Sonino, 1987). Angeli and Frairia (1985) described clinical and biochemical improvement in women with Cushing's disease, given long-term daily (600–800 mg) ketoconazole treatment. Contreras et al. (1985) reported regression of metastatic adrenal carcinoma associated with a fall in serum cortisol level and clinical improvement following treatment with a daily dose of ketoconazole varying from 600 to 1200 mg depending on the patient's tolerance. It has also produced symptomatic improvement in a patient with ectopic adrenocorticotropin production from a small cell carcinoma of the lung (Shepherd et al., 1985).

Ketoconazole has also been shown to inhibit renal production of 1,25-dihydroxyvitamin D in vitro, reduce serum levels of 1,25-dihydroxyvitamin D in normal volunteers, patients with hyperparathyroidism, and decrease elevated 1,25-dihydroxyvitamin D levels in patients with sarcoidosis. However, the effect on serum hypercalcemia has varied from none to 15% decrease in calcium levels (Glass *et al.*, 1990, Adams *et al.*, 1990).

4 Miscellaneous side-effects

A great variety of other side-effects have been reported in association with ketoconazole therapy, but none seem to be common. These include pruritus, rash, (in 5–6%), headache, photophobia, dizziness, fatigue, arthralgia, myalgia, paresthesiae, tinnitus, fever and chills, insomnia, abnormal dreams, and somnolence (Heel, 1982; Sugar *et al.*, 1987). Bilateral papilloedema has been reported to develop in a woman who received ketoconazole 800 mg daily for 4 months, and then resolved on cessation of the drug (Or *et al.*, 1993).

Severe photosensitive dermatitis (Mohamed, 1988) and a fixed drug eruption induced by ketoconazole have been described (Bharija and Belhaj, 1988). A rash consistent with a drug eruption developed within 24 h of a single 200-mg dose of ketoconazole, which resolved with steroids over 1 week (Kahana *et al.*, 1984). Another patient developed a hypersensitivity reaction of generalized urticaria and facial angioedema after the first dose of ketoconazole (Gonzalez-Delgado *et al.*, 1994). Anaphylactic reactions occurred in two patients shortly after taking the first tablet of ketoconazole, and one may have been previously sensitized to the imidazole drugs by topical miconazole (Van Dijke *et al.*, 1983). Contact dermatitis from ketoconazole cream in two patients was reported by Santucci *et al.* (1992). Less than 5% patients using ketoconazole cream complain of local adverse reactions including pruritus, local irritation and stinging. Hair loss, dry skin, scalp pustules, pruritus have all been described in association with the use of ketoconazole shampoo.

5 Biochemical changes

In addition to the effects on testosterone and cortisol synthesis, ketoconazole has been shown to be a potent inhibitor of cholesterol synthesis. Transient lowering of serum cholesterol levels has been observed, and thought to be due to the inhibition of 14 alpha-demthylation of lanosterol by ketoconazole (Catanzaro *et al.*, 1982; Miettinen and Valtonen, 1984). High-dose ketoconazole caused a 30% reduction in total cholesterol levels in men with prostate cancer (Kraemer and Pont, 1986). After treatment with ketoconazole for several months, serum triglyceride levels may become elevated, and this is more common with daily doses above 200 mg (Catanzaro *et al.*, 1982; Dismukes *et al.*, 1983).

6 Hematological side-effects

Hemolytic anemia, leukopenia and thrombocytopenia have all been reported rarely. Transient mild leukopenia has been noted in a small number of patients (Catanzaro *et al.*, 1982). Ketoconazole can cause suppression of granulocyte progenitor cells in tissue culture. An immune-mediated hemolytic anemia was reported in a previously healthy 42-year-old man after a 3-week course of ketoconazole 200 mg daily (Umstead *et al.*, 1987).

7 Effects on the immune system

No immunotoxic effects of ketoconazole on neutrophil function were detected by Marmer *et al.* (1981). Others have shown that ketoconazole can increase neutrophil chemotaxis, without compromising other cellular and humoral immune functions, except a slight inhibition of lymphocyte transformation (Van Rensburg *et al.*, 1983; Manzell and Clark, 1984; Roilides *et al.*, 1990). The clinical significance of laboratory experiments which show that ketoconazole can inhibit various metabolic aspects of human lymphocyte function is unknown (Alford and Cartwright, 1983; Buttke and Chapman, 1983). Ketoconazole may be synergistic with host cells against fungi resulting in increased fungicidal activity (Roilides *et al.*, 1990).

8 Interaction with other drugs

The mechanism postulated for the drug interactions between ketoconazole and other drugs is inhibition or activation of the mixed-function oxidase system activity of hepatic microsomal enzymes through the P-450 system. Ketoconazole decreases the total clearance and significantly prolongs the half-life of antipyrine in normal volunteers (D'Mello *et al.*, 1985). Co-administration of ketoconazole with cyclosporine can cause dramatic increases in serum cyclosporine levels, due to inhibition of metabolism of the drug. Elevated cyclosporine levels result in renal insufficiency with increased serum creatinine levels. After discontinuation of ketoconazole the creatinine and cyclosporine levels return to baseline (Dieperink and Moller, 1982; Ferguson *et al.*, 1982; Morgenstern *et al.*, 1982, Cunningham *et al.*, 1982; Daneshmend, 1982). Ketoconazole inhibits cyclosporin hydroxylase and the potent inhibition of cyclosporine metabolism by human liver microsomes has been confirmed *in vitro* (Back and Tjia, 1991). Gomez *et al.* (1995), determined that the increase in cyclosporine biovailability was due to inhibition of both gastrointestinal and hepatic cytochrome P-450 enzymes. Many transplant units (renal, heart, and bone marrow) have utilized the drug interaction between ketoconazole and cyclosporine, to reduce the dose (and cost) of cyclosporine required to maintain therapeutic concentrations and reduce cyclosporin toxicity (Schroeder *et al.*, 1987; Charles *et al.*, 1989; First *et al.*, 1991, 1993; Butman *et al.*, 1991). The ketoconazole-cyclosporine combination has been used for almost 4 years in a heart transplant patient, and some investigators recommend a reduction in ketoconazole dose by 50% (Girardet *et al.*, 1989).

Serum ketoconazole levels in a patient who received rifampicin, isoniazid and ketoconazole for 5 months were reduced 10-fold compared with levels obtained before the antituberculous drugs were initiated. This suggests that rifampicin can induce more rapid metabolism of ketoconazole (Brass *et al.*, 1982). When either rifampicin or isoniazid was added to treatment with ketoconazole, ketoconazole serum concentrations decreased by 70%, irrespective of whether the drugs were taken concurrently or 12 h apart. Moreover, serum concentrations of rifampicin were undetectable when the drug was given simultaneously with isoniazid and ketoconazole. Rifampicin concentrations were approximately halved when ketoconazole was given concurrently with rifampicin, but they were virtually unchanged if rifampicin was given 12 h after ketoconazole (Engelhard *et al.*,1984; Doble *et al.*, 1985). This drug interaction, when unrecognized has led to treatment failures of tuberculosis and blastomycosis (Engelhard *et al.*, 1984; Abadie-Kemmerly *et al.*, 1988). Doble *et al.* (1988) evaluated the interaction of rifampicin and ketoconazole in male volunteers, and found a 65% reduction in peak serum ketoconazole concentrations and 81% reduction in AUC when the drugs were taken simultaneously. Unlike other reports they found no effect on rifampicin levels. It is recommended that serum antibiotic levels are regularly monitored in those patients receiving both antituberculous medication and ketoconazole.

Ketoconazole reduces the clearance of methylprednisolone by about 50%, and oral prednisolone by 25%. The decrease in methylprednisolone clearance results in an additional cortisol suppressive effect, so the dose of methylprednisolone should be halved if co-administered with ketoconazole (Kandrotoas *et al.*, 1987). Although ketoconazole appears to reduce both the metabolic and renal clearance of prednisolone, there is a negligible effect on adrenal suppression, and therefore no clinical significance from the interaction is likely to occur (Zurcher *et al.*, 1989; Ludwig *et al.*, 1989; Yamashita *et al.*, 1991).

As discussed above (p. 1364), antacids, sucralfate and histamine H_2-receptor blockers (cimetidine, ranitidine) interfere with the absorption of ketoconazole and should be administered at least 2 h after the ketoconazole dose. Some authors recommend that ketoconazole be replaced by another antifungal agent if the patient has achlorhydria, or is receiving an agent that raises gastric pH, as the bioavailability of ketoconazole is dependent on gastric acidity (Blum *et al.*, 1991).

The effect on aminophylline pharmacokinetics was evaluated before and after 7 days of ketoconazole in normal volunteers. These authors suggested that no dosage adjustment for theophylline is necessary when concomitantly administered with ketoconazole, because of the lack of significant effect on clearance and half-life of theophylline (Heusner *et al.*, 1987). However, a potential drug interaction between theophylline and ketoconazole has been described in asthma patients in whom a 50% reduction in serum theophylline concentrations was noted after concomitant administration with ketoconazole, as well as a corresponding reduction in peak expiratory flow rate (Murphy *et al.*, 1987). Phenytoin appears to cause a significant reduction in the AUC for ketoconazole, so that double the dose of ketoconazole may be required for therapeutic effect (Brass *et al.*, 1982).

A disulfiram reaction (flushing, rash, nausea and headache) has been described in a patient who ingested alcohol while taking ketoconazole. The reaction occurred each time the woman consumed alcohol in the 14-day course (Magnasco and Magnasco, 1986). This is rarely reported, however.

In a limited study of two healthy volunteers, ketoconazole did not appear to potentiate the action of coumarin anticoagulant drugs (Brass *et al.*, 1982). However, potentiation of warfarin effect has been documented in at least one patient with an increase in anticoagulant effect of 3-fold. When ketoconazole was ceased the warfarin dose requirement returned to baseline in 3 weeks (Smith, 1984).

Ketoconazole inhibits the metabolism of terfenadine (a non-sedating antihistamine) which normally undergoes extensive first-pass metabolism to two metabolites. When these drugs are co-administered, the resulting high plasma levels of unchanged terfenadine cause a prolongation of the QT interval on the electrocardiogram (Matthews *et al.*, 1991). Prolongation of the QT interval is associated with a form of ventricular tachycardia called Torsades de Pointes, which requires different therapy to other forms of ventricular tachycardia. This syndrome has been reported in patients receiving both ketoconazole and terfenadine (Monahan *et al.*, 1990) and the electrocardiographic repolarization abnormalities confirmed in a study by Honig *et al.* (1993). Although ketoconazole causes a significant increase in peak plasma loratidine levels as well as an increase in plasma levels of the active metabolite of loratidine, no changes in the QT interval have been reported. The co-administration of ketoconazole and the non-sedating antihistamines (terfenadine and astemizole) is contraindicated. Torsades de Pointes and prolonged QT interval has also been reported after the concomitant administration of ketoconazole and cisapride. This combination is also contraindicated.

Ketoconazole appears to inhibit the glucuronidation of zidovudine in *in vitro* human liver microsomes to a minor extent, but is unlikely to cause any clinically significant effects (Sampol *et al.*, 1995).

Clinical Uses of the Drug

1 Dermatophyte infections

Ketoconazole is effective for the treatment of skin infections due to dermatophytes such as *Trichoplyton rubrum*, *T. mentagrophytes*, *T. tonsurans*, *Epidermophyton floccosum* and *Microsporum canis* (Heel, 1982; Heel *et al.*, 1982; Hay, 1983). Usually a daily dose of 200 mg has been used and most patients respond within 8 weeks (median time 4 weeks). Some trials have indicated that ketoconazole treatment results in more remissions and fewer relapses than treatment with griseofulvin. Comparative studies show that it has no clinical advantages over griseofulvin except in resistant cases (Hay *et al.*, 1985; Martinez-Roig *et al.*, 1988). In a randomized study comparing ketoconazole 200 mg daily and griseofulvin 250 mg for the treatment of tinea capitis in children aged 2–16 years, there was a trend to improved outcome for griseofulvin but no significant difference in the efficacy of the two treatments (73% versus 96%), but the time to culture negativity was greater for ketoconazole. It was also apparent from this study and others that the duration of therapy should be 12 weeks (Tanz *et al.*, 1988; Gan *et al.*, 1987). Patients with dermatophyte infections resistant to griseofulvin *in vitro* have responded to ketoconazole therapy (Robertson *et al.*, 1980). Segal *et al.* (1993) evaluated the efficacy of ketoconazole 400 mg given once-weekly for superficial fungal infections, and reported cure rates of 70% for tinea corporis, tinea cruris, and cutaneous candidiasis and 26% for tinea pedis. These results are comparable with studies reporting the efficacy of daily ketoconazole therapy, except the inferior results obtained for tinea pedis.

Despite this efficacy of ketoconazole against dermatophyte skin infections, it is preferable to use topical treatment for mild tinea corporis, tinea cruris (excluding scrotal involvement) or mild tinea pedis (Cohen, 1982). Topical imidazoles have the advantage of being effective against yeast infections. For extensive tinea and infections of the face, hair, nails and genital region, systemic therapy is preferred. Terbinafine is probably the drug of choice for this indication.

Ketoconazole is effective for some cases of onychomycosis due to *Trichophyton* spp. and *M. canis*; but response takes longer with a median time of 20–25 weeks. Once-weekly treatment with 400 mg ketoconazole gave disappointing results for onychomycosis, with no patients cured after a mean 36 weeks, but improvement noted in 43% of treated patients (Segal *et al.*, 1993). Nail infections unresponsive to griseofulvin have also responded, including some due to *T. rubrum* strains resistant to griseofulvin *in vitro*. Amorolfine is an effective alternative.

Ketoconazole is effective for the treatment of pityriasis versicolor. A single oral dose of 400 mg successfully clears 98% of patients after 4 weeks (Borelli, 1980; Rausch and Jacobs, 1984; Borelli *et al.*, 1991). Ketoconazole is a more convenient form of treatment for this infection than the topical use of agents such as 1% selenium sulfide, topical imidazoles, haloprogin and ciclopirox olamine, especially when the entire body is affected. Topical therapies are associated with a high relapse rate of 60–80% (Faergemann and Fredriksson, 1982). A controlled trial (terminated because of the risk of hepatotoxicity from ketoconazole) indicated that oral ketoconazole 400 mg daily for 1 month is effective in the treatment of scalp psoriasis (Farr *et al.*, 1985). Seborrheic dermatitis is thought to be caused by pityrosporum yeasts, and placebo-controlled trials of ketoconazole 2% shampoo have shown it to be an effective alternative to oral ketoconazole for scalp involvement (74% response rate) (Carr *et al.*, 1987). Ketoconazole 1% and 2% shampoo has been evaluated in controlled trials for the control of dandruff and response rates of 80–88% have been noted when used twice-weekly for 4 weeks

Peter and Richarz-Barthauer, 1995).The shampoo is massaged into the scalp and left for 3–5 minutes before rinsing with warm water (Cauwenbergh *et al.*, 1986, Go *et al.*, 1992). Relapse of symptomatic dandruff occurs within 1–3 weeks. In addition, ketoconazole 2% cream is an effective topical alternative for the treatment of seborrheic dermatitis of the face and trunk (Green *et al.*, 1987).

Ketoconazole 2% cream applied topically twice-daily was effective for the treatment of 'neonatal acne' (caused by *Malassezia furfur*). The erythema and papulopustules resolved in 1 week (Rapelanoro *et al.*, 1996).

2 Candidiasis

a Superficial infections Ketoconazole is effective for the treatment of cutaneous, oral and vaginal yeast infections (Heel, 1982; Heel *et al.*, 1982). Yeast infections of the skin tend to respond slightly more rapidly than those due to dermatophytes. Oral ketoconazole 200 mg daily was equally effective as topical econazole 2 ml four times daily for the treatment of chronic paronychia, and may be used for cases unresponsive to topical treatments (Wong *et al.*, 1984).

b Oropharyngeal and esophageal infections Doses of 200 mg for adults and 20 mg three times daily for children were successful for the treatment of a small number of patients with oral thrush, the median time to response being 1 week. Ketoconazole in a dose of 600 mg per day has proved effective in the treatment of thrush in non-neutropenic cancer patients (Meunier-Carpentier, 1983). A controlled study in which the drug was given in a dosage of 200 mg per m^2 of body surface daily for 14 days confirmed its efficacy for oral candidiasis in cancer patients, but clinical regression of lesions was only achieved in 72% of patients and eradication of culturable organisms in 36% (Hughes *et al.*, 1983). A randomized, double-blind study of ketoconazole 400 mg daily and fluconazole 100 mg daily for a median duration of 14 days in cancer patients with oropharyngeal candidiasis, revealed a 75% cure rate for both groups and an earlier time to relapse for ketoconazole-treated patients (Meunier, 1990).

De Wit *et al.* (1989) performed a randomized, double-blind study of oral fluconazole 50 mg daily and ketoconazole 200 mg daily for treatment of oropharyngeal candidiasis in HIV infection, and found fluconazole was more effective than ketoconazole (100% versus 75% response rate). Comparable efficacy between ketoconazole (7 mg per kg per day) and fluconazole (3 mg per kg per day) was reported in an open study of the treatment of oropharyngeal candidiasis in HIV-infected children. Higher clinical and mycological response rates were noted for fluconazole, and high rates of relapse following cessation of treatment were noted for both treatment groups (Hernandez-Sampelayo, 1994). In a randomized, controlled study of fluconazole 100 mg daily and ketoconazole 200 mg daily for esophageal candidiasis in patients with AIDS, fluconazole was significantly more effective than ketoconazole with endoscopic cure rates of 91% and 52%, and clinical sure rates of 85% and 65% respectively (Laine *et al.*, 1992). In contrast, Barchiesi *et al.* (1992) found no difference in efficacy of ketoconazole and fluconazole for oropharyngeal or esophageal candidiasis in AIDS patients. Ketoconazole 200 mg twice-daily for 4 weeks was found to be equivalent to itraconazole 200 mg daily for treatment of esophageal candidiasis in HIV-infected patients with 100% and 92% clinical resolution respectively (Smith *et al.*, 1991). Experience with six patients with AIDS, suggested that *Candida* esophagitis may not completely resolve with up to 6 months ketoconazole therapy, even though clinical symptoms abate after 5 days therapy. Resistance to ketoconazole was documented in two of the six treatment failures (Tavitian *et al.*, 1986). Fluconazole is preferred as initial treatment of oropharyngeal or esophageal candidiasis because of the high prevalence of gastric achlorhydria in HIV-infected patients. Chronic suppressive therapy is often recommended because of the high rate of relapse.

c Vaginal infections Various dosage schedules have been used to treat vaginal *Candida* infections. A dose of 200 mg once-daily for 6 days or twice-daily for 5 days appears to be effective. Topical treatment of superficial *Candida* infections with drugs, such as nystatin, amphotericin B, natamycin and other imidazole drugs (clotrimazole, econazole or miconazole) is successful in 85–90% of women. Bingham (1984) compared clotrimazole and ketoconazole in the treatment of vaginal candidiasis. Ketoconazole given orally 200 mg twice-daily for 5 days was as effective as clotrimazole 100 mg vaginal tablets inserted vaginally for 6 consecutive nights with the application of 1% clotrimazole cream to the vulval and perianal areas. However, there was a patient preference for oral treatment. Single-dose fluconazole 150 mg was also found to be as effective as ketoconazole 200 mg twice-daily for 5 days for vaginal candidiaisis. Clinical responses of 92% and 89% at short-term follow-up and similar relapse rates of 4–8% were noted (Kutzer *et al.*, 1988). Recurrent vulvovaginal candidiasis occurs in a small subset of women, and recurrent episodes can be prevented by treatment with cyclical ketoconazole (400 mg daily for 5 days at the onset of menses) or low-dose continuous ketoconazole 100 mg daily, which was significantly more effective in a prospective controlled trial (29% recurrence rate for cyclical ketoconazole versus 5% for low-dose continuous ketoconazole). Relapse remains common after withdrawl of treatment at 6 months (Sobel, 1986), and is not related to the development of resistance (Fong *et al.*, 1993). Concern over potential hepatotoxicity associated with ketoconazole use has led to the evaluation of fluconazole regimens for persistent or recurrent vulvovaginal candidiasis (Sobel, 1992).

d Chronic mucocutaneous candidiasis Many studies have confirmed the efficacy of ketoconazole in this disease (Heel *et al.*, 1982; Graybill *et al.*, 1980b). The drug has the added benefit of being effective against co-existent dermatophytosis, which is common in chronic mucocutaneous candidiasis (Horsburgh and Kirkpatrick, 1983). Usually ketoconazole has been prescribed in a dose of 200 mg daily for adults and in a median dose of 6.7 mg per kg per day, for children. Mucosal lesions usually healed within days to 2 months, skin lesions within 2 months, paronychiae within 3–4 months, while nail lesions took 4–14 months to resolve (Rosenblatt *et al.*, 1980; Graybill and Craven, 1983; Mobacken and Moberg, 1986).

e Prevention of systemic candidiasis in patients with hematological disorders Variable results have been obtained when ketoconazole has been used to prevent fungal colonization and infection in neutropenic patients with leukemia. Some failures may have been due to poor gastric absorption of the drug associated with antineoplastic chemotherapy and gastric achlorhydria. Higher doses (400 mg daily) have been efficacious in preventing fungal infections without affecting colonization rates with *C. albicans* (Young, 1982). Amphotericin B and ketoconazole both reduce the yield of *C. albicans* from surveillance stool, skin, urine and throat cultures of neutropenic patients (Meunier-Carpentier, 1984).

A trial comparing antifungal prophylaxis with oral ketoconazole (adults 400 mg and children 200 mg daily) and prophylaxis with oral amphotericin B and nystatin was carried out by Hann *et al.* (1982b). Patients with underlying hematological disease who developed neutropenia following induction therapy received non-absorbable antibiotics (neomycin and colistin), skin antisepsis, sterile food and oral co-trimoxazole. Protection against fungal infection was significantly superior in ketoconazole-treated patients. A similar comparison was made in patients who had received allogenic bone marrow transplants, and acute leukemic patients, but there was no significant difference between treatment groups in these patients (Donnelly *et al.*, 1984). Jones *et al.* (1984) showed that oral ketoconazole (200 mg daily) was more effective and better tolerated than oral nystatin (500 000 units four times daily) in reducing mucosal yeast infections in neutropenic patients. Shepp *et al.* (1985) compared ketoconazole (400 mg daily) and nystatin (3 million units four times daily) in the prevention of fungal infection in neutropenic patients undergoing bone marrow transplantation in a protective environment. Ketoconazole was better tolerated and more effective in reducing colonization due to *Candida* spp., but was associated with increased rates of colonization with *C. glabrata* in the rectum and vagina. However, ketoconazole did not significantly reduce the number of local mucosal infections.

Another placebo-controlled study of ketoconazole 400 mg daily for the prevention of fungal infections in cancer patients, showed it was effective in reducing the incidence of oral candidiasis, but did not appear to prevent esophagitis or vaginitis, reduce the number of febrile days or the requirement for amphotericin B (Hansen *et al.*, 1987). In the critical care surgical or trauma setting, the routine use of prophylactic ketoconazole was not associated with a significant reduction in yeast colonization or sepsis, when compared with placebo, clotrimazole or nystatin in one study (Savino *et al.*, 1994), but was found to be effective in another (Slotman and Burchard, 1987). There are problems in assessing the results of antifungal therapy in the prevention of candidiasis and no regimen has been uniformly accepted as effective (Meunier-Carpentier, 1984). With the introduction of fluconazole and itraconazole, the role of ketoconazole in antifungal prophylaxis in neutropenic patients has diminished (Working Party of the British Society for Antimicrobial Chemotherapy, 1993).

Walsh *et al.* (1991) compared high-dose ketoconazole (800 mg daily) with i.v. amphotericin B (0.5 mg per kg per day) for empiric antifungal therapy in persistently or recurrently febrile neutropenic cancer patients. Although there was no significant difference in the number of febrile days or the number of proven fungal infections, ketoconazole was inferior to amphotericin B for treatment of proven fungal infections. In addition, 20% patients were unable to swallow oral medication, and another 10% had refractory nausea. Another study compared ketoconazole 200 mg every 6 h with amphotericin B 1 mg per kg daily as empiric treatment of presumed or proven fungal infections in neutropenic cancer patients. There was no difference in response for either documented or presumed fungal infection, except for documented infection with *C. tropicalis* which did not respond to ketoconazole (Fainstein *et al.*, 1987).

f Systemic candidiasis A combination of amphotericin B and flucytosine is the preferred treatment for this infection (Graybill and Craven, 1983). Its use has resulted in improvement in *Candida* esophagitis, biliary candidiasis, musculoskeletal candidiasis and *Candida* fungemia (Heel *et al.*, 1982). The use of ketoconazole for *Candida* urinary tract infections is limited, because only a small amount of drug is excreted in the urine. Clinical experience with ketoconazole 200–400 mg daily for urinary tract infections reveal a 50% eradication rate. The drug is not useful for urinary tract infections due to *C. glabrata* (Wong-Beringer *et al.*, 1992; Gubbins *et al.*, 1993). An HIV-infected man with *C. albicans* epididymitis was successfully treated with ketoconazole 200 mg daily for 6 weeks (Swartz *et al.*, 1988).

Arthritis due to *C. tropicalis* in a cancer patient has responded to ketoconazole therapy (Fainstein *et al.*, 1982). *Candida* fungemia occurred in a woman following cesarean section, and responded to daily doses of 400–600 mg ketoconazole (Drouhet and Dupont, 1983). These authors also described encouraging results for the treatment of systemic candidiasis in i.v. drug users, with 15 of 18 patients with cutaneous involvement, six of six cases with ocular involvement and four of seven with osteoarticular involvement responding to ketoconazole. Systemic *Candida* infections which occur in i.v. drug users are different to the more fulminating infections seen in neutropenic patients with leukemia. Ketoconazole is not of proven therapeutic value in the latter (Graybill, 1983; Fainstein *et al.*, 1987). Short courses of i.v. miconazole followed by oral ketoconazole have been used successfully to treat three neonatal patients with systemic candidiasis (Tudehope and Rigby, 1983). The combination of ketoconazole and flucytosine eradicated *Candida lusitaniae* from the urinary tract of a newborn infant initially treated with amphotericin B for *C. lusitaniae* fungemia, then ketoconazole alone. A similar outcome may have been achieved if flucytosine had been added to amphotericin B (Yinnon *et al.*, 1992). The combination of ketoconazole and flucytosine has been used successfully for systemic fungal infections in neonates (Cotton and Ransome, 1989).

One patient with postoperative peritonitis due to *Saccharomyces cerivisiae* (baker's yeast) recovered with oral ketoconazole therapy (Canafax *et al.*, 1982).

3 Coccidioidomycosis

Treatment is indicated if there is progressive pulmonary disease or evidence of dissemination to bone, skin, soft tissue, or central nervous system and meninges. Immunosuppressed patients or those who experience more severe primary infections should receive immediate antifungal treatment. There have been a number of reports that ketoconazole caused improvement in this disease, including cases which failed to respond to amphotericin B (Catanzaro *et al.*, 1982; De Felice *et al.*, 1982; Heel *et al.*, 1982; Ross *et al.*, 1982). Most non-comparative studies show that the drug is moderately effective in non-meningeal forms of coccidioidomycosis and responses have been documented in skeletal (25–69% improvement), cutaneous (60–88% improvement), infiltrative and chronic pulmonary disease (41–83% improvement), and in disseminated disease (Catanzaro *et al.*, 1982; Stevens *et al.*, 1983; Knoper and Galgiani, 1988).

However, in most cases ketoconazole appears to suppress infection only, and frequent disease relapses occur when ketoconazole therapy is interrupted or discontinued (Catanzaro *et al.*, 1982; Graybill, 1983; Knoper and Galgiani, 1988). For this reason, duration of therapy with ketoconazole should be prolonged (minimum of 6–12 months), and some investigators question whether azole drugs can be stopped without a significant risk of relapse. There is some evidence that response may be better with higher daily doses of ketoconazole, even up to 2000 mg (Graybill *et al.*, 1982, 1988; Craven *et al.*, 1983; Graybill and Craven, 1983). However, a randomized study comparing 400 mg and 800 mg doses of ketoconazole for the treatment of progressive pulmonary, skeletal or soft tissue infections revealed minimal benefit for the majority of patients with non-meningeal disease. Response rates were generally poor (23% for 400 mg dose and 32% for the 800 mg dose. (Galgiani *et al.*, 1988). Higher daily doses result in higher serum levels and better penetration of the drug into the CSF, but are also associated with greater toxicity. Treatment results of meningeal coccidioidomycosis with high-dose ketoconazole have been similar to those seen with intrathecal amphotericin B (Graybill *et al.*, 1988). Limited experience suggests that a combination of oral ketoconazole and intrathecal amphotericin B may be useful in coccidioidal meningitis (Craven *et al.*, 1983; Graybill *et al.*, 1988). The optimum duration and dosage of ketoconazole in coccidioidomycosis, have yet to be determined. Itraconazole will probably replace ketoconazole for treatment or long-term suppression of this infection.

4 Paracoccidioidomycosis

The classic therapy for paracoccidioidomycosis was sulphonamides, which are inexpensive, effective in 70% of patients treated for 2–3 years and associated with a 35% relapse rate (Restrepo, 1994). Ketoconazole treatment with doses of 200–400 mg daily for 6–12 months is associated with a 90% response rate and 10% relapse rate. Ketoconazole therapy was also associated with a lower mortality rate (Restrepo et al., 1985a,b; Vargas and Recacoechea, 1988). Rapid healing of mucocutaneous lesions occurs within 2–6 months of treatment with ketoconazole, while the pulmonary and lymph node lesions require longer therapy (6 months) before improvement is noted. Pulmonary fibrosis often developed and was unaffected by treatment (Restrepo et al., 1985a; Brummer et al., 1993). Itraconazole is currently considered the drug of choice for paracoccidioidomycosis, because of a lower rate of adverse reactions, greater potency with dosing of 100 mg daily, shorter treatment period (6 months) and reduced relapse rate compared with ketoconazole. Patients who have relapsed on ketoconazole have been successfully treated with itraconazole (Restrepo, 1994).

5 Histoplasmosis

Ketoconazole has been shown to be effective for some patients with infections due to H. capsulatum and H. duboisii. In chronic pulmonary histoplasmosis, ketoconazole in doses of 400 mg daily for 6–12 months, is as effective as amphotericin B (Dismukes et al., 1985; Slama, 1983). Response rates of 84% were noted in a randomized study of ketoconazole 400 mg and 800 mg daily for chronic cavitatory pulmonary disease (National Institute of Allergy and Infectious Diseases Mycoses Study Group, 1985). Ketoconazole 400 mg daily for 6–12 months is also useful for treatment of chronic or subacute progressive disseminated histoplasmosis in the immunocompetent host, but it should not be used for treatment of acute progressive disseminated histoplasmosis in the immunocompromised host (including AIDS patients) and it is not recommended for chronic suppressive maintenance therapy, because of low success rates for induction treatment (10%) and 50% relapse rates (Wheat et al., 1990; Nightingale et al., 1990). Ketoconazole does not cross the blood–brain barrier and is therefore not recommended for treatment of histoplasma meningitis. The newer azoles, itraconazole and fluconazole will replace ketoconazole for this infection.

6 Blastomycosis

The National Institute of Allergy and Infectious Diseases Mycosis Study Group (1985) determined ketoconazole was effective for the treatment of non-life-threatening and non-meningeal blastomycosis with a cure rate of 89% of patients treated for at least 6 months. They found that 800 mg daily was significantly more effective than 400 mg daily (100% cure rate versus 79% cure rate), but was associated with greater adverse reactions. Bradsher et al. (1985) treated 43 patients with a dosage of 400 mg daily for at least 1 month. Of these, 35 patients (81%) were cured without relapse over a mean follow-up period of 17 months. Six patients relapsed (four due to non-compliance), and two had progressive disease despite adequate serum levels of the drug. It was concluded that ketoconazole replace amphotericin B as the initial treatment of blastomycosis, and therapy should be initiated with 400 mg daily and continued for 6 months with persistently negative cultures. The ketoconazole dose can be increased to 600–800 mg daily in those patients in whom disease progression occurs. There are several reports of neurologic relapse of blastomycosis after ketoconazole treatrment for pulmonary disease, probably due to progression of subclinical central nervous system infection due to inadequate penetration of ketoconazole across the blood–brain barrier (Bradsher et al., 1985; Pitrak and Andersen, 1989; Yancey et al., 1991). Patients with HIV infection and blastomycosis have more aggressive disease which is more rapidly fatal, especially in those who present with disseminated disease. These patients should receive amphotericin B as initial therapy to a total dose of 1 g, followed by chronic oral suppressive therapy with ketoconazole 400 mg daily or itraconazole (p. 1436) (Pappas et al., 1992). It is also recommended that treatment for blastomycosis in other immunocompromised hosts be initiated with amphotericin B (Greene et al., 1985). The optimal cumulative dose appears to be 1 g and this should be followed by a prolonged course of an oral azole, either ketoconazole or itraconazole, either for 6 months and until there is no evidence of disease. Primary therapy with ketoconazole or itraconazole is not currently recommended in the immunocompromised host (Pappas et al., 1993).

7 Chromoblastomycosis

A chronic fungal infection of the skin and subcutaneous tissues caused by dematiaceous fungi (most commonly *Fonsecaea pedrosoi*, *Philaophora verrucosa*, *Cladosporium carrionii*) which are found in soil and decomposing vegetation, and innoculated into skin by trauma. It is generally difficult to treat. Ketoconazole (200–400 mg daily) therapy for several months produced a moderate improvement in 30% of patients with mild disease. It is not effective in those with extensive disease (Restrepo, 1994). Cutaneous chromomycosis due to *F. pedrosoi* was reported in a renal transplant patient who required multiple excision biopsies and ketoconazole to effectively control her disease. Although residual skin lesions regressed over several months of treatment, they did not disappear and recurrent lessions developed while she was taking ketoconazole 200 mg daily. New crops of lesions were excised and the patient remained free of disease for 1 year on continued ketoconazole (Wackym *et al.*, 1985). Successful treatment with ketoconazole and flucytosine in combination has also been reported (Silber *et al.*, 1983).

8 Cryptococcosis

Ketoconazole does not appear to be useful in cryptococcosis (Heel, 1982). One patient with cryptococcal meningitis who had not completely responded to amphotericin B plus flucytosine treatment, relapsed while receiving ketoconazole alone in a daily dose of 600 mg (Perfect *et al.*, 1982). Cutaneous cryptococcosis without evidence of meningeal disease in a renal transplant recipient was successfully treated with ketoconazole 400 mg daily for 6 months without relapse or dissemination (Granier *et al.*, 1987).

9 Aspergillosis Improvement

Patients with allergic bronchopulmonary aspergillosis treated with ketoconazole 400 mg daily for 12 months experienced significant improvement in symptoms compared with placebo recipients in a small controlled trial (Shale *et al.*, 1987). Itraconazole, with its superior *in vitro* activity against *Aspergillus* species, is the preferred oral azole drug for management of non-invasive or invasive aspergillosis.

10 Pseudallescheria boydii infections

Ketoconazole has been used successfully to treat a small number of patients with bone, joint or subcutaneous infections due to *Pseudallescheria* (*Petriellidium*) *boydii* (Haapasaari *et al.*, 1982; Drouhet and Dupont, 1983). A combined medical and surgical approach appears essential for bone and soft tissue infections in non-immunocompromised patients. Ketoconazole has been used successfully in this situation (Sheftel *et al.*, 1987; Patterson *et al.*, 1990). *In vitro* susceptibility testing does not always correlate with clinical outcome as patients with resistant isolates have been successfully managed with ketoconazole. Four of seven patients with pulmonary disease due to *Pseudallescheria boydii* improved with ketoconazole 200–600 mg daily and two patients required surgical excision of pulmonary cavities, while one patient with osteomyelitis required surgery as well as ketoconazole (Galgiani *et al.*, 1984). Miconazole is the drug of choice for this infection, particularly in the immunocompromised host with disseminated disease (p. 1454).

11 Sporotrichosis

Several anecdotal case reports suggest that ketoconazole is effective for cutaneous sporotrichosis (including disseminated cutaneous and lymphocutaneous forms) in immunocompetent hosts. Treatment regimens of 400 mg daily for 6 weeks in adults, and 200 mg daily for 6 weeks in children were successful with no relapses in 6 months follow-up (Cullen *et al.*, 1992; Naqvi *et al.*, 1993). Calhoun *et al.* (1991) reported their experience with ketoconazole for invasive sporotrichosis (subcutaneous nodules, arthritis and soft tissue infection). Of those receiving 400–800 mg daily, 88% responded with resolution of symptoms, but half relapsed on cessation of ketoconazole. Sustained remission was achieved by longer duration of treatment (greater than 1 year). Others have reported unsuccessful treatment with ketoconazole for both systemic disease and pulmonary sporotrichosis (Pluss and Opal, 1986; Dall and Salzman, 1987; Purvis *et al.*, 1993). Itraconazole appears to have superior clinical efficacy for sporotrichosis (p. 1438).

12 Alternariosis

Cutaneous alternariosis is an uncommon, chronic localized skin infection which occurs in both immunocompetent and immunocompromised patients, often introduced by minor trauma. Several modes of therapy have been reported, including intralesional amphotericin B and miconazole, and oral ketoconazole. Mixed results have been obtained with ketoconazole and poor outcome is said to be associated with the presence of immunosuppression (including AIDS) and failure of previous therapy. Ketoconazole 400 mg daily for 4 months and cessation of oral corticosteroids was effective in the treatment of cutaneous alternariosis in an 80-year-old farmer (Aznar *et al.*, 1989).

13 Phaeohyphomycosis

A case of subcutaneous phaeohyphomycosis caused by *Exophiala jeanselmei* in a renal transplant patient manifesting as verrucous plaques on the thigh and anterior abdominal wall, was reported to be successfully treated with ketoconazole in doses of 400–800 mg daily for 2 years. The smaller lesion was surgically excised. The larger lesion had a 75% decrease in size by 7-months treatment and had resolved at 1 year (Sindhuphak *et al.*, 1985). A lower dose of ketoconazole (200 mg daily) has also been reported to be effective for subcutaneous phaeohyphomycosis (South *et al.*, 1981), and a patient with subcutaneous phaeohyphomycosis caused by *Exophiala spinifera* was cured with ketoconazole and flucytosine (Padhye *et al.*, 1984). Ketoconazole was not effective for subcutaneous *E. jeanselmei* in an immunosuppressed man (Allred, 1990). A review of phaeohyphomycosis caused by *Bipolaris* or *Exserohilum* species did not suggest a role for ketoconazole in these infections, and reported progressive disease in patients whose regimens were changed to ketoconazole (Adam *et al.*, 1986). *Curvularia lunata* pansinusitis with bone destruction and intracranial extension in an immunocompetent host was controlled with surgical debridement, i.v. amphotericin B to a total dose of 4 g and an 8-month course of ketoconazole 400 mg daily (Ismail *et al.*, 1993). Maxillary sinus fusariosis and a subcutaneous lesion due to *Fusarium solani* in immunocompetent hosts was successfully treated with ketoconazole 200 mg daily plus surgery (Hiemenz *et al.*, 1990; Kurien *et al.*, 1992).

14 Eumycetoma

This is a chronic destructive infection of the skin and subcutaneous tissue, caused by many different molds including *Madurella* spp., *Aspergillus* spp., *Acremonium* spp., and *Fusarium* spp. It is treated with surgical excision of small circumscribed lesions or amputation in extreme cases. Results of medical therapy have been disappointing; however, with the advent of the azole drugs, optimal medical therapy is yet to be determined. Of 12 patients with eumycetoma caused by *Madurella mycetomii* and treated with ketoconazole, three of four treated with 400 mg daily were cured in 3–7.5 months and the fourth patient improved on ketoconazole. Eight patients received 100–300 mg daily, and six showed no improvement or deterioration after treatment for 3–17 months (Maghoub and Gumaa, 1984). Eumycetoma due to *Madurella grisea* has responded to ketoconazole (Venugopal *et al.*, 1990). Cases of eumycetoma caused by *Pseudallescheria boydii* or *Acremonium* spp. have not responded to ketoconazole therapy (Restrepo, 1994), although a partial response was observed in a mycetoma of the foot caused by *P. boydii* after treatment with ketoconazole for 8 months (Stierstorfer *et al.*, 1988). Large necrotic ulcers over the dorsum of both feet with associated onycholysis of the toenails, due to *Fusarium oxysporum*, developed over 1 year in an immunocompetent man. Although biopsy specimens did not show evidence of tissue invasion, the ulcers completely healed after 4 weeks treatment with ketoconazole 200 mg daily (Landau and Srebenik, 1992).

15 Entomophthoromycosis

Caused by the molds *Conidiobolus* and *Basidiobolus* spp., entomophthoromycosis is manifest as a chronic inflammatory disease with a subcutaneous form involving the limbs, trunk and buttocks (basidiobolomycosis), or a mucocutaneous form localized to the face (conidiobolomycosis). A case of subcutaneous *Conidiobolus coronatus* infection involving the nose, forehead and neck present for 6 years, but initially improved with potassium iodide developed recurrent disease which resolved completely when treated with ketoconazole 200 mg twice-daily for 6 months. No relapse occurred during 3 years follow-up (Towersey *et al.*, 1988). Hay (1983) has reported a case that did not respond to 5 months treatment with ketoconazole. The number of cases reported in the literature are too small to make any recommendations concerning the efficacy of ketoconazole for this infection.

16 Acanthamoeba infections

In the immunocompromised host, *Acanthamoeba* infections present as disseminated infection with skin nodules or ulcers and spread to the brain (chronic granulomatous amebic encephalitis). Treatment results have been disappointing, although ketoconazole 400 mg daily may stabilize progression of the infection (Friedland *et al.*, 1992; Martinez , 1991). Successful treatment of disseminated *Acanthamoeba* infection in a renal transplant patient with an IgA deficiency was reported by Slater *et al.* (1994). The patient presented with cutaneous ulcers with black eschars, 2–6 cm in diameter, plus tender erythematous nodules with purulent drainage. He was treated with i.v. pentamidine isethionate 4 mg per kg daily and twice-daily topical therapy to the skin lesions with 2% ketoconazole cream after cleansing with chlorhexidine. Improvement of cutaneous disease was noted within 1 week.

17 Leishmaniasis

Cutaneous leishmaniasis due to *Leishmania major* was cured in 70% cases treated with ketoconazole 200–400 mg daily for 4–6 weeks. Response could not be predicted by duration of infection, duration of treatment, or the number and size of skin lesions (Weinrauch *et al.*, 1987). These clinical results are in contrast to the efficacy of ketoconazole for the treatment of *L. major* and *L. mexicana* in laboratory mice (Weinrauch and El-On, 1984). A randomized trial compared oral ketoconazole 600 mg daily with intramuscular antimony 20 mg per kg daily for 28 days for the treatment of cutaneous leishmaniasis due to *L. braziliensis*. Ketoconazole was equally as effective as antimony, which has been considered the agent of choice by the World Health Organization (76% cure rate compared with 68% for antimony) and was associated with fewer side-effects. The investigators noted that the majority of healing due to ketoconazole occurred after the end of the 28-day treatment period (Saenz *et al.*, 1990). Ketoconazole is effective in patients with cutaneous leishmaniasis who have not responded to antimony (Joliffe, 1986). Visceral leishmaniasis due to *L. donovani* which had not responded to antimony or relapsed after an initial response, did not respond to ketoconazole 400–800 mg daily (Sundar *et al.*, 1990), unlike eight of nine cases of antimony-resistant visceral leishmaniasis reported by Wali *et al.* (1990). In addition, two children with post kala-azar dermal leishmaniasis did not respond to ketoconazole (El Hassan *et al.*, 1992).

18 Blastocystis hominis

A case of *Blastocystis hominis* (protozoan infection) in a woman with chronic diarrhea was successfully treated with ketoconazole 200 mg daily after treatment failures with metronidazole, diphenoxylate, chloramphenicol, cotrimoxazole and sulfasalazine. A recurrence 14 months later also responded to a 2-week course of ketoconazole (Cohen, 1985).

References

Abadie-Kemmerly S, Pankey GA, Dalovisio JR (1988). Failure of ketoconazole treatment of *Blastomyces dermatitidis* due to interaction of isoniazid and rifampin. *Ann Intern Med* **109**: 844.

Adam RD, Paquin ML, Petersen EA *et al.* (1986). Phaeohyphomycosis caused by the fungal genera *Bipolaris* and *Exserohilum*. A report of 9 cases and review of the literature. *Medicine* **65**: 203.

Adams JS, Sharma OP, Diz MM, Endres DB (1990). Ketoconazole decreases the serum 1,25-dihydroxyvitamin D and calcium concentration in sarcoidosis-associated hypercalcemia. *J Clin Endocrinol Metab* **70**: 1090.

Alford RH, Cartwright BB (1983). Comparison of ketoconazole and amphotericin B in interference with thymidine uptake by and blastogenesis of lymphocytes stimulated with *Histoplasma capsulatum* antigens. *Antimicrob Ag Chemother* **24**: 575.

Allen JM, Kerle DJ, Ware H *et al.* (1983). Combined treatment with ketoconazole and luteinising hormone releasing hormone analogue: a novel approach to resistant prostatic cancer. *Brit Med J* **287**: 1766.

Allred BJ (1990). Subcutaneous phaeohyphomycosis due to *Exophiala jeanselmei* in an immunocompromised patient: case report. *New Z Med J* **103**: 321.

Angeli A, Frairia R (1985). Ketoconazole therapy in Cushing's disease. *Lancet* **i**: 821.

Aznar R, Marigil J, Puig de la Bellacasa J *et al.* (1989). Cutaneous alternariosis responding to ketoconazole. *Lancet* **i**: 667.

Back DJ, Tjia JF (1991). Comparative effects of the antimycotic drugs ketoconazole, fluconazole, itraconazole and terbinafine on the metabolism of cyclosporin by human liver microsomes. *Brit J Clin Pharmacol* **32**: 624.

Badcock NR, Bartholomeusz FD, Frewin DB *et al.* (1987). The pharmacokinetics of ketoconazole after chronic administration in adults. *Eur J Clin Pharmacol* **33**: 531.

Barchiesi F, Giacometti A, Arzeni D *et al.* (1992). Fluconazole and ketoconazole in the treatment of oral and esophageal candidiasis in AIDS patients. *J Chemother* **4**: 381.

Bardare M, Tortorano AM, Pietrogrande MC Viviani MA (1984). Pharmacokinetics of ketoconazole and treatment evaluation in candidal infections. *Arch Dis Child* **59**: 1068.

Beggs WH, Sarosi GA (1982). Combined activity of ketoconazole and 5-flurocytosine on potentially pathogenic yeasts. *Antimicrob Ag Chemother* **21**: 355.

Benson GD, Anderson PK, Combes B, Ishak KG (1988). Prolonged jaundice following ketoconazole-induced hepatic injury. *Dig Dis Sci* **33**: 240.

Bercoff E, Bernuau J, Degott C *et al.* (1985). Ketoconazole-induced fulminant hepatitis. *Gut* **26**: 636.

Berman JD (1981). Activity of imidazoles against *Leishmania tropica* in human macrophage cultures. *Amer J Trop Med Hyg* **30**: 566.

Bharija SC, Belhaj MS (1988). Ketoconazole-induced fixed drug eription. *Int J Dermatol* **27**: 278.

Bingham JS (1984). Single blind comparison of ketoconazole 200mg oral tablets and clotrimazole 100 mg vaginal tablets and 1% cream in treating acute vaginal candidosis. *Brit J Vener Dis* **60**: 175.

Blatchford NR, Emanuel MB, Cauwenbergh G (1982). Ketoconazole resistance. *Lancet* **ii**: 770.

Blum RA, D'Andrea DT, Florentino BM et al. (1991). Increased gastric pH and the bioavailability of fluconazole and ketoconazole. *Ann Intern Med* **114**: 755.

Borelli D (1980). Treatment of pityriasis versicolor with ketoconazole. *Rev Infect Dis* **2**: 592.

Borelli D, Jacobs PH, Nall L (1991). Tinea versicolor: Epidemiologic, clinical, and therapeutic aspects. *J Amer Acad Dermatol* **25**: 300.

Borgers M, De Brabander M, Van den Bossche H, Van Cutsem J (1979). Promotion of pseudomycelium formation of *Candida albicans* in culture: a morphological study of the effects of miconazole and ketoconazole. *Postgrad Med J* **55**: 687.

Borgers M, Van den Bossche H, De Brabander M (1983). The mechanism of action of the new antimycotic ketoconazole. *Amer J Med* **74**: 2.

Bradsher RW, Rice DC, Abernathy RS (1985). Ketoconazole therapy for endemic blastomycosis. *Ann Intern Med* **103**: 872.

Brass C, Galgiani JN, Blaschke TF et al. (1982). Disposition of ketoconazole, an oral antifungal, in humans. *Antimicrob Ag Chemother* **21**: 151.

Brummer E, Castaneda E, Restrepo A (1993). Paracoccidioidomycosis: an update. *Clin Microbiol Rev* **6**: 89.

Butman SM, Wild JC, Nolan PE et al. (1991). Prospective study of the safety and financial benefit of ketoconazole as adjunctive therapy to cyclosporine after heart transplantation. *J Heart Lung Transplant* **10**: 351.

Buttke TM, Chapman SW (1983). Inhibition by ketoconazole of mitogen-induced DNA synthesis and cholesterol biosynthesis in lymphocytes. *Antimicrob Ag Chemother* **24**: 478.

Calhoun DL, Waskin H, White MP et al. (1991). Treatment of sporotrichosis with ketoconazole. *Rev Infect Dis* **13**: 47.

Canafax DM, Mann HJ, Dougherty SH (1982). Postoperative peritonitis due to *Saccharomyces cerevisiae* treated with ketoconazole. *Drug Intell Clin Pharm* **16**: 698.

Carlson JA, Mann HJ, Canafax DM (1983). Effect of pH on disintegration and dissolution of ketoconazole tablets. *Amer J Hosp Pharm* **40**: 1334.

Carr MM, Pryce DM, Ive FA (1987). Treatment of seborrhoeic dermatitis with ketoconazole: I. Response of seborrhoeic dermatitis of the scalp to topical ketoconazole. *Brit J Dermatol* **116**: 213.

Carvalho D, Pignatelli D, Resende C (1985). Ketoconazole for hirsutism. *Lancet* **ii**: 560.

Carver PL, Berardi RR, Knapp MJ et al. (1994). *In vivo* interaction of ketoconazole and sucralfate in healthy volunteers. *Antimicrob Ag Chemother* **38**: 326.

Catanzaro A, Einstein H, Levine B et al. (1982). Ketoconazole for treatment of disseminated coccidioidomycosis. *Ann Intern Med* **96**: 436.

Cauwenbergh G, De Doncker P, Schrooten P, DeGreef H (1986). Treatment of dandruff with a 2% ketoconazole scalp gel. A double-blind placebo-controlled study. *Int J Dermatol* **25**: 541.

Chapman JR, Warnock DW (1983). Ketoconazole and fungal CAPD peritonitis. *Lancet* **ii**: 510.

Charles BG, Ravenscroft PJ, Rigby RJ (1989). The ketoconazole-cyclosporin interaction in an elderly renal transplant patient. *Aust N Z J Med* **19**: 292.

Chin TWF, Loeb M, Fong IW (1995). Effects of an acidic beverage (Coca-Cola) on absorption of ketoconazole. *Antimicrob Ag Chemother* **39**: 1671.

Church JA, Neff DN, Marbut C (1982). Resistance to ketoconazole. *Lancet* **ii**: 211.

Cohen AN (1985). Ketoconazole and resistant *Blastocystis hominis* infection. *Ann Intern Med* **103**: 480.

Cohen J (1982). Good antimicrobial prescribing. Antifungal chemotherapy. *Lancet* **ii**: 532.

Contreras P, Rojas A, Biagini L et al. (1985). Regression of metastatic adrenal carcinoma during palliative ketoconazole treatment. *Lancet* **ii**: 151.

Cook RA, McIntyre KA, Galgiani (1990). Effects of incubation temperature, inoculum size, and medium on agreement of macro- and microdilution broth susceptibility test results for yeasts. *Antimicrob Ag Chemother* **34**: 1542.

Cotton MF, Ransome OJ (1989). Oral ketoconazole and flucytosine for neonatal systemic candidiasis. *South Afr Med J* **75**: 388.

Craven PC, Graybill JR, Jorgensen JH et al. (1983). High-dose ketoconazole for treatment of fungal infections of the central nervous system. *Ann Intern Med* **98**: 160.

Cullen SI, Mauceri AA, Warner N (1992). Successful treatment of disseminated cutaneous sporotrichosis with ketoconazole. *J Amer Acad Dermatol* **27**: 463.

Cunningham C, Burke MD, Whiting PH et al. (1982). Ketoconazole, cyclosporin and the kidney. *Lancet* **ii**: 1464.

Dall L, Salzman G (1987). Treatment of pulmonary sporotrichosis with ketoconazole. *Rev Infect Dis* **9**: 795.

Daneshmend TK (1982). Ketoconazole-cyclosporin interaction. *Lancet* **ii**: 1342.

Daneshmend TK, Roberts CJC (1982). Ketoconazole. *Lancet* **i**: 517.

Daneshmend TK, Warnock DW (1988). Clinical pharmacokinetics of ketoconazole. *Clin Pharmacokinet* **14**: 13.

Daneshmend TK, Warnock DW, Turner A, Roberts CJC (1981). Pharmacokinetics of ketoconazole in normal subjects. *J Antimicrob Chemother* **8**: 299.

Daneshmend TK, Warnock DW, Ene MD et al. (1983). Multiple dose pharmacokinetics of ketoconazole and their effects on antipyrine kinetics in man. *J Antimicrob Chemother* **12**: 185.

Daneshmend TK, Warnock DW, Ene MD et al. (1984). Influence of food on the pharmacokinetics of ketoconazole. *Antimicrob Ag Chemother* **25**: 1.

De Felice R, Johnson DG, Galgiani JN (1981). Gynecomastia with ketoconazole. *Antimicrob Ag Chemother* **19**: 1073.

De Felice R, Galgiani JN, Campbell SC et al. (1982). Ketoconazole treatment of nonprimary coccidioidomycosis. *Amer J Med* **72**: 681.

De Wit S, Weerts D, Goossens H, Clumeck N (1989). Comparison of fluconazole and ketoconazole for oropharyngeal candidiasis in AIDS. *Lancet* **i**: 746.

Dieperink H, Moller J (1982). Ketoconazole and cyclosporin. *Lancet* **ii**: 1217.

Dismukes WE, Cloud G, Bowles C et al. (1985). Treatment of blastomycosis and histoplasmosis with ketoconazole. *Ann Intern Med* **103**: 861.

Dixon DM, Polak A (1987). *In vitro* and *in vivo* drug studies with three agents of central nervous system phaeohyphomycosis. *Chemotherapy* **33**: 129–140.

Doble N, Hykin P, Shaw R, Keal EE (1985). Pulmonary *Mycobacterium tuberculosis* in acquired immune deficiency syndrome. *Brit Med J* **291**: 849.

Doble N, Shaw R, Roland-Hill C et al. (1988). Pharmacokinetic study of the interaction between rifampicin and ketoconazole. *J Antimicrob Chemother* **21**: 633.

Doern GV, Tubert TA, Chapin K, Rinaldi MG (1986). Effect of medium composition on results of macrobroth dilution antifungal susceptibility testing of yeasts. *J Clin Microbiol* **24**: 507.

D'Mello AP, D'Souza MJ, Bates TR (1985). Pharmacokinetics of ketoconazole-antipyrine interaction. *Lancet* **ii**: 209.

Donnelly JP, Starke ID, Galton DAG et al. (1984). Oral ketoconazole and amphotericin B for the prevention of yeast colonization in patients with acute leukaemia. *J Hosp Infect* **5**: 83.

Drouhet E, Dupont B (1983). Laboratory and clinical assessment of ketoconazole in deep-seated mycoses. *Amer J Med* **74**: 30.

Duarte PA, Chow CC, Simmons F, Ruskin J (1984). Fatal hepatitis associated with ketoconazole therapy. *Arch Intern Med* **144**: 1069.

Dupont B, Drouhet E (1985). Cutaneous, ocular, and osteoarticular candidiasis in heroin addicts: new clinical and therapeutic aspects in 38 patients. *J Infect Dis* **152**: 577.

El Hassan AM, Ghalib HW, Zijlstra EE et al. (1992). Post kala-azar dermal leishmaniasis in the Sudan: clinical features, pathology and treatment. Trans Roy Soc Trop Med Hyg 86: 245.

Ene MD, Williamson PJ, Daneshmend TK, Blatchford NR (1984). Systemic absorption of ketoconazole from vaginal pessaries. Brit J Clin Pharmacol 17: 173.

Eng RHK, Person A, Mangura C et al. (1981). Susceptibility of Zygomycetes to amphotericin B, miconazole and ketoconazole. Antimicrob Ag Chemother 20: 688.

Engelhard D, Stutman HR, Marks MI (1984). Interaction of ketoconazole with rifampin and isoniazid. New Engl J Med 311: 1681.

Espinel-Ingroff A, Shadomy S, GebhartRJ (1984). In vitro studies with R 51,211. Antimicrob Ag Chemother 26: 5.

Faergemann J (1984). In vitro and in vivo activities of ketoconazole and itraconazole against Pityrosporum orbiculare. Antimicrob Ag Chemother 26: 773.

Faergemann J, Fredriksson T (1982). Tinea versicolor: some new aspects on etiology, pathogenesis, and treatment. Int J Dermatol 21: 8.

Fainstein V, Gilmore C, Hopfer RL et al. (1982). Septic arthritis due to Candida species in patients with cancer: report of five cases and review of the literature. Rev Infect Dis 4: 78.

Fainstein V, Bodey GP, Elting L et al. (1987). Amphotericin B or ketoconazole therapy of fungal infections in neutropenic cancer patients. Antimicrob Ag Chemother 31: 11.

Farr PM, Krause LB, Marks JM Shuster S (1985). Response of scalp psoriasis to oral ketoconazole. Lancet ii: 921.

Ferguson RM, Sutherland DER, Simmons RL, Najarian JS (1982). Ketoconazole, cyclosporin metabolism, and renal transplantation. Lancet ii: 882.

Fibbe WE, van der Meer JWM, Thompson J, Mouton RP (1980). CSF concentrations of ketoconazole. J Antimicrob Chemother 6: 681.

Firebrace DAJ (1981). Hepatitis and ketoconazole therapy. Brit Med J 283: 1058.

First MR, Schroeder TJ, Alexander JW et al. (1991). Cyclosporine dose reduction by ketoconazole administration in renal transplant recipients. Transplantation 51: 365.

First MR, Schroeder TJ, Michael A et al. (1993). Cyclosporine-ketoconazole interaction Long-term follow-up and preliminary results of a randomized trial. Transplantation 55: 1000.

Fong IW, Bannatyne RM, Wong P (1993). Lack of in vitro resistance of Candida albicans to ketoconazole, itraconazole and clotrimazole in women treated for recurrent vaginal candidiasis. Genitourin Med 69: 44.

Force RW, Nahata MC (1995). Salivary concentration of ketoconazole and fluconazole: implications for drug efficacy in oropharyngeal and esophageal candidiasis. Ann Pharmacother 29: 10.

Frazee LA, Neidig JA (1995). Ketoconazole to prevent acute respiratory distress syndrome in critically ill patients. Ann Pharmacother 29: 784.

Friedland LR, Raphael SA, Deutsch ES et al. (1992). Disseminated Acanthamoeba infection in a child with symptomatic human immunodeficiency virus infection. Pediatr Infect Dis J 11: 404.

Galgani JN, Stevens DA (1978). Turbidometric studies of growth inhibition of yeasts with three drugs: inquiry into inoculum-dependent susceptibility testing, time of onset of drug effect, and implications for current and newer methods. Antimicrob Ag Chemother 13: 249.

Galgiani JN, Stevens DA, Graybill JR et al. (1984). Pseudallescheria boydii infections treated with ketoconazole. Chest 86: 219.

Galgiani JN, Stevens DA, Graybill JR et al. (1988). Ketoconazole therapy of progressive coccidioidomycosis Comparison of 400– and 800-mg doses and observations at higher doses. Amer J Med 84: 603.

Gan VN, Petruska M, Ginsburg CM (1987). Epidemiology and treatment of tinea capitis: ketoconazole vs griseofulvin. Pediatr Infect Dis J 6: 46.

Gebhart RJ, Espinel-Ingroff A, Shadomy S (1984). In vitro susceptibility studies with oxiconazole (Ro 13–8996). Chemotherapy 30: 244.

Ghetti P, Patrone P, Tosti A (1986). Ketoconazole in the treatment of acne in women. Arch Dermatol 122: 629.

Ginsburg CM, McCracken GH Jr, Olsen K (1983). Pharmacology of ketoconazole suspension in infants and children. Antimicrob Ag Chemother 23: 787.

Girardet RE, Melo JC, Fox MS et al. (1989). Concomitant administration of cyclosporine and ketoconazole for three and a half years in one heart transplant recipient. Transplantation 48: 887.

Glass AR, Cerletty JM, Elliott W et al. (1990). Ketoconazole reduces elevated serum levels of 1,25-dihydroxyvitamin D in hypercalcemic sarcoidosis. J Endocrinol Invest 13: 407.

Go IH, Wientjens DP, Koster M (1992). A double-blind trial of 1% ketoconazole shampoo versus placebo in the treatment of dandruff. Mycoses 35: 103.

Gomez DY, Wacher VJ, Tomlanovich SJ et al. (1995). The effects of ketoconazole on the intestinal metabolism and bioavailability of cyclosporine. Clin Pharmacol Ther 58: 15.

Gonzalez-Delgado P, Florido-Lopez F, Saenz de San Pedro B et al. (1994). Hypersensitivity to ketoconazole. Ann Allergy 73: 326.

Goodman DF, Stern WH (1987). Oral ketoconazole and intraocular amphotericin B for treatment of postoperative Candida parapsilosis endophthalmitis. Arch Ophthalmol 105: 172.

Granier F, Kanitakis J, Hermier C et al. (1987). Localized cutaneous cryptococcosis successfully treated with ketoconazole. J Am Acad Dermatol 16: 243.

Graybill JR (1983). Summary: potential and problems with ketoconazole. Amer J Med 74: 86.

Graybill JR, Ahrens J (1983). Interaction of rifampin with other antifungal agents in experimental murine candidiasis. Rev Infect Dis 2 (Suppl 3): S620.

Graybill JR, Craven PC (1983). Antifungal agents used in systemic mycoses, activity and therapeutic use. Drugs 25: 41.

Graybill JR, Drutz DJ (1980). Ketoconazole: a major innovation for treatment of fungal disease. Ann Intern Med 93: 921.

Graybill JR, Williams DM, Cutsem EV et al. (1980a). Combination therapy of experimental histoplasmosis and cryptococcosis with amphotericin B and ketoconazole. Rev Infect Dis 2: 551.

Graybill JR, Herndon HJ, Kniker WT (1980b). Ketoconazole treatment of chronic mucocutaneous candidiasis. Arch Dermatol 111: 1137.

Graybill JR, Craven PC, Donovan W, Matthew EB (1982). Ketoconazole therapy for systemic fungal infections Inadequacy of standard dosage regimens. Amer Rev Respir Dis 126: 171.

Graybill JR, Galgiani JN, Jorgensen JH, Strandberg DA (1983). Ketoconazole therapy for fungal urinary tract infections. J Urol 129: 68.

Graybill JR, Stevens DA, Galgiani JN et al. (1988). Ketoconazole treatment of coccidioidal meningitis. Ann NY Acad Sci 544: 488.

Green CA, Farr PM, Shuster S (1987). Treatment of seborrhoeic dermatitis with ketoconazole: II Response of seborrhoeic dermatitis of the face, scalp and trunk to topical ketoconazole. Brit J Dermatol 116: 217.

Greene NB, Baughman RP, Kim CK, Roselle GA (1985). Failure of ketoconazole in an immunosuppressed patient with pulmonary blastomycosis. Chest 88: 640.

Grosso DS, Boyden TW, Pamenter RW et al. (1983). Ketoconazole inhibition of testicular secretion of testosterone and displacement of steroid hormones from serum transport proteins. Antimicrob Ag Chemother 23: 207.

Gubbins PO, Piscitelli SC, Danziger LH (1993). Candidal urinary tract infections: A comprehensive review of their diagnosis and management. Pharmacother 13: 110.

Haapasaari J, Essen RV, Kahapanaa A et al. (1982). Fungal arthritis simulating juvenile rheumatoid arthritis. Brit Med J 285: 923.

Hann IM, Prentice HG, Keaney M et al. (1982a). The pharmacokinetics of ketoconazole in severely immunocompromised patients. J Antimicrob Chemother 10: 489.

Hann IM, Prentice HG, Corringham R et al. (1982b). Ketoconazole versus nystatin plus amphotericin B for fungal prophylaxis in severely immunocompromised patients. Lancet i: 826.

Hansen RM, Reinerio N, Sohnle PG et al. (1987). Ketoconazole in the prevention of candidiasis in patients with cancer A prospective, randomized, controlled, double-blind study. Arch Intern Med 147: 710.

Haron E, Anaissie E, Dumphy F, McCredie K, Fainstein V (1988). *Hansenula anomala* fungemia. *Rev Infect Dis* **10**: 1182.

Harris R, Jones HE, Artis WM (1983). Orally administered ketoconazole: route of delivery to the human stratum corneum. *Antimicrob Ag Chemother* **24**: 876.

Hay RJ (1983). Ketoconazole in the treatment of fungal infection Clinical and laboratory studies. *Amer J Med* **74**: 16.

Hay RJ (1985). Ketoconazole: a reappraisal. *Brit Med J* **290**: 260.

Hay RJ, Clayton YM, Griffiths WA, Dowd PM (1985). A comparative double blind study of ketoconazole and griseofulvin in dermatophytosis. *Brit J Dermatol* **112**: 691.

Heel RC (1982). *Ketoconazole in the Management of Fungal Disease.* (Levine B, ed). New York: Adis Press.

Heel RC, Brogden RN, Carmine A *et al.* (1982). Ketoconazole ('Nizoral'): a new oral antifungal agent. *Curr Ther* **23**: 13.

Heeres J, Backx LJJ, Mostmans JH, Van Cutsem J (1979). Antimycotic imidazoles Part 4. Synthesis and antifungal activity of ketoconazole, a new potent orally active broad-spectrum antifungal agent. *J Med Chem* **22**: 1003.

Hegemann L, Toso SM, Lahijani KI, Webster GF, Uitto J (1993). Direct interaction of antifungal azole-derivatives with calmodulin: a possible mechanism for their therapeutic activity. *J Invest Dermatol* **100**: 343.

Heiberg JK, Svejgaard E (1981). Toxic hepatitis during ketoconazole treatment. *Brit Med J* **283**: 825.

Hernandez Molina JM, Llosa J, Martinez Brocal A, Ventosa A (1992). *In vitro* activity of cloconazole, sulconazole, butoconazole, isoconazole, fenticonazole, and five other antifungal agents against clinical isolates of *Candida albicans* and *Candida* spp. *Mycopathologia* **118**: 15.

Hernandez-Sampelayo T, and a Multicentre Study Group (1994). Fluconazole versus ketoconazole in the treatment of oropharyngeal candidiasis in HIV-infected children. *Eur J Clin Microbiol Infect Dis* **13**: 340.

Heusner JJ, Dukes GE, Rollins DE *et al.* (1987). Effect of chronically administered ketoconazole on the elimination of theophylline in man. *Drug Intell Clin Pharm* **21**: 514.

Heykants JJP, Woestenborghs RJH, Bisschop MPJM, Merkus JMWM (1982). Distribution of oral ketoconazole to vaginal tissue. *Eur J Clin Pharmacol* **23**: 331.

Hiemenz JW, Kennedy B, Kwon-Chung KJ (1990). Invasive fusariosis associated with an injury by a stingray barb. *J Med Vet Mycol* **28**: 209.

Hoeprich PD, Merry JM (1984). *In vitro* activities of two new antifungal azoles. *Antimicrob Ag Chemother* **25**: 339.

Hoeprich PD, Merry JM (1985). Activity of Bay n 7133 and Bay 1 9139 *in vitro* and in experimental murine coccidioidomycosis. *Eur J Clin Microbiol* **4**: 400.

Holland FJ, Fishman L, Bailey JD *et al.* (1985). Ketoconazole in the management of precocious puberty not responsive to LHRH-analogue therapy. *New Engl J Med* **312**: 1023.

Honig PK, Wortham DC, Zamani K *et al.* (1993). Terfenadine-ketoconazole interaction Pharmacokinetic and electrocardiographic consequences. *JAMA* **269**: 1513.

Horsburgh CR Jr, Kirkpatrick CH (1983). Long-term therapy of chronic mucocutaneous candidiasis with ketoconazole: experience with twenty-one patients. *Amer J Med* **74**: 23.

Horsburgh CR Jr, Kirkpatrick CH, Teutsch CB (1982). Ketoconazole and the liver. *Lancet* **i**: 860.

Huang Y-C, Colaizzi JL, Bierman RH, Woestenborghs R Heykants J (1986). Pharmacokinetics and dose proportionality of ketoconazole in normal volunteers. *Antimicrob Ag Chemother* **30**: 206.

Hughes CE, Peterson LR, Beggs WH, Gerding DN (1986). Ketoconazole and flucytosine alone and in combination against *Candida* spp in a neutropenic site in rabbits. *J Antimicrob Chemother* **18**: 65.

Hughes WT, Bartley DL, Patterson GG, Tufenkeji H (1983). Ketoconazole and candidiasis: a controlled study. *J Infect Dis* **147**: 1060.

Hussain Qadri SMH, Fluornoy DJ, Qadri SGM, Ramirez EG (1986). Susceptibility of clinical isolates of yeasts to antifungal agents. *Mycopathologia* **95**: 183.

Ismail Y, Johnson RH, Wells MV *et al.* (1993). Invasive sinusitis with intracranial extension caused by *Curvularia lunata*. *Arch Intern Med* **153**: 1604.

Iwatsu T (1988). Cutaneous alternariosis. *Arch Dermatol* **124**: 1822.

Janssen PAJ, Symoens JE (1983). Hepatic reactions during ketoconazole treatment. *Amer J Med* **74**: 80.

Johnson EM, Richardson MD, Warnock DW (1983). Effect of imidazole antifungals on the development of germ tubes by strains of *Candida albicans*. *J Antimicrob Chemother* **12**: 303.

Johnson EM, Richardson MD, Warnock DW (1984). *In vitro* resistance to imidazole antifungals in *Candida albicans*. *J Antimicrob Chemother* **13**: 547.

Johnson EM, Warnock DW, Richardson MD, Douglas CJ (1986). *In-vitro* effect of itraconazole, ketoconazole and amphotericin B on the phagocytic and candidacidal function of human neutrophils. *J Antimicrob Chemother* **18**: 83.

Johnson RJ, Blair AD, Ahmad S (1985). Ketoconazole kinetics in chronic peritoneal dialysis. *Clin Pharmacol Ther* **37**: 325.

Joliffe DS (1986). Cutaneous leishmaniasis from Belize-treatment with ketoconazole. *Clin Exp Dermatol* **11**: 62.

Jones PG, Kauffman CA, McAuliffe LS *et al.* (1984). Efficacy of ketoconazole v nystatin in prevention of fungal infections in neutropenic patients. *Arch Intern Med* **144**: 549.

Jorgensen JH, Alexander GA, Graybill JR, Drutz DJ (1981). Sensitive bioassay for ketoconazole in serum and cerebrospinal fluid. *Antimicrob Ag Chemother* **20**: 59.

Kahana M, Levy A, Yaron-Shiffer O, Schewach-Millet M (1984). Drug eruption following ketoconazole therapy. *Arch Dermatol* **120**: 837.

Kandrotas RJ, Slaughter RL, Brass C, Jusko WJ (1987). Ketoconazole effects on methylprednisolone disposition and their joint suppression of endogenous cortisol. *Clin Pharmacol Ther* **42**: 465.

Knight TE, Shikuma CY, Knight J (1991). Ketoconazole-induced fulminant hepatitis necessitating liver transplantation. *J Amer Acad Dermatol* **25**: 398.

Knoper SR, Galgiani JN (1988). Coccidioidomycosis. *Infect Dis Clin N Amer* **2**: 861.

Kraemer FB, Pont A (1986). Inhibition of cholesterol synthesis by ketoconazole. *Amer J Med* **80**: 616.

Kurien M, Anandi V, Raman R, Brahmadathan KN (1992). Maxillary sinus fusariosis in immunocompetent hosts. *J Laryngol Otol* **106**: 733.

Kutzer E, Oittner R, Leodolter S, Brammer KW (1988). A comparison of fluconazole and ketoconazole in the oral treatment of vaginal candidiasis; report of a double-blind multicentre trial. *Eur J Obstet Gynecol Reprod Biol* **29**: 305.

Laine L, Dretler RH, Conteas CN *et al.* (1992). Fluconazole compared with ketoconazole for the treatment of *Candida* esophagitis in AIDS. A randomized trial. *Ann Intern Med* **117**: 655.

Lake-Bakaar G, Scheuer PJ, Sherlock S (1987). Hepatic reactions associated with ketoconazole in the UK. *Brit Med J* **294**: 419.

Lake-Bakaar G, Tom W, Lake-Bakaar D *et al.* (1988). Gastropathy and ketoconazole malabsorption in the acquired immunodeficiency syndrome (AIDS). *Ann Intern Med* **109**: 471.

Landau M, Srebrnik A (1992). Systemic ketoconazole treatment for *Fusarium* leg ulcers. *Int J Dermatol* **31**: 511.

Lefler E, Brummer E, Perlman AM, Stevens DA (1985). Activities of the modified polyene *N*-D-Ornithyl amphotericin methyl ester and the azoles ICI 153066, Bay n 7133, and Bay 1 9139 compared with those of amphotericin B and ketoconazole in the therapy of experimental blastomycosis. *Antimicrob Ag Chemother* **27**: 363.

Lelawongs P, Barone JA, Colaizzi JL *et al.* (1988). Effect of food and gastric acidity on absorption of orally administered ketoconazole. *Clin Pharmacol* **7**: 228.

Levine HB (1982). Resistance to ketoconazole. *Lancet* **ii**: 211.

Lewis JH, Zimmerman HJ, Benson GD, Ishak KG (1984). Hepatic injury associated with ketoconazole therapy Analysis of 33 cases. *Gastroenterol* **86**: 503.

Ludwig EA, Slaughter RL, Savliwala M *et al.* (1989). Steroid-specific effects of ketoconazole on corticosteroid disposition: unrelated prednisolone elimination. *DICP* **23**: 858.

Macnair AL, Gascoigne E, Heap J *et al.* (1981). Hepatitis and ketoconazole therapy. *Brit Med J* **283**: 1058.

Magnasco AJ, Magnasco LD (1986). Interaction of ketoconazole and ethanol. *Clin Pharmacol* **5**: 522.

Mahgoub ES, Gumaa SA (1984). Ketoconazole in the treatment of eumycetoma due to *Madurella mycetomii. Trans Roy Soc Trop Med Hyg* **78**: 376.

Maksymiuk AW, Levine HB, Bodey GP (1982). Pharmacokinetics of ketoconazole in patients with neoplastic diseases. *Antimicrob Ag Chemother* **22**: 43.

Maldonado RA, Molina J, Payares G, Urbina JA (1993). Experimental chemotherapy with combinations of ergosterol biosynthesis inhibitors in murine models of Chagas' disease. *Antimicrob Ag Chemother* **37**: 1353.

Mannisto PT, Mantyla R, Nykanen S *et al.* (1982). Impairing effect of food on ketoconazole absorption. *Antimicrob Ag Chemother* **21**: 730.

Manzell JP, Clark JK (1984). Effect of ketoconazole on the *in-vitro* lymphocyte transformation response to mitogen stimulation. *J Antimicrob Chemother* **14**: 669.

Marcon MJ, Durrell DE, Powell DA, Buesching WJ (1987). *In vitro* activity of systemic antifungal agents against *Malassezia furfur. Antimicrob Ag Chemother* **31**: 951.

Marmer DJ, Fields BT Jr, France GL, Steele RW (1981). Ketoconazole, amphotericin B, and amphotericin B methyl ester: comparative *in vitro* and *in vivo* toxicological effects on neutrophil function. *Antimicrob Ag Chemother* **20**: 660.

Martin E, Parras P, Lozano MC (1992). *In vitro* susceptibility of 245 yeast isolates to amphotericin B, 5-fluorocytosine, ketoconazole, fluconazole and itraconazole. *Chemotherapy* **38**: 335.

Martin M (1982). Ketoconazole and the actinomycetales. *Lancet* **i**: 807.

Martinez AJ (1991). Infection of the central nervous system due to *Acanthamoeba. Rev Infect Dis* **13** (Suppl 5): S399.

Martinez-Roig A, Torres-Rodriguez JM, Bartlett-Coma A (1988). Double blind study of ketoconazole and griseofulvin in dermatophytoses. *Pediatr Infect Dis J* **7**: 37.

Matthews DR, McNutt B, Okerholm R *et al.* (1991). Torsades de Pointes occurring in association with terfenadine use. *JAMA* **266**: 2375.

McCabe RE, Arauio FG, Remington JS (1983). Ketoconazole protects against infection with *Trypanosoma cruzi* in a murine model. *Amer J Trop Med Hyg* **32**: 960.

McCabe RE Remington JS, Araujo FG (1984). Ketoconazole inhibition of intracellular multiplication of *Trypanosoma cruzi* and protection of mice against lethal infection with the organism. *J Infect Dis* **150**: 594.

Meunier F (1990). Fluconazole treatment of fungal infections in the immunocompromised host. *Semin Oncol* **17** (Suppl 6): 19.

Meunier-Carpentier F (1983). Treatment of mycoses in cancer patients. *Amer J Med* **74**: 74.

Meunier-Carpentier F (1984). Chemoprophylaxis of fungal infections. *Amer J Med* **76**: 652.

Miettinen TA, Valtonen VV (1984). Ketoconazole and cholesterol synthesis. *Lancet* **ii**: 1271.

Minagawa H, Kitaura K, Nakamizo N (1983). Effects of pH on the activity of ketoconazole against *Candida albicans. Antimicrob Ag Chemother* **23**: 105.

Mobacken H, Moberg S (1986). Ketoconazole treatment in 13 patients with chronic mucocutaneous candidiasis. A prospective 3-year trial. *Dermatologica* **173**: 229.

Mohamed KN (1988). Severe photodermatitis during ketoconazole therapy. *Clin Exp Dermatol* **13**: 54.

Monahan BP, Ferguson CL, Killeavy ES *et al.* (1990). Torsades de Pointes occurring in association with terfenadine use. *JAMA* **264**: 2788.

Moody MR, Young VM, Morris MJ, Schimpff SC (1980). *In vitro* activities of miconazole, miconazole nitrate, and ketoconazole alone and combined with rifampin against *Candida* spp. and *Torulopsis glabrata* recovered from cancer patients. *Antimicrob Ag Chemother* **17**: 871.

Morace G, Manzara S, Dettori G (1991). *In vitro* susceptibility of 119 yeast isolates to fluconazole, 5-fluorocytosine, amphotericin B and ketoconazole. *Chemotherapy* **37**: 23.

Moretti ME, Ito S, Koren G (1995). Disposition of maternal ketoconazole in breast milk. *Amer J Obstet Gynecol* **173**: 1625.

Morgenstern GR, Powles R, Robinson B, McElwain TJ (1982). Cyclosporin interaction with ketoconazole and melphalan. *Lancet* **ii**: 1342.

Murphy E, Hannon D, Callaghan B (1987). Ketoconazole-theophylline interaction. *Ir Med J* **80**: 123.

Naqvi SH, Becherer P, Gudipati S (1993). Ketoconazole treatment of a family with zoonotic sporotrichosis. *Scand J Infect Dis* **25**: 543.

National Institute of Allergy and Infectious Diseases Mycoses Study Group (1985). Treatment of blastomycosis and histoplasmosis with ketoconazole. Results of a randomized clinical trial. *Ann Intern Med* **103**: 861.

Nightingale SD, Parks JM, Pounders SM *et al.* (1990). Disseminated histoplasmosis in patients witth AIDS. *South Med J* **83**: 624.

Nobre G, Mendes E, Charrua MJ, Cruz O (1989). Ketoconazole resistance in *Torulopsis glabrata. Mycopathologia* **107**: 51.

O'Connor M, Sobel JD (1986). Epidemiology of recurrent vulvovaginal candidiasis: Identification and strain differentiation of *Candida albicans. J Infect Dis* **154**: 358.

O'Day DM, Head WS, Robinson RD *et al.* (1985). Intraocular penetration of systemically administered antifungal agents. *Current Eye Res* **4**: 131.

Odds FC (1979). Problems of the laboratory assessment of antifungal activity. *Postgrad Med J* **55**: 677.

Odds FC (1982). Ketoconazole resistance. *Lancet* **ii**: 77.

Odds FC (1993). Resistance of yeasts to azole-derivative antifungals. *J Antimicrob Chemother* **31**: 463.

Okeke CN, Gugnani HC (1987). *In vitro* sensitivity of environmental isolates of pathogenic dematiaceous fungi to azole compounds and a phenylpropyl-morpholine derivative. *Mycopathologia* **99**: 175.

Or M, Akbatur H, Hasanerisoglu B *et al.* (1993). Ketoconazole induced papilloedema. *Acta Ophthalmol Copenh* **71**: 270.

Padhye AA, Kaplan W, Neuman MA *et al.* (1984). Subcutaneous phaeohyphomycosis caused by *Exophiala spinifera. Sabouraudia* **22**: 493.

Pappas PG, Pottage JC, Powderly WG *et al.* (1992). Blastomycosis in patients with the acquired immunodeficiency syndrome. *Ann Intern Med* **116**: 847.

Pappas PG, Threlkeld MG, Bedsole GD *et al.* (1993). Blastomycosis in immunocompromised patients. *Medicine* **72**: 311.

Patterson TF, Andriole VT, Zervos MJ *et al.* (1990). The epidemiology of pseudallescheriasis complicating transplantation: Nosocomial and community-acquired infection. *Mycoses* **33**: 297.

Perfect JR, Durack DT, Hamilton JD, Gallis HA (1982). Failure of ketoconazole in cryptococcal meningitis. *JAMA* **247**: 3349.

Pershing LK, Corlett J, Jorgensen C (1994). *In vivo* pharmacokinetics and pharmacodynamics of topical ketoconazole and miconazole in human stratum corneum. *Antimicrob Ag Chemother* **38**: 90.

Peter RU, Richarz-Barthauer U (1995). Successful treatment and prophylaxis of scalp seborrhoeic dermatitis and dandruff with 2% ketoconazole shampoo: results of a multicentre, double-blind, placebo-controlled trial. *Brit J Dermatol* **132**: 441.

Petersen EA, Alling DW, Kirkpatrick CH (1980). Treatment of chronic mucocutaneous candidiasis with ketoconazole. A controlled clinical trial. *Ann Intern Med* **93**: 791.

Pfaller MA, Krogstad DJ (1981). Imidazole and polyene activity against chloroquine-resistant *Plasmodium falciparum. J Infect Dis* **144**: 372.

Pillans Pl, Cowan P, Whitelaw D (1985). Hyponatremia and confusion in a patient taking ketoconazole. *Lancet* **i**: 821.

Piscitelli SC, Goss TF, Wilton JH, D'Andrea DT, Goldstein H, Schentag JJ (1991). Effects of ranitidine and sucralfate on ketoconazole bioavailability. *Antimicrob Ag Chemother* **35**: 1765.

Pitrak DL, Andersen BR (1989). Cerebral blastomycoma after ketoconazole therapy for respiratory tract blastomycosis. *Amer J Med* **86**: 713.

Pluss JL, Opal SM (1986). Pulmonary sporotrichosis: Review of treatment and outcome. *Medicine* **65**: 143.

Polak A, Dixon DM (1987). Fungistatic and fungicidal effects of amphotericin B, ketoconazole and fluconazole (UK 49,858) against *Histoplasma capsulatum in vitro* and *in vivo*. *Mykosen* **30**: 186.

Polak A, Scholer JJ, Wall M (1982). Combination therapy of experimental candidiasis, cryptococcosis and aspergillosis in mice. *Chemotherapy* **28**: 461.

Polak A, Odds FC, Ludin E, Scholer HJ (1985). Correlation of susceptibility test results *in vitro* with response *in vivo*: ketoconazole therapy in a systemic candidiasis model. *Chemotherapy* **31**: 395.

Pont A, Williams PL, Azhar S *et al.* (1983). Ketoconazole blocks testosterone synthesis. *Arch Intern Med* **142**: 2137.

Pont A, Graybill JR, Craven PC *et al.* (1984). High-dose ketoconazole therapy and adrenal and testicular function in humans. *Arch Intern Med* **144**: 2150.

Pont A, Goldman ES, Sugar AM *et al.* (1985). Ketoconazole-induced increase in estradiol-testosterone ratio. Probable explanation for gynecomastia. *Arch Intern Med* **145**: 1429.

Pottage JC, Kessler HA (1985). Inhibition of *in vitro* HBsAg production by amphotericin B and ketoconazole. *J Med Virol* **16**: 275.

Pottage JC, Kessler HA, Goodrich JM *et al.* (1986). *In vitro* activity of ketoconazole against herpes simplex virus. *Antimicrob Ag Chemother* **30**: 215.

Purvis RS, Diven DG, Drechsel RD *et al.* (1993). Sporotrichosis presenting as arthritis and subcutaneous nodules. *J Amer Acad Dermatol* **28**: 879.

Rapelanoro R, Morturex P, Couprie B *et al.* (1996). Neonatal *Malassezia furfur* pustulosis. *Arch Dermatol* **132**: 190.

Rausch LJ, Jacobs PH (1984). Tinea versicolor treatment and prophylaxis with monthly administration of ketoconazole. *Cutis* **34**: 470.

Restrepo A (1994). Treatment of tropical mycoses. *J Amer Acad Dermatol* **31** (Suppl): S91.

Restrepo A, Gomez I, Cano LE *et al.* (1985a). Treatment of paracoccidioidomycosis with ketoconazole: a three-year experience. *Amer J Med* **78**: 48.

Restrepo A, Gomez I, Cano LE *et al.* (1985b). Post-therapy status of paracoccidioidomycosis patients treated with ketoconazole. *Amer J Med* **78**: 53.

Reuben A, Anaissie E, Nelson PE *et al.* (1989). Antifungal susceptibility of 44 clinical isolates of *Fusarium* species determined by using a broth microdilution method. *Antimicrob Ag Chemother* **33**: 1647.

Robertson MH, Hanifin JM, Parker F (1980). Oral therapy with ketoconazole for dermatophyte infections unresponsive to griseofulvin. *Rev Infect Dis* **2**: 586.

Roilides E, Walsh TJ, Rubin M *et al.* (1990). Effects of antifungal agents on the function of human neutrophils *in vitro*. *Antimicrob Ag Chemother* **34**: 196.

Rosenblatt HM, Byrne W, Ament ME *et al.* (1980). Successful treatment of chronic mucocutaneous candidiasis with ketoconazole. *J Pediatr* **97**: 657.

Ross JB, Levine B, Catanzaro A *et al.* (1982). Ketoconazole for treatment of chronic pulmonary coccidioidomycosis. *Ann Intern Med* **96**: 440.

Saenz RE, Paz H, Berman JD (1990). Efficacy of ketoconazole against *Leishmania braziliensis panamensis* cutaneous leishmaniasis. *Amer J Med* **89**: 147.

Sampol E, Lacarelle B, Rajaonarison JF *et al.* (1995). Comparative effects of antifungal agents on zidovudine glucuronidation by human liver microsomes. *Brit J Clin Pharmacol* **40**: 83.

San-Blas G, Calcagno AM, San-Blas F (1993). A preliminary study of *in vitro* antibiotic activity of saperconazole and other azoles on *Paracoccidioides brasiliensis*. *J Med Vet Mycol* **31**: 169.

Santucci B, Cannistraci C, Cristaudo A, Picardo M (1992). Contact dermatitis from ketoconazole cream. *Contact Dermatitis* **27**: 274.

Savino JA, Agarwal N, Wry P *et al.* (1994). Routine prophylactic antifungal agents (clotrimazole, ketoconazole, and nystatin) in non-transplant/nonburned critically ill surgical and trauma patients. *J Trauma* **36**: 20.

Schroeder TJ, Melvin DB, Clardy CW *et al.* (1987). Use of cyclosporine and ketoconazole without nephrotoxicity in two heart transplant recipients. *J Heart Transplant* **6**: 84.

Schurmeyer T, Nieschlag E (1982). Ketoconazole-induced drop in serum and saliva testosterone. *Lancet* **ii**: 1998.

Sears SD, O'Hare J (1988). *in vitro* susceptibility of *Trichomonas vaginalis* to 50 antimicrobial agents. *Antimicrob Ag Chemother* **32**: 144.

Segal R, Trattner A, Alteras I *et al.* (1993). Once-weekly treatment with oral ketoconazole for superficial fungal infections. *J Amer Acad Dermatol* **28**: 126.

Sekhon AS, Padhye AA, Garg AK (1992). *In vitro* sensitivity of *Penicillium marneffei* and *Pythium insidiosum* to various antifungal agents. *Eur J Epidemiol* **8**: 427.

Shadomy S, White SC, Yu HP, Dismukes WE, NIAID Mycoses Study Group (1985). Treatment of systemic mycoses with ketoconazole: *in vitro* susceptibilities of clinical isolates of systemic and pathogenic fungi to ketoconazole. *J Infect Dis* **152**: 1249.

Shale DJ, Faux JA, Lane DJ (1987). Trial of ketoconazole in non-invasive pulmonary aspergillosis. *Thorax* **42**: 26.

Sheftel TG, Mader JT, Cierny G (1987). *Pseudallescheria boydii* soft tissue abscess. *Clin Orthop* **215**: 212.

Shepherd FA, Hoffert B, Evans WK *et al.* (1985). Ketoconazole: use in the treatment of ectopic adrenocorticotropic hormone production and Cushing's syndrome in small-cell lung cancer. *Arch Intern Med* **145**: 863.

Shepp DH, Klosterman A, Siegel MS, Meyers JD (1985). Comparative trial of ketoconazole and nystatin for prevention of fungal infection in neutropenic patients treated in a protective environment. *J Infect Dis* **152**: 1257.

Silber JG, Gombert ME, Green KM *et al.* (1983). Treatment of chromomycosis with ketoconazole and 5-fluorocytosine. *J Amer Acad Dermatol* **8**: 236.

Sindhuphak W, MacDonald E, Head E, Hudson RD (1985). *Exophiala jeanselmei* infection in a postrenal transplant patient. *J Amer Acad Dermatol* **13**: 877.

Slama TG (1983). Treatment of disseminated and progressive cavitary histoplasmosis with ketoconazole. *Amer J Med* **74**: 70.

Slater CA, Sickel JZ, Visvesvara GS, Pabico RC, Gaspari AA (1994). Successful treatment of disseminated *Acanthamoeba* infection in an immunocompromised patient. *New Engl J Med* **331**: 85.

Slotman GJ Burchard KW (1987). Ketoconazole prevents *Candida* sepsis in critically ill surgical patients. *Arch Surg* **122**: 147.

Smego RA, Durack DT (1984). *In vitro* susceptibility testing of *Naegleria fowleri* to ketoconazole, Bay n 7133, and allopurinol riboside. *J Parasitol* **70**: 317.

Smith AG (1984). Potentiation of oral anticoagulants by ketoconazole. *Brit Med J* **288**: 188.

Smith DE, Midgley J, Allan M *et al.* (1991). Itraconazole versus ketoconazole in the treatment of oral and oesophageal candidosis in patients infected with HIV. *AIDS* **5**: 1367.

Sobel JD (1986). Recurrent vulvovaginal candidiasis A prospective study of the efficacy of maintenance ketoconazole therapy. *New Engl J Med* **315**: 1455.

Sobel JD (1992). Fluconazole maintenance therapy in recurrent vulvovaginal candidiasis. *Int J Gynecol Obstet* **37** (Suppl 1): 17.

Sobel JD, Muller G (1984). Ketoconazole in the prevention of experimental candidal vaginitis. *Antimicrob Ag Chemother* **25**: 281.

Sonino N (1987). The use of ketoconazole as an inhibitor of steroid production. *New Engl J Med* **317**: 812.

South DA, Brass C, Stevens DA (1981). Chromohyphomycosis. Treatment with ketoconazole. *Arch Dermatol* **117**: 311.

Stevens DA (1984). Antifungal susceptibility testing. *Mycopathologia* **87**: 135.

Stevens D A, Stille R L, Williams P L, Sugar A M (1983). Experience with ketoconazole in three major manifestations of progressive coccidiodomycosis. *Amer J Med* **74**: 58.

Stierstorfer MB, Schwartz BK, McGuire JB, Miller AC (1988). *Pseudallescheria boydii* mycetoma in northern New England. *Int J Dermatol* **27**: 383.

Stockley RJ, Daneshmend TK, Bredow MT *et al.* (1986). Ketoconazole pharmacokinetics during chronic dosing in adults with haematological malignancy. *Eur J Clin Microbiol* 5: 513.

Stricker BH, Block APR, Bronkhorst FB *et al.* (1986). Ketoconazole associated hepatic injury. *J Hepatol* 3: 399.

Sugar AM (1995). Use of amphotericin B with azole antifungal drugs: What are we doing? *Antimicrob Ag Chemother* 39: 1907.

Sugar AM, Stevens DA (1985). *Candida rugosa* in immunocompromised infection. *Cancer* 56: 318.

Sugar AM, Alsip SG, Galgiani JN *et al.* (1987). Pharmacology and toxicity of high-dose ketoconazole. *Antimicrob Ag Chemother* 31: 1874.

Sugar EF, Sugar AM, Kreger BE (1992). Effect of common beverages on the dissolution of ketoconazole tablets. *AIDS* 6: 1221.

Sugarman B, Mummaw N (1988). Effects of antimicrobial agents on growth and chemotaxis of *Trichomonas vaginalis*. *Antimicrob Ag Chemother* 32: 1323.

Sundar S, Kumar K, Singh VP (1990). Ketoconazole in visceral leishmaniasis. *Lancet* 336: 1582.

Svedhem A (1984). Toxic hepatitis following ketoconazole treatment. *Scand J Infect Dis* 16: 123.

Swartz DA, Harrington P, Wilcox R (1988). Candidal epididymitis treated with ketoconazole. *New Engl J Med* 319: 1485.

Symoens J, Moens M, Dom J *et al.* (1980). An evaluation of two years of clinical experience with ketoconazole. *Rev Infect Dis* 2: 674.

Tanz RR, Herbert AA, Esterly NB (1988). Treating tinea capitis: Should ketoconazole replace griseofulvin? *J Pediatr* 112: 987.

Tavitian A, Raufman J P, Rosenthal LE *et al.* (1986). Ketoconazole-resistant *Candida* esophagitis in patients with acquired immunodeficiency syndrome. *Gastroenterol* 90: 443.

Tkach JR, Rinaldi MG (1983). Treatment of vaginal candidiasis with ketoconazole. *Amer J Obstet Gynecol* 144: 122.

Towersey L, Wanke B, Estrella RR *et al.* (1988). *Conidiobolus coronatus* infection treated with ketoconazole. *Arch Dermatol* 124: 1392.

Trachtenberg J, Pont A (1984). Ketoconazole therapy for advanced prostate cancer. *Lancet* ii: 433.

Tucker W S Jr, Snell B B, Island D P, Gregg C R (1985). Reversible adrenal insufficiency induced by ketoconazole. *JAMA* 253: 2413.

Tudehope DI, Rigby B (1983). Neonatal systemic candidiasis treated with miconazole and ketoconazole. *Med J Aust* 1: 480.

Umstead GS, Babiak LM, Tejwani S (1987). Immune hemolytic anemia associated with ketoconazole therapy. *Clin Pharmacol* 6: 499.

Urbina JA, Lazardi K, Marchan E *et al.* (1993). Mevinolin (Lovastatin), potentiates the antiproliferative effects of ketoconazole and terbinafine against *Trypanosoma (Schizotrypanum) cruzi*: *In vitro* and *in vivo* studies. *Antimicrob Ag Chemother* 37: 580.

Van Cutsem J (1983). The antifungal activity of ketoconazole. *Amer J Med* 74: 9.

Van der Meer J W M, Keunung J J, Scheijgrond HW *et al.* (1980). The influence of gastric acidity on the bio-availability of ketoconazole. *J Antimicrob Chemother* 6: 552.

Van Dijke C P H, Veerman F R, Haverkamp H Ch (1983). Anaphylactic reactions to ketoconazole. *Brit Med J* 287: 1673.

Van Parys G, Evenpoel C, van Damme B, Desmet VJ (1987). Ketoconazole-induced hepatitis: a case with a definite cause-effect relationship. *Liver* 7: 27.

Van Rensburg C E J, Anderson R, Joone G *et al.* (1983). The effects of ketoconazole on cellular and humoral immune functions. *J Antimicrob Chemother* 11: 49.

Van Tyle JH, (1984). Ketoconazole. Mechanism of action, spectrum of activity, pharmacokinetics, drug interactions, adverse reactions and therapeutic use. *Pharmacotherapy* 4: 343.

Vargas J, Recacoechea M (1988). Ketoconazole in the treatment of paracoccidioidomycosis (South American blastomycosis). Experience in 30 cases in Bolivia. *Mycoses* 31: 187.

Venugopal, PV, Venugopal TV, Laing WN *et al.* (1990). Black grain mycetoma caused by *Madurella grisea* in Saudi Arabia. *Int J Dermatol* 29: 434.

Venugopal, PV, Venugopal TV, Ramakrishna ES, Ilavarasi S (1993). Antimycotic susceptibility testing of agents of black grain eumycetoma. *J Med Vet Mycol* 31: 161.

von Recklinghausen G, di Maio C, Ansorg R (1992). Activity of the antimycotic ketoconazole against *Helicobacter pylori*. *J Antimicrob Chemother* 30: 238.

Wali JP, Aggarwal P, Gupta U, Saluja S, Singh S (1990). Ketoconazole in the treatment of visceral leishmaniasis. *Lancet* 336: 810.

Walsh TJ, Rubin M, Hathorn J *et al.* (1991). Amphotericin B vs high-dose ketoconazole for empirical antifungal therapy among febrile, granulocytopenic cancer patients. A prospective, randomized study. *Arch Intern Med* 151: 765.

Warnock DW, Johnson EM, Richardson MD *et al.* (1983). Modified response to ketoconazole of *Candida albicans* from a treatment failure. *Lancet* i: 642.

Wheat LJ, Connolly-Stringfield PA, Baker RL *et al.* (1990). Disseminated histoplasmosis in the acquired immune deficiency syndrome: Clinical findings, diagnosis and treatment, and review of the literature. *Medicine* 69: 361.

White M C, Kendall-Taylor P (1985). Adrenal hypofunction in patients taking ketoconazole. *Lancet* i: 44.

Wong PW, Ching WTW, Kwon-Chung KJ, Meyer RD (1989). Disseminated *Phialophora parasitica* infection in humans: Case report and review. *Rev Infect Dis* 11: 770.

Wong-Beringer A, Jacobs RA, Guglielmo J (1992). Treatment of funguria. *JAMA* 267: 2780.

Yamashita SK, Ludwig EA, Middleton E, Jusko WJ (1991). Lack of pharmacokinetic and pharmacodynamic interactions between ketoconazole and prednisolone. *Clin Pharmacol Ther* 49: 558.

Yancy RW, Perlino CA, Kaufman L (1991). Asymptomatic blastomycosis of the central nervous system with progression in patients given ketoconazole therapy: a report of two cases. *J Infect Dis* 164: 807.

Yangco B G, Okafor J I, TeStrake D (1984). *In vitro* susceptibilities of human and wild-type isolates of *Basidiobolus* and *Conidiobolus* species. *Antimicrob Ag Chemother* 25: 413.

Yinnon AM, Woodin KA, Powell KR (1992). *Candida lusitaniae* infection in the newborn: case report and review of the literature. *Pediatr Infect Dis J* 11: 878.

Young LS (1982). Leading article The outlook for antifungal prophylaxis in the compromised host. *J Antimicrob Chemother* 9: 338.

Wackym PA, Gray GF, Richie RE, Gregg CR (1985). Cutaneous chromomycosis in renal transplant recipients. Successful management in two cases. *Arch Intern Med* 145: 1036.

Weinrauch L, El-On J (1984). The effect of ketoconazole and a combination of rifampicin/amphotericin B on cutaneous leishmaniasis in laboratory mice. *Trans Roy Soc Trop Med Hyg* 78: 389.

Weinrauch L, Livshin R, El-on J (1987). Ketoconazole in cutaneous leishmaniasis. *Brit J Dermatol* 117: 666.

Wong ESM, Hay RJ, Clayton YM, Noble WC (1984). Comparison of the therapeutic effect of ketoconazole tablets and econazole lotion in the treatment of chronic paronychia. *Clin Exp Dermatol* 9: 489.

Working Party of the British Society for Antimicrobial Chemotherapy (1993). Chemoprophylaxis for candidosis and aspergillosis in neutropenia and transplantation: a review and recommendations. *J Antimicrob Chemother* 32: 5.

Yancy RW, Perlino CA, Kaufman L (1991). Asymptomatic blastomycosis of the central nervous system with progression in patients given ketoconazole therapy. A report of two cases. *J Infect Dis* 164: 807.

Zurcher RM, Frey BM, Frey FJ (1989). Impact of ketoconazole on the metabolism of prednisolone. *Clin Pharmacol Ther* 45: 366.

Fluconazole

Description

Fluconazole is a bis-triazole derivative, which has good therapeutic activity in several fungal infections. It differs from the other azole derivatives by the substitution of a triazole group for the imidazole group, the addition of a second triazole group and the insertion of two fluoride atoms in the phenyl ring. These changes make fluconazole highly water soluble, and hence give it a more favorable pharmacokinetic and toxicity profile, in comparison with the older imidazole agents. Fluconazole has a high bioavailability, and peak serum concentrations are similar following administration of equal doses by the oral or i.v. route. It has the chemical name 2-(2,4-difluorophenyl)-1,3-bis(1H-1,2,4-triazol-1-yl)-2-propanol.

Sensitive Organisms

1 Pathogenic yeast

Fluconazole is active against the majority of isolates of *Cryptococcus neoformans*. Isolates from HIV-infected individuals with recurrent cryptococcal meningitis showed no decrease in antifungal susceptibility relative to the initial isolate; however, there was a wide range of MICs for fluconazole ranging from <0.125 μg per ml to 20 μg per ml (Casadevall *et al.*, 1993). In the rabbit model of cryptococcal meningitis, i.v. fluconazole 80 mg per kg per day had little effect on yeast counts in CSF for the first 4 days of treatment, despite high CSF levels of fluconazole, but there was a significant reduction in colony counts during the last 10 days of treatment. At the end of 14 days treatment four of seven rabbits had sterile CSF cultures compared with 11 of 15 rabbits similarly treated with itraconazole (Perfect *et al.*, 1986). In the experimental model of subacute disseminated *Cryptococcus* infection in rats developed by Negroni *et al.* (1991), oral fluconazole was shown to be active against cryptococcosis. A dose reponse was demonstrated, with higher fluconazole doses (32 mg per kg per day) being significantly more effective (Negroni *et al.*, 1991).

Fluconazole is generally active against *Candida albicans*, *C. tropicalis* and *C. parapsilosis*, has some activity against *C. guilliermondii*, and no activity against *C. krusei*. The *in vitro* activity of fluconazole against many pathogens does not correlate with its activity in animal model infections with the same organisms. Fluconazole showed no postantifungal effect against *C. albicans* in the absence of human serum, but a concentration dependent postantifungal effect was demonstrated in the presence of 10% serum (Minguez *et al.*, 1994). Fluconazole pre-treatment of *C. albicans* increased the polymorphonuclear killing of yeasts, suggesting that fluconazole can damage the yeast rendering it more susceptible to intracellular killing by polymorphonuclear cells (Minguez *et al.*, 1994).

In normal mice with systemic *C. albicans* infection, 0.1–1.0 mg per kg fluconazole significantly prolonged survival, and 2.5–10 mg per kg fluconazole significantly improved survival in immunosuppressed mice with systemic *C. albicans* infection. This study reported that fluconazole was more than 20-fold as effective as ketoconazole (Troke *et al.*, 1985). Fluconazole (2.5–20 mg per kg orally twice daily) was found to be equally effective at reducing colony counts of *C. albicans* in the kidney of normal and neutropenic mice with disseminated candidiasis, but inferior to ampherotericin B (AMB) (van 't Wout *et al.*, 1989). These observations were confirmed by Van Etten *et al.* (1993) who also showed that prolonged treatment with fluconazole did not improve its efficacy, and treatment with high doses of fluconazole (64 mg per kg per day) failed to prevent relapse in both normal and immunosuppressed mice. The candidiasis model of subacute systemic infection in rats which mimics human infection more closely than the mouse models, was used to show that oral fluconazole at 10 mg per kg per day was as effective as AMB at the end of 7 days treatment. After 21 days treatment, fluconazole was less effective for kidney infection, and was equivalent to AMB for liver infection. This comparative efficacy was mirrored in the diabetic rat (Fisher *et al.*, 1989b). The efficacy of i.v. fluconazole (80 mg per kg per day) in the long-term treatment of *C. albicans* endophthalmitis in rabbits was inferior to AMB (1 mg per kg per day). Treatment with fluconazole was effective to 17 days with reduced fungal colony counts in the choroid-retina, but the treatment effect was lost by 24 days, despite the fact that fluconazole penetrates ocular tissues to reach high levels. The reasons for failure of prolonged fluconazole therapy in this model could be the fungistatic action of fluconazole, the development of resistance of the isolates, and that levels of fluconazole in ocular fluids may not correlate with efficacy (Filler *et al.*, 1991).

Fluconazole was ineffective at doses of 50–100 mg per kg for prophylaxis of *C. albicans* endocarditis, and was found to be inferior to AMB in the treatment of *C. albicans* endocarditis in the rabbit model, although outcome was directly related to dose and duration of treatment, and delay in iniation of treatment (Witt and Bayer, 1991). For the treatment of established endocarditis with *C. parapsilosis* fluconazole was equivalent to AMB, and while both agents were effective in the treatment of *C. tropicalis* endocarditis, AMB was more rapidly fungicidal (Witt *et al.*, 1993). Fluconazole (20 and 80 mg per kg per day) was found to be effective in reducing colony counts of *C. tropicalis* and *C. glabrata* in both liver and spleen of infected rats, but ineffective in the treatment of *C. krusei*. These *Candida* isolates had high MICs which did not correlate with *in vivo* efficacy (Fisher *et al.*, 1989a).

Fluconazole (5–20 mg per kg) is more active than AMB in murine infection with *Trichosporon beigelii*. Fluconazole exhibited fungistatic activity by reduced kidney fungal counts in a dose-dependent manner, but sterilization did not occur (Anaissie *et al.*, 1994a). Walsh *et al.* (1992) examined the effect of antifungal agents in the disseminated trichosporonosis model in persistently granulocytopenic rabbits using *T. beigelii*. They established that AMB 1.2 mg per kg per day and liposomal AMB 5 mg per kg per day were ineffective, and fluconazole 25 mg per kg per day was the most active agent, able to reduce tissue infection in lung, liver, spleen, and kidney by 10^2- to 10^5-fold.

2 Dimorphic fungi

Wide variation in susceptibilities for *Histoplasma capsulatum* have been reported. Early studies examining the efficacy of fluconazole given twice-daily, for murine histoplasmosis revealed it was as effective as intraperitoneal AMB in normal mice, but not as effective in immunosuppressed mice. Fluconazole did not result in cure in the immunosuppressed mice (Graybill *et al.*, 1986a; Kobayashi *et al.*, 1986, 1987). Oral fluconazole in doses up to 20 mg per kg given only once-daily, was significantly less effective than either intraperitoneal AMB or Sch 39304 in treating histoplasmosis in normal and leukopenic mice (Kobayashi *et al.*, 1990). This study also showed that *in vitro* susceptibility testing of fluconazole may not be predictive of *in vivo* activity against isolates of *H. capsulatum*.

For treatment of pulmonary *Blastomyces dermatitidis* infections in mice, fluconazole at doses of 25 mg per kg and 50 mg per kg produced survival rates of 30% and 100%; however fluconazole was unable to eradicate the fungus from the lungs of survivng mice. Fluconazole is less effective than AMB for this infection (Lyman *et al.*, 1986). Fluconazole was inferior to AMB in the murine model of coccidioidal meningitis, although it did have some activity with reduction in colony counts of *Coccidioides immitis* from brain, and improved survival (Graybill *et al.*, 1986b). Up to 73% of clinical isolates of *Penicillium marneffei* are borderline susceptible or resistant to fluconazole which is considered the least active azole drug for this infection (Supparatpinyo *et al.*, 1993).

3 Molds or filamentous fungi

Aspergillus species are generally resistant to fluconazole in *in vitro* assays. In the murine model of aspergillosis, oral fluconazole in doses ranging from 0.1 to 100 mg per kg was noted to have intermediate activity between ketoconazole (minimal activity) and AMB (Troke *et al.*,1987). Lack of activity against agents of mucormycosis was confirmed in a guinea pig model infected with either *Rhizopus microsporus* var. *rhizopodiformis* or *Rhizopus oryzae* (Van Cutsem *et al.*, 1989). *Scedosporium inflatum* is a mold increasingly isolated from subcutaneous infections, and is resistant to fluconazole (Salkin *et al.*, 1988). Medically significant species of *Fusarium* are resistant to fluconazole (Sekhon *et al.*, 1994).

4 Algae

Prototheca species are usually resistant to fluconazole (Gibb *et al.*, 1991).

5 Acanthamoeba

Fluconazole showed little activity against either trophozoites or cysts of *Acanthamoeba* with *in vitro* minimum trophozoite inhibitory concentrations of 7.8 μg per ml and minimum trophozoite amoebicidal concentrations of 62.5 μg per ml (Kilvington *et al.*, 1990).

6 Pneumocystis carinii

Pneumocystis carinii is now considered to be more closely related to fungi than protozoa. The target of most systemic antifungal drugs is inhibition of synthesis of ergosterol, which appears to be lacking in *P. carinii*. The main sterol present in cell membranes is cholesterol. Fluconazole (10 μg per ml) was found to be inactive in short-term culture and ineffective in the rat model at a dose of 40 mg per kg (Bartlett *et al.*, 1994).

7 Synergism with other drugs

The combination of fluconazole and flucytosine, both orally bioavailable antifungal agents, is currently being evaluated in a number of clinical settings. *In vitro* synergy between fluconazole and flucytosine has been demonstrated for 62% of 50 clinical isolates of *Cryptococcus neoformans* var. *neoformans* and antagonism not observed. The addition of flucytosine did not increase the *in vitro* activity of fluconazole if the initial fluconazole MIC for the isolate was >8 μg per ml (Nguyen *et al.*, 1995a). The combination of fluconazole and flucytosine was significantly superior to either drug alone in the murine model of intracerebral infection with *C. neoformans*. Delayed mortality and a significantly reduced tissue burden of *C. neoformans* occurred in mice receiving the combination (Allendoerfer *et al.*, 1991). In contrast, in a different murine model of systemic cryptococcosis, Polak (1987) observed indifference for the combination of fluconazole and flucytosine if treatment lasted 5 days, and antagonism when the treatment lasted more than 10 days. Synergy was also noted with fluconazole and flucytosine in systemic candidiasis with partially resistant flucytosine strains, but not with sensitive strains, while an additive effect was seen in wangiellosis, and indifference in aspergillosis (Polak, 1987). A synergistic postantifungal effect on *Candida albicans* has been demonstrated for fluconazole and flucytosine combinations at concentrations below the individual MICs. Postantifungal effects of 3.8–10.5 h were achieved with flucytosine and fluconazole combinations in a ratio of 1:16 and 1:32, and concentrations of 0.024–0.098 μg per ml for flucytosine and 0.78–1.56 μg per ml for fluconazole (Scalarone *et al.*, 1991).

In general, fluconazole and AMB are not considered synergistic or antagonistic (p. 1249). However, enhanced therapeutic activity of the combination of fluconazole and AMB for treatment of murine trichosporonosis was reported by Anaissie *et al.* (1994a).

8 Acquired resistance

It is becoming apparent that resistance to fluconazole is an increasing problem which develops during treatment or prophylaxis with fluconazole. It is more common in the immunocompromised patient, especially HIV-infected individuals, in whom fluconazole-resistance is related to the degree of immunodeficiency and the total cumulative dose of administered fluconazole (Rex *et al.*, 1995). In HIV-infected patients with oropharyngeal candidiasis, primary resistance in *Candida albicans* is rare, but secondary resistance occurs both *in vitro* and clinically in 5–10% of patients (Baily *et al.*, 1994; Ruhnke *et al.*, 1994a; Redding *et al.*, 1994; Sanguineti *et al.*, 1993). The resistant strain of *C. albicans* is generally the same as the initial infecting strain, but newly infecting resistant isolates have been identified by DNA genotyping (Bart-Delabesse *et al.*, 1993; Barchiesi *et al.*, 1995). Selection of resistant *Candida* spp. other than *C. albicans* (e.g. *C. krusei*, *C. glabrata*) following repeated short courses (5–21 days) of fluconazole is uncommon but has been described in HIV-infected patients receiving long-term fluconazole (Fox *et al.*, 1991; Smith *et al.*, 1991; Ruhnke *et al.*, 1994b; Baily *et al.*, 1994) and cancer patients on fluconazole prophylaxis (Wingard *et al.*, 1991; Casasnovas *et al.*, 1992; Hoppe *et al.*, 1994).

Hitchcock *et al.* (1993) reported a case of infection with *C. glabrata* in which the organism developed resistance to fluconazole during therapy, and became cross-resistant to ketoconazole and itraconazole. These authors suggested resistance was unrelated to changes in the P-450 dependent 14 alpha-sterol demethylase, but was related to permeability changes of fungal cells to fluconazole.

The development of fluconazole-resistance has also been reported in *Cryptococcus neoformans* in AIDS patients with meningitis (Coker *et al.*, 1991; Paugam *et al.*, 1994).

9 Antifungal susceptibility testing

Several review articles have examined the problems associated with antifungal susceptibility testing in general, and with azoles in particular, which include the difficulty in reproducing results and the unreliable prediction of *in vivo* activity of the drug (Rex *et al.*, 1993; Working Party of the British Society for Antimicrobial Chemotherapy, 1995). Quantitative tests can vary depending on the methodology selected. For example, activity of fluconazole can be affected by the composition of culture medium, the pH, inoculum size, incubation temperature and duration of culture. One problem is 'tailing', when there is no sharp end-point and discernible growth occurs at increasing concentrations of triazoles. This phenomenon has been attributed to the pH and the composition of the medium used (Odds, 1985; Galgiani, 1987). The revised National Committee for Clinical Laboratory Standards (NCCLS) guidelines for determining MICs by broth macrodilution have markedly improved reproducibility but are extremely cumbersome for laboratories. Broth microdilution assays and E tests have been shown to be comparable and less arduous, although the E test gave falsely elevated results for fluconazole against *Candida tropicalis*, *Candida glabrata* and *Cryptococcus neoformans* (Espinel-Ingroff *et al.*, 1992; Barchiesi *et al.*, 1994; Sewell *et al.*, 1994; Colombo *et al.*, 1995; Chen *et al.*, 1996). The results of published *in vitro* studies are included below, but caution should be exercised in using these to guide therapy, as no correlation between *in vitro* results and clinical response in man has been established.

The definition of a susceptibility/resistant endpoint has not been established, but is considered by some investigators to be ≥25 µg per ml for *Candida albicans* (Pfaller *et al.*, 1994; Ruhnke *et al.*, 1994a,b). *In vivo* data are considered more relevant than *in vitro* susceptibility testing for antifungal drugs. Only in the murine hematogenous candidiasis model, has Anaissie *et al.* (1994b) demonstrated a correlation between *in vitro* susceptibility to fluconazole and clinical outcome measured by survival and reduced tissue burden. *In vitro* resistance appears to predict lack of *in vivo* activity in this model. Also a significant correlation between *in vitro* antifungal testing based on the NCCLS method and *in vivo* response to fluconazole treatment in murine cryptococcosis has been shown (Velez *et al.*, 1993).

10 Minimum inhibitory concentrations

The MICs of fluconazole are shown in Table IV.10.

Mode of Administration and Dosage

Fluconazole may be administered intravenously or orally. The dose is unchanged for the different formulations or mode of administration.

Indications and recommended doses
Oropharyngeal candidiasis: the US recommendations are 200-mg loading dose, followed by 100 mg daily, for at least 2 weeks. The UK guidelines recommend a lower dose of 50 mg daily for 7–14 days.

Esophageal candidiasis: the US recommendations are 200-mg loading dose, followed by 100 mg daily for a minimum of 3 weeks or 2 weeks after resolution of symptoms. The UK guidelines suggest 50 mg daily for 14–30 days, although 100 mg may be required in some situations.

Systemic candidiasis: 400-mg loading dose, followed by 200–400 mg daily

Cryptococcal infections: 400-mg loading dose, followed by 200–400 mg daily for at least 6–12 weeks, followed by indefinite 100–200 mg daily maintenance therapy.

The recommended doses in children older than 4 weeks are 3 mg per kg per day for mucosal candidiasis, 6–12 mg per kg per day for systemic candidiasis and cryptococcosis, and 3–12 mg per kg per day for prophylaxis of fungal infections in neutropenic children after radiotherapy or chemotherapy. Neonates aged 2–4 weeks require the same dose but at 48 h intervals, and neonates under 2 weeks should receive the same dose at 72 h intervals.

1 Patients with renal failure

The pharmacokinetics of a single oral dose of fluconazole were evaluated in patients with renal impairment (Toon *et al.*,1990). Although the maximum plasma concentration was not altered, the elimination half-life and total body clearance were significantly changed by decreasing glomerular filtration rate (GFR). The half-life was 31 h in those with normal renal function, 59 h

Table IV.10

Compiled from data published by Dixon and Polak (1987), Grant and Clissold (1987, 1990), Faergemann (1988), Patterson *et al.* (1990a), Sands *et al.* (1991), Penn *et al.* (1992), Sekhon *et al.* (1992, 1993, 1994), Wood *et al.* (1992), Barchiesi *et al.* (1993), Dube *et al.* (1994), Lau *et al.* (1995), Espinel-Ingroff *et al.* (1996), Van Eldere *et al.* (1996)

Organism	MIC (µg per ml) range	
	Broth	Agar
Yeast		
Candida spp.		
C. albicans	0.12–256	
C. guilliermondii	16	
C. krusei	32–>64	
C. parapsilosis	0.25–4	
C. tropicalis	0.5–>256	
C. kefyr (pseudotropicalis)	0.5–1.0	
C. lusitaniae	2–8	
C. rugosa	2.5–20	
C. glabrata (Torulopsis glabrata)	0.5–>32	
Cryptococcus neoformans	<0.125–32	
Hansenula anomala	1.56	
Malassezia furfur		12.5–50
Rhodotorula rubra	>100	
Trichosporon beigelii	2.5–16	
Dimorphic fungi		
Histoplasma capsulatum	2.95–>100	
Paracoccidioides brasiliensis	0.1	
Penicillium marneffei	6.25–25 (yeast form)	
	25–50 (myceliel form)	
Sporothrix schenckii	>80	
Mold		
Aspergillus spp.		
A. fumigatus	>100	
A. flavus	>100	
A. niger	>100	
Dematiaceous fungi		
Bipolaris spp.		10
Cladosporium spp.		>100
Dactylaria spp.		>100
Fonsecaea pedrosoi		20
Wangiella dermatitidis		30–100
Hyphomycetes		
Acremonium spp.		>32
Fusarium spp.	>100	
Hendersonula spp.		0.78–1.56
Pseudallescheria boydii		50
Scedosporium prolificans (inflatum)		>100
Dermatophytes		
Trichophyton spp.		0.05–0.39
Microsporum spp.		0.10–0.39
Epidermophyton spp.		0.05–0.10
Scytalidium spp.		0.78–1.56
Algae		
Prototheca wickerhamii	>80	

in those with a GFR of 20–70 ml per min, and 98 h in those with a GFR of less than 20 ml per min. The total clearance was directly proportional to the GFR, and the renal clearance in those with a GFR less than 20 ml per min was 20% of that observed in normal volunteers (Toon *et al.*, 1990).

Similar decreases in renal clearance and increases in half-lives were observed with decreasing creatinine clearance in multiple-dose pharmacokinetics of fluconazole (Berl *et al.*, 1995). In patients with end-stage renal disease undergoing hemodialysis, a 48% reduction in fluconazole plasma levels was noted over a 3 h hemodialysis period. The amount of fluconazole removed from the body by hemodialysis is approximately 38% of the administered dose. Plasma fluconazole concentrations declined minimally over the subsequent post-dialysis period (Toon *et al.*, 1990). A patient with acute renal failure undergoing continuous arteriovenous hemodiafiltration (CAVH) was found to have a total body clearance, area under the curve and half-life for fluconazole similar to those expected in normal volunteers (Nicolau *et al.*, 1994), and continuous venovenous hemofiltration (CVVH) in a patient with anuria effectively removed fluconazole by clearance into the hemofiltrate of 21 ml per min (Scholz *et al.*, 1995). No reduction in dose of fluconazole is required when patients undergo CAVH or CVVH. In patients with renal failure undergoing continuous ambulatory peritoneal dialysis (CAPD), and no peritoneal infection, the half-life of fluconazole ranged from 72 to 85 h, and the renal clearance (0.04 liter per h) was lower than the peritoneal clearance rate (0.33 liter per h). Only 3% of the administered dose of fluconazole was recovered in the urine in 144 h and approximately 18% of the administered dose was recovered in the dialysate in the 48 h post-dose. Total clearance is less than that observed in healthy volunteers, but the mean renal and peritoneal clearances correspond to 65% of the total clearance (Debruyne *et al.*, 1990).

The recommended dosing period for fluconazole in patients with renal insufficiency is 24 h for those with a creatinine clearance of greater than 40 ml per min, 48 h for those with a clearance of 20–40 ml per min and 72 h for those with a clearance of 10–20 ml per min. For individuals undergoing hemodialysis, a dose of 100–200 mg after each dialysis period is recommended (Oono *et al.*, 1992) and a 150-mg dose in a 2-liter dialysate bag every 2 days is recommended by Debruyne and Ryckelynck (1992). For patients with acute renal failure managed with continuous arteriovenous hemodiafiltration, standard maintenance doses apply, with no requirement for supplementation or dose adjustment (Nicolau *et al.*, 1994).

2 Intraperitoneal

Administration of fluconazole 50 mg or 150 mg in 2 liters of dialysis fluid, resulted in 87% of the dose absorbed by the peritoneum. However, the resorption was slow with time to maximum concentration of 7 h, and 18% of the administered dose recovered in the dialysate fluid from 6–48 h after administration (Debruyne *et al.*, 1990). The recommended dose of fluconazole for fungal peritonitis is 150 mg in 2 liters of dialysate fluid infused intraperitoneally over 6 h, every 48 h (Debruyne *et al.*, 1990). Reuman and Kondor (1992) have reported the use of 6 mg per kg fluconazole in 340 ml of dialysate fluid infused over 6 h followed by continuous cycling peritoneal dialysis with 90 min dwell time of dialysate fluid containing 3 mg per liter fluconazole, in a 19-month-old infant with end-stage renal disease and fungal peritonitis. Serum concentrations of fluconazole of 5–9.5 μg per ml were obtained with this regimen.

3 Intravitreal

Intravitreal fluconazole has been evaluated in rabbits and doses up to 100 μg in 0.1 ml have been injected intravitreally with no evidence of any corneal, lenticular or retinal toxicity (Schulman *et al.*, 1987). Fluconazole may be a potential agent for intravitreal use in the treatment of exogenous fungal endophthalmitis, although there is excellent penetration of all ocular tissues following either oral or i.v. administration.

4 Topical

Aqueous fluconazole solution (2 mg per ml in 0.9% saline), one drop applied to the eye every hour, in rabbits with experimentally induced *C. albicans* keratitis, penetrates into the cornea and aqueous humor well, and was shown to be highly effective in reducing the complication rate of the fungal keratitis, and eliminating *C. albicans* from the cornea (Behrens-Baumann *et al.*, 1990).

Availability

Intravenous formulation: 200 mg dose in 100 ml of sterile saline solution; 400 mg dose in 200 ml of sterile saline solution.

Oral formulation: 50 mg, 100 mg, and 200 mg tablets.

Oral suspension: 10 mg per ml, 40 mg per ml (requires reconstitution) – not available in all countries.

The stability of fluconazole 1 mg per ml and 2 mg per ml was evaluated in several types of injectable solutions. Stability was established in 20 mEq per liter potassium chloride plus 5% dextrose for 72 h, and sodium heparin 100 units per ml in 5% dextrose, lactated Ringer's solution for 24 h (Hunt Fugate *et al.*, 1993). Fluconazole 0.5 mg per ml or 1.75 mg per ml was determined to be stable in parenteral nutrition solutions containing 25% dextrose and either 1.0%, 2.5% and 5% amino acid solutions for up to 2 h (Couch *et al.*, 1992).

Serum Levels in Relation to Dose

The pharmacokinetics of fluconazole are independent of administration route or formulation (Brammer *et al.*, 1990). Following a 30-min infusion of 50 mg and 100 mg fluconazole in healthy male volunteers, the maximum plasma concentrations achieved were 0.96 μg per ml and 2.14 μg per ml, respectively. Steady-state was reached by 7 days of daily infusion and the terminal half-life was 30 h (Foulds *et al.*, 1988a). A comparison of the pharmacokinetics of single-dose fluconazole administered by the oral and i.v. routes in healthy volunteers reveals rapid absorption of the drug with maximum levels achieved within 2 h for oral doses of 25–100 mg, a gradual decline in plasma concentration with a half-life of 31 h (Shiba *et al.*, 1990). Fluconazole capsules and suspension formulations are bioequivalent in healthy adults (Laufen *et al.*, 1995). The long plasma half-life and long-sustained high plasma concentrations permits once-daily dosing. Maximum plasma concentrations and area-under-the-concentration-time-curve (AUC) are dose-dependent and the bioavailability is 90%, that is, the AUC after oral dosing was 90% of that measured after i.v. administration (Shiba *et al.*, 1990). In addition the bioavailability of fluconazole tablets crushed and administered via a feeding tube with enteral feeds to intensive care patients with normal gastrointestinal motility was 97% (Nicolau *et al.*, 1995). Mean plasma concentration at steady-state was 0.85 μg per ml after 25 mg and 1.45 μg per ml after 50 mg (Shiba *et al.*, 1990). The maximum plasma concentration was 10.1 μg per ml after 200 mg of fluconazole orally and 18.9 μg per ml after 400 mg orally (Grant and Clissold, 1990). Multiple dosing achieves a 2.5-fold increase in peak plasma concentrations of fluconazole, compared with single dosing, with steady-state achieved generally within 6–10 days (Brammer *et al.*, 1990). The apparent volume of distribution of fluconazole administered orally was 55–59 liters, which was equivalent to 75% of body weight, and approaches the volume of total body water (Shiba *et al.*, 1990).

Binding to plasma proteins is low at 11–12% (Humphrey *et al.*, 1985) and there is minimal binding to tissue proteins and fat. Haubrich *et al.* (1994) measured steady-state serum concentrations of fluconazole after administration of 800 mg orally in HIV-infected patients and reported a mean level of 45 ± 15 μg per ml. Mean steady-state peak plasma concentrations of fluconazole after doses of 1200 mg, 1600 mg, and 2000 mg daily in cancer patients with invasive mould infections were 51.8 μg per ml, 74.4 μg per ml and 91.8 μg per ml respectively (Anaissie *et al.*, 1995).

The pharmacokinetics of fluconazole given by daily i.v. infusion in doses of 2–8 mg per kg was evaluated in children with cancer, aged 5–15 years by Lee *et al.* (1992). Peak serum concentrations of 3.9–9.5 μg per ml were achieved after single doses of 2–8 mg per kg, and at steady-state maximum concentrations of 5.4–14.3 μg per ml were achieved. The total clearance was 12–29 ml per min and the half-life was 15.5–20.3 h. The volume of distribution approximated that of total body water and varies with age, (1.18–2.25 liters per kg in neonates and 0.7 liter per kg in young adults) (Brammer and Coates, 1994). Thus the pharmacokinetics of fluconazole in children reveal a shorter elimination half-life, larger volume of distribution and lower AUCs than those measured after comparable doses in adults (Lee *et al.*, 1992; Seay *et al.*, 1995). The pharmacokinetics of fluconazole administered as a single i.v. dose of 6 mg per kg followed by daily oral 3 mg per kg doses for 7 days to ten children with hematologic disorders, revealed a mean elimination half-life of 15.6 h, volume of distribution at steady-state of 0.77 liter per kg, and oral bioavailability was 92%, with rapid oral absorption (Seay *et al.*, 1995). Neonates eliminate fluconazole slowly, with a mean elimination half-life of 88.6 h, which decreases 1 week after birth to 67.5 h and 55.2 h at 2 weeks of age (Brammer and Coates, 1994). The single-dose pharmacokinetics of 2 mg per kg and 8 mg per kg fluconazole suspension in HIV-infected children revealed comparable levels with non-infected children. At doses of 2 mg per kg and

8 mg per kg, the peak plasma concentration ranged from 2.3 to 4.4 μg per ml and 5.4 to 12.1 μg per ml, the AUC was 84.9–136 μg.h per ml and 330–684 μg.h per ml, and the respective half-lives were 19.8–34.8 h and 25.6–42.3 h (Nahata and Brady, 1995).

Single-dose pharmacokinetics of a 100-mg fluconazole i.v. dose were studied in nine patients with cirrhosis of the liver, and compared with ten normal volunteers. There was a significant increase in the AUC and decrease in the plasma clearance. These observations do not appear to warrant dose reduction in cirrhosis (Ruhnke *et al.*, 1995).

There was no difference in peak plasma concentration of fluconazole in patients who received high dose melphalan and total body irradiation and normal volunteers indicating that absorption was not impaired by gastrointestinal mucosal damage caused by preparation for autologous bone marrow transplantation. However, the renal excretion was decreased in comparison with normal volunteers (Milliken *et al.*, 1989).

Evaluation of the pharmacokinetics of fluconazole in HIV-infected patients revealed that the AUCs, and maximum concentrations increased proportionally over a dose range of 50–400 mg (Tett *et al.*, 1995). There was no significant difference in bioavailability or maximum concentration after oral dosing with 100 mg fluconazole and time to achieve maximum concentration of fluconazole between HIV-infected patients and normal volunteers. None of the HIV-infected patients had diarrhea or had abnormal liver function tests. However, the total plasma clearance and the volume of distribution was significantly lower in the HIV-infected patients with low CD4 cell counts (less than 200 per mm^3) and the elimination half-life was significantly longer in this group also (Tett *et al.*,1995; DeMuria *et al.*, 1993). A single case report of the CSF penetration of fluconazole in an AIDS patient with cryptococcal meningitis revealed a CSF:serum ratio of 0.7 at 4 h post-dose (Chin *et al.*, 1990).

The effect of food on the bioavailability of fluconazole was evaluated by Zimmerman *et al.* (1994), and no significant effect of a light or heavy meal was found. The peak serum concentration was not significantly influenced by food, while the bioavailability of fluconazole relative to the full meal was 110% pre-prandially and 102% after a light meal. The absorption and elimination of fluconazole administered to healthy male volunteers was not affected by the concomitant administration of antacid containing aluminum and magnesium hydroxide (Thorpe *et al.*, 1990). The maximum concentration following a single oral dose of 100 mg was 1.70 μg per ml without concomitant antacid and 1.71 μg per ml when administered with antacid, and the bioavailability was unchanged (Thorpe *et al.*, 1990). Intravenous cimetidine infused to maintain the gastric pH greater than 6.0, had no significant effect on the bioavailability of fluconazole (Blum *et al.*, 1991a). However, oral administration of cimetidine resulted in a non-clinically significant reduction in maximum serum concentration and AUC of fluconazole (Lazar and Wilner, 1990). A patient who had undergone a partial gastrectomy with resection of his duodenum and ileum was found to achieve serum concentrations after oral dosing to a degree comparable with those obtained in normal volunteers (Joe *et al.*, 1994).

Excretion

1 Urine

The major route of elimination of fluconazole is renal clearance with 80% of the drug excreted unchanged in the urine. In children, the urinary excretion rate after i.v. dosing was 65% (Lee *et al.*, 1992). After oral administration of fluconazole, high urine concentrations 9.5 μg per ml and 38.7 μg per ml were measured at 2 h after 50 mg and 100 mg doses, respectively. Recovery of the unchanged form of fluconazole in the urine by 120 h after oral dosing was 69–75%. Brammer *et al.* (1991) determined the disposition and metabolism of ^{14}C-fluconazole in three healthy male volunteers. Mean excretion of unchanged drug in urine was 80% of the administered dose and an additional 11% was excreted in the urine as the glucuronide conjugate of unchanged fluconazole and *N*-oxide metabolites (Brammer *et al.*, 1991).

2 Inactivation in body

Fluconazole undergoes minimal metabolism with no significant concentrations of metabolites circulating in plasma (Brammer *et al.*, 1991).

3 Feces

Up to 2% is recovered in the feces and there appears to be no first-pass effect following gastrointestinal absorption (Dudley,1990).

Distribution of the Drug in Body

In animal studies, extensive tissue penetration has been demonstrated. As 90% of fluconazole circulates in plasma as unbound drug, it has a large volume of distribution corresponding to total body water. Tissue concentrations of fluconazole decline more slowly than plasma concentrations. Penetration of drug into CSF, brain, liver, spleen, kidney and vitreous humor after a 25 mg per kg i.v. dose of fluconazole in rabbits was excellent (Walsh et al., 1989). Positron emission tomographic scanning was used to determine the distribution of fluconazole in tissues of healthy male volunteers following infusion of a tracer dose of ^{18}F-fluconazole (5–7mCi) plus 400 mg of unlabeled drug. Concentrations of drug 2 h after the 5 mg per kg single dose were $4.92 \pm 0.17 \, \mu g$ per g for brain, $6.98 \pm 0.20 \, \mu g$ per g for heart, $7.81 \pm 0.46 \, \mu g$ per g for lung, $12.94 \pm 0.24 \, \mu g$ per g for liver, 22.96 ± 2.5 for spleen, $11.23 \pm 0.61 \, \mu g$ per g for kidney, $8.24 \pm 0.58 \, \mu g$ per g for prostate, $1.24 \pm 0.29 \, \mu g$ per g for bone, and $3.76 \pm 0.30 \, \mu g$ per ml for blood (Fischman et al., 1993). All tissue concentrations except bone exceeded the 6 µg per g concentration level thought necessary for inhibition of most Candida species. As steady-state plasma concentrations are 2- to 2.5-fold those after a single dose, tissue concentrations at steady-state would also be predicted to be 2- to 2.5-fold those after the single dose (Fischman et al., 1993). The penetration of fluconazole into brain was determined after 4 days of oral ingestion of fluconazole 400 mg daily in four patients with cerebral tumors. The mean plasma concentration was 13.5 µg per ml and mean brain tissue concentration was 17.6 µg per g, with a resultant brain to plasma ratio of 1.33 (Thaler et al., 1995).

There is significant penetration (60–80%) of fluconazole into the CSF of rabbits (Perfect and Durack, 1985) and this has been confirmed in normal volunteers and patients with inflamed meninges. In healthy male volunteers who received either 50 mg per day or 100 mg per day of i.v. fluconazole, the CSF concentrations at steady-state (day 7) were 1.26 µg per ml and 2.74 µg per ml, respectively (Foulds et al., 1988b). The penetration of fluconazole into CSF after oral dosing with 200 mg fluconazole in patients with meningitis was 60–70%, achieving CSF levels of 2.2–4.4 µg per ml (Foulds et al., 1988b). In patients with coccidioidal meningitis, mean CSF concentrations of fluconazole were 74–88% of the serum concentration, and there was a slightly longer half-life in CSF (Tucker et al., 1988). Byers et al. (1992) have corroborated the extensive penetration of fluconazole into CSF in a child with Candida tropicalis meningitis. They demonstrated that trough concentrations of fluconazole can exceed the corresponding trough serum concentration (approximately 8 µg per ml). At i.v. doses of 6 mg per kg fluconazole, the peak serum concentration was 15 µg per ml and peak CSF concentration was 11 µg per ml. The serum half-life was 20.6 h and CSF half-life was 26.5 h (Byers et al., 1992).

Peak concentrations of fluconazole in bile after administration of 200 mg fluconazole i.v. were equivalent to peak serum concentrations (11.9 µg per ml and 11.6 µg per ml), and were generally 2 µg per ml greater than corresponding serum concentrations from 6 h after administration. Bile concentrations were also 2 µg per ml greater than serum concentrations 6 h after the drug was administered orally (Bozzette et al., 1992).

Penetration of fluconazole into sputum was evaluated after a single dose of 150 mg of fluconazole in bronchiectatic patients. Sputum was collected at 4 and 24 h after dosing and fluconazole concentrations compared with plasma concentration collected at the same time. The mean ratio of sputum:plasma was 1.06 ± 0.38 at 4 h and 0.92 ± 0.4 at 24 h, indicating similar levels in sputum as in plasma, throughout the dosing period (Ebden et al., 1989).

Fluconazole levels in saliva after a single 400-mg dose of fluconazole are approximately half those achieved in plasma in normal volunteers. The mean peak salivary concentration was 2.6 µg per ml at 3 h post-administration and at 24 h the mean salivary concentration was 1.4 µg per ml (Brammer et al., 1990; Force and Nahata, 1995). AIDS patients with oropharyngeal candidosis, were found to have salivary fluconazole levels (measured by a bioassay using paper discs) greater than corresponding plasma concentrations in the majority of cases, and the correlation between serum and saliva concentrations was generally poor (Garcia-Hermoso et al., 1995). These investigators found salivary concentrations were not influenced by xerostomia, and that salivary fluconazole levels were lower than the MIC of the Candida isolate in patients who failed treatment. Laufen et al. (1995) have shown salivary concentrations of fluconazole were considerably higher and maintained for 4 h post-dose, when the equivalent dose of fluconazole is administered as a suspension rather than a capsule, and the oral mucosa exposure to fluconazole was increased by 80%.

Ocular penetration has been studied in rabbits, and fluconazole was found to penetrate all ocular tissues well after both i.v. and oral administration, with greater concentrations in all the ocular tissues assayed compared with the corresponding plasma concentration. Fluconazole readily penetrates the cornea, aqueous humor, vitreous humor, the choroid and retina. The fluconazole levels in the aqueous humor were 65% and 28% of the serum concentrations in the presence or absence of ocular inflammation (Savani et al., 1987; O'Day et al., 1990).

The concentration of fluconazole in abscess fluid in a patient receiving i.v. fluconazole 800 mg daily for extrapulmonary coccidioidomycosis was 28.4 μg per ml and was comparable with plasma levels achieved with the same dose (Haubrich et al., 1994). Fluconazole penetrates well into joint fluid in the setting of inflamed synovium. O'Meeghan et al. (1990) measured simultaneous plasma and joint fluid levels of 15.9 μg per ml and 17.9 μg per ml in specimens collected 20 h after the last dose of 400 mg i.v. fluconazole. Penetration of fluconazole into epidermis, and blister fluid was evaluated after a 50-mg oral dose in normal male and female volunteers. The mean blister fluid concentrations were 1.03 μg per ml and 2.84 μg per ml on days 1 and 14 of dosing, and the mean epidermis concentrations on days 1 and 14 were 5.55 μg per g and 6.45 μg per g respectively, which exceeded corresponding plasma concentrations (Haneke, 1992). Concentrations of fluconazole in the stratum corneum after 12 days of 50 mg daily were 73 μg per g and were 5.8 μg per g 7 days after cessation of the drug. Fluconazole levels in sweat were 4.6 μg per ml and dermis-epidermis were 2.8 μg per ml. The elimination of fluconazole from stratum corneum is 2- to 3-fold slower than from plasma, and fluconazole remained detectable in hair and toenails 4–5 months after 5-day dosing (Faergemann and Laufen, 1993; Wildfeuer et al., 1994).

Mean peak concentrations of fluconazole of 2.43 μg per g in vaginal secretions and 2.82 μg per ml in plasma were achieved in women after a 150-mg single oral dose. Levels of 1 μg per g fluconazole (greater than the MIC of most strains of Candida albicans) persisted in vaginal secretions for up to 72 h after the maximum concentration was achieved 8 h after administration (Houang et al., 1990). Penetration of fluconazole into the prostate is important, as it has been proposed as a reservoir for persistent infection with Cryptococcus neoformans in the immunocompromised host. Fluconazole concentrations in the prostate were measured in patients with benign prostatic hypertrophy who received 5 days of 200 mg oral fluconazole daily, and underwent prostate resection. The mean total concentration of prostate fluconazole was 1.93 μg per g and was approximately 30% of the corresponding serum levels (Finley et al., 1995).

Pascual et al. (1993) evaluated the uptake and intracellular activity of fluconazole in human polymorphonuclear leukocytes, and found a rapid uptake of fluconazole so that cell-associated concentrations were twice the extracellular concentrations, but the activity of fluconazole against intracellular C. albicans was significantly lower than that of amphotericin B.

Mode of Action

The principal mechanism of action of fluconazole is inhibition of C-14 alpha demethylation. The azole ring nitrogen is thought to bind to the heme component of the fungal cytochrome P-450 enzyme lanosterol C-14 demethylase thereby preventing conversion of lanosterol to ergosterol, which results in depletion of normal fungal sterols (ergosterol) and accumulation of 14 alpha methyl sterols (lanosterol) (see Fig. IV.1, p. 1261). This results in increased membrane permeability, with leakage of essential elements (potassium, amino acids) and impaired uptake of purine and pyrimidine precursors of DNA synthesis, as well as altered membrane-bound enzyme activity. Fluconazole is generally fungistatic.

Fluconazole has a much lower affinity for mammalian cytochrome P-450 enzyme systems. The IC_{50} for mammalian demethylase from rat hepatic microsome is >300 μg per ml, compared with the IC_{50} for C. albicans C-14 demethylase of 0.015 μg per ml (Shaw et al., 1987). Despite the high affinity for fungal cytochrome P-450 enzymes, fluconazole at doses of 10 mg per kg per day for 7 days can significantly induce the mammalian cytochrome P-450 enzyme system responsible for drug metabolism (Lavrijsen et al., 1990).

In addition to the inhibitory effect on fungal replication, fluconazole has also been shown to significantly reduce the adherence of Candida species to the oral mucosa. This may be an additional mode of action in the prevention and treatment of mucosal candidal infections (Darwazeh et al., 1991). Odds and Webster (1988) examined the influence of fluconazole on some aspects of the host–parasite interactions in the setting of Candida infections, and found that few effects were exerted. Fluconazole had no effect on the ability of polymorphonuclear leukocytes to phagocytose and kill C. albicans, and had no effect on lymphoproliferative responses to mitogens in vitro. It is thought that C. albicans may resist intracellular killing by macrophages through the development of germ tubes, the initial stage of hypha formation. Fluconazole inhibited the formation of germ tubes in macrophages, but had only a minimal effect on the number of Candida organisms inside the macrophages, in experiments performed by van 't Wout et al. (1990).

Toxicity

The overall rate of adverse effects in manufacturer-sponsored trials was 16% in over 4000 patients treated with the drug for longer than 7 days. The most frequently reported events were nausea (3.7%), vomiting (1.7%), diarrhea (1.5%), abdominal pain (1.7%), headache (1.9%) and skin rash (1.8%) (Grant and Clissold, 1990). A significant proportion of these patients had severe underlying disorders. Early discontinuation of therapy occurred in 1.5% of patients because of adverse events and 1.3% due to significant laboratory abnormalities (usually liver function). There did not appear to be a dose-dependent increase in the adverse event rate over the dose range of 100–400 mg (Todd et al., 1990). However, Anaissie et al. (1995) summarized their experience with high-dose fluconazole (800–2000 mg daily) and reported a definite increase in toxicity for those receiving 2000 mg daily. Doses of 1600 mg daily appeared to be associated with an increase in hepatic toxicity.

1 Gastrointestinal side-effects

Nausea, vomiting, abdominal pain, and diarrhea have been reported in about 5% patients and rarely are severe enough to warrant discontinuation of the drug. Less frequently reported gastrointestinal effects include dyspepsia, heartburn, anorexia, dry mouth, dysgeusia, flatus and bloating.

2 Rash and hypersensitivity reactions

A diffuse maculopapular rash with or without pruritus has been reported in about 5% patients taking fluconazole. Stevens–Johnson syndrome has been reported in seven patients with AIDS; however, the role of other drugs in the etiology could not be ruled out, and this complication appears to be rare (Gussenhoven et al., 1991). In addition, fluconazole-induced toxic epidermal necrolysis involving 70% of the body and with severe mucosal involvement, has been described in an HIV-infected patient and confirmed on skin biopsy. This patient had started fluconazole 5 days before the onset of the rash and was not taking any other medication (Azon-Masoliver and Vilaplana, 1993). A fixed drug eruption to fluconazole has been described and challenge with fluconazole provoked an identical reaction demonstrated on skin biopsy, in a man self-administering intermittent doses of 150 mg for recurrent balanitis (Morgan and Carmichael, 1994). A well documented case of angioedema has been reported in a woman receiving 150 mg fluconazole twice-monthly (Abbott et al., 1991), and an anaphylactic reaction following oral fluconazole 150 mg was reported in a woman who had never received fluconazole previously. She had been treated with ketoconazole over 2 years earlier (Neuhas et al., 1991).

Fluconazole-induced alopecia was reported in a 72-year-old woman who received 200–300 mg fluconazole daily for 6 months prior to the onset of hair loss. New hair growth started within 3 weeks of discontinuing fluconazole (Weinroth and Tuazon, 1993). Alopecia was observed in 16% patients with sporotrichosis after 3–6 months of fluconazole 400–800 mg per day, and in 13–20% of patients in Mycoses Study Group patients. Hair loss was reversible when fluconazole was stopped, and resolved within 6 months. This adverse effect appears to be associated with high-dose fluconazole (Pappas et al., 1995; Kauffman et al., 1996).

3 Hepatic effects

Modest elevations of aminotransferase activity is the most frequently reported laboratory adverse event reported in association with fluconazole therapy (De Wit et al., 1989). Asymptomatic elevation of hepatic transaminases occurred in three of 22 (12%) children after 4 days of i.v. fluconazole 2–8 mg per kg. The liver function tests returned to normal rapidly after cessation of the drug (Lee et al., 1992). In an open trial of i.v. fluconazole at two doses, elevated liver function tests were observed in 25% patients. All values returned to normal within 7 days of ceasing fluconazole. There was no dose-related hepatotoxicity (Graninger et al., 1993). Patients infected with HIV appear to experience a greater rate of liver function test abnormalities in association with fluconazole therapy (47% in one study) (Gil et al., 1991).

Symptomatic elevations in liver function test abnormalities, including jaundice, are less frequent and are usually seen in association with pre-existing liver disease or other potentially hepatotoxic drugs. However, jaundice and abnormal liver function tests have been reported with temporal trends of resolution on stopping fluconazole (Franklin et al., 1989; Munoz et al., 1991; Gearhart et al., 1994). Wells and Lever (1992) reported a case of fluconazole-induced cholestatic liver damage and suggested a dose-responsive toxicity effect, with deterioration in liver function when the dose of fluconazole was increased from 100 mg alternate days to 200 mg daily. Recently, subacute mitochondrial liver damage manifested as mixed cholestatic and trans-aminase hepatic enzyme elevation which improved on cessation of chronic fluconazole maintenance therapy, and recurred on rechallenge was reported in an AIDS patient. Electron micoscopy revealed giant mitochondria with paracrystalline inclusions and enlarged smooth endoplasmic reticulum. The light microscopy changes of increased granularity of the cytoplasm reversed on cessation of fluconazole (Guillame et al., 1995). Fatal fluconazole hepatotoxicity is a rare complication, and has been reported in an AIDS patient within 3 weeks of starting fluconazole 400 mg daily. Postmortem examination excluded other potential causes of acute fulminant hepatic necrosis (Jacobson *et al.*, 1994).

4 Hematologic effects

Anemia, leukopenia, neutropenia and thrombocytopenia have all been reported (Mercurio and Elewski, 1995). Eosinophilia, often in association with skin rash, has also been observed. Severe symptomatic thrombocytopenia (platelet count of 25 000 per μl) was noted in a renal transplant recipient receiving fluconazole 200 mg daily. After cessation of fluconazole the platelet count gradually rose to normal within 2 weeks (Agarwal *et al.*, 1990). Agranulocytosis and thrombocytopenia have been reported in a patient receiving fluconazole, and resolved after withdrawal of the drug (Murakami *et al.*, 1992).

5 Central nervous system effects

Headache and dizziness are the most commonly reported nervous system effects and occur in up to 2% patients. Seizures, psychiatric disturbances, fatigue, malaise, paresthesias of hands and feet, are events reported rarely. Central nervous system toxicity was described in three patients receiving 2000 mg daily, and included insomnia, confusion, disorientation, hallucinations and nightmares (Anaissie *et al.*, 1995).

6 Endocrine effects

Devenport *et al.* (1989) studied the effect of oral fluconazole on the metabolic profile of women, half of whom were also taking the oral contraceptive. At a dose of 50 mg daily, there was no clinically significant, consistent effect on the endocrinological profile or on the carbohydrate or lipid metabolism in women. Plasma testosterone levels were increased by 33% in male volunteers given 400 mg fluconazole daily for 5 days. The mechanism and clinical significance of this increase is uncertain (Touchette *et al.*, 1992). Fluconazole, at a concentration of 10 μg per ml, was a weak inhibitor of testosterone production in rat Leydig cells (Hanger *et al.*, 1988). No effect on serum estradiol levels was observed in premenopausal women, but there was a small increase in testosterone levels in women not taking the oral contraceptive. An *in vitro* mild suppressive effect on steroidogenesis in rat adrenal cells has been shown (Eckhoff *et al.*, 1988), but fluconazole administration in humans had no effect on serum cortisol responses to corticotrophin provocation even at doses of 400 mg (Devenport *et al.*, 1989). A single case of acute adrenal insufficiency in an AIDS patient has been reported to implicate fluconazole, because of a temporal association with starting the drug. However, no postmortem examination was performed to exclude more common causes of this syndrome in AIDS patients (Gradon and Sepkowitz, 1991).

7 Other adverse effects

Hypokalemia has been described in three patients with acute myeloid leukemia, which resolved on cessation of fluconazole or reduction in dose (Kidd *et al.*, 1989). Increased serum creatinine and blood urea nitrogen levels have also been reported.

8 Effect on the fetus

No studies are available on the effects of fluconazole on the human fetus, although fluconazole administration to pregnant rats during organogenesis resulted in offspring with congenital abnormalities including cleft palate, abnormal craniofacial ossification, supernumerary ribs and renal pelvis dilatation. Lee *et al.* (1992) reported a single case of congenital malformations (bradycephaly, nasal bone hypoplasia, cleft palate, craniosynostosis, frontal cranioschisis, sagittal craniostenosis, femoral and tibial bowing, radiohumeral synostosis and upper- and lower-extremity contractures) in the female infant of a woman taking 400 mg fluconazole daily for chronic coccidioidal meningitis when she became pregnant and the drug was taken for 24 weeks of the pregnancy. The congenital abnormalities were also consistent with Antley–Bixler syndrome, an autosomal recessive genetic disorder. The contribution of fluconazole to the teratogenic effects in this case was unknown. Since the report by Lee *et al.* (1992) another two cases of congenital anomalies have been described in the offspring of women taking fluconazole 400–800 mg daily during first-trimester pregnancy. Both additional cases were of craniofacial and skeletal defects, with significant cardiac anomalies in one child. One infant was the sibling of the infant described initially by Lee *et al.* (1992) and was exposed to the same dose of fluconazole. The mother had delivered a normal healthy child between these two pregnancies when not taking fluconazole (Pursley *et al.*, 1996). A prescription event-monitoring study of the outcomes of 280 pregnancies, in patients who had taken a single 150-mg dose of fluconazole, revealed the drug was not associated with an increased spontaneous abortion rate, and there were no fetal abnormalities recorded in women who took the fluconazole dose after the last menstrual period. Fetal abnormalities were noted in six pregnancies in which the drug was administered up to 16 weeks prior to the last menstrual period, giving an overall rate of fetal abnormality among the 240 pregnancies whose outcome could be established of 2.5%. This compares with an approximate 2% fetal abnormality rate in the UK. There was no trend to selected fetal abnormalities (Rubin *et al.*, 1992). The descriptions by Pursley *et al.* (1996) suggest that fluconazole is a teratogen in humans. The drug is currently contraindicated in pregnancy.

Fluconazole pentrates well into breast milk and achieves concentrations that approach those observed in plasma. The manufacturer recommends that fluconazole is not used during lactation (Force, 1995)

9 Drug interactions

As fluconazole reversibly inhibits the hepatic cytochrome P-450 enzymes, (in particular the P-450 3A group of enzymes) albeit to a lesser degree than ketoconazole, competition for metabolism by the cytochrome P-450 enzymes results in predictable and reported drug interactions (Maurice *et al.*, 1992). However, because of its ability to induce the hepatic cytochrome P-450 enzyme, fluconazole exhibits a biphasic effect of an inhibitory phase followed by an induction phase on the cytochrome P-450 enzyme system (Debruyne and Ryckelynck, 1993). Purda and Back (1986) found that fluconazole at a dose of 50 mg per day did not alter antipyrine metabolism. As a marker of human cytochrome P-450 activity and therefore predictor of hepatic drug metabolism, the lack of effect of antipyrine metabolism suggested significant drug interactions were unlikely. However, metabolism of phenytoin was significantly reduced by the addition of fluconazole, with a 75% increase in the area-under-the-serum-concentration-time-curve of phenytoin, after fluconazole was administered to normal volunteers receiving phenytoin (Blum *et al.*, 1991b). Symptomatic phenytoin toxicity was reported within 2 days of starting fluconazole 400 mg in a patient stabilized on phenytoin (Mitchell and Holland, 1989) and within 7 days of commencing fluconazole at a dose of 200 mg daily (Howitt and Oziemski,1989).

Prolongation of the prothrombin time from 19 seconds to 65 seconds has been reported in a patient stabilized on warfarin, who had fluconazole added for management of a wound infection (Seaton *et al.*,1990). Crussell-Porter *et al.* (1993) have examined the pharmacodynamic effect of 100 mg fluconazole in patients on stable doses of warfarin. They noted a progressive increase in prothrombin times over 1 week, although the changes in prothrombin time (6–10 s) were not as exaggerated as the case reported by Seaton *et al.* (1990). It is appropriate to monitor closely prothrombin times and phenytoin concentrations in patients receiving either of these drugs who start fluconazole.

The effect of fluconazole on cyclosporin pharmacokinetics appears to vary according to the dose of fluconazole used. In a placebo-controlled trial of oral fluconazole 200 mg, in renal transplant patients on a constant dose of cyclosporin, a 100% increase in trough levels of cyclosporin and a 50% reduction in the clearance of cyclosporin were noted (Canafax *et al.*, 1991a,b). Torregrossa *et al.* (1992) described three patients who underwent renal transplantation and required a 50% reduction in their cyclosporin dose when fluconazole 200 mg was added to their regimen. However, in an uncontrolled trial in bone marrow transplant recipients on stable doses of cyclosporin, the addition of 100 mg fluconazole did not have a statistically significant effect on the peak or trough cyclosporin concentrations, although the levels were slightly increased (Kruger *et al.*, 1989). Monitoring serum cyclosporin levels and serum creatinine appears to be appropriate for the management of patients who receive concomitant fluconazole.

Rifampicin is a potent inducer of hepatic cytochrome P-450 enzyme system. Rifampicin causes a 22% decrease in the half-life of fluconazole and a 23% decrease in the mean AUC for fluconazole in normal volunteers. It is apparent that rifampicin enhances the elimination of fluconazole, probably by induction of the hepatic cytochrome P-450 system (Apseloff *et al.*, 1991), and clinical relapse of cryptococcal meningitis has been reported in three HIV-infected patients who had rifampicin added to their treament, suggesting a fluconazole-rifampicin interaction (Coker *et al.*, 1990). Fluconazole doses should be increased if the concurrent administration with rifampicin is planned.

Unlike rifampicin, rifabutin does not increase the elimination of fluconazole, and nor does it alter fluconazole pharmacokinetics in HIV-infected patients (Trapnall *et al.*, 1996). However, fluconazole does increase rifabutin levels by 80%, and there is a significant 200% increase in the 25-desacetyl metabolite of rifabutin when the two drugs are co-administered (Trapnall *et al.*,

1996) thereby increasing both the risk of rifabutin toxicity, including uveitis, and the prophylactic effectiveness in prevention of disseminated *Mycobacterium avium* complex infection (Narang *et al.*, 1994; Fuller *et al.*, 1994; Havlir *et al.*, 1994).

Co-administration of fluconazole 400 mg daily and zidovudine 200 mg three times daily in HIV-infected patients, resulted in a 43% reduction in apparent clearance of zidovudine, a 74% increase in the zidovudine AUC, 84% increase in the maximum concentration and 128% increase in the terminal half-life of zidovudine. The interaction is thought to be due to inhibition of glucuronidation of zidovudine by fluconazole, and this was confirmed *in vitro* in human liver microsomes (Sampol *et al.*, 1995). The clinical consequences of this interaction have not been evaluated (Sahai *et al.*, 1994). There does not appear to be any significant effect of fluconazole on the pharmacokinetics of didanosine (Bruzzese *et al.*, 1995).

An important interaction between fluconazole and midazolam was investigated in a placebo-controlled trial in normal volunteers. Fluconazole reduced the clearance of i.v. midazolam by 51% and increased the area under the midazolam concentration time curve 3.5-fold after oral administration of midazolam, associated with a marked decrease in performance of psychomotor tests (Olkkola *et al.*, 1996). However, Vanakoski *et al.* (1995) found that fluconazole did not significantly affect psychomotor tests of individuals given oral midazolam 10 mg, compared with performance of these tests on midazolam alone.

Fluconazole appeared to reduce the metabolism of nortriptyline resulting in elevated trough serum concentrations of the drug and clinically significant sedation (Gannon, 1992). This drug interaction has not been described for other tricyclic antidepressant agents. The clearance of the oral contraceptive is not affected by fluconazole (Purda and Back, 1986). The effect of fluconazole on the pharmacokinetics of oral hypoglycemic agents was evaluated in a placebo-controlled trial. Healthy volunteers received tolbutamide, glipizide or glyburide after a single 100-mg dose of fluconazole or 7 days of continuous dosing. Increases of 10–20% in peak serum concentration and 43–38% in the AUC of each sulfonylurea was noted in those who received fluconazole. In this study, 25% of the volunteers experienced either hypoglycemic symptoms or low blood glucose (Kowalsky, 1990). However, in a study of postmenopausal diabetic women with vulvovaginitis, randomized to fluconazole orally for 14 days or topical clotrimazole, no significant changes in blood glucose control or symptomatic hypoglycemia occurred in the fluconazole group (Rowe *et al.*, 1992).

An important drug interaction of fluconazole with FK506 (an immunosuppressive agent used in transplantation) has also been described. Fluconazole inhibits the metabolism of FK506, resulting in increased plasma concentrations and the half-life of FK506, causing nephrotoxicity. It is recommended that the dose of FK506 be reduced by half if fluconazole is co-administered (Manez *et al.*, 1994; Assan *et al.*, 1994).

Clinical Uses of the Drug

1 Cryptococcosis

As discussed in the amphotericin B (AMB) section (p. 1268) the recommended treatment for cryptococcal meningitis (and cryptococcosis) in the non-AIDS patient is AMB and flucytosine, which is associated with response rates of 75–85% (Dismukes *et al.*, 1987). Response rates in AIDS patients are considerably lower at 40–50% when AMB (0.3–0.5 mg per kg per day) with or without flucytosine is used (Kovacs *et al.*, 1985; Zuger *et al.*, 1986). Adverse effects associated with both AMB and flucytosine are common, often resulting in administration of inadequate doses. In a randomized trial comparing AMB and oral fluconazole for cryptococcal meningitis in AIDS patients, fluconazole at a dose of 200 mg daily was effective in 34% of patients, compared with a 40% success rate for AMB (0.4–0.5 mg per kg) treated patients. This difference in efficacy was not statistically significantly different. Mortality during the first 2 weeks of therapy was greater in the fluconazole group, which also had a longer median time to the first negative CSF culture (64 days versus 42 days for AMB-treated patients) (Saag *et al.*, 1992). The doses of both antifungal drugs used in this study appeared suboptimal, but the conclusion that fluconazole was an effective alternative to AMB for the primary treatment of cryptococcal meningitis in HIV-infected patients, has resulted in widespread adoption of this management approach. It is unclear why a significant proportion of patients do not respond to fluconazole given the excellent CSF penetration of 60–80% and the *in vitro* activity of fluconazole against *Cryptococcus neoformans*.

Coker and Harris (1991) documented CSF concentrations that were more than adequate to inhibit the *C. neoformans* isolate in one patient who failed to respond to fluconazole. A smaller comparative study utilizing higher doses of both agents, found AMB (0.7 mg per kg per day for 1 week, then 0.7 mg per kg three times weekly for 9 weeks) in combination with flucytosine 150 mg per kg per day had significantly superior clinical and mycological response rates to oral fluconazole (400 mg per day for 10 weeks, then 200 mg per day). The response rates were 43% for fluconazole and 100% for AMB combined with flucytosine (Larsen *et al.*, 1990). These authors recommend the use of AMB at the higher dose, with or without flucytosine as the initial treatment of cryptococcal meningitis in AIDS. High doses of fluconazole (800 mg per day) were used successfully as salvage therapy in five of eight patients who had failed or relapsed after primary therapy. No major toxicity was observed in this small series (Berry *et al.*, 1992). Another small study utilizing high-dose fluconazole (800 mg per day) as primary therapy for cryptococcal disease in eight AIDS patients reported a 100% mycological response rate and an 87% clinical response rate (Haubrich *et al.*, 1994). Fluconazole at a dose of 150 mg per day sterilized CSF cultures within 2 weeks in a patient who had persistently positive CSF cultures after 10 g AMB (Byrne and Wajszczuk,1988). Although no study has stratified patients according to prognostic factors previously identified for response, several open, non-comparative studies have reported response rates of 38–57% (Squires *et al.*,1990; Pietroski *et al.*, 1990) for fluconazole 400 mg daily, that are similar to those reported for AMB. In an open study of 32 AIDS patients, the combination of fluconazole 400 mg per day achieved clinical responses in 63% patients and mycological responses in 75% patients (Larsen *et al.*, 1994).

Retrospective studies in AIDS patients have reported relapse rates of 50% for those patients who did not receive chronic suppressive therapy (Zuger *et al.*, 1986; Kovacs *et al.*, 1985). There have been two pivotal studies examining the prevention of relapse in AIDS patients. In a placebo-controlled trial of maintenance therapy with fluconazole 100–200 mg per day, Bozzette *et al.* (1991a) observed that 19% of 'successfully' treated patients with AMB had evidence of silent persistent infection (three CSF cultures and 13 urine cultures positive for *C. neoformans*). These were excluded from the study. Recurrent cryptococcal infection (frequently prostate) was significantly reduced in the fluconazole group (3% versus 37% in the placebo group). The second was a controlled trial comparing the efficacy of fluconazole 200 mg daily with AMB 1 mg per kg per week in preventing relapse of infection after successful treatment with AMB. Fluconazole was superior to weekly AMB in the prevention of recurrent cryptococcal disease as observed by the rate of relapse in fluconazole recipients of 2% compared with 18% in the AMB group (Powderly *et al.*, 1992). The experience reported in additional open studies establish fluconazole as the ideal drug for the maintenance treatment of cryptococcal infection in the chronically immunocompromised patient at significant risk of recurrent disease after primary treatment (Stern *et al.*, 1988; Sugar and Saunders, 1988). Some have suggested there is a dose-response in the prophylactic efficacy of fluconazole, with the observation of development of cryptococcal meningitis in patients receiving lower doses of 50–100 mg for oral candidiasis (Coker *et al.*, 1992) and a differential relapse rate of meningitis with doses of 200 mg (five of seven patients) and 400 mg (three of 25 patients) (Nelson *et al.*, 1994). Several studies have identified the prostate gland as the site of persistent cryptococcal infection with up to 30% HIV-infected patients with positive urine cultures for *C. neoformans* after successful primary treatment (Bozzette *et al.*, 1991b; Larsen *et al.*, 1989). These authors have proposed the prostate as the souce of recurrent infection in many patients. Persistent prostatic infection has also been documented in a lymphoma patient (King *et al.*, 1990). Fluconazole successfully eliminated *C. neoformans* in 50% patients with prostatic infection (Bozzette *et al.*, 1991b), and persistent prostatic infection has been documented in a man receiving 400 mg fluconazole at 12 and 18 weeks of treatment (Bailly *et al.*, 1991). Relapse rates up to 30% are also encountered in other groups of immunocompromised patients, so it would seem logical to extend the recommendation for chronic suppressive therapy with fluconazole to other immune compromised patients.

Quagliarello *et al.* (1995), determined that fluconazole conferred a 92% protective efficacy as primary prophylaxis for cryptococcal meningitis in HIV-infected patients with fewer than 250 CD4 cells per μl. The optimum dose of fluconazole and time of initiation of fluconazole was not established. The prophylactic efficacy of fluconazole in reducing the incidence of cryptococcal meningitis was confirmed in a prospective, randomized, controlled comparison of fluconazole 200 mg daily with clotrimazole troches 10 mg five times per day. The most pronounced effect of fluconazole occurred in those with the most advanced immunodeficiency (less than 50 CD4 cells per μl), reducing the estimated 2-year risk from 9.9% to 1.6% (Powderly *et al.*, 1995). Concerns with this prophylaxis approach include the large number of individuals who will risk toxicity, drug interactions and cost to prevent a small number of invasive fungal infections and the potential development of fluconazole resistance in *Candida* isolates and other fungi.

Cryptococcal infection in children is infrequent; however there are anecdotal reports of the safety and efficacy of fluconazole in children (Moncino and Gutman, 1990). Oral fluconazole was also effective for the management of localized cutaneous cryptococcosis in an elderly man with renal impairment (Shuttleworth *et al.*, 1988).

2 Candidiasis

a Fungemia The optimal management of systemic fungal infections remains controversial. Although AMB has been considered the 'gold standard' for all systemic fungal infections in both the immunocompetent and immunocompromised patient, controlled trials and open non-comparative studies utilizing fluconazole are currently challenging this role for AMB, and place fluconazole as a good alternative. The efficacy of oral or i.v. fluconazole (50 mg daily) was evaluated in an open trial of 20 non-neutropenic patients with deep-seated fungal infections. Clinical cure or improvement was achieved in 82% of patients, and combined clinical and mycological cure was achieved in just over half the patients (van 't Wout *et al.*, 1988). In another open label study of i.v. fluconazole in patients admitted to intensive care units with *Candida albicans* fungemia, a two-dose comparison revealed a superior response both clinically and mycologically for those patients treated with 10 mg per kg (83% clinical response, 100% mycological eradication) compared with 5 mg per kg (60% clinical response, 94% mycological eradication). This is similar to results of AMB treatment in comparable patients. Improved survival, higher eradication rates of *Candida* spp. from secondary sites of infection, and reduced relapse rates of infection were associated with the higher fluconazole dose (Graninger *et al.*, 1993). Finally, in an open non-comparative trial of fluconazole administered at 200–400 mg daily for proven (22 patients) or suspected (18 patients) fungal infections, relatively low response rates of 53% overall were observed. For proven or probable infections, the clinical response was 62% and mycological eradication rate was 65% (Milatovic and Voss, 1992).

Rex *et al.* (1994) performed the first randomized comparative study of fluconazole 400 mg daily with AMB 0.5–0.6 mg per kg per day for the treatment of candidemia in 237 patients without neutropenia and no major immunodeficiency. Treatment was continued for at least 14 days after the last positive blood culture. They found that fluconazole and AMB were not significantly different in the efficacy for treatment of candidemia. In the AMB group, 79% patients were judged to have successful treatment, compared with 70% in the fluconazole group. Persistent candidemia occurred in 12 AMB-treated patients and 15 fluconazole-treated patients, and the organism most frequently associated with failure was *C. albicans*. The mortality was 40% in the AMB group and 33% in the fluconazole group (Rex *et al.*, 1994). Susceptibility testing of baseline isolates from this study could not predict treatment outcome (Rex *et al.*, 1995). The equivalent efficacy for fluconazole and AMB in the treatment of candidemia was also observed in a prospective observational study of over 400 patients. The comparable efficacy was maintained when patients were stratified by risk factors for mortality. Fluconazole-treated patients experienced significantly fewer adverse effects (Nguyen *et al.*, 1995b). It is clear from these studies that fluconazole can be considered a safe and effective alternative to AMB for the treatment of candidemia in non-neutropenic patients. The optimal duration of therapy and the need to remove intravascular catheters which are often the source of infection, are issues which remain to be assessed. Determination of the species of *Candida* is important because of the lack of efficacy observed with specific isolates such as *C. krusei* and *C. glabrata* (Goldman *et al.*, 1993; Case *et al.*, 1991; Roder *et al.*, 1991; Persons *et al.*, 1991; Siegman-Igra and Rabau, 1992).

The place of fluconazole in the treatment of candidemia in the immunocompromised (neutropenic) patient needs to be evaluated in large comparative trials. The efficacy of AMB in these individuals is often less than satisfactory. Anecdotal reports of treatment with fluconazole in immunocompromised patients have been conflicting (Kirk *et al.*, 1989; Conti *et al.*, 1989; Soutar, 1991; Colville and Wale, 1991). However, there have been two reports of series of patients with leukemia and chronic disseminated candidiasis or hepatosplenic candidiasis who failed AMB in doses up to 2 g, or experienced significant AMB toxicity, and responded to fluconazole. Mortality rates following prolonged treatment with AMB are consistently reported at 30–50%. Anaisse *et al.* (1991) reported a response rate of 88% (14 of 16 patients) for fluconazole in doses of 100–400 mg daily for a median of 30 weeks, and this included resolution in seven of nine patients (78%) in whom seemingly adequate doses of AMB had failed to control the infection. There were no relapses in 12 patients who underwent further cytotoxic chemotherapy. In another case series of six patients with leukemia and hepatosplenic candidiasis who had failed prior AMB treatment, improvement of the lesions in liver and spleen was documented on CT scan in all patients treated with 200–400 mg fluconazole daily. Total resolution of lesions occurred within 4 weeks for two patients, 4–5 months for three patients and 1 year for the last patient (Kauffman *et al.*, 1991). Additional case reports support the use of fluconazole for hepatosplenic candidiasis following failure with AMB (Jakab *et al.*, 1990; Flannery *et al.*, 1992), but until a comparative trial is performed, fluconazole is not recommended as initial therapy of disseminated candidiasis in immunocompromised patients.

Experience with fluconazole for the treatment of *Candida* sepsis in children is also limited. Fluconazole has been reported to be successful in the treatment of *C. albicans* sepsis in two premature neonates born at 28 weeks gestation. One neonate responded rapidly to i.v. fluconazole 6 mg per kg daily (Wiest *et al.*, 1991) and the other received 5 mg per kg daily orally (Bode *et al.*, 1992). Viscoli *et al.* (1991) evaluated fluconazole (6 mg per kg daily either orally or i.v.) in an open non-comparative study of 34 episodes of candidiasis in immunocompromised children. Clinical and microbiological cure was achieved in 88% of episodes. Relapses occurred in 10% of the episodes within 15 days of ceasing fluconazole, but most of these were oral candidiasis or urinary tract infection. Similar clinical response rates were observed in a second case series in pediatric patients. The dose of fluconazole in this study depended on the organism, severity of infection and the child's condition, and ranged from 3.5 to 19 mg per kg daily. The two mycological failures were infections caused by *C. albicans* and *C. parapsilosis* (Presterl *et al.*, 1994). Comparative trials are necessary to establish the optimal agent, dose and duration of therapy.

Combination fluconazole 600 mg daily given i.v. and flucytosine 10 g daily was used to treat an episode of *C. albicans* sepsis. Flucytosine was added to the fluconazole when the patient failed to respond to fluconazole alone. Despite clinical improvement, blood cultures remained positive for 2 weeks of combination therapy, then became sterile (Scheven *et al.*, 1992). The combination of fluconazole and flucytosine was used successfully to treat a low birthweight infant with *Candida* sepsis and meningitis (Marr *et al.*, 1994).

b   Endophthalmitis   Hematogenously acquired fungal endophthalmitis appears less difficult to treat than post-surgical exogenously acquired infection. In the rabbit model of hematogenous *C. albicans* endophthalmitis, i.v. AMB was superior to i.v. fluconazole in eradication of fungus from the vitreous and the choroid-retina (Filler *et al.*, 1991). Successful treatment with fluconazole 400 mg i.v. loading dose, followed by 200 mg i.v. or orally for 18–21 days was reported for three cases of fungal ocular infection (two cases of *Candida* chorioretinitis and one case of panuveitis). No relapse occurred in the 5–7 months follow-up after cessation of fluconazole (Cruciani *et al.*, 1990). A case of exogenous *C. parapsilosis* endophthalmitis was successfully treated with fluconazole 100 mg twice-daily for 4 months, after failure of treatment with intravitreal AMB and ketoconazole (Borne *et al.*, 1993). There was a rapid therapeutic response with marked reduction in inflammation, preservation of vision and sterilization of vitreous cultures. The standard treatment for *Candida* endophthalmitis associated with an infected lens implant involves vitrectomy and intravitreal AMB injections. *Candida parapsilosis* endophthalmitis following intraocular lens implantation failed to respond to intravitreal AMB and vitrectomy in four patients, and was successfully managed symptomatically with oral fluconazole 200–400 mg daily for 1 year. Three patients relapsed within 5 months of cessation of fluconazole. The remaining patient had the lens implant removed after failing intravitreal AMB and was cured with fluconazole (no relapse of the *C. parapsilosis* infection in 2 years follow-up) (Kauffman *et al.*, 1993). Fluconazole 200 mg daily for 2 months appears to be a safe and effective alternative to AMB for treatment of candidal endophthalmitis with over 90% efficacy (Akler *et al.*, 1995).

c   Endocarditis   The utility of fluconazole (a fungistatic agent) in fungal endocarditis has not been established. The mortality of *Candida* endocarditis is high (90%) without surgical intervention, and AMB penetrates poorly into fungal vegetations. In the rabbit model of endocarditis, intraperitoneal fluconazole at doses of 10 mg per kg and 20 mg per kg daily for 2 weeks eradicated *C. parapsilosis* and *C. albicans* from cardiac vegetations (Longman *et al.*, 1990). Penetration of fluconazole into vegetations has not been studied. Effective treatment with fluconazole has been reported anecdotally for both native valve endocarditis and prosthetic valve endocarditis. An episode of *C. tropicalis* aortic valve endocarditis resolved after 6 weeks treatment with 200 mg fluconazole twice-daily alone (Roupie *et al.*, 1991), and another episode of *C. parapsilosis* right-sided mural endocarditis in a neutropenic man persisted despite i.v. fluconazole 3 mg per kg daily, increased to 6 mg per kg daily. The fungemia resolved promptly following addition of granulocyte macrophage colony-stimulating factor and the mural vegetation disappeared after 3 months treatment with oral fluconazole (Martino *et al.*, 1990). Three reports of successful treatment of *C. parapsilosis* prosthetic valve endocarditis involved the life time administration of oral fluconazole after initial AMB and flucytosine treatment without valve replacement (Czwerwiec *et al.*, 1993; Isalska and Stanbridge, 1988; Wallbridge *et al.*, 1993).

d Bone and joint infections The treatment of choice remains AMB. There are no controlled studies examining the effectiveness of fluconazole for osteomyelitis or arthritis due to *Candida* spp. Vertebral osteomyelitis and fungemia due to *C. albicans* in a man with acute renal failure responded to i.v. fluconazole 200 mg daily for 4 weeks, then oral fluconazole 200 mg daily for 12 months (Tang, 1993). There are no clear guidelines for the appropriate duration of therapy for *Candida* osteomyelitis (Gathe *et al.*, 1987). Mycologic cure was achieved in a case of *C. parapsilosis* prosthetic arthritis of the knee, using oral fluconazole 200 mg daily for 4 months. This patient had failed treatment with AMB and resection arthroplasty prior to institution of fluconazole. Sterilization of synovial fluid was documented after 8 weeks treatment with fluconazole (Tunkel *et al.*, 1993). There are also reports of failure of fluconazole therapy 400 mg daily for sternal osteomyelitis due to *C. albicans* (Dan and Priel, 1994).

e Meningitis An AIDS patient with *C. albicans* fungemia and meningitis was successfully treated with fluconazole 10 mg per kg daily for 6 weeks. Mycological and clinical cure was maintained for at least 12 months following treatment (Graninger *et al.*, 1993). Although excellent CSF penetration by fluconazole makes it an ideal agent for this infrequent infection, caution should be exercised if there are foreign bodies in association with the candidal infection, as fluconazole is a fungistatic agent. Epelbaum *et al.* (1993) described a case of *C. albicans* meningitis in an immunocompetent child with hydrocephalus and a ventriculoperitoneal shunt. The child was treated with i.v. fluconazole 12.5 mg per kg daily initially with good response, and was continued on oral fluconazole at the same dose. However, after 4 weeks of oral fluconazole, there was a relapse of the *C. albicans* meningitis and hydrocephalus despite the presence of the ventriculoperitoneal shunt and demonstration of good CSF penetration of the drug. A premature infant with hydrocephalus and a ventriculoperitoneal shunt and *Candida albicans* meningitis, was treated successfully with fluconazole 6 mg per kg i.v. daily for 13 days. The shunt was removed on day 4 of treatment and the shunt tip was culture-negative for *C. albicans*. A new shunt was placed on day 13, and remained uninfected for at least 19 months follow-up (Cruciani *et al.*, 1992).

f Urinary tract infection Despite the fact that 80% of a fluconazole dose is excreted in the urine as unchanged drug, the role of fluconazole in the management of both complicated and uncomplicated funguria remains to be defined. There are no controlled trials evaluating its efficacy for fungal urinary tract infection. Voss *et al.* (1994) have reviewed the case reports and and open label studies of fluconazole. Anecdotal reports using doses of 100–200 mg daily administered both i.v. and orally, provide support for the effectiveness of fluconazole. The duration of treatment ranged from 7 days for uncomplicated cystitis, to 3 months maintenance for renal papillary candidiasis. Clinical response rates of 71–100% and mycological eradication rates of 64–86% were reported in the case series.

Lower eradication rates occurred in those patients with indwelling urinary catheters. In the two comparative studies of fluconazole 50 mg orally daily with i.v. AMB 0.4–0.5 mg per kg per day for candiduria associated with an indwelling catheter, and fluconazole 200 mg daily with AMB 50 mg per liter bladder irrigation for *Candida* cystitis, fluconazole was found to be as effective as the AMB regardless of the route of administration (Voss *et al.*, 1994). For patients with renal papillary candidosis, eradication of deep-seated infection is difficult and long-term suppression with fluconazole as an agent with ideal pharmacokinetic properties and safety may be most appropriate. Successful treatment using fluconazole for 4 weeks in an immunocompromised patient with chronic renal calculi resulting in a partially obstructed renal pelvis and renal failure, and chronic infection with *C. albicans*, was achieved after failure to control the infection with a course of AMB (Tacker, 1992). Multiple relapses following cessation of treatment with fluconazole have been described in a patient with idiopathic papillary necrosis complicated with *Candida* infection (Dave *et al.*, 1989). Fluconazole solution prepared as a bladder irrigant to a concentration of 1 mg per ml in normal saline, effectively eradicated *Candida* spp. in 85% of patients with permanent nephrostomy or suprapubic catheter-associated candiduria (Simsek *et al.*, 1995).

g   Vaginal candidiasis   Single-dose 150 mg fluconazole has been extensively evaluated for the treatment of vaginal candidiasis. Fluconazole effectively penetrates vaginal secretions and tissues, achieving a peak concentration of 2.5 μg per ml. The concentration of fluconazole remains above the IC_{50} of *C. albicans* for at least 72 h (Houang *et al.*, 1990). It has been compared with single- and multiple-dose intravaginal azole treatments and multiple-dose oral azole treatment. The overall clinical response rate from 28 clinical studies of single-dose 150-mg fluconazole was 94% and the mycological cure rate at short-term follow-up was 87% (Phillips *et al.*, 1990; de los Reyes *et al.*, 1992). Fluconazole (150-mg single-dose) was found to have equivalent mycological and clinical efficacy as ketoconazole 200 mg twice-daily for 5 days, single-dose intravaginal clotrimazole 500 mg, daily intravaginal clotrimazole 100 mg for 7 days, single-dose intravaginal econazole 150 mg, daily intravaginal econazole 50 mg for 6 days, or intravaginal miconazole pessaries 400 mg for 3 nights, and it was better tolerated (Kutzer *et al.*, 1988; Brammer and Feczko, 1988; Boag *et al.*, 1991; Herzog and Ansmann, 1989; Osser *et al.*, 1991; Timonen, 1992; Sobel *et al.*, 1995). At 1 month post-treatment, women treated with fluconazole had a significantly higher clinical and mycological cure rate than those given econazole. Another larger comparative study of fluconazole 150 mg single dose with single-dose econazole 150 mg intravaginally, demonstrated a significantly higher clinical and mycological cure rate for fluconazole at long-term follow-up (Westrom *et al.*, 1992). There appears to be reduced rates of recurrence in the fluconazole-treated women (de los Reyes, 1992).

Women with recurrent or chronic vulvovaginal candidiasis require long-term maintenance prophylaxis to reduce the rate of symptomatic episodes of vaginitis. Once-monthly dosing of fluconazole 150 mg given 1–4 days after menstruation, was evaluated in two placebo-controlled trials, and found to reduce the rate of recurrent vulvovaginal candidiasis from 68% and 53% in the placebo arm to 42% and 39% in the fluconazole arm, and prolong the time to recurrence (Sobel, 1992).

h   Oral and esophageal candidiasis   Oral candidiasis occurs in 90% of HIV-infected patients at some time during the course of their infection. Infections may be asymptomatic, severe and are usually recurrent. Many patients are initially treated with topical antifungal agents, however in the last 5 years the use of fluconazole for this infection has markedly increased. A number of studies have examined the comparative efficacy of oral fluconazole 100 mg daily and topical clotrimazole troches 10 mg five times daily for the treatment of oral candidiasis. The duration of treatment in each study was 14 days. The clinical cure rates were equivalent in two studies and significantly superior for fluconazole in one study (fluconazole 96–100%, clotrimazole 65–94%). Mycological eradication was greater for fluconazole-treated patients (49–75%) than clotrimazole-treated patients (20–48%), and patients treated with fluconazole were more likely to remain relapse free in the follow-up period (Koletar *et al.*, 1990; Pons *et al.*, 1993; Sangeorzan *et al.*, 1994). Fluconazole suspension 2–3 mg per kg daily was significantly more effective in the treatment of oropharyngeal candidiasis in immunocompromised children than nystatin suspension 400 000 units four times daily (Flynn *et al.*, 1995).

The efficacy and safety of fluconazole versus ketoconazole for the treatment of oropharyngeal candidiasis in HIV-infected patients has been evaluated, and cure rates of 76–100% for fluconazole and 75–80% for ketoconazole were similar (Barchiesi *et al.*, 1992; De Wit *et al.*,1989). The increased failure rate of both drugs in these studies was felt to be due to inclusion of a greater proportion of patients who had received prior fluconazole prophylaxis (Barchiesi *et al.*, 1992). Over 80% patients who have failed treatment with ketoconazole will respond to fluconazole 50–200 mg daily (Thorsen and Mathieson, 1990). In the study reported by De Wit *et al.* (1989), there was a higher relapse rate in the fluconazole-treated group (46%) than in the ketoconazole-treated group (11%).

Relapses of oropharyngeal thrush are so frequent that maintenance therapy (secondary prophylaxis) is usually required, especially with deteriorating immune function. The safety and efficacy of fluconazole in doses of 50–100 mg daily, or 150 mg as a single-dose weekly have clearly been established. in placebo controlled trials (Just-Nubling *et al.*, 1991; Marriott *et al.*, 1993; Leen *et al.*, 1990; Stevens *et al.*, 1991; Esposito *et al.*, 1990). When used as a single weekly dose, fluconazole prevented clinical relapse in 71% patients over 3 months and 58% patients over 6 months (Marriott *et al.*,1993). However, the increasing reports of fluconazole failure and resistance is of concern and the routine practice of secondary prophylaxis for oropharyngeal candidiasis is under question. In one of the studies, the fluconazole MIC_{90} for *Candida* spp. increased from 0.5 μg per ml prior to acute therapy, to 8 μg per ml after fluconazole prophylaxis for a mean of 4 months (Sangeorzan *et al.*, 1994). These authors also found that fluconazole-resistance in *C. albicans* occurs most frequently in patients with severe immunodeficiency who are taking fluconazole prophylaxis. Resistance occurs either through the acquisition of a resistant *Candida* species or strain, or the development of resistance in a previously sensitive strain. There is an anecdotal report of response to increasing dose fluconazole to 800 mg daily, in a patient that had failed on 200–400 mg daily, without adverse effects (Ansari *et al.*, 1990). Baily *et al.* (1994) performed a retrospective review of a cohort of HIV-infected patients and established that fluconazole-resistant candidiasis occurred at a rate of 6%, and the risk of developing fluconazole-resistant candidosis that fails on treatment with azoles was significantly greater prior fluconazole exposure. Powderly (1992) has documented an increasing incidence of infection with non-*albicans Candida* spp. (especially *C. krusei* and *C. glabrata*) in HIV-infected patients with the increasing use of chronic azole therapy, similar to the reports in other immune-compromised patients.

Fluconazole is a preferable agent for the treatment of esophageal candidiasis, as ketoconazole is associated with impaired gastrointestinal absorption in HIV-infected patients, in addition to problems of hepatotoxicity, drug interactions, and the non-availability of an i.v. formulation. The safety and efficacy of fluconazole 100 mg daily for 2–4 weeks has been established in two open non-comparative studies. High cure rates of 100% were observed (87% after 1 week treatment). In addition, Laine and Rebeneck (1995) have established the efficacy of a fluconazole suspension used as a 200-mg loading dose, followed by 100 mg daily continued until 2 weeks after resolution of symptoms in a small open, non-comparative study. De Wit *et al.* (1991) noted a 17.5% relapse rate of oropharyngeal candidiasis in 1 month with no prophylaxis, but Gil *et al.* (1991) noted no relapses when fluconazole 200 mg weekly was given. The natural history of esophageal candidiasis after successful treatment is 90% recurrence within 2–3 months of completion of therapy (Laine, 1994). A comparative study of fluconazole and ketoconazole for esophageal candidiasis, confirmed the superiority of fluconazole (endoscopic cure in 87% fluconazole group and 53% ketoconazole group) (Laine *et al.*, 1992).

i Peritonitis Anecdotal reports of the use of fluconazole for candidal peritonitis, suggest that this mode of therapy should be subjected to controlled trials for efficacy, to determine its place in the treatment of fungal peritonitis. Fluconazole achieves more than 60% penetration into the peritoneal dialysate. Levine *et al.* (1989) report two cases of *Candida* peritonitis in patients undergoing CAPD. A loading dose of oral fluconazole 200 mg followed by 100 mg daily for 5 and 12 days failed to eradicate the *Candida* spp. until the Tenckhoff catheter was removed. Prompt symptom resolution occurred in both cases and a 6-week course of fluconazole was administered without relapse. Hoch *et al.* (1993) described their experience of *C. albicans* peritonitis (two cases) and *C. tropicalis* peritonitis (three cases), initially successfully treated with fluconazole 50–200 mg daily in four of five patients with sterilization of dialysate cultures, but with recurrent peritonitis documented in all patients within 1 month. Complete cure of the candidal infection did not occur unless the Tenckhoff catheter was removed. An additional report of the successful eradication of *C. albicans* in a patient with fungal peritonitis complicating CAPD, treated with oral fluconazole 100 mg twice-daily for 2 weeks. The Tenckhoff catheter was not removed until 1 week after completion of fluconazole therapy (Corbella *et al.*, 1990). Chan *et al.* (1994) described their experience of 21 cases of fungal peritonitis (86% due to *Candida* spp.) and reported a cure rate of 10% when fluconazole was used alone, compared with 67% when fluconazole was combined with Tenckhoff catheter removal if no improvement occurred. The sequential approach allowed the successful re-introduction of CAPD because of a low rate of peritoneal adhesions.

j Other *Candida* infections Fluconazole 200 mg orally daily was effective in the treatment of the rare condition of candida epididymo-orchitis in a 65-year-old diabetic man. The clinical symptoms rapidly resolved within 2 weeks and the man completed a 6-week course, with no relapse after long-term follow-up (Gordon and Maddern, 1992). Single-dose treatment with 150 mg fluconazole was found to be safe and effective for the management of balanitis due to *C. albicans* (Kinghorn and Woolley, 1990).

k Prophylaxis Prevention of disseminated candidiasis and other opportunistic fungal infections during periods of neutropenia remains a priority, as these infections become increasingly common. Studies utilizing non-absorbable polyenes or clotrimazole and ketoconazole have yielded disappointing results. The efficacy of fluconazole in comparison with other antifungal agents was established for the prevention of disseminated candidiasis in neutropenic animal models prior to evaluation in human trials (Walsh *et al.*, 1990).

Goodman *et al.* (1992) reported that oral fluconazole 400 mg daily, significantly reduced fungal colonization (30% versus 67%), superficial fungal infections (8% versus 33%) and systemic fungal infections (3% versus 16%) in bone marrow transplant recipients enrolled in a large placebo-controlled trial. Fluconazole was started at the onset of the conditioning regimen for bone marrow transplantation and was continued until recovery of the neutrophil count to >1000 per μl, (mean duration of prophylaxis was <40 days). Although there was no difference in mortality between the two groups, deaths from fungal infection were significantly lower in the fluconazole-treated group. There was no increase in the colonization or incidence of infection with *C. krusei* in the fluconazole group compared with the placebo group; however, the three episodes of candidemia in the fluconazole treated group were due to *C. krusei*. The rate of empirical use of AMB was no different between the two groups but the time to starting such empirical therapy was shorter in the placebo group (Goodman *et al.*, 1992). The significant reduction in systemic fungal infections due to *C. albicans*, superficial fungal infections, fungal colonization and empiric AMB use, was confirmed by Slavin *et al.* (1995) in a placebo-controlled trial of fluconazole 400 mg daily in bone marrow transplant recipients. They also found no increase in *Candida* infections other than *C. albicans*. A significant increase in survival was also noted for fluconazole recipients.

Concern over the perceived increase in frequency of *C. krusei* infections since the introduction of fluconazole for antifungal prophylaxis during neutropenia, has been reviewed in several studies (Cassasnovas *et al.*, 1992). Wingard *et al.* (1991) in a retrospective study of all bone marrow transplant and leukemic patients determined that antifungal prophylaxis with fluconazole was associated with a 7-fold greater risk of *C. krusei* infection than those who did not receive fluconazole. Colonization with *C. krusei* was also significantly associated with fluconazole prophylaxis. After recognition of the increased colonization with *C. krusei* associated with fluconazole prophylaxis, and institution of early empiric AMB and flucytosine in febrile neutropenic patients colonized with *C. krusei*, the same authors found *C. glabrata* fungemias assumed a greater proportion of fungemias observed (Wingard *et al.*, 1993).

Adult patients with acute leukemia undergoing chemotherapy associated with episodes of neutropenia were enrolled in a placebo-controlled trial of fluconazole 400 mg daily for antifungal prophylaxis. In this patient population, fluconazole significantly reduced fungal colonization (29% versus 68%), and superficial fungal infections (6% versus 15%), but was not associated with a significant reduction in invasive fungal infections (4% versus 8%). Fluconazole was highly effective in eliminating colonization and infection with *Candida* spp. other than *C. krusei*; however, the rate of *C. krusei* colonization and infection was low in both groups. The overall mortality, the use of empiric AMB, and the incidence of drug-induced adverse events were no different between groups (Winston *et al.*, 1993). The results of this study were confirmed in a smaller study performed by Chandrasekar *et al.* (1994) who also reported an increase in the recovery of *C. glabrata* from rectal swabs in both placebo and fluconazole groups, and a larger study by Schaffner and Schaffner (1995) in which no difference in the incidence of deep fungal infections, and survival was found. Over 10% of the fluconazole 400 mg daily group developed infection with molds (*Aspergillus* zygomycetes).

Two comparative studies of fluconazole and oral polyenes for prevention of fungal infections in patients with acute leukemia or bone marrow transplantation, established that oral fluconazole 50 mg daily was more effective in the prevention of oropharyngeal *Candida* infection or colonization, but equivalent to AMB oral suspension or tablets 200 mg-1 g four times daily, in the prevention of severe local or invasive fungal disease. There was no difference in the use of empiric AMB between groups (Philpott-Howard *et al.*, 1993; Rozenberg-Arska *et al.*, 1991). A large multicenter study compared fluconazole 150 mg daily with AMB suspension 500 mg four times daily in neutropenic leukemic patients, and found the two regimens to be equally effective in preventing superficial and systemic fungal infections. There was no difference in the empiric use of AMB for suspected fungal infection, but the fluconazole was better tolerated (Menichetti *et al.*, 1994). An additional study in children with hematological or oncological malignancies compared the prophylactic efficacy of oral fluconazole 3 mg per kg per day, with oral polyenes (oral nystatin 50 000U per kg four times daily or oral AMB 25 mg per kg four times daily). It revealed no difference in the fungal colonization rate, but a significant reduction in confirmed mucosal fungal infections. There was no difference in the rate of systemic fungal infections (Ninane *et al.*, 1994). Oral fluconazole at a dose of 50 mg daily was found to effectively reduce oropharyngeal candidiasis in cancer patients without neutropenia (Samonis *et al.*, 1990). Although fluconazole has been shown to reduce colonization, and mucosal fungal infection in the immunocompromised host, especially during periods of neutropenia, only a minority of studies have established a role in the prevention of invasive fungal infection with *Candida* species. The optimal timing and duration of prophylaxis, and the optimal dose of fluconazole are yet to be determined. Lower doses of fluconazole (100–200 mg daily) may be as efficacious as the high dose employed in several of the studies.

Fluconazole 200 mg daily was compared with clotrimazole troches 10 mg five times daily, in a randomized trial for the prevention of fungal infections in over 400 patients with advanced HIV infection (less than 50 CD4 cells per mm³). Fluconazole was found to significantly reduce the rate of cryptococcal meningitis and esophageal candidiasis, although there was a 10% incidence of candidiasis in those receiving fluconazole. No information concerning resistance is available (Powderly *et al.*, 1995).

l Chronic mucocutaneous candidiasis Topical therapy is usually ineffective in these patients. Ketoconazole has produced cures or remissions in significant numbers of patients but relapse of infection is frequent. In a non-comparative trial of 50 mg fluconazole daily in eight patients with chronic mucocutaneous candidiasis and oral candidosis that was either chronic and refractory to ketoconazole treatment, or relapsing, rapid clinical and mycological remissions were attained in all patients in a mean of 10 days. Three of the eight patients relapsed, but all responded to a short course of fluconazole (3 days) (Hay and Clayton, 1988). These authors suggested that intermittent oral antifungal therapy is the most appropriate treatment after the induction of remission in patients with chronic mucocutaneous candidiasis. No controlled trials have been performed to evaluate the use of fluconazole in the management of infection confined to the skin and nails.

3 Dermatophytosis and superficial candidiasis

Fluconazole was found to be effective at a dose of 50 mg orally daily for 4–6 weeks, in the treatment of mycologically proven fungal infections of the skin, including tinea pedis, tinea cruris, pityriasis versicolor, and candidal infections. Clinical cure was noted in 70% and mycological cure in 81% of 284 infected sites in an open, non-comparative study. There was a 77% clinical cure rate and a 77% mycological cure for the management of tinea versicolor. Failure of treatment occurred most frequently (20%) for infections with *Trichophyton rubrum* and *T. mentagrophytes*. There was a rapid response with the median time to symptom relief of 8 days (De Cuyper *et al.*, 1992a). A dose-ranging study of fluconazole (5–50 mg orally) for the treatment of cutaneous mycoses established a significant dose-response relationship. The 50 mg dose was the most effective, with lower doses associated with unsatisfactory clinical and mycological response rates (De Cuyper *et al.*, 1992b). Another open non-comparative study in 70 adults established that oral fluconazole 150 mg once-weekly for up to four doses was highly effective for the treatment of tinea pedis, and was associated with a 77% cure rate and 78% mycological eradication at long-term follow-up 30 days after the last dose (Del Aguila *et al.*, 1992).

Fluconazole 100 mg daily was used successfully to treat recalcitrant, severe *Candida* intertrigo in a woman with poorly controlled diabetes. Maintenance treatment with 200 mg monthly has been required to prevent relapses (Coldiron and Manders, 1991). In another case report, 100 mg fluconazole daily effectively eradicated *C. albicans* and effected marked improvement within 2 weeks in a 12-year-old with chronic fungating cutaneous candidiasis associated with keratitis, icthyosis and deafness syndrome (KID) (Shiraishi *et al.*, 1994). Cardiac transplant patients with pityrosporum folliculitis (*Malassezia furfur*) were successfully treated with fluconazole 100 mg daily for 4 weeks (Henning *et al.*, 1991). Fluconazole 2% shampoo was evaluated for the treatment of seborrheic dermatitis in adults. Complete resolution was noted in 80% of individuals who were culture positive for *Pityrosporum ovale* and who applied the shampoo to the face and scalp twice-weekly for 4 weeks (Rigopoulos *et al.*, 1994).

Onychomycosis may be difficult to treat. Anecdotal reports of the successful use of oral fluconazole 100 mg alternate days for 4–8 months without relapse for recalcitrant toenail infection with *T. rubrum*, and 150 mg once-weekly for chronic fingernail infection suggest that fluconazole may play a role in the management of onychomycosis (Coldiron, 1992; Nahass and Sisto, 1993).

4 Aspergillosis

In animal models, fluconazole exhibited a significant lack of activity at concentrations normally achieved in humans, and in a rabbit model of invasive aspergillosis doses of greater than 800 mg per day would be required for activity against *Aspergillus* spp. (Patterson *et al.*, 1990b). Fluconazole at 60 or 120 mg per kg per day given prophylactically to immunosuppressed temporarily leukopenic rabbits did prevent dissemination of invasive aspergillosis, and early treatment with fluconazole at these high doses was shown to reduce mortality and significantly reduce the tissue burden of fungal organisms, but was unable to sterilize liver, kidney or lung tissue (Patterson *et al.*, 1991). Fluconazole therefore has not been studied in a controlled manner for a role in the management of aspergillosis. Several case reports and small series of patients with pulmonary aspergillosis or aspergilloma treated with fluconazole have been published. In the majority of these cases, the diagnosis of aspergillosis was not confirmed on biopsy, but based on the isolation of *Aspergillus* spp. from sputum or bronchial washings. Fluconazole 400 mg per day was reported to be effective in 49% cases with pulmonary aspergillus infection from one series (Quist and Tauris, 1990; Grant and Clissold, 1990). High-dose fluconazole (1200–2000 mg daily) was ineffective for invasive aspergillosis in neutropenic patients (Anaissie *et al.*, 1995). Fluconazole is not recommended for the treatment of mold infections, in severely immunocompromised patients.

In placebo-controlled studies of fluconazole 400 mg orally daily for prophylaxis against systemic fungal infections in patients undergoing intensive chemotherapy for hematological malignancies or bone marrow transplantation, no prophylactic effect against aspergillosis has been demonstrated, although the incidence of *Aspergillus* infections in both placebo and fluconazole arms was small (Slavin *et al.*, 1995; Schaffner and Schaffner, 1995).

5 Histoplasmosis

Interest in the use of fluconazole for disseminated histoplasmosis was generated by the increase in cases associated with the HIV epidemic, and the chronic severe immunodeficiency that results in frequent relapses after successful treatment. Comparative trials of primary treatment and maintenance regimens have not been performed. Treatment recommendations are currently based on small series and anecdotal case reports. Fluconazole would be considered as alternative therapy to AMB or itraconazole. In one series of ten patients, half the patients were initially treated with 100 mg daily, and the other five patients received 400–800 mg daily. In each group, three patients failed to respond to treatment, resulting in a 40% response rate overall (Sharkey-Mathis *et al.*, 1993). In a retrospective study of maintenance therapy after induction treatment with AMB, fluconazole 400 mg daily, prevented relapse in 69 of 76 patients (88%) treated (Norris *et al.*, 1994). Wheat (1994) recommends fluconazole 800 mg per day for induction and 400 mg per day for maintenance treatment in those patients unable to tolerate itraconazole.

6 Blastomycosis

Experience with the use of fluconazole for treatment of blastomycosis is limited. Under the auspices of the National Institutes of Health Mycoses Study Group, doses of fluconazole less than 400 mg per day have been associated with response rates inferior to those seen with ketoconazole or itraconazole. Progressive disease was noted in four of six patients treated with 200–400 mg daily, at one center (Bradsher, 1992). In a review of blastomycosis in immunocompromised patients seen at one center over a period of 35 years, good responses were documented in two patients who received initial i.v. AMB followed by 4 and 8 months of oral fluconazole 400 mg per day. One patient was switched to 400 mg fluconazole after 2 months treatment with ketoconazole, and the other patient received fluconazole 400 mg daily for the treatment of relapsed blastomycosis after treatment with ketoconazole was discontinued (Pappas *et al.*, 1993). An additional report of two cases of pulmonary blastomycosis, one of which had presumed central nervous system involvement, revealed successful treatment with fluconazole 200 mg twice-daily, after a 10-day course of AMB 0.5 mg per kg per day (Pearson *et al.*, 1992). Until more data are available, fluconazole cannot be recommended as first-line therapy for pulmonary or extrapulmonary blastomycosis.

7 Coccidioidomycosis

Experience with fluconazole for the treatment of coccidioidomycosis is limited to small non-comparative studies using historical control response rates for comparison. The initial experience using low doses of 50–100 mg daily for 2–23 months in non-meningeal disease resulted in improvement in 85% of 14 patients treated, but unacceptably high clinical and mycological relapse rates of 45% in the responders, from 9 days to 15 months after ceasing fluconazole (Catanzaro *et al.*, 1990). In another study of fluconazole in coccidioidomycosis, two patients treated with 100 mg daily either failed to respond or relapsed. Fourteen of 16 patients who were treated with fluconazole 400–600 mg daily for 11–24 months responded. It was the impression of these authors that the time to a clinical and mycological response to treatment with fluconazole for patients with coccidioidomycosis was longer than that observed in patients with other deep-seated mycoses (Diaz *et al.*, 1992). Higher doses of fluconazole (200–400 mg daily) were used in a second open study of chronic pulmonary and non-meningeal coccidioidomycosis by the NIAID Mycoses Study Group. Responses were noted in 85% of those with skeletal infection, 55% of those with chronic pulmonary disease and 76% of those with soft tissue disease. The relapse rate remained high at 37% (Catanzaro *et al.*, 1995). Although i.v. AMB has been recommended for treatment of diffuse reticulonodular disease in HIV-infected patients, milder disease may be managed with 400–800 mg fluconazole daily (Wheat, 1994) and chronic maintenance treatment with fluconazole 200–400 mg daily is indicated to prevent relapse.

Coccidioidal meningitis has traditionally been treated with intrathecal AMB. Fluconazole is a desirable alternative to this mode of therapy, because of its excellent CSF penetration, oral bioavailability and minimal toxicity, which makes it appropriate for long-term treatment. Galgiani *et al.* (1993) have reported their experience in 50 patients (including nine HIV-infected) with coccidioidal meningitis treated with oral fluconazole 400 mg daily or 6 mg per kg daily. Half the patients had received therapy with intrathecal AMB and had failed or relapsed prior to enrolment in the fluconazole study. A response (defined as at least a 40% reduction in CSF abnormalities without relapse) was achieved in 80% patients (88% of those previously treated and 70% who received fluconazole as initial therapy). Of the ten patients who did not respond to 400 mg fluconazole, four subsequently responded to an increased dose of 800 mg daily. There was no difference in response in the subset of patients with HIV infection or those with hydrocephalus. Most of the improvement occurred in the first 4–8 months of treatment and 75% of the responding patients had persistent low level CSF abnormalities for over 12 months. The authors recommend indefinite treatment with fluconazole because it may not be curative. A response to fluconazole at doses of 100–150 mg per day has been reported in two patients (Classen *et al.*, 1988). A randomized trial of intrathecal AMB and oral fluconazole would determine the role of fluconazole for this infection. The appropriate dose and duration of therapy are yet to be determined.

8 Paracoccidioidomycosis

Preliminary results from a Pan American study of fluconazole for treatment of deep mycoses in immunocompetent hosts, revealed 27 of 29 (93%) patients with pulmonary or extrapulmonary disease responded to fluconazole 200–400 mg daily. Improvement in clinical symptoms occurred within 2–4 weeks of treatment. Only one patient who received 2 months fluconazole treatment relapsed at 24 months of follow-up. Duration of treatment varied from 2 to 17 months, with the majority of patients receiving less than 6 months treatment (Diaz *et al.*, 1992).

9 Mucormycosis

Fluconazole is not active against any of the agents of mucormycosis, and its activity against experimental mucormycosis has not been evaluated. Disease caused by one of the agents of Mucorales has occurred in leukemia or bone marrow transplant patients taking fluconazole as antifungal prophylaxis.

An anecdotal report of reasonable efficacy of fluconazole for the treatment of infection with *Conidiobolus coronatus* suggests the azoles could play a role in this infection (Costa *et al.*, 1991).

10 Penicillium marneffei infections

This infection is common in South-East Asia, and is usually associated with HIV infection. However, progressive disseminated disease can occur in individuals with no recognized immunodeficiency. The treatment of choice is AMB or itraconazole for mild to moderate disease. However there are a number of reports of resolution of symptoms with fluconazole in children (5 mg per kg per day or 300 mg daily) and adults (Lau *et al.*, 1992; Liu *et al.*, 1994; Sirisanthana and Sirisanthana, 1993). Success with initial therapy of fluconazole occurred in 36% (four of 11) patients reported by Supparatpinyo *et al.* (1993), compared with 77% (27 of 35) patients treated with AMB, and 75% (three of 12) patients treated with itraconazole.

11 Chromoblastomycosis

A severe case of chronic chromoblastomycosis involving the extremities, caused by *Cladosporium carrioni* responded to fluconazole after failing treatment with potassium iodide, AMB, flucytosine, clotrimazole, miconazole and ketoconazole. The lesions, present for 12 years improved within 1 week of receiving fluconazole 200 mg i.v. Treatment was continued for 30 days, at which time there was clinical and mycological resolution of infection. Oral fluconazole was continued for 2 years without relapse (Yu and Gao, 1994). However, in a series of eight patients with *Fonsecaea pedrosoi* infection, only one responded to fluconazole and this patient relapsed (Diaz *et al.*, 1992). Fluconazole is not recommended for treatment of this infection.

12 Phaeohyphomycosis

This term encompasses a heterogeneous group of mycotic infections caused by dematiaceous fungi from many different genera and species. The most common cause is *Exophiala jeanselmei*. Disease is distinguished from chromoblastomycosis on histological appearances, and often the etiological agent is unable to be cultured. An anecdotal report of treatment success using 50–100 mg fluconazole orally in a man with cutaneous phaeohyphomycosis suggested that the higher dose is associated with more rapid improvement for the cutaneous and superficial forms of disease (Boustany Noel *et al.*, 1988). Chronic *Alternaria alternata* infection of the nasopharynx, sinuses and external soft tissues of the nose which had continued to relapse after treatment with AMB, nystatin, ketoconazole and itraconazole over a 16-year period, was improved and controlled with fluconazole 400–600 mg daily over 18 months (Diaz *et al.*, 1990). Systemic forms of disease caused by the dematiaceous fungi are less common and less susceptible to treatment. A man with malignant lymphoma developed a brain abscess due to *Ochronis gallopavum* which was fatal despite treatment with AMB, flucytosine and fluconazole (Sides *et al.*, 1991). A renal transplant recipient with a subcutaneous abscess caused by *Phialophora parasitica* had no improvement following 18 weeks treatment with fluconazole. The abscess resolved after surgical resection (Fincher *et al.*, 1988).

13 Fusarium infections

Fusarium spp. are generally resistant to the azole drugs. This infection develops in severely neutropenic patients with hematological malignancy or recipients of bone marrow transplants, and has been documented in patients receiving fluconazole 200 mg daily as prophylaxis against invasive fungal infections (Ellis *et al.*, 1994). Three patients with invasive *Fusarium* infections who remained neutropenic, did not respond to high-dose fluconazole (1200–2000 mg daily) (Anaissie *et al.*, 1995).

14 Sporotrichosis

There is insufficient experience of the use of fluconazole for the treatment of sporotrichosis to recommend it as first-line therapy for this indication. Twelve of 19 patients treated with doses of 200–400 mg fluconazole daily for at least 6 months were successfully managed (Diaz *et al.*, 1992). Castro *et al.* (1993) reported successful treatment with fluconazole for three cases of cutaneous and lymphangiitic sporotrichosis. Treatment doses up to 400 mg daily were required for 3–6 months to effect a cure. However, an AIDS patient with cutaneous sporotrichosis responded well to AMB, but developed *Sporothrix schenckii* meningeal infection when fluconazole 100 mg daily was substituted for the AMB. The patient did not respond to reinstitution of AMB (Penn *et al.*, 1992). Kauffman *et al.* (1996) reported their experience with fluconazole 200–800 mg per day for at least 1 month in 30 patients with sporotrichosis. Cure was achieved in 10 of 14 patients (70%) with lymphocutaneous sporotrichosis, but only five of 16 patients with visceral or osteoarticular sporotrichosis improved with fluconazole and only two patients were cured. These responses are inferior to those seen with itraconazole.

15 Trichosporonosis

Disseminated infection with *Trichosporon beigelii* or more rarely, *Blastoschizomyces capitatus* (*Geotrichum capitatum* or *Trichosporon capitatum*) are reported with increasing frequency as opportunistic invasive fungal infections in severely immunocompromised patients with hematologic malignancy or bone marrow transplantation. The treatment of choice has been AMB, but despite antifungal treatment, the infection is associated with a high mortality rate, particularly in those who remain profoundly neutropenic (Hoy *et al.*, 1986). Disseminated infection has been diagnosed antemortem in individuals who received fluconazole prophylaxis (150 mg daily) during neutropenic episodes (Liu *et al.*, 1990). Anaissie *et al.* (1992) reported successful treatment with fluconazole 100–400 mg daily (and 3.5–7 mg per kg in an infant) in four cancer patients with invasive trichosporonosis. Two patients were not neutropenic and the other two patients had short-lived neutropenia at the time of treatment.

Fluconazole 400 mg daily for 3 weeks was used successfully in an AIDS patient with *T. beigelii* fungemia from an endovascular catheter infection. The infected catheter was removed at the time of institution of fluconazole (Barchiesi *et al.*, 1993). Prosthetic valve endocarditis due to *T. beigelii* was managed and controlled over 4 years with courses of AMB and ketoconazole. During the fifth episode of septic embolism this patient was started on fluconazole 400 mg daily, but 1 month later while on fluconazole, the blood cultures remained positive for *T. beigelii* and the patient died of septic shock (Martinez-Lacasa *et al.*, 1991). Another patient with disseminated *T. beigelii* infection and neutropenia failed to respond to fluconazole 400 mg daily for 2 weeks, until neutrophil recovery occurred. During the next episode of neutropenia, and despite i.v. AMB

1 mg per kg alternate days, the patient developed an acute septic arthritis due to *T. beigelii* (McWhinney *et al.*, 1992). These reports and the animal model work done by Walsh *et al.* (1992) suggest that fluconazole should be considered for treatment of trichosporonosis. In patients with prolonged and profound neutropenia, it is unlikely that any currently available antifungal agent will be effective.

Fluconazole successfully suppressed meningeal infection with *Blastoschizomyces capitatus* in an allogeneic bone marrow transplant recipient with chronic graft-versus-host disease. Resolution of meningeal symptoms and eradication of *Blastoschizomyces capitatus* from CSF occurred during 11 months treatment. However, 3 months after discontinuation of fluconazole the patient died a respiratory death, and meningeal invasion of fungus consistent with *Blastoschizomyces capitatus* was found at autopsy (Girmenia *et al.*, 1991).

16 Prototheca infections

Despite *in vitro* resistance to *Prototheca*, fluconazole 200 mg daily for 2 days, then 200 mg after each hemodialysis for 6 weeks, was associated with resolution of peritonitis caused by this organism, and the successful re-introduction of CAPD (Gibb *et al.*, 1991).

17 Other fungal infections

Fungemia secondary to central venous catheter infection due to *Rhodotorula minuta* developed in an AIDS patient receiving daily fluconazole 100 mg as prophylaxis, and *in vitro* susceptibility tests confirmed the isolate was resistant to fluconazole with an MIC >100 μg per ml. The patient was successfully treated with amphotericin B (Goldani *et al.*, 1995).

References

Abbott M, Hughes DL, Patel R, Kinghorn GR (1991). Angio-oedema after fluconazole. *Lancet* **338**: 633.

Agarwal A, Sakhuja V, Chugh KS (1990). Fluconazole-induced thrombocytopenia. *Ann Intern Med* **113**: 899.

Akler ME, Vellend H, McNeely DM *et al.* (1995). Use of fluconazole in the treatment of candidal endophthalmitis. *Clin Infect Dis* **20**: 657.

Allendoerfer R, Marquis AJ, Rinaldi MG, Graybill JR (1991). Combined therapy with fluconazole and flucytosine in murine cryptococcal meningitis. *Antimicrob Ag Chemother* **35**: 726.

Anaissie EJ, Bodey GP, Kantarjian H *et al.* (1991). Fluconazole therapy for chronic disseminated candidiasis in patients with leukemia and prior amphotericin B therapy. *Amer J Med* **91**: 142.

Anaissie E, Gokaslan A, Hachem R *et al.* (1992). Azole therapy for trichosporonosis: Clinical evaluation of eight patients, experimental therapy for murine infection, and review. *Clin Infect Dis* **15**: 781.

Anaissie EJ, Hachem R, Karyotakis NC *et al.* (1994a). Comparative efficacies of amphotericin B, triazoles and combination of both as experimental therapy for murine trichosporonosis. *Antimicrob Ag Chemother* **38**: 2541.

Anaissie EJ, Karyotakis NC, Hachem R *et al.* (1994b). Correlation between *in vitro* and *in vivo* activity of antifungal agents against *Candida* species. *J Infect Dis* **170**: 3841.

Anaissie EJ, Kontoyiannis DP, Huls C *et al.* (1995). Safety, plasma concentrations, and efficacy of high-dose fluconazole in invasive mold infections. *J Infect Dis* **172**: 599.

Ansari AM, gould JM, Douglas JG (1990). High dose oral fluconazole for oropharyngeal candidosis in AIDS. *J Antimicrob Chemother* **25**: 720.

Apseloff G, Hilligoss DM, Gardner MJ *et al.* (1991). Induction of fluconazole metabolism by rifampin: *In vivo* study in humans. *J Clin Pharmacol* **31**: 358.

Assan R, Fredj G, Larger E *et al.* (1994). FK 506/fluconazole interaction enhances FK 506 nephrotoxicity. *Diabet Metab* **20**: 49.

Azon-Masoliver A, Vilaplana J (1993). Fluconazole-induced toxic epi-

dermal necrolysis in a patient with human immunodeficiency virus infection. *Dermatologia* **187**: 268.

Baily GG, Perry FM, Denning DW, Mandal BK (1994). Fluconazole-resistant candidosis in an HIV cohort. *AIDS* **8**: 787.

Bailly MP, Boibieux A, Biron F *et al.* (1991). Persistence of *Cryptococcus neoformans* in the prostate: Failure of fluconazole despite high doses. *J Infect Dis* **164**: 435.

Barchiesi F, Giacometti A, Arzeni D *et al.* (1992). Fluconazole and ketoconazole in the treatment of oral and esophageal candidiasis in AIDS patients. *J Chemother* **4**: 381.

Barchiesi F, Morbiducci V, Ancarani F *et al.* (1993). *Trichosporon beigelii* fungaemia in an AIDS patient. *AIDS* **7**: 139.

Barchiesi F, Colombo AL, McGough DA, Rinaldi MG (1994). Comparative study of broth macrodilution and microdilution techniques for *in vitro* antifungal susceptibility of yeasts by using the National Committee for Clinical Laboratory Standards' proposed guidelines. *J Clin Microbiol* **32**: 2494.

Barchiesi F, Hollis RJ, McGough DA *et al.* (1995). DNA subtypes and fluconazole susceptibilities of *Candida albicans* isolates from the oral cavities of patients with AIDS. *Clin Infect Dis* **20**: 634.

Bart-Delabesse E, Boiron P, Carlotti A, Dupont B (1993). *Candida albicans* genotyping in studies with patients with AIDS developing resistance to fluconazole. *J Clin Microbiol* **31**: 2933.

Bartlett MS, Queener SF, Shaw MM *et al.* (1994). *Pneumocystis carinii* is resistant to imidazole antifungal agents. *Antimicrob Ag Chemother* **38**: 1859.

Behrens-Baumann W, Klinge B, Ruchel R (1990). Topical fluconazole for experimental *Candida* keratitis in rabbits. *Brit J Ophthalmol* **74**: 40.

Berl T, Wilner KD, Gardner M *et al.* (1995). Pharmacokinetics of fluconazole in renal failure. *J Amer Soc Nephrol* **6**: 242.

Berry AJ, Rinaldi MG, Graybill JR (1992). Use of high-dose fluconazole as salvage therapy for cryptococcal meningitis in patients with AIDS. *Antimicrob Ag Chemother* **36**: 690.

Blum RA, D'Andrea DT, Florentino BM et al. (1991a). Increased gastric pH and the bioavailability of fluconazole and ketoconazole. Ann Intern Med 114: 755.

Blum RA, Wilton JH, Hilligoss DM et al. (1991b). Effect of fluconazole on the disposition of phenytoin. Clin Pharmacol Ther 49: 420.

Boag FC, Houang ET, Westrom R et al. (1991). Comparison of vaginal flora after treatment with a clotrimazole 500 mg vaginal pessary or a fluconazole 150 mg capsule for vaginal candidosis. Genitourin Med 67: 232.

Bode S, Pedersen-Bjergaard L, Hjelt K (1992). Candida albicans septicemia in a premature infant successfully treated with oral fluconazole. Scand J Infect Dis 24: 673.

Borne MJ, Elliott JH, O'Day DH (1993). Ocular fluconazole treatment of Candida parapsilosis endophthalmitis after failed intravitreal amphotericin B. Arch Ophthalmol 111: 1326.

Boustany Noel S, Greer DL, Abadie SM et al. (1988). Primary cutaneous phaeohyphomycosis. J Amer Acad Dermatol 18: 1023.

Bozzette SA, Larsen RA, Chiu J (1991a). A placebo-controlled trial of maintenance therapy with fluconazole after treatment of cryptococcal meningitis in the acquired immunodeficiency syndrome. New Engl J Med 324: 580.

Bozzette SA, Larsen RA, Chiu J (1991b). Fluconazole treatment of persistent Cryptococcus neoformans prostatic infection in AIDS. Ann Intern Med 115: 285.

Bozzette SA, Gordon RL, Yen A et al. (1992). Biliary concentrations of fluconazole in a patient with candidal cholecystitis: Case report. Clin Infect Dis 15: 701.

Bradsher RW (1992). Blastomycosis. Clin Infect Dis 14 (Suppl 1): S82–90.

Brammer KW, Coates PE (1994). Pharmacokinetics of fluconazole in pediatric patients. Eur J Clin Microbiol Infect Dis 13: 325.

Brammer KW, Feczko JM (1988). Single-dose oral fluconazole in the treatment of vaginal candidosis. Ann NY Acad Sci 544: 561.

Brammer KW, Farrow PR, Faulkner JK (1990). Pharmacokinetics and tissue penetration of fluconazole in humans. Rev Infect Dis 12 (Suppl 3): S318.

Brammer KW, Coakley AJ, Jezequel SG, Tarbit MH (1991). The disposition and metabolism of [14C]fluconazole in humans. Drug Metab Dispos Biol Fate Chem 19: 764.

Bruzzese VL, Gillum JG, Israel DS et al. (1995). Effect of fluconazole on pharmacokinetics of 2'3'-dideoxyinosine in persons seropositive for human immunodeficiency virus. Antimicrob Ag Chemother 39: 1050.

Byers M, Chapman S, Feldman S, Parent A (1992). Fluconazole pharmacokinetics in the cerebrospinal fluid of a child with Candida tropicalis meningitis. Ped Infect Dis J 11: 895.

Byrne WR, Wajszczuk CP (1988). Cryptococcal meningitis in the acquired immunodeficiency syndrome (AIDS): Successful treatment with fluconazole after failure of amphotericin B. Ann Intern Med 108: 384.

Canafax DM, Graves NM, Hilligoss DM et al. (1991a). Interaction between cyclosporine and fluconazole in renal allograft recipients. Transplantation 51: 1014.

Canafax DM, Graves NM, Hilligoss DM et al. (1991b). Increased cyclosporine levels as a result of simultaneous fluconazole and cyclosporin therapy in renal transplant recipients: a double-blind, randomized pharmacokinetic and safety study. Transplant Proc 23: 1041.

Casadevall A, Spitzer ED, Webb D, Rinaldi MG (1993). Susceptibilities of serial Cryptococcus neoformans isolates from patients with recurrent cryptococcal meningitis to amphotericin B and fluconazole. Antimicrob Ag Chemother 37: 1383.

Casasnovas R-O, Caillot D, Solary E et al. (1992). Prophylactic fluconazole and Candida krusei infections. New Engl J Med 326: 891.

Case CP, MacGowan AP, Brown NM et al. (1991). Prophylactic oral fluconazole and candida fungemia. Lancet 337: 790.

Castro LG, Belda W Jr, Cuce LC et al. (1993). Successful treatment of sporotrichosis with oral fluconazole: a report of three cases. Brit J Dermatol 128: 352.

Catanzaro A, Fierer J, Friedman PJ (1990). Fluconazole in the treatment of persistent coccidioidomycosis. Chest 97: 666.

Catanzaro A, Galgiani JN, Levine BE et al. (1995). Fluconazole in the treatment of chronic pulmonary and nonmeningeal coccidioidomycosis. NIAID Mycoses Study Group. Amer J Med 98: 249.

Chan TM, Chan CY, Cheng SW et al. (1994). Treatment of fungal peritonitis complicating continuous ambulatory peritoneal dialysis with oral fluconazole: a series of 21 patients. Nephrol Dial Transplant 9: 539.

Chandrasekar PH, Gatney CM, and the Bone Marrow Transplant Team (1994). The effect of fluconazole prophylaxis on fungal colonization in neutropenic cancer patients. J Antimicrob Chemother 33: 309.

Chen SC, O'Donnell ML, Gordon S, Gilbert GL (1996). Antifungal susceptibility testing using the E test: comparison with the broth macrodilution technique. J Antimicrob Chemother 37: 265.

Chin T, Fong IW, Vandenbroucke A (1990). Pharmacokinetics of fluconazole in serum and cerebrospinal fluid in a patient with AIDS and cryptococcal meningitis. Pharmacother 10: 305.

Classen DC, Burke JP, Smith CB (1988). Treatment of coccidioidal meningitis with fluconazole. J Infect Dis 158: 903.

Coker RJ, Harris JRW (1991). Failure of fluconazole treatment in cryptococcal meningitis despite adequate CSF levels. J Infect 23: 101.

Coker RJ, Tomlinson DR, Parkin J et al. (1990). Interaction between fluconazole and rifampin. Brit Med J 301: 818.

Coker RJ, Moulopoulos D, Main J et al. (1992). Cryptococcal meningitis in AIDS occurring despite systemic antifungal therapy. J Infect 24: 107.

Colombo ML, Barchiesi F, McGough DA, Rinaldi MG (1995). Comparison of E test and National Committee for Clinical Laboratory Standards broth macrodilution method for azole susceptibility testing. J Clin Microbiol 33: 535.

Coldiron B (1992). Recalcitrant onychomycosis of the toenails successfully treated with fluconazole. Arch Dermatol 128: 909.

Coldiron BM, Manders SM (1991). Persistent Candida intertrigo treated with fluconazole. Arch Dermatol 127: 165.

Colville A, Wale MCJ (1991). Fluconazole or amphotericin for candidemia in non-neutropenic patients. Lancet 337: 1605.

Conti DJ, Tolkoff-Rubin NE, Baker GP et al. (1989). Successful treatment of invasive fungal infection with fluconazole in organ transplant recipients. Transplantation 48: 692.

Corbella X, Sirvent JM, Carratala J (1991). Fluconazole treatment without catheter removal in Candida albicans peritonitis complicating peritoneal dialysis. Amer J Med 90: 277.

Costa AR, Porto E, Pegas JRP et al. (1991). Rhinofacial zygomycosis caused by Conidiobolus coronatus. A case report. Mycopathologia 115: 1.

Couch P, Jacobson P, Johnson CE (1992). Stability of fluconazole and amino acids in parenteral nutrient solutions. Amer J Hosp Pharm 49: 1459.

Cruciani M, Di Perri G, Concia E et al. (1990). Fluconazole and fungal ocular infection. J Antimicrob Chemother 25: 718.

Cruciani M, Di Perri G, Molesini M et al. (1992). Use of fluconazole in the treatment of Candida albicans hydrocephalus shunt infection. Eur J Clin Microbiol Infect Dis 11: 957.

Crussell-Porter LL, Rindone JP, Ford MA, Jaskar DW (1993). Low-dose fluconazole therapy potentiates the hypoprothrombinemic response of warfarin sodium. Arch Intern Med 153: 102.

Czwerwiec FS, Bilsker MS, Kamerman ML, Bisno AL (1993). Long-term survival after fluconazole therapy of candidal prosthetic valve endocarditis. Amer J Med 94: 545.

Dan M, Priel I (1994). Failure of fluconazole therapy for sternal osteomyelitis due to Candida albicans. Clin Infect Dis 18: 126.

Darwazeh AMG, Lamey P-J, Lewis MAO, Samaranayake LP (1991). Systemic fluconazole therapy and in vitro adhesion of Candida albicans to human buccal epithelial cells. J Oral Pathol Med 20: 17.

Dave J, Hickey MM, Wilkins EGL (1989). Fluconazole in renal candidosis. Lancet 336: 163.

Debruyne D, Ryckelynck J-P (1992). Fluconazole serum, urine, and dialysate levels in CAPD patients. Perit Dial Bull 12: 328.

Debruyne D, Ryckelynck J-P (1993). Clinical pharmacokinetics of fluconazole. *Clin Pharmacokinet* **24**: 10.

Debruyne D, Ryckelynck J-P, Moulin M *et al.* (1990). Pharmacokinetics of fluconazole in patients undergoing continuous ambulatory peritoneal dialysis. *Clin Pharmacokinet* **18**: 491.

De Cuyper C, Amblard P, Austad J *et al.* (1992a). Noncomparative study of fluconazole in the treatment of patients with common fungal infections of the skin. *Int J Dermatol* **31** (Suppl 2): 17.

De Cuyper C, de Bersaques J, Delescluse J *et al.* (1992b). Evaluation of four oral daily doses of fluconazole in the treatment of cutaneous mycoses. *Int J Dermatol* **31** (Suppl 2): 8.

Del Aguila R, Montero Gel F, Robles M *et al.* (1992). Once-weekly oral doses of fluconazole 150 mg in the treatment of tinea pedis. *Clin Exp Dermatol* **17**: 402.

de los Reyes C, Edelman DE, De Bruin MF (1992). Clinical experience with single-dose fluconazole in vaginal candidiasis. A review of the worldwide database. *Int J Gynecol Obstet* **37** (Suppl): 9.

DeMuria D, Forrest A, Rich *et al.* (1993). Pharmacokinetics and bioavailability of fluconazole in patients with AIDS. *Antimicrob Ag Chemother* **37**: 2187.

Devenport MH, Crook D, Wynn V, Lees LJ (1989). Metabolic effects of low-dose fluconazole in healthy female users and non-users of oral contraceptives. *Brit J Clin Pharmacol* **27**: 851.

De Wit F, Weerts D, Gooffens D, Clumeck N (1989). Comparison of fluconazole and ketoconazole for oropharyngeal candidiasis in AIDS. *Lancet* **i**: 746.

De Wit S, Urbain D, Rahir F *et al.* (1991). Efficacy of oral fluconazole in the treatment of AIDS associated oesophageal candidiasis. *Eur J Clin Microbiol Infect Dis* **10**: 503.

Diaz M, Puente R, Trevino MA (1990). Response of long-running *Alternaria alternata* infection to fluconazole. *Lancet* **336**: 513.

Diaz M, Negroni R, Montero-Gei F *et al.* (1992). A Pan-American 5-year study of fluconazole therapy for deep mycoses in the immunocompetent host. *Clin Infect Dis* **14** (Suppl 1): S68.

Dismukes WE, Cloud G, Gallis HA *et al.* (1987). Treatment of cryptococcal meningitis with combination amphotericin B and flucytosine for four as compared with six weeks. *New Engl J Med* **317**: 334.

Dixon DM, Polak A (1987). *In vitro* and *in vivo* drug studies with three agents of central nervous system phaeohyphomycosis. *Chemother* **33**: 129.

Dube MP, Heseltine PN, Rinaldi MG *et al.* (1994). Fungemia and colonization with nystatin-resistant *Candida rugosa* in a burn unit. *Clin Infect Dis* **18**: 77.

Dudley MN (1990). Clinical pharmacology of fluconazole. *Pharmacother* **10** (Suppl): S141.

Ebden P, Neill P, Farrow PR (1989). Sputum levels of fluconazole in humans. *Antimicrob Ag Chemother* **33**: 963.

Eckhoff C, Oelkeb W, Bahr V (1988). Effects of two antimycotics, ketoconazole and fluzconazole upon steroidogenesis in rat adrenal cells *in vitro*. *J Steroid Biochem* **31**: 819.

Ellis ME, Clink H, Younge D, Hainu B (1994). Successful combined surgical and medical treatment of *Fusarium* infection after bone marrow transplantation. *Scand J Infect Dis* **2**: 225.

Epelbaum S, Laurent C, Morin G *et al.* (1993). Failure of fluconazole treatment in *Candida* meningitis. *J Pediatr* **123**: 168.

Espinel-Ingroff A, Kish CW, Kerkering TM *et al.* (1992). Collaborative comparison of broth macrodilution and microdilution antifungal susceptibility tests. *J Clin Microbiol* **30**: 3138.

Espinel-Ingroff A, Pfaller M, Erwin ME, Jones RN (1996). Interlaboratory evaluation of Etest method for testing antifungal susceptibilities of pathogenic yeasts to five antifungal agents by using casitone agar and solidified RPMI 1640 medium with 2% glucose. *J Clin Microbiol* **34**: 848.

Esposito R, Castagna A, Foppa CU (1990). Maintenance therapy of oropharyngeal candidiasis in HIV-infected patients with fluconazole. *AIDS* **4**: 1033.

Faergemann J (1988). Activity of triazole derivatives against *Pityrosporum orbiculare in vitro* and *in vivo*. *Ann NY Acad Sci* **544**: 348.

Faergemann J, Laufen H (1993). Levels of fluconazole in serum, stratum corneum, epidermis-dermis (without stratum corneum) and eccrine sweat. *Clin Exp Dermatol* **18**: 102.

Filler SG, Crislip MA, Mayer CL, Edwards JE (1991). Comparison of fluconazole and amphotericin B for treatment of disseminated candidiasis and endophthalmitis in rabbits. *Antimicrob Ag Chemother* **35**: 288.

Fincher RM, Fisher JF, Padhye AA *et al.* (1988). Subcutaneous phaeohyphomycotic abscess caused by *Phialophora parasitica* in a renal allogreaft recipient. *J Med Vet Mycol* **26**: 311.

Finley RW, Cleary JD, Goolsby J, Chapman SW (1995). Fluconazole penetration into the human prostate. *Antimicrob Ag Chemother* **39**: 553.

Fischman AJ, Alpert NM, Livni E *et al.* (1993). Pharmacokinetics of ^{18}F-labeled fluconazole in healthy human subjects by positron emission tomography. *Antimicrob Ag Chemother* **37**: 1270.

Fisher MA, Shen S-H, Haddad J, Tarry WF (1989a). Comparison of *in vivo* activity of fluconazole with that of amphotericin B against *Candida tropicalis*, *Candida glabrata*, and *Candida krusei*. *Antimicrob Ag Chemother* **33**: 1443.

Fisher MA, Lee PG, Tarry WF (1989b). Fluconazole (UK-49,858). treatment of candidiasis in normal and diabetic rats. *Antimicrob Ag Chemother* **33**: 1042.

Flannery MT, Simmons DB, Saba H *et al.* (1992). Fluconazole in the treatment of hepatosplenic candidiasis. *Arch Intern Med* **152**: 406.

Flynn PM, Cunningham CK, Kerkering T *et al.* (1995). Oropharyngeal candidiasis in immunocompromised children: a randomized, multicenter study of orally administered fluconazole suspension versus nystatin. The Multicenter Fluconazole Study Group. *J Pediatr* **127**: 322.

Force RW (1995). Fluconazole concentrations in breast milk. *Pediatr Infect Dis J* **14**: 235.

Force RW, Nahata MC (1995). Salivary concentration of ketoconazole and fluconazole: implications for drug efficacy in oropharyngeal and esophageal candidiasis. *Ann Pharmacother* **29**: 10.

Foulds G, Wajszczuk C, Weidler DJ *et al.* (1988a). Steady state parenteral kinetics of fluconazole in man. *Ann NY Acad Sci* **544**: 427.

Foulds G, Brennan DR, Wajszczuk C *et al.* (1988b). Fluconazole penetration into cerebrospinal fluid in humans. *J Clin Pharmacol* **28**: 363.

Fox R, Neal KR, Leen CL, Ellis ME, Mandal BK (1991). Fluconazole-resistant candida in AIDS. *J Infect* **22**: 201.

Franklin IM, Elias E, Hirsch C (1990). Fluconazole-induced jaundice. *Lancet* **336**: 565.

Fuller JD, Stanfield LED, Craven DE (1994). Rifabutin prophylaxis and uveitis. *New Engl J Med* **330**: 1315.

Galgiani JN (1987). Antifungal susceptibility tests. *Antimicrob Ag Chemother* **21**: 1867.

Galgiani JN, Catanzaro A, Cloud GA *et al.* (1993). Fluconazole therapy for coccidioidal meningitis. *Ann Intern Med* **119**: 28.

Gannon RH, Anderson ML (1992). Fluconazole-nortriptyline drug interaction. *Ann Pharmacother* **26**: 1456.

Garcia-Hermoso D, Dromer F, Improvisi L *et al.* (1995). Fluconazole concentrations in saliva from AIDS patients with oro-pharyngeal candidosis refractory to treatment with fluconazole. *Antimicrob Ag Chemother* **39**: 656.

Gathe JC, Harris RL, Garland B *et al.* (1987). *Candida* osteomyelitis: report of five cases and review of the literature. *Amer J Med* **82**: 927.

Gearhart MO (1994). Worsening of liver function with fluconazole and review of azole antifungal hepatotoxicity. *Ann Pharmacother* **28**: 1177.

Gibb AP, Aggarwal R, Swainson CP (1991). Successful treatment of *Prototheca* peritonitis complicating continuous ambulatory peritoneal dialysis. *J Infect* **22**: 183.

Gil A, Lavilla P, Valencia E *et al.* (1991). Safety and efficacy of fluconazole treatment for *Candida* oesophagitis in AIDS. *Postgrad Med J* **67**: 548.

Girmenia C, Micozzi A, Venditti M *et al.* (1991). Fluconazole treatment of *Blastoschizomyces capitatus* meningitis in an allogeneic bone marrow transplant recipient. *Eur J Clin Microbiol Infect Dis* **10**: 752.

Goldani LZ, Craven DE, Sugar AM (1995). Central venous catheter infection with *Rhodotorula minuta* in a patient with AIDS taking suppressive doses of fluconazole. *J Med Vet Mycol* **33**: 267.

Goldman M, Pottage JC, Weaver DC (1993). *Candida krusei* fungemia: Report of 4 cases and review of the literature. *Medicine* **72**: 143.

Goodman JL, Winston DJ, Greenfield RA et al. (1992). A controlled trial of fluconazole to prevent fungal infections in patients undergoing bone marrow transplantation. *New Engl J Med* **326**: 845.

Gordon DL, Maddern J (1992). Treatment of candida epididymo-orchitis with oral fluconazole. *Med J Aust* **156**: 744.

Gordon MA, Lapa EW, Passero PG (1988). Improved method for azole antifungal susceptibility testing. *J Clin Microbiol* **26**: 1874.

Gradon JD, Sepkowittz DV (1991). Fluconazole-associated acute adrenal insufficiency. *Postgrad Med J* **67**: 1084.

Graninger W, Presteril E, Schneeweiss B et al. (1993). Treatment of *Candida albicans* fungaemia with fluconazole. *J Infection* **26**: 133.

Grant SM, Clissold SP (1990). Fluconazole: A review of its pharmacodynamic and pharmacokinetic properties, and therapeutic potential in superficial and systemic mycoses. *Drugs* **39**: 877.

Graybill JR, Palou E, Ahrens J (1986a). Treatment of murine histoplasmosis with UK 49,858 (Fluconazole). *Amer Rev Resp Dis* **134**: 768.

Graybill JR, Sun SH, Ahrens J (1986b). Treatment of murine coccidioidal meningitis with fluconazole (UK 49,858). *J Med Vet Mycol* **24**: 113.

Guillame MP, De Prez C, Cogan E (1995). Subacute mitochondrial liver disease in a patient with AIDS: poosible relationship to prolonged fluconazole administration. *Amer J Gastroenterol* **91**: 165.

Gussenhoven MJE, Haak A, Peereboom-Wynia JDR (1991). Stevens–Johnson syndrome after fluconazole. *Lancet* **338**: 120.

Haneke E (1990). Fluconazole levels in human epidermis and blister fluid. *Brit J Dermatol* **123**: 273.

Haneke E (1992). Pharmacokinetic evaluation of fluconazole in plasma, epidermis, and blister fluid. *Int J Dermatol* **31** (Suppl 2): 3.

Hanger DP, Jevons S, Shaw JTB (1988). Fluconazole and testosterone: In vivo and in vitro studies. *Antimicrob Ag Chemother* **32**: 646.

Haubrich RH, Haghighat D, Bozzette SA et al. (1994). High-dose fluconazole for treatment of cryptococcal disease in patients with human immunodeficiency virus infection. The California Collaborative Treatment Group. *J Infect Dis* **170**: 238.

Havlir D, Torriani F, Dube M (1994). Uveitis associated with rifabutin. *Ann Intern Med* **121**: 510.

Hay RJ, Clayton YM (1988). Fluconazole in the management of patients with chronic mucocutaneous candidosis. *Brit J Dermatol* **119**: 683.

Henning R, Twomey A, Smith L et al. (1991). Therapeutic efficacy of fluconazole in cardiac transplant recipients with *Malassezia* folliculitis. In *Program and Abstracts of the 31st Interscience Conference on Antimicrobial Agents and Chemotherapy, Chicago* (Abstr. 222). Washington, DC: American Society for Microbiology.

Herzog RE, Ansmann EB (1989). Treatment of vaginal candidosis with fluconazole. *Mycoses* **32**: 204.

Hitchcock CA, Pye GW, Troke PF et al. (1993). Fluconazole resistance in *Candida glabrata*. *Antimicrob Ag Chemother* **37**: 1962.

Hoch BS, Namboodiri NK, Banayat G et al. (1993). The use of fluconazole in the management of *Candida* peritonitis in patients on peritoneal dialysis. *Perit Dial Int* **13** (Suppl 2): S357.

Hoppe JE, Klingebiel T, Niethammer D (1994). Selection of *Candida glabrata* in pediatric bone marrow transplant recipients receiving fluconazole. *Pediatr Hematol Oncol* **11**: 207.

Houang ET, Chappatte O, Byrne D et al. (1990). Fluconazole levels in plasma and vaginal secretions of patients after a 150 mg single oral dose and rate of eradication of infection in vaginal candidiasis. *Antimicrob Ag Chemother* **34**: 909.

Howitt KM, Oziemski MA (1989). Phenytoin toxicity induced by fluconazole. *Med J Aust* **151**: 604.

Hoy J, Hsu KC, Rolston K et al. (1986). *Trichosporon beigelii* infection: a review. *Rev Infect Dis* **8**: 959.

Humphrey MJ, Jevons S, Tarbit MH (1985). Pharmacokinetic evaluation of UK-49,858, a metabolically stable triazole antifungal drug, in animals and humans. *Antimicrob Ag Chemother* **28**: 648.

Hunt Fugate AK, Hennessey CK, Kazarian CM (1993). Stability of fluconazole in injectable solutions. *Amer J Hosp Pharm* **50**: 1186.

Isalska BJ, Stanbridge TN (1988). Fluconazole in the treatment of candidal prosthetic valve endocarditis. *Brit Med J* **297**: 178.

Jacobson MA, Hanks DK, Ferrell LD (1994). Fatal acute hepatic necrosis due to fluconazole. *Amer J Med* **96**: 188.

Jakab K, Kelemen E, Prinz G, Torok I (1990). Amphotericin-resistant invasive candidiasis controlled by fluconazole. *Lancet* **335**: 473.

Joe LA, Jacobs RA, Guglielmo BJ (1994). Systemic absorption of oral fluconazole after gastrointestinal resection. *J Antimicrob Chemother* **33**: 1070.

Just-Nubling G, Gentschew G, Mei(ner K et al. (1991). Fluconazole prophylaxis of recurrent oral candidiasis in HIV-positive patients. *Eur J Clin Microbiol Infect Dis* **10**: 917.

Kauffman CA, Bradley SF, Ross SC,Weber DR (1991). Hepatosplenic candidiasis: Successful treatment with fluconazole. *Amer J Med* **91**: 137.

Kauffman CA, Bradley SF, Vine AK (1993). *Candida* endophthalmitis associated with intraocular lens implantation: efficacy of fluconazole therapy. *Mycoses* **36**: 13.

Kauffman CA, Pappas PG, McKinsey DS et al. (1996). Treatment of lymphocutaneous and visceral sporotrichosis with fluconazole. *Clin Infect Dis* **22**: 46.

Kidd D, Ranaghan EA, Morris TCM (1989). Hypokalemia in patients with acute myeloid leukemia after treatment with fluconazole. *Lancet* **334**: 1017.

Kiehn TE, Gorey E, Brown AE et al. (1992). Sepsis due to *Rhodotorula* related to use of indwelling central venous catheters. *Clin Infect Dis* **14**: 841.

King C, Finley R, Chapman SW (1990). Prostatic cryptococcal infection. *Ann Intern Med* **113**: 720.

Kinghorn GR, Woolley PD (1990). Single-dose fluconazole in the treatment of *Candida albicans* balanoposthitis. *Int J STD AIDS* **1**: 366.

Kirk AJB, Gould FK, Freeman R et al. (1989). Fluconazole and candidosis. *Lancet* **334**: 339.

Kilvington S, Larkin DFP, White DG, Beeching JR (1990). Laboratory investigation of *Acanthamoeba* keratitis. *J Clin Microbiol* **28**: 2722.

Kobayashi GS, Travis S, Medoff G (1986). Comparison of the in vitro and in vivo activity of the Bis-triazole derivative UK-49,858 with that of amphotericin B against *Histoplasma capsulatum*. *Antimicrob Ag Chemother* **29**: 660.

Kobayashi GS, Travis S, Medoff G (1987). Comparison of fluconazole and amphotericin B in treating histoplasmosis in immunosuppressed mice. *Antimicrob Ag Chemother* **31**: 2005.

Kobayashi GS, Travis S, Rinaldi MG,Medoff G (1990). In vitro and in vivo activities of Sch 39304, fluconazole, and amphotericin B against *Histoplasma capsulatum*. *Antimicrob Ag Chemother* **34**: 524.

Koletar SL, Russell JA, Fass RJ, Plouffe JF (1990). Comparison of oral fluconazole and clotrimazole troches as treatment for oral candidiasis in patients infected with human immunodeficiency virus. *Antimicrob Ag Chemother* **34**: 2267.

Kostiuk KA, Pons VG, Guglielmo BJ (1994). Penetration of fluconazole into abscess fluid. *J Antimicrob Chemother* **34**: 603.

Kovacs JA, Kovacs AA, Polis MA et al. (1985). Cryptococcosis in the acquired immunodeficiency syndrome. *Ann Intern Med* **103**: 533.

Kowalsky SF (1990). Drug interactions with fluconazole. *Pharmacother* **10** (Suppl 6): 170S.

Kruger HU, Schuler U, Zimmerman R, Ehninger G (1989). Absence of significant interaction of fluconazole with cyclosporin. *J Antimicrob Chemother* **24**: 781.

Kutzer E, Oittner R, Leodolter S, Brammer KW (1988). A comparison of fluconazole and ketoconazole in the oral treatment of vaginal candidiasis; report of a double-blind multicentre trial. *Eur J Obstet Gynecol Reproduct Biol* **29**: 305.

Laine L (1994). The natural history of esophageal candidiasis after successful treatment in patients with AIDS. *Gastroenterology* **107**: 744.

Laine L, Rabeneck L (1995). Prospective study of fluconazole suspension for the treatment of oesophageal candidiasis in patients with AIDS. *Aliment Pharmacol Ther* **9**: 553.

Laine L, Dretler RH, Conteas CN et al. (1992). Fluconazole compared with ketoconazole for the treatment of candida esophagitis in AIDS: a randomized trial. Ann Intern Med 117: 655.

Larsen RA, Bozzette S, McCutchan JA et al. (1989). Persistent Cryptococcus neoformans infection of the prostate after successful treatment of meningitis. Ann Intern Med 111: 125.

Larsen RA, Leal MAE, Chan LS (1990). Fluconazole compared with amphotericin B plus flucytosine for cryptococcal meningitis in AIDS. Ann Intern Med 113: 183.

Larsen RA, Bozzette SA, Jones BE et al. (1994). Fluconazole combined with flucytosine for treatment of cryptococcal meningitis in patients with AIDS. Clin Infect Dis 19: 741.

Lau GKK, Kumana CR, Wong KL et al. (1992). Disseminated Penicillium marneffei infection responding to treatment with oral fluconazole. J Hong Kong Med Assoc 44: 176.

Lau YL, Yuen KY, Lee CW, Chan CF (1995). Invasive Acremonium falciforme infection in a patient with severe combined immunodeficiency. Clin Infect Dis 20: 197.

Laufen H, Yeates RA, Zimmerman T, de los Reyes C (1995). Pharmacokinetic optimization of the treatment of oral candidiasis with fluconazole: studies with a suspension. Drugs Exp Clin Res 21: 23.

Lavrijsen KLM, Van Houdt JMG, Van Dyck DMJ et al. (1990). Induction potential of fluconazole toward drug-metabolizing enzymes in rats. Antimicrob Ag Chemother 34: 402.

Lazar JD, Wilner KD (1990). Drug interactions with fluconazole. Rev Infect Dis 12: 327.

Lee BE, Feinberg M, Abraham JJ, Murthy ARK (1992). Congenital malformations in an infant born to a woman treated with fluconazole. Ped Infect Dis J 11: 1062.

Lee JW, Seibel NL, Amantea M et al. (1992). Safety and pharmacokinetics of fluconazole in children with neoplastic diseases. J Paediatr 120: 987.

Leen CLS, Dunbar EM, Ellis ME, Mandal BK (1990). Once weekly fluconazole to prevent recurrence of oropharyngeal candidiasis in patients with AIDS and AIDS-related complex: a double-blind placebo-controlled study. J Infection 21: 55.

Levine J, Bernard DB, Idelson BA et al. (1989). Fungal peritonitis complicating Continuous Ambulatory Peritoneal Dialysis: Successful treatment with fluconazole, a new orally active antifungal agent. Amer J Med 86: 825.

Liu KL, Herbrecht R, Bergerat JP et al. (1990). Disseminated Trichosporon capitatum infection in a patient with acute leukemia undergoing bone marrow transplantation. Bone Marrow Transpl 6: 219.

Liu MT, Wong CK, Fung CP (1994). Disseminated Penicillium marneffei infection with cutaneous lesions in an HIV-positive patient. Brit J Dermatol 131: 280.

Longman LP, Hibbert SA, Martin MV (1990). Efficacy of fluconazole in prophylaxis and treatment of experimental Candida endocarditis. Rev Infect Dis 12: 294.

Lyman CA, Sugar AM, Diamond RD (1986). Comparative activities of UK-49,858 and amphotericin B against Blastomyces dermatitidis infections in mice. Antimicrob Ag Chemother 29: 161.

Manez R, Martin M, Raman V et al. (1994). Fluconazole therapy in transplant recipients receiving FK506. Transplantation 57: 1521.

Marr B, Gross S, Cunningham C, Weiner L (1994). Candidal sepsis and meningitis in a very-low-birth-weight infant successfully treated with fluconazole and flucytosine. Clin Infect Dis 19: 795.

Marriott DJE, Jones PD, Hoy JF et al. (1993). Fluconazole once a week as secondary prophylaxis against oropharyngeal candidiasis in HIV-infected patients. Med J Aust 158: 312.

Martinez-Lacasa J, Mana J, Niubo R et al. (1991). Long term survival of a patient with prosthetic valve endocarditis due to Trichosporon beigelii. Eur J Clin Microbiol Infect Dis 10: 756.

Martino P, Meloni G, Cassone A (1990). Candidal endocarditis and treatment with fluconazole and Granulocyte-Macrophage Colony Stimulating Factor. Ann Intern Med 112: 966.

Maurice M, Pichard L, Daujat M et al. (1992). Effects of imidazole derivatives on cytochrome p450 from human hepatocytes in primary culture. FASEB J 6: 752.

McWhinney PHM, Madgwick JCA, Hoffbrand AV et al. (1992). Successful surgical management of septic arthritis due to Trichosporon beigelii in a patient with acute myeloid leukemia. Scand J Infect Dis 24: 245.

Menichetti F, Del Favero A, Martino P et al. (1994). Preventing fungal infection in neutropenic patients with acute leukemia: fluconazole compared with oral amphotericin B. The GIMEMA Infection Program. Ann Intern Med 120: 913.

Mercurio MG, Elewski BE (1995). Thrombocytopenia caused by fluconazole therapy. J Amer Acad Dermatol 32: 525.

Milatovic D, Voss A (1992). Efficacy of fluconazole in the treatment of systemic fungal infections. Eur J Clin Microbiol Infect Dis 11: 395.

Milliken S, Powles R, Jones A, Helenglass G (1989). Pharmacokinetics of oral fluconazole in autologous bone marrow transplantation recipients given TBI and high-dose melphalan. Transpl Proc 21: 3067.

Minguez F, Chiu ML, Lima JE et al. (1994). Activity of fluconazole: postantifungal effect, effects of low concentrations and of pre-treatment on the susceptibility of Candida albicans to leukocytes. J Antimicrob Chemother 34: 93.

Mitchell AS, Holland JT (1989). Fluconazole and phenytoin: a predictable interaction. Brit Med J 298: 1315.

Moncino MD, Gutman LT (1990). Severe systemic cryptococcal disease in a child: review of prognostic indicators predicting treatment failure and an approach to maintenance therapy with oral fluconazole. Pediatr Infect Dis J 9: 363.

Morgan JM, Carmichael AJ (1994). Fixed drug eruption with fluconazole. Brit Med J 308: 454.

Munoz P, Moreno S, Berenguer J et al. (1991). Fluconazole-related hepatotoxicity in patients with acquired immunodeficiency syndrome. Arch Intern Med 151: 1020.

Murakami H, Katahira H, Matsushima T et al. (1992). Agranulocytosis during treatment with fluconazole. J Int Med Res 20: 492.

Nahass GT, Sisto M (1993). Onychomycosis: Successful treatment with once-weekly fluconazole. Dermatology 186: 59.

Nahata MC, Brady MT (1995). Pharmacokinetics of fluconazole after oral administration in children with human immunodeficiency virus infection. Eur J Clin Pharmacol 48: 291.

Narang PK, Trapnell CB, Schoenfelder JR et al. (1994). Fluconazole and enhanced effect of rifabutin prophylaxis. New Engl J Med 330: 1316.

Negroni R, de Elias Costa MRI, Finquelievich JL et al. (1991). Treatment of experimental cryptococcosis with SCH 39304 and fluconazole. Antimicrob Ag Chemother 35: 1460.

Nelson MR, Fisher M, Cartledge J et al. (1994). The role of azoles in the treatement and prophylaxis of cryptococcal disease in HIV infection. AIDS 8: 651.

Neuhas G, Pavic N, Pletscher M (1991). Anaphylactic reaction after oral fluconazole. Brit Med J 302: 1341.

Nguyen MH, Barchiesi F, McGough DA et al. (1995a). In vitro evaluation of combination of fluconazole and flucytosine against Cryptococcus neoformans var neoformans. Antimicrob Ag Chemother 39: 1691.

Nguyen MH, Peacock JE, Tanner DC et al. (1995b). Therapeutic approaches in patients with candidemia. Evaluation in a multicenter, prospective, observational study. Arch Intern Med 155: 2429.

Nicolau DP, Crowe H, Nightingale CH, Quintiliani R (1994). Effect of continuous arteriovenous hemodiafiltration on the pharmacokinetics of fluconazole. Pharmacother 14: 502.

Nicolau DP, Crowe H, Nightingale CH, Quintiliani R (1995). Bioavailability of fluconazole administered via a feeding tube in intensive care unit patients. J Antimicrob Chemother 36: 395.

Ninane J, and a Multicentre Study Group (1994). A multicentre study of fluconazole versus oral polyenes in the prevention of fungal infection in children with hematological and oncological malignancies. Eur J Clin Microbiol Infect Dis 13: 330.

Norris S, Wheat J, McKinsey D et al. (1994). Prevention of relapse of histoplasmosis with fluconazole in patients with the acquired immunodeficiency syndrome. Amer J Med 96: 504.

O'Day DM, Foulds G, Williams TE *et al.* (1990). Ocular uptake of fluconazole following oral administration. *Arch Ophthalmol* **108**: 1006.

Odds FC (1985). Laboratory tests for the activity of imidazole and triazole antifungal agents *in vitro*. *Semin Dermatol* **4**: 260.

Odds FC, Webster CE (1988). Effects of azole antifungals *in vitro* on host/parasite interactions relevant to candida infections. *J Antimicrob Chemother* **22**: 473.

Olkkola KT, Ahonen J, Neuvonen PJ (1996). The effects of the systemic antimycotics, itraconazole and fluconazole, on the pharmacokinetics and pharmacodynamics of intravenous and oral midazolam. *Anesthes Analges* **82**: 511.

O'Meeghan T, Varcoe R, Thomas M, Ellis-Pegler R (1990). Fluconazole concentration in joint fluid during successful treatment of *Candida albicans* septic arthritis. *J Antimicrob Chemother* **26**: 601.

Oono S, Tabei K, Tetsuba T, Asano Y (1992). The pharmacokinetics of fluconazole during hemodialysis. *Eur J Clin Pharmacol* **42**: 667.

Osser S, Haglund A, Westrom L (1991). Treatment of candidal vaginitis. A prospective randomized investigator-blind multicenter study comparing topically applied econazole with oral fluconazole. *Acta Obstet Gynecol Scand* **70**: 73.

Oyeka CA, Gugnani HC (1990). *In vitro* activity of seven azole compounds against some clinical isolates of non-dermatophytic filamentous fungi and some dermatophytes. *Mycopathologia* **110**: 157.

Pappas PG, Threlkeld MG, Bedsole GD *et al.* WE (1993). Blastomycosis in immunocompromised patients. *Medicine* **72**: 311.

Pappas PG, Kauffman CA, Perfect J *et al.* (1995). Alopecia associated with fluconazole therapy. *Ann Intern Med* **123**: 354.

Pascual A, Garcia I, Conejo C, Perea EJ (1993). Uptake and intracellular activity of fluconazole in human polymorphonuclear leukocytes. *Antimicrob Ag Chemother* **37**: 187.

Patterson TF, Andriole VT, Zervos MJ *et al.* (1990a). The epidemiology of pseudallescheriasis complicating transplantation: Nosocomial and community-acquired infection. *Mycoses* **33**: 297.

Patterson TF, Miniter P, Andriole VT (1990b). Efficacy of fluconazole in experimental invasive aspergillosis. *Rev Infect Dis* **12** (Suppl): S281.

Patterson TF, George D, Miniter P, Andriole VT (1991). The role of fluconazole in the early treatment and prophylaxis of experimental invasive aspergillosis. *J Infect Dis* **164**: 575.

Paugam A, Dupouy-Camet J, Blanche P *et al.* D (1994). Increased fluconazole resistance of *Cryptococcus neoformans* isolated from a patient with AIDS and recurrent meningitis. *Clin Infect Dis* **19**: 975.

Pearson GJ, Chin TWF, Fong IW (1992). Case report: Treatment of blastomycosis with fluconazole. *Amer J Med Sci* **303**: 313.

Penn CC, Goldstein E, Bartholomew WR (1992). *Sporothrix schenckii* meningitis in a patient with AIDS. *Clin Infect Dis* **15**: 741.

Perfect JR, Durack DT (1985). Penetration of imidazoles and triazoles into cerebrospinal fluid of rabbits. *J Antimicrob Chemother* **16**: 81.

Perfect JR, Savani DV, Durack DT (1986). Comparison of itraconazole and fluconazole in treatment of cryptococcal meningitis and *Candida* pyelonephritis in rabbits. *Antimicrob Ag Chemother* **29**: 579.

Persons DA, Laughlin M, Tanner D *et al.* (1991). Fluconazole and *Candida krusei* fungemia. *New Engl J Med* **325**: 1315.

Pfaller MA, Bale M, Buschelman B *et al.* (1994). Selection of candidate quality control isolates and tentative quality control ranges for *in vitro* susceptibility testing of yeast isolates by National Committee for Clinical Laboratory Standards proposed standard methods. *J Clin Microbiol* **32**: 1650.

Phillips RJM, Watson SA, McKay FF (1990). An open multicentre study of the efficacy and safety of a single dose of fluconazole 150 mg in the treatment of vaginal candidiasis in general practice. *Brit J Clin Pract* **44**: 219.

Philpott-Howard JN, Wade JJ, Mufti GJ *et al.*, for the Multicentre Study Group (1993). Randomized comparison of oral fluconazole versus oral polyenes for the prevention of fungal infection in patients at risk of neutropenia. *J Antimicrob Chemother* **31**: 973.

Pietroski N, Buckley RM, Braffman MN, Stern JJ (1990). Intravenous and oral fluconazole in treatment of acute cryptococcal meningitis. In *Program and Abstracts of the 30th Interscience Conference on Antimicrobial Agents and Chemotherapy, Atlanta* (Abstr. 135). Washington, DC: American Society for Microbiology.

Polak A (1987). Combination therapy of experimental candidiasis, cryptococcosis, aspergillosis and wangiellosis in mice. *Chemotherapy* **33**: 381.

Pons V, Greenspan D, Debruin M and the Multicenter Study Group (1993). Therapy for oropharyngeal candidiasis in HIV-infected patients: A randomized, prospective multicenter study of oral fluconazole versus clotrimazole troches. *J AIDS* **6**: 1311.

Powderly WG (1992). Mucosal candidiasis caused by non-albicans species of *Candida* in HIV-positive patients. *AIDS* **6**: 604.

Powderly WG, Saag MS, Cloud GA *et al.* (1992). A controlled trial of fluconazole or amphotericin B to prevent relapse of cryptococcal meningitis in patients with acquired immunodeficiency syndrome. *New Engl J Med* **326**: 793.

Powderly WG, Finlelstein DM, Feinberg J *et al.* (1995). A randomized trial comparing fluconazole with clotrimazole troches for the prevention of fungal infections in patients with advanced human immunodeficiency virus infection. *New Engl J Med* **332**: 700.

Presterl E, Graninger W and the Multicentre Study Group (1994). Efficacy and safety of fluconazole in the treatment of systemic fungal infections in pediatric patients. *Eur J Clin Microbiol Infect Dis* **13**: 347.

Purda HS, Back DJ (1986). Effect of fluconazole (UK-49,858). on antipyrine metabolism. *Brit J Clin Pharmacol* **21**: 603.

Pursley TJ, Blomquist IK, Abraham J *et al.* (1996). Fluconazole-induced congenital anomalies in three infants. *Clin Infect Dis* **22**: 336.

Quagliarello VJ, Viscoli C, Horwitz RI (1995). Primary prevention of cryptococcal meningitis by fluconazole in HIV-infected patients. *Lancet* **345**: 530.

Quist P, Tauris P (1990). Short-term curative treatment of *Aspergillus fumigatus* pneumonia with fluconazole. *Scand J Infect Dis* **22**: 749.

Redding S, Smith J, Farinacci G *et al.* (1994). Resistance of *Candida albicans* to fluconazole during treatment of oropharyngeal candidiasis in a patient with AIDS: documentation by *in vitro* susceptibility testing and DNA subtype analysis. *Clin Infect Dis* **18**: 240.

Redondo-Lopez V, Lynch M, Schmitt C *et al.* (1990). *Torulopsis glabrata* vaginitis: clinical aspects and susceptibility to antifungal agents. *Obstet Gynaecol* **76**: 651.

Reuman PD, Neiberger R, Kondor DA (1992). Intraperitoneal and intravenous fluconazole pharmacokinetics in a pediatric patient with end-stage renal disease. *Ped Infect Dis J* **11**: 132.

Rex, JH, Pfaller MA, Rinaldi MG *et al.* (1993). Antifungal susceptibility testing. *Clin Microbiol Rev* **6**: 367.

Rex JH, Bennett JE, Sugar AM *et al.* (1994). A randomized trial comparing fluconazole with amphotericin B for the treatment of candidemia in patients without neutropenia. *New Engl J Med* **331**: 1325.

Rex JH, Pfaller MA, Barry AL *et al.* (1995). Antifungal susceptibility testing of isolates from a randomized, multicenter trial of fluconazole versus amphotericin B as treatment of nonneutropenic patients with candidemia. NIAID Mycoses Study Group and the Candidemia Study Group. *Antimicrob Ag Chemother* **39**: 40.

Rigopoulos D, Katsambas A, Antoniou C *et al.* (1994). Facial seborrheic dermatitis treated with fluconazole 2% shampoo. *Int J Dermatol* **33**: 136.

Roder BL, Sonnenschein C, Hartzen SH (1991). Failure of fluconazole therapy in *Candida krusei* fungemia. *Eur J Clin Microbiol Infect Dis* **10**: 173.

Rogers TE, Galgiani JN (1986). Activity of fluconazole (UK-49,858). and ketoconazole against *Candida albicans in vitro* and *in vivo*. *Antimicrob Ag Chemother* **30**: 418.

Roupie E, Darmon J-Y, Brochard L *et al.* (1991). Fluconazole therapy of candidal native valve endocarditis. *Eur J Clin Microbiol Infect Dis* **10**: 458.

Rowe BR, Thorpe J, Barnett A (1992). Safety of fluconazole in women taking oral hypoglycemic agents. *Lancet* **339**: 255.

Rozenberg-Arska M, Dekker AW, Branger J, Verhoef J (1991). A randomized study to compare oral fluconazole to amphotericin B in the prevention of fungal infections in patients with acute leukemia. *J Antimicrob Chemother* **27**: 369.

Rubin PC, Wilton LV, Inman WHW (1992). Fluconazole and pregnancy: results of a prescription event-monitoring study. *Int J Gynecol Obstet* **37** (Suppl): S25.

Ruhnke M, Eigler A, Tennagen I *et al.* (1994a). Emergence of fluconazole-resistant strains of *Candida albicans* in patients with recurrent oropharyngeal candidosis and human immunodeficiency virus infection. *J Clin Microbiol* **32**: 2092.

Ruhnke M, Eigler A, Engelmann E *et al.* (1994b). Correlation between antifungal susceptibility testing of *Candida* isolates from patients with HIV infection and clinical results after treatment with fluconazole. *Infection* **22**: 132.

Ruhnke M, Yeates RA, Pfaff G *et al.* (1995). Single-dose pharmacokinetics of fluconazole in patients with liver cirrhosis. *J Antimicrob Chemother* **35**: 641.

Ryckelynck JP, Debruyne D, Hurault de Ligny B *et al.* (1990). Pharmacokinetics of fluconazole administered intraperitoneally (IP) and orally (O) in patients undergoing CAPD. *Fifth Congress of the International Society of Peritoneal Dialysis, Kyoto*. Abstract no SS-06–02.

Saag MS, Powderly WG, Cloud GA *et al.* (1992). Comparison of amphotericin B with fluconazole in the treatment of AIDS-associated cryptococcal meningitis. *New Engl J Med* **326**: 83.

Sahai J, Gallicano K, Pakuts A, Cameron DW (1994). Effect of fluconazole on zidovudine pharmacokinetics in patients infected with human immunodeficiency virus. *J Infect Dis* **169**: 1103.

Salkin IF, McGinnis MR, Dykstra MJ, Rinaldi MG (1988). *Scedosporium inflatum*, an emerging pathogen. *J Clin Microbiol* **26**: 498.

Samonis G, Rolston K, Karl C, Miller P, Bodey GP (1990). Prophylaxis of oropharyngeal candidiasis with fluconazole. *Rev Infect Dis* **12** (Suppl3): S369.

Sampol E, Lacarelle B, Rajaonarison JF, Catalin J, Durand A (1995). Comparative effects of antifungal agents on zidovudine glucuronidation by human liver microsomes. *Brit J Clin Pharmacol* **40**: 83.

Sands M, Poppel D, Brown R (1991). Peritonitis due to *Prototheca wickerhamii* in a patient undergoing chronic ambulatory peritoneal dialysis. *Rev Infect Dis* **13**: 376.

Sangeorzan JA, Bradley SF, He X *et al.* (1994). Epidemiology of oral candidiasis in HIV-infected patients: Colonization, infection, treatment and emergence of fluconazole resistance. *Amer J Med* **97**: 339.

Sanguineti A, Carmichael JK, Campbell K (1993). Fluconazole-resistant *Candida albicans* after long-term suppressive therapy. *Arch Intern Med* **153**: 1122.

Savani DV, Perfect JR, Cobo M, Durack DT (1987). Penetration of new azole compounds into the eye and efficacy in experimental *Candida* endophthalmitis. *Antimicrob Ag Chemother* **31**: 6.

Seay RE, Larson TA, Toscano JP *et al.* (1995). Pharmacokinetics of fluconazole in immune-compromised children with leukemia or other hematologic diseases. *Pharmacother* **15**: 52.

Scalarone GM, Mikami Y, Kurita N *et al.* (1991). *In vitro* comparative evaluations of the postantifungal effect: synergistic interaction between flucytosine and fluconazole against *Candida albicans*. *Mycoses* **34**: 405.

Schaffner A, Schaffner M (1995). Effect of prophylactic fluconazole on the frequency of fungal infections, amphotericin B use, and health care costs in patients undergoing intensive chemotherapy for haematologic neoplasias. *J Infect Dis* **172**: 1035.

Scheven M, Junemann K, Schramm H, Huhn W (1992). Successful treatment of a *Candida albicans* sepsis with a combination of flucytosine and fluconazole. *Mycoses* **35**: 315.

Scholz J, Schulz M, Steinfath M *et al.* (1995). Fluconazole is removed by continuous venovenous hemofiltration in a liver transplant patient. *J Mol Med* **73**: 145.

Schulman JA, Peyman G, Fiscella R *et al.* (1987). Toxicity of intravitreal injection of fluconazole in rabbits. *Can J Ophthalmol* **22**: 304.

Seaton TL, Celum CL, Black DJ (1990). Possible potentiation of warfarin by fluconazole. *DICP Ann Pharmacother* **24**: 1177.

Sekhon AS, Kowalewska-Grochowska J, Garg AK, Vaudry W (1992). *Hansenula anomala* fungemia in an infant with gastric and cardiac complications with a review of the literature. *Eur J Epidemiol* **8**: 305.

Sekhon AS, Garg AK Padhye AA, Hamir Z (1993). *In vitro* susceptibility of myceliel and yeast forms of *Penicillium marneffei* to amphotericin B, fluconazole, 5-fluorocytosine and itraconazole. *Eur J Epidemiol* **9**: 553.

Sekhon AS, Padhye AA, Garg AK *et al.* (1994). *In vitro* sensitivity of medically significant *Fusarium* species to various antimycotics. *Chemotherapy* **40**: 239.

Sewell D, Pfaller MA, Barry AL (1994). Comparison of broth macrodilution, broth microdilution and E test antifungal susceptibility tests for fluconazole. *J Clin Microbiol* **32**: 2099.

Sharkey-Mathis PK, Velez J, Fetchick R, Graybill JR (1993). Histoplasmosis in the Acquired Immunodeficiency Syndrome (AIDS): Treatment with itraconazole and fluconazole. *J AIDS* **6**: 809.

Shaw JTB, Tarbit MH, Troke PF (1987). Cytochrome P-450 mediated sterol synthesis and metabolism: differences in sensitivity to fluconazole and other azoles. In *Recent Trends in the Discovery, Development and Evaluation of Antifungal Agents* (Fromtling RA, ed), p. 125. Barcelona, Spain: JR Prous Science Publishers.

Shiba K, Saito A, Miyahara T (1990). Safety and pharmacokinetics of single oral and intravenous doses of fluconazole in healthy subjects. *Clin Ther* **12**: 206.

Shiraishi S, Murakami S, Miki Y (1994). Oral fluconazole treatment of fungating candidiasis in the keratitis, icthyosis and deafness (KID). syndrome. *Brit J Dermatol* **131**: 904.

Shuttleworth D, Philpot CM, Knight AG (1989). Cutaneous cryptococcosis: treatment with oral fluconazole. *Brit J Dermatol* **120**: 683.

Sides EH, Benson JD, Padhye AA (1991). Phaeohyphomycotic brain abscess due to *Ochronis gallopavum* in a patient with malignant lymphoma of a large cell type. *J Med Vet Mycol* **29**: 317.

Siegman-Igra Y, Rabau MY (1992). Failure of fluconazole in systemic candidiasis. *Eur J Clin Microbiol Infect Dis* **11**: 201.

Simsek U, Akinci H, Oktay B *et al.* (1995). Treatment of catheter-associated candiduria with fluconazole irrigation. *Brit J Urol* **75**: 75.

Sirisanthana V, Sirisanthana T (1993). *Penicillium marneffei* infection in children infected with human immunodeficiency virus. *Pediatr Infect Dis J* **12**: 12021.

Slavin MA, Osborne B, Adams R *et al.* (1995). Efficacy and safety of fluconazole prophylaxis for fungal infections after marrow transplantation – a prospective, randomized, double-blind study. *J Infect Dis* **171**: 1545.

Smith D, Boag F, Midgely J *et al.* (1991). Fluconazole resistant candida in AIDS. *J Infect* **23**: 345.

Sobel JD (1992). Fluconazole maintenance therapy in recurrent vulvovaginal candidiasis. *Int J Gynecol Obstet* **37** (Suppl 1): 17.

Sobel JD, Brooker D, Stein GE *et al.* (1995). Single dose fluconazole compared with conventional clotrimazole topical therapy of *Candida* vaginitis. Fluconazole Vaginitis Study Group. *Amer J Obstet Gynecol* **172**: 1263.

Soutar RL (1991). Fluconazole or amphotericin for candidosis in neutropenic patients. *Lancet* **337**: 181.

Squires K, Rowland V, Gassyuk E *et al.* (1990). Fluconazole as therapy for acute cryptococcal meningitis. In *Program and Abstracts of the 30th Interscience Conference on Antimicrobial Agents and Chemotherapy, October 21–24, Atlanta*. Washington, DC: American Society for Microbiology.

Stern JJ, Hartman BJ, Sharkey P *et al.* (1988). Oral fluconazole therapy for patients with acquired immunodeficiency syndrome and cryptococcosis: Experience with 22 patients. *Amer J Med* **85**: 477.

Stevens DA, Greene SI, Lang OS (1991). Thrush can be prevented in patients with acquired immunodeficiency syndrome and the acquired immunodeficiency syndrome related complex. *Arch Intern Med* **151**: 2458.

Sugar AM, Saunders C (1988). Oral fluconazole as suppressive therapy of disseminated cryptococcosis in patients with acquired immunodeficiency syndrome. *Amer J Med* **85**: 481.

Supparatpinyo K, Nelson KE, Merz WG *et al.* (1993). Response to antifungal therapy by human immunodeficiency virus-infected patients with disseminated *Penicillium marneffei* infections and *in vitro* susceptibilities of isolates from clinical specimens. *Antimicrob Ag Chemother* **37**: 2407.

Tacker JR (1992). Successful use of fluconazole for treatment of urinary tract fungal infections. *J Urol* **148**: 1917.

Tang C (1993). Successful treatment of *Candida albicans* osteomyelitis with fluconazole. *J Infect* **26**: 89.

Tett S, Moore S, Ray J (1995). Pharmacokinetics and bioavailability of fluconazole in two groups of males with human immunodeficiency virus (HIV) infection compared with those in a group of males without HIV infection. *Antimicrob Ag Chemother* **39**: 1835.

Thaler F, Bernard B, Tod M *et al.* (1995). Fluconazole penetration in cerebral parenchyma in humans at steady state. *Antimicrob Ag Chemother* **39**: 1154.

Thorpe JE, Baker N, Bromet-Petit M (1990). Effect of oral antacid administration on the pharmacokinetics of oral fluconazole. *Antimicrob Ag Chemother* **34**: 2032.

Thorsen S, Mathiesen LR (1990). Fluconazole for ketoconazole-resistant oropharyngeal candidiasis in HIV-1 infected patients. *Scand J Infect Dis* **22**: 375.

Timonen H (1992). Shorter treatment for vaginal candidosis: comparison between single-dose oral fluconazole and three-day treatment with local miconazole. *Mycoses* **35**: 317.

Toon S, Ross CE, Gokal R, Rowland M (1990). An assessment of the effects of impaired renal function and haemodialysis on the pharmacokinetics of fluconazole. *Brit J Clin Pharmacol* **29**: 221.

Torregrossa V, De la Torre M, Campistol JM *et al.* (1992). Interaction of fluconazole with cyclosporin. *Nephron* **60**: 125.

Touchette MA, Chandrasekar PH, Milad MA, Edwards DJ (1992). Contrasting effects of fluconazole and ketoconazole on phenytoin and testosterone disposition in man. *Brit J Clin Pharmacol* **34**: 75.

Trapnall CB, Narang PK, Li R, Lavelle JP (1996). Increased plasma rifabutin levels with concomitant fluconazole therapy in HIV-infected patients. *Ann Intern Med* **124**: 573.

Troke PF, Andrews RJ, Brammer KW *et al.* (1985). Efficacy of UK-49,858 (fluconazole) against *Candida albicans* experimental infections in mice. *Antimicrob Ag Chemother* **28**: 815.

Troke PF, Andrews RJ, Marriott MS, Richardson K (1987). Efficacy of fluconazole (UK-49,858) against experimental aspergillosis and crypto-coccosis in mice. *J Antimicrob Chemother* **19**: 663.

Tucker RM, Williams PL, Arathoon EG *et al.* (1988). Pharmacokinetics of fluconazole in cerebrospinal fluid and serum in human coccidioidal meningitis. *Antimicrob Ag Chemother* **32**: 369.

Tunkel AR, Thomas CY, Wispelwey B (1993). *Candida* prosthetic arthritis: Report of a case treated with fluconazole and review of the literature. *Amer J Med* **94**: 100.

Vanakoski J, Mattila MJ, Vainio P *et al.* (1995). 150 mg fluconazole does not substantially increase the effects of 10 mg midazolam or the plasma midazolam concentrations in healthy subjects. *Int J Clin Pharmacol Ther* **33**: 518.

Van Cutsem J, Van Gervan F, Fransen J, Janssen PA (1989). Treatment of experimental zygomycosis in guinea pigs with azoles and with AMB. *Chemotherapy* **35**: 267.

Van Eldere J, Jooston L, Verhaeghe A, Surmont I (1996). Fluconazole and amphotericin B antifungal susceptibility testing by National Committee for Clinical Laboratory Standards Broth Macrodilution method compared with E-test and semi-automated broth microdilution test. *J Clin Microbiol* **34**: 842.

Van Etten EWM, van den Heuvel-de Groot C, Bakker-Woudenberg IAJM (1993). Efficacies of amphotericin B-desoxycholate (Fungizone), liposomal amphotericin B (AmBisome). and fluconazole in the treatment of systemic candidosis in immunocompetent and leukopenic mice. *J Antimicrob Chemother* **32**: 723.

van 't Wout JW, Mattie H, van Furth R (1988). A prospective study of the efficacy of fluconazole (UK-49,858). against deep-seated fungal infection. *J Antimicrob Chemother* **21**: 665.

van 't Wout JW, Mattie H, van Furth R (1989). Comparison of the efficacies of amphotericin B, fluconazole, and itraconazole against a systemic *Candida albicans* infection in normal and neutropenic mice. *Antimicrob Ag Chemother* **33**: 147.

van 't Wout JW, Meynaar I, Linde I *et al.* (1990). Effect of amphotericin B, fluconazole and itraconazole on intracellular *Candida albicans* and germ tube development in macrophages. *J Antimicrob Chemother* **25**: 803.

Velez JD, Allendoerfer R, Luther M *et al.* (1993). Correlation of in vitro azole susceptibility with *in vivo* response in a murine model of cryptococcal meningitis. *J Infect Dis* **168**: 508.

Viscoli C, Castagnola E, Fioredda F *et al.* (1991). Fluconazole in the treatment of candidiasis in immunocompromised children. *Antimicrob Ag Chemother* **35**: 365.

Voss A, Meis JFGM, Hoogkamp-Korstanje (1994). Fluconazole in the management of fungal urinary tract infections. *Infection* **22**: 247.

Wallbridge DR, McCartney AC, Richardson MD (1993). Fluconazole in the treatment of *Candida* prosthetic valve endocarditis. *Mycoses* **36**: 259.

Walsh TJ, Foulds G, Pizzo PA (1989). Pharmacokinetics and tissue penetration of fluconazole in rabbits. *Antimicrob Ag Chemother* **33**: 467.

Walsh TJ, Aoki S, Mechinaud F *et al.* (1990). Effects of preventive, early, and late anti-fungal chemotherapy with fluconazole in different granulocytopenic models of experimental disseminated candidiasis. *J Infect Dis* **161**: 755.

Walsh TJ, Lee JW, Melcher GP *et al.* (1992). Experimental *Trichosporon* infection in persistently granulocytopenic rabbits: Implications for pathogenesis, diagnosis, and treatment of an emerging opportunistic mycosis. *J Infect Dis* **166**: 121.

Weinroth SE, Tuazon CU (1993). Alopecia associated with fluconazole treatment. *Ann Intern Med* **119**: 637.

Wells C, Lever AML (1992). Dose-dependent fluconazole hepatotoxicity proven on biopsy and rechallenge. *J Infection* **24**: 111.

Westrom L, Hagland A, Svensson L (1992). Fluconazole versus econazole in treating vaginal candidiasis. *Int J Gynecol Obstet* **37** (Suppl): 29.

Wheat J (1994). Histoplasmosis and coccidioidomycosis in individuals with AIDS. A clinical review. *Infect Dis Clin N Amer* **8**: 467.

Wiest DB, Fowler SL, Garner SS, Simons DR (1991). Fluconazole in neonatal disseminated candidiasis. *Arch Dis Childhood* **66**: 1002.

Wildfeuer A, Faergemann J, Laufen H *et al.* (1994). Bioavailability of fluconazole in the skin after oral medication. *Mycoses* **37**: 127.

Wingard JR, Merz WG, Rinaldi MG *et al.* (1991). Increase in *Candida krusei* infection among patients with bone marrow transplantation and neutropenia treated prophylactically with fluconazole. *New Engl J Med* **325**: 1274.

Wingard JR, Merz WG, Rinaldi MG *et al.* (1993). Association of *Torulopsis glabrata* infections with fluconazole prophylaxis in neutropenic bone marrow transplant patients. *Antimicrob Ag Chemother* **37**: 1847.

Winston DJ, Pranatharthi PH, Lazarus HM *et al.* (1993). Fluconazole prophylaxis of fungal infections in patients with acute leukemia. Results of a randomized placebo-controlled, double-blind multicenter trial. *Ann Intern Med* **118**: 495.

Witt MD, Bayer AS (1991). Comparison of fluconazole and amphotericin B for prevention and treatment of experimental *Candida* endocarditis. *Antimicrob Ag Chemother* **35**: 2481.

Witt MD, Imhoff T, Li C, Bayer AS (1993). Comparison of fluconazole and amphotericin B for treatment of experimental *Candida* endocarditis caused by non-*C albicans* strains. *Antimicrob Ag Chemother* **37**: 2030.

Wood GM, McCormack JG, Muir DB *et al.* (1992). Clinical features of human infection with *Scedosporium inflatum*. *Clin Infect Dis* **14**: 1027.

Working Party of the British Society for Antimicrobial Chemotherapy (1995). Antifungal drug susceptibility testing. *J Antimicrob Chemother* **36**: 899.

Yu RY, Gao L (1994). Chromoblastomycosis successfully treated with fluconazole. *Int J Dermatol* **33**: 716.

Zimmerman T, Yeates RA, Laufen H *et al.* (1994). Influence of concomitant food intake on the oral absorption of two triazole antifungal agents, itraconazole and fluconazole. *Eur J Clin Pharmacol* **46**: 147.

Zuger A, Louie E, Holzman RS *et al.* (1986). Cryptococcal disease in patients with the acquired immunodeficiency syndrome: diagnostic features and outcome of treatment. *Ann Intern Med* **104**: 234.

Itraconazole

Description

Itraconazole is a synthetic triazole drug developed by Janssen Pharmaceutica as an alternative to ketoconazole with reduced toxicity, better pharmacokinetics, and broader spectrum of antifungal activity. It was synthesized in 1980 as the first orally bioavailable triazole agent. However, it is highly lipophilic and essentially insoluble in aqueous solutions at neutral pH. There is no intravenous formulation available. It was the first orally active agent against aspergillosis and sporotrichosis.

The chemical name of itraconazole is (±)-cis-4-[4-[4-[4-[[2-(2,4-dichlorophenyl)-2-(1H-1, 2,4-triazol-1-ylmethyl)-1,3-dioxolan-4-yl]methoxy]phenyl]-1-piperazinyl]phenyl]-2,4-dihydro-2-(1-methylpropyl)-3H-1,2,4-triazol-3-one. It is a racemic mixture of 4 diastereomers (two enantiomeric pairs)

Sensitive Organisms

1 Pathogenic yeast

Cryptococcus neoformans is highly susceptible to itraconazole in both agar and broth dilution testing (Espinel-Ingroff *et al.*, 1984; Van Cutsem *et al.*, 1987). There is one report of an itraconazole-resistant isolate of *C. neoformans* (Denning *et al.*, 1989a). In animal models of cryptococcal meningitis, itraconazole effectively sterilized CSF cultures in 50% of mice, and 75% of rabbits despite undetectable CSF itraconazole levels (Grant and Clissold, 1989; Perfect *et al.*, 1986).

Candida spp. are variably susceptible to itraconazole depending on the *in vitro* methodology used to evaluate its activity. Espinel-Ingroff *et al.* (1984) using agar dilution determined many strains of *Candida albicans*, *C. parapsilosis*, *C. tropicalis* and *C. glabrata* were resistant to itraconazole, while in broth dilution assays, the majority of isolates of *Candida* spp. were inhibited by concentrations of itraconazole ranging from 0.001 to 10 µg per ml (Van Cutsem *et al.*, 1987). Martin *et al.* (1992), revealed that most strains of *Candida* spp. were susceptible to itraconazole using an agar dilution method. Van 't Wout *et al.* (1989), determined that itraconazole in concentrations up to 100 µg per ml had a minimal effect on the growth of *C. albicans in vitro*, compared with amphotericin B which was fungicidal. In the murine systemic candidiasis model, itraconazole activity was inferior to amphotericin B and fluconazole and it was equally effective in normal and neutropenic mice. Itraconazole concentrates poorly in the main target organ of *Candida* infection in this model, the kidney (Van 't Wout *et al.*, 1989). Itraconazole significantly inhibited germ tube formation of *C. albicans* in intracellular macrophages, which may assist host defenses (Van 't Wout *et al.*, 1990a). The guinea pig model of superficial candidiasis revealed cure rates of 63–96% using 0.063%-2.5% itraconazole ointment for vaginal candidosis, and similar cure rates using 3 days of oral treatment. In systemic candidiasis in guinea pigs and mice, parenteral and oral treatment were equally effective (Van Cutsem *et al.*, 1987; Grant and Clissold, 1989). Dose-dependent clinical and mycological responses were observed. At 5 mg per kg itraconazole, 50% of animals had negative cultures on day 14 of treatment. This increased to 100% of animals at day 21.

Malassezia furfur (Pityrosporum orbiculare) is highly susceptible to itraconazole *in vitro*, and 5 mg per kg protected 80% of rabbits from experimental infection with this organism (Faergemann, 1988). *Trichosporon* spp. are also sensitive (Van Cutsem, 1989).

2 Dimorphic fungi

Blastomyces dermatitidis, Coccidioides immitis, Paracoccidioides brasiliensis and *Histoplasma capsulatum* are all very sensitive to itraconazole *in vitro* and efficacy in an *in vivo* animal model infection has been established for *H. capsulatum* and *P. brasiliensis* (Espinel-Ingroff *et al.*, 1984; Van Cutsem *et al.*, 1987; Graybill *et al.*, 1990; San-Blas *et al.*, 1993). *Penicillium marneffei* is highly susceptible to itraconazole with an MIC range of 0.002–0.78 μg per ml (Van Cutsem, 1989; Sekhon *et al.*, 1992; Supparatpinyo *et al.*, 1993). The excellent *in vitro* activity has been confirmed in an immunosuppressed guinea pig model of experimental systemic penicilliosis with low doses of itraconazole (Sekhon *et al.*, 1992).

Sporothrix schenckii requires a higher concentration of itraconazole for growth inhibition than the other dimorphic fungi at >1 μg per ml (Van Cutsem *et al.*, 1987). In the guinea pig model of sporotrichosis, itraconazole 40 mg per kg administered on the day of inoculation, was able to eliminate organisms from liver and testicle cultures (Van Cutsem *et al.*, 1987). However, itraconazole was unable to protect mice from disseminated sporotrichosis in the murine model, although it was associated with improved survival (Kan and Bennett, 1988).

3 Molds or filamentous fungi

Itraconazole has significant activity against *Aspergillus* spp. whether measured by MIC or relative inhibition factors (Espinel-Ingroff *et al.*, 1984; Odds *et al.*, 1984; Van Cutsem *et al.*, 1987; Denning *et al.*, 1992). Over 95% of isolates had an MIC <6.3 μg per ml (Denning *et al.*, 1992). Complete inhibition of spore germination of *Aspergillus* strains was achieved at itraconazole concentrations of 6.25–12.5 μg per ml (Grant and Clissold, 1989). The activity of itraconazole was confirmed in guinea pig, murine and rabbit models of aspergillosis, as well as an immunocompromised guinea pig model (Van Cutsem, 1987; Grant and Clissold, 1989). In the rabbit model of invasive pulmonary aspergillosis, the antifungal activity of itraconazole correlated strongly with plasma concentrations of itraconazole. At doses of itraconazole of 40 mg per kg orally daily, amphotericin B was significantly more effective than itraconazole. When plasma levels of >6 μg per ml were achieved, a significantly greater antifungal effect equivalent to that of amphotericin B was observed (Berenguer *et al.*, 1994). Also, the itraconazole-cyclodextrin solution administered at a dose of 40 mg per kg orally to immunocompromised rabbits with invasive aspergillosis, was as effective as amphotericin B in eradication of *A. fumigatus* from tissues and improved survival (Patterson *et al.*, 1993). However, the efficacy of itraconazole solubilized in hydroxypropyl-beta-cyclodextrin at a dose of 10 mg per kg administered i.v. to rats with invasive pulmonary aspergillosis was equivalent to amphotericin B 1 mg per kg (Miyazaki *et al.*, 1993). Itraconazole 5 mg per kg successfully eradicated *A. fumigatus* from cardiac vegetations in the rabbit model of endocarditis (Longman and Martin, 1987).

The dermatophytes, *Trichophyton, Microsporum* and *Epidermophyton* spp. are all susceptible to itraconazole with 95% of isolates inhibited by 0.1 μg per ml (Van Cutsem *et al.*, 1987). Espinel-Ingroff *et al.* (1984) reported a wide range of MICs for *Trichophyton* spp. from 0.063 to 64 μg per ml. In the guinea pig model of dermatophyosis, topical itraconazole 0.063% and 0.125%, oral itraconazole 10 mg per kg and i.v. 1.25 and 2.5 mg per kg were all effective therapy if given for 14 days (Van Cutsem *et al.*, 1987). Of the Zygomycetes, *Mucor* spp., *Rhizopus* spp. and *Mortiella* spp. are generally resistant to clinically achievable levels of itraconazole. Whereas *Absidia corymbifera, Rhizomucor* spp. and the entomophthorales are all susceptible to itraconazole (Van Cutsem, 1989). The *Fusarium* spp. are also generally resistant. One quarter of the *Fusarium* spp. tested by broth dilution were sensitive to itraconazole in one study (Sekhon *et al.*, 1994); however, itraconazole showed poor inhibitory and fungicidal activiy against 44 clinical isolates of *Fusarium* spp. in another study (Reuben *et al.*, 1989). *Madurella* spp. with MICs of 0.001–0.1 μg per ml, and other causative agents of black grain eumycetoma are susceptible to itraconazole (Van Cutsem *et al.*, 1987; Venugopal, *et al.*, 1993). Contradictory results were obtained for the causative agents of chromomycosis, *Fonsecaea pedrosoi,* and *Phialophora verrucosa* when susceptibility tests were performed by agar dilution (resistant) or broth (highly sensitive), while *Cladosporium* spp. were sensitive in both media (Espinel-Ingroff *et al.*, 1984; Van Cutsem *et al.*, 1987). *Scedosporium inflatum* is generally resistant to amphotericin B, ketoconazole, miconazole and fluconazole; however, four of 14 isolates were found to be susceptible to itraconazole (Salkin *et al.*, 1988).

4 Actinomycetales

Nocardia spp. and *Actinomyces israeli*, which are aerobic bacteria, are also resistant to itraconazole (Van Cutsem *et al.*, 1987).

5 Algae

Some isolates of the achloric algae *Prototheca wickerhamii* are partially susceptible to itraconazole with an MIC of 10 μg per ml (Van Cutsem *et al.*, 1987).

6 Trypanosomes

Itracaonazole has excellent activity against *Trypanosoma cruzi in vitro*, and in the murine model of trypanosomiasis both as a prophylactic agent and as treatment. Itraconazole concentrations of 0.001 μg per ml inhibited intracellular replication of amastigotes (McCabe *et al.*, 1986).

7 Synergism with other drugs

In vitro susceptibility testing of the combination of amphotericin B and itraconazole against several *Candida* species including *C. albicans* revealed the combination was antagonistic for these yeast (Petrou and Rogers, 1991). For isolates of *Aspergillus* spp., the combination of amphotericin B and itraconazole was shown to be either synergistic, additive or antagonistic (Denning *et al.*, 1992). Polak (1987, 1989) reported that amphotericin B and triazoles were antagonistic *in vitro* against most species when they were added simultaneously to the test system. However, if the triazole was added to the fungal culture after the amphotericin B, synergy could be demonstrated. Pre-exposure to itraconazole in a macrophage model reduced subsequent amphotericin B activity against intracellular *C. albicans* (Ponce and Pechere, 1990). In animal models, the combination of amphotericin B and itraconazole was antagonistic in its effect on candidosis and aspergillosis in immunosuppressed mice, albeit to a lesser degree than the antagonism seen with ketoconazole and amphotericin B. Antagonism of itraconazole and amphotericin B could not be demonstrated in murine histoplasmosis (Polak, 1989). Finally, antagonism of the amphotericin B effect was seen with both sequential and concurrent administration of the two drugs to immunosuppressed mice with aspergillosis (Schaffner and Bohler, 1993).

The combination of itraconazole and flucytosine is synergistic in the animal model of systemic candidosis and indifferent in cryptococcosis. The combination also had a synergistic effect in aspergillosis when the *Aspergillus* strain was flucytosine-sensitive, but indifference occurred when the strain was flucytosine-resistant (Polak, 1989). Kerkering and Espinel-Ingroff (1987) showed the combination of itraconazole and flucytosine was synergistic for 50% of *A. fumigatus* and 30% of *A. flavus* isolates and the synergy was independent of the flucytosine susceptibility. Synergistic or additive effects were also noted for the triple combination of amphotericin B, flucytosine and itraconazole against cryptococcosis, but mild antagonism was demonstrated for candidosis and aspergillosis (Polak, 1989).

In vitro synergy between itraconazole and rifampicin was demonstrated against *Cryptococcus neoformans* isolates and the myceliel phase (arthroconidia) of *Coccidioides immitis*, but *in vitro* synergy was much weaker for the pathogenic endospore phase of *C. immitis* (Tucker *et al.*, 1992). Synergy was demonstrated between itraconazole and low doses of quinolones (nalidixic acid, enoxacin, ciprofloxacin and norfloxacin) against *Candida* spp., but antagonism occurred when high doses of ciprofloxacin and norfloxacin were combined with itraconazole (Petrou and Rogers, 1988). The clinical significance of these observations is unknown.

8 Acquired resistance

There have been occasional reports of acquired resistance to itraconazole published in the literature to date (Le Guennec *et al.*, 1995). An attempt to induce resistance or decreased susceptibility to itraconazole in a strain of *Cryptococcus neoformans* in the laboratory was unsuccessful (Grant and Clissold, 1989). The isolated cases of acquired ketoconazole-resistance in *C. albicans* following long-term treatment with ketoconazole for chronic mucocutaneous candidiasis, were also cross-resistant with other azole drugs including itraconazole (Smith *et al.*, 1986). The development of resistance to itraconazole during prolonged therapy (more than a few months) in immunocompromised patients would not be unexpected given the mechanism of action and similarity with fluconazole to which reduced susceptibilities on therapy has been documented. Three mechanisms of azole-resistance have been described to date and include alterations in the sterol composition of the fungal cell membrane thereby reducing permeability to the azole drug, mutation of the 14-alpha demethylase enzyme with decreased binding affinity for azole drugs, and overproduction of the same fungal target cell membrane 14-alpha demethylase (Odds, 1993). Azole drug cross-resistance can be anticipated from these observations.

Johnson *et al.* (1995) investigated the *in vitro* susceptibilities of over 1000 *Candida* spp. and reported that cross-resistance between fluconazole and itraconazole does exist. Of fluconazole-resistant isolates, 18% of *C. albicans* were cross-resistant with itraconazole, and 55–61% of *C. glabrata* and *C. tropicalis* isolates were also cross-resistant with itraconazole. The MICs of itraconazole for fluconazole-susceptible isolates were markedly lower than the itraconazole MIC for fluconazole-resistant isolates. The demonstration of increasing itraconazole MICs for *C. albicans* during therapy with fluconazole and the emergence of clinical itraconazole-resistance was documented in HIV patients by Le Guennec *et al.* (1995).

9 Minimum inhibitory concentrations

Although the National Committee for Clinical Laboratory Standards (NCCLS) has now developed standardized guidelines for antifungal susceptibility testing for yeasts, the published studies of *in vitro* susceptibilities utilize various methods making comparisons between studies questionable. There are no guidelines for susceptibility testing of filamentous fungi. In addition to the problems of assessment of *in vitro* efficacy, there is no correlation with clinical efficacy. The following susceptibility data in Table IV.11 have been compiled from studies that have not necessarily used the NCCLS guidelines.

Mode of Administration and Dose

Indications and recommended doses
Superficial dermatomycosis: Tinea corporis, tinea cruris – 100 mg daily for 2 weeks; tinea pedis, tinea manus – 100 mg daily for 4 weeks.

Vulvovaginal candidiasis: 200 mg 12 h apart in one day, or 200 mg daily for 3 days.

Fungal keratitis: 200 mg daily for 3 weeks.

Pityriasis versicolor: 200 mg daily for 1 week.

Oral candidiasis in immunocompromised patients: 100–200 mg daily for 2 weeks; 20 ml oral solution for 1 week.

Fluconazole-resistant oral and/or esophageal candidiasis: 200–400 mg daily for 2 weeks, as capsules or oral solution.

1 Patients with renal failure

Itraconazole is not dialyzable by either hemodialysis or continuous ambulatory peritoneal dialysis (CAPD) (Boelaert *et al.*, 1988). Plasma protein binding remains high (99%) in patients with renal insufficiency. The dose of itraconazole does not need to be modified for patients with renal impairment, patients on hemodialysis or CAPD.

2 Patients with hepatic insufficiency

Serum concentrations of itraconazole may be increased in the presence of liver failure due to a decrease in first-pass metabolism. Whether dose adjustment is required in the presence of hepatic insufficiency remains to be elucidated.

3 Intravitreal

Ocular toxicity studies in rabbits determined that no substantial retinal toxicity occurred following intravitreal injection of itraconazole 10 μg (Schulman *et al.*, 1991). No human experience has been reported.

Availability

Oral formulation: 100 mg capsules.

Oral solution: (10 mg per ml) in hydroxypropyl-beta-cyclodextrin.

Serum levels in Relation to Dose

Healthy male volunteers received a single i.v. dose of itraconazole 100 mg followed 2 weeks later with a single dose of 100 mg administered orally. Peak plasma itraconazole levels at the end of the 1 h infusion of 100 mg were 0.66 μg per ml, compared with the maximum plasma concentration 5 h after oral administration of 0.13 μg per ml. The terminal half-life was similar after both i.v. and oral dosing at 21 h. The absolute bioavailability for itraconazole was 55% (Heykants *et al.*, 1989). Steady-state pharmacokinetics were evaluated in five healthy male

Table IV.11

Compiled from data published by Espinel-Ingroff *et al.* (1984), Faergemann (1984), Ganer *et al.* (1987), Van Cutsem *et al.* (1987, 1989), Haron *et al.* (1988), Reuben *et al.* (1989), Wong *et al.* (1989), Patterson *et al.* (1990), Martin *et al.* (1992), Sekhon *et al.* (1992), Tucker *et al.* (1992), Supparatpinyo *et al.* (1993), Naqvi *et al.* (1993), Venugopal *et al.* (1993), Lau *et al.* (1995)

Organism	MIC (μg per ml) range	
	Broth	Agar
Yeast		
Candida spp.		
C. albicans	0.001–100	≤0.05–50
C. guilliermondii	0.1–1	≤0.05–0.2
C. krusei	0.001–100	≤0.05–3.2
C. parapsilosis	0.01–10	≤0.05
C. tropicalis	0.001–1	≤0.05–100
C. kefyr (pseudotropicalis)	0.01–0.1	
C. lusitaniae	0.01–0.1	≤0.05–6.4
C. glabrata (Torulopsis glabrata)	0.001–100	≤0.05–0.2
Cryptococcus neoformans	0.01–0.1	0.063–0.13
Hansenula anomala	12.5	
Malassezia furfur	0.01–1	
Rhodotorula rubra	0.1–100	
Trichosporon beigelii	0.01–1	
Dimorphic fungi		
Histoplasma capsulatum	0.001–0.01	0.063–0.13
Blastomyces dermatitidis	0.001–0.1	0.13
Coccidioides immitis	0.018	
Paracoccidioides brasiliensis	0.001–0.1	
Penicillium marneffei	≤0.002–0.078	
Mold		
Aspergillus spp.		
A. fumigatus	0.01–10	0.063–2
A. flavus	0.1	0.063–0.13
A. niger	10–100	
Dematiaceous fungi		
Alternaria alternata	0.1	
Bipolaris spp.	0.01–0.1	
Drechslera spp.	3.13	
Cladosporium spp.	0.001–0.1	0.13
Cladosporium carrionii	0.001	
Curvularia spp.	0.1	
Exophiala jeanselmei	0.001–5	0.13
Fonsecaea pedrosoi	0.001–1	0.063–>128
Phialophora parasitica	50	
Phialophora verrucosa	0.01	0.063–>128
Sporothrix schenckii	0.1–1	1–4
Wangiella dermatitidis	0.78	0.13
Agents of zygomycosis		
Absidia corymbifera	0.1–1	
Rhizomucor pusillus	0.1	
Mucor spp.	1–100	>128
Rhizopus spp.	100	>128
Mortierella spp.	100	
Conidiobolus spp.	1	
Basidiobolus spp.	0.1–1	

Table IV.11
continued

Organism	MIC (μg per ml) range	
	Broth	Agar
Hyphomycetes		
Acremonium spp.	0.1–>100	0.05
Fusarium spp.	8–>32	
Paecilomyces spp.	0.1	
Pseudallescheria boydii	0.01–1	6.25
Scopulariopsis brevicaulis	100–>100	
Phaeoannellomyces wernickii	0.1	
Piedraia hortae	0.001	
Pythium insidiosum	25–50	
Scytalidium spp.	0.1	
Dermatophytes		
Trichophyton spp.	0.001–10	0.063–64
Microsporum spp.	0.01–0.1	0.063–0.25
Epidermophyton spp.	0.001–0.1	0.063
Algae		
Prototheca spp.	>50	

volunteers given itraconazole capsules 100 mg daily, 200 mg daily or 200 mg twice-daily with a standard meal for 15 days. The mean peak itraconazole concentration after a 100-mg single dose was 0.11 μg per ml, after a 200-mg single dose was 0.27 μg per ml, and after two doses of 200 mg 12 h apart was 0.55 μg per ml. The trough concentrations of itraconazole gradually increased over the dosing period, with steady-state reached on day 13. The mean peak itraconazole plasma concentration reached on day 15 was 0.41 μg per ml for 100 mg daily, 1.07 μg per ml for 200-mg daily and 1.98 μg per ml for the 200-mg twice-daily regimen. There was wide intersubject variation in itraconazole steady-state levels. The half-life was 15–20 h after a single dose and increased to 34–42 h after 15 days dosing. There was a non-linear increase in the area-under-the-concentration-time-curve (AUC) values with increased doses suggesting the pharmacokinetics are dose-dependent (Hardin *et al.*, 1988). The non-linear pharmacokinetics was confirmed by Van Peer *et al.* (1989), using single doses of 50 mg, 100 mg and 200 mg. Pharmacokinetics of itraconazole are no different in the elderly (Heykants *et al.*, 1989).

A major metabolite of itraconazole is hydroxyitraconazole, which has equipotent antifungal activity against some pathogens compared with itraconazole, both *in vitro* and in selected animal models (Heykants *et al.*, 1989; Hostetler *et al.*, 1993a). Peak plasma concentrations of hydroxyitraconazole tend to be 70% higher than itraconazole after administration of a single dose and steady-state mean plasma levels of hydroxyitraconazole range from 0.4–0.79 μg per ml. At steady-state, the mean plasma levels of hydroxyitraconazole are about twice the the mean plasma concentration of itraconazole (0.19–0.62 μg per ml), and the half-life of the biologically active metabolite was shorter at 18 h than that of itraconazole at 28 h (Heykants *et al.*, 1989; Hostetler *et al.*, 1993a). Bioassay determinations of itraconazole concentrations have consistently measured higher itraconazole levels than high-performance liquid chromotography (HPLC) methods, because the bioassay measures the additive activity of itraconazole and hydroxyitraconazole, whereas the HPLC can distinguish between the two compounds. This difference can explain the discrepancies in 'itraconazole' levels obtained in different laboratory studies (Warnock *et al.*, 1988; Hostetler *et al.*, 1993a).

Administration of itraconazole in the fasting state reduces the systemic bioavailability of itraconazole. Several investigators have confirmed the enhanced absorption of itraconazole when taken with food, with increases of the mean maximum plasma concentration of itraconazole from 0.14 μg per ml in the fasting state to 0.24 μg per ml after a standard meal with a 200 mg itraconazole capsule, and increased mean bioavailability relative to a full meal from 54–59% fasting to 86% after a light meal. High intersubject variability was reported again (Wishart, 1987; Barone *et al.*, 1993; Zimmerman *et al.*, 1994). Itraconazole is slowly absorbed from the gastrointestinal tract and peak plasma concentrations occur between 4 and 6 h post-dose. There was no difference in the rate of absorption of itraconazole between the fasting and fed states. These investigators used the current commercially available itraconazole capsules which contain itraconazole-coated sugar spheres. Hydroxyitraconazole plasma levels were also decreased when itraconazole was administered fasting, albeit to a lesser degree than the effect on itraconazole levels in plasma, and the ratio of hydroxyitraconazole to itraconazole AUC was not affected by food (Barone *et al.*, 1993).

Although mean peak plasma concentrations of itraconazole were slightly lower than baseline levels after co-administration of itraconazole and cimetidine or ranitidine in healthy volunteers, the difference was not statistically significant. The authors concluded that H_2-receptor antagonists do not modify the single-dose pharmacokinetics of itraconazole (Stein *et al.*, 1988). However, the absorption of itraconazole is significantly reduced in the presence of gastric hypochlorhydria with plasma itraconazole concentrations reduced to 50% in the presence of famotidine-induced hypochlorhydria (Lim *et al.*, 1993). Smith *et al.* (1992) evaluated the pharmacokinetics of oral itraconazole in AIDS patients. Mean peak plasma levels of itraconazole occurred 4 h after administration of 200 mg orally, and were 0.20, 0.45 and 0.53 µg per ml on days 1, 8 and 15 respectively. These compared with levels obtained in healthy volunteers given 100 mg daily (Hardin *et al.*, 1988) and suggest that the absorption of itraconazole is reduced by at least 50% in AIDS patients. This observation is in keeping with reports of high prevalence of gastric hypochlorhydria in AIDS patients.

Large individual variations in plasma itraconazole concentrations have been noted for patients with acute leukemia and neutropenic patients undergoing bone marrow transplantation, and as for AIDS patients, the levels are inferior to those achieved by normal volunteers (Remmel *et al.*, 1988; Persat *et al.*, 1992; Bradford *et al.*, 1991). Steady-state was generally achieved within 7 days of dosing with either 400 mg or 600 mg once-daily in neutropenic patients, with levels of 0.273 and 0.311 µg per ml respectively. Differences between the two dose levels in neutropenic patients with leukemia were less clear than the differences in neutropenic bone marrow transplant patients who achieved higher trough itraconazole levels (>0.25 µg per ml) with 600 mg daily (Persat *et al.*, 1992). Two studies in neutropenic patients receiving long-term prophylaxis with itraconazole, determined that patients who maintained a plasma itraconazole concentration >0.25 µg per ml were significantly less likely to develop invasive fungal infections (Boogaerts *et al.*, 1989; Tricot *et al.*, 1987).

Boelaert *et al.* (1988) examined the pharmacokinetics of single-dose oral itraconazole 200 mg in a group of patients who were either uremic, undergoing hemodialysis or CAPD. Again, a high interindividual variability in pharmacokinetics was noted for this group of patients. The mean peak plasma itraconazole concentration of 0.21 µg per ml, time to peak plasma level of 4.0 h and elimination half-life of 25.1 h observed in the uremic patients, were similar to the values obtained for normal volunteers. Plasma protein binding was 99.8%. The hemodialysis patients had non-significant lower mean maximum plasma concentrations both on a hemodialysis day and between dialysis days, compared with the non-dialyzed uremic patients. It was apparent, by comparison of plasma concentration time curves, that little if any itraconazole is removed through the dialyzer. The mean peak plasma itraconazole concentration in CAPD patients was one-third that of the uremic patients, suggesting decreased gastrointestinal absorption or increased first-pass metabolism. The peritoneal dialysate did not contain detectable itraconazole.

In a group of 12 cirrhotic patients given a single dose of itraconazole 100 mg, mean peak plasma itraconazole levels of 0.087 µg per ml were slightly lower than those seen in normal volunteers, but the half-life was prolonged to 37 h. The longer half-life would result from a reduced first-pass hepatic metabolism which might be expected in these patients (Heykants *et al.*, 1989).

The use of beta-cyclodextrin as a carrier molecule for the lipophilic itraconazole improves its oral bioavailability. Itraconazole formulated in hydroxypropyl-beta-cyclodextrin has improved solubility. Peak plasma concentrations and AUCs of itraconazole in hydroxypropyl-beta-cyclodextrin were 24- and 121-fold higher respectively, than a corresponding dose administered in the usual formulation of polyethylene glycol in mice (Hostetler *et al.*, 1992a). There are no data published on the comparative pharmacokinetics of the itraconazole solution versus the capsule formulation. Multiple-dose pharmacokinetics of the oral solution of 10 mg per ml in 40% hydroxypropyl-beta-cyclodextrin were determined in two studies, one in leukemic patients undergoing remission-induction chemotherapy and the second in patients receiving chemotherapy followed by autologous bone marrow transplantation. Doses of 5 mg per kg once-daily, 2.5 mg per kg twice-daily, or 2.5 mg per kg once-daily and 1.25 mg per kg twice-daily were evaluated in a small open randomized study. Marked interpatient variation was again noted. The peak serum concentration achieved on day 8 was 0.59–0.66 μg per ml for the patients receiving 5 mg per kg once-daily and 2.5 mg per kg twice-daily, and 0.33–0.63 μg per ml for those receiving 2.5 mg once-daily and 1.25 mg twice-daily. The mean itraconazole serum concentration on day 8 for those receiving a total dose of 5 mg per kg was 0.49–0.50 μg per ml and for those on 2.5 mg per kg per day was 0.11–0.44 μg per ml. The mean AUC was significantly higher for the 5 mg per kg group but the AUCs for the once-daily and twice-daily dosing were not significantly different. Steady-state appeared to have been achieved by day 15 of dosing. These studies established that serum levels of itraconazole required for prophylacyic efficacy (0.25 μg per ml) are achieved by the time of development of neutropenia (Prentice *et al.*, 1994, 1995). Improved efficacy of this formulation has been shown for the animal model of murine cryptococcosis, invasive aspergillosis in rats and rabbits, and human experience with oropharyngeal and esophageal candidiasis unresponsive to other antifungals (Patterson *et al.*, 1993; Miyazaki *et al.*, 1993; Hostetler *et al.*, 1993b; Cartledge *et al.*, 1994). The solution formulation of itraconazole complexed in hydroxypropyl-beta-cyclodextrin is now available commercially.

Excretion

1 Urine

Following a single oral dose of ³H-itraconazole in an aqueous dimethyl-beta-cyclodextrin solution in healthy volunteers, 35% of the radioactivity was excreted in the urine over 1 week. Unchanged itraconazole was not detected in the urine of these volunteers, nor was it detected in the urine of volunteers administered oral doses of 100–200 mg once- or twice-daily for 15 days (Hardin *et al.*, 1988; Heykants *et al.*, 1989).

2 Inactivation in the body

Itraconazole is almost completely absorbed and extensively metabolized in the liver. Metabolism involves oxidative scission of the azole ring, oxidative degradation of the piperazine ring and *N*-dealkylation, with a large number of metabolites formed. The primary route of elimination of the metabolites is the biliary tract. One of the major metabolites produced by (ω-1) oxidation at the 1-methylpropyl substituent is hydroxyitraconazole (Heykants *et al.*, 1989). The elimination of itraconazole and hydroxyitraconazole appears to be saturable (Barone *et al.*, 1993).

3 Feces

Fecal excretion of radioactivity following a single oral dose of ³H-itraconazole represented 54% of the administered dose, and 3–18% of the dose was unchanged itraconazole (Heykants *et al.*, 1989).

Distribution of the Drug in Body

Plasma protein binding of itraconazole is 99.8%, and binding to albumin predominates (Heykants *et al.*, 1989). Because only 0.2% of itraconazole in the plasma is free for distribution, and itraconazole has a relatively high molecular weight, there is very low concentration of the drug in CSF. The poor penetration of itraconazole across the blood–CSF barrier has been documented in rabbits with 2–5% penetration into CSF with uninflamed meninges and 9% penetration with inflamed meninges (Perfect and Durack, 1985) and humans (de Gans *et al.*, 1992). Patients with chronic coccidioidal meningitis on itraconazole 400 mg daily and mean serum itraconazole concentrations of 3.4–15.4 μg per ml, had undetectable levels of itraconazole in CSF at steady-state (Tucker *et al.*, 1990a). Tissue concentrations of itraconazole in lung, liver, bone, muscle, spleen, esophagus and stomach are 2- to 3-fold higher than plasma and adipose tissue concentrations are up to 20-fold more than those of plasma after a single 200-mg dose (Heykants *et al.*, 1987; Darouiche *et al.*, 1995). The distribution of itraconazole after repeated dosing in rats reveals higher concentrations in brain, liver, lung, kidney and skin than corresponding plasma levels (Van Cauteren *et al.*, 1987). There is rapid and extensive intracellular uptake of itraconazole by alveolar macrophages *in vitro* (Perfect *et al.*, 1993), and the intracellular accumulation of intraconazole may explain the *in vivo* efficacy of itraconazole despite relatively low concentrations in biological fluids. Itraconazole was detected in reasonably high concentrations from bronchial washings, lavage and biopy specimens from a man with allergic bronchopulmonary aspergillosis receiving itraconazole 100 mg on alternate days (Watkins *et al.*, 1992).

Intraocular penetration of itraconazole was evaluated by bioassay in rabbits given 80 mg orally. Serum levels were 2.13 μg per ml, and levels of 0.05 μg per g in the cornea, 0.92 μg per ml in aqueous humor, and 0.22 μg per ml in the vitreous body were obtained in the inflamed eye. Itraconazole was not detected in the tissues of the uninflamed eye, apart from 0.05 μg per g in the cornea. Despite the poor penetration into ocular tissues, itraconazole was as effective as fluconazole (excellent penetration) in the treatment of experimental *Candida* endophthalmitis (Savani *et al.*, 1987). Subconjunctival injection of itraconazole 2.5 mg per ml into rabbits with either intact or debrided corneal epithelium revealed peak itraconazole levels occurred in the cornea at 2 h, and persisted in the cornea for 24 h (Klippenstein *et al.*, 1993).

Itraconazole penetration into the female genital tract was evaluated in women given a single 200-mg dose prior to hysterectomy, and tissue concentrations throughout the genital tract were 4- to 10-fold higher than the corresponding plasma concentration (Larosa *et al.*, 1986; Heykants *et al.*, 1989). In addition, itraconazole levels in the vaginal mucosa are 5- 6-fold more than the corresponding plasma levels after administration of 400 mg (given as 200 mg 12 h apart) and therapeutic levels remain in the vaginal mucosa for 4 days compared with just 1 day in plasma (Heykants *et al.*, 1989). Levels of 500 μg per g are achieved in cervical mucus after a single dose of 200 mg itraconazole (Van Cauteren *et al.*, 1987).

The penetration of itraconazole into skin, hair, nails and sweat was evaluated in healthy volunteers after administration of 100–200 mg itraconazole daily for 4 weeks. The mean peak plasma and tissue levels of itraconazole at steady-state were 0.34–0.50 μg per ml for plasma, 0.07–0.13 μg per g for stratum corneum of palms, 1.47 μg per g for stratum corneum of the beard area, 0.59 μg per g for stratum corneum of the back, 0.04 μg per g for hair tip, 0.13 μg per g for nails, 4.64 μg per g for sebum and 0.07 μg per g for sweat. Sebum concentrations were 6-fold greater than those of plasma, while sweat concentrations were 20% of plasma levels. Sebum, and not sweat appears to deliver high concentrations of itraconazole to the stratum corneum, and itraconazole levels in sebum persist for 1–2 weeks after the end of treatment. Tissue levels persist in stratum corneum for 2–4 weeks after cessation of the drug (Cauwenbergh *et al.*, 1988). Skin blistering techniques were used by Schafer-Korting *et al.* (1990) to evaluate itraconazole pharmacokinetics in the skin. They determined that free itraconazole trough concentrations in blister fluid were significantly lower than corresponding plasma levels, and below the MIC for *Candida* spp. and dermatophytes.

Penetration of itraconazole into nails was examined after 3 months treatment with itraconazole 100 mg daily, and concentrations of 0.1 μg per g itraconazole persisted for 6 months in toenails after cessation of treatment (Heykants *et al.*, 1989). Pulse-therapy for 1 week with 400 mg daily of itraconazole administered monthly for 3 or 4 months, resulted in mean itraconazole concentrations in the distal ends of the nail of 67 and 103 ng per g for toenails and fingernails respectively at 1 month, and 471 and 424 ng per g at 6 months. Concentrations of 186 ng per g were still present in nails 7–8 months after ceasing treatment (De Doncker, 1996). Itraconazole does not appear to redistribute back to plasma at the end of treatment, as evidenced by persistent concentrations of drug in skin, hair and nails. It is eliminated from the skin, hair and nails by natural shedding.

Mode of Action

The mechanism of action is similar to the other imidazole and triazole antifungal agents. The primary mechanism of action involves binding of a nitrogen atom (N-4) in the triazole ring to the heme iron of cytochrome P-450 thereby inhibiting activation and function of the cytochrome enzyme. Because 14 alpha-demethylation of the precursor of ergosterol, lanosterol, is dependent on P-450 activation, these sterols accumulate and ergosterol biosynthesis and therefore cell division is inhibited. Accumulation of ^{14}C-methylated sterols in the fungal cell membrane causes increased membrane permeability and 'leakiness', altered membrane-bound enzyme function, interference with cell division and ultimately cell death (see Fig IV.1, p. 1261). Itraconazole has a high affinity for fungal P-450 cytochrome enzymes and binds weakly to mammalian cytochrome P-450 enzymes (Vanden Bossche *et al.*, 1986; Vanden Bossche *et al.*, 1990, 1993). Azoles also have a direct interaction with membrane phospholipids which may produce fungicidal effects at high drug concentrations (Sud *et al.*, 1979; Sud and Feingold, 1981).

Toxicity

1 Gastrointestinal side-effects

Nausea with or without vomiting occurred in 10% of patients receiving chronic therapy with itraconazole 400 mg daily, and diarrhea and flatulence occurred in 2% of patients (Tucker *et al.*, 1990b). Anorexia and abdominal pain have also been described in about 1% of patients. But in immunocompromised patients receiving 400–600 mg daily for cryptococcosis, gastrointestinal adverse events occurred in 40% of patients (Hostetler *et al.*, 1992b), and nausea occurred in 25% of AIDS patients on 400 mg daily (de Gans *et al.*, 1992).

2 Rash and hypersensitivity reactions

Rash complicated the therapy of 2% of patients receiving chronic therapy with 400 mg itraconazole daily. Maculopapular rashes resolved on cessation of itraconazole. One recurred on rechallenge (Tucker *et al.*, 1990b). Rash and pruritus have been reported in several series of patients treated with itraconazole (Graybill *et al.*, 1990). An urticarial reaction to itraconazole occurred on day 8 of treatment with 100 mg daily for dermatophytosis (Katsambas *et al.*, 1993). Angioedema, Stevens–Johnson syndrome and toxic epidermal necrolysis, and an acute exanthemic pustulosis have been reported (Heymann and Manders, 1995).

3 Hepatic effects

Hepatotoxicity appears to be uncommon. Abnormal liver function tests were noted in 7% patients in one series of patients given 400 mg daily. Elevation of hepatic transaminases was the most common abnormality and was mild in the majority (Tucker *et al.*, 1990b). Others report mild reversible increases in hepatic transaminases in 1–2% patients (Restrepo *et al.*, 1986; Legendre and Esola-Macre, 1990). Three cases of symptomatic hepatic injury induced by itraconazole have been reported by Lavrijsen *et al.* (1992). The patients developed a mixed hepatocellular-cholestatic liver function test abnormality, with alanine aminotransferase levels 10 times normal in two cases and four times normal in the third after treatment for at least 1 month with 200 or 400 mg daily, and all abnormalities resolved on cessation of itraconazole. Reversible intraconazole-induced cholestatic hepatitis was reported by Gearhart (1994) and Hann *et al.* (1993).

4 Hematologic effects

Thrombocytopenia without evidence of bleeding in a diabetic patient with chronic hepatitis, and neutropenia in AIDS patients were reported by Denning *et al.* (1989a). Leukopenia has also been reported as a possible toxicity of itraconazole (Graybill *et al.*, 1990).

5 Central nervous system effects

Paresthesias, tinnitus, headache, and dizzinesss were reported as adverse events in one study of non-meningeal histoplasmosis (Dismukes *et al.*, 1992), and headaches, dizziness, photophobia, blurred vision, hallucinations and somnolence were reported in another series of non-meningeal coccidioidomycosis (Graybill *et al.*, 1990). Confusion, visual hallucinations and weakness developed 2 h after administration of itraconazole 200 mg, and resolved 8 h later in a 75-year-old woman. These symptoms recurred on another two occasions after taking a single dose of itraconazole (Cleveland and Campbell, 1995). Bohme *et al.* (1995) reported a more severe vincristine-induced neurotoxicity involving paresthesia and muscle weakness of both extremities, laryngeal nerve paresis requiring artificial ventilation and paralytic ileus in patients on the combination of vincristine and itraconazole. The neurotoxicity occurred earlier, after the first or second vincristine administration.

6 Endocrine effects

A reduced cortisol response to ACTH stimulation noted in an AIDS patient 2 weeks after starting itraconazole 600 mg daily, became increasingly blunted 2 weeks later, at which time the patient had symptomatic adrenal insufficiency. After a reduction in dose of itraconazole to 400 mg daily, there was a resolution of symptoms of adrenal insufficiency and an improvement of the cortisol response. Seven other patients receiving high dose itraconazole did not experience blunted cortisol responses to prolonged courses of itraconazole 600 mg daily (Sharkey *et al.*, 1991). Adrenal suppression did not appear to be associated with itraconazole doses of 400 mg daily in ten patients with invasive mycoses who were tested both pre- and post-treatment with itraconazole (Phillips *et al.*, 1987a). *In vitro* and *in vivo* studies in rats and observations in humans suggest that high dose itraconazole has a higher affinity for the 11–beta-hydroxylase enzyme thereby inhibiting cortisol synthesis, and little affinity for the C17–20 lyase enzymes and therefore has minimal effect on androgen synthesis (Sharkey *et al.*, 1991). One AIDS patient receiving high dose itraconazole (600 mg daily) developed breast tenderness in the setting of a normal serum testosterone level (Sharkey *et al.*, 1991). Reversible painful gynecomastia has also been noted in another male patient receiving 400 mg daily (Tucker *et al.*, 1990). Plasma testosterone and cortisol levels in healthy male volunteers were not affected by the administration of itraconazole 50–100 mg daily (Van Cauteren *et al.*, 1987). Itraconazole-associated impotence and diminished libido were reported by several patients receiving 200–400 mg daily (Graybill *et al.*, 1990; Dismukes *et al.*, 1992).

7 Other adverse effects

Hypokalemia was noted in five of eight AIDS patients receiving 600 mg daily itraconazole. In addition, five patients had mild hypertension and most were also edematous (Sharkey *et al.*, 1991). Hypertension and edema was also noted in mildly immunocompromised patients (Graybill *et al.*, 1990; Diaz *et al.*, 1991; Denning *et al.*, 1994), and non-immunocompromised patients (Tailor *et al.*, 1996). Progressive ankle edema and impressive weight gain developed in a patient on 200 mg daily, which resolved completely on cessation of the drug (Dismukes *et al.*, 1992). Rarely, the edema may become debilitating (Rosen, 1994). Hypokalemia has also been noted in up to 6% of patients in other studies of itraconazole (Borelli, 1987; Graybill *et al.*, 1990; Tucker *et al.*, 1990b). Severe hypokalemia secondary to itraconazole was associated with several episodes of ventricular fibrillation which responded to cardioversion and i.v. potassium in an AIDS patient on itraconazole 800 mg daily (Nelson *et al.*, 1993). Hypertriglyceridemia was noted in 9% patients receiving chronic itraconazole, but not all were definitely drug-related (Tucker *et al.*, 1990b). Alopecia has been reported to be attributable to itraconazole therapy (Moller Heilesen, 1986; van 't Wout *et al.*, 1990b; Graybill *et al.*, 1990).

8 Effect on the fetus

Studies in pregnant rats reveal limited transfer of itraconazole across the placenta, with 0.4% of a maternal dose recovered from the fetus (Grant and Clissold, 1989). Itraconazole in high doses produces both embryotoxic and teratogenic effects (usually musculoskeletal malformations) in rats (Van Cauteren *et al.*, 1989). There are no studies examining the safety of itraconazole in pregnant women. A report of inadvertent use of itraconazole 100 mg daily for 5 months during pregnancy that did not result in any adverse outcome, complements a recent report of the use of itraconazole in the first trimester and from weeks 12 to 16 of pregnancy in a woman with cryptococcal meningitis, who delivered a normal baby (Lavalle *et al.*, 1987; Chotmongkol and Sookprasert, 1992).

9 Drug interactions

Both *in vitro* and *in vivo* studies have confirmed itraconazole is a weak reversible inhibitor of rat microsomal enzyme activities by interaction with cytochrome P-450. In rats, single doses and repetitive dosing did not inhibit the metabolism of cyclosporin, a coumarin derivative, phenytoin or tolbutamide (Lavrijsen *et al.*, 1986; Heykants *et al.*, 1989). However, itraconazole has been shown to inhibit the metabolism of cyclosporin by human liver microsomes *in vitro*, presumably by inhibition of the hepatic cytochrome P-450 3A4 isoenzyme. Itraconazole is more potent than fluconazole but less potent than ketoconazole in its ability to inhibit cyclosporin metabolism (Back and Tjia, 1991). A 2-fold increase in cyclosporin levels was observed in the rabbit model of invasive pulmonary aspergillosis when itraconazole was combined with cyclosporin (Berenguer *et al.*, 1994). There are several reports of increased cyclosporin plasma levels with concomitant itraconazole treatment at 200 mg daily (Kwan *et al.*, 1987; Trenk *et al.*, 1987; Kramer *et al.*, 1990) but there is also a report of 13 patients simultaneously treated with cyclosporin and itraconazole 200 mg daily without elevation of cyclosporin blood levels (Novakava *et al.*, 1987).

Potentiation of the action of warfarin was reported in a woman who had been stable on 5 mg of warfarin for 12 months. Within 4 days of starting itraconazole 200 mg twice-daily, she developed generalized bruising, recurrent epistaxis and intractable bleeding associated with an international normalized ratio greater than 8 (Yeh *et al.*, 1990).

Itraconazole can inhibit metabolism of drugs that are metabolized by the cytochrome P-450 3A group. An extremely important drug interaction can occur with concomitant treatment with terfenadine (a non-sedating antihistamine available over the counter in some countries) and itraconazole. Symptomatic torsades de pointes ventricular tachycardia, preceded by lengthening of the QT interval on the electrocardiogram was documented in a patient with impaired hepatic metabolism of terfenadine due to concurrent itraconazole treatment (Pohjola-Sintonen et al., 1993). Another report of prolonged QT interval and bursts of ventricular fibrillation due to impaired metabolism of terfenadine because of an interaction with itraconazole was documented with markedly elevated blood levels of terfenadine (Crane and Shih, 1993). These cases are similar to the ketoconazole-terfenadine interactions causing torsades de pointes and syncope (Monahan et al., 1990). There may also be prolonged sedation following administration of i.v. midazolam in patients receiving itraconazole. Itraconazole reduces the clearance of midazolam and increases the AUC for midazolam by 6- to 15-fold, plasma concentrations by 3- to 4-fold, and the elimination half-life 2-fold, and the combination results in a statistically significant adverse performance in psychomotor tests when compared with midazolam and placebo (Ollkola et al., 1994; Ahonen et al., 1995). The addition of itraconazole to patients stable on digoxin, can result in decreased clearance of digoxin, with increased blood levels and symptoms of digoxin toxicity. Reduction in digoxin dose to 25% of the original dose may be required (Rex, 1992; Kauffman and Bagnasco, 1992; Alderman and Jersmann, 1993; Sachs et al., 1993, McClean and Sheehan, 1994).

Itraconazole does not induce hepatic drug metabolizing enzyme activites (cytochrome P-450 dependent activiy, NADPH-cyt c-reductase, UDP-glucuronosyltransferase) in rats or mice, nor does it affect the hepatic cytochrome P-450 content (Heykants et al., 1989). The metabolic clearance of antipyrine was not altered in humans given 200 mg daily for over 4 weeks, and from these observations it was concluded that itraconazole was devoid of hepatic microsomal enzyme induction properties (Heykants et al., 1989). Itraconazole does not appear to alter the bioavailability of the oral contraceptive, as plasma ethinylestradiol and norethisterone levels remain unchanged (Heykants et al., 1989). However, clinical observations suggest that other potent inducers of the hepatic metabolizing enzymes can adversely affect itraconazole pharmacokinetics. The concurrent administration of a single dose of rifampicin and itraconazole results in an initial increase in the AUC of itraconazole (inhibited metabolism), followed 3 days later by a marked reduction to 20% of the original AUC (rifampicin-induced increased clearance of itraconazole). Negligible plasma levels of itraconazole have been reported in patients treated with itraconazole and rifampicin (Blomley et al., 1990; Drayton et al., 1994). Tucker et al. (1992) reported a series of patients in whom serum itraconazole concentrations became substantially lower or undetectable when combination itraconazole and rifampicin was administered. Decreases in the serum itraconazole concentration occurred on initiation of concurrent therapy, but it took several weeks for increases in the itraconazole concentration to occur when rifampicin was discontinued. In some cases, the rifampicin-induced reduction of itraconazole can result in treatment failure (Tucker et al., 1992; Denning et al., 1994). Decreased itraconazole levels have also been noted in patients receiving phenobarbitone, carbamazepine and phenytoin in combination with itraconazole, and the combinations were often associated with clinical treatment failure (Hay et al., 1988; de Gans et al., 1992; Tucker et al., 1992; Denning et al., 1994). Co-administration of phenytoin and itraconazole resulted in a 90% decrease of the AUC of itraconazole and a decrease in the half-life of itraconazole from 22 h to 4 h, and these observations were mirrored for hydroxyitraconazole pharmacokinetics. Itraconazole decreased the AUC of phenytoin by 10% (Ducharme et al., 1995).

Itraconazole does not appear to inhibit in vitro glucuronidation of zidovudine by human liver microsomes, unlike ketoconazole and fluconazole (Sampol et al., 1995). When didanosine is administered simultaneously with ketoconazole, the dihydroxyaluminum sodium carbonate, sodium citrate, and magnesium hydroxide buffers coating the didanosine to prevent gastric acid destruction of the didanosine, reduce the absorption of ketoconazole, and it is recommended ketoconazole is given at least 2 h prior to didanosine. Moreno et al. (1993) report a potentially similar interaction between itraconazole and didanosine, with clinical failure and delayed itraconazole absorption with mildly decreased peak itraconazole levels in a patient on combination treatment. Simultaneous administration of didanosine and itraconazole was shown to significantly decrease the absorption of itraconazole in normal volunteers, to the extent that itraconazole is not detectable in plasma during therapy with didanosine (May et al., 1994). It would seem prudent to recommend the separation of didanosine and itraconazole administration by 2 h.

Clinical Uses of the Drug

1 Cryptococcosis

In the animal model of cryptococcosis in rabbits, itraconazole was not detectable in CSF and had no significant effect on the cryptococcal yeast count during the first few days of treatment, but at the end of 2 weeks treatment, there was a significant decrease in yeast count with sterilization of CSF in 75% of itraconazole-treated rabbits, and treatment efficacy with itraconazole was similar to fluconazole (Perfect et al., 1986). In uncontrolled series, itraconazole has been shown to be effective treatment for cryptococcosis (Viviani et al., 1987, 1989; Denning et al., 1989a). The efficacy of itraconazole for treatment of cryptococcosis was reviewed by Denning et al. (1989a). Of 33 patients who received itraconazole 200 mg twice-daily, 32 were immunocompromised (26 AIDS patients), 24 had cryptococcal meningitis, and six had prior antifungal therapy. Itraconazole treatment produced a complete response in 65% patients with meningitis, and a further 25% had clinical improvement but persistent positive CSF cultures. Of the 20 assessable cryptococcal meningitis patients, 10% failed treatment, 15% relapsed during treatment, and a further 15% relapsed when itraconazole was discontinued (poor compliance). There was a 100% response rate for extrameningeal cryptococcosis (cryptococcemia, osteomyelitis, pulmonary and soft-tissue infection). These results compare favorably with those achieved by amphotericin B with or without flucytosine, and fluconazole (p. 1268 and p. 1398).

Patients with cryptococcal meningitis who have persistent positive CSF cultures despite a good clinical response are more likely to have serum itraconazole concentrations <1 µg per ml than patients who successfully sterilize the CSF (Tucker et al., 1992). In a series of 57 immunocompromised patients with cryptococcal meningitis, Hostetler et al. (1992b), reported a complete response following treatment with itraconazole 400–600 mg daily in 69% of previously untreated or partially treated patients, and clinical improvement in 24%. In those who received amphotericin B for the first 7 days, a 91% complete response was seen. Despite serum itraconazole concentrations >1.0 µg per ml, 40% of those patients who responded to itraconazole had recrudescent infection while on itraconazole. However, itraconazole (200 mg twice-daily) was shown to be less effective than amphotericin B (0.3 mg per kg daily) and flucytosine (150 mg per kg daily) for cryptococcal meningitis in AIDS patients in a prospective randomized trial. A complete response was seen in 42% of itraconazole-treated patients compared with 100% amphotericin B and flucytosine-treated patients who completed 6 weeks therapy. Itraconazole-treated patients also had a significantly higher rate of recrudescence of infection (50%) during maintenance therapy with itraconazole 200 mg daily, and all patients who recrudesced had positive CSF cultures at 6 weeks when the dose of itraconazole was halved (de Gans et al., 1992).

Maintenance therapy is essential in AIDS patients to prevent relapse of disease. In several series itraconazole has been shown to be effective for maintenance treatment of cryptococcal meningitis in AIDS, although recrudescence rates on treatment with 200–400 mg daily ranged from 19 to 50% (Viviani et al., 1987; de Gans et al., 1988, 1992; Denning et al., 1989a). In a randomized, double-blind comparison of itraconazole 200 mg daily and fluconazole 200 mg daily as maintenance therapy for cryptococcal meningitis in AIDS patients, fluconazole was significantly superior to itraconazole in the prevention of relapse with 23.8% relapse in the itraconazole group and 3.8% in the fluconazole group (Saag et al., 1995). Staib et al. (1990) have hypothesized that the prostate gland may act as a niche for persistent *Cryptococcus neoformans* organisms and recrudescence and relapse of infection occur despite treatment with itraconazole.

Viviani et al. (1990) compared treatment with itraconazole 200–400 mg daily and itraconazole at the same dose plus flucytosine (150–200 mg per kg daily) for cryptococcal meningitis in HIV-infected patients, in a small non-randomized study. Nine of 12 itraconazole-treated patients and eight of ten itraconazole plus flucytosine-treated patients had symptomatic improvement and sterilization of CSF cultures. There was no apparent difference in the time to CSF sterilization or symptom resolution. Similar response rates were seen by Chotmongkol and Jitpimolmard (1994) in an open study of ten cases treated with itraconazole plus flucytosine.

2 Candidiasis

Published studies evaluating the therapeutic efficacy of itraconazole for systemic candidiasis, and in particular randomized comparative trials, are limited.

a Fungemia In a small randomized study of itraconazole 200 mg twice-daily versus amphotericin B for the treatment of proven or highly probable systemic fungal infections in neutropenic patients, no significant difference between the efficacies of the two treatments was found (63% versus 56% respectively). However, itraconazole was ineffective for proven candidiasis including candidemia (three patients) while two of three itraconazole-treated patients with possible candidiasis responded. Problems identified with itraconazole in this patient population included inability to tolerate oral medication secondary to side-effects of cytotoxic therapy (20%), and variable absorption of the drug. Patients with low plasma concentrations of itraconazole tended to have poorer response to therapy (van 't Wout et al., 1991). Recommendations for treatment of invasive candidiasis (including fungemia, acute disseminated candidiasis, chronic disseminated candidiasis and peritonitis) in neutropenic patients, do not currently include itraconazole (Walsh et al., 1996).

Itraconazole in hydroxypropyl-beta-cyclodextrin solution (5 mg per kg daily) for 21 days was used successfully in the treatment of C. albicans septicemia in a preterm neonate (van den Anker, 1992).

b   Vaginal candidiasis   Itraconazole is effective for the treatment of acute vulvovaginal candidiasis, with clinical response rates of 85–96% and mycological eradication rates of 85–95% following a course of 200 mg daily for 3 days (Sanz Sanz and del Palacio Hernanz, 1987; Silva Cruz et al., 1991; Stein and Mummaw, 1993). A comparison of itraconazole 200 mg administered 12 h apart in 1 day, with 200 mg daily for 2 days and 200 mg daily for 3 days for acute vulvovaginal candidiasis revealed no significant difference in cure rates, and this observation could be explained by persistent therapeutic itraconazole levels in vaginal epithelium for 4 days after discontinuation of the drug (Wesel, 1990). Clinical and mycological efficacy was not significantly different in women treated with a single clotrimazole vaginal tablet compared with those treated with itraconazole 200 mg 12 h apart in 1 day (Tobin et al., 1992). Itraconazole 200 mg for 3 days produced a significantly better mycological eradication rate than econazole 150 mg vaginal tablet inserted nightly for 3 nights, but the clinical response was similar (Timonen et al., 1992). In a comparative study of a single dose of fluconazole 150 mg with two doses of itraconazole 200 mg given 12 h apart, the short-term clinical response rates were similar at 94% and 93% respectively, but the fluconazole mycological response rate of 81% was significantly better than that for itraconazole (71%). At long-term follow-up, fluconazole-treated patients had a significantly greater sustained clinical and mycologocal response rates of 84% and 85% versus 59% and 49% for itraconazole-treated patients (Rees and Phillips, 1992). The 3-day course of itraconazole 200 mg daily was associated with a sustained clinical response rate of 83% at 4 weeks follow-up (Stein and Mummaw, 1993). Persistent vulvovaginal candidiasis not responding to prolonged courses of itraconazole may be due to itraconazole-resistant C. glabrata, a situation in which speciation and antifungal susceptibility testing is recommended to help guide therapy (White et al., 1993).

The efficacy of chronic suppressive therapy with itraconazole 200 mg twice-weekly was compared with intravaginal clotrimazole 200 mg twice-weekly for 6 months in a prospective randomized study in women with recurrent vaginal candidiasis. During suppressive therapy clotrimazole was significantly more effective than itraconazole (33% of itraconazole-treated women had recurrent candidal vaginitis compared with no failures of suppressive treatment in the clotrimazole-treated women), but there was no difference in the recurrence rate after the 6-month treatment period (48% in the itraconazole group and 64% in the clotrimazole group). Itraconazole was better tolerated (Fong, 1992).

c   Oral and esophageal candidiasis   Itraconazole 100–200 mg daily for 14 days is significantly more effective than placebo for the treatment of oropharyngeal candidiasis and equivalent to clotrimazole troches 10 mg five times daily. Itraconazole-treated patients had a significantly more rapid response to itraconazole (Blatchford, 1990). Itraconazole 200 mg daily was found to be as effective as ketoconazole 200 mg twice-daily for 4 weeks as treatment for oropharyngeal and esophageal candidiasis in a controlled trial in HIV-infected patients, with clinical response rates of 75% and 82% respectively at 7 days and 93% for both groups at 28 days. Ketoconazole-treated patients had a significantly more rapid mycological response with the 7-day response rates of 92% for ketoconazole and 68% for itraconazole. The mycological eradication rate at 28 days was 85%. Over 80% patients in both groups had recurrent oropharyngeal candidiasis at 3 months follow-up (Smith et al., 1991). Itraconazole 200 mg daily administered as 100 mg capsules twice-daily was significantly less effective for the treatment of esophageal candidiasis in HIV-infected patients than fluconazole 200 mg daily (Barbaro and Di Lorenzo, 1995).

Itraconazole-cyclodextrin solution (200 or 400 mg daily) was reported to be an effective treatment for oral and esophageal candidiasis in HIV-infected patients, who had failed therapy with two or more of ketoconazole, fluconazole or itraconazole capsules in the previous month. After 14 days treatment 18 of 25 (72%) responded to itraconazole solution, including six who had not responded to the itraconazole capsules. For those who continued itraconazole solution, the median relapse-free time was significantly greater in those taking the higher secondary prophylaxis dose of 400 mg (93 days) compared with 200 mg daily (52.5 days) (Cartledge et al., 1994). Two multicenter randomized double-blind double-dummy trials compared the efficacy of fluconazole with itraconazole solution for the treatment of oral and esophageal candidiasis in HIV-infected patients. Itraconazole oral solution in hydroxypropyl-beta-cyclodextrin was found to be at least as effective as fluconazole for the treatment of oral candidiasis (Graybill et al., 1995; Darouiche et al., 1996), and esophageal candidiasis (Moskovitz et al., 1996) with clinical and mycological response rates of 75–90%. The oral solution is licensed for the treatment of oropharyngeal and esophageal candidiasis in HIV-infected patients and other immunocompromised hosts. The recommended dose is 200 mg daily for 7–14 days. The dose should be doubled for the treatment of fluconazole-resistant candidosis and treatment should continue for 2–4 weeks.

d Prophylaxis A non-randomized comparison of prophylaxis with ketoconazole 200 mg twice-daily or itraconazole 200 mg twice-daily in patients with hematological malignancies and cytotoxic chemotherapy-induced prolonged neutropenia, revealed a significant reduction in mortality due to fungal infections and infection due to *Aspergillus* spp. in the itraconazole-treated patients (Tricot et al., 1987). This study also revealed that 50% of itraconazole-treated patients had inadequate plasma itraconazole concentrations and were at greater risk of development of invasive fungal infection. Boogaerts et al. (1989) established a significant correlation between plasma itraconazole levels and prophylactic efficacy of itraconazole. There was a significant reduction in the incidence of systemic mycoses and fungal pneumonia in neutropenic patients who received itraconazole 400 mg daily and nystatin suspension as a mouthwash (1.1%), compared with that observed in an historical control group (11.3%) who received nystatin tablets and mouthwash (Thunnissen et al., 1991). In a non-randomized comparison in neutropenic children, itraconazole was no more effective than ketoconazole in the prevention of mucosal candidiasis (Ninane et al., 1988). A small prospective randomized, placebo-controlled trial of itraconazole 200 mg twice-daily in neutropenic patients with hematological malignancies determined that itraconazole was not significantly better than placebo in the prevention of fungal infections or improved survival (Vreugdenhil et al., 1993). There have been no prospective randomized trials comparing the efficacy and safety of fluconazole and itraconazole. The Working Party of the British Society for Antimicrobial Chemotherapy (1993) has recommended that itraconazole should be substituted for other antifungal prophylaxis in patients neutropenic for more than 20 days, and not in HEPA-filtered air, because of the increased risk of invasive aspergillosis.

e Chronic mucocutaneous candidiasis Itraconazole 100 mg daily for 5 months resulted in marked improvement in a patient with chronic mucocutaneous candidiasis that responded poorly to ketoconazole, but no complete resolution of skin lesions occurred. Increased dosing to 200 mg daily for 6 months resulted in almost complete resolution of lesions (Phillips et al., 1987b).

3 Dermatophytosis and superficial candidiasis

Superficial candidiasis did not respond clinically to itraconazole 50 mg daily in a small number of patients treated in an open study, and *C. albicans* was not eradicated (Saul et al., 1987). Much greater efficacy of itraconazole (50–100 mg daily) was demonstrated for the treatment of dermatophytoses with response rates of 80–96%, and more rapid improvement was noted with the 100 mg dose (Degreef et al., 1987; De Doncker and Cauwenbergh, 1992; Katsambas et al., 1993). Itraconazole has also been found to be highly effective in the treatment of tinea capitis with a 94% response rate in 50 patients treated with 25–100 mg daily for 3–10 weeks (Legendre and Esola-Macre, 1990). Three placebo-controlled trials of itraconazole have been performed for the treatment of superficial dermatophytoses, including tinea corporis, tinea cruris, tinea pedis and tinea manum. The first, using doses of 50 mg confirmed that this dose is insufficient for the management of dermatophytoses (Cauwenbergh and De Doncker, 1987) and the other two trials, using 100 mg daily for 2 or 4 weeks, established a significant benefit over placebo (clinical response in 96% versus 39%, mycological cure rates of 79% for itraconazole and 40% for placebo) (Roseeuw et al., 1990; Pariser et al., 1994). Itraconazole 100 mg daily for 15 days was compared with griseofulvin 500 mg daily in several double-blind studies for treatment of tinea corporis or tinea cruris, and itraconazole was found to be significantly superior with clinical response rates 2–3 weeks after cessation of therapy (88% versus 69% respectively) and mycological eradication (81% versus 65%) (Bourland et al., 1989; Panagiotidou et al., 1992).

Results of two trials comparing itraconazole 100 mg daily for 30 days with griseofulvin 500 mg daily for treatment of tinea pedis and tinea manus revealed 82% of itraconazole-treated patients and 83% of griseofulvin-treated patients had a clinical response at follow-up; however, itraconazole had a significantly better mycological eradication rate of 77% (Lachapelle et al., 1992). For the treatment of tinea capitis in children, itraconazole 100 mg daily was as effective as griseofulvin 500 mg daily for 6 weeks, with an 88% cure rate in each group (Lopez-Gomez et al., 1994). Double-blind randomized studies comparing itraconazole 100 mg daily with terbinafine 250 mg daily for treatment of dermatophyte infections have established the superior clinical and mycological cure rates and significantly reduced relapse rates for terbinafine-treated patients (Budimulja et al., 1994; De Keyser et al., 1994).

A pilot study examining the optimal dose and duration of itraconazole for tinea versicolor, established that a total dose of 1000 mg given as 200 mg daily for 5 days or 100 mg daily for 10 days was associated with a sustained clinical and mycological response rate of 60–70%. Twenty patients with widespread tinea versicolor were treated with 100 mg itraconazole daily for 15 days and 19 (95%) had a sustained clinical and mycological response at the 40 week follow-up assessment (Robertson, 1987).

Itraconazole in doses of 100–200 mg daily for 3–6 months is effective for the treatment of onychomycosis with cure rates of 55–100% for fingernail onychomycosis and 60–80% for toenail onychomycosis (Difonzo et al., 1990; Wals(e et al., 1990, Rongioletti et al., 1992). Itraconazole 100 mg daily effectively eradicated C. albicans and induced complete clinical remission in all patients treated (Hay et al., 1988). For dermatophyte onychomycosis, response rates of 64% for fingernail infections and 73% for toenail infections were achieved with itraconazole 100–200 mg daily. Patients with infections due to Hendersonula toruloidea did not respond to itraconazole (Hay et al., 1988).

Itraconazole was found to be as effective as griseofulvin in a randomized single-blind study comparing itraconazole 100 mg daily with griseofulvin 500 mg daily for 6–9 months in patients with dermatophyte onychomycosis. There was no statistically significant difference in outcome with cure or marked improvement noted at the end of treatment in 100% of itraconazole-treated patients compared with 85% of griseofulvin-treated patients. Relapse occurred in a similar proportion of responders (27% of itraconazole patients and 25% of griseofulvin patients). Itraconazole-treated patients continued to improve during the follow-up period as would be expected from the pharmacokinetics of itraconazole in the nail with therapeutic concentrations persisting for up to 6 months after cessation of treatment (Piepponen et al., 1992). In another comparison of itraconazole 100 mg daily with medium and high dose ultramicrosize griseofulvin given for 18 months as treatment of toenail onychomycosis, cure or partial cure was achieved in 19% of the itraconazole group, 14% of the 990 mg griseofulvin group and 6% of the 660 mg griseofulvin group. No statistical difference in the markedly improved outcome was observed between treatment groups either. However, itraconazole was better tolerated than griseofulvin (Korting et al., 1993). Willemson et al. (1992) established that response rates were significantly higher when itraconazole 200 mg daily was used, with 10-fold higher nail concentrations of itraconazole compared with 100 mg itraconazole dosing. Pulse therapy with itraconazole 400 mg daily for 1 week for 3–4 consecutive months clinically cured 93% of patients with toenail onychomycosis, with a sustained cure rate to 2 years of follow-up (De Doncker et al., 1995).

Itraconazole 200 mg daily for 12 weeks was significantly less effective than terbinafine 250 mg daily for the treatment of toenail onychomycosis, with mycological eradication rates of 67% for itraconazole and 92% for terbinafine, and clinical and mycological cure achieved in 63% of itraconazole-treated patients and 81% of terbinafine-treated patients (Brautigam et al., 1995).

4 Aspergillosis

Itraconazole is a suitable oral agent for invasive aspergillosis. Limited data is available from controlled trials of therapy for aspergillosis, and published reports of efficacy are biased by the exclusion of cases with early failure of therapy resulting in inflated estimates of successful treatment. Moreover, comparative efficacy with amphotericin B is essentially unknown. In the extensive review of published cases of aspergillosis, Denning and Stevens (1990) reported that itraconazole was effective in about 75% of cases, particularly invasive pulmonary aspergillosis and bone and joint disease. An international open-label treatment program of itraconazole 50–400 mg daily in 35 patients of whom 25 had received prior amphotericin B, revealed a 60% response rate (cure and improved, mycological eradication) for invasive aspergillosis, 66%

response rate for chronic necrotizing pulmonary aspergillosis, and a 56% rate of improvement in patients with chronic pulmonary aspergilloma but only 30% radiological improvement (De Beule *et al.*, 1988). Dupont (1990) reported a 70% response rate (cure and improved) for itraconazole treatment of invasive aspergillosis.

The National Institutes of Allergy and Infectious Diseases performed a prospective, non-comparative trial of itraconazole 600 mg per day for 4 days followed by 400 mg daily for the treatment of invasive aspergillosis in patients who had either no previous treatment or those who had failed prior therapy. Of the 76 patients enrolled, only six were immunocompetent, 51 had pulmonary aspergillosis and 25 had extrapulmonary aspergillosis (sinus, central nervous system or other site). Response rates varied according to type of invasive aspergillosis and host factors. After 12 weeks treatment, the overall response rate was 32%; however, those with pulmonary aspergillosis had a response rate of 44% compared with the 12% response rate in those with extrapulmonary disease. The highest itraconazole failure rate occurred in the subgroup of central nervous system aspergillosis (50%). AIDS patients had an itraconazole failure rate of 25%, neutropenic, bone marrow transplant patients and cancer patients had a 19% itraconazole failure rate. The end of treatment response rates were slightly higher with an overall response rate of 39%, 49% for pulmonary aspergillosis, 61% for neutropenic cancer patients and 57% for solid organ transplant patients; however, the failure rate in AIDS patients increased to 44% for an end of treatment response. The overall failure rate was 56% at the end of study, with 26% attributed to itraconazole failure. Long-term follow-up revealed a 12% relapse rate in those who completed therapy and a 40% relapse rate who did not complete a full course of treatment. Patients who failed treatment were more likely to have low or undetectable serum itraconazole concentrations, but a threshold concentration for response was not identified (Denning *et al.*, 1994). In a small randomized comparative study of itraconazole 200 mg twice daily with amphotericin B 0.6 mg per kg daily for the treatment of systemic fungal infections in neutropenic patients, 13 patients had *Aspergillus* spp. isolated. Response was documented in six of eight itraconazole-treated patients and only two of five amphotericin B-treated patients, which was not statistically different (van 't Wout *et al.*, 1991).

Most patients with invasive aspergillosis, especially neutropenic patients, are treated initially on an empiric basis following a presumptive daignosis. Initial treatment is usually with amphotericin B at a dose of 1.0–1.25 mg per kg daily (p. 1275). Sequential therapy with oral itraconazole, allows for a longer duration of therapy following discharge from hospital. There was no difference in response rate in those patients who received itraconazole following amphotericin B treatment and those who received primary therapy with itraconazole in the NIAID Mycoses Study Group trial (Denning *et al.*, 1994). The duration of therapy for those who respond to itraconazole is unclear. Denning (1994) suggests that treatment should continue for years in patients with AIDS, chronic granulomatous disease, aplastic anemia and allogeneic bone marrow transplant recipients. Immunocompromised patients should remain on therapy until a complete response has been documented and immune system recovery has occurred. Secondary prohylaxis is also required for patients who discontinue antifungal treatment and receive further cycles of chemotherapy or bone marrow transplantation to prevent recurrent disease. The efficacy of itraconazole has not been evaluated in this setting. There is one case-report of failure of amphotericin B treatment for aspergillosis in a patient who had received prior therapy with itraconazole, and together with the *in vitro* and murine model data, this observation raises caution about the sequential use of itraconazole and amphotericin B (Schaffner and Bohler, 1993).

Pulmonry aspergillosis in HIV infection generally occurs at advanced stages of immunodeficiency, and presents either as invasive aspergillosis or obstructing bronchial aspergillosis. In a series reported by Kriesel *et al.* (1991), itraconazole produced an 82% cure rate for invasive pulmonary aspergillosis. These authors suggested optimal therapeutic efficacy was obtained by early presumptive diagnosis. Denning *et al.* (1991a) reviewed their experience with aspergillosis in AIDS and reported that four of six patients treated with itraconazole responded (low serum itraconazole levels may have been responsible for the two failures); however, one of the responders relapsed while on itraconazole therapy, and another died of active aspergillosis without autopsy confirmation. This response rate is similar to that reported in other immunocompromised patients, treated with 200–400 mg daily.

Dupont (1990) reported a 70% response rate (cure and improved) for pulmonary aspergilloma, and a 90% response rate for chronic necrotizing pulmonary aspergillosis. However, Campbell *et al.* (1991) were unable to document clinical or mycological improvement in seven of nine patients with pulmonary aspergilloma treated with itraconazole 200 mg daily for a minimum of 6 months. Deep mucosal tracheobronchial ulceration caused by *Aspergillus* infection in heart-lung transplant recipients was successfully treated by itraconazole in five of six patients (Kramer *et al.*, 1991). Two cases of pleural aspergillosis successfully treated with itraconazole have been reported (Denning *et* al., 1989b; Dupont and Drouhet, 1987). Itraconazole may have an adjunctive role in the management of allergic bronchopulmonary aspergillosis. In a small series of six patients treated with 200 mg twice-daily, improvement in lung function, reduction in steroid dose and mean total serum IgE levels was noted in all patients (Denning et al., 1991b).

Itraconazole 300–400 mg daily resulted in complete resolution of Aspergillus osteomyelitis in patients with chronic granulomatous disease, and rheumatoid arthritis and diabetes, following moderate improvement only or poor response with amphotericin B. These patients continued on maintenance doses of itraconazole for a minimum of 1–3 years (Sachs et al., 1990; van 't Wout et al., 1990b). Invasive otitis externa with bone involvement has also been successfully controlled in AIDS patients treated with itraconazole (Reiss et al., 1991). A case of postoperative lumbar discitis due to Aspergillus fumigatus was treated with surgical debridement and itraconazole 200 mg twice-daily for 10 weeks. However, a clinical and mycological relapse occurred 4 weeks after cessation of the itraconazole, and treatment was reinstituted with amphotericin B for 1 week only followed by a prolonged course of itraconazole without further relapse (Peters-Christodoulou et al., 1991). A child with chronic granulomatous disease and invasive pulmonary aspergillosis which invaded his chest wall failed to respond to liposomal amphotericin B and was switched to the itraconazole suspension initiated at 5 mg per kg daily and increased to 14 mg per kg daily (100 mg twice-daily). On this regimen he had a continued reduction in size of the external chest wall mass and the pulmonary mass over 8 months treatment (Spencer et al., 1994). Invasive otitis externa due to Aspergillus spp. in an immunocompromised patient failed to respond to i.v. amphotericin B (2 g) but resolved following a 3-month course of itraconazole (Phillips et al., 1990). Paranasal Aspergillus granuloma is managed with surgical excision and has been associated with an 80% relapse rate. Using itraconazole 200–300 mg daily postoperatively for a mean period of 5 months, 12 of 19 patients (62%) remained in complete remission for a mean duration of 17 months after the end of therapy (Gumaa et al., 1992).

Two non-randomized studies comparing the efficacy of ketoconazole as an historical control group with itraconazole for prophylaxis in patients with hematological malignancy and prolonged neutropenia, suggested that itraconazole 200 mg twice-daily effectively reduced the incidence of invasive aspergillosis from 36% to 12%, and was most effective in those patients who achieved adequate serum levels of itraconazole (p. 1424) (Tricot et al., 1987; Boogaerts et al., 1989). However, at least 25% of patients in the latter study had inadequate plasma itraconazole levels. Todeschini et al. (1993) reported a significant reduction in the incidence of invasive aspergillosis in neutropenic patients with hematological malignancies following the introduction of prophylaxis with itraconazole 200 mg daily plus nasal amphotericin B 10 mg daily from 11.7% to 4.9%. The comparison in this study was an historical control group who received no aspergillosis prophylaxis. The interpretation of results from these non-randomized studies utilizing historical control groups is always difficult. Clearly, itraconazole is a potential agent for prophylaxis of aspergillosis in the neutropenic patient. Large, prospective, randomized, controlled studies are required to define the role of this drug as either prophylaxis or pre-emptive treatment in neutropenic and other immunocompromised patients at risk of invasive aspergillosis. The Working Party of the British Society for Antimicrobial Chemotherapy (1993) has recommended that those patients neutropenic for more than 20 days and not nursed in HEPA-filtered air should receive itraconazole prophylaxis.

5 Histoplasmosis

Itraconazole is effective therapy for histoplasmosis. Treatment of subacute or chronic disseminated histoplasmosis with 100 mg daily for 2 months followed by 50 mg daily for 4 months was associated with cure or marked improvement in 94–97% of treated patients (Negroni et al., 1987, 1989). An open-phase II clinical trial of itraconazole 200–400 mg daily for a minimum 3 months for treatment of non-meningeal non-life-threatening histoplasmosis reported successful treatment in 86% of 35 patients treated for more than 2 months. Cure was achieved in 65% of 20 patients with chronic cavitary histoplasmosis treated for a median of 9 months, 100% of those with mediastinal or nodular parenchymal disease, and 100% of those with extrapulmonary disseminated histoplasmosis. Patients classified as failures had either persistent infection on itraconazole or relapsed when itraconazole was discontinued, and one patient experienced drug toxicity (Dismukes et al., 1992). Itraconazole appears to be an effective treatment for disseminated histoplasmosis in AIDS patients. A pilot study utilizing doses of 400 mg daily was associated with a 75% response rate (nine of 12 patients) of which seven patients were classified as remission on chronic suppressive therapy with itraconazole (Sharkey-Mathis et al., 1993a). Daily itraconazole doses of 200 mg for 6 months produced clinical improvement in 78% of 23 AIDS patients (Negroni et al., 1992), and 85% of AIDS patients with disseminated histoplasmosis that was non-life threatening and not involving the central nervous system, responded to itraconazole 300 mg twice-daily for 3 days followed by 200 mg twice-daily for 12 weeks (Wheat *et al.*, 1995). Wheat (1994) has recommended the use of itraconazole 400 mg daily for mild to moderate histoplasmosis in AIDS, reserving amphotericin B for moderate to severe disease. Because itraconazole does not reach detectable concentrations in CSF, its role in central nervous system disease has not been established.

Maintenance therapy is required for histoplasmosis in HIV-infected individuals as the relapse rate without maintenance antifungal therapy is 35–80% (Wheat *et al.*, 1990; Wheat, 1994). Itraconazole 200 mg twice-daily effectively prevented relapse of histoplasmosis in patients with AIDS who successfully completed induction treatment with amphotericin B, in an open-label non-comparative trial. Two of 42 patients relapsed during a median follow-up of 98 weeks, only one of which had proven recurrent histoplasmosis. Itraconazole maintenance therapy was also associated with clearance of *Histoplasma capsulatum* var. *capsulatum* antigen from blood in 75% of antigen-positive patients at baseline and from urine in 43% of patients (Wheat *et al.*, 1993). Randomized comparative studies are required to evaluate the role of itraconazole for induction and maintenance treatment of histoplasmosis. Itraconazole is currently the drug of choice for maintenance therapy of histoplasmosis following successful induction treatment in AIDS (Wheat, 1994).

Histoplasma capsulatum var. *duboisii* causes 'African histoplasmosis' often manifest as chronic localized skin nodules, or psoriaform, ulcerative skin lesions. Multiple skeletal lesions and disseminated disease is less common. Itraconazole 100 mg daily for 7 weeks resulted in resolution of a single skin lesion which had been present for 6 months in an Angolan patient, and no relapse occurred in 10 months follow-up (Abrucio Neto *et al.*, 1993)

6 Blastomycosis

A phase II open study of itraconazole 200–400 mg daily for non-meningeal, non-life-threatening blastomycosis was performed by the National Institutes for Allergy and Infectious Diseases. Successful treatment occurred in 43 of 48 (90%) patients, and 95% of 40 patients treated for greater than 2 months (median of 6 months). Only one patient relapsed after successful treatment (Dismukes *et al.*, 1992). No randomized controlled trials have been performed to support the recommendation that itraconazole 200 mg daily is the azole drug of choice for blastomycosis in the immunocompetent patient, and there is limited information published of its use in immunocompromised patients. Amphotericin B remains the drug of choice as initial therapy in immunocompromised patients (Pappas *et al.*, 1993).

7 Coccidioidomycosis

Itraconazole has been evaluated in several open, non-randomized, non-comparative studies for the treatment of coccidioidomycosis. Graybill *et al.* (1990) reported response rates of 57% for itraconazole treatment of 49 patients with non-meningeal coccidioidomycosis (pulmonary, osteoarticular and skin or soft tissue involvement). Of these 60% had relapsed following prior antifungal treatment with ketoconazole or amphotericin B. The majority of patients received 400 mg itraconazole daily, while 25% received 100–200 mg daily. Most patients required more than 10 months treatment before clinical improvement occurred, and slow clinical responses were associated with doses less than 400 mg daily. In addition, four of the 25 patients who achieved remission subsequently relapsed. The failure rate of 43% comprised 16 clinical failures and three patients with drug intolerance. Another open study of itraconazole at doses of 200 mg twice-daily for pulmonary coccidioidomycosis, revealed that 15 of 16 patients achieved remission after 12 months treatment; however, there was a 25% relapse rate in the 14 months after cessation of treatment (Diaz *et al.*, 1991).

Ten patients with chronic coccidioidal meningitis for 5–194 months, which was refractory to standard therapy, were treated with itraconazole 400 mg daily in a prospective non-randomized open trial. Of these, five were treated with itraconazole alone and five received a combination of itraconazole and intrathecal amphotericin B. Eight of the ten patients were evaluable for efficacy, and all patients receiving intrathecal amphotericin B discontinued this mode of treatment without activation of disease. Four of five patients receiving itraconazole alone had reductions in CSF titers of coccidioidal antibody and a clinical remission, despite undetectable levels of itraconazole in three patients tested and the known poor penetration of itraconazole into CSF (Tucker *et al.*, 1990a). No comparative studies have been performed to determine the optimal dose, duration of therapy or choice of antifungal agent in the setting of non-meningeal or meningeal coccidioidomycosis. In addition, the efficacy of itraconazole for treatment of coccidioidomycosis in HIV-infected patients has not been examined.

8 Paracoccidioidomycosis

Itraconazole 100 mg daily was established as a safe and effective treatment for both the chronic adult form of paracoccidioidomycosis and the juvenile form (Naranjo et al., 1990). In an open non-comparative study of 57 patients, treated for a mean duration of 6 months (range of 3–24 months), complete resolution of disease occurred in only one patient; however, marked improvement occurred in 89% of treated patients. No patient deteriorated on itraconazole, and no relapse occurred in 15 patients followed for 12 months post-therapy. Others have reported a relapse rate of 3–5% following itraconazole therapy (Restrepo, 1994). No formal comparative study has been performed, but the results are similar to those obtained with ketoconazole therapy (Restrepo et al., 1983).

9 Mucormycosis

As the majority of the zygomycetes are resistant to itraconazole, it is unlikely this drug will have a role in the treatment of mucormycosis. An unusual case of necrotic pyoderma gangrenosum of the upper arm due to Rhizopus arrhizus was successfully treated with itraconazole (Liao et al., 1995).

10 Penicillium marneffei infections

Itraconazole 200 mg twice-daily for 8–12 weeks was used as initial therapy in 16 AIDS patients and 9 (56%) responded both clinically and microbiologically. Five of the nine responders relapsed within 4 months of completion of treatment (Supparatpinyo et al., 1993). In an open study to assess the efficacy of itraconazole 200 mg twice-daily for 2 months followed by 100 mg daily for 1 month as treatment for previously untreated P. marneffei infection in ten patients, clinical improvement was noted in eight patients and the median time for cultures to become negative was 57 days in seven patients. Nine of the ten patients were HIV co-infected and two patients died during therapy. Five of seven patients relapsed within 4 months of cessation of itraconazole underscoring the importance of long-term suppressive therapy for this infection in AIDS patients (Supparatpinyo et al., 1992).

11 Chromoblastomycosis

This chronic infection of skin and subcutaneous tissue is often difficult to treat. Itraconazole 200 mg daily produces response rates of about 60%, with infections due to Cladosporium carrionii responding within 2–3 months while those due to Fonsecaea pedrosoi requiring longer duration of treatment for a clinical response. Relapse rates of 10% have been noted (Restrepo, 1994; Yu, 1995). In a non-comparative trial of itraconazole 200–400 mg daily in 19 patients with F. pedrosoi infection, clinical improvement was noted in all patients. In those with mild to moderate disease, eight of ten patients had a clinical and mycological cure after a mean duration of treatment for 11.6 months, but no mycological cures were noted in those with severe disease. Clinical cures were noted in six of nine patients with severe disease and clinical improvement noted in the rest after treatment for a mean duration of 22.6 months (Queiroz-Telles et al., 1992). In patients who had responded poorly to itraconazole monotherapy, the addition of flucytosine 100 mg per kg daily to itraconazole 100 mg per day appeared to effect a clinical response in 50% of patients (Bayles, 1992). Subsequently, eight patients with extensive disease due to F. pedrosoi received itraconazole and flucytosine combination therapy for 3–31 months with cure noted in two patients and marked clinical improvement in five patients (Bayles, 1992). These observations suggest itraconazole monotherapy or combination with flucytosine offer therapeutic efficacy not observed with other antifungal or surgical modes of therapy.

Rapidly progressive cutaneous lesions due to Phialophora richardsiae and Exophiala jeanselmei in an immunosuppressed man were successfully treated with itraconazole 100 mg daily for 3 months (Tam and Freeman, 1989). Itraconazole 200 mg twice-daily for 4 months resulted in complete resolution of subcutaneous phaeohyphomycosis due to E. jeanselmei (Whittle and Kominos, 1995; Chuan and Wu, 1995). Extensive cutaneous disease due to Phialophora verrucosa failed to respond to ketoconazole in an AIDS patient, but regressed when treatment with itraconazole was instituted (Duggan et al., 1995).

12 Phaeohyphomycosis

Cutaneous phaeohyphomycosis caused by Alternaria infection was cured with itraconazole 100 mg daily in an immunocompetent elderly woman who received treatment for 1 month (Lanigman, 1992) and an immunocompromised elderly man with post-traumatic ulcers over the hand and spreading eczematous rash over the hand and forearm (Duffill and Coley, 1993).

13 Fusarium infections

Fusarium spp. are generally resistant to itraconazole, which does not play a role in the treatment of this infection in immunocompromised hosts.

14 Sporotrichosis

Itraconazole in doses of 100–600 mg daily for 3–18 months produced an 80% response rate in 30 courses of treatment for sporotrichosis. In this open-label study in which the majority of patients received 200–400 mg daily, response rates of 100% (ten of ten) for lymphocutaneous sporotrichosis, 75% (three of four) for pulmonary sporotrichosis, 76% (10 of 13) for articular or osseus sporotrichosis, and 66% (two of three) for multifocal systemic sporotrichosis were observed. Seven of 25 responders (28%) relapsed within 1–7 months of ceasing treatment with itraconazole, three patients continued on long-term treatment and 14 remained disease-free for 6–42 months. These patients had received treatment for 6–18 months prior to classification as a responder (Sharkey-Mathis *et al.*, 1993b).

The efficacy of itraconazole 100 mg daily for the treatment of lymphocutaneous sporotrichosis has been demonstrated in other small series, with sustained response rates in up to 90% patients treated for at least 3–4 months (Restrepo *et al.*, 1986; Lavalle *et al.*, 1987; Bayles, 1992). For systemic sporotrichosis with pulmonary or bone involvement, higher doses of itraconazole (200–400 mg daily) are recommended, and is a reasonable alternative to amphotericin B. Osseus and articular sporotrichosis is more difficult to treat with significant risk of permanent joint damage. Itraconazole successfully eradicated *Sporothrix schenckii* in a patient with polyarticular sporotrichosis who relapsed after amphotericin B treatment (Lesperance *et al.*, 1988). Baker *et al.* (1989) reported a case of amphotericin B-resistant *S. schenckii* fungemia and cutaneous lesions which responded slowly to amphotericin B, but persistent isolation of *S. schenckii* from new subcutaneous nodules precipitated a change to azole therapy. Itraconazole 200 mg daily produced a complete remission within 7 days of treatment initiation, but relapse occurred within 3 months of completing 7 months treatment. This responded promptly to itraconazole again and after 18 months of chronic suppression with itraconazole, the patient remained asymptomatic. Recommendations for the treatment of sporotrichosis have been developed by Kauffman (1995). These include itraconazole 100–200 mg daily administered for 3–6 months for localized lymphocutaneous sporotrichosis, and itraconazole 200 mg twice-daily for 1–2 years for osteoarticular, pulmonary and disseminated sporotrichosis.

15 Acanthamoeba infections

Three patients with *Acanthamoeba* keratitis responded to oral itraconazole, topical 0.1% miconazole eyedrops administered hourly during the day and surgical debridement. Clinical resolution occurred in 5–9 weeks and was associated with marked improvement in visual acuity (Ishibashi *et al.*, 1990).

16 Pseudallescheria boydii infections

Only case-reports have been published describing a therapeutic response to itraconazole for this infection. Itraconazole 100 mg daily effectively controlled arthritis and osteomyelitis of the knee caused by *Scedosporium apiospermum* (the asexual structure of *Pseudallescheria boydii*) in a 6-year-old immunocompetent child with progressive disease on treatment with miconazole. Improvement was noted after 1 month of treatment, regression of osteolytic lesions occurred and normal bone growth and function ensued (Piper *et al.*, 1990). Itraconazole 400 mg daily produced marked clinical improvement in chronic pulmonary pseudallescheriasis in an immunocompetent man (Stolk-Engelaar and Cox, 1993), and pulmonary pseudallescheriasis in immunocompromised patients (Walsh *et al.*, 1992; Goldberg *et al.*, 1993).

17 Leishmaniasis

Several case-reports suggested a role for itraconazole in the treatment of leishmaniasis at a dose of 100 mg daily for 1–2 months (Borelli, 1987; Albanese *et al.*, 1989). An open randomized trial of pentamidine, meglumine antimonate, itraconazole 200 mg twice-daily for 4 weeks or no treatment in 80 males with cutaneous leishmaniasis in Colombia, established that itraconazole was no better than no treatment with a 75% failure rate (Soto-Mancipe *et al.*, 1993). Contrasting results were obtained in a randomized, placebo-controlled trial of itraconazole 200 mg twice-daily for 6–8 weeks for treatment of cutaneous leishmaniasis in Kuwait. The 75% response rate achieved by itraconazole treatment compared with response in one of nine patients randomized to placebo (Al-Fouzan *et al.*, 1991). The difference in response rates may be due to predominance of different species of *Leishmania* (*L. panamensis*, *L. mexicana* and *L. braziliensis* in Colombia, and *L. tropica* and *L. major* in Kuwait) or the duration of treatment.

Visceral leishmaniasis caused by *L. donovani* occurs as an opportunistic infection in HIV-infected individuals, and antimonial agents often are ineffective in HIV patients. Itraconazole 400 mg daily, has been shown to be an effective treatment, as well as maintenance therapy for visceral leishmaniasis in HIV-infected patients (Pialoux *et al.*, 1990; Lafeuillade *et al.*, 1992). A case report of an HIV-infected patient initally effectively treated with a combination of itraconazole 400 mg daily and allopurinol 21 mg per kg daily. Rapid resolution of clinical symptoms and negative blood smears for *Leishmania* spp., were achieved after 1 month of treatment. However, bone marrow aspirates remained positive for amastigotes and the patient relapsed 7 months later (Raffi *et al.*, 1995).

18 Other rare mycoses

Paecilomyces varioti soft tissue infection of the foot initiated by minor trauma in a child with chronic granulomatous disease was successfully managed by amphotericin B for 7 weeks followed by itraconazole 100 mg daily for 1 year. Itraconazole therapy resulted in resolution of all signs of inflammation that persisted despite amphotericin B treatment (Williamson *et al.*, 1992).

A septic arthritis due to *Scedosporium inflatum* developed in an immunocompetent boy following trauma resulting in a marine soil contaminated laceration. Initial treatment with amphotericin B (0.85 mg per kg per day for 6 weeks) caused minimal clinical response, but after institution of itraconazole rapid clinical improvement occurred. The child completed 5 months treatment with 100 mg twice-daily resulting in complete resolution (Wood *et al.*, 1992).

Eumycetoma caused by *Madurella mycetomatis* has been reported to respond in about 40% of cases, but itraconazole is less effective than ketoconazole (Restrepo, 1994). Cutaneous infection with *Prototheca wickerhamii* producing chronic ulcerated papules and plaques on the legs responded to itraconazole with gradual resolution of the ulcers (Tang *et al.*, 1995). Itraconazole 200 mg daily for 2 months cured a chronic subcutaneous infection of the hand due to *Acremonium recifei* which developed after local trauma in an immunocompetent woman, and a mycetoma on the right temple region due to *Acremonium falciforme* (Zaitz *et al.*, 1995; Lee *et al.*, 1995).

References

Abrucio Neto L, Takahashi MD, Salebian A, Cuce LC (1993). African histoplasmosis. Report of the first case in Brazil and treatment with itraconazole. *Rev Inst Med Trop Sao Paulo* **35**: 295.

Albanese G, Giorgetti P, Santagostino L *et al.* (1989). Cutaneous leishmaniasis. Treatment with itraconazole. *Arch Dermatol* **125**: 1540.

Ahonen J, Olkkola KT, Neuvonen PJ (1995). Effect of itraconazole and terbinafine on the pharmacokinetics and pharmacodynamics of midazolam in healthy volunteers. *Brit J Clin Pharmacol* **40**: 270.

Alderman CP, Jersmann HPA (1993). Digoxin-itraconazole interaction. *Med J Aust* **159**: 838.

Al-Fouzan AS, Al Saleh QA, Najem NM, Rostom AI (1991). Cutaneous leishmaniasis in Kuwait. Clinical experience with itraconazole. *Int J Dermatol* **30**: 519.

Back DJ, Tjia JF (1991). Comparative effects of the antimycotic drugs ketoconazole, fluconazole, itraconazole and terbinafine on the metabolism of cyclosporin by human liver microsomes. *Brit J Clin Pharmacol* **32**: 624.

Baker JH, Goodpasture HC, Kuhns HR, Rinaldi MG (1989). Fungemia caused by an amphotericin B-resistant isolate of *Sporothrix schenckii*. Successful treatment with itraconazole. *Arch Pathol Lab Med* **113**: 1279.

Barbaro G, Di Lorenzo G (1995). Comparison of therapeutic activity of fluconazole and itraconazole in the treatment of oesophageal candidiasis in AIDS patients: a double-blind, randomized, controlled clinical study. *Ital J Gastroenterol* **27**: 175.

Barone JA, Koh JG, Bierman RH *et al.* (1993). Food interaction and steady-state pharmacokinetics of itraconazole capsules in healthy male volunteers. *Antimicrob Ag Chemother* **37**: 778.

Bayles MAH (1992). Tropical mycoses. *Chemotherapy* **38** (Suppl 1): S27.

Berenguer J, Ali NM, Allende MC *et al.* (1994). Itraconazole for experimental pulmonary aspergillosis: Comparison with amphotericin B, interaction with cyclosporin A, and correlation between therapeutic response and itraconazole concentrations in plasma. *Antimicrob Ag Chemother* **38**: 1303.

Blatchford NR (1990). Treatment of oral candidosis with itraconazole: a review. *J Amer Acad Dermatol* **23**: 561.

Blomley M, Teare EL, de Belder A *et al.* (1990). Itraconazole and anti-tuberculosis drugs. *Lancet* **336**: 1255.

Boelaert J, Schurgers M, Matthys E *et al.* (1988). Itraconazole pharmacokinetics in patients with renal dysfunction. *Antimicrob Ag Chemother* **32**: 1595.

Bohme A, Ganser A, Hoelzer D (1995). Aggravation of vincristine-induced neurotoxicity by itraconazole in the treatment of adult ALL. *Ann Hematol* **71**: 311.

Boogaerts MA, Verhoef GE, Zachee P *et al.* (1989). Antifungal prophylaxis with itraconazole in prolonged neutropenia: correlation with plasma levels. *Mycoses* **32** (Suppl 1): 103.

Borelli D (1987). A clinical trial of itraconazole in the treatment of deep mycoses and leishmaniasis. *Rev Infect Dis* **9** (Suppl 1): S57.

Bourlond A, Lachapelle JM, Aussems J *et al.* (1989). Double-blind comparison of itraconazole with griseofulvin in the treatment of tinea corporis and tinea cruris. *Int J Dermatol* **28**: 410.

Brautigam M, Nolting S, Schopf RE, Weidinger G (1995). Randomised double blind comparison of terbinafine and itraconazole for treatment of toenail infection. Seventh Lamisil German Onychomycosis Study Group. *Brit Med J* **311**: 919.

Bradford CR, Prentice AG, Warnock DW, Copplestone JA (1991). Comparison of the multiple dose pharmacokinetics of two formulations of itraconazole during remission induction for acute myeloblastic leukemia. *J Antimicrob Chemother* **28**: 555.

Budimulja U, Kuswadji K, Bramono S et al. (1994). A double-blind, randomized, stratified controlled study of the treatment of tinea imbricata with oral terbinafine or itraconazole. *Brit J Dermatol* **130** (Suppl 43): 29.

Campbell JH, Winter JH, Richardson MD et al. (1991). Treatment of pulmonary aspergilloma with itraconazole. *Thorax* **46**: 839.

Cartledge JD, Midgley J, Youle M, Gazzard BG (1994). Itraconazole cyclodextrin solution – effective treatment for HIV-related candidosis unresponsive to other azole therapy. *J Antimicrob Chemother* **33**: 1071.

Cauwenbergh G, De Doncker P (1987). The clinical use of itraconazole in superficial and deep mycoses In *Recent Trends in the Discovery, Development and Evaluation of Antifungal Agents* (Fromtling RA ed), p. 273. Barcelona: JR Prous Science Publishers.

Cauwenbergh G, Degreef H, Heykants J et al. (1988). Pharmacokinetic profile of orally administered itraconazole in human skin. *J Amer Acad Dermatol* **18**: 263.

Chotmongkol V, Jitpimolmard S (1994). Treatment of cryptococcal meningitis with combination itraconazole and flucytosine. *J Med Assoc Thai* **77**: 253.

Chotmongkol V, Sookprasert A (1992). Itraconazole in cryptococcal meningitis in pregnancy: a case report. *J Med Assoc Thai* **75**: 606.

Chuan MT, Wu MC (1995). Subcutaneous phaeohyphomycosis caused by *Exophiala jeanselmei*: successful treatment with itraconazole. *Int J Dermatol* **34**: 563.

Cleveland KO, Campbell JW (1995). Hallucinations associated with itraconazole therapy. *Clin Infect Dis* **21**: 456.

Crane JK, Shih H-T (1993). Syncope and cardiac arrhythmia due to an interaction between itraconazole and terfenadine. *Amer J Med* **95**: 445.

Darouiche RO, Setoodeh A, Anaissie EJ (1995). Potential use of a simplified method for determination of itraconazole levels in plasma and esophageal tissue by using high-performance liquid chromatography. *Antimicrob Ag Chemother* **39**: 757.

Darouiche RO, Graybill JR, Vazquez J et al. (1996). Itraconazole oral solution (IS). for the treatment of oropharyngeal candidiasis (OC): Results of two randomized, blinded studies. *Proc XI International Conference on AIDS, Vancouver, Canada.* (Abstr. MoB117).

De Beule K, De Doncker P, Cauwenbergh G et al. (1988). The treatment of aspergillosis and aspergilloma with itraconazole, Clinical results of an open international study (1982–1987). *Mycoses* **9**: 476.

De Doncker P, Cauwenbergh G (1992). Management of fungal skin infections with 15 days of itraconazole treatment: a worldwide review. *Brit J Clin Pract* **71** (Suppl): S118.

De Doncker P, Van Lint J, Dockx P, Roseeuw D (1995). Pulse therapy with one-week itraconazole monthly for three or four months in the treatment of onychomycosis. *Cutis* **56**: 180.

De Doncker P, Decroix J, Pierard GE et al. (1996). Antifungal pulse therapy for onychomycosis. A pharmacokinetic and pharmacodynamic investigation of monthly cycles of 1-week pulse therapy with itraconazole. *Arch Dermatol* **132**: 34.

de Gans J, Eeftinck Schattenkerk JKM, van Ketel RJ (1988). Itraconazole as maintenance treatment for cryptococcal meningitis in the acquired immunodeficiency syndrome. *Brit Med J* **296**: 339.

de Gans J, Portegies P, Tiessens G et al. (1992). Itraconazole compared with amphotericin B plus flucytosine in AIDS patients with cryptococcal meningitis. *AIDS* **6**: 185.

Degreef H, Marien K, De Veylder H et al. (1987). Itraconazole in the treatment of dermatophytoses: A comparison of two daily dosages. *Rev Infect Dis* **9** (Suppl 1): S104.

De Keyser P, De Backer M, Massert DL, Westelinck KJ (1994). Two-week oral treatment of tinea pedis, comparing terbinafine (250 mg per day) with itraconazole (100 mg per day): a double-blind, multicentre study. *Brit J Dermatol* **130** (Suppl 43): 22.

Denning DW (1994). Treatment of invasive aspergillosis. *J Infect* **28** (Suppl 1): 25.

Denning DW, Stevens DA (1990). Antifungal and surgical treatment of invasive aspergillosis: Review of 2121 published cases. *Rev Infect Dis* **12**: 1147.

Denning DW, Tucker RM, Hanson LH et al. (1989a). Itraconazole therapy for cryptococcal meningitis and cryptococcosis. *Arch Intern Med* **149**: 2301.

Denning DW, Tucker RM, Hanson LH, Stevens DA (1989b). Treatment of invasive aspergillosis with itraconazole. *Amer J Med* **86**: 791.

Denning DW, Follansbee SE, Scolaro M et al. (1991a). Pulmonary aspergillosis in the acquired immunodeficiency syndrome. *New Engl J Med* **324**: 654.

Denning DW, Van Wye JE, Lewiston NJ, Stevens DA (1991b). Adjunctive therapy of allergic bronchopulmonary aspergillosis with itraconazole. *Chest* **100**: 813.

Denning DW, Hanson LH, Perlman AM, Stevens DA (1992). *In vitro* susceptibility and synergy studies of *Aspergillus* species to conventional and new agents. *Diagn Microbiol Infect Dis* **15**: 21.

Denning DW, Lee JY, Hostetler JS et al. (1994). NIAID Mycoses Study Group Multicenter trial of oral itraconazole therapy for invasive aspergillosis. *Amer J Med* **97**: 135.

Diaz M, Puente R, de Hoyos LA, Cruz S (1991). Itraconazole in the treatment of coccidioidomycosis. *Chest* **100**: 682.

Difonzo EM, Panconesi E, Cilli P (1990). Itraconazole in dermatophyte infections: clinical experience in Italy. *Brit J Clin Pract* **44** (Suppl 9): 115.

Dismukes WE, Bradsher RW, Cloud GC et al. (1992). Itraconazole therapy for blastomycosis and histoplasmosis. *Amer J Med* **93**: 489.

Drayton J, Dickinson G, Rinaldi M (1994). Coadministration of rifampin and itraconazole leads to undetectable levels of serum itraconazole. *Clin Infect Dis* **18**: 266.

Ducharme MP, Slaughter RL, Warbasse LH et al. (1995). Itraconazole and hydroxyitraconazole serum concentrations are reduced more than tenfold by phenytoin. *Clin Pharmacol Ther* **58**: 617.

Dupont B (1990). Itraconazole therapy in aspergillosis: Study in 49 patients. *J Amer Acad Dermatol* **23**: 607.

Dupont B, Drouhet E (1987). Early experience with itraconazole *in vitro* and in patients: Pharmacokinetic studies and clinical results. *Rev Infect Dis* **9** (Suppl 1): S71.

Duffill MB, Coley KE (1993). Cutaneous phaeohyphomycosis due to *Alternaria alternata* responding to itraconazole. *Clin Exp Dermatol* **18**: 156.

Duggan JM, Wolf MD, Kauffman CA (1995). *Phialophora verrucosa* infection in an AIDS patient. *Mycoses* **38**: 215.

Espinel-Ingroff A, Shadomy S, Gebhart RJ (1984). *In vitro* studies with R51,211 (itraconazole). *Antimicrob Ag Chemother* **26**: 5.

Faergemann J (1984). *In vitro* and *in vivo* activities of ketoconazole and itraconazole against *Pityrosporum orbiculare*. *Antimicrob Ag Chemother* **26**: 773.

Faergemann J (1988). Activity of triazole derivatives against *Pityrosporum orbiculare in vitro* and *in vivo*. *Ann NY Acad Sci* **544**: 348.

Fong IW (1992). The value of chronic suppressive therapy with itraconazole versus clotrimazole in women with recurrent vaginal candidiasis. *Genitourin Med* **68**: 374.

Ganer A, Arathoon E, Stevens DA (1987). Initial experience in therapy for progressive mycoses with itraconazole, the first clinically studied triazole. *Rev Infect Dis* **9** (Suppl 1): S77.

Gearhart MO (1994). Worsening of liver function with fluconazole and review of azole antifungal hepatotoxicity. *Ann Pharmacother* **28**: 1177.

Goldberg SL, Geha DJ, Marshall WF et al. (1993). Successful treatment of simultaneous pulmonary *Pseudallescheria boydii* and *Aspergillus terreus* infection with oral itraconazole. *Clin Infect Dis* **16**: 803.

Grant SM, Clissold SP (1989). Itraconazole A review of its pharmacodynamic and pharmacokinetic properties, and therapeutic use in superficial and systemic mycoses. *Drugs* **37**: 310.

Graybill JR, Stevens DA, Galgiani JN et al. (1990). Itraconazole treatment of coccidioidomycosis. *Amer J Med* **89**: 282.

Graybill JR, Vazquez J, Darouiche RO et al. (1995). Itraconazole oral solution (IS). versus fluconazole (F). treatment of oropharyngeal candidiasis (OC). In *Abstracts and Program of the 35th Interscience Conference on Antimicrobial Agents and Chemotherapy, San Francisco, California* (Abstr. 1220), p. 224. Washington, DC: American Society for Microbiology.

Gumaa SA, Mahgoub ES, Hay RJ (1992). Post-operative responses of paranasal *Aspergillus granuloma* to itraconazole. *Trans Roy Soc Trop Med Hyg* **86**: 93.

Hann SK, Kim JB, Im S *et al.* (1993). Itraconazole-induced acute hepatitis. *Brit J Dermatol* **129**: 500.

Hardin TC, Graybill JR, Fetchick R *et al.* (1988). Pharmacokinetics of itraconazole following oral administration to normal volunteers. *Antimicrob Ag Chemother* **32**: 1310.

Haron E, Anaissie E, Dumphy F *et al.* (1988). *Hansenula anomala* fungemia. *Rev Infect Dis* **10**: 1182.

Hay R, Clayton Y, Moore M, Midgeley G (1988). An evaluation of itraconazole in the management of onychomycosis. *Brit J Dermatol* **119**: 359.

Heykants J, Michiels M, Meuldermans W *et al.* (1987). The pharmacokinetics of itraconazole in animals and man: an overview. In *Recent Trends in the Discovery, Development and Evaluation of Antifungal Agents* (Fromtling RA, ed), p. 223. Barcelona: JR Prous Science Publishers.

Heykants J, Van Peer A, Van de Velde V *et al.* (1989). The clinical pharmacokinetics of itraconazole: an overview. *Mycoses* **32** (Suppl 1): 67.

Heymann WR, Manders SM (1995). Itraconazole-induced acute generalized exanthemic pustulosis. *J Amer Acad Dermatol* **33**: 130.

Hostetler JS, Hanson LH, Stevens DA (1992a). Effect of cyclodextrin on the pharmacology of antifungal oral azoles. *Antimicrob Ag Chemother* **36**: 477.

Hostetler JS, Denning DW, Stevens DA (1992b). US experience with itraconazole in *Aspergillus*, *Cryptococcus* and *Histoplasma* infections in the immunocompromised host. *Chemotherapy* **38** (Suppl 1): 12.

Hostetler JS, Heykants J, Clemons KV *et al.* (1993a). Discrepancies in bioassay and chromatography determinations explained by metabolism of itraconazole to hydroxyitraconazole: Studies of interpatient variations in concentrations. *Antimicrob Ag Chemother* **37**: 2224.

Hostetler JS, Hanson LH, Stevens DA (1993b). Effect of hydroxypropyl-β-cyclodextrin on efficacy of oral itraconazole in disseminated murine cryptococcosis. *J Antimicrob Chemother* **32**: 459.

Ishibashi Y, Matsumoto Y, Kabata T *et al.* (1990). Oral itraconazole and topical miconazole with debridement for *Acanthamoeba* keratitis. *Amer J Ophthalmol* **109**: 121.

Johnson EM, Davey KG, Szekely A, Warnock DW (1995). Itraconazole susceptibilities of fluconazole susceptible and resistant isolates of five *Candida* species. *J Antimicrob Chemother* **36**: 787.

Kan VL, Bennett JE (1988). Efficacies of four antifungal agents in experimental murine sporotrichosis. *Antimicrob Ag Chemother* **32**: 1619.

Katsambas A, Antoniou C, Frangouli E *et al.* (1993). Itraconazole in the treatment of tinea corporis and tinea cruris. *Clin Exp Dermatol* **18**: 322.

Kauffman CA (1995). Old and new therapies for sporotrichosis. *Clin Infect Dis* **21**: 981.

Kauffman CA, Bagnasco FA (1992). Digoxin toxicity associated with itraconazole therapy. *Clin Infect Dis* **15**: 886.

Kerkering TM, Espinel-Ingroff A (1987). *In vitro* synergistic activity of itraconazole and 5-flourocytosine against *Aspergillus fumigatus* and *Aspergillus flavus*. In *Recent Trends in the Discovery, Development and Evaluation of Antifungal Agents* (Fromtling RA, ed), p. 61. Barcelona: JR Prous Science Publishers.

Klippenstein K, O'Day DM, Robinson RD *et al.* (1993). The qualitative evaluation of the pharmacokinetics of subconjunctivally injected antifungal agents in rabbits. *Cornea* **12**: 512.

Korting HC, Schafer-Korting M, Zienicke H *et al.* (1993). Treatment of tinea unguium with medium and high doses of ultramicrosize griseofulvin compared with that with itraconazole. *Antimicrob Ag Chemother* **37**: 2064.

Kramer MR, Marshall SE, Denning DW *et al.* (1990). Cyclosporine and itraconazole interaction in heart and lung transplant recipients. *Ann Intern Med* **113**: 327.

Kramer MR, Denning DW, Marshall SE *et al.* (1991). Ulcerative tracheobronchitis after lung transplantation. A new form of invasive aspergillosis. *Amer Rev Resp Dis* **144**: 552.

Kriesel W, Kochling G, von Schilling C *et al.* (1991). Therapy of invasive aspergillosis with itraconazole: improvement of therapeutic efficacy by early diagnosis. *Mycoses* **44**: 385.

Kwan J, Foxall P, Davidson D *et al.* (1987). Interaction of cyclosporin and itraconazole. *Lancet* **ii**: 282.

Lachapelle JM, De Doncker P, Tennstedt D *et al.* (1992). Itraconazole compared with griseofulvin in the treatment of tinea corporis/cruris and tinea pedis/manus: An interpretation of the clinical results of all completed double-blind studies with respect to the pharmacokinetic profile. *Dermatol* **184**: 45.

Lafeuillade A, Chaffanjon P, Delbeke E, Quilichini R (1992). Maintenance itraconazole for visceral leishmaniasis in HIV infection. *Amer J Med* **92**: 449.

Lanigman SW (1992). Cutaneous *Alternaria* infection treated with itraconazole. *Brit J Dermatol* **127**: 39.

Larosa F, Cauwenbergh G, Cilli P *et al.* (1986). Itraconazole pharmacokinetics in the female genital tract: plasma and tissue levels in patients undergoing hysterectomy after a single dose of 200 mg itraconazole. *Eur J Obstet Gynecol* **23**: 85.

Lau YL, Yuen KY, Lee CW, Chan CF (1995). Invasive *Acremonium falciforme* infection in a patient with severe combined immunodeficiency. *Clin Infect Dis* **20**: 197–198.

Lavalle P, Suchil P, De Ovando F, Reynoso S (1987). Itraconazole for deep mycoses: preliminary experience in Mexico. *Rev Infect Dis* **9** (Suppl 1): S64.

Lavrijsen K, Van Houdt J, Thijs D *et al.* (1986). Induction potential of antifungals containing an imidazole or triazole moiety: miconazole and ketoconazole, but not itraconazole, are able to induce hepatic drug metabolizing enzymes of male rats at high doses. *Biochem Pharmacol* **35**: 1867.

Lavrijsen APM, Balmus KJ, Nugteren-Huying WM *et al.* (1992). Hepatic injury associated with itraconazole. *Lancet* **340**: 251.

Lee MW, Kim JC, Choi JS *et al.* (1995). Mycetoma caused by *Acremonium falciforme*: successful treatment with itraconazole. *J Amer Acad Dermatol* **32**: 897.

Legendre R, Esola-Macre J (1990). Itraconazole in the treatment of tinea capitis. *J Amer Acad Dermatol* **23**: 559.

Le Guennec R, Reynes J, Mallie M *et al.* (1995). Fluconazole- and itraconazole-resistant *Candida albicans* from AIDS patients: multilocus enzyme electrophoresis analysis and antifungal susceptibilities. *J Clin Microbiol* **33**: 2732.

Lesperance M, Baumgartner D, Kauffman CA (1988). Polyarticular arthritis due to *Sporothrix schenckii*. *Mycoses* **31**: 599.

Liao WQ, Yao ZR, Li ZQ *et al.* (1995). Pyoderma gangrenosum caused by *Rhizopus arrhizus*. *Mycoses* **38**: 75.

Lim SG, Sawyerr AM, Hudson M *et al.* (1993). The absorption of fluconazole and itraconazole under conditios of low intragastric acidity. *Aliment Pharmacol Ther* **7**: 317.

Longman LP, Martin MV (1987). A comparison of the efficacy of itraconazole, amphotericin B and 5-fluorocytosine in the treatment of *Aspergillus fumigatus* endocarditis in the rabbit. *J Antimicrob Chemother* **20**: 719.

Lopez -Gomez S, Del palacio A, Van Cutsem J *et al.* (1994). Itraconazole versus griseofulvin in the treatment of tinea capitis: a double-blind randomized study in children. *Int J Dermatol* **33**: 743.

Martin E, Parras P, Lozano MC (1992). *In vitro* susceptibility of 245 yeast isolates to amphotericin B, 5-fluorocytosine, ketoconazole, fluconazole and itraconazole. *Chemotherapy* **38**: 335.

May DB, Drew RH, Yedinak KC, Bartlett JA (1994). Effect of simultaneous didanosine administration on itraconazole absorption in healthy volunteers. *Pharmacother* **14**: 509.

McCabe RE, Remington JS, Araujo FG (1986). *In vitro* and *in vivo* effects of itraconazole against *Trypanosoma cruzi*. *Amer J Trop Med Hyg* **35**: 280.

McClean KL, Sheehan GJ (1994). Interaction between itraconazole and digoxin. *Clin Infect Dis* **18**: 259.

Miyazaki HM, Kohno S, Miyazaki Y *et al.* (1993). Efficacy of intravenous itraconazole against experimental pulmonary aspergillosis. *Antimicrob Ag Chemother* **37**: 2762.

Moller Heilesen A (1986). Hair loss during itraconazole treatment. *Brit Med J* **293**: 823.

Monahan BP, Ferguson CL, Killeavy ES *et al.* (1990). Torsades de pointes occurring in association with terfenadine use. *JAMA* **264**: 2788.

Moreno F, Hardin TC, Rinaldi MG, Graybill JR (1993). Itraconazole-didanosine interaction. *JAMA* **269**: 1506.

Moskovitz BL, Wilcox CM, Darouiche R *et al.* (1996). Itraconazole oral solution (IS). compared with fluconazole (F) for treatment of esophageal candidiasis. *Proc XI International Conference on AIDS, Vancouver, Canada* (Abstr. MoB116).

Naqvi SH, Becherer P, Gudipati S (1993). Ketoconazole treatment of a family with zoonotic sporotrochosis. *Scand J Infect Dis* **25**: 543.

Naranjo MS, Trujillo M, Munera MI *et al.* (1990). Treatment of paracoccidioidomycosis with itraconazole. *J Med Vet Mycol* **28**: 67.

Negroni R, Palmieri O, Koren F *et al.* (1987). Oral treatment of paracoccidioidomycosis and histoplasmosis with itraconazole in humans. *Rev Infect Dis* **1987** (Suppl 1): S47.

Negroni R, Robles AM, Arechavala A, Taborda A (1989). Itraconazole in human histoplasmosis. *Mycoses* **32**: 123.

Negroni R, Taborda A, Robies AM, Archevala A (1992). Itraconazole in the treatment of histoplasmosis associated with AIDS. *Mycoses* **35**: 281.

Nelson MR, Smith D, Erskine D, Gazzard BG (1993). Ventricular fibrillation secondary to itraconazole induced hypokalemia. *J Infect* **26**: 348.

Ninane J, Sluysmans T, Vermylen C *et al.* (1988). Itraconazole versus ketoconazole for the prophylaxis of fungal infection in neutropenic children. Results of two non-randomised studies. *Pediatr Hematol Oncol* **6**: 349.

Novakava L, Donelly P, De Witte T *et al.* (1987). Itraconazole and cyclosporin nephrotoxicity. *Lancet* **ii**: 920.

Odds FC (1993). Resistance of yeasts to azole-derivative antifungals. *J Antimicrob Chemother* **31**: 463.

Odds FC, Webster CE, Abbott AB (1984). Antifungal relative inhibition factors: Bay 1–9319, bifonazole, butoconazole, isoconazole, itraconazole (R 51,211), oxiconazole, RO 14–4767/002, sulconazole, terconazole and vibunazole (Bay n-7133) compared *in vitro* with nine established antifungal agents. *J Antimicrob Chemother* **14**: 105.

Olkkola KT, Backman JT, Neuvonen PJ (1994). Midazolam should be avoided in patients receiving the systemic antimycotics ketoconazole and itraconazole. *Clin Pharmacol Ther* **55**: 481.

Olkkola KT, Ahonen J, Neuvonen PJ (1996). The effects of the systemic antimycotics, itraconazole and fluconazole, on the pharmacokinetics and pharmacodynamics of intravenous and oral midazolam. *Anesthes Analges* **82**: 511.

Panagiotidou D, Kousidou T, Chaidemenos G *et al.* (1992). A comparison of itraconazole and griseofulvin in the treatment of tinea corporis and tinea cruris: a double-blind study. *J Int Med Res* **20**: 392.

Pappas PG, Threlkeld MG, Bedsole GD *et al.* (1993). Blastomycosis in immunocompromised patients. *Medicine* **72**: 311.

Pariser DM, Pariser RJ, Ruoff G, Ray TL (1994). Double-blind comparison of itraconazole and placebo in the treatment of tinea corporis and tinea cruris. *J Amer Acad Dermatol* **31**: 232.

Patterson TF, Andriole VT, Zervos MJ *et al.* (1990). The epidemiology of pseudallescheriasis complicating transplantation: Nosocomial and community-acquired infection. *Mycoses* **33**: 297.

Patterson TF, Fothergill AW, Rinaldi MG (1993). Efficacy of itraconazole solution in a rabbit model of invasive aspergillosis. *Antimicrob Ag Chemother* **37**: 2307.

Perfect JR, Durack DT (1985). Penetration of imidazole and triazoles into cerebrospinal fluid in rabbits. *J Antimicrob Chemother* **16**: 81.

Perfect JR, Savani DV, Durack DT (1986). Comparison of itraconazole and fluconazole in treatment of cryptococcal meningitis and candida pyelonephritis in rabbits. *Antimicrob Ag Chemother* **29**: 579.

Perfect JR, Savani DV, Durack DT (1993). Uptake of itraconazole by alveolar macrophages. *Antimicrob Ag Chemother* **37**: 903.

Persat F, Marzullo C, Guyotat D *et al.* (1992). Plasma itraconazole concentrations in neutropenic patients after repeated high-dose treatment. *Eur J Cancer* **28A**: 838.

Peters-Christodoulou MN, de Beer FC, Bots GTAM *et al.* (1991). Treatment of postoperative *Aspergillus fumigatus* spondylodiscitis with itraconazole. *Scand J Infect Dis* **23**: 373.

Petrou MA, Rogers TR (1988). *In-vitro* activity of antifungal agents in combination with four quinolones. *Drugs Exp Clin Res* **14**: 9.

Petrou MA, Rogers TR (1991). Interactions *in vitro* between polyenes and imidazoles against yeast. *J Antimicrob Chemother* **27**: 491.

Phillips P, Graybill JR, Fetchick R, Dunn JF (1987a). Adrenal responses to corticotropin during therapy with itraconazole. *Antimicrob Ag Chemother* **31**: 647.

Phillips P, Fetchick R, Weisman I *et al.* (1987b). Tolerance to and efficacy of itraconazole in treatment of systemic mycoses: Preliminary results. *Rev Infect Dis* **9** (Suppl 1): S87.

Phillips P, Bryce G, Shepherd J, Mintz D (1990). Invasive external otitis caused by *Aspergillus*. *Rev Infect Dis* **12**: 277.

Pialoux G, Hennequin C, Dupont B, Ravisse P (1990). Cutaneous leishmaniasis in an AIDS patient: cure with itraconazole. *J Infect Dis* **102**: 1221.

Piepponen T, Blomqvist K, Brandt H *et al.* (1992). Efficacy and safety of itraconazole in the long-term treatment of onychomycosis. *J Antimicrob Chemother* **29**: 195.

Piper JP, Golden J, Brown D, Broestler J (1990). Successful treatment of *Scedosporium apiospermum* suppurative arthritis with itraconazole. *Pediatr Infect Dis J* **9**: 674.

Pohjola-Sintonen S, Viitasalo M, Toivonene L, Neuvonen P (1993). Torsades de pointes after terfenadine-itraconazole interaction. *Brit Med J* **306**: 186.

Polak A (1987). Combination therapy of experimental candidiasis, cryptococcosis, aspergillosis and wangiellosis in mice. *Chemotherapy* **33**: 381.

Polak A (1989). Combination therapy for systemic mycosis. *Infection* **17**: 203.

Ponce E, Pechere JC (1990). Activity of amphotericin B and itraconazole against intraphagocytic *Candida albicans*. *Eur J Microbiol Infect Dis* **9**: 738.

Prentice AG, Warnock DW, Johnson SA *et al.* (1994). Multiple dose pharmacokinetics of an oral solution of itraconazole in autologous bone marrow transplant recipients. *J Antimicrob Chemother* **34**: 247.

Prentice AG, Warnock DW, Johnson SA *et al.* (1995). Multiple dose pharmacokinetics of an oral solution of itraconazole in patients receiving chemotherapy for acute myeloid leukemia. *J Antimicrob Chemother* **36**: 657.

Queiroz-Telles F, Purim KS, Fillus JN *et al.* (1992). Itraconazole in the treatment of chromoblastomycosis due to *Fonsecaea pedrosoi*. *Int J Dermatol* **31**: 805.

Raffi F, Merrien D, Le Page P, Reliquet V (1995). Use of an itraconazole/allopurinol combination for the treatment of visceral leishmaniasis in a patient with AIDS. *Clin Infect Dis* **21**: 1338.

Rees T, Phillips R (1992). Multicenter comparison of one-day oral therapy with fluconazole or itraconazole in vaginal candidiasis. *Int J Gynecol Obstet* **37** (Suppl): 33.

Reiss P, Hadderingh R, Schot LJ, Danner SA (1991). Invasive external otitis caused by *Aspergillus fumigatus* in two patients with AIDS. *AIDS* **5**: 605.

Remmel RP, Dombrovskis D, Canafax DM (1988). Assay of itraconazole in leukemic patients plasma by reverse phase small-bore liquid chromatography. *J Chromatogr Biomed Appl* **432**: 388.

Restrepo A. (1994). Treatment of tropical mycoses. *J Amer Acad Dermatol* **31**: 591.

Restrepo A, Gomez I, Cano LE *et al.* (1983). Treatment of paracoccidioidomycosis with ketoconazole: a 3-year experience. *Amer J Med* **74** (Suppl 1B): 48.

Restrepo A, Robledo J, Gomez I *et al.* (1986). Itraconazole therapy in lymphangitic and cutaneous sporotrichosis. *Arch Dermatol* **122**: 413.

Reuben A, Anaissie E, Nelson PE *et al.* (1989). Antifungal susceptibility of 44 clinical isolates of *Fusarium* species determined by using a broth microdilution method. *Antimicrob Ag Chemother* **33**: 1647.

Rex J (1992). Itraconazole-digoxin interaction. *Ann Intern Med* **116**: 525.

Robertson LI (1987). Itraconazole in the treatment of widespread tinea versicolor. *Clin Exp Dermatol* **12**: 178.

Rongioletti F, Robert E, Tripodi S *et al.* (1992). Treatment of onychomycosis with itraconazole. *J Dermatol Treatm* **2**: 155.

Roseeuw D, Willemsen M, 'T Kint R *et al.* (1990). Itraconazole in the treatment of superficial mycoses – a double-blind study vs placebo. *Clin Exp Dermatol* **15**: 101.

Rosen T (1994). Debilitating edema associated with itraconazole. *Arch Dermatol* **130**: 260.

Saag MS, Cloud GC, Graybill JR *et al.* (1995). Comparison of fluconazole (FLU) versus itraconazole (ITRA) as maintenance therapy of AIDS-associated cryptococcal meningitis. In *Abstracts and Program of the 35th Interscience Conference on Antimicrobial Agents and Chemotherapy, San Francisco, California* (Abstr. 1218), p. 244. Washington, DC: American Society for Microbiology.

Sachs MK, Paluzzi RG, Moore JH *et al.* (1990). Amphotericin-resistant aspergillus osteomyelitis controlled by itraconazole. *Lancet* **335**: 1475.

Sachs MK, Blanchard LM, Green PJ (1993). Interaction of itraconazole and digoxin. *Clin Infect Dis* **16**: 400.

Salkin IF, McGinnis MR, Dykstra MJ, Rinaldi MG (1988). *Scedosporium inflatum*, an emerging pathogen. *J Clin Microbiol* **26**: 498.

Sampol E, Lacarelle B, Rajaonarison JF *et al.* (1995). Comparative effects of antifungal agents on zidovudine glucuronidation by human liver microsomes. *Brit J Clin Pharmacol* **40**: 83.

San-Blas G, Calcagno AM, San-Blas F (1993). A preliminary study of *in vitro* antibiotic activity of saperconazole and other azoles on *Paracoccidioides brasiliensis*. *J Med Vet Mycol* **31**: 169.

Sanz Sanz F, del Palacio Hernanz A (1987). Randomized comparative trial of three regimens of itraconazole for treatment of vaginal mycoses. *Rev Infect Dis* **9** (Suppl 1): S139.

Saul A, Bonifaz A, Arias I (1987). Itraconazole in the treatment of superficial mycoses: An open trial of 40 cases. *Rev Infect Dis* **9** (Suppl 1): S100.

Savani DV, Perfect JR, Cobo M, Durack DT (1987). Penetration of new azole compounds into the eye and efficacy in experimental *Candida* endophthalmitis. *Antimicrob Ag Chemother* **31**: 6.

Schafer-Korting U, Korting HC, Lukacs A *et al.* (1990). Levels of itraconazole in skin blister fluid after a single oral dose and during repetitive administration. *J Amer Acad Dermatol* **22**: 211.

Schaffner A, Bohler A (1993). Amphotericin B refractory aspergillosis after itraconazole – evidence for significant antagonism. *Mycoses* **36**: 421.

Schulman JA, Peyman GA, Dietlein J, Fiscella R (1991). Ocular toxicity of experimental intravitreal itraconazole. *Int Ophthalmol* **15**: 21.

Sekhon AS, Padhye AA, Garg AK (1992). *In vitro* sensitivity of *Penicillium marneffei* and *Pythium insidiosum* to various antifungal agents. *Eur J Epidemiol* **8**: 427.

Sekhon AS, Padhye AA, Garg AK *et al.* (1994). *In vitro* sensitivity of medically significant *Fusarium* species to various antimycotics. *Chemotherapy* **40**: 239.

Sharkey PK, Rinaldi MG, Dunn JF *et al.* (1991). High-dose itraconazole in the treatment of severe mycoses. *Antimicrob Ag Chemother* **35**: 707.

Sharkey-Mathis PK, Velez J, Fetchick R, Graybill JR (1993a). Histoplasmosis in the acquired immunodeficiency syndrome (AIDS): Treatment with itraconazole and fluconazole. *J AIDS* **6**: 809.

Sharkey-Mathis PK, Kauffman CA, Graybill JR *et al.* (1993b). Treatment of sporotrichosis with itraconazole. *Amer J Med* **95**: 279.

Silva Cruz A, Andrade L, Sobral L, Francisca A (1991). Itraconazole versus placebo in the management of vaginal candidiasis. *Int J Gynecol Obstet* **36**: 229.

Smith DE, Midgley J, Allan M *et al.* (1991). Itraconazole versus ketoconazole in the treatment of oral and oesophageal candidosis in patients infected with HIV. *AIDS* **5**: 1367.

Smith D Van de Velde V, Woestenborghs R, Gazzard BG (1992). The pharmacokinetics of oral itraconazole in AIDS patients. *J Pharm Pharmacol* **44**: 618.

Smith KJ, Warnock DW, Kennedy CTC *et al.* (1986). Azole resistance in *Candida albicans*. *J Med Vet Mycol* **24**: 133.

Soto-Mancipe J, Grogl M, Berman JD (1993). Evaluation of pentamidine for the treatment of cutaneous leishmaniasis in Colombia. *Clin Infect Dis* **16**: 417.

Spencer DA, John P, Ferryman SR *et al.* (1994). Successful treatment of invasive pulmonary aspergillosis in chronic granulomatous disease with orally administered itraconazole suspension. *Amer J Respir Crit Care Med* **149**: 239.

Staib F, Seibold M, L'Age M (1990). Persistence of *Cryptococcus neoformans* in seminal fluid and urine under itraconazole treatment. The urogenital tract (prostate) as a niche for *Cryptococcus neoformans*. *Mycoses* **33**: 369.

Stein A, Daneshmend T, Warnock D *et al.* (1988). The effects of H2-receptor antagonists on the pharmacokinetics of itraconazole, a new oral antifungal. *Brit J Clin Pharmacol* **27**: 105P.

Stein GE, Mummaw N (1993). Placebo-controlled trial of itraconazole for treatment of acute vaginal candidiasis. *Antimicrob Ag Chemother* **37**: 89.

Stolk-Engelaar MV, Cox NJ (1993). Successful treatment of pulmonary pseudallescheriasis with itraconazole. *Eur J Clin Microbiol Infect Dis* **12**: 142.

Sud IJ, Feingold DS (1981). Mechanisms of action of the antimycotic imidazoles. *J Invest Dermatol* **76**: 438.

Sud IJ, Chou DL, Feingold DS (1979). Effect of free fatty acids on liposome susceptibility to imidazole antifungals. *Antimicrob Ag Chemother* **16**: 660.

Supparatpinyo K, Chiewchanvit S, Hirunsri P *et al.* (1992). An efficacy study in the treatment of *Penicillium marneffei* infection. *J Med Assoc Thai* **75**: 688.

Supparatpinyo K, Nelson KE, Merz WG *et al.* (1993). Response to antifungal therapy by human immunodeficiency virus-infected patients with disseminated *Penicillium marneffei* infections and *in vitro* susceptibilities of isolates from clinical specimens. *Antimicrob Ag Chemother* **37**: 2407.

Tailor SA, Gupta AK, Walker SE, Shear NH (1996). Peripheral edema due to nidefipine-intraconazole interaction: a case report. *Arch Dermatol* **132**: 350.

Tam M, Freeman S (1989). Phaeohyphomycosis due to *Phialophora richardsiae*. *Australas J Dermatol* **30**: 37.

Tang WY, Lo KK, Lam WY *et al.* (1995). Cutaneous protothecosis: report of a case in Hong Kong. *Brit J Dermatol* **133**: 479.

Thunnissen PLM, Sizoo W, Hendriks WDH (1991). Safety and efficacy of itraconazole in prevention of fungal infections in neutropenic patients. *Neth J Med* **39**: 84.

Timonen H, Hartikainen-Vahtera P, Kivijarvi A *et al.* (1992). A double-blind comparison of the effectiveness of itraconazole capsules to econazole vaginal capsules in the treatment of vaginal candidosis. *Drug Invest* **4**: 515.

Tobin JM, Loo P, Granger SE (1992). Treatment of vaginal candidosis: a comparative study of the efficacy and acceptability of itraconazole and clotrimazole. *Genitourin Med* **68**: 36.

Todeschini G, Murari C, Bonesi R *et al.* (1993). Oral itraconazole plus nasal amphotericin B for prophylaxis of invasive aspergillosis in patients with hematological malignancies. *Eur J Clin Microbiol Infect Dis* **12**: 614.

Trenk D, Brett W, Jahnchen E, Birnbaum D (1987). Time course of cyclosporin/itraconazole interaction. *Lancet* **ii**: 1335.

Tricot G, Joosten E, Boogaerts MA *et al.* (1987). Ketoconazole vs itraconazole for antifungal prophylaxis in patients with severe granulocytopenia: Preliminary results of two nonrandomized studies. *Rev Infect Dis* **9** (Suppl 1): S94.

Tucker RM, Denning DW, Dupont B, Stevens DA (1990a). Itraconazole therapy for chronic coccidioidal meningitis. *An Intern Med* **112**: 108.

Tucker RM, Haq Y, Denning DW, Stevens DA (1990b). Adverse events associated with itraconazole in 189 patients on chronic therapy. *J Antimicrob Chemother* **26**: 561.

Tucker RM, Denning DW, Hanson LH *et al.* (1992). Interaction of azoles with rifampin, phenytoin, and carbamazepine: *In vitro* and clinical observations. *Clin Infect Dis* **14**: 165.

Van Cauteren H, Heykants J, De Coster R, Cauwenbergh G (1987). Itraconazole: Pharmacological studies in animals and humans. *Rev Infect Dis* **9** (Suppl 1): S43.

Van Cauteren H, Lampo A, Vandenberghe J *et al.* (1989). Toxicological profile and safety evaluation of antifungal azole derivatives. *Mycoses* **32** (Suppl 1): 60.

Van Cutsem J (1989). The *in-vitro* antifungal spectrum of itraconazole. *Mycoses* **32** (Suppl 1): 7.

Van Cutsem J, Van Gerven F, Janssen PAJ (1987). Activity of orally, topically, and parenterally administered itraconazole in the treatment of superficial and deep mycoses: Animal models. *Rev Infect Dis* **9** (Suppl 1): S15.

van den Anker JN (1992). Treatment of neonatal *Candida albicans* septicemia with itraconazole. *Pediatr Infect Dis J* **11**: 684.

Vanden Bossche H, Bellens D, Cools W *et al.* (1986). Cytochrome P-450: target for itraconazole. *Drug Dev Res* **8**: 287.

Vanden Bossche H, Marichal P, Gorrens J, Coene M-C (1990). Biochemical basis for the activity and selectivity of oral antifungal drugs. *Brit J Clin Pract* **71** (Suppl). 41.

Vanden Bossche H, Marichal P, le Jeune L *et al.* (1993). Effects of itraconazole on cytochrome P-450-dependent sterol 14 demethylation and reduction of 3-ketosteroids in *Cryptococcus neoformans. Antimicrob Ag Chemother* **37**: 2101.

Van Peer A, Woestenborghs R, Heykants J *et al.* (1989). The effects of food on the oral systemic availability of itraconazole in healthy subjects. *Eur J Clin Pharmacol* **36**: 423.

van 't Wout JW, Mattie H, Van Furth R (1989). Comparison of the efficacies of amphotericin B, fluconazole, and itraconazole against a systemic *Candida albicans* infection in normal and neutropenic mice. *Antimicrob Ag Chemother* **33**: 147.

van 't Wout JW, Meynaar I, Linde I *et al.* (1990a). Effect of amphotericin B, fluconazole and itraconazole on intracellular *C. albicans* and germ tube development in macrophages. *J Antimicrob Chemother* **25**: 803.

van 't Wout JW, Raven EJM, van der Meer JWM (1990b). Treatment of invasive aspergillosis with itraconazole in a patient with chronic granulomatous disease. *J Infect* **20**: 147.

van 't Wout JW, Novakova I, Verhagen CAH *et al.* (1991). The efficacy of itraconazole against systemic fungal infections in neutropenic patients: a randomised comparative study with amphotericin B. *J Infect* **22**: 45.

Venugopal, PV, Venugopal TV, Ramakrishna ES, Ilavarasi S (1993). Antimycotic susceptibility testing of agents of black grain eumycetoma. *J Med Vet Mycol* **31**: 161.

Viviani MA, Tortorano AM, Giani PC *et al.* (1987). Itraconazole for cryptococcal infection in the acquired immunodeficiency syndrome. *Ann Intern Med* **106**: 166.

Viviani MA, Tortorano AM, Langer M *et al.* (1989). Experience with itraconazole in cryptococcosis and aspergillosis. *J Infect* **18**: 151.

Viviani MA, Tortorano AM, Pagano A *et al.* (1990). European experience with itraconazole in systemic mycoses. *J Amer Acad Dermatol* **23**: 587.

Vreugdenhil G, Van Dijke BJ, Donnelly JP *et al.* (1993). Efficacy of itraconazole in the prevention of fungal infections among neutropenic patients with hematologic malignancies and intensive chemotherapy. A double-blind, placebo controlled study. *Leuk Lymphoma* **11**: 353.

Walsh M, White L, Atkinson K, Enno A (1992). Fungal *Pseudallescheria boydii* lung infiltrates unresponsive to amphotericin B in leukaemic patients. *Aust NZ J Med* **22**: 265.

Walsh TJ, Hiemenz JW, Anaissie E (1996). Recent progress and current problems in treatment of invasive fungal infections in neutropenic patients. *Infect Dis Clin N Amer* **10**: 365.

Walsøe I, Stangerup M, Svejgaard E (1990). Itraconazole in onychomycosis. Open and double-blind studies. *Acta Derm Venereol* **70**: 137.

Warnock DW, Turner A, Burke J (1988). Comparison of high performance liquid chromatographic and microbiological methods for determination of itraconazole. *J Antimicrob Chemother* **21**: 93.

Watkins DN, Badcock NR, Thompson PJ (1992). Itraconazole concentrations in airway fluid and tissue. *Brit J Clin Pharmacol* **33**: 206.

Wesel S (1990). Itraconazole: a single-day oral treatment for acute vulvovaginal candidosis. *Brit J Clin Pract Symp* **71** (Suppl): 77.

Wheat J (1994). Histoplasmosis and coccidioidomycosis in individuals with AIDS. A clinical review. *Infect Dis Clinics N Amer* **8**: 467.

Wheat J, Hafner R, Wulfsohn M *et al.* (1993). Prevention of relapse of histoplasmosis with itraconazole in patients with the acquired immunodeficiency syndrome. *Ann Intern Med* **118**: 610.

Wheat J, Hafner R, Korzun AH *et al.* (1995). Itraconazole treatment of disseminated histoplasmosis in patients with the acquired immunodeficiency syndrome. AIDS Clinical Trial Group. *Amer J Med* **98**: 336.

Wheat LJ, Connolly-Stringfield PA, Baker RL *et al.* (1990). Disseminated histoplasmosis in the acquired immunodeficiency syndrome: Clinical findings, diagnosis and treatment, and review of the literature. *Medicine* **69**: 361–374.

White DJ, Johnson EM, Warnock DW (1993). Management of persistent vulvovaginal candidosis due to azole-resistant *Candida glabrata. Genitourin Med* **69**: 112.

Whittle DI, Kominos S (1995). Use of itraconazole for treating subcutaneous phaeohyphomycosis caused by *Exophiala jeanselmei. Clin Infect Dis* **21**: 1068.

Willemson M, De Doncker P, Willems J *et al.* (1992). Posttreatment itraconazole levels in the nail: new implications for treatment of onychomycosis. *J Amer Acad Dermatol* **26**: 731.

Williamson PR, Kwon-Chung KJ, Gallin JI (1992). Successful treatment of *Paecilomyces varioti* infection in a patient with chronic granulomatous disease and a review of *Paecilomyces* species infection. *Clin Infect Dis* **14**: 1023.

Wishart JM (1987). The influence of food on the pharmacokinetics of itraconazole in patients with superficial fungal infection. *J Amer Acad Dermatol* **17**: 220.

Wong PW, Ching WTW, Kwon-Chung KJ, Meyer RD (1989). Disseminated *Phialophora parasitica* infection in humans: Case report and review. *Rev Infect Dis* **11**: 770.

Wood GM, McCormack JG, Muir DB *et al.* (1992). Clinical features of human infection with *Scedosporium inflatum. Clin Infect Dis* **14**: 1027.

Working Party of the British Society for Antimicrobial Chemotherapy (1993). Working Party Report: Chemoprophylaxis for candidosis and aspergillosis in neutropenia and transplantation: a review and recommendations. *J Antimicrob Chemother* **32**: 5.

Yeh J, Soo S-C, Summerton C, Richardson C (1990). Potentiation of action of warfarin by itraconazole. *Brit Med J* **301**: 669.

Yu R (1995). Successful treatment of chromoblastomycosis with itraconazole. *Mycoses* **38**: 79.

Zaitz C, Porto E, Heins-Vaccari EM *et al.* (1995). Subcutaneous hyalohyphomycosis caused by *Acremonium recifei*: case report. *Rev Inst Med Trop Sao Paulo* **37**: 267.

Zimmerman T, Yeates RA, Laufen H *et al.* (1994). Influence of concomitant food intake on the oral absorption of two triazole antifungal agents, itraconazole and fluconazole. *Eur J Clin Pharmacol* **46**: 147.

Miconazole

Description

Miconazole is a phenethyl imidazole derivative, and was synthesized at Janssen Pharmaceutica Research Laboratories in Belgium (Godefroi et al., 1969). It is practically insoluble in water, needs to be solubilized in polyethoxylated castor oil (1% 'Cremophor' EL) and ethanol (10%) for i.v. administration, and has the chemical formula of 1-(2-(2,4-dichlorophenyl)-2-[(2,4-dichlorophenyl)methoxy)ethyl]-1H- imidazole. The topical preparations including vaginal preparations are miconazole nitrate and have the chemical name 1-[2,4-dichloro-beta-(2,4-dichloro-benzyloxy)phenethyl]imidazole nitrate.

This drug is used topically to treat superficial fungal and dermatophyte infections and by the i.v. route to treat certain deep mycoses, in particular *Pseudallescheria boydii* infections and refractory cryptococcal meningitis. Although it has a wide antifungal spectrum of activity *in vitro*, the toxicity associated with its use, limited therapeutic efficacy and lack of comparative trials with amphotericin B, has assigned miconazole to a second-line antifungal agent.

Sensitive Organisms

Miconazole has a wide range of antifungal activity *in vitro* (Brugmans et al., 1972; Van Cutsem and Thienpont, 1972).

1 Pathogenic yeasts

Cryptococcus neoformans is usually sensitive to miconazole, but for the treatment of murine cryptococcosis it is much less effective than amphotericin B (Graybill et al., 1978). Reported results of sensitivity testing of *Candida albicans* show considerable variation within strains, and also between different studies. Reported MICs for *C. albicans* have been in the range 0.5–32 μg per ml (Holbrook and Kippax, 1979). This may be attributable to the difficulty in obtaining reproducibility in different test procedures (Shadomy et al., 1977). When large numbers of isolates were tested, a high degree of susceptibility of *C. albicans* to miconazole has been demonstrated (Bannatyne and Cheung, 1978; Moody et al., 1980). More than 85% of 315 strains of *C. albicans* were susceptible to 0.5 μg per ml of the drug, with only a few strains requiring 2–4 μg per ml for inhibition (Moody et al., 1980). They also found MICs of 24 μg per ml for *C. tropicalis* and 1 μg per ml for *C. krusei*. Miconazole is efficacious for the treatment of disseminated candidiasis in rats (Balk et al., 1978). The majority of strains of *C. glabrata* are inhibited by a concentration of 4.0 μg per ml (Moody et al., 1980). *Pityrosporum orbicularis* (*Malassezia furfur*), the causative agent of tinea versicolor, is quite sensitive.

2 Dimorphic fungi

Histoplasma capsulatum, *Paracoccidioides brasiliensis* and *Blastomyces dermatitidis* are very sensitive. *Coccidioides immitis* is less sensitive to miconazole but, in experimental murine coccidioidomycosis, it has a marked therapeutic effect protecting all mice from 50 and 100% lethal doses (Levine et al., 1975). *Sporothrix schenckii* is usually only moderately sensitive.

3 Molds or filamentous fungi

The *Cladosporium* spp. and the *Phialophora* spp. are usually sensitive. *Aspergillus* spp. vary in susceptibility to miconazole, with 39% of isolates with an MIC less than 5 μg per ml (Denning et al., 1992). However, miconazole was not effective in the experimental model of aspergillosis (Fromtling, 1988). Miconazole has good activity against *Penicillium marneffei* (Sekhon et al., 1992). Miconazole has variable activity against *Fusarium* spp. (Reuben et al., 1989). Some of the agents which cause fungal mycetoma, such as *Madurella mycetomii*, are quite sensitive. Lutwick *et al.* (1976) showed that some clinical isolates of *Pseudallescheria boydii* (*Petriellidium boydii, Monosporium apiospermum*) were very sensitive (MIC < 0.25 µg per ml). Miconazole is very active against the dermatophytes, particularly *Trichophyton mentagrophytes*, *T. rubrum* and *Epidermophyton floccosum* and *in vivo* efficacy with topical miconazole has been demonstrated in guinea pigs with cutaneous infections with *T. mentagrophytes and Microsporum canis* (Van Cutsem and Thienpont, 1972). In the presence of 0.5 µg per ml miconazole *in vitro*, complete inhibition .of germ tube elongation of hyphae of *T. mentagrophytes* occurred, which was completely irreversible (Scott *et al.*, 1985). Species of the genera *Mucor, Rhizopus* and *Absidia* are resistant (Eng *et al.*, 1981), but those of the genera *Basidiobolus* and *Conidiobolus* are sensitive (Yangco *et al.*, 1984a).

4 Actinomycetes

Bacteria of the *Nocardia* and *Actinomadura* spp. which cause actinomycetoma are quite sensitive.

5 Other bacteria

Some Gram-positive cocci and bacilli are sensitive to miconazole. The MIC of miconazole for *Streptococcus pyogenes* is 0.01 µg per ml (Van Cutsem and Thienpont, 1972) and that for *Strep. agalactiae* is 2.8 µg per ml (De Louvois, 1980). Miconazole is also bactericidal against *Staphylococcus aureus* (Sud and Feingold, 1982).

6 Prototheca spp

Some species of these achloric algae which cause human infection (protothecosis) are sensitive (Segal *et al.*, 1976).

7 Naegleria

The growth of *Naegleria fowleri*, the cause of primary amebic meningoencephalitis in humans, is suppressed in culture by miconazole (Thong *et al.*, 1977).

8 Acanthamoebae

Fresh water amebae such as *Acanthamoeba polyphaga* and *A. castellanii* can cause suppurative corneal and intraocular infections resembling those due to fungi. These protozoa may be susceptible *in vitro* to miconazole, but there are reports of little or no activity of miconazole against trophozoites or cysts of *Acanthamoebae* (Nagington and Richards, 1976; Kilvington *et al.*, 1990).

9 Trichomonas vaginalis

Miconazole inhibitied the growth of *Trichomonas vaginalis*, to a similar degree to ketoconazole and metronidazole, and it also caused some chemorepulsion (Sugarman and Mummaw, 1988).

10 Malaria

Miconazole is active against chloroquine-sensitive and chloroquine-resistant *Plasmodium falciparum* parasites (Pfaller and Krogstad, 1981).

11 Synergism with other drugs

Variable results have been obtained when miconazole has been combined with amphotericin B and tested against various fungi and *N. fowleri*. Petrou and Rogers (1991) evaluated *in vitro* interactions between polyenes and imidazoles against yeast, and found that antagonism was the main interaction, and the degree of antagonism varied according to the methodology. Miconazole activity was minimally affected by amphotericin B, but miconazole antagonized the activity of amphotericin B. There is a single report of *in vivo* antagonism between miconazole and amphotericin B against *C. albicans* (Schacter *et al.*, 1976). Synergy has been observed with a miconazole-rifampicin combination when tested against various *Candida* spp., but it was not observed with a ketoconazole/rifampicin combination (Moody *et al.*, 1980). The combination of miconazole and lovastatin was demonstrated to be synergistic against *Leishmania* spp. *in vitro* (Haughan *et al.*, 1992).

Table IV.12

Compiled from data published by Dixon et al. 1978, Stevens et al. (1978), Gebhart et al. (1984), Hughes et al. (1984), Kusunoki and Harada, (1984), Yangco et al. (1984a,b), Adam et al. (1986), Bassiouny et al. (1986), Hussain Qadri et al. (1986), Walsh et al. (1986), Marcon et al. (1987), Okeke and Gugnani, (1987), Haron et al. (1988), Salkin et al. (1988), Reuben et al. (1989), Wong et al. (1989), Patterson et al. (1990), Hernandez Molina et al. (1992), Sekhon et al. (1992), Supparatpinyo et al. (1993), Venugopal et al. (1993)

Organism	MIC (µg per ml) range	
	Broth	Agar
Yeast		
Candida spp.		
C. albicans	0.1–2	0.25–32
C. guilliermondii	0.1–1	0.25–1
C. krusei	0.5–4	2–4
C. parapsilosis	0.1–2	0.12–0.5
C. tropicalis	0.5–>8	0.5–16
C. kefyr (pseudotropicalis)	0.1–1	0.12–0.25
C. lusitaniae	0.1–1	
C. glabrata (Torulopsis glabrata)	0.1–2	0.5–8
Cryptococcus neoformans	0.5–2	0.06–1
Hansenula anomala	>50	
Malassezia furfur		0.4–1.5
Rhodotorula rubra	1–4	
Trichosporon beigelii	0.125–2	
Dimorphic fungi		
Histoplasma capsulatum		<0.125
Blastomyces dermatitidis		<0.125–2
Coccidioides immitis		1–4
Paracoccidioides brasiliensis		0.001–0.005
Penicillium marneffei	<0.195	<0.002–0.156
Sporothrix schenckii		0.25–2
Mold		
Aspergillus spp.	0.1–100	
A. fumigatus	1.6–3.1	0.5–4
A. flavus	3.1	0.25–2
A. niger	1.6–3.1	
Dematiaceous fungi		
Alternaria alternata	1	
Bipolaris spp.	<0.06–4.79	
Cladosporium spp.	0.1–4	
Cladosporium carrionii		0.05–0.1
Exophiala jeanselmei	2.5–100	0.2
Exserohilum spp.	0.06	
Fonsecaea pedrosoi		0.05–0.39
Phialophora spp.	<0.05–0.5	
Phialophora verrucosa		0.05
Zygomycetes		
Mucor spp.		0.12–16
Rhizopus spp.		0.12–8
Conidiobolus spp.	0.098–3.1	
Basidiobolus spp.	<0.098–12.5	
Dermatophytes		
Trichophyton spp.	0.03–3	
Microsporum spp.	0.25–>6	
Epidermophyton spp.	0.06–0.25	
Hyphomycetes		
Fusarium spp.	8–32	
Paecilomyces spp.	0.1–40	
Pseudallescheria boydii	<0.016–4	0.2
Scedosporium prolificans (inflatum)	>20	
Madurella spp.	1–10	
Madurella mycetomatis	1–5	
Pythium insidiosum	0.39–3.12	

12 Acquired resistance

Holt and Azmi (1978) reported the emergence of resistance to miconazole of *C. albicans* during prolonged therapy for urinary candidiasis. The strain was cross-resistant to clotrimazole and econazole.

13 Minimum inhibitory concentrations

Table IV.12 shows MICs of miconazole against selected fungi. Serum concentrations of 2.4 μg per ml can be fairly easily attained by i.v. administration of the drug. Organisms with a MIC of 1.25 μg per ml have been regarded as sensitive (Plempel, 1979). Tests for the *in vitro* activity of antifungal agents were not standardized until recently, and many problems exist for reproducibility of results between laboratories, as well as a lack of correlation between *in vitro* activity and *in vivo* efficacy.

Mode of Administration and Dosage

1 Intravenous administration

Orally administered miconazole produces low serum levels with wide individual differences (Plempel, 1979), so that i.v. administration is necessary for the treatment of systemic infections. Optimal dosage schedules and duration of therapy have not been determined by clinical trials. The total daily dose is usually given in three divided doses and recommended doses vary from 200 to 1200 mg per infusion. The maximum total daily dose recommended is 3.6 g for adults and this has been used for months to treat coccidioidomycosis (Stevens *et al.*, 1976). For children, a total daily dose of about 20–40 mg per kg is generally adequate, but a dose of 15 mg per kg body weight per infusion should not be exceeded. An i.v. dose of 15 mg per kg body weight, twice-daily, has been used in babies (Symoens, 1977). A dose of 10 mg per kg has been used in a neonate, given in two divided doses infused over 2 h, but this was associated with intermittent ventricular tachycardia between infusions (Clarke *et al.*, 1980). Depending on the infection, treatment may be required for 3 weeks or more than 20 weeks, and repeated courses may be required for relapse or reinfection.

Miconazole should be diluted by adding at least 200 ml of either 0.9% sodium chloride or 5% dextrose; a maximum concentration of miconazole is 1200 mg (six ampoules) to 200 ml diluent. The i.v. infusion should be slowly administered over a period of 30–60 min. At 37°C, miconazole is stable in 5% dextrose for 7 days (Hoeprich and Huston 1978).

2 Intrathecal or intraventricular administration

Undiluted injectable miconazole may be given directly into the CSF (lumbar, cisternal or ventricular) in a 20 mg dose. Such therapy may be indicated in the treatment of cryptococcal or coccidioidal meningitis. A maximum total dose of 465 mg has been used in this way (Deresinski *et al.*, 1976). After this form of administration (20 mg maximum individual dose), CSF concentrations were 1.4 and 0.25 μg per ml, respectively, after 24 and 48 h. The drug was well tolerated by these routes. Arachnoiditis may complicate this route of administration.

3 Patients with renal failure

The serum half-life of miconazole in patients with renal failure or in those undergoing hemodialysis is not significantly different from that in subjects with normal renal function. Some patients with renal failure not undergoing hemodialysis may have elevated serum levels in the first 4 h due to a reduction in the apparent volume of distribution (Lewi *et al.*, 1976). Dosage modification is therefore unnecessary in patients with renal insufficiency.

4 Bladder instillation

Miconazole for injection has been used in a dose of 50 mg in 1 liter of normal saline for irrigation into the bladder continuously for 5 days to treat uncomplicated funguria (Wise *et al.*, 1987).

5 Use in pregnancy

Although miconazole does not appear to be teratogenic in animals, its safety when administered by the i.v. route in human pregnancy has not been established by controlled trials. Small amounts of miconazole are absorbed from the vagina, and although there have been no reports of resultant harm to the developing fetus, use of topical vaginal preparations is not recommended in the first trimester of pregnancy (Ainsworth, 1987). A prescription study of miconazole exposure in the first trimester of pregnancy revealed no statistical association for overall frequency of birth defects, but a slightly elevated risk (estimated relative risk of 1.4, with 95% confidence limits of 1.2–1.5) for spontaneous abortion (Rosa *et al.*, 1987). There is no information regarding the excretion of miconazole or its metabolites into breast milk.

6 Topical therapy

Miconazole is available as vaginal pessaries or vaginal cream for the treatment of vulvovaginal candidiasis. It is also available as a skin cream, lotion, powder, spray powder and tincture for the treatment of cutaneous dermatophytosis and candidiasis. Undiluted miconazole solution can be used for mouth washing or for wound infiltration.

7 Intraocular administration

The recommended dose is 40 μg for the treatment of fungal endophthalmitis (Tolentino *et al.*, 1982). No toxicity has been noted following doses of 10 μg and 25 μg in humans, or 100 μg in rabbits (Kattan and Pflugfelder, 1989).

8 Stability of miconazole

McGookin *et al.* (1987), examined the sorption of miconazole onto the plastic of infusion bags and i.v. administration sets and observed only a low rate of sorption which was felt unlikely to cause significant loss of clinical efficacy. The stability of miconazole mixed with peritoneal dialysis fluid to a final concentration of 20 mg per ml and stored in either glass ampoules or 2 liter polyvinyl chloride bags was examined. More than 10% of the initial concentration of miconazole was lost within 4 h and up to 30% in 3 days when miconazole was stored in the polyvinyl bags, whereas there was no appreciable loss in glass containers. It is recommended that admixtures of miconazole be prepared immediately prior to administration (Holmes and Aldous, 1991).

Availability

Intravenous preparation: 20 ml vials containing 10 mg per ml of miconazole in a colloidal suspension, stabilized with 'Cremophor' EL and ethanol.

Topical preparations: Miconazole nitrate gel for application to buccal mucosa containing 20 mg miconazole per ml.

Miconazole nitrate cream 2% in 15 g tubes

Miconazole nitrate 2% aerosol, 2% aerosol powder, 2% powder, 2% lotion, 2% tincture are available with and without prescription.

Vaginal pessaries/ovules: 100 mg and 200 mg.

Miconazole nitrate 2% vaginal cream. Vaginal pessaries and cream available without prescription in some countries.

Serum Levels in Relation to Dosage

1 Oral administration

Miconazole is poorly absorbed from the gastrointestinal tract. Peak serum levels are reached 4 h after administration (Brugmans *et al.*, 1972). After oral doses of 200 mg and 1 g, serum levels of 0.07–0.1 and 0.5–1.0 μg per ml, respectively, are reached and these persist for about 8 h. The serum half-life after oral administration is about 24 h. The oral formulation of miconazole is no longer available because of poor oral bioavailability.

2 Intravenous administration

After a 200-mg dose is infused i.v. over a period of 1 h, a peak serum level of about 1.6 μg per ml is reached at the end of the infusion (Shadomy *et al.*, 1977). When higher doses of 10–12 mg per kg body weight are given, short-term peak serum levels of 5–13 μg per ml are reached which fall to 2.5 and 0.5 μg per ml, after approximately 30 min and 12 h, respectively (Plempel, 1979). Serum levels resulting from various miconazole doses given by 1 h infusion were studied in 14 adult patients by Stevens *et al.* (1976). After the initial peak serum level, there is a rapid early decay period with a half-life of approximately 30 min, and this is followed by a late flat phase with a serum half-life of about 20 h. Doses above 9 mg per kg body weight produce peak serum levels above 1.0 μg per ml in 71% of patients, and levels of up to 7.5 μg per ml could be achieved in some.

3 Topical administration

In vivo pharmacokinetics and pharmacodynamics of miconazole 2% cream in human stratum corneum was evaluated by Pershing *et al.* (1994). In comparison with 2% ketoconazole cream, topical miconazole produced 7- to 14-fold lower drug concentrations in the stratum corneum from 1–8 h after a single dose, but were similar 24 h after drug removal. The miconazole concentration was 1.49 μg per cm^2 at 1 h and 1.58 μg per cm^2 at 24 h, however the bioactivity of miconazole decreased 8-fold over the 24 h period, while that of ketoconazole remained the same. Miconazole was 2- to 10-fold less potent (reported as bioactivity per amount of drug in stratum corneum) relative to ketoconazole.

Miconazole is minimally absorbed following intravaginal insertion of miconazole pessaries. Systemic absorption of miconazole after insertion of a 1200 mg vaginal pessary was examined in healthy volunteers. The mean maximum serum concentration was 10.4 μg per liter (<0.5% achieved after an i.v. dose of miconazole) and this low but detectable concentration persisted for 3 days, and the estimated systemic bioavailability of the vaginal pessary was 1.4%. There was a large intervolunteer variability in all pharmacokinetic parameters (Daneshmend, 1986). Similar rates of systemic absorption from the vagina have been noted with smaller dose pessaries (100 mg) or vaginal cream with about 1% of the administered dose in radioactive form, recovered in the urine and feces (Abrams and Weintraub, 1983). Miconazole persists in vaginal secretions for at least 48 h after a single application of 100 mg vaginal pessary (Odds and McDonald, 1981; Daneshmend, 1986).

Salivary concentrations of miconazole after administration of 3 g miconazole gel (equivalent 60 mg miconazole nitrate) peaked within minutes at 92–100 μg per ml and remained above the MIC for *C. albicans* (5 μg per ml) for a mean of 20 min. This compared with administration of a bioadhesive slow-release buccal tablet containing 10 mg miconazole nitrate, with a mean peak salivary concentration of 130 μg per ml which remained above the MIC for *C. albicans* for 10 h. The bioadhesive tablet is therefore a preferable drug delivery system for the oral cavity which would improve patient compliance (Bouckaert *et al.*, 1992).

The pharmacokinetics of subconjunctivally injected miconazole 10 mg per ml was evaluated in rabbits with both normal and debrided corneas. The corneal concentration of miconazole peaked at 2 h in both the normal and debrided corneas, and no drug was detectable after 4–8 h (Klippenstein *et al.*, 1993).

Excretion

1 Urine

After oral administration about 10% of the dose is excreted in the urine, largely as metabolites, only 1% being in the form of the unchanged drug (Brugmans *et al.*, 1972). In four volunteers given 200 mg i.v. no active drug was detected in the urine, but about one-quarter of the dose was present as a metabolite (Hoeprich and Goldstein, 1974).

2 Inactivation in body

Miconazole is inactivated in the body to produce a number of metabolites; O-dealkylation and oxidative N-dealkylation may be the metabolic pathway involved. This is the most important method by which miconazole is eliminated from the body. Metabolism of the drug or possible excretion in the feces appears to account for the fall of serum concentrations after i.v. administration (Lewi *et al.*, 1976). In man, even after prolonged i.v. administration, miconazole, unlike clotrimazole, does not cause induction of liver enzymes (Plempel, 1979).

3 Feces

Following oral administration about 50% of miconazole is excreted in the feces, mainly as the unchanged drug.

Distribution of the Drug in Body

Penetration of miconazole into the CSF is poor (Hoeprich and Goldstein, 1974; Shadomy *et al.*, 1977). When a dosage of 1 g every 12 h was given i.v. to an adult patient with disseminated coccidioidomycosis and meningitis, the miconazole concentration in the lumbar CSF rose to only 0.25 μg per ml despite a peak serum level of 5.1 μg per ml (Hoeprich and Goldstein, 1974). In a patient whose peak serum level was 2.5 μg per ml, cisternal and lumbar CSF taken 15–30 min later showed levels of 0.4 and 0.27 μg per ml, respectively (Stevens *et al.*, 1976). They also described another patient without meningitis who had a CSF level of 0.1 μg per ml 30 min after a peak serum level of 2.0 μg per ml.

Penetration into sputum also appears to be poor. Miconazole was undetectable in the sputum of a patient on two occasions 30 min after the peak serum levels were 6.7 and 4.5 μg per ml, respectively (Stevens *et al.*, 1976). One estimation of the concentration of the drug in the vitreous humor of a patient 2.25 h after an infusion of 1 g miconazole was 0.6 μg per ml (Lutwick *et al.*, 1976), and the plasma and vitreous levels of miconazole 1 h after i.v. administration of 800 mg were 1.11 and 0.058 μg per ml, respectively (Gallo *et al.*, 1985). The drug diffuses well into infected joints (Deresinski and Stevens, 1979). Serum protein binding of miconazole is approximately 90% (Stevens *et al.*, 1976).

Mode of Action

Miconazole has a fungistatic effect on susceptible fungi by inhibiting sterol C-14 demethylation of lanosterol resulting in ergosterol depletion in the fungal cell membrane (Pye and Marriott, 1982). Both the accumulation of 14 alpha-methyl sterols and the reduced ergosterol content affects the membrane fluidity and permeability and the activity of membrane-bound enzymes of fungi (Van den Bossche *et al.*, 1983) (see Fig. IV.1, p. 1261). At higher concentrations the drug may be fungicidal and bactericidal due to a direct damage to cell membranes (Taylor *et al.*, 1983). Miconazole also binds strongly to erythrocyte membrane lipoproteins and can induce hemolysis of mammalian erythrocytes (Sreedhara Swamy *et al.*, 1976).

Miconazole and other azole derivatives at low micromolar concentrations competitively inhibit calmodulin activity, which is involved in fungal infections as well as inflammatory skin diseases. Inhibition of calmodulin activity may explain the therapeutic activity of these agents in inflammatory skin disorders (Hegemann *et al.*, 1993).

Toxicity

In early studies when miconazole was given orally, there was no significant toxicity (Brugmans *et al.*, 1972). Diarrhea, sometimes necessitating cessation of treatment, has been observed with oral doses of 1 g three times daily (Lima *et al.*, 1977). The following side-effects have been observed with i.v. administration of the drug.

1 Gastrointestinal side-effects

In one large clinical study, nausea, vomiting, or both, occurred in 25% of patients. This appeared to be influenced by the infusion rate, being less severe during slower infusions (Jordan *et al.*, 1979). Nausea (20–45%) is more common than vomiting (<10%). In one patient described by Stevens *et al.* (1976), attempts to increase the dose above 600 mg once-daily resulted in malaise, chills, nausea and vomiting.

2 Neurotoxicity

Central nervous system side-effects, such as tremors, confusion, dizziness, and hallucinations occurred in 16% of patients studied by Jordan *et al.* (1979), as well as three cases of grand mal seizures preceded by tremors for several days. Inadvertent overdose with delivery of 500 mg miconazole instead of 50 mg infused over 1 h in a 4-month-old baby resulted in a generalized tonic–clonic convulsion. When the dose of 50 mg was re-instituted 36 h later, no further seizures occurred (Coulthard *et al.*, 1987). Symptomatic ventriculitis has been reported following intraventricular treatment with miconazole 20 mg every 72 h. The patient developed headaches, nausea, vomiting and fevers within 30 min of the intraventricular administration and symptoms lasted 24 h. On cessation of the drug, CSF pleocytosis and symptoms resolved (Perez *et al.*, 1988).

3 Cardiorespiratory toxicity and anaphylaxis

There were only isolated reports of such complications until Fainstein and Bodey (1980) described this toxicity in seven patients. During miconazole infusion two patients had a cardiac arrest, another had respiratory arrest and four others anaphylactic reactions (dyspnea, choking, hypotension, cyanosis and laryngeal edema), and all recovered. The authors emphasized the importance of administering miconazole over a period of no less than 60 min, and diluting it in at least 200 ml of fluid. Ventricular tachycardia has also been reported during miconazole therapy. A premature neonate experienced cardiotoxicity after receiving miconazole 50 mg per kg every 8 h, instead of once-daily. This was manifest as bradycardia, rhythm and conduction disturbances (Kanarek and Williams, 1986).

4 Hematological side-effects

In three patients with coccidioidomycosis treated by Stevens et al. (1976), a fall in hematocrit values was observed during treatment. These values returned to normal when the drug was stopped, and hematological investigations were unrevealing. Marmion et al. (1976) also recorded hematological changes in patients with active coccidioidomycosis treated by i.v. miconazole. All six patients developed a normocytic, normochromic anemia and progressive thrombocytosis with increasing doses of miconazole. Changes were first observed after a total dose ranging from 1.8 to 12.6 g had been administered. The lowest hemoglobin values (7.8–9.6 g per dl) coincided with maximal thrombocytosis (515 000–990 000 per cm^3) and they were observed after miconazole had been administered for periods ranging from 5 to 23 days. Bone marrow studies in three patients showed erythroid hypoplasia and increased or active platelet production. Other hematological investigations were normal, except for a prolonged clotting time in one patient. Total miconazole doses given to these patients were in the range of 21.4–74.0 g. The hematological changes appeared to be dose-related and reversible on cessation of the drug. About 45% of patients develop a transient normocytic anemia and 30% can develop thrombocytosis (Heel et al., 1980).

Other blood changes appear to be caused by the vehicle in which miconazole is available for i.v. use. Patients receiving i.v. miconazole therapy may develop high serum concentrations of cholesterol and triglycerides, and this is associated with an unusual pattern on paper lipoprotein electrophoresis. This hyperlipemic state has been attributed to the carrier solution of miconazole, 'Cremophor' EL (polyethoxylated castor oil) (Bagnarello et al., 1977; Rose et al., 1979). Another unusual side-effect noted in patients receiving i.v. miconazole is marked rouleaux formation in peripheral blood smears (Stevens et al., 1976). This may also be due to an unusual surface active phenomenon related to the carrier solution 'Cremophor' EL (Niell, 1977). It is also possible that the anemia and thrombocytosis described with i.v. miconazole is due to 'Cremophor' EL (Marmion et al., 1976).

Thrombocytopenia and leukopenia have been reported in a small percentage of patients. Miconazole can suppress granulocyte progenitor cells grown in tissue culture. Hematological monitoring should be carried out regularly in all patients receiving miconazole by the i.v. route.

5 Thrombophlebitis

This was the most common side-effect, occurring in 10 of 14 patients treated by i.v. miconazole, described by Stevens et al. (1976) and 30–35% patients with peripheral lines (Heel et al., 1980). Infusion via central venous catheters reduced this problem. Reformulation of the vehicle in which the drug is supplied has also reduced the frequency of phlebitis.

6 Other side-effects

Pruritus is a common complication (20–35% of patients) but rash occurs in less than 10%. Pruritus is usually controlled with antihistamines. Allergic rashes occur and sometimes may be severe enough to necessitate cessation of treatment (Marmion et al., 1976; Stevens et al., 1976; Fischer et al., 1977). Contact allergic dermatitis has been reported in a few patients using miconazole cream, and presents as an acute papulovesicular dermatitis (Aldridge and Main, 1984; Perret and Happle, 1988). Patch testing for cross-reactivity with other imidazole agents used topically reveal cross-reactions with clotrimazole and econazole in several cases (Raulin and Frosch, 1988). Dryness of the eyes and knee arthralgias were recorded in one patient (Stevens et al., 1976). Of five patients including three children treated by Fisher et al. (1975), some developed fever, sometimes with pruritus, and others showed transient mild rises in transaminases (AST and ALT). Experience with one patient who had received a renal transplant suggested that miconazole may occasionally be nephrotoxic (Lai et al., 1981). Drowsiness, flushes, anorexia and hyponatremia have been reported rarely. Corneal toxicity manifest as pinpoint vesicles with surrounding superficial punctate keratitis in the corneal epithelium has been described, and resolved on cessation of miconazole (Zaidman, 1991). Vulvovaginal burning, itching or irritation has been uncommonly associated with the use of miconazole cream.

7 Endocrine effects

Like ketoconazole, miconazole inhibits cytochrome P-450 enzymes, 17 alpha-hydroxylase and C17,20-lyase but has less affinity and reduced inhibitory potency than the former drug. Testosterone serum levels decrease by 16% following miconazole 200 mg i.v. and return to baseline after 5 h, indicating a minor alteration to testosterone biosynthesis (Morita *et al.*, 1990).

8 Immunosuppression

Miconazole in concentrations of 1–10 μg per ml inhibits mitogen-induced lymphocyte proliferative responses (Thong and Rowan-Kelly, 1978). The inhibition was confirmed in human mixed lymphocyte cultures and the effect was less than that observed with itraconazole and ketoconazole (Pawelec *et al.*, 1991). The drug can also inhibit granulocyte progenitor cells in tissue culture. The clinical significance of these observations is not known.

9 Interaction with other drugs

There is an enhanced anticoagulant effect noted when warfarin and miconazole are co-administered, and this is due to inhibition of hepatic P-450 enzymes (especially P-450 2C9 enzymes) responsible for the metabolism of warfarin, reduced total body clearance of warfarin and inhibition of oxidation of warfarin to phenolic metabolites (O'Reilly *et al.*, 1992). Since systemic absorption from the buccal mucosa after topical application of miconazole is minimal, interaction between warfarin and miconazole gel had not been considered to be problematic. However, clinically evident hemorrhage has been reported in two patients stabilized on warfarin, who were prescribed miconazole gel and 11 days later the international normalized ratio (INR) had increased from therapeutic (2.1 and 2.5) to 13.1 and 17.9 (Colquhoun *et al.*, 1987; Shenfield and Page,1991). There is also a report of apparent phenytoin intoxication as a result of concomitant treatment with miconazole due to inhibition of phenytoin metabolism (Rolan *et al.*, 1983). Increases in cyclosporine plasma concentration during concomitant therapy with miconazole was observed in a heart transplant patient, underscoring the importance of monitoring drug levels (Horton *et al.*, 1992). Co-administration of tobramycin and i.v. miconazole results in significant decreases of peak serum tobramycin levels, increases in the volume of distribution and clearance, but no change in trough concentrations. These pharmacologic changes paralleled changes in serum triglyceride levels. Tobramycin concentrations should be monitored when this drug is administered with miconazole (Hatfield *et al.*, 1986).

Clinical Uses of the Drug

1 Cryptococcosis

There have been numerous reports (e.g. Morgans *et al.*, 1979; Weinstein and Jacoby, 1980; De Wytt, 1981) describing improvement or cure of systemic cryptococcosis, cryptococcal meningitis and cerebral cryptococcoma following treatment with i.v. miconazole, sometimes supplemented by direct instillation of the drug into the CSF. Because most of the patients described had previously received amphotericin B and 5-flucytosine and their CSF was not shown to be negative for *C. neoformans* culture 12 months after therapy with miconazole (a common criterion of cure), there is insufficient data to conclude that miconazole is effective in this infection (Bennett and Remington, 1981). Miconazole is not a first-line drug for cryptococcosis, but it may have a place for treatment of patients with infections not responding to amphotericin B and flucytosine, or for others who cannot tolerate these drugs.

Miconazole administered as 6-mg intraventricular doses was used successfully in patients with cryptococcal meningitis who had failed to respond to amphotericin B. It was noted that intraventricular administration of miconazole did not result in distribution of miconazole into the lumbar CSF space (Graybill and Levine, 1978).

2 Candidiasis

a   Systemic infections   Miconazole has been used effectively to treat systemic infections due to various *Candida* spp. (Scheef *et al.*, 1974; Katz and Cassileth, 1977; Wust and Lennartz, 1977; Jordan *et al.*, 1979, Morison *et al.*, 1988). Similar to cryptococcosis, Bennett and Remington (1981) advise caution in assessing these reports, because criteria for the diagnosis of this infection are debatable and the natural history of the disease is variable. Although miconazole has been effective for the treatment of systemic candidiasis, its exact cure rate is not known.

Combination miconazole (1200–3000 mg per day) plus flucytosine treatment was used in 8 i.v. heroin users who presented with *C. albicans* endophthalmitis. The progression of intraocular disease was immediately halted, but the visual acuity improved in only half the patients. Improved responses were seen with higher doses of miconazole (2400 mg per day) (Gallo *et al.*, 1985). Several reports of failure of miconazole for systemic candidiasis in neonates (including a neonatal patient with *C. albicans* meningitis who failed to respond to miconazole, but the infection resolved when amphotericin B was used) have cautioned the use of miconazole in this age group (De Mol *et al.*, 1982; Sutton, 1983; McDougall *et al.*, 1982).

The efficacy of miconazole irrigation (continuous irrigation of 50 mg miconazole in 1 liter normal saline for 5 days) for uncomplicated *Candida* spp. funguria was examined in ten elderly patients with indwelling urinary catheters or suprapubic cystotomy tubes. Fungus was eradicated from urine within 3 days in seven of ten patients (Wise *et al.*, 1987). No comparative studies have been performed, and the current recommendation for treatment of uncomplicated funguria is local instillation of amphotericin B (Gubbins *et al.*, 1993).

b Superficial infections Miconazole vaginal cream (2%) given by an applicator in a 5 g dose each night for 14 days, is effective for the treatment of vaginal candidiasis (Morris and Sugrue, 1975). Results are comparable with those obtained with nystatin (Hilton *et al.*, 1978), clotrimazole pessaries (Clayton, 1979), terconazole cream (0.4% or 0.8%) (Corson *et al.*, 1991) and butoconazole cream (Bradbeer *et al.*, 1985). Miconazole-coated tampons inserted twice-daily for 5 days are also an acceptable and effective way of treating vaginal candidiasis (Baldson, 1981). Similar cure rates (>80%) for vaginal candidosis have also been obtained when single-dose oral fluconazole 150 mg was compared with vaginal miconazole pessaries 100 mg for 3 days (Timonen, 1992) or a single intravaginal dose of 1200 mg miconazole (van Heusden *et al.*, 1990). Ketoconazole 400 mg daily for 5 days was as effective as a single intravaginal dose of 1200 mg miconazole (van der Meijden, *et al.*, 1986). Treatment preference by the women was for oral therapy. Miconazole cream (2%) is useful for the treatment of cutaneous candidiasis (Zaias, 1975).

The drug has been used to treat oral candidiasis in immunosuppressed infants and adults, and was effective administered as a tablet (250 mg four times daily) retained in the mouth until dissolved, and then swallowed. This dose has been shown to achieve serum levels of 1 μg per ml miconazole which is active against most *C. albicans* strains (Brincker, 1976). Miconazole oral gel (20 mg miconazole per g gel) at a dose of 50 mg four times daily for 10 days was compared with ketoconazole 200 mg daily for esophageal candidiasis in a small study of 12 AIDS patients. All miconazole-treated patients had symptomatic relief within 3–5 days, and endoscopically normal esophageal mucosa at the end of therapy, while four of the six ketoconazole-treated patients responded (Deschamps *et al.*, 1988).

Intravenously administered miconazole has been used effectively to control chronic mucocutaneous candidiasis (Fischer *et al.*, 1977).

c Prevention of candidiasis in cancer patients Miconazole has been given i.v. 2 days a week, as part of antimicrobial prophylaxis for patients with lung malignancy undergoing intensive cancer chemotherapy. Several patients developed *Candida* esophagitis, suggesting that this use of the drug was ineffective (Bodey *et al.*, 1982). In a placebo-controlled trial, miconazole oral gel significantly reduced the prevalence of fungal rectal colonization (from 36.2% to 19.5%) in neonates in the neonatal intensive care unit, but did not reduce the incidence of systemic fungal infections. The use of miconazole oral gel for prophylaxis of neonatal systemic fungal infections is not recommended (Wainer *et al.*, 1992).

In a placebo-controlled trial of i.v. miconazole 5 mg per kg initiated with antibiotics as empiric treatment of cytotoxic-induced neutropenia and unexplained fever, there was a significant reduction in fungal sepsis in the miconazole group, but no significant reduction in death due to fungal sepsis or the use of amphotericin B for persistent unexplained fever (Wingard *et al.*, 1987).

3 Pseudallescheria boydii infections

This fungus is usually resistant to amphotericin B and flucytosine, and the clinical response to these antifungal agents is generally poor (Lutwick *et al.*, 1976). Isolates are generally susceptible to miconazole which has been used with success to treat pseudallescheriasis, and is considered the drug of choice for this infection (Lutwick *et al.*, 1979). Anecdotal reports of successful treatment with i.v. miconazole 600 mg every 8 h (or 10 mg per kg every 8 h in children) include a patient with sphenoidal sinusitis (Mader *et al.*, 1978), a heart transplant patient with a soft tissue infection secondary to trauma surgically debrided (Patterson *et al.*, 1990), pansinusitis with meningeal involvement (Schiess *et al.*, 1984), and orbital and brain abscess secondary to penetrating trauma (Anderson *et al.*, 1984). Perez *et al.* (1988) reported the successful treatment of a brain abscess due to *P. boydii,* with surgery, i.v. miconazole 600–800 mg every 8 h and intraventricular miconazole 20 mg every 3 days for 3 months.

Fungal endophthalmitis due to *P. boydii* can occur exogenously (superficial infection secondary to traumatic implantation of the fungus) or endogenously (secondary to hematogenous dissemination). McGuire *et al.* (1991) reviewed the 17 cases of ocular pseudallescheriasis reported and found similar efficacy for amphotericin B and miconazole. A variety of treatments including intravitreal and i.v. miconazole, either as initial treatment or after amphotericin B therapy and intravitreal and i.v. amphotericin B for varied ocular diagnoses made a meaningful comparison of efficacy difficult. However, three of seven patients on miconazole died of systemic infection (all had prior amphotericin B), none of the amphotericin B alone patients died. Others have reported progressive disease despite intravitreal instillation of 25 μg miconazole and systemic therapy with fluconazole for endogenous endophthalmitis (Pfeifer *et al.*, 1991).

4 Coccidioidomycosis

Amphotericin B is the drug of choice for the treatment of this disease (p. 1279). There have been reports of patients with various forms of coccidioidomycosis responding to treatment with miconazole. However, when recorded experience with the comparatively few patients (<100) is critically reviewed, results are disappointing. In disseminated coccidioidomycosis, miconazole has an unacceptable high rate of initial failure to respond (up to 70%) and a high frequency of early relapse when the drug is ceased (Stevens,1983). It is therefore not recommended for primary treatment of this disease (Hoeprich *et al.*, 1980). Miconazole may have a minor role for treatment of patients with non-meningeal coccidioidomycosis who cannot receive amphotericin B (Bouza *et al.*, 1981). Shehab *et al.* (1988) reported their experience of intraventricular miconazole and oral ketoconazole for the treatment of coccidioidal meningitis in eight children aged 2–10 years. Half the children had failed therapy with amphotericin B. Miconazole 3–5 mg was diluted in 1 ml of either 5% dextrose or normal saline, and injected over 30–60 seconds into a ventriculoperitoneal shunt Ommaya reservoir with the shunt valve closed. Treatment was initially daily, then decreased to once-weekly within 2–6 months. When coccidioidal complement fixation antibodies became negative in the CSF, miconazole intraventricular injections were decreased to every second week, then monthly, before cessation. All CSF cultures became negative and no child relapsed on oral ketoconazole therapy.

5 Paracoccidioidomycosis

Several reports from South America indicate that miconazole is an effective alternative to sulphonamides or amphotericin B. However, ketoconazole (p. 1375) and itraconazole (p. 1437) have demonstrated significant efficacy, with low relapse rates, and should be used for primary therapy. *Paracoccidioides brasiliensis* is very sensitive (MIC 0.001– 0.005 μg per ml) to miconazole *in vitro* (Stevens *et al.*, 1978). Paracoccidioidomycosis has responded to oral, i.v. or a combination of oral and i.v. treatment with miconazole. Lima *et al.* (1977) used a dose of 1 g three times daily orally for 3–8 months and Negroni *et al.* (1977) used 200–600 mg i.v. plus 2.5–3.0 g orally per day, for 60 days, followed by 1.5 g orally per day for up to 2 years. Relatively short courses of i.v. miconazole (0.6–1.2 g daily for 25–44 days) have also been quite effective in the short-term, but longer courses are required to prevent relapse (Stevens *et al.*, 1978). The oral form of miconazole is no longer available.

6 Blastomycosis

Amphotericin B is the recommended treatment (p. 1278). Miconazole has been successfully used to treat two patients whose pulmonary disease relapsed after prior response to amphotericin B (Rose and Varkev, 1978). Lopez *et al.* (1994) report a case of intraocular blastomycosis manifest as iritis with an iris mass and choroidal lesions, in association with disseminated disease. The iris mass and visual acuity did not respond to i.v. amphotericin B, but completely resolved with subconjunctival miconazole 5 mg per 0.5 ml injections.

7 Histoplasmosis

Miconazole has been used as an alternate to amphotericin B for the treatment of both localized and disseminated histoplasmosis (Nicholls *et al.*, 1980).

8 Sporotrichosis

Rohwedder and Archer (1976) reported the successful treatment of a patient with pulmonary sporotrichosis by miconazole. The drug was used when drug-resistance and treatment failure occurred, after initial treatment with amphotericin B and then with amphotericin B and 5-flucytosine in combination. Miconazole was used in a dose of 0.6–1.0 g three times daily i.v., and this produced clinical improvement despite serum drug levels which were below or only transiently in excess of the MIC of the strain of *Sporothrix schenckii* isolated from the patient.

9 Mycetoma

Surgical treatment is often required for these fungal infections, but amphotericin B and miconazole have been useful in some cases (Hay, 1979; Lutwick *et al.*, 1979).

10 Keratomycosis

Topically applied miconazole is recommended for this eye infection. In the rabbit model of keratomycosis, miconazole 1% in ointment base was more effective than 1% miconazole eye drops at healing fungal ulcers (Gupta, 1986).

11 Dermatophyte infections

Various forms of tinea due to *Trichophyton rubrum*, *T. mentagrophytes* and *Epidermophyton floccosum* respond well to 2% miconazole cream, applied twice-daily for 2–4 weeks (Fulton, 1975). Clinical response rates of 84% and mycological cure rates of 81% at week 4 of treatment with 2% miconazole cream applied twice-daily, were similar to those achieved with 1% naftifine cream or 2% fenticonazole cream (El Darouti and Kalinka, 1990; Athow Frost *et al.*, 1986). Tinea versicolor (caused by *Pityrosporum orbicularis,* also called *Malassezia furfur*) also responds well to treatment with 2% miconazole cream (Zaias, 1975). Tinea nigra palmaris (superficial infection of the palms caused by *Phaeoannellomyces werneckii*) resolved with topical miconazole 2% cream (Hughes *et al.*, 1993). An immunosuppressed woman developed a chronic cutaneous and subcutaneous infection due to *Microsporum canis* which was initially stabilized on griseofulvin and ketoconazole, but resolved with intralesional miconazole 20 mg in 1 ml injected into one nodule at a time, every second day (Barson, 1985).

12 Aspergillosis

Although some isolates of *Aspergillus* spp. will be susceptible to miconazole *in vitro* (Denning *et al.*, 1992), and a report of some *in vivo* activity of miconazole has been published (Denning and Stevens, 1990), itraconazole has greater activity against *Aspergillus* spp. and has a principal role in the management of this disease (p. 1433). Hammoto *et al.* (1983) reported successful treatment of a symptomatic pulmonary aspergilloma in a patient unable to undergo surgery, by endocavitary instillation of miconazole 5 or 10 mg in 20 ml normal saline infused eight times in 50 days. The patient experienced transient headache, nausea and mild fever within 1 h of several treatments. Sputum cultures became negative after four infusions and the fungus ball resolved on chest roentgenograms within 2 months.

13 Other fungal infections

Trichosporon beigelii septic arthritis occurred in a leukemic patient and was successfully treated with i.v. miconazole 600 mg 8-hourly, with flucytosine and rifampin. The knee joint was irrigated with miconazole 100 mg (3 g per liter normal saline) hourly for 48 h (McWhinney *et al.*, 1992). Anaissie *et al.* (1992) reviewed experience with azoles as treatment for trichosporonosis, and miconazole 1800 mg per day (for 2 weeks in three cases and 3 months in one case) was associated with a clinical response in all cases treated. However, it is important to note that all the patients had recovery from neutropenia, an important prognostic marker for this infection.

References

Abrams LS, Weintraub HS (1983). Disposition of radioactivity following intravaginal administration of ³H-miconazole nitrate. *Amer J Obstet Gynecol* **147**: 970.

Adam RD, Paquin ML, Petersen EA *et al.* (1986). Phaeohyphomycosis caused by the fungal genera *Bipolaris* and *Exserohilum*. A report of nine cases and review of the literature. *Medicine* **65**: 203.

Ainsworth RE (1987). Use and safety of miconazole during pregnancy. *West J Med* **147**: 599.

Aldridge RD, Main RA (1984). Contact dermatitis due to a combined miconazole nitrate/hydrocortisone cream. *Contact Derm* **10**: 58.

Anaissie E, Gokaslan A, Hachem R *et al.* (1992). Azole therapy for trichosporonosis: Clinical evaluation of eight patients, experimental therapy for murine infection, and review. *Clin Infect Dis* **15**: 781.

Anderson RL, Carroll TF, Harvey JT, Myers MG (1984). *Petrillidium (Allescheria) boydii* orbital and brain abscess treated with intravenous miconazole. *Amer J Ophthalmol* **97**: 771.

Athow Frost TA, Freeman K, Mann TA *et al.* (1986). Clinical evaluation of fenticonazole cream in cutaneous fungal infections: a comparison with miconazole cream. *Curr Med Res Opin* **10**: 107.

Bagnarello AG, Lewis LA, McHenry MC *et al.* (1977). Unusual serum lipoprotein abnormality induced by the vehicle of miconazole. *New Engl J Med* **296**: 497.

Baldson MJ (1981). Comparison of miconazole-coated tampons with clotrimazole vaginal tablets in the treatment of vaginal candidosis. *Brit J Vener Dis* **57**: 275.

Balk MW, Crumnne MH, Fischer GW (1978). Evaluation of miconazole therapy in experimental disseminated candidiasis in laboratory rats. *Antimicrob Ag Chemother* **13**: 321.

Bannatyne RM, Cheung R (1978). Susceptibility of *Candida albicans* to miconazole. *Antimicrob Ag Chemother* **13**: 1040.

Barson WJ (1985). Granuloma and pseudogranuloma of the skin due to *Microsporum canis*. *Arch Dermatol* **121**: 895.

Bassiouny A, Kamel T, Moawad MK, Hindawy DS (1986). Broad spectrum antifungal agents in otomycosis. *J Laryngol Otol* **100**: 867–873.

Bennett JE, Remington JS (1981). Miconazole in cryptococcosis and systemic candidiasis: a word of caution. *Ann Intern Med* **94**: 708.

Bodey GP, Rosenbaum B, Valdivieso M, Bolivar R (1982). Effect of systemic antimicrobial prophylaxis on microbial flora. *Antimicrob Ag Chemother* **21**: 367.

Bouckaert S, Schautteet H, Lefebvre RA *et al.* (1992). Comparison of salivary miconazole concentrations after administration of a bioadhesive slow-release buccal tablet and an oral gel. *Eur J Clin Pharmacol* **43**: 137.

Bouza E, Dreyer JS, Hewitt WL, Meyer RD (1981). Coccidioidal meningitis. An analysis of thirty-one cases and review of the literature. *Medicine* **60**: 139.

Bradbeer CS, Mayhew SR, Barlow D (1985). Butoconazole and miconazole in treating vaginal candidiasis. *Genitourin Med* **61**: 270.

Brincker H (1976). Treatment of oral candidiasis in debilitated patients with miconazole – a new potent antifungal drug. *Scand J Infect Dis* **8**: 117.

Brugmans J, Van Cutsem J, Heykants J *et al.* (1972). Systemic antifungal potential, safety, biotransport and transformation of miconazole nitrate. *Eur J Clin Pharmacol* **5**: 93.

Clarke M, Davies DP, Odds F, Mitchell C (1980). Neonatal systemic candidiasis treated with miconazole. *Brit Med J* **281**: 354.

Clayton YM (1979). Dermatophyte infections. *Postgrad Med J* **55**: 605.

Colquhoun MC, Daly M, Stewart P, Beeley L (1987). Interaction between warfarin and miconazole oral gel. *Lancet* **i**: 695.

Corson SL, Kapikian RR, nehring R (1991). Terconazole and miconazole cream for treating vulvovaginal candidiasis. A comparison. *J Reprod Med* **36**: 561.

Coulthard K, Martin J, Matthews N (1987). Convulsions after miconazole overdose. *Med J Aust* **146**: 57.

Daneshmend TK (1986). Systemic absorption of miconazole from the vagina. *J Antimicrob Chemother* **18**: 507.

De Louvois J (1980). Activity of miconazole against *Streptococcus agalactiae*. *J Antimicrob Chemother* **6**: 798.

De Mol P, Laureys W, Dorchy H (1982). Neonatal meningitis due to *Candida albicans* associated with osteomyelitis; failure to respond to miconazole. *J Infect* **5**: 195.

Denning DW Stevens DA (1990). Antifungal and surgical treatment of invasive aspergillosis: Review of 2,121 published cases. *Rev Infect Dis* **12**: 1147.

Denning DW, Hanson LH, Perlman AM, Stevens DA (1992). *In vitro* susceptibility and synergy studies of *Aspergillus* species to conventional and new agents. *Diagn Microbiol Infect Dis* **15**: 21.

Deresinski SC, Stevens DA (1979). Bone and joint coccidioidomycosis treated with miconazole. *Amer Rev Respir Dis* **120**: 1101.

Deresinski SC, Lilly RB, Levine HB *et al.* (1976). Treatment of fungal meningitis with miconazole. *Amer Rev Respir Dis* **113** (Suppl): 71.

Deschamps MH, Pape JW, Verdier RI *et al.* (1988). Treatment of *Candida* esophagitis in AIDS patients. *Amer J Gastroenterol* **83**: 20.

De Wytt CN (1981). Cryptococcal meningitis. Treatment of three patients with miconazole. *Med J Aust* **1**: 525.

Dixon D, Shadomy S, Shadomy HJ *et al.* (1978). Comparison of the *in vitro* antifungal activities of miconazole and a new imidazole, R41, 400. *J Infect Dis* **138**: 245.

El Darouti MA, Kalinka P (1990). Naftifine cream 1% compared with miconazole cream 2% in dermatophytosis. *Int J Dermatol* **29**: 521.

Eng RHK, Person A, Mangura C *et al.* (1981). Susceptibility of Zygomycetes to amphotericin B, miconazole and ketoconazole. *Antimicrob Ag Chemother* **20**: 688.

Fainstein V, Bodey GP (1980). Cardiorespiratory toxicity due to miconazole. *Ann Intern Med* **93**: 432.

Fischer TJ, Klein RB, Kershnar HE *et al.* (1977). Miconazole in the treatment of chronic mucocutaneous candidiasis: a preliminary report. *J Pediatr* **91**: 815.

Fisher JF, Duma RJ, Markowitz SM *et al.* (1975). Therapeutic failures with miconazole. *Antimicrob Ag Chemother* **13**: 965.

Fromtling RA (1988). Overview of medically important antifungal azole derivatives. *Clin Microbiol Rev* **1**: 187.

Fulton JE Jr (1975). Miconazole therapy for endemic fungal disease. *Arch Dermatol* **111**: 596.

Gallo J, Playfair J, Gregory-Roberts J *et al.* (1985). Fungal endophthalmitis in narcotic abusers Medical and surgical therapy in 10 patients. *Med J Aust* **142**: 386.

Gebhart RJ, Espinel-Ingroff A, Shadomy S (1984). *In vitro* susceptibility studies with oxiconazole (Ro 13–8996). *Chemotherapy* **30**: 244.

Godefroi EF, Heeres J, Van Cutsem J, Janssen PAJ (1969). The preparation and antimycotic properties of derivatives of l-phenethylimidazole. *J Med Chem* **12**: 784.

Graybill JR, Levine HB (1978). Successful treatment of cryptococcal meningitis with intraventricular miconazole. *Arch Intern Med* **138**: 814.

Graybill JR, Mitchell L, Levine HB (1978). Treatment of experimental murine cryptococcosis: A comparison of miconazole and amphotericin B. *Antimicrob Ag Chemother* **13**: 277.

Gubbins PO, Piscitelli SC, Danziger LH (1993). Candidal urinary tract infections: A comprehensive review of their diagnosis and management. *Pharmacotherapy* **13**: 110.

Gupta SK (1986). Efficacy of miconazole in experimental keratomycosis. *Aust NZ J Ophthalmol* **14**: 373.

Hammoto T, Watanabe K, Ikemoto H (1983). Endobronchial miconazole for pulmonary aspergilloma. *Ann Intern Med* **98**: 1030.

Haron E, Anaissie E, Dumphy F, McCredie K, Fainstein V (1988). *Hansenula anomala* fungemia. *Rev Infect Dis* **10**: 1182.

Hatfield SM, Crane LR, Duman K *et al.* (1986). Miconazole-induced alteration in tobramycin pharmacokinetics. *Clin Pharm* **5**: 415.

Haughan PA, Chance ML, Goad LJ (1992). Synergism *in vitro* of lovostatin and miconazole as anti-leishmanial agents. *Biochem Pharmacol* **44**: 2199.

Hay RJ (1979). Mycoses imported from the West Indies. A report of three cases. *Postgrad Med J* **55**: 603.

Heel RC, Brogden RN, Pakes GE *et al.* (1980). Miconazole: a preliminary review of its therapeutic efficacy in systemic fungal infections. *Drugs* **19**: 7.

Hegemann L, Toso SM, Lahijani KI *et al.* (1993). Direct interaction of antifungal azole-derivatives with calmodulin: a possible mechanism for their therapeutic activity. *J Invest Dermatol* **100**: 343.

Hernandez Molina JM, Llosa J, Martinez Brocal A, Ventosa A (1992). *In vitro* activity of cloconazole, sulconazole, butoconazole, isoconazole, fenticonazole, and five other antifungal agents against clinical isolates of *Candida albicans* and *Candida* spp. *Mycopathologia* **118**: 15.

Hilton AL, Warnock DW, Milne JD, Scott AJ (1978). Treatment of vaginal candidosis with miconazole. *Curr Med Res Opin* **5**: 295.

Hoeprich PD, Goldstein E (1974). Miconazole therapy for coccidioidomycosis. *JAMA* **230**: 1153.

Hoeprich PD, Huston AC (1978). Stability of four antifungal antimicrobics *in vitro*. *J Infect Dis* **137**: 87.

Hoeprich PD, Lawrence RM, Goldstein E (1980). Treatment of coccidioidomycosis with miconazole. *JAMA* **243**: 1923.

Holbrook WP, Kippax R (1979). Sensitivity of *Candida albicans* from patients with chronic oral candidiasis. *Postgrad Med J* **55**: 692.

Holmes SE, Aldous S (1991). Stability of miconazole in peritoneal dialysis fluid. *Amer J Hosp Pharm* **48**: 286.

Holt RJ, Azmi A (1978). Miconazole-resistant *Candida*. *Lancet* **1**: 50.

Horton CM, Freeman CD, Nolan PE, Copeland JG (1992). Cyclosporine interactions with miconazole and other azole-antimycotic: a case report and review of the literature. *J Heart Lung Transplant* **11**: 1127.

Hughes CE, Harris C, Moody JA *et al.* (1984). *In vitro* activities of amphotericin B in combination with four antifungal agents and rifampin against *Aspergillus* spp. *Antimicrob Ag Chemother* **25**: 560.

Hughes JR, Moore MK, Pembroke AC (1993). Tinea nigra palmaris. *Clin Exp Dermatol* **18**: 481.

Hussain Qadri SMH, Flournoy DJ, Qadri SGM, Ramirez EG (1986). Susceptibility of clinical isolates of yeasts to anti-fungal agents. *Mycopathologia* **95**: 183.

Jordan WM, Bodey GP, Rodriguez J *et al.* (1979). Miconazole therapy for treatment of fungal infections in cancer patients. *Antimicrob Ag Chemother* **16**: 792.

Kanarek KS, Williams PR (1986). Toxicity of intravenous miconazole overdosage in a preterm infant. *Pediatr Infect Dis* **5**: 486.

Kattan H, Pfugfeller SC (1989). Complications of intraocular antimicrobial agents. *Int Ophthalmol Clin* **29**: 188.

Katz ME, Cassileth PA (1977). Disseminated candidiasis in a patient with acute leukaemia. Successful treatment with miconazole. *JAMA* **237**: 1124.

Kilvington S, Larkin DFP, White DG, Beeching JR (1990). Laboratory investigation of *Acanthamoeba* keratitis. *J Clin Microbiol* **28**: 2722.

Klippenstein K, O'Day DM, Robinson RD *et al.* (1993). The qualitative evaluation of the pharmacokinetics of subconjunctivally injected antifungal agents in rabbits. *Cornea* **12**: 512.

Kusunoki T, Harada S (1984). Comparison of the *in vitro* antifungal activities of clotrimazole, miconazole, econazole and exalamide against clinical isolates of dermatophytes. *J Dermatol* **11**: 277–284.

Lai KN, Newton M, Seymour A *et al.* (1981). Miconazole treatment after renal transplantation. *Lancet* **ii**: 48.

Levine HB, Stevens DA, Cobb JM, Gebhardt AE (1975). Miconazole in coccidioidomycosis, l. Assay of activity in mice and *in vitro*. *J Infect Dis* **132**: 407.

Lewi PJ, Boelaert J, Daneels R *et al.* (1976). Pharmacokinetic profile of intravenous miconazole in man. Comparison of normal subjects and patients with renal insufficiency. *Eur J Clin Pharmacol* **10**: 49.

Lima NS, Teixeira G, Miranda J, de Valle ACF (1977). Treatment of South American blastomycosis (Paracoccidioidomycosis) with miconazole by the oral route: an on-going study. *Proc Roy Soc Med* **70** (Suppl 1): 35.

Lopez R, Mason JO, Parker JS, Pappas PG (1994). Intraocular blastomycosis: case report and review. *Clin Infect Dis* **18**: 805.

Lutwick Ll, Galgiani JN, Johnson RH, Stevens DA (1976). Visceral fungal infections due to *Petriellidium boydii* (*Allescheria boydii*). *In vitro* drug sensitivity studies. *Amer J Med* **61**: 632.

Lutwick LI, Rytel MW, Yanez JP *et al.* (1979). Deep infections from *Petriellidium boydii* treated with miconazole. *JAMA* **241**: 272.

Mader JT, Ream RS, Heath PW (1978). *Petriellidium boydii* (*Allescheria boydii*) sphenoidal sinusitis. *JAMA* **239**: 2368.

Marcon MJ, Durrell DE, Powell DA, Buesching WJ (1987). *In vitro* activity of systemic antifungal agents against *Malassezia furfur*. *Antimicrob Ag Chemother* **31**: 951.

Marmion LC, Desser KB, Lilly RB, Stevens DA (1976). Reversible thrombocytosis and anemia due to miconazole therapy. *Antimicrob Ag Chemother* **10**: 447.

McDougall PN, Fleming PJ, Speller DC *et al.* (1982). Neonatal systemic candidiasis: a failure to respond to intravenous miconazole in two neonates. *Arch Dis Child* **57**: 884.

McGookin AG, Millership JS, Scott EM (1987). Miconazole sorption to intravenous infusion sets. *J Clin Pharm Ther* **12**: 433.

McGuire TW, Bullock JD, Bullock JD Jr *et al.* (1991). Fungal endophthalmitis An experimental study with a review of 17 human ocular cases. *Arch Ophthalmol* **109**: 1289.

McWhinney PHM, Madgwick CA, Hoffbrand AV *et al.* (1992). Successful surgical management of septic arthritis due to *Trichosporon beigelii* in a patient with acute myeloid leukemia. *Scand J Infect Dis* **24**: 245.

Moody MR, Young VM, Morris MJ, Schimpff SC (1980). *In vitro* activities of miconazole, miconazole nitrate, and ketoconazole alone and combined with rifampin against *Candida* spp. and *Torulopsis glabrata* recovered from cancer patients. *Antimicrob Ag Chemother* **17**: 871.

Morgans ME, Thomas MEM, Mackenzie DWR (1979). Successful treatment of systemic cryptococcosis with miconazole. *Brit Med J* **2**: 100.

Morison A, Erasmus DS, Bowie MD (1988). Treatment of *Candida albicans* meningitis with intravenous and intrathecal miconazole. *S Afr Med J* **74**: 235.

Morita K, Ono T, Shimakawa H (1990). Inhibition of testosterone biosynthesis in testicular microsomes by various imidazole drugs. Comparative study with ketoconazole. *J Pharmacobiodyn* **13**: 336.

Morris DF, Sugrue DL (1975). Miconazole nitrate compared with chlordantoin in the treatment of vaginal candidiasis. *Brit J Vener Dis* **51**: 123.

Nagington J, Richards JE (1976). Chemotherapeutic compounds and *Acanthamoebae* from eye infection. *J Clin Path* **29**: 648.

Negroni R, Rubinstein P, Herrmann A, Gimenez A (1977). Results of miconazole therapy in twenty-eight patients with paracoccidioidomycosis (South American blastomycosis). *Proc Roy Soc Med* **70** (Suppl 1): 24.

Nicholls M, Robertson Tl, Jennis F (1980). Oral histoplasmosis treated with miconazole. *Aust NZ J Med* **10**: 563.

Niell HB (1977). Miconazole carrier solution, hyperlipidemia and hematologic problems. *New Engl J Med* **296**: 1479.

Odds FC, McDonald F (1981). Persistence of miconazole in vaginal secretions after single applications. Implications for the treatment of vaginal candidosis. *Brit J Vener Dis* **57**: 400.

Okeke CN, Gugnani HC (1987). *In vitro* sensitivity of environmental isolates of pathogenic dematiaceous fungi to azole compounds and a phenylpropyl-morpholine derivative. *Mycopathologia* **99**: 175.

O'Reilly RA, Goulart DA, Kunze KL *et al.* (1992). Mechanisms of the stereoselective interaction between miconazole and racemic warfarin in human subjects. *Clin Pharmacol Ther* **51**: 656.

Patterson TF, Andriole VT, Zervos MJ *et al.* (1990). The epidemiology of pseudallescheriasis complicating transplantation: Nosocomial and community-acquired infection. *Mycoses* **33**: 297.

Pawelec G, Ehninger G, Rehbein A, Schaudt K, Jaschonek K (1991). Comparison of the immunosuppressive activities of the antimycotic agents itraconazole, fluconazole, ketoconazole and miconazole on human T-cells. *Int J Immunopharmacol* **13**: 299.

Perez RE, Smith M, McClendon J *et al.* (1988). *Pseudallescheria boydii* brain abscess. Complication of an intravenous catheter. *Amer J Med* **84**: 359.

Perret CM, Happle R (1988). Contact allergy to miconazole. *Contact Derm* **19**: 75.

Pershing LK, Corlett J, Jorgensen C (1994). *In vivo* pharmacokinetics and pharmacodynamics of topical ketoconazole and miconazole in human stratum corneum. *Antimicrob Ag Chemother* **38**: 90.

Petrou MA, Rogers TR (1991). Interactions *in vitro* between polyenes and imidazoles against yeasts. *J Antimicrob Chemother* **27**: 491.

Pfaller MA, Krogstad DJ (1981). Imidazole and polyene activity against choroquine-resistant *Plasmodium falciparum*. *J Infect Dis* **144**: 372.

Pfeifer JD, Grand G, Thomas MA *et al.* (1991). Endogenous *Pseudallescheria boydii* endophthalmitis. Clinicopathologic findings in two cases. *Arch Ophthalmol* **109**: 1714.

Plempel M (1979). Pharmacokinetics of imidazole antimycotics. *Postgrad Med J* **55**: 662.

Pye GW, Marriott MS (1982). Inhibition of sterol C14 demethylation by imidazole-containing antifungals. *Sabouraudia* **20**: 325.

Raulin C, Frosch PJ (1988). Contact allergy to imidazole antimycotics. *Contact Derm* **18**: 76.

Reuben A, Anaissie E, Nelson PE *et al.* (1989). Antifungal susceptibility of 44 clinical isolates of *Fusarium* species determined by using a broth microdilution method. *Antimicrob Ag Chemother* **33**: 1647.

Rohwedder JJ, Archer G (1976). Pulmonary sporotrichosis: treatment with miconazole. *Amer Rev Respir Dis* **114**: 403.

Rolan PE, Somogyi AA, Drew MJR *et al.* (1983). Phenytoin intoxication during treatment with parenteral miconazole. *Brit Med J* **287**: 1760.

Rosa FW, Baum C, Shaw M (1987). Pregnancy outcomes after first trimester vaginitis drug therapy. *Obstet Gynecol* **69**: 751.

Rose HD, Varkey B (1978). Miconazole treatment of relapsed pulmonary blastomycosis. *Amer Rev Respir Dis* **118**: 403.

Rose HD, Roth DA, Barboriak JJ (1979). Hyperlipidemia related to miconazole therapy. *Ann Intern Med* **91**: 491.

Salkin IF, McGinnis MR, Dykstra MJ, Rinaldi MG (1988). *Scedosporium inflatum*, an emerging pathogen. *J Clin Microbiol* **26**: 498.

Schacter LP, Owellen RJ, Rathbun HK, Buchanan B (1976). Antagonism between miconazole and amphotericin B. *Lancet* **ii**: 318.

Scheef W, Symoens J, van Camp K *et al.* (1974). Chemotherapy of candidiasis. *Brit Med J* **1**: 78.

Schiess RJ, Coscia MF, McClellan GA (1984). *Petriellidium boydii* pachymeningitis treated with miconazole and ketoconazole. *Neurosurgery* **14**: 220.

Scott EM, Gorman SP, McGrath SJ (1985). Inhibition of hyphal development in *Trichophyton mentagrophytes* arthroconidia by ketoconazole and miconazole. *J Antimicrob Chemother* **15**: 405.

Segal E, Padhye AA, Ajello L (1976). Susceptibility of *Prothotheca* species to antifungal agents. *Antimicrob Ag Chemother* **10**: 75.

Sekhon AS, Padhye AA, Garg AK (1992). *In vitro* sensitivity of *Penicillium marneffei* and *Pythium insidiosum* to various antifungal agents. *Eur J Epidemiol* **8**: 427.

Shadomy S, Paxton L, Espinel-Ingroff A, Shadomy HJ (1977). *In vitro* studies with miconazole and miconazole nitrate. *J Antimicrob Chemother* **3**: 147.

Shehab ZM, Britton H, Dunn JH (1988). Imidazole therapy for coccidioidal meningitis in children. *Pediatr Infect Dis J* **7**: 40.

Shenfield GM, Page M (1991). Potentiation of warfarin action by miconazole oral gel. *Aust NZ J Med* **21**: 928.

Sreedhara Swamy KH, Joshi A, Ramananda Rao G (1976). Mechanism of action of miconazole: labilization of rat liver lysosomes *in vitro* by miconazole. *Antimicrob Ag Chemother* **9**: 903.

Stevens DA (1983). Miconazole in the treatment of coccidioidomycosis. *Drugs* **26**: 347.

Stevens DA, Levine HB, Deresinski SC (1976). Miconazole in coccidioidomycosis. II. Therapeutic and pharmacologic studies in man. *Amer J Med* **60**: 191.

Stevens DA, Restrepo A, Cortes A *et al.* (1978). Paracoccidioidomycosis (South American blastomycosis): treatment with miconazole. *Amer J Trop Med Hyg* **27**: 801.

Sud IJ, Feingold DS (1982). Action of antifungal imidazoles on *Staphylococcus aureus*. *Antimicrob Ag Chemother* **22**: 470.

Sugarman B, Mummaw N (1988). Effects of antimicrobial agents on growth and chemotaxis of *Trichomonas vaginalis*. *Antimicrob Ag Chemother* **32**: 1323.

Supparatpinyo K, Nelson KE, Merz WG *et al.* (1993). Response to antifungal therapy by human immunodeficiency virus-infected patients with disseminated *Penicillium marneffei* infections and *in vitro* susceptibilities of isolates from clinical specimens. *Antimicrob Ag Chemother* **37**: 2407.

Sutton A (1983). Miconazole in systemic candidiasis. *Arch Dis Child* **58**: 319.

Symoens J (1977). Clinical and experimental evidence on miconazole for the treatment of systemic mycosis: a review. *Proc Roy Soc Med* **70** (Suppl 1): 4.

Taylor FR, Rodriguez RJ, Parks LW (1983). Relationship between antifungal activity and inhibition of sterol biosynthesis in miconazole, clotrimazole and 15-azasterol. *Antimicrob Ag Chemother* **23**: 515.

Thong YH, Rowan-Kelly B (1978). Inhibitory effect of miconazole on mitogen -induced lymphocyte proliferative responses. *Brit Med J* **1**: 149.

Thong YH, Rowan-Kelly B, Shepherd C, Ferrante A (1977). Growth inhibition of *Naegleria fowleri* by tetracycline, rifamycin, and miconazole. *Lancet* **ii**: 876.

Timonen H (1992). Shorter treatment for vaginal candidosis: comparison between single-dose oral fluconazole and three-day treatment with local miconazole. *Mycosis* **35**: 317.

Tolentino FI, Foster S, Lahav M *et al.* (1982). Toxicity of intravitreal miconazole. *Arch Ophthalmol* **100**: 1504.

Van Cutsem JM, Thienpont D (1972). Miconazole, a broad-spectrum antimycotic agent with antibacterial activity. *Chemotherapy* **17**: 392.

Van den Bossche H, Williamsens G, Cools W *et al.* (1983). Hypothesis on the molecular basis of the antifungal activity of N-substituted imidazoles and triazoles. *Biochem Soc Trans* **11**: 665.

van der Meijden WI, van der Hoek JC, Staal HJ *et al.* (1986). Double-blind comparison of 200 mg ketoconazole oral tablets and 1200 mg miconazole vaginal capsule in the treatment of vaginal candidosis. *Eur J Obstet Gynecol Reprod Biol* **22**: 133.

van Heusden AM, Merkus HM, Corbeij RS *et al.* (1990). Single-dose oral fluconazole versus single-dose topical miconazole for the treatment of acute vulvovaginal candidosis. *Acta Obstet Gynecol Scand* **69**: 417.

Venugopal, PV, Venugopal TV, Ramakrishna ES, Ilavarasi S (1993). Antimycotic susceptibility testing of agents of black grain eumycetoma. *J Med Vet Mycol* **31**: 161.

Wainer S, Cooper PA, Funk E *et al.* (1992). Prophylactic miconazole oral gel for the prevention of neonatal fungal rectal colonization and systemic infection. *Pediatr Infect Dis J* **11**: 713.

Walsh TJ, Newman KR, Moody M *et al.* (1986). Trichosporonosis in patients with neoplastic disease. *Medicine* **65**: 268.

Weinstein L, Jacoby I (1980). Successful treatment of cerebral cryptococcoma and meningitis with miconazole. *Ann Intern Med* **93**: 569.

Wingard JR, Vaughan WP, Braine HG *et al.* (1987). Prevention of fungal sepsis in patients with prolonged neutropenia: A randomized, double-blind, placebo-controlled trial of intravenous miconazole. *Amer J Med* **83**: 1103.

Wise GJ, Goldman WM, Golgberg PE, Rothenberg RG (1987). Miconazole: a cost-effective antifungal genitourinary irrigant. *J Urol* **138**: 1413.

Wong PW, Ching WTW, Kwon-Chung KJ, Meyer RD (1989). Disseminated *Phialophora parasitica* infection in humans: Case report and review. *Rev Infect Dis* **11**: 770–775.

Wust HJ, Lennartz H (1977). Miconazole in systemic candidiasis. *Proc Roy Soc Med* **70** (Suppl 1): 18.

Yangco BG, Okafor JI, TeStrake D (1984a). *In vitro* susceptibilities of human and wild-type isolates of *Basidiobolus* and *Conidiobolus* species. *Antimicrob Ag Chemother* **25**: 413.

Yangco BG, TeStrake D, Okafor J (1984b). *Phialophora richardsiae* isolated from infected bone: Morphological, physiological and antifungal susceptibility studies. *Mycopathologia* **86**: 103.

Zaias N (1975). Clotrimazole and miconazole. PAHO and WHO: Proceedings of the Third International Conference on the Mycoses, Sao Paulo, Brazil, 27–29 August 1974 Scientific Publication No 304, p. 241.

Zaidman GW (1991). Miconazole corneal toxicity. *Cornea* **10**: 90.

Bifonazole

Description

Bifonazole is a substituted imidazole, structurally related to clotrimazole, econazole and miconazole. It has the chemical name of 1-(alpha-biphenyl-4-ylbenzyl)imidazole. Bifonazole has a broad spectrum of antifungal activity *in vitro* and has been shown to be an effective topical antifungal agent for the management of superficial fungal infections of the skin, particularly dermatophytoses, cutaneous candidiasis and tinea versicolor.

Sensitive Organisms

1 Pathogenic yeast

Cryptococcus neoformans is susceptible to bifonazole (Yamaguchi *et al.*, 1983). Most *Candida* species were less susceptible to bifonazole than to clotrimazole or miconazole (Yamaguchi *et al.*, 1983); however, more than 90% of strains of *C. albicans*, *C. glabrata* and *C. parapsilosis* were inhibited by bifonazole concentrations less than 4 μg per ml (Plempel *et al.*, 1983). *Candida krusei* was less susceptible with 40% of strains resistant. *Pityrosporum* spp. are susceptible to bifonazole concentrations of 1–2 μg per ml (Lackner and Clissold, 1989). Odds *et al.* (1987) in an attempt to overcome the difficulty in interpretation of *in vitro* MIC tests for the azole drugs in particular, due to lack of standardization and marked variability with methodology, growth medium, incubation temperature, pH and inoculum size (p. 1388) developed a method which measures the relative inhibition factor (RIF). This enables a comparison of antifungal activity between the plethora of azole drugs. The RIF data confirmed the MIC results for bifonazole, suggesting a lower potency against yeast pathogens, and a comparable RIF (mean of 56–77) for the topical azoles against the *Candida* spp. The systemic azoles tended to have lower RIF reflecting greater activity.

2 Dimorphic fungi

Species of dimorphic fungi other than *Sporothrix schenckii* are very sensitive to bifonazole with MICs less than 2 μg per ml (Plempel *et al.*, 1983; Yamaguchi *et al.*, 1983). Strains of *S. schenckii* have higher MICs and there are reports of resistance in 40% of strains (Shadomy, 1984, Yamaguchi *et al.*, 1983).

3 Molds or filamentous fungi

Bifonazole exhibits excellent *in vitro* activity against the dermatophytes, with over 95% of strains inhibited by bifonazole concentrations less than 2 μg per ml.It has been demonstrated that bifonazole is fungicidal against *Trichophyton rubrum*, *T. mentagrophytes*, and *Microsporum canis* (Shadomy *et al.*, 1982; Plempel *et al.*, 1983). Odds *et al.*, (1987), confirmed the potent activity against dermatophytes by measurement of RIF. *In vivo* efficacy in the guinea pig model of dermatophytosis, using *T. mentagrophytes,* was confirmed using 1% bifonazole cream or lotion once-daily for 5 days, and comparable efficacy with 1% clotrimazole and ciclopirox olamine was established (Plempel *et al.*, 1983; Yamaguchi and Uchida, 1984; Hanel *et al.*, 1988a). However, Hanel *et al.*, (1988b) determined in an *in vitro* pig skin model of *T. mentagrophytes* infection, bifonazole inhibitory and fungicidal activity was inferior to ciclopirox olamine. Against isolates of pathogenic non-dermatophyte filamentous fungi (*Hendersonula toruloidea*, *Scytalidium* spp.) bifonazole exhibited good *in vitro* activity but the MICs were higher (range of 0.39–3.1 μg per ml), than those for dermatophytes (Oyeka and Gugnani, 1990).

Aspergillus species are also readily inhibited by bifonazole, as are the agents of chromomycosis (*Fonsecaea pedrosoi, Phialophora verrucosa, Cladosporium carrionii*), *Madurella* spp., and *Pseudallescheria boydii* (Plempel *et al.*, 1983; Yamaguchi *et al.*, 1983; Okeke and Gugnani, 1987).

4 Bacteria

Bifonazole has antibacterial activity against Gram-positive cocci (*Staphylococcus aureus, Staph. epidermidis*, streptococci), *Corynebacterium* spp., and *Propionobacterium acnes* (Plempel *et al.*, 1983). It has no activity against Gram-negative bacteria or enterococcus.

Mode of Administration and Dose

Indications and recommended doses
Dermatophytoses:
Tinea pedis, tinea pedis interdigitalis – 1% cream once-daily for 21 days
Tinea corporis, tinea cruris, tinea manuum – 1% cream once-daily for 14–21 days
Pityriasis versicolor – 1% cream once-daily for 14 days

Superficial candidiasis:
1% cream once-daily for 14–28 days.

Availability

Topical formulations: 1% cream, 1% solution, 1% gel and 1% powder.

There have been no randomized, controlled trials to evaluate differences in efficacy of the different formulations of bifonazole. Comparable efficacy was reported from a large trial involving over 1000 patients and demonstrated clinical reponses in 79% of those treated with cream, 81% of solution-treated patients and 84% of those treated with gel (Lackner and Clissold, 1989).

Absorption of the Drug

Bifonazole is formulated only for topical use. Pharmacokinetic data in humans are limited to a study of the i.v. administration of 0.016 mg per kg ^{14}C-labeled bifonazole to four healthy volunteers. This study revealed rapid metabolism of bifonazole (95% within 4 h), and undetectable plasma bifonazole at 8 h post-infusion. The drug is distributed rapidly and the elimination is biphasic. The half-life of unchanged drug was 1.4 h, and the half-life of metabolic products of bifonazole is 8.9 h and 42 h. About 85% of the administered dose is recovered in urine and feces over 5 days (Patzschke *et al.*, 1983; Lackner and Clissold, 1989).

Radiolabeled bifonazole 1% cream was used to determine the percutaneous absorption of drug through healthy skin. Less than 1% of the dose is absorbed in 6 h (Patzschke *et al.*, 1983). The percutaneous absorption of bifonazole through inflamed skin is 3–4% (Ritter and Siefert, 1987). Bifonazole was not detected in plasma after daily application of 1% bifonazole solution for 2 weeks in healthy volunteers; however, in patients with pityriasis versicolor, dermatomycoses and neonates with *Candida* napkin rash, plasma bifonazole concentrations varied from <1–16 ng per ml, confirming the negligible systemic absorption from topical application (Ritter and Siefert, 1987).

Bifonazole penetrates the stratum corneum and 0.34% of a dose of ^{14}C radiolabeled bifonazole is retained on healthy skin, maintaining concentrations of bifonazole greater than the MIC for dermatophytes in the epidermis and stratum corneum (Patzschke *et al.*, 1983). The mean half-life of bifonazole in stratum corneum is 19–32 h, supporting the once-daily dosing recommendation (Ritter and Siefert, 1987).

Bifonazole does not appear to penetrate into the cornea and aqueous humor after topical application of bifonazole 1% drops in rabbits (Behrens-Baumann *et al.*, 1990).

Mode of Action

The primary mechanism of action, similar for all the imidazoles, is inhibition of cytochrome P-450 dependent C-14 alpha demethylation of lanosterol, preventing conversion to ergosterol, which results in depletion of normal fungal sterols (ergosterol) and accumulation of 14 alpha methyl sterols (lanosterol) in the fungal cell membrane (Lackner and Clissold, 1989) (see Fig. IV.1, p. 1261). Berg *et al.*, (1984), have also shown that bifonazole inhibits microsomal HMG-CoA-reductase an early step in the ergosterol biosynthesis pathway, and suggested that inhibition of this enzyme may be responsible for the relative enhanced fungicidal activity. Irreversible morphological changes and structural damage occur in *Pityosporum ovale*, *C. albicans*, *T. rubrum*, and *M. canis* following exposure to bifonazole (Lackner and Clissold, 1989).

Toxicity

Local adverse effects are experienced by about 4% of patients (4.1% for the cream, and 4.5% for the solution). Itching, burning, skin discomfort, redness and rash were reported in the clinical trials. These reactions were limited to the area of application, were generally mild and reversible (Lackner and Clissold, 1989).

Clinical Uses of the Drug

1 Dermatophytoses

Open non-comparative trials of 1% bifonazole applied once-daily for 14–21 days have consistently reported efficacy rates of 80–90% (Galimberti *et al.*, 1984; Belli *et al.*, 1985a; Earl *et al.*, 1986; Wheatley *et al.*, 1988; Lackner and Clissold, 1989). Placebo-controlled trials of bifonazole have shown significantly superior reponses for patients randomized to bifonazole 1% cream, gel or powder (Bagatell, 1986a,b; Coffey, 1986; Goffe, 1986; Lackner and Clissold, 1989).

In small comparative studies with other topical antifungal agents, bifonazole produced clinical and mycological cure rates in 65–100% of patients with a variety of superficial dermatomycoses. Bifonazole 1% cream, solution or gel applied once-daily had equivalent efficacy with econazole 1% cream or solution applied twice-daily for tinea pedis, tinea corporis or tinea cruris (Lackner and Clissold, 1989), sulconazole 1% cream applied twice-daily for tinea pedis or tinea cruris, miconazole 2% cream applied twice-daily for tinea pedis, tinea corporis and tinea cruris, amorolfine 0.5% cream, naftifine 1% cream, oxiconazole nitrate 1% cream and ciclopirox-olamine 1% cream (Roberts *et al.*, 1985; Wagner and Reckers-Czaschka, 1987; del Palacio-Hernanz *et al.*, 1989; Hanel *et al.*, 1988a; Lackner and Clissold, 1989; del Palacio *et al.*, 1992). A larger study compared bifonazole 1% cream with three different concentrations of amorolfine cream (0.125%, 0.25% and 0.5%) applied once-daily for 4 weeks and rates of mycological efficacy were not statistically different between the groups. Bifonazole 1% achieved negative cultures in 87% of patients compared with 91–92% for the three concentrations of amorolfine (Nolting *et al.*, 1992).

2 Cutaneous candidiasis

Bifonazole 1% is an effective agent for superficial candidiasis, with clinical and mycological response rates documented in 73–88% of treated patients (Belli *et al.*, 1985b; Lackner and Clissold, 1989). Lalosevic *et al.* (1984) established that application of bifonazole 1% cream was significantly superior to placebo, and that once-daily versus twice-daily application produced equivalent responses. It has been used effectively to treat candidal intertrigo, candidal balanitis and candidal napkin rash.

3 Pityriasis versicolor

Bifonazole 1% cream, solution or gel has been established as an effective agent for pityriasis versicolor in open non-comparative studies, placebo-controlled trials and comparative trials with other topical antifungal drugs. Clinical cure was achieved in 50–100% of patients treated once-daily for 14 days (Mora and Greer, 1984; Galimberti *et al.*, 1985; Goffe, 1986; Greer *et al.*, 1986; VanDersal, 1986; Lackner and Clissold, 1989). Approximately 60% of patients experience clinical resolution with a single topical application of bifonazole, but the response rate increases to 90% if 14 days treatment is applied. There is no significant difference in mycological and clinical response rates with 1 or 2 weeks treatment (Hernandez-Perez, 1986). Bifonazole 1% cream was found to be as effective as econazole 1% cream, miconazole 2% cream, 1% terbinafine cream and fenticonazole 1% lotion in controlled studies (Aste *et al.*, 1988; Lackner and Clissold, 1989; Aste *et al.*, 1991).

4 Other skin disorders

A placebo-controlled trial of bifonazole shampoo used for washing the scalp three times weekly for 6 weeks established the efficacy of bifonazole for the treatment of seborrheic dermatitis of the scalp (Segal *et al.*, 1992). Bifonazole 1% cream effectively cleared facial seborrheic dermatitis in 84% of patients treated once-daily for 4 weeks (Faergemann, 1989). It has also been reported to be effective in the management of inflammatory skin disorders, including psoriasis and rosacea. Hegemann *et al.* (1993), has postulated a possible mechanism for this activity by demonstrating that bifonazole, like other azole derivatives, competitively inhibits calmodulin activity which is implicated in the pathogenesis of both fungal infections and inflammatory skin disorders.

5 Onychomycosis

The effect of a 1% bifonazole/40% urea combination ointment was examined ex vivo using scanning electron microscopy and demonstrated effective penetration of the nail plate (Fritsch *et al.*, 1992). The urea paste causes a chemical nail avulsion and using the combination, mycological eradication has been achieved in 62% of patients 3 months after completion of treatment (Korting and Schafer-Korting, 1992). Torres-Rodriguez *et al.* (1991) used 1% bifonazole and 40% urea combination cream applied to infected nails until the nail softened and was removed, and then 1% bifonazole cream alone. With this regimen, mycological eradication occurred within 3 weeks and clinical cure was maintained in 89–94% of nails at 6–12 months. A similar open study of bifonazole 1%/urea 40% cream for 2 weeks followed by bifonazole 1% cream for 4 weeks caused nail avulsion in 97% and regrowth of a normal nail in 92%. The recurrence rate was 12% in the 12-week follow-up period (Hardjoko *et al.*, 1990).

References

Aste N, Pau M, Cordaro CI, Biggio P (1988). Double-blind study with fenticonazole or bifonazole in pityriasis versicolor. *Int J Pharmacol Res* **8**: 271.

Aste N, Pau M, Pinna AL *et al.* (1991). Clinical efficacy and tolerability of terbinafine in patients with pityriasis versicolor. *Mycoses* **34**: 353.

Bagatell FK (1986a). Elimination of dermatophytes causing tinea pedis interdigitalis with once-daily application of bifonazole 1% solution. *Adv Ther* **3**: 265.

Bagatell FK (1986b). A prospective study of bifonazole 1% cream in the once-daily management of tinea corporis/cruris. *Adv Ther* **3**: 294.

Behrens-Baumann W, Klinge B, Uter W (1990). Clotrimazole and bifonazole in the topical treatment of *Candida* keratitis in rabbits. *Mycoses* **33**: 567.

Belli L, Galimberti R, Negroni R *et al.* (1985a). Treatment of tinea corporis or tinea cruris with bifonazole 1% gel: an open, multicenter study. *Pharmatherapeutica* **4**: 106.

Belli L, Galimberti R, Negroni R *et al.* (1985b). Treatment of superficial candidiasis with bifonazole 1% gel. *Pharmatherapeutica* **4**: 102.

Berg D, Regel E, Harenberg HE, Plempel M (1984). Bifonazole and clotrimazole: their mode of action and the possible reason for the fungicidal behaviour of bifonazole. *Arzneim Forsch* **34**: 139.

Coffey W (1986). Management of tinea pedis interdigitalis with bifonazole 1% cream: double-blind study. *Adv Ther* **3**: 301.

del Palacio-Hernanz AD, Lopez-Gomez S, Moreno-Plancar P *et al.* (1989). A clinical double-blind trial comparing amorolfine cream 05% (Ro 14–4767) with bifonazole cream 1% in the treatment of dermatomycoses. *Clin Exp Derm* **14**: 141.

del Palacio A, Lopez-Gomez S, Garcia-Bravo M *et al.* (1992). Experience with amorolfine in the treatment of dermatomycoses. *Dermatologica* **184** (Suppl 1): 25.

Earl D, Allenby L, Richards H, Wright CM (1986). Bifonazole 1% gel in the treatment of superficial dermatophytoses and erythrasma of the feet and groin. *Pharmatherapeutica* **4**: 532.

Faergemann J (1989). Treatment of seborrheic dermatitis with bifonazole. *Mycoses* **32**: 309.

Fritsch H, Stettendorf S, Hegemann L (1992). Ultrastructural changes in onychomycosis during treatment with bifonazole/urea ointment. *Dermatologica* **185**: 32.

Galimberti RL, Belli L, Negroni R *et al.* (1984). Treatment of tinea pedis interdigitalis with bifonazole 1% gel. *Dermatologica* **169** (Suppl 1): 107.

Galimberti R, Belli L, Gatti JC *et al.* (1985). An open, multicentre assessment of the effectiveness of bifonazole in the treatment of tinea (pityriasis) versicolor. *Pharmatherapeutica* **4**: 109.

Goffe BS (1986). Response of tinea corporis-cruris and tinea (pityriasis) versicolor to once daily topical treatment with bifonazole cream: a safety and efficacy study. *Adv Ther* **3**: 289.

Greer DL, Mora RG, Jolly HW (1986). Assessment of bifonazole 1% solution in the eradication of organisms causing tinea (pityriasis) versicolor. *Adv Ther* **3**: 256.

Hanel H, Abrams B, Dittmar W, Ehlers G (1988a). A comparison of bifonazole and ciclopiroxolamine: in vitro, animal, and clinical studies. *Mycoses* **31**: 632.

Hanel H, Raether W, Dittmar W (1988b). Evaluation of fungicidal action *in vitro* and in a skin model considering the influence of penetration kinetics of various standard antimycotics. *Ann NY Acad Sci* **544**: 329.

Hardjoko FS, Widyanto S, Singgih I, Susilo J (1990). Treatment of onychomycosis with a bifonazole-urea combination. *Mycoses* **33**: 167.

Hegemann L, Toso SM, Lahijani KI *et al.* (1993). Direct interaction of antifungal azole-derivatives with calmodulin: a possible mechanism for their therapeutic activity. *J Invest Dermatol* **100**: 343.

Hernandez-Perez E (1986). A comparison between one- and two weeks treatment with bifonazole in pityriasis versicolor. *J Amer Acad Dermatol* **14**: 561.

Korting HC, Schafer-Korting M (1992). Is tinea unguim still widely incurable? A review three decades after the introduction of griseofulvin. *Arch Dermatol* **128**: 243.

Lackner TE, Clissold SP (1989). Bifonazole A review of its antimicrobial activity and therapeutic use in superficial mycoses. *Drugs* **38**: 204.

Lalosevic J, Rojas R, Astorga E, Gip L (1984). Bifonazole cream in the treatment of superficial candidosis. A double-blind comparative study. *Dermatologica* **169** (Suppl 1): 99.

Mora RG, Greer DL (1984). Comparative efficacy and tolerance of 1% bifonazole cream and bifonazole cream vehicle in patients with tinea versicolor. *Dermatologica* **169** (Suppl 1): 87.

Nolting S, Semig G, Friedrich HK *et al.* (1992). Double-blind comparison of amorolfine and bifonazole in the treatment of dermatomycoses. *Clin Exp Derm* **17** (Suppl 1): 56.

Odds FC, Webster CE, Abbott AB (1984). Antifungal relative inhibition factors; BAY 1–9139, bifonazole, butoconazole, isoconazole, itraconazole (R 51211), oxiconazole, Ro 14–4767/002, sulconazole, terconazole and vibunazole (BAY n-7133) compared with nine established antifungal agents. *J Antimicrob Chemother* **14**: 105.

Okeke CN, Gugnani HC (1987). *In vitro* sensitivity of environmental isolates of pathogenic dematiaceous fungi to azole compounds and a phenylpropyl-morpholine derivative. *Mycopathologia* **99**: 175.

Oyeka CA, Gugnani HC (1990). *In vitro* activity of seven azole compounds against some clinical isolates of non-dermatophyte filamentous fungi and some dermatophytes. *Mycopathologia* **110**: 157.

Patzschke K, Ritter W, Siefert HM *et al.* (1983). Pharmacokinetic studies following systemic and topical administration of radiolabeled bifonazole in man. *Arzneim Forschung* **33**: 745.

Plempel M, Regel E, Buchel KH (1983). Antimycotic efficacy of bifonazole *in vitro* and *in vivo*. *Arzneim Forschung* **33**: 517.

Ritter W, Siefert HM (1987). Biological disposition and percutaneous absorption of bifonazole in animals and man. In *Recent Trends in the Discovery, Development and Evaluation of Antifungal Agents* (Fromtling RA ed), p. 383. Barcelona: Prous Science Publishers.

Roberts DT, Adriaans B, Gentles JC (1985). A comparative study of once daily bifonazole cream versus twice daily miconazole cream in the treatment of tinea pedis. *Mykosen* **28**: 550.

Segal R, David M, Ingber A *et al.* (1992). Treatment with bifonazole shampoo for seborrhea and seborrheic dermatitis: a randomized, double-blind study. *Acta Dermato-Venereologica* **72**: 454.

Shadomy S, Dixon DM, May R (1982). A comparison of bifonazole (BAY H 4502) with clotrimazole *in vitro*. *Sabouraudia* **20**: 313.

Shadomy S, Espinel-Ingroff A, Kerkering TM (1984). *In-vitro* studies with four new antifungal agents: Bay n 7133, bifonazole (BAY h 4502), ICI 153,066 and Ro-14–4767/002. *Sabouraudia* **22**: 7.

Torres-Rodriguez JM, Madrenys N, Nicolas MC (1991). Non-traumatic topical treatment of onychomycosis with urea associated with bifonazole. *Mycoses* **34**: 499.

VanDersarl JV (1986). Evaluation of 1% bifonazole solution in patients with tinea corporis/cruris or tinea (pityriasis) versicolor infections. *Adv Ther* **3**: 281.

Wagner W, Reckers-Czaschka R (1987). Oxiconazole in dermatomycosis – a double-blind, randomized comparison with bifonazole. *Mykosen* **30**: 484.

Wheatley D, Richardson MD, Scott EM (1988). Tinea infections treated with bifonazole gel. *Mycoses* **31**: 471.

Yamaguchi H, Uchida K (1984). *In vivo* activity of bifonazole in guinea pigs: its characteristic features and comparison with clotrimazole. *Dermatologica* **169** (Suppl 1): 33.

Yamaguchi H, Hiratani T, Plempel M (1983). *In vitro* studies of a new imidazole antimycotic, bifonazole, in comparison with clotrimazole and miconazole. *Arzneim Forschung* **33**: 546.

Butoconazole

Description

Butoconazole nitrate is a synthetic imidazole derivative, which is structurally related to miconazole, and has the chemical name of 1-[4-(4-chlorophenyl)-2-(2,6-dichlorophenylthio)butyl]imidazole mononitrate. It has a broad spectrum of antifungal activity, but has been developed for use as a topical agent for vaginal candidiasis.

Sensitive Organisms

The first description of the synthesis and broad spectrum of activity of butoconazole which includes yeasts and dermatophytes in particular, was published by Walker *et al.* (1978). It has good *in vitro* activity against *Trichophyton mentagrophytes*, *T. rubrum*, *Epidermophyton floccosum* and *Microsporum canis* at concentrations less than 5 µg per ml. Butoconazole has potent activity against *Candida* spp. with an MIC range of 0.12–8 µg per ml. For *C. albicans* the MIC range is 0.12–8 µg per ml with 50% of isolates inhibited by 1 µg per ml (Hernandez Molina, 1992). Using the relative inhibition factor evaluation, Odds *et al.* (1984), determined butoconazole had moderately good activity against *Candida* spp., excellent activity against the dermatophytes and poor activity against *Aspergillus* spp. In the murine model of vaginal candidiasis, the activity of butoconazole was found to be superior to that of miconazole (Walker *et al.*, 1978; Matthews, 1986). Butoconazole also has good *in vitro* activity against some Gram-positive bacteria, including *Staphylococcus aureus* (MIC of 6.25 µg per ml), *Streptococcus pyogenes* (MIC of 0.0016 µg per ml) and *Strep. faecalis* (MIC of 3.12 µg per ml) (Matthews, 1986).

Mode of Administration and Dose

Indications and recommended doses
Vaginal candidiasis: 5 g of 2% butoconazole nitrate cream (100 mg butoconazole nitrate) intravaginally for 3 days in non-pregnant women, and for 6 days in pregnant women (second and third trimester).

Availability

Topical formulation of butoconazole nitrate: 100 mg vaginal pessary; 2% cream for vaginal use

Absorption of the Drug

Percutaneous absorption of the drug after vaginal application is minimal and amounts to about 5% of an intravaginal dose. In healthy volunteers, the peak plasma concentration of butoconazole after intravaginal administration of 5 g of radiolabeled butoconazole 2% cream (about 100 mg dose) was 19–44 ng per ml and occurred at 24 h. The radiolabeled drug first began to appear in plasma 2–8 h after administration and was detected for 4 days after a single dose. The plasma half-life of the absorbed drug has been estimated to be 21–24 h. The distribution of the absorbed drug into tissues has not been studied, but it is apparent that the drug is extensively metabolized in the liver and excreted in the urine and feces in equal amounts as metabolites (Droegemueller *et al.*, 1984; Fromtling, 1988).

Mode of Action

The exact mechanism of action of butoconazole has not been established. It is likely that it produces its antifungal activity in a similar manner as the other imidazole drugs, by binding to the heme iron of cytochrome P-450 thereby inhibiting the enzyme C14-demethylase (see Fig. IV.1, p. 1261). The resultant inhibition of the conversion of lanosterol to ergosterol and depletion of ergosterol in the fungal cell membrane gives rise to the fungistatic activity of the drug. A butoconazole concentration of 20 nmol is able to reduce the synthesis of C-4,14-desmethyl sterols in *Candida albicans* by 50%, and this activity is superior to ketoconazole, clotrimazole and miconazole. Butoconazole does not affect the carbohydrate composition of treated cells (Pye and Marriott, 1982; Pfaller *et al.*, 1990). At high concentrations, butoconazole has a growth-phase dependent fungicidal activity against *C. albicans* which is thought to be due to direct fungal cell membrane damage (Beggs, 1985).

Toxicity

Local reactions include vaginal burning, itching, soreness and stinging, vaginal bleeding and discharge occurred in about 2% of women in clinical trials. Up to 20% of women complain of an objectionable odor (Bradbeer *et al.*, 1985). Headache has also been reported rarely during butoconazole administration (Jacobson *et al.*, 1985).

Butoconazole nitrate cream and suppositaries do not compromise the barrier property of contraceptive devices (condom, cervical cap or diaphragm) after close contact for 3 days (Wong, 1988).

Butoconazole nitrate 2% cream has been used safely in the second and third trimesters of pregnancy without reports of adverse effect on the pregnancy or fetal abnormalities in the offspring. However, no such safety data is available for the use of butoconazole in the first trimester of pregnancy.

A case of severe reversible thrombocytopenia associated with hemorrhage possibly induced by butaconazole has been reported. It developed 1 week after starting treatment with butoconazole nitrate cream. No recurrence of the event occurred after rechallenge with the woman's other medication, but no rechallenge with butoconazole was performed (Maloley *et al.*, 1990)

Clinical Uses of the Drug

1 Vulvovaginal candidiasis

Randomized comparative studies of butaconazole nitrate 2% cream applied for 3 or 6 days for treatment of vulvovaginal candidiasis produce clinical cures in approximately 75–80% of women and mycological eradication in 80–95% of episodes treated in both pregnant and non-pregnant women. There has also been no difference in response for women taking the oral contraceptive (Adamson, 1988). Weisberg (1986) has suggested that butoconazole is significantly inferior to miconazole for the treatment of vaginal candidiasis in pregnant women.

The first clinical trial to examine the efficacy of butaconazole for vaginal candidosis compared 6-day regimens with either butoconazole nitrate 1% cream, butoconazole nitrate 2% cream and miconazole 2% cream. Although there was no statistical difference between the groups for mycological or clinical response, the butoconazole-treated women had a higher mycological rate eradication at 1 week post-treatment (91–98%) than the miconazole treated women (83%). Persistence of mycological response occurred in 80% and 82% of the butoconazole groups and 68% of the miconazole group (Jacobson *et al.*, 1985). Others have confirmed the comparable efficacy for butoconazole and miconazole. Bradbeer *et al.* (1985) demonstrated cure rates of 83% at short-term follow-up and 77% at long-term follow-up for women treated with butoconazole nitrate 2% cream for 3 days, and 85% at short-term and 76% at long-term follow-up for women treated with miconazole nitrate 2% cream for 7 days. Brown *et al.* (1986), determined that a 3-day course of butoconazole nitrate 2% cream produced equivalent results as a 6-day course, and the clinical and mycological response rates were comparable with a miconazole 2% cream regimen. Equivalent efficacy and safety were also established for a 3-day course of butoconazole nitrate 2% cream and a 7-day course of miconazole 2% cream in a large randomized study (Kaufman *et al.*, 1989).

Butoconazole nitrate 2% cream administered once-daily for 3 days was as effective as clotrimazole 200 mg vaginal tablets once-daily for 3 days although there was a trend to greater rates of mycological cure at 1 week after the end of treatment (95% versus 91%), clinical response (82% versus 72%) and persistence of clinical and mycological response (80% versus 74%) at 30 day follow-up (Droegemueller *et al.*, 1984; Fleury, 1986). Butoconazole nitrate 2%

cream applied for 3 days appeared more effective than clotrimazole 1% cream applied for 6 days, but the differences in clinical and mycological response was not statistically significant (Fleury, 1986; Hajman, 1988). Finally, a comparison of butaconazole nitrate vaginal suppositaries 100 mg daily for 3 days compared with clotrimazole 200 mg vaginal tablets revealed no significant difference in clinical or long-term mycological response, but butoconazole produced a significantly higher rate of mycological eradication (92% versus 74%) at 1 week after treatment (Adamson *et al.*, 1986).

A 3-day course of butoconazole nitrate 2% cream was also found to be more effective than a 7-day course of econazole 1% cream in producing sustained clinical and mycological responses, however the differences were not statistically different in this small study (Ruf and Vitse, 1990).

References

Adamson GD (1988). Three-day treatment of vulvovaginal candidiasis. *Amer J Obstet Gynecol* **158**: 1002.

Adamson GD, Brown D, Standard JV, Henzl MR (1986). Three-day treatment with butoconazole vaginal suppositaries for vulvovaginal candidiasis. *J Reprod Med* **31**: 131.

Beggs WH (1985). Influence of growth phase on the susceptibility of *Candida albicans* to butoconazole, oxiconazole, and sulconazole. *J Antimicrob Chemother* **16**: 397.

Bradbeer CS, Mayhew SR, Barlow D (1985). Butoconazole and miconazole in treating vaginal candidiasis. *Genitourin Med* **61**: 270.

Brown D, Henzl MR, LePage ME *et al.* (1986). Butoconazole vaginal cream in the treatment of vulvovaginal candidiasis. Comparison with miconazole nitrate and placebo. *J Reprod Med* **31**: 1045.

Droegemueller W, Adamson DG, Brown D *et al.* (1984). Three-day treatment with butoconazole nitrate for vulvovaginal candidiasis. *Obstet Gynecol* **64**: 530.

Fleury F (1986). A comparative study of butoconazole vs clotrimazole. *J Reprod Med* **31**: 664.

Fromtling RA (1988). Overview of medically important antifungal azole derivatives. *Clin Microbiol Rev* **1**: 187.

Hajman AJ (1988). Vulvovaginal candidosis: comparison of 3-day treatment with 2% butoconazole nitrate cream and 6-day treatment with 1% clotrimazole cream. *J Int Med Res* **16**: 367.

Hernandez Molina JM, Llosa J, Martinez Brocal A, Ventosa A (1992). *In vitro* activity of cloconazole, sulconazole, butoconazole, isoconazole, fenticonazole, and five other antifungal agents against clinical isolates of *Candida albicans* and *Candida* spp. *Mycopathologia* **118**: 15.

Jacobson JB, Hajman AJ, Wiese J *et al.* (1985). A new vaginal antifungal agent – butoconazole nitrate. *Acta Obstet Gynecol Scand* **64**: 241.

Kaufman RH, Henzl MR, Brown D *et al.* (1989). Comparison of a three-day butoconazole treatment with seven-day miconazole treatment for vulvovaginal candidiasis. *J Reprod Med* **34**: 479.

Maloley PA, Nelson E, Montgomery HA, Campbell JR (1990). Severe reversible thrombocytopenia resulting from butoconazole cream. *DICP* **24**: 143.

Matthews T (1986). Butoconazole. Pharmacologic considerations, chemistry and microbiology. *J Reprod Med* **31**: 655.

Odds FC, Webster CE, Abbott AB (1984). Antifungal relative inhibition factors; BAY 1–9139, bifonazole, butoconazole, isoconazole, itraconazole (R 51211), oxiconazole, Ro 14–4767/002, sulconazole, terconazole and vibunazole (BAY n-7133) compared with nine established antifungal agents. *J Antimicrob Chemother* **14**: 105.

Pfaller MA, Riley J, Koerner T (1990). Effects of terconazole and other azole antifungal agents on the sterol and carbohydrate composition of *Candida albicans*. *Diagn Microbiol Infect Dis* **13**: 31.

Pye GW, Marriott MS (1982). Inhibition of sterol C14 demethylation by imidazole-containing antifungals. *Sabouraudia* **20**: 325.

Ruf H, Vitse M (1990). A comparison of butoconazole nitrate cream with econazole nitrate cream for the treatment of vulvovaginal candidiasis. *J Int Med Res* **18**: 389.

Walker KAM, Braemer AC, Hitt S *et al.* (1978). 1-[4-(4-chlorophenyl).-2-(2,6-dichlorophenylthio).-n-butyl]-1-H-imidazole nitrate, a new potent antifungal agent *J Med Chem* **21**: 840.

Weisberg M (1986). Treatment of vaginal candidiasis in pregnant women. *Clin Ther* **8**: 563.

Wong AB (1988). Effect of butoconazole nitrate cream and wax insert on the barrier property of contraceptive devices. *Amer J Obstet Gynecol* **158**: 1011.

Croconazole

Description

Croconazole (cloconazole, 710674-S) is an imidazole derivative with the chemical name 1-(1-[o-{(m-chlorobenzyl)oxy]phenyl}vinyl)imidazole hydrochloride. It has been developed as a topical formulation and marketed in Japan in 1986, where it is indicated for the treatment of dermatomycoses and candidiasis (Fromtling, 1988).

Sensitive Organisms

Croconazole has potent antifungal activity against the dermatophytes, with MICs for *Trichophyton mentagrophytes*, *T. rubrum*, *Epidermophyton flocossum* and *Microsporum canis* in the range of 0.16–1.25 μg per ml. In addition the filamentous fungi, *Aspergillus* spp. and *Penicillium* spp. are susceptible with MICs of 0.63–5 μg per ml. The *in vitro* activity of croconazole compared with econazole, clotrimazole and miconazole was equivalent for isolates of *T. mentagrophytes*, but greater than the other imidazoles when tested against *T. rubrum* (Ogata *et al.*, 1983). In a guinea pig model of dermatomycoses due to *T. asteroides*, croconazole hydrochloride 1% cream was as effective as clotrimazole 1% cream, but the 1% gel formulation of croconazole appeared to be more effective than clotrimazole tincture in this model (Ogata *et al.*, 1983). Croconazole appears to be less active against *Candida albicans*, *Candida* spp., and *Cryptococcus neoformans*, with MICs in the range of 0.12–32 μg per ml (Ogata *et al.*, 1983; Hernandez Molina, 1992).

Availability

Topical formulation: croconazole hydrochloride 1% cream and 1% gel.

Absorption of the Drug

There is no published information on the absorption of croconazole after topical application, or the fate of any absorbed drug.

Mode of Action

The primary mehanism of action of croconazole has not been studied but is assumed to be similar to the other imidazoles, that is, inhibition of cytochrome P-450 dependent C-14 alpha demethylation of lanosterol, preventing conversion to ergosterol The resulting depletion of normal fungal sterols (ergosterol) and accumulation of 14 alpha methyl sterols (lanosterol) in the fungal cell membrane induces the damage to the cell. Ogata *et al.* (1983) established that croconazole concentrations of 80 μg per ml and 40 μg per ml were fungicidal for *C. albicans* and *T. rubrum* respectively.

Toxicity

Although croconazole did not produce phototoxicity, photoallergy or contact sensitivity after topical application in the guinea pig (Takechi and Harada, 1984), allergic contact dermatitis has been reported in at least 12 cases from Japan. Patch-testing confirmed the sensitization to croconazole down to a concentration of 0.1–0.5%. Cross-sensitization to sulconazole occurred in half those with contact dermatitis to croconazole (Shono *et al.*, 1989).

Clinical Uses of the Drug

There are no published reports of clinical efficacy either in clinical trials or open studies of croconazole for the treatment of superficial dermatomycoses.

References

Fromtling RA (1988). Overview of medically important antifungal azole derivatives. *Clin Microbiol Rev* **1**: 187.

Hernandez Molina JM, Llosa J, Martinez Brocal A, Ventosa A (1992). *In vitro* activity of cloconazole, sulconazole, butoconazole, isoconazole, fenticonazole, and five other antifungal agents against clinical isolates of *Candida albicans* and *Candida* spp. *Mycopathologia* **118**: 15.

Ogata M, Matsumoto H, Hamada Y *et al.* (1983). 1-[1-[2-[(3-chloro-benzyl)oxy]phenyl]vinyl]-1H-imidazole hydrochloride, a new potent antifungal agent. *J Med Chem* **26**: 768.

Shono M, Hayashi K, Sugimoto R (1989). Allergic contact dermatitis from croconazole hydrochloride. *Contact Derm* **21**: 225.

Takechi M, Harada M (1984). Antigenicity of 1-[1-[o-[(m-chlorobenzyloxy] phenyl]vinyl]-1H-imidazole hydrochloride (710674-S) in the guinea pig. *Pharmacometrics* **28**: 898.

Econazole

Description

Econazole, like clotrimazole and miconazole, is an imidazole derivative which was developed at Janssen Pharmaceutica Research Laboratories in Belgium (Godefroi *et al.*, 1969). It has an identical structure to miconazole with the absence of one chlorine atom on one benzene ring (Fromtling, 1988). Econazole is unsuitable for the treatment of systemic infections and its use is therefore restricted to treatment of superficial dermatophyte and candidal infections. Econazole has the chemical formula 1-[2,4-dichloro-beta-(ρ-chlorobenzyloxy)- penethyl]-imidazole nitrate.

Sensitive Organisms

1 Fungi

The drug has a wide range of antifungal activity (Thienpont *et al.*, 1975). It has a high degree of activity against the dermatophytes such as *Microsporum canis*, *Trichophyton* spp. and *Epidermophyton floccosum* (Kusunoki and Harada, 1984). Of the filamentous fungi, *Cladosporium* spp. and most *Aspergillus* spp. are quite sensitive. *Madurella mycetomii* is sensitive, but the Mucoraceae, such as *Absidia*, *Mucor* and *Rhizopus*, are resistant.

The dimorphic fungi, *Histoplasma capsulatum*, *Blastomyces dermatitidis*, *Sporothrix schenckii* and *Paracoccidioides brasiliensis* are very sensitive. The drug has an inhibitory effect on *Coccidioides immitis in vitro* and *in vivo* in mice (Levine, 1978). Pathogenic yeasts, such as *Cryptococcus neoformans* and *Candida* spp., are much less sensitive. *Pityrosporum orbicularis* (*Malassezia furfur*) is sensitive (Heel *et al.*, 1978; Schar *et al.*, 1976).

2 Bacteria

Econazole is quite active against some bacteria. Of the actinomycetes, it is active against *Actinomadura* (*Streptomyces*) *madurae*, *A. pelletierii*, *Streptomyces somaliensis* and *Nocardia asteroides*. It has no activity against Gram-negative bacteria, but it is highly active against some Gram-positive cocci and bacilli, including *Streptococcus pyogenes* and some strains of *Staphylococcus aureus*. It is also active against *Trichomonas vaginalis* (Schar *et al.*, 1976; Heel *et al.*, 1978).

3 Minimum inhibitory concentrations

The spectrum of activity of econazole resembles miconazole. *In vitro* susceptibility testing has not been standardized (see p. 1388). Table IV.13 is a compilation of published MICs for fungi that can cause cutaneous disease.

Availability

Vaginal preparations
Ovules: 150 mg
Cream: 1.5%, for delivery by an applicator (5 g cream contains 75 mg econazole nitrate)

Topical preparations
Cream, powder, lotion, foaming solution: 1% econazole nitrate

Table IV.13
Compiled from Bergan and Vangdal (1983), Kusunoki and Harada (1984), Bassiouny *et al.* (1986), Okeke and Gugnani (1987), Shadomy *et al.* (1988), Hernandez Molina *et al.* (1992), Venugopal *et al.* (1993)

Organism	MIC (μg per ml) range	
	Broth	Agar
Yeast		
Candida species		
C. albicans		0.25–32
C. guilliermondii		0.5–4
C. krusei		4–8
C. parapsilosis		0.25–4
C. tropicalis		0.5–16
C. kefyr (pseudotropicalis)		0.25–0.5
C. glabrata (Torulopsis glabrata)		0.25–0.5
Malassezia furfur		0.063–128
Trichosporon beigelii		1.0
Mold		
Aspergillus spp.	0.1–4	
A. fumigatus	1	
A. flavus	1	
A. niger	0.4	
Dematiaceous fungi		
Cladosporium carrionii		0.2–0.39
Exophiala jeanselmei	0.5–10	0.2–0.39
Fonsecaea pedrosoi		0.05–0.39
Phialophora verrucosa		0.1–0.39
Dermatophytes		
Trichophyton spp.	0.03–3	0.063–1.0
Microsporum spp.	0.03–>6	0.063–0.13
Epidermophyton spp.	0.01	0.063
Geotrichum capitatum		1.0
Phaeoannellomyces wernickii	0.063–2	

Serum Levels in Relation to Dosage and Excretion

About 3–7% of the dose of econazole nitrate cream administered intravaginally is absorbed (Heel *et al.*, 1978). Following intravaginal administration of a 5 g dose of radiolabeled 1% or 2% econazole nitrate cream to normal volunteers, the mean cumulative recovery over 96 h in both urine and feces was 2% and 8% respectively. Over half the administered dose leaked from the vagina (Vukovich *et al.*, 1977).

After application of 1% econazole nitrate ointment, the concentration of econazole in the epidermis at 100 min was 20 μg per ml and at 5 h was 5 μg per ml, and the levels in the stratum corneum ranged from 0.2–0.5 μg per ml at 100 min and at 5 h respectively. In addition, 0.6% of the applied dose was recovered in urine (Stuttgen and Bayer, 1982). The penetration of econazole nitrate 1% ointment into the nail plate and nail plate was compared with econazole nitrate 1% lotion in 99% dimethyl-sulfoxide (DMSO), or 49% DMSO. The level of econazole in the nail plate and nail bed was 10 μg per ml after application of 1% ointment, and was significantly higher after application of 1% lotion in 49% DMSO (70 μg per ml and 20 μg per ml for the nail plate and bed respectively) and 99% DMSO (50 μg per ml and 70 μg per ml respectively). Hence DMSO increases the rate of penetration of econazole into the nail plate (Stuttgen and Bauer, 1982).

The nature of metabolism and excretion of econazole is unknown. Only 1% of a topically administered dose of econazole is excreted in urine and feces.

Mode of Action

The mode of action of econazole is not well defined. Like other imidazoles, it binds to cytochrome P-450 inhibiting sterol C-14 demethylation of lanosterol and resulting in ergosterol depletion in the fungal cell membrane (see Fig. IV.1, p. 1261). The ensuing increase in cell membrane permeability may allow econazole to enter the cell to interfere with RNA and protein synthesis. There is disagreement over the finding of mitochondrial damage by econazole (Preusser and Rostek,1978; Mazabrey *et al.*, 1985). Georgopapadakou *et al.*, (1987) suggested that econazole causes direct membrane damage to *C. albicans*. Significant reduction in adherence of *C. albicans* occurred after 2 h incubation with econazole, and this may contribute to the antifungal effect of econazole (Vuddhakul *et al.*, 1988).

Toxicity

Local reactions following vaginal administration of cream or pessaries have been associated with itching, redness, irritation and burning in less than 5% of treated patients. It has been suggested that these reactions are due to the release of histamine from local mast cells, as histamine release induced by econazole has been documented in rat mast cells (Hanada and Oga, 1991).

Topical 1% econazole nitrate lotion used for the treatment of otomycosis can be associated with a burning sensation at the start of treatment in some cases, and a local allergic reaction was noted in one case. (Bassiouny *et al.*, 1986), and a slight stinging sensation was noted by patients in a trial of 1% econazole nitrate lotion for chronic paronychia (Wong *et al.*, 1984).

Contact allergic dermatitis has been described (Valsecchi *et al.*, 1982; Raulin and Frosch, 1988).

Safety of econazole in pregnancy has not been established. There is no evidence of teratogenicity in pregnant rats administered econazole. It is unknown whether econazole is excreted in breast milk, but as the systemic absorption of econazole is extremely low after topical or vaginal application of the drug, excretion into breast milk is likely to be negligible. In an open study of econazole treatment of vaginal candidiasis in pregnancy, there were no congenital abnormalities observed or adverse events in the neonates; however, the majority of women received therapy in the last trimester of pregnancy (Goormans *et al.*, 1985).

Clinical Uses of the Drug

1 Vulvovaginal candidiasis

Vaginal ovules and cream are effective in treating vulvovaginal candidiasis (90% response rates). One vaginal ovule (150 mg) inserted into the vagina on 3 consecutive nights or one applicator dose of 1% econazole nitrate cream (75 mg econazole nitrate in 5 g cream) is inserted intravaginally twice-daily for 3 days (Balmer, 1976; Bingham and Steele, 1981; Csonka *et al.*, 1981; Rana *et al.*, 1984). Such treatment is as effective as clotrimazole vaginal tabs (200 mg) used for 3 days (Benijts *et al.*, 1980; Gabriel and Thin, 1983) and a 14-day course with nystatin pessaries (Bingham and Steel, 1981). A single-dose 150-mg vaginal pessary was also as effective as single-dose application of 10% clotrimazole cream, with short- and long-term efficacy of 63–77% clinical response rates and 67–84% mycological eradication rates (Robinson *et al.*, 1989). Single-dose econazole (two 150-mg pessaries) was as effective as single-dose isoconazole (two 300-mg pessaries) with cure rates of 64% at 28 days (Bradbeer and Thin, 1985). Comparable results were obtained in a study of single-dose fluconazole with topical econazole 50 mg daily for 6 days (Herzog and Ansmann, 1989). However, a single oral dose of fluconazole 150 mg was significantly superior to a single intravaginal dose of econazole 150 mg for the treatment of acute candidal vaginitis. Statistically significantly higher clinical and mycological cure rates were noted at days 7 (100% versus 84%) and 28 (79% versus 56%), and at 3 months (62% versus 45%). The oral treatment was preferred by the participants (Osser *et al.*, 1991). These results were confirmed in a similar study by Westrom *et al.* (1992) with a combined clinical and mycological cure rate of 81% for fluconazole and 67% for econazole.

Pregnant women with vaginal candidiasis were treated with econazole vaginal pessaries, 150 mg on 3 consecutive nights. Clinical and mycological cure rates of 80% were no different to those reported in other studies, with a relapse rate of 13% (Goormans *et al.*, 1985).

2 Dermatophyte infections and cutaneous candidiasis

Econazole nitrate cream and lotion are effective for the treatment of cutaneous dermatophytosis and candidiasis. Econazole nitrate 1% cream was as effective as tioconazole 1% cream when applied twice-daily for a mean of 40 days for the treatment of cutaneous candidiasis or dermatophytosis, with over 90% clinical and mycological response rates in both groups (Grigoriu and Grigoriu, 1983). A similar double-blind study revealed comparable efficacies (90% clinical and mycological response rate) for econazole and oxiconazole for the treatment of cutaneous candidiasis, dermatophyte infections and tinea versicolor (Gip, 1984), and econazole also appears comparable with sulconazole for the treatment of dermatophytosis (Lassus and Forsstrom, 1984). Econazole nitrate 1% cream applied twice-daily for 4 weeks was inferior to naftifine 1% cream for the treatment of tinea cruris or tinea corporis, but overall cure rates of about 80% were the same for both groups 2 weeks after the end of treatment (Millikan et al., 1988). Clinical cure occurred in 86% of patients with tinea pedis after 4 weeks treatment with econazole nitrate 1% cream and 63% of cured patients remained relapse free at 3 months (Cullen et al., 1986).

In a comparative study of the treatment of chronic paronychia due to *Candida* species, econazole nitrate lotion administered topically to the nail fold at 2 ml four times daily, resulted in a cure rate of 58% and improvment in 42%. This cure and improved rate was comparable to treatment with oral ketoconazole 200 mg daily (Wong et al., 1984). Once daily administration of 1% econazole nitrate cream to areas of skin affected by tinea versicolor (infected with *Pityrsporum orbiculare*) was associated with a 76% cure rate and 21% improvement in clinical symptoms by 3 weeks of treatment, and was extremely well tolerated (Vicik et al., 1984)

3 Other fungal infections

Econazole nitrate as a 1% solution is effective for the treatment of otomycosis. It has *in vitro* activity against the majority of fungi causing otomycosis in the range of 0.1–4 μg per ml. (Bassiouny et al., 1986). As a 1% solution, econazole nitrate has been used by irrigation to treat facial maxillary sinusitis due to *Aspergillus fumigatus* (Grigoriu et al., 1979).

References

Balmer J (1976). Three day therapy of vulvovaginal candidiasis with econazole: a multicentric study comprising 996 cases. *Amer J Obstet Gynecol* **126**: 436.

Bassiouny A, Kamel T, Moawad MK, Hindawy DS (1986). Broad spectrum antifungal agents in otomycosis. *J Laryngol Otol* **100**: 867.

Benijts G, Vignalli M, Kreysing W, Stettendorf S (1980). Three-day therapy of vaginal candidiasis with clotrimazole vaginal tablets and econazole ovules: a multicentre comparative study. *Curr Med Res Opin* **7**: 55.

Bergan T, Vangdal M (1983). *In vitro* activity of antifungal agents against yeast species. *Chemotherapy* **29**: 104.

Bingham JS, Steele CE (1981). Treatment of vaginal candidosis with econazole nitrate and nystatin. A comparative study. *Brit J Vener Dis* **57**: 204.

Bradbeer CS, Thin RN (1985). Comparison of econazole and isoconazole as single dose treatment for vaginal candidosis. *Genitourin Med* **61**: 396.

Csonka GW, Sugrue DL, Kinsey RM et al. (1981). Econazole nitrate: a clinical study of three day therapy in vaginal candidiasis. *Brit J Sex Med* **8**: 43.

Cullen SI, Millikan LE, Mullen RH (1986). Treatment of tinea pedis with econazole nitrate cream. *Cutis* **37**: 388.

Fromtling RA (1988). Overview of medically important antifungal azole derivatives. *Clin Microbiol Rev* **1**: 187.

Gabriel G, Thin RN (1983). Clotrimazole and econazole in the treatment of vaginal candidosis. A single-blind comparison. *Brit J Vener Dis* **59**: 56.

Gip L (1984). Comparison of oxiconazole (Ro 13–8996) and econazole in dermatomycoses. *Mykosen* **27**: 295.

Godefroi EF, Heeres J, van Cutsem J, Janssen PAJ (1969). The preparation and antimycotic properties of derivatives of l-phenethylimidazole. *J Med Chem* **12**: 784.

Georgopapadakou NH, Dix BA, Smith SA et al. (1987). Effect of antifungal agents on lipid biosynthesis and membrane integrity in *Candida albicans*. *Antimicrob Ag Chemother* **31**: 46.

Goormans E, Beek JM, Declercq JA et al. (1985). Efficacy of econazole ('Gyno-Pevaryl' 150) in vaginal candidosis during pregnancy. *Curr Med Res Opin* **9**: 371.

Grigoriu D, Grigoriu A (1983). Double-blind comparison of the efficacy, toleration and safety of tioconazole base 1% and econazole nitrate 1% creams in the treatment of patients with fungal infections or erythrasma. *Dermatologica* **166** (Suppl 1): 8.

Grigoriu D, Bambule J, Delacretaz J (1979). Aspergillus sinusitis. *Postgrad Med J* **55**: 619.

Hanada S, Oga S (1991). Histamine release from rat mast cells induced by econazole. *Gen Pharmacol* **22**: 511.

Heel RC, Brogden RN, Speight TM, Avery GS (1978). Econazole: A review of its antifungal activity and therapeutic efficacy. *Drugs* **16**: 177.

Hernandez Molina JM, Llosa J, Martinez Brocal A, Ventosa A (1992). *In vitro* activity of cloconazole, sulconazole, butoconazole, isoconazole, fenticonazole, and five other antifungal agents against clinical isolates of *Candida albicans* and *Candida* spp. *Mycopathologia* **118**: 15.

Herzog RE, Ansmann EB (1989). Treatment of vaginal candidosis with fluconazole. *Mycoses* **32**: 204.

Kusunoki T, Harada S (1984). Comparison of the *in vitro* antifungal activities of clotrimazole, miconazole, econazole and exalamide against clinical isolates of dermatophytes. *J Dermatol* **11**: 277–284.

Lassus A, Forsstrom S (1984). A double-blind parallel study of sulconazole with econazole in the treatment of dermatophytoses. *Mykosen* **27**: 592.

Levine HB (1978). Econazole in experimental coccidioidomycosis. In *Proceedings of the 10th International Congress of Chemotherapy, Zurich/Switzerland, 1977* (Siegenthaler W, Luthy R, eds), p. 233. Washington, DC: American Society for Microbiology.

Mazabrey D, Nadel J, Seguel J-P, Linas M-D (1985). Scanning and transmission electron microscopy: study of the effects of econazole on *Microsporum canis*. *Mycopathologia* **91**: 151.

Millikan LE, Galen WK, Gewirtzman GB et al. (1988). Naftifine cream 1% versus econazole cream 1% in the treatment of tinea cruris and tinea corporis. *J Amer Acad Dermatol* **18**: 52.

Okeke CN, Gugnani HC (1987). *In vitro* sensitivity of environmental isolates of pathogenic dematiaceous fungi to azole compounds and a phenylpropyl-morpholine derivative. *Mycopathologia* **99**: 175.

Osser S, Haglund A, Westrom L (1991). Treatment of candidal vaginitis. A prospective randomized investigator-blind multicenter study comparing topically applied econazole with oral fluconazole. *Acta Obstet Gynecol Scand* **70**: 73.

Preusser HJ, Rostek H (1978). Econazole effects on *Trichophyton rubrum* and *Candida albicans*. Electron microscopic and cytochemical studies. *Mykosen* **21** (Suppl 1): 314.

Rana C, Appleton B, Williams R (1984). Three day treatment of vaginitis with econazole nitrate cream. *Aust Family Physician* **13**: 292.

Raulin C, Frosch PJ (1988). Contact allergy to imidazole antimycotics. *Contact Derm* **18**: 76.

Robinson AJ, Wilson JD, Spencer RS, Kinghorn GR (1989). Econazole nitrate (150 mg) single dose vaginal pessary compared with clotrimazole (10%) single dose vaginal cream to treat women with vaginal candidiasis. *Genitourin Med* **65**: 201.

Schar G, Keyer FH, Dupont MC (1976). Antimicrobial activity of econazole and miconazole *in vitro* and in experimental candidiasis and aspergillosis. *Chemotherapy* **22**: 221.

Shadomy S, Wang H, Shadomy HJ (1988). Further *in vitro* studies with oxiconazole nitrate. *Diagn Microbiol Infect Dis* **9**: 231.

Stuttgen G, Bauer E (1982). Bioavailability, skin- and nail penetration of topically applied antimycotics. *Mykosen* **25**: 74.

Thienpont D, van Cutsem J, van Nueten JM *et al.* (1975). Biological toxicological properties of econazole, a broad-spectrum antimycotic. *Arzneim Forsch (Drug Res)* **25**: 3.

Valsecchi R, Tornaghi A, Tribbia G (1982). Contact dermatitis from econazole. *Contact Derm* **8**: 422.

Venugopal, PV, Venugopal TV, Ramakrishna ES, Ilavarasi S (1993). Antimycotic susceptibility testing of agents of black grain eumycetoma. *J Med Vet Mycol* **31**: 161.

Vicik GJ, Mendiones M, Quinones CA, Thorne EG (1984). A new treatment for tinea versicolor using econazole nitrate 1.0 percent cream once a day. *Cutis* **33**: 570.

Vuddhakul V, McCormack JG, Seow WK *et al.* (1988). Inhibition of *Candida albicans* by conventional and experimental antifungal drugs. *J Antimicrob Chemother* **21**: 755.

Vukovich A, Heald A, Darragh A (1977). Vaginal absorption of two imidazole antifungal agents, econazole and miconazole. *Clin Pharmacol Ther* **21**: 121.

Westrom L, Haglund A, Svensson L (1992). Fluconazole versus econazole in treating vaginal candidiasis. *Int J Gynecol Obstet* **37** (Suppl): 29.

Wong ESM, Hay RJ, Clayon YM, Noble WC (1984). Comparison of the therapeutic effect of ketoconazole tablets and econazole lotion in the treatment of chronic paronychia. *Clin Exp Derm* **9**: 489.

Fenticonazole

Description

Fenticonazole is a synthetic imidazole derivative, with the chemical name of (±)-1-[2.4-dichloro-beta-{[p-(phenylthio)benzyl]oxy}phenethyl]imidazole mononitrate. It has a broad spectrum of antifungal activity, but is most potent against dermatophytes. The presence of serum significantly reduces its activity, so it has been developed for topical use (Fromtling, 1988).

Sensitive Organisms

Fenticonazole has potent activity against the dermatophytes (*Trichophyton* spp., *Epidermophyton* spp., and *Microsporum* spp.), and pathogenic yeast. It also possesses potent antibacterial activity (Veronese *et al.*, 1981a; Costa, 1982; Jones *et al.*, 1989). Against *Candida albicans* and other *Candida* spp., fenticonazole demonstrated comparable activity with econazole, miconazole or ketoconazole, with MICs in the range of 0.25–32 μg per ml. This activity was inferior to some of the other imidazole derivatives (Hernandez Molina *et al.*, 1992). The *in vitro* activity was noted to decrease significantly in the presence of serum (because of high levels of protein binding) and in an alkaline pH medium (Fromtling, 1988; Jones *et al.*, 1989). The activity of fenticonazole in the guinea pig model of candidiasis and dermatomycosis was comparable with the activity of miconazole and clotrimazole (Veronese *et al.*, 1981b). *Bacteroides* spp. associated with bacterial vaginosis and *Gardnerella vaginalis* are extremely susceptible to fenticonazole (MICs of less than 0.03–0.5 μg per ml), but the *Bacteroides fragilis* group of organisms are resistant. Skin pathogens such as *Staphylococcus aureus*, *Streptococcus pyogenes* and *Corynebacterium* spp. are all susceptible to fenticonazole (Jones *et al.*, 1989).

Mode of Administration and Dose

Indications and recommended doses

Superficial dermatomycoses: Fenticonazole nitrate 2% cream, lotion or spray, applied once- or twice-daily for tinea corporis, tinea cruris, tinea pedis, and tinea (pityriasis) versicolor.

Vaginal candidiasis: Fenticonazole nitrate 2% vaginal cream or vaginal ovules (100 mg, 200 mg).

Bacterial vaginosis: Fenticonazole nitrate vaginal ovules 600–1000 mg in a single dose.

Availability

Fenticonazole nitrate: 2% *cream, lotion*

Fenticonazole nitrate: 2% *vaginal cream*

Vaginal ovule: 100 mg, 200 mg, 600 mg

Absorption of the Drug

The absorption of fenticonazole after vaginal administration is minimal, and has been investigated in normal women, women with recurrent vulvovaginal candidiasis, and women with cervical cancer. A single administration of 1000 mg of radiolabeled ^{3}H-fenticonazole was followed with a vaginal wash at 12 h. There was no detectable radioactivity in the plasma of women with recurrent vaginal candidiasis or normal volunteers, while 80% of women with cervical cancer had detectable radioactivity which peaked at 8 h. About 0.4–1.5% of the administered dose was recovered from the urine over the ensuing 5 days and 0.18–0.32% was recovered from feces. Based on the amount of radioactivity excreted, it was estimated that 0.6%

of the dose was absorbed by women with normal vaginal mucosa, 1.8% was absorbed by women with vaginal candidiasis and 1.1% was absorbed by women with cervical cancer and amounts to about 0.4 mg per kg of fenticonazole (Novelli *et al.*, 1991).

Mode of Action

The exact mechanism of action of fenticonazole has not been established. It is likely that it produces its antifungal activity in a similar manner as the other imidazole drugs, by binding to the heme iron of cytochrome P-450 thereby inhibiting the enzyme C14-demethylase. The resultant inhibition of the conversion of lanosterol to ergosterol and depletion of ergosterol in the fungal cell membrane gives rise to to the fungistatic activity of the drug (see Fig. IV.1, p. 1261). Morphological changes produced by increasing concentrations of fenticonazole on *Candida albicans* have been documented by scanning electron microscope. At concentrations below the MIC, alterations in the plasma membrane architecture were noted, as well as the inhibition of formation of pseudohyphae. At concentrations of the MIC and higher, filamentous formation of *C. albicans* was completely prevented (Costa *et al.*, 1984).

Toxicity

Topical application of either the 2% cream or lotion are rarely associated with side-effects (Athow-Frost *et al.*, 1986). Local reactions include mild desquamation with the lotion, itching and erythema (Aste *et al.*, 1988). Fenticonazole had no photosensitizing capacity in animal studies, and there was no evidence of irritation after application to normal volunteers and no contact-sensitization was noted (Graziani and Cazzulani, 1981; Pigatto *et al.*, 1990).

Vaginal application is very well tolerated (Brewster *et al.*, 1986). Mild and transient vaginal irritation and burning was noted with single-dose treatment with fenticonazole 600 mg ovules (Wiest and Ruffmann, 1987; Lawrence *et al.*, 1990). No evidence of significant treatment-related laboratory abnormalities have been noted in the comparative studies (Jung *et al.*, 1988).

Clinical Uses of the Drug

1 Superficial dermatomycoses

An open study evaluating the efficacy of fenticonazole nitrate 2% cream for superficial mycoses revealed it was successful treatment in 85% of patients treated twice-daily for up to 5 weeks (Aste *et al.*, 1987). Fenticonazole nitrate 2% cream was found to be more active than econazole 1% cream and clotrimazole 1% cream (Kokoschka *et al.*, 1986; Finzi *et al.*, 1986), and to have comparable activity (90% clinical and mycological response at 4 weeks) with miconazole 2% cream (Athow-Frost *et al.*, 1986; Clerico and Ribuffo, 1987). A comparison of fenticonazole nitrate 2% cream applied once-daily for up to 4 weeks with bifonazole 1% cream determined fenticonazole was as effective as bifonazole, and fenticonazole treatment produced a statistically significant more rapid theraputic effect, with 71% of fenticonazole patients with a clinical and mycological cure at 3 weeks of treatment compared with 35% of bifonazole-treated patients (Jung *et al.*, 1988). Comparable efficacy of fenticonazole nitrate 2% spray applied once-daily for 2–4 weeks and ciclopirox olamine 1% spray was established in a double-blind trial with clinical responses achieved in 92% and 90% of patients respectively. Clinical relapse occurred in 30% of fenticonazole-treated patients compared with 21% of ciclopirox olamine-treated patients (Altmeyer *et al.*, 1990). The mycological and clinical therapeutic efficacy of fentaconazole nitrate 2% spray was also equivalent to that of naftifine 1% spray (94% versus 90%) for the treatment of cutaneous mycoses (including cutaneous candidiasis) with low rates of relapse of 3% for fenticonazole (Leiste *et al.*, 1989).

2 Tinea (pityriasis) versicolor

In an open study evaluating the efficacy of fenticonazole nitrate 2% lotion applied twice-daily for up to 5 weeks, there was a 100% response rate (Aste *et al.*, 1987). Fenticonazole nitrate 2% lotion applied once-daily for 3 weeks was as effective as bifonazole 1% lotion administered in the same regimen for the treatment of tinea versicolor (Aste *et al.*, 1988).

3 Vulvovaginal candidiasis

Comparative studies have demonstrated that fenticonazole is an effective and safe agent for the treatment of vulvovaginal candidiasis. Application of fenticonazole nitrate 2% cream for 7 days produced a 95% mycological and clinical response rate which was similar to that obtained in the clotrimazole-treated women. Relapses occurred in four fenticonazole-treated women and none of those given clotrimazole (Brewster *et al.*, 1986). Another study determined fenticonazole 100-mg vaginal pessaries administered twice-daily was as effective as miconazole 100-mg pessaries administered twice-daily with all women achieving cure in this small study. However, those treated with fenticonazole experienced a much more rapid response than the miconazole-treated women (Gastaldi, 1985).

Wiest and Ruffmann (1987) compared three regimens of fenticonazole nitrate ovules for treatment of vaginal candidiasis, 200 mg daily for 3 days, single administration of 600 mg, and a single administration of 1000 mg. The three treatment regimens were equally effective and produced clinical and mycological cures in 75–85% of women. A single dose of fenticonazole nitrate ovule 600 mg is as effective as a single dose of clotrimazole 500 mg tablet with mycological efficacy of 92% for fenticonazole and 89% for clotrimazole 1 week after administration of the treatment. At 1 month, clinical and mycological therapeutic efficacy was sustained in 84% of fenticonazole-treated women compared with 69% of the clotrimazole group (Lawrence *et al.*, 1990). Similar results from two other studies confirmed this observation (Studd *et al.*, 1989, Wiest *et al.*, 1989).

References

Altmeyer P, Nolting S, Kuhlwein A *et al.* (1990). Effect of fenticonazole spray in cutaneous mycoses: a double-blind clinical trial versus cyclopyroxolamine spray. *J Int Med Res* **18**: 61.

Aste N, Pau M, Zucca M, Biggio P (1987). Clinical experience with fenticonazole 2% formulation in the treatment of dermatomycoses and pityriasis versicolor. *Int J Pharmacol Res* **7**: 503.

Aste N, Pau M, Cordaro CI, Biggio P (1988). Double-blind study with fenticonazole or bifonazole in pityriasis versicolor. *Int J Pharmacol Res* **8**: 271.

Athow-Frost TA, Freeman K, Mann TA *et al.* (1986). Clinical evaluation of fenticonazole cream in cutaneous fungal infections: a comparison with miconazole cream. *Curr Med Res Opin* **10**: 107.

Brewster E, Preti PM, Ruffmann R, Studd J (1986). Effect of fenticonazole in vaginal candidiasis A double-blind clinical trial versus clotrimazole. *J Int Med Res* **14**: 306.

Clerico R, Rubiffo A (1987). Efficacy and tolerance of fenticonazole versus miconazole cream. *Int J Pharmacol Res* **7**: 77.

Costa AL (1982). "*In vitro*" antimycotic activity of fenticonazole (Rec 15/1476). *Mykosen* **27**: 29.

Costa AL, Valenti A, Veronese M (1984). Study of the morphofunctional alterations induced by fenticonazole on strains of *Candida albicans*, using the scanning electron microscope (SEM). *Mykosen* **27**: 29.

Gastaldi A (1985). Treatment of vaginal candidiasis with fenticonazole and miconazole. *Curr Ther Res* **35**: 489.

Finzi A, Fioroni A, Preti PM, Mounari M (1986). A double-blind evaluation of fenticonazole cream 2% and clotrimazole 1% in dermatomycoses. *Mykosen* **29**: 41.

Fromtling RA (1988). Overview of medically important antifungal azole derivatives. *Clin Microbiol Rev* **1**: 187.

Graziani G, Cazzulani P (1981). Irritation and toxicity studies with fenticonazole applied topically to the skin and mucous membranes. *Arneim Forsch* **31**: 2152.

Hernandez Molina JM, Llosa J, Martinez Brocal A, Ventosa A (1992). *In vitro* activity of cloconazole, sulconazole, butoconazole, isoconazole, fenticonazole, and five other antifungal agents against clinical isolates of *Candida albicans* and *Candida* spp. *Mycopathologia* **118**: 15.

Jones BM, Geary I, Lee ME, Duerden BI (1989). Comparison of the *in vitro* activities of fenticonazole, other imidazoles, metronidazole, and tetracycline against organisms associated with bacterial vaginosis and skin infections. *Antimicrob Ag Chemother* **33**: 970.

Jung EG, Bisco A, Azzollini E *et al.* (1988). Fenticonazole cream once-daily in dermatomycosis, a double-blind controlled trial versus bifonazole. *Dermatologica* **177**: 104.

Kokoschka EM, Miebauer G, Mounari M, Preti PM (1986). Treatment of dermatomycoses with fenticonazole and econazole. *Mykosen* **29**: 45.

Lawrence AG, Houang ET, Hiscock E *et al.* (1990). Single dose therapy of vaginal candidiasis: a comparative trial of fenticonazole vaginal ovules versus clotrimazole vaginal tablets. *Curr Med Res Opin* **12**: 114.

Leiste D, Braun W, Fegeler W *et al.* (1989). A double-blind clinical trial of fenticonazole (2%) spray versus naftifine (1%) spray in patients with cutaneous mycoses. *Curr Med Res Opin* **11**: 567.

Novelli A, Periti E, Massi GB *et al.* (1991). Systemic absorption of ^{3}H-fenticonazole after vaginal administration of 1 gram in patients. *J Chemother* **3**: 23.

Pigatto P, Colli E, Scatagna M, Finzi A (1990). Evaluation of skin irritation and contact sensitizing potential of fenticonazole. *Arneim Forsch* **40**: 329.

Studd JW, Dooley MM, Welch CC *et al.* (1989). Comparative clinical trial of fenticonazole ovule (600 mg) versus clotrimazole vaginal tablet (500 mg). in the treatment of symptomatic vaginal candidiasis. *Curr Med Res Opin* **11**: 477.

Veronese M, Salvaterra M, Barzaghi D (1981a). Fenticonazole, a new imidazole derivative with antibacterial and antifungal activity. *Arneim Forsch* **31**: 2133.

Veronese M, Barzaghi D, Bertoncini A (1981b). Antifungal activity of fenticonazole in experimental dermatomycosis and candidiasis. *Arneim Forsch* **31**: 2137.

Wiest W, Ruffmann R (1987). Short-term treatment of vaginal candidiasis with fenticonazole ovules: a three-dose schedule comparative trial. *J Int Med Res* **15**: 319.

Wiest W, Azzollini E, Ruffmann R (1989). Comparison of single administration with an ovule of 600 mg fenticonazole versus a 500 mg clotrimazole vaginal pessary in the treatment of vaginal candidiasis. *J Int Med Res* **17**: 369.

Isoconazole

Description

Isoconazole is an imidazole derivative, structurally related to clotrimazole, econazole and miconazole. It has the chemical name of 1-[2,4-dichloro-beta-(2,6-dichlorobenzyloxy)phenethyl] imidazole nitrate. Isoconazole has a broad spectrum of antifungal activity *in vitro* and has been shown to be an effective agent for the management of vaginal candidiasis.

Sensitive Organisms

Broad spectrum activity has been observed *in vitro* against dermatophytes, pathogenic fungi, filamentous fungi, some Gram-positive bacteria and trichomonads (Fromtling, 1988). *Candida* spp. are highly susceptible to isoconazole with MICs in the range of 0.12–4 μg per ml. *Candida albicans* susceptibility varied from an MIC of 0.12 to 4 μg per ml and 50% of isolates were inhibited by 1 μg per ml (Hernandez Molina *et al.*, 1992). Moderate activity for isoconazole was measured by relative inhibition factors and this drug had comparatively less activity than terconazole and butoconazole (Odds *et al.*, 1984). Systemic administration of isoconazole either orally or i.v. does not result in *in vivo* activity, and this was emphasized in the murine model of gastrointestinal candidiasis (Fromtling, 1988). Isoconazole showed potent *in vitro* activity against dermatophytes with MICs in the range of 0.05–0.39 μg per ml (Oyeka and Gugnani, 1990). Isoconazole also has good activity against *Hendersonula* spp. and *Scytalidium* spp. (Oyeka and Gugnani, 1990).

Mode of Administration and Dose

Indication and recommended dose
Vaginal candidiasis: single vaginal application of 600 mg (two 300 mg pessaries).

Availability

Topical formulation: Vaginal pessary 300 mg; 1% isoconazole cream.

Absorption of the Drug

There is little information regarding percutaneous or mucosal absorption of isoconazole after topical application. Negligible systemic absorption of isoconazole is said to occur following intravaginal insertion of two 300-mg pessaries. Fungicidal concentrations of isoconazole persist in the vagina for 3 days after a single dose of 600 mg inserted intravaginally (Tauber *et al.*, 1984; Fromtling, 1988).

Mode of Action

The mechanism of action of isoconazole is assumed to be similar to that of the other N-substituted imidazole derivatives (see Fig. IV.1, p. 1261).

Toxicity

Local reactions include vaginal burning and itching. Contact dermatitis has been reported (Frenzel and Gutekunst, 1983).

Clinical Uses of the Drug

1 Vaginal candidiasis

An 80–90% clinical and mycological cure rate was achieved with intravaginal administration of 600 mg isoconazole nitrate in women with vaginal candidiasis, and an open comparative study of isoconazole and oral ketoconazole revealed there was no difference in efficacy between the two treatments (Fromtling, 1988). Comparable efficacy was shown for isoconazole nitrate 600 mg and econazole 300 mg given as a single dose as treatment for vaginal candidosis with cure rates of 78% and 70% at 14 days after intravaginal administration, and sustained cure rates of 65% and 64% respectively at 4 weeks (Bradbeer and Thin, 1985). Equivalent mycological and clinical efficacy was also established for isoconazole administered as a single dose of 600 mg and clotrimazole 500 mg single dose (Cohen, 1984).

2 Dermatomycosis

An evaluation was made of 1% isoconazole nitrate cream in an open study of 27 patients with tinea versicolor, 23 patients with tinea cruris/corporis or tinea pedis, and intertriginous candidosis, and a localized infection due to *Trichsporon beigelii*, and *Geotrichum candidum*. Response was achieved with 3–4 weeks treatment in 60% of patients and 90% response occurred at 6 weeks treatment (Gugnani *et al.*, 1994).

References

Bradbeer CS, Thin RN (1985). Comparison of econazole and isoconazole as single dose treatment for vaginal candidosis. *Genitourin Med* **61**: 396.

Cohen L (1984). Single dose treatment of vaginal candidosis: comparison of clotrimazole and isoconazole. *Brit J Vener Dis* **60**: 42.

Frenzel UH, Gutekunst A (1983). Contact dermatitis to isoconazole nitrate. *Contact Derm* **9**: 74.

Fromtling RA (1988). Overview of medically important antifungal azole derivatives. *Clin Microbiol Rev* **1**: 187.

Gugnani HC, Akpata LE, Gugnani MK, Srivastava R (1994). Isoconazole nitrate in the treatment of tropical dermatomycosis. *Mycoses* **37**: 39.

Hernandez Molina JM, Llosa J, Martinez Brocal A, Ventosa A (1992). *In vitro* activity of cloconazole, sulconazole, butoconazole, isoconazole, fenticonazole, and five other antifungal agents against clinical isolates of *Candida albicans* and *Candida* spp. *Mycopathologia* **118**: 15.

Odds FC, Webster CE, Abbott AB (1984). Antifungal relative inhibition factors; BAY 1–9139, bifonazole, butoconazole, isoconazole, itraconazole (R 51211), oxiconazole, Ro 14–4767/002, sulconazole, terconazole and vibunazole (BAY n-7133) compared with nine established antifungal agents. *J Antimicrob Chemother* **14**: 105.

Oyeka CA, Gugnani HC (1990). *In vitro* activity of seven azole compounds against some clinical isolates of non-dermatophyte filamentous fungi and some dermatophytes. *Mycopathologia* **110**: 157.

Tauber U, Rach P, Lachnit U (1984). Persistence of isoconazole in vaginal secretion after single application. *Mykosen* **27**: 97.

Oxiconazole

Description

Oxiconazole is a substituted imidazole derivative, with the chemical name 2',4'-dichloro-2-imidazol-1-ylacetophenonel-O-(2,4-dichlorobenzyl)-oxime nitrate. It is structurally distinct from miconazole, econazole, clotrimazole and ketoconazole, because it is an acetophene-oxime derivative. It has a broad spectrum of antifungal activity including yeasts, dermatophytes and *Aspergillus* species. Oxiconazole is marketed as a topical formulation for the treatment of superficial dermatophyte infections.

Sensitive Organisms

As with all the azole derivatives, the results of *in vitro* activity by susceptibility testing vary considerably with method utilized, culture medium, pH, incubation temperature and inoculum size.

1 Pathogenic yeast

Cryptococcus neoformans is susceptible to oxiconazole with an MIC range of 0.001–0.3 μg per ml (Polak, 1982; Hiratani *et al.*, 1984). However, in the murine model of cryptococcosis, oral oxiconazole had no activity (Polak, 1982). The *in vitro* activity of oxiconazole against *Candida albicans* was less than miconazole with MIC ranges of 0.12–128 μg per ml. Other *Candida* species appear to be susceptible to oxiconazole with MICs of 0.06–64 μg per ml (Polak, 1983; Gebhart *et al.*, 1984). However, the activity of oxiconazole against *Candida* spp. was comparable with miconazole and clotrimazole when evaluated by relative inhibition factors (Odds *et al.*, 1984). Oxiconazole displayed poor activity when administered orally in the murine model of systemic candidiasis; however, it was the most potent imidazole drug in the rat model of vaginal candidiasis (Polak, 1982). Another important skin pathogen, *Malassezia furfur*, is usually susceptible to oxiconazole with MIC of 0.063 μg per ml, but three strains were resistant (Shadomy *et al.*, 1988).

2 Molds or filamentous fungi

Oxiconazole has potent activity against *Trichophyton mentagrophytes*, *T. rubrum*, *Microsporum canis*, and *Epidermophyton floccosum* with an MIC range of 0.03–3 μg per ml, and fungicidal activity at concentrations of 0.03–10 μg per ml (Gebhart *et al.*, 1984; Hiratani *et al.*, 1984; Shadomy *et al.*, 1988; Oyeka and Gugnani, 1990; Jegasothy and Pakes, 1991). Oxiconazole is active against other non-dermatophyte filamentous fungi, such as *Hendersonula toruloidea*, and *Scytalidium hyalinum* with MICs of 0.39–1.56 μg per ml (Oyeka and Gugnani, 1990). Good *in vitro* activity for *Aspergillus* spp. (MIC 0.25–4 μg per ml), *Mucor* spp. (MIC 0.06–8 μg per ml), and *Rhizopus* spp. (MIC 0.1–4 μg per ml), was also demonstrated (Gebhart *et al.*, 1984), but this was in contrast to the activity determined by Polak (1982). In addition, there was no *in vivo* activity of orally administered oxiconazole in the murine model of aspergillosis (Polak, 1982). *Sporothrix schenckii* is susceptible (MIC 0.5–4 μg per ml), but *Pseudallescheria boydii* is resistant (Gebhart *et al.*, 1984). *Exophiala werneckii* was shown to be susceptible to oxiconazole *in vitro* with an MIC of 0.063–0.5 μg per ml (Shadomy *et al.*, 1988).

3 Bacteria

Oxiconazole has been shown to have some *in vitro* activity against Gram-positive bacteria. *Nocardia asteroides*, *N. brasiliensis*, *Actinomadura madurae* and *Corynebacterium* spp. are susceptible *in vitro* (Polak, 1982).

4 Resistance

Isolates of *Candida albicans* that were resistant to oxiconazole were cross-resistant to ketoconazole and other imidazoles, and isolates of *Malassezia furfur* found to be resistant to oxiconazole were also resistant to econazole (Gebhart *et al.*, 1984; Shadomy *et al.*, 1988). There are no reports of development of resistance on treatment.

Mode of Administration and Dose

Indications and recommended doses
Dermatomycosis
Tinea corporis, tinea cruris: 1% oxiconazole nitrate cream applied once-daily for 2 weeks.
Tinea pedis: 1% oxiconazole nitrate cream applied once-daily for 4 weeks.

Availability

Topical formulation: 1% oxiconazole nitrate cream.

Absorption of the Drug

Negligible systemic absorption of oxiconazole occurs following topical application of the drug. In normal volunteers, 150 mg of ^{14}C-labeled oxiconazole ointment was applied as a single dose. A total of 94.5% of the administered dose was recovered, the majority in the stratum corneum and 0.3% recovered in urine over 5 days. It could not be detected in feces, and plasma levels of radioactivity were about 0.3 ng per ml (Jegasothy and Pakes, 1991).

The percutaneous absorption of the drug was evaluated after application of 2.5 mg per cm^2 ^{14}C-labeled oxiconazole cream to unabraded skin. Within 5 h, concentrations of oxiconazole in the epidermis, upper corneum, and lower corneum were 7.96 μg per ml, 1.79 μg per ml and 0.64 μg per ml (Stuttgen and Bauer, 1985). Inhibitory concentrations of oxiconazole in the epidermis and stratum corneum, and hair follicle persist for at least 16 h (Jegasothy and Pakes, 1991). Oxiconazole was compared with amorolfine and bifonazole in the guinea pig model, and it had the most potent activity at 48 h after application of the drugs (Fromtling, 1988).

Mode of Action

The exact mode of action of oxiconazole has not been established, but it is likely to produce its fungistatic and fungicidal activity through inhibition of C14 demethylation of lanosterol, thereby preventing conversion to ergosterol, which results in depletion of normal fungal sterols (ergosterol) and accumulation of 14 alpha methyl sterols (lanosterol) in the fungal cell membrane (Polak-Wyss *et al.*, 1985, Hiratani and Yamaguchi, 1985) (see Fig. IV.1, p. 1261). Depletion of ergosterol in the fungal cell membrane results in increased membrane permeability and leakage of essential cellular components. In addition, subinhibitory concentrations of oxiconazole inhibit synthesis of DNA and reduce intracellular concentrations of ATP (Odds *et al.*, 1985). Oxiconazole was fungistatic against both early stationary phase and early logarithmic phase cells of *C. albicans*, but did exhibit fungicidal activity against resting phase *C. parapsilosis* cells, supporting the notion of direct cell damage (Beggs, 1985).

Toxicity

Less than 2% of patients treated with oxiconazole nitrate 1% cream report adverse events. Itching, burning, erythema, maceration and fissuring are the most commonly reported side-effects (Jegasothy and Pakes, 1991). No significant differences in tolerability were noted in the comparative studies with econazole and bifonazole (Gip, 1984; Wagner and Reckers-Czaschka, 1987). Several women have noted intense vaginal burning following application of oxiconazole for the treatment of vaginal candidiasis (Gouveia and Jones da Silva, 1984). Contact allergic dermatitis was reported in 0.4% patients in oxiconazole clinical trials (Raulin and Frosch, 1987). The local reactions to oxiconazole are mild, and transient and resolve on cessation of the drug.

Clinical Uses of the Drug

1 Superficial dermatomycosis

Oxiconazole nitrate 1% cream is an effective topical treatment for superficial dermatomycoses. In two placebo-controlled trials, oxiconazole nitrate 1% cream applied either once- or twice-daily for 4 weeks as treatment for tinea pedis was significantly more effective than placebo in producing clinical (87–93% versus 61%) and mycological responses (82–83% versus 32%).

There was no significant difference in either clinical or mycological efficacy between the once-daily and twice-daily application groups in the placebo-controlled studies or other comparative studies (Wagner, 1986; Ramelet and Walker-Nasir, 1987; Ellis *et al.*, 1989; Lebwohl *et al.*, 1989). A subset analysis of individuals with plantar-type tinea pedis revealed mycological efficacy in 71–74% of oxiconazole-treated patients compared with 19% of placebo patients (Jegasothy and Pakes, 1991). Similar placebo-controlled studies of oxiconazole nitrate 1% cream applied once- or twice-daily for 2 weeks in the treatment of tinea corporis and tinea cruris determined mycological eradication rates of 83% versus 28% for placebo. Clinical cure (70–74%) was also significantly higher in the oxiconazole groups (Jegasothy and Pakes, 1991). Again, there was equivalent efficacy between the once-daily and twice-daily regimens (Wagner, 1986; Ramelet and Walker-Nasir, 1987).

Comparative studies of 1% oxiconazole nitrate cream with other topical azole drugs in the treatment of dermatomycoses are summarized by Jegasothy and Pakes (1991). In general, oxiconazole nitrate cream was applied twice-daily for periods of 3–6 weeks, and the clinical and mycological efficacy was equivalent to miconazole 2% cream, econazole 1% cream, clotrimazole 1% cream, bifonazole 1% cream and tolnaftate 2% cream (Gip, 1984; Wagner and Reckers-Czaschka, 1987; Jegasothy and Pakes, 1991). In only one open randomized study, 1% oxiconazole nitrate cream was found to be superior to 2% tolnaftate ointment and 2% miconazole cream for the treatment of superficial dermatomycosis (Jegasothy and Pakes, 1991). The overall clinical efficacy of 1% oxiconazole nitrate cream in these randomized studies ranged from 64% to 90%.

2 Tinea (pityriasis) versicolor

Placebo-controlled trials of oxiconazole nitrate 1% cream applied once- or twice-daily for 2 weeks in the treatment of tinea versicolor caused by *Malassezia furfur*, established the significantly superior clinical and mycological efficacy of oxiconazole with mycological eradication rates 2 weeks after the end of treatment of 88% and clinical cure achieved in 82–83%. There was no significant difference in efficacy between the once-daily or twice-daily applications of oxiconazole (Jegasothy and Pakes, 1991).

3 Cutaneous candidiasis

In a randomized, double-blind study of 1% oxiconazole nitrate cream applied twice daily for 3–6 weeks and econazole 1% cream for the treatment of cutaneous candidiasis, there was no significant difference in mycological or clinical efficacy between the two regimens. Rates of clinical cure and mycological eradication for oxiconazole were 85% and 90% respectively (Gip, 1984).

4 Vaginal candidiasis

A single dose of oxiconazole nitrate (600-mg vaginal tablet) was compared with a 3-day course of econazole 150-mg ovule inserted once-daily for vaginal candidiasis, and produced identical response rates of 92% (Gouveia and Jones da Silva, 1984).

References

Beggs WH (1985). Influence of growth phase on the susceptibility of *Candida albicans* to butaconazole, oxiconazole, and sulconazole. *J Antimicrob Chemother* **16**: 397.

Ellis CN, Gammon WR, Goldfarb MT *et al.* (1989). A placebo-controlled evaluation of once-daily versus twice-daily oxiconazole nitrate (1%) cream in the treatment of tinea pedis. *Curr Ther Res* **46**: 269.

Fromtling RA (1988). Overview of medically important antifungal azole derivatives. *Clin Microbiol Rev* **1**: 187.

Gebhart RJ, Espinel-Ingroff A, Shadomy S (1984). *In vitro* susceptibility studies with oxiconazole (Ro 13–8996) *Chemotherapy* **30**: 244.

Gip L (1984). Comparison of oxiconazole (Ro 13–8996) and econazole in dermatomycoses. *Mykosen* **27**: 295.

Gouveia DC, Jones da Silva C (1984). Oxiconazole in the treatment of vaginal candidiasis: single dose versus 3-day treatment with econazole. *Pharmatherapeutica* **3**: 682.

Hiratani T, Yamaguchi H (1985). Mode of antifungal action of oxiconazole nitrate toward *Candida albicans*. *Chemotherapy* **33**: 215.

Hiratani T, Uchida K, Yamaguchi H (1984). Oxiconazole nitrate, a new imidazole-antimycotic: Evaluation of antifungal activity *in vitro*. *Chemotherapy* **30**: 244.

Jegasothy BV, Pakes GE (1991). Oxiconazole nitrate: Pharmacology, efficacy, and safety of a new imidazole antifungal agent. *Clin Ther* **13**: 126.

Lebwohl M, Rex IH, Tschen E *et al.* (1989). Oxiconazole nitrate cream, 1%, once or twice daily in the treatment of tinea pedis. *Clin Res J* **92**: 468.

Odds FC, Webster CE, Abbott AB (1984). Antifungal relative inhibition factors; BAY 1–9139, bifonazole, butoconazole, isoconazole, itraconazole (R 51211), oxiconazole, Ro 14–4767/002, sulconazole, terconazole and vibunazole (BAY n-7133) compared with nine established antifungal agents. *J Antimicrob Chemother* **14**: 105.

Odds FC, Cheesman SL, Abbott AB (1985). Suppression of ATP in *Candida albicans* by imidazole and derivative antifungal agents. *Sabouraudia* **23**: 415.

Oyeka CA, Gugnani HC (1990). *In vitro* activity of seven azole compounds against some clinical isolates of non-dermatophyte filamentous fungi and some dermatophytes. *Mycopathologia* **110**: 157.

Polak A (1982). Oxiconazole, a new imidazole derivative. *Arneim Forsch* **32**: 17.

Polak A, (1983). Antifungal activity *in vitro* of Ro 14–4767/002, a phenylpropyl-morpholine. *Sabouraudia* **21**: 205.

Polak-Wyss A, Lengsfeld H, Oesterhelt G (1985). Effect of oxiconazole and Ro 14–4767/002 on sterol pattern in *Candida albicans*. *Sabouraudia* **23**: 433.

Raulin C, Frosch PJ (1987). Contact allergy to oxiconazole. *Contact Derm* **16**: 39.

Ramelet AA, Walker-Nasir E (1987). Once daily application of oxiconazole cream is sufficient for treating dermatomycoses. *Dermatologica* **175**: 293.

Shadomy S, Wang H, Shadomy HJ (1988). Further *in vitro* studies with oxiconazole nitrate. *Diagn Microbiol Infect Dis* **9**: 231.

Stuttgen G, Bauer E (1985). Permeation of labelled oxiconazole. *Mykosen* **28**: 138.

Wagner W (1986). Comparison of the clinical efficacy and tolerability of oxiconazole, one dose versus two doses daily. *Mykosen* **29**: 280.

Wagner W, Reckers-Czaschka R (1987). Oxiconazole in dermatomycosis – a double-blind, randomized comparison with bifonazole. *Mykosen* **30**: 484.

Sulconazole

Description

Sulconazole is a substituted imidazole, structurally related to clotrimazole, econazole and miconazole. It has the chemical name of 1-[2,4-dichloro-beta-(4-chlorobenzyl)thiophenethyl] imidazole nitrate. Sulconazole has a broad spectrum of antifungal activity *in vitro* and has been shown to be an effective topical antifungal agent for the management of superficial fungal infections of the skin, particularly dermatophytoses, and tinea versicolor.

Sensitive Organisms

1 Pathogenic yeast

Cryptococcus neoformans is susceptible *in vitro* to sulconazole with an MIC of 0.16–0.63 μg per ml (Benfield and Clissold, 1988). Sulconazole is active against *Candida* spp.. Hernandez Molina *et al.* (1992), determined that 97% of strains of *Candida albicans* were inhibited by 2 μg per ml, but had comparatively moderate activity against *C. krusei*, *C. parapsilosis*, *C. tropicalis* and *C. guilliermondi*. The moderate activity against *Candida* species was confirmed in the relative inhibition factor (RIF) model produced by Odds *et al.*, and was comparable with econazole, isoconazole and miconazole (1984). Beggs (1985) demonstrated a growth phase-dependent fungicidal effect for *C. albicans* and *C. parapsilosis*, where sulconazole was fungistatic at concentrations of 80 μg per ml for early stationary-phase fungi and fungicidal at concentrations of 20 μg per ml for late phase exponential growth cells.

2 Dimorphic fungi

Sulconazole possesses good *in vitro* activity against *Histoplasma capsulatum*, *Blastomyces dermatitidis*, and *Paracoccidioides brasiliensis* with MICs less than 0.4 μg per ml. *Sporothrix schenckii* is susceptible with an MIC of less than 4 μg per ml (Benfield and Clissold, 1988).

3 Molds or filamentous fungi

Sulconazole has good *in vitro* activity against the dermatophyte fungi with MICs ranging from less than 0.4 to 2.5 μg per ml (Benfield and Clissold, 1988). By RIF evaluation, sulconazole had excellent activity against the dermatophytes (Odds *et al.*, 1984). In the guinea pig model of trichophytosis caused by *Trichophyton mentagrophytes*, the *in vivo* activity of sulconazole 1% cream applied topically for 5 days was comparable with miconazole (Yoshida *et al.*, 1984a). In addition, *Aspergillus* spp. and the demitaceous fungi, including *Fonsacaea* spp. and *Phialophora verrucosa* are susceptible (Benfield and Clissold, 1988).

4 Bacteria

Antibacterial activity *in vitro* has been demonstrated for Gram-positive bacteria such as *Staphylococcus aureus*, *Staph. epidermidis*, *Microsporum* spp. and *Bacillus* spp, but there is no activity against Gram-negative bacteria (Yoshida *et al.*, 1984b).

Mode of Administration and Dose

Indications and recommended doses
Superficial dermatomycosis
Tinea corporis, tinea cruris: 1% sulconazole nitrate cream or solution applied twice-daily for 3 weeks.
Tinea pedis: 1% sulconazole nitrate cream or solution applied twice-daily for 4 weeks.
Tinea (pityriasis) versicolor: 1% sulconazole nitrate cream or solution applied twice-daily for 3 weeks.
Cutaneous candidiasis: 1% sulconazole nitrate cream or solution applied twice-daily for 3 weeks.

Availability

Topical formulation: 1% sulconazole nitrate cream; 1% sulconazole nitrate solution.

Absorption of the Drug

The percutaneous absorption of radiolabeled sulconazole has been examined in healthy male volunteers and animals. In human volunteers, application of 1 g ^{3}H-sulconazole to intact and abraded skin which was subsequently occluded, resulted in 80% of the dose recovered from stratum corneum after 8 h, and 12% of the dose recovered in the feces. The systemic absorption (9–12% of the dose) was similar for those with intact skin and abraded skin. Percutaneous absorption through shaved skin of animals varied according to species from 5–7% for dogs, 12–13% for rats, 6% for guinea pigs and 30–40% for rabbits (Benfield and Clissold, 1988; Franz and Lehman, 1988).

Concentrations of sulconazole achieved in epidermis and stratum corneum, hair follicles and sebum or sweat have not been published. In rats (which have a similar rate of absorption as man), tissue concentrations of radioactivity 24 h after a single application of radiolabeled 1% sulconazole cream, revealed high concentration in the adrenal glands, and moderate radioactivity in spleen, brain, blood and muscle (Benfield and Clissold, 1988).

Mode of Action

The mechanism of action of sulconazole has not been studied well, but is thought to be similar to the other imidazole derivatives. Inhibition of the sterol C-14 demethylation of lanosterol and resultant depletion of ergosterol in the fungal cell membrane is likely to explain part of its antifungal effect (see Fig. IV.1, p. 1261). The ensuing increase in cell membrane permeability with release of essential intracellular ions, and interference with RNA and DNA synthesis have been studied (Benfield and Clissold, 1988). There is also some evidence for direct cell membrane damage from the growth phase-dependent fungicidal activity demonstrated by Beggs (1985).

Toxicity

Topical sulconazole is well tolerated with a reported local reaction rate of 3.4% (Benfield and Clissold, 1988). Local reactions tend to occur after 1–2 weeks treatment and comprise irritation with pruritus, erythema and contact dermatitis.

Clinical Uses of the Drug

1 Superficial dermatomycoses

Open studies of sulconazole nitrate 1% solution applied two or three times daily for 1–6 weeks for the treatment of dermatophyte infections revealed mycological eradication occurred in 2 weeks in those with tinea corporis and tinea cruris, but up to 4 weeks treatment was often required for tinea pedis (Benfield and Clissold, 1988). Sulconazole nitrate 1% cream applied twice-daily was significantly more effective than placebo for chronic moccasin-type tinea pedis due to *T. rubrum* in 92% of cases, with a 57% cure rate. However, there was a 27% relapse rate 2 weeks after the end of treatment with sulconazole (Akers *et al.*, 1989). Comparative studies with other imidazole derivatives revealed comparative activity for sulconazole in the majority, with mycological eradication rates of 72–100%. Sulconazole nitrate 1% cream applied twice-daily for 4 weeks as treatment for tinea pedis was significantly superior to clotrimazole 1% cream in two studies and equivalent in another (Lassus *et al.*, 1983; McVie *et al.*, 1986; Benfield and Clissold, 1988). For treatment of tinea corporis and tinea cruris, sulconazole nitrate 1% cream once- or twice-daily for 2–3 weeks had equivalent activity as 1% clotrimazole cream, even in hot humid conditions (McVie *et al.*, 1986; Benfield and Clissold, 1988; Tanenbaum *et al.*, 1989). Sulconazole nitrate 1% cream applied twice-daily for 3 weeks was generally comparable with miconazole 2% cream, but was associated with significantly fewer side-effects and produced a more rapid clinical response (Avila, 1985; Gip and Forsstrom, 1983; Tanenbaum *et al.*, 1982). In two studies superior activity for sulconazole 1% cream was demonstrated for the treatment of tinea pedis (Tanenbaum *et al.*, 1982; Woscoff and Carabeli, 1986). Two small studies comparing econazole 1% cream with sulconazole revealed equivalent efficacy (Lassus and Forsstrom, 1984; Qadripur, 1984). Short-term relapse rates are very low for sulconazole-treated patients, and in one comparative study there was no relapses in sulconazole-treated patients compared with 19% of econazole-treated patients (Lassus and Forsstrom, 1984).

2 Tinea (pityriasis) versicolor

Equivalent activity with clotrimazole 1% cream or 1% solution and 2% miconazole cream was demonstrated in comparative studies with sulconazole nitrate 1% cream and solution (Benfield and Clissold, 1988; Tanenbaum et al., 1984; Tham, 1984). In the comparison with miconazole, mycological and clinical cures were observed in 93% and 89% of sulconazole-treated patients compared with 87% and 82% of miconazole-treated patients. Eradication of *Malassezia furfur* generally occurs within 2 weeks of treatment and response rates of 75% are seen.

3 Cutaneous candidiasis

Sulconazole nitrate 1% cream applied twice-daily for 3 weeks is an effective treatment for cutaneous candidiasis as demonstrated by the results of a placebo-controlled trial. The overall clinical and mycological cure was 96% compared with 10% for placebo (Tanenbaum et al., 1983). Comparative studies revealed sulconazole nitrate 1% cream had equivalent activity as 1% clotrimazole cream administered for 2 weeks (Rajan and Thirumoorthy, 1983; Benfield and Clissold, 1988), and 2% miconazole cream administered for 3 weeks (Tanenbaum et al., 1983). Fungal eradication usually occurs with 2 weeks treatment in 62–96% of treated patients.

4 Impetigo and ecthyema

Sulconazole nitrate 1% cream applied twice-daily for 14 days to patients with pyoderma caused by *Streptococcus pyogenes* and *Staphylococcus* spp., was extremely effective with mycological eradication in 100% of patients by day 7 of treatment and rapid clinical resolution. Sulconazole produced a more rapid mycological response than miconazole nitrate 2% cream but was equally effective at day 14 (Nolting and Strauss, 1988).

References

Akers WA, Lane A, Lynfield Y et al. (1989). Sulconazole nitrate 1% cream in the treatment of chronic moccasin-type tinea pedis caused by *Trichophyton rubrum. J Amer Acad Dermatol* **21**: 686.

Avila JM (1985). Treatment of dermatomycoses with sulconazole 1% nitrate cream or miconazole nitrate 2% cream. *Curr Ther Res* **38**: 328.

Beggs WH (1985). Influence of growth phase on the susceptibility of *Candida albicans* to butaconazole, oxiconazole, and sulconazole. *J Antimicrob Chemother* **16**: 397.

Benfield P, Clissold SP (1988). Sulconazole A review of its antimicrobial activity and therapeutic use in superficial dermatomycoses. *Drugs* **35**: 143.

Franz TJ, Lehman P (1988). Percutaneous absorption of sulconazole nitrate in humans. *J Pharm Sci* **77**: 489.

Gip L, Forsstrom S (1983). A double-blind parallel study of sulconazole nitrate 1% cream compared with miconazole nitrate 2% cream in dermatophytoses. *Mykosen* **26**: 231.

Hernandez Molina JM, Llosa J, Martinez Brocal A, Ventosa A (1992). *In vitro* activity of cloconazole, sulconazole, butoconazole, isoconazole, fenticonazole, and five other antifungal agents against clinical isolates of *Candida albicans* and *Candida* spp. *Mycopathologia* **118**: 15.

Lassus A, Forsstrom S (1984). A double-blind parallel study comparing sulconazole with econazole in the treatment of dermatophytoses. *Mykosen* **27**: 582.

Lassus A, Forsstrom S, Salo O (1983). A double-blind comparison of sulconazole nitrate 1% cream with clotrimazole 1% cream in the treatment of dermatophytoses. *Brit J Dermatol* **108**: 195.

McVie DH, Littlewood S, Allen BR et al. (1986). Sulconazole versus clotrimazole in the treatment of dermatophytosis. *Clin Exp Derm* **11**: 613.

Nolting S, Strauss WB (1988). Treatment of impetgo and ecthyema. A comparison of sulconazole with miconazole. *Int J Dermatol* **27**: 716.

Odds FC, Webster CE, Abbott AB (1984). Antifungal relative inhibition factors; BAY 1–9139, bifonazole, butoconazole, isoconazole, itracona-

zole (R 51211), oxiconazole, Ro 14–4767/002, sulconazole, terconazole and vibunazole (BAY n-7133) compared with nine established antifungal agents. *J Antimicrob Chemother* **14**: 105.

Qadripur S-A (1984). Double-blind parallel comparison of sulconazole nitrate 1% cream and powder with econazole 1% cream and powder, in the treatment of cutaneous dermatophytoses. *Curr Ther Res* **35**: 753.

Rajan VS, Thirumoorthy T (1983). Treatment of cutaneous candidiasis: a double blind comparison of sulconazole nitrate 1% cream and clotrimazole 1% cream. *Aust J Dermatol* **24**: 33.

Tanenbaum L, Anderson C, Rosenberg MJ et al. (1982). Sulconazole nitrate 1% cream: a comparison with miconazole in the treatment of tinea pedis and tinea cruris/corporis. *Cutis* **30**: 105.

Tanenbaum L, Anderson C, Rosenberg M, Dorr A (1983). A new treatment for cutaneous candidiasis: sulconazole nitrate cream 1%. *Int J Dermatol* **22**: 318.

Tanenbaum L, Anderson C, Rosenberg MJ, Akers W (1984). 1% sulconazole cream v 2% miconazole cream in the treatment of tinea versicolor. *Arch Dermatol* **120**: 216.

Tanenbaum L, Taplin D, Lavelle C et al. (1989). Sulconazole nitrate cream 1 percent for treating tinea cruris and corporis. *Cutis* **44**: 344.

Tham SN (1987). Treatment of pityriasis versicolor: comparison of sulconazole nitrate 1% solution and clotrimazole 1% solution. *Austr J Dermatol* **28**: 123.

Woscoff A, Carabeli S (1986). Treatment of tinea pedis with sulconazole nitrate 1% cream or miconazole nitrate 2% cream. *Curr Ther Res* **39**: 753.

Yoshida H, Kasuga T, Yamaguchi T et al. (1984a). Studies on the antifungal activities of sulconazole. 2. Therapeutic effect of the cream formulation on experimental *Trichophyton mentagrophytes* infection of guinea pig. *Chemotherapy* **32**: 485.

Yoshida H, Kasuga T, Yamaguchi T (1984b). Studies on the antifungal activities of sulconazole. I. *In vitro* antimicrobial activity. *Chemotherapy* **32**: 477.

Terconazole

Description

Terconazole was synthesized and developed by Janssen Pharmaceutica in 1983. It was the first triazole antifungal agent marketed (Fromtling, 1988). It has the chemical name of 1-{4-[[2-(2,4-dichlorophenyl)-*r*-2-(1*H*-1,2,4-triazol-1-ylmethyl)-1,3-dioxalan-*c*-4-yl]methoxy]phenyl}-4-isopropylpiperazine. It has a broad spectrum of activity against dermatophytes, pathogenic yeast and *Candida* species. It is marketed for topical use only.

Sensitive Organisms

The potent *in vitro* activity of terconazole against *Candida* species was demonstrated by Van Cutsem (1991), Pfaller and Gerarden, (1989) and Tolman *et al.* (1986). Depending upon the broth medium used for susceptibility testing, 100% of *Candida albicans* were sensitive to terconazole at a concentration of 0.1 μg per ml and was the most potent agent when compared with miconazole, clotrimazole and sulconazole. In addition, using the relative inhibition factor methodology, terconazole was the most active topical azole drug against *Candida* spp. (Odds *et al.*, 1984). In the rat model of vaginal candidiasis, topical administration of 0.5% and 1% terconazole creams twice-daily for 3 days produced cure rates of 76% and 97%. In contrast, oral administration of terconazole at a dose of 10 mg per kg produced a cure rate of 50%, which was inferior to those produced by ketoconazole (Van Cutsem *et al.*, 1983).

Terconazole also possesses potent *in vitro* activity against dermatophytes (Odds *et al.*, 1984). In the guinea pig model of dermatomycoses, topical terconazole 0.5% achieved 100% mycological and clinical cures for models infected with *Trichophyton mentagrophytes* and *Microsporum canis* (Heeres *et al.*, 1983; Fromtling, 1988).

Mode of Administration and Dose

Indications and recommended dose
Vulvovaginal candidiasis: 80 mg vaginal pessary or 5 g of 0.8% vaginal cream inserted once-daily for 3 consecutive nights; 5 g (1 applicator) of 0.4% vaginal cream administered intravaginally for 7 consecutive nights.

Availability

Topical formulation: 80 mg vaginal pessary; 0.4%, 0.8% vaginal cream.

Absorption of the Drug

Approximately 5–16% of terconazole administered intravaginally is absorbed into the systemic circulation. In normal healthy volunteers, mean peak serum terconazole levels of 0.01 μg per ml were measured at 7 h after administration. Peak levels are similar after multiple dosing, and in women with vaginitis. Systemically absorbed drug is rapidly metabolized by the liver and excreted in the urine and feces (Product information Terconazole, 1994).

Mode of Action

Terconazole binds to the heme iron component of the fungal cytochrome P-450 enzyme lanosterol C-14 demethylase, inhibiting the conversion of lanosterol to ergosterol (Isaacson *et al.*, 1988). The resultant membrane depletion of ergosterol causes an increase in membrane permeability and altered membrane enzyme activity (Weisberg 1989). Terconazole has a significantly greater affinity for the fungal cytochrome P-450 enzyme compared with mammalian cytochrome P-450. Because of this, there is a decreased tendency for the drug to induce hepatic cytochrome P-450 enzyme activity, and consequent induction of metabolism of the drug in vaginal tissue or epithelium (Cauwenbergh and Vanden Bossche, 1989). Terconazole also causes a significant increase in chitin in *C. albicans* cell walls which may contribute to the toxicity of the drug (Pfaller *et al.*, 1990).

Toxicity

Local reactions such as irritation, itching and burning are reported after vaginal administration of terconazole in women (Thomason, 1989). Skin rash has also been described rarely.

A flu-like syndrome has been described in patients who received 160 mg as a single intravaginal dose. Chills and fever begin about 1 h after administration and are associated with headache and hypotension. Symptoms resolve in 10–48 h (Geiger, 1988; Moebius, 1988; Hyder *et al.*, 1994). Over 100 cases have been reported and it has been hypothesized the symtoms may be a Herxheimer reaction (Weisberg, 1989). Approximately 30% of women complain of headache which subsides spontaneously. It occurs after administration of both the vaginal cream and the suppository, and may be a mild manifestation of the flu-like reaction.

Clinical Uses of the Drug

1 Vaginal candidiasis

Terconazole is an effective agent for vaginal candidiasis. Weisberg (1989) has summarized the results of the majority of clinical trials of terconazole. Regimens of 80-mg vaginal pessary inserted daily for 3 consecutive nights, and 7 consecutive days treatment with 0.4% cream were established as the optimal regimens producing mycological cure rates of 88% and 93% respectively (Hirsch, 1989). Placebo-controlled studies of terconazole 80 mg for 3 days were associated with clinical cure rates of 89–92% and mycological eradication rates of 80–85% (Thomason, 1989; Thomason *et al.*, 1990). There was no significant difference in clinical or mycological efficacy between terconazole 0.8% cream and 1.6% cream (Schmitt *et al.*, 1990).

Comparative trials of terconazole 80-mg pessary with clotrimazole vaginal tablets revealed equivalent mycological efficacy (95% and 85%), and a more rapid onset of symptomatic relief for terconazole-treated women (Kjaeldgaard and Larsson, 1985). In addition, the administration of the 80-mg pessary for 3 days had superior long-term efficacy than a single-dose 240 mg terconazole (Kjaeldgaard, 1986). A comparison of the 0.4% terconazole cream and 1% clotrimazole cream applied for 7 days in both pregnant and non-pregnant women showed a non-significant trend to higher mycological eradication rates in terconazole-treated women. At 1-month follow-up, there was no difference in the mycological eradication rate between the two treatment groups for pregnant women. The relapse rate for the terconazole group was 3% compared with 17% for clotrimazole-treated women (Weisberg, 1989).

In comparative studies comparing 0.4% terconazole cream with 2% miconazole, terconazole treatment produced a statistically significantly superior mycological eradication rate at 97–100%. There was also a significantly lower relapse rate of 0% in the terconazole group compared with 18% in the miconazole group in one study, but this observation was reversed in another smaller study (Weisberg, 1989). However, no confirmation of this observation occurred in comparative studies of terconazole 0.4% cream and miconazole 2% cream perfomed in the USA. Equivalent efficacy with mycological and clinical cure rates of 88% and 94% for terconazole and 83% and 91% for miconazole were demonstrated. Relapse rates for the two regimens were also comparable at 19% and 17% (Thomason, 1989; Weisberg, 1989).

Intravaginal insertion of terconazole 80 mg for 3 days was shown to have equivalent clinical and mycological efficacy as a single oral dose of 150 mg fluconazole at short-term evaluation with clinical response rates of 95% and 93% respectively and mycological cure rates of 91% and 82% respectively. At the long-term follow-up, topical terconazole was found to be significantly more effective than single dose fluconazole with clinical and mycological response rates of 93% and 91% for the terconazole group and 74% and 74% for the fluconazole group. De los Reyes (1992), who reported these results, suggested they should be interpreted in the light of an uneven distribution of previous episodes of vaginal candidiasis between the two treatment groups.

References

Cauwenbergh G, Vanden Bossche H (1989). Terconazole: Pharmacology of a new antimycotic agent. *J Reprod Med* **34**: 588.

de los Reyes C, Edelman DE, Bruin MF (1992). Clinical experience with single-dose fluconazole in vaginal candidiasis. A review of the worldwide database. *Int J Gynecol Obstet* **37** (Suppl): 9.

Fromtling RA (1988). Overview of medically important antifungal azole derivatives. *Clin Microbiol Rev* **1**: 187.

Geiger AJ (1988). Influenza-like syndrome after terconazole. *Lancet* **ii**: 1192.

Heeres J, Hendrickx R, Van Cutsem J (1983). Antimycotic imidazoles. 6. Synthesis and antifungal properties of terconazole, a novel triazole ketal. *J Med Chem* **26**: 611.

Hirsch HA (1989). Clinical evaluation of terconazole. European experience. *J Reprod Med* **34** (Suppl). 593.

Hyder SS, Manjon JE, Gantz NM (1994). Fever and leukocytosis related to terconazole vaginal suppository. *South Med J* **87**: 762.

Isaacson DM, Tolman EL, Tobia AJ *et al.* (1988). Selective inhibition of 14 alpha-desmethyl sterol synthesis in *Candida albicans* by terconazole, a new triazole antimycotic. *J Antimicrob Chemother* **21**: 333.

Kjaeldgaard A (1986). Comparison of terconazole and clotrimazole vaginal tablets in the treatment of vulvovaginal candidosis. *Pharmatherapeutica* **4**: 525.

Kjaeldgaard A, Larsson B (1985). Single-blind comparative trial of short-term therapy with terconazole versus clotrimazole vaginal tablets in vulvovaginal candidiasis. *Curr Ther Res* **38**: 939.

Moebius UM (1988). Influenza-like syndrome after terconazole. *Lancet* **ii**: 966.

Odds FC, Webster CE, Abbott AB (1984). Antifungal relative inhibition factors; BAY 1–9139, bifonazole, butoconazole, isoconazole, itraconazole (R 51211), oxiconazole, Ro 14–4767/002, sulconazole, terconazole and vibunazole (BAY n-7133) compared with nine established antifungal agents. *J Antimicrob Chemother* **14**: 105.

Pfaller MA, Gerarden T (1989). Susceptibility of clinical isolates of *Candida* spp to terconazole and other azole antifungal agents. *Diagn Microbiol Infect Dis* **12**: 467.

Pfaller MA, Riley J, Koerner T (1990). Effects of terconazole and other azole antifungal agents on the sterol and carbohydrate composition of *Candida albicans. Diagn Microbiol Infect Dis* **13**: 31.

Schmitt C, Sobel J, Meriwether C (1990). Comparison of the 0.8% and 1.6% terconazole cream in severe vulvovaginal candidiasis. *Obstet Gynecol* **76**: 414.

Thomason JL (1989). Clinical evaluation of terconazole: United States experience. *J Reprod Med* **34** (Suppl): 597.

Thomason JL, Gelbart SM, Kellett AV *et al.* (1990). Terconazole for the treatment of vulvovaginal candidiasis. *J Reprod Med* **35**: 992.

Tolman EL, Isaacson DM, Rosenthale ME *et al.* (1986). Anticandidal activities of terconazole, a broad spectrum antimycotic. *Antimicrob Ag Chemother* **29**: 986.

Van Cutsem J (1991). The *in vitro* activity of terconazole against yeasts: Its topical long-acting therapeutic efficacy in experimental vaginal candidiasis in rats. *Amer J Obstet Gynecol* **165**: 1200.

Van Cutsem J, Van Gerven F, Zaman R, Janssen PAJ (1983). Terconazole – a new, broad-spectrum antifungal. *Chemotherapy* **29**: 322.

Weisberg M (1989). Terconazole – a new antifungal agent for vulvovaginal candidiasis. *Clin Ther* **11**: 659.

Tioconazole

Description

Tioconazole is a substituted imidazole derivative, structurally related to econazole, clotrimazole and miconazole, with the chemical name 1-[2,4-dichloro-beta-(2-chloro-3-thenyloxy)-phenethyl] imidazole. It has a broad spectrum of antifungal activity including pathogenic yeasts, dermatophytes and *Aspergillus* species, as well as *Trichomonas vaginalis*. Tioconazole is marketed as a topical formulation for the treatment of superficial dermatophyte infections and vaginal candidiasis. It is available without prescription in some countries.

Sensitive Organisms

1 Pathogenic yeast

Tioconazole has good *in vitro* activity against *Candida* species and *Cryptococcus neoformans*, with MICs in the range of 0.12–2 µg per ml for *Candida albicans*, 0.12–0.5 µg per ml for *C. glabrata*, and 0.12 µg per ml for *C. neoformans*. The activity of tioconazole against other species of *Candida*, *Tricosporon* spp., *Rhodotorula* spp., and *Geotrichum candidum* was also potent and superior to other antifungal agents (Bergan and Vangdal, 1983; Jevons *et al.*, 1979; Odds, 1980; Marriott *et al.*, 1983). Fungicidal activity was demonstrated for *C. albicans* at tioconazole concentrations four times the MIC (Lefler and Stevens, 1984). *In vivo* activity of tioconazole administered by the i.v. and oral routes has been confirmed in the murine model of systemic candidiasis (Jevons *et al.*, 1979).

2 Molds or filamentous fungi

Tioconazole has potent activity against the common dermatophytes with MICs in the range of less than 0.1 to 1.0 µg per ml (Jevons *et al.*, 1979; Marriott *et al.*, 1983), and is rapidly fungicidal against *Trichophyton rubrum* and *T. mentagrophytes* (Clissold and Heel, 1986). This activity was confirmed in the guinea pig model of trichophytosis using topical application of tioconazole (Marriott *et al.*, 1983).

3 Bacteria

In vitro evaluation of tioconazole has revealed good *in vitro* activity against Gram-positive bacteria, such as *Staphylococcus aureus*, *S. epidermidis*, *Streptococcus pyogenes* and Group B *Streptococcus* (Clissold and Heel, 1986). Moderate activity against *Trichomonas vaginalis* and *Chlamydia trachomatis* has also been identified (Clissold and Heel, 1986).

Mode of Administration and Dose

Indications and recommended dose
Superficial fungal infections: 1% cream, lotion, powder, and spray solution.
   Dermatomycosis: once-daily application 2–4 weeks.
   Severe tinea pedis: once- or twice-daily application for up to 6 weeks.
   Cutaneous candidiasis: once-daily application for 2–4 weeks.
   Tinea (pityriasis) versicolor: once-daily application for 7 days.

Onychomycosis: 28% tioconazole solution applied twice-daily for 6 months.

Vaginal candidiasis: 300 mg (pessary or 5 g 6% ointment) as single dose; 100 mg (pessary or 5 g 2% cream) once at night for 3 days.

Availability

Topical formulation: 1% tioconazole cream, lotion, powder, and spray solution.

Vaginal formulations: 100 mg, 300 mg pessaries; 2% cream, 6.5% ointment.

Absorption of the Drug

Only minimal systemic absorption of tioconazole has been demonstrated in both animal and human studies. Following application of 0.1 g of ^{14}C-labeled tioconazole 2% cream in the rat, percutaneous absorption was slow with maximal plasma concentration achieved at 12 h, and elimination of unchanged drug and metabolites was by urine (2.9%) and feces (16.8%) over 120 h (Marriott *et al.*, 1983).

Tioconazole was negligibly absorbed following topical application of the 2% cream or 28% nail solution to the skin twice-daily for 14 days in a small number of patients. Plasma tioconazole levels were undetectable in half the patients and were 5–10 ng per ml in the remainder who applied the cream, and were undetectable in half the patients or detected at levels of 12–31 ng per ml in the remainder of those who applied the solution (Clissold and Heel, 1986).

Absorption of tioconazole was also extremely low following intravaginal application of 2% cream daily for 30 days (peak plasma tioconazole concentration of 4–14 ng per ml), or a single 300 mg pessary (10–36 ng per ml). There was no detectable plasma tioconazole 24 h after administration of the last dose. Mean concentrations of tioconazole in the vaginal fluid after a single application of 5 ml 6% vaginal ointment (300 mg) were 104 µg per ml at 24 h, 27 µg per ml at 48 h and 15 µg per ml at 72 h. After intravaginal administration of a 300 mg pessary, the mean vaginal fluid tioconazole concentrations were 21.2 µg per ml at 24 h and remained detectable in the majority of women at 48 h, but not at 72 h (Houang and Lawrence, 1985; Clissold and Heel, 1986).

Mode of Action

In a similar manner to the other imidazole agents, tioconazole inhibits sterol biosynthesis, by inhibition of cytochrome P-450 dependent C-14 alpha demethylation of lanosterol, preventing conversion to ergosterol, which results in depletion of normal fungal sterols (ergosterol) and accumulation of 14 alpha methyl sterols (lanosterol) in the fungal cell membrane (see Fig. IV.1, p. 1261). This inhibition is thought to produce fungistatic activity (Marriott, 1982; Pye and Marriott, 1982). At higher concentrations, tioconazole appears to produce direct cell membrane damage resulting in leakage of essential intracellular components and cell death (Ansehn and Nilson, 1984). Fungicidal activity has been demonstrated during stationary phases of growth in *Candida* spp. which supports the hypothesis of direct cell membrane damage (Beggs, 1984).

Toxicity

No systemic or laboratory adverse events have been noted in the clinical trials reported in the literature. Local skin reactions occur at a rate of 4–7% of patients. These are generally mild, transient and include erythema, itching, and burning. Contact dermatitis, confirmed with patch testing has been reported (Kuokkanen, 1982; Jones and Kennedy, 1990; Izu *et al.*, 1992; Gibson *et al.*, 1994; Quirino and Barros, 1994).

Intravaginal application of tioconazole whether in pessary, cream or ointment formulation results in leakage from the vagina. A minority of women did not tolerate the leakage (2.5%) and no staining of clothing was reported (Clissold and Heel, 1986). Reports of side-effects following intravaginal application are generally infrequent, and include mild burning, stinging and pruritus. However, 30% of tioconazole-treated patients experienced local irritation or itching in one comparative study (Stein *et al.*, 1986).

Tioconazole vaginal formulations have been used in the second and third trimester of pregnancy without evidence of drug-related complications (Akuse, 1984).

Clinical Uses of the Drug

1 Superficial dermatomycoses

Tioconazole 1% or 2% cream is an effective treatment for dermatomycoses, including tinea corporis, tinea cruris and tinea pedis, with clinical and mycological cure rates of 75–95%. Efficacy (80% cure rate) was demonstrated in a placebo-controlled trial of tioconazole 2% cream applied twice-daily for 4 weeks (Kuokkanen, 1982), and in open non-comparative studies. Kashin *et al.* (1985) established that application of the 1% cream once-daily was as effective as twice-daily application with mycological eradication rates of 85–95%. Controlled trials of tioconazole 1% or 2% cream with econazole 1% cream (Grigoriu and Grigoriu, 1983), miconazole 2% cream (Clayton *et al.*, 1982; Fredriksson, 1983;Vander Ploeg and De Villez, 1984) and clotrimazole (Clissold and Heel, 1986) revealed comparative efficacy, with a trend to enhanced activity for tioconazole compared with miconazole and clotrimazole (O'Neill East *et al.*, 1983).

2 Tinea (pityriasis) versicolor

Tioconazole 1% or 2% cream or lotion is an effective treatment for tinea versicolor with cure rates of 85%. It is more effective than miconazole 2% cream and 1% clotrimazole (Clayton *et al.*, 1982; O'Neill East *et al.*, 1983; Clissold and Heel, 1986; Alchorne *et al.*, 1987). Treatment with tioconazole lotion twice-daily for 2 weeks is associated with 94% mycological eradication and clinical response (Alchorne *et al.*, 1987).

3 Cutaneous candidiasis

Tioconazole 1% cream applied two or three times daily for 2 weeks, was significantly more effective than 1% clotrimazole cream with clinical and mycological cure rates of 71% (Clissold and Heel, 1986). A placebo-controlled evaluation of 1% tioconazole cream for the treatment of napkin dermatitis (mixed bacterial and *C. albicans* infection) confirmed tioconazole is an effective agent for this clinical entity with clinical and mycological cure rates of 78%. There was no relapse in 86% of children 6 weeks later (Clissold and Heel, 1986; Gibbs *et al.*, 1987).

4 Onychomycosis

An uncontrolled study examining the safety and efficacy of tioconazole 28% nail solution applied twice-daily for periods of 2–18 months, revealed some improvement in 70% of finger and toe nail infections (Clissold and Heel, 1986). In addition, Hay *et al.* (1985) reported clinical cure in 28% patients treated with 28% tioconazole solution for 3 months in a small study.

5 Vaginal candidiasis

Tioconazole is an effective treatment for vulvovaginal candidiasis. In non-comparative studies, intravaginal administration of tioconazole as a 300-mg pessary or 5 g of 6% ointment as a single dose appeared comparable with treatment regimens of 100-mg pessary or 5 g of 2% cream administered nightly for 3–6 days, and produced clinical and mycological cure rates of 70–90% (Akuse, 1984; Clissold and Heel, 1986).The response rate following a single dose of tioconazole can be increased to 100% by the administration of a second 300-mg vaginal pessary (Akuse, 1984). Leegaard (1985) noted mycological cure rates of 89% after two courses of tioconazole 2% cream administered daily for 3 days, 1 week apart. Relapse rates of less than 15% at 4–6 weeks have been reported for these regimens. Comparative studies have established significantly superior clinical and mycological cure rates for tioconazole compared with placebo.

Variable results have been obtained in other small comparative studies with clotrimazole, econazole, and miconazole, but tioconazole has equivalent efficacy to these agents at a minimum, and may have superior efficacy to econazole and clotrimazole (Clissold and Heel, 1986). Stein *et al.* (1986) showed a single dose of 5 g 6.5% tioconazole ointment was equivalent to clotrimazole 200 mg once at night for 3 consecutive nights. In a meta-analysis of the clinical trials of tioconazole for vaginal candidiasis, the pessary and cream formulations had comparable efficacy with an overall cure rate of 84%, and the pooled data suggested that tioconazole was significantly more effective than econazole and clotrimazole after 3 days treatment, than clotrimazole after 6 days treatment and better than miconazole and econazole after 14 days treatment. Relapse rates were similar for all the imidazole agents (Clissold and Heel, 1986).

Comparable efficacy of a single 5-g dose of tioconazole 6% vaginal ointment and 5 days treatment with oral ketoconazole 400 mg per day was demonstrated in an open, randomized study. The women treated with tioconazole had a more rapid onset of improvement in clinical symptoms and tolerated therapy better than those treated with oral ketoconazole (Rohde Werner, 1984).

6 Vaginal trichomoniasis

Tioconazole 2% vaginal cream effectively cured 95% of women with *Trichomonas vaginalis* infection, and mycological eradication was maintained in 95% (Donadio, 1986).

References

Akuse JT (1984). Assessment of the efficacy of tioconazole (Trosyd). 300 mg ovules in vaginal candidosis. *Curr Ther Res* **36**: 409.

Alchorne MM, Paschoalick RC, Forjaz MH (1987). Comparative study of tioconazole and clotrimazole in the treatment of tinea versicolor. *Clin Ther* **9**: 360.

Ansehn S, Nilsson L (1984). Direct membrane-damaging effect ketoconazole and tioconazole on *Candida albicans* demonstrated by bioluminescent assay of ATP. *Antimicrob Ag Chemother* **26**: 22.

Beggs WH (1984). Fungicidal activity of tioconazole in relation to growth phase of *Candida albicans* and *Candida parapsilosis*. *Antimicrob Ag Chemother* **26**: 699.

Bergan T, Vangdal M (1983). *In vitro* activity of antifungal agents against yeast species. *Chemotherapy* **29**: 104.

Clayton YM, Hay RJ, McGibbon DH, Pye RJ (1982). Double blind comparison of the efficacy of tioconazole and miconazole for the treatment of fungal infection of the skin or erythrasma. *Clin Exp Dermatol* **7**: 543.

Clissold SP, Heel RC (1986). Tioconazole A review of its antimicrobial activity and therapeutic use in superficial mycoses. *Drugs* **31**: 29.

Donadio C (1986). Tioconazole 2% cream in the treatment of *Trichomonas vaginalis* or mixed vaginal infections. *J Int Med Res* **14**: 50.

Fredriksson T (1983). Treatment of dermatomycoses with topical tioconazole and miconazole. *Dermatologica* **166** (Suppl 1): 14.

Gibbs DL, Kashin P, Jevons S (1987). Comparative and non-comparative studies of the efficacy and tolerance of tioconazole 1% cream versus another imidazole and/or placebo in neonates and infants with candidal diaper rash and/or impetigo. *J Int Med Res* **15**: 23.

Gibson G, Buckley A, Murphy GM (1994). Allergic contact dermatitis from tioconazole without cross-sensitivity to other imidazoles. *Contact Derm* **30**: 308.

Grigoriu D, Grigoriu A (1983). Double-blind comparison of the efficacy, toleration and safety of tioconazole base 1% and econazole nitrate 1% creams in the treatment of patients with fungal infections of the skin or erythrasma. *Dermatologica* **166** (Suppl 1): 8.

Hay RJ, Mackie RM, Clayton YM (1985). Tioconazole nail solution – an open study of its efficacy in onychomycosis. *Clin Exp Dermatol* **10**: 111.

Houang ET, Lawrence AG (1985). Systemic absorption and persistence of tioconazole in vaginal fluid after insertion of a single 300 mg tioconazole ovule. *Antimicrob Ag Chemother* **27**: 964.

Izu R, Aguirre A, Gonzalez M, Diaz-Perez JL (1992). Contact dermatitis from tioconazole with cross-sensitivity to other imidazoles. *Contact Derm* **26**: 130.

Jevons S, Gymer GE, Brammer KW *et al.* (1979). Antifungal activity of tioconazole (UK-20,349), a new imidazole derivative. *Antimicrob Ag Chemother* **15**: 597.

Jones SK, Kennedy CT (1990). Contact dermatitis from tioconazole. *Contact Derm* **22**: 122.

Kashin P, Phyfferoen MC, Gibbs DL (1985). A comparative study of once versus twice daily treatment of superficial dermatophyte and yeast infections with tioconazole (1%) cream. *J Int Med Res* **13**: 85.

Kuokkanen K (1982). Topical tioconazole in dermatomycosis. *Mykosen* **25**: 274.

Leegaard M (1985). Treatment of vaginal candidosis with tioconazole 2% vaginal cream. *Acta Obstet Gynecol Scand* **64**: 127.

Lefler E, Stevens DA (1984). Inhibition and killing of *Candida albicans in vitro* by five imidazoles in clinical use. *Antimicrob Ag Chemother* **25**: 450.

Marriott MS (1980). Inhibition of sterol biosynthesis in *Candida albicans* by imidazole-containing antifungals. *J Gen Microbiol* **117**: 253.

Marriott MS, Baird JRC, Brammer KW *et al.* (1983). Tioconazole, a new imidazole-antifungal agent for the treatment of dermatomycoses. Antifungal and pharmacologic properties. *Dermatologica* **166** (Suppl 1): 1.

Odds FC (1980). Laboratory evaluation of antifungal agents: a comparative study of five imidazole derivatives of clinical importance. *J Antimicrob Chemother* **6**: 749.

O'Neill East M, Henderson JT, Jevons S (1983). Tioconazole in the treatment of fungal infections of the skin. *Dermatologica* **166** (Suppl 1): 20.

Pye GW, Marriott MS (1982). Inhibition of sterol C14 demethylation by imidazole-containing antifungals. *Sabouraudia* **20**: 325.

Quirino AP, Barros MA (1994). Contact dermatitis from tioconazole. *Contact Derm* **30**: 240.

Rohde Werner H (1984). Topical tioconazole versus systemic ketoconazole treatment of vaginal candidiasis. *J Int Med Res* **12**: 298.

Stein GE, Gurwith D, Mummaw N, Gurwith M (1986). Single-dose tioconazole compared with 3-day clotrimazole treatment in vulvovaginal candidiasis. *Antimicrob Ag Chemother* **29**: 969.

Vander Ploeg DE, De Villez L (1984). A new topical antifungal drug: Tioconazole. *Int J Dermatol* **23**: 681.

Saperconazole

Description

Saperconazole (R 66905) is a synthetic difluorinated triazole derivative of itraconazole developed by Janssen Pharmaceutica, Belgium for systemic use, and has potent *in vitro* activity against *Aspergillus* spp., dermatophytes and *Candida* spp. It is lipophilic, and enhanced bioavailability was noted in mice when the drug was complexed with hydroxypropyl-beta-cyclodextrin (Hostetler *et al.*, 1992). It has been temporarily withdrawn from drug development because of the development of ovarian tumors in some animal models (Graybill and Sharkey-Mathis, 1992).

Sensitive Organisms

1 Pathogenic yeasts

Saperconazole has potent *in vitro* activity against *Candida* spp. with an MIC range from 0.045 to >100 μg per ml (Otcenasek, 1992). It was more potent than amphotericin B and fluconazole against *Candida albicans,* and more active than fluconazole against other *Candida* spp. (Fu *et al.*, 1992a). The *in vivo* activity of saperconazole has been evaluated in the rat model of vaginal candidiasis and it correlated well with the *in vitro* activity. Intravaginal administration of saperconazole produced equivalent efficacy to intravaginal fluconazole, but a single oral dose of saperconazole was 7-fold more effective than a single dose of fluconazole in achieving a mycological cure in 90–100% of animals (Fu *et al.*, 1992a). In the murine model of disseminated candidiasis, saperconazole caused a reduction in the colony count of *C. albicans* in the kidneys, and improved survival, but the activity was inferior to amphotericin B (Sugar *et al.*, 1994). *Trichosporon* spp. are susceptible to saperconazole with an MIC range of 0.09–0.39 μg per ml (Otcenasek, 1992).

2 Dimorphic fungi

Excellent *in vitro* activity of saperconazole against *Paracoccidioides brasiliensis* has been documented *in vitro* (San Blas *et al.*, 1993).

3 Molds and filamentous fungi

Saperconazole has potent activity against *Aspergillus* spp. with MICs of less than 0.1 μg.ml in one study, and 0.8–12.5 μg per ml in another study (Otcenasek, 1992; Denning *et al.*, 1991). Odds (1989) demonstrated very low relative inhibition factors for saperconazole against dermatophytes (5–10%) and *Aspergillus* spp. (6–18%) predictive of strong activity against these fungi. Saperconazole is extremely active against dermatophytes with MICs of 0.002–0.25 μg per ml for *Trichophyton* spp., 0.002–0.25 μg per ml for *Epidermophyton* spp., and 0.001–0.1 μg per ml for *Microsporum* spp. (Fu *et al.*, 1992b; Otcenasek, 1992). In the guinea pig model of trichophytosis 75% cure rate was achieved with topical administration of 0.25% saperconazole (Fu *et al.*, 1992b). *Fusarium* spp. and *Scopulariopsis brevicaulis* are resistant (Otcenasek, 1992). Saperconazole is not active against the Zygomycetes, except for *Absidia* spp. (Otcenasek, 1992).

Animal models of invasive aspergillosis confirmed the excellent *in vitro* activity of saperconazole. In a guinea pig model, oral doses of saperconazole of 2.5 mg per kg and greater were associated with almost 100% survival and eradication of *Aspergillus* from tissues. The activity of saperconazole was superior to that of amphotericin B (Van Cutsem *et al.*, 1989). In the immunosuppressed rabbit model of invasive aspergillosis, Patterson *et al.* (1992) established the dose response effect of orally administered saperconazole, and doses of 10 and 15 mg per kg significantly reduced the fungal tissue burden, as did the i.v. treatment which eradicated *Aspergillus* from tissues.

4 Synergism with other drugs

The combination of saperconazole and flucytosine was found to be synergistic against *C. albicans* and *C. tropicalis*, while the combination produced either a synergistic or additive interaction against *C. parapsilosis* and *C. glabrata* (Fu *et al.*, 1992a).

Serum Levels in Relation to Dose

Solubilization of saperconazole in hydroxypropyl-beta-cyclodextrin (HPCD) produced significantly higher plasma concentrations after oral dosing in mice compared with oral administration of saperconazole solubilized in polyethylene glycol (PEG). The peak serum concentration of saperconazole when administered in PEG in doses from 25 mg per kg to 200 mg per kg were <2 µg per ml, compared with peak serum concentrations of 3 µg per ml with 25 mg per kg, 10 µg per ml with 50 mg per kg and 18–19 µg per ml with 100 and 200 mg per kg doses delivered in HPCD (Hostetler *et al.*, 1992).

O'Day *et al.* (1992) studied the ocular pharmacokinetics of saperconazole administered either topically or orally in rabbits. Oral administration produced subtherapeutic concentrations in ocular tissues; however, following topical administration of either 0.25% saperconazole, corneal levels ranged from 2.32 -13.1 µg per g in normal and debrided corneas. Subconjunctival injection of saperconazole produced corneal concentrations that were twice those achieved by sustained topical administration.

Mode of Action

The mode of action of saperconazole is similar to that of the other azole drugs. It inhibits ergosterol biosynthesis by binding to the heme iron of cytochrome P-450 and preventing its activation. Inhibition of 14 alpha-demethylation of lanosterol, which is dependent on P-450 activation, results in accumulation of ^{14}C-methylated sterols in the fungal cell membrane and ergosterol depletion (Vanden Bossche *et al.*, 1990) (see Fig. IV.1, p. 1261). This alters the membrane properties and enzyme functions resulting in disturbed fungal metabolism and cell growth. The consequent ultrastructural changes are similar to those produced by the other azoles, and include thickened cell membranes with deposition of dense vesicles, and inhibition of hyphal outgrowth in *C. albicans* (Jansen *et al.*, 1991).

Toxicity

In doses of 100–200 mg once-daily for treatment durations of up to 6 months, no clinical or laboratory adverse effects were noted in an open study in 30 patients (Franco *et al.*, 1992).

Clinical Uses of the Drug

1 Sporotrichosis

Thirteen patients with sporotrichosis received oral saperconazole 100 mg once-daily for a mean period of 3.5 months (2–6 months). Clinical symptoms of ulcers, nodules and suppuration resolved in 2 months and infiltrations took up to 6 months to resolve. Cultures were negative at 2 months in 92% of patients (Franco *et al.*, 1992).

2 Paracoccidioidomycosis

Seven patients with paracoccidioidomycosis received oral saperconazole 100 mg once-daily and two patients with the juvenile form received 200 mg once-daily, for 3–6 months. Clinical improvement with resolution of fever and weakness was rapid, and mucosal ulcers resolved in 1–2 months. Pulmonary lesions on chest X-ray resolved in 3–6 months. Cultures became negative at 1–2 months treatment in all patients (Franco *et al.*, 1992).

3 Chromoblastomycosis

Saperconazole was used in doses of 200 mg once-daily in eight patients with chromoblastomycosis due to *Fonsecaea pedrosoi* for 5–12 months. Clinical and mycological improvement was slower, requiring 5–6 months treatment for improvement in clinical symptoms and mycological eradication (Franco *et al.*, 1992). The ulcerative, desquamating and exudative lesions resolved in 3–6 months, and nodular and verrucous lesions required 6–9 months treatment (Restrepo,1994).

4 Vaginal candidiasis

Saperconazole administered as a single oral dose of 200 mg, 100 mg twice-daily for 1 day, and 200 mg once-daily for 2 days produced clinical cure rates of 75%, and mycological eradication rates of 71%, 85%, and 92% 1 week after treatment (De Beule *et al.*, 1991).

References

De Beule K, Dhondt A, Van Cutsem J, Cauwenbergh G (1991). Phase II trial; an evaluation of oral saperconazole in acute vaginal candidiasis: a comparison of three dosage schedules. *Eur J Obstet Gynecol Reprod Biol* **41**: 231.

Denning DW, Hanson LH, Perlman AM, Stevens DA (1991). *In vitro* susceptibility and synergy studies of *Aspergillus* species to conventional and new agents. *Diagn Microbiol Infect Dis* **15**: 21.

Franco L, Gomez I, Restrepo A (1992). Saperconazole in the treatment of systemic and subcutaneous mycoses. *Int J Dermatol* **31**: 725.

Fu KP, Isaacson D, Foleno B, LoCoco J (1992a). Saperconazole: *In vitro* and *in vivo* anticandidal activity. *Chemotherapy* **38**: 174.

Fu KP, Isaacson DM, Lococo *et al.* (1992b). *In vitro* and *in vivo* antidermatophytic activity of saperconazole, a new fluorinated triazole. *Drugs Exp Clin Res* **18**: 443.

Graybill JR, Sharkey-Mathis PK (1992). New antifungal agents. *Curr Opin Infect Dis* **5**: 773.

Jansen T, Borgers M, Van de Ven M-A *et al.* (1991). The effects of saperconazole on the morphology of *Candida albicans*, *Pityrosporum ovale* and *Trichophyton rubrum in vitro*. *J Med Vet Mycol* **29**: 293.

Hostetler JS, Hanson LH, Stevens DA (1992). Effect of cyclodextrin on the pharmacology of antifungal oral azoles. *Antimicrob Ag Chemother* **36**: 477.

O'Day DM, Head S, Robinson RD *et al.* (1992). Ocular pharmacokinetics

of saperconazole in rabbits. *Arch Ophthalmol* **110**: 550.

Odds FC (1989). Antifungal activity of saperconazole (R 66 905) *in vitro*. *J Antimicrob Chemother* **24**: 533.

Otcenasek M (1992). Susceptibility of clinical isolates of fungi to saperconazole. *Mycopathologia* **118**: 179.

Patterson TF, George D, Miniter P, Andriole VT (1992). Saperconazole therapy in a rabbit model of invasive aspergillosis. *Antimicrob Ag Chemother* **36**: 2681.

Restrepo A (1994). Treatment of tropical mycoses. *J Amer Acad Dermatol* **31**: S91.

San Blas G, Calcagno AM, San Blas F (1993). A preliminary study of *in vitro* antibiotic activity of saperconazole and other azoles on *Paracoccidioides brasiliensis*. *J Med Vet Mycol* **31**: 169.

Sugar AM, Salibian M, Goldani LZ (1994). Saperconazole therapy of murine disseminated candidiasis: efficacy and interactions with amphotericin B. *Antimicrob Ag Chemother* **38**: 371.

Van Cutsem J, Ven Gerven F, Janssen AJ (1989). Oral and parenteral therapy with saperconazole (R 66905) of invasive aspergillosis in normal and immunocompromised animals. *Antimicrob Ag Chemother* **33**: 1063.

Vanden Bossche H, Marichal P, Willemsens G *et al.* (1990). Saperconazole: a selective inhibitor of the cytochrome P-450 dependent ergosterol synthesis in *Candida albicans*, *Aspergillus fumigatus* and *Trichophyton mentagrophytes*. *Mycoses* **33**: 335.

Genaconazole

Description

Genaconazole (SCH 39304) is a racemic difluorophenyl triazole antifungal agent, structurally related to fluconazole, which has poor aqueous solubility. Genaconazole is a racemate comprising 50% *RR* (active) and 50% *SS* (inactive) enantiomers (Lin *et al.*, 1996). Like fluconazole, it is a fungistatic agent. It is currently withdrawn from drug development.

Sensitive Organisms

Candida spp. are susceptible to genaconazole, with an MIC range of 0.25–>32 μg per ml. *Candida albicans* was variably susceptible to a similar extent as other azole drugs, and *C. glabrata* was least susceptible with MICs of ≥32 μg per ml (McIntyre and Galgiani, 1989; Fu *et al.*, 1992). The *in vivo* efficacy in treatment and prevention of systemic candidiasis has been established in animal models (Perfect *et al.*, 1989; Walsh *et al.*, 1990; Cacciapuoti *et al.*, 1992). *Trichosporon beigelii* is susceptible to genaconazole with an MIC of 4 μg per ml, and *in vivo* activity has been demonstrated in a murine model (Anaissie *et al.*, 1992). The *in vitro* susceptibility of *Histoplasma capsulatum* varies from an MIC of 2.95 to >1000 μg per ml; however, the *in vivo* efficacy of orally administered genaconazole in the murine model of disseminated histoplasmosis was significantly superior to fluconazole and equivalent to amphotericin B for both normal and leukopenic mice (Kobayashi *et al.*, 1990). Genaconazole also demonstrated superior *in vivo* activity in the murine model of coccidioidal meningitis and paracoccidioidomycosis (Clemons *et al.*, 1990; Defaveri *et al.*, 1990; Restrepo *et al.*, 1992), and has good *in vivo* activity in the murine and rabbit models of cryptococcosis and murine pulmonary blastomycosis (Restrepo *et al.*, 1989; Perfect *et al.*, 1989; Sugar *et al.*, 1990; Brummer *et al.*, 1991). *Aspergillus* spp. are resistant to genaconazole *in vitro* with MICs >12.5 μg per ml. However, the *in vivo* activity of genaconazole in an animal model of bronchopulmonary aspergillosis was superior to itraconazole (Schmitt *et al.*, 1992).

Serum Levels in Relation to Dose

The pharmacokinetics of genaconazole in healthy volunteers appear to be independent of the route of administration. A 100-mg genaconazole 30-min i.v. infusion produced identical parameters as the oral administration of 100 mg. The area-under-the-concentration-time-curve (AUC) was 136 μg.h per ml, and the half-life was long at 50 h. The absolute bioavailability was 100% (Mojaverian *et al.*, 1994). Following a single oral genaconazole dose of 200 mg, containing 100 mg of the *RR* enantiomer and 100 mg of the *SS* enantiomer, the mean serum concentration time curves and pharmacokinetics parameters for the two enantiomers were found to be identical. The mean peak serum concentration after a 100-mg dose was 1.7 μg per ml and after a 200 mg dose was 3.8 μg per ml, and dose proportionality was observed. The pharmacokinetics following administration of 100 mg of the *RR* enantiomer were identical to those obtained after administration of 200 mg genaconazole (which contains 100 mg of the *RR* enantiomer). The half-life after 200 mg dosing was 73–83 h, and allowed twice-weekly dosing (Lin *et al.*, 1996).

There was no evidence of metabolism of genaconazole (similar to the negligible biotransformation of fluconazole) and unchanged drug accounted for 64% of drug excreted in a radiolabeled drug study. After administration of ^{14}C-genaconazole, 67% of the dose was excreted in urine and 9% was excreted in feces (Lin *et al.*, 1996).

Distribution of the Drug in Body

Effective penetration of genaconazole into the central nervous system has been documented in a number of animal models (Perfect *et al.*, 1989; Restrepo *et al.*, 1989; Lee *et al.*, 1989). The steady-state serum and cerebrospinal fluid genaconazole concentrations after 200-mg doses were 18.3 and 15.4 µg per ml, after 300-mg doses were 37.5 and 27.5 µg per ml, and after 600 mg per week doses were 3.47 and 2.8 µg per ml respectively, in a study in cryptococcal meningitis patients. The mean CSF concentration of genaconazole was 79% of the plasma concentration (Lee *et al.*, 1992).

Toxicity

Skin rash, minor nausea, and asymptomatic hepatotoxicity has been reported (Lee *et al.*, 1992).

Clinical Uses of the Drug

1 Cryptococcal meningitis

Genaconazole has been used as primary therapy and salvage therapy in patients who have failed treatment, as well as maintenance treatment of cryptococcal meningitis in AIDS patients. The regimen used for primary therapy was i.v. amphotericin B for 2 weeks, followed by genaconazole 200 mg once-daily for 12 weeks. Genaconazole was effective and sterilized the CSF in two of three patients with mild cryptococcal meningitis. However, genaconazole was not useful as salvage treatment and it was no more effective than other antifungal agents in this setting. The maintenance regimen of genaconazole 600 mg once-weekly successfully prevented relapse of cryptococcal meningitis in four of four patients for a mean of 20 weeks (Lee *et al.*, 1992).

2 Coccidioidomycosis

Genaconazole in doses of 100 and 200 mg orally daily were administered to 54 patients with progressive coccidioidomycosis, of which 35% had failed alternative therapy. The 12-month response rate was 77% for pulmonary disease, 62% for skin and soft tissue disease, and 31% for bone and joint disease. The failure rate was 28% (Hostetler *et al.*, 1994).

3 Trichosporonosis

A patient with leukemia who became neutropenic after chemotherapy developed disseminated aspergillosis and *T. beigelii* fungemia. He was treated with genaconazole 200 mg daily for 5 weeks until his death. At autopsy, there was no evidence of trichosporonosis, but disseminated aspergillosis was evident (Anaisie *et al.*, 1992).

References

Anaissie E, Gokaslan A, Hachem R *et al.* (1992). Azole therapy for trichosporonosis: Clinical evaluation of eight patients, experimental therapy for murine infection, and review. *Clin Infect Dis* **15**: 781.

Brummer E, Hanson LH, Stevens DA (1991). SCH 39304 in the treatment of acute or established murine pulmonary blastomycosis. *Antimicrob Ag Chemother* **35**: 788.

Cacciapuoti A, Loebenberg D, Parmegiani R *et al.* (1992). Comparison of SCH 39304, fluconazole, and ketoconazole for treatment of systemic infections in mice. *Antimicrob Ag Chemother* **36**: 64.

Clemons KV, Hanson LH, Perlman AM, Stevens DA (1990). Activity of SCH 39304 and fluconazole in a murine model of disseminated coccidioidomycosis. *Antimicrob Ag Chemother* **34**: 928.

Defaveri J, Sun SH, Graybill JR (1990). Treatment of murine coccidioidal meningitis with SCH 39304. *Antimicrob Ag Chemother* **34**: 663.

Fu KP, Isaacson D, Foleno B, LoCoco J (1992). Saperconazole: *In vitro* and *in vivo* anticandidal activity. *Chemotherapy* **38**: 174.

Hostetler JS, Catanzaro A, Stevens DA *et al.* (1994). Treatment of coccidioidomycosis with SCH 39304. *J Med Vet Mycol* **32**: 105.

Kobayashi GS, Travis SJ, Rinaldi MG, Medoff G (1990). *In vitro* and *in vivo* activities of SCH 39304, fluconazole and amphotericin B against *Histoplasma capsulatum*. *Antimicrob Ag Chemother* **34**: 524.

Lee JA, Lin C, Loebenberg D, Rubin M, Pizzo PA, Walsh TJ (1989). Pharmacokinetics and tissue penetration of SCH 39304 in granulocytopenic and nongranulocytopenic rabbits. *Antimicrob Ag Chemother* **33**: 1932.

Lee BL, Padula AM, Tauber MG, Chambers HF, Sande MA (1992). Oral SCH 39304 as primary, salvage, and maintenance therapy for cryptococcal meningitis in AIDS. *J AIDS* **5**: 600.

Lin C, Kim H, Radwanski E, Affrime M, Brannan M, Cayen MN (1996). Pharmacokinetics and metabolism of genaconazole, a potent antifungal drug, in men. *Antimicrob Ag Chemother* **40**: 92.

McIntyre KA, Galgiani JN (1989). *In vitro* susceptibilities of yeasts to a new antifungal triazole, SCH 39304: Effects of test conditions and relation to *in vivo* efficacy. *Antimicrob Ag Chemother* **3**: 1095.

Mojaverian P, Radwanski E, Affrime MB *et al.* (1994). Pharmacokinetics of the triazole antifungal agent genaconazole in healthy men after oral and intravenous administration. *Antimicrob Ag Chemother* **38**: 2758.

Perfect JR, Wright KA, Hobbs MM, Durack DT (1989). Treatment of experimental cryptococcal meningitis and disseminated candidiasis with SCH 39304. *Antimicrob Ag Chemother* **33**: 1735.

Restrepo B, Ahrens J, Graybill JR (1989). Efficacy of SCH39304 in murine cryptococcosis. *Antimicrob Ag Chemother* **33**: 1242.

Restrepo S, Tabares AM, Restrepo A (1992). Activity of two different triazoles in a murine model of paracoccidioidomycosis. *Rev Inst Med Trop Sao Paulo* **34**: 171.

Schmitt HJ, Edwards F, Andrade J *et al.* (1992). Comparison of azoles against aspergilli *in vitro* and in an experimental model of pulmonary aspergillosis. *Chemother* **38**: 118.

Sugar AM, Picard M, Noble L (1990). Treatment of murine pulmonary blastomycosis with SCH 39304, a new triazole antifungal agent. *Antimicrob Ag Chemother* **34**: 896.

Walsh TJ, Lee JW, Lecciones J *et al.* (1990). SCH 39304 in prevention and treatment of disseminated candidiasis in persistently granulocytopenic rabbits. *Antimicrob Ag Chemother* **34**: 1560.

Cilofungin

Description

Cilofungin (LY 121019) is a semibiosynthetic lipopeptide antifungal analog of echinocandin B, with the chemical name *N*-ρ-octyloxybenzoylechinocandin B nucleus. It has a narrow spectrum of activity *in vitro* against yeast, in particular, *Candida* albicans, and is fungicidal against clinically relevant *Candida* species. It has currently been withdrawn from human clinical trials in its current formulation because of a possible association with acute renal failure and anion gap acidosis (Smith *et al.*, 1991).

Sensitive Organisms

Cilofungin possesses potent *in vitro* activity against *Candida* spp. It has equivalent activity to amphotericin B against *Candida albicans,* superior activity against *C. tropicalis,* and was less active than amphotericin B against *C. glabrata, C. parapsilosis* and other species of *Candida* (Odds, 1988; Meunier *et al.*, 1989; Pfaller *et al.*, 1989a). The MICs for clinical specimens of *Candida* spp. ranged from 0.125 to 16 µg per ml, but there was marked variation with susceptibility test media and inoculum size used (Hall *et al.*, 1988; Villareal *et al.*, 1994). *Candida parapsilosis* is relatively resistant to cilofungin with MIC of 10–>40 µg per ml, while other *Candida* spp. were inhibited by <5 µg per ml (Smith *et al.*, 1991). Results from *in vivo* studies have been varied, but may relate to the pharmacokinetics of cilofungin in the different animal species. In the rabbit endocarditis model, cilofungin did not reduce the fungal load in cardiac vegetations (Padula and Chambers, 1989; Perfect *et al.*, 1989), but when cilofungin was administered by continuous i.v. infusion its efficacy was similar to amphotericin B in rabbits. In this model a direct correlation between tissue concentration of cilofungin and antifungal activity was established (Walsh *et al.*, 1991; Rouse *et al.*, 1992). In the murine model of systemic candidiasis cilofungin had inferior activity to amphotericin B in sterilizing the kidneys and preventing death (Smith *et al.*, 1990; Morrison and Stevens, 1990), but in another study of disseminated candidiasis in both normal and neutropenic mice, cilofungin was superior to amphotericin B. Cilofungin was able to eliminate fungus from the kidneys, spleen and liver, but not from the brain (Khardori *et al.*, 1993). *In vivo* synergy or additive effects were demonstrated for cilofungin and amphotericin B in the murine model of disseminated candidiasis (Sugar *et al.*, 1991; Hanson *et al.*, 1991).

Cilofungin is not active against *Cryptococcus neoformans, Paracoccidioides brasiliensis, Blastomyces dermatitidis,* and *Aspergillus* spp. *in vitro* (Hanson and Stevens, 1989; Meunier *et al.*, 1989). However, Denning and Stevens (1991) demonstrated that cilofungin was at least as effective as amphotericin B in the murine model of disseminated aspergillosis. *Aspergillus fumigatus* cell wall contains (1,3)-beta-D-glucan synthase which has been shown to be more susceptible to cilofungin than the same enzyme in *C. albicans* (Beaulieu *et al.*, 1994).

Combinations of cilofungin with amphotericin B, flucytosine, ketoconazole or itrconazole were either additive or indifferent against most *Candida* spp. No antagonism was identified with combinations of amphotericin B or itraconazole with cilofungin (Smith *et al.*, 1991).

Mode of Action

Cilofungin is a specific, non-competitive inhibitor of (1,3)-beta-D-glucan synthase, the membrane-bound enzyme that catalyzes the synthesis of beta(1 → 3) glucan, a major cell wall component of *Candida* spp. This results in a 55–60% reduction in ergosterol and a 4–13% reduction in lanosterol. It does not have an effect on chitin synthetase. Inhibition of glucan synthesis results in inhibition of fungal cell growth, cell lysis and cell death (Taft *et al.*, 1988; Pfaller *et al.*, 1989b; Tang and Parr, 1991; Angiolella *et al.*, 1994).

Toxicity

Cilofungin has currently been withdrawn from drug development because of a possible association of acute renal failure and anion gap acidosis.

Clinical Uses of the Drug

Cilofungin was used in 14 patients with esophageal candidiasis or candidemia, prior to its withdrawal due to toxicity concerns. Of the 14 patients, 71% improved, and included six patients with esophagitis and four with fungemia. There was a suggestion of poorer outcome for those patients with isolates that had higher MICs (Villereal *et al.*, 1994).

References

Angiolella L, Simonetti N, Cassone A (1994). The lipopeptide antimycotic, cilofungin modulates the incorporation of glucan-associated proteins into the cell wall of *Candida albicans*. *J Antimicrob Chemother* **33**: 1137.

Beaulieu D, Tang J, Yan SB *et al.* (1994). Characterization and cilofungin inhibition of solubilized *Aspergillus fumigatus* (1,3)-β-D-glucan synthase. *Antimicrob Ag Chemother* **38**: 937.

Denning DW, Stevens DA (1991). Efficacy of cilofungin alone and in combination with amphotericin B in a murine model of disseminated aspergillosis. *Antimicrob Ag Chemother* **35**: 1329.

Hall GS, Myles C, Pratt KJ, Washington JA (1988). Cilofungin (LY121019), an antifungal agent with specific activity against *Candida albicans* and *Candida tropicalis*. *Antimicrob Ag Chemother* **32**: 1331.

Hanson LH, Stevens DA (1989). Evaluation of cilofungin, a lipopeptide antifungal agent, *in vitro* against fungi isolated from clinical specimens. *Antimicrob Ag Chemother* **33**: 1391.

Hanson LH, Perlman AM, Clemons KV, Stevens DA (1991). Synergy between cilofungin and amphotericin B in a murine model of candidiasis. *Antimicrob Ag Chemother* **35**: 1334.

Khardori N, Nguyen H, Stephens C *et al.* (1993). Comparative efficacies of cilofungin (LY121019) and amphotericin B against disseminated *Candida albicans* infection in normal and granulocytopenic mice. *Antimicrob Ag Chemother* **37**: 729.

Meunier F, Lambert C, Van der Anwera P (1989). *In-vitro* activity of cilofungin (LY121019) in comparison with amphotericin B. *J Antimicrob Chemother* **24**: 325.

Morrison CJ, Stevens DA (1990). Comparative effects of cilofungin and amphotericin B on experimental murine candidiasis. *Antimicrob Ag Chemother* **34**: 746.

Odds, FC (1988). Activity of cilofungin (LY121019) against *Candida* species *in vitro*. *J Antimicrob Chemother* **22**: 891.

Padula A, Chambers HF (1989). Evaluation of cilofungin (LY121019) for treatment of experimental *Candida albicans* endocarditis in rabbits. *Antimicrob Ag Chemother* **33**: 1822.

Perfect JR, Hobbs MM, Wright KA, Durack DT (1989). Treatment of experimental disseminated candidiasis with cilofungin. *Antimicrob Ag Chemother* **33**: 1811.

Pfaller MA, Wey S, Gerarden T *et al.* (1989a). Susceptibility of nosocomial isolates of *Candida* species to LY121019 and other antifungal agents. *Diagn Microbiol Infect Dis* **12**: 1.

Pfaller M Riley J, Koerner T (1989b). Effects of cilofungin (LY 121019) on carbohydrate and sterol composition of *Candida albicans*. *Eur J Clin Microbiol Infect Dis* **8**: 1067.

Rouse MS, Tallan BM, Steckelberg JM *et al.* (1992). Efficacy of cilofungin therapy administered by continuous intravenous infusion for experimental disseminated candidiasis in rabbits. *Antimicrob Ag Chemother* **36**: 56.

Smith KR, Lank KM, Cobbs CG *et al.* (1990). Comparison of cilofungin and amphotericin B for therapy of murine candidiasis. *Antimicrob Ag Chemother* **34**: 1619.

Smith KR, Lank KM, Dismukes WE, Cobbs CG (1991). *In vitro* comparison of cilofungin alone and in combination with other antifungal agents against clinical isolates of *Candida* species. *Eur J Clin Microbiol Infect Dis* **10**: 588.

Sugar AM, Goldiani LZ, Picard M (1991). Treatment of murine invasive candidiasis with amphotericin B and cilofungin: Evidence for enhanced activity with combination therapy. *Antimicrob Ag Chemother* **35**: 2128.

Taft CS, Stark T, Selitrennikoff CP (1988). Cilofungin (LY121019) inhibits *Candida albicans* (1–3)-β-D-glucan synthase activity. *Antimicrob Ag Chemother* **32**: 1901.

Tang J, Parr TR (1991). W-1 solubilization and kinetics of inhibition by cilofungin of *Candida albicans* (1–3)-β-D-glucan synthase. *Antimicrob Ag Chemother* **35**: 99.

Villereal KM, Cook RA, Galgiani JN *et al.* (1994). Comparative analysis of three antifungal susceptibility test methods against prospectively collected *Candida* species. *Diagn Microbiol Infect Dis* **18**: 89.

Walsh TJ, Lee JW, Kelly P *et al.* (1991). Antifungal effects of the nonlinear pharmacokinetics of cilofungin, a 1,3-β-glucan synthetase inhibitor, during continuous and intermittent intravenous infusions in treatment of experimental disseminated candidiasis. *Antimicrob Ag Chemother* **35**: 1321.

Vibunazole

Description

Vibunazole (BAY-n-7133) is a triazole derivative, with the chemical name of (1-(4-chlorophenoxy)-3_S3^1-dimethyl-2(1,2,4-triazol-1-yl)methyl-2-butanol which has been under development for 10 years. There is no information concerning clinical trial data available.

Sensitive Organisms

Vibunazole has activity against *Candida* spp., and the dermatophytes, but poor *in vitro* activity against *Aspergillus* spp., Zygomycetes, *Scopulariopsis* spp., and *Sporothrix schenckii* (Fromtling *et al.*, 1983, 1984; Yamaguchi *et al.*, 1983). The inhibitory activity of vibunazole against *Candida* spp. was inferior to that of itraconazole (Odds *et al.*, 1984). It has demonstrable activity against *Fusarium* spp., but the dematiaceous fungi, including *Fonsecaea pedrosoi* and *Phialophora verrucosa* are relatively resistant (Fromtling *et al.*, 1983; Okeke and Gugnani, 1987). It was the least active of seven azole compounds against the dermatophytes and other filamentous fungi that cause skin and nail disease, with MICs of 0.39–1.56 μg per ml for the dermatophytes, and 1.56–6.25 μg per ml for the filamentous fungi (Oyeka and Gugnani, 1990).

The *in vivo* animal data on the efficacy of vibunazole in experimental systemic and topical infections in various animal species is quite varied. Vibunazole was an effective agent in the animal model of aspergillosis and its activity was comparable with itraconazole and amphotericin B (Graybill *et al.*, 1983a). Contrasting results have been found for the treatment of coccidioidomycosis in mice (Hoeprich and Merry, 1985; Levine, 1984), and candidiasis (Plempel, 1984; Lefler and Stevens, 1985). In the animal models of blastomycosis (Lefler *et al.*, 1985a), cryptococcosis (Graybill *et al.*, 1983b), paracoccidioidomycosis (Lefler *et al.*, 1985b), vibunazole had inferior activity to ketoconazole.

Serum Levels in Relation to Dose

The mean peak plasma concentration of vibunazole after oral administration of a single 400-mg dose to healthy volunteers was 2.76 μg per ml, and this was not affected by co-administration with acid or cimetidine. The half-life was 2.3 h (van Gulpen *et al.*, 1985).

In animal pharmacokinetic studies, vibunazole was found to be absorbed well after oral dosing, with an oral bioavailability of 70%. The plasma half-life of the drug began to decrease after the fifth dose, suggestive of metabolic enzyme induction by vibunazole (Ritter and Plempel, 1984). This phenomenon may explain the divergent *in vivo* efficacy results in the animal models. In addition vibunazole poorly penetrates the blood–brain barrier in rabbits (Perfect and Durack, 1985).

Mode of Action

Vibunazole is a fungistatic agent which inhibits sterol biosynthesis, by inhibition of cytochrome P-450 dependent C-14 alpha demethylation of lanosterol, preventing conversion to ergosterol.

Clinical Uses of the Drug

Phase II and III clinical trials have been performed, but there is no information on safety and efficacy of this drug in humans published in the literature to date.

Voriconazole

Description

Voriconazole (UK-109,496) is a synthetic triazole derivative, that is structurally related to fluconazole. It has a broader spectrum of antifungal activity and is more potent than fluconazole against some fungal species. It is being developed in both an oral formulation and an i.v. preparation.

Sensitive Organisms

Voriconazole has potent activity against pathogenic yeasts, and its activity was superior to that of fluconazole. The susceptibility of voriconazole against *Candida albicans* (MIC $\leq$0.06–16 μg per ml), *C. krusei* (MIC $\leq$0.06–2 μg per ml), *C. parapsilosis* (MIC $\leq$0.06–0.25 μg per ml), and *C. tropicalis* (MIC $\leq$0.06–1 μg per ml) is at least 10-fold greater than fluconazole (Barry and Brown, 1996). Voriconazole has shown good *in vitro* inhibitory and fungicidal activity against *Aspergillus* spp. (MIC 0.19–0.58 μg per ml), and equivalent activity to amphotericin B in the rabbit model of invasive aspergillosis. Fungicidal activity against *Aspergillus* spp. is achieved at a concentration that is twice the MIC. The efficacy of voriconazole in reducing fungal burden in tissues was dose-dependent (Denning *et al.*, 1995a; McGinnis *et al.*, 1995; George *et al.*, 1996).

Mode of Administration and Dose

The oral formulation for phase III studies is a tablet in 50-mg and 200-mg sizes, and the i.v. preparation consists of voriconazole 10 mg per ml complexed with sulphobutyl ether-beta-cyclodextrin for infusion.

Mode of Action

Like the other azole drugs, the primary mode of action of voriconazole is inhibition of fungal cytochrome P-450 dependent C14-alpha sterol demethylase, thereby inhibiting ergosterol biosynthesis. Voriconazole is a potent inhibitor of this enzyme in both *C. albicans* and *Aspergillus fumigatus*.

Toxicity

From the open non-comparative studies, 15% of patients reported visual disturbances (increased brightness, or blurred vision) that are transient and reversible, and are associated with both the oral and i.v. route of administration. Investigations to date have not identified a cause for this phenomenon.

Elevated liver function tests occurred in about 10% of patients and are usually indicative of potential hepatic cholestasis. Skin rash has been associated with treatment with voriconazole in about 3% of patients.

Clinical Uses of the Drug

Voriconazole in doses of 200 mg twice-daily orally or i.v. voriconazole 3 mg per kg 12-hourly for up to 4 weeks followed by oral voriconazole for up to 6 months, have been evaluated in phase II, open non-comparative studies as treatment for acute aspergillosis in immunocompromised patients, and chronic aspergillosis in non-neutropenic patients.

D0870

Description

D0870 is the mycologically active enantiomer of ICI 195,739 and has the chemical name (*R*)-2-(2,4-difluorophenyl)-1-(3-[(*E*)-4-(2,2,3,3-tetra-fluoropropoxy)-styryl]-1H-1,2,4,-triazol-1-yl)-3-(1H-1,2,4-triazol-1-yl)propan-2-ol.

Sensitive Organisms

D0870 has good to excellent *in vitro* and *in vivo* activity against *Candida* spp. (MICs for *C. albicans* of 0.0037–0.06 μg per ml, *C. lusitaniae*, *C. parapsilosis*, and *C. tropicalis* of 0.015–2 μg per ml, and for *C. glabrata* and *C. krusei* of 0.125–4 μg per ml), *Cryptococcus neoformans* (MIC 0.037–0.125 µg per ml), *Histoplasma capsulatum, Blastomyces dermatitidis* and *Coccidioides immitis* (Clemons *et al.*, 1993; Peng and Galgiani, 1993; Yamada *et al.*, 1993). D0870 has inhibitory activity against *Aspergillus* spp.; however, this activity was inferior to both amphotericin B and itraconazole (Moore *et al.*, 1993; Yamada *et al.*, 1993), and in the murine model of invasive aspergillosis D0870 was inferior to amphotericin B in the non-immunocompromised model. In the neutropenic pulmonary model, D0870 administered in higher doses with serum levels of greater than 4 µg per ml, the drug was shown to have useful activity and was superior to amphotericin B and itraconazole in preventing death (Denning *et al.*, 1995b). D0870 also possesses inhibitory activity against dermatophytes and other filamentous fungi (Yamada *et al.*, 1993).

Mode of Action

Like the other triazoles, ICI 195,739 (and therefore D0870) inhibit ergosterol biosynthesis by inhibiting the activity of the cytochrome P-450 dependent C14 alpha demethylase (Fromtling, 1988).

Clinical Uses of the Drug

D0870 has been administered with good effect for the treatment of oropharyngeal candidiasis, including fluconazole-resistant disease (Cartledge *et al.*, 1994; De Wit *et al.*, 1994). No other clinical trial data are available currently.

References

Barry AL, Brown SD (1996). *In vitro* studies of two triazole antifungal agents (voriconazole (UK-109,496) and fluconazole against *Candida* species. *Antimicrob Ag Chemother* **40**: 1948.

Cartledge JD, Denning D, Dupont B *et al.* (1994). Treatment of fluconazole resistant oral candidosis with D0870 in patients with AIDS. In *Program and Abstracts of the 34th Interscience Conference on Antimicrobial Agents and Chemotherapy, Orlando* (Abstr. M89), p. 248. Washington, DC: American Society for Microbiology.

Clemons KV, Hanson LH, Stevens DA (1993). Activities of the triazole D0870 *in vitro* and against murine blastomycosis. *Antimicrob Ag Chemother* **37**: 1177.

Denning D, del Favero A, Gluckman E *et al.* (1995a). UK-109,496, a novel, wide-spectrum triazole derivative for the treatment of fungal infections: clinical efficacy in acute invasive aspergillosis In *Program and Abstracts of the 35th Interscience Conference on Antimicobial Agents and Chemotherapy, San Francisco* (Abstr. F80), p. 126. Washington, DC: American Society for Microbiology.

Denning DW, Hall L, Jackson M, Hollis S (1995b). Efficacy of D0870 compared with those of itraconazole and amphotericin B in two murine models of invasive aspergillosis. *Antimicrob Ag Chemother* **39**: 1809.

De Wit S, Dupont B, Cartledge JD *et al.* (1994). Pilot study of a new triazole derivative (D0870) in HIV patients with oral candidiasis. In *Program and Abstracts of the 34th Interscience Conference on Antimicrobial Agents and Chemotherapy, Orlando* (Abstr, MI225), p. 213. Washington, DC: American Society for Microbiology.

Fromtling RA (1988). Overview of medically important antifungal azole derivatives. *Clin Microbiol Rev* **1**: 187.

Fromtling RA, Yu H-P, Shadomy S (1983). *In vitro* inhibitory activities of 2 new orally absorbable imidazole derivatives: Bay n 7133 and Bay l 9139. *Sabouraudia* **21**: 179.

Fromtling RA, Yu H-P, Shadomy S (1984). *In vitro* antifungal activities of Bay N 7133 and Bay L 9139, two new orally absorbable antifungal imidazole derivatives, against pathogenic yeasts. *Mycopathologia* **86**: 45.

George D, Miniter P, Andriole VT (1996). Efficacy of UK-109496, a new azole antifungal agent, in an experimental model of invasive aspergillosis. *Antimicrob Ag Chemother* **40**: 86.

Graybill JR, Kaster SR, Drutz DJ (1983a). Treatment of experimental murine aspergillosis with Bay n7133. *J Infect Dis* **148**: 898.

Graybill JR, Kaster SR, Drutz DJ (1983b). Comparative activities of Bay n7133, ICI 153,066, and ketoconazole in murine cryptococcosis. *Antimicrob Ag Chemother* **24**: 829.

Hoeprich PD, Merry JM (1985). Activity of BAY n 7133 and BAY l 9139 *in vitro* and in experimental murine coccidioidomycosis. *Eur J Clin Microbiol* **4**: 400.

Lefler E, Stevens DA (1985). New azole compounds: vibunazole (Bay n7133). and Bay l9139, compared with ketoconazole in the therapy of systemic candidosis and in pharmacokinetic studies in mice. *J Antimicrob Chemother* **15**: 69.

Lefler E, Brummer E, Perlman AM, Stevens DA (1985a). Activities of the modified polyene *N*-D-ornithyl amphotericin methyl ester and the azoles ICI 153,066, Bay n 7133, and Bay l 9139 compared with those of amphotericin B and ketoconazole in the therapy of blastomycosis. *Antimicrob Ag Chemother* **27**: 363.

Lefler E, Brummer E, McEwen G, Hoyos GL, Restrepo A, Stevens DA (1985b). Study of current and new drugs in a murine model of acute paracoccidioidomycosis. *Amer J Trop Med Hyg* **34**: 134.

Levine HB (1984). A direct comparison of oral treatments with BAY-n-7133, BAY-l-9139 and ketoconazole in experimental murine coccidioidomycosis. *Sabouraudia* **22**: 37.

McGinnis MR, Pasarell L, Cooper CR (1995). *In vitro* susceptibility of clinical mould isolates to UK0109,496, amphotericin B, fluconazole, and itraconazole In *Program and Abstracts of the 35th Interscience Conference on Antimicobial Agents and Chemotherapy, San Francisco* (Abstr. E76), p. 99. Washington, DC: American Society for Microbiology.

Moore CB, Law D, Denning DW (1993). *In-vitro* activity of the new triazole D0870 compared with amphotericin B and itraconazole against *Aspergillus* spp. *J Antimicrob Chemother* **32**: 831.

Odds FC, Webster CE, Abbott AB (1984). Antifungal relative inhibition factors; BAY l–9139, bifonazole, butoconazole, isoconazole, itraconazole (R 51211), oxiconazole, Ro 14–4767/002, sulconazole, terconazole and vibunazole (BAY n-7133) compared with nine established antifungal agents. *J Antimicrob Chemother* **14**: 105.

Okeke CN, Gugnani HC (1987). *In vitro* sensitivity of environmental isolates of pathogenic dermatiaceous fungi to azole compounds and a phenylpropyl-morpholine derivative. *Mycopathologia* **99**: 175.

Oyeka CA, Gugnani HC (1990). *In vitro* activity of seven azole compounds against some clinical isolates of non-dermatophyte filamentous fungi and some dermatophytes. *Mycopathologia* **110**: 157.

Peng T, Galgiani JN (1993). *In vitro* studies of a new antifungal triazole, D0870, against *Candida albicans*, *Cryptococcus neoformans*, and other pathogenic yeasts. *Antimicrob Ag Chemother* **37**: 2126.

Perfect JR, Durack DT (1985). Penetration of imidazoles and triazoles into cerebrospinal fluid in rabbits. *J Antimicrob Chemother* **16**: 81.

Plempel M (1984). Antimycotic activity of BAY N 7133 in animal experiments. *J Antimicrob Chemother* **13**: 447.

Ritter W, Plempel M (1984). Pharmacokinetics of the oral triazole antimycotic vibunazole in animals. *J Antimicrob Chemother* **14**: 243.

Shadomy S, Espinel-Ingroff A, Kerkering TM (1984). *In vitro* studies with four new antifungal agents: BAY n 7133, bifonazole (BAY h 4502), ICI 153,066 and Ro 14–4767/002. *Sabouraudia* **22**: 7.

van Gulpen C, Kelder O, Mattie H *et al.* (1985). Pharmacokinetics of vibunazole (BAY n 7133). administered orally to healthy subjects. *J Antimicrob Chemother* **16**: 75.

Yamada H, Tsuda T, Watanabe T *et al.* (1993). *In vitro* and *in vivo* antifungal activities of D0870, a new triazole agent. *Antimicrob Ag Chemother* **37**: 2412.

Yamaguchi T, Hiratani T, Plempel M (1983). *In vitro* studies of a new oral azole antimycotic, BAY N 7133. *J Antimicrob Chemother* **11**: 135.

Part V

Antiviral Drugs

Aciclovir

Description

Aciclovir is an acyclic nucleoside analogue of guanine used predominantly for the treatment of herpesvirus infections. The discovery of aciclovir demonstrated for the first time the potential of compounds selectively to prevent the replication of DNA within a DNA virus without inhibiting cellular DNA synthesis (Elion, 1993).

Formerly known as acycloguanosine and having the chemical formula of 9-(2-hydroxyethoxymethyl) guanine, aciclovir was marketed under the trade name of 'Zovirax' initially by Burroughs Wellcome and now by GlaxoWellcome. Aciclovir, similar to idoxuridine (p. 1627) and adenine arabinoside (p. 1620), is a deoxynucleoside analog (Fig. V.1). It was selected from a number of analogs in which the cyclic carbohydrate moiety was replaced by an acyclic side-chain. In aciclovir the deoxyribose component of deoxyguanosine has been replaced by a hydroxyethoxymethyl substituent on the purine ring (Elion et al., 1977; Schaeffer et al., 1978). Concentrations of aciclovir are reported in both μg per ml and μM, but these can be approximately converted to μg per ml by dividing μM concentrations by 4 (1 μg per ml = 4.44 μM).

The most important prodrug of aciclovir that has been developed and is now in clinical use is valaciclovir (p. 1552). Ganciclovir (p. 1557) is closely related to aciclovir and differs by having an additional CH_2OH on the side-chain.

Antiviral Activity

Drug sensitivity testing systems for viruses are still poorly standardized. The plaque reduction assay is the most widely accepted method but is laborious to perform and results are often not available in time to alter clinical management. Antiviral assay results are usually reported as the 50% inhibitory dose or concentration (ID_{50} or IC_{50}) which differs from the 90% or 95% inhibitory concentration (IC_{90} or IC_{95}) which is the accepted bacteriological MIC; this is considered to be more clinically relevant (Safrin et al., 1994c) and the difference could be significant in immunocompromised patients (Dekker et al., 1983). Because in vitro sensitivity testing to aciclovir can be influenced by a number of factors, the results of sensitivity tests may vary between different laboratories. Rapid screening tests have been developed for the detection of antiviral susceptibility to aciclovir within 3 days (Safrin et al., 1994a; Tebas et al., 1995), but are not widely validated.

1 Herpesviruses

Aciclovir is active against human herpesviruses in vitro, and against some infections produced in animals by these viruses. Viruses which show the greatest sensitivity to aciclovir are herpes

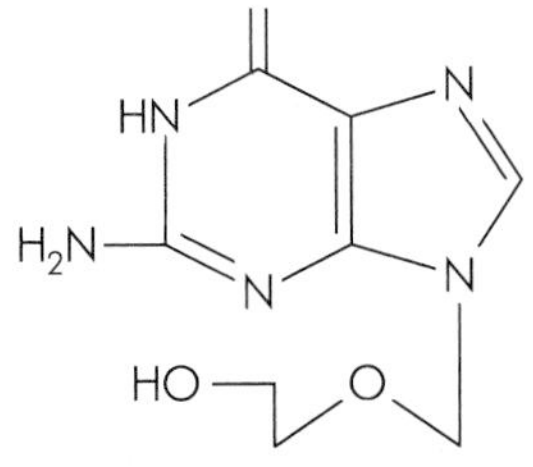

Fig. V.1.
Chemical structure of aciclovir.

simplex types 1 and 2, against which the drug is about equally active (Collins and Bauer, 1979; Crumpacker et al., 1979; McLaren et al., 1982). In one study with herpes simplex type 1, aciclovir was 160-fold more active than adenine arabinoside and 10-fold more active than idoxuridine (Schaeffer et al., 1978). Concentrations of aciclovir necessary to reduce plaques by 50% in tissue culture are in the range of 0.02–0.8 μg per ml for herpes simplex type 1, and 0.03–2.2 μg per ml for herpes simplex type 2 (Schaeffer et al., 1978; Crumpacker et al., 1979; Weinberg et al., 1992; Andrei et al., 1992). Barry and colleagues at Wellcome Research Laboratories (Barry et al., 1985) tested aciclovir-sensitivity of 1417 herpes simplex clinical isolates (two-thirds of which were type 2); the IC_{90} of type 1 isolates was 0.9 μg per ml and IC_{50} was 0.2 μg per ml; the respective values for type 2 isolates were 2.2 and 0.7 μg per ml.

A number of early studies performed in animals provided very useful safety and efficacy data. There have been numerous reports describing the value of aciclovir, given topically or systemically, for the protection against, or the treatment of, various experimental herpes simplex type 1 and 2 infections in animals. Mice are protected by aciclovir against infection following intracerebral inoculation (Schaeffer et al., 1978; Park et al., 1979a; Kern et al., 1982; Collins and Oliver 1982). Prophylactic and therapeutic aciclovir is also useful for cutaneous and genital infections (Klein et al., 1979; Park et al., 1979b, 1980; Kern 1982; Kern et al., 1983), and prevents recurrent infections (Hill et al., 1982). Penciclovir when administered subcutaneously as a single dose to mice infected intraperitoneally with herpes simplex type 1 was active at a 10-fold lower dose than aciclovir (Sutton and Boyd, 1993). When human immune globulin is combined with aciclovir, there is enhanced protection against herpes simplex virus in mice (Cho and Feng, 1980). In rabbits, it is effective topically and systemically for keratitis (Schaeffer et al., 1978; Bauer, 1982; Trousdale and Nesburn, 1982) and it is protective against neonatal infection (Sicher and Oh, 1981). However, chronic oral administration of aciclovir does not prevent recurrence of viral shedding or clinical corneal disease in rabbits with experimental herpes simplex keratitis (Kaufman et al., 1983). In guinea pigs, aciclovir has a prophylactic effect in genital herpes (Alenius et al., 1982; Kern, 1982; Landry et al., 1982) and it protects against neural disease in hamsters (Van Ekdom and Versteeg, 1982). The use of aciclovir may prevent latent herpes simplex infection in animals (Klein et al., 1979; Park et al., 1979b, 1980; Kern et al., 1983) and continuous aciclovir therapy can prevent in vitro reactivation of herpes simplex virus of latently infected murine and human ganglia, but it is not effective in eradicating latent virus (Klein et al., 1979, 1981; Lewis et al., 1983).

Varicella-zoster virus is susceptible to aciclovir with an IC_{50} ranging from 0.36 to 1.1 μg per ml, but less so than herpes simplex virus which in comparative studies had an IC_{50} of 0.01–0.45 μg per ml (Crumpacker et al., 1979; Biron and Elion, 1980; Nusinoff-Lehrman et al., 1993). The selectivity index of aciclovir for varicella-zoster virus clinical isolates is lower than that for sorivudine (BV-araU), but higher than that for cidofovir (HPMPC), ganciclovir and adefovir (PMEA) and equivalent for penciclovir (Andrei et al., 1995; Machida et al., 1995). Vaccine strains of varicella-zoster virus are susceptible to aciclovir (Preblud et al.,1984). Cell-associated varicella-zoster has been shown by plaque reduction assay to be about 8-fold more resistant to the antiviral effects of aciclovir than cell-free virus (Shiraki et al., 1992).

Aciclovir inhibits Epstein–Barr virus replication with an IC_{50} of 0.01–2.2 μg per ml (Van der Horst et al., 1987; Nusinoff-Lehrman et al., 1993; Bacon and Boyd, 1995), but it has no effect on latent cellular infection (Pagano and Datta, 1982), and does not inhibit the development of Epstein–Barr virus-associated B cell lymphoma in infected mice (Boyle et al., 1992).

Human cytomegalovirus is more resistant in vitro than other members of the herpesvirus group with an IC_{50} value ranging from 2.25 to >50 μg per ml (Crumpacker et al., 1979; Tyms et al., 1981; Nusinoff-Lehrman et al., 1993; Elion 1993). The drug is not useful in the treatment of guinea pigs infected with guinea-pig cytomegalovirus (Lucia et al., 1984). The mean IC_{50} concentration of aciclovir required to inhibit is approx 40 μM (Fletcher et al., 1991).

2 Other viruses or microorganisms

Aciclovir does not inhibit replication of vaccinia virus (De Clercq et al., 1980). It has little effect on adenoviruses and RNA viruses such as rhinovirus, yellow fever, measles, respiratory syncytial virus and influenza (Schaeffer, 1978). Aciclovir has been found to inhibit the replication of hepatitis B virus in cell lines, possibly related to the increase in HLA class I molecules induced on the surface of the cells following exposure to aciclovir (Takehara et al., 1992). Turkey herpesvirus and Marek's disease virus are inhibited by aciclovir in vitro (Samorek et al., 1987). If aciclovir is given i.v. early after infection with herpesvirus simiae, it protects rabbits against fatal disease (Boulter et al., 1980). Aciclovir has no effect on Pneumocystis carinii in the rat model (Walzer et al., 1992), or against Salmonella species in vitro (Sperber et al., 1993).

3 Synergy

In vitro, human interferon alpha has been found to be synergistic with aciclovir against herpes simplex virus; the inhibitory effects of interferon alpha on thymidine kinase (TK) activity may only be transient, however (Stanwick *et al.*, 1981; Hammer *et al.*, 1982; O'Brien *et al.*, 1990; Taylor *et al.*, 1994). Synergy between interferon alpha and aciclovir has also been demonstrated against cytomegalovirus (Smith *et al.*, 1983). A combination of aciclovir and adenine arabinoside given topically or systemically was more effective than the individual drugs in diminishing development of herpes simplex infection in hairless mice; given systemically, the combination also reduced the frequency of development of latent infection (Park *et al.*, 1984). Adenine arabinoside and aciclovir are also synergistic when tested against mice infected intravaginally with herpes simplex virus type 2 (Crane *et al.*, 1984). A combination of adenine arabinoside and aciclovir may be synergistic against varicella-zoster virus (Biron and Elion, 1982) and is synergistic against most isolates of human cytomegalovirus (Spector and Kelley 1985).

In one *in vitro* study, additive to synergistic inhibition of cytomegalovirus has been found using aciclovir and zidovudine (Snoeck *et al.*, 1992). This has been partially confirmed by a small clinical study (Sha *et al.*, 1991), although in this author's own clinical experience if this effect is present it is not clinically noticeable. Ribavirin has been found to potentiate the effect of aciclovir against herpes simplex type 1 in cell culture and in rabbits (Pancheva, 1991). Inhibitors of thymidylate synthetase and dihydrofolate reductase have been reported to potentiate the antiviral activity of aciclovir *in vitro* (Pritchard *et al.*, 1993a,b). Although inhibitors of the ribonucleotide reductase of herpes simplex viruses have been found *in vitro* and in mice to potentiate the activity of aciclovir, this combination has been associated with a lack of response in humans (Safrin *et al.*, 1993a,b).

4 Acquired resistance

There are two major mechanisms underlying the development of resistance of herpes simplex strains to aciclovir, involving the TK and DNA polymerase enzymes of herpes simplex virus (Table V.1). The first is the development of mutants with insertions or deletions usually resulting in premature termination of the TK gene and leading to the production of a truncated protein (TK negative mutants). Nucleotide substitutions within the TK gene can also result in the production of a premature stop-codon, and thus a truncated TK protein (TK negative mutant). More commonly, such substitutions lead to deficient activity of the virus-encoded TK in its ability to phosphorylate aciclovir, or a TK with altered substrate specificity in that the virus can phosphorylate thymidine but not aciclovir (TK altered mutants) (Ellis *et al.*, 1987). Mutations have been described within codons 105, 217, 336, 520, 668 within the TK gene associated with the development of resistance (Kit *et al.*, 1987; Chatis and Crumpacker, 1991; Palu *et al.*, 1992; Rechtin *et al.*, 1995).

Secondly, resistance to aciclovir may develop due to mutations that arise within the DNA polymerase (Field *et al.*, 1980; Knopf *et al.*, 1981; Coen *et al.*, 1982; Crumpacker, 1988; Collins *et al.*, 1989; Collins and Darby, 1991). A single point mutation within the DNA polymerase gene has been detected in a clinical isolate of herpes simplex that resulted in resistance to both aciclovir and foscarnet (Hwang *et al.*, 1992).

Mutants of herpes simplex virus that are resistant to aciclovir can be produced by serial passage of the virus in the presence of the drug. Strains resistant to aciclovir can also develop *in vivo* in mice with cutaneous herpes infection, after treatment with suboptimal therapeutic doses of the drug (Field, 1982). Resistant mutants seem to be less virulent in mice (Field and

Table V.1

Mechanisms of resistance of herpes simplex virus to aciclovir

Target gene	Mutation	Result
Thymidine kinase	Insertions/deletions	Truncated TK protein (TK deficient)
	Substitutions	Truncated TK protein (TK negative)
	Substitutions	Altered substrate specificity (TK altered)
DNA polymerase	Insertion/deletions	Decreased DNA polymerase sensitivity to ACV

Darby, 1980; Oliver *et al.*, 1989; Erlich *et al.*, 1989a), although other investigators have reported TK defective mutants of herpes simplex type 2 virus, and sometimes those of type 1 mutants, which retain virulence in animals (Sibrack *et al.*, 1982a; Sakuma *et al.*, 1988; Tanaka *et al.*, 1993).

Cultures often contain heterogeneous populations of sensitive and resistant herpes simplex virus (Parris and Harrington, 1982; Christophers *et al.*, 1987; Nugler *et al.*, 1992). Moreover, strains of herpes simplex virus have been detected among clinical isolates that are resistant to high concentrations of aciclovir prior to exposure to the drug; these are resistant possibly due to alterations in the DNA polymerase gene locus (Parris and Harrington, 1982). Variation in sensitivity of herpes simplex virus (types 1 and 2) to aciclovir among clinical isolates prior to exposure to the drug has been confirmed by larger studies (Dekker *et al.*, 1983; McLaren *et al.*, 1983).

There are now numerous reports of the emergence of strains of herpes simplex virus that are resistant to aciclovir associated with both i.v. and oral treatment with the drug, in both adults and children (Burns *et al.*, 1982; Wade *et al.*, 1982a,1983a; Crumpacker *et al.*, 1982; Sibrack *et al.*, 1982b; McLaren *et al.*, 1983; Straus *et al.*, 1984). It is now clear that in immunocompetent patients receiving aciclovir therapy the incidence of aciclovir-resistance is extremely rare (Barry *et al.*, 1985). In persons with immunodeficiency, resistant strains of herpes simplex were initially identified with increasing frequency (although this has now appeared to reach a plateau) and are associated with clinical lack of response to the drug (Collins and Ellis, 1993).

The low incidence of aciclovir-resistance associated with chronic therapy has been confirmed by more recent studies (Mertz *et al.*, 1988a; Englund *et al.*, 1990). No laboratory evidence of resistance was found in a study of more than 1100 immunocompetent individuals receiving up to 6 years of aciclovir for suppression of recurrent genital herpes (Baker, 1994). In another study of similar individuals taking aciclovir for 6 years, the median sensitivity of the participants' isolates to aciclovir following cessation of therapy was 0.79 µg per ml, with only 3.5% of isolates considered resistant, defined as an IC_{50} of ≥ 3 µg per ml (Fife *et al.*, 1994). Even in an immunocompromised population the incidence of aciclovir-resistance is low (Englund *et al.*, 1990; Tang and Shepp, 1992; Boivin *et al.*, 1993).

There is cross-resistance between aciclovir and penciclovir (Safrin and Phan, 1993) although this does not universally occur (see penciclovir p. 1544), as well as between aciclovir and bromovinyl desoxyuridine. Although there are reports of isolates with resistance to both foscarnet and aciclovir (Birch *et al.*, 1990; Hwang *et al.*, 1992; Safrin *et al.*, 1994b), cross-resistance is generally not observed between aciclovir-resistant TK mutants and adenine arabinoside or foscarnet, the latter being compounds that do not require phosphorylation for their antiviral activity (Fardeau *et al.*, 1993). Aciclovir-resistant TK mutants of herpes simplex are often cross-resistant to ganciclovir, whereas aciclovir-resistant polymerase mutants more commonly retain sensitivity to ganciclovir (Coen, 1991).

Aciclovir-resistant mutants of varicella-zoster virus can be selected by serial passage of the virus in tissue culture in the presence of the drug; this resistance also results from qualitative or quantitative alterations in virus-specified TK or DNA polymerase (Biron *et al.*, 1982). Early investigators were unable to detect the development of *in vivo* resistance to aciclovir in varicella-zoster virus isolates from patients receiving the drug for acute herpes zoster (Cole and Balfour, 1986). In subsequent studies, especially in patients with advanced HIV infection with chronic varicella-zoster, aciclovir-resistant isolates with deficient TK or with a TK with altered substrate specificity have been identified (Boivin *et al.*, 1994). Multiple mutations within TK have been associated with aciclovir-resistance of varicella-zoster virus. These include single nucleotide substitutions within highly conserved binding sites resulting in the introduction of a premature termination codon and the production of a truncated TK protein, as well as random nucleotide deletions and insertions resulting in amino acid substitutions within the TK protein (Talarico *et al.*, 1993; Boivin *et al.*, 1994) or DNA polymerase (Sawyer *et al.*, 1988a). Cross-resistance of aciclovir-resistant strains of varicella-zoster virus to penciclovir has been reported, but similarly to aciclovir-resistant strains of herpes simplex, the development of cross-resistance is not universal (see penciclovir p. 1544) (Hasegawa *et al.*, 1995).

5 Gene therapy

Aciclovir has been used *in vitro* to kill tumor cells transfected with the TK of herpes simplex type 1 as part of a gene therapy strategy (see also ganciclovir p. 1561) (Caruso and Klatzmann, 1992; Golumbek *et al.*, 1992).

Mode of Administration and Dosage

1 Intravenous administration

Following reconstitution of the 250 mg vial of aciclovir (p. 1515) the compound may be administered by i.v. injection in a solution containing 25 mg per ml of aciclovir using an infusion pump, or further diluted in a minimum of 50–100 ml (maximum concentration 5 mg of aciclovir per ml) for i.v. infusion. The solution should be given over 1 h to prevent renal tubular damage (Campos *et al.*, 1992). A number of solutions are recommended by GlaxoWellcome for the delivery of aciclovir, including Hartmann's solution, sodium chloride (0.18% w/v) and dextrose (4% w/v), sodium chloride (0.45% w/v) and dextrose (2.5% w/v) (see Aciclovir Product Information, GlaxoWellcome). The recommended doses and respective indications are summarized in Table V.2.

Table V.2
Indications for aciclovir therapy. (Reproduced with modification from Whitley and Gnann, 1992, with permission.)

Type of infection	Route and dosage[a]	Comments
Genital HSV		
Initial episode	200 mg orally 5 times per day for 10 days	Preferred route in normal host
	5 mg per kg i.v. every 8 h for 5 days	Reserved for severe cases
	5% ointment topically every 6 h for 7 days	Much less effective than oral therapy
Recurrent episode	200 mg orally 5 times per day for 5 days	Limited clinical benefit
Suppression	400 mg orally twice-daily	Titrate dose as required (see pp, 1514, 1523)
Mucocutaneous HSV		
In an immunocompromised patient	200–400 mg orally 5 times per day	
	5 mg per kg i.v. every 8 h for 7–10 days[b]	
	5% ointment topically every 6 h for 7 days	For minor lesions only
HSV encephalitis	10 mg per kg i.v. every 8 h for 10–14 days[c]	Alternative therapy: vidarabine
Neonatal HSV[d]	10 mg per kg i.v. every 8 h for 10–14 days[c]	Alternative therapy: vidarabine
Varicella		
Normal host	20 mg per kg orally 4–5 times per day for 5 days (maximal dose, 800 mg, 5 times per day)	
Immunocompromised patient	10 mg per kg i.v. every 8 h for 7–10 days[c]	
Herpes zoster		
Normal host	800 mg orally 5 times per day for 7 days	Preferably initiate within 48 h of onset of rash
Immunocompromised patient	10–12 mg per kg i.v. every 8 h for 7–10 days	Alternative therapy: foscarnet

[a] The doses are for adults with normal renal function unless otherwise noted.
[b] A dose of 250 mg per m^2 of body-surface area should be given to children under 12 years of age.
[c] A dose of 500 mg per m^2 of body-surface area should be given to children under 12 years of age.
[d] Aciclovir has not been approved by the Food and Drug Administration for this indication.

a   Herpes simplex   The adult dosage recommended for mucosal and cutaneous herpes simplex virus infections in patients with normal or compromised immune status is 5 mg per kg body weight, given i.v. every 8h for 5 days. The dosage for children aged 1–12 years is 250 mg per m^2 (square metre of body surface) (about 5 mg per kg body weight) every 8 h. Oral formulations of aciclovir or related compounds are more usually prescribed, with i.v. therapy being reserved for severe cases of primary herpes simplex in immunocompetent persons or for the treatment of more complicated cases of recurrent disease in immunocompromised patients (p. 1524). For herpes simplex encephalitis, the dosage for adults is 10mg per kg body weight given i.v. every 8h given for at least 10 days, and for children is 500 mg per m^2 administered 8-hourly. For other serious herpes infections in infants and children requiring i.v. administration of aciclovir, the dose is 250 mg per m^2 given 8-hourly.

b   Varicella-zoster   For non-immunocompromised adults with severe shingles the dose of aciclovir is 5 mg per kg i.v. every 8 h for 5 days, although again oral aciclovir is more frequently used. In the case of primary or recurrent varicella-zoster virus infection in an immunocompromised adult, a dose of 10 mg per kg of aciclovir i.v. every 8 h is recommended. Based on limited clinical experience, Gould *et al.* (1982) suggested that a dosage of 10 mg per kg 8-hourly for neonates and one of 250 mg per m^2 8-hourly for children over 1 month of age were effective and safe. Currently a dose of 500 mg per m^2 (or 10 mg per kg) given 8-hourly i.v. is recommended for infants and children.

2 Oral administration

The recommended doses and respective indications are summarized in Table V.2.

a   Herpes simplex   For initial episodes of genital herpes, the recommended dose of aciclovir is 200 mg 4-hourly during waking hours (i.e. five tablets per day) for 10 days. For persons with frequent recurrences, the recommended daily suppressive dose of aciclovir is 200 mg three times daily, or 400 mg twice-daily or 800 mg once-daily. The dose of aciclovir used to treat recurrent outbreaks is 200 mg five times per day, although 400 mg three times daily or 800 mg twice-daily are sanctioned alternatives (CDC, 1993). In a dose-ranging study, Mindel and colleagues (Mindel *et al.*, 1988) found that efficacy was increased by the frequency of administration and by daily dose. A dose of 400 mg twice-daily was less effective in suppressing recurrences of genital herpes than 200 mg taken four times per day. However, the convenience of twice-daily dosage for most patients results in greater compliance than four times daily therapy. After 6 months of therapy, aciclovir should be discontinued and the patient observed to ascertain whether further suppressive therapy is warranted. Patient-initiated therapy is commonly used to manage recurrent disease, with the patient commencing aciclovir 200 mg five times per day at the earliest symptom or sign and continuing therapy for 5 days.

b   Varicella-zoster   For patients with shingles, especially elderly patients with moderate to severe manifestations, aciclovir should be commenced as soon as possible (definitely within 72 h) after the onset of rash using a dose of 800 mg five times per day, and continued for a period of 7 days. Although not yet universally licensed for the following indications, aciclovir is used by a number of clinicians to treat adults with primary varicella who are well enough to take oral therapy, commencing treatment within the first 24 h, children older than 12 months with a chronic cutaneous or pulmonary disorder (American Academy of Pediatrics Committee on Infectious Diseases, 1993) and for some immunocompromised children with varicella (although i.v. therapy is usually preferred).

3 Patients with renal failure

Renal excretion of the drug is impaired in patients with severe renal dysfunction, and there is a fairly good correlation between total body clearance of aciclovir and the creatinine clearance value. For adult patients with creatinine clearance values of 25–50 ml per min, and 10–25 ml per min respectively, a dose of 5mg or 10 mg per kg i.v. should be administered at intervals of 12 and 24 h, respectively. For patients with a creatinine clearance of 0–10 ml per min, a dose of 2.5 or 5 mg per kg (i.e. half of the recommended dose) is given every 24h (Blum *et al.*, 1982; Aciclovir Product Information GlaxoWellcome; see Table V.3). The half-life of aciclovir during hemodialysis is 5.4 h (Krasny *et al.*, 1982), and there is a 45–60% decrease in plasma concentrations after a 3–6 h dialysis period; a dose should therefore be administered after each dialysis (Laskin *et al.*, 1982a; Leikin *et al.*, 1995; Almond *et al.*, 1995). There is negligible removal of the drug by peritoneal dialysis (Davenport *et al.*, 1992).

Table V.3
Aciclovir. (Reproduced from Zovirax Product Information, GlaxoWellcome, Australia, with permission.)

Creatinine clearance	Dosage
25–50 ml per min	The recommended dose (5 or 10 mg per kg) every 12 h
10–25 ml per min	The recommended dose (5 or 10 mg per kg) every 24 h
0 (anuric)–10 ml per min	The recommended dose should be halved (2.5 or 5 mg per kg) every 24 h and after dialysis

For patients with a creatinine clearance of less than 10 ml per min, an oral regimen of 200 or 800 mg five times daily should be reduced to 200 or 800 mg twice-daily (de Miranda and Blum 1983). However, results from a small open study suggest that even 800 mg twice-daily may result in neurotoxicity due to high aciclovir plasma concentrations in dialysis-dependent individuals, and the authors of this report recommend a 400-mg loading dose followed by 200 mg twice-daily in order to maintain mean plasma levels of greater than 6 μM; a further loading dose of 400 mg should be given following dialysis (Almond et al., 1995). For patients with moderate renal impairment (creatinine clearance 10–25 ml per min) the regimen of 800 mg administered five times per day should be reduced to 800 mg given three times per day. Dose adjustment is not required for patients with mild renal failure because, although their area-under-the-curve (AUC) values will be increased, these values will still not be greater than levels achieved by i.v. doses of 5 mg per kg three times daily (de Miranda and Blum, 1983).

4 Pregnant patients

Aciclovir is not teratogenic in animals (Tucker, 1982). The safety of aciclovir in pregnant women has not been established through controlled clinical trials, although the drug has been given to large numbers of pregnant women and published data do not indicate increased adverse effects related to its use in pregnancy (Brown and Baker, 1989; Andrews et al., 1992; Horowitz and Hankins, 1992; Spangler et al., 1994). If the potential benefit to the mother outweighs possible risks to the infant the drug may be administered to women during pregnancy. Limited data suggest that aciclovir is excreted in human milk. In one report, a lactating woman was treated with 800 mg of aciclovir for 7 days. On days 6 and 7 aciclovir concentrations in random breast milk samples ranged from 4.2 μg per ml to 5.8 μg per ml. The infant was estimated to ingest 1% of the maternal dose (approximately 0.7 mg per kg per day (Taddio et al., 1994). In another report, breast milk concentrations were 3.2-fold higher than serum levels in a lactating mother receiving oral aciclovir (Meyer et al., 1988). Thus the drug should be administered to nursing mothers if the benefit to the mother is considered to clearly outweigh any potential risk to her infant.

5 Children

In infants and children aged less than 2 years with herpes simplex infections, the commonly used dose of aciclovir is 100–200 mg five times per day; in children older than 2 years the dose is 200 mg five times per day. For varicella-zoster infections in children the dose is 20 mg per kg given four to five times per day.

6 Topical use

Aciclovir has been used as a 5% ointment in polyethylene glycol (Spruance et al., 1982), and a 5% cream in propylene glycol (Fiddian et al., 1983) for the treatment of herpes labialis. Topical preparations have also been used to treat genital herpes. The drug is given as an ointment (3%) to treat and prevent herpes keratitis.

Availability

Vials: These contain lyophilized aciclovir sodium (equivalent to 250 mg or 500 mg aciclovir) for i.v. administration. Each 250- or 500-mg vial should be reconstituted by adding 10 or 20 ml respectively of sterile water or normal saline suitable for use in injections. The final concentration is 25 mg aciclovir per ml.

Tablets: Tablets are available containing 200 mg or 400 mg of aciclovir.

Ophthalmic ointment: Each gram of ophthalmic ointment contains 30 mg of aciclovir (3% aciclovir).

Topical cream for mucocutaneous infections. Aciclovir is available as a 5% w/w cream in a water miscible base containing propylene glycol.

Serum Levels in Relation to Dosage

Serum levels can readily be measured by high-performance liquid chromatographic (HPLC) methods (Mascher *et al.*, 1992).

1 Intravenous administration

The following data were compiled by pooling results from ten small pharmacokinetic studies (Blum *et al.*, 1982). After administration of single doses of 0.5, 1.0, 2.5, 5.0, 10.0 and 15.0 mg aciclovir per kg body weight to adults, by constant infusion over a period of 1 h, the peak serum level was reached at the end of the infusion and was in proportion to the dose; mean peak levels for these doses were 1.0, 2.1, 4.2, 8.8, 14.6 and 22.7 μg per ml, respectively. High intersubject variation at some of these doses generally reflected a variability of renal function among the patients. When the same doses were given to adults every 8 h, steady-state peak serum concentrations (C_{max}) occurred which were similar to those after single dosing, indicating that there is little accumulation at these doses. For doses of 2.5, 5.0, 10.0 and 15.0 mg per kg every 8 h, the steady-state peak serum concentrations with trough levels in parenthesis were 5.1 (0.5), 9.8 (0.7), 20.7 (2.3) and 23.6 (2.0) μg per ml, respectively. In children given 250 mg per m^2 (about 5 mg per kg) and 500 mg per m^2 (about 10 mg per kg) every 8 h, mean steady-state C_{max} of 10.3 and 20.7 μg per ml, respectively, were nearly identical to those of adults.

2 Oral administration

Gastrointestinal absorption of aciclovir is generally fairly poor (15–20% with 200–400 mg given 4-hourly) and quite erratic, with a generally lower proportion absorbed with higher doses. About 10–15% of the drug is excreted unchanged in the urine and 15–25% is excreted unchanged in the feces (Straus *et al.*, 1982). Consequently, serum levels after oral administration are lower than those reached after i.v. aciclovir. When an oral dose of 200 mg is given to adults, a C_{max} of 0.35–1.0 (mean 0.6) μg per ml occurs 1.5–1.75 h later. Serum levels then fall in a linear fashion with a half-life of about 3 h (Van Dyke *et al.*, 1982).

Serum levels reach a steady-state after 1 day of multiple dosing; mean peak concentrations of 0.5, 1.2 and 1.3 μg per ml and trough levels of 0.3, 0.6 and 0.8 μg per ml occur on day 6 after 200, 400 and 600 mg doses every 4 h, respectively. Mean peak aciclovir levels after one dose were 58–77% of the steady-state peak level and steady-state trough levels were 50–62% of the peak levels. It appears that the net absorption of the drug is nearly proportional to dose in the 200–600 mg dose range (de Miranda and Blum, 1982).

When aciclovir is infused after a 1-g oral dose of probenecid, enhanced serum concentrations occur and the serum half-life of aciclovir is slightly prolonged, probably because probenecid inhibits its tubular secretion (Laskin *et al.*, 1982b). Gluckman *et al.* (1983) showed that oral absorption was unaltered in patients receiving chemotherapy; after a 200-mg dose, mean serum levels at 2, 4 and 6h were 0.37, 0.25 and 0.16 μg per ml, respectively.

3 Renal dysfunction

Since renal clearance is the major route for elimination of aciclovir higher serum levels of the drug are obtained and its serum half-life is prolonged in patients with renal failure (Laskin *et al.*, 1982a; Krasny *et al.*, 1982).

After a single i.v. dose of aciclovir, resultant serum levels decline in a biphasic manner, suggesting that the drug is distributed as in a two-compartment model. The half-life of its terminal elimination (beta phase) is about 3 h and this increases to about 18 h in anuric patients (Lietman, 1982). After an oral dose of 800 mg, administered to patients with end-stage oliguric renal failure, peak plasma levels of 12.54 ± 1.76 μM were achieved at 3 h, with a half-life of 20.2 h and a mean plasma level of 6.29 μM after 18 h (Almond *et al.*, 1995).

The mean half-life of aciclovir during hemodialysis has been variably reported to range from 5.7 to 10 h, and is also considerably prolonged in patients on continuous ambulatory peritoneal dialysis (CAPD) (13.2 ± 4.7 h) (Aciclovir Product Information GlaxoWellcome; Burgess and

Gill, 1990). Intraperitoneal dosing has been found to provide approximately 60% bioavailability (Burgess and Gill, 1990). In a small study plasmapheresis did not significantly alter aciclovir pharmacokinetics (Chavanet et al., 1990a).

4 Pregnancy

When aciclovir was given to 15 pregnant women in a dose of 200 mg or 400 mg every 8 h from week 38 of gestation until delivery, the drug was found to have similar pharmacokinetics to those found in other studies of non-pregnant adults, and there was no accumulation in the fetus (mean maternal/infant plasma ratio at delivery was 1.3) (Frenkel et al., 1991).

5 Pediatrics

In neonatal patients (aged 4 days-2 months) given aciclovir by 1 h infusion in dosages of 5, 10 and 15 mg per kg every 8 h, predictable and consistent serum levels are obtained; mean peak serum levels (trough levels in parenthesis) for these regimens were 7.5 (1.3), 15.3 (2.5) and 21.5 (3. 4) μg per ml, respectively (Hintz et al., 1982). Another study suggested that peak and trough serum levels in infants may vary considerably and change with chronological age (Yeager, 1982). In a more recent study, aciclovir was found to accumulate in premature neonates, and in those with hepatic or renal dysfunction (Englund et al., 1991).

When oral aciclovir in a dose of 400 mg (250–650 mg per m^2) five times daily was given to ten children (aged 3–15 years), peak serum levels were 0.79–3. 4 μg per ml and trough levels were 0.5–3.1 μg per ml (Novelli et al., 1984) and levels did not differ whether the drug was taken with or without food (Novelli et al., 1985). These data are supported by a second study in which the mean peak serum level in children receiving 600 mg per m^2 (aged 6 months to 6.9 years) or 300 mg per m^2 (less than 2 months of age) of an oral aciclovir suspension was 0.99 ± 0.38 μg per ml or 1.88 ± 1.11 μg per ml respectively, with the mean AUC being 5.56± 2.17 μg.h per ml and 6.54 ± 4.32 μg.h per ml respectively (Sullender et al., 1987).

6 Elderly

In a study of 32 patients over 60 years of age receiving oral aciclovir, 800 mg five times per day, trough plasma concentrations of aciclovir were considerably higher than reported values for younger subjects, and were higher even in patients with normal renal function. However, there was no evidence of accumulation of aciclovir. Diuretic use was associated with significantly higher concentrations, likely to be due to competition between aciclovir and the diuretic for active renal secretion sites (Wood et al., 1994a).

7 Topical administration

This method of administration does not produce detectable levels of aciclovir in the serum unless it is applied to large areas of skin (Whitley et al., 1984). Topical application to external genital lesions does not result in detectable levels in cervicovaginal secretions (Corey et al., 1982a).

Excretion

1 Urine

This is the principal route for the clearance of aciclovir after i.v. administration and the mean urinary recovery of the unchanged drug is 60% (Whitley et al., 1982a). Urinary elimination of aciclovir occurs rapidly; about 60% of the drug is excreted by 6 h, and over 99% by 24 h (Spector et al., 1981). Renal clearance of aciclovir greatly exceeds creatinine clearance indicating that tubular secretion of the drug is contributory (de Miranda et al., 1982).

2 Inactivation in the body

In anuric patients, aciclovir is slowly cleared from the body by non-renal routes. Studies in humans using radioactive aciclovir i.v. show that 71–99% of an administered dose is excreted in the urine. Up to 14.1% of the dose is excreted in the urine as the inactive metabolite, 9-carboxymethoxymethylguanine. Unchanged urinary aciclovir ranges from 62 to 91% of the dose (de Miranda et al., 1982).

3 Feces

Less than 2% of an i.v. dose is excreted in feces and only trace amounts are found in expired air (de Miranda et al., 1982).

Distribution of the Drug in Body

Aciclovir appears to be widely distributed in tissues and body fluids. Wade *et al.* (1982b) studied tissue aciclovir concentrations obtained at autopsy in five patients. The average level in lung was 131% of the simultaneous serum level and in one patient the drug was still detectable in lung tissue 6 days after discontinuation of treatment. Levels in heart and liver were similar to those in lung, but levels in the renal medulla and cortex were 10-fold higher than the serum level. Aciclovir concentrations in brain and spinal cord were variable, being 25–70% of the simultaneous serum level.

In limited studies of cerebrospinal fluid (CSF) from adults and children concentrations of aciclovir ranging from 0.2 to 4 μg per ml have been detected, which were about 13–50% of the simultaneous serum level (Blum *et al.*, 1982; Lycke *et al.*, 1989). Higher CSF penetration has been reported in patients receiving probenecid with aciclovir (Chavanet *et al.*, 1990b).

Following a 200-mg oral dose of aciclovir, a mean salivary level of 0.1 μg per ml was found after 2.2–2.5 h, being about 13% of concomitant serum levels. There was poor correlation between aciclovir levels in vaginal secretions and simultaneous serum levels, but they were about 76% of those in the serum (Van Dyke *et al.*, 1982). After an i.v. dose of 5 mg per kg every 8 h, aciclovir could not be detected in salivary or vaginal wash samples during the first 24 h of therapy; thereafter it was found in virtually all samples. The mean concentration in saliva was 0.27 μg per ml and that in cervicovaginal fluid 0.43 μg per ml. Aciclovir was often present in saliva and vaginal fluid up to 24 h after discontinuing the drug (Corey *et al.*, 1983a). Semen to plasma ratios after twice- and five-times daily dosing have been reported as 1:4 and 4:2 respectively (Douglas *et al.*, 1988).

Concentrations of aciclovir of 1.7 μg per ml have been detected in the aqueous humor of patients after topical administration to the eye (Collum *et al.*, 1982). The drug also reaches the aqueous humor after oral administration (Brigden *et al.*, 1983).

During i.v. infusion and oral dosing with aciclovir, concentrations of the drug in varicella-zoster vesicle fluid are approximately equal to serum levels (Spector *et al.*, 1982; de Miranda and Blum, 1983). Topical administration of aciclovir 5% ointment and cream have been found to provide 48-fold higher levels of the drug within the epidermis than those found after oral administration. However, at the basal level of the epidermis (the target site of infection) oral therapy provides 2- to 3-fold higher concentrations than topical therapy (Parry *et al.*, 1992). The binding of aciclovir to serum proteins is 9–22% (mean 15.4%) (Blum *et al.*, 1982).

Aciclovir given to women late in the third trimester of pregnancy accumulates in the amniotic fluid (Frenkel *et al.*, 1991). The level of aciclovir in breast milk of a lactating mother receiving oral aciclovir has been reported to be 3.2-fold higher than serum levels (Meyer *et al.*, 1988).

Mode of Action

Aciclovir is a potent inhibitor of the DNA polymerases of herpes simplex virus types 1 and 2, and varicella-zoster virus, but it has low toxicity for normal host cells. The inhibition of cellular DNA polymerases alpha, delta and epsilon by aciclovir is significantly weaker than the inhibition of the viral DNA polymerase by the drug (Ilsley *et al.*, 1995). A number of selective actions account for the 300- to 3000-fold difference between toxicity of aciclovir for herpes viruses and the host cell (Elion, 1982). These viruses encode a specific TK enzyme (Fig. V.2) which phosphorylates the drug to a monophosphate (Fyfe *et al.*, 1978); host cellular TK is unable to do this (although phosphorylation does occur to a small extent by some other enzymes, possibly through the action of 5' nucleotidase) (Cioe *et al.*, 1992). A similar but distinct TK is specified by varicella-zoster and this enzyme is responsible for monophosphorylation of aciclovir in cells

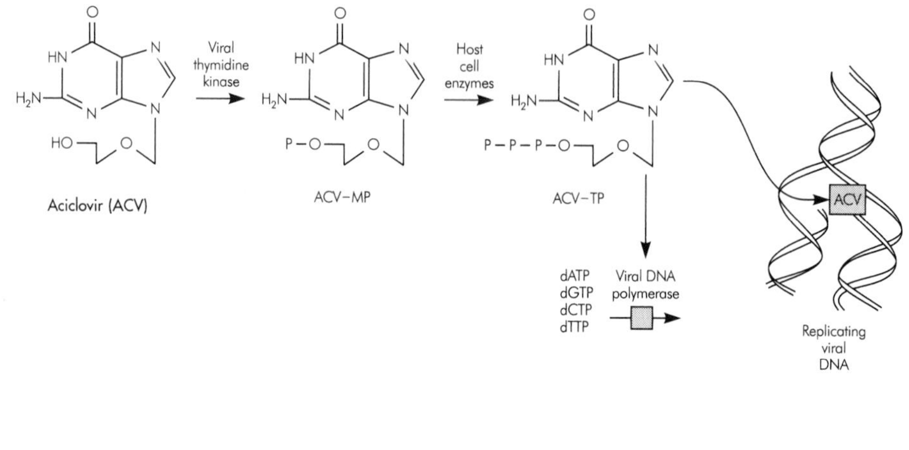

Fig. V.2.

Activity of aciclovir against herpes simplex virus. Aciclovir is metabolized to the monophosphate (MP) in herpes simplex infected cells by virus-specified thymidine kinase aciclovir monophosphate is converted to the triphosphate (TP) by cellular enzymes. Aciclovir triphosphate inhibits herpes simplex DNA polymerase and is incorporated into replacing DNA, resulting in chain termination. (Reproduced from Balfour *et al.*, 1983b, with permission.)

infected with this virus (Biron and Elion, 1980). Aciclovir monophosphate is then converted to aciclovir diphosphate and triphosphate by cellular enzymes in virus infected cells. Guanylate kinase is responsible for converting aciclovir monophosphate to the diphosphate derivative, an efficient process as the monophosphate form does not accumulate within the cell (Miller and Miller, 1980). A number of cellular enzymes, including phosphoglycerate kinase, nucleoside diphosphate kinase and phosphoenol pyruvate kinase, can convert aciclovir diphosphate to the active triphosphate form (Miller and Miller, 1982). The amount of aciclovir triphosphate formed in herpes simplex virus infected cells is 40- to 100-fold greater than the amount formed in uninfected cells.

Viral polymerase is necessary for the virus to replicate its own DNA genome. Aciclovir triphosphate competes with deoxyguanosine triphosphate as a substrate for the viral DNA polymerase, but in a non-linear fashion (reviewed in Elion, 1993). As the aciclovir triphosphate lacks the 3-hydroxyl group necessary for accepting the incoming nucleotide and subsequent DNA chain elongation, virus synthesis is thus terminated. The virus DNA polymerase becomes inactivated as a result of its complexing with the terminated DNA chain. Aciclovir triphosphate tends to persist in cells because cell membranes are permeable to the unphosphorylated drug, but they are impermeable to aciclovir triphosphate (Pagano and Datta, 1982). Aciclovir is effective only against virus which is actively replicating and does not eliminate latent viral genomes.

The antiviral activity of aciclovir is restricted to viruses that specify a TK capable of recognizing aciclovir as a substrate. Although vaccinia virus infection induces TK activity, this particular enzyme does not phosphorylate aciclovir (St Clair *et al.*, 1980).

Toxicity

Aciclovir appears to be relatively free from serious toxicity (Keeney *et al.*, 1982), even when taken regularly for many years (Mertz *et al.*, 1988b; Kaplowitz *et al.*, 1991; Tilson *et al.*, 1993).

1 Nephrotoxicity

In animals, a rapid i.v. bolus injection of aciclovir results in precipitation of the drug in the lower nephron of the kidney, causing transient impairment of renal function; this is due to the relatively low solubility of aciclovir in urine (Tucker, 1982).

Aciclovir nephrotoxicity is one of the most serious potential complications of the drug. In one review, 10% of patients who had been given the drug by rapid (bolus) i.v. injections developed rises in blood urea or serum creatinine (Keeney *et al.*, 1982). Risk of renal impairment is reduced if the drug is infused i.v. over a period of 1 h, adequate hydration of the patient is maintained and the dosage regimen is adjusted for renal function (p. 1515) (Brigden *et al.*, 1982). Adverse renal effects can be prevented by maintenance of adequate hydration to allow a urine output of approximately 1 liter per g of aciclovir administered (solubility in water 1–3 mg per ml) (Keeney *et al.*, 1982). Findings by Bean and Aeppli (1985) suggest that elevated serum creatinine levels are more frequent if the peak serum aciclovir level exceeds 25 μg per ml. Rapidly progressive, non-oliguric acute renal failure responding to cessation of the drug has been reported in patients taking oral aciclovir for zoster or herpes simplex encephalitis (Rashed *et al.*, 1990; Johnson *et al.*, 1994). In a study of children receiving high dose i.v. aciclovir for herpes simplex encephalitis, fluid restriction was associated with non-oliguric renal insufficiency which resolved within 1 week of cessation of the drug. Intratubular aciclovir crystalluria was considered to be the likely underlying pathology (Bianchetti *et al.*, 1991). Birefringent, needle-shaped crystals of aciclovir have been described in the urine of some patients with aciclovir-induced nephrotoxicity (Sawyer *et al.*, 1988b; Peterslund *et al.*, 1988), but are not present in other patients with aciclovir-induced acute tubular necrosis (Becker *et al.*, 1993).

2 Neurotoxicity

Neurotoxicity has been described in association with aciclovir therapy for patients with end-stage renal disease (Johnson *et al.*, 1985; Gill and Burgess, 1990; Davenport *et al.*, 1992). The development of neurotoxicity has been closely linked with high serum concentrations of aciclovir, usually developing with a delay of 24–48 h after peak serum concentrations (Feldman *et al.*, 1988; Rashiq *et al.*, 1993; Haefeli *et al.*, 1993). Neurologic symptoms associated with parenteral aciclovir treatment include lethargy, agitation, tremor, disorientation, dysarthria, seizures, ataxia, myoclonus, hyperesthesia, hyperacusis and transient hemiparesthesias (Wade and Myers, 1983; Johnson *et al.*, 1985, 1994). Improvement or resolution of symptoms occurs within 2 weeks after cessation of aciclovir therapy. An abnormal electroencephalogram is a consistent feature. Tomson *et al.* (1985) described psychiatric side-effects, including hallucinations and depression, in adult patients with chronic renal failure following the use of aciclovir in doses higher than those recommended.

3 Gastrointestinal side-effects

Of 23 patients given i.v. aciclovir for zoster, nearly half had two or more of the following symptoms: nausea, vomiting, abdominal pain and light-headedness. These appeared to be associated with peak serum aciclovir levels in excess of 25 μg per ml (Bean and Aeppli, 1985). In a more recent study, adverse gastrointestinal symptoms developed in 8% of patients with genital herpes who were treated with a high dose (4 g per day) of oral aciclovir (Wald *et al.*, 1994). There is one report of aciclovir-associated colitis (Moshkowitz *et al.*, 1993).

4 Hemopoietic side-effects

In vitro, aciclovir has little effect on human bone marrow in concentrations less than 50 μg per ml (McGuffin *et al.*, 1980; Parker *et al.*, 1982). Bean and Fletcher (1985) described neutropenia in three immunocompromised patients who were given high-dose aciclovir therapy and who also had received myelotoxic agents within the previous 30 days; more recently neutropenia has been well-described in association with aciclovir therapy (30 mg per kg per day) in an infant (Feder *et al.*, 1995). Megaloblastic hemopoiesis without detectable changes in the peripheral blood may occur (Amos and Amess, 1983). A child developed transient leukopenia and erythroblastopenia during i.v. aciclovir therapy that responded promptly to cessation of therapy (Tuncer *et al.*, 1989).

5 Effects on immune response

Aciclovir has minimal effects on human lymphocytic cell responses *in vitro* (Wingard *et al.*, 1983). Systemic treatment with aciclovir diminishes the humoral antibody response to herpes simplex virus in patients with genital herpes (Corey *et al.*, 1983b; Bernstein *et al.*, 1984); it also appears to delay the development and diminish the peak of *in vitro* lymphocyte transformation responses to inactivated herpes simplex virus antigens in such patients (Lafferty *et al.*, 1984). These alterations probably occur because aciclovir treatment reduces the duration of viral shedding and hence antigenic stimulation. Clinical presentation and subsequent immunological response of the first recurrences of genital herpes after aciclovir treatment are unaltered, but the immunological response in patients with an existing compromised immune response is unknown (Lafferty *et al.*, 1984).

6 Dermatologic side-effects

Allergic contact dermatitis attributed to aciclovir or the propylene glycol in aciclovir cream has been infrequently reported (Valsecchi *et al.*, 1990; Goday *et al.*, 1991; Kim and Kim, 1994). Cutaneous vesicular eruptions may occur in patients receiving aciclovir (Buck *et al.*, 1993). Successful aciclovir desensitization has been reported in a patient with recurrent mucocutaneous herpes simplex virus infection who developed angioedema with oral aciclovir therapy (Henry *et al.*, 1993). Topical aciclovir may cause transient burning when applied to genital lesions; this is more frequent with first episodes of genital herpes than with recurrent episodes, and is more frequent in women than men (Corey *et al.*, 1982a). In general, topical application to genital lesions is well tolerated (Fiddian *et al.*, 1983). Mild superficial punctate epithelial staining can occur after treatment with the ophthalmic ointment, but this disappears a few days after the drug is discontinued (Laibson *et al.*, 1982).

7 Embryotoxicity

Administration of very high doses (50–100 mg per kg) of aciclovir to pregnant rats can result in a high rate of resorptions of fetuses, and malformations of the skull, vertebral column and tail (Chahoud *et al.*, 1988; Stahlmann *et al.*, 1988). Lower doses of aciclovir have been associated with abnormal development of the fetal thymus (Foerster *et al.*, 1992; Stahlmann *et al.*, 1992). The Burroughs Wellcome Registry contains reports of pregnancy outcomes following prenatal maternal exposure to aciclovir between 1984 and 1993. Of 611 cases, 425 exposures to the drug occurred within the first trimester. Only 4% of infants had a birth defect (similar to surveillance data with no aciclovir exposure) and no specific pattern was noted (MMWR, 1993). Although virtually all reports of the use of aciclovir during pregnancy suggest no toxicity, fetal diastematomyelia, a rare spinal condition, was diagnosed in a pregnancy exposed to aciclovir at the time of implantation (Gubbels *et al.*, 1991).

8 Overdose

In reported cases of aciclovir overdose, including in neonates, no toxicity has been observed (McDonald *et al.*, 1989). The major exception is when aciclovir levels accumulate due to poor renal function; there have been a number of cases of neurotoxicity associated with elevated aciclovir plasma levels in patients with renal failure (Gill and Burgess, 1990; Davenport *et al.*, 1992; Leikin *et al.*, 1995).

9 Other side-effects

Since aciclovir for injection has a relatively high pH (9–11), local irritation occurs if it is extravasated into the tissues (Keeney *et al.*, 1982; Robbins *et al.*, 1993). Experience in one patient indicated that infusion of high concentrations (12 mg per ml) may cause vesiculation at the infusion site (Sylvester *et al.*, 1986). Fever, pulmonary infiltrates and a pleural effusion have been described in an elderly man following commencement of aciclovir; cessation of the drug resulted in clinical improvement (Pusateri and Muder, 1990).

10 Drug interactions

A minimal increase in the risk of toxicity has been reported when aciclovir is used in combination with zidovudine (Cooper *et al.*, 1991), although in this author's experience these drugs are commonly co-prescribed without the development of clinical problems. No pharmacokinetic interaction has been demonstrated between these two drugs (Hollander *et al.*, 1989; Rajaonarison *et al.*, 1992).

Clinical Uses of the Drug

Aciclovir is indicated as i.v. therapy for the treatment of severe primary mucocutaneous herpes simplex infections in immunocompetent persons, for primary or recurrent mucocutaneous infections in immunocompromised patients, for treatment of varicella-zoster in immunocompromised patients, and for herpes simplex encephalitis, and for life-threatening infections in neonates. Oral aciclovir is indicated for the treatment of primary or recurrent genital herpes and for non-ophthalmic zoster in the elderly (Aciclovir Product Information GlaxoWellcome).

1 Herpes simplex infections

a Mucocutaneous herpes simplex infections

i Genital infections Aciclovir is effective when administered i.v. to treat initial episodes of genital herpes (Corey *et al.*, 1983a; see Fig. V.4). The dosage is 5 mg per kg every 8 h for periods of 4–5 days (Mindel *et al.*, 1982; Corey *et al.*, 1983a; Peacock *et al.*, 1988). The duration of viral shedding, duration for healing of lesions and duration of local and systemic symptoms, were all significantly decreased by aciclovir. The frequency of new genital lesions was also reduced as

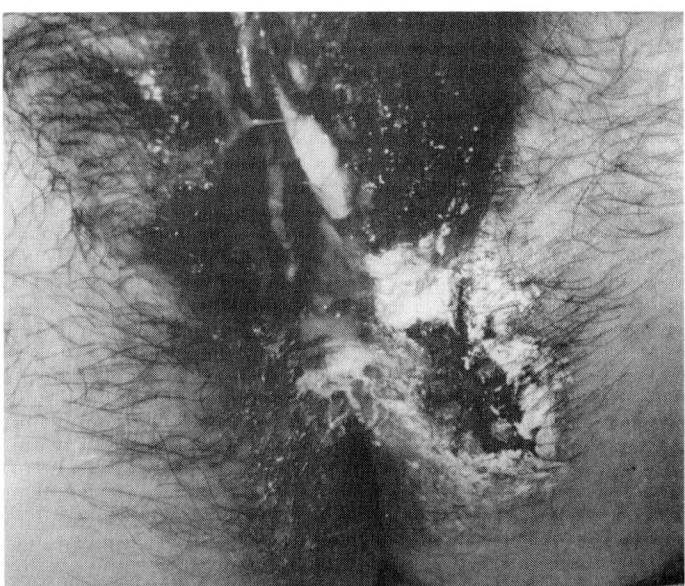

Fig. V.3.
Extensive local disease in female genitalia due to aciclovir-resistant herpes simplex. (From the library of the former Fairfield Hospital, Melbourne.)

Fig. V.4.

Clearance of herpes simplex virus from patients with primary genital lesions who are treated with aciclovir. (Reproduced from Corey *et al.*, 1983b, with permission.)

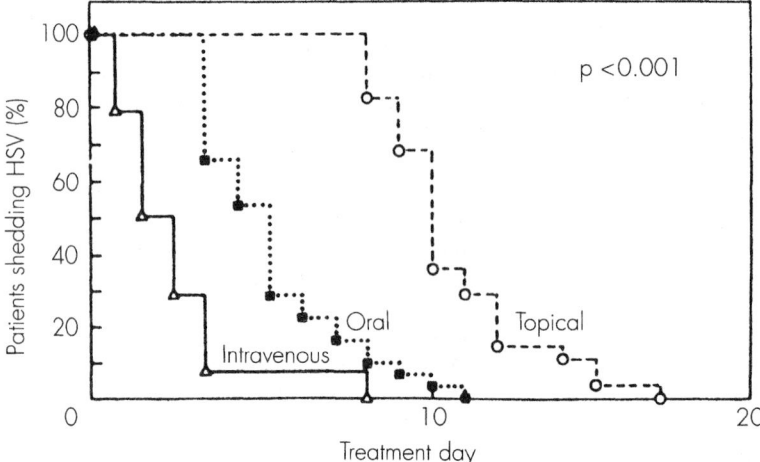

were complications of the disease. Aciclovir therapy does not influence the natural history of recurrent herpes simplex infection. Neither the interval between recurrences nor their severity is altered by previous treatment with aciclovir, however administered.

For primary genital herpes, oral aciclovir is used in a dosage of 200 mg five times per day for 10 days or until the lesions have resolved. This recommendation is based on efficacy data from a number of early studies (Nilsen *et al.*, 1982; Bryson *et al.*, 1983; Salo *et al.*, 1983; Mertz *et al.*, 1984). In first episodes of genital herpes, aciclovir therapy was associated with reduced duration of viral shedding, shorter duration of symptoms and signs of the disease and reduced occurrence of new lesions. All herpes simplex-associated genital lesions including proctitis respond to aciclovir (Rompalo *et al.*, 1988). In one study the mean time to seroconversion was longer in patients treated with aciclovir than in controls (Ragab *et al.*, 1989), although other investigators have not detected any alteration in antibody response by aciclovir therapy.

There are now good data regarding the benefit of aciclovir therapy in preventing transmission of herpes simplex at the time of delivery. In a small study of pregnant women given aciclovir late in the third trimester, aciclovir prevented transmission of the virus to the neonate in four of five cases (Haddad *et al.*, 1993). In a larger study, in which 46 pregnant women with first episodes of genital herpes during pregnancy were randomized to receive oral aciclovir 400 mg three times per day or placebo from week 36 of pregnancy until delivery, none of the 21 aciclovir recipients and nine of the 25 placebo recipients had clinical evidence of recurrent genital herpes at delivery. Cesarean section was required in 36% of the placebo-treated group for recurrent genital herpes and in none of the aciclovir group; there was no evidence of herpes infection in any neonate (Scott *et al.*, 1996).

Recurrent genital herpes is invariably less severe than the initial attack, and usually the period of treatment is shorter (5 days or until lesions resolve). The traditionally recommended regimen for treatment of a recurrent episode of genital herpes is 200 mg, five times per day for 5 days or until the lesions have resolved. However, a double-blind study comparing 800 mg twice-daily with conventional doses has demonstrated equal efficacy (Goldberg *et al.*, 1988). Similarly, the dose of 400 mg three times daily is an acceptable alternative.

Controlled studies have demonstrated that oral aciclovir is also useful for the suppression of frequently recurring genital herpes (Douglas *et al.*, 1984; Mindel *et al.*, 1984; Reichman *et al.*, 1984; Straus *et al.*, 1984; Kinghorn *et al.*, 1985; Thin *et al.*, 1985). Prolonged continuous therapy with aciclovir is better than intermittent oral therapy in preventing recurrences (Mattison *et al.*, 1988; Mertz *et al.*, 1988b). Aciclovir does not completely suppress asymptomatic shedding of herpes simplex virus (Bowman *et al.*, 1990; Wald *et al.*, 1996), and thus the virus may be transmitted to sexual partners in the absence of symptoms. In a double-blind study of 34 women with less than a 2-year history of genital herpes, placebo recipients shed herpes simplex on 83 of 1439 days (5.8%) compared with six of 1611 (0.37%) in aciclovir recipients (Wald *et al.*, 1996). In recurrent infections, treatment with oral aciclovir shortens the period of viral shedding and the time to complete healing of genital lesions; the frequency of new lesion formation is also reduced. However, these findings often translate to only subtle clinical improvement in the individual patient. The dose of 400 mg twice-daily is most commonly recommended, but 200 mg three times daily and 800 mg once-daily are acceptable alternatives. Mindel and colleagues

(Mindel *et al.*, 1988) performed a dose-ranging study evaluating aciclovir suppressive therapy in patients with frequently recurring genital herpes and found that 200 mg twice-daily appears to be almost as effective as the conventional dose of 400 mg twice-daily. They further reported that there was a decrease in the time to recurrence associated with reduction of the total daily dose and frequency of administration. Mostow *et al.* (1988) found that 800 mg of aciclovir in a single daily dose prevented 28% of recipients from developing any recurrence over a 2-year period. In a separate study, an oral regimen of 400 mg three times daily for 2 days a week was less effective than a daily regimen in preventing genital herpes (Straus *et al.*, 1986). Although recurrences were markedly reduced, they were not always completely prevented by suppressive treatment. These dose schedules were well tolerated, and the safety of long-term medication has now been established.

Continuous aciclovir therapy administered to large numbers of patients with frequently recurrent genital herpes for periods in excess of 5 years has provided evidence that the drug is well tolerated and not associated with serious adverse reactions or cumulative toxicity (Goldberg *et al.*, 1993; Mertz *et al.*, 1988a; Kaplowitz *et al.*, 1991; Baker 1994; Fife *et al.*, 1994). A progressive decrease in the number of recurrences per year has been reported with long-term suppressive therapy (Goldberg *et al.*, 1993), but this may just reflect the natural history of the disease, as there was no placebo arm beyond the first year of this study. Patients with HIV infection with recurrent genital herpes should be offered prophylactic aciclovir therapy if warranted by the frequency of their recurrences, similar to the non-HIV-infected patient.

Patient-initiated therapy, commencing aciclovir at the first recognition of symptoms or signs of recurrence, is an alternative to chronic suppressive therapy (Goldberg *et al.*, 1986; Whatley and Thin, 1991). This is the treatment of choice for persons with less frequent (less than six) recurrences of genital herpes per year.

A polyethylene glycol ointment containing 5% aciclovir was used in several controlled trials (Corey *et al.*, 1982a,b; Reichman *et al.*, 1983; Thin *et al.*, 1983). This ointment was applied to lesions four to six times daily, but not to the vagina or cervix. Although treatment reduced local symptoms and signs of primary genital herpes in some cases, and the duration of viral shedding was less, it is less effective than oral or i.v. therapy. In recurrent episodes of genital herpes, topical aciclovir used shortly after onset of lesions reduced viral shedding, but had no effect in reducing new lesion formation. In a controlled trial, Corey *et al.* (1982b) studied the effects of topical aciclovir in patients with primary or recurrent genital herpes. The cream was applied liberally five times per day for up to 10 days or until healing had occurred, treatment beginning within 48 hours after onset of symptoms in patients with recurrent genital herpes and within 6 days for patients with primary infection. In aciclovir-treated patients with initial infections, the duration of viral shedding, formation of new lesions, times to crusting and healing, and severity of symptoms were reduced. In patients with recurrent lesions, aciclovir treatment reduced the time to crusting of lesions in men but did not alter the symptoms or time to healing in women. Topical treatment with aciclovir has no effect on the time to first clinical recurrence with either herpes simplex virus type 1 or type 2 infections (Corey *et al.*, 1982a; Barton *et al.*, 1984).

ii Herpes labialis Treatment of patients during the prodromal phase with oral aciclovir (200 mg or 400 mg five times per day) for 5 days reduces the pain of the lesions and the time they take to crust by about 30% (Raborn *et al.*, 1987; Spruance *et al.*, 1990). There are a large number of studies supporting the use of suppressive therapy to prevent recurrences of herpes labialis (Thomas *et al.*, 1985; Green *et al.*, 1985; Spruance *et al.*, 1991; Rooney *et al.*, 1993). Aciclovir is also useful for recurrent herpes simplex infection that is induced by ultraviolet light exposure (Rooney *et al.*, 1992). A dose of 400 mg twice-daily appears to be effective.

In patients with recurrent herpes labialis, studies of suppressive therapy using aciclovir ointment or creams have provided mixed but predominantly disappointing results. Spruance *et al.* (1982) used 5% aciclovir ointment with polyethylene glycol as the vehicle in a controlled trial; reduced excretion of virus from lesions only occurred in patients who started treatment within 8 h of the onset of lesions, and no clinical benefit was observed. Spruance *et al.* (1984) showed in another trial that topical 10% aciclovir in polyethylene glycol was of no benefit in recurrent herpes labialis despite initiation of treatment in the prodrome or erythema stage of the disease. These findings showing lack of efficacy were confirmed by the same group in a more recent study, when 5% aciclovir was applied eight times daily without evidence of suppression (Spruance *et al.*, 1991). Somewhat better results were obtained by Fiddian and Ivanyi (1983) using a 5% ointment for recurrent herpes labialis; although treatment only shortened the duration of lesions by about 1 day, it greatly increased the number of abortive lesions. The poor results obtained using the polyethylene glycol ointment are probably due to the poor skin penetration of this formulation (Freeman et al., 1986). A 5% aciclovir cream using propylene glycol, which allows better penetration of the skin, produced better results in other controlled trials (Fiddian et al., 1983; Van Vloten et al., 1983). When treatment was started early in the course of the infection, the time for healing of ulcers was shortened, and the percentage of lesions progressing beyond the papular stage was reduced. The drug had no effect on the development of new lesions. In contrast, Shaw et al. (1985) found that 5% aciclovir cream had no therapeutic benefit over placebo 40% propylene glycol cream in patients with recurrent herpes labialis; they speculated whether the cream base itself may be beneficial.

iii Herpetic whitlow Herpetic whitlow responds to aciclovir suppressive therapy and treatment (Laskin, 1985; Schwandt et al., 1987).

iv Mucocutaneous herpes simplex in immunocompromised patients Controlled studies have demonstrated that treatment with aciclovir decreases the duration and severity of mucocutaneous herpes simplex infections in immunocompromised patients; these reactivation infections cause considerable morbidity and occasionally result in death due to dissemination. In most studies, the drug was given in an i.v. dosage of either 5 or 10 mg per kg every 8 h for 5–7 days. Termination of viral shedding was reduced in parallel with clinical response. Later recurrences of herpes simplex infections were not prevented. Trials involved patients with underlying malignancy or blood disease or recipients of bone marrow, cardiac or renal transplants (Chou et al., 1981; Mitchell et al., 1981; Meyers et al., 1982; Straus et al., 1982; Wade et al., 1982a). The currently recommended dose for treatment of mucocutaneous herpes simplex in immunocompromised patients is 5 mg per kg body weight, three times daily, given i.v.

An aciclovir dosage of about 5 mg per kg i.v. every 8–12 h for several weeks has also been highly effective in controlled trials to prevent herpes simplex infections in immunosuppressed patients (Saral et al., 1981, 1983; Hann et al., 1983; Prentice and Hann, 1983; Anderson et al., 1984). However, when a lower dose of i.v. aciclovir (250 mg per m² once-daily) was given for 4 weeks to bone marrow transplant recipients, although there was some delay in the appearance of herpetic lesions, protection was incomplete; this was clinically unacceptable compared with the above regimens (Shepp et al., 1985a). Mild clinical infections or viral shedding may occur after discontinuation of prophylaxis (Saral et al., 1981, 1983).

A well controlled study demonstrated that oral aciclovir, given in a dose of 400 mg five times daily for 10 days to marrow transplant recipients with recurrent mucocutaneous herpes simplex ulceration, was effective in shortening the period of viral shedding, new lesion formation, pain and time to healing; the results compared well with previous data from i.v. studies (Shepp et al., 1985b).

Oral aciclovir has also been used with some success to prevent mucocutaneous herpes simplex infections in immunosuppressed patients (Straus et al. 1982; Prentice and Hann, 1983). Better results were obtained by Gluckman et al. (1983) who used an oral dose of 200 mg 6-hourly in a controlled study of 39 bone marrow transplant recipients. Treatment was given from 8 days before to 35 days after transplantation. Protection against herpes simplex infection was complete in the treated group but 13 of 19 placebo-treated patients developed infection. There was no difference between these groups in the frequency of herpetic infection after cessation of treatment (days 35 to 100). In another controlled trial of bone marrow transplant recipients a dose of 400 mg of aciclovir was used every 4 h five times daily and treatment was begun 1 week before transplantation and was continued for a total of 5 weeks; five of 24 patients receiving aciclovir developed herpes simplex infection during prophylaxis (two of these were asymptomatic and the other three were not compliant), compared with 17 infections in 25 patients receiving placebo (Wade et al., 1984). Oral aciclovir (200 mg four times daily) has been used successfully to prevent herpes simplex infections in renal transplant recipients (Pettersson et al., 1985). Aciclovir does not appear to influence the development of graft-versus-host-disease (Saral, 1993).

A combination of i.v. and orally administered aciclovir was used by Lundgren et al. (1985) as prophylaxis against herpes virus infections in bone marrow transplant recipients. An i.v. dosage of 250 mg per m² twice-daily for 5 days was given before transplantation. By 5 weeks after transplantation, 400 mg orally three times daily (children less than 6 years, 200 mg three times daily) was substituted and continued until 6 months after transplantation. Of 22 placebo-treated patients, there were ten acute herpes simplex infections and five bouts of varicella-zoster. Among aciclovir-treated patients there was only one episode of herpes simplex infection.

Topical aciclovir ointment (5% in polyethylene glycol) was used to treat mucocutaneous herpes simplex infections in immunocompromised patients; the time for total healing of lesions was not altered, but the duration of viral shedding and pain was reduced (Whitley *et al.*, 1982b). Results from a later trial using the same ointment for a similar patient population were more encouraging; compared with a placebo-treated group, aciclovir recipients had accelerated clearance of virus and more rapid resolution of pain and enhanced healing (Whitley *et al.*, 1984). In a small trial, the topical use of a 5% aciclovir cream (40% propylene glycol) was ineffective in preventing recurrent herpes simplex infection with and without erythema multiforme (Fawcett *et al.*, 1983). Topical therapy is only recommended for the treatment of extremely minor lesions in immunocompromised patients (Whitley and Gnann, 1993).

v Aciclovir-resistant herpes simplex virus In adult and pediatric patients with HIV infection and other causes of immune suppression including bone marrow transplantation and hematological malignancy, resistance of herpes simplex to aciclovir can result in chronic lesions unresponsive to aciclovir therapy, but responsive to foscarnet (Erlich *et al.*, 1989b; Chatis *et al.*, 1989; Englund *et al.*, 1990; Safrin *et al.*, 1990, 1991a; Ljungman *et al.*, 1990; Hardy, 1992; Verdonck *et al.*, 1993; Balfour *et al.*, 1994). Aciclovir-resistant herpes simplex in HIV-infected patients is predominantly due to type 2 (90%), and usually causes extensive local disease (Fig. V.3) rather than cutaneous or visceral dissemination in patients with an advanced stage of immune suppression (CD4 count of less than 100 cells per μl) (Safrin 1993). Meningoencephalitis and esophagitis due to aciclovir-resistant herpes simplex have been reported (Sacks *et al.*, 1989; Gateley *et al.*, 1990).

Isolates that are both aciclovir- and foscarnet-resistant have been identified in HIV-infected patients with chronic clinically significant disease (Safrin *et al.*, 1994b). Topical trifluorothymidine with or without interferon alpha has also been found to benefit some patients with aciclovir-resistant herpes simplex (Birch *et al.*, 1992; Murphy *et al.*, 1992; Kessler *et al.*, 1996). Cidofovir (p. 1599) has resulted in clinical response in one patient with aciclovir-resistant herpes genitalis, although renal toxicity prevented completion of therapy (Lalezari *et al.*, 1994). There are no data to suggest benefit from the use of ribonucleotide reductase inhibitors in the treatment of aciclovir-resistant herpes simplex virus (Safrin *et al.*, 1993b).

Shedding of aciclovir-resistant herpes simplex by immunocompetent patients has been noted (Kost *et al.*, 1993). Aciclovir-resistant isolates of herpes simplex have been identified in persons receiving long-term suppressive therapy for genital herpes, but are generally not considered to be of any clinical significance and are not usually associated with treatment failure. However, there are rare case reports which indicate the potential of these resistant isolates to be clinically relevant (reviewed in Pottage and Kessler, 1995). An otherwise healthy young man developed recurrent genital herpes that was not suppressed by aciclovir therapy (Kost *et al.*, 1993). There is another report of a young man who had no prior history of genital herpes who presented with cutaneous and visceral dissemination of aciclovir-resistant herpes simplex type 2 infection developing 2 weeks after unprotected sexual intercourse. After failing to improve with i.v. aciclovir he responded to foscarnet therapy (Jones and Paul, 1995a). Transmission of aciclovir-resistant herpes simplex virus has also been reported in a neonate who subsequently developed stridor due to laryngeal infection (Nyquist *et al.*, 1994).

b Eye infections due to herpes simplex Aciclovir, used as a 3% ophthalmic ointment, is effective for herpes simplex keratitis (Jones *et al.*, 1979; Shiota, 1982). In controlled studies, aciclovir has been equally or more effective than adenine arabinoside (Laibson *et al.*, 1982; Young *et al.*, 1982), superior to idoxuridine (Collum *et al.*, 1982) and equally effective as trifluorothymidine (La Lau *et al.*, 1982). Aciclovir ophthalmic ointment has been used successfully to treat herpetic keratitis caused by viral strains clinically resistant to adenine arabinoside and idoxuridine (McGill and Tormey 1982). Aciclovir, because it penetrates the cornea and is of low toxicity, may be useful for deeper stromal eye infections, which require long-term medication (Collum *et al.*, 1982; Falcon, 1983).

c Herpes simplex encephalitis and disseminated infection

i Encephalitis Aciclovir is the drug of choice for the treatment of herpes simplex encephalitis. Despite therapy, neurologic sequelae are likely (Gordon *et al.*, 1990). Therapy should begin as soon as the diagnosis is suspected clinically and even before diagnostic investigations have been completed. Because of the low toxicity of aciclovir and the development of less invasive diagnostic procedures, the need for a brain biopsy to confirm the diagnosis is small. Results of two early trials, comparing aciclovir and adenine arabinoside, one Swedish and one American, have demonstrated that aciclovir is the most effective drug for herpes simplex encephalitis.

Fig. V.5.

Comparison of survival in patients with herpes simplex encephalitis treated with vidarabine or aciclovir. (Reproduced from Whitley *et al.*, 1986, with permission.)

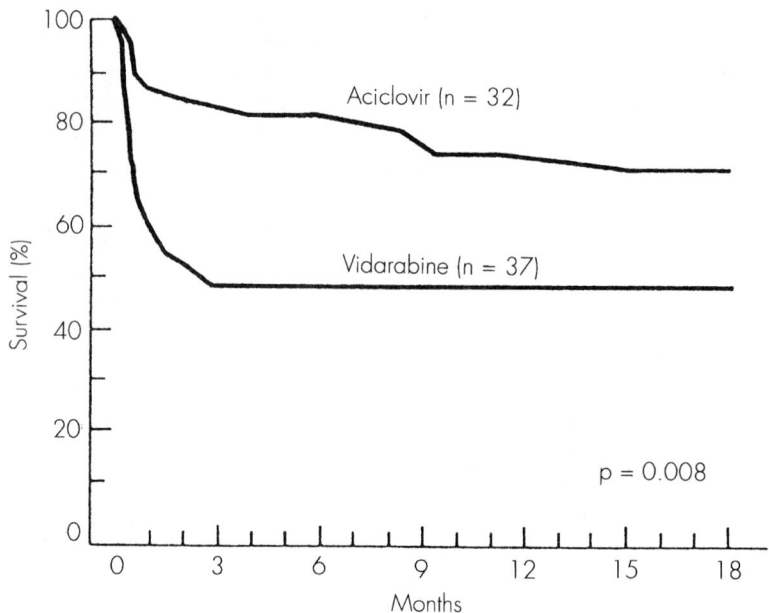

In the Swedish trial (Skoldenberg *et al.*, 1984) of 53 confirmed cases of herpes simplex encephalitis, 27 were treated with aciclovir (10 mg per kg 8-hourly) and 24 with adenine arabinoside (15mg per kg daily) for 10 days. Mortality was 19% in the aciclovir-treated group versus 50% in the adenine arabinoside group; after 6 months of observation 56% of the aciclovir-treated patients had returned to normal life compared with 13% of adenine arabinoside-treated patients; and the percentages who died or had severe sequelae were 33 and 76% respectively. In the American study (Whitley *et al.*, 1986) all cases were confirmed by brain biopsy whereas in Sweden various methods were used to confirm herpes simplex encephalitis. Nevertheless, results were very similar. Whitley *et al.* (1986) treated 37 patients with adenine arabinoside and 32 with aciclovir, using the same dosage regimens as used in Sweden. Mortality in adenine arabinoside recipients was 54%, compared with 28% in aciclovir recipients (Fig. V.5). A second course of aciclovir therapy is recommended for patients who relapse (Nicolaidou *et al.*, 1993).

ii Neonatal infections Approximately 80% of infants with neonatal herpes simplex virus infection will have typical mucocutaneous infections; the remainder will develop encephalitis or evidence of disseminated infection with hepatitis and pneumonia. Both aciclovir and vidarabine have been found to be of benefit in the treatment of these neonatal infections. In a multicenter, randomized blinded study of i.v. aciclovir (30 mg per kg per day) versus vidarabine for the treatment of neonatal herpes simplex infection (encephalitis in 71 babies and disseminated disease in 46), no difference was found in outcome in terms of morbidity or mortality between these two drugs (Whitley *et al.*, 1991). Laryngitis and tracheitis causing stridor and respiratory distress in a neonate with herpes simplex type 2 infection resolved following a prolonged course of aciclovir (Vitale *et al.*, 1993).

iii Disseminated herpes simplex infection in adults Presentation with fever and symptoms or signs of mucocutaneous dissemination, and/or visceral involvement, especially fulminant hepatitis, in pregnant women or other more profoundly immunocompromised patients is often fatal despite aciclovir therapy (Johnson *et al.*, 1992; Wolfsen *et al.*, 1993; Mudido *et al.*, 1993; Greenspoon *et al.*, 1994).

d   Other   Woolfson (1984) attributed clinical response in two young men with eczema herpeticum to treatment with oral aciclovir in a dosage of 100–200mg five times daily. Robinson *et al.* (1984) described two patients with genital herpes complicated by eczema herpeticum who responded to oral treatment with aciclovir. There have subsequently been a number of other reports supporting the use of aciclovir in this clinical setting (Niimura and Nishikawa, 1988; Parker and Guin, 1993). Erythema multiforme is often precipitated by preceding herpes simplex virus infection, and may be prevented by long-term suppressive therapy with aciclovir or by patient-initiated aciclovir therapy at the onset of recurrence of infection (Schofield *et al.*, 1993; Choy *et al.*, 1995). This has been recently confirmed by results from a randomized, double-blind placebo-controlled study of 20 patients with more than four episodes of herpes simplex-induced erythema multiforme per year, in whom continuous aciclovir suppressive therapy completely abolished recurrences (Tatnall *et al.*, 1995). Occasionally, erythema multiforme may be precipitated by Epstein–Barr virus infection; successful treatment with oral aciclovir has been described (Drago *et al.*, 1992). Aciclovir has also been found to be of clinical benefit in patients with Stevens–Johnson syndrome preceded by herpes simplex infection (Detjen *et al.*, 1992).

There is a report of two toddlers with atypical croup due to herpes simplex type 1 that responded promptly to aciclovir therapy (Inglis, 1993). Pharyngitis and esophagitis due to both herpes simplex types 1 and 2 in both adults and children with no evidence of underlying immune suppression respond to therapy with aciclovir (Lambert and Eastham, 1987; Galbraith and Shafran, 1992; McMillan *et al.*, 1993). Meningitis complicating either primary or recurrent herpes simplex type 2 responds well to aciclovir (Bergstrom and Alestig, 1990). Although extremely rare, herpes simplex virus pneumonia responsive to aciclovir therapy has been reported in young adults who have no evidence of immune deficiency (Martinez *et al.*, 1994).

2 Varicella-zoster virus infections

a Herpes zoster in the immunocompetent host Aciclovir is effective in the treatment of herpes zoster in normal adults; debate continues regarding who should receive treatment. This author generally offers treatment to all adults who present within 72 h of onset of lesions.

Intravenously administered aciclovir was found to be of benefit in the treatment of herpes zoster in early open clinical studies (Selby *et al.*, 1979; Spector *et al.*, 1982; Van der Meer and Versteeg, 1982; Ackland *et al.*, 1983). Results of controlled trials have confirmed these clinical impressions. In otherwise normal patients with herpes zoster, i.v. doses of 5–10 mg per kg, or 500 mg per m^2 (8.6–14.9 mg per kg), every 8 h have been employed for periods of about 5 days. Most trials demonstrated increased rate of healing of skin lesions, shortened period of pain in the acute phase, prevention of development of new lesions and reduction in duration of viral shedding, without reduction in post-herpetic neuralgia (Peterslund *et al.*, 1981; Bean *et al.*, 1982; Esmann *et al.*, 1982; McGill *et al.*, 1983; Huff *et al.*, 1988).

Orally administered aciclovir is more commonly used to treat herpes zoster in the immunocompetent host than intravenous therapy. Early experience with 19 otherwise healthy adults with herpes zoster suggested that an oral dosage of aciclovir of 200 mg five times daily for 5 days may arrest the infection if given within 24 h of the rash appearing (Finn and Smith, 1984). McKendrick *et al.* (1984) were sceptical as to whether this dose was adequate, and reported on their controlled trials in which higher oral doses were used; in 41 otherwise healthy adult patients entered within 72 h of the onset of rash, a dose of 400mg five times daily for 5 days suppressed new lesion formation but differences in other indices did not achieve significance. In another trial in which 41 similar patients were given 800 mg five times daily for 7 days, there was a reduction in the duration of vesicles, time to first and full crusting and pain severity during the first week. Supported by the results of a number of randomized trials (Wood *et al.*, 1988; Huff *et al.*, 1988) the recommended dose is 800 mg given five times per day. Therapy should be commenced as early as possible after the development of rash (within 48 h) and little effect is observed if therapy is delayed beyond 72 h (Wood *et al.*, 1988).

Whilst it is clear from controlled studies that aciclovir therapy can reduce both the severity and duration of acute pain associated with zoster, studies on the efficacy of aciclovir in preventing post-herpetic neuralgia have produced conflicting results (Van den Broek *et al.*, 1984; Wood *et al.*, 1988; McKendrick *et al.*, 1989; Benoldi *et al.*, 1991), suggesting that if an effect is present it is only marginal. When acute and chronic pain are considered as a continuum (zoster-associated pain) aciclovir has been reported to reduce the duration, when compared with placebo (Huff *et al.*, 1993). In a recent trial, 400 patients who had herpes zoster for less than 72 h were randomized to receive aciclovir in a dose of 800 mg five times per day for 7 or 21 days together with either prednisolone or placebo. Only slight benefits were observed with either longer therapy or the addition of prednisolone when compared with standard treatment of 7 days of aciclovir alone (Wood *et al.*, 1994b). Whitley and colleagues (1996) have recently published results from a randomized, placebo-controlled study involving 208 immunocompetent patients aged older than 50 years with localized herpes zoster who were enrolled within 72 h of onset. Patients randomized to receive aciclovir and prednisolone had accelerated time to cessation of acute neuritis compared with those who received aciclovir alone or no active therapy, although resolution of chronic pain was not significantly different to that in other groups.

b **Herpes zoster ophthalmicus** There is considerable debate regarding the optimum treatment of ophthalmic zoster and its complications. Intraocular complications, predominantly uveitis and keratitis, occur in about 50% of cases. Oral aciclovir treatment of herpes zoster ophthalmicus has been found to reduce the risk of complications including uveitis and keratitis, particularly if commenced within 48 h of onset of rash (Cobo *et al.*, 1986; Harding and Porter, 1991; Whitley and Gnann, 1992). However, treatment as late as 7 days after onset of lesions may still be of benefit (Cobo, 1988).

In one early study, topical administration of aciclovir to the eye controlled ocular complications of zoster, whereas i.v. therapy did not have an effect (McGill *et al.*, 1983). In a double-blind, randomized comparison of topical aciclovir versus topical betamethasone, these investigators found that aciclovir therapy was superior to glucocorticoids, as it shortened the duration of treatment, and was associated with fewer recurrences. However, although the time to resolution of corneal epithelial disease was shorter in aciclovir recipients, this benefit was not seen in patients with uveitis or scleritis (McGill and Chapman, 1983). These findings are not supported by the study of Marsh and Cooper (1991) who, on the basis of their findings that topical aciclovir alone was ineffective in controlling ocular inflammation, suggested the use of combination therapy. Current opinion favors the use of topical aciclovir monotherapy .

c **Herpes zoster in the immunocompromised host** Intravenous aciclovir significantly reduces the frequency of cutaneous dissemination and of the development of visceral complications of herpes zoster in immunocompromised patients (Whitley *et al.*, 1982c; Balfour *et al.*, 1983a). The currently recommended dose of i.v. aciclovir for the treatment of zoster or varicella in immunocompromised patients is 10 mg per kg of body weight administered three times per day. The benefits of oral therapy in immunocompromised adults with herpes zoster are not clear, and thus oral aciclovir should not be used in patients with profound immunosuppression, including bone marrow transplant recipients (Whitley and Gnann, 1992). In addition, aciclovir prophylaxis in bone marrow transplant recipients has been found in some studies to lower the risk of varicella-zoster virus infection and mortality (Perren *et al.*, 1988; Sempere *et al.*, 1992; Masaoka *et al.*, 1993), but not in others (Han *et al.*, 1994).

When aciclovir was compared with adenine arabinoside to treat varicella-zoster virus infections in severely immunocompromised patients, aciclovir was more effective than adenine arabinoside in preventing dissemination of infection, and promoting cutaneous healing and relief of pain (Shepp *et al.*, 1986). In another study, in which patients had disseminated herpes zoster at entry, aciclovir and vidarabine had similar efficacy (Whitley *et al.*, 1992). Aciclovir was effective for the treatment of immunocompromised patients with varicella-zoster meningoencephalitis; clinical response was noted by the third day of therapy and virus could not be cultured from vesicles and CSF at the end of 7 days of treatment (Steele *et al.*, 1983).

Patients with advanced HIV infection with varicella-zoster virus retinopathy require chronic suppressive therapy to prevent recurrences (Johnston *et al.*, 1993). Treatment of progressive outer retinal necrosis (thought to be due to varicella-zoster virus in patients with AIDS) has met with only limited success (Pinnolis *et al.*, 1995). The condition may be unilateral or bilateral, and is rapidly progressive with widespread retinal involvement and often retinal detachment with ultimately complete loss of vision. Very high dose aciclovir is considered the best option, but the condition has a poor prognosis (Pavesio *et al.*, 1995).

d **Aciclovir-resistant varicella-zoster virus infection** In both adult and pediatric patients with advanced HIV infection, chronic, hyperkeratotic papules due to aciclovir-resistant varicella-zoster virus have been reported (Pahwa *et al.*, 1988; Linnemann *et al.*, 1990; Lokke-Jensen *et al.*, 1993; Colebunders *et al.*, 1994; Lyall *et al.*, 1994). Meningoradiculoneuritis due to aciclovir-resistant varicella-zoster virus has also been reported in a patient with AIDS (Snoeck *et al.*, 1994). Foscarnet is the drug of choice for aciclovir-resistant zoster (Safrin *et al.*, 1991b). Trifluorothymidine alone or in combination with interferon alpha may also be of benefit in cases of aciclovir-resistance (Rossi *et al.*, 1995).

e **Congenital or neonatal varicella** Congenital varicella syndrome is associated with cutaneous and neuropathic damage, and is not usually associated with active viral replication. Thus aciclovir therapy is rarely useful in this situation (Arvin, 1993). Infants with varicella lesions or who develop varicella within the first 5 days of life as a result of maternal varicella late in pregnancy rarely develop severe varicella and rarely require aciclovir therapy. In contrast, if maternal varicella occurs close to delivery (4–5 days before, to 2 days after), the infant is at risk of fatal varicella infection, and varicella-zoster immune globulin should be administered at birth and i.v. aciclovir given if there is evidence of varicella with complications such as pneumonia, encephalitis, hepatitis or coagulation disorder (Arvin, 1993). Although varicella-zoster immune globulin reduces the risk of complications, in one study administration of this prophylaxis at birth to 118 infants with perinatal exposure failed to prevent severe varicella in 14% (Miller et al., 1989).

f   Varicella or herpes zoster in the pediatric immunocompromised host   Aciclovir therapy, administered by the i.v. route, substantially decreases morbidity and mortality in immunocompromised children with varicella. The recommended dose in children under 12 years of age is 500 mg per m^2 (about 12 mg per kg) every 8 h for 5 days (Whitley and Gnann, 1993). Although there are studies supporting its use (Novelli et al., 1984; Meszner et al., 1993), oral aciclovir therapy is not indicated for the treatment of varicella in immunocompromised children.

In an early open trial in four immunocompromised children who developed herpes zoster after bone marrow transplantation, aciclovir was administered in a dosage of 500 mg per m^2 every 8 h for 5 days; there was rapid improvement in the lesions and rapid relief of pain (Serota et al., 1982). The same regimen was used in a controlled trial to treat localized and disseminated herpes zoster in immunocompromised patients. Progression of lesions was halted even in patients whose therapy was delayed for 3 days after the onset of rash. However, there were fewer complications if the drug was given within the first 3 days of development of lesions, and there was accelerated clearance of virus from lesions (Balfour et al., 1983a).

The efficacy of i.v. aciclovir was further described in reports of two controlled trials in immunosuppressed children with varicella when a dose of 500 mg per m^2 (about 12 mg per kg) every 8 h for 7 days was used (Prober et al., 1982; Nyerges et al., 1988). However, administration of aciclovir together with varicella-zoster immune globulin to children with organ transplants following their exposure to varicella did not provide complete protection in one report (Lynfield et al., 1992). There is a case-report describing the efficacy of i.v. aciclovir therapy in an immunosuppressed adolescent with disseminated multifocal leukoencephalitis due to varicella-zoster virus (Herrold and Hahn, 1994).

g   Varicella in immunocompetent children and adolescents   A well-controlled study from the University of Minnesota provided data showing the safety of aciclovir at a dose of 20 mg per kg and the superior efficacy of this dose, when compared with 10 or 15 mg per kg, in terms of decreasing the number of skin lesions, their time to healing, the severity and duration of fever and other constitutional symptoms (Balfour et al., 1990; Balfour, 1993). In subsequent studies it became apparent that morbidity and mortality are higher in adolescents than in young children with varicella, and in secondary and tertiary cases within a household. In one of these studies, aciclovir was given at a dose of 20 mg per kg for children and 800 mg for adolescents, four times per day for 5 days commencing within 24 h of onset of rash; there was no alteration in antibody response as a result of therapy (Dunkle et al., 1991; Balfour et al., 1992). Aciclovir does not decrease the risk of transmission of the virus within the household (Feldman, 1993), nor reduce the duration of absence from school (American Academy of Pediatric Committee on Infectious Diseases, 1993).

Oral aciclovir has been given in an open multicenter study to children aged 3 months to 2 years in doses of 80 mg per kg per day in four divided doses for 4–6 days. When administered any time within the first 24 h, aciclovir resulted in a rapid defervescence, resolution of itch and other constitutional symptoms and cessation of new lesions with acceleration of healing of existing lesions; however, there was no placebo group for comparison (Chiodo et al., 1995).

There is no clear recommendation regarding the use of aciclovir in immunocompetent children and adolescents with varicella. The recent approval of the varicella vaccine will no doubt change the need for therapy. However, in this author's opinion aciclovir therapy should currently be considered in those with the highest risk of morbidity, namely all young children and infants, all adolescents and in all secondary and tertiary cases within a household. Other clinicians would treat all cases.

In one unrandomized study, post-exposure prophylaxis of family members using aciclovir (40 or 80 mg per kg per day in four divided doses for 7 days) was successful in preventing or modifying varicella, even when administered late in the incubation period. In 25 exposed children or infants who received aciclovir 7–9 days after exposure to the index case in the family, 16% developed varicella and 4% had fever, compared with 25 controls all of whom developed disease and over two-thirds developed fever; 84% of aciclovir recipients seroconverted (Asano et al., 1993).

h   Varicella in immunocompetent adults   Several controlled studies have found that both i.v. and oral aciclovir therapy if commenced early following the onset of rash can decrease the time to healing, the duration of fever, the maximum number of lesions, virus titer within the vesicles and severity of symptoms (Al-Nakib *et al.*, 1983; Feder, 1990; Wallace *et al.*, 1992). Treatment must be initiated within the first 24 h for aciclovir to be efficacious (Wallace *et al.*, 1992).

Although there are no controlled studies to prove efficacy, treatment of adults with varicella complicated by pneumonia using i.v. aciclovir is strongly supported by case reports and uncontrolled studies (Schlossberg and Littman, 1988; Haake *et al.*, 1990). Varicella pneumonia in a pregnant woman should be regarded as potentially life-threatening and treated with i.v. aciclovir (Smego and Asperilla, 1991; Boyd and Walker, 1988; Arvin, 1993; Haake *et al.*, 1990).

Oral aciclovir is not recommended for the treatment of uncomplicated varicella in pregnant women because risks and benefits to mother and fetus are not known (United States Pharmacopeia Drug Information, 1997).

3 Cytomegalovirus infections

Because cytomegalovirus is less sensitive to aciclovir than either herpes simplex or varicella-zoster virus, this drug is not effective for the treatment of cytomegalovirus infections (Wade *et al.*, 1982b, 1983b; Shepp *et al.*, 1984; Plotkin *et al.*, 1982). However, it has been found in some studies to decrease the frequency of symptomatic cytomegalovirus infections post-transplantation including in heart, renal and bone-marrow transplant recipients (Gluckman *et al.*, 1983; Meyers *et al.*, 1988; Balfour *et al.*, 1989; Fletcher *et al.*, 1991; Elkins *et al.*, 1993; Legendre *et al.*, 1993; Mollison *et al.*, 1993; Dunn *et al.*, 1994), but has not been successful in preventing cytomegalovirus infection or disease in all studies, especially in liver transplant recipients (Wong *et al.*, 1993; Bailey *et al.*, 1993; Bacigalupo *et al.*, 1994; Singh *et al.*, 1994; Boeck *et al.*, 1995; Winston *et al.*, 1995). Aciclovir is generally considered to be inferior to ganciclovir as prophylaxis against cytomegalovirus infection or disease in this patient population (p. 1577) (Martin *et al.*, 1994; Duncan *et al.*, 1994). In a study of 93 patients with symptomatic HIV infection, high-dose aciclovir failed to suppress the excretion of cytomegalovirus in urine; of potential importance in this patient population, aciclovir therapy was not associated with the development of ganciclovir-resistant strains of cytomegalovirus (Drew *et al.*, 1995). In a small, open-label study of patients with HIV-related cytomegalovirus retinitis who were treated with i.v. aciclovir (10 mg per kg of body weight every 8 h) following a course of ganciclovir induction therapy there was a median time to disease progression of only 32 days, suggesting that aciclovir is better than no therapy but inferior to ganciclovir or foscarnet (Sha *et al.*, 1991).

Oral aciclovir has also been used in a number of studies of patients undergoing solid organ transplantation as prophylactic therapy against cytomegalovirus infection and disease (Pay *et al.*, 1993; Prentice *et al.*, 1994). The data from these studies suggest that although in some cases aciclovir can prevent infection or delay the development of disease, it is inferior in efficacy to ganciclovir (p. 1579).

4 Epstein–Barr virus infection

Epstein–Barr virus which infects and replicates in B lymphocytes is a cause of lymphoproliferative disorders in immunodeficient hosts. Hanto *et al.* (1982) reported a patient with Epstein–Barr virus associated polyclonal B cell lymphoproliferative disease following renal transplantation, whose disease underwent regression on two occasions after treatment with i.v. aciclovir, before finally succumbing to the illness. However, i.v. aciclovir was of no apparent benefit in other reported cases of life-threatening Epstein–Barr virus infection (Sullivan *et al.*, 1982; Sakamoto *et al.*, 1992). In studies of patients with infectious mononucleosis, the use of i.v. aciclovir transiently interrupted virus excretion in the oropharynx, but clinical features of the disease were largely unaffected (Pagano *et al.*, 1983; Andersson *et al.*, 1985). Similarly, in patients with asymptomatic HIV infection, treatment with high-dose oral aciclovir did not eliminate persistent Epstein–Barr virus infection from the oropharynx (Luxton *et al.*, 1993). Oral therapy was found to be ineffective in the treatment of infectious mononucleosis (Van der Horst *et al.*, 1991). Oral hairy leukoplakia may respond to oral aciclovir (Resnick *et al.*, 1988; Lozada-Nur and Costa, 1992; Laskaris *et al.*, 1995), although patients frequently develop recurrences after cessation of therapy (Herbst *et al.*, 1989).

5 Hepatitis B virus infection

In early uncontrolled trials, aciclovir (10–15 mg per kg 8-hourly) given to patients with hepatitis B virus-related chronic liver disease, resulted in a decrease in hepatitis B virus-DNA polymerase and hepatitis B virus-DNA in some patients (Weller *et al.*, 1983). Similarly DNA polymerase activity was reduced in one patient with chronic hepatitis associated with hepatitis B virus when i.v. doses of aciclovir varying from 15 to 45 mg per kg daily were used (Smith *et al.*, 1982). Schalm *et al.* (1985, 1986) found that a combination of i.v. aciclovir and interferon in a small number of patients was more effective in depressing hepatitis B virus-DNA polymerase and HBe antigenemia than aciclovir or interferon alone. However, two large multicenter, randomized trials failed to demonstrate any benefit of aciclovir alone or any enhancement by aciclovir of the effects of interferon alpha on HBe antigen seroconversion in patients with chronic hepatitis B infection (Alexander *et al.*, 1986; Alexander *et al.*, 1987; Berk *et al.*, 1992).

6 Human immunodeficiency virus

Oral aciclovir therapy in doses of 800 mg four times per day has been used in conjunction with zidovudine in patients with HIV infection and, although not associated with a reduced risk of cytomegalovirus disease, in some studies the combination therapy has been associated with improved survival (Cooper *et al.*, 1993; Youle *et al.*, 1994; Stein *et al.*, 1994; Apolonio *et al.*, 1995). However, a recent observational study of over 1000 persons with advanced HIV infection failed to confirm these data (Gallant *et al.*, 1995). A new human herpes virus has been identified as the putative cause of AIDS-associated Kaposi's sarcoma. Examination of a large data-base revealed that the risk for Kaposi's sarcoma was lower in patients who had been treated with foscarnet but not with aciclovir (Jones *et al.*, 1995).

6 Other viruses

Intravenous aciclovir was administered to patients with chronic non-A, non-B hepatitis or to patients with chronic delta virus hepatitis without any appreciable long-term beneficial effect (Pappas *et al.*, 1985; Berk *et al.*, 1991). Herpes virus simiae may respond to aciclovir (Holmes *et al.*, 1990). Aciclovir therapy has been reported to provide no benefit in children with juvenile respiratory papillomatosis (Morrisson and Evans, 1993), although when combined with surgery, other investigators have found that a 6-month course of aciclovir (400 mg per day in patients under 5 years and 800 mg per day in those over 5 years) resulted in clinical remission in 75% of children during a mean follow-up period of 18 months (Kiroglu *et al.*, 1994). Neither orogenital ulceration associated with Behçet's syndrome nor idiopathic aphthous stomatitis are responsive to aciclovir therapy (Wormser *et al.*, 1988; Davies *et al.*, 1988). However, patients with acute myeloid leukemia who were receiving induction chemotherapy and who received oral aciclovir 800 mg per day had significantly fewer intraoral ulcers excluding the soft palate and less acute necrotizing ulcerative gingivitis than placebo-treated control patients (Bergmann *et al.*, 1995). In a double-blind, placebo-controlled trial treatment with aciclovir of 27 patients with symptoms attributable to chronic fatigue syndrome did not result in clinical benefit (Straus *et al.*, 1988).

Acknowledgement   The author would like to thank Sharon Safrin of Gilead Sciences Inc. for her critical review of this chapter.

References

Ackland SP, Bishop JF, Whiteside MG (1983). Acyclovir therapy in patients with malignant disease and disseminated herpes zoster. *Med J Aust* **1**: 637.

Alenius S, Berg M, Broberg F *et al.* (1982). Therapeutic effects of foscarnet sodium and acyclovir on cutaneous infection due to herpes simplex virus type I in guinea pigs. *J Infect Dis* **145**: 569.

Alexander GJ, Fagan EA, Hegarty JE *et al.* (1986). A controlled trial of acyclovir in stable chronic HBsAg, HEeAg positive carriers. *J Hepatology* **3**: S123.

Alexander GJ, Fagan EA, Hegarty JE *et al.* (1987). Controlled clinical trial of acyclovir in chronic hepatitis B virus infection. *J Med Virol* **21**: 81.

Almond MK, Fan S, Dhillon S *et al.* (1995). Avoiding acyclovir neurotoxicity in patients with chronic renal failure undergoing haemodialysis. *Nephron* **69**: 428.

Al-Nakib W, Al-Kandari S, El-Khalik DMA, El-Shirbiny AM (1983). A randomised controlled study of intravenous acyclovir (Zovirax) against placebo in adults with chickenpox. *J Infect* **6**: 49.

American Academy of Pediatrics Committee on Infectious Diseases (1993). The use of oral acyclovir in otherwise healthy children with varicella. *Pediatrics* **91**: 674.

Amos RJ, Amess JAL (1983). Megaloblastic haemopoiesis due to acyclovir. *Lancet* i: 242.

Anderson H, Scarffe JH, Sutton RNP *et al.* (1984). Oral acyclovir, prophylaxis against herpes simplex virus in non-Hodgkin lymphoma and acute lymphoblastic leukaemia patients receiving remission induction chemotherapy. A randomised double-blind, placebo controlled trial. *Brit J Cancer* **50**: 45.

Andersson J, Skoldenberg B, Ernberg I *et al.* (1985). Acyclovir treatment in primary Epstein-Barr virus infection. A double-blind placebo-controlled study. *Scand J Infect Dis* **47**: 107.

Andrei G, Snoeck R, Goubau P *et al.* (1992). Comparative activity of various compounds against clinical strains of herpes simplex virus. *Eur J Clin Microbiol Infect Dis* **11**: 143.

Andrei G, Snoeck R, Reymen D *et al.* (1995). Comparative activity of selected antiviral compounds against clinical isolates of varicella zoster virus. *Eur J Clin Microbiol Infect Dis* **14**: 318.

Andrews EB, Yankaskas BC, Cordero JF et al. (1992). Acyclovir in pregnancy registry; six years' experience. The Acyclovir in Pregnancy Registry Advisory Committee. *Obstet Gynecol* **79**: 7.

Apolonio EG, Hoover DR, He Y et al. (1995). Prognostic factors in human immunodeficiency virus positive patients with a CD4+ lymphocyte count <50/microL. *J Infect Dis* **171**: 829.

Arvin AM (1993). Management of varicella zoster virus infections complicating pregnancy. *Antiviral Chemother* **3**: 117.

Asano Y, Yoshikawa T, Suga S et al. (1993). Postexposure prophylaxis of varicella in family contact by oral acyclovir. *Pediatrics* **92**: 219.

Bacigalupo A, Tedone E, Van Lint MT et al. (1994). CMV prophylaxis with foscarnet in allogeneic bone marrow transplant recipients at high risk of developing CMV infections. *Bone Marrow Transplant* **13**: 783.

Bacon TH, Boyd MR (1995). Activity of penciclovir against Epstein-Barr virus. *Antimicrob Ag Chemother* **39**: 1599.

Bailey TC, Ettinger NA, Storch GA et al. (1993). Failure of high-dose oral acyclovir with or without immune globulin to prevent primary cytomegalovirus disease in recipients of solid organ transplants. *Amer J Med* **95**: 273.

Baker DA (1994). Long-term suppressive therapy with acyclovir for recurrent genital herpes. *J Int Med Res* **22**: 24A.

Balfour HH (1993). Treatment of varicella in immunocompetent children. *Antiviral Chemother* **3**: 125.

Balfour HH Jr, Bean B, Laskin OL et al. (1983a). Acyclovir halts progression of herpes zoster in immunocompromised patients. *New Engl J Med* **308**: 1448.

Balfour HH et al. (1983b). Resistance of herpes simplex to acyclovir. *Ann Intern Med* **98**: 404.

Balfour HH, Chace BA Stapleton JT et al. (1989). A randomized, placebo-controlled trial of oral acyclovir for the prevention of cytomegalovirus disease in recipients of renal allografts. *New Engl J Med* **320**: 1381.

Balfour HH, Kelly JM, Suarez CS et al. (1990). Acyclovir treatment of varicella in otherwise healthy children. *J Pediatr* **116**: 633.

Balfour HH Rotbart HA, Feldman S et al. (1992). Acyclovir treatment of varicella in otherwise healthy adolescents. The Collaborative Acyclovir Varicella Study Group. *J Pediatr* **120**: 627.

Balfour HH, Benson C, Braun J et al. (1994). Management of acyclovir-resistant herpes simplex and varicella zoster virus infections. *J AIDS* **7**: 254.

Barry DW, Nusinoff-Lehrman S, Nixon Ellis M et al. (1985). Viral resistance, clinical experience. *Scand J Infect Dis* **47**: 155.

Barton IG, Kinghorn GR, Rowland M et al. (1984). Recurrences after first episodes of genital herpes in patients treated with acyclovir cream. *Antiviral Res* **4**: 293.

Bauer DJ (1982). Acyclovir treatment of experimental herpetic keratitis in the rabbit eye. *Amer J Med* **73**: 109.

Bean B, Aeppli D (1985). Adverse effects of high-dose intravenous acyclovir in ambulatory patients with acute herpes zoster. *J Infect Dis* **151**: 362.

Bean B, Fletcher C (1985). Neutropenia in immunocompromised patients receiving intravenous acyclovir. In *Program and Abstract of the 25th Interscience Conference on Antimicrobial Agents and Chemotherapy, Minneapolis* (Abst No 786). Washington, DC: American Society for Microbiology.

Bean B, Braun C, Balfour HH Jr (1982). Acyclovir therapy for acute herpes zoster. *Lancet* **ii**: 11.

Becker BN, Fall P, Hall C et al. (1993). Rapidly progressive acute renal failure due to acyclovir; case report and review of the literature. *Amer J Kidney Dis* **22**: 611.

Benoldi D, Mirizzi S, Zucchi A, Allegra F (1991). Prevention of post-herpetic neuralgia Evaluation of treatment with oral prednisolone, oral acyclovir, and radiotherapy. *Int J Dermatol* **30**: 288.

Bergmann OJ, Ellermann-Eriksen S, Mogensen SC, Ellegaard J (1995). Acyclovir given as prophylaxis against oral ulcers in acute myeloid leukaemia; randomised, double blind, placebo controlled trial. *Brit Med J* **310**: 1169.

Bergstrom T, Alestig K (1990). Treatment of primary and recurrent herpes simplex virus type 2 induced meningitis with acyclovir. *Scand J Infect Dis* **22**: 239.

Berk L, de Man RA, Housset C et al. (1991). Alpha lymphoblastoid interferon and acyclovir for chronic hepatitis delta. *Prog Clin Biol Res* **364**: 411.

Berk L, Schalm SW, de Man RA et al. (1992). Failure of acyclovir to enhance the antiviral effect of alpha lymphoblastoid interferon on HBe-seroconversion in chronic hepatitis B. A multicentre randomised trial. *J Hepatol* **14**: 305.

Bernstein DI, Lovett MA, Bryson YJ (1984). The effects of acyclovir on antibody response to herpes simplex virus in primary genital herpetic infections. *J Infect Dis* **150**: 7.

Bianchetti MG, Roduit C, Oetliker OH (1991). Acyclovir-induced renal failure: course and risk factors. *Pediatr Nephrol* **5**: 238.

Birch CJ, Tachedjian G, Doherty RR et al. (1990). Altered sensitivity to antiviral drugs of herpes simplex virus isolates from a patient with the acquired immunodeficiency syndrome. *J Infect Dis* **162**: 731.

Birch CJ, Tyssen DP, Tachedjian G et al. (1992). Clinical effects and in vitro studies of trifluorothymidine combined with interferon-alpha for treatment of drug resistant and sensitive herpes simplex virus infections. *J Infect Dis* **166**: 108.

Biron KK, Elion GB (1980). *In vitro* susceptibility of varicella-zoster virus to acyclovir. *Antimicrob Ag Chemother* **18**: 443.

Biron KK, Elion GB (1982). Effect of acyclovir combined with other antiherpetic agents on varicella zoster virus in vitro. *Amer J Med* **73**: 54.

Biron KK, Fyfe JA, Noblin JE, Elion GB (1982). Selection and preliminary characterization of acyclovir-resistant mutants of varicella zoster virus. *Amer J Med* **73**: 383.

Blum MR, Liao SHT, De Miranda P (1982). Overview of acyclovir pharmacokinetic disposition in adults and children. *Amer J Med* **73**: 186.

Boeckh M, Gooley TA, Reusser P et al. (1995). Failure of high-dose acyclovir to prevent cytomegalovirus disease after autologous marrow transplantation. *J Infect Dis* **172**: 939.

Boivin G, Erice A, Crane DD et al. (1993). Acyclovir susceptibilities of herpes simplex virus strains isolated from solid organ transplant recipients after acyclovir or ganciclovir prophylaxis. *Antimicrob Ag Chemother* **37**: 357.

Boivin G, Edelman CK, Pedneault L et al. (1994). Phenotypic and genotypic characterisation of acyclovir-resistant varicella zoster viruses isolated from persons with AIDS. *J Infect Dis* **170**: 68.

Boulter EA, Thornton B, Bauer DJ, Bye A (1980). Successful treatment or experimental B virus (herpes virus simiae) infection with acyclovir. *Brit Med J* **280**: 681.

Bowman CA, Woolley PD, Herman S et al. (1990). Asymptomatic herpes simplex virus shedding from the genital tract whilst on suppressive doses of oral acyclovir. *Int J STD AIDS* **1**: 174.

Boyd K, Walker E (1988). Use of acyclovir to treat chickenpox in pregnancy. *Brit Med J* **296**: 393.

Boyle TJ, Tamburini M, Berend KR et al. (1992). Human B-cell lymphoma in severe combined immunodeficient mice after active infection with Epstein-Barr virus. *Surgery* **112**: 378.

Brigden D, Rosling AE, Woods NC (1982). Renal function after acyclovir intravenous injection. *Amer J Med* **73**: 182.

Brigden D, Keeney RE, King DH (1983). The present and future of acyclovir. *J Antimicrob Chemother* **12**: 195.

Brown ZA, Baker DA (1989). Acyclovir therapy during pregnancy. *Obstet Gynecol* **73**: 526.

Bryson YJ, Dillon M, Lovett M et al. (1983). Treatment of first episodes of genital herpes simplex virus infection with oral acyclovir. *New Engl J Med* **308**: 916.

Buck ML, Vittone SB, Zaglul HF (1993). Vesicular eruptions following acyclovir administration. *Ann Pharmacother* **27**: 1458.

Burgess ED, Gill MJ (1990). Intraperitoneal administration of acyclovir in patients receiving continuous ambulatory peritoneal dialysis. *J Clin Pharmacol* **30**: 997.

Burns WH, Saral R, Santos GW *et al.* (1982). Isolation and characterisation of resistant herpes simplex virus after acyclovir therapy. *Lancet* i: 421.

Campos SB, Seguro AC, Cesar KB, Rocha AS (1992). Effects of acyclovir on renal function. *Nephron* 62: 74.

Caruso M, Klatzmann D (1992). Selective killing of CD4+ cells harboring a human immunodeficiency virus inducible suicide gene prevents viral spread in an infected cell population. *Proc Natl Acad Sci USA* 89: 182.

CDC (Centers for Disease Control and prevention) (1993). Sexually transmitted diseases treatment guidelines. *MMWR* 42 (No RR-14):19.

Chahoud I, Stahlmann R, Bochert G *et al.* (1988). Cross-structural defects in rats after acyclovir application on day 10 of gestation. *Arch Toxicol* 62: 8.

Chatis PA, Crumpacker CS (1991). Analysis of the thymidine kinase gene from clinically isolated acyclovir resistant herpes simplex viruses. *Virology* 180: 793.

Chatis PA, Miller CH, Schrager LE, Crumpacker CS (1989). Successful treatment with foscarnet of an acyclovir-resistant mucocutaneous infection with herpes simplex virus in a patient with acquired immunodeficiency syndrome. *New Engl J Med* 320: 297.

Chavanet PY, Bailly F, Mousson C *et al.* (1990a) Acyclovir pharmacokinetics in plasmapheresis. *J Clin Apheresis* 5: 68.

Chavanet P, Lokiec F, Portier H (1990b) Meningeal diffusion of high doses of acyclovir given with probenecid. *J Antimicrob Chemother* 26: 294.

Chiodo F, Manfredi R, Antonelli P *et al.* (1995). Varicella in immunocompetent children in the first two years of life; role of treatment with oral acyclovir. Italian Acyclovir-Chickenpox Study Group. *J Chemother* 7: 62.

Cho CT, Feng KK (1980). Combined effects of acycloguanosine and humoral antibodies in experimental encephalitis due to herpes virus hominis. *J Infect Dis* 142: 451.

Chou S, Gallagher JG, Merigan TC (1981). Controlled clinical trial of intravenous acyclovir in heart-transplant patients with mucocutaneous herpes simplex infections. *Lancet* i: 1392.

Choy AC, Yarnold PR, Brown JE *et al.* (1995). Virus induced erythema multiforme and Stevens-Johnson syndrome. *Allergy Proc* 16: 157.

Christophers J, Sutton RN (1987). Characterisation of acyclovir-resistant and sensitive clinical herpes simplex virus isolates from an immunocompromised patient. *J Antimicrob Ag Chemother* 20: 389.

Cioe L, Mukhopadhyay S, Rovera G (1992). Selective inhibition of proliferation in v-abl and bcr-abl- transformed cells by nucleoside analog. *J Biol Chem* 267: 22178.

Cobo LM (1988). Reduction of the ocular complications of herpes zoster ophthalmicus by oral acyclovir. *Amer J Med* 85: 90.

Cobo LM, Foulks GN, Liesegang T *et al.* (1986). Oral acyclovir in the treatment of acute herpes zoster ophthalmicus. *Ophthalmol* 93: 763.

Coen DM (1991). the implications of resistance to antiviral agents for herpesvirus drug targets and drug therapy. *Antivir Res* 15: 282.

Coen DM, Schaffer PA, Furman PA *et al.* (1982). Biochemical and genetic analysis of acyclovir-resistant mutants of herpes simplex virus type 1. *Amer J Med* 73: 351.

Cole NL, Balfour HH Jr (1986). Varicella-zoster virus does not become more resistant to acyclovir during therapy. *J Infect Dis* 153: 605.

Colebunders R, Van Damme L, Van den Abbeele K *et al.* (1994). Atypical varicella zoster infection in persons with HIV infection. *Acta Clin Belg* 49: 104.

Collins P, Bauer DJ (1979). The activity *in vitro* against herpes virus of 9-(2-hydroxyethoxymethyl) guanine (acycloguanosine), a new antiviral agent. *J Antimicrob Chemother* 5: 431.

Collins P, Darby G (1991). Laboratory studies of herpes simplex virus strains resistant to acyclovir. *Rev Med Virol* 1: 19.

Collins P, Ellis NM (1993). Sensitivity monitoring of clinical isolates of herpes simplex virus to acyclovir. *J Med Virol* 1: 58.

Collins P, Oliver NM (1982). Acyclovir treatment of cutaneous herpes in guinea pigs and herpes encephalitis in mice. *Amer J Med* 73: 96.

Collins P, Larder BA, Oliver NM *et al.* (1989). Characterisation of a DNA polymerase mutant of herpes simplex virus from a severely immunocompromised patient receiving acyclovir. *J Gen Virol* 70: 375.

Collum LMT, Logan P, Hillary IB, Ravenscroft T (1982). Acyclovir in herpes keratitis. *Amer J Med* 73: 290.

Cooper DA, Pedersen C, Aiuti F *et al.* (1991). The efficacy and safety of zidovudine with or without acyclovir in the treatment of patients with AIDS-related complex. The European Australian Collaborative Group. *AIDS* 5: 933.

Cooper DA Pehrson PO, Pedersen C *et al.* (1993). The efficacy and safety of zidovudine alone or as cotherapy with acyclovir for the treatment of patients with AIDS and AIDS-related complex; a double-blind randomized trial. European-Australian Collaborative Group. *AIDS* 7: 197.

Corey L, Benedetti JK, Critchlow CW *et al.* (1982a) Double-blind controlled trial of topical acyclovir in genital herpes simplex virus infections. *Amer J Med* 73: 326.

Corey L, Nahmias AJ, Guinan ME *et al.* (1982b) A trial of topical acyclovir in genital herpes simplex virus infections. *New Engl J Med* 306: 1313.

Corey L, Fife KH, Benedetti JK *et al.* (1983a) Intravenous acyclovir for the treatment of primary genital herpes. *Ann Intern Med* 98: 914.

Corey L, Benedetti J, Critchlow C *et al.* (1983b) Treatment of primary first episode genital herpes simplex virus infections with acyclovir, results of topical, intravenous and oral therapy. *J Antimicrob Ag Chemother* 12: 79.

Crane LR, Milne DA, Sunstrum JC, Lerner AM (1984). Comparative activities of selected combinations of acyclovir, vidarabine, arabinosyl hypoxanthine, interferon, and polyriboinosinic acid-polyribocytidylic acid complex against herpes simplex virus type 2 in tissue culture and intravaginally inoculated mice. *Antimicrob Ag Chemother* 26: 557.

Crumpacker CS (1988). Significance of resistance of herpes simplex virus to acyclovir. *J Amer Acad Dermatol* 18: 190.

Crumpacker CS, Schnipper LE, Zaia JA, Levin MJ (1979). Growth inhibition by acycloguanosine of herpes viruses isolated from human infections. *Antimicrob Ag Chemother* 15: 642.

Crumpacker CS, Schnipper LE, Marlowe SI *et al.* (1982). Resistance to antiviral drugs of herpes simplex virus isolated from a patient treated with acyclovir. *New Engl Med* 306: 343.

Davenport A, Goel S, Mackenzie JC (1992). Neurotoxicity of acyclovir in patients with end-stage renal failure treated with continuous ambulatory peritoneal dialysis. *Amer J Kidney Dis* 20: 647.

Davies UM, Palmer RG, Denman AM (1988). Treatment with acyclovir does not affect orogenital ulcers in Behcet's syndrome; a randomized double-blind trial. *Brit J Rheumatol* 27: 300.

De Clercq E, Descamps J, Verheist G *et al.* (1980). Comparative efficacy of anti herpes drugs against different strains of Herpes simplex virus. *J Infect Dis* 141: 563.

Dekker C, Ellis MN, McClaren C *et al.* (1983). Virus resistance in clinical practice. *J Antimicrob Chemother* 12: 137.

de Miranda P, Blum MR (1983). Pharmacokinetics of acyclovir after intravenous and oral administration. *J Antimicrob Chemother* 12: 29.

de Miranda P, Good SS, Krasny HC *et al.* (1982). Metabolic fate of radioactive acyclovir in humans. *Amer J Med* 215.

Detjen PF, Patterson R, Noskin GA *et al.* (1992). Herpes simplex virus associated with recurrent Stevens-Johnson syndrome. A management strategy. *Arch Intern Med* 152: 1513.

Douglas JM, Critchlow C, Benedetti J *et al.* (1984). A double-blind study of oral acyclovir for suppression of recurrences of genital herpes simplex virus infection. *New Engl J Med* 310: 1551.

Douglas JM, Critchlow C, Benedetti J *et al.* (1988). A double blind, placebo-controlled trial of the effect of chronically administered oral acyclovir on sperm production in men with frequently recurrent genital herpes. *J Infect Dis* 157: 588.

Drago F, Romagnoli M, Loi A, Rebora A (1992). Epstein Barr virus related persistent erythema multiforme in chronic fatigue syndrome. *Arch Dermatol* 128: 217.

Drew WL, Anderson R, Lang W *et al.* (1995). Failure of high dose oral acyclovir to suppress CMV viruria or induce ganciclovir resistant CMV in HIV antibody positive patients. *J AIDS Hum Retrovirol* 8: 289.

Duncan SR, Grgurich WF, Iacono AT *et al.* (1994). A comparison of ganciclovir and acyclovir to prevent cytomegalovirus after lung transplantation. *Amer J Respir Crit Care Med* 150: 146.

Dunkle LM, Arvin AM, Whitley RJ *et al.* (1991). A controlled trial of acyclovir for chickenpox in normal children. *New Engl J Med* **325**: 1539.

Dunn DL, Gillingham KJ, Kramer MA *et al.* (1994). A prospective randomized study of acyclovir versus ganciclovir plus human immune globulin prophylaxis of cytomegalovirus infection after solid organ transplantation. *Transplant* **57**: 876.

Elion GB (1982). Mechanism of action and selectivity of acyclovir. *Amer J Med* **73**: 7.

Elion GB (1993). Acyclovir, discovery, mechanism of action and selectivity. *J Med Virol* **1**: 2.

Elion GB, Furman PA, Fyfe JA *et al.* (1977). Selectivity of action of an antiherpetic agent, 9-(2-hydroxyethoxymethyl) guanine. *Proc Natl Acad Sci USA* **74**: 5716.

Elkins CC, Frist WH, Dummer JS *et al.* (1993). Cytomegalovirus disease after heart transplantation; is acyclovir prophylaxis indicated? *Ann Thorac Surg* **56**: 1267.

Ellis MN, Keller PM, Fyfe JA *et al.* (1987). Clinical isolate of herpes simplex virus type 2 that induces a thymidine kinase with altered substrate specificity. *Antimicrob Ag Chemother* **31**: 1117.

Englund JA, Zimmerman ME, Swierkosz EM *et al.* (1990). Herpes simplex virus resistant to acyclovir. A study in a tertiary care center. *Ann Intern Med* **112**: 416.

Englund JA Fletcher CV, Balfour HH (1991). Acyclovir therapy in neonates. *J Pediatr* **119**: 129.

Erlich KS, Mills J, Chatis P *et al.* (1989a) Acyclovir-resistant herpes simplex virus infections in patients with the acquired immunodeficiency syndrome. *New Engl J Med* **320**: 293.

Erlich KS, Jacobson MA, Koehler JE *et al.* (1989b) Foscarnet therapy for severe acyclovir resistant herpes simplex virus type 2 infections in patients with the acquired immunodeficiency syndrome (AIDS). An uncontrolled trial. *Ann Intern Med* **110**: 710.

Esmann V, Ipsen J, Peterslund NA *et al.* (1982). Therapy of acute herpes zoster with acyclovir in the nonimmunocompromised host. *Amer J Med* **73**: 320.

Falcon MG (1983). Herpes simplex virus infections of the eye and their management with acyclovir. *J Antimicrob Chemother* **12**: 39.

Fardeau C, Langlois M, Nugier F *et al.* (1993). Cross-resistances to antiviral drugs of IUdR-resistant HSV-1 in rabbit keratitis and *in vitro*. *Cornea* **12**: 19.

Fawcett HA, Wansbrough-Jones MH, Clark AE, Leigh IM (1983). Prophylactic topical acyclovir for frequent recurrent herpes simplex infection with and without erythema multiforme. *Brit Med J* **287**: 798.

Feder HM (1990). Treatment of adult chickenpox with oral acyclovir. *Arch Intern Med* **150**: 2061.

Feder HM, Goyal RK, Krause PJ (1995). Acyclovir induced neutropenia in an infant with herpes simplex encephalitis case report. *Clin Infect Dis* **20**: 1557.

Feldman S (1993). Acyclovir therapy for varicella in otherwise healthy children and adolescents. *J Med Virol* **1**: 85.

Fiddian AP, Ivanyi L (1983) Topical acyclovir in the management of recurrent herpes labialis. *Brit J Derm* **109**: 321.

Fiddian AP, Yeo JM, Stubbings R, Dean D (1983). Successful treatment of labialis with topical acyclovir. *Brit Med J* **286**: 1699.

Field HJ (1982). Development of clinical resistance to acyclovir in herpes simplex virus-infected mice receiving oral therapy. *Antimicrob Ag Chemother* **21**: 744.

Field HJ, Darby G (1980). Pathogenicity in mice of strains of herpes simplex virus which are resistant to acyclovir *in vitro* and *in vivo*. *Antimicrob Ag Chemother* **17**: 209.

Field HJ, Darby G, Wildy P (1980). Isolation and characterization of acyclovir resistant mutants of herpes simplex virus. *J Gen Virol* **49**: 115.

Feldman S, Rodman J, Gregory B (1988). Excessive serum concentrations of acyclovir and neurotoxicity. *J Infect Dis* **157**: 385.

Fife KH, Crumpacker CS, Mertz GJ *et al.* (1994). Recurrence and resistance patterns of herpes simplex virus following cessation of > or = 6 years of chronic suppression with acyclovir Acyclovir Study Group. *J Infect Dis* **169**: 1338.

Finn R, Smith MA (1984). Oral acyclovir for herpes zoster. *Lancet* **ii**: 575.

Fletcher CV, Englund JA, Edelman CK *et al.* (1991). Pharmacologic basis for high-dose oral acicyclovir phrophylaxis of cytomegalovirus disease in renal allograft recipients. *Antimicrob Ag Chemother* **35**: 938.

Foerster M, Kastner U, Neuert R (1992). Effect of six virustatic nucleoside analogues on the development of fetal rat thymus in organ culture. *Arch Toxicol* **66**: 688.

Freeman DJ, Sheth NV, Spruance SL (1986). Failure of topical acyclovir in ointment to penetrate human skin. *Antimicrob Ag Chemother* **29**: 730.

Frenkel LM, Brown ZA, Bryson YJ *et al.* (1991). Pharmacokinetics of acyclovir in the term human pregnancy and neonate. *Amer J Obstet Gynacol* **164**: 569.

Fyfe JA, Keller PM, Furman PA *et al.* (1978). Thymidine kinase from herpes simplex virus phosphorylates the new antiviral compound 9-(2-hydroxyethoxymethyl)guanine. *J Biol Chem* **253**: 8721.

Galbraith JC, Shafran SD (1992). Herpes simplex esophagitis in the immunocompetent patient; report of our cases and review. *Clin Infect Dis* **14**: 894.

Gallant JE, Moore RD, Keruly J *et al.* (1995). Lack of association between acyclovir use and survival in patients with advanced human immunodeficiency virus disease treated with zidovudine. Zidovudine Epidemiology Study Group. *J Infect Dis* **172**: 346.

Gateley A, Gander RM, Johnson PC *et al.* (1990). Herpes simplex virus type 2 meningoencephalitis resistant to acyclovir in a patient with AIDS. *J Infect Dis* **161**: 711.

Gill MJ, Burgess E (1990). Neurotoxicity of acyclovir in end stage renal disease. *J Antimicrob Chemother* **25**: 300.

GlaxoWelcome Aciclovir Drug Information.

Gluckman E, Lotsberg J, Devergie A *et al.* (1983). Prophylaxis of herpes infections after bone-marrow transplantation by oral acyclovir. *Lancet* **ii**: 706.

Goday J, Aguirre A, Ibarra NG, Eizaguirre X (1991). Allergic contact dermatitis from acyclovir. *Contact Dermatitis* **24**: 380.

Goldberg LH, Kaufman R, Conant MA *et al.* (1986). Oral acyclovir for episodic treatment of recurrent genital herpes. *J Amer Acad Dermatol* **15**: 256.

Goldberg LH, Kaufman R, Conant MA *et al.* (1988). Episodic twice-daily treatment for recurrent genital herpes. *Amer J Med* **85**: 10.

Goldberg LH, Kaufman RH, Kurtz TO *et al.* (1993). Continuous five-year treatment of patients with frequently recurring genital herpes simplex virus infection with acyclovir. *J Med Virol* **1**: 45.

Golumbek PT, Hamzeh FM, Jaffee EM *et al.* (1992). Herpes simplex-1 virus thymidine kinase gene is unable to completely stimulate live nonimmunogenic tumor cell vaccines. *J Immunother* **12**: 224.

Gordon B, Selnes OA, Hart J *et al.* (1990). Long-term cognitive sequelae of acyclovir treated herpes simplex encephalitis. *Arch Neurol* **47**: 646.

Gould JM, Chessells JM, Marshall WC, McKendrick GDW (1982). Acyclovir in herpes virus infections in children: experience in an open study with particular reference to safety. *J Infect Dis* **5**: 283.

Green JA, Spruance SL, Wenerstrom G, Piepkorn MW (1985). Post-herpetic erythema multiforme prevented with prophylactic oral ACV. *Ann Int Med* **102**: 632.

Greenspoon JS, Wilcox JG, McHutchison LB, Rosen DJ (1994). Acyclovir for disseminated herpes simplex virus in pregnancy. A case report. *J Reprod Med* **39**: 311.

Gubbels JL, Gold WR, Bauserman S (1991). Prenatal diagnosis of fetal diastematomyelia in a pregnancy exposed to acyclovir. *Reprod Toxicol* **5**: 517.

Haake DA, Zakowski PC, Haake DL, Bryson YJ (1990). Early treatment with acyclovir for varicella pneumonia in otherwise healthy adults; retrospective controlled study and review. *Rev Infect Dis* **12**: 788.

Haddad J, Langer B, Astruc D *et al.* (1993). Oral acyclovir and recurrent genital herpes during late pregnancy. *Obstet Gynecol* **82**: 102.

Haefeli WE, Schoenenberger RA, Weiss P *et al.* (1993). Acyclovir-induced neurotoxicity; concentration-side effect relationship in acyclovir overdose. *Amer J Med* **94**: 212.

Hammer SM, Kaplan JC, Lowe BR, Hirsch M (1982). Alpha interferon and acyclovir treatment of herpes simplex virus in lymphoid cell cultures. *Antimicrob Ag Chemother* **21**: 634.

Han CS, Miller W, Haake R, Weisdorf D (1994). Varicella zoster infection after bone marrow transplantation; incidence, risk factors and complications. *Bone Marrow Transplant* **13**: 277.

Hann IM, Prentice HG, Blacklock HA *et al.* (1983). Acyclovir prophylaxis against herpes virus infections in severely immunocompromised patients: randomised double blind trial. *Brit Med J* **6**: 384.

Hanto DW, Frizzera G, Gajl-Peczalska KJ *et al.* (1982). Epstein-Barr virus induced B-cell lymphoma after renal transplantation. Acyclovir therapy and transition from polyclonal to monoclonal B-cell proliferation. *New Engl J Med* **306**: 913.

Harding SP, Porter SM (1991). Oral acyclovir in herpes zoster ophthalmicus. *Curr Eye Res* **10**: 177.

Hardy WD (1992). Foscarnet treatment of acyclovir-resistant herpes simplex virus infection in patients with acquired immunodeficiency syndrome; preliminary results of a controlled, randomized, regimen-comparative trial. *Amer J Med* **92**: 30S.

Hasegawa T, Kurokawa M, Yukawa TA *et al.* (1995). Inhibitory action of acyclovir (ACV) and penciclovir (PCV) on plaque formation and partial cross-resistance of ACV-resistant varicella-zoster virus to PCV. *Antiviral Res* **27**: 271.

Henry RE, Wegmann JA, Hartle JE, Christopher GW (1993). Successful oral acyclovir desensitization. *Ann Allergy* **70**: 386.

Herbst JS, Morgan J, Raab-Traub N, Resnick L (1989). Comparison of the efficacy of surgery and acyclovir therapy in oral hairy leukoplakia. *J Amer Acad Dermatol* **21**: 753.

Herrold JM, Hahn JS (1994). Disseminated multifocal herpes zoster leukoencephalitis and subcortical hemorrhage in an immunosuppressed child. *J Child Neurol* **9**: 56.

Hill TJ, Blyth WA, Harbour DA (1982). Recurrent Herpes simplex in mice: topical treatment with acyclovir cream. *Antiviral Res* **2**: 135.

Hintz M, Connor JD, Spector SA *et al.* (1982). Neonatal acyclovir pharmacokinetics in patients with herpes virus infections. *Amer J Med* **73**: 210.

Hollander H, Lifson AR, Maha M *et al.* (1989). Phase I study of low-dose zidovudine and acyclovir in asymptomatic human immunodeficiency virus seropositive individuals. *Amer J Med* **87**: 628.

Holmes GP, Hilliard JK, Klontz KC *et al.* (1990). B virus herpes virus simiae infection in human, epidemiologic investigation of a cluster. *Ann Intern Med* **112**: 833.

Horowitz GM, Hankins GD (1992). Early second trimester use of acyclovir in treating herpes zoster in a bone marrow transplant patient. *J Reprod Med* **37**: 280.

Huff JC, Bean B, Balfour HH *et al.* (1988). Therapy of herpes zoster with oral acyclovir. *Amer J Med* **85**: 84.

Huff JC, Drucker JL, Clemmer A *et al.* (1993). Effect of oral acyclovir on pain resolution in herpes zoster; a reanalysis. *J Med Virol* **1**: 93.

Hwang CB, Ruffner KL, Coen DM (1992). A point mutation within a distinct conserved region of the herpes simplex virus DNA polymerase gene confers drug resistance. *J Virol* **66**: 1774.

Ilsley DD, Lee SH, Miller WH, Kuchta RD (1995). Acyclic guanosine analogs inhibit DNA polymerases alpha, delta, and epsilon with very different potencies and have unique mechanisms of action. *Biochem* **34**: 2504.

Inglis AF (1993). Herpes simplex virus infection A rare cause of prolonged croup. *Arch Otolaryngol Head Neck Surg* **119**: 551.

Johnson GL, Limon L, Trikha G, Wall H (1994). Acute renal failure and neurotoxicity following oral acyclovir. *Ann Pharmacother* **28**: 460.

Johnson R, Douglas J, Corey L, Krasney H (1985). Adverse effects with acyclovir and meperidine. *Ann Intern Med* **103**: 962.

Johnson JR, Egaas S, Gleaves CA *et al.* (1992). Hepatitis due to herpes simplex virus in marrow-transplant recipients. *Clin Infect Dis* **14**: 38.

Johnston WH, Holland GN, Engstrom RE, Rimmer S (1993). Recurrence of presumed varicella zoster virus retinopathy in patients with acquired immunodeficiency syndrome. *Amer J Ophthalmol* **116**: 42.

Jones BR, Coster DJ, Fison PN *et al.* (1979). Efficacy of acycloguanosine (Welcome 248U) against Herpes-simplex corneal ulcers. *Lancet* i: 243.

Jones JL, Hanson DL, Chu SY *et al.* (1995) AIDS associated Kaposi's sarcoma. *Science* **267**: 1078.

Jones TJ, Paul R (1995). Disseminated acyclovir-resistant herpes simplex virus type 2 treated successful with foscarnet. *J Infect Dis* **171**: 508.

Kaplowitz LG, Baker D, Gelb L *et al.* (1991). Prolonged continuous acyclovir treatment of normal adults with frequently recurring genital herpes simplex virus infection. The Acyclovir Study Group. *JAMA* **265**: 747.

Kaufman HE, Varnell ED, Centifanto-Fitzgerald YM *et al.* (1983). Oral antiviral drugs in experimental herpes simplex keratitis. *Antimicrob Ag Chemother* **24**: 888.

Keeney RE, Kirk LE, Bridgen D (1982). Acyclovir tolerance in humans. *Amer J Med* **73**: 76.

Kern ER (1982). Acyclovir treatment of experimental genital herpes simplex virus infections. *Amer J Med* **73**: 100.

Kern ER, Richards JT, Glasgow LA *et al.* (1982). Optimal treatment of herpes simplex virus encephalitis in mice with oral acyclovir. *Amer J Med* **73**: 125.

Kern ER, Richards JT, Overall JC Jr, Glasgow LA (1983). Acyclovir treatment of experimental genital herpes simplex virus infections I Topical therapy of type 2 and type I infections of mice. *Antiviral Res* **3**: 253.

Kessler HA, Hurwitz S, Farthing *et al.* (1996). Pilot study of topical trifluridine for the treatment of aciclovir-resistant mucocutaneous herpes simplex disease in patients with AIDS (ACTG 172). *J AIDS Hum Retrovirol* **12**: 147.

Kim YJ, Kim JH (1994). Allergic contact dermatitis from propylene glycol in Zovirax cream. *Contact Dermatitis* **30**: 119.

Kinghorn GR, Jeavons M, Rowland M *et al.* (1985). Acyclovir prophylaxis of recurrent genital herpes: randomised placebo controlled crossover study. *Genitourin Med* **61**: 387.

Kiroglu M, Cetik F, Soylu L *et al.* (1994). Acyclovir in the treatment of recurrent respiratory papillomatosis; a preliminary report. *Amer J Otolaryngol* **15**: 212.

Kit S, Sheppard M, Ichimura H *et al.* (1987). Nucleotide sequence changes in thymidine kinase gene of herpes simplex virus type 2 clones from an isolate of a patient treated with acyclovir. *Antimicrob Ag Chemother* **31**: 1483.

Klein RJ, Friedman-Kien AE, De Stefano E (1979). Latent herpes simplex virus infections in sensory ganglia of hairless mice prevented by acycloguanosine. *Antimicrob Ag Chemother* **15**: 723.

Klein RJ, De Stefano E, Friedman-Kien AE, Brady E (1981). Effect of acyclovir on latent herpes simplex virus infections in trigeminal ganglia of mice. *Antimicrob Ag Chemother* **19**: 937.

Knopf KW, Kaufman ER, Crumpacker C (1981). Physical mapping of drug resistance mutations defines an active center on the herpes simplex virus DNA polymerase enzyme. *J Virol* **39**: 746.

Kost RG, Hill EL, Tigges M, Straus SE (1993). Brief report; recurrent acyclovir-resistant genital herpes in an immunocompetent patient. *New Engl J Med* **329**: 1777.

Krasny HC, Liao SHT, De Miranda P *et al.* (1982). Influence of hemodialysis on acyclovir pharmacokinetics in patients with chronic renal failure. *Amer J Med* **73**: 202.

Lafferty WE, Brewer LA, Corey L (1984). Alteration of lymphocyte transformation response to herpes simplex virus infection by acyclovir therapy. *Antimicrob Ag Chemother* **26**: 887.

Laibson PR, Pavan-Langston D, Yeakley WR, Lass J (1982). Acyclovir and vidarabine for the treatment of Herpes simplex keratitis. *Amer J Med* **73**: 281.

La Lau C, Oosterhuis JA, Versteeg J *et al.* (1982). Multicenter trial of acyclovir and trifluorothymidine in herpetic keratitis. *Amer J Med* **73**: 305.

Lalezari JP, Drew WL, Glutzer E *et al.* (1994). Treatment with intravenous (S)-1-[3-hydroxy-2-(phosphonylmethoxy)methoxy)propyl]-cytosine of acyclovir-resistant mucocutaneous infection with herpes simplex virus in a patient with AIDS. *J Infect Dis* **170**: 570.

Lambert H, Eastham EJ (1987). Herpes oesophagitis in a healthy 8 year old. *Arch Dis Childhood* **62**: 301.

Landry ML, Lucia HL, Hsiung AD *et al.* (1982). Effect of acyclovir on genital infection with herpes simplex virus types I and 2 in the guinea pig. *Amer J Med* **73**: 143.

Laskaris G, Laskaris M, Theodoridou M (1995). Oral hairy leukoplakia in a child with AIDS. *Oral Surg Oral Med Oral Pathol Oral Radiol Endod* **79**: 570.

Laskin OL (1985). Acyclovir and suppression of frequently recurring herpetic whitlow. *Ann Intern Med* **102**: 494.

Laskin OL, Longstreth JA, Whelton A *et al.* (1982a) Effect of renal failure on the pharmacokinetics of acyclovir. *Amer J Med* **73**: 197.

Laskin OL, De Miranda P, King DH *et al.* (1982b) Effects of probenecid on the pharmacokinetics and elimination of acyclovir in humans. *Antimicrob Ag Chemother* **21**: 804.

Legendre C, Ducloux D, Ferroni A *et al.* (1993). Acyclovir in preventing cytomegalovirus infection in kidney transplant recipients; a case controlled study. *J Med Virol* **1**: 118.

Leikin JB, Shicker L, Orlowski J *et al.* (1995). Hemodialysis removal of acyclovir. *Vet Hum Toxicol* **37**: 233.

Lewis ME, Warren KG, Jeffrey VM, Tyrell DLJ (1983). Effects of prolonged cultivation in the presence of acyclovir on recovery of latent herpes simplex virus from human trigeminal ganglia. *Antimicrob Ag Chemother* **23**: 487.

Lietman PS (1982). Acyclovir clinical pharmacology An overview. *Amer J Med* **73**: 193.

Linnemann CC, Biron KK, Hoppenjans WG, Solinger AM (1990). Emergence of acyclovir resistant varicella zoster virus in an AIDS patient on prolonged acyclovir therapy. *AIDS* **4**: 577.

Ljungman P, Ellis MN, Hackman RC *et al.* (1990). Acyclovir-resistant herpes simplex virus causing pneumonia after marrow transplantation. *J Infect Dis* **162**: 244.

Lokke-Jensen B, Weismann K, Mathiesen L, Klem-Thomsen H (1993). Atypical varicella zoster infection in AIDS. *Acta Derm Venereol* **73**: 123.

Lozada-Nur F, Costa C (1992). Retrospective findings of the clinical benefits of podophyllum resin 25% sol on hairy leukoplakia. Clinical results in 9 patients. *Oral Surg Oral Med Oral Pathol* **73**: 555.

Lucia HL, Griffith BP, Hsiuing GD (1984). Effect of acyclovir and phosphonoformate on Cytomegalovirus infection in guinea pigs. *Inter Virology* **21**: 141.

Lundgren G, Wilczek H, Lonnqvist B *et al.* (1985). Acyclovir prophylaxis in bone marrow transplant recipients. *Scand J Infect Dis* **47**: 137.

Luxton JC, Williams I, Weller I, Crawford DH (1993). Epstein Barr virus infection of HIV-seropositive individuals is transiently suppressed by high dose acyclovir treatment. *AIDS* **7**: 1337.

Lyall EG, Ogilvie MM, Smith NM, Burns S (1994). Acyclovir resistant varicella zoster and HIV infection. *Arch Dis Child* **70**: 133.

Lycke J, Andersen O, Svennerholm B *et al.* (1989). Acyclovir concentrations in serum and cerebrospinal fluid at steady state. *Antimicrob Ag Chemother* **24**: 947.

Lynfield R, Herrin JT, Rubin RH (1992). Varicella in pediatric renal transplant recipients. *Pediatrics* **90**: 216.

Machida H, Nishitani M, Watanabe Y *et al.* (1995). Comparison of the selectivity of anti-varicella zoster virus nucleoside analogues. *Microbiol Immunol* **39**: 201.

Marsh RJ, Cooper M (1991). Double-masked trial of topical acyclovir and steroids in the treatment of herpes zoster ocular inflammation. *Brit J Ophthalmol* **75**: 542.

Martin M, Manez R, Linden P, Estores D (1994). A prospective randomised trial comparing sequential ganciclovir high dose acyclovir to high dose acyclovir for prevention of cytomegalovirus disease in adult liver transplant recipients. *Transplant* **58**: 779.

Martinez E, de Diego A, Paradis A *et al.* (1994). Herpes simplex pneumonia in a young immunocompetent man. *Eur Respir J* **7**: 1185.

Masaoka T, Hiraoka A, Teshima H, Tominaga N (1993). Varicella zoster virus infection in immunocompromised patients. *J Med Virol* **1**: 82.

Mascher H, Kikuta C, Metz R, Vergin H (1992). New high sensitivity high performance liquid chromatographic method for the determination of acyclovir in human plasma, using fluorometric detection. *J Chromatogr* **583**: 122.

Mattison HR, Reichman RC, Benedetti J *et al.* (1988). Double-blind placebo-controlled trial comparing long-term suppressive with short-term oral acyclovir therapy for management of recurrent genital herpes. *Amer J Med* **85**: 20.

McDonald LK, Tartaglione TA, Mendelman PM *et al.* (1989). Lack of toxicity in two cases of neonatal acyclovir overdose. *Pediatr Infect Dis J* **8**: 529.

McGill J, Chapman C (1983). A comparison of topical acyclovir with steroids in the treatment of herpes zoster keratouveitis. *Brit J Ophthalmol* **67**: 746.

McGill J, Tormey P (1982). Use of acyclovir in herpetic ocular infection. *Amer J Med* **73**: 286.

McGill J, Macdonald DR, Fall D (1983). Intravenous acyclovir in acute herpes zoster infection. *J Infect Dis* **6**: 157.

McGuffin RW, Shiota FM, Meyers JD (1980). Lack of toxicity of acyclovir to granulocyte progenitor cells *in vitro*. *Antimicrob Ag Chemother* **18**: 471.

McKendrick MW, McGill JI, Bell AM *et al.* (1984). Oral acyclovir for herpes zoster. *Lancet* **ii**: 925.

McKendrick MW, McGill JI, Wood MJ (1989). Lack of effect of acyclovir on postherpetic neuralgia. *Brit Med J* **298**: 431.

McLaren C, Sibrack CD, Barry DW (1982). Spectrum of sensitivity to acyclovir of herpes simplex virus clinical isolates. *Amer J Med* **73**: 376.

McLaren C, Corey L, Dekket C, Barry DW (1983). *In vitro* sensitivity to acyclovir in genital herpes simplex viruses from acyclovir-treated patients. *J Infect Dis* **148**: 868.

McMillan JA, Weiner LB, Higgins AM, Lamparella VJ (1993). Pharyngitis associated with herpes simplex virus in college students. *Pediatr Infect Dis J* **12**: 280.

Mertz GJ, Critchlow CW, Benedetti J *et al.* (1984). Double-blind placebo controlled trial of oral acyclovir in first-episode genital herpes simplex virus infection. *JAMA* **2S2**: 1147.

Mertz GJ, Jones CC, Mills J *et al.* (1988a) Long term acyclovir suppression of frequently recurring genital herpes simplex virus infection. A multicenter double-blind trial. *JAMA* **260**: 201.

Mertz GJ, Eron L, Kaufman R *et al.* (1988b) Prolonged continuous versus intermittent oral acyclovir treatment in normal adults with frequently recurring genital herpes simplex virus infection. *Amer J Med* **85**: 14.

Meszner Z, Nyerges G, Bell AR (1993). Oral acyclovir to prevent dissemination of varicella in immunocompromised children. *J Infect* **26**: 9.

Meyer LJ, de Miranda P, Sheth N, Spurance S (1988). Acyclovir in human breast milk. *Amer J Obstet Gynecol* **158**: 586.

Meyers JD, Wade JC, Mitchell CD *et al.* (1982). Multicenter collaborative trial of intravenous acyclovir for treatment of mucocutaneous herpes simplex virus infection in the immunocompromised host. *Amer J Med* **73**: 229.

Meyers JD, Reed EC, Shepp DH *et al.* (1988). Acyclovir for prevention of cytomegalovirus infection and disease after allogeneic marrow transplantation. *New Engl J Med* **318**: 70.

Miller WH, Miller RL (1980). Phosphorylation of acyclovir (acycloguanosine) monophosphate by GMP kinase. *J Biol Chem* **255**: 7204.

Miller WH, Miller RL (1982). Phosphorylation of acyclovir diphosphate by cellular enzymes. *Biochem Pharmacol* **31**: 3879.

Miller E, Cradock-Watson JE, Ridehalgh MK (1989). Outcome in newborn babies given anti-varicella zoster immunoglobulin after perinatal maternal infection with varicella zoster virus. *Lancet* **ii**: 371.

Mindel A, Adler MW, Sutherland S, Fiddian AP (1982). Intravenous acyclovir in genital herpes An interim report. *Amer J Med* **73**: 347.

Mindel A, Weller IVD, Faherty A *et al.* (1984). Prophylactic oral acyclovir in recurrent genital herpes. *Lancet* **ii**: 57.

Mindel A, Faherty A, Carney O et al. (1988). Dosage and safety of long-term suppressive acyclovir therapy for recurrent genital herpes. Lancet i: 926.

Mitchell CD, Bean B, Gentry SR et al. (1981). Acyclovir therapy for mucocutaneous herpes simplex infections in immunocompromised patients. Lancet i: 1389.

MMWR (1993). Pregnancy outcomes following systemic prenatal acyclovir exposure June 1 1984–June 30th 1993. MMWR 42: 806.

Mollison LC, Richards MJ, Johnson PD et al. (1993). High-dose oral acyclovir reduces the incidence of cytomegalovirus infection in liver transplant recipients. J Infect Dis 168: 721.

Morrison GA, Evans JN (1993). Juvenile respiratory papillomatosis; acyclovir reassessed. Int J Pediatr Otorhinolaryngol 26: 193.

Moshkowitz M, Konikoff FM, Arber N et al. (1993). Acyclovir-associated colitis. Amer J Gastroenterol 88: 2110.

Mostow SR, Mayfield JL, Marr JJ, Drucker JL (1988). Suppression of recurrent genital herpes by single daily dosages of acyclovir. Amer J Med 85: 30.

Mudido P, Marshall GS, Howell RS et al. (1993). Disseminated herpes simplex virus infection during pregnancy. A case report. J Reprod Med 38: 964.

Murphy M, Morley A, Eglin RP, Monteiro E (1992). Topical trifluridine for mucocutaneous acyclovir- resistant herpes simplex II in AIDS patients. Lancet 340: 1040.

Nicolaidou P, Lacovidou N, Youroukos S et al. (1993). Relapse of herpes simplex encephalitis after acyclovir therapy. Eur J Pediatr 152: 737.

Niimura M, Nishikawa T (1988). Treatment of eczema herpeticum with oral acyclovir. Amer J Med 85: 49.

Nilsen AE, Aasen T, Halsos AM et al. (1982). Efficacy of oral acyclovir in the treatment of initial and recurrent genital herpes. Lancet ii: 571.

Novelli VM, Marshall WC, Yeo J, McKendrick GD (1984). Acyclovir administered perorally in immunocompromised children with varicella-zoster infections. J Infect Dis 3: 478.

Novelli VM, Marshall WC, Yeo J McKendrick GD (1985). High-dose oral acyclovir for children at risk of disseminated herpes virus infections. J Infect Dis 151: 372.

Nugler F, Colin JN, Aymard M, Langlois M (1992). Occurrence and characterisation of acyclovir-resistant herpes simplex virus isolates; report on a two-year sensitivity screening survey. J Med Virol 36: 1.

Nusinoff-Lehrman S, Smiley L, Szczech G (1993). Update on acyclovir prodrugs. In Antiviral Chemotherapy. New Directions for Clinical Applications and Research Vol. 3 (Mills J, Corey L, eds), p. 97. New Jersey: Prentice Hall Publishers.

Nyerges G, Meszner Z, Gyarmati E, Kerpel-Fronius S (1988). Acyclovir prevents dissemination of varicella in immunocompromised children. J Infect Dis 157: 309.

Nyquist AC, Rotbart HA, Cotton M et al. (1994). Acyclovir-resistant neonatal herpes simplex virus infection of the larynx. J Pediatr 124: 967.

O'Brien WJ, Coe EC, Taylor JL (1990). Nucleoside metabolism in herpes simplex virus-infected cells following treatment with interferon and acyclovir, a possible mechanism of synergistic antiviral activity. Antimicrob Ag Chemother 34: 1178.

Oliver NM, Collins P, Van der Meer J, Van't Wout JW (1989). Biological and biochemical characterisation of clinical isolates of herpes simplex virus type 2 resistant to acyclovir. Antimicrob Ag Chemother 33: 635.

Pagano JS, Datta AK (1982). Perspectives on interactions of acyclovir with Epstein-Barr and other herpes viruses. Amer J Med 73: 18.

Pagano JS, Sixbey JW, Lin JC (1983). Acyclovir and Epstein-Barr virus infection. J Antimicrob Chemother 12: 113.

Pahwa S, Biron K, Lim W et al. (1988). Continuous varicella zoster infection associated with acyclovir resistance in child with AIDS. JAMA 260: 2879.

Palu G, Gerna G, Bevilacqua F, Marcello A (1992). A point mutation in the thymidine kinase gene is responsible for acyclovir resistance in herpes simplex virus type 2 sequential isolates. Virus Res 25: 133.

Pancheva SN (1991). Potentiating effect of ribavirin on the anti-herpes activity of acyclovir. Antiviral Res 16: 151.

Pappas SC, Hoofnagle JH, Young N et al. (1985). Treatment of chronic non-A, non-B hepatitis with acyclovir: pilot study. J Med Virol 15: 1.

Park NH, Pavan-Langston D, McLean SL (1979a) Acyclovir in oral and ganglionic herpes simplex virus infections. J Infect Dis 140: 802.

Park NH, Pavan-Langston D, McLean SL, Albert DM (1979b) Therapy of experimental herpes simplex encephalitis with acyclovir in mice. Antimicrob Ag Chemother 15: 775.

Park NH, Pavan-Langston D, Hettinger ME et al. (1980). Topical therapeutic of 9-(2-hydroxyethoxymethyl) guanine and 5-iodo 5'-amino-2',5'-dideoxyuridine on oral infection with herpes simplex virus in mice. J Infect Dis 141: 575.

Park NH, Callahan JG, Pavan-Langston, D (1984). Effect of combined acyclovir and vidarabine on infection with herpes simplex virus in vitro and in vivo. J Infect Dis 149: 757.

Parker LM, Lipton JM, Binder N et al. (1982). Effect of acyclovir and interferon on human hematopoietic progenitor cells. Antimicrob Ag Chemother 21: 146.

Parker RK, Guin JD (1993). Hand eczema herpeticum. Cutis 52: 227.

Parris DS, Harrington JE (1982). Herpes simplex virus variants resistant to high concentrations of acyclovir exist in clinical isolates. Antimicrob Ag Chemother 22: 71.

Parry GE, Dunn P, Shah VP, Pershing LK (1992). Acyclovir bioavailability in human skin. J Invest Dermatol 98: 856.

Pavesio CE, Mitchell SM, Barton K et al. (1995). Progressive outer retinal necrosis (PORN) in AIDS patients; a different appearance of varicella-zoster retinitis. Eye 9: 271.

Pay CV, Marin E, Keating M et al. (1993). Solid organ transplantation; results and implications of acyclovir use in liver transplants. J Med Virol 1: 123.

Peacock JE, Kaplowitz LG, Sparling PF et al. (1988). Intravenous acyclovir therapy of first episodes of genital herpes; a multicenter double-blind, placebo controlled trial. Amer J Med 85: 301.

Perren TJ, Powles RL, Easton D et al. (1988). Prevention of herpes zoster in patients by long-term oral acyclovir after allogeneic bone marrow transplantation. Amer J Med 85: 99.

Peterslund NA, Seyer-Hansen K, Ipsen J et al. (1981). Acyclovir in herpes zoster. Lancet ii: 827.

Peterslund NA, Larsen ML, Mygind H (1988). Acyclovir crystalluria. Scand J Infect Dis 20: 225.

Pettersson E, Eklund B, Hockerstedt K et al. (1985). Acyclovir and renal transplantation. Scand J Infect Dis 47: 145.

Pinnolis MK, Foxworthy D, Kemp B (1995). Treatment of progressive outer retinal necrosis with sorivudine. Amer J Ophthalmol 119: 516.

Plotkin SA, Starr SE, Bryan CK (1982). In vitro and in vivo responses of cytomegalovirus to acyclovir. Amer J Med 73: 257.

Pottage JC, Kessler HA (1995). Herpes simplex virus resistance to acyclovir; clinical relevance. Infect Ag Dis 4: 115.

Preblud SR, Arbeter AM, Proctor, EA et al. (1984). Susceptibility of vaccine strains of varicella-zoster virus to antiviral compounds. Antimicrob Ag Chemother 25: 417.

Prentice HG, Hann IM (1983). Prophylactic studies against herpes infections in severely immunocompromised patients with acyclovir. J Infect 6: 17.

Prentice HG, Gluckman E, Powles RL et al. (1994). Impact of long term acyclovir on cytomegalovirus infection and survival after allogeneic bone marrow transplantation. Lancet 343: 749.

Pritchard MN, Pritchard LE, Shipman C (1993a) Inhibitors of thymidylate synthase and dihydrofolate reductase potentiate the antiviral effect of acyclovir. Antiviral Res 20: 249.

Pritchard MN, Prichard LE, Shipman C (1993b) Strategic design and three-dimensional analysis of antiviral drug combinations. Antimicrob Ag Chemother 37: 540.

Prober CG, Kirk LE, Keeney RE (1982). Acyclovir therapy of chickenpox in immunosuppressed children: a collaborative study. J Pediatr 101: 622.

Pusateri DW, Muder RR (1990). Fever, pulmonary infiltrates, and pleural effusion following acyclovir therapy for herpes zoster ophthalmicus. *Chest* **98**: 754.

Raborn GW, McGaw WT Grace M *et al.* (1987). Oral acyclovir and herpes labialis; a randomised, double-blind, placebo-controlled study. *J Amer Dental Assoc* **115**: 38.

Ragab NF, Habib MA, Ghozzi MY (1989). Serological assessment of acyclovir treatment of herpes genitalis. *Arch Androl* **23**: 147.

Rajaonarison JF, Lacarelle B, Catalin J *et al.* (1992). 3'-Azido-3'-deoxythymidine drug interactions. Screening for inhibitors in human liver microsomes. *Drug Metab Dispos* **20**: 578.

Rashed A, Azadeh B, Abu-Romeh SH (1990). Acyclovir induced acute tubulo interstitial nephritis. *Nephron* **56**: 436.

Rashiq S, Briewa L, Mooney M *et al.* (1993). Distinguishing acyclovir neurotoxicity from encephalomyelitis. *J Intern Med* **234**: 507.

Rechtin TM, Black ME, Mao F *et al.* (1995). Purification and photoaffinity labelling of herpes simplex virus type 1 thymidine kinase. *J Biol Chem* **270**: 7055.

Reichman RC, Badger GJ, Guinan ME *et al.* (1983). Topically administered acyclovir in the treatment of recurrent Herpes simplex genitalis: a controlled trial. *J Infect Dis* **147**: 336.

Reichman RC, Badger GJ, Mertz GJ *et al.* (1984). Treatment of recurrent genital herpes simplex infections with oral acyclovir: a controlled trial. *JAMA* **251**: 2103.

Resnick L, Herbst JS, Ablashi DV *et al.* (1988). Regression of oral hairy leukoplakia after orally administered acyclovir therapy. *JAMA* **259**: 384.

Robbins MS, Stromquist C, Tan LH (1993). Acyclovir pH-possible cause of extravasation tissue injury. *Ann Pharmacother* **27**: 238.

Robinson GE, Underhill GS, Forster GE *et al.* (1984). Treatment with acyclovir of genital herpes simplex virus infection complicated by eczema herpeticum. *Brit J Vener Dis* **60**: 241.

Rompalo AM, Mertz GJ, Davis LG *et al.* (1988). Oral acyclovir for treatment of first-episode herpes simplex virus proctitis. *JAMA* **259**: 2879.

Rooney JF, Straus SE, Mannix ML *et al.* (1992). UV light-induced reactivation of herpes simplex virus type 2 and prevention by acyclovir. *J Infect Dis* **166**: 500.

Rooney JF, Straus SE, Mannix ML *et al.* (1993). Oral acyclovir to suppress frequently recurrent herpes labialis. A double-blind, placebo controlled trial. *Ann Intern Med* **118**: 268.

Rossi S, Whitfeld M, Berger TG (1995). The treatment of acyclovir resistant herpes zoster with trifluorothymidine and interferon alfa. *Arch Dermatol* **131**: 24.

Sacks SL, Wanklin RJ, Reece DE *et al.* (1989). Progressive esophagitis from acyclovir-resistant herpes simplex. *Ann Int Med* **111**: 893.

Safrin S (1993). Treatment of patients with acyclovir-resistant herpes simplex virus infections. *Antiviral Chemother* **3**: 51.

Safrin S, Phan L (1993). *In vitro* activity of penciclovir against clinical isolates of acyclovir-resistant and foscarnet-resistant herpes simplex virus. *Antimicrob Ag Chemother* **37**: 2241.

Safrin S, Assaykeen T, Follansbee S, Mills J (1990). Foscarnet therapy for acyclovir-resistant mucocutaneous herpes simplex virus infection in 26 AIDS patients; preliminary data. *J Infect Dis* **161**: 1078.

Safrin S, Crumpacker C, Chatis P *et al.* (1991a) A controlled trial comparing foscarnet with vidarabine for acyclovir-resistant mucocutaneous herpes simplex in the acquired immunodeficiency syndrome. The AIDS Clinical Trials Group. *New Engl J Med* **325**: 551.

Safrin S, Berger TG, Gilson I *et al.* (1991b) Foscarnet therapy in five patients with AIDS and acyclovir-resistant varicella-zoster virus infection. *Ann Intern Med* **115**: 19.

Safrin S, Schacker T, Delehanty J *et al.* (1993a) Potential for combined therapy with 348U87, a ribonucleotide reductase inhibitor and acyclovir as treatment for acyclovir-resistant herpes simplex virus infection. *J Med Virol* **1**: 146.

Safrin S, Schacker T, Delehanty J *et al.* (1993b) Topical treatment of infection with acyclovir-resistant mucocutaneous herpes simplex virus with the ribonucleotide reductase inhibitor 348U87 in combination with acyclovir. *Antimicrob Ag Chemother* **37**: 975.

Safrin S, Elbeik T, Mills J (1994a) A rapid screen test for *in vitro* susceptibility of clinical herpes simplex virus isolates. *J Infect Dis* **169**: 879.

Safrin S, Kemmerly S, Plotkin B *et al.* (1994b) Foscarnet-resistant herpes simplex virus infection in patients with AIDS. *J Infect Dis* **169**: 193.

Safrin S, Elbeik T, Phan L *et al.* (1994c) Correlation between response to aciclvori and foscarnet therapy and *in vitro* susceptibility result for isolates of herpes simplex virus from human immunodeficiency virus-infected patients. *Antimicrob Ag Chemother* **38**: 1246.

Sakamoto T, Uemura M, Fukui H *et al.* (1992). Chronic active Epstein-Barr virus infection in an adult. *Intern Med* **31**: 1190.

Sakuma S, Yamamoto M, Kumano Y, Mori R (1988). An acyclovir-resistant strain of herpes simplex virus type 2 which is highly virulent for mice. *Arch Virol* **101**: 169.

Salo OP, Lassus A, Hovi T, Fiddian AP (1983). Double-blind placebo-controlled trial of oral acyclovir in recurrent genital herpes. *Eur J Sex Transm Dis* **1**: 95.

Samorek SE, Cakala A, Wijaszka T (1987). Effect of acyclovir on the replication of turkey herpes virus and Marek's disease virus. *Res Vet Sci* **42**: 334.

Saral R (1993). Acyclovir influence on graft versus host disease. *J Med Virol* **1**: 112.

Saral R, Burns WH, Laskin OL *et al.* (1981). Acyclovir prophylaxis of herpes simplex virus infections. *New Engl J Med* **305**: 63.

Saral R, Ambinder RF, Burns WH *et al.* (1983). Acyclovir prophylaxis against herpes simplex virus infection in patients with leukemia A randomized, double blind, placebo-controlled study. *Ann Intern Med* **99**: 773.

Sawyer MH, Inchauspe G, Biron KK *et al.* (1988a) Molecular analysis of the pyrimidine deoxyribonucleoside kinase gene of wild-type acyclovir-resistant strains of varicella-zoster virus. *J Gen Virol* **69**: 2585.

Sawyer MH, Webb DE, Balow JE, Straus SE (1988b) Acyclovir-induced renal failure; clinical course and histology. *Amer J Med* **84**: 1067.

Schaeffer HJ, Beauchamp L, De Miranda P *et al.* (1978). 9-(2-hydroxyethoxy-methyl) guanine activity against viruses of the herpes group. *Nature* **272**: 583.

Schalm SW, Heytink RA, van Burren HR *et al.* (1985). Acyclovir enhances the antiviral effect of interferon in chronic hepatitis B. *Lancet* **ii**: 358.

Schalm SW, Heytink RA, Van VH, De Man RA (1986). Acyclovir, oral, intravenous and combined with interferon for chronic HBeAg positive hepatitis. *J Hepatology* **3**: S137.

Schlossberg D, Littman M (1988). Varicella pneumonia. *Arch Int Med* **148**: 1630.

Schofield JK, Tatnall FM, Leigh IM (1993). Recurrent erythema; clinical features and treatment in a large series of patients. *Brit J Dermatol* **128**: 542.

Schwandt NW, Mjos DP, Lubow RM (1987). Acyclovir and the treatment of herpetic whitlow. *Oral Surg Oral Med Oral Pathol* **64**: 255.

Scott LL, Sanchez PJ, Jackson GL *et al.* (1996). Acyclovir suppression to prevent cesarean delivery after first-episode genital herpes. *Obstet Gynecol* **87**: 69.

Selby PJ, Powles RL, Jameson B *et al.* (1979). Parenteral acyclovir therapy for herpes virus infections in man. *Lancet* **ii**: 1267.

Sempere A, Sanz GF, Senent L *et al.* (1992). Long term acyclovir prophylaxis for prevention of varicella zoster virus infection after autologous blood stem cell transplantation in patients with acute leukemia. *Bone Marrow Transplant* **10**: 495.

Serota F T Starr SE, Bryan CK *et al.* (1982). Acyclovir treatment of herpes zoster infections Use in children undergoing bone marrow transplantation. *JAMA* **7**: 2132.

Sha BE, Benson CA, Deutsch TA *et al.* (1991). Suppression of cytomegalovirus retinitis in persons with AIDS with high-dose intravenous acyclovir. *J Infect Dis* **164**: 777.

Shaw M, King M, Best JM *et al.* (1985). Failure of acyclovir cream in treatment of recurrent herpes labialis. *Brit Med J* **291**: 7.

Shepp DH, Newton BA, Meyers JD (1984). Intravenous lymphoblastoid interferon and acyclovir for treatment of cytomegaloviral pneumonia. *J Infect Dis* **150**: 776.

Shepp DH, Dandliker PS, Flournoy N, Meyers JD (1985a) Once-daily intravenous acyclovir for prophylaxis of herpes simplex virus reactivation after marrow transplantation. *J Antimicrob Chemother* **16**: 389.

Shepp DH, Newton BA, Dandliker PS *et al.* (1985b) Oral acyclovir therapy for mucocutaneous herpes simplex virus infections in immunocompromised marrow transplant recipients. *Ann Intern Med* **102**: 783.

Shepp DH, Dandliker PS, Meyers JD (1986). Treatment of varicella-zoster virus infection in severely immunocompromised patients A randomized comparison of acyclovir and vidarabine. *New Engl J Med* **314**: 208.

Shiota H (1982). Clinical evaluation of acyclovir in the treatment of ulcerative herpetic keratitis. *Amer J Med* **73**: 307.

Shiraki K, Ochiai H, Namazue J *et al.* (1992). Comparison of antiviral assay methods using cell-free and cell-associated varicella-zoster virus. *Antiviral Res* **18**: 209.

Sibrack CD, McClaren C, Barry DW (1982a) Disease and latency characteristics of clinical herpes simplex virus isolates after acyclovir therapy. *Amer J Med* **73**: 372.

Sibrack CD, Gutman LT, Wilfert CM *et al.* (1982b) Pathogenicity of acyclovir resistant herpes simplex virus type I from an immunodeficient child. *J Infect Dis* **146**: 673.

Sicher SE, Oh JO (1981). Acyclovir therapy of neonatal herpes simplex virus type 2 infections in rabbits. *Antimicrob Ag Chemother* **20**: 503.

Singh N, Yu VL, Mieles L *et al.* (1994). High dose acyclovir compared with short course preemptive ganciclovir therapy to prevent cytomegalovirus disease in liver transplant recipients. A randomised trial. *Ann Intern Med* **120**: 375.

Skoldenberg B, Forsgren M, Alestig K *et al.* (1984). Acyclovir versus vidarabine in herpes simplex encephalitis. Randomised multicentre study in consecutive Swedish patients. *Lancet* **ii**: 707.

Smego RA, Asperilla MO (1991). Use of acyclovir for varicella pneumonia during pregnancy. *Obstet Gynecol* **78**: 1112.

Smith CI, Scullard GH, Gregory PB *et al.* (1982). Preliminary studies of acyclovir in chronic hepatitis B. *Amer J Med* **73**: 267.

Smith CA, Wigdahl B, Rapp F (1983). Synergistic antiviral activity of acyclovir and interferon on human cytomegalovirus. *Antimicrob Ag Chemother* **24**: 325.

Snoeck R, Andrei G, Schols D *et al.* (1992). Activity of different antiviral drug combinations against human cytomegalovirus replication *in vitro*. *Eur J Clin Microbiol Infect Dis* **11**: 1144.

Snoeck R, Gerard M, Sadzot-Delvaux C *et al.* (1994). Meningoradiculoneuritis due to acyclovir-resistant varicella zoster virus in an acquired immune deficiency syndrome patient. *J Med Virol* **42**: 338.

Spangler JG, Kirk JK, Knudson MP (1994). Uses and safety of acyclovir in pregnancy. *J Fam Pract* **38**: 186.

Spector SA, Kelley E (1985). Inhibition of human cytomegalovirus by combined acyclovir and vidarabine. *Antimicrob Ag Chemother* **27**: 600.

Spector SA, Connor JD, Hintz M *et al.* (1981). Single-dose pharmacokinetics of acyclovir. *Antimicrob Ag Chemother* **19**: 608.

Spector SA, Hintz M, Wyborny C *et al.* (1982). Treatment of herpes virus infections in immunocompromised patients with acyclovir by continuous intravenous infusion. *Amer J Med* **73**: 275.

Spector SA, Connor JA, McCutchan JA *et al.* (1985). 9-(2-hydroxy-1-(hydroxymethyl) ethoxymethyl) guanine (DHPG, BW759U) Treatment of AIDS patients with serious cytomegalovirus infections. In *Program and Abstracts of the 25th Interscience Conference on Antimicrobial Agents and Chemotherapy, Minneapolis* (Abstr 441). Washington, DC: American Society for Microbiology.

Sperber SJ, Feibusch EL, Damiani A, Weinstein MP (1993). *In vitro* activities of nucleoside analog antiviral agents against salmonellae. *Antimicrob Ag Chemother* **37**: 106.

Spruance SL, Schnipper LE, Overall JC Jr *et al.* (1982). Treatment of herpes simplex labialis with topical acyclovir in polyethylene glycol. *J Infect Dis* **146**: 85.

Spruance SL, Crumpacker CS, Schnipper LE *et al.* (1984). Early, patient-initiated treatment of herpes labialis with topical 10% acyclovir. *Antimicrob Ag Chemother* **25**: 553.

Spruance SL, Stewart JC, Rowe NH *et al.* (1990). Treatment of recurrent herpes simplex labialis with oral acyclovir. *J Infect Dis* **161**: 185.

Spruance SL, Freeman DJ, Stewart JCB *et al.* (1991). The natural history of UVR-induced herpes simplex labialis and response to therapy with peroral and topical formulations of ACV. *J Infect Dis* **163**: 728.

St Clair MH, Furman PA, Lubbers CM, Elion GB (1980). Inhibition of cellular alpha and virally induced deoxyribonucleic acid polymerases by the triphosphate of acyclovir. *Antimicrob Ag Chemother* **18**: 741.

Stahlmann R, Klug S, Lawandowski C *et al.* (1988). Prenatal toxicity of acyclovir in rats. *Arch Toxicol* **61**: 468.

Stahlmann R, Korte M, Van Loveren H *et al.* (1992). Abnormal thymus development and impaired function of the immune system in rats after prenatal exposure to acyclovir. *Arch Toxicol* **66**: 551.

Stanwick TL, Schinazi RF, Campbell DE, Nahmias AJ (1981). Combined antiviral effect of interferon and acyclovir on herpes simplex virus types I and 2. *Antimicrob Ag Chemother* **19**: 672.

Steele RW, Keeney RE, Bradsher RW *et al.* (1983). Treatment of varicella-zoster meningoencephalitis with acyclovir-demonstration of virus in cerebrospinal fluid by electron microscopy. *Amer J Clin Path* **80**: 57.

Stein DS, Graham NM, Park LP *et al.* (1994). The effect of the interaction of acyclovir with zidovudine on progression to AIDS and survival. Analysis of data in the Multicenter AIDS Cohort Study. *Ann Intern Med* **121**: 100.

Straus SE, Smith HA, Brickman C *et al.* (1982). Acyclovir for chronic mucocutaneous herpes simplex virus infection in immunosuppressed patients. *Ann Intern Med* **96**: 270.

Straus SE, TakiffHE, Seidlin M *et al.* (1984). Suppression of frequently recurring genital herpes. A placebo-controlled double-blind trial of oral acyclovir. *New Engl J Med* **310**: 1545.

Straus SE, Seidlin M, Takiff HE *et al.* (1986). Double-blind comparison of weekend and daily regimens of oral acyclovir for suppression of recurrent genital herpes. *Antiviral Res* **6**: 151.

Straus SE, Dale JK, Tobi M *et al.* (1988). Acyclovir treatment of the chronic fatigue syndrome lack of efficacy in a placebo controlled trial. *New Engl J Med* **319**: 1692.

Sullender WM, Arvin AM, Diaz PS *et al.* (1987). Pharmacokinetics of acyclovir suspension in infants and children. *Antimicrob Ag Chemother* **31**: 1722.

Sullivan JL, Byron KS, Brewster FE *et al.* (1982). Treatment of life-threatening Epstein-Barr virus infections with acyclovir. *Amer J Med* **73**: 262.

Sutton D, Boyd MR (1993). Comparative activity of penciclovir and acyclovir in mice infected intraperitoneally with herpes simplex virus type 1 SC16. *Antimicrob Ag Chemother* **37**: 642.

Sylvester RK, Ogden WB, Draxler CA, Lewis FB (1986). Vesicular eruption A complication of concentrated acyclovir infusions. *JAMA* **255**: 385.

Taddio A, Klein J, Koren G (1994). Acyclovir excretion in human breast milk. *Ann Pharmacother* **28**: 585.

Takehara T, Hayashi N, Katayama K *et al.* (1992). Enhanced expression of HLA class 1 by inhibited replication of hepatitis B virus. *J Hepatol* **14**: 232.

Talarico CL, Phelps WC, Biron KK (1993). Analysis of the thymidine kinase genes from acyclovir- resistant mutants of varicella-zoster virus isolated from patients with AIDS. *J Virol* **67**: 1024.

Tanaka S, Toh Y, Mohri R (1993). Molecular analysis of a neurovirulent herpes simplex virus type 2 strain with reduced thymidine kinase activity. *Arch Virol* **131**: 61.

Tang IT, Shepp DH (1992). Herpes simplex virus infection in cancer patients; prevention and treatment. *Oncology Huntingt* **6**: 101.

Tatnall FM, Schofield JK, Leigh IM (1995). A double-blind, placebo-controlled trial of continuous acyclovir therapy in recurrent erythema multiforme. *Brit J Dermatol* **132**: 267.

Taylor JL, Tom P, Guy J *et al.* (1994). Regulation of herpes simplex virus thymidine kinase in cells treated with a synergistic antiviral combination of alpha interferon and acyclovir. *Antimicrob Ag Chemother* **38**: 853.

Tebas P, Stabell EC, Olivo PD (1995). Antiviral susceptibility testing with a cell line which expresses beta galaclosidase after infection with herpes simplex virus. *Antimicrob Ag Chemother* **39**: 1287.

Thin RN, Nabarro JM, Davidson Parker J, Fiddian AP (1983). Topical acyclovir in the treatment of initial genital herpes. *Brit J Vener Dis* **59**: 116.

Thin RN, Jeffries DJ, Taylor PK *et al.* (1985). Recurrent genital herpes suppressed by oral acyclovir: a multicentre double blind trial. *J Antimicrob Chemother* **16**: 219.

Thomas RHM, Dodd HJ, Yeo JM, Kirby JTD (1985). Oral ACV in the suppression of recurrent non- genital herpes simplex virus infection. *Brit J Dermatol* **113**: 731.

Tilson HH, Engle CR, Andres EB (1993). Safety of acyclovir; a summary of the first 10 years experience. *J Med Virol* **1**: 67.

Tomson CR, Goodship THJ, Rodger RSC (1985). Psychiatric side-effects of acyclovir in patients with chronic renal failure. *Lancet* **ii**: 385.

Trousdale MD, Nesburn AB (1982). Evaluation of the antiherpetic activity of acyclovir in rabbits. *Amer J Med* **73**: 155.

Tucker WE Jr (1982). Preclinical toxicology of acyclovir: an overview. *Amer J Med* **73**: 27.

Tuncer AM, Evis B, Kunak B *et al.* (1989). Erythroblastopenia and leukopenia in the patient with severe herpes zoster treated with intravenous acyclovir. *Turk J Pediatr* **31**: 317.

Tyms AS, Scamans EM, Naim HM (1981). The *in vitro* activity of acyclovir and related compounds against cytomegalovirus infections. *J Antimicrob Chemother* **8**: 65.

United States Pharmacopeia Drug Information (1997). The United States Pharmacopeial Convention, Inc. April.

Valsecchi R, Imberti G, Cainelli T (1990). Contact allergy to acyclovir. *Contact Dermatitis* **23**: 372.

Van den Broek PJ, van der Meer JW, Mulder JD *et al.* (1984). Limited value of acyclovir in the treatment of uncomplicated herpes zoster; a placebo controlled study. *Infection* **12**: 338.

Van der Horst C, Lin JC, Raab TN *et al.* (1987). Differential effects of acyclovir and 9-(1,3-dihydroxy-2-propoxymethyl)guanine on herpes simplex virus and Epstein Barr virus in a dually infected human lymphoblastoid cell line. *J Virology* **61**: 607.

Van der Horst C, Joncas J, Ahronheim G *et al.* (1991). Lack of effort of peroral acyclovir for the treatment of acute infectious mononucleosis. *J Infect Dis* **164**: 788.

Van der Meer JWM, Versteeg J (1982). Acyclovir in severe herpes virus infections. *Amer J Med* **73**: 271.

Van Dyke RB, Connor JD, Wyborny C *et al.* (1982). Pharmacokinetics of orally administered acyclovir in patients with herpes progenitalis. *Amer J Med* **73**: 172.

Van Ekdom LTS, Versteeg J (1982). Preventive and curative effects of acyclovir on central nervous system infections in hamsters inoculated with Herpes simplex virus. *Amer J Med* **73**: 161.

Van Vloten WA, Swart RNJ, Pot F (1983). Topical acyclovir therapy in patients with recurrent orofacial herpes simplex infections. *J Antimicrob Chemother* **12**: 89.

Verdonck LF, Cornelissen JJ, Smit J *et al.* (1993). Successful foscarnet therapy for acyclovir-resistant mucocutaneous infection with herpes simplex virus in a recipient of allogeneic BMT. *Bone Marrow Transplant* **11**: 177.

Vitale VJ, Saiman L, Haddad J (1993). Herpes laryngitis and tracheitis causing respiratory distress in a neonate. *Arch Otolaryngol Head Neck Surg* **119**: 239.

Wade JC, Meyers lD (1983). Neurologic symptoms associated with parenteral acyclovir treatment after marrow transplantation. *Ann Intern Med* **98**: 921.

Wade JC Newton B, McLaren C *et al.* (1982a). Intravenous acyclovir to treat mucocutaneous herpes simplex virus infection after marrow transplantation. *Ann Intern Med* **96**: 265.

Wade JC, Hintz M, McGuffin RW *et al.* (1982b) Treatment of cyto-megalovirus pneumonia with high-dose acyclovir. *Amer J Med* **73**: 249.

Wade JC, McLaren C, Meyers JD (1983a) Frequency and significance of acyclovir-resistant herpes simplex virus isolated from marrow transplant patients receiving multiple courses of treatment with acyclovir. *J Infect Dis* **148**: 1077.

Wade JC, McGuffin RW, Springmeyer SC *et al.* (1983b) Treatment of cytomegaloviral pneumonia with high-dose acyclovir and human leuko-cyte interferon. *J Infect Dis* **148**: 557.

Wade JC, Newton B, Flournoy N, Meyers JD (1984). Oral acyclovir for prevention of herpes simplex virus reactivation after marrow transplanta-tion. *Ann Intern Med* **100**: 823.

Wald A, Benedetti J, Davis G *et al.* (1994). A randomised double-blind comparative trial comparing high and standard dose oral acyclovir for first-episode genital herpes infections. *Antimicrob Ag Chemother* **38**: 174.

Wald A, Zeh J, Barnum G *et al.* (1996). Suppression of subclinical shedding of herpes simplex virus type 2 with acyclovir. *Ann Intern Med* **124**: 8.

Wallace MR, Bowler WA, Murray NB, (1992). Treatment of adult varicella with oral acyclovir. A randomized, placebo-controlled trial. *Ann Intern Med* **117**: 358.

Walzer PD, Foy J, Steele P *et al.* (1992). Activities of antifolate, antiviral and other drugs in an immunosuppressed rat model of *Pneumocystis carinii* pneumonia. *Antimicrob Ag Chemother* **36**: 1935.

Weinberg A, Bate BJ, Masters HB *et al.* (1992). *In vitro* activities of penciclovir and acyclovir against herpes simplex virus types 1 and 2. *Antimicrob Ag Chemother* **36**: 2037.

Weller lVD, Carreno V, Fowler MJF *et al.* (1983). Acyclovir in hepatitis B antigen-positive chronic liver disease: inhibition of viral replication and transient renal impairment with iv bolus administration. *J Antimicrob Chemother* **11**: 223.

Whatley JD Thin RN (1991). Episodic acyclovir therapy to abort recurrent attacks of genital herpes simplex infection. *J Antimicrob Chemother* **27**: 677.

Whitley RJ, Gnann JW (1992). Drug therapy; acyclovir; A decade later. *New Engl J Med* **327**: 782.

Whitley RJ, Gnann JW, (1993). Acyclovir; a model for future antiviral drugs Acyclovir. *The Landmark Papers* **ix**.

Whitley RJ, Blum MR, Barton N, de Miranda P (1982a) Pharmacokinetics of acyclovir in humans following intravenous administration. A model for the development of parenteral antivirals. *Amer J Med* **73**: 165.

Whitley RJ, Barton N, Collins E *et al.* (1982b) Mucocutaneous herpes simplex virus infections in immunocompromised patients A model for evaluation of topical antiviral agents. *Amer J Med* **73**: 236.

Whitley RJ, Soong SJ, Dolin R *et al.* (1982c) Early vidarabine therapy to control the complications of herpes zoster in immunosuppressed patients. *New Engl J Med* **307**: 971.

Whitley RJ, Levin M, Barton N *et al.* (1984). Infections caused by herpes simplex virus in the immunocompromised host: natural history and topical acyclovir therapy. *J Infect Dis* **150**: 323.

Whitley RJ, Alford CA, Hirsch MS *et al.* (1986). Vidarabine versus acyclovir therapy in herpes simplex encephalitis. *New Engl J Med* **314**: 144.

Whitley RJ, Arvin A, Prober C *et al.* (1991). A controlled trial comparing vidarabine with acyclovir in neonatal herpes simplex virus infection. Infectious Diseases Collaborative Antiviral Study Group. *New Engl J Med* **324**: 444.

Whitley RJ, Gnann JW, Hinthorn D *et al.* (1992). Disseminated herpes zoster in the immunocompromised host; a comparative trial of acyclovir and vidarabine. The NIAID Collaborative Antiviral Study Group. *J Infect Dis* **165**: 450.

Whitley RJ, Weiss H, Gnann JW *et al.* (1996). Acyclovir with and without prednisolone for the treatment of herpes zoster. *Ann Intern Med* **125**: 376.

Wingard JR, Hess AD, Stuart RK *et al.* (1983). Effect of several antiviral agents on human lymphocyte functions and marrow progenitor cell proliferation. *Antimicrob Ag Chemother* **23**: 593.

Winston DJ, Wirin D, Shaked A, Busuttil RW (1995). Randomised comparison of ganciclovir and high dose acyclovir for long-term cytomegalovirus prophylaxis in liver-transplant recipients. *Lancet* **346**: 69.

Wolfsen HC, Bolen JW, Bowen JL, Fenster LF (1993). Fulminant herpes hepatitis mimicking hepatic abscesses. *J Clin Gastroenterol* **16**: 61.

Wong T, Lavaud S, Toupance O *et al.* (1993). Failure of acyclovir to prevent cytomegalovirus infection in renal allograft recipients. *Transpl Int* **6**: 285.

Wood MJ, Ogan PH, McKendrick MW (1988). Efficacy of oral acyclovir treatment of acute herpes zoster. *Amer J Med* **85**: 79.

Wood MJ, McKendrick MW, Freris MW *et al.* (1994a) Trough plasma acyclovir concentrations and safety of oral acyclovir, 800mg five times daily for 7 days in elderly patients with herpes zoster. *J Antimicrob Chemother* **33**: 1245.

Wood MJ, Johnson RW, McKendrick MW *et al.* (1994b) A randomised trial of acyclovir for 7 days or 21 days with and without prednisolone for treatment of acute herpes zoster. *New Engl J Med* **330**: 896.

Woolfson H (1984). Oral acyclovir in eczema herpeticum. *Brit Med J* **288**: 531.

Wormser GP, Mack L, Lednox T *et al.* (1988). Lack of effect of oral acyclovir on prevention of aphthous stomatitis. *Otolaryngol Head Neck Surg* **98**: 14.

Yeager AS (1982). Use of acyclovir in premature and term neonates. *Amer J Med* **73**: 205.

Youle MS, Gazzard BG, Johnson MA *et al.* (1994). Effects of high dose oral acyclovir on herpes virus disease and survival in patients with advanced HIV disease; a double-blind, placebo-controlled study. European-Australian Acyclovir Study Group. *AIDS* **8**: 641.

Young B, Patterson A, Ravenscroft T (1982). Double-blind clinical trial of acyclovir and adenine arabinoside in herpetic corneal ulceration. *Amer J Med* **73**: 311.

Famciclovir and Penciclovir

Description

The limited oral absorption of the acyclic guanine derivative, penciclovir (9-(4-hydroxy-3-hydroxymethylbut-1-yl)guanine; BRL 39123), prompted a search for orally bioavailable prodrugs. Famciclovir (9-(4-acetoxy-3 acetoxymethylbut-1-yl)-2-aminopurine, originally known as BRL 42810) is a well-absorbed oral prodrug of penciclovir. It is the diacetate ester of 6-deoxy penciclovir. BRL 42359 is the 6-deoxy precursor of penciclovir. Famciclovir is marketed by SmithKline Beecham Pharmaceuticals under the trade name of 'Famvir'. Its main clinical application is in the treatment of varicella-zoster virus infections, particularly herpes zoster. The drug is now licensed in many countries.

The molecular weight of famciclovir is 321.3. The molecular formula is $C_{14}H_{19}N_5O_4$. The chemical structures of penciclovir and famciclovir are shown in Fig. V.6. The concentration of penciclovir can be expressed either as µg per ml or µM; 1 µg per ml is equivalent to 3.9 µM.

Antiviral Activity

Famciclovir has activity against herpes simplex types 1 and 2, varicella-zoster virus and Epstein–Barr virus *in vitro* (Smith Kline Beecham, personal communication; Bacon and Boyd, 1995) with very limited activity against cytomegalovirus (Boyd and Safrin, 1993).

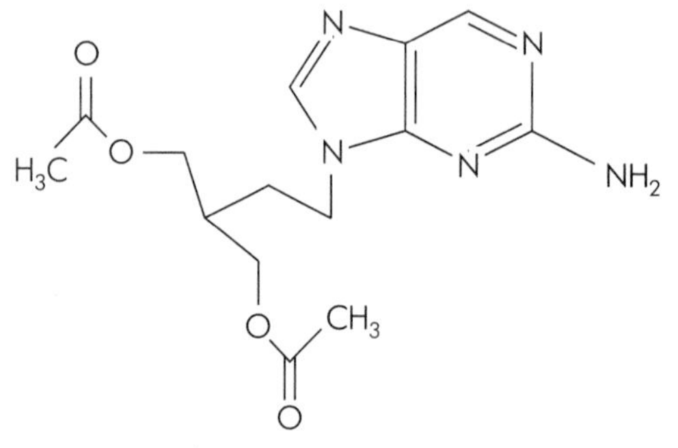

Famciclovir

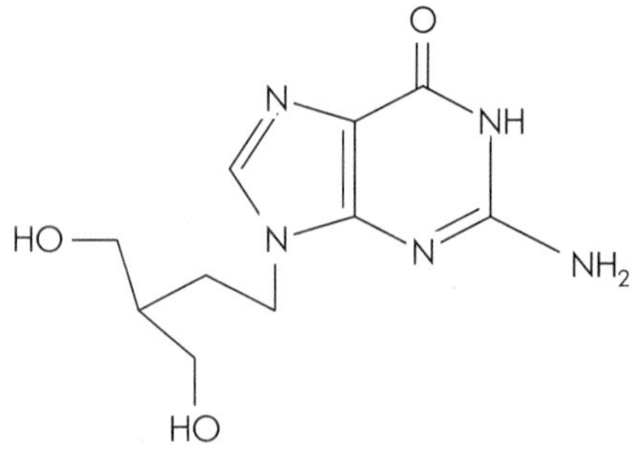

Penciclovir

Fig. V.6.
Chemical structures of famciclovir and penciclovir. (Reproduced from Perry and Wagstaff, 1995, with permission.)

1 Herpes simplex virus

In a comparative study, Safrin and her colleague (Safrin and Phan, 1993) found that the IC_{50} values for penciclovir against herpes simplex strains paralleled those of aciclovir, although the values for penciclovir are about twice as high as those for aciclovir; for aciclovir-sensitive strains the range of IC_{50} values for aciclovir and penciclovir were 0.12–0.9 µg per ml, and 0.21–2.3 µg per ml respectively. These results are supported by more recent reports (Ertl and Snowden, 1995; Bacon and Howard, 1996; Bacon et al., 1996a). There may be marked differences in antiviral sensitivity results of penciclovir when plaque reduction assays are conducted in different cell types (Bacon and Schinazi, 1993). In human amnion cell lines penciclovir was found to be more active than aciclovir against replication of herpes simplex types 1 and 2; in human lung cell lines, the reverse was found with aciclovir having better in vitro activity than penciclovir against both herpes simplex types 1 and 2 (Boyd, 1993). Other investigators report very similar in vitro sensitivities of herpes simplex type 1 to aciclovir and penciclovir, with IC_{50} concentrations of 0.5–0.8 µg per ml using several methods of analysis (Weinberg et al., 1992).

Oral famciclovir and penciclovir administered by oral, i.v., subcutaneous and topical routes have demonstrated efficacy against herpes simplex types 1 and 2 in murine and guinea pig models of infection reviewed by (Sutton and Kern, 1993). Topical penciclovir was as effective as aciclovir for the treatment of cutaneous herpes simplex type 1 infection and genital type 2 infection in guinea pigs (Boyd et al., 1988). In an immunosuppressed murine model of herpes simplex type 1 infection oral famciclovir and valaciclovir were both effective in clearing infection, famciclovir achieving virus clearance faster than valaciclovir (Field et al., 1995; Field and Thackray, 1995). Famciclovir has also been found to be superior to aciclovir in mice infected via the intraperitoneal route with herpes simplex type 1 (Ashton et al., 1994). A single subcutaneous injection of penciclovir given to mice infected intraperitoneally with herpes simplex type 1 administered 24 h post-infection was active at a 10-fold lower concentration than aciclovir, likely to be due to the relatively higher stability of intracellular penciclovir triphosphate compared with that of aciclovir (Sutton and Boyd, 1993). Equine herpes virus type 2 is inhibited by penciclovir in vitro with an IC_{50} of 1.6 µg per ml (de la Fuente et al., 1992).

2 Varicella-zoster virus

Penciclovir is more active in vitro against herpes simplex types 1 and 2 than varicella-zoster virus, with a mean IC_{50} for each virus of approximately 0.4, 1.5 and 3.1 µg per ml respectively (Boyd et al., 1987; Perry and Wagstaff, 1995). Other investigators have reported slightly lower IC_{50} values (1.2 µg per ml) of penciclovir for varicella-zoster virus (Shiraki et al., 1993). Intramuscular penciclovir treatment of African Green monkeys infected with simian varicella virus resulted in therapeutic effects on rash and viremia (Soike et al., 1993).

3 Cytomegalovirus

Laboratory strains of cytomegalovirus such as AD-169 are relatively resistant to penciclovir, with an IC_{50} of 51 µg per ml (Boyd et al., 1987; Perry and Wagstaff, 1995). Clinical isolates may be more susceptible with reported IC_{50} values of about 18 µg per ml (Bacon, 1996).

4 Epstein–Barr virus

Penciclovir has some activity against Epstein–Barr virus, with an IC_{50} value of 10 µg per ml (Boon and Griffin, 1996; Boyd et al., 1987; Bacon and Boyd, 1994; Bacon et al., 1996a,b). Unlike aciclovir, the antiviral activity of penciclovir persists after the removal of the drug, reflecting the stability of intracellular penciclovir triphosphate (Boyd, 1993).

5 Hepatitis B virus

In vitro antiviral activity of penciclovir has been reported against duck hepatitis B virus, with an IC_{50} of 0.7 ± 0.1 µM. Persistence of activity continued following the removal of extracellular penciclovir (Shaw et al., 1994). Oral famciclovir has inhibited duck hepatitis B virus DNA in ducklings infected in vivo (Tsiquaye et al., 1994). Chronically infected ducks treated with either famciclovir or penciclovir had evidence of suppression of hepatitis B virus replication as measured by plasma viral DNA and DNA polymerase. Following cessation of treatment there was a delay of only 2–8 days before plasma levels of these markers of hepatitis B replication began to increase again (Tsiquaye et al., 1996).

6 Resistance to penciclovir and cross-resistance with other drugs

Thymidine kinase (TK)-deficient strains of herpes simplex that are resistant to aciclovir are cross-resistant to penciclovir. However, there are differences between aciclovir and penciclovir in terms of interactions with TK. Thus, TK-altered strains of aciclovir (which have an altered substrate specificity) may remain sensitive to penciclovir (Boyd *et al.*, 1987). When clinical isolates of herpes simplex virus that were resistant to aciclovir or foscarnet were tested for their susceptibility to penciclovir *in vitro*, penciclovir remained relatively active against foscarnet-resistant strains (Safrin and Phan, 1993; Boyd and Safrin, 1993). Similarly, aciclovir-resistant strains of varicella-zoster virus generally show cross-resistance to penciclovir (Hasegawa *et al.*, 1995), although aciclovir-resistant strains due to altered specificty of TK may remain sensitive to penciclovir (Talarico *et al.*, 1993).

7 Synergism and antagonism

Penciclovir and either aciclovir or ganciclovir demonstrate additive antiviral interactions *in vitro* against herpes simplex types 1 and 2. Penciclovir was found to demonstrate synergism with foscarnet against herpes simplex type 1 but not type 2 (Sutton and Taylor, 1992). Human interferons (particularly alpha, but also beta and gamma) were highly synergistic with penciclovir against herpes simplex types 1 and 2. High concentrations of zidovudine (10μg per ml) were antagonistic to the antiviral effects of penciclovir in this study (Sutton and Taylor, 1992).

Mode of Administration and Dosage

The currently recommended dose of famciclovir for the treatment of herpes zoster is 500 mg three times daily for 7 days in the USA, and 250 mg three times daily in the UK, commencing within 72 h (and preferably within 48 h) after the development of rash. The recommended dose for the treatment of the first episode of genital herpes is 250 mg three times daily for 5 days commencing as soon as possible after the onset of symptoms or signs; the dose for recurrent genital herpes is 125 mg twice-daily for 5 days. The minimum dose for the treatment of herpes zoster or genital herpes has not been established.

1 Renal dysfunction

Because the drug is excreted by the kidneys, the dose should be reduced to 500 mg every 12 h in patients with a creatinine clearance of 40–59 ml per min, and to 500 mg once-daily in patients with a creatinine clearance of 20–39 ml per min (United States Pharmacopeia Drug Information, 1995). These data are based on results from studies in patients with renal impairment. Alternatively, it is suggested by the UK division of the company that the time interval between 250-mg doses of famciclovir could be increased from 8 to 12 or 24 h in patients with herpes zoster of primary genital herpes with mild (creatinine clearance 30–39 ml per min per 1.73m^2) or moderate (creatinine clearance 10–29 ml per min per 1.73m^2) renal impairment respectively reviewed in Perry and Wagstaff, 1995). For recurrent genital herpes, no dosage adjustment is necessary for patients with mild renal impairment, but for those with moderate reduction in creatinine clearance a dose of 125 mg of famciclovir daily is recommended. For patients requiring hemodialysis a dosage interval of 48 h is recommended, with the dose administered at the end of dialysis.

2 Hepatic dysfunction

The dose of famciclovir does not need to be altered in patients with well-compensated chronic liver disease. In two studies, a single dose of 500 mg of famciclovir administered to patients with chronic liver disease did not alter the area-under-the-curve (AUC), although the mean peak famciclovir plasma level was reduced by 43% in one report (SmithKline Beecham Pharmaceuticals, 1994; Boike *et al.*, 1994a,b; Pue *et al.*, 1994).

3 Elderly patients

Current evidence suggests that the dose of famciclovir does not need to be adjusted for elderly patients (provided renal function is not impaired). When a single dose of 750 mg of famciclovir was administered orally to 18 healthy but elderly subjects, the AUC was increased in those with reduced renal function (Fowles and Pue 1993). In another study, oral famciclovir (500 mg every 8 h) administered to persons with herpes zoster infection for 6 days, was associated with a higher peak plasma concentration and AUC in patients with reduced renal function in the elderly participants (Pratt, 1993). However, these age-dependent effects of renal function do not appear to be sufficient to require dose-adjustment (reviewed in Perry and Wagstaff, 1995).

Table V.4
Summary of clinically relevant pharmacokinetics of famciclovir

Good bioavailability of penciclovir after oral administration of famciclovir (41–75%).
May be taken with food.
Plasma levels increase in patients with renal dysfunction, requiring dose adjustment.
Famciclovir is metabolized in the liver and excreted predominantly in the urine.

Availability

Famciclovir is available for oral administration in 125 and 250 mg *tablets*.

Serum Levels in Relation to Dosage

1 Healthy adults

Penciclovir is limited in its clinical application by its poor oral bioavailability of only 5% (Easterbrook and Wood, 1994). However, the absorption of its prodrug famciclovir within the upper intestinal wall, and subsequent metabolism within the liver, allows the efficient conversion of famciclovir to penciclovir by deacetylation and then oxidation. The bioavailability of penciclovir after oral administration of famciclovir is between 41 and 75% (Pue and Benet, 1993; Vere Hodge, 1993; Filer *et al.*, 1994), and is not significantly altered by food (reviewed in Perry and Wagstaff, 1995) although the time to peak serum levels of penciclovir may be delayed when famciclovir is taken with food or just after a meal (Vere Hodge *et al.*, 1989; United States Pharmacopeia Drug Information, 1995; reviewed in Perry and Wagstaff, 1995) (Table V.4).

Penciclovir shows linear pharmacokinetics over famciclovir oral doses ranging from 125 to 750 mg. This was demonstrated in a study of the pharmacokinetics of penciclovir following administration of a single oral dose of famciclovir ranging from 125 to 750 mg, in which the AUCs and the peak plasma levels increased linearly with dose of famciclovir, with no alteration in time to peak serum level or elimination half-life (Pue *et al.*, 1994). Similar linear pharmacokinetics have been described when i.v. penciclovir was administered over a 1-h infusion in doses of 10, 15 and 20 mg per kg (Fowles *et al.*, 1992).

The time to achieve peak plasma levels following oral administration is 0.7 to 0.9 h. In two separate studies a single dose of 500 mg produced a mean peak plasma level of 3.3 and 3.6 μg per ml, with the AUC of 8.8 μg.h per ml (Filer *et al.*, 1994; Fowles *et al.*, 1994). When doses of 500 or 1000 mg of famciclovir are administered every 8 h for 5 days, the mean steady-state peak plasma concentration with the 500 mg dose was 13.2 ± 2.4 μM (3.4 ± 0.6 μg per ml), and 22.8 ± 2.4 μM (5.8 ± 0.6 μg per ml) with the 1000 mg dose. The mean serum half-life was 1.9 h, and the mean steady-state AUC for the 500- and 1000-mg doses were 29.6 ± 6.4 (7.6 ± 1.7 μg.h per ml) and 50.0 ± 2.8 μM.h (12.7 ± 0.7 μg.h per ml) respectively (Boyd, 1993). There is no difference in serum levels between males and females (Pratt and Pue, 1994).

To date there is no evidence that the dose of famciclovir should differ in geriatric populations when compared with that in younger adults. However, age-related decreases in renal function should be considered.

2 Renal impairment

In one study, 18 patients with mild, moderate and severe renal impairment and nine volunteers with normal renal function were treated with a single oral dose of 500 mg of famciclovir in an open-label study. The mean AUC was about 10-fold higher and the plasma elimination rate constant was approximately 4-fold lower in patients with a creatinine clearance of less than 30 ml per min, compared with normal volunteers (Boike *et al.*, 1994b). In patients with severe renal dysfunction (creatinine clearance of less than 30 ml per min) the half-life is prolonged (range 10–13 h).

3 Pediatrics and pregnancy

The pediatric dose has not yet been established. Until further data are available the drug is not recommended for use in pregnant or breast-feeding females.

Excretion and Distribution of the Drug in Body

Famciclovir undergoes extensive first-pass metabolism (Vere Hodge, 1993). The metabolic conversion of famciclovir to penciclovir is primarily through deacetylation within the intestinal wall producing the 6-deoxy derivative of penciclovir followed by oxidation at the 6-position in the purine base by aldehyde oxidase within the liver to produce penciclovir (Vere Hodge et al., 1989; reviewed in Bacon, 1996) (Fig. V.7).

Penciclovir is excreted primarily by the renal route, by glomerular filtration as well as tubular secretion, with little or none of the parent compound famciclovir being measured in the urine or blood (Pue and Benet, 1993). The terminal phase elimination half-life of penciclovir is approximately 2 h (Fowles and Pue, 1993). When multiple doses of 500 or 1000 mg of famciclovir were administered to normal humans every 8 h for 5 days, penciclovir was the major metabolite present in blood or urine (60%), with 6-deoxy-penciclovir also being detected as a minor metabolite (5%) (Boyd, 1993; Filer et al., 1994; Pue et al., 1994). Over a 3-day period approximately 25% of the administered dose of famciclovir will be recovered unchanged in the feces; penciclovir and 6-deoxy-penciclovir are present in faeces in lower quantities (less than 5% within 48 h) (Filer et al., 1994). There are no data as to whether penciclovir is removed from the blood by hemodialysis. It is not known whether penciclovir is distributed in breast milk following oral administration (United States Pharmacopeia Drug Information, 1995).

The steady-state volume of distribution of penciclovir has been reported to be 1.5 liters per kg, with a mean total plasma clearance of 39.3 liters per h and a mean terminal half-life of 2.0 h (Fowles et al., 1992). Unchanged famciclovir is virtually not detectable in the urine following an oral dose. Inactive metabolites detected in very small quantities (less than 1.5% of the dose) include 6-deoxy penciclovir, monoacetylated and diacetylated penciclovir, and monoacetylated 6-deoxypenciclovir (Vere Hodge et al., 1993; Boyd, 1993; United States Pharmacopeia Drug Information, 1995).

Mode of Action

Famciclovir is a prodrug of penciclovir, the latter being the active antiviral compound upon its triphosphorylation within the infected cell (Harnden et al., 1989; Vere Hodge et al., 1989; Earnshaw et al., 1992). Famciclovir is the diacetyl 6-deoxy analog of penciclovir. Penciclovir is phosphorylated by virus-specified TK to the monophosphate derivative (Fig. V.8); cellular kinases then convert penciclovir monophosphate to the di- and triphosphate forms (Vere Hodge and Perkins, 1989). Phosphorylation of penciclovir occurs more rapidly in infected cells than aciclovir (Vere Hodge and Perkins, 1989). The mode of action of penciclovir is very similar to that of aciclovir (p. 1518) (Balzarini et al., 1994). The level of penciclovir triphosphate in infected cells is approximately 100-fold more than that of aciclovir triphosphate, although the affinity of penciclovir triphosphate for the DNA polymerases of herpes simplex types 1 or 2 is of the order of 100-fold less than that of aciclovir triphosphate (Boyd, 1993). The half-life of penciclovir triphosphate within herpes simplex type 2 and varicella-zoster infected cells is 20 and 7 h respectively; in cells infected with herpes simplex type 1 it is approximately 10 h (Earnshaw

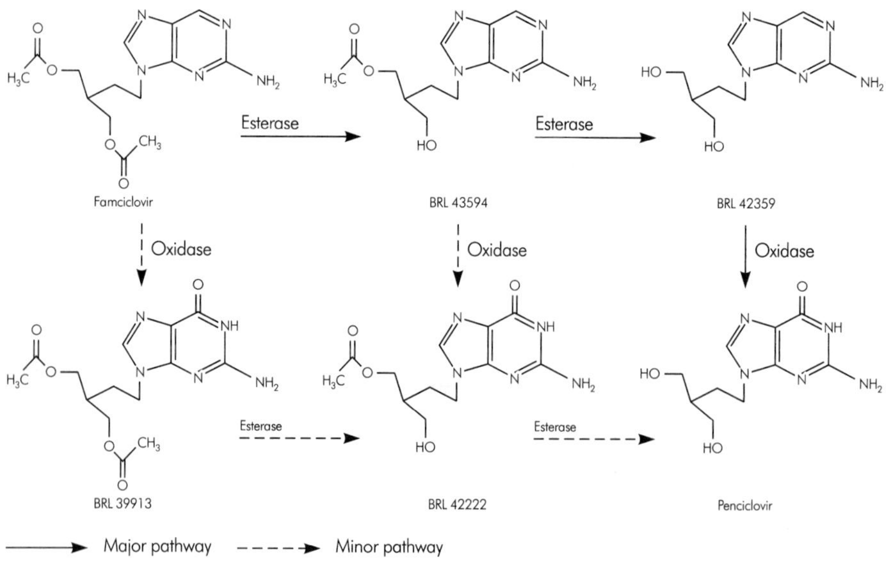

Fig. V.7.
Biotransformation of famciclovir in man. (Reproduced from Vere Hodge et al., 1989, with permission.)

Fig. V.8.
Schematic representation of inhibition of the viral DNA synthetic pathway by penciclovir in a herpesvirus-infected cell. (Reproduced from Perry and Wagstaff, 1995, with permission.)

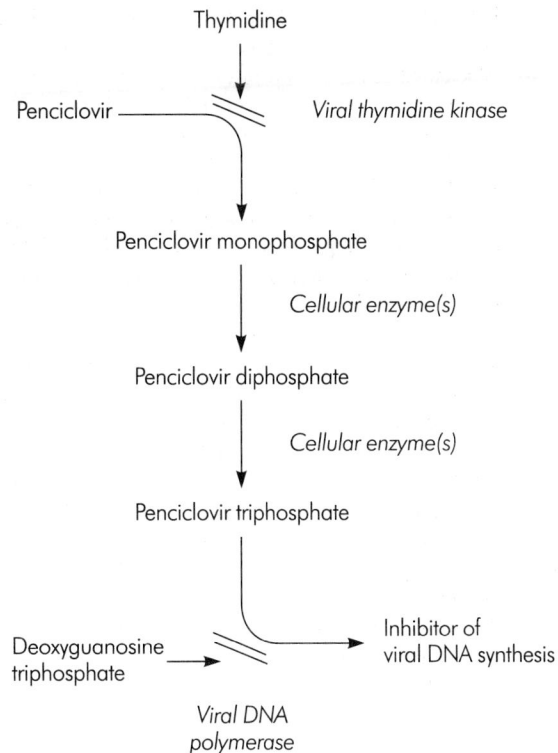

et al., 1992; United States Pharmacopeia Drug Information, 1995). The affinity of penciclovir triphosphate for host cell DNA polymerases is much weaker than for viral DNA polymerases (Iisley and Lee, 1995). Inhibition of herpes simplex types 1 and 2, and varicella-zoster DNA polymerases by the triphosphate derivative of penciclovir is competitive with deoxyguanosine triphosphate (Earnshaw *et al.*, 1992; Bacon, 1996). Aciclovir triphosphate, through its lack of a 3'-hydroxyl group on the acyclic side-chain that is necessary for extension of the viral DNA chain, results in DNA chain termination. However, penciclovir possesses two hydroxyl groups on the acyclic side-chain and thus can be incorporated into the viral DNA potentially allowing limited elongation (Earnshaw *et al.*, 1992).

Table V.5
Patients reporting adverse experiences related[a] to study medication in aciclovir-controlled herpes-zoster trials. (Reproduced from Salzman *et al.*, 1994, with permission.)

Adverse experience	No. (%) of patients in treatment group reporting adverse experience	
	Famiciclovir	Aciclovir
Headache	32 (6.0)	12 (4.6)
Nausea	20 (3.7)	7 (2.7)
Abdominal pain	9 (1.7)	6 (2.3)
Diarrhea	7 (1.3)	5 (1.9)
Vomiting	6 (1.1)	1 (0.4)
Dizziness	6 (1.1)	2 (0.8)
Constipation	6 (1.1)	1 (0.4)
Fatigue	4 (0.7)	6 (2.3)
Anorexia	1 (0.2)	5 (1.9)

[a] Includes categories of related, probably related, possibly related, and adverse experiences where the relationship was unassessable or not indicated. Of a total of 535 patients receiving famciclovir, 21.1% reported adverse experiences. Of a total of 263 patients receiving aciclovir, 20.2% reported adverse experiences.

Hepatitis B virus DNA polymerase is also sensitive to inhibition by penciclovir triphosphate. However, this virus dose not encode a TK. The enzyme(s) responsible for phosphorylation of penciclovir in hepatitis B infected hepatocytes is unknown, although cellular enzymes including cytoplasmic 5' nucleotidase may fulfil this function (reviewed in Bacon, 1996).

Toxicity

No serious toxicity has been observed with famciclovir. An analysis of safety data from 13 completed clinical trials involving 1600 patients has demonstrated that headache, nausea and diarrhea were the most common adverse experiences, with a frequency similar to that of placebo (Saltzman et al., 1994). The drug has a very similar safety profile to that of aciclovir (Table V.5).

1 Carcinogenicity and mutagenicity

The risk of mammary adenocarcinoma was found to be increased in female rats receiving 600 mg per kg of famciclovir (a dose that translates to 1.5-fold more than the human exposure when an oral dose of 500 mg three times daily is prescribed). Penciclovir caused chromosomal aberrations that were observed in unstimulated human lymphocytes. Famciclovir and penciclovir did not cause gene mutations when tested in vitro in bacteria (United States Pharmacopeia Drug Information, 1995).

2 Fertility

Dose-related testicular toxicity atrophy and abnormalities of spermatogenesis were noted in mice, rats and dogs treated on repeated occasions with either famciclovir or penciclovir for durations of up to 104 weeks (United States Pharmacopeia Drug Information, 1995). However, in experiments using human liver microsomes, incubation with famciclovir, penciclovir or BRL 42359 did not inhibit the 6-beta-hydroxylation of testosterone (Harrell et al., 1993). No embryo or fetal toxicity was observed in rats and rabbits treated with famciclovir in doses of up to 1000 mg per kg (3.6-fold the human exposure based on AUC concentrations) (United States Pharmacopeia Drug Information, 1995). Although there are no data to suggest embryotoxicity, it is recommended that famciclovir should only be prescribed to pregnant women if the estimated benefits are considered to outweigh potential risks of treatment.

3 Drug interactions

No clinically important drug interactions have been identified (Rolan, 1995). There is no evidence of any clinically significant interaction between famciclovir and allopurinol, cimetidine, theophylline or digoxin (Daniels and Schentag, 1993; Pratt et al., 1991; Pue et al., 1993; Fairless et al., 1992). Probenecid may compete with penciclovir for active tubular secretion in the kidney causing an increase in serum penciclovir levels. Allopurinol does not interfere with the pharmacokinetics of famciclovir (Fowles et al., 1994). Famciclovir and penciclovir do not inhibit cytochrome P-450 in the liver and are thus not considered likely to inhibit cyclosporin A or other substrates of cytochrome P-450 (Harrell et al., 1993).

Clinical Uses of the Drug

1 Herpes zoster

Famciclovir is indicated for the treatment of herpes zoster in immunocompetent adults who commence therapy within 72 h of onset of rash. Results of studies show that famciclovir has at least equivalent efficacy to that of aciclovir and a more favorable dosage regimen. Famciclovir decreases the duration of post-herpetic neuralgia and has similar efficacy to aciclovir in reducing the duration and intensity of acute pain (Perry and Wagstaff, 1995). Similar to aciclovir, efficacy depends on early administration of the drug following the onset of rash (best within 48 h).

In a randomized, double-blind, placebo-controlled multicenter trial, 419 immunocompetent hosts who presented with zoster within 72 h of onset of rash were randomized to receive famciclovir (either 500 mg or 750 mg three times daily) or placebo. The major finding was the shorter duration of post-herpetic neuralgia in famciclovir recipients (2 months less than in placebo recipients) with no significant difference between the two doses (Fig. V.9). There was no overall difference in the duration of acute pain between recipients of famciclovir or placebo. The times to full crusting of lesions and loss of vesicles were shorter for patients treated with famciclovir than placebo recipients. The 500-mg and 750-mg doses were equivalent (Tyring et al., 1995).

Fig. V.9.
Time to resolution of post-herpetic neuralgia in patients 50 years or older, treated with famciclovir 500 mg or 750 mg, compared with placebo (p = 0.005). (Reproduced from Tyring *et al.*, 1995, with permission.)

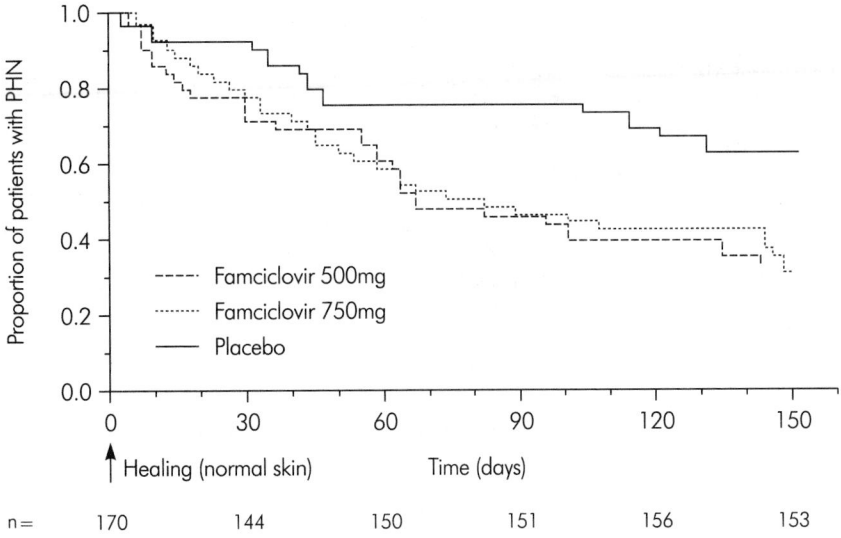

There have been several studies comparing the efficacy of famciclovir with aciclovir. A direct comparison of famciclovir and aciclovir in a clinical trial found similar efficacy in terms of healing of cutaneous lesions. Famciclovir was preferred because of the more favorable dosing schedule of three times daily compared with five times daily for aciclovir (Degreef and Famciclovir Herpes Zoster Clinical Study Group, 1994). A second study, only published in abstract form, generally confirmed these findings (Candaele and Candaele, 1994). There are currently no data on efficacy from trials in children, in patients with ophthalmic zoster, in immunocompromised hosts, or in patients with disseminated disease.

2 Genital herpes

Famciclovir has also been evaluated for the treatment of genital herpes, but to date the findings of these studies have only been published as abstracts. The drug is licensed in certain countries for the treatment of initial and recurrent episodes of genital herpes.

In a large, randomized, double-blinded study comparing famciclovir and aciclovir, famciclovir at a dose of 250, 500 or 750 mg three times daily for 5 days was as effective as aciclovir (200 mg five times daily) for the treatment of first episodes of genital herpes. A second, similar study compared a 10-day course of famciclovir (125, 250 and 500 mg three times daily) with aciclovir (200 mg five times daily) and also found there was no consistent difference between the two regimens. Thus the lowest effective dose of famciclovir has not yet been clearly established (Murphy *et al.*, 1991; Famciclovir Product Information).

Comparative studies of famciclovir and aciclovir for the treatment of recurrent genital herpes have not been performed. In a large multicenter placebo-controlled trial, the administration of famciclovir (125 or 250 mg once- or twice-daily, or 500 mg once-daily) for 120 days to 275 individuals with frequently recurring genital herpes resulted in a longer median time to recurrence when compared with placebo (Mertz *et al.*, 1994). In two studies, differing in that in the first medication was clinic-initiated and in the second patient-initiated, famciclovir (125–500 mg twice-daily) taken for 5 days was also shown to reduce the median time to healing of recurrent genital lesions, the median time of virus shedding and more rapid relief of pain and itch when compared with placebo, if commenced within 6 h of development of symptoms (Sacks and Martel, 1994; Sacks *et al.*, 1994; Sacks and Aoki, 1995).

3 Chronic hepatitis B infection

Following anecdotal evidence of potential efficacy for the treatment of chronic hepatitis B infection, famciclovir has undergone preliminary evaluation in clinical trials for the treatment of hepatitis B and has been found to reduce serum hepatitis B DNA to levels below 1 pg per ml within weeks of commencing therapy (reviewed in De Man *et al.*, 1995; Schalm *et al.*, 1995).

References

Ashton RJ, Abbott KH, Smith GM, Sutton D (1994). Antiviral activity of famciclovir and aciclovir in mice infected intraperitoneally with herpes simplex virus type 1 SC16. *J Antimicrob Chemother* 34: 287.

Bacon TH (1996). Famciclovir, from the bench to the patient, a comprehensive review of preclinical data. *Int J Antimicrob Ag* 7: 119.

Bacon TH, Boyd MR (1995). Activity of penciclovir against Epstein-Barr virus. *Antimicrob Chemother* 39: 15.

Bacon TH, Howard BA (1996). Further characterisation of the potent and prolonged inhibition of herpes simplex virus replication in human cell lines by penciclovir. *Antiviral Chem Chemother* 7: 128.

Bacon TH, Schinazi RF (1993). An overview of the further evaluation of penciclovir against herpes simplex virus and varicella-zoster virus in cell culture highlighting contrasts with aciclovir. *Antiviral Chem Chemother* 4: 25.

Bacon TH, Howard BA, Spencer LC, Boyd MR (1996a). Activity of penciclovir in antiviral assays against herpes simplex virus. *J Antimicrob Chemother* 37: 303.

Bacon TH, Gilbert JG, Howard BA, Standring-Cox R (1996b). Inhibition of varicella zoster virus by penciclovir in cell culture and mechanism of action. *Antiviral Chem Chemother* 7: 71.

Balzarini J, Bohman C, Walker RT, De Clercq E (1994). Comparative cytostatic activity of different antiherpetic drugs against herpes simplex virus thymidine kinase gene-transfected tumor cells. *Mol Pharmacol* 45: 1253.

Boike SC, Pue M, Audet PR et al. (1994a). Pharmacokinetics of famciclovir in subjects with chronic hepatic disease. *J Clin Pharmacol* 34: 1199.

Boike SC, Pue MA, Freed MI, et al (1994b). Pharmacokinetics of famciclovir in subjects with varying degrees of renal impairment. *Clin Pharmacol Ther* 55: 418.

Boon RJ, Griffith DR (1996). Famciclovir: Efficacy in zoster and issues in the assessment of pain. In *Antiviral Chemotherapy, New Directions for Clinical Application and Research* Vol. 4 (Mills J, Volberding PA, Corey L, eds), p. 17. New York: Plenum Press.

Boyd MR (1993). Update of famciclovir. In *Antiviral Chemotherapy, New Directions for Clinical Application and Research* Vol 3 (Mills J, Corey L, eds), p. 83. New Jersey: PTR Prentice Hall.

Boyd MR, Safrin S (1993). Penciclovir: a review of its spectrum of activity selectivity, and cross-resistance pattern. *Antiviral Chem Chemother* 4: 3.

Boyd MR, Bacon TH, Sutton D, Cole M (1987). Antiherpesvirus activity of 9-(4-hydroxy-3-hydroxy-methylbut-1-yl)guanine (BRL 39123). in cell culture. *Antimicrob Ag Chemother* 31: 1238.

Boyd MR, Bacon TH, Sutton D (1988). Antiherpesvirus activity of 9-(4-hydroxy-3-hydroxymethylbut-1-yl) guanine (BRL 39123). in animals. *Antimicrob Ag Chemother* 32: 358.

Candaele M, Candaele D (1994). Famciclovir, confirmed efficacy of 250mg tid for the treatment of herpes zoster infection. *Antiviral Res* 23: 98.

Daniels S, Schentag JJ (1993). Drug interaction studies and safety of famciclovir in healthy volunteers; a review. *Antiviral Chem Chemother* 4: 57.

de la Fuente R, Awan AR, Field HJ (1992). The acyclic nucleoside analogue penciclovir is a potent inhibitor of equine herpesvirus type 1 (EHV-1) in tissue culture and in a murine model. *Antiviral Res* 18: 77.

De Man RA, Heijtink RA, Niesters HG, Schalm SW (1995). New developments in antiviral therapy for chronic hepatitis B infection. *Scand J Gastroenterol* 212: 100.

Degreef H, Famciclovir Herpes Zoster Clinical Study Group (1994). Famciclovir, a new oral antiherpes drug; results of the first controlled clinical study demonstrating its efficacy and safety in the treatment of uncomplicated herpes zoster in immunocompetent patients. *Internat J Antimicrob Ag* 4: 241.

Earnshaw DL, Bacon TH, Darlison KE et al. (1992). Mode of antiviral action of penciclovir in MRC-5 cells infected with herpes simplex virus type 1 (HSV-1), HSV-2 and varicella zoster virus. *Antimicrob Ag Chemother* 36: 2747.

Easterbrook P, Wood MJ (1994). Successors to aciclovir. *J Antimicrobial Chemother* 34: 307.

Ertl P, Snowden W (1995). A comparative study of the *in vitro* and *in vivo* antiviral activities of aciclovir and penciclovir. *Antiviral Chem Chemother* 6: 89.

Fairless AJ, Pratt SK, Pue MA et al. (1992). An investigation into the potential interaction between theophylline and oral famciclovir in healthy male volunteers. *Proc Brit Pharmacol Soc* 8: 171P.

Field HH, Tewari D, Sutton D, Thackray AM (1995). Comparison of efficacies of famciclovir and valaciclovir against herpes simplex virus type 1 in a murine immunosuppression model. *Antimicrob Ag Chemother* 39: 1114.

Field HJ, Thackray AM (1995). The effects of delayed-onset chemotherapy using famciclovir or valaciclovir in a murine immunosuppression model for HSV-1. *Antiviral Chem Chemother* 6: 210.

Filer CW, Allen GD, Brown TA et al. (1994). Metabolic and pharmacokinetic studies following oral administration of 14C-famciclovir to healthy subjects. *Xenobiotica* 24: 357.

Fowles SE, Pue MA (1993). Pharmacokinetics of penciclovir in healthy elderly subjects following a single oral administration of 750mg famciclovir. *Brit J Clin Pharmacol;* 35: 450.

Fowles SE, Pierce DM, Prince WT et al. (1992). The tolerance to and pharmacokinetics of penciclovir (BRL 39,123A), a novel antiherpes agent, administered by intravenous infusion to healthy subjects. *Eur J Clin Pharmacol* 43: 513.

Fowles SE, Pratt SK, Laroche J, Prince WT (1994). Lack of a pharmacokinetic interaction between oral famciclovir and allopurinol in healthy volunteers. *Eur J Clin Pharmacol* 46: 355.

Harnden MR, Jarvest RL et al. (1989). Prodrugs of the selective antiherpes agent 9-[4-hydroxy-3- (hydroxymethyl)but-1-yl]guanine. *J Med Chem* 32: 1738.

Harrell AW, Wheeler SM, Pennick M et al. (1993). Evidence that famciclovir (BRL 42810). and its associated metabolites do not inhibit the 6 beta-hydroxylation of testosterone in human liver microsomes. *Drug Metab Dispos* 21: 18.

Hasegawa T, Kurokawa M, Yukawa TA et al. (1995). Inhibitory action of aciclovir (ACV) and penciclovir (PCV) on plaque formation and partial cross-resistance of ACT-resistant varicella zoster virus to PCV. *Antiviral Res* 27: 271.

Iisley DD, Lee SH (1995). Acyclic guanosine analogs inhibit DNA polymerases alpha, delta and epsilon with very different potencies and have unique mechanisms of action. *Biochemistry* 34: 2504.

Mertz GJ, Loveless MO, Kraus SJ et al. (1994). Famciclovir for suppression of recurrent genital herpes. In *Program and Abstracts of the 34th Interscience Conference on Antimicrobial Agents and Chemotherapy, Orlando* (Abstr. H3). Washington, DC: American Society for Microbiology.

Murphy SM, Ruck F et al. (1991). Oral famciclovir (FCV) a new antiherpes agent; comparative study with aciclovir in clinic initiated treatment of first episode genital herpes (FGH) [abstract]. *EADV/Triaena Congress; Athens.*

Perry CM, Wagstaff AJ (1995). Famciclovir A review of its pharmacological properties and therapeutic efficacy in herpesvirus infections. *Drugs* 50: 396.

Pratt SK (1993). The pharmacokinetics of penciclovir following oral administration of 500mg famciclovir to patients with uncomplicated herpes zoster infection. *3rd Congress of the European Academy of Dermatology and Venereology.*

Pratt SK, Fairless AJ et al. (1992). Linearity of the pharmacokinetics of penciclovir following oral administration of famciclovir over the therapeutic dose range 125 in 750mg. *Proc Brit Pharmacol Soc* 9: 80.

Pratt SK, Pue MA (1994). Lack of an effect of gender on the pharmacokinetics of penciclovir following single oral doses of famciclovir. *Proc Brit Pharmacol Soc:* 5: 493.

Pratt SK, Fowles SE, Pierce DM, Prince WT (1991). An investigation of the potential interaction between cimetidine and famciclovir in non patient volunteers *Proc Brit Pharmacol Soc* **10**: 656P.

Product Information SmithKline Beecham.

Pue MA, Benet LZ (1993). Pharmacokinetics of famciclovir in man. *Antiviral Chem* **4**: 47.

Pue MA, Boike SC (1994). Pharmacokinetics of penciclovir in subjects with hepatic insufficiency following oral famciclovir. *Proc Brit Pharmacol Soc* **5**: 494.

Pue MA, Saporito M, Laroche J *et al.* (1993). An investigation of the potential interaction between digoxin and oral famciclovir in healthy male volunteers. *Proc Brit Pharmacol Soc* **14**: 177P.

Pue MA, Pratt SK, Fairless AJ *et al.* (1994). Linear pharmacokinetics of penciclovir following administration of single oral doses of famciclovir 125, 250, 500 and 750mg to healthy volunteers. *J Antimicrob Chemother* **33**: 119.

Rolan P (1995). Pharmacokinetics of new antiherpetic agents. *Clin Pharmacokinet* **29**: 333.

Sacks SL, Aoki FY (1994). Patient initiated treatment (Tx) of recurrent genital herpes with oral famciclovir (FCV); a Canadian; multicenter, placebo-controlled, dose ranging study. In *Program and Abstracts of the 34th Interscience Conference of Antimicrobial Agents and Chemotherapy, Orlando* (Abstr. H4). Washington, DC: American Society for Microbiology.

Sacks SL, Aoki FY *et al.* (1995). Patient and clinic initiated treatment of recurrent genital herpes with twice daily oral famciclovir [Abstract 866A]. *7th European Congress of Clinical Microbiology and Infectious Diseases Vienna.*

Sacks SL, Martel A (1994). Early, clinical-initiated treatment of recurrent genital herpes using famciclovir; results of a Canadian, multicenter study [abstract]. *Clin Res* April: 300.

Safrin S, Phan L (1993). *In vitro* activity of penciclovir against clinical isolates of aciclovir-resistant and foscarnet-resistant herpes simplex virus. *Antimicrob Ag Chemother* **37**: 2241.

Saltzman R, Jurewicz R, Boon R (1994). Safety of famciclovir in patients with herpes zoster and genital herpes. *Antimicrob Ag Chemother* **38**: 2454.

Schalm SW, De Man RA, Heijtink RA, Niesters HG (1995). New nucleoside analogues for chronic hepatitis B. *J Hepatol* **22**: 52.

Shaw T, Amor P, Civitico G *et al.* (1994). *In vitro* antiviral activity of penciclovir, a novel purine nucleoside, against duck hepatitis B virus. *Antimicrob Ag Chemother* **38**: 719.

Shiraki K, Matsui S, Aiba N (1993). Susceptibility of Oka varicella vaccine strain in antiviral drugs. *Vaccine* **11**: 1380.

SmithKline Beecham Pharmaceuticals (1994). Famciclovir prescribing information. Philadelphia, Pennsylvania US.

Soike KF, Bohm R, Huang JL, Oberg B (1993). Efficacy of (-)-9-[4-hydroxy-2- (hydroxymethyl)butyl]guanine in African green monkeys infected with simian varicella virus. *Antimicrob Ag Chemother* **37**: 1370.

Sutton D, Boyd MR (1993). Comparative activity of penciclovir and aciclovir in mice infected intraperitoneally with herpes simplex virus type 1 SC16. *Antimicrob Ag Chemother* **37**: 642.

Sutton D, Kern ER (1993). Activity of famciclovir and penciclovir in HSV infected animals; a review. *Antiviral Chem Chemother* **4**: 37.

Sutton D, Taylor J (1992). Activity of penciclovir in combination with azidothymidine, ganciclovir, aciclovir, foscarnet and human interferons against herpes simplex virus replication in cell culture. *Antiviral Chem Chemother* **3**: 85.

Talarico CL, Phelps WC, Biron KK (1993). Analysis of the thymidine kinase genes from aciclovir- resistant mutants of varicella-zoster virus isolated from patients with AIDS. *J Virol* **87**: 1024.

Tsiquaye KN, Slomka MJ, Maung M (1994). Oral famciclovir against duck hepatitis B virus replication in hepatic and non hepatic tissues of ducklings infected *in vivo. J Med Virol* **42**: 306.

Tsiquaye KN, Sutton D, Mating M, Boyd MR (1996). Antiviral activity and pharmacokinetics of penciclovir and famciclovir in Pekin ducks chronically infected with duck hepatitis B virus. *Antiviral Chem Chemother* **7**: 153.

Tyring S, Barbarash RA, Nahlik JC *et al.* (1995). Famciclovir for the treatment of acute herpes zoster; Effects on acute disease and postherpetic neuralgia. *Ann Intern Med* **123**: 89.

United States Pharmacopeia Drug Information (1995). United States Pharmacopeial Convention Inc, January 1.

Vere Hodge RA (1993). Famciclovir and penciclovir. The mode of action of famciclovir including its conversion to penciclovir. *Antiviral Chem Chemother* **4**: 67.

Vere Hodge A, Perkins RM (1989). Mode of action of 9-(-hydroxy-3-hydroxymethylbut-2-yl)guanine (BRL 39123). against herpes simplex virus in MRC-5 cells. *Antimicrob Ag Chemother*; **33**: 223.

Vere Hodge RA, Sutton D, Boyd MR *et al.* (1989). Selection of an oral prodrug (BRL 42810; famciclovir) for the antiherpes agent BRL 39123). [9-(4-hydroxy-3-hydroxymethylbut-1-yl)guanine; penciclovir]. *Antimicrob Ag Chemother* **33**: 1765.

Vere Hodge RA, Darlison SJ, Readshaw SA (1993). Use of isotopically chiral [4'-^{13}C]famciclovir and ^{13}C NMR to identify the chiral monoacetylated intermediates in the conversion of famciclovir in penciclovir by human intestinal wall extract. *Chirality* **5**: 577.

Weinberg A, Bate BJ, Masters HB *et al.* (1992). *In vitro* activities of penciclovir and aciclovir against herpes simplex virus type 1 and 2. *Antimicrob Ag Chemother* **36**: 2037.

Valaciclovir

Description

Valaciclovir (also known as BW256U87, and marketed under the trade name of 'Valtrex' by GlaxoWellcome) is the hydrochloride salt of the l-valyl ester of aciclovir that was developed originally by Wellcome Research Laboratories. This prodrug is rapidly and virtually completely converted to aciclovir following oral administration. Valaciclovir has superior efficacy to aciclovir in the treatment of herpes zoster and equivalent efficacy to aciclovir in the treatment of recurrent genital herpes. The dosing regimen of valaciclovir is more favorable than that of aciclovir.

The chemical name of valaciclovir is 2-[2-amino-1,6-dihydro-6-oxo-9H-purin-9-yl)methoxy]-ethyl L-valinate hydrochloride. Aciclovir constitutes 69.4% of the molecular weight of valaciclovir base (Weller et al., 1993a; Fig. V.10). The molecular weight of valaciclovir is 324.34. A plasma concentration of valaciclovir of 1 μg per ml is equivalent to 4.4μM.

Antiviral Activity

This is expected to be identical to that of aciclovir (p. 1510).

Mode of Administration and Dosage

Based on limited data, a dose of valaciclovir of 1000 mg given three times daily for 7 days appears to be efficacious and safe for the treatment of herpes zoster. The drug should be administered as early as possible after the onset of lesions, although in one study there was no difference in zoster-associated pain in patients who commenced therapy within 48 h or between 48 and 72 h (Smiley et al., 1996); the less frequent dosing schedule of valaciclovir when compared with aciclovir favors the prodrug.

For the treatment of recurrent genital herpes, a dose of valaciclovir of 1000 mg administered orally twice-daily for 7 days, commencing within 24 h of onset of symptoms or signs, was found to be safe and as effective as aciclovir (Rockley et al., 1993). The dose used in clinical practice for recurrent herpes simplex infection is 500 mg administered orally twice-daily for 5 days. A dose of 500 mg twice-daily for 5–10 days is used for acute treatment of initial herpes simplex infections.

In patients with moderate or severe hepatic impairment, the rate of conversion of valaciclovir to aciclovir is reduced. However, there is no requirement to modify the dose of valaciclovir in

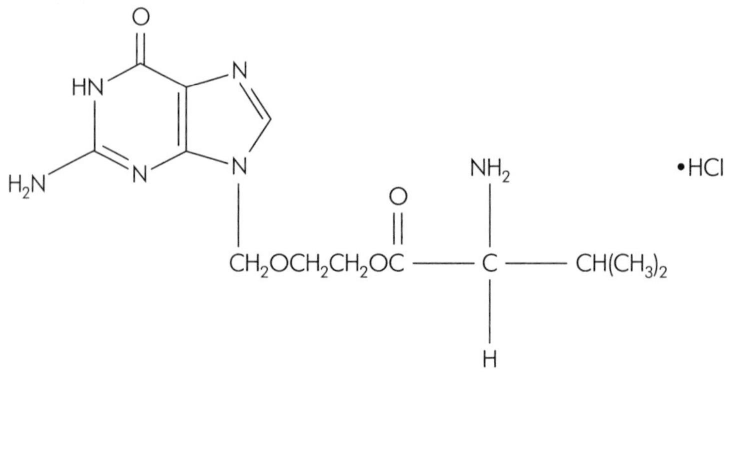

Fig. V.10.
Chemical structure of valaciclovir, the L-valyl ester of aciclovir (2-[2-amino-1, 6-dihydro-6-oxo-9H-purin-9-yl)methoxy]ethyl-L-valinate hydrochloride). Aciclovir constitutes 69.4% of the molecular weight of valaciclovir base. (Reproduced from Weller et al., 1993a, with permission.)

patients with cirrhosis. It is recommended that the dose of valaciclovir be reduced in patients with a creatinine clearance of less than 50 ml per min (Valaciclovir Product Information).

Availability

Valaciclovir is available as 500-mg *tablets*.

Serum Levels in Relation to Dosage

In monkeys, the bioavailability of aciclovir derived from oral valaciclovir is $67 \pm 13\%$ (de Miranda and Burnette, 1994). In humans, the bioavailability of aciclovir following oral administration of a 1000-mg dose of valaciclovir ranges from 51.3 to 54.2%. This is 3- to 5-fold more than the bioavailability of oral aciclovir (Wang *et al.*, 1993; Soul-Lawton *et al.*, 1995). Valaciclovir is extensively converted to aciclovir after oral administration by first-pass metabolism in either the liver or the intestine (Weller *et al.*, 1993a; Jacobson *et al.*, 1994). Aciclovir can be detected within plasma within 15 min of oral administration of valaciclovir (Jacobson *et al.*, 1994).

A single oral dose of 1000 mg results in a peak aciclovir plasma level (C_{max}) of 5–6 μg per ml (approximately 22.0 to 26.4μM), an area-under-the-curve (AUC) of 19 μg.h per ml, with the time to peak plasma concentration of 1– 2 h and a half-life of 2.8 h (Jacobson 1993, Table V.6). Multiple dosing of valaciclovir (2000 mg given four times daily for 10 days) resulted in a steady-state peak plasma level of 8.4 μg per ml, with the time to peak plasma concentration of 2.0 h, an AUC of 30.5 μg.h per ml and a half-life of 3.3 h (Jacobson, 1993). Multiple doses of 1000 mg four times daily in normal subjects resulted in systemic aciclovir exposure comparable with that of i.v. aciclovir at a dose of 5 mg per kg administered every 8 h (Weller *et al.*, 1993a). Multiple dosing studies have also been performed in persons with HIV infection. In 16 persons with advanced HIV infection who received 30 days oral administration of valaciclovir (either 1000 mg or 2000 mg four times daily), the peak plasma concentrations at the end of the study were 5.5 and 8.4 μg per ml, with a time to maximum plasma level of 2.0 h and a half-life in plasma of 3.1 and 3.3 h for the two dosing regimens respectively (Data on file, GlaxoWellcome).

The effect of food on the pharmacokinetics of valaciclovir was evaluated in 24 healthy males. A high fat breakfast increased the AUC of valaciclovir by 22% (Data on file, GlaxoWellcome).

In patients with reduced renal function, the peak plasma concentration and AUC of aciclovir are higher than in persons with normal renal function (Weller *et al.*, 1993b). Dosage adjustment is required in patients who have renal impairment (reviewed in Rolan, 1995). For geriatric patients, the mean AUC of aciclovir was 33–50% higher than in younger recipients (Smiley *et al.*, 1996).

Excretion

Aciclovir derived from valaciclovir is predominantly excreted by renal mechanisms. Following oral administration of valaciclovir to rats, the mean urinary excretion of aciclovir and valaciclovir was 57% and 2% of the dose respectively; other metabolites made up an additional

Table V.6

Aciclovir peak plasma concentrations (C_{max}) and AUC resulting from various dosing regimens of oral and i.v. aciclovir and valaciclovir. (Reproduced from Jacobson, 1993, with permission.)

Oral valaciclovir	Aciclovir	C_{max} (μg per ml)	Daily proj. AUC (h.μg per ml)
	Oral		
	200 mg 5 times per day	0.8	12
	800 mg 5 times per day	1.6	24
250 mg 4 times per day		2.1	23
500 mg 4 times per day		3.7	41
1000 mg 4 times per day		5.0	68
1500 mg 4 times per day		6.4	92
2000 mg 4 times per day		8.5	112
	Intravenous		
	5 mg per kg every 8 h	9.8	54
	10 mg per kg every 8 h	22.9	107

6%, resulting in a total of 65% excretion of the oral dose. The half-life of valaciclovir and aciclovir following oral administration of valaciclovir is 7 min and 1 h respectively in the rat (Burnette and de Miranda, 1994). Valaciclovir is more efficiently metabolized to aciclovir when given orally than by the i.v. route. Following i.v. administration, a total of 95% of the oral dose, with 65% and 23% comprising aciclovir and valaciclovir respectively, were found in the urine (Burnette and de Miranda, 1994).

Plasma levels of valaciclovir are extremely low (0.19 μM or 0.004 μg per ml) to undetectable 3 h following oral administration in humans (Jacobson *et al.*, 1994; Soul-Lawton *et al.*, 1995). Less than 1% of valaciclovir is recovered unchanged in urine, there is extensive first-pass metabolism in the liver. The aciclovir metabolite 9-[(carboxymethoxy)methyl]guanine represents up to 12% of the dose in urine, with between 80 and 85% comprising aciclovir (reviewed in Crooks and Murray, 1994).

Distribution of the Drug in Body

In the rat, a study of the distribution of aciclovir following oral administration of valaciclovir showed highest concentrations in that the stomach, small intestine, kidney, liver, lymph nodes and skin. Aciclovir was detected in all of these tissues within 20 min of oral administration of the prodrug (Burnette and de Miranda, 1994). For further details of the distribution of aciclovir (p. 1518).

Mode of Action

In order to improve on the poor oral bioavailability of aciclovir, 18 amino-acid esters of aciclovir were synthesized and tested (Beauchamp *et al.*, 1992). The L-valyl ester, valaciclovir hydrochloride, resulted in highest oral bioavailability of aciclovir (reviewed in Crooks and Murray, 1994).

Valaciclovir is converted to aciclovir and L-valine by hydrolysis, mediated by an enzyme associated with mitochondria within the liver that has been named valaciclovir hydrolase (Data on file, GlaxoWellcome; Burnette and de Miranda, 1994). Following this conversion, aciclovir is phophorylated to the mono-, di and triphosphate derivatives within infected cells and its mechanism of action is identical to that of aciclovir (p. 1518).

Toxicity

Bioassays performed in mouse and rat have not shown evidence of carcinogenesis (Smiley *et al.*, 1996). In a phase 1 study the main reported side-effects were gastrointestinal, with nausea, vomiting, diarrhea, and abdominal pain in up to one-third of patients; no renal or neurologic side-effects were noted, but two patients developed neutropenia (Jacobson *et al.*, 1994). During the AIDS Clinical Trials Group (ACTG) Trial 204, in which patients with advanced HIV infection were randomized to receive valaciclovir (2–4 g per day) or aciclovir prophylaxis against cytomegalovirus disease, nine cases of hemolytic uremic syndrome were reported in patients who were randomized to the valaciclovir arm. These patients were also receiving other drugs including fluconazole. An independent data and safety monitoring board for the trial considered that valaciclovir was associated with the development of the syndrome but allowed continuation of the study with modification to patient consent (Data on file, GlaxoWellcome). Another six cases of hemolytic uremic syndrome were reported in a double-blinded study of valaciclovir versus aciclovir in the suppression of cytomegalovirus infection and disease in bone marrow transplant recipients. There have been no reported cases in immunocompetent persons receiving valaciclovir (Data on file, GlaxoWellcome).

There is no apparent alteration in pharmacokinetics of valaciclovir in patients also taking thiazide diuretics (Smiley *et al.*, 1996). Cimetidine and probenecid have been associated with a slower conversion of valaciclovir to aciclovir, and to decrease the renal clearance of aciclovir, thus increasing the plasma aciclovir levels.

Clinical Uses of the Drug

1 Herpes zoster

A multicenter, double-blind, international trial in 1141 immunocompetent patients aged over 50 years, has compared the efficacy of valaciclovir, given in a dose of 1000 mg for 7 or 14 days, with that of aciclovir administered in a dose of 800 mg five times daily for 7 days. Only patients

Fig. V.11.

Plasma aciclovir concentrations during one dosing interval in patients with herpes zoster treated with oral valaciclovir or oral aciclovir VACV-7, valaciclovir at 1000 mg three times daily for 7 days; VACV-14, valaciclovir at 1000 mg three times daily for 14 days, ACV-7, aciclovir at 800 mg five times daily for 7 days. (Reproduced from Beutner *et al.*, 1995, with permission.)

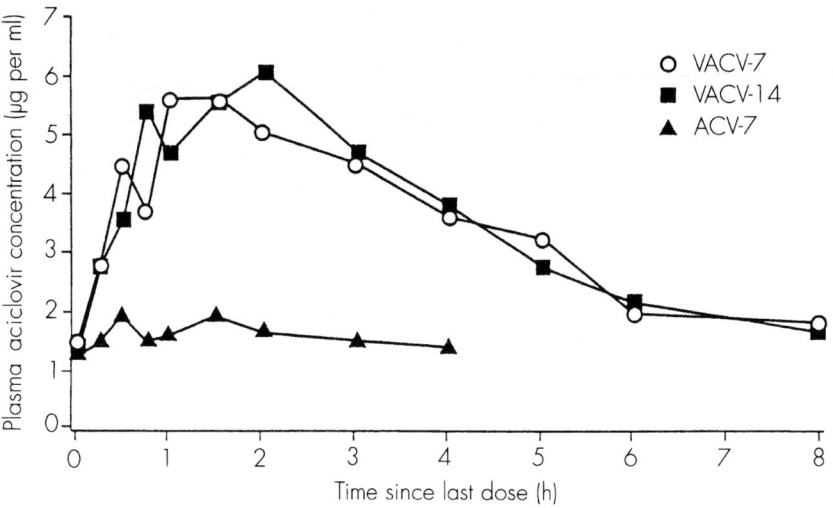

presenting within 72 h of onset of rash, and with localized zoster were included in the study. Valaciclovir was superior to aciclovir in accelerating loss of pain; the median times to cessation of acute pain in the 7- and 14-day valaciclovir recipients were statistically equivalent (38 and 44 days) compared with 51 days in the aciclovir arm. The proportion of patients with pain at 6 months was also lower in the valaciclovir group compared with aciclovir recipients (19.3% and 26% respectively). There was no difference between valaciclovir and aciclovir in time to cessation of new lesion formation (3 days) and time to more than 50% crusting of lesions (5 days). Those randomized to the valaciclovir arm used less analgesia and had less time away from work (Beutner *et al.*, 1995; Smiley *et al.*, 1996). Plasma concentrations of aciclovir were significantly higher throughout the dosing period in valaciclovir recipients compared with aciclovir (Beutner *et al.*, 1995; Fig. V.11).

2 Herpes simplex infection

Valaciclovir (1000 mg twice-daily for 5 days) has also been compared with aciclovir (200 mg five times daily for 5 days) and placebo for the treatment of recurrent genital herpes in another multicenter, double-blind, international trial. Over 1000 patients who presented within 24 h of developing symptoms or signs of recurrent disease were enrolled in the study. Valaciclovir was equivalent to aciclovir in reducing the median time to healing (116 and 115 h respectively), and both were superior to placebo (144 h) (Rockley *et al.*, 1993). Valaciclovir has also been shown to be effective in the treatment of initial episodes of genital herpes. In a randomized double-blind multicenter controlled trial of patients who presented within 3 days of an initial episode of genital herpes there was no clinically significant difference between valaciclovir (1000 mg twice daily) and standard aciclovir therapy in terms of time to healing and time of viral shedding (Data on file, GlaxoWellcome).

3 Cytomegalovirus infection

AIDS Clinical Trials Group phase III Trial 204 evaluated the efficacy of valaciclovir (2000 mg four times daily) versus oral aciclovir (800 mg four times daily or 400 mg twice-daily) in the prevention of cytomegalovirus end-organ disease in HIV and cytomegalovirus co-infected individuals with less than 100 CD4 cells per µl. A total of 1227 patients were enrolled, with a median CD4 count of 32 cells per µl, The median duration of follow-up was 13.2 months. The study was prematurely stopped after review of interim data by an independent monitoring board because survival was found to be lower in those randomized to receive valaciclovir than in the aciclovir group (p = 0.06). There were 184 confirmed end-points (79% retinitis and 15% gastrointestinal disease). A preliminary analysis of data suggests that there was a significant protective effect of valaciclovir in preventing end-organ disease (p = 0.03). Patients receiving valaciclovir were more likely to discontinue study medication than aciclovir recipients and there was a higher incidence of gastrointestinal side-effects in those receiving valaciclovir (Feinberg *et al.*, 1995).

References

Beauchamp LM, Orr GF, de Miranda P *et al.* (1992). Amino acid ester prodrugs of acyclovir. *Antiviral Res Chemother* **3**: 157.

Beutner KR, Friedman DJ, Forszpaniak C *et al.* (1995). Valaciclovir compared with aciclovir for improved therapy for herpes zoster in immunocompetent adults. *Antimicrob Ag Chemother* **39**: 546.

Burnette TC, de Miranda P (1994). Metabolic disposition of the acyclovir prodrug valaciclovir in the rat. *Drug Metab Dispos* **22**: 60.

Crooks RJ, Murray A (1994). Valaciclovir – a review of a promising new antiherpes agent. *Antiviral Chem Chemother* **5**: 31.

de Miranda P, Burnette TC (1994). Metabolic fate and pharmacokinetics of the acyclovir prodrug valaciclovir in cynomologus monkeys. *Drug Metab Dispos* **22**: 55.

Feinberg I, Cooper D, Horwitz S *et al.* (1995). Phase III study of valaciclovir (VACV) for cytomegalovirus (CMV) prophylaxis in patients with advanced HIV disease. ICCAC Conference, Vancouver.

Jacobson MA (1993). Valaciclovir (BW 256U87), the L-valyl ester of acyclovir. *J Med Virol* **1** (Suppl): 150.

Jacobson MA, Gallant J, Wang LH *et al.* (1994). Phase I trial of valaciclovir, the L-valyl ester of acyclovir, in patients with advanced human immunodeficiency virus disease. *Antimicrob Ag Chemother* **38**: 1534.

Rockley P, Tyring S, Smiley M and the International Valaciclovir HSV Study Group (1993). Valaciclovir is equally safe and effective for the treatment of recurrent genital herpes simplex virus infections as is acyclovir but with a more convenient dosing. *Clin Res* **41**: 778A.

Rolan P (1995). Pharmacokinetics of new antiherpetic agents. *Clin Pharmacokinet* **29**: 333.

Smiley L, Murray A, de Miranda, P (1996). Valacyclovir HC1 (Valaciclovir™) an acyclovir prodrug with improved pharmacokinetics and better efficacy for treatment of zoster. *Antiviral Chemother* **394**: 33.

Soul-Lawton J, Seaber E, On N *et al.* (1995). Absolute bioavailability and metabolic disposition of valaciclovir, the L-valyl ester of acyclovir, following oral administration in humans. *Antimicrob Ag Chemother* **39**: 2759.

Valaciclovir Product Information, GlaxoWellcome US September 1995.

Wang LH, Schultz M, Weller S *et al.* (1993). Pharmacokinetics and safety of valaciclovir An acyclovir prodrug, in geriatric volunteers with and without concomitant diuretic therapy. *Amer Ger Soc* **41**: SA23.

Weller S, Blum MR, Doucette M *et al.* (1993a). Pharmacokinetics of the acyclovir pro-drug valaciclovir after escalating single and multiple-dose administered to normal volunteers. *Clin Pharmacol Ther* **54**: 595.

Weller S, Blum MR, Smiley ML (1993b). Phase 1 pharmacokinetics of the acyclovir prodrug, valaciclovir. *Antiviral Res* **20**: 144.

Ganciclovir

Description

Ganciclovir (9-(1,3-dihydroxy-2-propoxymethyl)guanine, also known as DHPG, and in earlier studies as BW759 U (Burroughs Wellcome), BIOLF-62 (ENS Biologicals) and 2'NDG (Merck Sharpe and Dohme) is a synthetic acyclic nucleoside analog of guanine (Fig. V.12). It was marketed as 'Cymevene' and 'Cytovene' by Syntex initially and now by Roche. Ganciclovir and foscarnet (p. 1787) are currently the drugs of choice for management of cytomegalovirus disease, and cidofovir is becoming more widely used. Until recently, ganciclovir was given almost exclusively by i.v. infusion. Now it can also be administered by intravitreous injection, by intraocular implantation, and in an oral formulation.

The molecular formula for ganciclovir is $C_9H_{12}N_5NaO_4$. The molecular weight for the sodium salt is 277.21. Thus 1 μg per ml is approximately equal to 3.6 μM.

Antiviral Activity

Ganciclovir has activity against members of the herpes viruses and certain other DNA viruses (Martin et al., 1983) (Table V.7).

1 Cytomegalovirus

Whilst initial studies suggested that ganciclovir did not inhibit human cytomegalovirus even at high concentrations (Smith et al., 1982a), subsequent investigations confirmed that ganciclovir has excellent activity against this virus. The antiviral effects of ganciclovir only last for the duration of exposure of drug to infected cells, indicating the virustatic nature of inhibition of replication (Mar et al., 1983). When tested in vitro in viral plaque reduction assays, viral DNA synthesis or viral yield, ganciclovir inhibits the laboratory-adapted AD169 and Towne strains of cytomegalovirus as well as clinical isolates with IC_{50} values of sensitive strains ranging from 0.1 to 9 μM (0.025–2.28 μg per ml) (Tocci et al., 1984; Plotkin et al., 1985; Rush and Mills, 1987; Prichard et al., 1990; Andrei et al., 1991; Boivin et al., 1993; Hamzeh et al., 1993; Freitas et al., 1993a). The mean IC_{50} ranges from 1.7 to 5.9 μM, well within the concentrations of drug that can be achieved clinically (Plotkin et al., 1985; Cole and Balfour 1987; Boivin et al., 1993). Primary isolates have been reported to be less susceptible to ganciclovir than laboratory-adapted strains (Wahren et al., 1987), although this finding is not supported by other investigations (Rush and Mills, 1987; Shigeta et al., 1991). The IC_{90} for ganciclovir against the AD169 strain has been

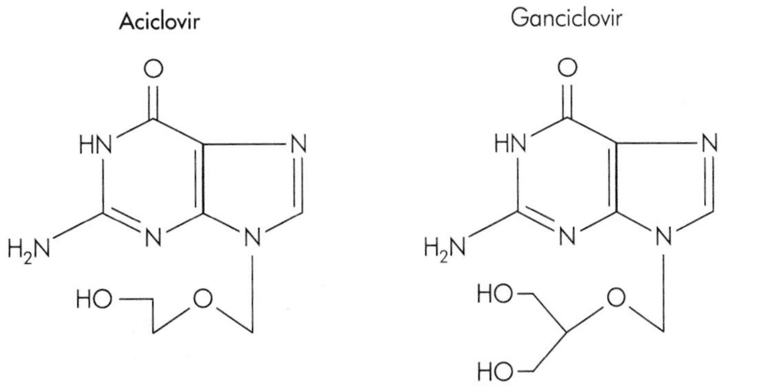

Fig. V.12.

Chemical structures of the antiviral drugs aciclovir and ganciclovir. (Reproduced from Crumpacker, 1996, with permission.)

Table V.7

Some viruses shown to be susceptible to
ganciclovir

Cytomegalovirus
Herpes simplex virus
Epstein–Barr virus
Varicella-zoster virus
Human herpes virus type 6
Adenovirus[a]
Hepatitis B virus[b]
Creutzfeldt-Jakob virus+

[a] Strain specific
[b] Limited data
(Refer to text for sources of data.)

variably reported to range from 0.5 to 19 μM (Neyts *et al.*, 1990; Freitas *et al.*, 1993a) and from 0.6 to 16 μM for clinical isolates (Plotkin *et al.*, 1985). Although the concentrations of ganciclovir that cause cellular toxicity are generally considerably higher than those required for antiviral activity, this is not true for bone marrow progenitor cells which appear to be especially sensitive to the drug. Fifty percent growth inhibition of bone marrow colony forming cells occurs at concentrations of ganciclovir of approximately $2.7 \pm 0.5 \mu$M (Somadossi and Carlisle, 1987). Ganciclovir is approximately 10- to 25-fold more active against cytomegalovirus compared with aciclovir using plaque reduction assays (Tyms, 1984; Cole and Balfour, 1987), but less effective against cytomegalovirus *in vitro* than cidofovir (HPMPC) (Shigeta *et al.*, 1991).

In mice infected with cytomegalovirus, daily administration of ganciclovir (up to 50 mg per kg) did not delay death by more than 21 days (Neyts *et al.*, 1993), although in a separate study the drug reduced lung titers of cytomegalovirus in mice following intranasal inoculation by over 90% (Debs *et al.*, 1988). In the murine model ganciclovir is inferior to cidofovir in terms of delaying the onset of disease and prolonging survival (de Castro *et al.*, 1991; Smee *et al.*, 1991; Neyts *et al.*, 1992). Ganciclovir was unable to suppress reactivation of virus in immunosuppressed mice with latent cytomegalovirus infection. In addition, the dose of ganciclovir required to reduce mortality in immunosuppressed mice who were lethally challenged with cytomegalovirus was 3-fold higher than the dose required to achieve the same survival in normal mice (Wilson *et al.*, 1987). In guinea pigs, treatment with ganciclovir prevented death but did not decrease virus load in blood (Aquino de Jesus and Griffith, 1989). These findings are supported by an earlier report in which the concentration of ganciclovir required to inhibit the replication of cytomegalovirus in guinea pig cell cultures was found to be as high as 71 μM (Fong *et al.*, 1987). Ganciclovir treatment of immunosuppressed rats infected with cytomegalovirus following allogeneic bone marrow transplant resulted in a decrease in virus titers in lungs and spleen, when compared with untreated animals (Stals *et al.*, 1993).

2 Herpes simplex

Although herpes viruses are inhibited by low concentrations of ganciclovir, there are differences in susceptibility among differing strains, and also different results obtained depending on the cell types and method used (Smith *et al.*, 1982a). Ganciclovir is more potent than aciclovir against herpes simplex types 1 and 2 *in vitro*. Collins and Oliver (1985) reported that the mean IC_{50} of ganciclovir was approximately 3-fold higher for herpes simplex virus type 2 compared with type 1 (1.67 and 0.57 μM respectively). Reported IC_{50} of ganciclovir for strains of herpes simplex virus type 1 and 2 as measured by plaque reduction assays range from 0.2 to 2.4 μM (Smee *et al.*, 1983, 1985a; Pulliam *et al.*, 1986), although the mean IC_{50} for herpes simplex virus type 2 has been as high as 10 μM in some reports (Faulds and Heel, 1990). The IC_{90} for ganciclovir against herpes simplex virus type 1 in a microtiter virus yield reduction assay was 0.7 μM (Prichard *et al.*, 1990). Other investigators have found marked reduction (up to 300 000-fold) in virus titer and viral DNA levels when herpes simplex virus type 1-infected Vero cells were cultured in the presence of 5–30 μM ganciclovir (Chun and Park, 1987; van der Horst *et al.*, 1987).

Intraperitoneal administration of ganciclovir to mice infected via the same route with herpes simplex virus type 2 provides moderate protection against systemic infection (Yang and Datema, 1991). Several groups have demonstrated the efficacy of ganciclovir in preventing herpetic lesions in a herpes simplex type 2 murine model at a dose of 5–10 mg per kg (Klein and

Friedman-Kien, 1985; Smee *et al.*, 1985a). In addition ganciclovir can prevent encephalitis due to murine herpes simplex type 1 in doses of less than 10 mg per kg, and herpetic vaginitis at a daily dose of 50 mg per kg (Smee *et al.*, 1983, 1985a). Early studies (Fraser-Smith *et al.*, 1983) showed that administration of ganciclovir to guinea-pigs commencing within 3 h of intravaginal inoculation of herpes simplex virus type 2 prevented the development of primary infection in 33% of animals, whereas delay to 24 h post-inoculation resulted in 100% infection rates. Ganciclovir given by intravitreal injection or by eye drops does not completely protect rabbits from retinitis caused by experimental herpes simplex virus type 1 infection (Naito *et al.*, 1991; Flores-Aguilar *et al.*, 1994), although in an earlier report 0.3% ganciclovir ointment given five times daily for 4 days to rabbits infected with herpes simplex virus was effective in preventing lesions (Shiota *et al.*, 1987). Equine herpesvirus type 1 has been reported to be sensitive to ganciclovir (Kit *et al.*, 1987).

3 Epstein–Barr virus

Ganciclovir is more active against Epstein–Barr virus than aciclovir (p. 1510). The IC_{50} of ganciclovir for Epstein–Barr virus is 0.05–1 μM, most commonly assessed by inhibition of genome replication, with an IC_{90} of 3–5 μM (Cheng *et al.*, 1983a; Lin *et al.*, 1984, 1986; Yao *et al.*, 1993). Ganciclovir has been found to suppress the replication of Epstein–Barr virus in human lymphoblastoid cells during 70 days of continuous exposure in culture without eradicating the infection; following removal of the drug the genome copy number returns to baseline (van der Horst *et al.*, 1987). Although ganciclovir has a prolonged inhibitory effect on active viral DNA replication, the drug does not affect the replication of episomal virus, which does not require a virus-encoded DNA polymerase (Lin *et al.*, 1984). Ganciclovir therapy can inhibit the development of B cell lymphomas in severe combined immunodeficiency (SCID) mice engrafted with human peripheral blood lymphocytes and subsequently infected with Epstein–Barr virus (Boyle *et al.*, 1992).

4 Varicella–zoster virus

Ganciclovir inhibits the replication of varicella-zoster virus, with mean IC_{50} values ranging from 0.6 to 8 μM (Field *et al.*, 1983; Collins and Oliver, 1985). Matthews and Boehme (1988) reported that ganciclovir had similar efficacy to aciclovir in inhibiting the replication of varicella-zoster virus. Ganciclovir improved the outcome of infection with simian varicella-zoster virus in African green monkeys when administered at a dose of 10 mg per kg twice-daily for 10 days (Soike *et al.*, 1987).

5 Human herpesvirus type 6

Ganciclovir has been reported to inhibit the replication of human herpesvirus type 6 *in vitro* with an IC_{50} of 1–4 μM (Agut *et al.*, 1989; Russler *et al.*, 1989; Burns and Sandford, 1990), although other investigators have found higher IC_{50} values around 25 μM (Akesson-Johansson *et al.*, 1990) with only partial inhibition of viral expression (Streicher *et al.*, 1988).

6 Adenovirus

The susceptibility of several strains of adenovirus (subgenus D) to ganciclovir has been demonstrated *in vitro*. However, the drug has only limited activity against other human adenoviruses. Ganciclovir has been reported to have some activity against human adenovirus type 5 that is associated with severe ocular disease. As assessed by plaque reduction, the ID_{50} was 47 μM. Three weeks of topical ganciclovir (3%) treatment of eyes of cotton rats inoculated with this strain resulted in a trend towards virus suppression, when compared with placebo (Trousdale *et al.*, 1994).

7 Other

Ganciclovir has no activity against the human immunodeficiency virus (Causey, 1991; Cox *et al.*, 1993). The replication of duck hepatitis B virus in primary hepatocytes has been found to be inhibited by ganciclovir during continuous short-term treatment of the cultures, but was less efficient in inhibiting replication during longer-term exposure to the drug (Shaw *et al.*, 1994). Ganciclovir treatment of ducks congenitally infected with duck hepatitis B resulted in a decrease in serum virus DNA levels (Wang *et al.*, 1991), although circulating duck hepatitis B virus surface antigen levels did not decline (Luscombe *et al.*, 1994). Markers of hepatitis B virus infection including hepatitis B virus DNA and viral DNA polymerase have been reported to fall to undetectable levels in patients during therapy with ganciclovir (Locarnini *et al.*, 1989). In ground squirrels chronically infected with hepatitis virus, ganciclovir at a dose of 50 mg per kg per day modestly decreased the levels of virion-associated DNA polymerase in serum during the course of treatment; post-therapy, levels returned to baseline (Smee *et al.*, 1985b). There has been one report that the human papovirus, Creutzfeldt-Jakob virus, the causative agent of progressive multifocal leukoencephalopathy, responds to ganciclovir *in vitro* when human fibroblasts are co-infected with cytomegalovirus (Heilbronn *et al.*, 1993). Aujeszky's disease virus (pseudorabies virus) is sensitive to ganciclovir *in vitro* with a mean IC_{50} in mouse embryo fibroblasts of 6 μM (Field, 1985). Ganciclovir is superior to aciclovir against pseudorabies virus *in vivo* (Rollinson and White, 1983); significant protection of mice from encephalitis caused by this virus occurred at a dose of 60 mg per kg per day (Rollinson, 1987). Herpesvirus simiae is relatively resistant to ganciclovir *in vitro*, with an IC_{50} of 36 μM (Zwartouw *et al.*, 1989). Available evidence suggests that ganciclovir has no activity against human papillomavirus, influenza virus or any RNA virus (Crumpacker, 1996).

8 Acquired resistance

Repeated passage of cytomegalovirus-infected cells in the presence of ganciclovir *in vitro* or the chronic administration of ganciclovir to patients may lead to the emergence of ganciclovir-resistant strains of cytomegalovirus. Exposure of infected cells to ganciclovir for up to 5 weeks does not alter the susceptibility of the isolate to ganciclovir (Cole and Balfour, 1987), but longer passage through increasing concentrations of ganciclovir up to 100 μM has permitted the development of resistant mutants (Biron *et al.*, 1986). Drew and colleagues (1991a) reported the lack of resistance in isolates from patients who had received less than 3 months of therapy; after this period of time 38% of isolates were ganciclovir-resistant. This is supported by earlier data in which ganciclovir-resistant strains of cytomegalovirus could be recovered after 60–131 days of ganciclovir therapy (Erice *et al.*, 1989). However, resistant strains of cytomegalovirus have reportedly also been isolated from persons who have never received ganciclovir (Lipson *et al.*, 1993). Ganciclovir-resistant strains of cytomegalovirus are defined by some investigators as having an IC_{50} of >4 μM (Safrin *et al.*, 1994), of >6 μM (Jacobson *et al.*, 1991; Lipson *et al.*, 1993), and by others as >12 μM (Drew *et al.*, 1991a; Slavin *et al.*, 1993) with reported IC_{50} levels of up to 200 μM (Lurain *et al.*, 1992; Slavin *et al.*, 1993). There appears to be no difference in the rates of development of resistance between oral and i.v. ganciclovir (Buhles *et al.*, 1994).

Resistance has been related to impaired monophosphorylation of ganciclovir in some reports (Lurain *et al.*, 1992; Baldanti *et al.*, 1995), although no impairment of phosphorylation by resistant isolates has also been reported (Tatarowicz *et al.*, 1992). Two separate mutations have been described within different parts of the viral genome (the UL97 gene of cytomegalovirus and the DNA polymerase gene of herpes simplex and cytomegalovirus) that can give rise to resistance (Crumpacker *et al.*, 1984; St Clair *et al.*, 1984; Sullivan *et al.*, 1992a). Mutations within the UL97 gene are more commonly associated with the development of resistance than mutations within DNA polymerase.

The UL97 gene of human cytomegalovirus is responsible for phosphorylation of ganciclovir within cytomegalovirus-infected cells; a mutation within the UL97 open reading frame causes resistance to ganciclovir (Sullivan *et al.*, 1992a). Mutations leading to substitutions at codons 460, 594 and 595 have been described in drug-resistant isolates (Lurain *et al.*, 1994; Baldanti *et al.*, 1995; Chou *et al.*, 1995a; Wolf *et al.*, 1995a). A mutation within codon 520 has also been reported (Chou *et al.*, 1995b). These substitutions have not been found in sensitive strains. Several reported mutations within the DNA polymerase gene of cytomegalovirus (glycine to alanine at amino acid position 987, and leucine to isoleucine at amino acid residue 501) can also confer ganciclovir-resistance. Phosphorylation of the drug was reported to be intact with the former mutation but impaired with the latter (Lurain *et al.*, 1992; Sullivan *et al.*, 1993). Mutations within the DNA polymerase of herpes simplex types 1 and 2 that map to a 2.2 kilobase-pair region are responsible for the development of resistance (Crumpacker *et al.*, 1984; St Clair *et al.*, 1984).

Treatment with aciclovir does not appear to induce ganciclovir-resistance (Drew *et al.*, 1995a). Although cross-resistance to cidofovir (Lurain *et al.*, 1992) and foscarnet (Tatarowicz *et al.*, 1992) have been described, other investigators have found that ganciclovir-resistant strains remain sensitive to these drugs, as well as to vidarabine, cidofovir, fialuridine and FIAC (Biron *et al.*, 1986; Biron, 1991; Stanat *et al.*, 1991; Drew *et al.*, 1991b). A recent report describes isolates with dual ganciclovir- and foscarnet-resistance from four AIDS patients treated with a combination of both drugs (Sarasini *et al.*, 1995).

Herpes simplex virus type 1 develops resistance to ganciclovir more slowly than to aciclovir, requiring continuous exposure *in vitro* to ganciclovir at a concentration of 30 μM for 70 days versus 14 days of aciclovir for resistant variants to emerge (van der Horst *et al.*, 1987). These ganciclovir-resistant isolates have been found to be cross-resistant to aciclovir, although this finding can be variable (McLaren *et al.*, 1985; van der Horst *et al.*, 1987).

9 Synergy

Foscarnet and ganciclovir are synergistic against human and murine cytomegalovirus and murine herpes virus type 2 both *in vitro* and *in vivo*, with up to 27-fold improvement in efficacy of ganciclovir when the two drugs are used in combination (Smith *et al.*, 1982b; Freitas *et al.*, 1989; Manischewitz *et al.*, 1990). A human neutralizing monoclonal antibody MSL-109 (Sandoz Pharmaceuticals) at concentrations of 1–10 μg per ml has been reported to have an additive effect when used in combination with ganciclovir (3–10 μM) in inhibiting replication of cytomegalovirus strain AD169 *in vitro* (Nokta *et al.*, 1994). Ganciclovir and nalidixic acid are more effective in inhibiting the replication of duck hepatitis B virus in the livers of infected ducks when used in combination compared with monotherapy (Wang *et al.*, 1995). Ampligen and ganciclovir have additive effects in inhibiting the replication of duck hepatitis B virus within the livers of infected ducks (Niu *et al.*, 1993). Recombinant human interferon beta and ganciclovir are strongly synergistic in their activity against simian varicella virus infection in monkeys, with up to 100-fold decrease in interferon beta and 10-fold less ganciclovir required to achieve an effective dose compared with monotherapy (Soike *et al.*, 1987). Recombinant human interferon alpha and ganciclovir were found to be highly synergistic against herpes simplex virus type 1 and type 2 *in vitro* in human fibroblasts (Moran *et al.*, 1985). Synergy has also been demonstrated between recombinant murine interferon alpha and ganciclovir both *in vitro* (Eppstein and Marsh, 1984) and when administered to mice infected with herpes simplex virus type 2, the effective dose of each drug being reduced 10-fold when given in combination (Fraser-Smith *et al.*, 1985).

10 Antagonism

Ganciclovir has been found to antagonize the antiretroviral activity of both zidovudine and didanosine *in vitro*, increasing the IC_{50} of the latter drugs by 3- to 6-fold; antagonism occurred at drug concentrations well below cytotoxic levels (Medina *et al.*, 1992). Furthermore, some investigators have found that zidovudine antagonizes the effects of ganciclovir against human cytomegalovirus *in vitro*; in this study, zidovudine also reduced the efficacy of ganciclovir in a guinea pig model (Feng *et al.*, 1993). However, this remains controversial as a number of other investigators have found the opposite: zidovudine has been reported to have an additive to synergistic effect with ganciclovir against laboratory-adapted strains and clinical isolates of cytomegalovirus *in vitro* (Snoeck *et al.*, 1992; Freitas *et al.*, 1993a; Data on file Roche) . There is no antagonism of the antiviral activity of ganciclovir by its use in combination with amphotericin B, ketoconazole, dapsone or co-trimoxazole (Pecyk *et al.*, 1989; Freitas *et al.*, 1993b).

11 Gene therapy

Gene therapy using cells transfected with a so-called 'suicide gene' followed by treatment with ganciclovir may become a future major strategy for the management of certain malignancies. Transfer of the herpes simplex thymidine kinase (TK) gene into tumor cells followed by treatment with ganciclovir has been found in a number of circumstances to provide selective killing of tumor cells. Examples include transfection of the TK gene into glioma cells by a retroviral vector followed by treatment of the cultures with ganciclovir which causes selective cytotoxicity of the TK-transfected cells, thus providing a possible therapeutic approach for patients with malignant glioma (Ezzeddine *et al.*, 1991; Oldfield *et al.*, 1993; Chen *et al.*, 1994, 1995b; Kato *et al.*, 1994). Similar findings have been obtained *in vitro* by transfecting certain other tumor cell lines, including carcinoembryonic antigen-secreting lung adenocarcinoma cells (Osaki *et al.*, 1994), mesiothelioma cell lines (Smythe *et al.*, 1995), small cell lung cancer cell lines (Kumagai *et al.*, 1996), hepatoma cell lines (Kaneko *et al.*, 1995) and others. This approach has also been successfully tested *in vivo*, in experimental gliomas in rats (Culver *et al.*, 1992), in severe combined immunodeficient mice engrafted with TK-transfected pancreatic carcinoma cells followed by intraperitoneal ganciclovir (DiMaio *et al.*, 1994), in BALB/c mice injected intrahepatically with TK-transfected colon carcinoma cell lines (Chen *et al.*, 1995a,b), in nude mice which were injected with TK-transfected gastric carcinoma cells (Yoshida *et al.*, 1995), and in nude mice in a model for human squamous cell carcinoma (O'Malley *et al.*, 1995). Ganciclovir treatment of T lymphocytes that have been transfected with a TK may also provide a means for selective depletion of these cells in bone marrow transplant patients who develop graft-versus-host-disease (Tiberghien *et al.*, 1994). Human granulocyte macrophage colony stimulating factor (GM-CSF) production can be regulated *in vitro* by transfecting TK into GM-CSF-producing cells, followed by ganciclovir treatment of the cultures (Aoki *et al.*, 1994). Smooth muscle cells transduced with TK have been found to be sensitive to ganciclovir *in vitro*, and in this way gene therapy can potentially be used to prevent accumulation of vascular smooth muscle following arterial injury (Ohno *et al.*, 1994).

Mode of Administration and Dosage

1 Intravenous administration

For induction therapy in patients with AIDS-related cytomegalovirus retinitis with normal renal function, ganciclovir is usually administered as a 1-h i.v. infusion of 5 mg per kg given twice-daily for 14–21 days. For maintenance therapy, the recommended dose is a 1-h i.v. infusion containing 5 mg per kg given once-daily on 7 days of the week, or 6 mg per kg daily on 5 days of the week (not weekends). For transplant recipients with normal renal function who are at risk of cytomegalovirus disease, a 1-h infusion of 5 mg per kg given twice-daily for 7–14 days is followed by maintenance therapy as outlined above. The length of time of maintenance therapy depends on the duration of immunosuppression, which in turn depends on the type of transplant. This is discussed in the section on Clinical Uses of the Drug. Permanent central venous lines (e.g. Hickman catheters) are often surgically inserted in patients requiring long-term therapy. Due to the high pH of the i.v. preparation of ganciclovir, tissue damage may occur if administered intramuscularly or subcutaneously. Frequent hematological monitoring is advised during the induction phase of therapy, and on a weekly basis during maintenance. Renal function should also be regularly measured.

A number of regimens have been examined in order to determine the optimum and most convenient dosage regimens for ganciclovir. A retrospective study of 45 patients with AIDS-related cytomegalovirus retinitis who received ganciclovir at a dose of 10 mg per kg per day three times weekly found they had a similar time to relapse (median of 5.4 months) as patients treated on 5–7 days weekly (Hall *et al.*, 1991). However, in a study of bone marrow transplant patients who had positive serology for cytomegalovirus prior to transplantation or who had seropositive donors, ganciclovir administered thrice-weekly at a dose of 5 or 6 mg per kg daily did not prevent cytomegalovirus reactivation (Przepiorka *et al.*, 1994).

Ganciclovir has been shown to be stable in parenteral nutrient solution containing 1–5% amino acids for at least 3 h (Johnson *et al.*, 1994). When reconstituted in normal saline or 5% dextrose in water to final drug concentrations of 1–10 mg per ml ganciclovir remains stable when stored at 4–25°C for 28–35 days (Silvestri *et al.*, 1991; Mole *et al.*, 1992; Parasrampuria *et al.*, 1992).

2 Oral administration

Based on studies that demonstrated efficacy at a dose of 3000 mg daily with no significant difference between administration of 500 mg six times daily and 1 g every 8 h, and on data demonstrating improved bioavailability when the drug is taken with a meal, the current dose of oral ganciclovir is 3000 mg daily given in three divided doses and taken with food.

3 Intravitreal injection

Ganciclovir can be given by intravitreal injection using a 30-gauge needle under topical anesthesia on an outpatient basis (Henry, 1987; Morlet *et al.*, 1993). Mercury bag decompression of the eye for 10–15 min prior to administration has been reported to reduce the elevation in intraocular pressure associated with the injection, and also reduce the level of discomfort (Morlet and Young, 1993). The usual dose of ganciclovir administered by intravitreal injection is 200–400 µg per 0.1 ml, given twice-weekly until resolution of acute disease, then once-weekly as maintenance therapy (Henry *et al.*, 1987; Ussery *et al.*, 1988; Cochereau-Massin *et al.*, 1991). In a small uncontrolled pilot study, intravitreal ganciclovir has been given at a dose of 2 mg per 0.1 ml for maintenance treatment of patients with AIDS-related cytomegalovirus retinitis and found to be effective in suppressing retinitis without evidence of retinal toxicity (Young *et al.*, 1992). A smaller volume of injection has also been used (350 µg in 50 µl) with similar efficacy to previous studies using volumes of 0.1 ml and with reportedly less associated discomfort (Baudouin and Gastaud, 1992).

4 Ganciclovir intraocular device

A sustained release device, containing a core of ganciclovir within layers of polymers, can be implanted subconjunctivally or intravitreally, maintaining local therapeutic concentrations for up to 8 months (Sanborn et al., 1992; Ashton et al., 1994). The average time to replacement has been reported to be 6 months (Morley et al., 1995), although the calculated efficacy is closer to 4 months duration (Anand et al., 1993a). Ganciclovir is released from these devices in a linear manner at rates of 1–5 μg per h (Smith et al., 1992; Anand et al., 1993a; Martin et al., 1994a). The device is surgically implanted.

5 Patients with renal failure

Dosage adjustments for both oral and i.v. administration of ganciclovir are required for patients with renal insufficiency, and recommendations are provided by the manufacturer with reductions in i.v. dose proportionate to impairment in creatinine clearance (see Table V.8). Hemodialysis has been reported to remove 50–60% of plasma concentrations following i.v. administration (Lake et al., 1988; Sommadossi et al., 1988; Swan et al., 1991; Combarnous et al., 1994), indicating that the drug should be administered by i.v. infusion at the end of dialysis. A reduction of 58% of the recommended i.v. dose (1.25 mg per kg at the end of dialysis, three times weekly) has been successfully used in an elderly anuric man requiring hemodialysis (Combarnous et al., 1994). The i.v. dose of ganciclovir in patients requiring hemodialysis should not exceed 1.25 mg per kg every 24 h. Measurement of drug levels in patients with renal failure receiving ganciclovir is recommended; although methodology is available (Hedaya and Sawchuk, 1990; Boulieu et al., 1991a,b), drug level monitoring may not be practical.

6 Patients with bone marrow suppression

The dose of ganciclovir should be withheld in patients whose neutrophil count falls below 500 cells per μl or who develop severe thrombocytopenia (platelet count of less than 25 000 per μl) until neutrophil count rises above 750 cells per μl, and the platelet count is higher than 50 000 per μl. Neutropenia caused by ganciclovir can be reversed in most patients by concomitant administration of granulocyte colony stimulating factor (G-CSF) in relatively low dose (Jacobson et al., 1992).

7 Pregnant patients

Ganciclovir is contraindicated in pregnancy.

8 Pediatric patients

There is still only very limited experience with ganciclovir therapy in children under 12 years of age, and the optimum dose of i.v. therapy has not been established. Daily doses of 7.5–10 mg per kg daily divided into two or three doses have been used for induction therapy, and doses of 2.5–5 mg per kg daily have been used for maintenance therapy (United States Pharmacopeia Drug Information, 1995). Although not indicated for the treatment of congenital infection, such infants have been treated with ganciclovir at a dose of 7.5 mg per kg by i.v. infusion over 1 h twice-daily for 2 weeks followed by 10 mg per kg three times weekly for 3 months, with good clinical results (Nigro et al., 1994). However, because of the long-term risks of carcinogenicity and gonadal toxicity, extreme caution should be exercised when considering treatment of children with ganciclovir.

9 Topical administration

Ganciclovir ophthalmic gel has been used in animal studies, in concentrations ranging from 0.0125% to 0.2% (Castela et al., 1994).

Table V.8
Dosage of ganciclovir for patients with renal insufficiency. (Adapted from Ganciclovir Product Information.)

Serum creatinine μM	Ganciclovir dose (mg per kg)	Dosing interval (h)
< 124	5.0	12
125 – 325	2.5	12
226 – 398	2.5	24
> 398	1.25	24

Availability

1 Intravenous use

The drug is packaged in glass *vials* in the form of *lyophilized powder* containing 500 mg of ganciclovir and 46 mg of sodium. The powder is reconstituted in 10 ml sterile water for injection (without preservatives) to achieve a final concentration of 50 mg per ml. Ganciclovir is then further diluted in normal saline, or 5% dextrose in water prior to infusion. Latex gloves and safety glasses are recommended to be worn during the preparation to prevent inhalation or direct contact with skin or mucous membranes.

2 Oral use

Oral ganciclovir is available as *capsules* containing 250 mg of active drug.

Serum and Tissue Levels in Relation to Dosage

1 Intravenous administration

A single i.v. dose of 5 mg per kg given over 1 h to adults with normal renal function results in a mean peak plasma level of $8.3 \pm 4.0 \,\mu g$ per ml, with a trough value of $0.56 \pm 0.66 \,\mu g$ per ml. The mean plasma half-life was 2.9 ± 1.3 h with a mean clearance of 3.64 ± 1.86 ml per min per kg. There is no accumulation of the drug in plasma with chronic administration. Following multiple doses of ganciclovir of 2.5 or 5 mg per kg given to adults with no renal impairment every 8 or 12 h by i.v. infusion over 1 h, the peak and trough serum levels were $4.0–6.2 \,\mu g$ per ml and less than $0.25–0.63 \,\mu g$ per ml respectively. The mean half-life of the drug ranged from 0.23 to 0.76 h, with a terminal elimination half-life ranging from 2.5 to 3.6 h (Fletcher *et al.*, 1986; Erice *et al.*, 1987; Sommadossi *et al.*, 1988).

Intravenous infusion of ganciclovir results in good intraocular penetration with the mean reported intravitreal concentration of ganciclovir in one study of $0.93 \pm 0.39 \,\mu g$ per ml ($3.6 \pm 1.5 \,\mu M$) (Kuppermann *et al.*, 1993a). In a study of 52 patients with cytomegalovirus retinitis and retinal detachment who were undergoing vitrectomy, the mean vitreous ganciclovir concentrations in patients receiving i.v. ganciclovir induction and maintenance therapy were $4.74 \pm 1.49 \,\mu M$ and $3.29 \pm 1.84 \,\mu M$ respectively (Arevalo *et al.*, 1995).

2 Oral administration

The absorption of oral ganciclovir is fairly poor (see Table V.9). Early studies demonstrated a 6% bioavailability following a single oral dose of 10 mg per kg or 1000 mg (de Miranda *et al.*, 1986). Taking the capsules with food was found to significantly increase the peak serum levels (by 13%) and area-under-the-curve (AUC) (by 20%). When oral ganciclovir is taken with a meal of approximately 600 calories and containing approximately 45% fat the steady-state AUC increased by a mean of 22% and the C_{max} increased from a mean of 0.85 to $0.96 \,\mu g$ per ml. In more recent studies, when oral ganciclovir was administered as a single oral dose of 1000 or 2000 mg the mean calculated bioavailability ranged from 5.6% to 13.4% and was not proportional to dose (Follansbee *et al.*, 1992; Anderson *et al.*, 1995). The poor oral bioavailability of the drug is supported by other studies in which oral bioavailability ranged from 2.6 to 7.3% (Spector *et al.*, 1995).

The mean steady-state peak and trough serum levels achieved with multiple dosing of 20 mg per kg every 6 h were 2.96 and $1.05 \,\mu M$ respectively, with a calculated absorption of 3% (Jacobson *et al.*, 1987). Steady-state serum levels are obtained 24 h after multiple dosing with

Table V.9

Summary of clinically relevant pharmacokinetics of oral ganciclovir

---

Mean oral bioavailability is 6%

Food increases peak plasma concentration and AUC

Mean half-life of oral ganciclovir to 5 h

Daily dose of 3000 mg results in serum levels of $>0.5 \,\mu g$ per ml (in range of IC_{50} of many clinical isolates)

Oral ganciclovir accumulates in patients with renal disfunction

---

mean peak serum concentrations for patients receiving a total daily dose of 3000 mg (either 1 g every 8 h or 500 mg six times daily) of 0.96 ±0.51 and 0.72 ± 0.40 μg per ml respectively (Oral ganciclovir investigational brochure, 1994). The mean trough plasma level with a 1000 mg three times daily regimen is 0.2 μg per ml (Oral ganciclovir investigational brochure, 1994; Spector *et al.*, 1995). The mean half-lives for oral ganciclovir (3000 mg per day) and i.v. ganciclovir (5 mg per kg daily) are 5.0 and 3.5 h respectively, with the AUC being 2-fold higher with i.v. therapy than with oral (26.8 versus 13.0 μg.h per ml respectively) (Oral ganciclovir investigational brochure 1994). This is similar to the findings of Anderson *et al.* (1995), where the AUC for oral ganciclovir (3 g per day) was 70% of that for i.v. administration of 5 mg per kg daily. Serum levels of greater than 0.5 μg.ml (2 μM) were achieved with a daily dose of 3000 mg, a concentration that approximates the IC_{50} of many clinical isolates (Data on file, Roche).

Preliminary data from an unpublished study of recipients of renal and liver allografts receiving oral ganciclovir suggest that there is significant accumulation of the drug in patients with creatine clearance levels of below 70 ml per min (Data on file, Roche).

3 Intravitreal injection

In rabbits, an intravitreal injection of 400 μg resulted in intravitreal levels that exceeded the IC_{50} of cytomegalovirus for over 60 h (Schulman *et al.*, 1986).

Intravitreal administration of 200 μg of ganciclovir to a patient with AIDS-related cytomegalovirus retinitis resulted in vitreous and aqueous humor levels of ganciclovir of 1.2 μg per ml and 0.66 μg per ml respectively, and no systemic absorption of the drug. The estimated elimination half-life of ganciclovir from the vitreous was 13.3 h, with the intravitreal level remaining above the IC_{50} of cytomegalovirus for approximately 62 h following a single dose (Henry *et al.*, 1987). The use of liposome-encapsulated ganciclovir has been reported to decrease the required number of intravitreal injections (Akula *et al.*, 1994).

4 Ganciclovir intraocular device

When sustained release devices containing ganciclovir are implanted into the vitreous of rabbits, mean intravitreal levels of ganciclovir of 9–16 μg per ml have been achieved, remaining at these levels for 42–80 days (Smith *et al.*, 1992).

5 Patients with renal failure

Intravenous administration of ganciclovir results in significantly different kinetics in patients with renal impairment than in those with normal renal function. In the former, there is a prolonged plasma half-life, an increase in peak plasma concentrations and a decrease in clearance of ganciclovir.

Administration of 5 mg per kg of ganciclovir in a 1 h i.v. infusion to a patient with renal failure resulted in a markedly elevated peak plasma level of 20 μg per ml, and a long elimination half-life of 6.3 h, with a decreased total body clearance of 35.5 ml per min (Swan *et al.*, 1991). The total body clearance of ganciclovir in patients requiring hemodialysis is approximately 5% of that calculated for individuals with normal renal function. In such patients the serum half-life ranges from 5 to 28 h, and the terminal half-life of ganciclovir is increased approximately 3-fold when compared with persons with normal renal function (Sommadossi *et al.*, 1988; United States Pharmacopeia Drug Information, 1995). In patients with renal failure dosages of ganciclovir of 5 mg per kg every 48 h resulted in peak and trough serum levels of 16.1 ± 2.4 and 5.5 ± 0.5 μg per ml, with a volume of distribution at steady-state of 0.64 ± 0.09 liters per kg (Bastien *et al.*, 1994). In a single case-report, decreasing the infusion dose to 1.25 mg per kg three times weekly at the end of dialysis resulted in a peak plasma level of 3.7 μg per ml, with a steady-state level of 2.6 μg per ml for nearly 40 h (Combarnous *et al.*, 1994). In such patients the terminal half-life of ganciclovir is increased approximately 3-fold when compared with persons with normal renal function (Sommadossi *et al.*, 1988; Combarnous *et al.*, 1994).

6 Pediatric patients

In neonates (2–49 days) with symptomatic cytomegalovirus infection who received a single i.v. infusion over 1 h of 4 or 6 mg per kg, ganciclovir was found to have linear pharmacokinetics. The apparent volume of distribution was 669 ± 70 ml per kg and 749 ± 59 ml per kg for the 4 mg per kg and 6 mg per kg doses respectively, and increased with increasing weight (Trang *et al.*, 1993).

In children after renal transplant with symptomatic cytomegalovirus infection and whose creatinine clearances were between 20 and 60 ml per min per 1.73 m^2, the clearance of ganciclovir ranged from 0.4 to 2.2 ml per min per kg, and the elimination half-lives were between 23.7 and 3.9 h (Jacqz-Aigrain *et al.*, 1992).

7 Race and gender

Based on only limited data, there appears to be a lower steady-state C_{max} and lower AUC of ganciclovir in blacks and Hispanics than in whites (Data on file, Roche).

8 Topical administration

Ganciclovir ophthalmic gel achieves corneal levels that are higher than the IC_{50} of ganciclovir for herpes simplex virus type 1 (Castela *et al.*, 1994).

Excretion

The major route of elimination of ganciclovir administered by i.v. infusion is via the kidneys, by both glomerular filtration and tubular secretion. In one report, the total clearance of the drug following i.v. infusion exceeded the creatinine clearance by a factor of 2.4 (Fletcher *et al.*, 1986). Virtually all of an i.v. dose of ganciclovir is excreted unchanged in the urine (Sommadossi *et al.*, 1988; Markham and Faulds, 1994).

When administered by i.v. infusion in a dose of 5 mg per kg every 48 h to anuric patients requiring hemodialysis, the elimination half-life is 18.9 ± 2.2 h, with a volume of distribution at steady-state of 0.68 ±0.10 liters per kg (Boulieu *et al.*, 1993). These observations are supported by a separate report of an anuric elderly patient requiring hemodialysis who was given 1.5 mg per kg daily of ganciclovir by i.v. infusion. The elimination half-life in this patient was 23.3 h (Rello, 1990). In another case-report of an anuric patient requiring hemodialysis the total plasma clearance was 0.05 ml per min per kg with an elimination half-life of 132 h (Combarnous *et al.*, 1994). In neonates after a single i.v. infusion of 4 or 6 mg per kg, the mean elimination half-life was 2.4 h, and the mean total body clearance was similar for the 4 mg per kg and 6 mg per kg dose groups, being 189 ± 28 ml per kg per h and 213 ± 21 ml per kg per h respectively, and increasing with age (Trang *et al.*, 1993).

In contrast to i.v. administered ganciclovir, only 5% of the oral form of the drug is excreted unchanged by the kidneys, and over 85% is eliminated unchanged in the feces (Data on file, Roche).

Distribution of the Drug in Body

Following i.v. administration ganciclovir is widely distributed in tissues, with good intraocular penetration, without evidence of accumulation (Fletcher and Balfour, 1989).

The volume of distribution at steady-state has been reported as 1.17 ± 0.54 liters per kg (Sommadossi *et al.*, 1988). There is minimal protein binding, in the range of 1–2%. Data obtained from sampling tissues at autopsy from patients who had received i.v. therapy have demonstrated highest concentrations of the drug in kidneys, with 10-fold lower levels in lung, liver, brain, testes and blood obtained from heart (Shepp *et al.*, 1985). The volume of distribution at steady-state is approximately 0.74 liters per kg. Sequential administration of ganciclovir (3.75 mg per kg daily) and foscarnet (60 mg per kg daily) did not alter the plasma clearance or volume of distribution of either drug (Aweeka *et al.*, 1995). Ganciclovir is able to cross the blood–brain barrier, with levels within the cerebrospinal fluid in the range of 24–67% of concomitant serum levels (Shepp *et al.*, 1985; Fletcher *et al.*, 1986).

Levels of ganciclovir within the vitreous fluid have been found to range from 44 to 65% of those in the serum (Daikos *et al.*, 1988). The half life of ganciclovir in vitreous fluid is approximately 13 h (United States Pharmacopeia Drug Information, 1995).

Following i.v. infusion ganciclovir crosses the placenta by simple diffusion (Gilstrap *et al.*, 1994). Using an *ex vivo* human placental cotyledon model with maternal concentrations of 4 and 40 μM of ganciclovir respectively the fetal concentrations were 17 and 19% respectively of maternal levels (Gilstrap *et al.*, 1994).

Mechanism of Action

Ganciclovir has a similar structure and mechanism of action to aciclovir (Figs V.12, V.13). The antiviral activity of ganciclovir is dependent upon its intracellular phosphorylation to the triphosphate derivative (Field *et al.*, 1983; Cheng *et al.*, 1983a). Initial phosphorylation to ganciclovir monophosphate is rate limiting. There are only minimal levels of the triphosphory-lated drug within uninfected cells.

Virus-induced TK is responsible for the initial phosphorylation of ganciclovir in cells infected with herpes simplex viruses type 1 or 2 (Smee *et al.*, 1983; Cheng *et al.*, 1983b). Herpes simplex virus-specified TK is an excellent substrate for ganciclovir (Ashton *et al.*, 1982). This knowledge

Fig. V.13.

Phosphorylation and mechanism of action of ganciclovir. [a] In herpes simplex virus and varicella-zoster virus infected cells; [b] in cytomegalovirus infected cells.

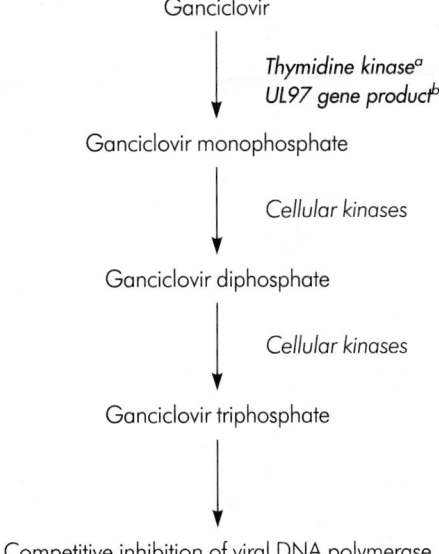

Ganciclovir

Thymidine kinase[a]
UL97 gene product[b]

Ganciclovir monophosphate

Cellular kinases

Ganciclovir diphosphate

Cellular kinases

Ganciclovir triphosphate

Competitive inhibition of viral DNA polymerase

has provided a new strategy for the treatment of tumors by gene therapy (Macri and Gordon, 1994) (p. 1561). Strains of herpes simplex types 1 and 2 with mutations within the virus-specified TK result in lack of susceptibility to ganciclovir (Elion *et al.*, 1977). There is no evidence to support the existence of a cytomegalovirus-encoded TK. However, the UL97 open reading frame contains sequences characteristic of protein kinases and encodes a protein that is capable of phosphorylating ganciclovir in cytomegalovirus-infected cells (Littler *et al.*, 1992; Sullivan *et al.*, 1992a,b). Although the enzyme responsible for phosphorylation of ganciclovir in Epstein–Barr virus-infected cells remains uncertain, it is clear that the drug is preferentially phosphorylated in infected versus uninfected cells, and that phosphorylation of ganciclovir is more efficient than aciclovir (Datta and Pagano, 1983; Lin *et al.*, 1986).

Cellular kinases are responsible for subsequent phosphorylation to di- and triphosphate derivatives, the latter being the active antiviral form of the drug. These kinases include cellular guanylate kinase, deoxyguanosine kinase and phosphoglycerate kinase, and are induced in cells infected with human cytomegalovirus (Boehme, 1984; Meijer *et al.*, 1984; Matthews and Boehme, 1988). Levels of ganciclovir triphosphate are 10- to 100-fold higher in cytomegalovirus infected versus uninfected cells (Biron *et al.*, 1985; Freitas *et al.*, 1985). *In vitro* experiments suggest that ganciclovir triphosphate is slowly catabolized in cytomegalovirus and herpes simplex virus infected cells, with 40–70% of original drug concentrations being detected 18–24 h after the drug is removed, and an intracellular half-life of >6 h (Biron *et al.*, 1985; Smee *et al.*, 1985c). Accumulation of ganciclovir triphosphate within infected cells contributes importantly to its superiority over aciclovir against cytomegalovirus.

The activity of ganciclovir triphosphate against cytomegalovirus is through inhibiting the replication of viral DNA by several mechanisms. Ganciclovir triphosphate competitively inhibits the incorporation of dGTP into DNA by potently inhibiting the action of viral DNA polymerase (see below). Second, ganciclovir triphosphate is incorporated internally into the growing chain of viral DNA, dramatically inhibiting its elongation and thus limiting viral DNA synthesis (Frank *et al.*, 1984; St Clair *et al.*, 1987). As ganciclovir contains hydroxyl groups similar to the 3' and 5' hydroxyl groups of endogenous nucleotides, chain elongation is not completely terminated but can continue very slowly following the incorporation of ganciclovir triphosphate into DNA (Frank *et al.*, 1984; Reardon 1989). The continuation of viral DNA synthesis results in the production of short DNA fragments of cytomegalovirus that accumulate within the nucleus but are not packaged or released as infectious virions (Hamzeh and Lietman, 1991). Chain-termination is apparently reversible: chain-elongation continues when the drug is removed (Matthews and Boehme, 1988).

Ganciclovir triphosphate is an excellent substrate for cytomegalovirus DNA polymerase, competitively inhibiting this enzyme with respect to dGTP with a K_i of 1.7 μM, with cellular DNA polymerases being inhibited with a significantly higher K_i of 17 μM (Freitas *et al.*, 1985). Ganciclovir triphosphate also selectively inhibits the DNA polymerases of herpes simplex virus types 1 and 2 with K_i values of 0.5–1 μM, with the K_i for cellular alpha DNA polymerase being 35- to 50-fold higher (Germershausen *et al.*, 1983; St Clair *et al.*, 1984). However, a recent study has found that ganciclovir triphosphate inhibits delta DNA polymerase at much lower drug concentrations than alpha DNA polymerase (K_is of 2 μM and 80 μM respectively) (Iisley *et al.*, 1995).

Toxicity

Most studies to date have been performed with patients receiving ganciclovir by i.v. infusion; adverse events related to oral ganciclovir and intraocular administration will be considered separately.

1 Bone marrow

The major toxicity of ganciclovir is bone marrow suppression, particularly neutropenia and to a lesser extent thrombocytopenia. Ganciclovir should not be administered to patients with fewer than 500 neutrophils per μl or with fewer than 25 000 platelets per μl. The prevalence of bone marrow suppression varies widely, and is dependent upon the route of administration, the dose, underlying illness, and the definition of neutropenia. The development of neutropenia has been reported to be independent of the duration of treatment, plasma drug levels or baseline neutrophil count (Reed *et al.*, 1988a), although other investigators have associated neutropenia in marrow transplant recipients with mean peak and trough plasma levels of ganciclovir exceeding 50 and 10 μM respectively (Shepp *et al.*, 1985). In an analysis of all adverse reactions reported from 655 patients treated with i.v. ganciclovir in the USA in clinical trials up until late 1990, neutropenia (defined as <1000 cells per μl) occurred overall in 42% of patients with AIDS, 41% of bone marrow transplant recipients, 7% of heart allograft recipients; thrombocytopenia (<50 000 per μl) was reported in 57% of bone marrow allograft recipients, in 13% of AIDS patients, and 8% of heart transplant patients (Data on file, Roche). These data are supported by smaller studies in which ganciclovir-associated neutropenia occurred more frequently in bone marrow transplant recipients than in other transplant patients (60% versus 35% respectively) (Erice *et al.*, 1987), and where neutropenia (<1000 cells per μl) was more commonly observed in AIDS patients (55%) than transplant recipients (20%) (Winston *et al.*, 1988).

In patients with AIDS-related cytomegalovirus gastrointestinal disease being treated with ganciclovir, receiving 5mg per kg every 12 h, moderate neutropenia (500–1000 cells per μl) or severe neutropenia (<500 cells per μl) have been reported in 13% and 3% respectively (Chachoua *et al.*, 1987). In other studies, neutropenia (<1000 cells per μl) requiring cessation of therapy occurred in 25% of AIDS patients with cytomegalovirus retinitis during induction therapy 7.5 mg per kg daily, and neutropenia (<800–1000 cells per μl) has also been reported in 31–36% of patients receiving long-term ganciclovir maintenance therapy, usually a dose of 5 mg per kg daily on 5 days per week (Holland *et al.*, 1986; Jacobson *et al.*, 1988a).

Neutropenia is more common in patients who receive combination therapy with ganciclovir and foscarnet than in patients treated with alternating therapy with these agents or with either drug alone (Dieterich *et al.*, 1993a; Jacobson *et al.*, 1994a). Neutropenia is usually reversible upon cessation of ganciclovir treatment (Jabs *et al.*, 1987; Reed *et al.*, 1988a), although cases of irreversible neutropenia and death have been reported (Data on file, Roche). Granulocytopenia most commonly develops during the second week of therapy, and is a risk factor for bacteremia, bacterial pneumonia and pulmonary aspergillosis (Miller *et al.*, 1994; Przepiorka *et al.*, 1994; Shepp *et al.*, 1994). There does not appear to be a higher incidence of indwelling catheter-related bacterial infections in patients who receive ganciclovir compared with foscarnet (Stanley *et al.*, 1994). Combination therapy using ganciclovir with recombinant GM-CSF or G-CSF has reduced the proportion of patients unable to continue ganciclovir due to severe neutropenia (Hardy, 1991; Miles *et al.*, 1991; Jacobson *et al.*, 1992; Hardy *et al.*, 1994).

In a study of bone marrow transplant recipients who received 6 mg per kg daily of ganciclovir or 5 days per week post-transplant as prophylaxis for cytomegalovirus, reversible neutropenia (<1000 cells per μl) developed in 58% of treated patients versus 28% in the placebo group (Winston *et al.*, 1993). In two studies of recipients of allogeneic marrow transplants 30% of those who received 5 mg per kg daily of ganciclovir as prophylactic therapy against cytomegalovirus infection post-transplant developed neutropenia (<750 cells per μl) compared with 0–8% of the patients receiving placebo (Goodrich *et al.*, 1991, 1993). Ganciclovir treatment of cytomegalovirus pneumonia in bone marrow transplant recipients (7.5 mg per kg daily for 14 days) was associated with dose-limiting neutropenia (<500 cells per μl), requiring cessation of treatment in 12% of patients (Reed *et al.*, 1988b). Ganciclovir appears to be less commonly associated with neutropenia in pediatric bone marrow transplant recipients than in adults (Roberts *et al.*, 1993).

Thrombocytopenia has been reported in 19% of AIDS patients receiving 7.5 mg per kg daily of ganciclovir as maintenance therapy (Buhles *et al.*, 1988). Anemia occurs in approximately 2% of treated patients.

2 Carcinogenesis and mutagenesis

In mice ganciclovir was carcinogenic following oral doses of 20–1000 mg per kg daily. At the highest doses ganciclovir caused malignancy of reproductive organs and liver. The drug was not found to be carcinogenic at doses of 1 mg per kg daily. Ganciclovir was teratogenic in rabbits at doses calculated to be similar to those recommended for humans (Data on file, Roche). Fetal resorptions occurred in approximately 85% of rabbits and mice when they received twice the human exposure based on AUC comparisons. There have been no controlled trials in pregnant women, thus potential risks and benefits must be considered prior to its use in this situation.

3 Gonadal toxicity

In preclinical studies ganciclovir was found to inhibit potently spermatogenesis in rats and dogs and to decrease fertility in male and female mice. In male patients (mostly with AIDS, many of whom had pre-existing hormonal abnormalities), there was no significant alteration in levels of serum testosterone, follicle stimulating hormone or luteinizing hormone associated with ganciclovir therapy. However, the manufacturer recommends that gonadal toxicity be assumed until further clinical data are available (Data on file, Roche).

4 Cytotoxicity

Dose-dependent inhibition of granulocyte-macrophage colony forming cells by ganciclovir has been observed *in vitro* with an IC_{50} of $2.7 \pm 0.5\ \mu M$ and IC_{90} of $35.7 \pm 3.6\ \mu M$ (Sommadossi and Carlisle, 1987). Although other investigators have reported higher IC_{50} values (approximately $40\ \mu M$) for ganciclovir-induced inhibition of colony forming units by human granulocyte-macrophage progenitor cells (Snoeck *et al.*, 1990), this value is still significantly lower than reports of ganciclovir cytotoxicity on non-bone marrow derived cells. Non-bone marrow derived cell lines are more resistant to ganciclovir cytotoxicity, with cell proliferation and cellular DNA synthesis being inhibited at drug concentrations 100- to 500-fold higher than concentrations required for antiviral efficacy (Neyts *et al.*, 1990). Stem cell factor enhances the number of granulocyte-macrophage colony forming units in the presence of ganciclovir *in vitro* (Scadden *et al.*, 1994). Ganciclovir has been reported to inhibit the proliferative responses of lymphocytes to phytohemagglutinin and cytomegalovirus antigens by more than 50% when the drug was tested at clinically relevant concentrations (Bowden *et al.*, 1987).

5 Central nervous system

In open-label compassionate-use trials of ganciclovir involving over 5000 patients, central nervous system toxicity was reported in 5% (de Armond and Doreman, 1990; Syndman, 1988). Seizures have been reported as a probable complication of ganciclovir therapy, commencing 1 month after initiation of the drug, resolving only on discontinuation of ganciclovir and recommencing with rechallenge (Barton *et al.*, 1992). In an analysis of toxicities in the foscarnet–ganciclovir cytomegalovirus retinitis trial, seizures were no more common in patients randomized to either drug (Studies of Ocular Complications of AIDS Research Group, 1995). There are several case reports of psychiatric disturbance possibly attributable to ganciclovir therapy in patients with renal insufficiency. Symptoms including nightmares, visual hallucinations, delirium and agitation, have been reported to cease on cessation of the drug and in one patient recurred with rechallenge (Davis *et al.*, 1990; Chen *et al.*, 1992). Psychosis with auditory and visual hallucinations has recently been observed in association with ganciclovir therapy in a patient without renal insufficiency (Hansen *et al.*, 1996).

6 Overdose

Reported toxicities associated with overdose with i.v. ganciclovir include irreversible pancytopenia, reversible neutropenia, hepatic and renal toxicity and seizures. Peritoneal dialysis, hemodialysis, hydration, exchange transfusion or treatment with colony stimulating factors may be useful and prevent the development of adverse events (Data on file, Roche).

7 Other

Abnormal liver function tests have been observed in approximately 2% of over 5000 patients who have received ganciclovir. Treatment of an AIDS patient with ganciclovir has been reported to cause a marked elevation of hepatic transaminases and alkaline phosphatase that recurred on rechallenge (Shea *et al.*, 1987). In a more recent report ganciclovir was again potentially linked with hepatotoxicity in five patients, although other drugs known to alter liver function had been administered in all cases (Figge *et al.*, 1992). Ventricular tachycardia has been reported in two patients with AIDS receiving ganciclovir, with recurrence of the arrhythmia on rechallenge with cardiac monitoring (Cohen *et al.*, 1990). Other adverse reactions that may be caused by ganciclovir include fever (6%), rash (6%), nausea, vomiting, diarrhea (4–6%) (Buhles *et al.*, 1988), impaired renal function, and hypotension (Keay *et al.*, 1988).

8 Ocular administration and related toxicity

Intravitreal ganciclovir was administered to rabbits one to three times weekly at a dose of up to 400 μg per injection without evidence of ganciclovir-induced toxicity (Data on file, Roche).

Although toxicity associated with intravitreal injections of ganciclovir in humans is relatively uncommon (Henry *et al.*, 1987b) a number of complications have been reported including retinal detachment (Ussery *et al.*, 1988; Cochereau-Massin *et al.*, 1991) and intravitreal hemorrhage (Cochereau-Massin *et al.*, 1991). In a single case report of accidental intravitreal administration of 40 mg per 0.1 ml of ganciclovir immediate surgery was unable to prevent permanent retinal damage and blindness (Saran and Maguire, 1994).

In 26 patients (30 eyes) treated for cytomegalovirus retinitis by a ganciclovir implant postoperative complications included retinal detachments (23%) and one retinal tear (Martin *et al.*, 1994a).

9 Oral administration and related toxicity

Preclinical studies in mice using doses of oral ganciclovir of up to 1000 mg per kg daily for 1 year demonstrated no drug-related events at a dose of 1 mg per kg daily. However, higher doses were associated with the development of testicular atrophy, with an increased incidence of abnormal morphology of spermatazoa (at a dose of 20–1000 mg per kg daily), tumors of the clitoris and stomach (1000 mg per kg daily). Longer therapy was associated with a range of epithelial, vascular and hemopoietic tumors. In dogs administered up to 6 mg per kg daily for 1 year, side-effects included low leukocyte counts (at a dose of 6 mg per kg daily), and at doses of 0.6–6 mg per kg daily a reduced cellularity of the bone marrow, testicular atrophy and decreased sperm counts, all of which were completely or partially reversible following cessation of the drug (Data on file, Roche).

Combined data from phase III studies in persons with HIV infection in the USA and Europe has predictably shown that there is less sepsis (less than 5% versus 8.5–15%) and less neutropenia (29% versus 41%) with oral ganciclovir when compared with i.v. administration of the drug (The Oral Ganciclovir European and Australian Co-operative Study Group, 1995; Drew *et al.*, 1995a,b) (Table V.10). In these studies, more patients developed rash with oral ganciclovir than with i.v. ganciclovir (10–15% versus less than 10% respectively), and diarrhea (33% versus 21%) (data on file Roche; The Oral Ganciclovir European and Australian Co-operative Study Group, 1995).

Table V.10
Reported toxicity of intravenous and oral ganciclovir. (Data from Drew *et al.*, 1995[1]; The Oral Ganciclovir European and Australian Co-operative Study Group, 1995[2], with permission.)

Adverse event	Intravenous (%)	Oral (%)
Neutropenia [a]	23–37	14–15
Thrombocytopenia[b]	2[1]–7[2]	3[1]–9[2]
Anemia[c]	24[1]–40[2]	15[1]–36[2]
Sepsis	8.5–19	3–8
Diarrhea	21–54	33–50
Rash	0	10
Nausea	29	34
Vomiting	15	15

[a] Defined as absolute neutrophil count <500 × 10⁶ per liter
[b] Defined as platelet count <50 × 10⁹ per liter
[c] Defined as hemoglobin <9.5g/dl[2] or <8g per liter[1]

10 Drug interactions

Ganciclovir and zidovudine are poorly tolerated because of bone marrow toxicity, with only five of 29 patients able to take zidovudine at a dose of 600 mg daily in conjunction with ganciclovir, and one of ten patients continuing zidovudine at a dose of 1200 mg daily in combination with ganciclovir (Hochster *et al.*, 1990; Jacobson *et al.*, 1993). Prolonged pancytopenia has been reported in an AIDS patient receiving both drugs (Jacobson *et al.*, 1988b). Synergistic cytotoxicity has been reported when physiologically relevant concentrations of zidovudine and ganciclovir were studied in human cell lines (Prichard *et al.*, 1991). Zidovudine should be dose-reduced or ceased depending on hematologic status in patients receiving ganciclovir (Causey, 1991). No alteration was found in pharmacokinetics of either ganciclovir or zidovudine when used in combination in one clinical trial (Hochster *et al.*, 1990), although i.v. ganciclovir has been reported to increase the apparent clearance of zidovudine (Burger *et al.*, 1994) and to possibly decrease the AUC and peak plasma concentrations of zidovudine (Jacobson *et al.*, 1988b). Oral ganciclovir has been found to increase the AUC for zidovudine by 14.5%. Co-administration of ganciclovir with other myelosuppressive drugs should be avoided or monitored carefully.

In a review of the tolerability of ganciclovir in patients taking didanosine under the Videx US Expanded Access Scheme, severe neutropenia (<500 cells per μl) was reported in only 12.5% of patients (Jacobson *et al.*, 1993). The pharmacokinetics of didanosine have previously been reported to be unaltered by concurrent ganciclovir therapy when the latter is administered by i.v. infusion (Hartman *et al.*, 1991). However, recent data suggest that both i.v. and oral administration of ganciclovir can markedly increase didanosine serum levels. Oral ganciclovir significantly increases the AUC of didanosine (by approximately 80–100%) thus potentially increasing the risk of didanosine-related toxicity; the AUC for ganciclovir is decreased by didanosine by 23% (Gaines *et al.*, 1994). Induction therapy with i.v. ganciclovir results in a mean increase in the AUC and maximal serum levels of didanosine of 70% and 49% respectively; maintenance therapy with ganciclovir increases these parameters by 50% and 26% (Frascino *et al.*, 1995). Additive cytotoxicity in T lymphoblastoid cell lines has been observed *in vitro* between didanosine and ganciclovir (Medina *et al.*, 1992).

Seizures have been reported in patients taking ganciclovir with imipenam (DeArmand, 1991). Ganciclovir does not alter cyclosporine serum levels in cardiac transplant patients (Cantarovich and Latter, 1994). To date no studies have formally addressed interactions between ganciclovir and other medications in transplant recipients.

Clinical Uses of the Drug

Since 1989 ganciclovir given by i.v. infusion has been indicated for both initial and maintenance treatment of cytomegalovirus retinitis in patients with AIDS. The drug is also indicated for the prophylaxis against cytomegalovirus disease in high-risk transplant recipients, and in the treatment of severe cytomegalovirus disease including disseminated infection, retinitis, pneumonia and gastrointestinal disease in immunocompromised patients. Clinical trials have demonstrated the efficacy of oral ganciclovir in secondary prophylaxis against cytomegalovirus retinitis in AIDS patients and the drug is now indicated for this use in the USA.

1 Cytomegalovirus infection in AIDS patients

a   Intravenous administration   Ganciclovir is effective in treating cytomegalovirus retinitis in this patient population. However, following stabilization, life-long maintenance therapy must be given using either oral, i.v. or local ganciclovir. Whilst there is less experience with intravitreal administration or the use of implants containing slowly-released ganciclovir, these

---

Table V.11
Interactions of nucleoside analogs with ganciclovir

Zidovudine co-administration
　　Poorly tolerated with ganciclovir due to bone marrow toxicity
　　Increase in zidovudine AUC by 14%
Didanosine co-administration
　　Increase in didanosine AUC by 70%[a] to >80%[b]
　　Decrease in ganciclovir AUC by 23%

Refer to text for sources of data.
[a] With i.v. ganciclovir induction therapy.
[b] With oral ganciclovir.

appear to be effective alternatives for maintenance administration of the drug. For other forms of cytomegalovirus disease in this patient population, ganciclovir therapy appears to have some efficacy and maintenance therapy may not be required. Details of clinical trials and reports upon which these generalizations are based are provided below. There are difficulties in making generalizations based on data from retinitis trials that did not utilize independent evaluation of retinal photographs as the basis for determining clinical endpoints, and there is a particular problem when describing results from studies that varied in use of objective standardized methodology.

An analysis of data from patients with severe cytomegalovirus disease including retinitis, and gastrointestinal disease, who were receiving the drug on a compassionate use basis showed that i.v. infusions of 10–15 mg per kg daily of ganciclovir for 14 days resulted in improvement or stabilization of disease in most patients, but that relapse occurred in over 75% of patients upon cessation of treatment (Collaborative DHPG Treatment Study Group, 1986). The time interval between cessation of ganciclovir and relapse of retinitis in two small studies was reported to be 19–35 days (Masur et al., 1986; Palestine et al., 1986), and it became clear that maintenance therapy must be used in all patients to prevent recurrence (Mills et al., 1988). An early dose-ranging open-label study of ganciclovir in 20 patients with AIDS and cytomegalovirus retinitis further demonstrated that ganciclovir treatment successfully halted disease progression in 95% of patients, and therapy was recommended for those with sight-threatening retinitis with central lesions at a dose of 2.5 mg per kg three times daily, followed by maintenance therapy of 5 mg per kg daily for 5 days per week (Holland et al., 1986). These findings were supported by another study in which improvement or stabilization occurred in 53% and 39% respectively of patients with cytomegalovirus retinitis treated with 7.5–15 mg per kg of ganciclovir daily; a dose of 1 mg per kg three times daily did not prevent progression of disease (Laskin et al., 1987). Independently-read fundoscopic photos were not used as a basis for time to progression in any of these studies. Ganciclovir may prolong survival, although this has not been formally tested in a controlled trial (Holland et al., 1990).

In the first randomized study, patients were treated with a 10-day induction course of ganciclovir (at a dose of 2.5 mg per kg three times daily) and then randomized to receive immediate maintenance therapy (5 mg per kg daily for 5 days per week) or no therapy until disease progression was observed referred to as deferred maintenance. The median time to progression was only 16 days in the deferred maintenance group, compared with 42–58 days when maintenance therapy was commenced immediately following the induction course (Jacobson et al., 1988e). Other studies have reported a median time to progression of 47 days in

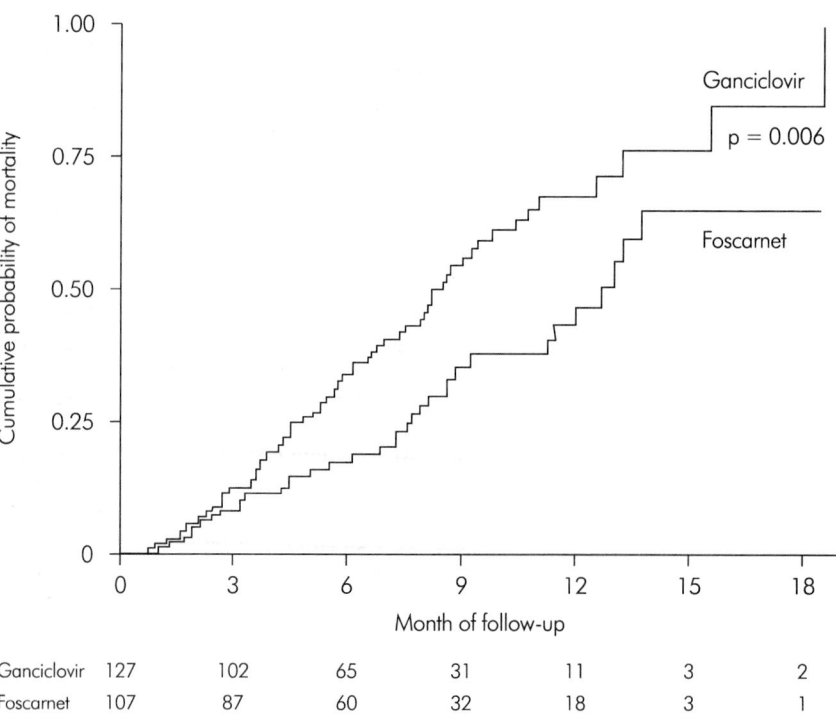

Fig. V.14.
Kaplan–Meier estimates of probability of mortality among patients with CMV retinitis randomized to receive ganciclovir or foscarnet (p = 0.006 by the log-rank test). (Reproduced from Studies of Ocular Complications of AIDS Research Group in collaboration with the AIDS Clinical Trials Group, 1992, with permission.)

	0	3	6	9	12	15	18
Ganciclovir	127	102	65	31	11	3	2
Foscarnet	107	87	60	32	18	3	1

patients not given maintenance therapy compared with 105 days in patients receiving maintenance therapy (Buhles *et al.*, 1988). Improvement in visual acuity may occur within 24 h of commencing therapy; and the rate of response may be dose-dependent (Masur *et al.*, 1986; Orellana *et al.*, 1987). In one study, maximum improvement in vision was reported to occur 21.5 days after commencing i.v. ganciclovir therapy (Orellana *et al.*, 1987). Relapse of retinitis usually responds to repeat induction therapy, although the possibility of ganciclovir-resistance should be considered (p.1582) Adjunctive therapy with cytomegalovirus i.v. immune globulin has not been found to improve the efficacy of ganciclovir in this patient population (Jacobson *et al.*, 1990). Again, none of these studies utilized independent evaluation of retinal photographs to determine clinical progression. The combination of GM-CSF together with ganciclovir therapy has been reported to delay progression of retinitis (Hardy *et al.*, 1994).

Although ganciclovir and foscarnet are equally efficacious in treating cytomegalovirus retinitis (Moyle *et al.*, 1992; Studies of Ocular Complications of AIDS (SOCA) Research Group, 1992), patients treated with foscarnet have been reported to survive longer than ganciclovir recipients (12.6 versus 8.5 months respectively) (Fig. V.14) (Studies of Ocular Complications of AIDS SOCA Research Group 1992; SOCA 1994). The SOCA study was one of the first to measure clinical progression based on fundoscopic photographs assessed by an independent investigator. In one study, patients treated with ganciclovir responded faster than those treated with foscarnet, although eventual rates of response did not differ (Moyle *et al.*, 1992).

Combination therapy using the two agents (ganciclovir at a dose of 5 mg per kg i.v. twice-daily and foscarnet at a dose of 60 mg per kg i.v. 8-hourly) is efficacious with complete or near-complete healing of all lesions (Kuppermann *et al.*, 1993b). However, in one prospective open trial the efficacy of combination therapy was found to be similar to monotherapy (Salzberger *et al.*, 1994). A recent multicenter, randomized, controlled trial was conducted to further evaluate combination foscarnet and ganciclovir therapy in a subset of patients who had persistently active cytomegalovirus retinitis or whose retinitis had relapsed on therapy. By fundoscopic photography, combination therapy was found to be the most effective therapy for controlling retinitis in this group, with median times to progression of 4.3 months for those randomized to receive combination therapy, compared with 1.3 and 2.0 months for those who received foscarnet induction and maintenance or ganciclovir induction and maintenance respectively (Studies on Ocular Complications of AIDS and AIDS Clinical Trials Group, 1996). Combination foscarnet and ganciclovir therapy is well tolerated, with no significant increase in renal, bone-marrow or other toxicity. Maintenance therapy again using these drugs in combination (ganciclovir 5 mg per kg i.v. once- or twice-daily and foscarnet 90–120 mg per kg daily) has also been found to be efficacious, and to have excellent *in vivo* antiviral activity, but the time involved for the sequential administration of both infusions causes difficulty for some patients (Kuppermann *et al.*, 1993b; Jacobson *et al.*, 1994a). Alternating therapy with these two drugs has also been found to be efficacious for either induction or maintenance therapy (Peters *et al.*, 1994). The time to progression appears to be much longer in patients with recurrent retinitis who receive combination therapy when compared with their previous records on monotherapy (Weinberg *et al.*, 1994). Foscarnet alone or in combination with ganciclovir has proved useful for patients with clinically resistant retinitis who have laboratory evidence of antiviral drug-resistance (Flores-Aguilar *et al.*, 1993; Jacobson *et al.*, 1994b). The safety and efficacy of alternating i.v. therapy for cytomegalovirus retinitis using ganciclovir (5 mg per kg) and foscarnet (120 mg per kg) on alternate days has been demonstrated; the median time to progression on this regimen was 105 days (Peters *et al.*, 1994).

Although the studies are small or not blind, lower doses of ganciclovir have been used for both induction and maintenance therapy with apparent success. In a randomized study involving 11 patients with cytomegalovirus retinitis, induction therapy using i.v. 5 mg per kg daily was found to be as effective as 10 mg per kg daily (Gaub *et al.*, 1988). Whilst maintenance therapy with i.v. ganciclovir is usually prescribed five times weekly, uncontrolled studies comparing the time to progression of retinitis in patients receiving ganciclovir three times weekly (10 mg per kg daily) with historical data of progression in patients receiving 5 mg per kg daily i.v. 5 times weekly suggest that thrice-weekly therapy is effective with a median time to clinical progression of 5.4 months (McCluskey *et al.*, 1990; Hall *et al.*, 1991).

The debate as to whether patients with peripheral, non sight-threatening cytomegalovirus retinitis would benefit from ganciclovir therapy continued until a clinical trial was designed to specifically address this question. Spector and colleagues (Spector *et al.*, 1993) found that patients with peripheral retinitis who were randomized to receive immediate therapy with ganciclovir 5 mg per kg twice-daily i.v. for 14 days followed by maintenance therapy of 5 mg per kg daily had a median time to progression of 49.5 days versus only 13.5 days in the group whose

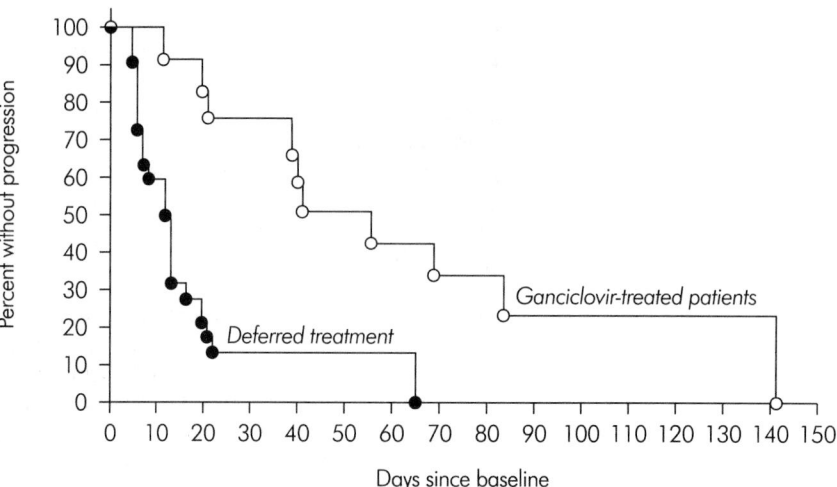

Fig. V.15.

Kaplan–Meier estimates of the proportion of patients with progression of retinitis when given immediate versus deferred ganciclovir therapy (p = 0.001 by the log-rank test). (Reproduced from Spector *et al.*, 1993, with permission.)

therapy was deferred until their disease progressed (Fig. V.15). This study also used independent assessments of fundus photography to determine time to progression. Thus all patients with AIDS-related cytomegalovirus retinitis, regardless of whether the lesions are peripheral or central, should be offered therapy. The median progression rates for patients receiving ganciclovir is 11.5 microns (μm) per day (range 0–25) and that for untreated patients is 24 μm per day (range 0–164) (Holland and Schuler, 1992).

There have been several reports of infants and children with cytomegalovirus retinitis who responded favorably to ganciclovir therapy (Salvador *et al.*, 1993; Peters *et al.*, 1995). Combination therapy using ganciclovir and foscarnet in a child with AIDS-related cytomegalovirus retinitis unresponsive to monotherapy with either drug has also been reported to be effective (Butler *et al.*, 1992).

Treatment of AIDS-related cytomegalovirus gastrointestinal disease with i.v. ganciclovir may be associated with a more lasting response than retinitis; in one report there was no evidence of clinical or colonoscopic relapse during a follow-up period of 200 days (Masur *et al.*, 1986). These data were supported by early, non-controlled studies by other investigators where there was a median time to relapse of 9 weeks post-induction therapy with no maintenance treatment (Chachoua *et al.*, 1987; Dieterich *et al.*, 1988) and in a subsequent controlled study in which recurrence of cytomegalovirus gastrointestinal disease, mostly colitis, only recurred in 25–30% of patients following a 14-day course of i.v. ganciclovir treatment (5 mg per kg twice-daily) with a median time to recurrence of 9 weeks from the start of therapy (Dieterich *et al.*, 1993b). A longer course of i.v. therapy (4 weeks) was considered to be more appropriate for the treatment of gastrointestinal cytomegalovirus disease than the 2-week course, although this was not evaluated in a double-blind manner (Dieterich *et al.*, 1993b). Esophagitis, gastritis, duodenitis and adrenalitis, which are less common presentations of cytomegalovirus disease in patients with AIDS, respond favorably to i.v. ganciclovir therapy and may be associated with prolonged periods of remission in the absence of maintenance therapy (Wilcox and Schwartz, 1992; Fujii *et al.*, 1994; Zucker *et al.*, 1994; Wilcox *et al.*, 1995; Sanhes *et al.*, 1995). Oropharyngeal ulceration due to cytomegalovirus responds well to ganciclovir and in one small series patients did not require maintenance therapy (French *et al.*, 1991).

Whilst the response to therapy in patients with gastrointestinal cytomegalovirus infection lasts longer than that in patients with retinitis, the proportion of patients who have a clinical response appears to be lower. In one retrospective analysis, ganciclovir therapy resulted in resolution of pain and diarrhea in only 73% and 64% respectively, whereas stabilization or improvement in retinitis occurred in 81.5% (Jacobson *et al.*, 1988a). A more recent study reported a good clinical response in 85% of ganciclovir recipients with symptomatic gastrointestinal infection (Blanshard *et al.*, 1995). A lower dose (1 mg per kg twice-daily) was found to be as effective in terms of leading to symptomatic improvement as conventional therapy of 5 mg per kg twice-daily in a randomized study (Heise *et al.*, 1993). Ganciclovir has also been used effectively to treat cytomegalovirus enterocolitis in young infants (Lim *et al.*, 1988). Wasting associated with disseminated cytomegalovirus infection has been reported to respond to ganciclovir with improvement in body cell mass, weight and energy (Kotler, 1991). In two reports, therapy with ganciclovir did not correct liver function test abnormalities in patients with cholestasis possibly attributable to cytomegalovirus infection (Jacobson *et al.*, 1988c; van der Ende *et al.*, 1992). Suspected cytomegalovirus pancreatitis and subsequent relapses have been successfully treated with ganciclovir (Colebunders *et al.*, 1994).

A small proportion of patients with AIDS develop myelitis due to cytomegalovirus infection. In one case report neither ganciclovir nor foscarnet therapy resulted in clinical improvement (Jacobson *et al.*, 1988d). Polyradiculopathy has been reported to improve following prolonged therapy with ganciclovir, providing the isolate is sensitive to the drug; however, the likelihood of success is low in advanced cases (de Gans *et al.*, 1990; Miller *et al.*, 1990; Kim and Hollander 1993; Cohen *et al.*, 1993a). In a recent study of 23 patients with lumbosacral polyradiculopathy, ganciclovir therapy was often associated with worsening of symptoms for the first couple of weeks of therapy, but was generally associated with clinical stabilization (So and Olney, 1994). Combination foscarnet and ganciclovir therapy has been infrequently reported for this condition (Karmochkine *et al.*, 1994). Ganciclovir is reported to have little beneficial effect in the treatment of cytomegalovirus ventriculoencephalitis, with some patients developing cerebral disease whilst receiving i.v. ganciclovir for other indications, and other patients dying of cerebral disease despite i.v. ganciclovir therapy (Schwarz *et al.*, 1990; Price *et al.*, 1992; Kalayjian *et al.*, 1993; Berman and Kim, 1994; Mastroianni *et al.*, 1994; Salazar *et al.*, 1995). Although viral replication in the central nervous system may be reduced by ganciclovir, complete suppression does not appear to be possible, based on data from a few patients (Cinque *et al.*, 1995). However, combination therapy using ganciclovir and foscarnet followed by alternating therapy with these agents as maintenance treatment resulted in clinical improvement in a patient with cytomegalovirus encephalitis that was resistant to ganciclovir alone (Peters *et al.*, 1992). There is an isolated report of successful treatment using ganciclovir in an AIDS patient with meningoencephalitis due to varicella-zoster virus (Poscher, 1994).

Cytomegalovirus pneumonitis, an uncommon condition in patients with AIDS, has been reported to respond to ganciclovir (Eng *et al.*, 1992). Similarly, cytomegalovirus infection of the larynx, an extremely rare condition in patients with AIDS, has been reported to respond slowly to ganciclovir therapy (Marelli *et al.*, 1992).

b   Intravitreal ganciclovir   A number of case-reports of intravitreal ganciclovir provided evidence of its potential use in the treatment of cytomegalovirus retinitis (Henry *et al.*, 1987; Heery and Hollows, 1989). In an early study by Heinemann (1989) stabilization of retinitis occurred in all of seven patients treated with intravitreal injections of ganciclovir (1200 μg in six divided doses) as induction therapy followed by 200 μg per week maintenance therapy. Success with this approach has also been observed in another study, in which treatment of 44 patients with unilateral cytomegalovirus retinitis (55%) or bilateral disease (45%) using intravitreal ganciclovir at a dose of 400 μg per injection led to cicatrization after a mean of 6.6 (range 4–14) injections per eye. After 8 weeks of maintenance therapy (one injection per week) the relapse rate was 53%. Involvement of the other eye occurred in 11% and systemic disease in 16% of patients (Cochereau-Massin *et al.*, 1991). Suppression of retinitis in 78% of treated eyes following intravitreal administration of ganciclovir has also been reported in patients who were unable to tolerate i.v. ganciclovir or who had retinitis unresponsive to i.v. ganciclovir therapy (Ussery *et al.*, 1988). However, (Orellana *et al.*, 1990) have reported that intravitreal therapy alone failed to improve cytomegalovirus retinitis.

c   Ganciclovir intraocular device   Efficacy of the device was established in several small studies. In all of seven patients with AIDS-related cytomegalovirus retinitis whose disease had progressed despite i.v. therapy, retinal lesions stabilized over a median follow-up period of 70 days following implantation of the ganciclovir introcular device (Anand *et al.*, 1993b). In a second study of 22 patients also with AIDS-related cytomegalovirus retinitis who were followed for a median of 125 days post-implantation, retinitis stabilized in 90%, with a mean time to progression of 133 days (Anand *et al.*, 1993a). Further analysis of the data from this study suggests that survival was shorter in those patients who did not receive i.v. ganciclovir at some time during the course of their treatment (Spaide, 1994). In one study the mean time before replacement of the implant was 6 months (Morley *et al.*, 1995). In a randomized trial of patients with peripheral retinitis, in which immediate therapy was compared with delayed treatment using an implant releasing 1 μg of ganciclovir per h, the median time to progression as judged by independently-assessed fundus photographs, in the immediate therapy group was 226 days, but the estimated risk of developing retinitis in the untreated eye at 6 months was 50% and visceral disease developed during this period of time in 31% of patients (Martin *et al.*, 1994a).

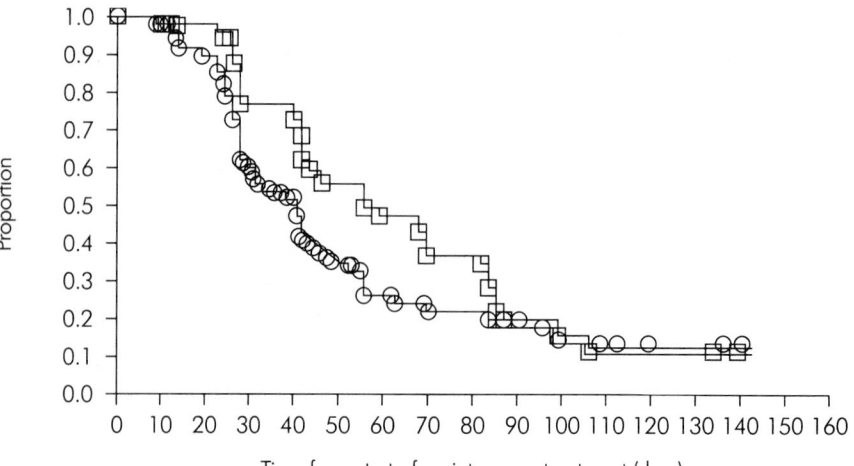

Fig. V.16.
Kaplan–Meier estimates a proportion of patients with CMV retinitis who remained free from progression when randomized to receive oral ganciclovir (o) or i.v. ganciclovir (□): (p = 0.15 by the log-rank test). (Reproduced from The Oral Ganciclovir European and Australian Co-operative Study Group, 1995, with permission.)

d Oral ganciclovir Oral ganciclovir appears to be effective in preventing recurrence of cytomegalovirus retinitis in patients with AIDS who have successfully completed induction therapy with i.v. ganciclovir. Whilst the drug is available for preventing disease, it has not yet been recommended by the US Department of Public Health and Human Services (MMWR, 1995). Oral therapy is convenient and has significant advantages in terms of reduced toxicity compared with i.v. therapy.

The European/Australian comparative study of i.v. versus oral ganciclovir assessed the efficacy and safety of these two forms of the drug in the prevention of recurrence of cytomegalovirus retinitis in AIDS patients. Patients with retinitis initially received induction therapy with i.v. ganciclovir (5 mg per kg 12-hourly) and were then randomized to receive maintenance therapy with either oral ganciclovir (500 mg six times daily) or i.v. ganciclovir (5 mg per kg daily). The mean time to progression as assessed by fundal photography was not statistically different between the two arms of the study, being 51 days with oral ganciclovir, and 62 days with i.v. therapy (Fig. V.16). There were also similar numbers of patients who progressed in both groups (The Oral Ganciclovir European and Australian Co-operative Study Group, 1995).

The findings of the Syntex Co-operative Oral Ganciclovir Study Group were similar. In a study of 117 subjects, the time to progression of cytomegalovirus retinitis (as assessed by examination of fundus photographs) in patients randomized to receive oral versus i.v. maintenance ganciclovir therapy following induction with i.v. ganciclovir was 62 versus 57 days respectively (Drew *et al.*, 1995b). More recent and as yet unpublished data suggest that the 3 g per day oral dose is less effective than i.v. ganciclovir (presented at the XI International Conference on AIDS in Vancouver 1996, abstract Th.B.305).

Preliminary data are available from the CPCRA 023 Trial, in which approximately 1000 patients with HIV infection and less than 100 CD4 cells per μl who were seropositive for cytomegalovirus without evidence of disease were randomized to receive prophylactic oral ganciclovir (1000 mg 8-hourly) or placebo. After a median follow-up time of 15 months it was found that oral ganciclovir did not prevent cytomegalovirus disease in this patient population (Brosgart *et al.*, 1995). A second study performed by the Roche Co-operative Oral Ganciclovir Study Group found that prophylactic treatment of patients with advanced HIV infection (CD4 count of less than 50 cells per μl or less than 100 cells per μl with a prior AIDS defining opportunistic infection) resulted in a 49% lower risk of developing cytomegalovirus disease. The dose of oral ganciclovir used in this randomized, placebo-controlled study was 1000 mg three times daily. Possible reasons for the discrepancy between the results from the two studies were provided: the CPCRA study enrolled patients with a mean CD4 count that was 67% higher than that of participants in the Roche study; the CPCRA study was of shorter duration; the CPCRA study did not require dilated eye examinations by an ophthalmologist at study entry or during the course of the study unless visual symptoms developed, thus potentially missed cases of asymptomatic cytomegalovirus retinitis either at baseline or during the study (Spector *et al.*, 1996).

2 Cytomegalovirus infection in bone marrow transplant recipients

a Prophylaxis against cytomegalovirus infection or disease Cytomegalovirus infection or reactivation can result in serious disease in bone marrow graft recipients, with the frequency being much higher in allogeneic than autologous graft recipients (Ljungman *et al.*, 1994). Prevention of cytomegalovirus infection in cytomegalovirus seronegative transplantation patients is possible by use of seronegative donors, blood-products and blood-filters (reviewed in Zaia, 1993). Prevention of reactivation of endogenous cytomegalovirus in seropositive bone marrow transplant recipients can be achieved by the judicious use of ganciclovir and immunoglobulin. Intravenous pooled immunoglobulin is used as prophylaxis against the development of cytomegalovirus disease although there are no convincing data that demonstrate its efficacy against cytomegalovirus infection (Guglielmo *et al.*, 1994), or even data to show that hyperimmune immunoglobulin inhibits replication of the virus *in vitro* (Jacobson *et al.*, 1990). Based on reports from over a dozen clinical studies, the recommended regimen is to administer i.v. immunoglobulin 500 mg per kg on alternate weeks starting 8 days prior to transplantation and continuing for 100 days post-transplantation (reviewed in Zaia, 1993).

A number of differing regimens of ganciclovir have met with success when used as prophylaxis against cytomegalovirus pneumonia in bone marrow transplant recipients who are seropositive for cytomegalovirus or who receive a transplant from a positive donor (Atkinson *et al.*, 1991; Yau *et al.*, 1991). In one regimen, prophylactic treatment of cytomegalovirus seropositive patients with i.v. ganciclovir (2.5 mg per kg 8-hourly) for 7 days prior to transplantation and then 6 mg per kg daily for 5 days per week following transplantation resulted in a significantly lower rate of infection being eight of 40 (20%) in treated patients versus 25 of 45 (56%) of placebo recipients and a trend towards a lower rate of disease (Winston *et al.*, 1993). Using a similar approach, ganciclovir prophylactic treatment, given prior to transplantation in a dose of 6 mg per kg to cytomegalovirus seropositive recipients and post-transplantation to bone marrow transplant patients who were seropositive or who had received a transplant from a seropositive donor, was found to significantly reduce the rate of symptomatic cytomegalovirus infection. Only one of 40 (2.5%) ganciclovir recipients developed symptoms, compared with untreated historical controls in whom 23 of 39 (59%) developed symptomatic disease (von Bueltzingsloewen *et al.*, 1993). In another approach, ganciclovir prophylaxis administered post-transplantation was shown to be superior to placebo in preventing the development of positive cytomegalovirus cultures (3% versus 45% respectively) and disease (0% versus 29% respectively) during the first 100 days post-transplant (Goodrich *et al.*, 1993). Administration of ganciclovir less frequently (three times weekly) has been found to be inadequate in the prevention of cytomegalovirus reactivation in this patient population (Przepiorka *et al.*, 1994).

However, although prophylactic ganciclovir therapy has significantly reduced the risk of early cytomegalovirus disease in this patient population, reactivation 1 year post-transplant is commonly seen, suggesting that T cell mediated responses to this virus are still suppressed (Li *et al.*, 1994).

b Treatment for cytomegalovirus disease Pre-emptive therapy of asymptomatic cytomegalovirus infection in bone marrow transplant recipients using ganciclovir has met with greater success than treating established symptomatic infection in several randomized controlled trials (Goodrich *et al.*, 1991; Schmidt *et al.*, 1991).

An early pre-emptive approach was studied by Schmidt and colleagues (Schmidt *et al.*, 1991) who randomized patients to commence ganciclovir therapy or no treatment if asymptomatic pulmonary infection was detected by routine bronchoscopy on day 35 post-bone-marrow transplant. Ganciclovir recipients had a lower incidence of pneumonitis or death (25%) compared with those randomized to no treatment (70%). Following this, in a randomized, double-blind, placebo-controlled study, patients were randomized to treatment with ganciclovir in a dose of 5 mg per kg every 12 h for 7 days then once-daily until day 100 post-transplant or to receive placebo commencing at the time any site became culture-positive for cytomegalovirus. Cytomegalovirus disease developed in 45% of placebo recipients and in 3% of the patients receiving ganciclovir; mortality was also significantly less in the ganciclovir group compared with placebo recipients, being 12% versus 19% respectively (Goodrich *et al.*, 1991) (Fig. V.17). Pre-emptive therapy following early detection of cytomegalovirus in blood or urine in asymptomatic bone marrow recipients is associated with lower mortality than treatment of established disease in both adults and children (Bacigalupo *et al.*, 1992, 1994; Locatelli *et al.*, 1994). A 3-week course of ganciclovir (10 mg per kg for 1 week, then 5 mg per kg for 2 weeks) was found to be adequate in preventing the development of cytomegalovirus disease in patients who were cytomegaloviremic after allogeneic bone marrow transplantation (Singhal *et al.*, 1995). Patients who develop diffuse alveolar hemorrhage have a high risk of subsequently

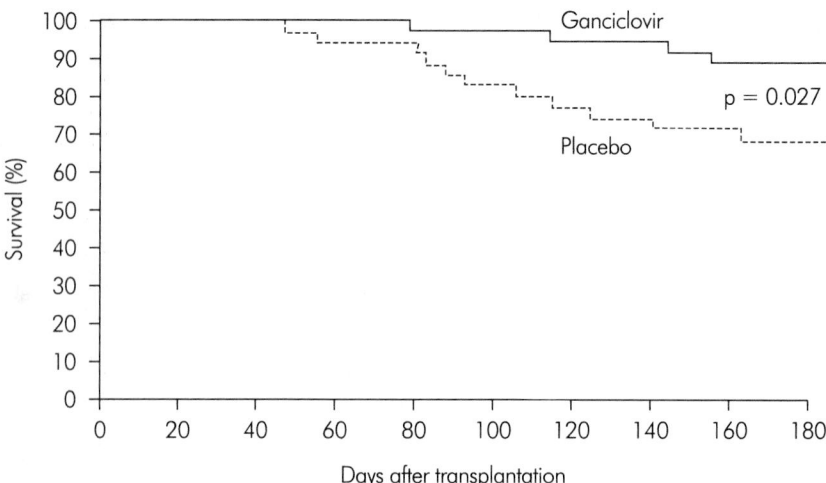

Fig. V.17.

Kaplan–Meier estimates of probability of survival during first 180 days following bone marrow transplantation in CMV seropositive patients who were randomized to receive ganciclovir or placebo (p = 0.027 by log-rank test). (Reproduced from Goodrich *et al.*, 1991, with permission.)

developing cytomegalovirus pneumonia and some investigators consider they warrant consideration for ganciclovir therapy (Mandanas *et al.*, 1996).

Once cytomegalovirus pneumonitis is established in bone marrow transplant recipients, ganciclovir either administered alone or with glucocorticoid therapy has resulted in only minor or no clinical benefit (Shepp *et al.*, 1985; Reed *et al.*, 1986, 1990; Aulitzky *et al.*, 1988; Winston *et al.*, 1988), despite evidence of virologic efficacy (Shepp *et al.*, 1985). This is in contrast to ganciclovir therapy for cytomegalovirus pneumonitis in patients following solid tissue transplants or other forms of immunosuppression (Winston *et al.*, 1988). Furthermore, other manifestations of cytomegalovirus disease following bone marrow transplantation, including gastrointestinal involvement, and disseminated disease without pneumonitis, are more responsive to ganciclovir monotherapy in both adults and children (Rosecan *et al.*, 1986; Reed *et al.*, 1988a, 1990; Gudnason *et al.*, 1989; Engelhard *et al.*, 1993), than those with respiratory disease.

Treatment with cytomegalovirus antibody-enriched immunoglobulin lessens the risk of cytomegalovirus infection but not disease (reviewed in Zaia, 1993). However, the combination of ganciclovir with hyperimmune immunoglobulin or pooled immunoglobulin has resulted in improved survival in bone marrow transplant patients who develop cytomegalovirus pneumonitis in some studies (Emanuel *et al.*, 1988; Schmidt *et al.*, 1988; Reed *et al.*, 1988b; Chow *et al.*, 1992), with reports of 35% response and a survival rate 30 days post-diagnosis of 31% (Ljungman *et al.*, 1992). This approach is considered especially useful if therapy is commenced prior to the development of respiratory failure (Enright *et al.*, 1993). In two early uncontrolled studies, patients with proven cytomegalovirus pneumonia after bone marrow transplantation were treated with ganciclovir induction therapy (2.5 mg per kg 8-hourly for 2 or 3 weeks) together with cytomegalovirus immunoglobulin, with or without subsequent combination maintenance therapy. These regimens resulted in 52–70% survival, significantly higher than that of <15% previously observed with ganciclovir monotherapy (Emanuel *et al.*, 1988; Reed *et al.*, 1988b).

Thus, due to the lack of efficacy of ganciclovir monotherapy, it is now generally recommended that i.v. immunoglobulin be used in combination with ganciclovir for the treatment of cytomegalovirus pneumonitis in bone marrow transplant recipients and that ganciclovir monotherapy be used for pneumonitis in other patient populations (reviewed in Zaia, 1993).

Retinitis, a rare manifestation of cytomegalovirus disease in bone marrow transplant recipients, has been reported to improve with ganciclovir therapy (Kaulfersch *et al.*, 1989).

3 Cytomegalovirus infection in renal transplant patients

a Prophylaxis against cytomegalovirus infection or disease The incidence of cytomegalovirus infection and symptomatic disease in cytomegalovirus seronegative recipients of renal transplants from positive donors is 70–90% and 50–60% respectively (Farrugia and Schwab, 1992). This mismatched subpopulation constitutes the major group at risk of cytomegalovirus disease in renal transplant recipients. There is no specific recommendation for strategies to prevent infection, and the general guidelines are similar to those described above for bone marrow transplant recipients. Most therapeutic approaches are designed to prevent cytomegalovirus disease in the short-term following transplantation when immunosuppression is maximum. However, the late development of cytomegalovirus disease (3–5 years post-transplantation) appears to be under-recognized (Boehler et al., 1994). Ganciclovir monotherapy is effective for the treatment for cytomegalovirus disease in renal transplant patients (Guerin et al., 1989; Buturovic-Ponikvar et al., 1992; de Koning et al., 1992; Jordan et al., 1992). Some of the major clinical trials are described below.

In an open-label, prospective study of ganciclovir prophylactic therapy (5 mg per kg i.v. 12-hourly for 14 days from day 14 post-transplant) versus no treatment in cytomegalovirus seronegative renal transplant recipients who had seropositive donors, the rate of cytomegalovirus infection and disease was similar in ganciclovir recipients (71% and 47% respectively) and untreated controls (80% and 73% respectively). However, disease was less severe and the time from transplantation to infection was significantly longer in the patients in the ganciclovir arm (Rondeau et al., 1993). Using a different strategy, Winston and colleagues examined prophylaxis using i.v. ganciclovir (2.5 mg per kg 8-hourly) given to cytomegalovirus seropositive patients for 7 days prior to transplantation and then 6 mg per kg daily for 5 days per week following transplantation. This approach was found to significantly lower the rate of infection to eight of 40 (20%) compared with placebo recipients (56%) and there was also a trend towards a lower rate of disease (Winston et al., 1993). Pre-emptive ganciclovir therapy given to renal transplant recipients who are positive for cytomegalovirus antibody has been found to reduce cytomegalovirus disease (Hibberd et al., 1995). Ganciclovir prophylactic therapy has also been reported to be of benefit in pediatric renal transplant patients (Prokurat et al., 1993).

Cytomegalovirus antibody-enriched immunoglobulin received approval by the Food and Drug Administration in the USA in 1990 for prophylaxis against cytomegalovirus infection in seronegative renal transplant recipients with seropositive donors (Snydman et al., 1993). When compared with ganciclovir as prophylactic therapy in cytomegalovirus seronegative renal transplant recipients who received grafts from positive donors, both therapies were associated with a lower incidence of serious cytomegalovirus disease (Conti et al., 1994).

b Treatment for cytomegalovirus disease Intravenous ganciclovir therapy given to renal transplantation patients and patients with cytomegalovirus pneumonia in one small uncontrolled study resulted in a favorable outcome in seven of the eight recipients (Stoffel et al., 1988). Similar results were obtained in other similar studies, in which a favorable clinical response was obtained in 99–100% of patients who developed severe cytomegalovirus disease including retinitis post-renal transplant, in 30% of ventilator-dependent patients with pneumonitis (Syndman, 1988; Jordan et al., 1992; Sawyer et al., 1993). Other studies have found that clinical improvement is more common in patients who are treated with ganciclovir for cytomegalovirus retinitis, hepatitis or gastrointestinal disease compared with cytomegalovirus pneumonitis (Winston et al., 1988). Ganciclovir therapy has been reported to be useful in the treatment of severe cytomegalovirus disease, even when administered during renal allograft rejection treatment (de Koning et al., 1992). Cultures for cytomegalovirus usually become negative within 3 days of commencing ganciclovir (van den Berg et al., 1992). Similar to heart transplant patients, renal allograft survival appears to be lower in patients who develop cytomegalovirus infection (Nevins and Dunn, 1992), although this is not found in all studies (Dunn et al., 1991). Quantitation of cytomegalovirus DNA in peripheral blood leukocytes by polymerase chain reaction (PCR) has provided a threshold value (≥1000 copies per ml) that is highly predictive for symptomatic infection (Kuhn et al., 1994).

4 Cytomegalovirus infection in heart/lung/liver/pancreas transplant patients

a Prophylaxis against cytomegalovirus infection or disease As donors of heart, lung or liver are scarce, matching of donor and recipient on the basis of cytomegalovirus serology prior to transplantation remains highly desirable but may in some cases not be feasible (Novick et al., 1990; Stratta et al., 1991a). Whilst the data strongly support the value of prophylactic ganciclovir in preventing cytomegalovirus-related disease in the high risk recipient, long courses of the drug have still been associated with failure and subsequent morbidity and mortality (Manez et al., 1995). Some of the trials are described below.

i Heart transplantation In a multicenter, randomized, placebo-controlled study of heart transplant patients, prophylactic treatment of the cytomegalovirus seropositive recipients with ganciclovir (5 mg per kg i.v. 12-hourly from days 1 to 14 post-transplant and then 6 mg per kg daily for 5 days per week for the next 2 weeks) resulted in a significant reduction in

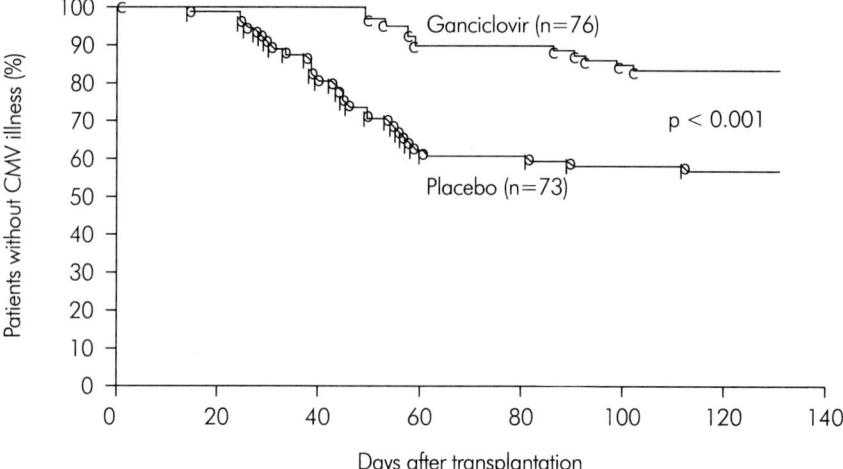

Fig. V.18.

Incidence of cytomegalovirus illness in heart transplant patients randomized to receive prophylactic ganciclovir or placebo. (Reproduced from Merigan *et al.*, 1992, with permission.)

cytomegalovirus disease compared with placebo (9% versus 46% respectively; Fig. V.18), although there was no difference in the frequency of illness in the seronegative recipients (Merigan *et al.*, 1992).

ii Lung transplantation Cytomegalovirus is a common opportunistic pathogen in this patient population, causing significant morbidity and mortality. Few prophylactic studies have been reported, and results to date have been conflicting (Ladurie *et al.*, 1991; Duncan *et al.*, 1992, 1994).

In a small uncontrolled study in which ganciclovir (2.5–5 mg per kg 12-hourly) was administered for the first 10–21 days post-transplantation in conjunction with i.v. immunoglobulin, followed by oral aciclovir, seven seronegative transplant recipients of organs from seropositive donors all developed pneumonitis (Bailey *et al.*, 1992). Other investigators have also found that ganciclovir prophylaxis in seronegative recipients has been associated with a high rate of failure. Adult transplant recipients who were randomized to receive ganciclovir (10 mg per kg daily i.v. from days 1 to 10 post-transplant were found in another study to have the same incidence of cytomegalovirus infection as untreated controls (86% in both) (Schmuth *et al.*, 1992). A third example of the failure of ganciclovir prophylaxis was demonstrated in a pediatric population in which symptomatic cytomegalovirus disease developed in 75% of patients despite 4 weeks of prophylactic ganciclovir following lung transplantation (Armitage *et al.*, 1995). However, Duncan and colleagues (Duncan *et al.*, 1994) have more recently completed a randomized trial of ganciclovir (5 mg per kg daily for 5 days per week) versus aciclovir (3200 mg daily) given for 90 days following an initial course of therapy with ganciclovir from weeks 1 to 3 post-transplantation. This study demonstrated that ganciclovir recipients had a significantly lower incidence of seroconversion during the first year post-transplantation.

Cytomegalovirus hyperimmune immunoglobulin has been used prophylactically for seronegative lung transplant recipients with a positive donor; however, over 50% developed cytomegalovirus pneumonitis and were treated with ganciclovir with moderate success (Gould *et al.*, 1993). When used in combination with ganciclovir, a delay in onset as well as a reduction in the incidence of disease, has been reported in a small number of seropositive lung transplant recipients (Zamora *et al.*, 1994).

iii Liver/pancreas transplantation Although prophylaxis against cytomegalovirus disease is undoubtedly also of value in this patient population, once again there is no recommended ideal regimen. Ganciclovir prophylaxis may decrease the incidence and morbidity of symptomatic cytomegalovirus infection, in terms of decreasing the rate of early rejection, development of bacterial and fungal infections, the requirement for OKT3, and rate of retransplantation in liver and pancreas transplant recipients (reviewed in Levy *et al.*, 1992; Hopt *et al.*, 1994; Markham and Faulds, 1994).

Liver transplant patients receiving OKT3 monoclonal antibodies who were treated prophylactically with ganciclovir had a lower incidence of cytomegalovirus disease compared with historical untreated controls (12% and 52% respectively) (Lumbreras *et al.*, 1993).

Ganciclovir has also been found to be superior to aciclovir in preventing symptoms of cytomegalovirus infection, both in liver and pancreas transplant recipients (Harland *et al.*, 1994; Martin *et al.*, 1994b). In a randomized study, treatment with ganciclovir (5 mg per kg 12-hourly for 2 weeks) followed by high-dose aciclovir for 3 months post-liver transplantation was found to be superior in preventing cytomegalovirus disease compared with high-dose aciclovir munotherapy (3200 mg daily) (Martin *et al.*, 1994b). A separate trial, comparing ganciclovir (6 mg per kg daily i.v. from days 1 to 30, then 6 mg per kg daily i.v. Monday to Friday until day 100) versus aciclovir (10 mg per kg i.v. 8-hourly from day 1 to discharge then 800 mg orally four times daily until day 100), found that cytomegalovirus infection occurred in 38% of aciclovir recipients and 5% of ganciclovir recipients; symptomatic disease occurred in 10% versus 0.8% of aciclovir and ganciclovir recipients respectively (Winston *et al.*, 1995). There are uncontrolled data to support the use of ganciclovir as prophylactic therapy in pediatric liver transplant recipients (Boudreaux *et al.*, 1993). However, ganciclovir monotherapy has not resulted in successful prophylaxis in all studies. Cohen and colleagues have reported a similar frequency of cytomegalovirus disease in liver transplant patients who were randomized to receive either ganciclovir prophylaxis from days 14 to 28 post-transplant or no therapy until the development of symptomatic disease (Cohen *et al.*, 1993a).

Prophylactic therapy using ganciclovir in combination with cytomegalovirus hyperimmune globulin is reportedly successful in decreasing the risk of cytomegalovirus disease in liver transplant patients (Nakazato *et al.*, 1993; Prian and Koep, 1994). Some clinicians consider that the expense of immunoglobulin is not justified in all solid organ transplant recipients, and this treatment should be limited to high-risk situations (Stratta *et al.*, 1994).

Pre-emptive therapy, starting ganciclovir upon development of a positive surveillance culture (from buffy coat or urine) in asymptomatic liver transplant recipients, has met with success. In a randomized controlled trial designed to compare the efficacy of prophylactic high-dose aciclovir with that of pre-emptive ganciclovir therapy (only given if surveillance cultures became positive), oral aciclovir was found to be ineffective prophylactic therapy against cytomegalovirus disease in this patient population, with disease developing in 29% of the aciclovir group and 4% of the ganciclovir group (Singh *et al.*, 1994).

b   Treatment for cytomegalovirus disease   Ganciclovir has been found to be effective in treating serious cytomegalovirus disease in liver (Paya *et al.*, 1988; Lumbreras *et al.*, 1992), kidney (Paya *et al.*, 1988) and heart and/or lung transplant patients (Keay *et al.*, 1988). The usual dose of ganciclovir is 5 mg per kg given twice-daily for 10–30 days, with an average duration of therapy of 14 days, although lower doses have been used (Harbison *et al.*, 1988; Paya *et al.*, 1988; Balfour and Heussner, 1993). Clinical response as measured by resolution of fever occurs within 2–9 (mean 5.3) days (Paya *et al.*, 1988). Relapses are usually successfully retreated with ganciclovir.

i   Liver transplantation   Ganciclovir therapy has a high success rate in liver transplant patients with cytomegalovirus disease (Stein *et al.*, 1988; Savage *et al.*, 1989; Stratta *et al.*, 1989; Lumbreras *et al.*, 1992). In one retrospective analysis, 74% of patients who developed cytomegalovirus disease responded to ganciclovir therapy, with one-fifth developing recurrent disease within 3 months. The 18-month survival after ganciclovir therapy was 76%, similar to that of patients who did not develop disease due to cytomegalovirus infection (Stratta *et al.*, 1991b). In a retrospective study of a small group of patients who received ganciclovir in combination with i.v. hyperimmune immunoglobulin for the treatment of cytomegalovirus pneumonitis following liver transplantation, data suggest that combination therapy may decrease the time required for intubation, and may increase long-term survival (George *et al.*, 1993).

ii   Heart/lung transplantation   Ganciclovir treatment is associated with approximately 80–90% survival in heart and heart/lung transplant recipients with serious cytomegalovirus disease, including pneumonitis, gastrointestinal disease, retinitis and disseminated infection (Keay *et al.*, 1988; Watson *et al.*, 1988; Cerrina *et al.*, 1991; Cooper *et al.*, 1991; Smythe *et al.*, 1991; Kirklin *et al.*, 1994). The onset of cytomegalovirus disease ranges from 3 weeks to 18 months post-heart transplantation (Cooper *et al.*, 1991). Whilst treatment often results in prompt resolution of symptoms, in up to 37% the disease recurs requiring repeated ganciclovir therapy (Arabia *et al.*, 1993), although others report a much lower incidence of relapse (Cooper *et al.*, 1991). Acute rejection is reportedly more common in patients who develop cytomegalovirus disease, despite ganciclovir therapy (Cooper *et al.*, 1991; Steinhoff *et al.*, 1991).

5 Ganciclovir-resistant cytomegalovirus infection

Cytomegalovirus strains that are both clinically and virologically resistant to ganciclovir have been described in different clinical settings including chronic lymphocytic leukemia and AIDS (Erice *et al.*, 1989). Clinical resistance of cytomegalovirus to ganciclovir has also been reported in bone marrow transplant recipients: (Razis *et al.*, 1994). The presence of mutations in UL97 associated with resistance to ganciclovir (codons 460, 594 and 595) were found in blood isolates of four patients who died from progressive disseminated cytomegalovirus disease (Boivin *et al.*, 1996). Ganciclovir-resistant isolates have been obtained from patients with cytomegalovirus central nervous system disease (Wolf *et al.*, 1995b). In patients who harbor ganciclovir-resistant strains causing disease, treatment with foscarnet is recommended.

6 Congenital cytomegalovirus infection

Although the drug is not licensed for this indication, improvement in neurologic function and clearance of cytomegalovirus has been observed in a study of 12 infants with symptomatic congenital cytomegalovirus disease treated with i.v. ganciclovir at a dose of 5 to 7.5 mg per kg 12-hourly. In addition, ganciclovir has been reported to be effective in treating cytomegalovirus pneumonitis in congenitally infected neonates in two case-reports (Vallejo *et al.*, 1994; Fukuda *et al.*, 1995). However, two other case reports suggest only minor or no improvement following the treatment with ganciclovir in three infants with congenital cytomegalovirus infection with persistent hepatosplenomegaly and developmental delay, and only temporary cessation of virus shedding (Reigstad *et al.*, 1992; Attard-Montalto *et al.*, 1993). More recently, data have emerged suggesting that a better outcome is associated with higher doses of ganciclovir given for longer periods of time (Nigro *et al.*, 1994).

7 Other infections

Herpesvirus simiae infection resulting in subtle features of brain stem encephalitis has been reported to respond to ganciclovir therapy (Davenport *et al.*, 1994). Combined therapy with ganciclovir and foscarnet has been reported to successfully control hepatitis B virus (HBV) replication in a patient with severe recurrence of hepatitis B virus infection following liver transplantation (Angus *et al.*, 1993). This report has been followed by a pilot study involving nine patients with post-transplant hepatitis B infection who were treated with ganciclovir for 3–10 months. Hepatitis B virus replication was reduced, as assessed by serum and hepatic HBV DNA levels and serum alanine aminotransferase levels (Gish *et al.*, 1996). Although exceedingly rare, cytomegalovirus encephalitis, esophagitis or pneumonitis have been reported in young adults with no apparent immune compromise; the disease has responded favorably to ganciclovir therapy (Pantoni *et al.*, 1991; Manian and Smith, 1993; Altman *et al.*, 1995; Lopez-Contreras *et al.*, 1995). Ganciclovir administered in combination with recombinant interleukin 2 to a young girl with chronic active Epstein–Barr virus infection resulted in clearance of the viral genome from her peripheral blood mononuclear cells, and symptomatic improvement (Ishida *et al.*, 1993). Successful treatment using ganciclovir of a bone marrow transplant patient with meningo-encephalitis due to Epstein–Barr virus has also been reported (Dellemijn *et al.*, 1995).

Acknowledgements The author would like to thank Mark Jacobson of San Francisco General Hospital, University of California San Francisco for his critical review of this chapter.

References

Agut H, Huraux JM, Collandre H, Montagnier L (1989). Susceptibility of human herpesvirus 6 to acyclovir and ganciclovir. *Lancet* **9**: 626.

Akesson-Johansson A, Harmenberg J, Wahren B, Linde A (1990). Inhibition of human herpesvirus 6 replication by 9-[4-hydroxy-2-(Hydroxymethyl) Butyl] guanine (2HM-HBG) and other antiviral compounds. *Antimicrob Ag Chemother* **34**: 2417.

Akula SK, Ma PE, Reyman GA *et al.* (1994). Treatment of cytomegalovirus retinitis with intravitreal injection of liposome encapsulated ganciclovir in a patient with AIDS. *Brit J Ophthalmol* **78**: 677.

Altman C, Bedossa P, Dussaix E, Buffet C (1995). Cytomegalovirus infection of esophagus in immunocompetent adults. *Dig Dis Sci* **40**: 606.

Anand R, Nightingale SD, Fish RH *et al.* (1993a). Control of cytomegalovirus retinitis using sustained release of intraocular ganciclovir. *Arch Ophthalmol* **111**: 223.

Anand R, Font RL, Nightingale SD *et al.* (1993b). Pathology of cytomegalovirus retinitis treated with sustained release intravitreal ganciclovir. *Ophthalmology* **100**: 1032.

Anderson RD, Griffy KG, Jung P *et al.* (1995). Ganciclovir absolute bioavailability and steady state pharmacokinetics after oral administration of two 3000 mg per day dosing regimens in human immunodeficiency virus and cytomegalovirus-seropositive patients. *Clin Ther* **17**: 425.

Andrei G, Snoeck R, Schols D *et al.* (1991). Comparative activity of selected antiviral compounds against clinical isolates of human cytomegalovirus. *Eur J Clin Microbiol Infect Dis* 10: 1026.

Angus P, Richards M, Bawden S *et al.* (1993). Combination antiviral therapy controls severe post-liver transplant recurrence of hepatitis B virus infection. *J Gastroenterol Hepatol* 8: 353.

Aoki Y, Tani K, Takahashi K *et al.* (1994). Regulation of recombinant human granulocyte colony-stimulation factor production using herpes simplex virus 1 thymidine kinase gene. *Biochem Biophys Res Commun* 200: 1245.

Aquino de Jesus MJ, Griffith BP (1989). Cytomegalovirus infection in immunocompromised guinea pigs: a model for testing antiviral agents *in vivo*. *Antiviral Res* 12: 181.

Arabia FA, Rosado LJ, Huston CL *et al.* (1993). Incidence and recurrence of gastrointestinal cytomegalovirus infection in heart transplantation. *Ann Thorac Surg* 55: 8.

Arevalo JF, Gonzalez C, Capparelli EV *et al.* (1995). Intravitreous and plasma concentrations of ganciclovir and foscarnet after intravenous therapy in patients with AIDS and cytomegalovirus retinitis. *J Infect Dis* 172: 051.

Armitage JM, Kurland G, Michaels M *et al.* (1995). Critical issues in pediatric lung transplantation. *J Thorac Cardiovasc Surg* 109: 60.

Ashton P, Blandford DL, Pearson PA *et al.* (1994). Review: Implants. *J Ocul Pharmacol* 10: 691.

Ashton WT, Karkas AK, Field AK, Tolman RL (1982). Activation by thymidine kinase and potent antiherpetic activity of 2'-nor-2'-deoxyguanosine (2'NDG). *Biochem Biophys Res Comm* 8: 16.

Atkinson K, Downs K, Golenia M *et al.* (1991). Prophylactic use of ganciclovir in allogeneic bone marrow transplantation: absence of clinical cytomegalovirus infection. *Brit J Haematol* 79: 57.

Attard-Montalto SP, English MC, Stimmler L, Snodgrass GJ (1993). Ganciclovir treatment of congenital cytomegalovirus infection; a report of two cases. *Scand J Infect Dis* 25: 385.

Aulitzky WE, Tilg H, Niederwieser G *et al* (1988). Ganciclovir and hyperimmunoglobulin for treating cytomegalovirus infection in bone marrow transplant recipients. *J Infect Dis* 158: 488.

Aweeka FT, Gamberloglio JG, Kramer F *et al.* (1995). Foscarnet and ganciclovir pharmacokinetics during concomitant or alternating maintenance therapy for AIDS related cytomegalovirus retinitis. *Clin Pharmacol Ther* 57: 403.

Bacigalupo A, Tedone E, Sanna MA *et al.* (1992). CMV infections following allogeneic BMT: risk factors, early treatment and correlation with transplant related mortality. *Haematologica* 77: 507.

Bacigalupo A, van Lint MT, Tedone E *et al.* (1994). Early treatment of CMV infections in allogeneic bone marrow transplant recipients with foscarnet of ganciclovir. *Bone Marrow Transplant* 13: 753.

Bailey TC, Trulock EP, Ettinger NA *et al.* (1992). Failure of prophylactic ganciclovir to prevent cytomegalovirus disease in recipients of lung transplants. *J Infect Dis* 165: 548.

Baldanti F, Silini E, Sarasini A *et al.* (1995). A three-nucleotide deletion in the UL97 open reading frame is responsible for the ganciclovir resistance of a human cytomegalovirus clinical isolate. *J Virol* 69: 796.

Balfour HH, Heussner RC (1993). Cytomegalovirus infections and liver transplantation; an overview. *Transplant Proc* 25: 2012.

Barton TL, Roush MK, Daver LL *et al.* (1992). Seizures associated with ganciclovir therapy. *Pharmacotherapy* 12: 413.

Bastien O, Boulieu R, Bleyzac N, Estanove S (1994). Clinical use of ganciclovir during renal failure and continuous haemodialysis. *Intensive Care Med* 20: 47.

Baudouin C, Gastaud P (1992). A modified procedure for intravitreal injections of ganciclovir in the treatment of cytomegalovirus retinitis. *Ophthalmology* 99: 1183.

Berman SM, Kim RC (1994). The development of cytomegalovirus encephalitis in AIDS patients receiving ganciclovir. *Amer J Med* 96: 415.

Biron KK (1991). Ganciclovir-resistant human cytomegalovirus clinical isolates; resistance mechanisms and *in vitro* susceptibility to antiviral agents. *Transplant Proc* 23: 162.

Biron KK, Stanat SC, Sorrell JB *et al.* (1985). Metabolic activation of the nucleoside analog 9-[(2-hydroxy-1-(hydroxymethyl)ethoxy]methyl)guanine in human diploid fibroblasts infected with human cytomegalovirus. *Proc Natl Acad Sci USA* 82: 2473.

Biron KK, Fyfe JA, Stanat SC *et al.* (1986). A human cytomegalovirus mutant resistant to the nucleoside analog 9-([2-hydroxy-1-(hydroxymethyl)ethoxy]methyl)guanine (BW B759U) induces reduced levels of BW B759U triphosphate. *Proc Natl Acad Sci USA* 83: 8769.

Blanshard C, Benhamou Y, Dohin E *et al.* (1995). Treatment of AIDS-associated gastrointestinal cytomegalovirus infection with foscarnet and ganciclovir; a randomised comparison. *J Infect Dis* 172: 622.

Boehler A, Schaffner A, Solomon F, Keusch G (1994). Cytomegalovirus disease of late onset following renal transplantation; a potentially fatal entity. *Scand J Infect Dis* 26: 369.

Boehme RE (1984). Phosphorylation of the antiviral precursor 9-(1,3-dihydroxy-2-propoxymethyl)guanine monophosphate by guanylate kinase isozymes. *J Biol Chem* 259: 12346.

Boivin G, Erice A, Crane DD *et al.* (1993). Ganciclovir susceptibilities of cytomegalovirus (CMV) isolates from solid organ transplant recipients with CMV viremia after antiviral prophylaxis. *J Infect Dis* 168: 332.

Boivin G, Chou S, Quirk MR *et al.* (1996). Detection of ganciclovir resistance mutations and quantitation of cytomegalovirus (CMV) DNA in leukocytes of patients with fatal disseminated CMV disease. *J Infect Dis* 173: 523.

Boudreaux JP, Hayes DH, Mizrahi S *et al.* (1993). Decreasing incidence of serious cytomegalovirus infection using ganciclovir prophylaxis in pediatric liver transplant patients. *Transplant Proc* 25: 1872.

Boulieu R, Bleyzac N, Ferry S *et al.* (1991a). High performance liquid chromatographic determination of ganciclovir in plasma. *J Chromatogr* 567: 481.

Boulieu R, Bleyzac N, Ferry S *et al.* (1991b). Modified high-performance liquid chromatographic method for the determination of ganciclovir in plasma from patients with severe renal impairment. *J Chromatogr* 571: 331.

Boulieu R, Bastien O, Bleyzac N *et al.* (1993). Pharmacokinetics of ganciclovir in heart transplant patients undergoing continuous venovenous haemodialysis. *Ther Drug Monit* 15: 105.

Bowden RA, Digel J, Reed EC, Meyers JP (1987). Immunosuppressive effects of ganciclovir on *in vitro* lymphocyte responses. *J Infect Dis* 156: 899.

Boyle TJ, Tamburini M, Berend KR *et al.* (1992). Human B-cell lymphoma in severe combined immunodeficient mice after active infection with Epstein–Barr virus. *Surgery* 112: 378.

Brosgart CL, Craig C, Hillman D *et al.* (1995). A randomised, placebo-controlled trial of the safety and efficacy of oral ganciclovir for prophylaxis of CMV retinal and gastrointestinal mucosal disease HIV-infected individuals with severe immunosuppression. In *Program and abstracts of the 35th Interscience Conference on Antimicrobial Agents and Chemotherapy, San Francisco.* Washington DC: American Society for Microbiology.

Buhles WC, Mastre BJ, Tinker AJ *et al.* (1988). Ganciclovir treatment of life or sight threatening cytomegalovirus infection; experience in 314 immunocompromised patients. *Rev Infect Dis* 10: S495.

Buhles WC, Drew WL, Minor D *et al.* (1994). Cytomegalovirus (CMV) resistance rates following treatment with IV and oral ganciclovir (GCV). In *Program and Abstracts of the 34th Interscience Conference on Antimicrobial Agents and Chemotherapy, Orlando.* Washington, DC: American Society for Microbiology.

Burger DM, Meenhorst PL, Ten-Napel CH *et al.* (1994). Pharmacokinetic variability of zidovudine in HIV-infected individuals: Subgroup analysis and drug interactions. *AIDS* 8: 1683.

Burns WH, Sandford GR (1990). Susceptibility of human herpesvirus 6 to antivirals *in vitro*. *J Infect Dis* 162: 634.

Butler KM, de Smet MD, Husson RN *et al.* (1992). Treatment of aggressive cytomegalovirus retinitis with ganciclovir in combination with foscarnet in a child infected with human immunodeficiency virus. *J Pediatr* **120**: 483.

Buturovic-Ponikvar J, Kandus A, Malovrh M *et al.* (1992). Ganciclovir treatment for cytomegalovirus infections in renal transplant recipients. *Transplant Proc* **24**: 1921.

Cantarovich M, Latter D (1994). Effect of prophylactic ganciclovir on renal function and cyclosporine levels after heart transplantation. *Transplant Proc* **26**: 2747.

Castela N, Vermerie N, Chast F *et al.* (1994). Ganciclovir ophthalmic gel in herpes simplex virus rabbit keratitis: intraocular penetration and efficacy. *J Ocul Pharmacol* **10**: 439.

Causey D (1991). Concomitant ganciclovir and zidovudine treatment for cytomegalovirus retinitis in patients with HIV infection: An approach to treatment. *J AIDS* **4**: S16.

Cerrina J, Bayoux E, Le Roy Ladurie F *et al.* (1991). Ganciclovir treatment of cytomegalovirus infection in heart-lung and double lung transplant recipients. *Transplant Proc* **23**: 1174.

Chachoua A, Dieterich D, Krasinski K *et al.* (1987). 9-(1,3-dihydroxy-2-propoxymethyl)guanine (ganciclovir) in the treatment of cytomegalovirus gastrointestinal disease with the acquired immunodeficiency syndrome. *Ann Intern Med* **107**: 133.

Chen JL, Brocavich JM, Lin AY *et al.* (1992). Psychiatric disturbances associated with ganciclovir therapy. *Ann Pharmacother* **26**: 193.

Chen SH, Shine HD, Goodman JC *et al.* (1994). Gene therapy for brain tumors: regression of experimental gliomas by adenovirus-mediated gene transfer *in vivo*. *Proc Natl Acad Sci USA* **91**: 3054.

Chen SH, Chen XH, Wang Y *et al.* (1995a). Combination gene therapy for liver metastasis of colon carcinoma *in vivo*. *Proc Natl Acad Sci USA* **92**: 2577.

Chen YC, Chang YN, Ryan P (1995b). Effect of herpes simplex virus thymidine kinase expression levels on ganciclovir mediated cytotoxicity and the 'bystander effect'. *Hum Gene Ther* **6**: 1467.

Cheng YC, Huang ES, Lin JC *et al.* (1983a). Unique spectrum of activity of 9-[(1,3-dihydroxy-2-propoxy)methyl]-guanine against herpesviruses *in vitro* and its mode of action against herpes simplex virus type 1. *Proc Natl Acad Sci USA* **80**: 2767.

Cheng YC, Grill SP, Dutschman GE *et al.* (1983b). Metabolism of 9-(1,3-dihydroxy-2-propoxymethyl)guanine, a new anti-herpes virus compound, in herpes simplex virus-infected cells. *J Biol Chem* **258**: 12460.

Chou S, Erice A, Jordan MC *et al.* (1995a). Analysis of the UL97 phosphotransferase coding sequence in clinical cytomegalovirus isolates and identification of mutations conferring ganciclovir resistance. *J Infect Dis* **171**: 576.

Chou S, Guentzel S, Michels KR *et al.* (1995b). Frequency of UL phosphotransferase mutations related to ganciclovir resistance in clinical cytomegalovirus isolates. *J Infect Dis* **172**: 239.

Chow JM, Lin MT, Chen YC *et al.* (1992). Successful treatment of cytomegalovirus pneumonitis with ganciclovir and high-dose intravenous immunoglobulin in a bone marrow transplant recipient. *J Formos Med Assoc* **91**: 996.

Chun YS, Park NH (1987). Effect of ganciclovir [9-(1,3-dihydroxy-2-propxymethyl)guanine] on viral DNA and protein synthesis in cells infected with herpes simplex virus. *Antimicrob Ag Chemother* **31**: 349.

Cinque P, Baldanti F, Vago L *et al.* (1995). Ganciclovir therapy for cytomegalovirus (CMV) infection of the central nervous system in AIDS patients. *J Infect Dis* **17**: 1603.

Cochereau-Massin I, Lehoang P, Lautier-Frau M *et al.* (1991). Efficacy and tolerance of intravitreal ganciclovir in cytomegalovirus retinitis in acquired immune deficiency syndrome. *Ophthalmology* **98**: 1348.

Cohen AJ, Weiser B, Afzal Q, Fuhrer J (1990). Ventricular tachycardia in two patients with AIDS receiving ganciclovir (DHPG). *AIDS* **4**: 807.

Cohen AT, O'Grady JG, Sutherland S *et al.* (1993a). Controlled trial of prophylaxis versus therapeutic use of ganciclovir after liver transplantation in adults. *J Med Virol* **40**: 5.

Cohen BA, McArthur JC, Grohman S *et al.* (1993b). Neurologic prognosis of cytomegalovirus polyradiculomyelopathy in AIDS. *Neurology* **43**: 493.

Cole NL, Balfour HH (1987). *In vitro* susceptibility of cytomegalovirus isolates from immunocompromised patients to acyclovir and ganciclovir. *Diagn Microbiol Infect Dis* **6**: 255.

Colebunders R, van den Abbeele K, Fleerackers Y *et al.* (1994). Two AIDS patients with life-threatening pancreatitis successfully treated, one with ganciclovir the other with foscarnet. *Acta Clin Belg* **49**: 229.

Collaborative DHPG Treatment Study Group (1986). Treatment of serious cytomegalovirus infections with 9-(1,3-dihydroxy-2-propoxymethyl) guanine in patients with AIDS and other immunodeficiencies. *New Engl J Med* **314**: 801.

Collins P, Oliver NM (1985). Comparison of the *in vitro* and *in vivo* antiherpes virus activities of the acyclic nucleosides, acyclovir (Zovirax) and 9-[(2-hydroxy-1-hydroxymethylethoxy)methyl)guanine (BWB7590). *Antiviral Res* **5**: 145.

Combarnous F, Fouque D, Bernard N *et al.* (1994). Pharmacokinetics of ganciclovir in a patient undergoing chronic haemodialysis. *Eur J Clin Pharmacol* **46**: 379.

Conti DJ, Freed BM, Gruber SA, Lempert N (1994). Prophylaxis of primary cytomegalovirus disease in renal transplant recipients. A trial of ganciclovir vs immunoglobulin. *Arch Surg* **129**: 443.

Cooper DK, Novitzky D, Schlegel V *et al.* (1991). Successful management of symptomatic cytomegalovirus disease with ganciclovir after heart transplantation. *J Heart Lung Transplant* **10**: 656.

Cox S, Vissgarden A, Wahren B *et al.* (1993). Effect upon the anti-HIV activity of 3'-azido-3'-deoxythymidine and 3'-fluoro-3'-deoxythymidine of combination with anti-herpes nucleoside analogues. *Antiviral Chem Chemother* **4**: 41.

Crumpacker CS, Kowalsky PN, Oliver SA *et al.* (1984). Resistance of herpes simplex virus to 9-{[2-hydroxy-1-(hydroxymethyl)ethoxy]methyl}guanine: Physical mapping of drug synergism within the viral DNA polymerase locus. *Proc Natl Acad Sci USA* **81**: 1556.

Crumpacker MD (1996). Ganciclovir. *New Engl J Med* **335**: 721.

Culver KW, Ram Z, Wallbridge S *et al.* (1992). *In vivo* gene transfer with retroviral vector-producer cells for treatment of experimental brain tumors. *Science* **256**: 1550.

Cytovene-iv and Cytovene Product Information (1995).

Daikos GL, Pulido J, Kathpalia SB *et al.* (1988). Intravenous and intra-ocular ganciclovir for CMV retinitis in patients with AIDS or chemotherapeutic immunosuppression. *Brit J Ophthalmol* **72**: 521.

Datta AK, Pagano JS (1983). Phosphorylation of acyclovir [9-(2-hydroxyethoxymethyl)guanine] *in vitro* in activated Burkitt's somatic cell hybrids. *J Antimicrob Ag Chemother* **24**: 10.

Davenport DS, Johnson DR, Holmes GP *et al.* (1994). Diagnosis and management of human B virus (Herpesvirus simiae) infections in Michigan. *Clin Infect Dis* **19**: 33.

Davis CL, Springmeyer S, Gmerek BJ *et al.* (1990). Central nervous system side effects of ganciclovir. *New Engl J Med* **322**: 933.

de Armond B, Doreman JS (1990). Central nervous system side effects of ganciclovir. *New Engl J Med* **322**: 934.

de Castro LM, Kern ER, De Clercq E *et al.* (1991). Phosphonylmethoxyalkyl purine and pyrimidine derivatives for treatment of opportunistic cytomegalovirus and herpes simplex virus infections in murine AIDS. *Antiviral Res* **16**: 191.

de Gans J, Portegies P, Tiessens G *et al.* (1990). Therapy for cytomegalovirus polyradiculomyelitis in patients with AIDS: Treatment with ganciclovir. *AIDS* **4**: 421.

de Koning J, van Dorp WT, van Es LA *et al.* (1992). Ganciclovir effectively treats cytomegalovirus disease after solid-organ transplantation, even during rejection treatment. *Nephrol Dial Transplant* **7**: 350.

de Miranda P, Burnette T, Cederberg D *et al.* (1986). In *Program and Abstracts of the 26th Interscience Conference on Antimicrobial Agents and Chemotherapy, New Orleans* (Abstr. 566). Washington, DC: American Society for Microbiology.

DeArmand B (1991). Safety consideration in the use of ganciclovir in immunocompromised patients. *Transplant Proc* **23**: 26.

Debs RJ, Montgomery AB, De Bruin M, Shanley JD (1988). Aerosol administration of antiviral agents to treat lung infection due to murine cytomegalovirus. *J Infect Dis* **157**: 327.

Dellemijn PL, Brandenburg A, Niesters HG *et al.* (1995). Successful treatment with ganciclovir of presumed Epstein–Barr meningo-encephalitis following bone marrow transplant. *Bone Marrow Transplant* **16**: 311.

Dieterich DT, Chachoua A, LaFleur F, Worrell C (1988). Ganciclovir treatment of gastrointestinal infections caused by cytomegalovirus in patients with AIDS. *Rev Infect Dis* **10**: S532.

Dieterich DT, Poles MA, Lew EA *et al.* (1993a). Concurrent use of ganciclovir and foscarnet to treat cytomegalovirus infection in AIDS patients. *J Infect Dis* **167**: 1184.

Dieterich DT, Kotler DP, Busch DF *et al.* (1993b). Ganciclovir treatment of cytomegalovirus colitis in AIDS: A randomised, double-blind, placebo-controlled multicenter study. *J Infect Dis* **167**: 278.

DiMaio JM, Clary BM, Via DF *et al.* (1994). Directed enzyme pro-drug gene therapy for pancreatic cancer *in vivo*. *Surgery* **116**: 205.

Drew WL, Miner RC, Lang W *et al.* (1991a). Prevalence of resistance in patients receiving ganciclovir for serious cytomegalovirus infection. *J Infect Dis* **163**: 716.

Drew WL, Miner R, King BD *et al.* (1991b). Antiviral activity of FIAU (1-[2'deoxy-2'-fluoro-1-beta-D-arabinofuranosyl)-5-iodo-uridine) on strains of cytomegalovirus sensitive and resistant to ganciclovir. *J Infect Dis* **163**: 1388.

Drew WL, Anderson R, Lang W *et al.* (1995a). Failure of high-dose oral acyclovir to suppress GMV viruria or induce ganciclovir-resistant CMV in HIV antibody positive patients. *J AIDS Retrovir* **8**: 289.

Drew L, Ives D, King BD *et al.* (1995b). Oral ganciclovir as maintenance treatment for cytomegalovirus retinitis in patients with AIDS. *New Engl J Med* **333**: 615.

Duncan SR, Paradis IL, Dauber JH *et al.* (1992). Ganciclovir prophylaxis for cytomegalovirus infections in pulmonary allograft recipients. *Amer Rev Respir Dis* **146**: 1213.

Duncan SR, Grgurich WE, Iacono AT *et al.* (1994). A comparison of ganciclovir and acyclovir to prevent cytomegalovirus after lung transplantation. *Amer J Respir Crit Care Med* **150**: 146.

Dunn DL, Mayoral JL, Gillingham KJ *et al.* (1991). Treatment of invasive cytomegalovirus disease in solid organ transplant patients with ganciclovir. *Transplantation* **51**: 98.

Elion GB, Furman PA, Fyfe JA *et al.* (1977). Selectivity of action of an antiherpetic agent, 9-(2-hydroxyethoxymethyl)guanine. *Proc Natl Acad Sci USA* **74**: 5716.

Emanuel D, Cunningham I, Jules-Elysee K *et al.* (1988). Cytomegalovirus pneumonia after bone marrow transplantation successfully treated with the combination of ganciclovir and high-dose intravenous immune globulin. *Ann Intern Med* **109**: 777.

Eng P, Allen DM, Chew SK *et al.* (1992). Cytomegalovirus pneumonitis in AIDS a case report. *Ann Acad Med Singapore* **21**: 843.

Engelhard D, Naparstek E, Or R *et al.* (1993). Ganciclovir for the treatment of disseminated CMV disease without pneumonia in allogeneic T-lymphocyte depleted bone marrow transplantation. *Leuk Lymphoma* **10**: 143.

Enright H, Haake R, Weisdorf D *et al.* (1993). Cytomegalovirus pneumonia after bone marrow transplantation. Risk factors and response to therapy. *Transplantation* **55**: 1339.

Eppstein DA, Marsh YV (1984). Potent synergistic inhibition of herpes simplex virus-2 by 9-[(1,3-dihydroxy-2-propoxy)methyl]guanine in combination with recombinant interferons. *Biochem Biophys Res Commun* **120**: 66.

Erice A, Jordan MC, Chace BA *et al.* (1987). Ganciclovir treatment of cytomegalovirus disease in transplant recipients and other immunocompromised hosts. *JAMA* **257**: 3082.

Erice A, Chou S, Biron KK *et al.* (1989). Progressive disease due to ganciclovir resistant cytomegalovirus in immunocompromised patients. *New Engl J Med* **320**: 289.

Ezzeddine ZD, Martuza RL, Platika D *et al.* (1991). Selective killing of glioma cells in culture and *in vivo* by retrovirus transfer of the herpes simplex virus thymidine kinase gene. *New Biol* **3**: 608.

Farrugia E, Schwab TR (1992). Management and prevention of cytomegalo-

virus infection after renal transplantation. *Mayo Clin Proc* **67**: 879.

Faulds D, Heel RC (1990). Ganciclovir A review of its antiviral activity, pharmacokinetic properties and therapeutic efficacy in cytomegalovirus infections. *Drugs* **39**: 597.

Feng JS, Crouch JY, Tian PV *et al.* (1993). Zidovudine antagonizes the antiviral effects of ganciclovir against cytomegalovirus infection in cultured cells and in guinea pigs. *Antiviral Chem Chemother* **4**: 19.

Field AK, Davies ME, De Witt C *et al.* (1983). 9-([2-hydroxy-1-(hydroxymethyl)ethoxylmethyl)guanine: A selective inhibitor of herpes group virus replication. *Proc Natl Acad Sci USA* **80**: 4139.

Field HJ (1985). Chemotherapy of Aujeszky's disease (pseudorabies) in the mouse by means of nucleoside analogues; bromovinyldeoxyuridine, acyclovir and dihydroxypropoxymethylguanine. *Antiviral Res* **5**: 157.

Figge HL, Bailie GR, Briceland LL, Kowalsky SF (1992). Possible ganciclovir induced hepatotoxicity in patients with AIDS. *Clin Pharm* **11**: 432.

Fletcher CV, Balfour HH (1989). Evaluation of ganciclovir for cytomegalovirus disease. *Drug Intell Clin Pharm* **23**: 5.

Fletcher C, Sawchuk R, Chinnock B *et al.* (1986). Human pharmacokinetics of the antiviral drug DHPG. *Clin Pharmacol Ther* **40**: 281.

Flores-Aguilar M, Kuppermann BD, Quiceno JI *et al.* (1993). Pathophysiology and treatment of clinically resistant cytomegalovirus retinitis. *Ophthalmology* **100**: 1022.

Flores-Aguilar M, Huang JS, Wiley CA *et al.* (1994). Long acting therapy of viral retinitis with (S)-1-(3-hydroxy-2-phosphonylmethoxypropyl) cystosine. *J Infect Dis* **169**: 642.

Follansbee S, Busch D, Conner CA, Mastie D (1992). Phase 1 study of the safety and pharmacokinetics of oral ganciclovir. *Eighth International Conference on AIDS, Amsterdam, The Netherlands.*

Fong CK, Cohen SD, McCormick S, Heiung GD (1987). Antiviral effect of 9-(1,3-dihydroxy-2-propoxymethyl)guanine against cytomegalovirus infection in a guinea pig model. *Antiviral Res* **7**: 11.

Frank KB, Chiou JF, Cheng YC *et al.* (1984). Interaction of herpes simplex virus-induced DNA polymerase with 9-(1,3-dihydroxy-2-propoxymethyl)guanine triphosphate. *J Biol Chem* **259**: 1566.

Frascino RJ, Anderson RD, Gaines Griffy K *et al.* (1995). Two multiple dose crossover studies of iv ganciclovir (GCV) and didanosine (ddI) in HIV infected persons. In *Program and Abstracts of the 35th Interscience Conference on Antimicrobial Agents and Chemotherapy, San Francisco.* Washington, DC: American Society for Microbiology.

Fraser-Smith EB, Smee DF, Matthews TR *et al.* (1983). Efficacy of the acyclic nucleoside 9-(1,3-dihydroxy-2-propoxymethyl)guanine against primary and recrudescent genital herpes simplex virus type 2 infections in guinea pigs. *Antimicrob Ag Chemother* **24**: 883.

Fraser-Smith EB, Eppstein DA, Marsh YV, Matthews TR (1985). Enhanced efficacy of the acyclic nucleoside 9-(1,3-dihydroxy-2-propoxymethyl-)guanine in combination with gamma interferon against herpes simplex virus type 2 in mice. *Antiviral Res* **5**: 137.

Freitas VR, Smee DE, Chernow M *et al.* (1985). Activity of 9-(1,3-dihydroxy-2-propoxymethyl)guanine compared with that of acyclovir against human, monkey and rodent cytomegaloviruses. *Antimicrob Ag Chemother* **28**: 240.

Freitas VR, Fraser-Smith EB, Matthews TR *et al.* (1989). Increased efficacy of ganciclovir in combination with foscarnet against cytomegalovirus and herpes simplex virus type 2 *in vitro* and *in vivo*. *Antiviral Res* **12**: 205.

Freitas VR, Fraser-Smith EB, Chin S *et al.* (1993a). Efficacy of ganciclovir in combination with zidovudine against cytomegalovirus *in vitro* and *in vivo*. *Antiviral Res* **21**: 301.

Freitas VR, Fraser-Smith EB, Matthews TR *et al.* (1993b). Efficacy of ganciclovir in combination with other antimicrobial agents against cytomegalovirus *in vitro* and *in vivo*. *Antiviral Res* **20**: 1.

French PD, Birchall MA, Harris JR *et al.* (1991). Cytomegalovirus ulceration of the oropharynx. *J Laryngol Otol* **105**: 739.

Fujii K, Morimoto I, Wake A *et al.* (1994). Adrenal insufficiency in a patient with acquired immunodeficiency syndrome. *Endocr J* **41**: 13.

Fukuda S, Miyachi M, Sugimoto S *et al.* (1995). A female infant successfully treated by ganciclovir for congenital cytomegalovirus infection. *Acta Paediatr Jpn* **37**: 206.

Gaines K, Wong R, Jung D *et al.* (1994). Pharmacokinetic interactions with oral ganciclovir: zidovudine, didanosine, probenecid. *Tenth International Conference on AIDS, Yokohama, Japan.*

Gaub J, Poulsen AG, Pedersen G *et al.* (1988). Efficacy and safety of two different dose levels of ganciclovir for the treatment of cytomegalovirus chorioretinitis in AIDS patients. *Scand J Infect Dis* **20**: 479.

George MJ, Snydman DR, Werner BC *et al.* (1993). Use of ganciclovir plus cytomegalovirus immune globulin to treat CMV pneumonia in orthotropic liver transplant recipients. The Boston Center for Liver Transplantation CMVIG-Study Group. *Transplant Proc* **25**: 22.

Germershausen J, Bostedor R, Field AK *et al.* (1983). A comparison of the antiviral agents 2'-nor'2'-deoxyguanosine and acyclovir: uptake and phosphorylation in tissue culture and kinetics of *in vitro* inhibition of viral and cellular DNA polymerase by their respective triphosphates. *Biochem Biophys Res Commun* **116**: 360.

Gilstrap LC, Bawdon RE, Roberts SW, Sobhi S (1994). The transfer of the nucleoside analog ganciclovir across the perfused human placenta. *Amer J Obstet Gynecol* **170**: 967.

Gish RG, Lau JY, Brooks L *et al.* (1996). Ganciclovir treatment of hepatitis B virus infection in liver transplant recipients. *Hepatology* **23**: 1.

Goodrich JM, Mori M, Gleaves CA *et al.* (1991). Early treatment with ganciclovir to prevent cytomegalovirus disease after allogeneic bone marrow transplantation. *New Engl J Med* **325**: 1601.

Goodrich JM, Bowden RA, Fisher L *et al.* (1993). Ganciclovir prophylaxis to prevent cytomegalovirus disease after allogeneic marrow transplant. *Ann Intern Med* **118**: 173.

Gould FK, Freeman R, Taylor CE *et al.* (1993). Prophylaxis and management of cytomegalovirus pneumonitis after lung transplantation; a review of experience in one center. *J Heart Lung Transplant* **12**: 695.

Gudnason T, Belani KK, Balfour HH *et al.* (1989). Ganciclovir treatment of cytomegalovirus disease in immunocompromised children. *Pediatr Infect Dis J* **8**: 436.

Guerin C, Pozzetto B, Broyet C *et al.* (1989). Ganciclovir therapy of symptomatic cytomegalovirus infection in renal transplant recipients. *Nephrol Dial Transplant* **4**: 906.

Guglielmo BJ, Wong-Beringer A, Linker CA *et al.* (1994). Immune globulin therapy in allogeneic bone marrow transplant; a critical review. *Bone Marrow Transplant* **13**: 499.

Hall AJ, Jennens ID, Lucas R *et al.* (1991). Low frequency maintenance ganciclovir for cytomegalovirus retinitis. *Scand J Infect Dis* **23**: 43.

Hamzeh FM, Lietman PS (1991). Intranuclear accumulation of subgenomic noninfectious human cytomegalovirus DNA in infected cells in the presence of ganciclovir. *Antimicrob Ag Chemother* **35**: 1818.

Hamzeh FM, Spector T, Lietman PS *et al.* (1993). 2-Acetylpyridine 5-[(dimethylamino)thiocarbonyl]-thiocarbonohydrazone (1110U81) potentially inhibits human cytomegalovirus replication and potentiates the antiviral effects of ganciclovir. *Antimicrob Ag Chemother* **37**: 602.

Hansen BA, Greenberg KS, Richter JA (1996). Ganciclovir-induced psychosis. *New Engl J Med* **335**: 1397.

Harbison MA, de Girolami PC, Jenkins RL, Hammer SM (1988). Ganciclovir therapy of severe cytomegalovirus infections in solid-organ transplant recipients. *Transplantation* **46**: 82.

Hardy D, Spector S, Polsky B *et al.* (1994). Combination of ganciclovir and granulocyte-macrophage colony stimulating factor in the treatment of cytomegalovirus retinitis in AIDS patients. The ACTG 073 team. *Eur J Clin Microbiol Infect Dis* **13**: S34.

Hardy WD (1991). Combined ganciclovir and recombinant human granulocyte-macrophage colony-stimulating factor in the treatment of cytomegalovirus retinitis in AIDS patients. *J AIDS* **4**: S22.

Harland RC, Vernon WB, Bunzendahl H *et al.* (1994). Ganciclovir/acyclovir prophylaxis reduces the incidence of cytomegalovirus infections in pancreas transplant recipients. *Transplant Proc* **26**: 432.

Hartman NR, Yarchoan R, Pluda JM *et al.* (1991). Pharmacokinetics of 2',3'-dideoxyinosine in patients with severe human immunodeficiency infection. II The effects of different oral formulations and the presence of other medications. *Clin Pharmacol Ther* **50**: 278.

Hedaya MA, Sawchuk RJ (1990). A sensitive and specific liquid-chromatographic assay for determination of ganciclovir in plasma and urine and its application to pharmacokinetic studies in the rabbit. *Pharm Res* **7**: 1113.

Heery S, Hollows F (1989). High dose intravitreal ganciclovir for cytomegaloviral (CMV) retinitis. *Aust NZ J Ophthalmol* **17**: 405.

Heilbronn R, Albrecht I, Stephen S *et al.* (1993). Human cytomegalovirus induces JC virus replication in human fibroblasts. *Proc Natl Acad Sci USA* **90**: 11406.

Heinemann MH (1989). Long-term intravitreal ganciclovir therapy for cytomegalovirus retinopathy. *Arch Ophthalmol* **107**: 1767.

Heise W, Nehm K, Skorde J *et al.* (1993). Ganciclovir in CMV gastrointestinal disease – a randomised double-blind study of two dose regimens in acute therapy. *Ninth International Conference on AIDS,6–11 June*: 441.

Henry K (1987). Intravenous ganciclovir for patients receiving zidovudine. *JAMA* **257**: 3066.

Henry K, Cantrill H, Fletcher C *et al.* (1987). Use of intravitreal ganciclovir (dihydroxy propoxymethyl guanine) for cytomegalovirus retinitis in a patient with AIDS. *Amer J Ophthalmol* **103**: 17.

Hibberd PL, Tolkoff-Rubin NE, Conti D *et al.* (1995). Preemptive ganciclovir therapy to prevent cytomegalovirus disease in cytomegalovirus antibody-positive renal transplant recipients. A randomized controlled trial. *Ann Intern Med* **123**: 18.

Hochster H, Dieterich D, Bozzette S *et al.* (1990). Toxicity of combined ganciclovir and zidovudine for cytomegalovirus disease associated with AIDS. An AIDS Clinical Trials Group Study. *Ann Intern Med* **113**: 111.

Holland GN, Schuler JD (1992). Progression rates of cytomegalovirus retinopathy in ganciclovir-treated and untreated patients. *Arch Ophthalmol* **110**: 1435.

Holland GN, Sakamoto MJ, Hardy D *et al.* (1986). Treatment of cytomegalovirus retinopathy in patients with acquired immunodeficiency syndrome Use of the experimental drug 9-[2-hydroxy-1-(hydroxymethyl) ethoxymethyl]guanine. *Arch Ophthalmol* **104**: 1794.

Holland GN, Sison RF, Jatulis DE *et al.* (1990). Survival of patients with the acquired immune deficiency syndrome after development of cytomegalovirus retinopathy. UCLA CMV Retinopathy Study Group. *Ophthalmology* **97**: 204.

Hopt UT, Pfeffer F, Schareck W *et al.* (1994). Ganciclovir for prophylaxis of CMV disease after pancreas/kidney transplantation. *Transplant Proc* **26**: 434.

Iisley DD, Lee SH, Miller WH, Kuchta RD (1995). Acyclic guanosine analogs inhibit DNA polymerases alpha, delta and epsilon with very different potencies and have unique mechanisms of action. *Biochemistry* **34**: 2504.

Ishida Y, Yokota Y, Tauchi H *et al.* (1993). Ganciclovir for chronic active Epstein-Barr virus infection. *Lancet* **341**: 560.

Jabs DA, Newman C, de Bustros S, Folk BF (1987). Treatment of cytomegalovirus retinitis with ganciclovir. *Ophthalmology* **94**: 824.

Jacobson MA, de Miranda P, Cederberg DM *et al.* (1987). Human pharmacokinetics and tolerance of oral ganciclovir. *Antimicrob Ag Chemother* **31**: 1251.

Jacobson MA, O'Donnell JJ, Porteous D *et al.* (1988a). Retinal and gastrointestinal disease due to cytomegalovirus in patients with the acquired immune deficiency syndrome: Prevalence, natural history, and response to ganciclovir therapy. *Quart J Med* **67**: 473.

Jacobson MA, de Miranda P, Gordon SM *et al.* (1988b). Prolonged pancytopenia due to combined ganciclovir and zidovudine therapy. *J Infect Dis* **158**: 489.

Jacobson MA, Cello JP, Brodie HR *et al.* (1988c). Cholestasis and disseminated cytomegalovirus disease in patients with the acquired immunodeficiency syndrome. *Amer J Med* **84**: 218.

Jacobson MA, Mills J, Rush J *et al.* (1988d). Failure of antiviral therapy for acquired immunodeficiency syndrome-related cytomegalovirus myelitis. *Arch Neurol* **45**: 1090.

Jacobson MA, O'Donnell JJ, Brodie HR *et al.* (1988e). Randomised prospective trial of ganciclovir maintenance therapy for cytomegalovirus retinitis. *J Med Virol* **35**: 339.

Jacobson MA, O'Donnell JJ, Rousell R *et al.* (1990). Failure of adjunctive cytomegalovirus intravenous immune globulin to improve efficacy of ganciclovir in patients with acquired immunodeficiency syndrome and cytomegalovirus retinitis: A phase I study. *Antimicrob Ag Chemother* **34**: 176.

Jacobson MA, Drew WL, Feinberg J *et al.* (1991). Foscarnet therapy for ganciclovir resistant cytomegalovirus retinitis in patients with AIDS. *J Infect Dis* **163**: 1348.

Jacobson MA, Stanley HD, Heard SE (1992).Ganciclovir with recombinant methionyl human granulocyte colony-stimulating factor for treatment of cytomegalovirus disease in AIDS patients (letter). *AIDS* **6**: 515.

Jacobson MA, Owen W, Campbell J *et al.* (1993). Tolerability of combined ganciclovir and didanosine for the treatment of cytomegalovirus disease associated with AIDS. *Clin Invest Dis* **16**: S69.

Jacobson MA, Kramer F, Bassiakos V *et al.* (1994a). Randomised phase 1 trial of two different combination foscarnet and ganciclovir chronic maintenance therapy regimens for AIDS patients with cytomegalovirus retinitis: AIDS clinical trials protocol 151. *J Infect Dis* **170**: 189.

Jacobson MA, Wulfsohn M, Feinberg JE *et al.* (1994b). Phase II dose-ranging trial of foscarnet salvage therapy for cytomegalovirus retinitis in AIDS patients intolerant of or resistant to ganciclovir (ACTG protocol 093). AIDS Clinical Trials Group of the National Institute of Allergy and Infectious Diseases. *AIDS* **8**: 451.

Jacqz-Aigrain E, Macher MA, Sauvageon-Marthe H (1992). Pharmacokinetics of ganciclovir in renal transplant children. *Pediatr Nephrol* **6**: 194.

Johnson CE, Jacobson PA, Chan E *et al.* (1994). Stability of ganciclovir sodium and amino acids in parenteral nutrient solutions. *Amer J Hosp Pharm* **51**: 503.

Jordan ML, Hrebinko RL, Dummer JS *et al.* (1992). Therapeutic use of ganciclovir for invasive cytomegalovirus infection in cadaveric renal allograft recipients. *J Urol* **148**: 1388.

Kalayjian RC, Cohen ML, Hayer C *et al.* (1993). Cytomegalovirus ventriculoencephalitis in AIDS. A syndrome with distinct clinical and pathologic features. *Medicine – Baltimore* **72**: 67.

Kaneko S, Hallenbeck P, Kotani T *et al.* (1995). Adenovirus mediated gene therapy of hepatocellular carcinoma using cancer specific gene expression. *Cancer Res* **55**: 5283.

Karmochkine M, Molina JM, Scieux C *et al.* (1994). Combined therapy with ganciclovir and foscarnet for cytomegalovirus polyradiculomyelitis in patients with AIDS. *Amer J Med* **97**: 196.

Kato K, Yoshida J, Mizuno M *et al.* (1994). Retroviral transfer of herpes simplex thymidine kinase gene into glioma cells causes targeting of ganciclovir cytotoxic effect. *Neurol Med Chir Tokyo* **34**: 339.

Kaulfersch W, Urban C, Hauer C *et al.* (1989). Successful treatment of CMV retinitis with ganciclovir after allogeneic marrow transplantation. *Bone Marrow Transplant* **4**: 587.

Keay S, Petersen E, Icenogle T *et al.* (1988). Ganciclovir treatment of serious cytomegalovirus infection in heart and heart-lung transplant recipients. *Rev Infect Dis* **10**: S563.

Kim YS, Hollander H (1993). Polyradiculopathy due to cytomegalovirus: Report of two cases in which improvement occurred after prolonged therapy and review of the literature. *Clin Invest Dis* **17**: 32.

Kirklin JK, Naftel DC, Levine TB *et al.* (1994). Cytomegalovirus after heart transplantation. Risk factors for infection and death; a multiinstitutional study. The Cardiac Transplant Research Database Group. *J Heart Lung Transplant* **13**: 394.

Kit S, Ichimura H, De Clercq E *et al.* (1987). Phosphorylation of nucleoside analogs by equine herpesvirus type 1 pyrimidine deoxyribonucleoside kinase. *Antiviral Res* **7**: 53.

Klein NJ, Friedman-Kien AE (1985). Effect of 9-(1,3-dihydroxy-2-propoxymethyl)guanine on the acute local phase of herpes simplex virus induced skin infections in mice and the establishment of latency. *Antimicrob Ag Chemother* **27**: 763.

Kotler DP (1991). Cytomegalovirus colitis and wasting. *J AIDS* **4**: S36.

Kuhn JE, Wendland T, Schafer P *et al.* (1994). Monitoring of renal allograft recipients by quantitation of human cytomegalovirus genomes in peripheral blood leukocytes. *J Med Virol* **44**: 398.

Kumagai T, Tanio Y, Osaki T *et al.* (1996). Eradication of Myc-overexpressing small cell lung cancer cells transfected with herpes simplex virus thymidine kinase gene containing Myc-Max response elements. *Cancer Res* **56**: 354.

Kuppermann BD, Quiceno JI, Flores-Aguilar M *et al.* (1993a). Intravitreal ganciclovir concentration after intravenous administration in AIDS patients with cytomegalovirus retinitis: implications for therapy. *J Infect Dis* **168**: 1506.

Kuppermann BD, Flores-Aguilar M, Quiceno JI *et al.* (1993b). Combination ganciclovir and foscarnet in the treatment of clinically resistant cytomegalovirus retinitis in patients with acquired immunodeficiency syndrome. *Arch Ophthalmol* **111**: 1359.

Ladurie FL, Cerrina J, Bavoux E *et al.* (1991). Ganciclovir for prevention of cytomegalovirus (CMV) infection in lung transplant (LT) recipients [abstract]. *Chest* **100**: 62.

Lake KD, Fletcher CV, Love KR *et al.* (1988). Ganciclovir pharmacokinetics during renal impairment. *Antimicrob Ag Chemother* **32**: 1899.

Laskin OL, Cederberg DM, Mills J *et al.* (1987). Ganciclovir for the treatment and suppression of serious infections caused by cytomegalovirus. *Amer J Med* **83**: 301.

Levy MF, Crippin JS, Gonwa TA *et al.* (1992). Cytomegalovirus (CMV) infections in liver transplant (Ltx) recipients; morbidity in the DHPG era [abstract no 9501]. *Hepatology* **16**: 282.

Li CR, Greenberg PD, Gilbert MJ *et al.* (1994). Recovery of HLA-restricted cytomegalovirus (CMV)-specific T-cell responses after allogeneic bone marrow transplant; correlation with CMV disease and effect of ganciclovir prophylaxis. *Blood* **83**: 1971.

Lim W, Kahn E, Gupta A *et al.* (1988). Treatment of cytomegalovirus enterocolitis with ganciclovir in an infant with acquired immunodeficiency syndrome. *Pediatr Infect Dis* **7**: 354.

Lin JC, Smith MC, Pagano JS *et al.* (1984). Prolonged inhibitory effect of 9-(1,3-dihydroxy-2-propoxymethyl)guanine against replication of Epstein-Barr virus. *J Virol* **50**: 50.

Lin JC, Nelson DJ, Lamb CU *et al.* (1986). Metabolic activation of 9([2-hydroxy-1-(hydroxymethyl)ethoxy]methyl)guanine in human lymphoblastoid cell lines infected with Epstein–Barr virus. *J Virology* **60**: 569.

Lipson SM, Tseng LF, Kaplan MH, Brondo FX (1993). Antiviral susceptibility testing of cytomegalovirus from primary culture using shell vial assay to detect the late viral antigen. *Diagn Microbiol Infect Dis* **17**: 283.

Littler E, Stuart AD, Chee MS *et al.* (1992). Human cytomegalovirus UL97 open reading frame encodes a protein that phosphorylates the antiviral nucleoside analogue ganciclovir. *Nature* **358**: 160.

Ljungman P, Engelhard D, Link D *et al.* (1992). Treatment of intravenous immune globulin; experience of European Bone Marrow Transplant Group. *Clin Infect Dis* **14**: 831.

Ljungman P, Biron P, Bosi A *et al.* (1994). Cytomegalovirus interstitial pneumonia in autologous bone marrow transplant recipients, Infectious Disease Working Party of the European Group for Bone Marrow Transplantation. *Bone Marrow Transplant* **13**: 209.

Locarnini S, Guo K, Lucas R, Gust ID (1989). Inhibition of HBV DNA replication by ganciclovir in patients with AIDS. *Lancet* **ii**: 1225.

Locatelli F, Percivalle E, Comoli P *et al.* (1994). Human cytomegalovirus (HCMV) infection in paediatric patients given allogeneic bone marrow transplantation; role of early antiviral treatment for HCMV antigenaemia on patients' outcome. *Brit J Haematol* **88**: 64.

Lopez-Contreras J, Ris J, Domingo P *et al.* (1995). Disseminated cytomegalovirus infection in an immunocompetent adult successfully treated with ganciclovir. *Scand J Infect Dis* **27**: 523.

Lumbreras C, Otero JR, Aguado JM *et al.* (1992). Prospective study of infection by cytomegalovirus in liver transplant recipients. *Med Clin* **99**: 401.

Lumbreras C, Otero JR, Herrero JA *et al.* (1993). Ganciclovir prophylaxis decreases frequency and severity of cytomegalovirus disease in seropositive liver transplant recipients treated with OKT3 monoclonal antibodies. *Antimicrob Ag Chemother* **37**: 2490.

Lurain NS, Thompson KD, Holmes EW, Read GS (1992). Point mutations in the DNA polymerase gene of human cytomegalovirus that result in resistance to antiviral agents. *J Virol* **66**: 7146.

Lurain NS, Spafford LE, Thompson KD (1994). Mutation in the UL97 open reading frame of human cytomegalovirus strains resistant to ganciclovir. *J Virol* **68**: 4427.

Luscombe C, Pedersen J, Bowden S, Locarini S (1994). Alterations in intrahepatic expression of duck hepatitis B viral markers with ganciclovir chemotherapy. *Liver* **14**: 182.

Macri P, Gordon JW (1994). Delayed morbidity and mortality of albumin/SV40 T-antigen transgenic mice after insertion of an alpha-fetoprotein/herpes virus thymidine kinase transgene and treatment with ganciclovir. *Hum Gene Ther* **5**: 175.

Mandanas RA, Saez RA, Selby GB, Confer DL (1996). Cytomegalovirus surveillance and prevention in allogeneic bone marrow transplantation; examination of a preemptive plan of ganciclovir therapy. *Amer J Hematol* **51**: 104.

Manez R, Kusne S, Green M *et al.* (1995). Incidence and risk factors associated with the development of cytomegalovirus disease after intestinal transplantation. *Transplantation* **59**: 1010.

Manian FA, Smith T (1993). Ganciclovir for the treatment of cytomegalovirus pneumonia in an immunocompetent host. *Clin Infect Dis* **17**: 137.

Manischewitz JF, Quinnan GV, Lane HC, Wittek AE (1990). Synergistic effect of ganciclovir and foscarnet on cytomegalovirus replication *in vitro. Antimicrob Ag Chemother* **34**: 373.

Mar EC, Cheng YC, Huang ES *et al.* (1983). Effect of 9-(1,3-dihydroxy-2-propoxymethyl)guanine on human cytomegalovirus replication *in vitro. Antimicrob Ag Chemother* **24**: 518.

Marelli RA, Biddinger PW, Gluckman JL *et al.* (1992). Cytomegalovirus infection of the larynx in the acquired immunodeficiency syndrome. *Otolaryngol Head Neck Surg* **106**: 296.

Markham A, Faulds D (1994). Ganciclovir: An update of its therapeutic use in cytomegalovirus infection. *Drugs* **48**: 455.

Martin JC, Dvorak CA, Smee DF *et al.* (1983). 9-{(1,3-Dihydroxy-2-propoxy)methyl]guanine: a new potent and selective antiherpes agent. *J Med Chem* **26**: 759.

Martin DF, Parks DJ, Mellow SD *et al.* (1994a). Treatment of cytomegalovirus retinitis with an intraocular sustained-release ganciclovir implant. A randomised controlled clinical trial. *Arch Ophthalmol* **112**: 1531.

Martin M, Manez R, Linden P *et al.* (1994b). A prospective randomized trial comparing sequential ganciclovir-high dose acyclovir to high dose acyclovir for prevention of cytomegalovirus disease in adult liver transplant recipients. *Transplantation* **58**: 779.

Mastroianni CM, Ciardi M, Folgori F *et al.* (1994). Cytomegalovirus encephalitis in two patients with AIDS receiving ganciclovir for cytomegalovirus retinitis. *J Infect Dis* **29**: 331.

Masur H, Lane HC, Palestine A *et al.* (1986). Effect of 9-(1,3-dihydroxy-2-propoxymethyl) guanine on serious cytomegalovirus disease in eight immunosuppressed homosexual men. *Ann Intern Med* **104**: 41.

Matthews T, Boehme R (1988). Antiviral activity and mechanism of action of ganciclovir. *Rev Infec Dis* **10**: S490.

McCluskey P, Wakefield D, Morgan M, Binneter R (1990). Cytomegalovirus retinopathy and the acquired immune deficiency syndrome: Results of treatment with ganciclovir. *Aust NZ J Ophthalmol* **18**: 385.

McLaren C, Chen MS, Ghazzouli I *et al.* (1985). Drug resistance patterns of herpes simplex virus isolates from patients treated with acyclovir. *Antimicrob Ag Chemother* **28**: 740.

Medina DJ, Hsiung GD, Mellors JW (1992). Ganciclovir antagonizes the anti-human immunodeficiency virus type 1 activity of zidovudine and didanosine *in vitro. Antimicrob Ag Chemother* **36**: 1127.

Meijer H, Bruggeman CA, Dormans PHJ, van Boven CP (1984). Human cytomegalovirus induces a cellular deoxyguanosine kinase, also interacting with acyclovir. *FEMS Microbiol Letters* **25**: 283.

Merigan TC, Renlund DG, Keay S *et al.* (1992). A controlled trial of ganciclovir to prevent cytomegalovirus disease after heart transplantation. *New Engl J Med* **326**: 1182.

Miles SA, Mitsuyasu RT, Moreno J *et al.* (1991). Combined therapy with recombinant granulocyte colony stimulating factor and erythropoietin decreases hematologic toxicity from zidovudine. *Blood* **77**: 2109.

Miller RG, Storey JR, Greco CM *et al.* (1990). Ganciclovir in the treatment of progressive AIDS-related polyradiculopathy. *Neurology* **40**: 569.

Miller WT, Sais GJ, Frank I *et al.* (1994). Pulmonary aspergillosis in patients with AIDS. Clinical and radiographic correlations. *Chest* **105**: 37.

Mills J, Jacobson MA, O'Donnell JJ *et al.* (1988). Treatment of cytomegalovirus retinitis in patients with AIDS. *Rev Infect Dis* **10**: S522.

MMWR (1995). Herpes simplex virus disease; Varicella zoster virus infection. *MMWR* **44**: 21.

Mole L, Oliva,C, O'Hanley P *et al.* (1992). Extended stability of ganciclovir for outpatient parenteral therapy for cytomegalovirus retinitis. *J AIDS* **5**: 354.

Moran DM, Kern ER, Overall JC *et al.* (1985). Synergism between recombinant human interferon and nucleoside antiviral agents against herpes simplex virus; examination with an automated microtiter plate assay. *J Infect Dis* **151**: 1116.

Morlet N, Young SH (1993). Prevention of intraocular pressure rise following intravitreal injection. *Brit J Ophthalmol* **77**: 572.

Morlet N, Young S, Strachan D, Coroneo MT (1993). Technique of intravitreal injection. *Aust NZ J Ophthalmol* **21**: 130.

Morley MG, Duker JS, Ashton P, Robinson MR (1995). Replacing ganciclovir implants. *Ophthalmology* **102**: 388.

Moyle G, Harman C, Mitchell S *et al.* (1992). Foscarnet and ganciclovir in the treatment of CMV retinitis in AIDS patients: A randomised comparison. *J Infect* **25**: 21.

Naito T, Nitta K, Kinouchi X *et al.* (1991). Effects of 9-(1,3-dihydroxy-2-propoxymethyl) guanine (DHPG) eye drops and cyclosporine eye drops in the treatment of herpetic stromal keratitis in rabbits. *Curr Eye Res* **10**: 201.

Nakazato PZ, Burns W, Moore P *et al.* (1993). Viral prophylaxis in hepatic transplantation; preliminary report of a randomized trial of acyclovir and ganciclovir. *Transplant Proc* **25**: 1935.

Nevins TE, Dunn DL (1992). Use of ganciclovir for cytomegalovirus infection. *J Amer Soc Nephrol* **2**: S270.

Neyts J, Snoeck R, Schols D *et al.* (1990). Selective inhibition of human cytomegalovirus DNA synthesis by (S)-1-J(3-dydroxy-2-phosphonyl-methoxyproyl)cytosine [(S)-HPMPC] and 9-(1,3-dihydroxy-2-propoxy-methyl)guanine (DHPG). *Virology* **179**: 41.

Neyts J, Balzarini J, Naesens L, De Clercq E (1992). Efficacy of (S)-1-(3-hydroxy-2-phosphonylmethoxypropyl) cytosine and 9-(1,3-dihydroxy-2-propoxymethyl) guanine for the treatment of murine cytomegalovirus infection in severe combined immunodeficiency mice. *J Med Virol* **37**: 67.

Neyts J, Sobis H, Snoeck R *et al.* (1993). Efficacy of (S)-1-(3-hydroxy-2-phosphonylmethoxypropyl)-cytosine and 9-(1,3-dihydroxy-2-propoxy-methyl)-guanine in the treatment of intracerebral murine cytomegalovirus infections in immunocompetent and immunodeficient mice. *Eur J Clin Microbiol Infect Dis* **12**: 269.

Nigro G, Scholz H, Bartmann U *et al.* (1994). Ganciclovir therapy for symptomatic congenital cytomegalovirus infection in infants; a two-regimen experience. *J Pediatr* **124**: 318.

Niu J, Wang Y, Dixon R *et al.* (1993). The use of ampligen alone and in combination with ganciclovir and coumermycin A1 for the treatment of ducks congenitally infected with duck hepatitis B virus. *Antiviral Res* **21**: 155.

Nokta M, Tolpin MD, Nadler PI, Pollard RB (1994). Human monoclonal anti-cytomegalovirus (CMV) antibody (MSL 109): enhancement of *in vitro* foscarnet and ganciclovir-induced inhibition of CMV replication. *Antiviral Res* **24**: 17.

Novick RJ, Menkis AH, McKenzie FN *et al.* (1990). Should heart-lung transplant donors and recipients be matched according to cytomegalovirus serologic status? *J Heart Transplant* **9**: 699.

O'Malley BW, Chen SH, Schwartz MR, Woo SL (1995). Adenovirus-mediated gene therapy for human head and neck squamous cell cancer in a nude mouse model. *Cancer Res* **55**: 1080.

Ohno T, Gordon D, San H *et al.* (1994). Gene therapy for vascular smooth muscle cell proliferation after arterial injury. *Science* **265**: 781.

Oldfield EH, Ram Z, Culver KW *et al.* (1993). Gene therapy for the treatment of brain tumors using intratumoral transduction with the thymidine kinase gene and intravenous ganciclovir. *Hum Gene Ther* **4**: 39.

Oral ganciclovir investigational brochure (1994). *Syntex* 7th Edition.

Orellana J, Teich SA, Friedman AH *et al.* (1987). Combined short and long-term therapy for the treatment of cytomegalovirus retinitis using ganciclovir (BW B759U). *Ophthalmology* **94**: 831.

Orellana J, Lieberman RM, Peairs R *et al.* (1990). Intravitreal therapy with ganciclovir for posterior pole cytomegalovirus retinitis in AIDS patients. *Brit J Ophthalmol* **14**: 511.

Osaki T, Tanio Y, Tachihana I *et al.* (1994). Gene therapy for carcinoembryonic antigen-producing human lung cancer cells by cell type-specific expression of herpes simplex virus thymidine kinase gene. *Cancer Res* **54**: 5258.

Palestine AG, Stevens G, Lane HC *et al.* (1986). Treatment of cytomegalovirus retinitis with dihydroxy propoxymethyl guanine. *Amer J Ophthalmol* **101**: 95.

Pantoni L, Inzitari D, Colao MG *et al.* (1991). Cytomegalovirus encephalitis in a non-immunocompromised patient; CSF diagnosis by *in situ* hybridization cells. *Acta Neurol Scand* **84**: 56.

Parasrampuria J, Li LC, Steimach AH *et al.* (1992). Stability of ganciclovir sodium in 5% dextrose injection and in 09% sodium chloride injection over 35 days. *Amer J Hosp Pharm* **49**: 116.

Paya CV, Hermans PE, Smith TF *et al.* (1988). Efficacy of ganciclovir in liver and kidney transplant recipients with severe cytomegalovirus infection. *Transplantation* **46**: 229.

Pecyk RA, Fraser-Smith EB, Matthews TR (1989). Lack of antiviral activity of ketoconazole alone or in combination with the acyclic nucleoside ganciclovir against a herpes virus type 2 infection in mice. *Acta Virol Praha* **33**: 569.

Peters M, Timm U, Schurmann D *et al.* (1992). Combined and alternating ganciclovir and foscarnet in acute and maintenance therapy of human immunodeficiency virus-related cytomegalovirus encephalitis refractory to ganciclovir alone. A case report and review of the literature. *Clin Invest* **70**: 456.

Peters M, Schurmann D, Dergmann F *et al.* (1994). Safety of alternating ganciclovir and foscarnet maintenance therapy in human immunodeficiency virus (HIV)-related cytomegalovirus infections. An open-labelled pilot study. *Scand J Infect Dis* **26**: 49.

Peters MJ, Moeller HU, Russell-Eggitt I, Novelli V (1995). Cytomegalovirus retinitis in AIDS. *Arch Dis Childhood* **72**: 54.

Plotkin SA, Drew WL, Felsenstein D, Hirsch MS (1985). Sensitivity of clinical isolates of human cytomegalovirus to 9-(1,3-dihydroxy-2-propoxymethyl)guanine. *J Infect Dis* **152**: 833.

Poscher ME (1994). Successful treatment of varicella zoster virus meningoencephalitis in patients with AIDS: Report of four cases and review. *AIDS* **8**: 1115.

Prian GW, Koep LJ (1994). Elimination of cytomegalovirus disease in liver transplant patients treated prophylactically with combination cytomegalovirus hyperimmune globulin and ganciclovir. *Transplant Proc* **26**: 54.

Price TA, Digioia RA, Simon GL *et al.* (1992). Ganciclovir treatment of cytomegalovirus ventriculitis in a patient infected with human immunodeficiency virus. *Clin Infect Dis* **15**: 606.

Prichard MN, Turk SR, Coleman LA *et al.* (1990). A microtiter virus yield reduction assay for the evaluation of antiviral compounds against human cytomegalovirus and herpes simplex virus. *J Virol Methods* **28**: 101.

Prichard MN, Prichard LE, Baguley WA *et al.* (1991). Three dimensional analysis of the synergistic cytotoxicity of ganciclovir and zidovudine. *Antimicrob Ag Chemother* **35**: 1060.

Prokurat S, Drabik E, Grenda R, Vogt E (1993). Ganciclovir in cytomegalovirus prophylaxis in high-risk pediatric renal transplant recipients. *Transplant Proc* **25**: 2577.

Przepiorka D, Ippoliti C, Panina A *et al.* (1994). Ganciclovir three times per week is not adequate to prevent cytomegalovirus reactivation after T cell-depleted marrow transplantation. *Bone Marrow Transplant* **13**: 461.

Pulliam L, Panitch HS, Baringer JR, Dix RD (1986). Effect of antiviral agents on replication of herpes simplex virus type 1 in brain culture. *Antimicrob Ag Chemother* **30**: 840.

Razis E, Cook,P, Mittelman A, Ahmed T (1994). Treatment of ganciclovir resistant cytomegalovirus with foscarnet; A report of two cases occurring after bone marrow transplantation. *Leuk Lymphoma* **12**: 477.

Reardon JE (1989). Herpes simplex virus type 1 and human RNA polymerase interactions with 2'=deoxyguanosine 5'-triphosphate analogues: Kinetics of incorporation into DNA and induction of inhibition. *J Biol Chem* **32**: 19039.

Reed EC, Dandliker PS, Meyers JD *et al.* (1986). Treatment of cytomegalovirus pneumonia with 9-[2-hydroxyl-1-(hydroxymethyl) ethoxymethyl] guanine and high dose corticosteroids. *Ann Intern Med* **105**: 214.

Reed EC, Shepp DH, Dandliker PS, Meyers JD (1988a). Ganciclovir treatment of cytomegalovirus infection of the gastrointestinal tract after marrow transplantation. *Bone Marrow Transplant* **3**: 199.

Reed EC, Bowden RA, Dandliker PS *et al.* (1988b). Treatment of cytomegalovirus pneumonia with ganciclovir and intravenous cytomegalovirus immunoglobulin in patients with bone marrow transplants. *Ann Intern Med* **109**: 783.

Reed EC, Wolford JL, Kopecky KJ *et al.* (1990). Ganciclovir for the treatment of cytomegalovirus gastroenteritis in bone marrow transplant patients A randomised, placebo-controlled trial. *Ann Intern Med* **112**: 505.

Reigstad H, Bjerknes R, Markestad T, Myrmel H (1992). Ganciclovir therapy of congenital cytomegalovirus disease. *Acta Paediatr* **81**: 707.

Rello J (1990). Effect of continuous arteriovenous hemodialysis on ganciclovir pharmacokinetics. *DICP. Ann Pharmacol* **24**: 544.

Roberts WD, Weinberg KI, Kohn DB *et al.* (1993). Granulocyte recovery in pediatric marrow transplant recipients treated with ganciclovir for cytomegalovirus infection. *Amer J Pediatr Hematol Oncol* **15**: 320.

Rollinson EA (1987). Comparative efficacy of three 2'-fluoropyrimidine nucleosides and 9-(1,3-dihydroxy-2-propoxymethyl)guanine (BW B759U) against pseudorabies and equine rhinopneumonitis virus infection *in vitro* and in laboratory animals. *Antiviral Res* **7**: 25.

Rollinson EA, White G (1983). Relative activities of acyclovir and BW759 against Aujeszky's disease and equine rhinopneumonitis viruses. *Antimicrob Ag Chemother* **24**: 221.

Rondeau E, Bourgeon B, Peraldi MN *et al.* (1993). Effect of prophylactic ganciclovir on cytomegalovirus infection in renal transplant recipients. *Nephrol Dial Transplant* **8**: 858.

Rosecan LR, Laskin OL, Kalman CM *et al.* (1986). Antiviral therapy with ganciclovir for cytomegalovirus retinitis and bilateral exudative retinal detachments in an immunocompromised child. *Ophthalmology* **93**: 1401.

Rush J, Mills J (1987). Effect of combinations of difluoromethylornithine (DFMO) and 9[(1,3-dihydroxy-2-propoxy) methyl]guanine (DHPG) on human cytomegalovirus. *J Med Virol* **21**: 269.

Russler SK, Tapper MA, Carrigan DR *et al.* (1989). Susceptibility of human herpesvirus 6 to acyclovir and ganciclovir. *Lancet* **12**: 382.

Safrin S, Kemmerly S, Plotkin B *et al.* (1994). Foscarnet resistant herpes simplex virus infection in patients with AIDS. *J Infect Dis* **169**: 193.

Salazar A, Podzamczer D, Rene R *et al.* (1995). Cytomegalovirus ventriculoencephalitis in AIDS patients. *Scand J Infect Dis* **27**: 165.

Salvador F, Blanco R, Colin A *et al.* (1993). Cytomegalovirus retinitis in pediatric acquired immunodeficiency syndrome report of two cases. *J Pediatr Ophthalmol Strabismus* **30**: 159.

Salzberger B, Stoehr A, Heise W *et al.* (1994). Foscarnet and ganciclovir combination therapy for CMV disease in HIV-infected patients. *Infection* **22**: 197.

Sanborn GE, Anand R, Torti RE *et al.* (1992). Sustained-release ganciclovir therapy for treatment of cytomegalovirus retinitis. Use of an intravitreal device. *Arch Ophthalmol* **110**: 188.

Sanhes L, Michez E, Essig M *et al.* (1995). Successful treatment of CMV-induced adrenal insufficiency by ganciclovir in a patient with the acquired immunodeficiency syndrome. *Nephrol Dial Transplant* **10**: 704.

Saran BR, Maguire AM (1994). Retinal toxicity of high dose intravitreal ganciclovir. *Retina* **14**: 248.

Sarasini A, Baldanti F, Furione M *et al.* (1995). Double resistance to ganciclovir and foscarnet of four human cytomegalovirus stains recovered from AIDS patients. *J Med Virol* **47**: 237.

Savage LH, Gonwa TA, Goldstein RM *et al.* (1989). Cytomegalovirus infection in orthotropic liver transplantation. *Transpl Int* **2**: 96.

Sawyer MD, Mayoral JL, Gillingham KJ *et al.* (1993). Treatment of recurrent cytomegalovirus disease in patients receiving solid organ transplants. *Arch Surg* **128**: 165.

Scadden DT, Wang A, Zeebo KM, Groopman JE (1994). *In vitro* effects of stem-cell factor or interleukin-3 on myelosuppression associated with AIDS. *AIDS* **8**: 193.

Schmidt GM, Kovacs A, Zaia JA *et al.* (1988). Ganciclovir immunoglobulin combination therapy for the treatment of human cytomegalovirus-associated interstitial pneumonia in bone marrow allograft recipients. *Transplantation* **46**: 905.

Schmidt GM, Horak DA, Niland JC *et al.* (1991). A randomised, controlled trial of prophylactic ganciclovir for cytomegalovirus pulmonary infection in recipients of allogeneic bone marrow transplants; The City of Hope-Stanford-Syntex CMV Study Group. *New Engl J Med* **324**: 1005.

Schmuth M, Grimm M, Wisser W *et al.* (1992). Perioperative ganciclovir-prophylaxis after lung transplantation does not reduce incidence of CMV-infection. *Chest* **102**: 18.

Schulman J, Peyman GA, Horton MB *et al.* (1986). Intraocular 9-([2-hydroxy-1-(hydroxymethyl) ethoxy] methyl) guanine levels after intravitreal and subconjunctival administration. *Ophthalmic Surg* **17**: 429.

Schwarz TF, Loeschke K, Hanus I *et al.* (1990). CMV encephalitis during ganciclovir therapy of CMV retinitis. *Infect* **18**: 289.

Shaw T, Amor P, Civitico G *et al.* (1994). *In vitro* antiviral activity of penciclovir, a novel purine nucleoside, against duck hepatitis B virus. *Antimicrob Ag Chemother* **38**: 719.

Shea BF, Hoffman S, Sesin GP, Hammer SM (1987). Ganciclovir hepatotoxicity. *Pharmacother* **7**: 223.

Shepp DH, Dandliker PS, de Miranda P *et al.* (1985). Activity of 9-[2-hydroxy-1-(hydroxymethyl]guanine in the treatment of cytomegalovirus pneumonia. *Ann Intern Med* **103**: 368.

Shepp DH, Tang IT, Ramundo MB *et al.* (1994). Serious *Pseudomonas aeruginosa* infection in AIDS. *J AIDS* **7**: 823.

Shigeta S, Konno K, Baba M *et al.* (1991). Comparative inhibitory effects of nucleoside analogues on different clinical isolates of human cytomegalovirus *in vitro*. *J Infect Dis* **163**: 270.

Shiota H, Naito T, Mimura Y *et al.* (1987). Anti-herpes simplex virus (HSV) effect of 9-(1,3-dihydroxy-2-propoxymethyl)guanine (DHPG) in rabbit cornea. *Curr Eye Res* **6**: 241.

Silvestri AP, Mitrano FP, Baptista RJ, Williams DA (1991). Stability and compatibility of ganciclovir sodium in 5% dextrose injection over 35 days. *Amer J Hosp Pharmacy* **48**: 2641.

Singh N, Yu VL, Mieles L *et al.* (1994). High-dose acyclovir compared with short-course preemptive ganciclovir therapy to prevent cytomegalovirus disease in liver transplant recipients. A randomised trial. *Ann Intern Med* **120**: 375.

Singhal S, Mehta J, Powles R *et al.* (1995). Three weeks of ganciclovir for cytomegaloviraemia after allogeneic bone marrow transplantation. *Bone Marrow Transplant* **15**: 777.

Slavin MA, Bindra RR, Gleaves CA *et al.* (1993). Ganciclovir sensitivity of cytomegalovirus at diagnosis and during treatment of cytomegalovirus pneumonia in marrow transplant recipients. *Antimicrob Ag Chemother* **37**: 1360.

Smee DF, Martin JC, Verheyden JP, Matthews TT (1983). Anti herpesvirus activity of the acyclic nucleoside 9-(1,3-hihydroxy-2-propoxymethyl) guanine. *Antimicrob Ag Chemother* **23**: 676.

Smee DF, Campbell NL, Matthews TR *et al.* (1985a). Comparative anti-herpesvirus activities of 9-(1,3-dihydroxy-2-propoxymethyl)guanine, acyclovir, and two 2'-fluoropyrimidine nucleosides. *Antiviral Res* **5**: 259.

Smee DF, Knight SS, Duke AE *et al.* (1985b). Activities of arabinosyladenine monophosphate and 9-(1,3-dihydroxy-2-propoxymethyl)guanine against ground squirrel hepatitis virus *in vivo* as determined by reduction in serum virion-associated DNA polymerase. *Antimicrob Ag Chemother* **27**: 277.

Smee DF, Boehme R, Chernow M *et al.* (1985c). Intracellular metabolism and enzymatic phosphorylation of 9-(1,3-dihydroxy-2-propoxymethyl-)guanine and acyclovir in herpes simplex virus-infected and uninfected cells. *Biochem Pharmacol* **34**: 1049.

Smee DF, Burger RA, Coombs J *et al.* (1991). Progressive murine cytomegalovirus disease after termination of ganciclovir therapy in mice immunosuppressed by cyclophosphamide treatment. *J Infect Dis* **164**: 958.

Smith KO, Galloway KS, Kennett WL *et al.* (1982a). A new nucleoside analog, 9-[[2-dydroxy-1-(hydroxymethyl) ethoxyl]guanine, highly active *in vitro* against herpes simplex virus type 1 and 2. *Antimicrob Ag Chemother* **22**: 55.

Smith KO, Galloway KS, Ogilvie EK, Cheriyan UO (1982b). Synergism among BIOLF-62, phosphonoformate, and other antiherpetic compounds. *Antimicrob Ag Chemother* **22**: 1026.

Smith TJ, Pearson PA, Blandford LK *et al.* (1992). Intravitreal sustained-release ganciclovir. *Arch Ophthalmol* **110**: 255.

Smythe RL, Scott JP, Borgsiewicz LK *et al.* (1991). Cytomegalovirus infection in heart-lung transplant recipients: Risk factors, clinical associations and response to treatment. *J Infect Dis* **164**: 1045.

Smythe WR, Hwang HC, Elshami AA *et al.* (1995). Differential sensitivity of thoracic malignant tumors to adenovirus-mediated drug sensitization gene therapy. *J Thorac Cardiovasc Surg* **109**: 626.

Snoeck R, Lagneaux L, Delforge A *et al.* (1990). Inhibitory effects of potent inhibitors of human immunodeficiency virus and cytomegalovirus on the growth of human granulocyte-macrophage progenitor cells. *Eur J Clin Microbiol Infect Dis* **9**: 615.

Snoeck R, Andrei G, Schols D *et al.* (1992). Activity of different antiviral drug combinations against human cytomegalovirus replication *in vitro*. *Eur J Clin Microbiol Infect Dis* **11**: 1144.

Snydman DR (1988). Ganciclovir therapy for cytomegalovirus disease associated with renal transplants. *Rev Infect Dis* **10**: S554.

Snydman DR, Rubin RH, Werner BG *et al.* (1993). New developments in cytomegalovirus prevention and management. *Amer J Kidney Dis* **21**: 217.

So YT, Olney RK (1994). Acute lumbosacral polyradiculopathy in acquired immunodeficiency syndrome: Experience in 23 patients *Ann Neurol* **35**: 53.

Soike KF, Eppstein DA, Gloff CA *et al.* (1987). Effect of 9-(1,3-dihydroxy-2-propoxymethyl)guanine and recombinant human beta-interferon alone and in combination on simian varicella virus infection in monkeys. *J Infect Dis* **156**: 607.

Sommadossi JP, Carlisle R (1987). Toxicity of 3'-azido-3'-deoxythymidine and 9-(1,3-dihydroxy-2-propoxymethyl)guanine for normal human hematopoietic progenitor cells *in vitro*. *Antimicrob Ag Chemother* **31**: 452.

Sommadossi JP, Bevan R, Ling T *et al.* (1988). Clinical pharmacokinetics of ganciclovir in patients with normal and impaired renal function. *Rev Infect Dis* **10**: S507.

Spaide RF (1994). Ganciclovir intraocular device and patient survival. *Arch Ophthalmol* **112**: 19.

Spector SA, Weingeist T, Pollard RB et al. (1993). A randomised controlled study of intravenous ganciclovir therapy for cytomegalovirus peripheral retinitis in patients with AIDS. AIDS Clinical Trials Group and Cytomegalovirus Co-operative Study Group. J Infect Dis 168: 557.

Spector SA, Busch DF, Follansbee S et al. (1995). Pharmacokinetic, safety and antiviral profiles of oral ganciclovir in persons infected with human immunodeficiency virus: A phase I/II study. J Infect Dis 171: 1431.

Spector SA, McKinley GF, Lalezari JP et al. (1996). Oral ganciclovir for the prevention of cytomegalovirus disease in persons with AIDS. New Engl J Med 334: 1491.

St Clair MH, Miller WH, Miller RL et al. (1984). Inhibition of cellular alpha DNA polymerase and herpes simplex virus induced by DNA polymerases by the triphosphate of BW759U. Antimicrob Ag Chemother 25: 191.

St Clair MH, Lambe CU, Furman PA et al. (1987). Inhibition by ganciclovir of cell growth and DNA synthesis of cells biochemically transformed with herpes virus genetic information. Antimicrob Ag Chemother 31: 844.

Stals FS, Zeytinoglu A, Havenith M et al. (1993). Rat cytomegalovirus induced pneumonitis after allogeneic bone marrow transplantation: effective treatment with (S)-1-(3-hydroxy-2-phosphonyl-methoxypropyl) cytosine. Antimicrob Ag Chemother 37: 218.

Stanat SC, Reardon JE, Erice A et al. (1991). Ganciclovir-resistant cytomegalovirus clinical isolates: mode of resistance to ganciclovir. Antimicrob Ag Chemother 35: 2191.

Stanley HD, Charlebois E, Harb G, Jacobson MA (1994). Central venous catheter infections in AIDS patients receiving treatment for cytomegalovirus disease. J AIDS 7: 272.

Stein DS, Verano AS, Levandowski RA et al. (1988). Successful treatment with ganciclovir of disseminated cytomegalovirus infection after liver transplantation. Amer J Gastroenterol 83: 684.

Steinhoff G, Behrend M, Wagner TO et al. (1991). Early diagnosis and effective treatment of pulmonary CMV infection after lung transplantation. J Heart Lung Transplant 10: 9.

Stoffel M, Pirson Y, Squifflet JP et al. (1988). Treatment of cytomegalovirus pneumonitis with ganciclovir in renal transplantation. Transpl Int 1: 181.

Stratta RJ, Shaefer MS, Markin RS et al. (1989). Clinical patterns of cytomegalovirus disease after liver transplantation. Arch Surg 124: 1443.

Stratta RJ, Shaefer MS, Cushing KA et al. (1991a). Successful prophylaxis of cytomegalovirus disease after primary CMV exposure in liver transplant recipients. Transplantation 51: 90.

Stratta R, Shaefer M, Markin RS et al. (1991b). Ganciclovir therapy for viral disease in liver transplant recipients. Transplant Proc 23: 1968.

Stratta RJ, Taylor RJ, Bynon JS et al. (1994). Viral prophylaxis in combined pancreas-kidney transplant recipients. Transplantation 57: 506.

Streicher HZ, Hung CL, Ablashi DV et al. (1988). In vitro inhibition of human herpesvirus-6 by phosphonoformate. J Virol Methods 21: 301.

Studies of Ocular Complications of AIDS Research Group in collaboration with the AIDS Clinical Trials Group (1992). Mortality in patients with acquired immune deficiency syndrome treated with either foscarnet or ganciclovir for cytomegalovirus retinitis. New Engl J Med 326: 213.

Studies of Ocular Complications of AIDS Research Group in collaboration with the AIDS Clinical Trials Group (1994). Foscarnet-ganciclovir cytomegalovirus retinitis trial. 4. Visual outcomes. Studies of ocular complications of AIDS Research Group in collaboration with the AIDS Clinical Trials Group. Ophthalmology 101: 1250.

Studies of Ocular Complications of AIDS Research Group, in collaboration with the AIDS Clinical Trials Group (1995). Morbidity and toxic effects associated with ganciclovir or foscarnet therapy in a randomised cytomegalovirus retinitis trial. Arch Intern Med 155: 74.

Studies of Ocular Complications of AIDS Research Group in collaboration with the AIDS Clinical Trials Group (1996). Combination foscarnet and ganciclovir therapy vs monotherapy for the treatment of relapsed cytomegalovirus retinitis in patients with AIDS. Arch Ophthalmol 114: 23.

Studies of Ocular Complications of AIDS SOCA Research Group (1992). Mortality in patients with the Acquired Immune Deficiency Syndrome treated with either foscarnet or ganciclovir for cytomegalovirus retinitis. New Engl J Med 326: 213.

Sullivan V, Talarico CL, Stanat SC et al. (1992a). A protein kinase homologue controls phosphorylation of ganciclovir in human cytomegalovirus-infected cells. Nature 358: 162.

Sullivan V, Talarico CL, Stanat SC et al. (1992b). A protein kinase homologue controls phosphorylation of ganciclovir in human cytomegalovirus-infected cells. Nature 359: 85.

Sullivan V, Biron KK, Talarico C et al. (1993). A point mutation in the human cytomegalovirus DNA polymerase gene confers resistance to ganciclovir and phosphonylmethoxyalkyl derivatives. Antimicrob Ag Chemother 37: 19.

Swan SK, Munar MY, Wigger MA, Bennett WM (1991). Pharmacokinetics of ganciclovir in a patient undergoing hemodialysis. Amer J Kidney Dis 17: 69.

Syndman DR (1988). Ganciclovir therapy for cytomegalovirus disease associated with renal transplants. Rev Infect Dis 10: S554.

Syntex Product Information (1995).

Tatarowic W Z, Lurain NS, Thompson KD et al. (1992). A ganciclovir-resistant clinical isolate of human cytomegalovirus exhibiting cross-resistance to other DNA polymerase inhibitors. J Infect Dis 166: 904.

The Oral Ganciclovir European and Australian Co-operative Study Group (1995). Intravenous versus oral ganciclovir: European/Australian comparative study of efficacy and safety in the prevention of cytomegalovirus retinitis recurrence in patients with AIDS. AIDS 9: 471.

Tiberghien P, Reynolds CW, Keller J et al. (1994). Ganciclovir treatment of herpes simplex thymidine kinase-transduced primary T lymphocytes; an approach for specific in vivo donor T-cell depletion after bone marrow transplantation. Blood 84: 1333.

Tocci MJ, Livelli TJ, Perry HC et al. (1984). Effects of the nucleoside analog 2'-nor-2'-deoxyguanosine on human cytomegalovirus replication. Antimicrob Ag Chemother 25: 247.

Trang JM, Kidd L, Gruber W et al. (1993). Linear single-dose pharmacokinetics of ganciclovir in newborns with congenital cytomegalovirus infections. NIAID Collaborative Antiviral Study Group. Clin Pharmacol Ther 53: 15.

Trousdale MD, Goldschmidt PL, Nobrega R et al. (1994). Activity of ganciclovir against human adenovirus type-5 infection in cell culture and cotton rat eyes. Cornea 13: 435.

Tyms AS (1984). BWB759U, an analogue of acyclovir, inhibits human cytomegalovirus in vitro. Lancet ii: 924.

United States Pharmacopeia Drug Information (1995).

Ussery FM, Gibson SR, Conklin RH et al. (1988). Intravitreal ganciclovir in the treatment of AIDS-associated cytomegalovirus retinitis. Ophthalmology 95: 640.

Vallejo JG, Englund JA, Garcia-Prats JA, Demmier GJ (1994). Ganciclovir treatment of steroid-associated cytomegalovirus disease in a congenitally infected neonate. Pediatr Infect Dis J 13: 239.

van den Berg AP, Tegzess AM, Schotten-Sampson A et al. (1992). Monitoring antigenemia is useful in guiding treatment of severe cytomegalovirus disease after organ transplantation. Transplant Int; 5: 101.

van der Ende ME, van Buuren AC, Kroes AC, ten Kate FJ (1992). Failure of antiviral therapy in AIDS-associated cytomegalovirus cholangitis. Infection 20: 6.

van der Horst CM, Lin JC, Raab-Traub N et al. (1987). Differential effects of acyclovir and 2-(1,3-dihdroxy-2-propoxymethyl)guanine on herpes simplex virus and Epstein-Barr virus in a dually infected human lymphoblastoid cell line. J Virol 61: 607.

von Bueltzingsloewen A, Bordigoni P, Witz F et al. (1993). Prophylactic use of ganciclovir for allogeneic bone marrow transplant recipients. Bone Marrow Transplant 12: 197.

Wahren B, Larsson A, Ruden U et al. (1987). Acyclic guanosine analogs as inhibitors of human cytomegalovirus. Antimicrob Ag Chemother 31: 317.

Wang Y, Bowden S, Shaw T et al. (1991). Inhibition of duck hepatitis B virus replication in vivo by the nucleoside analogue ganciclovir (9-[2-hydroxy-1-(hydroxymethyl) ethoxymethyl] guanine. Antiviral Chem Chemother; 2: 000.

Wang Y, Luscombe C, Bowden S *et al.* (1995). Inhibition of duck hepatitis B virus DNA replication by antiviral chemotherapy with ganciclovir-nalidixic acid. *Antimicrob Ag Chemother* **39**: 556.

Watson FS, O'Connell JB, Amber TJ *et al* (1988). Treatment of cytomegalovirus pneumonia in heart transplant recipients with 9(1,3-dihydroxy-2-proproxymethyl)-guanine (DHPG). *J Heart Transplant* **7**: 102.

Weinberg DV, Murphy R, Naughton K *et al.* (1994). Combined daily therapy with intravenous ganciclovir and foscarnet for patients with recurrent cytomegalovirus retinitis. *Amer J Ophthalmol* **117**: 776.

Wilcox CM, Schwartz DA (1992). Symptomatic CMV doudenitis. An important clinical problem in AIDS. *J Clin Gastroenterol* **14**: 293.

Wilcox CM, Straub RF, Schwartz DA *et al.* (1995). Cytomegalovirus esophagitis in AIDS: A prospective evaluation of clinical response to ganciclovir therapy, relapse rate, and long-term outcome. *Amer J Med* **98**: 169.

Wilson EJ, Medearis DN, Hansen LA, Rubin RH (1987). 9-(1–3-dihydroxy-2-propoxymethyl)guanine prevents death but not immunity in murine cytomegalovirus-infected normal and immunosuppressed BALB/c mice. *Antimicrob Ag Chemother* **31**: 1017.

Winston DJ, Ho WG, Bartoni K *et al.* (1988). Ganciclovir therapy for cytomegalovirus infections in recipients of bone marrow transplants and other immunosuppressed patients. *Rev Infect Dis* **10**: S547.

Winston DJ, Ho WG, Bartoni K *et al.* (1993). Ganciclovir prophylaxis of cytomegalovirus infection and disease in allogeneic bone marrow transplant recipients Results of a placebo controlled double blind trial. *Ann Intern Med* **118**: 179.

Winston DJ, Wirin D, Shaked A, Busuttil RW (1995). Randomised comparison of ganciclovir and high-dose acyclovir for long-term cytomegalovirus prophylaxis in liver transplant recipients. *Lancet* **346**: 69.

Wolf DG, Smith IL, Lee DJ *et al.* (1995a). Mutations in human cytomegalovirus UL97 gene confer clinical resistance to ganciclovir and can be detected directly in patient plasma. *J Clin Invest* **95**: 257.

Wolf DG, Lee DJ, Spector SA (1995b). Detection of human cytomegalovirus mutations associated with ganciclovir resistance in cerebrospinal fluid of AIDS patients with central nervous system disease. *Antimicrob Ag Chemother* **39**: 2552.

Yang H, Datema R (1991). Prolonged and potent therapeutic and prophylactic effects of (S)-1-[(3-hydroxy-2-phosphonylmethoxy)propyl)-cytosine against herpes simplex virus type 2 infections in mice. *Antimicrob Ag Chemother* **35**: 1596.

Yao GQ, Grill S, Egan W, Cheng YC (1993). Potent inhibition of Epstein–Barr virus by phosphorothioate oligodeoxynucleotides without sequence specification. *Antimicrob Ag Chemother* **37**: 1420.

Yau JC, Dimopoulos MA, Huan SD *et al.* (1991). Prophylaxis of cytomegalovirus infection with ganciclovir in allogeneic marrow transplantation. *Eur J Haematol* **47**: 371.

Yoshida K, Kawami H, Yamaguchi Y *et al.* (1995). Retrovirally transmitted gene therapy for gastric carcinoma using herpes simplex virus thymidine kinase gene. *Cancer* **75**: 1467.

Young SH, Morlet N, Heery S *et al.* (1992). High dose intravitreal ganciclovir in the treatment of cytomegalovirus retinitis. *Med J Aust* **157**: 370.

Zaia JA (1993). Prevention and treatment of cytomegalovirus pneumonia in transplant recipients. *Clin Infect Dis* **17**: S392.

Zamora MR, Fullerton DA, Campbell DN *et al.* (1994). Use of cytomegalovirus (CMV) hyperimmune globulin for prevention of CMV disease in CMV seropositive lung transplant recipients. *Transplant Proc* **26**: 49.

Zucker GM, Otis C, Korowski K, Navah F (1994). Cytomegalovirus gastritis associated with pseudolymphoma. *J Clin Gastroenterol* **18**: 222.

Zwartouw HT, Humphreys CR, Collins P *et al.* (1989). Oral chemotherapy of fatal B virus (herpesvirus simiae) infection. *Antiviral Res* **11**: 275.

Cidofovir

Description

Cidofovir (1-(S)-(3-hydroxy-2-phosphonylmethoxypropyl)cytosine or HPMPC, formerly known as GS-504) is a monophosphate nucleotide analog which, following conversion to the diphosphate derivative, has activity against a broad range of viruses, especially cytomegalovirus. It has been developed by Gilead Sciences Inc., under the trade name of 'Vistide'.

The molecular formula is $C_8H_{14}N_3O_6P.2H_2O$. The chemical structure is shown in Fig. V.19. The molecular weight is 315.2 (279.2 for anhydrous form). The concentration of the drug can be expressed as μg per ml or μM (1 μg per ml is equivalent to 3.6 μM).

Antiviral Activity

Cidofovir has excellent activity against herpes simplex types 1 and 2, including thymidine kinase (TK) deficient strains, varicella-zoster virus and cytomegalovirus infections when tested *in vitro* and in animal models (Bronson *et al.*, 1989; Snoeck *et al.*, 1988; De Clercq *et al.*, 1987; reviewed in Lalezari *et al.*, 1996). It is considered to be more active than either aciclovir or ganciclovir in the treatment and prophylaxis of herpes simplex virus types 1 and 2, varicella-zoster virus or cytomegalovirus infections in animal models (reviewed in De Clercq, 1993). It is the most potent and selective anti-cytomegalovirus compound identified so far, and has the longest duration of action. Cidofovir also has activity against human herpesvirus type 6, adenovirus, vaccinia, polyoma virus, hepatitis and papilloma viruses (Hitchcock *et al.*, 1996).

1 Cytomegalovirus

Cidofovir has a concentration-dependent, prolonged antiviral effect against cytomegalovirus *in vitro*, evident even with pretreatment of host cells and removal of drug from culture medium prior to infection (Neyts *et al.*, 1991; Otova *et al.*, 1992). The reported IC_{50} values, as assessed by inhibition of plaque formation, range from 0.1 to 0.25 μg per ml, with a selectivity index (ratio of the 50% inhibitory concentration for cellular growth to the 50% inhibitory concentration for virus plaque formation) of 300 to 1250 (Li *et al.*, 1990; Shigeta *et al.*, 1991; Snoeck *et al.*, 1991; Stals *et al.*, 1991). Cytomegalovirus DNA synthesis is completely inhibited at a concentration of cidofovir of 4 μg per ml (Neyts *et al.*, 1990). Cidofovir is about 5-fold more potent than ganciclovir *in vitro* against clinical and laboratory strains of cytomegalovirus (Andrei *et al.*, 1991).

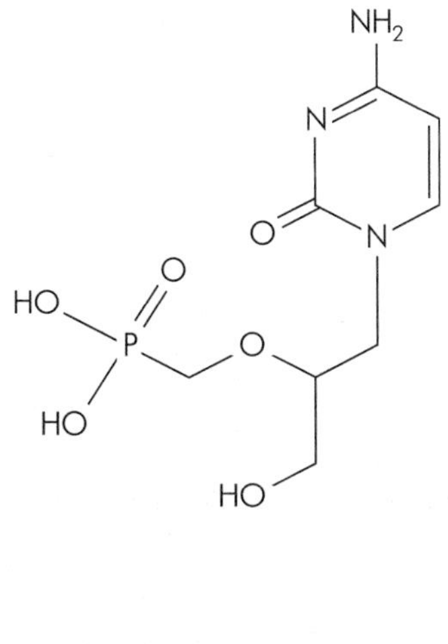

Fig. V.19.
Chemical structure of cidofovir.

Cytomegalovirus strains that are resistant to ganciclovir (due to a deficiency in ganciclovir phosphorylation because of mutations within UL97) remain sensitive in general to cidofovir (Stanat *et al.*, 1991). However, strains of cytomegalovirus with point mutations within the DNA polymerase gene rendering them resistant to ganciclovir have been found to be also cross-resistant to cidofovir (Sullivan *et al.*, 1993; Lurain *et al.*, 1992). Foscarnet-resistant strains of cytomegalovirus generally remain sensitive to both ganciclovir and cidofovir, although cross-resistance has recently been reported (reviewed in Hitchcock *et al.*, 1996). Cidofovir-resistant strains of cytomegalovirus have been selected by *in vitro* passage in the presence of increasing concentrations of the drug (Snoeck *et al.*, 1995). The IC_{50} of resistant strains ranges from 7 to 15 μM. Sequencing the DNA polymerase gene has identified a mutation within codon 513 (Lys$\rightarrow$Arg) which appears to be responsible for the development of resistance (reviewed in Hitchcock *et al.*, 1996).

Cidofovir has been shown in a number of studies to be more effective than ganciclovir in the treatment of intracerebral cytomegalovirus infection and interstitial pneumonitis in immunodeficient and immunocompetent mice and rats, in terms of delaying the onset of disease, improving survival and reducing virus titers in organs (De Castro *et al.*, 1991; Neyts *et al.*, 1992; Smee *et al.*, 1992; Stals 1993; Neyts *et al.*, 1993; Neyts and De Clercq, 1994a). Cidofovir has a relative therapeutic index that is 50-fold greater than that of ganciclovir (Smee *et al.*, 1992).

2 Herpes simplex virus

Cidofovir inhibits the replication of herpes simplex type 1 in Vero cells with reported IC_{50} to IC_{90} values of approximately 1–2 μg per ml (Chattergee *et al.*, 1992; Bravo *et al.*, 1993; Aduma *et al.*, 1995), although some investigators report that higher concentrations of cidofovir (5.6–25 μg per ml) are required for 50% inhibition (Andrei *et al.*, 1992). Similar to its effects on cytomegalovirus replication, exposure of cells to cidofovir for 12–24 h prior to the removal of drug and subsequent infection with herpes simplex results in long-lasting antiviral effects in excess of 7 days (Aduma *et al.*, 1995). Cidofovir also has potent and prolonged activity against herpes simplex type 2 (Yang and Datema, 1991; Bischofberger *et al.*, 1994).

Topical and systemic cidofovir therapy is efficacious in murine models of herpes simplex types 1 and 2 infection, including thymidine kinase (TK)-deficient strains (Maudgal and De Clercq, 1991a). Topical application of cidofovir (0.5%, 1% and 5% applied three times daily) was more effective than 5% acyclovir in treating primary genital herpes simplex types 1 and 2 infection of mice and guinea pigs (Bravo *et al.*, 1993). Intraperitoneal administration (100 or 250 mg per kg daily) suppresses the replication of herpes simplex type 1 in mice (De Clercq and Holy, 1991). Topical application of cidofovir (0.2%) also results in shorter healing times of herpes simplex type 1 dendritic keratitis in rabbits, lowers the virus titers within the eye, and shortens virus shedding in tears, with similar efficacy to trifluorothymidine (Maudgal and De Clercq, 1991b; Gordon *et al.*, 1994a). Intravitreal injection of cidofovir (100 μg per 0.1 ml) prior to intraocular infection with herpes simplex type 1 or within 7 days of viral inoculation protects rabbits from the development of retinitis for longer than 21 days (Flores-Aguilar *et al.*, 1994).

3 Varicella-zoster virus

Cidofovir is active *in vitro* against varicella-zoster virus, including TK-deficient aciclovir-resistant strains, with an IC_{50} value of 0.79 μM in human embryonic lung cells (De Clercq *et al.*, 1987; Snoeck *et al.*, 1992a, 1994a).

4 Epstein–Barr virus

Cidofovir has been reported to be active against Epstein–Barr virus with an IC_{50} for viral DNA replication of 0.03μM (Lin *et al.*, 1991). When compared with other antiviral compounds, cidofovir is more efficient than ganciclovir, adefovir (PMEA) and foscarnet and less efficient than sorivudine (BVaraU) in inhibiting clinical isolates and laboratory strains of varicella-zoster virus (Andrei *et al.*, 1995).

5 Human herpesvirus type 6

Cidofovir has activity against human herpesvirus type 6 (Reyman *et al.*, 1995).

6 Adenovirus

The earliest report of activity of cidofovir against three strains of adenovirus demonstrated an IC_{50} of 11 μM in human embryonic lung cells (De Clercq *et al.*, 1987). The mean IC_{50} of cidofovir against isolates of adenovirus type 8 is 0.47 μg per ml (range 0.02–0.82 μg per ml);

and 1.03 μg per ml (range 0.15–2.80 μg per ml) for adenovirus type 5 (Gordon *et al.*, 1994b). The range of IC_{50} values for laboratory strains and common clinical isolates of adenovirus (types 1, 5, 8 and 19) is 0.02–17.0 μg per ml with a high selectivity index (Gordon *et al.*, 1991; de Oliveira *et al.*, 1996). Topical administration of cidofovir inhibits replication of adenovirus type 5 in the New Zealand rabbit ocular model, resulting in reduced ocular viral titers and shortened duration of viral shedding (Gordon *et al.*, 1994b; De Oliveira *et al.*, 1996).

7 Other

The IC_{50} of cidofovir for equine herpesvirus type 1, as assessed by plaque reduction assay, is in the range of 0.03–0.07 μg per ml (Gibson *et al.*, 1992). A single subcutaneous dose of cidofovir (20 mg per kg) administered on the day prior to intranasal infection has been found to reduce clinical signs and virus replication, and also partially to protect mice from intracerebral inoculation of the virus (Gibson *et al.*, 1992). Cidofovir has been shown to prevent maternal transfer of equine herpesvirus type 1 to the fetus in a mouse model (Awan and Field, 1993). The drug also reduced replication of bovine herpesvirus type 1 and decreased clinical disease without preventing establishment of latency in calves treated with cidofovir 1 day prior to, or the day following virus inoculation (Gilliam and Field, 1993). Simian varicella infection can be inhibited *in vitro* and *in vivo* by cidofovir; a single 50 mg per kg i.v. dose prevents the development of rash, and improves survival in monkeys, even when administration is delayed for up to 4 days post-infection (Soike *et al.*, 1991).

The IC_{50} of cidofovir against one strain of vaccinia virus was found to be 13 μM (De Clercq *et al.*, 1987). Mortality associated with vaccinia virus infection of severe combined immunodeficient (SCID) mice is significantly delayed by cidofovir administration either prior to, coincident with, or post-infection (Neyts and De Clercq, 1993). Cidofovir inhibits the replication of African swine fever virus in Vero cells, with an IC_{50} of 1 μg per ml (Gil-Fernandez *et al.*, 1987). Cidofovir has also been reported to inhibit hepatitis B virus (Heijtink *et al.*, 1994).

8 Synergy and antagonism with other antiviral compounds

Foscarnet, ganciclovir and acyclovir demonstrate additive to synergistic inhibition of cytomegalovirus replication when combined with cidofovir *in vitro*. The synergism was more pronounced for clinical isolates of cytomegalovirus, compared with inhibition of activity against laboratory adapted strains (Snoeck *et al.*, 1992b). Depending on the ratios of the combined drugs, zidovudine and cidofovir may produce either a synergistic or antagonistic effect on inhibition of Epstein–Barr virus (Lin *et al.*, 1991). Zidovudine has also been reported to be synergistic with cidofovir against cytomegalovirus replication in a concentration-dependent manner (Snoeck *et al.* 1992b). Similarly, the concentration of ganciclovir used in combination with cidofovir may alter the inhibitory effect against cytomegalovirus: lower concentrations of ganciclovir are synergistic with cidofovir but higher concentrations of ganciclovir result in antagonism (Yang *et al.*, 1990).

Mode of Administration and Dosage

The long intracellular half-life of cidofovir with its subsequent prolonged antiviral effect allows infrequent dosing of cidofovir. The drug has been tested in phase I/II trials at doses of 0.5–10 mg per kg, administered i.v. once-weekly, but nephrotoxicity at doses of 3 mg per kg or greater was a dose-limiting factor. In an attempt to minimize nephrotoxicity, protocols then included probenecid and/ or concomitant hydration. The maximally tolerated weekly i.v. dose with probenecid is 5 mg per kg (Polis *et al.*, 1995). Cidofovir is currently administered in a modified regimen (Table V.12) including concomitant hydration (1 liter of saline over approximately 1 h immediately prior to cidofovir infusion) and administration of probenecid (2 g orally 3h prior to cidofovir infusion, 1 g 2 h post-infusion and 1 g 8 h post-infusion) in order to minimize renal toxicity (Lalezari *et al.*, 1994). The drug is administered via a peripheral vein over 1 h. For induction therapy, cidofovir is administered in a dose of 5 mg per kg in 100 ml of normal saline once-weekly for 2 weeks. The recommended dose for maintenance therapy is 5 mg per kg given i.v. in 100 ml of normal saline once every other week.The drug should be reduced to 3 mg per kg if serum creatine rises by 0.3–0.4 mg per dl above baseline, and should be discontinued if proteinuria (>3+) is documented or if serum creatinine increases more than 0.5 mg per dl above baseline (reviewed in Lalezari *et al.*, 1996).

Cidofovir has been encapsulated in liposomes and used as a delivery system in animal models of experimental retinitis (Besen *et al.*, 1995; Kuppermann *et al.*, 1996).

The effect of hemodialysis on cidofovir pharmacokinetics is not known. The drug is contraindicated in patients with a serum creatinine of greater than 1.5 mg per dl, or a creatinine clearance of less than 55 ml per min, or a urinary protein of greater than 100 mg per dl (2+ proteinuria).

Availability

The *i.v. preparation* of cidofovir is available in a 5ml *vial* containing 375 mg of cidofovir at a concentration of 75 mg per ml, formulated in water for injection and pH adjusted to 7.5.

Serum and Tissue Levels in Relation to Dose

1 Oral and subcutaneous administration

Oral bioavailability of cidofovir is less than 5% (Wachsman *et al.*, 1996). Subcutaneous administration is associated with good bioavailability (106%) but administration via this route is limited due to transient local fibrosis (Wachsman *et al.*, 1996).

2 Intravenous administration

Combined data from three phase I/II pharmacokinetic studies showed that serum levels of cidofovir following i.v. infusion were proportional to the dose over the range 1–10 mg per kg of body weight. Repeated dosing of cidofovir (3 or 10 mg per kg weekly) does not influence the pharmacokinetics of the drug (Cundy *et al.*, 1995). At doses of 3 and 5 mg per kg the peak plasma concentrations range from 7.3 to 20 μg per ml (approximately 26–72μM).

When administered with probenecid, cidofovir (5 mg per kg) has an AUC of 40.8 ± 9.0 μg.h per ml, with a C_{max} at the end of infusion of 19.6 ± 7.2 μg per ml (Cidofovir Product Information, 1996).

3 Intravitreal injection

The local half-life of cidofovir following intravitreal injection in rabbits is 24.4 h (Dolnak *et al.*, 1992). It is not available for intravitreal use in humans.

Excretion and Volume of Distribution in Body

Cidofovir is excreted largely by the kidney, by both glomerular filtration as well as active tubular secretion. Following i.v.infusion 90% of the dose of cidofovir is recovered unchanged in the urine within 24 h. The overall total clearance of cidofovir approximates renal clearance (Cundy *et al.*, 1995). The steady-state volume of distribution is approximately 500 ml per kg (Cundy *et al.*, 1995).

In preliminary studies, the CSF concentration of cidofovir (following i.v. infusion of 5 mg per kg) with co-administration of probenecid was undetectable (less than 0.1 μg per ml) whilst the corresponding plasma level was 8.7 μg per ml. Plasma protein binding of cidofovir is less than 6% (Cidofovir Product Information, 1996).

Mechanism of Action

Cidofovir is a member of a class of antiviral compounds known as phosphoryl-methylether nucleotide analogs (De Clercq *et al.*, 1986). It is a nucleotide analog of deoxycytidine monophosphate.

Within both infected and uninfected cells, cidofovir is phosphorylated by cellular enzymes to its mono- and then diphosphate derivative (Bronson *et al.*, 1990; Ho *et al.*, 1992; Neyts and De Clercq, 1994b). A third and major metabolite is the monophosphoryl-choline derivative. The diphosphate form corresponds to triphosphate analogs in terms of biologic activity. There is no significant difference in the concentration of cidofovir or its metabolites between infected and uninfected cells, suggesting that neither viral enzymes nor cellular enzymes induced by virus are required for its activation (Bronson *et al.*, 1990).

Cidofovir diphosphate acts as both an inhibitor of cytomegalovirus DNA polymerase as well as an alternate substrate for the enzyme, in competition with deoxycytidine triphosphate (Xiong *et al.*, 1995). The diphosphate form inhibits the viral DNA polymerase and thus viral DNA synthesis; the K_i for viral DNA polymerases being significantly lower (8- to 600-fold) than that for host cell DNA polymerases (Ho *et al.*, 1992). When it serves as an alternative substrate it can be incorporated into the growing DNA chain at the 3' end, resulting in chain-termination (reviewed in De Clercq, 1993). The antiviral activity of cidofovir is not reversed by the addition of cytidine or 2'-deoxycytidine suggesting that, unlike other deoxycytidine analogs, cidofovir does not depend on deoxycytidine kinase for its phosphorylation (Neyts *et al.*, 1991). The synthesis of cidofovir monophosphate is catalyzed by cellular pyrimidine nucleoside monophosphate kinase (Cihlar *et al.*,1992). The beta-oxygen atom of the phosphomethyl ether has been reported to be critical for the activity of cidofovir against herpes viruses (Kim *et al.*, 1991).

A limited exposure of infected cells to cidofovir results in pronounced and prolonged suppression of viral DNA synthesis and replication. The lasting antiviral effect of cidofovir (>7 days) can be attributed to the prolonged intracellular half-life of its metabolites (Moore *et al.*, 1994; Aduma *et al.*, 1995; reviewed in Hitchcock *et al.*, 1996). Cidofovir diphosphate accumulates within the cell, with a biphasic half-life (24 and 65 h) (Aduma *et al.*, 1995). The reported intracellular half-life of the active phosphodiester metabolite of cidofovir ranges from 48 to 87h (Ho *et al.*, 1992; Aduma *et al.*, 1995).

Toxicity

1 Pre-clinical studies

Cidofovir was reported to be embryotoxic in one study (Bila *et al.*, 1993), although in a separate study, when compared in mice with the related compound HPMPA, cidofovir was not found to be embryotoxic (Awan and Field, 1993). Cidofovir diphosphate is less inhibitory to human DNA polymerases beta and gamma than the triphosphate derivatives of zalcitabine and zidovudine (Cherrington *et al.*, 1994). At therapeutic concentrations cidofovir does not have a significant inhibitory effect on lymphocyte responses to T cell mitogens or on delayed type hypersensitivity responses (Simecka *et al.*, 1992). Similarly, cidofovir does not have any major inhibitory effect on colony forming unit formation by human granulocyte-macrophage progenitor cells (Snoeck *et al.*, 1990).

Nephrotoxicity (similar to Fanconi's syndrome) has been observed in animals exposed to cidofovir. Mild to moderate lesions resolve approximately 4 weeks after cessation of the drug. Cells within the proximal convoluted tubule are the principal targets of the drug. Monkeys given probenecid 1 h prior to cidofovir administration had less severe renal toxicity (reviewed in Hitchcock *et al.*, 1996).

2 Nephrotoxicity

The dose-limiting toxicity of cidofovir in clinical trials has been nephrotoxicity (Bischofberger *et al.*, 1994; Lalezari *et al.*, 1994). In phase I/II dose-escalation studies there was no nephrotoxicity in those receiving doses of less than 1.5 mg per kg twice-weekly. However, patients receiving doses of 3–5 mg per kg twice-weekly developed glycosuria and proteinuria, with elevated serum creatinine levels reported in some patients. Following the introduction of co-administration of probenecid and modifications to increase hydration (Table V.12), proteinuria was less frequently observed and creatinine levels remained within normal limits with doses of 3–7.5 mg per kg administered once-weekly (Polis *et al.*, 1995; Lalezari *et al.*, 1995). Probenecid

Table V.12
Cidofovir regimens used in phase I/II clinical trials. (Reproduced from Lalezari *et al.*, 1996, with permission.)

Dose (mg per kg)	Probenecid[a]	Dosing interval	Hydration [b]
Cidofovir alone			
0.5, 1.0, 3.0, 10.0	No	Once-weekly	±
Modified regimen			
3.0	Yes	Weekly	±
5.0	Yes	Weekly	±
5.0	Yes	Every 2 weeks[c]	±
7.5	Yes	Every 3 weeks	+

[a] Administered orally as 2 g (3 h pre-cidofovir), 1 g (2 h post-cidofovir), and 1 g (8 h post-cidofovir) (total dose = 4 g).
[b] Administered 1 liter normal saline over approximately 1 h immediately prior to cidofovir infusion.
[c] Administered every other week following two consecutive weekly doses.

is a benzoic acid derivative with a sulfa moiety. Probenecid hypersensitivity has been reported in approximately 16% of patients, all of whom were HIV- infected and had a past history of allergy to sulfa drugs. Not all patients with a history of sulfa intolerance develop hypersensitivity to probenecid. The symptoms of rash, nausea, vomiting and headache, usually develop 4–6 h after the third course of probenecid and recur with rechallenge. Probenecid desensitization has been successful (Lalezari et al., 1996). Administration of probenecid with doses of cidofovir greater than 3 mg per kg weekly results in reduced tubular secretion and clearance of cidofovir (Cundy et al., 1995).

3 Eye toxicity

Intravitreal injections of cidofovir have been found to be non-toxic to the retina in rabbits, even using concentrations up to 1000-fold higher than the effective dose (Dolnak et al., 1992). In clinical trials a significant decrease in intra-ocular pressure has been observed. A mild to moderate iritis has been found in about one-fifth of patients receiving a dose of 20 µg cidofovir administered intravitreally with oral probenecid (Kirsch et al., 1995a).

4 Other

Nausea, fever, alopecia, myalgia, neutropenia have been described in patients taking cidofovir (Lalezari et al., 1996).

5 Drug interactions

There is no apparent pharmacokinetic interaction between cidofovir and zidovudine (Cidofovir Product Information, 1996).

Clinical Uses of the Drug

1 Cytomegalovirus infection

There have now been a number of phase I and phase II/III studies of cidofovir which have been performed to determine the safety and efficacy of this drug in the treatment of AIDS-related cytomegalovirus retinitis.

In a phase I study, 75% of patients receiving 5 mg per kg twice-weekly and 50% of those receiving 5 mg per kg once-weekly or 7.5 mg per kg every 3 weeks had negative urine cultures for cytomegalovirus after 1–3 weeks of therapy, with evidence from sequential cultures of a prolonged antiviral effect (Polis et al., 1995). In a second study, cidofovir at doses of 3 and 10 mg per kg administered once-weekly demonstrated activity against cytomegalovirus with reduced titers in semen and urine (Lalezari et al., 1995). Overall, data from these studies show a virologic response rate of 93% and 74% for urine and semen cultures respectively (reviewed in Hitchcock et al., 1996). There was no loss of antiviral effect of cidofovir with concomitant probenecid (Lalezari et al., 1995), and no evidence of resistance to cidofovir emerging during treatment (Cherrington et al., 1996).

In an unblinded, uncontrolled study in a single center of patients with HIV-related active cytomegalovirus retinitis and no extraocular disease, a single intravitreal injection of cidofovir (20 µg) with concomitant oral probenecid resulted in a median time to disease progression of 55 days; following a repeat injection the subsequent time to progression was 63 days, indicating that prolonged suppression of disease can result from a single intravitreal injection of cidofovir (Kirsch et al., 1995a). A second unmasked, consecutive case study involving a similar population of patients with HIV-related cytomegalovirus retinitis were randomized to receive intravitreal cidofovir and i.v. ganciclovir or intravitreal cidofovir alone. The median times to progression of the two groups were 78 days and 63 days respectively, demonstrating the long duration of effect of cidofovir (Kirsch et al., 1995b).

In a phase II/III study HIV-infected patients with cytomegalovirus unresponsive to ganciclovir or foscarnet, or with intolerance to those drugs, were randomized to receive cidofovir at a dose of 5 mg per kg administered once-weekly for 2 weeks then 3 or 5 mg per kg administered every second week. Potential nephrotoxicity was minimized by co-administration of oral probenecid and normal saline. The median CD4 count at study entry was less than 10 cells per µl. The median times to progression were 115 and 49 days respectively in the 5 mg per kg and 3 mg per kg maintenance dose arms. Elevated creatinine levels developed in a total of four of 60 (7%) of patients, two in each arm of the study. Probenecid reactions occurred in 48% of patients and were mild to moderate and reversible; an additional two patients developed more serious but still reversible reactions (Lalezari *et al.*, 1996).

A study of 48 HIV-infected patients with untreated peripheral cytomegalovirus retinitis were randomized to receive either immediate cidofovir therapy (5 mg per kg weekly i.v for 2 weeks induction, and then once every 2 weeks for maintenance plus oral probenecid and i.v. saline hydration with each cidofovir infusion) or deferred therapy (no treatment until retinitis progressed). The study protocol enabled those on deferred therapy to obtain active drug if there was evidence of retinitis progression. The median times to progression for the deferred and immediate therapy groups were 22 days and 120 days respectively. Proteinuria developed in 23%, with discontinuation of drug in 13% due to proteinuria and in 5% because of elevation of serum creatinine. Probenecid reactions included rash and/or mild to moderate constitutional symptoms, and occurred in 55% of patients (reviewed in Hitchcock *et al.*, 1996).

2 Herpes simplex virus infection

A patient with HIV-related acyclovir-resistant herpes simplex perineal infection had prompt healing of lesions after four i.v. infusions of cidofovir (5 mg per kg weekly) with concomitant administration of probenecid and prehydration; recurrence was noted 2 weeks after cessation of therapy (Lalezari *et al.*, 1994). Similarly, topical cidofovir treatment of a bone marrow transplant recipient with orofacial herpes simplex infection that was resistant to aciclovir and foscarnet resulted in resolution of the lesions, with subsequent recurrence 1 week after cessation of therapy (Snoeck *et al.*, 1994b).

3 Papilloma infection

An elderly patient with squamous papilloma in the hypopharynx and esophagus that had been unresponsive to photocoagulation and interferon alpha therapy responded to weekly and then 3–5 once-weekly injections of cidofovir (1.25 mg per kg) into the tumor (Van Cutsem *et al.*, 1995).

Acknowledgements The author wishes to thank Sharon Safrin of Gilead Sciences Inc. for her critical review of this chapter.

References

Aduma P, Connelly MC, Srinivas RV, Fridland A (1995). Metabolic diversity and antiviral activities of acyclic nucleoside phosphonates. *Mol Pharmacol* **47**: 816.

Andrei G, Snoeck R, Schols D *et al.* (1991). Comparative activity of selected antiviral compounds against clinical isolates of human cytomegalovirus. *Eur J Clin Microbiol Infect Dis* **10**: 1026.

Andrei G, Snoeck P, Goubau J *et al.* (1992). Comparative activity of various compounds against clinical strains of herpes simplex virus. *Eur J Clin Microbiol Infect Dis* **11**: 143.

Andrei G, Snoeck R, Reymen D *et al.* (1995). Comparative activity of selected antiviral compounds against clinical isolates of varicella-zoster virus. *Eur J Clin Microbiol Infect Dis* **14**: 318.

Awan AR, Field HJ (1993). Effects of phosphonylmethoxyalkyl derivatives studied with a murine model for abortion induced by equine herpesvirus 1. *Antimicrob Ag Chemother* **37**: 2478.

Besen G, Flores-Aguilar M, Assil KK *et al.* (1995). Long-term therapy for herpes retinitis in an animal model with high-concentrated liposome-encapsulated HPMPC. *Arch Ophthalmol* **113**: 661.

Bila V, Otova B, Jelinek R *et al.* (1993). Antimitotic and teratogenic effects of acyclic nucleotide analogues 1-(S)-(-hydroxy-2-phosphonomethoxyethyl)cytosine (HPMPC) and 9-(2- phosphonomethoxyethyl) adenine (PMEA). *Folia Biol Praha* **39**: 150.

Bischofberger N, Hitchcock MJ, Chen MS *et al.* (1994). 1-[(S)-2-hydroxy-2-oxo-1,4,2- dioxaphosphorinan-5-yl)methyl] cytosine, an intracellular prodrug for (S)-1-(3-hydroxy-2- phosphonylmethoxypropyl)cytosine with improved therapeutic index *in vivo*. *Antimicrob Ag Chemother* **38**: 2387.

Bravo FJ, Stanberry LR, Kier AB *et al.* (1993). Evaluation of HPMPC therapy for primary and recurrent genital herpes in mice and guinea pigs. *Antiviral Res* **21**: 59.

Bronson JJ, Ghazzouli I, Hitchcock MJ *et al.* (1989). Synthesis and antiviral activity of the nucleotide analogue (S)-1-[3-hydroxy-2-(phosphonylmethoxy)propylicytosine. *J Medicinal Chemist* **32**: 1457.

Bronson JJ, Ho HT, De Boeck H *et al.* (1990). Biochemical pharmacology of acyclic nucleotide analogues. *Ann NY Acad Sci* **616**: 398.

Chatterjee S, Burns P, Whitley RJ, Kern ER (1992). Effect of (S)-1-[(3-hydroxy-2-phosphoryl methoxy) propyl] cytosine on the replication and morphogenesis of herpes simplex virus type 1. *Antiviral Res* **19**: 181.

Cherrington JM, Allen SJ, McKee BH, Chen MS (1994). Kinetic analysis of the interaction between the diphosphate of (S)-1-(3-hydroxy-2-phosphonylmethoxypropyl)cytosine, ddCTP, AZTTP and FIAUTP with human DNA polymerases beta and gamma. *Biochem Pharmacol* **48**: 1986.

Cherrington JM, Miner R, Hitchcock MJ et al. (1996). Susceptibility of human cytomegalovirus to cidofovir is unchanged after limited in vivo exposure to various regimens of drug. J Infect Dis 173: 987.

Cidofovir Product Information, Gilhead Sciences (1996).

Cihlar T, Votruba I, Horska K, Liboska R (1992). Metabolism of 1-(S)-(3-hydroxy-2-phosphonomethoxypropyl)cytosine (HPMPC) in human embryonic lung cells. Collect Czech Chem Commun 57: 661.

Cundy KC, Petty BG, Flaherty J et al. (1995). Clinical pharmacokinetics of cidofovir in human immunodeficiency virus-infected patients. Antimicrob Ag Chemother 39: 1247.

De Castro LM, Kern ER, De Clercq E et al. (1991). Phosphonylmethoxyalkyl purine and pyrimidine derivatives for treatment of opportunistic cytomegalovirus and herpes simplex virus infections in murine AIDS. Antiviral Res 16: 101.

De Clercq E (1993). Antivirals for the treatment of herpesvirus infection. J Antimicrob Chemother 32: S121.

De Clercq E, Holy A (1991). Efficacy of (S)-1-(3-hydroxy-2-phosphonylmethoxypropyl)cytosine in various models of herpes simplex virus infection in mice. Antimicrob Ag Chemother 35: 701.

De Clercq E, Holy A, Rosenberg I et al. (1986). A novel selective broad spectrum anti-DNA virus agent. Nature 323: 464.

De Clercq E, Sakuma T, Baba M et al. (1987). Antiviral activity of phosphonylmethoxyalkyl derivatives of purine and pyrimidines. Antiviral Res 8: 261.

De Oliveira CBR, Stevenson D, LaBree L et al. (1996). Evaluation of cidofovir (HPMPC, GS-504) against adenovirus type 5 infection in vitro and in a New Zealand rabbit ocular model. Antiviral Res 31: 165.

Dolnak DR, Munguia D, Wiley CA et al. (1992). Lack of retinal toxicity of the anticytomegalovirus drug (S)-1-(3-hydroxy-2-phosphonyimethoxypropyl) cytosine. Invest Ophthalmol Vis Sci 33: 1557.

Flores-Aguilar M, Huang JS, Wiley CA et al. (1994). Long-acting therapy of viral retinitis with (S)- 1-(3-hydroxy-2-phosphonylmethoxypropyl) cytosine. J Infect Dis 169: 642.

Gibson JS, Slater JD, Field HJ (1992). The activity of (S)-1-[(3-hydroxy-2-phosphoryl methoxy) propyl] cytosine (HPMPC) against equine herpesvirus-1 (EHV-1) in cell cultures, mice and horses. Antiviral Res 19: 219.

Gil-Fernandez C, Garcia-Villalon D, De Clercq E et al. (1987). Phosphonylmethoxyalkylpurines and – pyrimidines as inhibitors of African swine fever virus replication in vitro. Antiviral Res 8: 273.

Gilliam SE, Field HJ (1993). The effect of (S)-1-(3-hydroxy-2-phosphorylmethoxypropyl)cytosine (HPMPC) on bovine herpesvirus-1 (BHV-1) infection and reactivation in cattle. Antiviral Res 20: 21.

Gordon YJ, Romanowski E, Araullo-Cruz T et al. (1991). Inhibitory effect of (S)-HPMPM, (S)- HPMPA and 2'-nor-cyclic GMP on clinical ocular adenoviral isolates is serotype-dependent in vitro. Antiviral Res 16: 15213.

Gordon YJ, Romanowski EG, Araullo-Cruz T (1994a). HPMPC a broadspectrum topical antiviral agent, inhibits herpes simplex virus type 1 replication and promotes healing of dendritic keratitis in the New Zealand rabbit ocular model. Cornea 13: 516.

Gordon J, Romonowski EG, Araullo-Cruz T (1994b). Topical HPMPC inhibits adenovirus type 5 in the New Zealand rabbit ocular replication model. Invest Ophthalmol Vis Sci 35: 4135.

Heijtink RA, Kruining J, De Wilde GA et al. (1994). Inhibitory effects of acyclic nucleoside phosphonates on human hepatitis B virus and duck hepatitis B virus infections in tissue culture. Antimicrob Ag Chemother 38: 2180.

Hitchcock MJ, Jaffe HS, Martin JC, Stagg RJ (1996). Cidofovir, a new agent with potent anti- herpesvirus activity. Antiviral Chem Chemother 7: 115.

Ho HT, Woods KL, Bronson JJ et al. (1992). Intracellular metabolism of the antiherpes agent (S)- 1[3-hydroxy-2-(phosphonylmethoxy)propyl]cytosine. Mol Pharmacol 41: 197.

Kim CU, Misco PF, Luh BY et al. (1991). A new class of acyclic phosphonate nucleotide analogues; phosphonate isosteres of acyclovir and ganciclovir monophosphates as antiviral agents. J Med Chem 34: 2286.

Kirsch LS, Arevalo JF, Chavez de laPaz E et al. (1995a). Intravitreal cidofovir (HPMPC) treatment of cytomegalovirus retinitis in patients with acquired immune deficiency syndrome. Ophthalmology 102: 533.

Kirsch LS, Arevalo JF, De Clercq E et al. (1995b). Phase I/II study of intravitreal cidofovir for the treatment of cytomegalovirus retinitis in patients with the acquired immunodeficiency syndrome. Amer J Ophthalmol 119: 466.

Kuppermann BD, Assil KK, Vuong C et al. (1996). Liposome-encapsulated (S)-1-(3-hydroxy-2- phosphonylmethoxypropyl)cytosine for long-acting therapy of viral retinitis. J Infect Dis 173: 18.

Lalezari JP, Drew WL, Glutzer E et al. (1994). Treatment with intravenous (S)-1-[3-hydroxy-2- (phosphonylmethoxy)propyl]-cytosine of acyclovir-resistant mucocutaneous infection with herpes simplex virus in a patient with AIDS. J Infect Dis 170: 570.

Lalezari JP, Drew WL, Glutzer E et al. (1995). (S)-1-[3-Hydroxy-2-(Phosphonylmethoxy)propyl]cytosine (codofovir): results of a Phase I/II study of a novel antiviral nucleotide analogue. J Infect Dis 171: 788.

Lalezari JP, Stagg RJ, Jaffe HS et al. (1996). A preclinical and clinical overview of the nucleotide- based antiviral agent cidofovir (HPMPC). In Antiviral Chemotherapy Vol 4 (Mills J, Volberding P, Corey L, eds), p. 105. New York: Plenum Publishing Corporation.

Li SB, Yang ZH, Feng JS et al. (1990). Activity of (S)-1-(3-hydroxy-2-phosphonylmethoxypropyl)cytosine (HPMPC) against guinea pig cytomegalovirus infection in cultured cells and in guinea pigs. Antiviral Res 13: 237.

Lin JC, De Clercq E, Pagano JS (1991). Inhibitory effects of acyclic nucleoside phosphonate analogs, including (S)-1-(3-hydroxy-2-phosphonylmethoxypropyl)cytosine, on Epstein–Barr virus replication. Antimicrob Ag Chemother 35: 2440.

Lurain NS, Thompson KD, Holmes EW, Read GS (1992). Point mutations in the DNA polymerase gene of human cytomegalovirus that result in resistance to antiviral agents. J Virol 66: 7146.

Maudgal PC, De Clercq E (1991a). (S)-1-(3-hydroxy-2-phosphorylmethoxypropyl)cytosine in the therapy of thymidine kinase positive and deficient herpes simplex virus experimental keratitis. Invest Ophthalmol Vis Sci 32: 1816.

Maudgal PC, De Clercq E (1991b). Effects of phosphonylmethoxyalkylpurine and pyrimidine derivatives on TK+ and TK- HSV-1 keratitis in rabbits. Antiviral Res 16: 93.

Moore MR, Hamzeh FM, Lee FE, Lietman PS (1994). Activity of (S)-1-(3-hydroxy-2- phosphonylmethoxypropyl) cytosine against human cytomegalovirus when administered as single-bolus dose and continuous infusion in in vitro cell culture perfusion system. Antimicrob Ag Chemother 38: 2404.

Neyts J, De Clercq E (1993). Efficacy of (S)-1-(3-hydroxy-2-phosphonylmethoxypropyl)cytosine for the treatment of lethal vaccinia virus infections in severe combined immune deficiency (SCID) mice. J Med Virol 41: 242.

Neyts J, De Clercq E (1994a). New inhibitors of cytomegalovirus replication in vitro evaluation, mechanism of action and in vivo activity. Verh K Acad Geneeskd Belg 56: 561.

Neyts J, De Clercq E (1994b). Mechanism of action of acyclic nucleoside phosphonates against herpes virus replication. Biochem Pharmacol 47: 39.

Neyts J, Snoeck R, Schols D et al. (1990). Selective inhibition of human cytomegalovirus DNA synthesis by (S)-1-(3-hydroxy-2-phosphonylmethoxypropyl)cytosine [(S)-HPMPC] and 9-(1,3-dihydroxy- 2-propoxymethyl)guanine (DHPG). Virology 179: 41.

Neyts J, Snoeck R, Balzarini J, De Clercq E (1991). Particular characteristics of the anti-human cytomegalovirus activity of (S)-1-(3-hydroxy-2-phosphonylmethoxypropyl) cytosine (HPMPC) in vitro. Antiviral Res 16: 41.

Neyts J, Balzarini J, Naesens L, De Clercq E (1992). Efficacy of (S)-1-(3-hydroxy-2- phosphonylmethoxypropyl)cytosine and 9-(1,3-dihydroxy-2-propoxymethyl)guanine for the treatment for murine cytomegalovirus infection in severe combined immunodeficiency mice. J Med Virol 37: 67.

Neyts J, Sobis H, Snoeck R *et al.* (1993). Efficacy of (S)-1-(3-hydroxy-2-phosphonylmethoxypropyl)-cytosine and 9-(1,3-dihydroxy-2-propoxymethyl)-guanine in the treatment of intracerebral murine cytomegalovirus infections in immunocompetent and immunodeficient mice. *Eur J Clin Microbiol Infect Dis* **12**: 269.

Otova B, Votruba I, Holy A (1992). Pretreatment of the host cell with 1-(S)-(3-hydroxy-2-phosphonylmethoxypropyl)cytosine (HPMPC) is sufficient for its antiviral effect. *Acta Virol* **36**: 313.

Polis MA, Spooner KM, Baird BF *et al.* (1995). Anticytomegaloviral activity and safety of cidofovir in patients with human immunodeficiency virus infection and cytomegalovirus viruria. *Antimicrob Ag Chemother* **39**: 882.

Reyman D, Naesens L, Balzarini J *et al.* (1995). Antiviral activity of selected nucleoside analogues against human herpes virus type 6. *Antiviral Res* **26**: A326.

Shigeta S, Konno K, Baba M *et al.* (1991). Comparative inhibitory effects of nucleoside analogues on different clinical isolates of human cytomegalovirus *in vitro*. *J Infect Dis* **163**: 270.

Simecka JW, Patel P, Kern ER (1992). Immunotoxic potential of antiviral drugs; effects of ganciclovir and (S)-1-(3-hydroxy-2-phosphonyimethoxypropyl) cytosine on lymphocyte transformation and delayed type hypersensitivity responses. *Antiviral Res* **18**: 53.

Smee DF, Morris JL, Leonhardt JA *et al.* (1992). Treatment of murine cytomegalovirus infections in severe combined immunodeficient mice with ganciclovir, (S)-1-[3-hydroxy-2- (phosphonylmethoxy)propyl]cytosine, interferon, and bropirimine. *Antimicrob Ag Chemother* **36**: 1837.

Snoeck R, SakumaT, De Clercq E *et al.* (1988). (S)-1-(3-hydroxy-2-phosphonylmethoxypropyl)cytosine, a potent and selective inhibitor of human cytomegalovirus replication. *Antimicrob Ag Chemother* **32**: 1839.

Snoeck R, Lagneaux L, Delforge A *et al.* (1990). Inhibitory effects of potent inhibitors of human immunodeficiency virus and cytomegalovirus on the growth of human granulocyte-macrophage progenitor cells *in vitro*. *Eur J Clin Microbiol Infect Dis* **9**: 615.

Snoeck R, Schols D, Andrei G *et al.* (1991). Antiviral activity of anticytomegalovirus agents (HPMPC, HPMPA) assessed by a flow cytometric method and DNA hybridization technique. *Antiviral Res* **16**: 1.

Snoeck R, Schols D, Sadzot-Delvaux C *et al.* (1992a). Flow cytometric method for the detection of gp1 antigens of varicella zoster virus and evaluation of anti-VZV agents. *J Virol Methods* **38**: 243.

Snoeck R, Andrei G, Schols D *et al.* (1992b). Activity of different antiviral drug combinations against human cytomegalovirus replication *in vitro*. *Eur J Clin Microbiol Infect Dis* **11**: 1144.

Snoeck R, Gerard M, Sadzot-Delvaux C *et al.* (1994a). Meningoradiculoneuritis due to acyclovir- resistant varicella zoster virus in an acquired immune deficiency syndrome patient. *J Med Virol* **42**: 338.

Snoeck R, Andrei G, Gerard M *et al.* (1994b). Successful treatment of progressive mucocutaneous infection due to acyclovir and foscarnet-resistant herpes simplex virus with (S)-1-(3-hydroxy-2- phosphonylmethoxypropyl)cytosine (HPMPC). *Clin Infect Dis* **18**: 570.

Snoeck R, Andrei G, De Clercq E (1995). Human cytomegalovirus (HCMV) strains selected under selective pressure of phosphonoformate (PFA) are resistant for both PFA and phosphonylmethoxyethyl (PME) derivatives *in vitro*. *Antiviral Res* **26**: A320.

Soike KF, Huang JL, Zhang JY *et al.* (1991). Evaluation of infrequent dosing regimens with (S)-1- [3-hydroxy-2-(phosphonylmethoxy)propyl]-cytosine (S-HPMPC) on simian varicella infection in monkeys. *Antiviral Res* **16**: 17.

Stals FS, De Clercq E, Bruggeman CA (1991). Comparative activity of (S)-1-(3-hydroxy-2- phosphonylmethoxypropyl)cytosine and 9-(1,3-dihydroxy-2-propoxymethyl)guanine against rat cytomegalovirus infection *in vitro* and *in vivo*. *Antimicrob Ag Chemother* **35**: 2262.

Stals FS, Zeytinoglu A, Havenith M *et al.* (1993). Rat cytomegalovirus-induced pneumonitis after allogeneic bone marrow transplantation, effective treatment with (S)-1-(3-hydroxy-2-phosphoryl- methoxypropyl) cytosine. *Antimicrob Ag Chemother* **37**: 218.

Stanat SC, Reardon JE, Erice A *et al.* (1991). Ganciclovir-resistant cytomegalovirus clinical isolates; mode of resistance to ganciclovir. *Antimicrob Ag Chemother* **35**: 2191.

Sullivan V, Biron KK, Talarico C *et al.* (1993). A point mutation in the human cytomegalovirus DNA polymerase gene confers resistance to ganciclovir and phosphonylmethoxyalkyl derivatives. *Antimicrob Ag Chemother* **37**: 19.

Van Cutsem E, Snoeck R, Van Ranst M *et al.* (1995). Successful treatment of a squamous papilloma of the hypopharynx-esophagus by local injections of (S)-1-(3-hydroxy-2- phosphonylmethoxypropyl)cytosine. *J Med Virol* **45**: 230.

Wachsman M, Petty BG, Cundy KC *et al.* (1996). Pharmacokinetics, safety and bioavailability of HPMPC (cidofovir) in human immunodeficiency virus-infected subjects. *Antiviral Res* **29**: 153.

Xiong X, Smith JJ, Chen MS (1995). The consequence of incorporation of (S)-1-[(3-hydroxy-2- phosphoryl-methoxypropyl)cytosine by human cytomegalovirus DNA polymerase on DNA elongation. *Antiviral Res* **26**: A321.

Yang H, Datema R (1991). Prolonged and potent therapeutic and prophylactic effects of (S)-1-[(3- hydroxy-2-phosphonylmethoxy)propyl]cytosine against herpes simplex virus type 2 infections in mice. *Antimicrob Ag Chemother* **35**: 1596.

Yang ZH, Crouch JY, Feng JS *et al.* (1990). Combined antiviral effects of paired nucleosides against guinea pig cytomegalovirus replication *in vitro*. *Antiviral Res* **14**: 249.

Sorivudine

Description

Sorivudine (1-beta-D-arabinofuranosyl-5-(E-2-bromovinyl)uracil, also known as BV-araU, and YN-72, and marketed under the trade names of 'Brovavir' and 'Usevir') was co-developed in Japan by Yamasa Corporation and Nippon Shoji, and co-marketed by Nippon Shoji and Eisai. Outside Japan the drug has been licensed to Bristol-Myers Squibb. Sorivudine is a uracil derivative with activity against herpes simplex type 1 and is especially potent against varicella-zoster virus.

The chemical name of sorivudine is (+)-1-beta-D-arabinofuranosyl-5-[(E)-2-bromovinyl]-uracil. The molecular formula is $C_{11}H_{13}BrN_2O_6$. The chemical structure is shown in Fig. V.20. The molecular weight of sorivudine is 349.14. Sorivudine concentrations can be reported in μg per ml or μM (1 μg per ml is approximately equivalent to 3μM).

Antiviral Activity

1 Herpes simplex virus

Sorivudine has good *in vitro* activity against herpes simplex type 1 in murine and human cells (IC_{50} of 0.03 μg per ml) but not against herpes simplex type 2 (IC_{50} >20 μg per ml) or cytomegalovirus (Machida *et al.*, 1981; Machida, 1986, 1990a,b; Ashida *et al.*, 1994). The mean IC_{50} of sorivudine measured by plaque reduction assay against seven strains of herpes simplex type 1 has been reported as 0.2 μg per ml (Machida, 1990a). Concentrations of sorivudine as high as 1000 μg per ml did not impair the growth of human embryonic lung fibroblast cells used in these assays (Machida *et al.*, 1981). There is reported variation in the antiviral activity of sorivudine against herpes simplex when assayed in different cell types (Suzutani *et al.*, 1988a; Machida *et al.*, 1991; Rabasseda *et al.*, 1993).

A survival benefit has been observed in mice with intracerebral, intraperitoneal and cutaneous herpes simplex type 1 infections treated with an oral dose of 20–50 mg per kg twice-daily, in some cases even when treatment was delayed for several days post-infection (Machida *et al.*, 1990a, 1992a; Ijichi *et al.*, 1990; Ashida *et al.*, 1994). Intraperitoneal injections of sorivudine (200 mg per kg daily) and i.v. administration of the drug have also

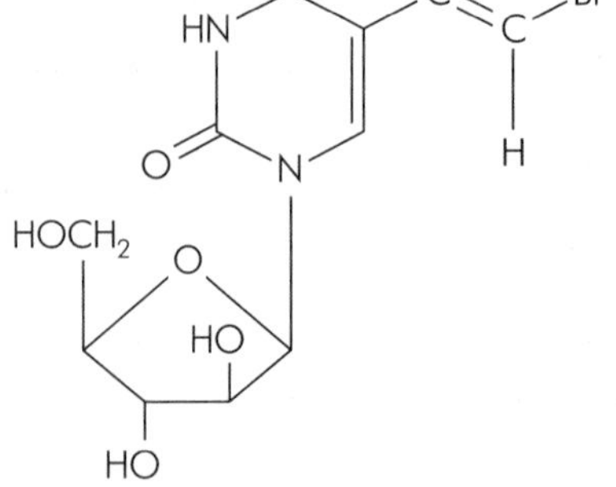

Fig. V.20.
Chemical structure of sorivudine.

Table V.13
Activity of selected antiviral compounds against varicella-zoster virus replication *in vitro*. (Adapted from Andrei *et al.*, 1995, with permission.)

Compound	IC$_{50}$ (μM)		
	Isolate 1	Isolate 2	Isolate 3
Aciclovir	1.7	1.0	2.4
Penciclovir	2.9	11.1	4.0
Sorivudine	0.0022	0.0016	0.0022
Foscarnet	100	50	57
Cidofovir	1.8	0.7	2.3

been reported to protect mice from lethal encephalitis due to herpes simplex type 1 infection (Machida and Sakata, 1984; Reefschlager *et al.*, 1986). However, some strains of herpes simplex type 1 are highly resistant to this drug (Machida and Takezawa, 1990). Topical treatment with sorivudine (5% cream) applied four times daily for 5 days post-infection of cutaneous herpes simplex infections in normal and immunosuppressed mice resulted in suppression of progression of lesions, again even if treatment were delayed for 48 h post-infection (Ijichi *et al.*, 1993). Sorivudine eyedrops (0.1%) can suppress the development of keratitis complicating experimental herpes simplex infection in rabbits, and reduce the virus titer in conjunctival swabs (Maudgal and De Clercq, 1985; Topke *et al.*, 1988; Rajcani and Reefschlager, 1987).

2 Varicella-zoster virus

Sorivudine has excellent activity against the Oka varicella vaccine virus as well as wild-type varicella-zoster virus, being about 1000–3000-fold more potent than aciclovir as assessed by plaque reduction assays; reported IC$_{50}$ values are 0.001–0.004 μg per ml (Machida *et al.*, 1990b, 1994; Shiraki *et al.*, 1993; Machida and Watanabe, 1991). Sorivudine is more potent than other antivirals that have reported activity against varicella-zoster virus including FIAC, aciclovir, penciclovir, ganciclovir and adefovir (PMEA) when tested in several different cell lines (Shigeta *et al.*, 1983; Baba *et al.*, 1986; Machida, 1986; Andrei *et al.*, 1995; Machida *et al.*, 1995a; Table V.13). Compared with aciclovir, the activity of sorivudine is about 1000–3000-fold greater against varicella-zoster virus (Machida, 1990b; Machida and Watanabe, 1991). The selectivity index for replication of varicella-zoster virus versus host cell DNA synthesis is 41 000 to 67 000 (Shigeta *et al.*, 1983). The IC$_{50}$ of sorivudine for cell-associated varicella-zoster virus has been reported to be higher than for cell-free virus (Shiraki *et al.*, 1992).

A mutation at position 18 (Asp –>Asn) of the varicella-zoster thymidine kinase (TK), as well as a single base pair deletion resulting in a frame-shift and premature termination of the viral DNA have been associated with development of resistance of varicella-zoster virus to sorivudine (Lacey *et al.*, 1991). Thymidine kinase-deficient strains of varicella-zoster virus that are resistant to aciclovir are not always cross-resistant to sorivudine; of nine aciclovir-resistant strains of varicella zoster, four were sensitive to sorivudine (Talarico *et al.*, 1993). Sorivudine-resistant strains are often but not always cross-resistant to 5-iododeoxyuridine and 5-bromodeoxyuridine (Sakuma, 1984).

3 Other

Sorivudine inhibits simian varicella virus with an IC$_{50}$ of approximately 0.05 μg per ml; when administered orally to African green monkeys in a dose of 0.1 mg per kg for 10 days or given by intramuscular injection, even when commenced up to 4 days post-infection with simian varicella virus, rash and viremia were suppressed (Soike *et al.*, 1984, 1992).

The replication of Epstein–Barr virus in superinfected Raji cells is inhibited by sorivudine with a similar IC$_{50}$ to that of aciclovir. There is however, a more prolonged antiviral effect following removal of sorivudine from culture when compared with aciclovir that has been observed in several studies (Farber *et al.*, 1987; Lin and Machida, 1988; Lin *et al.*, 1992).

Sorivudine has no activity against the human immunodeficiency virus (Machida *et al.*, 1992b).

Mode of Administration and Dosage

The optimal dosage is not clearly defined. A dose of 50 mg three times daily has been recommended, although this dose is associated with toxicity. Lower doses have been associated with efficacy in some clinical trials, as outlined below. A dose of 40 mg daily appears to be effective (R Whitley, personal communication, 1997).

A double-blind, placebo-controlled dose-ranging study (10–100 mg administered orally three times daily for 7 days) was performed to determine the optimum dose of sorivudine treatment in 226 immunocompetent patients with herpes zoster. Maximum efficacy was achieved with a dose of 150 mg daily (Niimura, 1990). A second study found that 30 mg per day was almost as effective as 150 mg per day, and both doses were considerably more effective than placebo, in terms of improvement of rash, duration of acute pain and eradication of virus (Niimura et al., 1990a). A third dose-ranging study was performed in immunosuppressed individuals with herpes zoster, and the findings suggested that a dose of 150 mg daily had superior efficacy to 30 mg daily (Hiraoka et al., 1991).

As sorivudine is excreted by the kidney, the dose should be carefully monitored in elderly patients and used with caution in patients with any renal dysfunction. The safety of sorivudine has not been established in pregnancy or lactation, and the drug should only be administered to pregnant women if the potential benefits outweigh possible risks to the fetus.

Availability

Tablets containing 50 mg of sorivudine.

Serum Levels in Relation to Dosage

Serum levels of sorivudine can be measured by high-performance liquid chromatography (HPLC) (Whigan and Cohen, 1991) or by radioassay (Jagoda et al., 1992).

Sorivudine is well absorbed in the rat intestine following oral administration, with a mean oral bioavailability of 63% (Ashida et al., 1994; Soike et al., 1990). In the rat, sorivudine has been found to be resistant to degradation by hepatic enzymes (Ashida et al., 1994), and degradation is apparently due to the action of enterobacteria (Machida et al., 1995b). The serum half-life in rats is about 4 h, with over 80% protein binding by the drug (Soike et al., 1990).

In humans, sorivudine is well absorbed and has good oral bioavailability, in the range of 50–70% (reviewed in Nikkels and Pierard, 1994). A single dose of 40 mg results in peak plasma concentrations (C_{max}) of 1.5–2 μg per ml, with trough levels at 24 h post-dose of 0.05 μg per ml (still significantly higher than the IC_{50} concentrations for varicella-zoster virus) (reviewed in Snoeck et al., 1994). The time to peak plasma concentration is approximately 12 h post-administration (Ogiwara et al., 1990). The mean peak serum level was found to be 1–2.5 μg per ml following repeated oral doses of 50 mg three times daily for 5 days; the level of the major metabolite E-5-(2-bromovinyl)uracil was about 0.4 μg per ml (Ogiwara et al., 1990).

Intravenous administration of 5, 10, or 20 mg of sorivudine once-daily for 10 days resulted in a dose-dependent peak serum concentration, and area-under-the-curve (AUC) concentration. The plasma levels of E-5-(2- bromovinyl)uracil were less than those found in blood following oral administration. An i.v. dose of sorivudine of 25 mg will result in approximately equivalent plasma concentrations as an oral dose of 40 mg (Olsen et al., 1991).

In elderly subjects a single oral dose of 40 mg of sorivudine was found to result in similar mean peak plasma concentrations and mean time to achieve peak plasma concentrations, steady-state volume of distribution and protein binding as in younger subjects; the AUC was slightly more prolonged, and elimination half-life higher in the older individuals. The mean serum level 24 h after administration was 0.16 and 0.10 μg per ml in the older and younger groups respectively (Sherman et al., 1990a).

Excretion and Distribution of the Drug in Body

Sorivudine is excreted in the urine (Sherman et al., 1990b). The major metabolite following oral administration of sorivudine is E-5-(2-bromovinyl)uracil, and 1–2% of the drug is excreted in urine as this derivative (Ogiwara et al., 1990; Ashida et al., 1993). The elimination half-life of sorivudine varies from 5 to 8 h, and is higher in elderly subjects compared with young adults (Snoeck et al., 1994).

In rabbits, there is very low intravitreal accumulation of sorivudine (0.1–0.2 μg per ml) 2 h after oral administration of a dose of 30 mg per kg. An intravitreal injection (100 μg) was associated with an intravitreal half-life of sorivudine of 2.4 h in rabbits (Mochizuki et al., 1994). Sorivudine is present in breast milk (Rabasseda et al., 1993).

Mode of Action

Sorivudine is selectively taken up by herpesvirus infected cells compared with uninfected cells (Suzutani *et al.*, 1988b; Yokota *et al.*, 1989; Machida, 1990a). Sorivudine is converted to the monophosphate derivative through the action of virus-specified TK (Yokota *et al.*, 1989), although cellular kinases have been reported by some investigators to catalyze this conversion (Kawai *et al.*, 1993); the monophosphate then inhibits thymidylate synthetase within the infected cell and suppresses viral replication (Kawai *et al.*, 1993), although other investigators report no inhibition of this enzyme by sorivudine in infected cells (Yokota *et al.*, 1993). The monophosphate is then converted into di- and triphosphate forms. There is competition between sorivudine and thymidine triphosphates for incorporation into DNA, mediated by viral and cellular DNA polymerases. It is clear that sorivudine triphosphate inhibits viral DNA polymerase, with a K_i value of $0.14\,\mu M$ which is significantly lower than values for cellular DNA polymerases (Descamps *et al.*, 1982), and although reported to also inhibit viral DNA synthesis by chain-termination, this mechanism of action has not been supported by the findings of others (reviewed in Gnann, 1994; Suzutani *et al.*, 1993; Yokota *et al.*, 1989). The poor activity of sorivudine against herpes simplex type 2 is due to the inability of type 2 kinases to effectively phosphorylate sorivudine in the infected cell (reviewed in Gnann, 1994). Di- and triphosphorylated derivatives of sorivudine are not found in herpes simplex type 2-infected cells (Ayisi *et al.*, 1987).

Toxicity

Pre-clinical animal studies found sorivudine to be safe, with no toxicity observed after single oral doses of 8000 mg per kg or 2000 mg per kg administered intraperitoneally or subcutaneously (Nagasaka *et al.*, 1990). At doses of 1000 and 4000 mg per kg daily administered for 4 weeks minor liver abnormalities were noted; a dose of less than 1000 mg per kg daily was non-toxic (Yoshifune *et al.*, 1993a). Longer-term therapy at doses of 80 mg per kg daily for 6 months were also not toxic to rats, although 400 mg per kg daily resulted in elevation of bilirubin and cholesterol levels (Yoshifune *et al.*, 1993b). Doses of up to 1000 mg per kg daily, prior to mating and during gestation and lactation, did not reduce fertility or cause fetal toxicity in rats (Ishida *et al.*, 1990).

Sorivudine has only a minor inhibitory effect on cell growth, with an IC_{50} value of 657 μg per ml; within the range of $1-800\,\mu g$ per ml there was no evidence of cellular mutagenesis (Suzutani and Machida, 1992).

In early phase I trials sorivudine was well tolerated, with the most frequent abnormality being an elevation of liver enzymes in between 4 and 7% of recipients (Hiraoka *et al.*, 1991). Caution should be used when administering sorivudine to any person with hepatic dysfunction. Other reported abnormalities include bone marrow suppression, gastrointestinal effects including vomiting, anorexia, diarrhea, and abdominal pain. In a small study, no clinically significant differences in safety were observed in HIV-infected patients taking zidovudine with either sorivudine or placebo (Olsen *et al.*, 1995).

When sorivudine was co-administered with 5-fluorouracil and related anticancer drugs in Japan, severe hematological and gastrointestinal toxicity was reported in 23 treated patients, resulting in at least 15 deaths (reviewed in Easterbrook and Wood, 1995; Fukushima, 1995). This is due to the inhibition of dihydropyrimidine dehydrogenase. This enzyme is rate-limiting in pyrimidine catabolism by a metabolite of sorivudine (5-(E-2- bromo-vinyl)uracil), and thus plasma levels of 5-fluorouracil are increased (Desgranges *et al.*, 1986; Machida *et al.*, 1995c). Subsequent treatment of two subjects with sorivudine (40 mg daily for 3 days) resulted in a decrease in the activity of dihydropyrimidine dehydrogenase in peripheral blood mononuclear cells by 90–100%, with recovery of activity occurring only 7–11 days following the last dose of sorivudine (Shahinian *et al.*, 1995). Sorivudine should not be administered to any person receiving fluorouracil derivatives (Whitley, 1995).

Sorivudine does not interfere with the antiretroviral activity of zidovudine and nor does zidovudine inhibit the antiviral activity of sorivudine (Machida *et al.*, 1992b).

Clinical Uses of the Drug

1 Varicella-zoster infection

Sorivudine was approved for the treatment of herpes zoster in Japan but was subsequently withdrawn from the market due to toxicity (reviewed in Easterbrook and Wood, 1995). The drug has not received approval in the USA. Trials of sorivudine for the treatment of herpes zoster are ongoing in other countries. Although sorivudine is a good substrate for the TK of herpes simplex type 1, it is not effective against type 2; as it is difficult to differentiate between these two viruses in clinical practice sorivudine is not regarded as useful for treating infections due to herpes simplex (Griffiths, 1994).

An early double-blind, placebo-controlled study of sorivudine (doses ranging from 10 to 50 mg three times daily) in immunocompetent patients with herpes zoster demonstrated clinical efficacy (Niimura *et al.*, 1990a,b). This was subsequently supported by the findings of a second randomized study in patients with hematologic malignancies and varicella-zoster virus infection, where treatment with sorivudine (30 or 150 mg daily) was also found to be of benefit (Hiraoka *et al.*, 1991).

In a double-blind study of sorivudine (40 mg once-daily) versus acyclovir (800 mg five times daily) for the treatment of herpes zoster in 170 patients with HIV infection (median CD4 169 cells per µl), the time to cessation of new vesicle formation was significantly shorter in sorivudine recipients than in placebo recipients (median 2.5 and 3.4 days respectively). Similarly the time to crusting of lesions was shorter in the sorivudine group, although the duration of acute pain was not different between the two groups (Gnann *et al.*, 1995).

A patient with advanced HIV infection who presented with progressive outer retinal necrosis that was presumed to be caused by varicella-zoster virus responded to therapy with combination sorivudine and ganciclovir (Pinnolis *et al.*, 1995). Two HIV-infected patients with complicated varicella-zoster (one with cutaneous dissemination, the other with progressive outer retinal necrosis, both progressing despite acyclovir and foscarnet therapy) responded to sorivudine at a dose of 40 mg daily for 14 days (Burdge *et al.*, 1995).

Acknowledgements The author would like to thank Richard Whitley, University of Alabama at Birmingham, for his critical review of this chapter.

References

Andrei G, Snoeck R, Reymen D (1995). Comparative activity of selected antiviral compounds against clinical isolates of varicella-zoster virus. *Eur J Clin Microbiol Infect Dis* **14**: 318.

Ashida N, Ijichi K, Watanabe Y, Machida H (1993). Metabolism of 5'-ether prodrugs of 1-beta-D- arabinofuranosyl-E-5-(2-bromovinyl)uracil in rats. *Biochem Pharmacol* **46**: 2201.

Ashida N, Sakata S, Kano F (1994). *In vitro* and *in vivo* anti-herpes viral activities and biological properties of CV-araU. *Antiviral Res* **25**: 179.

Ayisi NK, Wall RA, Wanklin RJ *et al.* (1987). Comparative metabolism of E-5-(2-bromvinyl)-2'-deoxyuridine and 1-beta-D-arabinofuranosyl-E-5-(2-bromovinyl)uracil in herpes simplex virus infected cells. *Molec Pharmacol* **31**: 422.

Baba M, Konno K, Shigeta S, De Clercq E (1986). Inhibitory effects of selected antiviral compounds on newly isolated clinical varicella zoster virus strains. *Tohoku J Exp Med* **148**: 275.

Burdge DR, Voigt R, Lindley JL (1995). Sorivudine (BV-ara-U) for the treatment of complicated refractory varicella zoster virus infection in HIV-infected patients. *AIDS* **9**: 810.

Descamps J, Sehgal RK, De Clercq E, Allaudeen HS (1982). Inhibitory effect of E-5-(2-bromovinyl)1- beta-D-arabinofuranosyluracil on herpes simplex virus replication and DNA synthesis. *J Virol* **43**: 332.

Desgranges S, Razaka G, DeClerq E (1986). Effect of (E)-5-(2-brono-vinyl) uracil on the catabolism and antitumour activity of 5-fluorouracil in rats and leukaemic mice. *Cancer Res* **46**: 1094.

Easterbrook P, Wood MJ (1995). Clinical experience with new drugs for the treatment of herpes viruses, particularly varicella-zoster virus. *Med Virol* **5**: 51.

Farber I, Klinger C, Wutzler JP *et al.* (1987). Effect of (E)-5-)2-bromovi-nyl)- and 5-vinyl-1-beta-D-arabinofuranoxyluracil on Epstein-Barr virus antigen expression in P3HR-1 cells, comparison with acyclovir. *Acta Virologica* **31**: 13.

Fukushima M (1995). Clinical trials in Japan. *Nature Med* **1**: 12.

Gnann C, Crumpacker R, Pollard G *et al.* (1995). Sorivudine (BV-araU) versus acyclovir for herpes zoster in HIV infected patients; results of a multi centre controlled trial. *J Invest Med* **43**: 369A.

Gnann JW (1994). New antivirals with activity against varicella-zoster virus. *Amer Neurol Assoc* **35**: S69.

Griffiths PD (1994). Spectrum of activity of antiherpesvirus drugs. *Antivir Chem Chemother* **5**: S17.

Hiraoka A, Masaoka T, Nagai K *et al.* (1991). Clinical effect of BV-araU on varicella-zoster virus infection in immunocompromised patients with haematological malignancies. *J Antimicrob Chemother* **27**: 361.

Ijichi K, Ashida N, Machida H (1990). Effect of 1-beta-D-arabinofuranosyl-E-5-(2-bromovinyl)uracil against herpes simplex virus type 1 infection in immunosuppressed mice. *Antimicrob Ag Chemother*; **34**: 2431.

Ijichi K, Ashida N, Varia S, Machida H (1993). Topical treatment with BV-araU of immunosuppressed and immunocompetent shaved mice cutaneously infected with herpes simplex virus type 1. *Antiviral Res* **21**: 47.

Ishida S, Ikatani M, Matsuoka T (1990). Perinatal and postnatal study in rats treated orally with YN-72 (brovavir). *Clin Rep* **24**: 987.

Jagoda E, Ogan M, Stouffer B *et al.* (1992). A radioimmunoassay for the new antiviral agent 1-beta-D-arabinofuranosyl-E-5-(2-bromovinyl)uracil. *Ther Drug Monit* **14**: 499.

Kawai H, Yoshida I, Suzutani T (1993). Antiviral activity of 1-beta-D-arabinofuranosyl-E-5-(2- bromovinyl)uracil against thymidine kinase negative strains of varicella-zoster virus. *Microbiol Immunol* **37**: 877.

Lacey SF, Suzutani T, Powell KL *et al.* (1991). Analysis of mutations in the thymidine kinase genes of drug-resistant varicella-zoster virus populations using the polymerase chain reaction. *J Gen Virol* **72**: 623.

Lin JC, Machida H (1988). Comparison of two bromovinyl nucleoside analogs 1-beta-D-arabinofuranosyl- E-5-(2-bromovinyl)uracil and E-5-J(2-bromovinyl)-2'-deoxyuridine. *Antimicrob Ag Chemother* **32**: 1068.

Lin JC, Reefschlager J, Herrmann G, Pagano JS (1992). Structure-activity relationship between (E)-5- (2-bromovinyl)- and 5-vinyl-1-beta-D-arabinofuranosyluracil (BV-araU, V-araU) in inhibition of Epstein–Barr virus replication. *Antiviral Res* **17**: 43.

Machida H (1986). Comparison of susceptibilities of varicella zoster virus and herpes simplex viruses to nucleoside analogs. *Antimicrob Ag Chemother* **29**: 524.

Machida H (1990a). *In vitro* anti-herpes virus action of a novel antiviral agent, brovavir (BV-araU). *Chemotherapy* **38**: 256.

Machida H (1990b). Drug susceptibilities of isolates of varicella zoster virus in a clinical study of oral brovavir. *Microbiol Immunol* **34**: 407.

Machida H, Sakata S (1984). *In vitro* and *in vivo* antiviral activity of 1-beta-D-arabinofuranosyl-E-5-(2-bromovinyl)uracil (BV-araU) and related compounds. *Antiviral Res* **4**: 136.

Machida H, Takezawa J (1990). Effect of 1-beta-D-arabinofuranosyl-E-5-(2-bromovinyl)uracil (brovavir) on experimental infections in mice with herpes simplex virus type 1 strains of different degrees of virulence. *Antimicrob Ag Chemother* **34**: 691.

Machida H, Watanabe Y (1991). Inhibition of DNA synthesis in varicella zoster virus infected cells by BV- araU. *Microbiol Immunol* **35**: 139.

Machida H, Sakata S, Kuninaka A, Yoshino H (1981). Antiherpesvirus and anticellular effects of 1-beta- D-arabinofuranosyl-[E-5-(2-halogenovinyl) uracils. *Antimicrob Ag Chemother* **20**: 47.

Machida H, Ikeda T, Ashida N (1990a). Comparison of antiviral efficacies of 1-beta-D-arabinofuranosyl- E-5-(2-bromovinyl)uracil (brovavir) and acyclovir against herpes simplex virus type 1 infections in mice. *Antiviral Res* **14**: 99.

Machida H, Ijichi K, Ohta A (1990b) Antiviral potencies of BV-araU and related nucleoside analogues against varicella-zoster virus in different cell lines. *Microbiol Immunol* **34**: 959.

Machida H, Nishitani M, Suzutani T, Hayashi K (1991). Different antiviral potencies of BV-araU and related nucleoside analogues against herpes simplex virus type 1 in human cell lines and Vero cells. *Microbiol Immunol* **35**: 963.

Machida H, Ijichi K, Takezawa J (1992a). Efficacy of oral treatment with BV-araU against cutaneous infection with herpes simplex type 1 in shaved mice. *Antiviral Res* **17**: 133.

Machida H, Ashida N, Ikeda T *et al.* (1992b). *In vitro* drug combination of 1-beta-D-arabinofuranosyl-E-5-(2-bromovinyl)uracil with anti-human immunodeficiency virus or anticancer nucleosides. *Antimicrob Ag Chemother* **36**: 214.

Machida H, Nishitani M, Ashida N (1994). Effect of BV-araU and acyclovir on varicella-zoster virus replication with various length and timing of drug exposure. *Microbiol Immunol* **38**: 109.

Machida H, Nishitani M, Watanabe Y *et al.* (1995a). Comparison of the selectivity of anti-varicella zoster virus nucleoside analogues. *Microbiol Immunol* **39**: 201.

Machida H, Watanabe Y, Kano F *et al.* (1995b). Deglycosylation of antiherpesviral 5-substituted arabinosyluracil derivatives by rat liver extract and enterobacteria cells. *Biochem Pharmacol* **49**: 763.

Machida H, Endo K, Watanabe Y *et al.* (1995c). Inhibition of dihydropyrimidine dehydorogenase by 5-(E-2-bromovinyl)uracil (BV-Ura) and recovery of rat liver DPD activity after administration of BV-Ura or sorivudine. *Antiviral Res* **26**: A341.

Maudgal PC, De Clercq E (1985). Evaluation of bromovinyldeoxyuridine-related compounds in the treatment of experimental herpes simplex keratitis. *Arch Ophthalmol* **103**: 1393.

Mochizuki K, Torisaki M, Yamashita Y *et al.* (1994). Retinal toxicity and ocular kinetics of 1-beta-D-arabinofuranosyl-E-5-(2-bromovinyl)uracil in rabbits. *Graetes Arch Clin Exp Ophthalmol* **232**: 503.

Nagasaka Y *et al.* (1990). Toxicological study of YN-72 (brovavir) (1) – Acute toxicity in rats. *Clin Rep* **24**: 873.

Niimura M (1990). A double-blind clinical study in patients with herpes zoster to establish YN-72 (Brovavir) dose. *Adv Exp Med Biol* **278**: 267.

Niimura M, Takahashi M, Nishikawa T *et al.* (1990a). Multicenter double blind study of YN-72 (BV-araU, brovavir) in patients with herpes zoster. *Jpn J Clin Dermatol* **44**: 447.

Niimura M, Nishikawa T, Ogawa H *et al.* (1990b). YN-72; dose-finding double-blind clinical study in patients with herpes zoster. The study of clinical efficacy. *Clin Virol* **18**: 115.

Nikkels AF, Pierard GE (1994). Recognition and treatment of shingles. *Drugs* **48**: 528–548.

Ogiwara T, Mikami H, Nakamanru M *et al.* (1990). Phase 1 clinical study of YN-72 (BV-araU), brovavir. *Jpn Pharmacol Ther* **18**: 255.

Olsen S *et al.* (1991). Ascending multiple-dose pharmacokinetic study of intravenous SQ 32, 756 (BV-araU) in healthy subjects. In *Program and Abstracts of the 31st Interscience Conference on Antimicrobial Agents and Chemotherapy, Chicago* (Abstr. 766). Washington, DC: American Society for Microbiology.

Olsen SJ, Saag M, Sommadossi JP (1995). Safety and pharmacokinetic interaction of sorivudine (BV- AraU) and zidovudine. In *Program and Abstracts of the 35th Interscience Conference on Antimicrobial Agents and Chemotherapy, San Francisco* (Abstr Aa58). Washington, DC: American Society for Microbiology.

Pinnolis MK, Foxworthy D, Kemp B (1995). Treatment of progressive outer retinal necrosis with sorivudine. *Amer J Ophthalmol* **119**: 516.

Rabasseda X, Mealy N *et al.* (1993). Sorivudine: A new antiviral drug specifically active against herpes simplex type 1 and varicella-zoster. *Drugs Today* **29**: 555.

Rajcani J, Reefschlager J (1987). Efficacy of (E)-5-(2-bromovinyl) and 5-vinyl-1-beta-D- arabinofuranosyluracil against acute herpes simplex virus keratitis and the establishment of latency; comparison with acyclovir and bromovinyldeoxyuridine. *Acta Virologica* **31**: 329.

Reefschlager J, Wutzler P, Thiel KD, Herrmann G (1986). Treatment of experimental herpes simplex virus type 1 encephalitis in mice with (E)-5-(2-bromovinyl- and 5-vinyl-1-beta-D-arabinofuranosyluracil comparison with bromovinyl-deoxyuridine and acyclovir. *Antiviral Res* **6**: 83.

Sakuma J (1984). Strains of varicella-zoster virus resistant to 1-beta-D-arabinofuranosyl-E-5-(2- bromovinyl)uracil. *Antimicrob Ag Chemother* **25**: 742.

Shahinian H, Amin G, Stewart M *et al.* (1995). Inhibition of peripheral blood mononuclear cell (PBMC) dihydropyrimidine dehydrogenase (DPD) activity by sorivudine (1-B-D-arabino-furanosyl-E-5-(2- bromovinyl)-uracil and its role in severe fluorouracil (F-Ura) toxicity. *Proc Asco* **14**: 169.

Sherman JW, Kassalow LM, Harkins JG *et al.* (1990a). SQ 32, 756 (BV-araU); characteristics and pharmacokinetic evaluation in healthy male volunteers. *Antiviral Res* (Suppl 1): Abst 117.

Sherman J, De Vault A, Natarajan M *et al.* (1990b). SQ 32756 (BV-araU) characteristics and pharmacokinetics in healthy young and elderly male volunteers. In *Program and Abstracts of the 30th Interscience Conference on Antimicrobial Agents and Chemotherapy, Atlanta* (Abstr. 1103). Washington, DC: American Society for Microbiology.

Shigeta S, Yokota T, Iwabuchi T *et al.* (1983). Comparative efficacy of antiherpes drugs against various strains of varicella zoster virus. *J Infect Dis* **147**: 576–584.

Shiraki K, Ochiai H, Namazue J *et al.* (1992). Comparison of antiviral assay methods using cell-free and cell-associated varicella-zoster virus. *Antiviral Res* **18**: 209.

Shiraki K, Matsui S, Aiba N *et al.* (1993). Susceptibility of Oka varicella vaccine strain to antiviral drugs. *Vaccine* **11**: 1380 .

Snoeck R, Andrei G, De Clercq E (1994). Chemotherapy of varicella zoster virus infections. *Antimicrob Ag* **4**: 211.

Soike KF, Baskin G, Cantrell C, Gerone P (1984). Investigation of antiviral activity of 1-beta-D- arabinofuranosylthymine (ara-1) and 1-beta-D-arabinofuranosyl-E-5-(2-bromovinyl)uracil (BV-ara-U) in monkeys infected with simian varicella virus. *Antiviral Res* **4**: 245.

Soike KF, Huang J, Tu J *et al.* (1990). Oral bioavailability and anti-simian varicella virus efficacy of BV-araU (brovavir) in monkeys. In *Program and Abstracts of the 30th Interscience Conference Antimicrobial Agents and Chemotherapy, Atlanta* (Abstr. 1102). Washington, DC: American Society for Microbiology.

Soike K, Huang JL, Tu JL *et al.* (1992). Oral bioavailability and anti-simian varicella virus efficacy of 1-beta-D-arabinofuranosyl-E-5-(2-bromovinyl)uracil (BV-araU) in monkeys. *J Infect Dis* **165**: 732.

Suzutani T, Machida H (1992). Analysis of toxic and mutagenic activities of antiherpesvirus nucleosides against HeLa cells and herpes simplex virus type 1. *Mutat Res* **267**: 125.

Suzutani T, Machida H, Sakuma T *et al.* (1988a). Efficacies of antiherpesvirus nucleosides against two strains of herpes simplex virus type 1 in vero and human embryo lung fibroblast cells. *Antimicrob Ag Chemother* **32**: 1046.

Suzutani T, Machida H, Sakuma T, Azuma M (1988b). Effects of various nucleosides on antiviral activity and metabolism of 1-beta-D-arabinofuranosyl-E-5-(2-bromovinyl)uracil against herpes simplex virus types 1 and 2. *Antimicrob Ag Chemother* **32**: 1547.

Suzutani T, Machida H, Honess RW (1993). Mechanism of inhibition of DNA synthesis by 1-beta-D- arabinofuranosyl-E-5-(2-bromovinyl)uracil. *Microbiol Immunol* **37**: 511.

Talarico CL, Phelps WC, Biron KK (1993). Analysis of the thymidine kinase genes from acyclovir- resistant mutants of varicella-zoster virus isolated from patients with AIDS. *J Virol* **67**: 1024.

Topke H, Graf M, Wutzler P *et al.* (1988). Evaluation of (E)-5-(2-bromovinyl) and 5-vinyl-1-beta-D-arabinofuranosyluracil (BrVaraU, VaraU) in the treatment of experimental herpes simplex virus type 1 keratitis in rabbits; comparison with (E)-5-(2-bromovinyl)-2'-deoxyuridine (BrVUdR). *Antiviral Res* **9**: 273.

Yokota T Konno K Mori S *et al.* (1989). Mechanism of selective inhibition of varicella zoster virus replication by 1-beta-D-arabinofuranosyl-E-5-(2-bromovinyl)uracil. *Molec Pharmacol* **36**: 312.

Yokota T, Konno K, Sigeta S (1993). Inhibition of thymidylate synthetase activity induced in varicella zoster virus infected cells by (E)-5-(2-bromovinyl)-2'-deoxyuridine. *Antiviral Res* **20**: (Suppl 1).

Yoshifune S *et al.* (1993a). Toxicological study of YN-72 (brovavir). 2. Subacute toxicity in rats. *Clin Rep* **27**: 3453.

Yoshifune S *et al.* (1993b). Toxicological study of YN-72 (brovavir). 3. Chronic toxicity in rats. *Clin Rep* **27**: 3475.

Whigan DB, Cohen AI (1991). High performance liquid chromatographic determination of 1-beta-D- arabinofuranosyl-E-5-(2-bromovinyl)uracil and its metabolite (E)-5-(2-bromovinyl)uracil in serum. *J Chromatogr* **568**: 85.

Whitley RJ (1995). Sorivudine, a promising drug for the treatment of varicella-zoster virus infection. *Neurology* **45**: S73.

Adefovir Dipivoxil

Description

Adefovir dipivoxil (9-[2-bis(pivaloyloxymethyl)-phosphonylmethoxyethyl]adenine, formerly known as bis-POM PMEA or GS-840) is the oral prodrug of the antiviral nucleotide parent compound adefovir (PMEA or GS-393). Adefovir has activity against retroviruses, herpesviruses and hepadnaviruses, and was developed by Gilead Sciences. No trade name has been assigned at this time.

The drug is a member of a class of compounds called phosphonomethylethers, in which the oxygen within the phosphodiester bond has been switched with the proximate carbon within the nucleotide in order to produce a stable nucleotide analog. The nucleotide is then phosphorylated to the active diphosphate derivative within lymphocytes and cells of macrophage lineage. As adefovir has low oral bioavailability, the orally bioavailable prodrug adefovir dipivoxil was selected for clinical development.

Adefovir dipivoxil has a molecular weight of 501.48. The chemical formula is $C_{20}H_{32}N_5O_8P$. The chemical structure of adefovir is shown in Fig. V.21.

Antiviral Activity

Adefovir and its prodrug are active *in vitro* against human immunodeficiency virus and a number of other animal retroviruses, all the members of the herpesviruses, and hepatitis B virus (Table V.14).

1 Retroviruses

Adefovir and its oral prodrug inhibit the replication of HIV-1 and HIV-2 in T cell lines at a concentration of 1.6–2 μM. The concentration that causes host cell toxicity is significantly higher (40–67 μM) (Balzarini *et al.*, 1989; Pauwels *et al.*, 1988). Adefovir also has activity against HIV in both monocyte-macrophages and T lymphocytes (Balzarini *et al.*, 1991a).

There is additive efficacy against HIV replication when adefovir is used in combination with didanosine, lamivudine, or the protease inhibitors ritonavir or saquinavir (Data on file, Gilead Sciences). There is modest synergy when adefovir is used in combination with zidovudine *in vitro* (Smith *et al.*, 1989). By continuous passage of HIV in increasing concentrations of the drug *in vitro*, resistant strains have been selected. Mutations within codons 65 and 70 have been identified in these resistant isolates.

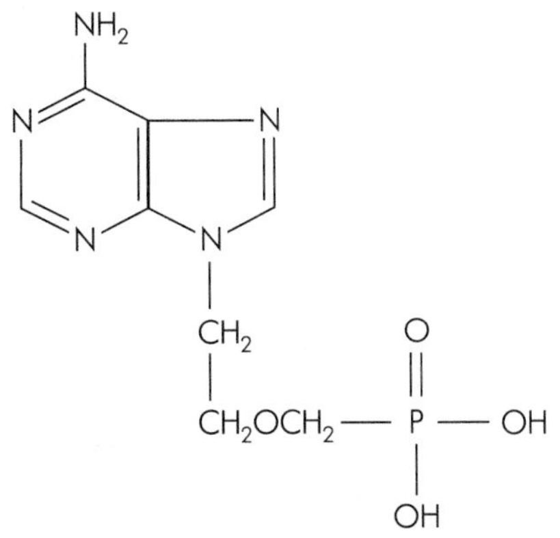

Fig. V.21.
Chemical structure of adefovir.

Table V.14

Human viruses which show *in vitro* dipivoxil susceptibility to adefovir

Human immunodeficiency virus
Cytomegalovirus
Herpes simplex virus type 1[a]
Herpes simplex virus type 2[a]
Human herpesvirus type 6
Epstein–Barr virus
Varicella-zoster virus
Hepatitis B virus

[a] Including both TK⁻ and TK⁺ strains. (See text for sources of data.)

2 Other retroviruses

Adefovir suppresses the replication of simian immunodeficiency virus (Balzarini *et al.*, 1990a, 1991b), Moloney murine sarcoma virus (Bronson *et al.*, 1989), Rauscher murine leukemia virus (Bronson *et al.*, 1989), feline leukemia virus (Hoover *et al.*, 1991), feline immunodeficiency virus (Egberink *et al.*, 1990; Hoover *et al.*, 1992) and visna virus (Thormor *et al.*, 1995a).

Adefovir (10 or 20 mg per kg daily) is effective for prophylaxis against infection with simian immunodeficiency virus when administered to macaques 48 h prior to inoculation and continued for 4 weeks post-exposure. In one study, five of 18 adefovir-treated monkeys developed infection over a 26-week follow-up period, compared with 17 of 18 control monkeys treated with zidovudine (100 mg per kg daily) starting 24 h prior to inoculation and continuing for 5 weeks after infection (Tsai *et al.*, 1993, 1994). Adefovir has also been shown to suppress simian immunodeficiency virus titers in chronically infected monkeys (Tsai *et al.*, 1995).

Lambs inoculated intracerebrally with visna virus and treated with adefovir (10 or 25 mg per kg) three times per week subcutaneously had lower recovery of virus from blood, CSF or brain tissue and less cerebral inflammation than untreated control animals (Thormor *et al.*, 1995b).

When administered via the intraperitoneal route to mice commencing at the time of infection with Rauscher murine leukemia virus or Moloney murine sarcoma virus and continuing post-infection on a daily regimen, adefovir suppresses virus replication with similar or greater efficacy than zidovudine (Bronson *et al.*, 1989). Other investigators have confirmed the activity of adefovir against Rauscher murine leukemia virus (Kunder *et al.*, 1995). The drug has also been shown to have greater efficacy in reducing tumors and mortality in mice infected with Moloney murine sarcoma virus when administered as a single high dose, compared with the same dose given in fractions over a weekly period, without increasing toxicity (Balzarini *et al.*, 1990b; Naesens *et al.*, 1991).

Subcutaneous administration of adefovir to cats commencing at the time of inoculation with feline leukemia virus and continuing for 7 weeks post-inoculation prevented infection as assessed by undetectable p27 antigen levels. Neutralizing antibody developed, and cats were protected from infection following rechallenge in so far as there was a lack of antigenemia (Hoover *et al.*, 1991). Suppression of infection occurred in cats given adefovir at the time of infection with feline immunodeficiency virus and treated for 5 weeks (Hoover *et al.*, 1992).

3 Herpesviruses

Adefovir dipivoxil has been found to inhibit replication of cytomegalovirus and both thymidine kinase (TK)-positive and -negative strains of herpes simplex virus type 1 and type 2 (De Clercq *et al.*, 1987, 1989; DeCastro *et al.*, 1991). Adefovir dipivoxil is 60-fold more active against herpes simplex virus type 2 than the parent compound , with IC_{50} values of 0.6 μM and 119 μM respectively (Starrett *et al.*, 1994). The activity of the adefovir prodrug is similar to that of ganciclovir, (Bronson *et al.*, 1989; De Clercq *et al.*, 1987). The IC_{50} of adefovir against human herpesvirus type 6 is 7 μg per ml (Reymen *et al.*, 1995). The drug also has activity against Epstein–Barr virus (Lin *et al.*, 1987), and against varicella-zoster virus (De Clercq *et al.*, 1987).

A strain of herpes simplex virus type 1 that was passaged in the presence of adefovir *in vitro* and developed resistance to this drug was found to be cross-resistant to foscarnet. Similarly, foscarnet-resistant strains of herpes simplex virus are cross-resistant to adefovir (Merta *et al.*, 1990).

Daily intraperitoneal administration of adefovir (50 or 100 mg per kg) to mice, commencing at the time of intracerebral inoculation of herpes simplex virus significantly reduced mortality due to encephalitis, compared with aciclovir-treated animals (Gangemi *et al.*, 1989). Adefovir (0.1% topical) has also been shown to suppress skin lesions and improve survival in mice inoculated with either TK-positive or TK-negative strains of herpes simplex, compared with treatment with 10% bromovinyldeoxyuridine (De Clercq *et al.*, 1989). Administered as a 0.2% solution, adefovir showed similar efficacy to 0.2% bromovinyldeoxyuridine in preventing herpes simplex keratitis due to infection with TK-positive strains of herpes simplex virus type 1, and superior efficacy with TK-negative strains (Maugdal and De Clercq, 1991). Treatment of mice with adefovir has also been shown to improve survival following infection with murine cytomegalovirus (DeCastro *et al.*, 1991).

4 Hepadnavirus

Adefovir inhibits replication of human hepatitis B virus in the HB611 hepatoma cell line *in vitro*, suppressing hepatitis B virus DNA synthesis with an IC_{50} value of 0.2 μM and a selectivity index of 300–500 (Yokota *et al.*, 1991). The replication of duck hepatitis B virus is suppressed by adefovir when assessed in primary duck hepatocytes, with an IC_{50} of 0.2 μM and a high selectivity index (Heijtink *et al.*, 1993).

Availability

Adefovir dipivoxil is available for oral administration in *tablets* of 60- and 120-mg strength.

Mode of Administration and Serum Levels in Relation to Dosage

Plasma concentrations of adefovir following i.v. administration of adefovir at a dose of 1 or 3 mg per kg were dose-proportional in phase I/II studies in HIV-infected individuals (Cundy *et al.*, 1995).

The oral bioavailability of adefovir was found in animal studies to be extremely low, probably due to poor intestinal permeability of the phosphonate. Oral bioavailability in HIV-infected persons receiving 3 mg per kg was less than 12% (Cundy *et al.*, 1995). Thus development of the i.v. compound, adefovir, was discontinued in favor of the oral prodrug, adefovir dipivoxil. When administered orally, the plasma concentrations of adefovir dipivoxil are 10- to 20-fold higher than those following administration of adefovir. There is rapid and complete conversion of adefovir dipivoxil to adefovir. The time to peak plasma concentration (C_{max}) of adefovir is 1–2 h (Data on file, Gilead Sciences).

In HIV-infected persons receiving adefovir dipivoxil in a phase I dose-escalation study (GS-94–401), the oral bioavailability of adefovir administered as granulated prodrug suspended in concentrated grape juice was 23.5 ± 9.2% to 28.6 ±8.8% for doses of 200 and 500 mg respectively. The mean oral bioavailability when the prodrug was administered as tablets to fasting subjects was 30.1±11.6%, and increased to 41.2±13.5% when taken with or following food (Data on file, Gilead Sciences).

In a phase I/II safety, tolerance and pharmacokinetics study (GS-94–402) of 14 days duration, HIV-infected persons with CD4 counts greater than 100 cells per μl received adefovir dipivoxil tablets in daily oral doses of 125, 250 or 500 mg under fed conditions. The oral bioavailability of the 250 mg dose was 39% on day 1 and 32% on day 14. The peak plasma concentration (C_{max}) of the 125 and 250 mg tablets were 0.21 ± 0.13 μg per ml and 0.44 ± 0.07 μg per ml respectively, with a time to peak plasma concentration (T_{max}) of 2.2 and 2.4 h respectively. There was a small decrease in oral bioavailability of the 500-mg dose after 14 days of treatment (88% of day 1 value), and this was reflected in a modest decrease in C_{max} and T_{max} for this dose (Data on file, Gilead Sciences).

During *in vivo* metabolism of adefovir dipivoxil to adefovir, pivalic acid is formed which can esterify free carnitine resulting in its renal excretion. As carnitine is required for transport of fatty acids across mitochondrial membranes, patients receiving adefovir in phase III studies also receive L-carnitine (200 mg daily) as an oral supplement.

Excretion and Distribution

The clearance of adefovir is largely by the renal route, with active tubular secretion of the drug by the kidney accounting for approximately 60% of its clearance (Cundy *et al.*, 1995). In phase I/II studies in HIV-infected individuals, the volume of distribution at steady-state was 418± 76 ml per kg, suggesting that the drug is distributed to total body water (Cundy *et al.*, 1995). Protein binding of i.v. adefovir is less than 3%. The majority of an i.v. dose of adefovir can be recovered unchanged in the urine within 24 h (Cundy *et al.*, 1995); no metabolites of adefovir are present in plasma or urine.

Mechanism of Action

The oral prodrug, adefovir dipivoxil, is rapidly metabolized within lymphocytes, and monocyte-macrophages to adefovir. Adefovir and adefovir dipivoxil are phosphorylated nucleosides (nucleotides) and are members of a class of drugs known as phosphonomethylethers.

Phosphorylation of adefovir to the diphosphate derivative is through the action of mitochondrial adenylate kinase and an uncharacterized cytoplasmic enzyme (Robbins et al., 1995). The diphosphate has a long intracellular half-life, ranging from 18 to 36 h (Data on file, Gilead Sciences). The phosphorylated derivative functions as a chain terminator of DNA synthesis following its incorporation into the growing DNA chain. The drug is a competitive inhibitor of human alpha, beta and gamma DNA polymerases as well as viral DNA polymerases. It inhibits the reverse transcriptase of HIV with a K_i of 0.012 μM, compared with the K_i of 0.008 for zidovudine (Cherrington et al., 1995). The K_i values for inhibition of human DNA polymerases by the phosphorylated derivative are considerably higher (1.2 μM, 70.4 μM and 1.0 μM for DNA polymerases alpha, beta and gamma respectively) than for viral reverse transcriptase, and as these values for DNA polymerase gamma also exceed the K_i values of stavudine and zalcitabine, less mitochondrial toxicity may be predicted (Cherrington et al., 1995).

The diphosphorylated drug also inhibits hepatitis B virus DNA polymerase with a K_i value of 0.1 μM (Yokota et al., 1994), and the DNA polymerases of human cytomegalovirus and herpes simplex virus with K_i values of 0.4 μM and 0.02 μM respectively (Data on file, Gilhead Sciences; Foster et al., 1991).

Toxicity

1 In vitro testing

The cytotoxicity of adefovir on human bone marrow progenitor cells is similar to that of zidovudine with IC_{50} values of 14 and 13 μM respectively (Balzarini et al., 1991c). The drug has been found to be cytostatic in cell culture using T lymphocyte cell lines (Starrett et al., 1992).

2 Animal studies

In rats, chronic high doses of adefovir (exceeding 10 mg per kg daily) resulted in bone marrow toxicity and nephrotoxicity; hair loss, exfoliation and erythema were observed with doses of greater than 25 mg per kg daily given over a 4-week period. No toxicity was observed below a dose of 2 mg per kg daily administered over 26 weeks. In monkeys, a dose-related increase in plasma hepatic aminotransaminases was observed with adefovir dipivoxil, and mild inflammation of the gastric epithelium and minimal dose-dependent nephropathy. No toxicity was observed with doses of less than 1 mg per kg daily given for 13 weeks. Embryotoxicity was not observed in animals receiving doses of less than 20 mg per kg daily (Data on file, Gilead Sciences).

3 Side-effects reported in clinical trials

Adefovir appears to be well tolerated with most adverse events being mild and reversible. Dose-related gastrointestinal symptoms were the most common side-effects observed in the GS-94–402 phase I/II study, with nausea occurring in 16% of patients, and diarrhea in 9%. Other reported adverse events which may or may not be related to adefovir include dysuria, atrial fibrillation, and muscle weakness. Mild dose-related increases in hepatic transaminases were observed in 5% or less of patients.

Dose-related decreases in serum carnitine levels were noted within 2 weeks of commencing adefovir dipivoxil therapy. Serum carnitine levels decreased by 18, 48, and 66% in those receiving 125, 250 and 500 mg daily. After 12 weeks of treatment with 125 or 250 mg per day, the mean decline in serum free carnitine was approximately 42% and 62% respectively. The decline in serum carnitine was reversible within 1 month of cessation of treatment and was not associated with symptoms relating to myopathy, cardiomyopathy, encephalopathy or hypoglycemia.

Clinical Uses of the Drug

Adefovir dipivoxil is currently in phase II/III trials in HIV-infected patients in the USA.

In the phase I/II randomized, double-blind, placebo-controlled GS-94–403 study, 72 HIV infected patients with more than 200 CD4 cells per μl, and not receiving other antiretroviral medication, were randomized to receive adefovir dipivoxil (125 mg escalating to 250 mg) or placebo. There was a significant improvement in CD4 counts and a modest (0.5 $\log_{10}$) decline in HIV RNA in adefovir recipients after 6 weeks of therapy. A subset of patients was evaluated for the effect of adefovir on cytomegalovirus levels in semen: there was a 0.7 $\log_{10}$ decline in plasma cytomegalovirus DNA in adefovir recipients. For both HIV and cytomegalovirus, the 125-mg dose provided more favorable effects on surrogate markers than the 250 mg dose (Data on file, Gilead Sciences).

A phase I/II randomized, double-blind, placebo-controlled trial (GS-94–404) evaluated the safety, tolerance and antiviral activity of adefovir dipivoxil in patients with chronic hepatitis B virus infection. This study is ongoing.

References

Balzarini J, Naesens L, Herdewun P et al. (1989). Marked *in vivo* antiretrovirus activity of 9-(2-phosphonylmethoxyethyl)adenine A selective anti-human immunodeficiency virus agent. *Proc Natl Acad Sci* **86**: 332.

Balzarini J, Naesens L, Slachmuylders J et al. (1990a). Potent anti-simian immunodeficiency virus (SIV) activity and pharmacokinetics of 9-(2-phosphonylmethoxyethyl)adenine (PMEA) in Rhesus monkeys. In *Animal Models in AIDS* (Schellekens H, Horzinek MC, eds), pp. 131–138. Amsterdam: Elsevier Science.

Balzarini J, Naesens L, De Clercq E (1990b). Anti-retrovirus activity of 9-(2-phosphonylmethoxyethyl)adenine (PMEA) *in vivo* increases when it is less frequently administered. *Int J Cancer* **46**: 340.

Balzarini J, Perno C, Schols D, De Clercq E (1991a). Activity of acyclic phosphonate analogues against human immunideficiency virus in monocytes/macrophages and peripheral blood lymphocytes. *BBRC* **178**: 329.

Balzarini J, Naesens L, Slachmuylders J et al. (1991b). 9-(2-Phosphonylmethoxyethyl)adenine (PMEA) effectively inhibits retrovirus replication *in vitro* and simian immunodeficiency virus infection in Rhesus monkeys. *AIDS* **5**: 21.

Balzarini J, Holy A, Jindrich J et al. (1991c). 9(2RS)-3-fluoro-2-phosphonomethoxypropyl) derivatives of purines; A class of highly selective antiretroviral agents *in vitro* and *in vivo*. *Proc Natl Acad Sci USA* **88**: 4961.

Bronson JJ, Kim CU, Ghazzouli J et al. (1989). Synthesis and antiviral activity of phosphonylmethoxyethyl derivatives of purine and pyrimidine bases. *Amer Chem Soc Symp* **401**: 72.

Cherrington JM, Allen SJW, McKee B et al. (1995). Kinetic interaction of the diphosphates of 9-(2-phosphonylmethoxyethyl)adenine and other anti-HIV active purine congeners with HIV reverse transcriptase and human DNA polymerases alpha, beta and gamma. *Antiviral Chem Chemother* **6**: 217.

Cundy KC, Barditch-Crovo P, Walker RE et al. (1995). Clinical pharmacokinetics of adefovir in human immunodeficiency virus type 1-infected patients. *Antimicrob Ag Chemother* **39**: 2401.

Data on File, Gilead Sciences.

DeCastro LM, Kern ER, De Clercq E et al. (1991). Phosphonylmethoxyalkyl purine and pyrimidine derivatives for treatment of opportunistic cytomegalovirus and herpes simplex virus infections in murine AIDS. *Antiviral Res* **16**: 101.

De Clercq E, Sakuma T, Baba M et al. (1987). Antiviral activity of phosphonylmethoxyalkyl derivatives of purines and pyrimidines. *Antiviral Res* **8**: 261.

De Clercq E, Holy A, Rosenberg I (1989). Efficacy of phosphonylmethoxyalkyl derivatives of adenine in experimental herpes simplex virus and vaccinia virus infections *in vivo*. *Antimicrob Ag Chemother* **33**: 185.

Egberink H, Borst M, Niphuis H et al. (1990). Suppression of feline immunodeficiency virus infection *in vivo* by 9-(2-phosphonyl-methoxyethyl)adenine. *Proc Natl Acad Sci USA* **87**: 3087.

Foster SA, Cerny J, Cheng Y (1991). Herpes simplex virus specified DNA polymerase is the target for the antiviral action of 9-(2-phosphonylmethoxyethyl)adenine. *J Biol Chem* **266**: 238.

Gangemi J, Cozens R, De Clercq E et al. (1989). 9-(2-phosphonylmethoxyethyl)adenine in the treatment of murine acquired immunodeficiency disease and opportunistic herpes simplex virus infections. *Antimicrob Ag Chemother* **33**: 1864.

Heijtink RA, De Wild GA, Kruining J et al. (1993). Inhibitory effect of 9-(2-phosphonylmethoxyethyl)adenine (PMEA) on human and duck hepatitis B virus infection. *Antiviral Res* **21**: 141.

Hoover EA, Enber JP, Zeidner NS, Mullins J (1991). Early therapy of feline leukemia virus infection (LeLV- FAIDS) with 9-(2-phosphonylmethoxyethyl)adenine (PMEA). *Antiviral Res* **16**: 77.

Hoover EA, Philpott MS, Ebner JP, Zeidner NS (1992). Experimental therapy of immunodeficiency inducing feline retroviruses with phosphonylmethoxyethyl adenine (PMEA). *Antiviral Res* **17**: 131.

Kunder S, Black P, Hall B, Ussery M (1995). PMEA has immunomodulatory activity and inhibits reverse transcriptase in the Rauscher murine leukemia virus (RMuLV) model. 8th ISAR Conference, Santa Fe, New Mexico, April 23–25. *Antiviral Res* **26**: 4276.

Lin J, De Clercq E, Pagano J (1987). Novel acyclic adenosine analogs inhibit Epstein–Barr virus replication. *Antimicrob Ag Chemother* **31**: 1431.

Maudgal PC, De Clercq E (1991). Effects of phosphonylmethoxyalkylpurine and pyrimidine derivatives on TK+ and TK-HSV-1 keratitis in rabbits. *Antiviral Res* **16**: 93.

Merta A, Votruba I, Rosenberg I et al. (1990). Inhibition of herpes simplex virus kDNA polymerase by diphosphates of acyclic phosphonylmethoxyalkyl nucleotide analogues. *Antiviral Res* **13**: 209.

Naesens L, Balzarini J, De Clercq E (1991). Single-dose administration of 9-(2- phosphonylmethoxyethyl)adenine (PMEA) and 9-(2-phosphonylmethoxyethyl)-2,6-diaminopurine (PMEDAP) in the prophylaxis of retrovirus infection *in vivo*. *Antiviral Res* **16**: 53.

Pauwels R, Balzarini J, Schols D et al. (1988). Phosphonylmethoxyethyl purine derivatives A new class of antihuman immunodeficiency virus agents. *Antimicrob Ag Chemother* **32**: 1025.

Reymen D, Naesens L, Balzarini J et al. (1995). Antiviral activity of selected nucleoside analogues against human herpes virus type 6. *Nucleosides Nucleotides* **14**: 567.

Robbins BI, Greenhaw JJ, Connelly MC, Fridland A (1995). Metabolic pathways for activation of the antiviral agent 9-(2-phosphonylmethoxyethyl)adenine in human lymphoid cells. *Antimicrob Ag Chemother* **39**: 2304.

Smith MS, Brian EL, De Clercq E, Pagano JS (1989). Susceptibility of human immunodeficiency virus type 1 replication *in vitro* to acyclic adenosine analogs and synergy of the analogs with 3'-azido-3'-deoxythymidine. *Antimicrob Ag Chemother* **33**: 1486.

Starrett SE, Tortolani DR, Hitchcock MJM et al. (1992). Synthesis and *in vitro* evaluation of a phosphonate prodrug, bis(pivaloyloxymethyl) 9-(2-phosphonylmethoxyethyl)adenine. *Antiviral Res* **19**: 267.

Starrett JE, Tortolani DR, Russell J *et al.* (1994). Synthesis, oral bioavailability determination, and *in vitro* evaluation of prodrugs of the antiviral agent 9-[2-(phosphonomethoxy)-ethyl]adenine (PMEA). *J Med Chem* **37**: 1857.

Thormor H, Balzarini J, Debyser Z *et al.* (1995a). Inhibition of visna virus replication and cytopathic effect in sheep choroid plexus cell cultures by selected anti-HIV agents. *Antiviral Res* **27**: 49.

Thormor H, Georgsson G, Palsson P *et al.* (1995b). Inhibitory effect of 9-(2-phosphonylmethoxyethyl)adenine on visna virus infections in lambs A model for *in vivo* testing of candidate anti-human immunodeficiency virus drugs. *Proc Natl Acad Sci USA* **92**: 3283.

Tsai CC, Follis KE, Grant RF *et al.* (1993). Effect of dosing frequency on AZT prophylaxis in macaques infected with simian immunodeficiency virus. *J AIDS* **6**: 1086.

Tsai CC, Follis KE, Sabo A *et al.* (1994). Pre-exposure prophylaxis with 9-(2-phosphonylmethoxyethyl) adenine (PMEA) against simian immunodeficiency virus infection in macaques. *J Infect Dis* **169**: 260.

Tsai CC, Follis K, Grant R, Bischofberger N (1995). Efficacy of 9-(2-phosphonylmethoxyethyl)adenine (PMEA) treatment against chronic simian immunodeficiency virus infection in macaques. *J Infect Dis* **171**: 1338.

Yokota T, Mochizuki S, Konno K *et al.* (1991). Inhibitory effects of selected antiviral compounds on human hepatitis B virus DNA synthesis. *Antimicrob Ag Chemother* **35**: 394.

Yokota T, Konno K, Shigeta S *et al.* (1994). Inhibitory effects of acyclic nucleoside phosphonate analogues on hepatitis B virus DNA synthesis in HB611 cells. *Antiviral Chem Chemother* **5**: 57.

Trifluorothymidine

Description

Trifluorothymidine, also known as trifluoridine, is a fluorinated pyrimidine nucleoside structurally related to thymidine and idoxuridine. It differs from thymidine in that there are three fluorine atoms in the place of three hydrogen atoms in the methyl group of the latter compound. It is marketed under the trade name 'Viroptic' by Glaxo Wellcome. The chemical name is 2'-deoxy-5-(trifluoromethyl)uridine. The drug is licensed for topical use for the treatment of keratoconjunctivitis and recurrent epithelial keratitis caused by herpes simplex virus types 1 and 2. The chemical formula is $F_3TdR.F_3T$. The chemical structure is shown in Fig. V.22.

Antiviral Activity

Trifluorothymidine has activity against herpes simplex virus types 1 and 2, cytomegalovirus, varicella-zoster virus, vaccinia virus and some strains of adenovirus.

1 Herpes simplex virus

Trifluorothymidine is effective in inhibiting the replication of herpes simplex virus, with variable results depending on the host cell used in the assay (Abghari et al., 1994). The antiviral index of trifluorothymidine against herpes simplex virus is between 10 and 100 (Wingard et al., 1983). Trifluorothymidine is synergistic with adenine arabinoside, and additive with aciclovir and foscarnet against herpes simplex types 1 and 2 (Schinazi and Nahmias, 1982).

Aciclovir-resistant strains of herpes simplex virus type-1 which are deficient in thymidine kinase (TK) activity are sensitive to trifluorothymidine (Field et al., 1981). Synergy between trifluorothymidine and interferon alpha has been demonstrated for clinical isolates that are resistant to aciclovir and foscarnet (Birch et al., 1992), although other investigators have reported a lack of synergy between these two drugs (Taylor et al., 1991). Strains of herpes simplex virus type 1 that are resistant to trifluorothymidine develop cross-resistance to other TK-dependent antiviral drugs (Fardeau et al., 1991).

Trifluorothymidine at a concentration of $0.01\,\mu g$ per ml inhibited bovid herpesvirus 1 in plaque reduction and in vitro yield reduction assays, in which aciclovir was inactive even at concentrations of $1000\,\mu g$ per ml (Babiuk et al., 1983). Similarly, topical aciclovir was superior to trifluorothymidine and adenine arabinoside in the treatment of guinea-pigs with cutaneous

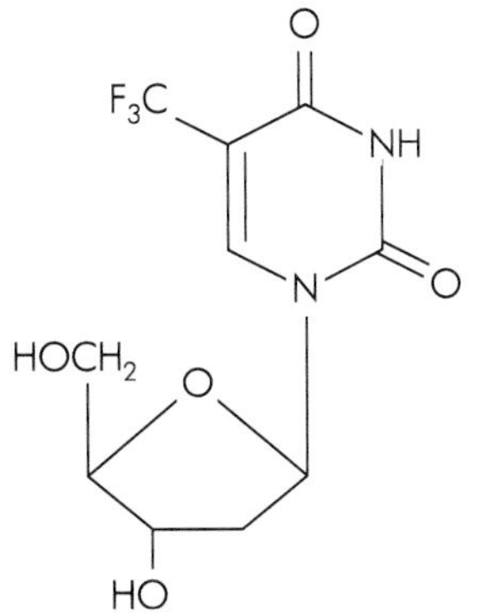

Fig. V.22.
Chemical structure of trifluorothymidine.

Table V.15

Treatment of aciclovir-resistant mucocutaneous herpes simplex with topical trifluorothymidine. (Adapted from Kessler *et al.*, 1996, with permission from Lippincott-Raven Publishers.)

Median duration of therapy (weeks)	5.3
Median time to complete resolution (weeks)	7.1
Median time to 50% healing (weeks)	2.4
Complete healing	29%
Complete resolution of pain post-therapy	45%
Median time to complete resolution of pain (weeks)	5

herpes simplex virus infection (Burkhardt and Wigand, 1983). In rabbits, trifluorothymidine was less effective than aciclovir in treating experimental herpetic keratitis (Bauer, 1982).

2 Cytomegalovirus

The IC_{50} values of trifluorothymidine for murine and human cytomegalovirus have been reported as 0.22 and 0.012 μM respectively, with an *in vitro* therapeutic ratio of 108 (Wingard *et al.*, 1981). However, there are large variances in the reported values. Other investigators have found that trifluorothymidine is ineffective in inhibiting the viral cytopathic effect of cytomegalovirus in a plaque reduction assay at concentrations below 50 μM (Lang and Cheung, 1982), and report a higher IC_{50} value of 0.57 μM against clinical isolates and 2.1 μM against the AD-169 laboratory-adapted strain (Spector *et al.*, 1983). Aciclovir and foscarnet have been found to be additive or synergistic when used in combination with trifluorothymidine against laboratory-adapted and clinical strains of human cytomegalovirus *in vitro* (Spector *et al.*, 1982, 1983).

3 Varicella-zoster virus

Bromovinyl-deoxyuridine is additive in its antiviral activity with trifluorothymidine against strains of varicella-zoster when assessed by plaque reduction or infectious center assays (Biron and Elion, 1982).

Mode of Administration and Dosage; Vitreous Levels in Relation to Dosage; Metabolism and Distribution

1 Ophthalmic administration

The recommended dose is one to two drops every 2 h (up to nine drops per day) while awake (although the conjunctival sac will usually only accommodate one drop). This should continue until re-epithelialization is complete. At this time the dose should be increased to one drop every 4 h while awake for an additional 7 days.

The half-life of trifluorothymidine in the vitreous following intravitreal injection (200 μg) in rabbits was 3.15 h, and the vitreous concentration remained above the IC_{50} for cytomegalovirus for about 30 h (Pang *et al.*, 1992).

Trifluorothymidine does not cross the blood–brain barrier (Rand *et al.*, 1986). Topical administration results in intraocular penetration which may be increased in the presence of reduced corneal integrity or local infection (United States Pharmacopeia Drug Information, 1996). Systemic absorption of trifluorothymidine after topical administration appears to be negligible. The major metabolite determined by *in vitro* perfusion studies, 5-carboxy-2'-deoxyuridine, is not detected in the aqueous humor or in plasma following topical administration.

2 Mucocutaneous administration

Trifluorothymidine has been used successfully to treat mucocutaneous herpes simplex (both genital and elsewhere on skin) and varicella-zoster that is resistant to aciclovir and foscarnet. The genital lesions are cleansed with hydrogen peroxide and a thin layer of trifluorothymidine ophthalmic solution (1%) is applied every 8 h to the entire surface of the affected area which is then covered with a non-adsorbable dressing containing polymyxin B-bacitracin ointment (Kessler *et al.*, 1996). An alternative method is to mix KY jelly containing 10% methyl cellulose with 1% trifluorothymidine ophthalmic solution in a ratio of 1:2, to achieve a final concentration of 0.67% trifluorothymidine (Mr Craig McArthur, Alfred Hospital Melbourne, personal communication; Birch *et al.*, 1992). The cutaneous lesions may also be treated with this mixture. Interferon alpha can also be included in this preparation at a concentration of 2 million units per ml (Mr Craig McArthur, Alfred Hospital Melbourne, personal communication; Birch *et al.*, 1992). Trifluorothymidine 1% solution has also been directly applied to cutaneous lesions four times daily with success (Rossi *et al.*, 1995).

Availability

A 1% trifluorothymidine *solution* is available for ophthalmic use.

Mode of Action

Trifluorothymidine is a thymidine analog. The drug inhibits thymidylic phosphorylase and thymidylate synthetase. Trifluorothymidine, and not thymidine, is incorporated into viral DNA during viral replication. The activity of trifluorothymidine against cytomegalovirus (and probably the other herpesviruses whose replication is inhibited by the drug) is dependent on host cell TK (Wingard *et al.*, 1981).

Toxicity

The most common adverse effect of trifluorothymidine is mild, transient stinging. Punctate keratopathy resulting in blurred vision and intense conjunctival hyperemia has been uncommonly reported in association with trifluorothymidine treatment in patients with dendritic keratitis (La-Lau *et al.*, 1981). Increased intraocular pressure and hypersensitivity with itch, redness and swelling have also been infrequently observed (United States Pharmacopeia Drug Information 1996). Cross-hypersensitivity between trifluorothymidine and idoxuridine or vidarabine is rare (Carmine *et al.*, 1982). Intraocular trifluorothymidine given by intravitreal injection (200 μg per 0.1 ml) to rabbits resulted in no evidence of toxicity (Pang *et al.*, 1986).

Trifluorothymidine has been found to be cytotoxic and mutagenic when assessed in a mammalian cell mutagenesis assay (Marquardt *et al.*, 1985). Adenocarcinomas, hemangiosarcomas and ovarian and prostate tumors developed with increased frequency in rats administered trifluorothymidine in doses of 1.5–15 mg per kg per day (United States Pharmacopeia Drug Information, 1996).

Trifluorothymidine has been administered topically to the eye concurrently with a number of ophthalmic preparations including chloramphenicol, dexamethosone, prednisolone, hydrocortisone, atropine sulfate, scopolamine hydrobromide, homatropine hydrobromide, pilocarpine, epinephrine hydrochloride without adverse interaction.

Clinical Uses of the Drug

1 Keratoconjunctivitis due to herpes simplex types 1 and 2 infection

Topical trifluorothymidine is indicated for the treatment of primary keratoconjunctivitis and recurrent epithelial keratitis due to herpes simplex viruses types 1 and 2. In comparative studies, predominantly in patients with dendritic ulcers, trifluorothymidine (1% solution) has been found to be efficacious in over 90% of cases, with activity comparable with vidarabine, bromovinyldeoxyuridine and idoxuridine (Van-Bijsterveld and Post, 1980; Carmine *et al.*, 1982; Power *et al.*, 1991). In a study of 34 patients, trifluorothymidine was found to be superior to debridement alone for the treatment of herpes simplex dendritic keratitis; debridement in combination with trifluorothymidine offered no advantage over the antiviral therapy alone (Parlato *et al.*, 1985).

A multicenter, double-blind trial compared aciclovir (3% ophthalmic ointment) with trifluorothymidine (2% ointment) in 59 patients with herpes keratitis. Healing occurred in 99% and 75% of the aciclovir-treated and trifluorothymidine-treated patients respectively within 14 days, with no significant difference in the rate of healing between the two treatment groups (La-Lau *et al.*, 1982). These data are supported by a subsequent trial in which treatment of herpes simplex keratitis with 3% aciclovir or 2% trifluorothymidine ophthalmic ointment resulted in healing in 6.7 and 5.9 days respectively (Hovding, 1989).

Human recombinant interferon alpha eye drops given in combination with trifluorothymidine eye drops resulted in no therapeutic advantage compared with trifluorothymidine monotherapy (Sundmacher *et al.*, 1987). The drug has been found in open studies to be useful for the treatment of patients with ulcers unresponsive to idoxuridine or vidarabine, when used alone or in combination with interferon (Carmine *et al.*, 1982; Soriano *et al.*, 1992).

2 Acyclovir- and foscarnet-resistant mucocutaneous herpes simplex and varicella-zoster virus infection

Trifluorothymidine is not licensed for this condition and there have been no placebo-controlled trials. However, single case-reports and a recently published pilot study support its use for these difficult to treat cases.

Trifluorothymidine has also been found to be clinically useful in treating severe cutaneous herpes simplex infection that was refractory to acyclovir and foscarnet due to resistance to the latter drugs (Birch *et al.*, 1992). The treatment has been used with success to treat both anogenital, facial and other cutaneous lesions (Birch *et al.*, 1992; Kessler *et al.*, 1996). Trifluorothymidine has been used in combination with interferon alpha (Birch *et al.*, 1992). Complete healing was reported in a pilot study of 24 patients in 30% of cases with an median time to complete healing of 7.1 weeks and an estimated time to 50% healing of 2.4 weeks (Kessler *et al.*, 1996).

Clinical improvement with topical trifluorothymidine therapy used in combination with intralesional interferon alpha-2b (given twice-weekly in a total dose of 10 million units per week) has also been reported in a patient with aciclovir-resistant varicella-zoster; the patient was intolerant of foscarnet. The hyperkeratotic lesions flattened after 5 weeks of therapy and cleared completely after 3 months of therapy with no recurrence in the 6 months following treatment (Rossi *et al.*, 1995).

References

Abghari SZ, Stulting RD, Zhu Z *et al.* (1994). Effect of genetically determined host factors on the efficacy of vidarabine, acyclovir and 5-trifluorothymidine in herpes simplex virus type 1 infection. *Ophthalmic Res* **26**: 95.

Babiuk LA, Acres SD, Misra V *et al.* (1983). Susceptibility of bovid herpesvirus 1 to antiviral drugs; *in vitro* versus *in vivo* efficacy of (E)-5-(2-bromovinyl)-2'-deoxyuridine *Antimicrob Ag Chemother* **23**: 715.

Bauer DJ (1982). Acyclovir treatment of experimental herpetic keratitis in the rabbit eye. *Amer J Med* **73**: 109.

Birch CJ, Tyssen DP, Tachedjian G *et al.* (1992). Clinical effects and *in vitro* studies of trifluorothymidine combined with interferon-alpha for treatment of drug-resistant and sensitive herpes simplex virus infections. *J Infect Dis* **166**: 108.

Biron KK, Elion GB (1982). Effect of acyclovir combined with other antiherpetic agents on varicella zoster virus *in vitro. Amer J Med* **73**: 54.

Burkhardt U, Wigand R (1983). Combined chemotherapy of cutaneous herpes simplex infection of the guinea pig. *J Med Virol* **12**: 137.

Carmine AA, Brogden RN, Heel RC *et al.* (1982). Trifluridine; a review of its antiviral activity and therapeutic use in the topical treatment of viral eye infections. *Drugs* **23**: 329.

Fardeau C, Langlois M, Mathys B *et al.* (1991). Emergence of cross-resistant herpes simplex virus following topical drug therapy in rabbit keratitis. *Curr Eye Res* **10**: 151.

Field H, McMillan A, Darby G (1981). The sensitivity of acyclovir-resistant mutants of herpes simplex virus to other antiviral drugs. *J Infect Dis* **143**: 281.

Hovding G (1989). A comparison between acyclovir and trifluorothymidine ointment in the treatment of epithelial dendritic keratitis A double-blind, randomised parallel group trial. *Acta Ophthalmol Copenh* **67**: 51.

Kessler HA, Hurwitz S, Farthing C *et al.* (1996). Pilot study of topical trifluridine for the treatment of acyclovir resistant mucocutaneous herpes simplex disease in patients with AIDS (ACTG 172). *J AIDS Hum Retrovirol* **12**: 147.

Lang DJ, Cheung KS (1982). Effectiveness of acycloguanosine and trifluorothymidine as inhibitors of cytomegalovirus infection *in vitro. Amer J Med* **73**: 49.

La-Lau C, Oosterhuis JA, Versteeg J *et al.* (1981). Acyclovir and trifluorothymidine in herpetic keratitis. Preliminary report of a multi-centered trial. *Doc Ophthalmol* **50**: 287.

La-Lau C, Oosterhuis JA, Versteeg J *et al.* (1982). Multicenter trial of acyclovir and trifluorothymidine in herpetic keratitis. *Amer J Med* **73**: 305.

Marquardt H, Westendorf J, De Clercq E, Marquardt H (1985). Potent antiviral 5-(2-bromovinyl) uracil nucleosides are inactive at inducing gene mutation in *Salmonella typhimurium* and V79 Chinese hamster cells and unscheduled DNA synthesis in primary rat hepatocytes. *Carcinogenesis* **6**: 1207.

Pang MP, Peyman GA, Nikoleit J *et al.* (1986). Intravitreal trifluor-othymidine and retinal toxicity. *Retina* **6**: 260.

Pang MP, Branchflower RV, Chang AT *et al.* (1992). Half-life vitreous clearance of trifluorothymidine after intravitreal injection in the rabbit eye. *Can J Ophthalmol* **27**: 6.

Parlato CJ, Cohen FJ, Sakauye CM *et al.* (1985). Role of debridement and trifluridine (trifluorothymidine) in herpes simplex dendritic keratitis. *Arch Ophthalmol* **103**: 673,.

Power WJ, Benedict-Smith A, Hillery M *et al.* (1991). Randomised double-blind trial of bromovinyldeoxyuridine (BVDU) and trifluorothymidine (TFT) in dendritic corneal ulceration. *Brit J Ophthalmol* **75**: 649.

Rand KH, Bodor N, el-Koussi AA *et al.* (1986). Potential treatment of herpes simplex virus encephalitis by brain specific delivery of tri-fluorothymidine using a dihydropyridine pyridinium salt type redox delivery system. *J Med Virol* **20**: 1.

Rossi S, Whitfeld M, Berger TG (1995). The treatment of acyclovir-resistant herpes zoster with trifluorothymidine and interferon alfa. *Arch Dermatol* **131**: 24.

Schinazi RF, Nahmias AJ (1982). Different *in vitro* effects of dual combinations of anti-herpes simplex virus compounds. *Amer J Med* **73**: 40.

Soriano JM, Funk J, Janknecht P, Matz B (1992). Recurrent herpetic keratitis during topical acyclovir application. *Eur J Ophthalmol* **2**: 155.

Spector SA, Tyndall M, Kelley E (1982). Effects of acyclovir combined with other antiviral agents on human cytomegalovirus. *Amer J Med* **20**: 36.

Spector SA, Tyndall M, Kelley E (1983). Inhibition of human cytomegalovirus by trifluorothymidine *Antimicrob Ag Chemother* **23**: 113.

Sundmacher R, Mattes A, Neumann-Haefelin D *et al.* (1987). The potency of interferon-alpha 2 and interferon-gamma in a combination therapy of dendritic hepatitis. A controlled clinical study. *Curr Eye Res* **6**: 273.

Taylor JL, Punda-Polic V, O'Brien WJ (1991). Combined anti-herpes virus activity of nucleoside analogs and interferon. *Curr Eye Res* **10**: 205.

United States Pharmacopeia Drug Information (1996).

Van-Bijsterveld OP, Post H (1980). Trifluorothymidine versus adenine arabinoside in the treatment of herpes simplex keratitis. *Brit J Ophthalmol* **64**: 33.

Wingard JR, Stuart KK, Saral R, Burns WH (1981). Activity of trifluorothymidine against cytomegalovirus *Antimicrob Ag Chemother* **20**: 286.

Wingard JR, Hess AD, Stuart RK *et al.* (1983). Effect of several antiviral agents on human lymphocyte functions and marrow progenitor cell proliferation *Antimicrob Ag Chemother* **23**: 593.

Vidarabine

Description

Vidarabine (also known as adenine arabinoside, or Ara-A) is a purine analog with virustatic activity against a wide range of DNA and some oncogenic RNA viruses (De Garilhe and Rudder, 1964). The chemical name is (9{beta-D-arabinofuranosyl}) adenine. The chemical structure is shown in Fig. V.23.

Vidarabine was originally developed as an anti-tumor agent in 1960 (Lee *et al.*, 1960). Activity against DNA viruses was recognized in 1964 (De Garilhe and Rudder, 1964). It was found to be naturally present in culture supernatants of *Streptomyces antibioticus* (Miller *et al.*, 1969) and was the first compound to have proven antiviral efficacy (Whitley *et al.*, 1976). In its parenteral form it is active against herpes simplex virus and varicella-zoster virus. The agent is now virtually obsolete in clinical practice, having been replaced by aciclovir. Until recently it was regarded as an important standard for comparative trials with new antivirals. In its topical form it has activity in the treatment of herpes keratitis. The ophthalmic preparation is marketed by Parke Davis under the brand name of 'Vira-A'.

Antiviral Activity

The reported activity of vidarabine against herpes simplex and vaccinia virus in 1964 (De Garilhe and Rudder, 1964) was subsequently followed by evidence of activity against cytomegalovirus and Rous sarcoma virus (Miller *et al.*, 1969; Schabel, 1968), strains of adenovirus (Wigand, 1979), and hepatitis B (Hess *et al.*, 1981) (reviewed in Schabel, 1968; Miller *et al.*, 1969; Hirsch and Swartz, 1980; Kitabayashi *et al.*, 1994).

1 Herpes simplex virus

The *in vitro* activity of vidarabine includes strains of herpes simplex virus types 1 and 2 which are resistant to idoxuridine (Shannon, 1975), bromovinyldeoxyuridine (Wilber and Docherty, 1994) and aciclovir (Schinazi, 1987). Vidarabine results in a dose-dependent reduction in virus titer in Vero cells (Pulliam *et al.*, 1986). The inhibitory activity of vidarabine against clinical strains of herpes simplex virus in cell culture has been compared with that of other antiviral agents. Vidarabine was less potent (IC_{50} 11 µg per ml) than aciclovir and bromovinyldeoxyuridine (IC_{50} ranging from 0.02 to 0.9 µg per ml) (Andrei *et al.*, 1992; Rabelais *et al.*, 1989). There

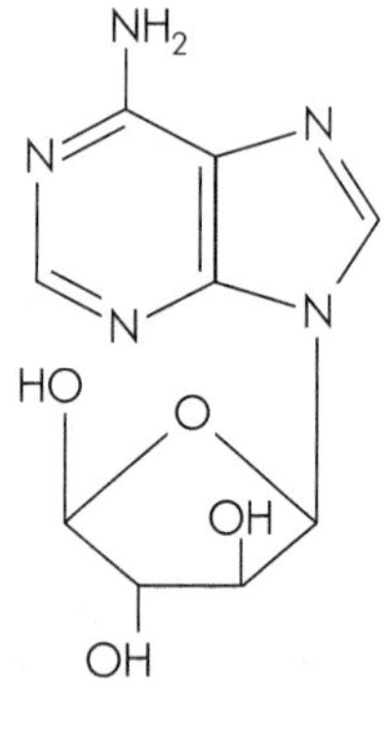

Fig. V.23.
Chemical structure of vidarabine.

is variation in sensitivity patterns depending on cell type used for the assay (Abghari *et al.*, 1994).

Mice injected intracerebrally with an aciclovir-resistant strain of herpes simplex virus responded to vidarabine (Schinazi 1987).

2 Varicella-zoster virus

By enzyme-linked immunosorbent assay performed directly on fixed varicella-zoster virus-infected human embryonic lung fibroblasts, vidarabine was more effective in inhibiting varicella-zoster virus (IC_{50} 1.0–3.5 μg per ml) than aciclovir (IC_{50} 2.5–50 μg per ml), of similar efficacy to trifluorothymidine (IC_{50} 1.2–5.0 μg per ml) and less effective than bromovinyldeoxyuridine (IC_{50} 0.02–0.5 μg per ml) (Berkowitz and Levin, 1985). Varicella-zoster virus is more susceptible to vidarabine than herpes simplex virus (Gephart and Lerner, 1981). Vidarabine has a lower selectivity index than aciclovir and penciclovir (Machida *et al.*, 1995). Aciclovir-resistant strains of varicella-zoster virus are sensitive to vidarabine with a mean IC_{50} of four clinical isolates being 1.4 μM (Jacobson *et al.*, 1990; Schinazi *et al.*, 1986).

3 Cytomegalovirus

Vidarabine potently inhibits cytomegalovirus replication *in vitro*, including foscarnet-resistant strains, with a narrow therapeutic margin (reviewed in Verheyden, 1988; Sullivan *et al.*, 1991).

4 Hepatitis B virus

The activity of vidarabine against hepatitis B virus has been demonstrated *in vitro* using a human hepatoblastoma cell line which continuously synthesizes hepatitis B viral DNA (Ueda *et al.*, 1989). In ducks chronically infected with hepatitis B virus, only high doses of vidarabine were shown to inhibit viral replication: a decrease in mature forms of viral DNA was accompanied by evidence of resistance of the supercoiled form of viral DNA to therapy (Hirota *et al.*, 1987; Omata *et al.*, 1986). More recent studies have failed to demonstrate an antiviral effect in woodchucks infected with woodchuck hepatitis virus (Fourel *et al.*, 1992).

5 Human immunodeficiency virus

The compound is not active against the human immunodeficiency virus (Balzarini *et al.*, 1986).

Mode of Administration and Dosage

1 Topical administration to eyes

Vidarabine is now only available commercially as an ophthalmic ointment called 'Vira-A Ophthalmic'. Approximately 1.5 cm of ointment is delivered into the lower conjunctival sac five times daily at 3-hourly intervals. After re-epithelialization has occurred (usually within 1–3 weeks), further treatment for an additional week, at reduced dosage (twice-daily), is recommended in order to prevent recurrence.

2 Parenteral administration

Intravenous preparations of vidarabine are no longer available in most countries, including the USA. In certain circumstances, the drug may be obtained to treat life-threatening, resistant infections for which no other suitable agent is available. The dosage recommended for treatment of chickenpox and disseminated varicella-zoster is 10 mg per kg daily for 5 days. For treatment of herpes simplex virus encephalitis the dose is 15 mg per kg daily for 10 days. The major metabolite arabinosyl hypoxanthine accumulates in patients with renal failure requiring dose adjustment for patients with renal impairment.

Availability

Ophthalmic ointment: each gram contains 30 mg adenine arabinoside monohydrate (28.1 mg adenine arabinoside) in a sterile, inert paraffin base.

Serum Levels, Excretion and Distribution in Body

Vidarabine is rapidly deaminated to arabinosyl hypoxanthine within erythrocytes by the enzyme adenosine deaminase (Kinkel and Buchanan, 1975). Levels of arabinosyl hypoxanthine in erythrocytes parallel those in serum and the CSF levels are approximately 35% of serum levels. During a 12-h infusion arabinosyl hypoxanthine levels are in the range of 3–6 μg per ml, and levels of the parent compound are less than 0.4 μg per ml. The predominant route of excretion is via the kidneys. There is no evidence of fecal excretion of the drug or its metabolite. As this drug is largely obsolete further details are not provided in this edition; refer to *The Use of Antibiotics*, 4th edition.

Mode of Action

Vidarabine exerts its antiviral effect by inhibiting DNA synthesis. The drug is a prodrug, requiring phosphorylation within the cell to mono-, di- and triphosphate derivatives in order to inhibit the viral DNA polymerase. In addition, vidarabine inhibits mammalian cell DNA polymerase, but to a lesser degree than for the viral-specified enzyme (Shannon, 1975; Le Page, 1973; Muller *et al.*, 1977). Vidarabine is also incorporated into both cellular and viral DNA during DNA synthesis (Muller *et al.*, 1977). *In vivo*, the major antiviral activity is mediated by arabinosyl hypoxanthine, which has considerably less activity than vidarabine (Shannon, 1975; Sloan, 1975; Bryson and Connor, 1976). Arabinosyl hypoxanthine is 30-fold less active against herpesvirus replication than vidarabine (Gephart and Lerner, 1981).

Studies in ducks infected with duck hepatitis B virus have shown that the mechanism of action of vidarabine against hepadna virus replication is through inhibition of the viral DNA polymerase, resulting in a decrease in the 'mature' forms of the viral DNA. There is, however, no effect on hepatitis B virus supercoiled DNA (Omata *et al.*, 1986).

Toxicity

In animals, vidarabine has low toxicity and does not appear to affect the hemopoietic system or the immune response (Le Page, 1973). It is teratogenic in rats and rabbits and oncogenic in some animals. Fibroblast proliferation is inhibited *in vitro* (Cheng *et al.*, 1995). Preliminary studies in humans indicated that in recommended doses it had virtually no effect on liver, kidneys and hemopoietic system, and its only consistent side-effect was nausea (Keeney, 1975). With increasing usage it became evident that vidarabine was associated with unacceptable toxicity.

Major effects are summerized below. For further details refer to *The Use of Antibiotics*, 4th edition, p. 1597.

1 Gastrointestinal toxicity

Dose-related gastrointestinal side-effects develop in approximately one-fifth of patients receiving the drug parenterally (Whitley *et al.*, 1976, 1982a,b,c). Symptoms include anorexia, nausea, vomiting and diarrhea. Severe hepatic failure has been reported following vidarabine therapy in combination with prednisolone in the treatment of chronic hepatitis B infection (Buti *et al.*, 1987).

2 Hematologic side-effects

At doses higher than 15 mg per kg daily pancytopenia and megaloblastic changes can occur. Changes in neutrophil counts may be paralleled by changes in bone marrow cellularity (Meyers *et al.*, 1982).

3 Neurotoxicity

Hallucinations, confusion, psychosis, tremors, ataxia, myoclonus, dysarthria, aphasia, neuralgia, seizures and coma have all been reported in association with vidarabine therapy (Meyers *et al.*, 1982; Sacks *et al.*, 1979, 1982; Lauter *et al.*, 1976; Ross *et al.*, 1976; Vilter, 1986; Feldman *et al.*, 1986; Safrin *et al.*, 1990, 1991). A severe and prolonged polyneuropathy was reported in association with a 12-week course of vidarabine in patients with chronic hepatitis B infection (Guardia *et al.*, 1986).

4 Other side-effects

Weakness, fatigue, weight loss, rash and thrombophlebitis at the i.v site can occur. Hyponatremia and the syndrome of inappropriate secretion of antidiuretic hormone have been related to vidarabine therapy (reviewed in Bevilacqua, 1994; Arzuaga *et al.*, 1994).

5 Ocular therapy

Lacrimation, conjunctivitis, burning, irritation, keratitis, pain, photophobia, punctal occlusion and hypersensitivity have been reported with vidarabine ointment.

Clinical Uses of the Drug

The efficacy of vidarabine has been established for the treatment of herpes simplex encephalitis, neonatal infection with herpes simplex, ocular herpes keratitis, and varicella-zoster in immunocompromised hosts.

1 Herpes simplex virus infections

Vidarabine has been shown in a number of controlled trials to reduce the death rate, and improve long-term outcome of treated individuals with herpes simplex encephalitis compared with no treatment (Whitley et al., 1977, 1981). In a randomized controlled study of patients with encephalitis, aciclovir was found to be superior to vidarabine in terms of survival and long-term morbidity (Whitley et al., 1986) (Fig. V.24). Early studies in neonates demonstrated lower mortality and sequelae in vidarabine recipients compared with those treated with placebo (Whitley et al., 1980). In neonates with severe herpes simplex virus infection no significant differences were observed between aciclovir and vidarabine in terms of both long-term morbidity and mortality (Whitley et al., 1991). Vidarabine has also been used successfully in the treatment of aciclovir-resistant herpes simplex virus in bone marrow transplant recipients (Ljungman et al., 1990). In a randomized trial in which foscarnet was compared with vidarabine for the treatment of aciclovir-resistant mucocutaneous herpes simplex in patients with AIDS, foscarnet therapy was superior to vidarabine in terms of a higher rate of healing, shorter time to healing and significantly less toxicity (Safrin et al., 1991).

2 Severe varicella-zoster virus infections

The clinical efficacy of vidarabine for the treatment of varicella-zoster virus infection in immunocompromised patients was demonstrated by a number of early studies (Whitley et al., 1976, 1982b,c). A randomized comparison of vidarabine and aciclovir for the treatment of varicella-zoster virus infections in immunocompromised patients who presented within 72 h of onset of symptoms demonstrated superior efficacy of aciclovir over vidarabine. Cutaneous dissemination did not develop in any of the ten aciclovir recipients compared with five of ten vidarabine recipients. There was also a shorter period of pain and less time to crusting of lesions in the aciclovir group compared with the vidarabine group (Shepp et al., 1986). These findings are supported by some studies (Vilde et al., 1986) although other investigators have found no significant difference between the two therapies when used to treat immunocompromised patients with disseminated varicella-zoster virus infection (Whitley et al., 1992). Thus i.v. vidarabine is probably not quite as efficacious and certainly associated with more toxicity than i.v. aciclovir for the treatment of severe varicella-zoster infections in immunocompromised patients (Whitley et al., 1992; reviewed in Wagstaff et al., 1994).

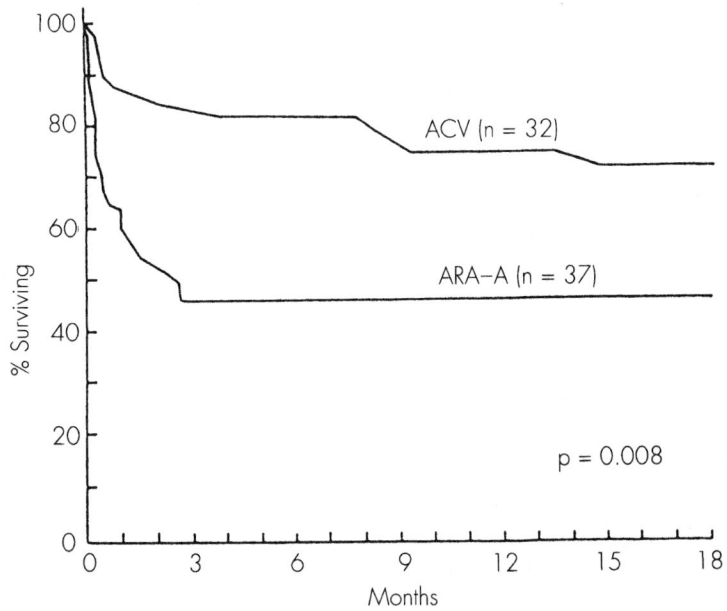

Fig. V.24.
Comparison of survival in patients with biopsy-proved herpes simplex encephalitis treated with vidarabine (ARA-A) or aciclovir (ACV) (p = 0.008). (Reproduced with permission from Whitley et al., 1986, with permission.)

3 Cytomegalovirus infection

Although vidarabine appeared to have efficacy in the treatment of cytomegalovirus retinitis in one early study (Pollard *et al.*, 1982), other investigators have reported lack of efficacy (Ch'ien *et al.*, 1974; Baublis *et al.*, 1975; Rytel and Kauffman, 1976; Marker *et al.*, 1980; Meyers *et al.*, 1982; Mills *et al.*, 1988).

4 Hepatitis B virus infection

Treatment of chronic hepatitis B with combination therapy using vidarabine alone or in combination with interferon alpha is not superior to interferon alpha monotherapy in terms of clinical outcome (Garcia *et al.*, 1987; Scully *et al.*, 1986; Schalm, 1994). There is a case report of successful treatment with vidarabine in an immunosuppressed patient who developed painful gross hematuria, renal dysfunction, thrombocytopenia with evidence of hemophagocytosis (Kitabayashi *et al.*, 1994).

As this drug is virtually obsolete now due to its toxicity, no further details will be given in this edition. This section has been extensively covered in *The Use of Antibiotics*, 4th edition, pp. 1597–1601.

Acknowledgements The author would like to thank Richard Whitley, of the University of Alabama at Birmingham for his critical review of this chapter.

References

Abghari SZ, Stulting RD, Zhu Z et al. (1994). Effect of genetically determined host factors on the efficacy of vidarabine, acyclovir and 5-trifluorothymidine in herpes simplex virus type 1 infection. *Ophthalmic Res* **26**: 95.

Andrei G Snoeck R, Goubau P et al. (1992). Comparative activity of various compounds against clinical strains of herpes simplex virus. *Eur J Clin Microbiol Infect Dis* **11**: 143.

Arzuaga JA, Estirado E, Roman F et al. (1994). Syndrome of inappropriate antidiuretic hormone secretion and herpes zoster infection; 1. Report of this association in a patient suffering from AIDS. *Nephron* **68**: 262.

Balzarini J, Mitsuya H, De CE et al. (1986). Comparative inhibitory effects of suramin and other selected compounds on the infectivity and replication of human T-cell lymphotropic virus (HTLV- III)/lymphadenopathy associated virus (LAV). *Int J Cancer* **37**: 451.

Baublis JV, Whitley RJ, Ch'ien LT, Alford CA (1975). Treatment of cytomegalovirus infection in infants and adults In *Adenine Arabinoside. An Antiviral Agent* (Pavan-Langston D, Buchanan RA, Alford CA Jr eds), p. 247. New York: Raven Press.

Berkowitz FE, Levin MJ (1985). Use of an enzyme linked immunosorbent assay performed directly on fixed infected cell monolayers for evaluating drugs against varicella zoster virus. *Antimicrob Ag Chemother* **28**: 207.

Bevilacqua M (1994). Hyponatraemia in AIDS. *Baillières Clin Endocrinol Metab* **8**: 837.

Bryson YJ, Connor JD (1976). *In vitro* susceptibility of varicella zoster virus to adenine arabinoside and hypoxanthine arabinoside. *Antimicrob Ag Chemother* **9**: 540.

Buti M, Esteban R, Esteban JI et al. (1987). Severe hepatic failure after ARA-A-prednisolone for chronic type B hepatitis. *Gastroenterol* **92**: 274.

Ch'ien LT, Cannon NJ, Whitley RJ et al. (1974). Effect of adenine arabinoside on cytomegalovirus infections. *J Infect Dis* **130**: 32.

Cheng Q, Shapourifar-Tehrani S, Lee DA (1995). Comparative efficacy of antiviral drugs on human ocular fibroblasts. *Exp Eye Res* **61**: 461.

De Garilhe P, De Rudder (1964). Effect de deux nucleosides de l'arabinose sur la multiplication des virus de herpes et de la vaccine en culture cellulaise. *CR Acad Sci* **259**: 2725.

Feldman S, Robertson PK, Lott L, Thornton D (1986). Neurotoxicity due to adenine arabinoside therapy during varicella zoster virus infections in immunocompromised children. *J Infect Dis* **154**: 889.

Fourel I, Li J, Hantz O et al. (1992). Effects of 2'-fluorinated arabinosylpyrimidine nucleosides on duck hepatitis B virus DNA level in serum and liver of chronically infected ducks. *J Med Virol* **37**: 122.

Garcia G, Smith CJ, Weissberg JI et al. (1987). Adenine arabinoside monophosphate (vidarabine phosphate) in combination with human leukocyte interferon in the treatment of chronic hepatitis B. A randomised, double-blinded, placebo-controlled trial. *Ann Intern Med* **107**: 278.

Gephart JF, Lerner AM (1981). Comparison of the effects of arabinosyladenine, arabinosylbypoxanthine, and arabinosyladenine 5'-monophosphate against herpes simplex virus, varicella zoster virus, and cytomegalovirus with their effects of cellular deoxyribonucleic acid synthesis. *Antimicrob Ag Chemother* **19**: 170.

Guardia J, Esteban R, Buti M et al. (1986). Prolonged inhibition of hepatitis B virus replication with vidarabine monophosphate in chronic active type B hepatitis. *Liver* **6**: 118.

Hess G, Arnold W, Meyer zum Buschenfelde KH (1981). Inhibition of hepatitis B virus deoxyribonucleic acid polymerase by the 5'-triphosphates of 9-beta-D-arabinofuranosyladenine and 1-beta-D-arabinofuranosylcytosine. *Antimicrob Ag Chemother* **19**: 44.

Hirota K, Sherker AH, Omata M et al. (1987). Effects of adenine arabinoside on serum and intrahepatic replicative forms of duck hepatitis B virus in chronic infection. *Hepatol* **7**: 24.

Hirsch MS, Swartz MN (1980). Antiviral agents. *Med Intelligence* **302**: 903.

Jacobson MA, Berger TG, Fikrig S et al. (1990). Acyclovir-resistant varicella zoster virus infection after chronic oral acyclovir therapy in patients with the acquired immunodeficiency syndrome (AIDS). *Ann Intern Med* **112**: 187.

Keeney RE (1975). Human tolerance of adenine arabinoside. In *Adenine Arabinoside. An Antiviral Agent* (Pavan-Langston D, Buchanan RA, Alford CA Jr eds), p.265. New York: Raven Press.

Kinkel AW, Buchanan RA (1975). Human pharmacology In *Adenine Arabinoside. An Antiviral Agent* (Pavan-Langston D, Buchanan RA, Alford CA Jr eds), p. 197. New York: Raven Press.

Kitabayashi A, Hirokawa M, Kuroki J et al. (1994). Successful vidarabine therapy for adenovirus type 11-associated acute hemorrhagic cystitis after allogeneic bone marrow transplantation. *Bone Marrow Transplant* **14**: 853.

Lauter CB, Bailey EJ, Lerner AM (1976). Microbiologic assays and neurological toxicity during use of adenine arabinoside in humans. *J Infect Dis* **134**: 75.

Le Page GA (1973). Purines and purine nucleoside antagonists. *Transplant Proc* **5**: 1157.

Lee WW, Benitez A, Goodman L, Baker BR (1960). Potential anticancer agents. XL Synthesis of the anomer of 9-(D-arabinofuranosyl)-adenine. *J Amer Chem Soc* **82**: 2648.

Ljungman P, Ellis MN, Hackman RC *et al.* (1990). Acyclovir resistant herpes simplex virus causing pneumonia after marrow transplantation. *J Infect Dis* **162**: 244.

Machida H, Nishitani M, Watanabe Y *et al.* (1995). Comparison of the selectivity of anti-varicella zoster virus nucleoside analogues. *Microbiol Immunol* **39**: 201.

Marker SC, Howard RJ, Groth KE *et al.* (1980). A trial of vidarabine for cytomegalovirus infection in renal transplant patients. *Arch Intern Med* **140**: 1441.

Meyers JD, McGuffin RW, Bryson YJ *et al.* (1982). Treatment of cytomegalovirus pneumonia after marrow transplant with combined vidarabine and human leukocyte interferon. *J Infect Dis* **146**: 80.

Miller FA, Dixon GJ, Ehrlich J *et al.* (1968). Antiviral activity of 9-beta-D-arabinofuranosyladenine. I Cell culture studies. *Antimicrob Ag Chemother* **8**: 136.

Mills J, Jacobson MA, O'Donnell JJ *et al.* (1988). Treatment of cytomegalovirus retinitis in patients with AIDS. *Rev Infect Dis* **10**: S522.

Muller WEG, Zahn RK, Bittlingmater K, Falke D (1977). Inhibition of herpes virus DNA synthesis by 9-beta-D-arabinofuranosyladenine in cellular and cell free systems. *Ann NY Acad Sci* **34**: 284.

Omata M, Hirota K, Yokosuka O (1986). *In vivo* study of the mechanism of action of antiviral agents against hepadna virus replication in the liver. Resistance of supercoiled viral DNA. *J Hepatol* **12**: S49.

Pollard RB, Egbert PR, Gallagher JG, Merigan TC (1982). cytomegalovirus retinitis in immunosuppressed hosts. 1. Natural history and effects of treatment with adenine arabinoside. *Ann Intern Med* **93**: 655.

Pulliam L, Panitch HS, Baringer JR, Dix RD (1986). Effect of antiviral agents on replication of herpes simplex virus type 1 in brain cultures. *Antimicrob Ag Chemother* **30**: 840.

Rabalais GP, Nusinoff LS, Arvin AM, Levin MJ (1989). Antiviral susceptibilities of herpes simplex virus isolates from infants with recurrent mucocutaneous lesions after neonatal infection. *Pediatr Infect Dis* **8**: 221.

Ross AH, Julia A, Balakrishnan C (1976). Toxicity of adenine arabinoside in humans. *J Infect Dis* **133**: 192.

Rytel WM, Kauffman HM (1976). Clinical efficacy of adenine arabinoside in humans. *J Infect Dis* **133**: 202.

Sacks SL, Smith JL, Pollard RB *et al.* (1979). Toxicity of vidarabine. *JAMA* **241**: 28.

Sacks SL, Scullard GH, Pollard RB *et al.* (1982). Antiviral treatment of chronic hepatitis B virus infection; pharmacokinetics and side effects of interferon and adenine arabinoside alone and in combination. *Antimicrob Ag Chemother* **21**: 93.

Safrin S, Assaykeen T, Follansbee S, Mills J (1990). Foscarnet therapy for acyclovir resistant mucocutaneous herpes simplex virus infection in 26 AIDS patients; preliminary data. *J Infect Dis* **161**: 1078.

Safrin S, Crumpacker C, Chatis P *et al.* (1991). A controlled trial comparing foscarnet with vidarabine for acyclovir resistant mucocutaneous herpes simplex in the acquired immunodeficiency syndrome The AIDS Clinical Trials Group. *New Engl J Med* **325**: 551.

Schabel FM (1968). The antiviral activity of 9-beta-D-arabinosuranosyladenine (Ara-A). *Chemother* **13**: 321.

Schalm SW (1994). Treatment of chronic hepatitis B. *Neth J Med* **44**: 103.

Schinazi RF, del BV, Scott RT, Dudley TJB (1986). Characterisation of acyclovir resistant and sensitive herpes simplex viruses isolated from a patient with an acquired immune deficiency. *J Antimicrob Chemother* **18**: 127.

Scully LJ, Lever AM, Yap I *et al.* (1986). Identification of factors influencing response rate to antiviral therapy of chronic hepatitis B virus infection A review of the efficacy of adenine; arabinoside and lymphoblastoid interferon in the Royal Free Hospital studies. *J Hepatol* **3**: S291.

Shannon WM (1975). Adenine arabinoside; antiviral activity *in vitro*. In *Adenine Arabinoside. An Antiviral Agent* (Payan-Langston D, Buchanan RA, Alford CA Jr, eds), p. 1. New York: Raven Press.

Shepp DH, Dandliker PS, Meyers JD (1986). Treatment of varicella zoster virus infection in severely immunocompromised patients A randomised comparison of acyclovir and vidarabine. *New Engl J Med* **314**: 208.

Shinazi RF. Drug combinations for treatment of mice infected with acyclovir-resistant herpes simplex virus. *Antimicrob Ag Chemother* **31**: 477.

Sloan BJ (1975). Adenine arabinoside; Chemotherapy studies in animals. In *Adenine Arabinoside. An Antiviral Agent* (Pavan-Langston D, Buchanan RA, Alford CA Jr eds), p. 45. New York: Raven Press.

Sullivan V, Coen DM (1991). Isolation of foscarnet-resistant human cytomegalovirus patterns of resistance and sensitivity to other antiviral drugs. *J Infect Dis* **164**: 781.

Ueda K, Tsurimoto T, Nagahata T *et al.* (1989). An *in vitro* system for screening anti-hepatitis B virus drugs. *Virology* **169**: 213.

Verheyden JP (1988). Evolution of therapy for cytomegalovirus infection. *Rev Infect Dis* **10**: S477.

Vilde JL, Bricaire F, Leport C *et al.* (1986). Comparative trial of acyclovir and vidarabine in disseminated varicella-zoster infections in immuno-compromised patients. *J Med Virol* **20**: 127.

Vilter RW (1986). Vidarabine associated encephalopathy and myoclonus. *Antimicrob Ag Chemother* **29**: 933.

Wagstaff AJ, Faulds D, Goa KL (1994). Aciclovir. A reappraisal of its antiviral activity, pharmacokinetic properties and therapeutic efficacy. *Drugs* **47**: 153.

Whitley RJ, Ch'ien LT, Dolin R *et al.* (1976). Adenine arabinoside therapy of herpes zoster in the immunosuppressed NIAID collaborative antiviral study. *New Engl J Med* **294**: 1193.

Whitley RJ, Soong SJ, Dolin R *et al.* (1977). Adenine arabinoside therapy of biopsy-proved herpes simplex encephalitis. National Institute of Allergy and Infectious Diseases collaborative antiviral study. *New Engl J Med* **297**: 289.

Whitley RJ, Nahmias AJ, Soong SJ *et al.* (1980). Vidarabine therapy of neonatal herpes simplex virus infection. *Pediatrics* **66**: 495.

Whitley RJ, Soong SJ, Hirsch MS *et al.* (1981). Herpes simplex encephalitis, vidarabine therapy and diagnostic problems. *New Engl J Med* **304**: 313.

Whitley RJ, Soong SJ, Linneman C *et al.* (1982a), Herpes simplex encephalitis. Clinical assessment. *JAMA* **247**: 317.

Whitley R, Hilty M, Haynes R *et al.* (1982b), Vidarabine therapy of varicella in immunosuppressed patients. *J Pediatr* **101**: 125.

Whitley RJ, Soong SJ, Dolin R *et al.* (1982c), Early vidarabine therapy to control the complications of herpes zoster in immunosuppressed patients. *New Engl J Med* **307**: 971.

Whitley RJ, Alford CA, Hirsch MS *et al.* (1986). Vidarabine versus acyclovir therapy to herpes simplex encephalitis. *New Engl J Med* **314**: 144.

Whitley R, Arvin A, Prober C *et al.* (1991). A controlled trail comparing vidarabine with acyclovir in neonatal herpes simplex virus infection. Infectious Diseases Collaborative Antiviral Study Group. *New Engl J Med* **324**: 445.

Whitley RJ, Gnann JWJ, Hinthorn D *et al.* (1992). Disseminated herpes zoster in the immunocompromised host; a comparative trial of acyclovir and vidarabine. The NIAID Collaborative Antiviral Study Group. *J Infect Dis* **165**: 450.

Wigand R (1979). Adenine arabinoside inhibition of adenovirus replication enhanced by an adenosine deaminase inhibitor. *J Med Virol* **4**: 59.

Wilber BA, Docherty JJ (1994). Analysis of the thymidine kinase of a herpes simplex virus type 1 isolate that exhibits resistance to (E)-5-(2-bromovinyl-2'-doexyuridine. *J Gen Virol* **75**: 1743.

Idoxuridine

Description

Idoxuridine (5-iodo-2'-deoxyuridine; IUdR; IDU) is an analog of the pyrimidine nucleoside thymidine. It was synthesized in 1959 as a possible anti-tumor agent (Prusoff 1959), and later shown to inhibit the growth of herpes simplex and vaccinia viruses in tissue culture (Herrman, 1961). Subsequently, it was reported to be useful for treatment of herpes simplex virus keratitis in man (Kaufman, 1962), and this remains its main clinical indication. Idoxuridine must be administered topically due to the severity of its systemic toxic effects. Idoxuridine is marketed with the trade names of 'Stoxil', 'Dendrid' and 'Herplex'. The molecular weight is 354.10. The chemical structure is shown in Fig. V.25.

Antiviral Activity

In vitro, idoxuridine inhibits the replication of DNA viruses including herpes simplex virus, varicella-zoster virus, cytomegalovirus and vaccinia (Marks, 1974; Baba *et al.*, 1986; reviewed in Verheyden, 1988)

1 Herpes simplex virus

Activity of idoxuridine against herpes simplex virus varies according to virus inoculum, tissue culture cell line and strain of the virus (Marks, 1974; Suzutani *et al.*, 1988). Idoxuridine has a low antiviral index (therapeutic efficacy/toxicity) of 27, like adenine arabinoside with an index of 16, compared with aciclovir with a value of 1250, when tested *in vitro* against herpes simplex virus type 1 (Park *et al.*, 1982).

In vitro activity does not necessarily reflect activity *in vivo*; varying results have been obtained when idoxuridine has been used to treat experimental viral infections in animals (Lefkowitz *et al.*, 1976; De Clercq *et al.*, 1976; Steffenhagen *et al.*, 1976). Idoxuridine has been reported to be five times less active against human keratinocytes infected with herpes simplex type 1 *in vitro* than guinea pig embryo cells, possibly attributable to the fact that the enzyme responsible for its catabolism, thymidine phosphorylase, has significantly greater activity in human compared with guinea pig embryo cells (Reuveni *et al.*, 1991). The drug has activity against both herpes simplex virus type 1 and type 2. Animals infected with equine herpes simplex virus type 2 resulting in ocular disease have responded to treatment with idoxuridine (Collinson *et al.*, 1994).

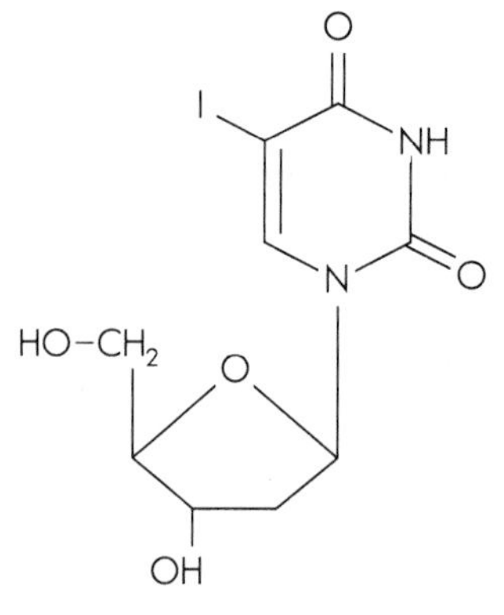

Fig. V.25.
Chemical structure of idoxuridine.

Idoxuridine is synergistic *in vitro* with human fibroblast interferon in inhibiting the replication of herpes simplex type 1 (Happonen *et al.*, 1990a).

Mutant viruses resistant to idoxuridine may develop both *in vitro* and *in vivo*. These strains are deficient in thymidine kinase (TK) activity (Renis and Buthala, 1965; Schabel and Montgomery, 1972). Herpes simplex virus type 1 resistant to idoxuridine has been identified following passage of virus through rabbits treated with the drug. Therapeutic failure was gradual. By the seventh passage, the resistant virus exhibited approximately 5% of TK activity compared with the parental strain, and was cross-resistant to bromovinyl deoxyuridine (0.5%) and aciclovir (3%) but not to adenine arabinoside (3%) or ganciclovir (3%) (Fardeau *et al.*, 1991, 1993). Evidence of resistance to both aciclovir and idoxuridine has been found in clinical isolates of herpes simplex virus type 1 from patients with herpes labialis who have had no prior antiviral exposure (Katz *et al.*, 1991).

2 Varicella-zoster virus

Idoxuridine has activity against varicella-zoster when tested in human embryonic fibroblast cell cultures (Baba *et al.*, 1986). Strains of varicella-zoster virus that are resistant to idoxuridine have been identified; these strains possess a deoxythymidine kinase that is inefficient at phosphorylating deoxythymidine (Shigeta *et al.*,1986).

Mode of Administration, Dosage and Distribution in Body

1 Systemic administration

Idoxuridine is no longer used systemically because of its toxicity and lack of clinical efficacy (Boston and NIAID Studies, 1975).

2 Topical administration

The topical use of idoxuridine for treatment of mucocutaneous infections due to herpes simplex and varicella-zoster viruses has been superseded by aciclovir (see aciclovir, pp. 1521, 1527).

3 Ocular administration

The drug may be applied to the cornea either as a 0.1% ophthalmic solution (1 mg per ml) or as a 0.5% ophthalmic ointment (5mg per g). If the solution is used, one drop is placed in the infected eye hourly during the day and every 2h during the night; the frequency of instillation may be halved as improvement occurs. The ointment, which is more convenient for the patient, should be instilled every 4 h during the day, with the last instillation at bedtime. Both forms of treatment should be continued for 3–5 days after healing becomes complete, but the total period of treatment should usually not exceed 21 days. Corticosteroids may be instilled into the eye with idoxuridine, but they are contraindicated in uncomplicated keratitis. Antibiotics and atropine may be instilled together with idoxuridine if necessary.

Idoxuridine has only limited penetration of the cornea, due to poor permeability of the polar drug across the lipoidal epithelial layer of the cornea (Narurkar and Mitra, 1989). Levels of idoxuridine in the stratum corneum of guinea pig skin peak 1–3 h after topical application and then gradually decline over the next 3–24 h (Sheth *et al.*, 1987). When glycyrrhizin gel is used as a carrier the idoxuridine preparation penetrates skin more effectively than the commercial ointment (Segal and Pisanty, 1987; Touitou *et al.*, 1988).

Mode of Action

Idoxuridine is phosphorylated in herpesvirus infected cells by a virus-specified TK. The drug is subsequently phosphorylated by cellular enzymes. Idoxuridine inhibits synthesis of DNA in normal human tissue cells and in DNA viruses. As idoxuridine triphosphate, it competes with thymidine, an essential constituent of DNA, and its phosphorylated derivatives inhibits thymidylic phosphorylase and the virus-coded DNA polymerases required for the incorporation of thymidine into viral DNA (reviewed in Kulikowski, 1994). Substitution of 0.1–1% of the thymidine residues in the DNA of varicella-zoster virus has been found to inhibit the replication of the virus (Yokota *et al.*, 1987). Idoxuridine is incorporated into both viral and mammalian DNA. The antiviral activity of idoxuridine is reversed by thymidine.

Toxicity

Instillation in the eye may occasionally cause allergy or inflammation with resultant pain and pruritus in the eye or eyelids (Pavan-Langston, 1975; Amon and Hanifin, 1976; Panda *et al.*, 1995). If idoxuridine is instilled more frequently than recommended, small defects may appear on the cornea, in which case the drug should be discontinued. Follicular conjunctivitis and punctate keratopathy have been reported (Naito *et al.*, 1987). Boric acid should not be used in the eye with idoxuridine because of interactions between boric acid and inert ingredients present in some formulations of idoxuridine resulting in precipitation (United States Pharmacopeia Drug Information, 1996).

Idoxuridine therapy is not recommended in pregnancy as fetal malformations and chromosomal aberrations have been reported in rabbits and mice .

Side-effects from mucosal therapy are reportedly minimal (Spruance *et al.*, 1990; Happonen *et al.*, 1990b).

Clinical Uses of the Drug

1 Ocular keratitis

Topical idoxuridine is an accepted form of treatment for keratitis due to herpes simplex virus (Patterson *et al.*, 1963; Laibson and Leopold, 1964). It is of some use for the treatment of acute dendritic ulcers, but is of no proven value for deep stromal ulcer or on corneal inflammation following herpetic keratitis. Other medications, particularly trifluorothymidine, appear to be more useful for the treatment of herpes keratitis. In cases of stromal keratitis or keratouveitis, either topical adenine arabinoside (Pavan-Langston 1975) or topical aciclovir is preferable. The 5-year recurrence rates for herpes simplex keratitis treated with aciclovir are significantly lower than those in patients treated with idoxuridine, being 17.5% and 52.9% respectively (Uchio *et al.*, 1993; Uchio *et al.*, 1994). In uncomplicated herpetic keratitis, 1% idoxuridine ointment has been found to be inferior to 2% trifluorothymidine ointment, 3% acyclovir ointment and 1% bromovinyl deoxyuridine in a randomized double-blind trial. The cure rates for idoxuridine, trifluorothymidine, aciclovir and bromovinyl deoxyuridine were 60%, 90%, 90%, and 95% respectively with average healing times of 13.4, 8.9, 8.5, and 7.5 days respectively (Panda *et al.*, 1995).

Idoxuridine is of no value for adenoviral keratoconjunctivitis, but it may be effective for herpes zoster keratitis (Pavan-Langston and McCulley, 1973). In these diseases, the rapid synthesis of viral DNA in the superficial part of the cornea is more sensitive to idoxuridine than DNA in the slowly proliferating corneal cells.

Prophylactic instillation of idoxuridine into the eye may be indicated if herpes lesions are adjacent to the eye, and sometimes when topical corticosteroids are used in the eye for other purposes. Herpes simplex virus strains may become resistant to idoxuridine *in vitro* and *in vivo* (Schabel and Montgomery, 1972), and this may explain the failure of this drug in the treatment of recurrent herpes simplex virus keratitis. Idoxuridine has no effect on herpes simplex virus within nerve ganglia serving the eye, thus allowing these ganglia, particularly the trigeminal ganglion, to become reservoirs for the virus to reinfect the cornea and conjunctiva. Bromovinyl deoxyuridine has been reported to be promote healing in ocular disease resistant to therapy with idoxuridine (Maudgal and De Clercq, 1991).

2 Herpes simplex labialis

Although all clinicians would choose to treat herpes simplex labialis with aciclovir or a related oral drug as first-line therapy, there is evidence for the use of idoxuridine in this clinical setting. In a double-blind, randomized, patient-initiated study involving 301 immunocompetent patients with recurrent herpes simplex labialis, topical treatment with 15% idoxuridine in dimethylsulfoxide was superior to control (dimethylsulfoxide solution in two concentrations) in shortening the mean duration of pain, and the mean time to crusting of lesions, particularly when treatment was commenced during the prodromal phase (Spruance *et al.*, 1990).

3 Genital condyloma acuminatum

Hasumi *et al.* (1984) used 0.25% idoxuridine in an ointment base to treat this sexually transmitted papillomavirus infection; treatment was effective in curing lesions in all six patients and there were no side-effects; in five patients treated with a placebo ointment there was no improvement. This open study was followed by a randomized, double-blind, placebo-controlled trial in which there was complete regression of lesions in 11 of 14 patients treated with idoxuridine ointment (0.25%) twice-daily for 14 days, but no regression in lesions in the ten who applied a placebo ointment (Hasumi, 1987). In a larger study, 40 patients with resistant penile warts with a mean of more than 12 months duration were treated with carbon dioxide laser plus 0.5% idoxuridine cream twice-daily. After 14 days of treatment complete healing occurred in 80% of patients; non-responders were retreated for another 14 days and after 4 and 12 weeks complete healing was observed in 87.5 and 85% of patients respectively (Happonen *et al.*, 1990a). In another study of 50 patients with genital warts of less than 3 months duration, 76% of those randomized to apply 0.5% cream twice-daily for 14 days compared with 36% of those randomized to apply 0.25% cream demonstrated complete healing (Happonen *et al.*, 1990b).

References

Amon RB, Hanifin JM (1976). Allergic contact dermatitis due to idoxuridine. *New Engl J Med* **294**: 956.

Baba M, Konno K, Shigeta S, De Clercq E (1986). Inhibitory effects of selected antiviral compounds on newly isolated clinical varicella zoster virus strains. *Tohoku J Exp Med* **148**: 275.

Boston Interhospital Virus Study Group and the NIAlD-Sponsored Cooperative Antiviral Clinical Study (1975). Failure of high dose 5-iodo-2'-deoxyuridine in the therapy of herpes simplex virus encephalitis. Evidence of unacceptable toxicity. *New Engl J Med* **292**: 600.

Collinson PN, O'Rielly JL, Ficorilli N, Studdert MJ (1994). Isolation of equine herpesvirus type 2 (equine gammaherpesvirus 2) from foals with keratoconjunctivitis. *J Amer Vet Med Assoc* **205**: 329.

De Clercq E, Luczak M, Shugar D *et al.* (1976). Effect of cytosine arabinoside, iododeoxyuridine, ethyldeoxyuridine, thiocyanatodeoxyuridine, and ribavirin on tail lesion formation in mice infected with Vaccinia virus (39241). *Proc Soc Exp Biol Med* **151**: 487.

Fardeau C, Langlois M, Mathys B *et al.* (1991). Emergence of cross-resistant herpes simplex virus following topical drug therapy in rabbit keratitis. *Curr Eye Res* **10**: 151.

Fardeau C, Langlois M, Nugler F *et al.* (1993). Cross-resistances to antiviral drugs of IUdR-resistant HSV-1 in rabbit keratitis and *in vitro*. *Cornea* **12**: 19.

Happonen HP, Lassus A, Santalahti J *et al.* (1990a) Combination of laser-therapy with 05% idoxuridine cream in the treatment of therapy-resistant genital warts in male patients; an open study. *Sex Transm Dis* **17**: 127.

Happonen HP, Lassus A, Santalahti J *et al.* (1990b) Topical idoxuridine for treatment of genital warts in males. A double-blind comparative study of 025% and 05% cream. *Genitourin Med* **66**: 254.

Hasumi K (1987). A trial of topical idoxuridine for vulvar condyloma acuminatum. *Brit J Obstet Gynaecol* **94**: 366.

Hasumi K, Kobayashi T, Ata M (1984). Topical idoxuridine for genital condyloma acuminatum. *Lancet* **i**: 968.

Herrman EC Jr (1961). Plaque inhibition test for detection of specific inhibitors of DNA containing viruses. *Proc Soc Exp Biol Med NY* **107**: 142.

Katz E, Rosenblat O, Pisanty S (1991). Isolation and characterisation of herpes simplex virus resistant to nucleoside analogs. *Oral Surg Oral Med Oral Pathol* **72**: 296.

Kaufman HE (1962). Clinical cure of herpes simplex keratitis by 5-iodo-2'-deoxyuridine. *Proc Soc Exp Biol Med NY* **109**: 251.

Kulikowski T (1994). Structure activity relationships and conformational features of antiherpetic pyrimidine and purine nucleoside analogues A review. *Pharm World Sci* **16**: 127.

Laibson PR, Leopold lH (1964). An evaluation of double-blind IDU therapy in 100 cases of herpetic keratitis. *Trans Amer Acad Ophthal Otolaryngol* **68**: 22.

Lefkowitz E, Worthington M, Conliffe McGA, Baron S (1976). Comparative effectiveness of six antiviral agents in herpes simplex type I infection of mice (39392). *Proc Soc Exp Biol Med* **152**: 337.

Marks MI (1974). Variables influencing the *in vitro* susceptibilities of herpes simplex viruses to antiviral drugs. *Antimicrob Ag Chemother* **6**: 34.

Maudgal PC, De Clercq E (1991). Bromovinyldeoxyuridine treatment of herpetic keratitis clinically resistant to other antiviral agents. *Curr Eye Res* **10**: 193.

Naito T, Shiota H, Mimura Y (1987). Side effects in the treatment of herpetic keratitis. *Curr Eye Res* **6**: 237.

Narurkar MM, Mitra AK (1989). Prodrugs of 5-iodo-2'-deoxyuridine for enhanced ocular transport. *Pharm Res* **6**: 887.

Panda A, Das GK, Khokhar S, Rao V (1995). Efficacy of four antiviral agents in the treatment of uncomplicated herpetic keratitis. *Can J Ophthalmol* **30**: 256.

Park NH, Pavan-Langston D, Boisjoly HM, De Clercq E (1982). Chemotherapeutic efficacy of E-5-(2-bromovinyl)-2-deoxyuridine for orofacial infection with herpes simplex virus type I in mice. *J Infect Dis* **145**: 909.

Patterson A, Fox AD, Davies G *et al.* (1963). Controlled studies of IDU in the treatment of herpetic keratitis. *Trans Ophthal Soc* **83**: 583.

Pavan-Langston D (1975). Clinical evaluation of adenine arabinoside and idoxuridine in the treatment of ocular herpes simplex. *Amer J Ophthalmol* **80**: 495.

Pavan-Langston D, McCulley JP (1973). Herpes zoster dendritic keratitis. *Arch Ophthalmol* **89**: 25.

Prusoff WH (1959). Synthesis and biological activities of iododeoxyuridine, an analogue of thymidine. *Biochem Biophys Acta* **32**: 295.

Renis HE, Buthala DA (1965). Development of resistance to antiviral drugs. *Ann NY Acad Sci* **130**: 343.

Reuveni H, Bull CO, Landry ML *et al.* (1991). Antiviral activity of 5-Iodo-2'-deoxyuridine and related drugs in human keratinocytes infected *in vitro* with herpes simplex virus type 1. *Skin Pharmacol* **4**: 291.

Schabel FM Jr, Montgomery JA (1972). Purines and pyrimidines. In *International Encyclopedia of Pharmacology and Therapeutics*. Section 61: *Chemother Virus Dis* Vol 1, p. 231. New York: Pergamon Press.

Segal R, Pisanty S (1987). Glycyrrhizin gel as a vehicle for idoxuridine-1. Clinical investigations. *J Clin Pharm Ther* **12**: 165.

Sheth NV, McKeough MB, Spruance SL (1987). Measurement of the stratum corneum drug reservoir to predict the therapeutic efficacy of topical iododeoxyuridine for herpes simplex virus infection. *J Invest Dermatol* **89**: 598.

Shigeta S, Mori S, Yokota T *et al.* (1986). Characterisation of a varicella zoster virus variant with altered thymidine kinase activity. *Antimicrob Ag Chemother* **29**: 1053.

Spruance SL, Stewart JC, Freeman DJ *et al.* (1990). Early application of topical 15% idoxuridine in dimethyl sulfoxide shortens the course of herpes simplex labialis; a multicenter placebo controlled trial. *J Infect Dis* **161**: 191.

Steffenhagen KA, Easterday BC, Galasso GJ (1976). Evaluation of 6-azauridine and 5-iododeoxyuridine in the treatment of experimental viral infections. *J Infect Dis* **133**: 603.

Suzutani T, Machida H, Sakuma T (1988). Efficacies of antiherpesvirus nucleosides against two strains of herpes simplex virus type 1 in vero and human embryo lung fibroblast cells. *Antimicrob Ag Chemother* **32**: 1046.

Touitou E, Segal R, Pisanty S, Milogoldzweig I (1988). Glycyrrhizin gel as vehicle for idoxuridine topical preparation; skin permeation behaviour. *Drug Des Deliv* **3**: 267.

Uchio E, Hatano H, Ohno S (1993). Altering clinical features of recurrent herpes simplex virus induced keratitis. *Ann Ophthalmol* **25**: 271.

Uchio E, Hatano H, Mitsui K *et al.* (1994). A retrospective study of herpes simplex keratitis over the last 30 years. *Jpn J Ophthalmol* **38**: 196.

United States Pharmacopeia Drug Information (1996).

Verheyden JP (1988). Evolution of therapy for cytomegalovirus infection. *Rev Infect Dis* **10**: S477.

Yokota T, Konno K, Shigeta S *et al.* (1987). Incorporation of (E)-5-(2-iodovinyl)-2'-deoxyuridine into deoxyribonucleic acids of varicella zoster virus (TK+ and TK- strains)-infected cells. *Mol Pharmacol* **31**: 493.

Foscarnet

Description

Phosphonoformate, also known as foscarnet, an inorganic pyrophosphate analog, was developed initially as a topical preparation for the treatment of herpesvirus infection. This drug is active against herpes simplex virus types 1 and 2, cytomegalovirus, varicella-zoster virus, Epstein–Barr virus, and human herpesviruses types 6 and 8 (Helgstrand *et al.*, 1984; Mesri *et al.*, 1996; reviewed in Wagstaff and Bryson, 1994). In addition, it can inhibit the DNA polymerase of hepatitis B, interferes with mRNA synthesis of influenza viruses (Stridh *et al.*, 1979; Oberg 1983; Strid *et al.* 1989) and inhibits the reverse transcriptase of HIV (Sandstrom, 1985; Sarin *et al.* 1985).

Foscarnet is used to treat immunosuppressed patients including organ transplant recipients and persons with the acquired immune deficiency syndrome (AIDS) with cytomegalovirus retinitis who cannot tolerate ganciclovir or who develop resistance to ganciclovir (p. 1571) or in combination with ganciclovir. In addition, foscarnet is useful for the treatment of those patients with aciclovir-resistant infection due to herpes simplex virus or varicella-zoster virus (pp. 1525, 1528).

Trisodium phosphonoformate hexahydrate, known as foscarnet, is marketed by Astra Pharmaceuticals under the brand name of 'Foscavir'. The molecular weight of foscarnet is 300.1. The chemical structure is shown in Fig. V.26. Foscarnet concentrations are reported in μM or μg per ml; the concentrations can be converted (1 μg per ml is approximately equivalent to 3.3 μM) (Hengge *et al.*, 1993).

Antiviral Activity

1 Herpesviruses

Foscarnet inhibits all classes of human herpesviruses including herpes simplex types 1 and 2, cytomegalovirus, human herpesviruses types 6 and 8, varicella-zoster virus and Epstein–Barr virus.

a Cytomegalovirus The concentration of foscarnet required to inhibit the DNA polymerase of cytomegalovirus by 50% (IC_{50}) has been reported as 0.3–0.8 μM (Oberg, 1983; Eriksson and Schinazi, 1989). The reported IC_{50} required to inhibit replication of human cytomegalovirus strain Ad-169 in cell culture is 102–130 μM, but this concentration is dependent upon the multiplicity of infection (Wahren, 1980; Manischewitz *et al.*, 1990). Others report lower IC_{50} concentrations ranging from 6 to 55 μM when measured by inhibition of plaque formation or

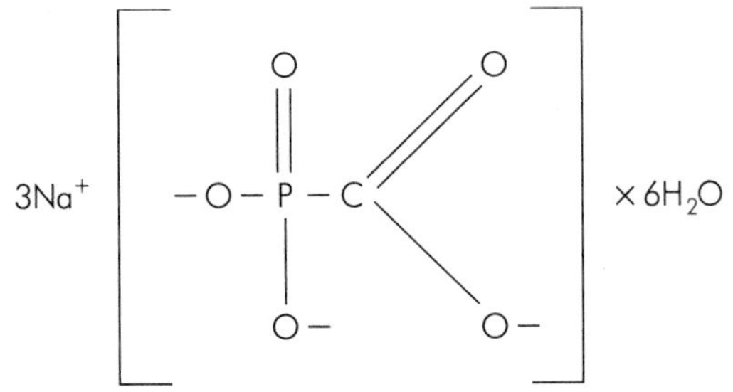

Fig. V.26.
Chemical structure of foscarnet.

Fig. V.27.

Dose isobologram for evaluation of the activity of ganciclovir and foscarnet in combination. Concentrations of ganciclovir and foscarnet which tested alone. The broken line joining the IC$_{50}$ of the individual drugs represents an isobol which indicates no interaction. The solid line represents the isobol of ganciclovir–foscarnet interactions. The bowing of the isobol towards the origin is indicative of a synergistic interaction. (Reproduced from Manischewitz *et al.*, 1990, with permission.)

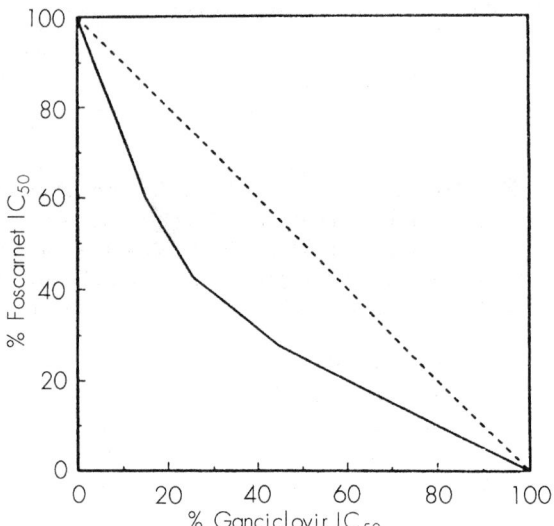

cytopathology using laboratory strains of cytomegalovirus (Andrei *et al.*, 1991; Wahren and Oberg, 1980; Neyts *et al.*, 1991). For clinical isolates of cytomegalovirus, the IC$_{50}$ for inhibition of replication is in the range of 108–270 μM, generally being 1.5- to 8-fold less sensitive than the laboratory strains (Oberg, 1989; Manischewitz *et al.*, 1990; Gerna *et al.*, 1994; reviewed in Chrisp and Clissold, 1991; reviewed in Wagstaff and Bryson, 1994). Synergistic inhibition of replication of cytomegalovirus *in vitro* by ganciclovir and foscarnet has been reported (Fig. V.27) (Manischewitz *et al.* 1990). Synergism against cytomegalovirus replication *in vitro* has also been found with combinations of foscarnet and trifluorothymidine (Spector *et al.*, 1983) and additive or synergistic interactions between foscarnet and zidovudine (Snoeck *et al.*, 1992; Eriksson and Schinazi, 1989; Koshida *et al.*, 1989).

Resistance of cytomegalovirus to foscarnet has been reported, both by culturing wild-type isolates in the presence of foscarnet *in vitro* (Sullivan and Coen, 1991), and in clinical isolates from patients treated with foscarnet (Knox *et al.* 1991; Leport *et al.*, 1993). Foscarnet-resistant isolates have also been reported to be resistant to ganciclovir (Tatarowicz *et al.*, 1992; Sarasini *et al.*, 1995), although generally ganciclovir-resistant strains remain sensitive to foscarnet. Foscarnet-resistant strains may also be cross-resistant to cidofovir. Similar patterns of cross-resistance have been observed with foscarnet-resistant strains of murine cytomegalovirus (Smee *et al.*, 1995).

b Herpes simplex virus Inhibition of the DNA polymerase of herpesvirus by 50% is in the range of 0.4–3.5 μM for herpes simplex type 1 and 0.6–22 μM for herpes simplex type 2 (Eriksson and Oberg 1979; Helgstrand *et al.*, 1978; Ostrander and Cheng 1980). Synergism against herpes simplex virus type 1 and an additive effect against type 2 has been demonstrated between foscarnet and penciclovir (Sutton *et al.*, 1992). Foscarnet is active against aciclovir-resistant strains of herpes simplex virus types 1 and 2 (Birch *et al.*, 1990; Verdonck *et al.*, 1993).

Resistance of herpes simplex virus to foscarnet has been defined by some investigators as reduced susceptibility (at IC$_{50}$ level) to concentrations of foscarnet of greater than 100 μg per ml (approximately 330 μM) (Safrin *et al.*, 1994a), whilst others use a cut-off of 400 μM (Drew 1996). It is generally agreed that these assays are difficult to perform, and results are not always predictive of the clinical response of the drug (reviewed in Wagstaff and Bryson, 1994). Examination of a drug-resistant mutant from a clinical isolate of herpes simplex virus has demonstrated a point mutation within a conserved region of the DNA polymerase gene, which conferred resistance to both aciclovir and foscarnet (Hwang *et al.*, 1992). Foscarnet-resistance is uncommonly found in herpes simplex isolates, accounting for 5% in a screen of 320 clinical isolates from 197 patients (Safrin *et al.*, 1994b). Clinical isolates have been obtained which are resistant to foscarnet and aciclovir (Birch *et al.*, 1992). Foscarnet-resistant clinical isolates of herpes simplex virus may retain susceptibility to penciclovir (Safrin and Phan, 1993), and to trifluorothymidine (Birch *et al.*, 1992). Foscarnet-resistant herpes simplex type 2 has been isolated from a patient treated with foscarnet and zidovudine whose strain of HIV remained sensitive to foscarnet (Tachedjian *et al.*, 1994).

c **Varicella-zoster virus** Foscarnet is active against strains of varicella-zoster, including aciclovir-resistant isolates deficient in thymidine kinase (TK) or with TK with altered substrate specificity (Boivin et al., 1994; Andrei et al., 1995). The IC_{50} of foscarnet required to inhibit the DNA polymerase of varicella-zoster virus is 0.4 μM (Oberg 1986).

2 Human immunodeficiency virus

Foscarnet inhibits the human immunodeficiency virus types 1 and 2 as well as the simian immunodeficiency virus (Sarin et al., 1985; Vrang et al., 1988). The concentration of foscarnet required to cause 50% inhibition of reverse transcriptase of HIV-1 is less than 2 μM (Sarin et al., 1985), and complete inhibition of enzyme activity has been achieved with 5 μM (Sandstrom, 1985). Replication of HIV in H9 T cell lines is inhibited by 50% by foscarnet in concentrations ranging from 10 to 25 μM (Sandstrom et al., 1985; Koshida et al., 1989). In peripheral blood mononuclear cells HIV is inhibited by a mean concentration of foscarnet of 29.7 μM (Cox et al., 1994). Replication of HIV is also inhibited by foscarnet in monocytes that are acutely infected but not in chronically infected cells (Crowe et al., 1991). Foscarnet reversibly inhibits cell growth by 50% at concentrations of approximately 1000 μM, significantly higher concentrations than those required for inhibition of virus replication (Stenberg, 1978). Synergistic inhibition of HIV replication in vitro has been reported using a combination of foscarnet and zidovudine (Eriksson and Schinazi, 1989; Chrisp and Clissold, 1991; Koshida et al., 1989), and an additive or synergistic effect has been found between foscarnet and interferon alpha (Degre and Beck, 1994; Hartshorn et al., 1986).

Strains of HIV with reduced sensitivity to foscarnet have been identified by passage in culture in the presence of increasing concentrations of drug and from a patient with AIDS on long-term foscarnet therapy (Tachedjian et al., 1995; Mellors et al., 1995). Foscarnet-resistant HIV has been shown by several investigators to be hypersensitive to zidovudine and nevirapine, with unaltered sensitivity to didanosine and zalcitabine (Tachedjian et al., 1995; Mellors et al., 1995). Mutations within codons 89 (Glu→Lys), 92 (Leu→Ile) and 156 (Ser→Ala) were found, and their role in foscarnet-resistance confirmed by site-directed mutagenesis (Tachedjian et al., 1995). Mutations within codons 88, 161 and 208 have also been described and demonstrated to be involved in foscarnet-resistance by site-directed mutagenesis (Mellors et al., 1995; Tachedjian et al., 1995). Other investigators have described foscarnet-resistant reverse transcriptase enzymes with mutations within codons 90 (Val→Ala/Thr/Gly) and 89 (Glu→Gly), that were cross-resistant to the active metabolites of zalcitabine, didanosine and zidovudine, but, at least in the case of the codon 90 (Val→Ala) mutation, which remained sensitive to nevirapine and other non-nucleoside reverse transcriptase inhibitors (Im et al., 1993; Prasad et al., 1991). Mutations that confer foscarnet-resistance can suppress zidovudine-resistance (Tachedjian et al.,1996).

Zidovudine and didanosine mutants of feline immunodeficiency virus have been selected in culture which showed cross-resistance to foscarnet and increased sensitivity to zalcitabine (Gobert et al., 1994).

3 Hepatitis B virus

Both human hepatitis B virus and the duck hepatitis B virus are sensitive to foscarnet (Sherker et al., 1986; Fourel et al., 1994). Hepatitis B DNA polymerase is inhibited by 10–100 μM of foscarnet (Oberg, 1983).

4 Other

Foscarnet, at a concentration of 20 μM, has been demonstrated to inhibit the RNA polymerase of influenza virus (Helgstrand, 1978; Stridh et al., 1979; Oberg, 1983; Strid et al., 1989). Replication of influenza virus is inhibited by 400 μM of foscarnet, (reviewed in Oberg, 1983). Rotavirus replication in MA104 cells is inhibited by foscarnet in a dose-dependent manner, with inhibition of both plus- and minus-strand RNA synthesis (Rios et al., 1995).

Mode of Administration and Dosage

1 Intravenous

As foscarnet has extremely poor oral absorption, it must be administered intravenously. Foscarnet is administered (preferably) via a central venous line or (if necessary) via a peripheral vein. Foscarnet should not be given by rapid injection, and is usually infused over 1–2 h (2 h for

Table V.16

Foscarnet dosing guide according to renal function. Induction therapy. (Reproduced from Foscarnet Product Information.)

CrCl (ml per min per kg)	HSV: Equivalent to		CMV: Equivalent to
	80 mg per kg per day total (40 mg per kg every 12h)	120 mg per kg per day total (40 mg per kg every 8h)	180 mg per kg per day total (60 mg per kg every 8h)
>1.4	40 every 12h	40 every 8h	60 every 8h
>1.0–1.4	30 every 12h	30 every 8h	45 every 8h
>0.8–1.0	20 every 12h	35 every 12h	50 every 12h
>0.6–0.8	35 every 24h	25 every 12h	40 every 12h
>0.5–0.6	25 every 24h	40 every 24h	60 every 24h
>0.4–0.5	20 every 24h	35 every 24h	50 every 24h
<0.4	Not recommended	Not recommended	Not recommended

doses of >60 mg per kg). The drug does not need to be diluted prior to administration via a central line, but must be diluted to 12 mg per ml if it is to be administered via a peripheral line. Superficial thrombophlebitis is a potential complication of foscarnet when administered through a peripheral vein. The incidence of central venous catheter-related sepsis is similar for ganciclovir and foscarnet (Stanley et al., 1994). The dosing schedule is dependent upon renal function (Table V.16). Adequate hydration must be provided during administration of foscarnet in order to minimize potential renal toxicity. In the absence of a contraindication, one liter of saline should be given i.v. prior to the administration of foscarnet during induction or maintenance therapy. In an uncontrolled study, Deray and colleagues found that a total of 2.5 liters of saline given during the night before foscarnet therapy and during the course of induction treatment appeared to prevent nephrotoxicity (Deray et al., 1989).

For patients with normal renal function, foscarnet can be administered at a dose of 200 mg per kg given continuously over 24 h. A bolus of 20 mg per kg given over 30 min is given at the start of therapy. More commonly, an intermittent infusion over 1 h of 60 mg per kg is given every 8 h, or 90–100 mg per kg over 2 h is given every 12 h. This high-dose induction therapy for the treatment of cytomegalovirus retinitis is continued for 14–21 days.

The optimum regimen for maintenance therapy for cytomegalovirus retinitis in patients with AIDS remains unknown and is the subject of ongoing clinical trials. However, for patients with normal renal function a once-daily infusion of 90–120 mg per kg administered over 2 h is effective in the prevention of relapse (Table V.17). A dose ranging study found that the median time to progression in patients receiving 120 mg per kg per day was more than 123 days. In those receiving 90 mg per kg daily this time decreased to 95 days, and to 90 days in those receiving 60 mg per kg daily (Jacobson, 1992a). In a second study of 32 patients with AIDS and previously untreated cytomegalovirus retinitis, maintenance doses of 90 and 120 mg per kg daily were compared. There was a significant survival advantage in the group randomized to receive the higher dose compared with the lower dose (mean of 157 and 336 days in the 90 and 120 mg per kg daily groups respectively). Furthermore, the time to progression of retinitis tended to be longer in the higher dose group than in the standard dose group (Jacobson et al., 1993). This was confirmed by a more detailed, retrospective analysis of data in which progression rates were determined by comparisons of baseline and follow-up photographs (Holland et al., 1995). However, a study by the same group of investigators has subsequently shown no difference in survival or time to retinitis progression in 156 patients with previously treated cytomegalovirus retinitis who received 60, 90 or 120 mg per kg of foscarnet per day as maintenance therapy (Jacobson et al., 1994).

Combination therapy using ganciclovir and foscarnet has been found to be of benefit in certain clinical situations (p. 1573). A number of different dosage regimens for induction have been evaluated. In general, foscarnet is administered at a dose of 60 mg per kg every 8 h or 90–100 mg per kg every 12 h with ganciclovir 5 mg per kg every 12 h. The dose of foscarnet for maintenance is 90–120 mg per kg daily, with 5 mg per kg of ganciclovir every 24 h (Kuppermann et al., 1993). The two drugs (foscarnet and ganciclovir) cannot be given together as they are incompatible. No other drug should be infused concomitantly with foscarnet.

Table V.17
Foscarnet dosing guide according to renal function. Maintenance therapy. (Reproduced from Foscarnet Product Information.)

CrCl (ml per min per kg)	CMV: Equivalent to	
	90 mg per kg per day (once-daily)	120 mg per kg per day (once-daily)
>1.4	90 every 24h	120 every 24h
>1.0–1.4	70 every 24h	90 every 24h
>0.8–1.0	50 every 24h	65 every 24h
>0.6–0.8	80 every 48h	105 every 48h
>0.5–0.6	60 every 48h	80 every 48h
≥0.4–0.5	50 every 48h	65 every 48h
<0.4	Not recommended	Not recommended

2 Renal insufficiency

The dosage of foscarnet is dependent upon renal function, and, based upon a weight-adjusted creatinine clearance, must be modified accordingly (Tables V.16 and V.17). Foscarnet should not be used in patients with severe renal dysfunction whose creatinine clearance is less than 0.4 ml per kg per min. Foscarnet has been successfully given to a patient undergoing renal dialysis, at an initial dosage of 60 mg per kg after each dialysis treatment. Thereafter, plasma concentrations of foscarnet were monitored weekly, and dosage adjusted to maintain peak plasma levels of 500–800 μM (MacGregor et al., 1991).

3 Children

Safety and efficacy in children have not yet been established.

4 Foscarnet cream

Clinic-initiated topical foscarnet was used for the treatment of recurrent genital herpes in early clinical trials. Compared with a placebo, topical foscarnet did not improve time to healing, but did shorten duration of viral shedding and resulted in a higher proportion of individuals who had no symptoms after 1 day of therapy (Sacks et al. 1987).

5 Intravitreal administration

Studies in animals have demonstrated the safety of intravitreal injections of foscarnet (Turrini et al., 1994; Berthe et al., 1994). Intravitreal foscarnet has been safely administered either alone or in combination with ganciclovir to persons with cytomegalovirus retinitis (Pearson et al., 1993; Lieberman et al., 1994). Intravitreal foscarnet has been associated with clinical improvement, no systemic absorption, and is well tolerated with no retinal toxicity (Diaz-Llopis, 1992). Doses of 2400 μg per injection given twice-weekly for 3 weeks during induction, and once-weekly for maintenance therapy have been reportedly effective in uncontrolled trials (Diaz-Llopis et al., 1994).

Availability

Foscarnet is available for *i.v. injection* as 1 ml (24 mg or 80 μM) of trisodium phosphonoformate hexahydrate and water, pH 7.4. Foscarnet *solution* is available for *i.v. infusion* in glass bottles containing 250 and 500 ml (24 mg per ml).

Serum Levels in Relation to Dosage

1 Intravenous administration

The pharmacokinetics of foscarnet with respect to plasma levels have been found to vary widely between patients following i.v. administration (Lietman, 1992; Taburet, 1992). It has been suggested that the variation in plasma levels of foscarnet may be partly attributed to interactions between phosphate and foscarnet resulting in variations in their sequestration in bone (Sjovall et *al.*, 1989; reviewed in Wagstaff and Bryson, 1994). Following a single infusion of foscarnet in a dose of 90 mg per kg the plasma concentrations varied from 297 to 1775 μg per ml (990–5920 μM) with a mean of 766 ± 400 μg per ml (Hengge *et al.*, 1993). During continuous administration of 230 mg per kg daily for 10–21 days, steady-state concentrations of foscarnet in plasma ranged between 75 and 529 μM (Sjovall *et al.*, 1988, 1989; Fanning, 1990). Steady-state concentrations of foscarnet during continuous i.v. administration are similar to those achieved with intermittent infusions.

In a study of AIDS patients with cytomegalovirus disease, who received 90 mg per kg of foscarnet twice-daily by i.v. infusion for 14 days, the mean peak and trough levels were 605±118 and 52±59 μM respectively (Taburet, 1992). The steady-state concentration of foscarnet in plasma was 218 ± 86 μM. In this same study the plasma half-life of foscarnet was 3.4 h. Due to this relatively short half-life, there is no accumulation of the drug in plasma.

2 Renal insufficiency

In an early study, foscarnet plasma levels above 400 μg per ml in a uremic patient were associated with hallucinations, tremor and abnormal liver function tests (Ringden *et al.*, 1986).

Excretion

Foscarnet is not significantly metabolized and is primarily excreted unchanged in urine, via both glomerular filtration and tubular secretion (Sjovall *et al.*, 1988, 1989). Plasma clearance of foscarnet following i.v. administration is 130–160 ml per min. Renal clearance is approximately 90 ml per min (Taburet, 1992). There is a long terminal-phase elimination half-life which may be attributed to slow release from bone (see below).

Distribution of the Drug in Body

Although the pattern of deposition of foscarnet in humans has not been studied, it is clear from studies in mice and from human pharmacokinetic studies that a significant proportion of the dose of foscarnet accumulates in bone and cartilage. In mice approximately 30% of foscarnet is retained in these tissues (Helgstrand *et al.*, 1978). Extrapolating from elimination and clearance values in humans it would appear that up to 22% of a dose is taken up into bone (reviewed in Wagstaff and Bryson, 1994).

The steady-state volume of distribution in patients receiving 90 mg per kg twice-daily was 0.5–0.6 liters per kg (Taburet, 1992). The diffusion of foscarnet into CSF has been examined in 27 patients with AIDS receiving i.v. foscarnet at various dosages. The median concentration of foscarnet was 80 μM with a median CSF to plasma ratio of 0.27 (Raffi *et al.*, 1993). A separate study in which 26 patients were given a single 90mg per kg i.v. infusion of foscarnet resulted in a mean CSF to plasma ratio of 0.23 ± 0.16 (Hengge *et al.*, 1993).

The reported levels of foscarnet in vitreous following intravitreal injection in two patients were 896 and 75 μM at approximately 23 and 43 h post-injection (Diaz-Llopis *et al.*, 1994). In a larger study where vitreous samples were obtained from 60 eyes (52 patients) the mean concentrations of foscarnet in the vitreous of patients receiving induction or maintenance therapy by intravitreal injection were 189 ± 177 and 163 ± 167 μM respectively; the mean vitreous to plasma ratio was 1.43 (Arevalo *et al.*, 1995).

Mode of Action

The antiviral effect of foscarnet is via inhibition of viral polymerases, without requiring phosphorylation of the drug by either viral or cellular enzymes.

Foscarnet inhibits the DNA polymerase of herpes viruses by binding at a site where pyrophosphate is removed during synthesis of nucleoside triphosphates (Sarin *et al.*, 1985). Viral DNA polymerase catalyzes the addition of deoxynucleoside triphosphates to the growing viral DNA chain resulting in its elongation, with the release of pyrophosphate during this process. Foscarnet selectively inhibits the viral DNA polymerase, without significantly inhibiting cellular enzymes (reviewed in Wagstaff and Bryson, 1994). Similarly, foscarnet inhibits the reverse transcriptase of the human immunodeficiency virus (Sarin *et al.*, 1985), and the DNA polymerase of hepadna viruses (Sherker *et al.*, 1986). This inhibition is reversed when the infected cells are no longer exposed to the compound. The hydrophobicity of the amino acid at position 90 of reverse transcriptase has been described as being critical for binding of foscarnet to the enzyme (Im *et al.*, 1993). However, this may not be correct, as codon 90 is not located within the dNTP binding site. The mechanism is most likely due to template binding repositioning, as described for mutations within codons 88, 92 and 156 (Tachedjian *et al.*, 1995).

Table V.18
Major toxicities associated with
foscarnet therapy

Nephrotoxicity	Tubulointerstitial nephritis
	Elevated serum creatinine
	Decrease in creatinine clearance
	Acute renal failure
Electrolyte	Low serum ionized calcium
	paresthesia
	tremor
	arrhythmias
	convulsions
	Hypo/hypercalcemia
	Hypo/hyperphosphatemia
	Hypomagnesemia
	Hypokalemia
Hematologic toxicity	Anemia
Genital ulceration	

Toxicity

The major toxicities of foscarnet are summarized in Table V.18.

1 Nephrotoxicity

This is the major adverse effect associated with foscarnet therapy. The most common abnormalities reported are an elevation in serum creatinine, a decrease in creatinine clearance and less commonly the development of acute renal failure due to a tubulointerstitial nephritis (Nyberg et al., 1989; Deray et al., 1989). Up to 25% of patients develop dose-limiting renal impairment when treated with intermittent i.v. foscarnet. Continuous infusion is associated with a higher risk (reviewed in Chrisp and Clissold, 1991). The incidence of renal toxicity can be reduced by frequent monitoring of creatinine clearance, dosage adjustment and careful hydration (Deray et al., 1989; Jacobson, 1992b). Renal impairment is usually reversible upon cessation of the drug (Seidel et al., 1993). Deposition of crystals of foscarnet within the glomerular capillaries and crescentic proliferation has been reported in patients with foscarnet-induced nephrotoxicity (Beaufils, 1990; Trolliet et al., 1995). If the creatinine clearance is below 0.4 ml per min per kg, it is recommended that foscarnet therapy be discontinued. The development of high fever in patients with foscarnet-induced renal dysfunction has been reported (Nyberg et al., 1989). Phosphaturia has been described (Loghman-Adham et al., 1993), caused by inhibition of renal tubular reabsorption of phosphate.

2 Electrolyte disturbances

A transient, dose-related decrease in the serum level of ionized calcium has been observed, and postulated as the underlying cause of paresthesias, tremors, arrhythmias, and convulsions in patients receiving foscarnet (Jacobson et al., 1989, 1992b; Ringden et al., 1986). The rate of infusion and dose have been implicated in the development of ionized hypocalcemia (Lor and Liu, 1994). The total serum calcium and 24-h urinary calcium excretion are often normal, despite low levels of ionized calcium in serum. It is likely that the low ionized serum calcium is due to complexing of foscarnet with ionized calcium (Jacobson et al., 1991, 1992b). Hypocalcemia and hypercalcemia have been reported in patients receiving foscarnet (Ringden et al., 1986; Youle et al., 1988; Palestine et al., 1991; Jacobson et al. 1989). Acute hypocalcemia developing during foscarnet administration may result in muscular spasms; reducing the flow rate of the infusion, or treating with calcium gluconate will usually alleviate symptoms (Gazzard, 1992). The concomitant administration of i.v. pentamidine and foscarnet has been associated with severe, potentially fatal hypocalcemia (Youle et al., 1988). Hypophosphatemia, hyperphosphatemia and hypomagnesemia have also been described, and again are usually transient and may be associated with muscle twitches, tremulousness and anxiety (Palestine et al., 1991; Jacobson et al., 1989; Gearhart and Sorg, 1993). Foscarnet-induced hypokalemia has been reported (Malin, 1992). Electrolytes must be monitored frequently during foscarnet induction and maintenance therapy.

3 Neurologic complications

Convulsions have been observed in patients receiving foscarnet (Lor and Liu, 1994). A decrease in ionized serum calcium (see above) has been postulated as the cause of the convulsions. Paresthesia may occur related to infusion, and in association with low serum ionized calcium (Jacobson, 1992b).

4 Hematologic abnormalities

The development of a mild, unexplained anemia has been observed in up to 33% of patients receiving foscarnet in clinical trials (Jacobson et al., 1989; Palestine et al., 1991; Studies of Ocular Complications of AIDS Research Group, in collaboration with AIDS Clinical Trials group, 1995b).

5 Genital ulceration

Genital irritation and ulceration have been described in men (glans penis) and women (vulva) (Lacey et al., 1992; Evans and Grossman, 1992; Gross and Dretler, 1993; Caumes et al., 1993; Brockmeyer, 1993). In some circumstances oral ulceration has also been observed. The ulceration resembles a fixed drug eruption, but this has not been supported by histological findings (Van der Pijl, 1990). There is a higher incidence of penile ulceration in uncircumcized males (Gazzard, 1992). The cause of ulceration associated with foscarnet therapy is not known. High concentrations of unmetabolized foscarnet in urine may cause irritation (Jacobson, 1992b); in addition, crystals of foscarnet in capillaries or arterioles may lead to the development of ulcers (Beaufils, 1990).

6 Superficial thrombophlebitis

The administration of foscarnet via a peripheral vein is associated with a high incidence of local irritation and development of thrombophlebitis. The incidence is increased if foscarnet is not diluted prior to administration.

7 Other

Nephrogenic diabetes insipidus has been associated with foscarnet therapy in the treatment of cytomegalovirus retinitis as well as in animal studies (Farese et al., 1990; Hoch et al., 1995). Nausea and other gastrointestinal symptoms often occur but do not usually require any modification of therapy (Palestine et al., 1991). Foscarnet has been associated with reversible cardiac dysfunction (Brown et al., 1993). Inhibition of vascular smooth muscle contraction by inhibition of calcium release from intracellular stores has been reported in animal models (Paspaliaris et al., 1993).

8 Drug interactions

No drugs should be infused simultaneously with foscarnet. Ganciclovir and foscarnet co-therapy do not alter the plasma clearance or volume of distribution of either drug (Aweeka et al., 1995). However, these drugs are not compatible and cannot be infused together. Concomitant therapy with foscarnet and zidovudine does not alter plasma clearance of foscarnet, nor peak plasma concentration or volume of distribution. Similarly, there was no alteration in pharmacokinetic parameters of zidovudine (Aweeka, 1992). Foscarnet should not be given to patients receiving i.v. pentamidine, as both drugs may cause hypocalcemia and renal insufficiency. Similarly, there is a recommendation that foscarnet should not be given to patients receiving amphotericin B, due to potential increase in risk of renal impairment (Reusser et al., 1992). There is no pharmacokinetic interaction between foscarnet and didanosine (Taburet et al., 1996).

Clinical Uses of the Drug

Foscarnet is licensed for the treatment of cytomegalovirus retinitis in patients with the acquired immune deficiency syndrome (see also ganciclovir, p. 1571). In many centers, ganciclovir is used as the drug of first choice, and foscarnet is reserved for patients who are intolerant of ganciclovir or who have developed ganciclovir-resistance.

1 Treatment of cytomegalovirus retinitis in patients with AIDS

Untreated, retinitis due to cytomegalovirus will usually progress rapidly, with a mean time to progression being 22 days (Fig. V.28), and a range of 2–6 weeks (Palestine et al., 1991). Therapy with foscarnet, given either as intermittent therapy of 60 mg per kg every 8 h or as a continuous infusion of 230 mg per kg daily following an initial bolus, results in clinical responses which are evident as early as the third day of therapy (Walmsley, 1988; Katlama et al., 1992). Without maintenance therapy, relapse will occur, often within a month of cessation of therapy (Walmsley, 1988). When treated with 60 mg per kg every 8 h for 2–3 weeks followed by maintenance

Fig. V.28.

Kaplan–Meier analysis of progression of CMV retinitis over time in patients receiving immediate foscarnet treatment or no (delayed) treatment. (Reproduced from Palestine *et al.*, 1991, with permission from the American College of Physicians.)

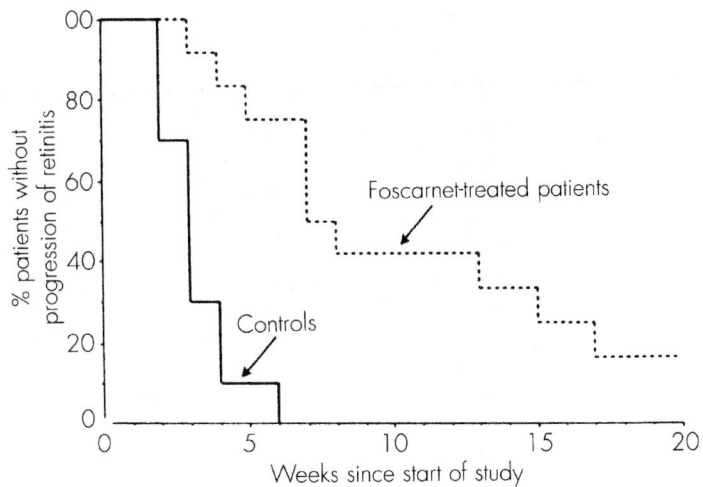

therapy of 90 mg per kg daily, the mean time to progression ranges from 6.7 to 13.3 weeks (Fig. V.28) (Palestine *et al.*, 1991; Jacobson 1992a,b).

Compared with ganciclovir (p. 1571) for the treatment of cytomegalovirus retinitis, foscarnet has certain advantages and disadvantages. A multicenter, randomized comparative trial of ganciclovir versus foscarnet, the Study for the Ocular Complications of AIDS (SOCA), found that both drugs had similar efficacy and were associated with similar times to progression of retinitis. However, there was a survival advantage for patients randomized to receive foscarnet (Fig. V.29) (Studies of Ocular Complications of AIDS Research Group, in collaboration with AIDS Clinical Trials Group, 1992, 1994). These findings were confirmed in a separate study (Polis, 1993), and may possibly be explained by the antiretroviral properties of foscarnet, which have been demonstrated in other studies *in vivo* (Jacobson *et al.*, 1988; Fletcher *et al.*, 1994; Studies of Ocular Complications of AIDS Research Group in collaboration with AIDS Clinical Trials Group 1995a; Kaiser *et al.*, 1995) as well as *in vitro* (Sandstrom, 1985; Sarin *et al.*, 1985). However, a recent study of

Fig. V.29.

Kaplan–Meier curves showing the cumulative probability of mortality among patients assigned to foscarnet or ganciclovir for CMV retinitis. Mortality was significantly higher in the ganciclovir group ($p = 0.006$ by the log-rank test). The numbers of patients at risk at each time point are shown at the bottom of the figure. (Reproduced from Studies of Ocular Complications of AIDS Research Group in Collaboration with the AIDS Clinical Trials Group, 1992, with permission.)

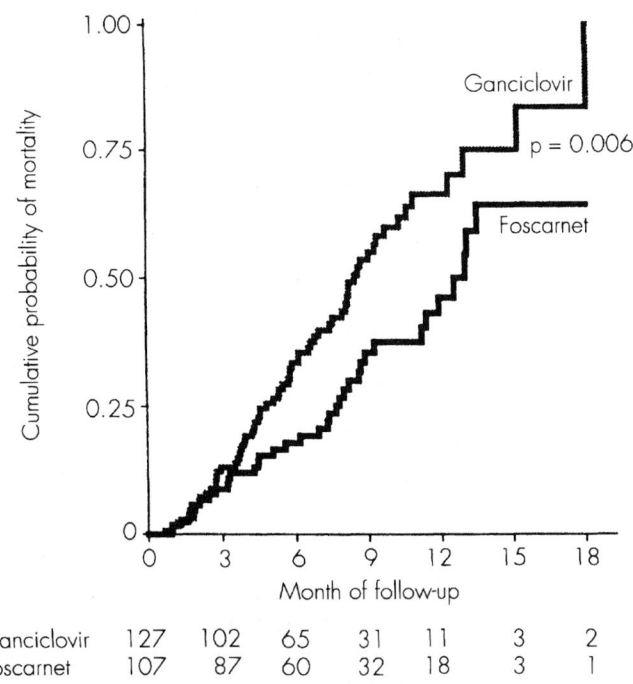

	0	3	6	9	12	15	18
Ganciclovir	127	102	65	31	11	3	2
Foscarnet	107	87	60	32	18	3	1

279 patients with persistently active or relapsed retinitis has found no survival advantage of foscarnet over ganciclovir or the combination of these two drugs (Studies of Ocular Complications of AIDS Research Group in collaboration with AIDS Clinical Trials Group, 1996). Practical disadvantages associated with foscarnet therapy are that the drug must be given daily for maintenance therapy, whereas ganciclovir may be given five times per week, or even three times per week (Hall *et al.*, 1991), and still be effective. The toxicity profiles of both drugs differ; however, dose-limiting toxicity is more likely with foscarnet administration and patients must be more closely monitored.

Combination therapy using ganciclovir and foscarnet has been found to be of benefit in patients with clinically resistant cytomegalovirus retinitis in a number of open and uncontrolled studies in adults and children (Coker *et al.*, 1991; Butler *et al.*, 1992; Flores-Aguilar *et al.*, 1993; Dieterich *et al.*, 1993a; Weinberg *et al.*, 1994), as well as in a recent randomized multicenter controlled trial of patients with persistently active or relapsed cytomegalovirus retinitis in which combination therapy was superior to either ganciclovir or foscarnet monotherapy in delaying time to progression as assessed by fundus photography (Studies of Ocular Complications of AIDS Research Group in collaboration with AIDS Clinical Trials Group, 1996). Cytomegalovirus replication appears also to be well controlled in patients receiving either combination or alternating therapy with ganciclovir and foscarnet when cumulative weekly doses of each drug are lower than standard monotherapy maintenance regimens, although this has not yet been tested in a large, multicenter randomized and controlled trial (Jacobson *et al.*, 1994; Peters *et al.*, 1994). Induction and maintenance regimens have varied (see above). Quality of life is less with combination therapy than with monotherapy, although some patients are opting for one drug to be given by i.v administration and the other drug to be received by intravitreal administration. Foscarnet and ganciclovir dually-resistant strains of cytomegalovirus have been isolated from patients with clinical resistance to both drugs (Lipson *et al.*, 1993). Intravitreal cidofovir is currently being evaluated for patients with ganciclovir and foscarnet-resistant strains (Kirsch *et al.*, 1995).

Intravitreal injections of foscarnet to date have generally been given to patients with catheter-related sepsis, renal toxicity, or who refuse i.v. therapy. In limited studies the response to therapy and the relapse rate appear to be acceptable (Diaz-Llopis *et al.*, 1994).

2 Foscarnet therapy for other cytomegalovirus disease in patients with AIDS

a Gastrointestinal disease Foscarnet has been used in clinical trials to treat patients with AIDS who have cytomegalovirus disease other than retinitis. Foscarnet has been found to be effective in the treatment of cytomegalovirus esophagitis, duodenitis, pancreatitis and colitis, with relapse following induction therapy being less common than with retinitis (Nelson *et al.*, 1991; Blanshard, 1992; Dieterich *et al.*, 1993b; Colebunders *et al.*, 1994; Wilcox *et al.*, 1995). Response to therapy usually occurs within 2 or 3 weeks of initiating therapy (Reusser *et al.*, 1992), and response rates are similar for ganciclovir and foscarnet (approximately 85% for each by endoscopic examination); maintenance therapy does not appear to prevent progression of disease (Blanshard *et al.*, 1995). Treatment of patients with acute cytomegalovirus hepatitis resulted in clinical and biochemical resolution of their disease within 3 weeks of therapy. Only a transient response was observed in patients in this same study who received foscarnet treatment for sclerosing cholangitis (Blanshard, 1992).

Combination therapy using ganciclovir and foscarnet was evaluated in an open study of 13 patients with colitis and esophagitis due to cytomegalovirus; five of seven patients responded clinically and histologically (Salzberger *et al.*, 1994).

b Neurological disease An AIDS patient who developed cytomegalovirus polyradiculitis whilst receiving ganciclovir did not respond to therapy with foscarnet (de Gans *et al.*, 1990), although there are other case reports where foscarnet has been used with success for this condition (Manji *et al.*, 1992; Domingo *et al.*, 1994). Cytomegalovirus ventriculoencephalitis has also been reported to respond poorly to foscarnet (Salazar *et al.*, 1995), although this may in part relate to difficulty in making the diagnosis thus delaying specific therapy until late in the course of the disease. In two case reports of patients with cytomegalovirus encephalitis which was refractory to ganciclovir alone, the patients received a 3–6 week combination of foscarnet and ganciclovir with documented success (Peters *et al.*, 1992; Enting *et al.*, 1992). Combination therapy with ganciclovir and foscarnet for cytomegalovirus polyradiculomyelitis has also been reported (Karmochkine *et al.*, 1994).

3 Foscarnet therapy for prevention or treatment of cytomegalovirus infection in bone marrow transplant patients

Foscarnet therapy has been evaluated for the prevention of cytomegalovirus infection in seropositive bone marrow transplant recipients. Patients received intermittent i.v. foscarnet at a dose of 40 mg per kg every 8 h from 7 days prior to 30 days post-transplant, then 60 mg per kg per day for another 45 days. No patient developed cytomegalovirus disease (Reusser *et al.*, 1992). This finding was supported by a more recent study in which foscarnet lowered the risk of cytomegalovirus infection compared with historic controls (Bacigalupo *et al.*, 1994a). A dose-ranging study of foscarnet for the treatment of cytomegalovirus infection in bone marrow and renal graft recipients found that there was clinical improvement in 70% of patients (Ringden *et al.*, 1986). A study designed to evaluate the efficacy of foscarnet for the treatment of cytomegalovirus infection in bone marrow transplant recipients, demonstrated a clinical improvement in approximately half of the patients. However, all patients with interstitial pneumonia died despite foscarnet therapy (Aschan *et al.*, 1992). Foscarnet has been found to be effective in clearing cytomegalovirus antigenemia in bone marrow transplant recipients (Bacigalupo *et al.*, 1994b). Bone marrow transplant recipients with ganciclovir-resistant cytomegalovirus infection have responded well to foscarnet therapy (Razis *et al.*, 1994).

4 Foscarnet treatment of aciclovir-resistant herpes simplex virus and varicella-zoster virus

Foscarnet is useful for the treatment of mucocutaneous herpes simplex virus infections or varicella-zoster virus in patients with AIDS who are resistant to aciclovir (Safrin *et al.*, 1990, 1991a). Treatment should commence within 7–10 days if aciclovir-resistant infection with herpes simplex virus or varicella-zoster virus is suspected and should continue for at least 10 days or until lesions are healed (Balfour *et al.*, 1994). Foscarnet-resistant multidermatomal zoster has been reported in a person with AIDS (Fillet *et al.*, 1995).

A controlled trial, comparing vidarabine with foscarnet for the treatment of patients with AIDS with aciclovir-resistant mucocutaneous herpes simplex infection, demonstrated superior efficacy of foscarnet (Safrin *et al.*, 1991b). Foscarnet has also been successful in the treatment of a bone marrow transplant recipient who developed extensive mucocutaneous infection due to an aciclovir-resistant strain of herpes simplex virus type 1 (Verdonck *et al.*, 1993). Foscarnet-resistant strains of herpes simplex virus type 2 have been isolated from patients unresponsive to foscarnet therapy or in whom lesions developed whilst undergoing foscarnet therapy. Interestingly in three patients treatment with aciclovir monotherapy or in combination with foscarnet resulted in healing (Safrin *et al.*, 1994c). Topical cidofovir (HPMPC) may be of use in patients with mucocutaneous lesions due to aciclovir and foscarnet-resistant herpes simplex virus (Snoeck *et al.*, 1994).

An open-label study found that foscarnet was effective in the treatment of TK-deficient or -altered strains of varicella zoster that were resistant to aciclovir (Safrin *et al.*, 1991a). There have been a number of case reports confirming the efficacy of foscarnet for the treatment of aciclovir-resistant varicella-zoster virus infection which presents with atypical keratotic papular skin lesions in patients with advanced HIV infection (Lokke-Jensen *et al.*, 1993).

5 Treatment of Kaposi's sarcoma

An open study of five patients with AIDS-related Kaposi's sarcoma demonstrated a response to foscarnet treatment (180 mg per kg daily for 10 days i.v.), with long periods of remission post-therapy (Morfeldt and Torssander, 1994).

6 Foscarnet therapy for hepatitis B

Patients in varying stages of coma due to fulminant hepatitis caused by hepatitis B infection have been reported to respond to foscarnet therapy with complete recovery in eight of ten cases (Hansson *et al.*, 1991). This success supports an earlier case report where a patient with fulminant hepatitis B received a loading dose of 20 mg per kg, followed by a continuous infusion of 24–41 mg per kg daily for 13 days resulting in clinical improvement (Price *et al.*, 1986).

In chronic carriers of hepatitis B virus, with HBeAg and HBV-DNA seropositivity, a continuous infusion of foscarnet at a dose of 216 mg per kg daily for 7 days then 60 mg per kg 8-hourly for 2 weeks resulted in only modest antiviral activity (Bain *et al.*, 1989). Foscarnet treatment of three additional patients with chronic hepatitis B infection resulted in only minor antiviral efficacy, although the dose may have been lower than optimum (Schvarcz *et al.*, 1994). There is a case report of a liver transplant patient with recurrence of severe hepatitis B infection who responded to foscarnet used in combination with ganciclovir (Angus *et al.*, 1993). However, a lack of sustained efficacy of combination ganciclovir and foscarnet for recurrent hepatitis B infection post-liver transplant has also been reported (Singh and Gayowski, 1995).

Acknowledgement The author would like to thank Gilda Tachedjian of Macfarlane Burnet Centre for Medical Research, Melbourne, and Mark Jacobson of San Francisco General Hospital, University of California San Francisco, for their critical review of the chapter.

References

Andrei G, Snoeck R, Schols D et al. (1991). Comparative activity of selected antiviral compounds against clinical isolates of human cytomegalovirus. Eur J Clin Microbiol Infect Dis 10: 1026.

Andrei G, Snoeck R, Reymen D et al. (1995). Comparative activity of selected antiviral compounds against clinical isolates of varicella zoster virus. Eur J Clin Microbiol Infect Dis 14: 318.

Angus P, Richards M, Bowden S et al. (1993). Combination antiviral therapy controls severe post-liver transplant recurrence of hepatitis B virus infection. J Gastroenterol Hepatol 8: 353.

Arevalo JF, Gonzalez C, Capparelli EV et al. (1995). Intravitreous and plasma concentrations of ganciclovir and foscarnet after intravenous therapy in patients with AIDS and cytomegalovirus retinitis. J Infect Dis 172: 951.

Aschan J, Ringden O, Ljungman P et al. (1992). Foscarnet for treatment of cytomegalovirus infections in bone marrow transplant recipients. Scand J Infect Dis 24: 143.

Aweeka F, Gambertoglio JG, van der Horst C et al. (1992). Pharmacokinetics of concomitantly administered foscarnet and zidovudine for treatment of human immunodeficiency virus infection (ACTG protocol 053); Antimicrob Ag Chemother 36: 1773.

Aweeka FT, Gambertoglio JG, Kramer F et al. (1995). Foscarnet and ganciclovir pharmacokinetics during concomitant or alternating maintenance therapy for AIDS related cytomegalovirus retinitis. Clin Pharmacol Ther 57: 403.

Bacigalupo A, Tedone E, Van Lint MT et al. (1994a). CMV prophylaxis with foscarnet in allogeneic bone marrow transplant recipients at high risk of developing CMV infections. Bone Marrow Transplant 13: 783.

Bacigalupo A, van Lint MT, Tedone E et al. (1994b). Early treatment of CMV infections in allogeneic bone marrow transplant recipients with foscarnet or ganciclovir. Bone Marrow Transplant 13: 753.

Bain VG, Daniels HM, Chanas A et al. (1989). Foscarnet therapy in chronic hepatitis B virus E antigen carriers. J Med Virol 29: 152.

Balfour HH, Benson C, Braun J et al. (1994). Management of acyclovir-resistant herpes simplex and varicella-zoster virus infections. J AIDS 7: 254.

Beaufils H, Deray G, Katlama C et al. (1990). Foscarnet and crystals in glomerular capillary lumens. Lancet 336: 755.

Berthe P, Baudouin C, Garraffo R et al. (1994). Toxicologic and pharmacokinetic analysis of intravitreal injections of foscarnet, either alone or in combination with ganciclovir. Invest Ophthalmol Vis Sci 35: 1038.

Birch CJ, Tachedjian GN, Doherty RR et al. (1990). Altered sensitivity to antiviral drugs of herpes siplex virus isolates from a patient with the acquired immune deficiency syndrome. J Inf Dis 162: 731.

Birch CJ, Tyssen DP, Tachedjian G et al. (1992). Clinical effects and in vitro studies of trifluorothymidine combined with interferon-alpha for treatment of drug-resistant and -sensitive herpes simplex virus infections. J Infect Dis 166: 108.

Blanshard C (1992). Treatment of HIV-related cytomegalovirus disease of the gastrointestinal tract with foscarnet. J AIDS 5: S25.

Blanshard C, Benhamou Y, Dohin E et al. (1995). Treatment of AIDS-associated gastrointestinal cytomegalovirus infection with foscarnet and ganciclovir; a randomised comparison. J Infect Dis 172: 622.

Boivin G, Edelman CK, Pedneault L et al. (1994). Phenotypic and genotypic characterisation of acyclovir-resistant varicella zoster viruses isolated from persons with AIDS. J Infect Dis 170: 68.

Brockmeyer NH, Hengge UR, Mertins L et al. (1993). Foscarnet treatment in various cytomegalovirus infections. Int J Clin Pharmacol Ther Toxicol 31: 204.

Brown DL, Sather S, Cheltlin MD (1993). Reversible cardiac dysfunction associated with foscarnet therapy for cytomegalovirus esophatitis in an AIDS patient. Amer Heart J 125: 1439.

Butler KM, De Smet MD, Husson RN et al. (1992). Treatment of aggressive cytomegalovirus retinitis with ganciclovir in combination with foscarnet in a child infected with human immunodeficiency virus. J Pediatr 120: 483.

Caumes E, Gatineau M, Bricaire F et al. (1993). Foscarnet induced vulvar erosion. J Amer Acad Dermatol 28: 799.

Chrisp P, Clissold SP (1991). Foscarnet A review of its antiviral activity, pharmacokinetic properties and therapeutic use in immunocompromised patients with cytomegalovirus retinitis. Drugs 41: 104.

Coker RJ, Tomlinson D, Horner P et al. (1991). Treatment of cytomegalovirus retinitis with ganciclovir and foscarnet. Lancet 338: 574.

Colebunders R, Van den Abbeele K, Fleerackers Y et al. (1994). Two AIDS patients with life-threatening pancreatitis successfully treated, one with ganciclovir the other with foscarnet. Acta Clin Belg 49: 229.

Cox SW, Aperia K, Sandstrom E et al. (1994). Cross resistance between AZT, ddI and other antiretroviral drugs in primary isolates of HIV-1. Antivir Chem Chemother 5: 7.

Crowe SM, Elbeik T, Ulrich PP et al. (1991). No evidence of occult human immunodeficiency virus in seronegative individuals at very high risk of infection. J Med Virol 35: 160.

de Gans J, Portegies P, Tiessens G et al. (1990). Therapy for cytomegalovirus polyradiculomyelitis in patients with AIDS: treatment with ganciclovir. AIDS 4: 421.

Degre M, Beck S (1994). Anti-HIV activity of dideoxynucleosides, foscarnet and fusidic acid is potentiated by human leukocyte interferon in blood derived macrophages. Chemother 40: 201.

Deray G, Martinez F, Katlama C et al. (1989). Foscarnet nephrotoxicity: mechanism, incidence and prevention. Amer J Nephrol 9: 316.

Diaz-Llopis M, Chipont, E, Sanchez S et al. (1992). Intravitreal foscarnet for cytomegalovirus retinitis in a patient with acquired immune deficiency syndrome. Amer J Ophthalmol 114: 742.

Diaz-Llopis M, Espana E, Munoz G et al. (1994). High dose intravitreal foscarnet in the treatment of cytomegalovirus retinitis in AIDS. Brit J Ophthalmol 78: 120.

Dieterich DT, Poles MA, Lew EA et al. (1993a). Concurrent use of ganciclovir and foscarnet to treat cytomegalovirus infection in AIDS patients. J Infect Dis 167: 1184.

Dieterich DT, Poles MA, Dicker M et al. (1993b). Foscarnet treatment of cytomegalovirus gastrointestinal infections in acquired immunodeficiency syndrome patients who have failed ganciclovir induction. Amer J Gastroenterol 88: 542.

Domingo P, Puig M, Iranzo A et al. (1994). Polyradiculopathy due to cytomegalovirus infection; report of a case in which an AIDS patient responded to foscarnet therapy. Clin Infect Dis 18: 1019.

Drew L (1996). Cytomegalovirus resistance to antiviral therapies. Amer J Hlth System Pharmacy 53 (Suppl 2): S17.

Enting R, De Gans J, Reiss K et al. (1992). Ganciclovir/foscarnet for cytomegalovirus meningoencephalitis in AIDS. Lancet 340: 559.

Eriksson B, Oberg B (1979). Characteristics of herpes virus mutants resistant to phosphonoformate and phosphonoacetate. Antimicrob Ag Chemother 15: 758.

Eriksson BF, Schinazi RF (1989). Combinations of 3'-azido-3'-deoxythymidine (zidovudine) and phosphonoformate (foscarnet) against human immunodeficiency virus type 1 and cytomegalovirus replication in vitro. Antimicrob Ag Chemother 33: 663.

Evans LM, Grossman ME (1992). Foscarnet-induced penile ulcer. J Amer Acad Dermatol 27: 124.

Fanning MM, Read SE, Benson M et al. (1990). Foscarnet therapy of cytomegalovirus retinitis in AIDS. J AIDS 3: 472.

Farese RVJ, Schambelan M, Hollander H et al. (1990). Nephrogenic diabetes insipidus associated with foscarnet treatment of cytomegalovirus retinitis. Ann Intern Med 112: 955.

Fillet AM, Visse B, Caumes E et al. (1995). Foscarnet resistant multidermatomal zoster in a patient with AIDS. Clin Infect Dis 21: 1348.

Fletcher CV, Collier AC, Rhame FS et al. (1994). Foscarnet for suppression of human immunodeficiency virus replication. Antimicrob Ag Chemother 38: 604.

Flores-Aguilar M, Kuppermann BD, Quiceno JI *et al.* (1993). Pathophysiology and treatment of clinically resistant cytomegalovirus retinitis. *Ophthalmology* **100**: 1022.

Fourel I, Saputelli J, Schaffer P, Mason WS (1994). The carbocyclic analog of 2'-deoxyguanosine induces a prolong inhibition of duck hepatitis B virus DNA synthesis in primary hepatocyte cultures and in the liver. *J Virol* **68**: 1059.

Gazzard BG (1992). Foscarnet therapy in persons with AIDS: clinical research and management considerations. *J AIDS* **5**: S1.

Gearhart MO, Sorg TB (1993). Foscarnet induced severe hypomagnesemia and other electrolyte disorders. *Ann Pharmacother* **27**: 285.

Gerna G, Baldanti F, Sarasini A *et al.* (1994). Effect of foscarnet induction treatment on quantitation of human cytomegalovirus (HCMV) DNA in peripheral blood polymorphonuclear leukocytes and aqueous humor of AIDS patients with HCMV retinitis. *Antimicrob Ag Chemother* **38**: 38.

Gobert JM, Remington KM, Zhu YQ, North TW (1994). Multiple drug resistant mutants of feline immunodeficiency virus selected with 2',3'-dideoxyinosine alone and in combination with 3'-azido-3'- deoxythymidine. *Antimicrob Ag Chemother* **38**: 861.

Gross AS, Dretler RH (1993). Foscarnet induced penile ulcer in an uncircumcised patient with AIDS. *Clin Infect Dis* **17**: 1076.

Hall AJ, Jennens ID, Lucas R *et al.* (1991). Low frequency maintenance ganciclovir cytomegalovirus retinitis. *Scand J Infect Dis* **23**: 43.

Hansson BG, Riesbeck K, Nordenfelt E *et al.* (1991). Successful treatment of fulminant hepatitis B and fulminant hepatitis B and D coinfection explained by inhibitory effect on the immune response? *Prog Clin Biol Res* **364**: 421.

Hartshorn KL, Sandstrom EG, Necimeger D *et al.* (1986). Synergistic inhibition of human T cell lymphotropic virus type III replication *in vitro* by phosphonoformate and recombinant alpha-A interferon. *Antimicrob Ag Chemother* **30**: 189.

Helgstrand E, Eriksson B, Johansson NG *et al.* (1978). Trisodium phosphonoformate, a new antiviral compound. *Science* **201**: 819.

Hengge UR, Brockmeyer NH, Malessa R *et al.* (1993). Foscarnet penetrates the blood barrier; rationale for therapy of cytomegalovirus encephalitis. *Antimicrob Ag Chemother* **37**: 1010.

Hoch BS, Shahmehdi SJ, Louis BM, Bipner HI (1995). Foscarnet alters antidiuretic hormone-mediated transport. *Antimicrob Ag Chemother* **39**: 2008.

Holland GN, Levinson RD, Jacobson MA (1995). Dose-related difference in progression rates of cytomegalovirus retinopathy during foscarnet maintenance therapy. AIDS Clinical Trials Group Protocol 915 Team. *Amer J Ophthalmol* **119**: 576.

Hwang CB, Ruffner KL, Coen DM (1992). A point mutation within a distinct conserved region of the herpes simplex virus DNA polymerase gene confers drug resistance. *J Virol* **66**: 1774.

Im GJ, Tramontano E, Gonzalez CJ, Cheng YC (1993). Identification of the amino acid in the human immunodeficiency virus type 1 reverse transcriptase involved in the pyrophosphate binding of antiviral nucleoside triphosphate analogs and phosphonoformate implications for multiple drug resistance. *Biochem Pharmacol* **46**: 2307.

Jacobson MA (1992a). Maintenance therapy for cytomegalovirus retinitis in patients with acquired immunodeficiency syndrome: foscarnet. *Amer J Med* **92**: (2A): .

Jacobson MA (1992b). Review of the toxicities of foscarnet. *J AIDS* **5**: S11.

Jacobson MA, Crowe S, Levy J *et al.* (1988). Effect of foscarnet therapy on infection with human immunodeficiency virus in patients with AIDS. *J Infect Dis* **158**: 862.

Jacobson MA, ODonnell JJ, Mills J (1989). Foscarnet treatment of cytomegalovirus retinitis in patients with the acquired immunodeficiency syndrome. *Antimicrob Ag Chemother* **33**: 736.

Jacobson MA, Gambertoglio JG, Aweeka FT *et al.* (1991). Foscarnet-induced hypocalcemia and effects of foscarnet on calcium metabolism. *J Clin Endocrinol Metab* **72**: 1130.

Jacobson MA, Causey D, Polsky B *et al.* (1993). A dose-ranging study of daily maintenance intravenous foscarnet therapy for cytomegalovirus retinitis in AIDS. *J Infect Dis* **168**: 444.

Jacobson MA, Wulfsohn M, Feinberg JE *et al.* (1994). Phase II dose ranging trial of foscarnet salvage therapy for cytomegalovirus retinitis in AIDS patients intolerant of or resistant to ganciclovir (ACTG protocol 093). AIDS Clinical Trials Group of the National Institute of Allergy and Infectious Diseases. *AIDS* **8**: 451.

Kaiser L, Perrin L, Hirschel B *et al.* (1995). Foscarnet decreases human immunodeficiency virus RNA. *J Infect Dis* **172**: 225.

Karmochkine M, Molina JM, Scieux C *et al.* (1994). Combined therapy with ganciclovir and foscarnet for cytomegalovirus polyradiculomyelitis in patients with AIDS. *Amer J Med* **97**: 196.

Katlama C, Dohin E, Caumes E *et al.* (1992). Foscarnet induction therapy for cytomegalovirus retinitis in AIDS: comparison of twice-daily and three-times-daily regimens. *J AIDS* **5**: S18.

Kirsch LS, Arevalo JF, De Clercq E *et al.* (1995). Phase I/II study of intravitreal cidofovir for the treatment of cytomegalovirus retinitis in patients with the acquired immunodeficiency syndrome. *Amer J Ophthalmol* **119**: 466.

Knox KK, Drobyski WR, Carrigan DR (1991). Cytomegalovirus isolate resistant to ganciclovir and foscarnet from a marrow transplant patient. *Lancet* **337**: 1292.

Koshida R, Vrang L, Gilljam G *et al.* (1989). Inhibition of human immunodeficiency virus *in vitro* by combinations of 3'-azido-3'-deoxythymidine and foscarnet. *Antimicrob Ag Chemother* **33**: 778.

Kuppermann BD, Flores-Aguilar M, Quiceno JI *et al.* (1993). Combination ganciclovir and foscarnet in the treatment of clinically resistant cytomegalovirus retinitis in patients with acquired immunodeficiency syndrome. *Arch Ophthalmol* **111**: 1359.

Lacey HB, Ness A, Mandal BK (1992). Vulval ulceration associated with foscarnet. *Genitourin Med* **68**: 182.

Leport C, Puget S, Pepin JM *et al.* (1993). Cytomegalovirus resistant to foscarnet; clinicovirologic correlation in a patient with human immunodeficiency virus. *J Infect Dis* **168**: 1329.

Lieberman RM, Orellana J, Melton RC (1994). Efficacy of intravitreal foscarnet in a patient with AIDS. *New Engl J Med* **330**: 868.

Lietman PS (1992). Clinical pharmacology: foscarnet. *Amer J Med* **92**: 8S.

Lipson SM, Tseng LF, Kaplan MH, Biondo FX (1993). Antiviral susceptibility testing of cytomegalovirus from primary culture using shell vial assay to detect the late viral antigen. *Diagn Microbiol Infect Dis* **17**: 283.

Loghman-Adham M, Levi M, Scherer SA *et al.* (1993). Phosphonoformic acid blunts adaptive response of renal and intestinal Pi transport. *Amer J Physiol* **265**: F756.

Lokke-Jensen B, Weismann K, Mathiesen L *et al.* (1993). Atypical varicella zoster infection in AIDS. *Acta Derm Venereol* **73**: 123.

Lor E, Liu YQ (1994). Neurologic sequelae associated with foscarnet therapy. *Ann Pharmacother* **28**: 1035.

MacGregor RR, Graziani AL, Weiss R *et al.* (1991). Successful foscarnet therapy for cytomegalovirus retinitis in an AIDS patient undergoing hemodialysis: rationale for empiric dosing and plasma level monitoring. *J Infect Dis* **164**: 785.

Malin A, Miller RF (1992). Foscarnet-induced hypokalaemia. *J Infect* **25**: 329.

Manischewitz JF, Quinnan GVJ, Lane HC *et al.* (1990). Synergistic effect of ganciclovir and foscarnet on cytomegalovirus replication *in vitro*. *Antimicrob Ag Chemother* **34**: 373.

Manji H, Malin A, Connolly S (1992). CMV polyradiculopathy in AIDS -suggestion for new strategies in treatment. *Genitourin Med* **68**: 192.

Mellors JW, Bazmi HZ, Schinazi RF *et al.* (1995). Novel mutations in reverse transcriptase of human immunodeficiency virus type 1 reduce susceptibility to foscarnet in laboratory and clinical isolates. *Antimicrob Ag Chemother* **39**: 1087.

Mesri EA, Cesarman E, Arvanitakis L *et al.* (1996). Human herpes virus-8/Kaposi's sarcoma-associated herpesvirus is a new transmissible virus that infects B cells. *J Exp Med* **183**: 2385.

Morfeldt L, Torssander J (1994). Long term remission of Kaposi's sarcoma following foscarnet treatment in HIV-infected patients. *Scand J Infect Dis* **26**: 749.

Nelson MR, Connolly GM, Hawkins DA et al. (1991). Foscarnet in the treatment of cytomegalovirus infection of the esophagus and colon in patients with the acquired immune deficiency syndrome. *Amer J Gastroenterol* **86**: 876.

Neyts J, Snoeck R, Schols D et al. (1991). Sensitive, reproducible and convenient fluorometric assay for the *in vitro* evaluation of anti-cytomegalovirus agents. *J Virol Meth* **35**: 27.

Nyberg G, Svalander C, Blohme I et al. (1989). Tubulointerstitial nephritis caused by the antiviral agent foscarnet. *Transpl Int* **2**: 223.

Oberg B (1983). Antiviral effect of phosphonoformate (PFA, Foscarnet sodium). *Pharmacol Ther* **19**: 387.

Oberg B (1986). Molecular basis of foscarnet action. In (Lopez & Roizman, eds), pp. 141–151. *Human Herpesvirus Infections*. New York: Raven Press.

Oberg B (1989). Antiviral effects of phosphonoformate (PFA, foscarnet sodium). *Pharmacol Ther* **40**: 213.

Ostrander M, Cheng YC (1980). Properties of herpes simplex virus type 1 and type 2 DNA polymerase. *Biochem Biophys Acta* **609**: 232.

Palestine AG, Polis MA, De SMD et al. (1991). A randomized, controlled trial of foscarnet in the treatment of cytomegalovirus retinitis in patients with AIDS. *Ann Intern Med* **115**: 665.

Paspaliaris V, Mai X, Leaver DD (1993). Foscarnet inhibits vascular smooth muscle contraction. *Life Sci* **53**: 1227.

Pearson PA, Jaffe GJ, Ashton P (1993). Intravitreal foscarnet for cytomegalovirus retinitis in a patient with acquired immunodeficiency syndrome. *Amer J Ophthalmol* **115**: 686.

Peters M, Timm U, Schurmann D et al. (1992). Combined and alternating ganciclovir and foscarnet in acute and maintenance therapy of human immunodeficiency virus-related cytomegalovirus encephalitis refractory to ganciclovir alone. A case report and review of the literature. *Clin Invest* **70**: 456.

Peters M, Schurmann D, Bergmann F et al. (1994). Safety of alternating ganciclovir and foscarnet maintenance therapy in human immunodeficiency virus (HIV) related cytomegalovirus infections. An open labeled pilot study. *Scand J Infect Dis* **26**: 49.

Polis M, de Smet MD, Baird BF et al. (1993). Increased survival of a cohort of patients with acquired immune deficiency syndrome and cytomegalovirus retinitis who received sodium phosphonoformate (foscarnet). *Amer J Med* **94**: 175.

Prasad VR, Lowry I, de Los Santos T et al. (1991). Isolation and characterization of dideoxyguanosine triphosphate-resistant mutant of human immunodeficiency virus reverse transcriptase. *Proc Natl Acad Sci USA* **88**: 11363.

Price JS, France AJ, Moaven LD et al. (1986). Foscarnet in fulminant hepatitis. *Lancet* **ii**: 1273.

Raffi F, Taburet AM, Ghaleh B et al. (1993). Penetration of foscarnet into cerebrospinal fluid of AIDS patients. *Antimicrob Ag Chemother* **37**: 1777.

Razis E, Cook P, Mittelman A, Ahmed T (1994). Treatment of ganciclovir resistant cytomegalovirus with foscarnet; a report of two cases occurring after bone marrow transplantation. *Leuk Lymphoma* **12**: 477.

Reusser P, Gambertoglio JG, Lilleby K et al. (1992). Phase I-II trial of foscarnet for prevention of cytomegalovirus infection in autologous and allogeneic marrow transplant recipients. *J Infect Dis* **166**: 473.

Ringden O, Lonnqvist B, Paulin T et al. (1986). Pharmacokinetics, safety and preliminary clinical experiences using foscarnet in the treatment of cytomegalovirus infections in bone marrow and renal transplant recipients. *J Antimicrob Chemother* **17**: 373.

Rios M, Munoz M, Spencer E (1995). Antiviral activity of phosphonoformate on rotavirus transcription and replication. *Antiviral Res* **27**: 71.

Sacks SL, Portnoy J, Lawee D et al. (1987). Clinical course of recurrent genital herpes and treatment with foscarnet cream: results of a Canadian multicenter trial. *J Infect Dis* **155**: 178.

Safrin S, Phan L (1993). *In vitro* activity of penciclovir against clinical isolates of acyclovir-resistant and foscarnet resistant herpes simplex virus. *Antimicrob Ag Chemother* **37**: 2241.

Safrin S, Assaykeen T, Follansbee S et al. (1990) Foscarnet therapy for acyclovir-resistant mucocutaneous herpes simplex virus infection in 26 AIDS patients: preliminary data. *J Infect Dis* **161**: 1078.

Safrin S, Berger TG, Gilson I et al. (1991a). Foscarnet therapy in five patients with AIDS and acyclovir-resistant varicella-zoster virus infection. *Ann Intern Med* **115**: 19.

Safrin S, Crumpacker C, Chatis P et al. (1991b). A controlled trial comparing foscarnet with vidarabine for acyclovir-resistant mucocutaneous herpes simplex in the acquired immunodeficiency syndrome. The AIDS Clinical Trials Group. *New Engl J Med* **325**: 551.

Safrin S, Elbeik T, Phan L et al. (1994a). Correlation between response to acyclovir and foscarnet therapy and *in vitro* susceptibility result for isolates of herpes simplex virus from human immunodeficiency virus-infected patients. *Antimicrob Ag Chemother* **38**: 1246.

Safrin S, Elbeik T, Mills J (1994b). A rapid screen test for *in vitro* susceptibility of clinical herpes simplex virus isolates. *J Infect Dis* **169**: 879.

Safrin S, Kemmerly S, Plotkin B et al. (1994c). Foscarnet-resistant herpes simplex virus infection in patients with AIDS. *J Infect Dis* **169**: 193.

Salazar A, Podzamczer D, Rene R et al. (1995). Cytomegalovirus ventriculoencephalitis in AIDS patients. *Scand J Infect Dis* **27**: 165.

Salzberger D, Stoehr A, Helse W et al. (1994). Foscarnet and ganciclovir combination therapy for CMV disease in HIV infected patients. *Infection* **22**: 197.

Sandstrom E, Kaplan J, Byington RE et al. (1985). Inhibition of human T-cell lymphotropic virus type III *in vitro* by phosphonoformate. *Lancet* **i**: 1480.

Sarasini A, Baldanti F, Furione M et al. (1995). Double resistance to ganciclovir and foscarnet of four human cytomegalovirus strains recovered from AIDS patients. *J Med Virol* **47**: 237.

Sarin PS, Taguchi Y, Sun D et al. (1985). Inhibition of HTLV-III/LAV replication by foscarnet. *Biochem Pharmacol* **34**: 4075.

Schvarcz R, Hansson BG, Lernestedt JO, Weiland O (1994). Treatment of chronic replicative hepatitis B virus infection with short term continuous infusion of foscarnet. *Infection* **22**: 330.

Seidel EA, Koenig S, Polis MA (1993). A dose-escalation study to determine the toxicity and maximally tolerated dose of foscarnet. *AIDS* **7**: 941.

Sherker AH, Hirota K, Omata M et al. (1986). Foscarnet decreases serum and liver duck hepatitis B virus DNA in chronically infected ducks. *Gastroenterology* **91**: 818.

Singh N, Gayowski T (1995). Lack of sustained efficacy of combination ganciclovir and foscarnet for hepatitis B virus recurrence after liver transplantation. *Transplant* **59**: 1629.

Sjovall J, Karlsson A, Ogenstad S et al. (1988). Pharmacokinetics and absorption of foscarnet after intravenous and oral administration to patients with human immunodeficiency virus. *Clin Pharmacol Ther* **44**: 65.

Sjovall J, Bergdahl S, Movin G et al. (1989). Pharmacokinetics of foscarnet and distribution to cerebrospinal fluid after intravenous infusion in patients with human immunodeficiency virus infection. *Antimicrob Ag Chemother* **33**: 1023.

Smee DF, Barnett BB, Sidwell RW et al. (1995). Antiviral activities of nucleosides and nucleotides against wild-type and drug-resistant strains of murine cytomegalovirus. *Antiviral Res* **26**: 1.

Snoeck R, Andrei G, Schols D et al. (1992). Activity of different antiviral drug combinations against human cytomegalovirus replication *in vitro*. *Eur J Clin Microbiol Infect Dis* **11**: 1144.

Snoeck R, Andrei G, Gerard M et al. (1994). Successful treatment of progressive mucocutaneous infection due to acyclovir and foscarnet resistant herpes simplex virus with (S)-1-(3-hydroxy-2- phosphonylmethoxypropyl)cytosine (HPMPC). *Clin Infect Dis* **18**: 570.

Spector SA, Tyndall M, Kelley E (1983). Inhibition of human cytomegalovirus by trifluorothymidine. *Antimicrob Ag Chemother* **23**: 113.

Stanley HD, Charlebois E, Harb G, Jacobson MA (1994). Central venous catheter infections in AIDS patients receiving treatment for cytomegalovirus disease. *J AIDS* 7: 272.

Stenberg K Larsson, A (1978). Reversible effects on cellular metabolism and proliferation by insodium phosphonoformate. *Antimicrob Ag Chemother* 14: 727.

Strid S, Ekstrom C, Datema R (1989). Comparison of foscarnet and foscarnet esters as anti-influenza virus agents. *Chemother* 35: 69.

Stridh S, Helgstrand E, Lannero B *et al.* (1979). The effect of pyrophosphate analogues on influenza virus RNA polymerase and influenza virus multiplication. *Archs Virol* 61: 245.

Studies of Ocular Complications of AIDS Research Group in collaboration with AIDS Clinical Trials Group (1992). Mortality in patients with the acquired immunodeficiency syndrome treated with either foscarnet or ganciclovir for cytomegalovirus retinitis. *New Engl J Med* 326: 213.

Studies of Ocular Complications of AIDS Research Group in collaboration with AIDS Clinical Trials Group (1994). Foscarnet-ganciclovir cytomegalovirus retinitis trial. 4. *Ophthalmology* 101: 1250.

Studies of Ocular Complications of AIDS Research Group in collaboration with AIDS Clinical Trials Group (1995a). Antiviral effects of foscarnet and ganciclovir therapy on human immunodeficiency virus p24 antigen in patients with AIDS and cytomegalovirus retinitis. *J Infect Dis* 172: 613.

Studies of Ocular Complications of AIDS Research Group in collaboration with AIDS Clinical Trials Group (1995b). Morbidity and toxic effects associated with ganciclovir or foscarnet therapy in a randomized cytomegalovirus trial. *Arch Int Med* 155: 65.

Studies of Ocular Complications of AIDS Research Group in Collaboration with the AIDS Clinical Trials Group (1996). Combination foscarnet and ganciclovir therapy vs monotherapy for the treatment of relapsed cytomegalovirus retinitis in patients with AIDS. The Cytomegalovirus Retreatment Trial. *Arch Ophthalmol* 114: 23.

Sullivan V, Coen DM (1991). Isolation of foscarnet-resistant human cytomegalovirus patterns of resistance and sensitivity to other antiviral drugs. *J Infect Dis* 164: 781.

Sutton D, Taylor J, Bacon TH *et al.* (1992). Activity of penciclovir in combination with azidothymidine, ganciclovir, acyclovir, foscarnet and human interferons against herpes simplex virus replication in cell culture. *Antivir Chem Chemother* 3: 85.

Taburet AM, Singlas E (1996). Drug interactions with antiviral drugs. *Clin-Pharmacokinet* 30: 385.

Taburet AM, Katlama C, Blanshard C *et al.* (1992). Pharmacokinetics of foscarnet after twice-daily administrations for treatment of cytomegalovirus disease in AIDS patients. *Antimicrob Ag Chemother* 36: 1821.

Tachedjian G, Hoy J, McGavin K, Birch C (1994). Long-term foscarnet therapy not associated with the development of foscarnet-resistant human immunodeficiency virus type 1 in an acquired immunodeficiency syndrome patient. *J Med Virol* 42: 207.

Tachedjian G, Hooker DJ, Gurusinghe AD *et al.* (1995). Characterisation of foscarnet-resistant strains of human immunodeficiency virus type 1. *Virology* 212: 58.

Tachedjian G, Mellows J, Bazmi H *et al.* (1996). Zidovudine resistance is suppressed by mutations conferring resistance of human immunodeficiency virus type 1 to foscarnet. *J Virol* 70: 7171

Tatarowicz WA, Lurain NS, Thompson KD (1992). A ganciclovir-resistant clinical isolate of human cytomegalovirus exhibiting cross-resistance to other DNA polymerase inhibitors. *J Infect Dis* 166: 904.

Trolliet P, Dijoud F, Cotte L *et al.* (1995). Crescentic glomerulonephritis and crystals within glomerular capillaries in an AIDS patient treated with foscarnet. *Amer J Nephrol* 15: 256.

Turrini B, Tognon MS, de Caro G, Secchi AG (1994). Intravitreal use of foscarnet; retinotoxicity of repeated injections in the rabbit eye. *Ophthalmic Res* 26: 110.

Van der Pijl J, Frissen PHJ, Reiss, P *et al.* (1990). Foscarnet and penile ulceration. *Lancet* 335: 286.

Verdonck LF, Cornelissen JJ, Smit J *et al.* (1993). Successful foscarnet therapy for acyclovir-resistant mucocutaneous infection with herpes simplex virus in a recipient of allogeneic BMT. *Bone Marrow Transplant* 11: 177.

Vrang L, Oberg B, Lower J *et al.* (1988). Reverse transcriptases from human immunodeficiency virus type 1 (HIV-1), HIV-2, and simian immunodeficiency virus (SIVMAC) are susceptible to inhibition by foscarnet and 3'-azido-3'-deoxythymidine triphosphate. *Antimicrob Ag Chemother* 32: 1733.

Wagstaff AJ, Bryson HA (1994). A reappraisal of its antiviral activity pharmacokinetic properties and therapeutic use in immunocompromised patients with viral infections. *Drugs* 48: 199.

Wahren B Oberg, B (1980). Reversible inhibition of cytomegalovirus replication by phosphonoformate. *Intervirology* 14: 7.

Walmsley S, Chew E, Read, SE *et al.* (1988). Treatment of cytomegalovirus retinitis with trisodium phosphonoformate hexahydrate (Foscarnet). *J Infect Dis* 157: 569.

Weinberg DV, Murphy R, Naughton K (1994). Combined daily therapy with intravenous ganciclovir and foscarnet for patients with recurrent cytomegalovirus retinitis. *Amer J Ophthalmol* 117: 776.

Wilcox CM, Straub RF, Schwartz DZ (1995). Cytomegalovirus esophagitis in AIDS; a prospective evaluation of clinical response to ganciclovir therapy. *Amer J Med* 98: 169.

Youle MS, Clarbour J, Gazzard B *et al.* (1988). Severe hypocalcaemia in AIDS patients treated with foscarnet and pentamidine. *Lancet* i: 1455

Soluble Recombinant CD4

Description

The human immunodeficiency virus (HIV) infects cells which bear the CD4 molecule on their surface. Virus binding occurs primarily through a high-affinity interaction between the CD4 molecule and the viral envelope glycoprotein, gp120. It is now clear that CC-CKR-5 (which is a receptor for the beta-chemokines RANTES, MIP-1alpha and MIP-1beta) mediates entry of macrophage-tropic strains of HIV-1 into CD4-expressing cells (Dragic *et al.*, 1996; Deng *et al.*, 1996) and that fusin, a seven-transmembrane, G-protein-coupled receptor mediates entry of syncytium-inducing strains (Feng *et al.*, 1996). A member of the immunoglobulin superfamily, CD4 contains four extracellular domains which have homology with immunoglobulin variable regions (Fig. V.30). Only the first of these variable domains (V1) of CD4 is required for HIV binding. Soluble forms of CD4, which lack the transmembrane domain of the CD4 molecule and which consist of either the full-length extracellular molecule or which are truncated to comprise only the V1 region, have been engineered by recombinant technology. These soluble, recombinant CD4 (soluble CD4) successfully compete for gp120 binding *in vitro* and block transmission of HIV in cell culture. Although soluble CD4 has been developed as a therapeutic agent it was found to have an unacceptably short plasma half-life. Second-generation compounds have combined the soluble CD4 with *Pseudomonas* exotoxin or CD4 linked to IgG_1 and IgG_2 (CD4-immunoadhesin) (Fig. V.30 and Fig. V.31) are currently being evaluated in clinical trials.

The molecular weight of CD4 is 55kDa, for soluble CD4 it is 41 kDa, for soluble CD4-*Pseudomonas* exotoxin it is 59 kDa, for soluble CD4-immunoadhesin it is 112 kDa.

Fig. V.30.
Structure of native CD4, soluble rCD4, and sCD4-PE40. The four domains of CD4 with disulfide bridges (S-S) are numbered 1–4. TM and CYT refer to the transmembrane and cytoplasmic domains of CD4, respectively. Approximate amino acid residue positions are indicated. For the sCD4-PE40 hybrid molecule, the truncated *Pseudomonas* exotoxin A moiety comprises the second and third domains responsible for movement across the cell membrane (translocase) and adenosine diphosphate-ribosylation (catalytic toxin), respectively. (Reproduced from Coombs, 1993, with permission.)

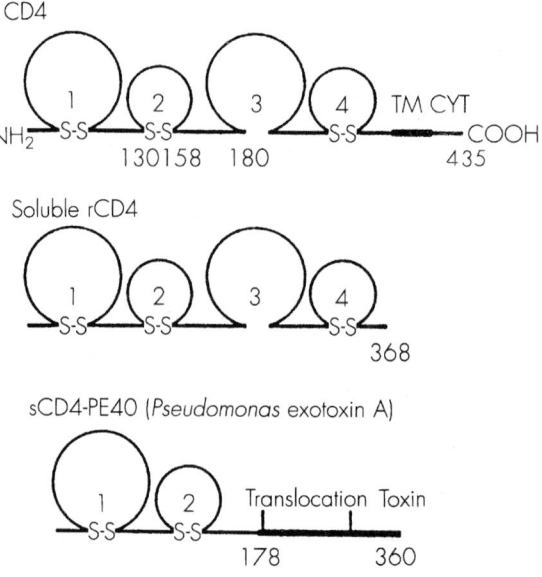

Fig. V.31.

Structure of CD4 immunoadhesin. CD4- and IgG1-derived sequences are indicated by shaded and unshaded regions, respectively. Soluble rCD4 is truncated after proline 368 of the mature CD4 polypeptide. The variable (V_H) and constant (C_H1, hinge, C_H2 and C_H3) regions of IgG1 heavy chain are shown. Disulfide bonds are indicated by S-S. CD4 immunoadhesin consists of residues 1–180 of the mature CD4 protein fused to IgG1 sequences beginning at aspartic acid 216 (taking amino acid 114 as the first residue of the heavy chain constant region) which is the first residue in the IgG1 hinge after the cysteine residue involved in heavy-light chain bonding. The CD4 immunoadhesin shown, which lacks a C_H1 domain, was derived from a C_H1 containing CD4 immunoadhesin by oligonucleotide-directed deletional mutagenesis, expressed in Chinese hamster ovary cells and purified to >99% purity using protein A sepharose chromatography. (Reproduced in part from Byrn *et al.*, 1990, with permission.)

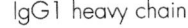

IgG1 heavy chain

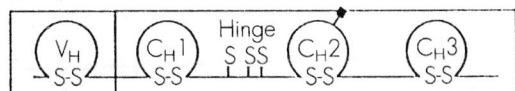

CD4 immunoadhesion

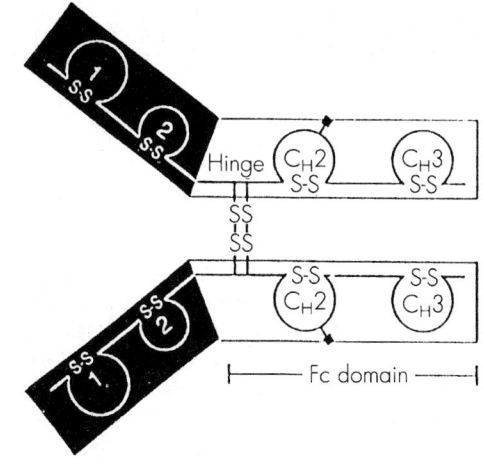

Antiviral Activity

Recombinant soluble CD4 has been purified from culture medium of a stably transfected Chinese hamster ovary cell line (Fisher *et al.*, 1988), using a baculovirus expression system (Hussey *et al.*, 1988; Webb *et al.*, 1989), expressed in *Escherichia coli* (Chao *et al.*, 1989; Garlick *et al.*, 1990; Rubino *et al.*, 1991), and by transfection of mammalian cells using a soluble CD4 expression vector (Smith *et al.*, 1987).

These forms of soluble CD4 usually have been found to inhibit HIV infection; enhancement of HIV and simian immunodeficiency virus (SIV) infection by soluble CD4 has also been reported.

1 Inhibition of HIV infection

Soluble CD4 has been shown to prevent HIV infection of peripheral blood mononuclear cells by diverse isolates of HIV-1 (Byrn *et al.*, 1989; reviewed in Daar and Ho, 1991). However, the concentration of soluble CD4 required to neutralize HIV-1 infection of peripheral blood mononuclear cells and transformed cell lines has been shown to vary greatly among different isolates of HIV. Laboratory strains of HIV-1 which have been passaged in transformed cell lines are more sensitive to neutralization with soluble CD4, with an IC_{90} of <0.1 μg per ml (O'Brien *et al.*, 1992; Turner *et al.*, 1992; Moore *et al.*, 1992). However, primary virus isolates require several hundred-fold to several thousand-fold higher concentrations of soluble CD4 for neutralization to occur with an IC_{90} ranging from 5 to 190 μg per ml (Table V.19) (O'Brien *et al.*, 1992; Daar *et al.*, 1990; Daar and Ho 1991; Chamow *et al.*, 1992).

Soluble CD4 has been found to block HIV-1 infection of peripheral blood monocyte-derived macrophages (Molina *et al.*, 1991) and to inhibit fusion and subsequent syncytium formation between HIV-infected macrophages and uninfected CD4-expressing T cell lines (Crowe *et al.*, 1990; Crowe *et al.*, 1992). Other investigators have described relative resistance of macrophage-tropic strains of HIV to neutralization by soluble CD4, compared with T cell tropic isolates (O'Brien *et al.*, 1994). Soluble CD4 inhibits HIV-1 entry into microglial cells, neuroglioma cells (Jordan *et al.*, 1991; Volsky *et al.*, 1992) and human placental trophoblastic cells (David *et al.*, 1992).

Table V.19
Inhibition of laboratory strains and primary isolates of HIV-1 *in vitro*. (Adapted from Daar *et al.*, 1990, with permission.)

Isolate		ID_{90} μg per ml
HIV-1$_{IIIB}$[a]		0.07
HIV-1$_{JR-FL}$[b]		110
HIV-1$_{JR-CSF}$[b]		180
Pt isolate	1	15
	2	18
	3	190
	4	110
	5	85
	6	30

[a] Laboratory adapted strains
[b] Well-characterized primary isolates.

2 Human immunodeficiency virus type 2 and simian immunodeficiency virus

The data are limited regarding the ability of soluble CD4 to inhibit HIV-1 or SIV entry into simian macrophages. In one study soluble (human) CD4 inhibited the interaction between surface SIV gp120 on monkey macrophages and CD4 on uninfected monkey T cells (McEntee *et al.*, 1991). Other investigators have reported that human soluble CD4 does not inhibit SIV replication in bone-marrow derived macrophages from rhesus monkeys (Watanabe *et al.*, 1991a). The treatment of SIV-infected rhesus monkeys with soluble (human) CD4 has resulted in a diminished ability to isolate SIV from the peripheral blood mononuclear cells and bone marrow macrophages of these animals (Watanabe *et al.*, 1989, 1991b).

Soluble CD4 has also been shown to have activity against HIV-2 (Byrn *et al.*, 1989). The concentration of soluble CD4 required to inhibit HIV-2 is 50- to 400-fold higher than that for HIV-1; the concentration of soluble CD4 required to inhibit SIV is 5- to 20-fold higher than needed for HIV-1 (Looney *et al.*, 1990). The ID_{90} of soluble CD4 for neutralization of HIV-2$_{(Rod)}$ in stimulated peripheral blood mononuclear cells from normal donors is 12 μg per ml (Daar *et al.*, 1990). In a separate study 100 μg per ml was required to completely block HIV-2 $_{(Rod)}$ and HIV-2 $_{(NIH-Z)}$ (Looney *et al.*, 1990). The affinity of the envelope glycoproteins of SIV and HIV-2 for soluble CD4 has been reported to be 70-fold and more than 280-fold respectively lower than that of a reference HIV-1 isolate (Ivey *et al.*, 1991).

3 Inhibition of HIV-1 using second-generation soluble CD4 compounds

The second-generation compounds include the genetically engineered hybrid toxin which contains the truncated CD4 molecule linked to active domains of *Pseudomonas aeruginosa* exotoxin A, or to ricin, and CD4-immunoglobulin hybrids.

The recombinant protein which contains CD4 and *Pseudomonas* exotoxin (CD4-PE) displays selective activity against cells which bear the HIV envelope glycoprotein on their surface (Chaudhary *et al.*, 1988). The *in vitro* potency of CD4-PE has been found to be determined by the length of the *Pseudomonas* exotoxin sequence (Winkler *et al.*, 1991). The hybrid toxin selectively kills cells infected with HIV-1, including lymphocytes and monocyte/macrophages (Ashorn *et al.*, 1991), with IC_{50} values of approximately 100 pM (Berger *et al.*, 1988). In addition, the compound inhibits the spread of HIV-1 in cell culture, as assessed by a marked suppression of free HIV production (Ashorn *et al.*, 1991; Berger *et al.*, 1988). Of interest the hybrid toxin inhibits primary strains of HIV-1 that are refractory to neutralization by soluble CD4 (Kennedy *et al.*, 1993). The hybrid toxin has been reported to kill SIV-infected cells which are expressing viral envelope glycoproteins (Ashorn *et al.*, 1992).

By recombinant technology, the first two immunoglobulin-like domains of CD4 have been fused to the entire constant region of the IgG heavy chain. In later developments, the hinge and Fc regions of the heavy chain of human immunoglobulin has been fused with the V1 and V2 regions of CD4 (Byrn *et al.*, 1990; Chamow *et al.*, 1992) (Fig. V.31). The CD4-immunoglobulin proteins (termed CD4-immunoadhesins) have similar *in vitro* activity to that of first-generation soluble CD4 as assessed by gp120 binding, and neutralization of laboratory and primary isolates of HIV-1 and HIV-2 (Byrn *et al.*, 1990; Daar *et al.*, 1990). Pretreatment of chimpanzees with CD4 immunoadhesin has also been found to inhibit HIV-1 infection (Ward *et al.*, 1991; Chamow *et al.*, 1992), although in two experiments involving SIV-infected macaques no beneficial effects were observed (Langner *et al.*, 1993).

Soluble CD4 conjugated to the deglycosylated A chain of the plant toxin ricin has been found to kill HIV-infected T cell lines, with less toxicity in uninfected cultures (Till *et al.*, 1988).

4 Enhancement of HIV and SIV infection

Soluble CD4 has been reported to induce or enhance cell fusion by a number of strains of HIV-2 (Clapham *et al.*, 1992). Incubation of soluble CD4 with SIV$_{(agm)}$ results in more rapid syncytium formation in T cell lines than when experiments are performed in the absence of soluble CD4. It has been postulated that this enhanced effect on SIV replication is due to modulation of gp120-CD4 binding, thus facilitating viral fusion and entry (Allan *et al.*, 1990).

5 Synergism

Zidovudine, didanosine or zalcitabine have all been shown to have synergy with soluble CD4 *in vitro* (Hayashi *et al.*, 1990; Johnson *et al.*, 1989). A three-drug regimen comprising zidovudine, soluble CD4 and recombinant interferon alpha also synergistically inhibits HIV-1 replication *in vitro* (Johnson *et al.*, 1990). This three-drug combination resulted in near-complete inhibition of HIV for 28 days in culture (2- to 3-fold longer than single-drug regimens). Other investigators have confirmed synergy between interferon alpha and soluble CD4 (Pan *et al.*, 1992). Reverse transcriptase inhibitors also have reported synergy with soluble CD4 linked to *Pseudomonas* exotoxin against spread of HIV-1 infection in T lymphocyte cultures (Ashorn *et al.*, 1990). There are conflicting data regarding antiviral interactions between soluble CD4 and HIV-1 antibody-containing human sera, with some investigators finding no evidence of antagonism or synergy (Kennedy *et al.*, 1991), and others reporting enhancement by soluble CD4 of antiviral activity of HIV antibody-containing serum (Smith-Burchnell *et al.*, 1991).

6 Antagonism

Dextran sulfate and soluble CD4 are antagonistic *in vitro* (Hayashi *et al.*, 1990), for the binding of gp120 from lymphocytes but not monocytes (Lynch *et al.*, 1994).

7 Acquired resistance

Passage of molecularly cloned HIV in the presence of soluble CD4 results in an 8- to 16-fold reduction in sensitivity to neutralization by soluble CD4 following *in vitro* exposure, with no loss in sensitivity to CD4-immunoadhesin (McKeating *et al.*, 1991).

Mode of Administration and Dosage

Soluble CD4 and CD4-immunoadhesin have been administered in clinical trials by i.v. infusion over a 10-min interval, by continuous i.v. infusion, and by intramuscular and subcutaneous injection (Kahn *et al.*, 1990; Hodges *et al.*, 1991; Husson *et al.*, 1992). Dosing regimens in phase I clinical trials have ranged from 0.001 to 10 mg per kg body weight (Hodges *et al.*, 1991; Schooley *et al.*, 1990; Kahn *et al.*, 1990; Schacker *et al.*, 1995; Meng *et al.*, 1995). The frequency of administration in these studies ranged from daily injection to once-weekly.

Serum Levels in Relation to Dosage

There have only been limited studies in humans addressing the relationship between route of administration of soluble CD4 and its related compounds, dosage and serum levels. In an NIAID-sponsored study, after a single i.v. infusion of 1 mg of soluble CD4, the peak plasma concentration of soluble CD4 was 100–300 ng per ml; with a single infusion of 10 mg of soluble CD4, the peak concentration rose to approximately 2000 ng per ml. This concentration greatly exceeds the IC$_{90}$ *in vitro* (Table V.19). A single intramuscular injection of 1 mg of soluble CD4 resulted in a serum level of 2–4 ng per ml 7 h after administration; when this dose was increased to 10 mg, the corresponding mean serum level was 23 ng per ml. In this clinical trial, intramuscular administration of 10 mg of soluble CD4 given 8-hourly resulted in a steady-state serum level of 50–300 ng per ml (Schooley *et al.*, 1990). The serum levels of CD4 in individuals randomized to receive 9 or 30 mg per day by intramuscular injection were within the reported range required to inhibit HIV-1 replication *in vitro* (Schooley *et al.*, 1990). The reported bioavailability of CD4 following intramuscular and subcutaneous injection is 51% and 45% respectively (Kahn *et al.*, 1990). Soluble CD4 has been found to demonstrate linear pharmacokinetics over a dose range of 1–10 mg per kg (Schacker *et al.*, 1995).

It is known that CD4-immunoadhesin has a significantly longer plasma half-life than soluble CD4, (Ward *et al.*, 1991; Chamow *et al.*, 1992), resulting in a 25-fold increase in levels of soluble CD4 in the blood (Ward *et al.*, 1991). The mean terminal half-life of CD4-immunoadhesin in a recent study was 50.2 h for persons receiving 1mg per kg i.v. (Chamow *et al.*, 1992). In a dose-escalating study of 41 HIV-infected patients with CD4 counts of less than 500 cells per μl who received combination therapy with soluble CD4 (300–3000 μg per kg twice-weekly) and oral zidovudine for 12 weeks, the serum half-life of CD4 immunoadhesin was approximately 32 h (Meng et al., 1995). Intravenous administration of CD4-immunoadhesin at 1 mg per kg dosage has resulted in peak serum concentrations 10 min after the infusion of 20–24 μg per ml (Hodges et al., 1991). Similar to soluble CD4, there appears to be considerable variation in the rate and extent of absorption of CD4-immunoadhesin following intramuscular administration. The bioavailability following intramuscular injection in this study ranged from 9 to 47% (Hodges et al., 1991). In another study intramuscular administration of 1 mg per kg of CD4-immunoadhesin resulted in a mean bioavailability of 21% (Chamow et al., 1992). The peak concentration following intramuscular administration of 1 mg per kg has been reported to be approximately 10-fold lower (mean: 2.7 μg per ml; range: 0.78–4.6 μg per ml) than when the compound is given by i.v. administration (Hodges et al., 1991).

Excretion and Distribution of the Drug in Body

Information from animal studies suggests that the major metabolic pathway of soluble CD4 is degradation to its constituent amino acids which subsequently become incorporated into endogenous proteins (Davis et al., 1992). In rats, soluble CD4 administered by i.v. injection results in rapid clearance from the plasma with an elimination $T_{1/2}$ of 7 min; low levels are found after subcutaneous injection (Davis et al., 1992).

Recombinant soluble CD4 is also rapidly cleared from human plasma after i.v. administration, with a plasma half-life of 45–60 min (Schooley et al., 1990; Kahn et al., 1990), and unpublished data suggesting that it may be as short as 15 min. The plasma half-life following intramuscular and subcutaneous administration was 9 and 11 h respectively (Kahn et al., 1990). Soluble CD4 is partially excreted as intact protein within the urine (Bugelski et al., 1992).

The steady-state volumes of distribution of CD4-immunoadhesin following a 1 mg per kg i.v. dose was only 76.5 ml per kg in the Genentech-sponsored phase I study. The clearance of the compound from the plasma was slow, 1.92 ml per h per kg (Hodges et al., 1991). Following intramuscular administration, the elimination half-life of CD4-immunoadhesin is 18.6–68.3 h, notably longer than that of 9.4 h for soluble CD4 (Hodges et al., 1991). In chimpanzees and pregnant rhesus monkeys, CD4-immunoadhesin is efficiently transferred across the placenta (Byrn et al., 1990; Chamow et al., 1992).

Mode of Action

The CD4 molecule is a 55 kDa glycoprotein found on the surface of the helper-inducer subset of T lymphocytes, peripheral blood monocytes and tissue macrophages. This molecule is the major receptor for HIV binding, although the importance of the chemokine receptors (see above) has been clearly demonstrated as cofactors for viral entry. Other molecules including galactosyl ceramide and Fc receptors have been reported to facilitate HIV entry into certain cells which do not express CD4. The binding of HIV envelope glycoprotein gp120 to the CD4 molecule is the first step involved in the entry of HIV into cells expressing the CD4 molecule on their surface. Several studies have confirmed that the gp120 binding site lies within the first 123 amino-terminal residues of CD4, comprising domain 1 and part of domain 2 of CD4 (Clayton et al., 1988; Rubino et al., 1991; Garlick et al., 1990; Berger et al., 1989; Chao et al., 1989; Autierio et al., 1991; Moore, 1993). There are discontinuous epitopes which comprise the binding site of CD4 on HIV gp120, with the CD4 binding domain predominantly residing towards the C terminus and mostly involving regions within the third (C3) and fourth conserved (C4) regions of gp120 (Wyatt et al., 1992; Cordell et al., 1991; Ho et al., 1991; McKeating et al., 1993). The variable V2 and to some extent V1 regions of gp120 also contribute to the efficiency of HIV-1 entry but are not absolutely required (Wyatt et al., 1995). Amino acids 257, 368, 370, 375 and 441 have been reported to be important for CD4 binding (McKeating et al., 1992, 1993; Morrison et al., 1995). Soluble recombinant CD4 binds to HIV gp120, thus preventing the virus from infecting the cell. In addition, soluble CD4 can bind to gp120 on infected cells and prevent cell to cell transmission of HIV. It has been found that with some strains of HIV the binding of gp120 to soluble CD4 results in cleavage of the envelope glycoprotein from the virus (Moore et al., 1990; Werner and Levy, 1993). This cleavage of gp120, however, exposes the fusogenic domain of gp41 and thus potentially could increase infectivity by facilitating cell to cell fusion (Sattentau and Moore, 1991; Hart et al., 1991; Moore et al., 1991). This mechanism may underlie the observed enhancement of infection with HIV-2 and SIV, described above.

The mechanisms underlying differences in sensitivity of primary isolates and laboratory strains of HIV to soluble CD4 are not clearly understood. The region of HIV gp120 which is important for macrophage and T cell line tropism includes the V3 region of gp120 but not the CD4 binding domain. The region of gp120 which determines resistance of primary isolates to soluble CD4 has been mapped to this same region (O'Brien *et al.*, 1992). The affinity of gp120 of these primary isolates for CD4 has been reported by some investigators to have lower affinity for soluble CD4. Other investigators have reported no differences in the CD4-binding affinities of different isolates for recombinant gp120 or gp120 derived from clinical isolates (Ashkenazi *et al.*, 1991; Brighty *et al.*, 1991; Turner *et al.*, 1992), although intact virions of patient isolates have 10- to 30-fold lower affinity for soluble CD4 than laboratory strains (Chamow *et al.*, 1992; Ashkenazi *et al.*, 1991; Moore *et al.*, 1992). These findings have also been observed using CD4-immunoadhesin (Moore *et al.*, 1992). Temperature-dependent changes in the affinity of soluble CD4 for gp120 on intact virions have been described (Moore *et al.*, 1991).

In addition to the extended plasma half-life of the CD4-immunoadhesins, these compounds have been reported to have other advantages over soluble CD4 including greater avidity for CD4 (Chamow *et al.*, 1992), and the ability to perform effector functions through Fc domains, including complement activation and antibody-dependent cell-mediated cytotoxicity (Zettlmeissl *et al*, 1990; Chamow *et al.*, 1992).

The immunotoxins (CD4-PE and CD4-ricin) provide targeted delivery of toxin to cells expressing viral envelope glycoproteins. Targeted cells are killed following uptake of the CD4-immunotoxin; CD4-PE contains the active translocation and ADP-ribosylation domains required for the penetration and killing of cells expressing gp120 (Chaudhary *et al.*, 1988).

Toxicity

In monkeys, i.v. administration of soluble CD4 with four daily doses of 100 mg per kg daily resulted in renal lesions involving the distal nephron, with protein casts containing soluble CD4 and Tamm-Horsfall protein (Bugelski *et al.*, 1992).

In humans, soluble CD4 has been associated with relatively few and minor side-effects. Approximately one-third of patients have developed mild to moderate local reactions at injection sites, consisting of mild and transient erythema. Other reported side-effects include fever, and a maculopapular rash which resolved on withdrawal of therapy. No hepatic, renal, or hematologic toxicity has been noted (Schooley *et al.*, 1990).

In clinical trials to date CD4-immunoadhesin has been associated with minimal toxicity. Mild to moderate symptoms have been reported in persons on study, but have been considered to be unrelated to study medication. These include esthenia, fever, sweating, dizziness, agitation, depression, paresthesia, tremor, short-term memory loss, myalgia, abdominal pain, nausea, vomiting, diarrhea, rhinitis and rash (Hodges *et al.*, 1991). Abnormal liver function tests and neutropenia have also been reported (Meng *et al.*, 1995).

The development of antibodies to soluble CD4 has been reported following 4 weeks of therapy; there was no associated change in the number of circulating CD4 T lymphocytes (Schooley *et al.*, 1990). In a pediatric study, two of 11 patients developed antibodies to CD4 (Husson *et al.*, 1992). Antibodies to CD4 linked to *Pseudomonas* exotoxin developed in 58% of patients, and these neutralized the effect of this compound *in vitro* (Davey *et al.*, 1994). Treatment of SIV-infected rhesus monkeys with soluble (human) CD4 has resulted in the development of anti-human CD4 as well as anti-rhesus monkey CD4 antibodies (Watanabe *et al.*, 1991b, 1992).

No drug interactions that affect the pharmacokinetics of soluble CD4 have been reported. There is no pharmacokinetic interaction between zalcitabine and soluble CD4 when these are co-administered (Qian *et al.*, 1992).

Clinical Uses of the Drug

1 Human immunodeficiency virus infection

Soluble CD4, CD4-immunoadhesin and CD4-PE are only available for treatment of HIV infection through clinical trials. The safety of soluble CD4, soluble CD4 *Pseudomonas* exotoxin and CD4-immunoadhesin have been established in patients with AIDS and AIDS-related complex. Unfortunately, there has not been a clear demonstration of efficacy in published studies to date (reviewed in Clumeck, 1993).

There was no evidence of antiviral activity in a phase I pediatric study continuous i.v. administration of soluble CD4 (100, 300 or 1000 µg per kg daily) to children with symptomatic HIV infection for 12 weeks (Husson *et al.*, 1992). However, i.v administration of single-dose boluses of soluble CD4 (2–10 mg per kg) demonstrated a dose-dependent reduction in plasma viremia in three of four adult subjects, with this inhibitory effect reflecting the IC_{90-95} values of the isolates (Schacker *et al.*, 1994, 1995).

In an open-label, multicenter phase I/II escalating dosage trial of soluble CD4 given by i.v. administration or intramuscular injection to patients with AIDS and AIDS-related complex, a modest decline in circulating HIV p24 antigen was only detected in persons receiving the highest dose of 30 mg per day (p = 0.02). The mean serum p24 antigen levels decreased from 1341 pg per ml to 789 pg per ml. There was no associated rise in CD4 lymphocyte counts, or in tests of T cell function (Schooley *et al.*, 1990).

In a dose-ranging, open-label phase I study in 18 persons with AIDS or AIDS-related complex who received 0.03 to 1 mg per kg of CD4-immunoadhesin either intravenously or via intramuscular injection there was no consistent change in either HIV p24 antigen levels or CD4 lymphocyte numbers (Hodges *et al.*, 1991). Other studies, using CD4-immunoadhesin, have similarly shown a lack of a convincing or sustained virologic response, and no immunologic improvement (Collier *et al.*, 1990).

Soluble CD4 *Pseudomonas* exotoxin was given to 17 patients in doses of 1–15 µg per kg once-monthly for 2 months then once-weekly for 6 weeks by i.v. bolus injection. No consistent evidence of immunologic or virologic efficacy was demonstrated (Davey *et al.*, 1994).

Soluble CD4 is present in normal plasma (Blasczyk *et al.*, 1993), and has been found to be elevated in patients with HIV infection, although the level did not correlate with stage of disease (Peakman *et al.*, 1992). This is not specific for HIV infection as elevated levels of soluble CD4 in plasma have also been described in patients with HTLV-1 infection, acute dengue hemorrhagic fever, measles and infectious mononucleosis (Tsukada *et al.*, 1991; Kurane *et al.*, 1991; Yoneyama *et al.*, 1995)

Acknowledgements The author would like to thank Damien Purcell, of Macfarlane Burnet Centre for Medical Research, Melbourne, for his critical review of this chapter.

References

Allan JS, Strauss J, Buck DW (1990). Enhancement of SIV infection with soluble receptor molecules. *Science* **247**: 1084.

Ashkenazi A, Smith DH, Marsters SA *et al.* (1991). Resistance of primary isolates of human immunodeficiency virus type 1 to soluble CD4 is independent of CD4-rgp-120 binding affinity. *Proc Natl Acad Sci USA* **88**: 7056.

Ashorn P, Moss B, Weinstein JN *et al.* (1990). Elimination of infectious human immunodeficiency virus from human T-cell cultures by synergistic action of CD4 *Pseudomonas* exotoxin and reverse transcriptase inhibitors. *Proc Natl Acad Sci USA* **87**: 8889.

Ashorn P, Englund G, Martin MA *et al.* (1991). Anti-HIV activity of CD4 *Pseudomonas* exotoxin on infected primary human lymphocytes and monocyte/macrophages. *J Infect Dis* **163**: 703.

Ashorn P, Moss B, Berger EA (1992). Activity of CD4-*Pseudomonas* exotoxin against cells expressing diverse forms of the HIV and SIV envelope glycoproteins. *J AIDS* **5**: 70.

Autiero M, Abrescia P, Dettin M *et al.* (1991). Binding to CD4 of synthetic peptides patterned on the principal neutralizing domain of the HIV-1 envelope protein. *Virology* **185**: 820.

Berger EA, Fuerst TR, Moss B (1988). A soluble recombinant polypeptide comprising the aminoterminal half of the extracellular region of the CD4 molecule contains an active binding site for human immunodeficiency virus. *Proc Natl Acad Sci USA* **85**: 2357.

Berger EA, Clouse KA, Chaudhary VK *et al.* (1989). CD4-*Pseudomonas* exotoxin hybrid protein blocks the spread of human immunodeficiency virus infection *in vitro* and is active against retroviruses. *Proc Natl Acad Sci USA* **86**: 9539.

Blasczyk R, Westhoff U, Grosse-Wilde H (1993). Soluble CD4, CD8 and HLA molecules in commercial immunoglobulin preparations. *Lancet* **341**: 789.

Brighty DW, Rosenberg M, Chen IS, Ivey-Hoyle M (1991). Envelope proteins from clinical isolates of human immunodeficiency virus type 1 that are refractory to neutralization by soluble CD4 possess high affinity for the CD4 receptor. *Proc Natl Acad Sci USA* **88**: 7802.

Bugelski PJ, Solleveld HA, Fong KL *et al.* (1992). Myeloma like cast nephropathy caused by human recombinant soluble CD4 (sCD4) in monkeys. *Amer J Pathol* **140**: 531.

Byrn RA, Sekigawa I, Chamow SM *et al.* (1989). Characterisation of *in vitro* inhibition of human immunodeficiency virus by purified recombinant CD4. *J Virol* **63**: 4370.

Byrn RA, Mordenti J, Lucas C *et al.* (1990). Biological properties of a CD4 immunoadhesion. *Nature* **344**: 667.

Chamow SM, Duliege AM, Ammann A *et al.* (1992). CD4 immunoadhesions in anti-HIV therapy; new developments. *Int J Cancer* **7**: 69.

Chao BH, Costopoulos DS, Curiel T *et al.* (1989). A 113-amino acid fragment of CD4 produced in *Escherichia coli* blocks human immunodeficiency virus-induced cell fusion. *J Biol Chem* **264**: 5812.

Chaudhary VK, Mizukami T, Fuerst TR *et al.* (1988). Selective killing of HIV-infected cells by recombinant human CD4 *Pseudomonas* exotoxin hybrid protein. *Nature* **335**: 369.

Clapham PR, McKnight A, Weiss RA (1992). Human immunodeficiency virus type 2 infection and fusion of CD4-negative human cell lines; induction and enhancement by soluble CD4. *J Virol* **66**: 3531.

Clayton LK, Hussey RW, Steinbrich R *et al.* (1988). Substitution of murine for human CD4 residues identifies amino acids critical for HIV gp120 binding. *Nature* **363**: 366.

Clumeck N (1993). Current use of anti-HIV drugs in AIDS. *J Antimicrob Ag Chemother* **32**: 133.

Collier A *et al.* (1990). Safety and pharmacokinetics of intravenous recombinant CD4 immunoadhesin (rCD4-IGG) (AIDS Clinical Trials Group Protocol 121). Int Conf AIDS; 6.

Coombs RW (1993). *Antiviral Chemotherapy. New Directions for Clinical Applications and Research* Vol. 3 (Mills J, Corey L, eds). Englewood Cliffs, New Jersey: Prentice Hall.

Cordell J, Moore JP, Dean CJ *et al.* (1991). Rat monoclonal antibodies to nonoverlapping epitopes of human immunodeficiency virus type 1 gp120 block CD4 binding *in vitro*. *Virology* **185**: 72.

Crowe SM, Mills J, Kirihara J *et al.* (1990). Full-length recombinant CD4 and recombinant gp120 inhibit fusion between HIV infected macrophages and uninfected CD4-expressing T- lymphoblastoid cells. *AIDS Res Hum Retrovir* **6**: 1031.

Crowe SM, Mills J, Elbeik T *et al.* (1992). Human immunodeficiency virus-infected monocyte derived macrophages express surface gp120 and fuse with CD4 lymphoid cells *in vitro* a possible mechanism of T-lymphocyte depletion *in vivo*. *Clin Immunol Immunopathol* **65**: 143.

Daar ES, Ho DD (1991). Relative resistance of primary HIV-1 isolates to neutralization by soluble CD4. *Amer J Med* **90**: 22S.

Daar ES, Li XL, Moudgil T, Ho DD (1990). High concentrations of recombinant soluble CD4 are required to neutralize primary human immunodeficiency virus type 1 isolates. *Proc Natl Acad Sci USA* **87**: 6574.

Davey RT, Boenning CM, Herpin BR *et al.* (1994). Use of recombinant soluble CD4 *Pseudomonas* exotoxin, a novel immunotoxin, for treatment of persons infected with human immunodeficiency virus. *J Infect Dis* **170**: 1180.

David FJ, Autran B, Tran HC *et al.* (1992). Human trophoblast cells express CD4 and are permissive for productive infection with HIV-1. *Clin Exp Immunol* **88**: 10.

Davis CB, Boyle KE, Urbanski JJ (1992). Disposition of metabolically labelled recombinant soluble CD4 (sT4) in male Sprague-Dawley rats following intravenous and subcutaneous administration. *Drug Metab Dispos* **20**: 695.

Deng H, Liu R, Ellmeier W *et al.* (1996). Identification of a major co-receptor for primary isolates of HIV-1. *Nature* **381**: 661.

Dragic T, Litwin V, Allaway G *et al.* (1996). HIV-1 entry inot CD4+ cells is mediated by chemokine receptor CC-CKR-5. *Nature* **381**: 668.

Feng Y, Broder CC, Kennedy PE *et al.* (1996). HIV-1 entry cofactor: functional cDNA cloning of a seven-transmembrane, G-coupled receptor. *Science* **272**: 872.

Fisher RA, Bertonis JM, Meter W *et al.* (1988). HIV infection is blocked *in vitro* by recombinant soluble CD4. *Nature* **331**: 76.

Garlick RL, Kirschner RJ, Eckenrode FM *et al.* (1990). *Escherichia coli* expression; purification and biological activity of a truncated soluble CD4. *AIDS Res Hum Retrovir* **6**: 465.

Hart TK, Kirsh R, Ellens H *et al.* (1991). Binding of soluble CD4 proteins to human immunodeficiency virus type 1 and infected cells induces release of envelope glycoprotein gp120. *Proc Natl Acad Sci USA* **88**: 2189.

Hayashi S, Fine RL, Chou TC *et al.* (1990). *In vitro* inhibition of the infectivity and replication of human immunodeficiency virus type 1 by combination of antiretroviral 2',3'-dideoxynucleosides and virus binding inhibitors. *Antimicrob Ag Chemother* **34**: 82.

Ho DD, Fung MS, Cao YZ *et al.* (1991). Another discontinuous epitope on glycoprotein gp120 that is important in human immunodeficiency virus type 1 neutralization is identified by a monoclonal antibody. *Proc Natl Acad Sci USA* **88**: 8949.

Hodges TL, Kahn JO, Kaplan LD *et al.* (1991). Phase 1 study of recombinant human CD4 immunoglobulin G therapy of patients with AIDS and AIDS-related complex. *Antimicrob Ag Chemother* **35**: 2580.

Hussey RE, Richardson NE, Kowalski M *et al.* (1988). A soluble CD4 protein selectively inhibits HIV replication and syncytium formation. *Nature* **331**: 78.

Husson RN, Chung Y, Mordenti J *et al.* (1992). Phase 1 study of continuous infusion soluble CD4 as symptomatic human immunodeficiency virus infection. *J Pediatr* **121**: 627.

Ivey HM, Culp JS, Chaikin MA *et al.* (1991). Envelope glycoproteins from biologically diverse isolates of immunodeficiency viruses have widely different affinities for CD4. *Proc Natl Acad Sci USA* **88**: 512.

Johnson VA, Barlow MA, Chou TC *et al.* (1989). Synergistic inhibition of human immunodeficiency virus type 1 (HIV-1) replication *in vitro* by recombinant soluble CD4 and 3'-azido- 3'-doexythymidine. *J Infect Dis* **159**: 837.

Johnson VA, Barlow MA, Merrill DP *et al.* (1990). Three drug synergistic inhibition of HIV-1 replication *in vitro* by zidovudine, recombinant soluble CD4, and recombinant interferon alpha A. *J Infect Dis* **161**: 1059.

Jordan CA, Watkins BA, Kufta C, Dubois-Dalcq M (1991). Infection of brain microglial cells by human immunodeficiency virus type 1 is CD4 dependent. *J Virol* **65**: 736.

Kahn JQ, Allan JD, Hodges TL *et al.* (1990). The safety and pharmacokinetics of recombinant soluble CD4 (rCD4) in subjects with the acquired immunodeficiency syndrome (AIDS) and AIDS- related complex. A phase 1 study. *Ann Intern Med* **112**: 254.

Kennedy MS, Orloff S, Ibegbu CC *et al.* (1991). Analysis of synergism/antagonism between HIV-1 antibody-positive human sera and soluble CD4 in blocking HIV-1 binding and infectivity. *AIDS Res Hum Retrovir* **7**: 975.

Kennedy PE, Moss B, Berger EA (1993). Primary HIV-1 isolates refractory to neutralization by soluble CD4 are potently inhibited by CD4-pseudomonas exotoxin. *Virology* **192**: 375.

Kurane I, Innis BL, Nimmannitya S *et al.* (1991). Activation of T lymphocytes in dengue virus infections. High levels of soluble interleukin 2 receptor, soluble CD4, soluble CD8, interleukin 2 and interferon-gamma in sera of children with dengue. *J Clin Invest* **88**: 1473.

Langner KD, Niedrig M, Fultz P *et al.* (1993). Antiviral effects of different CD4-immunoglobulin constructs against HIV-1 and SIV; immunological characterisation, pharmacokinetic data and *in vivo* experiments. *Arch Virol* **130**: 157.

Looney DJ, Hayashi S, Nicklas M *et al.* (1990). Differences in the interaction of HIV-1 and HIV-2 with CD4. *J AIDS* **3**: 649.

Lynch G, Low L, Li S *et al.* (1994). Sulfated polyanions prevent HIV infection of lymphocytes by disruption of CD4-gp120 interaction, but do not inhibit monocyte infection. *J Leuk Biol* **56**: 266.

McEntee MF, Sharma DP, Zink MC *et al.* (1991). Rhesus monkey macrophages infected with simian immunodeficiency virus cause rapid lysis of CD4-bearing lymphocytes. *J Gen Virol* **72**: 317.

McKeating J, Balfe P, Clapham P *et al.* (1991). Recombinant CD4-selected human immunodeficiency virus type 1 variants with reduced gp120 affinity for CD4 and increased cell fusion capacity. *J Virol* **65**: 4777.

McKeating JA, Thall M, Furman C *et al.* (1992). Amino acid residues of the human immunodeficiency virus type 1 gp120 critical for the binding of rat and human neutralizing antibodies that block the gp120 sCD4 interaction. *Virology* **190**: 134.

McKeating JA, Bennett J, Zolla-Pazner S *et al.* (1993). Resistance of a human serum-selected human immunodeficiency virus type 1 escape mutant to neutralization by CD4 binding site monoclonal antibodies is conferred by a single amino acid change in gp120. *J Virol* **67**: 5216.

Meng TC, Fischl MA, Cheeseman SH *et al.* (1995). Combination therapy with recombinant human soluble CD4 immunoglobulin G and zidovudine in patients with HIV infection; a phase I study. *J AIDS Hum Retrovir* **8**: 152.

Molina JM, Ferriani R, Amirault C, Groopman JE (1991). Purified recombinant CD4 inhibits HIV-1 infection of peripheral blood macrophages. *Pathol Biol Paris* **39**: 754.

Moore JP (1993). A monoclonal antibody to the CDR-3 region of CD4 inhibits soluble CD4 binding to virions of human immunodeficiency virus type 1. *J Virol* **67**: 3656.

Moore JP, McKeating JA, Weiss RA, Sattentau QJ (1990). Dissociation of gp120 from HIV-1 virions induced by soluble CD4. *Science* **250**: 1139.

Moore JP, McKeating JA, Norton WA, Sattentau QJ (1991). Direct measurement of soluble CD4 binding to human immunodeficiency virus type 1 virions; gp120 dissociation and its implications for virus-cell binding and fusion reactions and their neutralization by soluble CD4. *J Virol* **65**: 1133.

Moore JP, McKeating JA, Huang YX *et al.* (1992). Virions of primary human immunodeficiency virus type 1 isolates resistant to soluble CD4 (sCD4) neutralization differ in sCD4 binding and glycoprotein gp120 retention from sCD4-sensitive isolates. *J Virol* **66**: 235.

Morrison HG, Kirchhoff F, Desrosiers RC (1995). Effects of mutations in constant regions 3 and 4 of envelope of simian immunodeficiency virus. *Virology* **210**: 448.

O'Brien WA, Chen IS, Ho DD, Daar ES (1992). Mapping genetic determinants for human immunodeficiency virus type 1 resistance to soluble CD4. *J Virol* **66**: 3125.

O'Brien WA, Mao SH, Cao Y, Moore JP (1994). Macrophage tropic and T-cell line-adapted chimeric strains of human immunodeficiency virus type 1 differ in their susceptibilities to neutralization by soluble CD4 at different temperatures. *J Virol* **68**: 5264.

Pan XZ, Qiu ZD, Baron PA *et al.* (1992). Three drug synergistic inhibition of HIV-1 replication *in vitro* by 3'-fluoro-3'-deoxythymidine, recombinant soluble CD4, and recombinant interferon alpha. *AIDS Res Hum Retrovir* **8**: 589.

Peakman M, Senaldi G, Foote N *et al.* (1992). Naturally occurring soluble CD4 in patients with human immunodeficiency virus infection. *J Infect Dis* **165**: 799.

Qian M, Swagler AR, Fong KL *et al.* (1992). Pharmacokinetic evaluation of drug interactions with anti-human immunodeficiency virus drugs. V Effect of soluble CD4 on 2',3'dideoxycytidine kinetics in monkeys. *Drug Metab Dispos* **20**: 396.

Rubino KL, Tarpley WG, Nicholas JA (1991). Effects of a soluble CD4 and CD4-*Pseudomonas* exotoxin A chimeric protein on human peripheral blood lymphocytes: lymphocyte activation and anti- HIV activity *in vitro*. *Antiviral Res* **16**: 267.

Sattentau QJ, Moore JP (1991). Conformational changes induced in the human immunodeficiency virus envelope glycoprotein by soluble CD4 binding. *J Exp Med* **174**: 407.

Schacker T, Coombs RW, Collier AC *et al.* (1994). The effects of high-dose recombinant soluble CD4 on human immunodeficiency virus type 1 viremia. *J Infect Dis* **169**: 37.

Schacker T, Collier AC, Coombs R *et al.* (1995). Phase 1 study of high dose, intravenous rsCD4 in subjects with advanced HIV-1 infection. *J AIDS Hum Retrovir* **9**: 145.

Schooley RT, Merigan TC, Gaut P *et al.* (1990). Recombinant soluble CD4 therapy in patients with the acquired immunodeficiency syndrome (AIDS) and AIDS-related complex. A phase I-II escalating dosage trial. *Ann Intern Med* **112**: 247.

Smith DH, Byrn RA, Marsters SA *et al.* (1987). Blocking of HIV-1 infectivity by a soluble, secreted form of the CD4 antigen. *Science* **238**: 1704.

Smith-Burchnell C, Hussey L, Thomas D, Dalgleish A (1991). Soluble CD4 enhances antiviral activity of anti-HIV serum *in vitro*. *AIDS* **5**: 1030.

Till MA, Ghetie V, Gregory T *et al.* (1988). HIV infected cells are killed by rCD4-ricin A chain. *Science* **242**: 1166.

Tsukada N, Matsuda M, Miyagi K, Yanagisawa N (1991). Soluble CD4 and CD8 in the peripheral blood of patients with multiple sclerosis and HTLV-1 associated myelopathy. *J Neuroimmunol* **35**: 285.

Turner S, Tizard R, DeMarinis J *et al.* (1992). Resistance of primary isolates of human immunodeficiency virus type 1 to neutralization by soluble CD4 is not due to lower affinity with the viral envelope glycoprotein gp120. *Proc Natl Acad Sci USA* **89**: 1335.

Volsky B, Sakai K, Reddy MM, Volsky DJ (1992). A system for the high efficiency replication of HIV-1 in neural cells and its application to antiviral evaluation. *Virology* **186**: 303.

Ward RH, Capon DJ, Jett CM *et al.* (1991). Prevention of HIV-1 IIIB infection in chimpanzees by CD4 immunoadhesion. *Nature* **352**: 434.

Watanabe M, Reimann KA, KeLong PA *et al.* (1989). Effect of recombinant soluble CD4 in rhesus monkeys infected with simian immunodeficiency virus of macaques. *Nature* **337**: 267.

Watanabe M, Chen ZW, Tsubota H *et al.* (1991a). Soluble human CD4 elicits an antibody response in rhesus monkeys that inhibits simian immunodeficiency virus replication. *Proc Natl Acad Sci USA* **88**: 120.

Watanabe M, Levine CG, Shen L *et al.* (1991b). Immunization of simian immunodeficiency virus-infected rhesus monkeys with soluble human CD4 elicits an antiviral response. *Proc Natl Acad Sci USA* **88**: 4616.

Watanabe M, Boyson JE, Lord CJ, Letvin NL (1992). Chimpanzees immunized with recombinant soluble CD4 develop anti-self CD4 antibody responses with anti-human immunodeficiency virus activity. *Proc Natl Acad Sci USA* **89**: 5103.

Webb NR, Madoulet C, Tosi PP *et al.* (1989). Cell-surface expression and purification of human CD4 produced in baculovirus-infected insect cells. *Proc Natl Acad Sci USA* **86**: 7731.

Werner A, Levy JA (1993). Human immunodeficiency virus type 1 envelope gp120 is cleaved after incubation with recombinant soluble CD4. *J Virol* **67**: 2566.

Winkler G, Jakubowski A, Turner S *et al.* (1991). CD4-*Pseudomonas* exotoxin hybrid proteins; modulation of potency and therapeutic window through structural design and characterisation of cell internalization. *AIDS Res Hum Retrovir* **7**: 393.

Wyatt R, Thali M, Tilley S *et al.* (1992). Relationship of the human immunodeficiency virus type 1 gp120 third variable loop to a component of the CD4 binding site in the fourth conserved region. *J Virol* **66**: 6997.

Wyatt R, Moore J, Accola M *et al.* (1995). Involvement of the V1/V2 variable loop structure in the exposure of human immunodeficiency virus type 1 gp120 epitopes by receptor binding. *J Virol* **69**: 5723.

Yoneyama A, Nakahara K, Higashihara M, Kurokawa K (1995). Increased levels of soluble CD8 and CD4 in patients with infectious mononucleosis. *Brit J Haematol* **89**: 47.

Zettlmeissl G, Gregersen JP, Duport JM *et al.* (1990). Expression and characterisation of human CD4 immunoglobulin fusion proteins. *DNA Cell Biol* **9**: 347

Zidovudine

Description

Zidovudine, or 3'-azido-3'deoxythymidine, formerly known as azidothymidine (AZT; BW A509U), is an analog of the nucleoside thymidine. It is an inhibitor of the human immunodeficiency virus (HIV)-encoded enzyme reverse transcriptase. It was the first antiretroviral compound to be licensed for the treatment of persons infected with HIV. The compound was synthesized much earlier, however, by Horwitz and colleagues (Horwitz *et al.*, 1964) and subsequently used in anticancer research.

Zidovudine was developed by Burroughs Wellcome and is now marketed by GlaxoWellcome under the trade name of 'Retrovir', and is generally indicated for the treatment of patients with HIV infection.

The molecular weight of zidovudine is 267.24. The molecular formula is $C_{10}H_{13}N_5O_4$. The chemical structure is shown in Fig. V.32. The concentration of zidovudine can be expressed in either μM or μg per ml (1 μg per ml is equivalent to 3.7 μM).

Antiviral Activity

1 Human immunodeficiency virus

Zidovudine is active against HIV *in vitro*, with early reports suggesting that it exerted an antiviral effect at a concentration of 50–500 nM (Mitsuya *et al.*, 1985; Nakashima *et al.*, 1986). Both HIV-1 and HIV-2 are sensitive to zidovudine (Vrang *et al.*, 1988; Pauwels *et al.*, 1990), although the concentration of zidovudine required to inhibit HIV-2 in three human cell lines has been reported to be significantly higher than for HIV-1 (Richman, 1987c). HIV-1 is divided into group M (major) containing subtypes A-H, and group O (outlier) containing highly divergent strains of HIV-1 predominantly isolated from Cameroonian patients. Strains from group M and group O are sensitive to zidovudine (Descamps *et al.*, 1995).

From a number of reports it is evident that the concentration of the drug required to inhibit HIV-1 varies according to the assay used, the strain of HIV-1 and the multiplicity of infection used, with significant differences in drug potency also observed with differing cell lines (Balzarini *et al.*, 1988). Using the MT-4 T cell line, which is transformed with human T

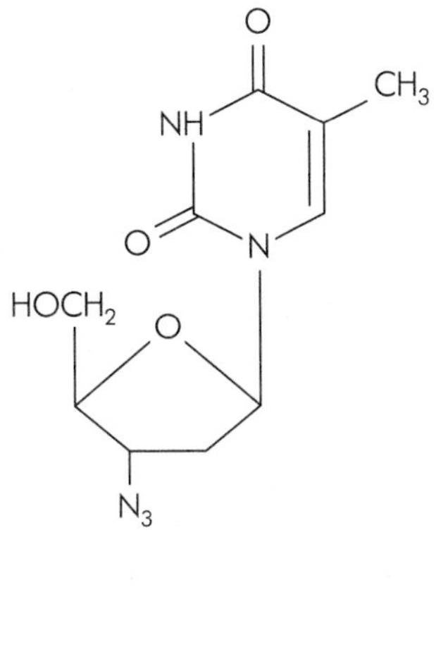

Fig. V.32.
Chemical structure of zidovudine.

lymphotropic virus type I, 0.004 µM of zidovudine inhibited the III$_B$ strain of HIV-1 by 50% when the multiplicity of infection was 0.0002, whereas at a 10-fold higher multiplicity of infection the IC$_{50}$ of zidovudine was 0.066 µM (Baba et al., 1987). Using a clone of the lymphoblastoid T cell line (H9) that was exposed to the HIV-1 isolate III$_B$, complete protection was achieved at concentration of 5 µM zidovudine, with approximately 50% inhibition still being evident when cells were cultured in the presence of 0.1 µM, as assessed by p24 assay (Mitsuya et al., 1985). Later studies demonstrated that concentrations of zidovudine of 1 µM, 0.25 µM and 0.0625 µM could inhibit HIV-1 replication in H9 cells by 97%, 86% and 71% respectively (Medina et al., 1992). Chronically infected lymphoblastoid cell lines are resistant to the effects of zidovudine, with 50 µg per ml achieving less than 60% inhibition of HIV-1 replication (Nakashima et al., 1986; Crowe et al., 1989). The effect of zidovudine in inhibiting HIV-1 replication in H9 cells in vitro is lost after 10–14 days in culture (Johnson et al., 1989a). Efficacy of the drug in inhibiting HIV-1 replication is still present even when zidovudine is added to infected cells 20 h after infection in vitro (Nakashima et al., 1986).

Inhibition of the viral-encoded reverse transcriptase by 50% is achieved with concentrations of 0.05 µM (0.013 µg per ml). Higher concentrations, in the range of 0.35 µM are required to reduce HIV core protein (p24) production by 50% in human T lymphocytes infected with laboratory-adapted isolates of HIV (reviewed in Furman and Barry, 1988).

Although the phosphorylation of zidovudine in monocytes and macrophages is 25% or less than that of T lymphocytes (Perno et al., 1988), zidovudine is more active in cells of macrophage lineage than in T lymphocytes or T lymphoblastic cell lines (Crowe et al., 1989; Perno et al., 1992a). Zidovudine at a concentration of 0.01 µg per ml inhibits acute infection of cultured monocytes with the DV strain of HIV-1 by over 90%. However, 50 µg per ml of zidovudine produced only 19–55% inhibition of HIV replication in chronically infected cells, as assessed by p24 assay (Crowe et al., 1989). When the Ba-L strain of HIV-1 is used, the IC$_{50}$ of zidovudine required to prevent infection of cells of macrophage lineage is 0.5 µM (Perno et al., 1989). Using the macrophage tropic strain HIV $_{Ada}$, pretreatment of monocyte-derived macrophages with zidovudine resulted in complete inhibition of cell-free infection (St Luce et al., 1993).

The susceptibility of HIV-1 isolates from patients prior to therapy (zidovudine-naive) has been reported to vary with IC$_{50}$ values ranging from 0.005 µM to 0.45 µM (Larder and Kemp, 1989; Land et al., 1990; Richman et al., 1990) and IC$_{90}$ values of 0.002–0.2 µM (Mohri et al., 1993; Shafer et al., 1993). A number of strains with differing genotype and phenotype are usually present in an infected person. These quasispecies will vary in their antiviral susceptibility (Richman et al., 1991a).

Strains of HIV that are resistant to non-nucleoside reverse transcriptase inhibitors which have mutations within codon 181 remain sensitive to zidovudine (Balzarini et al., 1993). Similarly strains of HIV that contain a mutation within codon 184 conferring resistance to lamivudine (p. 1747) remain sensitive to zidovudine (Tisdale et al., 1993). Isolates of HIV that are resistant to protease inhibitors including saquinavir, indinavir and ritonavir remain sensitive to zidovudine.

2 Other retroviruses

The reverse transcriptase of the simian immunodeficiency virus (SIV) is sensitive to zidovudine, with similar inhibition constants for zidovudine and other nucleoside analogs as the HIV-1 reverse transcriptase (Vrang et al., 1988; Wu et al., 1988). At a concentration of 4 µM zidovudine has been reported to completely inhibit SIV replication as assessed by syncytium formation, reverse transcriptase assay and viral antigen production (Tsai et al., 1988). The chimeric virus SHIV, in which the reverse transcriptase gene of simian immunodeficiency virus is replaced by the reverse transcriptase of HIV-1, is sensitive to both nucleoside and non-nucleoside reverse transcriptase inhibitors, unlike SIV which is inhibited only by nucleoside analogs including zidovudine and lamivudine (Balzarini et al., 1995).

By plaque-reduction assay using FG-10 cells, 50% inhibition is achieved with concentrations of zidovudine as low as 0.0037 µM (0.001 µg per ml) for the Friend murine leukemia virus and 0.0075 µM (0.002 µg per ml) for murine Harvey sarcoma virus (reviewed in Furman and Barry, 1988). Human T lymphotropic virus type 1, equine infectious anemia virus, avian leukosis virus, Moloney murine leukemia virus, avian myeloblastosis virus and feline leukemia virus are also sensitive to zidovudine (Krieg et al., 1978; reviewed in Olsen et al., 1987; Furman and Barry, 1988; Huang et al., 1990). The replication of visna virus is inhibited by zidovudine but this drug is significantly less potent than zalcitabine and didanosine and of similar potency to stavudine when replication is assessed in sheep choroid plexus cells (Thormar et al., 1993).

Table V.20
Additive to synergistic interactions between zidovudine and some other antiretroviral drugs. (See text for details.)

Didanosine and zidovudine[a]
Didanosine, lamivudine and zidovudine
Zalcitabine and zidovudine[a]
Zalcitabine, zidovudine and saquinavir
Stavudine and zidovudine[b]
Stavudine, zidovudine and nevirapine
Stavudine, zidovudine and saquinavir
Lamivudine and zidovudine
Lamivudine, zidovudine and saquinavir
Lamivudine, zidovudine and nevirapine
Lamivudine, zidovudine and stavudine
Non-nucleoside RT inhibitors and zidovudine[a]
Protease inhibitors and zidovudine[a]
Interferon alpha and zidovudine

[a] For both zidovudine-sensitive and-resistant strains of HIV.
[b] Some studies also show antagonism.

3 Synergism

There are a large number of antiretroviral compounds that have been shown to provide additive or synergistic inhibition of HIV replication when tested in combination with zidovudine in vitro (reviewed in Mazzulli and Hirsch, 1996) (Table V.20).

Using the MT-4 cell line, peripheral blood T lymphocytes and macrophages, didanosine and zidovudine have been demonstrated to synergistically inhibit zidovudine-sensitive and zidovudine-resistant HIV replication in vitro (Dornsife et al., 1991; Johnson et al., 1991). Such synergistic inhibition is evident against HIV-1 and HIV-2 (Cox et al., 1994). Even more potent is the combination of zidovudine, didanosine and lamivudine which can reduce the IC_{95} concentration by over 200-fold when compared with zidovudine alone in T cell lines (St Clair et al., 1995). In addition, zidovudine in combination with didanosine and nevirapine may result in combinations of mutations in the reverse transcriptase gene which lead to cessation of viral replication (Chow et al., 1993a), although these findings remain controversial, as other investigators have not been able to demonstrate evidence of 'replication incompatible' combinations of resistance mutations (Larder et al., 1993).

Similarly, zalcitabine is synergistic with zidovudine against zidovudine-sensitive and resistant isolates of HIV-1 (Eron et al., 1992; Mathez et al., 1993). Although not strictly synergism, a 3-day alternating regimen of zidovudine and zalcitabine in vitro resulted in more prolonged suppression of HIV in an infected T cell line than culture with zidovudine alone (Spector et al., 1989a). This synergy is unlikely to be due to synergistic inhibition of reverse transcriptase as the triphosphate derivatives of nucleoside analogs such as zidovudine, didanosine and zalcitabine cannot bind to reverse transcriptase simultaneously (White et al., 1993).

Sorensen and colleagues (Sorensen et al., 1993) have reported synergy between zidovudine and stavudine against laboratory-adapted strains of HIV in T cell lines. There is evidence of synergism between zidovudine and lamivudine in vitro (Mathez et al., 1993; Merrill et al., 1996). Three-drug combinations including lamivudine and zidovudine in combination with either saquinavir, nevirapine or stavudine, and stavudine and zidovudine in combination with either nevirapine or saquinavir have been found to be additive or synergistic against zidovudine-sensitive and some zidovudine-resistant strains of HIV (Merrill et al., 1996).

The dipyridodiazepinone class of non-nucleoside analog reverse transcriptase inhibitors (including nevirapine) acts synergistically with zidovudine to inhibit HIV-1 replication as assessed by the plaque reduction assay (Richman et al., 1991b). Other non-nucleoside reverse transcriptase inhibitors such as TIBO compounds, and bis-heteroarylpiperazine derivatives such as delavirdine and atevirdine, are also additive or synergistic with zidovudine against HIV replication in CD4-expressing T cell lines and peripheral blood lymphocytes; (Buckheit et al., 1993; Pauwels et al., 1994; Chong et al., 1994); some of these drugs have been tested with both zidovudine-sensitive and zidovudine-resistant variants of HIV (Campbell et al., 1993).

Additive to synergistic interactions against both zidovudine-sensitive and zidovudine-resistant strains of HIV-1 have been shown between zidovudine and several protease inhibitors including saquinavir (Craig et al., 1990; Johnson et al., 1992; Kageyama et al., 1992; Lambert et al., 1993). Triple-drug combinations with zidovudine, saquinavir and either lamivudine or zalcitabine have also demonstrated additive to synergistic inhibition of HIV replication (Craig *et al.*, 1994; Merrill *et al.*, 1996). Indinavir is synergistic with zidovudine *in vitro* (Vacca *et al.*, 1994). The Tat inhibitor Ro 24–7429 is synergistic with zidovudine in inhibiting syncytium formation and HIV antigen production (Connell *et al.*, 1994).

Recombinant interferon alpha, when added to zidovudine, or to zidovudine and didanosine in culture synergistically inhibits HIV replication in peripheral blood mononuclear cells, monocytes or in human bone marrow progenitor cells (Hartshorn *et al.*, 1987; Berman *et al.*, 1989; Johnson *et al.*, 1991; Degre and Beck, 1994). Of interest, recombinant interferon alpha has been reported to inhibit replication of cells that are chronically infected with HIV-1 (Poli *et al.*, 1989). Multidrug regimens combining zidovudine, interferon alpha, didanosine and saquinavir resulted in better inhibitory effect against HIV than single drug or fewer combined drugs *in vitro* (Mazzulli *et al.*, 1994). The addition of recombinant interferon beta to zidovudine also results in synergy, reducing by 4- to 1000-fold the amount of zidovudine required to maintain maximum inhibition of HIV p24 antigen synthesis (Williams and Colby, 1989).

Aciclovir has been reported to exert synergism with zidovudine in protecting cells from HIV-related cell death (Mitsuya and Broder, 1987), but the antiretroviral effect of aciclovir with or without zidovudine has not been confirmed subsequently. Synergism or at least an additive effect has also been demonstrated between zidovudine and foscarnet in inhibiting HIV replication in MT-4 cells and against the HIV reverse transcriptase (Eriksson and Schinazi, 1989; Koshida *et al.*, 1989; Jacobson *et al.*, 1991; Kong *et al.*, 1991). Three-drug synergism against HIV replication has been demonstrated between zidovudine, recombinant soluble CD4 and recombinant interferon alpha (Johnson *et al.*, 1990). Carbovir has also been demonstrated to act synergistically with zidovudine in inhibiting HIV replication in Jurkat cells and peripheral blood mononuclear cells (Smith *et al.*, 1993a). The phosphorothioate oligonucleotide (ISIS 5320) demonstrates additive to slightly synergistic inhibition with zidovudine *in vitro* against HIV (Buckheit *et al.*, 1994). Dipyridamole in micromolar concentrations synergistically improved the antiretroviral efficacy of zidovudine (Hendrix *et al.*, 1994). Recombinant, soluble CD4, either alone or when linked to *Pseudomonas aeruginosa* exotoxin A, and zidovudine are synergistic in limiting fusion between HIV-infected T lymphocytes with uninfected cells (Johnson *et al.*, 1989a, 1990; Ashorn *et al.*, 1990). There is synergistic inhibition of both HIV-1 and HIV-2 by castinospermine and zidovudine in T cell lines (Johnson *et al.*, 1989b).

Granulocyte-macrophage colony stimulating factor but not macrophage colony stimulating factor has demonstrated synergism with zidovudine in inhibiting HIV-1 replication in monocyte cell lines (Hammer and Gillis, 1987) and in macrophages (Perno *et al.*, 1992b).

4 Antagonism

Several antiretroviral compounds have been reported to show antagonism with zidovudine against HIV replication *in vitro* (Table V.21). Ribavirin has been demonstrated to antagonize the effect of zidovudine on HIV replication in a variety of primary cells and cell lines *in vitro* (Vogt *et al.*, 1987). The underlying mechanism was considered to be inhibition of phosphorylation of zidovudine by ribavirin. The level of reverse transcriptase activity when the drugs were used in combination was 1.5- to 5-fold higher than when zidovudine was used alone; antagonism was detected at all time points tested up to 18 days in culture (Vogt *et al.*, 1987). Stavudine and zidovudine have been found to be antagonistic when tested against zidovudine-resistant strains of HIV-1 (Merrill *et al.*, 1996). Ganciclovir has also been observed to antagonize the effects of zidovudine in H9 cells *in vitro*, resulting in an increase in the IC_{50} of zidovudine for III_B strain of HIV-1 by 3- to 6-fold (Medina *et al.*, 1992). Zidovudine has been reported to antagonize pyrimethamine in mice infected with *Toxoplasma gondii* (Israelski *et al.*, 1989). There is no evidence of synergism or antagonism between zidovudine and rifabutin in terms of antiretroviral efficacy (Birch *et al.*, 1988; Gallicano *et al.*, 1995) or between zidovudine and fluoroquinolones in terms of antibacterial activity (Lewin *et al.*, 1990). Intracellular phosphorylation of zidovudine is not inhibited by either didanosine or zalcitabine (Veal *et al.*, 1994).

Table V.21

Antagonistic *in vitro* interactions between zidovudine and other antiretroviral drugs

Ribavirin and zidovudine
Stavudine and zidovudine[a,b]

[a] Some studies show synergism.
[b] Using zidovudine–resistant strains of HIV.

5 Resistance of HIV to zidovudine

a Definition   There are a number of working definitions describing phenotypic sensitivity or resistance of HIV to zidovudine, the most commonly employed being the definition of sensitive strains being inhibited with an IC_{50} of less than 0.2 μM zidovudine, resistant strains being inhibited with an IC_{50} of 0.2–1 μM and highly resistant strains with an IC_{50} of greater than 1 μM zidovudine for inhibition (D'Aquila et al., 1995).

b Development of resistance *in vitro*   By culturing HIV in increasing concentrations of zidovudine *in vitro*, resistant strains emerge. Resistant strains of HIV-1 selected by passage in cell culture developed high-level resistance by the twelfth passage, with an IC_{50} of 2.5 μM or higher (Larder et al., 1991).

c *In vivo* development of resistance   The original report of zidovudine-resistance described reduced susceptibility of isolates from patients with advanced HIV infection who had been treated with zidovudine for periods in excess of 6 months. Sequential analysis of isolates from individual patients revealed a progressive loss of susceptibility. These isolates were not cross-resistant to zalcitabine or foscarnet (Larder et al., 1989). Further studies have confirmed the emergence of resistant strains during zidovudine therapy (Rooke et al., 1989; Land et al., 1990). When compared with non-nucleoside reverse transcriptase inhibitors zidovudine-resistance emerges after a considerably longer duration of therapy (Medina et al., 1995). Montaner and colleagues (Montaner et al., 1993) have reported that HIV isolates from 27 of 74 patients remained susceptible to zidovudine after 3.75 years. Zidovudine-resistance has also been identified in viral isolates from HIV-infected children treated with zidovudine, as well as with isolates cultured in the presence of zidovudine *in vitro* (Larder et al., 1991; Ogino et al., 1993; Dimitrov et al., 1993).

d Factors associated with the development of resistance *in vivo*   The time to the development of resistance after starting zidovudine therapy is at least in part related to the CD4 lymphocyte number and the stage of disease (Fig. V.33). After 12 months of zidovudine therapy, 89% of persons with late-stage HIV infection and a CD4 count of less than 100 cells per μl develop resistance compared with 27% of persons with early-stage infection and CD4 count greater than 400 cells per μl (Richman et al., 1990; Montaner et al., 1993). The dose of zidovudine does not conclusively influence the development of resistance (Richman et al., 1990). The IC_{90} of isolates of HIV-1 obtained from persons after institution of therapy ranges from 0.007 to >10 μM of zidovudine (Shafer et al., 1993).

e Isolation of resistant strains of HIV from plasma, cells and other body fluids   Virus isolates from plasma and peripheral blood mononuclear cells can differ in sensitivity to zidovudine. In one study, plasma virus had evidence of mutations in three codons of the reverse transcriptase gene whilst the cellular isolates remained genotypically and phenotypically sensitive, suggesting that zidovudine-resistant HIV may arise earlier in plasma than in leukocytes (Smith et al., 1993b). Other investigators have also found that mutations associated with zidovudine (or other antiretroviral drug)-resistance are detected earlier in plasma than in proviral DNA within peripheral blood mononuclear cells (Kozal et al., 1993; Anderson et al., 1994). The mean delay between detecting mutations in plasma RNA versus cellular DNA in one study was

Fig. V.33.
Relationship between development of zidovudine-resistance to HIV, stage of disease and CD4 count after 1 year of therapy. (Adapted from Moyle, 1995, with data from Richman et al., 1990, with permission.)

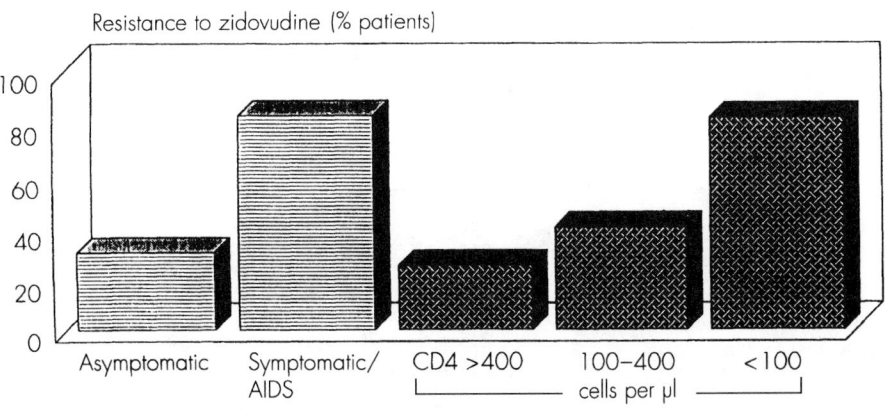

25 days (Kaye *et al.*, 1995). Zidovudine-resistant strains of HIV have also been recovered from genital fluids, with similar IC_{50} levels to that of virus isolated from blood at the same time (Wainberg *et al.*, 1993). However, mutations associated with zidovudine-resistance can be detected earlier in semen (coincident with plasma) than in proviral DNA in peripheral blood or seminal mononuclear cells (Kroodsma *et al.*, 1994).

f   Cross-resistance of zidovudine-resistant strains of HIV   Zidovudine-resistant strains of HIV generally remain sensitive to zalcitabine, didanosine, stavudine and lamivudine, although some reports of cross-resistance have emerged. There is no cross-resistance to phosphonoformate, and most cross-resistance is to structurally similar compounds such as 3'-azido-2',3'-dideoxyuridine (Larder and Kemp, 1989; Meng *et al.*, 1990). Although it was intially reported that there was no cross-resistance between stavudine and zidovudine, there has been a report in which two of 11 zidovudine-resistant isolates were cross-resistant to stavudine (Rooke *et al.*, 1991). Similarly, whilst it is generally found that there is no cross-resistance between didanosine and zidovudine, in one study of HIV from patients receiving only zidovudine therapy a correlation was shown between zidovudine-resistance and reduced susceptibility to didanosine and zalcitabine. For each 10-fold decline in zidovudine susceptibility, there was a 2.2-fold decline in susceptibility to zalcitabine and didanosine (Mayers *et al.*, 1994). There is also a case-report of a patient receiving didanosine monotherapy with no prior history of antiretroviral therapy who developed mutations in HIV isolates that are associated with zidovudine-resistance (Demeter *et al.*, 1995).

Zidovudine-resistant strains of HIV are not cross-resistant to bisheteroarylpiperazine derivatives including atevirdine (Campbell *et al.*, 1993; Dueweke *et al.*, 1993). Protease inhibitors appear to be equally effective against zidovudine-sensitive and -resistant strains of HIV (Otto *et al.*, 1993). Passage of zidovudine-resistant HIV in the presence of a protease inhibitor (Ro 31–8959) generated a dually resistant (reverse transcriptase and protease) variant (Tisdale *et al.*, 1995). Zidovudine-resistant mutants of feline immunodeficiency virus are cross-resistant to 3'-azido-2',3'-dideoxyuridine and 3'-azido-2',3'-dideoxyguanosine, but retain sensitivity to 2',3'- dideoxyinosine (Remington *et al.*, 1991; Gobert *et al.*, 1994).

g   Mutations conferring zidovudine-resistance   The emergence of zidovudine-resistant strains of HIV is due to mutations developing within the reverse transcriptase gene (Larder *et al.*, 1987; Mayers *et al.*, 1992; Sheehy and Desselberger, 1993). This is aided by the error-prone nature of the reverse transcriptase enzyme itself (Smith *et al.*, 1994a). At least seven amino acid substitutions within the reverse transcriptase have been shown to occur in the setting of a resistant phenotype (Table V.22). These are Met-41→Leu; Asp-67→Asn; Lys-70→Arg; Thr-215→Tyr or Thr-215→Phe; Lys-219→Arg; Leu-210→Trp (Larder and Kemp, 1989; Kellam *et al.*, 1992; Boucher *et al.*, 1993a; Hooker *et al.*, 1996; Harrigan *et al.*, 1996).

Table V.22

Major mutations conferring resistance of HIV to zidovudine. (Adapted from Moyle, 1995, with permission.)

Substitutions in codons

41	Met→Leu
67	Asp→Asn
70	Lys→Arg
210	Leu→Trp
215	Thr→Tyr/Phe
219	Lys→Arg

Mutation	Reduction in zidovudine susceptibilities (fold increase in IC_{50}) in zidovudine
70	8
215	16
215 + 41	60–70
215 + 67 + 70	31
215 + 67 + 70 + 41	179
215 + 67 + 70 + 219	166

Mutations signalling the development of resistance may be detected as early as 25 days after commencing zidovudine therapy, but more commonly develop after months of treatment (Loveday *et al.*, 1995). The pattern of emergence of mutations occurs generally in an ordered manner (Fig. V.34). The first mutation to appear is commonly at codon 70. The subsequent appearance of a mutation within codon 215 is often associated with disappearance of the codon 70 mutation (Boucher *et al.*, 1992). The mutation at codon 70 may then reappear, followed by mutations within codons 67 and 219. The codon 41 mutation has been described in 12 of 16 patients who had received 76 weeks of zidovudine therapy, and in combination with other mutations results in high levels of resistance (Kellam *et al.*, 1992). The rate of appearance of the mutation at codon 215 has been reported to correlate with CD4 number (Boucher *et al.*, 1990). The 215 (Thr→Phe) mutant is less resistant to zidovudine than the 215 (Thr→Tyr) variant (Lacey and Larder, 1994). Isolates with mutations only at codons 70 and 215 are partially resistant; highly resistant isolates usually have substitutions also at codons 67 and 219 (Larder *et al.*, 1991). A combination of mutations within codons 215, 70 and 41 result in additive resistance (Lacey and Larder, 1994). Mutations at codons 41, or 70 or 215 confer approximately a 4-fold, or 8-fold, or 16-fold decrease in susceptibility respectively. The presence of mutations within codons 70 and 215 together result in about a 6-fold decrease in susceptibility, and mutations at 41 and 215 result in a 60–70-fold reduction in sensitivity. The presence of mutations at each of codons 41, 67, 70, 215 and 219 decreases susceptibility about 180-fold (Fig. V.34) (Larder, 1994). The presence of the codon 215 mutation has been found to correlate with subsequent decline in CD4 count and thus disease progression. The importance of all of these mutations in conferring resistance to zidovudine has been confirmed by site-directed mutagenesis. Susceptibility to zidovudine can be reduced by increasing the bulk of amino acid side-chains at position 215 (Moyle, 1995). Of interest, both wild-type virus as well as mutated strains can be present in the one clinical sample, suggesting that the development of mutations is a gradual process. Similarly HIV species can contain various combinations of resistance mutations, particularly early in the course of zidovudine therapy (Kellam *et al.*, 1994). A similar order has been reported for the sequential appearance of mutations produced by selective pressure with zidovudine *in vitro* (Larder *et al.*, 1991). Other mutations conferring resistance have been reported including those at codons 44 (Glu→Asp), 210 (Leu→Trp), and 369

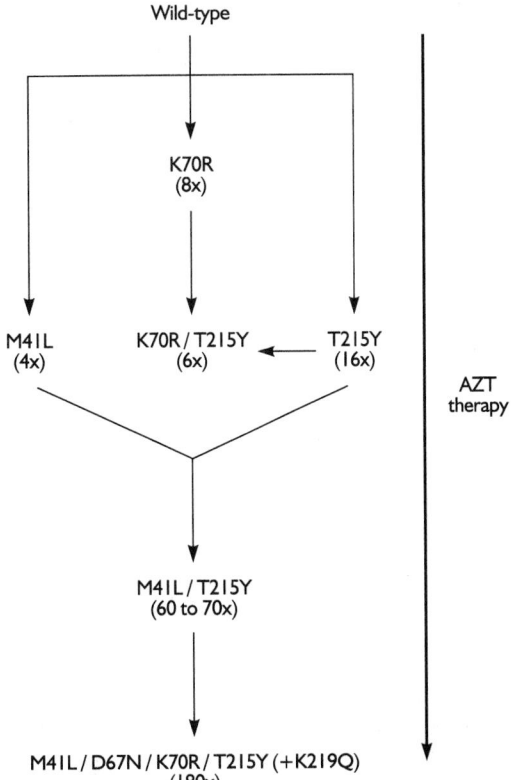

Fig. V.34.

Cumulative development of mutations within HIV reverse transcriptase conferring resistance to zidovudine during treatment; fold decrease in susceptibility is shown in parentheses. (Reproduced from Larder, 1994, with permission.)

(Thr→Ile) (Gurusinghe *et al.*, 1995), and at codons 125 (Leu→Trp), 142 (Ile→Val), and 294 (Pro→Thr) (Japour *et al.*, 1991). The 210 mutation is a late mutation, and is almost always found in combination with a mutation at 215 and usually 41 (Larder *et al.*, 1995b; Hooker *et al.*, 1996; Harrigan *et al.*, 1996).

Rapid assays have been developed to detect mutations within the *pol* gene that confer zidovudine-resistance (Anderson *et al.*, 1994; Frenkel *et al.*, 1995a; Richman *et al.*, 1991a). However these assays will only detect resistance if known mutations at specific sites are present, and it is clear that mutations at other sites may be responsible for zidovudine-resistance (Sheehy and Desselberger, 1993).

h Isolation of zidovudine-resistant strains from zidovudine-naive individuals Although some investigators have only found evidence of zidovudine-resistance in individuals who have been treated with the drug (Rooke *et al.*, 1989; Richman *et al.*, 1990, 1991a), more recent reports demonstrate the isolation of zidovudine-resistant HIV from individuals who are zidovudine naive, with genotypic confirmation of mutations within the reverse transcriptase gene (Mohri *et al.*, 1993; Najera *et al.*, 1994). In one report, the IC_{50} of an HIV-1 isolate obtained from a zidovudine-naive individual infected with a genotypically proven resistant strain (mutation at codon 215 of the reverse transcriptase) was $0.86\,\mu M$ (Erice *et al.*, 1993). Transmission of zidovudine-resistant variants of HIV (containing a mutation within codon 215 or 70) by heterosexual and homosexual contact, vertically and by injection of HIV-infected blood has been reported (Kuritkes *et al.*, 1994; Siegrist *et al.*, 1994; Conlon *et al.*, 1994; Veenstra *et al.*, 1995).

i Reversion of zidovudine-resistant strains to zidovudine-susceptible strains Following cessation of zidovudine, phenotypic and genotypic resistance may resolve. In several reported studies, reversion of mutations was slow, with mutations persisting 8–22 months after cessation of zidovudine therapy (Albert *et al.*, 1992; Boucher *et al.*, 1993a; Smith *et al.*, 1994b; Gurusinghe *et al.*, 1995). Institution of didanosine therapy in patients with zidovudine-resistant HIV who have ceased zidovudine, with the subsequent development of a mutation at codon 74 (Leu→Val), has been associated with increased zidovudine sensitivity in some but not all studies (St Clair *et al.*, 1991; Eron *et al.*, 1993). Similarly, suppression of zidovudine-resistance may follow the development of a mutation at codon 181 which confers HIV-1 resistance to non-nucleoside reverse transcriptase inhibitors (Larder, 1992). In one study of HIV isolates obtained from patients with advanced HIV infection who switched from zidovudine to didanosine therapy, the proportion of patients whose isolates had a mutation within codon 215 decreased from 84% to 59% after 24 weeks of didanosine therapy (Kozal *et al.*, 1994a). Zidovudine-resistant isolates of feline immunodeficiency virus revert rapidly to a zidovudine-sensitive phenotype when passaged in the absence of drug; however, genotypic reversion dose not occur (Remington *et al.*, 1994). Some mutations which may confer resistance to non-nucleoside reverse transcriptase inhibitors (such as substitutions within codons 100 and 181) may in fact suppress resistance to zidovudine when co-expressed with mutations that specifically confer resistance to zidovudine (Byrnes *et al.*, 1994).

j Effect of combination therapy on development of resistance Combination therapy has not prevented the emergence of resistant strains of HIV (Richman *et al.*, 1994), although some investigators have found that resistance is less likely to occur in the presence of two nucleoside analogs (Gao *et al.*, 1992). It is likely that up until now the available drugs have been unable completely to suppress HIV replication, thus allowing resistance to develop. It is possible that combination therapy using protease inhibitors such as indinavir or ritonavir in combination with zidovudine may prevent emergence of zidovudine-resistant strains by profound suppression of viral replication.

In persons with advanced HIV disease who have not previously received antiretroviral therapy and who commence combination therapy with zidovudine and zalcitabine, resistance to zidovudine has been found to develop in three-quarters of the individuals within 24–48 weeks of therapy (IC_{50} ranging from 0.45 to $2.0\,\mu M$), although no changes in phenotypic sensitivity to zalcitabine were observed (Richman *et al.*, 1994). Shafer and colleagues (Shafer *et al.*, 1994) have also found that combination therapy with didanosine and zidovudine for 1 year did not alter the emergence of zidovudine-resistant strains of HIV compared with those receiving zidovudine-monotherapy (10 of 24 and 8 of 26 patients respectively) although the incidence of didanosine-resistant variants was significantly lower in patients on combination therapy than in patients receiving didanosine monotherapy (2 of 24 versus 17 of 26 patients respectively). *In vitro* studies using site mutagenesis of infectious molecular clones with mutations conferring both zidovudine-resistance and resistance to the non-nucleoside reverse transcriptase inhibitors (Tyr-181→ Cys) resulted in the restoration of zidovudine sensitivity in a virus that maintained resistance to nevirapine (Larder, 1992). Similarly zidovudine-resistant strains of HIV became phenotypically sensitive when the mutant acquired a mutation within codon 184 conferring resistance to lamivudine; in this study zidovudine-lamivudine co-resistant strains of HIV were not observed (Larder *et al.*, 1995a). When zidovudine is given in combination with the non-nucleoside reverse transcriptase inhibitor L- 697,661, there is a delay in the appearance of the mutation at codon 181 and thus in the development of the high level resistance that is associated with monotherapy with L-697,661 (Staszewski *et al.*, 1995; Schooley *et al.*, 1996). Mutations that confer foscarnet-resistance (codons 88, 89, 92, 156, and 161) can phenotypically reverse zidovudine-resistance (Tachedjian *et al.*, 1995, 1996).

k Multiple-drug resistance Multiple-drug resistant variants of HIV can emerge during culture with nucleoside and non-nucleoside drug combinations. Combination therapy in some individuals with didanosine and zidovudine has been reported to select for multidrug-resistant strains containing novel *pol* mutations (within codons 62, 75, 77, 116, and 151), as well as for zidovudine-resistant strains lacking the codon 74 mutation associated with didanosine-resistance (Shafer *et al.*, 1994). The mutation within codon 151 conferred partial resistance to zidovudine, didanosine, zalcitabine and stavudine; combinations of mutations resulted in higher levels of resistance (Iversen *et al.*, 1996). Other investigators have reported similar findings in patients receiving combination therapy with zidovudine and either didanosine or zalcitabine, resulting in the development of multiple mutations in the *pol* gene, with the change in codon 151 being the first to develop *in vivo*, coincident with a rise in plasma viral load, and followed by the appearance of mutations in codons 116 and 77 (Shirasaka *et al.*, 1995).

6 Zidovudine hypersensitivity

Foscarnet-resistant strains of HIV (with substitutions within the reverse transcriptase encoding *pol* gene at codons 89, 92 or 156, and the dual mutations at 16 and 208) were hypersensitive to zidovudine (Tachedjian *et al.*, 1995, 1996; Mellors *et al.*, 1995).

7 Animal studies

In an early report, mice infected with Rauscher murine leukemia virus and treated with zidovudine did not develop splenomegaly, and had lower levels of viremia, with prolongation of life (Ruprecht *et al.*, 1986). Zidovudine therapy, 1 mg per ml in drinking water commencing 24 h prior to infection, has been reported to delay the progression of murine acquired immunodeficiency syndrome in mice infected with murine leukemia virus (Bilello *et al.*, 1992).

Immediate oral zidovudine treatment of newborn macaques who have been injected i.v. with SIV_{mac} has been found to prevent infection or reduce viral load and delay disease progression compared with untreated control animals (Van Rompay *et al.*, 1995). However, in other studies, zidovudine, even when administered to macaques prior to SIV inoculation or within 1 h of infection, has not prevented SIV infection, although, similar to the findings of Van Rompay and colleagues, peak levels of viremia were lower and later in zidovudine-treated animals than controls (Martin *et al.*, 1993; Le Grand *et al.*, 1994).

Zidovudine therapy, administered through drinking water, was initially reported to prevent disease in mice if commenced within 4 h after exposure to Friend virus, but not if delayed to 6 days post-infection. However, methods used to detect virus in this study were not sufficiently sensitive to detect low levels of viral infection (Morrey *et al.*, 1990). It was subsequently shown that, although mice inoculated with Friend leukemia virus and treated as early as 10 min post-infection with intraperitoneal injections of zidovudine three times per day for 20 days did not develop splenomegaly or die (compared with 38% of untreated controls), low levels of retrovirus were persistently present in splenocytes (Morrey *et al.*, 1991). Continuous subcutaneous infusion of zidovudine (40 mg per kg daily) to mice infected with Friend leukemia virus has been found to be more effective in inhibiting splenomegaly than subcutaneous administration (Sinet *et al.*, 1992).

Suppression of HIV infection in SCID-hu mice treated with zidovudine has been reported (McCune *et al.*, 1990; Shih *et al.*, 1991). Post-exposure prophylaxis of SCID-hu mice with administration of zidovudine (125–250 mg per kg daily) in drinking water for 1 day before or given by intraperitoneal bolus injection within 2 h of intravenous virus challenge followed by oral administration resulted in suppression of HIV in all animals when assessed at 2 weeks. Control mice all showed signs of HIV replication at this time. When zidovudine was given 48 h post-infection no protection was observed (Shih *et al.*, 1991). In a more recent study, lower doses (50 mg per kg daily) of zidovudine administered to SCID-hu mice for 1 week commencing after infection with a large inoculum of HIV reduced HIV p24 antigen burden in spleen by 95%, with doses of 5 and 0.5 mg per kg per day resulting in 52% and 18% reduction respectively (Alder *et al.*, 1995).

Recombinant interferon alpha and zidovudine have been reported to be highly synergistic in mice and, when administered 4 h after exposure to Rauscher leukemia virus protected against viremia and disease and led to protective immunity (Ruprecht *et al.*, 1990a).

Prophylactic zidovudine (30mg per kg daily) given by continuous subcutaneous infusion for 28 days to feline immunodeficiency virus-inoculated cats 48 h prior to viral inoculation prevented the development of early viremia (none of six zidovudine-treated cats examined 2 weeks post-inoculation compared with six of six untreated cats). However, by 10–14 weeks low levels of viral antigen were detected in plasma of two of the treated cats (Hayes *et al.*, 1993).

8 Herpesviruses

An early report suggests that Epstein–Barr virus is sensitive to zidovudine, with an IC_{50} of 1–10 μM (Lin *et al.*, 1988). However, zidovudine has no effect on the replication of cytomegalovirus, varicella-zoster virus and herpes simplex viruses types I and 2, the IC_{50} for each being in excess of 100 μM. When combined with aciclovir, ganciclovir and foscarnet, potentiation of effect against cytomegalovirus replication is additive to synergistic (Snoeck *et al.*, 1992).

9 Hepatitis B virus

Zidovudine triphosphate has been reported to inhibit the DNA polymerase of human hepatitis B virus by 50% at a concentration of 0.3 μM (Berk *et al.*, 1992). In another study, zidovudine had less efficacy in inhibiting hepatitis B virus replication in a Hep-G2 hepatoblastoma cell line (Aoki-Sei *et al.*, 1991), confirming data generated from patients treated with zidovudine in whom serum hepatitis B virus DNA levels did not alter (Haritani *et al.*, 1989).

10 Mycoplasma

Inhibition of growth of *Mycoplasma* spp. by zidovudine has been reported by some investigators (Lafeuillade *et al.*, 1992; Papierok *et al.*, 1992) but not others (Taylor-Robinson and Furr, 1992), using the metabolism-inhibition technique to determine sensitivity.

Mode of Administration and Dosage

1 Oral administration

The current oral dose of zidovudine is 500–600 mg per day, with the recommendation being 200 mg every 8 h (600 mg per day) or 100 mg every 4 h (600 mg per day) or omitting the dose during the night (500 mg per day). However, a number of clinicians prescribe 250 mg 12-hourly in order to improve patient compliance. The twice-daily dosage schedule has been compared with a four times daily schedule in a double-blind, randomized study of asymptomatic persons and shown to have similar virologic efficacy (Gill *et al.*, 1991). The current oral dose has been derived from the results of a number of clinical trials.

The first clinical trial of zidovudine in patients with the acquired imunodeficiency syndrome (AIDS) or AIDS related complex (ARC) commenced with intravenous therapy and then oral regimens of 2 mg per kg 8-hourly up to 10 mg per kg 4-hourly (Yarchoan *et al.*, 1986). As these dosages were found to be well absorbed from the gastrointestinal tract and associated only with mild side-effects, headache being the most common, clinical trials commenced to determine the optimal oral dose. In subsequent clinical trials regimens of 1200–1500 mg daily in six divided doses were used, demonstrating antiviral, immunologic and clinical efficacy but associated with significant side-effects (described below) (Fischl *et al.*, 1987, 1990a; Richman *et al.*, 1987a; Yarchoan *et al.*, 1987).

In persons with a previous diagnosis of AIDS (*Pneumocystis carinii* pneumonia), in whom the effects of 250 mg of zidovudine 4-hourly were compared with therapy of 100 mg 4-hourly, the lower dose was at least as effective as the higher dose over a median follow-up period of 25 months, but was associated with less toxicity (Fischl *et al.*, 1990b). In a randomized, multicenter, placebo-controlled trial of zidovudine comparing 500 mg per day with 1500 mg per day in persons with asymptomatic HIV infection and less than 500 CD4 cells per μl, the lower dose was found to be equally efficacious as the higher dose and was associated with less toxicity (Volberding *et al.*, 1990). At about the same time, in a phase II open-label dose-escalating study aimed to determine clinical and antiviral efficacy of zidovudine at concentrations of 300 mg per day, 600 mg per day and 1500 mg per day in symptomatic persons who had not developed an AIDS-defining illness, the three doses were found to result in similar antiviral and immunologic benefit, with the highest dose, resulting in greatest toxicity (Collier *et al.*, 1990). A daily oral dose of 150 mg has been reported to be associated with suboptimal virologic and immunologic efficacy (Meng *et al.*, 1992).

2 Intravenous administration

The recommended dose of zidovudine for i.v. administration is 1.9 mg per kg body weight every 4 h, or approximately 800 mg per day for a patient who weighs about 70 kg. (This corresponds to an oral dose of zidovudine of 1200 mg per day which is higher than the currently recommended dose.) The dose should be administered slowly over a 1-h period (Retrovir IV Product Information).

Intravenous therapy has been used in a small number of clinical trials in both adults (Yarchoan *et al.*, 1986) and children (Balis *et al.*, 1989a,b), and on very rare occasions in health care workers in an attempt to protect against infection following accidental exposure to HIV. The dose that has been administered by this route to adults has ranged from 1mg per kg 8-hourly up to 5 mg per kg 4-hourly, each dose being administered over 1 h for 14 days (Yarchoan *et al.*, 1986). It has been predicted that an i.v. dose of 5 mg per kg infused over 1 h is needed to achieve plasma concentrations greater than 1 μM (Balis *et al.*, 1989a). Recently high-dose zidovudine has been studied in cancer patients, with doses ranging from 2 to 20 g per m^2 daily as a continuous i.v. infusion over 48 h (Marchbanks *et al.*, 1995).

3 Pediatric patients

Limited studies in neonates suggest that elimination of zidovudine is delayed. In babies less than 2 weeks of age the oral dose of 2 mg per kg 6-hourly results in appropriate plasma levels and is well tolerated (Connor *et al.*, 1994). For babies older than 2 weeks the dose can be safely increased to 3 mg per kg 6-hourly (Boucher *et al.*, 1993b).

Zidovudine appears to be safe in children, with similar pharmacokinetics in children over 1 year of age and adults (McKinney *et al.*, 1990; Balis *et al.*, 1991). The recommended oral dose for children over 3 months of age is 180 mg per m^2 6-hourly (Balis *et al.*, 1991). Over a 24-week period, oral zidovudine therapy at a dose of 180 mg per m^2 in children with advanced HIV disease has been found to be well tolerated and demonstrated clinical efficacy (see below) (McKinney *et al.*, 1991).

In an early study, zidovudine was administered by continuous i.v. administration to children with symptomatic HIV disease. This study recommended the i.v. dose of zidovudine of 0.9–1.4 mg per kg per h (Pizzo *et al.*, 1988). In a subsequent phase I study of children with symptomatic HIV infection, doses of up to 120 mg per m^2 administered by the i.v. route (or 180 mg per m^2 given orally 6-hourly) were well tolerated apart from myelosuppression (Balis *et al.*, 1989a,b; McKinney *et al.*, 1990).

4 Pregnant women

Although the safety of zidovudine in pregnant women has not been completely established, the current data suggest that this drug is well tolerated by both mother and infant, with no alteration in pharmacokinetics as a result of pregnancy (Chavanet *et al.*, 1989; Lopez-Anaya *et al.*, 1991). No dose reduction is required because of pregnancy (Watts *et al.*, 1991). The drug crosses the placenta, thus similar concentrations of the drug will be present in both mother and fetus (Chavanet *et al.*, 1989; Schenker *et al.*, 1990; Watts *et al.*, 1991). In a retrospective study of 43 pregnant women who were prescribed oral zidovudine in doses ranging from 300 to 1200 mg per day the drug was not associated with teratogenic effects, even with exposure to zidovudine during the first trimester (Sperling *et al.*, 1992a). In a follow-up study of the offspring of seven pregnant women who were prescribed 18 mg per kg of zidovudine after the 16th week of gestation, all infants developed macrocytosis and two developed anemia, both of which resolved within the second month of life (Ferrazin *et al.*, 1993). In the pivotal ACTG 076 study of safety and efficacy of zidovudine in reducing maternal–infant transmission of HIV, infected pregnant mothers received 100 mg five times per day antepartum, and 2 mg per kg i.v. over 1 h followed by 1 mg per kg per h i.v intrapartum. Adverse effects were of similar nature and prevalence in zidovudine and placebo groups (Connor *et al.*, 1994).

5 Patients with renal failure

Pharmacokinetics of zidovudine can be significantly altered in persons with renal failure (described below). In one report, three patients with end-stage renal disease requiring hemodialysis three times per week and a fourth patient with chronic renal failure (creatinine clearance 20 ml per min) were treated with zidovudine 100 mg thrice-daily maintaining optimal plasma concentrations over an 8-month period (Paoli *et al.*, 1992). This dose has also been used successfully in other patients (Pachon *et al.*, 1992).

6 Patients with liver disease

Although not validated yet by clinical trials it has been proposed that dosage adjustment should be considered in persons with hepatic dysfunction, based on alterations in the pharmacokinetics of zidovudine (described below) (Taburet *et al.*, 1990; Child *et al.*, 1991). In a small study of three patients with AIDS and hepatic dysfunction who received a single oral dose of zidovudine, the clearance of the drug was reduced by a mean of 63% and the area-under-the-curve (AUC) was increased, compared with AIDS patients with no evidence of hepatic disease (Fletcher *et al.*, 1992).

Availability

Capsules containing 100 mg, and in some countries including Australia capsules containing 250 mg of zidovudine.

The drug is also formulated as a syrup, in bottles containing 200 ml at a concentration of 10 mg per ml.

Zidovudine is available for i.v. administration. It is provided as a 1% solution in a vial containing 10 mg per ml of zidovudine. Each 20 ml vial contains 200 mg zidovudine. The contents of the vial should be diluted prior to administration using Glucose Intravenous Infusion BP (5% w/v) to give a final concentration of zidovudine of 2 or 4 mg per ml. It cannot be administered by i.m. injection.

Serum Levels in Relation to Dosage

1 Intravenous infusion

A single i.v. infusion of 1 mg per kg, 2.5 mg per kg or 5 mg per kg over 1 h results in peak plasma concentrations of 1.5–2 μM, 4–6 μM and 6–10 μM respectively, with a half-life of 1 h (Yarchoan *et al.*, 1986). In adults who have received 0.5 mg per kg or 2.5 mg per kg of zidovudine i.v. in a 1 h infusion every 4 h, the mean serum levels of the drug are 0.3 μM and 2.9 μM respectively, with blood being obtained from 15 min to 4 h after the infusion (Lane *et al.*, 1989). Recent studies of high dose zidovudine (2–20 g per m^2 daily) found that zidovudine exposure increased proportionately with increasing dose although total drug clearance was reduced in patients receiving the highest dose (Marchbank *et al.*, 1995).

In pediatric populations, a continuous i.v. infusion of 320 mg per m^2 daily was found to maintain the plasma concentration of zidovudine above 1 μM throughout the dosing interval (Balis *et al.*, 1991). Intravenous administration of zidovudine to children results in an age-dependent clearance of the drug, being more rapid in younger children even when normalized for body weight (Balis *et al.*, 1989a,b).

2 Oral administration

Clinically relevant pharmacokinetics are summarized in Table V.23. No significant differences have been observed in persons with differing stages of HIV disease, or in smokers versus non-smokers, in terms of half-life of zidovudine, maximum concentration or time to maximum plasma concentration, or AUC (Child *et al.*, 1991). Gastrointestinal absorption of zidovudine, didanosine and zalcitabine is rapid with a reported bioavailability of zidovudine ranging from 46% to 69% (Yarchoan *et al.*, 1989; Morse *et al.*, 1992, 1993). Low bioavailability has been reported in association with a mild alteration in bowel habit (up to four unformed or semi-solid motions per day) and in patients with low CD4 counts (Macnab *et al.*, 1993).

The drug has been reported to exhibit dose-dependent kinetics up to an oral dose of 10 mg per kg (Cload 1989; Collier *et al.*, 1991). Peak plasma levels attained 1 h after a single oral dose of 2 mg per kg, 5 mg per kg or 10 mg per kg range from 1.5 to 2 μM, 4 to 6 μM and 6 to 10 μM respectively (Yarchoan *et al.*, 1986). These plasma concentrations are equivalent to those attained by half of each dose infused i.v. over 1 h. Following a 300-mg dose, peak zidovudine

Table V.23
Summary of clinically relevant
pharmacokinetcs of zidovudine

Good oral bioavailability (46–69%)
May be taken with food without significant alteration to pharmacokinetics
Pharmacokinetics are not altered during pregnancy
Zidovudine crosses the placenta
Consider dose modification in patients with hepatic dysfunction
Major route of metabolism is via hepatic glucuronidation
Good central nervous system penetration (approximately 60%)

Refer to text for sources of data.

levels occur between 0.5 and 1 h, with a rapid decay over 1–4 h (Morse *et al.*, 1992). In a population of HIV-infected men, a single oral dose of 400 mg of zidovudine resulted in a peak plasma level (C_{max} of 7.3 ± 4.7 μM, achieved after a mean of 1.2 ± 0.5 h (Child *et al.*, 1991).

Under steady-state conditions with an oral dose of 200 mg 4-hourly, the mean plasma concentration of zidovudine at 0.5, 1 and 4 h in symptomatic HIV-infected persons has been reported as 4.3, 2.5, and 0.3 μM respectively (Laskin *et al.*, 1989). The trough level occurs at 4 h, and the peak serum level at 0.5–1.5 h, with concentrations ranging from 2.8 to 8.3 μM (Laskin *et al.*, 1989; Morse *et al.*, 1989; Yarchoan *et al.*, 1989).

Similar to many other antiretroviral compounds, the concentrations of the triphosphate derivative of zidovudine within cells rather than in plasma is likely to correlate best with the drug's activity and toxicity (Stretcher, 1995). Zidovudine has a plasma half-life of about 1 h (Balis *et al.*, 1991) and an intracellular half-life of about 3–4 h (Furman *et al.*, 1986; Stretcher *et al.*, 1992, 1994a). As a result, the ideal interval between oral doses is 4 h. There are methods to measure levels of phosphorylated zidovudine derivatives in peripheral blood mononuclear cells (Robbins *et al.*, 1994; Barry *et al.*, 1994). Measurements of intracellular zidovudine and its mono-, di- and triphosphate derivatives in peripheral blood mononuclear cells from six HIV-infected patients 2 h following a 300-mg capsule were 0.15 μM, 1.4 μM, 0.08 μM, 0.08 μM respectively (Slusher *et al.*, 1992). In a separate study, the intracellular concentrations of phosphorylated zidovudine in peripheral blood mononuclear cells have been reported to range from 0.33 to 3.54 pmol per 10^6 cells and to be unrelated to the plasma concentrations. During a 4 h dosing interval the intracellular concentration of phosphorylated zidovudine did not vary, although plasma levels declined. Also of interest in this report was the observation that there was a decline in intracellular levels of the phosphorylated derivatives of zidovudine in the study population with increasing duration of therapy (Stretcher *et al.*, 1991, 1994a). In one report zidovudine was phosphorylated to a greater extent in HIV-infected patients than in healthy volunteers (Barry *et al.*, 1994). The intracellular AUC of total phosphorylated zidovudine, but not the plasma AUC of zidovudine, correlates with CD4 percentage, beta-2-microglobulin and neopterin responses after initiation of zidovudine therapy (Stretcher *et al.*, 1994b).

Absorption of zidovudine has been found to be greater in the upper gastrointestinal tract than in the lower jejunum, ileum and colon in the rat model (Park and Mitra, 1992). Several studies have examined the effect of food on zidovudine absorption. A high-fat meal has been shown to significantly prolong the time to reach maximum steady-state concentration and to reduce the peak serum level in patients with AIDS as well as in asymptomatic HIV-infected individuals, although the AUC, and thus the systemic exposure, was unaltered (Unadkat *et al.*, 1990; Shelton *et al.*, 1994). In contrast, a 25 g protein meal has been reported to significantly decrease the maximum serum drug concentration, and increase the time to peak plasma concentration without altering the extent of absorption, the terminal half-life or the renal clearance of zidovudine (Sahai *et al.*, 1992).

3 Children

In newborn macaques less than 1 week of age treated with zidovudine, the total plasma clearance of zidovudine, and hepatic glucuronidation of the compound were reduced when compared with corresponding estimates at 4 months of age (Lopez-Anaya *et al.*, 1990b).

Zidovudine is rapidly absorbed in children following oral administration, with approximately 68% bioavailability. Oral administration of the recommended pediatric dose of 180 mg per m^2 every 6 h results in plasma concentrations of 1 μM for less than half the dosing interval (Balis *et al.*, 1991).

There are only limited data available in neonates. Infant cord blood levels of zidovudine have been reported to be slightly higher than maternal levels, and there is a slower elimination half-life (Watts *et al.*, 1991). In a phase I study, the half-life of zidovudine was found to be 10-fold higher in neonates than their mothers (O'Sullivan *et al.*, 1993). From these reports, zidovudine clearance may be delayed during the first month of life, compared with adults (Chavanet *et al.*, 1989; Watts *et al.*, 1991). This has been postulated to be due to decreased glucuronide conjugation and renal excretion which form the major mechanisms of elimination of the drug (Balis *et al.*, 1991). Total body clearance of zidovudine has been found to increase significantly with age, with a mean of 10.9 ml per min per kg in infants less than 14 days of age increasing to 19 ml per min per kg in older infants. This is associated with a decrease in serum half-life of the drug from 3.12 h in newborns to 1.87 h in babies 14 days or older. Bioavailability decreased from a mean of 89% in infants less than 14 days old to 61% in older infants (Boucher *et al.*, 1993b).

4 Pregnancy

In the macaque model, the plasma clearance, steady-state volume of distribution and terminal half-life of zidovudine have been assessed and found to be not significantly altered by pregnancy (Lopez-Anaya *et al.*, 1991). In pregnant baboons treated with zidovudine there was accumulation of the glucuronide form of the drug in amniotic fluid, although maternal zidovudine levels and that of its metabolite were unchanged (Hankins *et al.*, 1990).

In HIV seropositive women receiving zidovudine at a dose of 200 mg 4-hourly from weeks 19 to 39 of pregnancy, C_{max} values and AUC of zidovudine were lower during pregnancy than post partum (Watts *et al.*, 1991). However, in another report, the C_{max} of zidovudine in a woman receiving zidovudine in the third trimester was found to be comparable with levels in non-pregnant women (Sperling *et al.*, 1992b). In a phase I study of the pharmacokinetics and safety of zidovudine in asymptomatic HIV infected patients who were in the third trimester of pregnancy, the total body clearance of zidovudine, mean terminal elimination phase half-life and recovery of zidovudine in urine were similar to those in non-pregnant women (O'Sullivan *et al.*, 1993). As T_{max} values do not vary during pregnancy, this suggests that gastric absorption of zidovudine does not alter during pregnancy (Watts *et al.*, 1991; Sperling *et al.*, 1992b). Umbilical cord serum levels have been reported to range from 113% to 127% of maternal serum concentrations (Watts *et al.*, 1991).

Following termination of pregnancy at 13 weeks fetal tissues were examined in an HIV-infected woman who had received zidovudine 100 mg four times daily (and methadone) for the preceding 6 weeks. At 4 h post-last dose the maternal plasma concentration of zidovudine was $0.35\,\mu M$ with similar amniotic fluid levels ($0.31\,\mu M$). Concentrations of zidovudine within fetal liver, muscle and central nervous system were $0.14\,\mu M$, $0.26\,\mu M$ and $0.01\,\mu M$ respectively (Lyman *et al.*, 1990).

5 Patients with end-stage renal disease or undergoing hemodialysis or continuous ambulatory peritoneal dialysis (CAPD)

Plasma levels of the inactive glucuronide conjugate (the major renal metabolite of zidovudine), are markedly increased in patients with renal dysfunction, being reported to range from 20 to 440 times the zidovudine concentration (Balis *et al.*, 1991; Garraffo *et al.*, 1989; Tartaglione *et al.*, 1990; Pachon *et al.*, 1992). The clinical effect of markedly elevated levels of the glucuronide conjugates of zidovudine within the kidney is not known. The half-life of zidovudine in patients undergoing hemodialysis for chronic renal failure has been reported to be prolonged in one study (normalized by hemodialysis) (Pachon *et al.*, 1992) and unaltered in another report (Stellbrink *et al.*, 1993). In the latter study, hemodialysis was not found to significantly alter the plasma concentration of zidovudine (Stellbrink *et al.*, 1993). However, renal dialysis has been found to efficiently clear the glucuronide derivative (Garraffo *et al.*, 1989). Although there is great variation between patients, the effect of peritoneal dialysis on the clearance of zidovudine is reportedly negligible, and suggest that no supplementary doses of the drug are required in patients undergoing CAPD (Gallicano *et al.*, 1992; Kremer *et al.*, 1992).

6 Liver disease

The peak zidovudine concentration in plasma, the AUC and half-life have been found to be increased in patients with HIV infection who have liver disease including mild liver disease as well as cirrhosis, largely attributable to a marked drop in oral clearance (Taburet *et al.*, 1990; Bareggi *et al.*, 1994; Moore *et al.*, 1995). Thus a modified dosage should be considered in patients with liver dysfunction. In three AIDS patients with hepatic disease and serum transaminase levels ranging from 79 to 170 IU per liter, a dosage of 0.7 mg per kg of zidovudine orally 6-hourly resulted in peak and trough levels of zidovudine which are equivalent to those in patients with normal liver function receiving 100 mg five times daily (Fletcher *et al.*, 1992).

Excretion

1 Urine

Less than 20% of the oral dose of zidovudine is recovered unchanged in the urine (Cload, 1989). As the renal clearance of zidovudine exceeds that of creatinine, zidovudine is thought to undergo both glomerular filtration and renal tubular secretion in the kidney. Renal clearance is estimated to be 400 ml per min per 70 kg. Following i.v. administration, 18 ± 5% of the dose is excreted unchanged by the kidney, and 60% is converted to the glucuronide, the latter being rapidly cleared from the plasma with a half-life of 1 h (Cload, 1989). The apparent clearance of zidovudine varies considerably among different patient populations. In a useful study by Burger and colleagues, the clearance of zidovudine was found to be significantly reduced in patients with a lower body weight, in women, and in patients with advanced HIV infection, but did not seem to alter with age, or duration of zidovudine use (Burger *et al.*, 1994c).

Extrahepatic glucuronidation has been demonstrated *in vitro* in human renal microsomes (Howe *et al.*, 1992).

2 Bile

Studies in cynomolgus monkeys found that approximately 60% of a given dose of zidovudine was glucuronidated in the liver (Ayers, 1988). In humans, the major route of elimination is also by hepatic glucuronidation to form 3'-azido-3'-deoxy-5'-O-beta-D-glucopyranuronosylthymidine (GAZT) followed by excretion of this inactive metabolite in the urine (reviewed in Dudley, 1995). The glucuronide derivative has no antiviral activity.

Distribution of the Drug in Body

1 General disposition

Zidovudine is widely distributed throughout the body, and is present in virtually all tissues and fluids (Good and de Miranda, 1992). The estimated steady-state volume of distribution in humans is 1.4–1.6 liters per kg (Klecker *et al.*, 1987; Blum *et al.*, 1988), with a higher value (2.72 liters per kg) obtained in one study where high dose zidovudine was administered by i.v.infusion (Marchbanks *et al.*, 1995). Protein binding has been reported to range from 18 to 38% (Good and de Miranda, 1992; Luzier and Morse, 1993). There is no difference in protein binding of the drug in plasma compared with serum. The level of binding to albumin is low (Luzier and Morse, 1993). Drug clearance has been estimated at 1.3 ± 0.3 liters per kg per h, with a volume of distribution of 1.4 ± 0.4 liters per kg (Gitterman *et al.*, 1990).

2 Cerebrospinal fluid

In cynomolgus monkeys, the concentration of zidovudine in brain tissue following a 25 mg per kg subcutaneous injection was found to be approximately one-third of that in blood and muscle (Ljungdahl *et al.*, 1992). In monkeys, the glucuronide metabolite of zidovudine has been found to poorly cross the blood–brain-barrier (Cretton *et al.*, 1991).

Zidovudine is able to cross from blood into cerebrospinal fluid (CSF) in humans (Klecker *et al.*, 1987), although it would appear that it is not measurably transported across the blood–brain barrier (Terasaki and Pardridge, 1988). Thus entry of zidovudine into brain interstitial fluid is thought to occur by transport of the drug from the choroid plexus into CSF, diffusion across the ependymal lining of the ventricle and subsequent diffusion into brain tissue. The penetration of zidovudine into CSF in humans has been reported to be 60–75% in adults, calculated under non steady-state conditions and based on a single specimen taken 2–4 h after oral administration or 4 h after commencing an i.v. infusion (Yarchoan *et al.*, 1986; Cload, 1989; Yarchoan *et al.*, 1989). In a study of patients with AIDS who had received a minimum of 2 weeks of zidovudine therapy at a dose of 200–250 mg 4-hourly, the median CSF concentration of the drug was 0.47 µg per ml, with serum concentrations ranging from 0.017 to 1.37 µg per ml, and highly variable CSF: serum ratios (ranging from 8.8% to 120%) (Tartaglione *et al.*, 1991a,b). In a similar patient population receiving similar oral doses of zidovudine, the mean CSF concentration was found to be 0.43 µM; following i.v. administration of 0.5 mg per kg or 2.5 mg per kg the CSF levels were

0.25 μM and 0.58 μM respectively (Lane *et al.*, 1989). Other investigators have found that penetration of zidovudine into CSF is independent of the plasma concentration, and that levels in CSF show little fluctuation over time whereas plasma concentrations of the drug vary widely (Burger *et al.*, 1993b). In children receiving zidovudine by continuous i.v. infusion, the CSF penetration of the drug in one study has been found to be 24% of plasma concentration (Balis *et al.*, 1991a). Zidovudine levels are approximately twice as high on a molar basis compared with didanosine (Burger *et al.*, 1995).

3 Placenta

It has been shown that zidovudine crosses the placenta of pregnant mice following intraperitoneal injection (Ruprecht *et al*, 1990b), resulting in embryonic levels of approximately 50% of the maternal serum concentration. In pregnant women, zidovudine rapidly crosses the placenta by simple diffusion (Bawdon *et al.*, 1992; Dancis *et al.*, 1993). Extensive metabolism of the drug to one or more currently unidentified metabolites occurs within the placenta. The amount of zidovudine which is transferred to the fetal circulation is proportional to the level in the maternal blood (Liebes *et al.*, 1990). Neither zidovudine nor its glucuronide conjugate accumulate in the fetus (Bawdon *et al.*, 1992; Good and de Miranda, 1992).

4 Semen

As the blood–testes barrier may limit the penetration of zidovudine into the testes it is likely that seminal levels of zidovudine are derived from prostatic fluid rather than seminal fluid (Henry *et al.*, 1988; Sikka *et al.*, 1991; Good and de Miranda, 1992). In six symptomatic, HIV-infected persons who received an oral dose of 200 mg zidovudine, semen levels obtained 0.75–1.25 h post-dose were 3.63–7.19 μM. Semen levels in samples obtained 3–4.5 h post-dose were 1.68–6.43 μM (Henry *et al.*, 1988). In persons on long-term zidovudine therapy, who were receiving 600–1200 mg daily, seminal zidovudine concentrations ranged from 0 to 5 μM (median: 1.1 μM) (Anderson *et al.*, 1992).

5 Breast milk

In mice who receive an intraperitoneal injection of zidovudine, drug levels 0.5 h later are up to 5.5 times the serum concentration, with more rapid elimination subsequently (Ruprecht *et al.*, 1990b).

6 Lymph node

Zidovudine is distributed throughout the lymphatic system when administered by the i.v. or oral route to mice, and there is greater distribution of the drug to axillary lymph nodes compared with neck and mesenteric nodes (Manouilov *et al.*, 1995).

Mode of Action

Zidovudine is an analog of thymidine in which the 3'-hydroxy group is replaced by an azido group. Zidovudine requires phosphorylation in order for it to exert antiretroviral activity (Fig. V.35). In the triphosphate form it is a potent inhibitor of reverse transcriptase and terminates DNA chain synthesis (St Clair *et al.*, 1987).

Transport of zidovudine into cells is by simple diffusion (Kong *et al.*, 1992). Much of the important work on the mechanism of action of zidovudine was performed by Furman and his colleagues early after the discovery of its antiretroviral activity (Furman *et al.*, 1986). In contrast with aciclovir, cellular thymidine kinase (TK) phosphorylates ziduvudine to the monophosphate derivative. Furthermore, again in contrast with aciclovir, phosphorylation occurs in both uninfected and HIV-infected cells (Furman *et al.*, 1986). The herpes simplex specified TK cannot substitute for cellular TK in the phosphorylation of zidovudine (Lowy *et al.*, 1994). This phosphorylation of zidovudine by TK occurs as efficiently as phosphorylation of its native substrate, thymidine (K_m values for zidovudine and thymidine are 3.0 μM and 2.9 μM respectively) and is totally inhibited by addition of thymidine to the cellular extracts (Furman *et al.*, 1986). Macaque and human peripheral blood mononuclear cells convert zidovudine to its monophosphate derivative with similar speed, with levels of the phosphorylated compound in human cells increasing 7.7-fold when the extracellular concentration is increased approximately 30-fold (Qian *et al.*, 1994a). Subsequent phosphorylation to the diphosphate derivative is catalyzed by cellular thymidylate kinase and is less efficient than the initial phosphorylation step. Because of poor substrate-specificity of zidovudine monophosphate for thymidylate kinase, zidovudine monophosphate accounts for more than 95% of intracellular zidovudine (Furman *et al.*, 1986; Agarwal and Mian, 1991). Other cellular

Fig. V.35.

Phosphorylation of zidovudine in infected and uninfected cells.

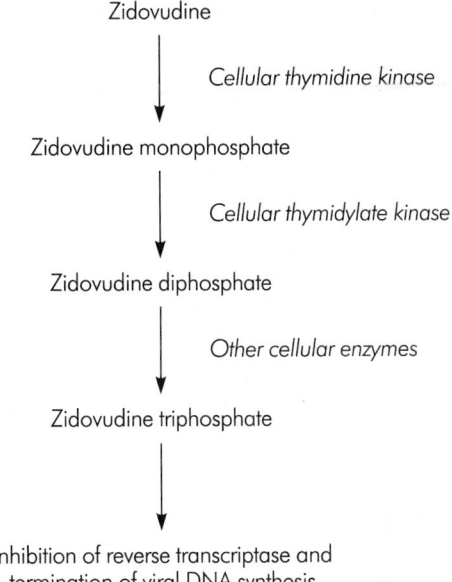

Zidovudine

Cellular thymidine kinase

Zidovudine monophosphate

Cellular thymidylate kinase

Zidovudine diphosphate

Other cellular enzymes

Zidovudine triphosphate

Inhibition of reverse transcriptase and termination of viral DNA synthesis

enzymes catalyze the conversion of di- to triphosphate. There is considerable variability between individuals in the ability of their peripheral blood mononuclear cells to phosphorylate zidovudine (Veal *et al.*, 1994). Inhibition of the reverse transcriptase by zidovudine triphosphate is at least moderately selective; inhibition of cellular DNA polymerase alpha and beta by zidovudine triphosphate is approximately 100-fold less (Furman *et al.*, 1986; Matthes *et al.*, 1987; Konig *et al.*, 1989). However, significant inhibition of DNA polymerase gamma (Konig *et al.*, 1989), delta and epsilon occurs (Nickel *et al.*, 1992).

In lymphocytes and T lymphoblastoid cells TK activity is greater than that in macrophages (Richman *et al.*, 1987b), but when the difference in cellular size and volume is taken into account the difference between the two cell lineages in kinase activity is only marginal (1.3-fold higher in lymphocytes) (Arner *et al.*, 1992), and may also be influenced by the stage of differentiation of the monocyte-macrophage (reviewed in Perno *et al.*, 1988). The fact that zidovudine is more effective in inhibiting HIV replication in acutely infected macrophages compared with lymphocytes is due to the increased ratio of dideoxynucleoside-triphosphate/deoxynucleoside-triphosphate in macrophages (Perno *et al.*, 1992a). However, these data appear to conflict with studies by Gao and colleagues who propose that zidovudine is preferentially phosphorylated and more active in activated cells than resting cells (Gao *et al.*, 1994). There need to be further studies comparing phosphorylation and potency of zidovudine in resting lymphocytes, activated lymphocytes and macrophages. The mitochondrial thymidine kinase (TK2) is thought to phosphorylate thymidine in macrophages, compared with the cytosolic enzyme (TK1) which is responsible for this activity in lymphocytes (Arner *et al.*, 1992). Some cells may be refractory to the antiretroviral effects of zidovudine, due to decreased accumulation of zidovudine triphosphate, or increased phosphorylation of thymidine to its triphosphate derivative (Medina *et al.*, 1995). In placental trophoblastic cells and Hofbauer (fetal macrophage) cells zidovudine has been reported to be 50- 100-fold less efficiently phosphorylated to the triphosphate derivative than in activated peripheral blood lymphocytes. Zidovudine di- and triphosphate constitute less than 4% of the total intracellular pool of phosphorylated zidovudine (Qian *et al.*, 1994b).

The HIV genome consists of *gag*, *pol*, and *env* genes and a number of accessory genes which encode the structural and regulatory proteins of HIV. The *pol* gene encodes a precursor polyprotein which is cleaved to form the reverse transcriptase, protease and endonuclease enzymes. In the replicative cycle of HIV, viral RNA is transcribed by reverse transcriptase initially into single-stranded and subsequently into double-stranded cDNA (Varmus and Swanstrom, 1982). During this process deoxynucleotides are incorporated into the growing strand of DNA and thus, in the triphosphate form, the thymidine analog zidovudine will be incorporated in place of the cellular deoxynucleotide and result in premature DNA chain termination (St Clair *et al.*, 1987).

The reverse transcriptase of HIV has been crystallized (Kohlstaedt *et al.*, 1992). Zidovudine binds to a site distinct to that of the non-nucleoside reverse transcriptase inhibitors (p. 1772).

Table V.24
Toxicity associated with zidovudine therapy

Major	
Bone marrow	
anemia	
neutropenia	
leukopenia	
Musculoskeletal	
myopathy	
Hepatic	
hepatitis	
lactic acidosis	
Less severe	
nausea, anorexia	
headache	
mood disturbance	
pigmentation of nails, skin	

Toxicity

The major toxic reactions reported in association with zidovudine therapy are summarized in Table V.24.

1 Hemopoietic toxicity

Using erythroid and granulocyte-macrophage progenitor colony forming assays it is clear that zidovudine can inhibit colony formation in both of these lineages *in vitro*. This inhibition by zidovudine occurs to a greater extent than with didanosine and stavudine but according to one study less potently than with zalcitabine (Dornsife *et al.*, 1991; Faraj *et al.*,1994). Pluripotent CD34+ cells when purified from bone marrow and cells in early phases of differentiation are less affected by zidovudine than more mature erythroid progenitor cells (Faraj *et al.*, 1994).

Significant hematologic toxicity occurred in early clinical trials in which patients with symptomatic HIV infection were administered high doses of zidovudine (in the range of 1000–1500 mg daily (Richman *et al.*, 1987a; Walker *et al.*, 1988; Moore *et al.*, 1991a,b; Cooper *et al.*, 1991). The main side-effects were bone marrow suppression, with up to 45% of treated individuals developing anemia, leukopenia or neutopenia and requiring dose-reduction (Richman *et al.*, 1987a). Toxicity was greater in persons with more advanced disease (Richman *et al.*, 1987a; Volberding *et al.*, 1990; Cooper *et al.*, 1993a). Similar findings have been observed in adults and children (Blanche *et al.*, 1988). Bone marrow hypoplasia or aplasia associated with severe pancytopenia has rarely been observed, and although it is usually associated with at least partial recovery following cessation of treatment, recovery may be markedly delayed (Gill *et al.*, 1987; Richman *et al.*, 1987a). Pure red cell aplasia with a maturation arrest of erythroid precursors has also been reported to occur within the first 3 months of zidovudine therapy (Walker *et al.*, 1988; Cohen *et al.*, 1989).

In asymptomatic individuals receiving more than 1000 mg daily of zidovudine there is a lower rate of anemia and neutropenia (<10%) than in patients with more advanced disease (Volberding *et al.*, 1990; Koch *et al.*, 1992; Cooper *et al.*, 1993a). In patients without symptoms receiving the currently recommended dose of 500–600 mg daily significant hematologic toxicity is rare, with the estimated risk of severe anemia after 18 months of continuous therapy being 2% (Gelmon *et al.*, 1989; Volberding *et al.*, 1990; Koch *et al.*, 1992). An intermittent regimen of zidovudine treatment for symptomatic patients who develop severe anemia comprising 4 weeks of zidovudine therapy (600–1000 mg daily) followed by 2 weeks without therapy has been associated with hematologic benefit with no evidence of virology deterioration (Williams *et al.*, 1993). This approach is not recommended by the author because of the potential to develop resistance.

Macrocytosis develops within weeks of commencing therapy (Richman *et al.*, 1987a; Weber *et al.*, 1991) with megaloblastic changes observed in the bone marrow in most patients within 18 weeks of commencing therapy; these changes are reversible upon cessation of treatment (Gelmon *et al.*, 1989). In some urban hospitals, zidovudine is now the most common cause of macrocytosis (Snower and Weil, 1993). The mean corpuscular volume slowly increases over the first 5–12 months of zidovudine therapy to a mean volume of 110 per μm^3, and subsequently stabilizes (Graham et al., 1991a); a gradual fall in hemoglobin occurs over the same period of time (Cooper et al., 1993a). The decline in hemoglobin may be observed as early as 1–2 weeks after commencing the drug, but more commonly develops within 1–3 months (Richman et al., 1987a; Cooper et al., 1991). These findings are supported by observations in cynomolgus monkeys who develop a dose-related macrocytic anemia within 3–6 months of commencing zidovudine therapy (Ayers, 1988). The increase in mean corpuscular volume predominantly occurs in patients who do not develop anemia, and remains stable or marginally increased in those in whom anemia develops (Walker et al., 1988). Red-cell transfusions are extremely rarely required as a result of zidovudine-induced anemia in asymptomatic persons receiving 500–600 mg daily. In earlier trials when doses of 1000 mg daily or higher were employed, 2–4 units were required every 3–4 weeks in up to 30% persons with advanced disease (Richman et al., 1987a; Cooper et al., 1991). A transient decline in the reticulocyte count may occur shortly after initiation of therapy. HIV-associated hemolytic anemia, in which zidovudine may have played an exacerbating role, has been reported (Telen et al., 1990). Vitamin B_{12} is usually not altered by zidovudine although there are some reports of persons with reduced levels (Richman et al., 1987a; Baum et al., 1991). Red cell folate is unchanged or even increased (Baum et al., 1991). Serum immunoreactive erythropoietin levels are increased in persons receiving zidovudine; however the bone marrow appears to be refractory to its effects (Spivak et al., 1989). Of interest, zidovudine has been found to down-regulate erythropoietin receptor expression on bone marrow progenitor cells, providing a potential explanation for this refractory response (Gogu et al., 1992). This results in a decrease in erythropoietin-responsive progenitor cells within bone marrow (Gallicchio and Hughes, 1992). Decreased levels of serum zinc and copper have been reported in association with zidovudine therapy (Baum et al., 1991).

Leukopenia, primarily due to neutropenia, may complicate zidovudine therapy, but is usually restricted to persons with advanced disease on high-dose zidovudine. Severe neutropenia (<750 x 10^6 per liter) has been reported in persons treated with 1000 mg per day or higher, and generally appears within the first 4 weeks of therapy (Cooper et al., 1991; Koch et al., 1992). In a study of hemophiliacs with asymptomatic HIV infection a dose of 1000 mg of zidovudine daily only resulted in a neutrophil count of less than 750 x 10^6 per liter in 5% of recipients (Mannucci et al., 1994). A lower dose of zidovudine (500–600 mg daily) is generally not associated with neutropenia (Koch et al., 1992; Cooper et al., 1993b; Volberding et al., 1990).

Infrequently, thrombocytopenia may occur in persons treated with zidovudine (Richman et al., 1987a; Cooper et al., 1991; Moore et al., 1991a), although an increase in platelet count associated with therapy is much more likely to occur (Cooper et al., 1991; Chow et al., 1993b; Cinque et al., 1993).

2 Musculoskeletal toxicity

An early placebo-controlled study reported the development of myalgias with higher frequency in persons receiving zidovudine than in those randomized to placebo (Richman et al., 1987a). Since then it has become apparent that zidovudine can also cause muscular weakness. As HIV itself can produce inflammatory myopathies including polymyositis, and proximal muscle weakness due to nemaline myopathy, it is sometimes difficult to distinguish these clinical entities from zidovudine-induced myopathy (Till and MacDonell, 1990; Espinoza et al., 1991). The development of zidovudine-induced myopathy is invariably associated with chronic therapy (mean 12 months), does not appear to be dose-related, usually results in improvement within about 8 weeks after cessation of therapy and recurs with rechallenge (Gertner et al., 1989; Dalakas et al., 1990; Till and MacDonell, 1990; Peters et al., 1993). The prevalence is up to 20% in long-term zidovudine-treated patients (Lewis and Dalakas, 1995). Serum creatinine kinase and aspartate aminotransferase levels may be normal, but are usually elevated from about 5–25 weeks prior to the onset of symptoms and return to normal when zidovudine is withdrawn (Gertner et al., 1989; Mhiri et al., 1991; Peters et al., 1993). Approximately 10–20% of persons who receive zidovudine for 6 months or longer develop an elevated serum creatinine kinase level (Till and MacDonell, 1990). The patient usually describes proximal weakness and wasting of slow onset, with pain being present in about half the cases (Helbert et al., 1988; Gertner et al., 1989). Many of the reported cases have been in persons with less than 200 CD4 cells per μl, suggesting that the development of zidovudine-induced myopathy is more common in persons with more advanced disease (Till and MacDonell, 1990). Non-steroidal anti-inflammatory agents and prednisolone (40–60 mg daily) may relieve symptoms in mild cases, however cessation of zidovudine is usually necessary for patients with moderate to severe symptoms (Dalakas et al., 1990; Till and MacDonell, 1990; Mhiri et al., 1991).

Little evidence of inflammation is present in histologic sections from muscle biopsy of patients with zidovudine- associated myopathy, although this is not universally observed. The main distinguishing features are the presence of ragged-red fibers suggesting abnormal mitochondria (Dalakas *et al.*, 1990) and striking cytoarchitectural changes (Gonzales *et al.*, 1988). Electron microscopic findings confirm muscle mitochondrial changes, with evidence of swelling, degeneration, paracrystalline inclusions, glycogen-packed sarcoplasm and lipid droplets (Till and MacDonell, 1990; Chen *et al.*, 1992; Peters *et al.*, 1993). Similar findings are present in the rat model (Lamperth *et al.*, 1991; Lewis *et al.*, 1992). There is a clinical correlation between the number of ragged-red fibers and severity of clinical symptoms (Dalakas *et al.*, 1990). Analysis of mitochondrial enzymes, including succinate-cytochrome c reductase, cytochrome coxidase and citrate synthase, indicates a decline in respiratory chain capacity with altered oxidation-phosphorylation coupling (Lamperth *et al.*, 1991; Mhiri *et al.*, 1991), although normal enzyme activity has been by other investigators (Herzberg *et al.*, 1992). Subsequently it has been shown that zidovudine inhibits mitochondrial DNA polymerase-gamma, resulting in inhibition of mitochondrial synthesis and function (Konig *et al.*, 1989; Izuta *et al.*, 1991; Schroder *et al.*, 1992). Other nucleoside analogs, including zalcitabine, didanosine, and stavudine, have also been shown to inhibit mitochondrial DNA synthesis (pp. 1719, 1737, 1763) (Chen *et al.*, 1991). Reduced muscle carnitine levels have been found in patients with zidovudine-induced mitochondrial myopathy (Dalakas *et al.*, 1994). It has been found that L-carnitine prevents zidovudine-associated mitochondrial destruction *in vitro* (Semino-Mora *et al.*, 1994a), and enhances recovery of zidovudine-associated myotubular destruction as well as aiding the restoration of mitochondrial structure (Semino-Mora *et al.*, 1994b; reviewed in Mintz, 1995).

A zidovudine-induced cardiomyopathy has been reported in rats (Lamperth *et al.*, 1991; Lewis *et al.*, 1991). Furthermore, there are a small number of reported cases of patients who have developed cardiac dysfunction with evidence of a cardiomyopathy whilst receiving zidovudine; cessation of therapy has resulted in clinical improvement (Herskowitz *et al.*, 1992). Cardiac mitochondrial DNA polymerase-gamma is inhibited competitively and non-competitively by zidovudine triphosphate *in vitro* (Lewis *et al.*, 1994).

3 Hepatic toxicity

Zidovudine may rarely cause acute hepatitis; the exact mechanism is not known (Dubin and Braffman, 1989; Gradon *et al.*, 1992). Fever has been associated with abdominal discomfort and nausea in reported cases. Liver function tests show a markedly elevated alkaline phosphatase (>10-fold the upper normal limit), and an elevated bilirubin, aspartate aminotransferase and alanine aminotransferase (>3–6-fold the upper normal limits) (Dubin and Braffman, 1989). Liver biopsy revealed that the patient had disseminated infection with *Mycobacterium intracellulare*, which may have contributed to the cholestatic picture. In other reports the alkaline phosphatase has been within the normal range, and the predominant abnormalities have been markedly increased aspartate and alanine aminotransferases (Gradon *et al.*, 1992). An HIV-infected hemophiliac with chronic hepatitis B infection developed hepatic failure with markedly elevated transaminase levels shortly after commencing zidovudine and subsequently died (Shintaku *et al.*, 1993). A syndrome comprising potentially fatal lactic acidosis, with or without massive hepatomegaly and steatosis has been described in a small number of persons receiving zidovudine. Most of these individuals were HIV-infected females with mild to moderate obesity who had not had an AIDS-defining illness (Chattha *et al.*, 1993; Freiman *et al.*, 1993). A similar case has been reported in a person who was receiving didanosine (p. 1720) but who had previously been prescribed zidovudine (Lai *et al.*, 1991). Fatal lactic acidosis and pancreatitis have been reported in a patient receiving zidovudine and didanosine combination therapy (Yarchoan *et al.*, 1994) .

4 Gastrointestinal toxicity

Nausea occurs in up to half of those taking zidovudine and is usually maximal in the first 6 weeks of therapy. Anorexia occurs less commonly (in 10–12% of persons). Altered taste, whilst reported, occurs with equal frequency in persons taking zidovudine and placebo (Richman *et al.*, 1987a). Non-specific mid-esophageal ulceration has been reported in persons with advanced disease who were taking zidovudine in a recumbent position without fluids (Edwards *et al.*, 1990).

5 Neuropsychiatric toxicity

Mood disturbances have been reported in up to 30% of those taking zidovudine (Gelmon *et al.*, 1989). Zidovudine has been reported to induce mania in individuals with no previous psychiatric history (Wright *et al.*, 1989). Sleep disturbances induced by zidovudine have been reported (Richman *et al.*, 1987a), although not confirmed by formal studies (Moeller *et al.*, 1992). Although acute meningo-encephalitis was attributed to dose-reduction of zidovudine in an early report this also has not been substantiated by others (Helbert *et al.*, 1988). Headache and focal seizures commencing 48 h after initiation of zidovudine (200 mg 4-hourly) ceasing with drug withdrawal and returning with drug rechallenge have been reported (Hagler and Frame, 1986). Somnolence and coma have been described in persons taking zidovudine (Richman *et al.*, 1987a; Riedel *et al.*, 1989).

6 Mucocutaneous side-effects

Initially described in blacks, progressive pigmentation of finger-nails and toe-nails has since been reported to also occur in Hispanics and whites as a result of zidovudine therapy (Furth and Kazakis, 1987; Grau *et al.*, 1990; Rahav and Maayan, 1992). The initial appearance is a bluish appearance of the lunulae of nails, progressing distally at a rate of 2 mm per week. Typically the onset is within 2–4 weeks after commencing zidovudine therapy (Furth and Kazakis, 1987; Greenberg and Berger, 1990). It is unclear whether nail pigmentation is related to dosage of zidovudine or stage of HIV disease (Tosti *et al.*, 1990; Rahav and Maayan, 1992). Hyperpigmentation of oral mucosa, including the lateral margins of the tongue, may occur in association with the nail changes (Merenich *et al.*, 1989; Greenberg and Berger, 1990; Tadini *et al.*, 1991). The pigmentation is due to melanin deposition; adrenal function is normal (Merenich *et al.*, 1989; Greenberg and Berger, 1990). Selective hyperpigmentation of footpads and tails has been observed in mice who receive zidovudine in their drinking water. Increased melanosomes are present within the epidermis and the pigmentation is reversible on cessation of therapy (Obuch *et al.*, 1992a).

Zidovudine has been reported to cause cutaneous hypersensitivity reactions including maculopapular eruptions associated with hepatic dysfunction which slowly resolve on cessation of therapy, and non-pruritic, blistering and erythematous lesions (Carr *et al.*, 1993). These lesions developed within 1–6 weeks of commencing the drug. Desensitization can be successful, permitting subsequent zidovudine therapy (Carr *et al.*, 1993). Cutaneous leukocytoclastic vasculitis has been reported in an AIDS patient taking zidovudine, and fluconazole, which resolved on cessation of zidovudine and redeveloped within 24 h following zidovudine challenge (Torres *et al.*, 1992).

7 Pregnancy, fetus, reproductive system

Zidovudine administration in high dose to pregnant mice has been associated with pregnancy failure in one study (Toltzis *et al.*, 1991), although these findings have not been supported in a subsequent report (Sieh *et al.*, 1992). There is *in vitro* evidence of embryonic toxicity, resulting from failure to develop to the blastocyst stage, when embryos are exposed to very high concentrations of zidovudine (Toltzis *et al.*, 1991; Sieh *et al.*, 1992). Similar effects have not been observed with other nucleoside analogs such as didanosine (p. 1720) (Sieh *et al.*, 1992). The adult pregnant mice were not adversely affected by exposure to zidovudine during gestation. Testicular and ovarian tissue from mice and rats receiving oral zidovudine show no reduction in spermatogenesis or follicular development respectively (Sikka *et al.*, 1991; Toltzis *et al.*, 1991). Zidovudine has been shown to reduce DNA synthesis of placental trophoblasts and also to inhibit secretion of progesterone by these cells (Bui *et al.*, 1993). In pigtailed macaques who received zidovudine during pregnancy, fetal growth was normal and there was no evidence of behavioral delay in infants (Ha *et al.*, 1994).

Pregnant HIV-infected women who received 300–1200 mg zidovudine daily for at least two trimesters had a very low incidence of side-effects (one hematologic and one gastrointestinal out of 43 women). Infants exposed to zidovudine in the first trimester had no teratogenic effects. Treatment was not associated with stillbirth, premature birth or fetal distress, and there was only a low incidence of intrauterine growth retardation (Sperling *et al.*, 1992a).

8 Carcinogenesis, mutagenesis

In studies of mice and rats using drug levels greater than 2- to 20-fold the estimated human exposure at the recommended dose of 500 mg per day, vaginal neoplasms (squamous cell carcinomas, papillomas and polyps) developed after 19 months of therapy (Zidovudine Product Information). Zidovudine was not mutagenic, as assessed by the Ames *Salmonella* mutagenicity assay. In an *in vitro* cytogenic assay using human lymphocytes chromosomal abnormalities were observed at concentrations of zidovudine of >3 μg per ml (Zidovudine Product Information).

Zidovudine at concentrations of 500 and 1000 μg per ml was found to damage DNA in human lymphocytes (Gonzalez and Larripa, 1994).

9 Health care workers following occupational exposure

Health care workers exposed to HIV who were prescribed 1000 mg or more of zidovudine daily for 4–6 weeks did not develop significant side-effects, with the risk of anemia, neutropenia and hepatic dysfunction being approximately 2.5%, 0.5% and 1% respectively (Puro et al., 1992). However, a higher proportion are likely to develop a reduction in hemoglobin or hematocrit (Tokars et al., 1993). Adverse side-effects including nausea, malaise, fatigue and headache are experienced by up to three-quarters of treated individuals (Tokars et al., 1993).

10 Overdose

An AIDS patient who intentionally ingested between 10 and 20 g (100–200 of the 100-mg capsules; 110–220 mg per kg body weight) with unknown quantities of phenobarbital and triazolam (Halcion) was found to have a serum zidovudine level of 24 μg per ml approximately 8 h post-ingestion. The level of zidovudine in CSF 16 h post-ingestion (0.34 μg per ml) exceeded the plasma concentration at the same time (0.12 μg per ml), which is consistent with slower clearance of the drug from the CSF. His only clinical signs were nystagmus and ataxia which resolved (Spear et al., 1988a). In a second report, ingestion of a month's supply of zidovudine, leading to serum levels of 340 μM 2 h post-ingestion, resulted in no acute myelotoxicity (Valentine et al., 1993).

A 27-month-old boy who ingested 130 mg zidovudine (10.2 mg per kg or 400 mg per m^2) was found to have plasma concentrations of zidovidine of 4.5 mg per ml (19 μM) 4 h post-ingestion, and approximately 3 h post-emesis (induced by ipecac syrup). There was no evidence of toxicity associated with this dose (Moore et al., 1990).

11 Other

There is no evidence that black or Hispanic patients differ in tolerance of zidovudine to white/non-Hispanic patients (Jacobson et al., 1995). Fatigue, malaise, loss of energy and headache are often particularly troublesome within the first 4–6 weeks of zidovudine therapy, and may sometimes be minimized by starting at 100 mg per day and gradually increasing the dose of zidovudine over several weeks up to the required level, although this is anecdotal and may possibly contribute to emergence of resistant strains. Zidovudine-induced fever which was confirmed by rechallenge has been described in association with IgM antibodies directed against a zidovudine-serum protein conformational determinant (Jacobson et al., 1989a). Hypertrichosis of the eyelashes has been described temporally related (within 2 weeks) to commencing zidovudine, without an increase in other body hair length (Klutman and Hinthorn, 1991). Symptomatic postural hypotension related to elevated zidovudine serum levels has been reported (Loke et al., 1990). Zidovudine-induced macular edema documented by fluorescein angiography has been reported in a patient with pre-existing but well-controlled uveitis. The macular edema commenced shortly after starting zidovudine and improved on cessation of the drug (Lalonde et al., 1991).

12 Drug interactions

The manufacturers recommend that co-administration of zidovudine with drugs that are nephrotoxic, cytotoxic or that suppress the bone marrow may increase the risk of toxicity and thus should be used with caution (Zidovudine Product Information).

No pharmacologic interaction has been observed between zidovudine and didanosine or between zidovudine and zalcitabine in adults (Qian et al., 1992; Wientjes and Au, 1992; Morse et al., 1995; Sahai et al., 1995). As the toxicities of the two drugs do not overlap, zidovudine and zalcitabine (and similarly, zidovudine and didanosine) are well-suited for combination therapy (p. 1681) (Merigan et al., 1991). Co-administration of zidovudine (200 mg per m^2) and didanosine (100 mg per m^2) in children does not significantly alter the pharmacokinetics of either drug. The elimination half-life of zidovudine was 1.4 $\pm$ 0.4 and 1.2 $\pm$ 0.2 h and the AUC was 14.2 $\pm$ 4.9 and 15.8 $\pm$ 7.2 μmol per h per liter in the presence and absence of didanosine respectively, with no alteration in the peak serum concentration, time to peak concentration or oral clearance (Mueller et al., 1994; Gibb et al., 1995).

Concurrent administration of zidovudine and foscarnet also does not alter the pharmacokinetic parameters of either drug (Aweeka et al., 1992). When zidovudine is co-administered with saquinavir there is no added toxicity over the individual profiles of these compounds, although formal pharmacokinetic data on their interactions are not yet available (Vella, 1994a). The co-administration of aciclovir and zidovudine does not affect hepatic glucuronidation of zidovudine, nor alter other pharmacokinetic parameters of zidovudine (Cload, 1989) (p. 1687). High-dose aciclovir (3200 mg per day) can be safely used with zidovudine, with reported side-effects being an increase in severity (but not incidence) of headaches and somnolence in patients receiving both medications compared with zidovudine alone (Cooper et al., 1991).

The combination of zidovudine (600–1200 mg daily) and ganciclovir (5–10 mg per kg daily; p. 1571) results in severe neutropenia which can be life-threatening and/or severe anemia in the majority of patients with HIV-related serious cytomegalovirus disease (Hochster et al., 1990; Causey, 1991). Zidovudine even at a dose of 500 mg per day is rarely tolerated with ganciclovir therapy, either induction or maintenance therapy (Hochster et al., 1990) and the zidovudine dose should be modified or the drug interrupted depending on the hematologic status of the patient (Causey, 1991). Other toxicities associated with zidovudine and ganciclovir co-therapy including severe vomiting, and severe hepatitis, are much less common.

Recombinant interferon alpha (10–20 million units per day) in combination with zidovudine has been reported to be well-tolerated in one study (Podzamczer et al., 1993); however, in most studies both hematologic and non-hematologic, dose-limiting toxicity (malaise, anorexia, fatigue and fever) have been dose-limiting (Krown et al., 1992a). In a phase I open-label study using daily subcutaneous injections of human lymphoblastoid interferon alpha (5–35 million units) in combination with zidovudine, neutropenia, thrombocytopenia and hepatic dysfunction occurred with higher frequency than had been anticipated, suggesting synergistic toxicity. Patients receiving 250 mg zidovudine were generally unable to tolerate 10 million units per day of interferon alpha, whereas the majority of patients receiving 100 mg per day of zidovudine tolerated 10–15 million units per day of interferon alpha (Kovacs et al., 1989). Neutropenia has also been the major dose-limiting toxicity in persons receiving interferon alpha 2a (4.5–18 million units per day) with hepatotoxicity, thrombocytopenia, anemia and fatigue also being significant side-effects; daily doses of 4.5 million units of interferon alpha 2a are tolerated by the majority of patients when given in combination with 200 mg zidovudine per day (Krown et al., 1990, 1992a,b). The addition of granulocyte-macrophage colony stimulating factor (GM-CSF) to zidovudine and interferon alpha combination therapy does not prevent the development of anorexia, fatigue and myalgia (Davey et al., 1991).

The enzymes required for glucuronidation of zidovudine may be inhibited by drugs which also undergo hepatic glucuronidation, resulting in prolongation of the half-life of zidovudine. These include probenecid, non-steroidal anti-inflammatory agents, narcotic analgesics, sulfonamide antibiotics (see below) (Yarchoan et al., 1989). Glucuronidation of zidovudine by human and animal microsomal preparations is also impaired by probenecid (Sim et al., 1991; Wong et al., 1992). In HIV-infected patients, zidovudine (100 mg) co-administered with probenecid (500mg) resulted in serum concentration time curves for zidovudine similar to those derived following 200 mg of zidovudine, but with a shorter time to T_{max} and a longer half-life (McDermott et al., 1992). Probenecid has also been reported to increase the amount of unmetabolized zidovudine from the urine in humans (Kornhauser et al., 1989). Atovaquone has been found to inhibit the glucuronidation of zidovudine, resulting in a significant increase in the AUC of zidovudine (Lee et al., 1996).

In the rat model, zidovudine has been found to inhibit completely glucuronidation of acetaminophen (paracetamol), whilst the latter only slightly inhibited glucuronidation of zidovudine (Ameer et al., 1992). Studies using human liver microsomes have demonstrated that acetaminophen does not inhibit zidovudine metabolism (Sim et al., 1991). Furthermore, neither zidovudine clearance nor production of the glucuronide conjugate was impaired in patients with AIDS who received acetaminophen and zidovudine every 4–6 h (Steffe et al., 1990; Sattler et al., 1991; Burger et al., 1994a). However, severe hepatotoxicity has been reported in a patient undergoing zidovudine therapy who received 3.3 g of acetaminophen over a 24 h period (Shriner and Goetz, 1992). Microsomal glucuronidation of zidovudine has been reported to be inhibited by chloramphenicol, indomethacin, naproxen, and ethinylestradiol, testosterone, codeine, morphine (Rajaonarison et al., 1992; Sim et al., 1991). Amphotericin B, ketoconazole, miconazole and fluconazole inhibit the formation of the glucuronide metabolite in vitro, whereas itraconazole and 5-fluorocytosine have no effect (Sampol et al., 1995). Ibuprofen and zidovudine co-therapy in hemophiliac men with HIV infection has been found to cause abnormal platelet aggregation with arachidonic acid, a low platelet adhesive index, a prolonged bleeding time and an increased frequency of spontaneous hemorrhages (Ragni et al., 1992a). It is unclear whether zidovudine alters phenytoin pharmacokinetics with early reports suggesting that zidovudine did interfere with phenytoin levels, and a more recent study suggesting that there is no interaction (Burger et al., 1994b). Until clarified, phenytoin levels should be carefully monitored in patients receiving zidovudine.

Zidovudine must be ceased or given in low dose and with extreme caution if used in conjunction with chemotherapeutic agents or other drugs which cause anemia or leukopenia, including high-dose co-trimoxazole, interferon (Tirelli *et al.*, 1992). In the murine model 5-fluorouracil enhances zidovudine cytotoxicity (Brunetti *et al.*, 1990). A number of cancer chemotherapeutic agents can inhibit the production of glucuronide metabolite of zidovudine *in vitro*. These include cyclophosphamide, methotrexate, etoposide, and vinblastine. However, the investigators considered that only cyclophosphamide should inhibit hepatic glucuronidation of zidovudine *in vivo* (Rajaonarison *et al.*, 1993).

Drugs that can significantly (by >50%) inhibit phosphorylation of zidovudine include ribavirin, and doxorubicin. Itraconazole, ganciclovir, and foscarnet have been found to modestly (by 10–15%) inhibit phosphorylation (Hoggard *et al.*, 1995).

Zidovudine therapy is well tolerated in patients also receiving isoniazid and rifampin for the treatment of *Mycobacterium tuberculosis* (Kavesh *et al.*, 1989; Antoniskis *et al.*, 1992). However, rifampin co-administration with zidovudine results in a higher clearance of zidovudine, and thus potentially lower zidovudine plasma levels, compared with these obtained with zidovudine therapy alone (Burger *et al.*, 1993a). Similarly, co-administration of clarithromycin may lower zidovudine levels. Rifabutin and zidovudine co-administration does not have any clinically significant pharmacokinetic interactions (Gallicano *et al.*, 1995).

No significant drug interaction has been observed between zidovudine and methadone, although in a study of nine patients the average AUC of zidovudine was 1.4-fold higher in methadone recipients than in controls (Schwartz *et al.*, 1992),

Clinical Uses of the Drug

A Zidovudine treatment of human immunodeficiency virus infection

The use of zidovudine in persons with advanced HIV infection has clearly been shown to be of benefit in delaying development of opportunistic infections and improving survival. In individuals with no symptoms and relatively well-preserved CD4 lymphocyte numbers, the benefits are less clear. However, data demonstrating the production of greater than 1 billion virions per day from the time of initial HIV infection has influenced most clinicians to commence therapy early in the course of HIV infection (arguments for early therapy are reviewed in Richman and Havlir, 1995 and Ho, 1995). Given the difficulties in interpreting the data from the clinical trials, the decision as to when to institute antiretroviral therapy usually depends on both the preference of the individual and the views of the physician. Zidovudine monotherapy is no longer acceptable therapy, based on the recent data showing the superiority of combination therapy using zalcitabine or didanosine with zidovudine over zidovudine monotherapy. Data from the use of double nucleoside analogs with a protease inhibitor have resulted in a radical change to the practise of many physicians. In addition, international recommendations regarding antiretroviral therapy suggest that the HIV RNA in plasma in conjunction with the CD4 count, should be used as a guide for treatment, and recommend that therapy should be offered to all patients whose viral load is greater than 5000–10 000 copies per ml (Carpenter *et al.*, 1996). The authors' current practice is to offer combination therapy that often includes zidovudine to all HIV-infected individuals with a CD4 count of less than 500 cells per μl (Crowe *et al.*, 1996), or for those whose plasma HIV RNA exceeds 500–10 000 copies per ml regardless of CD4 count. However, there are no data from prospective trials to support this latter recommendation. Currently, zidovudine is most commonly used in combination with another nucleoside analog (such as lamivudine, or didanosine, or zalcitabine), together with a protease inhibitor or a non-nucleoside reverse transcriptase inhibitor. Other issues such as lifestyle changes and compliance must be considered on an individual basis when commencing or changing treatment.

The evolution of the clinical use of zidovudine in clinical medicine can be seen from a chronological review of clinical trials with this drug.

1 Major clinical trials with zidovudine monotherapy

a Patients with advanced (symptomatic) HIV infection The first clinical trial was in 19 patients with AIDS or AIDS-related complex who received i.v. therapy for 2 weeks followed by oral treatment. Clinical, immunologic and virologic benefit was noted, with clearance of chronic fungal nailbed infections, weight gain, an increase in CD4 lymphocyte numbers in three-quarters of the patients, improved delayed type hypersensitivity reactions and reversion to negative viral culture of peripheral blood mononuclear cells (Yarchoan *et al.*, 1986).

As a result of the relative success of this pilot study, a phase II multicenter, double-blind, placebo-controlled trial (BW-02) was undertaken in 282 patients with AIDS or advanced AIDS-related complex who received 250 mg of zidovudine or placebo orally 4-hourly for 24 weeks. Mortality and the frequency and severity of opportunistic infections were significantly less in patients who were randomized to receive zidovudine than in the placebo group (Fig. V.36). Immunologic benefit was also more commonly observed in patients receiving zidovudine than placebo, with an increase in CD4 cell number and partial reversal of skin-test anergy (Fischl *et al.*, 1987). The increase in CD4 cell number was evident within the first 1–2 months in patients receiving zidovudine but thereafter declined; by week 20 CD4 number had often returned to base-line levels (Fischl *et al.*, 1987, 1989). Improvements in survival, however, were found to persist beyond 18 months of therapy (Creagh-Kirk *et al.*, 1988; Fischl *et al.*, 1989).

In a randomized, double-blind, placebo-controlled study (ACTG 016) of 711 mildly symptomatic persons with early AIDS-related complex (one or two symptoms) and a CD4 lymphocyte count of greater than 200 cells per μl who were followed for 9 months, zidovudine (200 mg every 4 h) delayed progression to advanced AIDS-related complex or AIDS and improved CD4 counts in those with CD4 counts of 200–500 cells per μl, but was of no obvious benefit in those with 500–800 cells per μl (there were too few events in this group for analysis). No difference in survival was observed, but only two deaths occurred during the trial (Fischl *et al.*, 1990a).

The Veterans Affairs Co-operative Study examined the effects of early versus deferred therapy in 338 patients with symptomatic AIDS-related complex and CD4 lymphocyte numbers of 200–500 cells per μl. Patients were randomized to receive zidovudine in a dose of 1500 mg per day on study entry (defined as 'early' therapy) or placebo until they developed an AIDS-defining illness or their CD4 number fell below 200 cells per μl ('late' therapy). Although 'early' therapy delayed disease progression, it did not improve survival (Hamilton *et al.*, 1992). Long-term follow-up (an additional 3 years beyond the 4-year trial) supported these initial results in that 'early' therapy delayed progression to AIDS but did not affect survival (Simberkoff *et al.*, 1996). Progression to AIDS strongly correlated with baseline CD4 counts and plasma HIV RNA (O'Brien *et al.*, 1996).

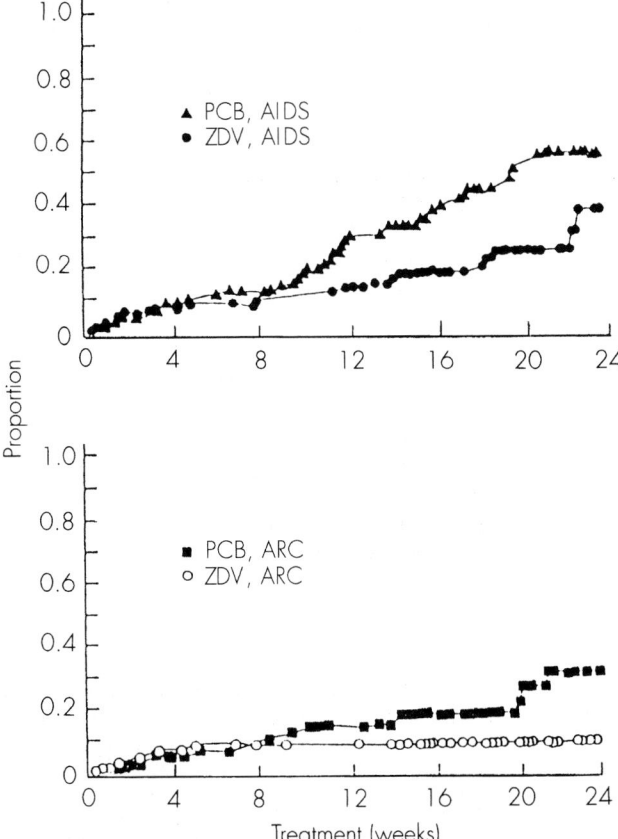

Fig. V.36.

Proportion of patients in whom opportunistic infections developed during the BW-02 study (Kaplan-Meier Product Limit Method). The upper panel shows infection among patients with AIDS who were receiving zidovudine (ZDV) or placebo (PCB), and the lower panel shows infection among those with AIDS- related complex (ARC). (Reproduced from Fischl *et al.*, 1987, with permission.)

A study of 2162 patients within the Multicenter AIDS Cohort found that regardless of presence or absence of symptoms, zidovudine therapy for HIV-infected individuals with CD4 lymphocyte numbers in the range of 200–350 cells per μl resulted in significantly reduced mortality. The effects of zidovudine in delaying progression to AIDS is often difficult to dissect within a population due to the concurrent and widespread use of primary prophylaxis for *Pneumocystis carinii* pneumonia, the latter having been shown to reduce the probability of developing *P. carinii* pneumonia (Graham *et al.*, 1991b). Adjusting for the effects of prophylaxis for *P. carinii* pneumonia, zidovudine therapy alone reduced mortality for up to 18 months (Graham *et al.*, 1992). Survival after a diagnosis of AIDS was longer in those who commenced zidovudine prior to the diagnosis compared with those who never received zidovudine, but was shorter than in those commencing zidovudine post-diagnosis (Saah *et al.*, 1994).

In 1102 patients with advanced HIV infection with fewer than 200 CD4 cells per μl, treatment with zidovudine and didnosine or zalcitabine was not superior to zidovudine monotherapy (Saravolatz *et al.*, 1996).

A number of additional studies of zidovudine therapy for patients with advanced, symptomatic HIV infection support the association between therapy and improved survival (Moore *et al.*, 1992; Vella *et al.*, 1992; Ragni *et al.*, 1992b; Dournon *et al.*, 1988; Stambuk *et al.*, 1989).

b Patients with early (asymptomatic) HIV infection The first randomized, multicenter, placebo-controlled clinical trial of zidovudine therapy in 1434 persons with asymptomatic HIV infection and fewer than 500 CD4 lymphocytes per μl compared two doses of zidovudine (1500 mg and 500 mg daily) with placebo (ACTG 019). The study was prematurely terminated after 24 weeks by an independent data and safety monitoring board when review of data showed that both doses of zidovudine delayed progression of disease compared with placebo. The rates of progression to AIDS or advanced AIDS-related complex were 7.6, 3.6 and 4.3 per 100 person-years in those receiving placebo, low-dose and high-dose respectively (Volberding *et al.*, 1990). An extended follow-up (mean duration 2.6 years) of patients enrolled in this study found that although zidovudine therapy was associated with a significant delay in clinical progression there was no survival benefit (Volberding *et al.*, 1994). Further follow-up (median 4.8 years) suggested that although the decline in CD4 cell numbers was delayed in the initial zidovudine-recipient group compared with those who commenced zidovudine 2 years later when open-label drug was offered to all participants, time to AIDS was not prolonged and, supporting the earlier analysis, there was no overall survival benefit (Fig. V.37) (Volberding *et al.*, 1995). Interestingly, a reduction in quality of life was associated with zidovudine treatment which approximated the improvement in life quality that was derived from the delay in disease progression (Lenderking *et al.*, 1994).

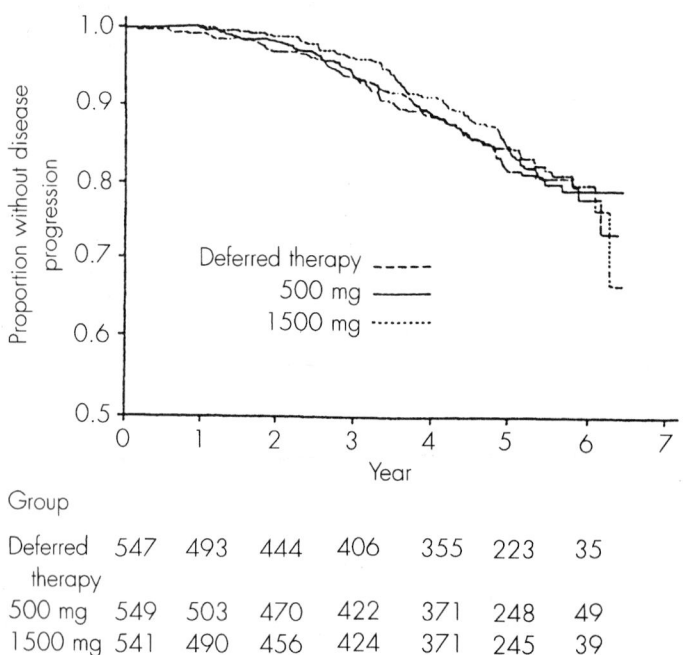

Fig. V.37.
Kaplan-Meier estimates of the progression to AIDS or death, according to treatment group. The number of subjects in the analysis each year is shown below the graph. (Reproduced from Volberding *et al.*, 1995, with permission.)

Group							
Deferred therapy	547	493	444	406	355	223	35
500 mg	549	503	470	422	371	248	49
1500 mg	541	490	456	424	371	245	39

In the European-Australian Collaborative Group placebo-controlled study (EACG 020) of 933 persons with asymptomatic infection and a CD4 lymphocyte number of greater than 400 per μl who were treated with zidovudine (500 mg twice-daily) zidovudine reduced the likelihood of developing symptomatic disease by 50% over a median duration of 2 years follow-up. There were too few end-points of progression to AIDS or death to comment on these parameters (Cooper *et al.*, 1993a).

In the European Concorde study of 1749 asymptomatically HIV-infected persons who were randomized in a double-blind fashion to receive zidovudine (1000 mg per day) on study entry ('immediate' therapy) or to remain on placebo until either the development of symptoms or a fall in the CD4 number to below 500 cells per μl ('deferred' therapy), the 'immediate' use of zidovudine was associated with an initial delay in disease progression but no sustained benefit. Although there was a significant improvement in CD4 lymphocyte numbers which was sustained for the duration of the 3 years of study, there was no significant difference in clinical progression or in survival benefit in those who were in the 'immediate' therapy arm compared with those in the 'deferred' group (Concorde Co-ordinating Committee, 1994).

The European-Australian Collaborative Group (EACG) study 017 compared treatment with zidovudine (500 mg twice-daily) with placebo in 329 individuals with asymptomatic HIV infection and CD4 counts between 200 and 400 cells per μl for a median treatment duration of approximately 60 weeks. Zidovudine therapy was found to significantly delay progression to symptomatic disease, and resulted in better preservation of the CD4 response than that in placebo recipients (Mulder *et al.*, 1994).

2 Major clinical trials using combination or alternating therapy of zidovudine and other nucleoside analogs

In a randomized pilot study in 41 patients with advanced HIV disease (AIDS or AIDS-related complex) and minimal prior antiretroviral treatment who were treated with alternating regimens of zidovudine and didanosine or combination therapy with both drugs, the combination therapy arm was associated with higher and more sustained CD4 counts and a significantly greater weight gain than patients in the group randomized to receive alternating therapy. The median CD4 count at study entry was 183 cells per μl in the simultaneous therapy arm and 202 cells per μl in the alternating therapy arm and the study follow-up was for 1 year (Yarchoan *et al.*, 1994).

A phase II study of complex design (ACTG 047) evaluated alternating and intermittent regimens of zidovudine and zalcitabine in 131 patients with advanced HIV infection, most (96%) of whom had not received zidovudine within 90 days prior to study entry. The data were analyzed for the first 48 weeks of therapy and it was concluded from this study that alternating zidovudine and zalcitabine reduced the toxicity associated with each drug alone whilst providing a sustained antiviral and immunologic benefit and a sustained weight gain over the 48 weeks of the study (Skowron *et al.*, 1993). Alternating therapy of zidovudine (180 mg per m^2 6-hourly for 3 weeks) with zalcitabine (0.015–0.04 mg per kg 6-hourly for 1 week) has also been employed in a clinical trial of children aged from 6 months to 13 years. This regimen was associated with an increase in weight, but no consistent immunologic or virologic benefit compared with monotherapy (Pizzo *et al.*, 1990).

In a dose-ranging trial (ACTG 106) comparing combination therapy of zidovudine (150–600 mg daily) and zalcitabine (0.015–0.03 mg per kg daily) with zidovudine monotherapy (150 mg daily) in 56 patients with advanced HIV infection (AIDS or AIDS-related complex and a CD4 count of less than 200 cells per μl), drug combinations including zidovudine at the 600 mg per day dose were associated with a sustained increase in CD4 number. A criticism in the study design was the low dose used in the zidovudine monotherapy arm which limited the ability to compare monotherapy and combination therapy. This study demonstrated clearly that 150 mg daily of zidovudine was suboptimal (Meng *et al.*, 1992).

In an open-label, partially randomized, dose-ranging study of 69 HIV-infected persons with less than 400 CD4 cells per μl and less than 4 months of prior zidovudine therapy combinations of zidovudine (150–600 mg per day) with didanosine (90–500 mg per day), were compared with zidovudine monotherapy (600 mg per day). The higher dose combinations were associated with a more sustained CD4 response and more frequent decreases in plasma HIV-1 RNA titers than the lower dose combinations or monotherapy (Collier *et al.*, 1993).

ACTG 155 was the first large study to evaluate combination therapy. A total of 1001 patients with advanced HIV infection (either symptomatic infection and CD4 count of less than 300 cells per μl, or asymptomatic infection with CD4 count of less than 200 cells per μl) who had previously tolerated zidovudine for a minimum of 6 months were randomized to receive zidovudine (600 mg per day) or zalcitabine (2.25 mg per day) or the combination of these drugs and followed for a median duration of 17.7 months. The primary endpoint was time to an AIDS-defining illness or death. No difference was found between any of the arms in terms of time to progression or death, with estimated 12-month event-free rates of 70%, 67% and 73% respectively. However, a subgroup analysis suggested that combination therapy may benefit those whose CD4 count was greater than 150 cells per μl at study entry, in terms of both disease progression and survival. There were concerns raised regarding this study in that 38% of patients withdrew for non-protocol-specified reasons, the subgroup analysis was unplanned, and there were frequent interruptions to study medications, particularly in the combination group (Fischl et al., 1995). Others considered, however, that the subgroup analysis was in fact valid and that the data supported findings from Delta, CPCRA 007 and ACTG 175 (D.Cooper, personal communication).

ACTG 175 was a randomized double-blind study comparing monotherapy with either zidovudine (600 mg per day) or didanosine (400 mg per day) with combination therapy using zidovudine with either zalcitabine (2.25 mg per day) or didanosine in patients with CD4 counts between 200 and 500 cells per μl and no prior AIDS defining illness except minimal Kaposi's sarcoma. The primary study endpoints were a 50% decline in CD4 count, progression to AIDS or death. The median duration of follow-up was 118 weeks. There was premature discontinuation of study treatment in 53% of participants. The majority of endpoints occurred in the antiretroviral experienced patients. The risk of progression to a primary endpoint was greatest in patients randomized to receive zidovudine monotherapy and was not significantly different between didanosine monotherapy or either of the combination therapy groups. For zidovudine-naive patients combination therapy with zidovudine and zalcitabine was significantly better than didanosine therapy. For experienced patients zidovudine and didanosine combination therapy was superior to either didanosine monotherapy or zalcitabine and zidovudine combination therapy (Table V.25) (Hammer et al,. 1996; Katzenstein et al., 1996).

Table V.25

Survival and disease progression. (Reproduced from Delta Co-ordinating Committee, 1996, with permission.)

	No of events/No at risk			Summary hazard ratios (95% CI)			p
	ZDV	ZDV + ddI	ZDV + ddC	ZDV + ddI vs ZDV alone	ZDV + ddC vs ZDV alone	ZDV + ddI vs ZDV + ddC	Global log rank test of 2 degrees of freedom
Deaths							
Delta 1	149/700	93/718	107/706	0.58 (0.45–0.75)	0.68 (0.53–0.88)	0.85 (0.64–1.12)	0.00006
Delta 2	126/355	103/362	121/366	0.77 (0.59–1.00)	0.91 (0.71–1.17)	0.84 (0.65–1.09)	0.14
All participants	275/1055	196/1080	228/1072	0.67 (0.56–0.80)	0.79 (0.66–0.94)	0.85 (0.70–1.02)	0.00006
AIDS or death							
Delta 1	211/620	145/627	182/615	0.64 (0.51–0.79)	0.83 (0.68–1.02)	0.76 (0.61–0.95)	0.0001
Delta 2	135/297	133/306	130/300	0.95 (0.75–1.21)	0.94 (0.74–1.20)	1.01 (0.79–1.28)	0.87
All participants	348/917	278/933	312/915	0.76 (0.65–0.89)	0.88 (0.75–1.02)	0.86 (0.73–1.01)	0.002
Advanced AIDS or death							
Delta 1	51/79	30/86	39/90	0.46 (0.30–0.73)	0.56 (0.37–0.86)	0.82 (0.51–1.33)	0.001
Delta 2	38/54	29/55	41/63	0.60 (0.37–0.98)	0.97 (0.62–1.51)	0.62 (0.39–1.01)	0.08
All participants	89/133	59/141	80/153	0.52 (0.38–0.73)	0.73 (0.54–0.98)	0.72 (0.52–1.01)	0.005
New AIDS event or death							
Delta 1	270/700	188/718	231/706	0.63 (0.53–0.76)	0.80 (0.67–0.76)	0.79 (0.65–0.96)	0.000008
Delta 2	178/355	165/362	175/366	0.87 (0.70–1.07)	0.95 (0.77–1.17)	0.92 (0.74–1.14)	0.43
All participants	448/1055	353/1080	406/1072	0.73 (0.63–0.84)	0.86 (0.75–0.98)	0.85 (0.73–0.98)	0.00004

ZDV: zidovudine; ddI: didanosine; ddC: zalcitabine.

The Delta study was a trial of zidovudine monotherapy or in combination with zalcitabine or didanosine in patients with AIDS or ARC or a CD4 count of less than 350 cells per µl. A total of 2124 zidovudine-naive patients were enrolled in Delta 1 and 1083 patients with a minimum of 3 months prior zidovudine treatment were enrolled into Delta 2. The primary endpoints were progression to AIDS or death. The mean CD4 counts at study entry for Delta 1 and Delta 2 were 213 cells per µl and 189 cells per µl espectively. Those enrolled in Delta 2 had received prior zidovudine for a median of 15–18 months (range 9–30 months). There was premature discontinuation of study medication in 71% of participants in Delta 1 and 80% of participants in Delta 2. The protocol was amended after study commencement to allow those patients who reached a clinical endpoint or who had participated for more than 2 years in the study to either change to open-label of the opposite study combination or to commence zidovudine plus lamivudine. The median follow up was 30 months. Analysis of data from Delta 1 provided strong evidence that combination therapy was superior to zidovudine monotherapy in terms of survival with an estimated reduction in mortality of 42% and 32% respectively for those treated with zidovudine and didanosine or zidovudine and zalcitabine versus zidovudine monotherapy. In Delta 2, addition of didanosine to zidovudiune resulted in a significant (23%) reduction in mortality, and although there was a trend in improved survival (9% reduction in mortality) in those who added zalcitabine to zidovudine therapy this was not significant (Table V.25) (Delta Co-ordinating Committee 1996).

The Community Programs for Clinical Research on AIDS study CPCRA 007 compared zidovudine alone with zidovudine and either didanosine or zalcitabine in 1102 patients with a diagnosis of AIDS or less than 200 CD4 cells per µl. After a median follow-up of 35 months, combination therapy with zidovudine and either didanosine or zalcitabine was not superior to zidovudine alone in terms of disease progression or survival, in this group or patients. It is important to note that 75% of the participants had received prior zidovudine treatment (Saravolatz *et al.*, 1996).

Treatment with lamivudine (300 mg twice-daily) or zidovudine (600 mg daily) mono-therapy or a combination of both drugs (300 mg twice-daily or 150 mg twice-daily of

Fig. V.38.

Mean (±SE) changes from baseline in the log concentration of HIV RNA, according to the week of the NUCA 3001 study. The number of patients shown for each week in each treatment group is the number who could be evaluated at that time. After week 24, the numbers of patients indicate the numbers available for study at each point in the analysis; the numbers do not indicate rates of withdrawal from the study. Some patients had not completed the extended phase of the study by the time of this analysis. (Reproduced from Eron *et al.*, 1995, with permission.)

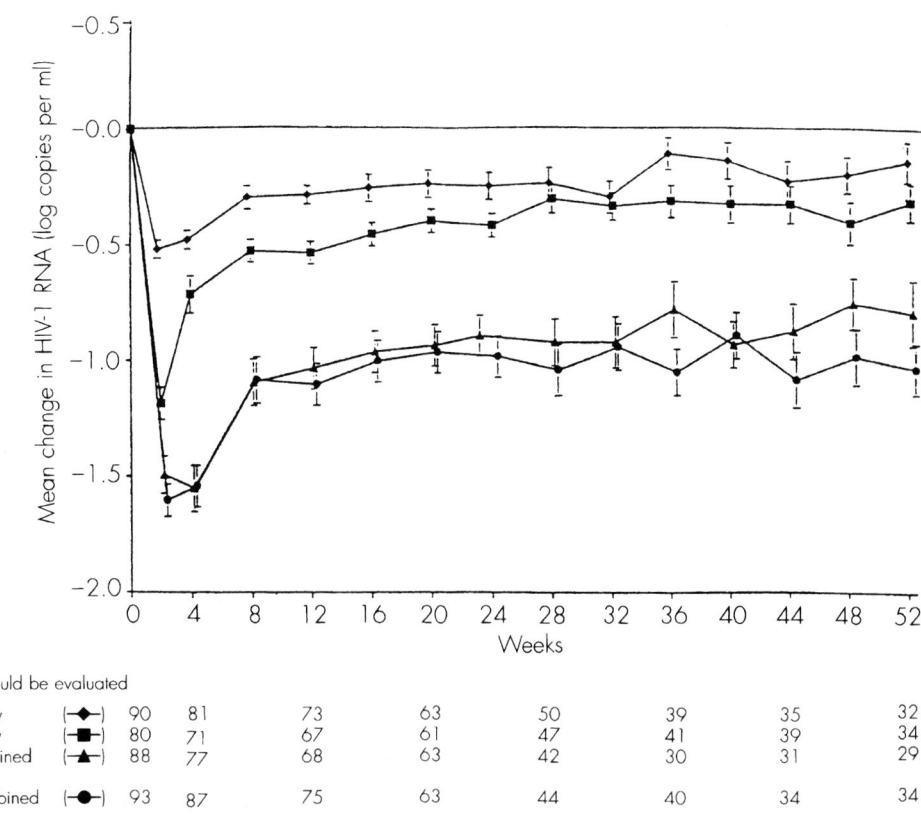

Patients who could be evaluated

Zidovudine only	(—◆—)	90	81	73	63	50	39	35	32
Lamivudine only	(—■—)	80	71	67	61	47	41	39	34
Low-dose combined therapy	(—▲—)	88	77	68	63	42	30	31	29
High-dose combined therapy	(—●—)	93	87	75	63	44	40	34	34

lamivudine, 600 mg of zidovudine daily) has been assessed in a randomized, double-blind trial conducted by the North American HIV Working Party in 366 HIV-infected patients with 200–500 CD4 cells per μl who had received up to 4 weeks of zidovudine prior to study entry (trial NUCA 3001). The study lasted 24 weeks with a 28-week extension phase. There was a sustained and higher increase in CD4 cell counts and a sustained and greater decline in HIV plasma RNA in the two combination therapy arms compared with either monotherapy group (Fig. V.38), persisting for the 52 weeks of follow-up (Eron *et al.*, 1995). This is despite the rapid emergence of lamivudine-resistant strains of HIV (Larder *et al.*, 1995a). A similar trial (NUCB 3001) was conducted in Europe, in which 129 HIV-infected persons with CD4 counts of 100–400 cells per μl and less than 4 weeks of prior zidovudine therapy were randomized to receive zidovudine as monotherapy or in combination with lamivudine 300 mg twice-daily for 24 weeks. Again, combination therapy was superior to monotherapy in terms of improvement in CD4 counts (an increase of 80 versus 20 cells per μl in those who received combination versus monotherapy respectively) and decline in HIV RNA (a decline of 1.33 log_{10} copies per ml compared with 0.57 log_{10} copies per ml in those who received combination and monotherapy respectively), with changes sustained for 48 weeks in those who elected to continue combination therapy (Katlama *et al.*, 1996).

In study NUCB 3002, conducted in Europe, HIV-infected patients with 100–400 CD4 cells per μl and a minimum of 24 weeks of prior zidovudine were randomized to receive lamivudine (either 150 mg twice-daily or 300 mg twice-daily) in combination with zidovudine versus zidovudine monotherapy for 24 weeks with an optional open-label 24-week extension phase in which participants all received combination therapy. Those who continued zidovudine monotherapy had no immunologic or virologic improvement as measured by CD4 counts or HIV RNA; those receiving combination therapy had a sustained decline in HIV RNA (0.59 and 1.06 log_{10} copies per ml for the lower and higher lamivudine groups respectively) and increase in CD4 counts (an increase of 40 and 30 cells per μl for the lower and higher lamivudine containing regimens respectively) (reviewed in Staszewski, 1995; Staszewski *et al.*, 1996). The NUCA 3002 study is described on p. 1754.

In another ACTG trial, 302 patients who had received prior zidovudine therapy for a median of 27 months and who had CD4 counts of 50–300 cells per μl were randomized to received saquinavir in combination wtih zidovudine and zalcitabine or zidovudine plus either zalcitabine or saquinavir for 24 weeks. The normalized AUC for CD4 and decline in plasma HIV RNA were significantly greater for the triple combination than for either of the double-combination regimens (Fig. V.39) (Collier *et al.*, 1996).

The ACTG 241 trial evaluated triple-combination therapy using nevirapine, zidovudine and didanosine versus zidovudine and didanosine in 398 HIV-infected, nucleoside-experienced patients with less than 350 CD4 cells per μl. Adding nevirapine to zidovudine and didanosine resulted in sustained higher CD4 counts and lower plasma HIV RNA levels than receiving the double combination (see p. 1774 for details) (D'Aquila *et al.*, 1996).

Fig. V.39.
Zidovudine-experienced, HIV-infected patients with < 350 CD4 cells per μl, receiving triple or double combination therapy (ACTG 229). Median plasma levels of HIV RNA in the study patients as determined by reverse transcriptase PCR, according to treatment group and study week. The numbers below the graphs are the numbers of patients studied in the weeks shown.
(Reproduced from Collier *et al.*, 1996, with permission.)

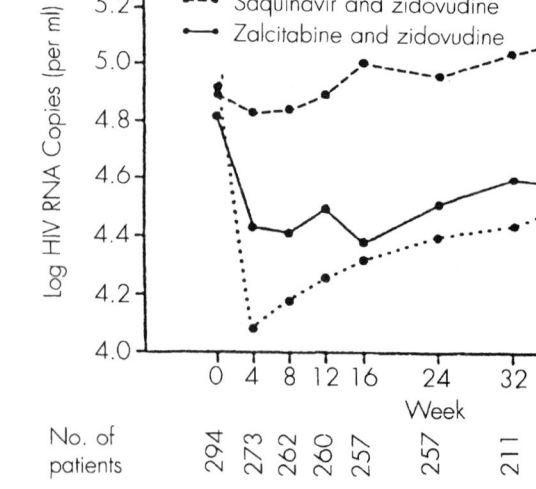

3 Clinical trials of didanosine or zalcitabine compared with zidovudine monotherapy in patients with zidovudine experience

A randomized double-blind trial compared monotherapy with zidovudine (1200 or 600 mg per day) or zalcitabine (0.75 mg three times daily) in 668 patients who were either zidovudine-naive or who had less than 3 months of zidovudine therapy and who had AIDS or ARC and less than 200 CD4 cells per µl (ACTG 114). Zidovudine was found to be more beneficial than zalcitabine in prolonging survival. It was concluded from this study that zidovudine was superior to zalcitabine as initial therapy in terms of clinical as well as functional outcomes, and monotherapy with zalcitabine is thus reserved only for patients intolerant of, or failing other therapies (reviewed in Murphy, 1995; Spooner et al., 1995; Bozzette et al., 1995) .

Zidovudine (600 mg per day) was compared with didanosine (500 or 750 mg per day) in a study of 617 patients with advanced HIV infection (AIDS or advanced ARC with less than 300 CD4 cells per µl or asymptomatic HIV infection and less than 200 CD4 cells per µl) and less than 16 weeks of prior zidovudine therapy (ACTG 116A). Primary endpoints were the development of a new AIDS defining illness or death. In the 380 patients who were zidovudine-naive, zidovudine was superior to didanosine in terms of progression to AIDS or a new opportunistic infection or death. However, in those who had been exposed to 1–8 weeks of prior zidovudine (n = 119) there was no difference between zidovudine and didanosine. For the 118 patients who had received 8–16 weeks of prior zidovudine therapy didanosine (500 mg daily dose) was associated with less progression than zidovudine, and the 750 mg daily dose of didanosine was associated with greater survival, although two patients in this arm died of pancreatitis. Overall there was no significant difference between the two doses of didanosine (Dolin et al., 1995).

In ACTG 116B/117, 913 patients with AIDS or ARC and a CD4 count of less than 300 cells per µl or asymptomatic HIV infection and a CD4 count of less than 200 cells per µl with greater than 16 weeks of prior zidovudine therapy were randomized to continue zidovudine (600 mg per day) or switch to didanosine (375 mg twice-daily or 250 mg twice-daily). At study entry the median duration of prior zidovudine was 13.9 months. There was no survival benefit seen with

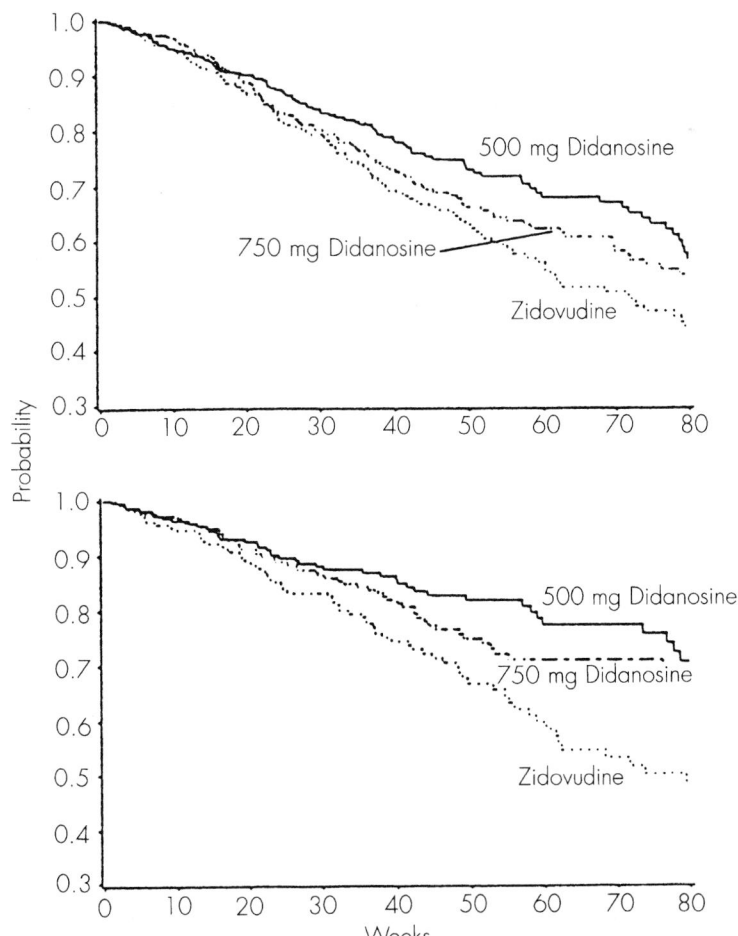

Fig. V.40.
Probability of a new, non-recurrent AIDS-defining event or death in the three study groups in ACTG 116B/117. The curves shown represent the entire study population of 913 subjects with AIDS, AIDS-related complex, or asymptomatic HIV infection. (Reproduced from Kahn et al., 1992, with permission.)

either therapy group, but patients randomized to didanosine had less progression than zidovudine recipients (Fig. V.40). The 500-mg daily dose was superior to the 750-mg daily dose of didanosine, and was less toxic (Kahn *et al.*, 1992). In a retrospective substudy analysis of 187 patients from whom baseline HIV-1 isolates had been stored it was found that the clinical benefit in switching from zidovudine to didanosine was not limited to patients with high-level zidovudine-resistance (D'Aquila *et al.*, 1995). Two-thirds of isolates obtained from participants at study entry contained mutations in codons 215 or 41 (Japour *et al.*, 1995).

A complementary study was performed by the Canadian HIV Trials Network Study Group (protocol 002) in which 246 HIV-infected patients with 200–500 CD4 cells per μl and a minimum of 6 months prior zidovudine therapy were randomized to remain on zidovudine therapy or to switch to didanosine. The primary endpoint was the development of a new AIDS-defining illness or death. At study entry 66% were asymptomatic, and 34% symptomatic including 4% with AIDS; the median CD4 count was 320 cells per μl, and median prior duration of zidovudine therapy was 471 days. Similar numbers (21% and 28% in the zidovudine and didanosine groups respectively) had evidence of high-level zidovudine-resistance at baseline. Eight zidovudine recipients and one didanosine recipient developed a new AIDS-defining illness; didanosine recipients had a significant increase in CD4 cell number that persisted for the 48-week duration of the study (Montaner *et al.*, 1995).

In the Bristol AI454–010 study, 312 patients with less than 300 CD4 cells per μl, evidence of clinical deterioration and a minimum of 6 months prior zidovudine therapy were randomized to zidovudine (600 mg per day) or didanosine (600 mg per day, adjusted for weight). The primary endpoints were a new AIDS-defining illness, development of two new or recurrent HIV-related symptoms and a 50% decline in CD4 cell count, or death. There was a 50% risk of reaching an endpoint in patients randomized to continue zidovudine monotherapy. However, switching to didanosine was associated with the development of fewer endpoints. There was no difference in survival between the two groups (Spruance *et al.*, 1994).

4 Other supportive studies of zidovudine monotherapy and combination therapy with didanosine or zalcitabine

In a retrospective study of persons who developed AIDS after April 1987 (when zidovudine became available in the USA), the median survival of patients who received zidovudine was 770 days compared with 190 days in untreated individuals (Moore *et al.*, 1991b). In a separate study, survival of patients with AIDS who were treated with zidovudine was greater than 73% after 44 weeks of therapy, and was positively influenced by pre-therapy hemoglobin of >120 g per liter, Karnofsky score of 90 or above and a diagnosis of *P. carinii* pneumonia within 90 days prior to commencing therapy (Creagh-Kirk *et al.*, 1988). A more recent study compared survival in patients treated and not treated with zidovudine and found that if zidovudine treatment is commenced following a diagnosis of AIDS, prognosis was improved, but for no longer than 2 years after initiating therapy (Lundgren *et al.*, 1994). In a study of patient survival, Easterbrook and colleagues (Easterbrook *et al.*, 1993) have found that the rate of CD4 decline during the first year of zidovudine treatment, rather than the occurrence of an initial increase in CD4 cell number, was predictive of survival.

There are data from the Italian Zidovudine Evaluation Group which suggest that zidovudine can delay clinical progression in asymptomatic patients for more than 2 years (Vella *et al.*, 1994a). In a prospective multicenter cohort study of patients with symptomatic HIV infection prior to an AIDS diagnosis doses of zidovudine in excess of 1000 mg per day were associated with more rapid progression (Vella *et al.*, 1995). The Italian Zidovudine Evaluation Group described an evaluation of zidovudine therapy in 936 asymptomatic HIV-infected individuals with less than 500 CD4 cells per μl (median CD4 at entry was 308 per μl). After a median follow-up of 55 weeks, the progression rate to AIDS was 3.2 events per 100 person-years, similar to that found in ACTG 019 (Vella *et al.*, 1994b). Zidovudine therapy has also been shown to reduce the incidence of heterosexual transmission of HIV in a study of 436 monogamous female partners of zidovudine-treated, HIV-infected males (Musicco *et al.*, 1994). The Australian Zidovudine Study group studied the efficacy and safety of zidovudine (1200 mg per day) in 235 patients with symptomatic HIV infection without an AIDS-defining illness, and found the median time to progression to AIDS was 61 weeks in those who received zidovudine, and 22 weeks in a small control group of 22 untreated patients (Swanson *et al.*, 1994).

5 Clinical trials of zidovudine alternating or in combination with other antiviral drugs

a Zidovudine and non-nucleoside reverse transcriptase inhibitors Ten antiretroviral-naive HIV-infected individuals were treated for 9–13 weeks with an alternating regimen of zidovudine (600 mg per day) for 3 weeks and nevirapine (200 mg per day) for 1 week, without evidence of preventing nevirapine-resistance or prolonging benefit from this drug (de Jong *et* *al.*, 1994). An open-label, phase I/II trial comparing zidovudine monotherapy (600 mg per day) with nevirapine (12.5, 50 and 200 mg per day) in combination with zidovudine in 62 patients with HIV infection and less than 400 CD4 cells per μl showed a reduction in HIV p24 antigen that persisted for more than 12 weeks despite rapid emergence of nevirapine-resistant strains of HIV (in all patients by 8 weeks of therapy) (Cheeseman *et al.*, 1995). A phase I combination study (ACTG 199) of atervidine and zidovudine in 15 antiretroviral-naive HIV-infected patients demonstrated immunologic improvement in 47% of patients with isolates from 62% of patients retaining sensitivity to atervidine after 24 weeks of therapy (Reichman *et al.*, 1995).

b   Zidovudine and protease inhibitors   A randomized, double-blind study of saquinavir compared monotherapy with saquinavir (600 mg three times daily), or zidovudine (200 mg three times daily), versus combination therapy with saquinavir in three doses (75, 200 or 600 mg three times daily) plus zidovudine (200 mg three times daily) was conducted in 92 HIV-infected, antiretroviral-naive patients with less than 300 CD4 cells per μl. The CD4 counts increased in all treatment groups, but were higher and more sustained in the combination therapy arms. The higher doses of saquinavir in combination with zidovudine were superior than the 75-mg dose, although inconsistencies were evident (200-mg dose superior in terms of CD4 response, 600-mg dose superior in terms of HIV RNA response) (Vella 1994a, 1996).

c   Zidovudine and interleukin-2   A good immunologic response with no significant change in viral burden was found in a phase I study of subcutaneous recombinant interleukin-2 (0.2–2 million units per m^2) given on 5 consecutive days in combination with oral zidovudine to 16 patients with advanced HIV infection (McMahon *et al.*, 1994). The safety and efficacy of polyethylene glycol (PEG)-modified interleukin 2 given by three-weekly infusions with continuous oral zidovudine to 19 HIV-infected persons was examined in a phase I/II dose-ranging study. Again, there were promising increases in CD4 numbers, natural killer cell activity and cytotoxic T cell responses without evidence of an increase in viral load (Wood *et al.*, 1993). These data were supported by results of a similar study in which PEG interleukin-2 was administered intradermally twice-weekly for 4 months to 13 HIV-infected patients also receiving zidovudine therapy (Teppler *et al.*, 1993).

d   Zidovudine and interferon alpha   Zidovudine with various sources of interferon alpha have been evaluated as combination therapy for the treatment of Kaposi's sarcoma in the setting of HIV infection (Kovacs *et al.*, 1989). In several studies of this combination, partial or complete tumor response occurred in about half of the participants (Kovacs *et al.*, 1989; Krown *et al.*, 1990), with best responses occurring in patients with more than 200 CD4 lymphocytes per μl (Podzamczer *et al.*, 1993). Both hematologic and non-hematologic dose-limiting toxicities have occurred in most trials (see Drug Interactions). A dose of 10 million units per day combined with zidovudine (500–800 mg per day) is relatively well-tolerated and still achieves a tumor response in over 40% of patients (Podzamczer *et al.*, 1993). Low-dose and long-term therapy with zidovudine and interferon alpha (3 million units three times per week administered to 17 patients with early but progressive Kaposi's sarcoma in combination with zidovudine resulted in a complete or partial remission in 11 (65%), all of whom had CD4 counts greater than 250 cells per liter, and lasting more than 2 years in four of the 11 patients (Mauss and Jablonowski, 1995).

Although some antiretroviral benefit has been observed in patients receiving the combination, this appears to be only short-term (Edlin *et al.*, 1992), and dependent on the doses that can be tolerated of both antivirals (Krown *et al.*, 1992a). The Zidon Study Group (Fernandez-Cruz *et al.*, 1995) reported on a comparison of zidovudine monotherapy with zidovudine and lymphoblastoid interferon alpha (3 million units given subcutaneously three times per week) in 402 HIV-infected persons in Europe, Australia and Canada with CD4 counts between 150 and 500 cells per μl. There was no advantage of the combination therapy over zidovudine monotherapy in terms of disease progression or CD4 decline.

e   Zidovudine and aciclovir   Combination therapy of zidovudine (600–1000 mg per day) and aciclovir (3200–4800 mg per day) has been well tolerated with some possible evidence for immunologic and virologic benefit (Surbone *et al.*, 1988; Cooper *et al.*, 1991). In addition, a survival advantage has been found in two randomized, placebo-controlled trials and one observational study of patients receiving aciclovir and zidovudine cotherapy compared with those receiving zidovudine alone (Cooper *et al.*, 1993b; Youle *et al.*, 1994; Stein *et al.*, 1994).

The absence of a proven mechanism has caused the results of these trials to be viewed by some clinicians with scepticism. In a multivariate analysis of prognostic factors for survival in a cohort of patients with CD4 counts of less than 50 cells per µl, longer survival was associated with concurrent aciclovir and zidovudine therapy (Apolonio et al., 1995). Although the dose required to provide this survival advantage has not been determined, it appears that 600–800 mg per day may be sufficient (Stein et al., 1994).

Other studies have not found an association with aciclovir and zidovudine cotherapy and survival. The Zidovudine Epidemiology Study Group performed an observational study of 1044 patients at all stages of HIV infection following commencement of zidovudine, 336 of whom also received regular aciclovir (800 mg per day). There was a trend towards increased mortality among aciclovir users versus non-users (Gallant et al., 1995). In a double-blind and randomized study involving 334 patients, aciclovir (4 g per day) as cotherapy with zidovudine was compared with zidovudine alone in persons with advanced HIV infection. There was no survival difference between the two groups (Collier et al., 1995).

f Zidovudine and foscarnet Patients with symptomatic HIV-infection who were treated with oral zidovudine (1200 mg per day) and i.v. foscarnet (30 mg per kg 8-hourly) were found to have a transient additive virologic effect compared with zidovudine alone (Jacobson et al., 1990).

g Zidovudine and colony stimulating factors In order to permit higher doses of interferon alpha and zidovudine therapy whilst limiting the hematologic toxicity, GM-CSF has been added to the combination regimens. This has successfully reduced the incidence of neutropenia but has not inhibited lymphokine-like side-effects (Krown et al., 1992a; Davey et al., 1991). GM-CSF (0.3–1 µg per kg daily) has been used to ameliorate zidovudine-associated neutropenia, although this is usually not necessary with the availability of other antiretroviral compounds which do not have hematologic toxicity (Levine et al., 1991; Hewitt et al., 1993). GM-CSF should be used with an antiretroviral when administered to patients with HIV infection as otherwise this growth factor can stimulate HIV replication (Kaplan et al., 1991; Perno et al., 1992b). However, when used in the presence of zidovudine, GM-CSF exerts synergistic inhibition of HIV replication (Hewitt and Morse, 1992). Similarly, granulocyte colony stimulating factor (G-CSF) allows both patients with neutropenia to receive zidovudine (Mueller et al., 1992), and has the advantage of not being associated with increased viral replication. Recombinant human erythropoietin can increase hematocrit levels and reduce transfusion requirements in HIV-infected patients with anemia who are being treated with zidovudine and who have low endogenous erythropoietin levels (less than 500 IU per liter) (Fischl et al., 1990c; Henry et al., 1992). Combinations of G-CSF, erythropoietin and zidovudine can be used in HIV-infected patients with neutropenia and anemia without altering the efficacy of zidovudine (Miles et al., 1991a,b).

h Zidovudine and alpha-glucosidase 1 inhibitors N-Butyl-deoxynojirimycin, an alpha-glucosidase 1 inhibitor, used in combination with zidovudine was well tolerated by a small number of patients with 200–500 CD4 lymphocytes per µl, but there was no evidence of virologic or immunologic benefit compared with zidovudine monotherapy (Fischl et al., 1994).

i Zidovudine and trichosanthin The efficacy of combination therapy with the ribosomal inhibitory protein trichosanthin in addition to another antiretroviral agent was studied in a phase II trial in 93 patients who were failing treatment. There was a significant increase in CD4 numbers after the addition of trichosanthin (Byers et al., 1994), although there is no convincing evidence of any antiretroviral efficacy.

6 The use of zidovudine in special HIV-related clinical conditions

a Primary HIV infection Zidovudine therapy for persons with primary HIV-1 infection in a dose of 1000 mg per day and maintained for a median period of 56 days was not found in a retrospective case-control study to prevent development of persistent HIV infection or result in earlier resolution of symptoms associated with the primary illness (Tindall et al., 1991). In addition, zidovudine therapy in persons with primary HIV-1 infection may dampen the CD8 lymphocyte response which is considered to be part of the host's attempts to control HIV replication (Tindall et al., 1993). A multicenter, randomized, double-blind, placebo-controlled trial of zidovudine was conducted in 77 patients with primary HIV infection who were enrolled into the study within a mean of 25.1 days from the time of onset of symptoms.

Zidovudine did not reduce the duration of the acute illness. However, disease progression was significantly less frequent and the CD4 count was better preserved in the zidovudine group over a 15-month follow-up period compared with the placebo group (Kinloch-De Loes *et al.*, 1995). In a third study, in which zidovudine was administered in combination with a non-nucleoside reverse transcriptase inhibitor (L-697–661) to four individuals for a period of 6 months, there was a reduction in viral load to low or undetectable levels in three of four patients and no response in the other participant. Cessation of therapy was associated with return of detectable HIV RNA within 10 days in the two patients whose viral load declined below baseline (Perrin and Kinloch-de Loes, 1995). Unpublished data suggest that combination therapy using zidovudine, lamivudine and a protease inhibitor such as ritonavir, indinavir or nelfinavir can reduce viral load to undetectable levels (less than 20 copies of HIV RNA per ml).

b HIV-related neurologic disease The benefits of zidovudine for the treatment of HIV-related neurologic disease were demonstrated shortly after the discovery of the virologic and immunologic benefits of zidovudine in persons with advanced HIV infection. In an open-label trial, the treatment of patients with AIDS-related dementia and peripheral neuropathy with zidovudine resulted in improvement as assessed clinically, by neuropsychometric testing, nerve conduction studies and positron emission tomography (Yarchoan *et al.*, 1987). These responses were sustained for up to 18 months (Yarchoan *et al.*, 1988a). Subsequently, a randomized, double-blind, placebo-controlled study demonstrated the efficacy of zidovudine (250 mg 4-hourly) in improving cognition of patients with AIDS, and to a lesser extent, those with AIDS-related complex (Schmitt *et al.*, 1988). A retrospective evaluation of 143 patients enrolled in a natural history study also provides supportive evidence that long-term zidovudine therapy is associated with improved cognitive function as assessed by standard neuropsychological and neurophysiological measures, in early as well as advanced HIV infection (Baldeweg *et al.*, 1995). In a neuropathologic study of 192 patients, the incidence of encephalitis was significantly lower in those who had been treated with zidovudine than in those who had never received zidovudine (Gray *et al.*, 1994). It has also been of interest to observe the decline in the incidence of AIDS-related dementia since the widespread availability of zidovudine therapy (Portegies *et al.*, 1989), with a subsequent reduction in the number of cases with neuropathological evidence of HIV-associated subacute encephalopathy at autopsy (Vago *et al.*, 1993; Maehlen *et al.*, 1995). However, another retrospective analysis suggests that the benefits of zidovudine are time-limited (Chiesi *et al.*, 1995).

Motor performance, as assessed by motor tests of index fingers, has been found to improve following commencement of zidovudine therapy (Arendt *et al.*, 1992). There have been reports of zidovudine-responsive acute encephalopathy due to HIV (Allworth and Kemp, 1989), and of responses within 2 weeks to zidovudine (1200 mg per day) in patients with biopsy-proven progressive multifocal leukoencephalopathy (Conway *et al.*, 1990; Singer *et al.*, 1994). Zidovudine does not appear to be of benefit for the treatment of HIV-related affective disorders (Schmitt *et al.*, 1988), although there is a report of an HIV-infected patient whose symptoms of depression diminished coincident with zidovudine therapy (Perkins and Evans, 1991).

In an uncontrolled study, children (3 months to 12 years) with AIDS or advanced AIDS-related complex with impaired cognitive function who were treated orally with zidovudine (180 mg per m^2 6-hourly) had improvement in function as assessed by cognitive test scores (McKinney *et al.*, 1991). Continuous i.v. infusion of zidovudine has also been associated with significant improvement in both cognitive and neurodevelopmental function in HIV-infected children aged 14 months to 12 years, although such an approach is not considered practical (Brouwers *et al.*, 1990). This enhancement of cognitive function is accompanied by improvement in CT brain scan, with reduction in mean ventricular area and ventricular:brain ratio (Brivio *et al.*, 1991). There is a report of a child with myelopathy who had a dramatic response to zidovudine, being able to walk again after 10 days of therapy (Blanche *et al.*, 1988). Resolution of HIV encephalopathy following the initiation of zidovudine therapy in a child has been described (Croft *et al.*, 1992). Zidovudine has also been reported to result in improvement in children with a moderate delay in developmental milestones (Blanche *et al.*, 1988). However, HIV-related neurologic disease in children does not always improve with zidovudine therapy (Blanche *et al.*, 1988).

There is a decline in beta-2-microglobulin and neopterin levels in CSF of HIV-infected patients with neurologic disease who have been treated with zidovudine for at least 45 days (Gulevich *et al.*, 1993). Levels of HIV p24 antigen in CSF also decline with zidovudine treatment (Portegies, 1995).

c Pregnancy There is now clear evidence that treatment of HIV-infected pregnant women with zidovudine can interrupt transmission of HIV to the fetus. In a preliminary report of 7 HIV-infected pregnant women who received zidovudine, starting from between weeks 16 and 30 of gestation, all women gave birth to infants who remained HIV seronegative for the duration of the study (mean: 22 months, range:16–32 months) (Ferrazin et al., 1993).

The pivotal study (Pediatric AIDS Clinical Trials Group Study 076) of the efficacy and safety of zidovudine in reducing the risk of transmission of HIV from mother to child was a randomized, double-blind, placebo-controlled study of 477 HIV-infected pregnant women between 14 and 34 weeks gestation (median at entry 26 weeks) with more than 200 CD4 cells per μl (median at entry 550 per μl) who had not received zidovudine during the pregnancy. The women were treated with zidovudine (100 mg five times daily prior to delivery, 2 mg per kg i.v. over 1 h and then 1 mg per kg i.v. intrapartum, and the neonate received 2 mg per kg orally every 4 h for 6 weeks. Approximately one-third of the women underwent cesarean section. The HIV status was known in 363 of the births. There were 13 of 180 in the zidovudine-group and 40 of 183 in the placebo-group with at least one positive HIV culture of peripheral blood mononuclear cells within the first 6 months of life. After 18 months, 8.3% of the zidovudine-group and 25.5% of the placebo-group were HIV infected. Thus the zidovudine regimen resulted in a 67.5% relative reduction in the risk of maternal–infant transmission of HIV (Connor et al., 1994).

Following analysis of AIDS Clinical Trials Group study 076 it has been recommended that all women with HIV infection should be offered zidovudine treatment, with therapy also given to the neonate (MMWR, 1994; Katz and Lim, 1995; Rouzioux, 1995). The full ACTG protocol 076 regimen should be used (MMWR, 1994) (Table V.26). In a separate study, zidovudine was shown to exert its protective effects by reducing maternal HIV RNA levels in plasma prior to delivery (Dickover et al., 1996). Vertical transmission of zidovudine-resistant HIV has been reported (Frenkel et al., 1995b), and thus the potential role for combination therapy, must also be considered. This author recommends that zidovudine should be used as part of combination therapy with other antiretroviral drugs. The timing of commencement of zidovudine for use in pregnancy has not been determined; de Santis and colleagues (de Santis et al., 1995) suggest that its use in the first trimester should be limited to those cases where it is absolutely indicated. Other ethical issues, such as compulsory testing for HIV infection of all pregnant women and unblinding heelstick surveys are under debate (Wilfert, 1994; Bayer, 1994; Minkoff and Willoughby, 1995; Hoffman and Munson, 1995).

A second non-randomized study of 63 pregnant HIV-infected women, 26 of whom received zidovudine therapy (mean CD4 370 cells per μl) during pregnancy and/or labor and delivery confirmed that zidovudine therapy can markedly reduce HIV transmission. Vertical transmission occurred in only one of 26 (4%) mothers receiving zidovudine versus 12 of 42 (29%) who did not receive the drug, suggesting that the findings of ACTG 076 may extend to pregnant women with lower CD4 cell numbers (Frissen et al., 1994). An observational study of 321 HIV-infected pregnant women also found no clear evidence that efficacy in interrupting transmission with zidovudine depended on the CD4 number of the mother (Matheson et al., 1995). Unpublished data indicate that there is also no clear correlation with viral load reduction, suggesting that the effect of zidovudine is by post-exposure prophylaxis of the infant. Zidovudine treatment does not appear to influence infant growth (Moye et al., 1996).

Table V.26
Eligibility criteria for HIV-infected pregnant women participating in AIDS Clinical Trials Group Protocol 076. (Reproduced from MMWR, 1994.)

Pregnancy at 14–24 weeks of gestation

No antiretroviral therapy during the current pregnancy

No clinical indications for antenatal antiretroviral therapy

CD4+ T lymphocyte count <200 cells per μl at the time of entry into the study

Zidovudine regimen from AIDS Clinical Trials Group Protocol 076

Oral administration of 100 mg of zidovudine (ZDV) five times daily, initiated at 14–34 weeks of gestation and continued throughout the pregnancy

During labor, i.v. administration of ZDV in a 1-h loading dose of 2 mg per kg of body weight, followed by a continuous infusion of 1 mg per kg of body weight per h until delivery

Oral administration of ZDV to the newborn (ZDV syrup at 2 mg per kg of body weight per dose every 6 h) for the first 6 weeks of life, beginning 8–12 h after birth

d Pediatric patients Zidovudine therapy (180 mg per m^2 6-hourly) can be safely given to children with advanced disease, with improvements in clinical, virologic and immunologic parameters which are similar to those observed in adults (McKinney *et al.*, 1991). Weight-for-age and rate of weight gain are useful prognostic indicators of survival in children with advanced HIV infection who are treated with zidovudine, but are less useful than CD4 percentage (McKinney and Wilfert, 1994). A phase I/II dose-ranging study of combination therapy with zidovudine (90–180 mg per m^2 6-hourly) and didanosine (90–180 mg per m^2 12-hourly) in 68 children who were either zidovudine-naive (54 children) or zidovudine-intolerant (14 children) showed that combination therapy resulted in a significant increase in CD4 cell number, from a median of 331–556 cells per μl (most pronounced in the naive group) and a decline in HIV p24 antigen in plasma (Husson *et al.*, 1994).

Table V.27
Provisional public health service recommendation of chemoprophylaxis after occupational exposure to HIV, by type of exposure and source material – 1996. (Reproduced from MMWR 1996.)

Type of exposure	Source material[a]	Antiretroviral prophylaxis[b]	Antiretroviral regimens[c]
Percutaneous	Blood[d]		
	Highest risk	Recommend	ZDV + 3TC plus IDV
	Increased risk	Recommend	ZDV + 3TC ±IDV[e]
	No increased risk	Offer	ZDV + 3TC
	Fluid containing visible blood, other potentially infectious fluid,[f] or tissue	Offer	ZDV + 3TC
	Other body fluid (e.g. urine)	Not offer	
Mucous membrane	Blood	Offer	ZDV + 3TC ±IDV[e]
	Fluid containing visible blood, other potentially infectious fluid,[f] or tissue	Offer	ZDV ±3TC
Skin, increased risks[g]	Blood	Offer	ZDV + 3TC, ±IDV[e]
	Fluid containing visible blood, other potentially infectious fluid,[f] or tissue	Offer	ZDV ±3TC
	Other body fluid (e.g. urine)	Not offer	

[a] Any exposure to concentrated HIV (e.g. in a research laboratory or production facility) is treated as percutaneous exposure to blood with highest risk.

[b] *Recommend* – Post-exposure prophylaxis (PEP) should be recommended to the exposed worker with counselling. *Offer* – PEP should be offered to the exposed worker with counselling *Not offer* – PEP should not be offered because these are not occupational exposures to HIV.

[c] Regimens: zidovudine (ZDV), 200 mg three times per day; lamivudine (3TC), 150 mg twice-daily, indinavir (IDV), 800 mg three times per day (if IDV is not available, saquinavir may be used, 600 mg three times per day). Prophylaxis is given for 4 weeks. For full prescribing information, see package inserts.

[d] *Highest risk* – BOTH larger volume of blood (e.g. deep injury with large diameter hollow needle previously in source patient's vein or artery, especially involving an injection of source-patient's blood) AND blood containing a high titer of HIV (e.g. source with acute retroviral illness or end-stage AIDS; viral load measurement may be considered, but its use in relation to PEP has not been evaluated). *Increased risk* – EITHER exposure to larger volume of blood OR blood with a high titer of HIV. *No increased risk* – NEITHER exposure to larger volume of blood NOR blood with a high titer of HIV (e.g. solid suture needle injury from source patient with asymptomatic HIV infection).

[e] Possible toxicity of additional drug my not be warranted.

[f] Includes semen; vaginal secretions; cerebrospinal, synovial, pleural, peritoneal, pericardial, and amniotic fluids.

[g] For skin, risk is increased for exposures involving a high titer of HIV, prolonged contact, an extensive area, or an area in which skin integrity is visibly compromised. For skin exposures without increased risk, the risk for drug toxicity outweighs the benefit of PEP.

e Prophylaxis for health care workers or others exposed to HIV Zidovudine is offered to health care workers who have significant occupational exposure to HIV through percutaneous injury or contact with mucous membranes or abraded skin (MMWR, 1990). One recommended prophylaxis schedule is 250 mg 4-hourly five times daily for 4 weeks, with an initial loading dose of 1000 mg. Therapy is recommended to commence as soon as possible after exposure (within 2 h) (Joint Working Party, 1992). Although zidovudine monotherapy has been the standard regimen provided to health care workers exposed to HIV, this has been changed in light of recent data demonstrating superior efficacy of combination therapy over monotherapy and new guidelines have been issued (Table V.27). Apart from offering prophylactic zidovudine therapy, the management of occupational exposures to HIV involves appropriate testing of blood and counseling (Gerberding and Henderson, 1992).

Studies of large numbers of health care workers who have been occupationally exposed to HIV through percutaneous injury suggest that the risk of HIV infection is low (approximately 0.3%) (McEvoy et al., 1987; Marcus and CDC Co-operative Needlestick Study Group, 1988; Beekmann et al., 1990; Tokars et al., 1993; MMWR, 1995). In health care workers enrolled in one multicenter study who were treated with zidovudine following exposure no hematologic or other toxicity sufficient to warrant dose-reduction was observed (Gerberding, 1993). In other studies hematochemical toxicity has been reported (anemia, neutropenia and increased serum transaminases in less than 2% of recipients) and 50–75% complain of constitutional symptoms (Puro et al., 1992; Tokars et al., 1993). In a prospective study of 113 health care workers in New York with occupational exposure to HIV-infected blood or body fluids who were offered zidovudine only 53% chose to take zidovudine and only 35% completed the 42-day course of 1200 mg per day; men were more likely to accept therapy and complete the course (Forseter et al., 1994). This supports results of a study of 14 health care workers who were treated with zidovudine following occupational exposure to HIV in whom seven (50%) prematurely ceased zidovudine, five due to severe subjective symptoms (Schmitz et al., 1994).

The US Centers for Disease Control, in collaboration with British and French public health authorities conducted a retrospective case-control study of health care workers after a documented occupational percutaneous exposure to HIV-infected blood resulting in seroconversion. The regimen was generally 1000 mg daily of zidovudine for 3–4 weeks. The findings suggest that post-exposure prophylaxis of health care workers using zidovudine reduced the risk of HIV transmission by 80% (MMWR, 1995, 1996; Gerberding, 1996).

There are however a number of reports of failed prophylaxis, despite high doses of zidovudine being administered within several minutes to hours of exposure (Looke and Grove, 1990; Miller, 1990; Durand et al., 1991; Jones, 1991; Anonymous, 1993; Palmer et al., 1994). Although not completely proven in humans, the situation is likely to be similar to that in mice infected with Rauscher murine leukemia virus, in which the success of chemoprevention has been found to critically depend on the virus titer in the inoculum (Ruprecht and Bronson, 1994). Zidovudine post-exposure prophylaxis failed to prevent HIV infection in a patient who accidentally received less than 200 μl of HIV-infected blood by the i.v. route. In this case-report, oral zidovudine therapy (500 mg 6-hourly) for the first 2 days, commencing 45 min after exposure, followed by i.v. administration (2.5 mg per kg 4-hourly) from days 3 to 20, and then oral zidovudine (500 mg 6-hourly) from day 21 to 37 failed to prevent infection (Lange et al., 1990). A prison officer who was stabbed in the buttock with a syringe containing HIV-infected blood was treated within 4 h with zidovudine 500 mg followed by 250 mg orally 6-hourly. Three weeks later he developed an acute illness consistent with primary HIV infection, and subsequently a positive virus culture (Jones, 1991).

Despite these failures, and given the recent data suggesting benefit as well as the fact that the number of infections which have been prevented is not known (and thus the failure-rate of prophylaxis cannot be determined), the current recommendation is to offer zidovudine in combination with lamivudine with or without indinavir to persons with significant exposure to HIV as soon as possible after exposure (preferably within 2 h) together with appropriate testing and counselling, and continue therapy for 4 weeks (Table V.27; MMWR, 1996). The potential benefit of zidovudine must also be considered in the light of increasing numbers of reports of transmission of zidovudine-resistant strains of HIV (Kuritkes et al., 1994; Siegrist et al., 1994; Conlon et al., 1994; Veenstra et al., 1995). Although there are currently no data regarding the use of combination therapy in the setting of occupational exposure it is obvious that the use of combinations of antiretroviral drugs is more appropriate than monotherapy.

Although there are also no data available it is considered appropriate to offer similar prophylaxis to persons incidentally (sexually) exposed to HIV.

f   HIV-related thrombocytopenia   Immunosuppressed mice with thrombocytopenia that are treated with zidovudine have sustained elevations in platelet count over a 120-day treatment period (Chow *et al.*, 1993b). Zidovudine can increase platelet counts in HIV-infected patients with normal platelet counts as well as those with HIV-related thrombocytopenia (Montaner *et al.*, 1990). In a small, placebo-controlled study, 8 weeks therapy with zidovudine resulted in a mean of a 2-fold increase in platelet count which was evident as early as 8 days after commencing therapy (The Swiss Group, 1988). However, the time to respond is highly variable and may be prolonged (median time 9–12 weeks) (Panzer *et al.*, 1989; Montaner *et al.*, 1990; Rarick *et al.*, 1991). Episodes of bleeding resolve with zidovudine therapy (Rarick *et al.*, 1991). The effects of zidovudine on platelet numbers can persist for periods of time in excess of 18 months (Cinque *et al.*, 1993). Following cessation of zidovudine, platelet counts usually decline; however, in one report elevated levels persisted for more than 4 weeks (The Swiss Group, 1988). With prolonged zidovudine therapy the platelet count may be sustained for 36 weeks (Montaner *et al.*, 1990). Two reports suggest that the response is related to the dose of zidovudine, with 1000 mg per day or higher being more effective in increasing platelet counts than 500–600 mg per day (Boyar and Beall, 1991; Landonio *et al.*, 1993). However, a dose-related response has not been reported by others (Montaner *et al.*, 1990). Zidovudine therapy is asociated with a decrease in the level of plasma glycocalicin, a platelet protein which correlates inversely with platelet survival, suggesting that zidovudine prolongs platelet survival (Panzer *et al.*, 1989; Boyar and Beall, 1991). A clinical response to zidovudine is not seen in all patients with HIV infection and thrombocytopenia (Oksenhendler *et al.*, 1989).

g   HIV-related psoriasis   Marked improvement in psoriatic dermatitis (plaque and pustular forms), nail lesions and arthritis has been observed in persons receiving zidovudine therapy (Kaplan *et al.*, 1989; Obuch *et al.*, 1992b). Withdrawal of zidovudine usually results in a relapse (Feeney and Frazer, 1988). In an open-label study of 19 patients with HIV-related psoriasis treated with a daily dose of 1200 mg of zidovudine, partial or complete improvement in psoriasis occurred during zidovudine treatment, although long-term relapses occurred and arthropathy was not improved (Duvic *et al.*, 1994).

h   Hemophiliacs   The efficacy of zidovudine in treatment of HIV infection in hemophiliacs is similar to those with other risk categories for HIV infection. In a controlled study of hemophiliacs with asymptomatic HIV infection treated with zidovudine (300 mg 4-hourly during waking hours) or placebo, there was a trend towards more rapid disease progression in those in the placebo arm compared with zidovudine therapy – similar findings to studies in asymptomatic non-hemophiliac patients (Merigan *et al.*, 1991). Hemophiliacs treated with zidovudine prior to an AIDS-defining illness have been found to take longer to progress to AIDS than those who do not receive zidovudine. Furthermore, the median survival after the diagnosis of AIDS is longer in those treated with zidovudine (either prior to or after diagnosis of AIDS) compared with patients who are not treated (Ragni *et al.*, 1992b). In a double-blind placebo-controlled trial of zidovudine in 143 hemophiliacs with asymptomatic infection and CD4 counts of 100–400 cells per μl there were no significant differences in the proportion of patients who developed clinical progression in the zidovudine and placebo arms (Mannucci *et al.*, 1994).

i   Lymphoma and other malignancies   As the role of zidovudine and other retroviral drugs as a risk factor for the development of lymphoma has been considered by some as being controversial, a case-control study of 112 HIV infected patients with lymphoma found that zidovudine therapy was not associated with an increased risk of development of lymphoma (Levine *et al.*, 1995). There is a case-report of a patient with pulmonary non-Hodgkins lymphoma that regressed whilst the patient was receiving zidovudine therapy alone (Baselga *et al.*, 1993). Two patients with HIV infection and neurologic manifestations associated with diffuse infiltrative CD8 lymphocytosis syndrome have been reported to respond to zidovudine (Bachmeyer *et al.*, 1995).

j   Other clinical uses of zidovudine   There is some evidence that HIV-associated nephropathy, characterized by nephrotic syndrome, and focal and segmental glomerulosclerosis on histology, with rapid progression to end-stage renal failure, is responsive to zidovudine (Ifudo *et al.*, 1995). Zidovudine has been reported to cause transient clinical improvement in HIV-associated nephropathy, with lowering of serum creatinine but not affecting levels of proteinuria (Lam and Park, 1990).

7 Impact of zidovudine on surrogate markers

a Immunologic Zidovudine monotherapy induces a transient increase in CD4 lymphocytes (absolute number as well as percentage) during the first 8–12 weeks of therapy in both adults and children; CD4 lymphocyte levels then usually decline to baseline levels within 20 weeks after starting therapy (Fischl *et al.*, 1987; Blanche *et al.*, 1988; Chaisson *et al.*, 1988; Richman and Andrews, 1988; Volberding *et al.*, 1990; Choi *et al.*, 1993). This increase in CD4 lymphocytes is also evident in persons with primary HIV infection who have normal CD4 counts (more than 600 cells per µl) at time of commencing zidovudine therapy (Tindall *et al.*, 1993). However, CD4 lymphocyte numbers are considered to be an imperfect marker for clinical progression in asymptomatic persons receiving zidovudine (Choi *et al.*, 1993). In approximately 75% of asymptomatic and symptomatic HIV-infected persons treated with zidovudine T helper cell function improves and this may be observed as early as 5 weeks after initiation of therapy (Clerici *et al.*, 1992).

Serum beta-2-microglobulin elevation is associated with progression of HIV disease. Zidovudine therapy reduces the concentration of beta-2-microglobulin in serum and CSF (Jacobson *et al.*, 1989b; Hagberg *et al.*, 1991). The zidovudine-induced decrease in serum beta-2-microglobulin and neopterin levels occurs within 1–2 weeks. The levels are not sustained; within 12 weeks beta-2-microglobulin concentrations have returned to baseline although neopterin levels remain depressed for at least 24 weeks (Bass *et al.*, 1992a,b). In another study, the zidovudine-induced reduction in beta-2-microglobulin and neopterin only lasted for 1 week (Liu *et al.*, 1994). The effects of zalcitabine on lowering serum beta-2-microglobulin and neopterin are smaller but more prolonged than for zidovudine (Liu *et al.*,1994).

French and colleagues in Australia have shown that the restoration of cellular immune responses against subclinical infection with *Mycobacterium avium* complex in patients treated with zidovudine can be measured by delayed type hypersensitivity testing (French *et al.*, 1992; Mallal *et al.*, 1994).

b Virologic Zidovudine decreases the titer of infectious virus in plasma as assessed by quantitative microculture (Ho *et al.*, 1989; Katzenstein *et al.*, 1992), reduces the level of plasma HIV RNA as assessed by quantitative competitive polymerase chain reaction (Piatek *et al.*, 1993) or branched DNA assay, and reduces the level of p24 antigen in plasma (Fischl *et al.*, 1987; Parks *et al.*, 1988; Volberding *et al.*, 1990). Plasma HIV RNA as well as HIV p24 antigen decrease significantly from baseline within 1 week of commencing therapy (Kappes *et al.*, 1995), with some investigators reporting a decline within 1–2 days of commencing treatment and maximum suppression within 7 days (Loveday *et al.*, 1995). The titer of HIV within peripheral blood mononuclear cells, however, is reportedly not altered by zidovudine therapy (Ho *et al.*, 1989).

In a study of 18 symptomatic, zidovudine-naive HIV-infected individuals with a median of 43 CD4 cells per µl, plasma viremia was found to be a useful short-term marker of antiretroviral efficacy but not to correlate with disease progression (Molina *et al.*, 1994). However, other investigators studying asymptomatically infected individuals have found that the decline in plasma HIV RNA levels after commencing zidovudine treatment was predictive of clinical outcome (Jurriaans *et al.*, 1995). Serum RNA may return to pretreatment levels within weeks of commencing therapy (Loveday *et al.*, 1995).

Asymptomatic patients receiving zidovudine have significantly less unintegrated HIV DNA in their peripheral blood mononuclear cells than asymptomatic persons not receiving therapy (Dickover *et al.*, 1992; Bush *et al.*, 1993). Institution of zidovudine results in decreases in HIV RNA copy number of up to 200-fold (Katzenstein *et al.*, 1992; Piatek *et al.*, 1993); in general a decline of 0.5–0.7 $\log_{10}$ copies of HIV RNA per ml can be expected with zidovudine monotherapy in a naive patient.

Zidovudine therapy of symptomatic children may dramatically decrease HIV titers in peripheral blood mononuclear cells as well as plasma (by 99%) (Srugo *et al.*, 1991), in contrast to some reports in adults (Ho *et al.*, 1989). Cessation of zidovudine is associated with a rebound increase in viral replication (Spear *et al.*, 1988b; Wainberg *et al.*, 1989). Zidovudine therapy reportedly does not alter the ability to recover HIV from semen (Krieger *et al.*, 1991; Hamed *et al.*, 1993) or peripheral blood (Spector *et al*, 1989a,b), although the time to positive culture from peripheral blood mononuclear cells is markedly increased in the zidovudine-treated patients (Parks *et al.*, 1988). Furthermore, ability to isolate HIV from patients receiving zidovudine therapy will also depend on whether the individual harbors a resistant strain.

A study of sequential HIV isolates from patients enrolled in the EACG 020 trial showed conclusively that zidovudine therapy dose not prevent the emergence of syncytium-inducing strains of HIV (Leal *et al.*, 1994). These data support the earlier findings of Koot and colleagues (Koot *et al.*, 1993) who similarly found that zidovudine did not inhibit the emergence of highly replicating syncytium-inducing strains of HIV. This group also demonstrated that clinical progression occurred in patients with this viral phenotype despite zidovudine therapy, suggesting that the benefit of zidovudine may be more useful in those patients with non-syncytium-inducing strains of HIV.

8 Correlation between zidovudine-resistance and clinical outcome

Although it is generally considered that the development of resistance of HIV to zidovudine is likely to be associated with clinical failure and disease progression, it has been difficult to prove this association. However, a body of circumstantial evidence is accumulating which supports this concept. The emergence of zidovudine-resistance (usually after 6 months of therapy) is temporally related to the decline in immunologic benefit which has been observed in clinical trials (Montaner et al., 1993). The survival of patients with AIDS receiving zidovudine therapy has been shown in one study, using a univariate Cox model, to be related to log IC_{90} of zidovudine (Gotzsche et al., 1992). The development of resistance of HIV to zidovudine in adult and pediatric patients representing various stages of HIV infection has been found to predict subsequent progression (Montaner et al., 1993; Ogino et al., 1993; Nielsen et al., 1995).

The appearance of a mutation at codon 215 within the pol gene has been associated with impending immunologic, virologic and clinical decline in HIV-infected adults, suggesting that the development of this mutation is associated with a loss of therapeutic efficacy (Kozal et al., 1993; Calderon et al., 1995). This mutation predicts progression independently of virus phenotype (Kozal et al., 1994b). A pediatric study has demonstrated that this mutation is strongly associated with clinical progression in children also (Principi et al., 1994). Mutations in both codons 41 and 215 reportedly confers a greater risk for clinical progression and shorter survival (Japour et al., 1995). Data from this study are supported by a case report of vertical transmission of a zidovudine-resistant strain resulting in rapid CD4 decline in the infant (Siegrist et al., 1994). There are also data from a pediatric study in which decreased sensitivity of HIV to zidovudine was highly correlated with poor clinical outcome (Tudor-Williams et al., 1992). However age-adjusted CD4 cell numbers were lower on study entry in children whose disease progressed, thus causing some concern regarding the validity of the findings. In a retrospective analysis of stored samples from 187 patients enrolled in ACTG study 116B/117 from whom there were baseline HIV isolates it was found that high-level zidovudine-resistance independently predicted more rapid clinical progression and death (D'Aquila et al., 1995). Transmission of zidovudine-resistant strains of HIV-1 have been reported (Veenstra et al., 1995).

B Zidovudine treatment of hepatitis B and C virus

Although there are reports of inhibition of the hepatitis B virus DNA polymerase by zidovudine triphosphate in vitro, no significant change in levels of hepatitis B virus DNA were evident in two studies in which patients with chronic hepatitis B virus and HIV infection were treated with zidovudine (Marcellin et al., 1989; Gilson et al., 1991). These findings are supported by a study of interferon alpha and zidovudine combination therapy in patients with dual infection with hepatitis B and HIV, in which zidovudine did not enhance the antiviral effect of interferon alpha (Janssen et al., 1993).

A pilot study examined therapy with interferon alpha (3 or 6 million units per day for 3 weeks and then thrice-weekly for 21 weeks, with oral zidovudine (500 mg per day) commencing in combination at the beginning of week 8 of interferon alpha therapy in 22 patients with chronic hepatitis C infection of the K1 type. In plasma HCV RNA was undetectable in 14.2% of the interferon-alone group and in 45.5% of the combination therapy group (Tsutsumi et al., 1995).

C Zidovudine treatment of other retroviruses

Treatment of human T cell leukemia-lymphoma virus (HTLV-1) with zidovudine (1000 mg per day) interferon alpha (5–10 million units subcutaneously daily) has been associated with clinical improvement in over 50% of treated patients, and complete remission in 26% (Gill et al., 1995). Other reports support these findings (Tobinai et al., 1995; Hermine et al., 1995).

Acknowledgements The author would like to thank David Cooper of the National Centre for HIV Epidemiology and Clinical Research, Sydney, and Gilda Tachedjian of Macfarlane Burnet Centre for Medical Research, Melbourne, for their critical review of this chapter.

References

Agarwal RP, Mian AM (1991). Thymidine and zidovudine metabolism in chronically zidovudine-exposed cells *in vitro*. *Biochem Pharmacol* **42**: 905.

Alder J, Hui YG, Clement J (1995). Efficacy of AZT therapy in reducing p24 antigen burden in a modified SCID mouse model of HIV infection. *Antiviral Res* **27**: 85.

Albert J, Wahlberg J, Lundeberg J *et al.* (1992). Persistence of azidothymidine-resistant human immunodeficiency virus type 1 RNA genotypes in post-treatment sera. *J Virol* **66**: 5627.

Allworth AM, Kemp RJ (1989). A case of acute encephalopathy caused by the human immunodeficiency virus apparently responsive to zidovudine. *Med J Aust* **151**: 285.

Ameer B, James MO, Saleh J (1992). Kinetic and inhibitor studies of acetaminophen and zidovudine glucuronidation in rat liver microsomes. *Drug Chem Toxicol* **15**: 161.

Anderson BD, Shirasaka T, Kojima E *et al.* (1994). Identification of drug related genotype changes in HIV-1 from serum using the selective polymerase chain reaction. *Antiviral Res* **25**: 245.

Anderson DJ, O'Brien TR, Politch JA *et al.* (1992). Effects of disease stage and zidovudine therapy on the detection of human immunodeficiency virus type 1 in semen. *JAMA* **267**: 2769.

Anderson BD, Shirasaka T, Kijima E *et al.* (1994). Identification of drug related genotype changes in HIV-1 from serum using the selective polymerase chain reaction. *Antiviral Res* **25**: 245.

Anonymous (1993). HIV seroconversion after occupational exposure despite early prophylactic zidovudine therapy. *Lancet* **341**: 1077.

Antoniskis D, Easley AC, Espina BM (1992). Combined toxicity of zidovudine and antituberculosis chemotherapy. *Amer Rev Respir Dis* **145**: 430.

Aoki-Sei S, O'Brien MC, Ford H (1991). *In vitro* inhibition of hepatitis B virus replication by 2',3'-dideoxyguanosine, 2',3'-dideoxyinosine, and 3'-azido-2',3'-dideoxythymidine in 2215 (PR) cells. *J Infect Dis* **164**: 843.

Apolonio EG, Hoover DR, He Y *et al.* (1995). Prognostic factors in human immunodeficiency virus-positive patients with a CD4+ lymphocyte count <50/microL. *J Infect Dis* **171**: 829.

Arendt G, Hefter H, Buescher L *et al.* (1992). Improvement of motor performance of HIV-positive patients under AZT therapy. *Neurology* **42**: 891.

Arner ES, Valentin A, Eriksson S (1992). Thymidine and 3'-azido-3'-deoxythymidine metabolism in human peripheral blood lymphocytes and monocyte-derived macrophages. A study of both anabolic and catabolic pathways. *J Biol Chem* **267**: 10968.

Ashorn P, Moss B, Weinstein JN *et al.* (1990). Elimination of infectious human immunodeficiency virus from human T-cell cultures by synergistic action of CD4-*Pseudomonas* exotoxin and reverse transcriptase inhibitors. *Proc Natl Acad Sci USA* **87**: 8889.

Aweeka FT, Gambertoglio JG, van der Horst C *et al.* (1992). Pharmacokinetics of concomitantly administered foscarnet and zidovudine for treatment of human immunodeficiency virus infection (AIDS Clinical Trials Group protocol 053). *Antimicrob Ag Chemother* **36**: 1773.

Ayers KM (1988). Preclinical toxicology of zidovudine. An overview. *Amer J Med* **85**: 186.

Baba M, Pauwels R, Balzarini J *et al.* (1987). Ribavirin antagonizes inhibitory effects of pyrimidine 2',3'-dideoxynucleosides but enhances inhibitory effects of purine 2,3'-dideoxynucleosides on replication of human immunodeficiency virus *in vitro*. *Antimicrob Ag Chemother* **31**: 1613.

Bachmeyer C, Dhote R, Blance P *et al.* (1995). Diffuse infiltrative CD8 lymphocytosis syndrome with predominant neurologic manifestations in two HIV-infected patients responding to zidovudine. *AIDS* **9**: 1101.

Baldeweg T, Catalan J, Lovett E *et al.* (1995). Long term zidovudine reduces neurocognitive deficits in HIV-1 infection. *AIDS* **9**: 589.

Balis FM, Pizzo PA, Eddy J *et al.* (1989a). Pharmacokinetics of zidovudine administered intravenously and orally in children with human immunodeficiency virus infection. *J Pediatr* **114**: 880.

Balis FM, Pizzo PA, Murphy RF *et al.* (1989b). The pharmacokinetics of zidovudine administered by continuous infusion in children. *Annl Intern Med* **110**: 279.

Balis FM, Blaney SM, Poplack DG (1991). Antiretroviral drug development and clinical pharmacology. *Pediatr Infect Dis* **10**: 849.

Balzarini J, Pauwels R, Baba M *et al.* (1988). The in vitro and in vivo antiretrovirus activity, and intracellular metabolism of 3'-azido-2',3'-dideoxythymidine and 2',3'-dideoxycytidine are highly dependent on the cell species. *Biochem Pharmacol* **37**: 897.

Balzarini J, Karlsson A, Perez-Perez MJ *et al.* (1993). Treatment of human immunodeficiency virus type 1 (HIV-1) infected cells with combinations of HIV-1 specific inhibitors results in a different resistance pattern than does treatment with single drug therapy. *J Virol* **67**: 5353.

Balzarini J, Weeger M, Camarasa MJ *et al.* (1995). Sensitivity/resistance profile of a simian immunodeficiency virus containing the reverse transcriptase gene of human immunodeficiency virus type 1 (HIV-1) toward the HIV-1 specific non-nucleoside reverse transcriptase inhibitors. *Biochem Biophys Res Commun* **211**: 850.

Bareggi SR, Cinque P, Mazzei M *et al.* (1994). Pharmacokinetics of zidovudine in HIV-positive patients with liver disease. *J Clin Pharmacol* **34**: 782.

Barry M, Wild M, Veal G *et al.* (1994). Zidovudine phosphorylation in HIV infected patients and seronegative volunteers. *AIDS* **8**: 1.

Baselga J, Krown SE, Telzak EE *et al.* (1993). Acquired immune deficiency syndrome-related pulmonary non-Hodgkin lymphoma regressing after zidovudine therapy. *Cancer* **71**: 2332.

Bass HZ, Hardy WD, Mitsuyasu RT *et al.* (1992a). The effect of zidovudine treatment on serum neopterin and beta 2-microglobulin levels in mildly symptomatic, HIV type 1 seropositive individuals. *J AIDS* **5**: 215.

Bass HZ, Hardy WD, Mitsuyasu RT *et al.* (1992b). Eleven lymphoid phenotypic markers in HIV infection: selective changes induced by zidovudine treatment. *J AIDS* **5**: 890.

Baum MK, Javier JJ, Mantero-Atienza E *et al.* (1991). Zidovudine-associated adverse reactions in a longitudinal study of asymptomatic HIV-1-infected homosexual males. *J AIDS* **4**: 1218.

Bawdon RE, Sobhi S, Dax J (1992). The transfer of anti-human immunodeficiency virus nucleoside compounds by the term human placenta. *Amer J Obstet Gynecol* **167**: 1570.

Bayer R (1994). Ethical challenges posed by zidovudine treatment to reduce vertical transmission of HIV. *New Engl J Med* **331**: 1223.

Beekmann SE, Fahey BJ, Gerberding JL, Henderson DK (1990). Risky business; using necessarily imprecise casualty counts to estimate occupational risks for HIV-1 infection. *Infect Control Hosp Epidemiol* **11**: 371.

Beitz JG, Damowski JW, Cummings FJ *et al.* (1995). Phase I trial of high-dose infused zidovudine combined with leucovorin plus fluorouracil. *Cancer Invest* **13**: 464.

Berk L, Schalm SW, Heijtink RA (1992). Zidovudine inhibits hepatitis B virus replication. *Antiviral Res* **19**: 111.

Berman E, Duigou OR, Krown SE *et al.* (1989). Synergistic cytotoxic effect of azidothymidine and recombinant interferon alpha on normal human bone marrow progenitor cells. *Blood* **74**: 1281.

Bilello JA, Kort J J, MacAuley C *et al.* (1992). ZDV delays but does not prevent the transmission of MAIDS by LP-BM5 MuLV-infected macrophage-monocytes. *J AIDS* **5**: 571.

Birch C, Tachedjian G, Lucas CR *et al.* (1988). *In vitro* effectiveness of a combination of zidovudine and ansamycin against human immunodeficiency virus. *J Infect Dis* **158**: 895.

Blanche S, Caniglia M, Fischer A *et al.* (1988). Zidovudine therapy in children with acquired immunodeficiency syndrome. *Amer J Med* **85**: 203.

Blum MR, Liao SH, Good SS, de Miranda P (1988). Pharmacokinetics and bioavailability of zidovudine in humans. *Amer J Med* **85**: 189.

Boucher CA (1992). Clinical significance of zidovudine-resistant human immunodeficiency viruses. *Res Virol* **143**: 134.

Boucher CA, Tersmette M, Lange JM et al. (1990). Zidovudine sensitivity of human immunodeficiency viruses from high-risk, symptom-free individuals during therapy. Lancet 336: 585.

Boucher CA, O'Sullivan E, Mulder JW et al. (1992). Ordered appearance of zidovudine resistance mutations during treatment of 18 human immunodeficiency virus-positive subjects. J Infect Dis 165: 105.

Boucher CA, Leeuwen RV, Kellam P et al. (1993a). Effects of discontinuation of zidovudine treatment on zidovudine sensitivity of human immunodeficiency virus type 1 isolates. Antimicrob Ag Chemother 37: 1525.

Boucher FD, Modlin JF, Weller S et al. (1993b). Phase I evaluation of zidovudine administered to infants exposed at birth to the human immunodeficiency virus. J Pediatr 122: 137.

Boyar A, Beall G (1991). HIV-seropositive thrombocytopenia: the action of zidovudine. AIDS 5: 1351.

Bozzette SA, Kanouse DD, Berry S, Duan N (1995). Health status and function with zidovudine or zalcitabine as initial therapy for AIDS A randomised controlled trial. Roche 3300/ACTG 114 Study Group. JAMA 273: 295.

Brivio L, Tornaghi R, Muscetti L et al. (1991). Improvement of auditory brainstem responses after treatment with zidovudine in a child with AIDS. Pediatr Neurol 7: 53.

Brouwers P, Moss H, Wolters P et al. (1990). Effect of continuous-infusion zidovudine therapy on neuropsychologic functioning in children with symptomatic human immunodeficiency virus infection. J Pediatr 117: 980.

Brunetti I, Falcone A, Calabresi P et al. (1990). 5-Fluorouracil enhances azidothymidine cytotoxicity: in vitro, in vivo, and biochemical studies. Cancer Res 50: 4026.

Buckheit RW, Germany-Decker J, Hollingshead MG et al. (1993). Differential antiviral activity of two TIBO derivatives against the human immunodeficiency and murine leukemia viruses alone and in combination with other anti-HIV agents. AIDS Res Hum Retrovir 9: 1097.

Buckheit RW, Roberson JL, Lackman-Smith C et al. (1994). Potent and specific inhibition of HIV envelope mediated cell fusion and virus binding by G quartet-forming oligonucleotide (ISIS 5320). AIDS Res Hum Retrovir 10: 1497.

Bui T, Bark D, Perkins M et al. (1993). Effect of zidovudine on human placental trophoblast and Hofbauer cell functions. J AIDS 6: 120.

Burger DM, Meenhorst PL, Koks CH, Beijnen JH (1993a). Pharmacokinetic interaction between rifampin and zidovudine. Antimicrob Ag Chemother 37: 1426.

Burger DM, Kraaijeveld CL, Meenhorst PL et al. (1993b). Penetration of zidovudine into the cerebrospinal fluid of patients infected with HIV. AIDS 7: 1581.

Burger DM, Meenhorst PL, Underberg WJ et al. (1994a). Short-term combined use of paracetamol and zidovudine does not alter the pharmacokinetics of either drug. Netherlands J Med 44: 161.

Burger DM, Meenhorst PL, Mulder JW et al. (1994b). Therapeutic drug monitoring of phenytoin in patients with the acquired immunodeficiency syndrome. Therapeutic Drug Monit 16: 616.

Burger DM, Meenhorst PL, ten Napel CH et al. (1994c). Pharmacokinetic variability of zidovudine in HIV infected individuals; subgroup analysis and drug interaction. AIDS 8: 1683.

Burger DM, Kraayeveld CL, Meenhorst PL et al. (1995). Study on didanosine concentrations in cerebrospinal fluid. Implications for the treatment and prevention of AIDS dementia complex. Pharm World Sci 17: 218.

Bush CE, Donovan RM, Smereck SM et al. (1993). Quantitation of unintegrated HIV-1 DNA in asymptomatic patients in the presence or absence of antiretroviral therapy. AIDS Res Hum Retrovir 9: 183.

Byers VS, Levin AS, Malvino A et al. (1994). A phase II study of effect of addition of trichosanthin to zidovudine in patients with HIV disease and failing antiretroviral agents. AIDS Res Hum Retrovir 10: 413.

Byrnes VW, Emini EA, Schleif WA et al. (1994). Susceptibilities of human immunodeficiency virus type 1 enzyme and viral variants expressing multiple resistance engendering amino acid substitutions to reserve transcriptase inhibitors. Antimicrob Ag Chemother 38: 1404.

Calderon EJ, Torres Y, Medrano FJ et al. (1995). Emergence and clinical relevance of mutations associated with zidovudine resistance in asymptomatic HIV-1 infected patients. Eur J Clin Microb Infect Dis 14: 512.

Campbell TB, Young RK, Eron JJ et al. (1993). Inhibition of human immunodeficiency virus type 1 replication in vitro by bisheteroarylpiperazine alevirdine (U-87201E) in combination with zidovudine or didanosine. J Infect Dis 168: 318.

Carpenter CC, Fischl MA, Hammer SM et al. (1996). Antiretroviral therapy for HIV infection in 1996. Recommendations of an International Panel. JAMA 276: 146.

Carr A, Penny R, Cooper DA (1993). Allergy and desensitization to zidovudine in patients with acquired immunodeficiency syndrome (AIDS). J Allergy Clin Immunol 91: 683.

Causey D (1991). Concomitant ganciclovir and zidovudine treatment for cytomegalovirus retinitis in patients with HIV infection: an approach to treatment. J AIDS 4: S16.

Chaisson RE, Leuther MD, Allain JP et al. (1988). Effect of zidovudine on serum human immunodeficiency virus core antigen levels. Arch Int Med 148: 2151.

Chattha G, Arieff AI, Cummings C, Tierney LM (1993). Lactic acidosis complicating the acquired immunodeficiency syndrome. Ann Int Med 118: 37.

Chavanet P, Diquet B, Waldner A, Portier H (1989). Perinatal pharmacokinetics of zidovudine [letter]. New Engl J Med 321: 1548.

Cheeseman SH, Havlir D, McLaughlin MM et al. (1995). Phase I/II evaluation of nevirapine alone and in combination with zidovudine for infection with human immunodeficiency virus. J AIDS 8: 141.

Chen CH, Vazquez PM, Cheng YC (1991). Effect of anti-human immunodeficiency virus nucleoside analogs on mitochondrial DNA and its implication for delayed toxicity. Mol Pharmacol 39: 625.

Chen SC, Barker SM, Mitchell DH et al. (1992). Concurrent zidovudine-induced myopathy and hepatoxicity in patients treated for human immunodeficiency virus (HIV) infection. Pathology 24: 109.

Chiesi A, Vella S, Dally LG et al. (1995). Epidemiology of AIDS dementia complex in Europe. AIDS in Europe Study Group. J AIDS Hum Retrovir 11: 39.

Child S, Montaner J, Tsoukas C (1991). Canadian multicenter azidothymidine trial: AZT pharmacokinetics. J AIDS 4: 865.

Choi S, Lagakos SW, Schooley R, Volberding PA (1993). CD4+ lymphocytes are an incomplete surrogate marker for clinical progression in persons with asymptomatic HIV infection taking zidovudine. Ann Intern Med 118: 674.

Chong KT, Pagano PJ, Hinshaw RR (1994). Bisheteroarylpiperazine reverse transcriptase inhibitor in combination with 3'-azido-3'-deoxythymidine or 2',3'-dideoxycytidine synergistically inhibits human immunodeficiency virus type 1 replication in vitro. Antimicrob Ag Chemother 38: 288.

Chow YK, Hirsch MS, Merrill DP (1993a). Use of evolutionary limitations of HIV-1 multidrug resistance to optimize therapy. Nature 361: 650.

Chow FP, Chen RB, Hamburger AW (1993b). Sustained elevation of platelet counts by long-term azidothymidine treatment of immunosuppressed mice. J Lab Clin Med 121: 562.

Cinque P, Landonio G, Lazzarin A (1993). Long-term treatment with zidovudine in patients with human immunodeficiency virus (HIV)-associated thrombocytopenia: modes of response and correlation with markers of HIV replication. Eur J Haematol 50: 17.

Clerici M, Landay AL, Kessler HA (1992). Reconstitution of long-term T helper cell function after zidovudine therapy in human immunodeficiency virus-infected patients. J Infect Dis 166: 723.

Cload PA (1989). A review of the pharmacokinetics of zidovudine in man. J Infect 1: 15.

Cohen H, Williams I, Matthey F et al. (1989). Reversible zidovudine-induced pure red-cell aplasia. AIDS 3: 177.

Collier AC, Bozzette S, Coombs RW (1990). A pilot study of low-dose zidovudine in human immunodeficiency virus infection. New Engl J Med 323: 1015.

Collier AC, Tartaglione T, Corey L (1991). To the editor: (letter). New Engl J Med 324: 996.

Collier AC, Coombs RW, Fischl MA (1993). Combination therapy with zidovudine and didanosine compared with zidovudine alone in HIV-1 infection. *Ann Int Med* **119**: 786.

Collier AC, Schoenfeld DA, Bourland D *et al.* (1995). Prospective comparative study of acyclovir (ACV) and zidovudine (ZDV) versus ZDV alone in patients with AIDS. *2nd National Conference Human Retrovir Related Infect* Abstract no. 383.

Collier AC, Coombs RW, Schoenfeld DA *et al.* (1996). Treatment of human immunodeficiency virus infection with saquinavir, zidovudine and zalcitabine AIDS Clinical Trials Group. *New Engl J Med* **334**: 1011.

Concorde Co-ordinating Committee (1994). MRC/ANRS randomised double-blind controlled trial of immediate and deferred zidovudine in symptom-free HIV infection. *Lancet* **343**: 871.

Conlon CP, Klenerman P, Edwards A *et al.* (1994). Heterosexual transmission of human immunodeficiency virus type 1 variants associated with zidovudine resistance. *J Infect Dis* **169**: 411.

Connell EV, Hsu MC, Richman DD (1994). Combinative interactions of a human immunodeficiency virus (HIV) Tat antagonist with HIV reverse transcriptase inhibitors and an HIV protease inhibitor. *Antimicrob Ag Chemother* **38**: 348.

Connor EM, Sperling RS, Gelber R *et al.* (1994). Reduction of maternal infant transmission of human immunodeficiency virus type 1 with zidovudine treatment Pediatric AIDS Clinical Trials Group Protocol 076 Study Group. *New Engl J Med* **331**: 1173.

Conway B, Halliday WC, Brunham RC (1990). Human immunodeficiency virus-associated progressive multifocal leukoencephalopathy: apparent response to 3'-azido-3'-deoxythymidine. *Rev Infect Dis* **12**: 479.

Cooper DA, Pedersen C, Aiuti F (1991). The efficacy and safety of zidovudine with or without acyclovir in the treatment of patients with AIDS-related complex. The European-Australian Collaborative Group. *AIDS* **5**: 933.

Cooper DA, Gatell JM, Kroon S (1993a). Zidovudine in persons with asymptomatic HIV infection and CD4+ cell counts greater than 400 per cubic millimeter. *New Engl J Med* **329**: 297.

Cooper DA, Pehrson PO, Pedersen C (1993b). The efficacy and safety of zidovudine alone or as cotherapy with acyclovir for the treatment of patients with AIDS and AIDS-related complex: a double-blind randomized trial European-Australian Collaborative Group. *AIDS* **7**: 197.

Cox SW, Aperia K, Albert J, Wahren B (1994). Comparison of the sensitivities of primary isolates of HIV type 2 and HIV type 1 to antiviral drugs and drug combinations. *AIDS Res Hum Retrovir* **10**: 1725.

Craig JC, Duncan IB, Whittaker L, Roberts NA (1990). Antiviral synergy between inhibitors of HIV proteinase and reverse transcriptase. *Antivir Chem Chemother* **4**: 161.

Craig JC, Whittaker L, Duncan IB, Roberts NA (1994). *In vitro* anti HIV and cytotoxicological evaluation of the triple combination; AZT and ddC with HIV proteinase inhibitor saquinavir (Ro 31–8959). *Antivir Chem Chemother* **5**: 380.

Creagh-Kirk T, Doi P, Andrews E *et al.* (1988). Survival experience among patients with AIDS receiving zidovudine. *JAMA* **260**: 3009.

Cretton EM, Schinazi RF, Mc Clure HM (1991). Pharmacokinetics of 3'-azido-3'-deoxythymidine and its catabolites and interactions with probenecid in rhesus monkeys. *Antimicrob Ag Chemother* **35**: 801.

Croft N, Yap PL, Mok JY (1992). Zidovudine therapy in combination with intravenous immunoglobulin in HIV infected children. *Scott Med J* **37**: 138.

Crowe SM, McGrath MS, Elbeik T *et al.* (1989). Comparative assessment of antiretrovirals in human monocyte-macrophages and lymphoid cell lines acutely and chronically infected with the human immunodeficiency virus. *J Med Virol* **29**: 176.

Crowe SM, Cooper DA, Chambers DE (1996). Antiretroviral therapies for HIV. *Med J Aust* **164**: 290.

D'Aquila RT, Johnson VA, Welles SL *et al.* (1995). Zidovudine resistance and HIV-1 disease progression during antiretroviral therapy. AIDS Clinical Trials Group Protocol 116B/117 Team and the Virology Committee Resistance Working Group. *Ann Int Med* **122**: 401.

D'Aquila RT, Hughes MD, Johnson VA (1996). Nevirapine, zidovudine and didanosine compared with zidovudine and didanosine in patients with HIV-1 infection. *Ann Intern Med* **124**: 1019.

Dalakas MC, Illa I, Pezeshkpour GH *et al.* (1990). Mitochondrial myopathy caused by long-term zidovudine therapy. *New Engl J Med* **322**: 1098.

Dalakas MC, Leon-Monzon ME, Bernardini I *et al.* (1994). Zidovudine induced mitochondrial myopathy is associated with muscle carniline deficiency and lipid storage. *Annl Neurol* **35**: 482.

Dancis J, Lee J, Mendoza S, Hebes L (1993). Nucleoside transport by perfused human placenta. *Placenta* **14**: 547.

Davey RT, Davey VJ, Metcalf JA (1991). A phase I/II trial of zidovudine, interferon-alpha, and granulocyte-macrophage colony-stimulating factor in the treatment of human immunodeficiency virus type 1 infection. *J Infect Dis* **164**: 43.

de Jong MP, Loewenthal M, Boucher CA *et al.* (1994). Alternating nevirapine and zidovudine treatment of human immunodeficiency virus type 1-infected persons does not prolong nevirapine activity. *J Infect Dis* **169**: 1346.

de Santis M, Noia G, Caruso A, Mancuso S (1995). Guidelines for the use of zidovudine in pregnant women with HIV infection. *Drugs* **50**: 43.

Degre M, Beck S (1994). Anti-HIV activity of dideoxynucleosides foscarnet and fusidic acid is potentiated by human leukocyte interferon in blood derived macrophages. *Chemother* **40**: 201.

Delta Coordinating Committee (1996). Delta; a randomised double blind controlled trial comparing combinations of zidovudine plus didanosine or zalcitabine with zidovudine alone in HIV infected individuals. *Lancet* **348**: 283.

Demeter LM, Nawaz T, Morse G *et al.* (1995). Development of zidovudine resistance mutations in patients receiving prolonged didanosine monotherapy. *J Infect Dis* **172**: 1480.

Descamps D, Collin G, Loussert-Ajaka I *et al.* (1995). HIV-1 group 0 sensitivity to antiretroviral drugs. *AIDS* **9**: 977.

Dickover RE, Donovan RM, Goldstein E *et al.* (1992). Decreases in unintegrated HIV DNA are associated with antiretroviral therapy in AIDS patients. *J AIDS* **5**: 31.

Dickover RE, Garratty EM, Herman SA *et al.* (1996). Identification of levels of maternal HIV-1 RNA associated with risk of perinatal transmission. Effect of maternal zidovudine treatment on viral load. *JAMA* **275**: 599.

Dimitrov DH, Hollinger FB, Baker CJ *et al.* (1993). Study of human immunodeficiency virus resistance to 2'-3'-dideoxyinosine and zidovudine in sequential isolates from pediatric patients on long-term therapy. *J Infect Dis* **167**: 818.

Dolin K, Amato DA, Fischl MA *et al.* (1995). Zidovudine compared with didanosine in patients with advanced HIV type 1 infection and little or no previous experience with zidovudine. AIDS Clinical Trials Group. *Arch Intern Med* **155**: 961.

Dornsife RE, St Clair MH, Huang AT *et al.* (1991). Anti-human immunodeficiency virus synergism by zidovudine (3'-azidothymidine) and didanosine (dideoxymosine) contrasts with their additive inhibition of normal human marrow progenitor cells. *Antimicrob Ag Chemother* **35**: 322.

Dournon E, Matheron S, Rozenbaum W *et al.* (1988). Effects of zidovudine in 365 consecutive patients with AIDS or AIDS-related complex. *Lancet* **ii**: 1297.

Dubin G, Braffman MN (1989). Zidovudine-induced hepatotoxicity. *Ann Intern Med* **110**: 85.

Dudley MN (1995). Clinical pharmacokinetics of nucleoside antiretroviral agents. *J Infect Dis* **171**: S99.

Dueweke TJ, Poppe SM, Romero DL *et al.* (1993). U-90152, a potent inhibitor of human immunodeficiency virus type 1 replication. *Antimicrob Ag Chemother* **37**: 127.

Durand E, Le JC, Hugues FC (1991). Failure of prophylactic zidovudine after suicidal self-inoculation of HIV-infected blood (letter). *New Engl J Med* **324**: 1062.

Duvic M, Crane MM, Conant M *et al.* (1994). Zidovudine improves psoriasis in human immunodeficiency virus-positive males. *Arch Dermatol* **130**: 447.

Easterbrook PJ, Emami J, Gozzard B (1993). Rate of CD4 cell decline and prediction of survival in zidovudine treated patients. *AIDS* **7**: 959.

Edlin BR, Weinstein RA, Whaling SM et al. (1992). Zidovudine-interferon-alpha combination therapy in patients with advanced human immunodeficiency virus type 1 infection: biphasic response of p24 antigen and quantitative polymerase chain reaction. *J Infect Dis* **165**: 793.

Edwards P, Turner J, Gold J, Cooper DA (1990). Esophageal ulceration induced by zidovudine. *Ann Intern Med* **112**: 65.

Erice A, Mayers DL, Strike DG et al. (1993). Brief report: primary infection with zidovudine-resistant human immunodeficiency virus type 1. *New Engl J Med* **328**: 1163.

Eriksson BF, Schinazi RF (1989). Combinations of 3'-azido-3'-deoxythymidine (zidovudine) and phosphonoformate (foscarnet) against human immunodeficiency virus type 1 and cytomegalovirus replication *in vitro*. *Antimicrob Ag Chemother* **33**: 663.

Eron JJ, Johnson VA, Merrill DP et al. (1992). Synergistic inhibition of replication of human immunodeficiency virus type 1, including that of a zidovudine-resistant isolate, by zidovudine and 2',3'-dideoxycytidine *in vitro*. *Antimicrob Ag Chemother* **36**: 1559.

Eron JJ, Chow YK, Caliendo AM et al. (1993). Pol mutations conferring zidovudine and didanosine resistance with different effects *in vitro* yield multiply resistant human immunodeficiency virus type 1 isolates *in vivo*. *Antimicrob Ag Chemother* **37**: 1480.

Eron JJ, Benoit SL, Jemsek J et al. (1995). Treatment with lamivudine, zidovudine or both in HIV positive patients with 200 to 500 CD4+ cells per cubic millimeter. North American HIV Working Party. *New Engl J Med* **333**: 1662.

Espinoza LR, Aguilar JL, Espinoza CG et al. (1991). Characteristics and pathogenesis of myositis in human immunodeficiency virus infection–distinction from azidothymidine-induced myopathy. *Rheum Dis Clin North Amer* **17**: 117.

Faraj A, Fowler DA, Bridges EG, Sommadossi JP (1994). Effects of 2',3'-dideoxynucleosides on proliferation and differentiation of human pluripotent progenitors in liquid culture and their effects on mitochondrial DNA synthesis. *Antimicrob Ag Chemother* **38**: 924.

Feeney GF, Frazer I (1988). AIDS-associated psoriasis responds to azidothymidine. *Med J Aust* **148**: 155.

Fernandez-Cruz E, Lang JM, Frissen J et al. (1995). Zidovudine plus interferon-alpha versus zidovudine alone in HIV-infected symptomatic or asymptomatic persons with CD4+ cell counts >150 x 10⁶/l. *AIDS* **9**: 1025.

Ferrazin A, De MA, Gotta C et al. (1993). Zidovudine therapy of HIV-1 infection during pregnancy: assessment of the effect on the newborns. *J AIDS* **6**: 376.

Fischl MA, Richman DD, Grieco MH et al. (1987). The efficacy of azidothymidine (AZT) in the treatment of patients with AIDS and AIDS-related complex. *New Engl J Med* **317**: 185.

Fischl MA, Richman DD, Causey DM et al. (1989). Prolonged zidovudine therapy in patients with AIDS and advanced AIDS-related complex. AZT Collaborative Working Group. *JAMA* **262**: 2405.

Fischl A, Richman DD, Hansen N et al. (1990a). The safety and efficacy of zidovudine (AZT) in the treatment of subjects with mildly symptomatic human immunodeficiency virus type 1 (HIV) infection; A double-blind, placebo-controlled trial. *Ann Int Med* **112**: 727.

Fischl M, Galpin JE, Levine JD et al. (1990b). Recombinant human erythropoietin for patients with AIDS treated with zidovudine. *New Engl J Med* **322**: 1488.

Fischl MA, Parker CB, Pettinelli C et al. (1990c). Reduced dose of zidovudine in treating AIDS. *New Engl J Med* **323**: 1009.

Fischl MA, Resnick L, Coombs R et al. (1994). The safety and efficacy of combination N-Butyl-deoxynojirimycin (SC-48334) and zidovudine in patients with HIV-1 infection and 200–500 CD4 cells/mm³. *J AIDS* **7**: 139.

Fischl MA, Stanley K, Collier AC et al. (1995). Combination and monotherapy with zidovudine and zalcitabine in patients with advanced HIV disease. The NIAID AIDS Clinical Trials Group. *Ann Int Med* **122**: 24.

Fletcher CV, Rhame FS, Beatty CC et al. (1992). Comparative pharmacokinetics of zidovudine in healthy volunteers and in patients with AIDS with and without hepatic disease. *Pharmacotherapy* **12**: 429.

Forseter G, Joline C, Wormser GP (1994). Tolerability, safety, and acceptability of zidovudine prophylaxis in health care workers. *Arch Int Med* **154**: 2745.

Freiman JP, Heifert KE, Hamrell MC, Stein DS (1993). Hepatomegaly with severe steatosis in HIV-seropositive patients. *AIDS* **7**: 370.

French MA, Mallal SA, Dawkins RL (1992). Zidovudine-induced restoration of cell-mediated immunity to mycobacteria in immunodeficient HIV-infected patients. *AIDS* **6**: 1293.

Frenkel LM, Wagner LE, Atwood SM et al. (1995a). Specific sensitive and rapid assay for human immunodeficiency virus type 1 pol mutations associated with resistance to zidovudine and didanosine. *J Clin Microb* **33**: 342.

Frenkel LM, Wagner LE, Demeter LM et al. (1995b). Effects of zidovudine use during pregnancy on resistance and vertical transmission of human immunodeficiency virus type 1. *Clin Infect Dis* **20**: 1321.

Frissen PH, van der Ende ME, ten Napel CH et al. (1994). Zidovudine and interferon-alpha combination therapy versus zidovudine monotherapy in subjects with symptomatic human immunodeficiency virus type 1 infection. *J Infect Dis* **169**: 1351.

Furman PA, Barry DW (1988). Spectrum of antiviral activity and mechanism of action of zidovudine. An overview. *Amer J Med* **85**: 176.

Furman PA, Fyfe JA, St Clair MH et al. (1986). Phosphorylation of 3'-azido-3'-deoxythymidine and selective interaction of the 5'-triphosphate with human immunodeficiency virus reverse transcriptase. *Proc Natl Acad Sci USA* **83**: 8333.

Furth PA, Kazakis AM (1987). Nail pigmentation changes associated with azidothymidine (zidovudine). *Ann Intern Med* **107**: 350.

Gallant JE, Moore RD, Keruly J et al. (1995). Lack of association between acyclovir use and survival in patients with advanced human immunodeficiency virus disease treated with zidovudine. Zidovudine Epidemiology Study Group. *J Infect Dis* **172**: 346.

Gallicano KD, Tobe S, Sahai J et al. (1992). Pharmacokinetics of single and chronic dose zidovudine in two HIV positive patients undergoing continuous ambulatory peritoneal dialysis (CAPD). *J AIDS* **5**: 242.

Gallicano K, Sahai J, Swick L et al. (1995). Effect of rifabutin on the pharmacokinetics of zidovudine in patients infected with human immunodeficiency virus. *Clin Infect Dis* **21**: 1008.

Gallicchio VS, Hughes NK (1992). Suppression of murine hematopoiesis *in vivo* after chronic administration of zidovudine: evidence that zidovudine-induced anemia is the result of decreased bone marrow-derived, erythropoietin-responsive progenitor cells. *Proc Soc Exp Biol Med* **199**: 459.

Gao Q, Gu ZX, Parniak MA et al. (1992). *In vitro* selection of variants of human immunodeficiency virus type 1 resistant to 3'-azido-3'-deoxythymidine and 2',3'-dideoxyinosine. *J Virol* **66**: 12.

Gao WY, Agbaria R, Driscoll JS, Mitsuya H (1994). Divergent anti-human immunodeficiency virus activity and anabolic phosphorylation of 2'-3'-dideoxynucleoside analogs in testing and activated human cells. *J Biol Chem* **269**: 12633.

Garraffo R, Cassuto VE, Barillon J et al. (1989). Influence of hemodialysis on zidovudine (AZT) and its glucuronide (GAZT) pharmacokinetics: two case reports. *Int J Clin Pharmacol Ther Toxicol* **27**: 535.

Gelmon K, Montaner JS, Fanning M et al. (1989). Nature, time course and dose dependence of zidovudine-related side effects; results from the multicenter Canadian azidothymidine trial. *AIDS* **3**: 555.

Gerberding J (1993). Is antiretroviral treatment after percutaneous HIV exposure justified? *Ann Int Med* **118**: 979.

Gerberding JL (1996). Prophylaxis for occupational exposure to HIV. *Ann Intern Med* **125**: 497.

Gerberding JL, Henderson DK (1992). Management of occupational exposures to bloodborne pathogens: hepatitis B virus, hepatitis C virus, and human immunodeficiency virus. *Clin Infect Dis* **14**: 1179.

Gertner E, Thurn JR, Williams DN *et al.* (1989). Zidovudine-associated myopathy. *Amer J Med* **86**: 814.

Gibb D, Barry M, Ormesher S *et al.* (1995). Pharmacokinetics of zidovudine and dideoxyinosine alone and in combination in children with HIV infection. *Brit J Clin Pharmacol* **39**: 527.

Gill PS, Rarick M, Brynes RK *et al.* (1987). Azidothymidine associated with bone marrow failure in the acquired immunodeficiency syndrome (AIDS). *Ann Int Med* **107**: 502.

Gill PS, Harringtoon W, Kaplan MH *et al.* (1995). Treatment of adult T-cell leukemia-lymphoma with a combination of interferon-alpha and zidovudine. *New Engl J Med* **332**: 1744.

Gill S, Tang A, Cordery M *et al.* (1991). The effects of twice and four times daily zidovudine on p24 antigenaemia in CDC stage II/III patients. *Genitourin Med* **67**: 15.

Gilson RJ, Hawkins AE, Kelly GK *et al.* (1991). No effect of zidovudine on hepatitis B virus replication in homosexual men with symptomatic HIV-1 infection. *AIDS* **5**: 217.

Gitterman SR, Drusano GL, Egorin MJ, Standiford HC (1990). Population pharmacokinetics of zidovudine. The Veterans Administration Cooperative Studies Group. *Clin Pharmacol Ther* **48**: 161.

Gobert JM, Remington KM, Zhu YG, North TW (1994). Multiple drug resistant mutants of feline immunodeficiency virus selected with 2',3'-dideoxyinosine alone and in combination with 3'-azido-3'- deoxythymidine. *Antimicrob Ag Chemother* **38**: 861.

Gogu SR, Malter JS, Agrawal KC (1992). Zidovudine-induced blockade of the expression and function of the erythropoietin receptor. *Biochem Pharmacol* **44**: 1009.

Gonzales CM, Larripa I (1994). Genatoxic activity of azidothymidine (AZT) in *in vitro* symptoms. *Pharmaceut Res* **32**: 113.

Gonzales MF, Olney RK, So YT *et al.* (1988). Subacute structural myopathy associated with human immunodeficiency virus infection. *Arch Neurol* **45**: 585.

Good SS, de Miranda P (1992). Species differences in the metabolism and disposition of antiviral nucleoside analogues: 2 zidovudine. *Antimicrob Ag Chemother* **3**: 65.

Gotzsche PC, Nielsen C, Gerstoft J *et al.* (1992). Trend towards decreased survival in patients infected with HIV resistant to zidovudine. *Scand J Infect Dis* **24**: 563.

Gradon JD, Chapnick EK, Sepkowitz DV (1992). Zidovudine-induced hepatitis. *J Intern Med* **231**: 317.

Graham NM, Zeger SL, Kuo V *et al.* (1991a). Zidovudine use in AIDS-free HIV-1-seropositive homosexual men in the Multicenter AIDS Cohort Study (MACS), 1987–1989. *J AIDS* **4**: 267.

Graham NM, Zeger SL, Park LP *et al.* (1991b). Effect of zidovudine and *Pneumocystis carinii* pneumonia prophylaxis on progression of HIV-1 infection to AIDS. The Multicenter AIDS Cohort Study. *Lancet* **338**: 265.

Graham NM, Zeger SL, Park LP *et al.* (1992). The effects on survival of early treatment of human immunodeficiency virus infection. *New Engl J Med* **326**: 1037.

Grau MM, Millan F, Febrer MI *et al.* (1990). Pigmented nail bands and mucocutaneous pigmentation in HIV-positive patients treated with zidovudine. *J Amer Acad Dermatol* **22**: 687.

Gray F, Belec L, Keohane C *et al.* (1994). Zidovudine therapy and HIV encephalitis; a 10 year neuropathological survey. *AIDS* **8**: 489.

Greenberg RG, Berger TG (1990). Nail and mucocutaneous hyperpigmentation with azidothymidine therapy. *J Amer Acad Dermatol* **22**: 327.

Gulevich SJ, McCutchan JA, Thal LJ *et al.* (1993). Effect of antiretroviral therapy on the cerebrospinal fluid of patients seropositive for the human immunodeficiency virus. *J AIDS* **6**: 1002.

Gurusinghe AD, Land SA, Birch C *et al.* (1995). Reverse transcriptase mutations in sequential HIV-1 isolates in a patient with AIDS. *J Med Virol* **46**: 238.

Ha JC, Nosbisch C, Conrad F (1994). Fetal toxicity of zidovudine (azidothymidine) in *Macaca nemestrina*: preliminary observations. *J AIDS* **7**: 154.

Hagberg L, Andersson M, Chiodi F *et al.* (1991). Effect of zidovudine on cerebrospinal fluid in patients with HIV infection and acute neurological disease. *Scand J Infect Dis* **23**: 681.

Hagler DN, Frame PT (1986). Azidothymidine neurotoxicity. *Lancet* **28**: 107.

Hamed KA, Winters MA, Holodniy M *et al.* (1993). Detection of human immunodeficiency virus type 1 in semen: effects of disease stage and nucleoside therapy. *J Infect Dis* **167**: 798.

Hamilton JD, Hartigan PM, Simberkoff MS *et al.* (1992). A controlled trial of early versus late treatment with zidovudine in symptomatic human immunodeficiency virus infection. Results of the Veterans Affairs Cooperative Study. *New Engl J Med* **326**: 437.

Hammer SM, Gillis JM (1987). Synergistic activity of granulocyte-macrophage colony-stimulating factor and 3'-azido-3'-deoxythymidine against human immunodeficiency virus *in vitro*. *Antimicrob Ag Chemother* **31**: 1046.

Hammer SM, Katzenstein DA, Hughes MD *et al.* (1996). A trial comparing nucleoside monotherapy with combination therapy in HIV-infected adults with CD4 cell counts from 200 to 500 per cubic millimeter. *New Engl J Med* **335**: 1081.

Hankins GD, Lowery CL, Scott RT *et al.* (1990). Transplacental transfer of zidovudine in the near-term pregnant baboon. *Amer J Obstet Gynecol* **163**: 728.

Haritani H, Uchida T, Okuda Y, Shikata T (1989). Effect of 3'-azido-3'-deoxythymidine on replication of duck hepatitis B virus *in vivo* and *in vitro*. *J Med Virol* **29**: 244.

Harrigan PR, Kinghorn I, Bloor S *et al.* (1996). Significance of amino acid variation at HIV-1 reverse transcriptase residue 210 for zidovudine susceptibility. *J Virol* **70**: 5930.

Hartshorn KL, Vogt MW, Chou TC *et al.* (1987). Synergistic inhibition of human immunodeficiency virus *in vitro* by azidothymidine and recombinant alpha A interferon. *Antimicrob Ag Chemother* **31**: 168.

Hayes KA, Lafrado LJ, Erickson JG *et al.* (1993). Prophylactic ZDV therapy prevents early viremia and lymphocyte decline but not primary infection in feline immunodeficiency virus-inoculated cats. *J AIDS* **6**: 127.

Helbert M, Robinson D, Peddle B *et al.* (1988). Acute meningo-encephalitis on dose reduction of zidovudine. *Lancet* **i**: 1249.

Hendrix CW, Flexner C, Szebeni J *et al.* (1994). Effect of dipyridamole on zidovudine pharmacokinetics and short term tolerance in asymptomatic human immunodeficiency virus infected subjects. *Antimicrob Ag Chemother* **38**: 1036.

Henry DH, Beall GN, Benson CA *et al.* (1992). Recombinant human erythropoietin in the treatment of anemia associated with human immunodeficiency virus (HIV) infection and zidovudine therapy. Overview of four clinical trials. *Ann Intern Med* **117**: 739.

Henry K, Chinnock BJ, Quinn RP *et al.* (1988). Concurrent zidovudine levels in semen and serum determined by radioimmunoassay in patients with AIDS or AIDS-related complex. *JAMA* **259**: 3023.

Herskowitz A, Willoughby SB, Baughman KL *et al.* (1992). Cardiomyopathy associated with antiretroviral therapy in patients with HIV infection: a report of six cases. *Ann Intern Med* **116**: 311.

Herzberg NH, Zorn I, Zwart R *et al.* (1992). Major growth reduction and minor decrease in mitochondrial enzyme activity in cultured human muscle cells after exposure to zidovudine. *Muscle Nerve* **15**: 706.

Hewitt RG, Morse GD (1992). Granulocyte-macrophage colony-stimulating factor and zidovudine in the treatment of neutropenia and human immunodeficiency virus infection. *Pharmacotherapy* **12**: 455.

Hewitt RG, Morse GD, Lawrence WD *et al.* (1993). Pharmacokinetics and pharmacodynamics of granulocyte-macrophage colony-stimulating factor and zidovudine in patients with AIDS and severe AIDS-related complex. *Antimicrob Ag Chemother* **37**: 512.

Ho DD (1995). A controlled trial of zidovudine in primary human immunodeficiency virus infection. *New Engl J Med* **333**: 408.

Ho DD, Moudgil T, Alam M (1989). Quantitation of human immunodeficiency virus type 1 in the blood of infected persons. *New Engl J Med* **321**: 1621.

Hochster H, Dieterich D, Bozzette S *et al.* (1990). Toxicity of combined ganciclovir and zidovudine for cytomegalovirus disease associated with AIDS. An AIDS Clinical Trials Group Study. *Ann Intern Med* **113**: 111.

Hoffman CA, Munson R (1995). Ethical issues in the use of zidovudine to reduce vertical transmission of HIV. *New Engl J Med* **332**: 891.

Hoggard PG, Veal GJ, Wild MJ *et al.* (1995). Drug interactions with zidovudine phosphorylation *in vitro*. *Antimicrob Ag Chemother* **39**: 1376.

Hooker DJ, Tachedjian G, Soloman AE *et al.* (1996). An *in vivo* mutation from leucine to tryptophan at position 210 in human immunodeficiency virus reverse transcriptase contributes to high-level resistance to AZT. *J Virol* **70**: 8010.

Horwitz JP, Chua J *et al.* (1964). The monomesylates of 1–(2'-deoxy-B-D-lyxofuranosyl) thymine. *J Org Chem* **29**: 2076.

Howe JL, Back DJ, Colbert J (1992). Extrahepatic metabolism of zidovudine. *Brit J Clin Pharmacol* **33**: 190.

Huang P, Farquhar D, Plunkett W (1990). Selective action of 3'-azido-3'-deoxythymidine 5'-triphosphate on viral reverse transcriptases and human DNA polymerases. *J Biol Chem* **265**: 11914.

Husson RN, Mueller BU, Farley M *et al.* (1994). Zidovudine and didanosine combination therapy in children with human immunodeficiency virus infection. *Pediatrics* **93**: 316.

Ifudu O, Rao TK, Tan CC *et al.* (1995). Zidovudine is beneficial in human immunodeficiency virus associated nephropathy. *Amer J Nephrol* **15**: 217.

Israelski DM, Tom C, Remington JS (1989). Zidovudine antagonizes the action of pyrimethamine in experimental infection with *Toxoplasma gondii*. *Antimicrob Ag Chemother* **33**: 30.

Iversen AK, Shafer RW, Wehrly K *et al.* (1996). Multidrug-resistant human immunodeficiency virus type 1 strains resulting from combination antiretroviral therapy. *J Virol* **70**: 1086.

Izuta S, Saneyoshi M, Sakurai T *et al.* (1991). Mechanisms of inhibitions of DNA polymerase gamma by nucleotide analogues having anti-HIV activities. *Nucleic Acids Symp Ser* **25**: 79.

Jacobson MA, McGrath MS, Joseph P *et al.* (1989a). Zidovudine-induced fever. *J AIDS* **2**: 382.

Jacobson MA, Abrams DI, Volberding PA, *et al* (1989b). Serum beta 2-microglobulin decreases in patients with AIDS or ARC treated with azidothymidine. *J Infect Dis* **159**: 1029.

Jacobson MA, van der Horst C, Causey DM *et al.* (1990). *In vivo* additive antiretroviral effect of combined zidovudine and foscarnet therapy for human immunodeficiency virus infection (ACTG Protocol 053). *J Infect Dis* **163**: 1219.

Jacobson MA, van der Horst C *et al.* (1991). *In vivo* additive antiretroviral effect of combined zidovudine and foscarnet therapy for human immunodeficiency virus infection (ACTG Protocol 053). *J Infect Dis* **163**: 1219.

Jacobson MA, Gundacker H, Hughes M *et al.* (1995). Zidovudine side effects as reported by black, hispanic and white/non-hispanic patients with early HIV disease; combined analysis of two multicenter placebo controlled trials. *J AIDS Hum Retrovir* **11**: 45.

Janssen HL, Berk L, Heijtink RA *et al.* (1993). Interferon-alpha and zidovudine combination therapy for chronic hepatitis B: results of a randomized, placebo-controlled trial. *Hepatology* **17**: 383.

Japour AJ, Chatis PA, Eigenrauch HA, Crumpacker CS (1991). Detection of human immunodeficiency virus type 1 clinical isolates with reduced sensitivity to zidovudine and dideoxyinosine by RNA-RNA hybridization. *Proc Natl Acad Sci USA*: **88**: 3092.

Japour AJ, Welles S, D'Aquila RT *et al.* (1995). Prevalence and clinical significance of zidovudine resistance mutations in human immunodeficiency virus isolated from patients after long term zidovudine treatment. AIDS Clinical Trials Group 1168/117 Study Team and the Virology Committee Resistance Working Group. *J Infect Dis* **171**: 1172.

Johnson VA, Barlow MA, Chou TC *et al.* (1989a). Synergistic inhibition of human immunodeficiency virus type 1 (HIV-1) replication *in vitro* by recombinant soluble CD4 and 3'-azido-3'-deoxythymidine. *J Infect Dis* **159**: 837.

Johnson VA, Walker BD, Barlow MA, *et al* (1989b). Synergistic inhibition of human immunodeficiency virus type 1 and type 2 replication *in vitro*

by castanospermine and 3'-azido-3'-deoxythymidine. *Antimicrob Ag Chemother* **33**: 53.

Johnson VA, Barlow MA, Morrill DP *et al.* (1990). Three-drug synergistic inhibition of HIV-1 replication *in vitro* by zidovudine, recombinant soluble CD4, and recombinant interferon-alpha A. *J Infect Dis* **161**: 1059.

Johnson VA, Merrill DP, Videler JA *et al.* (1991). Two-drug combinations of zidovudine, didanosine, and recombinant interferon-alpha A inhibit replication of zidovudine-resistant human immunodeficiency virus type 1 synergistically *in vitro*. *J Infect Dis* **164**: 646.

Johnson VA, Merrill DP, Chou TC, Hirsch MS (1992). Human immunodeficiency virus type 1 (HIV-1) inhibitory interactions between protease inhibitor Ro 31–8959 and zidovudine, 2',3'-dideoxycytidine, or recombinant interferon-alpha A against zidovudine-sensitive or -resistant HIV-1 *in vitro*. *J Infect Dis* **166**: 1143.

Joint Working Party of the Hospital Infection Society and the Surgical Infection Study Group (1992). Risks to surgeons and patients from HIV and hepatitis: guidelines on precautions and management of exposure to blood or body fluids. *Brit Med J* **305**: 1337.

Jones PD (1991). HIV transmission by stabbing despite zidovudine prophylaxis. *Lancet* **338**: 884.

Jurriaans S, Weverling GJ, Goudsmit J *et al.* (1995). Distinct changes in HIV type 1 RNA versus p24 antigen levels in serum during short-term zidovudine therapy in asymptomatic individuals with and without progression to AIDS. *AIDS Res Hum Retrovir* **11**: 473.

Kageyama S, Weinstein JN, Shirasaka T *et al.* (1992). *In vitro* inhibition of human immunodeficiency virus (HIV) type 1 replication by C2 symmetry-based HIV protease inhibitors as single agents or in combinations. *Antimicrob Ag Chemother* **36**: 926.

Kahn JO, Lagakos SW, Richman DD *et al.* (1992). A controlled trial comparing continued zidovudine with didanosine in human immunodeficiency virus infection The NIAID AIDS Clinical Trials Group. *New Engl J Med* **327**: 581.

Kaplan MH, Sadick NS, Wieder J *et al.* (1989). Antipsoriatic effects of zidovudine in human immunodeficiency virus-associated psoriasis. *J Amer Acad Dermatol* **20**: 76.

Kaplan MH, Sadick NS, Talmor M (1991). Acquired trichomegaly of the eyelashes: a cutaneous marker of acquired immunodeficiency syndrome. *J Amer Acad Dermatol* **25**: 801.

Kappes JC, Saag MS, Shaw GM *et al.* (1995). Assessment of antiretroviral therapy by plasma viral load testing; standard and ICD HIV-1 p24 antigen and viral RNA (QC-PCR) assays compared. *J AIDS Hum Retrovir* **10**: 139.

Katlama C, Ingrand D, Loveday C *et al.* (1996). Safety and efficacy of lamivudine-zidovudine combination therapy in antiretroviral-naive patients A randomized controlled comparison with zidovudine monotherapy. *JAMA* **276**: 118.

Katz VL, Lim W (1995). HIV infection in pregnancy, a review of current developments. *N Carolina Med J* **56**: 102.

Katzenstein DA, Holodniy M, Israelski DM *et al.* (1992). Plasma viremia in human immunodeficiency virus infection: relationship to stage of disease and antiviral treatment. *J AIDS* **5**: 107.

Katzenstein DA, Hammer SM, Hughes MD *et al.* (1996). The relation of virologic and immunologic markers to clinical outcomes after nucleoside therapy in HIV-infected adults with 200 to 500 CD4 cells per cubic millimeter. *New Engl J Med* **335**: 1091.

Kavesh NG, Holzman RS, Seidlin M *et al.* (1989). The combined toxicity of azidothymidine and antimycobacterial agents. A retrospective study. *Amer Rev Respir Dis* **139**: 1094.

Kaye S, Comber E, Tenant-Flowers M, Loveday C (1995). The appearance of drug resistance associated point mutations in HIV type 1 plasma RNA precedes their appearance in proviral DNA. *AIDS Res Hum Retrovir* **11**: 1221.

Kellam P, Boucher CA, Larder BA (1992). Fifth mutation in human immunodeficiency virus type 1 reverse transcriptase contributes to the development of high-level resistance to zidovudine. *Proc Natl Acad Sci USA* **89**: 1934.

Kellam P, Boucher CA, Tijnagel JM, Larder BA (1994). Zidovudine treatment results in the selection of human immunodeficiency virus type 1 variants whose genotypes confer increasing levels of drug resistance. *J Gen Virol* **75**: 341.

Kinloch-De Loes S, Hirschel BJ, Hoen B *et al.* (1995). A controlled trial of zidovudine in primary human immunodeficiency virus infection. *New Engl J Med* **333**: 408.

Klecker RW, Collins JM, Yarchoan R *et al.* (1987). Plasma and cerebrospinal fluid pharmacokinetics of 3'-azido-3'-deoxythymidine; a novel pyrimidine analog with potential application for the treatment of patients with AIDS and related diseases. *Clinical Pharmacol Ther* **41**: 407.

Klutman NE, Hinthorn DR (1991). Excessive growth of eyelashes in a patient with AIDS being treated with zidovudine. *New Engl J Med* **324**: 1896.

Koch MA, Volberding PA, Lagakos SW *et al.* (1992). Toxic effects of zidovudine in asymptomatic human immunodeficiency virus-infected individuals with CD4+ cell counts of 050 x 10(9)/L or less. Detailed and updated results from protocol 019 of the AIDS Clinical Trials Group. *Arch Intern Med* **152**: 2286.

Kohlstaedt LA, Wang J, Friedman JM *et al.* (1992). Crystal structure at 35 A resolution of HIV-1 reverse transcriptase complexed with an inhibitor. *Science* **256**: 1783.

Kong XB, Zhu QY, Ruprecht RM *et al.* (1991). Synergistic inhibition of human immunodeficiency virus type 1 replication *in vitro* by two-drug and three-drug combinations of 3'-azido-3'-deoxythymidine, phosphonoformate, and 2',3'-dideoxythymidine. *Antimicrob Ag Chemother* **35**: 2003.

Kong XB, Zhu QY, Vidal PM *et al.* (1992). Comparisons of anti-human immunodeficiency virus activities, cellular transport, and plasma and intracellular pharmacokinetics of 3'-fluoro-3'-deoxythymidine and 3'-azido-3'-deoxythymidine. *Antimicrob Ag Chemother* **36**: 808.

Konig H, Behr E, Lower J, Kurth R (1989). Azidothymidine triphosphate is an inhibitor of both human immunodeficiency virus type 1 reverse transcriptase and DNA polymerase gamma. *Antimicrob Ag Chemother* **33**: 2109.

Koot M, Schellekens PT, Mulder JW *et al.* (1993). Viral phenotype and T-cell reactivity in human immunodeficiency virus type 1-infected asymptomatic men treated with zidovudine. *J Infect Dis* **168**: 733.

Kornhauser DM, Petty BG *et al.* (1989). Probenecid and zidovudine metabolism. *Lancet* **ii**: 473.

Koshida R, Vrang L, Gilliam G *et al.* (1989). Inhibition of human immunodeficiency virus *in vitro* by combinations of 3'-azido-3'-deoxythymidine and foscarnet. *Antimicrob Ag Chemother* **33**: 778.

Kovacs JA, Deyton L, Davey R *et al.* (1989). Combined zidovudine and interferon-alpha therapy in patients with Kaposi Sarcoma and the acquired immunodeficiency syndrome (AIDS). *Ann Intern Med* **111**: 280.

Kozal MJ, Shafer RW, Winters MA *et al.* (1993). A mutation in human immunodeficiency virus reverse transcriptase and decline in CD4 lymphocyte numbers in long-term zidovudine recipients. *J Infect Dis* **167**: 526.

Kozal MJ, Kroodsma K, Winters MA *et al.* (1994a). Didanosine resistance in HIV infected patients switched from zidovudine to didanosine monotherapy. *Ann Intern Med* **121**: 263.

Kozal MJ, Shafer RW, Winters MA *et al.* (1994b). HIV-1 syncytium inducing phenotype virus burden, codon 215 reverse transcriptase mutation and CD4 cell decline in zidovudine treated patients. *J AIDS* **7**: 832.

Kremer D, Munar MY, Kohlhepp SJ *et al.* (1992). Zidovudine pharmacokinetics in five HIV seronegative patients undergoing continuous ambulatory peritoneal dialysis. *Pharmacotherapy* **12**: 56.

Krieg CJ, Ostertag W, Clauss U *et al.* (1978). Increase in intracisternal A-type particles in Friend cells during inhibition of Friend virus (SFFV) release by interferon or azidothymidine. *Exp Cell Res* **116**: 21.

Krieger JN, Coombs RW, Collier AC *et al.* (1991). Recovery of human immunodeficiency virus type 1 from semen: minimal impact of stage of infection and current antiviral chemotherapy. *J Infect Dis* **163**: 386.

Kroodsma KL, Kozal MJ, Hamed KA *et al.* (1994). Detection of drug resistance mutations in the human immunodeficiency virus type 1 (HIV-1) pol gene: differences in semen and blood HIV-1 RNA and proviral DNA. *J Infect Dis* **170**: 1292.

Krown SE, Gold JW, Neidwiecki D *et al.* (1990). Interferon-alpha with zidovudine: Safety, tolerance, and clinical and virologic effects in patients with Kaposi Sarcoma associated with the acquired immunodeficiency syndrome (AIDS). *Ann Intern Med* **112**: 812.

Krown SE, Paredes J, Bundow D *et al.* (1992a). Interferon-alpha, zidovudine, and granulocyte-macrophage colony-stimulating factor: a phase I AIDS Clinical Trials Group study in patients with Kaposi's sarcoma associated with AIDS. *J Clin Oncol* **10**: 1344.

Krown SE, Myskowski PL, Paredes J (1992b). Medical management of AIDS patients Kaposi's sarcoma. *Med Clin N Amer* **76**: 235.

Kuritzkes DR, Bell S, Bakhtiari M (1994). Rapid CD4+ cell decline after sexual transmission of a zidovudine resistant syncytium inducing isolate of HIV-1. *AIDS* **8**: 1017.

Lacey SF, Larder BA (1994). Mutagenic study of codons 74 and 215 of the human immunodeficiency virus type 1 reverse transcriptase which are significant in nucleoside analog resistance. *J Virol* **68**: 3421.

Lafeuillade A, Papierok G, Pautrat G *et al.* (1992). *In-vitro* activity of zidovudine against mycoplasma. *Lancet* **339**: 131.

Lai KK, Gang DL, Zawacki JK, Cooley TP (1991). Fulminant hepatic failure associated with 2',3' dideoxynosine (ddI). *Ann Intern Med* **115**: 283.

Lalonde RG, Deschenes JG, Seamone C (1991). Zidovudine-induced macular edema. *Ann Intern Med* **114**: 297.

Lam M, Park MC (1990). HIV-associated nephropathy-beneficial effect of zidovudine therapy (letter). *New Engl J Med* **323**: 1775.

Lambert DM, Bartus H, Fernandez AV *et al.* (1993). Synergistic drug interactions of an HIV-1 protease inhibitor with AZT in different *in vitro* models of HIV-1 infection. *Antiviral Res* **21**: 327.

Lamperth L, Dalakas MC, Dagani F *et al.* (1991). Abnormal skeletal and cardiac muscle mitochondria induced by zidovudine (AZT) in human muscle *in vitro* and in an animal model. *Lab Invest* **65**: 742.

Land S, Treloar G, McPhee D *et al.* (1990). Decreased *in vitro* susceptibility to zidovudine of HIV isolates obtained from patients with AIDS. *J Infect Dis* **161**: 326.

Landonio G, Cinque P, Nosari A *et al.* (1993). Comparison of two dose regimens of zidovudine in an open, randomized, multicentre study for severe HIV-related thrombocytopenia. *AIDS* **7**: 209.

Lane C, Falloon J, Walker RE *et al.* (1989). Zidovudine in patients with human immunodeficiency virus (HIV) infection and Kaposi sarcoma. A phase II randomized, placebo-controlled trial. *Ann Intern Med* **111**: 41.

Lange JM, Boucher CA, Hollak CE *et al.* (1990). Failure of zidovudine prophylaxis after accidental exposure to HIV-1. *New Engl J Med* **322**: 1375.

Larder BA (1992). 3'-Azido-3'-deoxythymidine resistance suppressed by a mutation conferring human immunodeficiency virus type 1 resistance to nonnucleoside reverse transcriptase inhibitors. *Antimicrob Ag Chemother* **36**: 2664.

Larder BA (1994). Interactions between drug resistance mutations in human immunodeficiency virus type 1 reverse transcriptase. *J Gen Virol* **75**: 951.

Larder BA, Kemp SD (1989). Multiple mutations in HIV-1 reverse transcriptase confer high-level resistance to zidovudine (AZT). *Science* **246**: 1155.

Larder BA, Purifoy DJ, Powell KL, Darby G (1987). Site-specific mutagenesis of AIDS virus reverse transcriptase. *Nature* **327**: 716.

Larder BA, Darby G, Richman DD (1989). HIV with reduced sensitivity to zidovudine (AZT) isolated during prolonged therapy. *Science* **243**: 1731.

Larder BA, Coates KE, Kemp SD (1991). Zidovudine-resistant human immunodeficiency virus selected by passage in cell culture. *J Virol* **65**: 5232.

Larder BA, Kellam P, Kemp SD (1993). Convergent combination therapy can select viable multidrug resistant HIV-1 *in vitro*. *Nature* **365**: 451.

Larder BA, Kemp SD, Harrigan PR (1995a). Potential mechanism for sustained antiretroviral efficacy of AZT 3TC combination therapy. *Science* **269**: 696.

Larder BA, Kinghorn I, Bloor S et al. (1995b). Significance of amino acid variation at RT codon 210 for AZT sensitivity. *J AIDS Hum Retrovir* **10**: S6.

Laskin OL, de MP, Blum MR (1989). Azidothymidine steady-state pharmacokinetics in patients with AIDS and AIDS-related complex. *J Infect Dis* **159**: 745.

Le Grand R, Clayette P, Noack O et al. (1994). An animal model for antilentiviral therapy; effect of zidovudine on viral load during acute infection after exposure of macaques to simian immunodeficiency virus. *AIDS Res Hum Retrovir* **10**: 1279.

Leal M, Torres Y, Medrano FJ et al. (1994). Does early zidovudine treatment prevent the emergency of syncytium inducing human immunodeficiency virus?. *J Infect Dis* **170**: 1041.

Lee BL, Tauber MG, Sadler B et al. (1996). Atovaquone inhibits the glucuronidation and increases the plasma concentrations of zidovudine. *Clin Pharmacol Ther* **59**: 14.

Lenderking WR, Gelber RD, Cotton DJ et al. (1994). Evaluation of the quality of life associated with zidovudine treatment in asymptomatic human immunodeficiency virus infection. *New Engl J Med* **330**: 738.

Levine AM, Bernstein L, Sullivan-Halley J et al. (1995). Role of zidovudine antiretroviral therapy in the pathogenesis of acquired immunodefiency syndrome-related lymphoma. *Blood* **86**: 4612.

Levine JD, Allan JD, Falcone N et al. (1991). Recombinant human granulocyte-macrophage colony-stimulating factor ameliorates zidovudine-induced neutropenia in patients with acquired immunodeficiency syndrome (AIDS)/AIDS-related complex. *Blood* **78**: 3148.

Lewin CS, Allen RA, Amyes SC (1990). Antibacterial activity of fluoroquinolones in combination with zidovudine. *J Med Microbiol* **33**: 127.

Lewis W, Dalakas MC (1995). Mitochondrial toxicity of antiviral drugs. *Nat Med* **1**: 417.

Lewis W, Papoian T, Gonzalez B et al. (1991). Mitochondrial ultrastructural and molecular changes induced by zidovudine in rat hearts. *Lab Invest* **65**: 228.

Lewis W, Gonzalez B, Chomyn A, Papioan T (1992). Zidovudine induces molecular, biochemical, and ultrastructural changes in rat skeletal muscle mitochondria. *J Clin Invest* **89**: 1354.

Lewis W, Simpson JF, Meyer RR (1994). Cardiac mitochondrial DNA polymerase gamma is inhibited competitively and noncompetitively by phosphorylated zidovudine. *Circulation Res* **74**: 344.

Liebes L, Mendoza S, Wilson D, Dancis J (1990). Transfer of zidovudine (AZT) by human placenta. *J Infect Dis* **161**: 203.

Lin JC, Zhang ZX, Smith MC et al. (1988). Anti-human immunodeficiency virus agent 3'-Azido-3'-deoxythymidine inhibits replication of Epstein-Barr virus. *Antimicrob Ag Chemother* **32**: 265.

Liu M, Fahey JL, Aziz N et al. (1994). Zidovudine and dideoxycytidine differ in their effects on human immunodeficiency virus induced pathologic activation of the immune system. AIDS Clinical Trial Res Group 047. *J Infect Dis* **170**: 1165.

Ljungdahl SE, Guzenda E, Bottiger D et al. (1992). Penetration of zidovudine and 3'-fluoro-3'-deoxythymidine into the brain, muscle tissue, and veins in cynomolgus monkeys: relation to antiviral action. *Antimicrob Ag Chemother* **36**: 2418.

Loke RH, Murray-Lyon IM, Carter GD (1990). Postural hypotension related to zidovudine in a patient infected with HIV. *Brit Med J* **300**: 163.

Looke DF, Grove DI (1990). Failed prophylactic zidovudine after needlestick injury. *Lancet* **335**: 1280.

Lopez-Anaya A, Unadkat JD, Schumann LA, Smith AL (1990a). Pharmacokinetics of zidovudine (azidothymidine). I Transplacental transfer. *J AIDS* **3**: 959.

Lopez-Anaya A, Unadkat JD, Schumann LA, Smith AL (1990b). Pharmaco-

kinetics of zidovudine (azidothymidine). II Development of metabolic and renal clearance pathways in the neonate. *J AIDS* **3**: 1052.

Lopez-Anaya A, Unadkat JD, Schumann LA, Smith AL (1991). Pharmacokinetics of zidovudine (azidothymidine). Effect of pregnancy. *J AIDS* **4**: 64.

Loveday C, Kaye S, Tenant-Flowers M et al. (1995). HIV-1 RNA serum load and resistant viral genotypes during early zidovudine therapy. *Lancet* **345**: 820.

Lowy I, Caruso M, Goff SP, Klatzmann D (1994). Cellular thymidine kinase activity is required for the inhibition of HIV-1 replication by AZT in lymphocytes. *Virology* **200**: 271.

Lundgren JD, Phillips AN, Pedersen C et al. (1994). Comparison of long term prognosis of patients with AIDS treated and not treated with zidovudine AIDS in Europe Study Group. *JAMA* **27**: 1088.

Luzier A, Morse GD (1993). Intravascular distribution of zidovudine: role of plasma proteins and whole blood components. *Antivir Res* **21**: 267.

Lyman WD, Tanaka KE, Kress Y et al. (1990). Zidovudine concentrations in human fetal tissue: implications for perinatal AIDS. *Lancet* **335**: 1280.

Macnab KA, Gill MJ, Sutherland LR et al. (1993). Erratic zidovudine bioavailability in HIV seropositive patients. *J Antimicrob Ag Chemother* **31**: 421.

Maehlen J, Dunlop O, Liestol K et al. (1995). Changing incidence of HIV-induced brain lesions in Oslo, 1983–1994; effects of zidovudine treatment. *AIDS* **9**: 1165.

Mallal SA, James IR, French MA (1994). Detection of subclinical *Mycobacterium avium–intracellulare* complex infection in immunodeficient HIV-infected patietns treated with zidovudine. *AIDS* **8**: 1263.

Mannucci PM, Gringeri A, Savidge G et al. (1994). Randomized double blind placebo controlled trial of twice-daily zidovudine in asymptomatic haemophillacs infected with the human immunodeficiency virus type 1. European Australian Haemophilla Collaborative Study Group. *Brit J Haematol* **86**: 174.

Manouilov KK, White CA, Boudinot FD et al. (1995). Lymphatic distribution of 3'-azido-3'-deoxythymidine and 3'-azido-2',3'-dideoxyuridine in mice. *Drug Metab Dispost* **23**: 658.

Marchbanks K, Dudley MN, Posner MR, Darnowski J (1995). Pharmacokinetics and pharmacodynamics of high dose zidovudine administered as a continuous infusion in patients with cancer. *Pharmacother* **15**: 451.

Marcellin P, Pialoux G, Girard PM et al. (1989). Absence of effect of zidovudine on replication of hepatitis B virus in patients with chronic HIV and HBV infection. *New Engl J Med* **321**: 1758.

Marcus R, CDC Co-operative Needlestick Study Group (1988). Surveillance of health-care workers exposed to blood from patients infected with the human immunodeficiency virus. *New Engl J Med* **319**: 1118.

Martin LN, Murphey-Corb M, Soike KF et al. (1993). Effects of initiation of 3'-azido, 3'-deoxythymidine (zidovudine) treatment at different times after infection of rhesus monkeys with simian immunodeficiency virus. *J Infect Dis* **168**: 825.

Matheson PB, Abrams EJ, Thomas PA et al. (1995). Efficacy of antenatal zidovudine in reducing perinatal transmission of human immunodeficiency virus type 1. The New York City Perinatal HIV Transmission Collaborative Study Group. *J Infect Dis* **172**: 353.

Mathez D, Schinazi RF, Liotta DC, Leibowitch J (1993). Infectious amplification of wild type human immunodeficiency virus from patients' lymphocytes and modulation by reverse transcriptase inhibitors *in vitro*. *Antimicrob Ag Chemother* **37**: 2206.

Matthes E, Lehmann CH, Scholz D et al. (1987). Inhibition of HIV-associated reverse transcriptase by sugar-modified derivatives of thymidine 5'-triphosphate in comparison to cellular DNA polymerases alpha and beta. *Biochem Biophys Res Commun* **148**: 78.

Mauss S, Jablonowski H (1995). Efficacy, safety, and tolerance of low-dose, long term interferon-alpha 2b and zidovudine in early-stage AIDS-associated Kapsoi's sarcoma. *J AIDS Hum Retrovir* **10**: 157.

Mayers DL, McCutchan FE, Sanders-Buell EE et al. (1992). Characterization of HIV isolates arising after prolonged zidovudine therapy. *J AIDS* **5**: 749.

Mayers DL, Japour AJ, Arduino JM et al. (1994). Dideoxynucleoside resistance emerges with prolonged zidovudine monotherapy. *Antimicrob Ag Chemother* **38**: 307.

Mazzulli T, Hirsch MS (1996). Combination therapy for HIV-1 infection. *Antiviral Chemother* **3**: 385.

Mazzulli T, Rusconi S, Merrill DP *et al.* (1994). Alternating versus continuous drug regimens in combination chemotherapy of human immunodeficiency virus type-1 infection *in vitro. Antimicrob Ag Chemother* **38**: 656.

McCune JM, Namikawa R, Shih CC *et al.* (1990). Suppression of HIV infection in AZT-treated SCID-hu mice. *Science* **247**: 564.

McDermott J, Kennedy J, Ellis-Pegler RB, Thomas MG (1992). Pharmacokinetics of zidovudine plus probenecid. *J Infect Dis* **166**: 687.

McEvoy M, Porter K, Mortimer P *et al.* (1987). Prospective study of clinical, laboratory, and anciliary staff with accidental exposures to blood or body fluids from patients infected with HIV. *Brit Med J* **294**: 1595.

McKinney RE, Wilfert C (1994). Growth as a prognostic indicator in children with human immunodeficiency virus infection treated with zidovudine. AIDS Clinical Trials Group Protocol 043 Study Group. *J Pediatr* **125**: 728.

McKinney RE, Pizzo PA, Scott GB *et al.* (1990). Safety and tolerance of intermittent intravenous and oral zidovudine therapy in human immunodeficiency virus-infected pediatric patients. Pediatric Zidovudine Phase I Study Group. *J Pediatr* **116**: 640.

McKinney RE, Maha MA, Connor EM *et al.* (1991). A multicenter trial of oral zidovudine in children with advanced human immunodeficiency virus disease. The Protocol 043 Study Group. *New Engl J Med* **324**: 1018.

McMahon DK, Armstrong JA, Huang XL *et al.* (1994). A phase 1 study of sub-cutaneous recombinant interferon-2 in patients with advanced HIV disease while on zidovudine. *AIDS* **8**: 59.

Medina DJ, Hsiung GD, Mellors JW (1992). Ganciclovir antagonizes the anti-human immunodeficiency virus type 1 activity of zidovudine and didanosine *in vitro. Antimicrob Ag Chemother* **36**: 1127.

Medina DJ, Tung PP, Lerner-Tung MB *et al.* (1995). Sanctuary growth of human immunodeficiency virus in the presence of 3'-azido-3'-deoxythymidine. *J Virol* **69**: 1606.

Mellors JW, Bazmi HZ, Schinazi RF *et al.* (1995). Novel mutations in reverse transcriptase of HIV-1 reduces susceptibility to foscarnet in laboratory and clinical isolates. *Antimicrob Ag Chemother* **39**: 1087.

Meng TC, Fischl MA, Richman DD (1990). AIDS Clinical Trials Group: phase I/II study of combination 2',3'-dideoxycytidine and zidovudine in patients with acquired immunodeficiency syndrome (AIDS) and advanced AIDS-related complex. *Amer J Med* **88**: S27.

Meng TC, Fischl MA, Boota AM *et al.* (1992). Combination therapy with zidovudine and dideoxycytidine in patients with advanced human immunodeficiency virus infection. A phase I/II study. *Ann Intern Med* **116**: 13.

Merenich JA, Hannon RN, Gentry RH, Harrison SM (1989). Azidothymidine-induced hyperpigmentation mimicking primary adrenal insufficiency. *Amer J Med* **86**: 469.

Merigan TC, Amato DA, Balsley J *et al.* (1991). Placebo-controlled trial to evaluate zidovudine in treatment of human immunodeficiency virus infection in asymptomatic patients with hemophilia. NHF-ACTG 036 Study Group. *Blood* **78**: 900.

Merrill DP, Moonis M, Chou TC, Hirsch MS (1996). Lamivudine or stavudine in two and three-drug combinations against human immunodeficiency virus type 1 replication *in vitro. J Infect Dis* **173**: 355.

Mhiri C, Baudrimont M, Bonne G *et al.* (1991). Zidovudine myopathy: a distinctive disorder associated with mitochondrial dysfunction. *Ann Neurol* **29**: 606.

Miles SA, Lee K, Hutlin L *et al.* (1991a). Potential use of human stem cell factor as adjunctive therapy for human immunodeficiency virus-related cytopenias. *Blood* **78**: 3200.

Miles SA, Mitsuyasu RT, Moreno J *et al.* (1991b). Combined therapy with recombinant granulocyte colony-stimulating factor and erythropoietin decreases hematologic toxicity from zidovudine. *Blood* **77**: 2109.

Miller RA (1990). Failure of zidovudine prophylaxis after exposure to HIV-1. *New Engl J Med* **323**: 915.

Minkoff H, Willoughby A (1995). Pediatric HIV disease, zidovudine in pregnancy and unblinding heelstick surveys. Reframing the debate on prenatal HIV testing. *JAMA* **274**: 1165.

Mintz M (1995). Carnitine in human immunodeficiency virus type 1 infection/acquired immune deficiency syndrome. *J Child Neurol* **10**: S40.

Mitsuya H, Broder S (1987). Strategies for antiviral therapy in AIDS. *Nature* **325**: 773.

Mitsuya H, Weinhold KJ, Furman PA *et al.* (1985). 3'-Azido-3'-deoxythymidine (BW A509U): an antiviral agent that inhibits the infectivity and cytopathic effect of human T-lymphotropic virus type III/lymphadenopathy-associated virus *in vitro. Proc Natl Acad Sci USA* **82**: 7096.

MMWR (1994). Recommendations of the US Public Health Service Task Force on the use of zidovudine to reduce perinatal transmission of human immunodeficiency virus. *MMWR* **43**: 1.

MMWR (1995). Case-control study of HIV seroconversion in health care workers after percutaneous exposure to HIV infected blood-France, United Kingdom and United States, Jan 1988 – Aug 1994. *MMWR* **44**: 929.

MMWR (1996). Provisional public health service recommendations for chemoprophylaxis after occupational exposure to HIV. *MMWR* **45**: 468.

Moeller AA, Wiegand M, Oechsner M *et al.* (1992). Effects of zidovudine on EEG sleep in HIV-infected men. *J AIDS* **5**: 636.

Mohri H, Singh MK, Ching WT, Ho DD (1993). Quantitation of zidovudine-resistant human immunodeficiency virus type 1 in the blood of treated and untreated patients. *Proc Natl Acad Sci USA* **90**: 25.

Molina JM, Ferchal F, Chevret S *et al.* (1994). Quantification of HIV-1 virus load under zidovudine therapy in patients with symptomatic HIV infection; relation to disease progression. *AIDS* **8**: 27.

Montaner JS, Le T, Fanning M *et al.* (1990). The effect of zidovudine on platelet count in HIV-infected individuals. *J AIDS* **3**: 565.

Montaner JS, Singer J, Schechter MT *et al.* (1993). Clinical correlates of *in vitro* HIV-1 resistance of zidovudine. Results of the Multicentre Canadian AZT Trial. *AIDS* **7**: 189.

Montaner JS, Schechter MT, Rachlis A *et al.* (1995). Didanosine compared with continued zidovudine therapy for HIV infected patients with 200 to 500 CD4 cells/mm3. A double-blind randomised, controlled trial. Canadian HIV Trials Network Protocol 002 Study Group. *Ann Int Med* **123**: 561.

Moore EC, Cohen F, Kauffman RE, Aravind MK (1990). Zidovudine overdose in a child. *New Engl J Med* **322**: 408.

Moore KH, Raasch RH, Brouwer KL *et al.* (1995). Pharmacokinetics and bioavailability of zidovudine and its glucuronidated metabolite in patients with human immunodeficiency virus infection and hepatic disease (AIDS Clinical Trials Group Protocol 062). *Antimicrob Ag Chemother* **39**: 2732.

Moore RD, Creagh KT, Keruly J *et al.* (1991a). Long-term safety and efficacy of zidovudine in patients with advanced human immunodeficiency virus disease. Zidovudine Epidemiology Study Group. *Arch Intern Med* 151: 981.

Moore RD, Hidalgo J, Sugland BW, Chaisson RE (1991b). Zidovudine and the natural history of the acquired immunodeficiency syndrome. *New Engl J Med* 324: 1412.

Moore RD, Keruly J, Richman DD *et al.* (1992). Natural history of advanced HIV disease in patients treated with zidovudine. The Zidovudine Epidemiology Study Group. *AIDS* **6**: 671.

Morrey JD, Warren RP, Okleberry KM *et al.* (1990). Effects of zidovudine on friend virus complex infection in Rfv-3r/s genotype-containing mice used as a model for HIV infection. *J AIDS* **3**: 500.

Morrey JD, Okleberry KM, Sidwell RW *et al.* (1991). Early-initiated zidovudine therapy prevents disease but not low levels of persistent retrovirus in mice. *J AIDS* **4**: 506.

Morse GD, Olson J, Portmore A *et al.* (1989). Pharmacokinetics of orally administered zidovudine among patients with hemophilia and asymptomatic human immunodeficiency virus (HIV) infection. *Antiviral Res* **11**: 57.

Morse GD, Portmore AC *et al.* (1992). Intravenous and oral zidovudine pharmacokinetics and coagulation effects in asymptomatic human immunodeficiency virus-infected hemophilia patients. *Antimicrob Ag Chemother* 36: 2245.

Morse GD, Shelton MJ, O'Donnel AM (1993). Comparative pharmacokinetics of antiviral nucleoside analogues. *Clin Pharmacokinet* 24: 101.

Morse GD, Shelton MJ, Ho M *et al.* (1995). Pharmacokinetics of zidovudine and didanosine during combination therapy. *Antiviral Res*: 27: 419.

Moye J, Rich KC, Kalish LA *et al.* (1996). Natural history of somatic growth born to women infected by human immunodeficiency virus. *J Pediatr* 128: 58.

Moyle GJ (1995). Resistance to antiretroviral compounds, implications for the clinical management of HIV infection. *Immunol Infect Dis* 5: 170.

Mueller BU, Jacobsen F, Butler KM *et al.* (1992). Combination treatment with azidothymidine and granulocyte colony-stimulating factor in children with human immunodeficiency virus infection. *J Pediatr* 121: 797.

Mueller BU, Pizzo PA, Farley M *et al.* (1994). Pharmacokinetic evaluation of the combination of zidovudine and didanosine in children with human immunodeficiency virus infection. *J Pediatr* 125: 142.

Mulder JW, Cooper DA, Mathiesen L *et al.* (1994). Zidovudine twice daily in asymptomatic subjects with HIV infection and a high risk of progression to AIDS; a randomised, double-blind placebo-controlled study. The European Australian Collaborative Group (Study 017). *AIDS* 8: 313.

Murphy R (1995). Clinical aspects of human immunodeficiency virus disease; clinical rationale for treatment. *J Infect Dis* 171: S81.

Musicco M, Lazzarin A, Nicolosi A *et al.* (1994). Antiretroviral treatment of men infected with human immunodeficiency virus type 1 reduces the incidence of heterosexual transmission. Italian Study Group on HIV Heterosexual Transmission. *Arch Int Med* 154: 1971.

Najera I, Richman DD, Olivares I *et al.* (1994). Natural occurence of drug resistance mutations in the reverse transcriptase of human immunodeficiency virus type 1 isolates. *AIDS Res Hum Retrovir* 10: 1479.

Nakashima H, Matsui T, Harada S *et al.* (1986). Inhibition of replication and cytopathic effect of human T cell lymphotropic virus type III/lymphadenopathy-associated virus by 3'-azido-3'-deoxythymidine *in vitro*. *Antimicrob Ag Chemother* 30: 933.

Nickel W, Austermann S, Bialek G, Grosse F (1992). Interactions of azidothymidine triphosphate with the cellular DNA polymerases alpha, delta, and epsilon and with DNA primase. *J Biol Chem* 267: 848.

Nielsen K, Wel LS, Sim MS *et al.* (1995). Correlation of clinical progression in human immunodeficiency virus-infected children with *in vitro* zidovudine resistance measured by a direct quantitative peripheral blood lymphocyte assay. *J Infect Dis* 172: 359.

O'Brien WA, Hartigan PM, Martin D *et al.* (1996). Changes in plasma HIV-1 RNA and CD4+ lymphocyte counts and the risk of progression to AIDS. Veterans Affairs Cooperative Study Group on AIDS. *New Engl J Med* 334: 426.

Obuch ML, Baker G, Roth RI *et al.* (1992a). Selective cutaneous hyperpigmentation in mice following zidovudine administration. *Arch Dermatol* 128: 508.

Obuch ML, Maurer TA, Becker B, Berger TG (1992b). Psoriasis and human immunodeficiency virus infection. *J Amer Acad Dermatol* 27: 667.

Ogino MT, Dankner WM, Spector SA (1993). Development and significance of zidovudine resistance in children infected with human immunodeficiency virus. *J Pediatr* 123: 1.

Oksenhendler E, Bierling P, Ferchal F *et al.* (1989). Zidovudine for thrombocytopenic purpura related to human immunodeficiency virus (HIV) infection. *Ann Int Med* 110: 365.

Olsen JC, Furman P, Fyfe JA *et al.* (1987). 3'-Azido-3'-deoxythymidine inhibits the replication of avian leukosis virus. *J Virol* 61: 2800.

O'Sullivan MJ, Boyer PJ, Scott GB *et al.* (1993). The pharmacokinetics and safety of zidovudine in the third trimester of pregnancy for women infected with human immunodeficiency virus and their infants; phase 1 acquired immunodeficiency syndrome clinical trials group study protocol 082. Zidovudine Collaborative Working Group. *Amer J Obst Gyn* 168: 1510.

Otto MJ, Reid CD, Garber S *et al.* (1993). *In vitro* anti-human immunodeficiency virus (HIV) activity of XM323, a novel HIV protease inhibitor. *Antimicrob Ag Chemother* 37: 2606.

Pachon J, Cisneros JM, Castillo JR *et al.* (1992). Pharmacokinetics of zidovudine in end-stage renal disease: influence of haemodialysis. *AIDS* 6: 827.

Palmer DL, Hjelle BL, Wiley CA *et al.* (1994). HIV-1 infection despite immediate combination antiviral therapy after infusion of contaminated white cells. *Amer J Med* 97: 289.

Panzer S, Stain C, Benda H, Mannhalter C (1989). Effects of 3-Azidothymidine on platelet counts, indium-iii-labelled platelet kinetics, and antiplatelet antibodies. *Vox Sang* 57: 120.

Paoli I, Dave M, Cohen BD (1992). Pharmacodynamics of zidovudine in patients with end-stage renal disease. *New Engl J Med* 326: 839.

Papierok G, Lafeuillade A, Dombrecht S *et al.* (1992). *In-vitro* activity of zidovudine against mycoplasma. *Lancet* 340: 1543.

Park GB, Mitra AK (1992). Mechanism and site dependency of intestinal mucosal transpor and metabolism of thymidine analogues. *Pharm Res* 9: 326.

Parks WP, Parks ES, Fischl MA *et al.* (1988). HIV-1 inhibition by azidothymidine in a concurrently randomized placebo-controlled trial. *J AIDS* 1: 125.

Pauwels R, Andries K, Desmyter S *et al.* (1990). Potent and selective inhibition of HIV-1 replication *in vitro* by a novel series of TIBO derivatives. *Nature* 343: 470.

Pauwels R, Andries K, Debyser Z *et al.* (1994). New tetrahydrolmidazo[4,5,l-jk] [1,4] benzodiazepin-2 [1H] one and thione derivatives are potent inhibitors of human immunodeficiency virus type 1 replication and are synergistic with 2',3'-dideoxynucleoside analogs. *Antimicrob Ag Chemother* 38: 2863.

Perkins D, Evans DL (1991). HIV-related major depression: response to zidovudine treatment. *Psychosomatics* 32: 451.

Perno CF, Yarchoan R, Cooney DA *et al.* (1988). Inhibition of human immunodeficiency virus (HIV-1/HTLV-IIIBa-L) replication in fresh and cultured human peripheral blood monocytes/macrophages by azidothymidine and related 2',3'-dideoxynucleosides. *J Exp Med* 168: 1111.

Perno CF, Yarchoan R, Cooney DA *et al.* (1989). Replication of human immunodeficiency virus in monocytes. *J Exp Med* 169: 933.

Perno CF, Yarchoan R, Balzarini J *et al.* (1992a). Different pattern of activity of inhibitors of the human immunodeficiency virus in lymphocytes and monocyte/macrophages. *Antiviral Res* 17: 289.

Perno CF, Cooney DA, Gao WY *et al.* (1992b). Effects of bone marrow stimulatory cytokines on human immunodeficiency virus replication and the antiviral activity of dideoxynucleosides in cultures of monocyte/macrophages. *Blood* 80: 995.

Perrin L, Kinloch-de Loes S (1995). Therapeutic interventions in primary HIV infection. *J AIDS Hum Retrovir* 10: S69.

Peters BS, Winer J, Landon DN *et al.* (1993). Mitochondrial myopathy associated with chronic zidovudine therapy in AIDS. *Quart J Med* 86: 5.

Piatek MJ, Saag MS, Yang LC *et al.* (1993). High levels of HIV-1 in plasma during all stages of infection determined by competitive PCR. *Science* 259: 1749.

Pizzo PA, Eddy J, Faloon J *et al.* (1988). Effect of continuous intravenous infusion of zidovudine (AZT) in children with symptomatic HIV infection. *New Engl J Med* 319: 899.

Pizzo PA, Butler K, Balis F *et al.* (1990). Dideoxycytidine alone and in an alternating schedule with zidovudine in children with symptomatic human immunodeficiency virus infection. *J Pediatr* 117: 799.

Podzamczer D, Bolao F, Clotet B *et al.* (1993). Low-dose interferon alpha combined with zidovudine in patients with AIDS-associated Kaposi's sarcoma. *J Intern Med* 233: 247.

Poli G, Orenstein JM, Kinter A *et al.* (1989). Interferon-alpha but not AZT suppresses HIV expression in chronically infected cell lines. *Science* 244: 575.

Portegies P (1995). Review of antiretroviral therapy in the prevention of HIV-related AIDS dementia complex (ADC). *Drugs* 49: 25.

Portegies P, de GJ, Cange JM *et al.* (1989). Declining incidence of AIDS dementia complex after introduction of zidovudine treatment [published erratum appears in BMJ 1989 Nov 4; 299(6708): 1141]. *Brit Med J* **299**: 819.

Principi N, Marchisio P, De Pasquale MP (1994). HIV-1 reverse transcriptase codon 215 mutation and clinical outcome in children treated with zidovudine. *AIDS Res Hum Retrovir* **10**: 721.

Product Information Burroughs Wellcome.

Puro V, Ippolito G, Guzzanti E *et al.* (1992). Zidovudine prophylaxis after accidental exposure to HIV: the Italian experience. The Italian Study Group on Occupational Risk of HIV Infection. *AIDS* **6**: 963.

Qian MX, Swagler AR, Mehta M *et al.* (1992). Pharmacokinetic evaluation of drug interactions with anti-human immunotrophic virus (HIV) Drugs III 2',3'-Dideoxycytidine (ddC) and zidovudine in monkeys. *Pharm Res* **9**: 224.

Qian M, Chandrasena G, Ho RJ, Unadkat JD (1994a). Comparison of rates of intracellular metabolism of zidovudine in human and primate peripheral blood mononuclear cells. *Antimicrob Ag Chemother* **38**: 2398.

Qian M, Bui T, Ho RJ, Unadkat JD (1994b). Metabolism of 3'-azido-3'-deoxythymidine (AZT) in human placental trophoblasts and Hofbauer cells. *Biochem Pharmacol* **48**: 383.

Ragni MV, Miller BJ *et al.* (1992a). Bleeding tendency, platelet function, and pharmacokinetics of ibuprofen and zidovudine in HIV(+) hemophilic men. *Amer J Hematol* **40**: 176.

Ragni MV, Kingsley LA, Zhou SJ (1992b). The effect of antiviral therapy on the natural history of human immunodeficiency virus infection in a cohort of hemophiliacs. *J AIDS* **5**: 120.

Rahav G, Maayan S (1992). Nail pigmentation associated with zidovudine: a review and report of a case. *Scand J Infect Dis* **24**: 557.

Rajaonarison JF, Lacarelle B, Catalin J *et al.* (1992). 3'-azido-3'-deoxythymidine drug interactions. Screening for inhibitors in human liver microsomes. *Drug Metab Dispos* **20**: 578.

Rajaonarison JF, Lacarelle B, Catalin J *et al.* (1993). Effect of anticancer drugs on the glucuronidation of 3'-azido-3'-deoxythymidine in human liver microsomes. *Drug Metab Dispos* **21**: 823.

Rarick MU, Espina B, Montgomery T *et al.* (1991). The long-term use of zidovudine in patients with severe immune-mediated thrombocytopenia secondary to infection with HIV. *AIDS* **5**: 1357.

Reichman RC, Morse GD, Demeter LM *et al.* (1995). Phase 1 study of atevirdine, a non-nucleoside reverse transcriptase inhibitor, in combination with zidovudine for human immunodeficiency virus type 1 infection. ACTG 199 Study Group. *J Infect Dis* **171**: 297.

Remington KM, Chesebro B, Wehrly K *et al.* (1991). Mutants of feline immunodeficiency virus resistant to 3'-azido-3'-deoxythymidine. *J Virol* **65**: 308.

Remington KM, Zhu YQ, Phillips TR, North TW (1994). Rapid phenotypic reversion of zidovudine resistant feline immunodeficiency virus without loss of drug resistant reverse transcriptase. *J Virol* **68**: 632.

Retrovir IV Product Information.

Richman DD (1987). Dideoxynucleosides are less inhibitory *in vitro* against human immunodeficiency virus type 2 (HIV-2) than against HIV-1. *Antimicrob Ag Chemother* **31**: 1879.

Richman DD, Andrews J (1988). Results of continued monitoring of participants in the placebo-controlled trial of zidovudine for serious human immunodeficiency virus infection. *Amer J Med* **85**: 208.

Richman DD, Havlir D (1995). Early versus of HIV infection Zidovudine should be given before symptoms develop. *Drugs* **49**: 9.

Richman DD, Fischl MA, Grieco MH *et al.* (1987a). The toxicity of azidothymidine (AZT) in the treatment of patients with AIDS and AIDS-related complex. A double-blind, placebo-controlled trial. *New Engl J Med* **317**: 192.

Richman DD, Kornbluth RS, Carson DA (1987b). Failure of dideoxynucleosides to inhibit human immunodeficiency virus replication in cultured human macrophages. *J Exp Med* **166**: 1144.

Richman DD, Grimes JM, Lagakos SW (1990). Effect of stage of disease and drug dose on zidovudine susceptibilities of isolates of human immunodeficiency virus. *J AIDS* **3**: 743.

Richman DD, Guatelli JC, Grimes J *et al.* (1991a). Detection of mutations associated with zidovudine resistance in human immunodeficiency virus by use of the polymerase chain reaction. *J Infect Dis* **164**: 1075.

Richman D, Rosenthal AS, Skoog M *et al.* (1991b). BI-RG-587 is active against zidovudine-resistant human immunodeficiency virus type 1 and synergistic with zidovudine. *Antimicrob Ag Chemother* **35**: 305.

Richman DD, Meng TC, Spector SA *et al.* (1994). Resistance to AZT and ddC during long-term combination therapy in patients with advanced infection with human immunodeficiency virus *J AIDS* **7**: 135.

Riedel RR, Clarenbach P, Reetz KP (1989). Coma during azidothymidine therapy for AIDS. *J Neurol* **236**: 185.

Robbins BL, Radman J, McDonald C *et al.* (1994). Enzymatic assay for measurement of zidovudine triphosphate in peripheral blood mononuclear cells. *Antimicrob Ag Chemother* **38**: 115.

Rooke R, Tremblay M, Soudeyns H, De Stephano L (1989). Isolation of drug-resistant variants of HIV-1 from patients on long-term zidovudine therapy. Canadian Zidovudine Multi-Centre Study Group. *AIDS* **3**: 411.

Rooke R, Parniak MA, Tremblay M *et al.* (1991). Biological comparison of wild-type and zidovudine resistant isolates of human immunodeficiency virus type 1 from the same subjects: susceptibility and resistance to other drugs. *Antimicrob Ag Chemother* **35**: 988.

Rouzioux C (1995). Prevention of maternal HIV transmission Practical guidelines. *Drugs* **49**: 17.

Ruprecht RM, Bronson R (1994). Chemoprevention of retroviral infection; success is determined by virus inoculum strength and cellular immunity. *DNA Cell Biol* **13**: 59.

Ruprecht RM, O'Brien LG, Rossoni LD *et al.* (1986). Suppression of mouse viraemia and retroviral disease by 3'-azido-3'-deoxythymidine. *Nature* **323**: 467.

Ruprecht RM, Chou TC, Chipty F *et al.* (1990a). Interferon alpha and 3'-Azido-3'deoxythymidine are highly synergistic in mice and prevent viremia after acute retrovirus exposure. *J AIDS* **3**: 591.

Ruprecht RM, Bernard LD, Gama-Sosa MA *et al.* (1990b). Murine models for evaluating antiretroviral therapy. *Cancer Res* **50**: 5618S.

Saah AJ, Hoover DR Lawrence YH *et al.* (1994). Factors influencing survival after AIDS: report from the multicenter AIDS cohort study (MACS). *J AIDS* **7**: 287.

Sahai J, Gallicano K, Garber G *et al.* (1992). The effect of a protein meal on zidovudine pharmacokinetics in HIV-infected patients. *Brit J Clin Pharmacol* **33**: 657.

Sahai J, Gallicano K, Garber G *et al.* (1995). Pharmacokinetics of simultaneously administered zidovudine and didanosine in HIV-seropositive male patients. *J AIDS Hum Retrovir* **10**: 54.

Sampol E, Lacarelle B, Rajaonarison JF *et al.* (1995). Comparative effects of antifungal agents on zidovudine glucuronidation by human liver microsomes. *Brit J Clin Pharmacol* **40**: 83.

Saravolatz LD, Winslow DL, Collins G *et al.* (1996). Zidovudine alone or in combination with didanosine or zalcitabine in HIV-infected patients with the acquired immunodeficiency syndrome or fewer than 200 CD4 cells per cubic millimeter. *New Engl J Med* **335**: 1091.

Sattler FR, Ko R, Antoniskis D *et al.* (1991). Acetaminophen does not impair clearance of zidovudine. *Ann Intern Med* **114**: 937.

Schenker S, Johnson RF, King TS *et al.* (1990). Azidothymidine (zidovudine) transport by the human placenta. *Amer J Med Sci* **299**: 16.

Schmitt FA, Bigley JW, McKinnis R *et al.* (1988). Neuropsychological outcome of zidovudine (AZT) treatment of patients with AIDS and AIDS related complex. *New Engl J Med* **319**: 1573.

Schmitz SH, Scheding S, Voliotis D *et al.* (1994). Side effects of AZT prophylaxis after occupational exposure to HIV-infected blood. *Annl Hematol* **69**: 135.

Schooley RT, Campbell TB, Kuritzkes DR *et al.* (1996). Phase 1 study of combination therapy with L-697,661 and zidovudine. The ACTG 184 protocol team. *J AIDS Hum Retrovir* **12**: 363.

Schroder JM, Bertram M, Schnabel R, Pfaff U (1992). Nuclear and mitochondrial changes of muscle fibers in AIDS after treatment with high doses of zidovudine. *Acta Neuropathol (Berl)* **85**: 39.

Schwartz EL, Brechbuhl AB, Kahl P *et al.* (1992). Pharmacokinetic interactions of zidovudine and methadone in intravenous drug-using patients with HIV infection. *J AIDS* **5**: 619.

Semino-Mora MC, Leon-Monzon ME, Dalakas MC (1994a). Effect of L-carnitine on the zidovudine induced destruction of human myotubes. Port L-carnitine prevents the myoloxicity of AZT *in vitro*. *Lab Invest* **71**: 102.

Semino-Mora MC, Leon-Monzon ME, Dalakas MC (1994b). The effect of L-carnitine on the AZT- induced destruction of human myotubes. Part II: Treatment with L-carnitine improves the AZT induced changes and prevents further destruction. *Lab Invest* **71**: 773.

Shafer RW, Kozal MJ, Katzenstein DA *et al.* (1993). Zidovudine susceptibility testing of human immunodeficiency virus type 1 (HIV) clinical isolates. *J Virol Meth* **41**: 297.

Shafer RW, Kozal MJ, Winters MA *et al.* (1994). Combination therapy with zidovudine and didanosine selects for drug resistant human immunodeficiency virus type 1 strains with unique patterns of pol gene mutations. *J Infect Dis* **169**: 722.

Sheehy N, Desselberger U (1993). Sequence analysis of reverse transcriptase genes of zidovudine (AZT)-resistant and -sensitive human immunodeficiency virus type 1 strains. *J Gen Virol* **74**: 223.

Shelton MJ, Portmore A, Blum MR *et al.* (1994). Prolonged but not diminished, zidovudine absorption induced by a high fat breakfast. *Pharmacother* **14**: 671.

Shih CC, Kaneshima H, Rabin L *et al.* (1991). Postexposure prophylaxis with zidovudine suppresses human immunodeficiency virus type 1 infection in SCID-hu mice in a time-dependent manner. *J Infect Dis* **163**: 625.

Shintaku M, Nasu K, Shimizu T *et al.* (1993). Fulminant hepatic failure in an AIDS patient: possible zidovudine-induced hepatotoxicity. *Amer J Gastroenterol* **88**: 464.

Shirasaka T, Kavlick MF, Ueno T *et al.* (1995). Emergence of human immunodeficiency virus type 1 variants with resistance to multiple dideoxynucleosides in patients receiving therapy with dideoxynucleosides. *Proc Natl Acad Sci USA* **92**: 2398.

Shriner K, Goetz MB (1992). Severe hepatotoxicity in a patient receiving both acetaminophen and zidovudine. *Amer J Med* **93**: 94.

Siegrist CA, Yerly S, Kaiser L *et al.* (1994). Mother to child transmission of zidovudine resistant HIV-1. *Lancet* **344**: 1771.

Sieh E, Coluzzi ML, Cusella-de Angelis MG *et al.* (1992). The effects of AZT and ddI on pre- and postimplantation mammalian embryos: an *in vivo* and *in vitro* study. *AIDS Res Hum Retrovir* **8**: 639.

Sikka SC, Gogu SR, Agrawal EC (1991). Effect of zidovudine (AZT) on reproductive and hematopoietic systems in the male rat. *Biochem Pharmacol* **42**: 1293.

Sim SM, Back DJ, Breckenridgee AM (1991). The effect of various drugs on the glucuronidation of zidovudine (azidothymidine; AZT) by human liver microsomes. *Brit J Clin Pharmacol* **32**: 17.

Simberkoff MS, Hartigan PM, Hamilton JD *et al.* (1996). Long-term follow-up of symptomatic HIV-infected patients originally randomized to early versus later zidovudine treatment; report of a Veterans Affairs Cooperative Study. VA Cooperative Study Group on AIDS Treatment. *J AIDS Hum Retrovir* **11**: 142.

Sinet M, Harcouet L, Desforges B *et al.* (1992). Efficacy of continuous zidovudine infusion at early stages of retroviral infection in mice. *J AIDS* **5**: 577.

Singer EJ, Stoner GL, Singer P *et al.* (1994). AIDS presenting as progressive multifocal leukoencephalopathy with clinical response to zidovudine. *Acta Neurol Scand* **90**: 443.

Skowron G, Bozzette SA, Lim L *et al.* (1993). Alternating and intermittent regimens of zidovudine and dideoxycytidine in patients with AIDS or AIDS-related complex. *Ann Intern Med* **118**: 321.

Slusher JT, Kuwahara SK, Hamzeh FM *et al.* (1992). Intracellular zidovudine (ZDV) and ZDV phosphates as measured by a validated combined high-pressure liquid chromatography-radioimmunoassay procedure. *Antimicrob Ag Chemother* **36**: 2473.

Smith MS, Kessler JA, Rankin CD *et al.* (1993a). Evaluation of synergy between carbovir and 3'-azido-2',3'-deoxythymidine for inhibition of human immunodeficiency virus type 1. *Antimicrob Ag Chemother* **37**: 144.

Smith MS, Koerber KL, Pagano JS (1993b). Zidovudine-resistant human immunodeficiency virus type 1 genomes detected in plasma distinct from viral genomes in peripheral blood mononuclear cells. *J Infect Dis* **167**: 445.

Smith M, Salomon H, Wainberg MA (1994a). Development and significance in nucleoside drug resistance to infection caused by the human immunodeficiency virus type 1. *Clin Invest Med* **17**: 226.

Smith MS, Koerber KL, Pagano JS (1994b). Long term persistence of zidovudine resistance mutations in plasma isolates of human immunodeficiency virus type 1 of dideoxyinosine treated patients removed from zidovudine therapy. *J Infect Dis* **169**: 184.

Snoeck R, Andrei G, Schols D *et al.* (1992). Activity of different antiviral drug combinations against human cytomegalovirus replication *in vitro*. *Eur J Clin Microbiol Infect Dis* **11**: 1144.

Snower DP, Weil SC (1993). Changing etiology of macrocytosis. Zidovudine as a frequent causative factor. *Amer J Clin Pathol* **99**: 57.

Sorensen AM, Nielsen C, Mathiesen LR *et al.* (1993). Evaluation of the combination effect of different antiviral compounds against HIV *in vitro*. *Scand J Infect Dis* **25**: 365.

Spear JB, Kessler HA, Lehrman SN *et al.* (1988a). Zidovudine overdosage. *Ann Intern Med* **109**: 76.

Spear JB, Benson CA, Pottage JC *et al.* (1988b). Rapid rebound of serum human immunodeficiency virus antigen after discontinuing zidovudine therapy. *J Infect Dis* **158**: 1132.

Spector SA, Ripley D, Hsia K *et al.* (1989a). Human immunodeficiency virus inhibition is prolonged by 3'-azido-3'-deoxythymidine alternating with 2',3'-dideoxycytidine compared with 3'-azido-3'-deoxythymidine alone. *Antimicrob Ag Chemother* **33**: 920.

Spector SA, Kennedy C, McCutchan JA *et al* (1989b). The antiviral effect of zidovudine and ribavirin in clinical trials and the use of p24 antigen levels as a virologic marker. *J Infect Dis* **159**: 822.

Sperling RS, Stratton P (1992). Treatment options for human immunodeficiency virus-infected pregnant women. Obstetric-Gynecologic Working Group of the AIDS Clinical Trials Group of the National Institute of Allergy and Infectious Diseases. *Obstet Gynecol* **79**: 443.

Sperling RS, Stratton P, O'Sullivan MJ *et al.* (1992a). A survey of zidovudine use in pregnant women with human immunodeficiency virus infection. *New Engl J Med* **326**: 857.

Sperling RS, Roboz J, Dische R *et al.* (1992b). Zidovudine pharmacokinetics during pregnancy. *Amer J Perinatol* **9**: 247.

Spivak JL, Barnes DC, Fuchs E, Quinn TC (1989). Serum immunoreactive erythropoietin in HIV-infected patients. *JAMA* **261**: 3104.

Spooner KM, Lane HC, Masur H (1995). Antiretroviral therapy; reference guide to major clinical trials in patients infected with human immunodeficiency virus. *Clin Infect Dis* **20**: 1145.

Spruance SL, Pavia AT, Peterson D *et al.* (1994). Didanosine compared with continuation of zidovudine in HIV infected patients with signs of clinical deterioration while receiving zidovudine. A randomised double blind clinical trial. The Bristol-Myers Squibb A1454 010 Study Group. *Ann Int Med* **120**: 360.

Srugo I, Brunell PA, chelyapou NV *et al.* (1991). Virus burden in human immunodeficiency virus type 1-infected children: relationship to disease status and effect of antiviral therapy. *Pediatrics* **87**: 921.

St Clair MH, Richards CA, Spector T *et al.* (1987). 3'-azido-3'-deoxythymidine triphosphate as an inhibitor and substrate of purified human immunodeficiency virus reverse transcriptase. *Antimicrob Ag Chemother* **31**: 1972.

St Clair MH, Martin JL *et al.* (1991). Resistance to ddI and sensitivity to AZT induced by a mutation in HIV-1 reverse transcriptase. *Science* **253**: 1557.

St Clair MH, Pennington KN, Rooney J, Barry DW (1995). *In vitro* comparison of selected triple drug combinations for suppression of HIV-1 replication: The Inter Company Collaboration Protocol. *J AIDS Hum Retrovir* **10**: S83.

St Luce, Arts E, Geleziunas R *et al.* (1993). Infection of human monocyte-derived macrophages by human immunodeficiency virus mediated by cell to cell transmission. *J Med Virol* **41**: 71.

Stambuk D, Hawkins D, Gazzard BG *et al.* (1989). Zidovudine treatment of patients with acquired immune deficiency syndrome and acquired immune deficiency syndrome-related complex, St Stephen's Hospital experience. *J Infect* **18**: 41.

Staszewski S (1995). Zidovudine and lamivudine; results of phase III studies. *J AIDS Hum Retrovir* **10**: S57.

Staszewski S, Massari FE, Kober A *et al.* (1995). Combination therapy with zidovudine prevents selection of human immunodeficiency virus type 1 variants expressing high level resistance to L-697,661 a non nucleoside reverse transcriptase inhibitor. *J Infect Dis* **171**: 1159.

Staszewski S, Loveday C, Picazo J *et al.* (1996). Safety and efficacy of lamivudine-zidovudine combination therapy in zidovudine-experienced patients. *JAMA* **276**: 111.

Steffe EM, King JH, Inciardi JF *et al.* (1990). The effect of acetaminophen on zidovudine metabolism in HIV-infected patients. *J AIDS* **3**: 691.

Stein DS, Graham NM, Park LP *et al.* (1994). The effect of the interaction of acyclovir with zidovudine on progression to AIDS and survival. Analysis of data in the Multicenter AIDS Cohort Study. *Ann Intern Med* **121**: 100.

Stellbrink HJ, Averdunk R, Stoehr A, Albrecht H (1993). Zidovudine half-life in haemodialysis patients. *AIDS* **7**: 141.

Stretcher BN (1995). Pharmacokinetic optimisation of antiretroviral therapy in patients with HIV infection. *Clin Pharmacokin* **29**: 46.

Stretcher BN, Pesce AJ, Murray JA *et al.* (1991). Concentrations of phosphorylated zidovudine (ZDV) in patient leukocytes do not correlate with ZDV dose or plasma concentrations. *Ther Drug Monit* **13**: 325.

Stretcher BN, Pesce AJ, Hurtubise PE Frame PT (1992). Pharmacokinetics of zidovudine phosphorylation in patients infected with the human immunodeficiency virus. *Ther Drug Monit* **14**: 281.

Stretcher BN, Pesce AJ, Frame PT, Stein DS (1994a). Pharmacokinetics of zidovudine phosphorylation in peripheral blood mononuclear cells from patients infected with human immunodeficiency virus. *Antimicrob Ag Chemother* **38**: 1541.

Stretcher BN, Pesce AJ, Frame PT *et al.* (1994b). Correlates of zidovudine phosphorylation with markers of HIV disease progression and drug toxicity. *AIDS* **8**: 763.

Surbone A, Yarchoan R, McAthee N *et al.* (1988). Treatment of the acquired immunodeficiency syndrome (AIDS) and AIDS-related complex with a regimen of 3'-azido-2',3'-diseoxythymidine (azidothymidine or zidovudine) and acyclovir. *Ann Intern Med* **108**: 534.

Swansonn CE, Tindall B, Cooper DA (1994). Efficacy of zidovudine treatment in homosexual men with AIDS-related complex: factors influencing development of AIDS, survival and drug intolerance. *AIDS* **8**: 625.

Swiss Group for Clinical Studies on the Acquired Immunodeficiency Syndrome (AIDS) (1988). Zidovudine for the treatment of thrombocytopenia associated with human immunodeficiency virus (HIV). A prospective study. *Ann Intern Med* **109**: 718.

Taburet AM, Naveau S, Zorza G *et al.* (1990). Pharmacokinetics of zidovudine in patients with liver cirrhosis. *Clin Pharmacol Ther* **47**: 731.

Tachedjian G, Hooker DJ, Gurusinghe AD *et al.* (1995). Characterisation of foscarnet resistant strains of human immunodeficiency virus type 1. *Virology* **212**: 58.

Tachedjian G, Mellors J, Basmi H *et al.*, (1996). Zidovudine-resistance is suppressed by mutations conferring resistance of HIV-1 to foscarnet. *J Virol* **70**: 7171–7181.

Tadini G, Dorso M, Cusini M, Alessi E (1991). Oral mucosa pigmentation: a new side effect of azidothymidine therapy in patients with acquired immunodeficiency syndrome. *Arch Dermatol* **127**: 267.

Tartaglione TA, Holeman E, Opheim K *et al.* (1990). Zidovudine disposition during hemodialysis in a patient with acquired immunodeficiency syndrome. *J AIDS* **3**: 32.

Tartaglione TA, Collier AC, Coombs RW *et al.* (1991a). Acquired immunodeficiency syndrome. Cerebrospinal fluid findings in patients before and during long-term oral zidovudine therapy. *Arch Neurol* **48**: 695.

Tartaglione TA, Collier AC, Opheim K *et al.* (1991b). Pharmacokinetic evaluations of low- and high-dose zidovudine plus high-dose acyclovir in patients with symptomatic human immunodeficiency virus infection. *Antimicrob Ag Chemother* **35**: 2225.

Taylor-Robinson D, Furr PM (1992). *In-vitro* activity of zidovudine against *Mycoplasma. Lancet* **339**: 686.

Telen MJ, Roberts KB, Bartlett JA (1990). HIV-associated autoimmune hemolytic anemia: report of a case and review of the literature. *J AIDS* **3**: 933.

Teppler H, Kaplan G, Smith KA *et al.* (1993). Prolonged immunostimulatory effect of low dose polyethylene glycol interleukin 2 in patients with human immunodeficiency virus type 1 infection. *J Exp Med* **177**: 483.

Terasaki T, Pardridge WM (1988). Restricted transport of 3'-azido-3'-deoxythymidine and dideoxynucleosides through the blood-brain barrier. *J Infect Dis* **158**: 630.

Thormar H, Balzarini J, Holy A *et al.* (1993). Inhibition of visna virus replication by 2',3'-dideoxynucleosides and acyclic nucleoside phosphonate analogs. *Antimicrob Ag Chemother* **37**: 2540.

Till M, MacDonell KB (1990). Myopathy with human immunodeficiency virus type 1 (HIV-1) infection: HIV-1 or zidovudine? *Annl Intern Med* **113**: 492.

Tindall B, Gaines H, Imrie A *et al.* (1991). Zidovudine in the management of primary HIV-1 infection. *AIDS* **5**: 477.

Tindall B, Carr A, Goldstein D *et al.* (1993). Administration of zidovudine during primary HIV-1 infection may be associated with a less vigorous immune response. *AIDS* **7**: 127.

Tirelli U, Errante D, Oksenhendler E *et al.* (1992). Prospective study with combined low-dose chemotherapy and zidovudine in 37 patients with poor-prognosis AIDS-related non-Hodgkin's lymphoma. French-Italian Cooperative Study Group. *Ann Oncol* **3**: 843.

Tisdale M, Kemp SD, Parry NR, Larder RA (1993). Rapid *in vitro* selection of human immunodeficiency virus type 1 resistant to 3'-thiacytidine inhibitors due to a mutation in the YMDD region of reverse transcriptase. *Proc Natl Acad Sci USA* **90**: 5653.

Tisdale M, Myers RE, Maschera B *et al.* (1995). Cross-resistance analysis of human immunodeficiency virus type 1 variants individually selected for resistance to five different protease inhibitors. *Antimicrob Ag Chemother* **39**: 1704.

Tobinai K, Kobayashi Y, Shimoyama M (1995). Interferon alpha and zidovudine in adult T-cell leukemia- lymphoma. Lymphoma Study Group of the Japan Clinical Oncology Group. *New Engl J Med* **333**: 1285.

Tokars JI, Marcus R, Culver DH *et al.* (1993). Surveillance of HIV infection and zidovudine use among health care workers after occupational exposure to HIV-infected blood. *Ann Intern Med* **118**: 913.

Toltzis P, Marx CM, Kleinman N *et al.* (1991). Zidovudine-associated embryonic toxicity in mice. *J Infect Dis* **163**: 1212.

Torres RA, Lin RY, Lee M *et al.* (1992). Zidovudine-induced leukocytoclastic vasculitis. *Arch Intern Med* **152**: 850.

Tosti A, Gaddoni G, Fanti PA *et al.* (1990). Longitudinal melanonychia induced by 3'-azidodeoxythymidine. Report of 9 cases. *Dermatologica* **180**: 217.

Tsai CC, Follis KE, Benveniste RE (1988). Antiviral effects of 3'-azido-3'-deoxythymidine, 2',3'-dideoxycytidine, and 2',3'-dideoxyadenosine against simian acquired immunodeficiency syndrome-associated type D retrovirus in vitro. *AIDS Res Hum Retrovir* **4**: 359.

Tsutsumi M, Takada A, Sawada M (1995). Efficacy of combination therapy with interferon and azidothymidine in chronic type C hepatitis; a pilot study. *J Gastroenterol* **30**: 485.

Tudor-Williams G, St Clair M *et al.* (1992). HIV-1 sensitivity to zidovudine and clinical outcome in children. *Lancet* **339**: 15.

Unadkat JD, Collier AC, Crosby SS *et al.* (1990). Pharmacokinetics of oral zidovudine (azidothymidine) in patients with AIDS when administered with and without a high-fat meal. *AIDS* **4**: 229.

Vacca JP, Dorsey BD, Schleif WA *et al.* (1994). L-735,524; an orally bioavailable human immunodeficiency virus type 1 protease inhibitor. *Proc Natl Acad Sci USA* **91**: 4096.

Vago L, Castagna A, Lazzarin A *et al.* (1993). Reduced frequency of HIV-induced brain lesions in AIDS patients treated with zidovudine. *J AIDS* **6**: 42.

Valentine C, Williams O, Davis A *et al.* (1993). Case study of zidovudine overdose. *AIDS* **7**: 436.

Van Rompay KK, Olsyula MG, Marthas ML *et al.* (1995). Immediate zidovudine treatment protects simian immunodeficiency virus infected newborn macaques against rapid onset of AIDS. *Antimicrob Ag Chemother* **39**: 125.

Varmus H, Swanstrom R (1982). Replication of retroviruses In *Molecular Biology of Tumor Viruses: RNA Tumor Viruses* (Weiss R, Teich N, Varmus H and Coffin J, eds), p. 369. New York: Cold Spring Harbor Laboratory, Cold Spring Harbor.

Veal GJ, Wild MJ, Barry MG, Back DJ (1994). Effects of dideoxyinosine and dideoxycytidine on the intracellular phosphorylation of zidovudine in human mononuclear cells. *Brit J Clin Pharmacol* **38**: 323.

Veenstra J, Schuurman R, Cornelissen M *et al.* (1995). Transmission of zidovudine-resistant human immunodeficiency virus type 1 variants following deliberate injection of blood from a patient with AIDS: characteristics and natural history of the virus. *Clin Infect Dis* **21**: 556.

Vella S (1994). HIV therapy advances. Update on a proteinase inhibitor. *AIDS* **8**: S25.

Vella S, Giuliano M, Pezzotti P *et al.* (1992). Survival of zidovudine-treated patients with AIDS compared with that of contemporary untreated patients. Italian zidovudine evaluation group. *JAMA* **267**: 1232.

Vella S, Giuliano M, Dally LG *et al.* (1994). Long-term follow-up of zidovudine therapy in asymptomatic HIV infection: Results of a multicenter cohort study. *J AIDS* **7**: 31.

Vella S, Giuliano M, Floridia M *et al.* (1995). Effect of sex, age and transmission category on the progression to AIDS and survival of zidovudine-treated symptomatic patients. *AIDS* **9**: 51.

Vella S, Galluzzo C, Giannini G *et al.* (1996). Saquinavir/zidovudine combination in patients with advanced HIV infection and no prior antiretroviral therapy: CD4 lymphocyte/plasma RNA changes, and emergence of HIV strains with reduced phenotypic sensitivity. *Antiviral Res* **29**: 91.

Vogt MW, Hartshorn KL, Furman PA *et al.* (1987). Ribavirin antagonizes the effect of azidothymidine on HIV replication. *Science* **235**: 1376.

Volberding PA, Lagakos SW, Koch MA *et al.* (1990). Zidovudine in asymptomatic human immunodeficiency virus infection. A controlled trial in persons with fewer than 500 CD4 positive cells per cubic millimeter. The AIDS Clinical Trials Group of the National Institute of Allergy and Infectious Diseases. *New Engl J Med* **322**: 941.

Volberding PA, Lagakos SW, Grimes JM *et al.* (1994). The duration of zidovudine benefit in persons with asymptomatic HIV infection. Prolonged evaluation of protocol 019 of the AIDS Clinical Trials Group. *JAMA* **272**: 437.

Volberding PA, Lagakos SW, Grimes JM *et al.* (1995). A comparison of immediate with deferred zidovudine therapy for asymptomatic HIV infected adults with CD4 cell counts of 500 or more per cubic millimeter. AIDS Clinical Trials Group. *New Engl J Med* **333**: 401.

Vrang L, Oberg B *et al.* (1988). Reverse transcriptase from human immunodeficiency virus type 1 (HIV-1), HIV-2, and simian immunodeficiency virus (SIVMAC) are susceptible to inhibition by foscarnet and 3'-azido-3'-deoxythymidine triphosphate. *Antimicrob Ag Chemother* **32**: 1733.

Wainberg MA, Falutz J, Fanning M *et al.* (1989). Cessation of zidovudine therapy may lead to increased replication of HIV-1. *JAMA* **261**: 865.

Wainberg MA, Beaulieu R, Tsoukas C, Thomas R (1993). Detection of zidovudine-resistant variants of HIV-1 in genital fluids. *AIDS* **7**: 433.

Walker RE, Parker RI, Kovacs JA *et al.* (1988). Anemia and erythropoiesis in patients with the acquired immunodeficiency syndrome (AIDS) and Kaposi Sarcoma treated with zidovudine. *Ann Int Med* **108**: 372.

Watts DH, Brown ZA, Tartaglione T *et al.* (1991). Pharmacokinetic disposition of zidovudine during pregnancy. *J Infect Dis* **163**: 226.

Weber R, Bonetti A, Jost J *et al.* (1991). Low-dose zidovudine in combination with either acyclovir or lymphoblastoid interferon-alpha in asymptomatic HIV-infected patients, a pilot study. *Infection* **19**: 395.

White EL, Parker WB, Ross LJ, Shannon WM (1993). Lack of synergy in the inhibition of HIV-1 reverse transcriptase by combinations of the 5'-triphosphates of various anti-HIV nucleoside analogs. *Antiviral Res* **22**: 295.

Wientjes MG, Au JL (1992). Lack of pharmacokinetic interaction between intravenous 2', 3'-dideoxyinosine and 3'-azido-3'-deoxythymidine in rats. *Antimicrob Ag Chemother* **36**: 665.

Wilfert CM (1994). Mandatory screening of pregnant women for the human immunodeficiency virus. *Clin Infect Dis* **19**: 664.

Williams GJ, Colby CB (1989). Recombinant human interferon-beta suppresses the replication of HIV and acts synergistically with AZT. *J Interferon Res* **9**: 709.

Williams IG, Tedder RS *et al.* (1993). Intermittent zidovudine regimen in patients with symptomatic HIV infection and previous haematological toxicity. *Antiviral Chem Chemother* **4**: 139.

Wong SL, Hedaya MA, Sawchuk RJ (1992). Competitive inhibition of zidovudine clearance by probenecid during continuous coadministration. *Pharm Res* **9**: 228.

Wood R, Montoya JG, Kundu SK *et al.* (1993). Safety and efficacy of polyethylene glycol-modified interleukin-2 and and zidovudine in human immunodeficiency virus type 1 infection; a phase I/II study. *J Infect Dis* **167**: 519.

Wright JM, Sachdev PS, Perkins RJ, Rodriguez P (1989). Zidovudine-related mania. *Med J Aust* **150**: 339.

Wu JC, Chernow M, Boehme RE *et al.* (1988). Kinetics and inhibition of reverse transcriptase from human and simian immunodeficiency viruses. *Antimicrob Ag Chemother* **32**: 1887.

Yarchoan R, Klecker RW, Weinhold KJ *et al.* (1986). Administration of 3'-azido-3'-deoxythymidine, an inhibitor of HTLV-III/LAV replication, to patients with AIDS or AIDS-related complex. *Lancet* **i**: 575.

Yarchoan R, Berg G, Brouwers P *et al.* (1987). Response of human-immunodeficiency-virus-associated neurological disease to 3'-azido-3'-deoxythymidine. *Lancet* **i**: 132.

Yarchoan R, Thomas RV, Grafman J *et al.* (1988a). Long-term administration of 3'-azido-2',3'-dideoxythymidine to patients with AIDS-related neurological disease. *Ann Neurol* **23**: S82.

Yarchoan R, Perno CF, Thomas RV *et al.* (1988b). Phase I studies of 2',3'-dideoxycytidine in severe human immunodeficiency virus infection as a single agent and alternating with zidovudine (AZT). *Lancet* **1**: 76.

Yarchoan R, Mitsuya H, Myers CE, Broder S (1989). Clinical pharmacology of 3'-azido-2',3'-dideoxythymidine (zidovudine) and related dideoxynucleosides [published erratum appears in *New Engl J Med* (1990) **322**: 280]. *New Engl J Med* **321**: 726.

Yarchoan R, Lietzau JA, Nguyen BY *et al.* (1994). A randomised pilot study of alternating or simultaneous zidovudine and didanosine therapy in patients with symptomatic human immunodeficiency virus infection. *J Infect Dis* **169**: 9.

Youle MS, Gazzard BG, Johnson MA *et al.* (1994). Effects of high-dose oral acyclovir on herpesvirus disease and survival in patients with advanced HIV disease; a double blind, placebo-controlled study. *AIDS* **8**: 641.

Didanosine

Description

Didanosine (2', 3'-dideoxyinosine, ddI) is a purine nucleoside analog that is active against HIV-1 and HIV-2, including strains of HIV that are resistant to zidovudine (Fig. V.41). The drug is marketed by Bristol-Myers-Squibb under the trade name 'Videx', and is used both as monotherapy (uncommonly) and in combination with other antiretroviral compounds for the treatment of HIV infection.

The molecular formula of didanosine is $C_{10}H_{12}N_4O_3$. It has a molecular weight of 236.2. The concentration can be expressed as μM or in μg per ml (1 μg per ml is approximately equivalent to 5 μM).

Antiviral Activity

1 Human immunodeficiency virus

Although didanosine has good efficacy against HIV *in vitro*, it has generally been found to be less potent as an inhibitor of HIV than zidovudine, lamivudine and zalcitabine (Hitchcock, 1993; Mathez *et al.*, 1993), but to have a much higher *in vitro* selectivity ratio (Coplan and Nolan, 1991). Didanosine is effective against both HIV-1 and HIV-2 and has *in vitro* activity against strains of HIV that are resistant to zidovudine (Richman, 1987; Mitsuya and Broder, 1988; Larder *et al.*, 1990; Connolly and Hammer, 1992).

A compound that is closely related to didanosine, 2'3'-dideoxyadenosine (ddA) was first synthesized in 1964 (Robins and Robins, 1964). In 1985, Mitsuya and Broder demonstrated the activity of both didanosine and ddA against HIV replication (Mitsuya and Broder, 1986, 1987). Both didanosine and ddA are able to inhibit HIV replication in T lymphocytes as well as macrophages that are exposed to the drug at the time of infection with HIV (Mitsuya and Broder, 1986; Perno *et al.*, 1988). In macrophages, the activity of didanosine against HIV is similar to, or greater than that of zidovudine, but less than that of zalcitabine (reviewed in Hitchcock, 1993). The IC_{50} of didanosine for HIV ranges from 2.5 to 10 μM (0.5–2 μg per ml) in activated T lymphocytes, and 0.001–0.1 μM in macrophages. These data are supported by the finding of Gao and colleagues (Gao *et al.*, 1994) who showed that didanosine is cell-activation independent and that activity is associated with higher cellular ratios of dideoxynucleoside triphosphate to deoxynucleoside triphosphate, and thus more potent antiviral activity in resting cells such as

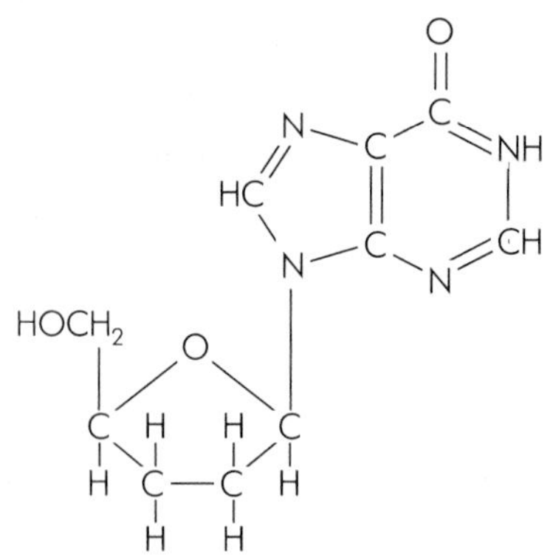

Fig. V.41.
Chemical structure of didanosine (2'-3'dideoxyinosine or ddI).

macrophages. Virtually 100% inhibition of HIV replication can be achieved in T lymphocytes and monocyte-macrophages at a concentration of 20 μM of didanosine (Hayashi *et al.*, 1990; Shirasaka *et al.*, 1990). At relatively high concentrations (10–100 μM) didanosine has been found to inhibit reverse transcription in resting T lymphocytes (Watson and Wilburn, 1992).

2 Other retroviruses

Didanosine and dideoxyadenosine, in contrast to zidovudine, do not inhibit replication of murine leukemia virus (Dahlberg *et al.*, 1987). Furthermore, compared with zidovudine, didanosine results in only modest inhibition of feline leukemia virus (Tavares *et al.*, 1989), including isolates that are resistant to zidovudine (Remington *et al.*, 1991), with reported IC_{50} values of 4.3 μM in a T cell line and 43.5 μM in a monocytoid cell line (Mukherji *et al.*, 1994). Simian immunodeficiency virus is also inhibited by didanosine (reviewed in Connolly and Hammer, 1992). Moloney murine sarcoma virus is inhibited *in vitro* and *in vivo* by didanosine (Balzarini *et al.*, 1990). Visna virus replication is inhibited by didanosine *in vitro*, although this drug is 10 to 30-fold less effective than zalcitabine in inhibiting virus-induced syncytium formation (Thormar *et al.*, 1993).

3 Hepatitis viruses

Didanosine has been reported to inhibit replication of hepatitis B and duck hepatitis B viruses *in vitro* (Fried *et al.*, 1992), although in general the antiviral effect has only been modest (Aoki-Sei *et al.*, 1991). Didanosine given by the i.v. route has been reported to suppress replication of the duck hepatitis B virus in chronically infected ducks (Martin *et al.*, 1989).

4 Other

Didanosine has antibacterial activity against non-typhoidal *Salmonella* spp., with an MIC of 2–125 μg per ml. *Escherichia coli* was less susceptible to didanosine with MICs ranging from 31 to >62.5 μg per ml (Sperber *et al.*, 1993). Didanosine has little or no activity against *Pneumocystis carinii in vitro* (Walzer *et al.*, 1992).

5 Synergism

Zidovudine and didanosine are synergistic against both HIV-1 and HIV-2 *in vitro* (Dornsife *et al.*, 1991; Johnson *et al.*, 1991; Cox *et al.*, 1994). Ribavirin has been shown by a number of investigators to enhance the antiretroviral activity of didanosine in lymphocytes and T cell lines (Balzarini *et al.*, 1990, 1991a,b; Hartman *et al.*, 1991a). Ribavirin stimulates the formation of the active form of didanosine, its triphosphate derivative, by inhibiting inosinate dehydrogenase (Hartman *et al.*, 1991a). Didanosine interacts synergistically when used in combination with interferon alpha *in vitro* (Dornsife *et al.*, 1991; Johnson *et al.*, 1991), although, in one study, synergism was only found at certain drug ratios (Schinazi *et al.*, 1990), and others have found only an additive effect between didanosine and interferon alpha (Degre and Beck 1994). Additive to synergistic interactions occur between protease inhibitors and didanosine against HIV-1 (Kageyama *et al.*, 1992). Soluble recombinant CD4 and didanosine have synergistic antiretroviral activity at clinically achievable concentrations (Hayashi *et al.*, 1990). *Pseudomonas exotoxin* linked to soluble recombinant CD4 has been shown to selectively kill cells infected with HIV *in vitro*, and inhibit spread of HIV to uninfected cells within the culture (Ashorn *et al.*, 1990). The combination of ampligen and didanosine results in additive inhibition of HIV replication (O'Marro *et al.*, 1992). Dextran sulfate, the Tat antagonist Ro 24–7429, and the TIBO derivative R86183 are each synergistic with didanosine in inhibiting HIV-1 *in vitro* (Hayashi *et al.*, 1990; Connell *et al.*, 1994; Pauwels *et al.*, 1994).

Zidovudine, didanosine and lamivudine in combination have greater antiviral activity *in vitro* than double-drug combinations or monotherapy (St Clair *et al.*, 1995).

6 Antagonism

Although granulocyte-macrophage colony stimulating factor (GM-CSF) stimulates the action of zidovudine, it reduces the antiretroviral activity of didanosine in macrophages and monocyte cell lines (Perno *et al.*, 1990a, 1992). Similarly macrophage colony stimulating factor (M-CSF) has been reported to decrease the *in vitro* antiviral efficacy of didanosine (Perno *et al.*, 1990b).

7 Resistance

During therapy HIV isolates from patients treated with didanosine have been shown to emerge with decreased sensitivity to didanosine. Didanosine-resistance appears to develop less readily than that to zidovudine, and when resistance does develop it is likely to be more modest than that

Table V.28

Mutations within HIV reverse transcriptase that confer resistance of HIV *in vitro* to didanosine

Codon	Mutation	Cross-resistance
65	Lys → Arg	Zalcitabine
74[a]	Leu → Val	Zalcitabine
75	Val → Thr	Stavudine, zalcitabine
184	Met → Val	Lamivudine, zalcitabine

[a] Major mutation conferring resistance.

observed with zidovudine. Patients who are treated with didanosine for up to 19 months may not develop resistance (Shirasaka *et al.*, 1993); HIV isolates from children treated with didanosine for 22–31 months has been associated with a 20-fold decrease in susceptibility (Dimitrov *et al.*, 1993).

In vitro culture of T cell lines with suboptimal concentrations of didanosine results in the generation of strains of HIV with diminished sensitivity to didanosine but without cross-resistance to zidovudine (Gao *et al.*, 1992). By similarly culturing cells in the presence of increasing concentrations of zalcitabine, variants of HIV that are resistant to both zalcitabine and didanosine, but not zidovudine, can also be generated (Gao *et al.*, 1993a). One group has reported that *in vitro* combinations of zidovudine, didanosine and nevirapine result in the development of mutations within the viral reverse transcriptase that are incompatible with viral replication (Chow *et al.*, 1993). This finding has not been supported by other studies.

Several mutations within HIV reverse transcriptase have been described in association with the development of resistance to didanosine (Table V.28). St Clair and colleagues were the first to describe reduced *in vitro* sensitivity of HIV to didanosine which developed in patients during 12 months of didanosine therapy, following cessation of zidovudine therapy (Fig. V.42). A mutation at position 74 (Leu –> Val) of the reverse transcriptase gene was found to confer reduced susceptibility to didanosine and was associated with cross-resistance to zalcitabine but not to zidovudine (St Clair *et al.*, 1991). In fact, development of this mutation has been reported by some investigators to result in improved susceptibility of zidovudine-resistant strains of HIV to zidovudine (St Clair *et al.*, 1991), but not by others (Eron *et al.*, 1993). The development of the mutation at codon 74 is independent of zidovudine-related mutations (Masquelier *et al.*, 1995).

A second mutation at amino acid site 184 (resulting in a substitution of Met → Val) has been found by some investigators to confer resistance to didanosine *in vitro* with cross-resistance to zalcitabine but again not to zidovudine (Gu *et al.*, 1992) or lamivudine (Boucher *et al.*, 1993). In addition this mutation has been detected in isolates from patients receiving long-term didanosine therapy (Gu *et al.*, 1992). Other investigators have found that this same mutation at codon 184 is associated with up to 1000-fold resistance to lamivudine with only a 4- to 8-fold

Fig. V.42.

The *in vitro* sensitivities (IC$_{50}$) to didanosine (O) and zidovudine (●) of sequential isolates of HIV from an individual with AIDS. At time zero zidovudine was ceased and didanosine therapy initiated. (Reproduced from St Clair *et al.*, 1991; *Science* **253**: 1557, with permission. Copyright 1991 American Association for the Advancement of Science.)

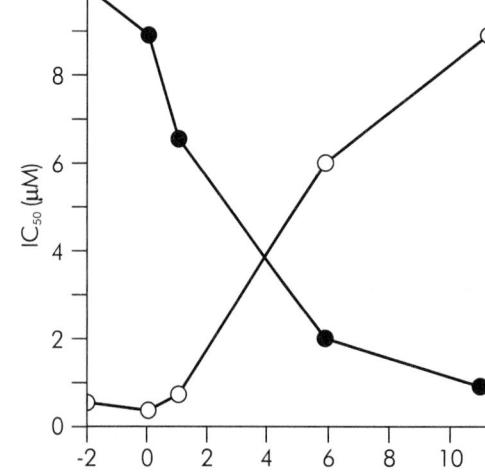

decrease in susceptibility to didanosine and zalcitabine (Gao *et al.*, 1993b; Tisdale *et al.*, 1993).

There are also reports of cross-resistance between zalcitabine and didanosine in association with a mutation at codon 65 (Lys → Arg) in strains of HIV selected by passage in the presence of increasing concentrations of zalcitabine *in vitro* as well as in isolates from patients treated with either zalcitabine or didanosine (Zhang *et al.*, 1994; Gu *et al.*, 1994). However, zalcitabine- and didanosine-resistance are not always present together, as a strain of HIV with a mutation at position 69 (Thr –> Asp) leading to zalcitabine-resistance did not confer resistance to didanosine (Fitzgibbon *et al.*, 1992).

Co-resistance to non-nucleoside reverse transcriptors has been reported in strains of HIV that develop the mutation at codon 74 (Leu-> Val) (Larder, 1992). In addition, a stavudine-resistant strain of HIV with a mutation at codon 75, altering Val to Thr resulted in co-resistance to didanosine and zalcitabine (Lacey and Larder, 1994). Foscarnet-resistant strains of HIV with mutations at codons 89, 92 and 156 remain sensitive to didanosine and zalcitabine (Tachedjian *et al.*, 1995).

Multiple mutations (within codons 62, 75, 77, 116, and 151) have been found in association with resistance to multiple dideoxynucleosides. These mutations have been detected in isolates from persons receiving combination therapy with zidovudine and zalcitabine or didanosine (Shirasaka *et al.*, 1995; Shafer *et al.*, 1995).

Strains of feline immunodeficiency virus cultured in the presence of both zidovudine and didanosine developed a 13-fold decrease in susceptibility to zidovudine but less than 2-fold decrease in susceptibility to didanosine (Gobert *et al.*, 1994).

Mode of Administration and Dosage

Didanosine is stable at neutral or slightly alkaline pH, but is rapidly destroyed by exposure to acid. Hydrolysis of didanosine at the C-N glycosidic bond results in the formation of hypoxanthine and deoxyribose with loss of antiretroviral activity (Mitsuya *et al.*, 1990). In hydrochloric acid at pH 2 the half-life of didanosine is only a few minutes (Marquez *et al.*, 1987).

1 Adults

The recommended dose for adults is dependent on weight (see Table V.29) with two tablets taken per dose and a 12 h dosing interval. This dosing interval is based on the finding that the intracellular half-life is prolonged when compared with plasma half-life (see below) (Ahluwalia *et al.*, 1987; Yarchoan *et al.*, 1989a). Two tablets contain sufficient antacid to prevent drug degradation and maximize bioavailability. The tablets should be taken on an empty stomach. They should be thoroughly chewed, manually crushed, or dispersed in at least 30 ml of water prior to consumption (Didanosine Product Information). The dosing schedule for tablets is approximately 25% lower than that for the buffered powder, as the former have higher bioavailability (Shelton *et al.*, 1992). Didanosine should always be taken on an empty stomach at least 30 min before a meal.

In a study of 913 adult patients with advanced HIV infection who were randomized to receive didanosine at a dose of either 500 mg per day or 750 mg per day, the clinical benefit was more

Table V.29
Didanosine dosing in adult and pediatric patients

Adults: body weight (kg)	Dose
>60	200 mg twice-daily
<60	125 mg twice-daily
Children: body surface area (m²)	Dose tablets (powder[a])
1.5–2	150 mg twice-daily (200 mg twice-daily)
1.0–1.4	100 mg twice-daily (150 mg twice-daily)
0.5–0.9	50 mg twice-daily (100 mg twice-daily)
<0.4	25 mg twice-daily (50 mg twice-daily)

[a] Pediatric powder for oral solution.

evident in those receiving the lower dose. Higher doses are more likely to be associated with adverse reactions (see below) (Kahn *et al.*, 1992). In phase I studies the maximum tolerated dose in patients treated for 28–44 weeks was 12 mg per kg daily (Cooley *et al.*, 1990a; Lambert *et al.*, 1990; Valentine *et al.*, 1990), although in another report in which patients were given the oral drug for a median of 12 weeks the maximum tolerated dose was as high as 20 mg per kg daily (Cooley *et al.*, 1990b). Preliminary findings of the European/Australian Alpha trial, which compared clinical efficacy of didanosine in two dosages in approximately 1900 patients with symptomatic HIV infection who were intolerant of zidovudine, suggest that there is no difference in high (750 mg per day if greater than 60 kg) and low-dose didanosine (200 mg per day) in terms of survival or disease progression, but that the lower dose is better tolerated (Darbyshire and Aboulker, 1992). In a study of patients with advanced disease (CD4 less than 50 cells per μl) the authors suggest that doses of less than 750 mg per day of didanosine be used in such patients, based on the high toxicity associated with doses of 750 mg per day compared with 200 mg per day (Jablonowski *et al.*, 1995).

2 Children

Pediatric dosing guidelines are based on the findings that for children over 6 months of age, a daily dose of 100–300 mg per m^2 is safe and effective. The pediatric dosing guidelines are based on average surface area (Table V.29). For children older than 1 year, a two-tablet dose should be taken on an empty stomach. Younger children should receive a one-tablet dose. Tablets should be chewed, crushed or dispersed as described for adults (Didanosine Product Information). Intravenous administration has been used in clinical trials (Balis *et al.*, 1992). There is currently insufficient information to provide a recommendation for the dose of didanosine in babies under 6 months of age.

3 Patients with renal failure

In a small study of HIV-infected patients with normal renal function and with renal failure requiring hemodialysis there was reduced clearance and a prolongation in serum half-life of didanosine in the uremic patients. Plasma concentrations were approximately 2-fold higher in patients with renal failure, reflecting reduced elimination (Singlas *et al.*, 1992). The extraction ratio of didanosine by hemodialysis was $53 \pm 8\%$, with a clearance of 107 ± 21 ml per min (Singlas *et al.*, 1992). Didanosine should thus be administered at the conclusion of hemodialysis. The dose should be reduced, with recommendations ranging from a daily dose of 150 mg given once-daily (a decrease in dose by a theoretical factor of 4.7, being the ratio of the area-under-the-curve (AUC) in uremic versus control patients) (Dettli 1976; Singlas *et al.*, 1992) to 375 mg per day (Faulds and Brogden, 1992). It should be remembered that didanosine tablets contain high levels of magnesium hydroxide, thus increasing the magnesium load to these patients with impaired renal function (Didanosine Product Information).

4 Pregnancy

In two women in their second trimester of pregnancy a single oral dose of 375 mg resulted in no alteration in pharmacokinetic parameters. Fetal blood concentrations were less than 20% of maternal serum concentration (Pons *et al.*, 1991). No dosage recommendations exist at present.

5 Geriatric patients and those with reduced hepatic dysfunction

Studies in the elderly and in patients with hepatic failure providing the basis for dosage recommendations in these clinical situations are not yet available. However, the manufacturers suggest that dose-reduction should be considered in persons with hepatic impairment due to altered drug metabolism (Didanosine Product Information).

Availability

Chewable/dispersible mint- or mandarin-flavored buffered tablets: available in the following strengths: 25, 50, 100 and 150 mg. Tablets may be dispersed in water and, if kept at room temperature, the dose remains stable for 1 h.

Buffered powder for oral solution: (100, 167, 250, and 375 mg). Powder should be reconstituted in water and used within 4 h (Shelton *et al.*, 1992).

Pediatric unbuffered powder for oral solution: supplied in 120 ml and 240 ml bottles containing 2 g and 4 g respectively. Bottles should be stored below 30°C. Prior to dispensing, the dry powder is reconstituted with purified water to an initial concentration of 20 mg per ml, and then immediately mixed with Mylanta II Liquid antacid to a final concentration of 5 or 10 mg per ml. This solution is stable for 30 days under refrigeration.

Serum Levels in Relation to Dosage

1 Animal studies

The drug can easily be measured in biological samples by high performance liquid chromatography (Carpen et al., 1990; Frijus-Plessen et al., 1990; Hartman et al., 1990). Comparisons of pharmacokinetic parameters obtained for didanosine in humans and monkeys indicates that the latter are suitable animal models for didanosine pharmacokinetic measurements in humans (Qian et al., 1991). Administration of didanosine to macaques at doses of 3–10 mg per kg by intravenous route results in similar mean plasma clearance (16.7 ml per kg per min), mean steady-state volume of distribution (1.5 liters per kg) and terminal plasma half-life (97 min). Subcutaneous injection of 20 mg per kg results in over 90% bioavailability and a peak plasma concentration within 30 min (Ravasco et al., 1992). Data from neonatal pig-tailed macaques suggest that the pharmacokinetics of didanosine change rapidly over the first few months of life, with significantly lower clearance and higher terminal half-life of didanosine in animals 1 week old compared with those aged 1 and 4 months (Pereira et al., 1994).

In dogs given dideoxyadenosine i.v., rapid deamination to didanosine occurs (McGowan et al., 1990). In these animals didanosine has a half-life of approximately 30 min following i.v. infusion; oral bioavailability ranges from 28 to 93% (Wientjes et al., 1991). The micropig has been studied as a model for didanosine pharmacokinetics in man but has been found to be unsuitable, based on differences in metabolism and excretion (Swagler et al., 1991).

2 Adults

The clinically relevant pharmacokinetic data are summarized in Table V.30. As didanosine is rapidly degraded by acid, there were initial serious concerns regarding its therapeutic potential. However, absorption after oral administration is sufficient to achieve appropriate blood levels when the drug is administered with antacid, although absorption can vary considerably depending on food ingestion and the presence of gastric abnormalities including achlorhydria (Shelton et al., 1992). Didanosine is rapidly absorbed (Knupp et al., 1991). Absorption of didanosine is greater in jejunum than in other parts of intestine (Mirchandani and Chien 1995); colorectal absorption has also been reported (Bramer et al., 1993). More metabolically stable analogs of didanosine have been reported (Masood et al., 1990; Shirasaka et al., 1990).

The mean oral bioavailability varies with different preparations and in early studies ranged from 17% to 43% (Hartman et al., 1991b; Knupp et al., 1991; Drusano et al., 1992a; Pai et al., 1992). When given to fasting patients as an oral solution with antacid, the bioavailability increases to 30–41%. When administered as buffered tablets the reported mean bioavailability is 33–37%, but dramatically declines if administered with a meal (Didanosine Product Information). When given as a powder containing buffer, and requiring reconstitution by the patient, the mean bioavailability of this 'sachet' preparation is 29%, decreasing to 17% when taken with food (Hartman et al., 1991b). A more recent study has compared pharmacokinetic parameters between sachets and chewable tablets of didanosine and found no significant

Table V.30
Summary of clinically relevant pharmacokinetic data relating to didanosine

Rapidly degraded by acid, therefore must be administered with antacid (present in formulation)

Mean bioavailability is approximately 35%; this decreases with food, so tablets should be taken prior to meals

Plasma half-life is approximately 2 h but intracellular half-life is 8–24 h.

Renal clearance is responsible for elimination of up to 50%

Placental metabolism may reduce fetal exposure

Modest central nervous system penetration (approximately 20% of plasma level)

Refer to text for sources of data.

difference in maximal plasma concentration (C_{max}), time to reach C_{max} (T_{max}) and the AUC between the two formulations (Burger et al., 1995).

The maximum serum concentration of didanosine has been shown to be significantly lower in persons who have recently eaten prior to taking didanosine compared with those who take didanosine in the fasted state (2.8 ±1.0 μg per ml and 1.3 ± 0.5 μg per ml respectively) (Shelton et al., 1992). There is reduced bioavailability of didanosine when given once-daily compared with twice-daily administration (27 versus 36%), probably because of saturation of the absorption process (Drusano et al., 1992a).

The reported plasma half-life ranges from 0.6 to 2.7 h (Yarchoan et al., 1989b; Knupp et al., 1991; Balis et al., 1992; Shelton et al., 1992). However, the intracellular half-life is much longer, in the range of 8–24 h, thus significantly exceeding that of zidovudine and providing the rationale for once- or twice-daily dosing regimens (Ahluwalia et al., 1987; Shelton et al., 1992). Linear pharmacokinetic behavior has been reported over dose ranges of 0.4–16.5 mg per kg given by the i.v. route and 0.8–10.2 mg per kg via oral administration (Knupp et al., 1991). The total body clearance ranges from 0.7 to 1 liter per kg per h (Shelton et al., 1992), with an elimination half-life of approximately 1.4 h (Knupp et al., 1991).

3 Pediatrics

Oral administration of 20–180 mg per m² given as a reconstituted powder in saline together with antacid, results in highly variable bioavailability, with an overall mean of 21% (Butler et al., 1991). In other reports bioavailability has also been found to be variable and limited, with a mean of 19% ± 17%, decreasing with increasing dose (Balis et al., 1992). Peak plasma levels generally occur within 30 min but again the levels are extremely variable; the mean peak plasma levels range from 0.45 μM with oral doses of 20 mg per m² to 4.2 μM with doses of 180 mg per m² (Butler et al., 1991). The i.v. administration over 1 h of 20–180 mg per m² results in a proportional increase in peak plasma concentration and area under the plasma concentration-time curve. The mean peak plasma concentration of didanosine ranges from 3.1 μM to 22 μM, with the mean AUC ranging from 3.4 to 32 μM per h per liter (Butler et al., 1991). The half-life of didanosine following intravenous infusion is 0.8 ± 0.4 h, with a total body clearance of approximately 490 ml per min per m² (Butler et al., 1991).

Excretion

Studies in dogs and using perfused rat livers in vitro have both confirmed extensive metabolism of didanosine, the major metabolites being hypoxanthine, xanthine, uric acid, and allantoin (Tay et al., 1991; Wientjes et al., 1991). Urinary excretion of unchanged didanosine in dogs accounts for approximately 20% of an administered dose (Wientjes et al., 1991).

Complete studies in humans have not been performed. However, it is presumed that metabolism of didanosine will be similar to that of other endogenous purines. Purine nucleoside phosphorylase metabolizes didanosine to hypoxanthine, the major metabolite; small amounts of uric acid are subsequently formed through the action of xanthine oxidase (Back et al., 1992).

Renal clearance accounts for the elimination of approximately 30–50% of an administered dose of didanosine (Knupp et al., 1991; Shelton et al., 1992), regardless of whether the drug is given i.v. or orally. Thus both tubular secretion and glomerular filtration both contribute to elimination of didanosine. The level of unchanged didanosine in the urine again depends on whether food is ingested shortly before taking didanosine, in one study falling from 21% to 11% in HIV-infected persons who took didanosine in the unfasted state (Shelton et al., 1992).

The proportion of an administered dose of didanosine that is cleared by further metabolism or by hepatobiliary excretion is not certain.

Distribution of the Drug in Body

The volume of distribution of didanosine is approximately 1 liter per kg (Hartman et al., 1990; Lambert et al., 1990; Knupp et al., 1991; Pai et al., 1992; Shelton et al., 1992; Drusano et al., 1992b). In rats, kidney concentrations of didanosine are approximately 10-fold greater than plasma concentrations, and significantly less drug can be detected in brain, spleen, lymph node, liver and pancreas (Kang et al., 1994).

1 Placenta

Didanosine appears to cross the placenta rapidly by simple diffusion, without accumulation (Bawdon et al., 1992). However, some investigators have documented extensive placental metabolism of the drug, with 15–50% of didanosine reaching the fetal circulation (Pons et al., 1991; Dancis et al., 1993; Henderson et al., 1994). This is significantly less than in the case of zidovudine, and suggests that treatment of an HIV-infected pregnant woman with didanosine will result in her fetus having lower exposure to this antiretroviral than if zidovudine were used (Dancis *et al.*, 1993).

2 Central nervous system

Didanosine has lower penetration into the central nervous system than zidovudine, (p. 1669) but similar to, or greater than zalcitabine (p. 1735) (Morgan *et al.*, 1992). The mean tissue to plasma concentration ratios of didanosine in CSF, and brain tissue have been reported to be less than 5% in rats (Anderson *et al.*, 1990; Hoesterey *et al.*, 1991) and up to 11% in dogs (Wientjes *et al.*, 1991). Animal studies suggest that co-administration of probenecid and didanosine can increase levels of the latter drug in CSF (Faulds and Brogden, 1992). In humans, approximately one-fifth of the plasma level of didanosine is present in CSF when measured 1 h after an i.v. infusion (Hartman *et al.*, 1990). In a pediatric study of patients receiving a single oral dose of 90 or 120 mg per m^2, the majority of CSF samples had undetectable levels of didanosine, with CSF from a minority of patients having less than 20% of serum concentrations (Balis *et al.*, 1992).

Liposome-encapsulated didanosine can be targeted to lymph nodes and macrophage-rich tissues including the spleen and liver (Harvie *et al.*, 1995). Higher didanosine levels in plasma have also been reported with a liposomal formulation administered orally to rats (Desormeaux *et al.*, 1994).

Mode of Action

Didanosine is the nucleoside analog of the naturally occurring purine inosine. Similar to zidovudine (see p. 1670) didanosine exerts its major action against HIV by inhibiting the enzyme reverse transcriptase and preventing elongation of the newly forming HIV DNA. Whilst there are indeed a number of similarities between didanosine and zalcitabine, sufficient differences exist to discuss the mode of action of this drug separately.

2',3'-Dideoxyadenosine (ddA) is the prodrug of didanosine and is rapidly converted into didanosine by adenosine deaminase (Fig. V.43). It is clear that both didanosine and ddA can diffuse into the cell without active transport; this is similar to zidovudine but differs to zalcitabine (McGowan *et al.*, 1990). Within the cell ddA may undergo several fates. It can be phosphorylated to form ddA monophosphate (ddAMP) by either deoxycytidine kinase or adenosine kinase; or it can be deaminated by adenosine deaminase to form didanosine, subsequently phosphorylated by 5'-nucleotidase to dideoxyinosine monophosphate (ddIMP) and

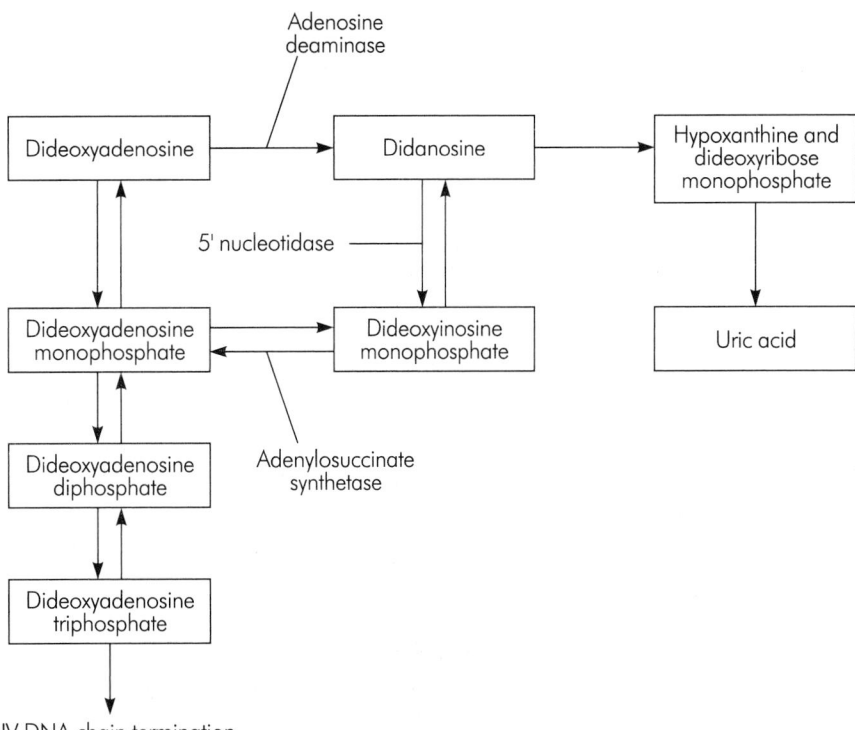

Fig. V.43.
Intracellular metabolism of didanosine.

then converted to ddAMP by adenylosuccinate synthetase and adenylosuccinate lyase (reviewed in Ahluwalia *et al.*, 1987; Cooney *et al.*, 1987; McGowan *et al.*, 1990; Carson *et al.*, 1991). Further phosphorylation of ddAMP is required to form the active compound, ddA triphosphate (ddATP) (Ahluwalia *et al.*, 1987). The dideoxyribose sugar moiety can also be cleaved from didanosine by the enzyme purine nucleoside phosphorylase, forming hypoxanthine and subsequently uric acid (Shelton *et al.*, 1992).

Similarly to zidovudine, the triphosphate analog of didanosine is able to compete with the naturally occurring purine for binding to HIV reverse transcriptase, and to a lesser extent cellular DNA polymerase. In addition to binding to the enzyme, didanosine triphosphate can become incorporated into the growing chain of viral DNA, preventing addition of further nucleotides through the $5' \rightarrow 3'$ phosphodiester linkages and thus causing premature termination of the DNA chain (Mitsuya *et al.*, 1987).

Unlike zidovudine and zalcitabine, the effects of didanosine are not reversed by the addition of the naturally occurring 2'-deoxynucleoside, even when added in 20-fold excess (Mitsuya *et al.*, 1985; McGowan *et al.*, 1990).

Toxicity

1 Pancreatitis

The most potentially serious toxicity is pancreatitis, which may be mild but has been fatal in some patients (Bouvet *et al.*, 1990; Yarchoan *et al.*, 1990; Bonacini, 1991; Maxson *et al.*, 1992). Didanosine-induced pancreatitis develops most frequently in persons receiving more than 9.6 mg per kg daily (Yarchoan and Mitsuya, 1992) and correlated in one study with cumulative dose (Seidlin *et al.*, 1992) (Table V.31). Although it has been reported to occur in 0.9–2% of patients receiving didanosine, in one study clinical pancreatitis developed in 23% of patients: it should be noted that these patients were being treated with 10–12 mg per kg daily (Maxson *et al.*, 1992).

In phase I clinical trials, three of 92 patients developed pancreatitis; the time of onset being between 13 and 19 weeks after initiating therapy (Rozencweig *et al.*, 1990). Other investigators have reported a higher incidence and earlier development of symptoms (Maxson *et al.*, 1992; Seidlin *et al.*, 1992). In the Didanosine Expanded Access Program involving over 21000 patients, those with advanced HIV disease (CD4 less than 50 cells per µl, and an AIDS diagnosis) had approximately a 5-fold higher estimated rate of pancreatitis than those with earlier stages of HIV infection (CD4 greater than 100 cells per µl and AIDS-related complex) (Schindzielorz *et al.*, 1994). These data support an earlier report in which advanced HIV infection, a prior history of pancreatitis, and concurrent ingestion of alcohol or co-administration of drugs that may cause pancreatitis appeared to increase the risk of didanosine-induced pancreatitis (Faulds and Brogden, 1992). Pancreatitis has been reported also in pediatric patients (Butler *et al.*, 1991, 1993).

The patient usually presents with abdominal pain that is accompanied by an increase in serum amylase. However, elevations in serum amylase, lipase or triglycerides may precede the development of pancreatic symptoms, and asymptomatic elevations have been frequently reported (Seidlin *et al.*, 1992; Shelton *et al.*, 1992). Some clinicians suggest that therapy should be discontinued if pancreatic amylase levels rise to 1.5- to 2-fold above normal (Yarchoan *et al.*, 1990). If a patient develops an elevated serum amylase levels in the absence of pancreatic symptoms, the author suggests that a pancreas-specific assay should be performed to guide clinical management.

Table V.31

Major toxicities of didanosine in phase I clinical trials. After Connolly *et al.* (1991), Cooley *et al.* (1990b), Lambert *et al.* (1990), Yarchoan *et al.* (1992). (Reproduced from Faulds and Brogden, 1992, with permission.)

Didanosine		Toxicity	
Dosage (mg per kg per day)	Duration (months)	Neuropathy (no/total)	Pancreatitis (no/total)
≤12.8	3–22	5/73	1/73
19–22	2–12	8/32	10/32
≥25	2–6	13/28	6/28
All patients	2–22	26/133	17/133

There are case-reports of didanosine-related hyperglycemia and diabetes mellitus (Munshi *et al.*, 1994; Chidiac *et al.*, 1995; Vittecoq *et al.*, 1994). In an *ex vivo* perfused canine pancreas preparation, lowered arterial pressure and pancreatic oxygen consumption followed the administration of didanosine (Nordback *et al.*, 1992), but in other animal studies didanosine has not been directly associated with pancreatic toxicity (Grady *et al.*, 1992).

2 Neurologic

A dose-related predominantly sensory, bilaterally symmetrical peripheral neuropathy is the most frequent major adverse reaction, and is generally reversible within 3–5 weeks of cessation of therapy (Cooley *et al.*, 1990b; Lambert *et al.*, 1990; Rozencweig *et al.*, 1990; Yarchoan *et al.*, 1990). Didanosine-associated peripheral neuropathy occurs less frequently than zalcitabine-induced neuropathy (Fichtenbaum *et al.*, 1995). In one phase I study, peripheral dysesthesia only occurred in patients receiving 19.2 mg per kg daily or more of didanosine, and generally appeared after a mean cumulative dose of 2600 mg per kg within the first 12 weeks of therapy (Yarchoan *et al.*, 1992; Kieburtz *et al.*, 1992), although lower mean cumulative doses have been reported (Rathbun and Martin, 1992). The time of onset appears to be related to the dose, with patients in phase I studies who received over 50 mg per kg daily developing symptoms within 4–7 weeks, those receiving 25–45 mg per kg daily developing symptoms generally around 10 weeks, and 22 weeks in a single patient who became symptomatic receiving only 12 mg per kg daily (Rozencweig *et al.*, 1990). The earliest symptoms are intermittent numbness, tingling, burning or pain involving the soles of the feet (and much less frequently the hands), that progress over 10–14 days to being present constantly and involving the legs (Yarchoan *et al.*, 1992; Kieburtz *et al.*, 1992). Distal vibration and pin-prick sensation, and ankle reflexes may be reduced or absent. Nerve conduction studies are frequently normal (reviewed in Shelton *et al.*, 1992), although a diminished sural sensory amplitude and slowed tibial nerve conduction in a symptomatic patient has been reported (Kieburtz *et al.*, 1992).

Some patients can tolerate reintroduction of didanosine in lower dose after resolution of symptoms (Kieburtz *et al.*, 1992). Although no predisposing factors were identified in one study of patients who developed didanosine-related peripheral neuropathy (Fichtenbaum *et al.*, 1995), the manufacturer recommends that patients with a history of peripheral neuropathy or those receiving potentially neurotoxic drugs should either not be treated with didanosine, or should be monitored very closely, as other studies have suggested that neuropathy occurs more frequently in these patients. Patients who develop peripheral neuropathy whilst receiving zalcitabine requiring cessation in therapy should not receive didanosine, as symptoms may worsen (LeLacheur and Simon, 1991).

Mitochondrial toxicity has been implicated as the cause of the delayed toxicity to peripheral nerves (Chen *et al.*, 1991). Compared with zalcitabine and stavudine, didanosine is the least toxic to mitochondria, as assessed by mitochondrial DNA content and morphology (Medina *et al.*, 1994; Tsai *et al.*, 1994).

In one early study of didanosine, approximately half of the patients experienced mild central nervous system side-effects, including irritability, insomnia, and headache (Yarchoan *et al.*, 1990). Didanosine has been reported to induce mania in one case report (Brouillette *et al.*, 1994).

3 Hematologic

Didanosine induces relatively less toxicity in human bone marrow progenitor cells compared with zidovudine, generally requiring a concentration of greater than 50–100 μM to inhibit 50% of cell growth compared with less than 5 μM for zidovudine (Molina and Groopman, 1989; Du *et al.*, 1990; Gallicchio *et al.*, 1993; reviewed in Hitchcock, 1993). These are similar data to those obtained in the canine model (Chan *et al.*, 1992). Didanosine also has insignificant effects on peripheral blood mononuclear cell mitogenesis, in contrast to zidovudine (Heagy *et al.*, 1991). Virtually no hematologic side-effects are associated with its use in patients (Connolly *et al.*, 1991). In fact, didanosine therapy has been reported to increase hemoglobin, white cell count and platelet numbers, compared with baseline estimations (Schacter *et al.*, 1992). In one phase I study, thrombocytopenia developed in two patients which may possibly be attributed to didanosine (Dolin *et al.*, 1990).

4 Gastrointestinal

Diarrhea is the most frequent adverse reaction to didanosine, reported in some early studies to occur in over 50% of patients (Rathbun and Martin, 1992), and possibly to have been related to the citrate-phosphate buffer in the earlier formulations (Didanosine Product Information).

Xerostomia has been reported in approximately 10% of patients enrolled in the Alpha Study of didanosine (Valentine *et al.*, 1992a), with elevations in the salivary component of serum amylase (Valentine *et al.*, 1992b). Other investigators who specifically measured salivary flow have documented reduced flow in up to one-third of patients receiving didanosine (Dodd *et al.*, 1992).

Elevation of hepatic transaminase levels was observed in phase I studies of didanosine (Cooley *et al.*, 1990a). Hepatitis has been reported in patients receiving didanosine (Yarchoan *et al.*, 1990), and fulminant hepatic failure with lactic acidosis (see p. 1674) has also been associated with didanosine therapy (Lai *et al.*, 1991). Hepatic toxicity, in some cases fatal, has also been reported in children receiving didanosine, although it must be noted that half of these children were co-infected with hepatitis C and all were receiving concurrent medications with known associated liver toxicity (Lacaille *et al.*, 1995).

5 Metabolic

Increased uric acid levels (resulting from metabolism of didanosine to hypoxanthine and then to uric acid) with no related clinical symptoms have been frequently observed in patients receiving doses of didanosine of 12.8 mg per kg daily or higher (Yarchoan *et al.*, 1992; Rozencweig *et al.*, 1990; Connolly *et al.*, 1991). Asymptomatic hypokalemia has been observed in association with didanosine therapy in three patients (Katlama *et al.*, 1991). Renal tubular dysfunction, with associated fluid, electrolyte and acid-base abnormalities, have been reported (Crowther *et al.*, 1993).

6 Visual disturbances

Didanosine has been implicated as the cause of abnormal vision and optic atrophy in a patient who presented with a scotoma and visual evoked potentials consistent with optic neuritis (Lafeuillade *et al.*, 1991). Retinal depigmentation has been reported in a small number of pediatric patients who were receiving high doses (>300 mg per m^2 daily) (Whitcup *et al.*, 1992, 1994), prompting the recommendation that children receiving didanosine should have examination of their retina every 6 months or if they develop visual symptoms (Didanosine Product Information).

7 Other

Potentially fatal rhabdomyolysis has been reported in three patients taking didanosine (Data on file, Bristol Myers Squibb). Didanosine has been implicated as a cofactor in the development of cardiac failure in four patients with AIDS (possibly due to the high salt content of the preparation used), although the contribution of the drug was not proven (de Jong and Borleffs, 1992; Willocks and Brettle *et al.*, 1992). In a study of 137 HIV-infected children with cardiac disease, didanosine therapy was not associated with the development of cardiomyopathy (Domanski *et al.*, 1995). Hypertension, thought to be secondary to the sodium content in the drug preparation, has been reported (Rathbun and Martin, 1992). Didanosine has been implicated but not proven in a patient who developed Stevens–Johnson syndrome whilst receiving the drug (Parneix-Spake *et al.*, 1992). Administration of didanosine to pregnant mice did not cause any detrimental effect or malformation in the embryos, nor alter postnatal development (Sieh *et al.*, 1992).

8 Drug interactions

As didanosine is so acid labile, drugs that potentially interfere with gastric acidity should be used with caution. Administration of ranitidine, an H_2-receptor antagonist, does not, however, consistently improve bioavailability (Hartman *et al.*, 1991b). The buffer in the didanosine formulations that neutralizes gastric acidity may interfere with absorption of (e.g. dapsone and ketoconazole). Thus it is recommended that these drugs be given 2 h prior to didanosine (Didanosine Product Information). Didanosine therapy given concurrently with dapsone has been associated with failure of prophylaxis for *Pneumocystis carinii* pneumonia (Metroka *et al.*, 1991), although plasma concentrations of dapsone were found in a separate study to be unaltered by administration of dapsone within 5 minutes of didanosine chewable tablets (Sahai *et al.*, 1995a). The aluminum component of the buffer in didanosine preparations precludes co-administration of didanosine with tetracyclines, and may also lower serum concentrations of quinolones (Didanosine Product Information). The absorption of ciprofloxacin is significantly reduced when it is administered with didanosine (Sahai *et al.*, 1993). Ciprofloxacin or other fluoroquinolones should be given 2 h before or more than 6 h after administration of didanosine or other antacids (Nix *et al.*, 1989; Sahai, 1995).

There is no change in the pharmacokinetics of patients receiving didanosine and ganciclovir (Hartman *et al.*, 1991b), although ganciclovir has been described as having potential pancreatic toxicity (reviewed in Shelton *et al.*, 1992), and thus should not be used – or used with extreme caution in patients receiving didanosine. Due to the potential pancreatic toxicity of didanosine, a number of other drugs that may cause pancreatitis, such as pentamidine, sulfonamides, ranitidine, cimetidine, and furosamide, should also be avoided or used with caution (Yarchoan *et al.*, 1992; Foisy *et al.*, 1994). The risk of pancreatitis is higher in individuals with high alcohol intake, and didanosine should be avoided in such patients.

Drugs known to cause peripheral neuropathy, including vincristine and zalcitabine, may increase the risk and should not be used concurrently with didanosine (LeLacheur and Simon, 1991).

Concurrent administration of zidovudine and didanosine to rats has not been associated with any pharmacokinetic interaction between the two drugs (Wientjes and Au, 1992). In humans co-administration of didanosine and zidovudine did not interfere with glucuronidation of zidovudine in one study (Rajaonarisone *et al.*, 1992), but resulted in a significant increase in renal clearance of the glucuronide metabolite (Sahai *et al.*, 1995b). In children, co-administration of zidovudine and didanosine does not significantly alter zidovudine pharmaco-kinetics, but the AUC of didanosine was reduced by 19% (Gibb *et al.*, 1995). Additive inhibition of human bone marrow progenitor cells *in vitro* by the two drugs has been reported (Dornsife *et al.*, 1991).

Co-administration of didanosine and stavudine does not alter the pharmacokinetics of either drug (Seifert *et al.*, 1994).

Human stem cell factor does not alter the efficacy of didanosine in inhibiting HIV replication within lymphocytes and monocytes (Miles *et al.*, 1991), in contrast to GM-CSF (Perno *et al.*, 1990a). A 7-day course of fluconazole (which inhibits cytochrome P-450 mediated drug metabolism) did not significantly alter the pharmacokinetics of didanosine in one study (Bruzzese *et al.*, 1995). However, other investigators have reported that itraconazole and didanosine co-administration results in a significant decrease in absorption of itraconazole (May *et al.*, 1994). Rifabutin, which can induce hepatic drug metabolism, does not interact pharmacokinetically with didanosine (Sahai *et al.*, 1995b).

Clinical Uses of the Drug

1 Human immunodeficiency virus infection

The specific indications for licensing didanosine currently vary from country to country. The drug in the past was generally limited to adults and children over 6 months of age who had advanced HIV infection and who were intolerant of zidovudine, or who had progressive disease on zidovudine therapy, or in whom zidovudine was contraindicated. In addition, didanosine was indicated for the treatment of patients with advanced HIV infection who had previously received 16 weeks of zidovudine therapy (Didanosine Product Information). However, based on data from ACTG 175 and the Delta Study (pp. 1682, 1683), many experts consider it appropriate to use didanosine in combination with zidovudine or certain other antiretroviral agents (such as stavudine or lamivudine, and a protease inhibitor). In many countries the indications have been changed accordingly. Data from ACTG 152 have enabled registration in some countries for the treatment of children.

a Clinical trials of didanosine monotherapy in adults A number of phase I studies collectively provided sufficient information for licensing of didanosine in the USA by the Federal Drug Administration, and by the relevant authorizing bodies in other countries. Many of these studies included an initial phase of i.v. administration, followed by oral therapy, and all were performed in patients with advanced HIV disease. Surrogate markers were the predominant criteria used to assess efficacy of the drug in each trial (Table V.32).

In the first dose-escalating phase I study of didanosine in 37 patients with AIDS or AIDS-related complex, there was a mild increase in CD4 lymphocyte numbers above baseline, a decline in HIV p24 antigen level in serum, and an increase in weight, appetite and energy levels (Hartman *et al.*, 1990; Yarchoan *et al.*, 1989b).

Another similar phase I dose-ranging trial of once-daily therapy in 36 patients with AIDS or AIDS-related complex resulted in over 85% of patients improving in terms of constitutional symptoms and weight, with a modest increase in CD4 lymphocyte counts evident within 2 weeks

Table V.32
Summary of phase I trials of didanosine. (Reproduced from Rozencweig *et al.* 1990, with permission.)

Patient group	No. of responders/no. evaluated (% responders)[a]			
	Weight gain	Improvement in clinical signs/ symptoms	Increase in CD4[+] cell count	Decrease in HIV p24 antigen
All patients	35/89 (39)	33/85 (39)	22/89 (25)	18/39 (46)
ARC	26/54 (48)[b]	23/51 (45)	16/54 (30)[c]	12/21 (57)
AIDS	9/35 (26)[b]	10/34 (29)	6/35 (17)[c]	6/18 (33)
Prior zidovudine	22/61 (36)	19/56 (34)	11/61 (18)[d]	11/28 (39)
No prior zidovudine	13/28 (46)	14/29 (48)	11/28 (39)[d]	7/11 (64)
CD4[+] <100 per mm^3	15/47 (32)	14/48 (29)[e]	6/47 (13)[f]	10/25 (40)
CD4[+] ≥100 per mm^3	20/42 (48)	19/37 (51)[e]	16/42 (38)[f]	8/14 (57)

[a] Not all patients were assessable for all parameters.
[b] $p = 0.046$; [c] $p = 0.085$; [d] $p = 0.038$; [e] $p = 0.045$; [f] $p = 0.007$.

of starting therapy, and in three-quarters of patients a decline in p24 antigen of at least 50% . The results were similar in patients who had received prior zidovudine therapy as well as those who were zidovudine-naive (Cooley *et al.*, 1990a,b).

A third phase I dose-escalation study in 37 patients with AIDS or AIDS-related complex using twice-daily administration found significant increases in CD4 numbers and decreases in plasma p24 titers as early as 2 weeks which were sustained to 20 weeks (Lambert *et al.*, 1990). In another phase I study of 30 patients, again who had AIDS or AIDS-related complex with a lower mean baseline CD4 number (mean of 48 cells per μl) than patients enrolled in previous studies, a decrease in plasma p24 antigen was observed in over 40% of patients who had detectable p24 antigen on study entry, with a non-sustained rise in CD4 number. A significant number of patients developed opportunistic infections during the study period (Connolly *et al.*, 1991).

In another report of a dose-escalating trial in 19 patients with AIDS or AIDS-related complex, serum levels of HIV p24 antigen decreased within 4 weeks in each of 16 patients. However, this was associated with only a modest increase in absolute CD4 numbers (and not in the percentage of CD4 lymphocytes) in less than one-third of the patients (Valentine *et al.*, 1990).

b   Clinical trials of switching from zidovudine to didanosine monotherapy   There have been a number of studies comparing the benefits of remaining on zidovudine versus switching to didanosine or zalcitabine in patients with prior zidovudine experience and generally with advanced disease.

In patients with AIDS, AIDS-related complex or a CD4 lymphocyte number below 200 per μl who had tolerated zidovudine therapy for at least 16 weeks, changing therapy from zidovudine to didanosine slowed disease progression, and improved immunologic and virologic markers (Kahn *et al.*, 1992). This study, ACTG 116B/117, provided the data in support of the early indication of didanosine therapy for adults with advanced HIV disease who had been previously treated for at least 16 weeks with zidovudine (Didanosine Product Information). However, 35% of patients voluntarily withdrew from the study medication (Saitz *et al.*, 1992), suggesting that caution should be exercised when interpreting the intention-to-treat analyses from this trial. The development of mutations within both codons 215 and 41 predicted disease progression and decreased survival, although the benefit of switching from zidovudine to didanosine was independent of the presence of these mutations (Japour *et al.*, 1995; D'Aquila *et al.*, 1995).

In the Bristol Myers Squibb study AI454–010, the benefits of switching to didanosine or continuing zidovudine were examined in 312 patients with CD4 counts of less than 300 cells per μl who had evidence of clinical deterioration and who had received at least 6 months of prior zidovudine therapy. Not surprisingly, those randomized to change to didanosine had fewer clinical or immunologic endpoints than those remaining on zidovudine therapy (Spruance *et al.*, 1994).

The Canadian HIV Trials Network Protocol 002 Study compared didanosine therapy with zidovudine therapy in 246 HIV-infected patients with 200–500 CD4 cells per μl who had received at least 6 months of prior zidovudine treatment. Switching to didanosine resulted in a decrease in rate of disease progression and a sustained increase in CD4 counts through the 48-week study duration (Montaner *et al.*, 1995).

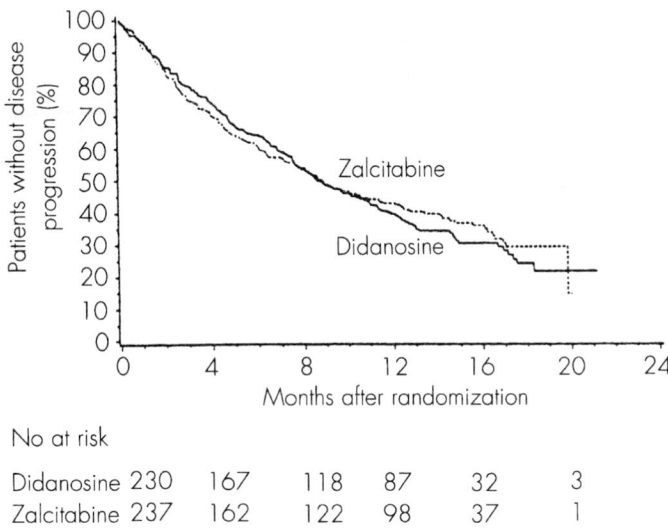

Fig. V.44.
Cumulative survival without disease progression in CPCRA Trial. (Reproduced from Abrams *et al.*, 1994, with permission.)

No at risk

Didanosine	230	167	118	87	32	3
Zalcitabine	237	162	122	98	37	1

A multicenter, open-label comparative study of didanosine or zalcitabine was performed by the Community Programs for Clinical Research on AIDS (CPCRA) involving 467 patients with prior zidovudine therapy (mean approximately 17 months) and CD4 lymphocyte numbers of less than 300 cells per μl (median approximately 40 cells per μl) or a diagnosis of AIDS (approximately 65% of participants). Patients were followed for a median of 16 months. Both zalcitabine and didanosine were similarly efficacious in delaying disease progression and preventing death (Fig. V.44) (Abrams *et al.*, 1994).

In an AIDS Clinical Trials Group trial zidovudine was compared with didanosine in 617 patients with advanced HIV infection and little or no (<16 weeks) prior zidovudine experience. In the 380 patient who were zidovudine-naive, zidovudine was more effective than didanosine; in those with 8–16 weeks of prior zidovudine therapy, didanosine was more effective than zidovudine, thus providing similar results to the earlier study of Kahn and colleagues (see above).

In ACTG 118 650 patients with symptomatic infection (AIDS or ARC) and CD4 counts of less than 300 cells per μl or asymptomatic HIV infection with less than 200 CD4 cells per μl with a history of hematologic intolerance to zidovudine were treated with didanosine in sachet formulation in doses of 200, 500 or 750 mg per day. These doses are equivalent to 160, 400 and 600 mg in tablet form. The median CD4 count on study entry was 33 cells per μl. Over the median follow-up period of 60.9 weeks there was no significant difference between the three groups in terms of progression to a new AIDS-defining illness or death. Nearly 10% (62) patients developed clinical pancreatitis, half of whom had no preceding elevation in serum amylase in the 2 weeks prior to illness (Data on file, Bristol-Myers Squibb).

c Clinical trials of didanosine combination therapy in adults The phase I/II ACTG 143 study of didanosine (500 mg daily) versus didanosine in combination with zidovudine (three arms, low dose (150 mg zidovudine and 134 mg didanosine daily), moderate dose (300 mg zidovudine and 334 mg didanosine daily) and high-dose (600 mg zidovudine and 500 mg didanosine daily) in 126 asymptomatic HIV-infected hemophiliac patients with 200–500 CD4 cells per μl resulted in no difference in clinical endpoints between the four arms (Ragni *et al.*, 1995).

Two important recent studies are ACTG 175 and Delta study (pp. 1682, 1683). Other combination studies with zidovudine are described (pp. 1681–1686). The ACTG 241 which evaluated nevirapine, zidovudine and didanosine in triple combination versus zidovudine and didanosine is described in the nevirapine chapter. The use of didanosine in combination with zidovudine in patients with advanced HIV infection (AIDS diagnosis or CD4 count of fewer than 200 cells per μl) is not superior to zidovudine monotherapy (Saravolatz *et al.*, 1996).

d Use of didanosine in children Didanosine is well-tolerated in children with symptomatic HIV infection, producing clinical, immunologic and virologic benefits (Pizzo, 1990). There is a significant decline in serum p24 antigen in children receiving didanosine. In addition, the median

CD4 lymphocyte number improves in children receiving didanosine, particularly those whose baseline CD4 is greater than 100 cells per μl (Butler *et al.*, 1991). Despite the reported low penetration of didanosine into CSF, neuropsychological improvement (increased IQ) of treated children was found to improve and to correlate with serum levels (Butler *et al.*, 1991; Balis *et al.*, 1992).

ACTG 152 enrolled 839 children and adults aged 3 months to 18 years in a comparison of zidovudine monotherapy, didanosine monotherapy or the two drugs in combination. They had less than 6 weeks of prior antiretroviral experience. The zidovudine monotherapy arm was closed in 1995 due to a significantly higher number of clinical endpoints in this group than the other arms. Final analysis of the study has shown no difference in progression rates in patients randomized to didanosine monotherapy or the combination. Over a median duration of treatment of 20 months the primary endpoint of disease progression or death was reached by 27% in the zidovudine monotherapy arm, 19% in the didanosine monotherapy arm and 18% in the combination arm. The risk of death or disease progression was significantly higher in the zidovudine montherapy group than either the didanosine monotherapy or the combination therapy arms. These results support the findings of ACTG 175 (Data on file, Bristol-Myers Squibb).

In a small study, stavudine (2 mg per kg per day) and didanosine (180 mg per m^2 per day) were co-administered in two divided doses to eight children whose mean age was 6.6 years and mean CD4 lymphocyte count was 42 cells per μl at baseline. Plasma HIV RNA declined by a median of 0.88 log$_{10}$, and there was no evidence of peripheral neuropathy or other adverse event over the 24-week duration of the study (Kline *et al.*, 1996).

e Use of didanosine as prophylaxis There are only limited data regarding the potential efficacy of didanosine in the setting of accidental exposure to HIV. One patient who received an i.v. inoculation of HIV was treated with zidovudine and later didanosine; HIV was recovered from the recipient 14 days later (Davis *et al.*, 1992).

f Surrogate markers and didanosine therapy A marked decrease in plasma HIV titer has been demonstrated in patients at various stages of HIV infection who are treated with didanosine (Aoki-Sei *et al.*, 1992). In over two-thirds of persons with advanced disease didanosine therapy leads to a 5-fold or higher decrease in plasma viremia (Shepp and Ashraf, 1993). In patients receiving didanosine therapy, changes in HIV RNA levels in plasma after 1 month of treatment predict survival independently of the CD4 count (Yerly *et al.*, 1995a,b). In ACTG 143, of the patients with 200–500 CD4 cells per μl who received combination therapy with zidovudine and didanosine for 2 years, those with a sustained decline in plasma viremia were more likely to maintain an increase in CD4 counts for the duration of the study and were less likely to develop drug-resistance (Shafer *et al.*, 1995).

In a retrospective analysis of patients with advanced symptomatic infection and a mean of 15 months of prior zidovudine therapy who received didanosine under the manufacturer's expanded access program, CD4 lymphocyte numbers increased above the level at entry by approximately 40%, returning to baseline after 5 months (Rathbun and Martin, 1992). An increase in total number of lymphocytes has been observed in didanosine-treated patients (Yarchoan *et al.*, 1990).

g Other Didanosine has been found to be useful for the treatment of some patients with zidovudine-resistant HIV who are deteriorating clinically (Bach, 1990). A small number of patients with impaired cognitive function related to HIV infection have been found to improve with didanosine therapy (Yarchoan *et al.*, 1990).

2 Hepatitis B virus infection

In two small studies of patients with both HIV infection and chronic hepatitis B virus infection, or chronic hepatitis B infection alone, therapy with didanosine was not associated with an appreciable change in hepatitis B virus DNA titers (Catterall *et al.*, 1992; Fried *et al.*, 1992).

References

Abrams DI, Goldman AI, Launer C et al. (1994). A comparative trial of didanosine or zalcitabine after treatment with zidovudine in patients with human immunodeficiency virus infection. New Engl J Med 330: 657.

Ahluwalia G, Cooney DA, Mitsuya H et al. (1987). Initial studies on the cellular pharmacology of 2',3'-dideoxyinosine, an inhibitor of HIV infectivity. Biochem Pharmacol 36: 3797.

Anderson BD, Hoesterey BL, Baker DG, Galinsky RE (1990). Uptake kinetics of 2',3'-dideoxyinosine into brain and cerebrospinal fluid of rats: intravenous infusion studies. J Pharmacol Exp Ther 253: 113.

Aoki-Sei S, O'Brien MC, Ford H et al. (1991). In vitro inhibition of hepatitis B virus replication by 2',3'-dideoxyguanosine 2',3'-dideoxyinosine, and 3'-azido-2',3'-dideoxythymidine in 2215 (PR) cells. J Infect Dis 164: 843.

Aoki-Sei S, Yarchoan R, Kageyama S et al. (1992). Plasma HIV-1 viremia in HIV-1 infected individuals assessed by polymerase chain reaction. AIDS Res Hum Retrovir 8: 1263.

Ashorn P, Moss B, Weinstein JN et al. (1990). Elimination of infectious human immunodeficiency virus from human T-cell cultures by synergistic action of CD4–Pseudomonas exotoxin and reverse transcriptase inhibitors. Proc Natl Acad Sci USA 87: 8889.

Bach MC (1990). Clinical response to dideoxyinosine in patients with HIV infection resistant to zidovudine. New Engl J Med 323: 275.

Back DJ, Ormesher S, Tjia JP, Macleod R (1992). Metabolism of 2',3'-dideoxyinosine (ddI) in human blood. Brit J Clin Pharmacol 33: 319.

Balis FM, Pizzo PA, Butler KM et al. (1992). Clinical pharmacology of 2',3'-dideoxyinosine in human immunodeficiency virus infected children. J Infect Dis 165: 99.

Balzarini J, Naesens L, Robins MJ, De Clercq E (1990). Potentiating effect of ribavirin on the in vitro and in vivo antiretrovirus activities of 2',3'-dideoxyinosine and 2',3'-dideoxy-2,6-diaminopurine riboside. J AIDS 3: 1140.

Balzarini J, Lee CK, Herdewijn P, De Clercq E (1991a). Mechanism of the potentiating effect of ribavirin on the activity of 2',3'-dideoxyinosine against human immunodeficiency virus. J Biol Chem 266: 21509.

Balzarini J, Lee CK, Schols D, De Clercq E (1991b). 1-beta-D-ribofuranosyl-1,2,4-triazole-3-carboxamide (ribavirin) and 5-ethynyl-1-beta-D-ribofuranosylimidazole-4-carboxamide (EICAR) markedly immunodeficiency virus in peripheral blood lymphocytes. Biochem Biophys Res Commun 178: 563.

Bawdon RE, Sobhi S, Dax L et al. (1992). The transfer of anti-human immunodeficiency virus nucleoside compounds by the term human placenta. Amer J Obstet Gynecol 167: 1570.

Bonacini M (1991). Pancreatic involvement in human immunodeficiency virus infection. J Clin Gastroenterol 13: 58.

Boucher CA, Cammack N, Schipper P et al. (1993). High level resistance to (-) enantiomeric 2'-deoxy-3'-thiacytidine in vitro is due to one amino acid substitution in the catalytic site of human immunodeficiency virus type 1 reverse transcriptase. Antimicrob Ag Chemother 37: 2231.

Bouvet E, Casalino E, Prevost MH, Vaction F (1990). Fatal case of 2',3'-dideoxyinosine-associated pancreatitis. Lancet 336: 1515.

Bramer SL, Wientjes MG, Au JL (1993). Absorption of 2',3'-dideoxyinosine from lower gastrointestinal tract in rats and kinetic evidence of different absorption rates in colon and rectum. Pharm Res 10: 763.

Bristol Myers Squibb Pharmaceutical Research Institute – letter to investigators.

Brouillette MJ, Chouinard G, Lalonde R (1994). Didanosine induced mania in HIV infection. Amer J Psychiat 151: 1839.

Bruzzese VL, Gillum JG, Israel DS et al. (1995). Effect of fluconazole on pharmacokinetics of 2',3'-dideoxyinosine in persons seropositive for human immunodeficiency virus. Antimicrob Ag Chemother 39: 1050.

Burger D, Meenhorst P, Mulder J et al. (1995). Substitution of didanosine sachets by chewable tablets; a pharmacokinetic study in patients with AIDS. J AIDS Hum Retrovir 10: 163.

Butler KM, Husson RN, Balis FM et al. (1991). Dideoxyinosine in children with symptomatic human immunodeficiency virus infection. New Engl J Med 324: 137.

Butler KM, Venzon D, Henry N et al. (1993). Pancreatitis in human immunodeficiency virus-infected children receiving dideoxyinosine. Pediatrics 91: 747.

Carpen ME, Poplack DG, Pizzo PA, Balis FM (1990). High performance liquid chromatographic method for analysis of 2',3'-dideoxyinosine in human body fluids. J Chromatogr 526: 69.

Carson DA, Carrera CJ, Wasson DB, Lizasa T (1991). Deoxyadenosine-resistant human T lymphoblasts with elevated 5'-nucleotidase activity. Biochem Biophys Acta 1091: 22.

Catterall AP, Moyle GJ, Hopes EA et al. (1992). Dideoxyinosine for chronic hepatitis B infection. J Med Virol 37: 307.

Chan TC, Boon GD, Shaffer L, Redmond P (1992). Antiviral nucleoside toxicity in canine bone marrow progenitor cells and its relationship to drug permeation. Eur J Haematol 49: 71.

Chen CH, Vazquez-Padua M, Cheng YC et al. (1991). Effect of anti-human immunodeficiency virus nucleoside analogs on mitochondrial DNA and its implication for delayed toxicity. Mol Pharmacol 39: 625.

Chidiac C, Alfandari S, Caron J, Mouton Y (1995). Diabetes mellitus following treatment of AIDS with didanosine. AIDS 9: 215.

Chow YK, Hirsch MS, Merrill DP et al. (1993). Use of evolutionary limitations of HIV-1 multidrug resistance to optimize therapy. Nature 361: 650.

Connolly KJ, Hammer SM (1992). Antiretroviral therapy: reverse transcriptase inhibition. Antimicrob Ag Chemother 36: 245.

Connolly KJ, Allan JD, Fitch H et al. (1991). Phase I study of 2'-3'-dideoxyinosine administered orally twice daily to patients with AIDS or AIDS-related complex and hematologic intolerance to zidovudine. Amer J Med 91: 471.

Connell EV, Hsu MC, Richman DD (1994). Combinative interactions of a human immunodeficiency virus (HIV) Tat antagonist with HIV reverse transcriptase inhibitors and an HIV protease inhibitor. Antimicrob Ag Chemother 38: 348.

Cooley TP, Kunches LM, Saunders CA et al. (1990a). Treatment of AIDS and AIDS-related complex with 2',3'-dideoxyinosine given once daily. Rev Infect Dis S5: S552.

Cooley TP, Kunches LM, Saunders CA et al. (1990b). Once-daily administration of 2',3'-dideoxyinosine (ddI) in patients with the acquired immunodeficiency syndrome or AIDS-related complex. Results of a Phase I trial. New Engl J Med 322: 1340.

Cooney DA, Ahluwalia G, Mitsuya H et al. (1987). Initial studies on the cellular pharmacology of 2',3'-dideoxyadenosine, an inhibitor of HTLV-III infectivity. Biochem Pharmacol 36: 1765.

Coplan PM, Nolan LL (1991). The selective toxicity of medications used in the treatment of AIDS on the CEM human leukemic CD4+ T-cell line. Drug Chem Toxicol 14: 257.

Cox SW, Aperia K, Albert J, Wahren B (1994). Comparison of the sensitivities of primary isolates of HIV type 2 and HIV type 1 to antiviral drugs and drug combinations. AIDS Res Hum Retrovir 10: 1725.

Crowther MA, Callaghan W, Hodsman AB, Mackie ID (1993). Dideoxyinosine-associated nephrotoxicity. AIDS 7: 131.

D'Aquila RT, Johnson VA, Welles SL et al. (1995). Zidovudine resistance and HIV-1 disease progression during antiretroviral therapy. AIDS Clinical Trials Group Protocol 116B/117 Team and the Virology Committee Resistance Working Group. Ann Intern Med 122: 401.

D'Aquila RT, Hughes MD, Johnson VA (1996). Nevirapine, zidovudine and didanosine compared with zidovudine and didanosine in patients with HIV-1 infection. Ann Intern Med 124: 1019.

Dahlberg JE, Mitsuya H, Blam SB et al. (1987). Broad spectrum antiretroviral activity of 2',3'-dideoxynucleosides. Proc Natl Acad Sci USA 84: 2469.

Dancis J, Lee JD, Mendoza S, Liebes L (1993). Transfer and metabolism of dideoxyinosine by the perfused human placenta. J AIDS 6: 2.

Darbyshire JH, Aboulker JP (1992). Didanosine for zidovudine-intolerant patients with HIV disease. *Lancet* **340**: 1346.

Davis LE, Hjelle BL, Miller VE *et al.* (1992). Early viral brain invasion in iatrogenic human immunodeficiency virus infection. *Neurology* **42**: 1736.

de Jong MD, Borleffs JC (1992). Didanosine and heart failure. *Lancet* **339**: 806.

Degre M, Beck S (1994). Anti-HIV activity of dideoxynucleosides, foscarnet and fusidic acid is potentiated by human leukocyte interferon in blood derived macrophages. *Chemother* **40**: 201.

Desormeaux A, Harvie P, Perron S *et al.* (1994). Antiviral efficacy, intracellular uptake and pharmacokinetics of free and liposome encapsulated 2',e'-dideoxyinosine. *AIDS* **8**: 1545.

Dettli L 1976 Drug dosage in renal disease. *Clin Pharmacokinet* **1**: 126.

Didanosine Product Information.

Dimitrov DH, Hollinger FB, Baker CJ *et al.* (1993). Study of human immunodeficiency virus resistance to 2'-3'-dideoxyinosine and zidovudine in sequential isolates from pediatric patients on long term therapy. *J Infect Dis* **167**: 818.

Dodd CL, Greenspan D *et al.* (1992). Reply to letter by Valentine. *Lancet* **340**: 1542.

Dolin R (1993). In *Antiviral Chemotherapy, New Directions for Clinical Applications and Research* Vol 3 (Mills J, Corey L, eds), p. 363. New York, London: PTR Prentice Hall.

Dolin R, Lambert JS, Morse GD *et al.* (1990). 2',3'-dideoxyinosine in patients with AIDS or AIDS-related complex. *Rev Infect Dis* **S5**: S540.

Domanski MJ, Sloas MM, Follmann DA *et al.* (1995). Effect of zidovudine and didanosine treatment on heart function in children infected with human immunodeficiency virus. *J Pediatr* **127**: 137.

Dornsife RE, St Clair MH, Huang AT *et al.* (1991). Anti-human immunodeficiency virus synergism by zidovudine (3'-azidothymidine) and didanosine (dideoxyinosine) contrasts with their additive inhibition of normal human marrow progenitor cells. *Antimicrob Ag Chemother* **35**: 322.

Drusano GL, Yuen GJ, Lambert JS *et al.* (1992a). Relationship between dideoxyinosine exposure, CD4 counts, and p24 antigen levels in human immunodeficiency virus infection. *Ann Int Med* **116**: 562.

Drusano GL, Yuen GJ, Morse G *et al.* (1992b). Impact of bioavailability on determination of the maximal tolerated dose of 2',3'-dideoxyinosine in phase I trials. *Antimicrob Ag Chemother* **36**: 1280.

Du DL, Volpe DA, Grieshaber CK, Murphy MJ (1990). *In vitro* myelotoxicity of 2',3'-dideoxynucleosides on human hematopoietic progenitor cells. *Exp Hematol* **18**: 832.

Eron JJ, Chow YK, Callendo AM *et al.* (1993). Pol mutations conferring zidovudine and didanosine resistance with different effects *in vitro* yield multiply resistant human immunodeficiency virus type 1 isolates *in vivo*. *Antimicrob Ag Chemother* **37**: 1480.

Faulds D, Brogden RN (1992). Didanosine, a review of its antiviral activity, pharmacokinetic properties and therapeutic potential in human immunodeficiency virus infection. *Drugs* **44**: 94.

Fichtenbaum CJ, Clifford DB, Powderly WG (1995). Risk factors for dideoxynucleoside induced toxic neuropathy in patients with the human immunodeficiency virus infection. *J AIDS Hum Retrovir* **10**: 169.

Fitzgibbon JE, Howell RM, Haberzettl CA *et al.* (1992). Human immunodeficiency virus type 1 pol gene mutations which cause decreased susceptibility to 2',3'-dideoxycytidine. *Antimicrob Ag Chemother* **36**: 153.

Foisy MM, Slayter KL, Hewitt RG, Morse GD (1994). Pancreatitis during intravenous pentamidine therapy in an AIDS patient with prior exposure to didanosine. *Ann Pharmacother* **28**: 1025.

Fried MW, Korenman JC, Di Bisceglie AM *et al.* (1992). A pilot study of 2'-3'-dideoxyinosine for the treatment of chronic hepatitis B. *Hepatology* **16**: 861.

Frijus-Plessen N, Michaelis HC, Foth H, Kahl GF (1990). Determination of 3'-azido-3'-deoxythymidine, 2',3'-dideoxycytidine, 3'-fluro-=3'-deoxythymidine and 2',3'-dideoxyinosine in biological samples by high-performance liquid chromatography. *J Chromatogr* **534**: 101.

Gallicchio VS, Hughes NK, Tse KF (1993). Comparison of dideoxynucleoside drugs (ddI and zidovudine) and induction of hematopoietic toxicity using normal human bone marrow cells *in vitro*. *Int J Immunopharmacol* **15**: 263.

Gao Q, Gu ZX, Parniak MA *et al.* (1992). *In vitro* selection of variants of human immunodeficiency virus type 1 resistance to 3'-azido-3'-deoxythymidine and 2',3'-dideoxyinosine. *J Virol* **66**: 12.

Gao Q, Gu Z, Hiscott J *et al.* (1993a). Generation of drug-resistant variants of human immunodeficiency virus type 1 b *in vitro* passage in increasing concentrations of 2',3'-dideoxycytidine and 2',3'-dideoxy-3'-thiacytidine. *Antimicrob Ag Chemother* **37**: 130.

Gao Q, Gu Z, Parniak MA *et al.* (1993b). The same mutation that encodes low-level human immunodeficiency virus type 1 resistance to 2',3'-dideoxyinosine and 2',3'-dideoxycytidine confers high level resistance to the (-) enantiomer of 2',3'dideoxy-3'-thiacytidine. *Antimicrob Ag Chemother* **37**: 1390.

Gao WY, Agbaria R, Driscoll JS, Mitsuya H (1994). Divergent anti-human immunodeficiency virus activity and anabolic phosphorylation of 2',3'-dideoxynucleoside analogs in testing and activated human cells. *J Biol Chem* **269**: 12633.

Gibb D, Barry M, Ormesher S *et al.* (1995). Pharmacokinetics of zidovudine and dideoxyinosine alone and in combination with HIV infection. *Brit J Clin Pharmacol* **39**: 527.

Gobert JM, Remington KM, Zhu YG, North TW (1994). Multiple drug resistant mutants of feline immunodeficiency virus selected with 2',3'-dideoxyinosine alone and in combination with 3'-azido-3'-deoxythymidine. *Antimicrob Ag Chemother* **38**: 861.

Grady T, Saluja AK, Steer ML *et al.* (1992). *In vivo* and *in vitro* effects of the azidothymidine analog dideoxyinosine on the exocrine pancreas of the rat. *J Pharmacol Exp Ther* **262**: 445.

Gu Z, Gao Q, Li X *et al.* (1992). Novel mutation in the human immunodeficiency virus type 1 reverse transcriptase gene that encodes cross-resistance to 2',3'-dideoxyinosine and 2',3'-dideoxycytidine. *J Virol* **66**: 7128.

Gu Z, Gao Q, Fang H *et al.* (1994). Identification of a mutation at codon 65 in the IKKK motif of reverse transcriptase that encodes human immunodeficiency virus resistance to 2',3'-dideoxycytidine and 2',3'-dideoxy-3'-thiacytidine. *Antimicrob Ag Chemother* **38**: 275.

Hartman NR, Yarchoan R, Pluda JM *et al.* (1990). Pharmacokinetics of 2',3'-dideoxyadenosine and 2',3'-dideoxyinosine in patients with severe human immunodeficiency virus infection. *Clin Pharmacol Ther* **47**: 647.

Hartman NR, Ahluwalia GS, Cooney DA *et al.* (1991a). Inhibitors of IMP dehydrogenase stimulate the phosphorylation of the anti-human immunodeficiency virus nucleosides 2',3'-dideoxyadenosine and 2',3'-dideoxyinosine. *Mol Pharmacol* **40**: 118.

Hartman NR, Yarchoan R, Pluda JM *et al.* (1991b). Pharmacokinetics of 2',3'-dideoxyinosine in patients with severe human immunodeficiency infection. II The effects of different oral formulations and the presence of other medications. *Clin Pharmacol Ther* **50**: 278.

Harvie P, Desormeaux A, Gagne N *et al.* (1995). Lymphoid tissues targeting of liposome encapsulated 2',3'-dideoxyinosine. *AIDS* **9**: 701.

Hayashi S, Fine RL, Chou JC *et al.* (1990). *In vitro* inhibition of the infectivity and replication of human immunodeficiency virus type 1 by combination of antiretroviral 2',3'-dideoxynucleosides and virus-binding inhibitors. *Antimicrob Ag Chemother* **34**: 82.

Heagy W, Crumpacker C, Lopez PA, Finberg RW (1991). Inhibition of immune functions by antiviral drugs. *J Clin Invest* **87**: 1916.

Henderson GI, Perez AB, Yang Y *et al.* (1994). Transfer of dideoxyinosine across the human isolated placenta. *Brit J Clin Pharmacol* **38**: 237.

Hitchcock MJ (1993). *In vitro* antiviral activity of didanosine compared with that of other dideoxynucleoside analogs against laboratory strains and clinical isolates of human immunodeficiency virus. *Clin Infect Dis* **1**: S16.

Hoesterey BL, Galinsky RE, Anderson BD *et al.* (1991). Dose dependence in the plasma pharmacokinetics and uptake kinetics of 2',3'-dideoxyinosine into brain and cerebrospinal fluid of rats. *Drug Metab Dispos Biol Fate Chem* **19**: 907.

Jablonowski H, Arasteh K, Staszewski S et al. (1995). A dose comparison study of didanosine in patients with very advanced HIV infection who are intolerant to or clinically deteriorate on zidovudine. German ddI Trial Group. AIDS 9: 463.

Japour AJ, Welles S, D'Aquilla RT et al. (1995). Prevalence and clinical significance of zidovudine resistance mutations in human immunodeficiency virus isolated from patients after long term zidovudine treatment. AIDS Clinical Trials Group 116B/117 Study Team and the Virology Committee Resistance Working group. J Infect Dis 171: 1172.

Johnson VA, Merrill DP, Videler JA et al. (1991). Two-drug combinations of zidovudine, didanosine, and recombinant immunodeficiency virus type 1 synergistically in vitro. J Infect Dis 164: 646.

Kageyama S, Weinstein JN, Shirasaka T et al. (1992). In vitro inhibition of human immunodeficiency virus (HIV) type 1 replication by C2 symmetry-based HIV protease inhibitors as single agents or in combinations. Antimicrob Ag Chemother 36: 926.

Kahn JO, Lagakos SW, Richman DD et al. (1992). A controlled trial comparing continued zidovudine with didanosine in human immunodeficiency virus infection. New Engl J Med 327: 581.

Kang HJ, Wientjes MG, Au JL (1994). Tissue pharmacokinetics of 2',3'-dideoxyinosine in rats. Biochem Pharmacol 48: 2109.

Katlama C, Tubiana R, Rosenheim M et al. (1991). Dideoxyinosine-associated hypokalaemia. Lancet 337: 183.

Kieburtz KD, Seidlin M, Lambert JS et al. (1992). Extended follow-up of peripheral neuropathy in patients with AIDS and AIDS-related complex treated with dideoxyinosine. J AIDS 5: 60.

Kline MW, Fletcher CV, Federici ME et al. (1996). Combination therapy with stavudine and didanosine in children with advanced human immunodeficiency virus infection: pharmacokinetics, safety, and immunologic and virologic effects. Pediatrics 97: 886.

Knupp CA, Shyu WC, Dolin R et al. (1991). Pharmacokinetics of didanosine in patients with acquired immunodeficiency syndrome or acquired immunodeficiency syndrome complex. Clin Pharmacol Ther 49: 523.

Lacaille F, Ortigao MB, Debre M et al. (1995). Hepatic toxicity associated with 2'-3'-dideoxyinosine in children with AIDS. J Pediatr Gastroenterol Nutr 20: 287.

Lacey SF, Larder BA (1994). Novel mutation (V751) in human immunodeficiency virus type 1 reverse transcriptase confers resistance to 2',3'-didehydro-2',3'dideoxythymidine in cell culture. Antimicrob Ag Chemother 38: 1428.

Lafeuillade A, Aubert L, Chaffanjon P, Quilichini R (1991). Optic neuritis associated with dideoxyinosine. Lancet 337: 615.

Lai KK, Gang DL, Zawacki JK, Cooley TP (1991). Fulminant hepatic failure associated with 2',3'-dideoxyinosine (ddI). Ann Int Med 115: 283.

Lambert JS, Seidlin M, Reichman RC et al. (1990). 2',3'-dideoxyinosine (ddI) in patients with the acquired immunodeficiency syndrome or AIDS-related complex A phase I trial. New Engl J Med 322: 1333.

Larder BA (1992). 3'-azido-3'-deoxythymidine resistance suppressed by a mutation conferring human immunodeficiency virus type 1 resistance to non-nucleoside reverse transcriptase inhibitors. Antimicrob Ag Chemother 36: 2664.

Larder BA, Chesebro B, Richman DD et al. (1990). Susceptibilities of zidovudine susceptible and resistant human immunodeficiency virus isolates to antiviral agents determined by using a quantitative plaque reduction assay. Antimicrob Ag Chemother 34: 436.

LeLacheur SF, Simon GL (1991). Exacerbation of dideoxycytidine-induced neuropathy with dideoxyinosine. J AIDS 4: 538.

Marquez VE, Tseng CK, Kelley JA et al. (1987). Dideoxy-2'-fluoro-ara-A: an acid-stable purine nucleoside active against human immunodeficiency virus. Biochem Pharmacol 36: 2719.

Martin P, Kassianides C, Korenman J et al. (1989). 2',3'-dideoxyinosine (ddI) and dideoxyguanosine (ddG) are potent inhibitors of hepadnaviruses in vivo [abstract]. Gastroenterol 96: A628.

Masood R, Ahluwalia G, Cooney DA et al. (1990). 2'-Fluro-2',3'-dideoxyarabinosyladenine: a metabolically stable analogue of the antiretroviral agent 2',3'-dideosyadenosine. Mol Pharmacol 37: 590.

Masqueller B, Pellegrin I, Ruffault A et al. (1995). Genotypic evolution of HIV-1 isolates from patients after a switch of therapy from zidovudine to didanosine. J AIDS 8: 330.

Mathez D, Schinazi RF, Liotta DC, Leibowitch J (1993). Infectious amplification of wild type human immunodeficiency virus from patients lymphocytes and modulation by reverse transcriptase inhibitors in vitro. Antimicrob Ag Chemother 37: 2206.

May DB, Drew RH, Yedinak KC, Bartlett JA (1994). Effect of simultaneous didanosine administration on itraconazole absorption in healthy volunteers. Pharmacother 14: 509.

Maxson CJ, Greenfield SM, Turner JL et al. (1992). Acute pancreatitis as a common complication of 2',3'-dideoxyinosine therapy in the acquired immunodeficiency syndrome. Amer J Gastroenterol 87: 708.

McGowan JJ, Tomaszewski JE, Cradock J et al. (1990). Overview of the preclinical development of an antiretroviral drug 2',3'-dideoxyinosine. Rev Infect Dis 12: S513.

Medina DJ, Tsai CH, Hsiung GD, Cheng YC (1994). Comparison of mitochondrial morphology, mitochondrial DNA content, and cell viability in cultured cells treated with three anti-human immunodeficiency virus dideoxynucleosides. Antimicrob Ag Chemother 38: 1824.

Metroka CE, McMechan MF, Andrada R et al. (1991). Failure of prophylaxis with dapsone in patients taking dideoxyinosine. New Engl J Med 325: 737.

Miles SA, Lee K, Hutlin L et al. (1991). Potential use of human stem cell factor as adjunctive therapy for human immunodeficiency virus-related cytopenias. Blood 78: 3200.

Mirchandani HL, Chien YW (1995). Intestinal absorption of dideoxynucleosides; characterisation using a multiloop in situ technique. J Pharm Sci 84: 44.

Mitsuya H, Broder S (1986). Inhibition of the in vitro infectivity and cytopathic effect of human T-lymphotropic virus type III/lymphadenopathy-associated virus (HTLV-III/LAV) by 2',3'-dideoxynucleosides. Proc Natl Acad Sci USA 83: 1911.

Mitsuya H, Broder S (1987). Strategies for antiviral therapy in AIDS. Nature 325: 773.

Mitsuya H, Broder S (1988). Inhibition of infectivity and replication of HIV-2 and SIV in helper T-cells by 2',3'-dideoxynucleosides in vitro. AIDS Res Hum Retrovir 4: 107.

Mitsuya H, Weinhold KJ, Furman PA, St Clair MH (1985). 3'-azido-3'-doexythymidine (BW A509U); an antiviral agent that inhibits the infectivity and cytopathic effect of human T-lymphotropic virus type III/ lymphadenopathy associated virus in vitro. Proc Natl Acad Sci USA 82: 7096.

Mitsuya H, Jarrett RF, Matsukura M et al. (1987). Long-term inhibition of human T-lymphotropic virus type III/lymphadenopathy-associated virus (human immunodeficiency virus) DNA synthesis and RNA expression in T cells protected by 2',3'-dideoxynucleosides in vitro. Proc Natl Acad Sci USA 84: 2033.

Mitsuya H, Yarchoan R, Broder S et al. (1990). Molecular targets for AIDS therapy. Science 249: 1533.

Molina JM, Groopman JE (1989). Bone marrow toxicity of dideoxyinosine. New Engl J Med 321: 1478.

Montaner JS, Schechter MT, Rachlis A et al. (1995). Didanosine compared with continued zidovudine therapy for HIV-infected patients with 200 to 500 CD4 cells/mm3. A double-blind, randomized trial. Canadian HIV Trials Network Protocol 002 Study Group. Ann Intern Med 123: 561.

Morgan ME, Chi SC, Murakami K et al. (1992). Central nervous system targeting of 2',3'-dideoxyinosine via adenosine deaminase-activated 6-halo-dideoxypurine prodrugs. Antimicrob Ag Chemother 36: 2156.

Mukherji E, Au JL, Mathes LE (1994). Differential antiviral activities and intracellular metabolism of 3'-azido-3'-deoxythymidine and 2',3'-dideoxyinosine in human cells. Antimicrob Ag Chemother 38: 1573.

Munshi MN, Martin RL, Fonseca VA (1994). Hyperosmolar nonketotic diabetic syndrome following treatment of human immunodeficiency virus infection with didanosine. Diabetes Care 17: 316.

Nix DE, Watson WA, Lener ME, Frost RW (1989). Effects of aluminum and magnesium antacids and rantidime on the absorption of ciprofloxacin. *Clin Pharmacol Ther* **46**: 700.

Nordback IH, Olson JL, Chaisson RE, Cameron JL (1992). Acute effects of a nucleoside analog dideoxyinosine (ddI) on the pancreas. *J Surg Res* **53**: 610.

O'Marro SD, Armstrong JA, Asuricion C et al. (1992). The effect of combinations of ampligen and zidovudine or dideoxyinosine against human immunodeficiency viruses in vitro. *Antiviral Res* **17**: 169.

Pai SM, Shukla UA, Grasela TH et al. (1992). Population pharmacokinetic analysis of didanosine (2',3'-dideoxyinosine) plasma concentrations obtained in phase I clinical trials in patients with AIDS or AIDS-related complex. *J Clin Pharmacol* **32**: 242.

Parneix-Spake A, Bastuji-Garin S, Levy Y et al. (1992). Didanosine as probable cause of Stevens-Johnson syndrome. *Lancet* **340**: 857.

Pauwels R, Andries K, Debyser Z et al. (1994). New tetrahydroimidazo[4,5,1-jk][1,4]-benzodiazepin-2(1H)-one and -thione derivatives are potent inhibitors of human immunodeficiency virus type 1 replication and are synergistic with 2',3'-dideoxynucleoside analogs. *Antimicrob Ag Chemother* **38**: 2863.

Perno CF, Yarchoan R, Cooney DA, Hartman NR (1988). Inhibition of human immunodeficiency virus (HIV-1/HTLV-III/Ba-L) replication in fresh and cultured human peripheral blood monocytes/macrophages by azidothymidine and related 2',3'-dideoxynucleosides. *J Exp Med* **168**: 1111.

Perno CF, Cooney DA, Currens MJ et al. (1990a). Ability of anti-HIV agents to inhibit HIV replication in monocyte/macrophages or U937 monocytoid cells under conditions of enhancement by GM-CSF or anti-HIV antibody. *AIDS Res Hum Retrovir* **6**: 1051.

Perno CF, Calio R et al. (1990b). In vitro modulation of the activity of anti-HIV drugs in monocytes by GM-CSF and other cytokines. *Antiviral Res* (Suppl 1): 94.

Perno CF, Cooney DA, Gao WY et al. (1992). Effects of bone marrow stimulatory cytokines on human immunodeficiency virus replication and the antiviral activity of dideoxynucleosides in cultures of monocyte/macrophages. *Blood* **80**: 995.

Pereira CM, Nosbisch C, Unadkat JD (1994). Pharmacokinetics of dideoxyinosine in neonatal pigtailed macaques. *Antimicrob Ag Chemother* **38**: 787.

Pizzo PA (1990). Considerations for the evaluation of antiretroviral agents in infants and children infected with human immunodeficiency virus. A perspective from the National Cancer Institute. *Rev Infect Dis* **12**: S561.

Pons JC, Boubon MC, Taburet AM et al. (1991). Fetoplacental passage of 2',3'-dideoxyinosine. *Lancet* **337**: 732.

Qian MX, Finco TS, Swagler AR, Gallo JM, (1991). Pharmacokinetics of 2',3'-dideoxyinosine in monkeys. *Antimicrob Ag Chemother* **35**: 1247.

Ragni MV, Amato DA, LoFaro ML et al. (1995). Randomized study of didanosine monotherapy and combination therapy with zidovudine in hemophilic and nonhemophilic subjects with asymptomatic human immunodeficiency virus-1 infection. AIDS Clinical Trial Groups. *Blood* **85**: 2337.

Rajaonarison JF, Lacarelle B, Catalin J et al. (1992). 3'-azido-3'-deoxythymidine drug interactions. Screening for inhibitors for human liver microsomes. *Drug Metab Dispos Biol Fate Chem* **20**: 578.

Rathbun RC, Martin ES (1992). Didanosine therapy in patients intolerant of or failing zidovudine therapy. *Ann Pharmacother* **26**: 1347.

Ravasco RJ, Unadkat JD, Tsai CC, Nosbisch C (1992). Pharmacokinetics of dideoxyinosine in pigtailed macaques (*Macaca nemestrina*) after intravenous and subcutaneous administration. *J AIDS* **5**: 1016.

Remington KM, Chesebro B, Wehrly K et al. (1991). Mutants of feline immunodeficiency virus resistant to 3'-azido-3'-deoxythymidine. *J Virol* **65**: 308.

Richman DD (1987). Dideoxynucleotides are less inhibitory in vitro against human immunodeficiency virus type 2 (HIV-2) than against HIV-1. *Antimicrob Ag Chemother* **31**: 1879.

Robins MJ, Robins RK (1964). The synthesis of 2',3'-dideoxyadenosine from 2'-deoxyadenosine. *J Amer Chem Soc* **86**: 3585.

Rozencweig M, McLaren C, Be Hangady M et al. (1990). Overview of phase I trials of 2',3'-dideoxyinosine (ddI) conducted on adult patients. *Rev Infect Dis* **12**: S570.

Sahai J (1995). Avoiding the ciprofloxacin didanosine interaction. *Ann Intern Med* **123**: 394.

Sahai J, Gallicano K, Oliveras L et al. (1993). Cations in the didanosine tablet reduce ciprofloxacin bioavailability. *Clin Pharmacol* **53**: 292.

Sahai J, Garber G, Gallicano K et al. (1995a). Effects of the antacids in didanosine tablets on dapsone pharmacokinetics. *Ann Intern Med* **123**: 8.

Sahai J, Gallicano K, Garber G et al. (1995b). Pharmacokinetics of simultaneously administered zidovudine and didanosine in HIV-seropositive male patients. *AIDS Hum Retrovir* **10**: 54.

Saitz R, Friedmann PD, roberts MS (1992). Continued zidovudine or didanosine for human immunodeficiency virus infection. *New Engl J Med* **327**: 1598.

Saravolatz LD, Winslow DL, Collins G et al. Zidovudine alone or in combination with didanosine or zalcitabine in HIV-infected patients with the acquired immunodeficiency syndrome or fewer than 200 CD4 cells per cubic millimeter. Investigators for the Terry Beirn Community Programs for Clinical Research on AIDS. *New Engl J Med* **335**: 1099.

Schacter BL, Rozencweig M, Beltangady M et al. (1992). Effects of therapy with didanosine on hematologic parameters in patients with advanced human immunodeficiency virus disease. *Blood* **80**: 2969.

Schinazi RF, Sommadossi JP, Saalmann V et al. (1990). Activities of 3'-azido-3'-deoxythymidine nucleotide dimers in primary lymphocytes infected with human immunodeficiency virus type 1. *Antimicrob Ag Chemother* **34**: 1061.

Schindzielorz A, Pike I, Daniels M et al. (1994). Rates and risk factors for adverse events associated with didanosine in the expanded access program. *Clin Infect Dis* **19**: 1076.

Seidlin M, Lambert JS, Dolin R, Valentine FT, (1992). Pancreatitis and pancreatic dysfunction in patients taking dideoxyinosine. *AIDS* **6**: 831.

Seifert RD, Stewart MB, Sramek JJ et al. (1994). Pharmacokinetics of co-administered didanosine and stavudine in HIV-seropositive male patients. *Brit J Clin Pharmacol* **38**: 405.

Shafer RW, Iversen AK, Winters MA et al. (1995). Drug resistance and heterogeneous long-term virologic responses of human immunodeficiency virus type 1 infected subjects to zidovudine and didanosine combination therapy. The AIDS Clinical Trials Group 143 Virology Team. *J Infect Dis* **172**: 70.

Shelton MJ, O'Donnell AM et al. (1992). Didanosine. *Ann Pharmacother* **26**: 660.

Shepp DH, Ashraf A (1993). Effect of didanosine on human immunodeficiency virus viremia and antigenemia in patients with advanced disease: correlation with clinical response. *J Infect Dis* **167**: 30.

Shirasaka T, Murakami K, Ford H et al. (1990). Lipophilic halogenated congeners of 2'-3'-dideoxypurine nucleosides active against human immunodeficiency virus in vitro. *Proc Natl Acad Sci USA* **87**: 9426.

Shirasaka T, Yarchoan R, O'Brien MC et al. (1993). Changes in drug sensitivity of human immunodeficiency virus type 1 during therapy with azidothymidine, dideoxycytidine, and dideoxyinosine: an in vitro comparative study. *Proc Natl Acad Sci USA* **90**: 562.

Shirasaka T, Kavlick MF, Ueno T et al. (1995). Emergence of human immunodeficiency virus type 1 variants with resistance to multiple dideoxynucleosides in patients receiving therapy with dideoxynucleosides. *Proc Natl Acad Sci USA* **92**: 2398.

Sieh E, Coluzzi ML, Cusella de Angelis MG et al. (1992). The effects of AZT and ddI on pre- and postimplantation mammalian embryos: an in vivo and in vitro study. *AIDS Res Hum Retrovir* **8**: 639.

Singlas E, Taburet AM, Borsa-Lebas F et al. (1992). Didanosine pharmacokinetics in patients with normal and impaired renal function: influence of hemodialysis. *Antimicrob Ag Chemother* **36**: 1519.

Sperber SJ, Feibusch EL, Damiani A, Weinstein MP (1993). In vitro activities of nucleoside analog antiviral agents against salmonellae. *Antimicrob Ag Chemother* **37**: 106.

Spruance SL, Pavia AT, Peterson D et al. (1994). Didanosine compared with continuation of zidovudine in HIV-infected patients with signs of clinical deterioration while receiving zidovudine. A randomised, double blind clinical trial. The Bristol Myers Squibb A1454–010 Study Group. *Ann Intern Med* **120**: 360.

St Clair MH, Martin JL, Tudor-Williams G *et al.* (1991). Resistance to ddI and sensitivity to AZT induced by a mutation in HIV-1 reverse transcriptase. *Science* **253**: 1557.

St Clair MH, Pennington KN, Rooney J, Barry DW (1995). *In vitro* comparison of selected triple drug combinations for suppression of HIV-1 replication the Inter-Company Collaboration Protocol. *J AIDS Hum Retrovir* **10**: S83.

Swagler AR, Qian MX, Gallo JM *et al.* (1991). Pharmacokinetics of anti-HIV nucleosides in microswine. *J Pharm Pharmacol* **43**: 823.

Tachedjian G, Hooker DJ, Gurusinghe AD *et al.* (1995). Characterisation of foscarnet resistant strains of human immunodeficiency virus type 1. *Virology* **212**: 58.

Tavares L, Roneker C, Postie L, de-Noronha F (1989). Testing of nucleoside analogues in cats infected with feline leukemia virus: a model. *Intervirology* **30**: 26.

Tay LK, Papp EA, Timoszyk J *et al.* (1991). Metabolism of 14C-2',3'-dideoxyinosine by the *in situ* perfused rat liver preparation. *Biopharm Drug Dispos* **12**: 285.

Tisdale M, Kemp SD, Parry NR, Larder BA (1993). Rapid *in vitro* selection of human immunodeficiency virus type 1 resistant to 3'-thiacytidine inhibitors due to a mutation in the YMDD region of reverse transcriptase. *Proc Natl Acad Sci USA* **90**: 5653.

Thormar H, Balzarini J, Holy A *et al.* (1993). Inhibition of visna virus replication by 2',3'-dideoxynucleosides and acyclic nucleoside phosphorate analogs. *Antimicrob Ag Chemother* **37**: 2540.

Tsai CH, Doong SL, Johns DG *et al.* (1994). Effect of anti-HIV 2'-beta-fluoro-2',3'-dideoxynucleoside analogs on the cellular content of mitochondrial DNA and on lactate production. *Biochem Pharmacol* **48**: 1477.

Valentine C, Deenmamode J, Sherwood R (1992a). Didanosine and amylase monitoring. *Lancet* **339**: 999.

Valentine C, Deenmamode J, Sherwood R (1992b). *Xerostomia* associated with didanosine. *Lancet* **340**: 1542.

Valentine FT, Seidlin M, Hochster H, Laverty M, (1990). Phase I study of 2',3'-dideoxyinosine: experience with 19 patients at New York University Medical Center. *Rev Infect Dis* **5**: S534.

Vittecoq D, Zucman D, Auperin I, Passeron J (1994). Transient insulin-dependent diabetes mellitus in an HIV-infected patient receiving didanosine. *AIDS* **8**: 1351.

Walzer PD, Foy J, Steele P *et al.* (1992). Activities of antifolate, antiviral, and other drugs in an immunosuppressed rat model of *Pneumocystis carinii* pneumonia. *Antimicrob Ag Chemother* **36**: 1935.

Watson AJ, Wilburn LM (1992). Inhibition of HIV infection of resting peripheral blood lymphocytes by nucleosides. *AIDS Res Hum Retrovir* **8**: 1221.

Whitcup SM, Butler KM, Caruso R *et al.* (1992). Retinal toxicity in human immunodeficiency virus-infected children treated with 2',3'-dideoxyinosine. *Amer J Ophthalmol* **113**: 1.

Whitcup SM, Dastgheib K, Nussenblatt RB *et al.* (1994). A clinicopathologic report of the retinal lesions associated with didanosine. *Arch Ophthalmol* **112**: 1594.

Wientjes MG, Au JL (1992). Lack of pharmacokinetic interaction between intravenous 2',3'-dideoxyinosine and 3'-azido-3'-deoxythymidine in rats. *Antimicrob Ag Chemother* **36**: 665.

Wientjes MG, Placke ME, Chang MJ *et al.* (1991). Pharmacokinetics of 2',3'-dideoxyadenosine in dogs. *Invest New Drugs* **9**: 159.

Willocks L, Brettle R, Keen J *et al.* (1992). Formulations of didanosine (ddI) and salt overload. *Lancet* **339**: 190.

Yarchoan R, Mitsuya H, Myers CE, Broder S (1989a). Clinical pharmacology of 3'-azido-2'-deoxythymidine (zidovudine) and related dideoxynucleosides. *New Engl J Med* **321**: 726.

Yarchoan R, Mitsuya H, Thomas RV *et al.* (1989b). *In vivo* activity against HIV and favorable toxicity profile of 2',3'-dideoxyinosine. *Science* **245**: 412.

Yarchoan R, Pluda JM, Thomas RV *et al.* (1990). Long-term toxicity/activity profile of 2',3'-dideoxyinosine in AIDS or AIDS-related complex. *Lancet* **336**: 526.

Yarchoan R, Mitsuya H *et al.* (1992). Study of 2',3'-dideoxyinosine administration in adults with AIDS or AIDS-related complex; analysis of activity and toxicity profiles. *Rev Infect Dis* (Suppl 5): S522.

Yerly S, Kaiser L, Mermillod B *et al.* (1995a). Response of HIV RNA to didanosine as a predictive marker of survival. *AIDS* **9**: 159.

Yerly S, Kaiser L, Baumberger G *et al.* (1995b). Early and prolonged decrease of viremia in HIV-1 infected patients treated with didanosine. *J AIDS Hum Retrovir* **8**: 358.

Zhang D, Callendo AM, Eron JJ *et al.* (1994). Resistance to 2',3'-dideoxycytidine conferred by a mutation in codon 65 of the human immunodeficiency virus type 1 reverse transcriptase. *Antimicrob Ag Chemother* **38**: 282

Zalcitabine

Description

The synthetic pyrimidine nucleoside analog zalcitabine (2',3'-dideoxycytidine, also known as ddC) was the third antiretroviral agent to be approved in the USA, Australia and Europe for the treatment of HIV infection. Zalcitabine is marketed by Roche under the trade name of 'Hivid'.

The chemical name of zalcitabine is 4-amino-1-beta-D-2',3'-dideoxyribofuranosyl-2-(1H)-pyrimidone, and it has the molecular formula $C_9H_{13}N_3O_3$. The molecular weight is 211.22. The chemical structure is shown in Fig. V.45. Concentrations of the drug and plasma levels may be expressed as either µg per ml or µM (1 µM is equivalent to 0.210 µg per ml).

Antiviral Activity

1 Human immunodeficiency virus

The antiretroviral activity of zalcitabine was first reported in 1986 by Mitsuya and colleagues (Mitsuya and Broder, 1986) and confirmed by Balzarini and colleagues in the same year (Balzarini *et al.*, 1986). The ability of zalcitabine to provide long-term protection of T cells against HIV infection through inhibiting retroviral DNA synthesis and mRNA expression was demonstrated shortly after (Mitsuya *et al.*, 1987). Both HIV-1 and HIV-2 are susceptible to zalcitabine (Mitsuya and Broder, 1988), including HIV subtype O, which is resistant to certain non-nucleoside reverse transcriptase inhibitors (Descamps *et al.*, 1995). Zalcitabine is more potent than didanosine on a molar basis (Jeffries, 1989; Hitchcock, 1993). In stimulated peripheral blood mononuclear cells the antiviral activities of zalcitabine and zidovudine are comparable (Sommadossi, 1993). There is complete antiviral protection of T cell lines at concentrations of 0.5–1 µM (Mitsuya and Broder, 1986) and significant antiviral activity is still present at concentrations of zalcitabine below 0.01 µM (Winslow *et al.*, 1994). The IC_{50} of zalcitabine for HIV is in the range of 30–500 nM. Viral expression is blocked even when zalcitabine is added up to 48 h post-infection (Pellegrino *et al.*, 1991). The antiretroviral activity of zalcitabine as well as other nucleoside analogs has been reported to be dependent upon the target cells used for assessment of efficacy (Balzarini *et al.*, 1989; Perno *et al.*, 1992a). Although an initial report suggested that zalcitabine did not inhibit HIV

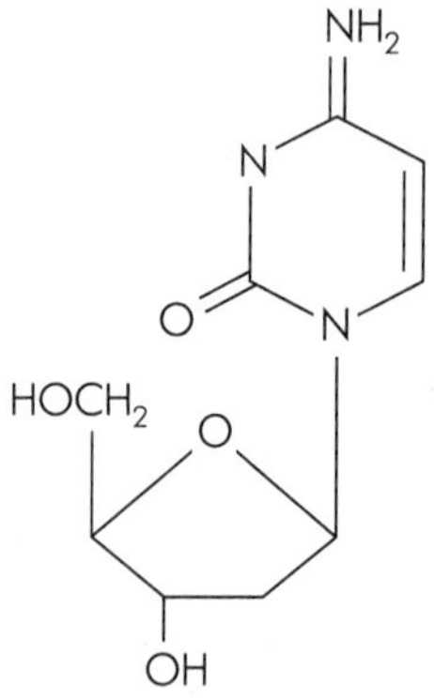

Fig. V.45.
Chemical structure of zalcitabine.

replication in human monocyte-derived macrophages even at concentrations of 100 μM (Richman *et al.*, 1987), this finding has not been confirmed by other investigators (Perno *et al.*, 1988, 1992a; Szebeni *et al.*, 1990). Chronically infected macrophages in which proviral DNA is already integrated, are not susceptible to zalcitabine (Perno *et al.*, 1994). The concentration of zalcitabine required to inhibit cell growth by 50% is in the range of 5 μM to >100 μM (Zalcitabine Product Information, 1992)

In the murine retrovirus-induced immunodeficiency model, LP-BM5, administration of oral zalcitabine (80 mg per kg daily), as either continuous monotherapy or alternating with zidovudine, has been found to prolong the survival of mice (Basham *et al.*, 1991), despite reports of poor phosphorylation of zalcitabine in murine cells *in vitro* (Richman, 1990a).

2 Other retroviruses

Zalcitabine, at concentrations as low as 0.5 μM, significantly decreases the expression of human T lymphotropic virus type 1 (HTLV-1) Gag proteins in T cell lines *in vitro*. Complete inhibition of Gag protein was observed in the presence of 2 μM zalcitabine (Matsushita *et al.*, 1987). The drug has activity against murine Moloney sarcoma virus *in vitro* and *in vivo* (Balzarini *et al.*, 1988a,b), and in the murine AIDS model (Rossi *et al.*, 1993). *In vitro* antiviral activity of zalcitabine against the feline leukemia virus has been reported to be dependent upon the target cell used for infection, with significantly higher concentrations of the drug being required to inhibit replication in primary bone marrow cells by 80% (43–384 μM) when compared with lymphoid cells (5–10 μM) (Polas *et al.*, 1990). In the cat model, zalcitabine-treated animals had equivalent levels of feline leukemia virus viremia to untreated control cats (Hoover *et al.*, 1989). Feline immunodeficiency virus is inhibited by zalcitabine (Gobert *et al.*, 1994). The simian type D retrovirus strain SAIDS-D/WA is sensitive to zalcitabine *in vitro* in Raji cells at concentrations of 1–10 μM without evidence of cellular toxicity (Tsai *et al.*, 1988). However, zalcitabine therapy of pig-tailed macaques naturally infected with the simian retrovirus serotype 2 (SRV-2) does not significantly inhibit virus replication, despite plasma concentrations of zalcitabine which inhibited virus replication *in vitro* (Tsai *et al.*, 1989).

3 Synergism with other drugs

Zidovudine and zalcitabine act synergistically to inhibit replication of both zidovudine-sensitive and zidovudine-resistant isolates of HIV-1 *in vitro* (Eron *et al.*, 1992; Mathez *et al.*, 1993). Alternating treatment of HIV-infected lymphoid cell lines *in vitro* with zidovudine and zalcitabine resulted in sustained inhibition of HIV replication (Spector *et al.*, 1989). The combination of zalcitabine and recombinant interferon alpha or human leukocyte interferon acts synergistically against HIV-1 replication *in vitro* when tested in human leukocytes as well as in T cell and monocyte cell lines (Vogt *et al.*, 1988; Degre and Beck, 1994). This combination has also demonstrated synergy against feline leukemia virus (Zeidner *et al.*, 1989). The HIV protease inhibitor saquinavir shows additive to synergistic anti-HIV-1 effect in combination with zalcitabine *in vitro* (Craig *et al.*, 1990; Martin *et al.*, 1991; Johnson *et al.*, 1992). Two derivatives of tetrahydroimidazo(4,5,1-jk)(1,4)-benzodiazepin-2(1H)-thione (TIBO) have been reported to show synergy with zalcitabine against HIV-1 (Buckheit *et al.*, 1993). Synergy also exists between bisheteroarylpiperazine compounds and zalcitabine (Chong *et al.*, 1994). Recombinant soluble CD4 is synergistic against HIV-1 in combination with zalcitabine (Hayashi *et al.*, 1990). Additive to synergistic interactions have also been demonstrated between the glucosidase inhibitor N-butyl deoxynojirimycin and zalcitabine (Ratner and Vander-Heyden, 1993). The coronary vasodilator dipyridamole has been reported to potentiate the activity of zalcitabine against HIV-1 in cells of macrophage lineage *in vitro* (Patel *et al.*, 1991).

4 Antagonism with other drugs

Although GM-CSF increases the antiretroviral activity of zidovudine in cells of macrophage lineage, the activities of both didanosine and zalcitabine are slightly diminished in the presence of GM-CSF (Perno *et al.*, 1992b). Tumor necrosis factor antagonizes the anti-HIV-1 activity of both zidovudine and zalcitabine (Ito *et al.*, 1990).

5 Resistance

a Development of zalcitabine-resistance *in vitro* HIV-1 develops reduced susceptibility to zidovudine more readily than to either didanosine or zalcitabine (Shirasaka *et al.*, 1993). Zalcitabine-resistant variants of HIV-1 have been generated by passaging the virus *in vitro* in increasing concentrations of zalcitabine. These resistant viruses have an IC$_{50}$ between 10- and 50-fold higher than that of the parenteral wild-type strains (Cinatl *et al.*, 1993; Gao *et al.*, 1993a).

b   Development of zalcitabine-resistance *in vivo*   Zalcitabine-resistant strains of HIV-1 have infrequently been recovered from patients who have received zalcitabine monotherapy for more than 1 year, and after prolonged therapy with alternating zidovudine and zalcitabine. In the latter, although all isolates that were studied had marked reduction in sensitivity to zidovudine, reduced susceptibility to both drugs was less common (Shirasaka *et al.*, 1993). A similar study of isolates from a small number of children receiving alternating therapy with zidovudine and zalcitabine failed to demonstrate any evidence of zalcitabine-resistance (Husson *et al.*, 1993). In addition, patients receiving combination therapy with zidovudine and zalcitabine developed high-level zidovudine-resistance with no changes in zalcitabine susceptibility, with isolates of HIV-1 from these patients having a median IC_{50} for zalcitabine of $0.2\,\mu M$ (Richman *et al.*, 1994).

c   Mutations which confer resistance to zalcitabine   A single mutation may be sufficient to confer resistance to zalcitabine (reviewed in Larder, 1995). Resistance to zalcitabine has been found in association with mutations at codons 65 (Lys → Arg or Asn), 74 (Leu → Val), 69 (Thr → Asp), 75 (Val → Thr), 184 (Met → Val), and according to some investigators 215 (Tyr → Cys) (Table V.33).

A mutation within the codon for reverse transcriptase at position 69 (Thr → Asp) results in a 5-fold reduction in sensitivity to zalcitabine compared with the wild-type (Fitzgibbon *et al.*, 1992). This variant may remain susceptible to zidovudine or didanosine (Fitzgibbon *et al.*, 1992; McLeod *et al.*, 1992).

Another mutation, within codon 65 (Lys → Arg), has been described in a zalcitabine-resistant variant of HIV-1 that was selected by sequential passage of the virus in increasing concentrations of zalcitabine *in vitro*, as well as in isolates from patients treated with zalcitabine or didanosine. Site-directed mutagenesis confirmed that this mutation resulted in a modest (4- to 10-fold) decrease in susceptibility of HIV to zalcitabine (Gu *et al.*, 1994a; Zhang *et al.*, 1994). The codon 65 mutation results in cross-resistance to lamivudine and didanosine but not zidovudine (Gu *et al.*, 1994b, 1995).

A mutation in the pol gene at amino acid site 184 (Met → Val) has been confirmed by site-directed mutagenesis to result in reduced sensitivity of the variant to both didanosine and zalcitabine when compared with wild-type virus (Gu *et al.*, 1992; Wainberg *et al.*, 1993).

A number of other mutations have been found in isolates from patients receiving combination therapy with zidovudine and either zalcitabine or didanosine. The development of a set of mutations at positions 62, 75, 77, 116, and 151 within the polymerase domain of reverse transcriptase confers resistance to multiple dideoxynucleosides, and the timing of these mutations has been linked with an increase in viral load in plasma (Shirasaka *et al.*, 1995a).

d   Cross-resistance between zalcitabine and other antiretroviral drugs   In general, zidovudine-resistant strains of HIV remain susceptible to zalcitabine and didanosine (Larder *et al.*, 1989; Richman 1990b,c; Rooke *et al.*, 1991). However, exceptions have been described. It has been found that HIV-1 passaged in the presence of zidovudine develops resistance to zidovudine and also reduced susceptibility to zalcitabine (Dianzani *et al.*, 1992). Isolates of HIV from zidovudine-naive individuals are more sensitive to zalcitabine than zidovudine-resistant strains from zidovudine-treated subjects, indicating partial cross-resistance occurs between these two compounds (Mathez *et al.*, 1993). In a study of patients treated only with zidovudine there was a correlation between zidovudine-resistance and reduced susceptibility to zalcitabine and

Table V.33

Mutations within reverse transcriptase conferring reduced susceptibility of HIV to zalcitabine. (Modified from Larder, 1995; Fitzgibbon *et al.*, 1992.)

Codon	Mutation	Confers decrease in susceptibility to
65	Lys → Arg/Asn	Didanosine, zalcitabine, lamivudine[a]
69	Thr → Asp	Zalcitabine[a]
74	Leu → Val	Didanosine, zalcitabine
75	Val → Thr	Stavudine, zalcitabine, didanosine
184	Met → Val	Zalcitabine[a], didanosine[a], lamivudine[b]

[a] Low level.
[b] High level.

didanosine with an approximate 2-fold decrease in dideoxynucleoside susceptibility for every 10-fold decline in zidovudine sensitivity (Mayers *et al.*, 1994). However, other studies of patients receiving zidovudine monotherapy have found preservation of susceptibility to zalcitabine despite the development of zidovudine-resistance (Rooke *et al.*, 1991).

Didanosine-resistant variants of HIV-1 have been reported to be cross-resistant to zalcitabine but not to zidovudine (St Clair *et al.*, 1991; Gao *et al.*, 1993a).

Rapid selection of HIV-1 resistance to lamivudine has been reported following limited passage *in vitro* (Tisdale *et al.*, 1993). Lamivudine-resistant strains of HIV-1, with a substitution of isoleucine for methionine at the second codon at position 184, have been reported to retain susceptibility to didanosine and zalcitabine (Boucher *et al.*, 1993), although other investigators have reported lamivudine-resistant variants of HIV-1 that have minimal to modest reduction in susceptibility to zalcitabine and didanosine without influencing zidovudine susceptibility (Gao *et al.*, 1993c; Schinazi *et al.*, 1993; Tisdale *et al.*, 1993; Kavlick *et al.*, 1995). A mutation involving codon 75 (Val → Thr) resulted in moderate resistance to stavudine and conferred cross-resistance to didanosine and zalcitabine (Lacey and Larder, 1994).

6 Hepatitis B virus

Zalcitabine inhibits replication of duck hepatitis B virus (DHBV) at concentrations significantly lower than those that are toxic to primary hepatocytes (Yokota *et al.*, 1990; Fourel *et al.*, 1994). Intravenous administration of zalcitabine to ducks chronically infected with DHBV resulted in a decline in serum DHBV DNA and DNA polymerase activity in all treated ducks in one study (Kassianides *et al.*, 1989), although these findings are not supported by other studies (Omata, 1989; Howe *et al.*, 1996). Infection of primary hepatocytes by woodchuck hepatitis B virus is inhibited by zalcitabine (Aldrich *et al.*, 1989). In addition, zalcitabine has been found to inhibit hepatitis B virus DNA synthesis with a high therapeutic index in a human hepatoblastoma cell line (Ueda *et al.*, 1989; Yokota *et al.*, 1991).

7 Other

Although zidovudine has antibacterial activity against a number of members of the enterobacteriaceae, there is no evidence of activity of zalcitabine against non-typhoidal salmonellae (Sperber *et al.*, 1993). *Mycoplasma* species and *Ureaplasma* species are resistant to zalcitabine *in vitro* (Ostashewski *et al.*, 1993).

Mode of Administration and Dosage

1 Oral administration

The current dosage of zalcitabine for adults is 0.75 mg given three times daily (total of 2.25 mg daily) as either monotherapy (although this is not recommended by the author) or concomitant with zidovudine (200 mg three times daily) (Zalcitabine Product Information, 1992). Phase I/II studies of oral and intravenous zalcitabine in adults with advanced HIV infection have demonstrated virologic efficacy with doses ranging in initial studies from 0.09 to 0.75 mg per kg daily (Yarchoan *et al.*, 1988). A later trial using lower doses (0.03 mg per kg daily) still demonstrated virologic efficacy but was associated with a lower incidence of toxicity (Merigan *et al.*, 1989). The minimum effective dose for zalcitabine when used in combination with zidovudine has not yet been established.

2 Intravenous therapy

Zalcitabine has been administered i.v. by infusion over 1 h in varying dosages ranging from 0.03 mg per kg 8-hourly to 0.25 mg per kg every 8 hours for 14 days (Yarchoan *et al.*, 1988).

3 Pediatric patients

The safety and efficacy of zalcitabine in HIV-infected infants and children under the age of 13 years has not yet been fully established. Children between 6 months of age and 13 years appear to tolerate dosages of zalcitabine of up to 0.04 mg per kg 6-hourly for a period of 8 weeks (Pizzo 1990; Pizzo *et al.*, 1990) and 0.01 mg per kg 8-hourly for 36 weeks (Spector, 1994). An oral suspension is available through a Compassionate Use Study conducted by Roche (Brady, 1994).

4 Pregnant women

Safe use in human pregnancy has not been established and effective contraception should be used whilst receiving zalcitabine.

5 Patients with liver impairment

Hepatic dysfunction may be exacerbated by zalcitabine. Thus patients with elevated liver enzymes or a history of liver disease or ethanol abuse should be carefully monitored whilst receiving zalcitabine, and dose-reduction or cessation considered (Zalcitabine Product Information).

6 Patients with renal failure

In patients with renal impairment, the clearance of zalcitabine may be reduced. The dose of zalcitabine should be decreased to 0.75 mg every 12 h if creatinine clearance is 10–40 ml per min, and 0.75 mg every 24 h for patients with a creatinine clearance of less than 10 ml per min (Zalcitabine Product Information).

7 Patients with pre-existing peripheral neuropathy

Zalcitabine should be used with caution in this patient population, and avoided in those individuals with moderate or severe symptoms or signs. If peripheral neuropathy develops, the dose of zalcitabine should be reduced or the drug ceased. The symptoms of neuropathy may worsen ('coasting') after cessation of therapy, prior to improvement. Reintroduction of zalcitabine may be considered at a dose of 0.375 mg three times daily provided symptoms have improved to only a mild level of discomfort (Zalcitabine Product Information).

8 Patients with a past history of pancreatitis

Zalcitabine should be used with caution in these individuals, with frequent monitoring of serum amylase and clinical symptoms. If symptoms of pancreatitis develop, including nausea and vomiting, or abdominal pain, therapy should be discontinued until the diagnosis is formed. Therapy should also be interrupted if there is a rising serum amylase level not associated with symptoms, but with concomitant rising triglyceride levels or abnormal blood glucose. An elevated serum amylase alone is of uncertain clinical significance. Zalcitabine should not be used concurrently with other medications known to cause pancreatitis. If clinical pancreatitis is diagnosed during zalcitabine therapy the drug should be permanently discontinued (Zalcitabine Product Information).

Availability

Zalcitabine is available in *tablet form* containing 0.37mg or 0.755 mg of the active compound.

Serum Levels in Relation to Dosage

Plasma zalcitabine levels can be measured by solid phase extraction-RIA (Kastrissios *et al.*, 1996).

1 Adults

Zalcitabine is stable at gastric pH (Shelton *et al.*, 1993), with high oral bioavailability, ranging from 70% to 88% in patients with advanced HIV infection (Klecker *et al.*, 1988; Yarchoan *et al.*, 1988; Broder, 1990). Absorption is greater from the jejunum than the ileum (Mirchandani and Chien, 1995). Administration of zalcitabine with food results in a mild reduction in bioavailability of about 14%, decreases the maximal plasma concentrations by 35% and may result in a 2-fold increase in the time to T_{max} (Gustavson *et al.*, 1990; Nazareno *et al.*, 1995).

Using a modified high performance liquid chromatography procedure, levels of zalcitabine as low as 0.1 μM (21 ng per ml) can be measured in urine and plasma (Klecker *et al.*, 1988). The plasma half life has been reported to be 1.2 h (range 0.5–2.2 h) when measured in patients with advanced HIV infection following an i.v. infusion of 0.03–0.25 mg per kg zalcitabine (Klecker *et al.*, 1988). The plasma half-life is very similar in some, but not all, other species, being 1.1 h in mice and 1.8 h in rhesus monkeys (Kelley *et al.*, 1987), but in excess of 7 h in neonatal goats (Williams *et al.*, 1989).

Over a dose range of 0.13–0.5 mg per kg, the kinetics of zalcitabine have been found to be linear (Klecker *et al.*, 1988). In patients with advanced HIV infection, the maximum plasma concentrations (C_{max}) following oral doses of 0.5 mg and 5 mg zalcitabine range from 5 to 12 ng per ml (0.25–0.6 μM) and 48–93 ng per ml (0.24–0.47 μM) respectively, occurring (T_{max}) within 0.8–1.6 h post-dose; extrapolated C_{max} values for zalcitabine following oral doses of

0.375 mg are approximately 0.03 μM (Klecker *et al.*, 1988). Peak serum levels of 0.5 μM have been reported following a 1 h i.v. infusion of 0.06 mg per kg or more (Yarchoan *et al.*, 1988). The mean plasma elimination half-life is 2 h.

Intracellular concentrations of zalcitabine triphosphate are in part related to plasma concentrations, although intracellular retention may result in higher concentrations within the cell than in plasma (Starnes and Cheng, 1987; Shelton *et al.*, 1993). There is a biphasic pattern of efflux of zalcitabine triphosphate from the cell, with an initial retention half-life of 2.6 h and a total intracellular half-life in fresh human leukocytes of 8–10 h (Starnes and Cheng, 1987; Zalcitabine Product Information, 1992). In duck hepatocytes the intracellular half-life is even longer than that in human cells, with zalcitabine accumulation reaching a maximum concentration after 24–26 hours (Kitos and Tyrrell, 1995). Liposomal preparations of zalcitabine are rapidly taken up by macrophages, with the free form of the drug accumulating more slowly in these cells (Makabi-Panuzu *et al.*, 1995).

2 Children

In a dose-ranging study involving children aged between 6 months and 13 years who were given zalcitabine at doses of 0.3 or 0.4 mg per kg orally or by i.v. infusion over 1 h, the mean total plasma clearance was found to be 150 ml per min per m^2, with a mean volume of distribution of 9.3 liters per m^2 at steady-state. The mean bioavailability was 54%, ranging from 29 to 100%, with a half-life of 0.8 h (Pizzo *et al.*, 1990b). When 23 children (mean age 4.2 years) were given a single oral dose of zalcitabine (0.02 mg per kg) zalcitabine was rapidly absorbed with a mean peak plasma concentration of 9.3 ng per ml, T_{max} of 1 h and a mean area-under-the-curve (AUC) of 25 ng per h per ml. The elimination half-life was 1.4 h. These data suggest that zalcitabine is cleared more rapidly in children than adults, as plasma concentrations are lower and the half-life of zalcitabine is shorter than in adults (Chadwick *et al.*, 1995).

3 Impaired renal function

As the kidneys are the main excretion pathway for zalcitabine, it is to be expected that renal failure results in prolonged elimination of the drug. In patients with an estimated renal clearance of less than 55 ml per min the half-life of zalcitabine has been found to be up to 8.5 h. It is not known whether zalcitabine is removed from plasma by renal or peritoneal dialysis (Zalcitabine Product Information).

4 Impaired liver function

In an expanded access program, 12% of patients with liver function test abnormalities at the time of commencing zalcitabine developed an exacerbation of hepatic impairment whilst receiving the drug. Thus zalcitabine should be used in caution in patients with pre-existing liver disease.

Excretion

Renal mechanisms (glomerular filtration as well as tubular secretion) are the predominant pathway for zalcitabine clearance (Klecker *et al.*, 1988). Following i.v. infusion, 75% of the parent drug has been found to be excreted unchanged in the urine; recovery following oral delivery was 62% (Klecker *et al.*, 1988). No metabolites of zalcitabine, including 2',3'-dideoxyuridine, were found in patient samples (Klecker *et al.*, 1988), although minor quantities of this urinary metabolite have been found in rhesus monkeys (Kelley *et al.*, 1987). These data are supported by the lack of detection of catabolites in macrophages exposed to zalcitabine for 24 h (Arner and Eriksson, 1993), although some investigators have detected phosphodiester metabolites (Hao *et al.*, 1993). The mean clearance following i.v. infusion has been reported to 5.6 ml per min per kg (Gustavson *et al.*, 1990).

Zalcitabine differs from zidovudine in that the latter drug undergoes considerable first-pass hepatic glucuronidation (p. 1669) whilst first-pass hepatic extraction of zalcitabine is very low (Terasaki and Pardridge, 1988; Morse *et al.*, 1993).

Distribution of the Drug in Body

Zalcitabine is not highly protein-bound (Morse *et al.*, 1993). The mean volume of distribution of zalcitabine at steady-state has been found to be 0.54–0.64 liters per kg, which is approximately the volume of total body water (Klecker *et al.*, 1988; Gustavson *et al.*, 1990).

Zalcitabine and zidovudine differ in their respective abilities to penetrate cerebrospinal fluid (CSF), with the reported mean CSF to plasma ratio for zalcitabine ranging from 0.14 to 0.20, when measured 2–3.5 h following administration. This level is approximately 3-fold less than that for zidovudine (Klecker *et al.*, 1988; Yarchoan *et al.*, 1988, 1989; Morse *et al.*, 1993). In

Table V.34

Summary of clinically relevant pharmacokinetic parameters of zalcitabine

Bioavailability of 70–88%
Mild reduction in bioavailability (14%) when taken with food
Absorption: jejunum greater than ileum
More rapid clearance in children than adults
Predominantly renal excretion
Minimal first-pass hepatic glucuronidation
Less than 5% binding to plasma proteins
CSF:plasma ratio about 0.20

patients with advanced HIV infection CSF levels were found to be between 0.03 and 0.05 µM 2 h after receiving zalcitabine (Klecker et al., 1988). In a rat model, the half-life for zalcitabine within CSF following intraventricular injection was found to be 1.1 h (Kim et al., 1990).

Zalcitabine crosses the placenta by simple diffusion (Bawden et al., 1992).

Mode of Action

Zalcitabine is an analog of the pyrimidine nucleoside deoxycytidine. The crystalline structures of both zalcitabine and didanosine have been resolved (Birnbaum et al., 1988; Silverton et al., 1988). Similar to zidovudine and didanosine, the antiretroviral activity of zalcitabine is dependent upon the intracellular phosphorylation of zalcitabine to the triphosphate derivative (Balzarini et al., 1987; Yarchoan et al., 1990). The phosphorylated form is a potent inhibitor of the HIV reverse transcriptase enzyme, binding to reverse transcriptase and preventing the conversion of HIV RNA to DNA, as well as resulting in premature termination of viral DNA chain elongation (Mitsuya et al., 1987). The nucleotide binding site of the reverse transcriptase has been localized to the lysine residue at position 73 (Cheng et al., 1993).

Zalcitabine enters the cell by both facilitated diffusion via the nucleoside carrier as well as by non-facilitated diffusion (Plageman et al., 1988; Domin et al., 1993). Following entry into the cell, zalcitabine is sequentially phosphorylated to the mono-, di- and triphosphate derivatives (Whittington and Brogden, 1992). The half-life of the triphosphate within cell lines and peripheral blood mononuclear cells ranges from 2.6 to 10 h. There is no significant difference in the ability of HIV-infected and uninfected T cell lines to phosphorylate zalcitabine (Cooney et al., 1986). Efficient phosphorylation of zalcitabine occurs through the action of deoxycytidine kinase in the cytoplasm of the human but not murine cells (Balzarini et al., 1988b; Chottiner et al., 1991; Habteyesus et al., 1991; Chen and Cheng, 1992; Kierdaszuk et al., 1992). Zalcitabine is not a substrate for thymidine kinases (Munch-Petersen et al., 1991). Phosphorylation of zalcitabine to its triphosphate derivative has been found to be less efficient in stimulated peripheral blood mononuclear cells than in resting cells (Gao et al., 1993b; Shirasaka et al., 1995b), although Perno and his colleagues have reported reduced phosphorylation of zalcitabine in macrophages compared with a T cell line (Perno et al., 1988). Both deoxycytidine and cytidine can competitively block the intracellular phosphorylation of zalcitabine, and reverse the antiretroviral activity of the drug (Balzarini et al., 1987; Johnson et al., 1987). GM-CSF and M-CSF can increase the intracellular levels of zalcitabine, didanosine and zidovudine triphosphate. However for zalcitabine and didanosine (but not zidovudine) there is also a parallel increase in the physiologic competitor deoxycytidine triphosphate. Thus there is no overall net improvement in antiretroviral activity of zalcitabine or didanosine in the presence of these colony stimulating factors, although these agents can potentiate the activity of zidovudine (Perno et al., 1992b).

Toxicity

1 Peripheral neuropathy

The major toxicity associated with zalcitabine therapy is the development of a dose-related peripheral neuropathy (Table V.35). Using the currently recommended dose of zalcitabine, up to 30% of patients develop peripheral neuropathy (Shelton et al., 1993), although results from other studies suggests that the incidence of neuropathy may be lower, as described below in data from ACTG 155.

Peripheral neuropathy has been reported in a number of early dose-ranging clinical trials of zalcitabine (Yarchoan et al., 1988; Dubinsky et al., 1989; Merigan et al., 1989). In a more

Table V.35

Features of peripheral neuropathy associated with zalcitabine therapy

Incidence is dose-related
Develops in up to 30% of patients taking 0.75 mg three times daily
Progression of symptoms is dose-related
Painful, predominantly sensory
May get worse initially after stopping zalcitabine ('coasting')
Due to inhibition of mitochondrial synthesis and function
    (zalcitabine > stavudine > didanosine > zidovudine)

detailed neurologic report of the clinical trial described by Merigan *et al.* (1989) involving 52 HIV-infected patients with advanced disease, all patients receiving zalcitabine in dosages of 0.03 and 0.06 mg per kg every 4 h developed a painful, predominantly sensory neuropathy, occurring a mean of 7.7 weeks after commencing therapy, and continuing at the same level or progressing in intensity for 2–3 weeks after cessation of therapy. Clinical symptoms were preceded by the development of abnormal vibration sense. Therapy with lower doses (0.01 and 0.005 mg per kg every 4 h) resulted in milder symptoms in a lower proportion of patients, which developed a mean of 9.3 and 26 weeks respectively after starting the drug. The progression of symptoms was slower in those receiving lower doses than in the higher dose groups (Berger *et al.*, 1993).

In another study of 131 patients with advanced HIV infection, weekly alternating zidovudine and zalcitabine therapy was still associated with high rates (41%) of peripheral neuropathy when a dose of zalcitabine of 0.03 mg per kg 4-hourly was used (Skowron *et al.*, 1993). In ACTG trial 155, HIV-infected patients with advanced disease who had received at least 6 months prior therapy with zidovudine were randomized to receive monotherapy with zidovudine or zalcitabine (0.75 mg 8-hourly) or combination therapy with the two drugs. Peripheral neuropathy of either moderate or severe intensity developed in 13% of patients randomized to remain on zidovudine, in 23% of those randomized to receive zalcitabine, and in 21% of those receiving the combination of both drugs (Fischl *et al.*, 1995). There is reported clinical evidence of additive or cumulative effects between zalcitabine and didanosine in the development of peripheral neuropathy (LeLacheur and Simon, 1991). Peripheral neuropathy does not appear to be a toxic effect of zalcitabine in children (Pizzo *et al.*, 1990).

In rabbits given zalcitabine, observed pathological changes include vacuolation and fragmentation of myelin sheaths, demyelination of axons, and intramyelinic edema (Feldman *et al.*, 1992). Zalcitabine causes toxicity to peripheral nerves by inhibiting mitochondrial synthesis and function. Chronic exposure of dorsal root ganglion cultures to low concentrations of zalcitabine resulted in a decrease in mitochondrial DNA levels (Werth *et al.*, 1994). Decreases in mitochondrial DNA content have been observed following exposure of T cells for 4 days to low concentrations (0.5 μM) of zalcitabine (Lewis *et al.*, 1992). Isolated mitochondrial preparations were more sensitive to inhibition by the triphosphate derivative of zalcitabine than to di-, mono- or unphosphorylated compound (Chen and Cheng, 1992). Inhibition of mitochondrial synthesis in T cell lines is more pronounced following exposure to zalcitabine than to stavudine, didanosine, or zidovudine (Chen *et al.*, 1991). Of interest, zalcitabine has been found to only inhibit the activity of DNA polymerase beta but not alpha or gamma (Ono *et al.*, 1989; see also zidovudine p 1674). The cell growth of mouse embryo fibroblasts is inhibited by zalcitabine in a concentration-dependent manner (Rossi *et al.*, 1992).

2 Other neurotoxicity

Ototoxicity due to VIIIth nerve damage has been reported in an HIV-infected person taking zalcitabine. The hearing defect recurred on rechallenge with the drug (Powderly *et al.*, 1990). Acoustic neuropathy considered to be related to zalcitabine therapy has also been reported in association with peripheral neuropathy (Martinez and French, 1993).

3 Pancreatitis

Zalcitabine-induced pancreatitis has been reported (Aponte-Cipriani *et al.*, 1993; Underwood and Frye, 1993) with an incidence of less than 1%, which is significantly lower than in didanosine recipients (Zalcitabine Product Information).

4 Other gastrointestinal and hepatic adverse reactions

Anorexia, nausea and vomiting are less commonly encountered in patients receiving zalcitabine than in recipients of didanosine or zidovudine (Yarchoan *et al.*, 1988; Merigan *et al.*, 1989). Potentially fatal lactic acidosis associated with hepatomegaly and steatosis has been rarely associated with zalcitabine (and zidovudine) therapy. There have also been rare cases of hepatic and renal failure. Thus zalcitabine should be used with caution in patients with pre-existing liver disease.

5 Hematologic toxicity

A reduction in the number of thymocytes within thymic lobes of rat fetuses has been observed in organ cultures exposed to zalcitabine (Foerster et al., 1992). Repeated administration of mice with very high doses of zalcitabine (1000 mg per kg per day) has been associated with the development of thymic lymphoma, due to suppression of a subpopulation of hemopoietic progenitor cells (Irons et al., 1995). No hemotoxicity was observed in canine bone marrow progenitor cells exposed to zalcitabine at concentrations of up to 80 μM (Chan et al., 1992). However, zalcitabine has been reported to be toxic to bone marrow progenitor cells (from normal persons and those with advanced HIV infection) and T cell lines with an IC_{50} of less than 5 μM (Johnson et al., 1988; Ullman et al., 1988; Ganser et al., 1989; Blakley et al., 1990; Lewis et al., 1992; Hitchcock, 1993; Faraj et al., 1994).

Although hematologic toxicity has not been a prominent feature of zalcitabine therapy, impaired thrombocytogenesis may occur at low concentrations (0.1 μM) of the drug (Inoue et al., 1989). Thrombocytopenia and neutropenia were observed in zalcitabine recipients in early clinical trials (Yarchoan et al., 1988; Merigan et al., 1989). Anemia occurred in less than 5% of treated patients in these trials. Zalcitabine appears to have no effect on polymorphonuclear leukocyte function, when chemotaxis, phagocytosis and superoxide production were studied in vitro using cells from HIV-infected and uninfected individuals (Roilides et al., 1990). Zalcitabine is more cytostatic to human than murine cell lines (Balzarini et al., 1988b), presumably due to reduced phosphorylation of the drug in the latter (see above).

6 Mucocutaneous reactions

Recurrent esophageal ulceration has been reported in a patient with advanced HIV infection taking zalcitabine (Indorf and Pegram, 1992). Apthous stomatitis has been reported, particularly in association with higher doses, in adults (McNeely et al., 1989; Yarchoan et al., 1988; Merigan et al., 1989) and children (Pizzo et al., 1990). The condition may improve without requiring cessation of therapy (Yarchoan et al., 1988; Merigan et al., 1989). A dose-related maculopapular eruption, occurring after 10 days of zalcitabine therapy in patients receiving 0.03 or 0.06 mg per kg of zalcitabine 4-hourly, has also been reported; in some instances this rash was associated with fever and mouth ulcers (McNeely et al., 1989; Merigan et al., 1989). In the early dose-finding studies, skin rash was a dose-limiting side-effect in 8–10% of patients (Yarchoan et al., 1988; Merigan et al., 1989).

7 Pregnancy

In rat embryos, zalcitabine exposure resulted in only very minimal interference with embryonic development with inhibition of blastocyst formation only occurring in two-cell embryos exposed to concentrations of 100 μM or greater (Klug et al., 1991; Toltzis et al., 1994).

8 Drug interactions

Zalcitabine does not inhibit glucuronidation of zidovudine when assessed by assays in human liver microsomes (Rajaonarison et al., 1992). Pharmacokinetic parameters measured in monkeys following intragastric administration of zalcitabine and zidovudine (Qian et al., 1992), and in HIV-infected patients enrolled in clinical trials of combination therapy with these drugs (Meng et al., 1992) revealed no significant interactions. There is no alteration of zalcitabine metabolism by lamivudine (Cammack et al., 1992).

Zalcitabine should be ceased in patients requiring drugs known potentially to cause pancreatitis, including i.v. pentamidine. In addition, the drug should be avoided in patients receiving therapy with drugs that have the potential to cause peripheral neuropathy, including dapsone, chloramphenicol, gold, metronidazole, isoniazid, phenytoin, ribavirin, vincristine, and didanosine. Amphotericin, foscarnet, and aminoglycosides should be used with caution in patients receiving zalcitabine, with frequent clinical and biochemical monitoring and consideration of dose adjustments (Zalcitabine Product Information). As zalcitabine is excreted predominantly by renal mechanisms, drugs that inhibit renal tubular function, such as probenecid may increase serum levels of zalcitabine (Morris, 1994).

Clinical Uses of the Drug

1 Human immunodefciency virus infection

Zalcitabine is indicated for use as monotherapy in patients with advanced HIV infection who are unable to tolerate zidovudine, or disease progression whilst taking zidovudine. Zalcitabine is also indicated in combination with zidovudine for the treatment of adults with HIV infection who have less than 300 CD4 cells per μl and who have not previously received zidovudine or who have taken zidovudine for less than 12 months (Zalcitabine Product Information). In many countries this indication is being replaced by the broader indication of treatment for HIV infection. This author has concerns regarding the use of zalcitabine monotherapy due to its poor penetration across the blood–brain barrier; it should only be used as monotherapy if no alternate combination is available.

Zalcitabine is regarded as a potent antiretroviral drug, but it has been shown to have only marginal clinical efficacy when used either as monotherapy or in combination with zidovudine in zidovudine-experienced patients (see below, ACTG 155). More recent data all demonstrate good virologic responses to zalcitabine in combination with zidovudine in naive patients that are either not seen in zidovudine-experienced patients (pp. 1679, 1680), or wane (with clinical decline) after 1 year (Schooley et al., 1996).

Zalcitabine is most commonly used in clinical practise in combination with another nucleoside analog (often zidovudine) and a protease inhibitor.

2 Clinical trials of zalcitabine monotherapy

The first clinical trial reported of zalcitabine therapy demonstrated modest immunologic and antiviral efficacy in a study of 20 HIV-infected patients with advanced disease, randomized to one of five dose regimens of i.v. zalcitabine for 2 weeks followed by oral therapy. The differing toxicity profiles of zidovudine and zalcitabine were demonstrated in this phase I trial (Yarchoan et al., 1988), and confirmed by results from a second, partially randomized, multicentered dose-ranging study of 61 patients, also with advanced HIV infection (Merigan et al., 1989).

In a double-blind, multicenter study of 635 adults with advanced HIV infection and CD4 counts of less than 200 cells per μl who had received less than 3 months of zidovudine therapy (ACTG 114), patients were randomized to receive zalcitabine 0.75 mg three times daily or zidovudine. The study was terminated after 1 year due to the finding of lower survival and higher progression to a new AIDS-defining illness in patients receiving zalcitabine compared with zidovudine. The health status and function of patients whose initial antiretroviral therapy was either zidovudine or zalcitabine was examined as a substudy of ACTG 114. It was concluded that recipients of zidovudine had better functional outcomes compared with zalcitabine recipients (Bozzette et al., 1995). A second, open-label study (ACTG 119) compared zalcitabine with zidovudine in 111 patients also with advanced HIV infection and CD4 counts of less than 200 cells per μl, but who had tolerated more than 48 weeks of prior zidovudine therapy. In this study there was no significant difference in survival or disease progression between the two groups, but the number of patients enrolled was smaller than planned (Fig. V.46) (Fischl et al., 1993).

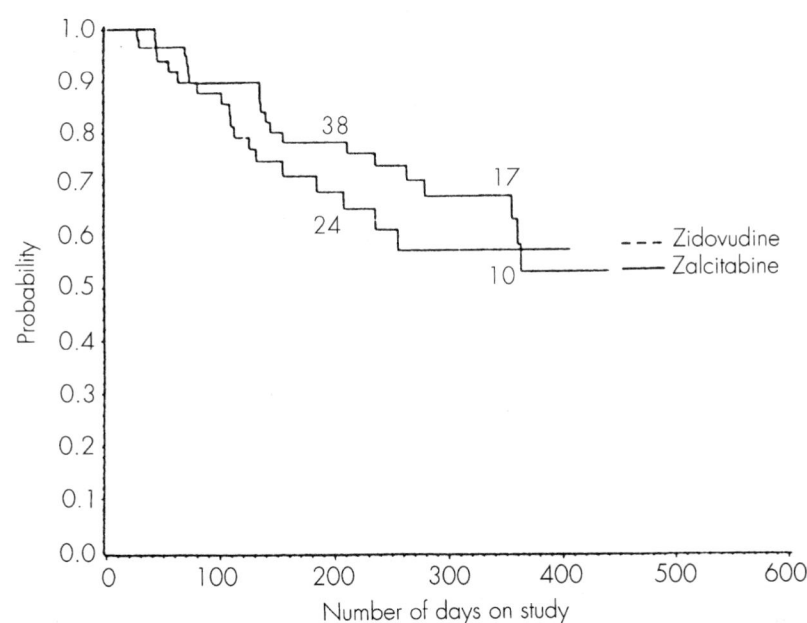

Fig. V.46.
ACTG 119 study. Kaplan–Meier estimation of time to AIDS-defining event or death p > 0.2. (Reproduced from Fischl et al. 1993, with permission from the American College of Physicians.)

A multicenter, open-label study was conducted by the Community Programs for Clinical Research on AIDS (CPCRA), comparing zalcitabine with didanosine in 467 patients with HIV infection and less than 300 CD4 cells per μl or with a prior AIDS defining illness. All patients had previously received zidovudine therapy. These patients had in fact very low CD4 counts (median of less than 50 cells per μl) and had been extensively pretreated with zidovudine (approximately 18 months); they were followed in this study for a median of 16 months. There was no significant difference between the two arms of the study in terms of survival or progression to a new AIDS defining event. However, there was some evidence of inequity between the treatment arms at baseline. When these baseline co-variates were controlled for, zalcitabine appeared to be possibly better than didanosine (Abrams et al., 1994).

3 Clinical trials of alternating therapy

Two open-label dose-ranging trials evaluated zalcitabine (0.01 and 0.03 mg per kg 4-hourly) and zidovudine in weekly and monthly alternating schedules compared with intermittent or continuous zidovudine therapy in zidovudine-naive individuals (ACTG 047) and in those with hematologic intolerance of zidovudine (ACTG 050). Alternating zidovudine and zalcitabine therapy was found to be less toxic than monotherapy with either zidovudine or zalcitabine, whilst maintaining good antiretroviral activity (Bozzette and Richman, 1990; Skowron et al., 1993).

4 Clinical trials of combination therapy

A phase I/II dose-ranging trial of combination therapy in 56 persons with advanced HIV infection and CD4 counts of less than 200 cells per μl (ACTG trial 106), compared six regimens of zidovudine and zalcitabine. This study demonstrated superior efficacy of combination therapy with zalcitabine and zidovudine in terms of producing greater and more durable virologic and immunologic benefit than monotherapy with either of these agents (Meng et al., 1990, 1992).

A double-blind phase II/III study sponsored by Burroughs Wellcome Co. (BW 34,225–02) compared zidovudine monotherapy in a dose of 600 mg per day with combination therapy of zalcitabine (2.25 mg per day) and zidovudine or didanosine and zalcitabine in patients with HIV infection and less than 300 CD4 cells per μl who had received prior therapy with zidovudine for less than 4 weeks. Results from an unscheduled study analysis revealed that the peak CD4 response was greater in patients receiving combination therapy, and was more prolonged, remaining higher than baseline throughout the initial 24-week period of study (McLeod and Hammer, 1992). This immunologic improvement was sustained through 72 weeks, and was associated with a significant and similarly sustained decline in HIV RNA in plasma. However, zidovudine therapy did not prevent the emergence of zidovudine-resistant strains of HIV (Schooley et al., 1996).

In a pilot study of 21 patients with advanced HIV infection sequential combination therapy given in 3-week cycles of zidovudine (200 mg 8-hourly) plus aciclovir (800 mg 8-hourly), or didanosine (3.5 mg per kg 12-hourly) or zalcitabine at a dose of 0.01 mg per kg 8-hourly (1 week of each combination) resulted in sustained elevation of CD4 lymphocyte numbers for beyond 40

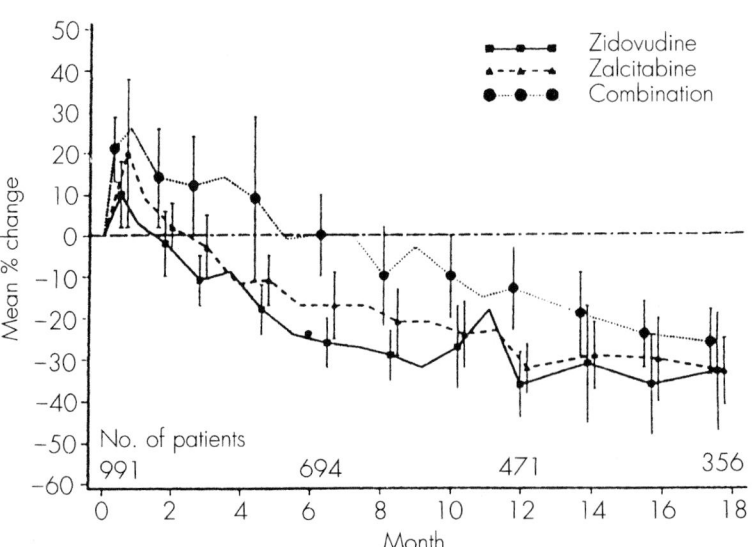

Fig. V.47.
Median changes in CD4 count from pretreatment values in patients enrolled in ACTG 115. (Reproduced from Fischl et al., 1995, with permission from the American College of Physicians.)

weeks of therapy, persistent decreases in serum p24 antigen levels and was well tolerated (Nguyen *et al.*, 1993).

The sequential evaluation of viral phenotype in antiretroviral-naive patients with advanced HIV infection who subsequently received zalcitabine and zidovudine combination therapy showed that the persistent elevation in CD4 count in patients receiving combination therapy compared with monotherapy was not due to delayed emergence of zidovudine-resistance (Richman *et al.*, 1994).

The AIDS Clinical Trials Group trial 155 was a randomized, double-blind study of 1001 patients with symptomatic HIV infection and less than 300 CD4 cells per µl, or asymptomatic infection with less than 200 CD4 cells per µl and who had tolerated zidovudine for a minimum of 6 months. The protocol compared zidovudine monotherapy (600 mg per day) and zalcitabine monotherapy (2.25 mg per day) with a combination of both drugs in the same dosages (Fig. V.47). After a median follow-up period of 17 months, slower disease progression and a survival benefit were found in patients with more than 150 CD4 cells per µl who were randomized to receive combination therapy compared with those receiving zidovudine alone. There were no differences between the three study arms in patients with less than 150 CD4 cells per µl (Fischl *et al.*, 1995).

The AIDS Clinical Trial Group also examined the efficacy of saquinavir in combination with zalcitabine and zidovudine versus saquinavir and zidovudine or zalcitabine and zidovudine in a 24-week study involving 302 patients with 50–300 CD4 cells per µl who had previously received zidovudine therapy for a median of 27 months. The triple combination was superior to either of the double combination arms in terms of sustained improvement in CD4 count and decline in plasma HIV RNA (Collier *et al.*, 1996).

When zalcitabine was given in combination with zidovudine to patients with advanced HIV infection (AIDS or fewer than 200 cells per µl), the relative risk of disease progression or death was similar to those who received zidovudine monotherapy (Saravolatz *et al.*, 1996).

5 Pediatric studies

A pilot study, in 15 children aged between 6 months and 13 years with symptomatic HIV infection, evaluated four dosage levels of zalcitabine (between 0.015 and 0.04 mg per kg every 6 hours). The majority of children had not received prior antiretroviral therapy. This study concluded that zalcitabine was safe and showed some virologic and immunologic benefit in children when treated for a short period of time (Pizzo *et al.*, 1990).

6 Prophylaxis

Prophylactic zalcitabine and alpha interferon have been used in the setting of exposure to HIV via a large needle-stick injury (Mildvan *et al.*, 1994). This is not regarded as optimal therapy (p. 1691), but might be considered by some clinicians if the index case had received long-term therapy with zidovudine, lamivudine and indinavir.

Acknowledgement   The author would like to thank Gail Skowron of Roger Williams Hospital, Brown University, Providence, USA for her critical review of this chapter.

References

Abrams DI, Goldman AI, Launer C *et al.* (1994). A comparative trial of didanosine or zalcitabine after treatment with zidovudine in patients with human immunodeficiency virus infection. The Terry Beirn Community Programs for Clinical Research on AIDS. *New Engl J Med* **330**: 657.

Aldrich CE, Coates L, Wu TT *et al.* (1989). *In vitro* infection of woodchuck hepatocytes with woodchuck hepatitis virus and ground squirrel hepatitis virus. *Virology* **172**: 247.

Aponte-Cipriani SL, Teplitz C, Yancovitz S (1993). Pancreatitis possibly related to 2'-3'-dideoxycytidine. *Ann Intern Med* **119**: 539.

Arner ES, Eriksson S (1993). Deoxycytidine and 2',3'-dideoxycytidine metabolism in human monocyte-derived macrophages A study of both anabolic and catabolic pathways. *Biochem Biophys Res Commun* **197**: 1499.

Balzarini J, Pauwels R, Herdewijn P *et al.* (1986). Potent and selective anti-HTLV-III/LAV activity of 2',3'-dideoxycytidinene, the 2',3'-unsaturated derivative of 2',3'-dideoxycytidine. *Biochem Biophys Res Commun* **140**: 735.

Balzarini J, Cooney DA, Dalal M *et al.* (1987). 2',3'-dideoxycytidine: regulation of the metabolism and anti-retroviral potency by natural pyrimidine nucleosides and by inhibitors of pyrimidine nucleotide synthesis. *Mol Pharmacol* **32**: 798.

Balzarini J, Baba M, Pauwels R *et al.* (1988a). Anti-retrovirus activity of 3'-fluoro- and 3'-azido-substituted pyrimidine 2',3'-dideoxynucleoside analogues. *Biochem Pharmacol* **37**: 2847.

Balzarini J, Pauwels R, Baba M *et al.* (1988b). The *in vitro* and *in vivo* anti-retrovirus activity, and intracellular metabolism of 3'-azido-2'-dideoxythymidine and 2',3'-dideoxycytidine are highly dependent on the cell species. *Biochem Pharmacol* **37**: 897.

Balzarini J, Matthes E, Meeus P *et al.* (1989). The antiretroviral and cytostatic activity and metabolism of 2',3'-dideoxycytidine are highly cell type dependent. *Adv Exp Med Biol* **253B**: 407.

Basham T, Holdener T, Merigan T (1991). Intermittent, alternating, and concurrent regimens of zidovudine and 2'-3'-dideoxycytidine in the LP-BM5 murine induced immunodeficiency model. *J Infect Dis* **163**: 869.

Bawden RE, Sobhi S, Dax J (1992). The transfer of anti-human immunodeficiency virus nucleoside compounds by the term human placenta. *Amer J Obstet Gynecol* **167**: 1570.

Berger AR, Arezzo JC, Schaumburg HH *et al.* (1993). 2',3'-dideoxycytidine (ddC) toxic neuropathy: A study of 52 patients. *Neurol* **32**: 358.

Birnbaum GI, Lin TS, Prusoff WH (1988). Unusual structural features of 2',3'-dideoxycytidine, an inhibitor of the HIV (AIDS) virus. *Biochem Biophys Res Commun* **151**: 608.

Blakley RL, Harwood FC, Huff KD (1990). Cytostatic effects of 2',3'-dideoxyribonucleosides on transformed human hemopoietic cell lines. *Mol Pharmacol* **37**: 328.

Boucher CA, Cammack N, Schipper P *et al.* (1993). High-level resistance to (-) enantiomeric 2'-deoxy-3'-thiacytidine *in vitro* immunodeficiency virus type 1 reverse transcriptase. *Antimicrob Ag Chemother* **37**: 2231.

Bozzette SA, Richman DD (1990). Salvage therapy for zidovudine-intolerant HIV-infected patients with alternating and intermittent regimens of zidovudine and dideoxycytidine. *Amer J Med* **88**: 24.

Bozzette SA, Kanouse DE, Berry S, Duan N (1995). Health status and function with zidovudine or zalcitabine as initial therapy for AIDS A randomized controlled trial Roche 3300/ACTG 114 Study Group. *J Amer Med Assoc* **273**: 295.

Brady MT (1994). Treatment of human immunodeficiency virus infection and its associated complications in children. *J Clin Pharmacol* **34**: 17.

Broder S (1990). Pharmacodynamics of 2',3'-dideoxycytidine: an inhibitor of human immunodeficiency virus. *Amer J Med* **88**: 2.

Buckheit RW, Germany-Decker J, Hollingshead MG *et al.* (1993). Differential antiviral activity of two TIBO derivatives against the human immunodeficiency and murine leukemia viruses alone and in combination with other anti-HIV agents. *AIDS Res Hum Retrovir* **9**: 1097.

Cammack N, Rouse P, Marr CL *et al.* (1992). Cellular metabolism of (-) enantiomeric 2'-deoxy-3'-thiacytidine. *Biochem Pharmacol* **43**: 2059.

Chadwick EG, Nazareno LA, Nieuwenhuis TJ *et al.* (1995). Phase 1 evaluation of zalcitabine administered to human immunodeficiency virus-infected children. *J Infect Dis* **172**: 1475.

Chan TC, Boon GD, Shaffer L, Redmond R (1992). Antiviral nucleoside toxicity in canine bone marrow progenitor cells and its relationship to drug permeation. *Eur J Haematol* **49**: 71.

Chen CH, Cheng YC (1992). The role of cytoplasmic deoxycytidine kinase in the mitochondrial effects of the antihuman immunodeficiency virus compound. *J Biol Chem* **267**: 2856.

Chen CH, Vazquez-Padua M, Cheng YC (1991). Effect of anti-human immunodeficiency virus nucleoside analogs on mitochondrial DNA and its implication for delayed toxicity. *Mol Pharmacol* **39**: 625.

Cheng N, Merrill BM, Painter GR *et al.* (1993). Identification of the nucleotide binding site of HIV-1 reverse transcriptase using dTTP as a photoaffinity label. *Biochem* **32**: 7630.

Chong KT, Pagano PJ, Hinshaw RR (1994). Bisheteroarylpiperazine reverse transcriptase inhibitor in combination with 3'-azido-3'-deoxythymidine or 2',3'-dideoxycytidine synergistically inhibits human immunodeficiency virus type 1 replication *in vitro*. *Antimicrob Ag Chemother* **38**: 288.

Chottiner EG, Shewach DS, Datta NS *et al.* (1991). Cloning and expression of human deoxycytidine kinase cDNA. *Proc Natl Acad Sci USA* **88**: 1531.

Cinatl J, Cinatl J, Weber B *et al.* (1993). Decreased anti-human immunodeficiency virus type-1 activities of 2',3'-dideoxynucleoside analogs in MOLT-4 cell sublines resistant to 2',3'-dideoxynucleoside analogs. *Acta Virol* **37**: 360.

Collier AC, Coombs RW, Schoenfeld DA *et al.* (1996). Treatment of human immunodeficiency virus infection with saquinavir, zidovudine and zalcitabine. AIDS Clinical Trials Group. *New Engl J Med* **334**: 1011.

Cooney DA, Dalal M, Mitsuya H *et al.* (1986). Initial studies on the cellular pharmacology of 2',3'-dideoxycytidine, an inhibitor of HTLV-III infectivity. *Biochem Pharmacol* **35**: 2065.

Craig JC, Duncan IB, Whittaker L, Roberts NA (1990). Antiviral synergy between inhibitors of HIV proteinase and reverse transcriptase. *Antivir Chem Chemother* **4**: 161.

Degre M, Beck S (1994). Anti-HIV activity of dideoxynucleosides, foscarnet and fusidic acid is potentiated by human leukocyte interferon in blood-derived macrophages. *Chemother* **40**: 201.

Descamps D, Collin G, Loussert-Ajaka S *et al.* (1995). Plasma HIV-1 load and nosocomial transmission in Romanian children. *AIDS* **9**: 977.

Dianzani F, Antonelli G, Turriziani O *et al.* (1992). *In vitro* selection of human immunodeficiency virus type 1 resistant to 3'-azido-3'-deoxythymidine. *Antiviral Res* **18**: 39.

Domin BA, Mahony WB, Zimmerman TP (1993). Membrane permeation mechanisms of 2',3'-dideoxynucleosides. *Biochemical Pharmacol* **36**: 725.

Dubinsky RM, Yarchoan R, Dalakas M, Broder S (1989). Reversible axonal neuropathy from the treatment of AIDS and related disorders with 2',3'-dideoxycytidine (ddC). *Muscle Nerve* **12**: 856.

Eron JJ, Johnson VA, Merrill DP *et al.* (1992). Synergistic inhibition of replication of human immunodeficiency virus type 1, including that of a zidovudine-resistant isolate, by zidovudine and 2',3'-dideoxycytidine *in vitro*. *Antimicrob Ag Chemother* **36**: 1559.

Faraj A, Fowler DA, Bridges EG, Sommadossi JP (1994). Effects of 2',3'-dideoxynucleosides on proliferation and differentiation of human pluripotent progenitors in liquid culture and their effects on mitochondrial DNA synthesis. *Antimicrob Ag Chemother* **38**: 924.

Feldman D, Brosnan C, Anderson TD (1992). Ultrastructure of peripheral neuropathy induced in rabbits by 2',3'-dideoxycytidine. *Lab Invest* **66**: 75.

Fischl MA, Olson RM, Follansbee SE *et al.* (1993). Zalcitabine compared with zidovudine in patients with advanced HIV-1 infection who received previous zidovudine therapy. *Ann Intern Med* **118**: 762.

Fischl MA, Stanley K, Collier AC *et al.* (1995). Combination and monotherapy with zidovudine and zalcitabine in patients with advanced HIV disease. *Ann Intern Med* **122**: 24.

Fitzgibbon JE, Howell RM, Haberzettl CA *et al.* (1992). Human immunodeficiency virus type 1 *pol* gene mutations which cause decreased susceptibility to 2',3'-dideoxycytidine. *Antimicrob Ag Chemother* **36**: 153.

Foerster M, Kastner U, Neubert R (1992). Effect of six virustatic nucleoside analogues on the development of fetal rat thymus in organ culture. *Arch Toxicol* **66**: 688.

Fourel I, Saputelli J, Schaffer P, Mason WS (1994). The carbocyclic analog of 2'-deoxyguanosine induces a prolonged inhibition of duck hepatitis B virus DNA synthesis in primary hepatocyte cultures and in the liver. *J Virol* **68**: 1059.

Ganser A, Greher J, Volkers B *et al.* (1989). Inhibitory effect of azidothymidine, 2'-3'-dideoxyadenosine, and 2'-3'-dideoxycytidine on *in vitro* growth of hematopoietic progenitor cells from normal persons and from patients with AIDS. *Exp Hematol* **17**: 321.

Gao Q, Gu Z, Dionne G, Wainberg MA (1993a). Generation of drug-resistant variants of human immunodeficiency virus type 1 *in vitro* passage in increasing concentrations of 2'-3'-dideoxycytidine and 2',3'-dideoxy-3'-thiacytidine. *Antimicrob Ag Chemother* **37**: 130.

Gao WY, Shirasaka T, Johns DG *et al.* (1993b). Differential phosphorylation of azidothymidine, dideoxycytidine, and dideoxyinosine in resting and activated peripheral blood mononuclear cells. *J Clin Invest* **91**: 3326.

Gao Q, Gu Z, Parniak MA *et al.* (1993c). The same mutation that encodes low-level human immunodeficiency virus type 1 resistance to 2',3'-dideoxyinosine and 2',3'-dideoxycytidine confers high-level resistance to the (-) enantiomer of 2',3'-dideoxy-3'-thiacytidine. *Antimicrob Ag Chemother* **37**: 1390.

Gobert JM, Remington KM, Zhu YQ, North TW (1994). Multiple drug resistant mutants of feline immunodeficiency virus selected with 2',3'-dideoxyinosine alone and in combination with 3'-azido-3'-deoxythymidine. *Antimicrob Ag Chemother* **38**: 861.

Gu Z, Gao Q, Li X *et al.* (1992). Novel mutation in the human immunodeficiency virus type 1 reverse transcriptase gene that encodes cross-resistance to 2',3'-dideoxycytidine. *J Virol* **66**: 7128.

Gu Z, Gao Q, Fang H *et al.* (1994a). Identification of novel mutations that confer drug resistance in the human immunodeficiency virus polymerase gene. *Leukemia* **1**: S166.

Gu Z, Gao Q, Fang H *et al.* (1994b). Identification of a mutation at codon 65 in the IKKK motif of reverse transcriptase that encodes human immunodeficiency virus resistance to 2',3'-dideoxycytidine and 2',3'-dideoxy-3'-thiacytidine. *Antimicrob Ag Chemother* **38**: 275.

Gu Z, Arts EJ, Parniak MA, Wainberg MA (1995). Mutated K65R recombinant reverse transcriptase of human immunodeficiency virus type 1 shows diminished chain termination in the presence of 2',3'-dideoxycytidine 5'-triphosphate and other drugs. *PNAS USA* **92**: 2760.

Gustavson LE, Fukuda EK, Rubio FA, Dunton AW (1990). A pilot study of the bioavailability and pharmacokinetics of 2',3'-dideoxycytidine in patients with AIDS or AIDS-related complex. *J AIDS* **3**: 28.

Habteyesus A, Nordenskjold A, Bohman C, Eriksson S (1991). Deoxynucleoside phosphorylating enzymes in monkey and human tissues show great similarities, while mouse deoxycytidine kinase has a different substrate specificity. *Biochem Pharmacol* **42**: 1829.

Hao Z, Stowe EE, Ahluwalia G *et al.* (1993). Characterisation of 2',3'-deoxycytidine diphosphocholine and 2',3'-dideoxycytidine diphosphoethanolamine. Prominent phosphodiester metabolites of the anti-HIV nucleoside 2',3'-dideoxycytidine. *Drug Metab Dispos Biol Fate Chem* **21**: 738.

Hayashi S, Fine RL, Chou TC *et al.* (1990). *In vitro* inhibition of the infectivity and replication of human immunodeficiency virus type 1 by combination of antiretroviral 2',3'-dideoxynucleosides and virus binding inhibitors. *Antimicrob Ag Chemother* **34**: 82.

Hitchcock MJ (1993). *In vitro* antiviral activity of didanosine compared with that of other dideoxynucleoside analogs against laboratory strains and clinical isolates of human immunodeficiency virus. *Clin Infect Dis* **16**: S16.

Hoover EA, Zeidner NS, Perigo NA *et al.* (1989). Feline leukemia virus-induced immunodeficiency syndrome in cats as a model for evaluation of antiretroviral therapy. *Intervirol* **30**: 12.

Howe AY, Robins MJ, Wilson JS, Tyrell DL (1996). Selective inhibition of the reverse transcription of duck hepatitis B virus by binding of 2',3'-dideoxyguanosine 5'-triphosphate to the viral polymerase. *Hepatology* **23**: 87.

Husson RN, Shirasaka T, Butler KM *et al.* (1993). High-level resistance to zidovudine but not to zalcitabine or didanosine in human immunodeficiency virus from children receiving antiretroviral therapy. *J Pediatr* **123**: 9.

Indorf AS, Pegram PS (1992). Esophageal ulceration related to zalcitabine (ddC). *Ann Intern Med* **117**: 133.

Inoue T, Tsushita K, Itoh T *et al.* (1989). *In vitro* bone marrow toxicity of nucleoside analogs against human immunodeficiency virus. *Antimicrob Ag Chemother* **23**: 576.

Irons RD, Le AT, Som DB, Stillman WS (1995). 2',3'-dideoxycytidine-induced thymic lymphoma correlates with species specific suppression of a subpopulation of primitive hematopoietic progenitor cells in mouse but not rat or human bone marrow. *J Clin Invest* **95**: 2777.

Ito M, Baba M, Mori S *et al.* (1990). Tumor necrosis factor antagonizes inhibitory effect of azidothymidine on human immunodeficiency virus (HIV) replication *in vitro*. *Biochem Biophys Res Commun* **166**: 1095.

Jeffries DJ (1989). The antiviral activity of dideoxycytidine. *J Antimicrob Chemother* **23**: 29.

Johnson MA, Johns DG, Fridland A (1987). 2',3'-dideoxynucleoside phosphorylation by deoxycytidine kinase from normal human thymus extracts: activation of potential drugs for AIDS therapy. *Biochem Biophys Res Commun* **148**: 1252.

Johnson M, Caiazzo T, Molina JM *et al.* (1988). Inhibition of bone marrow myelopoiesis and erythropoiesis *in vitro* by anti-retroviral nucleoside derivatives. *Brit J Haematol* **70**: 137.

Johnson VA, Merrill DP, Chou TC, Hirsch MS (1992). Human immunodeficiency virus type 1 (HIV-1) inhibitory interactions between protease inhibitor Ro 31–8959 and zidovudine, 2',3'-dideoxycytidine, or recombinant interferon-alpha A against zidovudine-sensitive or -resistant HIV *in vitro*. *J Infect Dis* **166**: 1143.

Kassianides C, Hoofnagle JH, Miller RH *et al.* (1989). Inhibition of duck hepatitis B virus replication by 2',3'-dideoxycytidine. A potent inhibitor of reverse transcriptase. *Gastroenterol* **97**: 1275.

Kastrissios H, Nakano M, Burton P, Blaschke T (1996). Improved combined solid phase extraction RIA method for quantifying zalcitabine in plasma. *Clin Chem* **42**: 465.

Kavlick MF, Shirasaka T, Kojima E *et al.* (1995). Genotypic and phenotypic characterisation of HIV-1 isolated from patients receiving (-)-2'-3'-dideoxy-3'-thiacytidine. *Antiviral Res* **28**: 133.

Kelley JA, Litterst CL, Roth JS *et al.* (1987). The disposition and metabolism of 2',3'-dideoxycytidine, an *in vitro* inhibitor of human T-lymphotrophic virus type III infectivity, in mice and monkeys. *Drug Metab Dispos Biol Fate Chem* **15**: 595.

Kierdaszuk B, Bohman C, Ullman B, Eriksson S (1992). Substrate specificity of human deoxycytidine kinase toward antiviral 2',3'-dideoxynucleoside analogs. *Biochem Pharmacol* **43**: 197.

Kim S, Scheerer S, Geyer MA, Howell SB (1990). Direct cerebrospinal fluid delivery of an antiretroviral agent using multivesicular liposomes. *J Infect Dis* **162**: 750.

Kitos TE, Tyrrell DL (1995). Intracellular metabolism of 2',3'-dideoxynucleosides in duck hepatocyte primary cultures. *Biochem Pharmacol* **49**: 1291.

Klecker RW, Collins JM, Yarchoan RC *et al.* (1988). Pharmacokinetics of 2',3'-dideoxycytidine in patients with AIDS and related disorders. *J Clin Pharmacol* **28**: 837.

Klug S, Lewandowski C, Merker HJ *et al.* (1991). *In vitro* and *in vivo* studies on the prenatal toxicity of five virustatic nucleoside analogues in comparison to acyclovir. *Arch Toxicol* **65**: 283.

Lacey SF, Larder MA (1994). Novel mutation (V75T) in human immunodeficiency virus type 1 reverse transcriptase confers resistance to 2',3-didehydro-2',3'-dideoxythymidine in cell culture. *Antimicrob Ag Chemother* **38**: 1428.

Larder BA (1995). Viral resistance and the selection of antiretroviral combinations. *J AIDS Hum Retrovir* **10**: S28.

Larder BA, Darby G, Richman DD (1989). HIV with reduced sensitivity to zidovudine (AZT) isolated during prolonged therapy. *Science* **243**: 1731.

LeLacheur SF, Simon GL (1991). Exacerbation of dideoxycytidine-induced neuropathy with dideoxyinosine. *J AIDS* **4**: 538.

Lewis LD, Hamzeh FM, Lietman PS (1992). Ultrastructural changes associated with reduced mitochondrial DNA and impaired mitochondrial function in the presence of 2',3'-dideoxycytidine. *Antimicrob Ag Chemother* **36**: 2061.

Makabi-Panuzu B, Lessard C, Beauchamp D *et al.* (1995). Uptake and binding of liposomal 2',3'-dideoxycytidine by RAW 264 7 cells: a three step process. *J AIDS Hum Retrovir* **8**: 227.

Martin JA, Mobberley MA, Redshawa S *et al.* (1991). The inhibitory activity of a peptide derivative against the growth of simian immunodeficiency virus in C8166 cells. *Biochem Biophys Res Commun* **178**: 180.

Martinez OP, French MA (1993). Acoustic neuropathy associated with zalcitabine-induced peripheral neuropathy. *AIDS* **7**: 901.

Mathez D, Schinazi RF, Liotta DC, Leibowitch J (1993). Infectious amplification of wild-type human immunodeficiency virus from patients' lymphocytes and modulation by reverse transcriptase inhibitors *in vitro*. *Antimicrob Ag Chemother* **37**: 2206.

Matsushita S, Mitsuya H, Reitz MS, Broder S (1987). Pharmacological inhibition of *in vitro* infectivity of human T lymphotropic virus type I. *J Clin Invest* **80**: 394.

Mayers DL, Japour AJ, Arduino JM et al. (1994). Dideoxynucleoside resistance emerges with prolonged zidovudine monotherapy. The RV43 Study Group. Antimicrob Ag Chemother 38: 307.

McLeod GX, Hammer SM (1992). Combination therapy. Hosp Pract 27: 14.

McLeod GX, McGrath JM, Ladd EA et al. (1992). Didanosine and zidovudine resistance patterns in clinical isolates of human immunodeficiency virus type 1 as determined by a replication endpoint concentration assay. Antimicrob Ag Chemother 36: 920.

McNeely MC, Yarchoan R, Broder S, Lawley TJ (1989). Dermatologic complications associated with administration of 2',3'-dideoxycytidine in patients with human immunodeficiency virus infection. J Amer Acad Dermatol 21: 1213.

Meng TC, Fischl MA, Richman DD (1990). AIDS Clinical Trials Group; phase I/II study of combination 2',3'-dideoxycytidine and zidovudine in patients with acquired immunodeficiency syndrome (AIDS) and advanced AIDS-related complex. Amer J Med 88: 27.

Meng TC, Fischl MA, Boota AM et al. (1992). Combination therapy with zidovudine and dideoxycytidine in patients with advanced human immunodeficiency virus infection. A phase I/II study. Ann Intern Med 116: 13.

Merigan TC, Skowron G, Bozzette SA et al. (1989). Circulating p24 antigen levels and responses to dideoxycytidine in human immunodeficiency virus (HIV) infections. A phase I and II study. Ann Int Med 110: 189.

Mildvan D, Berge P, Starrett S et al. (1994). Prophylactic zalcitabine and interferon-alpha for a large-bore needlestick exposure to human immunodeficiency virus. J AIDS 7: 416.

Mirchandani HL, Chien YW (1995). Intestinal absorption of dideoxynucleosides: characterisation using a multiloop in situ technique. J Pharmaceut Sci 84: 44.

Mitsuya H, Broder S (1986). Inhibition of the in vitro infectivity and cytopathic effect of human T-lymphotrophic virus type III/lymphadenopathy-associated virus (HTLV-III/LAV) by 2',3'-dideoxynucleosides. Proc Natl Acad Sci USA 83: 1911.

Mitsuya H, Broder S (1988). Inhibition of infectivity and replication of HIV-2 and SIV in helper T-cells by 2',3'-dideoxynucleosides in vitro. AIDS Res Hum Retrovir 4: 107.

Mitsuya H, Jarrett RF, Matsukura M et al. (1987). Long term inhibition of human T-lymphotropic virus type III/lymphadenopathy-associated virus (human immunodeficiency virus) DNA synthesis and RNA expression in T cells protected by 2',3'-dideoxynucleosides in vitro. Proc Natl Acad Sci USA 84: 2033.

Morris DJ (1994). Adverse effects and drug interactions of clinical importance with antiviral drugs. Drug Safety 10: 281.

Morse GB, Shelton MJ, O'Donnell AM (1993). Comparative pharmacokinetics of antiviral nucleoside analogues. Clin Pharmacokinet 24: 101.

Munch-Petersen B, Cloos L et al. (1991). Diverging substrate specificity of pure human thymidine kinase 1 and 2 against antiviral dideoxynucleosides. J Biol Chem 266: 9032.

Nazareno LA, Hotazo AA, Limjuco R et al. (1995). The effect of food on pharmacokinetics of zalcitabine in HIV positive patients. Pharm Res 12: 1462.

Nguyen BY, Shay LE, Wyvill KM et al. (1993). A pilot study of sequential therapy with zidovudine plus acyclovir, dideoxyinosine and dideoxycytidine in patients with severe human immunodeficiency virus infection. J Infect Dis 168: 810.

Omata M (1989). Liver diseases associated with hepadnavirus infection A study in duck model. Cancer Detect Prev 14: 231.

Ono K, Nakane H, Herdewijn P et al. (1989). Differential inhibitory effects of several pyrimidine 2',3'-dideoxynucleoside 5'-triphosphates on the activities of reverse transcriptase and various cellular DNA polymerases. Mol Pharmacol 35: 578.

Ostashewski PM, Houston SC, Robertson JA (1993). In vitro activity of zidovudine, zalcitabine and didanosine against mycoplasmas. Lancet 342: 1242.

Patel SS, Szebeni J, Wahl LM, Weinstein JN (1991). Differential inhibition of 2'-deoxycytidine salvage as a possible mechanism to potentiation of the anti-human immunodeficiency virus activity of 2'-3'-dideoxycytidine by dipyridamole. Antimicrob Ag Chemother 35: 1250.

Pellegrino MG, Li G, Potash MJ, Volsky DJ (1991). Contribution of multiple rounds of viral entry and reverse transcription to expression of human immunodeficiency virus type 1. J Biol Chem 266: 1783.

Perno CF, Yarchoan R, Cooney DA et al. (1988). Inhibition of human immunodeficiency virus (HIV-1/HTLV-IIIBa-L) replication in fresh and cultured human peripheral blood monocytes/macrophages by azidothymidine and related 2',3'-dideoxynucleosides. J Exp Med 168: 1111.

Perno CF, Yarchoan R, Balzarini J et al. (1992a). Different pattern of activity of inhibitors of the human immunodeficiency virus in lymphocytes and monocyte/macrophages. Antiviral Res 17: 289.

Perno CF, Cooney DA, Gao WY et al. (1992b). Effects of bone marrow stimulatory cytokines on human immunodeficiency virus replication and the antiviral activity of dideoxynucleosides in cultures of monocytes-macrophages. Blood 80: 995.

Perno CF, Aquaro S, Rosenwirth B et al. (1994). In vitro activity of inhibitors of late stages of the replication of HIV in chronically infected macrophages. J Leuk Biol 56: 381.

Pizzo PA (1990). Treatment of human immunodeficiency virus-infected infants and young children with dideoxynucleosides. Amer J Med 88: 16.

Pizzo PA, Butler K, Balis F et al. (1990). Dideoxycytidine alone and in an alternating schedule with zidovudine in children with symptomatic human immunodeficiency virus infection. J Paediatr 117: 799.

Plageman PGW, Wohlhueter RM, Woffendin C (1988). Nucleoside and nucleobase transport in animal cells. Biochim Biophys Acta 947: 405.

Polas PJ, Swenson CL, Sams R et al. (1990). In vitro and in vivo evidence that the antiviral activity of 2',3'-dideoxycytidine is target cell dependent in a feline retrovirus animal model. Antimicrob Ag Chemother 34: 1414.

Powderly WG, Klebert MK, Clifford DB (1990). Ototoxicity associated with dideoxycytidine. Lancet 335: 1106.

Qian MX, Swagler AR, Mehta M et al. (1992). Pharmacokinetic evaluation of drug interactions with anti-human immunotrophic virus (HIV) drugs: III 2',3'-dideoxycytidine (ddC) and zidovudine in monkeys. Pharm Res 9: 224.

Rajaonarison JF, Lacarelle B, Catalin J et al. (1992). 3'-azido-3'-deoxythymidine drug interactions: screening for inhibitors in liver microsomes. Drug Metab Dispos Biol Fate Chem 20: 578.

Ratner L, Vander-Heyden N (1993). Mechanism of action of N-butyl deoxynojirimycin in inhibiting HIV-1 infection and activity in combination with nucleoside analogs. AIDS Res Hum Retrovir 9: 291.

Richman DD (1990a). HIV and other human retroviruses In Antiviral Agents and Viral Diseases of Man 3rd ed (Galasso GJ, Whitley RJ, Merigan TC, eds.), pp. 581, 646. New York: Raven Press.

Richman DD (1990b). Zidovudine resistance of human immunodeficiency virus. Rev Infect Dis 5: S507.

Richman DD (1990c). Susceptibility to nucleoside analogues of zidovudine-resistant isolates of human immunodeficiency virus. Amer J Med 88: 8.

Richman DD, Kornbluth RS, Carson DA (1987). Failure of dideoxynucleosides to inhibit human immunodeficiency virus replication in cultured human macrophages. J Exp Med 166: 1144.

Richman DD, Meng TC, Spector SA et al. (1994). Resistance to AZT and ddC during long-term combination therapy in patients with advanced infection with human immunodeficiency virus. J AIDS 7: 135.

Roilides E, Venzon D, Pizzo PA, Rubin M (1990). Effects of antiretroviral dideoxynucleosides on polymorphonuclear leukocyte function. Antimicrob Ag Chemother 34: 1672.

Rooke R, Parniak MA, Tremblay M et al. (1991). Biological comparison of wild-type and zidovudine resistant isolates of human immunodeficiency virus type 1 from the same subjects: susceptibility and resistance to other drugs. Antimicrob Ag Chemother 35: 988.

Rossi L, Brandi G, Schiavano GF et al. (1992). In vitro and in vivo toxicity of 2',3'-dideoxycytidine in mice. Chem Biol Interact 85: 255.

Rossi L, Brandi G, Fraternale A et al. (1993). Inhibition of murine retrovirus-induced immunodeficiency disease by dideoxycytidine and dideoxycytidine 5'-triphosphate. J AIDS 6: 1179.

Saravolatz LD, Winslow DL, Collins G *et al.* (1996). Zidovudine alone or in combination with didanosine or zalcitabine in HIV-infected patients with the acquired immunodeficiency syndrome or fewer than 200 CD4 cells per cubic millimeter. Investigators for the Terry Beirn Community Programs for Clinical Research on AIDS. *New Engl J Med* **335**: 1099.

Schinazi RF, Lloyd RM, Nguyen MH *et al.* (1993). Characterisation of human immunodeficiency viruses resistant to oxathiolane-cytosine nucleosides. *Antimicrob Ag Chemother* **37**: 875.

Schooley RT, Ramirez-Ronda C, Lange JM *et al.* (1996). Virologic and immunologic benefits of initial combination therapy with zidovudine and zalcitabine or didanosine compared with zidovudine monotherapy. Wellcome Resistance Study Collaborative Group. *J Inf Dis* **173**: 1354.

Shelton MJ, O'Donnell AM, Morse GD (1993). Zalcitabine. *Ann Pharmacother* **27**: 480.

Shirasaka T, Yarchoan R, O'Brien MC *et al.* (1993). Changes in drug sensitivity of human immunodeficiency virus type 1 during therapy with azidothymidine, dideoxycytidine, and dideoxyinosine; an *in vitro* comparative study. *Proc Natl Acad Sci USA* **90**: 562.

Shirasaka T, Kavlick MF, Ueno T *et al.* (1995a). Emergence of human immunodeficiency virus type 1 variants with resistance to multiple dideoxynucleosides in patients receiving therapy with dideoxynucleosides. *PNAS USA* **92**: 6.

Shirasaka T, Chokekijchai S, Yamada A *et al.* (1995b). Comparative analysis of anti-human immunodeficiency virus type 1 activities of dideoxynucleoside analogs in resting and activated peripheral blood mononuclear cells. *Antimicrob Ag Chemother* **39**: 2555.

Silverton JV, Quinn FR, Haugwitz RD, Torado LJ (1988). Structures of two dideoxynucleosides: 2',3'-dideoxyadenosine and 2',3'-dideoxycytidine. *Acta Crystallogr C* **44**: 321.

Skowron G, Bozzette SA, Lim L *et al.* (1993). Alternating and intermittent regimens of zidovudine and dideoxycytidine in patients with AIDS or AIDS-related complex. *Ann Intern Med* **118**: 321.

Sommadossi JP (1993). Nucleoside analogs: similarities and differences. *Clin Infect Dis* **16**: S7.

Spector SA (1994). Pediatric antiretroviral choices. *AIDS* **8**: S15.

Spector SA, Ripley D, Hsia K (1989). Human immunodeficiency virus inhibition is prolonged by 3'-azido-3'-deoxythymidine alternating with 2',3'-dideoxycytidine compared with 3'-azido-3'-deoxythymidine alone. *Antimicrob Ag Chemother* **33**: 920.

Sperber SJ, Feibusch EL, Damiani A, Weinstein MP (1993). *In vitro* activities of nucleoside analog antiviral agents against salmonellae. *Antimicrob Ag Chemother* **37**: 106.

St Clair MH, Martin JL, Tudor-Williams G *et al.* (1991). Resistance to ddI and sensitivity to AZT induced by a mutation in HIV-1 reverse transcriptase. *Science* **253**: 1557.

Starnes MC, Cheng YC (1987). Cellular metabolism of 2',3'-dideoxycytidine, a compound active against human immunodeficiency virus *in vitro*. *J Biol Chem* **262**: 988.

Szebeni J, Wahl SM, Betageri GV *et al.* (1990). Inhibition of HIV-1 in monocyte/macrophage cultures by 2',3'-dideoxycytidine-5'-triphosphate, free and in liposomes. *AIDS Res Hum Retrovir* **6**: 691.

Terasaki T, Pardridge WM (1988). Restricted transport of 3'-azido-3'-deoxythymidine and dideoxynucleosides through the blood-brain barrier. *J Infect Dis* **158**: 630.

Tisdale M, Kemp SD, Parry NR, Larder BA (1993). Rapid *in vitro* selection of human immunodeficiency virus type 1 resistant to 3'-thiacytidine inhibitors due to a mutation in the YMDD region of reverse transcriptase. *Proc Natl Acad Sci USA* **90**: 5653.

Toltzis P, Mourton T, Magnuson T (1994). Comparative embryonic cytotoxicity of antiretroviral nucleosides. *J Infect Dis* **169**: 1100.

Tsai CC, Follis KE, Benveniste RE (1988). Antiviral effects of 3'-azido-3'-deoxythmidine, 2',3'-dideoxycytidine, and 2',3'-dideoxyadenosine against simian acquired immunodeficiency syndrome-associated type D retrovirus *in vitro*. *AIDS Res Hum Retrovir* **4**: 359.

Tsai CC, Follis KE, Yarnall M *et al.* (1989). Toxicity and efficacy of 2',3'-dideoxycytidine in clinical trials of pigtailed macaques infected with simian retrovirus type 2. *Antimicrob Ag Chemother* **33**: 1908.

Ueda K, Tsurimoto T, Nagahata T *et al.* (1989). An *in vitro* system for screening anti-hepatitis B virus drugs. *Virology* **169**: 213.

Ullman B, Coons T, Rockwell S, McCartan K (1988). Genetic analysis of 2',3'-dideoxycytidine incorporation into cultured human T lymphoblasts. *J Biol Chem* **263**: 12391.

Underwood TW, Frye CB (1993). Drug-induced pancreatitis. *Clin Pharm* **12**: 440.

Vogt MW, Durno AG, Chou TC *et al.* (1988). Synergistic interaction of 2',3'-dideoxycytidine and recombinant interferon-alpha-A on replication of human immunodeficiency virus type 1. *J Infect Dis* **158**: 378.

Wainberg MA, Gu Z, Gao Q *et al.* (1993). Clinical correlates and molecular basis of HIV drug resistance. *J AIDS* **1**: S36.

Werth JL, Zhou B, Nutter LM, Thayer SA (1994). 2',3'-dideoxycytidine alters calcium buffering in cultured dorsal root ganglion neurons. *Mol Pharmacol* **45**: 1119.

Whittington R, Brogden RN (1992). Zalcitabine. A review of its pharmacology and clinical potential in acquired immunodeficiency syndrome (AIDS). *Drugs* **44**: 656.

Williams RJ, Knight AP, Smith JA *et al.* (1989). Preliminary pharmacokinetics of 2',3'-dideoxycytidine in neonatal goats. *J Vet Pharmacol* **12**: 334.

Winslow DL, Mayers D, Scarnati H *et al.* (1994). *In vitro* susceptibility of clinical isolates of HIV-1 to XM323, a non-peptidyl HIV protease inhibitor. *AIDS* **8**: 753.

Yarchoan R, Perno CF, Thomas RV *et al.* (1988). Phase I studies of 2',3'-dideoxycytidine in severe human immunodeficiency virus infection as a single agent and alternating with zidovudine (AZT). *Lancet* **i**: 76.

Yarchoan R, Mitsuya H, Myers CE, Broder S (1989). Clinical pharmacology of 3'-azido-2',3'-dideoxythymidine (zidovudine) and related dideoxy-nucleosides. *New Engl J Med* **321**: 726.

Yarchoan R, Pluda JM, Perno CF *et al.* (1990). Initial clinical experience with dideoxynucleosides as single agents and in combination therapy. *Ann NY Acad Sci* **616**: 328.

Yokota T, Konno K, Chonan E *et al.* (1990). Comparative activities of several nucleoside analogs against duck hepatitis B virus *in vitro*. *Antimicrob Ag Chemother* **34**: 1326.

Yokota T, Mochizuki S, Konno K *et al.* (1991). Inhibitory effects of selected antiviral compounds on human hepatitis B virus DNA synthesis. *Antimicrob Ag Chemother* **35**: 394.

Zalcitabine Product Infomation.

Zeidner NS, Strobel JD, Perigo NA *et al.* (1989). Treatment of FeLV-induced immunodeficiency syndrome (FeLV-FAIDS) with controlled release capsular implantation of 2',3'-dideoxycytidine. *Antiviral Res* **11**: 147.

Zhang D, Callendo AM, Eron JJ *et al.* (1994). Resistance to 2',3'-dideoxycytidine conferred by a mutation in codon 65 of the human immunodeficiency virus type 1 reverse transcriptase. *Antimicrob Ag Chemother* **38**: 282.

Lamivudine

Description

Lamivudine is the negative enantiomer of 2'-deoxy-3'-thiacytidine, the racemic mixture of the two enantiomers being previously known as both BCH 189, and GR103365X. This dideoxynucleoside analog of cytidine is a potent inhibitor of the replication of HIV-1 and HIV-2 as well as hepatitis B virus. The drug was initially synthesized by Biochem Pharma Inc, Montreal Canada as GR103365X and the negative enantiomer (GR109714X) was subsequently developed by Glaxo Research and Development. Lamivudine is marketed by GlaxoWellcome under the trade names of '3TC' and 'Epivir'. Lamivudine is registered for the treatment of HIV infection in a number of countries including Australia, Europe and the USA. Registration has occurred rapidly through priority evaluation programs before publication of many of the relevant data, thus data on file with GlaxoWellcome and data provided in the company's Product Information have been supplied in this chapter.

The molecular weight of lamivudine is 229.3. The chemical name of lamivudine is (2R-*cis*)-4-amino-1- (2-hydroxymethyl-1,3-oxathiolan -5-yl)-(1H)-pyrimidin-2–1. The compound has the molecular formula of $C_8H_{11}N_8O_3S$. The chemical structure of lamivudine differs from that of zidovudine in that there is a sulphur atom that replaces the 3' carbon atom of the ribose (Fig. V.48). In addition lamivudine has a beta-L-sugar configuration and carries a cytosine base moiety. The concentration of the drug can be reported in μM or μg per ml (1 μM is approximately equivalent to 0.2 μg per ml).

Antiviral Activity

1 Human immunodeficiency virus

Lamivudine inhibits both HIV-1 and HIV-2 *in vitro*, including strains that are zidovudine-resistant. Depending on the strain of HIV, viral inoculum, cell type and assay used, the ranking order within the family of nucleoside analog reverse transcriptase inhibitors suggests that lamivudine has a potency similar or less than that of zidovudine (Coates *et al.*, 1992a; Mathez *et al.*, 1993; Schinazi *et al.*, 1992a), greater than didanosine (Mathez *et al.*, 1993) and similar or greater to that of zalcitabine (Coates *et al.*, 1992a,b). The positive and negative enantiomers of 2'-deoxy-3'-thiacytidine have equal potency against HIV but the negative enantiomer (lamivudine) is considerably less toxic (Coates *et al.*, 1992a). The IC$_{50}$ of lamivudine against HIV-1 in CD4-expressing T cell lines ranges from 4 nM to 0.67 μM, and in primary T

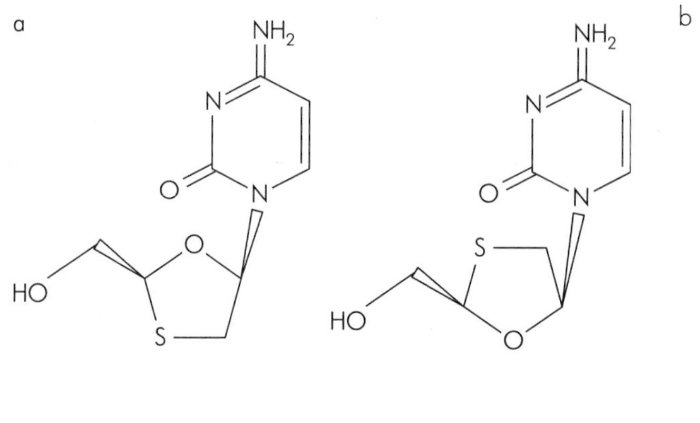

Fig. V.48.
Chemical structure of 2'-deoxy-3'-thiacytidine. (a) (+)-Enantiomer, (b) (−)-Enantiomer (lamivudine). (Reproduced from Hart *et al.*, 1992, with permission.)

lymphocytes the range is from 2.5 to 90 nM (Coates *et al.*, 1992b). The IC_{50} for cytotoxicity in these cells is 0.5–6 mM (Coates *et al.*, 1992b). The IC_{90} against HIV in peripheral blood lymphocytes has been reported to be 76 nM (Gray *et al.*, 1995). The IC_{50} and IC_{90} of lamivudine required to prevent HIV replication in monocyte cell lines (U937) are 120 and 1100 nM respectively (Coates *et al.*, 1992b). Lamivudine does not inhibit replication of HIV in chronically infected cells (Coates *et al.*, 1992b). Lamivudine has also been found to inhibit HIV replication in other primary cells including fetal brain macrophages, in which pretreatment of the cells with lamivudine at a concentration of 4.3 µM resulted in efficient block in the production of progeny virions (Geleziunas *et al.*, 1993).

2 Resistance

Lamivudine-resistant variants of HIV have been demonstrated following *in vitro* passage of HIV in the presence of increasing concentrations of lamivudine (Tisdale *et al.*, 1993; Boucher *et al.*, 1993) as well as in isolates of HIV from patients treated with lamivudine (Larder *et al.*, 1995). Passage of HIV in lamivudine-containing culture media results in the development of high-level resistance with IC_{50} values exceeding that of the wild-type by more than 100-fold (Boucher *et al.*, 1993). This has been reported for wild-type as well as zidovudine-resistant strains of HIV (Tisdale *et al.*, 1993). Resistance develops after as few as ten passages *in vitro*, with the resistant strain of HIV able to replicate in culture media containing more than 450 µM lamivudine (Boucher *et al.*, 1993).

Several mutations within the reverse transcriptase encoding region of the *pol* gene have been found to confer resistance of HIV to lamivudine (Table V.36). Substitution of methionine to valine or isoleucine at position 184 results in resistance to lamivudine (Boucher *et al.*,1993; Gao *et al.*, 1993; Gu *et al.*, 1992; Schinazi *et al.*, 1993; Faraj *et al.*, 1994), although these *in vitro*-derived isolates have been reported to remain susceptible to zalcitabine, didanosine and nevirapine (Tisdale *et al.*, 1993; Boucher *et al.*, 1993). Introduction of this mutation into an infectious clone of HIV caused more than 1000-fold reduction in susceptibility to lamivudine. The mutation at position 184 precedes the detection of phenotypic resistance (Wainberg *et al.*, 1995). The methionine 184 residue in the reverse transcriptase is part of the YXDD motif. Within this motif are three aspartic acid residues that make up the polymerase active site of the reverse transcriptase enzyme (Tantillo *et al.*, 1994; reviewed in Boyer and Hughes, 1995). Variants of HIV-1 that are resistant to lamivudine have lower reverse transcriptase activity than wild-type (Back *et al.*, 1996).

The introduction of an isoleucine substitution at codon 184 into zidovudine-resistant variants of HIV-1 that have mutations at codons 41 and 215 of reverse transcriptase results in reversing the susceptibility of the virus to zidovudine. The introduction of the mutation at position 184 improved the zidovudine susceptibility of the lamivudine-resistant HIV by 50-fold (Boucher *et al.*, 1993). Viral recombination following cellular fusion *in vitro* may also potentially give rise to variants of HIV that are dually resistant to both zidovudine and lamivudine (Gu *et al.*, 1995b), although co-resistance was not observed by other co-investigators during *in vitro* studies (Larder *et al.*, 1995). Strains of HIV that are resistant to both lamivudine and zidovudine have been isolated (Lamivudine Product Information). Lamivudine-resistant strains of HIV remain sensitive to nevirapine (Tisdale *et al.*, 1993).

The lysine-to-arginine substitution at amino acid 65 in HIV reverse transcriptase has also been reported in association with detection of resistance to lamivudine. This mutation appears to also confer cross-resistance to didanosine and zalcitabine *in vitro*. The mutation results in reduced chain-termination in the presence of these nucleoside analogs compared with wild-type virus (Gu *et al.*, 1994, 1995a).

Lamivudine monotherapy has been found to induce the rapid emergence of resistance, with evidence of resistance commencing as early as 1 week after onset of therapy (Schuurman *et al.*,

Table V.36

Drug-resistant mutations in HIV reverse transcriptase. (Adapted from Larder *et al.*, 1995, with permission.)

Drug	Codon within RT
Zidovudine	41, 67, 70, 210, 215, 219
Stavudine	75
Didanosine	65, 69, 74, 75, 184
Zalcitabine	65, 69, 74, 75, 184
Lamivudine	184, 65

1995; Wainberg *et al.*, 1995). High level resistance can develop following a single mutation at codon 184 (reviewed in Larder, 1995). In one study, after 4 weeks of therapy the IC_{50} of four of five patient isolates exceeded $100\,\mu M$. The emergence of resistant variants preceded an increase in viral RNA in plasma. Despite the detection of lamivudine-resistant variants of HIV in most patients, the viral load still remained below baseline for the duration of the study. This was considered by the investigators possibly to relate to continued partial susceptibility of the mutated virus to lamivudine, or to reduced replication potential of the HIV population following development of the mutation at codon 184 (Schuurman *et al.*, 1995). Methionine to isoleucine codon 184 mutants transiently appear in persons receiving lamivudine monotherapy prior to the development of methionine to valine mutants at position 184 (Wainberg *et al.*, 1995; Schuurman *et al.*, 1995). The methionine to valine mutant isolated from patients treated with lamivudine was found to be profoundly less susceptible to the drug (1800- to 5500-fold reduced susceptibility) compared with pre-therapy strains (Kavlick *et al.*, 1995). The strains were cross-resistant to zalcitabine (4.5- to 9-fold reduced susceptibility) and hypersensitive to zidovudine (2- to 14- fold) (Kavlick *et al.*, 1995).

Combination therapy with lamivudine and zidovudine does not prevent the emergence of lamivudine-resistant isolates, which are detected within 12 weeks of commencing therapy. However, combination therapy delays the emergence of zidovudine-resistant isolates (Lamivudine Product Information). *In vitro*, emergence of resistant strains of lamivudine could be delayed by combination with non-nucleoside inhibitors (Balzarini *et al.*, 1996).

3 Synergy and antagonism

Zidovudine and lamivudine have been found to interact synergistically against HIV-1 *in vitro* (Mathez *et al.*, 1993; Merrill *et al.*, 1996). Rarely, lamivudine and zidovudine have been found to act antagonistically rather than synergistically (Lamivudine Product Information). Zidovudine has no antagonistic effect on the phosphorylation of lamivudine, compared with stavudine (p. 1658) (Data on file, GlaxoWellcome). There is evidence of additive to synergistic activity between lamivudine and either zalcitabine, zidovudine, stavudine or didanosine (Merrill *et al.*, 1996; Bridges *et al.*, 1996). Lamivudine, zidovudine and didanosine used *in vitro* as a triple drug combination has been found to be more potent in inhibiting HIV replication than a number of other triple combinations including lamivudine, zidovudine and zalcitabine (St Clair *et al.*, 1995). Lamivudine is synergistic with stavudine, saquinavir, or nevirapine *in vitro*, and the three-drug combinations of lamivudine and zidovudine in combination with saquinavir or nevirapine have also been reported to be synergistic (Merrill *et al.*, 1996). Ganciclovir and ciprofloxacin have been found to reduce the antiviral potency of lamivudine *in vitro*, with a modest (2- to 3-fold) increase in IC_{50} (Data on file, GlaxoWellcome).

4 Hepatitis B virus

Duck hepatitis B virus replication in primary hepatocyte cultures is suppressed by lamivudine with an IC_{50} of $0.44\,\mu M$, through termination of viral DNA polymerase activity (Severini *et al.*, 1995). Lamivudine treatment of hepatitis B virus-transfected human hepatoma cell lines inhibits the production of hepatitis B virus DNA during the course of exposure; viral production rebounds on removal of drug (Data on file, GlaxoWellcome). The deoxycytidine deaminase-resistant (-) enantiomer is the active stereoisomer in inhibiting the replication of hepatitis B virus (Doong *et al.*, 1991; Chang *et al.*, 1992; Mansour *et al.*, 1995). Lamivudine also reduces DNA levels in the serum of hepatitis B infected chimpanzees and ducks (Tyrell *et al.*, 1993).

5 Other viruses

Simian immunodeficiency virus is sensitive to lamivudine (Balzarini *et al.*, 1995). Lamivudine has not been found to inhibit the replication of herpes simplex viruses types 1 and 2, varicella-zoster virus, human cytomegalovirus, Epstein–Barr virus, influenza virus types A and B, respiratory syncytial virus, human rhinoviruses types 2 and 14. The IC_{50} for each was greater than $400\,\mu M$ (Coates *et al.*, 1992b).

6 Other organisms

Lamivudine has no activity against a range of bacteria including *Staphylococcus aureus*, *Escherichia coli*, *Enterobacteria cloacae*, *Klebsiella aerogenes*, *Citrobacter* spp, *Proteus* spp, *Morganella morganii*, *Pseudomonas aeruginosa* and *Serratia marcescens* at concentrations of up to 62 µg per ml, *Mycobacteria avium* and *M. tuberculosis* at concentrations of up to 200 µg per ml, fungi including *Candida albicans*, *Candida glabrata*, *Cryptococcus neoformans* at concentrations of up to 125 µg per ml ($544\,\mu M$), *Pneumocystis carinii* and *Entamoeba histolytica* (Lamivudine Product Information, and Data on file, GlaxoWellcome).

7 Related compounds

In different cell lines and primary cell lines *in vitro* 2',3'-dideoxy-5-fluoro-3'-thiacytidine (FTC) is also an extremely potent inhibitor of HIV 1 and 2, simian immunodeficiency virus, feline immunodeficiency virus and hepatitis B virus. The (-) enantiomer is more potent than the (+) enantiomer (Schinazi *et al.*, 1992b; Furman *et al.*, 1992; Mansour *et al.*, 1995). Strains of HIV that are resistant to lamivudine are also cross-resistant to FTC (Tisdale *et al.*,1993).

Mode of Administration and Dosage

1 Adults and children with HIV infection

The recommended dose of lamivudine in adults is 4 mg per kg per day in two divided doses (for those weighing less than 50 kg), or 150 mg twice-daily, in combination with zidovudine. In children aged 3 months to 12 years the recommended dose is 8 mg per kg daily in two divided doses. There are no data on combination therapy using lamivudine and zidovudine in pediatric patients.

The mean oral bioavailability of lamivudine in adults was assessed in a phase I open-label study of 20 asymptomatic HIV infected individuals and found to be 82% (van Leeuwen *et al.*, 1992). In children the oral bioavailability is significantly lower (approximately 65%), thus the recommended dose in children is higher.

Although the systemic exposure (as assessed by AUC) is not significantly different, the C_{max} of oral lamivudine is 40% ± 23% lower and the time to C_{max} (T_{max}) is slower (3.2 ± 1.3 h versus 0.9 ± 0.3 h) when taken with food than in the fasted state (Lamivudine Product Information). Therefore, although absorption is delayed and the maximum concentration in the plasma is reduced, the amount of drug absorbed is not reduced and thus lamivudine can be taken without regard to food.

2 Adults with hepatitis B infection

The drug is not yet indicated for the treatment of hepatitis B but doses of 25–300 mg daily have been used with evidence of viral suppression and no serious adverse reactions in patients receiving 100 or 300 mg of lamivudine daily (Dienstag *et al.*, 1995).

3 Impaired renal function

In limited studies of adult patients with impaired renal function there is an increase in the AUC, C_{max} and half-life, proportional to the decrease in creatinine clearance. Thus the dosage of lamivudine should be modified in patients over 16 years of age with renal impairment (Table V.37).

4 Elderly

There have not been any pharmacokinetic studies in the elderly.

Availability

Oral tablets: containing 150 mg of lamivudine.

Oral solution: containing 10 mg of lamivudine per ml.

Table V.37
Adjustment of dosage of lamivudine in accordance with creatinine clearance. (Reproduced from Lamivudine Product Information GlaxoWellcome, with permission.)

Creatinine clearance (ml per min)	Recommended dosage of lamivudine
>50	150 mg twice-daily
30–49	150 mg once-daily
15–29	150 mg first dose, then 100 mg once-daily
5–14	150 mg first dose, then 50 mg once-daily
<5	50 mg first dose, then 25 mg once-daily

Serum Levels in Relation to Dose

The concentration of lamivudine in plasma and urine can be measured by an automated high performance liquid chromatography method (Hsyu and Lloyd, 1994; Harker *et al.*, 1994).

1 Oral therapy

Single oral doses of lamivudine show linearity over the dose-range 0.25–8 mg per kg. With chronic dosing, oral lamivudine (2 mg per kg twice-daily) results in a peak serum concentration (C_{max}) of $1.5 \pm 0.5 \mu g$ per ml, with both C_{max} and area-under-the-curve (AUC) increasing linearly over the dose range of 0.25–10 mg per kg. The T_{max} was 1–1.5 h in the majority of patients (Lamivudine Product Information and Data on file, GlaxoWellcome). Steady-state levels are achieved by day 15 of oral therapy. There is some accumulation of drug with time, with an accumulation ratio as measured by AUC on day 1 and day 15 ranging from 1.06 and 1.67, with the lower ratios occurring with higher dose levels (Data on file, GlaxoWellcome). Trough plasma levels have been reported as $0.7 \mu M$ ($0.14 \mu g$ per ml) (St Clair *et al.*, 1995).

The pharmacokinetics of lamivudine do not significantly alter when given in combination with zidovudine. Similarly, zidovudine pharmacokinetics are not altered appreciably by lamivudine co- therapy (Table V.38).

2 Intravenous therapy

In a dose-ranging pharmacokinetic study the C_{max} and AUC demonstrated linear pharmacokinetics over single doses of 0.25 mg per kg to 8 mg per kg administered i.v.

3 Pediatric patients

In pediatric patients with HIV infection (ages ranging from 4.8 months to 16 years, weight ranging from 5 to 66 kg), the absolute bioavailability was found to be lower than that in adults ($66\% \pm 26\%$ versus $86\% \pm 16\%$). The C_{max} is $1.1 \pm 0.6 \mu g$ per ml, and the half-life is lower than that in adults (2.0 ± 0.6 h and 3.7 ± 1 h respectively). The systemic clearance decreases with increasing age. The AUC for children receiving the recommended dose of 8 mg per kg daily and adults receiving the recommended adult dose of 4 mg per kg daily were similar.

4 Renal impairment

In a study of HIV-infected and uninfected individuals there was an increase in half-life from 11.5 h in those with normal renal function to 20.7 h in those with severe renal impairment. There was also a 2-fold increase in C_{max} (Data on file, GlaxoWellcome).

Excretion and Distribution

The majority (approximately 70%) of an oral dose of lamivudine is excreted unchanged in urine (van Leeuwen *et al.*, 1992). Following a single oral dose of lamivudine, the only identified metabolite was the *trans*-sulfoxide derivative which is also cleared by the kidneys, accounting for 5.2% of the dose excreted in the urine. There are no data regarding serum levels of this metabolite (Lamivudine Product Information).

The mean elimination half-life following a single oral dose of lamivudine ranges from 5 to 7 h, and is independent of the dose over the range 0.25–10 mg per kg (Lamivudine Product Information).

Table V.38
Pharmacodynamic parameters of lamivudine and zidovudine alone and in combination. (Adapted from Product Monograph, with permission.)

Drug	C_{max} (ng per ml)	AUC (ng.h per ml)	t_{max} (h)	$t_{1/2}$ (h)
Lamivudine				
Alone	588	1326	0.54	1.6
In combination	552	1326	0.34	0.8
Zidovudine				
Alone	695	383	0.25	0.6
In combination	690	564	0.14	0.56

In lactating rats, breast milk concentrations of lamivudine were slightly higher than plasma concentrations. There are no human data available. Nursing mothers are advised by the manufacturer to discontinue nursing if they are to receive lamivudine therapy (Lamivudine Product Information).

In animal studies the ratio of lamivudine in cerebrospinal fluid (CSF) compared with plasma is higher in lumbar CSF than ventricular CSF following an i.v. dose of 20 mg per kg (mean of 0.41 and 0.08 respectively) (Blaney *et al.*, 1995). The penetration of lamivudine into CSF in adults is poor (similar to that of didanosine and zalcitabine), with a reported CSF to plasma ratio of 0.06 (van Leeuwen *et al.*, 1995). In a study of eight pediatric patients receiving 8 mg per kg daily the CSF concentrations of lamivudine ranged from 5.6% to 30.9% of plasma concentrations (Lamivudine Product Information). Approximately one-fifth to one-third of lamivudine is bound to plasma proteins (Lamivudine Product Information).

The mean volume of distribution of lamivudine was assessed in 20 asymptomatic HIV-infected individuals and found to be 96 liters, with a mean clearance of 24 liters per h (Hussey *et al.*, 1994). The volume of distribution has been found to be independent of the dose of lamivudine and to not correlate with body weight (Lamivudine Product Information).

There are no available data as to whether lamivudine crosses the human placenta, although in a female pregnant rat the fetal plasma concentration of lamivudine ranged from 13 to 50% of maternal plasma concentrations 1 h post-dose, and 82% at 4 h (Data on file, Glaxo Wellcome).

Mode of Action

Lamivudine is a dideoxypyrimidine (analog of cytosine) that is a selective inhibitor of HIV replication. The compound lacks the hydroxyl group at the 3' carbon of the ribose, and the 3' carbon is replaced by a sulfur atom.

The mechanism of action for HIV is through competitive inhibition of HIV reverse transcriptase by lamivudine triphosphate. The phosphorylated compound then becomes incorporated into the growing DNA chain, resulting in chain-termination of reverse transcription (Hart *et al.*, 1992; Arts and Wainberg, 1994). Chain-termination occurs when lamivudine triphosphate is incorporated into the growing DNA chain in place of dCTP (Hart *et al.*, 1992). This mechanism of action is essentially similar to zidovudine (p. 1670), didanosine (p. 1717) and zalcitabine (p. 1736), although differences in phosphorylation exist. Like zalcitabine and didanosine, lamivudine produces higher ratios of dideoxycytidine triphosphate than deoxycytidine triphosphate in resting cells than in activated cells, and is thus more potent against HIV in resting cells (Gao *et al.*, 1994). Furthermore, lamivudine triphosphate is several orders of magnitude less efficient as a substrate for reverse transcriptase than zidovudine triphosphate (Data on file, GlaxoWellcome).

In studies where HIV-infected and uninfected peripheral blood lymphocytes were incubated with drug for 4 h, the triphosphate derivative of lamivudine was shown to comprise 40% of more of the total intracellular concentration of lamivudine (Cammack *et al.*, 1992). The intracellular half-life of lamivudine triphosphate ranges from 10.5 to 15.5 h (Cammack *et al.*, 1992). There is a linear relationship between the extracellular and intracellular concentrations of lamivudine up to an extracellular concentration of 10 μM (Gray *et al.*, 1995).

The mechanism of action of lamivudine against hepatitis B virus replication is by acting as a chain-terminator of DNA polymerase activity (Severini *et al.*, 1995).

Toxicity

The (-) enantiomer of racemic 2'-deoxy-3'-thiacytidine is considerably less toxic than the (+) enantiomer, although they are equipotent against HIV-1 and -2 (Coates *et al.*, 1992a). Lamivudine is associated with relatively few adverse reactions.

1 Main reported side-effects in clinical trials in adults

In an open-label phase I trial of lamivudine in 20 asymptomatic HIV infected persons, the main adverse event was mild headache (van Leeuwen *et al.*, 1992). In two phase I/II trials of lamivudine (0.5–20 mg per kg daily) in patients with AIDS or advanced HIV infection, as well as those at earlier stages of disease the only reported symptoms were mild headache, insomnia, nausea, diarrhea and abdominal pain, and a trend towards a lower neutrophil count in patients receiving the higher doses (Pluda *et al.*, 1995; van Leeuwin *et al.*, 1995). When used in combination with zidovudine in patients with predominantly asymptomatic HIV infection, adverse events were similar to those encountered with zidovudine monotherapy and of similar incidence (Eron *et al.*, 1995). When lamivudine has been used in adult patients with chronic hepatitis B infection, in doses of up to 300 mg per day, the drug is well tolerated, with only minor adverse reactions reported that were not dose-related, were asymptomatic and mainly resolved with continuation of therapy. These include elevations in serum lipase (in 12%) and amylase (in 6%) and transient elevations in creatinine kinase (in 12%). There were no reported cases of acidosis, anion gap, myopathy, hepatic decompensation, or renal impairment (Dienstag *et al.*, 1995).

2 Pancreatitis

The manufacturer recommends that HIV-infected pediatric patients with a history of pancreatitis or who have significant risk factors for the development of pancreatitis should only receive lamivudine if there is no acceptable alternative therapy, and should be monitored closely for symptoms or signs suggestive of pancreatitis. This is based on data from two studies. In the first, pancreatitis developed in 14% of 97 children receiving lamivudine monotherapy. In a second study of 47 children receiving open-label combination therapy with lamivudine and either zidovudine, didanosine or triple therapy with these drugs, 15% developed pancreatitis (Lamivudine Product Information).

3 Inhibition of cellular polymerases

Lamivudine triphosphate is a weak inhibitor of cellular alpha, beta and gamma DNA polymerases, less potent than zidovudine, zalcitabine or didanosine (Somadossi *et al.*, 1992; Hart *et al.*, 1992). Although lamivudine has been shown to inhibit mitochondrial DNA synthesis in T cell lines, this occurs only when cells are incubated with 500 μM lamivudine, 10-fold higher than the concentration required to inhibit mitochondrial DNA synthesis by zidovudine and didanosine (50 μM). The cytotoxicity of lamivudine in T cell lines and myeloid cells is lower than that of zidovudine, zalcitabine and didanosine (Somadossi *et al.*, 1992). An isolated case report describes an HIV-infected individual with a prior history of peripheral neuropathy that developed coincident with zidovudine and zalcitabine therapy and which partially resolved over 18 months post-therapy. Within 3 weeks of commencing lamivudine, painful burning and paresthesia developed in his lower limbs, with improvement following cessation of lamivudine and recurrence when rechallenged with the drug (Cupler and Dalakas, 1995).

4 Carcinogenicity and mutagenicity studies in animals

Data from long-term carcinogenicity studies are not yet available. Based upon disposition data, the rat is closest to the human, and thus most likely the most appropriate animal model for toxicity studies. Lamivudine was mutagenic in some *in vitro* studies, but did not induce chromosomal damage in bone marrow cells in rats receiving up to 2000 mg per kg. In reproduction studies in rats, lamivudine was not associated with teratogenic effects, or altered reproductive performance in doses of up to 130-fold more than the usual adult oral dose (Lamivudine Product Information). However, embryo deaths were observed in rabbits at significantly lower doses (5-fold more than the recommended adult human dose), and minor skeletal abnormalities were noted in rabbits receiving doses as low as 15 mg per kg daily (Data on file, GlaxoWellcome).

5 Acute toxicity data in animals

Acute toxicity studies in mouse and rat resulted in no deaths in mice at oral doses of up to 2000 mg per kg and less than 20% mortality in rats exposed to 2000 mg per kg i.v. During i.v. administration, animals developed hyperactivity, abnormal gait, rapid respiration and hunched posture (Data on file, GlaxoWellcome). In long-term dosing of lamivudine in the range of 1000–4000 mg per kg daily, mild decreases in hemoglobin, neutrophil and lymphocyte counts were observed and inflammatory changes developed in the cecum (Data on file, GlaxoWellcome).

6 Drug interactions

Trimethoprim-sulphamethoxazole co-administration with lamivudine results in an increase in the lamivudine AUC by 44% and reduced renal clearance of the drug (by 30%). There is no alteration to the pharmacokinetic properties of trimethoprim sulphamethoxazole (Lamivudine Product Information). There is an interaction between lamivudine and zidovudine when used in combination: lamivudine increases the AUC for zidovudine by 13% and the C_{max} for zidovudine by 28%; zidovudine only slightly increases the AUC and C_{max} for lamivudine. These interactions are regarded as being insignificant. There is no alteration in the AUC of lamivudine, or zidovudine or didanosine in children treated with lamivudine, zidovudine and didanosine triple combination (Data on file, GlaxoWellcome).

Clinical

1 Human immunodeficiency virus infection

Lamivudine is not indicated as monotherapy for the treatment of HIV infection, due to only limited efficacy and rapid development of resistance. Lamivudine is indicated in combination with zidovudine for the treatment of HIV infection, based on clinical trial surrogate endpoint data. In current clinical practise, lamivudine is often used in combination with a nucleoside analog, such as zidovudine or stavudine, together with a protease inhibitor.

In a phase I/II dose-ranging study of lamivudine in 97 patients with advanced HIV disease (median CD4 count at entry 128 per μl), lamivudine monotherapy (in doses of 8 mg per kg daily or greater) was associated with a transient immunologic and virologic benefit (Pluda et al., 1995). An open-label, multinational non-comparative escalating dose (0.5–20 mg per kg per day) phase I/II study conducted in Europe enrolled 104 patients. Sustained reductions in plasma HIV RNA were observed in those receiving the higher doses although these data did not achieve statistical significance (Ingrand et al., 1995). In a phase I/II substudy involving 20 patients with asymptomatic or mildly symptomatic HIV infection treated with lamivudine (0.5–20 mg per kg daily), there was approximately a 70% decline in HIV RNA and p24 antigen in plasma 3 days after commencing therapy, with a nadir (95% reduction in viral load or a more than 1.3 $\log_{10}$ reduction) recorded 1–2 weeks after commencing therapy (Schuurman et al., 1995). The non-sustained benefit is due to the rapid emergence of resistant variants of HIV-1 (p. 1747). In this study there was no consistent dose-response of surrogate markers to therapy, and improvement was detected only within the first 4 weeks of therapy (van Leeuwen et al., 1995).

There have been four pivotal studies in adults demonstrating efficacy of lamivudine (Table V.39).

The NUCA 3001 study was a randomized, double-blind multicentered study in 366 zidovudine-naive patients (defined in this study as up to 4 weeks of prior zidovudine therapy) in the USA with CD4 counts of 200–500 cells per μl. The patients were randomized to receive

Table V.39
Pivotal studies of lamivudine in combination with zidovudine in adults. (Reproduced from Lamivudine Product Information with permission.)

Protocol	Study design patients	Treatment doses	Number randomized	Duration of treatment	0–24 weeks Mean time-weighted change CD4	0–24 weeks Mean time-weighted change $\log_{10}$ HIV RNA	0–52 weeks 52 weeks change from baseline CD4	0–52 weeks 52 weeks change from baseline $\log_{10}$ HIV RNA
NUCA 3001	DB, MC ZDV-naive CD4 200–500	Lam 300 mg twice-daily ZDV 200 mg thrice-daily ZDV + Lam 150 mg ZDV + Lam 300 mg	87 93 92 94	24 weeks DB DB continuation	24 17 55 45	−0.59 −0.31 −1.12 −1.15	−11 −53 61 60	−0.32 −0.14 −0.80 −1.04
NUCA 3002	DB, MC ZDV-experienced CD4 100–300	ZDV + ddC 0.75 mg ZDV + Lam 150 mg ZDV + Lam 300 mg	86 84 84	24 weeks DB DB continuation	−2 38 39	−0.66 −0.80 −0.91	16 35 27	−0.50 −0.48 −0.55
NUCB 3001	DB, MC ZDV-naive CD4 100–400	ZDV 200 mg thrice-daily ZDV + Lam 300 mg	64 65	24 weeks DB OL continuation	18 75	−0.57 −1.33		
NUCB 3002	DB, MC ZDV-experienced CD4 100–400	ZDV 200 mg thrice-daily ZDV + Lam 150 mg ZDV + Lam 300 mg	73 75 75	24 weeks DB OL continuation	−18 38 32	−0.07 −0.96 −0.77		

Zidovudine given at a dose of 200 mg thrice-daily in all studies. Lamivudine dosed twice-daily in all studies.
ZDV: zidovudine; DB,MC: double-blind, multicenter; Lam: lamivudine; OL: open-label

lamivudine (300 mg twice-daily), zidovudine monotherapy (200 mg three times daily), or combination therapy with zidovudine and lamivudine (150 mg twice-daily or 300 mg twice-daily). The duration of treatment was initially for 24 weeks, with continuation in a double-blind fashion for an additional 28 weeks. Most (approximately 75%) of participants had asymptomatic HIV infection, with a median CD4 count at entry of 352 cells per μl. After 24 weeks the mean $\log_{10}$ declines in plasma HIV RNA in patients randomized to receive lamivudine monotherapy, zidovudine monotherapy, low-dose lamivudine combination therapy and high-dose lamivudine combination therapy were 0.59, 0.31, 1.12 and 1.15 respectively. After 52 weeks of therapy the only arm of the trial to maintain a mean of greater than a 1 $\log_{10}$ decline in plasma HIV RNA was the high-dose lamivudine combination group. Both combination arms and lamivudine monotherapy arms maintained a mean increase in CD4 counts above baseline after 52 weeks of therapy (Eron et al., 1995).

The NUCB 3001 trial was a second randomized, double-blind, multicentered study (Europe and Australia) in 129 zidovudine-naive patients with CD4 counts ranging from 100 to 400 cells per μl. Participants were randomized to receive zidovudine monotherapy (600 mg per day) or zidovudine in combination with lamivudine (300 mg twice-daily) for an initial duration of 24 weeks which was extended to continue in an open-label fashion with all participants offered combination therapy from week 24 to 48. Two-thirds of participants had asymptomatic HIV infection, and the median CD4 count at study entry was 260 cells per μl. After 4 weeks the decline in HIV RNA was significantly greater in those randomized to receive combination therapy versus monotherapy (greater than 1.7 and 0.7 $\log_{10}$ copies per ml respectively) (Harrigan, 1995). After 24 weeks of therapy, the mean $\log_{10}$ decline in plasma HIV RNA in monotherapy and combination therapy arms was 0.57 and 1.33 respectively. The increase in CD4 counts above baseline was significantly higher in the combination arm than in those randomized to receive zidovudine monotherapy (18 and 75 cells per μl respectively). Initial combination therapy was associated with better responses than initial monotherapy followed by a switch to combination therapy after 24 weeks (Staszewski, 1995; Katlama et al., 1996).

The NUCA 3002 trial was another randomized multicenter study in 254 zidovudine-experienced patients in the USA with CD4 counts in the range 100–300 cells per μl. The participants were randomized to receive zidovudine in combination with zalcitabine (0.75 mg three times daily), or zidovudine in combination with either high-dose lamivudine (300 mg twice-daily) or low-dose lamivudine (150 mg twice-daily). The median duration of prior zidovudine use was 24 months, with a median CD4 cell count at entry of 211 cells per μl; 58% of patients had asymptomatic HIV infection. After 24 weeks the mean $\log_{10}$ declines in patients receiving the zidovudine/zalcitabine, zidovudine/high-dose lamivudine and zidovudine/low-dose lamivudine combination therapies were 0.66, 0.80, and 0.91 respectively, with only the lamivudine combination therapies maintaining an increase in CD4 above baseline. After 52 weeks of therapy the three arms had similar mean $\log_{10}$ declines in plasma HIV RNA (0.50, 0.48, 0.55 respectively; Data on file, GlaxoWellcome). Dual zidovudine- and lamivudine-resistance was seen in isolates from 19% of participants (Johnson et al., 1995).

The NUCB 3002 trial was a randomized double-blind multicenter study in 223 zidovudine-experienced patients in Europe and Australia with CD4 counts ranging from 100 to 300 cells per μl who were randomized to receive zidovudine monotherapy or in combination with lamivudine (150 mg twice-daily or 300 mg twice-daily) for 24 weeks followed by open-label therapy of lamivudine plus optional zidovudine for a further 24 weeks. The median duration of prior zidovudine use was 23 months, and the median CD4 at entry was 211 cells per μl. After 24 weeks the mean $\log_{10}$ declines in plasma HIV RNA were 0.07, 0.96 and 0.77 in patients treated with zidovudine monotherapy, or low-dose lamivudine in combination with zidovudine, or high-dose lamivudine in combination with zidovudine respectively. Only patients receiving combination therapy maintained a mean CD4 count above baseline (Staszewski, 1995; Staszewski et al., 1996). By week 12 of study, virtually all of the tested samples from patients receiving combination therapy with zidovudine and lamivudine had evidence of mutation at codon 184 of reverse transcriptase (Harrigan et al., 1995).

The NUCB 3007 (Caesar) study was a randomized controlled double-blind trial to compare the efficacy and safety of lamivudine monotherapy versus lamivudine and loviride versus placebo in the treatment of persons with HIV infection with 25–250 CD4 cells per μl who were concurrently taking zidovudine either as monotherapy or in combination with either zalcitabine or didanosine. The duration of the study was for 52 weeks with a 52 week extension during which all patients were offered open-label lamivudine and loviride. A total of 1892 patients were enrolled into the study, with a median CD4 on study entry of 131 cells per μl. At baseline 62% were taking concurrent zidovudine monotherapy. A preliminary analysis of data has demonstrated that the time to progression to a new AIDS-defining illness or death was significantly lower in those receiving lamivudine (9%) or lamivudine/loviride (8%) than in those randomized to placebo (17%; p <0.0001) . The use of loviride did not provide any additional clinical benefit over the addition of lamivudine. In a subset of 332 patients CD4 counts and viral RNA were analyzed at 28 weeks. There was an increase of 28 CD4 cells per μl above baseline in the lamivudine arm (compared with a decrease of 18 cells per μl below baseline in the control arm) and 0.3 $\log_{10}$ reduction in plasma HIV RNA below baseline in the lamivudine arm (compared with an increase of 0.1 $\log_{10}$ above baseline levels in the control arm) (Data on file, GlaxoWellcome).

A dose-escalation monotherapy study of lamivudine (1–20 mg per kg daily) given for a duration of 24 weeks to antiretroviral-naive and -experienced children aged 3 months to 17 years demonstrated early resistance to lamivudine (Lewis *et al.*, 1996). There is also an ongoing open-label comparative study of lamivudine (8 mg per kg daily) in combination with zidovudine, didanosine or both, in HIV-infected children (3 months–18 years) for a duration of 24 weeks.

2 Hepatitis B virus infection

Phase I and II studies of lamivudine have demonstrated a potent antiviral effect in patients with chronic hepatitis B infection (Schalm *et al.*, 1995). Similarly lamivudine treatment (dose of 300 mg twice-daily) of 11 patients coinfected with hepatitis B and HIV (mean CD4 count of 73 cells per μl) was associated with a rapid reduction of HBV DNA in plasma to undetectable levels within 2 months of commencing therapy (Benhamou *et al.*, 1995). The drug has been tested in trials in the setting of hepatitis B requiring liver transplantation with preliminary evidence of success (Grellier *et al.*, 1995; Gutfreund *et al.*, 1995).

A double-blind trial of 32 patients with chronic hepatitis B infection including 17 prior non-responders to interferon alpha therapy were randomized to receive 25, 100 or 300mg of

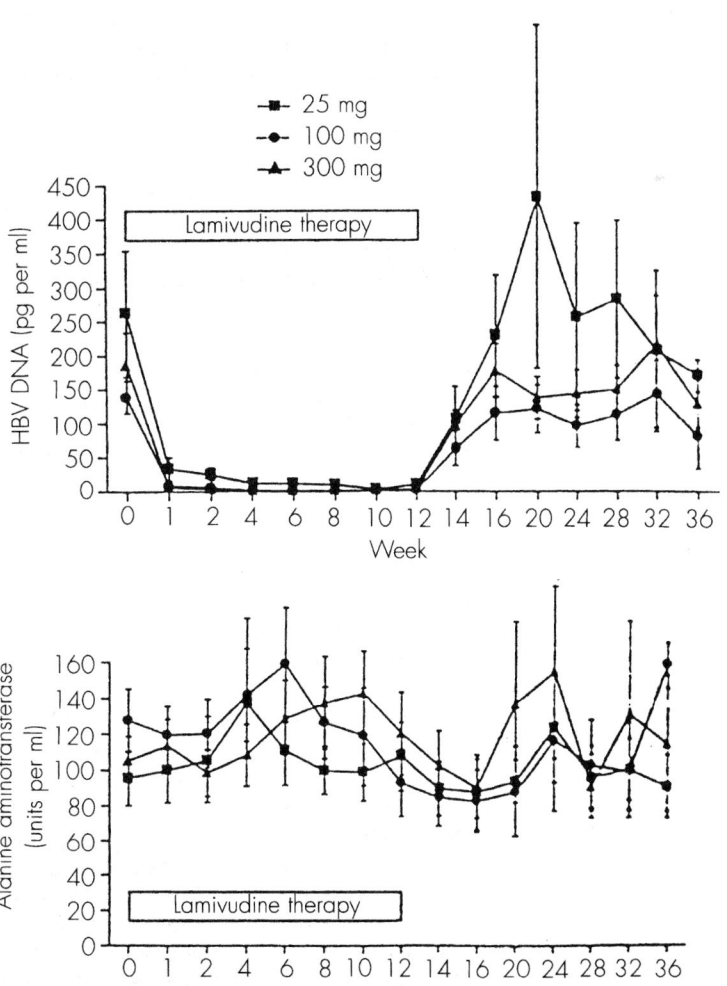

Fig. V.49.

Changes in mean (=SE) serum levels of HBV DNA (upper panel) and alanine aminotransferase (lower panels) during and after 12 weeks of therapy with 25, 100 or 300 mg of lamivudine. (Reproduced from Dienstag *et al.*, 1995, with permission. Copyright, 1995, Massachusetts Medical Society. All rights reserved.)

lamivudine daily for 12 weeks. Monitoring continued for an additional 24 weeks post-therapy. The two higher doses similarly suppressed plasma HBV DNA to undetectable levels in 100% of recipients, and this response was sustained in six of 32 (19%). Sustained suppression of HBV DNA was associated with a return of serum transaminases to normal values. In the rest of the participants levels of HBV DNA were again detected in plasma following cessation of therapy. Also HBV DNA fell to undetectable levels in 70% of the recipients of the lowest dose of lamivudine. Earlier suppression was achieved with the 300-mg daily dose. Prior non-responders to interferon alpha were responsive to lamivudine, and included five of the six sustained lamivudine responders. The level of HBV DNA in plasma was lower in those whose response to lamivudine was sustained than in transient responders (Dienstag *et al.*, 1995; Fig. V.49).

Acknowledgements The author wishes to thank Don Smith of the Community HIV Research Network, Sydney, for his critical review of this chapter.

References

Arts EJ, Wainberg MA (1994). Preferential incorporation of nucleoside analogs after template switching during human immunodeficiency virus reverse transcription. *Antimicrob Ag Chemother* **38**: 1008.

Back NK, Nijhuis M, Keulen N et al. (1996). Reduced replication of 3TC-resistant HIV variants in primary cells due to a processivity defect of the reverse transcriptase enzyme. *EMBO J* **15**: 4040.

Balzarini J, Weeger M, Camarasa MJ et al. (1995). Sensitivity-resistance profile of a simian immunodeficiency virus containing the reverse transcriptase gene of human immunodeficiency virus type 1 (HIV-1) toward the HIV-1 specific non-nucleoside reverse transcriptase inhibitors. *Biochem Biophy Res Commun* **211**: 850.

Balzarini J, Pelemans H, Perez-Perez MJ et al. (1996). Marked inhibitory activity of non- nucleoside reverse transcriptase inhibitors against human immunodeficiency virus type 1 when combined with (-)2'-3'-dideoxy-3'-thiacytidine. *Mol Pharmacol* **49**: 882.

Benhamou Y, Dohin E, Lunel-Fabiani F et al. (1995). Efficacy of lamivudine on replication of hepatitis B virus in HIV-infected patients. *Lancet* **345**: 396.

Blaney SM, Daniel MJ, Harker AJ et al. (1995). Pharmacokinetics of lamivudine and BCH-189 in plasma and cerebrospinal fluid of nonhuman primates. *Antimicrob Ag Chemother* **39**: 2779.

Boucher CA, Cammack N, Schipper P et al. (1993). High-level resistance to (-) enantiomeric 2'- deoxy-3'-thiacytidine in vitro is due to one amino acid substitution in the catalytic site of human immunodeficiency virus type 1 reverse transcriptase. *Antimicrob Ag Chemother* **37**: 2231.

Boyer PL, Hughes SH (1995). Analysis of mutations at position 184 in reverse transcriptase of human immunodeficiency virus type 1. *Antimicrob Ag Chemother* **39**: 1624.

Bridges EG, Detschman GE, Gullen EA Cheng YC (1996). Favourable interaction of beta-L(-) nucleoside analogues with clinically approved anti-HIV nucleoside analogues for the treatment of human immunodeficiency virus. *Biochem Pharmacol* **51**: 731.

Cammack N, Rouse P, Marr CL et al. (1992). Cellular metabolism of (-) enamtiomeric 2'-deoxy- 3'-thiacytidine. *Biochem Pharmacol* **43**: 2059.

Chang CN, Doong SL, Zhou JH et al. (1992). Deoxycytidine deaminase-resistant steroisomer is the active form of (±)-2',3'-dideoxy-3'-thiacytidine in the inhibition of hepatitis B virus replication. *J Biol Chem* **267**: 13938.

Coates JA, Cammack N, Jenkinson HJ et al. (1992a). The separated enantiomers of 2'-deoxy-3'- thiacytidine (BCH 189) both inhibit human immunodeficiency virus replication in vitro. *Antimicrob Ag Chemother* **36**: 202.

Coates JA, Cammack N, Jenkinson HJ et al. (1992b). (-)-2'-deoxy-3'-thiacytidine is a potent, highly selective inhibitor of human immuno-

deficiency virus type 1 and type 2 replication in vitro. *Antimicrob Ag Chemother* **36**: 733.

Cupler EJ, Dalakas MC (1995). Exacerbation of peripheral neuropathy by lamivudine. *Lancet* **345**: 460.

Data on file, GlaxoWellcome.

Dienstag JL, Perrillo RP, Schiff ER et al. (1995). A preliminary trial of lamivudine for chronic hepatitis B infection. *New Engl J Med* **333**: 1657.

Doong SL, Tsai CH, Schinazi RF et al. (1991). Inhibition of the replication of hepatitis B virus in vitro by 2',3'-dideoxy-3'-thiacytidine and related analogues. *Proc Natl Acad Sci USA* **88**: 8495.

Eron JJ, Benoit SL, Jemsek J et al. (1995). Treatment with lamivudine, zidovudine, or both in HIV-positive patients with 200 to 500 CD4+ cells per cubic millimetre. North American HIV Working Party. *New Engl J Med* **333**: 1662.

Faraj A, Agrofoglio LA, Wakefield JK et al. (1994). Inhibition of human immunodeficiency virus type 1 reverse transcriptase by the 5'-triphosphate beta enantiomers of cytidine analogs. *Antimicrob Ag Chemother* **38**: 2300.

Furman PA, Davis M, Liotta DC et al. (1992). The anti-hepatitis B virus activities, cytotoxicities, and anabolic profiles of the (-) and (+) enantiomers of cis-5-fluoro-1-[2-(hydroxymethyl)-1,3-oxathiolan-5yl]cytosine. *Antimicrob Ag Chemother* **36**: 2686.

Gao Q, Gu Z, Parniak MA et al. (1993). The same mutation that encodes low-level human immunodeficiency virus type 1 resistance to 2',3'-dideoxyinosine and 2',3'-dideoxycytidine confers high-level resistance to the (-) enantiomer of 2',3'-dideoxy-3'-thiacytidine. *Antimicrob Ag Chemother* **37**: 1390.

Gao WY, Agbaria R, Driscoll JS, Mitsuya H (1994). Divergent anti-human immunodeficiency virus activity and anabolic phosphorylation of 2',3'-dideoxynucleoside analogs in resting and activated human cells. *J Biol Chem* **269**: 12633.

Geleziunas R, Arts EJ, Boulerice F et al. (1993). Effect of 3'-azido-3'-deoxythymidine on human immunodeficiency virus type 1 replication in human fetal brain macrophages. *Antimicrob Ag Chemother* **37**: 1305.

Gray NM, Marr CL, Penn CR et al. (1995). The intracellular phosphorylation of (-)-2'-deoxy- 3'-thiacytidine (3TC) and the incorporation of 3TC 5'-monophosphate into DNA by HIV-1 reverse transcriptase and human DNA polymerase gamma. *Biochem Pharmacol* **50**: 1043.

Grellier L, Brown D, McPhillips A et al. (1995). Lamivudine prophylaxis A new strategy for prevention of reinfection in liver transplantation for hepatitis B DNA positive cirrhosis. *Hepatol* **22**: 224.

Gu Z, Gao Q, Li X et al. (1992). Novel mutation in the human immunodeficiency virus type 1 reverse transcriptase gene that encodes cross-resistance to 2',3'-dideoxyinosine and 2',3'- dideoxycytidine. *J Virol* **66**: 7128.

Gu Z, Fletcher RS, Arts EJ *et al.* (1994). The K65R mutant reverse transcriptase of HIV-1 cross- resistant to 2',3'-dideoxycytidine, 2',3'-dideoxy-3'-thiacytidine, and 2',3'-dideoxyinosine shows reduced sensitivity to specific dideoxynucleoside triphosphate inhibitors *in vitro*. *J Biol Chem* **269**: 28118.

Gu Z, Arts EJ, Parniak MA, Wainberg MA (1995a). Mutated K65R recombinant reverse transcriptase of human immunodeficiency virus type 1 shows diminished chain termination in the presence of 2',3'-dideoxycytidine 5'-triphosphate and other drugs. *Proc Natl Acad Sci USA* **92**: 2760.

Gu Z, Gao Q, Faust EA, Wainberg WA (1995b). Possible involvement of cell fusion and viral recombination in generation of human immunodeficiency virus variants that display dual resistance to AZT and 3TC. *J Gen Virol* **76**: 2601.

Gutfreund KS, Fischer KP, Tipples G *et al.* (1995). Lamivudine results in a complete and sustained suppression of hepatitis B virus replication in patients requiring orthotopic liver transplantation for cirrhosis secondary to hepatitis B. *Hepatol* **22**: 328A.

Harker AJ, Evans GL, Hawley AE, Morris DM (1994). High performance liquid chromatographic assay for 2'-deoxy-3'-thiacytidine in human serum. *J Chromatogr B Biomed Appl* **657**: 227.

Harrigan PR, Kinghorn I, Kohli A *et al.* (1995). Virological response to AZT\3TC combination therapy in AZT naive patients (Trial NUCB 3001). *J AIDS Hum Retrovir* **10**: S26.

Harrigan R (1995). Measuring viral load in the clinical setting. *J AIDS Hum Retrovir* **10**: S34.

Hart GJ, Orr DC, Penn CR *et al.* (1992). Effects of (-)-2'-deoxy-3'-thiacytidine (3TC) 5'- triphosphate on human immunodeficiency virus reverse transcriptase and mammalian DNA polymerases alpha, beta, and gamma. *Antimicrob Ag Chemother* **36**: 1688.

Hsyu PH, Lloyd TL (1994). Automated high performance liquid chromatographic analysis of (-)- 2'-deoxy-3'-thiacytidine in biological fluids using the automated sequential trace enrichment of dialysate systems. *J Chromatogr B Biomed Appl* **655**: 253.

Hussey EK, Donn KH, Daniel MJ *et al.* (1994). Interspecies scaling and pharmacokinetic parameters of 3TC in humans. *J Clin Pharmacol* **34**: 975.

Ingrand D, Weber J, Boucher CAB *et al.* (1995). Phase I/II study of 3TC (lamivudine) in HIV- positive, asymptomatic or mild AIDS-related complex patients; sustained reduction in viral markers. *AIDS* **9**: 1323.

Johnson VA, Overbay CB, Koel JL *et al.* (1995). Drug resistance, viral load, and SI phenotype in NUCA 3002: combined 3TC/ZDV therapy over a maximum of 52 weeks in ZDV-experienced (24 weeks) patients (CD4+ 100–300 cells/mm³). *5th International Workshop on HIV Drug Resistance*, Whistler, Canada 3rd-6th July.

Katlama C, Ingrand D, Loveday C *et al.* (1996). Safety and efficacy of lamivudine-zidovudine combination therapy in antiretroviral-naive patients. A randomized controlled comparison with zidovudine monotherapy. Lamuvidine European HIV Working Group. *J Amer Med Assoc* **276**: 118.

Kavlick MF, Shirasaka T, Kojima E *et al.* (1995). Genotypic and phenotypic characterisation of HIV-1 isolated from patients receiving (-) 2',3'-dideoxy-3'-thiacytidine. *Antiviral Res* **28**: 133.

Lamivudine Product Information.

Larder BA (1995). Viral resistance and the selection of antiretroviral combinations. *J AIDS Hum Retrovir* **10**: S28.

Larder BA, Kemp SD, Harrigan PR (1995). Potential mechanism for sustained antiretroviral efficacy of AZT-3TC combination therapy. *Science* **269**: 696.

Lewis LL, Venzon D, Church J *et al.* (1996). Lamivudine in children with human immunodeficiency virus infection: a phase I/II study. The National Cancer Institute Pediatric Branch – Human Immunodeficiency Virus Working Group. *J Infect Dis* **174**: 16.

Mansour TS, Jin H, Wang W *et al.* (1995). Anti-human immunodeficiency virus and anti- hepatitis B virus activities and toxicities of the enantiomers of 2'-deoxy-3'-oxa-4'-thiocytidine and their 5-fluoro analogues *in vitro*. *J Med Chem* **38**: 1.

Mathez D, Schinazi RF, Liotta DC, Leibowitch J (1993). Infectious amplification of wild-type human immunodeficiency virus from patients' lymphocytes and modulation by reverse transcriptase inhibitors *in vitro*. *Antimicrob Ag Chemother* **37**: 2206.

Merrill DP, Moonis M, Chou TC, Hirsch MS (1996). Lamivudine or stavudine in two and three drug combinations against human immunodeficiency virus type 1 replication *in vitro*. *J Infect Dis* **173**: 355.

Pluda JM, Cooley TP, Montaner JS *et al.* (1995). A phase I/II study of 2'-deoxy-3'-thiacytidine (lamivudine) in patients with advanced human immunodeficiency virus infection. *J Infect Dis* **171**: 1438.

Schalm SW, de Man RA, Heijtink RA, Niesters HG (1995). New nucleoside analogues for chronic hepatitis B. *J Hepatol* **22**: 52.

Schinazi RF, Chu CK, Peck A *et al.* (1992a). Activities of the four optical isomers of 2',3'- dideoxy-3'-thiacytidine (BCH-189) against human immunodeficiency virus type 1 in human lymphocytes. *Antimicrob Ag Chemother* **36**: 672.

Schinazi RF, McMillan A, Cannon D *et al.* (1992b). Selective inhibition of human immunodeficiency viruses by racemates and enantiomers of cis-5-fluoro-1-[2-(hydroxymethyl)-1,3- oxathiolan-5-yl]cytosine. *Antimicrob Ag Chemother* **36**: 2423.

Schinazi RF, Lloyd RM, Nguyen MH *et al.* (1993). Characterisation of human immunodeficiency viruses resistant to oxathiolane-cytosine nucleosides. *Antimicrob Ag Chemother* **37**: 875.

Schuurman R, Nijhuis M, van Leeuwen R *et al.* (1995). Rapid changes in human immunodeficiency virus type 1 RNA load and appearance of drug resistant virus populations in persons treated with lamivudine (3TC). *J Infect Dis* **171**: 1411.

Severini A, Liu XY, Wilson JS, Tyrrell DL (1995). Mechanism of inhibition of duck hepatitis B virus polymerase by (-)-beta-L-2',3'-dideoxy-3'-thiacytidine. *Antimicrob Ag Chemother* **39**: 1430.

Sommadossi JP, Schinazi RF, Chu CK *et al.* (1992). Comparison of cytotoxicity of the (-) and the (+) enantiomer of 2',3'-dideoxy-3'-thiacytidine in normal human bone marrow progenitor cells. *Biochem Pharmacol* **44**: 1921.

St Clair MH, Pennington KN, Rooney J, Barry DW (1995). *In vitro* comparison of selected triple-drug combinations for suppression of HIV-1 replication, the Inter-Company Collaboration Protocol. *J AIDS Hum Retrovir* **10**: S83.

Staszewski S (1995). Zidovudine and lamivudine; results of phase III studies. *J AIDS Hum Retrovir* **10**: S57.

Staszewski S, Loveday C, Picazo JJ *et al.* (1996). Safety and efficacy of lamuvidine-zidovudine combination therapy in zidovudine-experienced patients. A randomized controlled comparison with zidovudine monotherapy. Lamivudine European HIV Working Group. *JAMA* **276**: 111.

Tantillo CJ, Ding A, Jacobo-Molina RG *et al.* (1994). Rapid *in vitro* selection of human immunodeficiency virus type 1 resistant to 3'-thiacytidine inhibitors due to a mutation in the YMDD region of reverse transcriptase. *Proc Natl Acad Sci USA* **90**: 5653.

Tisdale M, Kemp SD, Parry NR, Larder BA (1993). Rapid *in vitro* selection of human immunodeficiency virus type 1 resistant to 3'-thiacytidine inhibitors due to a mutation in the YMDD region of reverse transcriptase. *Proc Natl Acad Sci USA* **90**: 5653.

Tyrrell DLJ, Fischer K, Savani K *et al.* (1993). Treatment of chimpanzees and ducks with lamivudine, 2',3'-dideoxy 3'-thiacytidine, results in a rapid suppression of hepaviral DNA in sera. *Clin Invest Med* **16**: B77 [abstract].

van Leeuwen R, Lange JM, Hussey EK *et al.* (1992). The safety and pharmacokinetics of a reverse transcriptase inhibitor, 3TC in patients with HIV infection; a phase 1 study. *AIDS* **6**: 1471.

van Leeuwen R, Katlama C, Kitchen V *et al.* (1995). Evaluation of safety and efficacy of 3TC (lamivudine) in patients with asymptomatic or mildly symptomatic human immunodeficiency virus infection; a phase I/II study. *J Infect Dis* **171**: 1166.

Wainberg MA, Salomon H, Gu Z *et al.* (1995). Development of HIV-1 resistance to (-)2'-deoxy- 3'-thiacytidine in patients with AIDS or advanced AIDS-related complex. *AIDS* **9**: 351.

Stavudine

Description

The nucleoside analog stavudine (2',3'-didehydro-2'3'-deoxythymidine, d4T) is a potent inhibitor of HIV reverse transcriptase *in vitro* and has received approval in a number of countries including Australia and the USA for the treatment of HIV infection. It was the fourth nucleoside inhibitor to become commercially available. It is marketed under the trade name of 'Zerit' by Bristol-Myers Squibb. Stavudine was first synthesized in 1966 by Horwitz and colleagues (Horwitz *et al.*, 1966).

The molecular weight of stavudine is 224.2. The molecular formula is $C_{10}H_{12}N_2O_4$. The chemical structure of stavudine is shown in Fig. V.50. Drug concentrations are described in μM or μg per ml (1 μM is approximately equivalent to 0.2 μg per ml).

Antiviral Activity

1 Human immunodeficiency virus

The antiretroviral activity of stavudine was first reported in 1987 (Lin *et al.*, 1987; Baba *et al.*, 1987; Hamamoto *et al.*, 1987). Stavudine inhibits the reverse transcriptase of HIV-1 *in vitro* with similar or lower potency compared with zidovudine (Inoue *et al.*, 1989; Mansuri *et al.*, 1989, 1990; Balzarini *et al.*, 1989a). The IC_{50} ranges from 0.009 to 4.1 μM (mean 0.24 μM) in peripheral blood lymphocytes and T cell lines (Friedland *et al.*, 1996), and between 0.04 and 0.3 μM in monocytes. The selectivity index in peripheral blood mononuclear cells is about 10 000 (Chu *et al.*, 1988). Stavudine has activity against both HIV-1 and HIV-2 (Balzarini *et al.*, 1989b). By plaque reduction assay, the IC_{50} for stavudine in HIV-2 infected T cells is 0.09 μM (Data on file, Bristol-Myers Squibb).

2 Other retroviruses

Stavudine has activity against Friend virus complex, with an IC_{50} of 1.2 μM, and evidence of *in vivo* activity with an oral dose of 375 mg per kg daily inhibiting disease progression in mice (Sidwell *et al.*, 1992). Moloney murine leukemia virus is also susceptible to stavudine, with an IC_{50} of 2.5 μM (100-fold higher than the concentration of zidovudine required to inhibit this virus in the same assay) (Lin *et al.*, 1987; Data on file, Bristol-Myers Squibb). Stavudine inhibits the replication of simian immunodeficiency virus, but is about 10-fold less potent than zidovudine (Tsai *et al.*, 1990). Although stavudine has activity against visna virus replication in

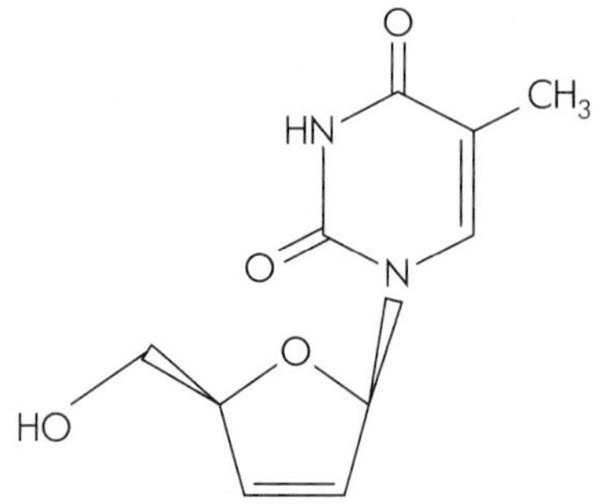

Fig. V.50
Chemical structure of stavudine.

sheep choroid plexus cells, it is less potent than zalcitabine, didanosine and equipotent to zidovudine. However, stavudine triphosphate is more inhibitory to the reverse transcriptase of visna virus than zalcitabine triphosphate. This discrepancy may possibly be due to less efficient phosphorylation of stavudine than zalcitabine in sheep choroid plexus cells (Thormar et al., 1993).

3 Resistance

Laboratory and clinical HIV-1 strains that have been sequentially passaged in T cell lines in vitro in the presence of increasing concentrations of stavudine have developed mutations conferring resistance, with IC_{50} values 20- to 30-fold greater than those of wild-type strains (Gao et al., 1994a). In vitro selection of mutations within codon 75 (Val → Thr) and codon 50 (Ile → Thr) of the reverse transcriptase gene have been described in association with stavudine-resistance, with a 7-fold and 30-fold increase in IC_{50} respectively (Lacey and Larder, 1994; Najera et al. 1994; Gu et al., 1994). Mutations associated with stavudine-resistance have also been identified in strains of HIV-1 from patients only exposed to zidovudine therapy (Najera et al., 1994).

The codon 75 mutation but not the codon 50 mutation has been detected in patients treated with stavudine. Phenotypic resistance to stavudine developed in less than 20% of tested isolates from patients treated with stavudine for 18–22 months, with 8- to 12-fold reduction in sensitivity (reviewed in Moyle, 1995). In one study, zidovudine-resistant isolates from patients previously treated with zidovudine remained sensitive to stavudine (Lin et al., 1994). This supports earlier studies in which zidovudine-resistant strains of HIV-1 failed to demonstrate evidence of cross-resistance to stavudine (Larder et al., 1989, 1990; Richman, 1990). However, clinical isolates with resistance to zidovudine and cross-resistance to stavudine have also been described (Rooke et al., 1991).

Cross-resistance to didanosine and zalcitabine has been reported with strains of HIV-1 that have the codon 75 mutation (Lacey and Larder, 1994); the mutation at codon 50 has not been associated with cross-resistance to other nucleoside analogs (Gu et al., 1994). Cross-resistance has not been demonstrated with stavudine and recombinant HIV encoding resistance to lamivudine or the non-nucleoside reverse transcriptase inhibitors (Mellors et al., 1992).

Multidrug-resistance has been reported in association with acquisition of mutations in codons 62, 75, 77, 116 and 151. These mutations have been reported to confer resistance to zidovudine, didanosine, zalcitabine, and stavudine (Iversen et al., 1996).

4 Synergy

Although antagonism has been reported between zidovudine and stavudine (p. 1658), in vitro synergy or additive effect against HIV replication has also been observed with this combination, and it may depend on the ratio of the drugs (Sorensen et al., 1993). Stavudine has been reported to be additive or synergistic with both zalcitabine and didanosine in vitro (reviewed in Friedland et al., 1996). Additive or synergistic interactions have also been found in a separate study between stavudine and lamivudine, saquinavir, nevirapine, zidovudine (with a zidovudine-sensitive isolate; see below) or didanosine (Merrill et al., 1996). GM-CSF has been found to enhance the activity of stavudine in monocyte-macrophage cultures infected with HIV-1 (Perno et al., 1989). Interferon alpha and stavudine show synergistic activity against Friend leukemia virus in vitro (Sidwell et al., 1995)

5 Antagonism

Zidovudine has been reported to inhibit the phosphorylation and thus the activity of stavudine in human lymphocytes (Ho and Hitchcock, 1989). This is attributed to the fact that thymidine kinase has significantly higher affinity for zidovudine than for stavudine. The drug combination resulted in only 3% of control levels of stavudine triphosphate. Merrill et al. (1996) have found antagonism between zidovudine and stavudine only when using a zidovudine-resistant strain of HIV.

6 Other viruses and bacteria

Stavudine has no antiviral efficacy against hepatitis B virus in vitro (Yokata et al., 1991; Lampertico et al., 1991) nor efficacy against a number of common bacteria (Hitchcock, 1991).

Table V.40
Recommended dose of stavudine for adults

Weight	Dose
≥60 kg	40 mg twice-daily
<60 kg	30 mg twice-daily

Mode of Administration and Dosage

1 Oral administration

The 5, 10, 20 and 40-mg capsules of stavudine are bioequivalent (Kaul *et al.*, 1995). The recommended doses are based on data from dose-ranging phase I studies. From two phase I dose-ranging studies it was determined that the maximum tolerated dose is 2 mg per kg daily, and the minimum effective dose is 1 mg per kg daily, based upon either a 50% decline in plasma p24 antigen level or a 50 cell per µl increase in CD4 count (Murray *et al.*, 1995; Browne *et al.*, 1993). This finding is supported by data from other phase I dose-ranging studies in which daily doses ranged from 0.1 to 12 mg per kg (reviewed in Skowron, 1995). In one of these trials, a dose of 0.5 mg per kg daily resulted in the most favorable therapeutic index (Petersen *et al.*, 1995).

The recommended dose of stavudine in patients weighing 60 kg or more is 40 mg twice-daily; for those weighing less than 60 kg the dose is 30 mg twice-daily (Anderson *et al.*, 1995; Stavudine Product Information, Bristol-Myers Squibb). The drug can be taken without regard to meals. The dosage interval should be 12 h.

No firm dosage guidelines can currently be given for children due to there being only limited data. Children between 7 months and 15 years of age have been treated with stavudine (doses ranging from 0.125 to 4 mg per kg daily) for up to 3 years, with peripheral neuropathy and elevated hepatic enzymes being the major adverse reactions. The oral bioavailability in this age group ranges from 61% to 78% (Kline *et al.*, 1995). Recently, a combination of didanosine (180 mg per m² per day in two divided doses) has been administered to eight children (median age 6.6 years, range 2.8–12 years) with advanced HIV infection (median CD4 count at baseline of 42 cells per µl). Over 24 weeks the drugs were well tolerated (Kline *et al.* 1996).

The drug should be ceased if symptoms of peripheral neuropathy develop, and may be reintroduced at half the original dose after symptoms resolve (Stavudine Product Information, Bristol-Myers Squibb). The manufacturer also recommends similar dose adjustments for patients who develop elevated serum transaminases whilst receiving stavudine therapy.

Based on preliminary data suggesting that the renal clearance of stavudine is impaired in patients with reduced creatinine clearance, the manufacturer has recommended that the dose of stavudine should be modified for patients with impaired renal function (see Table V.41). There are currently no recommendations regarding dose for patients who are undergoing hemodialysis; there are no available data as to whether stavudine is cleared by either peritoneal or hemodialysis.

There are no well-controlled data on the use of stavudine in pregnant women, and the manufacturer recommends that the drug should only be used in pregnant women if clearly needed. Similarly, due to lack of data, mothers are recommended to discontinue stavudine whilst nursing.

Table V.41
Dosage adjustments for stavudine in patients with renal dysfunction. (Reproduced from Stavudine Product Information, Bristol-Myers Squibb, with permission.)

Creatinine clearance (ml per min)	Recommended stavudine dose by patient weight	
	<60 kg	<60 kg
>50	40 mg every 12 h	30 mg every 12 h
26–50	20 mg every 12 h	15 mg every 12 h
10–25	20 mg every 24 h	15 mg every 24 h

Availability

Capsules are available in strengths of 15, 20, 30 and 40 mg of stavudine.

Serum Levels in Relation to Dosage

Serum levels of stavudine can be measured by reversed-phase high-performance liquid chromatography (Burger *et al.*, 1992; Janiszewski *et al.*, 1992). There is considerable patient to patient variation in plasma concentrations when each is administered the same dose of drug (Dudley, 1995).

1 Oral administration

Stavudine is rapidly absorbed after oral administration, with a mean bioavailability in adults following a 4 mg per kg oral dose ranging from 70 to 90% (Dudley *et al.*, 1992; Kaul and Dandekar, 1993; Cretton *et al.*, 1993; Neuzil, 1994; Kaul *et al.*, 1995). The mean oral bioavailability in HIV-infected pediatric patients is 70–80%. These values are consistent with the reported bioavailability of stavudine in mice and monkeys (Cretton *et al.*, 1993; Russell *et al.*, 1990). The high stability of stavudine at low pH and minimal pre-systemic metabolism of stavudine may account for the excellent oral bioavailability (Dudley, 1995).

Stavudine exhibits linear pharmacokinetics (Kaul *et al.*, 1995). Following oral administration of a single dose of 40 mg of stavudine the reported mean peak plasma concentration (C_{max}) of the drug is 603 ± 160 ng per ml with an area-under-the-curve (AUC) of 1246 ± 230 ng.h per ml (Seifert *et al.*, 1994). Peak plasma concentrations occur within 1 h of oral administration and increase in a dose-related manner (Kaul *et al.*, 1995) Plasma levels of stavudine decline to below 10% of C_{max} between 5 and 7 h after administration. Chronic dosing does not appreciably alter the pharmacokinetic parameters of stavudine (Dudley *et al.*, 1992).

The C_{max} of stavudine is approximately 2-fold lower when taken after a high-fat meal, and the time to C_{max} (T_{max}) is prolonged by approximately 2.5-fold (Stavudine Product Information, Bristol-Myers Squibb). However, the AUC of the drug is unaltered by food. Given the fact that the intracellular drug concentration of stavudine is more likely to reflect the AUC than the C_{max}, this author considers that this pharmacologic variation when stavudine is taken with food as opposed to fasting is unlikely to be of clinical significance.

In children, the C_{max} and AUC are lower than in adults receiving the same weight-adjusted dose, with faster elimination of stavudine (Kline *et al.*, 1995).

2 Intravenous administration

Intravenous administration of stavudine to 44 HIV-infected persons, in doses ranging from 0.06 to 1 mg per kg, resulted in a peak plasma concentration ranging from 0.09 to1.13 μg per ml, and a mean AUC ranging from 0.16 to 2.02 μg.h per ml, both increasing in proportion to dose (Data on file, Bristol-Myers Squibb).

Excretion and Distribution

Oral stavudine given to rats has a plasma half-life calculated from the terminal phase of 35.9 min and peak plasma concentration of 48.4 μM respectively (Hasegawa *et al.*, 1993). The plasma half-life of stavudine was found to be considerably less in macaques under 1 week of age compared with clearance in the same animals at 1 and 4 months (Keller *et al.*, 1995). In monkeys, the drug has a steady-state volume of distribution of 0.68 liters per kg, and a terminal half-life of 0.83 h (Kaul and Dandekar, 1993). In these animals, approximately 50% of the administered oral dose of stavudine is recovered unchanged in the urine and the rest is not recovered from either urine or feces (Kaul and Dandekar, 1993; Cretton *et al.*, 1993).

These findings are similar to humans, in whom between 34 and 40% of the dose of stavudine is excreted unchanged in the urine, and there is a plasma elimination half-life ranging from 1 to 1.6 h (Dudley *et al.*, 1992; Browne *et al.*, 1993). Renal clearance of stavudine is by both active tubular secretion as well as glomerular filtration. The fate of the rest of the dose of stavudine is probably cleaved to form thymine (Dudley, 1995). *In vitro* experiments using isolated hepatocytes to assess the metabolic fate of stavudine demonstrated that stavudine is rapidly

Table V.42
Clinically relevant pharmacokinetics of stavudine. (See text for sources of data).

Good oral bioavailability, ranging from 70 to 90%
May be taken with food
Up to 40% of oral dose of stavudine is excreted unchanged in urine
Good central nervous system penetration (30–55% of plasma level).

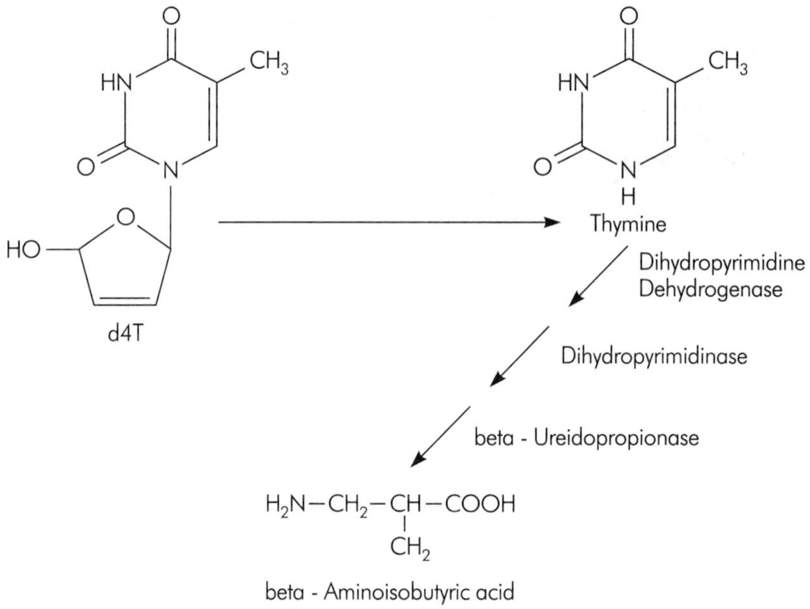

Fig. V.51.
Proposed catabolic pathway of
stavudine. (Reproduced from
Sommadossi, 1995, with permission.)

Thymine

Dihydropyrimidine
Dehydrogenase

Dihydropyrimidinase

beta - Ureidopropionase

$H_2N-CH_2-CH-COOH$
$\quad\quad\quad\quad |$
$\quad\quad\quad\quad CH_2$

beta - Aminoisobutyric acid

cleaved to thymine which is subsequently converted to beta-aminoisobutyric acid (Fig. V.51) (Cretton *et al.*, 1993; reviewed in Sommadossi, 1995).

The mean apparent volume of distribution in humans after a single oral dose is 66 liters, and there is minimal serum protein binding. There is equal distribution of stavudine between plasma and erythrocytes (Stavudine Product Information, Bristol-Myers Squibb).

The central nervous system penetration of stavudine in mice is low, although a single oral dose of 25 mg per kg resulted in levels of stavudine in the brain of greater than 0.01 μM, potentially sufficient to inhibit the replication of some strains of HIV (Russell *et al.*, 1990). In humans, limited studies suggest that stavudine penetrates the CSF to approximately the same extent as zidovudine. Within 3 h of oral administration of stavudine the CSF to plasma ratio ranges from 30 to 55%, at a dose of 1–2 mg per kg daily (Data on file, Bristol-Myers Squibb). Oral administration of stavudine in a dose of 1.3, 3, and 4 mg per kg resulted in CSF levels of 0.08, 0.20 and 0.48 μg per ml at 0.5, 1.75 and 5 h after the dose; plasma levels were not concurrently measured (Dudley *et al.*, 1992). In seven children participating in a dose-ranging study (0.125–4 mg per kg daily) the concentrations of stavudine within CSF varied from 16% to 97% of plasma values (Kline *et al.*, 1995).

Ex vivo maternal–fetal placental transfer studies suggest that stavudine crosses the placenta by simple perfusion, rapidly passing from the maternal to fetal circulation. There is a linear relationship between the mean concentration of the drug in the fetal and maternal circulations (Bawdon *et al.*, 1994). Plasma stavudine levels obtained from pregnant macaques receiving i.v. stavudine and their fetuses would suggest that exposure of the fetus to stavudine would be similar to that of the mother (Unadkat *et al.*, 1994). Stavudine is excreted in the milk of lactating rats; there are no data regarding excretion in human breast milk (Stavudine Product Information, Bristol-Myers Squibb).

Mode of Action

Stavudine, a synthetic pyrimidine (thymidine) analog, inhibits the replication of HIV following its phosphorylation in the cell to stavudine triphosphate. Stavudine triphosphate inhibits HIV reverse transcriptase by competing with endogenous deoxythymidine triphosphate, the natural substrate for the enzyme, as well as by causing premature HIV DNA chain-termination (due to the absence of a 3' hydroxyl group on the pentose ring necessary for 3'-5'phosphodiester linking) and thus inhibiting viral synthesis (Yarchoan *et al.*, 1989).

Stavudine has a different phosphorylation pattern to zidovudine. Both drugs are sequentially phosphorylated by cellular enzymes to the mono-, di-, and triphosphate derivatives. However, stavudine is phosphorylated intracellularly to its 5' monophosphate derivative by the cellular thymidine kinase about 300- to 600-fold less efficiently than zidovudine, with a K_m of 142 and 14 μM respectively in MT-4 cells (Balzarini *et al.*, 1989a). Stavudine does not accumulate in

Fig. V.52.

Occurrences of peripheral neuropathy, by dose, during 96 weeks of treatment with stavudine. (Reproduced by Skowron, 1995, with permission.)

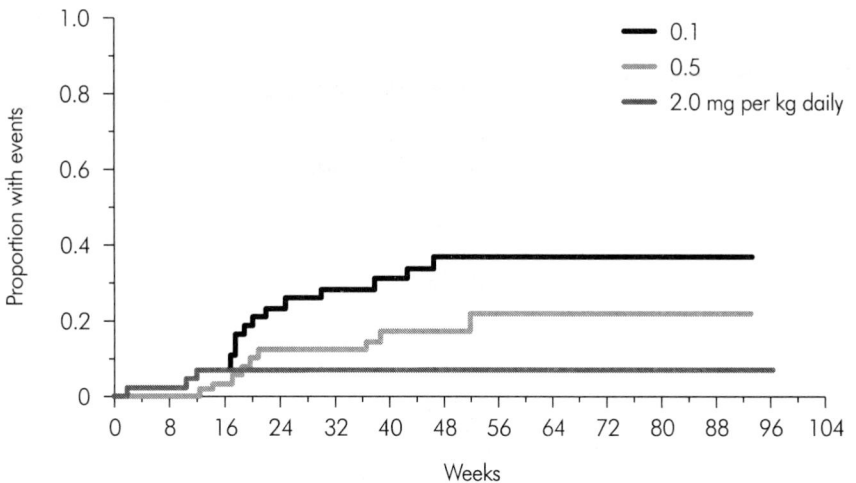

cells in its monophosphate form, again differing in this respect to zidovudine (August *et al.*, 1988; Balzarini, 1994). There are similar levels of each of the phosphorylated derivatives of stavudine, with the initial phosphorylation step being rate-limiting (Balzarini *et al.*, 1989a; Ho and Hitchcock, 1989). However, because the rate-limiting step in zidovudine intracellular metabolism is the phosphorylation to the diphosphate form, there is accumulation of zidovudine monophosphate (reviewed in Riddler *et al.*, 1995). Similar to zidovudine, stavudine is preferentially phosphorylated in activated cells rather than resting cells, differing to the cell-activation independent nucleoside analogs didanosine, zalcitabine and 3TC that exert more potent antiretroviral activity in resting cells (Gao *et al.*, 1994b). The intracellular half-lives of zidovudine triphosphate and stavudine triphosphate in peripheral blood mononuclear cells are similar, approximately 3.5 h (Ho and Hitchcock, 1989).

The steady-state levels of the triphosphate form of stavudine are 10- to 50-fold lower than zidovudine triphosphate (Zhu *et al.*, 1991). Cellular uptake, as demonstrated in experiments using the H9 T lymphocyte cell line, is by non-facilitated diffusion: intracellular and extracellular drug concentrations equilibrate within 2–3 min (August *et al.*, 1991).

Toxicity

Stavudine is generally well tolerated, with peripheral neuropathy being the major dose-limiting toxicity.

1 Peripheral neuropathy

Stavudine causes a dose-related, predominantly sensory peripheral neuropathy (Fig. V.52). In phase I trials of stavudine in patients with advanced HIV infection, the dose-limiting toxicity of the drug was the development of a sensory peripheral neuropathy which occurred in up to 55% of patients (Browne *et al.*, 1993). In another open-label, dose-ranging study in a similar population, the incidence of peripheral neuropathy in patients receiving 0.5 mg per kg daily was 17% after 1 year of therapy and 37% in those receiving 2 mg per kg daily (Petersen *et al.*, 1995). In a phase III trial dose-limiting peripheral neuropathy occurred in 15% of patients receiving stavudine and 6% of those randomized to zidovudine over an 80-week period (reviewed in Riddler *et al.*, 1995). The risk of stavudine-related peripheral neuropathy is higher in patients with a past history of neuropathy, and careful monitoring is advised if such patients are started on treatment with stavudine. The development of peripheral neuropathy is related to both dose and duration of treatment and generally resolves after discontinuation of stavudine (Skowron, 1995; Murray *et al.*, 1995). The time to resolution again is dependent on the prior dose, ranging from a median of 1 week for patients receiving 0.1 mg per kg per day to 3 weeks for those receiving 2 mg per kg daily (Petersen *et al.*, 1995). Some patients develop worsening of symptoms after stopping therapy, a phenomenon also seen with zalcitabine therapy and referred to as 'coasting'. Many patients can tolerate reinstitution of stavudine using half-dose after resolution of symptoms, for a duration in excess of 6 months (Petersen *et al.*, 1995). In a pediatric phase I/II dose-ranging study, there was a report of transient discomfort in the fingers of one participant who had neurologic abnormalities prior to study entry (Kline *et al.*, 1995).

Stavudine is more potent in reducing mitochondrial DNA content *in vitro* than didanosine and zidovudine, but less potent than zalcitabine (Chen *et al.*, 1991; Medina *et al.*, 1994). Inhibition of DNA polymerase gamma, and thus inhibition of mitochondrial synthesis and function is considered to be responsible for some of the chronic toxicity, including peripheral neuropathy, associated with some nucleoside analogs, although it has recently been postulated that the peripheral neuropathy associated with stavudine may be mediated by a different mechanism to that caused by zalcitabine and didanosine (Sommadossi, 1995). Inhibition of DNA polymerase alpha only occurs with high concentrations of stavudine triphosphate (Huang *et al.*, 1992).

2 Hepatotoxicity and pancreatitis

Although elevation of liver function tests has been reported in 11% of patients participating in a phase I trial of stavudine (Browne *et al.*, 1993), other studies suggest that this finding is most likely to reflect underlying liver disease rather than drug-related toxicity (Skowron, 1995). Pancreatitis was reported in 1% of patients in clinical trials and was associated with 14 deaths, five of which were considered drug-related (Stavudine Product Information, Bristol-Myers Squibb).

3 Bone marrow toxicity

Stavudine is generally regarded to be less myelotoxic to human bone marrow precursor cells *in vitro* than zidovudine (Mansuri *et al.*, 1989, 1990; Du *et al.*, 1992). Zidovudine and stavudine have similar effects on human progenitor erythrocytes (Mansuri *et al.*, 1989, 1990).

In a phase I trial of stavudine in patients with advanced HIV infection, 11% of participants developed anemia that required blood transfusion but not discontinuation of stavudine (Browne *et al.*, 1993). In several other studies there was no evidence of dose-related hematologic toxicity (Skowron, 1995).

4 Other

Stavudine does not appear to impair renal function (Petersen *et al.*, 1995). Decreased libido and impotence have been reported in one patient (Petersen *et al.*, 1995). Adult patients treated with up to 24 times the recommended daily dose did not develop any acute toxicity (Stavudine Product Information, Bristol-Myers Squibb). Embryotoxicity was demonstrated with inhibition of blastocyst formation from two cell embryos *in vitro* at concentrations of 100 μM or higher (Toltzis *et al.*, 1994). Stavudine is non-teratogenic in rats and rabbits with peak plasma concentrations in these animals being up to 400 times the human exposure (Schilling *et al.*, 1995).

5 Drug interactions

Co-administration of didanosine and stavudine does not result in any pharmacologic interaction and is well tolerated (Seifert *et al.*, 1994).

Clinical Uses of the Drug

Stavudine is indicated for the treatment of patients with HIV infection. In some countries various restrictions apply. Stavudine is used in combination with other nucleoside analogs (commonly didanosine or lamivudine) and often in combination with a protease inhibitor. Data regarding the efficacy of stavudine are provided from three phase I clinical trials, one phase II study and two phase III studies.

Studies 002 (AIDS Clinical Trials Group 089) and 003 were open-label, non randomized dose-ranging and safety studies of up to 3 years duration in HIV-infected persons with symptomatic infection, less than 500 CD4 cells per μl, and no active opportunistic infection. The daily dose of stavudine was escalated from 0.5 to 12 mg per kg daily using a twice-daily, three times daily or four times daily regimen until the maximally tolerated dose was determined and then reduced to determine the minimum effective dose. Stavudine was associated with a modest increase in CD4 counts and a decline in HIV p24 antigen, sustained in the 2 mg per kg daily dose group for 46 weeks. The dose of 0.5 mg per kg daily was less effective in maintaining immunologic and virologic responses over the study period. The maximum tolerated dose was 2 mg per kg daily, with the major dose-limiting toxicities being peripheral neuropathy and elevation of hepatic transaminases. A total of 41 subjects were enrolled in study 002 and 43 enrolled in 003, but a large number of patients prematurely withdrew from both studies (Browne *et al.*, 1993; Murray *et al.*, 1995). In a third phase I trial (004/005), 23 patients with symptomatic HIV infection, a CD4 count of less than 500 cells per μl (median CD4 at entry was 55 cells per μl) and hematologic intolerance to zidovudine, were randomized to receive stavudine in a dose of 0.5 or 1 mg per kg daily. Twenty (87%) of participants had previously developed dose-limiting anemia with zidovudine. Of these, only four developed severe recurrent anemia whilst receiving stavudine, and no patient required dose-reduction or cessation of drug for this condition (Skowron, 1995).

Study 006 was a multicenter, open-label randomized trial comparing three doses of stavudine (0.1 mg per kg daily, 0.5 mg per kg daily and 2 mg per kg daily) in 152 HIV-infected persons with less than 500 CD4 cells per μl. Of these, 41 had no prior exposure to zidovudine, and 110 had received prior zidovudine for a median duration of 69 weeks. Only 15 patients were asymptomatic (32 had a prior AIDS-defining illness, 105 were classified as having AIDS-related complex). The median CD4 count at study entry was 250 cells per μl. The study lacked power to detect differences in efficacy between the three dose groups; however, efficacy was evident on the basis of surrogate markers, with significant increases in CD4 numbers and decreases in HIV titer in peripheral blood mononuclear cells. Antiretroviral-naive patients had a greater CD4 response than pretreated patients (Petersen *et al.*, 1995).

Study 019 was a randomized, double-blind comparison of zidovudine (600 mg per day) versus stavudine (40 mg twice-daily for patients weighing at least 60 kg, or 30 mg twice-daily for those weighing less than 60 kg) in patients with HIV infection who had received at least 6 months of prior zidovudine, with a CD4 count of 50–500 cells per μl. The primary endpoints were the development of an AIDS-defining illness or death, or a decline in CD4 cell numbers of greater than 50%. A total of 822 patients were enrolled. Of these, 35–38% of patients were asymptomatic, the median CD4 count at baseline was 253 cells per μl and the median duration of prior zidovudine was 85 weeks. Stavudine was superior to zidovudine in this patient population in terms of CD4 cell response, survival (the relative risk (95% confidence interval) for death was 0.74 favoring stavudine over continued zidovudine treatment), and clinical progression or death (the relative risk (95% confidence interval) for first AIDS defining event or death was 0.82 (0.64 to 1.05) favoring stavudine over continued zidovudine treatment).

Study 009 was a parallel-track, compassionate-use program that enrolled over 13 000 patients with advanced HIV infection who were refractory to or intolerant of zidovudine and didanosine. Patients were randomized to receive 20 mg twice-daily or 40 mg twice-daily (approximating 0.5 and 1.0 mg per kg daily). The median CD4 count at study entry was 38 cells per μl. In patients receiving 40 mg twice-daily only marginal benefit was observed in comparison with the lower dose with respect to survival and development of AIDS-defining illnesses, with no evidence of benefit in Karnofsky scores or weight gain (Anderson *et al.*, 1995; Data on file, Bristol-Myers Squibb. As the incidence of peripheral neuropathy was higher in patients receiving 40 mg twice-daily, with no evidence of extra efficacy, the dose was decreased for all patients to 20 mg twice-daily (Simpson and Tagliati, 1995).

A phase I/II open and dose-ranging study was performed in 37 HIV-infected children ranging in age from 7 months to 15 years whose median CD4 count at baseline was 242 cells per μl. Thirty children had symptomatic HIV infection, and there was a previous history of zidovudine use in 29 participants. The dose of stavudine ranged from 0.125 to 4 mg per kg daily, in two divided doses. Although the study was not designed to measure efficacy, immunologic and virologic evidence of drug activity was noted (Kline *et al.*, 1995).

References

Anderson RE, Dunkle LM, Smaldone L *et al.* (1995). Design and implementation of the stavudine parallel-track program. *J Infect Dis* **171**: S118.

August EM, Maiongiu ME, Lin TS, Prusoff WH (1988). Initial studies on the cellular pharmacology of 3'-deoxythymidin-2'-ene (D4T): a potent and selective inhibitor of human immunodeficiency virus. *Biochem Pharmacol* **37**: 4419.

August EM, Birks EM, Prusoff WH (1991). 3'-deoxythymidin-2'-ene permeation of human lymphocyte H9 cells by nonfacilitated diffusion. *Mol Pharmacol* **39**: 246.

Baba M, Pauwels R, Herdewijn P *et al.* (1987). Both 2',3'-dideoxythymidine and its 2',3'-unsaturated derivative (2',3'-dideoxythymidinene) are potent and selective inhibitors of human immunodeficiency virus replication *in vitro*. *Biochem Biophys Res Commun* **142**: 128.

Balzarini J (1994). Metabolism and mechanism of antiretroviral action of purine and pyrimidine derivatives. *Pharm World Sci* **16**: 113.

Balzarini J, Herdewijn P, De Clercq E (1989a). Differential patterns of intracellular metabolism of 2',3'-didehydro-2'-3'-dideoxythymidine and 3'-azido-2',3'-dideoxythymidine, two potent anti-human immunodeficiency virus compounds. *J Biol Chem* **264**: 6127.

Balzarini J, Van Aerschot A, Herdewijn P, De Clercq E (1989b). 5-Chloro-substituted derivatives of 2',3'-didehydro-2',3'-dideoxyuridine 3'-fluoro-2',3'-dideoxyuridine and 3'-azido-2',3'-dideoxyuridine as anti-HIV agents. *Biochem Pharmacol* **38**: 869.

Bawdon RE, Kaul S, Sobhi S (1994). The *ex vivo* transfer of the anti-HIV nucleoside compound d4T in the human placenta. *Gynecol Obstet Invest* **38**: 1.

Browne MJ, Mayer KH, Chafee SB *et al.* (1993). 2',3'-didehydro-3'-deoxythymidine (d4T) in patients with AIDS or AIDS-related complex; a phase I trial. *J Infect Dis* **167**: 21.

Burger DM, Rosing H, van-Gijn R, *et al.*, (1992). Determination of stavudine, a new antiretroviral agent, in human plasma by reversed-phase high-performance liquid chromatography with ultraviolet detection. *J Chromatogr* **584**: 239.

Chen CH, Vazquez-Padua M, Cheng YC (1991). Effect of anti-human immunodeficiency virus nucleoside analogs on mitochondrial DNA and its implication for delayed toxicity. *Mol Pharmacol* **39**: 625.

Chu CK, Schinazi RF, Arnold BH *et al.* (1988). Comparative activity of 2',3'-saturated and unsaturated pyrimidine and purine nucleosides against human immunodeficiency virus type 1 in peripheral blood mononuclear cells. *Biochem Pharmacol* **37**: 3543.

Cretton EM, Zhou Z, Kidd LB *et al.* (1993). *In vitro* and *in vivo* disposition and metabolism of 3'-deoxy- 2',3'-didehydrothymidine. *Antimicrob Ag Chemother* **37**: 1816.

Data on file, Bristol-Myers Squibb.

Du DL, Volpe DA, Grieshaber CK, Murphy MJ (1992). *In vitro* toxicity of 3'-azido-3'-deoxythymidine, carbovir and 2',3'-didehydro-2',3'-dideoxythymidine to human and murine haematopoietic progenitor cells. *Brit J Haematol* **80**: 437.

Dudley MN (1995). Clinical pharmacokinetics of nucleoside antiretroviral agents. *J Infect Dis* **171**: S99.

Dudley MW, Graham KK, Kaul S *et al.* (1992). Pharmacokinetics of stavudine in patients with AIDS or AIDS-related complex. *J Infect Dis* **166**: 480.

Friedland G, Dunkle LW, Cross AP (1996). Stavudine (d4T, Zerit). *Antiviral Chemother* **4**: 271.

Gao Q, Gu Z, Salomon H *et al.* (1994a). Generation of multiple drug resistance by sequential *in vitro* passage of the human immunodeficiency virus type 1. *Arch Virol* **136**: 111.

Gao WY, Agbaria R, Driscoll JS, Mitsuya H (1994b). Divergent anti-human immunodeficiency virus activity and anabolic phosphorylation of 2',3'-dideoxynucleoside analogs in resting and activated human cells. *J Biol Chem* **269**: 12633.

Gu Z, Gao Q, Fang H, *et al*, (1994). Identification of novel mutations that confer drug resistance in the human immunodeficiency virus polymerase gene. *Leukemia* **8**: 5166.

Hamamoto Y, Nakashima H, Matsui T *et al.* (1987). Inhibitory effect of 2',3'-didehydro-2',3'- dideoxynucleosides on infectivity, cytopathic effects and replication of human immunodeficiency virus. *Antimicrob Ag Chemother* **31**: 907.

Hasegawa T, Seki T, Juni K *et al.* (1993). Prodrugs of 2',3'-didehydro-3'-deoxythymidine. *J Pharm Sci* **82**: 1232.

Hitchcock MJM (1991). 2',2'-didehydro-2',3'-dideoxythymidine, an anti-HIV agent. *Antiviral Chem Chemother* **2**: 125.

Ho HT, Hitchcock MJM (1989). Cellular pharmacology of 2',3'-didehydrothymidine, a nucleoside analog active against human immunodeficiency virus. *Antimicrob Ag Chemother* **33**: 844.

Horwitz JP, Chun J, Da Rooge MA *et al.* (1966). The formation of 2',3'-unsaturated pyrimidine nucleosides via a novel beta-elimination reaction. *J Org Chem* **31**: 205.

Huang P, Farquhar D, Plunkett W (1992). Selective action of 2',3'-didehydro-2',3'-dideoxythymidine triphosphate on human immunodeficiency virus reverse transcriptase and human DNA polymerases. *J Biol Chem* **267**: 2817.

Inoue T, Tsushita K, Itoh T *et al.* (1989). *In vitro* bone marrow toxicity of nucleoside analogs against human immunodeficiency virus. *Antimicrob Ag Chemother* **33**: 576.

Iversen AK, Shafer RW, Wehrly K, *et al.*, (1996). Multidrug resistant human immunodeficiency virus type 1 strains resulting from combination antiretroviral therapy. *J Virol* **70**: 1086.

Janiszewski JS, Mulvana DE, Kaul S *et al.* (1992). High-performance liquid chromatographic determination of 2',3'didehydro-3'-deoxythymidine; a new anti-human immunodeficiency virus agent, in human plasma and urine. *J Chromatogr* **577**: 151.

Kaul S, Dandekar KA (1993). Pharmacokinetics of the anti-human immunodeficiency virus nucleoside analog stavudine in cynomolgus monkeys. *Antimicrob Ag Chemother* **37**: 1160.

Kaul S, Mummaneni V, Barbhalya RH (1995). Dose proportionality of stavudine in HIV seropositive asymptomatic subjects, application to bioequivalence assessment of various capsule formulations. *Biopharm Drug Dispos* **16**: 125.

Keller RD, Nosbisch C, Unadkat JD (1995). Pharmacokinetics of stavudine (2'-3'-didehydro-3'- deoxythymidine) in the neonatal macaque (*Macaca nemestrina*). *Antimicrob Ag Chemother* **39**: 2829.

Kline MW, Dunkle LM, Church JA *et al.* (1995). A phase I/II evaluation of stavudine (D4T) in children with human immunodeficiency virus infection. *Pediatrics* **96**: 247.

Kline MW, Fletcher CV, Federici ME *et al.* (1996). Combination therapy with stavudine and didanosine in children with advanced human immunodeficiency virus infection: pharmacokinetic properties, safety, and immunologic and virologic effects. *Pediatrics* **97**: 886.

Lacey SF, Larder BA (1994). Novel mutation (V75T) in human immunodeficiency virus type 1 reverse transcriptase confers resistance to 2',3'-didehydro-2',3'-dideoxythymidine in cell culture. *Antimicrob Ag Chemother* **38**: 1428.

Lampertico P, Malter JS, Gerber MA (1991). Development and application of an *in vitro* model for screening anti-hepatitis B virus therapeutics. *Hepatology* **13**: 422.

Larder BA, Darby G, Richman DD (1989). HIV with reduced sensitivity to zidovudine (AZT) isolated during prolonged therapy. *Science* **243**: 1731.

Larder BA, Chesebro B, Richman DD (1990). Susceptibilities of zidovudine-susceptible and resistant human immunodeficiency virus isolates to antiviral agents determined by using a quantitative plaque reduction assay. *Antimicrob Ag Chemother* **34**: 436.

Lin TS Schinazi RF, Prusoff WH (1987). Potent and selective *in vitro* activity of 3'-deoxythymidin-2'-ene (3'-deoxy-2',3'-didehydrothymidine) against human immunodeficiency virus. *Biochem Pharmacol* **36**: 2713.

Lin PF, Samanta H, Rose RE *et al.* (1994). Genotypic and phenotypic analysis of human immunodeficiency virus type 1 isolates from patients on prolonged stavudine therapy. *J Infect Dis* **170**: 1157.

Mansuri MM, Starrett JE, Ghazzouli I *et al.* (1989). 1-(2,3-dideoxy-beta-D-glycero-pent-2-enofuranosyl)thymine A highly potent and selective anti-HIV agent. *J Med Chem* **32**: 461.

Mansuri MM, Hitchcock MJ, Buroker RA *et al.* (1990). Comparison of *in vitro* biological properties and mouse toxicities of three thymidine analogs active against human immunodeficiency virus. *Antimicrob Ag Chemother* **34**: 637.

Medina DJ, Tsai CH, Hsiung GD, Cheng YC (1994). Comparison of mitochondrial morphology, mitochondrial DNA content, and cell viability in cultured cells treated with three anti-human immunodeficiency virus dideoxynucleosides. *Antimicrob Ag Chemother* **38**: 1824.

Mellors JW, Dutschman GE, Im GJ *et al.* (1992). *In vitro* selection and molecular characterisation of human immunodeficiency virus-1 resistant to non-nucleoside inhibitors of reverse transcriptase. *Mol Pharmacol* **41**: 446.

Merrill DP, Moonis M, Chou TC, Hirsch MS (1996). Lamivudine or stavudine in two and three drug combinations against human immunodeficiency virus type 1 replication *in vitro*. *J Infect Dis* **173**: 355.

Moyle GJ (1995). Resistance to antiretroviral compounds for clinical management of HIV infection. *Immunol Infect Dis* **5**: 170.

Murray HW, Squires KE, Weiss W *et al.* (1995). Stavudine in patients with AIDS and AIDS-related complex; AIDS Clinical Trials Group 089. *J Infect Dis* **171**: S123.

Najera I, Richman DD, Olivares I *et al.* (1994). Natural occurrence of drug resistance mutations in the reverse transcriptase of human immunodeficiency virus type 1 isolates. *AIDS Res Hum Retrovir* **10**: 1479.

Neuzil KM (1994). Pharmacologic therapy for human immunodeficiency virus infection, a review. *Amer J Med Sci* **307**: 368.

Petersen EA, Ramirez-Ronda CH, Hardy WD (1995). Dose-related activity of stavudine in patients infected with human immunodeficiency virus. *J Infect Dis* **171**: S131.

Perno CF, Yarchoan R, Cooney DA *et al.* (1989). Replication of human immunodeficiency virus in monocytes. Granulocyte/macrophage colony-stimulating factor (GM-CSF) potentiates viral production yet enhances the antiviral effect mediated by 3'-azido-2'3'-dideoxythymidine (AZT) and other dideoxynucleoside congeners of thymidine. *J Exp Med* **169**: 933.

Richman DD (1990). Susceptibility to nucleoside analogues of zidovudine resistant isolates of human immunodeficiency virus. *Amer J Med* **88**: 8S.

Riddler SA, Anderson RE, Mellors JW (1995). Antiretroviral activity of stavudine (2',3'-didehydro-3'-deoxythymidine, DrT). *Antiviral Res* **27**: 189.

Rooke R, Parniak MA, Tremblay M *et al.* (1991). Biological comparisons of wild-type and zidovudine- resistant isolates of human immunodeficiency virus type 1 from the same subjects: susceptibility and resistance to other drugs. *Antimicrob Ag Chemother* **35**: 988.

Russell JW, Whiterock VJ, Marrero D, Klunk LJ (1990). Disposition in animals of a new anti-HIV agent: 2',3'-didehydro-3'-deoxythymidine. *Drug Metab Dispos Biol Fate Chem* **18**: 153.

Schilling BE, Nelson DR, Proctor JE *et al.* (1995). The nonclinical toxicologic profile of stavudine. *Curr Ther Res* **56**: 201.

Seifert RD, Stewart MB, Sramek JJ *et al.* (1994). Pharmacokinetics of co-administered didanosine and stavudine in HIV-seropositive male patients. *Brit J Clin Pharmacol* **38**: 405.

Sidwell RW, Hitchcock M, Okleberry KM *et al.* (1992). Suppression of murine retroviral disease by 2',3'-didehydro-2',3'-dideoxythymidine (D4T). *Antiviral Res* **19**: 313.

Sidwell RW, Warren RP, Okleberry K *et al.* (1995). Effect of the combination of interferon-alpha and stavudine on Friend virus infections in (B10,A x ABy)F1 mice. *J Infect Dis* **171**: S93.

Simpson DM, Tagliati M (1995). Nucleoside analogue associated peripheral neuropathy in human immunodeficiency virus infection. *J AIDS Hum Retrovir* **9**: 153.

Skowron G (1995). Biologic effects and safety of stavudine; overview of phase I and II clinical trials. *J Infect Dis* **171**: S113.

Sommadossi JP (1995). Comparison of metabolism and *in vitro* antiviral activity of stavudine versus other 2',3'- dideoxynucleoside analogues. *J Infect Dis* **171**: S88.

Sorensen AM, Nielsen C, Mathiesen LR *et al.* (1993). Evaluation of the combination effect of different antiviral compounds against HIV *in vitro*. *Scand J Infect Dis* **25**: 365.

Stavudine Product Information, Bristol-Myers Squibb.

Thomar H, Balzarini J, Holy A, *et al.* (1993). Inhibition of visna virus replication by 2',3'-dideoxynucleosides and acyclic nucleoside phosphonate analogs. *Antimicrob Ag Chemother* **37**: 2540.

Toltzis P, Mourton T, Magnuson T (1994). Comparative embryonic cytotoxicity of antiretroviral nucleosides. *J Infect Dis* **169**: 1100.

Tsai CC, Tollis KE, Yarnall M *et al.* (1990). *In vitro* screening for antiretroviral agents against simian immunodeficiency virus (SIV). *Antiviral Res* **14**: 87.

Unadkat JD, Keller Rd, Nosbisch C, *et al.*, (1994). Maternal fetal transfer of 2',3'-didehydro 3'-deoxythymidine (D4T). *Pharm Res* **11**: S451.

Yarchoan R, Mitsuya H, Myers CE, Broder S (1989). Clinical pharmacology of 3'-azido-2',3'-dideoxythymidine (zidovudine) and related dideoxynucleosides. *New Engl J Med* **321**: 726.

Yokota T, Mochizuki S, Konno K *et al.* (1991). Inhibitory effects of selected antiviral compounds on human hepatitis B virus DNA synthesis. *Antimicrob Ag Chemother* **35**: 394.

Zhu Z, Hitchcock MJ, Sommadossi JP (1991). Metabolism and DNA interaction of 2',3'-didehydro-2',3'-dideoxythymidine in human bone marrow cells. *Mol Pharmacol* **40**: 838.

Nevirapine

Description

The non-nucleoside nevirapine (previously known as BI-RG-587) is a dipyridodiazepinone derivative (Fig. V.53) and is a potent and highly specific inhibitor of the reverse transcriptase of HIV-1. It does not inhibit HIV-2 or any other retrovirus. It is a member of a class of structurally diverse non-nucleoside compounds that share part or all of the same binding site on the reverse transcriptase enzyme (Fig. V.53; Table V.43). A screening program at Boehringer Ingelheim Pharmaceuticals resulted in the discovery of nevirapine (Merluzzi *et al.*, 1990). It is marketed by Boehringer Ingelheim under the trade name 'Viramune'.

L-697,639

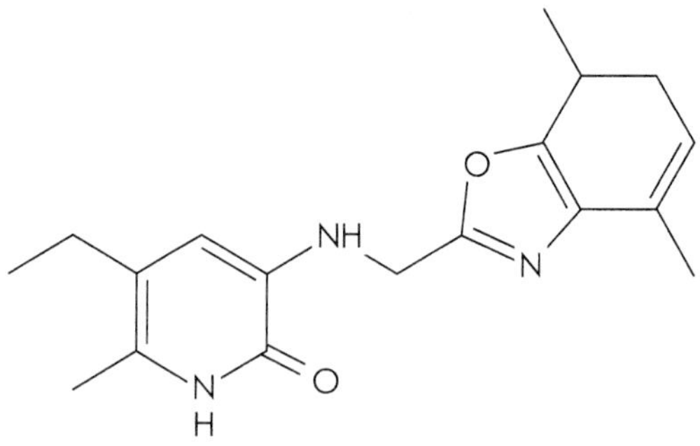

BI–RG–587
(Nevirapine)

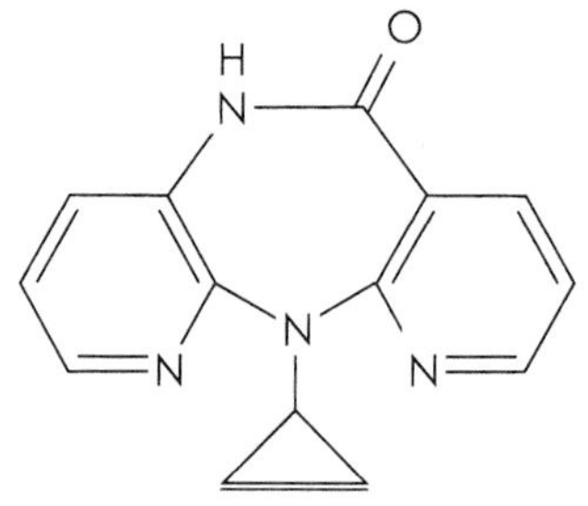

R82150
(TIBO)

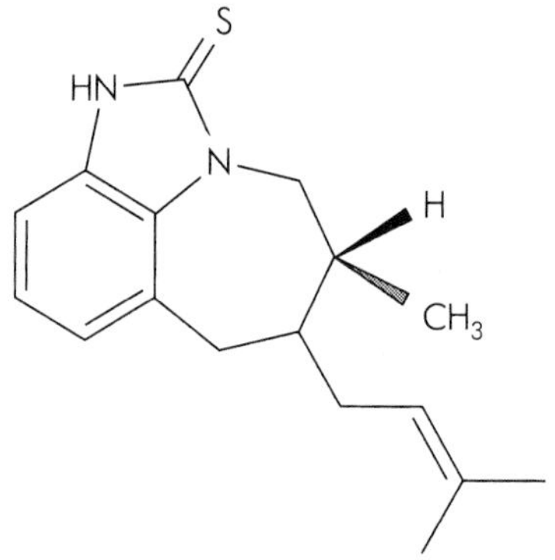

Fig. V.53.
Structure of three representatives of non-nucleoside reverse transcriptase inhibitors. (Reproduced from Condra *et al.*, 1992, with permission.)

Table V.43

Major classes of non-nucleoside reverse transcriptase inhibitors

Class and examples	Abbreviation

Bis(heteroaryl)piperazine derivatives (Romeo *et al.*, 1991, 1994)
    atevirdine (U87201E)
    delavirdine (U90152)
	BHAP

Alpha-anilinophenylacetamide derivatives (Pauwels *et al.*, 1993)
    R 89439
    R 95845
	Alpha-APA

Hydroxyethoxymethylphenylthiothymine derivatives (Miyasaka *et al.*, 1989; Yuasa *et al.*, 1993; Brennan *et al.*, 1995) MKC-442	HEPT

Tetrahydroimidazobenzodiazepinone derivatives (Pauwels *et al.*, 1990; Kukla *et al.*, 1991)
    R 82150
    R 82 913
	TIBO

Pyridinone derivatives (Goldman *et al.*, 1991, 1993)
    L 697,661
    L 697,639	

Tert-butyldimethylsilylspiroamine oxathioledioxide derivatives (Balzarini *et al.*, 1993a)	TSAO
Dipyridodiazepinone derivatives (Merluzzi *et al.*, 1990) Nevirapine	

The chemical name for nevirapine is 11-cyclopropyl-5,11-dihydro-4-methyl-6H-dipyrido[3,2-b:2',3'-e]- [1,4]diazepin-6–1. The molecular formula is $C_{15}H_{14}N_4 O$. The molecular weight of nevirapine is 266.3. The concentration of nevirapine can be expressed in μg per ml or μM (1 μg per ml is approximately 3.9 μM).

Antiviral Activity

1 Human immunodeficiency virus and other retroviruses

Nevirapine potently inhibits HIV-1 replication *in vitro* with IC_{50} values ranging from 15 to 40 nM against laboratory and clinical isolates, with low cytotoxicity and thus a high therapeutic index (Richman *et al.*, 1991a; Koup *et al.*, 1991; Grob *et al.*, 1992). The mean IC_{50} in enzyme assays ranges from 84 to 100 nM (Grob *et al.*, 1992; Borroto-Esoda and Boone, 1994). Nevirapine is active against both zidovudine-sensitive and -resistant strains of HIV-1 (Richman *et al.*, 1991a). Strains of HIV-1 that are resistant to lamivudine with mutations within codon 184 (Met–>Val) remain sensitive to nevirapine (Tisdale *et al.*, 1993), and HIV-1 strains resistant to TSAO derivatives also remain sensitive to nevirapine (Balzarini *et al.*, 1993b). The drug has no activity against HIV-2 (Richman *et al.*, 1991a; Koup *et al.*, 1991), although it inhibits replication of a chimeric HIV-1/-2 virus in which part of the HIV-2 reverse transcriptase gene (the region encoding for amino acids 176–190) is replaced with that of HIV-1 (Shih *et al.*, 1991).

Nevirapine is inactive against simian immunodeficiency virus. However, when the reverse transcriptase gene of SIV is replaced with that of HIV-1 to form a hybrid virus (RT-SHIV), nevirapine is active in inhibiting its replication *in vitro* (Balzarini *et al.*, 1995). The drug has no effect on the reverse transcriptase of feline reverse transcriptase enzymes (Merluzzi *et al.*, 1990).

2 Antagonism and synergy

Delavirdine and nevirapine in combination have been reported to have an antagonistic effect on HIV replication *in vitro* (Gu *et al.*, 1995). Additive to synergistic interactions have been reported for nevirapine when used in combination with zidovudine *in vitro* (Richman *et al.*, 1991a; Koup *et al.*, 1993), didanosine (Gu *et al.*, 1995), lamivudine (Gu *et al.*, 1995; Merrill *et al.*, 1996), stavudine (Merrill *et al.*, 1996), interferon alpha (Koup *et al.*, 1993), saquinavir (Data on file, Boehringer Ingelheim) and the tat antagonist Ro24–7429 (Connell *et al.*, 1994).

Fig. V.54
Susceptibility of HIV-1 passaged in presence of 1 μm nevirapine ■ passage 0, ● passage 12; ▲ passage 20. (Reproduced from Richman et al., 1991b, with permission. Copyright, 1991, National Academy of Sciences, USA.)

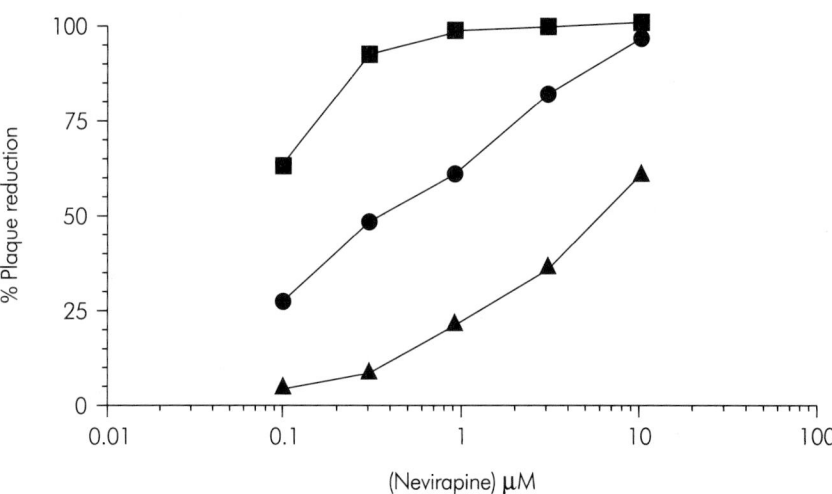

3 Resistance

After only one passage *in vitro* in the presence of nevirapine, mutant strains of HIV-1 resistant to the drug can be detected (Mellors *et al.*, 1992). The susceptibility of HIV-1 rapidly declines with subsequent passage in the presence of the drug (Fig. V.54).

The development of resistance results from rapid acquisition of one or more mutations that cluster in two regions of the reverse transcriptase gene, all within close proximity of the binding pocket for non-nucleoside reverse transcriptase inhibitors adjacent to the catalytic site. These clusters are in the vicinity of codons 180–188 and 100–110 (Nunberg *et al.*, 1991; Larder, 1992, 1995).

Nucleotide sequence analysis of resistant strains has identified a mutation within codon 181 (Tyr→ Cys) common to all nevirapine-resistant strains of HIV-1 and not present in sensitive isolates (Mellors *et al.*, 1992). This mutation results in a 100-fold or greater decrease in susceptibility to nevirapine (Richman *et al.*, 1991b), but has been reported to suppress the zidovudine-resistance phenotype (Tisdale *et al.*, 1993). A mutation within codon 188 also appears to be of major importance to the development of resistance to nevirapine, and, like codon 181 occupies a critical position within the nevirapine binding site of the reverse transcriptase (Richman *et al.*, 1991b; Grob *et al.*, 1992; Debyser *et al.*, 1993).

HIV-1 isolates from patients receiving nevirapine therapy who developed evidence of resistance to the drug as early as 1 week after initiation of therapy had mutations identified within codons 103, 106, 108, 181, 188, and 190 (Dueweke *et al.*, 1993; Richman *et al.*, 1994; reviewed in Nowak, 1995). Up to 80% of patients in phase I/II clinical trials develop a mutation within codon 181 by week 8 of nevirapine monotherapy. Co-administration of zidovudine with nevirapine prevented the emergence of the 181 mutation, and resulted in selection of other mutations within codons 103, 106, 188, and 190 (Richman *et al.*, 1994a). Nevirapine-resistance has been reportedly found in isolates of HIV-1 from patients who have only received zidovudine therapy (Najera *et al.*, 1994).

4 Cross-resistance

Mutations within codons 181 and 188 have been described in HIV-1 strains resistant to all non-nucleoside reverse transcriptase inhibitors including pyridinone derivatives, HEPT derivatives, BHAP derivatives and TIBO derivatives (Balzarini *et al.*, 1993c,d; Carroll *et al.*, 1994; Vandamme *et al.*, 1994; Taylor *et al.*, 1994; Fan *et al.*, 1995). In addition, mutations within codon 100 (Leu→ Ile) have also been reported in association with TIBO and BHAP-resistance, within codon 103 (Lys→ Asn) with pyridinone and TIBO-resistance, and within codon 138 (Glu→Lys) with TIBO and TSAO-resistance (Nunberg *et al.*, 1991; Mellors *et al.*, 1993; Balzarini *et al.*, 1993d,e; Goldman *et al.*, 1993). When BHAP or TIBO derivatives are used in combination with nevirapine, resistant HIV emerges as rapidly as with the single drug (Balzarini *et al.*, 1993e). A novel mutation at position 236 (Pro→ Leu) causing resistance to BHAP derivatives results in hypersensitivity to nevirapine (Dueweke *et al.*, 1993).

The nevirapine-resistant strains of HIV-1 are generally cross-resistant to other non-nucleoside reverse transcriptase inhibitors such as thiobenzimidazolone (TIBO) compounds, but remain sensitive to didanosine and zalcitabine and foscarnet (Mellors *et al.*, 1992, 1993). Conversely, foscarnet-resistant strains of HIV-1 remain sensitive, and even hypersensitive, to nevirapine (Tachedjian et al., 1995; Mellors et al., 1995). Cross-resistance between nevirapine and protease inhibitors is unlikely, given the different target enzymes of these compounds.

Mode of Administration and Dosage

The recommended dose of nevirapine is 200 mg daily for the first 14 days, then 200 mg twice-daily. The reason nevirapine is administered only in half-dose for the first 2 weeks is because this has been found to lessen the frequency of rash (from approximately 50% of treated individuals to approximately 30%) (see p. 1753). If rash develops during this 14-day period the manufacturer recommends continuing with the half-dose until the rash resolves. If the rash is severe or if Stevens–Johnson syndrome develops the drug should be discontinued. Nevirapine should only be commenced with at least one other antiretroviral drug as part of a new combination, as nevirapine monotherapy is associated with rapid emergence of resistance (Nevirapine Product Information).

There are no data currently available regarding dosages of nevirapine in patients with hepatic or renal dysfunction. As nevirapine is metabolized by the liver and excreted by the kidney, care should be taken if the drug is administered to any patient with significant hepatic or renal dysfunction. For patients with moderate or marked elevation of plasma aminotransaminases or alkaline phosphatase levels administration of nevirapine should be interrupted until liver function abnormalities return to baseline, and the drug should be ceased if there is a recurrence of moderate or marked plasma hepatic enzyme abnormalities. If interruption of nevirapine administration is or more than 1 week, recommencement of the drug should be at half-dose as described above.

The safety of nevirapine in pregnant women has also not been established, and, although teratogenicity has not been observed in animal studies, the manufacturer only recommends the use of nevirapine in pregnancy if it is considered that potential benefits outweigh potential risks.

The AIDS Clinical Trials Group has recently completed a study of nevirapine (120 mg per m^2, once-daily for 28 days, and then 200 mg per m^2 every 12 h) to infants with HIV infection aged 2–16 months. Nevirapine was administered orally, in combination with zidovudine and didanusine without any clinically important adverse events (Luziriaga et al., 1997).

Availability

Nevirapine is only available for oral administration in *tablets* containing 200 mg nevirapine.

Serum Levels in Relation to Dosage

Studies in chimpanzees have demonstrated good bioavailability of nevirapine (64%) and a long plasma half-life (11–24 h) (Hattox et al., 1992). In humans the absorption of nevirapine following single dose administration is 93 ± 9% (reviewed in Carr and Cooper, 1996).

In a pilot dose-ranging study to determine single-dose pharmacokinetics of nevirapine (2.5–400 mg) following administration to 21 HIV-infected persons, nevirapine was found to be rapidly absorbed, with the time to peak plasma concentrations (T_{max}) being within approximately 90 min of administration, and secondary peaks being observed between 3–12 or 24–28 h (higher doses were associated with later secondary peaks). Peak concentrations in plasma (C_{max}) and area-under-the-curve (AUC) increased in proportion to the dose up to 200 mg, but the AUC was less than proportional at the 400-mg dose (Cheeseman et al., 1993).

In a second dose-ranging phase I/II study performed through the AIDS Clinical Trials Group, 62 HIV- infected patients with CD4 counts of less than 400 cells per µl received nevirapine (12.5 mg, 50 mg or 200 mg per day) alone or in combination with zidovudine (600 mg per day). The mean steady-state trough levels were 0.23 µg per ml (approximately 0.95 µM), 1.1 µg per ml (approximately 4.4 µM) and 1.9 µg per ml (approximately 7.5 µM) respectively (Cheeseman et al., 1995). In a second study when the daily dose was increased to 400 mg nevirapine per day, administered over 12 weeks, the mean plasma trough level was 15.8 µM (4 µg per ml), exceeding the IC_{50} of resistant HIV (Havlir et al., 1995a).

Food has no apparent effect on absorption of nevirapine, nor is absorption significantly altered by concomitant administration of didanosine in alkaline buffer (Data on file, Boehringer Ingelheim).

Excretion

The drug is metabolized predominantly in the liver by the cytochrome P-450 pathway, and has a number of metabolites including hydroxymethyl-nevirapine. Metabolic autoinduction occurs with doses of nevirapine of 200 mg per day or greater. This results in a decrease in plasma levels of nevirapine that occur within 2 weeks of commencing the drug. During the first 2 weeks of therapy the plasma half-life decreases from 43 h to 23 h, thought to be due to autoinduction of hepatic cytochrome P-450 by nevirapine (reviewed in Carr and Cooper, 1996). After the enzymes have been induced by the drug the pharmacokinetics of nevirapine remain linear. Following cytochrome P-450 metabolism, many of the metabolites undergo glucuronidation, followed by urinary excretion (approximately 80% of an oral dose) with only 10% being excreted in feces. Less than 3% of the parent compound can be found in urine (Data on file, Boehringer Ingelheim).

Distribution of the Drug in Body

Nevirapine has been shown in rats and monkeys to cross the blood–brain barrier with CSF:plasma ratios of 0.04 when measured 2 h after oral administration of 20 mg per kg body weight, and plasma:brain ratios of 0.8 and 1.4 (Norris et al., 1992; Cheeseman et al., 1993). In humans, the ratio of CSF:plasma is approximately 0.45 (Data on file, Boehringer Ingelheim).

In humans the mean volume of distribution is 1.4 liters per kg, and the drug is fairly evenly distributed throughout most organs and tissues; protein binding is 62% (Cheeseman et al., 1993). Nevirapine is present in breast milk and crosses the placenta (Data on file, Boehringer Ingelheim).

Mode of Action

Nevirapine is a non-nucleoside inhibitor of the HIV-1 reverse transcriptase (Merluzzi et al., 1990). It does not require phosphorylation within the cell for its activity. Like delavirdine and other members of its class it is not a chain terminator of DNA synthesis (Gu et al., 1995). The infectivity of HIV virions declines dramatically in persons treated with nevirapine, suggesting that initial antiviral effects are on cell-free virions (Zhang et al., 1996).

Nevirapine is bound in a hydrophobic pocket created upon contact of the inhibitor with the enzyme in the p66 'palm' of reverse transcriptase, near but not overlapping the Pol active site, and in contact with the 'thumb' subdomain of reverse transcriptase (Kohlstaedt et al., 1992; Smerdon et al., 1994; Tantillo et al., 1994; Rodgers et al., 1995; reviewed in De Clercq, 1993).

Nevirapine acts non-competitively with respect to nucleoside triphosphates, template and primer. These findings suggest that nevirapine binds to a site distinct from the active site of the reverse transcriptase enzyme where nucleoside analogs such as zidovudine bind (Cohen et al., 1991). Nevirapine, and other structurally unrelated drugs with a similar site of activity are thus called 'second-site' reverse transcriptase inhibitors. The reported K_i is approximately 220 nM (Kopp et al., 1991; Grob et al., 1992). Nucleotide binding is not altered in the presence of nevirapine (Spence et al., 1995).

Complex tertiary folding of HIV-1 reverse transcriptase results in non-contiguous sites (such as amino acid residues 101, 103, 181 and 188) forming the binding site for nevirapine and other second site reverse transcriptase inhibitors (reviewed in Kilby and Saag, 1996). A number of investigators have demonstrated the importance of tyrosine amino acids within codons 181 and 188, that are located within the drug binding site of the reverse transcriptase, in determining the sensitivity of HIV-1 to nevirapine (Cohen et al., 1991; Shih et al., 1991; Grob et al., 1992; Bacolla et al., 1993; reviewed in De Clercq, 1993). This binding site is shared by all the non-nucleoside reverse transcriptase inhibitors including alpha-APA and TIBO derivatives which have been shown to roughly overlay each other in models of their interaction within the binding pocket (Wu et al., 1991; Kroeger-Smith et al., 1995). When nevirapine is not present, the pocket site is filled by the tyrosines of codons 181 and 188, and a pocket is only formed when these aromatic side-chains rotate (Tantillo et al., 1994). The amino acid at position 103 has been shown to functionally interact with the 181/188 region (Condra et al., 1992; Sardana et al., 1992). The non-nucleoside reverse transcriptase inhibitors as a group assume a butterfly shape and, although there are significant differences in the conformation of amino acids that form the binding pocket, computer modelling studies show that many of them (including alpha-APA, the pyridinone derivatives, and TIBO derivatives) bind to the reverse transcriptase in a manner similar to that of nevirapine (Ren et al., 1995; Kroeger-Smith et al., 1995; Ding et al., 1995).

Nevirapine-resistant variants of HIV-1 contain amino acid substitutions at positions within the reverse transcriptase that map to residues in close contact with nevirapine, and prevent the drug from making contact with the enzyme possibly due to steric hindrance, or by removing molecules that promote favorable enzyme–drug interactions (Smerdon et al., 1994; Emini et al., 1994). Nevirapine has a decreased affinity for the mutant compared with wild-type reverse transcriptase due to a faster inhibitor dissociation rate from the wild type enzyme (Spence et al., 1996).

Some investigators consider that both RNA- and DNA-dependent polymerase activities of reverse transcriptase are inhibited by nevirapine (Tramontano and Cheng, 1992), including altering the cleavage specificity of ribonuclease H (RNase H) and stimulating the activity of this enzyme (Palaniappan *et al.*, 1995). Others consider that only polymerase and not ribonuclease H function is affected by this group of compounds (Loya *et al.*, 1994). Nevirapine is specific for the polymerase activity of the reverse transcriptase of HIV-1; it does not affect that of HIV-2 (Loya *et al.*, 1994). Nevirapine has no effect on gp120/CD4 interaction, envelope glycoprotein processing or syncytia formation (Koup *et al.*, 1991).

Toxicity

1 General

The most frequent adverse reactions reported in patients receiving nevirapine include headache, rash, fever, mouth ulcers and somnolence. Many of these may be due to underlying disease or concomitant medication (reviewed in Carr and Cooper, 1996).

2 Rash

The most important adverse reaction is the development of rash, which has been described as severe in 3% of patients, and was part of Stevens–Johnson syndrome in 0.4% (reviewed in Carr and Cooper, 1996). The rash has been observed in up to 50% of patients who commence nevirapine therapy at a dose of 400 mg per day. However, this incidence has been reduced to about 20% when the drug is used at half-dose (i.e. 200 mg per day) for the first 14 days of therapy.

The rash usually develops between 1–4 weeks after commencing therapy, but may be delayed in onset and not be apparent until after 8 weeks of therapy (reviewed in Carr and Cooper, 1996). The rash may be associated with fever and elevated hepatic enzymes. The risk of rash is higher in patients with lower CD4 counts (48% in those in one study with a median CD4 count of 41 cells per μl) (Havlir *et al.*, 1995a).

3 Elevated liver enzymes

Serum gamma glutamyl transferase and alkaline phosphate levels may be elevated, especially during the first few weeks of therapy. This is considered to be in keeping with autoinduction of liver enzymes by the manufacturer, although there are also rare reports of liver toxicity with elevated serum alanine aminotransferases and bilirubin (Data on file, Boehringer Ingelheim). The frequency of elevated transaminase levels is only 1 or 2% greater than in patients receiving zidovudine.

4 Drug interactions

Concomitant administration of zidovudine with nevirapine has been reported to reduce the bioavailability of zidovudine by up to 20% (reviewed in Carr and Cooper, 1996). This interaction has not been found between nevirapine and didanosine or zalcitabine. As nevirapine induces cytochrome P-450 enzymes, the plasma level of any concomitant medications metabolized by this pathway may be decreased. Other medications such as rifabutin and rifampicin, known to induce cytochrome P-450, may require dose adjustments if administered with nevirapine, but this has not yet been conclusively shown. Studies of small numbers of patients have demonstrated a reduction in the trough plasma levels of nevirapine by 16% and 37% in patients taking nevirapine and either rifabutin or rifampicin respectively (Data on file, Boehringer Ingelheim). Ketoconazole has been shown to inhibit metabolism of nevirapine *in vitro*. Nevirapine decreases plasma levels of saquinavir by 17–70% (mean approximately 30%), and until more data are available the manufacturer recommends that nevirapine should not be administered in combination with antiretroviral drugs of this class (Data on file, Boehringer Ingelheim). As nevirapine may also decrease plasma levels of oral contraceptives, their concomitant use is not recommended (Data on file, Boehringer Ingelheim).

Clinical Uses of the Drug

1 Human immunodeficiency virus infection

Due to the rapid emergence of resistance with nevirapine monotherapy, this drug should be used only in combination with other antiretroviral drugs, specifically nucleoside analog reverse transcriptase inhibitors, for the treatment of HIV-1 infection. Insufficient data exist on combination with protease inhibitors at this time. Clinical trials outlining some of the trials demonstrating efficacy of nevirapine, and the antiretroviral drugs that have been studied in combination with nevirapine are outlined below.

In a European-Australian study (study 881) designed to evaluate whether alternating treatment with nevirapine and zidovudine would prolong the antiviral effect of nevirapine, ten patients with no prior history of antiretroviral therapy were treated with an alternating regimen of nevirapine (1 week, 200 mg per day) and zidovudine (3 weeks, 600 mg per day). Although virologic benefit was detected during the first week of therapy with decline of serum p24 antigen levels by a median of 59%, subsequent courses of nevirapine were associated with rising levels of p24 antigen. Following 8–12 weeks of therapy HIV isolates were 40- to 1000-fold less sensitive to nevirapine compared with pre-therapy strains (De-Jong et al., 1994). The rapid development of resistance to nevirapine monotherapy as well as in vitro data raised the point that nevirapine should be used as part of combination therapy for the treatment of HIV-1 infection (Grob et al., 1992). In support of this, five patients who received nevirapine in combination with zidovudine as part of the European-Australian study exhibited sustained antiviral responses (Carr and Cooper, 1996).

A number of studies were designed to determine whether higher doses of nevirapine would overcome the development of resistance. Of 21 HIV-infected patients with less than 400 CD4 cells per μl (median 41 cells per μl) who received open-label nevirapine for 24 weeks nevirapine-resistance still emerged rapidly, although there was suppression of HIV p24 antigen and HIV RNA in plasma for the duration of the study. The incidence of rash, particularly in the first 4 weeks was high in this group (see section on toxicity) (Havlir et al., 1995a).

The European-Australian study 1010 evaluated nevirapine in 20 antiretroviral-naive HIV-infected patients and CD4 counts of 100–400 cells per μl (median 195 per μl at study entry), and detectable p24 antigen in plasma (median 168 pg per ml). Most (15 of 20) had asymptomatic HIV infection. Following an initial regimen of 200 mg per day for the first 14 days (in an attempt to minimize the development of rash) all patients received 400 mg per day of nevirapine for 26 weeks. HIV p24 antigen levels declined by a mean of about 70% from baseline within 1 week, and suppression was maintained for the duration of the study with a mean of 50% decline from baseline at week 26. Despite an early increase in CD4 cell counts, these returned to baseline by week 12 (Carr and Cooper, 1996).

To examine whether the development of resistance was related to virus burden, asymptomatic HIV-infected persons with more than 500 CD4 cells per μl were enrolled in ACTG Protocol 208 and treated with nevirapine 400 mg per day and their viral load and susceptibility to nevirapine were monitored. The median decrease in plasma HIV RNA was 0.5 $\log_{10}$ copies per ml. By week 12 isolates from all participants were resistant to nevirapine. In some patients there was a sustained reduction in HIV RNA levels even in the presence of resistance (Havlir et al., 1995b). Thus although resistance develops early, there may be continuing activity with high doses despite emergence of resistant strains, although the underlying mechanism is difficult to imagine (Richman, 1994).

A third European-Australian study (study 1011) involved 49 patients with at least 6 months of prior zidovudine experience (median duration at baseline was 72 weeks) and CD4 counts of less than 500 cells per μl. Patients were randomized to receive nevirapine (200 mg per day for 14 days then 400 mg per day) in combination with zidovudine or to continue zidovudine monotherapy. Those randomized to receive zidovudine monotherapy were switched to nevirapine at week 28 or earlier if there was clear evidence of failure of therapy. There was rapid decrease in plasma p24 antigen levels only in those randomized to combination therapy, with a median decline of 67% by 4 weeks, and levels remained below baseline until week 28. There were unsustained mean increases in CD4 counts (37 cells per μl) and a decrease in viral load (0.6 $\log_{10}$) in those receiving combination therapy, maximal at week 4. The study was not powered to examine clinical endpoints (Carr and Cooper, 1996).

Study 1037 compared treatment with the combination nevirapine (200 mg per day for the first 14 days then 400 mg per day) and zidovudine versus zidovudine monotherapy in 60 HIV-infected patients with CD4 counts of 200–500 cells per μl (mean 373 per μl) and a mean plasma HIV RNA of 4.24 $\log_{10}$ copies per ml (17378 copies per ml) and between 3 and 24 months of prior zidovudine therapy (median 35 weeks). Those randomized to combination therapy had a sustained increase in CD4 counts over 24 weeks of study, with a mean maximal increase of approximately 55 cells per μl at week 8 and falling to baseline at week 28; those randomized to continue zidovudine monotherapy has a decline in CD4 counts (40 cells per μl below baseline at week 28). The mean maximal decline in HIV RNA in those receiving combination therapy was 1.6 $\log_{10}$ copies per ml at week 2, rising to 0.2 $\log_{10}$ copies below baseline by week 8 and then to baseline by week 16. There was no decline in HIV RNA in those continuing zidovudine monotherapy (Data on file, Boehringer Ingelheim).

The ACTG study 241, based on the *in vitro* convergent therapy hypothesis raised by findings of Chow and colleagues (Chow *et al.*, 1993), compared the triple combination of nevirapine (200 mg per day for 14 days followed by 400 mg per day) in combination with zidovudine and didanosine versus zidovudine and didanosine in 398 HIV-infected patients with CD4 counts of 350 cells per μl or less (median 136 per μl) and a mean plasma HIV RNA of 4.6 $\log_{10}$ copies per ml (38 905 copies per ml) with at least 6 months of prior nucleoside analog therapy (median 25 months). There was a significantly higher mean CD4 count in those randomized to receive triple therapy compared with those receiving the double combination. There was also a 0.25 $\log_{10}$ lower mean plasma HIV RNA in those receiving the triple versus double combination compared with the double combination recipients. There was no difference between the two groups in risk of disease progression, although this study was not powered to examine this as an endpoint (D'Aquila *et al.*, 1996).

Study 1046 compared treatment with nevirapine (200 mg per day for 14 days then 400 mg per day) in combination with zidovudine and didanosine versus nevirapine and zidovudine versus zidovudine and didanosine in 151 HIV-infected patients who were antiretroviral-naive with CD4 counts of 200–600 cells per μl (mean 376 per μl) and a mean plasma HIV RNA of 4.4 $\log_{10}$ copies per ml (25704 copies per ml) at baseline. After 24 weeks those randomized to receive triple therapy or zidovudine/didanosine had significantly higher mean CD4 cell increases over baseline (113 and 78 cells per μl respectively) compared with those randomized to receive zidovudine/nevirapine. By 12 months the triple therapy recipients had a continuing increase in CD4 cells that was significantly higher than in either of the double therapy arms. At week 28 the decline in plasma HIV RNA was greatest in the triple therapy arm (1.72 $\log_{10}$ copies per ml decline compared with baseline) versus 1.4 $\log_{10}$ in the zidovudine/didanosine arm and 0.5 $\log_{10}$ in the zidovudine/nevirapine arm. At week 28 approximately 70% of those receiving triple therapy and who were compliant with study medication had plasma RNA values below detectable levels, with no evidence of emerging nevirapine resistance (Data on file, Boehringer Ingelheim). The United States FDA and the Australian Therapeutic Goods Administration granted a provisional license for nevirapine on the basis of these data.

In an AIDS Clinical Trials Group Study of pediatric patients (p. 1771), nevirapine therapy in combination with zidovudine and didanosine resulted in sustained efficacy against HIV-1 (Luzuriaga *et al.*, 1997).

Acknowledgement   The author would like to thank Andrew Carr of St Vincent's Hospital, Sydney, for his critical review of this chapter.

References

Bacolla A, Shih CK, Rose JM *et al.* (1993). Amino acid substitutions in HIV-1 reverse transcriptase with corresponding residues from HIV-2 Effect on kinetic constants and inhibition by non-nucleoside analogs. *J Biol Chem* **268**: 16571.

Balzarini J, Velazquez S, San-Felix A *et al.* (1993a). Human immunodeficiency virus type 1-specific [2',5'-bis-0-(tert-butyidimethylsilyl)-beta-D-ribofuranosyl)-3'-spiro-5"-(4"-amino1",2"-oxathiole-2",2"- dioxide)- purine analogues show a resistance spectrum that is different from that of the human immunodeficiency virus type 1-specific non-nucleoside analogues. *Mol Pharmacol* **43**: 109.

Balzarini J, Karlsson A, Vandamme AM *et al.* (1993b). Human immunodeficiency virus type 1 (HIV-1) strains selected for resistance against the HIV-1 specific [2',5'-bis-0-(tert-butyldimethylsilyl)-3'-spiro-5'- (4'-amino-1'2'-oxathiole-2',2'-dioxide)]-beta-D-pentofurano syl (TSAO) nucleoside analogues retain sensitivity to HIV-1 specific nonnucleoside inhibitors. *Proc Natl Acad Sci USA* **90**: 6952.

Balzarini J, Karlsson A, De Clercq E (1993c). Human immunodeficiency virus type 1 drug-resistance patterns with different 1-[(2-hydroxyethoxy) methyl)-6-(phenylthio)thymine derivatives. *Mol Pharmacol* **44**: 694.

Balzarini J, Karlsson A, Perez-Perez MJ *et al.* (1993d) HIV-1 specific reverse transcriptase inhibitors show differential activity against HIV-1 mutant strains containing different amino acid substitutions in the reverse transcriptase. *Virology* **192**: 246.

Balzarini J, Karlsson A, Perez-Perez MJ *et al.* (1993e) Treatment of human immunodeficiency virus type 1 (HIV-1)-infected cells with combination of HIV-1-specific inhibitors results in a different resistance pattern than does treatment with single-drug therapy. *J Virol* **67**: 5353.

Balzarini J, Weeger M, Camarasa MJ *et al.* (1995). Sensitivity/resistance profile of a simian immunodeficiency virus containing the reverse transcriptase gene of human immunodeficiency virus type 1 (HIV-1) toward the HIV-1 specific non-nucleoside reverse transcriptase inhibitors. *Biochem Biophys Res Commun* **211**: 850.

Brennan TM, Taylor DL, Bridges CG *et al.* (1995). The inhibition of human immunodeficiency virus type 1 *in vitro* by a non-nucleoside reverse transcriptase inhibitor MKC-442, alone and in combination with other anti-HIV compounds. *Antiviral Res* **26**: 173.

Borroto-Esoda K, Boone LR (1994). Development of a human immunodeficiency virus-1 *in vitro* DNA synthesis system to study reverse transcriptase inhibitors. *Antiviral Res* **23**: 235.

Carr A, Cooper DA (1996). Current clinical experience with nevirapine for HIV infection *Antiviral Chemother, New Directions for Clinical Application and Research* Vol. 4, p. 299 (Mills J, Volberding PA, Corey L, eds). New York: Plenum Press.

Carroll SS, Geib J, Olsen DB *et al.* (1994). Sensitivity of HIV-1 reverse transcriptase and its mutants to inhibition by azidothymidine triphosphate. *Biochemistry* 33: 2113.

Cheeseman SH, Hattox SE, McLaughlin MM *et al.* (1993). Pharmacokinetics of nevirapine; initial single-rising-dose study in humans. *Antimicrob Ag Chemother* 37: 178.

Cheeseman SH, Havlir D, McLaughlin MM *et al.* (1995). Phase I/II evaluation of nevirapine alone and in combination with zidovudine for infection with human immunodeficiency virus. *J AIDS Hum Retrovir* 8: 141.

Chow YK, Hirsch MS, Merrill DP *et al.* (1993). Use of evolutionary limitations of HIV-1 multidrug resistance to optimise therapy. *Nature* 361: 650.

Cohen KA, Hopkins J, Ingraham RH *et al.* (1991). Characterisation of the binding site for nevirapine (BI-RG-587), a nonnucleoside inhibitor of human immunodeficiency virus type-1 reverse transcriptase. *J Biol Chem* 266: 14670.

Condra JH, Emini EA, Gotlib L *et al.* (1992). Identification of the human immunodeficiency virus reverse transcriptase residues that contribute to the activity of diverse nonnucleoside inhibitors. *Antimicrob Ag Chemother* 36: 1441.

Connell EV, Hsu MC, Richman DD (1994). Combinative interactions of a human immunodeficiency virus (HIV) Tat antagonist with HIV reverse transcriptase inhibitors and an HIV protease inhibitor. *Antimicrob Ag Chemother* 38: 348.

D'Aquila RT, Hughes MD, Johnson VA *et al.* (1996). Nevirapine, zidovudine and didanosine compared with zidovudine and didanosine in patients with HIV-1 infection. *Ann Intern Med* 124: 1019.

Data on file, Boehringer Ingelheim.

Debyser Z, De Vreese K, Knops-Gerrits PP *et al.* (1993). Kinetics of different human immunodeficiency virus type 1 reverse transcriptases resistant to human immunodeficiency virus type 1- specific reverse transcriptase inhibitors. *Mol Pharmacol* 43: 521.

De Clercq E (1993). HIV-1 specific RT inhibitors; highly selective inhibitors of human immunodeficiency virus type 1 that are specifically targeted at the viral reverse transcriptase. *Med Res Rev* 13: 229.

De Jong MD, Loewenthal M, Boucher CA *et al.* (1994). Alternating nevirapine and zidovudine treatment of human immunodeficiency virus type 1-infected persons does not prolong nevirapine activity. *J Infect Dis* 169: 1346.

Ding J, Das K, Moereels H *et al.* (1995). Structure of HIV-1 RT/TIBO 86183 complex reveals similarity in the binding of diverse nonnucleoside inhibitors. *Nat Struct Biol* 2: 407.

Dueweke TJ, Pushkarskaya T, Poppe SM *et al.* (1993). A mutation in reverse transcriptase of bis(heteroaryl)piperazine-resistant human immunodeficiency virus type 1 that confers increased sensitivity to other nonnucleoside inhibitors. *Proc Natl Acad Sci USA* 90: 4713.

Emini EA, Byrnes VW, Condra JH *et al.* (1994). The genetic and functional basis of HIV-1 resistance to nonnucleoside reverse transcriptase inhibitors. *Arch Virol* 9 (Suppl): 11.

Fan N, Rank KB, Evans DB *et al.* (1995). Simultaneous mutations at Tyr-181 in HIV-1 reverse transcriptase prevents inhibition of RNA-dependent DNA polymerase activity by the bisheteroarylpiperazine (BHAP) U-90152s. *FEBS Lett* 370: 59.

Goldman ME, Nunberg JH, O'Brien JA *et al.* (1991). Pyridinone derivatives; specific human immunodeficiency virus type 1 reverse transcriptase inhibitors with antiviral activity. *Proc Natl Acad Sci USA* 88: 6863.

Goldman ME, O'Brien JA Ruffing TL *et al.* (1993). A nonnucleoside reverse transcriptase inhibitor active on human immunodeficiency virus type 1 isolates resistant to related inhibitors. *Antimicrob Ag Chemother* 37: 947.

Grob PM, Wu JC, Cohen KA *et al.* (1992). Nonnucleoside inhibitors of HIV-1 reverse transcriptase; nevirapine as a prototype drug. *AIDS Res Hum Retrovir* 8: 145.

Gu Z, Quan Y, Li Z, Arts EJ, Wainberg MA (1995). Effects of non-nucleoside inhibitors of human immunodeficiency virus type 1 in cell-free recombinant reverse transcriptase assays. *J Biol Chem* 270: 31046.

Hattox SE, Cohn DL, Norris SH *et al.* (1992). Single and multiple dose pharmacokinetics of nevirapine, a novel nonnucleoside HIV-1 reverse transcriptase inhibitor, in chimpanzees. *Pharm Res* 9: S268.

Havlir D, Cheeseman SH, McLaughlin M *et al.* (1995a). High-dose nevirapine; safety, pharmacokinetics and antiviral effect in patients with human immunodeficiency virus infection. *J Infect Dis* 171: 537.

Havlir D, McLaughlin MM, Richman DD (1995b). A pilot study to evaluate the development of resistance to nevirapine in asymptomatic human immunodeficiency virus infected patients with CD4 cell counts of >500/mm3; AIDS Clinical Trials Group Protocol 208. *J Infect Dis* 172: 1379.

Kilby JM, Saag MS (1996). Clinical experience with non-nucleoside reverse transcriptase inhibitors: L- 697,661 and nevirapine. *Antiviral Chemotherapy, New Directions for Clinical Application and Research* Vol. 4, p. 291 (Mills J, Volberding PA, Corey L, eds). New York: Plenum Press.

Kohlstaedt LA, Wang J, Friedman JM *et al.* (1992). Crystal structure at 35 A resolution of HIV-1 reverse transcriptase complexed with an inhibitor. *Science* 256: 1783.

Kopp EB, Miglietta JJ, Shrutkowski AG *et al.* (1991). Steady state kinetics and inhibition of HIV-1 reverse transcriptase by a non-nucleoside dipyridodiazepinone, BI-RG-587, using a heteropolymeric template. *Nucleic Acids Res* 19: 3035.

Koup RA, Merluzzi VJ, Hargrave KD *et al.* (1991). Inhibition of human immunodeficiency virus type 1 (HIV-1) replication by the dipyridodiazepinone BI-RG 587. *J Infect Dis* 163: 966.

Koup RA, Brewster F, Grob P, Sullivan JL (1993). Nevirapine synergistically inhibits HIV-1 replication in combination with zidovudine, interferon or CD4 immunoadhesion. *AIDS* 7: 1181.

Kroeger-Smith MB,Rouzer CA, Taneyhill LA *et al.* (1995). Molecular modelling studies of HIV-1 reverse transcriptase nonnucleoside inhibitors; total energy of complexation as a predictor of drug placement and activity. *Protein Sci* 4: 2203.

Kukla MJ, Breslin HJ, Pauwels R *et al.* (1991). Synthesis and anti-HIV-1 activity of 4,5,6,7-tetrahydro-5-methylimidazo[4,5,1-jk][1,4]benzodiazepin-2(1H)-one (TIBO) derivatives. *J Med Chem* 34: 746.

Larder BA (1992). 3'-Azido-3'-deoxythymidine resistance suppressed by a mutation conferring human immunodeficiency virus type 1 resistance to nonnucleoside reverse transcriptase inhibitors. *Antimicrob Ag Chemother* 36: 2664.

Larder BA (1995). Viral resistance and the selection of antiretroviral combinations. *J AIDS Hum Retrovir* 10: S28.

Larder BA, Kellam P, Kemp SD (1993). Convergent combination therapy can select viable multidrug- resistant HIV *in vitro*. *Nature* 365: 451.

Loya S, Bakhanashvili M, Tal R *et al.* (1994). Enzymatic properties of two mutants of reverse transcriptase of human immunodeficiency virus type 1 (tyrosine 181-isoleucine and tyrosine 188-leucine), resistant to nonnucleoside inhibitors. *AIDS Res Hum Retrovir* 10: 939.

Luzuriaga K, Bryson Y, Krogstad P *et al.* (1996). Combination treatments with zidovudine, didanosine and nevirapine in infants with human immunodeficiency virus type 1 infection. *New Engl J Med* 336: 1343.

Mellors JW, Dutschman GE, Im GJ *et al.* (1992). In vitro selection and molecular characterisation of human immunodeficiency virus-1 resistant to non-nucleoside inhibitors of reverse transcriptase. *Mol Pharmacol* 41: 446.

Mellors JW, Im GJ, Tramontano E *et al.* (1993). A single conservative amino acid substitution in the reverse transcriptase of human immunodeficiency virus-1 confers resistance to (+)-(5S)-4,5,6,7-tetrahydro-5-methyl-6-(3-methyl-2-butenyl)imidzao[4,5 1-jk][1,4]benzodiazepin-2(1H)-thione (TIBO R82150). *Mol Pharmacol* 43: 11.

Mellors JW, Bazmi HZ, Schinazi RF *et al.* (1995). Novel mutations in reverse transcriptase of human immunodeficiency virus type 1 reduce susceptibility to foscarnet in laboratory and clinical isolates. *Antimicrob Ag Chemother* **39**: 1087.

Merluzzi VJ, Hargrave KD, Labadia M *et al.* (1990). Inhibition of HIV-1 replication by a nonnucleoside reverse transcriptase inhibitor. *Science* **250**: 1411.

Merrill DP, Moonis M, Chou TC, Hirsch MS (1996). Lamivudine or stavudine in two and three drug combinations against human immunodeficiency virus type 1 replication *in vitro. J Infect Dis* **173**: 355.

Miyasaka T, Tanake H, Baba M *et al.* (1989). A novel lead for specific anti-HIV-1 agents; 1-[(2-Hydroxyethoxy)methyl]-6-(phenylthio)thymine. *J Med Chem* **32**: 2507.

Najera I, Richman DD, Olivares I *et al.* (1994). Natural occurrence of drug resistance mutations in the reverse transcriptase of human immunodeficiency virus type 1 isolates. *AIDS Res Hum Retrovir* **10**: 1479.

Nevirapine Product Information.

Norris SH, Silverstein HH, St George RL, Johnstone JN (1992). Nevirapine, an HIV-1 reverse transcriptase inhibitor; absorption, distribution and excretion in rats. *Pharm Res* **9**: S263.

Nowak MA (1995). AIDS pathogenesis, from models to viral dynamics in patients. *J AIDS Hum Retrovir* **10**: S1.

Nunberg JH, Schleif WA, Boots EJ *et al.* (1991). Viral resistance to human immunodeficiency virus type 1-specific pyridinone reverse transcriptase inhibitors. *J Virol* **65**: 4887.

Palaniappan C, Fay PJ, Bambara RA (1995). Nevirapine alters the cleavage specificity of ribonuclease H of human immunodeficiency virus 1 reverse transcriptase. *J Biol Chem* **270**: 4861.

Pauwels R, Andries K, Desmyter J *et al.* (1990). Potent and selective inhibition of HIV-1 replication *in vitro* by a novel series of TIBO derivatives. *Nature* **343**: 470.

Pauwels R, Andries K, Debyser Z *et al.* (1993). Potent and highly selective human immunodeficiency virus type 1 (HIV-1) inhibition by a series of alpha-anilinophenylacetamide derivatives targeted at HIV-1 reverse transcriptase. *Proc Natl Acad Sci USA* **90**: 1711.

Ren J, Esnouf R, Hopkins A *et al.* (1995). The structure of HIV-1 reverse transcriptase complexed with 9-chloro-TIBO; lessons for inhibitor design. *Structure* **3**: 915.

Richman DD (1994). Resistance, drug failure, and disease progression. *AIDS Res Hum Retrovir* **10**: 901.

Richman D, Rosenthal AS, Skoog M *et al.* (1991a). BI-RG-587 is active against zidovudine-resistant human immunodeficiency virus type 1 and synergistic with zidovudine. *Antimicrob Ag Chemother* **35**: 305.

Richman D, Shih CK, Lowy I *et al.* (1991b). Human immunodeficiency virus type 1 mutants resistant to nonnucleoside inhibitors of reverse transcriptase arise in tissue culture. *Proc Natl Acad Sci USA* **88**: 11241.

Richman DD, Havlir D, Corbeil J *et al.* (1994). Nevirapine resistance mutations of human immunodeficiency virus type 1 selected during therapy. *J Virol* **68**: 1660.

Rodgers DW, Gamblin SJ, Harris BA *et al.* (1995). The structure of unliganded reverse transcriptase from the human immunodeficiency virus type 1. *Proc Natl Acad Sci USA* **92**: 1222.

Romero DL, Busso M, Tan CK *et al.* (1991). Nonnucleoside reverse transcriptase inhibitors that potently and specifically block human immunodeficiency virus type 1 replication. *Proc Natl Acad Sci USA* **88**: 8806.

Romero DL, Morge RA, Genin MJ *et al.* (1993). 5-chloro-3-(phenyl-sulfonyl)indole-2-carboxamide: a novel, non-nucleoside inhibitor of HIV-1 reverse transcriptase. *J Med Chem* **36**: 1291.

Romero DL, Morge RA, Biles C *et al.* (1994). Discovery, synthesis and bioactivity of bis(heteroaryl)piperazines I A novel class of non-nucleoside HIV-1 reverse transcriptase inhibitors. *J Med Chem* **37**: 999.

Sardana VV, Emini EA, Gotlib L *et al.* (1992). Functional analysis of HIV-1 reverse transcriptase amino acids involved in resistance to multiple nonnucleoside inhibitors. *J Biol Chem* **267**: 17526.

Shih CK, Rose JM, Hansen GL *et al.* (1991). Chimeric human immunodeficiency virus type 1/type 2 reverse transcriptases display reversed sensitivity to nonnucleoside analog inhibitors. *Proc Natl Acad Sci USA* **88**: 9878.

Smerdon SJ, Jager J, Wang J *et al.* (1994). Structure of the binding site for nonnucleoside inhibitors of the reverse transcriptase of human immunodeficiency virus type 1. *Proc Natl Acad Sci USA* **91**: 3911.

Spence RA, Kati WM, Anderson KS, Johnson KA (1995). Mechanism of inhibition of HIV-1 reverse transcriptase by nonnucleoside inhibitors. *Science* **267**: 988.

Spence RA, Anderson KS, Johnson KA (1996). HIV-1 reverse transcriptase resistance to nonnucleoside inhibitors. *Biochemistry* **35**: 1054.

Tachedjian G, Hooker DJ, Gurusinghe AD, (1995). Characterisation of foscarnet-resistant strains of human immunodeficiency virus type 1. *Virology* **212**: 58.

Tantillo C, Ding J, Jacob-Molina A *et al.* (1994). Locations of anti-AIDS drug binding sites and resistance mutations in the three dimensional structure of HIV-1 reverse transcriptase. Implications for mechanisms of drug inhibition and resistance. *J Mol Biol* **243**: 369.

Taylor PB, Culp JS, Debouck C *et al.* (1994). Kinetic and mutational analysis of human immunodeficiency virus type 1 reverse transcriptase inhibition by inophyllums, a novel class of nonnucleoside inhibitors. *J Biol Chem* **269**: 6325.

Tisdale M, Kemp SD, Parry NR, Larder BA (1993). Rapid *in vitro* selection of human immunodeficiency virus type 1 resistant to 3'-thiacytidine inhibitors due to a mutation in the YMDD region of reverse transcriptase. *Proc Natl Acad Sci USA* **90**: 5653.

Tramontano E, Cheng YC (1992). HIV-1 reverse transcriptase inhibition by a dipyridodiazepinone derivative; BI-RG-587. *Biochem Pharmacol* **43**: 1371.

Vandamme AM, Debyser Z, Pauwels R *et al.* (1994). Characterisation of HIV-1 strains isolated from patients with TIBO R82913. *AIDS Res Hum Retrovir* **10**: 39.

Wu JC, Warren TC, Adams J *et al.* (1991). A novel dipyridodiazepinone inhibitor of HIV-1 reverse transcriptase acts through a nonsubstrate binding site. *Biochemistry* **30**: 2022.

Yuasa S, Sadakata Y, Takashima H *et al.* (1993). Selective and synergistic inhibition of human immunodeficiency virus type 1 reverse transcriptase by a non-nucleoside inhibitor, MKC-442. *Mol Pharmacol* **44**: 895.

Zhang H, Domadula G, Wu Y *et al.* (1996). Kinetic analysis of intravirion reverse transcription in the blood plasma of human immunodeficiency virus type-1 infected individuals; direct assessment of resistance inhibitors *in vivo. J Virol* **70**: 628.

Delavirdine

Description

Delavirdine mesylate, formerly known as U-90152, is a member of the bisheteroarylpiperazine (BHAP) class of non-nucleoside reverse transcriptase inhibitors discovered at UpJohn Laboratories (Romero *et al.*, 1991). Like other members of its class, it is active against HIV-1 reverse transcriptase but not that of HIV-2 or other retroviruses. Atevirdine (U-87201E) is a closely related compound of the same class (Romero *et al.*, 1994). Delavirdine has in some countries received approval for treatment of HIV infection. It is marketed under the trade name 'Rescriptor'.

The chemical name of delavirdine is 1-[3-[(1-methylethyl)amino]-2-pyridinyl]-4-[[5-[(methylsulfonyl)amino]-1H-indol-2-yl]carbonyl]-piperazine, monomethanesulfonate. The molecular formula is $C_{22}H_{28}N_6O_3S.CH_4O_3S$. The molecular weight of delavirdine is 552.68. The chemical structure is shown in Fig. V.55.

Antiviral Activity

Delavirdine is active against HIV-1 but not HIV-2. The subtype O (outlier) of HIV-1 may not be inhibited by delavirdine. The antiretroviral activity of delavirdine has been evaluated in HIV-1 infected peripheral blood mononuclear cells, T cell lines and monocyte-derived macrophages. The IC_{50} of delavirdine against the reverse transcriptase of HIV-1 is 0.26–0.29 μM (Dueweke *et al.*, 1993a; Fan *et al.*, 1995a). Delavirdine inhibits replication of clinical isolates of HIV-1 (including isolates that are zidovudine and/or didanosine resistant) in peripheral blood mononuclear cells with a mean IC_{50} of 0.06 μM (range <0.001–0.69 μM), and an IC_{90} of 0.1 μM (Dueweke *et al.*, 1993a; Nottet *et al.*, 1994; reviewed in Freimuth, 1996). In macrophage cultures, delavirdine inhibits HIV replication with an IC_{50} ranging from 0.02 to 0.1 μM (Dueweke *et al.*, 1993a). Atevirdine has an IC_{50} against clinical isolates (including those which are zidovudine-resistant) ranging from 0.06 to 1.6 μM (Campbell *et al.*, 1993).

Delavirdine has greater activity against HIV-1 than the protease inhibitor U75875 in acutely infected microglial cells, but less activity than U75875 in chronically infected monocytic cell lines (Peterson *et al.*, 1994).

Delavirdine is synergistic against HIV-1 replication when tested in combination with the protease inhibitor U-75875 or interferon alpha *in vitro* (Pagano and Chong, 1995). Both

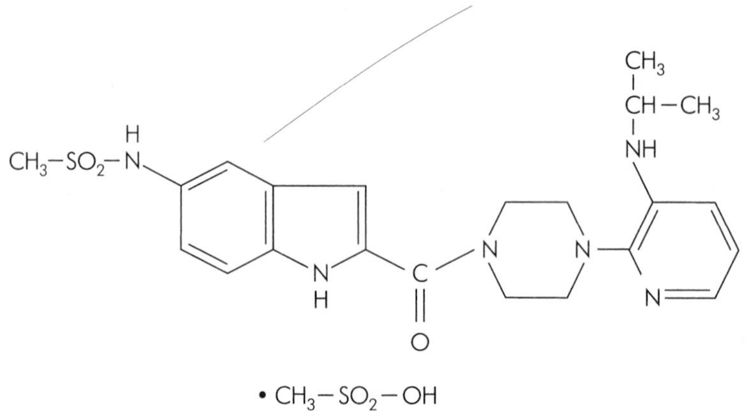

Fig. V.55.
Chemical structure of delavirdine. (Reproduced from Investigators Brochure, UpJohn Company, with permission.)

Table V.44
In vitro inhibition of recombinant HIV_IIIB RT mutants. (Reproduced from Dueweke *et al.*, 1993b, with permission. Copyright, 1993, National Academy of Sciences, USA.)

	IC$_{50}$ (μM) for indicated drug			
RT Mutant	Delavirdine (U-90152)	Nevirapine (BI-RG-587)	L-697–661	TIBO (R82913)
Wild type	0.26 ± 0.04	3.1 ± 0.32	0.80 ± 0.08	3.8 ± 0.6
Y181C	8.32 ± 0.70	>60[a]	>60[a]	38 ± 7
K103N	7.7 ± 0.6	>60[a]	15 ± 4.1	<60[a]
P236I	18.0 ± 2.1	0.32 ± 0.02	0.11 ± 0.01	0.34 ± 0.15
V181C/P236L	>60[a]	6 ± 1	10 ± 1.6	8.7 ± 1.1

[a] Highest concentration tested.

delavirdine and atevirdine show additive to synergistic effects with zidovudine against zidovudine-sensitive and -resistant strains of HIV-1 (Campbell *et al.*, 1993; Chong *et al.*, 1994). Didanosine is additive with atevirdine against didanosine-sensitive and resistant strains of HIV-1 (Campbell *et al.*, 1993). Three-drug combinations of delavirdine, and zidovudine with either didanosine or zalcitabine are synergistic in their inhibition of HIV-1 (Freimuth, 1996). The combination of delavirdine and nevirapine are antagonistic in their action on the inhibition of HIV reverse transcriptase activity (Gu *et al.*, 1995). There is synergistic activity between lamivudine and delavirdine (Delavirdine Product Information, 1997).

In vitro culture of cells infected with HIV-1 in the presence of delavirdine results in rapid emergence of resistance within three to four passages, with a 10- to 100-fold reduction in sensitivity to delavirdine (Balzarini *et al.*, 1993a,b). Combining delavirdine with nevirapine does not retard the development of mutations conferring resistance (Balzarini *et al.*, 1993b). A unique mutation at position 100 (Leu → Ile) has been reported in association with acquisition of resistance to delavirdine; this mutant remained sensitive to nevirapine (Balzarini *et al.*, 1993b,c). A mutation within amino acid 236 (Pro → Leu) results in a 70-fold decrease in susceptibility to delavirdine. An alteration in the shape of the binding pocket (p. 1772) preventing close interaction between delavirdine and the enzyme and thus conferring resistance of HIV-1 to delavirdine has been described in association with this mutation (Fan *et al.*, 1995b). The substitution results in sensitization of reverse transcriptase to nevirapine (Dueweke *et al.*, 1993b; Table V.44). Mutations within codons 228 and 273 have also been described (Dueweke *et al.*, 1993b), although they are not considered to be important in conferring resistance (Freimuth, 1996). Delavirdine only modestly inhibits strains of HIV-1 with the 181 mutation (Tyr → Cys), with an IC$_{50}$ of 8.3 μM, significantly higher compared with that of wild type (0.26 μM). Others have reported a greater than 150-fold reduction in sensitivity against recombinant reverse transcriptase mutants containing substitutions within both codons 181 and 188 (Fan *et al.*, 1995a), and in codons 103 and 181, suggesting that these residues contribute to the delavirdine binding site, and that there is a common binding site for nevirapine, delavirdine, the pyridinones and TIBO derivatives (Freimuth, 1996). Indeed, the IC$_{50}$ of nevirapine and pyridinone derivatives against a strain of HIV-1 with a mutation in codon 181 is greater than 60 μM for each drug) (Dueweke *et al.*, 1993b).

Phenotypic evidence of resistance has been observed in the majority of patients treated with delavirdine monotherapy within 8 weeks of commencing therapy. In a study of patients receiving delavirdine in combination with zidovudine, genotypic evidence of resistance was present in most patients within 24 weeks of treatment (Delavirdine Product Information, 1997).

In patients treated with delavirdine, the mutation at codon 103 has most frequently been observed. The 236 and 181 mutation have also been detected, but not mutations within codons 181 or 188 (Freimuth, 1996; Delavirdine Product Information, 1997).

Mode of Administration and Dosage

Delavirdine is administered orally in a dose of 400 mg three times daily. The drug may be administered with or without food. It should not be administered as monotherapy, due to rapid emergence of resistance. As delavirdine is metabolized mainly by the liver, the drug should be used with caution in patients with liver dysfunction (Delavirdine Product Information, 1997).

Availability

Delavirdine is available as 100-mg *tablets*.

Serum Levels in Relation to Dosage, Distribution of the Drug in Body and Excretion

Delavirdine is rapidly absorbed following oral administration, with a single-dose mean bioavailability of 85%. The peak in plasma concentration occurs in 1 h. In patients receiving 400 mg three times daily, the mean steady-state peak plasma concentration is 35 μM, with an area-under-the curve (AUC) of 180 μM (Delavirdine Product Information, 1997). Over total daily doses of 60–1200 mg the steady-state pharmacokinetics of delavirdine are non-linear, resulting in a 40-fold decrease in oral clearance and increase in apparent half-life as doses increase (reviewed in Freimuth, 1996). In dose-ranging studies, trough plasma levels of delavirdine in excess of 10 μM have readily been achieved, these being greater than 100-fold the IC_{90} of delavirdine. The mean plasma half-life of delavirdine is 5.8 h (range 2–11 h) following administration of 400 mg three times daily. Delavirdine is extensively bound to plasma proteins (approximately 98%) and is metabolized, at least partly, by the cytochrome P-450 enzymes (predominantly CYP3A, and possibly also CYP2D6) in the liver. Delavirdine decreases the activity of CYP3A and thus inhibits its own metabolism. Metabolism is mainly by N-desalkylation and pyridine hydroxylation. Steady-state concentrations of delavirdine in saliva and semen are 6% and 2% of plasma concentrations respectively in persons receiving 400 or 300 mg of delavirdine three times daily. The pharmacokinetics of delavirdine in children under the age of 16 years, or in patients with hepatic impairment have not been investigated. Women have a higher AUC (31%), with a dose of 400 mg three times daily, than men (Delavirdine Product Information, 1997).

Mode of Action

See chapter on nevirapine for details of mode of action of non-nucleoside reverse transcriptase inhibitors.

Similar to nevirapine, delavirdine and related BHAP compounds inhibit reverse transcriptase in a non-competitive fashion through binding to the enzyme at a site distinct from the nucleic acid binding site; they do not cause chain-termination (Dueweke *et al.*, 1992; Althaus *et al.*, 1993; Gu *et al.*, 1995).

Toxicity

From phase I/II clinical trials of delavirdine, the most frequent adverse reactions are a diffuse maculopapular rash, mild headache, nausea and fatigue.

1 Rash

The rash occurs in 30–45% of patients (although in some studies it was reported in less than 20%) and is more commonly seen in patients with lower CD4 counts (<100 cells per μl), than in those with CD4 counts >300 cells per μl. It usually develops between 1 and 2 weeks of initiating treatment, and is unrelated to dose or plasma concentration of drug. The rash is typically diffuse and maculopapular. Usually there are no associated symptoms although the rash may be pruritic. Treatment was interrupted in clinical trials of delavirdine in 43% of patients who developed rash. Generally patients were able to resume therapy after interruption. Dose titration does not significantly reduce the risk of rash. Stevens–Johnson syndrome has been rarely reported (one case in 1000) (Freimuth, 1996).

2 Other side-effects

Nausea is reported in a slightly higher proportion of patients receiving delavirdine in combination with didanosine or zidovudine than in those receiving either zidovudine or didanosine monotherapy. Similarly there are slightly more patients who experience increases in ALT or AST when receiving delavirdine in combination with zidovudine (about 2.5%) or didanosine (about 5%) than in those receiving either nucleoside as monotherapy (about 1–3%). Delavirdine Product Information, 1997).

3 Drug interactions

Co-administrations of a single dose of didanosine or antacid decreases the absorption and AUC of delavirdine (which is a weak base with low solubility at pH >3) by 37% and 48% respectively (Freimuth, 1996). In steady-state, however, co-administration of didanosine or taking delavirdine with food had no effect on the pharmacokinetics of the drug. However, the manufacturer recommends separating administration of delavirdine and didanosine by at least 1 h, based on other data which show a 20% decrease in both didanosine and delavirdine AUCs with simultaneous administration of these antiviral compounds. From phase I studies, there is no apparent pharmacokinetic interaction between delavirdine and zidovudine. Co-administration of delavirdine with either rifabutin or rifampicin, inducers of cytochrome P-450, resulted in 5- and 27-fold increases respectively in the clearance of delavirdine; rifampicin decreased trough plasma concentrations of delavirdine to less than $0.05\,\mu M$ (Freimuth, 1996). The rifabutin AUC was increased by 100% by co-administration with delavirdine. Antacids containing aluminum and magnesium result in a decrease in the AUC of delavirdine of approximately 41% (Delavirdine Product Information, 1997). Co-administration of clarithromycin in a dose of 500 mg twice-daily results in a 44% increase in the AUC of delavirdine (Delavirdine Product Information, 1997). Preliminary data suggest that co-administration of indinavir results in a 40% increase in AUC of indinavir with no effect on delavirdine pharmacokinetics. There appears to be no significant interaction between ritonavir and delavirdine but a study has not been performed using the currently recommended doses of these drugs. Delavirdine co-administration with saquinavir increases the AUC of saquinavir 5-fold, and also appears modestly to increase that of delavirdine (by about 15%) (Delavirdine Product Information, 1997). Ketoconazole increases the plasma trough concentration of delavirdine by 80%, although there appears to be no interaction with fluconazole. Fluoxetine increases the trough plasma concentration of delavirdine by about 50% (Delavirdine Product Information, 1997). Benzodiazepines, antihistamines such as terfenadine and astemizole, antimotility agents such as cisapride may all have increased plasma levels if co-administered with delavirdine. Anticonvulsants such as phenytoin and phenobarbital are predicted to lower delavirdine plasma levels (Delavirdine Product Information, 1997).

Clinical Uses of the Drug

Delavirdine has recently been aproved in some countries for the treatment of HIV infection, based on surrogate marker studies. Clinical benefit has not been demonstrated in a study comparing delavirdine monotherapy with delavirdine in combination with didanosine (Delavirdine Product Information, 1997). Like nevirapine, delavirdine should always be used in combination with other antiretroviral drugs.

Two phase I/II dose-escalation studies have been performed. Triple therapy with delavirdine (100–300 mg four times daily), didanosine and zidovudine was compared with didanosine and zidovudine in HIV- infected patients with CD4 counts of 100–300 cells per μl (mean 212 per μl at baseline) for a 24-week duration. The patients were a heavily pretreated group, with over 90% of participants receiving prior zidovudine therapy for a mean duration of 23 months, and over 70% receiving prior didanosine or zalcitabine for a mean duration of 10 months. Within 1 week, those randomized to receive triple therapy had a significant increase in CD4 counts and decline in both plasma p24 and HIV RNA levels. Strains of HIV resistant to delavirdine were present in some patients within 12 weeks of starting therapy, and this was reflected by a return towards baseline of surrogate markers. However, at week 24, a greater proportion of patients randomized to receive triple therapy than double therapy had a 5-fold or greater decline in plasma HIV RNA (44% versus 13% respectively) and a greater than 1 $\log_{10}$ decline in HIV RNA titer (77% versus 25% respectively) (reviewed in Freimuth, 1996).

In a second study 34 patients with 200–500 CD4 cells per μl (mean 390 per μl) and prior zidovudine experience for a mean duration of 17 months prior to study entry were given different doses of delavirdine (from 100 mg four times daily to 400 mg three times daily) in combination with zidovudine for 12 weeks. A rise in CD4 counts of greater than 50 cells per μl was evident in about half the participants; a decline in plasma p24 antigen occurred in approximately one-quarter of enrolled patients (reviewed in Freimuth, 1996).

In the randomized, double-blind study 0021, 718 patients with a mean baseline CD4 count of 334 cells per μl and a mean baseline plasma HIV RNA of 5.25 $\log_{10}$ copies per ml who had received less than 6 months of prior zidovudine therapy were randomized to receive either zidovudine of delavirdine (200 or 300 or 400 mg three times daily). There was no significant difference in CD4 count in dual therapy versus monotherapy recipients at week 24 of therapy. Recipients of delavirdine and zidovudine had a greater decline in HIV RNA than zidovudine monotherapy recipients (1 $\log_{10}$ versus 0.5 $\log_{10}$) at week 4 but there was little difference observed at 24 weeks, with those randomized to receive combination therapy having approximately a 0.6 $\log_{10}$ level below baseline and monotherapy group being about 0.5 $\log_{10}$ below baseline (Delavirdine Product Information, 1997).

In study 0017, delavirdine and didanosine combination therapy was compared with didanosine monotherapy in a randomized double-blind trial that enrolled 1190 HIV-infected patients who had a mean baseline CD4 count of 142 cells per µl and a mean baseline plasma HIV RNA of 5.77 $\log_{10}$ copies per ml. After 6 months of treatment there was no significant difference between the two arms in terms of survival or progression to AIDS (Delavirdine Product Information, 1997).

In the AIDS Clinical Trials Group (ACTG) 261 study, a total of 544 HIV-infected patients were enrolled who were nucleoside treatment-naive or who had less than 6 months experience with either zidovudine or didanosine. Two-thirds were antiretroviral-naive at entry. They had a mean baseline CD4 count of 296 cells per µl (range: 55–640 cells per µl) and were randomized to receive either delavirdine plus didanosine, delavirdine plus zidovudine, zidovudine plus didanosine or triple therapy with these drugs. The mean baseline plasma HIV RNA was 28 260 copies per ml. Preliminary data suggest that there is no difference in CD4 count or HIV RNA levels between the recipients of triple therapy or zidovudine and didanosine recipients (Delavirdine Product Information, 1997).

References

Althaus IW, Chou JJ, Gonzales AJ *et al.* (1993). Kinetic studies with the non-nucleoside HIV-1 reverse transcriptase inhibitor U-88204E. *Biochemistry* **32**: 6548.

Balzarini J, Karlsson A, Perez-Perez MJ, *et al.*, (1993a). Knocking out concentrations of HIV-1 specific inhibitors completely suppress HIV-1 infection and prevent the emergence of drug-resistant virus. *Virology* **196**: 576.

Balzarini J, Karlsson A, Perez-Perez MJ *et al.* (1993b). Treatment of human immunodeficiency virus type 1 (HIV-1)-infected cells with combinations of HIV-1 specific inhibitors results in a different resistance pattern than does treatment with single drug therapy. *J Virol* **67**: 5353.

Balzarini J, Karlsson A, De Clercq E (1993c). Human immunodeficiency virus type 1 drug-resistance patterns with different 1-[2-hydroxyethoxy) methyl]-6-(phenylthio)thymine derivatives. *Mol Pharmacol* **44**: 694.

Campbell TB, Young RK, Eron JJ *et al.* (1993). Inhibition of human immunodeficiency virus type 1 replication *in vitro* by the bisheteroaryl-piperazine atevirdine (U-87201E) in combination with zidovudine or didanosine. *J Infect Dis* **168**: 318.

Chong KT, Pagano PJ, Hinshaw RR (1994). Bisheteroarylpiperazine reverse transcriptase inhibitor in combination with 3'-azido-3'-deoxythymidine or 2',3'-dideoxyctidine synergistically inhibits human immunodeficiency virus type 1 replication *in vitro*. *Antimicrob Ag Chemother* **38**: 288.

Dueweke TJ, Kezdy FJ, Waszak GA *et al.* (1992). The binding of a novel bisheteroarylpiperazine mediates inhibition of human immunodeficiency virus type 1 reverse transcriptase. *J Biol Chem* **267**: 27.

Dueweke TJ, Poppe SM, Romero DL *et al.* (1993a). U-90152S, a potent inhibitor of human deficiency virus type 1 replication. *Antimicrob Ag Chemother* **37**: 1127.

Dueweke TJ, Pushkarskaya T, Poppe SM *et al.* (1993b). A mutation in reverse transcriptase of bisheteroaryl piperazine-resistant human immunodeficiency virus type 1 that confers increased sensitivity to other nonnucleoside inhibitors. *Proc Natl Acad Sci USA* **90**: 4713.

Fan N, Rank KB, Evans DT *et al.* (1995a). Simultaneous mutations of Tyr-181 and Tyr-188 in HIV-1 reverse transcriptase prevents inhibition of RNA-dependent DNA polymerase activity by the bisheteroarylpiperazine (BHAP) U-90152S. *FEBS Lett* **370**: 59.

Fan N, Evans DB, Rank KB *et al.* (1995b). Mechanism of resistance to U-90152S and sensitization to L-697,661 by a proline to leucine change at reside 236 of human immunodeficiency virus type 1 (HIV-1) reverse transcriptase. *FEBS Lett* **359**: 233.

Freimuth W (1996). Delavirdine mesylate, a potent non-nucleoside HIV-1 reverse transcriptase inhibitor. *Antiviral Chemotherapy, New Directions for Clinical Application and Research* Vol. 4, p. 279 (Mills J, Volberding P, Corey L, eds). New York: Plenum Press.

Gu Z, Quan Y, Li Z *et al.* (1995). Effects of non-nucleoside inhibitors of human immunodeficiency virus type 1 in cell-free recombinant reverse transcriptase assays. *J Biol Chem* **270**: 31046.

Nottet H, Oteman M, Visser MR *et al.* (1994). Anti-HIV-1 activities of novel non-nucleoside reverse transcriptase inhibitors. *J Antimicrob Ag Chemother* **33**: 366.

Pagano PJ, Chong KT (1995). *In vitro* inhibition of human immunodeficiency virus type 1 by a combination of delavirdine (U-90152) with protease inhibitor U-75875 or interferon-alpha. *J Infect Dis* **171**: 61.

Peterson PK, Gekker G, Hu S, Chao CC (1994). Anti-human immunodeficiency virus type 1 activities of U-90152 in human brain cell cultures. *Antimicrob Ag Chemother* **38**: 2465.

Romero DL, Busso M, Tan CK *et al.* (1991). Nonnucleoside reverse transcriptase inhibitors that potently and specifically block human immunodeficiency virus type 1 replication. *Proc Natl Acad Sci USA* **88**: 8806.

Romero DL, Morge RA, Biles C *et al.* (1994). Discovery, synthesis and bioactivity of bis(heteroaryl)piperazines 1 A novel class of non-nucleoside HIV-1 reverse transcriptase inhibitors. *J Med Chem* **37**: 999.

Saquinavir

Description

The HIV protease inhibitors are a novel and diverse group of compounds with activity against the aspartic class of proteases encoded by retroviruses. During replication of HIV, the structural Gag and Gag-Pol precursor proteins are proteolytically cleaved by the HIV protease (or proteinase) into smaller functional proteins necessary for structural integrity, maturation and infectivity of HIV. Inhibition of this enzyme results in the production of immature, non-infectious virions lacking the dense core structure characteristic of HIV virions. A number of inhibitors of the HIV protease have received approval for the treatment of HIV infection in certain countries. They include saquinavir mesylate (initially synthesized by S Redshaw of J A Martin's group at Roche Welwyn, previously called XVII:26, or Ro 31–8959), which is now marketed under the trade name 'Invirase' by Roche Pharmaceuticals, indinavir (previously called MK-639, or L-735,524), which is now marketed by Merck Sharpe and Dohme under the trade name of 'Crixivan' (p. 1800), ritonavir (previously called ABT-538), now marketed by Abbott under the trade name of 'Norvir' (p. 1795), and nelfinavir (previously known as AG1313), now marketed by Agouron under the trade name of 'Viracept' (p. 1806).

A number of other protease inhibitors are in basic or preclinical development or clinical trial. These include VX-478 developed by Vertex and currently under development by Glaxo-Wellcome (p. 1809), DG17 developed by Narhex and currently in early clinical trials in Australia, aminodiol protease inhibitors such as BMS 186,318 (Patick *et al.*, 1995), non-peptide cyclic urea protease inhibitors such as DMP323 (Erickson-Viitanen *et al.*, 1994) and XM323 developed by Du Pont-Merck (Winslow *et al.*, 1994). Others such as the penicillin-derived protease inhibitors (Kitchin *et al.*, 1994) have been found to have poor pharmacokinetic properties and have thus been suspended from clinical development.

Saquinavir is a peptide-based asymmetric hydroxyethylene mimetic of the transition state that occurs during peptide bond cleavage by aspartic proteases. It has a molecular weight of 766.96. The chemical name for saquinavir is *cis*-N-tert-butyl-decahydro-2[2(R)-hydroxy-4-phenyl-3(S)-[[N-(2-quinolylcarbonyl)-L-asparginyl]amino]butyl]-(4aS,8aS)-isoquinoline-3(S)-carboxyamide methanesulfonate. The molecular formula is $C_{38}H_{50}N_6O_51:1CH_4O_3S$. The chemical structure is shown in Fig. V.56.

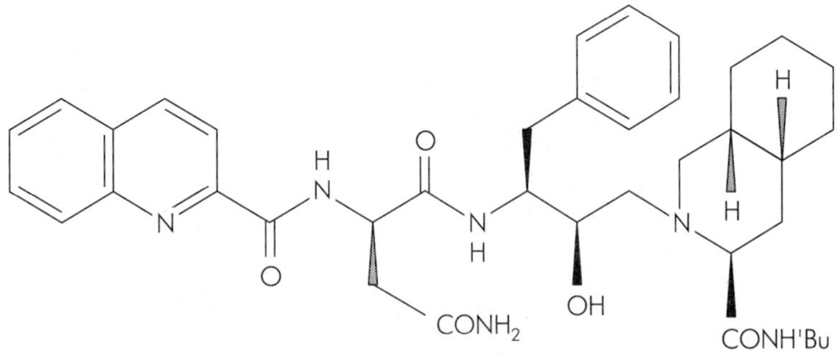

Fig. V.56.
Chemical structure of saquinavir.

Antiviral Activity

1 Human immunodeficiency virus

Saquinavir inhibits HIV-1 with an IC_{50} of 0.5–6 nM and an IC_{90} of 6–30 nM (Craig et al., 1991a; Eberle et al., 1995), with production of HIV markedly reduced in the presence of concentrations of saquinavir of 10 nM (Krausslich, 1992). Saquinavir is effective even when added to cultures post-infection (Craig et al., 1991a; Galpin et al., 1994), consistent with its activity late in the replicative cycle (assembly and maturation). In experiments in HIV-infected MT-4 T cell lines, addition of saquinavir at high concentration (100 nM) 1 h post-infection, with subsequent maintenance of the cells in the presence of this concentration of drug for 87 days resulted in clearance of detectable infection (Nitschko et al., 1994). Saquinavir is active against both zidovudine-sensitive and zidovudine-resistant strains of HIV (Galpin et al., 1994). Clinical isolates and reference strains from HIV-1 clades A, B, D and E have all been shown to be susceptible to saquinavir, as well as other protease inhibitors (Winslow et al., 1995). Although HIV-1 and HIV-2 proteases have different cleavage recognition sequences and only 50% homology at the amino acid level (Le Grice et al., 1989; Galpin et al., 1994), saquinavir is also active at nanomolar concentrations against HIV-2 protease and that of simian immunodeficiency virus SIV_{mac251} (Martin et al., 1991). Saquinavir poorly inhibits the protease of HTLV-1 (Daenke et al., 1994).

Antiretroviral efficacy of saquinavir at a concentration of 10 nM has also been demonstrated against HIV-1 replication in both acute and chronically infected cells in vitro (Craig et al., 1991a). This effect on chronically infected cells is to be expected given the activity of protease inhibitors at a site in the replicative cycle of HIV that is post-integration (pp. 1787–1790).

2 Animal studies

Oral or subcutaneous saquinavir therapy is effective in treating severe combined immunodeficiency (SCID) mice that were injected with human T cell lines infected with HIV-1 (Sato et al., 1995).

3 Synergy

Additive to synergistic interactions occur between saquinavir and zidovudine, against both zidovudine-sensitive and -resistant strains of HIV-1, and between saquinavir and zalcitabine (Craig et al., 1990; Johnson et al., 1992). The triple combination of zidovudine, saquinavir and zalcitabine produces at least the same level of synergistic inhibition of HIV in vitro as the double combinations (Craig et al., 1994). Lamivudine and saquinavir, and these two drugs in combination with zidovudine, have demonstrable additive or synergistic interactions. Similarly stavudine and saquinavir and these two drugs in combination with zidovudine are additive to synergistic against zidovudine sensitive strains of HIV-1 (Merrill et al., 1996). In vitro additive antiretroviral effect has been demonstrated between saquinavir and non-nucleoside inhibitors of HIV-1 (Brennan et al., 1995). Additive to synergistic activity has been demonstrated for the combination of interferon alpha and saquinavir (Johnson et al., 1992).

4 Acquired resistance

Resistance to saquinavir arises relatively slowly and to a modest degree compared with reverse transcriptase inhibitors such as lamivudine in which resistance develops rapidly. Strains of HIV-1

Table V.45

Resistance to protease inhibitors. Modified from Eberle et al., (1995), Condra et al., (1995), Tisdale et al. (1995).

Protease inhibitor	Major mutations		Cross-resistance[a]
Saquinavir	48	Gly→ Val	Nelfinavir[c] indinavir[c],
	90[b]	Leu→ Met	Ritonavir[a]
Indinavir	82[a]	Val→ Ala/Phe	Ritonavir, nelfinavir
	46	Met→ Ile	XM-412, saquinavir
	63	Leu→ Phe	VX-478
Ritonavir	82[b]	Val→ Ala/Phe	Indinavir
	54	Ile→ Val	
	36	Ile→ Leu	
	71	Ala→ Val/Thr	

[a] Data are based on studies of very small numbers of isolates; see text for sources of data.
[b] Key mutation in vivo.
[c] Infrequently reported to date.

(but not HIV-2) have been reported to develop resistance to saquinavir during *in vitro* passage in the presence of the drug; as few as five passages has been found to generate resistant strains (Dianzani *et al.*, 1993; Jacobsen *et al.*, 1995; Eberle *et al.*, 1995).

The development of resistance occurs as a result of a series of step-wise mutations (Table V.45). The initial mutation occurs at position 48 (Gly→ Val), and subsequently at position 90 (Leu→ Met) and/or 54 (Ile→ Val) (Turriziani *et al.*, 1994; Jacobsen *et al.*, 1995; Eberle *et al.*, 1995; Tisdale *et al.*, 1995). The individual mutations at position 48 and 90, and mutations at both these sites result in successively less processing of Gag and Gag-Pol polyproteins *in vitro*, as demonstrated by Western blot. Proteases from these mutants are 220-, 20-, and 720-fold less sensitive to saquinavir and resulting in a 4- to 6-fold, a 2-fold and an 8- to 10-fold increase in IC_{50} respectively (Maschera *et al.*, 1995). These results are supported by other investigators who found that mutations at positions 48, 90 and 54 caused a 50-fold increase in IC_{90} (from 20 to >1000 nM) (Eberle *et al.*, 1995). The mutation at position 48 occurs at the hinge of the beta ribbon strands near the active site of the protease, potentially sterically hindering entry of the inhibitor to the active site (Eberle *et al.*, 1995).

A study of sequences of HIV following intermediate passage of infected T-cell lines in the presence of increasing concentrations of saquinavir suggest that positions 12, 36, 57 and 63 contribute to the development of resistance (Jacobsen *et al.*, 1995). Mutations within codons 84 and 71, in the presence of changes in codons 48 and 90, have also been reported in association with saquinavir-resistance, and mutant HIV strains with all 4 of these mutations demonstrate cross-resistance to other protease inhibitors including VX-478, indinavir, ritonavir, and XM323 (Tisdale *et al.*, 1995). The mutation at position 84 occurs rarely (reviewed in Roberts, 1995).

Mutations conferring resistance have been shown to arise in 45% of patients treated with saquinavir (1800 mg per day) alone or in combination with zidovudine for 8–12 months. Of those receiving combination therapy with saquinavir, zalcitabine and zidovudine, protease-resistant strains of HIV-1 were detected in 22%. The most common mutation observed was within codon 90 (Leu→ Met), with mutations within codon 48 rarely observed (Jacobsen *et al.*, 1996).

5 Cross-resistance

As may be expected, there is no cross-resistance between the reverse transcriptase inhibitors and protease inhibitors including saquinavir. There is, however, evidence of cross-resistance between saquinavir-resistant strains of HIV and other protease inhibitors, although based on limited data broad cross-resistance to other protease inhibitors is not a feature of saquinavir-resistant isolates. Strains of HIV that are resistant to VX-478 and the aminodiol protease inhibitor BMS 186,318 remain sensitive to saquinavir (Partaledis *et al.*, 1995; Patick *et al.*, 1995).

Condra and colleagues (Condra *et al.*, 1995) reported that ritonavir-resistant strains of HIV obtained from patients treated with ritonavir demonstrated cross-resistance to saquinavir only after development of multiple mutations (at positions 10, 46, 63, 82 and 84 within the HIV protease). Current data suggest that HIV isolates from 80–90% of patients who take saquinavir for 1 year will retain sensitivity to indinavir and ritonavir (Data on file, Hoffman La Roche). Cross-resistance between saquinavir and nelfinavir has been observed (Jacobsen *et al.*, 1996).

Mode of Administration and Dosage

1 Oral administration

The recommended dose of saquinavir is 600 mg three times daily, each dose being taken within 2 h of eating (see below). This recommendation is based on dose-ranging studies in which higher doses (200 to 600 mg three times per day) were associated with somewhat better responses than lower doses in terms of surrogate markers (immunologic and virologic), although no clear cut evidence of benefit was shown (Kitchen *et al.*, 1995a).

2 Hepatic failure

Although there are no available data for patients regarding pharmacokinetics of saquinavir in patients with severe hepatic impairment, it would be prudent to monitor such patients closely during saquinavir therapy, and to consider dose-reduction.

Availability

Saquinavir is available as hard gelatin *capsules* containing 228.7 mg of saquinavir mesylate, which is equivalent to 200 mg saquinavir free base.

Serum Levels in Relation to Dosage

Data currently available relate to the hard gelatin capsule. The pharmacokinetics of the soft gelatin capsule are currently being evaluated. Plasma and urinary levels of saquinavir can be measured by high-performance liquid chromatography (Woolf *et al.*, 1995).

1 Oral administration

The doses of saquinavir for the first dose-ranging study were chosen to achieve a plasma concentration of 12 ng per ml, based on *in vitro* estimates of the IC_{90}. For patients receiving the 600 mg three times daily dose, steady-state plasma concentrations were five times the target concentration in 11 of 12 patients, remaining above this value for the entire dosing interval in 10 of 12 patients. For those receiving 200 mg three times daily, saquinavir was detectable in plasma for the duration of the dose interval in the majority of patients, but not in those receiving 25 mg three times daily (Kitchen *et al.*, 1995a). The drug has non-linear pharmacokinetics when measured in doses of 75, 200 and 600 mg administered three times daily (Noble and Faulds, 1996). There was evidence of drug accumulation (2- to 3-fold) over a period of 4 weeks (Kitchen *et al.*, 1995b).

The mean oral bioavailability of a 600 mg dose when taken following food is very low, in the range of 4% (18-fold greater than in the fasted state) (Table V.46) (Noble and Faulds, 1996). This is partly because only 30% is absorbed, and also due to considerable first-pass metabolism of the drug (Williams *et al.*, 1992). The absorption of saquinavir is rapid when administered after fasting (T_{max} 2.4 h), and is delayed when taken with food (T_{max} approximately 3.8 h) (Muirhead *et al.*, 1992). The extent of absorption is also markedly increased when taken following food (the area-under-the curve (AUC) increases from 24 ng per h per ml in the fasted state to 161 ng per h per ml when taken anytime from 5 min to 2 h following food). Unrefined grapefruit juice also increases absorption of saquinavir. Steady-state concentrations of saquinavir appear to be higher in HIV-infected patients than in healthy volunteers (Data on file, Hoffman-La Roche).

2 Liver dysfunction

As saquinavir is extensively metabolized in the liver, the drug should be used with caution in patients with evidence of hepatic impairment. An increase in saquinavir plasma concentrations could be expected in patients with moderate to severe liver disease, although formal studies have not been performed in this patient population.

3 Renal dysfunction

Saquinavir has not been formally assessed in patients with renal insufficiency. However, patients with mild to moderate renal dysfunction participated in phase I/II trials, and from these studies there are no data to suggest that the dose of saquinavir needs to be modified in this patient population (Data on file, Hoffman La Roche).

4 Pregnancy

Although saquinavir appears to be safe in animals in that there is no embryotoxicity or teratogenicity in animals when the drug is administered in high dose, caution should be used in prescribing saquinavir to pregnant women, and the manufacturer recommends that the drug should not be given to breast-feeding women.

5 Pediatric use

There are no data available on the pharmacokinetics of saquinavir in children under 12 years of age.

Table V.46
Clinically relevant pharmacokinetic data

Extremely low oral bioavailability in fasted state, increasing to 4% when taken with food
Plasma concentrations of saquinavir are increased by grapefruit juice
Extensive metabolism in liver by CYP 3A4 isoenzyme of cytochrome P-450
Less than 4% renal excretion
Very low central nervous system penetration

---

6 Elderly

There are no data on pharmacokinetics of saquinavir in patients over 60 years of age.

Excretion

Metabolism of saquinavir is predominantly by the liver, with the specific isoenzyme CYP3A4 of cytochrome P-450 mediating more than 90% of hepatic metabolism. The drug is metabolized to a number of inactive mono- and di-hydroxylated derivatives (Farrar et al., 1994). Of interest, saquinavir does not appear to be a potent inhibitor of the cytochrome P-450 system. The kidneys are responsible for less than 4% of the excretion of saquinavir; 96% of an i.v. dose appears in the feces within 48 h (Data on file, Hoffman La Roche).

Distribution of the Drug in Body

The mean steady-state volume of distribution was estimated to be 700 liters following i.v. administration of a 12-mg dose of saquinavir. The drug is distributed widely throughout the body, and is very highly protein bound (approximately 98%), the latter contributing to the very low levels found in CSF (<0.06% of plasma concentration). Intracellular concentrations are unknown.

Mode of Action

The HIV protease is a homodimer characterized by C2 symmetry, with each of the identical subunits containing the 99 amino acids of the protease gene product (reviewed in Leonard, 1996). The HIV-1 and HIV- 2 proteases, and those of other lentivirus proteases studied thus far, are similar in terms of gross structure (Mulichak et al., 1993) (Fig. V.57).

The development of many protease inhibitors was based on mimics of the transition state that occurs during peptide bond cleavage by aspartic proteases, with statine representing the lead structure. Importantly, the inhibitors of HIV protease were designed to contain a non-cleavable peptide bond (McQuade et al., 1990; reviewed in Debouck and Metcalf, 1990). Using this approach, the synthesis of peptide inhibitors with an optimum length of six to seven amino acids was initially adopted, despite prior knowledge of suboptimal properties of the peptide-based drugs, including proteolytic degradation resulting in reduced activity, rapid hepatic metabolism and poor oral bioavailability (Hadar and McGowan, 1993). These transition state mimics are sub-classified as reduced amides or aminomethylene isosteres (Dreyer et al., 1989), statine analogs (Hui et al., 1991), dihydroxyethylene, hydroxyethylene and hydroxyethylamine isosteres such as indinavir (Rich et al., 1990; Dreyer et al., 1989; Vacca et al., 1991; Roberts et al., 1990), alpha-difluoroketones (Dreyer et al., 1989) and phosphinate derivatives (Grobelny et al., 1990) (Fig. V.58). A second group of inhibitors are the C2-symmetric inhibitors such as ritonavir (Kempf et al., 1990; Erickson et al., 1990; Kort et al., 1993; Ho et al., 1994; Martin, 1993). Other classes of protease inhibitors are dimerization inhibitors, non-peptide cyclic urea inhibitors (Otto et al., 1993; Erickson-Viitanen et al., 1994) and natural products such as cerulenin (reviewed in Debouck, 1992).

Saquinavir was designed as a peptide-like structural mimetic of the transition state which occurs during cleavage of the Gag and Gag-Pol precursor proteins. These sites are only cleaved

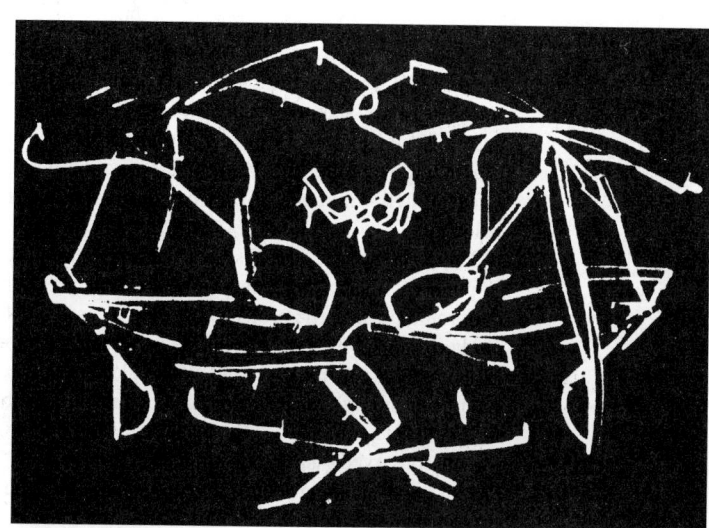

Fig. V.57.
Structure of HIV protease with an inhibitor that stabilizes the enzyme in an inactive configuration. (Reproduced from Coleman and Scheife, 1994, with permission.)

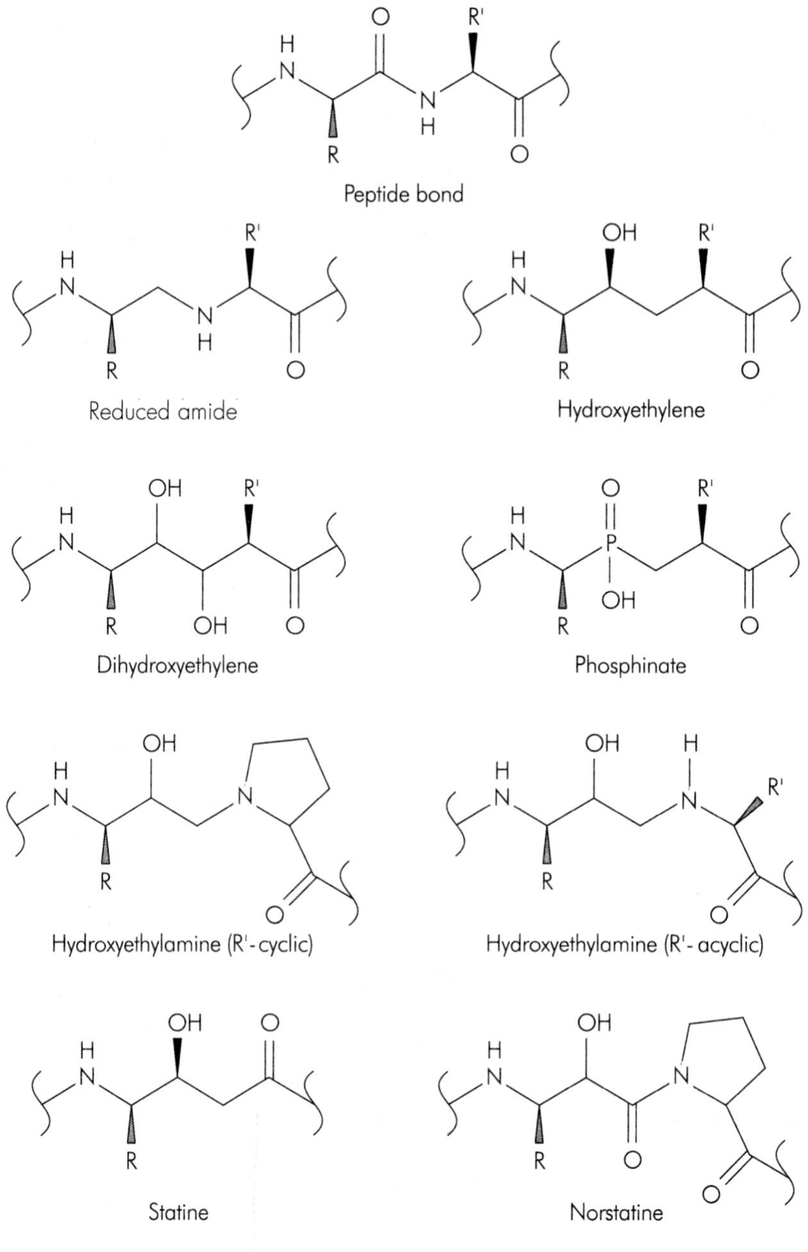

Fig. V.58.

Structural formulae of chemical groups that can replace a peptide in a proteinase inhibitor. (Reproduced from Wlodawer, 1994, with permission.)

Peptide bond

Reduced amide

Hydroxyethylene

Dihydroxyethylene

Phosphinate

Hydroxyethylamine (R'-cyclic)

Hydroxyethylamine (R'-acyclic)

Statine

Norstatine

by the HIV protease although a common amino acid sequence at each cleavage site is not apparent. Thus saquinavir can sit within the active site of the HIV protease and inhibit the activity of the enzyme. Unlike the reverse transcriptase inhibitors, protease inhibitors including saquinavir do not require metabolic activation within the cell in order to exert their inhibitory effects on HIV replication. The mechanism of action of saquinavir is described in more detail below.

The HIV protease belongs to the family of aspartic proteases, which includes cathepsin D and E, pepsin, renin and gastricsin (Darke *et al.*, 1989), and which can be inhibited in cell culture by the prototypic aspartic protease inhibitor pepstatin (Nutt *et al.*, 1988; Von der Helm *et al.*, 1989; Darke *et al.*, 1989). The HIV protease is a dimer, whereas the non-viral proteases of this class are monomeric (Gustchina and Weber, 1990). The active site is formed at the dimer interface, with one aspartyl residue from each subunit contributing to protease activity (Lapatto *et al.*, 1989; Miller *et al.*, 1989; Navia *et al.*, 1989; Weber *et al.*, 1989; Wlodawer *et al.*, 1989). The highly conserved Asp-Thr(Ser)-Gly sequence (DGT motif) within the HIV protease has been shown to be homologous to the catalytic site of proteases of the aspartic family, resulting in the inclusion of the HIV protease in this class of enzymes (Toh *et al.*, 1985; Pearl and Taylor, 1987).

Saquinavir is specific for HIV protease, and therefore does not inhibit renin, pepsin, cathepsins D or E and gastricsin at 10 μM concentration, or any of the serine or cysteine proteases (Martin, 1991). Pepstatin was the first aspartyl protease that demonstrated activity against HIV, as well as bovine leukemia virus, Moloney murine leukemia virus and HTLV-1 (Katoh *et al.*, 1987). Unlike cell-derived aspartic proteases, HIV proteases do not cleave at all of these expected sites in all proteins and are specific for their own precursor proteins (Skalka, 1989).

The critical role of proteolytic processing in retroviral replication is dependent on intact HIV protease function (Fig. V.59). The *gag* gene of HIV is translated as a 55kDa fusion protein, Pr55^{gag}, which is subsequently cleaved by HIV protease into the structural proteins matrix, capsid and nucleocapsid proteins. The *pol* gene is translated into the Gag-Pol polyprotein Pr60$^{gag-pol}$ which is processed by HIV protease to produce the reverse transcriptase, integrase, and RNase H (reviewed in Huff, 1991; Hirsch and D'Aquila, 1993). The cleavage by HIV protease within the Gag and Gag-Pol polyproteins is frequently between the hydrophobic Phe or Tyr and Pro peptides (four of the eight cleavage sites) (Kotler *et al.*, 1988; Roberts *et al.*, 1990), which is unusual in that other proteases cannot cut peptide bonds in front of a proline residue (Wlodawer, 1994). The precursor polyproteins are synthesized on cytoplasmic ribosomes and then accumulate at sites of virion assembly at the plasma membrane, associating with the membrane via myristoylation sequences on Gag and Gag-Pol. At this stage the immature virion separates from the host cell by a process of budding. The processing of these precursor polyproteins occurs during or soon after the budding of the new virion from the host cell membrane (reviewed in Wlodawer, 1994). Although most of the processing is membrane or virion associated, protease activity has also been observed within the cytoplasm: processing is blocked in both compartments by protease inhibitors (Kaplan and Swanstrom, 1991). From electron microscopic studies the activity of protease is associated with condensation of the retroviral core (Hockley *et al.*, 1988). Inhibition of HIV protease results in inhibition of particle assembly and the production of immature, non-infectious virions without a condensed core (Kohl *et al.*, 1988; Schatzl *et al.*, 1991). This inhibition can be demonstrated *in vitro* by Western blot analysis by an observed reduction in p24 and other Gag proteins in the culture supernatants of infected cells due to inhibition of processing of the Pr55^{Gag} precursor (Nutt *et al.*, 1988; McQuade *et al.*, 1990; Craig *et al.*, 1991b).

Solving the crystal structure of the HIV protease in 1989 (Navia *et al.*, 1989; Wlodawer *et al.*, 1989; Lapatto *et al.*, 1989), and HIV protease complexed with an inhibitor (Miller *et al.*, 1989; Fitzgerald *et al.*, 1990; Swain *et al.*, 1990) has provided a significant impetus for the rational design of protease inhibitors. Based on the symmetry afforded by the homodimeric structure of the HIV protease and its active site, symmetric inhibitors have been developed (Kempf *et al.*,

Fig. V.59.
Organization of the HIV-1 genome. Viral RNS is initially translated into the gag polyprotein or, through a translational frame shift, the gag-pol polyprotein. Protease is believed to begin the cascade of protein processing by autocatalytically cleaving itself out of gag-pol polyprotein. Protease is then free to process the remainder of the gag and gag-pol plyproteins into the proteins shown in the figure. RT = reverse transcriptase; RNaseH = ribonuclease H; IN = integrase. (Reproduced from Robins and Plattner, 1993, with permission from Lippencott–Raven Publishers.)

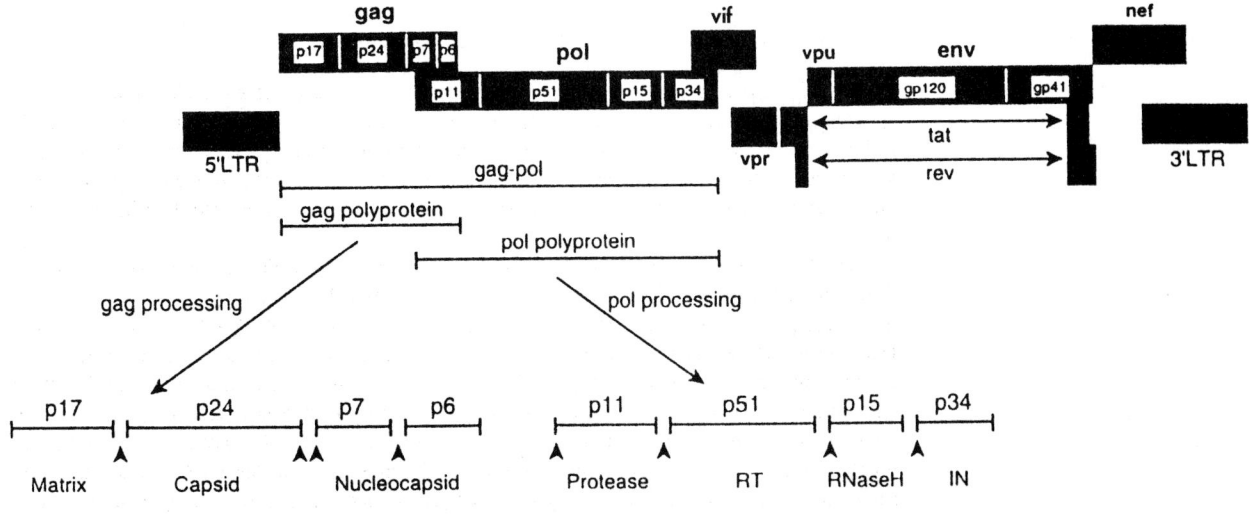

1990), as well as asymmetric inhibitors based upon Phe.Pro transition state analogs (Roberts *et al.*, 1990). These inhibitors can be peptidic (such as saquinavir) or non-peptidomimetic inhibitors. A prominent beta-strand hairpin loop from each monomer projects over, and encloses, the active site (Rodriguez *et al.*, 1993). These beta hairpins or 'flaps' of the protease are mobile and move by as much as 15–20 Angstroms to generate a completely open conformation in order to allow the natural substrate or the inhibitor gain access to the active site of the protease. Up to seven residues can be accommodated within this binding site (Weber *et al.*, 1989). After binding, the flaps close and catalytic action is initiated, directed by two essential aspartic acids contained within the active site (Gustchina and Weber, 1990; reviewed in Wlodawer, 1994). Although there is great structural diversity among the various HIV protease inhibitors, a common feature of protease-inhibitor complexes is the presence of a water molecule that forms a bridge between the two flaps of the protease and the inhibitor. The two hydrogen bonds between the conserved water and carbonyl oxygen atoms of the protease inhibitor are predicted to be important for the tight binding of the inhibitors within the active site (Gustchina *et al.*, 1994).

The cleavage of the peptide bond by aspartyl-type proteases occurs by a number of steps, the main one of which is the formation of a transition state analog. Following initial deprotonation of a water molecule by one of the aspartate carboxylates within the active site of the protease, an unstable tetrahydral transition state is formed when the donated proton binds to the scissile P_1-P'_1 peptide bond of the substrate, with the second aspartyl residue within the active site of the protease serving to stabilize this intermediate prior to final stages of catalysis (reviewed in Debouck and Metcalf, 1990; Debouck, 1992). Saquinavir and other transition state analogs mimic the natural recognition sites within the transition state for HIV protease but are resistant to proteolytic cleavage. The transition state binds to the protease more tightly than the substrate, thereby providing a strategy for the design of the transition state analog protease inhibitors (reviewed in Redshaw, 1994). As an example, the hydroxylethylamine group of saquinavir replaces the peptide bond within the transition state, thus preventing proteolytic cleavage. All the transition state mimetics have tetrahedral geometry at the position that would have formed the carbonyl centre of the scissile bond.

The synthesis of saquinavir has been described elsewhere (Martin 1991; Parkes *et al.*, 1994).

Toxicity

1 Adverse reactions reported in clinical trials

Saquinavir is extremely well tolerated, with no major reported adverse reactions. Some nausea, diarrhea and abdominal discomfort have been reported in less than 5% of study participants. Modest elevation of hepatic transaminases has been noted in some patients. In a randomized double-blind dose-ranging study in 49 HIV-infected asymptomatic individuals who were zidovudine-naive, doses of saquinavir of up to 600 mg three times daily for 16 weeks was not associated with any serious adverse events (Kitchen *et al.*, 1995). In a phase II trial saquinavir was not associated with any severe adverse reactions (Collier *et al.*, 1996).

2 Animal studies

Saquinavir was not mutagenic and did not induce DNA damage in animal toxicity studies. There was no evidence of impairment of fertility and no embryotoxicity or teratogenicity in rats although maternotoxicity and abortions were observed in pregnant rabbits (Data on file, Hoffman La Roche).

Table V.47

Some important drug interactions with saquinavir

Terfenanide[a]
Astemizole[a]
Cisapride[a]
Ketoconazole[b]
Rifampicin[c]
Rifabutin[c]
Ritonavir[b]

[a] Increases plasma concentration of this drug
[b] Increases plasma concentration of saquinavir
[c] Decreases plasma concentration of saquinavir

3 Drug interactions
(Table V.47)

Saquinavir should not be co-administered with terfenadine, astemizole, and cisapride because of potential elevations of plasma concentrations of the latter drugs and thus potential cardiac arrhythmias. Ketoconazole, which inhibits cytochrome P-450 enzymes, increases the plasma concentration of saquinavir approximately 3-fold. Rifampicin and rifabutin, both inducers of cytochrome P-450, significantly lower saquinavir levels (80% and 40% respectively). Ritonavir has been found to significantly increase saquinavir plasma concentrations, although ritonavir levels do not significantly alter (Data on file, Hoffman La Roche). There is no apparent pharmacokinetic interaction between saquinavir and zidovudine. There are a number of other potential interactions (see Saquinavir Product Information).

Clinical Uses of the Drug

1 Human immuodeficiency virus infection

In many countries, saquinavir is approved for use in the treatment of HIV infection in combination with nucleoside analog antiretroviral therapies. In general, therapy with saquinavir can be expected to increase CD4 counts in peripheral blood and reduce HIV RNA levels in plasma. Some of the studies demonstrating efficacy of saquinavir and its use in combination with other antiretroviral compounds are outlined below.

Three clinical studies have been performed in Europe. The antiviral activity, tolerability and pharmacokinetics of saquinavir were evaluated in a randomized, double-blind, dose-ranging study in the UK of 49 antiretroviral-naive, HIV-infected persons with asymptomatic or minimally symptomatic disease and CD4 counts of <500 cells per μl. Saquinavir was administered orally in doses of 25, 75, 200 or 600 mg three times daily after food for a duration of 16 weeks (Kitchen et al., 1995). The investigators concluded that the highest dose of saquinavir showed a trend towards improvement in CD4 counts, maximally occurring at about week 4 of treatment. The plasma HIV culture did not become negative in any of the eight individuals with detectable plasma viremia at baseline. Higher dose regimens of saquinavir were associated with a trend towards lowering of HIV RNA and DNA and decreased likelihood of isolation of virus from peripheral blood mononuclear cells. Adverse events were mild and mostly considered to be unrelated to treatment (Kitchen et al., 1995).

A similar phase I/II dose-ranging study was performed in France, in 61 HIV-infected participants who were antiretroviral-experienced and who had advanced disease with CD4 counts of 50–250 cells per μl. The median CD4 count at study entry was 153 cells per μl, and the median duration of prior zidovudine therapy was approximately 400 days. There was a trend towards improvement in CD4 counts with the 600-mg dose, with a median maximum change of 56 cells per μl occurring on average 2 weeks after commencing therapy. There was a significant difference in the change in the CD4 count in the 600-mg arm compared with the lower dosage regimens. At the end of the 16-week study, the median CD4 count was 5.5 cells per μl above baseline. The drug was also found to be very well tolerated in this trial (reviewed in Vella, 1994, 1995; Data on file, Hoffman La Roche).

In a third phase I/II trial in Italy, saquinavir, in doses of 75 mg, 200 mg and 600 mg given orally three times per day for 16 weeks, was evaluated in combination with zidovudine (600 mg per day), and compared with zidovudine and saquinavir (600 mg three times daily) monotherapies. The study participants were 92 antiretroviral-naive HIV-infected males and females with advanced infection (CD4 counts of less than 300 cells per μl). The toxicity profile of saquinavir was not altered by combination therapy with zidovudine, although the incidence of adverse events was greater in those receiving combination therapy than monotherapy. The mean increase in CD4 across all arms of the study during treatment was 22 cells per μl. Combination therapy with 200- and 600-mg doses of saquinavir was associated with higher and more sustained increases in CD4 counts than observed in either monotherapy arm, and the 600-mg dose in combination with zidovudine was associated with the greatest reduction in plasma viremia (reviewed in Vella, 1994, 1995; Pollard, 1994).

AIDS Clinical Trial Group study 229 was a randomized double-blind phase II trial of 24 weeks duration in 302 participants with 50–300 CD4 cells per μl who had received at least 4 months of prior zidovudine therapy. Patients were randomized to receive saquinavir (600 mg three times daily) in combination with zalcitabine (0.75 mg three times daily) and zidovudine (200 mg three times daily), or saquinavir and zidovudine, or zalcitabine and zidovudine. The study was later extended providing participants with an additional optional 3–8 months of unblinded therapy. These patients had extensive prior antiretroviral experience with a median duration of prior zidovudine therapy of 27 months. The median CD4 count at study entry was 145 cells per μl. Surrogate markers of CD4 count and quantitative virus culture in PBMCs were used as primary endpoints. The triple combination was found to be superior to either of the double-combination regimens. After 24 weeks of therapy, CD4 counts had returned to baseline in 31% of triple

Fig. V.60.
CD4+ T cell counts and plasma human immunodeficiency virus (HIV) RNA levels over time in patients receiving saquinavir, 3600 mg per day or 7200 mg per day. **Top:** Patients receiving 3600 mg per day. Open squares = CD4+ T cell counts; open circles = plasma HIV-1 RNA levels. **Bottom:** Patients receiving 7200 mg per day. Solid squares = CD4+ T cell counts; solid circles = plasma HIV-1 RNA levels. Bars indicate 95% CIs. (Reproduced from Schapiro, 1996, with permission from the American College of Physicians.)

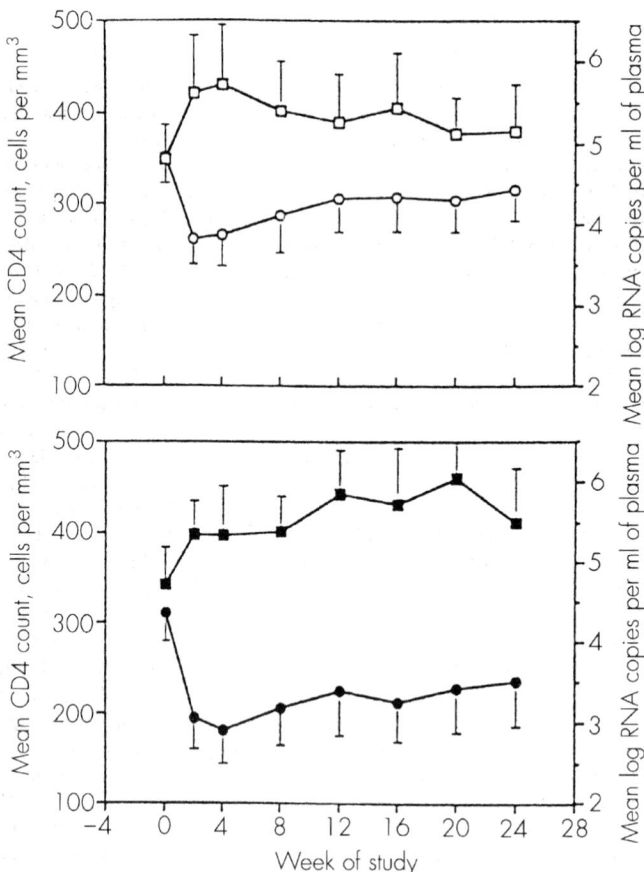

combination recipients, 37% receiving saquinavir and zidovudine, and 55% receiving zalcitabine and zidovudine. Similarly, greater reductions in viral burden were observed in those randomized to receive the triple-combination than the double-combination therapies. There was an approximate 0.8 $\log_{10}$ reduction in HIV RNA copies per ml plasma in triple combination recipients at week 4, with HIV RNA levels not returning to baseline in this arm over 48 weeks. There was no sustained decline in HIV RNA in saquinavir/zidovudine recipients, and a 0.4 $\log_{10}$ reduction in HIV RNA in zalcitabine/zidovudine recipients, maintained for 16 weeks, and not returning to baseline over 48 weeks. There was no significant difference in adverse events between the treatment arms (Collier *et al.*, 1996).

NV14256 was a randomized placebo-controlled trial of saquinavir monotherapy, versus zalcitabine monotherapy, versus the combination of both drugs in 1086 participants with a median CD4 count of 160–180 cells per μl, and approximately 72 weeks of prior zidovudine therapy. In this study, combination therapy was associated with fewer new opportunistic infections and significantly improved survival (Data on file, Hoffman La Roche).

The efficacy and safety of high dose saquinavir have recently been evaluated. In an open-label study, 40 HIV-infected patients with CD4 counts between 200 and 500 cells per μl were treated with either 3600 or 7200 mg of saquinavir per day for 24 weeks. The high-dose regimen was superior to the low-dose regimen (Fig. V.60) resulting in greater and more prolonged reduction in plasma HIV RNA than the low-dose regimen, with a mean maximum decline in plasma HIV RNA of 1.34 $\log_{10}$ and 1.06 $\log_{10}$ copies per ml respectively. The mean maximum increase in CD4 cells was higher in the high-dose than in the low-dose regimens, being 121 and 72 cells per μl respectively. The mean decline in plasma HIV RNA after 24 weeks of treatment was still greater in the high-dose than the low-dose group, being 0.85 and 0.48 $\log_{10}$ copies per ml respectively; similarly CD4 counts were 82 and 31 cells per μl above baseline in the high and low dose groups respectively (Schapiro *et al.*, 1996).

Acknowledgements The author would like to thank Christopher Birch, Victorian Infectious Diseases Reference Laboratory, Melbourne, for his critical review of this chapter.

References

Brennan TM, Taylor DL, Bridges CG et al. (1995). The inhibition of human immunodeficiency virus type 1 in vitro by a non-nucleoside reverse transcriptase inhibitor MKC-442, alone and in combination with other anti-HIV compounds. Antiviral Res 26: 173.

Coleman R, Scheife RT (1994). Proteinase inhibitors; the result of rational drug design. Pharmacotherapy 14: 1S.

Collier AC, Coombs RW, Schoenfeld DA (1996). Treatment of human immunodeficiency virus infection with saquinavir, zidovudine and zalcitabine. New Engl J Med 334: 1011.

Condra JH, Schleif WA, Blahy OM et al. (1995). In vivo emergence of HIV-1 variants resistant to multiple protease inhibitors. Nature 374: 569.

Craig JC, Duncan IB, Whittaker L, Roberts NA (1990). Antiviral synergy between inhibitors of HIV proteinase and reverse transcriptase. Antiviral Chem Chemother 4: 161.

Craig JC, Duncan IB, Hockley D et al. (1991a). Antiviral properties of Ro 31–8959, an inhibitor of human immunodeficiency virus (HIV) proteinase. Antiviral Res 16: 295.

Craig JC, Grief C, Mills JS et al. (1991b). Effects of a specific inhibitor of HIV proteinase (Ro 31–8959) on virus maturation in a chronically infected promonocytic cell line (U1). Antiviral Chem Chemother 2: 181.

Craig JC, Whittaker L, Duncan IB, Roberts NA (1994). In vitro anti-HIV and cytotoxicological evaluation of the triple combination; AZT and ddC with HIV proteinase inhibitor saquinavir (Ro 31–8959). Antiviral Chem Chemother 5: 380.

Daenke S, Schramm HJ, Bangham CR (1994). Analysis of substrate cleavage by recombinant protease of human T cell leukaemia virus type 1 reverse preferences and specificity of binding. J Gen Virol 75: 2233.

Darke PL, Leu CT, Davis LJ et al. (1989). Human immunodeficiency virus protease. Bacterial expression and characterisation of the purified aspartic protease. J Biol Chem 264: 2307.

Debouck C, Metcalf BW (1990). Human immunodeficiency virus protease. A target for AIDS therapy. Drug Develop Res 21: 1.

Debouck C (1992). The HIV-1 protease as a therapeutic target for AIDS. AIDS Res Hum Retrovir 8: 153.

Dianzani F, Antonelli G, Turrizianl O et al. (1993). In vitro selection of human immunodeficiency virus type 1 resistant to Ro 31–8959 proteinase inhibitor. Antiviral Chem Chemother 4: 329.

Data on file, Hoffman La Roche.

Dreyer GB, Metcalf BW, Tomaszek TA et al. (1989). Inhibition of human immunodeficiency virus 1 protease in vitro rational design of substrate analogue inhibitors. Proc Natl Acad Sci USA 86: 9752.

Eberle J, Bechowsky B, Rose D et al. (1995). Resistance of HIV type 1 to proteinase inhibitor Ro 31–8959. AIDS Res Human Retrovir 11: 671.

Erickson J, Neidhart DJ, Van Drie J et al. (1990). Design, activity and 28 A crystal structure of a C2 symmetric inhibitor complexed to HIV-1 protease. Science 249: 527.

Erickson-Viitanen S, Klabe RM, Cawood PG et al. (1994). Potency and selectivity of inhibition of human immunodeficiency virus protease by a small nonpeptide cyclic urea DMP 323. Antimicrob Ag Chemother 38: 1628.

Farrar G, Mitchell AM, Hopper H et al. (1994). Prediction of potential drug interactions of saquinavir (Ro 31–8959) from in vitro data. Brit J Clin Pharmacol 38: 162.

Fitzgerald PM, McKeever BM, Van Middlesworth JF et al. (1990). Crystallographic analysis of a complex between human immunodeficiency virus type 1 protease and acetyl-pepstatin at 20-A resolution. J Biol Chem 265: 14209.

Galpin S, Roberts NA, O'Connor T et al. (1994). Antiviral properties of the HIV-1 proteinase inhibitor Ro 31–8959. Antiviral Chem Chemother 5: 43.

Grobelny D, Wondiuk EM, Garlady RE et al. (1990). Selective phosphinate transition state analogue inhibitors of the protease inhibitor L-687, 908 a potent hydroxyethylene-containing HIV protease inhibitor. J Med Chem 34: 1111.

Gustchina A, Weber IT (1990). Comparison of inhibitor binding in HIV-1 protease and in non-viral aspartic proteases; the role of the flap. FEBS Lett 269: 269.

Gustchina A, Sansom C, Prevost M et al. (1994). Energy calculations and analysis of HIV-1 protease inhibitor crystal structures. Protein Eng 7: 309.

Hadar M, McGowan JJ (1993). Promising drugs in preclinical development for therapy of HIV infection. Antiviral Chemotherapy, New Directions for Clinical Application and Research Vol. 3, p. 275 (Mills J, Corey L, eds). New Jersey: PTR Prentice Hall.

Hirsch MS, D'Aquila RT (1993). Therapy for human immunodeficiency virus infection. New Engl J Med 328: 1686.

Ho DD, Toyoshima T, Mo H et al. (1994). Characterisation of human immunodeficiency virus type 1 variants with increased resistance to a C2-symmetric protease inhibitor. J Virol 66: 2016.

Hockley DJ, Wood RD, Jacobs JP, Garrett AJ (1988). Electron microscopy of human immunodeficiency virus. J Gen Virol 69: 2455.

Huff JR (1991). HIV proteases; A novel chemotherapeutic target for AIDS. J Med Chem 34: 2305.

Hui KY, Manetta JV, Gygi T et al. (1991). A rational approach in the search for potent inhibitors against HIV proteinase. FASEB J 5: 2606.

Jacobsen H, Yasargil K, Winslow DL et al. (1995). Characterisation of human immunodeficiency virus type 1 mutants with decreased sensitivity to proteinase inhibitor Ro 31–8959. Virology 206: 527.

Jacobsen H, Hanggi M, Ott M et al. (1996). In vivo resistance to a human immunodeficiency virus type 1 proteinase inhibitor; mutations, kinetics and frequencies. J Infect Dis 173: 1379.

Johnson VA, Merrill DP, Chou TC, Hirsch MS (1992). Human immunodeficiency virus type 1 (HIV-1) inhibitory interactions between protease inhibitor Ro 31 8959 and zidovudine, 2'3'-dideoxycytidine, or recombinant interferon-alpha A against zidovudine-sensitive or resistant HIV-1 in vitro. J Infect Dis 166: 1143.

Kaplan AH, Swanstrom R (1991). Human immunodeficiency virus type 1 Gag proteins are processed in two cellular compartments. Proc Natl Acad Sci USA 88: 4528.

Katoh I, Yasunaga T, Ikawa Y, Yoshinaka Y (1987). Inhibition of retroviral protease activity by an aspartyl proteinase inhibitor. Nature 329: 654.

Kempf DJ, Norbeck DW, Codacovi LM et al. (1990). Structure based C2 symmetric inhibitors of HIV protease. J Med Chem 33: 2687.

Kitchin J, Bethell RC, Cammack N et al. (1994). Synthesis and structure-activity relationships of a series of penicillin-derived HIV proteinase inhibitors; heterocyclic ring systems containing P1' and P2' substituents. J Med Chem 37: 3707.

Kitchen VS, Skinner C, Ariyoshi K et al. (1995a). Safety and activity of saquinavir in HIV infection. Lancet 345: 952.

Kitchen V, Stewart F, Bragman K, Weber J (1995b). Emerging proteinase inhibitors. Lancet 345: 1512.

Kohl NE, Emini EA, Schleif WA et al. (1988). Active human immunodeficiency virus protease is required for viral infectivity. Proc Natl Acad Sci USA 85: 4686.

Kort JJ, Bilello JA, Bauer G, Drusano GL (1993). Preclinical evaluation of antiviral activity and toxicity of Abbott A77003 an inhibitor of the human immunodeficiency virus type 1 protease. Antimicrob Ag Chemother 37: 115.

Kotler M, Katz RA, Danho W et al. (1988). Synthetic peptides as substrates and inhibitors of a retroviral protease. Proc Natl Acad Sci USA 85: 4185.

Krausslich HG (1992). Specific inhibitor of human immunodeficiency virus proteinase prevents the cytotoxic effects of a single chain proteinase dimer and restores particle formation. J Virol 66: 567.

Lapatto R, Blundell T, Hemmings A et al. (1989). X-ray analysis of HIV-1 proteinase at 27 A resolution confirms structural homology among retroviral enzymes. Nature 342: 299.

Le Grice SF, Ette R, Mills J, Mous J (1989). Comparison of the human immunodeficiency virus type 1 and 2 protease by hybrid gene construction and trans-complementation. J Biol Chem 264: 14902.

Leonard JM (1996). Perspectives in HIV protease inhibitors *Antiviral Chemotherapy, New Directions for Clinical Application and Research* Vol. 4, p. 319 (Mills J, Volberding PA, Corey L, eds). New York: Plenum Press.

Martin JA (1991). Ro 31–8959/003. *Drugs of the Future* **16**: 210.

Martin JA (1993). Recent advances in the design of HIV proteinase inhibitors. *Antiviral Res* **17**: 265.

Martin JA, Mobberley MA, Redshaw S *et al.* (1991). The inhibitory activity of a peptide derivative against the growth of simian immunodeficiency virus in CB166 cells. *Biochem Biophy Res Commun* **176**: 180.

Maschera B, Furfine E, Blair ED (1995). Analysis of resistance to human immunodeficiency virus type 1 protease inhibitors by using matched bacterial expression and proviral infection vectors. *J Virol* **69**: 5431.

McQuade TJ, Tomasselli AG, Lui L *et al.* (1990). A synthetic HIV-1 protease inhibitor with antiviral activity arrests HIV-like particle maturation. *Science* **247**: 454.

Merrill DP, Moonis M, Chou TC, Hirsch MS (1996). Lamivudine or stavudine in two and three drug combinations against human immunodeficiency virus type 1 replication *in vitro*. *J Infect Dis* **173**: 355.

Miller M, Schneider J, Sathyanarayana BK *et al.* (1989). Structure of complex of synthetic HIV-1 protease with a substrate based inhibitor at 23 A resolution. *Science* **246**: 1149.

Muirhead GJ, Shaw T, Williams PEO *et al.* (1992). Pharmacokinetics of the HIV proteinase inhibitor, RO-31–8959, after single and multiple oral doses in healthy volunteers. *Brit J Clin Pharmacol* **34**: 170.

Mulichak AM, Hui JO, Tomasselli AG *et al.* (1993). The crystallographic structure of the protease from human immunodeficiency virus type 2 with two synthetic peptide transition state analog inhibitors. *J Biol Chem* **268**: 13103.

Navia MA, Fitzgerald PMD, McKeever BM *et al.* (1989). Three dimensional structure of aspartyl protease from human immunodeficiency virus HIV-1. *Nature* **337**: 615.

Nitschko H, Lindhofer H, Schatzl H *et al.* (1994). Long-term treatment of HIV-infected MT-4 cells in culture with HIV proteinase inhibitor Ro 31–8959 leads to complete cure of infection. *Antiviral Chem Chemother* **5**: 236.

Noble S, Faulds D (1996). Saquinavir A review of its pharmacology and clinical potential in the management of HIV infection. *Drugs* **52**: 93.

Nutt RF, Brady SF, Darke PL *et al.* (1988). Chemical synthesis and enzymatic activity of a 99-residue peptide with a sequence proposed for the human immunodeficiency virus protease. *Proc Natl Acad Sci USA* **85**: 7129.

Otto MJ, Reid CD, Garber S *et al.* (1993). *In vitro* anti-human immunodeficiency virus (HIV) activity of XM323, a novel HIV protease inhibitor. *Antimicrob Ag Chemother* **37**: 2606.

Parkes K, Bushnell DJ, Crackett PH *et al.* (1994). Studies toward the large scale synthesis of the HIV proteinase inhibitor Ro 31–8959. *J Org Chem* **69**: 3656.

Partaledis JA, Yamaguchi K, Tisdale M *et al.* (1995). *In vitro* selection and characterisation of human immunodeficiency virus type 1 (HIV-1) isolates with reduced sensitivity to hydroxyethylamino sulfonamide inhibitors of HIV-1 aspartyl protease. *J Virol* **69**: 5228.

Patick AK, Rose R, Greytok J *et al.* (1995). Characterisation of a human immunodeficiency virus type 1 variant with reduced sensitivity to an aminodiol protease inhibitor. *J Virol* **69**: 2148.

Pearl IH, Taylor WR (1987). A structural model for the retroviral proteases. *Nature* **329**: 351.

Pollard RB (1994). Use of proteinase inhibitors in clinical practice. *Pharmacotherapy* **14**: 21S.

Redshaw S (1994). Inhibitors of HIV proteinase. *Expert Opinion Invest Drugs* **3**: 273.

Rich DH, Green J, Toth MW *et al.* (1990). Hydroxyethylamine analogues of the p17/p24 substrate cleavage site are tight-binding inhibitors of HIV protease. *J Med Chem* **33**: 1285.

Roberts NA (1995). Drug resistance patterns of saquinavir and other HIV proteinase inhibitors. *AIDS* **9** (Suppl 2): 27.

Roberts NA, Martin JA, Kinehington D *et al.* (1990). Rational design of peptide based HIV proteinase inhibitors. *Science* **248**: 358.

Robins T, Plattner J (1993). HIV proteinase inhibitors: their anti-HIV activity and potential role in treatment. *J AIDS* **6**: 162

Rodriguez EJ, Debouck C, Deckman IC *et al.* (1993). Inhibitor binding to the Phe53Trp mutant of HIV-1 protease promotes conformational changes detectable by spectrofluorometry. *Biochem* **32**: 3557.

Sato A, Kodama M, Abe K *et al.* (1995). A simple and rapid method for preliminary evaluation of *in vivo* efficacy of anti-HIV compounds in mice. *Antiviral Res* **27**: 151.

Schapiro JM, Winters MA, Stewart F *et al.* (1996). The effect of high dose saquinavir on viral load and CD4+ T-cell counts in HIV infected patients. *Ann Intern Med* **124**: 1039.

Schatzl H, Gelderblom HR, Nitschko H, von der Helm K (1991). Analysis of non infectious HIV particles produced in presence of HIV proteinase inhibitor. *Arch Virol* **120**: 71.

Skalka AM (1989). Retroviral proteases; first glimpses at the anatomy of a processing machine. *Cell* **55**: 911.

Swain AL, Miller MM, Green J *et al.* (1990). X-ray crystallographic structure of a complex between a synthetic protease of human immunodeficiency virus 1 and a substrate based hydroxyethylamine inhibitor. *Proc Natl Acad Sci USA* **87**: 8805.

Toh H, Ono M, Saigo K, Miyata T (1985). Retroviral protease-like sequence in the yeast transposon Ty1. *Nature* **315**: 691.

Tisdale M, Myers RE, Maschera B *et al.* (1995). Cross-resistance analysis of human immunodeficiency virus type 1 variants individually selected for resistance to five different protease inhibitors. *Antimicrob Ag Chemother* **39**: 1704.

Turriziani O, Antonelli G, Jacobsen H *et al.* (1994). Identification of an amino acid substitution involved in the reduction of sensitivity of HIV-1 to an inhibitor of viral proteinase. *Acta Virologica* **38**: 297.

Vacca JP, Guare JP, De Solms SJ, (1991). L-687,908 a potent hydroxy-ethylene-containing HIV protease inhibitor. *J Med Chem* **34**: 1225.

Vella S (1994). Update on a proteinase inhibitor. *AIDS* **8**: S25.

Vella S (1995). Rationale and experience with reverse transcriptase inhibitors and protease inhibitors. *J AIDS Hum Retrovir* **10**: S58.

Von der Helm K, Gurtler L, Eberle J, Deinhardt F (1989). Inhibition of HIV replication in cell culture by the specific aspartic protease inhibitor pepstatin A. *FEBS Lett* **247**: 349.

Weber IT, Miller M, Jaskolski M *et al.* (1989). Molecular modelling of the HIV-1 protease and its substrate binding site. *Science* **243**: 928.

Williams PEO, Sampson AP, Green CP *et al.* (1992). Disposition and bioavailability of the HIV proteinase inhibitor Ro 31–8959, after single doses in healthy volunteers. *Brit J Clin Pharmacol* **34**: 155.

Winslow DL, Mayers D, Scarnati H *et al.* (1994). *In vitro* susceptibility of clinical isolates of HIV-1 to XM323, a non-peptidyl HIV protease inhibitor. *AIDS* **6**: 753.

Winslow DL, Stack S, King R *et al.* (1995). Limited sequence diversity of the HIV type 1 protease gene from clinical isolates and *in vitro* susceptibility to HIV protease inhibitors. *AIDS Res Hum Retrovir* **11**: 107.

Wlodawer A (1994). Rational drug design; the proteinase inhibitors. *Pharmacotherapy* **14**: 9S.

Wlodawer A, Miller M, Jaskolski M *et al.* (1989). Conserved folding in retroviral proteases; crystal structure of a synthetic HIV-1 protease. *Science* **245**: 616.

Woolf E, Au T, Haddix H, Matuszewski B (1995). Determination of L-735 524, an human immunodeficiency virus protease inhibitor, in human plasma and urine via high performance liquid chromatography with column switching. *J Chromatog* **692**: 45.

Zhao B, Winborne E, Minnich MD *et al.* (1993). Three-dimensional structure of a simian immunodeficiency virus protease/inhibitor complex Implications for the design of human immunodeficiency virus type 1 and 2 protease inhibitors. *Biochem* **32**: 13054.

Ritonavir

Description

Ritonavir, (formerly known as ABT-538), is a peptidomimetic inhibitor of HIV-1 and HIV-2 proteases. It is marketed by Abbott under the brand name of 'Norvir'. The drug was developed as a modification of compounds A-77003 and A-80987, resulting in improved bioavailability.

The chemical name is 10-hydroxy-2-methyl-5-(1-methylethyl)-1-[2-(1-methylethyl)4-thiazolyl]-3,6-dioxo-8,11-bis(phenylmethyl)-2,4,7,12-tetraazatridecan-13-oicacid,5-thiazolylmethyl ester. The chemical formula is $C_{37}H_{48}N_6O_5S_2$. The molecular weight is 720.95. The chemical structure is shown in Fig. V.61. The concentration of the drug can be expressed as either μM or μg per ml, and 1 μM of ritonavir is approximately equivalent to 0.7 μg per ml.

Antiviral Activity

The IC_{50} of ritonavir against clinical and laboratory-adapted strains of HIV-1 in T cell lines is 22–130 nM and 160 nM against HIV-2 (Kempf *et al.*, 1995). The IC_{50} against clinical isolates of HIV-1 is approximately 22nM (Data on file, Abbott). The IC_{90} of ritonavir against HIV-1 when cells are cultured in medium containing 10% serum is approximately 100 nM (Kempf *et al.*, 1995). As ritonavir is virtually completely bound to plasma proteins (see below), the functional IC_{90} after adjusting for plasma protein binding is likely to be significantly higher, in the vicinity of 300 nM (approximately 2.1 μg per ml) (Danner *et al.*, 1995). Ritonavir is active against reverse-transcriptase-resistant strains of HIV (Leonard, 1996). The compound has low cytotoxicity, with greater than 20 μM of ritonavir required to inhibit cellular growth by 50%, resulting in an *in vitro* therapeutic index of at least 1000 (Data on file, Abbott).

Ritonavir is additive with the protease inhibitor VX-478 in inhibiting HIV replication *in vitro* (St Clair *et al.*, 1996).

Strains of HIV that have reduced susceptibility to ritonavir (or related compound A-77003) emerge rapidly during serial passage of virus in the presence of increasing concentrations of drug (Ho *et al.*, 1994; Kaplan *et al.*, 1994; Markowitz *et al.*, 1995b). After passaging 20 times *in vitro*, mutant strains of HIV have been reported with up to 16-fold increase in IC_{90} (Markowitz *et al.*, 1995b). Sequence analysis of isolates with a resistant phenotype revealed substitutions within codons 46 (Met→ Ile), 82 (Val→ Phe) and 84 (Ile→ Val). Computer modeling suggests that these changes destabilize the inhibitor-protease complex through either steric hindrance or by altering amino acid side-chains required for direct interactions (Leonard, 1996).

During treatment with ritonavir, strains of HIV-1 have been isolated which have decreased sensitivity to ritonavir *in vitro*. Genotypic analysis has revealed mutations within the HIV protease, including within codons 82 (Val→ Ala or Phe), 52 (Ile→ Val), 71(Ala→ Val), 84 (Ile→ Val) (Molla *et al.*, 1995; Norbeck *et al.*, 1995). In phase I/II trials, there appeared to be a stepwise development of mutations, with changes at positions 82 (Val→ Ala or Phe), 54 (Ile→Val), 71

Fig. V.61.
Structure of ritonavir (ph = phenyl). (Reproduced from Norvir (ritonavir capsules) Product Information, Abbott Australasia Pty Limited, with permission.)

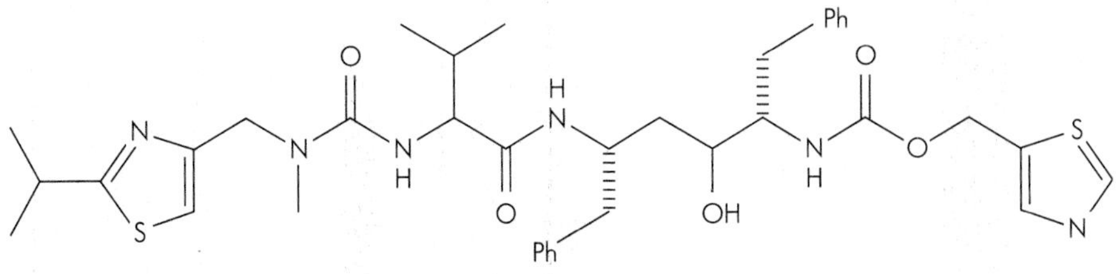

(Ala→ Val or Thr), and 36 (Ile→ Leu), followed by other combinations of mutations (see Table V.41, p. 1784). The mutation within codon 82 appears to be necessary for the development of phenotypic resistance, but this alone is insufficient to confer measurable resistance, and phenotypic changes usually also require the presence of at least one additional mutation (Molla et al., 1996). Higher plasma levels of ritonavir were associated with slower development of mutations conferring resistance (Molla et al., 1996).

Studies on cross-resistance are limited. Preliminary data suggest that ritonavir-resistant strains of HIV may also have reduced susceptibility to indinavir (Data on file, Abbott). Similarly, cross-resistance between indinavir-resistant strains of HIV and A-80987 (an inhibitor closely related to ritonavir) has been reported (Tisdale et al., 1995; reviewed in Emini et al., 1996). The ritonavir-resistant strains of HIV appear to remain sensitive to saquinavir and nelfinavir (Data on file, Abbott). There is no evidence of cross-resistance to reverse transcriptase inhibitors.

Mode of Administration and Dosage

Ritonavir is administered orally in a dose of 600 mg every 12 h, based on data from phase I/II studies. The dose-related side-effects suggest that the 600-mg regimen is approaching the maximum tolerated dose (Danner et al., 1995). It is recommended that ritonavir is taken with food.

The manufacturer recommends caution when using ritonavir in patients with impaired hepatic function as the drug is mainly metabolized by the liver.

Availability

Ritonavir is available in *capsules* containing 100 mg ritonavir, and *solution* containing 80 mg per ml.

Serum Levels in Relation to Dosage, Excretion and Distribution of the Drug in Body

Plasma concentrations of ritonavir in HIV-infected subjects receiving greater than 400 mg every 12 h exceed 2.1 μg per ml, the estimated IC_{90} after adjusting for plasma protein binding. In phase I studies, the time to peak plasma concentration (T_{max}) ranged from 2.2 h when ritonavir was administered every 12 h in a dose of 300 mg, to 3.3 h for doses of 500 or 600 mg administered every 12 h. The peak plasma concentration (C_{max}) at steady-state increased with the administered dose, being 5.7 $\pm$2.5 μg per ml for those given 300 mg twice-daily to 11.2 $\pm$3.6 μg per ml in those given 600 mg twice-daily. The area-under-the-curve (AUC) also increased in a similar fashion, being 29.7 $\pm$14.6 and 60.8 $\pm$ 23.4 μg per h per ml for the 300-mg and 600-mg doses respectively. Trough plasma concentrations were 3.7$\pm$ 2.6 μg per ml at steady-state with a dose of 600 mg every 12 h. The half-life ranged from 2.7 to 3.2 h (Danner et al., 1995; Kempf et al., 1995).

The absolute bioavailability of ritonavir has not been determined. The absorption of ritonavir capsules is approximately 15% higher when administered with a meal (Table V.48). Under non-fasting conditions the oral administration of ritonavir solution resulted in a reduction of plasma ritonavir levels by 23% (Data on file, Abbott).

Ritonavir is 99% bound to plasma proteins (Leonard, 1996), with alpha-1-acid glycoprotein being the principal binding protein (Data on file, Abbott).

The cytochrome P-450 pathway is the major pathway of metabolism of ritonavir, with CYP3A being the predominant iso-enzyme involved (this pathway is described in Slaughter and Edwards, 1995). Metabolites have been identified, with the isopropylthiazole oxidation derivative being the principal metabolite. Although this derivative has antiviral potency similar to that of the parent compound, the plasma levels are low and preliminary evidence suggests that it does not contribute significantly to the antiviral activity of ritonavir.

In individuals taking ritonavir solution, approximately 11% of the drug is excreted in urine, with about 3% of the oral dose being excreted unchanged. Fecal excretion comprises about 86%, with 33% of the dose eliminated as unchanged parent drug (Data on file, Abbott). The

Table V.48
Clinically relevant pharmacokinetics of ritonavir

Absorption of ritonavir increases when taken with food by about 15%
Ritonavir is highly bound to plasma proteins (99%)
The hepatic cytochrome P-450 pathway is the major metabolic pathway
Urinary excretion provides route of elimination for approximately 11% of the oral dose of ritonavir
There is minimal central nervous system penetration

pharmacokinetics of ritonavir have not yet been studied in patients with renal or hepatic insufficiency. As renal clearance is minimal there are no anticipated alterations in clearance in patients with renal dysfunction. The central nervous system penetration of ritonavir is minimal (Data on file, Abbott).

Mode of Action

As the HIV protease acts as a homodimer with near (or approximate) C2 symmetry, researchers at Abbott Laboratories considered that a symmetrical protease inhibitor should be able to be accommodated at the active site (Kempf et al., 1990). They developed and evaluated a series of compounds (Kempf et al., 1991; Reedijk et al., 1995; Kort et al., 1993) and chose ritonavir for clinical development based on its antiviral potency and favorable pharmacokinetics. Ritonavir is a C2-symmetry based thiazole inhibitor (Kempf et al., 1990, 1995).

Ritonavir is a competitive inhibitor of the purified aspartic acid proteases of both HIV-1 and HIV-2, with K_i values of 0.36 nM and 3.7 nM respectively (Data on file, Abbott). At concentrations of 40 μM there is no significant inhibition of mammalian aspartic acid proteases, thus ritonavir is specific for the viral enzyme. Through inhibition of the HIV protease enzymes, ritonavir causes defective processing of the HIV Gag-Pol polyprotein precursor, and thus leads to the production of non-infectious (immature) HIV particles (see chapter on saquinavir (p. 1787) for further details).

Toxicity

The most frequently experienced adverse events are nausea, vomiting, diarrhea, taste perversion and circumoral paresthesia. The gastrointestinal side effects of ritonavir are almost universally experienced. The most common laboratory abnormalities are elevated serum aminotransferase levels, and elevated cholesterol and triglyceride levels, which are reversible on cessation of treatment (Danner et al., 1995; Markowitz et al., 1995a). Approximately 15% of patients receiving ritonavir therapy for 4 weeks or longer develop elevated serum bilirubin levels; in general, treatment with ritonavir has been continued in these patients, who normally experience a gradual decline in bilirubin levels. Uric acid levels have been elevated in some patients (Data on file, Abbott).

Nephrolithiasis has also been reported in a small number of patients, associated with hematuria with or without flank pain, and in about two-thirds of these patients, passage of a stone or gravel. Most of these patients either did not cease therapy, or else interrupted therapy during acute symptoms. Recurrence of symptoms after recommencing treatment has been reported (Data on file, Abbott).

As ritonavir is metabolized by the hepatic cytochrome P-450 pathway, particularly the CYP3A enzyme, drugs that increase activity of this enzyme such as rifampicin, rifabutin, phenobarbitone and phenytoin would be predicted to reduce plasma concentrations of ritonavir, due to more rapid clearance (Table V.49). Ritonavir increases the AUC of clarithromycin by 77%. In patients with normal renal function the dose of clarithromycin does not need to be altered. However, if the creatinine clearance is between 30 and 60 ml per min, the dose of clarithromycin should be reduced by 50%, and if creatinine clearance is less than 30 ml per min the dose should be reduced by 75%. Consideration should be given to reducing the dose of desipramine in patients receiving ritonavir, as the AUC of desipramine is significantly increased with co-administration of these

Table V.49
Some important drug interactions with ritonavir

Rifampicin[a]
Rifabutin[a]
Phenobarbitone[a]
Phenytoin[a]
Clarithromycin[b]
Desipramine[b]
Saquinavir[b]
Ethinylestradiol[c]
Theophylline[c]

---

[a] Reduces plasma levels of ritonavir
[b] Increases plasma levels of this drug
[c] Decreases plasma levels of this drug.

drugs. As ritonavir contains alcohol in its formulation, disulfuram or drugs that produce disulfuram-like reactions including metronidazole should be used with caution. Ritonavir inhibits the metabolism of saquinavir, resulting in elevated saquinavir plasma levels. Recent, unpublished data suggest that ritonavir and indinavir co-administration increases plasma concentrations of indinavir. The AUCs of both ethinylestradiol and theophylline are reduced by approximately 40% when either is co-administered with ritonavir (see Ritonavir Product Information). There are a number of other potential drug interactions with ritonavir (refer to Product Information).

Clinical Uses of the Drug

Ritonavir is indicated for the treatment of HIV-infected persons, usually in combination with nucleoside analogs or, possibly in very rare circumstances, as monotherapy. This indication is based on surrogate marker data and not on evidence of efficacy in slowing clinical progression or improving survival.

A dramatic decline in viral load in patients treated with ritonavir has been demonstrated in several studies examining the dynamics of HIV replication. Ritonavir, when administered to HIV infected persons with fewer than 500 CD4 cells per μl and more than 15 000 HIV RNA copies per ml, resulted in an exponential decrease in plasma HIV RNA during the first 2 weeks of treatment (Ho et al., 1995). In a separate study in patients with fewer than 260 CD4 cells per μl and plasma HIV RNA levels of up to 7 $\log_{10}$ copies per ml, virus titers declined by up to 4 $\log_{10}$ copies per ml within 2–4 weeks of starting therapy (Wei et al., 1995). This viral load response has been shown in other studies to be associated with a significant increase in both CD4 and CD8 lymphocyte subsets (Kelleher et al., 1996).

In a preliminary study to assess efficacy and safety, ritonavir in four dosages (300, 400, 500, or 600 mg every 12 h) or placebo was administered to 62 HIV-infected patients with more than 50 CD4 cells per μl and no prior treatment with protease inhibitors. Participants were treated for 12 weeks in an initial 4-week double-blind study followed by an 8-week dose-blind phase. Of the 52 patients who completed the 12-week trial, there was an overall mean maximal decline of 1.7 $\log_{10}$ plasma HIV RNA copies per ml that was partly maintained for the 12-week duration of the study; CD4 counts rose by a median of 83 cells per μl at week 12 (Markowitz et al., 1995a).

The efficacy and safety of four regimens of ritonavir (300, 400, 500, or 600 mg every 12 h) were compared with placebo in a double-blind, randomized phase I/II trial in 84 HIV-infected patients with 50 or more CD4 cells per μl. More than two-thirds of patients had received prior antiretroviral treatment. The median CD4 counts at baseline of patients in the placebo groups were 98 and 86 cells per μl respectively, notably lower than the median CD4 counts in the four ritonavir arms (143, 100, 170 and 130 cells per μl respectively). Over the first 4 weeks of the study increases in CD4 count and reductions in plasma HIV RNA $\log_{10}$ copy number per ml were similar among the four dosage groups of ritonavir. By 16 weeks, the three lower dose groups had returned to baseline levels. In the seven patients who received the highest dose, the median increase in CD4 count after 32 weeks was 230 cells per μl above baseline. In this same group the median decline in plasma HIV RNA was 0.8 $\log_{10}$ copies per ml, but the assay used to obtain this data had a cut-off of 10 000 RNA equivalents per ml. Using a more sensitive assay, the mean maximal decline in HIV RNA in a subgroup of patients who received the two highest doses was 1.94 $\log_{10}$ copies per ml at week 8 of treatment (Danner et al., 1995).

Acknowledgements The author would like to thank Christopher Birch, of the Victorian Infectious Diseases Reference Laboratory, Melbourne, for his critical review of this chapter.

References

Danner SA, Carr A, Leonard JM et al. (1995). A short term study of the safety, pharmacokinetics and efficacy of ritonavir an inhibitor of HIV-1 protease. European Australian Collaborative Ritonavir Study Group. New Engl J Med **333**: 1528.

Data on file, Abbott.

Emini EA, Schleif WA, Deutsch P, Condra JH (1996). In vivo selection of HIV-1 variants with reduced susceptibility to the protease inhibitor L-735,524 and related compounds. Antiviral Chemotherapy, New Directions for Clinical Application and Research Vol. 4, p. 327 (Mills J, Volberding PA, Corey L, eds). New York: Plenum Press.

Ho DD, Toyoshima T, Mo H et al. (1994). Characterisation of human immunodeficiency virus type 1 variants with increased resistance to a C2-symmetric protease inhibitor. J Virol **68**: 2016.

Ho DD, Neumann AU, Perelson AS *et al.* (1995). Rapid turnover of plasma virions and CD4 lymphocytes in HIV-1 infection. *Nature* **373**: 123.

Kaplan AH, Michael SF, Wehbie RS *et al.* (1994). Selection of multiple human immunodeficiency virus type 1 variants that encode viral proteases with decreased sensitivity to an inhibitor of the viral protease. *Proc Natl Acad Sci USA* **91**: 5597.

Kelleher AD, Carr A, Zaunders J, Cooper DA (1996). Alterations in the immune response of human immunodeficiency virus (HIV)-infected subjects treated with an HIV specific protease inhibitor, ritonavir. *J Infect Dis* **173**: 321.

Kempf DJ, Norbeck DW, Codacosi I *et al.* (1990). Structure based C2 symmetric inhibitors of HIV protease. *J Med Chem* **33**: 2687.

Kempf DJ, Marsh KC, Paul DA *et al.* (1991). Antiviral and pharmacokinetic properties of C2 symmetric inhibitors of the human immunodeficiency virus type 1 protease. *Antimicrob Ag Chemother* **35**: 2209.

Kempf DJ, Marsh KC, Denissen JF *et al.* (1995). ABT-538 is a potent inhibitor of human immunodeficiency virus protease and has high oral bioavailability in humans. *Proc Natl Acad Sci USA* **92**: 2484.

Kort JJ, Bilello JA, Bauer G, Drusano GL (1993). Preclinical evaluation of antiviral activity and toxicity of Abbott A77003 an inhibitor of the human immunodeficiency virus type 1 protease. *Antimicrob Ag Chemother* **37**: 115.

Leonard JM (1996). Perspectives in HIV protease inhibitors. *Antiviral Chemotherapy, New Directions for Clinical Application and Research* Vol. 4, p. 319 (Mills J, Volberding PA, Corey L, eds). New York: Plenum Press.

Markowitz M, Saag M, Powderly WG *et al.* (1995a). A preliminary study of ritonavir, an inhibitor of HIV-1 protease, to treat HIV-1 infection. *New Engl J Med* **333**: 1534.

Markowitz M, Mo H, Kempf DJ *et al.* (1995b). Selection and analysis of human immunodeficiency virus type 1 variants with increased resistance to ABT-538, a novel protease inhibitor. *J Virol* **69**: 701.

Molla A, Boucher C, Korneyeva M *et al.* (1995). Evolution of resistance to protease inhibitor ritonavir (ABT-538) in HIV infected patients. *J AIDS Hum Retrovir* **10**: S34.

Molla A, Korneyeva M, Gao Q *et al.* (1996). Ordered accumulation of mutations in HIV protease confers resistance to ritonavir. *Nature Med* **2**: 760.

Norbeck D, Hsu A, Granneman R, Denissen J *et al.* (1995). Virologic and immunologic response to ritonavir (ABT-538), an inhibitor of HIV protease. *J AIDS Hum Retrovir* **10**: S34.

Reedijk M, Boucher CA, van Bommel T *et al.* (1995). Safety, pharmacokinetics and antiviral activity of A77003, a C2 symmetry based human immunodeficiency virus protease inhibitor. *Antimicrob Ag Chemother* **39**: 1559.

Slaughter RL, Edwards DJ (1995). Recent advances; the cytochrome p450 enzymes. *Ann Pharmacother* **29**: 619.

St Clair MH, Millard J, Rooney J *et al.*, (1996). *In vitro* antiviral activity of 141 W94 (VX-478) in combination with other antiretroviral agents. *antiviral res* **29**: 53.

Tisdale M, Myers RE, Maschera B *et al.* (1995). Cross resistance analysis of human immunodeficiency virus type 1 variants individually selected for resistance to five different protease inhibitors. *Antimicrob Ag Chemother* **39**: 1704.

Wei X, Ghosh SK, Taylor ME *et al.* (1995). Viral dynamics in human immunodeficiency virus type 1 infection. *Nature* **373**: 117.

Indinavir

Description

Indinavir sulfate (formerly known as L-735,524 and MK-639) is an inhibitor of HIV protease of the hydroxyaminopentane amide class of peptidomimetics. The drug prevents protease-mediated cleavage of HIV precursor polyproteins, resulting in the production of immature, non-infectious virus particles. Indinavir sulfate is marketed by Merck, Sharp and Dohme under the trade name 'Crixivan' for the treatment of HIV infection.

The chemical name for indinavir sulfate is [1(1S,2R),5(S)-2,3,5-trideoxy-N-(2,3-dihydro-2-hydroxy-1H-inden-1-yl)-5-[2-[[(1,1-dimethylethyl)amino]carbonyl]-4-(3-pyridinylmethyl)-1-piperazinyl]-2- (phenylmethyl)-D-erythro-pentanamide sulfate (1:1)salt. The chemical formula is $C_{36}H_{47}N_5O_4.H_2SO_4$. The structure of indinavir sulfate is shown in Fig. V.62. The molecular weight is 711.88

Antiviral Activity

1 Human immunodeficiency virus

Similar to saquinavir and other protease inhibitors, indinavir inhibits both HIV-1 and HIV-2 proteases (Dorsey et al., 1994). The IC_{95} values of indinavir in human T lymphoid cultures infected with laboratory strains of HIV range from 50 to 100 nM; the IC_{50} concentrations are 0.4 and 2.1 nM for HIV-1 and HIV-2 respectively. Indinavir is also active against primary strains of HIV with most isolates being inhibited by 20–50 nM (Dorsey et al., 1994). The IC_{95} of indinavir is 12 nM in monocyte–macrophage cultures infected with macrophage tropic strains of HIV-1. Indinavir at concentrations ranging from 0.4 to 12 μM inhibits the processing of the viral core precursor protein Pr55[Gag] to mature core protein p24.

As would be expected from its mechanism of action, indinavir is active against reverse-transcriptase-resistant strains of HIV (Data on file, Merck, Sharp and Dohme). Strains of HIV that are resistant to the hydroxyethylamino sulfonamide class of protease inhibitors (e.g. VX-478), with mutations in codons 10, 46, 47 and 50, remain sensitive to indinavir (Partaledis et al., 1995). Preliminary data from Hoffman La Roche suggest that saquinavir-resistant strains remain sensitive to indinavir in approximately 80% of cases (p. 1785).

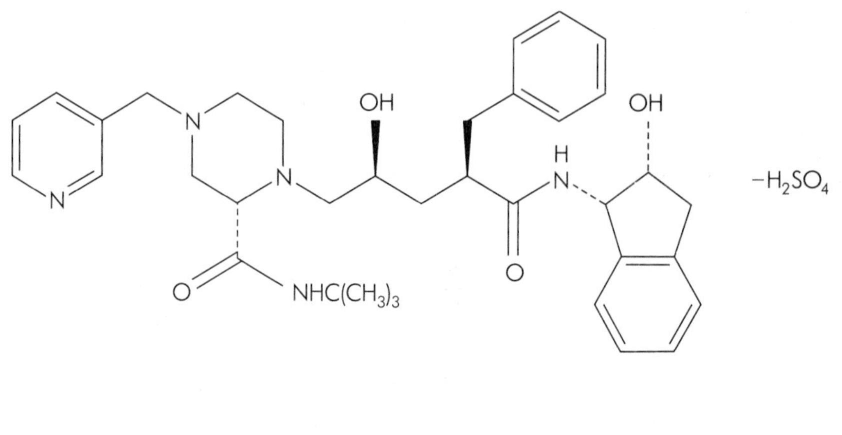

Fig. V.62.
Chemical structure of indinavir. (Reproduced from Merck, Sharp and Dohme Product Information, with permission.)

2 Synergy

Indinavir is reportedly synergistic when used with nucleoside analog reverse transcriptase inhibitors including zidovudine and didanosine, as well as several non-nucleoside reverse transcriptase inhibitors (Vacca *et al.*, 1994).

3 Resistance

Within six to eight passages of culturing HIV-infected cells in the presence of increasing concentrations of indinavir, drug-resistant variants have been detected by some investigators (Tisdale *et al.*, 1995), although others have found it considerably more difficult to produce resistant HIV during *in vitro* passage (Vacca *et al.*, 1994). A large number of mutations have been reported in association with resistance, and these may appear in any order and combination. It is clear that multiple mutations within the HIV protease are needed for the development of significant resistance (Tisdale *et al.*, 1995). The mutations reported in one *in vitro* study occur within codons 82, 46, 32, and 71 (Tisdale *et al.*, 1995). The mutation at position 82 (in combination with other mutations) appears to be necessary for phenotypic expression of resistance (Emini *et al.*, 1996). Other mutations derived *in vitro* occur within codons 8, 32, 47, 48, 84 (Ridky and Leis, 1995). There is no gross alteration in the structure of the protease resulting from mutations within codons 46 (Met→ Ile), 63 (Leu→ Phe), and 84 (Ile→ Val). However, the codon 84 substitution results in the development of a cavity unoccupied by water that is predicted to inhibit contact between the protease and indinavir (see below) (Chen *et al.*, 1995). Mutations within codons 46, 63, 82 and 84 appear to be the minimum alteration within the HIV protease for cross-resistance to develop (Condra *et al.*, 1995a). Cross-resistance to saquinavir and VX-478 requires the presence of the codon 84 mutation (reviewed in Moyle, 1995).

In patients, particularly those treated with suboptimal doses of indinavir, resistant variants of HIV-1 with multiple mutations within the protease have been reported after about 3–6 months of therapy (Condra *et al.*, 1995a,b). Mutations can be detected immediately following the start of therapy, although phenotypic reduction in susceptibility is not always observed (reviewed in Emini *et al.*, 1996). These mutations develop within codons 10, 46, 63, 82, 90, but with up to 15 amino acid substitutions in different combinations and order of appearance in each patient (Condra *et al.*, 1995a,b). Indinavir-resistant strains of HIV usually demonstrate cross-resistance with structurally diverse protease inhibitors including XM-412, nelfinavir and ritonavir. Cross-resistance variably occurs with saquinavir (indinavir-resistant strains are cross-resistant to saquinavir in up to 66% of cases, whilst 80% of saquinavir-resistant strains remain susceptible to indinavir), VX-478 (Vertex) and the Monsanto-Searle compound SC-52151 (Tisdale *et al.*, 1995; Condra *et al.*, 1995a,b). In another study, mutations within codons 82 or 90 (described as genetic signatures of indinavir-resistance) developed in three-quarters of treated patients receiving low-dose indinavir (1600 mg per day or less) (Mellors *et al.*, 1995).

Mode of Administration and Dosage

The recommended dose of indinavir is 800 mg every 8 h, based on data from dose-ranging studies. When indinavir therapy is commenced at doses lower than the recommended dose, resistant strains of HIV can emerge resulting in reduced suppression of viral replication. Thus it is recommended that therapy with indinavir should commence and be maintained at full dose.

For optimal absorption, indinavir is best administered in the fasted state, as light meals can result in variable plasma concentrations, and a heavy, fatty meal significantly decreases absorption. It is suggested by the manufacturer that at least 1.5 liters of liquid be consumed every 24 h to ensure adequate hydration.

Availability

Indinavir is available as capsules containing 100, 200, 300 and 400 mg indinavir (corresponding to 125, 250, 375 and 500 mg of indinavir sulfate respectively).

Serum Levels in Relation to Dosage

The absorption of indinavir in animal studies was found to be dependent on solubility, and this increased in the presence of acid (Kwei *et al.*, 1995). The absorption increases significantly in animals when administered after a meal, in contrast to that observed in humans (Lin *et al.*, 1995).

In humans, indinavir sulfate is absorbed rapidly in the fasted state. Light meals have no significant effect on the extent of absorption of the drug, although the rate of absorption is reduced (Table V.50). However, a high fat meal significantly and consistently decreases the area-under-the-curve (AUC) by about 56% and the peak plasma concentration (C_{max}) by about 77%, and increases the mean time to peak plasma concentration (T_{max}) from 0.9 to 2.8 h. The oral

Table V.50
Summary of clinically relevant pharmacokinetics of indinavir

Oral bioavailability is approximately 60%, light meals do not significantly alter absorption

Plasma levels of indinavir are increased in patients with mild to moderate hepatic impairment

Indinavir is metabolized by the liver (cytochrome P-450 enzyme CYP 3A4)

Urinary excretion accounts for 20% of indinavir excretion; adequate hydration is required to prevent indinavir nephrolithiasis.

No data regarding central nervous system penetration in humans, but it is low in animals.

bioavailability from preliminary studies is approximately 60%. In a dose of 600 mg three times daily the steady-state C_{max} and C_{min} of indinavir were 4.9 and 0.3 μM, levels which are approximately 50-fold and 3-fold greater than the IC_{95} for clinical isolates respectively (Stein *et al.*, 1996). When administered in the recommended dose of 800 mg every 8 h, C_{max} is 11 μM, and the trough plasma concentration (C_{min}) is 0.2 μM, resulting in plasma concentrations that exceed the IC_{95} for HIV *in vitro* throughout the dosing interval. The mean AUC is 23 μM per h. These values were similar for single dose or after multiple dosing when steady-state was achieved (Data on file, Merck, Sharp and Dohme).

There are data on plasma and breast milk levels of indinavir associated with its use in pregnancy in animals but not humans. In animals fetal plasma levels were less than 20% of maternal levels. The mean concentrations of indinavir in breast milk in animals was higher than plasma levels; it is not known whether indinavir is excreted in human milk (Data on file, Merck, Sharp and Dohme).

Hepatic impairment would be expected to impair indinavir metabolism, and in patients with mild to moderate hepatic insufficiency with features of cirrhosis, the AUC and C_{max} of indinavir are increased, compared with values in healthy controls (Data on file, Merck, Sharp and Dohme).

Excretion and Distribution of the Drug in Body

Hepatic metabolism followed by biliary excretion is the major route of elimination of indinavir. In humans, cytochrome CYP3A4 is the major isoenzyme of P-450 involved in its oxidative metabolism (Data on file, Merck, Sharp and Dohme).

Urinary excretion is less important, and accounts for approximately 19% of the excretion of the drug, with about 60% of this representing intact indinavir. Renal clearance exceeds glomerular filtration rate, suggesting that there is tubular secretion (Data on file, Merck, Sharp and Dohme). In a study of HIV seronegative persons who were administered a single oral dose of 1000 mg of indinavir, the major component in urine was intact parent compound, with a number of metabolites also present. The latter contribute very little to the inhibitory activity of the drug (Balani *et al.*, 1995). Plasma protein binding is 44–61%.

In animals there is wide distribution of indinavir in tissues, although there is only limited penetration of the blood–brain barrier, with a brain:plasma ratio of 0.18 (Data on file, Merck Sharp and Dohme). There are no data regarding the penetration of indinavir into the central nervous system in humans.

Mode of Action

Indinavir inhibits the proteases of HIV-1 and HIV-2 with K_i values of 0.5 and 3.3 nM respectively, by a mechanism involving competitive inhibition (Dorsey *et al.*, 1994). The inhibition prevents cleavage of the viral precursor Gag and Gag-Pol polyproteins, resulting in production of immature, non- infectious virions. Like saquinavir and other protease inhibitors, indinavir does not inhibit mammalian proteases of the aspartic acid class (for more general details of mode of actions of protease inhibitors).

The three-dimensional structure of indinavir complexed to the HIV-2 protease has been resolved at 1.9 Angstroms (Chen *et al.*, 1994). Indinavir is a member of a series of protease inhibitors known as hydroxyaminopentane amide compounds. These drugs incorporate a basic amino group into a hydroxyethylene transition state isostere (reviewed in Emini *et al.*, 1996).

Similar to saquinavir indinavir binds to the active site of the protease, with the flaps of the protease closing over the drug following its binding. One of the hydroxyl groups within indinavir binds to the carboxyl moiety of Asp-25 residues of the protease dimer. The amide oxygens of indinavir bind via a hydrogen bond to the backbone amide nitrogen of isoleucine of the HIV protease via an intervening water molecule. Other bridging water molecules also contribute to binding (Chen *et al.*, 1994).

Toxicity

1 General side-effects

From phase I/II studies, indinavir appears to be well tolerated, with few significant toxicities. The most commonly reported clinical adverse events include headache, fatigue, nausea, diarrhea, dry skin and taste disturbance. These adverse experiences are also common in patients receiving zidovudine, and only dry skin and taste disturbance were present with a higher incidence than in zidovudine recipients.

2 Nephrolithiasis

This is the major potentially serious side-effect of indinavir. In phase I/II trials, the incidence of nephrolithiasis (defined as flank pain, and/or hematuria, or demonstration of stones) was 3.6%; 16% of these patients had a past history of ureteric stones. High urinary concentrations of indinavir may exceed the saturation point of indinavir, resulting in the formation of stones composed of the drug. Crystalluria has also been demonstrated on microscopic examination of urine sediment in animals treated with indinavir; the crystals are consistent with parent drug (Data on file, Merck, Sharp and Dohme).

3 Cholestasis and elevated transaminases

These have been observed in rats and dogs respectively during treatment with indinavir (Lin *et al.*, 1992). In phase I/II trials, the most common laboratory adverse event was an elevated unconjugated bilirubin level (10% of recipients).

4 Major drug interactions

The cytochrome P-450 isoform CYP3A4 is responsible for most of the oxidative metabolism of indinavir. Inhibitors of cytochrome P-450 include cimetidine, ketoconazole, quinidine, grapefruit juice, ethinyl estradiol and norethindrone components of the oral contraceptive pill, and clarithromycin (Slaughter and Edwards, 1995; Ketter *et al.*, 1995). However, of these, only ketoconazole has been found to significantly increase the AUC of indinavir (Table V.51). Of note, grapefruit juice (which increases the plasma concentrations of saquinavir, also metabolized by cytochrome P-450) significantly decreased both the AUC and C_{max} when co-administered with indinavir (Data on file, Merck, Sharp and Dohme). Inducers of cytochrome P-450 include rifabutin and rifampicin. The AUC of indinavir was reduced by about 33%, and that of rifabutin was increased significantly when indinavir and rifabutin were given in combination. A dosage reduction of rifabutin is necessary when given to patients receiving indinavir (Data on file, Merck, Sharp and Dohme). No data are currently available with regard to rifampicin and indinavir co-administration, but the manufacturer does not recommend their use in combination due to the potential decrease in plasma concentration of indinavir. Any drug metabolized by the cytochrome P-450 isoenzyme CYP3A4 should be used with caution in patients receiving indinavir, including terfenadine, astemizole, cisapride, triazolam, midazolam and alprazolam, as co-administration may result in competitive inhibition of their metabolism and thus increase their plasma levels.

There is no significant interaction between indinavir and zidovudine or stavudine or fluconazole. Didanosine is rapidly degraded by gastric acid, whereas a normal gastric pH may be required for optimum absorption of indinavir. Thus indinavir and didanosine should be administered at least 1 h apart. Cotrimoxazole (two double-strength tablets per day) had no effect

Table V.51
Some of the major drug interactions with indinavir

Ketoconazole[a]
Grapefruit juice[b]
Rifabutin[c]
Rifampicin[c]
Terfenadine[c]
Astemizole[c]
Cisapride[c]
Alprazolam[c]
Triazolam[c]
Midazolam[c]

[a] Increases in plasma concentration of indinavir.
[b] Decreases in plasma concentration of indinavir.
[c] Increases in plasma concentration of this drug or is expected to do so.

on the AUC of indinavir; the AUC of both trimethoprim and sulfamethoxazole increased (Data on file, Merck, Sharp and Dohme). A small study has also provided data suggesting that indinavir may increase the AUC and C_{max} of isoniazid (Data on file, Merck, Sharp and Dohme).

Clinical Uses of the Drug

1 Human immunodeficiency virus infection

Indinavir is approved for treatment of adults with HIV infection. Although active as monotherapy, this author considers that indinavir should be used in combination with nucleoside analog reverse transcriptase inhibitors unless these cannot be tolerated. So far, efficacy has been based on only surrogate marker data.

Study 004 was a randomized, double-blind trial comparing indinavir monotherapy (400 mg 6-hourly) with zidovudine monotherapy in 12 patients. Over the 12-day study duration, indinavir-treated patients had an increase in CD4 counts (median 76 cells per μl) and a decline in plasma HIV RNA (median 1.4 $\log_{10}$ copies per ml). An open-label extension of this study in which all patients received 600 mg of indinavir 6-hourly for 2 weeks and then 400 mg for 4 weeks showed that indinavir had an antiviral effect over 8 weeks. The reduction of the dose from 600 to 400 mg resulted in a weakening of the antiviral effect.

Study 006 was a randomized, double-blind study comparing indinavir safety, tolerability and efficacy of monotherapy (initially 200 mg or 400 mg 6-hourly, then 600 mg 6-hourly) with zidovudine monotherapy in 72 patients with less than 500 CD4 cells per μl, and most with prior zidovudine experience. There was a modest rise in CD4 counts (44 cells per μl), and reduction in HIV RNA (0.4 $\log_{10}$ copies per ml) in the lowest dose group at the end of 24 weeks: those initially randomized to the 400 mg dose had better responses (a 71 CD4 cell per μl increment above baseline, and 0.7 $\log_{10}$ copies per ml reduction in HIV RNA). Of importance, the maximal decline in HIV RNA (1.3 $\log_{10}$) occurred at week 4 in those receiving the 400 mg dose, and then started to return towards baseline (Data on file, Merck, Sharp and Dohme).

Treatment of HIV-infected persons with suboptimal doses of indinavir results in the selection of variants of HIV with reduced susceptibility to the drug. At least three amino acid substitutions are required for a demonstrable decline in susceptibility. The development of mutations within codons 82 or 90 of the HIV protease during treatment with indinavir has been associated with a rise in HIV RNA towards pretreatment levels (Mellors et al., 1995).

Study 019 was a randomized, double-blind phase I/II study comparing safety, tolerability and efficacy of combination therapy with indinavir (600 mg 6-hourly) and zidovudine (600 mg per day) versus monotherapy with either indinavir or zidovudine in 73 zidovudine-naive subjects with CD4 counts of less than 500 cells per μl and HIV RNA levels of greater than 20 000 copies per ml at study entry. The median CD4 at study entry was 183 cells per μl. In the indinavir monotherapy group, CD4 counts rose by a median of 53 cells per μl over the 24 weeks study duration, with the peak increase occurring at 8 weeks (80 cells per μl) and then returning towards baseline. There was no increase in CD4 counts in those randomized to receive zidovudine monotherapy. Combination therapy resulted in a median increase of 87 cells per μl over 24 weeks, with the maximal increase observed at week 24 (103 cells per μl). Indinavir monotherapy resulted in a median decline of 1.5 $\log_{10}$ copies per ml at week 2, sustained over the 24 weeks duration. Zidovudine monotherapy was associated with a maximal median decline of 0.6 $\log_{10}$ copies per ml at week 2, and then a drift back towards baseline by week 24 (decrease at this time of 0.25 $\log_{10}$ copies per ml). Combination therapy resulted in the greatest decline in viral load, with a 2.6 $\log_{10}$ decline at week 12 maintained through week 24. By week 24, there were 9%, 0% and 50% of indinavir monotherapy, zidovudine monotherapy and combination therapy recipients whose HIV RNA levels were less than 200 copies per ml (below the limit of detection of the assay) (Data on file, Merck, Sharp and Dohme).

Protocol 020 was an open-labeled, randomized study of 24 weeks duration comparing efficacy and safety of indinavir, zidovudine and didanosine combination therapy with zidovudine and didanosine therapy or indinavir monotherapy in 70 evaluable patients who were predominantly antiretroviral-naive, with fewer than 500 CD4 cells at baseline (median of 150 cells per μl), and more than 20 000 copies HIV RNA per ml (median baseline HIV RNA of 5 $\log_{10}$ copies per ml). The CD4 counts increased in all treatment groups, with a maximal median increase at week 12 for indinavir monotherapy (90 cells per μl), week 24 for the triple therapy recipients (95 cells per μl) and week 8 for those randomized to receive zidovudine/didanosine therapy (80 cells per μl). Levels of HIV RNA also declined, with maximal median decreases at week 8 for indinavir monotherapy recipients (2 $\log_{10}$ copies per ml), week 20 for triple therapy recipients (2.9 $\log_{10}$ reduction) and week 4 for double therapy recipients (1.6 $\log_{10}$ reduction). By week 24 the declines in HIV RNA for indinavir monotherapy, triple therapy, and double-therapy recipients were 0.9, 2.3 and 1.0 $\log_{10}$ copies per ml respectively.

Indinavir monotherapy has also been compared with indinavir in a triple combination with zidovudine and lamivudine, and with zidovudine/lamivudine double-combination therapy in 97 HIV-infected patients with at least 6 months of prior zidovudine therapy. The median baseline CD4 was 142 cells per μl and median baseline HIV RNA was 4.6 $\log_{10}$ copies per ml. The maximal viral load reduction for the triple combination was greater than 2 $\log_{10}$ copies per ml, compared with a 1.6 and 1.4 log reduction in those treated with indinavir monotherapy and zidovudine/lamivudine combination therapy. After 24 weeks, 86% of individuals receiving the triple combination had undetectable HIV RNA, compared with 44% on indinavir monotherapy and 0% on zidovudine and lamivudine (Gulick et al., 1996).

A number of other studies are nearing completion. Preliminary data from ACTG 320 suggest that combination therapy using indinavir, zidovudine and lamivudine has a significant impact on clinical progression and survival.

Acknowledgements The author would like to thank Christopher Birch of the Victorian Infectious Diseases Reference Laboratory, Melbourne, for his critical review of this chapter.

References

Balani SK, Arison BH, Mathai L et al. (1995). Metabolites of L-735,524, a potent HIV-1 protease inhibitor, in human urine. *Drug Metabol Disposit* **23**: 266.

Chen Z, Li Y, Chen E et al. (1994). Crystal structure at 19–A resolution of human immunodeficiency virus (HIV) II protease complexed with L-735,524, an orally bioavailable inhibitor of the HIV proteases.. *J Biol Chem* **269**: 26344.

Condra JH, Schleif WA, Blahy OM et al. (1995a). *In vivo* emergence of HIV-1 variants resistant to multiple protease inhibitors. *Nature* **374**: 569.

Condra JH, Schleif WA, Blahy OM et al. (1995b). Dynamics of acquired HIV-1 clinical resistance to the protease inhibitor MK-639. *J AIDS Hum Retrovir* **10**: S35.

Data on file, Merck, Sharp and Dohme.

Dorsey BD, Levin RB, McDaniel SL et al. (1994). L-735,524; the design of a potent and orally bioavailable HIV protease inhibitor. *J Med Chem* **37**: 3443.

Emini EA, Schleif WA, Deutsch P, Condra JH (1996). *In vitro* selection of HIV-1 variants with reduced susceptibility to the protease inhibitor L-735,524 and related compounds. *Antiviral Chemotherapy, New Directions for Clinical Application and Research* Vol. 4, p. 327 (Mills J, Volberding PA, Corey L, eds). New York: Plenum Press.

Gulick R, Mellors J, Havlir D et al. (1996). Potent and sustained antiretroviral activity of indinavir in combination with zidovudine and lamivudine. *3rd Conference on Retroviruses and Opportunistic Infections*. Washington DC: Abstract no. LB7.

Ketter TA, Flockhart DA, Post RM et al. (1995). The emerging role of cytochrome p450 3A in psychopharmacology. *J Clin Psychopharm* **15**: 387.

Kwei GY, Novak LB, Hettrick LA et al. (1995). Regiospecific intestinal absorption of the HIV protease inhibitor L-735,524 in beagle dogs. *Pharmaceut Res* **12**: 884.

Lin JH, Chen IW, King J (1992). Dose-dependent toxicokinetics of L-689,502, a potent human immunodeficiency virus protease inhibitor, in rats and dogs. *J Pharmacol Exp Ther* **263**: 105.

Lin JH, Chen IW, Vastag KJ, Ostovic D (1995). PH-dependent oral absorption of L-735,524, a potent HIV protease inhibitor, in rats and dogs. *Drug Metab Disp* **23**: 730.

Mellors JW, Mahon DK, Chodakewitz JA et al. (1995). Correlation between genotypic evidence of HIV-1 resistance to the protease inhibitor MK-639 and loss of antiretroviral effect in treated patients. *J AIDS Hum Retrovir* **10**: S35.

Moyle GJ (1995). Resistance to antiretroviral compound for clinical management of HIV infection. *Immunol Infect Dis* **5**: 170.

Partaledis JA, Yamaguchi K, Tisdale M et al. (1995). *In vitro* selection and characterisation of human immunodeficiency virus type 1 (HIV-1) isolates with reduced sensitivity to hydroxyethylamino sulfonamide inhibitors of HIV-1 aspartyl protease. *J Virol* **69**: 5228.

Ridky T, Leis J (1995). Development of drug resistance to HIV-1 protease inhibitors. *J Biol Chem* **270**: 29621.

Slaughter RL, Edwards DJ (1995). Recent advances: The cytochrome p450 enzymes. *Ann Pharmacother* **29**: 619.

Stein DS, Fish DG, Bilello JA et al. (1996). A 24 week open label phase I/II evaluation of the HIV protease inhibitor MK 639 (indinavir). *AIDS* **10**: 485.

Tisdale M, Myers RE, Maschera B et al. (1995). Cross-resistance analysis of human immunodeficiency virus type 1 variants individually selected for resistance to five different protease inhibitors. *Antimicrob Ag Chemother* **39**: 1704.

Vacca JP, Dorsey BD, Schleif WA et al. (1994). L-735,524: an orally bioavailable human immunodeficiency virus type 1 protease inhibitor. *Proc Natl Acad Sci USA* **91**: 4096

Nelfinavir

Description

Nelfinavir mesylate (previously known as AG1343) is a non-peptidic protease inhibitor with potent activity against HIV-1 and HIV-2. It has been developed by Agouron and given the trade name of 'Viracept'.

The chemical name is [3S-[2(2S*,3S*),3alpha,4abeta,8abeta]]-N-(1,1-dimethylethyl)decahydro-2-[2-hydroxy-3- [(3-hydroxy-2-methylbenzoyl)amino]-4-(phenylthio)butyl]-3-isoquinoline-carboxamide monomethanesulfonate. It has the molecular formula of $C_{32}H_{45}N_3O_4S.CH_4O_3S$. The chemical structure is shown in Fig. V.63. Nelfinavir has a molecular weight of 663.90

Antiviral Activity

Nelfinavir inhibits HIV-1 replication *in vitro*, with IC_{50} values ranging from 9 to 60 nM against laboratory strains and clinical isolates of HIV-1, including strains that are resistant to zidovudine and non-nucleoside reverse transcriptase inhibitors. The drug is also active against HIV-2. Like other protease inhibitors, nelfinavir has a favorable therapeutic index of 526 to 926 when examined in T cell lines. The K_i against the HIV-1 protease is approximately 2 nM compared with a K_i of 3150 nM for pepstatin A. The *in vitro* activity of nelfinavir continues for up to 36 h after the inhibitor is removed from the culture, again similar to other protease inhibitors. Nelfinavir has demonstrated activity against HIV-1 in chronically infected T cell lines as well as protecting cells against acute infection (Patick *et al.*, 1996).

Nelfinavir inhibits processing of the $Pr55^{Gag}$ precursor polyprotein to p24 in chronically infected T cell lines (Data on file, Agouron).

Nelfinavir has synergistic anti-HIV activity when combined with lamivudine or zalcitabine, and additive to synergistic activity with didanosine and stavudine (Data on file, Agouron).

Resistance to nelfinavir has been described following continuous passage of HIV-1 in increasing concentrations of the drug *in vitro*. A 30-fold reduction in susceptibility could be demonstrated after 28 passages. Mutations at codon 46 (Met→ Ile) and within codon 84 (Ile→ Val/Ala) were identified (Patick *et al.*, 1996). Substitutions have also been observed in codons 48, 63, 71, 82 and 90. Single point mutations within codons 66, 48 and 82 have not been associated with decreased susceptibility. Single point mutations within codons 84 and 90 resulted in 4- to 5-fold decrease in sensitivity (Moyle, 1995). Significant levels of resistance (>10-fold

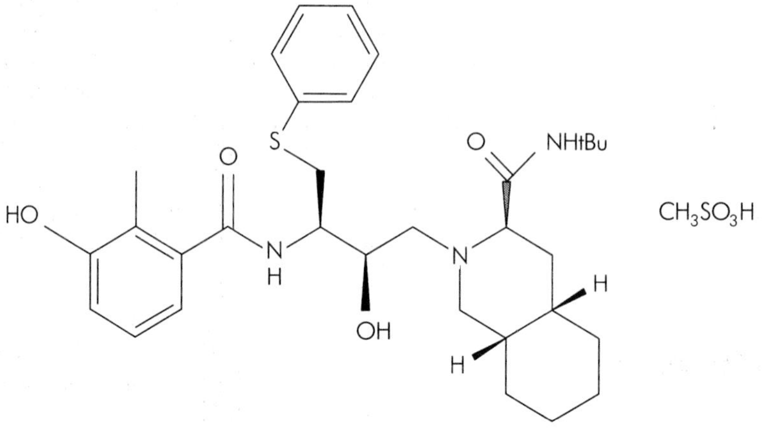

Fig. V.63.

Chemical structure of nelfinavir mesylate. (Reproduced from Shetty *et al.*, 1996, with permission.)

decrease in susceptibility) requires the presence of multiple mutations (Data on file, Agouron). Nelfinavir remains active against strains of HIV with mutations within codons 32, 82 and 48 of the protease (Data on file, Agouron). Resistance to nelfinavir in isolates of HIV-1 from patients participating in clinical trials of the drug has not yet been reported (Moyle, 1995).

Dosage and Mode of Administration

Administration of nelfinavir in fasted state results in a 27–54% decrease in the area-under-the-curve (AUC). Thus it is recommended that nelfinavir is taken with food (Data on file, Agouron; Quart *et al.*, 1995). When administered for 28 days at doses of up to 750 mg twice- or three times daily, nelfinavir was well tolerated, and its use was associated with a decline in viral load of at least 1 $\log_{10}$ during the first 14 days of therapy. Doses of 1000 mg twice-daily were associated with mild to moderate diarrhea. The optimum dose of nelfinavir is still being determined. Current clinical trials are evaluating nelfinavir in doses of 500 and 750 mg three times daily.

Availability

Nelfinavir is available as oral *tablets* containing 100 mg, 200mg, 250 mg.

Serum Levels in Relation to Dose

In animals the drug is slowly absorbed, resulting in high plasma concentrations for up to 7 h after a single oral dose. The oral bioavailability in animals ranges from 17 to 47% (Shetty *et al.*, 1996).

A phase I study in humans demonstrated that plasma concentrations after a single oral dose of 100 mg exceeded the IC_{95} for several hours; when a 400-mg tablet was administered, plasma concentrations remained above the IC_{95} for greater than 12 h. In the fed state, the mean peak plasma concentration obtained (C_{max}) with 100 mg, 200 mg, 400 mg and 800 mg doses was 313, 440, 1351 and 3165 ng per ml respectively, with a mean time to peak plasma concentration (T_{max}) of 2.75–4.00 h (mean 3.4 h). The respective AUCs for the 100-mg, 200-mg, 400-mg and 800-mg doses were 1140, 1754, 7820 and 23 212 ng per h per ml (Data on file, Agouron; Quart *et al.*, 1995).

Excretion and Distribution of the Drug in Body

In animal studies the total volume of distribution was greater than the total volume of body water indicating extensive tissue distribution. Drug elimination is via feces, with total recovery of the dose at 48 h. There is very high plasma protein binding (Shetty *et al.*, 1996).

Mechanism of Action

Nelfinavir was discovered using knowledge of the three-dimensional structure of the active site of HIV-1 protease to create a lead compound. The lead compound was then modified using X-ray crystallographic data to produce nelfinavir, the latter being 60 000-fold more active against HIV protease (K_i 1 nM) than the lead compound (Redshaw, 1994). The mesylate salt was chosen for development based on favorable preformulation studies (Longer *et al.*, 1995). For further details see saquinavir (p. 1787).

Toxicity

The most common side-effect observed in up to 70% of patients is a dose-related mild to moderate diarrhea, usually two to six bowel actions per day. Raised serum transaminases have been observed although it is not yet clear as to whether this can be attributed to nelfinavir. Other reported side-effects include fatigue, poor concentration, hypertension and nausea (Moyle *et al.*, 1996).

As nelfinavir is metabolized by cytochrome P-450, there are a number of potential drug interactions (see Nelfinavir Product Information). Nelfinavir should not be co-administered with terfenadine, astemizole, cisapride, trizolam or midazolam, as life-threatening cardiac arrhythmias or prolonged sedation may occur.

Nelfinavir has been approved for the treatment of HIV infection in adults and children in the USA, based on surrogate market data only. It should be administered in combination with other antiretroviral drugs.

Clinical Use of the Drug

Four phase II studies of nelfinavir administered as monotherapy (studies 503 and 504) and in combination with zidovudine and lamivudine (study 509) or in combination with stavudine (study 510) have been completed.

In the monotherapy studies, administration of nelfinavir produced dose-related declines in plasma HIV RNA levels of between 1.4 and 2 $\log_{10}$ and mean increases in CD4 cell counts of 37–100 cells per μl. These studies involved 50 HIV-infected patients with CD4 counts of greater than 200 cells per μl and HIV RNA levels in plasma of greater than 20,000 copies per ml (Conant et al., 1996; Youle et al., 1995).

When nelfinavir (750 mg three times daily) was given in combination with lamivudine and zidovudine in a phase II pilot study to 12 HIV infected, antiretroviral-naive persons who had a mean CD4 cell count of 258 cells per μl, there was a mean increase in CD4 cells of 109 cells per μl at week 12 and a mean decline in viral load of 2.6 $\log_{10}$ copies per ml. By week 16 of therapy the fall in viral load had increased to a mean of 3.9 $\log_{10}$ copies per ml, with 11 of 12 patients having undetectable viral load measurements (less than 25 copies per ml) (Data on file, Agouron; Markowitz et al., 1996).

Nelfinavir (500, 750 or 1000 mg three times daily) in combination with stavudine results in a greater decline in viral load than that observed with stavudine monotherapy (greater than 2 $\log_{10}$ copies per ml and 0.9 $\log_{10}$ respectively) after 28 days of therapy in those patients who elected to continue therapy. There was a decrease in viral load of 1.3 to 1.9 $\log_{10}$ copies per ml after 20 weeks of combination treatment (Data on file, Agouron; Gathe et al., 1996).

Acknowledgement The author would like to thank Christopher Birch of the Victorian Infectious Disease Reference Laboratory, Melbourne, for his critical review of this chapter.

References

Conant M, Markowitz M, Hurley A et al. (1996). A randomised phase II dose range-finding study of the HIV protease inhibitor Viracept as monotherapy in HIV positive patients [abstract TuB2129]. XI International Conference on AIDS. Vancouver: International AIDS Society.

Data on file, Agouron.

Gathe J, Burkhardt J, Hawley P et al. (1996). A randomised phase II study of Viracept, a novel HIV protease inhibitor, used in combination with stavudine vs stavudine alone [abstract MoB413]. XI International Conference on AIDS. Vancouver: International AIDS Society.

Longer M, Shetty B, Zamansky I, Tyle P (1995). Preformation studies of a novel HIV protease inhibitor, AG1343. J Pharmaceutic Sci 84: 1090.

Markowitz M, Cao Y, Hurley A et al. (1996). Triple therapy with AZT and 3TC in combination with nelfinavir mesylate in 12 antiretroviral naive subjects chronically infected with HIV-1 [abstract LBB6031]. XI International Conference on AIDS. Vancouver: International AIDS Society.

Moyle GJ (1995). Resistance to antiretroviral compound for clinical management of HIV infection. Immunol Infect Dis 5: 170.

Moyle GJ, Youle M, Higgs C et al. (1996). Extended follow up of safety and activity of Agouron's HIV proteinase inhibitor AG1343 (viracept) in virological responders from the UK Phase I/II dose finding study [abstract MoB1731]. XI International Conference on AIDS. Vancouver: International AIDS Society.

Patick AK, Mo H, Markowitz M et al. (1996). Antiviral and resistance studies of AG1343, an orally bioavailable inhibitor of human immunodeficiency virus protease. Antimicrob Ag Chemother 40: 292.

Quart BD, Chapman SK, Peterkin J et al. (1995). Phase I safety, tolerance, pharmacokinetics and food effect studies of AG1343 – a novel HIV protease inhibitor [abstract LB3]. 2nd National Conference on Human Retroviruses. Washington DC.

Redshaw S (1994). Inhibitors of HIV proteinase. Exp Opin Invest Drugs 3: 273.

Shetty BV, Kosa MB, Khalil DA, Webber S (1996). Preclinical pharmacokinetics and distribution to tissue of AG1343, an inhibitor of human immunodeficiency virus type 1 protease. Antimicrob Ag Chemother 40: 110.

Youle M, Moyle G, Chapman S et al. (1995). Phase I/II study of AG1343 – a novel HIV protease inhibitor [abstract]. 19th International Congress of Chemotherapy. Montreal.

Vertex Protease Inhibitor

Description

The GlaxoWellcome-Vertex protease inhibitor VX-478 is a protease inhibitor of the hydroxyethylamino sulfonamide class.

Similar to other protease inhibitors, VX-478 is a potent inhibitor of HIV replication *in vitro*. VX-478 has an IC_{50} of 0.08 μM against HIV-1$_{IIIB}$, and a mean IC_{50} of 0.012 μM against six clinical isolates (St Clair *et al.*, 1996).

Isolates of HIV-1 with reduced sensitivity (greater than 100-fold) to this compound have been selected *in vitro* by serial passage in the presence of increasing drug concentrations. This strategy has resulted in the accumulation of point mutations within codons 10 (Leu→Phe), 46 (Met→Ile), 47 (Ile→ Val), 50 (Ile→ Val), with the codon 50 mutation arising first, followed by the codon 46 mutation (Partaledis *et al.*, 1995; Tisdale *et al.*, 1995). The codon 50 mutation appears to be unique to this subclass of protease inhibitors. As a single mutation it results in a 2- to 3-fold reduction in susceptibility, and an 80-fold reduction in affinity for the inhibitor compared with that between the inhibitor and the parent enzyme. When mutations are present within codons 46, 47 and 50 there is a 14- to 20-fold reduction in susceptibility to the drug and up to a 270-fold reduction in inhibitor binding by the mutant enzyme compared with wild-type enzyme (Partaledis *et al.*, 1995). These mutations may occur individually, or in combination (double mutations within codons 10 and 50, or triple mutations involving codons 46, 47 and 50) (Pazhanisamy *et al.*, 1996). Preliminary data suggest that there is no evidence of cross-resistance between VX-478 and saquinavir or indinavir (Partaledis *et al.*, 1995) but cross-resistance between it and A-77003 (a developmental precursor of ritonavir) occurs (Tisdale *et al.*, 1995).

Synergy against HIV-1 with VX-478 has been demonstrated for zidovudine, didanosine and saquinavir, with additive interactions between VX-478 and indinavir or ritonavir (St Clair *et al.*, 1996).

VX-478 is currently in clinical trials and has shown promise in early phase I and phase I/II studies. The results of larger studies are not available.

Acknowledgement The author would like to thank Christopher Birch, of the Victorian Infectious Diseases Reference Laboratory, Melbourne, for his critical review of this chapter.

References

Partaledis JA, Yamaguchi K, Tisdale M *et al.* (1995). *In vitro* selection and characterisation of human immunodeficiency virus type 1 (HIV-1) isolates with reduced sensitivity to hydroxyethyamino sulfonamide inhibitors of HIV-1 aspartyl protease. *J Virol* **69**: 5228.

Pazhanisamy S, Stuver CM, Cullinam AB *et al.* (1996). Kinetic characterization of human immunodeficiency virus type 1 protease-resistant variants. *J Biol Chem* **271**: 17979.

St Clair MH, Millard J, Rooney J *et al.* (1996). *In vitro* antiviral activity of HIW94 (VX-478) in combination with other antiretroviral agents. *Antiviral Res* **29**: 53.

Tisdale M, Myers RE, Maschera B *et al.* (1995). Cross resistance analysis of human immunodeficiency virus type 1 variants individually selected for resistance to five different protease inhibitors. *Antimicrob Ag Chemother* **39**: 1704

Fialuridine

Description

Fialuridine also known as FIAU or 1-(2-deoxy-2-fluoro-beta-D-arabinofuranosyl)-5-iodouracil, is a 2'-fluoropyrimidine nucleoside analog (Fig. V.64). Fialuridine requires intracellular phosphorylation to the triphosphate derivative for its antiviral activity. The drug was developed by Oclassen Pharmaceuticals, in conjunction with Eli Lilly.

Fialuridine has activity against hepatitis B virus *in vitro*, with IC_{50} values of 0.9 μM, and a selectivity index of 382.6. (Staschke *et al.*, 1994). Virus replication is only temporarily halted by exposure to fialuridine *in vitro*, with resumption of DNA replication within 24 h of removing drug from the culture. The antiviral activity and cytotoxicity of fialuridine could be reversed *in vitro* by the addition of excess thymidine (Staschke and Colacino, 1994). Fialuridine also has activity against cytomegalovirus *in vitro* (Colacino and Lopez, 1983). Ganciclovir-sensitive and -resistant isolates of cytomegalovirus are inhibited by fialuridine with IC_{50} and IC_{90} concentrations of 2.05 and 5.5 μM respectively for ganciclovir-sensitive strains and 2.0 and 6.4 μM respectively for the ganciclovir-resistant strains (Drew *et al.*, 1991).

Pharmacokinetics of fialuridine were assessed in healthy volunteers. Absorption of fialuridine was rapid, with a mean peak plasma concentration in 0.5 h. The mean peak plasma concentration was 238 ± 75 ng per ml. The area-under-the-curve (AUC) calculated 24 h after a single 5-mg oral dose was 516 ± 127 ng.h per ml. Following this, there was a rapid decline in plasma concentration over the first 8 h, followed by a slower decline with a terminal beta half-life of approximately 29 h. The volume of distribution was 258 liters. Approximately 41% was excreted in urine within the first 24 h (Bowsher *et al.*, 1994).

Following encouraging results from early studies in patients with chronic hepatitis B virus infection, a further clinical trial of fialuridine was planned (reviewed in Schalm *et al.*, 1995). Of importance, whilst the larger study was under design, a patient who had been enrolled in an earlier study died of liver failure approximately 4 months after the end of the trial. His death was not attributed to fialuridine at that time. A second patient from the earlier study developed a painful peripheral neuropathy 90 days after cessation of fialuridine therapy (reported in Brahams, 1994).

In the National Institutes of Health-sponsored phase II trial which enrolled 15 patients with chronic hepatitis B infection, the drug was associated with fatal hepatic failure and lactic acidosis. The patients were randomized to receive either 0.1 or 0.25 mg per kg daily of fialuridine

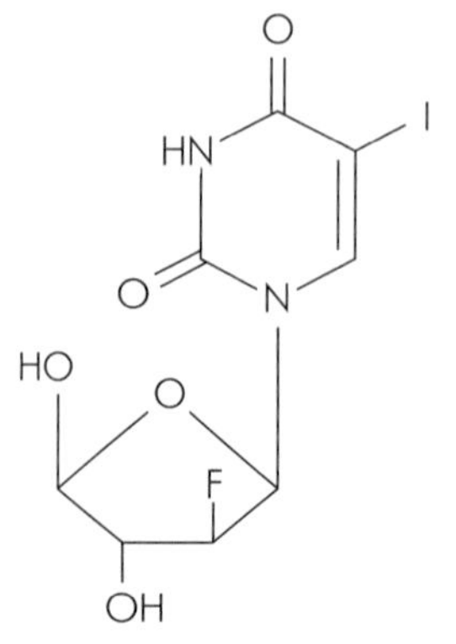

Fig. V.64.
Chemical structure of fialuridine.

for 24 weeks. During the 13th week of therapy, hepatic failure associated with lactic acidosis developed in one patient. Despite discontinuing treatment in all patients, another seven developed progressive liver failure (resulting in five deaths and two patients requiring liver transplantation), and three patients developed mild hepatic dysfunction. Pancreatitis, neuropathy and myopathy were also features of the severe toxicity (McKenzie *et al.*, 1995). The drug was found in a separate pharmacokinetic study to have a prolonged elimination half-life with a mean of 29.3 h (Bowsher *et al.*, 1994).

Mitochondrial abnormalities and hepatic fat accumulation were demonstrated in histologic tissue from treated patients using electron microscopy (McKenzie *et al.*, 1995). Although *in vitro* exposure of human hepatoma cell lines or T cell lines to fialuridine was not associated with a decrease in mitochondrial DNA content (Cui *et al.*, 1995; Colacino *et al.*, 1994), high levels of fialuridine were incorporated into mitochondria, and lactic acid production was increased, consistent with mitochondrial dysfunction (Cui *et al.*, 1995; Colacino *et al.*, 1994). In addition fialuridine was found to accumulate to high concentrations in genomic liver DNA (Richardson *et al.*, 1994) and as the monophosphate derivative to accumulate in mitochondrial DNA (Lewis *et al.*, 1994).

No further studies are likely to proceed with this drug.

References

Bowsher RR, Compton JA Kirkwood JA *et al.* (1994). Sensitive and specific radioimmunoassay for fialuridine: initial assessment of pharmacokinetics after single oral doses to health volunteers. *Antimicrob Ag Chemother* **38**: 2134.

Brahams D (1994). Deaths in US fialuridine trial. *Lancet* **343**: 1494.

Colacino JM, Lopez C (1983). Efficacy and selectivity of some nucleoside analogs as antihuman cytomegalovirus agents. *Antimicrob Ag Chemother* **24**: 505.

Colacino JM, Malcolm SK, Jaskunas SR (1994). Effect of fialuridine on replication of mitochondrial DNA in CEM cells and in human hepatoblastoma cells in culture. *Antimicrob Ag Chemother* **38**: 1997.

Cui L, Yoon S, Schinazi RF, Sommadossi JP (1995). Cellular and molecular events leading to mitochondrial toxicity of 1-(2-deoxy-2-fluoro-1-beta-D-arabinofuranosyl-5-iodouracil in human liver cells. *J Clin Invest* **95**: 55.

Drew WL, Miner R, King D (1991). Antiviral activity of EIAU (1-[2'deoxy-2'-fluro-1-beta-D- arabinofuranosyl]-5-iodo-uridine) on strains of cytomegalovirus sensitive and resistant to ganciclovir. *J Infect Dis* **163**: 1388.

Lewis W, Meyer RR, Simpson JF *et al.* (1994). Mammalian DNA polymerases alpha, beta, gamma, delta and epsilon incorporate fialuridine (FIAU) monophosphate into DNA and are inhibited competitively by FIAU triphosphate. *Biochemistry* **33**: 14620.

McKenzie R, Fried MW, Sallie R *et al.* (1995). Hepatic failure and lactic acidosis due to fialuridine (FIAU), an investigational nucleoside analogue for chronic hepatitis B. *New Engl J Med* **333**: 1099.

Richardson FC, Engelhardt JA, Bowsher RR (1994). Fialuridine accumulates in DNA of dogs, monkeys, and rats following long-term oral administration. *Proc Natl Acad Sci USA* **91**: 12003.

Schalm SW, de-Man RA, Heijtink RA, Niesters HG (1995). New nucleoside analogues for chronic hepatitis B. *J Hepatol* **22**: 52.

Staschke KA, Colacino JM (1994). Priming of duck hepatitis B virus reverse transcription *in vitro* premature termination of primer DNA induced by the 5'-triphosphate of fialuridine. *J Virol* **68**: 8265.

Staschke KA, Colacino JM, Mabry TE, Jones CD (1994). The *in vitro* anti-hepatitis B virus activity of FIAU. *Antiviral Res* **23**: 45.

Ribavirin

Description

Ribavirin (also known as ICN-1229, RTCA, tribavirin), an analog of guanosine, has an unusually wide spectrum of antiviral activity *in vitro*, perhaps the broadest spectrum against both DNA and RNA viruses of any known antiviral agent.

The drug was first described in 1972 (Sidwell *et al.*, 1972) and was approved by the Food and Drug Administration of the USA in 1986 for the treatment of children with severe respiratory syncytial virus infection, although the clinical use of ribavirin for this indication remains controversial (American Academy of Pediatrics Committee on Infectious Diseases, 1996). Past and ongoing clinical trials have demonstrated varying degrees of efficacy of ribavirin when used for the treatment of other viral infections including influenza A and B, parainfluenza, Lassa fever virus, the human immunodeficiency virus, hepatitis C, Junin virus, Hantaan virus and a number of animal and plant viruses. Furthermore, concerns remain regarding the teratogenic, carcinogenic and mutagenic potential of ribavirin (Hebert and Guglielmo, 1990).

The drug was synthesized at the ICN Nucleic Acid Research Institute in the USA in 1972. It is marketed by Viratek and is available under the trade names of 'Virazole', 'Virazide', 'Viramid' and 'Virazid'.

The chemical name of ribavirin is 1-beta-D-ribofuranosyl-1,2,4-triazole-3-carboxamide. The chemical formula is $C_8H_{12}N_4O_5$. The drug differs from guanosine in that the D-ribose of the nucleoside is attached to a 1,2,4-triazole-3-carboxamide moiety rather than a purine ring (Fig. V.65). The molecular weight is 244.2. The concentration of the drug is reported in either μM or μg per ml (1 μg per ml is approximately equivalent to 4.2 μM).

Antiviral Activity

1 Paramyxoviridae

Ribavirin inhibits the replication of respiratory syncytial virus with an IC_{50} of 1.38–5.82 μg per ml, concentrations well below the threshold for cellular toxicity (Hruska *et al.*, 1980; Browne, 1981; Kawana *et al.*, 1987; Shigeta *et al.*, 1988, 1992; Watanabe *et al.*, 1994). Some

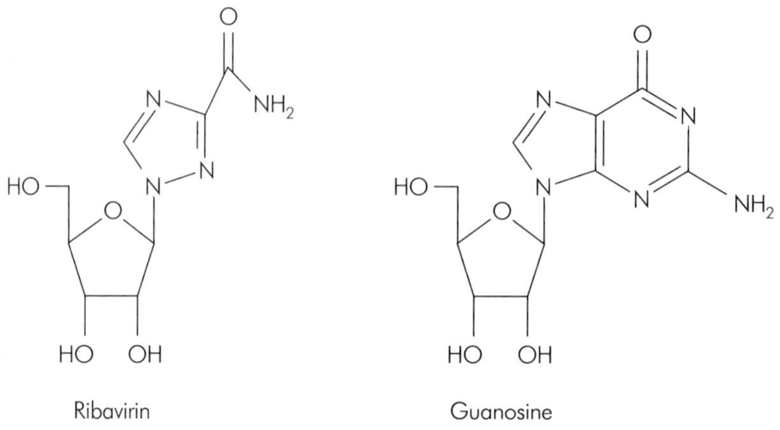

Fig. V.65.
Molecular structure of ribavirin.
(Reproduced from Johnson 1993, with permission from PTR Prentice Hall publishers, New Jersey.)

Ribavirin

Guanosine

strains are less susceptible, with IC_{50} values as high as $16 \mu g$ per ml (Johnson 1993; Table V.52). The activity of ribavirin against measles virus was first reported in 1978 (Murphy, 1978). In general, parainfluenza virus, measles and mumps virus are relatively less susceptible to ribavirin *in vitro* compared with respiratory syncytial virus with IC_{50} values in one study of $8.6–67 \mu g$ per ml determined by plaque reduction in HeLa or Vero cell lines (Shigeta *et al.*, 1992) and $21–32 \mu g$ per ml as assessed by inhibition of cytopathic effect in the same cell lines in an earlier report (Kirsi *et al.*, 1984). However some strains of measles virus are inhibited by $0.003 \mu g$ per ml of ribavirin (Ribavirin Product Information). Ribavirin inhibits subacute sclerosing pan encephalitis (SSPE)-related strains of measles virus *in vitro* (Hosoya *et al.*, 1989) at concentrations of $10–50 \mu g$ per ml, and although the drug did not improve survival of hamsters when administered intraperitoneally, it improved survival in a dose-dependent manner when given by the intracranial route (Honda *et al.*, 1994). Equine morbillivirus is moderately sensitive to ribavirin *in vitro* when tested in a variety of cell lines with IC_{50} values of approximately $188 \mu M$ ($45 \mu g$ per ml) (personal communication, Dr C Birch Victorian Infectious Diseases Reference Laboratory, Melbourne). Mumps virus is inhibited by $0.1–10 \mu g$ per ml (Ribavirin Product Information). Aerosolized ribavirin protects cotton-tail rats from respiratory syncytial virus and influenza B virus infections (Wyde *et al.*, 1987). Actinomycin D has been reported to inhibit the production of ribavirin triphosphate and to antagonize the antiviral effect of ribavirin against respiratory syncytial virus (Smee and Matthews, 1986). Resistance to ribavirin has not been observed in isolates from persons treated with ribavirin for up to 55 days (Hall *et al.*, 1983b, 1985; McIntosh *et al.*, 1984). Resistance of respiratory syncytial virus cultured in the presence of ribavirin has similarly not been detected (Hruska *et al.*, 1980).

Table V.52

Activity of ribavirin against selected viruses *in vitro*. (Modified from Johnson, 1993, with permission.)

DNA Viruses		RNA Viruses	
Virus	IC_{50} (μg per ml)	Virus	IC_{50} (μg per ml)
Herpesvirus		**Paramyxoviruses**	
HSV-1	0.32–100	RSV	1.3–16
HSV-2	1–100	Parainfluenza	3.2–67
CMV	10–100	Measles	0.003–67
		Equine morbillivirus	45
Adenoviruses	3–200	Mumps	0.1–10
Pox viruses		**Orthomyxoviruses**	
Vaccinia	3–320	Flu A, flu B	0.05–12
		Retrovirus	
		HIV	50
		Arenaviruses	
		Lassa	10–32
		Junin	3–32
		Bunyaviruses	
		Hantaan	15
		Crimean Congo	4–10
		Rift Valley	76–80
		Sandfly	75–80
		Punto Toro	2–10
		Toga viruses	
		Dengue	2–5
		Filoviruses	
		Ebola	>500

2 Orthomyxoviridae

The inhibitory concentration of ribavirin against influenza viruses varies according to the method used and the cell lines in which antiviral susceptibility is tested. Influenza A and B are inhibited by ribavirin in Madin-Darby canine kidney (MDCK) cells *in vitro* with IC_{50} values of 3.6–5 μg per ml and 1.3–3.8 μg per ml respectively (Sidwell *et al.*, 1985, 1995; Shigeta *et al.*, 1992; Hosoya *et al.*, 1993). Other investigators have found higher concentrations of ribavirin are required, with reported IC_{50} values of ribavirin for influenza A and B being 10–12 and 7 μg per ml respectively (Wray *et al.*, 1986a; Hayden *et al.*, 1994). Clinical and laboratory strains of influenza A and B are equally susceptible to ribavirin (Wray *et al.*, 1985a). Ribavirin has been found to be less active than amantadine in inhibiting influenza A using a plaque reduction assay. The IC_{50} for ribavirin against three strains of influenza A in this study was 3.6–8.5 μg per ml, compared with 0.2–0.5 μg per ml for amantadine (Browne *et al.*, 1983). More recent studies by Sidwell *et al.* (1995) have confirmed these findings and showed that amantadine is approximately 10-fold more active than ribavirin against influenza A *in vitro*. Rimantadine and human interferon alpha both act synergistically with ribavirin to inhibit the replication of influenza A and B (Hayden *et al.*, 1984). Selenazofurin and ribavirin have additive efficacy against the replication of influenza A or B (Wray *et al.*, 1986a).

In early studies, ribavirin was found to be effective in treating influenza infection of mice, ferrets and squirrel monkeys (Durr *et al.*, 1975; Schofield *et al.*, 1975; Fenton and Potter, 1977; Stephen *et al.*, 1977; Wyde *et al.*, 1986b). The treatment of mice experimentally infected with influenza A with ribavirin was equally successful as amantadine therapy when the drugs were given within 72 h of infection. Ribavirin treatment commencing later post-infection was less effective than amantadine. Only ribavirin was effective for mice infected with influenza B (Wilson *et al.*, 1980).

3 Retroviridae

Ribavirin, at concentrations of 50 μg per ml or greater, was found to suppress the replication of the human immunodeficiency virus in peripheral blood lymphocytes (McCormick *et al.*, 1984). In other studies ribavirin was not inhibitory to HIV (Balzarini *et al.*, 1986), and concentrations of ribavirin as high as 1 mM reduced the replication of visna virus by less than 50% (Frank *et al.*, 1987). Ribavirin has been reported to potentiate the activity of didanosine in primary lymphocyte cultures and T cell lines against the human immunodeficiency virus (p. 1711) and Moloney murine sarcoma virus; this effect is reversed by guanosine (Balzarini *et al.*, 1990, 1991). It is likely that this potentiation of didanosine activity is due at least in part to the ribavirin-induced increase in cellular levels of inosine 5'-monophosphate, the phosphate donor for the conversion of 2',3'-dideoxyinosine to 2',3'-dideoxyinosine monophosphate, and thus to the pharmacologically active metabolite dideoxyadenosine triphosphate (Balzarini *et al.*, 1991; Hartman *et al.*, 1991). Stimulation of the 5'-phosphorylation of 2',3'-dideoxyinosine results in enhanced antiretroviral activity of the parent compound (Johns *et al.*, 1993). Ribavirin and didanosine have also been shown to have synergistic efficacy against Rauscher murine leukemia virus (Allen *et al.*, 1995). Ribavirin has been reported by one group to enhance the efficacy of zidovudine against the human immunodeficiency virus *in vitro* (Fernandez-Larsson and Patterson, 1990), whilst most other investigators have found that ribavirin antagonizes the inhibitory effects of zidovudine, with a 1.5 to 5-fold increase in HIV replication when the drugs are used in combination (p. 1658) (Baba *et al.*, 1987; Vogt *et al.*, 1987; Hoggard *et al.*, 1995). The mechanism underlying antagonism appears to be the inhibition of phosphorylation of zidovudine, through a ribavirin-induced increase in levels of nucleoside triphosphate which subsequently feed back to inhibit thymidine kinase (TK) in the initial phosphorylation step of zidovudine to its monophosphate derivative (Vogt *et al.*, 1987). In the presence of ribavirin, there is a mean of 76% inhibition of zidovudine phosphorylation (Hoggard *et al.*, 1995).

4 Arenaviridae

Lassa fever virus and Junin virus (the etiological agent of Argentine hemorrhagic fever) are inhibited by ribavirin *in vitro* with an IC_{50} of 20–22 μg per ml (Huggins, 1989). Ribavirin at concentrations of 25 μg per ml reduces the yield of Junin virus in Vero cells to undetectable levels, with significant inhibition of cytopathic effect even at concentrations as low as 3.12 μg per ml (Rodriguez *et al.*, 1986). Tacaribe virus, another member of the arenavirus family, is inhibited by ribavirin *in vitro* at concentrations well below the cytotoxic threshold (Andrei and de Clercq, 1990). Early treatment (within 4 days of infection) of Lassa fever virus-infected cynomolgus and rhesus monkeys with ribavirin protected them from disease (Jahrling *et al.*, 1980, 1984). Early animal studies in which guinea pigs infected with Junin virus either intraperitoneally or intracerebrally were treated with subcutaneous ribavirin, survival was prolonged but not enhanced, compared with untreated control animals (Kenyon *et al.*, 1986). Intramuscular injection of ribavirin in rhesus macaques at the time of infection with Junin virus has been reported to protect the animals from clinical disease (McKee *et al.*, 1988). However, marmosets which were infected with Junin virus and given ribavirin therapy commencing 6 days post-infection, were initially protected from illness and then developed neurologic disease culminating in the death of five of the seven treated animals (Weissenbacher *et al.*, 1986). When ribavirin was given 2 h prior to intracerebral infection of rats the animals received partial protection (Remesar *et al.*, 1988). The prolonged treatment of strain 13 guinea pigs infected with Pichinde virus with ribavirin (25 mg per kg daily for 28 days) results in a decrease in mortality from 100% to 25% (Lucia *et al.*, 1989). Improved survival and up to 10 000-fold reduction of viral titers in liver, spleen, brain, and blood occurs even when ribavirin therapy commences 24 h after Pichinde virus challenge (Smee *et al.*, 1993).

5 Bunyaviridae

As assessed by plaque reduction assay, Korean hemorrhagic fever virus (Hantaan virus) is inhibited *in vitro* by ribavirin with an IC_{50} of 15 µg per ml (Huggins, 1989). Using the Hantaan virus-infected suckling mouse model, treatment with ribavirin, started 10 days after infection at the onset of clinical symptoms, resulted in improved survival (11 of 20 treated animals survived, compared with 0 of 70 untreated controls) (Huggins *et al.*, 1986). Other hantaviruses, including Muerto Canyon virus which is the cause of the hantavirus pulmonary syndrome, are also sensitive to ribavirin. The IC_{50} of ribavirin for Crimean-Congo hemorrhagic fever virus by plaque reduction assay in African green monkey kidney (Vero) cells is 4–10 µg per ml (Huggins, 1989; Watts *et al.*, 1989). Ribavirin treatment of infant mice infected intraperitoneally with this virus significantly reduced mortality, and decreased virus replication within the liver without, however, preventing viremia (Tignor and Hanham, 1993). Rift Valley fever virus and sandfly fever virus are less sensitive than other bunyaviridae, with IC_{50} by plaque reduction of 75–80 µg per ml (Huggins, 1989; Watts *et al.*, 1989). However, in rodents and monkeys infected with Rift Valley fever virus, ribavirin therapy has shown survival benefit (Huggins, 1989), and has been efficacious in preventing disease in hamsters (Peters *et al.*, 1986). Punto Toro virus is inhibited by ribavirin with an IC_{50} of 2 µg per ml as assessed by plaque reduction assay (Huggins, 1989), and 4–10 µg per ml as assessed by inhibition of cytopathic effect in LLC-MK2 cells (Sidwell *et al.*, 1988). Subcutaneous or oral administration of ribavirin to Punto Toro virus-infected mice resulted in increased survival, less hepatic dysfunction, and lower plasma viral titers. However, subcutaneous administration was not effective when mice were infected intracerebrally (Sidwell *et al.*, 1988).

6 Togaviidae

Ribavirin has been reported to significantly reduce the replication of dengue virus types 1–4 in monkey kidney cells, but not in human peripheral blood leukocytes (Koff *et al.*, 1982). The antiviral effects are completely reversed by the addition of guanosine. In more recent studies, dengue virus has been reported to be sensitive to ribavirin *in vitro* with an IC_{50} as assessed by plaque reduction in BHK-C15 cell line of 2–5 µg per ml (Huggins, 1989). However, the drug has proven to be ineffective when used for prophylaxis against dengue virus infection in monkeys, despite achieving peak plasma levels of 7 µg per ml (Malinoski *et al.*, 1990).

7 Filoviridae

Ebola is not sensitive to ribavirin *in vitro*, with IC_{50} values of greater than 500 µg per ml (Huggins, 1989). Similarly ribavirin is not effective against Marburg virus (Andrei and de Clercq, 1993).

8 Picornaviridae

Replication of coxsackie B on human amnion cell layers is inhibited by ribavirin, as assessed by plaque reduction assay; recombinant human leukocyte interferon alpha acts synergistically with ribavirin against this virus (Okada *et al.*, 1992). Myocardial titres of coxsackie B3 have been reported to be significantly lower in mice treated with ribavirin either commencing at the time of infection, or up to 4 days post-infection (Kishimoto *et al.*, 1988). Ribavirin is inactive against poliovirus.

9 Adenoviridae

Ribavirin has been found to inhibit the replication of adenoviruses in HeLa cells (Scheffler *et al.*, 1975; Murphy *et al.*, 1993).

10 Herpesviridae

Herpes simplex virus types 1 and 2 is variably inhibited by ribavirin with IC_{50} values ranging from 0.32 to 100 µg per ml (Johnson, 1993). Ribavirin has been reported to potentiate the antiviral effect of aciclovir (p. 1511) based on inhibition of cytopathic effect and viral yield reduction. The synergistic effect of the two drugs is reversed by guanosine (Pancheva, 1991). Although ribavirin inhibits cytomegalovirus with an IC_{50} of 10–100 µg per ml (Johnson, 1993), the drug is considered ineffective against this virus (Verheyden, 1988).

11 Other

Cytopathology caused by Simliki Forest virus is inhibited by ribavirin with an IC_{50} of 10 µM (Smee et al., 1988). Murine interferon and ribavirin are additive in their inhibitory efficacy against this virus (Harmsen et al., 1994). Cell cultures persistently infected with foot and mouth disease virus (a picornavirus) have been reportedly eliminated of infection by ribavirin (de la Torre et al., 1987). The replication of reovirus is inhibited by ribavirin at a concentration of 12.5 µM (Rankin et al., 1989). Cytopathic effects induced by growth of vaccinia virus in Vero cells is inhibited by ribavirin with an IC_{50} of 19 µg per ml (Kirsi et al., 1984), although other reports suggest less sensitivity, with an IC_{50} ranging from 3.2 to 320 µg per ml (Johnson, 1993). The in vitro activity of ribavirin against feline calicivirus (Povey, 1978a) is of interest, since the drug has also recently been found beneficial for the treatment of a related human virus, hepatitis C, in a pilot study (see below) (Di-Bisceglie et al., 1992). Oral ribavirin therapy commenced 1 to 4 days post-infection of cats with calicivirus failed to show clinical or virologic benefit (Povey, 1978b). Although there are no published data regarding the efficacy of ribavirin against human papillomavirus in vitro, ribavirin administered intradermally has been found to reduce the growth of warts in rabbits at early stages of infection with cottontail rabbit papillomavirus (Ostrow et al., 1992). Early reports found no activity of ribavirin when administered subcutaneously or orally against rotavirus-induced gastroenteritis of infant mice (Schoub and Prozesky, 1977). However, more recent studies have found that ribavirin is effective in vitro in inhibiting replication of rotavirus on embryonic rhesus monkey kidney monolayers, with an IC_{90} of 20 µg per ml (Kitaoka et al., 1986). The replication of vesicular stomatitis virus in Chinese hamster ovary cells is inhibited by high concentrations of ribavirin (200 µg per ml) (Toltzis and Huang, 1986). Although all three phosphorylated forms of ribavirin inhibit replication of this virus, the mono- and diphosphate derivatives are 2- to 3-fold more efficacious than ribavirin triphosphate (Toltzis et al., 1988).

Ribavirin has modest efficacy against hepatitis A virus at a concentration of approximately 24 µg per ml (Widell et al., 1986; Crance et al., 1990). Ribavirin has no effect against rabies infection in mice (Bussereau et al., 1988). The replication of hepatitis D virus in primary woodchuck hepatocytes is inhibited by ribavirin at a concentration of 10 µg per ml, even when added to the culture up to 3 days post-infection (Choi et al., 1989). Productive infection of L929 cells with lymphocytic choriomeningitis virus is inhibited by ribavirin at a low multiplicity of infection but increased in the presence of ribavirin when a high multiplicity of infection is used (Gessner and Lother, 1989). Incubation of rat pituitary cell lines infected with this virus in vitro with ribavirin reportedly eliminates the infection (de la Torre and Oldstone, 1992).

Mode of Administration and Dosage

Ribavirin is a water-soluble colorless substance which can be administered to humans by aerosol, oral and intravenous routes.

1 Aerosol administration

Ribavirin at a recommended concentration of 20 mg per ml is administered via an aerosol generator which produces small particles of mean diameter 1.3 µm (range 1–5 µm) in a mist containing about 190 µg of ribavirin per liter (Knight and Gilbert, 1988; Newth and Clark, 1989). The small particle aerosol generator (model SPAG-2) is the recommended nebuliser (Ribavirin Product Information). The drug is conventionally given at a rate of 12.5 liters of ribavirin in air per min continuously for 12–18 h per day for 3–7 days, via an oxygen tent, a mist-mask, an oxygen hood attached to the SPAG-2 aerosol generator or through a mechanical ventilator in conjunction with the SPAG-2 generator (Fig. V.66 and V.67; MMWR, 1988). Administration via an endotracheal tube in mechanically ventilated patients may result in reduced ventilation as a result of crystallization of ribavirin within tubing (Hicks et al., 1986; Hebert and Guglielmo, 1990). Timed circuit valve and tubing changes have been employed to avoid obstruction of tubing with precipitated ribavirin (Frankel et al., 1987; Outwater et al., 1988). Critical attention

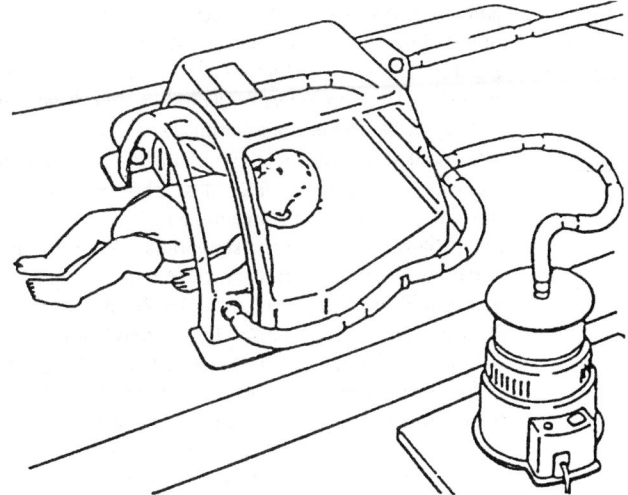

Fig. V.66.
Aerosol delivery hood (ICN Pharmaceuticals Inc). (Reproduced from Bradley, 1990, with permission.)

to the respiratory function of the patient and the apparatus is required. Tracheal intubation results in high pulmonary drug delivery with no deposition of the drug in the nasopharynx (Knight *et al.*, 1988).

A number of exhaust ventilation systems have been developed to capture and contain aerosolized particles of ribavirin during drug administration, in order to reduce the levels of ribavirin in rooms of patients receiving aerosolized ribavirin therapy, and thus minimize exposure of health care workers to the drug. Within the traditional hood, the breathing zone concentration of ribavirin can vary from 566 µg per m^3 to 58 000 µg per m^3 (Torres *et al.*, 1991; Arnold and Alonso, 1993). The installation of efficient scavenging systems is advised. These include over-the-head hoods connected to a filtered exhaust air system, which reduces the leak of aerosolized particles from 98% (with a conventional head hood) to less than 1% (Bradley, 1990; Matlock *et al.*, 1991), double tent containment systems with circulating mist and suction applied between the tents, reducing the general air concentration of exposed health care workers to between 37 and 64 µg per m^3 that is, a 5- to 20-fold decrease in ambient ribavirin concentrations compared with a single oxyhood (Torres *et al.*, 1991; Arnold and Alonso, 1993). Delivery of aerosolized ribavirin via a ventilator is associated with less exposure to health care personnel than when ribavirin is

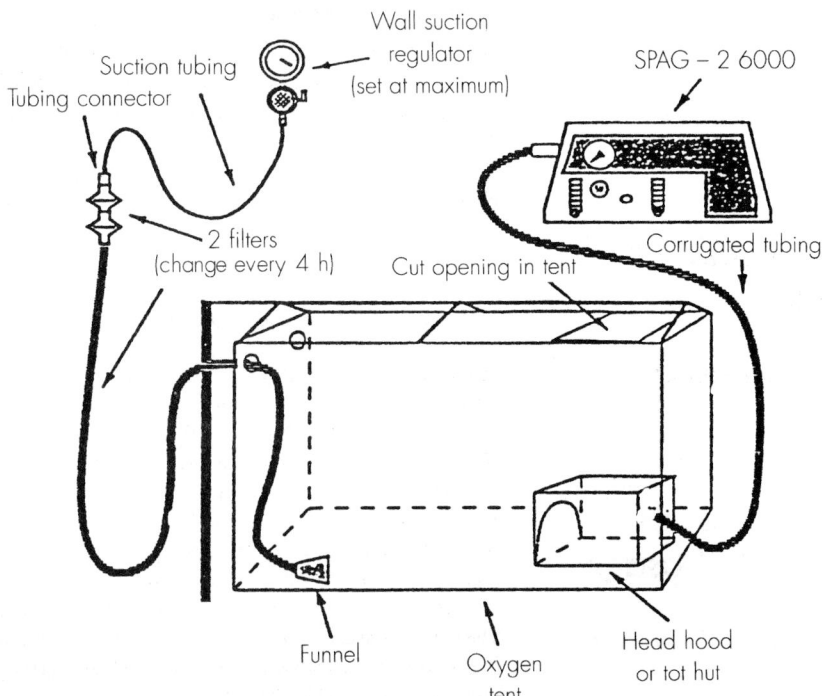

Fig. V.67.
Ribavirin scavenging equipment for head hood, tot hut or face mask. (Reproduced from Bradley, 1990, with permission.)

administered via an oxygen hood in adequately ventilated rooms (Bradley *et al.*, 1990). The level of ribavirin in the air calculated to be safe for occupational exposure during an 8-h shift has been calculated to be 91 μg per m^3 (Arnold and Alonso, 1993).

In infants with severe respiratory syncytial virus infection who required mechanical ventilation, the continuous administration of aerosolized ribavirin (20 mg per ml) was associated with clinical improvement (Smith *et al.*, 1991). Similar results were obtained in a prospective study directly comparing high-dose, short-duration therapy (60 mg per ml administered over 2 h three times daily) with conventional therapy (20 mg per ml administered over 18 h) (Englund *et al.*, 1990, 1994). These data support earlier animal studies in which rats and mice were protected from respiratory syncytial virus and influenza B virus infections with aerosolized ribavirin generated from reservoirs containing 60 mg per ml administered for 2 h twice-daily. However, aerosols generated form reservoirs containing lower doses (20–40 mg per ml administered once-daily) were associated with lower rates of success (Wyde *et al.*, 1987).

Elderly patients with chronic obstructive pulmonary disease tolerated ribavirin aerosol administered for 2 or 6 h with 6 h between therapy, with only minor drug-related changes in pulmonary function (Liss and Bernstein, 1988).

2 Oral administration

For prophylaxis for Lassa fever, the usual oral dose for adults and children aged 10 years of age and older is 500 mg every 6 h for 7–10 days. In children aged 6–9 years of age the recommended dose is 400 mg every 6 h for 7–10 days. The dose has not been established in younger children (United States Pharmacopeia Drug Information, 1996).

Although not approved for this indication, in early studies in patients with HIV infection, oral ribavirin therapy was used at a dose of 800–1000 mg per day (The Ribavirin ARC Study Group, 1993; Spanish Ribavirin Trial Group). For chronic hepatitis C infection the dose of ribavirin most commonly used is 600 mg twice-daily (Reichard *et al.*, 1991; James, 1995; Di Bisceglie *et al.*, 1995).

3 Intravenous administration

The drug should be infused over 15–20 min. For the treatment of hemorrhagic fever with renal syndrome, success has been achieved with i.v. ribavirin given in a loading dose of 33 mg per kg, followed by 16 mg per kg every 6 h for 4 days and then 8 mg per kg every 8 h for 3 days (Huggins *et al.*, 1991).

The recommended dose for the treatment of Lassa fever is 30 mg per kg of body weight loading dose, then 16 mg per kg every 6 h for 4 days, then 8 mg per kg every 8 h for 6 days for a total treatment duration of 10 days (United States Pharmacopeia Drug Information, 1996).

4 Other

In rabbits, intradermal administration of ribavirin in doses of up to 30 mg per kg daily mitigated the growth of warts caused by the cotton-tail rabbit papillomavirus (Ostrow *et al.*, 1992). There are no recommendations or indications for intradermal administration in humans.

Availability

Ribavirin in a sterile lyophilized powder (6g ribavirin) can be reconstituted for aerosol administration by adding sterile water for injections to the recommended volume of 300 ml (final concentration 20 mg per ml), pH approximately 5.5.

Oral ribavirin may be obtained by application to the company for individual patient use in capsules containing 200 mg of ribavirin.

Vials for i.v. infusion, containing 1g per 10ml, may be obtained by application to the company for individual patient use.

Serum Levels and Respiratory Tract Secretion Levels in Relation to Dosage

Serum, plasma or CSF levels of ribavirin can be quantified by high-performance liquid chromatography (Granich *et al.*, 1989).

1 Aerosolized administration

The concentration of ribavirin in respiratory secretions of mice after they received 15 min treatment with high-dose aerosolized ribavirin (60 mg per ml) fell below the ED$_{50}$ for influenza virus after about 9 h (Gilbert *et al.*, 1992).

In infants and children with suspected respiratory syncytial virus infection receiving aerosolized ribavirin (60 mg per ml for 2 h) either by endotracheal tube or oxygen hood, the mean peak concentration of ribavirin in respiratory secretions after the first dose was 1725 μM and 3.8 μM in plasma. The level in respiratory secretions rapidly declined, with a mean half-life of 1.9 h (Englund *et al.*, 1990). This estimate of half-life in respiratory secretions of children is supported by the findings of other investigators (Conner, 1990). The steady-state plasma concentration of ribavirin during therapy was between 5 and 10 μM, regardless of whether the drug was administered by endotracheal tube or via an oxygen hood.

Women have less respiratory tract deposition of ribavirin than males, and there is about 2-fold higher deposition of the drug in infants than in adults (Knight *et al.*, 1988). Fever has been shown to increase the deposition of ribavirin within respiratory tract secretions by 9% for every degree Centigrade above normal (Knight *et al.*, 1988a).

2 Oral administration

Following a single oral dose of 600, 1200 or 2400 mg of ribavirin, the mean peak plasma concentrations of ribavirin in asymptomatic HIV-infected persons were 5.1 μM, 9.9 μM and 12.6 μM respectively (Laskin *et al.*, 1987). Peak plasma concentrations were observed 1.5 h after oral administration. The mean oral bioavailability of ribavirin was 45% (Laskin *et al.*, 1987; Lertora *et al.*, 1991), which is similar to the reported value of 32.6 ± 16.7% in persons without HIV infection (Paroni *et al.*, 1989). More than 3-fold accumulation of ribavirin occurs with 6–8 h dosing regimens, necessitating longer dosage intervals (Laskin *et al.*, 1987). In asymptomatic HIV-infected individuals, the mean peak concentration at steady-state was 10 μM. With continued oral therapy at doses of 400 mg twice-daily there was considerable accumulation of ribavirin, with a steady-state reached in plasma and red blood cells in 2–4 weeks. The concentration of ribavirin within erythrocytes was 60-fold higher than in plasma. Trough levels at steady-state following therapy at a dose of 400 mg twice-daily were 10- to 14-fold higher than those following a single dose (Lertora *et al.*, 1991). In healthy normal adults the plasma half-life of 30.4–60 h and oral bioavailability of 32 ± 17%, is not significantly different to that reported in HIV-infected persons (Paroni *et al.*, 1989) (see Table V.53).

In children aged 1–10 years with symptomatic HIV infection treatment with 6 or 10 mg per kg body weight resulted in peak plasma concentrations of 2.5 μM and 3 μM respectively. The time to peak plasma concentration was 90 min, and oral bioavailability was 42.3%. Mean plasma trough concentrations after 60 days of chronic dosing with 6 or 10 mg per kg were found to be 2.6 μM and 4.1 μM respectively (Connor *et al.*, 1993).

3 Intravenous administration

The pharmacokinetics of ribavirin in HIV-infected persons has been studied by several groups (Laskin *et al.* 1987; Roberts *et al.*, 1987; Lertora *et al.*, 1991). The mean 1 h post-infusion plasma concentrations of ribavirin following i.v. administration of single doses of 600, 1200 or 2400 mg were 8 μM, 19.7 μM and 37.1 μM respectively (Laskin *et al.*, 1987).

4 Renal failure

Ribavirin is not significantly removed from plasma by hemodialysis. In one patient, the maximum amount of ribavirin removed during a dialysis session was 79 mg (Kramer *et al.*, 1990).

5 Elderly

In a study of elderly men (average age 63 years), oral ribavirin (600 mg every 8 h for 48 h, then 200 mg every 8 h for 72 h) with a total dose of 5.4 g resulted in a mean peak plasma level of

Table V.53
Summary of ribavirin pharmacokinetics[a]

Mean oral bioavailability	32–45%
Steady state C_{max}	1.2–3.0 μg per ml
T_{max}	1.5 h
Renal excretion	35–39%
Plasma half-life	27–61 h
Elimination half-life	approximately 2 weeks
CSF penetration	69–70%

[a] Data relate to adults following oral administration, compiled from references in text.

5.3 μM after 18 h of therapy. The mean peak plasma concentration in those receiving 800 mg every 8 h for 24 h then 400 mg every 12 h for 96 h (total dose 4.1 g) after 18 h of therapy was 11.8 μM (Bernstein et al., 1989).

Excretion

In rats, only 3% of i.v.-injected ^{14}C ribavirin is detected in expired CO_2 (Ferrara et al., 1981).

Studies of the renal clearance of ribavirin in HIV-infected persons found renal clearance exceeded creatinine clearance and accounted for 35% to 39% of the total body clearance (Lertora et al., 1991). Unaltered ribavirin has a long plasma half-life, with reported values of 30.4–61 h in normal volunteers and 27.1 h in asymptomatic HIV-infected individuals (Paroni et al., 1989; Lertora et al., 1991). There is some fecal excretion and modest retention in erythrocytes and CSF. The major metabolite of ribavirin is 1,2,3-triazole-3-carboxamide, and the plasma concentration of the metabolite is significantly higher after oral administration than following i.v. therapy (Paroni et al., 1989). Total body clearance is in the range of 26 liters per h in adults with a mean weight of 86.3 kg; taking weight into account ribavirin clearance in adults is 0.3 liters per kg per h (Barnes and Dourson, 1988; Ito and Koren, 1993). The elimination half-life of ribavirin is approximately 2 weeks (Roberts et al., 1987).

Distribution of the Drug in Body

In mice, ribavirin administered by aerosol has been detected in brain in concentrations which should be sufficient for antiviral efficacy. With prolonged aerosol administration, the concentrations of ribavirin in brain tissue increase, and the level within the CSF may reach 150 μM (Gilbert et al., 1991). Aerosol administration has been found to achieve higher concentrations of ribavirin within brain, serum and lungs than administration via intraperitoneal injection (Gilbert et al., 1991). Other studies in mice, comparing administration of liposome-encapsulated ribavirin with free ribavirin have demonstrated 5-fold higher concentrations of ribavirin in liver with the encapsulated drug (Kende et al., 1985).

In humans, most of the studies have been performed in HIV-infected individuals with early stage of disease. In these persons the mean volume of distribution has been reported as 802 liters, with a mean total plasma clearance of 26 liters per h (Lertora et al., 1991). Red cell concentrations are estimated to be 10- to 60-fold higher than plasma concentrations following long-term oral therapy (Conner, 1990; Lertora et al., 1991). This is most likely due to less efficient dephosphorylation by phosphatases in erythrocytes, leading to drug accumulation (Conner, 1990). This hypothesis is supported by in vitro data in which phosphorylation of ribavirin within erythrocytes, lymphoblasts and fibroblasts was associated with a significantly longer half-life of ribavirin nucleotides within erythrocytes compared with the other cell types (Page and Connor, 1990).

Ribavirin has been measured in the CSF of four HIV-infected persons with advanced disease (with and without neurological symptoms), who received several weeks of oral therapy. More than 67% of plasma levels of ribavirin were detected in all of the CSF samples (Crumpacker et al., 1986). Similar penetration (70% of plasma concentration) has been reported in the CSF of children treated with 6 or 10 mg per kg of oral ribavirin for 60 days (Connor et al., 1993). Ribavirin is not bound to plasma protein (Laskin et al., 1987).

Mode of Action

The mechanism by which ribavirin, an analog of guanosine, exerts its antiviral effects remains controversial, and may be virus specific (Table V.54). The drug exhibits broad-spectrum activity against both DNA and RNA viruses, as described above. Ribavirin enters cells by facilitated diffusion (Patterson et al., 1975). The drug then rapidly undergoes phosphorylation, and is primarily present in the triphosphate form, with mono- and diphosphate derivatives comprising 12 and 4% of the drug (Smee and Matthews, 1986). A number of mechanisms for the antiviral action of ribavirin have been proposed (Patterson and Fernandez-Larsson, 1990).

First, ribavirin therapy reduces intracellular pools of guanosine triphosphate, thus indirectly causing viral nucleic acid production to be suppressed (Streeter et al., 1973). Ribavirin monophosphate competitively inhibits inosine monophosphate dehydrogenase, an enzyme which is specific for the de novo synthesis of guanosine triphosphate (Streeter et al., 1973; Robins et al., 1985). Intracellular pools of guanosine triphosphate have been reported to be reduced by up to 60% in ribavirin-treated cells infected with influenza virus. Restoration of the inhibitory effects caused by ribavirin is only partly successful with the use of exogenous guanosine (Wray et al., 1985b).

A second mechanism involves the prevention of capping of mRNA by ribavirin, resulting in inefficient translation of viral transcripts (Goswami et al., 1979). Early studies were performed

Table V.54
Mechanisms of action of ribavirin

Broad spectrum activity against RNA and DNA viruses

Reduces intracellular GTP synthesis
→ indirectly suppresses viral replication

Prevents capping of mRNA
→ inefficient translation of viral mRNA

Inhibits viral polymerase
→ inhibits viral transcription

using vaccinia virus and a variety of plant viruses (Lerch, 1987). More recently, loss of cap structure has been demonstrated in cells infected with equine infectious anemia virus which were treated with ribavirin, as well as in ribavirin-treated cells infected with the human immunodeficiency virus (Fernandez-Larsson and Patterson, 1990). Other studies do not support interference with mRNA cap formation as a mechanism for antiviral activity (Browne, 1981; Rankin *et al.*, 1989).

Third, ribavirin has been reported to inhibit viral polymerase of influenza virus, vesicular stomatitis virus, visna virus and thus inhibit viral transcription (Eriksson *et al.*, 1977; Frank *et al.*, 1987). Work performed *in vitro* using vesicular stomatitis virus suggests that not only the triphosphate form of ribavirin is capable of inhibiting this enzyme: all three phosphorylated species inhibit viral transcription (Fernandez-Larsson *et al.*, 1989; Patterson and Fernandez-Larsson, 1990). Similarly, ribavirin-5'-diphosphate was approximately 40% more inhibitory to the reverse transcriptase enzyme of HIV than the triphosphate derivative. No chain-termination of HIV DNA was observed in association with the inhibition of the viral enzyme (Fernandez-Larsson *et al.*, 1989). It is important to note that, as a nucleoside analog, ribavirin has a modified base and thus differs to the reverse transcriptase inhibitor and viral DNA chain terminator zidovudine which has a modified sugar moiety.

The inhibition of the transcriptase of reovirus is proposed to occur predominantly through inhibiting transcription of reovirus genomic RNA into single-stranded RNA. Following binding of ribavirin triphosphate to a region close to the catalytic site of the enzyme, the compound inhibits the helicase function of the transcriptase, thus preventing the double-stranded RNA from unwinding. This in turn lowers the affinity of the enzyme for the viral template and prevents elongation by causing premature termination (Rankin *et al.*, 1989).

In addition to its antiviral effects, ribavirin has been reported to reduce wheezing associated with bronchiolitis, possibly by decreasing the production of respiratory syncytial virus-specific IgE, and mast cell release of inflammatory mediators (Snell, 1990).

Toxicity

In many clinical trials ribavirin, administered by oral or aerosol routes over a short duration, has been well tolerated and is considered as being a reasonably safe drug for infants, adults including the elderly, and health care workers (Uylangco *et al.*, 1981; Hall *et al.*, 1983a,b, 1995; Gilbert *et al.*, 1985; Knight and Gilbert, 1987; Janai *et al.*, 1990) (Table V.55).

1 Immunologic effects

Early studies demonstrated the effects of ribavirin in inhibiting cellular DNA and RNA synthesis (Drach and Shipman, 1977; Larsson *et al.*, 1978; Peavy *et al.*, 1980) and causing cytostasis in mouse and rat cell lines (Muller *et al.*, 1977; Jenkins and Chen, 1981). These antiproliferative effects are caused by the inhibition of inosine 5'-monophosphate dehydrogenase by ribavirin monophosphate, thus reducing the cellular pools of guanosine triphosphate. Ribavirin has been reported to cause a significant reduction in lymphocyte numbers (Roberts *et al.*, 1990a). Although ribavirin has been shown to exhibit immunosuppressive activity, the drug does not impair granulocyte functions including chemotaxis, opsonization and phagocytosis (Steele *et al.*, 1988). *In vitro*, ribavirin inhibits both IgE-stimulated and non-IgE-stimulated mast cell mediator secretion (Marquardt *et al.*, 1987).

2 Teratogenic effects

Ribavirin has also been associated with teratogenic effects in hamster and rat embryos. Developmental malformations involving the limbs, eyes and brain have been observed after administration of ribavirin to pregnant animals (Ferm *et al.*, 1978; Kochhar *et al.*, 1980).

Table V.55
Major adverse effects of ribavirin. (See text for sources of data.)

Respiratory[a]
  worsening of respiratory function
  dyspnea
  bronchospasm

Cardiovascular[a]
  arrhythmias
  hypotension

Hematologic
  anemia
  hemolysis
  potential teratogenic effects

Other
  transient rash[b]
  conjunctivitis[b]
  eye irritation, headache[b]
  elevation of serum aminotransferases
  seizures[c]
  potentially teratogenic

[a] Only associated with aerosol administration
[b] Predominantly associated with exposure of health care workers
[c] Only associated with i.v. administration

Ribavirin has also been reported as being mutagenic to bone marrow cells of mice (Rao and Rahiman, 1989). Tubular atrophy of testes in rats treated with ribavirin has been described (MMWR, 1988). Impairment of trophoblast development in female mice treated with ribavirin was associated with an increase in rate of abortion and retarded rate of embryo development (Clark et al., 1993).

3 Potential toxicity from environmental exposure

The environmental exposure of health care workers to ribavirin aerosol during the treatment of infants with respiratory disease appears to be low, but has required careful evaluation due to the teratogenic potential of the drug in animals. It has been calculated that a pregnant woman can safely work in a room used for ribavirin treatment for over 10 h per day if the ribavirin is administered through semi-closed circuits of ventilators. If, however, ribavirin is administered via oxygen hoods without appropriate room ventilation, pregnant health care workers should not care for these patients as the permissible exposure time has been calculated as being less than 15 min per day (Ito and Koren, 1993). Health care workers who are pregnant or who may become pregnant should be informed of risks associated with ribavirin exposure and alternative work responsibilities should be considered (MMWR, 1988). In one study over a 3-day period with exposure of 20–35 h, no toxic or adverse effects of ribavirin were observed in female health care workers and ribavirin was not detected in their erythrocytes, plasma or urine (Rodriguez et al., 1987a). In a separate study, trace levels of ribavirin have been reported in erythrocytes of a nurse who provided direct care to an infant receiving ribavirin via an oxygen tent (MMWR, 1988). In health care workers exposed to ribavirin aerosol, bronchospasm, nausea, headache, eye, nasal and throat irritation, and contact lens damage have been reported (Diamond and Dupuis, 1989; Hunt-Fugate and Murray, 1990).

4 Hematologic effects

Although usually well-tolerated, ribavirin can cause a decrease in red blood cell survival and can inhibit red cell release from the bone marrow (Canonico et al., 1984a,b) and is thus associated with the development of anemia. The anemia is dose-related, progressive and, although reversible, has been described as being most likely to occur 1–2 weeks post-ribavirin therapy (American Hospital Formulary Service Drug Information, 1995). It has been described following aerosol administration as well as following oral therapy (American Hospital Formulary Service Drug Information, 1995). If therapy is limited to 3–5 days there is insufficient accumulation of ribavirin to cause red cell toxicity. With longer duration of therapy the risk of hematologic toxicity rises (Conner, 1990). The red cell half-life of ribavirin is about 40 days (Conner, 1990). In the bone marrow, erythroid hypoplasia, vacuolization of erythroid precursors and megakaryocyte hyperplasia have been noted (Cosgriff *et al.*, 1984). In a multicenter clinical trial of ribavirin in HIV-infected persons, the most prominent adverse effect of ribavirin therapy during the 24-week study was the development of a mild hemolytic anemia which was reversible on cessation of therapy (The Ribavirin ARC Study Group, 1993). Other studies in HIV-infected patients have reported reductions in hemoglobin ranging from 0.8 to 3 g, which were generally well tolerated (Lertora *et al.*, 1991). Similarly in a pilot study of 24 weeks oral therapy of ribavirin for the treatment of hepatitis C virus infection, mild hemolysis was noted (Di Bisceglie *et al.*, 1992). In a later study in liver transplant recipients with chronic hepatitis C infection, ribavirin treatment was associated with hemolysis in approximately 40% of patients requiring a reduction in daily dose from 1.2 g to 0.2 g (Gane *et al.*, 1995). An increase in iron stores has also been reported in patients with chronic hepatitis C infection being treated with ribavirin (Di Bisceglie *et al.*, 1994). Mild reversible hemolysis was a side-effect of ribavirin therapy in patients with chronic hepatitis B. Thrombocytosis has also been reported in Junin virus- infected macaques receiving ribavirin (McKee *et al.*, 1988).

5 Respiratory and cardiovascular effects

Cardiac lesions were observed in mice and rats after receiving doses of 30 mg per kg or higher by aerosol for 4 weeks, and in monkeys and rats when given oral ribavirin in doses exceeding 100 mg per kg for 1–6 months (Ribavirin Product Information). Inflammatory changes developed in the lungs of ferrets receiving aerosolized ribavirin at a dose of 60 mg per kg for 10–30 days (Ribavirin Product Information).

Ribavirin has been reported to be temporally associated with a deterioration in patients who had respiratory syncytial virus infection as well as congenital heart disease, although it is unclear as to whether ribavirin actually caused the clinical decompensation (Eisenberg, 1990). Similar worsening of respiratory function during ribavirin inhalation therapy has also been observed in adults with chronic obstructive lung disease, and asthma, as well as minor pulmonary function disturbances in otherwise normal adults receiving ribavirin by inhalation (American Hospital Formulary Service Drug Information, 1995). Refractory congestive cardiac failure in infants with respiratory syncytial virus infection and congenital heart disease has also been reported. It is unknown whether ribavirin or the viral infection is responsible for the development of pulmonary edema in these cases (Martin *et al.*, 1990). Serious adverse reactions including hypotension, bradycardia, cyanosis, apnea, ventilator dependence and cardiac arrest have also been reported (American Hospital Formulary Service Drug Information, 1995).

6 Other effects

Uncommonly reported side-effects of ribavirin therapy in animals include focal alopecia and a decrease in body growth during prolonged treatment (Gillett *et al.*, 1990; Ostrow *et al.*, 1992). In humans, a rash and reversible skin irritation has been reported in infants receiving ribavirin (Janai *et al.*, 1990); a transient increase in serum bilirubin has been associated with ribavirin therapy when the oral dose was in the range of 600–1000 mg per day (Smith *et al.*, 1980). Aerosolized ribavirin at concentrations of 20 mg per ml does not impair ciliary function of human nasal epithelia *in vitro*, and although slowing of ciliary beating and ciliary stasis have been demonstrated at concentrations greater than 50 mg per ml, nasal inhalation of ribavirin at concentrations of 60 mg per ml for 20 min did not impair nasal ciliary function *in vivo* (Han *et al.*, 1990). Exacerbation of bronchospasm may occur more frequently than previously considered, being reported to occur in over 90% of patients in a recent questionnaire completed by pediatric critical care physicians (Zucker and Meadow, 1995).

7 Drug interactions

The potential pharmacokinetic interactions between ribavirin and other drugs such as digoxin, bronchodilators and antibiotics have not been evaluated.

Clinical Uses of the Drug

In 1986 the Food and Drug Administration in the USA approved ribavirin for the aerosolized treatment of infants and young children with severe respiratory syncytial virus infection.

1 Respiratory syncytial virus infection

Ribavirin aerosol may be effective in reducing symptoms due to respiratory syncytial virus in neonates, children and young adults (Conner, 1984); however, its use remains controversial. Although there are a number of studies providing data in support of the use of ribavirin for this condition, there are also a number of studies whose data have indicated lack of efficacy. The most recent recommendations from the American Academy of Pediatricians suggest that therapy with ribavirin may be considered in the treatment of certain infants who are at high risk of serious respiratory syncytial virus disease, including those infants with severe respiratory syncytial virus pneumonitis with or without mechanical ventilation, and infants who are at risk of developing more severe disease. Such infants include those with underlying congenital heart disease, bronchopulmonary dysplasia, chronic lung disease including cystic fibrosis, premature infants, those less than 6 weeks of age, infants with underlying immune deficiency, infants with hypoxemia (P_aO_2 <65 mmHg) and/or hypercapnia, and those with multiple congenital or neurologic or metabolic anomalies (American Academy of Pediatrics Committee on Infectious Diseases, 1996) (Table V.56). These guidelines are a change from previous recommendations from this committee which stated that ribavirin should be used (rather than considered) in the above circumstances, and which were not supported by a number of pediatric critical care physicians (Zucker and Meadow, 1995). Current information suggests a lack of effectiveness of ribavirin in the treatment of infants with respiratory syncytial virus disease (American Academy of Pediatrics Committee on Infectious Diseases, 1996).

In some studies, the clinical response to ribavirin has also been associated with a decrease in virus shedding (Hall *et al.*, 1983b, 1985). However, ribavirin has not consistently been observed to reduce respiratory syncytial virus load in respiratory secretions (Taber *et al.*, 1983). Most of the studies have been performed in spontaneously-breathing infants with respiratory syncytial virus infection, and FDA approval of the drug is limited to this group. Ribavirin has also been shown to be of clinical benefit in infants requiring mechanical ventilation due to infection with respiratory syncytial virus. In these babies ribavirin therapy (20 mg per ml administered continuously) decreased the duration of mechanical ventilation, requirement for oxygen therapy and duration of hospitalization (Smith *et al.*, 1991). However, other investigators have concluded from randomized double-blind trials that ribavirin therapy has not appeared to alter immediate clinical outcome in mechanically ventilated children with respiratory syncytial virus pneumonitis (Wheeler *et al.*, 1993; Meert *et al.*, 1994).

Groothius and colleagues (Groothius *et al.*, 1990) describe a study of 47 infants with underlying broncho-pulmonary dysplasia or congenital heart disease who developed mild respiratory syncytial virus infection and were treated with ribavirin or placebo within 72 h of developing symptoms. It was concluded on the basis of lower oxygen requirements, rate of clinical improvement and oxygen saturation levels that early administration of ribavirin could help to reduce morbidity associated with the infection. There are several other reports of placebo-controlled studies in infants with severe respiratory syncytial virus pneumonitis in which ribavirin treatment has been reportedly associated with improvement in clinical symptoms, in arterial blood gases and in the amount of virus in secretions (Rodriguez *et al.*, 1987b; Hall *et al.*, 1985).

In young adults, ribavirin has also been demonstrated to reduce viral shedding and reduce systemic symptoms and fever associated with experimental respiratory syncytial virus infection,

Table V.56

Indications for ribavirin in respiratory syncytial virus infections. (Adapted from American Academy of Pediatrics Committee on Infectious Diseases, 1996, with permission.)

Ribavirin aerosol therapy may be considered in the following infants and children who are at high risk for serious disease due to respiratory syncytial virus infection.

Congenital heart disease
Bronchopulmonary dysplasia
Cystic fibrosis
Other chronic lung disease
Premature infants (<37 weeks)
Infants <6 weeks of age
Underlying immunosuppression
  AIDS
  severe combined immunodeficiency
  organ transplantation
Severe respiratory syncytial virus infection based on PaO_2 <65 mmHg
Multiple congenital abnormalities, neurologic or metabolic diseases

compared with volunteers who received placebo (Hall *et al.*, 1983a). Aerosolized ribavirin treatment of previously healthy adults who develop severe respiratory syncytial virus pneumonitis requiring mechanical ventilation has been successful resulting in complete recovery (Aylward and Burdge, 1991). Similarly, aerosolized ribavirin therapy has also been used successfully to treat immunocompromised adults (after bone marrow or renal transplantation) with respiratory syncytial virus pneumonitis, resulting in full recovery in some patients (Peigue-Lafeuille *et al.*, 1990; Win *et al.*, 1992; van Dissel *et al.*, 1995) and possible benefit in others in whom therapy was commenced early in the course of infection (Harrington *et al.*, 1992). However, in general, mortality is still high (70%) in adult bone marrow transplant recipients who develop respiratory syncytial virus pneumonitis who are treated with aerosolized ribavirin alone. Combination of aerosolized ribavirin (20 mg per ml for 18 h daily) with i.v. immunoglobulin with respiratory syncytial virus neutralization antibody titers of >1:2048 (500 mg per kg on alternate days) was associated with lower mortality if initiated prior to the onset of respiratory failure (Whimbey *et al.*, 1995).

An infant with syncytial giant cell hepatitis associated with inclusions seen on electron microscopy of liver biopsy material which were indistinguishable from paramyxovirus capsids has been reported to respond to i.v. ribavirin therapy given for 10 days (Roberts *et al.*, 1993). Combined infection with respiratory syncytial virus and parainfluenza virus type 3 in an immunodeficient infant responded to ribavirin therapy delivered by small-particle aerosol (McIntosh *et al.*, 1984). Ribavirin has failed to eradicate respiratory syncytial virus from the respiratory secretions of a child co-infected with human immunodeficiency virus (King *et al.*, 1993).

2 Influenza virus infection

There have been a number of placebo-controlled clinical trials designed to assess the efficacy of prophylactic ribavirin therapy against influenza A and B infection. In general, prophylactic therapy with ribavirin (600–1000 mg per day) has not been found to prevent development of symptoms associated with experimental challenge with influenza A virus (H3N2) and influenza B in healthy volunteers, or to be associated with only marginal success (Cohen *et al.*, 1976; Togo and McCracken, 1976; Magnussen *et al.*, 1977). Ribavirin therapy given orally (1000 mg per day) and commenced within 48 h of the development of symptoms due to influenza A (H1N1) was reported to have no clinical or virologic benefit in a placebo-controlled study of naturally infected college students (Smith *et al.*, 1980). In a pediatric population hospitalized with influenza, a randomized trial of ribavirin versus placebo showed that the only advantage of ribavirin over placebo was in accelerating loss of fever (Rodriguez *et al.*, 1994). And in a randomized, placebo-controlled trial of aerosolized ribavirin for the treatment of influenza B infection, the drug was not associated with significant improvement in symptoms or fever compared with placebo (Bernstein *et al.*, 1988).

There are, however, a number of reports describing efficacy of ribavirin against influenza A or B. Ribavirin therapy has been reportedly associated with shorter duration of symptoms and a trend towards more rapid recovery in college students infected with influenza A (H1N1), with variable evidence of virologic benefit (Knight *et al.*, 1981; Wilson *et al.*, 1984; Gilbert *et al.*, 1985). Ribavirin therapy administered by small-particle aerosol was reported to be associated with clinical benefit in the treatment of influenza B in early studies (McClung *et al.*, 1983; Gilbert *et al.*, 1985). Stein *et al.* (1987) describe symptomatic improvement in patients with influenza A or B infection who were treated with a loading dose followed by short-term administration of oral ribavirin.

3 Hemorrhagic fevers

Experimental infection with Lassa fever virus has been successfully treated with ribavirin (Stephen and Jahrling, 1979). In persons living in Sierra Leone who developed Lassa fever, i.v. therapy with ribavirin for 10 days, begun at any stage during the illness, was associated with improved survival (McCormick *et al.*, 1986). Oral therapy has also been beneficial as treatment. Treatment is most likely to be effective if commenced within 6 days after onset of symptoms. Ribavirin is considered the drug of choice for both treatment and prevention of Lassa fever. High-risk contacts are those who have mucous membrane contact (kissing or sexual intercourse) with a patient with Lassa fever within 3 weeks of diagnosis, or who have needle-stick or other serious occupational exposure to blood or body fluids of a patient with Lassa fever (American Hospital Formulary Service Drug Information, 1995).

A prospective double-blind placebo controlled study of i.v. ribavirin for the treatment of hemorrhagic fever with renal syndrome in the People's Republic of China has found that i.v.

ribavirin (loading dose 33 mg per kg, 16 mg per kg every 6 h for 4 days then 8 mg per kg every 8 h for 3 days) was associated with a 7-fold reduction in mortality, and less risk of developing oliguria and hemorrhage (Huggins *et al.*, 1991). Ribavirin also reduces the proportion of patients with hemorrhagic fever with renal syndrome who are viremic, the duration of viremia and resulted in lower levels of specific IgG production (Yang *et al.*, 1991). Ribavirin has been designated an orphan drug by the US Food and Drug Administration for the treatment of this condition (American Hospital Formulary Service Drug Information, 1995).

Hantavirus pulmonary syndrome is caused by a hantavirus named Sin Nombre (Muerto Canyon) virus. The role of ribavirin in the treatment of hantavirus pulmonary syndrome remains to be elucidated although it is considered more likely to be beneficial if commenced early after onset of symptoms (Hart and Bennett, 1994; Levy, 1995; Morrison and Rathbun, 1995). Review of data derived from open-label use of the drug in the USA found no clear evidence of clinical efficacy in terms of outcome of infection (American Hospital Formulary Service Drug Information, 1995).

The length of time of survival was prolonged in patients with Argentinian fever who were treated with ribavirin more than 8 days after onset of symptoms (Enria *et al.*, 1987).

Three health care workers infected with Crimean-Congo hemorrhagic fever who were treated with oral ribavirin (4000 mg daily for 4 days then 2400 mg for 6 days) all made a complete recovery when the expected mortality rate was 90% (Fischer-Hoch *et al.*, 1995).

4 Measles

Ribavirin, in a double-blind placebo-controlled study has been reported to be of benefit in reducing severity of disease and reducing complications as a result of measles infection (Uylangco *et al.*, 1981). In oncology patients and patients with human immunodeficiency virus infection who acquired measles therapy with ribavirin has resulted in rapid defervescence and recovery (Gururangan *et al.*, 1990; Kaplan *et al.*, 1992). Early ribavirin treatment (days 2–5 of illness) at a dose of 20–35 mg per kg daily in six adults with life-threatening measles pneumonitis, four of whom required mechanical ventilation, resulted in prompt improvement in five of the six patients (Forni *et al.*, 1994). A case report describes rapid improvement in an HIV-infected patient who developed respiratory failure secondary to measles pneumonitis after commencing therapy with aerosolized ribavirin and i.v. immune globulin (Stogner *et al.*, 1993).

Ribavirin treatment of subacute measles encephalitis in two young immunocompromised patients resulted in survival in the patient in whom treatment was commenced early in the course of disease, but not in the patient who commenced i.v. therapy after several weeks of seizures when the patient was comatose (Mustafa *et al,*. 1993).

5 Adenovirus infection

Treatment of refractory adenovirus-associated hemorrhagic cystitis following bone-marrow transplantation with ribavirin has been reported to be successful, with resolution of hematuria and urinary symptoms and resolution of adenovirus excretion (Cassano, 1991; Murphy *et al.*, 1993; Liles *et al.*, 1993; Jurado *et al.*, 1995). However, there is also a case report in which a bone marrow transplant recipient failed to clear adenovirus infection with ribavirin therapy (Hromas *et al.*, 1994). Two children with adenovirus pneumonia (diagnosed by detectable adenovirus in sputum by immunofluorescence with raised titers by adenovirus CFT or by culture) were successfully treated with a 3-day course of nebulized ribavirin (Buchdahl *et al.*, 1985). An immunosuppressed elderly woman with adenoviral pneumonitis responded clinically and radiologically to treatment with nebulized and i.v. ribavirin used in combination with i.v. pooled normal human immunoglobulin (Sabroe *et al.*, 1995).

6 Human immunodeficiency virus infection

Ribavirin has been investigated for oral use in the management of human immunodeficiency virus infections. A phase I study of oral ribavirin therapy (1200 mg twice-daily for 3 days followed by 300 mg twice-daily for up to 12 months) for persons with advanced HIV infection was found to be safe and associated with at least transient virologic and immunologic improvement in six of nine patients (Crumpacker *et al.*, 1987). A second phase I study of ribavirin (1200 and 1600 mg per day) for the treatment of early HIV infection was associated with a reduction in CD4 lymphocyte numbers in persons randomized to the higher dose, presumably reflecting a direct lymphotoxic effect of ribavirin (Roberts *et al.*, 1990a). Following this, three large studies were performed to further evaluate the efficacy of ribavirin for the treatment of HIV. A multicenter placebo-controlled trial of 1000 mg per day showed no clinical or immunologic benefit in persons with CDC group III disease treated with ribavirin for a mean of 39 weeks with a dose of 15 mg per kg daily (average daily dose 1000 mg) (Spanish Ribavirin Trial Group, 1991). In a second multicenter placebo-controlled clinical trial of ribavirin (600 and 800 mg per day) for the treatment of symptomatic, HIV-infection, ribavirin was not shown to affect the rate of progression to AIDS, or have a significant effect on immunologic or virologic parameters (The Ribavirin ARC Study Group, 1993). A double-blind randomized, placebo-controlled trial comparing two doses of ribavirin (600 mg per day and 800 mg per day) with placebo for 24 weeks in 164 asymptomatic HIV-infected individuals showed that therapy with ribavirin did not significantly suppress HIV (Roberts et al., 1990b). However, the time to progression to AIDS in this study was significantly longer in the patients receiving 800 mg per day of ribavirin than the lower dose or placebo (Roberts et al., 1990c). In a European study in which patients with symptomatic HIV infection were treated with 3000 mg per day for the first week, 2000 mg per day for the second week and 1000 mg per day for the following 22 weeks, some symptomatic improvement was observed in patients with AIDS-related complex but not those with AIDS; no immunologic efficacy was noted (Crocchiolo et al., 1989). Thus there have been a number of studies addressing the efficacy of ribavirin against human immunodeficiency virus. None has shown substantial beneficial effects.

7 Herpes simplex virus infection

In a double-blind, placebo-controlled study ribavirin therapy (800 mg per day) reduced disease severity and was associated with more rapid recovery than placebo (Bierman et al., 1981). These results are supported by a second placebo-controlled study in patients with recurrent oral or genital herpes simplex infection who were treated with ribavirin (800–1600 mg per day for 7 days) or placebo. The efficacy of ribavirin compared with placebo was more marked if treatment were commenced as soon as possible after the development of symptoms or signs (Palmiero et al., 1987).

8 Hepatitis

It appears from current data that ribavirin produces only a transient response in patients with chronic hepatitis C infection, without altering serum hepatitis C RNA levels (Fig. V.68).

Four uncontrolled pilot studies of ribavirin therapy (1000–1200 mg per day in two divided doses for 4–12 weeks) for the treatment of chronic hepatitis C infection suggested a beneficial effect, in that biochemical parameters improved and titers of hepatitis C RNA in serum declined during therapy (Reichard et al., 1991, 1993; Di Bisceglie et al., 1992; Tong et al., 1994). However, within 6 weeks of stopping therapy there was a return in liver enzyme levels to pretreatment values (Reichard et al., 1991; Tong et al., 1994).

In a randomized, double-blind, placebo-controlled trial of ribavirin therapy for the treatment of chronic hepatitis C, 29 patients were randomized to receive either ribavirin (600 mg twice-daily) or placebo for 12 months. Although there was a prompt decline in liver transaminases, these were not sustained after stopping treatment and there was no change in hepatitis C RNA levels in plasma during therapy (Di Bisceglie et al., 1995). In a placebo-controlled Anglo-Swedish study ribavirin therapy did not reduce HCV RNA titers (Dusheiko et al., 1994). Thus ribavirin is unlikely to be of therapeutic value in the treatment of chronic hepatitis C.

Several uncontrolled studies of ribavirin therapy in liver transplant recipients with chronic hepatitis C infection have found that ribavirin improves symptoms of lethargy, nausea and anorexia within 2 weeks of commencing therapy. Although liver transaminases decline during therapy, and histologic improvement has been observed, there is invariably no decline in hepatitis C RNA levels in plasma (Gane et al., 1995).

Treatment of patients chronically infected with hepatitis C virus (who have previously failed to respond to interferon therapy) with interferon alpha and ribavirin for 60 days and then interferon alpha alone for 4 months has shown a reduction in transaminase levels during combination therapy in 40% of patients with return to pretreatment values during the phase of interferon monotherapy (Scotto et al., 1995). More promising results were obtained in another small study of ten patients with chronic hepatitis C infection, four of whom had a non-sustained response to prior interferon alpha therapy. In these four patients combination therapy with ribavirin (1000 mg–1200 mg per day) and subcutaneous interferon alpha therapy resulted in a sustained decrease in serum aminotransferases and, in three of four patients, a loss of serum hepatitis C RNA (Schvarcz et al., 1995).

In a controlled trial of ribavirin therapy in combination with interferon alpha versus interferon alpha alone for 6 months in patients with chronic hepatitis C infection who had previously failed therapy with interferon, a sustained loss of hepatitis C RNA in plasma and normalization of

Fig. V.68a.
Serum alanine aminotransferase levels in patients with chronic hepatitis C who were treated with ribavirin or placebo. (Reproduced from Di Bisceglie, 1995, with permission from the American College of Physicians.)

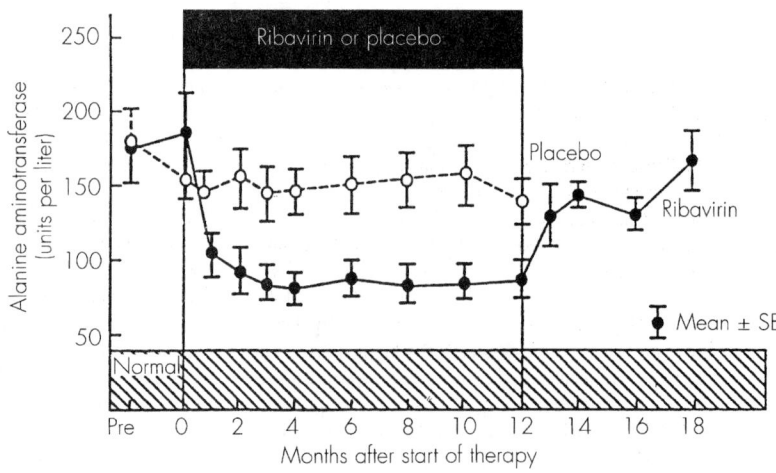

Fig. V.68b.
Hepatitis C RNA levels in patients with chronic hepatitis C treated with ribavirin or placebo. (Reproduced from Di Bisceglie, 1995, with permission from the American College of Physicians.)

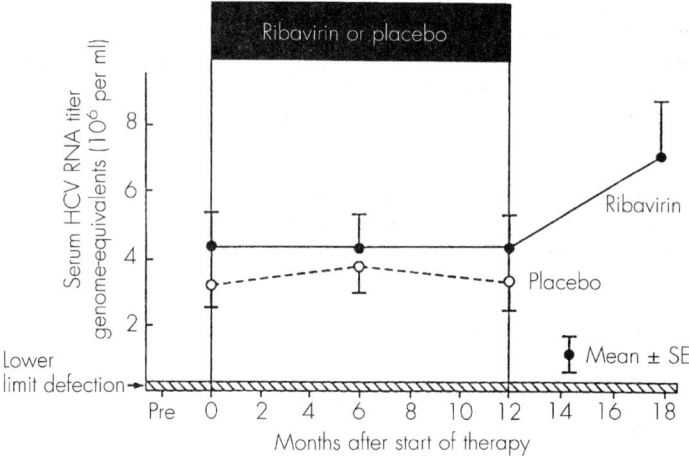

aminotransferase levels was reported in 40% of patients receiving combination therapy and none in those randomized to interferon monotherapy (Brillanti *et al.*, 1994).

A pilot study of ribavirin therapy (800–1000 mg per day) was performed in 24 patients with chronic hepatitis B infection versus interferon beta monotherapy (3 million units three times per week intravenously) or in combination with ribavirin. Ribavirin monotherapy or in combination with interferon beta resulted in suppression of hepatitis B replication, but was less effective than interferon beta monotherapy (Kakumu *et al.*, 1993). Ribavirin treatment of patients with chronic hepatitis B infection at a dose of 800, or 1000 or 1200 mg per day for 24 weeks resulted in a similar response across all three dose regimens with a decline in serum hepatitis B DNA (peak decline at week 20), and a non-sustained but marked decline in serum aminotransferase levels, that returned to baseline within 4 weeks of cessation of therapy (Fried *et al.*, 1994).

Chronic delta hepatitis infection appears unresponsive to ribavirin therapy (Rosina and Cozzolongo, 1994; Garripoli *et al.*, 1994).

9 Other

In one case report, a patient with rabies virus encephalitis failed to respond to treatment with ribavirin (Warrell *et al.*, 1989). An uncontrolled study of four patients laryngeal papillomatosis treated with oral ribavirin (23 mg per kg per day for 6 months) resulted in a remission in two patients lasting for 2 months, with only minimal recurrent disease after a further 2 months, and a partial response in the other two patients (McGlennen *et al.*, 1993). Aerosolized ribavirin (6g per 150ml over 9 h on 3 consecutive nights every 2 weeks for 7 weeks) in conjunction with oral ribavirin (15 mg per kg daily) has also been described in a single case report to result in significant regression of disease (Morrison *et al.*, 1993).

References

Allen LB, Quenelle DC, Westbrook L *et al.* (1995). *In vitro* and *in vivo* enhancement of ddI activity against Rauscher murine leukemia virus by ribavirin. *Antiviral Res* **27**: 317.

American Academy of Pediatrics Committee on Infectious Diseases (1996). Reassessment of the indications for ribavirin therapy in respiratory syncytial virus infections. *Pediatrics* **97**: 137.

American Hospital Formulary Service (AHFS) (1995). *Drug Information* (McEvoy GK, ed). Bethesda USA: American Society Health-System Pharmacists Inc.

Andrei G, De Clercq E (1990). Inhibitory effect of selected antiviral compounds on arenavirus replication *in vitro. Antiviral Res* **14**: 287.

Andrei G, De Clercq E (1993). Molecular approaches for the treatment of hemorrhagic fever virus infections. *Antiviral Res* **22**: 45.

Arnold SD, Alonso R (1993). Ribavirin aerosol; methods for reducing employee exposure. *AAOHN J* **41**: 382.

Aylward RB, Burdge DR (1991). Ribavirin therapy of adult respiratory syncytial virus pneumonitis. *Arch Int Med* **151**: 2303.

Baba M, Pauwels R, Balzarini J *et al.* (1987). Ribavirin antagonizes inhibitory effects of pyrimidine 2′,3′-dideoxynucleosides but enhances inhibitory effects of purine 2′,3′-dideoxynucleosides on replication of human immunodeficiency virus *in vitro. Antimicrob Ag Chemother* **31**: 1613.

Balzarini J, Mitsuya H, De Clercq E, Broder S (1986). Comparative inhibitory effects of suramin and other selected compounds on the infectivity and replication of human T-cell lymphotropic virus (HTLV- III)/lymphadenopathy-associated virus (LAV). *Int J Cancer* **37**: 451.

Balzarini J, Naesens L, Robins MJ, De Clercq E *et al.* (1990). Potentiating effect of ribavirin on the *in vitro* and *in vivo* antiretrovirus activities of 2′,3′-dideoxyinosine and 2′,3′-dideoxy-2,6-diamthopurine riboside. *J AIDS* **3**: 1140.

Balzarini J, Lee CK, Herdewijn P, De Clercq E *et al.* (1991). Mechanism of the potentiating effect of ribavirin on the activity of 2′,3′-dideoxyinosine against human immunodeficiency virus. *J Biol Chem* **266**: 21509.

Barnes DG, Dourson M (1988). Reference dose: description and use in health risk assessments. *Reg Toxicol Pharmacol* **8**: 471.

Bernstein DI, Reuman PD, Sherwood JR *et al.*, (1988). Ribavirin small particle aerosol treatment of influenza B virus infection. *Antimicrob Ag Chemother* **32**: 761.

Bernstein JM, Liss H, Erk SD *et al.* (1989). Comparison of oral and aerosol ribavirin regimens in the high risk elderly. *J Clin Pharmacol* **29**: 1128.

Bierman SM, Kirkpatrick W, Fernandez H *et al.* (1981). Clinical efficacy of ribavirin in the treatment of genital herpes simplex virus infection. *Chemotherapy* **27**: 139.

Bradley J (1990). Environmental exposure to ribavirin aerosol. *Pediatr Infect Dis J* **9**: S95.

Bradley JS, Connor JD, Compogiannis LS, Eiger LL *et al.* (1990). Exposure of health care workers to ribavirin during therapy for respiratory syncytial virus infections. *Antimicrob Ag Chemother* **34**: 668.

Brillanti S, Garson J, Foli M *et al.*, (1994). A pilot study of combination therapy with ribavirin plus interferon alpha for interferon alpha-resistant chronic hepatitis C. *Gastroenterol* **107**: 812.

Browne MJ (1981). Comparative inhibition of influenza and parainfluenza virus replication by ribavirin in MDCK cells. *Antimicrob Ag Chemother* **19**: 712.

Browne MJ, Moss MY, Boyd MR *et al.* (1983). Comparative activity of amantadine and ribavirin against influenza virus *in vitro*: Possible clinical relevance. *Antimicrob Ag Chemother* **23**: 503.

Buchdahl RM, Taylor P, Warner JO (1985). Nebulised ribavirin for adenovirus pneumonia. *Lancet* **9**: 1071.

Bussereau F, Picard M, Blancou J *et al.* (1988). Treatment of rabies in mice and foxes with antiviral compounds. *Acta Virologica* **32**: 33.

Canonico PG, Kastello MD, (1984a). Haematological and bone marrow effects of ribavirin in rhesus monkeys. *Toxicol Appl Pharmacol* **74**: 163.

Canonico PG, Kastello MD *et al.* (1984b). Effects of ribavirin on red blood cells. *Toxicol Appl Pharmacol* **74**: 155.

Cassano WF (1991). Intravenous ribavirin therapy for adenovirus cystitis after allogeneic bone marrow transplantation. *Bone Marrow Transplant* **7**: 247.

Choi SS, Rasshofer R, Roggendorf M (1989). Inhibition of hepatitis delta virus RNA replication in primary woodchuck hepatocytes. *Antiviral Res* **12**: 213.

Clark DA, Banwatt D, Croy BA (1993). Murine trophoblast failure and spontaneous abortion. *Amer J Reprod Immunol* **29**: 199.

Cohen A, Togo Y, Khakoo R *et al.* (1976). Comparative clinical and laboratory evaluation of the prophylactic capacity of ribavirin, amantadine hydrochloride, and placebo in induced human influenza Type A. *J Infect Dis* **133**: A114.

Conner CS (1984). Ribavirin. *Drug Intell Clin Pharm* **18**: 137.

Conner J (1990). Ribavirin pharmacokinetics. *Pediatr Infect Dis* **9**: S91.

Connor E, Morrison S, Lane J *et al.*, (1993). Safety, tolerance and pharmacokinetics of systemic ribavirin in children with human immunodeficiency virus infection. *Antimicrob Ag Chemother* **37**: 532.

Cosgriff TM, Hodgson LA, Canonico PG *et al.* (1984). Morphological alterations in blood and bone marrow of ribavirin treated monkeys. *Acta Haematol* **72**: 195.

Crance JM, Biziagos E, Passagot J *et al.* (1990). Inhibition of hepatitis A virus replication *in vitro* by antiviral compounds. *J Med Virol* **31**: 155.

Crocchiolo P, Pristera R, Lazzarin A *et al.* (1989). A trial with ribavirin in patients with AIDS or AIDS- related complex. *Boll del Sierot Milanese* **68**: 185.

Crumpacker C, Bubley G, Lucey D *et al.* (1986). Ribavirin enters cerebrospinal fluid. *Lancet* **ii**: 45.

Crumpacker C, Heagy W, Bubley G *et al.* (1987). Ribavirin treatment of the acquired immunodeficiency syndrome (AIDS) and the acquired-immuno-deficiency-syndrome-related complex (ARC). A phase I study shows transient clinical improvement associated with suppression of the human immunodeficiency virus and enhanced lymphocyte proliferation. *Ann Intern Med* **107**: 664.

de la Torre JC, Oldstone MB (1992). Selective disruption of growth hormone transcription machinery by viral infection. *Proc Natl Acad Sci USA* **89**: 9939.

de la Torre JC, Alarcon B, Martinez-Salas E *et al.* (1987). Ribavirin cures cells of a persistent infection with foot-and-mouth disease virus *in vitro. J Virol* **61**: 233.

Di Bisceglie AM, Shindo M, Fong TSE *et al.* (1992). A pilot study of ribavirin therapy for chronic hepatitis C. *Hepatology* **16**: 649.

Di Bisceglie AM, Bacon BR, Kleiner DE *et al.* (1994). Increase in hepatic iron stores following prolonged therapy with ribavirin in patients with chronic hepatitis C. *J Hepatol* **21**: 1109.

Di Bisceglie AM, Conjeevaram HS, Freid MW *et al.* (1995). Ribavirin as therapy for chronic hepatitis C A randomised double-blind placebo-controlled trial. *Ann Intern Med* **123**: 897.

Diamond SA, Dupuis LL (1989). Contact lens damage due to ribavirin exposure. *Drug Intell Clin Pathol* **23**: 428.

Drach JC, Shipman C (1977). The selective inhibition of viral DNA synthesis by chemotherapeutic agents: an indicator of clinical usefulness. *Ann NY Acad Sci* **284**: 396.

Durr FE, Lindh HF, Forbes M *et al.* (1975). Efficacy of 1-beta-D-ribofuranosyl-1,2,4-triazole-3-carboxamide against influenza virus infections in mice. *Antimicrob Ag Chemother* **7**: 582.

Dusheiko G, Weiland O, Thomas H *et al.* (1994). Results of a placebo-controlled study of ribavirin in patients with chronic hepatitis C. *Hepatology* **20**: 206A.

Eisenberg J (1990). Hemodynamic alterations in patients with ribavirin. *Pediatr Infect Dis J* **9**: S95.

Englund JA, Piedra PA, Jefferson LS *et al.* (1990). High-dose, short duration ribavirin aerosol therapy in children with suspected respiratory syncytial virus infection. *J Pediatr* **117**: 313.

Englund JA, Piedra PA, Ahn YM *et al.* (1994). High dose, short duration ribavirin aerosol therapy compared with standard ribavirin therapy in children with suspected respiratory syncytial virus infection. *J Pediatr* **125**: 635.

Enria DA, Briggiler AM, Levis S *et al.* (1987). Tolerance and antiviral effect of ribavirin in patients with Argentine hemorrhagic fever. *Antiviral Res* **7**: 353.

Eriksson B, Helgstrand E, Johansson NG *et al.* (1977). Inhibition of influenza virus ribonucleic acid polymerase by ribavirin triphosphate. *Antimicrob Ag Chemother* **11**: 946.

Fenton RJ, Potter CW (1977). Dose-response activity of ribavirin against influenza virus infection in ferrets. *J Antimicrob Chemother* **3**: 263.

Ferm VH, Willhite C, Kilham L *et al.* (1978). Teratogenic effects of ribavirin on hamster and rat embryos. *Teratology* **17**: 93.

Fernandez-Larsson R, Patterson JL (1990). Ribavirin is an inhibitor of human immunodeficiency virus reverse transcriptase. *Mol Pharmacol* **38**: 766.

Fernandez-Larsson R, O'Connell K, Koumans E, Patterson JL (1989). Molecular analysis of the inhibitory effect of phosphorylated ribavirin on the vesicular stomatitis virus *in vitro* polymerase reaction. *Antimicrob Ag Chemother* **33**: 1668.

Ferrara EA, Oishi JS, Wannemacher RW, Stephen EL (1981). Plasma disappearance, urine excretion and tissue distribution of ribavirin in rats and rhesus monkeys. *Antimicrob Ag Chemother* **19**: 1042.

Fisher-Hoch SP, Khan JA, Rehman S *et al.* (1995). Crimean Congo-hemorrhagic fever treated with oral ribavirin. *Lancet* **346**: 472.

Forni AL, Schluger NW, Roberts R (1994). Severe measles pneumonitis in adults. Evaluation of clinical characteristics and therapy with intravenous ribavirin. *Clin Infect Dis* **19**: 454.

Frank KB, McKernan PA, Smith RA, Smee DF (1987). Visna virus as an *in vitro* model for human immunodeficiency virus and inhibition by ribavirin, phosphonoformate, and 2',3'-dideoxynucleosides. *Antimicrob Ag Chemother* **31**: 1369.

Frankel LR, Wilson CW, Demers RR *et al.* (1987). A technique for the administration of ribavirin to mechanically ventilated infants with severe respiratory syncytial virus infection. *Crit Care Med* **15**: 1051.

Fried MW, Fong TL, Swain MG *et al.* (1994). Therapy of chronichepatitis B with a 6 month course of ribavirin. *J Hepatol* **21**: 145.

Gane EJ, Tibbs CJ, Ramage J K *et al.* (1995). Ribavirin therapy for hepatitis C infection following liver transplantation. *Transplant Int* **8**: 61.

Garripoli A, Di Marco V, Cozzolango R *et al.* (1994). Ribavirin treatment for chronic hepatitis D. A pilot study. *Liver* **14**: 154.

Gessner A, Lother H (1989). Homologous interference of lymphocytic choriomeningitis virus involves ribavirin susceptible block in virus replication. *J Virol* **63**: 1827.

Gilbert BE, Wilson SZ, Knight V *et al.* (1985). Ribavirin small-particle aerosol treatment of infections caused by influenza virus strains A/Victoria/7/83 (H1N1) and B/Texas/1/84. *Antimicrob Ag Chemother* **27**: 309.

Gilbert BE, Wyde PR, Wilson S, Robins R (1991). Aerosol and intraperitoneal administration of ribavirin and ribavirin triacetate: pharmacokinetics and protection of mice against intracerebral infection with influenza A/WSN virus. *Antimicrob Ag Chemother* **35**: 1448.

Gilbert BE, Wyde PR, Ambrose MW *et al.* (1992). Further studies with short duration ribavirin aerosol for the treatment of influenza virus infection in mice and respiratory syncytial virus infection in cotton rats. *Antiviral Res* **17**: 33.

Gillett CS, Gunther R, Ostrow RS, Faras AJ (1990). Alopecia associated with ribavirin administration in rabbits. *Lab Anim Care* **40**: 207.

Goswami BB, Borek E, Sharma OK *et al.* (1979). The broad spectrum antiviral agent ribavirin inhibits capping of mRNA. *Biochem Biophys Res Commun* **89**: 830.

Granich GG, Krogstad DJ, Connor JD (1989). High-performance liquid chromatography (HPLC) assay for ribavirin and comparison of the HPLC assay with radioimmunoassay. *Antimicrob Ag Chemother* **33**: 311.

Groothuis JR, Woodin KA, Katz R (1990). Early ribavirin treatment of respiratory syncytial viral infection in high risk children. *J Pediatr* **117**: 792.

Gururangan S, Stevens RF, Morris DJ (1990). Ribavirin response in measles pneumonia. *J Infect* **30**: 219.

Hall CB, Walsh EE, Hruska JF *et al.* (1983a). Ribavirin treatment of experimental respiratory syncytial viral infection. A controlled double-blind study in young adults. *JAMA* **249**: 2666.

Hall CB, McBride JT, Walsh EE *et al.* (1983b). Aerosolized ribavirin treatment of infants with respiratory syncytial viral infection. A randomised double-blind study. *New Engl J Med* **308**: 1443.

Hall CB, McBride JT, Gala CL *et al.* (1985). Ribavirin treatment of respiratory syncytial viral infection in infants with underlying cardiopulmonary disease. *JAMA* **254**: 3047.

Han LY, Wilson R, Slater S *et al.* (1990). *In vitro* and *in vivo* effects of ribavirin on human respiratory epithelium. *Thorax* **45**: 100.

Harmsen T, van Veenendaal D, Kraaijeveld, CA (1994). Inhibition of Scmliki Forest virus multiplication in L-cells by combinations of interferon and ribavirin as measured by plaque titration and direct enzyme immunoassay. *Int J Med Microbiol, Virol Paristol Infect Dis* **280**: 386.

Harrington RD, Hooton TM, Hackman RC *et al.* (1992). An outbreak of respiratory syncytial virus in a bone marrow transplant center. *J Infect Dis* **165**: 987.

Hart CA, Bennett M (1994). Hantavirus an increasing problem? *Ann Trop Med Paristol* **88**: 347.

Hartman NR, Ahluwalia GS, Cooney DA *et al.* (1991). Inhibitors of IMP dehydrogenase stimulate the phosphorylation of the anti-human immunodeficiency virus nucleosides 2',3'-dideoxyadenosine and 2',3'- dideoxyinosine. *Mol Pharmacol* **40**: 118.

Hayden FG, Schlepushkin AN, Pushkarskaya NL *et al.* (1984). Combined interferon-alpha 2, rimantadine hydrochloride, and ribavirin inhibition of influenza virus replication *in vitro*. *Antimicrob Ag Chemother* **25**: 53.

Hayden FG, Rollins DS, Madren, LK *et al.* (1994). Anti-influenza virus activity of the neuraminidase inhibitor 4-guanidino-Neu5Ac2en in cell culture and in human respiratory epithelium. *Antiviral Res* **25**: 123.

Hebert MF, Guglielmo BJ (1990). What is the clinical role of aerosolized ribavirin? *Drug Intell Clin Pharmacol* **24**: 735.

Hicks RA, Olson LC, Jackson MA, Burry VF (1986). Precipitation of ribavirin causing obstruction of a ventilation tube. *Ped Infect Dis* **5**: 707.

Hoggard PG, Veal GJ, Wild MJ *et al.* (1995). Drug interactions with zidovudine phosphorylation *in vitro*. *Antimicrob Ag Chemother* **39**: 1376.

Honda Y, Hosoya M, Ishii T *et al.* (1994). Effect of ribavirin on subacute sclerosing panencephalitis virus infections in hamsters. *Antimicrob Ag Chemother* **38**: 653.

Hosoya M, Shigeta S, Nakamura K, De Clercq E (1989). Inhibitory effect of selected antiviral compounds on measles (SSPE) virus replication *in vitro*. *Antiviral Res* **12**: 87.

Hosoya M, Shigeta S, Ishii T *et al.* (1993). Comparative inhibitory effects of various nucleoside and non- nucleoside analogues on replication of influenza virus types A and B *in vitro* and *in vivo*. *J Infect Dis* **168**: 641.

Hromas R, Clark C, Blanke, C *et al.* (1994). Failure of ribavirin to clear adenovirus infections in T cell depleted allogenic bone marrow transplantation. *Bone Marrow Transplant* **14**: 663.

Hruska JF, Bernstein JM, Douglas RG, Hall CB (1980). Effects of ribavirin on respiratory syncytial virus *in vitro*. *Antimicrob Ag Chemother* **17**: 770.

Huggins JW (1989). Prospects for treatment of viral hemorrhagic fevers with ribavirin, a broad-spectrum antiviral drug. *Rev Infect Dis* **11**: S750.

Huggins JW, Kim GR, Brand DM, McKee KT, (1986). Ribavirin therapy for Hantaan virus infection in suckling mice. *J Infect Dis* **153**: 489.

Huggins JW, Hsiang CM, Cosgriff TM *et al.* (1991). Prospective, double-blind, concurrent placebo-controlled clinical trial of intravenous ribavirin therapy of hemorrhagic fever with renal syndrome. *J Infect Dis* **164**: 1119.

Hunt-Fugate A, Murray DL (1990). Adverse reactions to ribavirin. *Pediatr Infect Dis J* **9**: 680.

Ito S, Koren G (1993). Exposure to pregnant women to ribavirin-contaminated air: Risk assessment and recommendations. *Pediatr Infect Dis J* 12: 2.

Jahrling PB, Hesse RA, Stephen EL *et al.* (1980). Lassa virus infection of rhesus monkeys: Pathogenesis and treatment with ribavirin. *J Infect Dis* 141: 580.

Jahrling PB, Peters CJ, Stephen EL (1984). Enhanced treatment of Lassa fever by immune plasma combined with ribavirin in cynomolgus monkeys. *J Infect Dis* 149: 420.

James DG (1995). Treatment options for chronic hepatitis C infection. *J Antimicrob Chemother* 36: 591.

Janai HK, Marks MI, Zaleska M, Stutman MR (1990). Ribavirin; adverse drug reactions, 1986 to 1988. *Pediatr Infect Dis J* 9: 209.

Jenkins FJ, Chen, YC (1981). Effect of ribavirin on Rous sarcoma virus transformation. *Antimicrob Ag Chemother* 19: 364.

Johns DG, Ahluwalia GS, Cooney DA *et al.* (1993). Enhanced stimulation to ribavirin of the 5'- phosphorylation and anti-human immunodeficiency virus activity of purine 2'-beta-fluoro-2'3'-dideoxynucleosides. *Mol Pharmacol* 44: 519.

Johnson KM (1993). Ribavirin treatment of arenavirus, hantavirus, pneumovirus and paramyxovirus disease: tropical and systemic therapy. *Antiviral Chemotherapy, New Directions for Clinical Application and Research* Vol. 3, p. 229 (Mills J, Corey L, eds). New Jersey: PTR Prentice Hall.

Jurado M, Navarro JM, Hernandez T *et al.* (1995). Adenovirus associated haemorrhagic cystitis after bone marrow transplantation successfully treated with intravenous ribavirin. *Bone Marrow Transplant* 15: 651.

Kakumu S, Yoshioka K, Wakita T *et al.* (1993). Pilot study of ribavirin and interferon-beta for chronic hepatitis B. *Hepatology* 18: 258.

Kaplan LJ, Daum RS, Smaron M, McCarthy CA (1992). Severe measles in immunocompromised patients. *JAMA* 267: 1237.

Kawana F, Shigeta S, Hosoya M *et al.* (1987). Inhibitory effects of antiviral compounds on respiratory syncytial virus replication *in vitro*. *Antimicrob Ag Chemother* 31: 1225.

Kende M, Alving CR, Rill WL *et al.* (1985). Enhanced efficacy of liposome-encapsulated ribavirin against Rift Valley fever virus infection in mice. *Antimicrob Ag Chemother* 27: 903.

Kenyon RH, Canonico PG, Green DE, Peters GJ (1986). Effect of ribavirin and tributylribavirin on argentine hemorrhagic fever (Junin virus) in guinea pigs. *Antimicrob Ag Chemother* 29: 521.

King JC, Burke AR, Clemens JD *et al.* (1993). Respiratory syncytial virus illnesses in human immunodeficiency virus and noninfected children. *Pediatr Infect Dis J* 12: 733.

Kirsi JJ, McKernan PA, Burns NJ *et al.* (1984). Broad-spectrum synergistic antiviral activity of selenazofurin and ribavirin. *Antimicrob Ag Chemother* 26: 466.

Kishimoto C, Crumpacker CS, Abelmann WH *et al.* (1988). Ribavirin treatment of murine coxsackie virus B3 myocarditis with analyses of lymphocyte subsets. *J Amer Coll Cardiol* 12: 1334.

Kitaoka S, Konno T, De Clercq E *et al.* (1986). Comparative efficacy of broad spectrum antiviral agents as inhibitors of rotavirus replication *in vitro*. *Antiviral Res* 6: 57.

Knight V, Gilbert B E (1987). Ribavirin aerosol treatment of influenza. *Infect Dis Clin N Amer* 1: 441.

Knight V, Gilbert B (1988). Antiviral therapy with small-particle aerosols. *Eur J Clin Microbiol Infect Dis* 7: 721.

Knight V, McClung HW, Wilson SZ *et al.* (1981). Ribavirin small-particle aerosol treatment of influenza. *Lancet* ii: 945.

Knight V, Yu CP, Gilbert BE *et al.* (1988). Estimating the dosage of ribavirin aerosol according to age and other variables. *J Infect Dis* 158: 443.

Kochhar DM, Penner JD, Knudsen TB *et al.* (1980). Embryotoxic, teratogenic, and metabolic effects of ribavirin in mice. *Toxicol Appl Pharmacol* 52: 99.

Koff WC, Elm JL, Halstead SB *et al.* (1982). Antiviral effects if ribavirin and 6-mercapto-9-tetrahydro-2-furylpurine against dengue viruses *in vitro*. *Antiviral Res* 2: 69.

Kramer TH, Gaar GG, Ray CJ *et al.* (1990). Hemodialysis clearance of intravenously administered ribavirin. *Antimicrob Ag Chemother* 34: 489.

Larsson A, Stenberg K, Oberg B *et al.* (1978). Reversible inhibition of cellular metabolism by ribavirin. *Antimicrob Ag Chemother* 13: 154.

Laskin OL, Longstreth JA, Hart CC *et al.* (1987). Ribavirin disposition in high-risk patients for acquired immunodeficiency syndrome. *Clin Pharmacol Ther* 41: 546.

Lerch B (1987). On the inhibition of plant virus multiplication by ribavirin. *Antiviral Res* 7: 257

Lertora JJ, Rege AB, Lacour JT *et al.* (1991). Pharmacokinetics and long-term tolerance to ribavirin in asymptomatic patients infected with human immunodeficiency virus. *Clin Pharmacol Ther* 50: 442.

Levy DL (1995). Hantavirus pulmonary syndrome Outbreak of a new disease caused by a new virus. *Postgrad Med* 97: 127.

Liles WC, Cushing H, Hoit S *et al.* (1993). Severe adenoviral nephritis following bone marrow transplantation successful treatment with intravenous ribavirin. *Bone Marrow Transplant* 12: 409.

Liss HP, Bernstein J (1988). Ribavirin aerosol in the elderly. *Chest* 93: 1239.

Lucia HL, Coppenhaver DH, Baron S *et al.* (1989). Arenavirus infection in the guinea pig model: antiviral therapy with recombinant interferon-alpha, the immunomodulator CL246 738 and ribavirin. *Antiviral Res* 12: 279.

Magnussen RC, Douglas GR, Betts RF *et al.* (1977). Double-blind evaluation of oral ribavirin (Virazole) in experimental influenza A virus infection in volunteers. *Antimicrob Ag Chemother* 12: 498.

Malinoski FJ, Hasty SE, Ussery MA, Dalrumple JM (1990). Prophylactic ribavirin treatment of dengue type 1 infection in rhesus monkeys. *Antiviral Res* 13: 139.

Marquardt DL, Gruber HE, Walker LL, (1987). Ribavirin inhibits mast cell mediator release. *J Pharmacol Exp Ther* 240: 145.

Martin JT, Kugler JD, Gumbiner CH *et al.* (1990). Refractory congestive heart failure after ribavirin in infants with heart disease and respiratory syncytial virus. *Nebr Med J* 75: 23.

Matlock D, Buchan RM, Tillery M (1991). A local exhaust ventilation system to reduce airborne ribavirin concentrations. *Amer Ind Hyg Assoc J* 52: 428.

McClung HW, Knight V, Gilbert BE *et al.* (1983). Ribavirin aerosol treatment of influenza B virus infection. *Trans Assoc Amer Physicians* 96: 284.

McCormick JB, Getchell JP, Mitchell SW, Hicks DR (1984). Ribavirin suppresses replication of lymphadenopathy-associated virus in cultures of human adult T lymphocytes. *Lancet* ii: 1367.

McCormick JB, King IJ, Webb PA *et al.* (1986). Lassa fever. Effective therapy with ribavirin. *New Engl J Med* 314: 20.

McGlennen RC, Adams GL, Lewis CM *et al.* (1993). Pilot trial of ribavirin for the treatment of laryngeal papillomatosis. *Head Neck* 15: 504.

McIntosh K, Kurachek SC, Cairns LM *et al.* (1984). Treatment of respiratory viral infection in an immunodeficient infant with ribavirin aerosol. *Amer J Dis Child* 138: 305.

McKee KT, Huggins JW, Trahan CJ, Mahlandi BG (1988). Ribavirin prophylaxis and therapy for experimental argentine hemorrhagic fever. *Antimicrob Ag Chemother* 32: 1304.

Meert KL, Sarnaik AP, Gelmini MJ, Lieh-Lai MW (1994). Aerosolized ribavirin in mechanically ventilated children with respiratory syncytial virus lower respiratory tract disease; a prospective double-blind randomized trial. *Crit Care Med* 22: 566.

MMWR (1988). Assessing exposures of health-care personnel to aerosols of ribavirin – California. *MMWR* 37: 560.

Morrison GA, Kotecha B, (1993). Ribavirin treatment for juvenile respiratory papillomatosis. *J Laryngol Otol* 107: 423.

Morrison YY, Rathbun RC (1995). Hantavirus pulmonary syndrome; the Four Corners disease. *Ann Pharmacother* 29: 57.

Muller WEG, Maidhof A, Taschner H, Zahn RK, (1977). Virazole, a cytostatic agent. *Biochem Pharmacol* 26: 1071.

Murphy MF (1978). *In vitro* inhibition of subacute sclerosing pan-encephalitis virus by the antiviral agent ribavirin. *J Infect Dis* 138: 249.

Murphy GF, Wood DP, McRoberts JW, Henslee-Downey PJ (1993). Adenovirus-associated hemorrhagic cystitis treated with intravenous ribavirin. *J Urol* **149**: 565.

Mustafa MM, Weitman SD, Winick NJ *et al.* (1993). Subacute measles encephalitis in the young immunocompromised host; report of two cases diagnosed by polymerase chain reaction and treated with ribavirin and review of the literature. *Clin Infect Dis* **16**: 654.

Newth CJ, Clark AR (1989). *In vitro* performance of the small particle aerosol generator (SPAG-2). *Ped Pulmonol* **7**: 183.

Okada I, Matsumori A, Matoba Y *et al.* (1992). Combination treatment with ribavirin and interferon for coxsackie virus B3 replication. *J Lab Clin Med* **120**: 569.

Ostrow RS, Forslund KM, McGlennen RC *et al.* (1992). Ribavirin mitigates wart growth in rabbits at early stages of infection with cottontail rabbit papillomavirus. *Antiviral Res* **17**: 99.

Outwater KM, Meissner HC, Peterson MB *et al.* (1988). Ribavirin administration to infants receiving mechanical ventilation. *Amer J Dis* **142**: 512.

Palmieri G, Ambrosi G, Ferraro G *et al.* (1987). Clinical and immunological evaluation of oral ribavirin administration in recurrent herpes simplex infections. *J Int Med Res* **15**: 264.

Page T, Connor JD (1990). The metabolism of ribavirin in erythrocytes and nucleated cells. *Int J Biochem* **22**: 379.

Pancheva SN (1991). Potentiating effect of ribavirin on the anti-herpes activity of acyclovir. *Antiviral Res* **16**: 151.

Paroni R, Del-Puppo M, Borghi C *et al.* (1989). Pharmacokinetics of ribavirin and urinary excretion of the major metabolite 1,2,4-triazole-3-carboxamide in normal volunteers. *Int J Clin Pharmacol Ther Toxicol* **27**: 302.

Patterson AR, Kim SC *et al.* (1975). Transport of nucleosides. *Ann NY Acad Sci* **255**: 402.

Patterson JL, Fernandez-Larsson R (1990). Molecular mechanisms of action of ribavirin. *Rev Infect Dis* **12**: 1139.

Peavy DL, Koff WC, Hyman DS, Knight V (1980). Inhibition of lymphocyte proliferative responses by ribavirin. *Infect Immun* **29**: 583.

Peigue-Lafeuille Gazuy N, Mignoi P, Deteix P *et al.* (1990). Severe respiratory syncytial virus pneumonia in an adult renal transplant recipient successful treatment with ribavirin. *Scand J Infect Dis* **22**: 87.

Peters CJ, Reynolds JA, Stone TW *et al.* (1986). Prophylaxis of Rift Valley fever with antiviral drugs. Immune serum, an interferon inducer and a macrophage activator. *Antiviral Res* **6**: 285.

Povey RC (1978a). *In vitro* antiviral efficacy of ribavirin against feline calicivirus, feline viral rhinotracheitis virus, and canine parainfluenza virus. *Amer J Vet Res* **39**: 175.

Povey RC (1978b). Effect of orally administered ribavirin on experimental feline calicivirus infection in cats. *Amer J Vet Res* **39**: 1337.

Product Information, Viratek.

Rankin JT, Eppes SB, Antezak JB, Joklik WK (1989). Studies on the mechanism of the antiviral activity of ribavirin against reovirus. *Virology* **168**: 147.

Rao KP, Rahiman MA (1989). Cytogenetic effects of ribavirin on mouse bone marrow. *Mutat Res* **224**: 213.

Reichard O, Andersson J, Schvarcz R, Weiland O, (1991). Ribavirin treatment for hepatitis C. *Lancet* **337**: 1058.

Reichard O, Yun ZB, Sonnerborg A, Weiland O (1993). Hepatitis C viral RNA titers in serum prior to during and after oral treatment with ribavirin for chronic hepatitis C. *J Med Virol* **41**: 99.

Remesar MC, Blejer JL, Weissenbacher MC, Nejamkis MR (1988). Ribavirin effect on experimental Junin virus-induced encephalitis. *J Med Virol* **26**: 79.

Roberts RB, Laskin OL, Laurence J *et al.* (1987). Ribavirin pharmacodynamics in high-risk patients for acquired immunodeficiency syndrome. *Clin Pharmacol Ther* **42**: 365.

Roberts RB, Jurica K, Meyer WA (1990a). A phase I study of ribavirin in human immunodeficiency virus-infected patients. *J Infect Dis* **162**: 638.

Roberts RB, Hollinger FB, Parks WP *et al.* (1990b). A multicenter clinical trial of oral ribavirin in HIV infected people with lymphadenopathy virologic observations. Ribavirin LAS Collaborative Group. *AIDS* **4**: 67.

Roberts RB, Dickinson GM, Haseltine PN (1990c). A multicenter clinical trial of oral ribavirin in HIV- infected patients with lymphadenopathy. The Ribavirin LAS Collaborative Group. *J AIDS* **3**: 884.

Roberts E, Ford-Jones EL, James Phillips M (1993). Ribavirin for syncytial giant cell hepatitis. *Lancet* **341**: 640.

Robins RK, Revankar GR, McKernan PA *et al.* (1985). The importance of IMP dehydrogenase inhibition in the broad spectrum antiviral activity of ribavirin and selenazofurin. *Adv Enzyme Reg* **24**: 29.

Rodriguez M, McCormick JD, Weissenbacher MC (1986). Antiviral effect of ribavirin on Junin virus replication *in vitro*. *Rev Argentina Microbiol* **18**: 69.

Rodriguez WJ, Bui RH, Connor JD *et al.* (1987a). Environmental exposure of primary care personnel to ribavirin aerosol when supervising treatment of infants with respiratory syncytial virus infections. *Antimicrob Ag Chemother* **31**: 1143.

Rodriguez WJ, Kim HW, Brandt CD *et al.* (1987b). Aerosolized ribavirin in the treatment of patients with respiratory syncytial virus disease. *Pediatr Infect Dis J* **6**: 159.

Rodriguez WJ, Hall CB, Welliver R *et al.* (1994). Efficacy and safety of aerosolized ribavirin in young children hospitalized with influenza a double blind, multicenter, placebo controlled trial. *J Pediatr* **125**: 129.

Rosina F, Cozzolongo R (1994). Interferon in HDV infection. *Antiviral Res* **24**: 165.

Sabroe I, McHale J, Tait DR *et al.* (1995). Treatment of adenoviral pneumonitis with intravenous ribavirin and immunoglobulin. *Thorax* **50**: 1219.

Scheffler R, Haghchenas D, Wigand R *et al.* (1975). The effect of purine and pyrimidine analogues and virazole on adenovirus replication. *Acta Virol (Praha)* **19**: 106.

Schofield KP, Potter CW, Coley D *et al.* (1975). Antiviral activity of ribavirin on influenza infection in ferrets. *J Antimicrob Chemother* **1**: 63.

Schvarcz R, Yun ZB, Sonnerborg A, Wetland G (1995). Combined treatment with interferon alpha-2b and ribavirin for chronic hepatitis C in patients with a previous non-response or non-sustained response to interferon alone. *J Med Virol* **46**: 43.

Schoub BD Prozesky OW (1977). Antiviral activity of ribavirin in rotavirus gastroenteritis of mice. *Antimicrob Ag Chemother* **12**: 543.

Scotto G, Ferrara S, Mangano A *et al.* (1995). Treatment with ribavirin+alpha interferon in HCV chronic active hepatitis non-responders to interferon alone, preliminary results. *J Chemother* **7**: 58.

Shigeta S, Konno K, Yokota T *et al.* (1988). Comparative activities of several nucleoside analogs against influenza A, B and C viruses *in vitro*. *Antimicrob Ag Chemother* **32**: 906.

Shigeta S, Mori S, Baba M *et al.* (1992). Antiviral activities of ribavirin, 5-ethynyl-1-beta-D-ribofuranosylimidazole-4-carboxamide, and 6'-(R)-6' -C-methylneplanocin A against several ortho- and paramyxoviruses. *Antimicrob Ag Chemother* **36**: 435.

Sidwell RW, Huffman JH, Call EW *et al.* (1972). Broad-spectrum antiviral activity of virazole: 1-beta-D- ribofuranosyl-1,2,4-trizole-3-carboxamide. *Science* 177, 705–706.

Sidwell RW, Huffman JH, Call EW *et al.* (1985). Activity of sclenazofurin against influenza A and B viruses *in vitro*. *Antimicrob Ag Chemother* **28**: 375.

Sidwell RW, Huffman JH,Barnett DB, Pifat DY (1988). *In vitro* and in vivo Phlebovirus inhibition by ribavirin. *Antimicrob Ag Chemother* **32**: 331.

Sidwell RW, Bailey, KW, Wong MH, Huffman JH (1995). *In vitro* and in vivo sensitivity of a non-mouse adapted influenza A (Beijing) virus infection to amantadine and ribavirin. *Chemotherapy* **41**: 455.

Smee DF, Matthews TR (1986). Metabolism of ribavirin in respiratory syncytial virus-infected cells and uninfected cells. *Antimicrob Ag Chemotherapy* **30**: 117.

Smee DF, Alaghamanda HA, Kini GD, Robins RK, (1988). Antiviral activity and mode of action of ribavirin 5'-sulfamate against Semliki Forest virus. *Antiviral Res* **10**: 253.

Smee DF, Gilbert, J, Leonhardt JA *et al.* (1993). Treatment of lethal Pichinde virus infections in weanling LVG/Lak hamsters with ribavirin, ribamidine, selenazefurin and ampligen. *Antiviral Res* **20**: 57.

Smith CB, Charette R P, Fox JP *et al.* (1980). Lack of effect of oral ribavirin in naturally occurring influenza A virus (H1N1) infection. *J Infect Dis* **141**: 548.

Smith DW, Frankel LR, Mathers CH *et al.* (1991). A controlled trial of aerosolized ribavirin in infants receiving mechanical ventilation for severe respiratory syncytial virus infection. *New Engl J Med* **325**: 24.

Snell NJ (1990). Economic and long-term benefits of ribavirin therapy on respiratory syncytial virus infection. *Lung* **168**: 422.

Spanish Ribavirin Trial Group, (1991). Comparison of ribavirin and placebo in CDC group III human immunodeficiency virus infection. *Lancet* **338**: 6.

Steele RW, Crosby DL, Steele RW *et al.* (1988). Effects of ribavirin on neutrophil function. *Amer J Med Sci* **295**: 503.

Stein DS, Creticos CM, Jackson GG *et al.* (1987). Oral ribavirin treatment of influenza A and B. *Antimicrob Ag Chemother* **31**: 1285.

Stephen EL, Jahrling PB (1979). Experimental Lassa fever virus infection successfully treated with ribavirin. *Lancet* **i**: 268.

Stephen EL, Walker JS, Dominik JW *et al.* (1977). Aerosol therapy of influenza infections of mice and primates with rimantadine, ribavirin, and related compounds. *Ann NY Acad Sci* **284**: 264.

Stogner SW, King, JW, Black-Pane C, Bocchim J (1993). Ribavirin and intravenous immune globulin therapy for measles pneumonia in HIV infection. *Southern Med J* **86**: 1415.

Streeter DG, Witkowski JT, Khare GP *et al.* (1973). Mechanism of action of virazole, a new broad-spectrum antiviral agent. *PNAS* **70**: 1174.

Taber LH, Knight V, Gilbert PC *et al.* (1983). Ribavirin aerosol treatment of bronchiolitis associated with respiratory syncytial virus infection in infants. *Pediatrics* **72**: 613.

The Ribavirin ARC Study Group (1993). Multicenter clinical trial of oral ribavirin in symptomatic HIV-infected patients. *J AIDS* **6**: 32.

Tignor GH, Hanham, CA (1993). Ribavirin efficacy in an *in vivo* model of Crimean-Congo hemorrhagic fever virus (CCHF) infection. *Antiviral Res* **22**: 309.

Togo Y, McCracken, E A (1976). Chemoprophylaxis and therapy of respiratory viral infections. *J Infect Dis* **133**: A109.

Toltzis P, Huang AS (1986). Effect of ribavirin on macromolecular synthesis in vesicular stomatitis virus-infected cells. *Antimicrob Ag Chemotherapy* **29**: 1010.

Toltzis P, O'Connell, K Patterson JL (1988). Effect of phosphorylated ribavirin on vesicular stomatitis virus transcription. *Antimicrob Ag Chemother* **32**: 492.

Torres A, Krilov, LR, Jacobson JM *et al.* (1991). Reduced environmental exposure to aerosolized ribavirin using a simple containment system. *Pediatr Infect Dis J* **10**: 217.

Tong MJ, Hwang, SJ, Lefkowitz M *et al.* (1994). Correlation of serum HCV RNA and alanine aminotransferase levels in chronic hepatitis C patients during treatment with ribavirin. *J Gastroent Hepatol* **9**: 587.

United States Pharmacopeia Drug Information, 16th edn (1996).

Uylangco CV, Beroy GJ, Santiago LT *et al.* (1981). A double-blind, placebo-controlled evaluation of ribavirin in the treatment of acute measles. *Clin Ther* **3**: 389.

van Dissel JT, Zijlmans, JM, Kroes AC, Fibbe WE (1995). Respiratory syncytial virus, a rare cause of severe pneumonia following bone marrow transplantation. *Ann Hematol* **71**: 253.

Verheyden JP (1988). Evolution of therapy for cytomegalovirus infection. *Rev Infect Dis* **10**: S477.

Vogt M W, Hartshorn KL, Furman PA *et al.* (1987). Ribavirin antagonizes the effect of azidothymidine on HIV replication. *Science* **235**: 1376.

Warrell,MJ, White, NJ, Looareesuwan S *et al.* (1989). Failure of interferon alfa and ribavirin in rabies encephalitis. *Brit Med J* **299**: 830.

Watanabe W, Konno, K, Ijichi K *et al.* (1994). MTT colorimetric assay system for the screening of anti-orthomyxo- and anti-paramyxoviral agents. *J Virol Meth* **48**: 257.

Watts DM, Ussery MA, Nash D, Peters CJ (1989). Inhibition of Crimean-Congo hemorrhagic fever viral infectivity yields *in vitro* by ribavirin. *Amer J Trop Med Hyg* **41**: 581.

Weissenbacher MC, Calello, MA, Merani MS *et al.* (1986). Therapeutic effect of the antiviral agent ribavirin in Junin virus infection of primates. *J Med Virol* **20**: 261.

Wheeler JG, Wofford, J, Turner RB (1993). Historical cohort evaluation of ribavirin efficacy in respiratory syncytial virus infection. *Pediatr Infect Dis J* **12**: 209.

Whimbey E, Champlin, RE, Englund JA *et al.* (1995). Combination therapy with aerosolized ribavirin and intravenous immunoglobulin for respiratory syncytial virus disease in adult bone marrow transplant recipients. *Bone Marrow Transplant* **16**: 393.

Widell A, Hansson, BG, Oberg B, Nordenfelt E (1986). Influence of twenty potentially antiviral substances on *in vitro* multiplication of hepatitis A virus. *Antiviral Res* **6**: 103.

Wilson SZ, Knight V, Wyde PR *et al.* (1980). Amantadine and ribavirin aerosol treatment of influenza A and B infection in mice. *Antimicrob Ag Chemother* **17**: 642.

Wilson SZ, Gilbert BE, Quarles JM *et al.* (1984). Treatment of influenza A (H1N1) virus infection with ribavirin aerosol. *Antimicrob Ag Chemother* **26**: 200.

Win N, Mitchell, D, Pugh S, Russell NH (1992). Successful therapy with ribavirin of late onset respiratory syncytial virus pneumonitis complicating allogeneic bone transplantation. *Clin Lab Haematol* **14**: 29.

Wray SK, Gilbert BE, Knight V (1985a). Effect of ribavirin triphosphates on primer generation and clongation during influenza virus transcription *in vitro*. *Antiviral Res* **5**: 39.

Wray S K, Gilbert, B E, Noall MW, Knight V (1985b). Mode of action of ribavirin: Effect of nucleotide pool alterations on influenza virus ribonucleoprotein synthesis. *Antiviral Res* **5**: 29.

Wray SK, Smith, RH, Gilbert RE, Knight V (1986a). Effects of selenazofurin and ribavirin and their 5'-triphosphates on replicative functions of influenza A and B viruses. *Antimicrob Ag Chemother* **29**: 67.

Wray PR, Wilson, SZ, Gilbert, BE, Smith, RH (1986b). Protection of mice from lethal influenza virus infection with high dose-short duration ribavirin aerosol. *Antimicrob Ag Chemother* **30**: 942.

Wyde PR, Wilson, SZ, Petrella, R, Gilbert, BE (1987). Efficacy of high dose-short duration ribavirin aerosol in the treatment of respiratory syncytial virus infected cotton rats and influenza B virus infected mice. *Antiviral Res* **7**: 211.

Yang ZQ, Zhang, TM, Zhang MV *et al.*, (1991). Interruption study of viremia of patients with hemorrhagic fever with renal syndrome in the febrile phase. *Chinese Med J* **104**: 149.

Zucker AR, Meadow, WL (1995). Pediatric critical care physicians attitudes about guidelines for the use of ribavirin in critically ill children with respiratory syncytial virus pneumonia. *Crit Care Med* **23**: 767

Amantadine and Rimantadine

Description

Amantadine (1-adamantanamine hydrochloride) is a tricyclic amine compound that was first synthesized from its precursor adamantane in 1941. The drug is useful for seasonal chemoprophylaxis, and prophylaxis in institutionalized populations, and to a lesser extent therapeutic agent against infection with all strains of influenza A virus, but has no activity against influenza B. Amantadine was initially licensed in the USA in 1966 for prophylaxis against only influenza A/H2N2 and 10 years later for prophylactic and therapeutic use against all influenza A subtypes. A closely related derivative, rimantadine, (alpha-methyl-l-adamantane-methylamine hydrochloride) has a similar antiviral spectrum *in vitro* and *in vivo* to amantadine (WHO, 1985), but it is more active than amantadine on a molar concentration basis, equally effective clinically and less toxic. It has been approved for use in the former Soviet Union (Zlydnikov *et al.*, 1981) and more recently in 1993 for use in the USA.

Amantadine is also used for treatment of Parkinson's disease and drug-induced extrapyramidal symptoms. Amantadine is marketed under the trade name of 'Symmetrel' (Geigy). Rimantadine is marketed by Forest Pharmaceuticals as 'Flumadine'.

The chemical structure of amantadine and rimantadine are shown in Fig. V.69.

Antiviral Activity

1 Influenza virus

Amantadine has activity against strains of influenza A virus at low concentrations (<1 μg per ml), although influenza B virus isolates are resistant. Susceptibility of sensitive viruses varies according to the strain studied and the *in vitro* test system employed (Oxford, 1975). Hayden *et al.* (1980a) showed that clinical isolates of A/H1N1, A/H2N2, A/H3N2 were sensitive to amantadine, but the highly passaged classical strain A/PR/8/34/H0N1 was over 15-fold more resistant to amantadine (and rimantadine). By plaque inhibition, the 50% inhibitory concentrations of amantadine and rimantadine for influenza viruses are in the range of 0.01–<1.0 μg per ml (Hayden *et al.*, 1980a, 1989; Browne *et al.*, 1983; Hay *et al.*, 1985; Sidwell *et al.*, 1995).

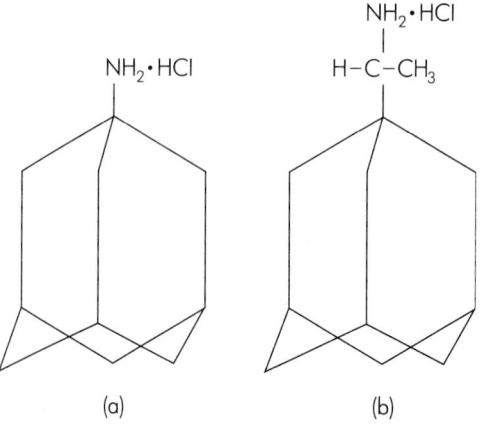

Fig. V.69.

Chemical structures of amantadine hydrochloride (a) and rimantadine hydrochloride (b).

Table V.57

Antiviral activity of amantadine and rimantadine *in vitro*

Sensitive viruses	Resistant viruses
Influenza A[a]	Influenza B
Influenza C	Measles
Parainfluenza[b]	Mumps
Respiratory syncytial virus[b]	Human immunodeficiency virus
Rubella[b]	Polio
Dengue[b]	Herpes simplex
Junin[b]	Rota virus
Lassa[b]	
Pichinde[b]	
Rabies[b]	

[a] High sensitivity (less than 1 μg per ml)
[b] Intermediate sensitivity (10–50 μg per ml, not clinically useful concentrations)
For sources of data refer to text.

Rimantadine is 4- to 8-fold more active than amantadine when tested at low concentrations against influenza A/H3N2 in tracheal-organ cultures (Burlington *et al.*, 1982). This has been subsequently shown by other investigators to be true also for H1N1 and H3N2 strains of influenza A (Belshe *et al.*, 1989).

In experimental mouse infections, oral or injected amantadine protects against the same spectrum of viruses as in tissue culture (Davies *et al.*, 1964; Cochran *et al.*, 1965; Wood, 1965). Amantadine does not provide complete protection of mice; it only reduces the mortality or increases survival time. Avian (chicken) strains of influenza A/H5N2 are susceptible to amantadine (Webster *et al.*, 1985). The drugs are most effective when a relatively low infecting dose of virus is used and when treatment is begun at the time of the infection, with marked decrease in efficacy when added to cultures 24 h or longer post-infection (Burlington *et al.*, 1982). Mice in whom treatment with rimantadine was delayed for more than 8 h after infection had no significant reductions in pulmonary virus titers of influenza A, when infected experimentally with influenza A/H3N2 virus (Herrmann *et al.*, 1989, 1990).

Amantadine has been reported to have activity also against influenza C (Davies *et al.*, 1964).

2 Other viruses

Amantadine has activity against a number of other viruses, mostly enveloped RNA viruses, but usually at higher concentrations (10–50 μg per ml) than required to inhibit influenza A (Couch and Howard, 1986). However, such concentrations are considered to be clinically irrelevant, particularly as concentrations of >10–20 μg per ml are cytotoxic in most cell systems when careful studies have been performed (F Hayden, personal communication).

a Paramyxoviridae Amantadine has no appreciable activity against measles virus *in vitro* (Hosoya *et al.*, 1989). Parainfluenza viruses and respiratory syncytial virus may be inhibited *in vitro* with high concentrations of amantadine and rimantadine, although there have been differing reports (Couch and Howard, 1986). Mumps virus is resistant.

b Togaviridae Early studies by Maassab and Cochran (1964) demonstrated that amantadine could inhibit rubella *in vitro*. Sindbis virus is resistant (Cassell *et al.*, 1984), although other investigators report that sindbis virus is susceptible to both amantadine and rimantadine (Couch and Howard, 1986). There are conflicting reports regarding the susceptibility of Semliki Forest virus, with documentation of greater than 90% inhibition by amantadine at high concentration (0.5mM) (Helenius *et al.*, 1982) as well as resistance (Couch and Howard, 1986).

c Flaviviridae Amantadine at concentrations of 50 μg per ml has been reported to inhibit replication by 90% of all four types of dengue virus in tissue culture (Koff *et al.*, 1980), although rimantadine, administered within minutes of infection via the intraperitoneal route, had no effect on survival of mice infected with dengue virus type 2 (Koff *et al.*, 1983).

d Retroviridae Murine leukemia virus is inhibited by amantadine (McClure *et al.*, 1990) but this drug appears to have no activity against human immunodeficiency virus (McClure *et al.*, 1988).

e Arenaviridae The entry of a number of viruses into cells is dependent on pH and thus can be inhibited by amantadine. This is the likely mechanism of action underlying the efficacy of amantadine against viruses including Junin virus (Castilla *et al.*, 1994), Lassa and Pichinde viruses (Glushakova and Lukashevich, 1989).

f Picornaviridae Amantadine does not inhibit the cellular entry of poliovirus (Perez and Carrasco, 1993). Moderate inhibition of hepatitis A virus antigen expression by amantadine at a concentration of 100 μM (and stronger inhibition at higher doses of up to 500 μM which are too toxic for use) has been reported *in vitro* (Widell *et al.*, 1986; Superti *et al.*, 1987a; Crance *et al.*, 1990).

g Rhabdoviridae Amantadine has been reported to block early events in the replication of several rhabdoviruses (rabies, infectious hematopoietic necrosis virus and vesicular stomatitis virus) *in vitro* (Schlegel *et al.*, 1982; Superti *et al.*, 1985; Fukuhara *et al.*, 1987; Superti *et al.*, 1987b; Hudson *et al.*, 1988). However the intramuscular administration of amantadine to mice experimentally infected with rabies was associated with no therapeutic effect (Bussereau *et al.*, 1988).

h Herpesviridae Although amantadine itself has no activity against herpes simplex virus type 1 (Wittels and Spear, 1991), its derivative tromantadine (N-1-adamantyl-N-(2-(dimethylamino)ethoxy) acetamide hydrochloride) can inhibit herpes simplex virus type 1 *in vitro* when used at high concentration (ranging from 25 to 500 μg per ml) (Rosenthal *et al.*, 1982; Ickes *et al.*, 1990).

i Miscellaneous African swine fever virus is susceptible to high concentrations of amantadine (Alcami *et al.*, 1989). Amantadine has been reported to have activity against simian virus 40 infection of rat and monkey cells (Shimura *et al.*, 1987). Rift Valley fever virus, a member of the Bunyaviridae, is resistant to rimantadine (Peters *et al.*, 1986). Amantadine has little inhibitory effect on human rotavirus infection *in vitro* (Fukuhara *et al.*, 1987)

3 Other microorganisms

Amantadine at a concentration of 1 μg per ml can increase the pH within the phagolysosomes in which *Coxiella burnetti* replicates and, when used in combination with doxycycline, can significantly reduce the numbers of viable organisms (Raoult *et al.*, 1990; Maurin *et al.*, 1992). Probably also due to its lysosomotropic properties, amantadine has *in vitro* activity against *Plasmodium falciparum*; chloroquine-resistant strains are most susceptible (Evans and Havlik, 1993). However, it exerts no activity against *Pneumocystis carinii* (Walzer *et al.*, 1992) or *Chlamydia trachomatis* (Ward and Murray, 1984).

4 Resistance

Early studies showed that strains of influenza A virus could quickly develop resistance to amantadine and rimantadine *in vitro* (Cochran *et al.*, 1965; Grunert *et al.*, 1965; Oxford *et al.*, 1970; Webster *et al.*, 1985). Resistant isolates of influenza A are defined as those that have a threshold EC_{50} of 1 μg per ml for rimantadine or amantadine (Pemberton *et al.*, 1986; Hall *et al.*, 1987; Mast *et al.*, 1991; Valette *et al.*, 1993). This resistance threshold value is arbitrary but is relevant to achievable plasma and respiratory secretion concentrations of the drugs (reviewed in Hayden, 1996). Single amino acid changes within a critical transmembrane region of the M_2 protein are sufficient to confer resistance. The development of resistance of influenza A to both amantadine and rimantadine can also develop during therapy or prophylactic treatment of patients (Belshe *et al.*, 1989; Degelau *et al.*, 1992). These resistant viruses that emerge during treatment of patients with amantadine or rimantadine appear to have no alteration in virulence (Sweet *et al.*, 1991), although shedding may be prolonged (Klimov *et al.*, 1995). There is clear evidence that resistant strains of influenza A can be transmitted from infected to uninfected chickens (Webster *et al.*, 1985; Beard *et al.*, 1987) as well as from infected humans to family members and other contacts (Hayden *et al.*, 1989). Resistant strains of influenza A (with a consistent mutation Ser31$\rightarrow$ Asp documented within the M_2 protein) have been recovered from persons without exposure to either amantadine or rimantadine and from persons treated with amantadine for less than 48 h (Houck *et al.*, 1995).

Resistance is genetically controlled (Tuckova *et al.*, 1973), and amantadine-resistant mutations appears to be similar or identical in both avian and human strains (Bean *et al.*, 1989). Genetic characterization of both rimantadine- and amantadine-resistant isolates has shown that resistance to these drugs can emerge as a result of a single change in the nucleotide sequence coding for the transmembrane domain of M_2 protein, resulting in substitutions in amino acids 27, 30, 31 or 34 (Hay *et al.*, 1985, 1986; Belshe *et al.*, 1988, 1989; Hayden *et al.*, 1989). Amantadine and rimantadine appear to have a similar risk of inducing resistance (Hayden *et al.*, 1989). There are no changes in M_1 protein (Galabov *et al.*, 1994). Resistant strains appear to be genetically stable with no evidence of reversion to wild type even following multiple passage *in vivo* (Bean *et al.*, 1989). Rimantadine-resistant isolates of influenza A are cross-resistant to amantadine (Hayden *et al.*, 1989; Manchand *et al.*, 1990).

5 Synergy

Early studies showed that interferon from allantoic fluid when used in combination with amantadine resulted in synergy against influenza AperWSN in chick embryo cultures (Lavrov *et al.*, 1968). Treatment of chicken and human trachea organ cultures with amantadine in combination with chicken or human leukocyte interferon results in *in vitro* synergy against replication of influenza virus (Lukacsi *et al.*, 1985). Combination of rimantadine and human interferon alpha show additive to synergistic activity against influenza A/H3N2 or /H1N1 subtypes (Hayden *et al.*, 1984). Amantadine and ribavirin have been reported to have additive to synergistic activity against influenza A *in vitro* (Hayden *et al.*, 1980c; Burlington *et al.*, 1983). Similarly, combination therapy using rimantadine and ribavirin can prolong survival in influenza A/H3N2-infected mice (Hayden, 1986). The nucleoside analog 2'-deoxy-2'- fluoroguanosine, and the sialidase inhibitor 4'guanidino-2',4'-deoxy-2',3'-dehydro-N-acetylneuraminic acid both show additive activity with rimantadine against influenza A *in vitro* (Madren *et al.*, 1995; reviewed in Hayden, 1996).

Mode of Administration and Dosage

1 Oral administration

Amantadine and rimantadine are both well absorbed from the gastrointestinal tract, and thus suitable for oral administration. Amantadine has a mean relative oral bioavailability reportedly ranging from 55 to 94% (Aoki *et al.*, 1979; Aoki and Sitar, 1985, 1988). The oral bioavailability of rimantadine in mice and dogs ranges from 60 to 99% (Hoffman *et al.*, 1988), and in healthy adults is 90–96% (Wills *et al.*, 1987b; Wintermeyer and Nahata, 1995). The relative bioavailability of rimantadine syrup is also high (96%) (Wills *et al.*, 1987b). Absorption of neither drug is affected by food.

The recommended dosage of both amantadine and rimantadine for prophylaxis and treatment of adults under 65 years of age is 100 mg given twice-daily, usually at breakfast and lunch (Table V.58). However, in a study of healthy adults aged between 18 and 55 years, prophylactic efficacy of amantadine was maintained with a lower dose of 100 mg per day (Reuman *et al.*, 1989). The normal serum half-life of amantadine has been variously reported to range from 7 to 24 h (mean about 12–16 h) (Soung *et al.*, 1980; Horadam *et al.*, 1981; Hayden *et al.*, 1985). The half-life of rimantadine is considerably longer, ranging from 25 to >36 h in adults and children (Hayden *et al.*, 1985; Anderson *et al.*, 1987; Tominack *et al.*, 1988).

Experience with amantadine and rimantadine suggests that for greatest efficacy therapy should be commenced within 48 h of onset of symptoms (Mostow, 1987). Therapy with amantadine or rimantadine is recommended to continue for 24–48 h after the disappearance of symptoms and signs, generally providing 3–5 days of treatment (CDC,1996).

2 Pregnant women

Amantadine is contraindicated during pregnancy and, as it is secreted in breast milk, it should not be administered to nursing mothers. One case-report suggests that amantadine may be teratogenic in humans (Nora *et al.*, 1975).

Table V.58

Recommended dosage for amantadine and rimantadine treatment and prophylaxis. (Reproduced from CDC, 1996.)

Antiviral	Age			
	1–9 years	10–13 years	14–64 years	≥65 years
Amantadine[a]				
Treatment	5 mg per kg per day up to 150 mg[b] in two divided doses	100 mg twice-daily[c]	100 mg twice-daily	≤100 mg per day
Prophylaxis	5 mg per kg per day up to 150 mg[b] in two divided doses	100 mg twice-daily[c]	100 mg twice-daily	≤100 mg per day
Rimantadine[d]				
Treatment	NA	NA	100 mg twice-daily	100 or 200[e] mg per day
Prophylaxis	5 mg per kg per day up to 150 mg[b]	100 mg twice-daily	100 mg twice-daily	100 or 200[e] mg per day

[a] The drug package insert should be consulted for dosage recommendations for administering amantadine to persons with creatine clearance ≤50 ml per min.

[b] 5 mg per kg of amantadine or rimantadine syrup = 1 tsp per 22 lbs.

[c] Children ≥10 years of age who weigh <40 kg should be administered amantadine or rimantadine at a dose of 5 mg per kg per day.

[d] A reduction in dose to 100 mg per day of rimantadine is recommended for persons who have severe hepatic dysfunction or those with creatine clearance ≤10 ml per min. Other persons with less severe hepatic or renal dysfunction taking >100 mg per kg per day should be observed closely, and the dosage should be reduced or the drug discontinued, if necessary.

[e] Elderly nursing-home residents should be administered only 100 mg per day of rimantadine. A reduction dose to 100 mg per day should be considered for all persons ≥65 years of age if they experience possible side-effects when taking 200 mg per day.

NA: Not applicable.

3 Children

For children aged 1–9 years the recommended dosage of amantadine for prophylaxis or therapy is 5 mg per kg daily (approved dose is 4.4–8.8 mg per kg daily) up to 150 mg per day in two divided doses. For children 10–13 years the full adult dose of both drugs of 100 mg twice-daily is used, although if the weight of the child is less than 40 kg a dose of 5 mg per kg daily is recommended (CDC, 1996). The dose of rimantadine for prophylaxis is 5 mg per kg daily not to exceed 150 mg per day. Rimantadine is not approved for treatment of influenza A in children. Rimantadine syrup in a dose of 3 mg per kg daily has been given to infants aged 1–10 months with apparent safety (Nahata and Brady, 1986).

4 Elderly persons

Reduced dosages of amantadine are indicated for persons aged over 65 years, as serum half-life is increased and renal drug clearance is diminished (Aoki and Sitar, 1985a). For both prophylaxis and treatment of elderly persons amantadine and rimantadine are recommended to be given at a dose of 100 mg once-daily. This dose of amantadine may still need to be reduced in some elderly persons. However, a study of six young (mean age 27 years) and ten elderly (mean age 71.5 years) adults found no significant age-related differences in pharmacokinetics of rimantadine (Hayden *et al.*, 1985). Thus for healthy persons aged over 65 years some clinicians prescribe rimantadine at the full dose of 100 mg twice-daily and reduce this to 100 mg per day if side-effects are experienced (CDC, 1996).

5 Hepatic dysfunction

There is no increase in side-effects in patients with liver disease who receive amantadine. The dose of rimantadine is recommended by the manufacturer to be reduced to 100 mg per day in patients with severe hepatic dysfunction, as the apparent clearance of rimantadine has been reported to be reduced by 50% (CDC, 1996), although in a study of six persons with moderate chronic liver disease the pharmacokinetics of rimantadine were not significantly altered (Wills et al., 1987d).

6 Renal dysfunction

The dose of amantadine should be reduced to 100 mg per day in patients whose creatinine clearance is less than 50 ml per min, as a result of increased serum half-life (Wu et al., 1982; Capparelli et al., 1988; CDC, 1996). The serum half-life of amantadine in patients with renal failure has been reported to be prolonged for as long as 33 days (Horadam et al., 1981). These authors suggested a dosage regimen of amantadine for patients with renal failure, which was designed to yield serum concentrations at a steady-state of 0.7–1.0 μg per ml. Renal function should be closely monitored with dosage adjustments made as necessary. Rimantadine has not yet been fully evaluated in patients with renal dysfunction. Based on limited data, renal clearance of this drug appears to be reduced in persons with severe renal dysfunction and a reduction in dose to 100 mg per day is recommended in persons with a creatinine clearance of <10 ml per min (CDC, 1996).

7 Seizure disorders

As increases in seizures have been reported in patients with a past history of convulsions who take amantadine (Atkinson et al., 1986), such persons should be monitored closely during amantadine therapy (CDC, 1996). The effects of rimantadine on seizure activity has not been studied.

8 Aerosol administration

Small-particle aerosol administration of amantadine has been effective for the treatment of experimental influenzal infection in mice; both amantadine and rimantadine have also been administered as a small-particle aerosol to humans (Hayden et al., 1979; Knight et al., 1979; Tominack and Hayden, 1987). Rimantadine was well tolerated at concentrations of 20 μg per liter of air administered via a continuous-flow, modified Collison nebulizer (Atmar et al., 1990). Both amantadine and rimantadine have been administered by simpler aerosol methods. Hayden et al. (1980b) gave amantadine hydrochloride (1.0 g per 100 ml of distilled water) in a nebulized form by means of a face mask for periods of 20 min, three times per day for 4 days. Rimantadine has been administered in a similar manner in solution (25 mg in 3 ml saline) over periods of 10 min, twice-daily for 5 days (Hayden et al., 1982).

9 Parenteral administration

An infusion of amantadine sulfate (200 mg per day) has been used in the treatment of Parkinson's disease (Brenner et al., 1989). There is no parenteral formulation of the hydrochloride derivatives of amantadine or rimantadine.

Availability

Amantadine is available as 100-mg *capsules*, and as a *syrup*. Rimantadine is available as a 100-mg *tablet* and as a *syrup* containing 50 mg of rimantadine per 5 ml. Both should be stored at room temperature.

Serum Levels in Relation to Dosage

1 Healthy young adults

The peak serum level of amantadine is usually reached 1– 4h after an oral dose, with maximal levels of 0.3 μg per ml after a dose of 2.5 mg per kg and of 0.6 μg per ml when the dose is 5mg per kg (Couch and Jackson, 1976). Serum levels may be measured by high-performance liquid chromatography (Zhou et al., 1993), or by gas chromatography-mass spectrometry (Rubio et al., 1989). Regular monitoring of serum levels is not considered practical.

Patients with normal renal function, who have taken 200 mg amantadine daily for 4–7 days, have steady-state serum concentrations of 0.2–0.9 μg per ml (Pacifici et al., 1976). Similar results were obtained by Hayden et al. (1983) when they administered amantadine to healthy adult volunteers; the mean serum level at 4 h after an oral dose of 100 mg was 0.3ug per ml, and when the drug was continued in this dose twice-daily, the mean value 4 h after the ninth dose was 0.7 μg per ml. The corresponding value 4 h after a single 200mg dose was 0.6 μg per ml and when the drug was continued in two daily doses of 200 and 100 mg, the serum level 4 h after the ninth dose was 1.4 μg per ml.

After aerosol administration of amantadine, only low concentrations are attained in serum, but high levels are reached in nasal washings. By 1 h after a 30 min aerosol administration (1 g per 100 ml), levels of the drug in nasal wash samples were 1.7–108 (mean 30.3) μg per ml, and the peak serum level 2–3 h after the aerosol was 0.02 μg per ml (Hayden *et al.*, 1979). Later studies confirmed that aerosol administration of amantadine in the same dosage produces concentrations of >20 μg per ml in respiratory secretions (Hayden *et al.*, 1980b). Nasal wash levels are much higher than those obtained with oral amantadine; these were 0.02–0.2 μg per ml after an oral dose of 200 mg daily (Smith *et al.*, 1967). Aerosol administration of rimantadine results in mean peak plasma levels that are about 10-fold less than those achieved after oral administration of 200 mg (0.03 and 0.25 μg per ml respectively) with nasal wash levels that are approximately 100-fold higher (6.6 and 0.07 μg per ml respectively) (Atmar *et al.*, 1990).

Intravenous infusions of amantadine sulphate (200 mg per day) in patients with Parkinson's disease have been reported to produce serum concentrations during the infusion of between 0.5 and 1 μg per ml (Brenner *et al.*, 1989).

Rimantadine takes longer to achieve maximum plasma concentration than amantadine, generally peaking 2–6 h after oral absorption (Wills *et al.*, 1987b,c). Hayden *et al.* (1983) studied serum levels after oral rimantadine administration to healthy adult volunteers; the mean serum concentration 4 h after a dose of 100 mg was 0.14 μg per ml and when the drug was continued in this dose twice-daily, the value 4 h after the ninth dose was 0.4 μg per ml. The corresponding value after a single 200 mg dose was 0.3 μg per ml, and when the drug was continued in two daily doses of 200 and 100 mg, the level 4h after the ninth dose was 0.9 μg per ml. After multiple doses of 100 mg twice-daily given to healthy young adults steady-state peak and trough concentrations of rimantadine in plasma are in the range of 0.4–0.5 μg per ml and 0.2–0.4 μg per ml respectively (Wills *et al.*, 1987a). In infants receiving 3 mg per kg daily the steady-state plasma concentrations of rimantadine range from 0.1 to 2.6 μg per ml (Wintermeyer and Nahata, 1995).

2 Elderly persons

Hayden *et al.* (1985) gave 200 mg single oral doses of amantadine after overnight fasting to six young and six elderly adults; the latter had a lower mean creatinine clearance. Peak serum levels occurred at about 2 h in both groups and the elimination half-lives (mean 14.4 h and 19.0 h for young and elderly groups, respectively) were not significantly different. However, peak serum levels in the elderly were 1.5-fold higher (0.8 versus 0.5 μg per ml) and the area-under-the-curve (AUC) was 1.7-fold greater. Serum levels obtained from residents in a nursing home who received amantadine prophylaxis (100 mg per day) for 35 days ranged from 0.1 to 0.7 μg per ml (Arden *et al.*, 1988), similar to levels in healthy young adults receiving 200 mg per day (Hayden *et al.*, 1983). In another study, the same dose of amantadine in a population whose mean age was 87 years resulted in serum levels ranging from 0.1 to 5.8 μg per ml suggesting that this dose may still be too high in some nursing home residents (Degelau *et al.*, 1990). However, a dose of 50 mg per day of amantadine administered to elderly nursing home residents (mean age 85 years) failed to achieve adequate mean steady-state trough serum levels, defined in a previous study as 0.3 μg per ml (Aoki and Sitar, 1985; Aoki *et al.*, 1985; Somani *et al.*, 1991).

Prolonged administration of rimantadine in a dose of 200 mg per day to elderly residents of nursing homes resulted in a mean serum level of 1.2 μg per ml, 2- to 3-fold higher than in young adults (Patriarca *et al.*, 1984). However, in a study of persons older than 60 years who received a single 200-mg dose of rimantadine, Hayden and colleagues found the peak serum concentration to be 0.25 μg per ml, and the peak elimination half-life was doubled when compared with that of amantadine (36.5 versus 16.7 h respectively). In contrast to the findings with amantadine, there was no differences in rimantadine pharmacokinetics in these two age groups (Hayden *et al.*, 1985). In a third study, the mean peak concentrations of rimantadine in plasma of healthy adults aged 50–60 years, 61–70 years, and 71–79 years treated with 200 mg per day for 9.5 days were 0.4 μg per ml, 0.4 μg per ml and 0.5 μg per ml respectively. The peak elimination half-life was also similar in the three groups, again suggesting no major difference in pharmacokinetics of rimantadine in this population (Tominack *et al.*, 1988). There may be difficulties in interpreting data from rimantadine pharmacokinetic studies in the elderly, as some were performed in ambulatory, generally healthy individuals and are not necessarily predictive of findings in infirm, nursing home residents (F Hayden, personal communication).

3 Renal dysfunction and hemodialysis

In patients with reduced creatinine clearance the plasma half-life of amantadine has been reported to range from 27 to 144 h, correlating with serum creatinine levels (Wu *et al.*, 1982). Renal amantadine clearance is also reduced in patients with diminished creatinine clearance (Wu *et al.*, 1982). Negligible amounts (2–5%) of amantadine and rimantadine are removed by hemodialysis (Horadam *et al.*, 1981; Capparelli *et al.*, 1988). The plasma half-life of rimantadine in patients with end-stage renal failure who received two 100-mg doses was 43.6 h, significantly longer than that of age-matched healthy subjects (27.5 h).

4 Hepatic dysfunction

Patients with chronic liver disease who received a single dose of two 100-mg tablets of rimantadine were found to have similar peak serum levels, elimination half-life, AUC, and renal clearance of rimantadine when compared with healthy controls (Wills *et al.*, 1987d).

5 Children

In infants aged 1–10 months administered rimantadine (3 mg per kg per day), steady-state peak serum concentrations were obtained 2.5–6 h post-dose, ranging from 0.1 to 0.6 µg per ml, (Nahata and Brady, 1986). In children aged 5–8 years the mean serum half-life of rimantadine was 25 h (Anderson *et al.*, 1987).

6 Overdosage

Intoxication resulting from renal failure and excessive amantadine plasma concentrations has been reported to contribute to unexpected death (Hartshorne *et al.*, 1995).

Excretion

Amantadine is not metabolized and elimination is almost entirely by renal clearance (both glomerular filtration and tubular secretion) (Aoki and Sitar, 1988). After a single oral dose, an average of 86% of the drug is excreted in the urine within 4 days (average urinary excretion within 24 h is 56%) (Bleidner *et al.*, 1965). After a single 200-mg dose, the proportion of this dose recovered from the urine in the first 24 h as the parent drug was 51.7% for young adults and 39.7% for elderly adults (Hayden *et al.*, 1985). Amantadine is not efficiently removed from plasma during hemodialysis and supplemental doses are not usually given.

Rimantadine is extensively metabolized in the liver to produce ortho-, para-, and meta-hydroxylated metabolites. After a single 200-mg dose of rimantadine, the proportion of this dose recovered from the urine in the first 24 h as the parent drug is less than 1%, reportedly being 0.8% for young adults and 0.5% for elderly subjects (Hayden *et al.*, 1985). Subsequent studies using improved methodology suggest that up to 16% of rimantadine is excreted unchanged in urine (Capparelli *et al.*, 1988). The total urinary recovery of rimantadine and its hydroxylated metabolites was found to be approximately 18% in young adults and 20% in elderly subjects (Hayden *et al.*, 1985). Similar to amantadine, rimantadine is not efficiently removed by hemodialysis.

Table V.59
Pharmacokinetic parameters of rimantadine and amantadine. (Reproduced from Rimantadine Product Monograph, with permission.)

	Rimantadine	Amantadine
Time to peak serum concentration (h)	3.6	2.4
Excreted unchanged in urine (%)	<10	>90
Peak steady-state plasma concentration (µg per ml)	0.20–0.40	0.50–0.70
Volume of distribution (liter per kg)	10–15	4–10
Protein binding (%)	40	67
Maximum nasal mucus concentration (µg per g)	0.42	0.45
Ratio of maximum nasal mucus concentration to maximum plasma concentration	1.73	0.71

Distribution of the Drugs in Body

In the recommended doses, maximal concentrations of amantadine are achieved in tissues (particularly lungs, heart and brain) in about 48 h. The apparent volume of distribution of amantadine and rimantadine is large; the volume of distribution for rimantadine is about 2.5-fold larger than that of amantadine (Soung *et al.*, 1980; Hayden *et al.*, 1985). In a study of healthy young adults the volume of distribution was significantly higher in smokers than non-smokers (Wong *et al.*, 1995). A high degree of tissue binding explains their low serum levels and the small amounts of drug removed by hemodialysis. In an experimental model, approximately two-thirds of amantadine added to plasma samples becomes protein bound (Liu *et al.*, 1984).

Hayden *et al.* (1985) estimated concentrations of amantadine and rimantadine in nasal mucus after 200-mg single oral doses of each drug. Nasal mucus levels of the drug rose over 8 h, despite a decline in plasma concentration. The maximum concentrations of rimantadine and amantadine in nasal secretions were found to be similar (mean of 0.42 and 0.45 μg per g respectively). However, the mucus:plasma ratio of drug was 1.75 for rimantadine and 0.95 for amantadine, suggesting that rimantadine may be concentrated within respiratory secretions.

In the rat model, between 26 and 88% of amantadine and rimantadine is transported across the blood–brain barrier (Spector, 1988). In humans, amantadine concentrations in the CSF are about 60% of those in the serum.

Mode of Action

Work is continuing to define the precise mechanism of action of these drugs. Both amantadine and rimantadine can act at several stages in the replicative cycle of influenza A. Most strains of the virus are inhibited early in the replicative cycle, at a stage subsequent to attachment and entry; some strains are blocked at the level of virion protein maturation, assembly and release (Oxford and Schild, 1967; Kato and Eggers, 1969; Pinto, 1992). Inhibition of replication is mediated through preventing the function of proton channels by the influenza A M_2 protein (Hay *et al.*, 1985; Duff and Ashley, 1992; Duff *et al.*, 1994).

The influenza A virus enters the cell by initial binding to surface sialic residues followed by receptor-mediated endocytosis (Matlin, 1982; Marsh and Helenius, 1989). These processes do not appear to be altered by the presence of amantadine or rimantadine (Couch and Howard, 1986; Richman *et al.*, 1986). Similarly, amantadine does not appear to act at this step in the replicative cycle of other viruses that are susceptible to the drug in higher concentrations (Superti *et al.*, 1985; Perez and Carrasco, 1993).

In order for the virus to reach the cytosol, the viral envelope must fuse with the membranes of the endosome in which it is contained through a low pH-induced conformational change of the viral hemagglutinin. Fusion enables the release of uncoated virion nucleic acids and proteins into the cytosol. At high concentration, this uncoating is inhibited by amantadine and rimantadine by

Table V.60

Comparison of the properties of amantadine and rimantadine. (Reproduced from Arruda and Hayden, 1996, with permission from Plenum Press, New York.)

Shared features
Similar chemical structure (adamantanamines)
Spectrum limited to influenza A virus
M_2 protein as target of antiviral action
Cross-sensitivity or resistance *in vitro*
Excellent oral bioavailability (>90%)
Good penetration into respiratory secretions
Prolonged elimination half-life (rimantadine > amantadine)

Distinguishing features
Risk of central nervous system side-effects (amantadine > rimantadine)
Peak plasma concentrations (amantadine > rimantadine)
Major route of elimination
amantadine - renal
rimantadine - metabolism
Dose reduction for renal insufficiency
amantadine – Cl_{cr} < 80 ml per min
rimantadine – Cl_{cr} < 10–20 ml per min

preventing acidification of the endosome (Koff and Knight, 1979; Bukrinskaya et al., 1980, 1982; Daniels et al., 1985; Richman et al., 1986). As the inhibition of fusion only occurs in the presence of high concentrations of amantadine, this is unlikely to be the primary target of the drug (Bron et al., 1993). The hemagglutinins of amantadine-resistant strains of influenza A have been found to participate in fusion at a higher pH than wild-type virus (Daniels et al., 1985). Uncoating is the likely target of amantadine for some viruses such as vesicular stomatitis virus which are susceptible to the drug at higher concentrations (Superti et al., 1985).

The M_2 membrane protein of influenza A provides an ion channel that transports protons into the virion and facilitates uncoating. Lower concentrations of amantadine and rimantadine inhibit this process (Hay et al., 1985; Kendal and Klenk, 1991; Holsinger et al., 1994; Wharton et al., 1994). The pH of activation of the M_2 ion channel is similar for human, swine, equine and avian strains of influenza A (Wang et al., 1993).

Within the cytosol, the viral ribonucleoproteins are transported to the nucleus for viral transcription and replication, a process not found to be inhibited by amantadine (Kemler et al., 1994), although an earlier report indicated that amantadine prevented the import of ribonucleoproteins into the nucleus by blocking the dissociation of the viral matrix protein M_1 and the ribonucleoproteins.

Assembly of newly formed viral nucleoproteins commences in the nucleus. Newly synthesized viral proteins are then transported to the cell surface via the acidic trans-Golgi. The M_2 membrane protein of influenza A facilitates these processes by functioning as an ion channel (Pinto, 1992). Amantadine has been reported to inhibit the release of influenza A virions from the surface of cells infected with the Rostock (H7N1) strain (Sugrue et al., 1990; Ruigrok et al., 1991). This is thought to occur as a result of an M_2-mediated conversion of the influenza A hemagglutinin to its low pH conformation within the trans-Golgi compartment (Sugrue et al., 1990; Ciampor et al., 1992). The M_2 protein regulates pH gradients across membranes within the trans-Golgi (Grambas et al., 1992), and is itself pH regulated (Pinto, 1992). Mutations that result in resistance to amantadine and rimantadine are solely contained within hydrophobic regions of the M_2 protein, suggesting that the membrane-associated part of this molecule is the major target of these drugs (Hay et al., 1986). No difference in matrix protein M_1 have been observed in rimantadine-resistant and sensitive strains of influenza A (H3N2) (Galabov et al., 1994).

Toxicity

1 Amantadine

a Nervous system The most commonly encountered side-effects of amantadine are nervous system symptoms, such as nervousness, difficulty in concentration, insomnia, light-headedness, dizziness, tremor, slurred speech, ataxia, drowsiness, depression, confusion, hallucinations and headache; these symptoms are reported by 11–33% of young adults who take amantadine at a dose of 100 mg twice-daily (Bryson et al., 1980; Hayden et al., 1981; Snoey and Bessen, 1990). Convulsions and mania have only rarely been reported (Rego and Giller, 1989). There is a case report of pathologic jealousy (Othello syndrome) in a patient receiving amantadine that was ascribed to the drug (McNamara and Durso, 1991).

A placebo-controlled study of 476 healthy adults aged 18–55 years found that side-effects were comparable in those receiving prophylaxis with 100 mg per day and placebo, but were significantly higher in the group receiving 200 mg per day (Reuman et al., 1989). During a trial of amantadine for prophylaxis (200 mg daily) against influenza A virus infection in young adults, Bryson et al. (1980) found that side-effects (dizziness, nervousness and insomnia) occurred in 33% of those receiving the drug compared with 10% of those receiving placebo; they also noted some decrease in performance of sustained attention tasks.

Hayden et al. (1981) in a larger controlled study in healthy adults showed that amantadine was well tolerated at a dose of 200 mg daily, but central nervous system symptoms were more frequent with a daily dose of 300 mg; nervousness, difficulty in concentration, light-headedness and insomnia were the most common side-effects. Amantadine has no effects on psychomotor function at a dosage of 200 mg daily, but the performance of attentional tasks is decreased with a dose of 300 mg daily (Hayden et al., 1981; Millet et al., 1982). Central nervous system side-effects occur more frequently in patients with renal failure in whom the drug accumulates. These effects may be more likely with serum concentrations of 1.5–2.0 μg per ml or higher (Ing et al., 1980; Soung et al., 1980; Arden et al., 1988; Degelau et al., 1990; Strong et al., 1991). Coma has been reported in a patient with renal failure (Macchio et al., 1993). The drug should be used with care in elderly patients (Strange et al., 1991) and those with a history of seizures or psychosis (Atkinson *et al.*, 1986; Nestelbaum *et al.*, 1986). There have been two case reports of the successful use of physostigmine in the treatment of amantadine neurotoxicity (Casey, 1978; Berkowitz, 1979).

b Gastrointestinal tract Symptoms of anorexia, nausea and vomiting may occur. All these side-effects usually develop within the first 24 h, plateau on the second day and may then improve despite continued treatment (Hayden *et al.*, 1981).

c Other Uncommon side-effects of amantadine are rashes, postural hypotension and leukopenia (Van den Berg and Van Ketel 1983). Anticholinergic effects may complicate amantadine therapy, such as transient blurring of vision, mouth dryness and palpitations, and the drug should be used with caution in patients with glaucoma or prostatic enlargement. Progressive muscular weakness ultimately requiring ventilatory support has been reported in a woman who received 200 mg per day of amantadine for 3 days (Miller and Miller, 1994). Corneal lesions have been reported in association with amantadine therapy (Fraunfelder *et al.*, 1990). These lesions include the development of superficial punctate keratitis and corneal abrasion (Gaudry *et al.*, 1993) and corneal edema (Blanchard, 1990). There have been single-case reports of heart failure (Vale and Maclean, 1977), and temporary diminution of visual acuity (Pearlman *et al.*, 1977) associated with amantadine therapy. Ventricular arrhythmias have been reported, in one patient associated with attempted suicide by amantadine overdose (Sartori *et al.*, 1984; Pimentel and Hughes, 1991). Prolonged use of amantadine over periods of months, as in the treatment of Parkinson's disease, may be associated with the development of livedo reticularis and peripheral edema; both resolve on cessation of the drug. Hyponatremia has been reported in a patient who was taking amantadine and L-dopa (Lammers and Roos, 1993). A woman treated with amantadine during the first trimester of pregnancy gave birth to an infant at 29 weeks with tetralogy of Fallot and tibial hemimelia: the relationship between the development of these abnormalities and amantadine administration has not been proven (Pandit *et al.*, 1994). Amantadine has been reported to inhibit lymphocyte proliferation *in vitro* (Clark *et al.*, 1991).

In clinical studies using amantadine for prophylaxis and in volunteer studies, minimal toxicity occurs when the drug is used in a dose of 200 mg daily (Hayden *et al.*, 1981). At this dosage the frequency of side-effects has been in the order of 7–10% (Couch and Jackson, 1976; Delker *et al.*, 1980; Hayden *et al.*, 1981).

Amantadine aerosol treatment is usually well tolerated when a solution of 1.0 g per 100 ml is used; with solutions of 1.5 or 2.5 g per 100 ml, during and up to 1 h after aerosol exposures, nasal irritation, rhinorrhea or dysgeusia may occur (Hayden *et al.*, 1979). A trial of amantadine aerosol (1 g per 100 ml) in naturally occurring influenza, produced a greater frequency of rhinorrhea and nasal irritation than placebo aerosol (Hayden *et al.*, 1980b).

2 Rimantadine

Side-effects of this analog are the same as with amantadine, but the relative frequency with each drug differs. Rimantadine appears to cause fewer central nervous system symptoms than amantadine, but has a similar frequency of gastrointestinal symptoms (Hayden *et al.*, 1981; Dolin *et al.*, 1982; Guay, 1994).

Both amantadine and rimantadine were well tolerated when given in a daily dose of 200 mg (Hayden *et al.*, 1981; Millet *et al.*, 1982). At 300 mg per day, Hayden *et al* (1981) found that there were more central nervous system side-effects with amantadine than with rimantadine; amantadine recipients did not perform tests requiring sustained attention and problem-solving as well as volunteers receiving rimantadine. Further pharmacokinetic studies by Hayden *et al.* (1983) provided an explanation for this difference. When daily doses of 200 or 300 mg are given to healthy adults, rimantadine produces lower serum levels than amantadine. There was a low correlation between the serum concentrations of either drug and the occurrence of side-effects, but serum levels of toxic and non-toxic subjects overlapped extensively. These studies indicated that amantadine and rimantadine have differing pharmacokinetics, but they have a similar potential to cause side-effects at comparable serum levels. Patriarca *et al.* (1984) used rimantadine in a dose of 100 mg twice-daily in 18 elderly patients for a mean period of 80 days; compared with patients given placebo treatment, a greater proportion of the rimantadine group developed anxiety and/or nausea; these side-effects usually lasted less than 9 days, but they necessitated cessation of treatment in three patients. In 14 of the rimantadine-treated patients tested, high serum levels were detected.

Rimantadine is well tolerated in children with nausea and vomiting being reported in only a few recipients (Hall *et al.*, 1987; Crawford *et al.*, 1988). Central nervous system effects have been reported in 3.2% of treated children under 10 years of age (about 2.5-fold less frequently than in adults), and gastrointestinal adverse effects in 8.4% (Wintermeyer and Nahata, 1995).

Rimantadine administered as a small particle aerosol at a concentration of 40 μg per liter of air has been associated with nasal burning and irritation; at a concentration of 20 μg per liter of air it was better tolerated with only mild nasal irritation in two of 13 recipients (Atmar *et al.*, 1990).

When tested *in vitro* on the ciliated epithelium of organ cultures of ferret tracheal rings, rimantadine produced comparable damage at concentrations of only one-third those of amantadine (Burlington *et al.*, 1981).

3 Drug interactions

Concomitant administration of antihistamines seems to enhance some amantadine side-effects (Millet *et al.*, 1982). Cotherapy with amantadine and anticholinergics in elderly patients may result in visual hallucinations and delirium. Drugs that have a stimulant effect on the central nervous system should not be taken with amantadine. There has been a report of acute mental confusion when trimethoprim sulfamethoxazole was given to a patient with amantadine, due to reduced renal tubular secretion of amantadine (Speeg *et al.*, 1989; Guay, 1994). There is no interaction between ethanol and amantadine in humans (Alkana *et al.*, 1982). However, nicotine (at concentrations found in the plasma of chronic smokers) has been reported to interfere with the proximal tubular transport of amantadine in the kidneys (Wong *et al.*, 1992). Cimetidine when given simultaneously with rimantadine has no clinically significant interaction (Holazo *et al.*, 1989). The renal clearance of amantadine has been reported to be significantly inhibited by quinine and quinidine, but curiously only in male patients (Gaudry *et al.*, 1993). No alteration in the recommended dose of amantadine is required in patients taking this drug concurrently with acetaminophen (Aoki and Sitar, 1992a). There is a reported interaction between amantadine and one of the components of the diuretic 'Dyazide' (hydrochlorothiazide and triamterene), resulting in reduced renal clearance of amantadine (Wilson and Rajput, 1983).

In cell culture amantadine significantly slows the excretion of digoxin (Griffiths *et al.*, 1983). There have been no reports of clinically significant drug interactions with rimantadine.

Clinical Uses of the Drugs

Amantadine and rimantadine are efficacious chemoprophylactic agents against artificial and naturally acquired uncomplicated influenza A virus infections of all subtypes, preventing 70–90% of symptomatic infections (O'Donoghue *et al.*, 1973; Atkinson *et al.*, 1986; Mostow, 1987; Wiselka, 1994). Amantadine is indicated for the treatment and prophylaxis of adults and children over 1 year of age. Rimantadine received approval in 1993 for the same indications as amantadine in adults, but only for prophylaxis in children (CDC, 1996). The drugs have no prophylactic or therapeutic effect in influenza B virus infections (Smorodintsev *et al.*, 1970a).

Although studies dating back to 1964 have consistently shown that amantadine and, more recently rimantadine, are effective chemoprophylactic agents in influenza A virus infections, these drugs have not been widely used because of the clinical difficulty in recognizing influenza (Bennett, 1973) and the absence of facilities for rapid virological diagnosis in many areas. There is also concern regarding the frequency of side-effects of amantadine, particularly in the elderly (especially if there is occult impaired renal function), and the rapid emergence and potential transmission of resistant strains with both rimantadine and amantadine treatment.

1 Recommendations for use of amantadine and rimantadine

Amantadine or rimantadine are not substitutes for influenza vaccination. The drugs are however of use in certain circumstances, and guidelines have been established and revised for amantadine and rimantadine by the World Health Organisation (WHO, 1986) and the Centers for Disease Control in Atlanta (CDC, 1996).

Chemoprophylaxis should be considered in residents of nursing homes and chronic care institutions during epidemics of influenza A, as an adjunct to seasonal or late influenza immunization. In particular chemoprophylaxis should be considered in adults at high risk of serious morbidity and mortality due to influenza because of underlying diseases, which include pulmonary, cardiovascular, metabolic, neuromuscular, or immunodeficiency diseases. The adjunctive administration of amantadine or rimantadine to high-risk, previously vaccinated persons can enhance prophylaxis. Chemoprophylaxis may also be considered for home carers of high-risk persons including household members, volunteers and district nurses who have not been vaccinated during community outbreaks of influenza A. Immunodeficient patients who do not mount an adequate immune response to influenza immunization or those for whom influenza vaccination is contraindicated may benefit from amantadine or rimantadine during community outbreaks (WHO, 1985; CDC, 1996). Chemoprophylaxis is also considered for children aged 6 months to 18 years receiving long-term aspirin therapy and who may be at risk for Reye syndrome as a complication of influenza (CDC, 1996). It remains controversial whether unvaccinated hospital medical, nursing and pharmacy staff should receive prophylaxis during community outbreaks, and side-effects and cost are important considerations (Cox, 1991). If an epidemic is caused by a subtype of influenza A not covered by the vaccine, chemoprophylaxis may be considered for all health care personnel (CDC, 1996).

For maximum efficacy the drug is taken for the duration of the epidemic; a more cost-effective approach is for administration only during the peak of influenza activity within the community (CDC, 1996). Non-immunized persons who commence amantadine at the same time as receiving influenza vaccine would need to take prophylaxis to protect against influenza A for the period required for the vaccine-induced immune response to be established, usually 2 weeks in adults and up to 6 weeks in children (Mostow, 1987; CDC, 1996).

These drugs should also be considered for the treatment of high-risk patients who develop influenza during a known influenza A outbreak within the community. Administration should commence within 24–48 h of onset of symptoms and continue for 48 h following resolution of illness (CDC, 1996).

2 Amantadine prophylaxis

Controlled trials in which protection was judged by artificial challenge with influenza virus have been conducted (Jackson et al., 1963; Stanley et al., 1965; Schiffet et al., 1966; Hornick et al., 1967; Togo et al., 1968; Bloomfield et al., 1970; Likar, 1970; Smorodintsev et al., 1970a; Sears and Clements, 1987). All but one (Tyrell et al., 1965), demonstrated the prophylactic value of amantadine. Although the earlier trials used higher doses, 100 mg per day has been shown to have similar prophylactic efficacy (Sears and Clements, 1987; Reuman et al., 1989).

Many studies have been carried out on the protective value of amantadine in naturally occurring influenza (Wendel, 1964; Quilligan et al., 1966; Finklea et al., 1967; Galbraith et al., 1969a, b; Knight et al., 1969; Nafta et al., 1970; Oker-Blom et al., 1970; Smorodintsev et al., 1970b; O'Donoghue et al., 1973; Monto et al., 1979; Pettersson et al., 1980; Dolin et al., 1982; Payler and Purdham, 1984; Atkinson et al., 1986; Peters et al., 1989). These trials were carried out on a variety of population groups including university students, military personnel, prison volunteers, schoolboys, children in institutions, family groups, nursing home residents and general hospital patients. With the exception of one report by Galbraith et al. (1969b), all confirmed the efficacy of amantadine in protecting contacts against natural influenza A virus infections. Subclinical infections have been reported to occur in up to 30% of amantadine recipients (Karlsson et al., 1987). Immune responses may develop in such persons that will confer subsequent protection against related viruses (CDC, 1996). Various degrees of protection have been reported, but it seems that under field conditions amantadine provides about 50% protection against influenzal infection and 60–70% protection against illness (Couch and Jackson, 1976; Delker et al., 1980). Protective value is evident after 48 h treatment with the drug, but it ceases when amantadine is stopped (Muldoon et al., 1976).

Amantadine administered prophylactically to institutionalized children during naturally occurring epidemics has resulted in less illness and reduced incidence of household spread (Quilligan et al., 1966; Finklea et al., 1967; Galbraith et al., 1969b). In a boys boarding school where annual influenza vaccination was routine, amantadine therapy or placebo were given during an influenza A (H1N1) epidemic. Of 267 boys, three receiving amantadine and 29 in the placebo group developed proven infection (Payler and Purdham, 1984).

3 Rimantadine prophylaxis

Rimantadine prophylaxis (100 mg per day) was found to be effective in a randomized, double-blind study of adults aged 18–55 years who were administered the drug or placebo during the influenza season; influenza virus was only isolated from placebo recipients (Brady et al., 1990). Rimantadine was given to 145 children during an outbreak of influenza A (H1N1) in a randomized blind trial. Laboratory-confirmed influenza occurred in 31.7% receiving placebo and in 2.9% of children in the rimantadine group. No rimantadine recipients developed clinical illness compared with 17% receiving placebo (Clover et al., 1986). Crawford et al. (1988) confirmed the efficacy of rimantadine in children aged 1–18 years when used as prophylaxis against infection with a different subtype of influenza A (H3N2) during a naturally occurring outbreak. Laboratory-confirmed influenza occurred in 31% of children in the placebo group and in only 7.4% of rimantidine recipients. There was also a lower incidence of influenza in households of rimantidine-treated children (Crawford et al., 1988).

4 Amantadine therapy

Used therapeutically, amantadine will reduce the duration of fever and shorten illness by up to 50% (Hornick et al., 1969, 1970; Wingfield et al., 1969; Togo et al., 1970; Galbraith et al., 1971; Wink, 1975; Younkin et al., 1983). Others have confirmed that amantadine has a therapeutic effect in influenza when administered within 48 h of onset of clinical disease (Van Voris et al., 1981; Younkin et al., 1983). This effect is on generalized symptoms particularly, but it also reduces localized respiratory symptoms; amantadine shortens the duration of illness by 24 h or roughly 33% of the illness duration. Moreover, Younkin et al. (1983) demonstrated that this therapeutic effect could also be obtained with a dose of 100 mg amantadine daily in adults; control subjects given 3.25 g of aspirin daily had more side-effects than volunteers receiving daily doses of 100 or 200 mg amantadine. Although aspirin therapy results in shorter time to defervescence there is subsequently greater symptomatic improvement in amantadine recipients (Younkin et al., 1983). In natural influenza A virus infection in students, amantadine therapy appeared to be associated with resolution of peripheral airways dysfunction which occurs in uncomplicated influenza (Little et al., 1976).

Effects of amantadine on virus shedding are inconsistent; no effect was found by Togo et al. (1970), but in later studies a reduction in the frequency and quantity of virus shedding in nasal washes has been demonstrated (Van Voris et al., 1981; Younkin et al., 1983). Sears et al. (1987) reported that amantadine recipients shed 100-fold less influenza following experimental challenge, and for half as many days when compared with a placebo group. There is no significant difference in the level of viral shedding in patients taking 100 or 200 mg of amantadine per day (Reuman et al., 1989).

There are no studies which provide data regarding the efficacy of amantadine or rimantadine in preventing serious complications of influenza. In one report amantadine treatment did not prevent the death of two patients with myocarditis due to influenza A (Ray et al., 1989). However, a woman with respiratory failure due to influenza pneumonia in the third trimester of pregnancy had a favorable outcome following amantadine therapy (Kirshon et al., 1988). In bone marrow transplant patients with influenza A complicated by pneumonia, amantadine treatment has been associated with a survival of over 80% (Whimbey et al., 1994).

Amantadine administered by aerosol has been used in a controlled trial to treat patients with naturally acquired influenza A virus infections (either H1N1 or H3N2). Treated patients had more rapid resolution of clinical signs and symptoms, but fever and frequency of virus isolation were unaffected (Hayden et al., 1980b).

5 Rimantadine therapy

There have been several studies of rimantadine for the treatment of patients with proven influenza A. Hayden et al. (1986) demonstrated the efficacy of rimantadine in a placebo-controlled, double-blind study of patients with uncomplicated influenza A (H3N2). When treated with 200 mg per day for 5 days, those randomized to receive rimantadine had lower virus titers in nasal secretions, less systemic symptoms and more rapid defervescence (mean 37 h shorter) than placebo recipients (Hayden and Monto, 1986). In a more recent randomized, double-blind study, Hayden et al. (1991) studied children and adults with laboratory confirmed influenza A (H3N2) who were treated with rimantadine (200 mg per day) or placebo for 10 days, commencing within 2 days of onset of illness. Patients who received rimantadine had a significantly shorter duration of symptoms (mean difference in time to a 50% reduction of 2.5 days) than placebo recipients. The number of days of fever was shortened by a mean of 1.6 days, and there were fewer days missed from work or school and overall days of restricted activity (means of 1.0 and 1.5 days respectively) in the rimantadine group. By day 5, drug-resistant strains were recovered from 33% of rimantadine recipients, but not from those receiving placebo. Those with resistant virus recovered more slowly than those whose strains remained sensitive, the mean time to a 50% reduction in symptom score being 5.1 and 3.4 days respectively (Hayden et al., 1991) (Fig. V.70). When rimantadine is prescribed for both treatment of index cases and post-exposure prophylaxis to their family members, the drug is not effective in preventing infection in household contacts, due to the rapid emergence and transmission of resistant strains (Hayden et al., 1989).

Children with laboratory proven influenza A (H3N2) were randomized to treatment with rimantadine or acetaminophen for 5 days. Rimantadine recipients had greater reduction in fever and more rapid symptomatic improvement during the first 3 days compared with the placebo group. Rimantadine resistance rapidly emerged (Hall et al., 1987). However, another study comparing the same therapies in children with proven influenza (H1N1) found no difference in clinical resolution between the two groups, although virus shedding during the first two days was lower in rimantadine recipients (Thompson et al., 1987).

Fig. V.70.

Resolution of symptoms in rimantadine-treated, influenza A infected patients who shed resistant virus, and those who had no detectable resistant virus. The symptom scores in the placebo group are indicated for comparison.
(Reproduced from Hayden *et al.*, 1991, with permission.)

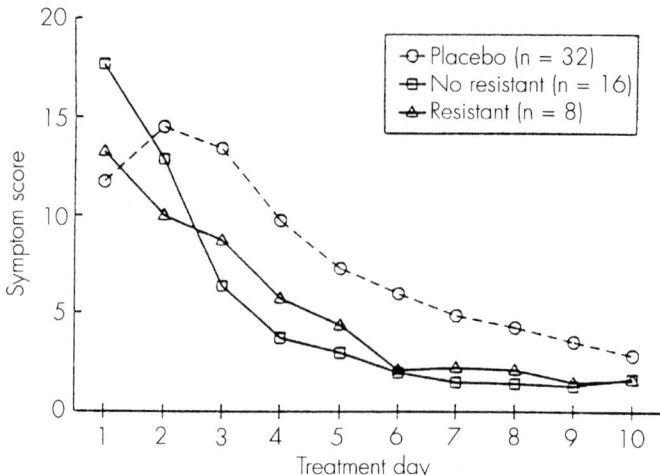

Aerosolized rimantadine (p. 1839) has been used therapeutically in volunteers infected with attenuated influenza A (HINI) virus; this produced a clinical benefit comparable with that found with low dose (50 mg per day) oral rimantadine, but no effect on virus shedding occurred (Hayden *et al.*, 1982). Aerosol treatment of influenza by amantadine or rimantadine by the method employed in these trials is unlikely to have a clinical application because it is cumbersome and time-consuming.

6 Comparison of amantadine versus rimantadine

The comparative efficacy of amantadine and rimantadine has been evaluated in naturally occurring influenza infections. Rimantadine is equally effective and less toxic when compared with amantadine for both prophylactic (Dolin *et al.*, 1982) and therapeutic (Van Voris *et al.*, 1981) use against influenza A.

When both drugs were used for therapy of influenza A (HINI) virus infection in a dose of 200 mg daily, amantadine seemed to have a slight advantage over rimantadine (Van Voris *et al.*, 1981). During an influenza epidemic (both HINI and H3N2 subtypes), when each drug was given in a daily dose of 200 mg, they were both highly effective in preventing influenza, and there was no difference between the rates of illness or infection in the two drug-treated groups; but more side-effects occurred in amantadine recipients (Dolin *et al.*, 1982). It is likely that the marginal therapeutic advantage and higher frequency of side-effects with amantadine is because it produces higher serum levels than rimantadine at comparable doses (Hayden *et al.*, 1983). That rimantadine penetrates better into nasal mucus than amantadine may be a factor in its clinical efficacy despite lower resultant serum levels at comparable dosage.

7 Resistance to amantadine and rimantadine

Strains of influenza A resistant to amantadine and rimantadine have been recovered from about 30% of patients receiving treatment, and less frequently in those receiving prophylactic therapy (Hayden and Hay, 1992). Resistance to amantadine and rimantadine has been reported in the absence of exposure to either drug (Houck *et al.*, 1995). Resistance may develop within 48 h of commencing therapy (Houck *et al.*, 1995). These drug-resistant strains can be transmitted to contacts (Belshe *et al.*, 1989; Hayden *et al.*, 1989; Mast *et al.*, 1991), and cause typical symptoms of influenza (Hayden *et al.*, 1991; Sweet *et al.*, 1991).

8 Effect of amantadine or rimantadine on immune response

There are differing data regarding the effects of amantadine and rimantadine therapy on production of influenza-specific antibody. The consensus is that treatment of established infection using these drugs does not interfere with antibody responses to influenza (Sears and Clements, 1987; CDC, 1996), although some reduction in local immune responses has been described in pediatric cases (Clover *et al.*, 1991).

Table V.61

Influenza-like illness: laboratory documented influenza, and infection with influenza A virus among volunteers receiving placebo, rimantadine or amantadine. (Reproduced from Dolin *et al.* 1982, with permission.)

Treatment group (no. of subjects)	No. with influenza-like illness[a]	No. with laboratory-documented influenza[b]	No. infected with influenza A virus[c]
Placebo (132)	54 (41%)	27 (21%)	32 (24%)
Rimantadine (133)	19 (14%)[d]	4 (3%)[d]	11 (8%)[d]
efficacy rate (%)[e]	65	85	66
Amantadine (113)	10 (9%)[d]	2 (2%)[d]	7 (6%)[d]
efficacy rate (%)	78	91	74

[a] Defined as a cough or an oral temperature of $>37.7°C$, or both, and at least two of the following: sore throat, headache, and myalgia. Figures in parenthesis indicate percentages of subjects with indicated finding.

[b] Defined as influenza-like illness along with virus isolation or a rise in serum antibody to influenza A virus.

[c] Defined as influenza A virus isolation or a rise in serum antibody to influenza A virus, irrespective of the presence of illness.

[d] $p < 0.001$ compared with placebo by χ^2 analysis.

[e] Efficacy rates are calculated by the expression:

$$\frac{\text{rate in placebo recipients} - \text{rate in rimantadine or amantadine recipients}}{\text{rate in placebo recipients}} = 100$$

9 Other potential clinical uses of amantadine

Persistent hiccup has been reported to respond to amantadine therapy at a dose of 100 mg per day; interruption of therapy resulted in resumption of hiccups within 24 h (Askenasy *et al.*, 1988). Amantadine may be useful in the management of post-herpetic neuralgia due to herpes zoster if given in the acute phase (Robertson and George, 1990). In a double-blind, placebo-controlled trial, therapy with amantadine at a dose of 100 mg twice-daily for 1 month reduced zoster-associated pain (Watson, 1989). However, this finding has not been put into clinical practice. The related compound tromantadine has been assessed in the treatment of genital herpes. Administered as a 1% ointment there was no difference when compared with placebo in time to healing or subjective discomfort (Petersen *et al.*, 1993). Amantadine (and presumably rimantadine) has no beneficial effects in human experimental parainfluenza type I virus infection (Smith *et al.*, 1967).

Acknowledgements The author would like to thank Frederick Hayden, University of Virginia, Charlottesville, for his critical review of this chapter.

References

Alcami A, Carrascosa AL, Vinuela E *et al.* (1989). The entry of African swine fever virus into vero cells. *Virology* **171**: 68.

Alkana RL, Parker, ES, Malcolm RD *et al.* (1982). Interaction of apomorphine and amantadine with ethanol in men. *Alcohol Clin Exp Res* **6**: 403.

Anderson EL, Van Vori LP, Bartram J *et al.* (1987). Pharmacokinetics of a single dose of rimantadine in young adults and children. *Antimicrob Ag Chemother* **31**: 1140.

Aoki FY, Sitar DS (1985). Amantadine kinetics in healthy elderly men; implications for influenza prevention. *Clin Pharmacol Ther* **37**: 137.

Aoki FY, Sitar DS (1988). Clinical pharmacokinetics of amantadine hydrochloride. *Clin Pharmacokinet* **14**: 35.

Aoki FY, Sitar DS (1992). Effects of chronic amantadine hydrochloride ingestion on its and acetaminophen pharmacokinetics in young adults. *J Clin Pharmacol* **32**: 24.

Aoki FY, Sitar DS, Ogilvie RI (1979). Amantadine kinetics in healthy young subjects after long-term dosing. *Clin Pharmacol Ther* **26**: 729.

Aoki FY, Stiver HG, Sitar DS *et al.* (1985). Prophylactic amantadine dose and plasma concentration-effect relationships in healthy adults. *Clin Pharmacol Ther* **37**: 128.

Arden NH, Patriarca PA, Fosano MB *et al.* (1988). The roles of vaccination and amantadine prophylaxis in controlling an outbreak of influenza A (N3N2) in a nursing home. *Arch Intern Med* **148**: 865.

Arruda E, Hayden FG (1996). In *Antiviral chemotherapy: New Directions for Clinical Application and Research* Vol 4, p.175 (Mills J, Volberding Carey L, eds) New York: Plenum Press.

Askenasy JJ, Boiangiu M, Davidovitch S *et al.* (1988). Persistent hiccup cured by amantadine. *New Engl J Med* **318**: 711.

Atkinson WL, Arden NH, Patriarca PA *et al.* (1986). Amantadine prophylaxis during an institutional outbreak of type A (H1N1) influenza. *Arch Intern Med* **146**: 1751.

Atmar RL, Greenberg SB, Quarles JM *et al.* (1990). Safety and pharmacokinetics of rimantadine small-particle aerosol. *Antimicrob Ag Chemother* **34**: 2228.

Bean WJ, Threlkeld SC, Webster RG *et al.* (1989). Biologic potential of amantadine-resistant influenza A virus in an avian model. *J Infect Dis* **159**: 1050.

Beard CW, Brugh M, Webster RG (1987). Emergence of amantadine-resistant N5N2 avian influenza virus during a simulated layer flock treatment program. *Avian Dis* **31**: 533.

Belshe RB, Smith MH, Hall CB *et al.* (1988). Genetic basis of resistance to rimantadine emerging during treatment of influenza virus infection. *J Virol* **62**: 1508.

Belshe RB, Burk B, Newman F *et al.* (1989). Resistance of influenza A virus to amantadine and rimantadine: results of one decade of surveillance. *J Infect Dis* **159**: 430.

Bennett NM (1973). Diagnosis of influenza. *Med J Aust* (Spec Suppl): 19.

Berkowitz CD (1979). Treatment of acute amantadine toxicity with physostigmine. *J Pediatr* **95**: 144.

Blanchard DL (1990). Amantadine caused corneal edema. *Cornea* **9**: 181.

Bleidner WE, Harmon JB, Hewes T *et al.* (1965). Absorption, distribution and excretion of amantadine hydrochloride. *J Pharmacol Exp Ther* **150**: 484.

Bloomfield SS, Gaffney TE, Schiff GM (1970). A design for the evaluation of antiviral drugs in human influenza. *Amer J Epid* **91**: 568.

Brady MT, Sears SD, Pacini DL *et al.* (1990). Safety and prophylactic efficacy of low-dose rimantadine in adults during an influenza A epidemic. *Antimicrob Ag Chemother* **34**: 1633.

Brenner M, Haass A, Jacobi P, Schimrigk K (1989). Amantadine sulphate in treating Parkinson's disease: Clinical effects, psychometric tests and serum concentrations. *J Neurol* **236**: 153.

Bron R, Kendal AP, Klenk HD, Wilschut J (1993). Role of the M_2 protein in influenza virus membrane fusion; effects of amantadine and monensin on fusion kinetics. *Virology* **195**: 808.

Browne MJ, Moss MY, Boyd MR *et al.* (1983). Comparative activity of amantadine and ribavirin against influenza virus *in vitro*: possible clinical relevance. *Antimicrob Ag Chemother* **23**: 503.

Bryson YJ, Monahan C, Pollack M, Shields WD (1980). A prospective double-blind study of side effects associated with the administration of amantadine for influenza A virus prophylaxis. *J Infect Dis* **141**: 543.

Bukrinskaya AG, Vorkunova NK, Narmanbetora RA (1980). Rimantadine hydrochloride blocks the second step of influenza virus uncoating. *Archives Virol* **66**: 275.

Bukrinskaya AG, Vorkunova NK, Pushkarskaya NL *et al.* (1982). Uncoating of a rimantadine-resistant variant of influenza virus in the presence of rimantadine. *J Gen Virol* **60**: 61.

Burlington DB, Meiklejohn G, Mostow SR (1981). Toxicity of amantadine and rimantadine for the ciliated epithelium of ferret tracheal rings. *J Infect Dis* **144**: 77.

Burlington DB, Meiklejohn G, Mostow SR (1982). Anti-influenza A virus activity of amantadine hydrochloride and rimantadine hydrochloride in ferret tracheal ciliated epithelium. *Antimicrob Ag Chemother* **21**: 794.

Burlington DB, Meiklejohn G, Mostow SR (1983). Anti-influenza A activity of combinations of amantadine and ribavirin in ferret tracheal ciliated epithelium. *J Antimicrob Chemother* **11**: 7.

Bussereau F, Picard M, Blancou J, Sureau P (1988). Treatment of rabies in mice and foxes with antiviral compounds. *Acta Virol Prah* **32**: 33.

Capparelli EV, Stevens RC, Chow MS *et al.* (1988). Rimantadine pharmacokinetics in healthy subjects and patients with end-stage renal failure. *Clin Pharmacol Ther* **43**: 536.

Casey DE (1978). Amantadine intoxication reversed by physostigmine. *New Engl J Med* **298**: 516.

Cassell S, Edwards J, Brown DT (1984). Effects of lysosomotropic weak bases on infection of BHK-21 cells by Sindbis virus. *J Virol* **52**: 857.

Castilla V, Mersich SE, Candurra NA, Damonte EB (1994). The entry of Junin virus into vero cells. *Arch Virol* **136**: 363.

CDC (Centres for Disease Control and Prevention) (1996). Prevention and control of influenza: recommendations of the Advisory Committee on Immunization Practices (ACIP). *MMWR* **45** (RR-5): 1.

Ciampor F, Bayley PM, Nermut MV *et al.* (1992). Evidence that the amantadine-induced, M_2-mediated conversion of influenza A virus hemagglutinin to the low pH conformation occurs in an acidic *trans* Golgi compartment. *Virol* **188**: 14.

Clark C, Woodson MM, Nagasawa HT (1991). Inhibition of lymphocyte proliferation by amantadine and its isomer, 2-aminoadamantane; impact on Lyt-2+ T cells while sparing L3T4+ T cells. *Immunopharmacol* **21**: 41.

Clover RD, Crawford SA, Becker L, Davis A (1986). Effectiveness of rimantadine prophylaxis of children within families. *Amer J Dis Child* **140**: 706.

Clover RD, Waner JL, Becker L, Davis A (1991). Effect of rimantadine on the immune response to influenza A infections. *J Med Virol* **34**: 68.

Cochran KW, Maasab HF, Tsunoda A, Berlin BS (1965). Studies on the antiviral activity of amantadine hydrochloride. *Ann NY Acad Sci* **130**: 432.

Couch RB, Howard R (1986). The antiviral spectrum and mechanism of action of amantadine and rimantadine. *Anti Chemother New Direct Clin Applic Res* 50.

Couch RB, Jackson GG (1976). Antiviral agents in influenza; Summary of influenza workshop VIII. *J Infect Dis* **134**: 516.

Cox RA (1991). Amantadine prophylaxis for health care workers' unanswered questions. *J Antimicrob Chemother* **27**: 1.

Crance JM, Biziago E, Passagot J *et al.* (1990). Inhibition of hepatitis A virus replication *in vitro* by antiviral compounds. *J Med Virol* **31**: 155.

Crawford SA, Clover RD, Abell TD *et al.* (1988). Rimantadine prophylaxis in children; a follow-up study. *Pediatr Infect Dis J* **7**: 379.

Daniels, R S, Downie, J C, Hay AJ *et al.* (1985). Fusion mutants of the influenza virus hemagglutinin glycoprotein. *Cell* **40**: 431.

Davies WL, Grunert RR, Haff RF *et al.* (1964). Antiviral activity of l-adamantanamine HCl. *Science NY* **144**: 862.

Degelau J, Somani S, Cooper SL, Irvine PW (1990). Occurrence of adverse effects and high amantadine concentrations with influenza prophylaxis in the nursing home. *J Amer Geriatr Soc* **38**: 428.

Degelau J, Somani SK, Cooper SL *et al.* (1992). Amantadine-resistant influenza A in a nursing facility. *Arch Intern Med* **152**: 390.

Delker LE, Moser RH, Nelson JD *et al.* (1980). Amantadine: does it have a role in the prevention and treatment of influenza? A National Institutes of Health Consensus Development Conference. *Ann Intern Med* **92**: 256.

Dolin R, Reichman RC, Madore HP *et al.* (1982). A controlled trial of amantadine and rimantadine in the prophylaxis of influenza A infection. *New Engl J Med* **307**: 580.

Duff KC, Ashley RH (1992). The transmembrane domain of influenza A M_2 protein forms amantadine-sensitive proton channels in planar lipid bilayers. *Virology* **190**: 485.

Duff KC, Gilchrist PJ, Saxena AM, Bradshaw JP (1994). Neutron diffraction reveals the site of amantadine blockade in the influenza A M_2 ion channel. *Virology* **202**: 287.

Evans SG, Havlik I (1993). Plasmodium falciparum; effects of amantadine, an antiviral, on chloroquine-resistant and sensitive parasites *in vitro* and its influence on chloroquine activity. *Biochem Pharmacol* **45**: 1168.

Finklea JF, Hennessy AV, Davenport FM *et al.* (1967). A field trial of amantadine prophylaxis in naturally occurring acute respiratory illness. *Amer J Epid* **85**: 403.

Fraunfelder FT, Coster DJ, Drew R, Fraunfelder FW (1990). Ocular injury induced by methyl ethyl ketone peroxide. *Amer J Ophthalmol* **110**: 635.

Fukuhara N, Yoshie O, Kitaoka S *et al.* (1987). Evidence for endocytosis-independent infection by human rotavirus. *Arch Virol* **97**: 93.

Galabov AS, Khristova ML, Uzunov S *et al.* (1994). Alteration in the antigenic structure of M1 protein of influenza A virus mutant resistant to a new antiviral compound mopyridone. *Acta Virol* **38**: 5.

Galbraith AW, Oxford JS, Schild GC, Watson GI (1969a). Protective effect of 1-adamantanamine hydrochloride on influenza A2 infection in the family environment. *Lancet* **ii**: 1026.

Galbraith AW, Oxford JS, Schild GC, Watson GI (1969b). Study of 1-adamantanamine hydrochloride used prophylactically during the Hong Kong influenza epidemic in the family environment. *Bull Wld Hlth Org* **41**: 677.

Galbraith AW, Oxford JS, Schild GC et al. (1971). Therapeutic effect of l-adamantanamine hydrochloride in naturally occurring influenza A Aper Hong Kong infection. A controlled double-blind study. *Lancet* **ii**: 113.

Gaudry SE, Sitar DS, Smyth DD et al. (1993). Gender and age as factors in the inhibition of renal clearance of amantadine by quinine and quinidine. *Clin Pharmacol Ther* **54**: 23.

Glushakova SE, Lukashevich IS (1989). Early events in arenavirus replication are sensitive to lysosomotropic compounds. *Arch Virol* **104**: 157.

Grambas S, Bennett MS, Hay AJ et al. (1992). Influence of amantadine resistance mutations on the pH regulatory function of the M2 protein of influenza A viruses. *Virology* **191**: 541.

Griffiths N, Lamb JF, Ogden P (1983). The effects of chloroquine and other weak bases on the accumulation and efflux of digoxin and ouabain in HeLa cells. *Brit J Pharmacol* **79**: 877.

Grunert RR, McGahen JW, Davies WL (1965). The *in vivo* antiviral activity of l-adamantanamine. 1 Prophylactic and therapeutic activity against influenza. *Virology* **26**: 262.

Guay DR (1994). Amantadine and rimantadine prophylaxis of influenza A in nursing homes. A tolerability perspective. *Drugs Aging* **5**: 8.

Hall CB, Dolin R, Gala CL et al. (1987). Children with influenza A infection: treatment with rimantadine. *Pediatrics* **80**: 275.

Hartshorne NJ, Harruff RC, Logan BK (1995). Unexpected amantadine intoxication in the death of a trauma patient. *Amer J Forensic Med Pathol* **16**: 340.

Hay AJ, Wolstenholme AJ, Skehel JJ, Smith MH (1985). The molecular basis of the specific anti-influenza action of amantadine. *EMBO J* **4**: 3021.

Hay AJ, Zambon MC, Wolstenholme AJ et al. (1986). Molecular basis of resistance of influenza A viruses to amantadine. *J Antimicrob Chemother* **18**: 19.

Hayden FG (1986). Combinations of antiviral agents for treatment of influenza virus infections. *J Antimicrob Chemother* **18**: 177.

Hayden FG (1996). Amantadine and rimantadine – clinical aspects. In *Antiviral Drug Resistance* (Richman DD, ed). Chichester: John Wiley and Sons Ltd.

Hayden FG, Hay AJ (1992). Emergence and transmission of influenza A viruses resistant to amantadine and rimantadine. *Curr Top Microbiol Immunol* **176**: 119.

Hayden FG, Monto AS (1986). Oral rimantadine hydrochloride therapy of influenza A virus H3N2 subtype infection in adults. *Antimicrob Ag Chemother* **29**: 339.

Hayden FG, Hall WJ, Douglas RG, Speers DM (1979). Amantadine aerosols in normal volunteers; pharmacology and safety testing. *Antimicrob Ag Chemother* **16**: 644.

Hayden FG, Cote KM, Douglas RG (1980a). Plaque inhibition assay for drug susceptibility testing of influenza viruses. *Antimicrob Ag Chemother* **17**: 865.

Hayden FG, Hall WJ, Douglas RG (1980b). Therapeutic effects of aerosolized amantadine in naturally acquired infection due to influenza A virus. *J Infect Dis* **141**: 535.

Hayden FG, Douglas RG, Simmons R (1980c). Enhancement of activity against influenza viruses by combinations of antiviral agents. *Antimicrob Ag Chemother* 18: 536.

Hayden FG, Gwaltney JM, Van de Castle RL, et al (1981). Comparative toxicity of amantadine hydrochloride and rimantadine hydrochloride in healthy adults. *Antimicrob Ag Chemother* **19**: 226.

Hayden FG, Zylidnikov DM, Iijenko VI, Padolka YV (1982). Combined therapeutic effect of aerosolized and oral rimantadine HCl in experimental human influenza A virus infection. *Antiviral Res* **2**: 147.

Hayden FG, Hoffman HE, Spyker DA et al. (1983). Differences in side-effects of amantadine hydrochloride and rimantadine hydrochloride relate to differences in pharmacokinetics. *Antimicrob Ag Chemother* **23**: 458.

Hayden FG, Schlepushkin AN, Pushkarskaya NL (1984). Combined interferon-alpha 2, rimantadine hydrochloride, and ribavirin inhibition of influenza virus replication *in vitro*. *Antimicrob Ag Chemother* **25**: 53.

Hayden FG, Minocha A, Spyker DA, Hoffman HE (1985). Comparative single-dose pharmacokinetics of amantadine hydrochloride and rimantadine hydrochloride in young and elderly adults. *Antimicrob Ag Chemother* **28**: 216.

Hayden FG, Belshe RB, Clover RD et al. (1989). Emergence and apparent transmission of rimantadine-resistant influenza A virus in families. *New Engl J Med* **321**: 1696.

Hayden FG, Sperber SJ, Belshe RB et al. (1991). Recovery of drug resistant influenza A virus during therapeutic use of rimantadine. *Antimicrob Ag Chemother* **35**: 1741.

Helenius A, Marsh M, White J (1982). Inhibition of Semliki forest virus penetration by lysosomotropic weak bases. *J Gen Virol* **58**: 47.

Herrmann JE, Bruns M, West K, Ennis FA (1989). Efficacy of rimantadine hydrochloride in the treatment of influenza infection of mice. *Antiviral Res* **11**: 127.

Herrmann JE, West K, Bruns M, Ennis FA (1990). Effect of rimantadine on cytotoxic T lymphocyte responses and immunity to reinfection in mice infected with influenza A virus. *J Infect Dis* **161**: 180.

Hoffman HE, Gaylord JC, Blasecki JW et al. (1988). Pharmacokinetics and metabolism of rimantadine hydrochloride in mice and dogs. *Antimicrob Ag Chemother* **32**: 1699.

Holazo AA, Choma N, Brown SY et al. (1989). Effect of cimetidine on the disposition of rimantadine in healthy subjects. *Antimicrob Ag Chemotherapy* **13**: 820.

Holsinger LJ, Nichani D, Pinto LH, Lamb RA (1994). Influenza A virus M2 ion channel protein; a structure-function analysis. *J Virol* **68**: 1551.

Horadam VW, Sharp JG, Smilack JD et al. (1981). Pharmacokinetics of amantadine hydrochloride in subjects with normal and impaired renal function. *Ann Intern Med* **94**: 454.

Hornick RB, Togo Y et al. (1967). Clinical evaluation of amantadine HCl in the prophylaxis of induced influenza. *von Viruskrankungen* 272.

Hornick RB, Togo Y, Mahler S, Iezzoni D (1969). Evaluation of amantadine hydrochloride in the treatment of A2 influenzal disease. *Bull Wld Hlth Org* **41**: 671.

Hornick RB, Togo Y et al. (1970). Evaluation of amantadine hydrochloride in the treatment of A2 influenzal disease. *Ann NY Acad Sci* **173**: 10.

Hosoya M, Shigeta S, Nakamura K, De Clercq E (1989). Inhibitory effect of selected antiviral compounds on measles (SSPE) virus replication *in vitro*. *Antiviral Res* **12**: 87.

Houck P, Hemphill M, LaCroix S et al. (1995). Amantadine resistant influenza A in nursing homes. Identification of a resistant virus prior to drug use. *Arch Intern Med* **155**: 533.

Hudson JB, Graham EA, Simpson MF (1988). The efficacy of amantadine and other antiviral compounds against two salmonid viruses *in vitro*. *Antiviral Res* **9**: 379.

Ickes DE, Venetta TM, Phonphok Y, Rosenthal KS (1990). Tromantadine inhibits a late step in herpes simplex virus type 1 replication and syncytium formation. *Antiviral Res* **14**: 75.

Ing TS, Daugirdas JT, Soung LS (1980). The posology of amantadine: a note of caution. *JAMA* **243**: 1844.

Jackson GG, Muldoon RL, Akers LW (1963). Serologic evidence for prevention of influenza illness in volunteers by an antiinfluenzal drug amantadine hydrochloride. *Antimicrob Ag Chemother* 703.

Karlsson M, Reichard O, Linda A et al. (1987). Amantadine for prophylaxis against influenza A. *Scand J Infect Dis* **19**: 141.

Kato N, Eggers, HJ (1969). Inhibition of uncoating of fowl plague virus by 1-adamantanamine hydrochloride. *Virology* **37**: 632.

Kemler I, Whittaker G, Helenius A et al. (1994). Nuclear import of microinjected influenza virus ribonucleoproteins. *Virology* **202**: 1028.

Kendal AP, Klenk HD (1991). Amantadine inhibits an early, M2 protein-dependent event in the replication cycle of avian influenza (H7) viruses. *Arch Virol* **119**: 265.

Klimov AI, Rocha F, Hayden FG et al. (1995). Prolonged shedding of amantadine-resistant influenzae A viruses by immunodeficient patients; detection by polymerase chain reaction-restriction analysis. *J Infect Dis* **172**: 1352.

Kirshon B, Faro S, Zurowin RK et al. (1988). Favourable outcome after treatment with amantadine and ribavirin in a pregnancy complicated by influenza pneumonia. A case report. *J Reprod Med* **33**: 399.

Knight V, Fedson D, Baldini J et al. (1969). Amantadine therapy of epidemic influenza A2 Hong Kong. *Antimicrob Ag Chemother* **9**: 370.

Knight V, Bloom K, Wilson SZ, Wilson RK (1979). Amantadine aerosol in humans. *Antimicrob Ag Chemother* **16**: 572.

Koff WC, Knight V (1979). Inhibition of influenza virus uncoating by amantadine hydrochloride. *J Virol* **31**: 261.

Koff WC, Elm JL, Halstead SB et al. (1980). Inhibition of dengue virus replication by amantadine hydrochloride. *Antimicrob Ag Chemother* **18**: 125.

Koff WC, Pratt RD, Elm JL et al. (1983). Treatment of intracranial dengue virus infections in mice with a lipophilic derivative of ribavirin. *Antimicrob Ag Chemother* **24**: 134.

Lammers GJ, Roos RA (1993). Hyponatraemia due to amantadine hydrochloride and L-dopapercarbidopa. *Lancet* **342**: 439.

Lavrov SV, Eremkina E, Orlova TG et al. (1968). Combined inhibition of influenza virus reproduction in cell culture using interferon and amantadine. *Nature* **217**: 856.

Likar M (1970). Effectiveness of amantadine in protecting vaccinated volunteers from an attenuated strain of influenza AperHong Kong virus. *Ann NY Acad Sci* **173**: 108.

Little JW, Hall WJ, Douglas RG et al. (1976). Amantadine effect on peripheral airways abnormalities in influenza. *Ann Intern Med* **85**: 177.

Liu P, Cheng PJ, Ing TS et al. (1984). *In vitro* binding of amantadine to plasma proteins. *Clin Neuropharmacol* **7**: 149.

Lukacsi K, Molnar M, Siroki O, Rosztoszy I (1985). Combined effects of amantadine and interferon on influenza virus replication in chicken and human embryo trachea organ culture. *Acta Microbiol Hung* **32**: 357.

Maassab HF, Cochran KW (1964). Rubella virus: inhibition *in vitro* by amantadine HCL. *Science* **145**: 1443.

Macchio GJ, Ito V, Sahgal V et al. (1993). Amantadine-induced coma. *Arch Phys Med Rehabil* **74**: 1119.

Madren LK, Shipman C, Hayden FG (1996). *In vitro* inhibitory effects of combinations of anti-influenza agents. *Antivir Chem Chemother*; **6**: 109

Manchand PS, Cerruti RL, Martin JA, et al (1990). Synthesis and antiviral activity of metabolites of rimantadine. *J Med Chem* **23**: 1992.

Marsh M, Helenius A (1989). Virus entry into animal cells. *Adv virus Res* **36**: 107

Martin K, Helenius A (1991). Nuclear transport of influenza virus ribonucleoproteins; the viral matrix protein (M1) promotes export and inhibits import. *Cell* **67**: 117.

Mast EE, Harmon MW, Gravenstein S, et al. (1991). Emergence and possible transmission of amantadine-resistant viruses during nursing home outbreaks of influenza A (H3N2). *Amer J Epidemiol* **134**: 988.

Matlin KS (1982). The entry of enveloped viruses into an epithelial line. *Prog Clin Biol Res* **91**: 599.

Maurin M, Benoliel AM, Bongrand P, Baoult D (1992). Phagolysosomal alkalinization and the bactericidal effect of antibiotics: the *Coxiella burnetti* paradigm. *J Infect Dis* **166**: 1097.

McClure MO, Marsh M, Weiss RA (1988). Human immunodeficiency virus infection of CD4-bearing cells occurs by a pH-independent mechanism. *EMBO* **7**: 513.

McClure MO, Sommerfelt MA, Marsh M, Weiss RA (1990). The pH independence of mammalian retrovirus infection. *J Gen Virol* **71**: 767.

McNamara P, Durso R (1991). Reversible pathologic jealousy (Othello syndrome) associated with amantadine. *J Geriat Psychiat Neurol* **4**: 157.

Miller KS, Miller JM (1994). Toxic effects of amantadine in patients with renal failure. *Chest* **105**: 1630.

Millet VM, Dreisbach M, Bryson YJ (1982). Double-blind controlled study of central nervous system side effects of amantadine, rimantadine, and chlorpheniramine. *Antimicrob Ag Chemother* **21**: 1.

MMWR (1987). Prevention and control of influenzae. Recommendations of the Immunization Practises Advisory Committee (ACIP). *MMWR* **36**: 373.

MMWR (1994). Prevention and control of influenza: Part II, antiviral agents. Recommendations of the Advisory Committee on Imunization Practises (ACIP). *MMWR* **43**: 1.

Monto AS, Gunn RA, Bandyk MG, King CL (1979). Prevention of Russian influenza by amantadine. *JAMA* **241**: 1003.

Mostow SR (1987). Prevention, management and control of influenza. Role of amantadine. *Amer J Med* **82**: 35.

Muldoon RL, Stanley ED, Jackson GG (1976). Use and withdrawal of amantadine chemoprophylaxis during epidemic influenza A. *Amer Rev Respir Dis* **113**: 487.

Nafta I, Turcanu AG, Braun I et al. (1970). Administration of amantadine for the prevention of Hong Kong influenza. *Bull Wld Hlth Org* **42**: 423.

Nahata MC, Brady MT, (1986). Serum concentrations and safety of rimantadine in paediatric patients. *Eur J Clin Pharmacol* 30: 719.

Nestelbaum Z, Siris SG, Rifkin A et al. (1986). Exacerbation of schizophrenia associated with amantadine. *Amer J Psychiat* **143**: 1170.

Nora JJ, Nora AH, Way GL (1975). Cardiovascular maldevelopment associated with maternal exposure to amantadine. *Lancet* **ii**: 607.

O'Donoghue JM, Ray GG, Terry DW, Beaty HN (1973). Prevention of nosocomial influenza infection with amantadine. *Amer J Epid* **97**: 276.

Oker-Blom N, Hovi T, Leinikki P et al. (1970). Protection of man from natural infection with influenza A2 Hong Kong virus by amantadine; a controlled field trial. *Brit Med J* **3**: 676.

Oxford JS (1975). Specific inhibitors of influenza virus replication as potential chemoprophylactic agents. *J Antimicrob Ag Chemother* **1**: 7.

Oxford JS, Schild GC (1967). Inhibition of the growth of influenza and rubella viruses by amines and ammonium salts. *Brit J Exp Path* **48**: 235.

Oxford JS, Logan IS, Potter CW (1970). Passage of influenza strains in the presence of animoadamantane. *Ann NY Acad Sci* **173**: 300.

Pacifici GM, Nardini M, Ferrari P et al. (1976). Effect of amantadine on drug induced parkinsonism; relationship between plasma levels and effect. *Brit J Clin Pharmacol* **3**: 883.

Pandit PB, Chitayat D, Jeffries AL et al. (1994). Tibial hemimelia and tetralogy of fallot associated with first trimester exposure to amantadine. *Reprod Toxicol* **8**: 89.

Patriarca PA, Kater NA, Kendal AP et al. (1984). Safety of prolonged administration of rimantadine hydrochloride in the prophylaxis of influenza A virus infections in nursing homes. *Antimicrob Ag Chemother* **26**: 101.

Payler DK, Purdham PA (1984). Influenza A prophylaxis with amantadine in a boarding school. *Lancet* **1**: 502.

Pearlman JT, Kadish AH, Ramseyer JC et al. (1977). Vision loss associated with amantadine hydrochloride use. *JAMA* **237**: 1200.

Pemberton RM, Jennings R, Potter CW, Oxford JS (1986). Amantadine resistance in clinical influenza A (H1N1) virus isolates. *J Antimicrob Chemother* **18**: 135.

Perez L, Carrasco L (1993). Entry of poliovirus into cells does not require a low-pH step. *J Virol* **67**: 4543.

Peters CJ, Reynolds JA, Slone TW et al. (1986). Prophylaxis of rift valley fever with antiviral drugs, immune serum, an interferon inducer, and a macrophage activator. *Antiviral Res* **6**: 285.

Peters NL, Oboler S, Hair C et al. (1989). Treatment of an influenza A outbreak in a teaching nursing home. Effectiveness of a protocol for prevention and control. *J Amer Geriatr Soc* **37**: 210.

Petersen CS, Weismann K, Avnstorp C et al. (1993). Topical tromantadine in the treatment of genital herpes. A double-blind placebo controlled study. *Dan Med Bull* **40**: 506.

Pettersson RF, Hellstrom PE, Penttinen K *et al.* (1980). Evaluation of amantadine in the prophylaxis of influenza A (H1N1) virus infection; a controlled field trial among young adults and high-risk patients. *J Infect Dis* **142**: 377.

Pimentel L, Hughes B (1991). Amantadine toxicity presenting with complex ventricular ectopy and hallucinations. *Pediatr Emerg Care* **7**: 89.

Pinto LH (1992). Influenza virus M2 protein has ion channel activity. *Cell* **69**: 517.

Quilligan JJ, Hirayama M, Baernstein HD *et al.* (1966). The suppression of A2 influenza in children by the chemoprophylactic use of amantadine. *J Pediatr* **69**: 572.

Raoult D, Drancourt M, Vestris G *et al.* (1990). Bactericidal effect of doxycycline associated with lysosomotropic agents on *Coxiella burnetii* in P388D1 cells. *Antimicrob Ag Chemother* **34**: 1512.

Ray CG, Icenogle TB, Minnich LL *et al.* (1989). The use of intravenous ribavirin to treat influenza virus-associated acute myocarditis. *J Infect Dis* **159**: 829.

Rego MD, Giller EL (1989). Mania secondary to amantadine treatment of neuroleptic induced hyperprolactinemia. *J Clin Psychiat* **50**: 143.

Reuman PD, Bernstein,DI, Eefer MC *et al.* (1989). Efficacy and safety of low dosage amantadine hydrochloride as prophylaxis for influenza A. *Antiviral Res* **11**: 27.

Richman DD, Hostetler KY, Yazaki PJ, Clark S (1986). Fate of influenza A virion proteins after entry into subcellular fractions of LLC cells and the effect of amantadine. *Virology* **151**: 200.

Rimantadine Product Monograph.

Robertson DR, George CF (1990). Treatment of post herpetic neuralgia in the elderly. *Brit Med Bull* **46**: 113.

Rosenthal KS, Sokol MS, Ingram RL *et al.* (1982). Tromantadine: inhibitor of early and late events in herpes simplex virus replication. *Antimicrob Ag Chemother* **22**: 1031.

Rubio FA, Choma N, Fukuda EK *et al.* (1989). Determination of rimantadine and its hydroxylated metabolites in human plasma and urine. *J Chromatogr* **497**: 147.

Ruigrok RW, Hirst EM, Hay AJ (1991). The specific inhibition of influenza A virus maturation by amantadine: an electron microscopic examination. *J Gen Virol* **72**: 191.

Sartori M, Pratt CM, Young JB *et al.* (1984). Malignant cardiac arrhythmia induced by amantadine poisoning. *Amer J Med* **77**: 388.

Schiffet G, Bloomfield S, Gaffney T (1966). The effects of amantadine HCL on experimental human influenza. Annual meeting of the America Federation for Clinical Research. *Clin Res* **14**: 343.

Schlegel R, Dickson RB, Willingham MC, PastanIH (1982). Amantadine and dansylcadaverine inhibit vesicular stomatitis virus uptake and receptor-mediated endocytosis of alpha 2-macroglobulin. *PNAS USA* **79**: 9291.

Sears SD, Clements ML (1987). Protective efficacy of low dose amantadine in adults challenged with wild-type influenza A virus. *Antimicrob Ag Chemother* **31**: 1470.

Shimura H, Umeno Y, Kimura G (1987). Effects of inhibitors of the cytoplasmic structures and functions on the early phase of infection of cultured cells with simian virus 40. *Virology* **158**: 34.

Sidwell RW, Bailey KW, Wong MH, Huffman JH (1995). *In vitro* and *in vivo* sensitivity of a non-mouse adapted influenza A (Beijing) virus infection to amantadine and ribavirin. *Chemother* **41**: 455.

Smith CB, Purcell RH, Chanock RM (1967). Effect of amantadine hydrochloride on parainfluenza type 1 virus infections in adult volunteers. *Amer Rev Respir Dis* **95**: 689.

Smorodintsev AA, Zlydnikov DM, Kiseleva AM *et al.* (1970a). Evaluation of amantadine in artificially induced A2 and B influenza. *JAMA* **213**: 1448.

Smorodintsev AA, Karpuchin GI, Zlydnikov SM *et al.* (1970b). The prospect of amantadine for prevention of influenza A2 in humans (effectiveness of amantadine during influenza A2 Hong Kong epidemics in Jan-Feb 1969 in Leningrad). *Ann NY Acad Sci* **173**: 44.

Snoey ER, Bessen HA (1990). Acute psychosis after amantadine overdose. *Ann Emerg Med* **19**: 668.

Somani SK, Degelau J, Cooper SL *et al.* (1991). Comparison of pharmacokinetic and safety profiles of amantadine 50- and 100mg daily doses in elderly nursing home residents. *Pharmacother* **11**: 460.

Soung L S, Ing TS, Daugirdas JT *et al.* (1980). Amantadine hydrochloride pharmacokinetics in hemodialysis patients. *Ann Intern Med* **93**: 46.

Spector R (1988). Transport of amantadine and rimantadine through the blood-brain barrier. *J Pharmacol Exp Ther* **244**: 516.

Speeg KV, Leighton JA, Maldonado AL (1989). Toxic delirium in a patient taking amantadine and trimethoprim sulfamethoxazole. *Amer J Med Sci* **298**: 410.

Stanley ED, Muldoon RE, Akers LW, Jackson GG (1965). Evaluation of antiviral drugs; the effect of amantadine on influenza in volunteers. *Ann NY Acad* **130**: 44.

Strange KC, Little DW, Blatnik B (1991). Adverse reactions to amantadine prophylaxis of influenza in a retirement home. *J Amer Geriatr Soc* **39**: 700.

Strong DK, Elsenstat DD, Bryson SM, *et al* (1991). Amantadine neurotoxicity in a pediatric patient with renal insufficiency. *DICP* **25**: 1175.

Sugrue RJ, Bahadur G, Zambori MC *et al.* (1990). Specific structural alteration of the influenza haemagglutinin by amantadine. *EMBO* **9**: 3469.

Superti F, Seganti L, Pana A, Orsi N (1985). Effect of amantadine on rhabdovirus infection. *Drugs Exp Clin Res* **11**: 69.

Superti F, Seganti L, Orsi N *et al.* (1987a). The effect of lipophilic amines on the growth of hepatitis A virus in Frpper3 cells. *Arch Virol* **96**: 289.

Superti F, Seganti L, Ruggeri FM *et al.* (1987b). Entry pathway of vesicular stomatitis virus into different host cells. *J Gen Virol* **68**: 387.

Sweet C, Hayden FG, Jakeman KJ *et al.* (1991). Virulence of rimantadine-resistant human influenza A (H3N2) viruses in ferrets. *J Infect Dis* **164**: 969.

Thompson J, Fleet W, Lawrence E *et al.* (1987). A comparison of acetaminophen and rimantadine in the treatment of influenza A infection in children. *J Med Virol* **21**: 249.

Togo Y, Hornick RB, Dawkins AT *et al.* (1968). Studies on induced influenza in man. 1 double-blind studies designed to assess prophylactic efficacy of amantadine hydrochloride against A2perRockvilleper1per65 strain. *JAMA* **203**: 1089.

Togo Y, Hornick RB, Felitti VJ *et al.* (1970). Evaluation of therapeutic efficacy of amantadine in patients with naturally occurring A2 influenza. *JAMA* **211**: 1149.

Tominack RL, Hayden FG (1987). Rimantadine hydrochloride and amantadine hydrochloride use in influenza A virus infections. *Infect Dis Clin N Amer* **1**: 459.

Tominack RL, Wills RJ, Gustavson LE, Hayden FG (1988). Multiple-dose pharmacokinetics of rimantadine in elderly adults. *Antimicrob Ag Chemother* **32**: 1813.

Tuckova E, Vonka V, Zavadova H, Kutinova L (1973). Sensitivity to l-adamantanamine as a marker in genetic studies with influenza viruses. *J Biol Stand* **1**: 341.

Tyrell DAJ, Bynoe ML, Hoorn B (1965). Studies on antiviral activity of 1-adamantanamine. *Brit J Exp Path* **46**: 370.

Vale JA, Maclean KS (1977). Amantadine induced heart failure. *Lancet* **i**: 548.

Valette M, Allard JP, Aymard M, Millet V (1993). Susceptibilities to rimantadine of influenza A/H1N1 and A/H3N2 viruses isolated during the epidemics of 1988 to 1989 and 1989 to 1990. *Antimicrob Ag Chemother* **37**: 2239.

Van den Berg WH, Van Ketel WG (1983). Photosensitization by amantadine (Symmetrel). *Contact Dermatitis* **9**: 165.

Van Voris LP, Betts RF, Hayden FG *et al.* (1981). Successful treatment of naturally occurring influenza A/USSR/77 H1N1. *JAMA* **2A5**: 1128.

Walzer PD, Foy J, Steele P *et al.* (1992). Activities of antifolate, antiviral, and other drugs in an immunosuppressed rat model of *Pneumocystis carinii* pneumonia. *Antimicrob Ag Chemother* **36**: 1935.

Wang C, Takeuchi K, Pinto LH, Lamb RA (1993). Ion channel activity of influenza A virus M2 protein; characterisation of the amantadine block. *J Virol* **67**: 5585.

Ward ME, Murray A (1984). Control mechanisms governing the infectivity of *Chlamydia trachomatis* for HeLa cells; mechanisms of endocytosis. *J Gen Microbiol* **130**: 1765.

Watson CP (1989). Postherpetic neuralgia. *Neurol Clin* **7**: 231.

Webster RG, Kawaoka Y, Bean WJ *et al.* (1985). Chemotherapy and vaccination: a possible strategy for the control of highly virulent influenza virus. *J Virol* **55**: 173.

Wendel HA (1964). Clinical and serologic effects in influenza of 1-adamantanamine HCl: a double-blind study. *Fed Proc* **23**: 387.

Wharton SA, Belshe RB, Skehel JJ, Hay AJ (1994). Role of virion M2 protein in influenza virus uncoating; specific reduction in the rate of membrane fusion between virus and liposomes by amantadine. *J Gen Virol* **75**: 945.

Whimbey E, Elting LS, Couch RB *et al.* (1994). Influenza A virus infections among hospitalized adult bone marrow transplant recipients. *Bone Marrow Transplant* **13**: 437.

WHO (World Health Organisation) (1985). Current status of amantadine and rimantadine as anti-influenza-A agents: memorandum from a WHO meeting. *Bull Wld Hlth Org* **63**: 51.

Widell A, Hansson BG, Oberg B, Nordenfelt E (1986). Influence of twenty potentially antiviral substances on *in vitro* multiplication of hepatitis A virus. *Antiviral Res* **6**: 103.

Wills RJ, Farolino DA, Choma N *et al.* (1987a). Rimantadine pharmacokinetics after single and multiple doses. *Antimicrob Ag Chemother* **31**: 826.

Wills RJ, Choma N, Buonpane G, *et al.* (1987b). Relative bioavailability of rimantadine HCl tablet and syrup formulations in healthy subjects. *J Pharm Sci* **76**: 886.

Wills RJ, Rodriguez LC, Choma N *et al.* (1987c). Influence of a meal on the bioavailability of rimantadine HCl. *J Clin Pharmacol* **27**: 821.

Wills RJ, Belshe R, Tomlinsin D *et al.* (1987d). Pharmacokinetics of rimantadine hydrochloride in patients with chronic liver disease. *Clin Pharmacol Ther* **42**: 449.

Wilson TW, Rajput AH (1983). Amantadine dyazide interaction. *Can Med Assoc J* **129**: 974.

Wingfield WL, Pollac, D, Grunert RR (1969). Therapeutic efficacy of amantadine HCl and rimantadine HCl in naturally occurring influenza A2 respiratory illness in man. *New Engl J Med* **281**: 579.

Wink CAS (1975). *Symmetrel in Virology*: Macclesfield. Geigy Pharmaceuticals.

Wintermeyer SM, Nahata MC (1995). Rimantadine; a clinical perspective. *Ann Pharmacother* **29**: 299.

Wiselka, M (1994). Influenza; diagnosis, management, and prophylaxis. *Brit Med J* **308**: 1341.

Wittels M, Spear PG (1991). Penetration of cells by herpes simplex virus does not require a low pH-dependent endocytic pathway. *Virus Res* **18**: 271.

Wong LT, Smyth DD, Sitar DS (1992). Interference with renal organic cation transport by (-)- and (+)-nicotine at concentrations documented in plasma of habitual tobacco smokers. *J Pharmacol Exp Ther* **261**: 21.

Wong LT, Sitar DS, Aoki FY (1995). Chronic tobacco smoking and gender as variables affecting amantadine disposition in healthy subjects. *Brit J Clin Pharmacol* **39**: 81.

Wood TR (1965). Methods useful in evaluating 1-adamantanamine hydrochloride-a new orally active synthetic antiviral agent. *Ann NY Acad Sci* **130**: 419.

Wu MJ, Ing TS, Soung LS *et al.* (1982). Amantadine hydrochloride pharmacokinetics in patients with impaired renal function. *Clin Nephrol* **17**: 19.

Younkin SW, Betts RF, Roth FK, Douglas RG (1983). Reduction in fever and symptoms in young adults with influenza AperBrazilper78 H1N1 infection after treatment with aspirin or amantadine. *Antimicrob Ag Chemother* **23**: 577.

Zhou FX, Krull IS, Feibush B *et al.* (1993). Direct determination of adamantanamine in plasma and urine with automated solid phase derivatization. *J Chromatogr* **619**: 93.

Zlydnikov DM, Kubar OI, Kovaleva TP, Kamforin LE (1981). Study of rimantadine in the USSR; a review of the literature. *Rev Infect Dis* **3**: 408.

Interferon Alpha

Description

Interferons are naturally occurring proteins which have a wide variety of antiviral, antiproliferative and immunomodulatory effects. They act in a non-specific manner to inhibit viral infection. There are three classes of interferons: interferon alpha (multiple subtypes), interferon beta and interferon gamma.

The earliest form of interferon discovered was human leukocyte interferon, produced by exposing peripheral blood mononuclear cells to mouse parainfluenza virus (Sendai) with subsequent partial purification of the pooled subtypes of alpha interferon (Strander and Cantell, 1966). Following this, immortalized lymphoblastoid cell lines were used instead of peripheral blood mononuclear cells; these cells secrete multiple subtypes of human interferon alpha and the lymphoblastoid product is then highly purified (marketed under the trade name of 'Wellferon' by GlaxoWellcome) (Johnston, 1985; Zoon et al., 1989). The beta and gamma interferons are glycosylated whilst the alpha interferons are generally not; their molecular weights vary up to 37 kDa.

In the early 1980s recombinant technology was used to produce a number of recombinant interferons for commercial use (Goeddel et al., 1980; Nagata et al., 1980). Interferon alpha-2a (marketed under the trade name of 'Roferon-A', by Roche) is produced by recombinant technology in which human interferon alpha cDNA is transfected into *Escherichia coli* which expresses the human interferon protein. The highly purified protein contains 165 amino acids and has a molecular weight of approximately 19 kDa. Interferon alpha-2b (marketed under the trade name of 'Intron A', by Schering-Plough) and interferon alpha-2c (marketed under the trade name of 'Berefor' by Boehringer Ingelheim) are produced by similar recombinant DNA procedures. The non-glycosylated recombinant proteins differ from each other by a single amino acid; interferon alpha-2a and -2b differ only in the residue at position 23 (arginine and lysine respectively).

The main viral infections in which treatment with interferon alpha has been found to be clinically useful are hepatitis B, hepatitis C, and condyloma acuminata. Interferon alpha is also useful in the treatment of HIV-related Kaposi's sarcoma.

Antiviral Activity

1 Hepatitis B virus

Interferon alpha transiently inhibits hepatitis B virus replication, when assessed using a hepatoblastoma cell line transfected with hepatitis B DNA (Caselmann et al., 1992) or a hepatocarcinoma cell line (Ueda et al., 1989). Suppression is maintained during treatment but replication recommences as soon as I day after removal of interferon from cultures (Caselmann et al., 1992). Activity of 2'5'oligoadenylate synthetase activity increases up to 18-fold during interferon treatment, and expression of MHC class I molecules is likewise increased (Caselmann, 1994).

Mismatched double-stranded RNA can induce interferon and inhibit duck hepatitis B virus replication *in vitro* with an associated increase in activity of the interferon-induced enzyme 2'5'-oligoadenylate synthetase (Ijichi et al., 1994).

2 Hepatitis A, D and C virus

Interferon alpha results in a concentration-dependent reduction in expression of hepatitis A virus antigens and hepatitis A virus replication in a human hepatoma cell line when added prior to infection or even after the first round of viral replication (Crance *et al.*, 1995). Hepatitis D virus replication is not inhibited by interferon alpha (McNair *et al.*, 1994). Interferon alpha inhibits replication of hepatitis C virus RNA in chimpanzee hepatocytes *in vitro* (Lanford *et al.*, 1994).

3 Human immunodeficiency virus

The envelope glycoprotein of HIV (gp120) induces interferon alpha in uninfected peripheral blood mononuclear cells and monocytes *in vitro* following interaction with the surface CD4 molecule (Capobianchi *et al.*, 1992; Francis and Meltzer, 1993). However, productive infection of monocytes results in impaired synthesis of interferon alpha (Gendelman *et al.*, 1990a). Interferon alpha suppresses HIV replication *in vitro* in monocytes (Crowe *et al.*, 1991; Meltzer *et al.*, 1991; Perno *et al.*, 1994), monocyte cell lines (Fernie *et al.*, 1991), peripheral blood mononuclear cells (Ho *et al.*, 1985) and CD4-expressing T cells (Yamamoto *et al.*, 1986; Hartshorn *et al.*, 1987). Natural interferon alpha has been found to be more effective than recombinant interferon alpha-2a or -2b in inhibiting HIV replication in monocytes (Fan *et al.*, 1993). Other investigators have reported that a concentration of 100 international units (IU) per ml suppresses HIV replication by more than 50% with 77–99% inhibition at concentrations of 500 IU per ml using leukocyte and recombinant preparations of interferon alpha (Yamamoto *et al.*, 1986). Replication of HIV is inhibited in both acute and chronically infected cells (Poli *et al.*, 1989), although maximal inhibition is seen in *de novo* infection with less efficient inhibition in chronically infected cells (Crowe *et al.*, 1991; Michaelis and Levy, 1989; Kornbluth *et al.*, 1989; reviewed in Pitha, 1994).

Interferon alpha is synergistic with zidovudine and zalcitabine against HIV *in vitro* (Dubreuil *et al.*, 1990; Degre and Beck, 1994), and additive to synergistic when used in combination with either didanosine or foscarnet (Johnson *et al.*, 1991; Degre and Beck, 1994). Zidovudine, recombinant soluble CD4 and interferon alpha synergistically inhibit HIV replication in both peripheral blood mononuclear cells and T cell lines (Johnson *et al.*, 1990). Delavirdine and interferon alpha demonstrate *in vitro* synergy against HIV replication in T cell lines (Pagano and Chong, 1995).

4 Other retroviruses

The replication of simian immunodeficiency virus in CD4-expressing T cell lines is markedly inhibited by interferon alpha (Agy *et al.*, 1995). Post-exposure treatment using interferon alpha in combination with zidovudine prevents viremia and disease due to infection with Rauscher leukemia virus in mice (Ruprecht *et al.*, 1990; Ruprecht and Bronson, 1994). However, the combination of zidovudine and interferon alpha has not been successful when used as post-exposure prophylaxis in preventing infection with simian immunodeficiency virus (Fazely *et al.*, 1991). Zidovudine and interferon alpha are additive in inhibiting feline immunodeficiency virus *in vitro* (Zeidner *et al.*, 1990).

5 Human papillomavirus

Certain subtypes of interferon alpha have been found to be effective in inhibiting human papillomavirus proliferation in human papillomavirus type 16-immortalized human keratinocytes at concentrations of 100 IU per ml (Gangemi *et al.*, 1994; Khan *et al.*, 1993). Following transfection interferon also inhibited human papillomavirus-mediated immortalization of normal human keratinocytes. Continuous treatment of HeLa cells containing human papillomavirus type 18 genome with interferon alpha (200 IU per ml) for 42 days resulted in a decrease in viral mRNA expression (Lopez *et al.*, 1993).

6 Other

Interferon alpha treatment has been reported to be effective in inhibiting Epstein–Barr virus-induced transformation of B cells using both laboratory strains of virus and clinical isolates (Garner *et al.*, 1984). Growth of vesicular stomatitis virus is inhibited in tissue culture by interferon alpha at low concentration (Olcszak and Stewart, 1985). Interferon alpha treatment of rat prostatic carcinoma cells prior to infection with Sindbis virus reduces viral replication without protecting against cell death (Despres *et al.*, 1995). Interferon alpha transiently inhibits herpes simplex virus thymidine kinase (TK) (Taylor *et al.*, 1994). African swine virus is synergistically inhibited by interferon alpha and gamma (Paez *et al.*, 1990). Mice infected with lethal doses of Coxsackie B had improved survival when treated with interferon alpha concomitant with infection or shortly after, compared with untreated controls (Capobianchi *et al.*, 1991). Pseudorabies virus replication in epithelial cells is reduced in the presence of interferon alpha

(Pol *et al.*, 1991). Puumala virus, a causative agent of hemorrhagic fever with renal syndrome, is sensitive to interferon alpha *in vitro* (Temonen *et al.*, 1995).

Availability

Each vial of interferon alpha-2a contains 3, 4.5, 9, or 18 million IU, with a specific activity of 2×10^8 IU per mg protein. Interferon alpha-2b is available in vials containing 1, 3, 5, 9, 10, and 30 million IU.

Mode of Administration and Dosage

Interferon alpha is most commonly administered either by the subcutaneous or intramuscular route. Subcutaneous administration is particularly useful for patients with thrombocytopenia or other risk factors for bleeding. A continuous subcutaneous infusion can be administered via a portable syringe pump (Carreno *et al.*, 1992). There appears to be little difference in efficacy between interferon alpha-2a and -2b, although interferon alpha-2b is more widely used in certain countries. The dose regimens of the two forms of interferon alpha are largely interchangeable. There are still insufficient data to be confident in recommending doses for individual diseases, and the following are the current recommendations based on knowledge at this time (Table V.62).

Table V.62
Recommended dose of interferon alpha for specific viral infections or related conditions

Indication	Dose	Route	Duration
Chronic active hepatitis B	5–10 million IU × 3 times per week	s.c.	6 months
Chronic hepatitis C	3 million IU × 3 times per week	s.c.	12–18 months
AIDS-related Kaposi's sarcoma			
induction	36 million IU	i.m.	4 weeks (longer if tolerated)
maintenance	36 million IU	i.m.	indefinitely
Condyloma acuminata	1 million IU × 3 times per week (max. 15 million IU per week)	intralesional injection	3 weeks

IU: International units; s.c.: subcutaneous; i.m.: intramuscular.
See text for further details and source of data.

1 AIDS-related Kaposi's sarcoma

The recommended dose for HIV-related Kaposi's sarcoma is an induction phase of 36 million IU daily for 4 weeks administered by intramuscular injection, which may be extended to 12 weeks if tolerated, followed by maintenance treatment at a dose of 36 million IU three times weekly (Roche Product Information). The optimal duration of treatment has not been established. Treatment is recommended to continue until there is no clinical evidence of tumor.

2 Chronic hepatitis B

The recommended dose of interferon alpha-2a for chronic active hepatitis B is 4.5 or 5 million IU (2.5 million IU per m^2) three times weekly by subcutaneous injection for 4–6 months. The dose should be increased (incrementally, up to a maximum of 18 million IU three times per week) if genomic markers of hepatitis B virus replication or HBeAg in the serum do not decline after 1 month of therapy. Best responses have been observed with a dose of 10 million IU three times weekly or 5 million IU administered daily. Regardless of the starting dose of interferon, the dose will usually require modification based on tolerance and markers of efficacy (particularly hepatitis B DNA). Monthly measurement of serum liver transaminases, hepatitis B DNA and HBeAg is recommended to monitor therapeutic success (Ryff, 1993). Therapy should be ceased if no response is observed 3–4 months after starting therapy (reviewed in Haria and Benfield, 1995). Treatment is recommended for those with stable chronic hepatitis B infection with detectable HBsAg, HBeAg and hepatitis B DNA in serum, with serum alanine aminotransferase levels at least twice the upper normal limit, with histologically proven chronic hepatitis and without evidence of cirrhosis on biopsy, ascites, encephalopathy variceal hemorrhage (Roche Product Information; and reviewed in Haria and Benfields, 1995).

In one study a dose of 4.5 million IU three times weekly given to patients with chronic hepatitis B infection for only 4 months was not associated with a significantly higher rate of serologic or clinical response than with controls (Fattovich et al., 1989).There are data from other studies that suggest that higher doses (10 million IU three times per week) result in more consistent virologic, serologic, histologic and/or clinical improvement than lower doses (Porres et al., 1988; Thomas et al., 1990).

Although not currently recommended, if interferon therapy is used in patients with compensated cirrhosis due to chronic hepatitis B infection the patient should be carefully monitored and treatment undertaken with caution using relatively low doses of 2 to 5 million IU three times weekly (Hoofnagle et al., 1993), with access to a liver transplant center.

There are no recommendations as yet for dosage in children. Dose regimens of 5 to 10 million IU per m^2 of body surface area administered three times per week intramuscularly or subcutaneously for up to 6 months have been used with clinical success in Caucasian children (Moreno et al., 1990).

3 Chronic hepatitis C

Although the optimal treatment regimen is not yet clear, the currently recommended dose for chronic hepatitis C infection is 3 million IU three times per week for up to 12–18 months in patients who respond to treatment. In patients who fail to respond after 12–16 weeks of treatment, discontinuation of treatment is recommended. Treatment should be considered for patients with well-compensated laboratory-proven chronic hepatitis C infection with evidence of chronic hepatitis on liver biopsy. Although there are no recommendations regarding interferon therapy in elderly patients with chronic hepatitis C, data from one study suggest that doses of 5 million IU administered three times per week for 6 months in patients aged over 65 years was not associated with any increase in adverse events compared with younger individuals (Van Thiel et al., 1995a). However, most clinicians would treat for longer than 6 months even in elderly patients provided there was evidence of a response and side-effects were acceptable.

4 Condyloma acuminata

The recommended dose of interferon alpha-2b for condylomata acuminata is 1 million IU administered intralesionally three times per week using a tuberculin syringe for 3 weeks with the maximum total dose not exceeding 15 million IU per week. The needle should be directed into the dermal core of the wart to prevent deep tissue or subcutaneous administration (Dorr, 1993). Doses of less than 1 million IU have been found to be less beneficial (Vance et al., 1986a).

Serum Levels in Relation to Dosage

There is good absorption of interferon alpha (approximately 80%) when administered by either intramuscularly or subcutaneously injection (Wills 1990). Intramuscular and subcutaneous administration of interferon alpha results in similar peak plasma concentrations with the time to T_{max} being longer following subcutaneous compared with intramuscular injection (reviewed in Bocci, 1994). A dose of 36 million IU administered by subcutaneously and intramuscular routes results in peak plasma concentrations of 1.7 and 2.0 μg per ml respectively, occurring 7.3 and 3.8 h post-administration (Wills et al., 1984). The area-under-the-curve following this dose when administered by intravenous, subcutaneous, and intramuscular routes is 17.6, 15.9 and 14.6 μg per liter per h respectively, suggesting good bioavailability following subcutaneous and intramuscular injection (Wills et al., 1984). Single intramuscular doses of up to 198 million IU result in dose-proportional increases in serum concentrations (Roche Product Information). The plasma half-life ranges from 5 to 8.2 h (Gutterman et al., 1982; Bornemann et al., 1985).

Excretion

From animal studies it is evident that interferon alpha is filtered through the glomeruli and then rapidly degraded during tubular reabsorption, resulting in negligible parent compound in the systemic circulation (Bino et al., 1982; Bocci et al., 1981, 1982). Liver metabolism and biliary excretion are minor pathways of elimination (Roche Product Information).

Distribution of the Drug in Body

The volume of distribution of interferon alpha-2a at steady-state is 31.4 liters (Wills *et al.*, 1984). There is little distribution of interferon alpha into cerebrospinal fluid (CSF) unless doses of 50 million IU are administered (Smith *et al.*, 1985). There is evidence from *in vitro* studies that interferon alpha does not cross the human placenta and there are currently no data regarding secretion into breast milk (reviewed in Haria and Benfield, 1995).

Mechanism of Action

Interferons are naturally occurring glycoproteins, discovered in 1957 (Isaacs and Lindenmann, 1957) that are produced by the immune system early in the course of viral infection, prior to the production of specific antibodies (Gresser *et al.*, 1976a,b). They exert their antiviral effects by inhibiting viral entry into susceptible cells, interfering with uncoating of the virus following entry, inducing cellular enzymes and other proteins that inhibit viral replication and impairing viral assembly. All peripheral blood mononuclear cells constitutively produce interferon alpha (Greenway *et al.*, 1995). There are about 15 genes encoding different subtypes of interferon alpha, with 70% homology at the amino acid level but which differ in biologic properties (Finter, 1991). There is a single human interferon beta, sharing 30% homology with interferon alpha and binding to the same cellular receptor (Novick *et al.*, 1994; Hertzog *et al.*, 1994a). The biologic effects of interferon are species-restricted (Sutton and Tyrrell, 1961), because the receptor is species-specific.

1 General overview of mechanism of action of interferon alpha

Interferon alpha induces a non-specific state of cellular resistance to viral infections and modulates the host immune response in an attempt to neutralize virus or eliminate virus-infected cells (Roferon Product Information). Human chromosome 21 is important for interferon responses as it contains the genes encoding the components of the interferon receptor (Lutfalla *et al.*, 1990; Langer *et al.*, 1990; Hertzog *et al.*, 1994a). The role of the interferon system in antiviral defence was demonstrated in mice with a mutation in the gene encoding a component of the receptor. This resulted in mice which were non-responsive to interferons alpha and beta, and highly susceptible to viral infections with unrestricted replication of virus in organs (Hwang *et al.*, 1995).

Following the binding of interferon to its surface receptors (Uze *et al.*, 1990; Novick *et al.*, 1994), a complex sequence of intracellular events is initiated (reviewed in Hertzog *et al.*, 1994b). Within minutes of binding, the tyrosine kinases Tyk-2 and JAK-1 are activated to phosphorylate specific proteins called signal transducers and activators of transcription (STAT 2 and 1) respectively (Barbieri *et al.*, 1994; Darnell *et al.*, 1994). The Tyk-2 and JAK-1 kinases are physically associated with components of the interferon receptor (Novick *et al.*, 1994; Colamonici *et al.*, 1994), and binding of interferon draws the receptor components together, allowing subsequent activation of the kinases, phosphorylation of STAT 1 and 2 and phosphorylation of the receptor (Platanias *et al.*, 1994; Colamonici *et al.*, 1994). JAK-1 but not JAK-2 is required for the response to interferon alpha (and also interferon beta) (Watling *et al.*, 1993). Phosphorylated STAT 1 and 2 dimerize after they leave the receptor, and as such are known as interferon- stimulated gene factor 3-alpha (ISGF3-alpha). ISGF3-alpha recruits another protein called ISGF3-gamma (p48) to comprise the cytoplasmic transcription factor ISGF3 (Imam *et al.*, 1990; Fu *et al.*, 1990; Improta *et al.*, 1994). ISGF3 moves to the nucleus where it stimulates the expression of interferon alpha stimulated genes (ISGs) through binding to the interferon sensitive response element (ISRE) present within these genes (Kessler *et al.*, 1990; Kessler and Levy, 1991; Stark and Kerr, 1992; Schindler *et al.*, 1992; Veals *et al.*, 1991; Darnell *et al.*, 1994) (Fig. V.71).

The binding of ISGF3 to the ISRE initiates transcription and synthesis of a number of proteins including 2'5'oligoadenylate synthetase (2'5'OAS), a double-stranded RNA-dependent protein kinase, Mx proteins, MHC class 1 antigens and others (Rubinstein and Orchansky, 1986; Pestka *et al.*, 1987; Samuel, 1988; Hovanessian, 1989; Decker *et al.*, 1991; Haque and Williams, 1994). Interferon can also suppress expression of certain genes including a number of proto-oncogenes and receptors for cellular growth factors (reviewed in Hertzog *et al.*, 1994b). In addition to this pathway there are other mechanisms by which interferon inducible genes are regulated, involving other transcription factors.

2'5'-Oligoadenylate synthetase is one of the best characterized interferon-induced proteins. It is a double-stranded RNA-dependent protein which activates the intracellular ribonuclease RNase L, also double-stranded RNA-dependent, resulting in the degradation of viral mRNA (Faltynek and Kung, 1988; reviewed in Davis, 1993; reviewed in Muller, 1991). The interferon-induced double-stranded RNA-dependent protein kinase (PKR) decreases translation of viral

Fig. V.71.
Regulation of interferon inducible genes. (Figure kindly provided by Dr P Hertzog, Molecular Genetics and Development Group, Institute of Reproduction and Development, Monash University, Melbourne, Australia.)

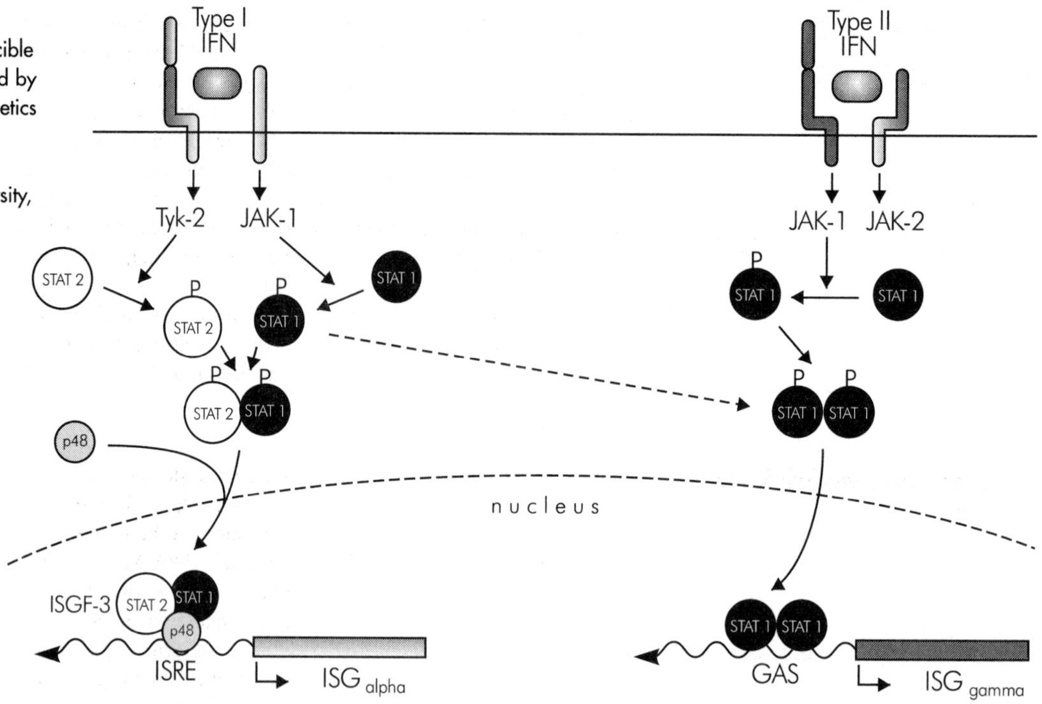

proteins by phosphorylating the alpha subunit of the translation initiation factor 2, and prevents initiation of protein synthesis (Pestka *et al.*, 1987; Tanaka and Samuel 1994; reviewed in Baron and Dianzani, 1994). The activity of 2'5'OAS and protein kinase within cells correlate with antiviral activity and resistance to viral infection respectively. Other proteins with more specific viral activity have been reported to be induced by interferon, including the murine Mx proteins and their human homologs which inhibit production of influenza virus and vesicular stomatitis virus mRNA in the nucleus of the infected cell (Horisberger *et al.*, 1983; Arnheiter and Meier, 1990; Horisberger and Gunst, 1991; Pavlovic *et al.*, 1993). Interferon regulatory factor-1 (IRF-1) is a transcriptional activator induced by interferon and is necessary for the antiviral action of interferon against some viruses (Kimura *et al.*, 1994). The antiviral state peaks about 6 h after exposure to interferon but then declines slowly over many hours (reviewed in Finter *et al.*, 1991).

In addition, interferon alpha enhances immunologic defence mechanisms, such as activation of effector cells and the expression of HLA class I antigen on the cellular surface both *in vitro* and *in vivo* (Chorvath *et al.*, 1991a; Hayata *et al.*, 1991), leading to enhanced recognition by, and activity of, cytotoxic T cells and natural killer cells (Cai *et al.*, 1990; Actis *et al.*, 1991; reviewed in Reiter, 1993). HLA class II expression is not altered by interferon alpha (Chorvath *et al.*, 1991b). The production of oxygen radicals by neutrophils is enhanced by interferon alpha (Kasimir *et al.*, 1991).

2 Hepatitis B and C infection

Treatment of patients with chronic hepatitis with interferon therapy results initially in inhibition of viral replication, by inhibiting synthesis of viral RNA and by activating enzymes and proteins as described above. This is associated with a decline in serum hepatitis B DNA. However, this response is insufficient to eliminate the virus. The second phase of activity of interferon alpha against hepatitis B virus is through stimulation of the immune response against infected hepatocytes by increasing the expression of MHC class I molecules on their cell surface and thus stimulating cytotoxic and natural killer cell activity. This is reflected several months after commencing therapy with interferon by a transient increase in liver damage (reflected by elevations in serum aminotransferases) due to immunologically mediated lysis of infected cells, which may precede viral elimination (reviewed in Foster and Thomas, 1994). There is also a non-cytolytic mechanism by which interferon can induce non-specific immune regulation of hepatitis B virus replication (Romero and Levine, 1996).

There is evidence that there is inadequate interferon production during acute and chronic hepatitis B infection, enabling persistence of infection (reviewed in Muller, 1991). However, it is important to note that in adults, chronic infection occurs in less than 5% of infected persons. In patients with acute but not chronic hepatitis B infection, levels of 2'5'oligoadenylate synthetase (see above) are elevated (Poitrine et al., 1985). There is reduced interferon alpha production by lymphocytes from patients with chronic hepatitis B infection when they are stimulated in vitro (Tolentino et al., 1975; Kata et al., 1982; Abb et al., 1985). Monocytes from patients with chronic hepatitis B do not possess the characteristic tubuloreticular inclusion bodies associated with exposure to interferon resulting in their stimulation (Grimley et al., 1985; Schaff et al., 1986).

Interferon therapy in patients with hepatitis C virus infection results in a purely antiviral effect without evidence of immune enhancement. Levels of 2'5'-oligoadenylate synthetase are elevated in patients with chronic hepatitis C infection (Pawlotsky et al., 1995).

3 Human immunodeficiency virus

It is likely that interferon alpha acts at multiple steps of the replicative cycle of HIV (Kornbluth et al., 1989; Gendelman et al., 1990b; Pitha, 1994). Both transcription from proviral DNA and translation of HIV proteins have been reported to be inhibited by interferon alpha (Gendelman et al., 1990b; Ho et al., 1985; Kornbluth et al., 1989; Meyelan et al., 1993). In addition, assembly and release of progeny virions are impaired (Poli et al., 1989; Smith et al.,1991; Yasuda et al., 1990). Other investigators have reported inhibition of preintegration events including reverse transcription (Shirazi and Pitha, 1992; Baca-Regen et al., 1994).

The effects of interferon alpha on HIV replication appear to differ somewhat depending on the cell type, with assembly and release being predominantly affected in chronically infected T cells rather than synthesis of viral RNA and protein (Dolei et al., 1986; Poli et al., 1989) and decreased levels of transcription and/or degradation of viral RNAs being reported to be the major effect in chronically infected macrophages (Gendelman et al., 1991a; Kornbluth et al., 1989, 1990). In acutely infected T cell lines and primary T cells, suppression of HIV is also at the post-translational level (Ho et al., 1985; Michaelis and Levy 1989; Yamamoto et al., 1986; Brinchman et al., 1991; Shirazi and Pitha, 1992). However, in acute infection of monocytes, interferon decreases levels of integrated provirus (Kornbluth et al., 1989, 1990). Recently interferon-induced deregulation of viral protein processing and reduced protein stability in acutely infected T cell lines has been reported, with no alteration in levels of virus-specific RNAs (Agy et al., 1995).

4 Other

Natural killer cellular activity is enhanced when human rhinovirus serotype 2 is incubated with healthy peripheral blood mononuclear cells, associated with the production of interferon alpha production (Levandowski and Horohov, 1991).

Toxicity

1 General

On starting therapy, flu-like symptoms are very common and include general malaise, myalgia, fever, and headache (reviewed in Haria and Benfield, 1995). These symptoms are often most pronounced 4–6 h after the first few injections, continue during the first few weeks of therapy, decrease with time and can be relieved with paracetamol, or aspirin (Hendrix et al., 1995). Leucopenia occurs frequently, and, uncommonly, elevation of serum alanine aminotransferase; fatal hepatic decompensation has been reported in association with interferon alpha therapy, particularly in patients with cirrhosis (Janssen et al., 1992). The more delayed side-effects including depression, emotional lability, irritability, and fatigue can be more troublesome and require dose-reduction.

2 Neuro-psychological side-effects

Apart from symptoms described above, acute paranoia, attempted suicide, depression and mood disorders, seizures, cognitive dysfunction and delirium may occur, usually in the setting of pre-existing psychological problems (Janssen et al., 1990; Reichen et al., 1994; Morris, 1994; Poutiainen et al., 1994; Goldman, 1994).

3 Autoimmune disease

A number of autoimmune diseases can be induced or exacerbated by interferon therapy (Conlon et al., 1990; Roonbloom et al., 1991). Autoimmune thyroid disease has been reported in up to 8% of patients who receive interferon alpha, with those who have microsome antibodies prior to therapy being at highest risk (Watanabe et al., 1994). Other autoantibodies including antithyrotropin receptor antibodies and antithyroglobulin antibodies also develop in up to 50% of treated patients (Fonseca et al., 1991; Carella et al., 1995; Matsuda et al., 1995). In one study in which 2.5% of 237 patients treated with interferon alpha developed overt thyroid disease, symptoms did not revert with cessation of therapy (Lisker-Melman et al., 1992). Although a number of patients treated with interferon alpha may develop laboratory evidence of thyroid dysfunction, normalization of tests generally occurs when therapy is ceased (Jacobs et al., 1991). Both hyperthyroidism and hypothyroidism have been observed (Fonseca et al., 1991; Jacobs et al., 1991; Uchida et al., 1996). Autoimmune hepatitis may become manifest during interferon alpha therapy for chronic hepatitis C infection, particularly in female patients (Garcia-Buey et al., 1995). Primary biliary cirrhosis has been reported to develop in a woman with no pre-existing evidence of autoimmune disease during treatment with interferon alpha-2a (D'Amico et al., 1995). Exacerbation of ulcerative colitis has also been reported in a patient with chronic hepatitis C who was treated with interferon alpha therapy; cessation of treatment improved his symptoms (Mitoro et al., 1993). Interferon alpha can induce type 1 diabetes in transgenic mice (Stewart et al., 1993) and there have been several case reports of patients receiving interferon alpha therapy for chronic hepatitis who develop diabetes (Waguri et al., 1994; Lopes et al., 1994). Hemolytic anemia, thrombocytopenia, and arthritis have also been reported, often in patients with underlying autoimmune disease prior to interferon therapy (Nadir et al., 1994; Maccari et al., 1991). Interferon treatment has been associated with the development of an antibody inhibitor of factor VIII coagulant protein resulting in a fatal hemorrhagic diathesis (Stricker et al., 1994). Raynaud's phenomenon and exacerbation of psoriasis have been described in association with interferon alpha treatment; the severity of psoriasis appears to be dose-related (Funk et al., 1991; Arslan et al., 1994; Pauluzzi et al., 1993).

4 Development of antibodies to interferon alpha

A proportion of patients who are treated with interferon alpha for many months develop antibodies which can neutralize interferon alpha, and, if in sufficiently high concentration, may abrogate clinical benefits from this therapy. The prevalence of antibodies varies with different interferon preparations. In one study, neutralizing antibodies directed against interferon alpha were detected in 20.2% of patients treated with interferon alpha-2a, but only 6.9% of those treated with interferon alpha-2b and 1.2% of those treated with lymphoblastoid interferon alpha (Antonelli et al., 1991). Cross-reactivity of these antibodies between interferons-2a and -2b has been demonstrated (reviewed in Antonelli, 1994). Cross-reactivity between interferon alpha-2a and lymphoblastoid interferon has not been evident in some studies (Lok and Lai, 1991; Antonelli, 1994) although other investigators report cross- resistance between these different preparations (Brand et al., 1993). Naturally occurring antibodies of IgG class directed against interferon alpha-2a have been reported in patients with acute viral hepatitis (Ikeda et al., 1991). The development of antibodies directed against interferon have very clearly been associated with treatment failure in some patients receiving interferon alpha-2a therapy for chronic hepatitis C; switching to lymphoblastoid interferon restored a complete response in all of 12 treated patients (Roffi et al., 1995). Although clinical relevance of antibodies to interferon has not been clearly established in all studies (Gianelli et al., 1994), a relationship between development of antibodies directed against interferon alpha and failure of therapy has been demonstrated by other investigators in the treatment of both hepatitis B and C (Antonelli et al., 1993; Bonetti et al., 1994; Lok et al., 1990a).

5 Hematological reactions

Neutropenia is common in patients treated with interferon alpha but is rarely dose-limiting. Transient lymphopenia (reaching a nadir 12–24 h after subcutaneously administration) and neutrophilia have been reported after administration of interferon alpha (Aulitzky et al., 1991). Thrombocytopenia is also often observed but only rarely requires cessation of therapy (Coppens et al., 1990). Interferon alpha also inhibits erythropoiesis both in vitro and in vivo (Tarumi et al., 1995).

6 Other

Pneumonitis has been described in three patients with chronic hepatitis C who received interferon alpha (Chin et al., 1994), and in a patient who developed hemolytic anemia and cholestatic liver dysfunction in association with interferon alpha treatment (Hizawa *et al.*, 1994). Cardiac toxicity, resulting in heart failure, may occur rarely during therapy. Interferon alpha can stimulate hepatic fatty acid synthesis thus altering lipid metabolism. Hypertriglyceridemia has been reported in association with interferon alpha therapy, although this is uncommon in patients who have normal levels at baseline (Grunfeld *et al.*, 1991; Sunderkotter *et al.*, 1993; Picciotto *et al.*, 1995). Plasma ACTH and cortisol levels have been found to increase in patients receiving interferon alpha (Muller, 1991). Acute axonal polyneuropathy has been reported to develop during interferon alpha-2a therapy in a patient with chronic hepatitis C (Negoro *et al.*, 1994). Interstitial nephritis and minimal change nephropathy have been attributed to interferon alpha therapy in one case report (Traynor *et al.*, 1994). A disturbance of water and electrolyte balance has been reported to occur during high-dose interferon alpha therapy (Farkkila *et al.*, 1990). Sudden hearing loss and/or tinnitus has been reported in up to 45% of patients whilst receiving interferon alpha therapy (Kanda *et al.*, 1994). Ocular complications of interferon therapy have also been reported (Yamada *et al.*, 1994).

7 Drug interactions

Interferon alpha therapy has been reported to cause significant and transient inhibition of cytochrome P-450 activity, which may potentially affect the metabolism of a large number of drugs (Moochhala and Renton, 1991; Stanley *et al.*, 1991; Horsmans *et al.*, 1994; Anari *et al.*, 1995). When interferon alpha-2a and theophylline are co-administered, the clearance of theophylline decreases approximately 4-fold and the half-life of theophylline increases from 4.7 h to 11.6 h (Roche Product Information).

Clinical Uses of the Drug

There are a number of indications of interferon alpha that are not within the scope of this text. Virus-related indications are included below including chronic active hepatitis B, chronic hepatitis C infection, and condylomata acuminata. Interferon alpha is also indicated for the treatment of HIV-related Kaposi's sarcoma. Comparative studies of the different preparations of interferon have not been performed and therefore their clinical effects and toxicities cannot be directly compared. It is assumed that the different preparations have similar biologic activity.

1 Chronic hepatitis C infection

Interferon alpha is approved for the treatment of patients with chronic hepatitis C infection at a dose of 3 million IU three times per week administered subcutaneously for up to 18 months. A number of studies have confirmed that a dose of 3 million IU three times per week is the optimal dose, given that higher doses (although sometimes associated with a higher response rate) are accompanied by an unacceptably higher incidence of side-effects. The optimal duration of treatment has still not been defined. However, 18 months has been found to be superior to shorter courses, in terms of decreasing the relapse rate. Shorter courses (up to 6 months) were associated with response in 40–50% of patients, but about half of these relapsed on cessation of therapy, resulting in a sustained response in only about 20–25% of the total treated population (Davis *et al.*, 1989; Di Bisceglie *et al.*, 1989). Others estimate relapse in approximately 70% of responding patients (reviewed in Davis, 1994). Recurrences usually occur within 6 months after stopping therapy, but may occur even 3 years later (Saracco and Rizetto, 1995).

The earliest reported trial of interferon therapy was performed at the National Institutes of Health in the USA in 1986 (Hoofnagle *et al.*, 1986). In this study, ten patients with chronic non-A-non-B hepatitis who were treated with low-dose interferon had a sharp decline in serum amino transaminase levels, without the classical 'flare' seen in patients with chronic hepatitis B infection who receive interferon therapy. Since this time there has been a huge number of clinical trials, many small and uncontrolled, with some more recent pivotal studies.

A multicenter study enrolled 168 patients (over 80% of whom had a history of blood transfusion, and 78– 90% of whom were seropositive for hepatitis C) who were randomized to receive 1 million IU, 3 million IU both administered three times weekly by subcutaneous injection, or no therapy for 24 weeks. There were dose-dependent responses in normalization of serum aminotransaminases, improvement in liver histology, and development of toxicity. Improvement in serum aminotransaminases occurred early in the course of treatment: all patients who had a complete response had a decline in serum alanine transaminase levels to normal values within the first 8 weeks. This has provided the basis for the recommendation that patients whose serum aminotransaminase levels do not fall to normal within the first 12 weeks of therapy should have treatment with interferon discontinued. Approximately 50% of those receiving the

3 million IU dose responded to treatment, with 50% of these relapsing within 24 weeks of cessation of therapy (mostly within the first 12 weeks) (Davis *et al.*, 1989; reviewed in Sherlock, 1994; reviewed in Hoofnagle, 1994). Patients who relapse will usually respond to retreatment with interferon alpha (Hess *et al.*, 1991).

A second study designed to examine response to therapy over a 24-week duration enrolled 41 patients with chronic hepatitis C infection, 90% of whom were seropositive for hepatitis C. They were randomized to receive either placebo or interferon-2b (initially 1 million IU per day for 7 days then 2 million IU three times weekly for 23 weeks). There was normalization of serum alanine transaminase levels in 48% of interferon recipients and significant improvement in liver histology but again a high relapse rate (Di Bisceglie *et al.*, 1989).

The results from these trials were supported by two other similar studies conducted in France, in which treatment with 3 million IU three times per week resulted in a complete response in 43% and 39% of patients (Causse *et al.*, 1991; Marcellin *et al.*, 1991).

Treatment for longer periods was initially investigated in a pilot study of ten patients who received 5 million IU daily for 1 year. This resulted in an initial response rate of 80%, with sustained remission in 60% (Koretz *et al.*, 1985), and provided a basis for extending the duration of treatment in larger studies.

In an open-label, randomized, multicenter study performed in France a total of 303 patients with hepatitis C were treated initially for 6 months with 3 million IU of interferon alpha, and then randomized to continue 3 million IU three times weekly for another 48 weeks (total 18 months), or continue at a reduced dose of 1 million IU for 48 weeks or discontinue therapy, and restart at a dose of 3 million IU only if serum alanine transaminase levels were elevated for 3 consecutive months. At the end of the study the response in the group treated for 18 months with the 3 million IU dose was significantly better than either the 1 million IU dose group or the group who discontinued treatment after 6 months (44.7% versus 26.7% versus 12.1% respectively). Liver histology at the end of treatment also showed more significant improvement in the group treated for 18 months with 3 million IU dose compared with the lower dose (Poynard *et al.*, 1995).

The multicenter, randomized open-label Australian study compared treatment with interferon alpha-2b in dosage regimens of 3 million IU three times weekly for 6 months versus 5 million IU three times weekly for 6 months versus 3 million IU three times weekly for 24 months in 230 patients, predominantly injecting drug users, all of whom were seropositive for hepatitis C. The relapse rate documented 6 months after ceasing treatment was 73% in those treated for 6 months and 46% in those treated for 2 years. There was significantly greater histologic improvement in those treated for 2 years than in either of the groups treated for 6 months (which were not significantly different from each other) (Lin *et al.*, 1995).

Other studies have supported the extra benefit of longer duration of therapy. Treatment for 52 weeks of 21 patients with chronic hepatitis C was associated with a normalization of serum alanine aminotransferase levels in 67% and in 43% undetectable hepatitis C RNA over a 3-year follow-up period (Yokosuka *et al.*, 1995) and 42% of patients with chronic hepatitis C infection in Sweden who were treated with 3 million IU three times per week for 60 weeks had evidence of clearance of virus at a 24-week follow-up after cessation of therapy (Reichard *et al.*, 1994).

Continuing treatment in patients with chronic hepatitis C who have failed to respond to an initial course has not been found to have favorable results. with normalization of serum aminotransferase levels in only 14% of patients who are given a further 6 months of therapy (Bresci *et al.*, 1995). Increasing the dose of interferon alpha to 6 million IU three times per week does not improve outcome in initial non-responders to interferon (Cimino *et al.*, 1991). Patients with normal or near normal alanine aminotransferase levels (up to 1.5 times the upper limit of normal) may have histologically advanced liver disease and have been found in an uncontrolled trial to respond to interferon alpha resulting in clearance of hepatitis C RNA from serum with an overall response rate of 65% (Van Thiel *et al.*, 1995b). However, in another small study, standard interferon therapy for 6 months of patients with normal liver function tests despite chronic hepatitis on biopsy resulted in no sustained virologic or histologic response (Serfaty *et al.*, 1996).

Approximately 40% of patients with chronic hepatitis C who failed to respond to interferon alpha were found in a pilot study to achieve a sustained decline in serum aminotransferase levels, with loss of hepatitis C RNA when treated with ribavirin in combination with interferon alpha (Brillanti *et al.*, 1994). Ribavirin therapy alone has also been found to provide evidence of a biochemical response (but no effect on viremia) in one study in about half of the 12 patients with chronic hepatitis C who were unresponsive to a prior 6–12 month course of interferon alpha therapy (Camps *et al.*, 1993a).

In a pilot study of 18 patients with hepatitis C infection after liver transplantation, interferon alpha treatment resulted in lack of response in 72% in terms of persistent elevation of serum aminotransferases and no significant improvement in histology (Wright *et al.*, 1994). Using a different patient population, in a multicenter, randomized controlled trial of interferon alpha-2b involving 38 patients with acute transfusion-associated hepatitis C infection, 53% of the 22 treated patients and none of the 16 untreated patients had normal serum alanine transferase levels and undetectable hepatitis C RNA at the end of treatment (Lampertico *et al.*, 1994).

Patients with hepatitis C and HIV co-infection have been reported to respond to interferon alpha therapy (Makris *et al.*, 1991).

Children with thalassemia and chronic hepatitis C infection respond to interferon therapy with the response being inversely related to liver iron burden (Clemente *et al.*, 1994). The inverse relationship between hepatic iron content and response to interferon therapy has also been reported for adult patients (Van Thiel *et al.*, 1994).

a Factors predictive of response to interferon in patients with chronic hepatitis C infection Pretreatment RNA levels and genotype are the main factors which predict response to interferon therapy in patients with chronic hepatitis C infection.

Viral genotype has been found to be an important predictor of response to interferon alpha therapy in patients with chronic hepatitis C infection (Tsubota *et al.*, 1994). In general, non-genotype 1 is associated with better response rates, based on data from a number of studies. Patients with hepatitis C genotype 3 appear to respond to interferon alpha therapy better than those with genotypes 1, 2 or 4 (Okada *et al.*, 1992; Weiland *et al.*, 1995; Chemello *et al.*, 1995; Yamada *et al.*, 1995; Hino *et al.*, 1994). In one study 69% of patients with genotype 3 had undetectable hepatitis C RNA at the end of a 24-week course of interferon alpha therapy (Kanai *et al.*, 1995). Genotypes 1 and 2 appear to be the most resistant to interferon alpha therapy, with only 8% of genotypes 1a and 1b and 20% of genotypes 2 responding to treatment (Weiland *et al.*, 1995; Okamoto *et al.*, 1992; Kanai *et al.*, 1992; Trepo *et al.*, 1994). The paucity of response in association with genotypes 1a and 1b has been confirmed by other investigators (Craxi *et al.*, 1995), but may in part relate to higher viral load in patients harboring genotype I compared with other genotypes (Craxi *et al.*, 1995; Kohara *et al.*, 1995). Mutations within the non-structural protein 5A gene may predict a response to interferon in patients infected with the 1b genotype of hepatitis C: mutations within this region are associated with response to therapy, whereas wild-type correlates with a lack of response (Enomoto *et al.*, 1994, 1996).

In a number of studies, patients with low hepatitis C viral load prior to therapy, variably defined as less than 350 000 RNA copies per ml, less than 2×10^6 RNA equivalents per ml and as 10^7 RNA copies per ml, have been found to be more likely to respond to interferon alpha therapy, independent of genotype (Lau *et al.*, 1993; Yamada *et al.*, 1995; Hagiwara *et al.*, 1993; Negro *et al.*, 1995). Lower pretreatment viral load is also associated with a lower incidence of relapse in initial responders (Lau *et al.*, 1993). Alcohol has been found to increase hepatitis C RNA levels in serum and to reduce efficacy of interferon alpha treatment (Oshita *et al.*, 1994).

More severe liver disease based on histology, including cirrhosis, has been associated with poor response to interferon alpha therapy (Lin *et al.*, 1991; Camps *et al.*, 1993b; Chemello *et al.*, 1995; Sieck *et al.*, 1993). Chronic co-infection with hepatitis B and C, or hepatitis B and D has been associated with a poor response to interferon alpha compared with hepatitis C infection alone (Weltman *et al.*, 1995). In one study, a patient age of less than 45 years was significantly associated with a sustained response (Chemello *et al.*, 1995). However, other investigators have failed to find an association between age and response to therapy and in one study elderly (over 65 years) and younger (under 45 years) adults had a similar rate of response to interferon therapy (Marcellin *et al.*, 1991; Van Thiel *et al.*, 1995a). A duration of infection of less than 5 years has been associated with a sustained response, although again this is controversial with other investigators not finding duration of disease to predict response (Farrell *et al.*, 1991). Other variables that may predict a response include lower pre-therapy serum alanine transferase levels and gamma glutamyltranspeptidase levels, normalization of serum alanine aminotransferase levels within 4 weeks of commencing interferon, female sex (Battezzati *et al.*, 1992; Laurent-Puig *et al.*, 1995; reviewed in Gibas, 1993; reviewed in Weiland, 1994), acquisition of hepatitis C infection by injecting drug use than blood transfusion (Lin *et al.*, 1991), all of which are controversial (Marcellin *et al.*, 1991). The persistence of hepatitis C RNA in plasma, peripheral blood mononuclear cells or liver at the end of therapy predicts relapse, although its absence is not necessarily a reliable indicator of cure (Berenguer *et al.*, 1995; Shindo *et al.*, 1995). The persistence of hepatic hepatitis C RNA at the end of therapy is the most important predictor of

Fig. V.72.
Probability of maintaining normal serum alanine aminotransferase levels at long-term follow-up (Kaplan-Meier curves). The line with asterisks represents patients who were negative for hepatitis C virus RNA and the solid line represents patients who were positive and had a sustained biochemical response to interferon alpha as long as 12 months after discontinuation of therapy. In viremic patients, the estimated probability of hepatitis relapse is 53% 4 years after therapy; in HCV RNA-negative patients, the probability is 0% (log-rank test; p<0.001). (Reproduced from Chemello et al., 1996, with permission.)

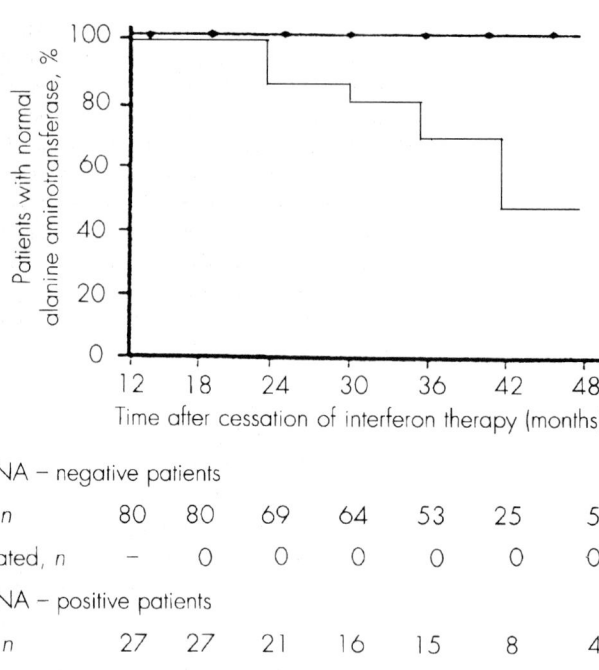

HCV RNA − negative patients							
At risk, n	80	80	69	64	53	25	5
Reactivated, n	−	0	0	0	0	0	0
HCV RNA − positive patients							
At risk, n	27	27	21	16	15	8	4
Reactivated, n	−	0	3	1	2	2	0

relapse (Shindo et al., 1995; Chemello et al 1996) (Fig. V.72). Higher body weight has also been associated with macrovesicular steatosis on liver biopsy and lower response rates to interferon alpha (Schvarcz et al., 1991). Activity of 2'5'OAS in peripheral blood mononuclear cells has been found to correlate with response to interferon therapy, with higher pre-therapy levels being associated with a lower response rate (Okuno et al., 1991). Schistosomiasis is associated with a lower complete response rate in patients with concomitant chronic infection with hepatitis C who are treated with interferon alpha (el-Shazly et al., 1994).

It has been recommended that certain subgroups of patients with chronic hepatitis C should not receive interferon therapy, including those with decompensated cirrhosis, associated autoimmune disease, psychiatric disorders or significant bone marrow suppression, due to potential adverse reactions (reviewed in Davis, 1994). However, with continuing reports it is clear that in some patients with the above conditions cautious therapy with interferon alpha can be of benefit without aggravating underlying conditions. Human lymphoblastoid interferon has been administered to patients with compensated cirrhosis associated with chronic hepatitis C infection, in doses of 1 or 3 million IU daily for the first 2 weeks and then three times per week for 24 weeks with no serious adverse effects. There was normalization of serum alanine transaminase levels in 40% of patients who were randomized to receive the higher dose interferon therapy (3 million IU three times per week) but in no patients receiving the lower dose. At follow-up 24 weeks after stopping treatment 10% of patients who received the 3 million IU dose remained in remission (Saito et al., 1994). Patients with co-existent psychiatric illness and chronic hepatitis C can safely receive interferon with active participation of the psychiatrist and appropriate antidepressant therapy (Van Thiel et al., 1995c).

Interferon alpha has been reported to ameliorate necrotizing vasculitis, arthralgia and fatigue caused by type II cryoglobulinemia associated with hepatitis C infection (Lunel et al., 1994; Durand et al., 1994; Levey et al., 1994; Sepp et al., 1995), although there are also reports of exacerbation of cryoglobulinemia associated with interferon therapy (Harle et al., 1995).

2 Hepatitis B infection

Interferon should not be used to treat patients with uncomplicated acute hepatitis B infection, as most cases resolve with clearance of the virus and no long-term hepatic damage (Dusheiko and Zuckerman, 1991). Interferon alpha therapy is also not considered useful following liver transplantation (Perillo, 1993), but treatment prior to liver transplantation has been shown to reduce hepatitis B reinfection in those in whom interferon therapy resulted in undetectable hepatitis B DNA, being 17% versus 78% in PCR-positive transplant recipients in one study (Marcellin et al., 1994).

The standard treatment of a patient with chronic hepatitis B who has detectable hepatitis B DNA and HBeAg is a 16-week course of interferon alpha, administered three times per week (De Man *et al.*, 1995). Remission, as defined by clearance of hepatitis B DNA and HBeAg from plasma and normalization of serum alanine aminotransferase levels, occurs in approximately 30–45% of patients with chronic hepatitis B who are treated with interferon alpha-2a or -2b in doses of 5–10 million IU three times per week for 4–6 months; the rate of spontaneous remission in untreated persons is 5–15% per year (Haria and Benfield, 1995).

The earliest study was in the 1970s when Greenberg *et al.*, used human leukocyte interferon to treat chronic hepatitis B, and demonstrated that a 10-day course resulted in a decline in HBsAg and DNA polymerase activity (Greenberg *et al.*, 1976). Since then, there have been a large number of trials, both controlled and uncontrolled, mainly including only patients with evidence of chronic hepatitis on liver biopsy and without evidence of cirrhosis, with stable elevated levels of serum aminotransaminases, circulating hepatitis B DNA and HBeAg in serum, and no complicating illness.

In a randomized study 45 patients with symptomatic chronic hepatitis B infection (27% of whom also had AIDS) received either no treatment or interferon alpha-2b in a dose of 5 million IU daily or 10 million IU every second day by subcutaneous injection. After 4 months of treatment one-third of treated patients (10 of 31) became HBeAg negative and hepatitis B DNA negative, with corresponding normalization of serum alanine transaminase; nine of these ten patients also had improvement in liver histology (Hoofnagle *et al.*, 1988).

Following promising results in a small randomized controlled study which found that a short-term course of prednisolone followed by treatment with recombinant interferon alpha-2b in 39 patients was effective in sustaining loss of HBeAg and hepatitis B DNA in selected patients (Perillo *et al.*, 1988), a study was conducted by the Hepatitis Interventional Therapy Group to further examine the effect of pretreatment with oral prednisolone followed by interferon alpha-2b in 169 patients with chronic hepatitis B infection who had circulating HBeAg and detectable hepatitis B DNA in serum. Patients were randomized to receive no therapy, or either oral prednisolone 60 mg per day decreasing to 20 mg per day over 6 weeks or placebo. Prednisolone-treated patients then received interferon alpha-2b in a dose of 5 million IU per day for 4 months; placebo-treated patients were randomized to receive either 5 or 1 million IU per day for 4 months. The overall response rate was higher in those who received the 5 million IU dose of interferon alpha with or without prednisolone than in the 1 million IU dose group or the untreated group, with a loss of HBeAg and hepatitis B DNA in 36%, 37%, 17% and 7% respectively. Thus 'prednisolone priming' did not improve the response rates (Table V.63) (Perillo *et al.*, 1990). These data have been confirmed by the results of a randomized controlled trial which differed in design in that concomitant prednisolone was administered with interferon alpha-2b rather than prior to interferon therapy to patients with chronic hepatitis C. The combination did not improve

Table V.63

Responses to treatment in the multicenter trial of patients with chronic hepatitis B. (Reproduced from Perillo *et al.*, 1990, with permission.)

Characteristic	Prednisone plus interferon	Interferon alone		Untreated controls
		5 million IU	1 million IU	
No. of patients	44	41	41	43
	Number (%)			
Loss of HBV DNA and HBeAg	16 (36)	15 (37)	7 (17)	3 (7)
Indeterminate response at 24-week follow-up	4 (9)	3 (7)	4 (10)	2 (5)
Loss of HBsAg	5 (11)	5 (12)	1 (2)	0
ALT, AST normal at last follow-up	19 (43)	18 (44)	11 (27)	8 (19)
Reactivation of HBeAg or HBV DNA during follow-up	1 (2)	0	1 (2)	0

IU: International units.

response rates when compared with interferon alpha alone (Zarski *et al.*, 1994), and the only deaths occurred in the prednisolone group.

A cohort of 23 patients with chronic hepatitis B who lost HBeAg and DNA after treatment with interferon alpha were followed for 3–7 years (mean 4.3 years) to examine the long-term therapeutic benefit. Only data from five patients were available at the end of the study. During treatment three patients relapsed, all within the first year following therapy. Another 13 patients lost HBsAg at a mean of 3 years post-treatment, and 11 of these also had undetectable hepatitis B DNA by PCR; the seven remaining patients had detectable hepatitis B DNA and remained HBsAg seropositive. Thus treatment-induced remissions are of long duration and associated with loss of markers of viral replication in approximately 50% (Korenman *et al.*, 1991).

a Prognostic features for response to therapy with chronic hepatitis B The most useful predictors of a response to interferon therapy are a low pre-therapy hepatitis B DNA and high pre-therapy serum alanine transferase level (Perillo, 1993). Other reported predictors of response to therapy include short duration of hepatitis B infection prior to therapy (Christensen, 1987), development of hepatitis B in adult life (Thomas *et al.*, 1991), active liver disease on liver biopsy (Perillo *et al.*, 1990), female sex, lack of HIV infection or other immunosuppression including renal disease and diabetes, Caucasian race, and presence of IgM anti-HBc (Brook *et al.*, 1989; Perillo *et al.*, 1990; reviewed in Hoofnagle, 1990; reviewed in Thomas *et al.*, 1991). Responders to interferon alpha have higher levels of 2'5'oligoadenylate synthetase and an increase in serum beta-2-microglobulin (Perillo *et al.*, 1990; Pignatelli *et al.*, 1986). The prevalence of more than 20% of precore mutant hepatitis B virus within the circulating virus pool is associated with resistance to interferon therapy (Brunetto *et al.*, 1993), or, more commonly, lack of a durable response (Brunetto *et al.*, 1989). The appearance of pre-core mutants during therapy with interferon alpha usually predicts failure to clear hepatitis B (Fattovich *et al.*, 1995).

Patients who have chronic hepatitis B infection with circulating HBeAg who respond to interferon alpha treatment often have a 'flare' in serum aminotransaminases with 2- to 4-fold increases in levels occurring within 6–12 weeks of starting interferon therapy, associated with a decline in hepatitis B DNA and followed by seroconversion to anti-HBeAg several weeks to months later, with normalization of serum aminotransferases and sustained resolution of liver disease (Sherlock and Thomas, 1985; Greenberg *et al.*, 1986; Williams and Alexander, 1986).

b Immunosuppressed patients with chronic hepatitis B A lack of response to interferon therapy has been observed in homosexual men and patients with human immunodeficiency virus infection (Novick *et al.*, 1984; Perillo *et al.*, 1988; McDonald *et al.*, 1987).

c Asian patients with chronic hepatitis B The rates of seroconversion of HBeAg in Asian pediatric and adult chronic hepatitis B carriers who are treated with interferon alpha is lower than in Caucasians, possibly due to reduced immunologic response to the virus and immune tolerance (Lai *et al.*, 1987; Lok *et al.*, 1988) or due to higher prevalence of neutralizing antibodies against interferon alpha (Lok *et al.*, 1990a). Poor responses are particularly common in Asian patients with relatively normal serum aminotransaminases; those with higher levels are more likely to respond (Lok *et al.*, 1990b; Lok, 1991). Prednisone pretreatment followed by interferon alpha was found to improve the likelihood of persistent loss of HBeAg and hepatitis B DNA in Asian children compared with untreated patients and those treated with interferon alpha alone, by increasing viral replication and breaking immune tolerance (Lai *et al.*, 1991; Table V.64). Asian patients are also more likely to suffer a relapse after successful therapy when compared with Caucasians (Lok *et al.*, 1989). In one study, in which 128 Chinese adults were treated with interferon alpha and then followed for a median of 41 months (range 19–79 months), 29 patients lost HBeAg and two also lost HBsAg within 1 year of treatment. Of the responders reactivation of disease occurred in 24%, and only 21% had sustained clearance of hepatitis B DNA in serum (Lok *et al.*, 1993).

Table V.64

Antiviral response to interferon alpha with and without prior prednisone in Chinese children; results at 12 months. (Reproduced from Lok *et al.* 1989, with permission.)

Treatment	No. treated	No. HBeAg negative	No. HBsAg negative
Prednisone/interferon	31	4 (13%)	1 (3%)
Placebo/interferon	29	1 (3%)	1 (3%)
Control	30	0 (0%)	0 (0%)

d Chronic hepatitis B and decompensated liver disease Interferon treatment of patients with chronic hepatitis B and mild clinically apparent cirrhosis has been studied in patients without evidence of decompensation (jaundice, ascites, variceal hemorrhage or hepatic encephalopathy) but who had active cirrhosis on liver biopsy and raised serum aminotransferase levels, and detectable hepatitis B DNA; 15 of 18 were HBeAg seropositive. Treatment with interferon alpha was effective in a selected population, resulting in sustained loss of HBeAg (if present at baseline), loss of hepatitis B DNA and decrease in serum aminotransferase levels in 33%, with resolution of clinical symptoms in these patients (Hoofnagle *et al.*, 1993). Low-dose regimens titrated in each patient are safer than previously considered in patients with mild to moderate hepatic decompensation (Perillo *et al.*, 1995). Many patients with liver disease and chronic hepatitis B who respond to interferon therapy experience a rapid and clinically overt elevation in serum hepatic transaminases associated with a decrease in hepatitis B DNA prior to clinical and biochemical improvement (Hoofnagle, 1990). Adverse reactions are more common in these patients (Renault *et al.*, 1987; Kassianides *et al.*, 1988).

e Treatment of patients with chronic hepatitis B and normal transaminases Asian patients and children frequently have normal serum liver enzymes but high levels of hepatitis B DNA (that is, they are tolerant to hepatitis B virus). The response rate to interferon therapy in patients with relatively normal serum aminotransaminases has been found in several studies to be relatively poor (Perillo *et al.*, 1990; Brook *et al.*, 1989).

f Pediatric chronic hepatitis B infection Although some studies suggest that interferon alpha is less effective in children than adults, in general therapy has been shown to hasten seroconversion to anti HBeAg and accelerate the rate of spontaneous clearance of hepatitis B in children with low viral burden and high baseline serum alanine transferase levels with similar response rates to adults (Barbera *et al.*, 1994; reviewed in Maggiore, 1995). There is a different response according to age at infection, with better responses in those with horizontally transmitted infection when compared with the response of those infected vertically (Bruguera *et al.*, 1993). Interferon therapy (5 to 10 million IU per m^2 three times per week for up to 24 weeks) in Caucasian children with chronic hepatitis B infection, particularly when administered before 3 years of age, can result in a complete response of similar frequency to that observed in treated adults (Narkewwicz *et al.*, 1995; Ruiz-Moreno *et al.*, 1990, 1991). In a small prospective randomized controlled trial of 20 children aged 6–14 years, interferon alpha treatment was associated with only slightly greater response rate than untreated controls (Utili *et al.*, 1991). Prednisolone treatment followed by interferon alpha therapy (3 million IU per m^2 three times per week for 12 months) was evaluated in a randomized controlled study of 43 children with chronic hepatitis B and found to be safe. Clearance of HBeAg occurred in 75% of children who had low baseline hepatitis B DNA levels (Utili *et al.*, 1994).

3 Hepatitis D infection

The role of interferon alpha in the treatment of hepatitis D remains unclear. However, it is generally considered to be of marginal use with only a minority of patients appearing to benefit even transiently (reviewed in Muller, 1991). Available data suggest that if interferon alpha is used, benefit is more likely in patients with recent infection who receive high doses (9 to 10 million IU three times per week) for at least 12 months (reviewed in Rosina and Cozzolongo, 1994).

In one study the beneficial effects of interferon alpha were modest, resulting in normalization of serum transaminases in 31% of patients receiving high-dose interferon alpha (18 million IU per day) and 12% in those receiving 3 million IU per day. Hepatitis D RNA was undetectable in only two of 32 patients at the end of treatment, and levels returned to baseline during follow-up (Madejon *et al.*, 1994; Hadziyannis, 1991). In another study in which patients with chronic hepatitis D were randomized to receive interferon alpha for 12 months or no therapy levels of serum hepatitis D RNA and intrahepatic delta antigen were similar in treated and untreated patients, although alanine aminotransferase levels were lower in interferon alpha recipients (Rosina *et al.*, 1991). Interferon alpha has also been used together with standard immunosuppressive therapy following liver transplantation of four patients co-infected with hepatitis B and D in an uncontrolled study. Reinfection with hepatitis D occurred in all patients. Treatment with interferon alpha resulted in a transient decline in viral replication (Hopf *et al.*, 1991).

4 Fulminant acute hepatitis

Interferon alpha has also not generally been considered by experienced clinicians to be of benefit in the treatment of fulminant hepatitis B infection (Dusheiko and Zuckerman, 1991) although there are case reports where therapy has been successful (Halevy *et al.*, 1990). In one study of 32 patients with fulminant hepatitis (including hepatitis A, B, and non-differentiated non-A-non-B infections) interferon alpha therapy resulted in recovery in 50% including 40% of those who were in coma of grade III or IV at institution of therapy. Adult patients were treated with 3 million IU per day for a mean of 8 days; infants received 70 000 IU per kg per day. In those who responded, improvement was noted on approximately day 5 of therapy. There was a poor recovery rate in children under the age of 4 years. The investigators demonstrated that in some of their patients there was a profound lack of endogenous interferon production and they concluded that interferon therapy may be of greatest benefit in these patients (Levin *et al.*, 1989). However, the usual treatment is open liver transplantation.

5 Human immunodeficiency virus infection

There are conflicting reports in the literature regarding production of interferon alpha in patients with HIV infection. Elevated levels of interferon alpha have been detected in plasma of HIV-infected individuals, paradoxically in association with disease progression (Krown *et al.*, 1991; Grunfeld *et al.*, 1991; Francis *et al.*, 1992), despite reports that the synthesis of interferon alpha mRNA and protein is defective (Voth *et al.*, 1990). This may be explained by the production of acid-labile interferon, a dysfunctional form that inhibits the normal production or activity of interferon (Hess *et al.*, 1991); acid-labile interferon has been detected in plasma of HIV-infected individuals (reviewed in Poli *et al.*, 1994) and is produced by HIV-infected monocytes (Szebeni *et al.*, 1991). It is likely that acid-labile interferon is identical to or closely related to interferon omega (Kontsek *et al.*, 1991). Other investigators report deficient production of interferon alpha by AIDS patients (Howell *et al.*, 1994), supported by *in vitro* data suggesting that there is a markedly reduced capacity of HIV-infected monocytes to produce interferon alpha (Gendelman *et al.*, 1990a, 1991b).

A blinded pilot study of low dose oral interferon alpha (150 IU daily for 6 weeks) was not associated with any clinical, or immunologic benefit in patients with HIV infection and CD4 counts of 150 to 600 cells per μl (Sperber *et al.*, 1993). When administered by subcutaneously injection at a mean dose of 17.5 million IU per day for 12 weeks or more in a randomized placebo controlled double-blind study involving 34 patients with asymptomatic HIV infection and more than 400 CD4 cells per μl, there was a higher incidence of negative viral culture, sustained or increased CD4 counts and lower incidence of development of an AIDS-related opportunistic infection in the interferon treated group compared with placebo recipients. However, it must be considered unusual that five of 17 patients in the placebo group with this early stage of HIV infection developed AIDS-defining opportunistic infections during the course of this short study (Lane *et al.*, 1990).

When interferon alpha was combined with zidovudine there appeared to be no additional advantage over zidovudine alone in patients with advanced HIV infection (Berglund *et al.*, 1991), although other phase I studies demonstrated clinical improvement with this combination (Fischl *et al.*, 1991). A lack of effect was confirmed by the findings of a larger randomized trial in Europe, Australia and Canada (Zidon) comparing treatment with interferon (3 million IU three times per week subcutaneously) in combination with zidovudine versus zidovudine alone in 402 HIV-infected patients with symptomatic infection and CD4 counts of 150–500 cells per μl or asymptomatic infection and CD4 counts of 150–350 cells per μl. There was no clinical, immunologic or virologic benefit of the combination therapy compared with zidovudine monotherapy (Fernandez-Cruz *et al.*, 1995). Other investigators report a beneficial effect of combination therapy using zidovudine in combination with interferon alpha when compared with zidovudine monotherapy (Frissen *et al.*, 1994).

a HIV-related Kaposi's sarcoma In general, high doses of interferon alpha are required to maximize response rates. It is suggested that there should be cautious dose escalation from 3 to 9 to 18 to 36 million IU administered three times per week, with most patients requiring in excess of 20 million IU per day to achieve a response (Krown, 1987; Dorr, 1993). The response rate at this dose is approximately 30% (reviewed in Mitsuyasu, 1991). Remission is more likely if treatment at high dose is instituted prior to waning CD4 count or the development of fever, night sweats and weight loss (Krown, 1987). There is little additional benefit to be obtained by combining interferon alpha with cytotoxic agents such as vinblastine, etoposide or doxorubicin (Dorr, 1993). However, zidovudine (500 mg per day) in combination with interferon alpha (up to 18 million IU per day) results in suppression of the tumor in about 40–46% whilst also suppressing HIV infection (Krown *et al.*, 1990; Podzamczer *et al.*, 1993). Other investigators have found no benefit in combining interferon alpha (up to 18 million IU per day for 4 weeks) with zidovudine for the treatment of AIDS-associated Kaposi's sarcoma (de Wit *et al.*, 1991). Greater myelotoxicity is observed with this combination (Groopman, 1987).

b   Primary HIV infection   Combination therapy using zidovudine and interferon alpha has been used as prophylaxis against HIV infection following needle-stick exposure (Mildvan *et al.*, 1994; Palmer *et al.*, 1994), but this is superseded by combination with zidovudine, lamivudine and a protease inhibitor (see zidovudine, p. 1655).

c   Other HIV-associated conditions   Interferon alpha (three million IU three times weekly) given for 16 weeks resulted in significant improvement in platelet counts in an uncontrolled study of 16 HIV-infected patients with immune thrombocytopenic purpura who had failed to respond to zidovudine (Northfelt *et al.*, 1995). These data confirm results from earlier case reports (Northfelt *et al.*, 1991) and a randomized placebo controlled double-blind study conducted in Europe (Marroni *et al.*, 1994). Interferon alpha was successful in treating recalcitrant molluscum contagiosum in HIV-infected patients using one million IU weekly injected into the lesions for 4 weeks (Nelson *et al.*, 1995).

6 Condyloma acuminata

Human papilloma viruses, usually types 6 and 11, cause genital warts. Interferon alpha-2b given intralesionally at a dose of 1 million IU three times weekly has been approved for the treatment of warts (see above). Responses usually occur within 8 weeks; if necessary treatment courses can be repeated after 3–4 months (Dorr, 1993).

There were a number of early studies which examined the efficacy of topical interferon alpha in the treatment of cervical and vulval warts, with some studies suggesting benefit (Ikic *et al.*, 1975a,b; reviewed in Cirelli and Tyring, 1994) and others showing no improvement over placebo (Keay *et al.*, 1988).

Human leukocyte interferon cream (2×10^6 IU per g) has been compared with 0.5% podophyllotoxin cream and placebo for the treatment of genital warts in a double-blind, randomized trial involving 60 patients. The interferon cream was found to be superior to podophyllotoxin and placebo in terms of progression of lesions (90%, 55% and 15% respectively) (Syed *et al.*, 1995a).

Intralesional use of interferon alpha has been generally associated with remission in 45–62% of patients, compared with rates of 17–22% in placebo recipients (Friedman-Kein *et al.*, 1988; Reichman *et al.*, 1988), although other investigators report virtually no benefit above placebo (Vance *et al.*, 1986b; Condylomata International Collaborative Study Group, 1993).

A placebo-controlled study involving 296 patients examined the efficacy of interferon alpha-2b at a dose of 1 million IU injected intralesionally three times weekly for 3 weeks. The mean wart area decreased by 62% in the interferon-treated patients after 1 week of therapy, with only a 1.2% decrease in placebo-treated controls. After 12 weeks, the mean wart area had decreased by 40% in the interferon-treated group and increased by 46% in the placebo group (Eron *et al.*, 1986).

Trials of systemic therapy for condyloma acuminata have again produced conflicting results. In a randomized placebo-controlled trial in which 3 million IU of interferon alpha given by intramuscular injection on alternate days for 4 weeks, approximately 45% of the 22 treated patients had a complete recovery compared with 10% of spontaneous recovery in the untreated group (Gentile *et al.*, 1994). This is supported by another study in which patients who had received laser treatment for genital warts were then randomized to receive interferon alpha-2b (5 million IU subcutaneously three times per week for 4 weeks) or placebo. A significantly higher cure rate was observed in interferon alpha-treated patients than in placebo recipients (52% versus 23% respectively) (Petersen *et al.*, 1991). However, in a study in which patients received 1.5 million IU three times per week subcutaneously for the first week then the dose increased to 3 million IU no significant therapeutic effect was observed (Yliskoski *et al.*, 1991).

A multicenter, randomized clinical trial has examined the benefit of human leukocyte interferon treatment of recurrent respiratory papillomavirus infection in 123 patients who received surgery plus interferon (2 million IU per m^2 per day for 1 week then three times per week for 1 year) or surgery alone. Interferon recipients had a non-sustained reduced rate of growth of papillomas during the first 6 months of therapy, leading the investigators to conclude that interferon treatment was of no substantial value in the management of these patients (Healy *et al.*, 1988). However, a subsequent study which analyzed the long-term benefit of treatment suggested that there was a sustained or repeated response to treatment with lymphoblastoid interferon when used in a dose of 2 million IU per m^2 per day or 4 million IU per m^2 on alternate days administered by intramuscular injection (Leventhal *et al.*, 1991).

7 Respiratory virus infections

Treatment of infants who were infected with respiratory syncytial virus for a maximum of 5 days with interferon alpha in doses of 10 000 to 70 000 IU per day by intramuscular injection resulted in improvement in 3–5 days without toxic effects (Portnoy *et al.*, 1988). In a double-blind placebo-controlled study, self-administered interferon alpha-2a prior to challenge reduced the incidence and severity of respiratory syncytial virus infection compared with placebo (Higgins *et al.*, 1990). Symptoms of colds due to coronavirus infections can be shortened and reduced in severity by the prophylactic administration of interferon alpha when administered by the intranasal route (Turner *et al.*, 1986). Similarly symptoms due to parainfluenza virus can be prevented by the administration of interferon alpha-2b (1.5 million IU given intranasally twice-daily) although infection itself is not prevented (Monto *et al.*, 1986). Prevention of rhinovirus infections has been demonstrated in a number of randomized placebo-controlled studies with prophylactic interferon alpha-2b with a protective efficacy in one study of 76%, and resulting in reduced symptoms in those who commenced treatment after they had developed infection (Hayden *et al.*, 1986; Monto *et al.*, 1986; Douglas *et al.*, 1986). However, other studies have found that commencing interferon treatment within 48 h of developing a cold (proven subsequently to be due to rhinovirus) the median duration of symptoms was in fact longer than in those who received placebo (Hayden *et al.*, 1988). When interferon alpha is applied intranasally prior to challenge with influenza virus there was no significant difference between placebo and interferon recipients in terms of viral shedding although there was a reduction in duration of shedding in interferon recipients and possibly some reduction in the severity of illness (Treanor *et al.*, 1987).

8 Herpesvirus infections

Several randomized double-blind placebo controlled trials have demonstrated success using topical interferon alpha for the treatment of genital herpes. In one study, patients with recurrent genital herpes were randomized to receive patient-initiated topical interferon alpha (1 million IU per g with 1% nonoxynol-9, or 1000 IU per g with 0.1% nonoxynol-9, or placebo three times per day for 5 days. High-dose recipients had a shorter time to negative virus culture (2.5 days versus 3.9 days respectively), and a shorter median duration of symptoms (2.7 days versus 3.7 days respectively) compared with placebo recipients (Sacks *et al.*, 1990). Human leukocyte interferon alpha in a hydrophilic cream (2 x 10^6 IU per g used three times daily for 5 days) has been used with reported success for the treatment of herpes simplex in a double-blind, placebo-controlled trial of patients with first episode of genital herpes, resulting in a shorter mean duration of healing (mean 5.9 days) compared with placebo recipients (mean 15 days) (Syed *et al.*, 1995b). Treatment with prophylactic interferon alpha commencing prior to renal transplantation and then continuing for 14 weeks post-surgery was associated with reduced clinical signs of cytomegalovirus disease compared with placebo recipients (Hirsch *et al.*, 1983). In immunocompromised children with varicella treatment with interferon was found in an early study to reduce the number of patients with life-threatening dissemination of infection (Arvin *et al.*, 1982). Human lymphoblastoid interferon alpha therapy has been reported to be of benefit in a case of common variable immunodeficiency complicated by chronic Epstein–Barr virus infection with severe thrombocytopenia (Toraldo *et al.*, 1995) and in X-linked lymphoproliferative syndrome when used in combination with immunoglobulin (Okano *et al.*, 1990).

9 Other

Intraventricular administration of interferon alpha has been reported to improve the clinical course of subacute sclerosing panencephalitis, and to reduce levels of antibodies to measles virus within CSF (Steiner *et al.*, 1989; Cianchetti *et al.*, 1994) although other neurologic pathology developed during therapy in some cases (Cianchetti *et al.*, 1994). A small series of patients with bilateral mumps orchitis received systemic treatment with interferon alpha (3 million IU per day for 1 week) resulting in complete resolution of clinical symptoms within 2–4 days and no evidence of testicular atrophy on long-term follow-up (Erpenbach, 1991). Treatment of five patients with human T lymphotropic virus type-1 (HTLV-1) associated myelopathy with interferon alpha resulted in clinical improvement in four of five patients (Nakamura *et al.*, 1990). In a second uncontrolled study of 17 patients with HTLV-1-associated myelopathy who were treated with 1.5 to 8 million IU of interferon alpha daily for 4 weeks, a moderate or marked clinical response was observed in 11 patients (Shibayama *et al.*, 1991). Hemorrhagic fever with renal syndrome due to Hantaan virus does not respond to interferon alpha therapy (Gui *et al.*, 1987).

Acknowledgements The author wishes to thank William Sievert, Monash Medical Centre, Melbourne, and Paul Hertzog of Monash University Institute of Reproduction and Development, Melbourne, for their critical review of this chapter.

References

Abb J, Zachoval R, Eisenburg J *et al.* (1985). Production of interferon alpha and interferon gamma by peripheral blood leukocytes from patients with chronic hepatitis B virus infection. *J Med Virol* **16**: 171.

Actis GC, Ponzetto A, D'Urso N *et al.* (1991). Chronic active hepatitis B interferon-activated natural killer-like cells against a hepatoma cell line transfected with the hepatitis B virus nucleic acid. *Liver* **11**: 106.

Agy MB, Acker RL, Sherbert CH, Katze MG (1995). Interferon treatment inhibits virus replication in HIV-1 and SIV-infected CD4+ T-cell lines by distinct mechanisms, evidence for decreased stability and aberrant processing of HIV-1 proteins. *Virology* **214**: 379.

Anari MR, Cribb AE, Renton KW (1995). The duration of induction and species influences the down regulation of cytochrome P450 by the interferon inducer polyinosinic acid polycytidylic acid. *Drug Metab Dis* **23**: 536.

Antonelli G (1994). Development of neutralizing and binding antibodies to interferon (IFN) in patients undergoing IFN therapy. *Antiviral Res* **24**: 235.

Antonelli G, Currenti M, Turriziani O, Dianzani F (1991). Neutralizing antibodies to interferon alpha, relative frequency in patients treated with different interferon preparations. *J Infect Dis* **163**: 882.

Antonelli MM, Currenti ST, Mariano ML *et al.* (1993). Neutralising antibodies to recombinant alpha interferon and response to therapy in chronic hepatitis C virus infection. *Liver* **13**: 146.

Arnheiter H, Meier E (1990). Mx proteins; antiviral proteins by chance or by necessity. *New Biol* **2**: 851.

Arslan M, Ozyilkan E, Keyhan B, Telatar H (1994). Decreased frequency of functional natural interferon-prodrug cells in peripheral blood of patients with the acquired immune deficiency syndrome. *Clin Immunol Immunopathol* **71**: 223.

Arvin AM, Kushner JH, Feldman S *et al.* (1982). Human leukocyte interferon for the treatment of varicella in children with cancer. *New Engl J Med* **306**: 761.

Aulitzky WE, Tilg H, Vogel W *et al.* (1991). Acute hematologic effects of interferon alpha, interferon gamma tumor necrosis factor alpha and interleukin 2. *Ann Hematol* **62**: 25.

Baca-Regen L, Heinzinger N, Stevenson M, Gendelman HE (1994). Alpha interferon-induced antiretroviral activities; restriction of viral nucleic acid synthesis and progeny virion production in human immunodeficiency virus type 1 infected monocytes. *J Virol* **68**: 7559.

Barbera C, Bortolotti F, Crivellaro C *et al.* (1994). Recombinant interferon alpha 2a hastens the rate of HBeAg clearance in children with chronic hepatitis B. *Hepatology* **20**: 287.

Barbieri G, Velazquez L, Scrobogna M *et al.* (1994). Activation of the protein tyrosine kinase tyk2 by interferon alpha/beta. *Eur J Biochem* **223**: 427.

Baron S, Dianzani F (1994). The interferons: a biological system with therapeutic potential in viral infections. *Antiviral Res* **24**: 97.

Battezzati PM, Podda M, Bruno S *et al.* (1992). Factors predicting early response to treatment with recombinant interferon alpha-2a in chronic non-A, non-B hepatitis. *Ital J Gastroenterol* **24**: 481.

Berenguer M, Olaso V, Cordoba J *et al.* (1995). Genome detection in liver and peripheral blood mononuclear cells; predictor factors of sustained response in patients with chronic hepatitis C. *Eur J Gastroenterol* **7**: 899.

Berglund O, Engman K, Ehrnst A *et al.* (1991). Combined treatment of symptomatic human immunodeficiency virus type 1 infection with native interferon alpha and zidovudine. *J Infect Dis* **163**: 710.

Bino T, Edery H, Gertler A, Rosenberg H (1982). Involvement of the kidney in catabolism of human leukocyte interferon. *J Gen Virol* **59**: 39.

Bocci V (1994). Pharmacology and side effects of interferons. *Antiviral Res* **24**: 111.

Bocci V, Pacini A, Muscettola M *et al.* (1981). Renal filtration, absorption and catabolism of human alpha interferon. *J Interfer Res* **1**: 347.

Bocci V, Pacini A, Muscettola M *et al.* (1982). The kidney is the main site of interferon catabolism. *J Interfer Res* **2**: 309.

Bonetti P, Diodati G, Drago C *et al.* (1994). Interferon antibodies in patients with chronic hepatitic C virus infection treated with recombinant interferon alpha-2 alpha. *J Hepatol* **20**: 416.

Bornemann LD, Spiegel HE, Dziewanowska ZE *et al.* (1985). Intravenous and intramuscular pharmacokinetics of recombinant leukocyte A interferon. *Eur J Clin Pharmacol* **28**: 469.

Brand CM, Ledbeater L, Bellati G *et al.* (1993). Antibodies developing against a single recombinant interferon protein may neutralize many other interferon alpha subtypes. *J Interfer Res* **13**: 121.

Bresci G, Parisi G, Banti S, Capzia A (1995). Re-treatment of interferon-resistant patients with chronic hepatitis C with interferon-alpha. *J Virol Hepat* **2**: 155.

Brillanti S, Garson J, Foli M *et al.* (1994). A pilot study of combination therapy with ribavirin plus interferon alfa for interferon alfa-resistant chronic hepatitis C. *Gastroenterology* **107**: 812.

Brinchmann JE, Gaudernack G, Varidal F (1991). *In vitro* replication of HIV-1 in naturally infected CD4+ T cells is inhibited by rIFN-alpha2 and by a soluble factor secreted by activated CD8+ T cells, but not by rIFN-beta, rIFN-gamma or recombinant tumor necrosis factor-alpha. *J AIDS* **4**: 480.

Brook MG, Karayiannis P, Thomas HC (1989). Which patients with chronic hepatitis B virus infection will respond to alpha interferon therapy? A statistical analysis of predictive factors. *Hepatology* **10**: 761.

Bruguera M, Amat L, Garcia O *et al.* (1993). Treatment of chronic hepatitis B in children with recombinant alfa interferon. Different response according to age at infection. *J Clin Gastroenterol* **17**: 296.

Brunetto MR, Oliveri F, Rocca G *et al.* (1989). Natural course and response to interferon of chronic hepatitis B accompanied by antibody to hepatitis B e antigen. *Hepatology* **10**: 198.

Brunetto MR, Giarin M, Saracco G *et al.* (1993). Hepatitis B virus unable to secrete e antigen and response to interferon in chronic hepatitis B. *Gastroenterology* **195**: 845.

Cai Q, Huang XL, Rappocciolo G, Rinaldo CR (1990). Natural killer cell responses in homosexual men with early HIV infection. *J AIDS* **3**: 669.

Camps J, Garcia N, Riezu-Boj JI *et al.* (1993a). Ribavirin in the treatment of chronic hepatitis C unresponsive to alfa interferon. *J Hepatol* **19**: 408.

Camps J, Crisoslomo S, Garcia-Granero M *et al.* (1993b). Prediction of the response of chronic hepatitis C to interferon alfa; a statistical analysis of pretreatment variables. *Gut* **34**: 1714.

Capobianchi MR, Matteucci D, Giovannetti A *et al.* (1991). Role of interferon in lethality and lymphoid atrophy induced by Coxsackievirus B3 infection in mice. *Virol Immunol* **4**: 103.

Capobianchi MR, Ankel H, Ameglio F *et al.* (1992). Recombinant glycoprotein 120 of human immunodeficiency virus is a potent interferon inducer. *AIDS Res Hum Retrovir* **8**: 575.

Carella C, Amato G, Biondi B *et al.* (1995). Longitudinal study of antibodies against thyroid in patients undergoing interferon-alpha therapy for HCV chronic hepatitis. *Horm Res* **44**: 110.

Carreno V, Tapia L, Ryff JC *et al.* (1992). Treatment of chronic hepatitis C by continuous subcutaneous infusion of interferon alpha. *J Med Virol* **37**: 215.

Caselmann WH (1994). HBV and HDV replication in experimental models; effect of interferon. *Antiviral Res* **24**: 121.

Caselmann WH, Meyer M, Scholz S *et al.* (1992). Type 1 interferons inhibit hepatitis B replication and induce hepatocellular gene expression in cultured liver cells. *J Infect Dis* **166**: 966.

Causse X, Godinot H, Chevallier M *et al.* (1991). Comparison of 1 or 3 MU of interferon alfa-2b and placebo in patients with chronic non-A, non-B hepatitis. *Gastroenterology* **101**: 497.

Chemello L, Cavalletto L, Noventa F *et al.* (1995). Predictors of sustained response, relapse and no response in patients with chronic hepatitis C treated with interferon alpha. *J Virol Hepat* **2**: 91.

Chemello L, Cavalletto L, Casarin C *et al.* (1996). Persistent hepatitis C viremia predicts late relapse after sustained response to interferon alpha in chronic hepatitis C. In *Veneto Viral Hepatitis Group. Ann Intern Med* **124**: 1058.

Chin K, Tabata C, Sataka N *et al.* (1994). Pneumonitis associated with natural and recombinant interferon alfa therapy for chronic hepatitis C. *Chest* **105**: 939.

Chorvath B, Sediak J, Fuchsberger N (1991a). Interferon alpha-induced modulation of leukocyte cell surface antigens; immunocytofluorometric study with human leukaemia/lymphoma cell lines. *Acta Virol* **35**: 7.

Chorvath B, Sediak J, Dubovsky P, Pleskova I (1991b). Differential modulation of leucocyte surface antigens by various inducers on the T-cell line MOLT-4. *Fola Biol Praha* **37**: 27.

Christensen E (1987). Multivariate survival analysis using Cox's regression model. *Hepatology* **7**: 1346.

Cianchetti C, Fratta AL, Muntoni F *et al.* (1994). Toxic effect of intraventricular interferon alpha in subacute sclerosing panencephalitis. *Ital J Neurol Sci* **15**: 153.

Cimino L, Nardone G, Citarella C *et al.* (1991). Treatment of chronic hepatitis C with recombinant interferon alfa. *Ital J Gastroenterol* **7**: 399.

Cirelli R, Tyring SK (1994). Interferons in human papillomavirus infections. *Antiviral Res* **24**: 191.

Clemente MG Congia M, Lai ME *et al.* (1994). Effect of iron overload on the response to recombinant interferon-alfa treatment in transfusion dependent patients with thalassemia major and chronic hepatitis C. *J Pediatr* **125**: 123.

Colamonici OR, Uyttendaele H, Domanski P *et al.* (1994). p135tyk2, an interferon-alpha activated tyrosine kinase, is physically associated with an interferon-alpha receptor. *J Biol Chem* **269**: 3518.

Condylomata International Collaborative Study Group, (1993). Recurrent condylomata acuminata treated with recombinant interferon alpha 2A. A multicentre double blind placebo controlled clinical trial. *Acta Derm Venereol* **73**: 223.

Conlon KC, Urba WJ, Smith JW *et al.* (1990). Exacerbation of symptoms of autoimmune disease in patients receiving alpha interferon therapy. *Cancer* **65**: 2237.

Coppens JP, Cornu C, Lens E *et al.* (1990). Prospective trial of recombinant leucocyte interferon in chronic hepatitis B; a long-term follow up study. *J Hepatol* **11**: S126.

Crance JM, Leveque F, Chousterman S *et al.* (1995). Antiviral activity of recombinant interferon alpha on hepatitis A virus replication in human liver cells. *Antiviral Res* **28**: 69.

Craxi A, Magrin S, Fabiano C *et al.* (1995). Host and viral features in chronic HCV infection; relevance to interferon responsiveness. *Res Virol* **146**: 273.

Crowe SM, Elbeik T, Ulrich PP *et al.* (1991). No evidence of occult human immunodeficiency virus in seronegative individuals at very high risk of infection. *J Med Virol* **35**: 160.

D'Amico E, Paroli M, Fratelli V *et al.* (1995). Primary biliary cirrhosis induced by interferon-alpha therapy for hepatitis C virus infection. *Dig Dis Sci* **40**: 2113.

Darnell JE, Kerr IM, Stark GR (1994). Jak-STAT pathways and transcriptional activation in response to IFNs and other extracellular signalling proteins. *Science* **264**: 1415.

Davis GL (1993). Treatment of chronic hepatitis C. *Antiviral Chemotherapy, New Directions for Clinical Application and Research* Vol 3, p. 267 (Mills J, Corey L, eds). New Jersey: Prentice Hall.

Davis GL (1994). Interferon treatment of chronic hepatitis C. *Amer J Med* **96**: 41S.

Davis GL, Balart LA, Schiff ER *et al.* (1989). Treatment of chronic hepatitis C with recombinant interferon alfa A multicenter randomised controlled trial. *New Engl J Med* **321**: 1501.

De Man RA, Heijtink RA, Neisters HG Schalm SW (1995). New developments in antiviral therapy for chronic hepatitis B infection. *Scand J Gastroenterol* **212**: 100.

De Wit R, Danner SA, Bakker PJ *et al.* (1991). Combined zidovudine and interferon alpha treatment in patients with AIDS associated Kaposi's sarcoma. *J Intern Med* **229**: 35.

Decker T, Lew DJ, Darnell JE (1991). Two distinct alpha interferon dependent signal transduction pathways may contribute to activation of transcription of the guanylate binding protein gene. *Mol Cell Biol* **11**: 5147.

Degre M, Beck S (1994). Anti-HIV activity of dideoxynucleosides, foscarnet and fusidic acid is potentiated by human leukocyte interferon in blood-derived macrophages. *Chemother* **40**: 201.

Despres P, Griffin JW, Griffin DE (1995). Antiviral activity of alpha interferon in Sindbis virus-infected cells is restored by anti-E2 monoclonal antibody treatment. *J Virol* **69**: 7345.

Di Bisceglie AM, Martin P, Kassianides C *et al.* (1989). Recombinant interferon alfa therapy for chronic hepatitis C, A randomised double-blind placebo-controlled trial. *New Engl J Med* **131**: 1506.

Dolei A, Fattorossi A, D'Amelio R *et al.* (1986). Direct and cell-mediated effects of interferon-alpha and gamma on cells chronically infected with HTLV-III. *J Interfer Res* **6**: 543.

Dorr RT (1993). Interferon-alpha in malignant and viral diseases. A review. *Drugs* **45**: 177.

Douglas RM, Moore BW, Miles HB *et al.* (1986). Prophylactic efficacy of intranasal alpha interferon against rhinovirus infections in the family setting. *New Engl J Med* **314**: 65.

Dubreuil M, Sportza L, D'Addario M *et al.* (1990). Inhibition of HIV-1 transmission by interferon and 3'-azido-3'-deoxythymidine during *de novo* infection of promonocytic cells. *Virology* **179**: 388.

Durand JM, Gretel E, Kaplanski G *et al.* (1993). Long term results of therapy with interferon alpha for cryoglobulinemia associated with hepatitis C virus infection. *Clin Rheumatol* **13**: 123.

Dusheiko GM, Zuckerman AJ (1991). Therapy for hepatitis B. *Curr Opin Infect Dis* **4**: 785.

Dusheiko GM, Zuckerman AJ (1993). Treatment of chronic viral hepatitis. *J Antimicrob Chemother* **32**: 107.

el-Shazly Y, Abdel-Salam AF, Abdel-Ghaffar A *et al.* (1994). Schistosomiasis as an important determining factor for the response of Egyptian patients with chronic hepatitis C to therapy with recombinant human alpha-2 interferon. *Trans Roy Soc Trop Med Hyg* **88**: 229.

Enomoto N, Sato C, Kurosaki M, Marumo F (1994). Hepatitis C virus after interferon treatment has the variation in the hypervariable region of envelope 2 gene. *J Hepatol* **20**: 252.

Enomoto N, Sakuma I, Asahina Y *et al.* (1996). Mutations in the nonstructural protein 5A gene and response to interferon in patients with chronic hepatitis C virus 1b infection. *New Engl J Med* **334**: 77.

Eron LJ, Judson F, Tucker S *et al.* (1986). Interferon therapy for condylomata acuminata. *New Engl J Med* **315**: 1059.

Erpenbach KH (1991). Systemic treatment with interferon alpha 2b; an effective method to prevent sterility after bilateral mumps orchitis. *J Urol* **146**: 54.

Faltynek CR, Kung H (1988). The biochemical mechanisms of action of the interferons. *BioFactors* **1**: 227.

Fan SX, Skillman DR, Liao MJ *et al.* (1993). Increased efficacy of human natural interferon alpha (IFN-alpha n3) versus human recombinant IFN-alpha 2 for inhibition of HIV-1 replication in primary human monocytes. *AIDS Res Hum Retrovir* **9**: 1115.

Farkkila AM, Iivanainen MV, Farkkila MA (1990). Disturbance of the water and electrolyte balance during high dose interferon treatment. *J Interfer Res* **10**: 221.

Farrell GC, Lin R, Coverdale S (1991). Prediction of response to interferon in patients with chronic active hepatitis C, and evidence that this improves hepatic metabolic function. *Gastroenterology* **26**: 243.

Fattovich G, Brollo L, Boscaro S *et al.* (1989). Long-term effect of low dose recombinant interferon therapy in patients with chronic hepatitis B. *J Hepatol* **9**: 331.

Fazely F, Haseltine WA, Rodger RF, Ruprecht RM (1991). Postexposure chemoprophylaxis with ZDV or ZDV combined with interferon-alpha failure after inoculating rhesus monkeys with a high dose of SIV. *J AIDS* **4**: 1093.

Fernandez-Cruz E, Lang JM, Frissen J *et al.* (1995). Zidovudine plus interferon-alpha versus zidovudine alone in HIV-infected symptomatic of asymptomatic persons with CD4+ cell counts > 150 x 10(6)/L; results of the Zodon Trial Study Group. *AIDS* **9**: 1025.

Fernie BF, Poli G, Fauci AS (1991). Alpha interferon suppresses virion but not soluble human immunodeficiency virus antigen production in chronically infected T-lymphocytic cells. *J Virol* **65**: 3968.

Finter NB (1991). Why are there so many subtypes of alpha-interferons? *J Interfer Res* (Special edn): 185.

Finter NB, Chapman S, Dowd P *et al.* (1991). The use of interferon-alpha in virus infections. *Drugs* **42**: 749.

Fischl MA, Uttamchandani RB, Resnick L *et al.* (1991). A phase I study of recombinant human interferon alpha 2a or human lymphoblastoid interferon alpha n1 and concomitant zidovudine in patients with AIDS related Kaposi's sarcoma. *J AIDS* **4**: 1.

Fonseca V, Thomas M, Dusheiko G (1991). Thyrotropin receptor antibodies following treatment with recombinant alpha-interferon in patients with hepatitis. *Acta Endocrinol Copenh* **125**: 491.

Foster GR, Thomas HC (1994). Effects of hepatitis B and hepatitis C virus replication on the actions of interferon. *Antiviral Res* **24**: 131.

Francis ML, Meltzer MS (1993). Induction of INF-alpha by HIV-1 in monocyte-enriched PBM requires gp120-CD4 interaction but not virus replication. *J Immunol* **151**: 2208.

Francis ML, Meltzer MS, Gendelman HE (1992). Interferons in the persistence, pathogenesis and treatment of HIV infection. *AIDS Res Hum Retrovir* **8**: 199.

Friedman-Kien AE, Eron LJ, Conani M *et al.* (1988). Natural interferon alfa for treatment of condylomata acuminata. *JAMA* **259**: 533.

Frissen PH, van der Ende ME, ten-Napel CH *et al.* (1994). Zidovudine and interferon alpha combination therapy versus zidovudine monotherapy in subjects with symptomatic human immunodeficiency virus type 1 infection. *J Infect Dis* **169**: 1351.

Fu XY, Kessler DS, Veals SA *et al.* (1990). ISGF3, the transcriptional activator induced by interferon alpha, consists of multiple interacting polypeptide chains. *Proc Natl Acad Sci USA* **87**: 8555.

Funk J, Langeland T, Schrumpf E, Hanssen LE (1991). Psoriasis induced by interferon alpha. *Brit J Dermatol* **125**: 463.

Gangemi JD, Pirisi L, Angell M, Kreider JW (1994). HPV replication in experimental models; effects of interferon. *Antiviral Res* **24**: 175.

Garcia-Buey L, Garcia-Monzon C, Rodriguez S *et al.* (1995). Latent autoimmune hepatitis triggered during interferon therapy in patients with chronic hepatitis C. *Gastroenterology* **108**: 1770.

Garner JG, Hirsch MS, Schooley RT (1984). Prevention of Epstein-Barr virus-induced B-cell outgrowth by interferon alpha. *Infect Immun* **43**: 920.

Gendelman HE, Friedman RM, Joe S *et al.* (1990a). A selective defect of interferon a production in human immunodeficiency virus-infected monocytes. *J Exp Med* **172**: 1433.

Gendelman HE, Baca LM, Turpin J *et al.* (1990b). Regulation of HIV replication in infected monocytes by IFN-alpha. Mechanisms for viral restriction. *J Immunol* **145**: 2669.

Gendelman HE, Friedman RM, Silverman R, Meltzer MS (1991a). The role of interferon in the persistence and pathogenicity of human immunodeficiency viral (HIV) disease. *J Interferon Res* **11**: S73.

Gendelman HE, Friedman RM, Joe S *et al.* (1991b). Interferon induced proteins; identification of Mx proteins in various mammalian species. *Virology* **180**: 185.

Gentile G, Formelli G, Busacchi P, Pelusi G (1994). Systemic interferon therapy for female florid genital condylomata. *Clin Exp Obstet Gynecol* **21**: 198.

Giannelli G, Antonelli G, Fera G *et al.* (1994). Biological and clinical significance of neutralising and binding antibodies to interferon alpha (INF-alpha) during therapy for chronic hepatitis C. *Clin Exp Immunol* **97**: 4.

Gibas AL (1993). Use of interferon in the treatment of chronic viral hepatitis. *Gastroenterology* **1**: 129.

Goeddel DV, Yelverton E, Ullrich A *et al.* (1980). Human leukocyte interferon produced by *E. coli* is biologically active. *Nature* **287**: 411.

Goldman LS (1994). Successful treatment of interferon alfa-induced mood disorder with nortriptyline. *Psychosomatics* **35**: 412.

Greenberg HBV, Pollard RB, Lutwick LJ *et al.* (1976). Effect of human leukocyte interferon on hepatitis B virus infection in patients with chronic active hepatitis. *New Engl J Med* **295**: 517.

Greenberg HB, Pollard RB, Lutwick LI *et al.* (1986). Effect of human leukocyte interferon on hepatitis B virus infection in patients with chronic active hepatitis. *J Infect Dis* **143**: 772.

Greenway AL, Hertzog PJ, Devenish RJ, Linnane AW (1995). Constitutive and virus induced interferon production by peripheral blood leukocytes. *Exp Hematol* **23**: 229.

Gresser I, Tovey MG, Bandu TM *et al.* (1976a). Role of interferon in the pathogenesis of virus diseases as demonstrated by the use of anti-interferon serum. I. Rapid evolution of encephalomyocarditis virus infection. *J Exp Med* **144**: 1305.

Gresser I, Tovey MG, Maury C, Bandu MT (1976b). Role of interferon in the pathogenesis of virus disease as demonstrated by the use of anti-interferon serum. II. Studies with herpes simplex, moloney sarcoma, vesicular stomatitis Newcastle disease and influenza viruses. *J Exp Med* **144**: 1316.

Grimley PM, David GL, Kang Y *et al.* (1985). Tubuloreticular inclusions in peripheral blood mononuclear cells related to systemic therapy with alpha interferon. *Lab Invest* **52**: 638.

Groopman JE (1987). Neoplasms in the acquired immune deficiency syndrome: a multidisciplinary approach to treatment. *Semin Oncol* **14**: 1.

Grunfeld G, Kotler DP, Shigenaga JK *et al.* (1991). Circulating interferon-alpha levels and hypertriglyceridemia in the acquired immunodeficiency syndrome. *Amer J Med* **90**: 154.

Gui XE, Ho M, Cohes MS *et al.* (1987). Hemorrhagic fever with renal syndrome; treatment with recombinant alpha interferon. *J Infect Dis* **155**: 1047.

Gutterman JU, Fine S, Quesada J *et al.* (1982). Recombinant leukocyte A interferon; pharmacokinetics, single-dose tolerance, and biologic effects in cancer patients. *Ann Intern Med* **96**: 549.

Hadziyannis SJ (1991). Use of alpha interferon in the treatment of chronic delta hepatitis. *J Hepatol* **13**: S21.

Hagiwara H, Hayashi N, Mita E *et al.* (1993). Quantitative analysis of hepatitis C virus RNA in serum during interferon alfa therapy. *Gastroenterology* **104**: 877.

Halevy J, Achiron A, Spiegel D *et al.* (1990). Recombinant alpha interferon may be efficacious in acute hepatitis B. *Amer J Gastroenterol* **85**: 210.

Haque SJ, Williams BR (1994). Identification and characterisation of an interferon (IFN) stimulated response element IFN stimulated gene factor 3-independent signalling pathway for IFN-alpha. *J Biol Chem* **269**: 19523.

Haria M, Benfield P (1995). Interferon-alpha 2a. A review of its pharmacological properties and therapeutic use in the management of viral hepatitis. *Drugs* **50**: 873.

Harle JR, Disdier P, Pelletier J *et al.* (1995). Dramatic worsening of hepatitis C virus related cryoglobulinemia subsequent to treatment with interferon alfa. *JAMA* **274**: 126.

Hartshorn KL, Neumeyer D, Yogt MW *et al.* (1987). Activity of interferons alpha, beta, and gamma against human immuno-deficiency virus replication *in vitro*. *AIDS Res Hum Retrovir* **3**: 125.

Hayata T, Nakano Y, Yoshizawa K *et al.* (1991). Effects of interferon on intrahepatic human leukocyte antigens and lymphocyte subsets in patients with chronic hepatitis B and C. *Hepatology* **13**: 1022.

Hayden FG, Albrecht JK, Kaiser DL *et al.* (1986). Prevention of natural colds by contact prophylaxis with intranasal alpha₂ interferon. *New Engl J Med* **314**: 71.

Hayden FG, Kaiser DI, Albrecht JK (1988). Intranasal recombinant alfa-2b interferon treatment of naturally occurring common colds. *Antimicrob Ag Chemother* **32**: 224.

Healy GB, Gelber RD, Trowbridge AI, (1988). Treatment of recurrent respiratory papillomatosis with human leukocyte interferon. *New Engl J Med* **319**: 401.

Hendrix CW, Petty BG, Woods A *et al.* (1995). Modulation of alpha-interferon's antiviral and clinical effects by aspirin, acetaminophen, and prednisone in healthy volunteers. *Antiviral Res* **28**: 121.

Hertzog PJ, Hwang SY, Holland KA et al. (1994a). A gene on human chromosome 21 located in the region 21q222 to 21q223 encodes a factor necessary for signal transduction and antiviral response to type 1 interferons. *J Biol Chem* **269**: 14088.

Hertzog PJ, Hwang SY, Kola I (1994b). Rofle of interferons in the regulation of cell proliferation, differentiation and development. *Mol Reprod Develop* **39**: 226.

Hess G (1991). Treatment of chronic hepatitis C. *J Hepatol* **1**: S17.

Hess G, Rossol S, Rossol R et al. (1991). Tumor necrosis factor and interferon as prognostic markers in human immunodeficiency virus (HIV) infection. *Infection* **2**: 93.

Higgins PG, Barrow GI, Tyrrell DA et al. (1990). The efficacy of intranasal interferon alpha-2a in respiratory syncytial virus infection in volunteers. *Antiviral Res* **14**: 3.

Hino K, Sainokami S, Shimoda K et al. (1994). Genotypes and titers of hepatitis C virus for predicting response to interferon in patients with chronic hepatitis C. *J Med Virol* **42**: 299.

Hirsch MS, Schooley RT, Cosimi B et al. (1983). Effects of interferon alpha on cytomegalovirus reactivation syndromes in renal transplant recipients. *New Engl J Med* **308**: 1489.

Hizawa N, Kojima J, Kojima T et al. (1994). A patient with chronic hepatitis C who simultaneously developed interstitial pneumonia, hemolytic anaemia and cholestatic liver dysfunction after alpha-interferon administration. *Intern Med* **33**: 337.

Ho D, Rota T, Kaplan SC (1985). Recombinant human interferon-alpha suppresses HTLV-III replication *in vitro. Lancet* **ii**: 602.

Hoofnagle JH (1990). Alpha interferon therapy of chronic hepatitis B. Current status and recommendations. *J Hepatol* **11**: S100.

Hoofnagle JH (1994). Therapy of acute and chronic viral hepatitis. *Adv Intern Med* **39**: 241.

Hoofnagle JH, Mullen KD, Jones DB et al. (1986). Treatment of chronic non-A, non-B hepatitis with recombinant human alpha interferon; a preliminary report. *New Engl J Med* **315**: 1575.

Hoofnagle JH, Peters M, Mullen KD et al. (1988). Randomized, controlled trail of recombinant human alpha-interferon in patients with chronic hepatitis B. *Gastroenterology* **95**: 1318.

Hoofnagle JH, Di Bisceglie AM, Waggoner JG, Park Y (1993). Interferon alfa for patients with clinically apparent cirrhosis due to chronic hepatitis B. *Gastroenterology* **104**: 1116.

Hopf U, Neghaus P, Lobeck H et al. (1991). Follow up of recurrent hepatitis B and delta infection in liver allograft recipients after treatment with recombinant interferon alpha. *J Hepatol* **13**: 339.

Horisberger MA, Gunst MC (1991). Interferon-induced proteins; identification of Mx proteins in various mammalian species. *Virology* **180**: 185.

Horisberger MA, Stacheli P, Haller O (1983). Interferon induces a unique protein in mouse cells bearing a gene for resistance to influenza virus. *Proc Natl Acad Sci USA* **80**: 1910.

Horsmans Y, Brenard R, Geubel AP (1994). Short report; interferon-alpha decreases 14C-aminopyrine breath lest values in patients with chronic hepatiits C. *Aliment Pharmacol Ther* **8**: 353.

Hovanessian AG (1989). The double stranded RNA-activated protein kinase induced by interferon; ds RNA-PK. *J Interfer Res* **9**: 641.

Howell DM, Feldman SB, Kloser P, Fitzgerald-Bocarsly P (1994). Decreased frequency of functional natural interferon producing cells in peripheral blood of patients with acquired immune deficiency syndrome. *Clin Immunol Immunopathol* **71**: 223.

Hwang SY, Hertzog PJ, Holland KA et al. (1995). A null mutation in the gene encoding a type 1 interferon receptor component eliminates antiproliferative and antiviral responses to interferons alpha and beta and alters macrophage responses. *Proc Natl Acad Sci USA* **92**: 11284.

Ikeda Y, Toda G, Hashimoto N et al. (1991). Naturally occurring anti interferon alpha 2a antibodies in patients with acute viral hepatitis. *Clin Exp Immunol* **85**: 80.

Isaacs A, Lindenmann J (1957). *Interferon Proc Roy Soc Ser B* **147**: 258.

Ijichi K, Mitamura K, Ida S et al. (1994). *In vivo* antiviral effects of mismatched double-stranded RNA on duck hepatitis B virus. *J Med Virol* **43**: 161.

Ikic D, Bosnic N, Smerdel S et al. (1975a). Double blind clinical study with human leukocyte interferon in the therapy of condylomata acuminata. *Proc Symp Clin Use Interferon*, p. 229. Zagreb: Yugoslav Acad Sci Arts.

Ikic D, Orescanin M, Krusic J, Cestar Z (1975b). Preliminary study of the effect of human leukocyte interferon on condyloma acuminata in women. *Proc Symp Clin Use Interferon*, p. 223. Zagreb: Yugoslav Acad Sci Arts.

Imam AM, Ackrill AM, Dale TC et al. (1990). Transcription factors induced by interferons alpha and gamma. *Nucleic Acid Res* **18**: 6573.

Improta T, Schindler C, Horvath CM et al. (1994). Transcription factor ISGF-3 formation requires phosphorylated Stat91 protein, but Stat113 protein is phosphorylated independently of Stat91 protein. *Proc Natl Acad Sci USA* **91**: 4776.

Jacobs EL, Clare-Salzler MJ, Chopra IJ Figlin RA (1991). Thyroid function abnormalities associated with the chronic outpatient administration of recombinant interleukin-2 and recombinant interferon-alpha. *J Immunother* **10**: 448.

Janssen HL, Berk L, Vermeulen M, Schalm SW (1990). Seizures associated with low-dose alpha-interferon. *Lancet* **336**: 1580.

Janssen HLA, Brouwer JT, Nevens F et al. (1992). Fatal hepatic decompensation associated with interferon alfa. *Brit Med J* **306**: 107.

Johnson VA, Barlow MA, Merrill DP et al. (1990). Three drug synergistic inhibition of HIV-1 replication *in vitro* by zidovudine, recombinant soluble CD4, and recombinant interferon alpha A. *J Infect Dis* **161**: 1059.

Johnson VA, Merrill DP, Videler JA et al. (1991). Two-drug combinations of zidovudine, didanosine and recombinant interferon-alpha A inhibit replication of zidovudine-resistant human immunodeficiency virus type 1 synergistically *in vitro. J Infect Dis* **164**: 646.

Johnston MD (1985). Sources of interferon for clinical use; alpha-interferons from human lymphoblastoid cells In *Interferon 4: In vivo and Clinical Studies* (Finter NB, Oldham RK, eds), pp. 81–87. Amsterdam: Elsevier.

Kanai K, Kako M, Okamoto H (1992). HCV genotypes in chronic hepatitis C and response to interferon. *Lancet* **339**: 1543.

Kanai K, Kako M, Aikawa T et al. (1995). Clearance of serum hepatitis C virus RNA after interferon therapy in relation to virus genotype. *Liver* **15**: 185.

Kanda Y, Shigeno K, Kinoshita N et al. (1994). Sudden hearing loss associated with interferon. *Lancet* **343**: 1134.

Kanda Y, Shigeno K, Matsuo H et al. (1995). Interferon induced sudden hearing loss. *Audiology* **34**: 98.

Kasimir S, Brom J, Konig W (1991). Effect of interferon-alpha on neutrophil functions. *Immunology* **74**: 271.

Kassianides C, Di Bisceglie AM, Hoofnagle JH et al. (1988). Alpha interferon therapy in patients with decompensated chronic type B hepatitis. In *Viral Hepatitis and Liver Disease* (Zuckerman AJ, ed), pp. 840–843. New York: Alan R Liss.

Kata Y, Nakagawa H, Kobayashi K et al. (1982). Interferon production by peripheral lymphocytes in HbsAg positive liver diseases. *Hepatology* **2**: 789.

Keay S, Teng N, Eisenberg M et al. (1988). Topical interferon for treating condyloma acuminata in women. *J Infect Dis* **158**: 934.

Kessler DS, Levy DE (1991). Protein kinase activity required for an early step in interferon alpha signalling. *J Biol Chem* **266**: 23471.

Kessler DS, Veals SA, Fu XY, Leve DE (1990). Interferon-alpha regulates nuclear translocation and DNA binding affinity of ISGF3, a multimeric transcriptional activator. *Genes Dev* **4**: 1753.

Khan MA, Tolleson WH, Gangemi JD, Pirisi L (1993). Inhibition of growth transformation and expression of human papillomavirus type 16 E7 in human keratinocytes by alpha interferons. *J Virol* **67**: 3396.

Kimura T, Nakayama K, Penninger J et al. (1994). Involvement of the IRF-1 transcription factor in antiviral responses to interferons. *Science* **264**: 1921.

Kohara M, Tanaka T, Tsukiyama-Kohara K et al. (1995). Hepatitis C virus genotypes 1 and 2 respond to interferon-alpha with different virologic kinetics. *J Infect Dis* **172**: 934.

Kontsek P, Borecky L, Novak M (1991). Are the acid-labile interferon alpha and interferon omega-1 identical?. *Virology* **181**: 416.

Korenman J, Baker B, Waggoner J *et al.* (1991). Long term remission of chronic hepatitis B after alpha-interferon therapy. *Ann Intern Med* **114**: 629.

Koretz RL, Stone O, Mousa M *et al.* (1985). Non-A, non-B post transfusion hepatiits – a decade later. *Gastroenterology* **88**: 1251.

Kornbluth RS, Oh PS, Munis JR *et al.* (1989). Interferons and bacterial lipopolysaccharide protect macrophages from productive infection by human immunodeficiency virus *in vitro*. *J Exp Med* **169**: 1137.

Kornbluth RS, Oh PS, Munis JR *et al.* (1990). The role of interferons in the control of HIV replication in macrophages. *Clin Immunol Immunopath* **43**: 200.

Krown SE (1987). the role of interferon in the therapy of epidemic Kaposi's sarcoma. *Sem Oncol* **14**: 27.

Krown SE, Gold JW, Neidzwiecki D *et al.* (1990). Interferon alpha with zidovudine, safety, tolerance, and clinical and virologic effects in patients with Kaposi sarcoma associated with the acquired immunodeficiency syndrome (AIDS). *Ann Intern Med* **112**: 812.

Krown SE, Neidzwiecki D, Bhalkla RB *et al.* (1991). Relationship and prognostic value of endogenous interferon alpha, beta-2 microglobulin, and neopterin serum levels in patients with Kaposi's sarcoma and AIDS. *J AIDS* **4**: S871.

Lai CL, Lok ASF, Lin HJ *et al.* (1987). Placebo controlled trial of recombinant alpha-interferon in Chinese HBsAg carrier children. *Lancet* **ii**: 877.

Lai CL, Lin HJ, Lau JN *et al.* (1991). Effect of recombinant alpha-2 interferon with or without prednisone in Chinese HBsAg carrier children. *Quart J Med* **78**: 155.

Lampertico P, Rumi M, Romero R *et al.* (1994). A multicentre randomized controlled trial of recombinant interfreon-alpha 2b in patients with acute transfusion-associated hepatitis C. *Hepatology* **19**: 19.

Lane HC, Davey V, Kovacs JA *et al.* (1990). Interferon alpha in patients with asymptomatic human immunodeficiency virus (HIV) infection. A randomised, placebo controlled trial. *Ann Intern Med* **112**: 805.

Lanford RE, Sureau C, Jacob JR *et al.* (1994). Demonstration of *in vitro* infection of chimpanzee hepatocytes with hepatitis C virus using strand-specific RT/PCR. *Virology* **202**: 606.

Langer JA, Rashidbaigi A, Lai LW *et al.* (1990). Sublocalization on chromosome 21 of human interferon alpha receptor gene and the gene for an interferon gamma response protein. *Somat Cell Mol Genet* **16**: 231.

Lau JY, Davis GL, Kniffen J *et al.* (1993). Significance of serum hepatitis C virus DNA levels in chronic hepatitis C. *Lancet* **341**: 1501.

Laurent-Puig P, Dussaix E *et al.* (1995). Host and viral characteristics affecting the response to interferon therapy in chronic hepatitis C. *Eur J Gastroenterol Hepatol* **7**: 335.

Levandowski RA, Horohov DW (1991). Rhinovirus induces natural killer-like cytotoxic cells and interferon alpha in mononuclear leukocytes. *J Med Virol* **35**: 116.

Levey JM, Bjornsson B, Banner B *et al.* (1994). Mixed cryoglobinemia in chronic hepatitis C infection. A clinicopathologic analysis of 10 cases and review of recent literature. *Med Baltimore* **73**: 53.

Levin F, Leibowitz J, Torten J, Hahn T (1989). Interferon treatment in acute progressive and fulminant hepatitis. *J Med Sci* **25**: 364.

Leventhal BG, Kashma HK, Mounts P *et al.* (1991). Long term response of recurrent respiratory papillomatosis to treatment with lymphoblastoid interferon alfa-n1. *New Engl J Med* **325**: 613.

Lin R, Schoeman MN, Craig PI *et al.* (1991). Can the response to interferon treatment be predicted in patients with chronic active hepatitis C? *Aust NZ J Med* **21**: 387.

Lin R, Roach E, Zimmerman M *et al.* (1995). Interferon alfa-2b for chronic hepatitis C; effects of dose increment and duration of treatment on response rates. *J Hepatol* **23**: 487–496.

Lisker-Melman M, Di Bisceglie AM, Usala SJ *et al.* (1992). Development of thyroid disease during therapy of chronic viral hepatitis with interferon Alfa. *Gastroenterology* **6**: 2155.

Lok AS (1991). Alpha interferon therapy for chronic hepatitis B virus infection in children and Oriental patients. *J Gastroenterol Hepatol* **6**: 15.

Lok AS, Lai CL (1991). Incidence, neutralizing activity and clinical significance of interferon antibodies in chronic hepatitis B patients receiving recombinant alpha interferons. In *Viral Hepatitis and Liver Disease* (Int Symp Viral Hepatitis and Liver Disease, 4–8 Apr 1990, Houston, Texas, USA), (Hollinger FB *et al.*, eds), p.643. Baltimore: Williams and Wilkins.

Lok ASF, Lai CL, Wu PC *et al.* (1988). Long term follow up in a randomised controlled trial of recombinant alpha-interferon in Chinese patients with chronic hepatitis B virus infection. *Lancet* **ii**: 298.

Lok ASF, Lai CL, Wu PC *et al.* (1989). Treatment of chronic hepatitis B with interferon; experience in Asian patients. *Semin Liver Dis* **9**: 249.

Lok AS, Lai CL, Leung EK (1990a). Interferon antibodies may negate the antiviral effects of recombinant alpha interferon treatment in patients with chronic hepatitis B virus infection. *Hepatology* **12**: 1266.

Lok AS, Lai CL, Wu PC *et al.* (1990b). Alpha interferon treatment in Chinese patients with chronic hepatitis B. *J Hepatol* **11**: S121.

Lok ASF, Chung HT, Liu VWS *et al.* (1993). Long-term follow up of chronic hepatitis B patients treated with interferon alfa. *Gastroenterology* **105**: 1833.

Lopes EPA, Oliveira PM, Silva AE *et al.* (1994). Exacerbation of type 2 diabetes mellitus during interferon-alfa therapy for chronic hepatitis B. *Lancet* **343**: 244.

Lopez-Ocejo O, Perea SE, Reyes A *et al.* (1993). Partial phenotypic reversion of HeLa cells by long term interferon-alpha treatment. *J Interferon Res* **13**: 369.

Lunel F, Musset L, Cacoub P *et al.* (1994). Cryoglobulinemia in chronic liver diseases; role of hepatitis C virus and liver damage. *Gastroenterology* **106**: 1291.

Lutfalla G, Roeckel N, Mogensen KE *et al.* (1990). Assignment of the human interferon-alpha receptor gene to chromosome 21q221 by *in situ* hybridisation. *J Interfer Res* **10**: 515.

Maccari S, Bassi C, Giovannini AG, Plancher AC (1991). A case of arthropathy and hypothyroidism during recombinant alpha interferon therapy. *Clin Rheumatol* **10**: 452.

Madejon A, Colonal T, Bartolome J *et al.* (1994). Treatment of chronic hepatitis D virus infection with low and high doses of interferon alpha 2a; utility of polymerase chain reaction in monitoring antiviral response. *Hepatology* **19**: 1331.

Maggiore G (1995). Chronic hepatitis in children. *Curr Opin Pediatr* **7**: 539.

Makris M, Preston FE, Triger DR *et al.* (1991). A randomised controlled trial of recombinant interferon-alpha in chronic hepatitis C in hemophiliacs. *Blood* **78**: 1672.

Marcellin P, Boyer N, Giostra E *et al.* (1991). Recombinant human alpha-interferon in patients with chronic non-A, non-B hepatitis; a multicenter randomized controlled trial from France. *Hepatology* **13**: 393.

Marcellin P, Samuel D, Areias J *et al.* (1994). Pretransplantation interferon treatment and recurrence of hepatitis B virus infection after liver transplantation for hepatitis B related end-stage liver disease. *Hepatology* **19**: 6.

Marroni M, Gresele P, Landonio G *et al.* (1994). Interferon alpha is effective in the treatment of HIV-1 related, severe zidovudine resistant thrombocytopenia. A prospective placebo controlled, double blind trial. *Ann Intern Med* **121**: 423.

Matsuda J, Saitoh N, Gotoh M *et al.* (1995). High prevalence of anti-phospholipid antibodies and anti-thyroglobulin antibody in patients with hepatitis C virus infection treated with interferon-alpha. *Amer J Gastroenterol* **90**: 1138.

McDonald JA, Caruso L, Karayiannis P *et al.* (1987). Diminished responsiveness of male homosexual chronic hepatitis B virus carriers with HTLV III antibodies to recombinant alpha interferon. *Hepatology* **7**: 719.

McNair AN, Cheng D, Monjardino J *et al.* (1994). Hepatitis delta virus replication *in vitro* is not affected by interferon alpha or gamma despite intact cellular responses in interferon and dsRNA. *J Gen Virol* **75**: 1371.

Meltzer MS Baca L, Turpin JA *et al.* (1991). Regulation of cytokine and viral gene expression in monocytes infected with the human immunodeficiency virus. *Pathobiology* **59**: 209.

Meyelan PR, Guatelli JC, Munis JR *et al.* (1993). Mechanisms for the inhibition of HIV replication by interferons-alpha, beta, and gamma in primary human macrophages. *Virology* **193**: 138.

Michaelis B, Levy JA (1989). HIV replication can be blocked by recombinant human interferon beta. *AIDS* **3**: 27.

Mildvan D, Berge P, Starrett S *et al.* (1994). Prophylactic zalcitabine and interferon alpha for a large bore needlestick exposure to human immunodeficiency virus. *J AIDS* **7**: 416.

Mitoro A, Yoshikawa M, Yamamoto K *et al.* (1993). Exacerbation of ulcerative colitis during alpha-interferon therapy for chronic hepatitis C. *Intern Med* **32**: 327.

Mitsuyasu RT (1991). Interferon alpha in the treatment of AIDS-related Kaposi's sarcoma. *Brit J Haematol* **79**: 69.

Monto AS, Shope TC, Schwartz SA, Albrecht JK (1986). Intranasal interferon alpha 2b for seasonal prophylaxis of respiratory infection. *J Infect Dis* **154**: 128.

Moochhala S, Renton KW (1991). The effect of IFN-alpha-Con 1 on hepatic cytochrome P-450 and protein synthesis and degradation in hepatic microsomes. *Int J Immunopharmacol* **13**: 903.

Moreno MR, Jimenez J, Porres JC *et al.* (1990). A controlled trial of recombinant interferon alpha in Caucasian children with chronic hepatitis B. *Digestion* **45**: 26.

Morris DJ (1994). Adverse effects and drug interactions of clinical importance with antiviral drugs. *Drug Saf* **10**: 281.

Muller R (1991). Interferons in chronic viral hepatitis. *Hepato Gastroent* **38**: 4.

Muller H, Hammes E, Hiemke C, Hess G (1991). Interferon alpha-2-induced stimulation of ACTH and cortisol secretion in man. *Neuroendocrinology* **54**: 499.

Nadir F, Fagiuoli S, Wright HI *et al.* (1994). Rheumatoid arthritis; a complication of interferon therapy. *J Oklahom State Med Assoc* **87**: 228.

Nagata S, Taira H, Hall A *et al.* (1980). Synthesis in *E. coli* of a polypeptide with human leucocyte interferon activity. *Nature* **284**: 316.

Nakamura T, Shibayama K, Nagasato K *et al.* (1990). The efficacy of interferon alpha treatment in human T-lymphotropic virus type 1 associated myelopathy. *Jpn J Med* **29**: 362.

Narkewicz MR, Smith D, Silverman A *et al.* (1995). Clearance of chronic hepatitis B virus infection in young children after alpha interferon treatment. *J Pediatr* **127**: 815.

Negoro K, Fukusako T, Morimatsu M, Liao CM (1994). Acute axonal polyneuropathy during interferon alpha 2A therapy for chronic hepatitis type C. *Muscle Nerve* **17**: 1351.

Negro F, Abate ML, Mondardini A *et al.* (1995). The fluctuations of hepatitis C virus RNA and IgM anti-HCV (core) serum levels correlate with those of alanine aminotransferases during the hepatitis relapses of patients treated with interferon. *J Viral Hepatitis* **2**: 171.

Nelson MR, Chard S, Barton SE (1995). Intralesional interferon for the treatment of recalcitrant molluscum contagiosum in HIV antibody positive individuals: a preliminary report. *Int J STD AIDS* **6**: 351.

Northfelt DW, Kaplan LD, Abrams DI (1991). Continuous, low dose therapy with interferon alpha for human immunodeficiency virus (HIV)-related immune thrombocytopenic purpura. *Amer J Hematol* **38**: 238.

Northfelt DW, Charlebois ED, Mirda MI *et al.* (1995). Continuous low dose interferon alpha therapy for HIV-related immune thrombocytopenic purpura. *J AIDS Hum Retrovir* **8**: 45.

Novick DM, Lok AS, Thomas HC (1984). Diminished responsiveness of homosexual men in antiviral therapy for HB$_3$Ag-positive chronic liver disease. *J Hepatol* **1**: 29.

Novick D, Cohen B, Rubinstein M (1994). The human interferon alpha/beta receptor; characterisation and molecular cloning. *Cell* **77**: 391.

Okada SI, Akahane Y, Suzuki H *et al.* (1992). The degree of variability in the amino terminal region of the E2/NS1 protein of hepatitis C virus correlated with responsiveness to interferon therapy in viremic patients. *Hepatology* **16**: 619.

Okamoto H, Sugiyama Y, Okada S *et al.* (1992). Typing hepatitis C virus by polymerase chain reaction with type specific primers, application to clinical surveys and tracing infectious sources. *J Gen Virol* **73**: 673.

Okano M, Pirruccello SJ, Grierson HL *et al.* (1990). Immunovirological studies of fatal infectious mononucleosis in a patient with X-linked lymphoproliferative syndrome treated with intravenous immunoglobulin and interferon alpha. *Clin Immunol Immunopathol* **54**: 410.

Okuno T, Shindo M, Arai K *et al.* (1991). 2',5' Oligoadenylate synthetase activity in peripheral blood mononuclear cells and serum during interferon treatment of chronic non-A, non-B hepatitis. *Gastroenterology* **26**: 603.

Olcszak E, Stewart EW (1985). Potentiation of the antiviral and anticellular activities of interferons by mixtures of HuIFN-gamma or HuINF-beta. *J Interfer Res* **5**: 361.

Oshita M, Hayashi N, Kasahara A *et al.* (1994). Increased serum hepatitis C virus RNA levels among alcoholic patients with chronic hepatitis C. *Hepatology* **20**: 1115.

Paez C, Garcia F, Gil-Fernandez C (1990). Interferon cures cells lytically and persistently infected with African swine fever virus *in vitro*. *Arch Virol* **112**: 115.

Pagano PJ, Chong KT (1995). *In vitro* inhibition of human immunodeficiency virus type 1 by a combination of delavirdine (U-90152) with protease inhibitor U-75875 or interferon-alpha. *J Infect Dis* **171**: 61.

Palmer DL, Hjelle BL, Wiley CA *et al.* (1994). HIV-1 infection despite immediate combination antiviral therapy after infusion of contaminated white cells. *Amer J Med* **97**: 289.

Pauluzzi P, Kokelj F, Perkan V *et al.* (1993). Psoriasis exacerbation induced by interferon alpha. Report of two cases. *Acta Derm Venerol* **73**: 395.

Pavlovic J, Schroder A, Blank A *et al.* (1993). Mx proteins; GTPases involved in the interferon-induced antiviral state. *Ciba Foundat Symp* **176**: 233.

Pawlotsky JM, Hovanessian A, Roudot-Thoraval F *et al.* (1995). Activity of interferon-induced 2',5'-oligoadenylate synthetase in patients with chronic hepatitis C. *J Interfer Cytok Res* **15**: 857.

Perno CF, Aquaro S, Rosenwirth B *et al.* (1994). *In vitro* activity of inhibitors of late stages of the replication of HIV in chronically infected macrophages. *J Leukoc Biol* **56**: 381.

Perrillo RP (1990). Factors influencing response to interferon in chronic hepatitis B; implications for Asian and Western populations. *Hepatology* **12**: 1433.

Perrillo RP (1993). Interferon in the management of chronic hepatitis B. *Digest Dis Sci* **38**: 577.

Perrillo RP, Fredric G, Regenstein FG, (1988). Prednisone withdrawal followed by recombinant alpha interferon in the treatment of chronic type B hepatitis. *Ann Intern Med* **109**: 95.

Perrillo RP, Schiff ER, Davis GL *et al.* (1990). A randomised, controlled trail of interferon alfa-2b alone and after prednisone withdrawal for the treatment of chronic hepatitis B. *New Engl J Med* **323**: 295.

Perrillo R, Tamburro C, Regenstein P *et al.* (1995). Low dose, titratable interferon alfa in decompensated liver disease caused by chronic infection with hepatitis B virus. *Gastroenterology* **109**: 908.

Pestka S, Langer JA, Zoon KC, Samuel CE (1987). Interferons and their actions. *Ann Rev Biochem* **56**: 727.

Petersen CS, Bjerring P, Larsen J *et al.* (1991). Systemic interferon alpha 2b increases the cure rate in laster treated patients with multiple persistent genital warts; a placebo-controlled study. *Genitourin Med* **67**: 99.

Picciotto A, Bertolini S, Bardellini E *et al.* (1995). Serum lipid levels during interferon therapy in patients with chronic hepatitis C. *J Interferon Cytok Res* **15**: 703.

Pignatelli I, Waters J, Brown D *et al.* (1986). HLA class 1 antigens on the hepatocyte membrane during recovery from acute hepatitis B virus infection and during interferon therapy in chronic hepatitis B virus infection. *Hepatology* **6**: 349.

Pitha PM (1994). Multiple effects of interferon on the replication of human immunodeficiency virus type 1. *Antiviral Res* **24**: 205.

Platanias LC, Uddin S, Colamonici OR (1994). Tyrosine phosphorylation of the alpha and beta subunits of the type 1 interferon receptor. Interferon-beta selectively induces tyrosine phosphorylation of an alpha subunit associated protein. *J Biol Chem* **269**: 17761.

Podzamczer D, Bolao F, Clotet B et al. (1993). Low dose interferon alpha combined with zidovudine in patients with AIDS associated Kaposi's sarcoma. *J Intern Med* **233**: 247.

Poitrine A, Chousterman S, Chousterman M et al., 1985) Lack of *in vivo* activation of the interferon system in HBsAg positive chronic active hepatitis. *Hepatology* **5**: 171.

Pol JM, Broekhuysen-Davies JM, Wagenaar F, La Bonnardiere C (1991). The influence of porcine recombinant interferon-alpha 1 on Pseudorabies virus infection in porcine nasal mucosa *in vitro*. *J Gen Virol* **72**: 933.

Poli G, Orenstein JM, Kinter A et al. (1989). Interferon-alpha but not AZT suppresses HIV expression in chronically infected cell lines. *Science* **244**: 575.

Poli G, Biswas P, Fauci AS (1994). Interferons in the pathogenesis and treatment of human immunodeficiency virus infection. *Antiviral Res* **24**: 221.

Porres JC, Mora CL, Gutlez J et al., 1988) Different doses of recombinant alpha interferon in the treatment of chronic hepatitis B patients without antibodies against the human immunodeficiency virus. *Hepato Gastroenterol* **35**: 300.

Portnoy J, Hicks R, Pacheco F, Olson L (1988). Pilot study of recombinant interferon alpha-2a for treatment of infants with bronchiolitis induced by respiratory syncytial virus. *Antimicrob Ag Chemother* **32**: 589.

Poutiainen E, Hokkanen L, Niemi ML, Farkkila M (1994). Reversible cognitive decline during high dose alpha-interferon treatment. *Pharmacol Biochem Behav* **47**: 901

Poynard T, Bedossa P, Chevallier M et al. (1995). A comparison of three interferon alfa-2b regimens for the long term treatment of chronic non-A, non-B hepatitis. Multicenter Study Group. *New Engl J Med* **332**: 1457.

Reichard O, Foberg U, Fryden A et al. (1994). High sustained response rate and clearance of viremia in chronic hepatitis C after treatment with interferon-alpha for 60 weeks. *Hepatology* **19**: 280.

Reichen J, Bianchi L, Frei PC et al. (1994). Efficacy of steroid withdrawal and low dose interferon treatment in chronic active hepatitis B. Results of a randomized multicenter trial. Swiss Association for the Study of the Liver. *J Hepatol* **20**: 168.

Reichman RC, Oakes D, Bonnez W et al. (1988). Treatment of condyloma acuminatum with three different interferons administered intralesionally. A double blind, placebo controlled trial. *Ann Intern Med* **108**: 675.

Reiter Z (1993). Interferon a major regulator of natural killer cell mediated cytotoxicity. *J Interfer Res* **13**: 247.

Renault PF, Hoofnagle JH, Park Y et al. (1987). Psychiatric complications of long term interferon alfa therapy. *Arch Intern Med* **147**: 1577.

Roche Product Information.

Roffi L, Mels GC, Antonelli G et al. (1995). Breakthrough during recombinant interferon alfa therapy in patients with chronic hepatitis C virus infection. Prevalence, etiology and management. *Hepatology* **31**: 645.

Romero R, Levine JE (1996). Cytokine inhibition of the hepatitis B virus core promoter. *Hepatology* **23**: 17.

Roonbloom LE, Alm GV, Oberg KE (1991). Autoimmunity after alpha-interferon therapy for malignant carcinoid tumors. *Ann Intern Med* **115**: 178.

Rosina F, Cozzolongo R (1994). Interferon in HDV infection. *Antiviral Res* **24**: 165.

Rosina F, Pintus C, Meschievits C, Rizzetto M (1991). A randomised controlled trial of a 12 month course of recombinant human interferon alpha in chronic delta (type D) hepatitis; a multicenter Italian study. *Hepatology* **13**: 1052.

Rubinstein M, Orchansky P (1986). The interferon receptors. *CRC Crit Rev Biochem* **121**: 249.

Ruiz-Moreno M, Jimenez J, Porres JC et al. (1990). A controlled trail of recombinant interferon alpha in Caucasian children with chronic hepatitis B. *Digestion* **45**: 26.

Ruiz-Moreno M, Rua MJ, Molina J et al. (1991). Prospective, randomized controlled trial of interferon alpha in children with chronic hepatitis B. *Hepatology* **13**: 1035.

Ruprecht RM, Bronson R (1994). Chemoprevention of retroviral infection; success is determined by virus inoculum strength and cellular immunity. *DNA Cell Biol* **13**: 59.

Ruprecht RM, Chou TC, Chipty F et al. (1990). Interferon-alpha and 3'-azido-3'-deoxythymidine are highly synergistic in mice and prevent viremia after acute retrovirus exposure. *J AIDS* **3**: 591.

Ryff JC (1993). The judicious use of interferon-alpha-2a for the treatment of chronic hepatitis B. *J Hepatol* **17**: S42.

Sacks SL, Varner TL, Davies KS et al. (1990). Randomised double-blind placebo-controlled, patient-initiated study of topical high and low dose interferon alpha with nonoxynol-9 in the treatment of recurrent genital herpes. *J Infect Dis* **161**: 692.

Saito T, Shinzawa H, Kuboki M et al. (1994). A randomized, controlled of human lymphoblastoid interferon in patients with compensated type C cirrhosis. *Amer J Gastroenterol* **89**: 681.

Samuel CE (1988). Mechanisms of the antiviral action of interferons. *Proc Nucl Acid Res* **35**: 27.

Saracco G, Rizzetto M (1995). The long term efficacy of interferon alfa in chronic hepatitis C patients: a clinical review. *J Gastroneterol Hepatol* **10**: 668.

Schaff Z, Hoofnagle JH, Grimly PM (1986). Hepatic inclusions during interferon therapy in chronic viral hepatitis. *Hepatology* **6**: 966.

Schindler C, Fu XY, Improta T et al. (1992). Proteins of transcription factor ISGF-3: One gene encodes the 91 and 84-kDs ISGF-3 proteins that are activated by interferon alpha. *Proc Natl Acad Sci USA* **89**: 7836.

Schvarcz R, Glaumann H, Weiland O et al. (1991). Interferon alpha 2b treatment of chronic post transfusion non-A, non-B/C hepatitis; long-term outcome and effect of increased interferon doses in non responders. *Scand J Infect Dis* **23**: 413.

Sepp NT, Umlauft F, Illersperger B et al. (1995). Necrotizing vasculitis associated with hepatitis C virus infection; successful treatment of vasculitis with interferon alpha despite persistence of mixed cryoglobulinemia. *Dermatology* **191**: 43.

Serfaty L, Chazouilleres O, Pawlotsky JM et al. (1996). Interferon alfa therapy in patients with chronic hepatitis C and persistently normal aminotransferase activity. *Gastroenterology* **110**: 291.

Sherlock DS (1994). Chronic hepatitis C. *Dis Mon* **40**: 117.

Sherlock S, Thomas HC (1985). Treatment of chronic hepatitis due to hepatitis B virus. *Lancet* **ii**: 1343.

Shibayama K, Nakamura T, Nagasato K et al. (1991). Interferon alpha treatment in HTLV-1 associated myelopathy. Studies of clinical and immunological aspects. *J Neurol Sci* **106**: 186.

Shindo M, Arai K, Sokawa Y, Okuno T (1995). Hepatic hepatitis C virus RNA as a predictor of a long-term response to interferon alpha therapy. *Ann Intern Med* **122**: 586.

Shirazi Y, Pitha PM (1992). Alpha interferon inhibits early stages of the human immunodeficiency virus type 1 replication cycle. *J Virol* **66**: 1321.

Sieck JO, Ellis ME, Alfurayh O, (1993). Histologically advanced chronic hepatitis C treated with recombinant alpha-interferon; a randomised placebo controlled double-blind cross over study. *J Hepatol* **19**: 418.

Smith MS, Thresher RJ, Pagano JS (1991). Inhibition of human immunodeficiency virus type 1 morphogenesis in T cells by alpha interferon. *Antimicrob Ag Chemother* **35**: 62.

Smith RA, Norris F, Palmer D et al. (1985). Distribution of alpha interferon in serum and cerebrospinal fluid after systemic administration. *Clin Pharmacol Ther* **37**: 85.

Sperber SJ, Gocks DJ, Haberzettl CA, Pestka S (1993). Low dose oral recombinant interferon alpha A in patients with HIV-1 infection; a blinded pilot study. *AIDS* **7**: 693.

Stanley LA, Adams DJ, Balkwill FR et al. (1991). Differential effects of recombinant interferon alpha on constitutive and inducible cytochrome P450 isozymes in mouse liver. *Biochem Pharmacol* **42**: 311.

Stark GR, Kerr IM (1992). Interferon dependent signalling pathways DNA elements, transcription factors, mutations, and effects of viral proteins. *J Interf Res* **12**: 147.

Steiner I, Wirguin I, Morag A, Abramsky O (1989). Intraventricular interferon treatment for subacute sclerosing panencephalitis. *J Child Neurol* **4**: 20.

Stewart TA, Hultgren B, Huang X *et al.* (1993). Induction of type 1 diabetes by interferon-alpha in transgenic mice. *Science* **260**: 1942.

Strander H, Cantell K (1996). Production of interferon by human leucocytes *in vitro. Ann Med Exp Biol Fennae* **44**: 265.

Stricker RB, Barlogie B, Kiprov DD (1994). Acquired factor VIII inhibitor associated with chronic interferon alpha therapy. *J Rheumatol* **21**: 350.

Sunderkotter C, Luger T, Kolde G (1993). Severe hypertiglyceridaemia and interferon-alpha. *Lancet* **342**: 1111.

Sutton RNP, Tyrrell DAJ (1961). Some observations on interferon prepared in tissue cultures. *Brit J Exp Pathol* **42**: 99.

Syed TA, Cheema KM, Khayyami M *et al.* (1995a). Human leukocyte interferon alpha versus podophyllotoxin in cream for the treatment of genital warts in males. A placebo controlled, double blind, comparative study. *Dermatology* **191**: 129.

Syed TA, Cheema KM, Kahlon BM *et al.* (1995b). Human leukocyte interferon alpha in cream for the treatment of genital herpes in Asian males. A placebo controlled double blind study. *Dermatology* **191**: 32.

Szebeni J, Dieffenbach C, Wahl SM *et al.* (1991). Induction of alpha interferon by human immunodeficiency virus type 1 in human monocyte macrophage cultures. *J Virol* **65**: 6362.

Tanaka H, Samuel CE (1994). Mechanism of interferon action; structure of the mouse PKR gene encoding the interferon-inducible RNA dependent protein kinase. *Proc Natl Acad Sci USA* **91**: 7995.

Tarumi T, Sawada K, Sato N *et al.* (1995). Interferon alpha induced apoptosis in human erythroid progenitors. *Exp Hematol* **23**: 1310.

Taylor JL, Tom P, Guy J *et al.* (1994). Regulation of herpes simplex virus thymidine kinase in cells treated with a synergistic antiviral combination of alpha interferon and acyclovir. *Antimicrob Ag Chemother* **38**: 853.

Temonen M, Lankinen H, Vapalahti O *et al.* (1995). Effect of interferon-alpha and cell differentiation on Putimala virus infection in human monocyte/macrophages. *Virology* **206**: 8.

Thomas HC, Dusheiko GM, Lok ASF *et al.* (1990). Comparative study of three doses of interferon alpha-2A in chronic active hepatitis B. In *Viral Hepatitis and Liver Disease* (Int Symp Viral Hepatitis and Liver Disease, 4–8 Apr, 1990, Houston, Texas) (Hollinger FB *et al.*, eds), p. 644. Baltimore: Williams and Wilkins.

Thomas HC, Karaylannis P, Brook G (1991). Treatment of hepatitis B virus infection with interferon. Factors predicting response to interferon. *J Hepatol* **13**: S4.

Tolentino DF, Dianzani M, Zucca M, Giacchino R (1975). Decreased interferon response by lymphocytes from children with chronic hepatitis. *Infect Dis* **132**: 459.

Toraldo R, D'Avanzo M, Tolone C *et al.* (1995). Effect of interferon alpha therapy in a patient with common variable immunodeficiency and chronic Epstein–Barr virus infection. *Pediatr Hematol Oncol* **12**: 489.

Traynor A, Kuzel T, Samuelson E, Kanwar Y (1994). Minimal change glomerulopathy and glomerular visceral epithelial hyperplasia associated with alpha interferon therapy for cutaneous T-cell lymphoma. *Nephron* **67**: 94.

Treanor JJ, Betts RF, Erb SM *et al.* (1987). Intranasally administered interferon as prophylaxis against experimentally induced influenza A virus infection in humans. *J Infect Dis* **156**: 379.

Trepo C, Habersetzer F, Bailly F *et al.* (1994). Interferon therapy for hepatitis C1. *Antiviral Res* **24**: 155.

Tsubota A, Chayama K, Ikeda K *et al.* (1994). Factors predictive of response to interferon alpha therapy in hepatitis C virus infection. *Hepatology* **19**: 1088.

Turner RB, Felton A, Kosak K *et al.* (1986). Prevention of experimental coronavirus colds with intranasal alpha-2b interferon. *J Infect Dis* **154**: 443.

Uchida K, Matsui A, Nakano S *et al.* (1996). Painless thyroiditis occurring during long-term treatment with interferon alfa in a patient with chronic active hepatitis C. *South Med J* **89**: 81.

Ueda K, Tsurimoto T, Nagahata T *et al.* (1989). An *in vitro* system for screening anti-hepatitis B virus drugs. *Virology* **169**: 213.

Utili R, Sagnelli E, Galanti B *et al.* (1991). Prolonged treatment of children with chronic hepatitis B with recombinant alpha 2a interferon; a controlled randomized study. *Amer J Gastroenterol* **86**: 327.

Utili R, Sagnelli E, Gaeta GB *et al.* (1994). Treatment of chronic hepatitis B in children with prednisone followed by alfa-interferon; a controlled randomized study. *J Hepatol* **20**: 163.

Uze G, Lutfalla G, Gresser I (1990). Genetic transfer of a functional human interferon alpha receptor into mouse cells; cloning and expression of its cDNA. *Cell* **60**: 225.

Van Thiel DH, Friedlander L, Fagiuoli S *et al.* (1994). Response to interferon alpha therapy is influenced by the iron content of the liver. *J Hepatol* **20**: 410.

Van Thiel DH, Friedlander L, Caraceni P *et al.* (1995a). Treatment of hepatitis C virus in elderly persons with interferon alpha. *J Gerontol* **50**: M330.

Van Thiel DH, Caraceni P, Molloy PJ *et al.* (1995b). Chronic hepatitis C in patients with normal or near normal alanine aminotransferase levels; the role of interferon alpha 2b therapy. *J Hepatol* **23**: 503.

Van Thiel DH, Friedlander L, Molloy PJ *et al.* (1995c). Interferon alpha can be used successfully in patients with hepatitis C virus-positive chronic hepatitis who have a psychiatric illness. *Eur J Gastroenterol Hepatol* **7**: 165.

Vance JC, Bart BJ, Hansen RC *et al.* (1986a). Intralesional recombinant alpha-2 interferon for the treatment of patients with condyloma acumunaium or verruca plantaris. *Arch Dermatol* **122**: 272.

Vance JC, Bart BJ, Bart B *et al.* (1986b). Effectiveness of intralesional human recombinant alfa-2b interferon (intron-A) for the treatment of patients with condyloma acuminatum. *Clin Res* **34**: 993A.

Veals SA, Kessler DS, Jesiah S *et al.* (1991). Signal transduction pathway activating interferon-alpha stimulated gene expression. *J Infect Dis* **132**: 459.

Voth R, Rossol S, Klein K *et al.* (1990). Differential gene expression of IFN-alpha and tumor necrosis factor-alpha in peripheral blood mononuclear cells from patients with AIDS related complex and AIDS. *J Immunol* **144**: 970.

Waguri M, Hanafusa T, Itoh N *et al.* (1994). Occurrence of IDDM during interferon therapy for chronic viral hepatitis. *Diabet Res Clin Pract* **23**: 33.

Watanabe U, Hashimoto E, Hisamitsu T *et al.* (1994). The risk factor for development of thyroid disease during interferon-alpha therapy for chronic hepatitis C. *Amer J Gastroenterol* **89**: 399.

Watling D, Guschin D, Mufler M *et al.* (1993). Complementation by the protein tyrosine kinase JAK2 of a mutant cell line defective in the interferon-gamma signal transduction pathway. *Nature* **366**: 166.

Weiland O (1994). Interferon therapy in chronic hepatitis C virus infection. *FEMS Microbiol Rev* **14**: 279.

Weiland O, Chen M, Lindh G *et al.* (1995). Efficacy of human leucocyte alpha interferon treatment for chronic hepatitis C virus infection. *Scand J Infect Dis* **27**: 319.

Weltman MD, Brotodihardji A, Crewe EB *et al.* (1995). Coinfection with hepatitis B and C or B, C and delta viruses results in severe chronic liver disease and responds poorly to interferon-alpha treatment. *J Viral Hepatitis* **2**: 39.

Williams R, Alexander GJM (1986). Natural history of chronic hepatitis B virus related liver disease and its relationship to serum markers of viral replication. *J Hepatology* **3**: S3.

Wills RJ (1990). Clinical pharmacokinetics of interferons. *Clin Pharmacokinet* **19**: 390.

Wills RJ, Dennis S, Spiegel HE *et al.* (1984). Interferon kinetics and adverse reactions after intravenous intramuscular, and subcutaneous injection. *Clin Pharmacol Ther* **35**: 722.

Wright TL, Combs C, Kim M *et al.* (1994). Interferon-alpha therapy for hepatitis C virus infection after liver transplantation. *Hepatology* **20**: 773.

Yamada H, Mizobuchi K, Isogai Y (1994). Acute onset of ocular complications with interferon. *Lancet* **343**: 914.

Yamada G, Takatani M, Kishi F *et al.* (1995). Efficacy of interferon alfa therapy in chronic hepatitis C patients depends primarily on hepatitis C virus RNA level. *Hepatology* **22**: 1351.

Yamamoto JK, Barre-Sinoussi F, Bolton Y *et al.* (1986). Human alpha and beta-interferon but not gamma-suppress the *in vitro* replication of LAV,HTLV-III and ARV-2. *J Interferon Res* **6**: 143.

Yasuda Y, Miyake S, Kato S *et al.* (1990). Interferon-alpha treatment leads to accumulation of virus particles on the surface of cells persistently infected with the human immunodeficiency virus type 1. *J AIDS* **3**: 1046.

Yliskoski M, Syrjanen K, Syrjanen S *et al.* (1991). Systemic alpha interferon (Wellferon) treatment of genital human papillomavirus (HPV) type 6, 11, 16 and 18 infections; double blind, placebo controlled trial. *Gynecol Oncol* **43**: 55.

Yokosuka O, Kato N, Hosoda K *et al.* (1995). Efficacy of long term interferon treatment in chronic liver disease evaluated by sensitive polymerase chain reaction assay for hepatitis C virus RNA. *Gut* **37**: 721.

Zarski JP, Causse X, Cohard M *et al.* (1994). A randomised controlled trail of interferon alfa-2b alone and with simultaneous prednisone for the treatment of chronic hepatitis B. French Multicenter Group. *J Hepatol* **20**: 735.

Zeidner NS, Rose LM, Mathason-DuBard CK *et al.* (1990). Zidovudine in combination with alpha interferon and interleukin-2 as prophylactic therapy for FeLV-induced immunodeficiency syndrome (FeLV- FAIDS). *J AIDS* **3**: 787.

Zoon KC, Miller D, Bekisz J *et al.* (1989). Chemical characterisation of human lymphoblastoid interferon-alpha species. *J Inter Res* **9**: S184

Index